Bonica's
MANAGEMENT OF PAIN

Bonica's MANAGEMENT OF PAIN

Editors

Scott M. Fishman, MD
Chief, Division of Pain Medicine
Professor of Anesthesiology
Department of Anesthesiology and Pain
   Medicine
University of California, Davis School of
   Medicine
Sacramento, California

Jane C. Ballantyne, MD, FRCA
Professor of Anesthesiology
   and Critical Care
University of Pennsylvania
Philadelphia, Pennsylvania

James P. Rathmell, MD
Chief, Division of Pain Medicine
Department of Anesthesia, Critical Care and
   Pain Medicine
Massachusetts General Hospital
Associate Professor of Anaesthesia
Harvard Medical School
Boston, Massachusetts

Wolters Kluwer | Lippincott Williams & Wilkins
Health

Philadelphia · Baltimore · New York · London
Buenos Aires · Hong Kong · Sydney · Tokyo

Acquisitions Editor: Frances DeStefano
Marketing Manager: Angela Panetta
Manufacturing Manager: Benjamin Rivera
Product Manager: Nicole Dernoski
Design Coordinator: Teresa Mallon
Production Service: Absolute Service, Inc./MDC

Library of Congress Cataloging-in-Publication Data

Library of Congress Cataloging-in-Publication Data

Bonica's management of pain. — 4th ed. / editors, Jane C. Ballantyne, Scott M. Fishman.
    p. ; cm.
  Includes bibliographical references and index.
  ISBN 978-0-7817-6827-6
 1. Pain—Treatment. 2. Analgesia. 3. Chronic pain—Treatment. I. Ballantyne, Jane,
1948- II. Fishman, Scott, 1959- III. Bonica, John J., 1917–1994. IV. Title: Management of
pain.
  [DNLM: 1. Pain—therapy. WL 704 B715 2010]

RB127.B685 2010
616′.0472—dc22

                        2009028543

   *The publishers have made every effort to trace the copyright holders for borrowed ma-
terial. If they have inadvertently overlooked any, they will be pleased to make the necessary arrangements at the first opportunity.*
   To purchase additional copies of this book, call our customer service department at
(800) 638-3030 or fax orders to **(301) 223-2320**. International customers should call **(301)
223-2300**.
   Visit Lippincott Williams & Wilkins on the Internet: http://www.LWW.com. Lippincott Williams & Wilkins customer service representatives are available from 8:30 am to
6:00 pm, EST.

                        06 07 08 09 10
                      1 2 3 4 5 6 7 8 9 10

TO THE LASTING MEMORY OF JOHN BONICA AND HIS ENDURING QUEST
TO END NEEDLESS PAIN.

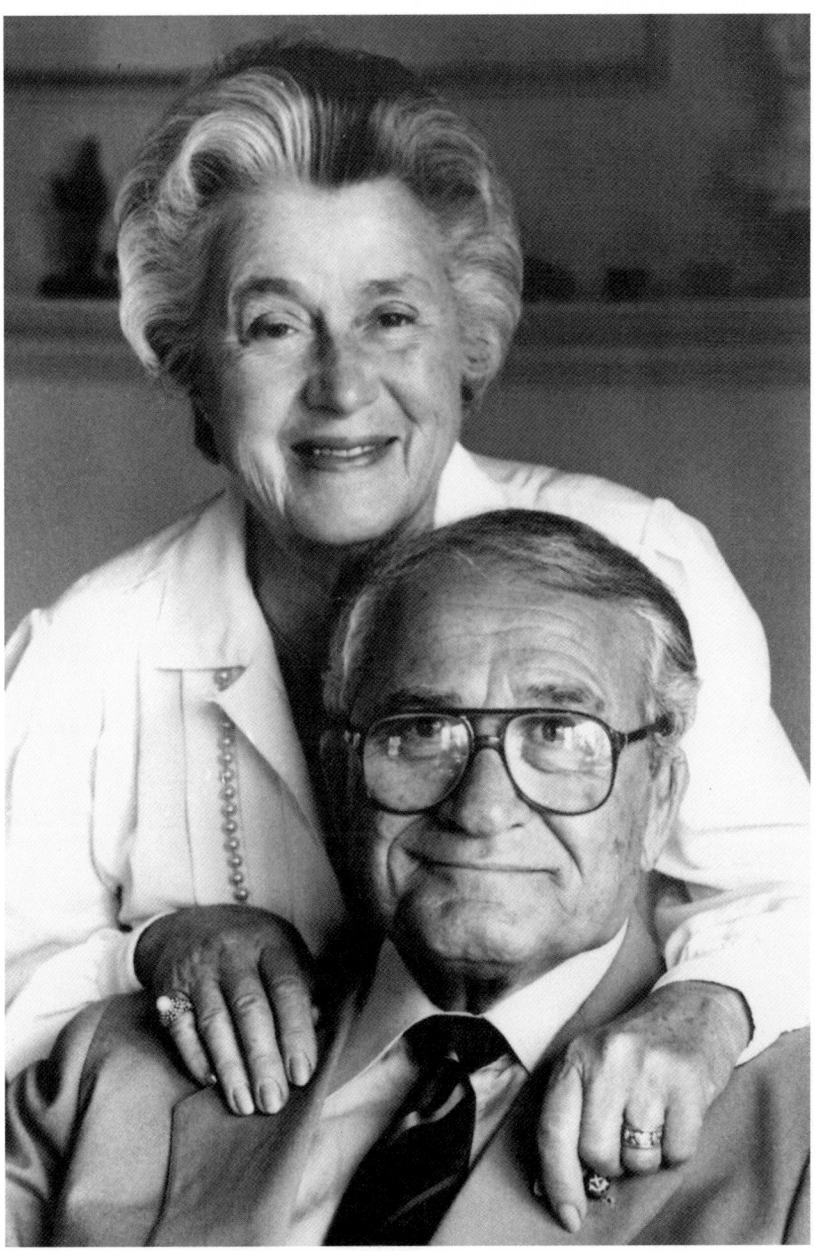

John and Emma L. Bonica

CONTRIBUTING AUTHORS

Janet Abrahm, MD
Associate Professor, Medicine
Harvard Medical School
Director, Pain and Palliative Care Program
Dana-Farber Cancer Institute and Brigham and Women's
    Hospital
Boston, Massachusetts

Ajit S. Ahluwalia, MD, MHA
Capital Hospice and Palliative Care
Falls Church, Virginia

Roger J. Allen, BS, BSPT, MS, PhD
Professor
Department of Physical Therapy
University of Puget Sound
Tacoma, Washington

Charles E. Argoff, MD
Professor of Neurology
Albany Medical College
Director, Comprehensive Pain Program
Albany Medical Center
Albany, New York

Paul M. Arnstein, RN, PhD
Clinical Nurse Specialist for Pain Relief
Director, MGH Cares About Pain Relief Project
Massachusetts General Hospital
Boston, Massachusetts

Wael F. Assad, MD
Department of Brain and Cognitive Sciences
Center for Learning and Memory
Massachusetts Institute of Technology
Boston, Massachusetts

Misha-Miroslav Backonja, MD
Professor of Neurology
University of Wisconsin
Madison, Wisconsin

Zahid H. Bajwa, MD
Director, Education and Clinical Pain Research
Beth Israel Deaconess Medical Center
Harvard Medical School
Boston, Massachusetts

Samir K. Ballas, MD, FACP, FASCP, DABPM
Professor of Medicine and Pediatrics
Cardeza Foundation for Hematologic Research
Department of Medicine
Jefferson Medical College
Philadelphia, Pennsylvania

Andrew Baranowski, MBBS, FRCA, MD, FFPMRCA
Honorary Senior Lecturer
The Institute for Neurology
University College London
Consultant in Pain Medicine
The Pain Management Centre
The National Hospital for Neurology and Neurosurgery
London, England

David Barnard, PhD, JD
Professor of Medicine
Director, Institute to Enhance Palliative Care
Director of Palliative Care Education, Center for Bioethics
    and Health Law
University of Pittsburgh
Pittsburgh, Pennsylvania

Allan J. Belzberg, MD, FRCSC
Associate Professor of Neurosurgery
Johns Hopkins School of Medicine
Attending Neurosurgeon
Johns Hopkins Hospital
Baltimore, Maryland

Charles B. Berde, MD, PhD
Sara Page Mayo Chair in Pediatric Pain Medicine
Chief, Division of Pain Medicine
Department of Anesthesiology, Perioperative and Pain
    Medicine
Children's Hospital
Professor of Anaesthesia (Pediatrics)
Harvard Medical School
Boston, Massachusetts

Prabhat K. Bhama, MD
Resident
Department of Otolaryngology—Head & Neck Surgery
University of Washington School of Medicine
Seattle, Washington

Andrew R. Block, PhD
Director of Pain Programs
Texas Back Institute
Plano, Texas

Nikolai Bogduk, MD, PhD
Conjoint Professor of Pain Medicine
University of Newcastle
Head, Department of Clinical Research
Royal Newcastly Centre
Newcastle, New South Wales
Australia

William S. Breitbart, MD
Chief, Psychiatry Service
Memorial Sloan-Kettering Cancer Center
New York, New York

Gary J. Brenner, MD, PhD
Assistant Professor
Harvard Medical School
Program Director, MGH Pain Medicine Fellowship
Department of Anesthesia, Critical Care and Pain Medicine
Massachusetts General Hospital
Boston, Massachusetts

Shane E. Brogan, MB, BCh
Assistant Professor
Department of Anesthesiology
University of Utah Health Sciences Center
Salt Lake City, Utah

David L. Brown, MD
Professor and Chair
Institute of Anesthesiology
Cleveland Clinic Foundation
Cleveland, Ohio

Stephen P. Bruehl, PhD
Department of Anesthesiology
Vanderbilt University School of Medicine
Nashville, Tennessee

Luis F. Buenaver, PhD
Department of Psychiatry & Behavioral Sciences
Center for Mind-Body Research
Johns Hopkins University School of Medicine
Baltimore, Maryland

Asokumar Buvanendran
Associate Professor of Anesthesiology
Department of Anesthesiology
Director, Orthopedic Anesthesia
Rush University Medical Center
Chicago, Illinois

Cynthia Campbell, MD
Swedish Medical Center
Seattle, Washington

Claudia M. Campbell
Department of Psychiatry & Behavioral Sciences
Center for Mind-Body Research
Johns Hopkins University School of Medicine
Baltimore, Maryland

James N. Campbell, MD
Professor of Neurosurgery
Department of Neurosurgery
Johns Hopkins University School of Medicine
Baltimore, Maryland

Jacqueline Casillas, MD, MSHS
Assistant Professor of Pediatrics
Division of Hematology/Oncology
Department of Pediatrics
David Geffen School of Medicine at UCLA
Los Angeles, California

Douglas G. Chang, MD, PhD
Chief, Physical Medicine and Rehabilitation
Department of Orthopaedic Surgery
University of California, San Diego
San Diego, California

C. Richard Chapman, PhD
Professor and Director
Department of Anesthesia
Pain Research Center
University of Utah
Salt Lake City, Utah

Ming L. Cheng, MD
Department of Neurosurgery
Rhode Island Hospital
Brown Medical School
Providence, Rhode Island

Gary P. Chimes, MD, PhD
Assistant Professor
Department of Physical Medicine and Rehabilitation
Director, Jackson T. Stephens Spine Clinic
Assistant Residency Program Director
University of Arkansas for Medical Sciences
Little Rock, Arkansas

Roger Chou, MD
Oregon Health & Science University
Associate Professor of Medicine
Department of Medicine and Department of Medical
    Informatics and Clinical Epidemiology
Portland, Oregon

Michael R. Clark, MD, MPH
Associate Professor and Director
Chronic Pain Treatment Programs
Department of Psychiatry & Behavioral Sciences
Johns Hopkins Medical Institutions
Baltimore, Maryland

Daniel J. Clauw, MD
Professor of Anesthesiology and Medicine
Associate Dean for Clinical and Translational Research
The University of Michigan
Ann Arbor, Michigan

Steven P. Cohen, MD
Associate Professor
Department of Anesthesiology & Critical Care Medicine
Johns Hopkins School of Medicine
Baltimore, Maryland
Associate Professor
Department of Anesthesiology
Uniformed Services University of the Health Sciences
Colonel, US Army
Walter Reed Army Medical Center
Washington, DC

Doris K. Cope, MS, MD
Professor and Vice Chairman of Pain Medicine
Department of Anesthesiology
University of Pittsburgh School of Medicine
Pittsburgh, Pennsylvania

Alberto Cortes-Ladino, MD
Chief Fellow, Department of Psychiatry and Behavioral
  Sciences
Memorial Sloan-Kettering Cancer Center
Weill Cornell Medical College
New York, New York

Michele Curatolo, MD, PhD
Professor
Department of Anaesthesia
Division of Pain Therapy
Bern University Hospital
Bern, Switzerland

Elaine S. Date, MD
Associate Professor
Division Head and Program Director
Physical Medicine and Rehabilitation
Department of Orthopaedic Surgery
Stanford University
Stanford, California

Richard A. Deyo, MD, MPH
Kaiser Permanente Professor of Evidence-Based Family
  Medicine
Director, OCTRI Community and Practice-Based Research
Departments of Family Medicine and Internal Medicine
Oregon Health & Science University
Portland, Oregon

Jan Dommerholt, PT, MPS, FAAPM
Bethesda Physiocare, Inc/Myopain Seminars, LLC
Bethesda, Maryland

Michael J. Dorsi, MD, FRCSC
Neurosurgical Resident
Department of Neurosurgery
Johns Hopkins Hospital
Baltimore, Maryland

Robert H. Dworkin, PhD
Professor of Anesthesiology, Neurology, Oncology, and
  Psychiatry
Vice-Chair for Clinical Research, Department of
  Anesthesiology
Director, Anesthesiology Clinical Research Center
University of Rochester School of Medicine and Dentistry
Rochester, New York

Elon Eisenberg
Director, Pain Relief Unit
Rambam Medical Center
Haifa, Israel

Joyce M. Engel, PhD, OT
Professor
Department of Rehabilitation Medicine
University of Washington School of Medicine
Seattle, Washington

Joel B. Epstein, DMD, MSD, FRCD(C)
Professor and Head
Department of Oral Medicine and Diagnostic Sciences
Director of Interdisciplinary Program in Oral Cancer
Chicago Cancer Center
College Medicine
University of Illinois at Chicago
Chicago, Illinois

Emad N. Eskandar, MD
Assistant Professor
Harvard Medical School
Director of Stereotactic and Functional Neurosurgery
Massachusetts General Hospital
Boston, Massachusetts

Ronnie Fass, MD
Professor of Medicine
Section of Gastroenterology
University of Arizona School of Medicine
Head, Neuroenteric Clinical Research Group
Southern Arizona VA Health Care System
University of Arizona Health Sciences Center
Tucson, Arizona

Roger B. Fillingim, PhD
Professor
University of Florida College of Dentistry
Staff Psychologist
Malcom Randall VA Medical Center
Gainesville, Florida

Ezekiel Fink, MD
Clinical Instructor
Departments of Neurology and Physical Medicine and
  Rehabilitation
University of California
Los Angeles, California

Scott M. Fishman, MD
Professor of Anesthesiology
Chief, Division of Pain Medicine
Department of Anesthesiology and Pain Medicine
University of California, Davis School of Medicine
Sacramento, California

Dermot R. Fitzgibbon, MB, BCh
Associate Professor of Anesthesiology
Adjunct Associate Professor of Medicine
University of Washington School of Medicine
Director of Pain Services
University of Washington Medical Center
Director, Cancer Pain Services
University of Washington Medical Center and Seattle Cancer
  Care Alliance
Seattle, Washington

Rollin M. Gallagher, MD, MPH
Clinical Professor of Psychiatry and Anesthesiology and
  Critical Care
University of Pennsylvania
Director of Pain Management
Philadelphia Veteran Affairs Medical Center
Philadelphia, Pennsylvania

Gregory C. Gardner, MD, FACP
Professor of Medicine
Division of Rheumatology
Adjunct Professor of Orthopaedics and Rehabilitation
  Medicine
University of Washington School of Medicine
Seattle, Washington

Robert J. Gatchel, PhD, ABPP
Professor and Chairman
Department of Psychology
College of Science
University of Texas at Arlington
Arlington, Texas
Clinical Research Director
Eugene McDermott Center for Pain Management
University of Texas Southwestern Medial Center at Dallas
Dallas, Texas

Gerald F. Gebhart, PhD
Director, Center for Pain Research
University of Pittsburgh
Pittsburgh, Pennsylvania

Youssef Ghabrial
Area Director
Department of Orthopaedics
Newcastle Bone and Joint Institute
Newcastle, New South Wales
Australia

Christopher Gilligan, MD, MBA
Staff Physician
Center for Pain Medicine
Massachusetts General Hospital
Instructor in Anaesthesia and Emergency Medicine
Harvard Medical School
Boston, Massachusetts

Aaron M. Gilson, MS, MSSW, PhD
Associate Director for US Policy Research
Pain and Policy Studies Group
Paul P. Carbone Comprehensive Cancer Center
University of Wisconsin School of Medicine and Public
  Health
Madison, Wisconsin

Peter J. Goadsby, MD, PhD, DSc, FRACP, FRCP
Professor of Neurology
Headache Group, Department of Neurology
University of California
San Francisco, California

Michael S. Gold, PhD
Associate Professor
Department of Anesthesiology
University of Pittsburgh School of Medicine
Pittsburgh, Pennsylvania

Douglas L. Gourlay, MD, MSc, FRCPC, FASAM
Centre for Addiction and Mental Health
Toronto, Ontario
Canada

Jayantilal Govind†, MBChB, MMed, FAFOM
Director and Senior Staff Specialist
Occupational and Pain Medicine
Canberra Hospital and Australian National University
Canberra, Australian Capital Territory
Conjoint Senior Lecturer
University of Newcastle
Newcastle, New South Wales
Australia

Christine Greco, MD
Department of Anesthesiology, Perioperative and Pain
  Medicine
Children's Hospital
Boston, Massachusetts

Joel D. Greenspan, PhD
Professor
Department of Biomedical Sciences
University of Maryland Dental School
Program in Neuroscience
University of Maryland
Baltimore, Maryland

Robert S. Griffin, MD, PhD
Department of Anesthesia and Critical Care
Massachusetts General Hospital
Boston, Massachusetts

Narasimha R. Gundamaraj, MD
Assistant Professor of Clinical Anesthesiology
Keck School of Medicine
University of Southern California
Staff Physician
University of Southern California Pain Clinic
Los Angeles, California

Neil A. Hagen, MD, FRCP
Head, Division of Palliative Medicine
University of Calgary
Calgary, Alberta
Canada

R. Norman Harden, MD
Associate Professor
Northwestern University
Director, Center for Pain Studies
Rehabilitation Institute of Chicago
Chicago, Illinois

Michael Hauck
Department of Neurophysiology and Pathophysiology
University Medical Center Hamburg-Eppendorf
Hamburg, Germany

Jennifer A. Haythornthwaite, PhD
Professor
Department of Psychiatry & Behavioral Sciences
Center for Mind-Body Research
Johns Hopkins University School of Medicine
Baltimore, Maryland

Michael L. Hearndon, DO
Department of Physical Medicine and Rehabilitation
University of Arkansas for Medical Sciences
Little Rock, Arkansas

Howard A. Heit, MD, FACP, FASAM
Assistant Clinical Professor of Medicine
Georgetown University School of Medicine
Washington, DC

†Deceased

Jeanne Hernandez, PhD, MSPH
Assistant Professor
Department of Anesthesiology
University of North Carolina
Director of Behavioral Medicine
Anesthesia Pain Clinic
Spine and Pain Center, UNC Hospitals
Chapel Hill, North Carolina

Keela A. Herr, PhD, RN, FAAN, AGSF
Professor and Chair, Adult and Gerontology
RWJ Executive Nurse Fellow
College of Nursing
University of Iowa
Iowa City, Iowa

Stanley A. Herring, MD
Clinical Professor
Director, UW Medicine Spine Center
University of Washington
Seattle, Washington

Anita H. Hickey, MD, CAPT, USN
Head, Pain Research
Department of Anesthesiology
Naval Medical Center San Diego
San Diego, California

Robert W. Hurley, MD, PhD
Associate Professor
Chief of Pain Medicine
Department of Anesthesiology
University of Florida
Gainesville, Florida

Charles E. Inturrisi, PhD
Professor
Department of Pharmacology
Weill Cornell Medical College
New York, New York

Gordon A. Irving, MBBS, MSc, MMed, FFA(SA)
Clinical Associate Professor
Department of Anesthesia
University of Washington School of Medicine
Medical Director, Swedish Pain and Headache Center
Seattle, Washington

Kenneth C. Jackson II, BSc Pharmacy, PharmD
Associate Professor
Pacific University School of Pharmacy
Hillsboro, Oregon

Robert N. Jamison, PhD
Associate Professor
Harvard Medical School
Brigham and Women's Hospital
Boston, Massachusetts

Nora A. Janjan, MD, MPSA
Professor
Department of Radiation Oncology
University of Texas M.D. Anderson Cancer Center
Houston, Texas

Mark P. Jensen, PhD
Professor
Department of Rehabilitation Medicine
University of Washington School of Medicine
Seattle, Washington

Kaj H. Johansen, MD, PhD
Clinical Professor of Surgery
George I. Thomas, MD, Clinical Professor of Surgery (Emeritus)
University of Washington School of Medicine
Swedish Heart and Vascular Institute
Seattle, Washington

David E. Joranson, MSSW
Distinguished Scientist
Director, Pain and Policy Studies Group
Paul P. Carbone Comprehensive Cancer Center
University of Wisconsin School of Medicine and Public Health
Madison, Wisconsin

David A. Keith, BDS, FRDSCS, DMD
Professor
Department of Oral and Maxillofacial Surgery
Massachusetts General Hospital
Harvard School of Dental Medicine
Director, Dental/Oral and Maxillofacial Surgery
Harvard Vanguard Medical Associates
Boston, Massachusetts

Joel L. Kent, MD
Associate Professor
Department of Anesthesiology
Director, Division of Pain Management
University of Rochester School of Medicine and Dentistry
Rochester, New York

Kenneth L. Kirsh, PhD
Assistant Professor
Pharmacy Practice and Science
University of Kentucky College of Pharmacy
Clinical Psychologist
The Pain Treatment Center of the Bluegrass
Lexington, Kentucky

Nancy D. Kishino, OTR, CVE
Director, West Coast Spine Restoration Center
Riverside, California

Robert J. Klickovich, MD
Department of Anesthesiology, Pain and Perioperative Medicine
Brigham and Women's Hospital
Boston, Massachusetts

Ronald J. Kulich, PhD
Associate Professor
The Craniofacial Pain and Headache Center
Tufts University School of Dental Medicine
Lecturer, Department of Anesthesia and Critical Care
Division of Pain Medicine
Massachusetts General Hospital
Harvard Medical School
Boston, Massachusetts

Irfan Lalani, MD
Assistant Professor
Department of Anesthesiology and Pain Medicine
University of Texas M.D. Anderson Cancer Center
Houston, Texas

Joseph C. Langlois, MD
Clinical Professor of Dermatology
University of Washington School of Medicine
Seattle, Washington

Frederick A. Lenz, MD
Professor of Neurosurgery
Johns Hopkins University School of Medicine
Baltimore, Maryland

Bengt Linderoth, MD, PhD
Department of Neurosurgery
Karolinska Hospital
Stockholm, Sweden

Arthur G. Lipman, PharmD
Professor, Department of Pharmacotherapy
College of Pharmacy
Adjunct Professor, Department of Anesthesiology
School of Medicine
Director of Clinical Pharmacology, Pain Management Center
University of Utah Health Sciences Center
Salt Lake City, Utah

Spencer S. Liu, MD
Clinical Professor of Anesthesiology
Director of Acute Pain Service
Hospital for Special Surgery
Weill Cornell Medical Center
New York, New York

David Loomba, MD
Assistant Professor
Director of Resident Education
Department of Anesthesiology and Pain Medicine
University of California
UC Davis Health System
Sacramento, California

Jürgen Lorenz, MD
Faculty of Life Sciences
Hamburg University of Applied Sciences
Human Physiology and Biology Lab
Hamburg, Germany

Raymond J. Maciewicz, MD, PhD
Director, PBS Medical Consulting
Boston, Massachusetts

Gagan Mahajan, MD
Assistant Professor
Director, Fellowship in Pain Medicine
Department of Anesthesiology and Pain Medicine
University of California, Davis School of Medicine
UC Davis Medical Center
Sacramento, California

Kenneth R. Maravilla, MD
Professor, Radiology
Neurological Surgery Director
MR Research Laboratory
University of Washington
Seattle, Washington

Martha A. Maurer, MSSW, MPH
Pain and Policy Studies Group
World Health Organization Collaborating Center for Policy
    and Communications in Cancer Care
University of Wisconsin School of Medicine and Public
    Health
Paul P. Carbone Comprehensive Cancer Center
Madison, Wisconsin

Emeran Mayer
Professor, Departments of Medicine, Physiology, Psychiatry,
    and Biobehavioral Sciences
David Geffen School of Medicine at UCLA
Director, UCLA Center for Neurovisceral Sciences &
    Women's Health
UCLA Division of Digestive Diseases
Los Angeles, California

Bill McCarberg, MD
Founder, Chronic Pain Management Program
Kaiser Permanente
Assistant Clinical Professor (voluntary)
University of California, San Diego
San Diego, California

Regina McConley, MA
Doctoral Graduate Student
Medical Psychology
University of Alabama at Birmingham
Birmingham, Alabama

Lance M. McCracken, PhD
Consultant Clinical Psychologist and Clinical Lead
Pain Management Unit
Royal National Hospital for Rheumatic Diseases
Visiting Fellow, Pain Management Unit
Department of Psychology
University of Bath
Bath, United Kingdom

Ellen McGough, PT, MEd
Lecturer
Department of Rehabilitation Medicine
University of Washington
Seattle, Washington

**Brian E. McGuirk, MBBS, DPH(OH),
    FAFOM(RACP), FAFOM**
Senior Staff Specialist, Occupational (Musculoskeletal)
    Medicine
Hunter New England Area Health Service
New Castle, New South Wales
Australia

James P. McLean[†], MD
Assistant Professor
Department of Physical Medicine and Rehabilitation
University of Kansas Medical Center
Kansas City, Kansas

Noshir R. Mehta, DMD, MDS, MS
Professor and Director
The Craniofacial Pain and Headache Center
Tufts University
Chairman
Department of General Dentistry
Tufts University School of Dental Medicine
Boston, Massachusetts

M. Stephen Melton, MD
Assistant Professor
Department of Anesthesiology
Duke University Medical Center
Durham, North Carolina

[†]Deceased

James R. Miner, MD, FACEP
Associate Professor of Emergency Medicine
University of Minnesota Medical School
Department of Emergency Medicine
Hennepin County Medical Center
Minneapolis, Minnesota

Asako Miyakoshi, MD
Assistant Professor of Neuroradiology
Department of Radiology
University of Washington School of Medicine
Seattle, Washington

Jane Moore, MBBS, MSc
Honorary Consultant Gynaecologist
Nuffield Department of Obstetrics and Gynaecology
John Radcliffe Hospital
Oxford, England

David B. Morris, PhD
University Professor
University of Virginia
Charlottesville, Virginia

Cameron Muir, MD
Executive Vice President, Quality and Access
Capital Hospice and Palliative Care
Falls Church, Virginia

Richard A. Mularski, MD, MSHS, MCR, FCCP
Clinical Assistant Professor
Departments of Medicine, Pulmonary and Critical Care
    Medicine
Senior Scholar, Center for Ethics in Health Care
Oregon Health & Science University
Clinical Investigator, The Center for Health Research
Pulmonary/Critical Care Medicine
Kaiser Permanente Northwest
Portland, Oregon

Timothy Ness, MD, PhD
Professor of Anesthesiology
University of Alabama at Birmingham
Birmingham, Alabama

Carl E. Noe, MD
Medical Director
Baylor Center for Pain Management
Baylor University Medical Center
Dallas, Texas

Richard B. North, MD
Professor of Neurosurgery, Anesthesiology and Critical Care
    Medicine (ret.)
Johns Hopkins University School of Medicine
LifeBridge Brain & Spine Institute
Baltimore, Maryland

Donna D. Ohnmeiss, PhD
President
Texas Back Institute Research Foundation
Plano, Texas

Akiko Okifuji, PhD
Professor
Department of Anesthesiology
University of Utah
Salt Lake City, Utah

John E. Olerud, MD
Professor of Medicine
Head, Division of Dermatology
Department of Medicine
University of Washington School of Medicine
Seattle, Washington

Richard K. Osenbach, MD
Assistant Professor
Division of Neurosurgery
Duke University Medical Center
Durham, North Carolina

Judith A. Paice, PhD, RN, FAAN
Research Professor of Medicine
Director, Cancer Pain Program
Division of Hematology-Oncology
Feinberg School of Medicine, Northwestern University
Full Member, Robert H. Lurie Comprehensive Cancer
    Center
Chicago, Illinois

Tonya M. Palermo, PhD
Associate Professor
Anesthesiology & Peri-Operative Medicine/Pain and
    Regional Anesthesia Research
Oregon Health & Science University
Portland, Oregon

Steven D. Passik, PhD
Associate Attending Psychologist
Memorial Sloan-Kettering Cancer Center
Associate Professor of Psychiatry
Weill Cornell Medical College
New York, New York

Parag G. Patil, MD, PhD
Department of Neurosurgery
University of Michigan Hospitals and Heath Centers
Ann Arbor, Michigan

David R. Patterson, PhD, ABPP, ABPH
Professor, Department of Psychology
Department of Rehabilitation Medicine
University of Washington School of Medicine
Seattle, Washington

David Peterson, MD
Drug Information Specialist
University of Utah Hospital
Drug Information Service
Salt Lake City, Utah

Joel M. Press, MD
Reva and David Logan Distinguished Chair of
    Musculoskeletal Rehabilitation
Associate Professor of Physical Medicine and Rehabilitation
Feinberg/Northwestern School of Medicine
Rehabilitation Institute of Chicago
Chicago, Illinois

Alan Randich, PhD
Professor and Director, Behavioral Neuroscience Program
Department of Psychology
University of Alabama at Birmingham
Birmingham, Alabama

Ralph F. Rashbaum, MD
Texas Back Institute
Plano, Texas

James P. Rathmell, MD
Chief, Division of Pain Medicine
Department of Anesthesia, Critical Care and Pain Medicine
Massachusetts General Hospital
Associate Professor of Anaesthesia
Harvard Medical School Boston
Boston, Massachusetts

Ben A. Rich, JD, PhD
Professor of Bioethics
University of California, Davis School of Medicine
Department of Internal Medicine
Department of Anesthesiology and Pain Medicine
UC Davis Health System
Sacramento, California

Steven Richeimer, MD
Chief, Division of Pain Medicine
Associate Professor of Anesthesiology
Keck School of Medicine
University of Southern California
Los Angeles, California

James P. Robinson, MD, PhD
Clinical Associate Professor
Department of Rehabilitation Medicine
University of Washington
Seattle, Washington

Lauren J. Rogak
Department of Psychiatry and Behavioral Sciences
Memorial Sloan-Kettering Cancer Center
New York, New York

Edgar Ross, MD
Director, Pain Management Center
Brigham and Women's Hospital
Assistant Professor of Anesthesia
Harvard Medical School
Boston, Massachusetts

Karen M. Ryan, MA
Associate Director for International Policy Research
Pain and Policy Studies Group
Paul P. Carbone Comprehensive Cancer Center
University of Wisconsin School of Medicine and Public
   Health
Madison, Wisconsin

Andrew J. Saxon, MD
Professor, Department of Psychiatry & Behavioral Sciences
University of Washington
Director, Addiction Patient Care Line
Center of Excellence in Substance Abuse Treatment and
   Education
VA Puget Sound Health Care System
Seattle, Washington

Michael E. Schatman, PhD
Research Director
Pain and Addiction Study Foundation
Bellevue, Washington

Neil L. Schechter, MD
Director, Pain Relief Program
Connecticut Children's Medical Center
Hartford, Connecticut
Professor of Pediatrics
University of Connecticut School of Medicine
Farmington, Connecticut

Gregory A. Schmidt, MD, FCCP
Professor of Medicine
Director of Critical Care
Division of Pulmonary Diseases, Critical Care, and
   Occupational Medicine
Carver College of Medicine
University of Iowa
Iowa City, Iowa

Jerome Schofferman, MD
SpineCare Medical Group
San Francisco Spine Institute
Daly City, California

Mark M. Schubert, DDS, MSD
Professor, Department of Oral Medicine
University of Washington School of Dentistry
Director of Oral Medicine
Seattle Cancer Care Alliance and Fred Hutchinson Cancer
   Research Center
Seattle, Washington

Steven J. Scrivani, DDS, DMedSc
Professor
The Craniofacial Pain and Headache Center
Tufts University
Research Associate
Pain and Analgesia Imaging and Neuroscience (P.A.I.N.)
   Group
Brain Imaging Center
McLean Hospital
Harvard Medical School
Boston, Massachusetts

Curtis N. Sessler, MD, FCCP, FCCM
Orhan Muren Professor of Medicine
Pulmonary and Critical Care Medicine
Virginia Commonwealth University
Medical Director
Critical Care, MRICU
Medical College of Virginia Hospitals
Richmond, Virginia

Jay P. Shah, MD
Staff Physiatrist
Rehabilitation Medicine Department
Clinical Research Center
National Institutes of Health
Washington, DC

Sam R. Sharar, MD
Professor
Department of Anesthesiology
University of Washington School of Medicine
Harborview Medical Center
Seattle, Washington

Donald C. Shields, MD, PhD
Department of Neurosurgery
Massachusetts General Hospital
Harvard Medical School
Boston, Massachusetts

Philip J. Siddall, MBBS MM (Pain Mgt), PhD, FFPMANZCA
Clinical Associate Professor
Pain Management Research Institute
University of Sydney
Royal North Shore Hospital
Sydney, Australia

Charles A. Simpson, DC, DACBO
Vice President, Medical Director
Complementary Healthcare Plans, Inc
Beaverton, Oregon

Howard S. Smith, MD
Associate Professor & Academic Director of Pain
    Management
Department of Anesthesiology
Albany Medical College
Albany, New York

Pamela L. Squire, MD, CCFP
North Vancouver, British Columbia
Canada

Steven P. Stanos, Jr, DO
Medical Director
Chronic Pain Care Center
Rehabilitation Institute of Chicago
Assistant Professor
Department of Physical Medicine and Rehabilitation
Assistant Program Director
Multidisciplinary Pain Fellowship
Northwestern University Medical School
Feinberg School of Medicine
Chicago, Illinois

Tatiana D. Starr, MA
Department of Psychiatry and Behavioral Sciences
Memorial Sloan-Kettering Cancer Center
New York, New York

M. Alan Stiles, DMD
Facial Pain Management
Department of Oral and Maxillofacial Surgery
Thomas Jefferson University
Philadelphia, Pennsylvania

Milan P. Stojanovic, MD
Spine & Pain Institute of New England
Dedham, Massachusetts

Mark D. Sullivan, MD, PhD
Department of Rehabilitation Medicine
University of Washington
Seattle, Washington

Kimberly S. Swanson, PhD
Licensed Clinical Psychologist
The Everett Clinic
Everett, Washington

Karen L. Syrjala, PhD
Member and Director of Behavioral Sciences
Clinical Research Division
Fred Hutchinson Cancer Research Center
Associate Professor
Department of Psychiatry and Behavioral Sciences
University of Washington School of Medicine
Seattle, Washington

Raymond C. Tait, PhD
Professor, Department of Neurology and Psychiatry
St. Louis University
St. Louis, Missouri

Ronald R. Tasker, MD, MSc, FRCS(C)
Professor Emeritus of Neurosurgery
University of Toronto
Division of Neurosurgery
Toronto Western Hospital
Toronto, Canada

Rajbala Thakur, MD
Associate Professor of Anesthesiology
Medical Director, Anesthesia Clinical Research Center
University of Rochester School of Medicine and Dentistry
Rochester, New York

Brian R. Theodore, MS
Department of Psychology
University of Texas at Arlington
Arlington, Texas

George I. Thomas, MD
Clinical Professor of Surgery
University of Washington School of Medicine
Seattle, Washington

Beverly E. Thorn, PhD, ABPP
Editor, Journal of Clinical Psychology
Professor of Psychology
University of Alabama
Tuscaloosa, Alabama

Knox H. Todd, MD, MPH
Professor of Emergency Medicine
Albert Einstein College of Medicine
Director, Pain and Emergency Medicine Institute
Beth Israel Medical Center
New York, New York

Rolf-Detlef Treede, MD
Professor of Neurophysiology
Center for Biomedicine and Medical Technology, Mannheim
Ruprecht Karls University, Heidelberg
Mannheim, Germany

Dennis C. Turk, PhD
John and Emma Bonica Professor of Anesthesiology & Pain
    Research
University of Washington
Seattle, Washington

Katy Vincent, MBBS, BSc
Pelvic Pain Fellow and Honorary Registrar
Nuffield Department of Obstetrics and Gynaecology
John Radcliffe Hospital
Oxford, England

Gary A. Walco, PhD
Director, The David Center for Children's Pain and
    Palliative Care
Hackensack University Medical Center
Hackensack, New Jersey
Professor of Pediatrics
University of Medicine and Dentistry of New Jersey—
    New Jersey Medical School
Newark, New Jersey

David Walk, MD
Associate Professor or Neurology
University of Minnesota
Minneapolis, Minnesota

Barbara B. Walker, PhD
Clinical Professor
Department of Psychological and Brain Sciences
Indiana University
Bloomington, Indiana

Anthony C. Wang, MD
Department of Neurosurgery
University of Michigan Medical School
Ann Arbor, Michigan

Ajay D. Wasan, MD
Assistant Professor of Anesthesiology and Psychiatry
Harvard Medical School and Brigham and Women's
    Hospital
Boston, Massachusetts

Ernest A. Weymuller, Jr., MD
Allison T. Wanamaker Professor and Chair
Department of Otolaryngology – Head & Neck Surgery
University of Washington School of Medicine
Seattle, Washington

Stuart E. Willick, MD
Associate Professor
Division of Physical Medicine and Rehabilitation
University of Utah
Salt Lake City, Utah

Hilary D. Wilson, PhD
Senior Fellow
Anesthesiology
University of Washington
Seattle, Washington

Ann M. Wilson, PT, MEd
Clinical Associate Professor
Department of Physical Therapy
University of Puget Sound
Tacoma, Washington

Cynthia A. Wong, MD
Associate Professor
Department of Anesthesiology
Northwestern University Feinberg School of Medicine
Chicago, Illinois

Heng Yu Wong, BM BCh, FRCP, FAMS, MA
Gastroenterologist
Mount Elizabeth Hospital
Singapore

Joshua Wootton, Mdiv, PhD
Director of Pain Psychology
Arnold Pain Management Center
Beth Israel Deaconess Medical Center
Assistant Professor
Department of Aneasthesia
Harvard Medical School
Boston, Massachusetts

**Paul J. Wrigley, MBBS MM (Pain Mgt), PhD,
    FFPMANZCA**
Clinical Senior Lecturer and Senior Staff Specialist in Pain
    Medicine
University of Sydney
Royal North Shore Hospital
Sydney, Australia

Christopher L. Wu, MD
Associate Professor
Department of Anesthesiology
The Johns Hopkins University
Baltimore, Maryland

Jean C. Yi, PhD
Senior Fellow
Biobehavioral Sciences, Clinical Research Division
Fred Hutchinson Cancer Research Center
Seattle, Washington

Way Yin, MD
Medical Director
Bellingham Spine Pain Specialists,
Bellingham, Washington
Clinical Assistant Professor
Department of Anesthesiology
University of Washington School of Medicine
Seattle, Washington

Lonnie K. Zeltzer, MD
Director, Pediatric Pain Program
Mattel Children's Hospital at UCLA
Professor of Pediatrics, Anesthesiology, Psyciatry and
    Biobehavioral Sciences
David Geffen School of Medicine at UCLA
Los Angeles, California

Michael Zenz, MD
Professor of Anaesthesiology and Director of
    Anaesthesiology, Intensive Care, Palliative Medicine and
    Pain Therapy
University Hospital Bergmannsheil
Bochum, Germany

Nikolai Bogduk, MD, PhD
Conjoint Professor of Pain Medicine
University of Newcastle
Head, Department of Clinical Research
Royal Newcastle Centre
Newcastle, New South Wales, Australia
Spinal Pain/Interventional Pain Treatment

C. Richard Chapman, PhD
Professor and Director
Pain Research Center
Department of Anesthesiology
University of Utah
Salt Lake City, Utah
Psychology

Emad N. Eskandar, MD
Director of Stereotactic and Functional Neurosurgery
Massachusetts General Hospital
Assistant Professor
Harvard Medical School
Boston, Massachusetts
Neurosurgical Approaches to Pain

Perry G. Fine, MD
Professor, Department of Anesthesiology
Pain Research Center
School of Medicine
University of Utah
Salt Lake City, Utah
Vice President for Medical Affairs
National Hospice and Palliative Care Organization
Alexandria, Virginia
Cancer Related Pain

Gerald F. Gebhart, PhD
Director, Center for Pain Research
University of Pittsburgh
Pittsburgh, Pennsylvania
Visceral Pain

Arthur G. Lipman, PharmD
Professor
Department of Pharmacotherapy, College of Pharmacy
Adjunct Professor
Department of Anesthesiology, School of Medicine
Director of Clinical Pharmacology
Pain Management Center, University Hospitals and Clinics
University of Utah Health Sciences Center
Salt Lake City, Utah
Pharmacology

Timothy Ness, MD, PhD
Professor of Anesthesiology
University of Alabama at Birmingham
Birmingham, Alabama
Basic Science

Ben A. Rich, JD, PhD
Professor of Bioethics
University of California, Davis School of Medicine
Department of Internal Medicine
Department of Anesthesiology and Pain Medicine
UC Davis Health System
Sacramento, California
Legal and Ethical Issues

James P. Robinson, MD, PhD
Clinical Associate Professor
Department of Rehabilitation Medicine
University of Washington
Seattle, Washington
Musculoskeletal Pain/Pain Rehabilitation

Mark S. Wallace, MD
Professor of Clinical Anesthesiology
Program Director
Center for Pain Medicine
University of California, San Diego
San Diego, California
Neuropathic Pain/Pain Evaluation

Christopher L. Wu, MD
Associate Professor
Department of Anesthesiology
The Johns Hopkins University
Baltimore, Maryland
Acute Pain

This, the fourth edition of *Bonica's Management of Pain*, continues the tradition that John J. Bonica, M.D., started with the publication of the first edition in 1953. That was a herculean endeavor and monumental achievement, as no one had ever attempted to comprehensively describe all that was known about pain and how to diagnose and treat it. The first edition was almost exclusively the work of Dr. Bonica; only minor sections were contributed by his colleagues. It took him 30 years to bring out the second edition, which was the product of not only Dr. Bonica but also of a long list of contributors who, in fact, wrote more than half of the pages. This edition was characterized by extensive consideration of the anatomy and physiology underlying pain and by the discussion of multidisciplinary pain management and pain clinics.

The field of pain management, launched by Dr. Bonica's own practice and teaching and by his founding of the International Association for the Study of Pain, had flourished by the time of the second edition. The field of pain medicine developed rapidly, and Bonica knew that another edition of the *Management of Pain* would have to be written to keep his textbook current. Unfortunately, his health limited his ability to undertake this task. Shortly before he died, I promised him that there would be a third edition that I would edit with the help of colleagues at the University of Washington. The third edition was published in 2000, firmly based upon the format of the prior editions but expanding the content to keep up with developments in both basic science and clinical pain management.

Another decade has passed; the sciences basic to pain and clinical practice have continued to rapidly expand. It is time for a new edition of this great book; I am thrilled by the job that the new editors have done in assembling an all-star group of contributors to continue what Dr. Bonica began over 50 years ago. This latest edition of *Bonica's Management of Pain* will again set the pace for the coming decade of pain research, teaching, and patient care.

Whereas everyone active in pain research or patient care knew John Bonica in the last 30 years of the twentieth century, we now have spawned a generation or two of workers in this field who know him only through his publications or the occasional prophetic story. Although this is an understandable reality, it is unfortunate. Dr. Bonica was a truly great man whose efforts almost single handedly caused pain to be put on the road maps of both basic science and health care. As I wrote in his obituary published in *Pain*[1]:

"He cared about his patients for whom he tirelessly worked. He cared about the research that scientists undertook to understand the mechanisms of pain. He cared about those who suffered in far-away places; he wanted their doctors to learn about pain management. He cared about how governments impacted the delivery of pain management services. He cared about his students, trainees and colleagues. He really cared about those who attempted to continue what he had started. He cared about his children and his wife, although his career took time away from them." [(p2)]

More than an inscription on his gravestone, the continued life of *Bonica's Management of Pain* tells us of his accomplishments. It was a true privilege to have known him and his family, worked for and with him, and to have carried on the traditions that he launched. JJB, as he was known to all who worked alongside him, would have been gratified to see the advances that he inspired. His greatness will live on through the publication of this fourth edition.

John D. Loeser, M. D.
March, 2009

1. Loeser, JD: Obituary: John J Bonica, M.D., and Emma B. Bonica. Pain. 1994;59:1–3.

PREFACE TO THE FOURTH EDITION (2009)

This book was first introduced 56 years ago, a time that many believe marks the beginning of the multidisciplinary field of pain management. The idea for a clinical textbook devoted to the management of pain came from John Bonica, and in its first edition he wrote that the book offers a synthesis of information from disparate disciplines to form a complete discussion on pain and its management. Such a book, he believed, would strengthen the pain field by assimilating new insights and growing knowledge from many interested disciplines. Since the first edition in 1953, the purpose of the book has remained essentially the same, despite extraordinary growth in the science and practice of pain management, and the emergence of pain medicine as its own discipline. The book has remained a key reference for clinicians through all its editions, largely because of the high quality of the original book, and the ability to attract world-class experts to engage in his project, even years after Dr. Bonica's death in 1994. It was with trepidation and pride that we, the three chief editors, accepted the task of shepherding the next edition of this essential book to publication. We quickly realized that we were no match for Bonica, who formulated and wrote large parts of the original book himself and from the start, we solicited help from expert subeditors. As an editorial group, we made several key decisions: that we would keep the book near its original manageable size, that understanding anew the key role played by central mechanisms in pain, that we would shift the book's emphasis from its focus on peripheral (anatomically-based) mechanisms to one with a greater focus on neural (global) mechanisms, and that we would include new or updated chapters on issues that impact clinical pain management such as pain training, regulatory and political issues, and conducting clinical trials.

In his first edition, John Bonica tells us that he was called to write his book out of of the ". . . deep feeling for those who are afflicted with intractable pain, and by an intense desire to contribute something toward the alleviation of their suffering." This commitment originated from his experiences in treating wounded soldiers with intractable pain during the Second World War. It is sad and ironic that this fourth edition is now published at a time when undertreated pain is more widely recognized than ever and, in part, informed by wounded soldiers returning from the wars in Iraq and Afghanistan. In the year just prior to publishing this, the fourth edition, the U.S. Congress passed, and the President of the United States signed into law, two bills that aim to improve pain care for our active military personnel and veterans respectively. More than 50 years after Bonica began to raise awareness about the plight of those in pain, our society increasingly values safe and effective control of pain, and this trend echoes Bonica's vision of a world free of suffering from treatable pain.

The fourth edition of the textbook remains faithful to Bonica's original intent that his book should provide a comprehensive reference for practicing clinicians across all disciplines. In 1953, Bonica was one of few experts in the new field of pain medicine, and he almost single-handedly undertook the task of producing the first clinical textbook. Now, there are many experts with a remarkable depth of knowledge. It is a testament to Bonica that the many leading authorities contributing to the present edition as authors and section editors feel sincerely indebted to him, and they have willingly given of their time to maintain his legacy. Through its second and third editions, the book maintained a structure and organization similar to the 1st edition. In this new edition, every chapter has been revised, substantially rewritten, or represents a completely new chapter and or topic. With the addition of new material, there will undoubtedly be overlap between chapters. With a text of such broad scope, some degree of overlap is inevitable; indeed, we often allowed significant overlap, so that each chapter would stand on its own during independent perusal or study.

This book is divided into 6 parts: (1) Basic Considerations, (2) Economic, Political, Legal, and Ethical Considerations, (3) Evaluation of the Pain Patient, (4) Pain Conditions, (5) Methods for Symptomatic Control, and (6) Provisions of Pain Treatment. Basic Considerations offers an orientation to the history of pain management and the concepts and paradigms fundamental to this field, including taxonomy, basic science, anatomy, physiology, psychology, and social science. Economic, Political, Legal, and Ethical Considerations represents new content for this textbook, reflecting the emerging social impact of pain and pain management. Evaluation of the Pain Patient covers physical and psychological assessment, use of imaging and other technology-based testing, as well as special assessment for function, disability, addiction, and multidisciplinary care. Pain Conditions is the largest single part of the text, comprising 9 sections and 53 chapters. These sections include neuropathic pain syndromes; psychological contributions to pain; vascular, cutaneous, and musculoskeletal pain disorders; pain due to cancer; acute pain; pain in special populations; visceral pain disorders; regional pain; and low back pain. The section on pain in special populations addresses populations such as children, older persons, and those with pain and addiction. The regional pain section is a holdover from past editions and covers pain disorders that are associated with discrete parts of the body such as facial pain, cranial neuralgias, and pain syndromes associated with upper or lower extremities. Methods of Symptomatic Control is another large part of the text which is partitioned into the following 6 sections: pharmacologic therapies, psychological techniques, physical and other noninterventional modalities, implanted electrical stimulators, interventional pain management, and surgical approaches. Provision of Pain Treatment is the final part of this text, addressing systems for delivery of care and means for training pain specialists. Special areas of medicine in which pain has a prominent role are addressed, including primary care, end of life care, intensive care, and emergency care. The text concludes with a brief view toward the future of pain management.

This book would not be possible without the extensive contributions of the section editors and particularly the efforts of the chapter authors; the success of this work is directly attributable to these individuals. The editors are indebted to Brian Brown and Francis DeStefano of Lippincott, Williams &

Wilkins who served critical roles in shepherding this project into existence, and to Keith Donnellan of Dovetail Content Solutions who managed its development with skill and diplomacy.

As the field of pain medicine has evolved, so has this text. Despite much that is new or revised, the text remains incomplete, a reflection of an emerging field that awaits profound discoveries and development. Through the many chapters and pages of this new edition of his classic text, we hope that John Bonica's passion for an integrated, coherent, and compassionate field will live on. Like Bonica, our central purpose is to assist students and practitioners across all medical disciplines, advance their knowledge of pain medicine, and relieve suffering.

PREFACE TO THE FIRST EDITION (1953)

The purpose of this book is to present within one volume a concise but complete discussion of the fundamental aspects of pain, the various diseases and disorders in which pain constitutes a major problem, and the methods employed in its management, with special emphasis on the use of analgesic block as an aid in the diagnosis, prognosis, and therapy. Although several books dealing with certain phases of this problem are available, none is complete from the standpoint of the practitioner; for it is necessary for him to consult several texts in order to obtain information regarding the cause, characteristics, mechanisms, effects, diagnosis, and therapy of pain and management of its intractable variety with analgesic block and certain adjuvant methods. The present volume is the product of the author's desire to facilitate the task of the busy practitioner and to supply him easily accessible information with the conviction that this will induce more clinicians to employ these methods of diagnosis and therapy.

One need not elaborate on the reasons for writing on the management of pain, for reflection emphasized that this age-old problem is still one of the most difficult and often vexing phases of medical practice—a fact well appreciated by most physicians. This fact, as well as other reasons, are presented in the introduction and are emphasized throughout the book, particularly in Chapter 5.

I have been motivated to write this volume by a deep feeling for those who are afflicted with intractable pain, and by an intense desire to contribute something toward the alleviation of their suffering. The plan for its writing was germinated almost a decade ago during the Second World War, while I was Chief of the Anesthesia Section of a large Army hospital, where I was afforded the opportunity to observe and manage an unusually large number of patients with severe intractable pain. The gratifying results obtained with analgesic block in some instances impressed me with the efficacy of this method in selected cases. In addition, the fact that these procedures effected relief which frequently was not only dramatic, but outlasted by hours and days the transient physiochemical interruption of nerve impulses, fascinated me and aroused my interest. Perusal of the literature revealed a paucity of material on this subject—a situation which has not changed much since then and which clearly indicated an obvious need for a practical source of information about this perplexing phenomenon and the application of analgesic block to its management.

This book is composed of three parts. *The first part* includes a discussion of the fundamental aspects of pain. While some of the material, on superficial thought, might be considered too detailed or entirely unnecessary, it has been included because of my conviction that in order to manage pain properly its anatomical, physiological and psychological bases must be understood. As is true in all fields of endeavor, a thorough knowledge of fundamental principles is an essential prerequisite without which optimal results are precluded. In order to diagnose and treat it properly, the physician must know the course of pain from its place of origin to the apperception centers in the brain and must be well versed in all the essentials and components of which pain consists; he must know its causes, mechanisms, characteristics, varieties, its localizations and significance, and the mental and physical effects it produces.

The second part deals with methods and techniques of managing pain. It was originally planned to include only the method which is the central theme of the book—analgesic block. However, it was soon realized that while this important phase is, to be sure, here treated in a comprehensive manner, it does not present the complete story of the management of pain; because frequently other adjuvant methods are employed in conjunction with nerve blocking. To illustrate the point, trigeminal neuralgia is frequently treated with neurolytic blocks, but sometimes this does not afford sufficiently long relief, and neurotomy is resorted to. The pain associated with malignancy is managed with alcohol nerve block, but roentgen therapy is frequently employed as an adjuvant. Moreover physical and/or psychiatric therapy constitute integral phases of the management of pain without which optimal results cannot be hoped for. After careful consideration, it was decided to include another section in Part II in which are presented methods that are frequently employed in conjunction with analgesic block. It is hoped that such inclusion will give the book a wider scope and greater usefulness.

In the third part are presented various diseases or disorders with painful syndromes which have been and can be managed with analgesic block with or without the aid of other methods. The arrangement of this part is explained in detail on page 671. It is suggested that the reader refer to that page before proceeding further to read any on the pain syndromes. Though the material in this part mainly represents my observations, clinical impressions, and opinions, obtained or developed from experience with, and statistical analysis of, many thousands of cases, it also includes unpublished data of several outstanding authorities who have kindly placed them at my disposal. Moreover, it includes the published views and clinical experiences of others, with credit given where it is due.

In writing this comprehensive treatise, which has involved no small amount of time and effort, the one principle which has always been kept in mind and adhered to has been to present the fundamental considerations and principles of the problem before the practical aspects are discussed.

I have endeavored to make this book as complete as possible, and to this end have thoroughly searched the literature, both English and foreign, and have taken from it all that I thought might be valuable to the reader. In order to comply with the aim of completeness and still keep the book concise and within reasonable size, the material has been selected with care and discretion. In a field so vast and complex as pain, it is unavoidable that what might be thought sufficiently important to deserve detailed discussion is presented in an abbreviated manner or entirely omitted. In other instances, mere mention or omission represents a reluctant compliance with the requirements dictated by the size of the volume. Nonetheless, I believe thoroughness and important detail have not been sacrificed. The bibliography represents the most important references, and many excellent articles on each subject were also reluctantly omitted for that reason.

The book is intended for practitioners of every field of medicine, because pain is universal and provides the main reason why patients seek the aid of the doctor. It is hoped that it will prove useful, not only to the anesthesiologist, neurologist, neurosurgeon, orthopedist, and physiatrist to whom especially is relegated the task of caring for patients with intractable pain, but also to the general practitioner, surgeon, internist, psychiatrist, and any other physician who may be confronted with this problem. It is especially intended for general practitioners, particularly those practicing in smaller communities where the services of a specialist in analgesic blocking are not available. With this aim in mind the techniques of analgesic block are presented in such a manner that most of them may be effectively accomplished by any physician, even though he may be a novice with regional analgesia. In order to facilitate the task of the busy reader, less relevant facts—material which has been included because of its academic importance, for the sake of completeness, or for consumption by students and those who wish to delve deeper into the problem—are presented in small type. These can be omitted without losing continuity of thought. In this manner, while completeness, detail, and thoroughness are not sacrificed, emphasis is laid on the practical aspects of the problem at hand.

The unusually large number of illustrations, many of which are original and composed from dissected material or clinical cases, have been included with the conviction that these frequently tell the story much better than words.

A book of this nature is made possible only by the contribution of many individuals. The information set forth in the first part of the volume represents the fruition of the joint effort of anatomists, physiologists, pharmacologists, neurologists, neurosurgeons, anesthesiologists, psychiatrists, and many other laboratory and clinical investigators who have spent untold time, labor, and effort to discover the mystery of pain. I am grateful for their elucidating knowledge. To clinicians who have reported their experiences, and to others who have placed at my disposal unpublished data, observations, and opinions, my sincere thanks. I am particularly obliged to General Maxwell Keeler, and Col. Clinton S. Lyter, of Madigan Army Hospital for their continuous cooper-

ation in obtaining much of the clinical data embraced in this volume. I want to express my gratitude to Mr. Harold Woodworth for his friendship, sympathetic understanding and devotion to the cause of medicine. I also want to thank the other members of the Board of Trustees of Tacoma General Hospital, but particularly Mr. Alex Babbit, and Mr. Walter Heath and John Dobyns, Directors of the hospital. Their continuous cooperation has facilitated the activities of the Department of Anesthesia, Nerve Block Clinic, and Pain Clinic.

I am very grateful to Dr. Robert Johnson, Associate Professor of Anatomy of the University of Washington School of Medicine, for his encouragement and criticism of some parts of the manuscript; to Doctor Frederick Haugen for his assistance, criticism and suggestion.

My collaborators, Professor Robert Ripley, Doctors Wendell Peterson, Frank Rigos, John T. Robson, Col. Clark Williams, M.C., and Lieut. Col. Walter Lumpkin, M.D., have my heartfelt thanks for their contributions and cooperation.

My appreciation is extended to Miss Joy Polis, Miss Virginia Coleman, and other artists for the illustrations and to Mr. Kenneth Ollar for the photography; to Mrs. Louise Cameron for her cooperation in obtaining the roentgenograms; to Mrs. Katherine Rogers Miller, Miss Eleanor Ekberg and the late Mrs. Blanch DeWitt of Tacoma, Miss Bertha Hallam, Portland, and Mr. Alderson Fry, Seattle—all librarians whose cooperation has facilitated a difficult task, and to Mr. John Morrison for editorial work.

This preface would be incomplete if I did not acknowledge my indebtedness to my secretaries, Miss Katherine Stryker and Mrs. Dorothy Richmond, for the inestimable aid they have given me in the preparation of the manuscript.

My appreciation is extended to my publishers for their courtesy, cooperation, and considerateness throughout the preparation of this volume.

John J. Bonica
Tacoma, Washington

■ ACKNOWLEDGMENTS

Jane C. Ballantyne and James P. Rathmell thank Tina Toland for editorial assistance and Dr. Warren Zapol, immediate past Chair of the Department of Anesthesiology and Critical Care at Massachusetts General Hospital, for his encouragement and support.

Scott M. Fishman thanks Mureen Darrington, Marnie Livingston, and Katherine Chu for editorial assistance and the faculty of the Division of Pain Medicine and Dr. Peter Moore, Chair of the Department of Anesthesiology and Pain Medicine at the University of California, Davis, for encouragement and support.

CONTENTS

PART I ▪ BASIC CONSIDERATIONS

PART II ▪ ECONOMIC, POLITICAL, LEGAL, AND ETHICAL CONSIDERATIONS

PART III ■ EVALUATION OF THE PAIN PATIENT

PART IV ■ PAIN CONDITIONS

SECTION A ■ NEUROPATHIC PAIN SYNDROMES

SECTION B ■ PSYCHOLOGICAL CONTRIBUTIONS TO PAIN

PART V ■ METHODS FOR SYMPTOMATIC CONTROL

PART VI ■ PROVISION OF PAIN TREATMENT

CHAPTER 1 ■ INTELLECTUAL MILESTONES IN OUR UNDERSTANDING AND TREATMENT OF PAIN

DORIS K. COPE

In order to treat something we first must learn to recognize it.
—Sir William Osler[1]

Through the ages, pain and suffering have been the primary reason that patients have sought medical care. What is pain? It is both a personal emotional experience as well as the result of complex physiological adaptations of molecular and biological function. This chapter will discuss this duality of concepts, the familiar mind-body dilemma in the context of how our mental constructs shape our understanding, and then treatment of this complex phenomenon we call pain. The chapter will close with a discussion of how the medical subspecialty is evolving within the broader context of medical specialization and thoughts for future development.[2]

PAIN UNDERSTOOD AS PART OF A LARGER PHILOSOPHY OR WORLD VIEW

Since the beginning of time, humans are born through a painful process and the experience of suffering remains universal. The meaning of pain reflects the contemporary spirit of the age and, therefore, has changed over recorded history with changing world views. Among the earliest systems of pain management, dating back to the Stone Age, was Chinese acupuncture, theoretically based on the philosophy of imbalances of between yin and yang affecting qi and blood flow. Thousands of years ago, Egyptians considered the experience of pain to be a god or disincarnate spirit afflicting the heart, which was conceptualized as the center of emotion. Galen, and later Aristotle (Fig. 1.1), described pain as an emotional experience, or "a passion of the soul."[3]

An important concept dating from antiquity that persisted until the 19th century was the theory of importance of the four humors. This world view was espoused by Greek philosophers in approximately 400 BC and later applied to medicine by Hippocrates (Fig. 1.2) who described humors as related to one of the four constitutions, shown in Table 1.1. Seasonal changes evoked pain and certain disorders, such as migraine, were associated with specific humors (e.g., excessive cold humors thought to result in a mucus discharge requiring application of "hot effusions" to the head).

Consistent with this ideology was the custom of treating pain by applying "opposites" such as hot applications to the head to counterbalance and evacuate "cold" humors of headaches.[5] Again, based on the humor theory and treatment via "opposites," was the technique called cupping. Warm suction cups were applied to the skin that on cooling resulted in raised reddened welts thought to "draw out" any unbalanced humors.[6]

Later, during the Middle Ages, coincident with the spread of Christianity, pain, not surprisingly, was explained in a spiritual, religious context. Medieval life has been described as short, cheap, and brutish, especially for the lower classes, with pain accepted as the universal lot of mankind. Little is known of how pain was actually treated during this period, but a suffering

Christ, martyred saints, and the concept of physical pain in purgatory originated around the 12th century AD.[6,7] Commonly revered was the iconography of tortured saints with ecstatic faces depicting pain as a spiritual discipline bringing the saints closer to God, relieved primarily by prayer and meditation. A clear example of pain as ennobling was St. Ignatius Loyola's habit of wearing ropes and chains cutting into the skin and encouraging other humiliations of the flesh to enhance his spiritual development.[3]

An interesting example of pain as a function of the sociological concepts of the day is the rise and fall of the diagnosis of hysteria, common in the 17th century and virtually nonexistent today. Thomas Sydenham (Fig. 1.3), in 1681, wrote, "Of all chronic diseases hysteria—unless I err—is the commonest."[8] The one cardinal symptom of this condition was unexplained pain. In mid-19th century Europe and America, hysteria was virtually

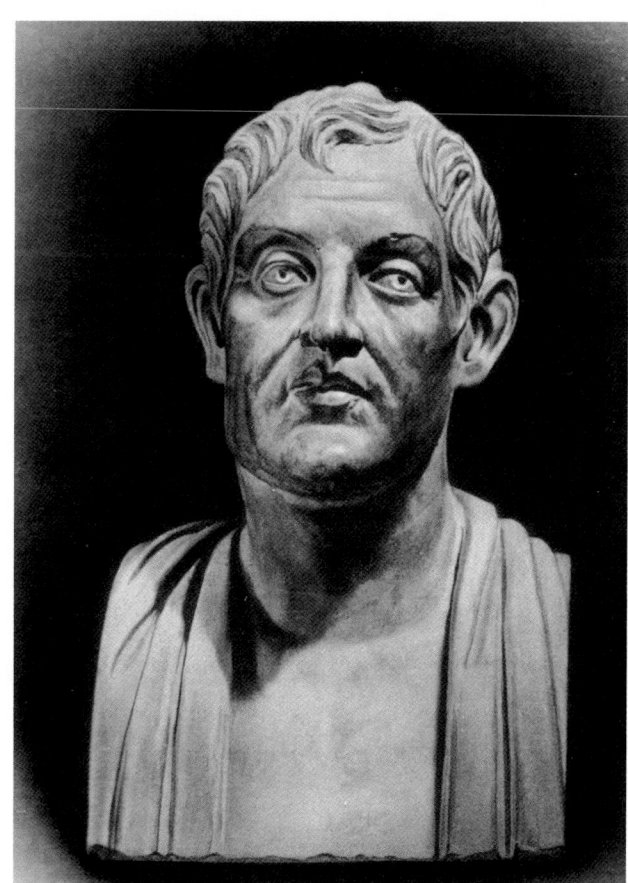

FIGURE 1.1 Aristotle. (Courtesy of the National Library of Medicine.)

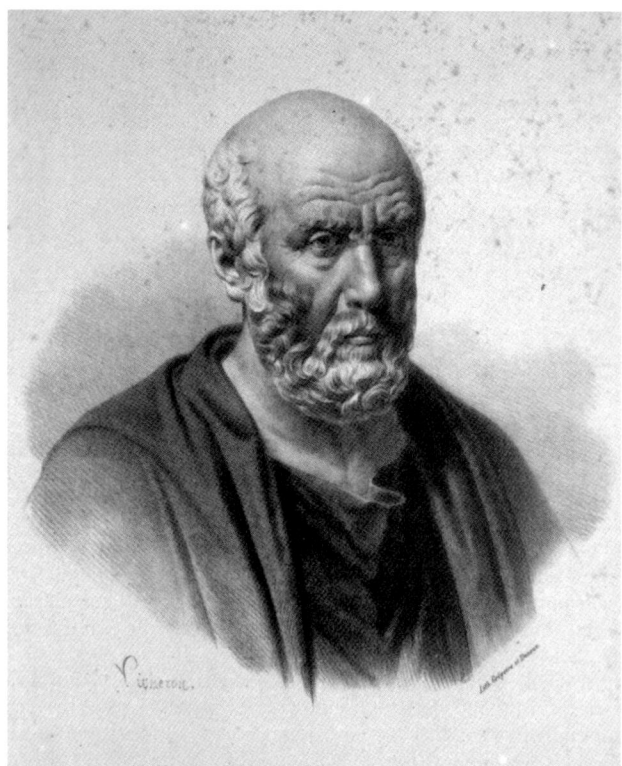

FIGURE 1.2 Hippocrates. (Courtesy of the National Library of Medicine.)

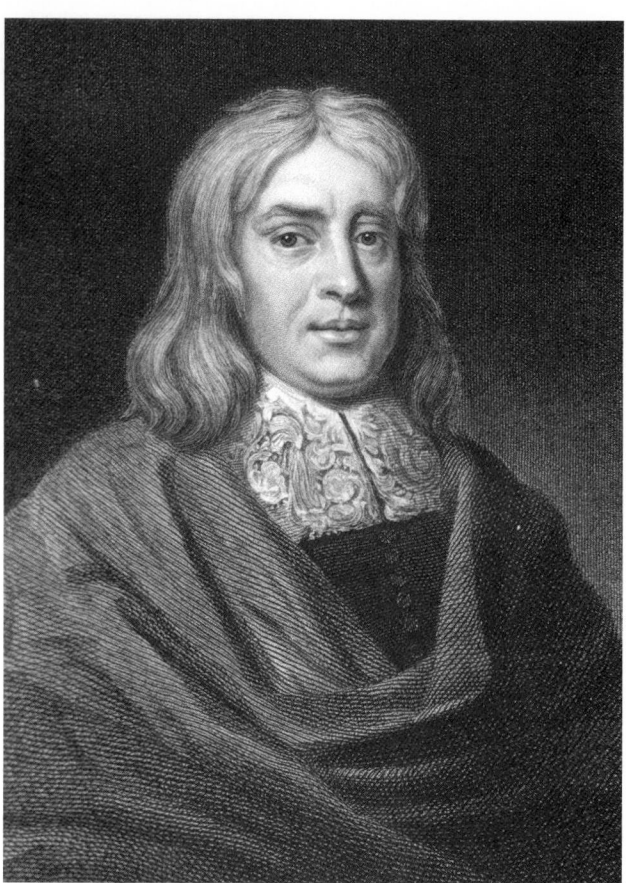

FIGURE 1.3 Thomas Sydenham. (Courtesy of the National Library of Medicine.)

everywhere, found in every community. Invalids, mostly females, filled homes, spas, and convalescent facilities at the turn of the 19th century. This mysterious syndrome, afflicting only middle and upper class females, was treated by complete social isolation, bed confinement, and a total prohibition on any form of intellectual activity, even sewing or reading.[9] As the social situation and educational opportunities for women improved, this disorder almost totally disappeared, a public health success on the order of magnitude of the eradication of influenza or yellow fever. In the 21st century, fibromyalgia, while a commonly diagnosed condition in western countries, interestingly enough, is either underreported or not significantly present in Asian and developing country populations.

Another very clear link between mental state and the perception and control of pain can be seen in the work of the German physician Franz Anton Mesmer (Fig. 1.4). In 1766, he published his doctoral dissertation entitled "On the Influence of the Planets on the Human Body," describing animal (or life spirit) magnetism as a force to cure many ills.[10] He used iron magnets to treat various diseases, amplifying the magnetic fields with room-sized Leyden jars. His demonstrations of his technique, combining hypnotism with spectacle, included the wearing of brightly colored

TABLE 1.1

RELATIONSHIPS IN ANTIQUITY BETWEEN THE FOUR HUMORS, ELEMENTS, CONSTITUTIONS, AND SEASONS[4]

Black Bile	Blood	Phlegm	Yellow Bile
Earth	Air	Water	Fire
Dry, cold	Hot, wet	Cold, wet	Hot, dry
Autumn	Spring	Winter	Summer

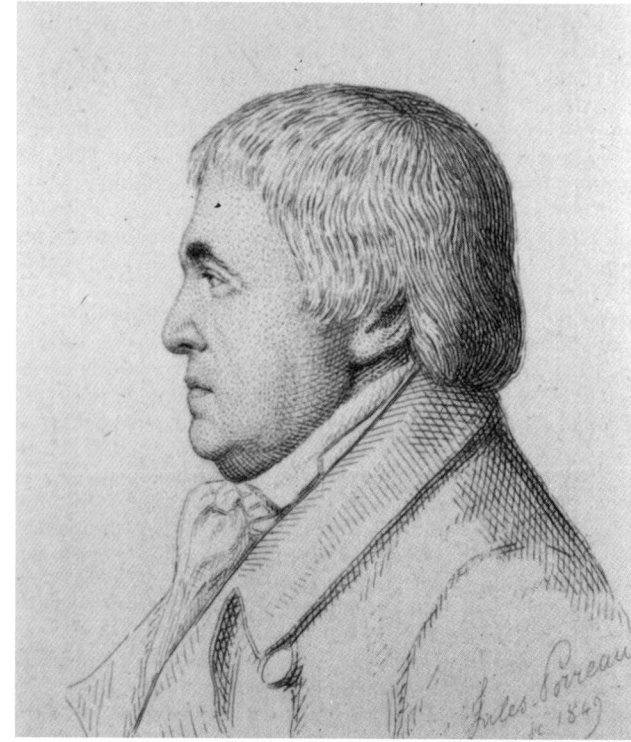

FIGURE 1.4 Franz Anton Mesmer. (Courtesy of the National Library of Medicine.)

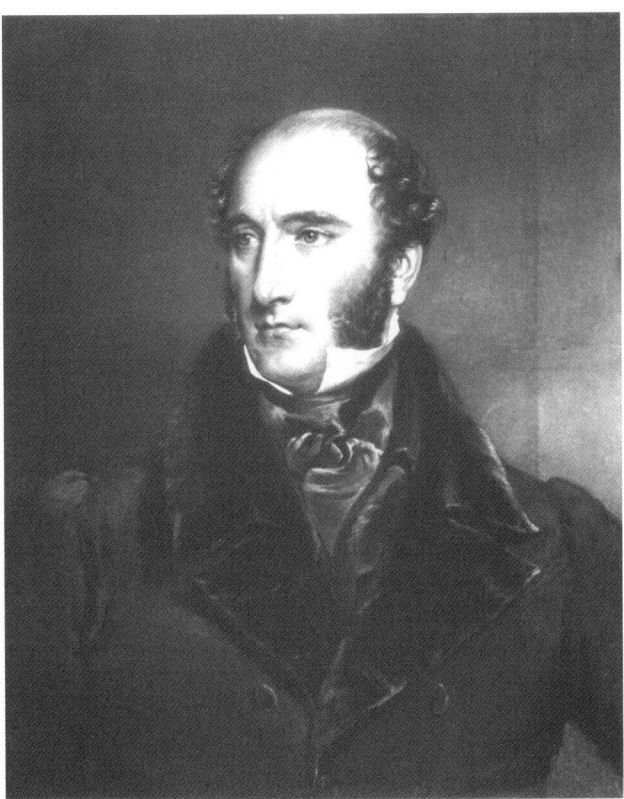

FIGURE 1.5 Robert Liston, Esquire. (Courtesy of the National Library of Medicine.)

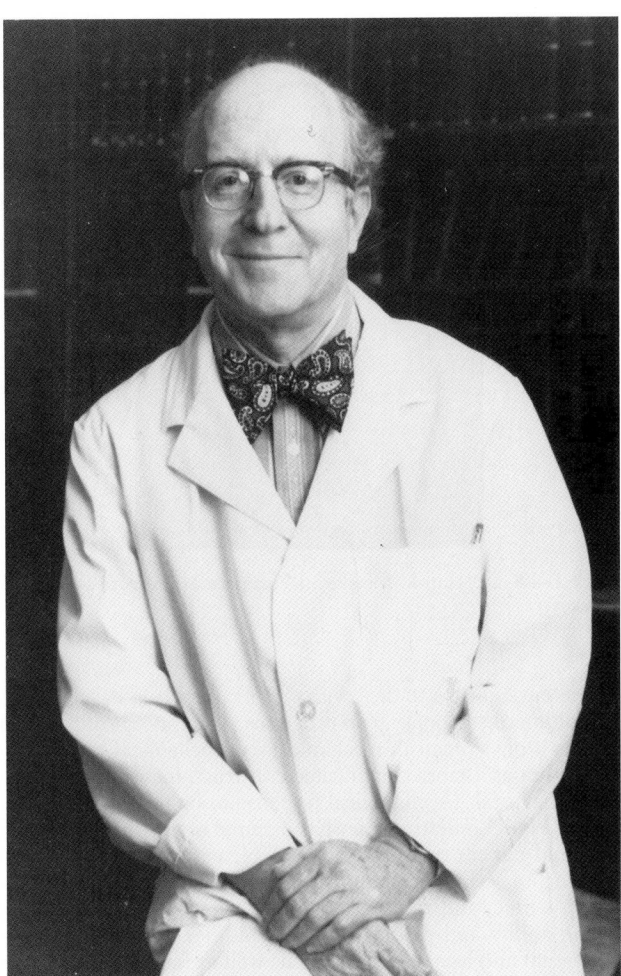

FIGURE 1.6 George L. Engel, MD. (With permission from the Edward G. Miner Library, University of Rochester Medical Center, NY)

robes in dimly lit ritualistic séances, with soft music playing from a glass harmonium. He invoked magnetic power with poles either held or waved over the patient and his techniques were an early rival to ether anesthesia as a way to relieve pain during surgical procedures.[11] Mesmerism was such a common form of pain therapy during his day that Robert Liston (Fig. 1.5) reportedly exclaimed after the successful administration of ether anesthesia in an early above-knee operation, "This Yankee Dodge beats mesmerism hollow."[12] Mesmerism was based on the larger, generally accepted, vitalism theory which posited that every part of a living thing was endowed with sensibility. The energy or force which animated a living organism was capable of being stimulated or consumed. In disease, pain was necessary to produce a "crisis" which rid the patient of original pain by stimulating the diminishing energy.[13]

A further development of the link between mind and body and the understanding of pain was the landmark development of Freudian theory in understanding the subconscious influences on pain perception and behavior. The link between the unconscious mind and physical sensation in hysterical conversion disorders was posited as an explanation for psychogenic pain and continues to be influential today. This conceptual paradigm was expanded in the 1970s by the psychiatrist George L. Engel (Fig. 1.6) who demonstrated the link between chronic pain and psychiatric illness.[14] Later psychiatrists, psychologists, and social scientists, including Thomas Szasz (Fig.1.7),[15] Allan Walters,[16] and Harold Merskey (Fig. 1.8),[17] explored social situations, psychological character traits, and the effects of past life experiences in understanding chronic pain in patients. Depression, stress, and personality, in addition to physiological mechanisms, have proved to be critical grounds for investigation and therapy. From these early studies investigating the mind-body interface of pain grew the cognitive-behavioral school of pain therapy in the 1980s that is widely employed today, emphasizing the development of

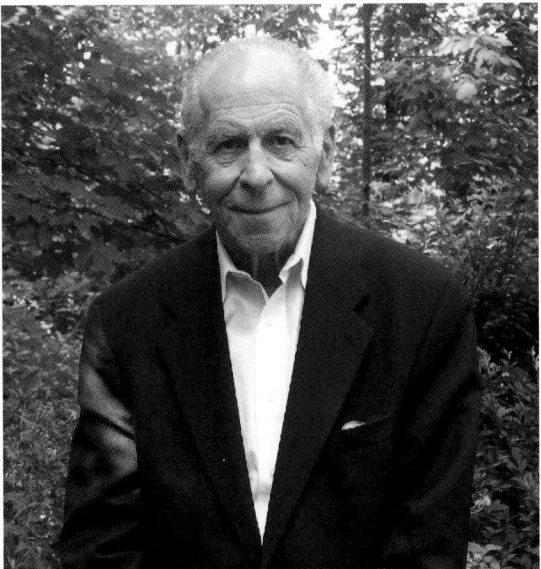

FIGURE 1.7 Thomas S. Szasz, MD. (With permission from Dr. Thomas Szasz. Photo courtesy of J. A. Schaler.)

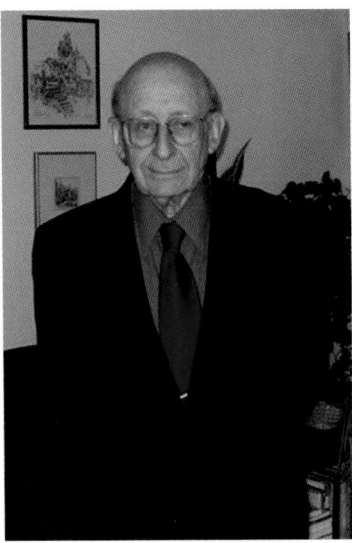

FIGURE 1.8 Dr. Harold Merskey. (With permission from Dr. Harold Merskey.)

coping mechanisms to deal with chronic pain as a basic component of interdisciplinary pain programs. The concept of pain, not only as a physiological, mechanical, neurochemical response to stimuli but as a more complicated construct, incorporating a social, behavioral, psychological response to unpleasant stimuli, is an intellectual milestone that has inspired a wealth of investigations and patient treatment options. New areas of investigation now include pain in relationship to social setting, gender, national, ethnic, and racial background, as well as differences in coping ability and psychiatric comorbidities. Considerations of vocational and legal environment as well as family and interpersonal dynamics are also relevant to the understanding and care of individual patients.

This global philosophy of pain as only part of an entire life experience can best be summed up in the words of Alexander Pope in his *Essay on Man*, 1733:

> Say what the use, were finer optics giv'n,
> T' inspect a mite, not comprehend the heav'n?
> Or touch, if tremblingly alive all o'er,
> To smart and agonize at ev'ry pore?
> Or, quick effluvia darting thro' the brain,
> Die of a rose in aromatic pain?[18]

MECHANISTIC VIEWS OF PAIN

In counterpoint to the holistic philosophical consideration of pain was mechanism, the philosophical mind set suggesting that the human body functions as a simple machine with pain being the result of its malfunction.[19] This viewpoint is clearly seen in Descartes' *Passions of the Soul* in 1649 where he compares a human being to a watch:

> [T]he difference between the body of a living man and that of a dead man is just like the difference between, on the one hand, a watch or other automaton (that is, a self-moving machine) when it is wound up and contains in itself the corporeal principle of the movements for which it is designed . . . ; and, on the other hand, the same watch or machine when it is broken and the principle of its movement ceases to be active.[20]

How did the mechanistic view of the body develop and even supersede traditional theological and philosophical explanations for pain? Early anatomical studies were conducted beginning

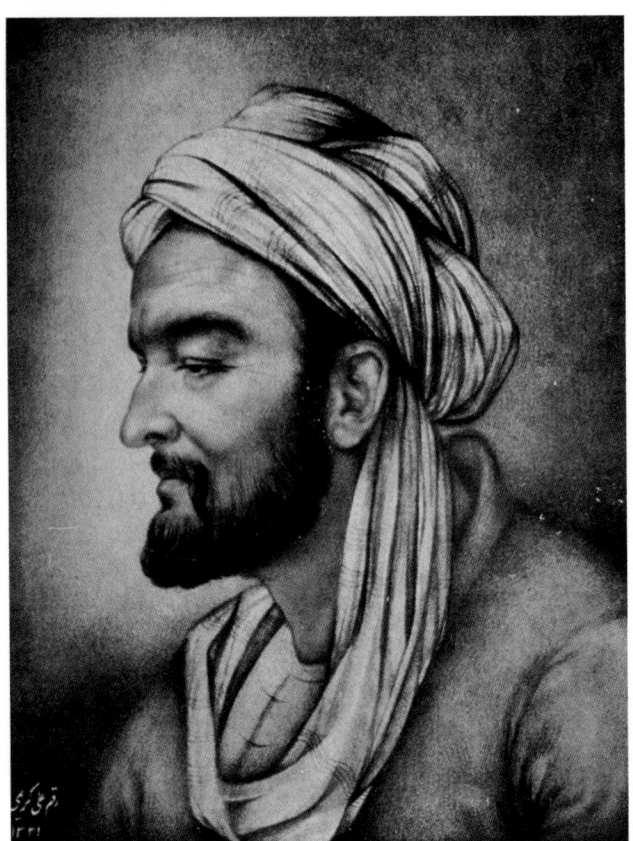

FIGURE 1.9 Avicenna. (Courtesy of the National Library of Medicine.)

with Galen of Pergamum (130–201 AD) and Avicenna (Fig. 1.9), the Persian Muslim polymath (980–1037), forming an intellectual basis for pain as an actual physical sensation rather than as a mental, spiritual dilemma. Later, in the 14th through 17th centuries, the Renaissance cultural movement questioned the basis of all knowledge including ideas about the human body and the experience of pain. Empiricism and the development of scientific inquiry with direct observation into the mysteries of life became the basis for advances in both medical understanding and treatment, including the now commonly accepted neurological basis of pain. Extended wars on the continent between France and Spain resulted in bullet and musket ball injuries, with bullets and musket balls tearing the skin, forcing surgical removal and amputation. Wounds were bound and foreign bodies extracted, originally posited to prevent leakage of the "vital force" or to inhibit the entrance of animal spirits into the injured body. Gradually, direct observation of the circulation of the blood by William Harvey (Fig. 1.10) in 1628[21] and the direct anatomical studies of Descartes (Fig. 1.11) in 1662[22] elucidating sensory physiology became the theoretical basis for further exploration in the 18th and 19th centuries.

In this era of scientific discovery, mechanism based theories of pain (e.g., specificity theory, pattern theory, summation theory, and gate control theory) developed.

Specificity Theory

While there were many very important milestones leading to this transformation, the work of Charles Bell (Fig. 1.12) in Scotland in 1811 was a significant turning point. The specificity theory, the seminal concept that pain had a truly physical basis that could be dissected out by individual sensory nerves which are special-

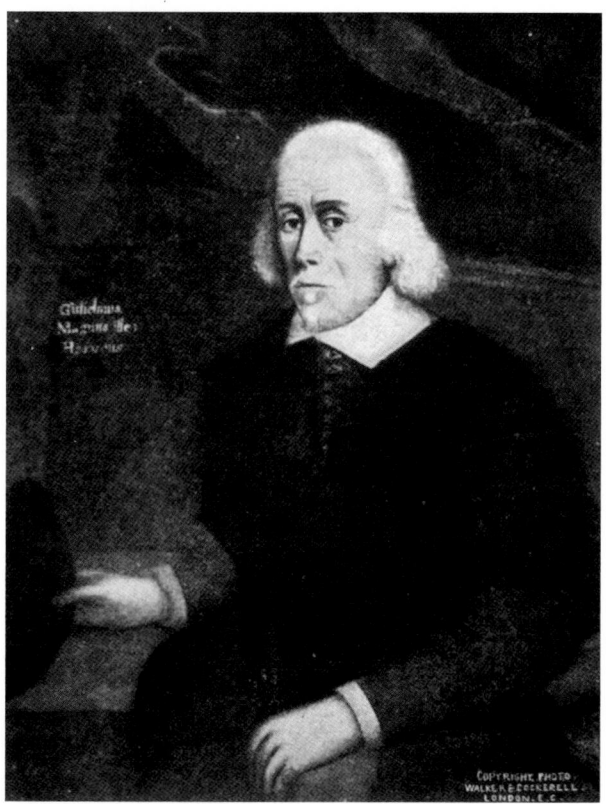

FIGURE 1.10 William Harvey. (Courtesy of the National Library of Medicine.)

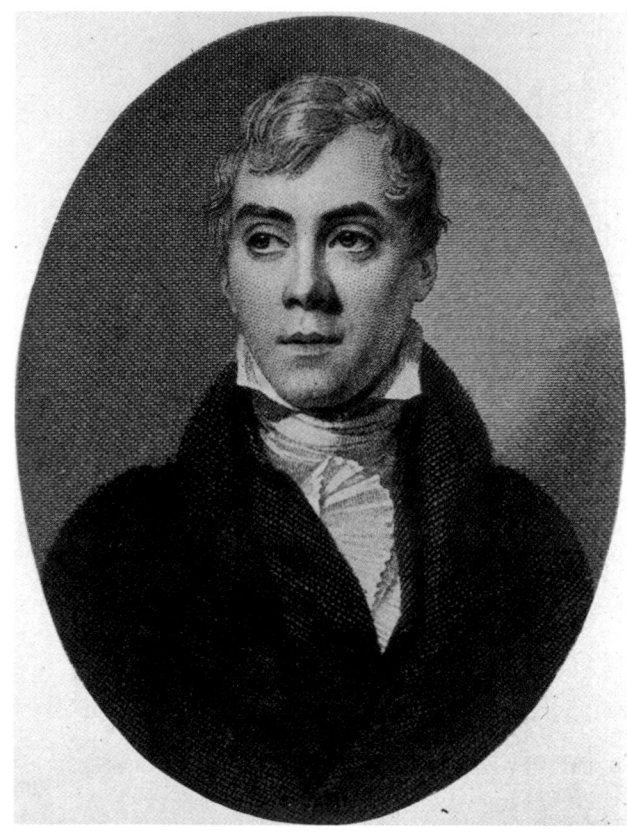

FIGURE 1.12 Sir Charles Bell. (Courtesy of the National Library of Medicine.)

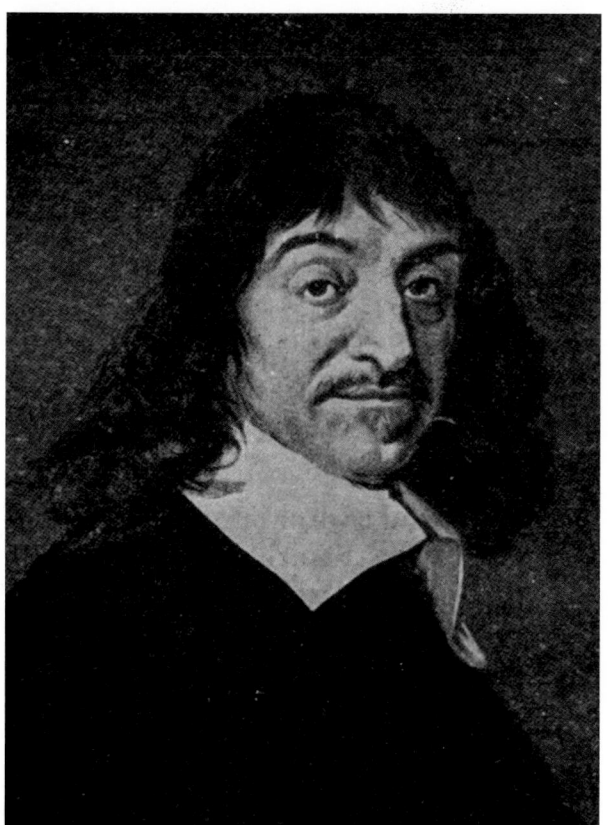

FIGURE 1.11 René Descartes. (Courtesy of the National Library of Medicine.)

ized to perceive and transmit information from an individual stimulus type, opened the way for much more subsequent experimentation.[23] Although, in the early 1800s, anatomical dissection was still considered distasteful to Charles Bell, later anatomists expanded on his theoretical anatomical deductions by their own direct observations. For example, Charles Bell's discovery of ventral root stimulation controlling muscle contraction led the way for François Magendie's (Fig. 1.13) 1882 demonstration of sensory function via stimulation of dorsal nerve roots based on his experiments on puppies where surgically sectioning posterior nerve roots resulted in paralysis and insensibility of the corresponding limbs.[23,24] In 1839, Johannes Müller (Fig. 1.14) advanced the important idea of specialization of nerve fibers linked to the idea of vitalism. For example, he considered the sensation of sound to be the "specific energy" of the acoustic nerve, as the sensation of light the particular "energy" of the visual nerve.[25] Charles-Édouard Brown-Séquard (Fig. 1.15) and Sir William Richard Gowers (Fig. 1.16) expanded these concepts and, in this investigative climate, the physiological study of pain flourished. As Galen, Avicenna, Descartes, and Müller had theorized, specificity advanced the idea of specific pathways and specific receptors for pain.

In 1858, Moritz Schiff demonstrated that particular lesions of the spinal cord produced a reproducible loss of tactile and painful sensation. It was over 50 years later that a surgeon in Philadelphia applied these findings with the introduction of spinal cordotomy in a human patient.

Max von Frey (Fig. 1.17) continued investigations based on the specificity model, expanding Müller's concept of specific receptors, by defining specialized end organ receptors to detect cold and warmth. In 1896, he used horsehairs of various diameters and described "pain spots" in human patients observing sensitivity in a wider distribution than the injured site alone.[26] This ex-

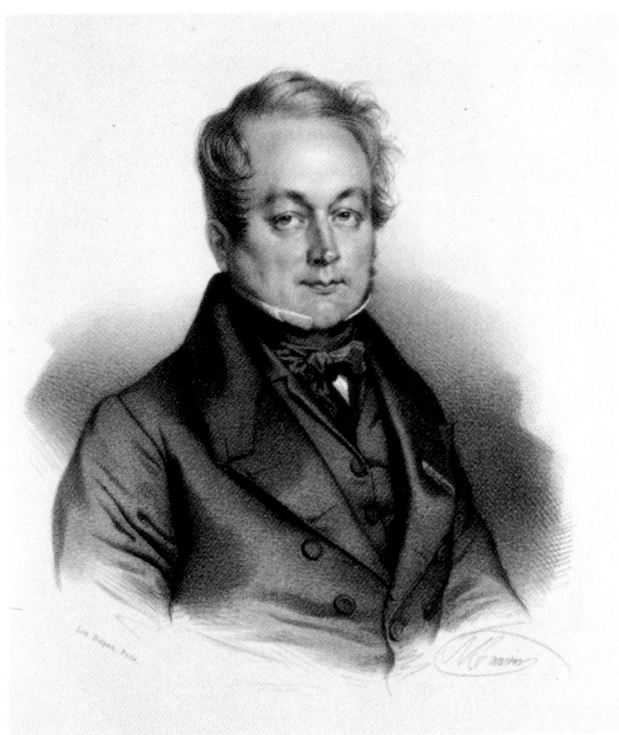

FIGURE 1.13 François Magendie. (Courtesy of the National Library of Medicine.)

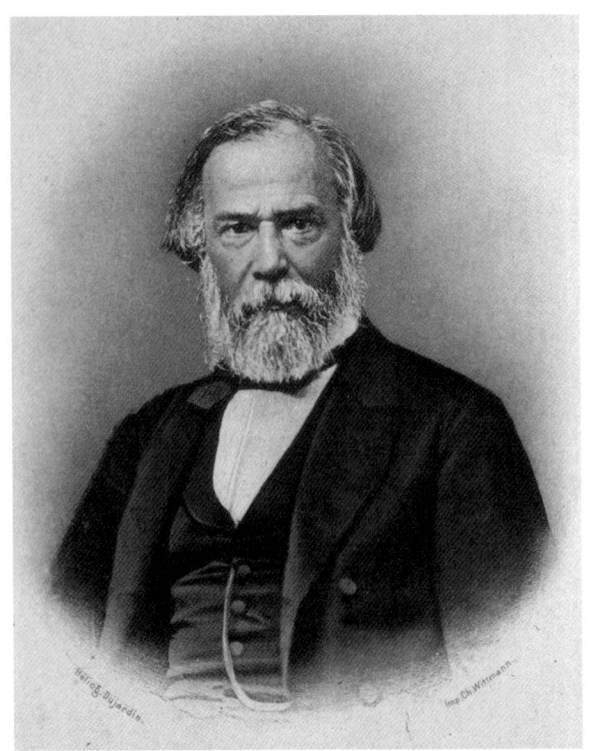

FIGURE 1.15 Charles-Édouard Brown-Séquard. (Courtesy of the National Library of Medicine.)

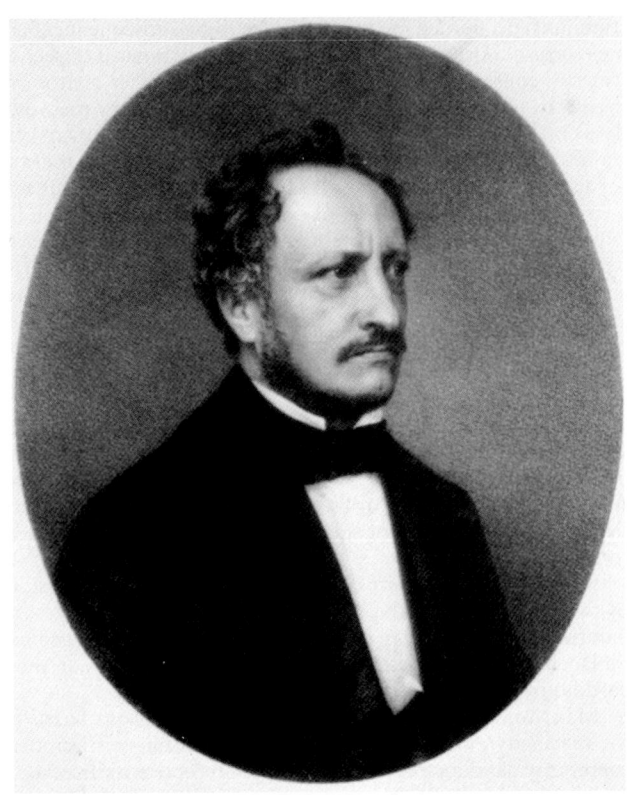

FIGURE 1.14 Johannes Müller. (Courtesy of the National Library of Medicine.)

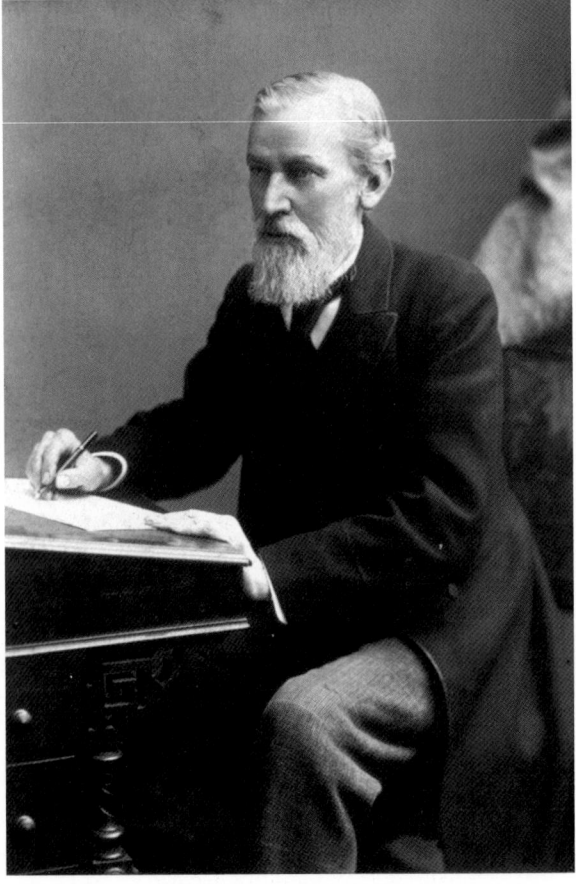

FIGURE 1.16 Sir William Richard Gowers. (Courtesy of the National Library of Medicine.)

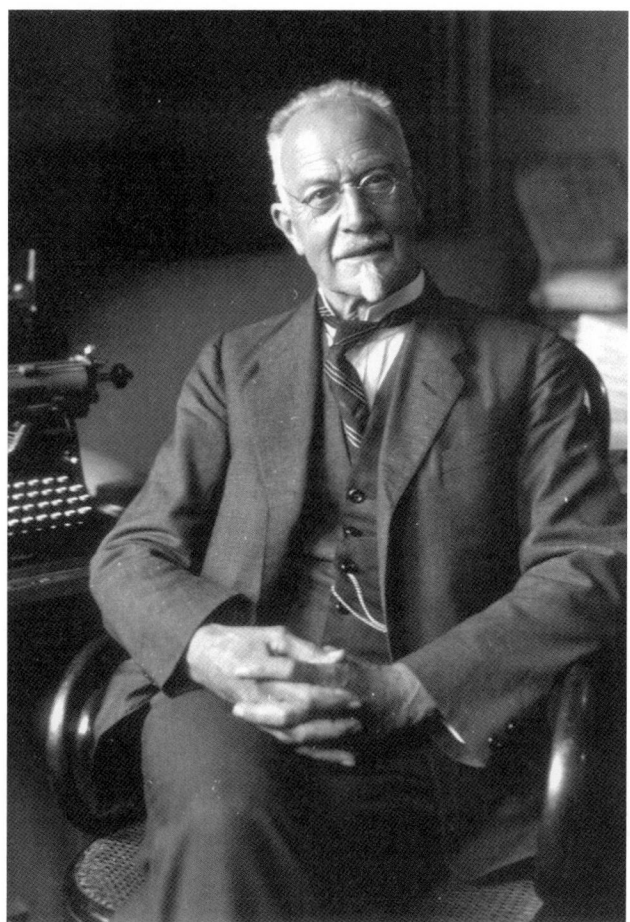

FIGURE 1.17 Max von Frey. (Courtesy of the National Library of Medicine.)

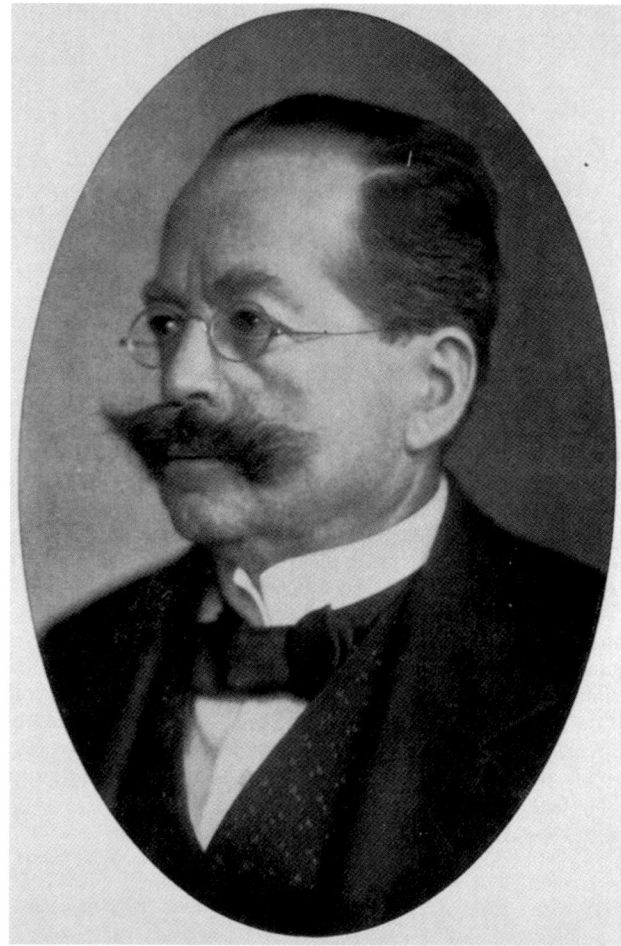

FIGURE 1.18 Dr. Alfred Goldscheider. (Courtesy of the National Library of Medicine.)

perimental determination of painful skin receptor areas continues today with von Frey filaments still used in animal and human models.

Other important findings demonstrating specific receptors of pain were the microscopic anatomical observations of the corpuscles of Pacini and Meissner-Wagner, the demonstration of free nerve endings, and the later discovery of the bulbous corpuscles of Krause in 1860 and Golgi-Mazzoni.[27]

Pattern Theory

The origin of the another dominant pain theory, the pattern theory, was introduced in 1894 by Alfred Goldscheider (Fig. 1.18), a German army physician, who posited that certain patterns of nerve activation were produced by the summation of sensory input from the skin in the dorsal horn. Before his research, the skin had been commonly regarded as an organ endowed with only one kind of sensation. He demonstrated that skin contains instead a number of different perceptive organs, being a mosaic of a complicated pattern, in which each item represents a particular kind of sensibility. He found three kinds of sensitive areas in the skin (pressure, warmth, and cold) and was able to prove that each localized point reacted only to the appropriate stimulus and each point had a specific function.[28] Nafe further formalized this theory by expanding the concept that all sensation is the result of patterns spatially and temporally of nerve impulses rather than the result of individual or specific receptors of pathways.[29] In 1955, Sinclair and Weddell expanded the pattern concept empha-

sizing that all fiber endings, except those innervating hair follicles, are similar and it is only the pattern that is important in sensory discrimination.[30,31]

Summation Theory

William K. Livingstone, J. D. Hardy, and H. G. Wolff demonstrated the importance of interactions between various neurons and internuncial activity, the sympathetic nervous system, and the somatic nervous system in developing secondary hyperalgesia, a forerunner to the later concept of central sensitization. They based their ideas on their observations of discontinuous pain fields, which were not adequately explained by the earlier theories. They clinically noted the exacerbation of pain with repeated stimuli (hyperalgesia). Pressure sensation over time resulted in painful sensation and pressure points responded differently to stimulation than adjacent areas.[32] Thus, a summation theory was proposed to explain these clinical phenomena. Another clear milestone in the understanding of pain as a science was the work of Dr. Charles S. Sherrington, often described as the father of pain physiology. In 1932 he was awarded the Nobel Prize in Medicine for developing the concept of the motor-unit, comprising receptor, conductor, and effector. This theoretical framework of transmission integrated earlier findings as explained in his book, *The Integrative Action of the Nervous System*, published in 1906. His further experiments in noxious stimulus in skin resulted in the novel and still relevant concepts of nonselective (polymodal) receptors and selective excitability.[33]

Gate Theory

The complexity of pain, however, could not be explained as simply a specific pathway, pattern, or summation of stimuli with a behavioral response; rather, it is a more complex interaction between the central and peripheral nervous systems. At least partial resolution of somewhat conflicting paradigms was reconciled to a degree in 1965 by the groundbreaking published theories of the Canadian psychologist Ronald Melzack (Fig. 1.19) and the British physiologist Patrick Wall (Fig. 1.20).[34] This challenge to the specificity theory gave at least a theoretical, conceptual framework to meld the old mind-body dichotomy with pain considered as an intersection between both physiology and psychology. Melzack and Wall introduced the theory that the information coming in over C fibers is modulated through presynaptic inhibition from incoming beta-fibers in the substantia gelatinosa. This "gating" mechanism depends on the relative quantity of information coming in over the larger fibers versus the smaller fibers. Two major pathways in which pain "gets through" the gate is either through damage to the beta-fibers, allowing spontaneous pain or activation of the C fibers by excessive stimulation through inflammation of pressure on the C fibers. While many specifics of the gate control theory have been since discounted, the importance of pain modulation by central mechanisms and competing stimuli at the spinal cord level has allowed a more complex understanding of pain.

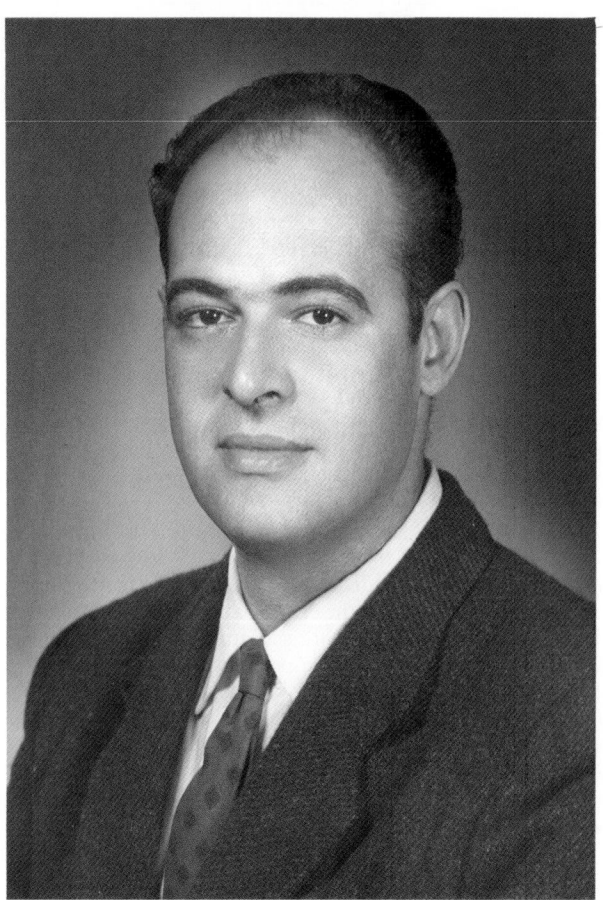

FIGURE 1.19 Ronald Melzack, PhD. (Courtesy MIT Museum.)

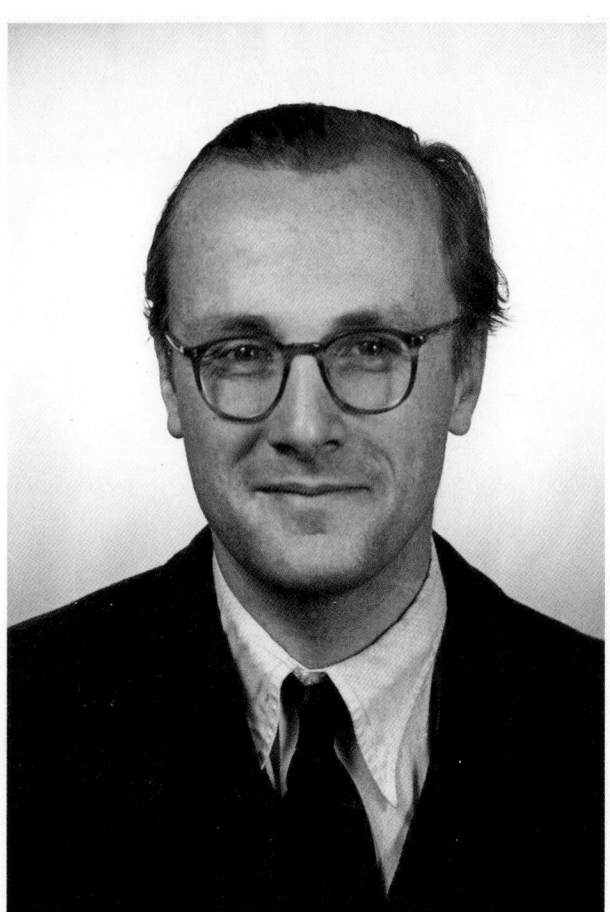

FIGURE 1.20 Patrick D. Wall, MD. (Courtesy MIT Museum.)

NEURAL PLASTICITY AND CENTRAL SENSITIZATION

More recently, the explosion of research into the transmission and transduction of pain has focused on molecular, biochemical, and genetic alterations. A key tenet and basis for many of these studies has been the concept of neural plasticity and hyperexcitability in the spinal cord early elucidated by Clifford Woolf (Fig. 1.21). He defined neural plasticity as "the capacity of neurons to change their structure, function, or chemical profile via activation, modulation, and modification . . . contributing to pain hypersensitivity."[35] Many more advances, primarily in cellular biology, have described various neuroactive proinflammatory cytokines, a variety of growth factors, microglial cells, and even changes in genetic transcription as active participants in the pain response, further explored in the later chapters of this textbook.

TREATMENTS FOR PAIN

The rationale for choosing one form or pain treatment over another more often reflects the philosophical world view of the physician more than the patient's presenting condition. Physicians who are focused on the patient's adaptation to life might focus on issues of lifestyle, stress, and emotional upheaval and assist the patient to work toward more adaptive behavioral responses to their pain. Physicians who see pain in mechanistic terms most likely will look for the anatomic foci of pain and be confounded if the source of the suffering is unclear. In the first

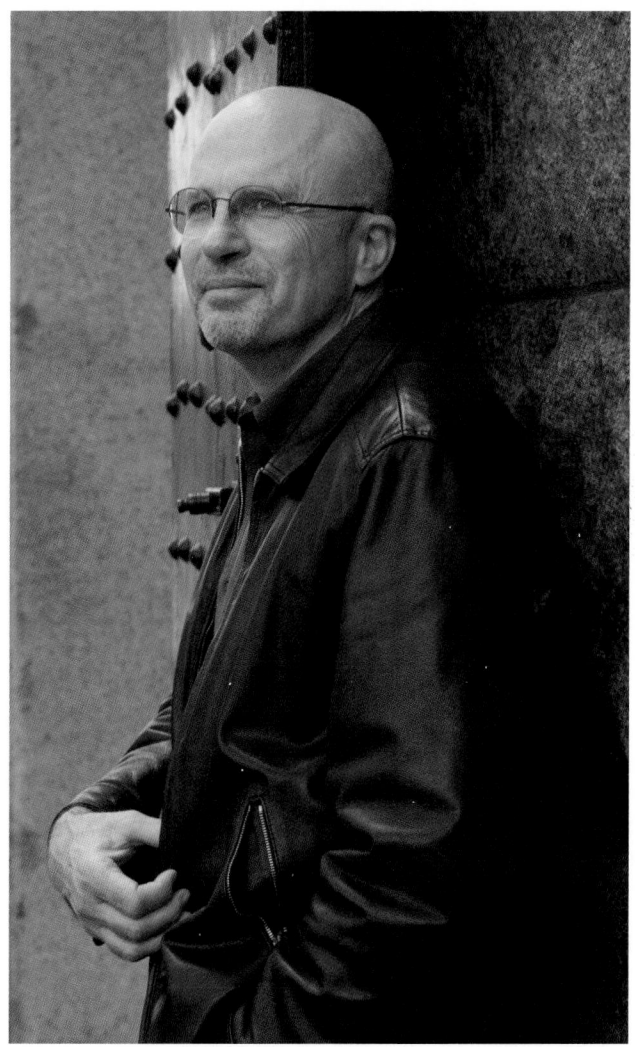

FIGURE 1.21 Clifford Woolf, MD, PhD. (With permission from Clifford Woolf, MD, PhD.)

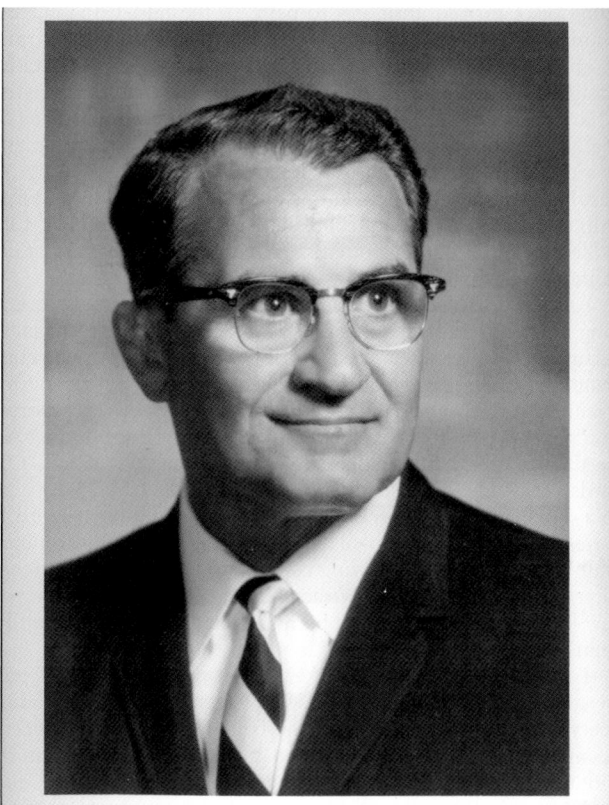

FIGURE 1.22 Dr. John J. Bonica. (Courtesy of the Wood Library-Museum of Anesthesiology.)

older, historical paradigm, pain is a part of an entire life and the enhancing adaptation to life is also needed to manage painful conditions. In the second, a specific anatomical or physiological lesion is sought with therapy specifically directed toward the underlying pathology.

COGNITIVE TREATMENT FOR PAIN

The fundamental significance of the word "pain" in English is derived from the Latin word *poena*, meaning punishment, and its relief was through prayer.[36] This reflects the supposed cause of the pain being harm inflicted by the powers above for putative wrongdoing. Prior to the 18th century, nonspecific therapies were employed for many types of pain, including acupuncture, the application of humoral opposites, bloodletting, purging, topical and oral herbal compounds, and distraction by creating a competing, more severe pain. To better define why patients experienced pain and, presumably, how to treat it, physicians attempted classification by causes. However, treatment options were still limited. During the Roman emperor Trajan's time, a noted physician recorded 13 causes of pain. Avicenna, a noted Muslim healer in the early 11th century, described 15 separate causes. And Hah-

nemann, the founder of homeopathy, listed 75.[37] However, nonspecific treatments such as mesmerism and hypnotism, and even general anesthetics, were based on a whole body cure rather than a mechanistic view of pain. Later, cognitive behavioral therapy and palliative care focused on the care of the whole person as a human being in need of adaptive coping skills. Early work in the 1950s by Engel, based on Freud's theoretical ideals, explored the link between suffering from pain and psychiatric diagnosis. Merskey and Spear, in the mid 1960s, confirmed that chronic pain patients also often had coexisting psychiatric morbidity.[38] Henry Beecher, in the battlefields of World War II, observed that seriously wounded soldiers reported less pain than civilian patients in the Massachusetts General Hospital recovery room. Their injury may have been subjectively interpreted as a cause of removal from harm and their return home as a war survivor. Later, however, these same patients would complain loudly about a minor insult such as venous puncture, causing Beecher to conclude that the experience of pain was derived from a complex interaction between physical sensation, cognition, and an emotional reaction.[39]

Dame Cicely Saunders, mother of the hospice movement in Great Britain and throughout the world, championed the idea of "total pain" emphasizing the holistic concept of patient-centered pain management.[40] John Bonica (Fig. 1.22) also treated World War II veterans with complex multifocal persistent pain and organized an early multidisciplinary conference in Seattle, attended by 300 clinicians and researchers of various disciplines, which eventually became the International Association for the Study of Pain.[41]

PHARMACOLOGICAL TREATMENT OF PAIN

The development of pharmacology as a science parallels the treatment of painful conditions by medications. Alcohol and morphine were proven antidotes to pain. In the mid-17th century, Thomas Sydenham concocted laudanum, the ubiquitous mix combining sherry, wine, opium, saffron, cinnamon, and clove and used to treat everything from dysentery to hysteria and gout. In South America, cocoa leaves were in common use, both as an orally chewed remedy for altitude sickness and physical pain and as a topical treatment. The alkaloid cocaine was isolated by Albert Niemann in his 1860s auto-experimentation and was originally touted as a cure for alcohol and morphine addiction.[42] Carl Koller, in 1884, demonstrated the local anesthetic effects of cocaine in reducing corneal movement during eye surgery.[43]

As chemical analysis became more sophisticated, opium, a long known treatment for pain, was studied by the pharmacist Serturner who isolated "the soporific principle" from the compound in 1806. Despite being well-known to herbalists, the first scientific report of the power of willow derivatives was reported in a paper to the Royal Society of Medicine in London in 1763 by the Reverend Edmund Stone from Chipping Norton, Oxfordshire.[44] The overuse of quinine in the early 19th century led to a shortage of the Peruvian cinchona trees and, therefore, there were increased efforts to isolate, characterize, and then commercially synthesize pain-relieving compounds. In 1829, the French pharmacist Henri Leroux extracted the active compound in willow leaves and bark that had been used in application to painful joints.

Later, in 1873, Charles von Gerhardt prepared salicylic acid by combining sodium salicylate with acetyl chloride to produce acetylsalicylic acid or aspirin. The benefit of adding the acetyl group was decreased irritation to mucous membranes of the mouth, esophagus, and stomach and avoidance of the bitter alkaloid taste.[45] Clinically, the benefits of this newly synthesized product were reported in treating acute rheumatism by Thomas J. Mac Lagan in 1876, over a century after Rev. Stone's first report.[46]

Two other landmarks that marked clear leaps forward in the pharmacological treatment of pain were the development of the hypodermic needle by Rynd[47] and the syringe by Wood,[48] permitting injection of analgesics and anesthetics. Morton's 1846 landmark demonstration of ether anesthesia, following Crawford Long's earlier application of ether anesthesia in 1843, marked a new era of surgical anesthesia.

ANATOMICALLY SPECIFIC TREATMENTS FOR PAIN

In contrast, the majority of the treatment options for pain in the last two centuries have been inspired by specificity theory and its refined derivatives. Surgical cures have been employed for pain relief by interruption of specific sensory tracts in neurotomies, division of the anterolateral column of the spinal cord, dorsal roots excision, thalamectomy, mesencephalic lesioning, psychosurgical lobotomies, and other procedures that specifically alter the anatomy of the central nervous system. This paradigm shift developed over time, paralleling the scientific advances in understanding the mechanisms of pain transmission.

As knowledge of the importance of the central nervous system in the transmission of pain increased, cures based on this new science proliferated. An early treatment, neurocompression, was developed by James Moore, a Glasgow-born London surgeon. He demonstrated that compression of specific nerves provided anesthesia in patients via clamps in both upper and lower limbs inducing reversible neurapraxia to anesthetize a limb.[49]

Before his time, Ambroise Paré (Fig.1.23) (1510–1590), the great French surgeon of the Renaissance and "physician to the kings of France," linked observable injury to the development of chronic pain. He not only sustained a prolific medical practice but wrote 10 books of surgery (*Dix Livres de la Chirugie*). These

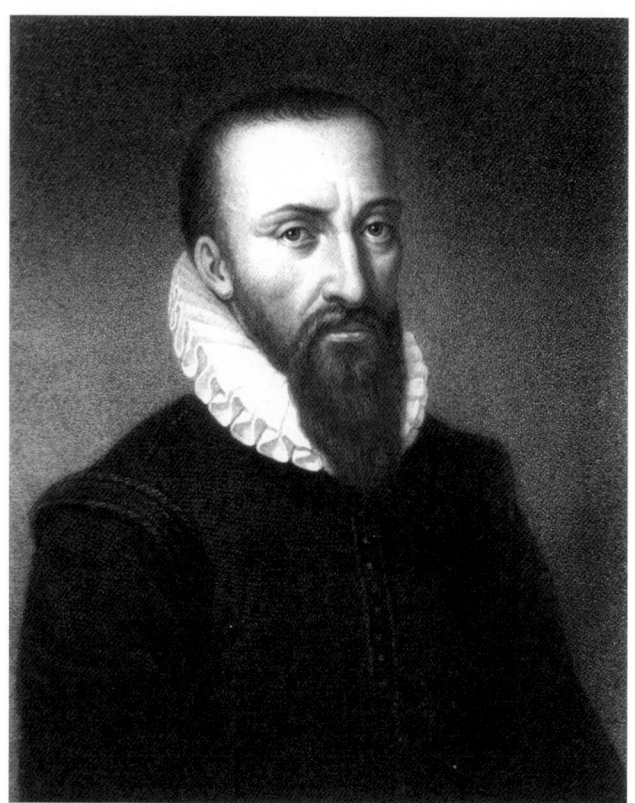

FIGURE 1.23 Ambroise Paré, MD. (Courtesy of the National Library of Medicine.)

books were based on his extensive experience in treating gun and sword wounds and the pain that attended them.[50] He was the first to describe pain after the amputation of limbs, 300 years before the conceptualization of "phantom limb pain" was ever expressed. Remarkably, contrary to the current philosophy of his time, he resisted the prevailing wisdom that pain was either inevitable and to be passively tolerated or in some way the will of God to be accepted by man as a path to holiness by actively treating pain in his suffering patients. Some of his innovations included the development of prosthetic devices for missing limbs, a steam bath chair for urethral stone pain, and combinations, called "allodynes," of opium and other drugs to treat the symptoms of pain.[51]

Other compassionate physicians observing their tormented pain patients, primarily as a result of catastrophic war injuries, continued to develop options to treat pain out of necessity. The U.S. Civil War resulted in untold numbers of soldiers who suffered damaged nerves after amputation and injury, with resultant chronic "nerve" disease. The persistent burning pain long after the initial injury was first called *reflex paralysis* by Silas Weir Mitchell (Fig. 1.24) in 1864. Dr. Mitchell, born in Philadelphia as the seventh physician within three generations, was told at an early age by his physician father, "you are wanting in nearly all the qualities that go to make a success in medicine." Despite this, he graduated from Jefferson Medical College in 1848 and, at the outbreak of hostilities in 1861, was placed in charge of Turner's Lane Hospital in Philadelphia, a 400-bed hospital for nervous diseases. With colleagues, William Williams Keen, Jr. (Fig. 1.25) and George Read Morehouse (Fig. 1.26), he personally transported railroad cars full of wounded soldiers from the Gettysburg battlefield and undertook their care. Based on daily patient observation and review of literally thousands of pages of careful clinical notes, he described causalgia for the first time in 1864 in the work *Gunshot Wounds and Other Injuries of Nerves.*[52–54]

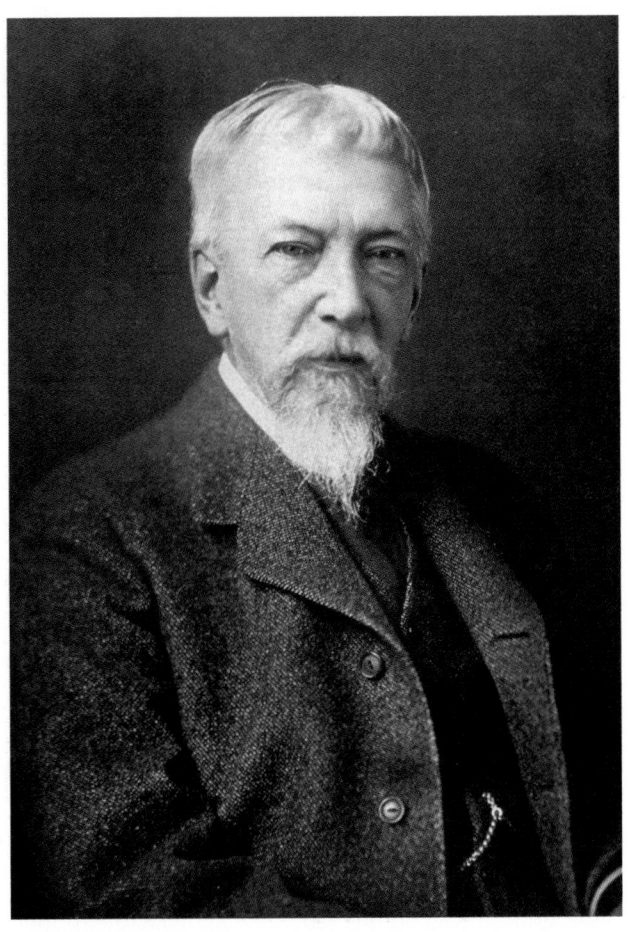

FIGURE 1.24 Silas Weir Mitchell, MD. (Courtesy of the National Library of Medicine.)

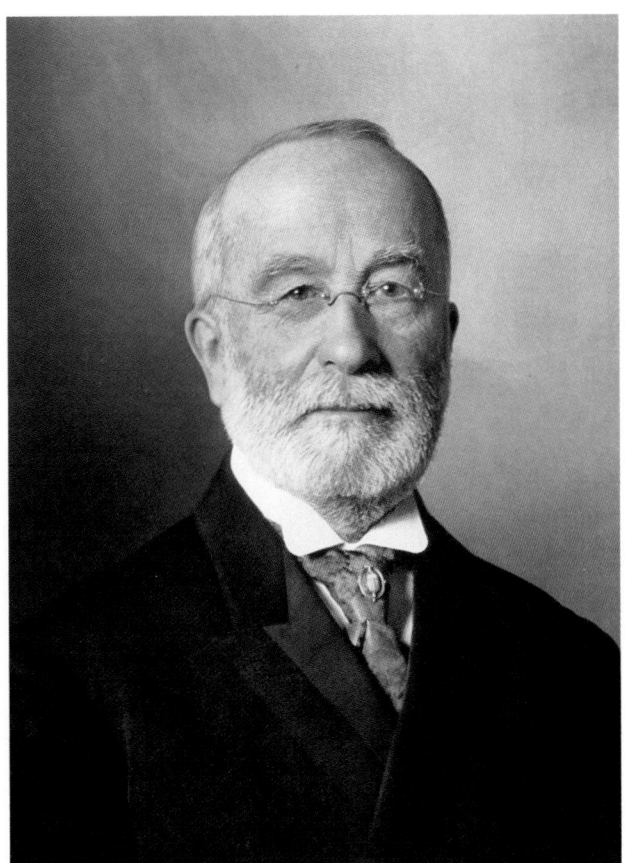

FIGURE 1.25 William Williams Keen, Jr., MD. (Courtesy of the National Library of Medicine.)

An early example of injecting specific nerves to produce analgesia was the work of Schloesser in 1903. He injected alcohol to produce long-lasting interruption of neural conduction in patients with convulsive facial tics, obtaining paralysis that lasted from days to a month. He recommended lytic injections for the patients with clinical supraorbital neuralgia and tic douloureux.[55]

Later, war injuries in World War I soldiers inspired a practical surgeon, René Leriche, to study pain and its treatment in various forms of pathology. He identified patients with sympathetic nerve injuries—his "pariahs of pain"—that he treated by injecting the local anesthetic procaine and surgical sympathectomy, which later became standard therapy in the 1930s. He was a clinician's clinician, describing pain from direct personal observation: "Physical pain is not a simple affair of an impulse, traveling at a fixed rate along a nerve. It is the resultant of a conflict between a stimulus and the whole individual."[56]

Following the theory of pain arising from specific nerve injuries, surgeons in the 1920s performed nerve ablation procedures for chronic unexplained pain syndromes. Following this model, anesthesiologists experimented with various local anesthetic nerve blocks to provide analgesia for surgery. The first nerve block clinic for pain relief was started by Emery Rovenstine (Fig. 1.27) at Bellevue Hospital in New York City, New York, in 1936.[57] Eleven years later, the first nerve block clinic in the UK was established at University College Hospital in London in 1947.[58]

Current therapies based on central nervous system plasticity modulating input from peripheral nerves include spinal cord stimulation, sympathetic nerve blocks, radiofrequency modulation

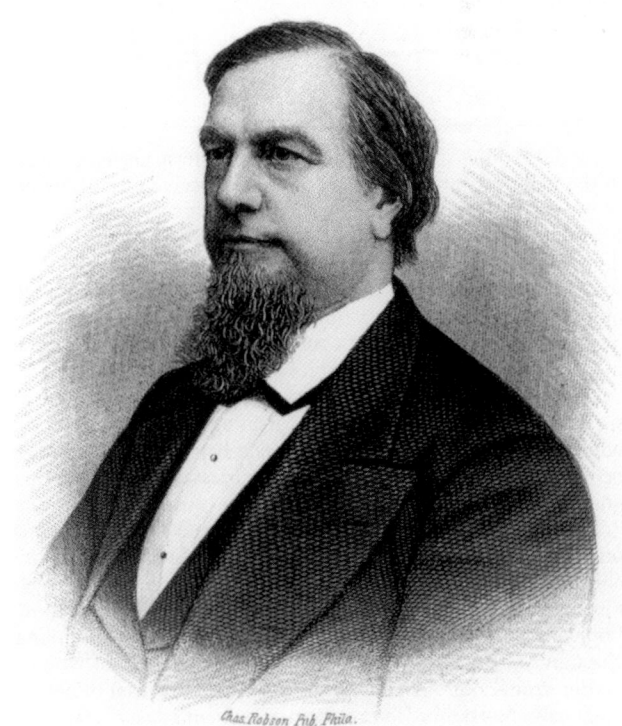

FIGURE 1.26 George Read Morehouse, MD. (Courtesy of Thomas Jefferson University, Philadelphia, PA.)

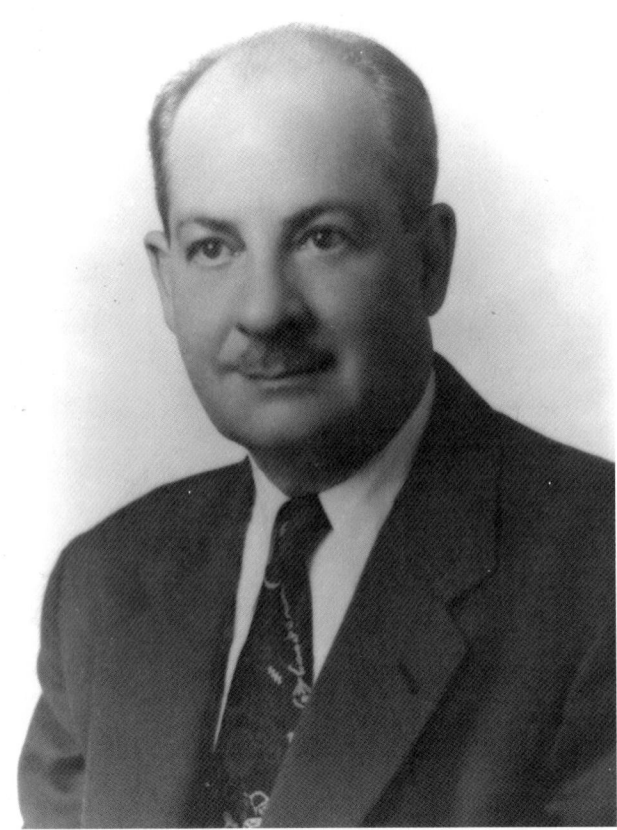

FIGURE 1.27 Emery A. Rovenstine, MD. (Courtesy of the Wood Library-Museum of Anesthesiology.)

(both pulsed and lesioning), and cognitive therapies and are now commonly available in modern pain practice.

THE SPECIALTY OF PAIN MEDICINE

How did pain as a medical specialty and physicians specializing in the diagnosis and treatment of pain conceive of chronic pain as an original and new field of clinical practice? A sociologist, Isabelle Baszanger, observed two clinics in Paris that had very different constructs of pain and pain treatment, which she described as the two poles of pain. The first "curing through techniques" considers pain as a function of physiological abnormalities, with diagnosis aimed at confirming the pathology and using medication and technical therapies to treat it. As more technological possibilities develop, the treatments become more focused and sophisticated. The second pole is "healing through adaptation," which considers pain a poorly adaptive behavior and, therefore, behavior and cognitive therapies are necessary to alleviate pain and suffering.[59]

Earlier, in 1936, Emery A. Rovenstine (1895–1960) set up one of the first outpatient clinics devoted to the treatment of chronic pain in Bellevue Hospital in New York City.[60] However, the founding father of interdisciplinary pain care was John J. Bonica (1917–1994), who established the first multidisciplinary clinic in Seattle in 1947 to treat the pain problems of wounded World War II veterans. He published the first edition of his comprehensive textbook, *Management of Pain*, in 1953.[61] His clinical practice increased and gained support after aligning with the University of Washington in Seattle in 1960. As his reputation grew, he encouraged other centers to recognize and treat pain as an

integral part of health care.[62] He then proceeded to work internationally to foster the study and treatment of pain. He was the prime mover in hosting the first International Symposium on Pain in Issaquah, Washington, on May 21–26, 1973, and the subsequent establishment of the International Association for the Study of Pain as their first president. This association currently represents over 60 scientific disciplines in active research and clinical practice in a wide variety of pain related fields. The journal, *Pain*, supported by this organization, foreshadowed the numerous peer reviewed scholarly publications now focused on all levels of pain research.[63] The American Board of Anesthesiology (ABA) approved a Certificate of Added Qualification in Pain Management in 1991, followed by subspecialty certification from the American Board of Psychiatry and Neurology (ABPN) and the American Board of Physical Medicine and Rehabilitation (ABPMR) in 2000.[64]

It is an exciting time for the study and treatment of pain. Many scientific investigations are now possible with the probes of molecular biology for microneurographic stimulation and the ability to elucidate genetic codes. Newly developing technologies to study pain, such as positron emission tomography (PET) and functional magnetic resonance imaging (fMRI), and more sophisticated constructs of neural plasticity will result in ever more intriguing questions and hypotheses being developed. Advances in understanding of the interactions between the peripheral and central nervous system, the thalamus and cerebral cortex, and the limbic system continue to increase our understanding of pain processing. Enhanced imaging techniques such as PET and fMRI allow in vivo, real time investigation of information processing evoked by pain stimuli. Identification of newer molecular receptors for opioid compounds and genetic variability in pain expression provide the hope more pain syndromes can be defined and treated in a much more specific manner. And the role of cognition, personality, and memory in descending modulation of spinal mechanisms of pain affords better and more holistic treatment of the patient in pain. The complexity of the field is fertile ground for the ingenuity and persistent questioning of future pain scientists and clinicians. Therefore, the history of pain as science and pain medicine as a focused clinical specialty is only beginning to be written.

References

1. Weiner RS. *Innovations in Pain Management: A Practical Guide for Clinicians.* Orlando, FL: Paul M. Deutsch Press, Inc., 1990.
2. Benedelow GA, Williams SJ. Transcending the dualisms toward a study of pain. *Sociology of Health & Illness* 1995;17(2):139–165.
3. Birk RK. The history of pain management. *History of Anesthesia Society Proceedings* 2006;36:37–46.
4. Keirsey D. *Please Understand Me II: Temperament, Character, Intelligence.* Del Mar, CA: Prometheus Nemesis Book Co, Inc., 1998.
5. King H. The early anodynes: pain in the ancient world. In: Mann RD, ed. *The History of the Management of Pain.* Lancaster, UK: Parthenon Publishing Group Ltd., 1988:51–60.
6. Rey R. Christianity and pain in the Middle Ages. In: Rey R. *The History of Pain.* Cambridge, MA: Harvard University Press, 1955:48–49.
7. Bonica JJ. *The Management of Pain.* Philadelphia, PA: Lea & Febiger, 1953:23.
8. Epistolary Dissertation (1681). In: RG Latham, trans-ed. *The Works of Thomas Sydenham, M.D.*, 2 vols. London: Sydenham Society, 1848–1850;2:85.
9. Charlotte Perkins Gilman as quoted in Rey R. The History of Pain. Gilman CP. *The Living of Charlotte Perkins Gilman: An Autobiography.* New York and London: D. Appleton-Century Co., 1935:96.
10. J. C. Colquhoun, ed. *Report of the Experiments on Animal Magnetism Made by a Committee of the Medical Section of the French Royal Academy of Sciences, Paris, France, 21st and 28th of June 1831.* Edinburgh: R. Cadell; London: Whittaker, 1833.
11. Zimmermann M. The history of pain concepts and treatment before IASP. In: Merskey H, Loeser JD, Dubner R, eds. *The Paths of Pain,1975–2005.* Seattle, WA: IASP Press, 2005:9.
12. Squire WW. On the introduction of ether inhalation as an anesthetic in London. *Lancet* 1888;22:1220–1221.

13. Rey R. Christianity and pain in the Middle Ages. In: Rey R. *The History of Pain*. Cambridge, MA: Harvard University Press, 1955.
14. Engel GL. Psychogenic pain. *Med Clin North Am* 1958;42(6):1481–1496.
15. Szasz TS. *Pain and Pleasure: A Study of Bodily Feelings*. London: Taistock, 1957.
16. Walters A. Psychogenic regional pain alias hysterical pain. *Brain* 1961;84:1–18.
17. Merskey H. Psychiatric patients with persistent pain. *J Psychosom Res* 1965;9:299–309.
18. Pope A. *An Essay on Man Epistle I. An Essay on Man In Four Epistles*. Whitefish, MT: Kessinger Publishing, LLC, 2004.
19. Sawday J. *Engines of the Imagination: Renaissance Culture and the Rise of the Machine*. London: Routledge, 2007.
20. Descartes R. *L'Homme*. Paris: C. Angot, 1664.
21. Harvey W. *Exercitatio Anatomica de Motu Cordis et Sanguinis in Animalibus*, 1628.
22. Cranefield PF. *The Way In and the Way Out: François Magendie, Charles Bell and the Roots of the Spinal Nerves*. Mount Kisco, NY: Futura Publishing Company, 1974.
23. Bell C. *Idea of a New Anatomy of the Brain; Submitted for the Observations of His Friends*. London: Strahan & Preston, 1811.
24. Magendie F. Experiments on the spinal nerves. *Journal of Experimental Physiology and Pathology* 1822;2:276–279.
25. Müller J. *Handbuch der Physiologie des Menschen*, Vol 2. In: Baly W, trans-ed. London: Raylor & Walton, 1839
26. Rey R. Von Frey and the theory of specificity. In: Rey R. *The History of Pain*. Cambridge, MA: Harvard University Press, 1955:215–218.
27. Rey R. Von Frey and the theory of specificity. In: Rey R. *The History of Pain*. Cambridge, MA: Harvard University Press, 1955:215.
28. Goldscheider A. Die spezifische Energie der Gefühlsnerven der Haut. *Prakt Derm* 1884;3:283.
29. Nafe JP. A quantitative theory of feeling. *J Gen Psychol* 1929;2:199–211.
30. Sinclair DC. Cutaneous sensation and the doctrine of specific energy. *Brain* 1955;78:584–614.
31. Weddell G. Somesthesis and the chemical senses. *Ann Rev Psychol* 1955;6:119–136.
32. Perl ER. Ideas about pain, a historical review. *Nature Reviews Neuroscience* 2007;8:72.
33. Sherrington CS. *The Integrative Action of the Nervous System*. Cambridge, UK: Cambridge University Press, 1906.
34. Melzack R, Wall PD. Pain mechanisms: a new theory. *Science* 1965;150:971–979.
35. Woolf CJ, Salter MW. Neuronal plasticity: increasing the gain in pain. *Science* 2000;288(5472):1765–1769.
36. Parris W. The history of pain medicine. In: Raj PP, ed. *Practical Management of Pain*. 3rd ed. St. Louis, MO: Mosby, Inc., 2000:4.
37. Fülöp-Miller R. *Triumph Over Pain*. In: Paul E, Paul C, trans-eds. New York: Literary Guild of America, 1938:396.
38. Engel GL. Psychogenic pain. *Med Clin North Am* 1959;42:1481–1496.
39. Beecher HK. Pain in men wounded in battle. *Ann Surg* 1946;123:96–105.
40. Clark D. Total pain: Disciplinary power and the power in the work of Cicely Saunders, 1958–1967. *Social Science and Medicine* 1999;49:727–736.
41. Liebeskind JC, Meldrum ML. John J. Bonica. World champion of pain. In: Jensen TS, Turner JA, Wiesenfeld-Hallin Z, eds. *Proceedings of the Eighth World Congress on Pain: Progress in Pain Research and Management*, Vol. 8. Seattle, WA: International Association for the Study of Pain Press, 1997:19–32.
42. Niemann A. Über einer organische Base in der Coca. *Annalen Chemie* 1860;114:213.
43. Koller C. On the use of cocaine for producing anaesthesia on the eye. *Lancet* 1884;2:990.
44. Leake CD. *An Historical Account of Pharmacology to the Twentieth Century*. Springfield, IL: CC Thomas, 1975:160.
45. Fairley P. *The Conquest of Pain*. London: Michael Joseph, 1978.
46. Andermann AAJ. Physicians, fads, and pharmaceuticals: A history of aspirin. *McGill J Med* 1996;2(2).
47. Rynd F. Neuralgia—Introduction of fluid to the nerve. *Dublin Med Press* 1845;13:167.
48. Mann RD. The history of the non-steroidal anti-inflammatory drugs. In: Birk RK. The history of pain management. *History of Anesthesia Society Proceedings*. September 2006:43.
49. Moore J. *A Method of Preventing or Diminishing Pain in Several Operations of Surgery*. London: T. Cadell, 1784.
50. Malgaigne JF. Oeuvres completes d'Ambroise Paré. 3 vols, Paris: Baillière, 1840–1841.
51. Zimmermann M. The history of pain concepts and treatment before IASP. In: Merskey H, Loeser JD, Dubner R, eds. *The Paths of Pain, 1975–2005*. Seattle, WA: IASP Press, 2005:4.
52. Mitchell SW, Morehouse GR, Keen WW. *Gunshot Wounds and Other Injuries of Nerves*. Philadelphia: J. B. Lippincott & Co., 1864.
53. Mitchell SW. Civilization and pain. *JAMA* 1892;18:108.
54. Mitchell SW. *Injuries to Nerves and Their Consequences*. Philadelphia: J. B. Lippincott & Co., 1872.
55. Schloesser. Heilung peripharer Reizzustände sensibler und motorischer Nerven. *Klin Monatsbl Augenheilkd* 1903;41:244.
56. Leriche R. *La Chirurgie de la Douleur*. Paris: Masson, 1937.
57. Rovenstine EA, Wertheim HM. Therapeutic nerve block. *JAMA* 1941;117:1599–1603.
58. Swerdlow M. The early development of pain relief clinics in the UK. *Anaesthesia* 1992;47:977–980.
59. Baszanger I. Deciphering chronic pain. *Society of Health and Illness* 1992;14(2):181–215.
60. Cousins M. History of neural blockade and pain management. In: Cousins MJ, Bridenbaugh PO, eds. *Neural Blockade in Clinical Anesthesia and Management of Pain*. 3rd ed. Philadelphia: Lippincott-Raven, 1998:21–22.
61. Bonica JJ. *The Management of Pain*. Philadelphia: Lea & Febiger, 1953:23.
62. Bonica JJ. Basic principles in managing chronic pain. *Arch Surg* 1977;112(6):783.
63. Bond MR, Dubner R, Jones LE, et al. The history of the IASP: progress in pain since 1975. In: Merskey H, Loeser JD, Dubner R, eds. *The Paths of Pain, 1975–2005*. Seattle, WA: IASP Press, 2005:23–32.
64. Fishman S, Gallager, RM, Carr DB, et al. The case for pain medicine. *Medicine* 2004;5(3):281–286.

CHAPTER 2 ■ PAIN TERMS AND TAXONOMIES OF PAIN

DENNIS C. TURK AND AKIKO OKIFUJI

INTRODUCTION

The inherent subjectivity of pain presents a fundamental impediment to increased understanding of its mechanisms and control. The language used by any two individuals attempting to describe a similar injury and their pain experience often varies markedly. Similarly, clinicians and clinical investigators commonly use multiple terms that at times have idiosyncratic meanings. Needless to say, appropriate communication requires a common language and a classification system that is used in a consistent fashion. Thus, we have two primary goals in this chapter: (1) to provide definitions for many commonly used terms in the pain literature, in an effort to bring about consistency and thereby improve communication, and (2) to describe and discuss different classification systems or taxonomies that have been used or proposed, in an attempt to improve communication and bring consistency to research and treatment of patients reporting pain.

DEFINITION OF COMMONLY USED PAIN TERMS

Discussions of pain involve many terms. The meaning and connotation of these different terms may vary widely. For example, some authors use the term "pain" to relate to a stimulus, others to a thing, and still others to a response. Such inconsistent usage creates difficulties in communication. As Merskey[1] noted, it would be most convenient and helpful if there were some consensus on technical meanings and usage. Based on this belief, the editors of the two editions of the International Association for the Study of Pain (IASP) Classification of Chronic Pain included a set of definitions of commonly used pain terms[2,3] (note that a third edition is currently in preparation). In the second edition of this text, Bonica reproduced a list of the terms and in some cases provided annotations. We adopt a similar strategy. We follow the convention of IASP; we begin with the definition of pain and then proceed alphabetically. Terms preceded by an asterisk come directly from the IASP descriptions of pain terms.[3]

> *Pain*: An unpleasant sensory *and* emotional experience associated with *actual or potential* tissue damage, or described in terms of such damage (emphasis added).

> *Pain, acute/chronic*[1]: Definitions of acute, chronic, recurrent, and cancer pain are not specifically included in the IASP list of pain terms. We believe, however, that it is important to clarify these because they are commonly used in the literature.

> Traditionally, the distinction between acute and chronic pain has relied upon a single continuum of time, with some interval since the onset of pain used to designate the onset of acute pain or the transition point when acute pain becomes chronic. The two most commonly used chronological markers used to denote chronic pain have been 3 months and 6 months since the initiation of pain; however, these distinctions are arbitrary.

> Another criterion for chronic pain is "pain that extends beyond the expected period of healing." This is relatively independent of time because it considers pain as chronic even when it has persisted for a relatively brief duration. Unfortunately, how long the expected process of healing will (or should) take is ambiguous.

> Some hold that pain that persists for long periods of time in the presence of ongoing pathology should be considered an extended "acute" pain state. In this case, treatment targets the underlying pathology. This is not to encourage a Cartesian dualistic perspective of pain that treats mind and body as independent entities with distinctive functions. Historically, such distinction led to a faulty assumption of acute pain as "real" whereas chronic pain without known pathology was suspect and viewed as being merely "functional." As the IASP definition clearly states, any pain, acute or chronic, regardless of the presence of identifiable tissue damage, is an unpleasant experience, inherently influenced by various cognitive, affective, and environmental factors. We hold that the weighing of psychological and environmental factors is often greater in chronic pain than acute pain, and the importance of these factors escalates over time, contributing to the experience of pain and associated disability.

> We propose conceptualizing acute and chronic pain on two

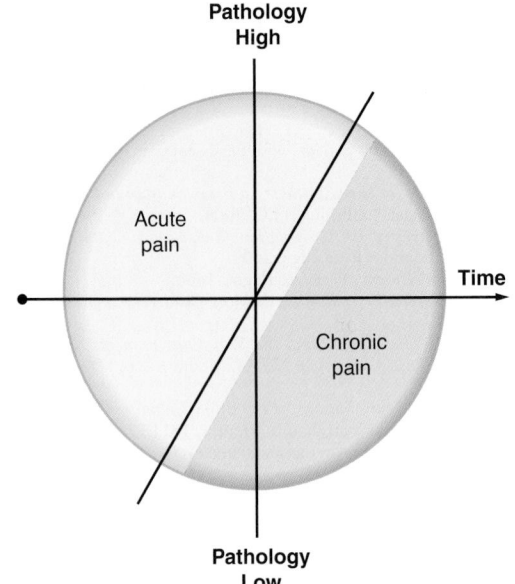

FIGURE 2.1 Pictorial representation of acute and chronic pain.

dimensions: time and physical pathology. Figure 2.1 schematically depicts this two-dimensional conceptualization of acute and chronic pain. From this perspective, any case falling above the diagonal line (short duration or high physical pathology) is acute pain; whereas cases falling below the diagonal line (low physical pathology or long duration) suggest chronic pain. The perspective presented in Figure 2.1 leads to the following definitions of acute and chronic pain.

> *Acute pain*: Pain elicited by the injury of body tissues and activation of nociceptive transducers at the site of local tissue damage. The local injury alters the response characteristics of the nociceptors and perhaps their central connections and the autonomic nervous system in the region. In general, the state of acute pain lasts for a relatively limited time and remits when the underlying pathology resolves (however, see definition of central sensitization below). This type of pain often serves as the impetus to seek health care and it occurs following trauma, some disease processes, and invasive interventions.

> *Chronic pain*: May be elicited by an injury or disease but is likely to be perpetuated by factors that are both pathogenetically and physically remote from the originating cause. Chronic pain extends for a long period of time and/or represents low levels of underlying pathology that does not explain the presence and extent of pain (e.g., mechanical back pain, fibromyalgia syndrome [FM]). Recently, there have been suggestions that chronic pain in the apparent absence of pathology may be attributable to modification of nerves and sensitization of the peripheral or central nervous system. There have also been suggestions that genetic factors and prior life experiences might predispose some to develop chronic pain problems following an initiating insult that resolves in others who do not have the predisposition. Just as the brain is modified by experience, especially in early life, the brain may alter the way noxious information is processed to reduce or augment its impact on subjective awareness.

> Chronic pain frequently is the impetus for people to seek health care. Currently available treatments are rarely capable of totally eliminating the noxious sensations and thereby "curing" chronic pain. Because the pain persists, it is likely that environmental, emotional, and cognitive factors will interact with the already sensitized nervous system, contributing to the persistence of pain and associated illness behaviors (see

---

[1]The discussion describing the distinction between acute and chronic pain reflects on deliberations among the editors of the previous edition of this volume.

description of pain behaviors below). It is also possible that, just as the brain is modified by experience, especially in early life, the brain may alter the way noxious information is processed to reduce or augment its impact on subjective awareness.

Cancer pain: Pain associated with cancer includes pain associated with disease progression as well as treatments (e.g., chemotherapy, radiotherapy, surgery) that may damage the nervous system. Although some contend that pain associated with neoplastic disease is unique, in the majority of instances we view it as fitting within our description of acute and chronic pain, as depicted in Figure 2.1. Moreover, pain associated with cancer can have multiple causes, namely, disease progression, treatment, and co-occurring diseases (e.g., arthritis). Regardless of whether the pain associated with cancer stems from disease progression, treatment, or a co-occurring disease, it may be either acute or chronic. Thus, we do not advocate a separate classification of cancer pain as distinct from acute and chronic pain.

Some concerns have also been raised regarding the common usage of malignant and benign pain[4]; often, pain unrelated to cancer is referred to as "benign" to distinguish it from cancer-related pain. Certainly, people who have pain associated with neoplastic disease experience a unique and disease-specific situation, but from a mechanistic perspective there may be little to substantiate continued use of this dichotomy. Moreover, patients who have chronic non–cancer pain who are told that their pain is "benign" may feel denigrated because, from their perspective, the inference is that their pain is not a serious concern.

Recurrent pain: Episodic or intermittent occurrences of pain, with each episode lasting for a relatively short period of time but recurring across an extended period of time (e.g., migraine headaches, tic douloureux, sickle cell crisis). Our distinction between acute and chronic pain using the integration of the dimensions of time and pathology does not specifically include recurrent pain. In the case of recurrent pain, patients may experience episodes of pain interspersed with periods of being completely pain free. Although recurrent pain may seem acute because each pain episode (e.g., sickle cell crisis) is of short duration, the pathophysiology of many recurrent pain disorders (e.g., migraine) is not well understood. Syndromes characterized by recurrent acute pain share features in common with both acute and chronic pain. The fact that these syndromes extend over time, however, suggests that psychosocial and behavioral factors, not only physical pathology, may be major contributors to illness behavior.

Transient pain: Pain elicited by activation of nociceptors in the absence of any significant local tissue damage. This type of pain is ubiquitous in everyday life and is rarely a reason to seek heath care. It is seen in the clinical setting and only in incidental or procedural pain, such as during a venipuncture or injection. This type of pain ceases as soon as the stimulus is removed. There are situations where sources of transient pain may be treated by providers with preventive analgesic or topical medication.

Addiction: A behavioral pattern of substance, including prescribed medication, abuse characterized by overwhelming involvement with the use of a drug (i.e., compulsive use), the securing of its supply, and a high tendency to relapse. The compulsive use of the drug results in physical, psychological, and/or social harm to the user and use continues despite this harm. See also Physical Dependency.

*Alloydnia: Pain due to a stimulus that does not normally provoke pain.

Analgesia: Absence of the spontaneous report of pain or pain behaviors in response to stimulation that would normally be expected to be painful. The term implies a defined stimulus and a defined response. Analgesic responses can be tested in animals as well as humans.

*Anesthesia dolorosa: Spontaneous pain in an area or region that is anesthetic.

Breakthrough pain: A transient increase in pain to greater than moderate intensity superimposed on an otherwise stable pattern or level of pain of mild to moderate intensity. Breakthrough pain includes (1) incident pain that may arise from some activity or physical function (e.g., coughing, standing up), (2) pain that routinely increases as the duration of analgesic medication in reaching its limit (end-of-dose failure), and (3) spontaneous exacerbation of a stable level of pain for nonspecific reasons.

Catastrophizing: A cognitive and emotional process that involves magnification of pain-related stimuli, feelings of helplessness, and a negative orientation to pain and life circumstances. Catastrophizing has been shown to be an important predictor of response to both acute and chronic pain.[5]

*Central pain: Pain initiated or caused by a primary lesion or dysfunction in the central nervous system.

Central sensitization: Increase in the excitability and responsiveness of neurons in the spinal cord.

*Complex regional pain syndrome type 1 (formerly reflex sympathetic dystrophy): A syndrome that usually develops after an initiating noxious event, is not limited to the distribution of a single peripheral nerve, and is apparently disproportionate to the inciting event. It is associated at some point with evidence of edema, changes in skin blood flow, abnormal pseudomotor activity in the region of the pain, or allodynia or hyperalgesia.

*Complex regional pain syndrome type 2 (formerly causalgia): A syndrome of sustained burning pain, allodynia, and hyperpathia following a traumatic nerve lesion, often combined with vasomotor dysfunction and later trophic changes.

Cost–benefit analysis: Evaluation of the costs and effects of an intervention in a common, usually monetary unit. The standardization of unit has an advantage because it permits comparisons across dissimilar intervention programs. On the other hand, the conversion of treatment effects to monetary units may not always be feasible. Estimation of the cost to outcome ratio is possible, as are comparisons between interventions using the rates of improvement (e.g., return to work) with common denominators.

Cost-effectiveness analysis: Estimation of treatment outcome entails criteria other than monetary terms, such as lives saved or return to work. An intervention is cost-effective when it satisfies one of the following conditions:

1. It is more effective than an alternative modality at the same cost;
2. it is less costly and at least as effective as an alternative modality;
3. it is more effective and more costly than an alternative treatment, but the benefit exceeds the added cost; or
4. it is less effective and less costly, but the added benefit of the alternative is not worth the additional cost.

Diffuse noxious inhibitory control: Inhibition of wide dynamic range neurons in the dorsal horn of the spinal cord by heterosegmental noxious afferent input.

Disability: Any restriction or loss of capacity to perform an activity in the manner or within the range considered normal for a human being, such as climbing stairs, lifting groceries, or talking on a telephone. It is a task-based concept that involves both the person and the environment. Disability is essentially a social and not a medical term or classification. Level of disability should be determined only after a patient has reached maximum medical improvement following appropriate treatment and rehabilitation.

Dysesthesia: An unpleasant abnormal sensation, whether spontaneous or evoked.

Hyperalgesia: An increased response to a stimulus that is normally painful.

Hyperesthesia: Increased sensitivity to stimulation, excluding special senses.

Hyperpathia: A painful syndrome characterized by an abnormally painful reaction to a stimulus, especially a repetitive stimulus, as well as an increased threshold.

Hypoalgesia: Diminished pain in response to a normally painful stimulus.

Hypochondriasis: An excessive preoccupation with bodily sensations and fears that they represent serious disease despite reassurance to the contrary.

Impairment: Any loss of use of, or abnormality of, psychological, physiological, or anatomical structure or function that is quantifiable. It is not equivalent to disability. Impairment is to disability as disease is to illness.

Malingering: A conscious and willful feigning or exaggeration of a disease or effect of an injury in order to obtain a specific external gain. It is usually motivated by external incentives such as financial compensation, avoiding work, or obtaining drugs.

Maximum medical improvement: The state beyond which additional medical treatment is unlikely to produce an improvement in function.

Minimum clinically important difference (MCID): The magnitude of reduction in pain or related problems that a patient would consider minimally important. In considering the determination of clinically important differences, two different aspects of the interpretation of clinical trial results must be distinguished. One is establishing the difference in the magnitude of response between the treatment and control groups that will be considered large enough to establish the scientific or therapeutic importance of the results. The other is establishing what change in the outcome measure represents a meaningful difference for patients. This later consideration has come to be referred to as the minimum clinically important difference. The development of criteria for determining what are important changes in an individuals' scores on the outcome measures used in chronic pain trials would provide clinicians and researchers with essential methods for evaluating treatment responses of individuals in clinical trials and clinical practice. Such individual-level criteria make it possible to conduct responder analyses that classify each trial participant as "improved," "stable," or "worse" on the basis of validated criteria of important change. (See description of patient global impression of change.)

Multidisciplinary (interdisciplinary) pain center: An organization of health care professionals and basic and applied scientists that includes research, teaching, and patient care related to acute and chronic pain. It includes a wide array of health care professionals including physicians, psychologists, nurses, physical therapists, occupational therapists, and other specialty health care providers. Multiple therapeutic modalities are available. These centers provide evaluation and treatment and are usually affiliated with major health science institutions.

Neuralgia: Pain in the distribution of a nerve or nerves.

Neuritis: Inflammation of a nerve or nerves.

Neurogenic pain: Pain initiated or caused by a primary lesion, dysfunction, or transitory perturbation in the peripheral or central nervous system.

Neuropathic pain: Pain arising as a direct consequence of a lesion or disease affecting the somatosensory system.[6]

Neuropathy: A disturbance of function or pathological change in a nerve: in one nerve, mononeurapathy; in several nerves, mononeuropathy multiplex; if diffuse and bilateral, polyneuropathy.

Nocebo: Negative treatment effects induced by a substance or procedure containing no toxic or detrimental substance.

Nociceptor: A receptor preferentially sensitive to tissue trauma or to a stimulus that would damage tissue if prolonged.

Nociception: Activation of sensory transduction in nerves by thermal, mechanical, or chemical energy impinging on specialized nerve endings. The nerve(s) involved conveys information about tissue damage to the central nervous system.

Noxious stimulus: A stimulus that is capable of activating receptors for tissue damage.

Pain behavior: Verbal or nonverbal actions understood by observers to indicate that a person may be experiencing pain and suffering. These actions may include audible emissions (e.g., signs, moans), facial expressions, abnormal postures or gait, use of prosthetic devices, avoidance of activities, and verbal indications of pain, distress, and suffering.

Pain clinic: Facilities focusing on diagnosis and management of patients with pain problems. It may specialize in specific diagnoses or pain related to a specific area of the body.

Pain relief: Report of reduced pain after a treatment. It does not require reduced response to a noxious stimulus and is not a synonym for analgesia. The term applies only to humans.

Pain threshold: The least level of stimulus intensity perceived as painful. In psychophysics, this is defined as a level of stimulus intensity that a person recognizes as painful 50% of time.

Pain tolerance level: The greatest level of noxious stimulation that an individual is willing to tolerate.

Pain sensitivity range: The difference between the pain threshold and the pain tolerance level.

Paresthesia: An abnormal sensation whether spontaneous or evoked.

Patient global impression of change (PGIC): Patients' overall evaluation of improvement or worsening of symptoms over the course of treatment. This measure is often a single-item rating by patients on a 7-point scale that ranges from "very much improved" to "very much worse" with "no change" as the midpoint.

Peripheral neurogenic pain: Pain initiated or caused by a primary lesion or dysfunction or transitory perturbation in the peripheral nervous system.

Physical dependence: A pharmacological property of a drug (e.g., opioid) characterized by the occurrence of an abstinence syndrome following abrupt discontinuation of the substance or administration of an antagonist. It does not imply an aberrant psychological state or behavior or addiction.

Placebo: A substance or procedure without therapeutic effect that is provided as a treatment. It is frequently used to control patients' expectations for the efficacy in testing a treatment intervention.

Placebo effects: Refers to the positive benefit(s) from a placebo (i.e., inert) preparation or procedure when such benefit is generally achieved only with an active treatment intervention. Active treatments also are likely to have a placebo component that augments the active component associated with the treatment.

Plasticity, neural: Nociceptive input leading to structural and functional changes that may cause altered perceptual processing and contribute to pain chronicity.

Pseudoaddiction: Refers to drug-seeking behavior or misuse by patients who have severe pain and are under-medicated or who have not received other effective pain treatment interventions. Such patients may appear preoccupied with obtaining opioids, but the preoccupation reflects a need for pain relief and not drug addiction. Pseudoaddictive behavior differs from true addictive behavior because when higher doses of opioid are provided, the patient does not use these in a manner that persistently causes sedation or euphoria, the level of function is increased rather than decreased, and the medications are used as prescribed without loss of control over use.

Psychogenic pain: Report of pain attributable primarily to psychological factors usually in the absence of any objective physical pathology that could account for pain. This term is commonly used in a pejorative sense. It often suggests a Cartesian dualism and is not usually a helpful method of describing a patient.

Quality of life/health-related quality of life: Quality of life (QOL) refers to an individual's perception of his or her position in life in the context of the culture and value systems in which they live and in relation to their goals, expectations, standards, and concerns. Concerns with this all-encompassing description have led a number of investigators to use a more circumscribed construct, *health-related quality of life* (HRQOL). Although HRQOL has been used interchangeably with terms such as health status and functional status, HRQOL is a narrower term than QOL because it does not include aspects of work, environmental conditions, housing, and other variables that are often considered relevant to QOL but that do not involve health directly.[7]

Rehabilitation: Restoration of an individual to maximal physical and mental functioning in light of his or her impairment.

Residual functional capacity: The capacity to perform specific social and work-related physical and mental activities following rehabilitation related to impairment or when a condition has reached a point of maximum medical improvement.

Summed pain intensity difference (SPID): A strategy for combining relief magnitude and duration in a single score. It is calculated by the sum of the time-weighted pain intensity difference (difference between current pain and pain at baseline) multiplied by the interval between ratings.

Symptom magnification: Conscious or unconscious exaggeration of symptom severity in an attempt to convince an observer that one is truly experiencing some level of pain. It differs from malingering as it is an effort to be believed, not necessarily to achieve a positive outcome (i.e., secondary gain) such as financial compensation.

Suffering: Reaction to the physical or emotional components of pain with a feeling of uncontrollability, helplessness, hopelessness, intolerability, and interminability. Suffering implies a threat to the intactness of an individual's self-concept, self-identify, and integrity.

Tolerance, drug: A physiological state in which a person requires an increased dosage of a psychoactive substance to sustain a desired effect.

Total pain relief (TOPAR): Is used in clinical trials to assess pain relief over time. It is a cumulative measure that is comprised of the sum of time-weighted pain relief score multiplied by the interval between ratings. TOPAR is frequently used in clinical trials of medications designed to ameliorate pain.

Wind-up: Slow temporal summation of pain mediated by C-fibers due to repetitive noxious stimulation at a rate faster than 1 stimulus every 3 seconds. May cause the person to experience a gradual increase in the perceived magnitude of pain.

TAXONOMIES

The lack of a classification of chronic pain syndromes that is used on a consistent basis inhibits the advancement of knowledge and treatment of chronic pain and makes it hard for investigators as well as practitioners to compare observations and results of research. Bonica[8] referred to this language ambiguity as "a modern tower of Babel."

In order to identify target groups, conduct research, prescribe treatment, evaluate treatment efficacy, and for policy and deci-

sion-making, it is essential that some consensually-validated criteria are used to distinguish groups of individuals who share a common set of relevant attributes. The primary purpose of such a classification is to describe the relationships of constituent members based upon their equivalence along a set of basic dimensions that represent the structure of a particular domain. Infinite classification systems are possible, depending upon the rationale about common factors and the variables believed to discriminate among individuals. The majority of the current taxonomies of pain are "expert-based" classifications.

Expert-Based Classifications of Pain

Classifications of disease are usually based on a preconceived combination of characteristics (e.g., symptoms, signs, results of diagnostic tests), with no single characteristics being both necessary and sufficient for every member of the category, yet the group as a whole possesses a certain unity.[9] Most classification systems used in pain medicine (e.g., International Classification of Diseases [ICD],[10] Classification and Diagnostic Criteria for Headache Disorders, Cranial Neuralgias, and Facial pain,[11] International Association for the Study of Pain Classification of Chronic Pain[2]) and dentistry (i.e., Research Diagnostic Criteria for Temporomandibular Disorders[12]) are based on the consensus arrived at by a group of "experts." In this sense they reflect the inclusion or elimination of certain diagnostic features depending on agreement.

"Expert-based" classification tends to result in preconceived categories and "force" individuals into the most appropriate one even if not all characteristics defining the category are present. Expert-based classification systems do not explicitly state the mathematical rules that should exist among the variables used in order to assign a case to a specific category.

In an ideal classification, the categories comprising the taxonomy should be mutually exclusive and completely exhaustive for the data to be incorporated. Every element in a classification should fit into one, and only one, place and no other element should fit into that place. An example of such an ideal, natural taxonomy is the periodic table in chemistry. We can also develop artificial classifications such as a telephone directory. The criterion for the classification, namely, the sequence of letters in the alphabet, bears no relation to the people, addresses, and telephone numbers being classified; but it is quite satisfactory for the intended purpose.[3] No classification in medicine or dentistry has achieved such aims. For example, the Research Diagnostic Criteria (RDC) for Temporomandibular Disorders[12] includes eight different diagnoses. In one study, over 50% of the sample received three or more RDC diagnoses.[13] Thus, the classifications or diagnoses are not mutually exclusive.

The most commonly used classification system of pain is the International Classification of Diseases published by the World Health Organization. In the most recent edition, the ICD-10,[10] conditions are classified along a number of different dimensions including causal agent, body system involved, pattern and type of symptoms, and whether or not they are related to the artificial intervention of an operation, time of occurrence or grouped as signs, symptoms, and abnormal clinical and laboratory findings. Within major groups there are subdivisions by symptom pattern, the presence of hereditary or degenerative disease, extrapyramidal and movement disorders, location, and etiology. Overlapping occurs repeatedly in such approaches to categorization; thus, they are not ideal even if they serve a useful function.

Further complications arise when clinicians require a separate coding system. In the United States, for example, in addition to the ICD codes a clinician must select current procedural terminology (CPT) coding schemes for the billing purpose. This has created a tendency where the fulfillment of the CPT coding may dictate the ICD selections to justify the procedures. Such practices often needlessly create diagnoses and additional treatments for billing purposes only.

It is clear that the classification of pain cannot approach the ideal found in chemistry or telephone books, but this is not unique to pain; it characterizes medical classification systems in general. Classification in medicine, dentistry, and psychology is pragmatic. It does not provide absolute truth but rather provides categories with which we can work to identify individuals with similar phenomena, prognoses, or causes.[3] Currently, the majority of pain classifications in pain medicine rely upon various parameters of pain experience such as anatomy, system, severity, duration, and etiology.

Classification Based on Anatomy

Several pain syndromes are classified by body location. For example, low back pain, pelvic pain, and headache each refer to the specific location of symptoms. However, the extent to which the anatomy-based classification of pain is clinically meaningful is limited, at least partially, due to the lack of anatomically defined specificity in the neurophysiology of pain.

Classification Based on Duration

As previously discussed, one common way to classify pain is to consider it along a continuum of duration. Thus, pain associated with tissue damage, inflammation, or a disease process that is of relatively brief duration (i.e., hours, days, or even weeks), regardless of how intense, is frequently referred to as acute pain (e.g., postsurgical pain). Many pain problems can be classified as chronic. For example, pain that persists for extended periods of time (i.e., months or years), accompanies a disease process (e.g., rheumatoid arthritis), or is associated with an injury that has not resolved within an expected period of time (e.g., low back pain, phantom limb pain) are all referred to as chronic. As noted, however, a single dimension of duration is inadequate because pathological factors may be relatively independent of duration.

Classification Based on the Etiology of Pain

Another way to classify pain is based on etiology. The crudest classification of this kind is to simply distinguish somatogenic pain from psychogenic pain (pain of psychological origin). Simply put, when a range of physical examination, diagnostic imaging, and laboratory tests fail to identify the physical basis for the report of pain, pain is attributed to psychic conflict or psychopathology. Variations on the dichotomous somatogenic versus psychogenic classification exist. For example, Portenoy[14] proposed that three primary categories of pain be used: nociceptive, neuropathic, and psychogenic. In this system, somatogenic pain is subdivided into two subtypes that contrast with psychogenic pain.

The processes by which clinicians determine whether pain is somatogenic or psychogenic are distinctive. The classification of somatogenic pain is established by identification of positive organic findings, whereas psychogenic pain is indicated only in the absence of positive signs. We question the utility of such a classification scheme.

Classification Based on Body System

Classification may focus on the body system involved. For example, Fricton[15] proposed the use of five categories; namely, myofascial, rheumatic, causalgic, neurologic, or vascular. In this case patients are assigned to one of five rather than two or three categories as proposed by Portenoy.[14] However, the decision regarding classification is still based on a single dimension system for the experience of pain.

Classification Based on Severity

Frequently, pain is classified unidimensionally on the basis of severity (0- to 10-point scale with 0 = no pain and 10 = the worst pain that can be imagined). That is, regardless of the scale's level of measurement—nominal, ordinal, or interval—the construct involves a single dimension. When pain is classified on the basis of severity, it is dependent on the subjective report of patients. Assuming pain threshold is normally distributed, there will be significant variability among patients' rating severity of what might be objectively the same nociceptive stimulation.

Ratings of pain severity will be anchored to how questions are asked and responses may vary widely depending on the question. For example, if the ratings associated with "pain right now," "over the past week?" "usual severity," "severity at its worst," "severity at its lowest," "during specific movements," or "at rest?" Pain severity may be very useful in evaluating individual patients but less so for comparison among groups.

Classification Based on Functioning

The International Classification of Functioning Disability and Health (ICF)[16] aims to provide a standard framework for the comparison and understanding of health outcomes. For any given health outcome, including chronic pain, the ICF identified three main outcomes: impairment, activity limitations, and participation restrictions. To date, the efforts of the ICF have been largely focused on identification of common domains across measures that can be used to evaluate patients and treatment outcomes. It has less emphasis on classification of patients but it can be used for this purpose. The empirical approach described below can be readily applied to the ICF conceptual model.

Mechanism-Based Classification of Pain

The conventional classifications of pain disorders based upon anatomy, duration, and systems have drawn criticism for their deficiency in sensibility for guiding treatment or research.[17] Woolf et al.[17] support developing a mechanism-based classification of pain, proposing a potential list of pain mechanisms (Table 2.1). They argue that the list needs to include affective, behavioral, and cognitive factors relevant to pain, although they do not specify what these factors may be, or how they would be incorporated within the proposed classification system.

The mechanism-based classifications of pain differ from the conventional classification in that the former frees pain from diseases that may accompany reports of pain. Mechanism-based classification groups patients who are homogeneous in pain mechanisms but heterogeneous in disease conditions or diagnoses. Woolf et al.[17] emphasize that their proposal is not to replace but rather to supplement the current system.

The basic premise underlying the mechanism-based classification of pain is helpful, both in guiding treatment and in bridging research to clinical practice in pain medicine. However, such a system is still at the conceptual stage. Ongoing efforts to synthesize findings from various areas of pain research will help to formulate this new classification system.

This approach contrasts with our description of the use of two dimensions, time and severity, to distinguish acute and chronic pain (Fig. 2.1). An explication of attempts to develop multidimensional classification systems incorporating features of several of the classifications is reviewed in the next section.

TABLE 2.1

CATEGORIES OF PAIN AND POSSIBLE MECHANISMS

TRANSIENT PAIN
Nociceptor specialization

TISSUE INJURY PAIN
Primary Afferent
Sensitization
Recruitment of silent nociceptors
Alteration in phenotype
Hyperinnervation

CNS Mediated
Central sensitization recruitment, summation, amplification

NERVOUS SYSTEM INJURY PAIN
Primary Afferent
Acquisition of spontaneous and stimulus-evoked activity by
   nociceptor axons and somata at loci other than peripheral
   terminals
Alteration in phenotype

CNS Mediated
Central sensitization
Deafferentation of 2nd order neurons
Disinhibition
Structural reorganization

(Adapted with permission from Woolf CJ, Bennett GJ, Doherty M, et al. Toward a mechanism-based classification of pain (editorial). *Pain* 1998;77: 227–229.)

Multidimensional Classification of Pain: International Association for the Study of Pain Taxonomy

An alternative to the unidimensional approaches is a multidimensional approach that uses several relevant rather than a single dimension as the basis for developing the classification system and for assigning patients to a particular subgroup or diagnosis. The IASP has published an expert based multiaxial classification of chronic pain[1,2] intended to standardize descriptions of relevant pain syndromes and to provide a point of reference. The published taxonomy classifies chronic pain patients according to five axes based upon the best published information and consensus:

1. **Region** of the body (Axis I),
2. **System** whose abnormal functioning could conceivably produce the pain (Axis II),
3. **Temporal characteristics** of pain and pattern of occurrence (Axis III),
4. **Patient's statement of intensity** and time since onset of pain (Axis IV), and
5. Presumed **Etiology** (Axis V)(see Table 2.2).

This system establishes a five-digit code that assigns to each chronic pain diagnosis, a unique number. For example, the code for carpal tunnel syndrome is 204.X6. Thus,

   200 = REGION: upper shoulder and upper limbs
   00 = SYSTEM: the abnormal functioning is attributed to the nervous system
   4 = TEMPORAL CHARACTERISTICS: symptoms occur irregularly
   X = PATIENTS STATEMENT OF INTENSITY AND TIME SINCE ONSET: this will vary by patient
   06 = ETIOLOGY: degenerative, mechanical

Table 2.3 contains the IASP scheme developed for the coding of chronic pain diagnoses.

The IASP classification is the most comprehensive approach to classification of chronic pain syndromes. By design the IASP classification is a heuristic, multiaxial guide that emphasizes the consideration of both signs and symptoms. Unfortunately, it excludes assessment of psychosocial or behavioral data. Moreover, to be useful, any classification system must be reliable and valid, but as yet little published research has evaluated the reliability, validity, or utility of the IASP classification. What little evidence is available[18] indicates that, although Axis 1 (body region) demonstrated reliable coding across examiners, Axis 5 (etiology) failed to achieve acceptable inter-rater reliability. The consistency (test–retest reliability) of the IASP taxonomy has yet to be established. Further research is needed in order to evaluate the psychometric properties of the classification system and to facilitate refinements of the system. The classifications we have described are only a few examples and are definitely not exhaustive. Specialists can arrive at classification categories based on clinical experience, published data, and consensus [e.g., 6]. There is no single system for classifying pain patients that is universally accepted by clinicians or researchers. Furthermore, several problems associated with the current classification systems have generated debate and research concerning an alternative classification of pain. We provide several examples to illustrate different attempts to devise alternative taxonomies of pain and chronic pain patients.

Empirically-Based Classifications of Pain

Those who advocate the use of empirically-derived taxonomies maintain that quantitative analysis should define the relationships of contiguity and similarity among individuals. That is, the taxonomic system must reflect clinically relevant characteristics that exist in nature, defined by empirical methods rather than based on expert judgment and consensus.

The American College of Rheumatology provides an empirical diagnosis for the classification of FM. In a multicenter study,[19] a group of FM experts from several medical centers collected FM-related variables and used those variables in an attempt to differentiate FM patients from patients with other types of chronic pain syndromes. The acceptable sensitivity and specificity were achieved by two criteria: presence of widespread pain (i.e., above and below the waist, right and left side of the body, and along the midline) and at least 11 of 18 positive tender points upon palpation. Other symptoms commonly reported by FM patients, such as fatigue and stiffness, did not differentiate between FM and other types of chronic pain. Since publication, most subsequent research seems to conform to this classification system, making it a bit easier to compare results across studies. Nonetheless, debate remains about the extent that this classification contributes to clinical practice and the meaning of tender points and the necessity of the tender point criterion.[20]

Several statistical methods (e.g., cluster analysis) can be used to empirically identify categories that share relationships derived directly from data rather than hypothesized relationships. This is the case with more traditional consensus-based deductive systems. The results of identification analyses can lead to explicit, mathematically-derived categories. This permits physicians and clinical investigators to assign patients to specific categories on an objective basis.

Although quantification, replication, and objectivity are the hallmarks of the inductive approach, it is important to acknowledge that all relevant factors cannot be measured by a single classification system. The use of an inductive approach depends on what the investigator chooses to include within the statistical analysis. Thus, in practice, the inductive approach to classification is not a totally objective process that is completely atheoretical. In light of this notion, some advocate the dual-diagnostic approach, using the two loosely defined domains biophysiologic

TABLE 2.2

INTERNATIONAL ASSOCIATION FOR THE STUDY OF PAIN: SCHEME FOR CODING CHRONIC PAIN SYNDROMES

Axis I: Regions

Head, face, and mouth	000
Cervical region	100
Upper shoulder and upper limbs	200
Thoracic region	300
Abdominal region	400
Lower back, lumbar spine, sacrum, & coccyx	500
Lower limbs	600
Pelvic region	700
Anal, perineal, & genital region	800
More than three major sites	900

Axis II: Systems

Nervous system (central, peripheral, and autonomic) and special senses; physical disturbance or dysfunction	00
Nervous system (psychological and social)	10
Respiratory & cardiovascular systems	20
Musculoskeletal system and connective tissue	30
Cutaneous and subcutaneous and associated glands (breast, apocrine, etc)	40
Gastrointestinal system	50
Genito-urinary system	60
Other organs or viscera (e.g., thyroid, lymphatic hemopoietic)	70
More than one system	80
Unknown	90

Axis III: Temporal Characteristics of Pain: Pattern of Occurrence

Not recorded, not applicable, or not known	0
Single episode, limited duration (e.g., ruptured aneurysm, sprained ankle)	1
Continuous or nearly continuous, nonfluctuating (eg, low back pain)	2
Continuous or nearly continuous, fluctuating (eg, ruptured intervertebral disc)	3
Recurring irregularly (e.g., headache, mixed type)	4
Recurring regularly (e.g., premenstrual pain)	5
Paroxysmal (e.g., tic douloureux)	6
Sustained with superimposed paroxysms	7
Other combinations	8
None of the above	9

Axis IV: Patient's Statement of Intensity: Time Since onset of Pain

Not recorded, not applicable, or not known	.0
Mild—1 month or less	.1
Mild—1 month to 6 months	.2
Mild—more than 6 months	.3
Medium—1 month or less	.4
Medium—1 month to 6 months	.5
Medium—more than 6 months	.6
Severe—1 month or less	.7
Severe—1 month to 6 months	.8
Severe—more than 6 months	.9

Axis V: Etiology

Genetic or congenital disorders (e.g., congenital dislocations)	.00
Trauma, operation, burns	.01
Infective, parasitic	.02
Inflammatory (no known infective agent), immune reaction	.03
Neoplasm	.04
Toxic, metabolic (e.g., alcoholic neuropathy) anoxia, vascular, nutritional, endocrine, radiation	.05
Degenerative, mechanical	.06
Dysfunctional (including psychophysiological)	.07
Unknown or other	.08
Psychological origin (e.g., conversion hysteria, depressive hallucination)	.09

IASP Chronic Pain Syndromes

A. Relatively generalized syndromes

B. Relatively localized syndromes of the head and neck
  I. Neuralgias of the head and face
  II. Craniofacial pain of musculoskeletal origin
  III. Lesions of the ear, nose, and oral cavity
  IV. Primary headache syndromes, vascular disorders, and cerebrospinal fluid syndromes
  V. Pain of psychological origin in the head, face, and neck
  VI. Suboccipital and cervical musculoskeletal disorders
  VII. Visceral pain in the neck

C. Spinal pain—spinal and radicular pain syndromes

D. Spinal pain—spinal and radicular pain syndromes of the cervical and thoracic regions

E. Local syndromes of the upper limbs and relatively generalized syndromes of the upper and lower limbs
  I. Pain in the shoulder, arm, and hand
  II. Vascular disease of the limbs
  III. Collagen disease of the limbs
  IV. Vasodilating functional disease of the limbs
  V. Arterial insufficiency in the limbs
  VI. Pain of psychological origin in the lower limbs

F. Visceral and other syndromes of the trunk apart from spinal and radicular pain
  I. Visceral and other chest pain
  II. Chest pain of psychological origin
  III. Chest pain referred from abdomen or gastrointestinal tract
  IV. Abdominal pain of neurological origin
  V. Abdominal pain of visceral origin
  VI. Abdominal pain syndromes of generalized diseases
  VII. Abdominal pain of psychological origin
  VIII. Diseases of the bladder, uterus, ovaries, and adnexa
  IX. Pain in the rectum, perineum, and external genitalia

G. Spinal pain—spinal and radicular pain syndromes of the lumbar, sacral, and coccygeal regions
  I. Lumbar spinal or radicular pain syndromes
  II. Sacral spinal or radicular pain syndromes
  III. Coccygeal pain syndromes
  IV. Diffuse or generalized spinal pain
  V. Low back pain or psychological origin with referral

H. Local syndromes of the lower limbs
  I. Local syndromes in the leg or foot: pain of neurological origin
  II. Pain syndromes of the hip and thigh of musculoskeletal origin
  III. Musculoskeletal syndromes of the leg

TABLE 2.3

LIST OF DESCRIPTIONS IN EACH SYNDROME IN THE IASP CLASSIFICATION

Definition
Site
System(s) involved
Main features of the pain including its prevalence, age of onset, sex ratio if known, duration, severity, and quality
Associated features; aggravating and relieving agents
Signs
Laboratory findings
Natural course
Complications
Social and physical disability
Pathology or other contributing factors
Essential features and diagnostic criteria
Differential diagnosis
Code based on the five axes
References (optional)

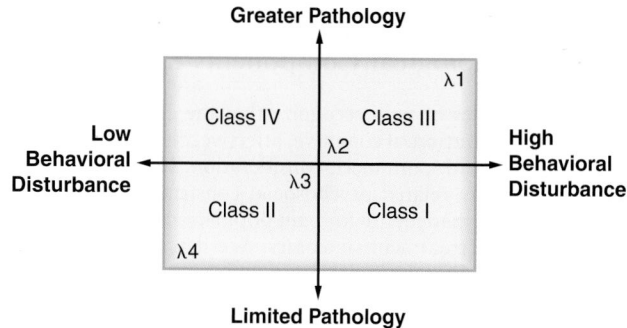

FIGURE 2.2 The Emory pain estimate model. (Redrawn after Turk DC, Rudy TE. Classification logic and strategies in chronic pain. In: Turk DC, Melzack R, eds. *Handbook of Pain Assessment.* New York: Guilford: 1992:409–428.)

and psychosocial.[12,21] In this framework, physiologically homogeneous patients exhibit a range of psychosocial heterogeneity.

Multiaxial Classification of Pain

Ever since the gate control model underscored the importance of cognitive–evaluative and motivational–affective factors in the process of pain experience, the importance of integrating the psychosocial domains in the classification of pain has been proposed by a number of clinical investigators. However, as in other domains of pain medicine, the psychosocial classifications of pain have largely depended upon the traditionally defined diagnosis system, in this case, identification of psychopathology. Although the psychiatrically-defined classification of pain patients may help identify patients with specific psychiatric disorders thereby directing treatments for those disorders, psychological classification systems to identify the specific psychological components (affective, evaluative, motivational) of pain have been introduced.

The Emory Pain Estimate Model

The Emory Pain Estimate Model (EPEM) was the first attempt to integrate the biophysiologic and psychosocial domains in classifying pain patients.[22,23] Brena and colleagues arbitrarily labeled the dimensions "pathology" and "behavior." The pathology dimension included the quantification of physical examination procedures (e.g., ratings of joint mobility, muscle strength) as well as assigning numerical indices to reflect the extent of abnormalities determined from diagnostic procedures such as radiographic studies. The behavioral dimension comprises a composite of activity levels, pain verbalizations, drug use, and measures of psychopathology based on the elevations of scales of the Minnesota Multiphasic Personality Inventory (MMPI).

Using median divisions on the pathology and behavior dimensions, the EPEM defines four classes of chronic pain patients (see Fig. 2.2). Class I patients are characterized by higher scores on the behavior dimension and lower scores on the pathology dimension. The EPEM describes these patients as displaying low activity levels, high verbalizations of pain, prominent social and psychological malfunctions, and frequent misuse of medications. Class II patients are those who display lower scores on both the pathology and behavioral dimensions. These patients are described as displaying dramatized pain complaints with ill-defined anatomical patterns. However they do not display significant behavioral

dysfunction. Class III represents patients with higher scores on both dimensions, characterized as showing clear evidence of physical pathology and high intensity illness behavior. Finally, Class IV patients are those who have higher scores on the pathology dimension and a lower score on the behavior dimension, thus demonstrating competent coping in the presence of a physical pathological condition.

Although Brena and his colleagues[22,23] appropriately emphasized the importance of integrating physical and psychological data in order to develop a classification system for chronic pain patients, some of the basic theoretical and quantitative characteristics of the EPEM are problematic. We see this framework as a conceptual model rather than an adequately operationalized empirical one. For example, from a theoretical standpoint, the inclusion of activity levels, pain verbalizations, and measures of psychopathology under a single dimension labeled "behavioral" is troubling because research shows that there is little association between pain behaviors and psychopathology. Thus, the behavioral dimension is most likely not unidimensional and, therefore, cannot measure behavior directly.

Examination of the empirical aspects of the scoring and classification system used in the EPEM identifies additional problems. For example, the weights assigned to specific medical–physical findings are a priori and were not empirically derived. Moreover, applying median divisions to the two dimensions, although intuitively appealing, artificially creates four classes of patients. That is, there is no statistical demonstration that four nonoverlapping groups of pain patients naturally exist in these data or that, in fact, the pathology and behavioral dimensions are independent. Review of the 2 × 2 grid displayed in Figure 2.2 reveals that within the EPEM extreme, scores are treated the same as scores near the medians. For example, the scores of patients 1 and 2, depicted as points in Figure 2.2, would both be assigned to Class III, whereas those of patients 3 and 4 would be classified in Class II. In reality, however, the scores of patients 2 and 3 are more similar than they are with the scores of patient 1 or patient 4. Thus, this method of establishing classification rules may lead to erroneous or nonindependent patient assignments because it is derived from artificial and external mathematical criteria rather than from divisions or clustering of groups that occur naturally within patients' scores. Von Korff and colleagues[24] developed a similar model, the Chronic Pain Grade, which integrates the conceptual approach of the EPEM but adds greater emphasis of empirical determination of criteria for subgroup classification and empirical validation. The Chronic Pain Grade classifies patients into one of five categories: (1) pain free, (2) low pain intensity and low disability, (3) high pain intensity and low disability, (4) low pain intensity and high disability, and (5) high pain severity and high disability.

Empirically-Based Classification of the Psychological Components of Pain

Many taxonomies of pain recognize that the conceptualization and operationalization of cognitive, affective, and behavioral factors associated with pain merit consideration. Numerous instruments assess pain-related psychosocial constructs but most are unidimensional, inadequate for pain populations, or lack predictive validity for treatment outcomes. We describe one specific multidimensional psychosocial classification system used primarily with patients with chronic pain conditions.

The Multidimensional Pain Inventory[25] consists of a set of empirically-derived scales designed to assess chronic pain patients' (1) reports of pain severity and suffering; (2) perceptions of how pain interferes with their lives, including interference with family and marital functioning, work, and social and recreational activities; (3) their dissatisfaction with present levels of functioning in family, marriage, work, and social life; (4) appraisals of support received from significant others; (5) perceived life control incorporating perceived ability to solve problems and feelings of personal mastery and competence; (6) their affective distress, including depressed mood, irritability, and tension; and (7) activity levels. Using the MPI, Turk and Rudy[26] were able to group patients within three relatively homogeneous sets.

Turk and Rudy[26] performed cluster analyses on a heterogeneous sample of chronic pain patients' responses on the MPI scales. Three distinct profiles were identified: (1) dysfunctional (DYS), patients who perceived the severity of their pain to be high, reported that pain interfered with much of their lives, reported a higher degree of psychological distress due to pain, and reported low levels of activity; (2) interpersonally distressed (ID), patients with a common perception that significant others were not very supportive of their pain problems; and (3) adaptive copers (AC), patients who reported high levels of social support, relatively low levels of pain and perceived interference, and relatively high levels of activity. Reliable, external scales supported the uniqueness of each of the three subgroups of patients. Performing a 12-dimension Bayesian calculation to test goodness of fit can identify the profile that best fits a patient.

In addition to categorical classification that assigns an individual patient to a specific diagnosis, the empirical–statistical approach permits judgments about how well a patient matches the central features of that diagnosis. This is especially useful in complex pain syndromes that involve various clinical characteristics with rather large individual variability, even within a single diagnostic group. Using an empirical method, one can not only establish whether a patient fits the diagnostic classification but also determine how good a fit the diagnosis is to the patient. For example, based on a set of patient characteristics, signs, and symptoms, a prototype for a diagnosis is established. It is possible to statistically determine how close an individual case matches that prototype. Assume that a perfect match to a prototype is 0.99. A particular case may fit within the diagnosis but not be a perfect fit, thus the fit might be 0.80. Some statistical rule can decide the minimum fit to the characteristics of the diagnosis; for example, 0.67. Thus, any two individuals with the same diagnosis must share certain characteristics but not necessarily all; the similarity of two patients with the same diagnosis has a statistical definition.

Subsequent testing of the MPI profiles across various pain disorders suggests that the MPI psychosocial classification is independent of the conventionally defined pain syndromes, such as low back pain, TMD, migraine headaches, FMS, and pain associated with cancer. In other words, two patients whose pain pathologies are likely to differ (cancer and migraine headaches, for example) could have a homogeneous psychological classification of pain. On the other hand, two patients, both having same type of TMD based upon the RDC[12] for comparable duration, may fare

differently in the psychological classification of pain. Clinical trials using the MPI-based classification have yielded differential responses to a cognitive–behavioral approach.[27,28] Such results strongly suggest that the psychosocial treatment components need to conform to the psychological classification of pain.

We suggest that disease classification should reflect physical assessment and treatment [e.g., 2] and that a psychosocial–behavioral taxonomy should determine complementary psychological treatment strategies. Both physical and psychosocial diagnoses are important in the person with a chronic pain syndrome. Several groups[12,21,29] have proposed the use of a dual-diagnostic approach, whereby two diagnoses are assigned concurrently: physical and psychosocial–behavioral. Treatment could then target both simultaneously. A chronic pain patient might have diagnoses on two different but complementary taxonomies; for example, IASP and MPI-based classification. Thus, a patient might be classified as having complex regional pain Type 1 of the upper extremity (203.X1, Axis 1 Region = upper shoulder and upper limbs, Axis II System = nervous, Axis III Temporal Characteristics of Pain: Pattern of Occurrence = none of the codes listed, Axis IV Intensity and Time of Onset = based on patient report, Axis V Aetiology = trauma) on the IASP taxonomy and be classified DYS on the MPI-based taxonomy. Note that not all CRPS-1 patients would be classified as DYS and not all DYS patients would have CRPS-1. A second patient might have the same IASP diagnosis, CRPS-1, but be ID on the MPI-based classification. Conversely, patients might have quite different classifications on the IASP system but have an identical MPI-based classification. The most appropriate treatment for these different groups might vary, with different complementary components of treatments addressing the physical diagnosis (IASP) and the psychosocial diagnosis (MPI-based).

Psychometric Considerations

The general utility of any proposed empirical taxonomy links closely to the psychometric properties (i.e., reliability, validity, and utility) of the measures, scales, or instruments used to derive the classification system. Because these are the building blocks used to generate profiles or clusters, the reliability and validity of the classification system depends, in part, on the psychometric quality of the measures used. Because reliability and validity coefficients are generic terms, the specific psychometric techniques used to evaluate a measure's "psychometric properties" require consideration. There are multiple ways to demonstrate the reliability and validity of measures. Therefore, the more psychometric support there is for a measure, the more likely it will perform well when used in taxometric identification and classification procedures. Additionally, replication of classification accuracy on new samples and demonstrating substantial, statistically significant differences across patient profiles for conceptually related measures *external* to the measures used to develop the profiles are some of the best ways to demonstrate the reliability and validity of empirically derived profiles. Evaluation of any classification should demonstrate reliability, validity, and utility prior to widespread adoption.

CONCLUSION

Pain management specialists have witnessed rapid advances in the basic sciences and clinical arenas of pain medicine over the past 3 decades. Many pain-related terms, once a major source of confusion, have received clear definitions, aiding efficient and productive communication among researchers and clinicians. The classification systems that direct our research and clinical practice need to reflect the progress in our understanding of mechanisms,

TABLE 2.4

TAXONOMY OF PAIN BASED UPON MULTI-FACTORIAL ASSESSMENT: A PROPOSAL

Pain Parameters:
Anatomy/System
Duration/Intensity/Quality
Associated Abnormality (physical/psychological)

Underlying Diseases:
Signs/Symptoms

Pain Mechanisms:
NEUROPHYSIOLOGICAL
   Primary afferent involvement
   CNS involvement

PSYCHOLOGICAL
Cognitive–Affective–Behavioral Involvement
   Cognitive appraisal of pain
   Coping
   Affect/mood
   Environment

multifactorial integration, and outcome predictability of classification criteria. In this chapter, we have reviewed several conventional classifications as well as emerging classification systems that can supplement the conventional ones. The review of various classification systems suggests that the comprehensive taxonomy of pain require multifactorial assessments (See Table 2.4).

The multiaxial approach to the assessment of pain and dysfunction described earlier appears to be a reasonable strategy to adopt. Given a comprehensive set of physical, psychosocial, and behavioral measures, the strategy of matching patients to existing classification systems could provide a basis for treatment decisions. The use of the dual-diagnostic approach holds promise because it incorporates biomedical, psychosocial, and behavioral data in the assignment of patients to empirically derived categories. Future research needs to relate patient classification to performance on standardized physical capacity assessment protocols, rehabilitation, and ability to engage in gainful employment and regular homemaking activities.

The utility of any classification system depends upon application. The important question is whether assignment of an individual to a class truly facilitates treatment decisions or predictions of future behavior. Few of the taxometric systems have demonstrated their utility to predict treatment outcome.[21] Preliminary results on the MPI-based classification demonstrate the potential of such an approach. Research efforts to evaluate the predictive value of any classification of pain need to demonstrate the validity of that classification system or taxonomy.

Acknowledgment

Support for preparation of this manuscript was provided by a grant from the National Institutes of Health/National Institute of Arthritis and Musculoskeletal and Skin Disorders (R01AR044724).

References

1. Merskey H. Classification of chronic pain. Descriptions of chronic pain syndromes and definitions. *Pain* 1986;(Suppl3):345–356.
2. Merskey H, Bogduk N. *Classification of Chronic Pain: Descriptions of Chronic Pain Syndromes and Definitions of Pain Terms*. 2nd ed. Seattle, WA: IASP Press; 1994.
3. Merskey H. Classification and diagnosis of fibromyalgia. *Pain Res Manage* 1996;1:42–44.
4. Turk DC. Remember what you learned about the distinction between malignant and benign pain? Well, forget it. *Clin J Pain* 2002;18:75–76.
5. Sullivan MJ, Thorn B, Haythornthwaite JA, et al. Theoretical perspectives on the relation between catastrophizing and pain. *Clin J Pain* 2001;17:52–64.
6. Treede RD, Jensen TS, Campbell JN, et al. Neuropathic pain: redefinition and a grading system for clinical and research purposes. *Neurology* 2008;70(18):1630–1635.
7. Turk DC, Dworkin RH. The initiative on methods, measurement, and pain assessment in clinical trials [IMMPACT]: process and recommendations. In: Wittink H, Carr D, eds. *Evidence, Outcomes and Quality of Life: A Handbook*. New York: Elsevier; 2008:287–304.
8. Bonica JJ. The need of a taxonomy. *Pain* 1979;6:247–248.
9. Baron DN, Fraser PM. Medical applications of taxonomic methods. *Br Med Bull* 1968;24:236–240.
10. World Health Organization, ed. *ICD-10: International Statistical Classification of Diseases and Related Health Problems*. 10th rev., Vol 1. Geneva, Switzerland: World Health Organization; 1992.
11. Classification and diagnostic criteria for headache disorders, cranial neuralgias and facial pain. Headache Classification Committee of the International Headache Society. *Cephalalgia* 1988;8(Suppl 7):1–96.
12. Dworkin SF, LeResche L. Research diagnostic criteria for temporomandibular disorders: review, criteria, examinations and specifications, critique. *J Craniomandib Disord* 1992;6:301–355.
13. Zaki H, Rudy T, Turk D, et al. Reliability of Axis I research diagnostic criteria for TMD (abstract). *J Dent Res* 1994;73:186.
14. Portenoy RK. Mechanisms of clinical pain. Observations and speculations. *Neurol Clin* 1989;7:205–230.
15. Friction J. Medical evaluation of patients with chronic pain. In: Barber J, Adrian C, eds. *Psychological Approaches to the Management of Pain*. New York: Brunner/Mazel; 1982:37–61.
16. World Health Organization. *International Classification of Functioning, Disability and Health: ICF*. Geneva, Switzerland: World Health Organization, 2001.
17. Woolf C, Bennett G, Doherty M, et al. Towards a mechanism-based classification of pain? *Pain* 1998;77:227–229.
18. Turk DC, Rudy TE. Towards a comprehensive assessment of chronic pain patients. *Behav Res Ther* 1987;25:237–249.
19. Wolfe F, Smythe HA, Yunus MB, et al. The American College of Rheumatology 1990 Criteria for the Classification of Fibromyalgia. Report of the Multicenter Criteria Committee. *Arthritis Rheum* 1990;33(2):160–172.
20. Clauw DJ. Fibromyalgia: update on mechanisms and management. *J Clin Rheumatol* 2007;13:102–109.
21. Turk DC. Customizing treatment for chronic pain patients: who, what, and why. *Clin J Pain* 1990;6:255–270.
22. Brena S, Koch D. A "pain estimate" model for quantification and classification of chronic pain states. *Anesth Rev* 1975;2:8–13.
23. Brena S, Koch D, Moss R. Reliability of the "pain estimate" model. *Anesth Rev* 1976;3:28–29.
24. Von Korff M, Ormel J, Keefe FJ, et al. Grading the severity of chronic pain. *Pain* 1992;50:133–149.
25. Kerns RD, Turk DC, Rudy TE. The West Haven-Yale Multidimensional Pain Inventory (WHYMPI). *Pain* 1985;23(4):345–356.
26. Turk DC, Rudy TE. Toward an empirically derived taxonomy of chronic pain patients: integration of psychological assessment data. *J Consult Clin Psychol* 1988;56:233–238.
27. Turk DC, Okifuji A, Sinclair JD, et al. Differential responses by psychosocial subgroups of fibromyalgia syndrome patients to an interdisciplinary treatment. *Arthritis Care Res* 1998;11:397–404.
28. Turk DC, Rudy TE, Kubinski JA, et al. Dysfunctional patients with temporomandibular disorders: evaluating the efficacy of a tailored treatment protocol. *J Consult Clin Psychol* 1996;64:139–146.
29. Scharff L, Turk DC, Marcus DA. Psychosocial and behavioral characteristics in chronic headache patients: support for a continuum and dual-diagnostic approach. *Cephalalgia* 1995;15:216–223.

CHAPTER 3 ■ PERIPHERAL PAIN MECHANISMS AND NOCICEPTOR SENSITIZATION

MICHAEL S. GOLD AND GERALD F. GEBHART

INTRODUCTION TO PERIPHERAL PAIN MECHANISMS AND NOCICEPTOR SENSITIZATION

Pain has been categorized by duration (acute vs. chronic), location (superficial or deep; cutaneous, bone/joint, muscle, or viscera) and cause or type (inflammatory, neuropathic, cancer). Generally, activation of and/or ongoing activity in nociceptors underlies the experience of pain regardless of how it is categorized. Accordingly, nociceptors are key players in understanding mechanisms of and managing pain.

Sherrington anticipated by many decades the existence of nociceptors (sensory receptors that respond to noxious stimuli) and provided for us the operational definition of stimuli that are noxious (i.e., stimuli that damage or threaten damage of tissue). Two considerations are important to this discussion. First, Sherrington's definition of the nociceptor is a functional definition, meaning that the response to its activation by a noxious stimulus (e.g., a nociceptive withdrawal reflex, pain) defines the receptor. Second, the definition of an applied stimulus as noxious is based on response to stimuli applied to skin and subcutaneous structures.

Sherrington's definition of a nociceptor continues to the present day, although the term has undergone change and challenge over the past 100 years. It is therefore important to consider, within the context of our current knowledge, how a nociceptor is defined, identified, and studied. The importance of these issues relates to management of pain that is based on understanding mechanisms of pain. Nociceptors underlie important features of those mechanisms. All would agree that a nociceptor is a sensory receptor which, when activated or active, can contribute to the experience of pain. Nociceptors are present in skin, muscle, joints, and viscera, although the density of innervation (i.e., the number and distribution of sensory endings) varies between as well as within tissues. Strictly speaking, a nociceptor is the peripheral sensory terminal (i.e., the site of energy transduction, see following section), although commonly the term is used to also include the cell body (either in a dorsal root, trigeminal, or nodose ganglion) and its central termination in the spinal cord or brainstem. Beyond this, agreement about important features of nociceptors is less uniform. Because stimuli adequate for activation of nociceptors differ between tissues (e.g., tissue damage is not always required), defining a noxious stimulus has become a challenge. For example, some nociceptors in skin and joints and most nociceptors in the viscera have low thresholds for mechanical activation that do not conform to the condition that stimulus intensity must be either damaging or threaten damage. Further, so-called "silent" or "sleeping" nociceptors are unresponsive to intense mechanical stimulation (and are better denoted as mechanically insensitive nociceptors), but develop spontaneous activity and mechanosensitivity after exposure to inflammatory and other endogenous mediators. These types of nociceptors—low threshold and sleeping—are considered further in discussion of sensitization below.

As indicated above, nociceptors are defined classically in a functional context. However, in experimental situations where function cannot be assessed, other criteria to classify a cell as a nociceptor have been advanced. These include the presence or absence of axon myelination, cell size and/or cell content (e.g., peptide or ion channel), or central termination pattern. Sensory neurons commonly identified as nociceptors are those with unmyelinated (C-fiber) axons and small cell body diameters (<20 or 25 µm). More recently, the presence or absence of certain markers (e.g., the tetrodotoxin-resistant sodium channel NaV1.8, the transient receptor potential vanilloid receptor TRPV1, etc.) have been used to identify subsets of nociceptors. With respect to cell body size and myelination, it should be appreciated that there exist some large diameter cells with heavily myelinated and rapidly conducting axons that have been documented functionally to be nociceptors. Conversely, many non-nociceptors have unmyelinated axons and thus axon myelination or cell diameter cannot be applied as reliable criteria to define a nociceptor. Similarly, identifying nociceptors by content or what they express has limitations. For example, cells other than nociceptors express TRPV1 and the subset of nociceptors that stain positive for the isolectin B4 does not apply to the visceral innervation. These and other markers have been advanced as characteristics of nociceptive sensory neurons, but the extent to which any one or several reliably reveals a cell's function remains to be established.

The fact that no single criterion can be used to identify all nociceptors highlights another important point: this population of afferents is extremely heterogeneous. In addition to the anatomical, biochemical, and physiological heterogeneity in the afferent population generally referred to as nociceptors, there is functional heterogeneity. As will be discussed below, this functional heterogeneity is manifest both within the context of nociceptive signaling (i.e., subpopulations of nociceptors may underlie distinct "types" of pain such as cold allodynia or thermal hyperalgesia) and in the context of non-nociceptive function (i.e., such as the maintenance of tissue integrity).

That said, there are two functional properties common to all nociceptors: they encode stimulus intensity into the noxious range and they sensitize. Given our current understanding of the complexity of peripheral pain mechanisms, it seems unlikely that the range of intensities within any one modality (thermal, mechanical) that is encoded by a nociceptor and initiates nociceptive transmission involves only a single voltage- or ligand-gated channel. Though the ability to sensitize is one means of functionally defining a peripheral neuron as a nociceptor, the endogenous mediators and factors that contribute to an increase in the excitability of nociceptors (i.e., sensitization) are numerous, synergetic, and differ in different pain conditions (e.g., inflammation, nerve injury, etc.). A sampling of the complexities and contributors to sensitization are discussed in the following section.

Why include in a clinical textbook of pain management a chapter on peripheral pain mechanisms and nociceptors? There are many reasons. First, in most cases blockage of peripheral nociceptor activity removes the "drive" for the experience of pain. Further, if a primary goal is to develop mechanism-based strategies for pain management, it is critical that characteristics of a key player—the nociceptor—are fully understood. Finally, nociceptor characteristics change as the local environment in which they reside changes (inflammation, nerve injury, etc.). We discuss below how nociceptors are activated, differ in different tissues, contribute to the experience of pain, and how their behavior changes when they become sensitized. Where possible, we have added relevant clinical examples and have inserted text boxes to elaborate on key issues.

NOCICEPTOR CHARACTERISTICS

Anatomy of the Nociceptor

As stated above, nociceptors are sensory neurons with a cell body located in dorsal root, trigeminal, or nodose ganglia. All sensory neurons arising from these ganglia are pseudounipolar neurons with a central process terminating in the central nervous system (e.g., spinal dorsal horn) and a peripheral process terminating in a peripheral target such as the skin, muscle, or viscera. Both central and peripheral processes terminate in a branching pattern referred to as a terminal arbor. The extent of the peripheral arbor depends on the afferent type and site of innervation with the general rule that the higher the spatial resolution for sensory discrimination, the smaller the terminal arbor. In contrast to low threshold afferents that are responsive to non-noxious stimuli, such as brush or vibration, and which terminate in specialized structures, such as Rufinni endings or Merkel discs,[1,2] nociceptors are said to have "free" (unencapsulated) nerve endings because peripheral terminals of these afferents do not appear to be associated with any specific cell type.[3]

Both light and electron micrographic analyses of peripheral nociceptor terminals reveal complex anatomical structures. As suggested above, the structure of the terminal arbor varies with target of innervation. There is also evidence that subpopulations of nociceptive afferents have distinct terminal arbor patterns within the same structure. For example, the terminal arbor morphology of cutaneous C-fibers varies according to whether the C-fiber is peptidergic (i.e., expresses substance P or calcitonin gene-relative peptide) or expresses the Mas-related gene, MrgD.[4] Recent evidence suggests that these distinct but overlapping subpopulations of nociceptors may signal distinct aspects of the painful experience (i.e., sensory/discriminative versus emotional/motivational),[5] suggesting that it may someday be possible to selectively treat the suffering associated with chronic pain while still enabling patients to appropriately respond to noxious stimuli in their environment.

Four distinct events are necessary for a nociceptor to convey information to the central nervous system about noxious stimuli impinging on peripheral tissues (Fig. 3.1—the events are discussed fully in the following paragraphs). First, "energy" from the stimulus (mechanical, thermal, or chemical) must be converted into an electrical signal. This process, referred to as signal transduction, results in a generator potential or depolarization of the peripheral terminal. Second, the generator potential must initiate an action potential, the rapid "all or nothing" change in membrane potential that constitutes the basic unit of electrical activity in the nervous system. This process is sometimes referred to as transformation. Third, the action potential must be successfully propagated from the peripheral terminal to the central terminal. And fourth, the propagated action potential invading the central terminal must drive a sufficient increase in intracellular calcium ions to enable release of enough transmitters to initiate the whole process once again in the second order neuron. Distinct sets of proteins underlie each of these processes, and are therefore the targets of a wide variety of therapeutic interventions.

Stimulus Transduction

An important implication of the fact that nociceptive afferents terminate in "free nerve endings" is that they are not dependent on other cell types for the transduction of a noxious stimulus. That is, proteins responsible for transduction should be intrinsic to the nociceptor. Consistent with this suggestion, isolated sensory neurons are responsive to thermal (both heating[6,7] and cooling[8,9]), mechanical,[10] and a wide variety of chemical stimuli, including both endogenous[11,12] and exogenous[13,14] compounds that activate nociceptors in vivo. Proteins involved in the transduction of each stimulus modality have been identified.[15]

With the exception of transient receptor potential (TRP) channels (see below), and possibly the acid sensing ion channels (ASICs), chemotransducers are, in general, only activated by chemical stimuli (and not also mechanical or thermal stimuli) and encompass various families of proteins that respond to specific molecules such as adenosine triphosphate (ATP)[16] and protons.[17] There is also compelling evidence to support the suggestion that different members of the TRP superfamily underlie thermal transduction of temperatures ranging from the very cold (TRPA1[18]) to the very hot (TRPV2[19]), with receptors for cool,[20] warm,[21,22] and hot,[23] in between. Subsequent research, however, suggests that in contrast to traditional chemoreceptors, TRP family members are not modality specific, as all are activated by specific chemicals,[24] and several contribute to mechanical transduction.[25,26]

Because the only sensation associated with TRPV1 activation is pain, this receptor has received considerable attention from pain researchers. Cloned in 1997, data from an array of studies paint a picture of TRPV1 as an excellent example of a polymodal receptor; it is activated by exogenous compounds such as capsaicin and resiniferatoxin, endogenous compounds ranging from protons to lipids, and noxious heat.[24] Recent evidence suggests that TRPV1 is present on the central terminals of nociceptive afferents where it also facilitates transmission of noxious mechanical stimuli.[27] Furthermore, excessive activation of the receptor with compounds such as capsaicin results in desensitization of the nociceptive terminal to all modes of stimuli, a process that underlies the therapeutic efficacy of topical capsaicin application.[28] More recently, intrathecal application of resiniferatoxin has been used to selectively ablate the central terminals of TRPV1 containing nerve terminals, resulting in a sustained block of nociceptive transmission.[29] There is also evidence that TRPV1 receptor antagonists may have analgesic efficacy, although the therapeutic potential of these compounds may be limited by a small but significant hyperthermia associated with systemic administration of blood-brain barrier permeable analogs.[28]

Of the three modalities of noxious stimuli, molecular mechanisms of mechanotransduction remain the most elusive. Many mechanically sensitive proteins have been identified,[30] but none appear to be both necessary and sufficient for mechanotransduction in nociceptive afferents. Data from null mutant mice, where the deletion of a single putative mechanotransducer results in an increase in mechanosensitivity in one population of afferents and a decrease in others,[31,32] suggests that several different proteins are likely to work together in specific subpopulations of afferents to enable responses to specific forms of mechanical stimuli (e.g., stretch or compression). That even these more specialized forms of mechanosensitivity reflect intrinsic properties of afferents is suggested by the emergence of mechanosensitivity at the severed ends of a subpopulation of axons within hours of transection.[33] Despite the lack of success in this area, identification of a nociceptor specific mechanotransducer blocker remains an active area of investigation because of its therapeutic potential in light of the fact that mechanical hypersensitivity is the primary complaint associated with the vast majority of chronic pain syndromes.[34]

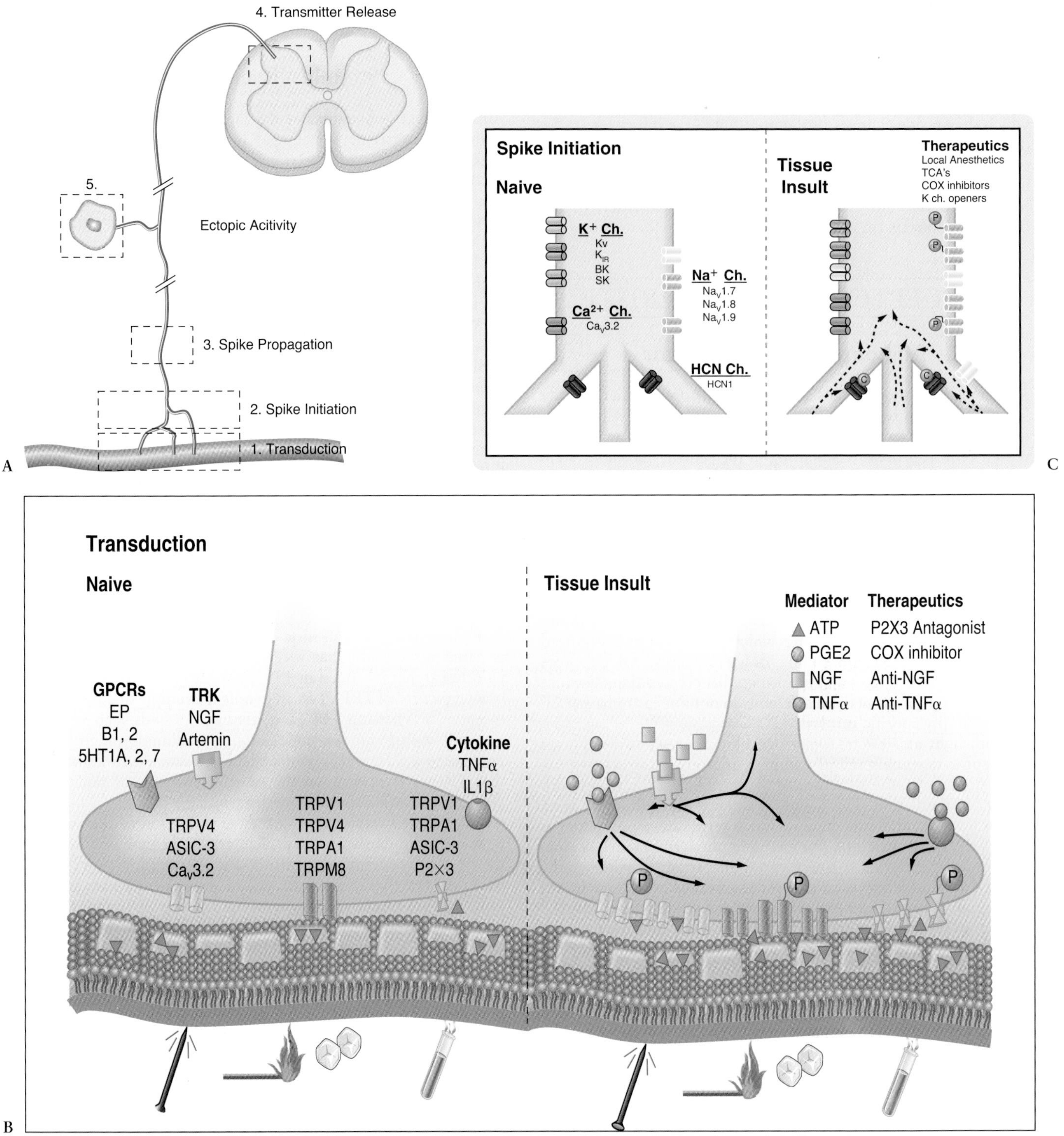

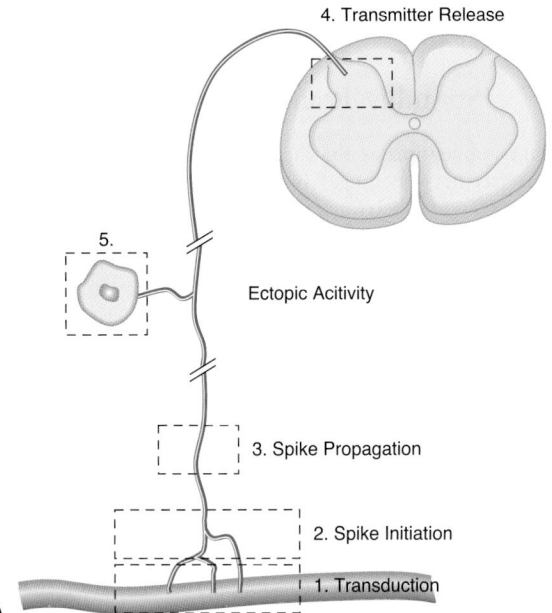

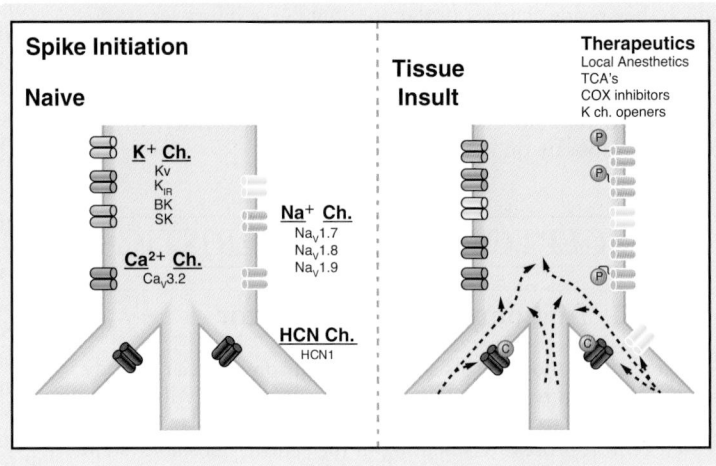

FIGURE 3.1 Nociceptive afferents terminate as free nerve endings in skin and other tissues. **A.** Their principal sensory functions consist of: (1) transduction of external or internal chemical or physical stimuli into generator potentials, (2) transformation of a generator potential into an action potential, (3) propagation of the action potential toward the central nervous system, and (4) release of neurotransmitters and neuromodulators into the superficial dorsal horn of the spinal cord or brainstem. Nociceptive afferents also release transmitters in the periphery, a process that contributes a neurogenic component to inflammation (not shown). The sensory neuron cell body (soma, 5) appears to be a site critical for the integration of neural activity. Proteins and signaling molecules are delivered to the soma via axonal transport mechanisms (not shown) under normal conditions, which may contribute to aberrant or ectopic activity under pathological conditions. Many of the proteins responsible for each of these processes, both under normal and pathological conditions, have been identified. While not a complete list, several lines of data implicate each of the proteins and mediators illustrated in each subpanel. **B. Transduction:** In naïve tissue, proteins thought to play a role in mechanotransduction include transient receptor potential vanilloid type 4 (TRPV4), acid sensing ion channel type 3 (ASIC-3) and the low threshold voltage-gated calcium channel (VGCC) CaV3.2. Several different classes of TRP channels are involved in transduction of changes in temperature from noxious cold (TRPA1, ankyrin type 1), cool (TRPM8, melastatin type 8), warm (TRPV4), and hot (TRPV1, vanilloid type 1). Many chemoreceptors are present in nociceptive afferents including those involved in the response to tissue acidosis (TRPV1 and ASIC-3), noxious organic compounds (e.g., aldehydes at TRPA1) and endogenous chemicals (e.g., ATP at P2X3, the ionotropic purine receptor type 3). A wide variety of other receptors for both pro- and anti-inflammatory (not shown) mediators are also present on the terminals of nociceptive afferents. These include G-protein

(*continues*)

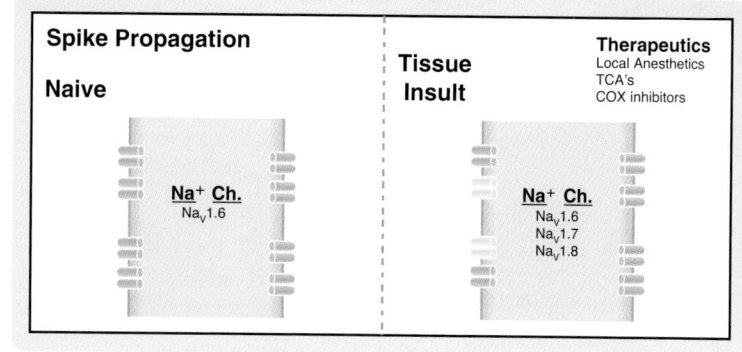

D

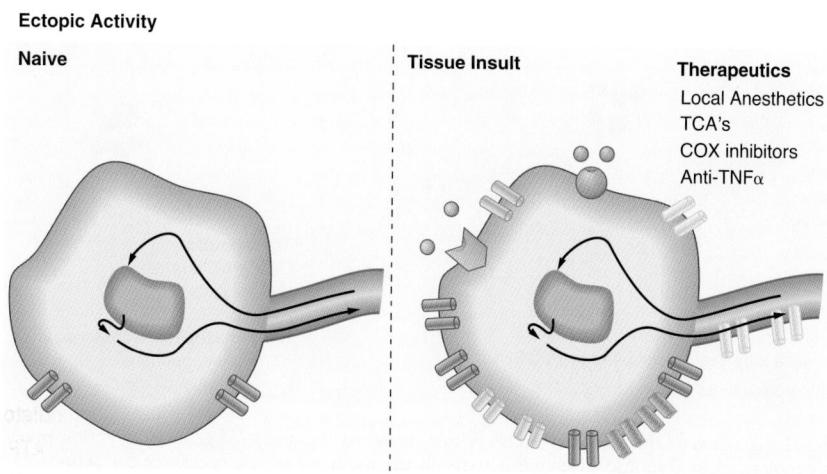

E

FIGURE 3.1 (*continued*) coupled receptors (GPCRs) responsive to E-type prostaglandins (EP), bradykinin (B) types 1 and 2, and serotonin (5HT) types 1A, 2, and 7. Tyrosine receptor kinases (TRK), responsive to trophic factors such as nerve growth factor (NGF) and artemin, are present as are receptors for cytokines such as TNF-α and interleukin 1-β. Also depicted are transmitters such as ATP stored in epithelial cells. Following tissue insult, there are changes in nociceptive terminals that result in both an increase in sensitivity to noxious stimuli as well as the emergence of membrane depolarization. There are increases in the density of several transducers as well as posttranslational modifications (depicted as phosphorylation, P) that increase channel activity or sensitivity such that the transducers are activated by lower intensity stimuli. These changes are brought about by actions of inflammatory mediators such as ATP, prostaglandin E2, NGF, and TNF-α that can directly depolarize nociceptive terminals, drive posttranslational changes via the activation of second messenger cascades and/or alter the expression of transducers via influencing transcription and/or translation. All of these processes may be facilitated as a result of an increase in the release of mediators from epithelial cells, resident (mast) cells and recruited (macrophages) immune cells. Several therapeutics currently in use or in development act via suppressing the actions of proinflammatory mediators. The specific pattern of changes and mediators depends on many factors, including the type and site of injury, time after injury, previous history of the injured tissue, as well as age and sex, which also influence the relative efficacy of the therapeutic intervention. **C. Spike Intiation:** The appropriate anatomical distribution of ion channels is critical for normal function. A number of ion channels play an important role in determining the threshold for spike initiation and upstroke of the spike. Action potential threshold appears to be critically regulated by K$^+$ channels, which include voltage-gated K$^+$ channels (K$_V$), inward rectifying K$^+$ channels (K$_{IR}$), 2-pore K$^+$ channels (K2P), large-conductance calcium modulated K$^+$ channels (BK), and small conductance calcium dependent K$^+$ channels (SK). The nonselective inward rectifying cation channel (HCN) also contributes to action potential threshold. In some cases, the low-threshold calcium channel (CaV3.2) may contribute to action potential threshold, but when present, CaV3.2 appears to play a more prominent role in mediating burst activity. The voltage-gated sodium channel (VGSC) NaV1.9 may also contribute to establishing action potential threshold. Finally, the channels responsible for the upstroke of the action potential include the VGSCs NaV1.7 and NaV1.8. As with transduction, there are a number of changes in ion channels that affect action potential threshold and spike initiation to increase in the excitability of nociceptive afferents in the presence of insult. These changes include a decrease in K$^+$ channel density and/or current and an increase in CaV3.2, HCN, and NaV channel density and/ or activity. These changes are the result of both posttranslational modifications and/or changes in transcription driven by the same inflammatory mediators that influence transduction. Thus, several of the therapeutics listed under transduction may also act by inhibiting changes in channels underlying spike initiation. Other drugs may act via direct inhibition of the ion channels underlying spike initiation (which include local anesthetics, tricyclic antidepressants [TCAs], and several cyclooxygenase inhibitors). K$^+$ channel openers such as retigabine may also have efficacy in increasing the threshold for spike initiation. **D. Action Potential Propagation:** The ion channels underlying action potential propagation are distinct from those underlying spike initiation. The channel most prominently implicated in action potential propagation is the VGSC NaV1.6. In myelinated axons, NaV1.6 is clustered at nodes of Ranvier, while in unmyelinated axons, the channel is distributed throughout the axon. Following insult, however, the pattern of channel expression can change, including redistribution of VGSCs NaV1.7 and/or NaV1.8 to the cell membrane. The dependence of action potential propagation on VGSCs confers the therapeutic efficacy of sodium channel blocking compounds such as local anesthetics, TCAs, and some COX inhibitors. **E. Ectopic Activity:** As is true for all neurons in the absence of tissue insult, the soma serves as the supply depot for the rest of the neuron, synthesizing and packaging the proteins, transmitters, and lipids that will be used

(continues)

Transmitter Release

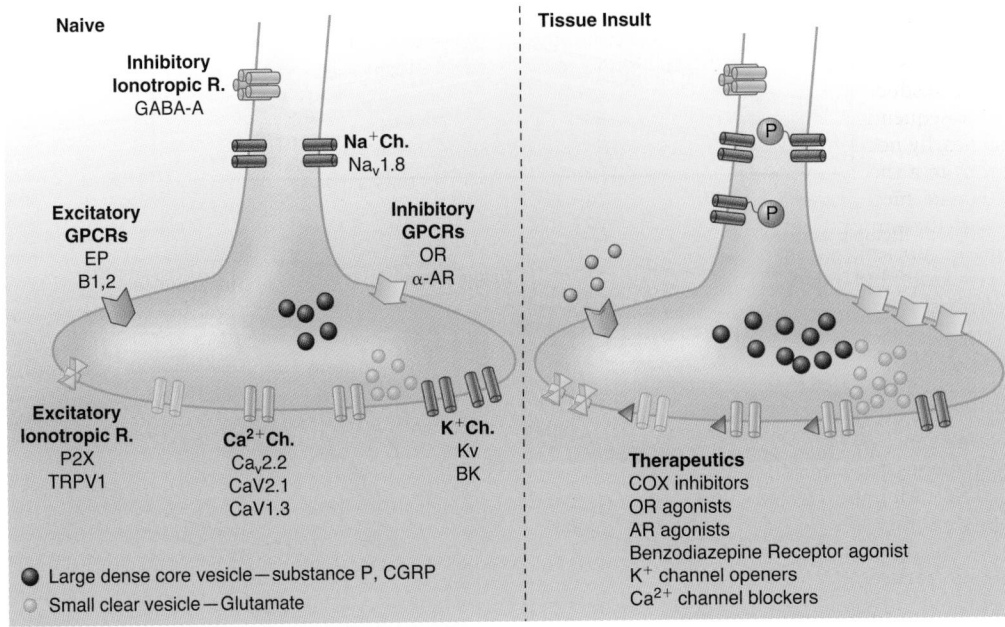

FIGURE 3.1 (*continued*) throughout the cell. While the soma is capable of generating action potentials and is likely depolarized in response to neural activity in the axons, it is not necessary for action potentials to invade the soma for information to propagate from the periphery to the central nervous system. In nociceptive afferents, the VGSC NaV1.8 can be the primary, if not the only sodium channel in the cell underlying action potential generation. In the presence of nerve injury, however, changes in the soma and/or proximal axon can include an increase in transducer proteins that may make the soma responsive to mechanical, thermal, and chemical stimuli, an increase in sodium channels that may lead to membrane instability (manifesting as oscillatory behavior) and an increase in inflammatory mediators and their receptors. The result of such changes is that the soma and/or proximal axon may become a source of aberrant or ectopic activity. An important implication of this activity is that local administration of therapeutic agents to block activity arising from peripheral terminals may not provide pain relief. Given the source of much of this activity, therapeutic interventions designed to block sodium channels and/or inhibit the actions of inflammatory mediators are predicted to have the greatest efficacy. **F. Transmitter Release:** The release of transmitter at the central terminals of nociceptive afferents is essential for transmission of nociceptive information to the central nervous system. This process is calcium dependent—extracellular calcium enters the central terminal generally via high threshold VGCCs that are activated following invasion of the action potential into the central terminals. N-type channels (CaV2.2) are the most abundant, but P/Q-type (CaV2.1) and L-type (CaV1.3) are also present. CaV2.2 is most readily modulated following activation of inhibitory GPCRs, serving as the primary mechanism for the therapeutic efficacy of intrathecal opioid receptor and alpha adrenergic receptor (α-AR) agonists. Transmitters present in nociceptive afferents are generally packaged in vesicles referred to as small clear vesicles, which generally contain the excitatory amino acid glutamate, and large dense core vesicles, which contain, among other things, neuropeptides such as substance P and calcitonin gene-related peptide (GRP). There are a number of excitatory ionotropic receptors, including P2X3 and TRPV1, that appear to facilitate transmitter release from the central terminals. Inhibition of the central terminal may involve activation of voltage gated (K_V) and calcium modulated (BK) K^+ channels. Under normal conditions, presynaptic ionotropic γ-aminobutyric acid (GABA) receptors (GABA-A) play a major role in mediating presynaptic inhibition of the central terminals of nociceptive afferents. The VGSC that appears to play a major role in enabling spike invasion of the central terminals of nociceptive afferents is NaV1.8. Finally, excitatory GPCRs (e.g., EP and B1,2 receptors) are also present. As with other steps in the process, a number of changes occur in the central terminals of nociceptive afferents after tissue insult that contribute to the transmission of nociceptive information. These include an increase in the alpha2delta1 subunit in VGSCs. This subunit is important for trafficking channels to the membrane and, importantly, is a binding site for gabapentin and pregabalin. There is also an increase in neuropeptide expression, the emergence of additional excitatory receptors, modulation of ion channels such as NaV1.8 and a decrease in K^+ currents that facilitate nociceptive signaling. Interestingly, there is a growing body of evidence suggesting that there may be changes in GABA-A receptor signaling as well such that activation of these receptors may become excitatory secondary to changes in the regulation of intracellular chloride. This issue is complicated by the fact that benzodiazepine receptor agonists may have therapeutic efficacy in the presence of tissue insult which appears to involve, at least in part, activation of presynaptic receptors. From the therapeutic perspective, it is important to note that following tissue insult, in particular that associated with inflammation, there may be an increase in the expression of inhibitory receptors, ultimately facilitating the therapeutic efficacy of opioid and adrenergic receptor agonists. Additional therapeutic interventions may also involve inhibitors of VGCCs, K^+ channel openers, and inhibitors to inflammatory mediators.

Whereas mechanotransduction is an intrinsic property of many nociceptors, there is evidence that epithelial cells may also be mechanosensitive.[35] Because these cells may store and release transmitters such as ATP, it has been suggested that afferent activity evoked with mechanical stimulation of peripheral structures such as the bladder,[35] gastrointestinal tract,[36] and skin[37] may be secondary to the transduction event that has occurred in the epithelial cell that subsequently releases a chemical mediator capable of activating nearby nociceptor terminals. The implication of this mechanism from a therapeutic perspective is that it may be possible to attenuate mechanical hypersensitivity in several peripheral tissues with the appropriate antagonist of the responsible chemoreceptors on nociceptive afferents.[38] Consistent with this idea, there is evidence that mechanical hypersensitivity observed in several visceral structures can be attenuated with ATP receptor antagonists.[39]

Aberrant expression of transducers may play a significant role in chronic pain associated with tissue injury. The presence of a functional transducer at a site other than the peripheral terminal may underlie the emergence of ectopic activity and contribute to ongoing or spontaneous pain. Such changes have been most extensively detailed following nerve injury, where, as mentioned above, mechanical sensitivity is detectable in cut axons within hours of injury[33] and may persist in neuromas indefinitely. Similarly, chemosensitivity, particularly to adrenergic agonists, develops at both the cut ends of nociceptive afferents[40] as well as within the ganglia itself,[41] contributing to ectopic activity arising from both the site of injury and from the ganglia. The emergence of ectopic activity arising from sites distant to the site of injury may explain why interventions targeting the site of injury are unsuccessful.

Action Potential Generation

A generator potential at a primary afferent terminal ending is not equivalent to an action potential propagated along that afferent's axon. The generator potential decays over distance from the point of origin as a function of membrane resistance, membrane capacitance, and internal resistance of the nerve terminal and may or may not be propagated beyond the terminal ending. Generally considered stable properties, there is evidence for dynamic remodeling of the terminal arbor of central nervous system neurons[42] which may influence both membrane capacitance and internal resistance; it remains to be determined whether such changes may also impact passive conduction of generator potentials in peripheral terminals. In contrast, a number of ion channels have been identified that may establish resting membrane resistance and therefore the spread of the generator potential within the terminal arbor.[43] This issue is important to nociceptive signaling because action potential initiation does not always occur at the site of stimulus transduction.[44] Consequently, the magnitude of the generator potential at the site of action potential initiation must be greater than or equal to action potential threshold. Thus, at least in some fiber types, it may be possible to block nociceptor signaling, and therefore pain with manipulations such as the local administration of potassium (K^+) channel openers[45,46] that decrease membrane resistance and therefore the spread of the generator potential.

Voltage-gated sodium channels (VGSCs) are responsible for the upstroke of the action potential in virtually all excitable tissue. As their name implies, these channels are gated (opened and closed) by changes in membrane potential. VGSCs are generally composed of an alpha subunit and up to two beta subunits. The alpha subunit is a large molecule (~200 kD) that contains all features necessary for a functional channel including voltage sensor, ion selectivity filter, channel pore, and inactivation gate.[47]

Ten alpha subunits have been identified, nine of which form functional channels in heterologous expression systems. The channels encoded by each of these subunits can be distinguished by a combination of pharmacological and biophysical properties. Eight of these nine alpha subunits are present in the nervous system, all eight of which are present in nociceptive afferents.[15] Beta subunits influence channel gating properties as well as trafficking and localization in the plasma membrane.[48] Four beta subunits have been identified, at least three of which are present in nociceptive afferents.[15]

The VGSC alpha subunit primarily responsible for action potential initiation in the majority of nociceptors is NaV1.8. This subunit is unique in several ways. First, it is normally only expressed in primary afferents[49,50] where it is primarily expressed in nociceptors.[51] This unique pattern of distribution, in combination with its primary function in spike initiation, makes it an ideal target for novel therapeutics.[52] Second, NaV1.8 has a relatively high threshold for activation. Whereas many other VGSCs begin to activate at membrane potentials between -50 and -40 mV, a depolarization to -30 mV or greater is necessary to activate NaV1.8.[53] This feature may explain, at least in part, why greater intensity stimuli are generally needed for nociceptor activation. Third, NaV1.8 is relatively resistant to steady-state inactivation, a voltage-dependent process whereby channels residing in a closed or resting state transition to an inactive state before they ever get a chance to open. Recovery from the inactivated state requires membrane hyperpolarization; thus, inactivated channels cannot contribute to the upstroke of the action potential. Even a small sustained depolarization to -50 mV can inactivate virtually all other VGSCs. However, NaV1.8 is still fully available for activation at this membrane potential.[53] Fourth, NaV1.8 recovers from inactivation rapidly.[54] These last two features enable the channel to underlie sustained activity in the face of a persistent depolarization that might be observed in the presence of inflammatory mediators. Fifth, NaV1.8 is resistant to cooling-induced inactivation.[55] Other VGSCs are completely inactivated at temperature at or below 18° C. However, NaV1.8 is still functional at temperatures down to 4° C, enabling the burning pain associated with noxious cold stimuli. Sixth, in contrast to all but one other VGSC alpha subunit (NaV1.9), NaV1.8 is resistant to tetrodotoxin (TTX), and is therefore referred to as a TTX-resistant channel.

Whereas NaV1.8 is critical for action potential initiation in nociceptors, in many of these afferents this alpha subunit appears to work in concert with another VGSC alpha subunit, NaV1.7.[56] The NaV1.7 subunit has unique features enabling it to play a significant role in spike initiation.[57] That this channel plays a critical role in nociceptor activity is highlighted by the recent discovery of individuals possessing both gain-of-function and loss-of-function point mutations in this subunit. Strikingly, two distinct pain syndromes—primary erythermalgia (PE) and paroxysmal extreme pain disorder (PEPD)—reveal the specific impact of gain-of-function mutations.[58] PE is associated with burning pain in the hands and feet, and PEPD is associated with pain in the rectum at early stages, ultimately progressing to trigeminal structures including the eye and jaw. The unique distribution of these pain syndromes, in light of the widespread distribution of NaV1.7 in the peripheral nervous system as well as neuroendocrine tissues, highlights the importance of other channels in sculpting the response properties of sensory neurons. Furthermore, in contrast to the impact of the gain-of-function mutations, loss-of-function mutations that result in nonfunctional channels are associated with a complete insensitivity to pain.[59]

Recent evidence suggests that low voltage activated, or T-type, calcium channels may also contribute to spike initiation in the periphery.[60] Whereas there is compelling evidence that these channels are present in high density in low threshold D-hair afferents,[61] there is also evidence that they may be present in a subpopulation of nociceptors as well.[62] The biophysical properties of these channels enable them to play a particularly important role in mediating bursting activity, as the channels underlie a sustained membrane depolarization after a single action potential that provides the driving force for the initiation of subsequent action potentials.[63] This feature has led some to speculate that selective T-Type channel blockers may be particularly effective for treating paroxysmal pain[62] such as that associated with trigeminal neuralgia.

Whereas the focus on NaV1.8 has been on its role in action potential initiation in the periphery, there is also evidence that the channels are present and functional at central nociceptor terminals.[64,65] At the central terminal, the channel appears to facilitate the spread of the invading action potential throughout the terminal arbor and consequently the release of transmitter from the primary afferent. There is also a growing body of evidence suggesting that action potentials may also be initiated at the central terminals of nociceptors, where they are conducted antidromically to the periphery.[66] This activity, referred to as the dorsal root reflex, appears to play a significant role in the neurogenic inflammation that develops following tissue injury.

Action Potential Propagation

Whereas NaV1.8 and NaV1.7 underlie action potential generation and even propagation over the first 5–10 mm of peripheral axon, a different set of VGSCs underlies action potential propagation into the central nervous system in the absence of tissue injury. NaV1.6 is the subunit primarily responsible for propagation in both myelinated and unmyelinated axons of both nociceptive and non-nociceptive afferents,[67] although other subunits may contribute as well. Unfortunately, the distribution of NaV1.6 in the peripheral nervous system in combination with its widespread expression in the central nervous system precludes selective block of propagation in nociceptors via a NaV1.6 specific mechanism. Nevertheless, block of these channels with local anesthetics and/or TTX remains an effective means of blocking input into the central nervous system.

Transmitter Release

Voltage-gated calcium channels (VGCCs) are primarily responsible for the initial influx of calcium necessary for initiation of machinery underlying the release of neurotransmitters. Like VGSCs, these channels consist of a large alpha subunit that contains all of the features necessary for a functional channel. Ten alpha subunits have been identified, encoding channels that are commonly defined by their threshold for activation or pharmacological properties.[68] T-type channels (CaV3.1–3.3), as mentioned above, have a low threshold for activation while all others have a high threshold for activation. The high threshold channels are further subdivided based on their sensitivity to specific channel blockers: L-type channels (CaV1.1–1.4) are blocked by dihydropyridines such as nimodipine, N-type channels (CaV2.2) are blocked by the snail toxin ω-conotoxin GVIA, P/Q-type channels (CaV2.1) are blocked by the spider toxin ω-agatoxin IVA, and R-type channels (CaV2.3) are blocked by the spider toxin SNX-482. In contrast to VGSCs, VGCCs are not effectively targeted to the plasma membrane in the absence of the alpha2delta-subunit complex.[69] A single beta subunit also appears to be important for efficient gating.[70] All VGCC subtypes are present in nociceptors. And whereas there is evidence that all high-threshold calcium channels may contribute to transmitter release, N-type channels appear to play a dominant role in the release of transmitter from nociceptors.[71]

The dominant role N-type channels play in mediating transmitter release from nociceptive afferent terminals makes them an ideal target for both endogenous and exogenous analgesics. Opioid and adrenergic receptor agonists act through inhibitory G-protein coupled receptors which enable inhibition of VGCCs via two major intracellular pathways. The first is a rapid, membrane delimited pathway involving G-protein βγ-subunit displacement of the VGCC β-subunit, resulting in a "sleepy" or "unwilling" channel that requires a larger membrane depolarization for channel opening.[70] The second pathway involves more traditional second messenger-kinase dependent signaling with a slower onset and offset.[72] Interestingly, neither pathway results in complete VGCC block, yet both result in a dramatic inhibition of transmitter release. This amplification effect reflects the fact that there is considerable cooperativity of calcium in mediating vesicle fusion to the cell membrane that is necessary for transmitter release: 4–5 calcium ions are needed to trigger vesicle fusion.[73] This amplification effect is also likely to facilitate the use of relatively low concentrations of the N-type channel blocker SNX-111 (ziconotide), enabling the block of transmitter release from nociceptive afferent terminals in the superficial dorsal horn while minimizing side effects associated with block of channels at more distant sites. Finally, while it remains to be determined exactly how gabapentin and pregabalin block high VGCC, the fact that it binds to the α2δ-subunit complex critical for membrane targeting of the alpha subunit puts the compound in a good position to interfere with ion flux through the channel.[74]

NOCICEPTOR SENSITIZATION

Sensitization is a characterizing feature of nociceptors; non-nociceptors do not sensitize following tissue insult. Sensitization represents an increase in nociceptor excitability, which is expressed and defined as an increase in response to a noxious stimulus. Sensitization is also typically accompanied by a reduction in the threshold for activation and occasionally by the development of ongoing, spontaneous activity. Nociceptor sensitization is the cause of primary hyperalgesia (i.e., increased pain produced by stimulation at the site of tissue insult) and is important because nociceptor sensitization is the trigger for initiation of an increase in excitability of central neurons in the nociceptive pathway, an event termed "central sensitization."

An increase in nociceptor excitability is a reflection of changes in the behavior of nociceptor voltage- and/or ligand-gated ion channels produced by actions of endogenous substances either released or synthesized at the site of tissue insult or attracted there. Endogenous substances considered classically to contribute to sensitization include products of arachidonic acid metabolism (e.g., prostaglandin E2), histamine, serotonin, protons, and ATP, but the list has grown quite extensively and now also includes cytokines, chemokines, growth factors, peptides, etc., some of which are released from immune competent cells attracted to the site of insult (e.g., macrophages), released from nearby cells (e.g., mast cells), or from nociceptor (and other) nerve terminals (e.g., peptides). Interestingly, despite the variety of mediators capable of producing nociceptor sensitization, several appear to play particularly important roles. This list includes prostanoids, as evidenced by the antihyperalgesic efficacy of nonsteriodal anti-inflammatory drugs (NSAIDs) that act via inhibition of cyclo-oxygenase and thus prostanoid synthesis. More recently, the importance of tumor necrosis factor alpha (TNF-α) in chronic inflammatory conditions has been highlighted by the antinociceptive efficacy of compounds such as entanercept, which are designed to absorb TNF-α released at sites of inflammation. Finally, nerve growth factor appears to play a major role in orchestrating a variety of signaling cascades necessary for an inflammatory response and therefore has also been targeted with antibody based strategies.[75–78]

The mechanisms that trigger changes in nociceptor excitability are not fully known. A growing body of evidence suggests that despite what appears to be a bewildering assortment of mediators and membrane receptors, there are only a few common intracellular pathways that are ultimately accessed and influenced by what appear to be disparate extracellular or membrane mechanisms that initiate common intracellular pathways. For example, both prostaglandins and bradykinin, which are among the most extensively studied inflammatory mediators, act at G-protein coupled receptors. Two major G-protein dependent pathways have been implicated. One involves a stimulatory G-protein, Gs, which drives activation of adenylate cyclase, resulting in an increase in cyclic adenosine monophosphate and the activation of protein kinase A (PKA).[79,80] The other involves a Gq-dependent pathway, resulting in the activation of phospholipase C, the liberation of diacyl glycerol (DAG) and IP3, and the subsequent activation of protein kinase C (PKC).[81,82] The PKC-epsilon isoform appears to play a particularly important role in nociceptor sensitization. Other mediators that appear to play important roles in nociceptor sensitization, such as TNF-α and interleukin 1β, utilize a mitogen-activated protein kinase (MAPK)-dependent pathway ultimately resulting in the activation of p38.[83] Channels underlying transduction and spike initiation, in particular TRPV1 and NaV1.8, respectively, appear to be final common targets for this diverse array of mediators and second messenger pathways.[84] Phosphorylation of specific residues on the channel or associated proteins results in increases in channel density and/or increases in channel function.

Still other mediators directly activate ion channels. For example, protons (which increase in concentration during inflammation) act at TRPV1 and acid-sensing ion channels (ASICs). ASIC-3 is important to pain associated with ischemia, such as occurs during angina, and deep muscle pain where protons and lactic acid accumulate. In contrast, ATP and its metabolites act at ionotropic P2X and metabotropic P2Y receptors to modulate nociceptor excitability.

Types of Nociceptors

To this point, we have discussed nociceptors only in a general context, but there are in fact many types of nociceptors, our knowledge of which has been advanced by human psychophysical studies while recording from afferent fibers (Box 3-1). In human skin, for example, there exist nociceptors that respond only to mechanical, only to cold thermal, or only to hot thermal stimuli as well as those that are insensitive to both mechanical and heat stimuli (mechanically insensitive or sleeping nociceptors). The most abundant nociceptor is the polymodal nociceptor, which responds to mechanical, thermal, and chemical stimuli. In general, nociceptors that innervate skin have the broadest range of modality-selectivity whereas nociceptors innervating deeper structures tend to be less modality-selective and more polymodal in character. For example, mechanical sensitivity is a prominent feature of visceral and joint nociceptors because stimuli adequate for their activation include hollow organ distension and overrotation, respectively. Many of these nociceptors also respond to chemical and/or thermal stimuli as well, although the functional significance of thermal sensitivity in deep tissues in uncertain. An important characteristic of polymodal nociceptors, whether the modalities of stimulation to which they respond is two or all three, is that when sensitized, (e.g., by an inflammatory insult) responses to the other modality(ies) of stimuli to which it responds are all increased. That is, it is not only the mechanosensi-

---

BOX 3.1

MICRONEUROGRAPHY

The development of a method to record from human nerve fibers in situ,[85] termed microneurography, provided a unparalleled opportunity to expand our knowledge about peripheral sensory receptors, including nociceptors. The method involves percutaneous insertion of the tip of a sharp, insulated metal microelectrode into a nerve (e.g., peroneal or radial nerve) and the application of search stimuli to sites distal to the electrode. In earlier work, mechanical search stimuli (e.g., von Frey filaments) were used and, accordingly, only mechanosensitive afferents were studied. An electrical search stimulus (surface electrode), however, has become favored because the electrical stimulus identifies afferent fibers independent of sensitivity to natural stimulation. After an afferent fiber is isolated, the innervation territory can be drawn on the skin and the adequate, natural stimulus/stimuli determined.

Because microneurography can be easily coupled with a psychophysical approach, human subjects are able to describe stimulus-produced experiences (e.g., pain) while recording from single afferent fibers. Microneurography has also been expanded to include intraneural electrical stimulation of the fiber through the recording electrode, providing additional insight into the qualities of sensation produced, for example, by low- and high-frequency stimulation in addition to qualities associated with natural stimulation. Microneurography has confirmed in psychophysical experiments sensations associated with activation of rapidly adapting (flutter, vibration) and slowly adapting (pressure) cutaneous mechanoreceptors, Aδ-mechanonociceptors (AM$_{[mechano]}$; sharp pain), C-polymodal nociceptors (CM$_{[mechano]}$H$_{[heat]}$; dull, burning [heat] pain), and group IV muscle nociceptors (cramping pain).

Electrical search strategies have revealed a wider range of nociceptors, including[86]: A-mechanoheat (AMH), which have similar heat thresholds as CMH (C-polymodal) fibers and also typically respond to chemical stimuli; C-mechanonociceptors (CM), C-heat (CH); C-mechano- and heat-insensitive (CM$_i$H$_i$, or sleeping nociceptors); and C-mechano-insensitive-histamine responsive (CM$_i$His+, or itch fibers[87];). Microneurography has also been extended to psychophysical study of pathological pain states in humans. In a study of patients suffering from erythromelalgia, a condition characterized by painful, red, and hot extremities, a proportion of CM$_i$H$_i$ fibers were found to be spontaneously active or sensitized to mechanical stimuli. Because CM$_i$H$_i$ fibers also mediate the axon flare reflex, their hyperexcitability was considered to contribute to the patients' ongoing pain and tenderness as well as the redness and warming in this pain syndrome. In patients with painful peripheral neuropathy, Ochoa et al.[88] reported hyperexcitability in CMH and CM$_i$H$_i$ fibers. Signs of hyperexcitability included reduced thresholds to mechanical and heat stimuli, spontaneous activity, and increased responses to stimulation. In diabetic neuropathic pain patients, Ørstavik et al.[89] found that the ratio of CMH to CM$_i$H$_i$ fibers was reduced by about 50%, apparently due to loss of mechanical and heat responsiveness in CMH fibers.

These and future studies will help to understand which nociceptors (and perhaps non-nociceptors) in which conditions contribute to spontaneous, ongoing pain as well as stimulus-evoked pain, and what therapeutic strategies are most effective.

tive modality, for example, that becomes sensitized, but other modalities to which it responds are sensitized as well.

With respect to mechanosensitivity, nociceptors at the opposite extremes of sensitivity are most interesting. Nociceptors with low mechanical thresholds for response and those with very high mechanical thresholds for response (i.e., sleeping nociceptors) are both clinically important. Mechanosensitive sensory neurons with low thresholds for response have long been classed as non-nociceptors because it was considered that nociceptors had to have response thresholds in the noxious range. Some mechanosensitive skin, joint, and many visceral sensory neurons have low thresholds for response (i.e., in the non-noxious range), but possess characteristics that suggest an important role in pain. First, they encode stimulus intensity well into the noxious range and, moreover, typically give greater responses to all intensities of stimulation than do nociceptors with high mechanical thresholds for response. Second, they sensitize after tissue insult. The mechanically-insensitive, sleeping nociceptors, on the other hand, normally provide no information to the central nervous system but after tissue insult become spontaneously active and mechanosensitive.

Clinical Implications of Nociceptor Function

As researchers have begun to explore the basis for chronic pain syndromes generally associated with specific body regions and/or organs (e.g., temporomandibular joint disorder [TMJD], inflammatory bowel disease [IBD], irritable bowel syndrome [IBS] or painful bladder syndrome [formerly interstitial cystitis, IC]), a number of common themes have emerged that are likely to impact future treatment approaches. First, specific mechanisms underlying injury-induced sensitization of nociceptors vary as a function of target of innervation. For example, inflammation-induced sensitization of masseter muscle afferents appears to reflect a decrease in a specific subpopulation of voltage-gated potassium channels.[90] The same channels do not appear to contribute to the sensitization of TMJ afferents.[91] Similarly, inflammation-induced increases in the excitability of bladder sensory neurons appear to reflect one pattern of changes in voltage-gated[92] or ligand-gated[93] ion channels whereas the inflammation-induced increase in sensory neurons innervating the stomach,[94–96] ileum,[97,98] or colon[99] reflect other patterns. While tissue-specific patterns of inflammation may contribute to these differences between subpopulations of afferents, differences persist when the response to inflammatory mediators is studied in vitro.[100] The implication of these observations is that it may be possible, if not necessary, to treat pain arising from a specific structure with a specific intervention. Second, specific mechanisms underlying in-

sult-induced sensitization of nociceptors also varies as a function of the type of insult. For example, acute phosphorylation-dependent modulation of the VGSC NaV1.8[101] results in an increase in current which contributes to an inflammation-induced increase in nociceptor excitability.[102] In contrast, following traumatic nerve injury, redistribution of NaV1.8 to the axons of uninjured afferents appears to be necessary for the expression of mechanical hypersensitivity associated with nerve injury.[103] The dynamic allodynia that often develops after nerve injury, however, likely represents more than only a redistribution of NaV1.8 (Box 3-2). With respect to the viscera, because each organ receives innervation from two nerves, the effect of organ insult can be different in the two groups of sensory neurons that innervate the organ.[93] These observations underscore the importance of developing diagnostic criteria that enable identification of the factors primarily responsible for ongoing pain. Third, the history of the nociceptor influences the response to subsequent challenge. For example, in naïve tissue, peripheral injection of prostaglandin E2 produces a PKA-dependent sensitization of nociceptors that lasts approximately 90 minutes, whereas the same manipulation in previously inflamed tissue results in a PKC-dependent sensitization that lasts for more than 24 hours.[82] This "memory" of a previous insult lasts for at least 21 days in the adult. Furthermore, there is evidence of a developmental window within which injury may produce permanent changes in nociceptors.[104] With the development of more specific therapeutic tools, patient history may become a critical factor in the identification of the most appropriate intervention. Fourth, there is evidence for sex differences in both the excitability of different groups of nociceptors[105] as well as the response to tissue injury.[106] These differences appear to be mediated, at least in part, through the actions of gonadal hormones and may contribute to sex differences in the manifestation of a number of chronic pain syndromes. Finally, there is recent evidence for age-dependent changes in nociceptor function.[107] With the aging of society, this particular issue in is need of further investigation.

As indicated above, the consequences of tissue insult are not limited only to changes in the excitability of nociceptors and the awakening of sleeping nociceptors. Because sensitization leads to an increased response to noxious stimuli and a decrease in response threshold, previously non-noxious intensities of stimulation also are now able to activate nociceptors. In addition, spontaneous activity may develop. In the aggregate, central nervous system input from sensitized nociceptors, awakened sleeping nociceptors, and spontaneously active nociceptors is significantly increased. For example, approximately 15% of human cutaneous C-fibers are sleeping nociceptors,[86] comprising significant new input to the central nervous system if awakened. Consequently,

BOX 3.2

AFFERENT CONTRIBUTIONS TO NEUROPATHIC PAIN AND ALLODYNIA

One of the most striking positive symptoms of neuropathic pain is dynamic mechanical allodynia, a term used to describe pain resulting from light tactile stimuli that would never be considered noxious in the absence of nervous system injury. This phenomenon can be recapitulated with a subcutaneous injection of capsaicin.[108] Data from detailed psychophysical analysis in combination with microneurography[109] and dorsal horn recording in animal models[110] all suggest that dynamic mechanical allodynia reflects activity in low-threshold afferents that signal pain as a result of changes in the central nervous system. The exact nature of these changes, generally referred to as central sensitization, is still debated,[111,112] but it is clear that they depend on

activity in nociceptive afferents. Another possibility, however, is that low threshold afferents undergo a phenotypic switch such that they begin to transmit information to the central nervous system as if they were nociceptive afferents. Consistent with this possibility, there is evidence following peripheral nerve injury that a subpopulation of putative non-nociceptive afferents begins to express the neuropeptide, substance P,[113] although this change does not appear to be necessary for the expression of allodynia.[114] Evidence of a third possibility, which would involve sprouting of non-nociceptive afferents into more superficial layers of the dorsal horn to enable low threshold drive of nociceptive dorsal horn neurons,[115] remains largely unsubstantiated.[116–118]

the amount of neurotransmitters (as well as perhaps their relative proportions) released onto central neurons is increased, which in turn alters the excitability of central neurons. The increase in excitability of central neurons is manifest as an increase in the size of the cutaneous receptive field (i.e., secondary hyperalgesia) or area of tenderness referred from deep structures, particularly the viscera. Although the principal focus of study of mechanisms of central sensitization has been the spinal cord, it should be appreciated that nociceptor-driven changes in central excitability extend throughout the central nervous system.

References

1. Johnson KO. The roles and functions of cutaneous mechanoreceptors. *Curr Opin Neurobiol* 2001;11(4):455–461.
2. Mearow KM, Diamond J. Merkel cells and the mechanosensitivity of normal and regenerating nerves in Xenopus skin. *Neuroscience* 1988;26(2):695–708.
3. Kruger L, Kavookjian AM, Kumazawa T, et al. Nociceptor structural specialization in canine and rodent testicular "free" nerve endings. *J Comp Neurol* 2003;463(2):197–211.
4. Zylka MJ, Rice FL, Anderson DJ. Topographically distinct epidermal nociceptive circuits revealed by axonal tracers targeted to Mrgprd. *Neuron* 2005;45(1):17–25.
5. Braz JM, Nassar MA, Wood JN, et al. Parallel "pain" pathways arise from subpopulations of primary afferent nociceptor. *Neuron* 2005;47(6):787–793.
6. Cesare P, McNaughton P. A novel heat-activated current in nociceptive neurons and its sensitization by bradykinin. *Proc Natl Acad Sci USA* 1996;93:15435–15439.
7. Reichling DB, Levine JD. Heat transduction in rat sensory neurons by calcium-dependent activation of a cation channel. *Proc Natl Acad Sci USA* 1997;94(13):7006–7011.
8. Reid G, Flonta ML. Physiology. Cold current in thermoreceptive neurons. *Nature* 2001;413(6855):480.
9. Thut PD, Wrigley D, Gold MS. Cold transduction in rat trigeminal ganglia neurons in vitro. *Neuroscience* 2003;119(4):1071–1083.
10. McCarter GC, Reichling DB, Levine JD. Mechanical transduction by rat dorsal root ganglion neurons in vitro. *Neurosci Lett* 1999;273(3):179–182.
11. Bevan S, Yeats J. Protons activate a cation conductance in a sub-population of rat dorsal root ganglion neurones. *J Physiol (Lond)* 1991;433:145–161.
12. Krishtal OA, Marchenko SM, Obukhov AG. Cationic channels activated by extracellular ATP in rat sensory neurons. *Neuroscience* 1988;27(3):995–1000.
13. Heyman I, Rang HP. Depolarizing responses to capsaicin in a subpopulation of rat dorsal root ganglion cells. *Neurosci Lett* 1985;56(1):69–75.
14. Bautista DM, Jordt SE, Nikai T, et al. TRPA1 mediates the inflammatory actions of environmental irritants and proalgesic agents. *Cell* 2006;124(6):1269–1282.
15. Gold MS. Ion channels: recent advances and clinical applications. In: Flor H, Kaslo E, Dostrovsky JO, eds. *Proceedings of the 11th World Congress on Pain.* Seattle: IASP Press; 2006:73–92.
16. Burnstock G. Physiology and pathophysiology of purinergic neurotransmission. *Physiol Rev* 2007;87(2):659–797.
17. Wemmie JA, Price MP, Welsh MJ. Acid-sensing ion channels: advances, questions and therapeutic opportunities. *Trends Neurosci* 2006;29(10):578–586.
18. Story GM, Peier AM, Reeve AJ, et al. ANKTM1, a TRP-like channel expressed in nociceptive neurons, is activated by cold temperatures. *Cell* 2003;112(6):819–829.
19. Caterina MJ, Rosen TA, Tominaga M, et al. A capsaicin-receptor homologue with a high threshold for noxious heat. *Nature* 1999;398(6726):436–441.
20. McKemy DD, Neuhausser WM, Julius D. Identification of a cold receptor reveals a general role for TRP channels in thermosensation. *Nature* 2002;416(6876):52–58.
21. Xu H, Ramsey IS, Kotecha SA, et al. TRPV3 is a calcium-permeable temperature-sensitive cation channel. *Nature* 2002;418(6894):181–186.
22. Guler AD, Lee H, Iida T, et al. Heat-evoked activation of the ion channel, TRPV4. *J Neurosci* 2002;22(15):6408–6414.
23. Caterina MJ, Schumacher MA, Tominaga M, et al. The capsaicin receptor: a heat-activated ion channel in the pain pathway. *Nature* 1997;389(6653):816–824.
24. Venkatachalam K, Montell C. TRP channels. *Annu Rev Biochem* 2007;76:387–417.
25. Kwan KY, Allchorne AJ, Vollrath MA, et al. TRPA1 contributes to cold, mechanical, and chemical nociception but is not essential for hair-cell transduction. *Neuron* 2006;50(2):277–289.
26. Alessandri-Haber N, Joseph E, Dina OA, et al. TRPV4 mediates pain-related behavior induced by mild hypertonic stimuli in the presence of inflammatory mediator. *Pain* 2005;118(1–2):70–79.
27. Honore P, Wismer CT, Mikusa J, et al. A-425619 (1-isoquinolin-5-yl-3-[4-trifluoromethyl-benzyl]-urea), a novel transient receptor potential type V1 receptor antagonist, relieves pathophysiological pain associated with inflammation and tissue injury in rats. *J Pharmacol Exp Ther* 2005;314(1):410–421.
28. Wong GY, Gavva NR. Therapeutic potential of vanilloid receptor TRPV1 agonists and antagonists as analgesics: recent advances and setbacks. *Brain Res Rev* 2009;60(1):267–277.
29. Karai L, Brown DC, Mannes AJ, et al. Deletion of vanilloid receptor 1-expressing primary afferent neurons for pain control. *J Clin Invest* 2004;113(9):1344–1352.
30. Hermanstyne TO, Fan L, Markowitz K, et al. Mechanotransducers in rat pulpal afferents. *J Dent Res* 2008;87(9):834–838.
31. Price MP, Lewin GR, McIlwrath SL, et al. The mammalian sodium channel BNC1 is required for normal touch sensation. *Nature* 2000;407(6807):1007–1011.
32. Shin JB, Martinez-Salgado C, Heppenstall PA, et al. A T-type calcium channel required for normal function of a mammalian mechanoreceptor. *Nat Neurosci* 2003;6(7):724–730.
33. Michaelis M, Blenk KH, Vogel C, et al. Distribution of sensory properties among axotomized cutaneous C-fibres in adult rats. *Neuroscience* 1999;94(1):7–10.
34. Drew LJ, Rugiero F, Cesare P, et al. High-threshold mechanosensitive ion channels blocked by a novel conopeptide mediate pressure-evoked pain. *PLoS ONE* 2007;2(6):e515.
35. Birder LA. More than just a barrier: urothelium as a drug target for urinary bladder pain. *Am J Physiol Renal Physiol* 2005;289(3):F489–F495.
36. Wynn G, Rong W, Xiang Z, et al. Purinergic mechanisms contribute to mechanosensory transduction in the rat colorectum. *Gastroenterology* 2003;125(5):1398–1409.
37. Mizumoto N, Mummert ME, Shalhevet D, et al. Keratinocyte ATP release assay for testing skin-irritating potentials of structurally diverse chemicals. *J Invest Dermatol* 2003;121(5):1066–1072.
38. Burnstock G. Purinergic P2 receptors as targets for novel analgesics. *Pharmacol Ther* 2006;110(3):433–454.
39. Xu GY, Shenoy M, Winston JH, et al. P2X receptor-mediated visceral hyperalgesia in a rat model of chronic visceral hypersensitivity. *Gut* 2008;57(9):1230–1237.
40. Korenman EMD, Devor M. Ectopic adrenergic sensitivity in damaged peripheral nerve axons in the rat. *Exp Neurol* 1981;72:63–81.
41. Devor M, Janig W, Michaelis M. Modulation of activity in dorsal root ganglion neurons by sympathetic activation in nerve-injured rats. *J Neurophysiol* 1994;71(1):38–47.
42. Mantyh PW, DeMaster E, Malhotra A, et al. Receptor endocytosis and dendrite reshaping in spinal neurons after somatosensory stimulation. *Science* 1995;268(5217):1629–1632.
43. Gold MS. Molecular basis of receptors. In: Merskey H, Loeser JD, Dubner R, eds. *The Paths of Pain 1975–2005.* Seattle: IASP Press; 2005:49–67.
44. Carr RW, Pianova S, Brock JA. The effects of polarizing current on nerve terminal impulses recorded from polymodal and cold receptors in the guinea-pig cornea. *J Gen Physiol* 2002;120(3):395–405.
45. Zhang XF, Gopalakrishnan M, Shieh CC. Modulation of action potential firing by iberiotoxin and NS1619 in rat dorsal root ganglion neurons. *Neuroscience* 2003;122(4):1003–1011.
46. Passmore GM, Selyanko AA, Mistry M, et al. KCNQ/M currents in sensory neurons: significance for pain therapy. *J Neurosci* 2003;23(18):7227–7236.
47. Catterall WA, Hulme JT, Jiang X, et al. Regulation of sodium and calcium channels by signaling complexes. *J Recept Signal Transduct Res* 2006;26(5–6):577–598.
48. Isom LL. Sodium channel beta subunits: anything but auxiliary. *Neuroscientist* 2001;7(1):42–54.
49. Sangameswaran L, Delgado SG, Fish LM, et al. Structure and function of a novel voltage-gated, tetrodoxtoxin-resistant sodium channel specfic to sensory neurons. *J Biol Chem* 1996;271(11):5953–5956.
50. Akopian AN, Sivilotti L, Wood JN. A tetrodotoxin-resistant voltage-gated sodium channel expressed by sensory neurons. *Nature* 1996;379(6562):257–262.
51. Djouhri L, Fang X, Okuse K, et al. The TTX-resistant sodium channel Nav1.8 (SNS/PN3): expression and correlation with membrane properties in rat nociceptive primary afferent neurons. *J Physiol* 2003;550(Pt 3):739–752.
52. Jarvis MF, Honore P, Shieh CC, et al. A-803467, a potent and selective Nav1.8 sodium channel blocker, attenuates neuropathic and inflammatory pain in the rat. *Proc Natl Acad Sci USA* 2007;104(20):8520–8525.
53. Elliott AA, Elliott JR. Characterization of TTX-sensitive and TTX-resistant sodium currents in small cells from adult rat dorsal root ganglia. *J Physiol (Lond)* 1993;463(39):39–56.
54. Gold MS, Zhang L, Wrigley DL, et al. Prostaglandin E(2) modulates TTX-R I(Na) in rat colonic sensory neurons. *J Neurophysiol* 2002;88(3):1512–1522.
55. Zimmermann K, Leffler A, Babes A, et al. Sensory neuron sodium channel Nav1.8 is essential for pain at low temperatures. *Nature* 2007;447(7146):855–858.
56. Rush AM, Dib-Hajj SD, Liu S, et al. A single sodium channel mutation produces hyper- or hypoexcitability in different types of neurons. *Proc Natl Acad Sci USA* 2006;103(21):8245–8250.
57. Cummins TR, Dib-Hajj SD, Waxman SG. Electrophysiological properties of mutant Nav1.7 sodium channels in a painful inherited neuropathy. *J Neurosci* 2004;24(38):8232–8236.
58. Waxman SG. Channel, neuronal and clinical function in sodium channelopathies: from genotype to phenotype. *Nat Neurosci* 2007;10(4):405–409.
59. Cox JJ, Reimann F, Nicholas AK, et al. An SCN9A channelopathy causes congenital inability to experience pain. *Nature* 2006;444(7121):894–898.

60. Zamponi GW, Lewis RJ, Todorovic SM, et al. Role of voltage calcium channels in ascending pain pathway. *Brain Res Rev* 2009;60(1):84–89.

61. Dubreuil AS, Boukhaddaoui H, Desmadryl G, et al. Role of T-type calcium current in identified D-hair mechanoreceptor neurons studied in vitro. *J Neurosci* 2004;24(39):8480–8484.

62. Todorovic SM, Jevtovic-Todorovic V. The role of T-type calcium channels in peripheral and central pain processing. *CNS Neurol Disord Drug Targets* 2006;5(6):639–653.

63. White G, Lovinger DM, Weight FF. Transient low-threshold Ca^{2+} current triggers burst firing through an afterdepolarizing potential in an adult mammalian neuron. *Proc Natl Acad Sci* 1989;86(17):6802–6806.

64. Gu JG, MacDermott AB. Activation of ATP P2X receptors elicits glutamate release from sensory neuron synapses. *Nature* 1997;389(6652):749–753.

65. Jeftinija S. The role of tetrodotoxin-resistant sodium channels of small primary afferent fibers. *Brain Res* 1994;639(1):125–134.

66. Willis WD Jr. Dorsal root potentials and dorsal root reflexes: a double-edged sword. *Exp Brain Res* 1999;124(4):395–421.

67. Wittmack EK, Rush AM, Craner MJ, et al. Fibroblast growth factor homologous factor 2B: association with Nav1.6 and selective colocalization at nodes of Ranvier of dorsal root axons. *J Neurosci* 2004;24(30):6765–7675.

68. Catterall WA, Perez-Reyes E, Snutch TP, et al. International Union of Pharmacology. XLVIII. Nomenclature and structure-function relationships of voltage-gated calcium channels. *Pharmacol Rev* 2005;57(4):411–425.

69. Davies A, Hendrich J, Van Minh AT, et al. Functional biology of the alpha(2)-delta subunits of voltage-gated calcium channels. *Trends Pharmacol Sci* 2007;28(5):220–228.

70. Ikeda SR. Voltage-dependent modulation of N-type calcium channels by G-protein beta gamma subunits. *Nature* 1996;380(6571):255–258.

71. Rycroft BK, Vikman KS, Christie MJ. Inflammation reduces the contribution of N-type calcium channels to primary afferent synaptic transmission onto NK1 receptor-positive lamina I neurons in the rat dorsal horn. *J Physiol* 2007;580(Pt.3):883–894.

72. Ewald DA, Matthies HJ, Perney TM, et al. The effect of down regulation of protein kinase C on the inhibitory modulation of dorsal root ganglion neuron Ca2+ currents by neuropeptide Y. *J Neurosci* 1988;8(7):2447–2451.

73. Schneggenburger R, Neher E. Presynaptic calcium and control of vesicle fusion. *Curr Opin Neurobiol* 2005;15(3):266–274.

74. Li CY, Zhang XL, Matthews EA, et al. Calcium channel alpha2delta1 subunit mediates spinal hyperexcitability in pain modulation. *Pain* 2006;125(1–2):20–34.

75. Jimenez-Andrade JM, Martin CD, Koewler NJ, et al. Nerve growth factor sequestering therapy attenuates non-malignant skeletal pain following fracture. *Pain* 2007;133(1–3):183–196.

76. Koewler NJ, Freeman KT, Buus RJ, et al. Effects of a monoclonal antibody raised against nerve growth factor on skeletal pain and bone healing after fracture of the C57BL/6J mouse femur. *J Bone Miner Res* 2007;22(11):1732–1742.

77. Sabsovich I, Wei T, Guo TZ, et al. Effect of anti-NGF antibodies in a rat tibia fracture model of complex regional pain syndrome type I. *Pain* 2008;138(1):47–60.

78. Wild KD, Bian D, Zhu D, et al. Antibodies to nerve growth factor reverse established tactile allodynia in rodent models of neuropathic pain without tolerance. *J Pharmacol Exp Ther* 2007;322(1):282–287.

79. Gold MS, Levine JD, Correa AM. Modulation of TTX-R INa by PKC and PKA and their role in PGE2-induced sensitization of rat sensory neurons in vitro [In Process Citation]. *J Neurosci* 1998;18(24):10345–10355.

80. Taiwo YO, Bjerknes LK, Goetzl EJ, et al. Mediation of primary afferent peripheral hyperalgesia by the cAMP second messenger system. *Neuroscience* 1989;32(3):577–580.

81. Ahlgren SC, Levine JD. Protein kinase C inhibitors decrease hyperalgesia and C-fiber hyperexcitability in the streptozotocin-diabetic rat. *J Neurophysiol* 1994;72(2):684–692.

82. Aley KO, Messing RO, Mochly-Rosen D, et al. Chronic hypersensitivity for inflammatory nociceptor sensitization mediated by the epsilon isozyme of protein kinase C. *J Neurosci* 2000;20(12):4680–4685.

83. Jin X, Gereau RWt. Acute p38-mediated modulation of tetrodotoxin-resistant sodium channels in mouse sensory neurons by tumor necrosis factor-alpha. *J Neurosci* 2006;26(1):246–255.

84. Gold MS, Caterina MJ. Molecular biology of nociceptor transduction. In: Basbaum AI, Bushnell MC, eds. Science of Pain. Oxford: Academic Press; 2009:43–74.

85. Hagbarth KE, Vallbo AB. Mechanoreceptor activity recorded percutaneously with semi-microelectrodes in human peripheral nerves. *Acta Physiol Scand* 1967;69(1):121–122.

86. Torebjörk HE, Schmelz M, Hankwerker HO. Functional properties of human cutaneous nociceptors and their role in pain and hyperalgesia. In: Belmonte C, Cervero F, eds. Neurobiology of Nociceptors. Oxford: Oxford University Press; 1996.

87. Schmelz M, Schmidt R, Weidner C, et al. Chemical response pattern of different classes of C-nociceptors to pruritogens and algogens. *J Neurophysiol* 2003;89(5):2441–2448.

88. Ochoa JL, Campero M, Serra J, et al. Hyperexcitable polymodal and insensitive nociceptors in painful human neuropathy. *Muscle Nerve* 2005;32(4):459–472.

89. Ørstavik K, Namer B, Schmidt R, et al. Abnormal function of C-fibers in patients with diabetic neuropathy. *J Neurosci* 2006;26(44):11287–11294.

90. Harriott AM, Dessem D, Gold MS. Inflammation increases the excitability of masseter muscle afferents. *Neuroscience* 2006;141(1):433–442.

91. Flake NM, Gold MS. Inflammation alters sodium and calcium excitability of temporomandibular joint afferents. *Neurosci Lett* 2005;384(3):294–299.

92. Yoshimura N, de Groat WC. Increased excitability of afferent neurons innervating rat urinary bladder after chronic bladder inflammation. *J Neurosci* 1999;19(11):4644–4653.

93. Dang K, Lamb K, Cohen M, et al. Cyclophosphamide-induced bladder inflammation sensitizes and enhances P2X receptor function in rat bladder sensory neurons. *J Neurophysiol* 2008;99(1):49–59.

94. Bielefeldt K, Ozaki N, Gebhart GF. Experimental ulcers alter voltage-sensitive sodium currents in rat gastric sensory neurons. *Gastroenterology* 2002;122(2):394–405.

95. Dang K, Bielefeldt K, Gebhart GF. Gastric ulcers reduce A-type potassium currents in rat gastric sensory ganglion neurons. *Am J Physiol Gastrointest Liver Physiol* 2004;286(4):G573–G579.

96. Sugiura T, Dang K, Lamb K, et al. Acid-sensing properties in rat gastric sensory neurons from normal and ulcerated stomach. *J Neurosci* 2005;25(10):2617–2627.

97. Moore BA, Stewart TM, Hill C, et al. TNBS ileitis evokes hyperexcitability and changes in ionic membrane properties of nociceptive DRG neurons. *Am J Physiol Gastrointest Liver Physiol* 2002;282(6):G1045–G1051.

98. Stewart T, Beyak MJ, Vanner S. Ileitis modulates potassium and sodium currents in guinea pig dorsal root ganglia sensory neurons. *J Physiol* 2003;552(Pt 3):797–807.

99. Beyak MJ, Ramji N, Krol KM, et al. Two TTX-resistant Na+ currents in mouse colonic dorsal root ganglia neurons and their role in colitis-induced hyperexcitability. *Am J Physiol Gastrointest Liver Physiol* 2004;287(4):G845–G855.

100. Gold MS, Traub RJ. Cutaneous and colonic rat DRG neurons differ with respect to both baseline and PGE2-induced changes in passive and active electrophysiological properties. *J Neurophysiol* 2004;91(6):2524–2531.

101. Fitzgerald EM, Okuse K, Wood JN, et al. cAmp-dependent phosphorylation of the tetrodotoxin-resistant voltage-dependent sodium channel Sns. *J Physiol (Lond)* 1999;516(Pt 2):433–446.

102. Gold MS, Reichling DB, Shuster MJ, et al. Hyperalgesic agents increase a tetrodotoxin-resistant Na+ current in nociceptors. *Proc Natl Acad Sci USA* 1996;93(3):1108–1112.

103. Gold MS, Weinreich D, Kim CS, et al. Redistribution of Na(V)1.8 in uninjured axons enables neuropathic pain. *J Neurosci* 2003;23(1):158–166.

104. Ruda MA, Ling QD, Hohmann AG, et al. Altered nociceptive neuronal circuits after neonatal peripheral inflammation. *Science* 2000;289(5479):628–631.

105. Cairns BE, Hu JW, Arendt-Nielsen L, et al. Sex-related differences in human pain and rat afferent discharge evoked by injection of glutamate into the masseter muscle. *J Neurophysiol* 2001;86(2):782–791.

106. Flake NM, Hermanstyne TO, Gold MS. Testosterone and estrogen have opposing actions on inflammation-induced plasma extravasation in the rat temporomandibular joint. *Am J Physiol Regul Integr Comp Physiol* 2006;291(2):R343–R348.

107. Wang S, Davis BM, Zwick M, et al. Reduced thermal sensitivity and Nav1.8 and TRPV1 channel expression in sensory neurons of aged mice. *Neurobiol Aging* 2006;27(6):895–903.

108. Baumann TK, Simone DA, Shain CN, et al. Neurogenic hyperalgesia: the search for primary cutaneous afferent fibers that contribute to capsaicin-induced pain and hyperalgesia. *J Neurophysiol* 1991;66(1):212–227.

109. Torebjörk HE, Lundberg LE, LaMotte RH. Central changes in processing of mechanoreceptive input in capsaicin-induced secondary hyperalgesia in humans. *J Physiol (Lond)* 1992;448:765–780.

110. Weng HR, Dougherty PM. Response properties of dorsal root reflexes in cutaneous C fibers before and after intradermal capsaicin injection in rats. *Neuroscience* 2005;132(3):823–831.

111. Polgár E, Todd AJ. Tactile allodynia can occur in the spared nerve injury model in the rat without selective loss of GABA or GABA(A) receptors from synapses in laminae I–II of the ipsilateral spinal dorsal horn. *Neuroscience* 2008;156(1):193–202.

112. Schoffnegger D, Ruscheweyh R, Sandkuhler J. Spread of excitation across modality borders in spinal dorsal horn of neuropathic rats. *Pain* 2008;135(3):300–310.

113. Noguchi K, Dubner R, De Leon M, et al. Axotomy induces preprotachykinin gene expression in a subpopulation of dorsal root ganglion neurons. *J Neurosci Res* 1994;37(5):596–603.

114. Hughes DI, Scott DT, Riddell JS, et al. Upregulation of substance P in low-threshold myelinated afferents is not required for tactile allodynia in the chronic constriction injury and spinal nerve ligation models. *J Neurosci* 2007;27(8):2035–2044.

115. Woolf CJ, Shortland P, Coggeshall RE. Peripheral nerve injury triggers central sprouting of myelinated afferents. *Nature* 1992;355(6355):75–78.

116. Hughes DI, Scott DT, Todd AJ, et al. Lack of evidence for sprouting of Abeta afferents into the superficial laminas of the spinal cord dorsal horn after nerve section. *J Neurosci* 2003;23(29):9491–9499.

117. Shehab SA, Spike RC, Todd AJ. Do central terminals of intact myelinated primary afferents sprout into the superficial dorsal horn of rat spinal cord after injury to a neighboring peripheral nerve? *J Comp Neurol* 2004;474(3):427–437.

118. Woodbury CJ, Kullmann FA, McIlwrath SL, et al. Identity of myelinated cutaneous sensory neurons projecting to nociceptive laminae following nerve injury in adult mice. *J Comp Neurol* 2008;508(3):500–509.

CHAPTER 4 ■ SUBSTRATES OF SPINAL CORD NOCICEPTIVE PROCESSING

TIMOTHY NESS AND ALAN RANDICH

INTRODUCTION

The spinal cord and brainstem nuclei are home to second order neurons, the first step of central nervous system (CNS) processing. The first site of sensory integration and modulation, second order neurons are more than a simple relay and any plan for the treatment of nociception must understand the critical role these neurons play in the formation of painful sensation. The second order neuron converts afferent input from multiple sites and often multiple modalities into an encoded message that is sent to other parts of the CNS. Those other parts of the CNS, in turn, modify the second order neuron through both excitatory and inhibitory mechanisms. These modifying influences are the subject of the next chapter whereas the present chapter will focus on the neuro-anatomical and neurochemical characteristics of these spinal substrates.

Although it seems like a simple statement that pain-related second order neurons are the neurons which receive primary afferent input related to tissue damage (nociceptors), it must be accepted that this statement may or may not be wholly true since in certain pathological states pain can be evoked by non–tissue-damaging stimuli (allodynia). It is unfortunate that there has been a tendency in pain-related research to turn common observations into over-generalizations and so an attempt will be made in this chapter to be precise when possible. Sometimes "assumptions" related to neuronal substrates of sensation have been necessarily used as "premises" on which to build scientific logic. The primary premise on which this chapter is based is that all nociceptive second order neurons receive nociceptive primary afferent input as *one* of their excitatory modalities. If one can accept that premise, then one can identify where the neurons receiving such input are located and can further identify where these neurons send the information.

DEFINING NOCICEPTIVE SYSTEMS

Models of Pain Processing

Pain is both a sensation and responses to that sensation. The sensory component of pain is described in terms of tissue damage (e.g., cutting, burning, rending) even when tissue damage is not occurring and so the sensation of pain is defined as nociception. The sensory systems of our body which encode for nociception can be modeled in two main ways: (1) as a system which is specific for pain (Specificity Theory) or (2) as a system that requires a pattern of neuronal activation to occur for the experience of pain to be generated (Pattern Theory). The simplest and oldest of the pattern theories is that which suggests pain is due to high intensities of input that is independent of modality (Intensity Theory). Each of these theories (or the multiple variants thereof) has prominent proponents who can make persuasive arguments that focus on subsets of data that support their particular view. Each knowledgeable person must derive their own model system which is ideally based on characterized human phenomena and which must clearly go beyond simple models.

As is apparent from the preceding chapter, primary afferent neurons with sensory endings have been characterized using electrophysiological and immunohistochemical methods. A subset of these primary afferents with sensory endings in cutaneous tissues are only activated by (and so *specific* for) pain-producing stimuli. Although these afferents may be polymodal (i.e., encode for multiple different stimuli), the stimuli which excite these primary afferents have in common the potential for producing tissue damage. They have therefore been defined as nociceptors. Primary afferent nociceptors are thinly myelinated or nonmyelinated and so fall into the Aδ- and C-fiber classes. Human psychophysical data support that when Aδ- and/or C-fiber function is disrupted by ischemia or pharmacological agents, then cutaneous sensations associated with immediate (first) or briefly delayed (second) pains are similarly disrupted. Unfortunately (for sake of easy logic), there are also many primary afferents that do not encode for tissue-damaging stimuli (e.g., "warm" receptors) but which are also of the Aδ- and C-fiber classes. Hence, it is a flawed logic that interprets all Aδ- and C-fiber–related input to second order neurons as nociceptive. Existent literature constrains further definition of specific nociceptor neurochemical and localization characteristics except on an anecdotal (single unit) basis. With that caveat, there are basic patterns that appear common to most Aδ- and C-fibers and generalizations related to these fiber groups have some validity as being representative of nociceptor localization and neurochemical content.

Methods of Neuronal Characterization

To definitively describe the structure and function of CNS structures is a daunting task. Standard histological, ultrastructural, and immunohistochemical methods used to examine CNS structure have allowed for precise definition of axons, dendrites, and neurotransmitter content but, unfortunately, they do not allow for the precise definition of function. Studies of neuronal function typically utilize electrophysiological techniques to measure the real-time electrochemical activity of single neuronal units (e.g., action potentials) which may be evoked by multiple manipulations. These neurophysiological measures utilize electrodes placed either extracellularly or intracellularly. When the former technique is utilized, correlative anatomic localization is possible but little more. Electrophysiological techniques such as retrograde activation of axonal extensions can define some of the neuronal anatomy, but true morphology is only certain with the intracellular injection of a dye. Immunohistochemical characterization of intracellularly labeled neurons is methodologically feasible and so it is possible to quantitatively define sensory elements. However, such studies are sufficiently tedious and subject to interpretive concerns related to sampling error and preparation effects (i.e., anesthesia) that, to date, have only been performed at a rudimentary level. A compromise microscopic analysis technique is that which uses c-*fos* gene induction in response to neuronal activation to functionally identify neurons excited by a tissue-damaging stimulus. A proto-oncogene, c-*fos*, is activated after potentially tissue-damaging stimuli are applied to most tissues. The expressed product, Fos protein, is immunohistochemically identifiable within hours of stimulation. As a consequence, mapping of gene induction or Fos protein in the nucleus of activated neurons can be used to functionally define these neurons as "nociceptive."[1] Labelled neurons can then be co-labelled with antibodies against neurotransmitters or important cell proteins or specific histological stains to further characterize the neurons. Analgesic pharmacological manipulations such as systemic morphine reduce both the total number of labeled neurons and the total Fos content of the spinal cord following a noxious stimulus. Even newer technologies have been able to identify a changed form of receptors following neuronal activation by noxious stimuli. For example, the internalization of neurokinin (NK) 1 receptors following activation by substance P[2] or the phosphorylation of glutamate receptor subtypes[3] have been used as surrogates for neuronal excitation. Macroscopic examination of CNS activation sites using magnetic resonance imaging technologies have allowed confirmation of microscopic techniques and further demonstrated the functional complexity of spinal and supraspinal connections. At a microscopic level, "tracer" dyes which are taken up by the terminal endings of axons of neurons and transported back to the neurons' cell bodies allow for a histological identification of axonal projections of spinal neurons that is dependent on the site of dye injections (e.g., spinothalamic neurons are back-labelled to the spinal cord by injections in the thalamus). Such labeling techniques, when coupled together with functional techniques, have made it possible to construct a quantitative but nonspecific "global" neuroanatomic view of spinal cord nociceptive processing that appears to agree with anecdotal definitive evidence generated by single-unit studies.

Defining Nociceptive Second Order Neurons

Strict proponents of Specificity Theory state that all discussion related to pain should only involve CNS neurons excited *exclusively* by primary afferent nociceptors. Such specific second order neurons are a small but obviously important minority of the total sample of spinal neurons receiving input from primary afferent nociceptors. One can also argue that the presence of primary afferent neurons with specificity for pain-producing stimuli does not necessitate that the second order neurons responsible for pain sensation have a similar specificity. For purposes of the present discussion, the primary premise of the rest of this chapter is that such excitatory input is a *necessary* requirement of pain-related second order neurons, but it is notable that most second order neurons receiving such input receive other types of sensory input. Excitation of second order neurons may come from primary afferent pathways or from segmental (interneurons), propriospinal (nonsegmental intraspinal), and supraspinal sources. Inhibition arises from the same CNS sources. Inhibition can promote neuronal specificity by selectively reducing responsiveness to nonnociceptive inputs. It is for this reason that proponents of Pattern Theory argue that all second order neurons receiving nociceptive inputs should be considered as candidates for inclusion in pain-processing pathways.

Development of Sensory Systems

The embryological development of the nervous system suggests reasons that differences can exist between peripheral and central phenomena since excitatory systems develop before inhibitory systems. The edges of the neural plate that come together to form the neural tube split off to become the migratory cells of the neural crest. These cells spread to form the sensory components of the peripheral nervous system. At a spinal cord level, substances from the ventrally located notochord induce the formation of motoneurons with axonal extensions extending to the periphery. The dorsal aspect of the spinal cord, lacking effects of the notochord, forms short connections (local connectivity) or develops axonal projections attracted to distant spinal cord and/or brainstem sites. Sensory structures that develop from the neural crest send axonal projections both to the periphery as well as into the dorsal aspect of the spinal cord and contain neurotransmitters that are predominantly excitatory. At birth, sensory systems have very little inhibitory connectivity. This changes during development until inhibitory connections become the predominant form of CNS communication.

In humans, the precise timing of both excitatory and inhibitory system maturation is not fully known, but based on experiments in nonhuman animals these systems appear highly plastic with cell death processes as important as cell growth processes in relation to the final product.[4] Specific transcriptional factor expression has been used to track neuronal subgroup development and has demonstrated a profound role for pathological modification of nociceptive circuitry.[5] The general phenomenon of use-dependent growth (or preservation) appears to hold in multiple sensory systems ranging from taste to vision with the nociceptive systems notwithstanding. Ruda and colleagues[6] have demonstrated that injury during critical periods of development, such as the neonatal period, can have profound effects on the subsequent development of nociceptive systems. In humans, critical periods of neuronal outgrowth and myelination occur in childhood, during puberty, and following events that injure nervous system structures.

TARGETS OF PRIMARY AFFERENT INPUT

Gross Anatomy of the Spinal Cord

The spinal cord is segregated into areas that, on gross examination, appear as white and grey matter, and which consist of predominantly myelinated nerve fiber tracts and cell bodies, respectively. Wrapped in protective pial, arachnoid, and dural meninges, the spinal cord is continually being penetrated by centrally directed axons of primary afferent neurons whose cell bodies reside within the neighboring dorsal root ganglia. These axons enter as the dorsal roots and may traverse several spinal segments rostrally or caudally in the dorsolaterally located Lissauer's tract before entering the grey matter for synaptic contact. The spinal cord white matter is divided into multiple subdivisions with component "tracts" consisting of ascending or descending axonal fibers of various origins and destinations. There is significant overlap of these tracts such that any lesion of white matter is likely to interrupt fibers of passage with multiple origins and multiple sites of termination. The white matter gets larger as one ascends the spinal cord from sacral to cervical levels as additional ascending fibers to the brain add to the white matter and progressive numbers of descending fibers to spinal targets drop out to form synaptic connection. Grey matter is largest at the cervical and lumbar enlargements due to association with sensation and motor control of the limbs. The most notable divisions of the white matter that are important to pain sensation are the dorsal columns, the dorsolateral fasciculus, and the ventrolateral (anterolateral) fasciculus and their associated subdivision into tracts (Fig. 4.1).

Spinal Laminae

The morphology of neurons in the grey matter of the spinal cord differs depending on location. Using Rexed's classification system, there are at least 10 different layers or laminae of neu-

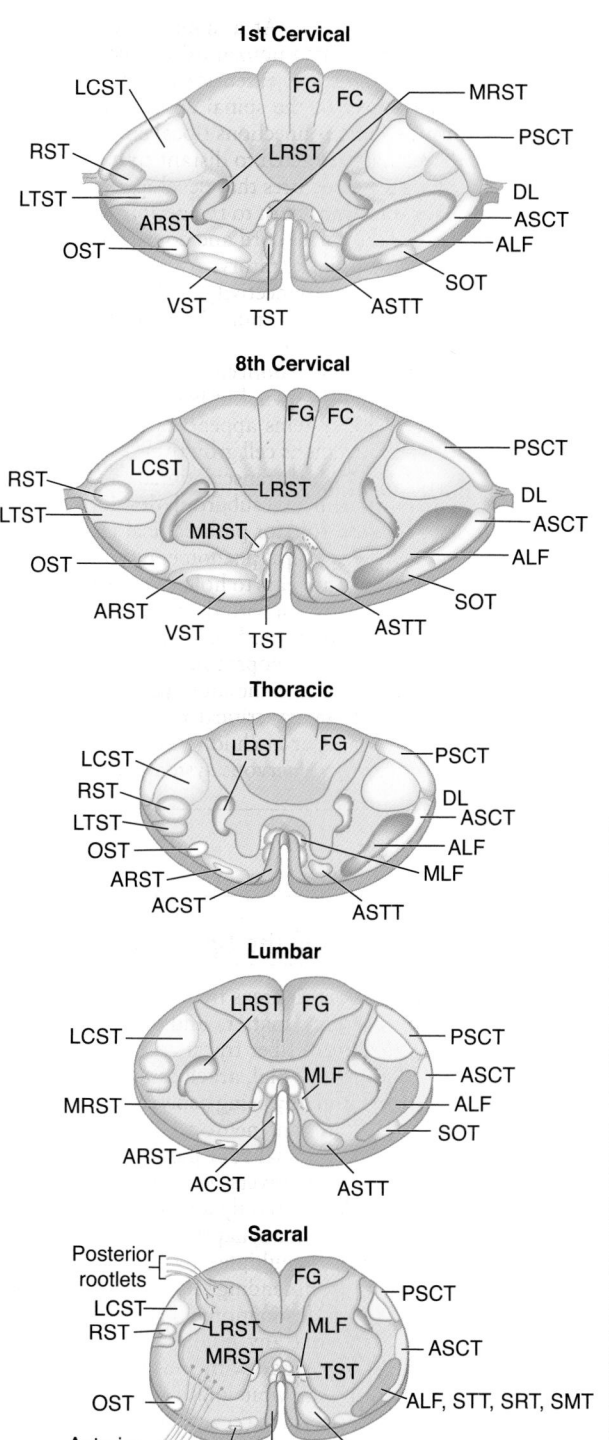

1st Cervical

8th Cervical

Thoracic

Lumbar

Sacral

MLF	Medial longitudinal fasciculus
ARST	Anterior reticulospinal tract
MRST	Medial reticulospinal tract
ACST	Anterior corticospinal tract
LRST	Lateral reticulospinal tract
LCST	Lateral corticospinal tract
FG	Fasciculus gracilis
FC	Fasciculus cuneatus
PSCT	Posterior spinocerebellar tract
DL	Dentate ligament
ASCT	Anterior spinocerebellar tract
ALF	Anterolateral fasciculus
SOT	Spino-olivary tract
ASTT	Anterior spinothalamic tract
TST	Tectospinal tract
VST	Vestibulospinal tract
OST	Olivospinal tract
LTST	Lateral tegmentospinal tract
RST	Reciculospinal tract

FIGURE 4.1 Diagram of the white matter of the spinal cord. The ascending tracts are emphasized on the right side and the descending tracts on the left side. The anterolateral (ventrolateral) funiculus, which is composed of the anterolateral fasciculus (ALF), composed of the spinothalamic (STT), spinoreticular (SRT), and spinomesencephalic (SMT) tracts in the spinal cord. As it ascends, the ALF becomes progressively larger, the largest part being in the upper cervical region. This is not only because the STT continues to add axons but also because there are more SRT cell bodies (and hence axons) in the cervical enlargement than in the lumbosacral enlargement. Throughout the course of the ALF in the spinal cord, the three nociceptive pathways are situated medial to the anterior (ventral) spinocerebellar tract, lateral to the ventrolateral and ventral horns, and posterolateral to the spinoolivary tract. The anterior spinothalamic tract (ASTT), which may be an alternate nociceptive pathway, is separate from the three tracts of the ALF. Because a cordotomy lesion in the upper thoracic or cervical segments, usually extends from the dentate ligament medially the ASTT and some of the descending tracts are likely to be interrupted with the operation. In the cervical region, the ALF is shaped as a somewhat flat triangle with the apex medial and the base lateral. At successively higher cervical levels there is a gradual dorsolateral shift of the ALF.

rons—the first six of which (I–VI) are termed the dorsal horn of the spinal cord (Fig. 4.2). These laminae, plus the area around the central canal (lamina X), receive a bulk of primary afferent inputs. Spinal dorsal horn neurons receiving excitatory inputs from nociceptive afferents have been demonstrated to be present throughout the dorsal horn, but with particular localization to laminae I, II, V, VI, and X. One must remember that laminar assignment is based on the central location of the neuronal soma. However, dendritic extensions of these neurons may extend throughout numerous laminae such that the immunohistochemi-

cal demonstration of primary afferent neuron terminations in specific laminae does not limit connectivity to just neurons of those laminae. Mapping of individual C-fiber primary afferents encoding for cutaneous nociception have demonstrated sites of connectivity that are highly localized into tight "baskets" typically located in superficial laminae of a single spinal segment. In contrast, single primary C-fiber afferents from deep, visceral structures have been demonstrated to travel via Lissauer's tract to reach multiple spinal segments and multiple laminae (I, V, X, and even contralateral sites)[7] (Fig. 4.3). Fine muscle afferents and

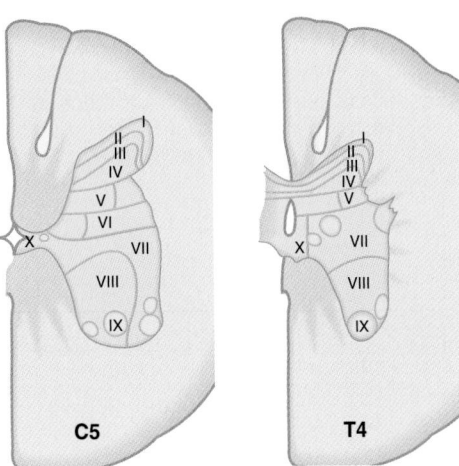
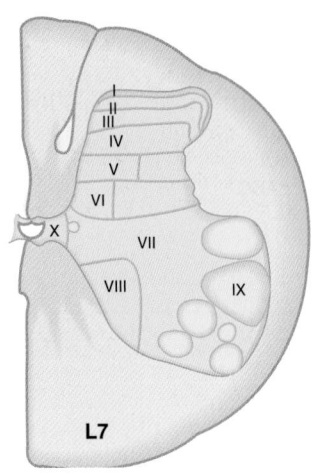

FIGURE 4.2 Diagrams showing Rexed's laminar histologic organization of the cat spinal cord grey matter at three levels. The dorsal horn corresponds to laminae I through VI inclusive. (Redrawn after Rexed B. The cytoarchitectonic organization of the spinal cord in the cat. *J Comp Neurol* 1952;96: 415–495, with permission.)

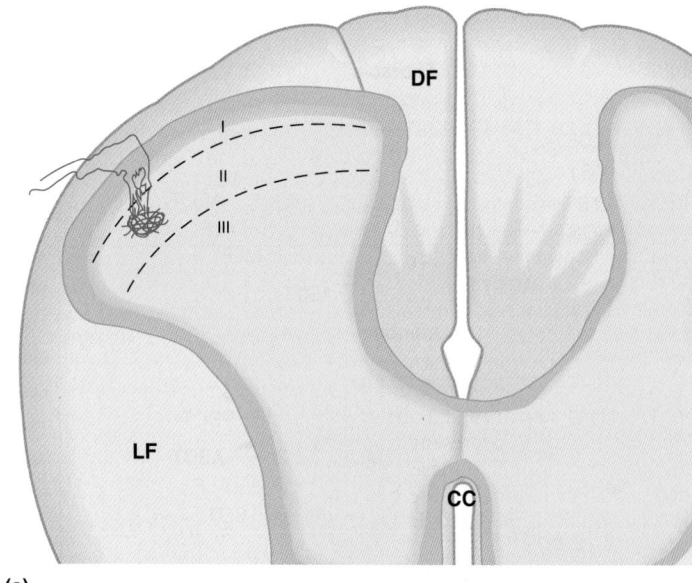

(a)

FIGURE 4.3 The different extents of central terminal fields are shown here for an individual somatic C-fiber primary afferent (**A**) and a visceral C-fiber primary afferent (**B**) from guinea pigs that were injected with phaseolus vulgaris leucoagglutinin after functional identification. The visceral C-fiber afferent had many more central branches and numerous arbors that include contralateral projections, whereas the somatic C-fiber afferent had a more limited terminal field (*CC*, central canal; *Df*; dorsal funiculus; *LF*, lateral funiculus.) (Redrawn after Sugiura Y, Terui N, Hosoya Y. Difference in distribution of central terminals between visceral and somatic unmyelinated (C) primary afferent fibers. *J Neurophysiol* 1989;62:834–840, with permission.)

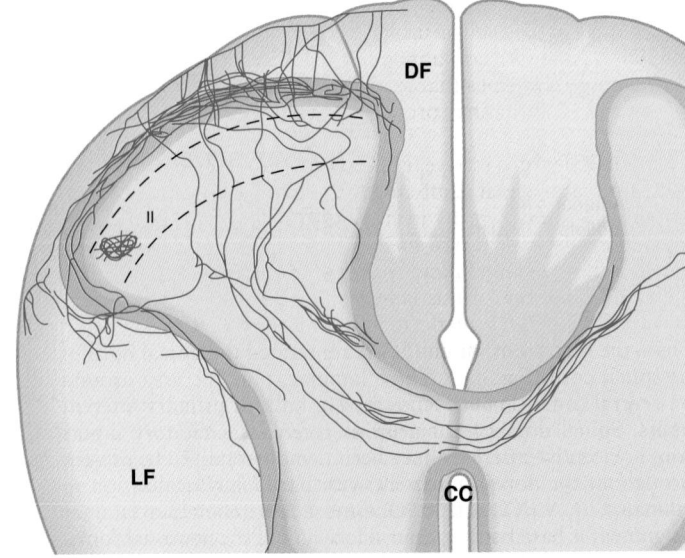

(b)

articular afferents have sites of termination similar to those of visceral afferents. By using intracellular recording and labeling techniques it has been possible to determine that nociceptive afferents connect with second order neurons that have many different morphologies—some of which correlate with electrophysiological characteristics (see Morris et al.[8]). The morphology and neurotransmitter content of each lamina will be briefly discussed.

Lamina I is termed the marginal zone as it forms the outermost layer of the dorsal horn. This single lamina contains a heterogenous population of neurons with morphological studies identifying neurons with pyramidal, fusiform, and multipolar shapes, some with smooth dendrites, some with spiny dendrites. Lamina I and the adjoining Lamina II are the predominant location of excitatory neuropeptide input from primary afferent neurons with heavy immunohistochemical labeling for substance P and calcitonin gene-related peptide (CGRP). Axonal projections of a subset of lamina I neurons extend to supraspinal structures such as the medulla, midbrain, and/or thalamus. Fos induction in response to noxious stimuli has consistently been reported to occur in lamina I with double-labeling noted in association with antibodies to preproenkephalin, dynorphin, glutamate, N-methyl-D-aspartate (NMDA) receptors, gamma amino butyric acid (GABA), glycine, GABA-B receptors, NK1 receptors, calbindin, glucocorticoid receptors, and estrogen receptor-α[1].

Lamina II is called the substantia gelatinosa due to its gross appearance in fresh cut tissue. The neurons of this lamina are generally small with four or more distinct morphologies, two of which are viewed as important to the local processing of nociceptive information: stalked and islet cells (using the terminology of Gobel[9]). Stalked cells have soma at the outer edge of lamina II with centrally arborizing dendrites and axons that synapse with lamina I projection neurons. Islet cells have fusiform cell bodies with extensive dendritic and axonal arborizations containing inhibitory neurotransmitters such as GABA or enkephalin.[10,11] Axodendritic, dendrodendritic, and axoaxonic synapses are manifest throughout lamina II on ultrastructural analysis demonstrating a profound potential for neuronal interaction and signal processing. Primary afferent input from both nociceptive and nonnociceptive neurons has been noted and descending axonal connections are also present with evidence of serotonergic and noradrenergic inputs to these neurons. A distinction is frequently made between lamina II-outer (II$_o$) and lamina II-inner (II$_i$) with II$_o$ commonly combined with lamina I in discussions of the superficial dorsal horn.

Lamina III and **Lamina IV** are known as the nucleus proprius as both receive highly myelinated low-threshold primary afferent neuronal inputs that include proprioceptors. Whereas lamina III consists mainly of small neurons with morphologies similar to lamina II, lamina IV has a subpopulation of large cells with extensive dendritic extensions that reach superficially. Lamina IV also has neurons with axonal projections extending up the dorsal columns.

Lamina V neurons receive input from Aδ- and C-fiber nociceptors as well as myelinated afferents carrying low threshold information. Cell bodies are frequently moderately sized pyramidal cells and may have dendritic extensions through the entire dorsal horn reaching to lamina I and II sites of synaptic contact as well as laterally. Neurons of this lamina have been demonstrated to receive input from all somatic, muscle, and visceral afferent types. Axonal projections of lamina V neurons to supraspinal sites are common.

Lamina VI neurons are small neurons present in the cervical and lumbar enlargements, but largely missing in the rest of the spinal cord. Low-threshold muscle afferents and both low- and high-threshold cutaneous afferents reach to this lamina.

Laminae VII–IX represent neurons of the ventral horn.

Lamina X neurons are arranged around the central canal of the spinal cord. They receive bilateral inputs of unmyelinated, poorly myelinated, and highly myelinated afferents. Cell bodies are of moderate size with local dendritic arborizations. Some neurons in the dorsal aspects of lamina X have axonal projections extending up the dorsal columns to reach medullary targets. Peptidergic inputs are extensive and immunohistochemical localization of noradrenergic and serotonergic inputs have been identified. Inhibitory neurons with immunohistochemical identification of glycinergic and GABAergic enzymes are locally present.

Functional Characterization of Nociceptive Neurons

In addition to morphological heterogeneity, the multiple laminae of the spinal cord also have functional heterogeneity.

Second order neurons have been characterized electrophysiologically according to their responsiveness to cutaneous and deep tissue stimuli. Most commonly, a distinction is made between excitatory responses that are produced by noxious (potentially tissue-damaging) stimuli such as high intensity mechanical or thermal stimuli and those produced by innocuous stimuli such as hair movement or vibration. Using these two criteria, the simplest nomenclature defines neurons as Class 1 if excited only by innocuous stimuli, Class 2 if excited by both innocuous and noxious stimuli, and Class 3 if excited only by noxious stimuli. Similar nomenclatures, but with additional subtle meanings implied by their original descriptions, include the use of terms such as *low threshold* for Class 1 neurons, *wide-dynamic-range*[12] or "convergent" neurons[13] for Class 2 neurons, and *high threshold* or *nociceptive-specific* neurons for Class 3 neurons. A fourth *nonresponder* group also must be factored in for neurons that fail to be excited by any of the employed stimuli. Despite the "clean" nature of this categorization, there unfortunately appears to be a spectrum of responses to all afferent input modalities with varying overlap that is somewhat dependent on the precise stimuli and definitions employed. The definition of neurons according to excitatory stimuli also appears to be preparation dependent as extracellular dorsal horn recordings of spinal neurons in cats have demonstrated that the classification of an individual neuron may change with the administration of anesthesia.[14]

The number of neuronal subgroups in any classification system is a function of the number of criteria employed for that classification. Despite this, it has been suggested that the use of inhibitory inputs as part of a classification criterion might actually simplify overall schema. One such inhibitory influence used in classification is known as *diffuse noxious inhibitory controls* (DNIC) which is proposed to be an endogenous inhibitory system activated by a nonsegmental noxious stimulus. DNIC produces inhibition of ongoing or evoked dorsal horn neuronal activity and according to its original description,[15,16] DNIC is specific for Class 2 (WDR, convergent) neurons and has no effect on Class 3 (nociceptive specific) neurons. Subsequent studies of DNIC would support the general statement that DNIC effects are highly *selective* for Class 2 neurons with lesser effect on Class 3 neurons. Nomenclatures using a combination of responses to excitatory and inhibitory inputs have not been universally accepted.

Classification According to Site of Projection

Second order nociceptive spinal dorsal horn neurons frequently have axonal extensions projecting to rostral (and caudal) sites of termination. These sites include other segments of the spinal cord and supraspinal structures such as the thalamus, the hypothalamus, the midbrain, the pons, and the medulla. These axons travel predominantly within the white matter of the spinal cord in two main sites: the ventrolateral quadrants and the dorsal midline. Ascending fiber tracts in the dorsolateral funiculus have also been described. Decussation of fibers to the contralateral ventrolateral white matter occurs for axons projecting to the thalamus and most other brainstem sites although many axons with sites of termination in "reticular" structures remain in the ipsilateral ventrolateral white matter. Dorsal column pathways have sites of termination in the gracile or cuneatus nucleus of the medulla. Intraspinal pathways that may stay within the grey matter have also been demonstrated as well as extensive collateralization of axons with multiple sites of termination at supraspinal and intraspinal sites.

TARGETS OF AXONAL PROJECTIONS

Intraspinal Pathways

Multiple interconnections occur between spinal neurons. On a segmental level this is referred to as interneuron connectivity. When connections are more distant, the pathways of connection are termed "propriospinal" based on the initial demonstration of a coordinating connectivity between the cervical and lumbar enlargements of quadrupeds that allowed for coordinated motion. Intraspinal connectivity has also been demonstrated in the case of neurons receiving afferent input from pelvic structures with a dual innervation through thoracolumbar sympathetic and sacral pelvic nerves. These intraspinal connections appear to coordinate autonomic functions related to the pelvic organs.[17,18] A precise white matter localization of the axonal extensions of propriospinal nociceptive neurons has not been performed but they are presumed to follow the paths of other propriospinal neurons which include dorsally located white matter paths and some within grey matter extensions. Collateral intraspinal extensions of ascending axons located within the ventrolateral white matter have also been demonstrated.

A separate system of intraspinal connections, the multisynaptic ascending system, may have particular relevance to chronic pain. In concepts championed by Noordenbos but first proposed by Goldscheider,[19] long chains or "webs" of neuronal connections extend through the length of the spinal cord and carry nociceptive information in a slow but progressive fashion to the brain by short "hops." Support for this concept is given by animal experiments in which opposing hemisections performed at differing spinal levels fail to block nociceptive behaviors, but total transections at a single level are effective.[20] Traditionally described as an ascending pathway, bidirectionality of signaling is possible with a potential for the generation of "reverberatory" circuits.

Spinothalamic Tract

Ventrolateral (Anterolateral) Axonal Pathways

The most studied spinal projection pathway is the spinothalamic tract which is located within the ventrolateral white matter of the spinal cord. Both ipsilateral and contralateral localization of axon pathways have been demonstrated en route to supraspinal sites, but the predominant path for axonal projections traveling to the ventrobasal thalamus resides on the contralateral side. Experiments utilizing lesions of the ventrolateral spinal white matter have demonstrated reduction or abolition of ventrobasal thalamic neuronal responses to most somatic noxious stimuli. Consistent with this observation, surgical or traumatic interruption of ventrolateral fiber pathways results in the lack of sensation to noxious cutaneous stimuli (i.e., pinprick) applied to the contralat-

eral side of the body at spinal segments below the level of the lesion. The second order neurons which project to the thalamus have been identified in rodent, feline, and primate models using neuroanatomical (retrograde dye labeling or chromatolytic responses to axonal section) and electrophysiological (antidromic activation) methods. Neurophysiological experiments have not always proven that the neurons of study had axonal projections that actually reach the thalamus, but have always demonstrated that neurons of interest have axons present within the ventrolateral spinal white matter and so the term "spinothalamic tract" neurons (STT) is generally employed to describe the neurons rather than the more specific term "spinothalamic."

Neospinothalamic versus Paleospinothalamic

There exist two different components of the spinothalamic tract—the neospinothalamic tract (nSTT) and the paleospinothalamic tract (pSTT), the former of which forms a direct, dedicated relay to the ventrobasal group of the thalamus and the latter of which has many neurons with one or more axonal bifurcations that form dichotomizing fibers ending in synaptic contact with medullary, pontine, midbrain, and medial thalamic structures. Ascending information transmitted through the pSTT produces activation of numerous limbic structures and has therefore been viewed as important to affective and motivational aspects of pain, whereas the nSTT, through relays in the ventrobasal and posterior thalamus, activates the somatosensory cortex and so has been viewed as important to localization and intensity coding of pain-related sensations. Axonal collateral branchings of pSTT neurons have been identified that correspond to multiple areas of limbic and autonomic activation which include medullary, pontine, mesencephalic, hypothalamic, and medial thalamic targets.

Laminar Distribution of Spinothalamic Tract Neurons

The cells of origin of the STT reside within all laminae of the spinal cord except motoneuronal layers and therefore can have multiple different morphologies. At lumbar levels in primates, the greatest number of nSTT neurons reside in laminae I and V, but also are highly represented in laminae IV, VI, IX, and X with additional representation in III, VII, and VIII. In contrast, the neurons of the pSTT have soma in deeper laminae (VI–VIII) with a lesser representation in I, IV, and V. The axons of STT neurons typically decussate to the contralateral side via the dorsal commissure within one to two spinal segments of the neuronal soma but at sacral and upper cervical levels, a significant number (up to 26%) of axons of STT neurons may remain ipsilateral.[21] A general somatotopic organization of the ascending fibers within the STT has been noted with an inner-to-outer progression of layers of fibers to the white matter from cervical to sacral levels (Fig. 4.4). A similar somatotopy is noted at medullary levels. The STT splits into two parts through the rostral medulla and pons to merge again at mesencephalic regions where an anterior-to-posterior somatotopic distribution is noted. Differences in conduction velocity of subsets of STT neurons has been identified (lamina I STT neurons have slower conduction velocities than lamina V STT neurons) suggesting differences in axonal diameter and myelination processes. That, in turn, suggests a potential for temporally different delivery of sensory information to brain structures and differential susceptibility to pathological processes.

Functional Characterization of Spinothalamic Tract Neurons

Quantitative electrophysiological characterization of STT neurons has demonstrated a predominance for neurons processing nociceptive information. However, approximately 20% of STT neurons encode exclusively for nonnoxious light touch sensa-

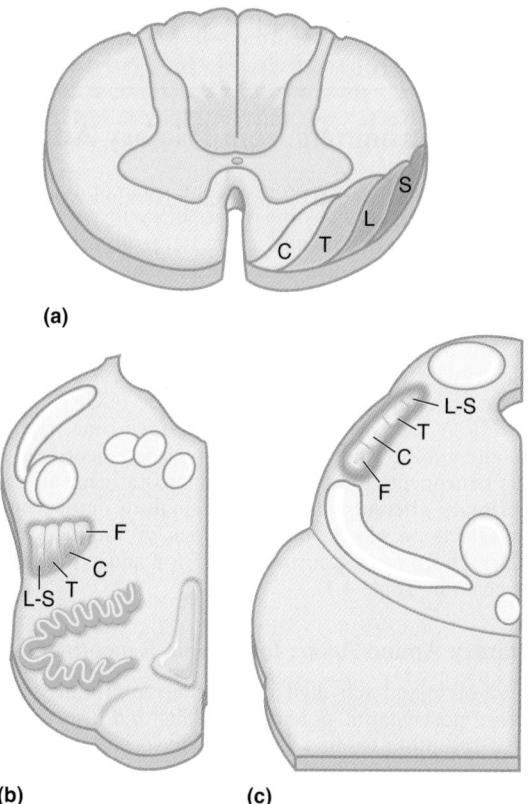

(a)

(b)   **(c)**

FIGURE 4.4 Schematic diagrams showing cross-section of the spinal cord, medulla, and midbrain, depicting the laminar arrangement of the ascending tracts in the ventrolateral funiculus in the upper part of the cervical spinal cord (**A**) and with the addition of the trigeminothalamic tract in the medulla (**B**) and midbrain (**C**). (*S*, sacral, *L*, lumbar, *T*, thoracic, *C*, cervical, *F*, face.)

and lateral thalamus appear similar to neurons with projections only to the lateral thalamus.

Dorsolateral and Ventromedial Axonal Pathways

Spinothalamic neurons with soma primarily located within lamina I have been demonstrated to send axonal projections to the contralateral posterior nuclei of the thalamus via a contralateral dorsolateral pathway.[25,26] Estimated to form up to a quarter of all spinothalamic neurons,[27] these neurons have been identified electrophysiologically to be primarily NS neurons with small cutaneous receptive fields. Deeper laminae neurons and WDR neurons are also represented in this pathway. Many axons of spinothalamic neurons also travel within the ventromedial white matter of the spinal cord with soma located within laminae I, IV, V, VI, and VII.[28] Functional characterization of spinothalamic neurons with axons in the ventromedial white matter suggest a mixture of nonnociceptive and nociceptive neurons with supraspinal targets in the mesencephalon and intralaminar nuclei of the thalamus.

Spinoreticular and Spinomesencephalic Tracts

Ventrolateral (Anterolateral) Axonal Pathways

As noted previously, ascending axonal fibers of nociceptive second order neurons traveling to the thalamus may frequently branch and send collaterals into brainstem structures including the medulla, pons, and mesencephalon. However, numerous ascending fibers travel to these brainstem structures without having collaterals to the thalamus and collectively are described as spinoreticular if they reach medullary and pontine sites or spinomesencephalic if they reach midbrain targets. Subsets of spinoreticular neurons, defined by known targets for the axons, include spinomedullary, spinopontine, spinoolivary, spinosolitary, spinoraphe, and spinoparabrachial neuronal groups. Identification of these subgroups has been possible using focal injections of retrogradely transported neuronal dyes at supraspinal sites or antidromic electrical activation of axonal extensions. Although the former technique has reasonable localization potential, the latter does not always discriminate axons of passage from final sites of termination. The presence of collateralization of axons to multiple targets has been identified but not quantitatively defined and so the overlap between the sampling of groups is not known. The spinal localization of spinoreticular and spinomesencephalic ascending axons overlap with those of the ventrolateral STT except for a greater propensity for remaining ipsilateral within the spinal cord and a slightly more medial line of passage upon entering the medulla. Spinomesencephalic neurons also utilize the dorsolateral funiculus for a subset of lamina I neurons in a fashion similar to that of similar spinothalamic neurons.

Features of Spinoreticular Neurons

The locations and functional characteristics of spinoreticular neurons in primates are virtually identical with the same features of STT neurons with projections to the medial thalamus. They demonstrate a predominant localization to deeper laminae of the spinal cord and tend to have large, sometimes whole body, receptive fields of the NS and WDR types. Synaptic targets include many areas of the medulla and brainstem highly involved in autonomic regulation as well as the regulation of nociceptive systems. The potential for feedback control of nociceptive processing is therefore anatomically present. An important relay site is the parabrachial nucleus in the pons[29] which has extensive projections to limbic subcortical structures such as the amygdala.

tions[11] and a small subset encode for proprioceptive information. Multiple subsets of nociceptive neurons have been identified that have selective laminar localization. Nociceptive specific (NS) STT neurons, with slow adapting responses to noxious pinch, heat, or chemical stimulation are commonly located in lamina I but are also present in deeper laminae. Noxious cold has been used as an additional characterizing stimulus[22] and allowed for the identification of additional subsets of lamina I NS STT neurons. Wide dynamic range (WDR) STT neurons, which demonstrate excitatory responses to multimodal sensory inputs (including both noxious and nonnoxious stimuli), are found extensively in lamina V but can also be found in all other laminae. Convergence of visceral, myofascial, articular, and cutaneous inputs is the rule rather than the exception when examining WDR STT neurons,[23] but similar convergence has been noted in NS STT neurons. Overall, with the possible exception of noxious cold inputs, the presence or absence of a particular group of sensory inputs has been of limited value in identifying lamina specific, morphological, functional, or projection-related neuronal subsets. However, there are important generalities that are apparent in quantitative analyses of neuronal subsets[24]: lamina I STT neurons tend to be NS neurons; lamina V (and other deep laminae) STT neurons tend to be WDR neurons; STT neurons with projections to the medial thalamus (pSTT) are more likely to be NS rather than WDR neurons and frequently have large receptive fields; STT neurons with projections to the lateral thalamus (nSTT) are more likely to be WDR rather than NS neurons and often have smaller receptive fields; and STT neurons with projections to both medial

Features of Spinomesencephalic Neurons

In contrast to spinoreticular neurons, the locations and functional characteristics of spinomesencephalic neurons in primates are similar to STT neurons with projections to the lateral thalamus although significant differences are present. They demonstrate a predominant localization of soma to laminae I and V of the spinal cord with a small scattering to other deep laminae. Electrophysiological characterization of spinomesencephalic neurons suggests a predominance of NS neurons. Synaptic targets include the periaqueductal gray, a site with known importance to the regulation of nociception, as well as the collicular and cuneiformis nuclei.

Postsynaptic Dorsal Column Neurons

Recently, there has been increasing evidence for the existence of a spinal pathway in the midline of the dorsal spinal cord that carries the rostral transmission of deep tissue nociception. Traditionally the dorsal columns have been viewed as transmitting information related to nonnociceptive information such as vibration or other light touch sensations. However, discrete neurosurgical lesions of this portion of the spinal cord have been demonstrated to relieve cancer-related pain in patients with pelvic visceral and deep muscle pathology.[30,31] Parallel studies in nonhuman animals have demonstrated that in this area of spinal white matter there exist axons of postsynaptic dorsal column (PSDC) neurons receiving noxious excitatory input from the colon, bladder, and/or uterus. Excitatory responses of neurons located in the ventrobasal thalamus to noxious deep tissue stimuli are attenuated/abolished with lesions of the dorsal midline region of the spinal cord[30] but are only minimally affected by lesions of the traditional spinothalamic pathways (ventrolateral quadrant).

The soma of PSDC neurons are located predominantly in lamina III, IV, and X and, in a limited number of studies, the neurons have been demonstrated to be responsive to both somatic and visceral nociceptive inputs. Both NS and WDR neuronal types have been reported and their role in nociception is linked more to the secondary effects of dorsal column lesions than inherent neuronal characteristics. Targets for synaptic contact include the gracile and cuneatus nuclei of the medulla (dorsal column nuclei) but it is notable that the presence or absence of collaterals to other ascending tracts or other supraspinal targets has not been performed.

Other Ascending Pathways

There exist other pathways to the brain apart from those noted. The spinocervicothalamic tract is important in other species but appears minimal or absent in humans. Direct projection pathways to the hypothalamus, amygdala,[29] and cerebellum have also been identified with presumed roles in autonomic function, affective-emotional modulation, and motor coordination, respectively. Extraspinal pathways for peripheral primary afferents exist and can sometime lend confusion to studies of central pathways. Vagal afferents can reach the brainstem carrying extensive information from visceral and other deep tissue structures leaving brainstem-mediated responses intact despite the interruption of spinal pathways. Similarly, primary afferents from deep structures including the viscera and peripheral vasculature can travel via the sympathetic chain to enter the spinal cord at levels much higher than expected and so can "bypass" selective spinal lesions of ascending pathways forming synaptic contact at levels above the lesions. Clinically, these other pathways sometimes prove important to consider, particularly in conditions of spinal cord injury.

NEUROCHEMISTRY OF SECOND ORDER NEURONS

Neurotransmitters from Primary Afferents

Excitatory neurotransmission of second order spinal neurons is produced predominantly by the release of excitatory amino acids (EEAs), such as glutamate and aspartate, from primary afferent neurons. Various other neurotransmitters lead to neuroexcitatory effects by channel activation or sometimes via second messenger systems but, in most cases, these other neurotransmitters appear to have the augmentation of EAA-induced excitatory responses as their primary function. Most notable of these neurotransmitters are calcitonin-gene-related polypeptide (CGRP), substance P, and NK-A, but roles for serotonin, adenosine triphosphate (ATP), and cholecystokinin (CCK) have been identified. The inhibitory neuropeptides galanin and somatostatin are also released from primary afferents, but they are small in number and with limited effects on second order neurons. A summary of spinal cord dorsal horn neurotransmitter location and associated receptors is given in Table 4.1.

Excitatory Amino Acids: Ionotropic Receptor/Channels

EAAs act on ligand-activated ion channels to produce immediate excitatory postsynaptic potentials (EPSPs) but also act at metabotropic receptors to alter intracellular second messenger systems (discussed later). Three different EEA-activated ion channels have been characterized: α-amino-3-hydroxy-5-methyl-4-isoxazoleproprionic acid (AMPA) receptors; N-methyl-D-aspartate (NMDA) receptors; and kainate (KA) receptors. These receptors have differential functions despite frequent co-localization on the same neurons due to differences in their regulation by baseline membrane potentials. As different receptors/channels, they are also differentially affected by the presence of other agonists and ions such as magnesium.

Activation of AMPA receptors immediately allows selective sodium ion flow through the extracellular membrane and is responsible for a majority of the "fast" transmission in nociceptive systems. AMPA receptors are unaffected by the baseline depolarization state of the second order neuron. In contrast, NMDA receptors are both voltage and ligand gated and allow permeability to both sodium and calcium ions. Magnesium ions act to block the channels of NMDA receptors which only become unblocked following a sustained depolarization of the extracellular membrane. Such a sustained alteration in membrane potential enables the magnesium ion to disengage intracellularly which then allows the opening and activation of the NMDA receptor-channel complex which, in turn, results in a *very* sustained depolarization. Since the NMDA receptor-channel is permeable to calcium, its sustained activation can produce alterations in intracellular second messenger functions of calcium.

Two phenomena have been clearly linked to NMDA receptor activation: "wind-up" (increasing responses to repeated stimuli of equal intensity) and "central sensitization" (decreased thresholds for response and/or increased vigor of responses due to a sensitizing event). NMDA antagonists will block/blunt both phenomena, but these phenomena can also be stopped prior to their development by pharmacological antagonists that block the initial event that led to the sustained depolarization that allowed the NMDA receptor activation. As a consequence, the antagonism of other excitatory systems (i.e., AMPA receptors) or the activation of endogenous inhibitory systems may also blunt or block these "hyperalgesic" phenomena. Clinical use of NMDA receptor antagonists such as ketamine or dextromethorphan has been demonstrated to produce prolonged analgesic effects when coadministered with opioids or as part of a perioperative regimen.

TABLE 4.1

LOCATION OF SUBSTRATES OF NOCICEPTION

Neurotransmitter (receptor)	Primary afferent neuron (presynaptic)	Second order neuron (postsynaptic)	Interneuron	Descending fibers
Glutamate/Aspartate	x	x	x	x
AMPA	+	+	+	
NMDA	+	+	+	
KA	+	+	+	
mGlu	+	+/−	+/−	
GABA			x	x
GABA-A	−	−	−	
GABA-B	−	−	−	
Glycine			x	x
strych-sensitive	−	−	−	
strych-insensitive	−	−	−	
NMDA bind site	+	+		
Substance P	x		x	x
NK1		+		
Neurokinin A	x			
NK2		+		
CGRP	x			
CGRP-R		+		
ATP	x		x	x
P2X	+	+		
Adenosine			x	
A1		−		
Serotonin			x	x
5HT2		−		
5HT3	+/−	+		
Norepinephrine				x
α1			+	
α2	−	−		
Acetylcholine			x	
nACh	−	+		
mACh	−			
Cholecystokinin	x		x	x
CCK-A		+		
CCK-B	+	+		
Galanin	x		x	
gal1	−			
gal2		−		
Somatostatin	x			
SSN-R2		−		
SSN-R4	−			
VIP	x			
VIP-R		+		
Enkephalin			x	x
Dynorphin			x	
MOR	−	−		
DOR	−	−		
KOR	−	+/−		
Nociceptin			x	
ORL1	+/−	−		
NPY	x		x	
NPY-1	−	−		

(continued)

TABLE 4.1

CONTINUED

Neurotransmitter (receptor)	Primary afferent neuron (presynaptic)	Second order neuron (postsynaptic)	Interneuron	Descending fibers
Bombesin			x	
NM	+			
Other neurotransmitters implicated in central modulation of nociception				
Dopamine				x (−)
Oxytocin				x (−)
CRF and urocortins			x (+/−)	x (+/−)
Nitric oxide			x (+)	
Neurotensin			x (−)	
NFF			x (+/−)	
TRH			x (+)	x (+)
Other receptors implicated in central modulation of nociception				
(TRPV1)	+			
(B2)	+			
(CB1)	−			

Pharmacological systems thought to contribute to the transmission and modulation of second order nociceptive neurons in the dorsal horn of the spinal cord. The various neurochemicals and receptors depicted each has its own pharmacological profile and may represent independent populations of neurons and fibers, but more commonly coexist and interact with each other at individual synapses. Interactions may take place at presynaptic terminals, dendrites, and somata.

x, origin of neurotransmitter; +, pronociceptive effect; −, antinociceptive effect; α1, α2, alpha adrenoceptors; A1, adenosine receptor 1; Ach, acetylcholine; mAChR and nAChR, muscarinic and nicotinic acetylcholine receptors; AMPA, α-amino-3-hydroxy-5-methyl-4-isoxazoleproprionate; ATP, adenosine triphosphate; CB1, cannabinoid receptor 1; CCK, cholecystokinin; CGRP, calcitonin gene-related peptide; CRF, corticotrophin releasing factor; 5HT, serotonin; GABA, gamma amino butyric acid; Gal1 and Gal2, galinin receptors types 1 and 2; KA, kainate receptors; mGlu, metabotropic glutamate receptor; MOR, DOR, and KOR, mu, delta, and kappa opioid receptors; NFF, neuropeptide FF; NK1 and NK2, neurokinin 1and 2 receptors; NM, neuromedin receptor; NPY, neuropeptide Y; ORL1, nociceptin/orphanin FQ peptide receptor; SSN-R2 and -R4, somatostatin receptor 2 and 4; TRH, thyrotropin-releasing hormone; TRPV1, transient receptor potential vanilloid-1; VIP, vasoactive intestinal polypeptide. (Supportive references: 2, 33, 35, 44–49, 51, 58–63.)

The third ligand-activated ion channel, the KA channel, is not well understood but is likely to affect nociceptive systems in a yet-to-be-defined fashion. Metabotropic effects (second messenger-mediated) of the KA receptor that are in addition to its primary ionotropic effects have been observed in CNS sites such as the hippocampus. Evidence of participation in intracellular signaling cascades and G protein activation that lead to the modulation of GABA release suggest that KA receptors could have a role in nociceptive processing.[32]

Metabotropic Glutamate Receptors

Acting via second messenger systems rather than channel activation, the eight different metabotropic glutamate receptors (mGluRs) can be classified into three groups on the basis of sequence similarity and whether they positively couple to the phospholipase C cascade or negatively couple to the adenyl cyclases.[33] Group I (mGluR1 and mGluR5) has been linked to nociceptive processing as these receptors produce alterations in NMDA receptor-channel opening. As such they have been implicated in processes of central sensitization and persistent pain. Group II (mGluR2 and mGluR3) has also been used to modify nociceptive behavioral responses in models of neuropathic and inflammatory pain. Group III (mGluR6, mGluR7, and mGluR8) has not yet had a clearly defined role in nociception.

Substance P

This neuropeptide has long been attributed a special role in pain processing as it is located in small diameter primary afferents and is released following cutaneous noxious stimuli.[34,35] Substance P acts by binding to NK1 receptors on second order neurons thereby affecting intracellular G-protein–related phosphorylation processes. It is often co-localized with, and so co-released with, glutamate from primary afferents and promotes membrane depolarization produced by glutamate. In this way it modifies the gain of nociceptive transmission. It is important in conditions of inflammation, particularly neurogenic inflammation, where it is released from peripheral axons and produces a local tissue effect. However, substance P may not be necessary for acute nociceptive transmission since the pharmacological or genetic "knock-out" of the NK1 receptor has minimal effect on acute responses to most nociceptive stimuli. Substance P is present in highest concentration is laminae I and II$_o$ as well as in laminae V and VI. Other neurokinin receptors also exist which bind other neuropeptides such as NK-A which has physiological effects similar to substance P. Neuropeptide antagonists such as the NK1 antagonists have proved to have disappointing results in clinical trials when pain was the clinical endpoint,[36] although efficacy has been noted in association with nausea therapy.

Calcitonin Gene-Related Peptide

The most commonly located neuropeptide in afferent systems, CGRP, has a poorly defined role in nociceptive processing with mixed results from depletion, augmentation, and antagonism studies.[37] At present, its most important effects appear to be related to peripheral vasodilation that is associated with the generation of headaches.[38] Electrophysiological studies of spinal WDR second order neurons have demonstrated an augmentation of nociceptive responses due to direct application of CGRP in a neuromodulatory fashion similar to substance P and NK1 receptor activation.[39] Like substance P, the knockout of CGRP synthesis has little effect on acute experimental models. CGRP localizes in primary afferent terminals in laminae I, II, and V. Human and nonhuman animal studies suggest that CGRP may be most important in relation to neurogenic inflammatory processes—particularly those associated with migraine headache.

There is a clear association between headache symptomatology and the peripheral release of CGRP and antagonists to the GCRP receptor have been reported as efficacious for the relief of acute migraine attacks.[40] For these reasons, CGRP may not be as important as a substrate for spinal cord processing as it is for the peripheral effects of nociceptor activation.

Cholecystokinin

A peptide present in primary afferent neurons, CCK has little effect in animals without pathology but the neuropeptide increases in content and its receptors in number following nerve injury.[41,42] Opioid receptor function and CCK receptor activation are also related in a complex fashion as CCK receptor antagonists may promote opioid analgesia and slow morphine tolerance development at spinal levels. Consistent with this, CCK receptor antagonists may be analgesic in neuropathic pain models and this analgesia is antagonized by naloxone. CCK is localized predominantly to lamina I, II, IV, and X and is a neurotransmitter present in both primary afferents and interneurons.

Other Neuropeptides

Multiple other neuropeptides that are in primary afferent neurons or which have receptors on the central terminals of primary afferent receptors have been implicated in nociceptive spinal processing. These include vasoactive intestinal polypeptide (VIP), bombesin, gastrin-releasing peptide, neuromedin B, neuromedin C, neuropeptide YY, and thyrotropin-releasing hormone. Action of most of these neurotransmitters on nociceptive systems appears to be predominantly a facilitatory presynaptic action on primary afferent neurotransmitter release. VIP has a presence in the ventral horn of the spinal cord, but the predominant source of VIP to the dorsal horn is primary afferents with strong localization in lamina I and a sparse representation in lamina V. Two neuropeptides located in primary afferent terminals, galanin and somatostatin, have inhibitory influences on second order neurons.[42,43] Trophic factors such as nerve growth factor and brain-derived neurotrophic factor also act as influences to the second order neurons particularly in conditions of nerve injury or death.

Adenosine Triphosphate

Present in many primary afferents, ATP, as a neurotransmitter, is known to activate the ligand-gated ion channels of the P2X family as well as the metabotropic P2Y family of receptors. P2X receptor activation both potentiates glutamatergic transmission and produces fast transmission related to nociceptor activation.[44,45] Ubiquitous as the compound used to drive most energy-requiring processes of metabolism, ATP also has breakdown products that may serve as agonists to other purinergic receptors (A1, A2) located both extracellularly and intracellularly on second order neurons.

Co-localization of Neurotransmitters

A combination of neurotransmitters released from primary afferent neurons is the typical rule rather than exception in relation to small diameter fibers. EAAs coexist with ATP, substance P, NK-A, CGRP, and other neuropeptides. These neuropeptides coexist in nerve terminals in varying combinations with each other with all possible mixtures described in overlap. CGRP is the most ubiquitous of the neurotransmitters located within C-fibers and so commonly co-localized with other neurotransmitters.

Neurotransmitters from Interneurons

Whereas the predominant effect of primary afferent neurotransmitter release upon second order spinal neurons is excitation, the predominant effect of interneuron neurotransmitter release is inhibition. Second order neurons may act as interneurons and at the same time may also be third, fourth, or higher order neurons responsible for excitatory and/or inhibitory effects on other second order neurons. This is apparent in intermediate laminae neurons which have complex cutaneous receptive fields that represent the total body when both excitatory and inhibitory influences are considered.[13] Interneurons utilize many of the same excitatory neurotransmitters as primary afferents but, in addition, utilize many other neurotransmitters to produce inhibitory influences. These fall mainly into the amino acid, neuropeptide, and small molecule groups. A listing of these neurotransmitters is also given in Table 4.1.

Inhibitory Amino Acids

GABA and glycine are the two main inhibitory amino acids of the CNS. GABAergic systems appear to be more predominant at supraspinal sites and glycine at spinal sites, but both are present throughout the CNS. GABA acts through a "fast" ligand-activated ion channel that allows chloride ion flow which in turn produces hyperpolarization of the neuronal membrane. Termed the $GABA_A$ receptor, it has associated structures that allow benzodiazepine or barbiturate binding to alter the GABA-affinity and channel activation characteristics of the receptor-channel complex. The "slow" metabotropic receptor for GABA, the $GABA_B$ receptor is the binding site for baclofen and works via G-protein–linked systems to alter potassium (promotes) and calcium (inhibits) ion channel flow. Via actions on motoneurons, $GABA_B$ receptor activation leads to decreased spasticity and muscle tone. At brainstem levels, in association with cranial nerve function, $GABA_B$ activation may be analgesic and so is indicated in the treatment of various cranial neuralgias. A putative $GABA_C$ receptor which is ionotropic has been described but with an uncertain role in sensory systems.

Glycine acts through both strychnine-sensitive and strychnine-insensitive receptors. The former, a ligand-gated anion channel very similar to the $GABA_A$ complex, is diffusely located but with particular effect in the ventral horn of the spinal cord such that the administration of strychnine can lead to spontaneous muscle contractions. Also present in spinal sensory systems, the antagonism of glycine effects with strychnine in animal models leads to motor and autonomic hyperreflexia. Paradoxically, glycine can also have excitatory effects via binding as a coagonist to a separate site of the NMDA receptor. Because of their multiple nonspecific effects, anti- or pro-glycinergic drugs have not been employed clinically although theoretical uses are present.

Opioids

Endogenous opioids form the most prominent family of inhibitory neuropeptides in the dorsal horn. Arising from intrinsic spinal interneurons, enkephalins, dynorphin, and β-endorphin bind to G-protein–related receptor complexes that fall into three major classes: the mu opioid receptors (MOR), the kappa opioid receptors (KOR), and the delta opioid receptors (DOR). Exogenously administered MOR agonists are the mainstay of analgesic therapy for severe pain today with actions at both spinal and supraspinal sites. Spinal effects arising from supraspinal actions of MOR agonists are via descending serotonergic and noradrenergic mechanisms. MOR agonists administered to spinal sites act both presynaptically on primary afferents to inhibit release of excitatory neurotransmitters and postsynaptically to directly inhibit second order neurons. KOR agonists, such as the endogenous dynorphins, have been demonstrated to be neurotoxic when administered in high concentrations. Peripherally, these same agents appear to produce analgesia particularly in the realm of deep tissue afferents. DOR agonists hold great promise with many of the favorable characteristics of MOR agonists. However, to date, study of selective DOR agonists have been hampered by the lack of highly selective, nontoxic drugs for use.

An opioid-receptor related neurotransmitter is the substance nociceptin and its receptor, the N/OFQ peptide receptor. Due to the technology of functional genomics this receptor, formerly known as the opioid receptor like orphan receptor-1, was the first of hundreds of G-protein coupled receptors identified which had no known endogenous ligand or function. Subsequently, nociceptin (orphanin FQ) was identified and functional pharmacology performed with agonists to the N/OFQ peptide receptor showing some promise in relation to the treatment of anxiety, stress-induced anorexia, cough, neurogenic bladder, edema, drug dependence, cerebral ischemia, and epilepsy.[46] The precise role of nociceptin in pain processing is still being determined with both antiopioid and opioid-potentiating modulatory properties demonstrated.[47]

Acetylcholine

A developing, novel pharmacology only increasing recognition for its importance to nociceptive processing is that involving the cholinergic systems. Numerous dorsal horn interneurons label positive for enzymes associated with acetylcholine synthesis and/ or degradation and pharmacological effects have been noted in relation to both nicotinic and muscarinic subtypes. Use of neuraxially delivered cholinesterase inhibitors, which lead to the increased activation of both nicotinic and muscarinic receptors, clearly produces analgesia in nonhuman animal models, but also produces intractable nausea in clinical studies (which reduces enthusiasm for their use). Cholinergic interneurons may act as intermediary steps for other analgesic treatments such as descending norepinephrine-related inhibitory systems.

Other Neurotransmitters Within Interneurons

Numerous other neuropeptides and small molecules have been localized to interneurons which include thyroid-stimulating hormone (TSH), neurotensin, neuropeptide FF, and neuropeptide Y. All of these have been demonstrated to have dorsal horn localization and all produce neuromodulatory effects, many with mixed excitatory/inhibitory interactions with opioid systems.

Neurotransmitters from Supraspinal Sources

Spinal transection leads to a depletion of the content of several neurotransmitters within the dorsal horn of the spinal cord. Most notable of these are the monoamines serotonin and norepinephrine. Spinal transection still leaves residual serotonin content within the ventral horn indicating some local production of neurotransmitter that may be in addition to that circulating in blood components. Any residual noradrenergic content appears to be of sympathetic origin. As will be discussed in the next chapter, descending noradrenergic and serotonergic fibers originating in the brainstem produce robust inhibitory effects on second order spinal neurons. It has also been recently appreciated that these same neurotransmitters may also produce excitatory effects and may therefore serve as the mechanisms of descending facilitation, another topic of the next chapter.

Serotonin (5-Hydroxytryptamine; 5-HT)

The pharmacological characterization of responses to the endogenous substance, serotonin, has identified a highly complex interaction of this substance with multiple receptors, some with multiple subtypes. At last count, four major groups of 5-HT receptors had been identified, some with inhibitory and some with excitatory effects. The receptor of relevance to pain production or excitatory phenomena is the 5-HT3 receptor, the only one of the receptors which is a ligand-gated ion channel.[48] Excitatory responses to serotonin administered peripherally suggest that it can directly activate nociceptive primary afferent neurons. Actions

on the dorsal roots have been postulated to be pronociceptive, antinociceptive, and pro-pruritic. Boutons with serotonin content have been noted throughout the dorsal horn and cell bodies with serotonin have been identified in the ventral horn. A co-localization within synaptic boutons with the neuropeptide substance P has been commonly noted.

Noradrenaline

Adrenoceptors important to the spinal processing of pain appear to be of the α_1 or α_2 subtypes based on the use of agonists (i.e., clonidine) and antagonists administered spinally. Descending from brainstem noradrenergic neuronal nuclei (primarily A5, A6, and A7), known pharmacological sites of action for norepinephrine include presynaptic terminals of nociceptive primary afferent neurons ($\alpha 2$ inhibitory), second order neurons ($\alpha 2$ inhibitory), and interneurons ($\alpha 1$ excitatory) and, as such, has been implicated in both descending inhibition and descending facilitation of nociceptive transmission.[49] Immunohistochemical localization of noradrenergic nerve fibers have found them widely dispersed throughout the dorsal horn and much of the release of neurotransmitter appears nonsynaptic in nature,[50] such that the neurotransmitter has to diffuse from its site of release to its site of action which may be neuronal or glial.[51] Extensive synaptic contact of noradrenergic nerve endings does occur within the ventral horn and intermediolateral grey.

Other Neurotransmitters in Descending Systems

Often co-localized with other neurotransmitters, certain neuropeptides and other monoamines are also in descending fibers that make contact with the spinal dorsal horn. These include substance P, CCK, corticotrophin releasing factor, urocortin 1, and thyrotropin-releasing hormone (TRH) which have excitatory neuromodulatory effects and dopamine, oxytocin, and endogenous opioids which have inhibitory neuromodulatory effects. These descending fibers modulate more than just nociceptive sensory information but when exogenously administered to the spinal cord can produce profound autonomic and motor effects. TSH has been noted to have effects that are like CCK in that it appears to inhibit opioid analgesia.

Neurotransmitters from Glia or Unknown Sources

Numerous substances alter the excitability of second order neurons to nociceptive input that are not from neural structures. For example, bradykinin, which is normally known for its peripheral nervous system effects, activates B2 receptors in the dorsal horn with the subsequent induction of hyperalgesia phenomena. Destruction of primary afferents results in the loss of two thirds of these receptors, but the source of the activating bradykinin is unknown. Likewise, other substances associated with inflammation, such as prostanoids and cytokines, have similar neuromodulatory effects and the spinal administration of prostaglandin receptor agonists such those associated with PGE2, PGD2, or PGI2 leads to hypersensitivity. Prostaglandin receptor activation may require other receptors for full expression of sensory phenomena as appears to be the case for PGE2 which needs an intact NMDA receptor and PGD2 which requires intact NK1 receptors. Cytokines such as IL-1B, IL-6, and tumor necrosis factor-α, which are released by activated microglia and other neuroimmunological cellular components of the CNS following nerve injury, have also been appreciated as having neurotoxicity effects on nociceptive neurons that involve purinergic mechanisms.[52,53] Growth factors such as nerve growth factor (NGF), glial-derived neurotrophic factor (GDNF), and brain-derived neurotrophic factor (BDNF) may come from multiple sources, including neural structures, and have obvious effects on central nervous system systems producing trophic and potentially phenotypic changes with resulting actions on pain-related structures.[54–56]

Other Important Receptors/Channels

Consideration needs to be given to the presence of receptors or channels that are either "universal" in that their pharmacological modulation seemingly affects all spinal cord neurons in a relatively nondiscriminative fashion or "selective" in that they are present in a subset and/or sub-site of neurons such as the end terminals of primary afferent neurons. A particular group of ion channels that are in the *selective* group are the N-type calcium channels found on primary afferent neurons.[57] Calcium influx into the intercellular space due to receptor activation (ligand-gated) or due to membrane depolarization (voltage-gated) results in both membrane depolarization effects and second messenger cascade activation. In primary afferents, this calcium influx is associated with the release of neurotransmitter at synapses. There exist at least 5 families of voltage-gated channels (L, N, P/Q, R, and T) with differing pharmacologies and localization within the spinal cord. Some of the families share auxiliary subunits such as the L- and N-type channels which both have an $\alpha 2\delta$ subunit. This subunit is the site to which the drugs gabapentin and pregabalin bind with a subsequent reduction, but not abolition of membrane excitability. The N-type calcium channels are located throughout the CNS, but at a spinal cord level have particular localization to the nerve terminals of small diameter primary afferents. The ω-conotoxin ziconitide binds to and blocks ion flow through this channel and has found clinical utility in the control of pain when administered intrathecally.

WHAT IS IMPORTANT TO THE CLINICIAN

The substrates of nociception that exist at a spinal level are as complex as the phenomenon of pain itself. More than 30 different neurotransmitters acting at more than 50 different receptors have been identified as present in the spinal cord and associated with some pain-related phenomenon. Sensory pathways connecting the spinal cord to the brain have been identified that result in rapid transmission of information that is highly organized and site-specific but similar pathways have also been identified which have slow transmission that is poorly organized and therefore resistant to attempts at ablation. The clinician must synthesize these diverse pieces of information into a general model of nociceptive processing and must accept that, at this point in time, the model is incomplete. The effectiveness of therapeutic interventions intended to treat pain is dependent on the modulation of these substrates of nociception which forms the topic of the next chapter.

Acknowledgments

The authors of this chapter are supported by DK51419, DK 73218, and DK78655.

Note: The present chapter is intended as a summary of information important to pain clinicians and as a presentation of new information coupled with a simplification of previous presentations of similar information in this text and other sources.[60–62] As such, referencing has been lessened, although many of the primary sources of information may be found in the previous reviews.

References

1. Coggeshall RE. Fos, nociception and the dorsal horn. *Prog Neurobiol* 2005; 77:299–352.
2. Mantyh PW. Neurobiology of substance P and NK1 receptor. *J Clin Psychiatry* 2002;63(suppl 11):6–10.
3. Guo W, Wei F, Zou S, et al. Group 1 metabotropic glutamate receptor NMDA receptor coupling and signaling cascade mediate spinal dorsal horn NMDA receptor 2B tyrosine phosphorylation associated with inflammatory hyperalgesia. *J Neurosci* 2004;24:9161–9173.
4. Pattinson D, Fitzgerald M. The neurobiology of infant pain: development of excitatory and inhibitory neurotransmission in the spinal dorsal horn. *Reg Anesth Pain Med* 2004;29:36–44.
5. Zhang X, Bao L. The development and modulation of nociceptive circuitry. *Curr Opin Neurobiol* 2006;16:460–466.
6. Ruda MA, Ling QD, Hohmann AG, et al. Altered nociceptive neuronal circuits after neonatal peripheral inflammation. *Science* 2000;289:628–631.
7. Sugiura Y, Terui N, Hosoya Y. Difference in distribution of central terminals between visceral and somatic unmyelinated C-primary afferent fibers. *J Neurophysiol* 1989;62:834–840.
8. Morris R, Cheunsuang O, Stewart A, et al. Spinal dorsal horn neurone targets for nociceptive primary afferents: do single neurone morphological characteristics suggest how nociceptive information is processed at the spinal level. *Brain Res Rev* 2004;46:173–190.
9. Gobel S. Golgi studies of the neurons in layer II of the dorsal horn of the medulla (trigeminal nucleus caudalis). *J Comp Neurol* 1978;180:395–413.
10. Gobel S. Neural circuitry in the substantia gelatinosa of Rolando: anatomical insights. In: Bonica JJ, Liebeskind J, Albe-Fessard D, eds. *Advances in Pain Research and Therapy.* Vol 3. New York: Raven Press; 1979:175–195.
11. Dubner R, Bennett GJ. Spinal and trigeminal mechanisms of nociception. *Ann Rev Neurosci* 1983;6:381–418.
12. Mendell LM, Wall PD. Responses of single dorsal cord cells to peripheral cutaneous unmyelinated fibres. *Nature* 1965;206:97–99.
13. LeBars D. The whole body receptive field of dorsal horn multireceptive neurons. *Brain Res Revs* 2002;40:29–44.
14. Collins JG, Ren K. WDR response profiles of spinal dorsal horn neurons may be unmasked by barbiturate anesthesia. *Pain* 1987;28:369–378.
15. LeBars D, Dickenson AH, Besson JM. Diffuse noxious Inhibitory Controls (DNIC): I Effects on dorsal horn convergent neurones in the rat. *Pain* 1979; 6:283–304.
16. LeBars D, Dickenson AH, Besson JM. Diffuse noxious Inhibitory Controls (DNIC): II Lack of effect on non-convergent neurons, supraspinal involvement and theoretical implications. *Pain* 1979;6:305–327.
17. McMahon SB, Morrison JF. Two groups of spinal interneurones that respond to stimulation of the abdominal viscera of the cat. *J Physiol* 1982;322:21–34.
18. McMahon SB, Morrison JF. Spinal neurones with long projections activated from the abdominal viscera of the cat. *J Physiol* 1982;322:1–20.
19. Noordenbos W. *Pain.* Amsterdam: Elsevier; 1959.
20. Basbaum AI. Conduction of the effects of noxious stimulation by short-fiber multisynaptic systems of the spinal cord in the rat. *Exp Neurol* 1973;40:699–716.
21. Willis WD, Kenshalo DR Jr, Leonard RB. The cells of origin of the primate spino-thalamic tract. *J Comp Neurol* 1979;188:543–573.
22. Han ZS, Zhang ET, Craig AD. Nociceptive and thermoreceptive lamina I neurons are anatomically distinct. *Nat Neurosci* 1998;1:218–225.
23. Willis WD, Westlund KN. Neuroanatomy of the pain system and the pathways that modulate pain. *J Clin Neurophysiol* 1997;14:2–31.
24. Giesler GJ Jr, Yezierski RP, Gerhart KD, et al. Spinothalamic tract neurons that project to medial and/or lateral thalamic nuclei: evidence for a physiologically novel population of spinal cord neurons. *J Neurophysiol* 1981;46:1285–1308.
25. Ralston HJ III, Ralston DD. The primate dorsal spinothalamic tract: evidence for a specific termination in the posterior nuclei (Po/SG) of the thalamus. *Pain* 1992;48:107–118.
26. Martin RJ, Apkarian AV, Hodge CJ Jr. Ventrolateral and dorsolateral ascending spinal cord pathway influence on thalamic nociception in cat. *J Neurophysiol* 1990;64:1400–1412.
27. Apkarian AV, Hodge CJ. Primate spinothalamic pathways: II. The cells of origin of the dorsolateral and ventral spinothalamic pathways. *J Comp Neurol* 1989;288:474–492.
28. Kerr F. Segmental circuitry and ascending pathways of the nociceptive systems. In: Beers RF, Bassett EJ, eds. *Mechanisms of Pain and Analgesic Compounds.* New York: Raven Press; 1979:113–141.
29. Bernard JF, Bester H, Besson JM. Involvement of the spino-parabrachio, -amygdaloid and -hypothalamic pathways in the autonomic and affective emotional aspects of pain. *Prog Brain Res* 1996;107:243–255.
30. Hirschberg RM, Al-Chaer ED, Lawand NB, et al. Is there a pathway in the posterior funiculus that signals visceral pain? *Pain* 1996;67:291–305.
31. Nauta HJ, Soukup VM, Fabian RH, et al. Punctate midline myelotomy for the relief of visceral cancer pain. *J Neurosurg* 2000;92(suppl 2):125–130.
32. Rodriguez-Moreno A, Sihra TS. Metabotropic actions of kainate receptors in the CNS. *J Neurochem* 2007;103:2121–2135.
33. Gerber U, Gee CE, Benquet P. Metabotropic glutamate receptors: intracellular signaling pathways. *Curr Opin Pharmacol* 2007;7:56–61.

34. Hill RG, Oliver KR. Neuropeptide and kinin antagonists. *Handb Exp Pharmacol* 2007;177:181–216.
35. Harrison S, Geppetti P. Substance P. *Int J Biochem Cell Biol* 2001;33:555–576.
36. Hill R. NK1 (substance P) receptor antagonists—why are they not analgesic in humans? *Trends Pharmacol Sci* 2000;21:244–246.
37. Van Rossum D, Hanisch UK, Quirion R. Neuroanatomical localization, pharmacological characterization and functions of CGRP, related peptides and their receptors. *Neurosci Biobehav Rev* 1997;21:649–678.
38. Brain SD, Cox HM. Neuropeptides and their receptors: innovative science providing novel therapeutic targets. *Br J Pharmacol* 2006;147:S202–S211.
39. Yu Y, Lundeberg T, Yu LC. Role of calcitonin gene-related peptide and its antagonist on the evoked discharge frequency of wide dynamic range neurons in the dorsal horn of the spinal cord in rats. *Regul Pept* 2002;103:23–27.
40. Edvinsson L, Petersen KA. CGRP-receptor antagonism in migraine treatment. *CNS Neurol Disord Drug Targets* 2007;6:240–246.
41. Wiesenfeld–Hallin Z, Xu XJ, Hökfelt T. The role of spinal cholecystokinin in chronic pain states. *Pharmacol Toxicol* 2002;91:398–403.
42. Wiesenfeld–Hallin Z, Xu XJ. Neuropeptides in neuropathic and inflammatory pain with special emphasis on cholecystokinin and galanin. *Eur J Pharmacol* 2001;429:49–59.
43. Pan HL, Wu ZZ, Zhou HY, et al. Modulation of pain transmission by G-protein-coupled receptors. *Pharmacol Ther* 2008;117:141–161.
44. Gu JG, MacDermott AB. Activation of ATP P2X receptors elicits glutamate release from sensory neuron synapses. *Nature* 1997;389:749–753.
45. Gu JG, Bardoni R, Magherini PC, et al. Effects of the P2-purinoceptor antagonists suramin and pyridoxal-phosphate-6-azophenyl-2′,4′-disulfonic acid on glutaminergic synaptic transmission in rat dorsal horn neurons of the spinal cord. *Neurosci Lett* 1998;253:167–170.
46. Chiou LC, Liao YY, Fan PC, et al. Nociceptin/orphanin FQ peptide receptors: pharmacology and clinical implications. *Curr Drug Targets* 2007;8:117–135.
47. Mollereau C, Roumy M, Zajac JM. Opioid-modulating peptides: mechanisms of action. *Curr Top Med Chem* 2005;5:341–355.
48. Färber L, Haus U, Späth M, et al. Physiology and pathophysiology of the 5-HT3 receptor. *Scand J Rheumatol Suppl* 2004;119:2–8.
49. Pertovaara A. Noradrenergic pain modulation. *Prog Neurobiol* 2006;80:53–83.
50. Rajaofetra N, Ridet JL, Poulat P, et al. Immunocytochemical mapping of noradrenergic projections to the rat spinal cord with an antiserum against noradrenaline. *J Neurocytol* 1992;21:481–494.
51. Ridet JL, Rajaofetra N, Teilhac JR, et al. Evidence for nonsynaptic serotonergic and noradrenergic innervation of the rat dorsal horn and possible involvement of neuron-glia interactions. *Neuroscience* 1993;52:143–157.
52. Tsuda M, Inoue K, Salter MW. Neuropathic pain and spinal microglia: a big problem from molecules in 'small' glia. *Trends Neurosci* 2005;28:101–107.
53. Inoue K. The function of microglia through purinergic receptors: neuropathic pain and cytokine release. *Pharmacol Ther* 2006;109:210–226.
54. Sah DW, Ossipov MH, Rossomando A, et al. New approaches for the treatment of pain: the GDNF family of neurotropic growth factors. *Curr Top Med Chem* 2005;5:577–583.
55. Bennett DL. Neurotrophic factors: important regulators of nociceptive function. *Neuroscientist* 2001;7:13–17.
56. Obata K, Noguchi K. BDNF in sensory neurons and chronic pain. *Neurosci Res* 2006;55:1–10.
57. Yaksh TL. Calcium channels as therapeutic targets in neuropathic pain. *J Pain* 2006;7:S13–S30.
58. Dickenson A. Pharmacology of pain. In: *Receptor and Ion Channel Nomenclature Supplement*, 4th ed. Cambridge: Elsevier; 1993.
59. Terman GW, Bonica JJ, Liebeskind JC. Spinal mechanisms and their modulation. In: Loeser JD, Butler SH, Chapman CR, Turk DC, eds. *Bonica's Management of Pain*. 3rd ed. New York: Lippincott Williams & Wilkins; 2001: 73–153.
60. Ness TJ, Brennan TJ. Sensory systems. In: Hemmings HC, Hopkins PM, eds. *Foundations of Anesthesia*. 2nd ed. London: Mosby Press; 2006.
61. Millan MJ. The induction of pain: an integrative review. *Prog Neurobio* 1999; 57:1–164.
62. Korosi A, Kozicz T, Richter J, et al. Corticotropin-releasing factor, urocortin 1, and their receptors in the mouse spinal cord. *J Comp Neurol* 2007;502: 973–989.
63. Vasconcelos LA, Donaldson C, Sita LV, et al. Urocortin in the central nervous sytem of a primate (Cebus apella): sequencing, immunohistochemical, and hybridization histochemical characterization. *J Comp Neurol* 2003;463:157–175.

CHAPTER 5 ■ MODULATION OF SPINAL NOCICEPTIVE PROCESSING

ALAN RANDICH AND TIMOTHY NESS

INTRODUCTION

The preceding chapter addressed the neuroanatomy and neurochemistry of neurons located within the spinal cord that process information related to pain-related sensation. These neurons are highly regulated components of the central nervous system (CNS) with inhibitory and excitatory feedback mechanisms. Pain may be a result of a failure of feedback regulation as much as it can be due to increased primary afferent input. Too much "gain" or inadequate "braking" can result in an excess of sensory transmission. In the normally functioning state, the responses of second order neurons can be suppressed or facilitated dependent on other events important to the organism. Some modulatory effects are relatively "hardwired" occurring in a reliable and predictable fashion. Other modulators are less predictable and may be dependent on psychic/cognitive processes that vary from organism to organism and may involve learning, motivation, or emotional factors. In most cases, modulatory systems are adaptive in that they help an organism to function optimally. Unfortunately, with disease, some of these same modulatory systems have become maladaptive and serve to impede both physiological and social processes of healing. The complex nature of these modulatory influences will be discussed in three parts beginning with a discussion of mechanisms based at spinal levels, followed by a discussion of mechanisms related to descending influences, and finally by a discussion of three particular "triggers" that may occur pathologically and/or iatrogenically: inflammation, nerve injury, and chronic opioid treatment. These triggers will be used as examples of the interactive nature of these modulatory forces. There is value in understanding endogenous modulatory systems because they are the systems which the clinician activates or suppresses by using exogenous modulators, such as electrical stimulation or pharmacological agents. Modulation occurs at each step of processing within the CNS, but the focus of the present discussion will be the modulation of the spinal second order nociceptive neuron.

SPINAL CORD-BASED MODULATORY MECHANISMS

Acute Segmental Modulatory Effects

Sensory inputs to the spinal cord and trigeminal nucleus begin to interact at the very first steps of transmission. Activation of large diameter afferents (Aβ) produces an inhibitory effect on the processing of signals from small diameter (Aδ & C-fiber) afferents. This effect has been documented since ancient times and is relearned by every child who rubs or massages injured parts of their bodies in order to achieve pain relief. The mechanism of this manipulation has been more difficult to explain than the time-honored efficacy of the effect.[1] What is clear is that second order neurons of the spinal cord have both excitatory and inhibitory "receptive fields." Namely, stimulation of different parts of the body using one or more types of stimuli (e.g., noxious heat, low threshold mechanical, high threshold mechanical) results in the depolarization or hyperpolarization of individual second order neurons. Inhibition of second order neurons which is produced by noxious stimuli can be evoked from heterosegmental sites and so is discussed separately later. Inhibition of second order neurons which is produced by nonnoxious stimulation appears to be predominantly segmentally organized. Theoretically formulated as the initial Gate Control Theory of Melzack and Wall,[2] this effect was hypothesized to occur because of a combination of presynaptic inhibition and the actions of inhibitory interneurons located in lamina II (substantia gelatinosa) of the spinal cord which are activated by large diameter afferents (Fig. 5.1). Although the specifics of this theory have evolved further to include nonsegmental effects, its general description has served as the theoretical underpinnings for the clinical effects of neuro-modulatory (electrostimulatory analgesic) techniques ranging from transcutaneous electrical nerve stimulation to spinal cord stimulation and aspects of acupuncture.

Numerous electrophysiological studies of second order neurons have observed that low intensity, high frequency electrical stimulation of nerves or somatic tissues located at the same segmental level as the neuron produces an inhibitory effect which is not reduced by naloxone (nonopioidergic) but which may involve GABAergic or glycinergic mechanisms. This phenomenon is present in both spinally transected and intact animals and so does not necessarily involve a brainstem mechanism. Dorsal column stimulation which produces retrograde activation of Aβ-fiber inputs to the spinal cord (but may also activate descending modulatory pathways) produces similar nonopioid, GABAergic, and/or glycinergic inhibition of spinal nociceptive processing.

Heterosegmental Modulatory Systems

Both excitatory and inhibitory effects can occur at one spinal level when stimuli are presented to distant portions of the body. Excitatory effects have generally been described in imprecise terms as "extended connectivity" or as "propriospinal" pathways. Some of these intraspinal networks serve to integrate both sensory and motor functions involving the upper and lower extremities with an example being crossed flexion-extension reflex responses to noxious stimuli. A coordination of pelvic organ function also relies on intraspinal excitatory and inhibitory connections that link processing of sensory information from afferents traveling in the pelvic nerve to the lumbosacral cord with that of afferents traveling in sympathetic nerves to the thoracolumbar spinal cord.[3,4] Intraspinal networks of neurons which form a reticular webwork in the deeper parts of the spinal dorsal horn have been described in the context of the multisynaptic ascending system of Noordenboos.[5] This same network could just as easily serve as the substrates for multisynaptic descending modulatory influences.

The most formally studied heterosegmental interaction related to nociception is the phenomenon known as diffuse noxious inhibitory controls (DNIC). This endogenous inhibitory system is activated by heterosegmental noxious stimuli which produce an inhibition of ongoing or evoked dorsal horn neuronal activity. The mechanisms of DNIC are postulated to involve the activation of brainstem nuclei that subsequently produce inhibition of spinal dorsal horn neurons through a descending modulatory mechanism, but it is notable that the neurophysiological phenomena associated with DNIC have been demonstrated in spinally transected preparations. These "propriospinal" phenomena represent a general inhibitory system activated by heterosegmental noxious conditioning stimuli which is either synonymous with or highly augmented by the presence of a brainstem and mechanisms of DNIC. According to its original description by Lebars et al.,[6,7] DNIC results in the inhibition of Class 2 (wide dynamic range; convergent) neurons and has no effect on Class 3 (nociceptive specific) neurons. A consistency of many studies related to DNIC (and propriospinal heterosegmental inhibition) is that they have identified that most spinal neurons responsive to noxious stimuli effectively have "total body" receptive fields in that noxious stimuli will produce excitation or inhibition that is dependent on precise body site.[8]

C-fiber Windup and Central Sensitization

Changes in excitability occur in second order neurons when repetitive or prolonged high intensity input is received from primary afferent C-fibers. One of these changes in excitability is termed C-fiber "wind-up." Noted by Mendell[9] when recording from ascending axons of spinal dorsal horn neurons, wind-up is the phenomenon whereby repeated electrical C-fiber activation at certain rates (i.e., ≥1 Hz) leads to a sequential increase in the number of action potentials evoked by each stimulus (Fig. 5.2). Slower stimulus rates do not produce progressive increases in activation. Mechanical and thermal stimuli at intensities sufficient to activate C-fibers also produce similar wind-up. This sequential increase in response can be blunted through use of N-methyl-D-aspartate (NMDA) receptor antagonists and the effect disappears after a few seconds of nonstimulation.

Another general category of increased neuronal excitability is termed "central sensitization." This term has been used in a focused manner to describe acute changes in the responsiveness of

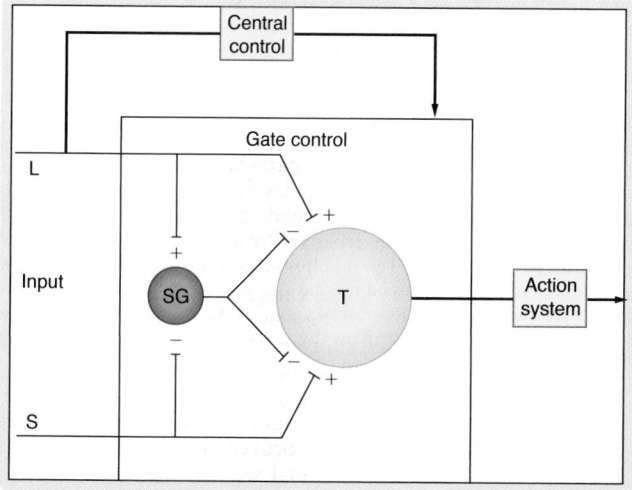

FIGURE 5.1 Gate control theory as originally schematically described by Melzack and Wall[2] where large-diameter (L) and small-diameter (S) primary afferent fibers project to substantia gelatinosa (SG) and second order transmission (T) neurons in the spinal dorsal horn. The inhibitory effect of SG neuronal activity is increased by L and decreased by S fiber activity. T neurons transmit information to the brain and other action sites. Activation of peripheral or central projections of L fibers using transcutaneous nerve stimulation, peripheral nerve stimulators, or dorsal column stimulators would all be expected to produce inhibition of S fiber input to the T cells.

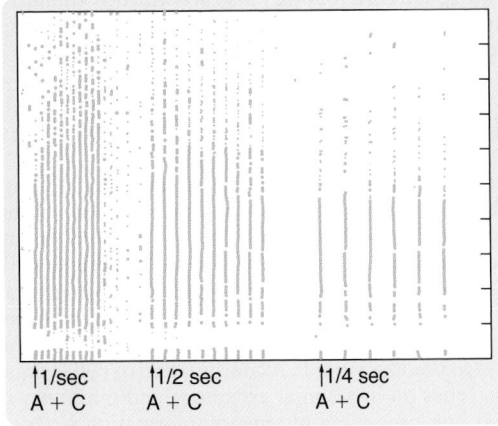

FIGURE 5.2 Wind-up responses of single dorsolateral column axon to repeated stimulation of the sural nerve at sufficient intensity to activate A and C fibers (no wind-up seen with A-fiber stimulation by itself). The vertical time markers on the far right represent 100 msec. Each mark at the bottom of the time line represents the stimulation artifact and the burst of activity immediately above each of these stimulations is the response to A-fiber stimulation (each dot represents an action potential). The more delayed responses are to the more slowly conducting C-fiber inputs. Response to stimulation shows increasing C-fiber wind-up responses on to 1 per second stimulation (not to 1 every 2 or 1 every 4 second stimulation rates at right). Wind-up lasts for only several seconds following the stimulation as seen by transient increase in spontaneous activity. (Redrawn from Mendell LM. Physiological properties of unmyelinated fiber projections to the spinal cord. *Exp Neurol* 1966;16:316–332.)

second order neurons following high intensity or prolonged stimuli such as occur with nonneuronal tissue injury and subsequent inflammation. The term has also been used to describe phenomena such as delayed-onset nerve injury-related hypersensitivity and, in that case, is more subacute or chronic in nature with a potential for morphological as well as biochemical alteration. For purposes of the present discussion, injury-induced central sensitization as described by Woolf[10] will be used as the archetype model of central sensitization (Fig. 5.3). Multiple studies have demonstrated that tissue injury produces an augmentation of nociceptive reflexes that is NMDA receptor dependent. In preclinical models, pharmacological treatment has the greatest effect if given prior to injury and a blocking of afferent input serves to delay the onset of development of hypersensitivity. Extrapolating from this data and coupling it with evidence of long-term potentiation (LTP) of synaptic efficacy in the spinal cord after even brief bouts of NMDA receptor activation,[11] some have further extrapolated these laboratory data to the clinical concept of "preemptive analgesia." Treating pain before (and after) it begins has a clear potential for clinical benefit although the true clinical significance of early intervention has proven difficult to define. On a neurophysiological basis, an expansion of cutaneous excitatory receptive fields has been noted following tissue injury which follows a similar pharmacology, but specific results have been model and species dependent.

SUPRASPINAL MODULATORY SYSTEMS

Tonic Descending Inhibition

A characteristic of spinal nociceptive systems is that they are under tonic descending inhibition such that a common effect of injury to spinal pathways is a release from this inhibition. Hyper-

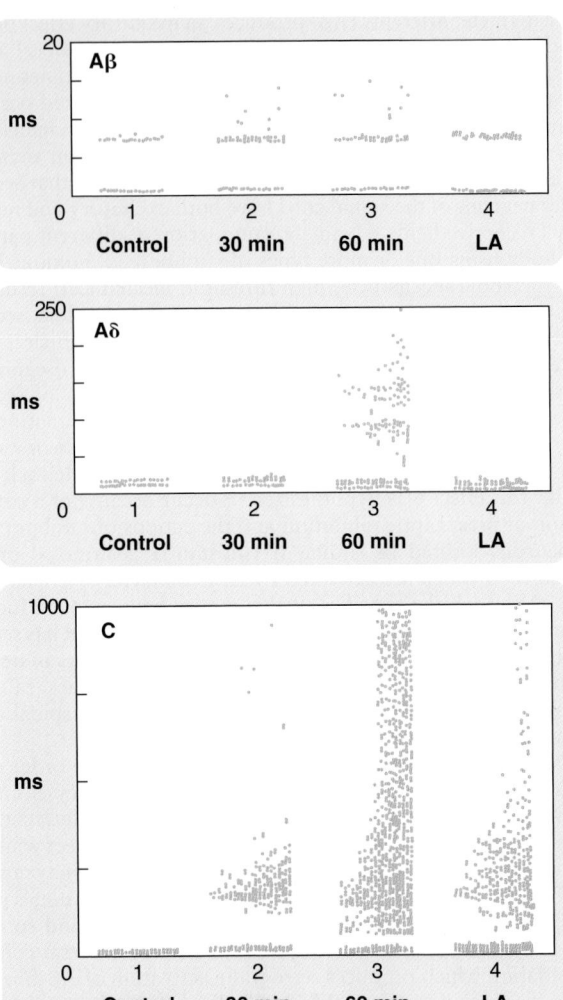

FIGURE 5.3 Raster dot displays of a single biceps femoris unit activated by stimulation of the sural nerve once every 2 seconds before an ipsilateral thermal injury (Control), 30 and 60 minutes postinjury, and 10 minutes after the injured foot has been completely anesthetized with local anesthetic (LA). Each dot represents a unit discharge. The vertical scale is the latency of the responses after sural nerve stimulation, and the stimulus artifact can be seen at time 0. Stimulation strengths were sufficient to activate Aβ, Aδ, and C-fibers. Note the different time scales used in the three panels to record the activity evoked by the three different fiber populations. In the preinjury state, only Aβ input was evoked. Thirty minutes after injury, a C-fiber response begins to occur; whereas, at 60 minutes both Aδ and C-fiber evoked responses are present (the C-fiber responses with wind-up). Ten minutes after LA, the C-fiber evoked responses remain higher than before the injury suggesting a central component of the sensitization. (Redrawn from Woolf CJ. Evidence for a central component of post-injury pain hypersensitivity. *Nature* 1983;306: 686–688.)

reflexive states with secondary spasticity and autonomic lability can occur. The precise neurophysiological circuits associated with this descending inhibition is of significant debate, but known inhibitory neurotransmitters such as norepinephrine (NE) and serotonin (SHT) are synthesized in the brainstem and transported to the spinal cord from multiple supraspinal sites. This role for supraspinal structures in providing descending influences on spinal reflexes has long been recognized. In 1915 Sherrington and Sowton[12] demonstrated enhanced flexion reflexes following spinal transection. Later in 1926, Fulton[13] suggested that this effect reflected removal of tonic descending inhibitory modulation of spinal interneurons mediating those reflexes. Descending

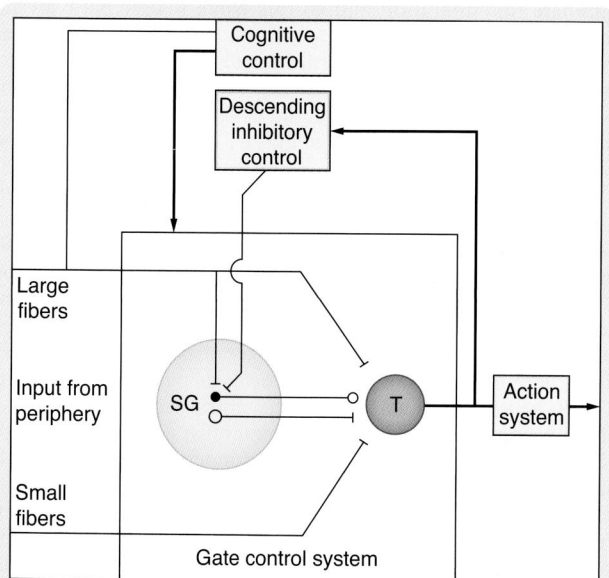

FIGURE 5.4 A modification of the gate control theory schematic models includes excitatory (*white circle*) and inhibitory (*black circle*) links form the substantia gelatinosa (SG) to the transmission (T) cells, as well as descending inhibitory control from brainstem systems. The round knob at the end of the inhibitory link indicates that its actions may be presynaptic, postsynaptic, or both. All connections are excitatory except the inhibitory link from SG to T cells. (Redrawn after Melzack R, Wall PD. *The Challenge of Pain.* New York: Basic Books; 1983.)

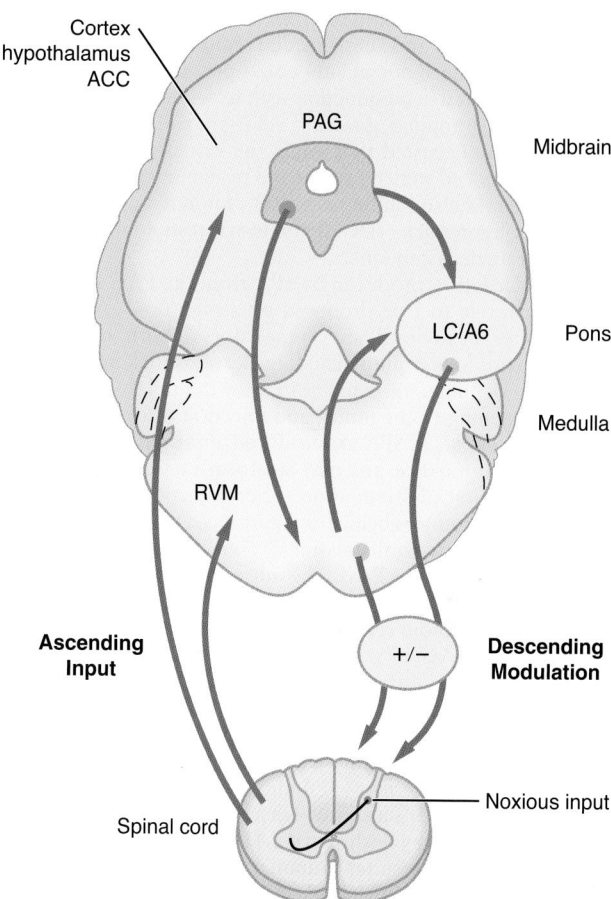

FIGURE 5.5 Schematic diagram of descending modulatory influences of spinal nociceptive processing. Multiple sites within the brain have been demonstrated to be of importance including the midbrain periaqueductal grey (PAG), locus coeruleus/A6 cell group (LC/A6), and the rostral ventromedial medulla (RVM). These sites are reciprocally interconnected, are activated by ascending nociceptive information, and serve as relays for other brain sites known to modulate spinal processing including the anterior cingulate cortex (ACC), other cortical sites (somatosensory, motor, insular, ventrolateral orbital), and the hypothalamus. Resultant modulatory effects on spinal dorsal horn processing can be inhibitory (−) or facilitatory (+) to nociceptive primary afferent input.

control of flexion reflexes was extensively studied in ensuing years,[14] but these studies did not target the issue of how the brain might specifically modulate incoming nociceptive signals from peripheral tissue.

A series of seminal events in the late 1960s and early 1970s led to a full-fledged appreciation and analysis of descending modulation of spinal nociceptive processing. These included a modification of the original Gate Control theory to include supraspinal systems (Fig. 5.4). This change was prompted by studies which showed that spinal dorsal horn neurons were subject to tonic descending inhibitory influences[15] and Reynolds' demonstration that electrical stimulation of the midbrain periaqueductal grey (PAG) produced analgesia sufficient to perform abdominal surgery in a rat.[16] This last phenomenon was referred to as "stimulation-produced analgesia" (SPA).[17,18] SPA can also be produced in humans[19] and it suggests the existence of endogenous systems that can selectively modulate pain. This served as the impetus for the extensive, formal analyses of supraspinal structures involved in descending modulation of spinal nociceptive processing that ensued during the next 35 years. Later, a number of investigators found that electrical or chemical stimulation of other brain regions could also promote *facilitation* of nociceptive processing,[20,21] suggesting the existence of similar descending facilitatory systems.

Brainstem Substrates Mediating the Descending Modulation of Pain

The midbrain PAG and the medullary nucleus raphe magnus (NRM) figured prominently in the original analyses of descending modulation of pain. Indeed, they are often viewed as the "backbone" of the pain modulatory system[22] and have been more extensively studied than any other brain regions. Yet, other brainstem nuclei/cell groups also serve in this role and include the nucleus gigantocellularis (NGC), nucleus reticularis gigantocellu-

laris pars alpha (NGCα), midbrain reticular formation, locus coeruleus/A6 cell group (LC/A6), lateral reticular nucleus (LRN), parabrachial/A7 and A5 cell groups, and the nucleus tractus solitarius (NTS). A limited amount of information has also become available on cortical and diencephalic systems that contribute to descending modulation. It is the investigation of these structures that has led to our current understanding of how descending pain modulatory systems affect pain perception. Each is described separately below and a summary of the most important components is described in Figure 5.5.

Periaqueductal Grey of the Mesencephalon

The PAG was the initial site of investigation for endogenous pain control systems and is still viewed as an integral component of these systems. Early studies of the PAG provided some evidence that the effects of SPA from this region were limited to nociceptive processing and could not be explained by more gross stimulation-produced deficits in sensory or motor function. Fardin et al.[23,24] performed an exhaustive analysis of the PAG of the rat and showed that a "pure" antinociceptive effect (i.e., with no side effects) could only be derived from sites of stimulation located in the ventrolateral and ventromedial regions of the PAG. Stimulation in other more dorsal sites could produce antinociception, but often occurred in conjunction with aversive reactions (vocalizations, flight, jumping), gnawing, rotation, and/or tremor. Other investigations suggested that while the primary effects of PAG stimulation indeed were on spinal and trigeminal nociceptive processing, it could also inhibit responses of nonnociceptive neurons in dorsal column nuclei (DCN) and low threshold neurons in the trigeminal nucleus caudalis.[25]

Antinociception produced by SPA from the PAG is profound and comparable to that produced by a high dose of morphine. It eliminates behavioral and spinal dorsal horn neuronal responses to noxious stimuli including electric shock applied to the tooth pulp or limbs, noxious heating of the tail and hind paws, noxious pinching of the limbs, and injection of irritants into the viscera. The effects of SPA are produced almost immediately after the onset of stimulation and may last from a few seconds to hours after termination of stimulation. Microinjection of opiates into the PAG also produces behavioral antinociception and inhibition of spinal nociceptive transmission[26,27] via disinhibition of inhibitory interneurons in the PAG. The subsequent discovery of endogenous opioid receptors[28] and peptides[29–31] and demonstration of the presence of opioid receptors in the PAG[32] further established a role for the PAG in pain modulation. Similarities were also observed between phenomena associated with PAG-derived inhibitory effects and opiate-induced analgesia, including tolerance and cross tolerance[33] and reversibility by the opiate receptor antagonist naloxone,[34,35] although the latter finding was not confirmed by all laboratories.[36] SPA and morphine induced antinociception from the PAG also involve a spinal release of 5-HT and NE, and mediation by both spinal 5-HT receptors and α_2 adrenoreceptors.[37–39] The resultant summary of these studies is that the PAG represents a brain site that provides descending influences on spinal and trigeminal nociceptive processing, utilizes several neurotransmitters in the production of their effects, can mediate the analgesic actions of exogenous opiates, and leads to multiple spinal neurochemical alterations.

Nucleus Raphe Magnus/Rostral Ventromedial Medulla

Anatomical studies reveal relatively few fibers that descend from the PAG directly to the spinal cord.[40] However the PAG does have strong projections to the NRM and adjacent areas of the rostral ventromedial medulla (RVM). Attention has therefore been focused on the NRM as the primary relay in mediating the antinociceptive effects of activation of PAG neurons. Studies of the NRM were performed in a manner analogous to those performed in the PAG, and often with comparable results.[40,41] Electrical stimulation of sites within the PAG or NRM produces inhibitory postsynaptic potentials (IPSPs) in dorsal horn neurons including those with ascending projections.[42] Acetylcholine (Ach), 5-HT, and NE all are implicated in mediating these effects in both trigeminal and spinal regions.[43] Electrical stimulation of the NRM produces strong antinociception that can be reversed by either naloxone[44] or intrathecal 5-HT receptor antagonists or α_2 adrenoreceptor antagonists.[45] Glutamate microinjection in either the NRM or adjacent NGCα produces antinociception[46,47] supporting the view that cell bodies located in these regions are responsible for producing the antinociception. The antinociception derived from the NRM, but not the NGCα, could be blocked by intrathecal administration of a δ_2 opioid receptor antagonist[48] confirming possible involvement of spinal opioid systems.

Electrical and chemical stimulation of the NRM inhibits responses of spinothalamic tract cells to noxious inputs in monkeys. Lesions of the dorsolateral funiculi (DLFs) of the spinal cord

eliminate this inhibition and so this white matter pathway has been viewed as the primary spinal locus for descending fibers from the NRM.[49] Ventrolateral funiculi (VLFs) have also been implicated as the spinal pathways by which descending systems access the spinal dorsal horn but there is greater evidence for these descending paths to promote facilitatory influences as opposed to inhibitory influences.

NRM neurons responsible for producing spinal mechanisms of antinociception may be part of a direct raphespinal system, but NRM neurons also relay to secondary sites in the brain prior to joining other descending systems to the spinal cord. Inhibitory effects from the NRM/RVM can be antagonized by systemic or intrathecal administration of not only 5-HT antagonists, but also NE antagonists and GABA antagonists. For example, SPA from the NRM and the nucleus reticularis paragigantocellularis (NRPG) can be attenuated by either intrathecal administration of the nonspecific 5-HT receptor antagonist methysergide or the NE antagonist phentolamine.[50,51] Antinociception produced by microinjection of morphine in the NRM is blocked by either systemic naloxone or a 5-HT receptor antagonist.[52] While some investigators viewed the NRM and NRPG as functioning separately in pain suppression, Hammond and Yaksh[51] argued against a selective involvement of 5-HT and NE bulbospinal systems in SPA derived from the NRM and NRPG, respectively. NRM innervation of the A7 cell group could explain the NE component of inhibitory influences produced by activation of NRM cells, and although sparser connections exist to A5 and A6 regions, both support antinociception.[53]

Detailed electrical stimulation mapping and intensity studies of the RVM, and the NGC and NGCα in particular, reveal that these regions not only support inhibition of nociceptive reflexes, but also facilitation or enhancement of those reflexes under certain conditions.[21] Inhibition of the tail flick reflex has been observed in the majority of sites tested, particularly in the NRM, and ventral and lateral regions of the NGC and NGCα, but a substantial number of other sites, located primarily in the NGCα or more dorsally, supported facilitation of the tail flick reflex at lesser intensities of electrical stimulation. In most cases, facilitatory effects were supplanted by inhibitory effects at a given site of stimulation when greater intensities of electrical stimulation were examined. The results of behavioral studies were paralleled by in-depth analyses of the effects of either electrical stimulation or glutamate microinjection into the NGC and NGCα on spontaneous activity and noxious heat-evoked activity of spinal dorsal horn neurons. The results are generally comparable in nature. Electrical stimulation or glutamate microinjection produce only spinal inhibitory effects at most sites or biphasic effects (i.e., facilitatory effects at low intensities of stimulation and inhibitory effects at greater intensities of stimulation) at most of the remaining sites. Facilitatory effects are observed as a parallel leftward shift in the stimulus-response functions (SRFs) to graded heat, whereas inhibition is manifested as a rightward shift or a decrease in the slope of the SRF to heat. Inhibitory effects were also bilateral, such that unilateral and bilateral transactions of the DLFs both had an influence on descending inhibitory effects in the rat, as was shown previously for the NRM in behavioral studies. However, DLF transactions did not affect facilitatory effects in the rat, presumably because the descending systems responsible for facilitation traveled in the ventrolateral funiculi (VLFs). Cumulative sum analyses, which are used to determine how rapidly an effect occurs, revealed that the latency for inhibitory effects was much shorter (approximately 80 msec) than facilitatory effects (approximately 231 msec) derived from the RVM.

These outcomes, in conjunction with the behavioral studies, reinforced the notion that that activation of cell bodies in the NGC/NGCα can produce direct descending inhibitory effects via pathways traveling in the DLFs, but that the facilitatory effects required at least another relay prior to passage in the VLFs of the spinal cord.[54] Electrophysiological studies performed in monkeys have been generally consistent with studies in rodents with a few exceptions.[20] Specifically, electrical stimulation of the NGC has been shown to either inhibit or facilitate spinothalamic projection neurons in the lumbosacral or cervical regions of primates. These effects are somewhat preferential for nociceptive input, but responses to all types of stimuli, including nonnoxious stimuli, were affected. There was no obvious topographic organization of sites in the NGC that supported inhibition or facilitation. Unlike studies in rat, both inhibitory and facilitatory influences in primates are apparently unaffected by lesions of the DLFs.

In the rat, facilitation involving descending projections in the VLFs was mediated by spinal 5-HT$_1$ receptors[55] and cholecystokinin (CCK)$_B$ receptors, whereas inhibition involved descending projections in the DLFs and spinal cholinergic and monoaminergic receptors.[54,56–58] In a series of studies, Urban and colleagues[57,58] reported that low dose neurotensin microinjected in the RVM facilitated nociceptive reflexes and responses of spinal dorsal horn neurons to noxious thermal stimuli, but high doses of neurotensin inhibited spinal nociceptive processing. Urban and Gebhart[57] found that a neurotensin receptor antagonist SR48692 was able to block the high-dose inhibitory, but not the low-dose facilitatory effects of neurotensin administration in the NRM. Neubert et al.[59] then showed that microinjection of low doses of neurotensin in the RVM selectively activated subpopulations of medullary neurons and facilitated the paw withdrawal response to noxious heat. Recent evidence[60] indicates that the activation of the NT receptor subtype 1 (NTR1) is responsible for producing facilitatory effects and is mediated by spinal release of both NE and 5-HT, whereas activation of the NT receptor subtype 2 (NTR2) produces antinociception and is mediated by spinal release of NE. The source of endogenous neurotensin to the RVM is not known, but may include the PAG, nucleus cuneiformis, PB, and/or the NCPG.

Brain-derived neurotrophic factor (BDNF) also may be part of the PAG-RVM facilitatory network. Guo et al.[61] reported that microinjection of BDNF in the RVM facilitated the paw withdrawal response to noxious heat and this effect was blocked by administration of AP5, suggesting mediation by NMDA receptors (NMDARs). They also showed that a BDNF efferent projection exists from the ventrolateral PAG to the RVM, PAG stimulation releases BDNF in the RVM, and PAG stimulation activates TrkB and its signaling cascade and produces facilitatory effects. However, this pathway does not appear to be tonically active and may be a system reactive to tissue injury. Specifically, peripheral inflammation increased levels of both BDNF in the PAG and TrkB in RVM neurons, and sequestration of BDNF and RNAi of TrkB in the RVM suppressed the inflammatory hyperalgesia. Finally, CCK release in the RVM may also play a significant role in producing pronociceptive influences and may play a unique role in mediating "antiopioid" effects and opioid tolerance.

Locus Coeruleus

Using the nomenclature of Dahlstrom and Fuxe[62] the noradrenergic nuclei of the central nervous system are designated as "A" nuclei numbered in ascending order from the caudal medulla near the lateral reticular nucleus (A1) to the lateral pons near the parabrachial nucleus (A7). One of the most important of these nuclei is the A6 nucleus which colocalizes with and is also ventral to the morphologic structure, the locus coeruleus (LC). This area has extensive direct axonal projections to the spinal cord. Electrical stimulation or glutamate microinjection in the LC/A6 region produces antinociceptive effects in animals. These treatments generally inhibit reflex responses to noxious somatic stimuli, noxious colorectal distention, and responses of both trigeminal caudalis and spinal dorsal horn neurons to noxious stimuli in the rat.[63–68] The LC in rats and primates is composed primarily of NE-containing neurons[69] which provide most of the noradrenergic

innervation of the spinal cord[70] and stimulation of the LC results in spinal release of NE.[71] The descending fibers mediating the antinociception travel in the ventrolateral funiculi. The spinal inhibitory effects related to LC stimulation are primarily mediated by spinal α$_2$ adrenoreceptors[63] and the α$_{2A}$ subtype may be critical. α$_{2A}$ adrenoreceptor labeling is heavy throughout the spinal dorsal horn[72] and immunohistochemical studies show localization on terminals of capsaicin-sensitive, substance P containing primary afferents.[73] Spinal administration of α$_2$ adrenoreceptor agonists, and particularly those with an affinity for the α$_{2A}$ subtype, produce antinociception in a wide variety behavioral assays of both somatic and visceral nociception.[74] There is some evidence that the α$_{2C}$ receptor also may play a role in mediating the antinociceptive effects of adrenoreceptor agonists under conditions of neuropathic pain,[75] but this may be specific to that state and not normal pain modulation.[76] The effects of LC/A6 descending inhibition are independent of midbrain or medullary mediation, although the reverse is not necessarily true.

Parabrachial Nucleus/A7/Kölliker-Fuse Area

The parabrachial nucleus (PB) and adjacent A7/Kölliker-Fuse area has also been examined in relation to descending pain modulation. The Kölliker-Fuse nucleus, which is lateral and ventral to the LC, is the principal source of descending NE-containing fibers in the cat and may play a comparable role to that of the LC noted above for rat and primate.[77] The parabrachial nucleus (PB) has long been known for its role in respiratory and cardiovascular function, taste and aversions, locomotion, and sleep. However, the PB, the Kölliker-Fuse nucleus, and nucleus cuneiformis may all have particular relevance to descending modulation of nociception.

Unilateral electrical stimulation of or glutamate microinjection into the A7 cell group produces antinociception; for example, as indexed by bilateral increases in paw withdrawal responses to noxious heat, although it is generally more effective on the side ipsilateral to the stimulation site.[78] A7-mediated antinociception can be significantly reduced or abolished by intrathecal administration of nonselective α adrenergic receptor antagonists or selective α$_2$ adrenergic receptor antagonists. NE containing neurons in the A7 cell group project via the DLFs to terminate primarily in the ipsilateral spinal dorsal horn[79] and it is likely that these descending pathways mediate the effects of A7 stimulation, rather than relaying to other NE-containing cell groups in the brainstem. It is also likely that some antinociceptive effects derived from activation of RVM neurons are relayed to the A7 NE-containing neurons to produce their effects in conjunction with direct descending influences from the RVM. Similarly, the antinociceptive effects of SPA derived from the ventrolateral PAG may be mediated, in part, by direct projections to the A7 cell group[80] which then send their projections to the spinal cord.

Electrical stimulation in or glutamate activation of the PB inhibits nociceptive responses of trigeminal neurons,[81] although these effects have also been observed in neurons responsive to low threshold mechanical input. Occasional facilitation of nonnociceptive and nociceptive response of trigeminal nociceptive neurons when stimulating in the PB has also been observed. These facilitatory effects may bear on those described previously in the RVM, but have not been systematically studied. The PB has few direct projections to spinal cord but has connections with PAG, NRM, nucleus paragigantocellularis, and the ventrolateral medulla.

A5 Cell Group

Electrical stimulation of the region of the A5 cell group in the ventrolateral pons produces antinociception that can be antagonized by intrathecal administration of NE receptor antagonists.[82,83] The A5 cells project to the spinal cord, although their overall contribution to the total NE innervation of the spinal cord is relatively small, and A5 neurons may exert their effects primarily on lamina X neurons.[84] Afferents to the A5 cell group arise from the RVM, NTS, LC, dorsal raphe and lateral hypothalamus, and these regions are innervated by ascending fibers from the spinal cord. SPA derived from the ventrolateral PAG may be mediated by direct projections to the A5 cell group.[80]

Lateral Reticular Nucleus

The LRN is a bilateral structure located in the ventrolateral medulla (VLM) and lies in close proximity to the A1 (norepinephrine-containing) and C1 (epinephrine-containing) cell groups. Electrical and glutamate stimulation of the LRN inhibits spinal nociceptive reflexes and responses of spinal dorsal horn neurons to noxious stimuli.[85–87] These effects can be antagonized by spinal administration of α_2 receptor antagonists.[87] The involvement of spinal adrenoreceptors in these antinociceptive effects suggests that the LRN relays to a NE containing cell group to produce these outcomes because little or no NE-containing fibers descend from the LRN. The A5 or A7 regions may be involved in this mediation since local anesthetic blockade of the LC does not affect antinociceptive effects of LRN activation.[86] The descending inhibitory effects of LRN activation are mediated by fibers traveling in the DLFs, not the VLFs, again suggesting potential involvement of A5 or A7 cell groups rather than the A6 cell group. The LRN is also innervated by the PAG, parabrachial nucleus, LC, and NRM regions suggesting complex reciprocal interactions exist between all these regions. The LRN has also played a role in the issue of tonic descending inhibitory influences on spinal nociceptive function. It was suggested that the LRN was the primary source of tonic descending inhibitory influence based on lesions studies of the cat but these outcomes were not reproduced in studies of the rat.[85,86]

Nucleus Tractus Solitarius

Several studies have demonstrated that the NTS is a region that is both capable of modulating pain and may serve as a relay site for peripheral cardiopulmonary afferent influences on nociception. Electrical stimulation of the NTS inhibits the nociceptive tail flick reflex evoked by noxious heat[88–90] and inhibits noxious heat-evoked, pinch-evoked, and C-fiber evoked responses of spinal dorsal horn neurons in rat and cat.[91,92] Systematic mapping studies indicated that lateral sites within the NTS supported antinociception, while medial sites evoke motor responses.[90,91] Glutamate microinjection in caudal, but not rostral, NTS produces antinociception[93] and inhibits responses of spinal dorsal horn neurons to noxious heat and stimulation of spinal afferents.[92,94] The NTS has few direct spinal projections suggesting that changes in nociception derived from the NTS involved secondary relays including the NRM, LC/A6, PAG, A5 cell groups, and other forebrain loops.[93,94] This view is consistent with the finding that antinociception produced by glutamate microinjection in the NTS can be antagonized in a dose-dependent manner by intrathecal administration of the combination of an α-adrenergic and 5-HT receptor antagonists, but is unaffected by intrathecal administration of either agent alone, or by the opioid receptor antagonist naloxone.

Diencephalon

Electrical stimulation of a variety of hypothalamic structures results in antinociception, although not necessarily with similar characteristics. The hypothalamus has connections with a variety of structures implicated in descending inhibitory influences including the PAG, NTS, and RVM and these sites may be necessary for the effects of the hypothalamus on nociception.[95–99] Electrical stimulation of the paraventricular nucleus of the hypothalamus inhibits both the tail flick reflex in lightly anesthetized rats and the paw lick response in the hot plate test in conscious rats[100] which is unaffected by naloxone administration. In contrast, electrical stimulation of the arcuate nucleus of the hypothalamus also inhibits the tail flick reflex and intrathecal administration of naloxone reverses this inhibitory effect.[101] Electrical stimulation of either the anterior hypothalamus or lateral hypothalamus (LH), or morphine microinjection into either the LH or posterior regions of the hypothalamus, inhibits a variety of responses to noxious input including the tail flick reflex to noxious heat, behavioral responses in the formalin test, and responses of wide dynamic range neurons to noxious heating of the skin.

Cerebral Cortex

Stimulation of both somatosensory cortex (SSC) and motor cortex (MC) have been used in the clinical treatment of neuropathic pain, central post stroke pain, and phantom limb pain. These have been achieved using either electrical stimulation or transcranial magnetic stimulation and, while spinal influences of such treatments have been reported, there is reason to believe most of their effects are mediated at the supraspinal level.[102] These factors notwithstanding, there is evidence for SSC and other cortical influences in producing descending inhibition of spinal nociceptive transmission via various brainstem sites. Senapati et al.[103] provided one of the stronger demonstrations of cortical influences on spinal nociceptive transmission. They showed that electrical stimulation of either the ipsilateral or contralateral primary SSC of rats inhibited responses of L5–L6 WDR neurons to noxious pressure and pinch, but not brush. In contrast, electrical stimulation of the secondary SSC has been reported to produce only a weak behavioral antinociception in the second phase of the formalin test, and was without effect on responses to noxious thermal and mechanical stimuli.[104] There are reports that electrical stimulation of or glutamate microinjections into the ventrolateral orbital cortex (VLO) can inhibit the tail flick reflex via the PAG,[105,106] but others have found pronociceptive effects of similar treatments.[107] Morphine administration in the VLO also has been reported to inhibit both the hot plate and paw withdrawal responses to noxious heat in intact rats, and the tactile allodynia, hot plate, and paw withdrawal responses in rats with peripheral mononeuropathy. The antinociceptive effects observed in neuropathic rats were reversed by naloxone while those observed in intact rats were not affected by naloxone. However, it cannot be ascertained from these studies whether descending inhibitory systems were activated by morphine since all of the response measures were are organized at the supraspinal level.[108] Morphine microinjection in the rostral agranular insular cortex (RAIS), a structure immediately caudal to the VLO, also has been reported to inhibit nociceptive responses in the formalin test, reduce c-Fos expression in the spinal cord ipsilateral to a formalin stimulus, and produce a naloxone-reversible inhibition of spinal dorsal horn neuronal responses to a noxious thermal stimulus.[109] The influence on the RAIS on descending inhibitory influences may critically depend on dopamine acting on neurons in this region.[110]

There is also evidence that some cortical regions can provide descending facilitatory influences. Electrical stimulation or chemical activation of metabotropic glutamate receptors (mGluRs) in the anterior cingulate cortex (ACC) produced significant facilitation of the tail flick reflex evoked by noxious heat in rats and could be blocked by local anesthesia of the RVM, whereas microinjection of either the mu-opioid receptor, DAMGO, or the delta-opioid receptor agonist, DPDPE, into the ACC inhibited paw lick responses in mice.[111] Similar evidence of hyperalgesia derived from activation of the ACC were obtained by Zhang et al.[112] They showed that high frequency electrical stimulation of the ACC produced long lasting increases in C-fiber field potentials evoked from the sciatic nerve, decreases in paw withdrawal latencies to noxious heating of the rat hind paw, and similar effects were obtained using microinjections of either NMDA or homocysteic acid into the ACC. These effects could be blocked by bilateral lesions of the dorsal reticular nucleus, a site often cited as a possible final common pathway for descending facilitatory influences. Interestingly, these effects were particularly long-lasting, with some lasting over an hour, and merit further research on possible stimulation-induced changes in the ACC itself.

Summary of Supraspinal Influences

There is overwhelming support for the structures discussed in the previous sections in mediating descending inhibitory and facilitatory influences on spinal nociceptive transmission. There is also overwhelming support that activation of most of these structures involves spinal release of *both* SHT and NE in producing inhibitory phenomena, but many other neurotransmitters including acetylcholine, GABA, glycine, substance P, corticotrophin releasing factor, urocortins, thyroid stimulating hormone, and oxytocin which have been described as part of both excitatory and inhibitory mechanisms.[113] Thus, "coactivation" or "recruitment" of more than a single system appears to be the rule rather than the exception.[114] Only the inhibitory effects derived from activation of the A5 and A6 cell groups appears to involve a single transmitter, NE, and a single spinal receptor system, α_2 adrenoreceptors. It is quite surprising, therefore, that while the discovery of endogenous opioids prompted the intense study of descending modulatory systems, endogenous opioids per se have not figured prominently in the "system" side of the analyses. Rather they appear far more critical in the local circuitries of specific brainstem or spinal regions that allow these systems to function. Furthermore, while the structures supplying these transmitters affecting spinal nociceptive transmission have been identified, for the most part, our general knowledge about how those structures interact in producing inhibitory and facilitatory effects is still not well understood.

On-, Off-, and Neutral Cells

With the identification of CNS sites that could be stimulated to produce inhibitory and/or facilitatory effects at the spinal cord level came theories related to the neuronal constituents of those sites. Studies performed by Fields and colleagues[115,116] demonstrated the existence of three types of neurons in the RVM that can be classified based on the neuron's response to noxious heat applied to the tail of a lightly anesthetized rat that elicited the tail flick reflex. ON cells were shown to increase their firing rate just before the occurrence of the tail flick, OFF cells decreased their firing rate just before the occurrence of the tail flick, and NEUTRAL cells showed no change in activity throughout the application of noxious heat. Importantly, the activity of ON and OFF cells, but not NEUTRAL cells, was shown to be affected by systemic administration of morphine. At doses of systemic morphine that inhibit the tail flick reflex, OFF cells became continuously active and failed to pause before reflex movements whereas ON cell activity decreased.[116,117] These and other findings led to the proposition that OFF cells exert descending inhibitory effects on spinal nociceptive transmission. ON cells were hypothesized to exert a pronociceptive or facilitatory influence. NEUTRAL cells were purported to have no role in nociception.

Extensive studies have examined the role of ON and OFF cells in relation to other descending modulation-related phenomena with a mixture of results, but the role of a subpopulation of these

neurons in pain modulation is firmly established. Neurons with the same characteristics as RVM ON and OFF cells have been identified in other CNS sites such as the PAG such that an exclusive role of the ON and OFF cells located in the RVM is unlikely. An exclusive association of ON and OFF cells with nociception is similarly unlikely. Mason[22] has argued that there is substantial evidence that these cells are involved in a variety of homeostatic control functions including micturition, arterial blood pressure control, and that they should be viewed as modulating a much broader spectrum of somatosensory inputs than nociception. Indeed, correlative data supporting a role of ON and OFF cells in control of arterial blood pressure is equally as compelling as for pain modulation. Whether different subsets of ON and OFF cells serve different functions, or whether individual ON and OFF cells can subserve or coordinate many different functions, remains to be determined.

TRIGGERS OF CLINICAL HYPERSENSITIVITY

Allodynia and Hyperalgesia

The terms allodynia and hyperalgesia are clinical terms that represent different forms of hypersensitivity. Defined using clinical terms, allodynia has been defined as "pain produced by a stimulus that does not normally cause pain." Similarly defined, hyperalgesia is "an increased response to a stimulus that is normally painful" which may mean either a lower threshold for evoking pain or a higher intensity of pain perception produced by a given intensity of a suprathreshold painful stimulus. Based on psychophysical experiments, hyperalgesia may be either "primary" when it is located at a site of injury such as a burn or "secondary" when altered sensations are evoked from uninjured tissue that typically surrounds the site of injury, but in some cases could be physically distant. Primary hyperalgesia has generally been relegated to mechanisms involving the primary afferents and secondary hyperalgesia to spinal second order neuron effects.

Both allodynia and hyperalgesia are normal physiological responses to injury but also occur in other conditions including neuropathic pain. Notably, when studying hypersensitivity in nonhuman animal models interpretive issues can be problematic, particularly when studying phenomena that have clinical definitions. For purposes of the present discussion hyperalgesia will be defined as augmented responses and/or lowered stimulus thresholds for response to a nociceptive stimulus. Allodynia will be defined as the evocation of responses that would have been called nociceptive (e.g., flexion-withdrawal responses) to clearly nonnociceptive stimuli (e.g., light brushing).

Inflammation-Induced Hypersensitivity

As noted previously, tissue damaging events can result in the peripheral sensitization of primary afferent nociceptors and the central sensitization of spinal dorsal horn neurons. Historically, these two phenomena have played a fundamental role in accounting for primary and secondary hyperalgesia, respectively. These phenomena were viewed as either increased input to or increased responsiveness of second order neurons with an emphasis on local spinal mechanisms. However, a role for brainstem descending control systems in both primary and secondary hyperalgesia phenomena are now receiving increasing attention and have led to a much better understanding of persistent pain states. There is now evidence that the RVM and the LC are responsible for exerting primarily descending inhibitory influences under conditions of primary hyperalgesia associated with either somatic or visceral tissue damage, and primarily descending facilitatory influences under conditions of secondary hyperalgesia. These processes are not well understood but spinobulbospinal loops are now being proposed to recognize that enhanced afferent input from the spinal dorsal horn ascends either directly or indirectly to the RVM, which in turn, changes this balance and ultimately, the perception of pain.

A wide variety of evidence supports a role for the RVM in both the development and maintenance of secondary hyperalgesia resulting from inflammation.[118,119] Similar results have been obtained in behavioral studies with various inflammatory agents including mustard oil, carrageen, and formalin. For example, topical application of mustard oil to the ankle of a rat produces tactile allodynia of the foot which can be prevented by either spinal transection or local anesthetic blockade of the RVM.[120] Lidocaine microinjection reversed or prior bilateral ibotenic acid lesions of the rostral medial medulla prevented secondary thermal hyperalgesia induced by either intraarticular administration of carrageenan or topical application of mustard oil to the hind leg, but did not affect primary hyperalgesia produced by intraplantar administration of carrageenan.[121] Interestingly, the ibotenic acid lesions in this study were highly restricted, localized only to the NGC and dorsal paragigantocellular nuclei, and none impinged on either the NGCα or the NRM. Yet, secondary thermal hyperalgesia was also eliminated using the same preparation and topical application of mustard oil to the hind leg with either spinal transection or extensive electrolytic lesions of the RVM that appeared more ventral to the ibotenic acid lesions, and included the NRM.[122] Thus, the NGC, dorsal paragigantocellular nuclei, NGCα, and NRM may all contribute to this phenomenon.

There is also substantial evidence that RVM ON cells, originally hypothesized to exert a pronociceptive effect, may be responsible for contributing to the descending facilitatory influences that result in secondary hyperalgesia in persistent pain states. Acute inflammation produced by ipsilateral topical application of mustard oil above the knee of a rat increases ongoing ON cell discharge and decreases ongoing discharge of OFF cells. These changes correlate with a decrease in the withdrawal latency of the ipsilateral, but not contralateral paw. Thus, mustard oil-induced inflammation caused a shift in the balance between ON and OFF cell firing, such that ON cells were more likely to be in an active phase and OFF cells in a quiescent phase.[123] This hyperalgesic effect could be blocked by either lidocaine infusion[123] or a local infusion of the NMDA-receptor antagonist APV[124] into the RVM suggesting the NMDA-receptor activation induced by inflammation contributes to the secondary hyperalgesia.

The spinobulbospinal loop engaged by peripheral cutaneous inflammation and mediating secondary hyperalgesia may involve spinal release of CCK because intrathecal administration of CCK antagonists block these effects.[122] These data suggest that at least one descending facilitatory system uses either intrinsic spinal CCK neurons, or descending medullospinal CCK projecting neurons in producing these effects. However, administration of these CCK receptor antagonists, and blockade of these facilitatory effects, also reveals an underlying descending inhibition that was engaged by the inflammatory treatment; supporting the view that concomitant activation of both facilitatory and inhibitory descending systems occurs under conditions of inflammation and the relative balance between the two dictates the type of pain state.

Inflammation-Induced Inhibitory Systems

Whereas secondary hyperalgesia may be augmented by descending facilitatory systems, primary hyperalgesia (increased primary afferent activity) associated with either acute or persistent inflammation may actively engage descending *inhibitory* influences. Schaible et al.[125] showed that a mixture of kaolin and carrageenan injected into the knee joint of the cat resulted in a progressive increase in both spontaneous activity and evoked activity of spinal dorsal horn neurons to innocuous and noxious stimuli. Reversible interruption of descending modulatory influences using spinal cold block further increased activity in a progressive fashion demonstrating that spinal descending inhibitory influences were being progressively engaged by inflammation. Ren and Dubner[126] showed that primary thermal hyperalgesia produced by carrageenan administration into the hind paw of the rat was increased by prior transactions of the DLFs, and that lidocaine microinjection in the RVM increased the spontaneous activity of nociceptive dorsal horn neurons, and their responses to mechanical and thermal stimulation of the inflamed hind paw.

In the RVM, this enhancement of descending inhibitory influences may reflect inflammation-induced increases in the synthesis of enkephalins and/or enhanced efficacy of endogenous opioids acting at mu- and delta-opioid receptors such that the effectiveness of opioids is increased.[127,128] Mechanistically, these changes would be consistent with opioid inhibition of pronociceptive ON cells and disinhibition of pro-inhibitory OFF cells; the net outcome of which should be enhanced descending inhibition. They also depend on RVM glutaminergic influences which apparently vary as a function of time after inflammation. At shorter times after inflammation, for example, 3 hours, an increase in glutaminergic descending facilitation tends to counteract the descending inhibitory influences, but then dissipates as a function of time over the next 24 hours.[129,130] There are corresponding spinal changes that accompany these changes in the RVM including increased sensitivity to both NE and opioidergic spinal inhibitory mechanisms.

Complete Freund's Adjuvant (CFA) injected into the hind paw of the rat has been reported to increase the NR1, NR2A, and NR2B NMDA receptor subunit expression in the RVM beginning at 5 hours after inflammation and persisting for up to 7 days.[131] These data suggest that inflammation can produce a prolonged upregulation of NMDA receptor subunit gene expression that could contribute to RVM excitability and be viewed as "brainstem central sensitization" following inflammation. CFA injected into the hind paw of the rat also induces increases in mRNA for spinal lumbar dynorphin and enkephalin, and therefore may be molecular markers of hyperalgesia associated with inflammation. These changes in mRNA expression are increased further in rats with thoracic spinal transection indicating that descending afferents inhibit responses of opioid-containing neurons to noxious stimulation.[132]

The LC/A6 region may play a comparable role to the RVM in attenuating the development of primary hyperalgesia induced by acute inflammatory pain, but not necessarily persistent inflammatory pain. For example, behavioral thermal hyperalgesia produced by subcutaneous injection of carrageenan resulted in a small, but significant enhancement by prior bilateral lesions of the LC.[133] However, this effect was only observed 4 hours after carrageenan injection, and not observed 7 days after carrageenan, even though edema and hyperalgesia were still present at 7 days.[134] Interestingly, recruitment of the descending LC inhibitory influence derived from unilateral hind paw inflammation was expressed only unilaterally, but both in the lumbar region innervating the inflamed paw and in the cervical region markedly distant from the area of primary inflammation.[135] Systemic naloxone administration produced a further decrease of the paw withdrawal latencies to noxious thermal stimulation at 4 hours after carrageenan administration in LC-lesioned, but not in sham-operated rats. Similar effects of bilateral LC lesions in enhancing thermally evoked noxious responses of spinal dorsal horn neurons in rats have been reported.[136] These data suggest that the development of hyperalgesia in the acute phase of inflammation might depend on the interaction between the descending modulation system from the LC and an opioid inhibitory system, and that an intact LC system suppresses the opioid influence. Upregulation of spinal α2 adrenoreceptors under conditions of inflammation may therefore enhance the potency of this descending inhibitory influence.

That descending inhibitory influences are recruited from both the RVM and LC under conditions of inflammation are supported by studies of spinal cord lesions. Wei et al.[137] observed that the c-fos expression observed in the L4–L5 spinal segments observed 24 hours after hind paw injection of CFA was significantly increased on the side ipsilateral, but not contralateral to the injection by either bilateral DLF or VLF lesions. The increases occurred in both superficial and deep laminae, as well as lamina III-IV, region of termination of mechanoreceptor afferents. Presumably, descending facilitatory influences accompanying the CFA-induced inflammatory state, and which should have been eliminated by these lesions, were masked by the descending inhibitory influences.

However, outcomes obtained with formalin are not as quite as clear with respect to descending inhibition and primary hyperalgesia. Vanegas and Schaible[119] argued that if the early phase (1–5 minutes) and late (15–60 minutes) phase responses to subcutaneous injection of formalin are viewed as a primary hyperalgesia, then the predominant formalin-activated descending influence is facilitation rather than inhibition. However, these views were based on a limited number of studies involving a spinal 5-HT3 antagonist (ondansetron) and RVM recordings of ON and OFF cells[138] that were not consistent with those obtained by Robinson et al.[139] Hence, additional work may be required before the role of descending influences can be stated for formalin-induced pain.

Neuropathic Pain

The injury of peripheral nerves has many consequences, one of which is an alteration in spinal dorsal horn neuron excitability. One of the recently identified mechanisms important to this is the activation of spinal microglia by substances such as fractaline released by the central processes of the injured nerves. Subsequent release of cytokines, purines, and growth factors result in the sensitization of second order nociceptive neurons[140] and subsequent increased excitability reflected as hyperalgesia and allodynia. These spinal mechanisms are not the whole phenomenon as there is clear evidence that supraspinal modulatory systems are also important to the development of hypersensitivity following nerve injury. In particular, the RVM is now believed to significantly contribute to neuropathic pain produced by such experimental treatments such as loose ligation of L5–L6 spinal and chronic sciatic nerve transection. For example, inactivation of the RVM with lidocaine injections both enhanced the withdrawal response and the thermal and tactile hypersensitivity produced by peripheral nerve injury.[141,142] Various lines of evidence suggest that RVM ON cells may be critical for sustaining neuropathic pain. Selective lesions of ON cells, produced by microinjection of demorphin conjugated to the cytotoxin saporin, blocks the thermal hyperalgesia and tactile hyperesthesias produced by peripheral nerve injury.[142] Other evidence suggests that the effect of ON cells in contributing to neuropathic pain may reside in spinal release of 5-HT and a presynaptic action on 5-HT3 receptors located on SP-containing terminals.[143] Similar effects may be responsible for selective effects on the mechanical allodynia that occurs in spinal cord injury (SCI). For example, administration of the 5-HT3 receptor antagonist ondansetron significantly attenuates mechanical allodynia in an SCI model and administration of m-chloropheynlbiguanide (m-CPBG), a 5-HT3 agonist, exaggerated pain behaviors.[144] Interestingly, however, similar studies conducted of inflammatory pain using carrageenan revealed little influence of a descending system using 5-HT3 receptors.[145] Yet, the precise details relating ON cell activation to spinal 5-HT release remain to be worked out since some studies have reported that neither ON nor OFF cells contain 5-HT.[146,147]

In neuropathic pain, the influence of the LC/A6 may be reduced. Following rhizotomy, the antinociceptive effect produced by LC stimulation is reduced.[148]

Opioid-Induced Hyperalgesia

Opiates remain the primary treatment for a wide variety of pain disorders in both acute and chronic clinical pain disorders. Prolonged administration of opiates can be associated with significant reactive processes including the development of tolerance to the analgesic effects of the drugs such that greater doses of drug are required to achieve adequate pain relief. Recently it has been recognized that exposure to opioids can also result in paradoxical pain including regions not described in the initial pain complaint,[149] a phenomenon commonly referred to as "opioid-induced hyperalgesia"[150] although the terms "opioid-abstinence hyperalgesia" and "opioid-withdrawal hyperalgesia" have also been used to describe similar, if not identical, phenomena. Many substances delivered spinally can reverse or block antinociceptive tolerance as well as opioid-induced hyperalgesia which include NMDA receptor antagonists, phosphokinase C inhibitors, cyclooxygenase inhibitors, and use of differing opioid receptor subtype agonists/antagonists.[150] It is also clear that there is an effect of chronic opioids on descending pain modulatory systems that is critical to the development of the spinal cord changes mediating paradoxical pain and antinociceptive tolerance with known neuroexcitatory effects arising within the RVM and PAG[151-154] when the effects of opioids are rapidly reversed by naloxone or other substances interacting with opioid systems. Additional evidence that supraspinal modulatory systems are involved in the mechanisms of opioid-induced hyperalgesia includes the demonstration that animals with lesions of the dorsolateral funiculi of the spinal cord do not appear to develop abnormal pain or antinociceptive tolerance that are normally a consequence of prolonged opiate administration.[155,156] Further, the effects of both acute and prolonged exposure to morphine (tactile hyperesthesia, thermal hyperalgesia, and antinociceptive tolerance) are abolished by local anesthesia blockade of the RVM.[155-157] Thus, opioid-induced pain and tolerance in these circumstances may be mediated in part by activation of descending facilitatory mechanisms arising in the RVM. This, in turn, has been suggested to act as a trigger for the upregulation of spinal dynorphin that serves to promote enhanced input from nociceptors.[158] An underlying assumption related to these studies has been that opioid-induced hyperalgesia requires the activation of opioid receptors. However, it is possible that opioid drugs may also be acting by nonopioid mechanisms to produce their physiological effects. The demonstration that opioid-induced hyperalgesia can be elicited in mice without functional mu-, kappa-, or delta-opioid receptors supports this possibility.[159] At this point in time, it is clear that the use of opioids for the treatment of pain leads to a series of complicated interactions in spinal pain processing systems such that the resultant physiological effects may be at times beneficial (analgesic) and at other times detrimental to the function of the organism.

CONCLUSION

The original proposition of Gate Control theory of Melzack and Wall[2] that nociceptive input to spinal dorsal horn neurons could be modulated by a number of systems prompted investigations of the systems that modulate our perception of pain. One could hardly have envisioned both the diversity and complexity of the systems that have been identified. The original notions of systems descending from supraspinal sites to the spinal cord to inhibit pain have been expanded to include descending systems that also enhance our perception of pain. At the present time, our analyses indicate these two systems are functionally and anatomically intertwined and appear to operate as a unit rather than as separate entities. The ultimate perception we develop following exposure to noxious events represents some balance between these two systems. It is possible that these systems attenuate or amplify responses to noxious stimuli in order to enhance our ability to localize and attend to peripheral stimuli that threaten us. Studies of stress, inflammation, neuropathic pain, drug-induced hypersensitivity, or other mechanisms leading to chronic pain states have begun to demonstrate that deficits in descending inhibition and/or activation of descending facilitation-related systems may also serve as mechanisms of pain generation or amplification.

Studies related to the neurotransmitters of modulation have consistently identified NE, SHT, and endogenous opioids to be key substances involved in the balance of inhibitory and excitatory influences. It should come as no small wonder then, that the drugs clinicians find useful in the treatment of hypersensitivity and pain are associated with noradrenergic, serotonergic, and opioidergic function within the CNS. It is the subtleties of the pharmacology that will define future refinements in therapeutics and many of these subtleties are only now being defined.

References

1. Terman GW, Bonica JJ. Spinal mechanisms and their modulation. In: Loeser JD, Butler SH, Chapman CR, Turk DC, eds. *Bonica's Management of Pain.* 3rd ed. Philadelphia: Lippincott Williams & Wilkins; 2001:73–153.
2. Melzack R, Wall PD. Pain mechanisms: a new theory. *Science* 1965;150(699): 971–979.
3. McMahon SB, Morrison JF. Two groups of spinal interneurones that respond to stimulation of the abdominal viscera of the cat. *J Physiol* 1982;322:21–34.
4. McMahon SB, Morrison JF. Spinal neurones with long projections activated from the abdominal viscera of the cat. *J Physiol* 1982;322:1–20.
5. Noordenbos W. *Pain.* Amsterdam: Elsevier; 1959.
6. Le Bars D, Dickenson AH, Besson JM. Diffuse noxious inhibitory controls (DNIC). I. Effects on dorsal horn convergent neurones in the rat. *Pain* 1979; 6:283–304.
7. Le Bars D, Dickenson AH, Besson JM. Diffuse noxious inhibitory controls (DNIC). II. Lack of effect on non-convergent neurons, supraspinal involvement and theoretical implications. *Pain* 1979;6:305–327.
8. LeBars D. The whole body receptive field of dorsal horn multireceptive neurons. *Brain Res Brain Res Rev* 2002;40:29–44.
9. Mendell LM. Physiological properties of unmyelinated fiber projections to the spinal cord. *Exp Neurol* 1966;16:316–332.
10. Woolf CJ. Evidence for a central component of post-injury pain hypersensitivity. *Nature* 1983;306:686–688.
11. Sandkühler J. Understanding LTP in pain pathways. *Mol Pain* 2007;3:9.
12. Sherrington CS, Sowton SC. Observations on reflex responses to single break-shocks. *J Physiol* 1915;49:331–348.
13. Fulton JF. *Muscular Contraction and the Reflex Control of Movement.* Baltimore: Williams & Wilkins; 1926.
14. Lundberg A. Supraspinal control of transmission in reflex paths to motoneurons and primary afferents. *Prog Brain Res* 1964;12:197–221.
15. Wall PD. The laminar organization of the dorsal horn and effects of descending impulses. *J Physiol* 1967;188:403–423.
16. Reynolds DV. Surgery in the rat during electrical analgesia induced by focal brain stimulation. *Science* 1969;164:444–445.
17. Mayer DJ, Liebeskind JC. Pain reduction by focal electrical stimulation of the brain: an anatomical and behavioral analysis. *Brain Res* 1974;68:73–93.
18. Mayer DJ, Wolfle TL, Akil H, et al. Analgesia from electrical stimulation in the brainstem of the rat. *Science* 1971;174:1351–1354.
19. Adams JE. Naloxone reversal of analgesia produced by brain stimulation in the human. *Pain* 1976;2:161–166.
20. Haber LH, Martin RF, Chung JM, et al. Inhibition and excitation of primate spinothalamic tract neurons by stimulation in the region of nucleus reticularis gigantocellularis. *J Neurophysiol* 1980;43:1578–1593.
21. Zhuo M, Gebhart GF. Characterization of descending inhibition and facilitation from the nuclei reticularis gigantocellularis and gigantocellularis pars alpha in the rat. *Pain* 1990;42:337–350.
22. Mason P. Ventromedial medulla: Pain modulation and beyond. *J Comp Neurol* 2005;493:2–8.
23. Fardin V, Oliveras JL, Besson JM. A reinvestigation of the analgesic effects induced by stimulation of the periaqueductal gray matter in the rat. I. The production of behavioral side effects together with analgesia. *Brain Res* 1984; 306(1–2):105–123.
24. Fardin V, Oliveras JL, Besson JM. A reinvestigation of the analgesic effects induced by stimulation of the periaqueductal gray matter in the rat. II. Differ-

25. ential characteristics of the analgesia induced by ventral and dorsal PAG stimulation. *Brain Res* 1984;306:125–139.
25. Dostrovsky JO. Raphe and periaqueductal gray induced suppression of non-nociceptive neuronal responses in the dorsal column nuclei and trigeminal sub-nucleus caudalis. *Brain Res* 1980;200:184–189.
26. Lewis VA, Gebhart GF. Evaluation of the periaqueductal central gray (PAG) as a morphine-specific locus of action and examination of morphine-induced and stimulation produced analgesia at coincident PAG loci. *Brain Res* 1977; 124:283–303.
27. Yaksh TL, Rudy TA. Narcotic analgesics: CNS sites and mechanisms of action as revealed by intracerebral injection techniques. *Pain* 1978;4:299–359.
28. Pert CB, Snyder SH. Opiate receptor: Demonstration in nervous tissue. *Science* 1973;179:1011–1014.
29. Cox BM, Opheim KE, Teschemacher H, et al. A peptide-like substance from pituitary that acts like morphine. 2. Purification and properties. *Life Sci* 1975; 16:1777–1782.
30. Hughes J, Smith TW, Kosterlitz HW, et al. Identification of two related penta-peptides from the brain with potent opiate agonist activity. *Nature* 1975; 258(5536):577–580.
31. Simantov R, Snyder SH. Morphine-like peptides in mammalian brain: Isolation, structure elucidation, and interactions with the opiate receptor. *Proc Natl Acad Sci U S A;*1976;73:2515–2519.
32. Atweh S, Kuhar MJ. Autoradiographic localization of opiate receptors in rat brain. II. The brain stem. *Brain Res* 1977;129:1–12.
33. Mayer DJ, Hayes RL. Stimulation-produced analgesia: development of tolerance and cross-tolerance to morphine. *Science* 1975;188(4191)961–962.
34. Akil H, Mayer DJ, Liebeskind JC. Antagonism of stimulation-produced analgesia by naloxone, a narcotic antagonist. *Science* 1976;191(4230):961–962.
35. Budai D, Fields HL. Endogenous opioid peptides acting at mu-opioid receptors in the dorsal horn contribute to midbrain modulation of spinal nociceptive neurons. *J Neurophysiol* 1998;79:677–687.
36. Yaksh TL, Yeung JC, Rudy TA. An inability to antagonize with naloxone the elevated nociceptive thresholds resulting from electrical stimulation of the mesencephalic central gray. *Life Sci* 1976;18:1193–1198.
37. Yaksh TL. Direct evidence that spinal serotonin and noradrenalin terminals mediate the spinal antinociceptive effects of morphine in the periaqueductal gray. *Brain Res* 1979;180–185.
38. Yaksh TL, Tyce GM. Microinjection of morphine into the periaqueductal gray evokes the release of serotonin from spinal cord. *Brain Res* 1979;171: 176–181.
39. Camarata PJ, Yaksh TL. Characterization of the spinal adrenergic receptors mediating the spinal effects produced by microinjection of morphine into the periaqueductal gray. *Brain Res* 1985;336:133–142.
40. Basbaum AI, Fields HL. Endogenous pain control systems: review and hypothesis. *Ann Neurol* 1978;4:451–462.
41. Basbaum AI, Fields HL. Endogenous pain control systems: Brainstem spinal pathways and endorphin circuitry. *Annu Rev Neurosci* 1984;7:309–338.
42. Gerhart KD, Wilcox TK, Chung JM, et al. Inhibition of nociceptive and non-nociceptive responses of primate spinothalamic cells by stimulation in medial brain stem. *J Neurophysiol* 1981;45:121–136.
43. Li P, Zhuo M. Cholinergic, noradrenergic, and serotonergic inhibition of fast synaptic transmission in the spinal lumbar dorsal horn of rat. *Brain Res Bull* 2001;54:639–647.
44. Oliveras JL, Hosobuchi Y, Redjemi F, et al. Opiate antagonist, naloxone, strongly reduces analgesia induced by stimulation of a raphe nucleus (centralis inferior). *Brain Res* 1977;129:221–229.
45. Barbaro NM, Hammond DL, Fields HL. Effects of intrathecally administered methysergide and yohimbine on microstimulation-produced antinociception in the rat. *Brain Res* 1985;23:223–229.
46. Jensen TS, Yaksh TL. Spinal monoamine and opiate systems partly mediate the antinociceptive effects produced by glutamate at brainstem studies. *Brain Res* 1984;321:287–297.
47. Sandkühler J, Gebhart GF. Relative contributions of the nucleus raphe magnus and adjacent medullary reticular formation to the inhibition by stimulation in the periaqueductal gray of a spinal nociceptive reflex in the pentobarbital-anesthetized rat. *Brain Res* 1984;305:77–87.
48. Hammond DL, Donahue BB, Stewart PE. Role spinal delta1 and delta2 opioid receptors in the antinociception produced by microinjection of L-glutamate in the ventromedial medulla of the rat. *Brain Res* 1997;765:177–181.
49. Basbaum AI, Clanton CH, Fields HL. Three bulbospinal pathways from the rostral medulla of the cat: an autoradiographic study of pain modulating systems. *J Comp Neurol* 1978;178:209–224.
50. Yaksh TL, Al-Rodhan NR, Jensen TS. Sites of action of opiates in production of analgesia. *Prog Brain Res* 1998;77:371–394.
51. Hammond DL, Yaksh TL. Antagonism of stimulation-produced antinociception by intrathecal administration of methysergide or phentolamine. *Brain Res* 1984;298:329–337.
52. Azami J, Llewelyn MB, Roberts MH. The contribution of nucleus reticularis paragigantocellularis and nucleus raphe magnus to the analgesia produced by systemically administered morphine, investigated with the microinjection technique. *Pain* 1982;12:229–246.
53. Clark FM, Proudfit HK. Projections of neurons in the ventromedial medulla to pontine catecholamine cell groups involved in the modulation of nociception. *Brain Res* 1991;540:105–115.
54. Zhuo M, Gebhart GF. Characterization of descending facilitation and inhibition of spinal nociceptive transmission from the nuclei reticularis gigantocellu-

laris and gigantocellularis pars alpha in the rat. *J Neurophysiol* 1992;67:1599–1614.

55. Zhuo M, Gebhart GF. Spinal serotonin receptors mediate descending facilitation of a nociceptive reflex from the nuclei reticularis gigantocellularis and gigantocellularis pars alpha in the rat. *Brain Res* 1991;550:35–48.

56. Zhuo M, Gebhart GF. Biphasic modulation of spinal nociceptive transmission from the medullary raphe nuclei in the rat. *J Neurophysiol* 1997;78:746–758.

57. Urban MO, Gebhart GF. Characterization of biphasic modulation of spinal nociceptive transmission by neurotensin in the rat rostral ventromedial medulla. *J Neurophysiol* 1997;78:1550–1562.

58. Urban MO, Smith DJ. Role of neurotensin in the nucleus raphe magnus in opioid induced antinociception from the periaqueductal grey. *J Pharmacol Exp Ther* 1993;265:580–586.

59. Neubert MJ, Kincaid W, Heinricher MM. Nociceptive facilitating neurons in the rostral ventral medulla. *Pain* 2004;110:158–165.

60. Buhler AV, Proudfit HK, Gebhart GF. Neurotensin-produced antinociception in the rostral ventromedial medulla is partially mediated by spinal cord norepinephrine. *Pain* 2008;135:280–290.

61. Guo W, Robbins MT, Wei F, et al. Supraspinal brain-derived neurotrophic factor signaling: a novel mechanism for descending pain facilitation. *J Neurosci* 2006;261:126–137.

62. Dahlstrom A, Fuxe K. Evidence for the existence of monoamine-containing neurons in the central nervous system. I. Demonstration of monoamines in the cell bodies of brainstem neurons. *Acta Physiol Scand Suppl* 1964;(Suppl 62):1–55.

63. Jones SL, Gebhart GF. Characterization of caerulospinal inhibition of the nociceptive tail flick reflex in the rat: mediation by spinal alpha 2-adrenoreceptors. *Brain Res* 1986;364:315–330.

64. Jones SL, Gebhart GF. Quantitative characterization of caerulospinal inhibition of nociceptive transmission in the rat. *J Neurophysiol* 1986;56:1397–1410.

65. Segal M, Sandberg D. Analgesia produced by electrical stimulation of catecholamine nuclei in the brainstem. *Brain Res* 1977;123:369–372.

66. Margalit D, Segal M. A pharmacologic study of analgesia produced by stimulation of the nucleus locus coeruleus. *Psychopharmacology (Berl)* 1979;62:169–173.

67. Tsuruoka M, Maeda M, Inoue T. Stimulation of the nucleus locus coeruleus/subcoeruleus suppresses visceromotor responses to colorectal distention in the rat. *Neurosci Lett* 2005;381:97–101.

68. Tsuruoka M, Matsutani K, Inoue T. Coeruleospinal inhibition of nociceptive processing in the dorsal horn during unilateral hindpaw inflammation in the rat. *Pain* 2003;104:353–361.

69. Ungerstedt U. Stereotaxic mapping of the monoamine pathways in the rat brain. *Acta Physiol Scand Suppl* 1971;367:1–48.

70. Bjorklund A, Skagerberg G. Descending monoaminergic projections to the spinal cord. In: Sjolund B, Bjorklund A., eds. *Brainstem Control of Spinal Mechanisms*. Amsterdam: Elsevier; 1982:55–88.

71. Crawley JN, Roth RH, Mass JW. Locus coeruleus stimulation increases noradrenergic metabolite levels in rat spinal cord. *Brain Res* 1979;166:180–184.

72. Shi TJ, Winer-Serhan U, Leslie F, Hokfelt T. Distribution of alpha2-adrenoreceptor mRNA in the rat lumbar spinal cord in normal and axotomized rats. *Neuroreport* 1999;10:2835–2839.

73. Stone LS, Broberger C, Vulchanova L, et al. Differential distribution of alpha2A and alpha2C adrenergic receptor immunoreactivity in the rat spinal cord. *J Neurosci* 1998;18:5298–5937.

74. Pertovaara A. Noradrenergic pain modulation. *Prog Neurobiol* 2006;80:53–83.

75. Duflo F, Li X, Bantel C, et al. Peripheral nerve injury alters the alpha2 adrenoreceptor subtype activated by clonidine for analgesia. *Anesthesiology* 2002;97:636–641.

76. Malberg AB, Hedley LR, Jasper JR, et al. Contribution of alpha(2) receptor subtypes to nerve injury-induced pain and its regulation by dexmedetomidine. *Br J Pharmacol* 2001;132:1827–1836.

77. Stevens RT, Hodge CJ Jr, Apkarian AV. Kölliker-Fuse nucleus: The principal source of pontine catecholaminergic cells projecting to the lumbar spinal cord of the cat. *Brain Res* 1982;239:589–594.

78. Yeomans DC, Clark FM, Paice JA, et al. Antinociception induced by electrical stimulation of spinally projecting noradrenergic neurons in the A7 catecholamine cell group of the rat. *Pain* 1992;48:449–461.

79. Clark FM, Proudfit HK. The projection of noradrenergic neurons to the spinal cord in the rat determined by anterograde tracing combined with immunocytochemistry. *Brain Res* 1991;538:231–245.

80. Proudfit HK. The challenge of defining brainstem pain modulation circuits. *J Pain* 2002;3:350–354.

81. Chiang CY, Hu JW, Sessle BJ. Parabrachial area and nucleus raphe magnus-induced modulation of nociceptive and nonnociceptive trigeminal subnucleus caudalis neurons activated by cutaneous or deep inputs. *J Neurophysiol* 1994;71:2430–2445.

82. Miller JF, Proudfit HK. Antagonism of stimulation-produced antinociception from ventrolateral pontine sites by intrathecal administration of α-adrenergic antagonists and naloxone. *Brain Res* 1990;530:20–34.

83. Burnett A, Gebhart GF. Characterization of descending modulation of nociception from the A5 cell group. *Brain Res* 1991;546:271–281.

84. Burstein R, Dado RJ, Giesler GJ Jr. The cells of origin of the spinothalamic tract of the rat: a quantitative reexamination. *Brain Res* 1990;551:329–337.

85. Janss AJ, Gebhart GF. Quantitative characterization and spinal pathway mediating inhibition of spinal nociceptive transmission from the lateral reticular nucleus in the rat. *J Neurophysiol* 1988;59:226–247.

86. Janss AJ, Gebhart GF. Brainstem and spinal pathways mediating descending inhibition from the medullary lateral reticular nucleus in the rat. *Brain Res* 1988;440:109–122.

87. Gebhart GR, Ossipov MH. Characterization of inhibition of the nociceptive tail flick reflex in the rat from the medullary lateral reticular nucleus. *J Neurosci* 1986;6:701–713.

88. Morgan MM, Sohn JH, Lohof AM, et al. Characterization of stimulation-produced analgesia from the nucleus tractus solitarius in the rat. *Brain Res* 1989;486:175–180.

89. Randich A, Aicher SA. Medullary substrates mediating antinociception produced by electrical stimulation of the vagus. *Brain Res* 1988;335:68–76.

90. Aicher S, Randich A. Antinociception and cardiovascular responses produced by electrical stimulation of the nucleus tractus solitarius, nucleus reticularis ventralis, and the caudal medulla. *Pain* 1990;42:103–119.

91. Ren K, Randich A, Gebhart GF. Modulation of spinal nociceptive transmission from nuclei tractus solitarii: a relay for effects of vagal afferent stimulation. *J Neurophysiol* 1990;63:971–986.

92. Randich A, Ren K, Gebhart GF. Electrical stimulation of cervical vagal afferents. II. Central relays for behavioral antinociception and arterial blood pressure decreases. *J Neurophysiol* 1990;64:1115–1124.

93. Randich A, Roose MG, Gebhart GF. Characterization of antinociception produced by glutamate microinjection in the nucleus tractus solitarius and the nucleus reticularis ventralis. *J Neurosci* 1988;8:4675–46584.

94. Ren K, Randich A, Gebhart GF. Electrical stimulation of cervical vagal afferents. I. Central relays for modulation of spinal nociceptive transmission. *J Neurophysiol* 1990;64:1098–1114.

95. Aimone LD, Gebhart GF. Serotonin and/or an excitatory amino acid in the medial medulla mediates stimulation-produced antinociception from the lateral hypothalamus in the rat. *Brain Res* 1988;450:170–180.

96. Behbehani MM, Park MR, Clement ME. Interactions between the lateral hypothalamus and the periaqueductal gray. *J Neurosci* 1988;8:2780–2787.

97. Carstens E. Hypothalamic inhibition of rat dorsal horn neuronal responses to noxious skin heat. *Pain* 1986;25:97–107.

98. Dafny N, Dong WQ, Prieto-Gomez C, et al. Lateral hypothalamus: site involved in pain modulation. *Neurosci* 1996;70:449–460.

99. Manning BH, Morgan MJ, Franklin KB. Morphine analgesia in the formalin test: Evidence for forebrain and midbrain sites of action. *Neurosci* 1994;63:289–294.

100. Yirmiya R, Ben-Eliyahu S, Shavit Y, et al. Stimulation of the hypothalamic paraventricular nucleus produces analgesia not mediated by vasopressin or endogenous opioids. *Brain Res* 1990;537:169–174.

101. Wang Q, Mao LM, Shi YS, et al. Lumbar intrathecal administration of naloxone antagonizes analgesia produced by electrical stimulation of the hypothalamic arcuate nucleus in pentobarbital-anesthetized rats. *Neuropharmacology* 1990;29:1123–1129.

102. Ohara PT, Vit JP, Jasmin L. Cortical modulation of pain. *Cell Mol Life Sci* 2005;62:44–52.

103. Senapti AK, Huntington PJ, LaGraize SC, et al. Electrical stimulation of the primary somatosensory cortex inhibits spinal dorsal horn neuron activity. *Brain Res* 2005;1057:134–140.

104. Kuroda R, Kawabata A, Kawao N, et al. Somatosensory cortex stimulation-evoked analgesia in rats: potentiation by NO synthase inhibition. *Life Sci* 2000;66:PL271–PL276.

105. Zhang YQ, Tang JS, Yuan G, et al. Inhibitory effects of electrically evoked activation of ventrolateral orbital cortex on the tail-flick reflex are mediated by the periaqueductal gray in rats. *Pain* 1997;72:127–135.

106. Zhang S, Tang JS, Yuan G, et al. Involvement of the frontal ventrolateral orbital cortex in descending inhibition of nociception mediated by the periaqueductal gray in rats. *Neurosci Lett* 1997;224:142–146.

107. Hutchinson WD, Harfa L, Dostrovsky JO. Ventrolateral orbital cortex and periaqueductal gray stimulation-induced effects on- and off-cells in the rostral medial medulla in the rat. *Neuroscience* 1996;70:391–407.

108. Al Amin HA, Atweh SF, Baki SA, et al. Continuous perfusion with morphine of the orbitofrontal cortex reduces allodynia and hyperalgesia in a rat model for mononeuropathy. *Neuroscience Lett* 2004;364:27–31.

109. Burkey AR, Carstens E, Wenniger JJ, et al. An opioidergic cortical antinociception triggering site in the agranular insular cortex of the rat that contributes to morphine antinociception. *J Neurosci* 1996;16:6612–6623.

110. Burkey AR, Carstens EJ. Dopamine reuptake inhibitor in the rostral agranular insular cortex produces antinociception. *J Neurosci* 1999;19:4169–4179.

111. Lee DE, Kim SJ, Zhuo M. Comparison of behavioral responses to noxious cold and heat in mice. *Brain Res* 1999;845:117–121.

112. Zhang L, Zhang Y, Zhao ZQ. Anterior cingulate cortex contributes to the descending facilitatory modulation of pain via dorsal reticular nucleus. *Eur J Neurosci* 2005;22:1141–1148.

113. Millan MJ. Descending control of pain. *Prog Neurobiol* 2002;66:355–474.

114. Gebhart GF, Randich A. Brainstem modulation of nociception. In: Klemm WR, Vertes RP, eds. *Brainstem Mechanisms of Behavior*. New York: John Wiley and Sons, Inc; 1990:315–352.

115. Fields HL, Bry J, Hentall I, et al. The activity of neurons in the rostral medulla of the rat during withdrawal from noxious heat. *J Neurosci* 1983;3:2545–2552.

116. Fields HL, Vanegas H, Hentall I, et al. Evidence that disinhibition of brain stem neurons contributes to morphine analgesia. *Nature* 1983;306:684–686.

117. Barbaro H, Heinricher M, Fields HL. Putative pain modulating neurons in the rostral ventral medulla: reflex-related activity predicts effects of morphine. *Brain Res* 1986;366:203–210.

118. Urban MO, Gebhart GF. Supraspinal contribution to hyperalgesia. *Proc Natl Acad Sci U S A* 1999;96:7687–7692.

119. Vanegas H, Schaible HG. Descending control of persistent pain: inhibitory or facilitatory? *Brain Res Brain Res Rev* 2004;46:295–309.

120. Mansikka H, Pertovaara A. Supraspinal influence on hindlimb withdrawal thresholds and mustard oil-induced secondary allodynia in rats. *Brain Res Bull* 1997;42:359–365.

121. Urban MO, Zahn PK, Gebhart GF. Descending facilitatory influences from the rostral medial medulla mediate secondary, but not primary hyperalgesia in the rat. *Neuroscience* 1999;90:349–352.

122. Urban MO, Jiang MC, Gebhart GF. Participation of central descending nociceptive facilitatory systems in secondary hyperalgesia produced by mustard oil. *Brain Res* 1996;737:83–91.

123. Kincaid W, Neubert MJ, Xu M, et al. Role for medullary pain facilitating neurons in secondary thermal hyperalgesia. *J Neurophysiol* 2006;95:33–41.

124. Urban MO, Coutinho SV, Gebhart GF. Involvement of excitatory amino acid receptors and nitric oxide in the rostral ventromedial medulla in modulating secondary hyperalgesia produced by mustard oil. *Pain* 1999;81:45–55.

125. Schaible HG, Neugebauer V, Cervero F, et al. Changes in tonic descending inhibition of spinal neurons with articular input during the development of acute arthritis in the cat. *J Neurophysiol* 1991;66:1021–1032.

126. Ren K, Dubner R. Enhanced descending modulation of nociception in rats with persistent hindpaw inflammation. *J Neurophysiol* 1996;76:3025–3037.

127. Hurley RW, Hammond DL. The analgesic effects of supraspinal mu and delta opioid receptor agonists are potentiated during persistent inflammation. *J Neurosci* 2000;20:1249–1259.

128. Hurley RW, Hammond DL. Contribution of endogenous enkephalins to the enhanced analgesic effects of supraspinal mu opioid receptor agonists after inflammatory injury. *J Neurosci* 2001;21:2536–2545.

129. Teryama R, Guan, Y, Dubner R, et al. Activity-induced plasticity in brain stem pain modulatory circuitry after inflammation. *Neuroreport* 2000;11:1915–1919.

130. Guan Y, Terayama R, Dubner R, et al. Plasticity in excitatory amino acid receptor-mediated descending pain modulation after inflammation. *J Pharmacol Exp Ther* 2002;300:513–520.

131. Miki K, Zhou QQ, Guo W, et al. Changes in gene expression and neuronal phenotype in brain stem pain modulatory circuitry after inflammation. *J Neurophysiol* 2002;87:750–760.

132. MacArthur L, Ren K, Pfaffenroth E, et al. Descending modulation of opioid-containing nociceptive neurons in rats with peripheral inflammation and hyperalgesia. *Neuroscience* 1999;887:499–506.

133. Tsuruoka M, Willis WD Jr. Bilateral lesions in the area of the nucleus coeruleus affect the development of hyperalgesia during carrageenan-induced inflammation. *Brain Res* 1996;726:233–236.

134. Tsuruoka M, Willis WD. Descending modulation from the region of the locus coeruleus on nociceptive sensitivity in rat model of inflammatory hyperalgesia. *Brain Res* 1996;743:86–92.

135. Tsuruoka M, Maeda M, Inoue T. Persistent hindpaw inflammation produces coeruleospinal antinociception in the non-inflamed forepaw of rats. *Neurosci Lett* 2004;367:66–70.

136. Tsuruoka M, Matsutani K, Maeda M, et al. Coeruleotrigeminal inhibition of nociceptive processing in the rat trigeminal subnucleus caudalis. *Brain Res* 2003;993:146–153.

137. Wei, F, Ren K, Dubner R. Inflammation-induced Fos protein expression in the rat spinal cord is enhanced following dorsolateral or ventrolateral funiculus lesions. *Brain Res* 1998;782:136–141.

138. Tortorici V, Salas R, Nogueira L, et al. Modulation of the formalin response by on- and off-cells of the rostral ventromedial medulla [abstract]. *Soc Neurosci* 2001;27(Prog No 161.166).

139. Robinson DA, Calejesan AA, Zhou M. Long-lasting changes in rostral ventral medulla neuronal activity after inflammation. *J Pain* 2002;3:292–300.

140. Scholz J, Woolf CJ. The neuropathic pain triad: neurons, immune cells and glia. *Nat Neurosci* 2007;10:1361–1368.

141. Kovelowski CJ, Ossipov MH, Sun H, et al. Supraspinal cholecystokinin may drive tonic descending facilitation mechanisms to maintain neuropathic pain in the rat. *Pain* 2000;87:265–273.

142. Burgess SE, Gardell LR, Ossipov MH, et al. Time-dependent descending facilitation from the rostral ventromedial medulla maintains, but does not initiate, neuropathic pain. *J Neurosci* 2002;22:5129–5136.

143. Suzuki R, Rygh LJ, Dickenson AH. Bad news from the brain: descending 5-HT pathway that control spinal pain processing. *Trends Pharm Sci* 2004;25(12):613–617.

144. Oatway M, Chen Y, Weaver LC. The 5-HT3 receptor facilitates at-level mechanical allodynia following spinal cord injury. *Pain* 2004;110:259–268.

145. Rahman W, Suzuki R, Rygh LJ, et al. Descending serotonergic facilitation mediated through rat spinal 5HT3 receptors is unaltered following carrageenan inflammation. *Neurosci Lett* 2004;361:229–231.

146. Potrebic SB, Field HL, Mason P. Serotonin immunoreactivity is contained in one physiological cell class in the rat rostral ventromedial medulla. *J Neurosci* 1994;14:1655–1665.

147. Gao K, Mason P. Serotonergic raphe magnus cells that respond to noxious tail heat are not ON or OFF cells. *J Neurophysiol* 2000;84:1719–1725.

148. Hodge CJ Jr, Apkarian AV, Owen MP, et al. Changes in the effects of stimulation of locus coeruleus and nucleus raphe magnus following dorsal rhizotomy. *Brain Res* 1983;288:325–329.

149. King T, Ossipov MH, Vanderah TW, et al. Is paradoxical pain induced by sustained opioid exposure an underlying mechanism of opioid antinociceptive tolerance? *Neurosignals* 2005;14:194–205.

150. Angst MS, Clark JD. Opioid-induced hyperalgesia: a qualitative systematic review. *Anesthesiology* 2006;104:570–587.

151. Bederson JB, Fields HL, Barbaro NM. Hyperalgesia during naloxone-precipitated withdrawal from morphine is associated with increased on-cell activity in the rostral ventral medulla. *Somatosens Mot Res* 1990;7:185–203.

152. Bie B, Fields HL, Williams JT, et al. Roles of alpha1- and alpha2-adrenoceptors in the nucleus raphe magnus in opioid analgesia and opioid abstinence-induced hyperalgesia. *J Neurosci* 2003;23:7950–7957.

153. Bie B, Pan ZZ. Presynaptic mechanism for anti-analgesic and anti-hyperalgesic actions of kappa-opioid receptors. *J Neurosci* 2003;23:7262–7268.

154. Burden TA, Graeff FG, Pelá IR. Opioid mediation of the antiaversive and hyperalgesic actions of bradykinin injected into the dorsal periaqueductal gray of the rat. *Physiol Behav* 1992;52:405–410.

155. Vanderah TW, Suenaga NM, Ossipov MH, et al. Tonic descending facilitation from the rostral ventromedial medulla mediates opioid-induced abnormal pain and antinociceptive tolerance. *J Neurosci* 2001;21:279–286.

156. Vanderah TW, Ossipov MH, Lai J, et al. Mechanisms of opioid-induced pain and antinociceptive tolerance: descending facilitation and spinal dynorphin. *Pain* 2001;92:5–9.

157. Kaplan H, Fields HL. Hyperalgesia during acute opioid abstinence: evidence for a nociceptive facilitating function of the rostral ventromedial medulla. *J Neurosci* 1991;11:1433–1439.

158. Ossipov MH, Lai J, King T, et al. Underlying mechanisms of pronociceptive consequences of prolonged morphine exposure. *Biopolymers* 2005;80:319–324.

159. Juni A, Klein G, Pintar JE, et al. Nociception increases during opioid infusion in opioid receptor triple knock-out mice. *Neuroscience* 2007;147:439–444.

CHAPTER 6 ■ SUPRASPINAL MECHANISMS OF PAIN AND NOCICEPTION

JÜRGEN LORENZ AND MICHAEL HAUCK

INTRODUCTION

The two preceding chapters addressed the peripheral and spinal mechanisms of nociceptive processing. Neither normal nor pathological pain can be understood without knowledge of supraspinal mechanisms. Supraspinal structures include the hindbrain (lower and upper brainstem and cerebellum) and the forebrain. The forebrain has two major divisions, the lower diencephalon involving hypothalamus and thalamus and the cerebrum involving the cortex, basal ganglia, and the limbic system (cingulate cortex, amygdala, hippocampus). The cerebrum has two hemispheres, each divided into frontal, parietal, temporal, and occipital lobes (Fig. 6.1). In humans, the forebrain anatomically dominates and physiologically controls much more than in other species' nociceptive processing. Because the human forebrain forms a large proportion of the entire central nervous system (CNS) volume (85%) when compared to the spinal cord (2%), descending modulatory influences from that site assume much greater importance than in the rat in which the forebrain comprises 44% and the spinal cord 35% of CNS volume.[1] Thus, the great variety of psychological phenomena characterizing normal and abnormal pain in humans are best studied in humans, although anatomical tracing and electrophysiological techniques and behavioral studies in rodents and primates have contributed significantly to our current knowledge about the pathways connecting the dorsal horn with supraspinal structures.

FUNCTIONAL IMAGING OF PAIN IN HUMANS

Since release of the last edition of this textbook, functional brain imaging in human volunteers and patients has addressed many questions pertaining to brain structures involved in pain processing. Before going into the details of supraspinal regions engaged in pain processing and perception, we will briefly describe the methodological basis of these technologies.

Methodologies of Noninvasive Functional Brain Imaging

Functional imaging techniques applied for the study of pain are positron emission tomography (PET), functional magnetic resonance imaging (fMRI), multi-channel electroencephalography (EEG), and magnetoencephalography (MEG).

PET measures cerebral blood flow, glucose metabolism, or neurotransmitter kinetics. A very small amount of a labeled compound (called the radiotracer) is intravenously injected into the patient or volunteer. During its uptake and decay in the brain, the radionuclide emits a positron, which, after traveling a short distance, "annihilates" with an electron from the surrounding environment. This event results in the emission of two gamma rays of 511 keV in opposite directions, the coincidence of which is detected by a ring of photo-multipliers inside the scanner. In

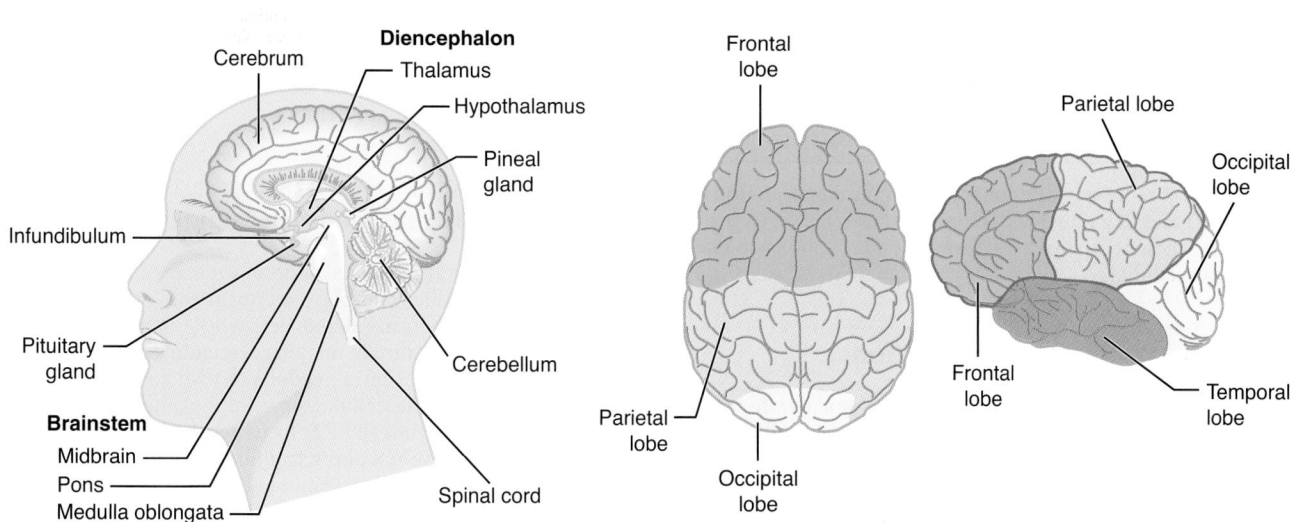

FIGURE 6.1 Structure of the brain.

case of the most common use of O^{15}-water injection, counting and spatial reconstruction of these occurrences within the brain anatomy allow visualization of the regional cerebral blood flow response (rCBF) as an indicator of neuronal activity. Usually scans during painful stimulation are statistically compared with scans during the resting state or nonpainful stimulation (blocked design) and plotted as 3-dimensional color-coded t- or Z-score statistical maps. Radio-labeled fluordeoxy-glucose (FDG) is applied to measure regional energy consumption as a function of metabolic rate. An interesting refinement of PET technology represents the use of neurotransmitters as tracers to investigate binding mechanisms and kinetics, for example in the opioidergic system.

FMRI images blood oxygenation, a technique called BOLD (blood oxygen level-dependent), which exploits the phenomenon that oxygenated and deoxygenated hemoglobin possess different magnetic properties resulting in different relaxation behavior following radio-frequency pulses inside the magnet. Both the rCBF using O^{15}-water PET and the BOLD technique rely on neurovascular coupling mechanisms that are not yet fully understood, but which overcompensate local oxygen consumption, thus causing a flow of oxygenated blood into neuronally active brain areas in excess of that utilized.[2]

EEG and MEG are noninvasive neurophysiological techniques that measure the respective electrical potentials and magnetic fields generated by neuronal activity of the brain and propagated to the surface of the skull where they are picked up with EEG-electrodes or, in the case of its magnetic counterpart, received by SQUID (supra conducting quantum interference device) sensors located outside the skull. Compared with PET and fMRI, EEG and MEG are direct indicators of neuronal activity and yield a higher temporal resolution of investigated brain function. The spatial distributions of EEG potentials and MEG fields at characteristic time points following noxious stimulation are analyzed using an inverse mathematical modeling approach called equivalent current dipole (ECD) reconstruction. An ECD evoked by painful stimuli hence represents a source model of pain-relevant activity within the brain. Similar approaches such as beamforming use spatial filtering techniques, firstly applied in antenna and ultrasound technologies. The spatial acuity of MEG is higher than that of EEG because the latter measures the extracellular volume currents that are distorted by the differentially conducting tissues such as grey and white matter, cerebrospinal fluid, dura mater, and bone. In contrast, MEG measures the magnetic field perpendicular to the intracellular currents undistorted by the surrounding tissue. Given the different geometry of electrical potentials and magnetic fields, MEG is predominantly sensitive to dipoles oriented tangentially to the head convexity, whereas EEG depends primarily on radial, but also on tangential dipoles.[3]

BRAINSTEM

The brainstem represents the connection of the diencephalon (hypothalamus and thalamus) with the spinal cord (Fig. 6.1). It comprises the mesencephalon (midbrain) and rhombencephalon (pons and medulla).

Reticular Formation

A major rhombencephalic structure is the reticular formation (RF) which encompasses a distributed network of small and large nerve fibers and extends from the medulla up to the level of the thalamus. It has a multitude of local interneuronal connections within the brainstem and contains both ascending and descending projecting systems. It is divided into three vertical zones. The medial magnocellular zone contains the ascending reticular activating system (ARAS), a major pathway to the thalamus, hypo-

thalamus, and basal forebrain (a group of structures at the base of the frontal lobe, including the nucleus basalis, diagonal band, medial septum, and substantia innominata). The median and paramedian zones contain the raphe nuclei of serotonergic projection neurons. The lateral parvocellular zone receives afferents from the amygdala and hypothalamus. The RF and basal forebrain have reciprocal connection with virtually all cortical and subcortical structures through cholinergic (from the basal forebrain), noradrenergic (from the locus ceruleus), dopaminergic (from the substantia nigra and ventral tegmentum), and serotoninergic (from the raphe) pathways. Reciprocal connections with the spinal cord mediate motor, respiratory, and cardiovascular functions and pain modulation.

The RF is an important mediator of consciousness. The stream of information about the outer world that reaches specific nuclei of the thalamus and cortex through the sensory pathways of vision, audition, gustation, and somatosensation is blocked when the activity of the mesencephalic RF that drives nonspecific thalamic sites drops below a critical level, such as during slow wave sleep or certain types of absence epilepsies.[4] Wakefulness and arousal are thus closely coupled to the RF, which acts as the "energetic supplier" of conscious perception and behavior. Widespread areas of the RF are responsive to noxious stimuli.[5] The gigantocellular and magnocellular fields of the medullary reticular formation, that is, the bulboreticular region, mediate escape behavior following acute painful stimuli[6,7] and respond neurochemically during persistent pain.[8] The close relationship of nociception and pain with arousal and consciousness guarantees optimal alertness and readiness to avoid bodily harm. Sleep is therefore disrupted by the awakening nature of pain through its influence upon the RF. Similarly, opioid-induced sedation is antagonized by residual pain. These aspects will be discussed in more detail later.

The view of a more or less unspecific role of RF in pain through enhancing arousal and escape behavior has been challenged by more recent research. The subnucleus reticularis dorsalis (SRD) represents a homogenous population of neurons in the caudal-dorsal medulla whose axons form both ascending and descending collaterals to the thalamus and spinal cord, respectively. SRD neurons are strongly activated by noxious cutaneous and visceral stimuli from any part of the body.[9] It is regarded as a medullary substrate of the link between nociceptive and motor activities. SRD has also been suggested as major supraspinal site mediating the "pain-inhibits-pain," or counterirritation, phenomenon as formulated in the concept of diffuse noxious inhibitory controls (DNIC).[10] As part of a spinal-bulbospinal feedback loop, SRD is proposed to facilitate the extraction of nociceptive information by increasing the signal-to-noise ratio between a pool of deep dorsal horn neurons activated by a tonic painful focus and the remaining population of such neurons, which are inhibited for simultaneous phasic noxious input.

Periaquaductal Grey Matter: A Key Structure of Endogenous Analgesia

The periaqueductal gray is a midbrain territory that surrounds the cerebral aqueduct and plays a critical role in the expression of a variety of emotion-related behaviors, including pain.[11] It represents a key structure in relaying descending pain modulation via nuclei of the rostroventral medulla (RVM; nucleus raphe magnus and nucleus gigantocellularis pars alpha) and of the dorsolateral pontine tegmentum (DLPT; locus ceruleus and A7 catecholamine cells) to the spinal and trigeminal dorsal horn. It receives input from both ascending spinomesencephalic and descending pathways, the latter originating in the limbic forebrain, namely medial prefrontal cortex, rostral anterior cingulate cortex, amygdala, and hypothalamus. Early systematic studies identified PAG and RVM as brainstem sites that elicit powerful surgical levels of analgesia through focal brain stimulation,[12] subsequently more elaborated and referred to as "stimulus-induced analgesia."[13–15] A milestone contribution to the understanding of the interaction between PAG and RVM and its role in opioid analgesia was delivered by Field's working group who identified two classes of pain modulatory cells in the RVM exerting inhibitory and facilitatory actions through respective off- and on-cells.[16] Off-cells are activated by local infusion of μ-opioid agonists and their activity inhibits nociceptive transmission. In contrast, on-cells facilitate nociceptive transmission, are inhibited by local μ-opioids, and are activated by naloxone and morphine abstinence. Approximately 15% of RVM neurons are serotonergic and are neither on- nor off-cells and do not respond to opioids.[17] Some respond to baroreceptor input integrating cardiovascular and nociceptive function.[18] Descending fibers from the RVM project to dorsal horn neurons via the dorsolateral funiculus.

The biological significance of endogenous pain control is generally seen in the context of behavioral conflicts in which the subject needs to disengage from pain in order to fight or escape at the presence of body injury. Analogous human life situations are sporting competition or combat, during which a subject may fail to be aware of even severe tissue damage, which becomes painful when the victim releases engagement in these activities. Thus, forebrain input to the PAG mediates contextual information from the prefrontal cortex, the amygdala, the anterior cingulate cortex, and the hypothalamus about momentary behavioral goals, past experience, and bodily needs. Evidence furthermore indicates that injury and inflammation causing increased sensitivity to painful stimuli (primary hyperalgesia) triggers the RVM pain modulating circuitry.[19]

Recently, using the expression of the immediate early gene, c-fos, as a marker of neuronal activation, an interesting regional distinction for deep versus cutaneous pain had been demonstrated within the midbrain PAG. Noxious stimulation of a range of deep somatic and visceral structures evoked a selective increase in Fos expression in the ventrolateral PAG column (vlPAG), whereas noxious cutaneous stimulation evoked Fos expression predominantly in the lateral PAG column (lPAG).[20] Ventrolateral and lateral PAG areas are suggested to represent different modes of behavioral adaptation characterizing inescapable and escapable types of pain, respectively. Earlier studies showed that both deep pain as well as microinjection of excitatory amino acids (EAA) into the vlPAG of freely moving animals evoked a response of quiescence, decreased vigilance, decreased reactivity, hypotension, and bradycardia. In contrast, cutaneous pain as well as activation of the lPAG evoked fight and flight behavior, increased vigilance, hyperreactivity, hypertension, and tachycardia. Lamb et al.[21,22] presented evidence that differential representation of escapable and inescapable pain in the PAG extends to distinct representations of "first" and "second" pain, as indicated by the columnar distribution of neurons activated by inputs from respective Aδ- and C-nociceptors. Furthermore, the functional organization of projections from circumscribed regions of the hypothalamus to the different columns of the PAG indicates that the behavioral significance of the pain signal is represented in brain regions other than the PAG. A PET study comparing brain activity of heat pain inflicted on normal skin of healthy volunteers with that of a normally warm stimulus, but perceived as equally painful on the same skin area when it was sensitized by topical capsaicin (heat allodynia), lends further support for the view that the brain represents different types (exteroceptive vs. interoceptive) or behavioral significances (escapable vs. inescapable) of pain in a region-specific manner.[23] This PET study demonstrates that in parallel with a unique recruitment of medial thalamus and frontal lobe structures, the midbrain encompassing the PAG exhibited significantly greater activation following heat allodynia after capsaicin-induced C-fiber sensitization than during normal heat pain that involves both C- and Aδ-nociceptor activation

(Fig. 6.2). It is therefore conceivable that different pathways inform the brain about the nature and significance of pain as coming from outside (normal heat pain) or inside the body (inflammatory heat hyperalgesia and allodynia) to engage highly elaborated forebrain structures that interact with region-specific output systems of the PAG. Such specificity may coordinate antinociception with adequate behavioral and autonomic responses to prevent damage, in case of an imminent threat, or promote healing when an injury is already manifest.

HYPOTHALAMUS

The hypothalamus occupies the ventral half of the diencephalon below the thalamus on either side of the third ventricle. It lies just above the pituitary gland with which it is intimately coupled for various neuroendocrine secretions subserving autonomic functions. Neurosecretory neurons are mainly located in periventricular and supraoptic nuclei. Fiber tracts to the pituitary gland are subdivided into two parts: (1) magnocellular secretory cells expressing vasopressin and oxytocin innervate the posterior pituitary gland and (2) parvocellular secretory cells which secrete factors related to the release and/or inhibition of other hormones from the anterior pituitary gland. The hypothalamus receives nociceptive inputs from the midbrain parabrachial nucleus, the ventrolateral medulla, and the spinal and trigeminal dorsal horn.[24,25] The nucleus of the solitary tract (NTS), a major relay of cardiorespiratory, visceral, and gustatory information, is also connected with the hypothalamus. Its role in nociception is not quite clear, but the convergence of autonomic, visceral, and nociceptive information in the hypothalamus underpins the importance of it for the control of homeostasis as part of the brain's defense system.

THALAMUS

The thalamus is the major structure of the diencephalon, which additionally contains, in relation to thalamus, basally the hypothalamus, laterally the globus pallidus and nucleus subthalamicus, and medially the third ventricle. With the exception of the olfactory system, all sensory systems send afferent input to the thalamus from where it is projected into the specific cortical representation areas. This is why the thalamus is often referred to as "the gate to consciousness." The intralaminar and ventral motor nuclei are the main sources of thalamic inputs to the striatum (putamen and caudate nucleus). Thalamostriatal and corticostriatal connections form the motor loop of the basal ganglia which is under control of dopaminergic input from the midbrain substantia nigra. The thalamic extension of the ascending reticular activating system contributes to arousal and wakefulness driven by the midbrain reticular formation (see previous text). The multidimensional nature of pain as composed of sensory-discriminative and affective-motivational determinants, first introduced by Melzack and Casey[26] four decades ago, formed a conceptual framework that guided many research groups studying supraspinal pain mechanisms. One of their postulates was that sensory and affective pain dimensions are anatomically represented by spinal pathways that differentially target respective lateral and medial nuclei of the dorsal thalamus.

The Lateral Pain System: The Sensory-Discriminative Pathway

The cell bodies of spinothalamic tract (STT) fibers are located in the most superficial layers, lamina I, the outer region of lamina II, and deeper laminae V–VI according to the Rexed scheme. STT axons cross via the anterior commissure to the anterolateral

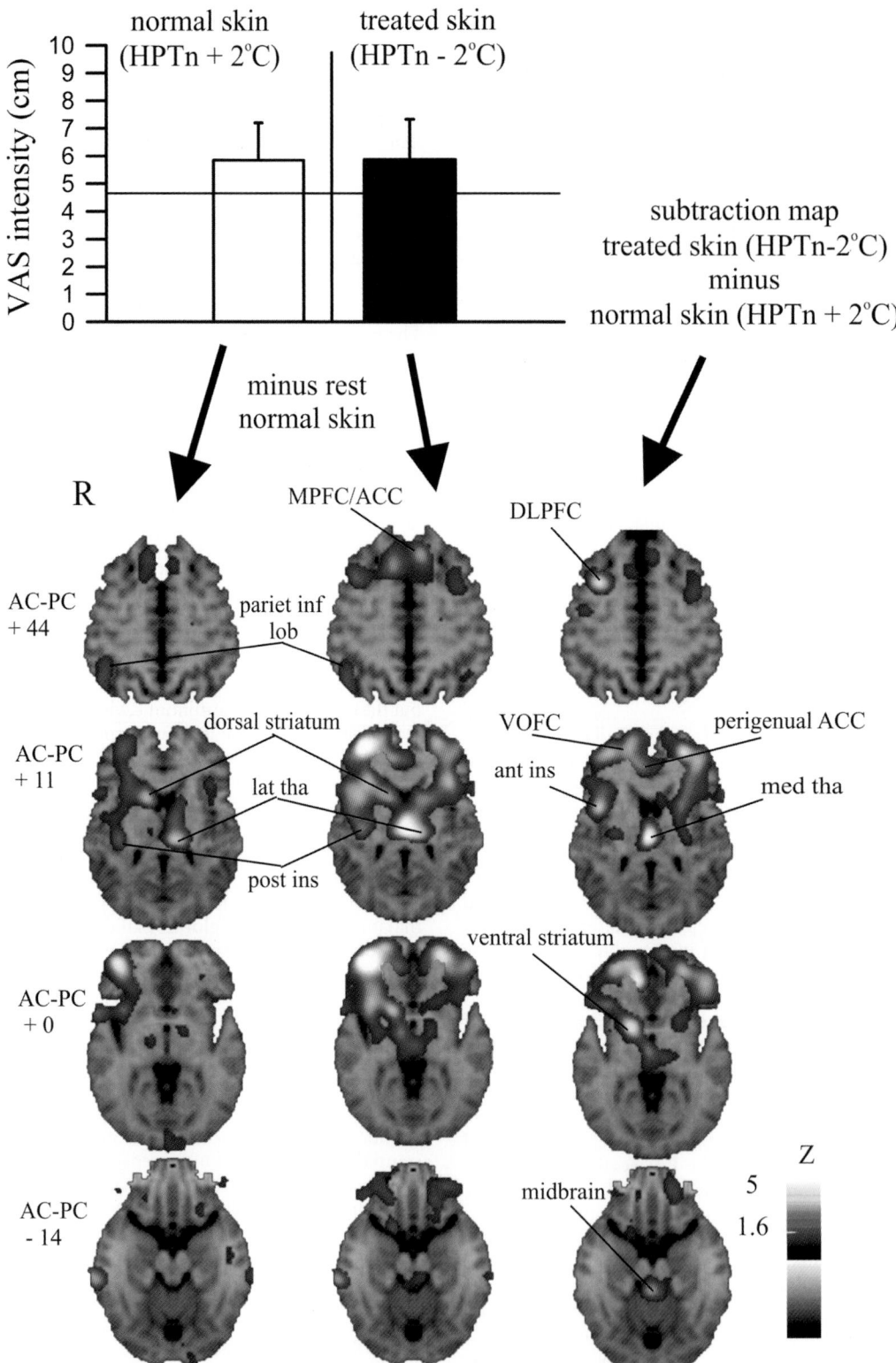

FIGURE 6.2 Regional brain activity during equally intense pains across normal and capsaicin-treated skin conditions. *Top*: Stimulation of the normal skin with the high intensity stimulus yields the same pain intensity as stimulation with the low intensity stimulus on capsaicin-treated skin. However, the O^{15}-water PET images during heat pain (*left*) and equally intense heat allodynia (*middle*) are different when compared against normal rest condition. Similar magnitudes of activity in the dorsal striatum, lateral thalamus (*lat tha*), and posterior insula (*post ins*) are removed in the image subtraction of heat allodynia minus heat pain (*right*) contrasting activity in the ventral striatum, medial thalamus (*med tha*), anterior insula (*ant ins*), midbrain, dorsolateral prefrontal cortex (DLPFC), medial prefrontal (MPFC) and ventral/orbitofrontal (VOFC), and perigenual anterior cingulate cortex (ACC) during heat allodynia. (Reproduced from Lorenz J, Minoshima S, Casey KL. Keeping pain out of mind: the role of the dorsolateral prefrontal cortex in pain modulation. *Brain* 2003;126: 1079–1091, with permission.)

portion of the contralateral hemisphere and have their main thalamic targets in lateral nuclei, namely ventral posterolateral (VPL; from the body) and posteromedial (VPM; from the face) nuclei, and the ventral posterior inferior (VPI) nucleus. These fibers contribute to thermal and pain sensation. The lateral thalamic nuclei have small receptive fields and mostly gradual stimulus response functions over nonnoxious and noxious intensities, representing the "wide-dynamic-range," or to a lesser extent, over noxious range only, representing the "nociceptive-specific" type of cells. These features render lateral thalamic targets of spinal nociceptive afferents ideally suited for the encoding of spatial localization and intensity of painful stimuli, similar to the properties of touch. The sensory-discriminative determinant of pain is thus governed by a spinal afferent pathway that mainly reaches lateral thalamic nuclei, from where neuronal activity is projected into the contralateral primary (SI) and bilateral secondary (SII) somatosensory cortices and mid and posterior sections of the insula (see later).

Spinal Connections to Brainstem and Medial Thalamus: The Affective Pathway

Although direct connections of lamina I STT cells exist with medial thalamic nuclei, namely the central lateral nucleus and intralaminar complex,[27–29] the major source of nociceptive input to the medial thalamus is likely indirect through the brainstem that relays spinoreticular, spinomesencephalic, and spino-parabrachial input from both superficial and deeper dorsal horn. Medial thalamic nuclei project densely into key structures of the limbic system, such as the anterior cingulate cortex, the amygdala, the hippocampus, the anterior insula, and prefrontal cortex which represent the perceived intrusion and threat by pain, referred to as affective-motivational and cognitive-evaluative determinants of pain.[26]

The concept of a nociceptive pathway that closely parallels or is partly convergent with that of touch at distinct sites of spinal cord, thalamus, and parietal lobe as a key element for the sensory-discriminative or exteroceptive function of pain has recently been challenged by Craig.[30] An important component of his hypothesis is the assumption that pain is a purely interoceptive perception like hunger, thirst, or itch. It originates in specific lamina I neurons which impinge upon specific thalamic nuclei, such as the posterior part of the ventral medial nucleus (VMpo) and the ventral caudal part of the mediodorsal nucleus (MDvc). These distinct thalamic nuclei relay afferent input to the dorsal posterior insula and caudal ACC respectively, and form separate pathways regarded as important elements of a hierarchical system subserving homeostasis, linking thermal sensation and pain contributing to the sense of the physiological condition of the body (interoception) with subjective feelings and emotion.

CORTEX

The human cortex is divided according to functional and anatomical criteria. The German neuroanatomist and psychiatrist Brodmann[31] introduced a systematic classification of the human cortex based on cytoarchitectonic properties, which, in refined modification, is still often referred to in the neuroimaging literature. Functional classifications consider the specific relevance of different cortical structures for motor, sensory, cognitive, emotional, or autonomic information processing. These functional areas can be divided into hierarchically organized subregions, for example, primary and secondary projection areas, or network systems consisting of distributed areas. The current view is that higher order projection areas and distributed networks rather than a unique "pain center" represent the cortical substrate of pain perception. This view is consistent with the multidimen-

sional definition of pain[26,32] which postulates differential projection of lateral and medial thalamic pathways to respective sensory and limbic cortical structures in addition to cortico-cortical as well as cortico-subcortical interactions for the composition of sensory-discriminative, affective-motivational, and cognitive-evaluative determinants (see previous text). According to this concept the primary (SI) and secondary somatosensory (SII) cortices receiving input from lateral thalamic nuclei are responsible for sensory-discriminative processing. Emotional content and aversive quality to noxious stimuli motivating escape and avoidance behavior are linked to limbic areas. The limbic system involves cortical and subcortical areas from the frontal, parietal, and temporal lobe that from a ring (limbus) around the upper brainstem and diencephalons, first regarded by Papez[33] as important for emotion. It includes the cingulate cortex, the insula, the prefrontal cortex, and, as subcortical structures, amygdala, hippocampus, medial thalamus, and hypothalamus.

Sensory Areas

Primary Somatosensory Cortex

The primary somatosensory cortex (SI) is located in the parietal lobe within the postcentral gyrus (Fig. 6.3). It includes the Brodmann areas 1, 2, 3a, and 3b, the latter two occupying the depth and the posterior wall of the central sulcus and generally considered to be the major recipient of cutaneous somatosensory input. Early studies of patients with cortical lesions reported controversial results. Whereas Head and Holmes[34] did not find deficits in pain sensitivity following cortical lesions, studies on World War I and II injury victims with lesions of SI (area 3a) reported loss of cutaneous pain sensibility.[35–37] Experimental data using single cell recordings in awake monkeys revealed a strong correlation between SI firing rate and stimulus intensity and duration of painful stimuli.[38] Patients with subdural electrodes implanted for surgical treatment of intractable epilepsy showed encoding of intensity of painful stimuli within SI.[39] Direct intracerebral electrical stimulation of SI in awake patients, however, failed to elicit painful sensations.[40,41] Thus, it appears that SI processes nociceptive input, but it is not sufficient to cause a pain sensation. Due to its spatial and intensity encoding properties, SI is regarded to contribute to discriminative analysis of painful stimuli but does obviously not cause the aversive nature of pain perception.

Consistent evidence for SI involvement in pain processing is derived from more recent functional neuroimaging studies in humans. SI is organized somatotopically; that is, neighboring peripheral skin areas are also represented by neighboring cortical sites. Human imaging studies established a somatotopic organization of SI for painful laser stimuli[42] (Fig. 6.4). Accordingly, laser stimuli at the foot and hand activated SI regions medially, near the interhemispheric gap, or more laterally, respectively. Ploner et al.[43] and Tran et al.[44] showed that laser-evoked MEG responses to Aδ- and C-fiber activation, respectively, appeared simultaneously in SI and SII, a finding which contrasts the sequential activation of SI and SII following tactile stimuli. Kanda et al.[45] confirmed these results by using implanted subdural electrodes. Yet, not all functional imaging studies revealed SI activation related to pain. PET and fMRI studies exhibited robust SI activity following painful stimuli when using contact heat,[46–48] laser radiant heat,[42,49] or electrical pain,[50,51] but less consistently during spontaneous or provoked clinical pain states.[52,53] Casey et al.[54] noted a clear temporal dynamic of SI activity following painful contact heat using PET. Notably, hypnotic suggestion of sensory pain quality enhanced SI activity following thermal stimulation,[55] whereas that of the affective pain quality did not.[56] This latter result with experimental pain stimuli fits with clinical observation that SI lesions alter sensory qualities but leave affective or cognitive aspects of pain, especially chronic pain, largely

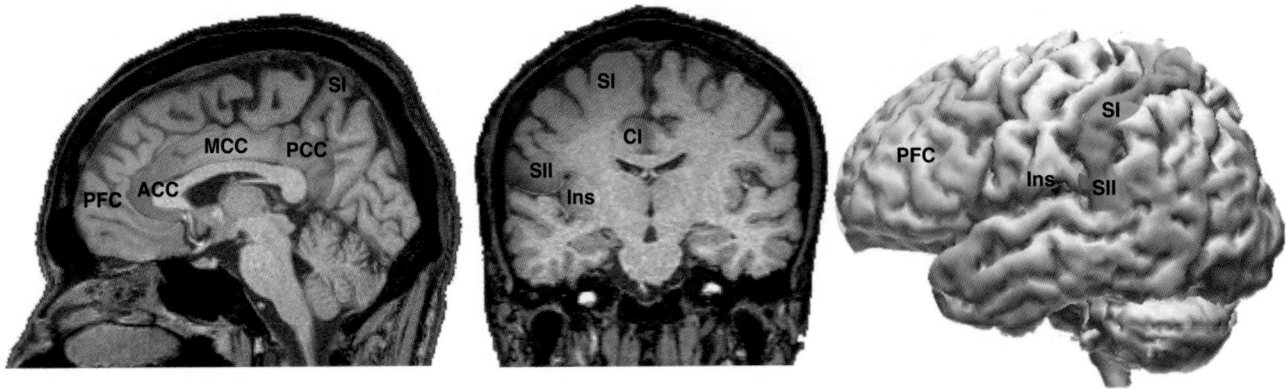

FIGURE 6.3 Schematic anatomical localization of cortical areas, which are regarded as important for pain processing. Somatosensory areas, which are responsible for sensory-discriminative pain processing such as intensity and stimulus decoding, are the primary (SI) and secondary somatosensory cortex (SII). Adjacent to SII is the insula (*Ins*), which belongs to the limbic system and is involved in emotional-affective pain processing. Other limbic structures include the cingulate gyrus with its subdivisions anterior cingulate cortex (ACC), midcingulate cortex (MCC), and posterior cingulate gyrus (PCC). Finally the prefrontal cortex (PFC) plays an important role in cognitive-evaluative pain processing especially for the organization of context-dependent pain behavior.

unchanged.[57] Collective evidence thus indicates that noninvasive imaging methods strongly support the participation of SI in sensory-discriminative aspects of pain perception although temporal aspects of the applied stimulus method and imaging technique and attentional and cognitive factors can significantly modify SI activity.[54,58,59]

Secondary Somatosensory Cortex

The existence of a secondary somatosensory cortex (SII) was introduced for the first time by Adrian[60] in the cat. SII is situated lateral and posterior to SI and occupies the posterior parietal operculum at the upper bank of the Sylvian fissure (Fig. 6.3), encompassing Brodmann areas 40 and 43.[61] Because SII receives input from the thalamus via the spinothalamic projection into lateral nuclei (VPI, VPL, VPM) and sends output to the adjacent insula, SII is in a position to link nociceptive information to limbic cortical regions, such as the anterior cingulate cortex and medial prefrontal cortex. Because of the robust generation of dipolar electric activity following noxious laser stimuli in SII that is oriented tangentially to the skull convexity, multichannel MEG re-

cordings became an important functional brain imaging method to study pain-related SII activity in humans at high temporal resolution. The activity starts between 90 and 150 ms after the painful laser stimulus, depending on the body site and activated nerve fiber spectrum[62–64] and coincides with parallel SI activation.[43] Selective C-fiber activation also activates SII.[65] PET and fMRI revealed SII as one of the most consistent structures activated by pain.[57,58,66,67] Although less precise than SI, SII is also organized somatotopically[41,42,59,68] (see also Fig. 6.4). Patients with lesions within the SII-cortex have been reported to exhibit elevated pain thresholds at contralateral sites,[69] sometimes associated with a central (neuropathic) pain syndrome.[70,71] Several authors point to the problem of differentiating SII from the adjacent posterior insula.[66] Recent evidence from intracerebral recording and stimulations in patients, however, indicates separate representations of nociceptive processing in SII and insula.[41,72] The functional role of SII is not clear. Given its coarse somatotopy, it is unlikely to represent a critical site for spatial discrimination, but rather supplements SI in the organization of spatially guided defensive

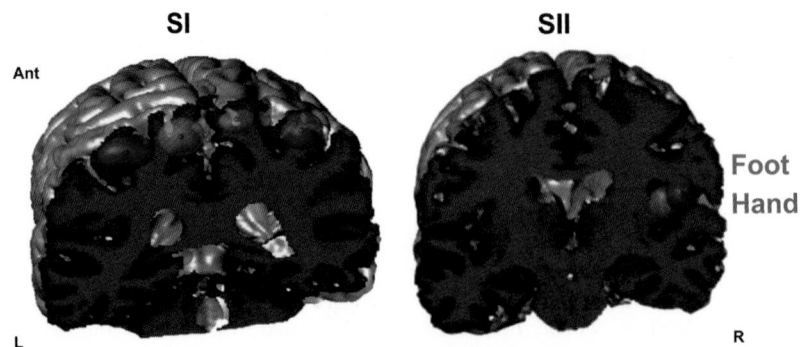

FIGURE 6.4 Somatotopic organization of somatosensory areas. Experimental pain was induced using an infrared laser, which elicits a short burning and pinprick-like pain sensation. Laser stimuli were given at both hands and feet, before pain-induced activation of the primary (SI) and secondary somatosensory (SII) areas were localized using functional magnetic resonance imaging (fMRI) technique. Pain induced activation after hand stimulation (*red*) was found in SI near the interhemispheric gap, whereas foot stimulation (*green*) elicits more lateral activation of SI. Pain induced localization in SII is less spatially separated between hand and foot stimulation. The center of the colored circles is the mean coordinate of the subjects, whereas the radius of the circle is the standard deviation. (Reproduced from Bingel U, Lorenz J, Glauche V, et al. Somatotopic organization of human somatosensory cortices for pain: a single trial fMRI study. *Neuroimage* 2004;23(1):224–232, with permission.)

and protective behavior against bodily threat. Accordingly, SII seems to be involved in recognition, memory, and learning of painful events[73] in that it links a primordial sensory representation of pain with further cognitive evaluation and affective appraisal.

Limbic Areas

Insular Cortex

As stated above, the insula belongs to the limbic system and is located adjacent to SII and can be divided cytoarchitectonically into Brodmann areas 13 (anterior insula) and 41 (posterior insula). Functionally, the anterior insula which lies rostral to the most lateral point of the central sulcus, mainly processes visceral autonomic (i.e., interoceptive) functions, and is closely linked to taste and smell, thus, proximal senses. In contrast, the posterior part is related to distal senses such as hearing, vision and somatosensation (i.e., exteroceptive functions). Craig[30] attributes a key role to the insular cortex in the integration of thermosensation and pain for homeostatic feelings and behavior. Despite the already cited evidence of distinct representations of pain in SII and posterior insula (see previous text), there are not enough data to clearly delineate SII and posterior insula functionally. However, the anterior part appears to represent separate functions from posterior insula and SII, from where it receives input. Further input comes from the amygdala and brainstem nuclei. Projections from the anterior insula go to various limbic structures such as the anterior cingulate cortex and the entorhinal cortex of the temporal lobe (amygdala and hippocampus).

Few lesion studies from patients have been conducted. Isolated anterior insula lesions without damage of the posterior insula and SII yield normal heat pain thresholds.[69] Others reported that damage of the anterior insula reduces pain affect and the ability to assign pain an appropriate meaning referred to as pain asymbolia.[74] Functional imaging studies strongly confirmed the engagement of the anterior insula in pain and the ability to manipulate anterior and posterior insula differentially.[75] Using PET, Casey et al.[54] demonstrated that anterior insula responds early, while posterior insula is activated late following painful contact heat stimuli. This result is consistent with the dissociation of anterior

and posterior insula according to respective anticipatory and real pain sensations.[76] Lorenz et al.[23] found stronger anterior insula activation with PET following heat stimuli applied on sensitized skin (heat allodynia) in comparison with equally intense heat stimuli applied on normal skin, whereas posterior insula and SII exhibited same activation across skin conditions (Fig. 6.2). This result may be partly related to the fact that heat allodynia is more unpleasant than normal heat pain. Consistent with this assumption, Schreckenberger et al.[77] found a significant positive correlation of unpleasantness ratings with regional glucose metabolization rate in bilateral insula following painful injections of an acidic solution into skin and muscle as measured with FDG-PET (Fig. 6.5). Thus, although both portions of the insula vary with pain intensity, anterior insula additionally represents subjective relevance and meaning of the pain in terms of its relation to an exteroceptive or interoceptive threat. This is also consistent with the role of the anterior insula in processing stimulus novelty.[78]

Cingulate Cortex

The cingulate cortex represents a key structure of the limbic system. Anatomically, it is located in the medial portion of both hemispheres above the corpus callosum. Cytoarchitectonically it is divided into distinct areas: the anterior cingulate cortex (ACC, area 24 and 25) and the posterior cingulate cortex (PCC, area 23). A more recent view additionally separates the midcingulate cortex (MCC, area 24) and the retrosplenial cortex (RSC). A major input to ACC comes from medial and intralaminar thalamic nuclei[79] which places the ACC into the center of the medial pain system subserving affective-motivational and cognitive-evaluative pain determinants.[26] Anatomically distinct regions are thought to relate to different functions, some more specifically related to pain, others to motor, autonomic, and cognitive functions[79,80] (Fig. 6.6). Whereas cingulotomy for intractable pain yielded only a modest relief from pain, it appeared that the degree to which pain interfered with other cognitive activities, behaviors, and social functions was significantly reduced.[81] Also, cingulate lesions in animals revealed minimal deficits in discriminative pain function but robust changes in pain-related behavior and learning.[82,83] A multimodal integrative rather than a specific nociceptive role of the ACC is also underlined by its large receptive fields and the absence of somatotopy.[79] MEG activity following laser radiant heat pain demonstrates a preferential response of the

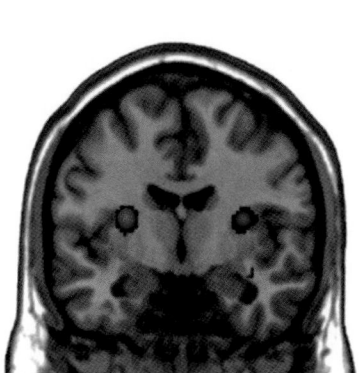
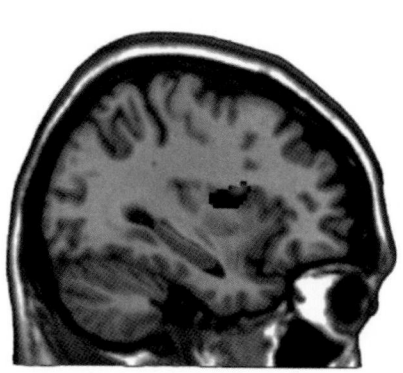
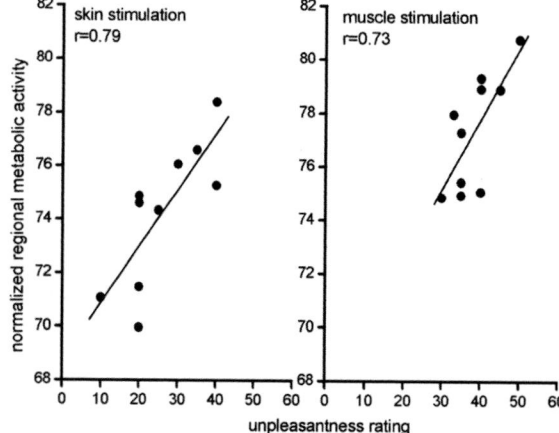

FIGURE 6.5 Correlation between unpleasantness rating and insula activation. Experimental pain was induced by infusion of low pH (5.2) solution in either the skin or the hand muscle. Subjects had to rate the unpleasantness of the painful stimulation, which was then correlated with regional metabolized activity within the insula using positron emission tomography (PET). Results show a strong significant ($p < 0.05$) correlation between unpleasantness ratings and insula activity for both skin and muscle pain. (Reproduced from Schreckenberger M, Siessmeier T, Viertmann A, et al. The unpleasantness of tonic pain is encoded by the insular cortex. *Neurology* 2005;64(7):1175–1183, with permission.)

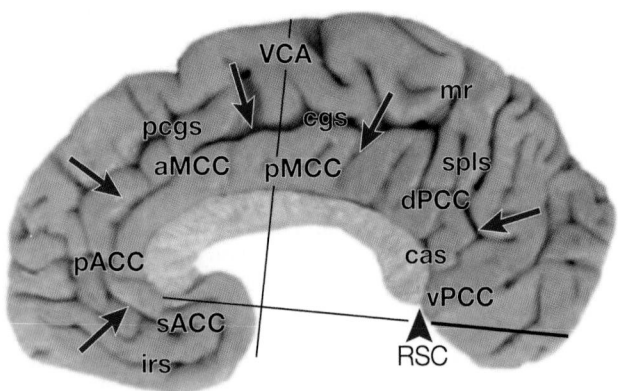

FIGURE 6.6 Region borders of the cingulate cortex according to Vogt. Subregions are marked with arrows and were determined based on postmortem cases that were coregistered to a stereotaxic atlas with the vertical plane at the anterior commissure (VCA) and the anteroposterior commissural line. A functional overview, derived from the analysis of a large volume of literature, is provided. This illustrates general regional function and, where known, subregional specializations. aMCC, anterior midcingulate cortex; cas, callosal sulcus; cgs, cingulate sulcus; dPCC, dorsal posterior cingulate cortex; irs, inferior rostral sulcus; mr, marginal ramus of cgs; pACC, pregenual anterior cingulate cortex; pcgs, paracingulate sulcus; pMCC, posterior midcingulate cortex; RSC, retrosplenial cortex; sACC, subgenual anterior cingulate cortex; spls, splenial sulci; vPCC, ventral posterior cingulate cortex. (Modified from Vogt BA. Pain and emotion interactions in subregions of the cingulate gyrus. *Nat Rev Neurosci* 2005;6(7):533–544, with permission.)

ACC to C-fiber input, regarded as important for the sustained "suffering" component of pain associated with C- rather than Aδ-fiber activity.[84] Together with SII and insula, ACC is the most consistent region activated by pain.[63,67,75] However, imaging of subjects engaged in a variety of cognitive, affective, and motor tasks also revealed ACC as the most consistent brain area.[85] The MCC is involved in response selection, fear avoidance, and motor function. Despite the diversity of perceptual, emotional, cognitive, motor, and autonomic processes harbored within distinct or overlapping cingulate cortex structures as revealed from numerous functional imaging studies, a common function to which all these processes converge may be seen in the awareness and monitoring of bodily threat or behavioral conflict demanding executive control. Such a view would explain why both detrimental effects of pain upon cognition as well as beneficial effects of cognitive distraction upon pain are represented in the anterior cingulate cortex.[86,87] Thus, the reciprocity of pain and cognitive processes at the level of the ACC might significantly determine the degree by which pain interrupts cognitive performance and is intrinsically difficult to ignore.[88]

Prefrontal Cortex

The prefrontal cortex (PFC) is the anterior part of the frontal lobe and contains numerous neurons and a large volume (30% of brain mass) and is furthest developed in humans compared to nonhuman species.[89] It can be divided into different subdivisions[85]: the mid-dorsal (area 9), dorsolateral (BA 46), ventrolateral, orbitofrontal, and medial frontal parts (BA 10, 11, 13, 14). All these frontal areas receive convergent input from different sensory modalities and again project to different associative sensory areas, motor areas, and limbic structures. The PFC is considered to be important for higher cortical functions that characterize the flexibility of human behavior, the ability to control attention, and the richness of intellectual and emotional competence. With respect to pain, PFC plays a major role in cognitive, attentional, and emotional processing of painful stimuli and recruitment of endogenous pain control. A particular part of the

PFC, the dorsolateral prefrontal cortex (DLPFC), is important for continuous monitoring of the external world, maintenance of information in short-term memory, and governing efficient performance control in the presence of distracting or conflicting stimuli.[90,91] In turn, orbital and medial portions of the prefrontal cortex are known to be important for mood and emotional behavior; for example, when guided by cues of reward or punishment, as well as for visceral and autonomic homeostasis related to eating and drinking behavior.[92] The famous case of Phineas Gage demonstrated that lesions of the PFC can strongly interfere with the maintenance of an individual's personality, socially appropriate behavior, and learning capabilities.[93,94] There is evidence of elevated pain thresholds in patients with frontal lobe lesions.[95]

The PFC is activated in several, not all, functional imaging studies using experimental painful stimuli or clinical pain states. It typically fails to show a clear pain-related stimulus-response function,[49,96] which led to the assumption that PFC activity mainly relates to the engagement of attention during pain processing.[66] Evidence indicates that the PFC, irrespective of pain intensity, integrates information about the psychological and bodily context of pain in order to allow disengagement from pain through activating endogenous pain control. Lorenz et al.[23,97] confirmed strong responses of dorsolateral PFC and orbitofrontal and medial PFC (OMPFC) during inflammatory pain as induced by topical capsaicin (see Fig. 6.2). Whereas DLPFC exhibited a negative relationship, OMPFC yielded a positive relationship to the unpleasantness of perceived pain. Furthermore, the interregional correlation of activity between midbrain and medial thalamus was significantly reduced during high compared to low left DLPFC activity, which could indicate a top-down mode of inhibition of effective synaptic connectivity between brainstem and medial thalamus as a cause for the inverse relationship of DLPFC activity to pain unpleasantness. A role of the DLPFC in the initiation of endogenous pain control is further supported by its participation in placebo analgesia. Wager et al.[98] demonstrated that DLPFC responds to cues that inform test participants about an expected analgesic effect in a placebo experiment. The analgesic effect itself, however, goes along with stronger rostral ACC activation[98,99] being stronger when coupled with the brainstem PAG.[100]

Recent clinical studies lend further support for the association of the DLPFC with pain suppression. Apkarian et al.[101] observed a reduction of the grey matter density determined by morphometry of magnetic resonance scans in bilateral DLPFC and right thalamus in chronic back pain patients that was strongly related to pain characteristics. In agreement with the suggested role of DLPFC in pain control, high-frequency transcranial magnetic stimulation (rTMS) over left DLPFC was able to ameliorate chronic migraine.[102] This is consistent with earlier studies in animals where electrical stimulation of fiber connections of the prefrontal cortex to the midbrain mediates antinociceptive effects in rodents.[103] In summary, collective evidence suggests that the PFC represents an important brain substrate for the human ability to actively disengage from pain.

Amygdala

The amygdala is an almond-shaped structure deep in the midtemporal lobe and belongs to the limbic system. The amygdala complex comprises about 13 nuclei, which are further divided into subregions.[104] These nuclei can also be grouped by functional properties in frontotemporal, autonomic, main, and accessory olfactory systems.[105] Tracer studies reveal that the amygdala gets multiple inputs from different cortical and subcortical structures and all sensory modalities. Cortical somatosensory and pain input arises directly from SI, SII and the insula,[102] whereas subcortical pain signals arise among others from the thalamus and the brainstem parabrachial nucleus. In addition, numerous projections from the amygdala go back to the brainstem, the hippocampus, and cortical areas such as the prefrontal cortex, whereas output connections to sensory areas are rare.[106] Numerous, but not all, imaging studies reveal amygdala activation during pain perception. There is no steady increase of activity in the amygdala with stimulus intensity, but rather a step-wise increase once stimulus intensity transits into pain.[49] This finding may point to learning following painful stimuli or to processing the emotional valence of pain stimuli.[107] Amygdala activation during pain might also reflect activation of a "defensive behavioral system," which controls transmission of nociceptive experience to the brain through descending modulatory circuits.[108] There are projections of the amygdala to the periaqueductal grey matter (PAG) that might initiate antinociceptive function during emotional stress or pain expectation.[109–111] Lesions in the amygdala, also known as Klüver-Bucy syndrome, lead to flattened emotional reactivity and loss of fear conditioning, but, as with ACC lesions, do not impair pain discrimination but change the behavioral response to pain. It is conceivable that the amygdala is important for the memory storage of past pain experiences and their context, in terms of the processes underlying fear conditioning to facilitate defensive autonomic reactions and behavior.

Hippocampus

The hippocampus forms, relative to the amygdala, the caudal extension of the deep medial temporal lobe (Fig. 6.5). It can be subdivided into the dentate gyrus and the cornu ammonis (CA1 and CA2). Its major input comes from the entorhinal cortex, a network including the DLPFC and parietal association cortex. Reports of Patient H. M.[112,113] highlight the role of the hippocampus in learning and explicit memory. Moreover, the importance for the involvement in pain processing and learning pain-related behavior is evident, because associations between pain and predictive cues have fundamental adaptive value.[114] Furthermore, learning adverse effects can play an important role in chronic pain and chronic pain-related avoidance behavior. Functional imaging revealed hippocampus activity during mild and moderate heat pain,[108,115] in a pain-learning paradigm when pain was not expected, and when pain stimuli were manipulated as to induce anxiety.[114] Together with the assumed role of the amygdala in pain, these findings show that medial temporal lobe structures participate in elaborating the experience of pain based on emotional state, expectation, and past experience.[57]

VIGILANCE, AROUSAL, AND ATTENTION

Attention is not a single neurophysiological entity. Many authors, including Parasuraman et al.,[116] describe different major components of attention that rely on a finite set of brain processes being hierarchically organized and interacting with each other. A basic component serves the maintenance of behavioral goals over time and is largely synonymous with arousal, vigilance, alertness, or sustained attention. It also involves the regulation of the sleep–wake cycle. Cholinergic and noradrenergic ascending systems originating in the reticular formation (see previous text) and the locus ceruleus and dopaminergic projections into the striatum are regarded as important for this function referred to as "the vigilance network" by Posner and Petersen.[117] Another component concerns the bias or filtering of task-relevant against irrelevant information. It serves to cope with capacity limits of central information processing which cannot deal with the huge amount of input from a large variety of sensors in different modalities at the same time. This component is often referred to as selective or focused attention and, according to Posner and Pertersen,[117] depends on the posterior attention network that includes brain structures such as the superior colliculus, thalamic pulvinar, and the posterior parietal cortex. Selective attention is often meta-phorically described by a "spotlight" or "cocktail party" effect, which emphasizes the phenomenon that the focus of awareness can momentarily fluctuate between sensory objects, features, or locations sometimes without overt orientation in the form of eye or head movements. It is believed that the gating of the afferent flow of information within attentional channels (i.e., the set of stimuli benefiting from selective attention) optimizes functional efficiency even at very early stages of modality-specific cortical processes. Closely linked to this function is a supervisory component of attention that temporarily intervenes into ongoing performance when called for by new relevant, unfamiliar, or potentially dangerous information; the detection of performance errors; or when internal representations need to be continuously updated, that is, during working memory operations. This component is often referred to as executive attention, largely governed by the anterior attention network *sensu*[117] that comprises the anterior cingulate, medial and lateral prefrontal cortex areas, and the supplementary motor area.

Long duration mental tasks yield a characteristic vigilance decrement that can be measured subjectively or by behavioral indicators such as reaction time.[116] Similarly, amplitudes of pain-relevant evoked potentials after electrical stimuli, painful chemical stimulation of the nasal mucosa, and laser stimulation are strongly attenuated by habituation and decreases of vigilance over time.[118] Although pain generally enhances arousal, the test situation for the recording of pain-relevant laser evoked potential (LEP) is characterized by short durations of single laser stimuli, presented at long inter-stimulus intervals in quite monotonous long-stimulus blocks, which contribute to reduced LEP amplitudes by vigilance decrements. Experimental pain studies therefore use study designs to avoid or control for habituation. Pain habituation can be observed during short-term pain experience but also during longer lasting pain after several days. FMRI experiments on the mechanisms of habituation revealed decreases of activation in major pain areas including the thalamus, insula, SII, and the putamen. Notably, an increase in activation was observed in the ACC.[119] One possible mechanism could be the involvement of the endogenous opioidergic pain control system (see previous text). In an animal model of habituation, naloxone sufficiently prevents habituation to repeated electrical pain stimuli.[120] There are important inter-individual differences regarding the strength of habituation that are not well understood. However, it is described that especially chronic pain patients show an impairment of habituation.[121–124]

Beydoun et al.[125] examined subjects who they allowed to fall asleep after one day of sleep deprivation to look for LEP during different sleep stages compared to normal wakefulness. They demonstrated the abolition of the major LEP component at the vertex position during sleep stage II, defined by the appearance of sleep spindles, and its strong amplitude attenuation during sleep stage I, defined by drop-out of alpha activity and appearance of lateral eye movements. It appears that there is a reciprocal relationship between sleep and pain, allowing sleep to reduce pain but also pain to reduce or disturb sleep.[126] Furthermore, decreases of pain sensitivity also accompany sedation and drowsiness when induced pharmacologically using benzodiazepines,[127] clonidine,[128] or subanesthetic isoflurane.[129] It is therefore often difficult to differentiate drowsiness or sedation from analgesia.

Given the profound role of attention for conscious perception, it significantly impacts behavior and pain experience.[88] Pain is a salient stimulus and draws attention for extended periods.[78] The manipulation of attention by distraction or focused attention has been used as a therapeutic intervention for several years[130,131] and reflects everyday life experience such as when a mother tries to distract her children when they are hurt. Clinical evidence suggests that attentional mechanisms may be also involved in the amplification of some chronic clinical pain stages.[132] Patients with chronic pain problems seem to selectively attend to pain and the degree by which pain distracts attention from concurrent tasks appears to depend on the evaluation of pain stimuli as threatening or worrying.[88] In tasks where attentional shifts are required, anxious patients exhibit difficulties disengaging from painful stimuli.[133]

The neural mechanisms underlying attentional modulation of pain are not fully understood, but various areas of the pain matrix appear to be involved.[134] More recent studies using EEG and MEG focused on cortical synchronization processes as indicators of attentional modulation of sensory input. Mainly derived from experiments with nonpainful stimuli, it is proposed that selective attention may act by modulating sub-threshold oscillations in sensory assemblies and by enhancing the gain of oscillatory responses to stimuli that match stored contextual information.[135,136] A recent study indicates that during selective attention to pain, bilateral somatosensory cortical sites yield enhanced oscillatory activity in the gamma bandwidth of MEG (120 Hz rhythms), and a stronger inter-regional degree of synchronization as sign of increased communication[137] (Fig. 6.7). One possible neuronal correlate of abnormal attentional amplification may therefore be suspected as an "over-synchronization" in pain-related cortical areas, leading to an uncontrolled spread of signals even in the case of weak or absent nociceptive input. Thus, the dynamic control of neuronal signal flow might be disturbed, preventing an appropriate context-dependent modulation of the gain of neural signals, and reducing the capacity for descending control of nociceptive afferent inputs. As assumed for states of chronic pain, such an "over-synchronization" might be viewed as the result of central neuroplastic changes underlying a learning process.[138]

PAIN PLASTICITY

The brain is an adaptive system, which has a high plasticity to change the excitability of its networks according to a variety of external and internal processes. The uniqueness of pain compared with other human senses is characterized by its enormous plasticity to adapt according to both the bodily and the psychological context in which pain occurs. Studies on acute pain models in animals and humans had long made clear that clinically important pains exhibit distinct neurophysiological and pharmacological properties due to alteration of impulse generation at the site of an injury and propagation into and through the central nervous system. Once tissue damage and inflammation occur, the production and release of chemical mediators excite and sensitize nociceptors, rendering their axons much more responsive and giving rise to tenderness and hyperalgesia as well as spontaneous pain.

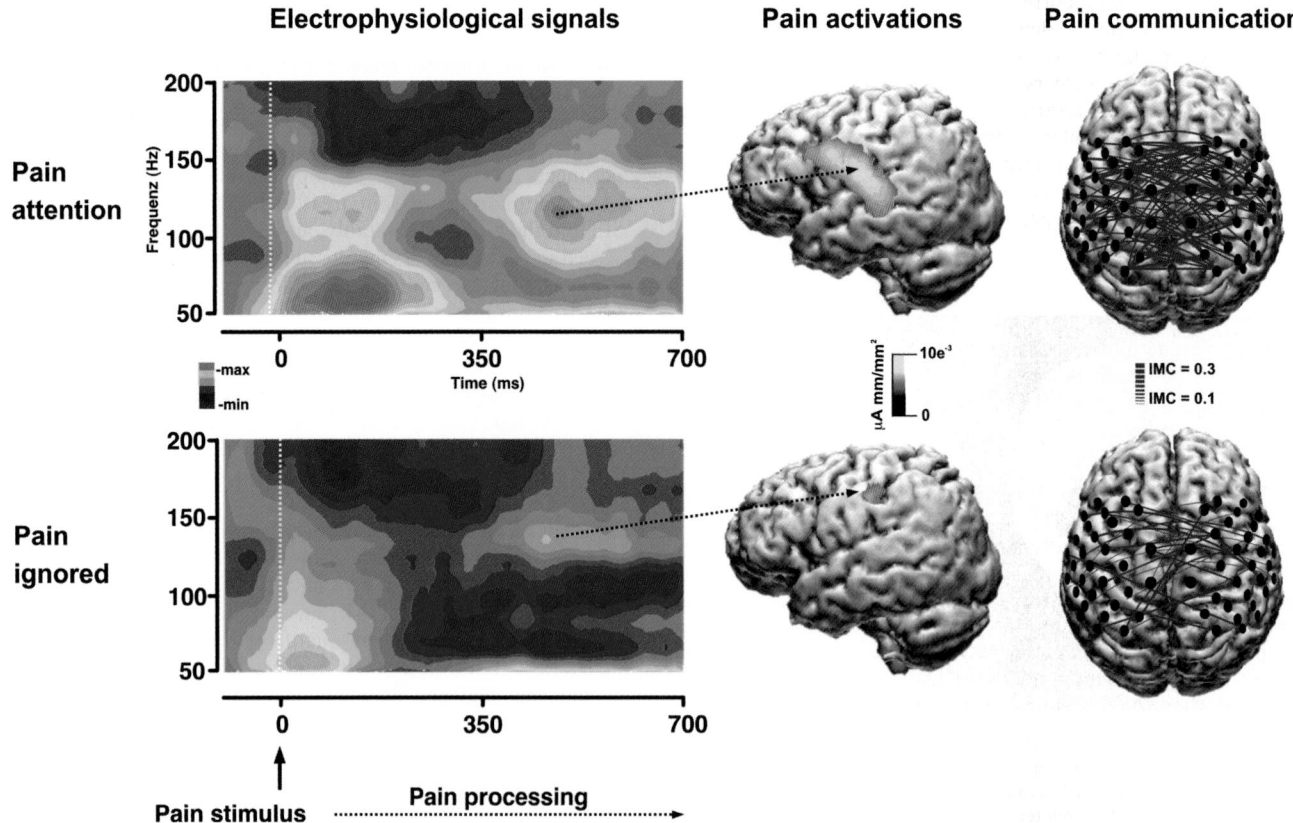

FIGURE 6.7 Pain modulation by attention. Attention to pain (pain attention) was induced by counting rare electrical pain stimuli at one finger, while ignoring frequent pain stimuli at the other finger (pain ignored) within a random series (oddball paradigm). Electrophysiological signals were recorded using magnetoencephalography (MEG). After time-frequency transformation, neuronal oscillations around 120 Hz (gamma band) and with latencies around 500 ms indicated a difference for attention. This effect was localized in sensory-motor areas. Furthermore, an increased communication (imaginary coherence, IMC) between both sensory-motor sites was observed during attention. (Modified from Hauck M, Lorenz J, Engel AK. Attention to painful stimulation enhances gamma-band activity and synchronization in human sensorimotor cortex. *J Neurosci* 2007;27(35): 9270–9277, with permission.)

Hyperexcitability also occurs at the level of the dorsal horn in the spinal cord following tissue damage and inflammation, further aggravating sensitization and even rendering innocuous tactile stimuli outside the lesion capable of producing pain through increase of synaptic efficacy of local interneurons, a phenomenon called allodynia. Thus, the bodily context of normal versus damaged tissue dramatically determines the perception of pain.

Several pain states, such as chronic pain or phantom pain, can induce central cortical changes in the pain matrix. Patients suffering from cancer with intractable unilateral pain developed a decrease in metabolism within the contralateral thalamus, which was abolished after blocking nociceptive input by surgical hemicordotomy.[139] A smaller representation of the affected hand was found in somatosensory areas (SI and SII) for nonpainful stimulation that correlated with symptom severity in patients suffering from complex regional pain syndrome (CRPS),[140] whereas representation for nociceptive input is extended in somatosensory areas in these patients.[141] Similarly, other chronic pain states yielded exaggerated activation and occupied larger areas in somatosensory cortex as demonstrated for low back pain,[142] fibromyalgia,[143] and neuropathic pain.[144] Anatomical changes in grey matter density can also be observed for chronic pain patients. Using MRI scans with voxel based morphometry analysis, changes in white and grey matter can be compared between groups and within subjects during different time points. Changes in different cortical areas were found for different pain syndromes. In chronic back pain patients,[101] atrophy in the thalamus and the prefrontal cortex were observed (Fig. 6.8). Interestingly, these grey matter density changes occur in pain-related regions such as the prefrontal cortex, thalamus, the insula, and the cingulate cortex. Others describe atrophy in the hippocampus, the midcingulate cortex, the frontal cortex, and the insula in fibromyalgia.[145] Similar findings were made in chronic headache.[146] Whether this is a result of the brain atrophy, or a consequence of ongoing pain, is still debated. Another possible explanation for the decreased grey matter density in these disorders might be atrophy secondary to excitotoxicity and/or exposure to inflammation-related agents, such as cytokines.[101]

CONCLUSION

Noninvasive functional neuroimaging of pain in human volunteers and patients has attracted enormous interest and activity in pain research and significantly enriched our knowledge about the contribution of the brain in processing and modifying peripheral and spinal nociceptive signals. Supraspinal mechanisms of nociception and pain rely on a multilevel organization of brain structures involving the brainstem (medulla, pons, midbrain), diencephalon (thalamus, hypothalamus), primary (SI) and secondary (SII) somatosensory cortices, and fronto-limbic circuits (prefrontal cortex, anterior cingulate cortex, insula, amygdala, hippocampus). Spinal nociceptive afferents that reach predominantly lateral thalamic nuclei convey nociceptive signals into the sensory cortex (SI, SII) and provide the individual with the capability to recognize intensity, location, and duration of noxious stimuli. This lateral pain system is therefore commonly referred to as the major brain anatomical substrate of the sensory-discriminative determinant of pain. Direct and multi-synaptic projections from the dorsal horn and brainstem into medial thalamic nuclei transmit nociceptive signals into the limbic system (insula, ACC, prefrontal cortex). This medial pain system predominantly comprises the affective-motivational determinant of pain. A pivotal role of the dorsolateral prefrontal cortex (DLPFC) in pain is its ability to coordinate nociceptive signals with momentary bodily needs and behavioral goals to account for the significance and threat value of pain. The numerous supra-modal connectivity of the DLPFC with sensory and motor systems allow the individual to maintain attention upon pain, but also to release it in favor of superior behavioral goals or in expectation of positive outcome through recruitment of endogenous pain control systems. A predominant feature of pain in comparison with other human senses is its enormous ability to adapt its response properties according to both the bodily and psychological context. This plasticity implies fundamental changes in the course of pathological processes underlying tissue damage and inflammation, or in the course of memory processes and learning from past pain experiences. Supraspinal mechanisms thus contribute to such plasticity by integrating information about the nature and behavioral significance of pain by recruiting unique pathways during normal or sensitized conditions and by facilitating learned pain behaviors. While in most instances such plasticity is adaptive to avoid actual bodily damage or promote the healing process, it also forms the basis for maladaptive consequences underlying chronic pain and neuropathic pain.

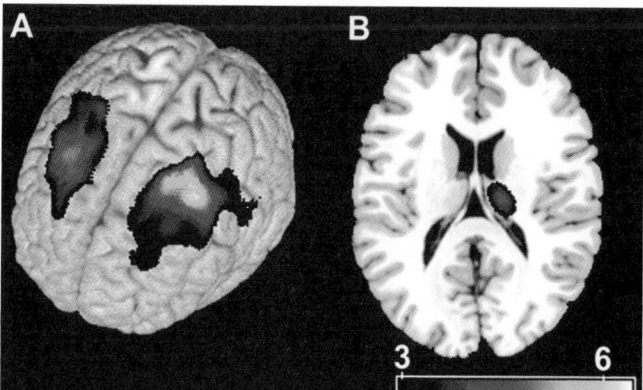

FIGURE 6.8 Regional grey matter density decreases in patients suffering from chronic back pain (CBP). A nonparametric comparison of voxel-based morphometry (VBM) between CBP and control subjects is shown. **(A)** Grey matter density is bilaterally reduced in the dorsolateral prefrontal cortex (DLPFC). The result is from a VBM permutation-based pseudo-*t* test and voxel-level contrasts when all brain grey matter voxels were compared between controls and CBP subjects. Pseudocolor highly positive values indicate regions where grey matter density was reduced in CBP subjects (controls, CBP). **(B)** A nonparametric comparison spatially limited to the thalami revealed a significant decrease in grey matter density in the right anterior thalamus. A slice at the peak of decreased thalamic grey matter is shown. Pseudo-*t* values are color coded; range is 3–6. (Reproduced from Apkarian AV, Sosa Y, Sonty S, et al. Chronic back pain is associated with decreased prefrontal and thalamic gray matter density. *J Neurosci* 2004;24(46):10410–10415, with permission.)

References

1. Casey KL. Forebrain mechanisms of nociception and pain: analysis through imaging. *Proc Natl Acad Sci U S A* 1999;96:7668–7674.
2. Gusnard DA, Raichle ME, Raichle ME. Searching for a baseline: functional imaging and the resting human brain. *Nat Rev Neurosci* 2001;2(10):685–694.
3. Bromm B, Lorenz J. Neurophysiological evaluation of pain. *Electroencephalogr Clin Neurophysiol* 1998;107:227–253.
4. Coenen AM. Neuronal phenomena associated with vigilance and consciousness: from cellular mechanisms to electroencephalographic patterns. *Conscious Cogn* 1998;7(1):42–53.
5. Bowsher D. Role of the reticular formation in responses to noxious stimulation. *Pain* 1976;2(4):361–378.
6. Casey KL, Morrow TJ. Effect of medial bulboreticular and raphe nuclear lesions on the excitation and modulation of supraspinal nocifensive behaviors in the cat. *Brain Res* 1989;501(1):150–161.
7. Casey KL. Somatosensory responses of bulboreticular units in awake cat: relation to escape-producing stimuli. *Science* 1971;173(991):77–80.
8. Wei F, Dubner R, Ren K. Nucleus reticularis gigantocellularis and nucleus raphe magnus in the brain stem exert opposite effects on behavioral hyperalgesia and spinal Fos protein expression after peripheral inflammation. *Pain* 1999;80:127–141.

9. Villanueva L, Bouhassira D, Le Bars D. The medullary subnucleus reticularis dorsalis (SRD) as a key link in both the transmission and modulation of pain signals. *Pain* 1996;67:231–240.

10. Villanueva L, Le Bars D. The activation of bulbo-spinal controls by peripheral nociceptive inputs: diffuse noxious inhibitory controls. *Biol Res* 1995;28(1):113–125.

11. Merker B. Consciousness without a cerebral cortex: a challenge for neuroscience and medicine. *Behav Brain Sci* 2007;30(1):63–81.

12. Reynolds DV. Surgery in the rat during electrical analgesia induced by focal brain stimulation. *Science* 1969;164(878):444–445.

13. Mayer DJ, Wolfle TL, Akil H, et al. Analgesia from electrical stimulation in the brainstem of the rat. *Science* 1971;174(16):1351–1354.

14. Oliveras JL, Redjemi F, Guilbaud G, et al. Analgesia induced by electrical stimulation of the inferior centralis nucleus of the raphe in the cat. *Pain* 1975;1(2):139–145.

15. Basbaum AI, Fields HL. Endogenous pain control mechanisms: review and hypothesis. *Ann Neurol* 1978;4(5):451–462.

16. Fields HL, Vanegas H, Hentall ID, et al. Evidence that disinhibition of brain stem neurones contributes to morphine analgesia. *Nature* 1983;306(5944):684–686.

17. Potrebic SB, Fields HL, Mason P. Serotonin immunoreactivity is contained in one physiological cell class in the rat rostral ventromedial medulla. *J Neurosci* 1994;14:1655–1665.

18. Lima D, Albino-Teixeira A, Tavares I. The caudal medullary ventrolateral reticular formation in nociceptive-cardiovascular integration. An experimental study in the rat. *Exp Physiol* 2002;87(2):267–274.

19. Ren K, Ruda MA. Descending modulation of Fos expression after persistent peripheral inflammation. *Neuroreport* 1996;7(13):2186–2190.

20. Keay KA, Bandler R. Deep and superficial noxious stimulation increases Fos-like immunoreactivity in different regions of the midbrain periaqueductal grey of the rat. *Neurosci Lett* 1993;154(1–2):23–26.

21. Lumb BM. Inescapable and escapable pain is represented in distinct hypothalamic-midbrain circuits: specific roles for Adelta- and C-nociceptors. *Exp Physiol* 2002;87(2):281–286.

22. Lumb BM. Hypothalamic and midbrain circuitry that distinguishes between escapable and inescapable pain. *News Physiol Sci* 2004;19:22–26.

23. Lorenz J, Cross, D, Minoshima S, Morrow TJ, Paulson PE, Casey K. A unique representation of heat allodynia in the human brain. *Neuron* 2002;35:393.

24. Bernard JF, Bester H, Besson JM. Involvement of the spino-parabrachio-amygdaloid and hypothalamic pathways in the autonomic and affective emotional aspects of pain. In: Holstege G, Bandler R, Saper CB, eds. *The Emotional Motor System*. Amsterdam: Elsevier; 1996:243–255.

25. Burstein R, Falkowsky O, Borsook D, et al. Distinct lateral and medial projections of the spinohypothalamic tract of the rat. *J Comp Neurol* 1996;373(4):549–574.

26. Melzack R, Casey KL. Sensory, motivational, and central control determinants of pain. In: Kenshalo DR, ed. *The Skin Senses*. Springfield, IL: Charles C Thomas; 1968:423–443.

27. Mehler WR, Feferman ME, Nauta WJ. Ascending axon degeneration following anterolateral cordotomy. An experimental study in the monkey. *Brain* 1960;83:718–750.

28. Willis WD, Kenshalo DR Jr, Leonard RB. The cells of origin of the primate spinothalamic tract. *J Comp Neurol* 1979;188(4):543–573.

29. Apkarian AV, Shi T. Squirrel monkey lateral thalamus. I. Somatic nociresponsive neurons and their relation to spinothalamic terminals. *J Neurosci* 1994;14(11 Pt 2):6779–6795.

30. Craig AD. How do you feel? Interoception: the sense of the physiological condition of the body. *Nat Rev Neurosci* 2002;3:655–660.

31. Brodmann K. Beiträge zur histologischen Lokalisation der Grosshirnrinde: dritte Mitteilung: Die Rindenfelder der niederen Affen. *Journal für Psychologie und Neurologie* 1905;4:177–226.

32. Price DD. Psychological and neural mechanisms of the affective dimension of pain. *Science* 2000;288:1769–1772.

33. Papez JW. A proposed mechanism of emotion. 1937. *J Neuropsychiatry Clin Neurosci* 1995;7:103–112.

34. Head H, Holmes G. Sensory disturbances from cerebral lesions. *Brain* 1911;34:102–254.

35. Kleist K. Kriegsverletzungen des Gehirns in ihrer Bedeutung für die Hirnlokalisation und Hirnpathologie. In: von Schjerning O, ed. *Handbuch der Ärztlichen Erfahrungen im Weltkriege 1914–1918. Geistes- und Nervenkrankheiten.* Vol. 4. Leipzig: Barth; 1934:1343–1393.

36. Russell WR. Transient disturbances following gunshot wounds of the head. *Brain* 1945;68:79–97.

37. Marshall J. Sensory disturbances of cortical wounds with special reference to pain. *J Neurol Neurosurg Psychiat* 1951;14:187–204.

38. Kenshalo DR Jr, Chudler EH, Anton F, et al. SI nociceptive neurons participate in the encoding process by which monkeys perceive the intensity of noxious thermal stimulation. *Brain Res* 1988;454(1–2):378–382.

39. Ohara S, Crone NE, Weiss N, et al. Amplitudes of laser evoked potential recorded from primary somatosensory, parasylvian and medial frontal cortex are graded with stimulus intensity. *Pain* 2004;110(1–2):318–328.

40. Penfield W, Boldrey E. Somatic motor and sensory representation in the cerebral cortex of man as studied by electrical stimulation. *Brain* 1937;60:389–443.

41. Mazzola L, Isnard J, Mauguière F. Somatosensory and pain responses to stimulation of the second somatosensory area (SII) in humans. A comparison with SI and insular responses. *Cereb Cortex* 2006;16(7):960–968.

42. Bingel U, Lorenz J, Glauche V, et al. Somatotopic organization of human somatosensory cortices for pain: a single trial fMRI study. *Neuroimage* 2004;23(1):224–232.

43. Ploner M, Schmitz F, Freund HJ, et al. Parallel activation of primary and secondary somatosensory cortices in human pain processing. *J Neurophysiol* 1999;81(6):3100–3104.

44. Tran TD, Inui K, Hoshiyama M, et al. Cerebral activation by the signals ascending through unmyelinated C-fibers in humans: a magnetoencephalographic study. *Neuroscience* 2002;113(2):375–386.

45. Kanda M, Nagamine T, Ikeda A, et al. Primary somatosensory cortex is actively involved in pain processing in human. *Brain Res* 2000;853(2):282–289.

46. Talbot JD, Marrett S, Evans AC, et al. Multiple representations of pain in human cerebral cortex. *Science* 1991;251(4999):1355–1358.

47. Coghill RC, Talbot JD, Evans AC, et al. Distributed processing of pain and vibration by the human brain. *J Neurosci* 1994;14(7):4095–4108.

48. Casey KL, Minoshima S, Morrow TJ, et al. Comparison of human cerebral activation pattern during cutaneous warmth, heat pain, and deep cold pain. *J Neurophysiol* 1996;76(1):571–581.

49. Bornhövd K, Quante M, Glauche V, et al. Painful stimuli evoke different stimulus-response functions in the amygdala, prefrontal, insula and somatosensory cortex: a single-trial fMRI study. *Brain* 2002;125:1326–1336.

50. Davis KD, Wood ML, Crawley AP, et al. fMRI of human somatosensory and cingulate cortex during painful electrical nerve stimulation. *Neuroreport* 1995;7(1):321–325.

51. Oshiro Y, Fujita N, Tanaka H, et al. Functional mapping of pain-related activation with echo-planar MRI: significance of the SII-insular region. *Neuroreport* 1998;9(10):2285–2289.

52. Rosen SD, Paulesu E, Frith CD, et al. Central nervous pathways mediating angina pectoris. *Lancet* 1994;344(8916):147–150.

53. Weiller C, May A, Limmroth V, et al. Brain stem activation in spontaneous human migraine attacks. *Nat Med* 1995;1(7):658–660.

54. Casey KL, Morrow TJ, Lorenz J, et al. Temporal and spatial dynamics of human forebrain activity during heat pain: analysis by positron emission tomography. *J Neurophysiol* 2001;85(2):951–959.

55. Rainville P, Duncan GH, Price DD, et al. Pain affect encoded in human anterior cingulate but not somatosensory cortex. *Science* 1997;277:968–971.

56. Hofbauer RK, Rainville P, Duncan GH, et al. Cortical representation of the sensory dimension of pain. *J Neurophysiol* 2001;86:402–411.

57. Casey KL. Cortical and limbic mechanisms mediating pain and pain-related behaviour. In: Schmidt R, Willis WD, eds. *Encyclopedic Reference of Pain*. Heidelberg: Springer; 2007:465–477.

58. Bushnell MC, Duncan GH, Hofbauer RK, et al. Pain perception: is there a role for primary somatosensory cortex? *Proc Natl Acad Sci U S A* 1999;96(14):7705–7709.

59. Ploner M, Platzen J, Pollok B, et al. Evoked response amplitudes from somatosensory cortices do not determine reaction times to tactile stimuli. *Eur J Neurosci* 2007;25(12):3734–3741.

60. Adrian ED. Double representation of the feet in the sensory cortex of the cat. *J Physiol* 1940;98:16–18.

61. Eickhoff SB, Grefkes C, Zilles K, et al. The somatotopic organization of cytoarchitectonic areas on the human parietal operculum. *Cereb Cortex* 2007;17(8):1800–1811.

62. Hari R, Kaukoranta E. Neuromagnetic studies of somatosensory system: principles and examples. *Prog Neurobiol* 1985;24(3):233–256.

63. Treede RD, Kenshalo DR, Gracely RH, et al. The cortical representation of pain. *Pain* 1999;79(2–3):105–111.

64. Bromm B. Brain images of pain. *News Physiol Sci* 2001;16:244–249.

65. Opsommer E, Weiss T, Plaghki L, et al. Dipole analysis of ultralate (C-fibres) evoked potentials after laser stimulation of tiny cutaneous surface areas in humans. *Neurosci Lett* 2001;298(1):41–44.

66. Peyron R, Frot M, Schneider F, et al. Role of operculoinsular cortices in human pain processing: converging evidence from PET, fMRI, dipole modeling, and intracerebral recordings of evoked potentials. *Neuroimage* 2002;17(3):1336–1344.

67. Tracey I, Mantyh PW. The cerebral signature for pain perception and its modulation. *Neuron* 2007;55(3):377–391.

68. Burton H, Fabri M, Alloway K. Cortical areas within the lateral sulcus connected to cutaneous representations in areas 3b and 1: a revised interpretation of the second somatosensory area in macaque monkeys. *J Comp Neurol* 1995;355(4):539–562.

69. Greenspan JD, Lee RR, Lenz FA. Pain sensitivity alterations as a function of lesion location in the parasylvian cortex. *Pain* 1999;81(3):273–282.

70. Schmahmann JD, Leifer D. Parietal pseudothalamic pain syndrome. Clinical features and anatomic correlates. *Arch Neurol* 1992;49(10):1032–1037.

71. Horiuchi T, Unoki T, Yokoh A, et al. Pure sensory stroke caused by cortical infarction associated with the secondary somatosensory area. *J Neurol Neurosurg Psychiatry* 1996;60(5):588–589.

72. Frot M, Magnin M, Mauguière F, et al. Human SII and posterior insula differently encode thermal laser stimuli. *Cereb Cortex* 2007;17(3):610–620.

73. Schnitzler A, Ploner M. Neurophysiology and functional neuroanatomy of pain perception. *J Clin Neurophysiol* 2000;17(6):592–603.

74. Berthier M, Starkstein S, Leiguarda R. Asymbolia for pain: a sensory-limbic disconnection syndrome. *Ann Neurol* 1988;24(1):41–49.

75. Apkarian AV, Bushnell MC, Treede RD, et al. Human brain mechanisms of pain perception and regulation in health and disease. *Eur J Pain* 2005;9(4):463–484.

76. Ploghaus A, Tracey I, Gati JS, Clare S, et al. Dissociating pain from its anticipation in the human brain. *Science* 1999;284:1979–1981.

77. Schreckenberger M, Siessmeier T, Viertmann A, et al. The unpleasantness of tonic pain is encoded by the insular cortex. *Neurology* 2005;64(7):1175–1783.

78. Downar J, Mikulis DJ, Davis KD. Neural correlates of the prolonged salience of painful stimulation. *Neuroimage* 2003;20(3):1540–1551.

79. Vogt BA. Pain and emotion interactions in subregions of the cingulate gyrus. *Nat Rev Neurosci* 2005;6(7):533–544.

80. Vogt BA, Laureys S. Posterior cingulate, precuneal and retrosplenial cortices: cytology and components of the neural network correlates of consciousness. *Prog Brain Res* 2005;150:205–217.

81. Cohen RA, Kaplan RF, Moser DJ, et al. Impairments of attention after cingulotomy. *Neurology* 1999;53(4):819–824.

82. Vaccarino AL, Melzack R. Analgesia produced by injection of lidocaine into the anterior cingulum bundle of the rat. *Pain* 1989;39(2):213–219.

83. Gabriel M, Kubota Y, Sparenborg S, et al. Effects of cingulate cortical lesions on avoidance learning and training-induced unit activity in rabbits. *Exp Brain Res* 1991;86(3):585–600.

84. Ploner M, Gross J, Timmermann L, et al. Cortical representation of first and second pain sensation in humans. *Proc Natl Acad Sci U S A* 2002;99(19):12444–12448.

85. Miller EK, Cohen JD. An integrative theory of prefrontal cortex function. *Annu Rev Neurosci* 2001;24:167–202.

86. Bingel U, Rose M, Gläscher J, et al. fMRI reveals how pain modulates visual object processing in the ventral visual stream. *Neuron* 2007;55(1):157–167.

87. Valet M, Sprenger T, Boecker H, et al. Distraction modulates connectivity of the cingulo-frontal cortex and the midbrain during pain—an fMRI analysis. *Pain* 2004;109(3):399–408.

88. Eccleston C, Crombez G. Pain demands attention: a cognitive-affective model of the interruptive function of pain. *Psychol Bull* 1999;125:356–366.

89. Casey KL. The imaging of pain: background and rationale. In: Casey KL, Bushnell MC, eds. *Pain Imaging*. Seattle, Wash: IASP Press; 2000:1–29.

90. Bunge SA, Ochsner KN, Desmond JE, et al. Prefrontal regions involved in keeping information in and out of mind. *Brain* 2001;124:2074–2086.

91. Sakai K, Rowe JB, Passingham RE. Active maintenance in prefrontal area 46 creates distractor-resistant memory. *Nat Neurosci* 2002;5:479–484.

92. Price JL, Carmichael ST, Drevets WC. Networks related to the orbital and medial prefrontal cortex; a substrate for emotional behavior? *Prog Brain Res* 1996;107:523–536.

93. Goodenough OR, Prehn K. A neuroscientific approach to normative judgment in law and justice. *Philos Trans R Soc Lond B Biol Sci* 2004;359(1451):1709–1726.

94. Damasio H, Grabowski T, Frank R, et al. The return of Phineas Gage: clues about the brain from the skull of a famous patient. *Science* 1994;264(5162):1102–1105.

95. Daum I, Braun C, Riesch G, et al. Pain-related cerebral potentials in patients with frontal or parietal lobe lesions. *Neurosci Lett* 1995;197(2):137–140.

96. Coghill RC, Sang CN, Maisog JM, et al. Pain intensity processing within the human brain: a bilateral, distributed mechanism. *J Neurophysiol* 1999;82:1934–1943.

97. Lorenz J, Minoshima S, Casey KL. Keeping pain out of mind: the role of the dorsolateral prefrontal cortex in pain modulation. *Brain* 2003;126:1079–1091.

98. Wager TD, Rilling JK, Smith EE, et al. Placebo-induced changes in FMRI in the anticipation and experience of pain. *Science* 2004;303(5661):1162–1167.

99. Petrovic P, Kalso E, Petersson KM, et al. Placebo and opioid analgesia—imaging a shared neuronal network. *Science* 2002;295: 1737–1740.

100. Bingel U, Lorenz J, Schoell E, et al. Mechanisms of placebo analgesia: rACC recruitment of a subcortical antinociceptive network. *Pain* 2006;120(1–2):8–15.

101. Apkarian AV, Sosa Y, Sonty S, et al. Chronic back pain is associated with decreased prefrontal and thalamic gray matter density. *J Neurosci* 2004;24(46):10410–10415.

102. Brighina F, Piazza A, Vitello G, et al. rTMS of the prefrontal cortex in the treatment of chronic migraine: a pilot study. *J Neurol Sci* 2004;227(1):67–71.

103. Hardy SG, Haigler HJ. Prefrontal influences upon the midbrain: a possible route for pain modulation. *Brain Res* 1985;339(2):285–293.

104. Sah P, Faber ES, Lopez De Armentia M, et al. The amygdaloid complex: anatomy and physiology. *Physiol Rev* 2003;83(3):803–834.

105. Swanson LW, Petrovich GD. What is the amygdala? *Trends Neurosci* 1998;21(8):323–331.

106. Shi CJ, Cassell MD. Cascade projections from somatosensory cortex to the rat basolateral amygdala via the parietal insular cortex. *J Comp Neurol* 1998;399(4):469–491.

107. Schneider F, Habel U, Holthusen H, et al. Subjective ratings of pain correlate with subcortical-limbic blood flow: an fMRI study. *Neuropsychobiology* 2001;43(3):175–185.

108. Bingel U, Quante M, Knab R, et al. Subcortical structures involved in pain processing: evidence from single-trial fMRI. *Pain* 2002;99(1–2):313–321.

109. Borszcz GS, Streltsov NG. Amygdaloid-thalamic interactions mediate the antinociceptive action of morphine microinjected into the periaqueductal gray. *Behav Neurosci* 2000;114(3):574–584.

110. Fields HL. Pain modulation: expectation, opioid analgesia and virtual pain. *Prog Brain Res* 2000;122:245–253.

111. Mena NB, Mathur R, Nayar U. Amygdalar involvement in pain. *Indian J Physiol Pharmacol* 1995;39(4):339–346.

112. Scoville WB, Milner B. Loss of recent memory after bilateral hippocampal lesions. 1957. *J Neuropsychiatry Clin Neurosci* 2000;12(1):103–113.

113. Neylan TC. Neuropsychiatric consequences of traumatic brain injury: observations from Adolf Meyer. *J Neuropsychiatry Clin Neurosci* 2000;12(3):406.

114. Ploghaus A, Tracey I, Clare S, et al. Learning about pain: the neural substrate of the prediction error for aversive events. *Proc Natl Acad Sci U S A* 2000; 97(16):9281–9286.

115. Derbyshire SW, Jones AK, Gyulai F, et al. Pain processing during three levels of noxious stimulation produces differential patterns of central activity. *Pain* 1997;73(3):431–445.

116. Parasuraman R, Warm, JS, See, JE. Brain systems of vigilance. In: Parasuraman R, ed. *The Attentive Brain*. Cambridge, Mass: MIT Press; 1998:221–256

117. Posner MI, Petersen SE. The attention system in the human brain. *Ann. Rev. Neurosci* 1990:13:25–42.

118. Lorenz J, Garcia-Larrea L. Contribution of attentional and cognitive factors to laser evoked brain potentials. *Neurophysiol Clin* 2003;33:293–301.

119. Bingel U, Schoell E, Herken W, et al. Habituation to painful stimulation involves the antinociceptive system. *Pain* 2007 Sep;131(1–2):21–30.

120. Janicki P, Libich J, Gumulka W. Lack of habituation of pain evoked potentials after naloxone. *Pol J Pharmacol Pharm* 1979;31(3):201–205.

121. Peters ML, Schmidt AJ, Van den Hout MA. Chronic low back pain and the reaction to repeated acute pain stimulation. *Pain* 1989;39(1):69–76.

122. Demirci S, Savas S. The auditory event related potentials in episodic and chronic pain sufferers. *Eur J Pain* 2002;6(3):239–244.

123. Valeriani M, de Tommaso M, Restuccia D, et al. Reduced habituation to experimental pain in migraine patients: a CO(2) laser evoked potential study. *Pain* 2003;105(1–2):57–64.

124. Flor H, Diers M, Birbaumer N. Peripheral and electrocortical responses to painful and non-painful stimulation in chronic pain patients, tension headache patients and healthy controls. *Neurosci Lett* 2004;361(1–3):147–150.

125. Beydoun A, Morrow TJ, Shen, JF, et al. Variability of laser-evoked potentials: attention, arousal and lateralized differences. *Electroencephalogr Clin Neurophysiol* 1993;88:173–181.

126. Moldofsky H. Sleep and pain. *Sleep Med Rev* 2001;5(5):385–396.

127. Zaslansky R, Sprecher E, Katz Y, et al. Pain-evoked potentials: what do they really measure? *Electroencephalogr Clin Neurophysiol* 1996;100(5):384–391.

128. Hauck M, Bischoff P, Schmidt G, et al. Clonidine effects on pain evoked SII activity in humans. *Eur J Pain* 2006;10(8):757–765.

129. Roth D, Petersen-Felix S, Bak P, et al. Analgesic effect in humans of subanaesthetic isoflurane concentrations evaluated by evoked potentials. *Br J Anaesth* 1996;76:38–42.

130. McCracken LM, Turk DC. Behavioral and cognitive-behavioral treatment for chronic pain: outcome, predictors of outcome, and treatment process. *Spine* 2002;27(22):2564–2573.

131. McCabe C, Lewis J, Shenker N, et al. Don't look now! Pain and attention. *Clin Med* 2005;5(5):482–486.

132. Vlaeyen JW, Linton SJ. Fear-avoidance and its consequences in chronic musculoskeletal pain: a state of the art. *Pain* 2000;85(3):317–332.

133. Van Damme S, Crombez G, Eccleston C, et al. Impaired disengagement from threatening cues of impending pain in a crossmodal cueing paradigm. *Eur J Pain* 2004;8:227–236.

134. Villemure C, Bushnell MC. Cognitive modulation of pain: how do attention and emotion influence pain processing? *Pain* 2002;95(3):195–199.

135. Engel AK, Fries P, Singer W. Dynamic predictions: oscillations and synchrony in top-down processing. *Nat Rev Neurosci* 2001;2(10):704–716.

136. Herrmann CS, Munk MH, Engel AK. Cognitive functions of gamma-band activity: memory match and utilization. *Trends Cogn Sci* 2004;8(8):347–355.

137. Hauck M, Lorenz J, Engel AK. Attention to painful stimulation enhances gamma-band activity and synchronization in human sensorimotor cortex. *J Neurosci* 2007;27(35):9270–9277.

138. Flor H, Diers M. Limitations of pharmacotherapy: behavioral approaches to chronic pain. *Handb Exp Pharmacol* 2007;(177):415–427.

139. Di Piero V, Jones AK, Iannotti F, et al. Chronic pain: a PET study of the central effects of percutaneous high cervical cordotomy. *Pain* 1991;46(1):9–12.

140. Pleger B, Ragert P, Schwenkreis P, et al. Patterns of cortical reorganization parallel impaired tactile discrimination and pain intensity in complex regional pain syndrome. *Neuroimage* 2006;32(2):503–510.

141. Maihöfner C, Forster C, Birklein F, et al. Brain processing during mechanical hyperalgesia in complex regional pain syndrome: a functional MRI study. *Pain* 2005;114(1–2):93–103.

142. Flor H, Braun C, Elbert T, et al. Extensive reorganization of primary somatosensory cortex in chronic back pain patients. *Neurosci Lett* 1997;224(1):5–8.

143. Montoya P, Pauli P, Batra A, et al. Altered processing of pain-related information in patients with fibromyalgia. *Eur J Pain* 2005;9(3):293–303.

144. Peyron R, Schneider F, Faillenot I, et al. An fMRI study of cortical representation of mechanical allodynia in patients with neuropathic pain. *Neurology* 2004;63(10):1838–1846.

145. Kuchinad A, Schweinhardt P, Seminowicz DA, et al. Accelerated brain gray matter loss in fibromyalgia patients: premature aging of the brain? *J Neurosci* 2007;27(15):4004–4007.

146. May A, Matharu M. New insights into migraine: application of functional and structural imaging. *Curr Opin Neurol* 2007;20(3):306–309.

CHAPTER 7 ■ PSYCHOLOGICAL ASPECTS OF PAIN

DENNIS C. TURK, KIMBERLY S. SWANSON, AND HILARY D. WILSON

INTRODUCTION

Advances in the knowledge of the neurophysiology of pain have resulted in the development of new pharmacological agents, sophisticated surgical interventions, and the use of advanced technologies (e.g., spinal cord stimulation, implantable drug delivery systems) for the treatment of pain. Despite these advances, the cure of pain remains elusive. Regardless of the treatment, the amount of pain reduction averages only about 35%, and fewer than 50% of persons treated with these interventions obtain this result. The extent of improvement in emotional, physical, and social functioning is often below these dissatisfying levels.[1]

Despite the poor track record of chronic pain treatments, chronic pain patients are often given an expectation for a cure. Although individuals with acute pain can often receive relief from primary health care providers, people with persistent pain become enmeshed in the medical system as they shuttle from doctor to doctor, diagnostic test to diagnostic, in a frustrating search to have their pain successfully treated. This experience of "medical limbo"—the presence of a painful condition that, in the absence of acceptable pathology, is either attributed to psychiatric causation or malingering on the one hand, or an undiagnosed but potentially progressive disease on the other—is itself a source of significant and chronic stress that can initiate emotional distress or aggravate a premorbid psychiatric condition.

The person who has a chronic pain condition resides in a complex and costly world that is populated not only by them but also by their significant others, health care providers, employers, and third–party payers. Family members feel increasingly hopeless and distressed as medical costs, disability, and emotional suffering increase while income and available treatment options decline. Health care providers grow increasingly frustrated and feel defeated and ineffective as available treatment options are exhausted, while the pain condition remains a mystery and may worsen. Employers, who are already resentful of growing worker's compensation benefits, pay higher costs while productivity suffers because the employee frequently calls out sick or is unable to perform at his or her usual level ("presenteeism"). Third-party payers watch as health care expenditures soar with repeated diagnostic testing, often with inconclusive results. In time, the legitimacy of the individual's report of pain may be questioned, since oftentimes a medical etiology fails to substantiate the cause of the symptoms.

People with chronic pain may begin to feel that their health care providers, employers, and even family members are blaming them when their condition does not respond to treatment. Some may suggest that the individual is complaining excessively in an attempt to receive attention, avoid undesirable activities, or be relieved from onerous obligations (e.g., gainful employment, household chores). Others may suggest that the pain is not real, they are feigning or exaggerating their symptoms, and is all in their head—"psychogenic." Third-party payers may even suggest that the individual is intentionally exaggerating his or her pain in order to obtain financial gain while others may attribute reported symptoms to the desire to obtain mood-altering medications. In this way they may come to be viewed as "whimps," "crocks," or "fakes." Patients may in turn come to view health care providers as "quacks," "hacks," or "thieves." Often, the result is an unfortunate and inappropriate adversarial relationship.

As a result of the attitudes, and in the absence of cure or even substantial relief described, individuals with chronic pain may withdraw from society, lose their jobs, alienate family and friends, and become more and more isolated, despondent, depressed, and, in general, demoralized. Their bodies, the health care system, and their significant other have all let them down; they may feel they have even let themselves down as they relinquish their usual activities and responsibilities due to symptoms that are intractable, yet often inscrutable when not validated by objective pathological findings. This emotional distress, however, can be exacerbated by a variety of other factors, including fear, inadequate or maladaptive support systems, inadequate personal and material coping resources, treatment-induced (iatrogenic) complications, overuse of potent drugs, inability to work, financial difficulties, prolonged litigation, disruption of usual activities, and sleep disturbance. Living with persistent pain conditions requires considerable emotional resilience and tends to deplete people's emotional reserves, taxing not only the individual sufferer but also the capacity of family, friends, coworkers, employers, and society to provide support.

Based on the evidence presented, two conclusions are obvious: (1) psychosocial and behavioral factors play a significant role in the experience, maintenance, and exacerbation of pain; and (2) since some level of pain persists in the majority of people with chronic pain regardless of treatment, self-management is an important complement to biomedical approaches. In this chapter we will emphasize a set of important psychological constructs including dispositional, cognitive, affective, and behavioral factors. We discuss them separately for ease of explication. It is important to note, however, that although we will describe these separately, there is considerable overlap and integration among them. We will conclude with a discussion of integrative models and treatments of chronic pain.

COGNITIVE FACTORS: PREDISPOSITIONS, APPRAISALS, BELIEFS, PERCEIVED CONTROL, AND SELF-EFFICACY

Predispositions

Temperament is putatively, at least partly, heritable and may show continuity throughout life. Personality in adulthood reflects the molding of underlying temperament by life experiences. Temperament and personality may predispose individuals toward misinterpretation of pain sensations and maladaptive pain beliefs, or they can have a protective role.

Potential vulnerability factors that have been proposed are negative affectivity, anxiety sensitivity (AS), and illness/injury sensitivity. Negative affectivity may be considered as heritable, stable, and promoting a tendency to experience a broad range of negative emotions and to view the world as threatening and distressing.[2] Negative affectivity has been associated with heightened vigilance to bodily sensations and interpretational biases toward ambiguous internal signals.[3,4] Studies in nonclinical populations found negative affectivity to predict lower pain tolerance.[5] However, studies in chronic pain populations have so far not provided consistent evidence for a role of trait negative affectivity. Thus, although negative affectivity has often been implicated as a vulnerability factor in chronic pain, convincing evidence is lacking.

More convincing has been the research on another potential vulnerability factor: AS. AS is defined as the fear of anxiety-related sensations, and is conceived as a partly heritable personality trait.[6] Individuals with high AS interpret unpleasant physical sensations (like rapid heart beating, feeling faint) more often as a sign of danger than individuals with low anxiety sensitivity. There is growing evidence that AS may also be a risk factor for the maintenance and exacerbation of chronic pain and disability.[7] AS has been shown to correlate with measures of fear-avoidance and is associated with distress, analgesic use, and physical and social functioning in patients across a wide range of different pain-related conditions.[8] Moreover, path analyses and mediation models suggest that anxiety sensitivity exacerbates fear-avoidance beliefs and the negative interpretation of bodily sensations, which in turn leads to enhanced pain experience and pain avoidance.[9,10] Studies examining the predictive value of AS in relation to cognitive and behavioral reactions to experimentally induced pain support a causal, negative biasing role of AS in maladaptive cognitive and behavioral pain response.

In contrast to the extensive search after negative predisposing factors described, there has been relatively little research on protective factors for chronic pain and disability. Three potential resilience factors will be discussed here: optimism, hope, and benefit finding. Review of the literature suggests that optimism may be one of the most important personality traits in relation to adjustment to chronic pain. Dispositional optimism is defined as "the tendency to believe that one will generally experience good outcomes in life"[11] and is distinguishable from neuroticism and trait anxiety.[12] In cross-sectional and prospective studies, optimism was found to be associated with better general health, adaptation to chronic disease, and recovery after various surgical procedures.[12-14]

Only a few studies have explored the role of dispositional optimism or hope in adaptation to chronic pain. Novy[15] found that optimism was related to less catastrophizing and more use of active coping strategies in chronic pain patients. Affleck and Tennen[16] reported that dispositional optimism predicts pleasant daily mood in fibromyalgia but that it is not related to daily pain. Finally, in studying rheumatoid arthritis patients, Treharne and colleagues[17] found that optimism was associated with less depression and pain, and higher life satisfaction for patients in the early and intermediate stages of disease.

The primary mechanism of the beneficial effect of optimism may be differences in coping behavior between optimistic and pessimistic people.[18] In general, pessimists turn to avoidant coping strategies and denial more often, while optimists employ more problem-focused coping strategies. When problem-focused coping is not possible, they turn to coping strategies such as acceptance, use of humor, and positive reframing of the situation.[12,13] Thus, it may not be the use of specific coping strategies, but flexibility of coping that protects against disability and distress.[14] Snyder has described a similar pathway for hope, with people with low hope showing a tendency to catastrophize, whereas people with high hope seek means to encounter future challenges and show flexibility in finding alternative life goals when their original goals are blocked.[19]

Appraisal and Beliefs

Specific appraisal and beliefs are largely shaped by an individual's learning history through direct experience, observational learning, or information from others. These experiences may interact with an individual's traits and their general outlook on the world. That is, personality factors may predispose some people to make certain kinds of appraisals and to be more susceptible to some beliefs than to others.

Pain appraisal refers to the meaning ascribed to pain by an individual.[20] In accordance with the transactional stress model,[21] a distinction can be made between primary appraisal (evaluation of the significance of pain in terms of threatening, benign, or irrelevant) and secondary appraisal (evaluation of the controllability of pain and one's coping resources). Beliefs refer to assumptions about reality that shape how one interprets events, and can thus be considered as determinants of appraisal. Pain beliefs develop during the lifetime as a result of an individual's learning history and cover all aspects of the pain experience (e.g., the causes of pain, its prognosis, suitable treatments).

Appraisal and beliefs about pain can have a strong impact on an individual's response to pain. If a pain signal is interpreted as harmful (threat), it may be perceived as more intense, more unpleasant, and evoke more escape or avoidance behavior. For instance, Smith and colleagues[22] demonstrated that cancer patients who attributed pain sensations after physiotherapy directly to cancer reported more intense pain than patients who attributed this pain to other causes. Perception of danger of an experimental pain stimulus may also lead to avoidance of this stimulus. Arntz and Claassens[23] experimentally manipulated the appraisal of a mildly painful stimulus (a very cold metal bar placed against the neck) by suggesting that it was either very hot or very cold. As expected, participants rated the stimulus as more painful in the condition where they were informed that it was hot. The effect appeared to be mediated by the belief that the stimulus would be harmful. These studies demonstrate the important role of people's interpretations regarding the meaning of the pain.

Pain appraisal and pain beliefs are also prominent determinants of adjustment to chronic pain.[24,25] Pain that is viewed as a signal of damage, leads to disability, is uncontrollable, and is a permanent condition has been shown to affect individuals' responses[25,26] and these beliefs are widespread.[27,28]

Catastrophizing and Fear-Avoidance Beliefs

Pain catastrophizing can be defined as an exaggerated negative orientation toward actual or anticipated pain experiences. Current conceptualizations most often describe it in terms of appraisal or as a set of maladaptive beliefs.[29-31] Cross-sectional studies have demonstrated that catastrophizing is associated with increased pain, increased illness behavior, and physical and psychological dysfunction across numerous clinical and nonclinical populations. Prospective studies indicated that catastrophizing might be predictive of the inception of chronic musculoskeletal pain in the general population,[32,33] and of more intense pain and slower recovery after surgical intervention.[34,35]

People with chronic pain often anticipate that certain activities will increase their pain or induce further injury. These fears may contribute to avoidance of activity and subsequently greater physical deconditioning, emotional distress, and, ultimately, greater disability. Their failure to engage in activities prevents them from obtaining any corrective feedback about the associations among activity, pain, and injury.

In addition to fear of movement, people with persistent pain may be anxious about the meaning of their symptoms for the future—will their pain increase, will their physical capacity diminish, will they have progressive disability where they ultimately end up in a wheelchair or bedridden? In addition to these sources of fear, pain sufferers may fear that on the one hand people will not believe that they are suffering and on the other they may be told that they are beyond help and will "just have to learn to live with it." Such fears can contribute to additional emotional distress and to increased muscle tension and physiological arousal that may directly exacerbate and maintain pain.

The role of catastrophizing and the belief that pain means harm and activity should be avoided has been most articulated in fear-avoidance models (FAMs) of chronic pain.[36,37] Although FAMs are multifaceted and include affective (fear) and behavioral (avoidance) components, cognitions are identified as the core determinants of entering into a negative pain cycle. The tenets of contemporary FAMs can be summarized as follows: When pain is perceived following injury, an individual's idiosyncratic beliefs will determine the extent to which pain is catastrophically interpreted. A catastrophic interpretation of pain gives rise to physiological (arousal), behavioral (avoidance), and cognitive fear responses. The cognitive shift that takes place during fear enhances threat perception (e.g., by narrowing of attention) and further feeds the catastrophic appraisal of pain.[36]

There is substantial evidence that fear-avoidance beliefs are associated with disability and impaired physical performance in chronic pain.[37–39] A systematic review of the literature on psychological risk factors in back and neck pain indicated that the evidence for the association between fear-avoidance beliefs and increased pain and disability was of the highest level.[37] In addition, prospective studies have shown that fear-avoidance beliefs in patients seeking care for acute pain may be predictive of pain persistence, disability, and long-term sick leave.[40–42]

Fear-avoidance beliefs of health care providers have also been found to be related to their treatment behavior and their recommendation for engaging in physical activities.[43–45] The beliefs of patients and health care providers may further interact with each other in a mutually reinforcing way because a patient's beliefs may guide the choice of which health care provider is visited.[46]

Perceived Control and Self-Efficacy

Perceived control over pain refers to the belief that one can exert influence on the duration, frequency, intensity, or unpleasantness of pain. Perceived controllability of a pain stimulus may modify the meaning of this stimulus and directly affect threat appraisal.[47] As a consequence, pain may be rated as less intense or less unpleasant, and pain tolerance may increase.

The belief that one has control over pain has a strong influence on disability in patients with chronic pain complaints,[25,48] and an increase in this belief after multidisciplinary pain treatment may predict pain reduction and decreases in disability[49–51] demonstrated that perceived control over the effects of pain was more strongly related to better adjustment and less disability than perceived control over pain itself.

Related to perceived control is the construct of self-efficacy. Self-efficacy is the conviction that one can successfully perform a certain task or produce a desirable outcome.[52] A major determinant of self-efficacy is prior mastery experience. In laboratory experiments, self-efficacy beliefs predict pain tolerance.[53,54] In chronic pain patients, self-efficacy positively affects physical and psychological functioning,[55,56] and improvements in self-efficacy after self-management and cognitive-behavioral interventions are associated with improvements in pain, functional status, and psychological adjustment.[57,58] Recent reviews of psychological factors in chronic pain have concluded that the evidence for the role of self-efficacy across a broad range of pain populations is impressive.[29,57] Moreover, self-efficacy also influences the prognosis after acute physical interventions like surgery. Prospective studies in patients who underwent surgery demonstrated that high self-efficacy before the start of rehabilitation and larger in-

creases over the course of rehabilitation speed recovery and predict better long-term outcome.[59,60] A preoperative intervention (an instruction video demonstrating movement and breathing skills) in hysterectomy patients was able to enhance preoperative self-efficacy and decrease pain associated with postoperative activities and promote earlier mobilization.[61] Perceived self-efficacy has been shown to have a direct effect on the body's opioid and immune systems[62] confirming the important association between psychological constructs and physiology.

STRESS AND AUTONOMIC RESPONSES: HYPOTHALAMIC-PITUITARY-ADRENAL AXIS DYSREGULATION

It is becoming clear that the pain experience is determined by a multitude of factors. Although the focus has historically been directed at sensory mechanisms, more attention is being placed on factors related to cognitive and homeostatic factors. The primary basis for including discussions of homeostatic factors is that chronic pain threatens the organism and produces a cascade of events that eventually contributes to the maintenance of such conditions. If one views pain as a primary threat to the organism, then mechanisms should be present to engage and motivate the organism to restore basic homeostatic function.[63] The major consequence of homeostatic imbalance is stress. Regardless of the source, stressors activate numerous systems such as the autonomic nervous system and the hypothalamic-pituitary-adrenal (HPA) axis. Prolonged activation of the stress system has disastrous effects on the body[64] and sets up a condition of a feedback loop between pain and stress reactivity.

During periods of short-term stress and homeostatic imbalance, the hypothalamus activates the pituitary gland to secrete adrenocorticotropic hormone, which acts on the adrenal cortex to secrete cortisol. Secretion of cortisol elevates blood sugar levels and enhances metabolism, an adaptive response that allows the organism to mobilize energy resources to deal with the threat and restore homeostatic balance (i.e., fight or flight response). The situation is much more serious during prolonged periods of stress and homeostatic imbalance that is associated with long-term psychological stress, chronic pain, and other pathological conditions. Prolonged, elevated levels of cortisol are related to the exhaustion phase of Selye's General Adaptation Syndrome.[64] The negative effects of this stage of the adaptation syndrome include atrophy of muscle tissue, impairment of growth and tissue repair, and immune system suppression which together might set up conditions for the development and maintenance of a variety of chronic pain conditions.[65,66] According to Melzack,[67] psychological stress, as well as sensory and cognitive events, modulates the neurosignature of the body-self neuromatrix which, as a consequence of altered neuromatrix output, is associated with chronic pain conditions. The concept of the neuromatrix has potentially important explanatory implications for brain function in general, and also provides a theoretical framework for the biopsychosocial perspective of chronic pain. As will be discussed later, there is a growing literature demonstrating the importance of psychosocial factors (emotion and cognition) in this neuromatrix conceptualization.

EMOTION

Pain is ultimately a subjective, private experience, but it is invariably described in terms of sensory and affective properties. As defined by the International Association for the Study of Pain: "[Pain] is unquestionably a sensation in a part or parts of the body but it is also always unpleasant and therefore also an *emotional experience*"[68] (emphasis added). The central and interactive roles of sensory information and affective state are supported by an overwhelming amount of evidence.[69] The affective component of pain incorporates many different emotions. Depression and anxiety have received the greatest amount of attention in chronic pain patients; however, anger has recently received considerable interest as a significant emotion in chronic pain patients. Additionally, the ability to maintain positive affect during times of stress has been investigated in relationship to pain.[70]

In addition to affect being one of the three interconnected components of pain, pain and emotions interact in a number of ways. Emotional distress may predispose people to experience pain, be a precipitant of symptoms, be a modulating factor amplifying or inhibiting the severity of pain, be a consequence of persistent pain, or a perpetuating factor. Moreover, these potential roles are not mutually exclusive and any number of them may be involved in a particular circumstance interacting with cognitive appraisals. For example, the literature is replete with studies demonstrating that current mood state modulates reports of pain as well as tolerance for acute pain.[71] Levels of anxiety have been shown to influence not only pain severity but complications following surgery and number of days of hospitalization.[72,73] Individual difference variables, such as anxiety sensitivity, have also been shown to play an important predisposing and augmenting role in the experience of pain.[74] Level of depression has been observed to play a significant role in premature termination from pain rehabilitation programs.[75]

Emotional distress is commonly observed in people with chronic pain. People with chronic and recurrent (episodic) acute pain often feel rejected by the medical system, believing that they are blamed or labeled as symptom magnifiers and complainers by their physicians, family members, friends, and employers when their pain condition does not respond to treatment. They may see multiple physicians and undergo numerous laboratory tests and imaging procedures in an effort to have their pain diagnosed and successfully treated. As treatments expected to alleviate pain are proven ineffective, pain sufferers may lose faith and become frustrated and irritated with the medical system. As their pain persists, they may be unable to work, have financial difficulties, difficulty performing everyday activities, sleep disturbance, or treatment-related complications. They may be fearful and have inadequate or maladaptive support systems and other coping resources available to them. They may feel hostility toward the health care system in its inability to eliminate their pain. They may also feel resentment toward their significant others who they may perceive as providing inadequate support. And, they are even angry with themselves for allowing their pain to take over their lives. These consequences of chronic pain can result in depression, anger, anxiety, self-preoccupation, and isolation—an overall sense of demoralization. Because chronic pain persists over long periods of time, affective state will continue to play a role as the impact of pain comes to influence all aspects of the pain sufferers' lives.

Although most of the literature has focused on the relationship between negative affect and pain, research has indicated the ability to maintain positive affect during stress is an important factor contributing to ongoing adaptation to chronic illness. Positive affect serves to decrease distress in chronic pain patients by broadening the individual's range of affective and cognitive responses permitting a wider range of experiences.[70,76,77] Positive affect can serve as psychological immunity in that chronic pain patients may experience more optimal functioning and improved quality of life while living with ongoing pain. There is some evidence suggesting that, specifically, patients with fibromyalgia report less positive affect, appear to have deficits in daily experiences with positive emotions, and are less able compared to others with chronic pain to maintain positive affect during stress.[70,76,77] This lack of positive emotional regulation heightens the vulnerability of fibromyalgia patients.

Although we will provide an overview of research on the predominant emotions—anxiety, depression, and anger—associated with pain individually, it is important to acknowledge that these emotions are not as distinct when it comes to the experience of pain. They interact and augment each other over time.

Anxiety

It is common for patients with symptoms of pain to be anxious and worried. This is especially true when the symptoms are unexplained, as is often the case for chronic pain syndromes. For example, in a large scale, multicentered study of fibromyalgia syndrome patients, between 44% and 51% of patients acknowledged that they were anxious.[78] People with persistent pain may be anxious about the meaning of their symptoms and for their futures—will their pain increase, will their physical capacity diminish, will their symptoms result in progressive disability where they ultimately end in a wheelchair or bedridden? In addition to these sources of fear, pain sufferers may be worried that, on the one hand, people will not believe that they are suffering and, on the other, they may be told that they are beyond help and will "just have to learn to live with it." Fear and anxiety will also relate to activities that people with pain anticipate will increase their pain or exacerbate whatever physical factors might be contributing to the pain. These fears may contribute to avoidance, motivate inactivity, and, ultimately, greater disability. Continual vigilance and monitoring of noxious stimulation and the belief that it signifies disease progression may render even low intensity aversive sensations less bearable. In addition, such fears will contribute to increased muscle tension and physiological arousal that may exacerbate and maintain pain.

Threat of intense pain captures attention from which it is difficult to disengage. The experience of pain may initiate a set of extremely negative thoughts, as noted previously, and arouse fears—fears of inciting more pain and injury, fear of their future impact.[37] Fear and anticipation of pain are cognitive-perceptual processes that are not driven exclusively by the actual sensory experience of pain, and can exert a significant impact on the level of function and pain tolerance.[79,80] People are motivated to avoid and escape from unpleasant consequences; they learn that avoidance of situations and activities in which they have experienced acute episodes of pain will reduce the likelihood of re-experiencing pain or causing further physical damage. They may become hypervigilant to their environment as a way of preventing the occurrence of pain.

Investigators[81,82] have suggested that fear of pain, driven by the anticipation of pain and not by the sensory experience of pain itself, produces strong negative reinforcement for the persistence of avoidance behavior, and the putative functional disability in pain patients. Avoidance behavior is reinforced in the short-term, through the reduction of suffering associated with noxious stimulation.[83] Avoidance, however, can be a maladaptive response if it persists and leads to increased fear, limited activity, and other physical and psychological consequences that contribute to disability and persistence of pain.

Studies have demonstrated that fear of movement and fear of (re)injury are better predictors of functional limitations than biomedical parameters or even pain severity and duration.[84,85] For example, Crombez, Vlaeyen, and Heuts[84] showed that pain-related fear was the best predictor of behavioral performance in trunk-extension, flexion, and weight lifting tasks, even after partitioning out the effects of pain intensity. Moreover, Vlaeyen and colleagues[86] found that fear of movement/(re)injury was the best predictor of self-reported disability among chronic back pain patients, and that physiological sensory perception of pain and biomedical findings did not add any predictive value. The importance of fear of activity appears to generalize to daily activities, as well as in the clinical experimental context. Approximately two-thirds of chronic nonspecific low back pain sufferers avoid back straining activities because of fear of (re)injury.[84] For example, fear-avoidance beliefs about physical demands of a job are strongly related to disability and work lost during the previous year, even more so than pain severity or other pain variables.[87,88] Interestingly, reduction in pain-related anxiety predicts improvement in functioning, affective distress, pain, and pain-related interference with activity.[83] Clearly, fear, pain-related anxiety, and concerns about harm-avoidance all play important roles in chronic pain and need to be assessed and addressed in treatment.

Pain-related fear and concerns about harm avoidance all appear to exacerbate symptoms.[82] Anxiety is an affective state that is greatly influenced by appraisal processes; to cite the stoic philosopher Epictetus, "There is nothing either bad or good but thinking makes it so." Thus, there is a reciprocal relationship between affective state and cognitive-interpretive processes. Thinking affects mood and mood influences appraisals and, ultimately, the experience of pain.

Depression

Research suggests that 40% to 50% of chronic pain patients suffer from depression.[89,90] Epidemiologic studies provide solid evidence for a strong association between chronic pain and depression, but do not address whether chronic pain causes depression or depression causes chronic pain. Prospective studies of patients with chronic musculoskeletal pain have suggested that chronic pain can cause depression,[91] that depression can cause chronic pain,[92] and that they exist in a mutually reinforcing relationship.[93]

One fact often raised to support the idea that pain causes depression is that the current depressive episode often began after the onset of the pain problem. The majority of studies appear to support this contention.[94] However, several studies have documented that many patients with chronic pain (especially those disabled patients seen in pain clinics) have often had prior episodes of depression that predated their pain problem by years.[95] A small longitudinal study[96] followed patients with herpes zoster for 1 year. They observed that those who developed more severe pain (i.e., postherpetic neuralgia) 3 months after the initial diagnosis scored higher on baseline levels of depressed mood. However, these results were not confirmed in a recent larger study conducted by this group.[97] One important prospective study[98] demonstrated that levels of depression predicted the development of low back pain 3 years following the initial assessment. Patients with depression were 2.3 times more likely to report back pain compared to those who did not report depression. Depression was a much stronger predictor of incident back pain then any clinical or anatomic risk factors. This has led some investigators to propose that there may exist a common trait of susceptibility to dysphoric physical symptoms (including pain) and negative psychological symptoms (including anxiety as well as depression). They conclude that "pain and psychological illness should be viewed as having reciprocal psychological and behavioral effects involving both processes of illness expression and adaptation."[99]

Given the scenario of chronic pain just described, it is hardly surprising that chronic pain patients are depressed. It is interesting, however, to ponder the flip side of the coin—why are not *all* chronic pain patients depressed? Turk and colleagues[93,100] examined this question and determined that two factors appear to mediate the pain-depression relationship: patients' appraisals of the effects of the pain on their lives, and appraisals of their ability to exert any control over their pain and lives. That is, those patients who believed that they could continue to function and that they could maintain some control despite their pain were less likely to become depressed. Here we see the interdependence of cognition and affect.

As noted previously, in the majority of cases depression appears to be reactive, although some have suggested that chronic pain is a form of "masked depression," whereby patients use pain to express their depressed mood because they feel it is more acceptable to complain of pain than to acknowledge that one is depressed. Once a person has a chronic pain diagnosis, it no longer matters which is the cause and which is the consequence—pain or depression. Both need to be treated.

Anger

Anger has been widely observed in people with chronic pain.[101] Even though chronic pain patients might present an image of themselves as even-tempered, Corbishley and colleagues[102] found that 88% acknowledged their feelings of anger when these were explicitly sought. Approximately 98% of the patients referred to a multidisciplinary pain rehabilitation center reported that they were feeling some degree of anger at the time of the assessment.[103] We must be cautious in interpreting data from patients recruited at pain centers, however, as there may be a referral bias such that the most distressed patients are sent to these facilities, and they do not represent the large number of people with persistent pain who are never evaluated in treatment facilities that specialize in pain management.

Since anger is frequently considered as socially undesirable, some patients in the studies cited previously may have found it difficult to admit that they were angry to the health care professionals. Thus, it is possible that the anger rates may actually be an underestimate. The high prevalence of anger observed is perhaps not surprising, given the frustrations related to persistence of symptoms, limited information on etiology, and repeated treatment failures along with anger toward others (employers, insurance companies, the health care system, family members), and anger toward themselves, perhaps, for their inability to alleviate their symptoms and to move on with their lives.[103] Several empirical studies provide preliminary support for the association between anger and pain intensity,[104,105] unpleasantness of pain,[106] affective component of pain,[107] and emotional distress in chronic pain patients,[108,109] as well as families of chronic pain patients.[101]

Anger in chronic pain has been considered by some to be attributable to enduring personality dispositions associated with unconscious conflicts,[110] whereas others have suggested that anger may be a reaction to the presence of recalcitrant symptoms that have been unsubstantiated by objective medical findings and unrelieved by medical treatments.[111] There is some evidence supporting the latter hypothesis. For example, a laboratory study[112] demonstrated that the mere anticipation of pain was sufficient to provoke angry behavioral responses in healthy individuals. Using the cross-lagged design with a clinical sample, Arena, Blanchard, and Andrasik[113] found that an increase in pain tends to precede anger, directly contradicting the anger-somatization association.

The relatively fruitless debate over the cause–effect relationship between anger and pain is reminiscent of the arguments on the associations between pain and depression.[114] In order to refine our understanding of the association between anger and pain beyond this debate, several investigators have begun to examine individual differences in how anger is expressed. In an early study, Pilowsky and Spence[115] found that chronic pain patients are less willing to express anger compared to outpatient medical patients. Similarly, individuals with chronic pain problems appear to inhibit their anger compared to pain-free, healthy persons.[116,117] Furthermore, inhibition of anger seems to contribute to aversion of the chronic pain experience. Inhibition of anger has been found to be related to pain severity and overt pain behaviors,[118] as well as to increased emotional distress.[108,119]

Denial of anger also appears to be common among chronic pain patients. However, awareness of anger should not be confused with anger expression. For example, Corbishely et al.[102] observed that chronic pain patients tend to show strong reservations about expressing socially undesirable emotions that could create interpersonal conflict. For these individuals, it seems that expression of the emotion is under conscious control. They are aware of their anger but choose not to express it. On the other hand, some chronic pain patients may lack awareness of their angry feelings and have increased difficulties in recognizing and reporting these feelings.[120]

Fernandez and Turk[111] proposed that the specificity of targets toward which patients experience angry feelings may be important in understanding of the relationship between pain and anger. When a pain sufferer is angry, there are a range of possible targets (e.g., employer, insurance company, health care providers). The presence or intensity of anger toward different targets may be differentially related to chronic pain experience. That is, there may be some targets of anger that are more relevant to the chronic pain experience than others. As will be discussed later, Okifuji et al.[103] found that anger directed toward oneself was particularly common among chronic pain patients evaluated at a pain rehabilitation facility.

Another important issue regarding anger concerns gender differences. There is a growing literature suggesting the presence of important differences in the ways that males and females respond to pain.[121] Moreover, in the Western cultures, there appear to be social conventions regarding the expression of anger. In general, it seems acceptable for men to display angry feelings, whereas women are socialized to avoid overt expression of anger. However, research investigating gender differences in anger expression has revealed unequivocal results. Some studies report that females report significantly higher levels of generalized anger than males,[122] some report the opposite results,[109,123,124] and still others report no gender differences in anger expression.[125,126] In the chronic pain population, some studies note that male patients seem to acknowledge angry feelings more readily than do female patients.[109,123] In contrast, other investigators[103,127,128] suggest that there may be substantial variability within groups of men and women. There seems to be a subgroup of females who do outwardly express anger, whereas some male patients may suppress their anger.

Although the effects of anger and frustration on exacerbation of pain and treatment acceptance has not received as much attention as anxiety and depression, Kerns et al.[118] found that the suppressed feelings of anger accounted for a significant portion of the variance in pain intensity, perceived interference, and frequency of pain behaviors. Furthermore, Summers et al.[105] found that anger and hostility were powerful predictors of pain severity in people with spinal cord injuries.

It is thus reasonable to expect that the presence of anger may serve as a complicating factor, increasing autonomic arousal and blocking motivation and acceptance of treatments oriented toward rehabilitation and disability management rather than cure, which are often the only treatments available for chronic pain.[71] It would be reasonable to expect that the presence of anger may serve as a complicating factor, increasing autonomic arousal and blocking motivation and acceptance of treatments oriented toward rehabilitation and disability management rather than cure.

Frustrations related to persistence of symptoms, unknown etiology, and repeated treatment failures, along with anger toward employers, insurers, the health care system, family, and themselves, all contribute to the general dysphoric mood of patients.[103] Okifuji et al.[103] reported that 60% of patients expressed anger toward health care providers, 39% toward significant others, 30% toward insurance companies, 26% toward employers, and 20% toward attorneys. The target of anger most commonly acknowledged, however, was anger toward themselves (endorsed by approximately 70% of the sample). Internalization of angry feelings is strongly related to measures of pain intensity, perceived interference, and frequency of pain behaviors.[118] Overall, corre-

lations between anger and pain severity have been shown to be statistically significant, ranging from 0.17 to 0.35.[118,127] Okifuji et al.[103] reported that anger was significantly correlated with pain intensity (correlations = 0.30–0.35). Okifuji et al.[103] also reported that anger was significantly correlated with disability ($r = 0.26$) and was highly associated with depression ($r = 0.52$).

The precise mechanisms by which anger and frustration exacerbate pain are not known. One reasonable possibility is that anger exacerbates pain by increasing autonomic arousal.[129,130] Anger may also interact with depression to modulate perceived severity of pain. In addition, anger may block motivation for, and acceptance of, treatments oriented toward rehabilitation and disability management rather than cure. Yet, rehabilitation and disability management are often the only treatments available for these patients.

In summary, it is important to be aware of the significant role of negative mood in chronic pain patients because it is likely to influence treatment motivation and compliance with treatment recommendations. For example, patients who are anxious may fear engaging in what they perceive as demanding activities; patients who are depressed and who feel helpless may have little initiative to comply; and patients who are angry with the health care system are not likely to be motivated to respond to recommendations from yet another health care professional. Thus, clinicians who are treating people with persistent pain must focus on their mood states, as well as physical pathology and somatic factors. Pain cannot be treated successfully without attending to the patient's emotional state. This is true for acute pain, such as pain associated with surgery, and persistent pain states.

PSYCHOGENIC CONCEPTUALIZATIONS OF CHRONIC PAIN

As a result of the multiple psychosocial factors involved in the onset and maintenance of chronic pain, a number of different psychological perspectives on chronic pain have evolved. Many of the psychological treatments for chronic pain are based on different psychological principles which at times compete and differ from one another. Thus, it is important to consider the varying perspectives.

Psychogenic View

Frequently in medicine, when physical explanations seem inadequate or when the results of treatment are inconsistent, reports of pain are attributed to a psychological etiology (and thus are "psychogenic"). Although psychogenic views of pain have been discussed since the formulation of psychodynamic theory, a psychodynamic perspective on chronic pain was first described systematically in the 1960s. During this time people with pain were viewed as having compulsive and masochistic tendencies, inhibited aggressive needs, and feelings of guilt—"pain-prone personalities."[131] It was commonly held that people with pain had childhood histories fraught with emotional abuse, family dysfunction (e.g., parental quarrels, separation, divorce), illness or death of a parent, early responsibilities, and high orientation toward achievement.[132] Some current research has reported associations between chronic pain and childhood trauma, although the research is not consistent.[133] Based on the psychogenic perspective, assessment of persons with chronic pain is directed toward identifying the psychopathological tendencies that instigate and maintain pain. Although the evidence to support this model is scarce, the American Psychiatric Association[134] has created a psychiatric diagnosis, Somatoform Pain Disorder. Diagnosis of a pain disorder requires that the person's report of pain must be either inconsistent with the anatomical distribution of the nervous system or, if it mimics a known disease entity, cannot, after extensive diagnostic evaluation, be adequately accounted for by organic pathology.[134] Even in the presence of a medical condition that may cause pain, psychological factors may be implicated and, thus, the person may receive a psychiatric diagnosis of "pain disorder associated with both psychological factors and a general medical condition."

It is assumed that reports of pain will cease once the psychogenic mechanisms are resolved. Treatment is geared toward helping patients gain "insight" into the underlying maladaptive psychological contributors.[133,135]

Empirical evidence supporting the psychogenic view is scarce. A number of chronic pain sufferers do not exhibit significant psychopathology. Furthermore, insight-oriented psychotherapy has not been shown to be effective in reducing symptoms for the majority of patients with chronic pain. Studies suggest that the emotional distress observed in patients with chronic pain more typically occurs in *response to* the persistence of pain and not as a causal agent[93,136] and may resolve once pain is adequately treated.[137] The psychogenic model has thus come under scrutiny, and may be flawed in its view of chronic pain.

BEHAVIORAL FORMULATIONS

Classical Conditioning

According to the classical or respondent conditioning model, if a painful stimulus is repeatedly paired with a neutral stimulus, the neutral stimulus will elicit a pain response. For example, a person who experienced pain after performing a treadmill exercise may become conditioned to experience a negative emotional response to the presence of the treadmill and to any stimulus associated with it (e.g., physical therapist, gym). The negative emotional reaction may instigate muscle tensing, thereby exacerbating pain, and further reinforcing the association between the stimulus and pain. Based on this, people with chronic pain may avoid activities previously associated with pain onset or exacerbation.

Operant Conditioning

In 1976, Fordyce[138] introduced an extension of operant conditioning to chronic pain. This view proposes that acute pain behaviors (such as avoidance of activity to protect a painful area from additional pain) may come under the control of external contingencies of reinforcement (responses increase or decrease as a function of their reinforcing consequences) and thus develop into a chronic pain problem. Fordyce underscored the fact that since there is no objective way to measure pain—no pain thermometer—the only way we can know of anyone's pain is by their behavior, whether verbal or nonverbal expressions. Overt pain behaviors include verbal reports, paralinguistic vocalizations (sighs, moans), motor activity, facial expressions, body postures and gesturing (limping, rubbing a painful body part, grimacing), functional limitations (reclining for extensive periods of time, inactivity), and behaviors designed to reduce pain (taking medication, use of the health care system).

The central features of pain behaviors are that they are (1) sources of communication and (2) observable. Observable behaviors are capable of eliciting a response and the consequences of behavior will influence subsequent behavior. Through a process of learning, responses that receive positive consequences, especially repeated desirable consequences, will more likely be maintained; behaviors that fail to activate positive consequences, or that receive negative consequences, will be less likely to occur (i.e., extinguished). Pain behaviors may be positively reinforced directly (e.g., attention from a spouse or health care provider, monetary compensation, avoidance of undesirable activity).[139] Pain behaviors may also be maintained by the escape from noxious stimulation through the use of drugs or rest, or the avoidance of undesirable activities such as work. In addition, "well behaviors" (e.g., activity, working) may not be positively reinforcing and the more rewarding pain behaviors may, therefore, be maintained.

The operant conditioning model considers pain an internal subjective experience that can be directly assessed and may be maintained even after an initial physical basis of pain has resolved rather than the initial causes. The pain behavior originally elicited by organic factors caused by injury or disease may later occur, totally or in part, in response to reinforcing environmental events.

It is important, however, not to make the mistake of viewing pain behaviors as being synonymous with malingering. Malingering involves consciously and purposely faking a symptom such as pain for some gain, usually financial or to gain attention. Contrary to the beliefs of many third-party payers, there is little support for the contention that outright faking of pain for financial gain is prevalent.

Social Learning

The *social learning model* emphasizes the point that behavior can be learned not only by actual reinforcement of the individual's behavior, but also by observation. This is a powerful way of learning especially when the others being observed are judged to be similar to the observer. For example, a middle-aged man might learn what to expect by observing how other middle-aged men with similar medical problems are treated. People can acquire responses that were not previously in their behavioral repertoire by the observation of others performing these activities. Expectancies and actual behavioral responses to nociceptive stimulation are based, at least partially, on prior social learning history.

Another example of social learning occurs in children. Children develop attitudes about health and health care and the perception and interpretation of symptoms and physiological processes from their parents and others they confront in their social environment. They learn how others respond to injury and disease and thus may be more or less likely to ignore or over-respond to symptoms they experience based on behaviors modeled in childhood. For example, children of chronic pain patients may make more pain-related responses during stressful times or exhibit greater illness behaviors (e.g., complaining, days absent, visit to school nurse) than children of healthy parents based on what they observed and learned at home.[140] Models can influence the expression, localization, and methods of coping with pain. Even physiological responses may be conditioned during observation of others in pain.[141]

A central construct of the social learning perspective is that of self-efficacy.[52] Self-efficacy is a personal expectation that is important in patients with chronic pain. A self-efficacy belief is defined as a personal conviction that one can successfully execute a course of action (perform required behaviors) to produce a desired outcome in a given situation.[52] Given sufficient motivation to engage in a behavior, it is a person's self-efficacy beliefs that determine the choice of activities that the he or she will initiate, the amount of effort that will be expended, and how long the individual will persist in the face of obstacles and aversive experiences. In this way, self-efficacy plays an important role in therapeutic change and compliance to psychological and medical regimes.[142]

Efficacy judgments are based on four sources of information regarding one's capabilities, listed in descending order of importance[52]: one's own past performance at the task or similar tasks, the performance accomplishments of others who are perceived to be similar to oneself, verbal persuasion by others that one is capable, and perception of one's own state of physiological arousal, which is, in turn, partly determined by prior efficacy estimation. Performance mastery can then be created by encouraging people to undertake sub-tasks that are initially attainable but become increasingly difficult, and subsequently approaching the desired level of performance. It is important to remember that coping behaviors are influenced by the person's beliefs that the demands of a situation do not exceed their coping resources.

How people interpret, respond to, and cope with illness is determined by cultural norms and perceptions of self-efficacy. These two sets of factors contribute to the marked variability in response to objectively similar degrees of physical pathology noted by health care providers.

Gate Control Model

Although not a psychological formulation itself, the *gate control model*[143] was the first to popularize the importance of central, psychological factors in pain perception. Perhaps the most important contribution of the gate control theory is the way it changed thinking about pain perception. Melzack and Casey[144] differentiate three systems related to the processing of nociceptive stimulation—sensory-discriminative, motivational-affective, and cognitive-evaluative—all thought to contribute to the subjective experience of pain. Thus the gate control theory specifically includes psychological factors as an integral aspect of the pain experience. It emphasizes the central nervous system (CNS) mechanisms and provides a physiological basis for the role of psychological factors in chronic pain.

The gate control model contradicts the notion that pain is *either* somatic *or* psychogenic. Instead, it postulates that both factors have potentiating and moderating effects. According to this model, both the central and peripheral nervous systems interact to contribute to the experience of pain. It is not only these physical factors that guide the brain's interpretation of painful stimuli that is at the center of this model; psychological factors (e.g., thoughts, beliefs, emotions) are also painful stimuli.

Prior to the Melzack and Wall[143] formulation of the gate control theory, psychological processes were largely dismissed as reactions to pain. Although the physiological details of the gate control model have been challenged,[145] it has had a substantial impact on basic research and can be credited as a source of inspiration for diverse clinical applications to control or manage pain, including neurophysiologically based procedures (e.g., neural stimulation techniques from peripheral nerves and collateral processes in the dorsal columns of the spinal cord, pharmacological advances, behavioral treatments, and those interventions that target modification of attentional and perceptual processes involved in the pain experience).

COGNITIVE-BEHAVIORAL PERSPECTIVE

The *cognitive-behavioral model*, perhaps the most commonly accepted model for the psychological treatment of individuals with chronic pain,[146,147] incorporates many of the psychological variables previously described—namely, anticipation, avoidance, and contingencies of reinforcement—but suggests that cognitive factors rather than conditioning factors are of central importance. The model suggests that conditioned reactions are largely self-activated on the basis of learned expectations rather than automatically evoked. The model suggests that behaviors and emotions are influenced by interpretations of events, and emphasis is placed on how peoples' beliefs and attitudes interact with physical, affective, and behavioral factors. It proposes that conditioned reactions are largely activated by learned *expectations* rather than automatically evoked. In other words, it is the person's information processing that result in anticipatory anxiety and avoidance. The critical factor, therefore, is that people learn to anticipate and predict events and to express appropriate reactions.[148]

From the cognitive-behavioral model, people with pain are viewed as having negative expectations about their own ability to control certain motor skills without pain. Moreover, people with chronic pain tend to believe they have limited ability to exert any control over their pain. Such negative, maladaptive appraisals about the situation and personal efficacy may reinforce the experience of demoralization, inactivity, and overreaction to nociceptive stimulation. These cognitive appraisals and expectations are postulated as having an effect on behavior leading to reduced efforts and activity, which may contribute to increased psychological distress (helplessness) and subsequent physical limitations. If one accepts that pain is a complex, subjective phenomenon that is uniquely experienced by each person, then knowledge about idiosyncratic beliefs, appraisals, and coping repertoires becomes critical for optimal treatment planning and for accurately evaluating treatment outcome.

People with chronic pain's beliefs, appraisals, and expectations about pain, their ability to cope, social supports, their disorder, the medicolegal system, the health care system, and their employers are all important because they may facilitate or disrupt the sufferer's sense of control. These factors also influence patients' investment in treatment, acceptance of responsibility, perceptions of disability, adherence to treatment recommendations, support from significant others, expectancies for treatment, and acceptance of treatment rationale.

Cognitive interpretations also affect how patients present symptoms to others, including health care providers. Overt communication of pain, suffering, and distress will enlist responses that may reinforce pain behaviors and impressions about the seriousness, severity, and uncontrollability of pain. That is, complaints of pain may induce physicians to prescribe more potent medications, order additional diagnostic tests, and, in some cases, perform surgery. Significant others may express sympathy, excuse the person with chronic pain from responsibilities, and encourage passivity, thereby fostering further physical deconditioning. It should be obvious that the cognitive-behavioral perspective integrates the operant conditioning emphasis on external reinforcement and respondent view of conditioned avoidance within the framework of information processing.

People with persistent pain often have negative expectations about their own ability and responsibility to exert any control over their pain. Moreover, they often view themselves as helpless. Such negative, maladaptive appraisals about their condition, situation, and their personal efficacy in controlling their pain and problems associated with pain reinforce their experience of demoralization, inactivity, and overreaction to nociceptive stimulation. These cognitive appraisals are posited as having an effect on behavior, leading to reduced effort, reduced perseverance in the face of difficulty, reduced activity, and increased psychological distress.

The cognitive-behavioral perspective on pain management focuses on providing the patient with techniques to gain a sense of control over the effects of pain on his or her life as well as actually modifying the affective, behavioral, cognitive, and sensory facets of the experience. Behavioral experiences help to show pain sufferers that they are capable of more than they assumed, increasing their sense of personal competence. Cognitive techniques (e.g., self-monitoring to identify relationships among thoughts, mood, and behavior, distraction using imagery, and problem solving) help to place affective, behavioral, cognitive, and sensory responses under the person's control.

The assumption is that long-term maintenance of behavioral changes will occur only if the person with pain has learned to attribute success to his or her own efforts. There are suggestions that these treatments can result in changes of beliefs about pain, coping style, and reported pain severity, as well as direct behavior changes. Treatment that results in increases in perceived control over pain and decreased catastrophizing also results in decreases in pain severity and functional disability. When successful rehabilitation occurs there is a major shift from beliefs about helplessness and passivity to resourcefulness and ability to function regardless of pain, and from an illness conviction to a rehabilitation conviction.

A number of studies have attempted to identify cognitive factors that contribute to pain and disability.[142,149] These studies have consistently demonstrated that a person's attitudes, beliefs, and expectancies about their plight, themselves, their coping resources, and the health care system affect reports of pain, activity, disability, and response to treatment. For example, people respond to medical conditions in part based on their subjective ideas about illness and their symptoms. When pain is interpreted as signifying ongoing tissue damage or a progressive disease, it is likely to produce considerably more suffering and behavioral dysfunction than if it is viewed as being the result of a stable problem that is expected to improve.

Once beliefs and expectancies are formed, they become stable and rigid and relatively impervious to modification. Pain sufferers tend to avoid experiences that could invalidate their beliefs (disconfirmations) and guide their behavior in accordance with these beliefs, even in situations where these beliefs are no longer valid. It is thus essential for people with chronic pain to develop adaptive beliefs about the relationships among impairment, pain, suffering, and disability, and to deemphasize the role of experienced pain in their regulation of functioning.

Distorted thinking can also contribute to the maintenance and exacerbation of pain. A particularly potent and pernicious thinking style that has been observed among people with chronic pain is catastrophizing (holding negative thoughts about one's situation and interpreting even minor problems as major catastrophes).[150] Research has indicated that people who spontaneously use more catastrophizing thoughts report more pain than those who do not catastrophize.[150]

Coping strategies, or a person's specific ways of adjusting to or minimizing pain and distress, act to alter both the perception of pain intensity and one's ability to manage or tolerate pain and continue everyday activities. Overt behavioral coping strategies include rest, medication, and use of relaxation, among others. Covert coping strategies include various means of distracting oneself from pain, reassuring oneself that the pain will diminish, seeking information, and problem solving, to list some of the most prominent.

Studies have found active coping strategies (efforts to function in spite of pain or to distract oneself from pain) to be associated with adaptive functioning, and passive coping strategies (depending on others for help with pain control, avoiding activities because of fear of pain/injury, self-medication, alcohol) to be related to greater pain and depression.[151] Regardless of the type of coping strategy, if people with chronic pain are instructed in the use of adaptive coping strategies, their rating of intensity of pain decreases and tolerance of pain increases.[151] Thus, the perspective on how people function and the emphasis on facilitating self-management are more important than any specific cognitive or behavioral techniques that are used to bring about change in thinking and changes in behavior.

BIOPSYCHOSOCIAL MODEL

Although the gate control model described previously introduced the role of psychological factors in the maintenance of pain symptoms, it focused primarily on the basic anatomy and neurophysiology of pain. The biopsychosocial model, which expands the cognitive-behavioral model of pain, views illness as a dynamic and reciprocal interaction between biological, psychological, and sociocultural variables that shape the person's response to pain.[85,151] What is unique about the model is that it takes into consideration the influence of higher order cognitions, including perception and appraisal. It accepts that people are active processors of information and that behavior, emotions, and even physiology are influenced by interpretations of events, rather than solely by physiological factors.[85,151] People with chronic pain may therefore have negative expectations about their own ability and responsibility to exert any control over their pain. Moreover, behaviors of people with pain elicit responses from significant others that can reinforce both adaptive and maladaptive modes of thinking, feeling, and behaving.

Loeser[152] originally formulated a general model that delineated four dimensions associated with the concept of pain: nociception, the stimulation of nerves that convey information about possible tissue damage to the brain; pain, the subjective perception that is the result of transduction, transmission, and modulation of sensory information; suffering, the emotional responses that are triggered by nociception or some other aversive event associated with it, such as fear or depression; and pain behavior, those things that people do when they are suffering or in pain, such as avoiding activities or exercise for fear of (re)injury. Subsequently, Waddell[153] emphasized that pain cannot be comprehensively evaluated without an understanding of the individual who is exposed to the nociception. Waddell also made a comparison between Loeser's[154] model of pain and the earlier discussed call by Engel[155] of the need for a new, more biopsychosocial model in medicine. Engel proposed the important dimensions of the physical problem, distress, illness behavior, and the sick role, which corresponded to Loeser's dimensions of nociception, pain, suffering, and pain behavior, respectively. Thus, with this general perspective, a diversity of pain or illness can be expected (including its severity, duration, and psychosocial consequences). In order to fully understand a person's perception and response to pain and illness, the interrelationships among biological changes, psychological status, and the sociocultural context all need to be considered. Any model that focuses on only one of these dimensions will be incomplete.

FAMILY SYSTEMS PERSPECTIVE

In *family systems* (and this could be expanded to significant others and not only traditional conceptualizations of nuclear families) the family is viewed as an interactional unit, and family members profoundly impact each other's emotions, thoughts, and behaviors. Thus, the functioning of family members is interdependent and family relationships are an important factor not only in psychological but also physical health.[156]

Increasingly, evidence supports family members contribute to behavioral risk factors such as smoking, lack of exercise, poor diet, to the development of numerous chronic illnesses, as well as compliance to treatment regimes.[157] Additionally, families influence the development of chronic pain via operant theory. For example, expressions of acute pain (reporting pain, grimacing, avoidance of activity, and use of pain medication), because they are overt and observable, may be reinforced through expressions of concern from family members. Furthermore, in support of this idea, a number of investigators[90,139] found that spousal attentiveness to expressions of pain was positively correlated with higher levels of reported pain, pain behavior frequency, and disability.

The experience of chronic stress within the family has also been hypothesized to contribute to the development of chronic illness.[158] Specifically, chronic stress within the family may play an important role in sympathetic nervous system and endocrine dysregulation often found in chronic pain patients.

As noted previously, pain does not take place in isolation but in a social context. Pain does not occur solely in people's bodies, nor does it occur solely in their brains, but, rather, it occurs in their lives. The emphasis on the role of significant others is important, as it reminds us that to successfully treat chronic pain patients requires that we not only assess and treat the patient, but must also target significant others that can either impede or facilitate rehabilitation.[159]

CONCLUSION

For the person experiencing chronic pain, there is a continuing quest for relief that often remains elusive, leading to feelings of helplessness, hopelessness, demoralization, and outright depression. Emotional distress may be attributed to a variety of factors, including inadequate or maladaptive coping resources, iatrogenic complications, overuse of medication, disability, financial difficulties, litigation, disruption of usual activities, lack of social support, and sleep disturbance. Thus, chronic pain is a demoralizing situation that confronts the person not only with the stress created by pain but with a cascade of ongoing stressors that compromise all aspects of the life of the sufferer. Living with chronic pain requires considerable emotional resilience and tends to deplete emotional reserve, and taxes not only the pain sufferer but also the capacity of significant others to provide support.

There is a large body of evidence to demonstrate that psychological factors can interfere with or hinder a person's ability to cope with the pain experience. As a result, psychological intervention in the assessment and treatment of chronic pain is becoming standard practice. Psychological treatments can focus on the emotional distress that accompanies chronic pain and provide education and training in the use of cognitive and behavioral techniques that may reduce perceptions of pain and related disability. Psychologists and psychological principles have played a major role in the understanding and treatment of people with pain, and psychologists have an important function in interdisciplinary pain rehabilitation program (IPRPs) as clinicians and researchers.

None of the treatments described are successful in eliminating pain completely, in fact, the same statement can be made in reference to the most commonly used pharmacological, medical, and surgical interventions[1]; consequently, the majority of people have to adapt to the presence of chronic pain and learn self-management in the face of persistent pain and accompanying symptoms. The various psychological interventions described in this chapter provide a general overview of different treatment strategies. By far, however, treatment with cognitive-behavioral therapy alone or within the context of an IPRP holds the greatest empirical evidence for success. There is a substantial and overwhelming body of research supporting the effectiveness of various psychological approaches. At point, it seems prudent to consider the use of psychological treatments in combination with traditional medical interventions.

Acknowledgment

Support for preparation of this manuscript was provided by a grant from the National Institutes of Health/National Institute of Arthritis and Musculoskeletal and Skin Disorders (R01AR044724).

References

1. Turk DC. Clinical effectiveness and cost-effectiveness of treatments for patients with chronic pain. *Clin J Pain* 2002;18(6):355–365.
2. Watson D, Clark LA, Harkness AR. Structures of personality and their relevance to psychopathology. *J Abnorm Psychol* 1994;103:18–31.
3. Stegen K, Van Diest I, Van de Woestijne KP, et al. Negative affectivity and bodily sensations induced by 5.5% CO-sub-2 enriched air inhalation: is there a bias to interpret bodily sensations negatively in persons with negative affect? *Psychol Heath* 2000;15:513–525.
4. Stegen K, Van Diest I, Van de Woestijne KP, et al. Do persons with negative affect have an attentional bias to bodily sensations? *Cogn Emot* 2001;15:813–829.
5. Fillingim RB, Hastie BA, Ness TJ, et al. Sex-related psychological predictors of baseline pain perception and analgesic responses to pentazocine. *Biol Psychol* 2005;69:97–112.
6. Reiss S, Peterson RA, Gursky DM, et al. Anxiety sensitivity, anxiety frequency and the predictions of fearfulness. *Behav Res Ther* 1986;24:1–8.
7. Asmundson GJG, Wright KD, Hadjistavropoulos HD. Anxiety sensitivity and disabling chronic health conditions: State of the art and future directions. *Scand J Behav Ther* 2000;29:100–117.
8. Keogh E, Asmundson GJG. Negative affectivity, catastrophizing and anxiety sensitivity, In: Asmundson GJG, Vlaeyen JWS, Crombez G, eds. *Understanding and Treating Fear of Pain.* Oxford: Oxford University Press; 2004.
9. Asmundson GJG, Taylor S. Role of anxiety sensitivity in pain-related fear and avoidance. *J Behav Med* 1996;19:577–586.
10. Keogh E, Hamid R, Hamid S, et al. Investigating the effect of anxiety sensitivity, gender and negative interpretative bias on the perception of chest pain. *Pain* 2004;111:209–217.
11. Scheier MF, Carver CS. Optimism, coping, and health: assessment and implications of generalized outcome expectancies. *Health Psychol* 1985;4:219–247.
12. Scheier MF, Carver CS, Bridges MW. Distinguishing optimism from neuroticism (and trait anxiety, self-mastery, and self-esteem): a reevaluation of the Life Orientation Test. *J Pers Soc Psychol* 1994;67:1063–1078.
13. Scheier MF, Carver CS. Effects of optimism on psychological and physical well-being: Theoretical overview and empirical update. *Cogn Ther Res* 1992;16:201–228.
14. Carver CS, Scheier MF. Optimism, In: Snyder CR, Lopez SJ, eds. *Handbook of Positive Psychology.* Oxford: Oxford University Press; 2005.
15. Novy DM. Psychological approaches for managing chronic pain. *J Psychopathol Behav Assess* 2004;26:279–288.
16. Affleck G, Tennen H. Construing benefits from adversity: adaptational significance and dispositional underpinnings. *J Pers* 1996;64:899–922.
17. Treharne GJ, Kitas GD, Lyons AC, et al. Well-being in rheumatoid arthritis: the effects of disease duration and psychosocial factors. *J Health Psychol* 2005;10:457–474.
18. Garofalo JP. Perceived optimism in chronic pain, In: Gatchel RJ, Weisberg JN, eds. *Personality Characteristics of Patients with Pain.* Washington, DC: American Psychological Association; 2000:203–217.
19. Snyder CR, Rand KL, Sigmond DR. Hope Theory: a member of the positive psychology family, In: Snyder CR, Lopez SJ, eds. *Handbook of Positive Psychology.* Oxford: Oxford University Press; 2005.
20. Sharp TJ. Chronic pain: A reformulation of the cognitive-behavioural model. *Behav Res Ther* 2001;39:787–800.
21. Lazarus RS, Folkman S. *Stress, appraisal, and coping,* New York: Springer; 1984.
22. Smith WB, Gracely RH, Safer MA. The meaning of pain: cancer patients' rating and recall of pain intensity and affect. *Pain* 1998;78:123–129.
23. Arntz A, Claassens L. The meaning of pain influences its experienced pain intensity. *Pain* 2004;109:20–25.
24. Stroud MW, Thorn BE, Jensen MP, et al. The relation between pain beliefs, negative thoughts, and psychosocial functioning in chronic pain patients. *Pain* 2000;84:347–352.
25. Turner JA, Jensen MP, Romano JM. Do beliefs, coping, and catastrophizing independently predict functioning in patients with chronic pain? *Pain* 2000;85:115–125.
26. Jensen MP, Turner JA, Romano JM, et al. Relationship of pain-specific beliefs to chronic pain adjustment. *Pain* 1994;57:301–309.
27. Balderson BHK, Lin EHB, Von Korff M. The management of pain-related fear in primary care, In: Asmundson GJG, Vlaeyen JWS, Crombez G, eds. *Understanding and Treating Fear of Pain.* Oxford: Oxford University Press; 2004.
28. Ihlebaek C, Erikson HR. Are the "myths" of low back pain alive in the general Norwegian population? *Scand J Public Health* 2003;31:395–398.
29. Geisser ME, Robinson ME, Miller QL, et al. Psychosocial factors and functional capacity evaluation among persons with chronic pain. *J Occup Rehabil* 2003;13:259–276.
30. Severeijns R, Vlaeyen JWS, van den Hout MA. Do we need a communal coping model of pain catastrophizing? An alternative explanation. *Pain* 2004;111:226–229.
31. Thorn BE, Rich MA, Boothby JL. Pain beliefs and coping attempts. *Pain Forum* 1999;8:169–171.
32. Picavet HS, Vlaeyen JWS, Schouten JS. Pain catastrophizing and kinesiophobia: Predictors of chronic low back pain. *Am J Epidemiol* 2002;156:1028–1034.
33. Severeijns R, Vlaeyen JWS, van den Hout MA, et al. Pain catastrophizing and consequences of musculoskeletal pain: a prospective study in the Dutch community. *J Pain* 2005;6:125–132.
34. Granot M, Ferber SG. The roles of pain catastrophizing and anxiety in the prediction of postoperative pain intensity: a prospective study. *Clin J Pain* 2005;21:439–445.
35. Pavlin DJ, Sullivan MJ, Freund PR, et al. Catastrophizing: a risk factor for postsurgical pain. *Clin J Pain* 2005;21:83–90.
36. Asmundson GJG, Norton PJ, Vlaeyen JWS. Fear-avoidance models of chronic

CHAPTER 8 ■ INDIVIDUAL DIFFERENCES IN PAIN: THE ROLES OF GENDER, ETHNICITY, AND GENETICS

ROGER B. FILLINGIM

INTRODUCTION

Abundant evidence clearly demonstrates that pain responses are characterized by substantial interindividual variability. In other words, an identical noxious stimulus produces vastly different experiences of pain in different people. Such individual differences in pain responses are inarguable; however, the contributing factors and clinical importance of individual differences in pain remain important topics of study. The purpose of this chapter is to discuss the nature of individual differences in responses to pain and its treatment. After a brief discussion of individual differences in clinical and experimental pain responses as well as interindividual variability in treatment outcomes, an overview of the role of demographic factors such as sex/gender and ethnicity will be provided as examples of variables influencing individual differences in pain. Also, the contribution of genetics to individual differences in pain will be reviewed. The chapter will conclude with consideration of the clinical relevance of individual differences, including implications for treatment tailoring.

In the clinical setting, individual differences across patients in the severity and impact of clinical pain are the rule. This variability is often attributed to differences in disease severity, based on the misguided assumption that the noxious stimulus itself is the primary determinant of the pain experience, despite considerable evidence suggesting otherwise. For example, the majority of individuals who show radiographic evidence of osteoarthritis are asymptomatic,[1] and, even in symptomatic patients, radiographic measures of disease severity in osteoarthritis account for a minimal proportion of the interindividual variability in pain and disability.[2–5] Likewise, physical and diagnostic findings have limited value in predicting the occurrence or severity of low back pain.[6,7] Moreover, in the acute pain setting, patients undergoing similar surgical procedures report vastly different amounts of pain.[8–12] Thus, for many forms of clinical pain, estimates of the intensity of the noxious clinical stimulus appear to be poor predictors of the degree of pain experienced.

Of course, a disadvantage in the clinical setting is that the noxious stimulus is not precisely quantified or controlled. Moreover, clinical pain reports are often influenced by previous or current therapies, which can contribute to interindividual variability. However, these issues can be overcome with the application of painful stimuli in the laboratory setting. Evidence from studies of experimentally induced pain also clearly demonstrates individual differences in pain perception.[13] For example, a recent study of 188 healthy adults reported pain intensity ratings ranging from 0 to 100 for an identical cold water stimulus, and ratings of the maximum heat stimulus delivered ranged from 0 to 95.2.[14] These authors estimated that stimulus intensity accounted for only 40% of the variance in pain ratings, while true individual differences accounted for the other 60%. Similarly, Diatchenko and colleagues[15] created a summary index of experimental pain

sensitivity by summing standardized (z-scores) scores across 16 individual pain measures, such that the group mean was set to 0 and negative values reflected lower pain sensitivity. Their findings revealed a normal distribution of summed z-scores, which ranged from −20 to greater than 30 across the sample of 202 healthy young females. Thus, even when the research setting and the noxious stimulus are highly controlled, dramatic individual differences in pain responses emerge (Fig. 8.1).

In addition to interindividual variability in clinical and experimental pain sensitivity, substantial individual differences in responses to pain treatments exist. For example, in a study of postoperative pain, the median number of morphine boluses required to achieve pain relief (Visual Analog Scale rating <30) was 4, but the number of boluses ranged from 1 to 20 across patients.[8] In a clinical trial of opioids for chronic neuropathic pain, treatment-related changes in pain ranged from a 100% decrease to a nearly 70% increase in pain.[16] Even in the context of experimentally induced pain, responses to opioids vary greatly across individuals.[17–19] Moreover, responses to nonpharmacologic pain treatments also show considerable variability across individuals. For example, a long-term (8–10 year) follow-up study of outcomes from surgical and nonsurgical management of spinal stenosis showed that approximately half of the patients in both treatment groups reported improvement in their symptoms over the follow-up period, while 20% to 25% reported no change and 20% to 25% reported that their symptoms had worsened.[20] Significant variability in analgesic responses to acupuncture have also been reported,[21] and responses to cognitive-behavioral interventions for pain vary robustly both within and between studies.[22] Indeed, the well-recognized variability in pain treatment responses has prompted some to recommend individual responder analyses of clinical trial outcomes as an alternative to analysis of group means to take advantage of these individual differences in treatment response.[23]

This brief discussion and the examples cited make it clear that responses to pain and its treatment are characterized by robust and consistent interindividual differences. While variability in pain responses has been studied for decades,[24,25] interest in individual differences in pain and responses to treatment has increased substantially in recent years, reinvigorated largely by the genomics revolution. However, variability in pain perception and responses to treatment is driven by complex interactions among multiple biopsychosocial factors, including, but certainly not limited to, genetic influences. Before embarking on a discussion of specific individual difference factors associated with variability in pain responses, a general framework for conceptualizing sources of individual differences in pain will be presented.

Individual differences in pain (and treatment) responses are typically manifested as between subject variability in a particular measure of interest, such as pain ratings or pain relief. Interestingly, considerable statistical and methodological effort is often

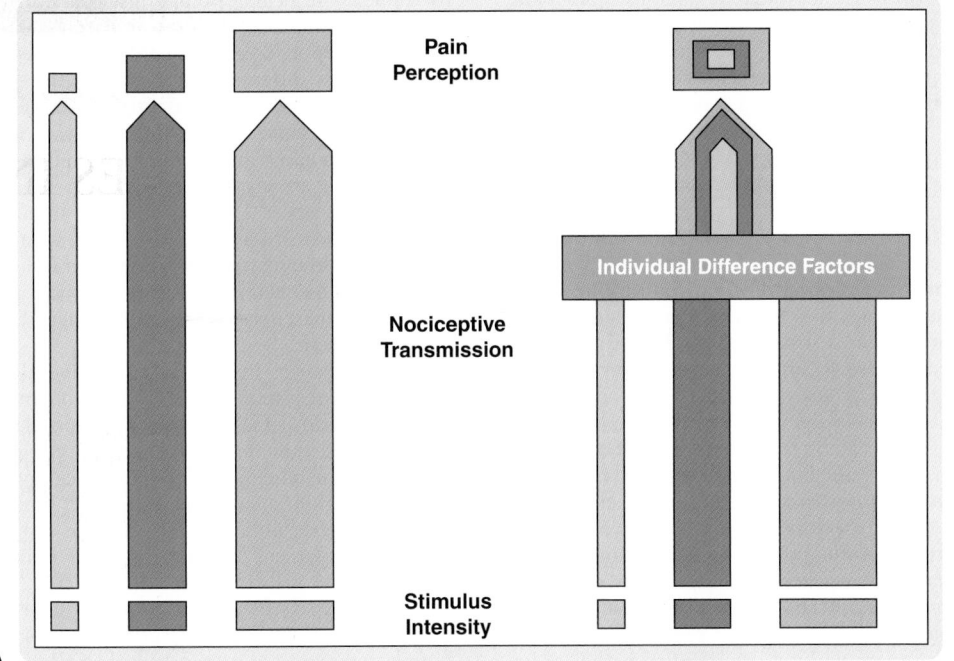

FIGURE 8.1 Schematic representation of the relatively poor association between stimulus intensity and perceived pain. (**A**) Traditional, and inaccurate, view that stimulus activity is strongly associated with pain sensitivity, which ignores the voluminous literature on individual differences in pain perception. (**B**) More valid view that while stimulus intensity may predict activation of nociceptive pathways, once filtered by individual difference factors, it becomes very difficult to predict the magnitude of perceived pain.

expended to minimize this variability, based on the assumption that it represents error variance. However, it is important to recognize that error variance is a general term, which refers not only to actual measurement error but also to sources of variance outside those of most interest to the investigator. For example, in a clinical trial investigating the pain relieving effects of a new medication, the proportion of change in clinical pain that is not attributable to the medication is defined as "error variance." While some percentage of this variance is actually associated with measurement error, multiple additional sources of variability are present (e.g., age, sex, ethnicity, genetics, environmental factors, etc.). In the context of most clinical trials, the investigator will try to reduce this "error variance" by statistically controlling for these factors, in hopes of increasing the probability of achieving statistical significance. However, in contrast to controlling away the influence of these factors to reduce error variance, investigators studying individual differences in pain would argue that there is scientific and clinical merit to elucidating the mechanisms whereby these various factors influence pain treatment responses. A graphical depiction of these sources of variability is presented in Figure 8.2.

An important goal of research on individual differences in responses to pain and its treatment is to develop the ability to generate accurate a priori predictions of a person's response to pain or pain treatment based on assessment of specific characteristics of that individual. For example, if sufficient knowledge were available, we might predict response to a pain medication based on a combination of body size, genetics, sex, ethnicity, and other factors. Of course, before this type of individualized pain medicine can be realized, a substantially better understanding of individual differences in responses to pain and pain treatment will be needed. The remainder of this chapter will discuss current knowledge of three important individual difference factors related to pain: sex/gender, race/ethnicity, and genetics.

SEX AND GENDER DIFFERENCES IN PAIN

Clinical Pain

Research regarding sex, gender, and pain has exploded over the past 15 years.[26,27] This interest in sex differences in pain is driven primarily by epidemiologic and clinical findings indicating that the burden of pain is substantially greater among women than

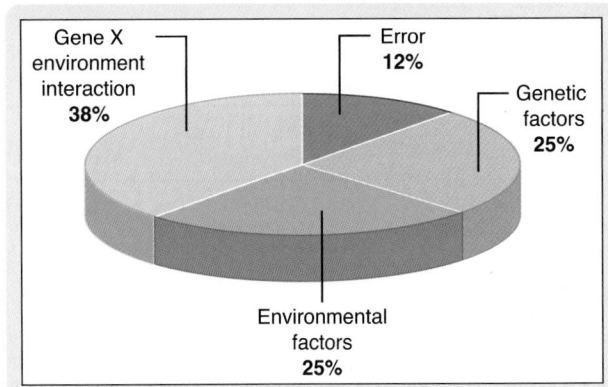

FIGURE 8.2 Graphical example of the sources of variability in pain perception or treatment response. The specific percentages are for illustrative purposes only and do not reflect actual proportions of variance accounted for. Indeed, the proportions of variance would be expected to vary depending on multiple factors, including the nature of the pain, the characteristics of the sample, the influence of longstanding and transient environmental influences, etc. . . .

men. Several population-based surveys have demonstrated higher frequencies of pain among women than men. The NUPRIN Pain Report was a telephone survey of 1254 adults in the United States, which queried respondents about seven types of pain: headache, backache, muscle pain, joint pain, stomach pain, dental pain, and perimenstrual pain.[28] Women reported more frequent headaches, stomach pain, joint pain, and back pain than men. In a Canadian household survey, women reported higher rates of both temporary and persistent pain,[29] and a mail survey of more than 3600 adults in Scotland found that women were significantly more likely than men to report chronic pain.[30] A postal survey in rural Sweden revealed that women reported pain in multiple body sites more often than men,[31] and in a Norwegian population-based survey women reported pain in a significantly higher number of body sites compared to men.[32] Similarly, in a survey of health maintenance organization enrollees in Seattle, Von Korff and colleagues[33] found that women were significantly more likely than men to report at least three of the following five pain conditions: headache, back pain, chest pain, abdominal pain, and facial pain. Numerous other population-based studies echo these findings,[34,35] and even among healthy young adults, women have been found to report pain with greater frequency than men.[36,37]

In addition to these data on general pain symptoms, considerable evidence suggests that specific pain conditions show sex differences in their prevalence.[34,38-42] Berkley[43] provided a thorough list of pain disorders separated by those showing higher prevalence among females, those with higher prevalence among males, and those showing no sex difference in prevalence. Substantially more disorders showed higher prevalence among females than males; however, many of the pain disorders listed are relatively uncommon. When restricting the list of pain disorders to those associated with the greatest frequency and most significant societal costs, the differences become even more dramatic[35] (see Table 8.1). Furthermore, these represent population prevalence rates, and because women are more likely to seek health care for pain,[44-47] females typically make up an even greater proportion of individuals in the clinical setting. Thus, the prevalence rates of the most common and costly pain conditions are generally higher among women than men, suggesting that the public health burden of pain is disproportionately distributed among women.

Additional clinical evidence of sex differences in pain comes from studies examining whether the severity of clinical pain and related symptoms differs among women and men. Several investigators have explored sex differences in postoperative pain.

In mixed surgical populations, inconsistent findings have emerged, with some reporting greater pain among women[48,49] and others reporting greater pain among men.[50] Studies have also examined sex differences in postoperative pain among patients undergoing specific surgical procedures. For example, women have reported more severe pain after oral surgery in several studies,[51-55] though others have reported no sex differences.[56] Greater pain among women has also been observed after orthopedic surgery,[57-61] cardiothoracic surgery,[62,63] and laparoscopic cholecystectomy.[11,64] Moreover, women report more pain than men following endoscopic colorectal cancer screening procedures.[65,66] On balance, studies of clinical pain associated with surgery or other invasive procedures suggest greater pain severity among women.

Sex differences in clinical pain have also been investigated among patients presenting for evaluation and treatment of ongoing chronic pain. One survey study reported that among individuals with pain that limited their activity, women reported more frequent pain, greater pain-related negative affect, and higher levels of disability compared to men.[67] Among patients with arthritis, evidence indicates that women report greater pain and disability than men,[68,69] including individuals undergoing imminent total hip arthroplasty.[70] In addition, pain among women with multiple sclerosis report more frequent and severe pain than men with this disease.[71] Also, in a heterogeneous chronic pain population recruited from a multidisciplinary pain clinic, women had higher pain severity than men.[72] George and colleagues found that pain ratings were similar across sex in a sample of patients with chronic musculoskeletal pain, but women indicated a greater area of pain based on their pain drawings. However, other investigators have reported minimal sex differences in pain severity in heterogeneous chronic pain populations.[73-75] Also, no sex differences in measures of clinical pain, experimental pain sensitivity, psychological/personality factors or illness behaviors were reported among patients with pain due to temporomandibular disorders.[76] A recent study found that men had higher levels of pain and poorer pain-related adjustment in a sample of patients seeking treatment primarily for myofascial pain in a multidisciplinary clinic.[77] Thus, the evidence regarding sex differences in the severity of chronic clinical pain is mixed.

Experimental Pain

The literature reviewed above suggests that women experience more frequent and more severe clinical pain than men, which has led some investigators to suggest that sex differences in nociceptive processing may contribute to the greater burden of clinical pain among women.[78,79] This possibility seems particularly plausible in light of findings that several female predominant pain disorders are characterized by enhanced sensitivity to experimentally induced pain.[80-85] One potential hypothesis is that enhanced pain sensitivity represents a preexisting risk factor for the development of certain pain conditions.[86] One corollary of this hypothesis states that if women show greater pain sensitivity than men, this that places women at greater risk for certain pain conditions.

As previously reviewed,[79,87-89] a large number of studies have examined sex differences in perceptual responses to experimentally evoked somatic pain. Taken together, the findings demonstrate lower pain thresholds and tolerances among women relative to men, across multiple stimulus modalities. While the direction of the findings is quite consistent, the magnitude of the sex difference varies across studies, with a previous meta-analysis showing that the average effect size was moderate.[87] Since the publication of this quantitative review, additional evidence has emerged addressing sex differences in the perception of laboratory-induced pain. For example, several studies have demonstrated greater temporal summation of pain among women compared to men.[90-92] Cairns and colleagues[93,94] reported that

TABLE 8.1

SEX DIFFERENCES IN THE PREVALENCE OF COMMON CHRONIC PAIN CONDITIONS

Condition	Overall Point Prevalence*	Female: Male Ratio*
Migraine headache	12%–20%	2–3:1
Chronic tension-type headache	2%–5%	2:1
Low back pain	4%–33%	1.2:1
Irritable bowel syndrome	15%–20%	1.5:1
Temporomandibular disorder	4%–12%	2:1
Fibromyalgia	2%–4%	6:1
Chronic widespread pain	10.6%–13%	1.5–2:1
Arthritis	21.6%	1.4–1.6:1

* Prevalence data and female:male ratios were estimated from several sources.[26,38,41] These estimates reflect the overall population rates, and it is important to recognize that both the prevalence and female:male ratio can vary greatly across the lifespan.[35]

injection of glutamate into the masseter muscle produced higher peak pain, longer lasting pain, and a greater area of pain among women compared to men. Similarly, muscle injections of hypertonic saline produced greater intensity of pain and greater areas of referred pain among females.[83] In contrast to these findings, another experimental model of muscle pain, delayed onset muscle soreness, has consistently failed to show sex differences.[95–97] Similarly, studies of visceral pain perception (e.g., rectal distention, esophageal stimulation) have revealed minimal sex differences.[98,99]

In addition to perceptual responses to laboratory pain stimuli, several investigators have examined sex differences in autonomic, electrophysiological, and cerebral responses to noxious stimuli. Maixner and Humphrey[100] reported that men exhibited more robust blood pressure responses to ischemic pain compared to women, despite higher ratings of pain among women. In contrast, women showed greater pupil dilation, a marker of autonomic reactivity, in response to pressure pain relative to men.[101] Further, the nociceptive flexion reflex, a pain-related muscle reflex, has been shown to occur at lower stimulus intensities among women than men.[102,103] Functional brain imaging has been used to explore sex differences in cerebral responses to evoked pain. In response to a painful (50° C) thermal stimulus, women provided higher pain ratings and showed greater activation in the contralateral prefrontal cortex, insula, and thalamus compared to men.[104] Using individually tailored laser stimuli to produce warmth, mild pain and moderate pain, Derbyshire and colleagues[105] found that males showed greater pain-related activation in bilateral parietal cortex and contralateral secondary somatosensory and prefrontal cortices. More recently, it was shown that in response to mild and moderate intensity visceral pressure, men showed greater activation in the anterior insular compared to women, whereas women showed greater deactivation in the midcingulate and thalamus.[106] Also, in a functional magnetic resonance imaging (fMRI) study using heat pain stimuli, Moulton and colleagues reported greater pain-related activation in men in several brain regions, including primary somatosensory, midanterior cingulate, and dorsolateral prefrontal cortices.[107] However, these authors then determined that these sex differences were primarily driven by greater negative blood oxygen level dependent (BOLD) signal changes in women, which may indicate greater pain-related deactivation in these brain regions among females. In a study of both cutaneous and muscle pain, fMRI revealed that females showed greater increases in BOLD activity in the mid-cingulate cortex and greater decreases in activity in the cerebellum and hippocampus, while men showed greater BOLD activity decreases in the dorsolateral prefrontal cortex.[108]

Responses to Pain Treatment

An expanding body of literature addresses whether women and men respond differently to a variety of pharmacologic and nonpharmacologic pain treatments. Several studies have compared females' and males' responses to mu-opioids. For example, some findings of patient controlled analgesia following surgery suggest that women generally consume significantly lower amounts of opioid medication for postoperative pain compared to men.[50,109] In contrast, the absence of sex differences in morphine analgesia has been reported following oral surgery[50,109,110] and among patients with chronic cancer pain.[111] Others have shown enhanced opioid analgesia among males. Cepeda and Carr[49] reported that for comparable analgesic efficacy, women required 30% more morphine than men, and in a mixed postsurgical sample women required significantly higher doses of morphine to achieve pain relief.[48] Other investigators assessing responses to kappa-agonist-antagonists using an oral surgery model have found that women showed more robust and/or longer lasting analgesic responses to pentazocine, nalbuphine, and butorphanol compared to

men.[56,112–114] Also, a study of trauma-related pain in the emergency room showed that butorphanol was more effective than morphine for women, and men showed marginally greater morphine analgesia women.[115] Using experimental pain models, one study has showed more robust morphine analgesia in women.[19] However, this study was not placebo controlled. This may be important, because Pud and colleagues[116] also found that while women showed greater morphine analgesia than men, when women's greater placebo response was controlled, the sex difference in morphine analgesia was not significant. Others report no sex differences in responses to morphine and other mu agonists,[18,117] and the only experimental studies examining kappa-agonist-antagonists revealed no sex differences in analgesic responses.[118,119] Overall, the conflicting nature of the evidence regarding sex differences in opioid analgesia can be attributed to a variety of factors, including the specific opioid and dose administered, the type of pain being treated, and characteristics of the study sample.

Sex differences in responses to nonpharmacologic pain treatments have also been investigated. Among patients with back pain, a conventional physical therapy intervention produced better outcomes for men, but women showed greater pain reduction in response to intensive dynamic back exercises.[120] Similarly, another investigation of back pain showed that women undergoing cognitive-behavioral treatment with or without physical therapy showed increased health-related quality of life and lower rates of disability, while men showed no such treatment responses.[121] In contrast, other investigators show no sex differences in the effectiveness of rehabilitation treatments for chronic low back pain.[122,123] Multidisciplinary treatment for pain due to temporomandibular disorder was associated with significant decreases in pain over a 2-year period in women, but not men.[124] More recently, Keogh and colleagues[125] found that women and men showed comparable initial responses to multidisciplinary pain treatment; however, men maintained their treatment gains over the 3-month follow-up period, while women regressed to their pretreatment levels. Thus, the literature on sex differences in responses to nonpharmacologic treatment yields conflicting results.

As reviewed elsewhere,[27,43,79,89,126,127] multiple biopsychosocial factors contribute to these sex differences in clinical and experimental pain responses. For example, several lines of evidence indicate that gonadal hormones can influence responses to pain and pain medications.[126,128,129] Several clinical pain syndromes show alterations in their severity across the female menstrual cycle.[129] Evidence from human studies indicates that females exhibit greater pain sensitivity during the late luteal (i.e., premenstrual) phase versus the follicular (i.e., postmenstrual) phase of their menstrual cycle; although, the effects are inconsistent across studies and are often small in magnitude.[130,131] Exogenous hormone use, especially hormone replacement among postmenopausal women, has been associated with increased risk for clinical pain[132–134] and experimental pain sensitivity,[135] though others have failed to show such an association.[136] While these findings support a pronociceptive role for estrogen, other results suggest that estrogen may be antinociceptive. For example, brain responses to heat pain, especially in regions associated with the affective component of pain, were lower during high versus low estrogen menstrual phases.[137] Moreover, exogenous administration of estrogen was associated with both reduced muscle pain sensitivity and enhanced pain-related brain mu-opioid receptor binding in healthy women,[138] suggesting that estrogen promotes pain endogenous opioid-mediated inhibition. Thus, while gonadal hormones can alter pain responses, a complete understanding of the pattern and direction of these effects remains elusive.

Psychosocial factors also contribute to sex differences in pain responses. For example, women and men differ in pain coping, which may partially account for sex differences in clinical and experimental pain.[139,140] In addition, sex differences in mood are commonly observed, and the association of affective variables to pain responses often differs for women versus men.[73,141–143] Further, stereotypic gender roles have been associated with responses to experimental pain, based on the assumption that traditional feminine roles may encourage reporting pain, while masculine roles promote stoicism. Indeed, both women and men describe women as more willing to report pain compared to men, and this willingness to report pain has accounted for sex differences in experimental pain responses.[91,144] Also, using traditional measures of gender roles, masculinity and femininity have been associated with lower and higher pain sensitivity, respectively,[145–149] and men who identified strongly with masculine gender norms had higher pain tolerance than men with low masculine identification.[150] The extent to which such gender roles contribute to sex differences in clinical pain has received little empirical attention.

ETHNIC GROUP DIFFERENCES IN PAIN

Ethnicity represents another demographic factor associated with individual differences in pain responses. Disparities in health status across ethnic and racial groups in the United States have been well documented, such that minority groups, especially African Americans and Hispanics, generally have poorer health status compared to non-Hispanic whites.[151] It has become increasingly clear that these ethnic/racial group differences extend to pain conditions.[152,153] In order to better frame the discussion of ethnic differences in pain, a brief consideration of some important methodologic and conceptual issues is warranted. Amidst the debate regarding terminology used to characterize population groups, one rare point of agreement is that the terms race and ethnicity have different definitions and their interchangeable and imprecise use has produced confusion and slowed the progress of research on differences in health and disease across population groups.[154] Historically, the term race was used to connote biological differences among groups of people who had distinguishing physical characteristics, while ethnicity referred to groups defined by a combination of cultural factors (e.g., language, religion, diet) typically associated with race.[155] The validity of race as a biological or genetic construct has been challenged by many experts,[156,157] while others point to well-documented differences in frequency of genetic variants across self-reported racial and ethnic groups, some of which may be relevant to health and disease.[158,159] The only firm conclusion is that race and ethnicity are poorly defined terms applied to complex and dynamic social constructs whose connection to biology is far from perfect. Given the lack of consensus, the author will generally use the combined term ethnic/racial.

Clinical Pain

An increasing clinical literature suggests that the experience of clinical pain varies across ethnic/racial groups in the United States. For example, greater pain among African Americans compared to non-Hispanic whites has been documented for several painful conditions, including cancer,[160] arthritis,[161–164] back pain,[165] and among children with temporomandibular disorders.[166] Also, one study demonstrated more widespread pain among African American women, while Caucasian women reported greater pain severity and increased tenderness to palpation.[167] Also, in studies of heterogeneous chronic pain populations, African Americans have shown higher levels of pain and poorer pain-related adjustment than non-Hispanic whites.[168–171] Evidence of racial/ethnic group differences also emerges from studies of Hispanics in the U.S. For example, among chronic pain patients, Hispanics reported the highest pain levels.[172] Also, one study showed that Hispanic workers were more likely to report musculoskeletal pain than non-Hispanic whites,[173] and another study reported a greater proportion of persistent symptoms among Hispanics versus non-Hispanic whites following an occupational injury.[174] In addition to these findings related to chronic painful conditions, ethnic differences have been reported for acute clinical pain and for reports of pain in nonclinical samples. "Latino" and "black American" patients reported greater pain after oral surgery compared to patients of European descent,[175] and African Americans reported greater pain than whites following spinal fusion.[176] Community-based surveys have also indicated a greater prevalence of severe pain among Hispanics and African Americans compared to whites,[177] and that whites report a longer duration of pain, while African Americans and Hispanics reported more severe pain.[178] Importantly, while these findings indicate ethnic/racial group differences in clinical pain, additional studies of ethnic/racial influences on pain prevalence or severity have reported no such group differences.[179–183]

Experimental Pain

These ethnic/racial group differences in clinical pain are inevitably driven by complex interactions among multiple system, provider, and patient level variables. For example, socioeconomic variables, such as education and income, are associated with increased risk for pain and poor health status and are likely to contribute to ethnic/racial disparities in pain.[164,178,184–186] Also, considerable evidence indicates that African American and Hispanic patients are at increased risk for undertreatment of pain,[153,187–190] which could obviously contribute to increased severity of pain in these groups. In addition to these system and provider level factors, ethnic/racial group differences in the actual experience of pain could contribute to the group differences in clinical pain characteristics. That is, if certain ethnic/racial groups expressed greater sensitivity to pain, this could translate into enhanced clinical pain. Evidence of ethnic/racial group differences in pain perception derives from studies using controlled laboratory pain stimuli.

The most frequent comparisons in experimental studies have been between African Americans and non-Hispanic whites. More than 60 years ago, Chapman and Jones[24] found that African Americans displayed significantly lower heat pain thresholds and tolerances compared to non-Hispanic Whites. In a large study involving more than 40,000 participants, African Americans showed lower pressure pain tolerance than whites.[191] Also, higher cold pain tolerance was observed in non-Hispanic whites compared to a combined group of Hispanics and African Americans.[192] Edwards and Fillingim[193] reported that while neither heat pain thresholds nor ratings of heat pain intensity differed across ethnic/racial groups, African Americans had lower heat pain tolerances and higher ratings of heat pain unpleasantness compared to whites, and similar findings were subsequently reported by others.[194] Several recent reports have demonstrated lower pain tolerances, but not pain thresholds, among African Americans compared to whites.[195–198] Weisse and colleagues found that African Americans provided higher ratings of cold pain intensity and unpleasantness; however, an interaction of participant ethnic/racial group and experimenter gender revealed that these higher ratings were only observed when the experimenter was female.[199] One study among patients with chronic pain revealed lower ischemic pain tolerance among African American compared to white patients,[200] while another study failed to show ethnic/racial group differences in ischemic pain responses among patients with chronic pain.[201]

Some additional studies have examined differences in laboratory pain responses among other ethnic/racial groups. Regarding Asian populations, "oriental" subjects provided higher ratings of cold pain than "occidental" subjects.[202] Another study compared

Japanese subjects tested in Japan to "American" subjects tested in America; however, the American group was comprised of half "Caucasians" and half second- or third-generation Japanese living in America (referred to as Nisei). Overall, the American group had higher pain threshold and required a higher stimulus intensity to achieve moderate pain, but this group difference was driven primarily by the Nisei participants who showed the lowest pain sensitivity of all three groups.[203] More recently, South Asian groups have been found more sensitive to heat pain[204] and capsaicin-induced pain[205] compared to Europeans. In contrast, others have reported no differences in pressure pain perception between "Afro-Asian" and white participants.[206] One study found that Asian Indians reported higher cold pain tolerance than Americans, and interestingly individuals in this study were tested in separate labs in their home countries.[207]

Responses to Pain Treatment

While ethnic/racial group differences in clinical and experimental pain responses have received considerable empirical attention, little research has addressed ethnic/racial group differences in responses to pain treatment. Multiple studies have demonstrated that African American and Hispanic patients are likely to receive analgesic interventions at lower doses or with lower frequency than their non-Hispanic white counterparts,[153,187–190,208,209] though some studies have shown no such disparity.[210–212] However, few studies have examined whether responses to of analgesics vary across ethnic/racial groups. Kaiko and colleagues[111] found that African Americans with chronic cancer pain showed greater analgesic responses to morphine than whites. Also, ethnic differences in respiratory responses to morphine have been reported, with native Indians (from Columbia) showing greater respiratory depression than whites,[213] while whites showed greater respiratory depression than Chinese patients.[214] Also, after administration of meperidine or morphine, white patients showed more nausea and vomiting than black patients.[214,215] Thus, the influence of ethnic/racial group on responses to pain medications warrants additional investigation.

As with sex differences, ethnic/racial group differences in pain are mediated by multiple biopsychosocial factors. Little research has directly investigated biological contributions to ethnic/racial group differences in pain. However, a recent study examined the association of stress-induced increases in blood pressure, norepinephrine, and cortisol on experimental pain responses in African Americans and whites.[197] Stress-induced physiological reactivity was more strongly associated with reduction of pain responses among white compared to African American participants. This research group also found that lower resting levels of allopregnanolone, higher cortisol, and higher beta-endorphin were associated with reduced pain sensitivity among non-Hispanic whites but not African Americans.[216] Thus, neuroendocrine factors may contribute to ethnic/racial group differences in pain perception. Regarding psychosocial factors, ethnic/racial group differences in pain coping have been observed. Among patients with rheumatoid arthritis, African Americans reported greater use of distraction and praying/hoping, while whites reported higher use of ignoring pain and coping statements and a greater perceived ability to control pain,[217] and others have also reported group differences in pain coping.[180,218] In a study of experimental pain perception, African Americans showed higher levels of passive coping and hypervigilance; however, these psychological variables did not account for group differences in pain perception.[195] Sociocultural factors also contribute to both variation in pain responses both within and between ethnic/racial groups.[219] Zborowski[220] proposed that expression of pain is culturally prescribed, based on attitudes toward pain behavior and expression that are inherent within cultural groups. In general, these hypotheses have not been empirically tested; however, a recent study

reported that higher levels of ethnic identification were associated with greater pain sensitivity among African American and Hispanic groups, but not among non-Hispanic whites.[198] Additional investigation of sociocultural contributions to clinical and experimental pain responses is needed.

GENETIC CONTRIBUTIONS TO PAIN

In recent years, research on individual differences in pain responses has increasingly involved consideration of genetic contributions. A comprehensive review of this literature is beyond the scope of this chapter[221–224]; rather, the author would like to highlight some relevant findings in the broader context of individual differences in pain, including interactions between genetics and other individual differences factors, such as sex and ethnic/racial group.

Clinical Pain

Increasing evidence from human research documents the importance of genetic influences in numerous clinical pain conditions. Significant familial aggregation has been demonstrated for several syndromes, including arthritis, fibromyalgia, irritable bowel syndrome, and migraine and tension-type headache.[225–229] This is consistent with a genetic contribution, but could also be explained by shared environmental influences. However, heritability estimates derived from large scale twin studies, comparing monozygotic to dizygotic twins, suggest that genetic factors account for a substantial proportion of the variance in multiple pain conditions, including chronic widespread pain, back pain, neck pain, arthritis, headache, and functional bowel disorders.[230–236] While one possibility is that genes associated with the pathophysiological processes of specific diseases may produce high heritability for a given condition, this is difficult to determine, because several of the pain conditions that show high heritability are not characterized by any known specific etiopathogenesis. An alternative possibility is that genetic influences on pain perception or endogenous pain modulation could potentially contribute to the heritability of chronic pain conditions. This possibility is bolstered by findings that many of these heritable pain syndromes are characterized by enhanced pain sensitivity and/or altered endogenous pain modulation.[237–239]

Experimental Pain

Considerable evidence from preclinical models suggests that both basal nociceptive sensitivity and antinociceptive responses to drugs show significant heritability,[240] and increasing research has addressed genetic contributions to experimental pain sensitivity in humans. Pressure pain threshold was assessed in monozygotic and dizygotic twins and showed a heritability of only 10%[241]; however, twin studies are typically underpowered for detecting genetic associations for multifactorial traits like pain sensitivity. Also, these investigators tested twin pairs together, which may have inflated any environmental contribution. Two more recent twin studies have examined additional laboratory pain phenotypes. Nielsen and colleagues[14] found a significant genetic contribution to both heat pain and cold pain ratings, with heritability estimates of 26% for the former and 60% for the latter. Also, another recent twin study reported significant heritability estimates ranging from 22% to 55% for several experimental pain phenotypes, including responses to heat pain and chemically induced pain.[242] Another approach to investigating genetic influences has been to examine genetic associations between single

TABLE 8.2

SUMMARY OF ASSOCIATIONS STUDIES LINKING SPECIFIC CANDIDATE GENES WITH EXPERIMENTAL PAIN PERCEPTION

Authors	Candidate Gene(s)	Pain Measures	Sample Size	Findings
Zubieta et al. 2003[248]	COMT (val158met)	Hypertonic saline in masseter muscle; brain mu-opioid receptor binding	18 healthy adults	val/val Ss showed greater mu-opioid activation and lower pain responses than met/met Ss
Diatchenko et al. 2005[15]	COMT (haplotypes)	Summed z-score across multiple pain measures	202 healthy females	LPS haplotype associated with lower summed z-score (reduced pain sensitivity) compared to HPS haplotype
Diatchenko et al. 2006[282]	COMT (haplotypes and val158met)	Heat, pressure, ischemic pain	202 healthy females	LPS haplotype showed lower sensitivity to heat pain compared to HPS; met/met showed lower temporal summation of heat pain compared to val/val; Associations with pressure and ischemic pain not significant
Kim et al. 2004[269]	COMT, TRPV1, OPRD1	Heat pain, cold pain	384 healthy adults	Among white females only, TRPV1 val585val higher cold pain tolerance compared to heterozygotes or ile585 homozygotes; Among males OPRD1 Phe27Cys heterozygotes report lower heat pain ratings than homozygotes; No association with COMT val158met
Kim et al. 2006[283]	COMT, TRPV1, TRPA1, TRPM8, FAAH	Heat pain, cold pain	368 healthy European American adults	In females, a TRPA1 SNP (rs11988795) was associated with cold pain tolerance, and a COMT SNP (rs6269) was associated with cold pain ratings. In males, 2 FAAH SNPs (rs932816 and rs4141964) were associated with cold pain responses
Fillingim et al. 2005[256]	OPRM1 (A118G)	Heat pain, pressure pain, ischemic pain	167 healthy adults	Ss with 1 or 2 rare alleles had higher pressure threshold than A118A Ss; Sex X genotype interaction emerged for heat pain ratings, as G allele was associated with lower ratings in men, but higher ratings in women
Lotsch et al. 2006[257]	OPRM1 (A118G)	ERP response to intranasal CO_2	45 healthy adults	N1 ERP response to CO_2 was lower in carriers of the rare (G) allele
Tegeder et al. 2006[246]	GCH (haplotype)	Thermal, pressure, ischemic pain	547 healthy adults	Significant association of haplotype with pressure pain thresholds
Kim and Dionne, 2007[247]	GCH (haplotype)	Cold pain, heat pain	735 healthy adults	No significant associations
Mogil et al. 2005[284]	MC1R (multiple SNPs)	Electrical pain	47 healthy adults	Ss with two or more variant alleles across 3 SNPs had significantly higher electrical pain tolerance than those with 0 or 1 variant alleles

ERP, event-related potential; HPS; high pain sensitive; LPS, low pain sensitive; SNPs, single nucleotide polymorphisms.

nucleotide polymorphisms (SNPs) of specific genes and responses to experimentally induced pain. Specific SNPs of several genes have been associated with various experimental pain phenotypes, as shown in Table 8.2. As is common in genetic association studies,[243–245] few of these associations have been replicated in more than one sample. Therefore genetic associations that have been examined across multiple cohorts will be discussed in more detail here, and readers are referred to other recent reviews for a more thorough presentation of the literature.[222–224]

One group of investigators implemented a translational approach to identifying a potential genetic marker of pain sensitivity.[246] First, they found that an enzyme (GT cyclohydrolase, or GCH) and its end product BH4 were upregulated in an animal model of neuropathic pain, and the importance of BH4 in neuropathic pain was demonstrated by blocking GCH, which reversed mechanical and cold hypersensitivity. A similar pattern of results

was shown for inflammatory pain, and BH4 injected intrathecally produced increased basal pain sensitivity in rats and heightened hypersensitivity in rats following nerve injury and inflammation. Next, the findings were translated into humans by identifying a haplotype of the GCH1 gene that was associated with lower levels of persistent pain following lumbar surgery for disc herniation. The authors also showed that this pain protective haplotype conferred reduced sensitivity to experimentally induced pain in a separate cohort of healthy adults. Another group of investigators has failed to replicate these results in a separate study, perhaps due to a different haplotypic structure in their population as well as differences in the pain models examined.[247]

Another gene that has been examined across multiple samples is the gene that encodes catechol-O-methyltransferase (COMT), an enzyme that metabolizes catecholamines. One functional COMT polymorphism that has received substantial attention involves the substitution of valine by methionine at codon 158 (*val158met*), which produces a thermally unstable enzyme and reduced enzymatic activity. Zubieta and colleagues[248] reported that the val158met SNP of *COMT* was associated with brain mu-opioid receptor binding in response to chemically-induced muscle pain, such that the *val/val* genotype group showed significantly greater pain-related mu-opioid activation. Moreover, *val/val* individuals required a greater amount of hypertonic saline to evoke moderate pain over the last 10 minutes of the pain induction period, suggesting lower pain sensitivity in this group. Subsequently, this same *COMT* SNP failed to show an association with ratings of cold pain.[249] Diatchenko and colleagues[15] constructed *COMT* haplotypes based on 4 SNPs and then examined associations with a pain phenotype created by computing a summary score of pain sensitivity across multiple stimulus modalities. *COMT* haplotype was associated with overall pain sensitivity as well as risk for subsequent development of temporomandibular pain. Associations of *COMT* with other clinical pain conditions have been reported by some investigators,[250,251] and a recent report suggests that *COMT* haplotype may interact with psychological factors to predict clinical pain severity in patients with shoulder pain.[252]

An additional candidate gene that has been examined for associations with pain responses is the mu-opioid receptor gene (*OPRM1*). The A118G SNP of *OPRM1* is a common polymorphism with potential functional effects, as the variant receptor showed higher binding affinity for beta-endorphin in one study[253] but not another,[254] and the G allele resulted in lower mRNA expression and protein yield compared to the A allele.[255] Carriers of at least one rare allele showed lower mechanical pain sensitivity compared to homozygotes for the consensus allele,[256] suggesting that the G allele may confer reduced pain sensitivity. Consistent with this finding, pain-related evoked potential responses were found to be reduced in carriers of the G allele compared to those carrying two consensus alleles.[257] Interestingly, the G allele showed lower frequency in a sample of chronic pain patients compared to a group of postsurgical patients.[258] In addition to these data regarding basal pain responses, several studies have investigated whether *OPRM1* is associated with responses to mu-opioid agonists. In a laboratory study, carriers of the G allele showed significantly reduced analgesic responses to alfentanil relative to individuals with two consensus alleles, and G homozygotes also showed significantly reduced respiratory depression, such that their therapeutic window was actually improved.[259] These investigators subsequently showed that alfentanil attenuated pain intensity-related cortical responses more strongly in A versus G homozygotes.[260] Another group showed that the rare allele was associated with reduced analgesic responses to another mu-opioid agonist, M6G, but A118G genotype was not related to respiratory depression.[261] Clinical evidence supports these laboratory findings, as homozygous carriers of the rare allele have shown increased morphine requirements for postoperative[262,263] and cancer pain.[264] Interestingly, the G allele showed lower frequency in a sample of chronic pain patients compared to a group of postsurgical patients, and among the chronic pain patients that consensus allele homozygotes were consuming higher opioid doses than those with one or two minor alleles.[258] While this runs counter to the above findings in postoperative pain, higher opioid doses may have been required in the major allele group due to enhanced clinical pain rather than poorer analgesic response.

INTERACTIONS AMONG INDIVIDUAL DIFFERENCE FACTORS

The previous discussion treats each individual difference factor separately, as though sex, race/ethnicity, and genetic factors each

exist in isolation. Obviously, these and many other individual difference variables coexist and have the potential to interactively influence pain responses. For example, little is known regarding whether sex differences vary as a function of racial/ethnic group, but it is conceivable that such sex by ethnicity interactions may occur. In contrast, some evidence has examined interactions between sex and genetic factors. For example, family history of pain has been more strongly associated with pain complaints and with experimental pain responses among women than men[265–267]; although, these findings could be explained by genetic or environmental factors. More direct evidence comes from a large twin study, in which the heritability of neck pain was significantly higher in females (51%) than males (33%).[230] Several laboratory studies also suggest sex by genotype interactions. Using a translational approach, Mogil and colleagues[268] identified a novel sex-dependent genetic association, such that the melanocortin-1-receptor gene (*MC1R*) was associated with analgesic responses to a kappa-opioid agonist in female but not male mice. They then examined pentazocine analgesia among humans as a function of *MC1R* status and found a sex by genotype interaction, with a significant genetic association among women but not men. In another study, while the sex X genotype interaction was not statistically significant, the association of *OPRM1* with pressure pain thresholds was only significant among men, and a frankly significant sex X genotype interaction emerged for ratings of heat pain.[256] Kim and colleagues[269] reported that the delta-opioid receptor gene (*OPRD1*) was associated with heat pain ratings only among men, which is consistent with previous murine evidence.[270] Thus, genetic contributions to pain and analgesic responses may differ across sexes, which indicates the importance of including both females and males in genetic studies.

Genetic contributions to pain and analgesia may also differ as a function of racial/ethnic group. Indeed, despite considerable genetic similarity across groups, it is well recognized that allele frequencies for many SNPs differ considerably across ethnic/racial population groups, which may contribute to group differences in health relevant phenotypes.[159,271–273] While little evidence has addressed this issue in pain research, it has been documented that allele frequencies for the A118G SNP of *OPRM1* differ across ethnic groups, with the rare allele occurring with significantly lower frequency among African Americans.[274,275] Given that the rare allele predicts reduced pain sensitivity[256,257] and higher morphine requirements,[262,263] it is tempting to speculate that this SNP may contribute to the previously reported increased pain sensitivity[195,198] and reduced morphine requirements[111] among African Americans. However, empirical confirmation of this speculation is required. Even when allele frequencies are similar across ethnic groups, genetic associations may differ. For example, preliminary data from our laboratory suggests that while Hispanic and non-Hispanic whites show similar allele frequencies of the A118G SNP of *OPRM1*, the rare allele is associated with reduced pain sensitivity among non-Hispanic whites, while Hispanics with the G allele show a tendency toward increased pain sensitivity. Another candidate pain gene, *COMT*, is also characterized by ethnic differences in allele frequency,[276] and COMT enzyme activity is significantly higher in African Americans compared to whites.[277] Thus, it is plausible to suggest that racial/ethnic group differences in allelic frequencies of pain-related SNPs, or differences in the association of SNPs with pain-related phenotypes could contribute to group differences in pain sensitivity and analgesic responses, but additional research is needed to directly support or refute this possibility.

CONCLUSION

Multiple factors contribute to the robust interindividual differences that characterize pain and analgesic responses, and the above discussion highlights the influences of sex, ethnic/racial group, and genetics. Relative to men, women are at greater risk for many forms of clinical pain, and they display significantly greater sensitivity to experimentally induced pain. Sex differences in analgesic responses have been investigated, but the results are complex and sometimes contradictory. Regarding ethnic differences, minority patients, specifically African Americans and Hispanics, have shown higher levels of pain and disability than non-Hispanic whites in several clinical populations. These minority groups also exhibit greater perceptual responses to experimental pain. Thus, both sex and racial/ethnic group are associated with variability in pain responses. Multiple biopsychosocial mechanisms contribute to these sex and racial/ethnic group differences. Despite these sometimes large and consistent group differences, it is important to remember that differences are always greater within than between groups. Moreover, the factors contributing to pain responses can differ substantially across groups. For example, several studies have demonstrated that anxiety is more strongly associated with both clinical and experimental pain responses among men than women.[73,278–281] Also, examples above show that genetic associations with pain or analgesia can be sex-specific. Thus, demographic group variables such as sex and ethnic/racial group not only represent individual differences factors themselves, but they may also moderate the effects of other pain-related individual difference factors.

One undeniable implication of this information regarding individual differences in pain is that measures of tissue damage will continue to be poor predictors of pain and disability. Hence, treatments based solely on biomedical findings or markers of disease or injury will continue to achieve suboptimal outcomes. Given the current state of the evidence, tailoring pain treatment based on sex, ethnic/racial group, or genetics may not be practical at this time; however, with enhanced understanding of the influences of these and other individual difference variables on pain, individualized treatment could become a reality in the future. Of particular importance will be large-scale studies that provide opportunity for modeling interactions among multiple individual difference factors. More widespread recognition of the importance of individual differences in pain along with additional research to illuminate the nature of mechanisms of these individual differences will ultimately lead to more effective pain diagnosis and treatment.

References

1. Lawrence RC, Felson DT, Helmick CG, et al. Estimates of the prevalence of arthritis and other rheumatic conditions in the United States. Part II. *Arthritis Rheum* 2008;58:26–35.
2. Hagglund KJ, Haley WE, Reveille JD, et al. Predicting individual differences in pain and functional impairment among patients with rheumatoid arthritis. *Arthritis Rheum* 1989;32:851–858.
3. Pells JJ, Shelby RA, Keefe FJ, et al. Arthritis self-efficacy and self-efficacy for resisting eating: Relationships to pain, disability, and eating behavior in overweight and obese individuals with osteoarthritic knee pain. *Pain* 2008; 136:340–347.
4. Summers MN, Haley WE, Reveille JD, et al. Radiographic assessment and psychologic variables as predictors of pain and functional impairment in osteoarthritis of the knee or hip. *Arthritis Rheum* 1988;31:204–209.
5. Szebenyi B, Hollander AP, Dieppe P, et al. Associations between pain, function, and radiographic features in osteoarthritis of the knee. *Arthritis Rheum* 2006;54:230–235.
6. Bigos SJ, Battie MC, Spengler DM, et al. A longitudinal, prospective study of industrial back injury reporting. *Clin Orthop Relat Res* 1992;21–34.
7. Carragee EJ, Alamin TF, Miller JL, et al. Discographic, MRI and psychosocial determinants of low back pain disability and remission: a prospective study in subjects with benign persistent back pain. *Spine J* 2005;5:24–35.
8. Aubrun F, Langeron O, Quesnel C, et al. Relationships between measurement of pain using visual analog score and morphine requirements during postoperative intravenous morphine titration. *Anesthesiology* 2003;98:1415–1421.
9. Bisgaard T, Klarskov B, Rosenberg J, et al. Characteristics and prediction of early pain after laparoscopic cholecystectomy. *Pain* 2001;90:261–269.
10. Perkins FM, Kehlet H. Chronic pain as an outcome of surgery. A review of predictive factors. *Anesthesiology* 2000;93:1123–1133.
11. Uchiyama K, Kawai M, Tani M, et al. Gender differences in postoperative pain after laparoscopic cholecystectomy. *Surg Endosc* 2006;20:448–451.
12. Werner MU, Duun P, Kehlet H. Prediction of postoperative pain by preoperative nociceptive responses to heat stimulation. *Anesthesiology* 2004;100: 115–119.
13. Fillingim RB. Individual differences in pain responses. *Curr Rheumatol Rep* 2005;7:342–347.
14. Nielsen CS, Stubhaug A, Price DD, et al. Individual differences in pain sensitivity: genetic and environmental contributions. *Pain* 2008;136:21–29.
15. Diatchenko L, Slade GD, Nackley AG, et al. Genetic basis for individual variations in pain perception and the development of a chronic pain condition. *Hum Mol Genet* 2005;14:135–143.
16. Edwards RR, Haythornthwaite JA, Tella P, et al. Basal heat pain thresholds predict opioid analgesia in patients with postherpetic neuralgia. *Anesthesiology* 2006;104:1243–1248.
17. Fillingim RB, Hastie BA, Ness TJ, et al. Sex-related psychological predictors of baseline pain perception and analgesic responses to pentazocine. *Biol Psychol* 2005;69:97–112.
18. Fillingim RB, Ness TJ, Glover TL, et al. Morphine responses and experimental pain: sex differences in side effects and cardiovascular responses but not analgesia. *J Pain* 2005;6:116–124.
19. Sarton E, Olofsen E, Romberg R, et al. Sex differences in morphine analgesia: an experimental study in healthy volunteers. *Anesthesiology* 2000;93:1245–1254.
20. Atlas SJ, Keller RB, Wu YA, et al. Long-term outcomes of surgical and nonsurgical management of lumbar spinal stenosis: 8 to 10 year results from the maine lumbar spine study. *Spine* 2005;30:936–943.
21. Chae Y, Park HJ, Hahm DH, et al. Individual differences of acupuncture analgesia in humans using cDNA microarray. *J Physiol Sci* 2006;56:425–431.
22. Hoffman BM, Papas RK, Chatkoff DK, et al. Meta-analysis of psychological interventions for chronic low back pain. *Health Psychol* 2007;26:1–9.
23. Dionne RA, Bartoshuk L, Mogil J, et al. Individual responder analyses for pain: does one pain scale fit all? *Trends Pharmacol Sci* 2005;26:125–130.
24. Chapman WP, Jones CM. Variations in cutaneous and visceral pain sensitivity in normal subjects. *J Clin Invest* 1944;23:81–91.
25. Hardy JD, Wolff HG, Goodell H. *Pain Sensation and Reactions.* Baltimore, Md: Williams and Wilkins; 1952.
26. Fillingim RB. *Sex, Gender, and Pain.* Seattle, WA: IASP Press; 2000.
27. Greenspan JD, Craft RM, LeResche L, et al. Studying sex and gender differences in pain and analgesia: A consensus report. *Pain* 2007;132S1:S26–S45.
28. Sternbach RA. Survey of pain in the United States: The Nuprin Pain Report. *Clin J Pain* 1986;2:49–53.
29. Crook J, Rideout E, Browne G. The prevalence of pain complaints in a general population. *Pain* 1984;18:299–314.
30. Elliott AM, Smith BH, Penny KI, et al. The epidemiology of chronic pain in the community. *Lancet* 1999;354:1248–1252.
31. Andersson HI, Ejlertsson G, Leden I, et al. Chronic pain in a geographically defined general population: studies of differences in age, gender, social class, and pain localization. *Clin J Pain* 1993;9:174–182.
32. Kamaleri Y, Natvig B, Ihlebaek CM, et al. Number of pain sites is associated with demographic, lifestyle, and health-related factors in the general population. *Eur J Pain* 2008;12:742–748.
33. Von Korff M, Dworkin SF, LeResche L, et al. An epidemiologic comparison of pain complaints. *Pain* 1988;32:173–183.
34. LeResche L. Gender considerations in the epidemiology of chronic pain. In: Crombie IK, ed. *Epidemiology of Pain.* Seattle, WA: IASP Press; 1999:43–52.
35. LeResche L. Epidemiologic perspectives on sex differences in pain. In: Fillingim RB, editor. *Sex, Gender, and Pain.* Seattle, WA: IASP Press; 2000: 233–249.
36. Fillingim RB, Wilkinson CS, Powell T. Self-reported abuse history and pain complaints among healthy young adults. *Clin J Pain* 1999;15:85–91.
37. Lester N, Lefebvre JC, Keefe FJ. Pain in young adults: I. Relationship to gender and family pain history. *Clin J Pain* 1994;10:282–289.
38. Crombie IK, Croft PR, Linton SJ, et al. *Epidemiology of Pain.* Seattle, WA: IASP Press; 1999.
39. Drangsholt M, LeResche L. Temporomandibular disorder pain. In: Crombie IK, Croft PR, Linton SJ, LeResche L, Von Korff M, eds. *Epidemiology of Pain.* Seattle, WA: IASP Press; 1999:203–233.
40. Mayer EA, Naliboff B, Lee O, et al. Review article: gender-related differences in functional gastrointestinal disorders. *Aliment Pharmacol Ther* 1999;13: 65–69.
41. Theis KA, Helmick CG, Hootman JM. Arthritis burden and impact are greater among U.S. women than men: intervention opportunities. *J Womens Health (Larchmt)* 2007;16:441–453.
42. Wolfe F, Ross K, Anderson J, et al. Aspects of fibromyalgia in the general population: sex, pain threshold, and fibromyalgia symptoms. *J Rheumatol* 1995;22:151–156.
43. Berkley KJ. Sex differences in pain. *Behav Brain Sci* 1997;20:371–380.
44. Barsky AJ, Peekna HM, Borus JF. Somatic symptom reporting in women and men. *J Gen Intern Med* 2001;16:266–275.
45. Kaur S, Stechuchak KM, Coffman CJ, et al. Gender differences in health care utilization among veterans with chronic pain. *J Gen Intern Med* 2007;22: 228–233.
46. Linton SJ, Hellsing AL, Halldén K. A population-based study of spinal pain among 35–45-year-old individuals. Prevalence, sick leave, and health care use. *Spine* 1998;23:1457–1463.
47. Verbrugge LM. Sex differentials in health. *Public Health Rep* 1982;97: 417–437.

48. Aubrun F, Salvi N, Coriat P, et al. Sex- and age-related differences in morphine requirements for postoperative pain relief. *Anesthesiology* 2005;103:156–160.

49. Cepeda MS, Carr DB. Women experience more pain and require more morphine than men to achieve a similar degree of analgesia. *Anesth Analg* 2003; 97:1464–1468.

50. Chia YY, Chow LH, Hung CC, et al. Gender and pain upon movement are associated with the requirements for postoperative patient-controlled iv analgesia: a prospective survey of 2,298 Chinese patients. *Can J Anaesth* 2002; 49:249–255.

51. Averbuch M, Katzper M. A search for sex differences in response to analgesia. *Arch Intern Med* 2000;11;160:3424–3428.

52. Averbuch M, Katzper M. Gender and the placebo analgesic effect in acute pain. *Clin Pharmacol Ther* 2001;70:287–291.

53. Faucett J, Gordon N, Levine J. Differences in postoperative pain severity among four ethnic groups. *J Pain Symptom Manage* 1994;9:383–389.

54. Grossi GB, Maiorana C, Garramone RA, et al. Assessing postoperative discomfort after third molar surgery: a prospective study. *J Oral Maxillofac Surg* 2007;65:901–917.

55. Phillips C, White RP, Jr., Shugars DA, et al. Risk factors associated with prolonged recovery and delayed healing after third molar surgery. *J Oral Maxillofac Surg* 2003;61:1436–1448.

56. Gear RW, Gordon NC, Heller PH, et al. Gender difference in analgesic response to the kappa-opioid pentazocine. *Neurosci Lett* 1996;205:207–209.

57. Shabat S, Folman Y, Arinzon Z, et al. Gender differences as an influence on patients' satisfaction rates in spinal surgery of elderly patients. *Eur Spine J* 2005;14:1027–1032.

58. Heyer EJ, Sharma R, Winfree CJ, et al. Severe pain confounds neuropsychological test performance. *J Clin Exp Neuropsychol* 2000;22:633–639.

59. Logan DE, Rose JB. Gender differences in post-operative pain and patient controlled analgesia use among adolescent surgical patients. *Pain* 2004;109: 481–487.

60. Rosseland LA, Stubhaug A. Gender is a confounding factor in pain trials: women report more pain than men after arthroscopic surgery. *Pain* 2004; 112:248–253.

61. Taenzer AH, Clark C, Curry CS. Gender affects report of pain and function after arthroscopic anterior cruciate ligament reconstruction. *Anesthesiology* 2000;93:670–675.

62. Ochroch EA, Gottschalk A, Augostides J, et al. Long-term pain and activity during recovery from major thoracotomy using thoracic epidural analgesia. *Anesthesiology* 2002;97:1234–1244.

63. Ochroch EA, Gottschalk A, Troxel AB, et al. Women suffer more short and long-term pain than men after major thoracotomy. *Clin J Pain* 2006;22: 491–498.

64. Uchiyama K, Tani M, Kawai M, et al. Clinical significance of drainage tube insertion in laparoscopic cholecystectomy: a prospective randomized controlled trial. *J Hepatobiliary Pancreat Surg* 2007;14:551–556.

65. Bytzer P, Lindeberg B. Impact of an information video before colonoscopy on patient satisfaction and anxiety - a randomized trial. *Endoscopy* 2007;39: 710–714.

66. Eloubeidi MA, Wallace MB, Desmond R, et al. Female gender and other factors predictive of a limited screening flexible sigmoidoscopy examination for colorectal cancer. *Am J Gastroenterol* 2003;98:1634–1639.

67. Müllersdorf M, Söderback I. The actual state of the effects, treatment and incidence of disabling pain in a gender perspective—a Swedish study. *Disabil Rehabil* 2000;22:840–854.

68. Affleck G, Tennen H, Keefe FJ, et al. Everyday life with osteoarthritis or rheumatoid arthritis: independent effects of disease and gender on daily pain, mood, and coping. *Pain* 1999;83:601–609.

69. Keefe FJ, Lefebvre JC, Egert JR, et al. The relationship of gender to pain, pain behavior, and disability in osteoarthritis patients: the role of catastrophizing. *Pain* 2000;87:325–334.

70. Holtzman J, Saleh K, Kane R. Gender differences in functional status and pain in a Medicare population undergoing elective total hip arthroplasty. *Med Care* 2002;40:461–470.

71. Warnell P. The pain experience of a multiple sclerosis population: a descriptive study. *Axone* 1991;13:26–28.

72. Fillingim RB, Doleys DM, Edwards RR, et al. Clinical characteristics of chronic back pain as a function of gender and oral opioid use. *Spine* 2003; 28:143–150.

73. Edwards RR, Augustson E, Fillingim RB. Differential relationships retween anxiety and treatment-associated pain reduction among male and female chronic pain patients. *Clin J Pain* 2003;19:208–216.

74. Robinson ME, Wise EA, Riley JLI. Sex differences in clinical pain: a multisample study. *J Clin Psychol Med Settings* 1998;5:413–423.

75. Turk DC, Okifuji A. Does sex make a difference in the prescription of treatments and the adaptation to chronic pain by cancer and non-cancer patients? *Pain* 1999;82:139–148.

76. Bush FM, Harkins SW, Harrington WG, et al. Analysis of gender effects on pain perception and symptom presentation in temporomandibular joint pain. *Pain* 1993;53:73–80.

77. Marcus DA. Gender differences in chronic pain in a treatment-seeking population. *J Gend Specif Med* 2003;6:19–24.

78. Cairns BE. The influence of gender and sex steroids on craniofacial nociception. *Headache* 2007;47:319–324.

79. Fillingim RB, Maixner W. Gender differences in the responses to noxious stimuli. *Pain Forum* 1995;4:209–221.

80. Maixner W, Fillingim R, Booker D, et al. Sensitivity of patients with painful temporomandibular disorders to experimentally evoked pain. *Pain* 1995;63: 341–351.

81. Maixner W, Fillingim R, Sigurdsson A, et al. Sensitivity of patients with temporomandibular disorders to experimentally evoked pain: evidence for altered temporal summation of pain. *Pain* 1998;76:71–81.

82. Ness TJ, Powell-Boone T, Cannon R, et al. Psychophysical evidence of hypersensitivity in subjects with interstitial cystitis. *J Urol* 2005;173:1983–1987.

83. Schmidt-Hansen PT, Svensson P, Bendtsen L, et al. Increased muscle pain sensitivity in patients with tension-type headache. *Pain* 2007;129:113–121.

84. Staud R, Vierck CJ, Cannon RL, et al. Abnormal sensitization and temporal summation of second pain (wind-up) in patients with fibromyalgia syndrome. *Pain* 2001;91:165–175.

85. Verne GN, Robinson ME, Price DD. Hypersensitivity to visceral and cutaneous pain in the irritable bowel syndrome. *Pain* 2001;93:7–14.

86. Diatchenko L, Nackley AG, Slade GD, et al. Idiopathic pain disorders—pathways of vulnerability. *Pain* 2006;123:226–230.

87. Riley JL 3rd, Robinson ME, Wise EA, et al. Sex differences in the perception of noxious experimental stimuli: a meta-analysis. *Pain* 1998;74:181–187.

88. Rollman GB, Abdel-Shaheed J, Gillespie JM, et al. Does past pain influence current pain: biological and psychosocial models of sex differences. *Eur J Pain* 2004;8:427–433.

89. Wiesenfeld-Hallin Z. Sex differences in pain perception. *Gend Med* 2005;2: 137–145.

90. Fillingim RB, Maixner W, Kincaid S, et al. Sex differences in temporal summation but not sensory-discriminative processing of thermal pain. *Pain* 1998; 75:121–127.

91. Robinson ME, Wise EA, Gagnon C, et al. Influences of gender role and anxiety on sex differences in temporal summation of pain. *J Pain* 2004 Mar;5:77–82.

92. Sarlani E, Grace EG, Reynolds MA, et al. Sex differences in temporal summation of pain and aftersensations following repetitive noxious mechanical stimulation. *Pain* 2004;109:115–123.

93. Cairns BE, Hu JW, Arendt-Nielsen L, et al. Sex-related differences in human pain and rat afferent discharge evoked by injection of glutamate into the masseter muscle. *J Neurophysiol* 2001;86:782–791.

94. Svensson P, Cairns BE, Wang K, et al. Glutamate-evoked pain and mechanical allodynia in the human masseter muscle. *Pain* 2003;101:221–227.

95. Dannecker EA, Hausenblas HA, Kaminski TW, et al. Sex differences in delayed onset muscle pain. *Clin J Pain* 2005;21:120–126.

96. Dannecker EA, Knoll V, Robinson ME. Sex Differences in Muscle Pain: Self-Care Behaviors and Effects on Daily Activities. *J Pain* 200;9:200–209.

97. Poudevigne MS, O'Connor PJ, Pasley JD. Lack of both sex differences and influence of resting blood pressure on muscle pain intensity. *Clin J Pain* 2002; 18:386–393.

98. Chang L, Mayer EA, Labus JS, et al. Effect of sex on perception of rectosigmoid stimuli in irritable bowel syndrome. *Am J Physiol Regul Integr Comp Physiol* 2006;291:R277–R284.

99. Kim HS, Rhee PL, Park J, et al. Gender-related differences in visceral perception in health and irritable bowel syndrome. *J Gastroenterol Hepatol* 2006; 21:468–473.

100. Maixner W, Humphrey C. Gender differences in pain and cardiovascular responses to forearm ischemia. *Clin J Pain* 1993;9:16–25.

101. Ellermeier W, Westphal W. Gender differences in pain ratings and pupil reactions to painful pressure stimuli. *Pain* 1995;61:435–439.

102. France CR, Suchowiecki S. A comparison of diffuse noxious inhibitory controls in men and women. *Pain* 1999;81:77–84.

103. Mylius V, Kunz M, Schepelmann K, et al. Sex differences in nociceptive withdrawal reflex and pain perception. *Somatosens Mot Res* 2005;22:207–211.

104. Paulson PE, Minoshima S, Morrow TJ, et al. Gender differences in pain perception and patterns of cerebral activation during noxious heat stimulation in humans. *Pain* 1998;76:223–229.

105. Derbyshire SW, Nichols T, Firestone L, et al. Gender differences in patterns of cerebral activation during equal experience of painful laser stimulation. *J Pain* 2002;3:401–411.

106. Berman S, Munakata J, Naliboff BD, et al. Gender differences in regional brain response to visceral pressure in IBS patients. *Eur J Pain* 2000;4: 157–172.

107. Moulton EA, Keaser ML, Gullapalli RP, et al. Sex differences in the cerebral BOLD signal response to painful heat stimuli. *Am J Physiol Regul Integr Comp Physiol* 2006;291:R257–R267.

108. Henderson LA, Gandevia SC, Macefield VG. Gender differences in brain activity evoked by muscle and cutaneous pain: A retrospective study of single-trial fMRI data. *Neuroimage* 2008;39:1867–1876.

109. Miaskowski C, Levine JD. Does opioid analgesia show a gender preference for females? *Pain Forum* 1999;8:34–44.

110. Gordon NC, Gear RW, Heller PH, et al. Enhancement of morphine analgesia by the GABAB agonist baclofen. *Neuroscience* 1995;69:345–359.

111. Kaiko RF, Wallenstein SL, Rogers AG, et al. Sources of variation in analgesic responses in cancer patients with chronic pain receiving morphine. *Pain* 1983; 15:191–200.

112. Gear RW, Miaskowski C, Gordon NC, et al. Kappa-opioids produce significantly greater analgesia in women than in men. *Nat Med* 1996;2:1248–1250.

113. Gear RW, Gordon NC, Heller PH, et al. Gender difference in analgesic response to the kappa-opioid pentazocine. *Neurosci Lett* 1996;205:207–209.

114. Gear RW, Miaskowski C, Gordon NC, et al. The kappa opioid nalbuphine produces gender- and dose-dependent analgesia and antianalgesia in patients with postoperative pain. *Pain* 1999 Nov;83:339–345.

115. Miller PL, Ernst AA. Sex differences in analgesia: a randomized trial of mu versus kappa opioid agonists. *South Med J* 2004;97:35–41.

116. Pud D, Yarnitsky D, Sprecher E, et al. Can personality traits and gender predict the response to morphine? An experimental cold pain study. *Eur J Pain* 2006;10:103–112.

117. Romberg R, Olofsen E, Sarton E, et al. Pharmacokinetic-pharmacodynamic modeling of morphine-6-glucuronide-induced analgesia in healthy volunteers: absence of sex differences. *Anesthesiology* 2004;100:120–133.

118. Fillingim RB, Ness TJ, Glover TL, et al. Experimental pain models reveal no sex differences in pentazocine analgesia in humans. *Anesthesiology* 2004;100: 1263–1270.

119. Zacny JP, Beckman NJ. The effects of a cold-water stimulus on butorphanol effects in males and females. *Pharmacol Biochem Behav* 2004;78:653–659.

120. Hansen FR, Bendix T, Skov P, et al. Intensive, dynamic back-muscle exercises, conventional physiotherapy, or placebo-control treatment of low-back pain. A randomized, observer-blind trial. *Spine* 1993;18:98–108.

121. Jensen IB, Bergström G, Ljungquist T, et al. A randomized controlled component analysis of a behavioral medicine rehabilitation program for chronic spinal pain: are the effects dependent on gender? *Pain* 2001;91:65–78.

122. Kankaanpää M, Taimela S, Airaksinen O, et al. The efficacy of active rehabilitation in chronic low back pain. Effect on pain intensity, self-experienced disability, and lumbar fatigability. *Spine* 1999;24:1034–1042.

123. Mannion AF, Junge A, Taimela S, et al. Active therapy for chronic low back pain: part 3. Factors influencing self-rated disability and its change following therapy. *Spine* 2001;26:920–929.

124. Krogstad BS, Jokstad A, Dahl BL, et al. The reporting of pain, somatic complaints, and anxiety in a group of patients with TMD before and 2 years after treatment: sex differences. *J Orofac Pain* 1996;10:263–269.

125. Keogh E, McCracken LM, Eccleston C. Do men and women differ in their response to interdisciplinary chronic pain management? *Pain* 2005;114: 37–46.

126. Fillingim RB, Ness TJ. Sex-related hormonal influences on pain and analgesic responses. *Neurosci Biobehav Rev* 2000;24:485–501.

127. Fillingim RB, Gear RW. Sex differences in opioid analgesia: clinical and experimental findings. *Eur J Pain* 2004;8:413–425.

128. Craft RM, Mogil JS, Aloisi AM. Sex differences in pain and analgesia: the role of gonadal hormones. *Eur J Pain* 2004;8:397–411.

129. Kuba T, Quinones-Jenab V. The role of female gonadal hormones in behavioral sex differences in persistent and chronic pain: clinical versus preclinical studies. *Brain Res Bull* 2005;66:179–188.

130. Riley JL 3rd, Robinson ME, Wise EA, et al. A meta-analytic review of pain perception across the menstrual cycle. *Pain* 1999;81:225–235.

131. Sherman JJ, LeResche L. Does experimental pain response vary across the menstrual cycle? A methodological review. *Am J Physiol Regul Integr Comp Physiol* 2006;291:R245–R256.

132. Brynhildsen JO, Björs E, Skarsğrd C, et al. Is hormone replacement therapy a risk factor for low back pain among postmenopausal women? *Spine* 1998; 23:809–813.

133. Musgrave DS, Vogt MT, Nevitt MC, et al. Back problems among postmenopausal women taking estrogen replacement therapy. *Spine* 2001;26:1606–1612.

134. Wise EA, Riley JL 3rd, Robinson ME. Clinical pain perception and hormone replacement therapy in post-menopausal females experiencing orofacial pain. *Clin J Pain* 2000;16:121–126.

135. Fillingim RB, Edwards RR. The association of hormone replacement therapy with experimental pain responses in postmenopausal women. *Pain* 2001;92: 229–234.

136. Macfarlane TV, Blinkhorn A, Worthington HV, et al. Sex hormonal factors and chronic widespread pain: a population study among women. *Rheumatology (Oxford)* 2002;41:454–457.

137. de Leeuw R, Albuquerque RJ, Andersen AH, et al. Influence of estrogen on brain activation during stimulation with painful heat. *J Oral Maxillofac Surg* 2006;64:158–166.

138. Smith YR, Stohler CS, Nichols TE, et al. Pronociceptive and antinociceptive effects of estradiol through endogenous opioid neurotransmission in women. *J Neurosci* 2006;26:5777–5785.

139. Edwards RR, Haythornthwaite JA, Sullivan MJ, et al. Catastrophizing as a mediator of sex differences in pain: differential effects for daily pain versus laboratory-induced pain. *Pain* 2004;111:335–341.

140. Unruh AM, Ritchie J, Merskey H. Does gender affect appraisal of pain and pain coping strategies? *Clin J Pain* 1999;15:31–40.

141. Haley WE, Turner JA, Romano JM. Depression in chronic pain patients: relation to pain, activity, and sex differences. *Pain* 1985;23:337–343.

142. Riley JL, III, Robinson ME, Wade JB, et al. Sex differences in negative emotional responses to chronic pain. *J Pain* 2001;2:354–359.

143. Robinson ME, Riley JL, III, Myers CD. Psychosocial contributions to sex-related differences in pain responses. In: Fillingim RB, ed. *Sex, Gender, and Pain.* Seattle, WA: IASP Press; 2000:41–68.

144. Robinson ME, Riley JL 3rd, Myers CD, et al. Gender role expectations of pain: relationship to sex differences in pain. *J Pain* 2001;2:251–257.

145. Myers CD, Robinson ME, Riley JL 3rd, et al. Sex, gender, and blood pressure: contributions to experimental pain report. *Psychosom Med* 2001;63:545–550.

146. Myers CD, Tsao JC, Glover DA, et al. Sex, gender, and age: contributions to laboratory pain responding in children and adolescents. *J Pain* 2006;7: 556–564.

147. Otto MW, Dougher MJ. Sex differences and personality factors in responsivity to pain. *Percept Mot Skills* 1985;61:383–390.

148. Sanford SD, Kersh BC, Thorn BE, et al. Psychosocial mediators of sex differences in pain responsivity. *J Pain* 2002;3:58–64.

149. Thorn BE, Clements KL, Ward LC, et al. Personality factors in the explanation of sex differences in pain catastrophizing and response to experimental pain. *Clin J Pain* 2004;20:275–282.

150. Pool GJ, Schwegler AF, Theodore BR, et al. Role of gender norms and group identification on hypothetical and experimental pain tolerance. *Pain* 2007; 129:122–129.

151. Smedley BD, Stith AY, Nelson AR. *Unequal Treatment.* Washington, DC: The National Academies Press; 2002.

152. Edwards CL, Fillingim RB, Keefe FJ. Race, ethnicity and pain. *Pain* 2001;94: 133–137.

153. Green CR, Anderson KO, Baker TA, et al. The unequal burden of pain: confronting racial and ethnic disparities in pain. *Pain Med* 2003;4:277–294.

154. Bhopal R. Race and ethnicity: responsible use from epidemiological and public health perspectives. *J Law Med Ethics* 2006;34:500–507, 479.

155. Bhopal R. Glossary of terms relating to ethnicity and race: for reflection and debate. *J Epidemiol Community Health* 2004;58:441–445.

156. Bhopal R. Is research into ethnicity and health racist, unsound, or important science? *BMJ* 1997;314:1751–1756.

157. Byrd WM, Clayton LA. Racial and ethnic disparities in health care: a background and history. In: Smedley BD, Stith AY, Nelson AR, eds. *Unequal Treatment.* Washington, DC: The National Academies Press; 2002:455–527.

158. Collins FS. What we do and don't know about 'race', 'ethnicity', genetics and health at the dawn of the genome era. *Nat Genet* 2004;36:S13–S15.

159. Mountain JL, Risch N. Assessing genetic contributions to phenotypic differences among 'racial' and 'ethnic' groups. *Nat Genet* 2004;36(11 Suppl): S48–S53.

160. Castel LD, Saville BR, Depuy V, et al. Racial differences in pain during 1 year among women with metastatic breast cancer: a hazards analysis of interval-censored data. *Cancer* 2008;112:162–170.

161. Creamer P, Lethbridge-Cejku M, Hochberg MC. Determinants of pain severity in knee osteoarthritis: effect of demographic and psychosocial variables using 3 pain measures. *J Rheumatol* 1999;26:1785–1792.

162. Ibrahim SA, Burant CJ, Siminoff LA, et al. Self-assessed global quality of life: a comparison between African-American and white older patients with arthritis. *J Clin Epidemiol* 2002;55:512–517.

163. Shih VC, Song J, Chang RW, et al. Racial differences in activities of daily living limitation onset in older adults with arthritis: a national cohort study. *Arch Phys Med Rehabil* 2005;86:1521–1526.

164. Bruce B, Fries JF, Murtagh KN. Health status disparities in ethnic minority patients with rheumatoid arthritis: a cross-sectional study. *J Rheumatol* 2007; 34:1475–1479.

165. Carey TS, Garrett JM. The relation of race to outcomes and the use of health care services for acute low back pain. *Spine* 2003;28:390–394.

166. Widmalm SE, Christiansen RL, Gunn SM, et al. Prevalence of signs and symptoms of craniomandibular disorders and orofacial parafunction in 4–6-year-old African-American and Caucasian children. *J Oral Rehabil* 1995;22: 87–93.

167. Gansky SA, Plesh O. Widespread pain and fibromyalgia in a biracial cohort of young women. *J Rheumatol* 2007;34:810–817.

168. Edwards RR, Doleys DM, Fillingim RB, et al. Ethnic differences in pain tolerance: clinical implications in a chronic pain population. *Psychosom Med* 2001;63:316–323.

169. Green CR, Baker TA, Smith EM, et al. The effect of race in older adults presenting for chronic pain management: a comparative study of black and white Americans. *J Pain* 2003;4:82–90.

170. Green CR, Baker TA, Sato Y, et al. Race and chronic pain: A comparative study of young black and white Americans presenting for management. *J Pain* 2003;4:176–183.

171. McCracken LM, Matthews AK, Tang TS, et al. A comparison of blacks and whites seeking treatment for chronic pain. *Clin J Pain* 2001;17:249–255.

172. Bates MS, Edwards WT, Anderson KO. Ethnocultural influences on variation in chronic pain perception. *Pain* 1993;52:101–112.

173. Wang PC, Rempel D, Harrison R, et al. Work-organizational and personal factors associated with upper body musculoskeletal disorders among sewing machine operators. *Occup Environ Med* 2007 May 23 [Epub ahead of print].

174. Welch LS, Hunting KL, Nessel-Stephens L. Chronic symptoms in construction workers treated for musculoskeletal injuries [see comments]. *Am J Ind Med* 1999;36:532–540.

175. Faucett J, Gordon N, Levine J. Differences in postoperative pain severity among four ethnic groups. *J Pain Sympt Manage* 1994;9:383–389.

176. White SF, Asher MA, Lai SM, et al. Patients' perceptions of overall function, pain, and appearance after primary posterior instrumentation and fusion for idiopathic scoliosis. *Spine* 1999;24:1693–1699.

177. Reyes-Gibby CC, Aday LA, Todd KH, et al. Pain in aging community-dwelling adults in the United States: non-Hispanic whites, non-Hispanic blacks, and Hispanics. *J Pain* 2007;8:75–84.

178. Portenoy RK, Ugarte C, Fuller I, et al. Population-based survey of pain in the United States: differences among white, African American, and Hispanic subjects. *J Pain* 2004;5:317–328.

179. Calvillo ER, Flaskerud JH. Evaluation of the pain response by Mexican American and Anglo American women and their nurses. *J Adv Nurs* 1993;18: 451–459.

180. Edwards RR, Moric M, Husfeldt B, et al. Ethnic similarities and differences in the chronic pain experience: a comparison of african american, Hispanic, and white patients. *Pain Med* 2005;6:88–98.

181. Hastie BA, Riley JL, Fillingim RB. Ethnic differences and responses to pain in healthy young adults. *Pain Med* 2005;6:61–71.

182. Pfefferbaum B, Adams J, Aceves J. The influence of culture on pain in Anglo and Hispanic children with cancer. *J Am Acad Child Adolesc Psychiatry* 1990; 29:642–647.

183. Todd KH, Lee T, Hoffman JR. The effect of ethnicity on physician estimates of pain severity in patients with isolated extremity trauma [see comments]. *JAMA* 1994;271:925–928.

184. Deyo RA, Mirza SK, Martin BI. Back pain prevalence and visit rates: estimates from U.S. national surveys, 2002. *Spine* 2006;31:2724–2727.

185. Fuentes M, Hart-Johnson T, Green CR. The association among neighborhood socioeconomic status, race and chronic pain in black and white older adults. *J Natl Med Assoc* 2007;99:1160–1169.

186. Volkers AC, Westert GP, Schellevis FG. Health disparities by occupation, modified by education: a cross-sectional population study. *BMC Public Health* 2007;7:196.

187. Ng B, Dimsdale JE, Rollnik JD, et al. The effect of ethnicity on prescriptions for patient-controlled analgesia for post-operative pain. *Pain* 1996;66:9–12.

188. Pletcher MJ, Kertesz SG, Kohn MA, et al. Trends in opioid prescribing by race/ethnicity for patients seeking care in US emergency departments. *JAMA* 2008;299:70–78.

189. Todd KH, Samaroo N, Hoffman JR. Ethnicity as a risk factor for inadequate emergency department analgesia. *JAMA* 1993;269:1537–1539.

190. Todd KH, Deaton C, D'Adamo AP, et al. Ethnicity and analgesic practice. *Ann Emerg Med* 2000;35:11–16.

191. Woodrow KM, Friedman GD, Siegelaub AB, et al. Pain tolerance: Differences according to sex and race. *Psychosom Med* 1972;34:548–556.

192. Walsh NE, Schoenfeld L, Ramamurthy S, et al. Normative model for cold pressor test. *Am J Phys Med Rehab* 1989;68:6–11.

193. Edwards RR, Fillingim RB. Ethnic differences in thermal pain responses. *Psychosom Med* 1999;61:346–354.

194. Sheffield D, Biles PL, Orom H, et al. Race and sex differences in cutaneous pain perception. *Psychosom Med* 2000;62:517–523.

195. Campbell CM, Edwards RR, Fillingim RB. Ethnic differences in responses to multiple experimental pain stimuli. *Pain* 2005;113:20–26.

196. Klatzkin RR, Mechlin B, Bunevicius R, et al. Race and histories of mood disorders modulate experimental pain tolerance in women. *J Pain* 2007;8: 861–868.

197. Mechlin MB, Maixner W, Light KC, et al. African Americans show alterations in endogenous pain regulatory mechanisms and reduced pain tolerance to experimental pain procedures. *Psychosom Med* 2005;67:948–956.

198. Rahim-Williams FB, Riley JL 3rd, Herrera D, et al. Ethnic identity predicts experimental pain sensitivity in African Americans and Hispanics. *Pain* 2007; 129:177–184.

199. Weisse CS, Foster KK, Fisher EA. The influence of experimenter gender and race on pain reporting: does racial or gender concordance matter? *Pain Med* 2005;6:80–87.

200. Edwards RR, Doleys DM, Fillingim RB, et al. Ethnic differences in pain tolerance: clinical implications in a chronic pain population. *Psychosom Med* 2001;63(2):316–323.

201. Lawlis GF, Achterberg J, Kenner L, et al. Ethnic and sex differences in response to clinical and induced pain in chronic spinal pain patients. *Spine* 1984;9:751–754.

202. Knox VJ, Shum K, McLaughlin DM. Response to cold pressor pain and to acupuncture analgesia in Oriental and Occidental subjects. *Pain* 1977;4: 49–57.

203. Chapman CR, Sato T, Martin RW, et al. Comparative effects of acupuncture in Japan and the United States on dental pain perception. *Pain* 1982;12: 319–328.

204. Watson PJ, Latif RK, Rowbotham DJ. Ethnic differences in thermal pain responses: a comparison of South Asian and White British healthy males. *Pain* 2005;118:194–200.

205. Gazerani P, Arendt-Nielsen L. The impact of ethnic differences in response to capsaicin-induced trigeminal sensitization. *Pain* 2005;117:223–229.

206. Merskey H, Spear FG. The reliability of the pressure algometer. *Br J Soc Clin Psychol* 1964;3:130–136.

207. Nayak S, Shiflett SC, Eshun S, et al. Culture and gender effects in pain beliefs and the prediction of pain tolerance. *Cross-Cult Res: J Comp Soc Sci* 2000; 34:135–151.

208. Chen I, Kurz J, Pasanen M, et al. Racial differences in opioid use for chronic nonmalignant pain. *J Gen Intern Med* 2005;20:593–598.

209. Cleeland CS, Gonin R, Baez L, et al. Pain and treatment of pain in minority patients with cancer. The Eastern Cooperative Oncology Group Minority Outpatient Pain Study. *Ann Intern Med* 1997;127:813–816.

210. Adams RJ, Armstrong EP, Erstad BL. Prescribing and self-administration of morphine in Hispanic and non Hispanic Caucasian patients treated with patient-controlled analgesia. *J Pain Palliat Care Pharmacother* 2004;18:29–38.

211. Fuentes EF, Kohn MA, Neighbor ML. Lack of association between patient ethnicity or race and fracture analgesia. *Acad Emerg Med* 2002;9:910–915.

212. Yen K, Kim M, Stremski ES, et al. Effect of ethnicity and race on the use of pain medications in children with long bone fractures in the emergency department. *Ann Emerg Med* 2003;42:41–47.

213. Cepeda MS, Farrar JT, Roa JH, et al. Ethnicity influences morphine pharmacokinetics and pharmacodynamics. *Clin Pharmacol Ther* 2001;70:351–361.

214. Zhou HH, Sheller JR, Nu H, et al. Ethnic differences in response to morphine. *Clin Pharmacol Ther* 1993;54:507–513.

215. Cepeda MS, Farrar JT, Baumgarten M, et al. Side effects of opioids during short-term administration: effect of age, gender, and race. *Clin Pharmacol Ther* 2003;74:102–112.

216. Mechlin B, Morrow AL, Maixner W, et al. The relationship of allopregnanolone immunoreactivity and HPA-axis measures to experimental pain sensitivity: Evidence for ethnic differences. *Pain* 2007;131:142–152.

217. Jordan MS, Lumley MA, Leisen JC. The relationships of cognitive coping and pain control beliefs to pain and adjustment among African-American and Caucasian women with rheumatoid arthritis. *Arthritis Care Res* 1998;11: 80–88.

218. Hastie BA, Riley JL 3rd, Fillingim RB. Ethnic differences in pain coping: factor structure of the coping strategies questionnaire and coping strategies questionnaire-revised. *J Pain* 2004;5:304–316.

219. Bates MS. *Biocultural Dimensions of Chronic pain: Implications for Treatment of Multiethnic Populations*. Albany, NY: State University of New York Press; 1996.

220. Zborowski M. Cultural components in response to pain. *J Soc Issues* 1952; 8:16–30.

221. Belfer I, Wu T, Kingman A, et al. Candidate gene studies of human pain mechanisms: methods for optimizing choice of polymorphisms and sample size. *Anesthesiology* 2004;100:1562–1572.

222. Diatchenko L, Nackley AG, Tchivileva IE, et al. Genetic architecture of human pain perception. *Trends Genet* 2007;23:605–613.

223. Edwards RR. Genetic predictors of acute and chronic pain. *Curr Rheumatol Rep* 2006;8:411–417.

224. Lötsch J, Geisslinger G. Current evidence for a modulation of nociception by human genetic polymorphisms. *Pain* 2007;132:18–22.

225. Arnold LM, Hudson JI, Hess EV, et al. Family study of fibromyalgia. *Arthritis Rheum* 2004;50:944–952.

226. Kalantar JS, Locke GR 3rd, Zinsmeister AR, et al. Familial aggregation of irritable bowel syndrome: a prospective study. *Gut* 2003;52:1703–1707.

227. Kirk KM, Bellamy N, O'Gorman LE, et al. The validity and heritability of self-report osteoarthritis in an Australian older twin sample. *Twin Res* 2002; 5:98–106.

228. Russell MB, Saltyte-Benth J, Levi N. Are infrequent episodic, frequent episodic and chronic tension-type headache inherited? A population-based study of 11 199 twin pairs. *J Headache Pain* 2006;7:119–126.

229. Stewart WF, Bigal ME, Kolodner K, et al. Familial risk of migraine: variation by proband age at onset and headache severity. *Neurology* 2006;66:344–348.

230. Fejer R, Hartvigsen J, Kyvik KO. Heritability of neck pain: a population-based study of 33,794 Danish twins. *Rheumatology (Oxford)* 2006;45:589–594.

231. Hestbaek L, Iachine IA, Leboeuf-Yde C, et al. Heredity of low back pain in a young population: a classical twin study. *Twin Res* 2004;7:16–26.

232. Kato K, Sullivan PF, Evengrd B, et al. Importance of genetic influences on chronic widespread pain. *Arthritis Rheum* 2006;54:1682–1686.

233. Leboeuf-Yde C. Back pain—individual and genetic factors. *J Electromyogr Kinesiol* 2004;14:129–133.

234. Macgregor AJ, Andrew T, Sambrook PN, et al. Structural, psychological, and genetic influences on low back and neck pain: a study of adult female twins. *Arthritis Rheum* 2004;51:160–167.

235. Morris-Yates A, Talley NJ, Boyce PM, et al. Evidence of a genetic contribution to functional bowel disorder. *Am J Gastroenterol* 1998;93:1311–1317.

236. Spector TD, Macgregor AJ. Risk factors for osteoarthritis: genetics. *Osteoarthritis Cartilage* 2004;(12 Suppl)A:S39–S44.

237. Edwards RR, Sarlani E, Wesselmann U, et al. Quantitative assessment of experimental pain perception: multiple domains of clinical relevance. *Pain* 2005;114:315–319.

238. Edwards RR. Individual differences in endogenous pain modulation as a risk factor for chronic pain. *Neurology* 2005;65:437–443.

239. Fillingim RB, Lautenbacher S. The importance of quantitative sensory testing in the clinical setting. In: Lautenbacher S, Fillingim RB, eds. *Pathophysiology of Pain Perception*. New York: Kluwer Academic Plenum Publishers; 2004.

240. Mogil JS, ed. *The Genetics of Pain*. Seattle, WA: IASP Press; 2004.

241. MacGregor AJ, Griffiths GO, Baker J, et al. Determinants of pressure pain threshold in adult twins: evidence that shared environmental influences predominate. *Pain* 1997;73:253–257.

242. Norbury TA, Macgregor AJ, Urwin J, et al. Heritability of responses to painful stimuli in women: a classical twin study. *Brain* 2007;130:3041–3049.

243. Lohmueller KE, Pearce CL, Pike M, et al. Meta-analysis of genetic association studies supports a contribution of common variants to susceptibility to common disease. *Nat Genet* 2003;33:177–182.

244. Hirschhorn JN, Lohmueller K, Byrne E, et al. A comprehensive review of genetic association studies. *Genet Med* 2002;4:45–61.

245. Ioannidis JP. Non-replication and inconsistency in the genome-wide association setting. *Hum Hered* 2007;64:203–213.

246. Tegeder I, Costigan M, Griffin RS, et al. GTP cyclohydrolase and tetrahydrobiopterin regulate pain sensitivity and persistence. *Nat Med* 2006;12: 1269–1277.

247. Kim H, Dionne RA. Lack of influence of GTP cyclohydrolase gene (GCH1) variations on pain sensitivity in humans. *Mol Pain* 2007;3:6.

248. Zubieta JK, Heitzeg MM, Smith YR, et al. COMT val158met genotype affects mu-opioid neurotransmitter responses to a pain stressor. *Science* 2003;299:1240–1243.
249. Kim H, Mittal DP, Iadarola MJ, et al. Genetic predictors for acute experimental cold and heat pain sensitivity in humans. *J Med Genet* 2006;43:e40.
250. Gürsoy S, Erdal E, Herken H, et al. Significance of catechol-O-methyltransferase gene polymorphism in fibromyalgia syndrome. *Rheumatol Int* 2003;23:104–107.
251. Hagen K, Pettersen E, Stovner LJ, et al. The association between headache and Val158Met polymorphism in the catechol-O-methyltransferase gene: the HUNT Study. *J Headache Pain* 2006;7:70–74.
252. George SZ, Wallace MR, Wright TW, et al. Evidence for a biopsychosocial influence on shoulder pain: Pain catastrophizing and catechol-O-methyltransferase (COMT) diplotype predict clinical pain ratings. *Pain* 2008;136:53–61.
253. Bond C, LaForge KS, Tian M, et al. Single-nucleotide polymorphism in the human mu opioid receptor gene alters beta-endorphin binding and activity: possible implications for opiate addiction. *Proc Natl Acad Sci U S A* 1998;95:9608–9613.
254. Beyer A, Koch T, Schröder H, et al. Effect of the A118G polymorphism on binding affinity, potency and agonist-mediated endocytosis, desensitization, and resensitization of the human mu-opioid receptor. *J Neurochem* 2004 May;89:553–560.
255. Zhang Y, Wang D, Johnson AD, et al. Allelic expression imbalance of human mu opioid receptor (OPRM1) caused by variant A118G. *J Biol Chem* 2005;280:32618–32624.
256. Fillingim RB, Kaplan L, Staud R, et al. The A118G single nucleotide polymorphism of the mu-opioid receptor gene (OPRM1) is associated with pressure pain sensitivity in humans. *J Pain* 2005;6:159–167.
257. Lötsch J, Stuck B, Hummel T. The human mu-opioid receptor gene polymorphism 118A > G decreases cortical activation in response to specific nociceptive stimulation. *Behav Neurosci* 2006;120:1218–1224.
258. Janicki PK, Schuler G, Francis D, et al. A genetic association study of the functional A118G polymorphism of the human mu-opioid receptor gene in patients with acute and chronic pain. *Anesth Analg* 2006;103:1011–1017.
259. Oertel BG, Schmidt R, Schneider A, et al. The mu-opioid receptor gene polymorphism 118A>G depletes alfentanil-induced analgesia and protects against respiratory depression in homozygous carriers. *Pharmacogenet Genomics* 2006;16:625–636.
260. Oertel BG, Preibisch C, Wallenhorst T, et al. Differential opioid action on sensory and affective cerebral pain processing. *Clin Pharmacol Ther* 2008;83:577–588.
261. Romberg RR, Olofsen E, Bijl H, et al. Polymorphism of mu-opioid receptor gene (OPRM1:c.118A>G) does not protect against opioid-induced respiratory depression despite reduced analgesic response. *Anesthesiology* 2005;102:522–530.
262. Chou WY, Yang LC, Lu HF, et al. Association of mu-opioid receptor gene polymorphism (A118G) with variations in morphine consumption for analgesia after total knee arthroplasty. *Acta Anaesthesiol Scand* 2006;50:787–792.
263. Chou WY, Wang CH, Liu PH, et al. Human opioid receptor A118G polymorphism affects intravenous patient-controlled analgesia morphine consumption after total abdominal hysterectomy. *Anesthesiology* 2006;105:334–337.
264. Klepstad P, Rakvåg TT, Kaasa S, et al. The 118 A > G polymorphism in the human mu-opioid receptor gene may increase morphine requirements in patients with pain caused by malignant disease. *Acta Anaesthesiol Scand* 2004;48:1232–1239.
265. Edwards PW, Zeichner A, Kuczmierczyk AR, et al. Familial pain models: the relationship between family history of pain and current pain experience. *Pain* 1985;21:379–384.
266. Fillingim RB, Edwards RR, Powell T. Sex-dependent effects of reported familial pain history on clinical and experimental pain responses. *Pain* 2000;86:87–94.
267. Neumann L, Buskila D. Quality of life and physical functioning of relatives of fibromyalgia patients. *Semin Arthritis & Rheum* 1997;26:834–839.
268. Mogil JS, Wilson SG, Chesler EJ, et al. The melanocortin-1 receptor gene mediates female-specific mechanisms of analgesia in mice and humans. *Proc Natl Acad Sci U S A* 2003;100:4867–4872.
269. Kim H, Neubert JK, San Miguel A, et al. Genetic influence on variability in human acute experimental pain sensitivity associated with gender, ethnicity and psychological temperament. *Pain* 2004;109:488–496.
270. Mogil JS, Richards SP, O'Toole LA, et al. Genetic sensitivity to hot-plate nociception in DBA/2J and C57BL/6J inbred mouse strains: possible sex-specific mediation by delta2-opioid receptors. *Pain* 1997;70:267–277.
271. Gower BA, Fernández JR, Beasley TM, et al. Using genetic admixture to explain racial differences in insulin-related phenotypes. *Diabetes* 2003;52:1047–1051.
272. Shriver MD. Ethnic variation as a key to the biology of human disease. *Ann Intern Med* 1997;127:401–403.
273. Shriver MD, Kennedy GC, Parra EJ, et al. The genomic distribution of population substructure in four populations using 8,525 autosomal SNPs. *Hum Genomics* 2004;1:274–286.
274. Gelernter J, Kranzler H, Cubells J. Genetics of two mu opioid receptor gene (OPRM1) exon I polymorphisms: population studies, and allele frequencies in alcohol- and drug-dependent subjects. *Mol Psychiatry* 1999;4:476–483.
275. Hastie BA, Kaplan L, Campbell CM, et al. Association of A118G single nucleotide polymorphism of the u opioid receptor gene (OPRM) with experimental pain in a multi-ethnic sample. *J Pain* 2006;7:S4.
276. Kunugi H, Nanko S, Ueki A, et al. High and low activity alleles of catechol-O-methyltransferase gene: ethnic difference and possible association with Parkinson's disease. *Neurosci Lett* 1997;221:202–204.
277. McLeod HL, Fang L, Luo X, et al. Ethnic differences in erythrocyte catechol-O-methyltransferase activity in black and white Americans. *J Pharmacol Exp Ther* 1994;270:26–29.
278. Edwards RR, Augustson E, Fillingim RB. Sex-specific effects of pain-related anxiety on adjustment to chronic pain. *Clin J Pain* 2000;16:46–53.
279. Fillingim RB, Keefe FJ, Light KC, et al. The influence of gender and psychological factors on pain perception. *J Gender Cult Health* 1996;1:21–36.
280. Jones A, Zachariae R, Arendt-Nielsen L. Dispositional anxiety and the experience of pain: gender-specific effects. *Eur J Pain* 2003;7:387–395.
281. Jones A, Zachariae R. Investigation of the interactive effects of gender and psychological factors on pain response. *Br J Health Psychol* 2004;9:405–418.
282. Diatchenko L, Nackley AG, Slade GD, et al. Catechol-O-methyltransferase gene polymorphisms are associated with multiple pain-evoking stimuli. *Pain* 2006;125:216–224.
283. Kim H, Mittal DP, Iadarola MJ, et al. Genetic predictors for acute experimental cold and heat pain sensitivity in humans. *J Med Genet* 2006;43:e40.
284. Mogil JS, Ritchie J, Smith SB, et al. Melanocortin-1 receptor gene variants affect pain and mu-opioid analgesia in mice and humans. *J Med Genet* 2005;42:583–587.

CHAPTER 9 ■ FUNCTIONAL NEUROANATOMY OF THE NOCICEPTIVE SYSTEM

ROBERT GRIFFIN, EZEKIEL FINK, AND GARY J. BRENNER

INTRODUCTION TO FUNCTIONAL NEUROANATOMY OF THE NOCICEPTIVE SYSTEM

From the standpoint of the physician, there are two perspectives from which to view pain. One is as a symptom of a disease process that will inform about the underlying pathophysiology. The other is as the primary cause for suffering that requires treatment in its own right. These two views of pain often coexist when the pain reveals pathology whose treatment will not resolve the pain rapidly enough for the patient to tolerate. For example, in acute myocardial ischemia, the pain is the cardinal symptom of the underlying illness but in itself can provide an ongoing stimulus for a catecholaminergic state that will increase myocardial demand and potentially worsen the ischemic state. Both of these perspectives, either using the pain as a clue or addressing it as the primary aim of treatment,[1] are enhanced by considering the patient's report of their pain in light of the specific anatomic structures that collect information about noxious stimuli and communicate this information to the central nervous system (CNS) where pain is perceived and a behavioral response is generated.

Pain may be described according to three major parameters: acute vs. chronic, physiologic (nociceptive) vs. pathologic (neuropathic), and somatic vs. visceral. Full understanding of the nature of any pain complaint requires knowledge of the anatomic structures involved and the functional status of these structures. Chronicity of pain is determined by the duration of the irritating stimulus and by the plastic response of the peripheral and CNS to injury or ongoing stimulus. Pain may be either nociceptive, induced by high-threshold sensory stimuli required for activation of peripheral nociceptors, or pathologic, induced by low-threshold stimuli due to a heightened state of nervous system excitability brought on by either inflammatory cell–cell signaling (i.e., inflammatory pain) and signal transduction or by the extensive anatomic and physiologic alterations brought on by nerve injury (i.e., neuropathic pain).[2] Finally, pain may be somatic, transmitted by the somatosensory nervous system, or visceral, transmitted by splanchnic sympathetic and pelvic nerve afferent fibers (or by specific cranial nerves in the case of the head and neck).[3,4] This chapter will touch on the specific anatomic structures that are involved in the transduction of physical stimuli into sensory responses, the conduction of sensory information to the CNS, the processing and relay of this sensory information within the spinal cord and brain, and will discuss some of the major perturbations in these structures as related to clinical pain phenomena.

ORGANIZATION OF THE PERIPHERAL NOCICEPTIVE SYSTEM

There are several major anatomic units involved in pain sensation. First, primary sensory neurons whose peripheral terminals respond to physical energy conduct action potentials along long axons bundled into peripheral nerves from the site of sensory stimulus to the CNS.[5] Next, nociceptive synaptic relay occurs at the dorsal horn of the spinal cord, where substantial sensory processing occurs.[6–8] Ascending fiber tracts carry this information to the brainstem and, from there, diverse brain regions. Descending fiber tracts project from the brainstem and brain to the dorsal horn of the spinal cord and regulate the processing of incoming sensory information.[9]

The peripheral nerves that carry sensory information from visceral organs, bone, muscle, joint, or skin to the CNS may be either cranial nerves or spinal nerves. Cranial nerves carry sensory information to the brainstem,[10] while spinal nerves carry sensory information to the spinal cord and may bear axons for neurons that synapse within the spinal cord or brainstem.[11,12] Spinal nerves are mixed nerves that carry general somatic afferent fibers, general visceral afferent fibers, general somatic efferent fibers, and general visceral efferent fibers. Somatic afferents primarily carry information from skin, muscle, tendon, and joint, whereas visceral afferents carry information from the other tissues. The cell bodies of both the somatic and the visceral afferent fibers carried by spinal nerves reside in the dorsal root ganglia (DRG) of the spinal cord, whereas those carried by cranial nerves reside in the brainstem cranial nerve nuclei.[12]

The ability to localize painful stimuli depends on the topographic organization of the nervous system. The somatic afferent system and the visceral afferent system are strikingly different in this regard, with precise stimulus position detected and encoded by the somatic nervous system but only relatively diffuse information coming to conscious awareness from the visceral afferent system.[4] In the clinical setting, precise localization of pain is often considered as evidence that the pain is detected by somatic afferents rather than visceral afferents. For example, knife-like well-localized pain associated with inspiration is likely detected by somatic fibers innervating the parietal pleura.[13] In the abdomen, well-localized lower right quadrant pain occurring late in the course of acute appendicitis is likely due to spread of the periappendiceal inflammation that irritates the somatic nerves innervating the abdominal wall overlying the appendix.[14]

In the somatic system, the spinal cord is segmentally organized, such that each spinal segment receives afferent information about a specific cutaneous band or dermatome (Fig. 9.1).[15] This organization arises during embryonic development when the embryonic neural tube and adjacent mesodermal tissues segment into a series of rostro-caudally adjacent somites.[16] Each spinal nerve innervates tissue developing from a single somite.[17] Spinal nerves from several different spinal segments, such as axons from neurons with cell bodies located in several different DRG, join to give rise to peripheral nerves with cutaneous fields of innervation that span multiple dermatomes (Fig. 9.2).[18] The innervation of specific peripheral cutaneous nerves, as compared to the organization of the cutaneous dermatomes, is illustrated (Fig. 9.3).

In contrast to cutaneous sensation, visceral pain is perceived as deep and is typically not well spatially localized. The clinical features of visceral as compared to somatic pain are summarized in Table 9.1. Visceral pain has a different quality than somatic pain. It is referred to structures or areas other than the organ being affected, such as the experience of arm pain with myocardial infarction.[19] The diffuse nature of the visceral pain is felt to be secondary to the large receptive field of the sensory fibers in the viscera which corresponds to the low density of sensory innervation.[20,21]

Although there are many anatomical similarities between the somatic and autonomic afferent fibers, there are significant differences in the clinical presentation of visceral pain and somatic pain. Pain symptoms resulting from visceral afferents are felt in a location different than the organ itself. This is felt to be as a result of convergence from somatic structures and viscera at multiple sites of the CNS. Convergence occurs in the dorsal horn neurons in lamina I, IV, and V as well as in the intermediate gray matter in lamina X (Fig. 9.4)[22] as well as other areas of the CNS including the brainstem, basal forebrain, thalamus, and cerebral cortex.[23] Functional neuroimaging studies have shown that regions of the cortex that are activated by noxious stimuli can also be activated by visceral stimuli.[24] A possible explanation for the clinical symptoms of referred pain is that peripheral nociceptors from somatic and visceral origin converge on a single projection neuron in the dorsal horn. As a result, higher levels of the CNS cannot distinguish the source of the signal input and attribute the sensation to somatic structures by default because somatic sensory representation predominates in the CNS. In the thorax, substernal chest pain may be due to any of the visceral sensory afferents from the T1 to T6 spinal segments and may arise from the heart and great vessels, esophagus, lungs, or chest wall. Visceral pain in the abdomen tends to follow the structure of endodermal embryonic development with pain due to foregut structures (stomach, proximal duodenum, liver, biliary system, and pancreas) perceived in the epigastrium or upper abdomen, pain due to midgut structures (distal duodenum, small bowel, cecum, appendix, ascending colon, and proximal transverse colon) perceived in the periumbilical region, and pain due to hindgut structures (distal transverse colon, descending colon, sigmoid, rectum, and urinary bladder) perceived in the lower abdomen.[14]

The central processes of the visceral fibers synapse extensively above and below the segment where they entered, thus activating spinothalamic cells at multiple levels. Clinically, noxious stimulation of the viscera elicits an autonomic spinal reflex reaction, with sympathetic activation that causes symptoms such as excessive sweating and pronounced changes in circulatory system resulting

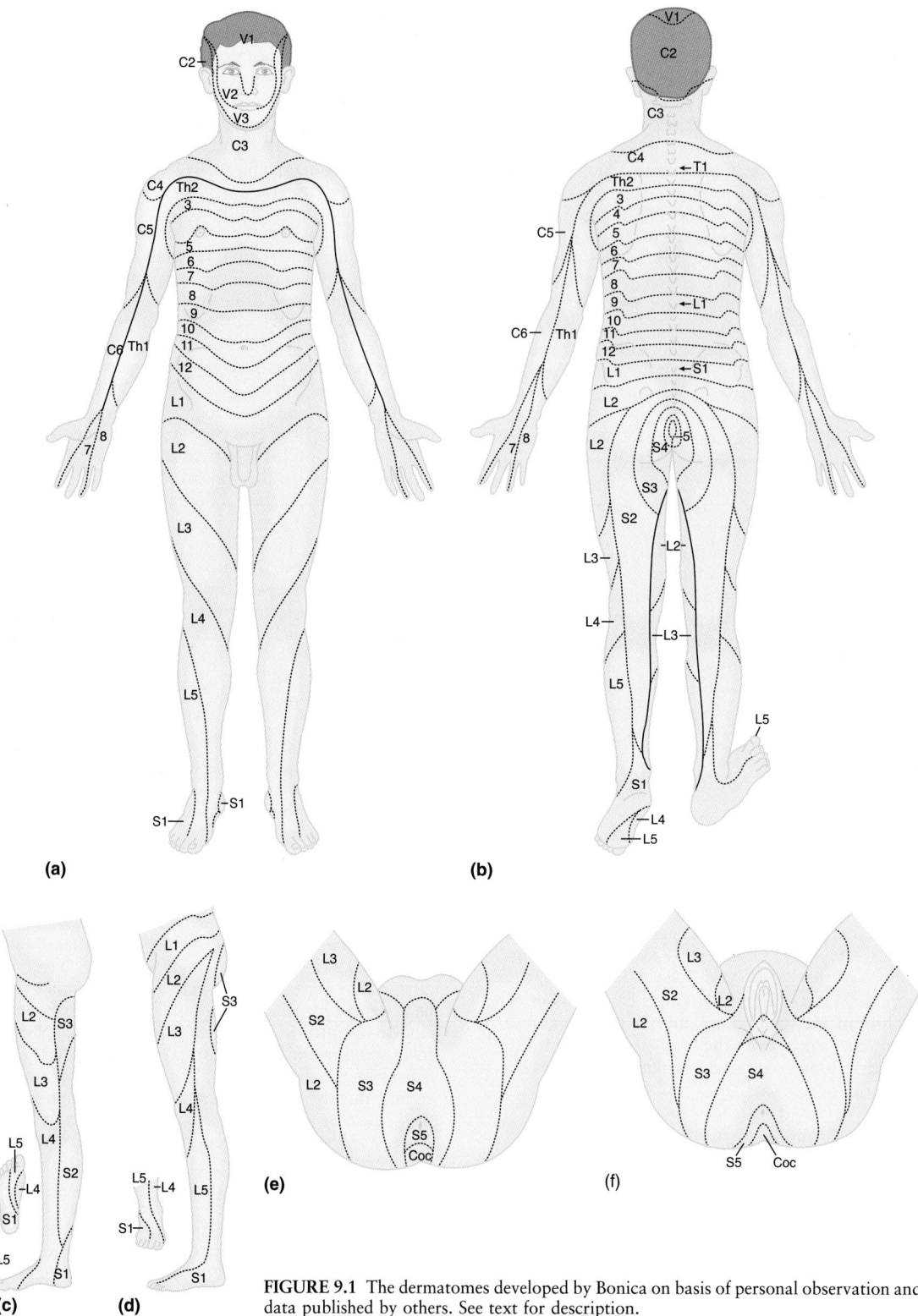

FIGURE 9.1 The dermatomes developed by Bonica on basis of personal observation and data published by others. See text for description.

in increased blood pressure. This reflex reaction tends to be more pronounced than what is seen with noxious stimulation of the skin. Noxious visceral stimulation can also result in hypotension and bradycardia by either reflex inhibition of sympathetic outflow or activation of the parasympathetic nervous system.[25] These reactions may be mediated by the periaqueductal gray matter (PAG) and the nucleus of the solitary tract. There are also protective reflexes that are directed toward reducing pain, such as the inhibition of visceral motility. Deregulation of this reflex as well as aberrant response by vagal afferents in the enteric system is thought to contribute to the pathophysiology of irritable bowel syndrome.[26] Coordination centers at higher levels of the CNS, such as the PAG, also mediate nausea and vomiting as well as complex somatic responses in the context of visceral pain.

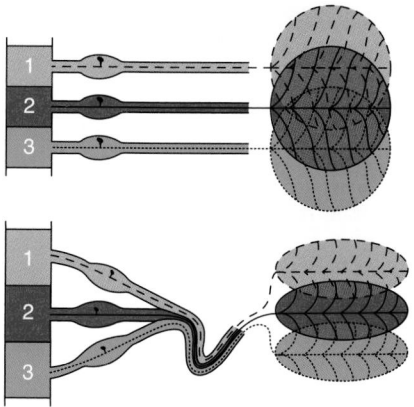

FIGURE 9.2 Simple diagrams to illustrate the overlap of cutaneous fields of segmental and peripheral nerves. In the upper figure, three intercostal (segmental) nerves extending from the periphery to the spinal cord are represented. The lower figure illustrates a somewhat analogous but less extensive overlap in the peripheral nerves.

PERIPHERAL NERVOUS SYSTEM STRUCTURES OF PAIN SENSATION

Within the DRG, there are several neuronal populations classified primarily according to caliber and myelination and secondarily according to the expression of chemical markers.[27] Large myelinated fibers comprise the A-beta (Aβ) population, which respond predominantly to low-energy, nonpainful mechanical stimuli and conduct action potentials rapidly. Small, thinly myelinated fibers make up the A-delta (Aδ) population, which respond to high-energy mechanical stimuli and have intermediate conduction velocity. Small, unmyelinated fibers are classified as the C-fiber population, and have slow conduction velocity.[28] In general, C-fibers can respond to chemical, thermal, and high-threshold mechanical stimuli, with several subclasses of C-fibers exhibiting responses to various combinations of these stimulus categories.[29] Typical of electrically excitable cells, the conduction of action potentials along the axons of primary afferent sensory neurons depends on voltage gated ion channels. The inward current of the action potential is carried by voltage-gated sodium ion channels. There are six types of these in the DRG neurons of which two,

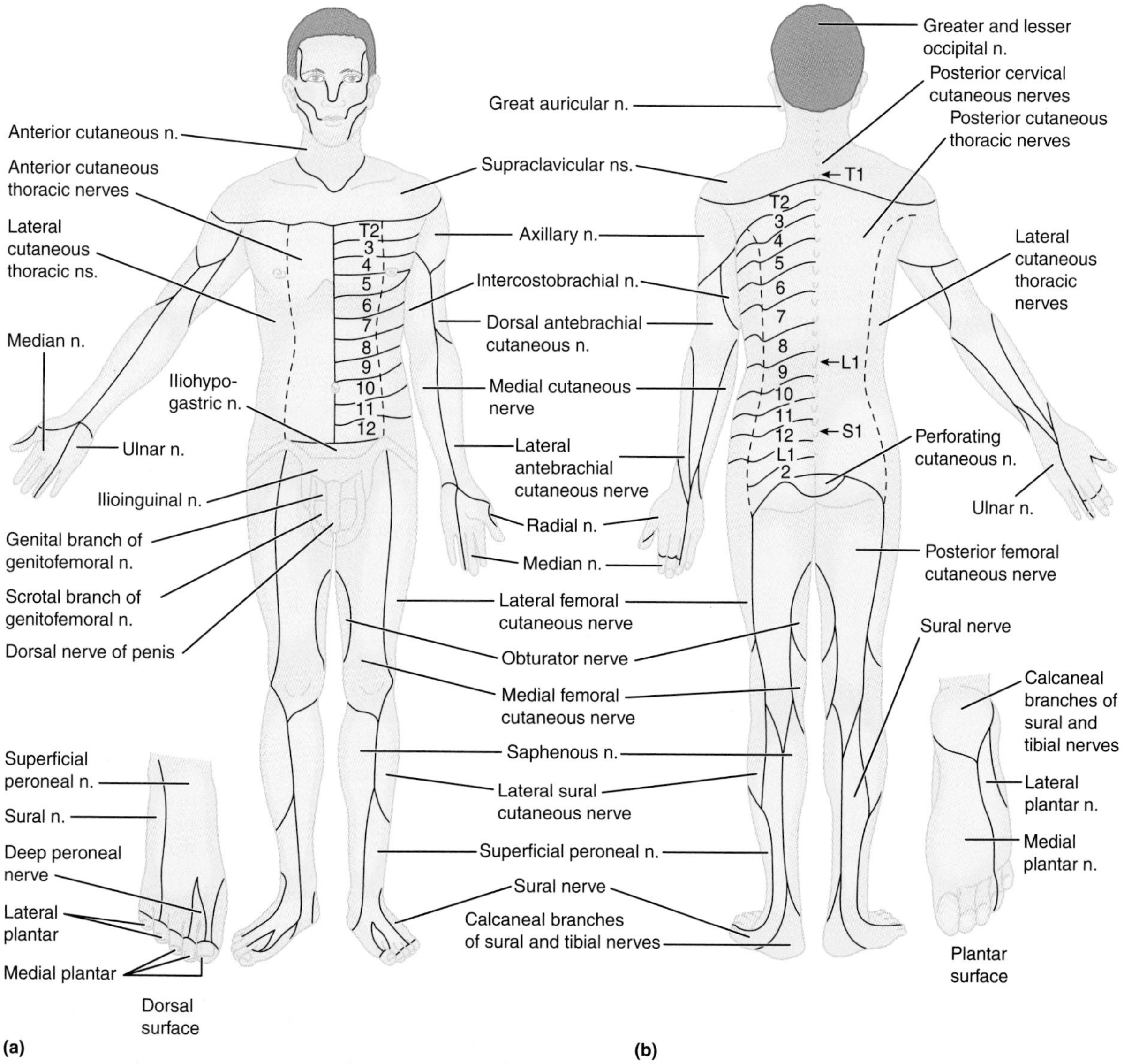

FIGURE 9.3 The cutaneous fields of peripheral nerves (n). **A.** Anterior view. **B.** Posterior view. In both figures, the numbers on the trunk refer to the intercostal nerves.

TABLE 9.1

COMPARISON OF SOMATIC AND VISCERAL NOCICEPTIVE PAIN

	Somatic nociceptive pain	Visceral nociceptive pain
Localization	More focused	More diffuse and poorly localized; pain felt in distribution innervated by the same spinal segment as organ; referred to other locations
Quality	Sharp, aching, burning, stabbing	Vague discomfort Hyperesthesia, hyperalgesia, allodynia
Associated symptoms	Accompanied by motor reflexes	Accompanied by motor and autonomic reflexes: associated muscle contraction/ spasm, nausea/vomiting, faint sensation, circulatory changes in the region, decreased pulse/blood pressure, cold sweat
Triggers	Tissue injury	Distention, contraction, ischemia, inflammation; pain not evoked from all viscera (organs such as liver and kidneys are not sensitive to pain)

Nav 1.8 and Nav 1.9, have expression pattern limited to sensory neurons, with Nav 1.8 limited to nociceptors.[30–32]

C-fiber neurons are further subdivided into two groups. One group expresses the nerve growth factor (NGF) receptor TrkA, as well as the neuropeptides substance P and calcitonin gene-related peptide (CGRP), while the other group of C-fibers expresses the glial derived neurotrophic factor receptor c-ret and binds to the isolectin B4 (IB4).[33,34] Interestingly, recent data has demonstrated that the free nerve endings in the epidermis are anatomically structured such that the peptidergic fibers terminate in the stratum spinosum, while the nonpeptidergic fibers terminate in the more superficial stratum granulosum.[35] This topographic separation is maintained at the level of the dorsal horn of the spinal cord, where the peptidergic and nonpeptidergic afferents terminate in distinct Rexed laminae.

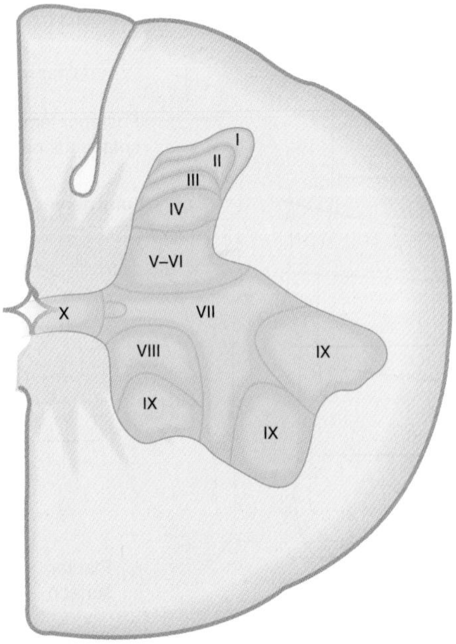

The peripheral terminals of DRG neurons are specialized to respond to thermal, mechanical, or chemical energy. Briefly, thermosensation depends on thermosensitive ion channels in the transient receptor potential (TRP) family, with TRPV1 and TRPV2 responsive to heat that is usually perceived as painful.[36,37] Recently, a specific inhibitor of TRPV1 has been identified that may eventually prove to have a role as a pain-specific local anesthetic agent.[38] Mechanosensation likely also depends on a set of mechanosensitive ion channels; however, the receptors responsible for transducing this information have yet to be unequivocally identified.[39–41] A wide range of chemical mediators can also act on the peripheral terminals of DRG neurons, acting either directly to activate nociceptors or indirectly by sensitizing the peripheral terminals to be activated at a lower stimulus threshold. Chemical mediators may be either exogenous (e.g., capsaicin, mustard oil, chemical acids, bee venom) or endogenous (e.g., many of the myriad inflammatory mediators). Endogenously released chemical mediators that cause pain directly are typically associated with tissue destruction that alters the chemical microenvironment, for example $H+$ ions and adenosine triphosphate, or causes an inflammatory response, such as bradykinin.[42,43]

FIGURE 9.4 Schematic drawing of a cross-section of the cervical spinal cord highlighting the lamina. (Modified from Kiernan JA. *Barr's: The Human Nervous System: an Anatomical Viewpoint*. 7th ed. Philadelphia: Lippincott Williams & Wilkins; 1998.)

FUNCTIONAL ANATOMY OF THE CENTRAL NERVOUS SYSTEM

Among the sensations that are transmitted from the periphery to the CNS for processing, pain is the most distinctive of all the sensory modalities. Unlike other senses, pain is defined by not only the physiologic perception of nociception but also the affective and emotional response to that perception. Pain is a highly individual and subjective experience to the extent that the same stimulus can produce different responses in different individuals under the same conditions. The CNS is both the processing center for the perception of noxious stimulation and the primary regulator of adaptive and modulatory mechanisms to produce a pain behavior. Pain is primarily categorized by duration of symptoms (acute vs. chronic) and the origin of the pain signal (visceral vs. somatic and nociceptive vs. neuropathic). Understanding the anatomy and function of the pain structures and pathways in the CNS is essential to understanding and managing the different categories of pain.

Dorsal Horn

The dorsal horn represents the termination point of the dorsal root in the CNS. There is a correspondence between the functional and anatomical organization of the dorsal horn. It is arranged into 10 laminae, and distinct sensory modalities from the periphery terminate in distinct laminae (see Fig. 9.4).[44] Signals conducting nociceptive signals (Aδ and C-fibers) terminate in the superficially located laminae I (also called the marginal layer) and II (also called the substantia gelatinosa). Many neurons from lamina I respond exclusively to noxious stimulation and project to higher levels of the CNS. Some neurons called wide dynamic range neurons respond in a stepwise fashion to peripheral stimulation. The neurons of lamina II are mostly interneurons and modulate nociceptive responses at the level of the dorsal horn. The Aδ fibers also terminate in lamina V which contains wide dynamic range neurons that project to higher levels of the CNS including the thalamus.[45] There is some convergence of somatic and visceral nociceptive input into lamina V, which may explain referred pain from visceral structures.[46] Single axons of all receptors give off ascending and descending branches after entering the spinal cord. In addition to synapsing at the level they enter, these branches give off multiple collaterals that end in the gray matter of the dorsal horns at one to two levels above and below where the axon entered the spinal cord.[47] Integration of signals from the periphery and higher levels of the CNS occur at the level of the dorsal horn through the dense network of dendrites and interneurons.

Synaptic transmission by nociceptive afferent neurons at the level of the dorsal horn is mediated primarily by the excitatory neurotransmitter glutamate. Both ionotropic and metabotropic glutamate receptors are located in high concentration in the substantia gelatinosa.[48] Many neuropeptides (e.g., substance P, vasoactive intestinal polypeptide, cholecystokinin, and CGRP) which are theorized to modulate synaptic action are present in the neurons in the dorsal horn. The receptors for most of these neuropeptides are concentrated in the substantia gelatinosa which suggests that they are involved in the transmission of pain. Among the neuropeptides, substance P and its receptor, neurokinin-1, are likely to be involved in the processing and modulating of pain signals in the dorsal horn. Substance P may increase the excitation from incoming sensory fibers by enhancing and prolonging the actions of glutamate. This has been demonstrated experimentally: substance P and CGRP have been found to increase the release of glutamate; substance P induces the N-methyl-D-aspartate (NMDA) receptors to become more sensitive to glutamate. This unmasks normally silent interneurons and sensitizes second order spinal neurons.[49] Blocking the neurokinin-1 receptors can prevent many of these effects. Substance P can also extend long distances within the spinal cord and sensitize dorsal horn neurons several segments away from the initial nociceptive signal. This results in an expansion of receptive fields and the activation of wide dynamic neurons by non-nociceptive afferent impulses.[50]

Sustained noxious stimulation or high-intensity nociceptive signals to the dorsal horn neurons may lead to increased neuronal responsiveness or central sensitization.[51] Hyperalgesia, which is an exaggerated perception of painful stimuli, is at least partially mediated through low-threshold mechanoreceptors (Aβ afferents) in the dorsal horn. Allodynia, which is a perception of innocuous stimuli as painful, is mediated through high threshold nociceptors (Aδ or C-fibers) in the dorsal horn. The factors that contribute to these hyperexcitable states include altered function of neurochemical and electrophysiological systems as well as changes in the anatomy in the dorsal horn.[52]

"Wind up" refers to a central spinal mechanism in which repetitive noxious stimulation results in a slow summation of these signals that is experienced as increased pain.[53] The amplification of the pain signal occurs in the spinal cord when nociceptive C-fibers synapse on the dorsal horn nociceptive neurons activating the NMDA receptors.[54] A cascade of events ensues with the activation of nitric oxide synthase.[55] This ultimately leads to enhance the release of sensory neuropeptides, including substance P, from presynaptic neurons, contributing to the development of hyperalgesia and maintenance of central sensitization.[56] Wind-up can be elicited if identical nociceptive stimuli are applied at a frequency of 3 seconds or less.[57]

Spinothalamic Tract

Prior to synapsing in the dorsal horn of the spinal cord, C- and Aδ fibers may ascend or descend one to two spinal levels, forming a tract dorsal to the dorsal horn called the tract of Lissauer (Fig. 9.5); Lissauer's tract also contains axons of interneurons that may travel for several spinal segments. Following synapsing of the central projections of C- and Aδ afferents, the axons of many of the second-order neurons cross the midline, forming the lateral spinothalamic tract which ascends without interruption from the dorsal horn through the brainstem to the thalamus. This somatotopically organized tract carries information from neurons about the location, intensity, and duration of nociceptive stimuli. This tract is also responsible for relaying the sensation of temperature and, to a lesser extent, it transmits touch and pressure sensation. A large proportion of the neurons that contribute fibers to the lateral spinothalamic tract originate in lamina I. There is also a dorsally located spinothalamic tract arising ipsilaterally from lamina I neurons, though this projection of second-order nociceptive neurons is less well described.

Lamina V also contributes a large group of neurons to the spinothalamic tract mostly comprised of Aδ fibers. The anterior spinothalamic tract, which conveys information about the location of nociception, is largely composed of fibers from lamina VII and VIII. Conversely, lamina II sends very few fibers to the spinothalamic tracts despite being the destination for many C-fibers. The fibers from lamina II modulate the spinothalamic cells in lamina I, V, VII, and VIII at the level of the nociceptive input as well as at spinal segments above and below via spinal interneurons that travel in the tract of Lissauer. This complex mesh of interneurons plays a significant role in determining whether signals from nociceptors will be propagated to higher levels of the nervous system or be inhibited. Spinal interneurons modulate the intensity of a stimulus and also establish connections with other spinal neurons to form somatic and autonomic reflex arcs at the level of the spinal cord. While interruption of the spinothalamic tract results in immediate loss of pain and temperature perception in the contralateral side of the body, injuries of the spinothalamic tract can develop into central pain syndromes.

Nociceptive afferents from visceral organs and somatic structures terminate in the same population of spinothalamic cells in the spinal cord, which in turn synapse in the thalamus. The convergence of nociceptive signals in the spinal cord is segmentally arranged and may account for pain from visceral organs being referred to somatic structures. This topic is discussed in more detail later in the chapter.

There are several other ascending tracts that supply nociceptive signals to higher levels of the CNS. The spinoreticular tract transmits nociceptive signals on the ipsilateral side of the spinal cord. This tract is clinically important as it may explain the persistence of pain after an anterior cordotomy.

Thalamus

The majority of the second order lateral spinothalamic tract fibers terminate in the lateral nuclear group of the thalamus which contains both the ventroposterior lateral (VPL) nucleus and the ventroposterior medial (VPM) nucleus. The VPL nucleus of the thala-

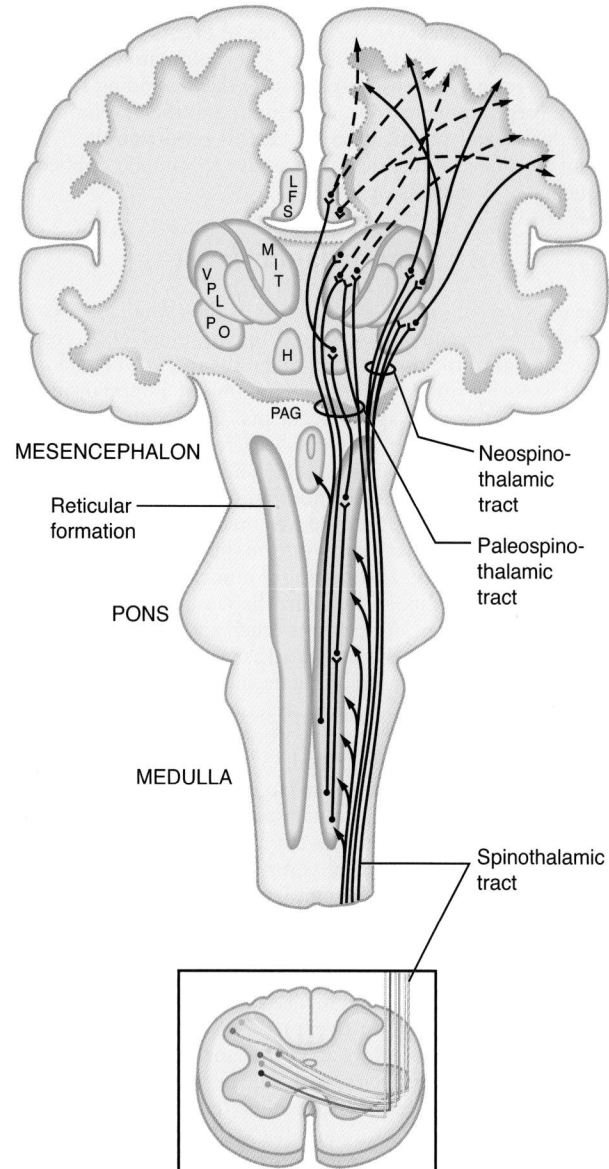

FIGURE 9.5 Simple diagram of the course and termination of the spinothalamic tract. Most of the fibers cross to the opposite side and ascend to the brainstem and brain, although some ascend ipsilaterally. The neospinothalamic part of the tract has cell bodies located primarily in laminae I and V of the dorsal horn, whereas the paleospinothalamic tract has its cell bodies in deeper laminae. The neospinothalamic fibers ascend in a more superficial part of the tract and project without interruption to the caudal part of the ventroposterolateral thalamic nucleus (VPLc), the oral part of this nucleus (VPLo), and the medial part of the posterior thalamus (POm). In these structures, they synapse with a third relay of neurons, which project to the somatosensory cortex (SI, SII, and retroinsular cortex) (*solid lines*). Some of the fibers of the paleospinothalamic tract pass directly to the medial/intralaminar thalamic nuclei, and others project to the nuclei and the reticular formation of the brainstem and thence to the PAG, hypothalamus (H), nucleus submedius, and medial/intralaminar thalamic nuclei. Once there, these axons synapse with neurons that connect with the limbic forebrain structure (LFS) via complex circuits and also send diffuse projections to various parts of the brain.

mus receives information from the lateral spinothalamic tract while the VPM nucleus receives sensory information from the spinal trigeminal nucleus, which transmits sensory information from the face (Fig. 9.6). Spinothalamic fibers also terminate in areas of the intralaminar nuclei and in the mediodorsal nucleus. These fibers transmit signals to the limbic system which integrates autonomic and arousal responses and attention to the perception of pain. Many of the fibers originating in lamina I terminate in the ventromedial (VM) nucleus. Most of the neurons in VM are activated by nociceptors. Lesions of the thalamus, such as stroke, can result in severe central pain syndromes on the contralateral side of the body.

With the exception of olfaction, all sensory pathways traveling from the periphery to the cerebral cortex synapse in the thalamus. The spinothalamic fibers terminate in multiple areas of the thalamus and subsequently are relayed to different areas of the cortex. VPL/VPM supplies the primary and secondary somatosensory cortex (S1, S2) with nociceptive signals. Spinothalamic fibers terminating in other areas of the thalamus influence other cortical areas, such as the insular cortex.

Sensory Cortex

Nociceptive signals from the thalamus terminate in multiple areas of the cerebral cortex and subcortical regions. The somatosensory cortex is somatotopically organized and has a laminated columnar structure. The thalamic fibers project primarily to layer IV of the primary somatosensory cortex (S1) to transmit information about limb position, sense of touch, and discriminative aspects of sensation. This area of the cortex makes a limited contribution to the perception of nociception. The cortical association areas and secondary somatic sensory cortex are connected with S1 and help further process tactile information necessary for object recognition and spatial relationships.

Functional imaging has demonstrated that the insula and anterior cingulate gyrus are the areas most consistently linked with nociceptive stimulation.[58] The insular cortex receives direct projections from the medial thalamic nuclei as well as from the lateral nuclear group. This area of the cortex processes nociceptive information on the internal state of the body and regulates the autonomic component of the pain response. Patients with lesions of the insular cortex do not display appropriate emotional responses to pain as part of a syndrome termed pain asymbolia.[59] The anterior cingulated gyrus integrates the affective component of pain. The anterior cingulate gyrus in particular is a target for ablation in some patients with chronic pain. This lesion separates the nociceptive perception from the affective/ motivational component of the pain behavior.

To a lesser extent, S1, the premotor cortex, the prefrontal cortex, and posterior parietal cortex are activated with nociception. In the subcortical region, the amygdala, hypothalamus, PAG, basal ganglia, and cerebellum are all activated with nociception. While there are multiple cortical regions that play significant roles in the perception of nociception, there is enough variability in the patterns of activation that, as of yet, there is not a defined area considered to be specific for nociceptive perception.

Descending Pathways of the Central Nervous System

There are descending pathways from the cortex that modulate sensory impulses. For example, somatotopically organized fibers from the S1 terminate in the thalamus, brainstem, and spinal cord which selectively modulate, both facilitating and inhibiting, sensory signals from specific receptors and/or areas of the body. The inhibitory effects are most common and are usually transmit-

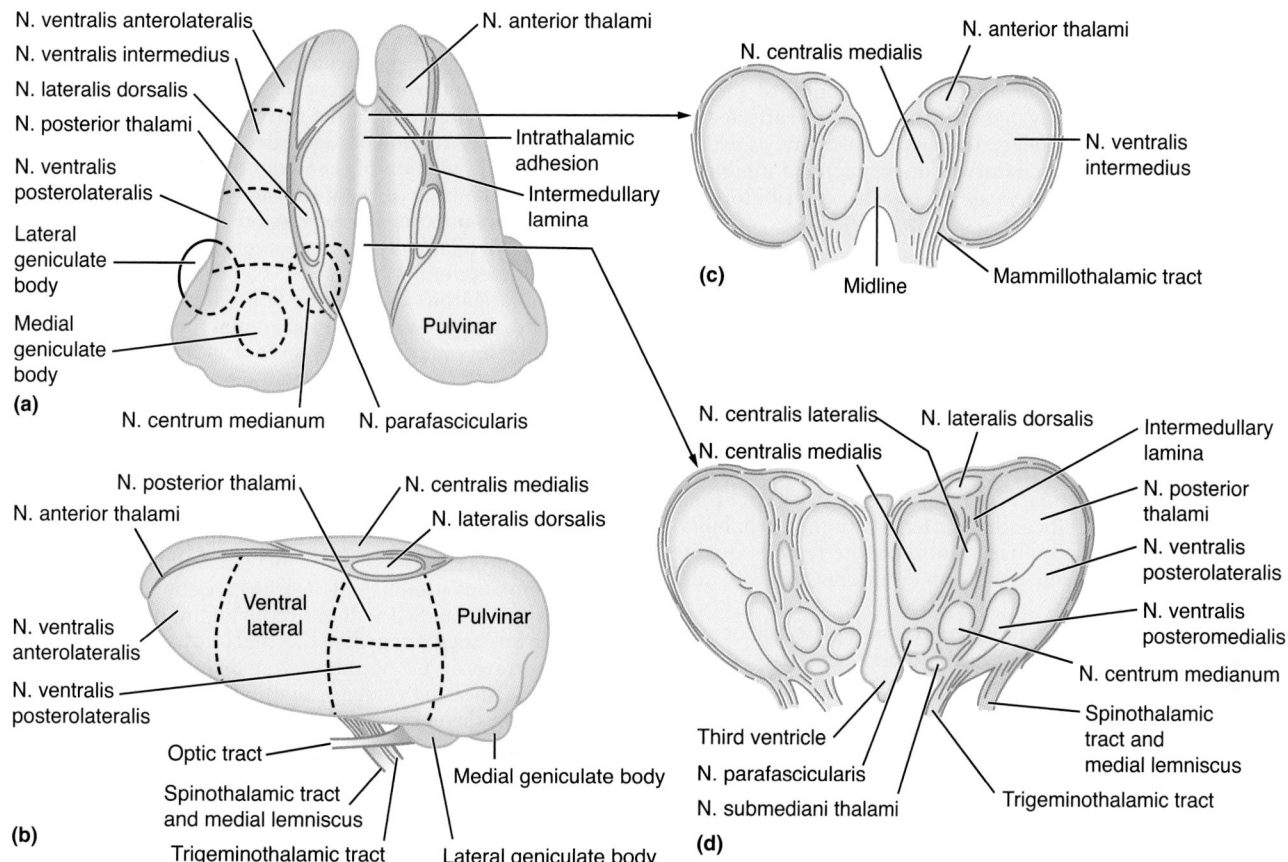

FIGURE 9.6 Schematic diagram of the human thalamus. **A.** Superior view. **B.** Lateral view shows the locations of the most important nuclei. **C.** Frontal section of the anterior part of the thalamus depicts the relationships of various nuclei. **D.** Frontal section of the middle part of the thalamus. Note that the spinothalamic tract and medial lemniscus terminate in nucleus (N.) ventralis posterolateralis, whereas the trigeminothalamic tract terminates in N. ventralis posteromedialis.

ted through inhibitor interneurons. The sensory system is designed to react to the dynamic nature of the environment. As a result, sensory signals are highly monitored at multiple levels of the nervous system.[60]

Collateral fibers from the PAG modulate both descending and ascending pain pathways. The PAG has been experimentally demonstrated to produce analgesia when stimulated and is felt to play a major role in modulating nociception at the level of the dorsal horn as well as at higher levels of the CNS.[61] The PAG receives signals from limbic and cortical centers involved in the affective component of pain. The descending signal from the PAG travels through the nucleus raphe magnus (NRM) in the medulla as well as the medullary reticular formation. The serotonergic NRM fibers descend to inhibit peripheral nociceptors in the dorsal horn in lamina I and II. Clinically, this descending system blocks the spinal withdrawal reflex at the level of the dorsal horn. The PAG has ascending connections which may modulate sensory signals at the level of the thalamus. The PAG also supplies the reticular activating system responsible for arousal to painful stimuli. Of note, there are a number of other pathways in the CNS which modulate the sensation of pain and the response to nociceptive input.

Central Pain

Central pain (CP) is a term that includes dysesthesias, paresthesias, and even pruritus[62] initiated by a lesion that interferes with the pathway of nociceptive signals within the CNS from the spinothalamic tract to the parietal somatosensory areas. CP remains an underdiagnosed condition that occurs with damage to the CNS. Studies suggest that up to 10% of all strokes,[63] up to two-thirds of SCIs,[64] 18% of patients with multiple sclerosis, and an undefined number of patients with other neurologic conditions suffer CP.[65]

CP is a complex complaint with several subtypes of pain that can be moderate to severe in intensity. Patients may complain of a constant pain often described as aching, burning, pricking, dysesthesias, paresthesias, or pruritus in isolation or in combination. The majority of patients with CP also complain of evoked pain with stimulus. Patients may complain of spontaneous episodic pain superimposed on their chronic symptoms that is most commonly characterized as lancinating.[61] These uncomfortable sensations are difficult to treat and are often poorly tolerated, which leads to a decrease in quality of life.

The neurologic examination usually reveals areas of hypoanesthesia to thermal and nociceptive stimulation. In the evaluation of the single patient, pain scales can be employed but these are most useful in the research setting. Pain with peripheral nerve injuries, such as a diabetic peripheral neuropathy, often has similar qualities to CP. Pain associated with muscle cramping or dystonia as a result of abnormal tone, posture, or muscle excitability is often seen after CNS damage and must be differentiated from CP.[66]

Central poststroke pain was first described by Dejerine and Roussy[67] in 1906 who found that thalamic stroke on one side of the brain can cause a pain syndrome affecting the contralateral half of the body. This syndrome may occur after a stroke in any location in the CNS. There are several theories as to the mechanism of central poststroke pain. Interruption of the descending inhibitory pathway, hyperexcitability of the affected afferent sensory pathways, denervation hypersensitivity, as well as loss of balance between excitatory (glutamergic) and inhibitory (GABAergic) neurotransmitters are all possible contributors.

Central Pain After Spinal Cord Injury

Chronic pain is a major complication of spinal cord injury (SCI), with approximately two-thirds of all SCI patients experiencing some type of chronic pain and up to one-third complaining of that their pain is severe.[68] The prevalence of pain after SCI often increases with time after injury.[68] There are an estimated 40 cases per million population in the United States, or approximately 11,000 new cases each year.[69] Research suggests that chronic pain in SCI patients significantly interferes with their rehabilitation and activities of daily living and therefore reduces quality of life. Attempts to manage these pain symptoms are costly and success is often limited.[70]

In addition to central pain, there are multiple types of pain that develop after SCI including musculoskeletal, visceral, and peripheral neuropathic pain. The etiology of pain in SCI is multifaceted and the various types of SCI pain differ with regard to clinical findings, pathophysiology, and therapy. The mechanisms involved in the development of CP after SCI are not fully elucidated but continuing research has identified possible mechanisms for pain generation. CP has been reported with injury to all levels of the spinal cord.[71]

CP is a common sequelae of SCI. It has many descriptors; it is often characterized by patients as a continuous burning, shooting, aching, and tingling. The distribution of pain is usually bilateral and can involve multiple adjacent dermatomes or be regional in nature. In addition, many patients with SCI report feeling the phantom phenomenon of their body below the lesion and it is described in a distorted fashion. This occurs despite most patients having no conscious appreciation of sensory input below the spinal cord lesion.[72] Central neuropathic pain after SCI has been categorized based on the location of the complaint as either at the level of the injury or below the level of the injury. Although it may be difficult to distinguish the two clinically (and both may be present in the same patient), CP that occurs at the level of injury is due to segmental spinal cord damage, not nerve root damage. CP that occurs at the level of injury can be within two dermatomal levels either above or below the level of injury.[73] CP associated with SCI may be caused by syringomyelia.[72]

Physiologic changes occur to the nociceptive neurons in the dorsal horn following SCI, including an increase in abnormal spontaneous and evoked discharges from dorsal horn cells.[74,75] Noxious stimulation causes primary afferent C-fibers to release excitatory amino acid neurotransmitters in the dorsal horn. Prolonged high-intensity noxious stimulation activates the NMDA receptors, which induces a cascade that may result in central sensitization.[76] The cascade includes upregulation of neurokinin receptors and activation of the intracellular cyclo-oxygenase-2, nitric oxide synthase, and protein kinase C enzymes.[77] Other neuroanatomic and neurochemical changes thought to impact CP in SCI include alteration in the activity of the neurotransmitter glutamate,[78] interruption of descending serotonin inhibitor pathways,[79] and dysfunction of the inhibitory GABAergic interneurons,[80] all at the level of the dorsal horn. On a molecular level, abnormal sodium channel expression within the dorsal horn (laminae I–VI) bilaterally has been implicated as a major contributor to hyperexcitability.

Thalamic neurons appear to undergo changes after SCI in both human and animal models. In the animal model, enhanced neuronal excitability in the VPL has been demonstrated directly[81] as well as indirectly; enhanced regional blood flow has been found in the rat VPL after SCI, suggesting increased neuronal activity.[82] There appears to be somatotopic maps as well as an increase in the peripheral receptive fields of VPL neurons.[83] Magnetic resonance spectroscopy studies have demonstrated changes in metabolism of the neurons in human thalamus associated with pain in SCI.[84] Much like the neurons in the dorsal horn, the thalamic neurons after SCI show increased activity with noxious and non-noxious stimuli. VPL neurons are spontaneously hyperexcitable following SCI without receiving input from the spinal cord neurons suggesting that the thalamus may act as a pain signal generator in CP accompanying SCI.[72]

There is emerging evidence that cortical reorganization may play a role in the development of phantom symptoms after loss of limbs, but little evidence of the cortical mechanisms at work with the development of phantom phenomena after SCI.[85] The full spectrum of anatomical, chemical, and physiologic changes contributing to central neuropathic pain after SCI is still being elucidated.

AUTONOMIC NERVOUS SYSTEM

At the turn of the 20th century, the Cambridge physiologist John Newport Langley coined the term "autonomic nervous system" (ANS) to describe the portion of the nervous system that mediated the unconscious function of the internal organs.[86] Soon afterward, the concept of two distinct components of the ANS, the sympathetic and parasympathetic systems, which antagonize each other to maintain homeostasis, was developed. The enteric system is also recognized as being a distinct part of the ANS. In addition to regulating the activity of visceral organs, vessels, and glands, the ANS has been found to play an active role in many pain states. Understanding the complexity of the pain–ANS interaction is essential to physicians managing all types of pain. The anatomy of the ANS with the current understanding of the interrelationship between these structures is shown in Figure 9.7. The ANS is composed of peripheral and central portions.

Peripheral Autonomic Nervous System

The peripheral efferent pathways of both the sympathetic and parasympathetic nervous system have two components: a pri-

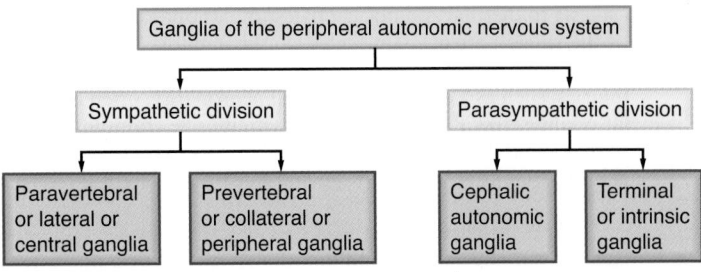

FIGURE 9.7 Ganglia of the peripheral autonomic nervous system.

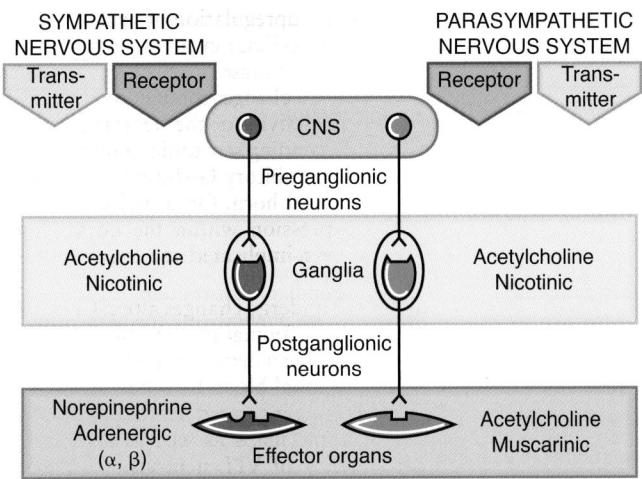

FIGURE 9.8 Transmitter substances in the peripheral autonomic nervous system. (Modified from Jänig W. The autonomic nervous system. In: Schmidt RF, Thews G, eds. *Human physiology.* Berlin: Springer-Verlag; 1983:111.)

mary presynaptic or preganglionic neuron and a secondary postsynaptic or postganglionic neuron. Unlike the somatic motor system which has its motor neurons in the CNS, the motor neurons of the ANS are located in the periphery. As such, the transmission of autonomic signals from the CNS synapses at ganglia in the periphery prior to reaching the target organ (Fig. 9.8). The different locations of the cell bodies of the primary preganglionic neurons of the different divisions of the ANS will be discussed later.

The cell bodies of the postganglionic neurons are arranged in aggregates known as ganglia, wherein the synapses between pre- and postganglionic neurons take place. The ganglia of the ANS are complex collections of nerve fibers regulating a host of vital functions. In addition to this, some ganglia receive sensory fibers from visceral organs and have interneurons suggesting that there is regulation of autonomic signaling at this level. As shown in Figure 9.7, there are four general groups of these ganglia, two with the sympathetic division and two with the parasympathetic division.

A typical feature of the ANS is that postganglionic fibers form nerve plexuses around their target organs composed of both sympathetic and parasympathetic fibers. Unlike their somatic efferent counterparts, the postganglionic fibers branch extensively, forming a network of varicosities in the vicinity of their effector cells allowing one fiber to act on several effector cells.

Parasympathetic Division

The parasympathetic preganglionic fibers travel from the CNS to synapse in ganglia located close to their target organs. In most areas, parasympathetic innervation tends to be more precise than sympathetic innervation. Parasympathetic fibers generally innervate visceral organs. Table 9.2 summarizes parasympathetic nerve supply to essential body structures.

Cranial Parasympathetics

The preganglionic parasympathetic neurons have their cell bodies in the gray matter of the brainstem, and their fibers travel with the oculomotor, facial, glossopharyngeal, and vagus nerves (Fig. 9.9). The preganglionic fibers from the oculomotor, facial, and glossopharyngeal nerves synapse in the ciliary, sphenopalatine, otic, and submaxillary ganglia, all of which are located in the

head. From these ganglia, the postganglionic fibers travel to the target organs (e.g., the lacrimal and salivary glands).

The preganglionic parasympathetic fibers in the vagus nerve travel out of the head to terminate in visceral organs. In the abdomen, many of these fibers synapse in a diffuse network of postganglionic neurons to form a plexus within the wall of the gastrointestinal tract. The postganglionic neurons within this plexus send short processes to innervate the smooth muscles and glands in the gastrointestinal tract. In the thorax, the vagus nerve supplies parasympathetic innervation to the heart (via the cardiac plexus) and airways. In the heart, the sinus node and atrioventricular node have significant parasympathetic innervation. This is in contrast to the ventricles, which are supplied with dense sympathetic innervation.[87]

Sacral Parasympathetics

The sacral portion of the parasympathetic system consists of preganglionic neurons which have their cell bodies in the intermediolateral column of the gray matter of the S2–S4 spinal segments (see Figs. 9.9 and 9.10). The preganglionic fibers travel via the ventral roots to the corresponding spinal nerves for a short distance and then form the pelvic splanchnic nerves. These nerves form the pelvic plexuses which are in close proximity to the target organs (rectum, bladder, prostate gland in the male, cervix in the female). Many of these preganglionic fibers synapse in the plexus while other fibers pass through the plexus without interruption and terminate in intramural ganglia of their target organs (e.g., urinary bladder, descending colon, sigmoid colon and rectum, and genital organs). All of the pelvic organs are innervated by postganglionic parasympathetic fibers. These fibers play an essential role in eliminating waste products from the bladder and rectum.[88]

Sympathetic (Thoracolumbar) Division

The peripheral sympathetic nervous system is composed of efferent and afferent fibers. The efferent portion of the sympathetic division of the ANS consists of preganglionic neurons, the two paravertebral (lateral) sympathetic chains, prevertebral and terminal ganglia, and postganglionic neurons (see Figs. 9.9 and 9.10).[89,90]

Sympathetic Preganglionic Neurons

The cell bodies of the efferent preganglionic neurons are located in the intermediolateral column in the spinal cord from T1–L2. The efferent fibers of these preganglionic neurons travel from the spinal cord into the periphery through the ventral roots accompanying the somatic fibers at these levels at the thoracolumbar spine. From this point, the preganglionic neurons diverge to provide inputs to ganglia in multiple locations. Each preganglionic fiber synapses on multiple postganglionic cells, thus serving to amplify the sympathetic outflow from the CNS.[91] Some of the sympathetic fibers leave the spinal nerve immediately after the ventral and dorsal roots fuse to form the white communicating ramus which synapses with postganglionic neurons in the sympathetic ganglia outside the neuraxis (see Fig. 9.10). The white rami are usually present only in the thoracic and upper two or three lumbar segments corresponding to the location of the intermediolateral column in the spinal cord (see Fig. 9.10). The white color of the rami is a result of the sympathetic fibers being myelinated.

The peripheral ganglia of the sympathetic nervous system are located close to the CNS. These paravertebral ganglia are segmentally arranged in two sympathetic trunks, each of which is a vertical row along the anterior margin of the vertebral column. Each trunk is comprised of a longitudinal network of ganglia connected

TABLE 9.2

SUMMARY OF PARASYMPATHETIC NERVE SUPPLY TO ESSENTIAL BODY STRUCTURES

	Parasympathetic nerve supply		Action
Region/structure/organ	Location of cell body/preganglionic neurons in the CNS	Site of synapse of the preganglionic with postganglionic neurons	
Head and neck			
Eye	Parasympathetic oculomotor nucleus/ Edinger Westphal Nucleus	Ciliary ganglion	Pupillary constriction, accommodation for near vision
Lacrimal gland	Superior salvatory nucleus	Pterygopalatine nucleus	Secretion
Parotid gland	Inferior salvatory nucleus	Otic ganglion	Secretion
Submandibular and sublingual glands	Superior salvatory nucleus	Submandibular ganglion	Secretion
Thoracic viscera			
Heart	Dorsal motor vagus nucleus	Cardiac plexus	Decreased heart rate and cardiac output
Trachea, bronchi, and lungs	Dorsal motor vagus nucleus	Pulmonary plexus	Constriction of bronchial muscles and increased glandular secretion
Abdominal viscera			
Stomach	Dorsal motor vagus nucleus	Gastric plexus	Increased motility and secretion, relaxed sphincter
Pancreas	Dorsal MVN	Periarterial plexus	Dilation of blood vessels and increased secretion
Pelvic viscera			
Ureter	Sacral cord S3–S4	Pelvic plexus	Increased tone and motility
Bladder	Sacral cord S3–S4	Pelvic plexus	Contracted detrusor muscle

to each other by ascending and descending nerve fibers that extend the entire length of the spinal column. As each spinal segment develops in the embryo, one sympathetic ganglion is formed for every level on each side. Some of these ganglia fuse, so the final number of ganglia is usually less than the number of spinal segments.[92] This is most prominent in the cervical region where only the superior, middle, intermediate, and inferior cervical ganglia are present for seven cervical vertebrae. The middle cervical ganglion is often not present, and the inferior cervical ganglion commonly fuses with the upper thoracic ganglion forming the stellate ganglion. The cephalic end of the paravertebral ganglia continues beyond the cervical spine, traveling along the carotid nerve to eventually distribute sympathetic fibers within the head. The caudal end of the two trunks converges and terminates in front of the coccyx as the ganglion impar.[89]

The paravertebral sympathetic ganglia are connected by interganglionic fibers forming the lateral sympathetic chain which extends from the skull to the coccyx. On entering the sympathetic chain, some preganglionic axons synapse in the ganglia at the spinal level they exited the neuraxis. Other preganglionic fibers pass uninterrupted cephalad or caudad within the sympathetic trunk before they synapse to ensure that preganglionic fibers synapse at all levels of the sympathetic trunk.

Some preganglionic sympathetic fibers pass uninterrupted through the sympathetic chain to form splanchnic nerves that synapse within one of the prevertebral ganglia that are found at the junction of the celiac and mesenteric arteries and the abdominal aorta. The postganglionic fibers that travel from the preverte-

bral ganglion tend to follow arteries within the abdomen to their target organs. The greater and lesser splanchnic nerves are formed from preganglionic fibers from the T6–T10 levels, pass through the sympathetic chain without synapsing, and terminate in ganglia that innervate the abdominal viscera in the upper and middle part of the abdomen. Splanchnic nerves also contribute preganglionic fibers to the adrenal medulla. These fibers synapse within chromaffin cells, which are homologous to postganglionic neurons but release epinephrine into the bloodstream with sympathetic stimulation.[93]

The DRG contains sympathetic efferent fibers. After an injury in the periphery, more sympathetic fibers grow into the DRG and predominantly surround the cell bodies of mechanoreceptors. This is of unclear clinical significance, but it may contribute to the augmentation of peripheral stimuli (allodynia, hyperalgesia, the wind-up phenomenon, and central sensitization) in painful conditions.[94]

Sympathetic Postganglionic Neurons

The axons of the postganglionic neurons travel via multiple pathways into the periphery. Some of the postganglionic neurons which have their cell bodies in the paravertebral chain re-enter the spinal nerves via the gray communicating ramus, which, in distinction to the white rami, has a gray color because most of these postganglionic fibers are unmyelinated. Postganglionic sympathetic neurons from gray rami communicans travel in all spinal nerves. These postganglionic sympathetic fibers follow the

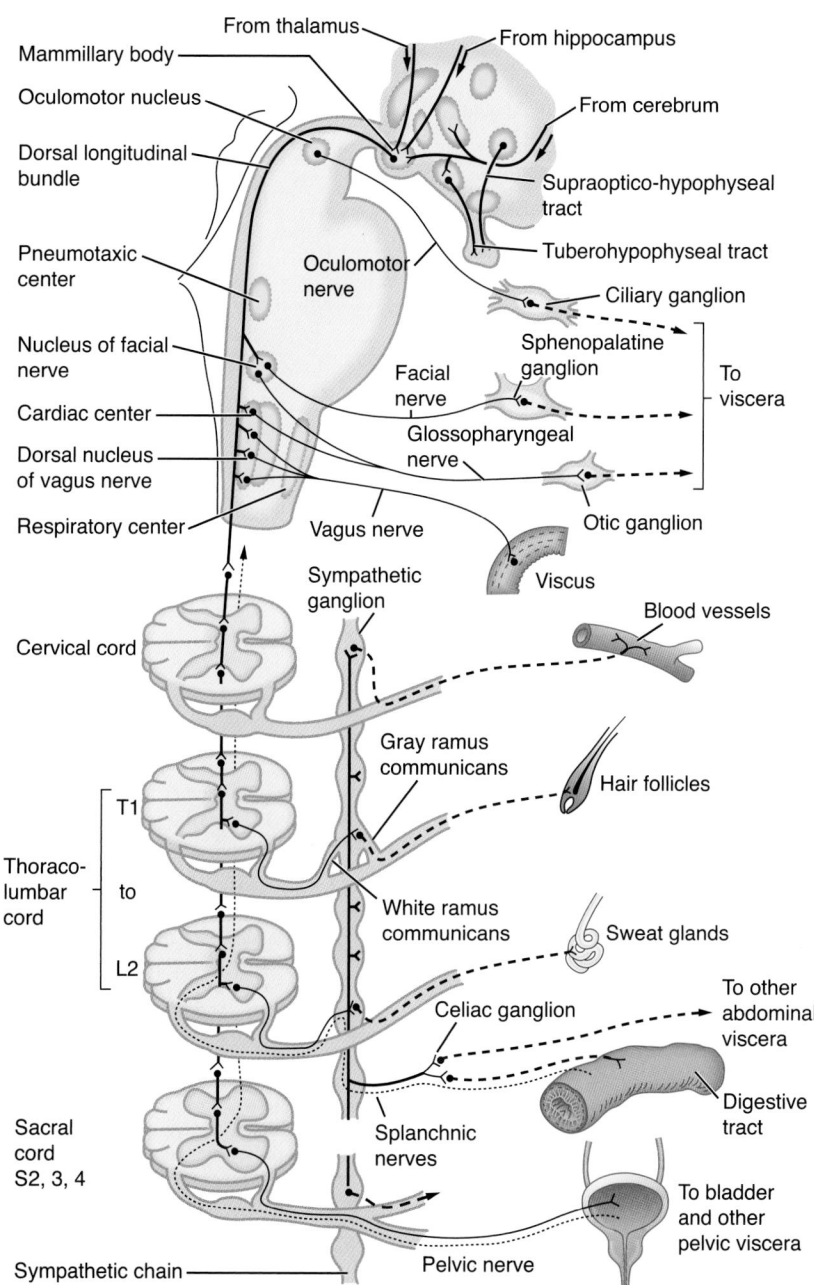

Labels in figure:
- From thalamus
- From hippocampus
- From cerebrum
- Mammillary body
- Oculomotor nucleus
- Dorsal longitudinal bundle
- Supraoptico-hypophyseal tract
- Tuberohypophyseal tract
- Pneumotaxic center
- Oculomotor nerve
- Ciliary ganglion
- Sphenopalatine ganglion
- Nucleus of facial nerve
- Facial nerve
- To viscera
- Cardiac center
- Glossopharyngeal nerve
- Dorsal nucleus of vagus nerve
- Respiratory center
- Vagus nerve
- Otic ganglion
- Viscus
- Sympathetic ganglion
- Blood vessels
- Cervical cord
- Gray ramus communicans
- Hair follicles
- T1
- Thoraco-lumbar cord
- to
- L2
- White ramus communicans
- Sweat glands
- Celiac ganglion
- To other abdominal viscera
- Digestive tract
- Sacral cord S2, 3, 4
- Splanchnic nerves
- To bladder and other pelvic viscera
- Sympathetic chain
- Pelvic nerve

FIGURE 9.9 Schematic representation of autonomic pathways in the neuraxis and the efferent peripheral pathways. Note the connection among the various hypothalamic nuclei and between these structures and the nuclei and important autonomic centers in the brainstem and spinal cord. The dorsal longitudinal fasciculus (DLF) passes from the hypothalamus caudad through the central and tegmental portion of the mesencephalon and the tegmental portion of the pons to terminate in the reticular formation, the autonomic centers and cranial nerve nuclei in the brainstem, and in the intermediolateral cell column of the spinal cord. The DLF is composed of both crossed and uncrossed fibers, including some long ones and an extensive system of short fibers, which are arranged in the gray matter in frequent relays. Note also that the cell bodies of preganglionic sympathetic neurons are located only in spinal cord segments T1 through L2, whereas the parasympathetic neurons are located in cranial nerves and in S2, S3, and S4. The solid lines represent preganglionic fibers, the dashed lines represent postganglionic fibers, and the dotted lines are afferent (sensory) fibers. Not shown are the sensory fibers contained in the facial, glossopharyngeal, and vagus nerves, which transmit nociceptive and other somatosensory information from the head.

spinal nerves into somatic areas innervating various somatic, sudomotor, and pilomotor structures, such as the sweat glands and smooth muscle fibers in hair follicles in the skin. The axons of other postganglionic neurons, which have their cell bodies in the paravertebral chain, travel largely along arteries to pass to the thoracic and pelvic viscera. This is in contrast to the preganglionic neurons that pass uninterrupted to the prevertebral ganglia via the greater and lesser splanchnic nerves and are distributed to the viscera in the upper and middle part of the abdomen. The visceral organs in the lower abdomen receive their sympathetic innervation from the lumbar splanchnic nerve which also synapses in prevertebral ganglia. The celiac ganglia is usually the largest of the prevertebral ganglia and it surrounds the celiac artery at its juncture with the aorta. The sympathetic innervation of the heart originates in the cervical and thoracic ganglia and travels via the cardiac nerves to the heart. Table 9.3 summarizes the autonomic and nociceptive pathways to various body structures.

In addition to the gray rami, the sympathetic trunks give off postganglionic rami that supply the viscera of the head, chest, and abdomen. These rami include the carotid nerve, the superior, middle, and inferior cardiac nerves, the superior, middle, and inferior thoracic splanchnic nerves, and the lumbar and sacral splanchnic nerves.

Some preganglionic fibers synapse in the intermediary ganglia in the white communicating rami, ventral nerve roots, or the spinal nerves outside of the sympathetic chain.[89,90] These anomalous sympathetic pathways are most commonly found in the sympathetic trunk at the cervicothoracic juncture and the thoracolumbar juncture.[95–97] These pathways explain why surgical interruption of the sympathetic chain may not completely block sympathetic outflow. Conversely, these anatomic variations often respond to sympathetic blockade with a local anesthetic solution because it diffuses locally to affect these pathways.[95] A sympathetic block can therefore be a poor predictor of the efficacy of surgical sympathectomy. In cases of incomplete sympathectomy,

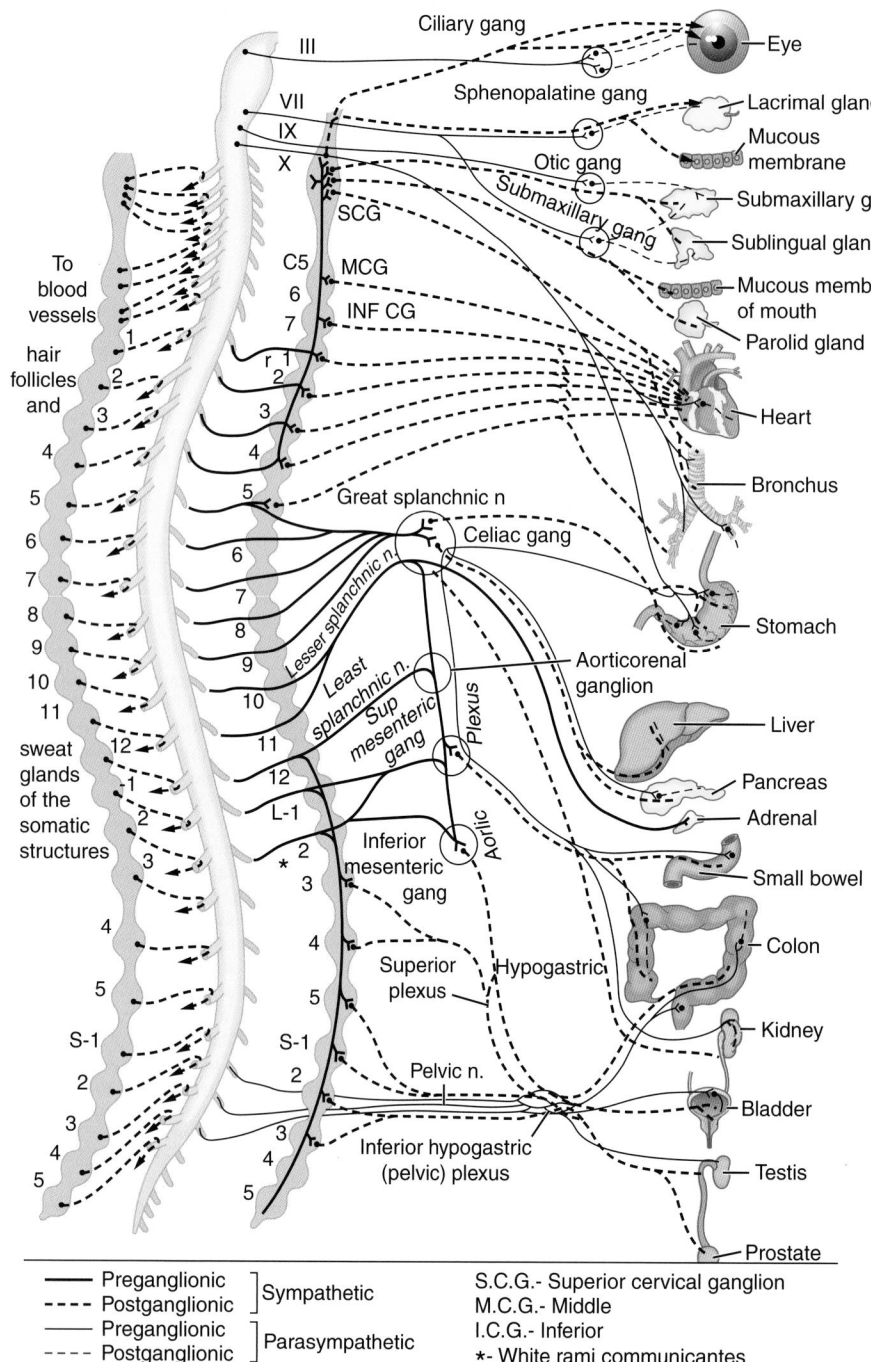

FIGURE 9.10 Distribution of peripheral autonomic nervous system to various structures of the body. On the reader's right are shown (from above downward) the four cranial nerves which contain preganglionic parasympathetic fibers, the axons of preganglionic sympathetic fibers (which pass from the anterior root to the paravertebral sympathetic chain), and the parasympathetic preganglionic axons in S2, S3, and S4. Note that the axons of all of the preganglionic sympathetic neurons pass via the white rami communicantes into the paravertebral chain, in which some synapse with postganglionic neurons, whereas others pass to the prevertebral sympathetic ganglia, in which they synapse with postganglionic fibers. On the reader's left are depicted the gray rami communicantes, containing postganglionic sympathetic fibers, which originate in the paravertebral chain and then pass to each of the spinal nerves to innervate blood vessels, hair follicles, and sweat glands in various parts of the body.

a postsurgical sympathetic block that produces complete interruption of sympathetic outflow and pain relief in sympathetically dependent pain syndromes may suggest the presence of anomalous sympathetic ganglia.[95,96]

Sympathetic postganglionic neurons may be involved in the generation of pain, hyperalgesia, and inflammation in disease. Depending on the extent of the peripheral nerve lesion, plastic changes can occur at multiple levels of the ANS. Release of mediators (e.g., epinephrine, norepinephrine) from efferent sympathetic nerves both locally and systemically and upregulation of adrenoreceptors in nociceptive afferents contribute to the increased excitability of nociceptors and changes in local vasomotor and sudomotor activity.[98] This reorganization of the peripheral neurons may lead to chemical coupling between sympathetic and afferent neurons. This may be responsible for sensitization and/or activation of primary afferent neurons by the sympathetic neurons.[99]

Sensation in Visceral Organs

Visceral afferent fibers convey sensory information from the internal organs to the CNS. Although these fibers do not establish direct connections with the peripheral autonomic neurons, sensory fibers from viscera follow autonomic nerves as they travel centrally; the majority of the fibers conducting nociceptive information travel along sympathetic nerves. The neurons of visceral afferent fibers are structurally similar to somatic afferent fibers and, like their somatic counterparts, have cell bodies in the DRG

TABLE 9.3

SUMMARY OF SYMPATHETIC AND NOCICEPTIVE NERVE SUPPLY TO MORE IMPORTANT BODY STRUCTURES

Region, structure	Sympathetic nerve supply			Nociceptive pathways	
	Location of cell body in spinal cord and course of preganglionic neurons	Site of synapse of preganglionic with postganglionic neurons	Course of postganglionic axons	Location of primary afferent pathway	Entrance into central nervous system
Head and neck					
Meninges and arteries of brain	T1, 2 (3)† To and through cervical sympathetic chain	All cervical sympathetic ganglia	Plexuses around internal carotid and vertebral arteries	Cranial nerves (CN) V, IX, X C-1–3	Trigeminal subnucleus caudalis C-1–3 spinal segments
Eye*	T1, 2, 3 (4) To and through cervical sympathetic chain	Superior cervical ganglion and ganglia in internal carotid plexus	Internal carotid and cavernous plexuses→ciliary ganglion or nasociliary nerve→ciliary nerves or along ophthalmic artery	Ophthalmic branch of CN V	Trigeminal subnucleus caudalis
Lacrimal gland*	T1, 2 To and through cervical sympathetic ganglia	Superior cervical sympathetic ganglion	Internal carotid plexus→vidian nerve→sphenopalatine ganglion→maxillary nerve→zygomatic/lacrimal nerves	Lacrimal nerve→ ophthalmic branch of CN V	As above
Parotid gland*	As above	All cervical sympathetic ganglia	External carotid plexus→internal maxillary and middle meningeal plexus→to auriculotemporal nerve and plexus and to the parotid arterial plexuses	Parotid nerve→ auriculotemporal nerve of mandibular division of CN V	As above
Submandibular and sublingual glands*	As above	As above	External carotid plexus→facial plexus→submandibular ganglion→direct glandular filaments or via lingual nerves or directly to glands along vessels	Submandibular branch of lingual nerve→ mandibular division of CN V	As above
Thyroid gland	As above	Middle and inferior cervical sympathetic ganglia	Perivascular sympathetic plexuses accompanying superior and inferior thyroid arteries	Afferents accompanying sympathetic pathways	T1 and 2 spinal cord segments
Blood vessels of skin and somatic structures Sweat glands Hair follicles	T1–4 To and through cervical sympathetic chain	All cervical sympathetic ganglia	In perivascular plexuses accompanying various branches of external and internal carotid arteries	Afferents accompanying sympathetic nerves CN V, IX, X C2–4	T1–4 spinal cord Subnucleus caudalis C2–4 spinal cord segments
Thoracic viscera					
Heart	T1–4 (5) To upper thoracic and cervical sympathetic chain	All cervical and upper four (5) thoracic ganglia	Superior, middle, and inferior cervical cardiac nerves and the four (5) thoracic cardiac nerves→cardiac plexuses	Afferents in middle and inferior cervical cardiac and the thoracic cardiac nerves	T1–4 (5)

(continued)

TABLE 9.3

CONTINUED

	Sympathetic nerve supply			Nociceptive pathways	
Larynx	T1, 2 To and through cervical sympathetic chain	Superior cervical ganglion	Laryngeal branch of superior cervical ganglion—superior laryngeal nerve	Superior laryngeal nerve	Trigeminal subnucleus caudalis
Trachea, bronchi, and lungs	T2–6 (7) To upper thoracic sympathetic chain	T2–6 (7) Sympathetic ganglia	Pulmonary branches from sympathetic trunk—pulmonary plexuses	Afferents with sympathetics / Afferents with vagus	T2–6 (7) / Nucleus tractus solitarius (medulla)
Esophagus Cervical	T2–4 To and through upper thoracic sympathetic chain	All cervical sympathetic ganglia and pharyngeal plexus	From cervical ganglia to recurrent laryngeal nerve	Afferents in vagus / Afferents with sympathetics	N. tractus solitarius / T2–4(?)
Thoracic	T3–6 To and through upper thoracic sympathetic chain	Stellate and upper thoracic ganglia	Direct esophageal branches and through cardiac sympathetic nerves	Afferents with vagus / Afferents with sympathetics	N. tractus solitarius / T3–6(?)
Abdominal	T5–8 To thoracic sympathetic chain—superior thoracic splanchnic nerve	Celiac ganglia	Via plexuses around left gastric and inferior phrenic arteries	Afferents with sympathetics / Afferents with vagus	T5–8 / N. tractus solitarius
Thoracic aorta	T1–5 (6) To thoracic sympathetic chain	Synapse upper five (six) thoracic sympathetic ganglia	Branches from cardiac sympathetic nerves and direct fibers from thoracic sympathetic chain	Afferents with sympathetic pathways	T1–5 (6)
Abdominal viscera Abdominal aorta	T5–L2 Some through splanchnic nerves and direct branches	Celiac ganglia and paravertebral sympathetic chain	Fibers that contribute to the aortic plexus	Afferents associated with sympathetics	T5–L2
Stomach and duodenum	T(5) 6–9 (10) (11) Superior (greater) and middle (lesser) thoracic splanchnic nerves and celiac plexus	Celiac ganglia	Right and left gastric and gastroepiploic plexuses	Afferents with sympathetics	T(5) 6–9 (10) (11)
Gallbladder and bile ducts	T(5) 6–9 (10) Superior thoracic (greater) splanchnic nerves and celiac plexus	Celiac ganglia	Hepatic and gastroduodenal plexuses	Afferents associated with sympathetics	T(5) 6–9 (10)
Liver	T(5) 6–9 (10) Superior thoracic (greater) splanchnic nerves and celiac plexus	Celiac ganglia	Hepatic plexus	Afferents associated with sympathetics	T(5) 6–9 (10)
Pancreas	T(5) 6–10 (11) Superior thoracic (greater) splanchnic nerves and celiac plexus	Celiac ganglia	Direct branches from celiac plexus and offshoots from splenic, gastroduodenal, and pancreaticoduodenal plexuses	Afferents associated with sympathetics	T5–10 (11)

Organ	Spinal segments / splanchnic nerves	Ganglia	Plexuses / nerves	Pathway	Referred segments
Small intestines	T8–12 right / T8–11 left / To superior (greater) and middle (lesser) thoracic splanchnic nerves to celiac plexus	Celiac and superior mesenteric ganglia	Superior mesenteric plexus→nerves alongside jejunal and ileal arteries	Follow sympathetic pathways through celiac and inferior mesenteric plexuses	T(8) 9, 10 / T10, 11
Cecum and appendix*	T10–12 / Superior (greater) and middle (lesser) thoracic splanchnic nerves→celiac and superior mesenteric plexuses	Celiac and superior mesenteric ganglia	Nerves alongside ileocolic artery	Accompanying sympathetic pathways	T10–12
Colon to splenic flexure*	T10–L1 / Middle (lesser) and inferior (least) thoracic and first lumbar splanchnic nerves	Superior and inferior mesenteric ganglia	Mesenteric plexus→nerves alongside right, middle, and superior left colic arteries	Associated with sympathetics, pass through superior and inferior mesenteric plexuses and splanchnic nerves and to spinal cord	T10–L1
Splenic flexure to rectum*	L1, 2 (left side) / S2–4 / Lumbar and sacral splanchnic nerves→inferior mesenteric and inferior hypogastric pelvic plexuses	Inferior mesenteric ganglion and ganglia in superior and inferior plexuses	Nerves alongside inferior left colic and rectal arteries	Afferents with parasympathetic nerves and pudendal nerves	S2–4
Suprarenal (adrenal) glands*	T(7) 8–L1 (2) / Superior (greater), middle (lesser), and inferior (least) thoracic splanchnic nerves and first (second) lumbar splanchnic nerves	Chromaffin cells of adrenal medulla	Within the gland		
Kidneys*	T10–12, L1 (2) / Middle (lesser) and inferior (least) thoracic splanchnic nerves and first (second) lumbar splanchnic nerves→celiac and renal plexuses	Celiac and aorticorenal ganglia	Along renal plexus	Accompanies sympathetic pathways	T10–12 (L1, 2)
Ureters* Upper two-thirds	T(10), 11, 12, L1, 2 / Middle and inferior thoracic splanchnic and upper two lumbar splanchnic nerves	Celiac and aorticorenal ganglia	Superior mesenteric and renal plexuses→superior and middle ureteric nerves	Associated with sympathetics	T10–12 (L1, 12)
Ureters Lower one-third	T11–L1, S2–4	Aorticorenal ganglion and sacral sympathetic ganglia	Aortic, superior hypogastric, and inferior hypogastric (pelvic) plexuses and sacral splanchnic nerves	Accompany sympathetic and parasympathetic nerves	T10–12

(continued)

TABLE 9.3

CONTINUED

	Sympathetic nerve supply			Nociceptive pathways	
Pelvic viscera					
Bladder	T(11), 12, L1, 2 Middle and inferior thoracic splanchnic nerves	Inferior mesenteric ganglion and sacral paravertebral ganglia	Superior and inferior hypogastric plexuses and sacral splanchnic nerves to vesical plexus	Predominantly afferents of parasympathetic nerves; also some sympathetic afferents	S2–4
Uterus	T(6–9) 10–12, L1 (2) Splanchnic nerves to aortic and ovarian plexuses and superior and inferior hypogastric plexuses	Celiac ganglion and various paravertebral ganglia	Lumbar and sacral splanchnic nerves; superior, middle, and inferior hypogastric plexuses→uterine plexus	Accompanying sympathetic pathways	T11–L2
Testes, ductus deferens, epididymis, seminal vesicles, prostate	T10–L1 inclusive Splanchnic nerves→aortic and superior hypogastric plexus	Prevertebral ganglia and inferior mesenteric ganglion	Follow various vascular plexuses in sacral splanchnic nerves	Testes (ovaries) Prostate Parasympathetic afferents	T10 S2–4
Trunks and limbs (Innervation of vessels, sweat glands, and hair follicles)					
Trunk	T1–12	T1–12 paravertebral sympathetic ganglia	Gray rami communicantes→thoracic spinal nerves	Primary afferents in spinal nerves	T2–L1
Upper extremities	T2–8 (9) To and through upper thoracic and lower cervical sympathetic chain	Middle and stellate ganglia; T-2 and 3 ganglia	Gray rami communicantes to roots of brachial plexus→brachial plexus and its major nerves; some directly to plexuses around subclavian, axillary, and upper brachial arteries	Brachial plexus and its branches	C5–T1
Lower extremities	T10–12, L1, 2 To and through lumbar and upper sacral sympathetic chain	L1–5, S1–3 paravertebral ganglia	Gray rami communicantes→lumbosacral plexus and its major nerves; direct branches to perivascular plexuses as far as upper femoral artery	Lumbosacral plexus	L1–S3

*Unilateral innervation.
†Segments in parentheses are inconstant.

of spinal nerves. Their central processes pass to the spinal dorsal horn, primarily in lamina I and V, and from there visceral information travel centrally via dorsal column pathways as well as by the spinothalamic and spinoreticular tracts. At the level of the dorsal horn, some primary afferents make synaptic connections with somatic motor neurons while others synapse with preganglionic neurons in the intermediolateral cell column, thus mediating complex visceral reflexes. These reflexes usually involve alteration of the function of the viscera, increase in skeletal muscle tension, and increased sympathetic activity.

Visceral afferent fibers mediate reflexes such as coughing, cardiopulmonary reflexes, and emptying of the bladder. Most of the visceral receptors are free nerve endings with large receptive fields that are able to respond to varied stimuli. The receptors responsible for transmitting nociceptive signals are largely chemoreceptors that are sensitive to changes that disrupt the internal milieu such as ischemia, inflammation, or the presence of an irritant (e.g., bile, blood). Indeed, in inflammatory diseases of the viscera, such as Crohn's disease or ulcerative colitis, the peripheral nerve endings may become essentially engulfed in the inflammatory infiltrate that invades the mucosa. The visceral afferent fibers are sensitive to distension and contraction, not cutting or tearing of tissue like the somatic afferents. Although visceral sensations are for the most part not consciously perceived, nociceptive information is transmitted. These fibers also transmit information about the immune system and contribute to the development of fever in the presence of infection.[91,100]

Cervical spinothalamic cells receive input from cardiothoracic afferent fibers and transmit the information to autonomic and nociceptive centers higher in the CNS; these afferent fibers also activate propriospinal pathways in the cervical spine that modulate visceral input from lower levels of the spine.[101]

Autonomic Centers in the Central Nervous System

Unlike the peripheral ANS, distinctions between the somatic and autonomic structures and pathways are often difficult in the CNS. The cortex is the central integration center for both somatic and vegetative functions. Multiple cortical structures have been identified as playing a role in the pain–ANS interaction. The insula, in addition to being associated with the limbic system, is the primary cortex for the viscerosensory system and is involved in the discriminative aspect of pain sensation. It plays a role in the subjective experience of pain and has connections with multiple centers (amygdala, lateral hypothalamus, etc.) involved with autonomic outflow.[102,103] The anterior cingulate cortex receives nociceptive inputs and maintains broad connections with multiple areas of the central autonomic network. In addition to being included as part of the limbic system and being involved in goal related behavior, it plays an essential role in affective and motivational components of pain.[104] Surgical stimulation of this region elicits a range of autonomic responses.[105] The amygdala is comprised of several nuclei with distinct functional properties. It plays an essential role in modulating the ANS and is closely linked to the hypothalamus. The amygdala plays a role in the subjective perception of pain as well as expression of emotional response to pain.[106] The PAG is a complex region of the CNS that has distinct anatomical and functional regions. Different areas of the PAG receive sensory information and help integrate and regulate autonomic responses to these signals and modulate the sympathetic nervous system in analgesia.[107] The PAG receives sensory signals from lamina I and V of the dorsal horn and helps regulate responses to cardiovascular and nociceptive input.

There are several autonomic centers in the brainstem that have been physiologically delineated. In addition to regulating vital functions such as breathing and circulation, aggregates of neurons in the medullary and pontine reticular formation regulate

TABLE 9.4

AUTONOMIC CENTERS (AC) IN SPINAL CORD

Structure	Location of AC in spinal cord
Head and neck	T1–4
Upper limb	T2–8/9
Upper trunk	T2–8
Lower trunk	T9–L2
Lower limb	T10–L2
Viscera	
Thoracic (sympathetic)	T1–5 (8)
Abdominal (sympathetic)	T5–L2
Pelvic (parasympathetic)	S2–4

the ANS through ascending and descending tracts. In the medulla, the nucleus of the solitary tract is a control center of vegetative functions and also appears to contribute antinociceptive input to the dorsal horn.[24] The parabrachial nucleus integrates nociceptive and visceral information through its extensive connections with the medulla, hypothalamus, and amygdala to maintain homeostasis. The autonomic centers in the brainstem give rise to the parasympathetic visceral efferent fibers of the cranial nerves.[108]

The spinal cord is a central area of integrating the somatic and autonomic functions. Through spinal reflexes, somatic nociception can exert a major impact on the autonomic system. Noxious stimulation to the skin induces a cascade of sympathetic responses, including increased sweat production and skin vasomotor responses.[109]

The location of the preganglionic neurons for the sympathetic and parasympathetic nervous systems in the CNS differ. The sympathetic preganglionic neurons are located in the T1 through L2 spinal segments of the spinal cord. The parasympathetic preganglionic neurons are located in the brainstem and the S2–S4 spinal segments (see Figs. 9.9 and 9.10). The locations of the cell bodies of preganglionic sympathetic and parasympathetic neurons, which mediate their function in various parts of the body, are listed in Table 9.4. There are essential differences between the ganglia these neurons form. The sympathetic ganglia are distributed widely throughout the body, are located close to the CNS, and use epinephrine as the primary neurotransmitter. In contrast, the parasympathetic ganglia largely innervate visceral organs, which they are in close proximity to, and use acetylcholine as a neurotransmitter. Figure 9.9 depicts the autonomic pathways that connect the preganglionic neurons in the intermediolateral horn of the spinal cord with the hypothalamus and other brainstem structures.

Transmission in the Peripheral Autonomic Nervous System

The majority of preganglionic neurons in the autonomic nervous system are cholinergic, as are some sympathetic postganglionic neurons, such as sweat glands. Acetylcholine binds nicotinic receptors in the membrane of postganglionic neurons. Postganglionic parasympathetic neurons also release acetylcholine, which binds to muscarinic receptors in effector organs (e.g., cardiac and smooth muscle, glandular cells). There are drugs that selectively block each of these receptors (see Fig. 9.8).

Norepinephrine is the transmitter substance in the majority of sympathetic postganglionic nerve endings. The response of the

TABLE 9.5

PHYSIOLOGIC RESPONSES TO AUTONOMIC STIMULATION

Structures/organs	Sympathetic stimulation	Adrenergic receptors	Parasympathetic stimulation
Eye			
Ciliary muscle	Relaxed for far vision	β	Contraction (accommodation for near vision)
Pupillary muscles			
Dilator	Dilated (mydriasis)	α	—
Sphincter	—		Contraction (miosis)
Lacrimal gland	—		Secretion
Salivary glands			
Parotid	Sparse, thick secretion	α	Profuse serous secretion
Sublingual			
Submaxillary			
Thyroid gland	Stimulated		—
Tracheobronchial tree			
Bronchial muscles	Relaxed	β	Contracted
Bronchial glands	—(?)		Secretion
Heart			
Rate	Increased	β	Decreased
Output	Increased	β	Decreased
Esophagus			
Motility	Decreased	α and β	Increased
Sphincters	Contracted	α	Relaxed
Stomach			
Motility	Decreased	α and β	Increased
Sphincters	Contracted	α	Relaxed
Secretion	Inhibited	α	Increased
Liver	Glycogenolysis, gluconeogenesis	β	—
Gallbladder and biliary ducts	Relaxed	β	Contracted
Pancreas			
Blood vessels	Constriction		Dilation
Insulin secretion	Reduced	α	Increased
Spleen	Contraction of capsule	α	—
Intestines			
Motility	Decreased	α and β	Increased
Sphincters	Relaxed	β	Contracted
Secretion	Decreased	α	Increased
Adrenal gland	Secretion of 80% epinephrine/ 20% norepinephrine	α	—
Kidneys			
Arterioles	Constriction	α	Dilation
Ureter			
Tone and motility	Decreased	α	Increased
Urinary bladder			
Detrusor muscles	Relaxed	β	Contracted
Trigone and sphincter	Contracted	α	Relaxed
Genital organs			
Seminal vesicles	Contraction	α	—(?)
Vas deferens	Contraction	α	—(?)
Uterus	Contraction	α	Depends on species and hormonal status
	Relaxation	β	
Blood vessels			
Coronary arteries	Constriction	α	—
	Dilation?	β	—
Arteries in skeletal muscles	Constriction	α*	—
	Dilation	β	
Arteries in penis or clitoris	—(?)		Dilation
All other arteries	Constriction	α	Dilation
Veins	Constriction	α	—

*By circulating epinephrine only.

effector cells is mediated by two types of receptors: the alpha and beta adrenergic receptors. These receptors have different effects at different organs. For example, in the heart norepinephrine binding to a beta receptor causes an increase in heart rate, while in the bladder and airways this same process causes a relaxation of smooth muscle cells. A variety of pharmacologic agents can either enhance or block the action of these receptor subtypes.

The cells in the adrenal medulla, which are homologues of the postganglionic neurons, mainly release epinephrine into the bloodstream with sympathetic stimulation. Though it has many of the same effects as norepinephrine, epinephrine stimulates the beta receptors in the fat and liver cells accelerating metabolism of fat and glucose.

There are other neurotransmitters in the ANS. Most preganglionic neurons contain neuropeptides (enkephalin, somatostatin) of unclear functional purpose in addition to acetylcholine. Some autonomic neurons do not contain either acetylcholine or norepinephrine. These are primarily located in the gastrointestinal tract.

Physiology of the Autonomic Nervous System

The ANS regulates activities that are required for maintenance of the internal environment of an organism but which are not normally under voluntary or conscious control. This includes modulating functions such as metabolism, circulation, respiration, body temperature, digestion, sweating, circadian rhythm, and endocrine secretion. The ANS coordinates these physiologic processes to maintain homeostasis,[110] such as the constancy of the internal environment.

The effects of stimulating either portion of the ANS and its impact on various organs, visceral structures, and effector cells are summarized in Table 9.5. The sympathetic nervous system is focused on catabolic function and mobilizing the body's resources. In contrast to the sympathetic nervous system, the parasympathetic function is anabolic and dedicated to regulating functions that maintain an organism over the long term. Through regulation of the enteric system, it conserves and stores energy, it plays a central role in coordinating the muscular contraction of the bladder and rectum to eliminate waste products, and it maintains the basal heart rate and respiration under normal conditions.[92]

The functional balance that is normally maintained by the two divisions of the ANS can be disturbed in disease. Linkages exist between the autonomic and immune systems that may be important in the production of disease states and the response to neoplasia and other chronic disease that may lead to pain.[111] Pain itself may alter the immune response and thereby alter the progression of a disease.[112] Animal and human physiologic and pharmacologic studies of visceral as well as somatic pain have demonstrated both plasticity and functional characteristics that are far more complex than the basic anatomy described in this chapter; entire books have been written, for example, on visceral pain.[113]

Enteric Nervous System

The enteric nervous system (ENS) is a highly dynamic division of the ANS often referred to as the "Little Brain" of the gut and contains as many neurons as the spinal cord. It controls gastrointestinal motility and secretion and is involved in visceral sensation. The digestive tract consists of two plexuses, the myenteric and submucous plexuses, formed from sympathetic and parasympathetic postganglionic neurons and a significant number of enteric neurons (Fig. 9.11).[114] Though these plexi interact with the ANS ganglia in the periphery as well as the spinal cord, brainstem,

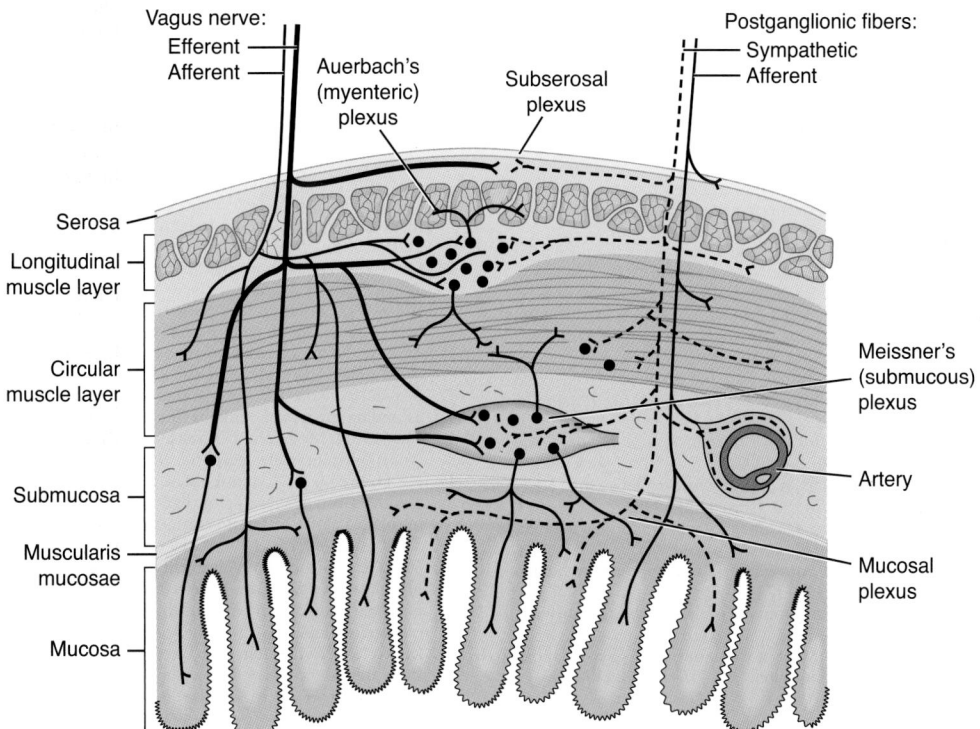

FIGURE 9.11 Arrangement of nerve cells and nerve fibers in the intramural plexuses in the intestine. The axonal endings of the parasympathetic preganglionic neurons synapse in the wall of the intestine, whereas the axonal endings of postganglionic sympathetic neurons are largely distributed to the intramural ganglia and the blood vessels. (Modified from Kuntz A. *Autonomic nervous system.* 4th ed. Philadelphia: Lea & Febiger; 1953:215.)

and cortex, the ENS can function autonomously without input from the sympathetic and parasympathetic systems or the CNS.[115] Enteric neurons were once felt to be postganglionic parasympathetic fibers but are now felt to comprise an independent system in the ANS. The ENS regulates the gastrointestinal system to maintain homeostasis through control of peristalsis, blood vessels, and glandular activity. The ENS also has extensive interaction with the immune system. Disruption of this delicate relationship may be the cause of functional bowel disorders such as irritable bowel syndrome.[26] Enteric neurons appear able to change their function and phenotype, a phenomenon called neuronal plasticity, which contributes to the pathogenesis of visceral hypersensitivity.[114]

CONCLUSION

Complete evaluation of individuals with persistent pain includes anatomic localization of the lesion or lesions responsible for both the initiation and maintenance of pain. It is necessary to distinguish between pain that is of peripheral, central, and mixed origin; it is necessary to determine whether pain is somatic or visceral. Thus, optimal evaluation and care of patients with persistent pain is dependent upon a thorough knowledge of the anatomy of nociceptive systems. Future advances in our understanding of the anatomy and physiology of pain in conjunction with improvements in evaluative and diagnostic technologies (e.g., imaging, genetic, etc.) will no doubt enhance the care of individual patients.

References

1. Woolf CJ, Mannion RJ. Neuropathic pain: aetiology, symptoms, mechanisms, and management. *Lancet* 1999;353(9168):1959–1964.
2. Woolf CJ, Costigan M. Transcriptional and posttranslational plasticity and the generation of inflammatory pain. *Proc Natl Acad Sci USA* 1999;96(14):7723–7730.
3. Al-Chaer ED, Traub RJ. Biological basis of visceral pain: recent developments. *Pain* 2002;96(3):221–225.
4. Cervero F, Laird JM. Visceral pain. *Lancet* 1999;353(9170):2145–2148.
5. Almeida TF, Roizenblatt S, Tufik S. Afferent pain pathways: a neuroanatomical review. *Brain Res* 2004;1000(1–2):40–56.
6. Craig AD. Pain mechanisms: labeled lines versus convergence in central processing. *Annu Rev Neurosci* 2003;26:1–30.
7. Woolf CJ. Evidence for a central component of post-injury pain hypersensitivity. *Nature* 1983;306(5944):686–688.
8. Woolf CJ, Fitzgerald M. The properties of neurones recorded in the superficial dorsal horn of the rat spinal cord. *J Comp Neurol* 1983;221(3):313–328.
9. Saadé NE, Jabbur SJ. Nociceptive behavior in animal models for peripheral neuropathy: spinal and supraspinal mechanisms. *Prog Neurobiol* 2008;86:22–47.
10. Laine FJ, Smoker WR. Anatomy of the cranial nerves. *Neuroimaging Clin N Am* 1998;8(1):69–100.
11. White JC. Sensory innervation of the viscera. *Res Publ Assoc Nerv Ment Dis* 1943;373–390.
12. Nolte J, Sundsten JW. *The Human Brain: An Introduction to its Functional Anatomy.* 5th ed. St. Louis, MO: Mosby; 2002.
13. DeGowin RL, DeGowin EL, Brown DD, et al. *DeGowin & DeGowin's Diagnostic Examination.* 6th ed. New York: McGraw-Hill; 1994.
14. Silen W, Cope Z. *Cope's Early Diagnosis of the Acute Abdomen.* 21st ed. New York: Oxford University Press; 2005.
15. Lee MW, McPhee RW, Stringer MD. An evidence-based approach to human dermatomes. *Clin Anat* 2008;21(5):363–373.
16. Dequéant ML, Pourquié O. Segmental patterning of the vertebrate embryonic axis. *Nat Rev Genet* 2008;9(5):370–382.
17. Tannahill D, Britto JM, Vermeren MM, et al. Orienting axon growth: spinal nerve segmentation and surround-repulsion. *Int J Dev Biol* 2000;44(1):119–127.
18. Netter FH. *Atlas of Human Anatomy.* 4th ed. Philadelphia, PA: Saunders/Elsevier; 2006.
19. Swap CJ, Nagurney JT. Value and limitations of chest pain history in the evaluation of patients with suspected acute coronary syndromes. *JAMA* 2005;294(20):2623–2629.
20. Cervero F, Laird JM, Pozo MA. Selective changes of receptive field properties of spinal nociceptive neurones induced by noxious visceral stimulation in the cat. *Pain* 1992;51(3):335–342.
21. Cervero F, Tattersall JE. Somatic and visceral inputs to the thoracic spinal cord of the cat: marginal zone (lamina I) of the dorsal horn. *J Physiol* 1987;388:383–395.
22. Foreman RD. Integration of viscerosomatic sensory input at the spinal level. *Prog Brain Res* 2000;122:209–221.
23. Saper CB. Pain as a visceral sensation. *Prog Brain Res* 2000;122:237–243.
24. Pappagallo M. *The Neurological Basis of Pain.* New York: McGraw-Hill; 2005.
25. Westlund KN. Visceral nociception. *Curr Rev Pain* 2000;4(6):478–487.
26. Bueno L. Neuroimmune alterations of ENS functioning. *Gut* 2000;47(suppl 4):iv63–65,discussion iv76.
27. Julius D, Basbaum AI. Molecular mechanisms of nociception. *Nature* 2001;413(6852):203–210.
28. Cain DM, Khasabov SG, Simone DA. Response properties of mechanoreceptors and nociceptors in mouse glabrous skin: an in vivo study. *J Neurophysiol* 2001;85(4):1561–1574.
29. Perl ER. Cutaneous polymodal receptors: characteristics and plasticity. *Prog Brain Res* 1996;113:21–37.
30. Wood JN, Akopian AN, Baker M, et al. Sodium channels in primary sensory neurons: relationship to pain states. *Novartis Found Symp* 2002;241:159–168, discussion 68–72,226–232.
31. Rush AM, Cummins TR, Waxman SG. Multiple sodium channels and their roles in electrogenesis within dorsal root ganglion neurons. *J Physiol* 2007;579(Pt 1):1–14.
32. Amaya F, Decosterd I, Samad TA, et al. Diversity of expression of the sensory neuron-specific TTX-resistant voltage-gated sodium ion channels SNS and SNS2. *Mol Cell Neurosci* 2000;15(4):331–342.
33. Fang X, Djouhri L, McMullan S, et al. Intense isolectin-B4 binding in rat dorsal root ganglion neurons distinguishes C-fiber nociceptors with broad action potentials and high Nav1.9 expression. *J Neurosci* 2006;26(27):7281–7292.
34. Luo W, Wickramasinghe SR, Savitt JM, et al. A hierarchical NGF signaling cascade controls Ret-dependent and Ret-independent events during development of nonpeptidergic DRG neurons. *Neuron* 2007;54(5):739–754.
35. Zylka MJ, Rice FL, Anderson DJ. Topographically distinct epidermal nociceptive circuits revealed by axonal tracers targeted to Mrgprd. *Neuron* 2005;45(1):17–25.
36. Jordt SE, McKemy DD, Julius D. Lessons from peppers and peppermint: the molecular logic of thermosensation. *Curr Opin Neurobiol* 2003;13(4):487–492.
37. Levine JD, Alessandri-Haber N. TRP channels: targets for the relief of pain. *Biochim Biophys Acta* 2007;1772(8):989–1003.
38. Binshtok AM, Bean BP, Woolf CJ. Inhibition of nociceptors by TRPV1-mediated entry of impermeant sodium channel blockers. *Nature* 2007;449(7162):607–610.
39. Lumpkin EA, Bautista DM. Feeling the pressure in mammalian somatosensation. *Curr Opin Neurobiol* 2005;15(4):382–388.
40. Wemmie JA, Price MP, Welsh MJ. Acid-sensing ion channels: advances, questions and therapeutic opportunities. *Trends Neurosci* 2006;29(10):578–586.
41. Christensen AP, Corey DP. TRP channels in mechanosensation: direct or indirect activation? *Nat Rev Neurosci* 2007;8(7):510–521.
42. Kohno T, Wang H, Amaya F, et al. Bradykinin enhances AMPA and NMDA receptor activity in spinal cord dorsal horn neurons by activating multiple kinases to produce pain hypersensitivity. *J Neurosci* 2008;28(17):4533–4540.
43. Wang H, Kohno T, Amaya F, et al. Bradykinin produces pain hypersensitivity by potentiating spinal cord glutamatergic synaptic transmission. *J Neurosci* 2005;25(35):7986–7992.
44. Cervero F. Dorsal horn neurons and their sensory inputs. In: Yaksh TL, ed. *Spinal Afferent Processing.* New York: Plenum Press; 1986.
45. Willis WD, Westlund KN. Neuroanatomy of the pain system and of the pathways that modulate pain. *J Clin Neurophysiol* 1997;14(1):2–31.
46. Jänig W. Neuronal mechanisms of pain with special emphasis on visceral and deep somatic pain. *Acta Neurochir Suppl (Wien)* 1987;38:16–32.
47. Brown AG, Fyffe RE. Form and function of dorsal horn neurones with axons ascending the dorsal columns in cat. *J Physiol* 1981;321:31–47.
48. Rustioni A. Modulation of sensory input to the spinal cord by presynaptic ionotropic glutamate receptors. *Arch Ital Biol* 2005;143(2):103–112.
49. Liu H, Brown JL, Jasmin L, et al. Synaptic relationship between substance P and the substance P receptor: light and electron microscopic characterization of the mismatch between neuropeptides and their receptors. *Proc Natl Acad Sci USA* 1994;91(3):1009–1013.
50. Staud R. Evidence of involvement of central neural mechanisms in generating fibromyalgia pain. *Curr Rheumatol Rep* 2002;4(4):299–305.
51. Baranauskas G, Nistri A. Sensitization of pain pathways in the spinal cord: cellular mechanisms. *Prog Neurobiol* 1998;54(3):349–365.
52. DeLeo JA, Winkelstein BA. Physiology of chronic spinal pain syndromes: from animal models to biomechanics. *Spine* 2002;27(22):2526–2537.
53. Gracely RH, Grant MA, Giesecke T. Evoked pain measures in fibromyalgia. *Best Pract Res Clin Rheumatol* 2003;17(4):593–609.
54. Bennett GJ. Update on the neurophysiology of pain transmission and modulation: focus on the NMDA-receptor. *J Pain Symptom Manage* 2000;19(1 suppl):S2–S6.
55. Meller ST, Gebhart GF. Nitric oxide (NO) and nociceptive processing in the spinal cord. *Pain* 1993;52(2):127–136.
56. Luo ZD, Cizkova D. The role of nitric oxide in nociception. *Curr Rev Pain* 2000;4(6):459–466.

57. Price DD, Hu JW, Dubner R, et al. Peripheral suppression of first pain and central summation of second pain evoked by noxious heat pulses. *Pain* 1977; 3(1):57–68.

58. Schnitzler A, Ploner M. Neurophysiology and functional neuroanatomy of pain perception. *J Clin Neurophysiol* 2000;17(6):592–603.

59. Masson C, Koskas P, Cambier J, et al. Left pseudothalamic cortical syndrome and pain asymbolia [in French]. *Rev Neurol (Paris)* 1991;147(10):668–670.

60. Vanegas H, Schaible HG. Descending control of persistent pain: inhibitory or facilitatory? *Brain Res Brain Res Rev* 2004;46(3):295–309.

61. Tasker R. Central pain states. In: Loeser JD, ed. *Bonica's Management of Pain*. 3rd ed. Philadelphia: Lippincott Williams & Wilkins; 2001:433–457.

62. Canavero S, Bonicalzi V, Massa-Micon B. Central neurogenic pruritus: a literature review. *Acta Neurol Belg* 1997;97(4):244–247.

63. Andersen G, Vestergaard K, Ingeman-Nielsen M, et al. Incidence of central post-stroke pain. *Pain* 1995;61(2):187–193.

64. Finnerup NB, Johannesen IL, Sindrup SH, et al. Pain and dysesthesia in patients with spinal cord injury: a postal survey. *Spinal Cord* 2001;39(5): 256–262.

65. Canavero S, Bonicalzi V. *Central Pain Syndrome: Pathophysiology, Diagnosis and Management*. Cambridge, New York: Cambridge University Press; 2007.

66. Siddall PJ, Yezierski RP, Loeser JD. Pain following spinal cord injury: clinical features, prevalence, and taxonomy. *IASP Newsletter* 2000;3.

67. Dejerine J, Roussy G. Le syndrome thalamique. *Rev Neurol (Paris)* 1906;14: 521–532.

68. Waxman SG, Hains BC. Fire and phantoms after spinal cord injury: Na + channels and central pain. *Trends Neurosci* 2006;29(4):207–215.

69. National Spinal Cord Injury Statistical Center. In.

70. Finnerup NB, Jensen TS. Spinal cord injury pain—mechanisms and treatment. *Eur J Neurol* 2004;11(2):73–82.

71. Siddall PJ, Loeser JD. Pain following spinal cord injury. *Spinal Cord* 2001; 39(2):63–73.

72. Todor DR, Mu HT, Milhorat TH. Pain and syringomyelia: a review. *Neurosurg Focus* 2000;8(3):E11.

73. Ragnarsson KT. Management of pain in persons with spinal cord injury. *J Spinal Cord Med* 1997;20(2):186–199.

74. Loeser JD, Ward AA Jr, White LE Jr. Chronic deafferentation of human spinal cord neurons. *J Neurosurg* 1968;29(1):48–50.

75. Hains BC, Johnson KM, Eaton MJ, et al. Serotonergic neural precursor cell grafts attenuate bilateral hyperexcitability of dorsal horn neurons after spinal hemisection in rat. *Neuroscience* 2003;116(4):1097–1110.

76. Davies SN, Lodge D. Evidence for involvement of N-methylaspartate receptors in 'wind-up' of class 2 neurones in the dorsal horn of the rat. *Brain Res* 1987;424(2):402–406.

77. Yaksh TL, Hua XY, Kalcheva I, et al. The spinal biology in humans and animals of pain states generated by persistent small afferent input. *Proc Natl Acad Sci USA* 1999;96(14):7680–7686.

78. Mills CD, Johnson KM, Hulsebosch CE. Group I metabotropic glutamate receptors in spinal cord injury: roles in neuroprotection and the development of chronic central pain. *J Neurotrauma* 2002;19(1):23–42.

79. Hains BC, Willis WD, Hulsebosch CE. Serotonin receptors 5-HT1A and 5-HT3 reduce hyperexcitability of dorsal horn neurons after chronic spinal cord hemisection injury in rat. *Exp Brain Res* 2003;149(2):174–186.

80. Drew GM, Siddall PJ, Duggan AW. Mechanical allodynia following contusion injury of the rat spinal cord is associated with loss of GABAergic inhibition in the dorsal horn. *Pain* 2004;109(3):379–388.

81. Hains BC, Saab CY, Waxman SG. Changes in electrophysiological properties and sodium channel Nav1.3 expression in thalamic neurons after spinal cord injury. *Brain* 2005;128(Pt 10):2359–2371.

82. Morrow TJ, Paulson PE, Brewer KL, et al. Chronic, selective forebrain responses to excitotoxic dorsal horn injury. *Exp Neurol* 2000;161(1):220–226.

83. Lenz FA, Kwan HC, Martin R, et al. Characteristics of somatotopic organization and spontaneous neuronal activity in the region of the thalamic principal sensory nucleus in patients with spinal cord transection. *J Neurophysiol* 1994; 72(4):1570–1587.

84. Pattany PM, Yezierski RP, Widerström-Noga EG, et al. Proton magnetic resonance spectroscopy of the thalamus in patients with chronic neuropathic pain after spinal cord injury. *AJNR Am J Neuroradiol* 2002;23(6):901–905.

85. Birbaumer N, Lutzenberger W, Montoya P, et al. Effects of regional anesthesia on phantom limb pain are mirrored in changes in cortical reorganization. *J Neurosci* 1997;17(14):5503–5508.

86. Langley JN. The autonomic nervous system. *Brain* 1903;26:1–26.

87. Longhurst JC. Cardiac receptors: their function in health and disease. *Prog Cardiovasc Dis* 1984;27(3):201–222.

88. Shefchyk SJ. Spinal cord neural organization controlling the urinary bladder and striated sphincter. *Prog Brain Res* 2002;137:71–82.

89. Mitchell GAG. *Anatomy of the Autonomic Nervous System*. Edinburgh: Livingstone; 1953.

90. Pick J. *The Autonomic Nervous System; Morphological, Comparative, Clinical, and Surgical Aspects*. Philadelphia: Lippincott; 1970.

91. Jänig W. Neurobiology of visceral afferent neurons: neuroanatomy, functions, organ regulations and sensations. *Biol Psychol* 1996;42(1–2):29–51.

92. Brodal P. *The Central Nervous System: Structure and Function*. 3rd ed. Oxford, New York: Oxford University Press; 2004.

93. Aunis D, Langley K. Physiological aspects of exocytosis in chromaffin cells of the adrenal medulla. *Acta Physiol Scand* 1999;167(2):89–97.

94. Chung K, Lee BH, Yoon YW, et al. Sympathetic sprouting in the dorsal root ganglia of the injured peripheral nerve in a rat neuropathic pain model. *J Comp Neurol* 1996;376(2):241–252.

95. Cho HM, Lee DY, Sung SW. Anatomical variations of rami communicantes in the upper thoracic sympathetic trunk. *Eur J Cardiothorac Surg* 2005;27(2): 320–324.

96. Murata Y, Takahashi K, Yamagata M, et al. Variations in the number and position of human lumbar sympathetic ganglia and rami communicantes. *Clin Anat* 2003;16(2):108–113.

97. Ramsaroop L, Partab P, Singh B, et al. Thoracic origin of a sympathetic supply to the upper limb: the 'nerve of Kuntz' revisited. *J Anat* 2001;199(Pt 6): 675–682.

98. Sato J, Perl ER. Adrenergic excitation of cutaneous pain receptors induced by peripheral nerve injury. *Science* 1991;251(5001):1608–1610.

99. Jänig W, Levine JD, Michaelis M. Interactions of sympathetic and primary afferent neurons following nerve injury and tissue trauma. *Prog Brain Res* 1996;113:161–184.

100. Joshi SK, Gebhart GF. Visceral pain. *Curr Rev Pain* 2000;4(6):499–506.

101. Hobbs SF, Oh UT, Chandler MJ, et al. Evidence that C1 and C2 propriospinal neurons mediate the inhibitory effects of viscerosomatic spinal afferent input on primate spinothalamic tract neurons. *J Neurophysiol* 1992;67(4):852–860.

102. Craig AD. Distribution of trigeminothalamic and spinothalamic lamina I terminations in the macaque monkey. *J Comp Neurol* 2004;477(2):119–148.

103. Craig AD. A new view of pain as a homeostatic emotion. *Trends Neurosci* 2003;26(6):303–307.

104. Vogt BA, Berger GR, Derbyshire SW. Structural and functional dichotomy of human midcingulate cortex. *Eur J Neurosci* 2003;18(11):3134–3144.

105. Oppenheimer SM, Gelb A, Girvin JP, et al. Cardiovascular effects of human insular cortex stimulation. *Neurology* 1992;42(9):1727–1732.

106. Davis M, Whalen PJ. The amygdala: vigilance and emotion. *Mol Psychiatry* 2001;6(1):13–34.

107. Benarroch EE. Pain-autonomic interactions. *Neurol Sci* 2006;27(suppl 2): S130–133.

108. Bernard JF, Bester H, Besson JM. Involvement of the spino-parabrachio-amygdaloid and -hypothalamic pathways in the autonomic and affective emotional aspects of pain. *Prog Brain Res* 1996;107:243–255.

109. Janig W. The sympathetic nervous system in pain. *Eur J Anaesthesiol Suppl* 1995;10:53–60.

110. Cannon WB. *The Wisdom of the Body*. Rev. and enl. ed. New York: Norton; 1939.

111. Ader R, Cohen N, Felten D. Psychoneuroimmunology: interactions between the nervous system and the immune system. *Lancet* 1995;345(8942):99–103.

112. Page GG, Ben-Eliyahu S. The immune-suppressive nature of pain. *Semin Oncol Nurs* 1997;13(1):10–15.

113. Gebhart GF. *Visceral Pain*. Seattle: IASP Press; 1995.

114. Boeckxstaens GE. Understanding and controlling the enteric nervous system. *Best Pract Res Clin Gastroenterol* 2002;16(6):1013–1023.

115. Hodgkiss JP. Intrinsic reflexes underlying peristalsis in the small intestine of the domestic fowl. *J Physiol* 1986;380:311–328.

CHAPTER 10 ■ CLINICAL TRIALS

ROGER CHOU AND RICHARD A. DEYO

Controversies abound in the clinical management of pain, and there are enormous geographic variations in care. Lumbar spine surgery rates vary fivefold among developed countries, with rates in the United States being highest and rates in the United Kingdom being among the lowest[1]—yet patient outcomes appear to be broadly similar across countries. In smaller geographic areas, variations are also striking. Within the United States, rates of lumbar fusion surgery among Medicare enrollees vary more than 20-fold between regions, from 4.6 per 1000 enrollees in Idaho Falls, Idaho, to 0.2 per 1000 in Bangor, Maine.[2] Within Washington state, county back surgery rates vary more than sevenfold, even after excluding the smallest counties.[3]

Another problem in pain management is the successive uptake of a series of fads in treatment. Research has eventually discredited many of these, but they enjoyed widespread use, with substantial costs and side effects, before they were found to be ineffective. Examples include sacroiliac joint fusion for the treatment of low back pain, coccygectomy for coccydynia, bed rest and traction for back pain, and many others.[4] This phenomenon is prominent in the field of pain medicine, but not unique to it. Examples of abandoned therapies from other areas of medicine include internal mammary artery ligation for treating angina pectoris, gastric freezing for duodenal ulcers, and vitamin E and hormone therapy for prevention of cardiovascular events.[5-7] Promoting such ineffective treatments drains resources from more useful interventions, produces side effects, and eventually damages professional credibility.

Despite welcome breakthroughs in basic science research on pain, increases in knowledge regarding optimal ergonomics of work tasks, and the development and use of more technologically advanced medical therapies, studies show an increasing prevalence of chronic back pain and disability. In the state of North Carolina, the prevalence of chronic, impairing back pain more than doubled from 3.9% in 1992 to 10.2% in 2006.[8] A large and steady rise in use of surgery and interventional therapies for low back pain has not been associated with improved health status, but appears to be an important factor contributing to increases in health care expenditures associated with back pain.[9,10] Thus, despite impressive gains in our understanding of the molecular and cellular origins of pain, there is an important gap in translating this knowledge into effective clinical management. One reason may be the widespread reliance on inadequate research designs that lead to conflicting, confusing, or misinterpreted results. Biostatistical and epidemiologic methods make it possible to substantially improve this situation, but many key principles are not widely appreciated.

UNCONTROLLED STUDIES PARADIGM

Historically, much of pain treatment research consisted simply of uncontrolled studies in which clinicians treated a group of patients, then reported mean pain scores or the proportion who improved. Such studies are often referred to as *case series*, though the alternative term *before-after study* may help distinguish them from studies that identify cases based on an outcome (such as

an adverse event) rather than an exposure (such as a medical intervention), and only assesses patients at one point in time.[11] The before-after study design remains popular in part because it usually does not require extensive resources, but is vulnerable to many pitfalls.[12]

First, many uncontrolled studies are retrospectively reported. After treating a certain number of patients, the clinician looks back at his or her experience and tries to summarize the characteristics, treatments, and outcomes of the patients studied. Unfortunately, in this retrospective approach, there is often incomplete baseline information on patient characteristics. For example, factors such as age, sex, previous surgery, disability compensation, neurological deficits, psychological comorbidities, and pain duration often have a major influence on the outcomes of back surgery. Yet, in a systematic review of outcome studies on surgery for spinal stenosis, 74 relevant articles were found, but less than 10% mentioned all of these patient characteristics.[7]

Another problem with the retrospective approach is that it can be difficult to identify an inception cohort of all patients (or a random sample) who met specified criteria and received the intervention. A systematic review of 72 uncontrolled studies of spinal cord stimulation for chronic low back pain or failed back surgery syndrome found that less than one-quarter clearly described evaluation of a consecutive or representative sample of patients.[13] In such studies, it is impossible to know if patients with poorer results were excluded for arbitrary reasons, or how many patients received the treatment but were lost to follow-up. If patients lost to follow-up were more likely to experience poor outcomes than those who were followed, this could result in serious overestimates of benefits.

A third problem with uncontrolled studies is that, even if the researcher collects data prospectively, there is typically no blinding of patient, therapist, or outcome assessor to the nature of the treatment provided. This allows important unconscious biases to creep into the assessments. This is particularly important with outcomes related to pain, which by nature are subjective. Most of us would not trust outcomes rated by a surgeon evaluating his or her own patients, and yet this is the norm in much of the literature.

By definition, uncontrolled studies do not include control groups for comparison. The assumption seems to be that patients with painful conditions, and especially chronic pain, will not improve unless effective treatment is given. However, there are many reasons why patients improve in the face of ineffective therapy, some of which are listed in Table 10.1. First, the natural

TABLE 10.1

WHY PATIENTS MAY IMPROVE WITH INEFFECTIVE THERAPY

Natural history of a condition to improve
Placebo effects
Regression to the mean
Nonspecific effects: concern, conviction, enthusiasm, attention

history of many painful conditions is to improve spontaneously. This may be true even for patients with long standing pain, who sometimes improve for unclear reasons. For conditions such as acute low back pain, rapid early improvement is the norm.[14] Second are placebo effects, which are not well understood but are consistently underestimated, and may be particularly important when assessing pain.[7] Several factors may mediate placebo effects, including patient expectations, learning and conditioning from previous treatments, reduction of anxiety, and endorphin effects.

Another poorly appreciated factor is *regression to the mean*.[15] This term was coined by statisticians who observed that in a group of patients who are assembled because of the extreme nature of some clinical condition, there is a tendency for the condition to return to some average level that is less severe over time. Figure 10.1 shows what we often assume to be the course of chronic pain problems, with a steady level of severity that falls after successful intervention. However, the second panel is more likely to represent the true natural history, with good days and bad days, and fluctuations being the norm.[16] Patients seek us out when their symptoms are most extreme. We might easily be misled into believing that improved outcomes are due to the intervention when, in fact, random fluctuations are why their symptoms have returned toward a more average level. As Sartwell et al. pointed out, "the term chronic has a tendency to conjure up ideas of stability and unchangeability . . . it is changeability and varia-

Imagined Course of LBP

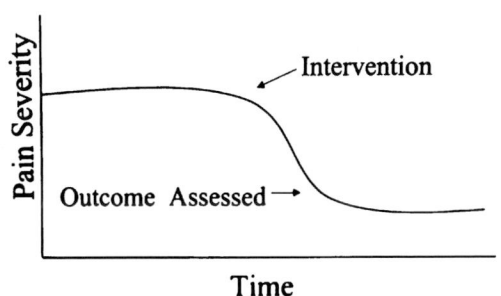

More Likely Course of LBP

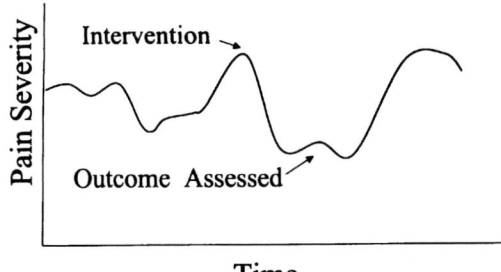

FIGURE 10.1 Hypothetical course of chronic low back pain. (From Deyo RA. Practice variations, treatment fads, rising disability. Do we need a new clinical research paradigm? *Spine* 1993;18:2153–2162, with permission.)

TABLE 10.2

THERAPEUTIC TRIAL FOR PATIENTS WITH CHRONIC LOW BACK PAIN: MEAN DURATION OF 4 YEARS, *n* = 31

Outcome measure	Score improvement Baseline to 1-month follow-up	*p* Value
Overall function (SIP)	32%	.002
Physical function	44%	.001
Pain severity (VAS)	33%	.006
Pain frequency (5-point scale)	20%	.000

Reprinted with permission from Deyo RA. Practice variations, treatment fads, rising disability. Do we need a new clinical research paradigm? *Spine* 1993;18:2153–2162.
SIP, Sickness Impact Profile; VAS, visual analog scale.

tion, not stability, that is in fact the dominant characteristic of most long-lived conditions."[17]

A host of other nonspecific effects also can affect assessments of patient improvement. Increased concern, conviction, enthusiasm, and attention of a therapist, a researcher, and a clinical staff may all have positive but nonspecific effects on patient outcomes. Table 10.2 shows a potential consequence of all these factors, using data from a clinical trial of patients with chronic low back pain.[16] The 31 patients in Table 10.2 had had back pain an average of 4 years. They received a clinical intervention that resulted in 20% to 44% improvements in pain frequency, severity, and function, all of which were highly statistically significant. However, this seemingly effective treatment for chronic pain was a sham transcutaneous electrical nerve stimulation (TENS) unit, along with hot packs twice a week. This was the control arm of a randomized trial, and illustrates the substantial improvements that may occur among those with long standing pain who receive ineffective treatments.

Finally, an issue that has begun to receive more attention is that uncontrolled studies are highly susceptible to publication bias.[18] There is little incentive for clinicians to publicize poor or even average results. Estimates of efficacy from uncontrolled studies that get published will therefore often over-represent the most positive results.

There is considerable room for improvement in the design and conduct of uncontrolled studies of pain interventions.[13,19] However, even when conducted well, the ability of uncontrolled studies to provide reliable information about treatment efficacy will always be limited. Exceptions can occur when the relationship between an intervention and outcomes is obvious, the effects are immediate, and the effects are so dramatic that that they cannot be explained by other factors.[20] Examples include surgery for appendicitis, eyeglasses for correction of refractive error, and cataract surgery. For nearly all pain conditions, however, there are many plausible explanations for the observed changes in outcomes, and reliable conclusions about treatment efficacy require the use of more rigorous study designs. There is simply too much noise to sort out whether outcomes are due to the treatment or to other factors.[21]

Control Groups: An Improvement Over the Case Series

Given the variety of factors that may produce improvement with ineffective therapy, it is incumbent on investigators to have a comparison group of subjects with the same likelihood for improvement as a treatment group, but who do not receive the active therapy. The goal should be to minimize the potential differences across groups in the effects of the various nonspecific causes for improvement that are listed in Table 10.1. With this goal in mind, the appropriate comparison group is unlikely to be one that receives no care at all. Patients in such a group would not experience placebo effects or the nonspecific effects of clinical concern and enthusiasm. The importance of having an adequate placebo is illustrated by a trial that found acupuncture more effective than no treatment for chronic low back pain, but no more effective than sham acupuncture.[22] Similarly, using a *waiting list* control group is usually not adequate because these patients experience none of the placebo or nonspecific effects of the intervention group. A preferable control group would be one that receives other credible, appropriate care that does not include the specific treatment under study. This might consist of usual care supplemented by a placebo of some sort. The placebo should be difficult to distinguish from the intervention under study so that it is perceived as being as likely to help as the active therapy. This is the reason for providing inactive pills in the control groups of drug trials; but, even for nondrug treatments, credible placebos should be provided when possible. Examples include the use of sham TENS units in trials of TENS, the use of sham injections in trials of interventional therapies, the use of subtherapeutic weight in trials of traction, or misplaced needling as a control for acupuncture.

In some cases, it may be unethical or impossible to provide a true placebo. Examples include many surgical interventions, psychological therapies, and rehabilitation interventions. In such situations, a reasonable alternative is to provide a placebo that creates some sense that patients are receiving an additional intervention and attention, but is not likely to have a strong effect on outcomes. One example might be a brief educational brochure.[23]

In addition to choosing an appropriate control intervention, it is also important to make the treatment and control groups as similar to each other as possible in other ways. Confounding is a critical concept that refers to variables associated with both the intervention being evaluated and the observed outcomes. A classic example of confounding is the association between alcohol consumption and lung cancer. This association is confounded by smoking, which is associated with alcohol consumption and is also an independent risk factor for lung cancer. Examples of common confounders in pain research include severity of baseline pain or functional deficits, psychological and medical comorbidities, age, and use of other therapies. The consequence of confounding is that the observed treatment effect is a poor estimate of the true effect. The modifying effect of the confounding variables result in either an overestimate or underestimate of treatment benefits, and can sometimes even result in a positive effect when the true effect is negative (or vice versa).

Selection of controls to minimize the potential for confounding is often a challenge. Control groups that are convenient to assemble are also, unfortunately, frequently associated with important pitfalls. For example, it would be unwise to choose patients who did not have adequate insurance coverage for the treatment being provided as a control group, because insurance coverage is related to important sociodemographic characteristics. Patients with the best insurance are typically those with the highest salaries and the most satisfying jobs, are happier with their insurance, and are more likely to practice healthy behaviors. Failure to adjust for socioeconomic status in observational studies could have resulted in the subsequently disproven belief in the positive cardiovascular benefits of hormone replacement therapy.[24] Similarly, selecting patients noncompliant with intended therapy as a control group is a flawed strategy. In a large-scale study of cholesterol-lowering therapy, control patients were divided among those who took more than 80% of their placebo tablets and those who took less than 80%.[25] Even after adjusting

for 40 coronary risk factors, there were enormous differences in mortality between the compliant and noncompliant groups. Patients who were compliant with their placebos had a 5-year mortality of only 16%, whereas those who were not compliant had a 5-year mortality rate of 26% ($p < 0.0001$). These findings were probably related to important differences between the groups that were not reflected in their coronary risk factors. These may have included other health habits, behaviors, attitudes toward risk, and occupations. Thus, noncompliant patients are often strikingly different from compliant patients, and we cannot assume that any differences in outcome are related only to treatment effects.

Sometimes the issues of proper selection of control patients and treatments are intertwined. A study that assigned patients with presumed discogenic low back pain to intradiscal electrothermal therapy (IDET) or rehabilitation therapy, based on their insurance coverage for IDET, reported an average 4.5 point improvement in pain scores.[26] Subsequent randomized trials found either no advantage of IDET, or only a 1 point difference between IDET and sham treatment.[27,28] In addition to potential socioeconomic differences related to differential insurance coverage, patients who were denied intradiscal electrothermal therapy probably had lower expectations about the likely benefits of rehabilitation therapy, particularly since some had previously received this treatment but had not responded.

Confounding by indication is particularly important in studies that assess treatment efficacy. It refers to the strong, natural (and appropriate) tendency for clinicians to selectively use therapies in patients most likely to benefit. A striking example of confounding by indication is a study of new users of nonsteroidal anti-inflammatory drugs (NSAIDs) that found use of ulcer-healing drugs associated with a tenfold *increase* in risk of gastrointestinal bleeding or perforations.[29] Obviously, ulcer-healing drugs don't cause ulcers. Rather, the increased risk of gastrointestinal complications in patients deemed appropriate for ulcer-healing drugs dwarfed any protective effect of the drugs.

There are ways to minimize or adjust for the effects of confounding. These include matching patient selection on the variables thought to be the most important potential confounders, restricting enrollment to patients defined by a narrow set of inclusion criteria, and statistical adjustment or analysis on known confounders.[30] Nonetheless, the effects of confounding can be dramatic even when one or more of these strategies are employed. For example, confounding by indication was strong in the study on ulcer-healing drugs, even though it attempted to restrict enrollment to lower-risk patients without a previous ulcer, or who had even been previously prescribed an ulcer-healing drug.[29]

Matching also may not be enough to overcome effects of confounding. Table 10.3 shows how one might assemble two groups of objects that are well matched on five different characteristics

---

TABLE 10.3

WHY NOT FIND "MATCHING" CONTROLS?

	Apples	Oranges
Shape	Round	Round
Source	Tree	Tree
Edible?	Yes	Yes
Size	Handheld	Handheld
Weight	½ lb.	½ lb.

Reprinted from Deyo RA. Practice variations, treatment fads, rising disability. Do we need a new clinical research paradigm? *Spine* 1993;18: 2153–2162, with permission.

TABLE 10.4

TWO COHORTS OF MEDICARE PATIENTS WITH LAMINECTOMY FOR STENOSIS (1985)

	Group A (n = 252)	Group B (n = 141)	Significance
% Women	57%	55%	NS
Mean age	71	72	NS
% Fusion	0	0	NS
4-Year reoperations	4%	15%	<.0005

Reprinted from Deyo RA. Practice variations, treatment fads, rising disability. Do we need a new clinical research paradigm? *Spine* 1993;18:2153–2162, with permission.
NS, not significant.

and yet literally be comparing apples and oranges.[16] Table 10.4 shows real data from a comparison of outcomes of two groups of Medicare patients who underwent low back surgery. They were matched on diagnosis (all had spinal stenosis), gender, age, insurance (all Medicare), and surgical procedure (all had a laminectomy without fusion). Despite being well matched on these five characteristics, the likelihood of reoperations differed almost fourfold between the two groups. Differences of this magnitude might easily be attributed to some dramatic advantage of the treatment used in group A. However, these groups were intentionally assembled in such a way that group A was composed of African American patients who had not had prior surgery, and group B was composed of white patients with prior surgery.[16] These two characteristics, which might have easily been overlooked, accounted entirely for the difference in reoperation rates. Unfortunately, it usually isn't as simple as matching on a few critical and easily measured variables. The cholesterol-lowering placebo study described previously shows how even matching (or adjusting) for 40 different risk factors may not capture important differences between two groups of patients.[25]

If waiting lists, patients with insufficient insurance coverage, noncompliant patients, or even carefully matched patients receiving appropriate placebo treatments make poor control groups, is there a better solution? Fortunately, the concept of random allocation provides an ideal method of establishing a comparison group that is likely to be similar in nearly all respects to an intervention group.

RANDOMIZED ALLOCATION OF TREATMENT AND CONTROL GROUPS

The term *randomized trial* has become familiar among clinicians and, yet, is often misunderstood. Some assume that a randomized trial is one in which patients are randomly selected from a population of interest. However, just the opposite may be true. Patients may be highly selected from a group of potential candidates based on specific characteristics that make the study treatment safe and likely to succeed. Randomization does not refer to the selection of patients to be studied, but rather to the patients' allocation to the treatment or the control group.

Why is randomization such a desirable way of creating a control group? It is attractive because the problem of confounding is largely eliminated.[31] Because it is never possible to completely understand or measure all confounders, residual confounding is always a potential issue in studies that are not randomized.[32] With random allocation, we may not even know the important

prognostic factors, but they will be equally distributed (given a fair randomization and enough patients) between the treatment and control groups. Effective randomization requires the generation of a truly unpredictable (random) allocation sequence, as well as its successful implementation via allocation concealment.[33]

There is sometimes confusion about what constitutes randomization. Randomization requires using a list of random numbers that may be published or determined by a computer program. Each successive subject has an equal likelihood of being assigned to each treatment arm, though the order in which they are assigned is unpredictable. Alternating assignment is not the same as randomization because it is predictable. Similarly, assigning patients without conscious bias, or haphazardly, is not the same as random allocation. Using hospital numbers, date of birth, or day of the week is also not randomization. If day of the week is used, a patient could simply come in (or be told to come in) on the day that the desired intervention will be offered. Allocation concealment means that the allocation sequence remains unknown until at least after patients have been assigned to therapy, thus preserving the actual randomization. A traditional method to help preserve allocation concealment is use of opaque sealed envelopes containing the treatment assignment. An increasingly common alternative is to have an off-site facility that keeps the random sequence, so research personnel cannot know the next assignment as a subject is enrolled.[34]

A dramatic example of the effects of randomization in pain research is a systematic review of TENS therapy for postoperative pain that found that 15 of 17 randomized trials of efficacy showed no benefit.[35] By contrast, 17 of 19 nonrandomized studies showed a substantial positive treatment effect. Some investigators have also quantified the magnitude of bias that occurs when allocation concealment is inadequate. One such study, shown in Table 10.5, compared randomization with adequate allocation concealment with randomization with inadequate allocation concealment and with nonrandom allocation of controls.[36] The investigators examined a series of treatments for acute myocardial infarction and, as Table 10.5 shows, demonstrated that maldistribution of prognostic factors was least with randomization with adequate allocation concealment and greatest with nonrandom allocation. Similarly, the likelihood of finding a substantial improvement in case fatality rate rose dramatically, from just 9% of trials with randomization and adequate allocation concealment to up to almost 60% of trials with nonrandom allocation. Other studies suggest that, on average, inadequate allocation concealment inflates results by about 40% compared to studies with adequate allocation concealment.[34,37]

Why is allocation concealment so important? There are probably several reasons. Failure to conceal allocation makes it easy

TABLE 10.5

BIAS IN STUDIES OF MYOCARDIAL INFARCTION

Allocation method	Prognostic maldistribution (%)	Difference found in case-fatality (%)
Blinded randomization	14	9
Unblinded randomization	27	24
Nonrandomized	58	58

Data from Chalmers T, Celano P, Sacks HS, Smith J. Bias in treatment assignment in controlled clinical trials. *N Engl J Med* 1983;309: 1358–1361; reprinted from Deyo RA. Practice variations, treatment fads, rising disability. Do we need a new clinical research paradigm? *Spine* 1993; 18:2153–2162, with permission.

to subvert the randomization process. If this occurs, confounding by indication can be as much of a problem as in nonrandomized studies.[34] Some overt methods that have been used to bypass randomization include adjusting treatment assignments based on posted allocation sequences, or ignoring allocation to treatments perceived as less desirable.[38] Inadequate allocation concealment can also have more subtle effects. If the investigator has a bias as to which treatment group is more effective—even a subconscious bias—he or she may approach the next subject differently if he or she can determine what the next treatment assignment will be. This may affect the way in which a clinical trial is presented to a patient, the enthusiasm with which consent is sought, or the rigor with which eligibility criteria are applied.

For certain interventions, it may be undesirable or unfeasible to randomly allocate individual patients to a treatment or a control group. For example, if one were testing a guideline that involved changes in clinic organization and changes in management by nurses or other ancillary staff, it might be extremely difficult to ensure that all involved gave one particular approach to some patients and not to others. Furthermore, individual physicians would have difficulty treating certain patients according to a guideline and others not according to the guideline. In such a circumstance, one might wish to allocate clusters of patients, such as entire clinics, to intervention or control arms. Such studies are referred to as cluster randomized trials.[39] When these designs are used, specific statistical methods are needed to account for the similarities among patients of a single physician or facility, which can inflate estimates of treatment effects. Analytic techniques, such as the cluster correlation correction for such studies, have been well described[40] and appropriate computer software is available to perform these analyses.

OTHER METHODS FOR REDUCING BIAS IN CLINICAL TRIALS

Randomization is a powerful method for minimizing the possibility of confounding, but does not protect against other types of bias, or systematic errors in measurement. The quality of a trial refers to how rigorously it employs measures to protect against bias. Table 10.6 lists criteria that have been proposed for critical readers to evaluate the quality of studies on treatment efficacy.[41,42] A lengthier and more detailed set of criteria for evaluating clinical trials has been developed by the back subgroup of the Cochrane Collaboration.[43] Additional guidance for clinical investigators includes recommendations on how to report the methods and results of randomized trials.[44] The list of criteria in Table 10.6 begins with random allocation, which was discussed in detail previously.

Baseline Similarity of Study Groups

Randomization usually provides the best way to produce groups with equivalent prognoses. However, randomization may not always work and investigators should present a comparison of baseline characteristics of patients in the treatment and control groups. In a properly randomized trial, any observed differences are chance occurrences, but may still be sufficiently large to compromise the validity of the study. When this occurs, investigators sometimes adjust for baseline differences using statistical techniques. However, such statistical adjustments should be based on how strongly the prognostic factor is thought to be associated with the outcomes and the clinical importance of baseline imbalances, not on the results of statistical tests for significant differences.[45] Statistical tests can be misleading, as small differences may be clinically trivial but statistically significant in large trials, and large differences may be clinically important but statistically nonsignificant in small trials.

TABLE 10.6

READERS' GUIDES FOR AN ARTICLE ABOUT THERAPY

Are the results of the study valid?
  Primary guides
    Was the assignment of patients to treatments randomized?
    Were all patients who entered the trial properly accounted for and attributed at its conclusion?
    Was follow-up complete?
      Were patients analyzed in the groups to which they were randomized?
  Secondary guides
    Were patients, health workers, and study personnel "blind" to treatment?
    Were the groups similar at the start of the trial?
    Aside from the experimental intervention, were the groups treated equally?

What were the results?
  How large was the treatment effect?
  How precise was the estimate of the treatment effect?

Will the results help me in caring for my patients?
  Can the results be applied to my patient care?
  Were all clinically important outcomes considered?
  Are the likely treatment benefits worth the potential harms and costs?

Reprinted from Guyatt GH, Sackett DL, Cook DJ. Users' guides to the medical literature II. How to use an article about therapy or prevention. A. Are the results of the study valid? *JAMA* 1993;270:2598–2601, with permission.

Even if adjustment is appropriate, it cannot control for differences in unmeasured confounders. It is also important to consider whether baseline imbalances could be due to intentional subversion of randomization.[46]

Blinding

The importance of blinding is that it helps to create similar expectations on the part of patients and similar enthusiasm by the therapists. Furthermore, it ensures that the same level of attention and concern is provided to both a treatment and a control group. Blinding is particularly important in studies that assess subjective outcomes such as pain. In one study, lack of blinding inflated estimates of treatment effects by 30% in trials with subjective outcomes, but had no effect on estimates in trials with objective outcomes.[47]

It is common to talk about *double-blind* trials, but the term is often used ambiguously.[48] Typically, it is meant to imply that the patient is unaware whether he or she is receiving active treatment or a placebo, and the person administering or prescribing the treatment is also unaware. In some cases, it may be impossible to blind patients or therapists, as in trials of surgical treatments or some rehabilitation interventions. There is also a third party that may be blinded—an independent assessor of outcomes. Maintaining such a blinded assessor should generally be feasible, even when it is impossible to blind patients and therapists. Trials should explicitly describe who was blinded, rather than use nonspecific jargon such as single-, double-, or even triple-blinded.[48]

As noted in the discussion of control groups, creativity can sometimes produce credible placebo or alternative treatments that at least help to maintain blinding. In many situations, it would be informative to test the success of blinding at the end of a study. This is not done frequently, but is important for certain drugs and other interventions that have side effects or other characteristics that can give the treatment away.[49] In a trial of TENS therapy for low back pain, for example, sham treatment does not produce the same sensation as active therapy, so patients could know they are receiving sham rather than active therapy. This would essentially result in an unblinded trial. In fact, one trial of TENS found that patients and physicians were able to guess better than random chance whether individual patients were in the treatment or control group, but the magnitude of blinding failure was sufficiently modest that the results could be presented with some confidence.[50]

In trials of drug therapy, crossover designs have commonly been used because they help to reduce the effects of interpatient variability in baseline and outcome measures. For many pain treatments, however, such designs may be undesirable because patients would experience both treatments and could determine with a high level of certainty whether they were receiving active treatment or placebo. For example, maintenance of blinding would be very difficult in a crossover study from sham TENS to true TENS, or from subtherapeutic weight to therapeutic weight with traction, or from mild exercise to strenuous exercise. Because of the potential for loss of blinding and other issues such as carryover effects and loss to follow-up during the first intervention period,[51] crossover trials may be undesirable for many types of pain therapy.

Were Groups Treated Equally Except for the Experimental Treatment?

Sometimes patients in a treatment group are given multiple interventions and, yet, the authors or readers are tempted to ascribe the results to a single feature of the treatment. For example, a patient who receives a sclerosant injection into the spinal ligaments, along with corticosteroids and spinal manipulation, might be said to have improved because of the sclerosant therapy, and yet much of the observed improvement might be due to the cotreatments.[52] Thus, it is important that any cotreatments also be given to the control group and that the intensity of the treatments is equal.[53]

Furthermore, use of multiple treatments for chronic painful conditions is common. Many patients obtain over-the-counter pain medications, visit multiple physicians, or seek alternative forms of therapy such as chiropractic care, acupuncture, or massage. In outpatient trials, it may be difficult to prevent patients from obtaining such cotreatments, and it may simply be necessary to inquire about these cointerventions and determine if they are roughly equivalent between two groups. Alternatively, investigators may make strenuous efforts to ensure that patients do not receive certain types of cointerventions. Even the nature of follow-up should be consistent between study groups. If one group has closer or more frequent follow-up, for example, more adverse events might be reported, or treatment might be given more intensively. Increased contact with a caring clinician can also have important nonspecific effects, as noted previously.

Low Loss to Follow-Up and Intention-to-Treat Analysis

The second item in the list in Table 10.6 concerns completeness of follow-up for patients who entered the trial. As discussed in the section on uncontrolled studies, investigators should attempt to follow-up on every patient who enters the study because those who drop out may be systematically different from patients who remain in the study, resulting in attrition bias. For example, disgruntled patients who have failed to improve may drop out of a trial, leaving an obvious bias in favor of the new treatment. On the other hand, patients with dramatic improvements may drop out because they are so much better they see no need for contin-

ued medical contact. Dropouts from clinical studies often differ systematically from those who remain with regard to their baseline characteristics.

In highly mobile societies, such as the United States, obtaining complete follow-up can be difficult. Strategies for maximizing follow-up include gathering multiple telephone numbers at the time of enrollment for the patient, relatives, and friends; excluding patients who are planning to move in the near future; excluding patients who have no telephone; multiple mailings of questionnaires; financial incentives to return data; maintaining contact with greeting cards or newsletters; using the briefest possible follow-up questionnaires; and even use of the Internet to track patients through public records.

A useful rule of thumb is that at least 85% of patients who enter a trial should be included at the end of the study. One way to ensure that the results are robust in the face of dropouts is to do a worst-case analysis, in which one assumes that all dropouts from the treatment group failed to improve, whereas all dropouts from the comparison group improved substantially. If this worst-case analysis does not change the conclusion, one can be confident in the findings.[41]

It is also important that patients be analyzed in the groups to which they were randomized (intention-to-treat analysis), regardless of whether they received the intended treatment, how well they adhered to the assigned therapy, and whether they completed the trial.[54] We have seen the hazards of assuming that patients who are noncompliant are otherwise the same as compliant patients. Indeed, patients who do not receive the intended therapy may be systematically different from those who do. The only way to maintain the benefits of randomization and to avoid a biased comparison is to keep patients, for analytic purposes, in the group to which they were assigned. Intention-to-treat analyses take into account the fact that patients in clinical practice are autonomous and do not always follow the trial protocol to the letter—or at all. In some cases, intention-to-treat analyses can be difficult to interpret. In the Spine Outcomes Research Trials of surgery, nearly 40% of patients crossed over from surgery to nonsurgical therapy, and vice versa.[55] The intention-to-treat analysis still provides information about patient outcomes when they are advised to undergo surgery or nonsurgical therapy, even though many patients decided not to proceed with the recommended therapy. An as-treated analysis provides additional information based on which therapy the patients actually received. This can also be informative, so long as potential confounders are adjusted for, and the high probability of some residual confounding is recognized.[56]

OTHER ISSUES IN CLINICAL TRIALS

Measurement of Outcomes

What outcomes should be measured in a clinical trial? In traditional clinical trials, investigators often seek the most objective possible outcomes for evaluation, such as joint range of motion, spinal fluid endorphins, or dynamometer measures of muscle strength. Although the search for objective outcome measures is appropriate for many medical conditions, pain is inherently a subjective phenomenon and one that often correlates only modestly with these physiologic measures. Table 10.7 illustrates several examples of dissociations between physiologic measures and pain or functioning.[57] Some researchers have argued that the essence of hard data is their reproducibility under the same circumstances.[58] Happily, many subjective phenomena can be measured in reproducible fashion. A good example is the use of visual analog pain scales and other ordinal rating scales for quantifying pain.

TABLE 10.7

EXAMPLES OF DISSOCIATIONS BETWEEN VARIOUS OUTCOME MEASURES

- Biofeedback reduces paraspinal electromyography activity but not pain.
- Tricyclic antidepressants relieve pain and depression but do not alter cerebrospinal fluid beta-endorphin levels or paraspinous electromyography activity.
- Statements of pain severity correlate poorly with medication use, health care use, and activity level.
- Reduced spinal mobility may be associated with improvement in pain and disability or lower risk of pain.
- Muscle function does not predict 10-year incidence of back symptoms.
- Correlations between lumbar spine mobility and modified Oswestry questionnaire are only .04–.17 (absolute value).
- In a clinical trial of rigid corset, improvements in symptoms with activity were observed but not in spine mobility or straight-leg raising.

Reprinted from Deyo RA. Measuring the functional status of patients with low back pain. *Arch Phys Med Rehabil* 1988;69:1044–1053, with permission.

For evaluation of therapies for chronic pain, trials should go beyond the self-report of pain to routinely examine patients' behavior and function in their daily lives.[59] Function should be considered a separate domain from pain and be measured separately because improvements in pain and function often correlate only loosely with one another.[60] For example, trials of opioids for chronic noncancer pain and exercise therapy for low back pain both found considerably smaller benefits according to measures of function compared to measures of pain.[61,62] So how should function be assessed? Performance measures such as a series of timed tasks or an obstacle course may have the attraction of seeming objectivity, but performance can be highly influenced by motivation, mood, setting, financial incentives, and other non-physical attributes of the patient and his or her environment. Such measures often do not correlate well with how a patient actually functions on a day-to-day basis. By contrast, a number of self-report measures of health status or functional status have been validated and are quite reproducible. Examples include the Sickness Impact Profile[63,64] and the Medical Outcomes Study Short-Form-36,[65] as well as condition-specific scales such as the Roland Morris Disability Questionnaire and Oswestry Disability Index for patients with back pain,[66] the Arthritis Impact Measurement Scale,[67] the Western Ontario and McMaster Universities Osteoarthritis Index physical function subscale,[68] and many others.

To provide a full picture of the effects of pain interventions, the Initiative on Methods, Measurement, and Pain Assessment in Clinical Trials (IMMPACT) recommends that clinical trials routinely measure outcomes in multiple core domains. In addition to pain, physical functioning, and emotional functioning, IMMPACT recommends assessment of participant ratings of global improvement and satisfaction with treatment, symptoms and adverse events, and participant disposition.[59]

Work status is often used as an outcome measure for chronic pain treatment because of its clear relevance to both patients and to society. However, it has a number of drawbacks as an outcome measure, most important of which is that it is influenced by many nonmedical factors. For example, studies have demonstrated that the likelihood of return to work in the face of a painful medical condition varies depending on job satisfaction, relationships with fellow employees and supervisors, regional unemployment rates, the presence of another breadwinner in the family, proximity to retirement age, and physical job demands. Similarly, the duration of pain-related disability is strongly associated with the patient's educational status, income,[69] and the generosity of disability benefits. For many members of our society, including students, homemakers, and retired persons, return to employment is simply not available as an indicator of outcome. Thus, although this measure of outcome is important in many settings, it should be interpreted in light of these potentially confounding factors.

Reporting the Results

Many clinical trials report mean outcome scores, or mean differences in scores compared to baseline values. This can be difficult to interpret clinically, as a 10-point mean improvement on a 100-point scale could indicate that nearly all patients experienced only very mild improvement, or that some proportion of patients experienced a clinically significant improvement while others did not. Reporting the proportion of patients that met a certain threshold for improvement can be very helpful for interpreting the clinical significance of results. The minimal important change, or the smallest change in outcome scores perceived by patients to be meaningful, is a key concept.[70] It refers to the smallest amount of improvement perceived by patients as being important. For low back pain, a consensus group recently proposed a 30% improvement from baseline in pain or function as the minimum important change.[71]

In some studies, actual outcome measurements are not reported. Rather, only the *p* values for the significance of results are provided. A *p* value tells us the probability of obtaining a result that is at least as extreme as the one actually observed, assuming that the null hypothesis of no difference between treatments is true. However, this gives a reader no idea what the magnitude of treatment effects may have been.[72] In a very large trial, a difference between groups may achieve statistical significance even though the difference is too trivial to be clinically relevant. On the other hand, in a very small trial, a large treatment effect might fail to achieve statistical significance. Thus, the magnitude of treatment effect is somewhat independent of statistical significance, and should be reported. An ideal way to present the results is to give the actual estimate of success rates or mean scores along with 95% confidence limits, which allow the reader to see the range of results that would be consistent with the study findings. The 95% confidence limits are closely related to *p* values, but give readers a better understanding of the potential range of effects compatible with the data.

Statistical Power

When a trial shows no statistically significant difference, it is often interpreted as meaning that it has proven that there is no difference between the intervention and control groups. However, this interpretation is often incorrect. In fact, most trials are too small to prove that there is no difference between groups—rather, they only show an absence of evidence of a difference.[73] This is a critical distinction. The likelihood that a true difference may not have been detected is referred to as Type II (or β) error, in contrast to Type I (or α) error (which is reflected in the *p* value).[74] Statistical power (calculated as $1 - \beta$) refers to the likelihood that a clinically relevant difference between groups will be identified. Larger sample sizes increase statistical power. On the other hand, statistical power decreases as the size of the clinical effect to be detected (typically the minimal important change) goes down. Nonstatistically significant results should always be interpreted in the context of the statistical power of the study.

Generalizability of Results and Efficacy Versus Effectiveness

Even if a clinical trial is internally valid, its results may not be applicable (generalizable) to other patients and settings. Patients who enroll in low back pain clinical trials, for example, tend to be better educated, more frequently employed, and different in other prognostically important ways from patients in everyday practice[75] Clinical trials often exclude patients with medical or psychological comorbidities, or use run-in periods to identify and exclude patients who experience adverse events before randomizing them. For example, older patients have often been excluded from trials of arthritis drugs, even though they are the most likely to receive such drugs in actual practice. Patients enrolled in clinical trials are usually recruited from tertiary care settings, and the resources available in clinical trials to help maximize patient compliance and follow-up are rarely available to most clinicians. A number of other threats to generalizability have been described.[76] It is important for patients, treatments, and study conditions to be adequately reported so readers can determine whether they would be likely to apply to their own situations.

Related to generalizability is the concept of efficacy versus effectiveness. Most clinical trials are designed to evaluate efficacy, or the benefits of an intervention in optimal populations and under ideal conditions. Such studies generally focus on narrow, short-term outcomes. Effectiveness studies, on the other hand, are designed to evaluate whether an intervention will actually work under conditions encountered in usual practice.[77] Of course, there is a continuum between efficacy and effectiveness, though most randomized trials fall squarely on the efficacy side of the spectrum. Factors that can enhance the ability of clinical trials to evaluate effectiveness are the use of less stringent eligibility criteria, enrollment of patients from primary care populations, evaluation of multiple clinically relevant outcomes, and longer duration of follow-up.[78] Observational studies can also be helpful for evaluating effectiveness, once efficacy has been established in randomized trials.

Subgroup Analyses

Sometimes, analyses are performed to examine whether the effects of an intervention differ in clinically relevant groups of patients defined by some factor (such as baseline pain score, sex, or age).[79] For example, a trial of glucosamine for osteoarthritis found no overall treatment benefit, but a subgroup analysis found that it was effective in patients with high baseline pain scores.[80] There is a great risk that subgroup analyses may be overinterpreted, as results could simply represent chance effects, particularly when data are mined to look for significant results. Confidence in subgroup analyses is enhanced if the treatment effects are large, are unlikely to have occurred by chance, occur in an analysis based on a prespecified and plausible hypothesis, come from a small number of subgroup analyses, and are replicated in other studies.

Effects of Funding Source

Commercially funded clinical trials are consistently more likely to report results that favor the funder than trials that are not commercially funded.[81,82] This appears to be true for devices, such as surgical implants, as well as drugs.[83,84] Why might this be? One reason is publication bias. This refers to the differential tendency for studies to be published depending on the strength and direction of results.[85] Generally, studies that report statistically significant and more strongly positive results are more likely to be published compared to those that report statistically insig-

nificant or less striking results. The result is inflated estimates of treatment effects. Publication bias can occur no matter what the source of funding is, but commercially funded clinical trials appear to be particularly susceptible, either due to overt or more subtle pressures.[82,86,87] A related situation is the selective reporting of outcomes.[88–90] This leads to bias because more favorable results tend to be reported and publicized, and there is often no indication to readers that other (less favorable) outcomes were even assessed. Results can also be spun to appear more favorable than they really are. One study found that of 36 industry-sponsored new drug approval trials of antidepressants viewed by the U.S. Food and Drug Administration (FDA) as having negative or questionable results, 22 had not been published, and another 11 were reported in a way that conveyed positive outcomes.[91] Another questionable strategy that has begun to receive increased scrutiny is the practice of *seeding* trials following new drug approvals.[92] Such trials are framed as scientific research but, in reality, are marketing tools designed to increase familiarity and use of the medication by experienced clinicians.

This is not to say that commercially funded trials cannot be conducted and reported rigorously. However, replication of results in noncommercially funded trials may be required to increase confidence in the findings of commercially funded trials, even when methodological shortcomings are not readily apparent. Statistical and graphical methods are available to formally assess for the likelihood of publication bias, though all have some limitations.[93] The FDA website can be a useful resource for identifying unpublished trials and unreported outcomes, but data are often incomplete or redacted. Ideally, publication and selective outcome reporting bias would not only be detected, but would not occur in the first place. The development of clinical trial registries and mandatory requirements for researchers to submit trial protocols and full results in order to be considered for journal publication, or for new drug approvals, may help reduce the effects of these biases.[94,95] However, the usefulness of clinical trial registries will depend on how assiduously and quickly researchers comply with reporting requirements.

Assessment of Harms

In order to generate balanced conclusions about an intervention, it is important to understand both its benefits and harms.[96] However, benefits have been accorded far greater prominence than harms when conducting and reporting clinical trials. In fact, most randomized trials lack prespecified hypotheses for harms. Rather, hypotheses are usually designed to evaluate beneficial effects, with assessment of harms a secondary consideration. As a result, the quality and quantity of harm reporting in clinical trials is often inadequate.[97]

There are other problems with relying solely on clinical trials to assess harms.[98] Few clinical trials have large enough sample sizes or are long enough in duration to adequately assess uncommon or long-term harms. For example, one systematic review found that trials of opioids for chronic noncancer pain averaged only 5 weeks in duration, even though patients frequently remain on these medications indefinitely.[61] In addition, patients who are more susceptible to adverse events are often excluded from clinical trials, though they may commonly receive the therapy in clinical practice. For example, all trials of opioids for chronic noncancer pain that reported information on history of drug addiction excluded such patients.[61] Harms may also be downplayed or misrepresented if there is a vested interest in doing so.[99] Aggressive promotion of unsubstantiated claims of lower abuse, diversion, and withdrawal risks of OxyContin (Purdue Pharma, Stamford, CT), a sustained-release formulation of oxycodone, eventually resulted in a criminal conviction and $634 million fine against the Purdue Frederick Company, Inc., along with three company executives.[100]

Assessment and reporting of harms in clinical trials can certainly be improved. This is also an area where observational studies can be a very useful source of information. Unlike assessments of treatment benefits, confounding by indication is usually not an issue with unexpected or unpredictable adverse events because such outcomes are not related to the decision to use the therapy.[31,101] An example would be the observational studies on risk of myocardial infarction associated with cyclo-oxygenase-2 selective NSAIDs. Those conducted prior to knowledge regarding the cardiovascular risks of rofecoxib were unlikely to be affected by confounding by indication related to the baseline risk of heart disease. Observational studies can also provide important information on rare or long-term adverse events and in populations under-represented in clinical trials (such as pregnant women, children, older adults, or those with important comorbidities). Even uncontrolled studies such as case reports have been invaluable for evaluating harms, and may be the first or primary signal of a rare adverse event.

Trial-based Cost-effectiveness Analysis

Even if the balance of benefits to harms of a treatment is acceptable, widespread implementation may not make sense if costs are very high. Clinical trials can also be designed to assess the question "Is it worth it?" by collecting cost data alongside clinical outcomes.[77] Unlike decision analytic studies that model costs and clinical outcomes, such trial-based cost-effectiveness analyses directly measure the cost per some increment of clinical utility (often a quality-adjusted life-year). One challenge with cost-effectiveness analyses of clinical trials is that cost data are often associated with large variability, so estimates can be imprecise unless sample sizes are large.[102] In addition, distributions of cost estimates are often quite skewed, which can pose a statistical challenge.

NEW DIRECTIONS IN CLINICAL TRIALS

Pragmatic Trials

With increased attention to effectiveness has come an increased demand for pragmatic trials that attempt to inform routine clinical practice better than traditional efficacy trials. Key features of pragmatic trials are that they are set in normal practice settings rather than highly specialized or controlled settings, apply few exclusion criteria, allow flexibility in use of treatment interventions, and assess key, patient-centered outcomes.[103] For example, a pragmatic trial of acupuncture for chronic low back pain was conducted in general practice and private acupuncture clinics in the UK, enrolled anyone aged 18 to 65 with nonspecific low back pain of 4 to 52 weeks' duration (with few exclusion criteria), allowed acupuncturists to determine the content and number of treatments, and evaluated bodily pain as well as outcomes related to use of analgesics and patient satisfaction.[104]

Expertise-based Trials

For nonpharmacological interventions, such as surgery, that are highly dependent on the skill and training of the clinician, expertise-based randomized controlled trials have been proposed.[105] In the traditional randomized controlled trial, participants are randomized to one of two interventions and individual clinicians provide intervention A to some patients and intervention B to others. In the expertise-based randomized trial, participants are randomized to individual clinicians with expertise in intervention

A or to clinicians with expertise in intervention B. Proposed advantages of expertise-based randomized trials are that they can reduce the effects of differential expertise bias. In the case of surgery this can be important because many procedures require considerable experience to gain proficiency. In addition, the expertise-based design reduces potential effects of differential enthusiasm or skepticism for the different procedures, as each surgeon provides only the procedure that he or she believes is the best. As yet, however, there is relatively little evidence on the validity of expertise-based randomized trials.

Comparative Effectiveness

Another direction in clinical trials is toward increased evaluations of not just effectiveness of interventions versus placebo, but comparative effectiveness of two or more interventions.[106] Head-to-head trials that compare two interventions are the most direct method for evaluating comparative effectiveness. However, head-to-head trials are not always available. An alternative method for evaluating comparative effectiveness is through indirect comparisons. This refers to assessments of the relative benefits and harms of competing interventions based on how well each performs against a common comparator (usually placebo). Methods are available for conducting indirect comparisons that preserve some of the benefits of randomization, as well as for more complex network analyses and mixed treatment comparisons that incorporate both indirect and direct evidence.[107] In all cases, the validity of indirect comparisons is based on the critical assumption that treatment effects are consistent across all trials. This assumption can be violated due to a number of factors, including differences in study quality, patient populations, settings, outcomes, and other factors. In fact, large discrepancies between indirect and direct studies have been reported. For example, in patients with neuropathic pain, an indirect comparison found tricyclic antidepressants associated with a much higher likelihood of achieving pain relief compared to gabapentin, but head-to-head trials found no significant difference.[108] Indirect comparisons should only be used when the critical assumption of similarity of treatment effects is met, and verified against results from head-to-head trials as they become available.

Equivalence and Noninferiority Trials

Traditional clinical trials are designed to determine whether an active treatment is superior to another treatment (often placebo). The null hypothesis is that there is no difference between the treatments being compared. In equivalence trials, on the other hand, the purpose is to determine whether one (typically new) intervention is therapeutically similar (equivalent) to another, usually established, treatment.[109] This requires testing of a different null hypothesis—specifically the null hypothesis that there *is* a difference being treatments. Noninferiority trials are similar to equivalence trials, but they are designed to focus on whether a new treatment is no worse than (rather than therapeutically similar to) an established treatment. For either type of trial, boundaries for what will be considered equivalent or noninferior must be defined in order to perform appropriate hypothesis testing. Unfortunately, many trials that report equivalence do not define these boundaries, or are based on misapplied or misinterpreted statistical analyses, often based on standard superiority hypotheses or inadequate sample sizes.[110] Guidance is available to help improve the conduct, reporting, and interpretation of equivalence and noninferiority trials.[109]

Factorial Design

In a factorial design, patients are simultaneously randomized to receive or not receive two different treatments.[111] In the UK Back

Pain Exercise and Manipulation (BEAM) trial, for example, patients were allocated to receive exercise therapy versus no exercise therapy and to receive spinal manipulation or no spinal manipulation.[112] Such factorial designs have important efficiencies if the dropout rate is low. If there is no statistical interaction between the two treatments (in this example, exercise therapy and spinal manipulation) then one has an unbiased assessment of the effect of each treatment. Such designs might be useful in studying combinations of therapy such as an analgesic plus a muscle relaxant, drug therapy plus physical therapy, and other clinically relevant combinations. Indeed, factorial designs may be the best way to evaluate the multicomponent therapy that is widely advocated for the treatment of chronic pain. If there is no synergy between treatments, the investigator essentially has two trials for the price of one. If there is synergy or additive effects between treatments, there is no other way to identify this effect. Factorial designs introduce analytical complexities that are avoided in simple parallel designs, but in some circumstances, the benefits may outweigh the disadvantages.[113]

Bayesian Statistical Inference and Adaptive Designs

Another direction in clinical trials is the use of Bayesian frameworks of statistical inference instead of the standard classical (frequentist) framework.[114] Although a full discussion of Bayesian statistical inference is beyond the scope of this chapter, in essence the Bayesian framework incorporates new evidence or observations to update probabilities that a hypothesis might be true. Bayesian adaptive trials use Bayesian methods to incorporate data collected during the course of a trial in order to inform decisions regarding the need to update, modify, or stop the trial.

SYSTEMATIC REVIEWS

The relatively rapid advances in other fields of medicine, such as oncology and cardiology, occur because a succession of large randomized trials, typically implemented in multiple centers, result in cumulative knowledge. Such large, multicenter trials are still the exception rather than the rule in pain treatment, perhaps in part because of lower research funding for nonfatal conditions. Nonetheless, more pain research trials are being conducted, resulting in an ever-growing body of literature. This growth has been exponential. Between 1950 and 1990, more than 8000 randomized controlled trials of pain research were published, with over 85% appearing during the last 15 years of that period.[115]

Given the amount of evidence, it is difficult for clinicians to keep up with the literature on even a circumscribed area of medicine. Review articles can be a useful way to summarize the evidence on a given topic. A systematic review is a particular type of review article that applies explicit methods to reduce bias and error when summarizing evidence.[116] This is in contrast with traditional or narrative reviews, which do not use explicit methods to identify, select, and assess evidence. Such review articles are relatively subjective and are apt to be based on incomplete, outdated, or flawed evidence. This increases the likelihood of incorrect or unsubstantiated conclusions.

A systematic review attempts to bring the same level of scientific rigor to the review article as should be used when conducting original research. Systematic reviews can be qualitative or quantitative. The latter are also referred to as meta-analyses even though, strictly speaking, a meta-analysis is not necessarily based on systematic methods. Potential advantages of systematic review

TABLE 10.8

POTENTIAL ADVANTAGES OF SYSTEMATIC REVIEWS OVER NARRATIVE REVIEWS

Designed to address a focused clinical question
Describes explicit methods used to identify as many of the relevant trials as possible
Reports literature search dates
Describes and applies predefined study inclusion criteria
Formally assesses characteristics of studies associated with biases
Follows explicit methods for weighing and synthesizing studies
Can pool studies quantitatively, leading to more precise estimates and increased statistical power
Can test for statistical heterogeneity and explore reasons for heterogeneity through subgroup, sensitivity, and other analyses
Research gaps and areas of uncertainty more clearly delineated
Can test for and estimate effects of publication bias on results
Conclusions more directly linked to data and analyses

Adapted from Chou R. Using evidence in pain practice. Part I. Assessing quality of systematic reviews and clinical practice guidelines. *Pain Medicine* 2008;9:518–530, with permission.

over traditional review articles are shown in Table 10.8. A high-quality systematic review minimizes bias and random error by using transparent, reproducible, and objective methods. In addition to summarizing existing data, systematic reviews can also increase statistical power for evaluating low frequency events, provide more precise estimates of treatment effects, permit formal comparisons between studies, permit formal assessments of publication bias, and help delineate areas of uncertainty.

Before trusting the results of systematic reviews, it is important to critically evaluate whether rigorous methods were used. In fact, results of lower quality reviews can be misleading, as they are more likely than higher quality reviews to produce positive conclusions about the effectiveness of interventions.[115,117] Table 10.9 lists some factors that can influence whether a systematic review is likely to be reliable. A number of other methods for assessing the quality of systematic reviews are available, including the more detailed list of criteria in the Assessment of Multiple Systematic Reviews (AMSTAR) tool.[118] All quality rating methods are based on the idea that systematic reviews that are comprehensive, up-to-date, and use appropriate methods to identify, select, assess, and synthesize the literature are more likely to provide a complete and unbiased picture than those that use suboptimal methods.

The Cochrane Collaboration is an international effort to systematically review the results of multiple randomized clinical

TABLE 10.9

FACTORS TO CONSIDER WHEN ASSESSING QUALITY OF SYSTEMATIC REVIEWS

Was the search comprehensive?
Was selection of studies unbiased?
Is the systematic review current?
Was quality of included studies appropriately assessed?
Was evidence combined and summarized appropriately?
Was publication bias assessed?
Are the conclusions justified?

From Chou R. Using evidence in pain practice. Part I. Assessing quality of systematic reviews and clinical practice guidelines. *Pain Medicine* 2008;9: 518–530, with permission.

trials and make the results widely available via the Internet. The number of Cochrane reviews on pain topics is rapidly expanding, and many have been published in conventional journals as well as in the Cochrane Library.

CONCLUSION

Despite the rapid growth of research literature on the treatment of pain, there remain wide variations in care and the successive use of fads that are later demonstrated to be ineffective when well-designed studies are performed. Both the prevalence of painful conditions and their associated disability are increasing, and there is only a limited professional consensus on optimal approaches to many painful conditions. The disappointing pace of progress may be partly the result of few comprehensive theories that would guide treatment innovations. However, an equally important factor may be the methodological inadequacy of the research used to justify the introduction of new or innovative therapies to clinical care. Flaws in research design jeopardize not only the internal validity of research results, but also their generalizability to routine clinical practice. Greater attention to scientific principles in the design of clinical research should accelerate progress in this area, lead to more consistent clinical practices, and improve patient care.

References

1. Cherkin DC, Deyo RA, Loeser JD, et al. An international comparison of back surgery rates. *Spine* 1994;19:1201–1206.
2. Weinstein JN, Lurie JD, Olson PR, et al. United States' trends and regional variations in lumbar spine surgery: 1992–2003. *Spine* 2006;31:2707–2714.
3. Volinn E, Mayer J, Diehr P, et al. Small area analysis of surgery for low-back pain. *Spine* 1992;17:575–579.
4. Deyo RA. Fads in the treatment of low back pain. *N Engl J Med* 1991; 325(14):1039–1040.
5. Eidelman RS, Hollar D, Hebert PR, et al. Randomized trials of vitamin E in the treatment and prevention of cardiovascular disease. *Arch Intern Med* 2004;164:1552–1556.
6. Herrington DM, Howard TD. From presumed benefit to potential harm—hormone therapy and heart disease. *New Engl J Med* 2003;349: 519–521.
7. Turner JA, Deyo RA, Loeser JD, et al. The importance of placebo effects in pain treatment and research. *JAMA* 1994;271:1609–1614.
8. Freburger JK, Holmes GM, Agans RP, et al. The rising prevalence of chronic low back pain. *Arch Intern Med* 2009;169:251–258.
9. Friedly J, Chan L, Deyo R. Increases in lumbosacral injections in the Medicare population. *Spine* 2007;32:1754–1760.
10. Martin BI, Deyo RA, Mirza SK, et al. Expenditures and health status among adults with back and neck problems. *JAMA* 2008;299:656–664.
11. Briss PA, Zaza S, Pappaioanou M, et al. Developing an evidence-based Guide to Community Preventive Services—methods. The Task Force on Community Preventive Services. *Am J Prev Med* 2000;18(suppl 1):35–43.
12. Carey TS, Boden SD. A critical guide to case series reports. *Spine* 2003;28: 1631–1634.
13. Taylor RS, Van Buyten J, Buscher E. Spinal cord stimulation for chronic back pain and leg pain and failed back surgery syndrome: a systematic review and analysis of progressive factors. *Spine* 2005;30(1):152–160.
14. Pengel LHM, Herbert RD, et al. Acute low back pain: systematic review of its prognosis. *BMJ* 2003;327:323–327.
15. Whitney CW, Von Korff M. Regression to the mean in treated versus untreated chronic pain. *Pain* 1992;50:281–285.
16. Deyo RA. Practice variations, treatment fads, rising disability. *Spine* 1993; 18(15):2153–2162.
17. Sartwell P, Merrell M. Influence of the dynamic character of chronic disease on the interpretation of morbidity rates. *Am J Public Health* 1952;42: 579–584.
18. Albrecht J, Meves A, Bigby M. Case reports and case series from Lancet had significant impact on medical literature. *J Clin Epidemiol* 2005;58: 1227–1232.
19. Hartz A, Benson K, Glaser J, et al. Assessing observational studies of spinal fusion and chemonucleolysis. *Spine* 2003;28:2268–2275.
20. Eddy DM. Medicine, money, and mathematics. *Bulletin of the American College of Surgeons* 1992;77:36–49.
21. Glasziou P, Chalmers I, Rawlins M, et al. When are randomised trials unnecessary? Picking signal from noise. *BMJ* 2007;334:349–351.
22. Brinkhaus B, Witt CM, Jena S, et al. Acupuncture in patients with chronic low back pain: a randomized controlled trial. *Arch Intern Med* 2006;166: 450–457.
23. Cherkin DC, Deyo RA, Street JH, et al. Pitfalls of patient education. Limited success of a program for back pain in primary care. *Spine* 1996;21(3): 345–355.
24. Humphrey LL, Chan BK, Sox HC. Postmenopausal hormone replacement therapy and the primary prevention of cardiovascular disease. *Ann Intern Med* 2002;137:273–284.
25. Coronary Drug Project Research Group. Influence of adherence to treatment and response of cholesterol on mortality in the coronary drug project. *N Engl J Med* 1980;303:1038–1041.
26. Bogduk N, Karasek M. Two-year follow-up of a controlled trial of intradiscal electrothermal anuloplasty for chronic low back pain resulting from internal disc disruption. *Spine J* 2002;2(5):343–350.
27. Freeman BJ, Fraser RD, Cain CM, et al. A randomized, double-blind, controlled trial: intradiscal electrothermal therapy versus placebo for the treatment of chronic discogenic low back pain. *Spine* 2005;30(21):2369–2377.
28. Pauza KJ, Howell S, Dreyfuss P, et al. A randomized, placebo-controlled trial of intradiscal electrothermal therapy for the treatment of discogenic low back pain. *Spine J* 2004;4(1):27–35.
29. McMahon AD. Observation and experiment with the efficacy of drugs: a warning example from a cohort of nonsteroidal anti-inflammatory and ulcer-healing drug users. *Am J Epidemiol* 2001;154:557–562.
30. Normand ST, Sykora K, Li P, et al. Readers guide to critical appraisal of cohort studies: 3. Analytical strategies to reduce confounding. *BMJ* 2005; 330:1021–1023.
31. Miettinen OS. The need for randomization in the study of intended effects. *Statistics in Medicine* 1983;2:267–271.
32. Psaty BM, Koepsell TD, Lin D, et al. Assessment and control for confounding by indication in observational studies. *J Am Geriatr Soc* 1999;47:749–754.
33. Schulz KF, Grimes DA. Allocation concealment in randomised trials: defending against deciphering. *Lancet* 2002;359:614–618.
34. Schulz KF, Chalmers I, Hayes RJ, et al. Empirical evidence of bias. Dimensions of methodological quality associated with estimates of treatment effects in controlled trials. *JAMA* 1995;273(5):408–412.
35. Carroll D, Trawer M, McQuay H, et al. Randomization is important in studies with pain outcomes: systematic review of transcutaneous electrical nerve stimulation in acute postoperative pain. *Br J Anaesth* 1996;77:798–803.
36. Chalmers TC, Celano P, Sacks HS, et al. Bias in treatment assignment in controlled clinical trials. *New Engl J Med* 1983;309:1358–1361.
37. Moher D, Pham B, Jones A, et al. Does quality of reports of randomised trials affect estimates of intervention efficacy reported in meta-analyses? *Lancet* 1998;352(9128):609–613.
38. Schulz KF. Subverting randomization in controlled trials. *JAMA* 1995;274: 1456–1458.
39. Campbell MK, Elbourne DR, Altman DG, for the CONSORT Group. CONSORT statement: extension to cluster randomised trials. *BMJ* 2004;328: 702–708.
40. Donner A, Birkett N, Buck C. Randomization by cluster: sample size requirement and analysis. *Am J Epidemiol* 1981;114:906–914.
41. Guyatt G. Users' guides to the medical literature: II. How to use an article about therapy or prevention. A. Are the results of the study valid? *JAMA* 1993;270(21):2598–2601.
42. Guyatt G. Users' guides to the medical literature: II. How to use an article about therapy or prevention. B. What were the results and will they help me in caring for my patients? *JAMA* 1994;271(1):59–63.
43. van Tulder M, Furlan AD, Bombardier C, Bouter L, the Editorial Board of the Cochrane Collaboration Back Review Group. Updated method guidelines for systematic reviews in the Cochrane Collaboration Back Review Group. *Spine* 2003;28(12):1290–1299.
44. Moher D, Schulz KF, Altman D, for the CONSORT group. The CONSORT statement: revised recommendations for improving the quality of reports of parallel-group randomized trials. *JAMA* 2001;285(15):1987–1991.
45. Assmann SF, Pocock SJ, Enos LE, et al. Subgroup analysis and other (mis)uses of baseline data in clinical trials. [see comment]. *Lancet* 2000;355(9209): 1064–1069.
46. Roberts C, Torgerson DJ. Baseline imbalance in randomised controlled trials. *BMJ* 1999;319:185.
47. Wood LE, Egger M, Gluud LL, et al. Empirical evidence of bias in treatment effect estimates in controlled trials with different interventions and outcomes: meta-epidemiological study. *BMJ* 2008;336:601–605.
48. Schulz KF, Chalmers I, Altman DG. The landscape and lexicon of blinding in randomized trials. *Ann Intern Med* 2002;136(3):254–259.
49. Machado LA, Kamper SJ, Herbert RD, et al. Imperfect placebos are common in low back pain trials: a systematic review of the literature. *Eur Spine J* 2008; 17:889–904.
50. Deyo RA, Walsh NE, Schoenfeld LS, et al. Can trials of physical treatments be blinded? The example of transcutaneous electrical nerve stimulation for chronic pain. *Am J Phys Med Rehabil* 1990;69(1):6–10 (comment 219–220).
51. Elbourne DR, Altman DG, Higgins JP, et al. A meta-analyses involving crossover trials: methodological issues. *Int J Epidemiol* 2002;31(1):140–149.
52. Ongley MJ, Klein RG, Dorman TA, et al. A new approach to the treatment of chronic low back pain. *Lancet* 1987;2(8551):143–146.
53. Klein R, Eek B, DeLong W, et al. A randomized double-blind trial of dextrose-glycerine-phenol injections for chronic, low back pain. *J Spinal Disord* 1993; 6(1):23–33.

54. Fisher LD, Dixon DO, Herson J, et al, eds. *Intention to Treat in Clinical Trials*. New York: Marcel Dekker; 1990.

55. Weinstein JN, Tosteson TD, Lurie JD, et al. Surgical vs nonoperative treatment for lumbar disk herniation: the Spine Patient Outcomes Research Trial (SPORT): a randomized trial. *JAMA* 2006;296(20):2441–2450.

56. Deyo RA. Back surgery—who needs it? *N Engl J Med* 2007;356:2239–2243.

57. Deyo RA. Measuring the functional status of patients with low back pain. *Arch Phys Med Rehabil* 1988;69:1044–1053.

58. Feinstein AR. Clinical biostatistics XLI. Hard science, soft data, and challenges of choosing clinical variables in research. *Clin Pharmacol Ther* 1977;22:485–498.

59. Dworkin RH, Turk DC, Farrar JT, et al. Core outcome measures for chronic pain clinical trials: IMMPACT recommendations. *Pain* 2005;113:9–19.

60. Carey TS, Mielenz TJ. Measuring outcomes in back care. *Spine* 2007;32(suppl 11):S9–S14.

61. Furlan AD, Sandoval JA, Mailis-Gagnon A, et al. Opioids for chronic noncancer pain: a meta-analysis of effectiveness and side effects. *CMAJ* 2006;174(11):1589–1594.

62. Hayden J, van Tulder M, Malmivaara A, et al. Exercise therapy for low-back pain. *Cochrane Database of Systematic Reviews* 2005;(3):CD000335.

63. Bergner M, Bobbitt RA, Carter WB, et al. The Sickness Impact Profile: development and final revision of a health status measure. *Med Care* 1981;19:787–805.

64. Follick MJ, Smith TW, Ahern DK. The Sickness Impact Profile: a global measure of disability in chronic low back pain. *Pain* 1985;21:67–76.

65. Ware JE, Sherbourne C. The MOS 36-item short-form survey (SF-36). I. Conceptual framework and item selection. *Med Care* 1992;30:473–483.

66. Roland M, Fairbank J. The Roland-Morris Disability Questionnaire and the Oswestry Disability Questionnaire. *Spine* 2000;25:3115–3124.

67. Meenan RF, Gertman PM, Mason JH. Measuring health status in arthritis: the Arthritis Impact Measurement Scales. *Arthritis Rheum* 1980;23:146–152.

68. Bellamy N, Buchanan WW, Goldsmith CH, et al. Validation study of WOMAC: a health status instrument for measuring clinically important patient relevant outcomes to antirheumatic drug therapy in patients with osteoarthritis of the hip or knee. *J Rheumatol* 1988;15:1833–1840.

69. Deyo RA, Tsui-Wu YJ. Functional disability due to back pain: a population-based study indicating the importance of socioeconomic factors. *Arthritis Rheum* 1987;30:1247–1253.

70. Dworkin RH, Turk DC, Wyrwich KW, et al. Interpreting the clinical importance of treatment outcomes in chronic pain clinical trials: IMMPACT recommendations. *J Pain* 2008;9:105–121.

71. Ostelo RW, Deyo RA, Stratford P, et al. Interpreting change scores for pain and functional status in low back pain: towards international consensus regarding minimal important change. *Spine* 2008;33:90–94.

72. Goodman SN. Toward evidence-based medical statistics. 1: The P value fallacy. *Ann Intern Med* 1999;130(12):995–1004.

73. Altman DG, Bland JM. Absence of evidence is not evidence of absence. *BMJ* 1995;311:485.

74. Freiman JA, Chalmers TC, Smith H Jr, et al. The importance of beta, the type II error and sample size in the design and interpretation of the randomized control trial. *N Engl J Med* 1978;299:690–694.

75. Deyo RA, Bass JE, Walsh NE, et al. Prognostic variability among chronic pain patients: implications for study design, interpretation, and reporting. *Arch Phys Med Rehabil* 1988;69:174–178.

76. Rothwell PM. External validity of randomised controlled trials: "to whom do the results of this trial apply?" *Lancet* 2005;365(9453):82–93.

77. Haynes B. Can it work? Does it work? Is it worth it? The testing of healthcare interventions is evolving. *BMJ* 1999;319:652–653.

78. Gartlehner G, Hansen RA, Nissman D, et al. A simple and valid tool distinguished efficacy from effectiveness studies. *J Clin Epidemiol* 2006;59(10):1040–1048.

79. Rothwell PM. Treating individuals 2. Subgroup analysis in randomised controlled trials: importance, indications, and interpretation. *Lancet* 2005;365(9454):176–186.

80. Clegg DO, Reda DJ, Harris CL, et al. Glucosamine, chondroitin sulfate, and the two in combination for painful knee osteoarthritis. *N Engl J Med* 2006;354:795–808.

81. Als-Nielsen B, Chen W, Gluud C, et al. Association of funding and conclusions in randomized drug trials: a reflection of treatment effect or adverse events. *JAMA* 2003;290(7):921–928.

82. Lexchin J, Bero LA, Djulbegovic B, et al. Pharmaceutical industry sponsorship and research outcome and quality: systematic review. *BMJ* 2003;326(7400):1167–1170.

83. Ezzet KA. The prevalence of corporate funding in adult lower extremity research and its correlation with reported results. *J Arthroplasty* 2003;18(7 suppl 1):138–145.

84. Shah RV, Albert TJ, Bruegel-Sanchez V, et al. Industry support and correlation to study outcome for papers published in Spine. *Spine* 2005;30:1099–1104.

85. Easterbrook PJ, Berlin JA, Gopalan R, et al. Publication bias in clinical research. *Lancet* 1991;337:867–872.

86. Bekelman JE, Li Y, Gross CP. Scope and impact of financial conflicts of interest in biomedical research: a systematic review. *JAMA* 2003;289:454–465.

87. Lee K, Bacchetti P, Sim I. Publication of clinical trials supporting successful new drug applications: a literature analysis. *PLoS Med* 2008;5:e191.

88. Chan AW, Hróbjartsson A, Haahr MT, et al. Empirical evidence for selective reporting of outcomes in randomized trials: comparison of protocols to published articles. *JAMA* 2004;291(20):2457–2465.

89. Melander H, Ahlqvist-Rastad J, Meijer G, et al. Evidence b(i)ased medicine—selective reporting from studies sponsored by pharmaceutical industry: review of studies in new drug applications. *BMJ* 2003;326(7400):1171–1173.

90. Rising K, Bacchetti P, Bero L. Reporting bias in drug trials submitted to the Food and Drug Administration: review of publication and presentation. *PLoS Med* 2008;5:e217.

91. Turner EH, Matthews AM, Linardatos E, et al. Selective publication of antidepressant trials and its influence on apparent efficacy. *N Engl J Med* 2008;358:252–260.

92. Hill KP, Ross JS, Egilman DS, et al. The ADVANTAGE seeding trial: a review of internal documents. *Ann Intern Med* 2008;149:251–258.

93. Sterne JA, Egger M, Smith GD. Systematic reviews in health care: Investigating and dealing with publication and other biases in meta-analysis. *BMJ* 2001;323:101–105.

94. Drazen JM, Morrissey S, Curfman GD. Open clinical trials. *N Engl J Med* 2007;357:1756–1757.

95. Laine C, Horton R, DeAngelis CD, et al. Clinical trial registration—looking back and moving ahead. *N Engl J Med* 2007;356:2734–2736.

96. Loke YK, Price D, Herxheimer A. Systematic reviews of adverse effects: framework for a structured approach. *BMC Med Res Methodol* 2007;7:32.

97. Ioannidis JP, Lau J. Completeness of safety reporting in randomized trials: an evaluation of 7 medical areas. *JAMA* 2001;285(4):437–443.

98. Chou R, Helfand M. Challenges in systematic reviews that assess treatment harms. *Ann Intern Med* 2005;142(12 Pt 2):1090–1099.

99. Golder S, Loke YK. Is there evidence for biased reporting of published adverse effects data in pharmaceutical industry-funded studies? *Brit J Clin Pharmacol* 2008;66:767–773.

100. Van Zee A. The promotion and marketing of oxycontin: commercial triumph, public health tragedy. *Am J Public Health* 2009;99:221–227.

101. Psaty BM, Koepsell T, Lin D, et al. Assessment and control for confounding by indication in observational studies. *J Am Geriatr Soc* 1999;47:749–754.

102. Barber JA, Thompson SG. Analysis and interpretation of cost data in randomised controlled trials: review of published studies. *BMJ* 1998;317:1195–2000.

103. Zwarenstein M, Treweek S, Gagnier JJ, et al. Improving the reporting of pragmatic trials: an extension of the CONSORT statement. *BMJ* 2008;337:a2390.

104. Thomas KJ, MacPherson H, Thorpe L, et al. Randomised controlled trial of a short course of traditional acupuncture compared with usual care for persistent non-specific low back pain. *BMJ* 2006;333(7569):623.

105. Devereaux PJ, Bhandari M, Clarke M, et al. Need for expertise based randomised controlled trials. *BMJ* 2005;330:88.

106. Lohr KN. Emerging methods in comparative effectiveness and safety: symposium overview and summary. *Med Care* 2007;45:S5–S8.

107. Glenny AM, Altman DG, Song F, et al. Indirect comparisons of competing interventions. *Health Technol Assess* 2005;9(26):1–134.

108. Chou R, Carson S, Chan BK. Gabapentin versus tricyclic antidepressants for diabetic neuropathy and post-herpetic neuralgia: discrepancies between direct and indirect meta-analyses of randomized controlled trials. *J Gen Intern Med* 2009;24:178–188.

109. Piaggio G, Elbourne DR, Altman DG, et al. Reporting of noninferiority and equivalence randomized trials: an extension of the CONSORT statement. *JAMA* 2006;295(10):1152–1160.

110. Greene WL, Concato J, Feinstein AR. Claims of equivalence in medical research: are they supported by the evidence? *Ann Intern Med* 2000;132(9):715–722.

111. Chalmers TC. A potpourri of RCT topics. *Control Clin Trials* 1982;3:285–298.

112. UK BEAM Trial Team. United Kingdom back pain exercise and manipulation (UK BEAM) randomised trial: effectiveness of physical treatments for back pain in primary care. *BMJ* 2004;329(7479):1377.

113. Brittain E, Wittes J. Factorial designs in clinical trials: the effects of non-compliance and subadditivity. *Stat Med* 1989;8:161–171.

114. Goodman SN. Toward evidence-based medical statistics. 2: The Bayes factor. *Ann Intern Med* 1999;130(12):1005–1013.

115. Jadad AR, Carroll D, Moore A, et al. Developing a database of published reports of randomised clinical trials in pain research. *Pain* 1996;66:239–246.

116. Cook DJ, Mulrow CD, Haynes RB. Systematic reviews: synthesis of best evidence for clinical decisions. *Ann Intern Med* 1997;126:376–380.

117. Furlan AD, Clarke J, Esmail R, et al. A critical review of reviews on the treatment of chronic low back pain. *Spine* 2001;26(7):E155–E162.

118. Shea BJ, Grimshaw JM, Wells GA, et al. Development of AMSTAR: a measurement tool to assess the methodological quality of systematic reviews. *BMC Med Res Methodol* 2007;7:10.

CHAPTER 11 ■ SOCIOCULTURAL DIMENSIONS OF PAIN MANAGEMENT

DAVID B. MORRIS

"Chronic pain is a transdermal phenomenon and the environment is always a player in the chronic pain patient's predicament."
—J. D. Loeser[1]

INTRODUCTION

"A threshold has been crossed," writes sociologist Nikolas Rose.[2] Rose is Director of the BIOS Centre for the Study of Bioscience, Biomedicine, Biotechnology and Society at the London School of Economics and Political Science. He wants to avoid what he calls "breathless epochalization"—a sense that history is undergoing an abrupt massive transformation—and he understands the present as the unfolding of "multiple histories" that emerge from the intersection of numerous "contingent pathways." Nonetheless, he also provides in *The Politics of Life Itself* (2007) an indispensable framework for considering how much has changed since the first edition of John Bonica's ground-breaking text *The Management of Pain* (1953). Pain too has changed, especially chronic pain, as pain has moved from the status of symptom to diagnosis, from the category of what humans passively endure (a mark of our changeless humanity) to what patients and health professionals together, as partnered agents of somatic change, now actively manage.

The single change that Rose sees as the embodiment of our unfolding multiple histories of the present and future is what he calls "a molecular vision of life." Contemporary medicine and the biotechnologies on which it relies increasingly understand life at a sub-cellular level and with consequences that extend far beyond the old categories of illness and health, of pathology and normality, of treatment and enhancement. The new techno-medicine, he argues, does not just cure disease or correct organic damage but, in its promise to refigure human vital processes at the molecular level, even changes "what it is to be a biological organism."

What it is to be a biological organism has always included vulnerability to pain. Not only has pain changed since 1953—including the volume of research devoted to eliminating it—but also pain patients. Today traditional patients have often been transformed into well-briefed self-educated medical consumers, relentlessly informed (or misinformed) by Internet sites and by ad campaigns. Often too (in addition to their newly self-aware status as proto-plaintiffs) patients accept a role implicit in the molecular gaze as they embrace a unique "genetic citizenship."[3] Test the fetus for Down syndrome. Regulate your cholesterol. Find the gene for pain and knock it out. Never mind that most researchers do not seek a single specific "gene for" but rather variations in multiple loci within multiple gene systems, with resulting wide distribution of phenotypes and of susceptibilities. Chronic pain, once a burden, is now a scandal. No longer a predictable companion of old age or a fact about the human condition, chronic pain represents an unaccountable failure of the molecular gaze to identify a local culprit neuron, a shameful lockout from the promise of somatic optimization. The damage that chronic pain inflicts on body, mind, and spirit leaves many patients not at the threshold of a shining future but in a futureless limbo.

What follows, then, is an effort to place the new understanding of pain within a conflict-rich field where sociocultural explanations often run counter to the expectations of a molecular gaze that extends far beyond medicine. Today the push for cellular microtherapies and extreme bioengineering may come less from doctors than from patients. ("Hey, doc, can't we inject some stem cells into it?") The dilemma that has developed over the past 50 years, clearer to physicians than to patients, is that chronic pain, in its numerous types from migraine to cancer, is often as amenable to sociocultural analysis and to psychosocial therapies as to biomedical cure. Clearly it is an advance to understand gout as a type of congenital arthritis—not, as in this 19th-century etching (Fig. 11.1), a moral punishment for aristocratic luxuriousness.

The pain of gout, however, clearly correlates not only with molecular processes affecting serum uric acid levels, but also with psychosocial forces underlying diet.[4] What most patients don't know about chronic pain—its links with beliefs, cultures, and social practices—is exactly what an evidence-based, best-practices pain treatment in the era of the molecular gaze cannot ignore.

WHAT IS TRANSDERMAL PAIN?

Pain, especially chronic pain, is a transdermal phenomenon in that it occurs not only within an individual nervous system, including the brain, but also within a social and cultural environment. "Our concepts of pain, impairment, and disability," writes Wilbert E. Fordyce, "must consider environmental factors as well as the person."[5] Clinical practice frequently reduces environmental factors to three main stressors—employment, family, and alcohol or drugs—but this trio can serve as placeholder for a more extensive mix of sociocultural variables. The fundamental question is whether the sociocultural environment merely *influences* pain that already exists as a purely biological phenomenon, simply modulating it, or does the sociocultural environment (beyond mere influence and modulation) help to *construct* and to *constitute* pain.

The difference between influence and construction is significant, with a possibly direct impact on treatment. A theory of influence understands pain as independent of environmental factors, which provide mere triggers or nuances. For influence theory, the individual nervous system alone generates pain, and pain is solely a somatic event, to which the social or cultural environment adds mere modifications. Modifications add local color—such as an honor-driven suppression of a mother's cries in childbirth—but the social environment does not help construct the pain. A theory of construction, by contrast, sees human pain as coming into existence *only* as an individual nervous system

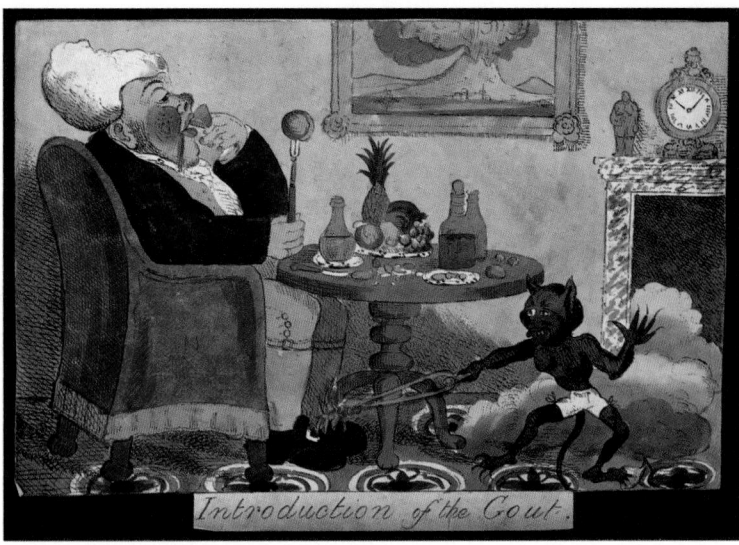

Introduction of the Gout.

FIGURE 11.1 George Cruikshank. *Introduction of the gout.* 1819 (This impression 1835). Colored etching. (Courtesy of the Wellcome Library, London.)

encounters a specific sociocultural environment. The environment does more than trigger, modify, or color pain—it helps to *constitute* pain. Minus a sociocultural context intrinsic to mental life, the transmission of nociceptive impulses may generate autonomic responses, the human equivalent of a tail flick, but nociception alone does not constitute human pain, which, according to the prestigious International Association for the Study of Pain (IASP) in its classification of pain terms, is "always a psychological state."[6]

Influence theory and construction theory both marshal strong arguments and persuasive evidence, and quick resolution seems unlikely, even unnecessary. The important point here is that most pain specialists today attribute a significant role to the sociocultural environment—a truly historic change in thinking about pain and pain management. This recent transformation in thinking about pain has important implications for pain management. "Prior to 1960," writes John Loeser, "there were no pain specialists. Only one pain textbook had been written—the first edition of *Bonica's Management of Pain*, published in 1953. It was mainly the work of one man. There were no journals devoted to pain, no dedicated research laboratories, and no funding programs aimed at pain research or training for clinicians. . . . Pain was always described as a byproduct of a disease state; the implication was that proper treatment of disease would relieve pain. The sensory nervous system was envisioned as a passive set of wires that conducted incoming impulses to the brain."[7] The molecular gaze, as it intensified its focus, provided not only a greatly revised picture of the human nervous system but also a new understanding of pain.

The Management of Pain, in its first edition, contained no discussion of sociocultural environment. Herbert S. Ripley contributed a brief chapter entitled "The Psychologic Basis of Pain," which came after far more substantial chapters on the anatomical, neurophysiological, and physiopathological basis of pain, but there was little follow-up beyond another chapter by Ripley, "Psychotherapeutic Methods in the Management of Pain." Pain, nonetheless, had decisively entered a new domain of medical management. It is largely due to Bonica and to his colleagues in the emerging field of pain medicine that patients today no longer regard pain as a mostly inescapable aspect of the human condition but rather—in the tradition of the molecular gaze—a treatable, manageable disorder. The transformations that followed *The Management of Pain*, however, consistently expanded an awareness of how far the molecular gaze alone is insufficient.

The new managers of pain, if a sociologist might highlight what doctors regard as self-evident, are now doctors and health care professionals. What matters in this truism is that medicine and health care now account for 16% of the U.S. gross domestic product and, in any nation, cannot be cordoned off from the surrounding culture and subcultures. The surrounding culture interpenetrates medicine and health care, just as cultures and subcultures today are inescapably medicalized. Pain too has been medicalized in the (once not obvious) sense of calling for scientific-technical knowledge—rather than, say, for trepanation, prayer, or home remedies. The medicalization of pain, which patients and doctors may both regard as necessary, is not without consequences, especially when medical care fails. A sociocultural perspective thus needs to emphasize that pain medicine is not a neutral byproduct of scientific knowledge. Pain medicine too belongs to a new sociocultural environment that influences and helps to construct pain. That is, many patients experience pain only within a context that includes pain specialists, both official and unofficial, from orthopedists, oncologists, and neurologists to acupuncturists and homeopaths. Pain specialists cannot excuse themselves from discussion as if they were mere impartial technicians, objective researchers, or altruistic caregivers—who analyze and treat pain but do not affect how patients understand or experience it. Pain specialists are among the players in the new sociocultural environment that helps constitute the chronic pain patient's predicament.

The new active role for pain specialists is certainly driven by patient demand, but not *solely* by patient demand, and it also cannot be ignored as inconsequential. When clinicians employ evidence-based practices, chart pain as a vital sign, or "game" insurance systems on behalf of patients, their actions contribute to the creation and maintenance of a significant new sociocultural environment within which patients experience pain. Although pain medicine did not invent insurance payers and disability systems, it operates today within a field of economic compensation that sets patients in an altered relationship to their pain. In a controversial recommendation, an IASP task force argues that chronic nonspecific low back pain in the workplace, in the absence of an organic lesion and under specified circumstances, should be reconceptualized not as a medical problem but as "activity intolerance."[8] *Activity intolerance* is less a diagnosis than a counter-narrative meant to contest the sociocultural script that redeems chronic low back pain for disability payments and for freedom from job obligations. From the patient's perspective, the not-inevitable passage from citizenship to patienthood—from person-in-pain to pain patient—involves an invisible phenomenology of forms to fill out, waiting rooms, secretaries, insurance companies, drugs, side effects, disability systems, referrals, more waiting rooms, indignities, task forces, protocols, and waiting rooms.[9] In short, it involves a web of sociocultural interrelations that reframe pain.

FROM INFLUENCE TO CONSTRUCTION: ETHNICITY, RACE, SEX, AND GENDER

The irony is that, while patients increasingly embody the expectations of a molecular gaze, pain medicine finds increasing evidence to support a nonmolecular and sociocultural understanding of pain. Culture and biology both contribute to pain, as a biopsychosocial model implies, interweaving distributed neural networks with rites of passage or disability payments. Although a sociocultural perspective cannot provide a full account of pain, even an openly lopsided account here helps illustrate how human pain is always intersubjective. It depends on social systems from family, church, and nation to jobs and prisons, just as it meshes with variable cultural practices from stoic dispassion to pharmaceutical trials. Of course, some people defy social systems and oppose cultural norms. Even exiles, immigrants, strangers, and renegades, however, cannot wholly live outside the social environments that help shape their resistances. Sociocultural environments are not places, not material locales that you might conceivably be outside of, but internalized subsets of a surrounding *lifeworld* experienced as a state of body, mind, and emotion. Such states remain accessible in memory even when people change locale. Chronic pain, as a mind/body state, is inextricable from the sociocultural lifeworlds that shape it.

There is no question that sociocultural environments shape pain. The relation, however, seldom reduces to a direct connection in which culture *causes* pain, in the sense that stress, say, triggers the biological cascade that produces a tension headache. (Cultures, however, certainly can cause stress.) Data are often conflicting or inconsistent, as in laboratory studies about racial tolerance for thermal pain,[10] especially where underlying categories such as race are poorly defined. Some links between pain and its sociocultural environments, however, are clear and correctible. In New York City, nonwhite patients (often blacks and Hispanics) who lived in disadvantaged neighborhoods had substantially less access to pharmacies than did white patients in affluent neighborhoods. Moreover, the pharmacies in disadvantaged areas did not maintain adequate stocks of pain medication.[11] A sociocultural environment that reduces access to medication indirectly but clearly has an impact on pain. Although reduced access did not directly cause pain, it surely *maintained* pain (pain *eliminated* in other communities) through unequal and unfair social practices.

The 1996 SUPPORT study demonstrated that 50% of hospitalized seriously ill or dying patients failed to receive adequate pain medication.[12] Hospitals, like doctors, belong to the larger sociocultural environment, an environment defined by drug abuse and opioid-phobia, and here too the environment indirectly but clearly influences pain. Researchers can disentangle pain from indirect environmental influences, at least theoretically or in the lab. Anesthesia erases pain, temporarily, by targeting the nervous system alone, not the environment. The paradox, however, is that anesthesia belongs to the sociocultural environment of the hospital, just as illegal street drugs belong to the sociocultural environment of the street. Pure pain—pain free from all direct or indirect sociocultural influence—is a pain that exists nowhere except in theory.

Race and ethnicity are frequently discussed in recent studies on pain, but discussion is often impeded by failures to clarify underlying concepts. Numerous researchers report ethnic differences in the prevalence and severity of pain, and they find interethnic differences in tolerance levels for clinical and experimentally induced pains.[13] Attitudes toward pain, for example, show sharp differences along ethnic lines among surgical patients in Australia.[14] Yet, just what *are* ethnicity and race? Ethnicity is traditionally defined as perceived cultural distinctiveness, while race refers to perceived physical and biogenetic characteristics. The medical literature on ethnicity and pain is extensive enough to have drawn several review articles.[15,16] One review concluded that racial and ethnic disparities in pain perception, assessment, and treatment are found in various medical settings and across all types of pain.[17] The crucial point, however, despite mixed data and questionable assumptions, is that both ethnicity and race affect pain mainly through sociocultural influences, not (with a few exceptions such as sickle cell pain) through specific common genetic traits.

Pain specialists need to engage with recent thinking about race and ethnicity. While a few single-gene defects are responsible for the handful of diseases typical of specific groups, such as Tay-Sachs disease among east European Jews, there is no genetic signature for race. Skin color is a surface similarity that links population groups as different as their languages: say, Italians and Swedes, Scots and Russians, Belgians and Croats. Blackness, as a racial category, includes both West Africans and the historically very different East Africans, as well as Haitians, African Americans, some Hispanics, and various hyphenated groups linked mainly by skin color. The census term "Asian" has a different meaning in Europe than in America, and census data in Western democracies make race and ethnicity a matter of self-identification. In general, there is more genetic variation within (so-called) races than across races, and biological anthropologists regard both race and ethnicity as social rather than genetic categories.[18] The recent turn in health care discussion tends to emphasize *population groups*, where biology and genetics are relevant but not determinative. Rose summarizes this recent movement away from reductive ideas of racial science: "Key, here, is not so much race, but the belief that a particular community has specific health needs that may have a genomic basis, and that research on the genomic basis is essential if these needs are to be met."[19] Population groups, once relatively stable, are now increasingly open to intermarriage and to health-related cultural differences between immigrants and their acculturated offspring.

Race and ethnicity, then, may correlate with the specific health needs of a population group based on genomic difference, but as social categories they are malleable, contentious, and open to historical forces, especially forces associated with discrimination and intolerance. Their influence on pain management is both indirect and direct. Over half of Hispanics who presented at emergency rooms with long bone fractures did not receive pain medication and were twice as likely as similar white patients to go without pain medicine.[20,21] Clearly, medical degrees do not confer immunity from conscious or unwitting acts of discrimination. Although many blacks carry a gene that puts people of African descent at risk for sickle cell disease, their need for pain relief too often runs up against medical suspicions of drug-seeking behavior.[22,23] The history of sickle cell pain warns, like the Tuskegee syphilis experiments on black airmen, about the danger of open or covert racist attitudes within medicine that can influence pain treatment and its absences.[24,25]

Race and ethnicity may one day indicate special needs for pain medication based on genomic discoveries, but today pain management needs to focus on failures of delivery. African American cancer patients in nursing homes were 63% more likely than whites to receive no pain treatment.[26] Other minorities with cancer pain also experience inadequate pain relief[27]—in disproportion to the generally inadequate relief for all cancer patients. The unequal worldwide distribution and consumption of morphine means that adequate medication for pain is far more available to white patients than to nonwhites.[28,29] This difference is not mainly a function of income. The U.S. campaign against illegal drug trafficking makes inadequate pain relief for Mexican patients largely political in origin, wired into the sociocultural environment.[30] Pain management, in confronting questions about clinical policy and research design, must recognize that race and ethnicity are ill-defined and socially explosive categories dangerously associated with patient stereotypes. The categories apply (and mis-apply) not only to patients but also to the attitudes, beliefs, and sociocultural environments of providers and of institutions.

Sex and gender raise additional complications in assessing sociocultural influences on pain. Animal studies indicate differences between male and female rodents in pain processing, including a greater efficacy of mu-opioids in males. In humans, kappa-opioids produce significantly greater analgesia in women than in men.[31] Red-haired women (in a study that did not test men) show increased sensitivity to thermal pain and reduced responsiveness to subcutaneous lidocaine, because of specific mutations of the melanocortin-1 receptor.[32,33] Biologically based sexual differences play a role in women's pain across a range of chronic pain conditions from migraine to irritable bowel syndrome, although the precise mechanisms are often unclear. Sex steroid hormones in men and women appear to modulate different nociceptive behaviors. Pregnancy, for example, whatever its sociocultural influences associated with pain, creates an antinociception that involves delta-opioid and kappa-opioid but not mu-opioid systems.[34]

Gender differences further complicate the analysis of pain, splintering the neat sexual male/female binary into a rainbow of orientations from gay and lesbian to transgender. While a number of pain researchers examine male and female differences, there are few reliable studies exploring gender as distinct from sexual difference. One persuasive argument holds that gender is largely performative: that is, gender—no matter how individual, eccentric, or dependent on hormone therapies—constitutes a quasi-public social role.[35] The women whom Charcot photographed in his famous hysteria wards in the 19th century clearly "performed" their illness for the camera, even if unknowingly, and today women tend to perform gender roles (as overextended caregivers, for example) that are sociocultural and not entirely unrelated to pain. The same observation applies to men. Pain differences in males and females are biological, but differences in men and women are *both* biological and sociocultural. A treatment program that recognizes the complicating roles of sex, gender, ethnicity, and race—including the openness of these categories to redefinition—is well equipped to understand the multiple lines of causation and of influence that so often converge in chronic pain.

The complex interrelations between biology and culture raise a crucial question for pain management programs. Is it necessary to distinguish biological processes from sociocultural influences? Yes, where possible and with caution, for two reasons. First, drugs and surgery can sometimes erase pain associated with clear organic sources. Back pain, however, especially chronic nonspecific low back pain, exposes the limits of drugs and surgery where sociocultural forces—such as family, job, and disability—are prominently involved. Furthermore, organic lesions do not map exactly onto pain. Most adults who complain of back pain have lumbar disk disease, but so do many adults without pain complaints.[36] In America, long-term functioning of patients treated for back pain is similar whether doctors prescribe medication and bed rest or self-care and education.[37] Pain simply does not provide an accurate report of tissue damage. "The truth is that pain is a very poor reporting system," writes Patrick Wall. He adds:

"The doctrine that pain is a useful signal needs heavy qualification."[38] The erroneous belief that pain is a reliable alarm system not only justifies countless unnecessary surgeries but also cannot begin to explain why the two strongest signs predicting that an American worker will develop chronic back pain are job dissatisfaction and unsatisfactory social relations in the workplace.[39,40] It is as if the American low back is wired directly into the sociocultural work environment.

Second, one benefit of separating out sociocultural influences lies in the possibility of system-wide change in pain management. In 1999, a memorandum directed to over 1200 sites required the entire U.S. Veterans Health Administration to make policy and procedural changes implicit in the new principle that pain is the *fifth vital sign*.[41] At one VA outpatient clinic this change produced no improvement in pain-management quality,[42] but the possibilities for system-wide change are impressive. A similar directive altered policies in pain management and in palliative medicine throughout all the hospitals in the vast southwest region of the U.S. Indian Health Service.[43] Such changes acknowledge that pain medicine belongs to a surrounding sociocultural environment that includes the changing subculture of medicine. Systemic changes in pain management thus can influence not only the experience of individual patients but also the wider sociocultural environments within which patients and also nonpatients experience pain.

Can systemic changes in the sociocultural environment of medicine alter individual experience and relieve pain? The IASP defines pain as "always subjective."[44] Pain, by implication, will change when a person's subjective state sufficiently changes. Suppose that a woman from a low-income neighborhood repeatedly fails to receive adequate pain medication from her local pharmacy. Repeated frustration, humiliation, and rage constitute a significant change in her subjective state. Such damaging psychological and emotional changes, along with changes in any presumed neurobiological substrates, arguably will alter her pain for the worse. Fear, as researchers consistently show, elevates pain intensity.[45] Pain specialist Mark Sullivan argues that pain *is* an emotion.[46] Quantitative and qualitative studies are needed to show if and how systemic changes might alter individual subjective experience and thereby alter pain. Patient education and improved access to care offer two promising areas for systemic change. Effective systemic changes in pain management generate additional evidence for the importance of sociocultural environments in shaping and reshaping the individual experience of pain.

ACROSS CULTURES: PAIN BELIEFS AND PAIN BEHAVIORS

Pain varies across individuals, cultures, and times. This strong claim contradicts the universalist view that pain is a changeless sensory signal, identical in everyone, everywhere. It has been demonstrated, at least in women, that sensitivity to a variety of experimental thermal, mechanical, and chemical pain-producing stimuli has a genetic contribution.[47] Universalists, however, cannot explain why individual variations in reported pain intensity produced by exposure to an identical noxious stimulus correlate directly, as functional magnetic resonance imaging (fMRI) studies indicate, with altered brain patterns.[48] Most researchers agree that pain includes both sensory and *affective* components. These affective components of pain show wide variation across individuals and cultures. Paid volunteers in an experiment were told that exposure to an electrical stimulator might possibly produce pain, but researchers deliberately did not explain that the stimulator was set to produce nothing beyond a harmless hum. Fully one half of the volunteers, on hearing the hum, reported pain.[49] Such significant variation in pain reports no doubt involves the biopsychology of expectation,[50,51] as well as at least a passing cultural familiarity with electronics. The fact that pain and its related brain states vary significantly among individuals exposed to a similar or identical sensory stimulus is nonetheless well established by various forms of quantitative data. True, it is reported that 1950s-era surgically lobotomized patients could still feel pain but said that the pain no longer *bothered* them. It may require a philosopher to decide whether pain that fails to bother us counts as pain. (It won't often show up at pain management centers.) Pain that is wholly affect-free, however, constitutes a self-contradiction.

Real world pain, then, is characterized by an affective quality of aversiveness open to wide modulation. This aversiveness depends on cortico-limbic networks, much as anxiety correlates with activity in the septo-hippocampal system, but emotions are also in part socially constructed and socially modified.[52] Stoic philosophers exalted the use of reason to modify normal pain behavior. "If you desire to master pain/ Unroll this book and read with care," wrote an unknown Byzantine poet in verses regularly copied with the *Meditations* of Roman emperor Marcus Aurelius.[53] Athletes, dancers, yogis, and religious celebrants continue to demonstrate how minds, emotions, and sociocultural environments help modify pain. Environments are not neutral containers for bodies in pain—like mere stage sets. Environmental toxins affect human biology, and sociocultural forces shape human pain. Pain is not *contained* by the environment but influenced and very possibly *constituted* by the social and cultural world. Even the clinic and research lab are sociocultural spaces. They help shape inchoate sensation into pain as surely as ancient religions shaped pain through doctrines of demonic possession. Aversiveness and affect are, in part, learned, and whatever we learn (including what we know and fear about pain) is open to wide variation, to personal modulation, and to targeted sociocultural re-education.

Cross-cultural studies of pain further demonstrate this inherent variation. Chronic low back pain patients in Japan were compared with a similar group in the United States and found significantly less impaired in psychological, social, vocational, and avocational function.[54] Pain evoked in a laboratory setting may differ from everyday pain experienced outside the lab,[55] and outside environments include not only tangible institutions such as families, schools, and workplaces but also intangible feelings and beliefs. Beliefs and feelings often intertwine, and the resulting synergy can affect pain. The general proposition that all men are mortal, for example, is less potent than if intertwined with the particular belief that my own pain signals a brain tumor. Pain beliefs thus are less general propositions than culturally specific, affect-rich, cognitive nodes of hope, fear, and expectation. Catastrophizing—a compound of extreme fear, belief, and expectation—proved the single most important predictor for quality of life in chronic pain patients.[56] Intertwined feelings and beliefs associated with pain are never wholly private, subjective, and inaccessible, as some claim, but, crucially, both personal and *intersubjective*.

Intersubjectivity, as a phenomenon in health care, is understudied, but recent findings about obesity, based on data from the Framingham Heart Study, offer a powerful indication of its importance to illness. Obesity, according to surprising research data, appears to spread through social ties—a finding, as researchers say, that has implication for clinical and public health interventions.[57] Chronic pain too is shaped by social ties. Specific cultures encourage distinctive beliefs about pain, which come to constitute social norms that underlie distinctive practices and behaviors. These normative practices and behaviors, like the beliefs that support them, prove amenable to observation. In fact, observation of pain beliefs (via questionnaire) is a robust sub-discipline within pain medicine.[58–60] Current studies of pain beliefs focus on the big three—catastrophizing, control, and disability—but researchers are beginning to study more diverse cognitive/emo-

tional states associated with religious faith and spiritual practices[61] as well as attitudes about personal identity and self-efficacy.[62] Future studies might well expand their methods and focus to include narrative data. Cultural and personal narratives, as a vehicle for the communication of complex beliefs and feelings, help shape the pain that we live out.[63]

Transdermal pain, then, is not a subclass of pain, but rather an encompassing tautology: all pain, especially chronic pain, is transdermal. It is shaped, invisibly, by sociocultural and intersubjective forces. This counterintuitive claim seems berserk to a weekend handyman who has just hammered his thumb. The common sense sequence is hammer, tissue damage, pain. Like vision, however, common sense is the product of a developmental process that takes place only within a cultural context. (Long-blind adults who recover their eyesight often cannot adjust to the flood of unedited visual information.[64]) Pain too depends on developmental learning and cultural editing. Ice packs on a throbbing thumb invoke an elementary cultural education, as does the limited belief that pain correlates directly with tissue damage. Chronic pain requires a personal and cultural re-education in which talk of neural pathways, genetic susceptibilities, and neurotransmitters is compatible with research into modulating sociocultural variables.[65] Even neuropathic pain in laboratory rats appears to show the impact of rodent-specific social variables.[66] While the literature on sociocultural variables is too vast to review here, future research needs to contemplate two large issues so far merely touched upon: globalization and narrative.

PAIN AND GLOBALIZATION: POWER, MONEY, SYSTEMS

In *Power & Illness* (1977), sociologist Elliott A. Krause shows how health and health care are "intimately involved with the political, economic, and social struggles of the present day."[67] Krause studied power as oppressive and coercive—a perspective that is relevant to current legal, military, and medical discussions of pain in torture, say, or in capital punishment.[68,69] Michel Foucault, however, moves beyond a focus on power as oppressive, top-down, and hegemonic, expressed in prohibitions and restraints. In his later work, Foucault views power as horizontal, distributed, even demotic, expressed as usable energies flowing within a social system, like electricity coursing through the walls.[70] This later perspective illuminates the recent ongoing transformation of patients from passive subjects of a colonizing biomedical gaze to active agents, whose limited but real powers range from noncompliance and litigation to undisclosed alternative, holistic self-care. Such changes, reflected in hospitals that openly post a patient's bill of rights to adequate pain relief, suggest the need to resituate the discussion of pain management within the vast social power shift known as globalization.

Globalization holds potent implications for pain that ripple through cultures directly and indirectly. An economic analysis might focus on corporate mergers and takeovers. For example, the publicly owned, family-run, Midwest-based U.S. pharmaceutical company Upjohn, which marketed ibuprofen and its over-the-counter spin-off, Motrin, merged in 1995 with European conglomerate Pharmacia, headquartered in Sweden; the merged company Pharmacia & Upjohn in 2000 merged with Monsanto and took the name Pharmacia Corporation; and in 2002 Pharmacia Corporation was bought by the international colossus Pfizer in pursuit of full rights to the (now disgraced) blockbuster pain drug Celebrex, previously acquired by Pharmacia. Marketplace dominance consolidated in a few transnational monoliths that underwrite activities and organizations in support of pain specialists justifies Foucault's concept of *biopower*, which describes a modern, medical, state-sponsored authority over health-related activities from sexuality to population control.[71] Nikolas Rose proposes the term *biopolitics* to describe a postmodern extension of biopower to far broader supra-state manipulations of human vitality, morbidity, and mortality.[72] Pain management, inseparable from a transnational pharmaceutical industry, cannot today be fairly represented as encounters between an individual patient and a caring doctor. A full sociocultural analysis of pain management would need to situate the doctor/patient encounter within a shaping globalized biopolitics as dominant (if dimly perceived) as the force of gravity.

Money and pain? Pain patients are, of course, cared for only within systems assuring that health care professionals are paid. Even indigenous medicine involves compensation, so the key issue is not payment but the particular systems of compensation that characterize the era of global pain management. Local compensation issues are often influenced by national or international forces, such as the traffic in illegal drugs and its effect on domestic licensing and disciplinary boards charged with regulating opioids.[73] Less dramatic questions are equally important. Who is eligible for treatment in a pain center or clinic? The answer may not involve the intensity of pain but matters of citizenship and insurance coverage. Is likelihood of improvement a criterion for enrolling patients? If insurance coverage is held to enhance the likelihood of improvement, then uninsured patients are excluded. Some 16% of the U.S. population has no health insurance, with percentages far higher among black and Latino minorities. These bland statistics expose how pain is silently enfolded within systems of biopower and of biopolitics.

Biopower and *biopolitics* are not mere concepts but realities that influence the profound inequalities (in access to care and in treatment of pain) that face individual patients as the consequences of race, socioeconomic status, and the fast-changing configuration of national and international health care systems.[74] In Haiti, for example, anthropologist-physician Paul Farmer struggles against global pharmaceutical companies and cost-driven policies of the World Health Organization to provide medication for HIV/AIDS patients with multiple drug-resistant tuberculosis.[75] Even national systems of universal health care cannot ignore cost in decisions about whom to treat and how. Among postoperative patients, patient-controlled analgesia (PCA) lessens pain, shortens hospital stays, and reduces pain medication, but it is also expensive, raising unresolved questions about cost-effectiveness, social justice, and access to care.[76] Who gets it? In a balancing act that weighs cost against temporary discomfort, many patients and systems cannot afford adequate pain control.[77] There is no mechanism for creating balance—indeed, no agreement about what constitutes balance. For HIV/AIDS patients in sub-Saharan Africa who may barely find enough to eat, pain medications and nondrug therapies alike are an unaffordable luxury.[78]

The impact of changing worldwide health systems shows up in pain management as patient concern for alternative and complementary medicine. Patients today pick the latest secularized healing art from a menu of eclectic, health-related therapies marketed like vitamin pills to late-capitalist consumers in what has been described as a new global "ethnomedicine."[79] In 1990 Americans made 425 million visits to providers of complementary and alternative medicine or, as it was first called, "unconventional therapy."[80] This figure startled many analysts because it exceeded the population of the United States. It did not express an outright rejection of biomedicine, as 83% of these patients also sought treatment for the same condition from a medical doctor: significantly, they also paid 75% of all costs out-of-pocket. A sense of the illicit nonetheless surrounded these excursions outside the biomedical model. The vast majority (72%) of patients who used unconventional therapies did not tell their physicians.

Official discourse and unofficial practice—including the practice and discourse of pain medicine—has begun to change in response to this new populist, eclectic self-care that draws its principles and therapies from around the globe. From 1990 to 1997 there was an almost 50% increase in visits to "alternative medicine practitioners,"[81] a number that soon exceeded visits to primary care physicians. This change, no mere lifestyle fad, extends even to cancer patients, who show a high prevalence of complementary and alternative medicine (CAM) use, especially among patients who are well-educated, well-off, young, and female. Three quarters of U.S. medical schools now require coursework in CAM, and CAM therapies crossover to pain medicine with surprising ease. Among people reporting back or neck pain within the last 12 months, a national telephone survey in the U.S. found that 54% used complementary therapies (especially chiropractic, massage, and relaxation techniques), compared with 37% who saw a conventional provider.[82] CAM research increasingly supports the use of nontraditional treatments for symptom control among seriously ill and elderly patients.[83] It demonstrates, for example, that mind-body therapies can both cut the number of physician visits and reduce arthritis pain.[84]

Today the U.S. National Center for Complementary and Alternative Medicine (NCCAM), with an annual budget over $100 million, represents a major institutional change in the history of mind-body relations, and pain is the focus of significant research into CAM therapies. The reports are mixed reports. In one study, CAM therapies for low back pain did not result in clinically significant improvements, while greater patient satisfaction for CAM therapies was offset by higher costs.[85] In less extensive samples, back pain was the most common reason for visits to acupuncturists, chiropractors, and massage therapists,[86] and most patients with chronic back pain expressed interest in CAM therapies.[87] CAM *mind-body* therapies, however, are not a popular treatment for pain. Mind/body therapies, one study found, were used infrequently for headaches and for back or neck pain[88] and not commonly used (at least in the U.S.) for prolonged musculoskeletal pain.[89] The inconclusive and scattered data boil down to a strong initial preference among back pain patients for acupuncture, chiropractic, and massage. Beyond individual therapies, a clearer conclusion is visible. Pain management now takes place in a globalized medical marketplace where drugs and surgery face competition from homeopaths, multicultural Internet remedies, mind/body meditation techniques, and CAM therapies. Consumer activism and global options are changing the culture of medicine, at least from a patient's perspective, and additional related changes are predictable for pain management.

The cultural system that has received most attention in its impact on chronic pain is disability insurance. Like most developed nations, for example, Scandinavian countries face rapidly mounting claims for pain associated with automobile accidents. Lithuania, however, which has no auto insurance, also shows no significant difference between accident victims and a control group in reports of headache and neck pain.[90] Chronic whiplash syndrome appears to be partly an artifact of social systems of accident and disability insurance. It is the systems, as much as neurons, that produce a call for pain treatment. This new post-1950s postmodern cash-driven disability narrative, however well intended, entails emotional costs for patients and big social costs for health care systems, and it often makes successful treatment more difficult.[91-94] Pain today, in short, exists inside cultures where national health care systems and third-party insurers establish potential careers for patients as damaging as hysteria in the 19th century. Even the decision to become a patient is a cultural artifact: in a small aboriginal community in Australia, back pain is not regarded as a health issue, people do not show recognizable public pain behaviors, and sorcery is a standard resource.[95] The development of health maintenance and managed care organizations in the U.S. has created new issues for pain management, especially as regards accreditation, regulatory initiatives, and drug costs.[96] Regulation of controlled substances may recast patients as adversaries suspected of drug-seeking behavior. Some organizations require pain patients to sign contracts that transform prescription drug abuse into legal grounds for denial of treatment. Employers too play a role in reframing pain, as monotonous jobs and lack of workplace autonomy are predictors of chronic pain disability.[97] The category of repetitive stress injury shows how sociocultural changes create new patterns of pain. Older employees with lower education and lower occupational status appear at increased risk for disabling chronic pain,[98] while women of "deprived" socioeconomic status both run higher risk of pain and experience pain as more severe and disabling.[99]

Families as a sociocultural system, like jobs, add significant complications to pain.[100] Large-scale changes in family structure create new challenges for clinicians, as postmodern families emerge reconfigured as nuclear units fractured by divorce, blended across multiple marriages, mixed in race, and marked by local or national demographic shifts. The family dynamics of chronic pain has so far yielded inconclusive data,[101] but researchers agree that pain and families exist in an intricate loop of reciprocal relations, such that the patient's pain affects the family and the family affects the patient's pain.[102] Among people with rheumatoid arthritis, spousal interaction has a complex influence on pain-related catastrophizing.[103] The precise family dynamics across specific disease conditions is less important here than identifiable links between family life and chronic pain patterns. As various predictable, almost scripted social roles and responses grow clearer, pain specialists have expressed new interest in narrative.

PAIN AND NARRATIVE: CULTURE, MEANING, PRESENCE, ETHICS

"When somebody comes in with 25 years of chronic pain, I might sit with them for 90 minutes to get the beginning of the story, to really understand what's happening," explains Scott Fishman, chief of pain medicine at the University of California at Davis. "The insurers would rather pay me $1,000 to do a 20-minute injection than pay me a fraction of that to spend an hour or two talking with a patient."[104] Rita Charon has described in the *Journal of the American Medical Association* a new clinical approach called "narrative medicine."[105] Narrative—from Latin *narro, to tell*—has been described as "*someone telling something to someone about something*,"[106] and narrative medicine sets out to reframe the everyday act of talking with patients. Charon also reframes narrative as a form of knowledge (not chitchat or entertainment). Philosopher Alasdair MacIntyre identifies the widest importance of narrative knowledge when he writes that "we all live out narratives in our lives" and "we understand our own lives in terms of the narratives that we live out."[107] Life, as the new discipline of narrative psychology puts it, is inherently "storied."[108,109] A sociocultural perspective, then, needs to include *narrative knowledge*—a complement to the molecular gaze and to what Charon calls biomedical *logicoscientific knowledge*—as it affects the understanding and experience of pain.[110]

Narrative offers distinctive insights into human pain. As a vehicle for the communication of cultural beliefs and social practices, narrative clearly plays a role in communicating beliefs and practices related to pain. Research concerning adult twins and pressure pain thresholds, for example, makes it clear that cultural patterns help determine perceived sensitivity to pain,[111] and cultural patterning begins early. By 2 months of age, Chinese and non-Chinese Canadian infants show significant differences in acute pain response.[112] Chronic pain requires a longer, more complex personal and cultural education, which for some individuals may amount to noneducation or the acquisition of erroneous beliefs. Pain narratives often encode mistaken beliefs, such as the dominant biomedical myth that regards pain as the invariable consequence and bona fide symptom of tissue damage. (The IASP

corrects this myth in asserting that many people report pain "in the absence of tissue damage or any likely pathophysiological cause."[113]) An attention to narrative thus helps to identify erroneous beliefs and harmful practices that may impede treatment. It can help uncover relevant cultural difference, such as the divergence among cancer patients in India and in America, for example, over the meaning of pain and over relations between pain and quality of life.[114] The personal narrative of a pain patient, as it conveys fine nuances of meaning and unaware self-contradiction, offers a significant tool for understanding treatment-related attitudes that may elude the coarse, broad grid of generic questionnaires.[115]

Meaning is intrinsic to human pain.[116] Even children and infants are enfolded in a web of cultural assumptions not of their making. In adults, chronic pain implies a continuous and co-extensive process of interpretation—conscious, nonconscious, personal, cultural—that both builds up and deconstructs meaning. Why me? Is it serious? Most important: will I get better? Such questions and the changing responses that they elicit, often subliminally, illustrate how meaning is not merely an add-on. Meaning is intrinsic to pain even at the zero degree where patients (consumers of the dominant biomedical myth) assert that pain is meaningless. We cannot name or discuss pain except in a natural language—English, Spanish, Farsi—that inevitably colors our understanding and shapes our experience.[117] Pain thus comes always already interpreted, and meanings silently infiltrate behavior through underlying implicit narratives, much as athletes often play out a script in which tolerance for pain affirms male courage, team loyalty, and physical strength. Pain in its social functions and in the tacit cultural narratives we act out regularly reverts to its Latin root meaning of punishment. Childhood discipline, spouse abuse, and even the self-punishments of guilt belong to a punitive narrative semantics of pain. While drugs temporarily stop pain and bypass meaning, meaning does not therefore die out. The brief pharmaceutical erasure perpetuates another cultural narrative—a myth backed by heavy narrative-based advertising—that drug therapies can buy you relief from pain. This promotional myth directly affects pain management when patients abuse chemical remedies to an extent that drug detoxification is often a necessary first step in effective treatment.

Meaning and belief in their power to reshape pain find an influential demonstration in the biblical narrative of Adam and Eve. Christian faithful over many generations associated their pain with Adam's original sin, much as today medicine has replaced theology as the main source of pain narratives. Pain beliefs now tend to focus on organic cause, control, duration, outcome, and blame.[118,119] A postmodern semantics of pain, however, is often less explicitly medical, evoking biocultural conditions from childbirth to disability[120,121] in media from feature films to podcasts, and such narratives give currency to a wide variety of pain beliefs—beliefs that extend from chronic pain to acute and even postoperative pain.[122] Moreover, narratized beliefs about pain often carry strong emotion: anger toward a negligent employer, fear of a catastrophic outcome, hope for financial compensation, any of which may complicate treatment. The good news about pain semantics: function is better in patients who believe that they have some control over their pain, who believe in the value of medical services, who believe that family members care for them, and who believe that they are not severely disabled.[123] Pain believed to mean catastrophe ahead or lifelong disability makes it much harder for patients to recover. Narrative meaning is important precisely because patients, often unknowingly, repeat or enact harmful emotional scripts that exacerbate pain as much as a raw nerve or errant neurotransmitter.

A narrative medicine for pain, as Rita Charon calls it, promises significant therapeutic benefits where other approaches fail or fall short.[124] As chronic pain often confronts patients with what anthropologists call damaged or spoiled identity, narrative offers an insight into a patient's experience of self and a means for patients to reconstruct selfhood as a step toward exiting the role of chronic pain sufferer.[125] The findings in a study of fibromyalgia patients, for example, suggest that narrative approaches both helped participants find their own coping strategies and helped them find identities other than as patients.[126] Narrative in written form also demonstrates, if not analgesic properties, at least an astonishing power to moderate pain. Rheumatoid arthritis patients who wrote in narrative form about stressful experiences showed significant symptom-reduction.[127] Indeed, writing about trauma is associated with various measurable health benefits[128,129]—but the beneficial writing takes a specific form. "Using our computer analyses as a guide," psychologist James Pennebaker explains, "we realized that the people who benefited from writing were constructing stories."[130]

Narrative, like any instrument, has limits to its uses as a therapy.[131] Pain can push both narrative and meaning to an extreme point of collapse, where nothing can be written or spoken, a black hole from which meaning cannot emerge. Victims of torture may undergo an experience so horrific and chaotic that it blocks any possible narration,[132] finding its only available idiom in somatization. Medical narrative offers the formula that a patient "presents" with symptoms. What does it mean to present? The act of "presenting" might be said to create what some theorists call "presence": a bodily, spatial, tangible, immediate, sensual material appearance that is utterly withdrawn from the grids of meaning—including medical meanings—that humans before or after superimpose on it.[133] There would seem to be an ethical obligation to respect the limits of narration, an extreme withdrawal of meaning, in a space where tools and therapies and language may seem as inadequate as squirt guns confronting a forest fire.

Stories hold an underground commerce with ethics. Narrative had no relevance to bioethics construed, at its modern beginnings in the 1970s, as a branch of analytic philosophy, wedded to a rationalist, universalist discourse of principles. From a sociocultural perspective, however, ethics is not a discourse of universal truths and timeless principles but, like medicine, an intersubjective project shot through with narrative.[134] Pain medicine has developed professional guidelines concerning an ethics of research, on animals and on humans, and guidelines are useful in promoting desired behavior, as well as in protecting the interests of professions that depend on public trust. There is room and need, however, for an ethics of pain that moves beyond professional guidelines and beyond principlism to engage contemporary philosophers outside the analytic tradition.[135] Pain, like love, calls into question the basis of our relations with others, including people or creatures who are *radically* other, nothing like us, enemies perhaps or aliens. Does their pain "call" us to act? What, if any, are the limits of empathy? The challenge of a narrative ethics is to understand pain as always embedded in the story of an individual life, where ethical choices are difficult because they fail to map precisely onto a universal logic of principles. A narrative ethics can also illuminate choices and contexts less with moral rules or right action than with human values.

Values, intricately layered with beliefs, have proven correlations with pain. Among adult patients in a pain management unit, success at living in accordance with one's values correlated with measures of disability, depression, and pain-related anxiety.[136] Differences in values often underlie conflict or misunderstanding, and narrative analysis helped researchers discover that patient autonomy (the gold standard in bioethics) meant something very different to Korean-Americans and Mexican-Americans than to their African American and Caucasian neighbors.[137] Religion and spirituality also engage value-based beliefs that narrative helps illuminate. Among predominantly white, Christian, Midwestern patients with chronic musculoskeletal pain, the religious and spiritual beliefs of patients turned out to differ from the beliefs of a healthy population. Surprisingly, private religious practices such as prayer and meditation were inversely related to physical health outcomes; long-time pain patients received less support than other patients from their church community; they tended to lose hope, become bitter, grow angry at themselves, at society, and at God.[138] Pain narratives turn especially complex when values clash or change. Should pain management now be understood as a basic human right?[139] The question is less likely to be resolved by invoking timeless principles or universal truths than by extended narrative discourse that ultimately hammers out an agreement on values. Even if declared a universal human right, pain management depends on values that situate human affliction within the modifying medico-socio-cultural environments of specific times and places.

BEYOND THE GATE: SOCIAL IMPLICATIONS OF THE MOLECULAR GAZE

The threshold leading into an era of the molecular gaze marks difficult new challenges for pain management. While insurers and peer-reviewers want hard evidence, chronic pain is characterized by multiple influences not easily reducible to quantitative data or amenable to cellular repair. Research on chronic low back pain is mostly restricted to high-income countries, for example, where rates of low back pain run 2 to 4 times higher than in low-income countries. Within low-income countries, rates of low back pain are higher in urban populations than in rural populations.[140] These variations suggest that low back pain—perhaps the signature representative of much chronic pain—is not a likely candidate for molecular cure. Multidisciplinary treatment programs now recognize the importance of psychosocial factors, but the question is whether the concept of "psychosocial factors" (typically contracted and enfolded within a still dominant biomedical model) is adequate to describe the ways in which chronic pain seems deeply rooted in the sociocultural environment.

The gate control theory, despite its advances, works better for acute pain than for chronic pain because it focuses on neural impulses blocked or transmitted at specific cerebral and spinal locales.[141] Some 21st century specialists find the gate control theory entirely adequate,[142] while others remain quiet or uneasy. Ronald Melzack has radically revised or possibly simply abandoned the theory he co-created in 1965, with its prominent dorsal horn gating mechanism, and he now emphasizes a cortical "neuromatrix."[143] Neuromatrix theory proposes numerous networked brain connections that, beyond nociception, call into play a range of human mental-emotional activity, often rooted in the sociocultural environment. A molecular gaze that focuses on a few "gates" may prove adequate for specific chronic conditions such as neuropathic pain, although (despite gate control theory) treatment for neuropathic pain remains extremely difficult.[144] A molecular gaze that reduces all chronic pain to neural impulses blocked or passing through a gate, however, risks ignoring the complex interrelations of a transdermal perspective.

An additional danger in an unrevised gate control theory is that it may excuse specialists from an opportunity—ethical or medical—to address pain-related conditions outside the nervous system. Pain specialists are not required to be social activists, although *Douleur Sans Frontièrs* (based on the Nobel-Prize winning organization Doctors Without Borders) offers one model of socially engaged care. Reflective practice, however, might encourage specialists to observe how far pain management programs belong to a larger process that sociologist Peter Conrad calls the "medicalization" of society: a transformation of human conditions into treatable disorders.[145] It is laudable work, of course, to assist patients who seek help. Nonetheless, pain management programs contribute inescapably to a medicalization of society that defines selected people in pain as pain patients and then enfolds them within a professional-economic structure that is never *simply* about compassionate care and rigorous science. It is a structure that redefines pain (as a treatable disorder) in addition to treating it, a structure that reframes people in pain (as patients) in addition to helping them, a structure that rarely encourages follow-up on patients whom it fails to help. Most important, it is a structure that bases much of its knowledge about chronic pain on the study of a subset of people who choose to enroll in research sponsored by pain management programs. Any community, however, includes—like Australian aboriginal communities—people who do not seek medical care for chronic pain but who lead, by their account, happy, productive, successful lives. How do they do it?

The study of chronic pain patients will not necessarily explain how some people not only "cope" (a medicalized concept) but also live successfully with chronic pain. The new field of positive psychology argues for shifting focus away from the study of dysfunction, in an effort to discover what specific practices, beliefs, and attitudes appear to promote effective function and personal happiness.[146] Positive psychology suggests that there is value in identifying "success stories" (another narrative genre relevant to medicine) drawn from people in pain who do not enter pain treatment programs or research protocols.[147] Even the *biopsychosocial* model, in practice, usually throws emphasis on its first syllable, reducing complex psychological states and tangled sociocultural environments to "factors" that affect human neurobiology. The concept of transdermal pain views sociocultural environments as something beyond a "factor" in otherwise mainly biological processes. It views chronic pain as always biological and as always cultural.

A STEP BACK: MOLAR IMAGES OF PAIN

The limitations of a molecular gaze for understanding chronic pain would seem clear in proposals that seek to reduce all pain to one organic cause; for example, to inflammation.[148] Neither inflammation nor any other single molecular process can wholly explain the peculiar difficulties of treating chronic pain in children, for example, where cognitive development, linguistic abilities, and family relations are central.[149] It cannot illuminate the challenges that face elderly chronic pain patients.[150] Or people with HIV/AIDS.[151,152] Or dying patients.[153] Pain, from a transdermal perspective, is never simply a matter of molecules, just as medicine is never merely the application of science. A final step back, into the 19th century, helps make this sociocultural perspective clearer as it applies to the present and future.

British satirist George Cruikshank depicted colic within a visual narrative where pain is the natural consequence of an irrational, fashion-crazed, upper-class, female lifestyle (Fig. 11.2).

Although today colic is a mysterious and usually passing affliction of infants, medical writers from the Middle Ages through the 19th century described colic as an adult affliction: "severe paroxysmal griping pains in the belly."[154] The Greek root of *colic* refers to the colon, especially to the lower part of the intestinal canal (or bowels), and colic may be a 19th century antecedent of irritable bowel syndrome (IBS). IBS, a disorder of the intestines that is associated with belly pain and other symptoms, affects 10% to 15% of people in North America[155] and is twice as common in women.[156] While inflammation, brain-to-muscle signals, and possibly genetics are involved in its painful episodes, IBS is characteristic of chronic pain syndromes in raising questions about the role of sociocultural environment. Biology and genes simply cannot explain all relations among chronic pain, sex, and gender.[157] Childhood sexual abuse, for example, is a sociocultural fact for some boys and girls, as well as a subject of fantasy. Women diagnosed with somatization disorder are more likely to report childhood sexual abuse than are women with mood disorders.[158,159] Chronic pelvic pain in women certainly correlates with sexual dysfunction.[160] Cruikshank's visual narrative, wholly lacking in medical knowledge, places colic within a sociocultural frame where pain is a punishment for sexualized female folly.

Cruikshank's narrative of colic repeats for women the same satiric moral (excess breeds pain) that his image of gout offers men. The framed picture above the sofa (hard to see in this reproduction) depicts an obese woman, at her bedside in a nightcap, drinking from a decanter. *Nightcap*, defined figuratively as an alcoholic drink taken before bed, dates exactly from this period. The obese tippler may not be the tortured woman on the sofa, but their caps and figures connect them. Cruikshank links colic with fashionable excess not only in private alcohol consumption but also in public styles that squeeze a full-bodied woman into

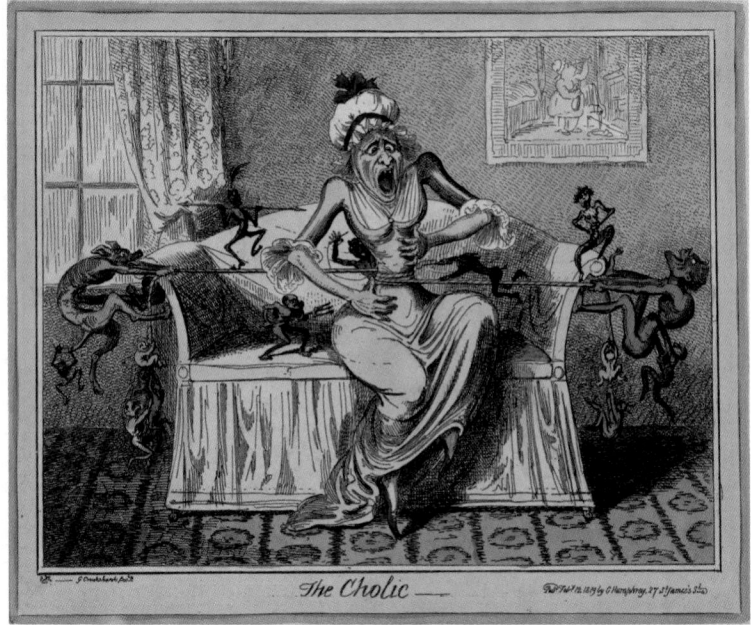

The Cholic —

FIGURE 11.2 George Cruikshank. *The Cholic*. 1835. Colored etching. (Courtesy of the Claude Moore Health Sciences Library, University of Virginia, Charlottesville, VA.)

an hourglass shape. The *sofa*—furniture associated with the decline of virtuous simplicity and the rise of luxury and vice[161]—is co-occupied by a devil engaged in sewing or lacing up the corsetlike garment, invoking religious traditions that understand pain as a hellish punishment for sin. Sin seems less evident than self-punitive folly, until we account for additional information within the image that links pain and sexuality.

A sexual subtext is hard to ignore because male admirers ultimately stand behind the woman's painful fashion choice. (She does not dress this way in private.) The constricting rope is pulled tight, at either end, by related parallel figures: an emaciated, hyperactive dog and a leering naked male. The naked figures on the tightrope, female and male, reinforce an aura of sexual tension, but here the sexual subtext connects with larger sociocultural contexts. The two figures also evoke British imperialism and its power over exotic local populations (represented here as free from the absurd repressions of Western fashion). Social historians have shown how medicine served as an instrument of empire.[162] Although individual doctors doubtless acted from altruistic motives, the extension of Western medical knowledge to the ends of empire was not pure philanthropy, a narrative about the white man's burden in carrying light into darkness. The *réal-biopolitick* of empire involved uprooting indigenous medical traditions and imposing institutional controls favorable to colonial power. A future transdermal perspective needs to ask whether a globalized pain management might, however laudable its intentions to extend care, included unintended consequences in uprooting local knowledge, securing commercial interests, and imposing favorable institutions of control.[163]

The central figure in Cruikshank's exploration of links between pain and its sociocultural environment raises the question of whether cultures might shape a distinctively female pain. Pain associated with somatization disorder, for example, runs at a 10 to 1 ratio of female-to-male.[164] Women are frequently overextended caregivers in chaotic families, just as women are no doubt overrepresented among battered spouses. A molecular gaze, while valuable in exploding harmful social myths of illness, creates its own limiting counter-myth if it represents pain as a purely internal state, unrelated to political and social contexts. Cruikshank (it goes without saying only if one is white) represents the fashionable woman suffering from colic as white, while the various punitive devils and sexualized figurines reflect a nonwhite realm. According to U.S. government figures, the amount of five major painkillers sold at retail stores rose 90% between 1997 and 2005.[165] Who bought them? Misuse of painkillers represents three-fourths of the overall problem of prescription drug abuse.[166] Who misused them? Between 2 million and 3 million doses of codeine, hydrocodone, and oxycodone are stolen annually.[167] Who stole them? Such questions, with their inevitable narrative response in individual cases, are not irrelevant to pain management programs and to the valuable work that they perform. Pain and pain-killing drugs belong not only to genetics, to neurobiology, and to a molecular gaze but also, for better or worse, to the transdermal texts and textures of human lives in particular places and in distinctive, even unparalleled, sociocultural histories.

CONCLUSION

There is no magic bullet for chronic pain. Maybe researchers will someday find one. S. Weir Mitchell, founder of modern neurology, on its 50th anniversary in 1896 celebrated the first surgical use of ether as heralding the "death of pain." Chronic pain, on the contrary, appears on the rise in industrial and postindustrial nations, and it does not respond well to ether-like strategies effective in controlling acute pain. The search for a magic bullet may be as misguided as unicorn hunts, which of course does not rule out fruitful byproducts of a fundamentally erroneous pursuit.

The absence of a magic bullet, even if temporary, invites other approaches to understanding and treating chronic pain. *Overdetermination*, in psychoanalytic theory, refers to the concept that multiple causes combine to produce a single behavior, emotion, symptom, or dream. The cumulative data cited in this chapter suggest that chronic pain is over-determined. It does not depend on a single, clear, independent cause that a magic bullet (or gene therapy) might knock out, but rather it appears to develop through multiple, intersecting, proliferating routes of transmission, like a rhizome.

Chronic pain, over-determined in spades, is often described today not as a symptom but as a disease, although it is less a classic disease state than a complex, changing, multivariate event staged within human consciousness. Consciousness—defined, arguably, as an emergent property of human brains—modifies and interprets nociceptive sensory input in ways that depend on cultural and social forces within an individual's environment. Thus, chronic pain is open to significant modification—for better or worse—from, for example, workplace, gender, ethnicity, belief, emotion, money, and narrative. Children, in part because of their distinctive cultural, social, and linguistic backgrounds, may experience pain differently than their parents do. First-generation immigrants may experience pain differently than their assimilated second-generation children do. Persons with HIV/AIDS may face a pain that is distinctive depending on how, in individual cases, a specific infectious disease engages the highly variable forces of geography, nation, social class, race, stigma, and access to care.

Chronic pain, in short, cannot be reduced to a diagram of cellular processes. Cellular processes are open to modification by cultural and social forces. This extracellular and nonmolecular dimension, as it manifests in patients with different personal, social, and cultural backgrounds, remains among the most difficult challenges that pain medicine in the 21st century needs to address effectively.

Acknowledgments

For his assistance, I am grateful to John Loeser, who attributes the phrase "transdermal pain" to his colleague Wilbert Fordyce. Many thanks as well to Daniel B. Carr.

References

1. Loeser JD. Economic implications of pain management. *Acta Anaesthesiol Scand* 1999;43(9):957–959.
2. Rose N. *The Politics of Life Itself: Biomedicine, Power, and Subjectivity in the Twenty-First Century.* Princeton: Princeton University Press; 2007.
3. Heath D, Rapp R, Taussig KS. Genetic citizenship. In: Nugent D, Vincent J, eds. *A Companion to the Anthropology of Politics.* Oxford: Blackwell; 2004: 152–167.
4. Choi HK, Curhan G. Gout: epidemiology and lifestyle choices. *Curr Opin Rheumatol* 2005;17(3):341–345.
5. Fordyce WE, ed. *Back Pain in the Workplace: Management of Disability in Nonspecific Conditions.* Seattle, WA: IASP Press; 1995:4.
6. Merskey H, Bogduk N, eds. *Classification of Chronic Pain: Descriptions of Chronic Pain Syndromes and Definitions of Pain Terms.* 2nd ed. Seattle, WA: IASP Press; 1994:210.
7. Loeser JD. The future: will pain be abolished or just pain specialists? *Minn Med* 2000;84:20–21.
8. Fordyce WE, ed. *Back Pain in the Workplace: Management of Disability in Nonspecific Conditions.* Seattle, WA: IASP Press; 1995:xiii.
9. Becker DM. Through the looking glass: the patient's point of view. In: Mills AE, Chen DT, Werhane PH, et al, eds. *Professionalism in Tomorrow's Healthcare System: Towards Fulfilling the ACGME Requirements for Systems-Based Practice and Professionalism.* Hagerstown, MD: University Publishing Group; 2005:169–177.
10. Foster JB. Racial, ethnic variables shape the experience of chronic pain. *Applied Neurology* 2006;2(11):19–22.
11. Morris RS, Wallenstein S, Natale DK, et al. "We don't carry that"—failure of pharmacies in predominantly nonwhite neighborhoods to stock opioid analgesics. *N Engl J Med* 2000;342(14):1023–1026.
12. SUPPORT Principal Investigators. A controlled trial to improve care for seriously ill hospitalized patients. *JAMA* 1995;274(20):1591–1598.

13. Bates MS, Edwards WT, Anderson KO. Ethnocultural influences on variation in chronic pain perception. *Pain* 1993;52(1):101–112.

14. Madjar I. Pain and the surgical patient: a cross-cultural perspective. *Aust J Adv Nurs* 1985;2(2):29–33.

15. Wolff BB. Ethnocultural factors influencing pain and illness behavior. *Clin J Pain* 1985;1(1):23–30.

16. Jordan JM. Effect of race and ethnicity on outcomes in arthritis and rheumatic conditions. *Curr Opin Rheumatol* 1999;11(2):98–103.

17. Green CR, Anderson KO, Baker TA, et al. The unequal burden of pain: confronting racial and ethnic disparities in pain. *Pain Med* 2003;4(3):277–294.

18. Morris DB. Ethnicity and pain. *Pain: Clin Updates* 2001;9(4):1–8.

19. Rose N. *The Politics of Life Itself: Biomedicine, Power, and Subjectivity in the Twenty-First Century.* Princeton: Princeton University Press; 2007:175.

20. Todd K, Samaroo N, Hoffman J. Ethnicity as a risk factor for inadequate emergency department analgesia. *JAMA* 1993;269(12):1537–1539.

21. Todd KH. Pain assessment and ethnicity. *Ann Emerg Med* 1996;27(4):421–423.

22. Maxwell K, Streetly A, Bevan D. Experiences of hospital care and treatment seeking for pain from sickle cell disease: qualitative study. *BMJ* 1999;318(7198):1585–1590.

23. Ballas SK. *Sickle Cell Pain.* Seattle, WA: IASP Press; 1998.

24. Jones JH. *Bad Blood: The Tuskegee Syphilis Experiment.* New York: Free Press; 1993.

25. Wailoo K. *Dying in the City of the Blues: Sickle Cell Anemia and the Politics of Race and Health.* Chapel Hill, NC: University of North Carolina Press; 2001.

26. Bernabei R, Gambassi G, Lapane K, et al. Management of pain in elderly patients with cancer. *JAMA* 1998;279(23):1877–1882.

27. Cleeland C, Gonin R, Baez L, et al. Pain and treatment of pain in minority patients with cancer: the Eastern Cooperative Oncology Group Minority Outpatient Pain Study. *Ann Intern Med* 1997;127(9):813–816.

28. Joranson DE. Global opioid consumption: trends, barriers, and diversion. *IASP Newsletter* 1994 September/October:4–5.

29. Pain & Policy Studies Group, University of Wisconsin Paul P. Carbone Comprehensive Cancer Center. Availability of morphine and pethidine in the world and Africa, with a special focus on Botswana, Ethiopia, Kenya, Malawi, Nigeria, Rwanda, Tanzania, Zambia [2006]. Available at http://www.painpolicy.wisc.edu/publicat/monograp/africa06.pdf.

30. DePalma A. For Mexicans, pain relief is both a medical and a political problem. *New York Times.* June 19, 1966:A4.

31. Gear RW, Miaskowski C, Gordon NC, et al. Kappa-opioids produce significantly greater analgesia in women than in men. *Nat Med* 1996;2(11):1248–1250.

32. Liem EB, Lin CM, Suleman MI, et al. Anesthetic requirement is increased in redheads. *Anesthesiology* 2004;101(2):279–283.

33. Liem EB, Joiner TV, Tsueda K, et al. Increased sensitivity to thermal pain and reduced subcutaneous lidocaine efficacy in redheads. *Anesthesiology* 2005;102(3): 509–514.

34. Berkley KJ. Female pain versus male pain? In: Fillingim RB, ed. *Sex, Gender, and Pain.* Seattle, WA: IASP Press; 2000:373–381.

35. Butler J. *Gender Trouble: Feminism and the Subversion of Identity.* New York: Routledge; 1990:25.

36. Jensen MC, Brant-Zawadzki MN, Obuchowski N, et al. Magnetic resonance imaging of the lumbar spine in people without back pain. *N Engl J Med* 1994;331(2):69–73.

37. Von Korff M, Barlow W, Cherkin D, et al. Effects of practice style in managing back pain. *Ann Intern Med* 1994;121(3):187–195.

38. Wall PD, Jones M. *Defeating Pain: The War Against a Silent Epidemic.* New York: Plenum Press; 1991:44.

39. Bigos SJ, Battié MC, Spengler DM, et al. A prospective study of work perceptions and psychosocial factors affecting the report of back injury. *Spine* 1991;16(1):1–6.

40. Dwyer T, Raftery AE. Industrial accidents are produced by social relations of work: a sociological theory of industrial accidents. *Appl Ergon* 1991;22(3):167–178.

41. Veterans Health Administration Memorandum. *Pain as the Fifth Vital Sign.* March 1, 1999.

42. Mularski RA, White-Chu F, Overbay D, et al. Measuring pain as the 5th vital sign does not improve quality of pain management. *J Gen Intern Med* 2006;21(6):607–612.

43. Kitzes JA. Palliative medicine: facing the challenge of care beyond cure. *IHS Prim Care Provid* 1999;24(2):23–25.

44. Merskey H, Bogduk N, eds. *Classification of Chronic Pain: Descriptions of Chronic Pain Syndromes and Definitions of Pain Terms.* 2nd ed. Seattle, WA: IASP Press; 1994:210.

45. Vlaeyen JWS, Crombez G. Fear and pain. *Pain: Clin Updates* 2007;15(6):1–4.

46. Sullivan MD. Pain as emotion. *Pain Forum* 1996;5(3):208–209.

47. Norbury TA, MacGregor AJ, Urwin J, et al. Heritability of responses to painful stimuli in women: a classical twin study. *Brain* 2007;130(11):3041–3049.

48. Coghill RC, McHaffie JG, Yen YF. Neural correlates of interindividual differences in the subjective experience of pain. *Proc Natl Acad Sci U S A* 2003;100(14):8538–8542.

49. Bayer TL, Baer PE, Early C. Situational and psychophysiological factors in psychologically induced pain. *Pain* 1991;44(1):45–50.

50. Koyama T, McHaffie JG, Laurienti PJ, et al. The subjective experience of pain: where expectations become reality. *Proc Natl Acad Sci U S A* 2005;102(36):12950–12955.

51. Keltner JR, Furst A, Fan C, et al. Isolating the modulatory effect of expectation on pain transmission: a functional magnetic resonance imaging study. *J Neurosci* 2006;26(16):4437–4443.

52. Gray JA. *The Neuropsychology of Anxiety: An Enquiry into the Functions of the Septo-Hippocampal System.* Oxford: Clarendon Press; 1982.

53. Hays G. Introduction. In: Aurelius M, ed. *Meditations: A New Translation.* New York: Modern Library; 2002:xlviii.

54. Brena SF, Sanders SH, Motoyama H. American and Japanese chronic low back pain patients: cross-cultural similarities and differences. *Clin J Pain* 1990;6(2):118–124.

55. Zeltner L. Innovative models for studying pain in children. Highlights of the 2nd joint scientific meeting of the American Pain Society and the Canadian Pain Society 2004. Available at http://www.medscape.com/viewprogram/3174.

56. Lamé IE, Peters ML, Vlaeyen JW, et al. Quality of life in chronic pain is more associated with beliefs about pain, than with pain intensity. *Eur J Pain* 2005;9(1):15–24.

57. Christakis NA, Fowler JH. The spread of obesity in a large social network over 32 years. *N Engl J Med* 2007;357(4):370–379.

58. Jensen MP, Keefe FJ, Lefebvre JC, et al. One- and two-item measures of pain beliefs and coping strategies. *Pain* 2003;104(3):453–469.

59. Williams DA, Keefe FJ. Pain beliefs and the use of cognitive-behavioral coping strategies. *Pain* 1991;46(2):185–190.

60. Shutty MS Jr, DeGood DE, Tuttle DH. Chronic pain patients' beliefs about their pain and treatment outcomes. *Arch Phys Med Rehabil* 1990;71(2):128–132.

61. Bowker JW. *Problems of Suffering in Religions of the World.* Cambridge: Cambridge University Press; 1970.

62. Eccleston C, Williams AC, Rogers WS. Patients' and professionals' understandings of the causes of chronic pain: blame, responsibility and identity protection. *Soc Sci Med* 1997;43(5):699–709.

63. Carr DB, Loeser JD, Morris DB, eds. *Narrative, Pain, and Suffering.* Seattle, WA: IASP Press; 2005.

64. Sacks O. To see and not see. In: *An Anthropologist on Mars: Seven Paradoxical Tales.* New York: Knopf; 1995:108–152.

65. Loeser J. Socioeconomic factors in pain. In: Cousins M, Bridenbaugh P, Carr D, Horlocker T, eds. *Cousins and Bridenbaugh's Neural Blockade in Clinical Anesthesia and Management of Pain.* 4th ed. Philadelphia: Lippincott Williams & Wilkins; 2008:644–650.

66. Raber P, Devor M. Social variables affect phenotype in the neuroma model of neuropathic pain. *Pain* 2002;97(1–2):139–150.

67. Krause E. *Power and Illness: The Political Sociology of Health and Medical Care.* New York: Elsevier; 1977:xi.

68. Scarry E. *The Body in Pain: The Making and Unmaking of the World.* New York: Oxford University Press; 1985.

69. Nutkiewicz M. Chronic pain patients and torture survivors: intersecting lines and lines of demarcation. *Newsletter of the IASP Special Interest Group on Pain from Torture, Organized Violence, and War* 2007 January 3–4.

70. Foucault M. *Power/knowledge: Selected Interviews and Other Writings 1972–1977.* New York: Pantheon Books; 1980:183–193. Gordon C, Marshall L, Mepham J, Soper K, translators.

71. Foucault M. *The History of Sexuality: vol 1, An Introduction.* New York: Random House; 1978:140–144. Hurley R, translator.

72. Rose N. *The Politics of Life Itself: Biomedicine, Power, and Subjectivity in the Twenty-First Century.* Princeton: Princeton University Press; 2007:54.

73. Hill CS Jr. The negative influence of licensing and disciplinary boards and drug enforcement agencies on pain treatment with opioid analgesics. *J Pharm Care in Pain Symptom Contrl* 1993;1(1):43–62.

74. Laurent S. No time to die. In: Carr DB, Loeser JD, Morris DB, eds. *Narrative, Pain, and Suffering.* Seattle, WA: IASP Press; 2005:243–248.

75. Viscusi ER, Schechter LN. Patient-controlled analgesia: finding a balance between cost and comfort. *Am J Health Syst Pharm* 2006;63(8 suppl 1):S3–13.

76. Green CR. Racial disparities in access to pain treatment. *Pain: Clin Updates* 2004;12(6):1–4.

77. Farmer P. *Pathologies of Power: Health, Human Rights, and the New War on the Poor.* Berkeley: University of California Press; 2003.

78. Jacox A, Carr DB, Mahrenholz DM, et al. Cost considerations in patient-controlled analgesia. *Pharmacoeconomics* 1997;12(2Pt1):109–120.

79. Herskovits EJ. *Sick at Heart: Modern Disease & Modern Therapeutics in Malaysia.* Dissertation. University of California San Francisco; 1999:14–19.

80. Eisenberg DM, Kessler RC, Foster C, et al. Unconventional medicine in the United States: prevalence, costs, and patterns of use. *N Engl J Med* 1993;328(4):246–252.

81. Eisenberg DM, Davis RB, Ettner SL, et al. Trends in alternative medicine use in the United States, 1990–1997: results of a follow-up national survey. *JAMA* 1998;280(18): 1569–1575.

82. Cassileth BR, Vickers AJ. High prevalence of complementary and alternative medicine use among cancer patients: implications for research and clinical care. *J Clin Oncol* 2005;23(12): 2590–2592.

83. Luskin FM, Newell KA, Griffith M, et al. A review of mind/body therapies in the treatment of musculoskeletal disorders with implications for the elderly. *Altern Ther Health Med* 2000;6(2):46–56.

84. Eisenberg DM, Post DE, Davis RB, et al. Addition of choice of complementary

therapies to usual care for acute low back pain: a randomized controlled trial. *Spine* 2007;32(2):151–158.

85. Wolsko PM, Eisenberg DM, Davis RB, et al. Patterns and perceptions of care for treatment of back and neck pain: results of a national survey. *Spine* 2003; 28(3):292–297.

86. Sherman KJ, Cherkin DC, Deyo RA et al. The diagnosis and treatment of chronic back pain by acupuncturists, chiropractors, and massage therapists. *Clin J Pain* 2006;22(3):227–234.

87. Sherman KJ, Cherkin DC, Connelly MT, Erro J, et al. Complementary and alternative medical therapies for chronic low back pain: what treatments are patients willing to try? *BMC Complement Altern Med* 2004;4(19):9.

88. Wolsko PM, Eisenberg DM, Davis DM, et al. Use of mind–body medical therapies. *J Gen Intern Med* 2004;19(1):43–50.

89. Tindle HA, Wolsko P, Davis RB, et al. Factors associated with the use of mind–body therapies among United States adults with musculoskeletal pain. *Complement Ther Med* 2005;13(3):155–164.

90. Schrader H, Obelieniene D, Bovim G, et al. Natural evolution of late whiplash syndrome outside the medicolegal context. *Lancet* 1996;347(9010): 1207–1211.

91. Teasell RW. Compensation and chronic pain. *Clin J Pain* 2001;17(4 suppl): S46–S64.

92. Mendelson G. Compensation and chronic pain. *Pain* 1992;48(2):121–123.

93. Guest GH, Drummond PD. Effect of compensation on emotional state and disability in chronic back pain. *Pain* 1992;48(2):125–130.

94. Rohling ML, Binder LM, Langhinrichsen–Rohling J. Money matters: a meta-analytic review of the association between financial compensation and the experience and treatment of chronic pain. *Health Psychol* 1995;14(6): 537–547.

95. Honeyman PT, Jacobs EA. Effects of culture on back pain in Australian aboriginals. *Spine* 1996;21(7):841–843.

96. Lande SD, Loeser JD. The future of pain management in managed care. *Manag Care Interface* 2001;14(5):69–75.

97. Teasell RW, Bombardier C. Employment-related factors in chronic pain and chronic pain disability. *Clin J Pain* 2001;17(4 suppl):S39–45.

98. Saastamoinen P, Leino–Arjas P, Laaksonen M, Lahelma E. Socio-economic differences in the prevalence of acute, chronic and disabling chronic pain among ageing employees. *Pain* 2005;114(3):364–371.

99. Jablonska B, Soares JJ, Sundin O. Pain among women: associations with socio-economic and work conditions. *Eur J Pain* 2006;10(5):435–447.

100. Payne B, Norfleet MA. Chronic pain and the family: a review. *Pain* 1986; 26(1):1–22.

101. Flor H, Turk DC, Rudy TE. Pain and families. II. assessment and treatment. *Pain* 1987;30(1):29–45.

102. The family and chronic pain: a special issue of the *International Journal of Family Therapy* 1985;7(4).

103. Holtzman S, DeLongis A. One day at a time: the impact of daily satisfaction with spouse responses on pain, negative affect and catastrophizing among individuals with rheumatoid arthritis. *Pain* 2007;131(1–2):202–213.

104. Fishman S. In: Wallis C. The right (and wrong) way to treat pain. *Time* 2005; 165(9):46–57.

105. Charon R. The patient–physician relationship. Narrative medicine: a model for empathy, reflection, profession, trust. *JAMA* 2001; 286(15):1897–1902.

106. Kearney R. *On Stories*. New York: Routledge; 2002:5.

107. MacIntyre A. *After Virtue: A Study in Moral Theory*. Notre Dame, IN: Notre Dame University Press; 1981:197.

108. Sarbin TR, ed. *Narrative Psychology: The Storied Nature of Human Conduct*. New York: Praeger; 1986.

109. Crossley ML. *Introducing Narrative Psychology: Self, Trauma and the Construction of Meaning*. New York: McGraw–Hill; 2000.

110. Carr DR, Loeser JD, Morris DB, eds. *Narrative, Pain, and Suffering*. Seattle, WA: IASP Press; 2005.

111. MacGregor AJ, Griffiths GO, Baker J, et al. Determinants of pressure pain threshold in adult twins: evidence that shared environmental influences predominate. *Pain* 1997;73(2):253–257.

112. Rosmus C, Johnston CC, Chan–Yip A, et al. Pain response in Chinese and non-Chinese Canadian infants: is there a difference? *Soc Sci Med* 2000;51(2): 175–184.

113. Mersky H, Bogduk N, eds. *Classification of Chronic Pain: Descriptions of Chronic Pain Syndromes and Definitions of Pain Terms*. 2nd ed. Seattle, WA: IASP Press; 1994:210.

114. Kodiath MF, Kodiath A. A comparative study of patients who experience chronic malignant pain in India and the United States. *Cancer Nurs* 1995; 18(3):189–196.

115. Kearney R. *On Stories*. New York: Routledge, 2002.

116. Morris DB. *The Culture of Pain*. Berkeley: University of California Press; 1991.

117. Sullivan MD. Pain in language: from sentience to sapience. *Pain Forum* 1995; 4(1):3–14.

118. Williams DA, Thorn BE. An empirical assessment of pain beliefs. *Pain* 1989; 36(3):351–358.

119. Jensen MP, Turner JA, Romano JM, et al. Coping with chronic pain: a critical review of the literature. *Pain* 1991;47(3):249–283.

120. Good M-JD, Brodwin PE, Good BJ, et al, eds. *Pain as Human Experience: An Anthropological Perspective*. Berkeley: University of California Press; 1992.

121. Moore R, Brødsgaard I. Cross-cultural investigations of pain. In: Crombie IK, Croft PR, Linton SJ, et al. eds. *Epidemiology of Pain*. Seattle, WA: IASP Press; 1999:53–80.

122. Williams DA. Acute pain management. In: Gatchel RJ, Turk DC, eds. *Psychological Approaches to Pain Management: A Practitioner's Handbook*. New York: Guilford Press; 1996:55–77.

123. Jensen MP. Pain-specific beliefs, perceived symptom severity, and adjustment to chronic pain. *Clin J Pain* 1992;8(2):123–130.

124. Charon R. Suffering, storytelling, and community: an approach to pain treatment from Columbia's Program in Narrative Medicine. In: Flor H, Kalso E, Dostrovsky JO, eds. *Proceedings of the 11th World Congress on Pain*. Seattle, WA: IASP Press; 2006:19–27.

125. Kelley P, Clifford P. Coping with chronic pain: assessing narrative approaches. *Soc Work* 1997;42(3):266–277.

126. Jackson JE. *Camp Pain: Talking with Chronic Pain Patients*. Philadelphia: University of Pennsylvania Press; 1999.

127. Smyth JM, Stone AA, Hurewitz A, et al. Effects of writing about stressful experiences on symptom reduction in patients with asthma or rheumatoid arthritis: a randomized trial. *JAMA* 1999; 281(14):1304–1309.

128. Pennebaker JW, Beall SK. Confronting a traumatic event: toward an understanding of inhibition and disease. *J Abnor Psychol* 1986;95(3):274–281.

129. Pennebaker JW, Seagal JD. Forming a story: the health benefits of narrative. *J Clin Psychol* 1999;55(10):1243–1254.

130. Pennebaker JW. *Opening Up: The Healing Power of Expressing Emotions*. Revised ed. New York: The Guilford Press; 1997:103.

131. Nelson HL, ed. *Stories and Their Limits: Narrative Approaches to Bioethics*. New York: Routledge; 1997.

132. Waitzkin H, Magaña H. The black box in somatization: unexplained physical symptoms, culture, and narratives of trauma. *Soc Sci Med* 1997;45(6): 811–825.

133. Gumbrecht HU. *The Production of Presence: What Meaning Cannot Convey*. Stanford: Stanford University Press; 2004.

134. Charon R, Montello M, eds. *Stories Matter: The Role of Narrative in Medical Ethics*. New York: Routledge; 2002.

135. Morris DB. Ethics beyond guidelines: culture, pain, and conflict. In: Dostrovsky JO, Carr DB, Koltzenburg M, eds. *Proceedings of the 10th World Congress on Pain*. Seattle, WA: IASP Press; 2003:37–48.

136. McCracken LM, Yang SY. The role of values in a contextual cognitive-behavioral approach to chronic pain. *Pain* 2006;123(1–2):137–145.

137. Blackhall LJ, Murphy ST, Frank G, et al. Ethnicity and attitudes toward patient autonomy. *JAMA* 1995;274(10):820–825.

138. Rippentrop AE, Altmaier EM, Chen JJ, et al. The relationship between religion/spirituality and physical health, mental health, and pain in a chronic pain population. *Pain* 2005;116(3):311–321.

139. Brennan F, Carr DB, Cousins M. Pain management: a fundamental human right. *Anesth Analg* 2007;105(1):205–221.

140. Volinn E. The epidemiology of low back pain in the rest of the world: a review of surveys in low- and middle-income countries. *Spine* 1997;22(15): 1747–1754.

141. Melzack R, Wall PD. Pain mechanisms: a new theory. *Science* 1965;150(699): 971–979.

142. Dickenson AH. Gate control theory of pain stands the test of time. *Br J Anaesth* 2002;88(6):755–757.

143. Melzack R. From the gate to the neuromatrix. *Pain* 1999;82(suppl 1): S121–S126.

144. Siniscalco D, Rossi F, Maione S. Molecular approaches for neuropathic pain treatment. *Curr Med Chem* 2007;14(16):1783–1787.

145. Conrad P. *The Medicalization of Society: On the Transformation of Human Conditions into Treatable Disorders*. Baltimore: Johns Hopkins University Press; 2007.

146. Snyder CR, Lopez SJ, eds. *Handbook of Positive Psychology*. New York: Oxford University Press; 2002.

147. Morris DB. Success stories: narrative, pain, and the limits of storylessness. In: Carr, DB, Loeser JD, Morris DB, eds. *Narrative, Pain, and Suffering*. Seattle, WA: IASP Press; 2005:269–285.

148. Omoigui S. The biochemical origin of pain—proposing a new law of pain: the origin of all pain is inflammation and the inflammatory response. *Med Hypotheses* 2007;69(1):70–82.

149. McGrath PJ, Finley GA, eds. *Pediatric Pain: Biological and Social Context*. Seattle, WA: IASP Press; 2003.

150. Gibson SJ, Weiner DK, eds. *Pain in Older Persons*. Seattle: IASP Press; 2005.

151. Breitbart W, Dibiase L. Current perspectives on pain in AIDS. *Oncology* 2002; 16(6):818–829, 834–835.

152. Breitbart W, Dibiase L. Current perspectives on pain in AIDS. *Oncology* 2002; 16(7):964–968, 972.

153. Giordana J, Gomez CF, Harrison C. On the potential role for interventional pain management in palliative care. *Pain Physician* 2007;10(3):395–398.

154. *Colic*, n[1]. *The Oxford English Dictionary*. 2nd ed. 1989, OED Online. Oxford University Press; 4 April 2000. Available at http://dictionary.oed.com/cgi/entry/00181778.

155. American College of Gastroenterology Functional Gastrointestinal Disorders Task Force. Evidence-based position statement on the management of irritable bowel syndrome in North America. *Am J Gastroenterol* 2002;97(11 suppl): S1–S5.

156. Jailwala J, Imperiale TF, Kroenke K. Pharmacologic treatment of the irritable bowel syndrome: a systematic review of randomized, controlled trials. *Ann Intern Med* 2000;133(2):136–147.

157. Fillingim RB, ed. *Sex, Gender, and Pain.* Seattle, WA: IASP Press; 2000.

158. Coryell W, Norten SG. Briquet's syndrome (somatization disorder) and primary depression: comparison of background and outcome. *Compr Psychiatry* 1981;22(3):249–256.

159. Morrison J. Childhood sexual histories of women with somatization disorder. *Am J Psychiatry* 1989;146(2):239–241.

160. Verit FF, Verit A, Yeni E. The prevalence of sexual dysfunction and associated risk factors in women with chronic pelvic pain: a cross-sectional study. *Arch Gynecol Obstet* 2006;274(5):297–302.

161. *Sofa,* n². *The Oxford English Dictionary.* 2nd ed. 1989, OED Online. Oxford University Press. Available at http://dictionary.oed.com/cgi/entry/50229920. Accessed April 4, 2000.

162. Arnold D. *Colonizing the Body: State Medicine and Epidemic Disease in Nineteenth-Century India.* Berkeley: University of California Press; 1993.

163. Lewis B. The new global health movement: R$_x$ for the world? *New Literary History* 2007;38(3):459–478.

164. Robins LN, Helzer JE, Weissman MM, et al. Lifetime prevalence of specific psychiatric disorders in three sites. *Arch Gen Psychiatry* 1984;41(10), 949–958.

165. Painkiller use rising at alarming rate. August 20, 2007. Available at http://www.msnbc.msn.com/id/20327132.

166. U.S. Drug Enforcement Administration. Fact sheet: prescription drug abuse—a DEA focus. August 11, 2007. Available at http://www.usdoj.gov/dea/good_medicine_bad_behavior_factsheet.doc.

167. Bass F. Pain medicine use has nearly doubled. *Associated Press* August 20, 2007. Available at http://www.washingtonpost.com/wp-dyn/content/article/2007/08/20/AR2007082000147.html.

CHAPTER 12 ■ ETHICAL ISSUES IN PAIN MANAGEMENT

BEN A. RICH

INTRODUCTION

The ethics of pain management is intricately intertwined with, and yet in certain essential aspects distinct from, traditional concepts and principles of patient care. The primary focus of this chapter will be those distinctive ways in which ethics has been interpreted and applied in pain management. It is important to note that in previous editions of this text there was no chapter devoted to ethics or any of the other topics covered in this section of the 4th edition. We can only speculate as to why that was so, but it is ironic because since early in the 1970s studies began to indicate that the phenomenon of undertreated pain was pervasive and inconsistent with available therapeutic options.

One can argue that the traditional view of the ethics of pain management, to the extent that it was articulated at all in the professional literature, provided a basis for undertreating pain, particularly if what was required to adequately relieve pain involved the administration of opioid analgesics. In that sense, during the last 15 to 20 years there has been a gradual but highly significant paradigm shift in the ethics of pain management. Until quite recently, as David Morris insightfully notes in his book *The Culture of Pain*: "The everyday medical dealings with pain conceal unacknowledged ethical questions." Even in the care of cancer patients, Morris continues, the clinical ethos has been tainted by "an unacknowledged moral code expressing half-baked notions about the evil of drugs and the duty to bear affliction." He concludes with the grim observation that "The ethics of pain management, unfortunately, may not receive proper attention until the first doctor is successfully sued for failing to provide adequate relief."[1] There was a remarkable prescience to Morris' suggestion, for in the very year in which his book was published, a jury awarded millions of dollars in both compensatory and punitive damages to the family of a patient whose terminal cancer pain was undertreated. That case is discussed in detail in Chapter 16 of this text. Similarly, the ethical issues pertaining to the care of the dying patient are discussed in depth in Chapter 14, and the laws and policies relating to opioid analgesia are surveyed in Chapter 17.

In the decade and a half since the publication of *The Culture of Pain*, the ethics of pain management has finally begun to receive the attention, discussion, and debate that had been so starkly absent before. Herein we will consider that process and the current state of affairs.

PAIN, SUFFERING, AND THE CORE VALUES OF HEALTH CARE

For centuries the core values of medicine and the other health professions never seemed to be in doubt. They were often, however, encapsulated in vague maxims of uncertain origin and authenticity such as "*primum non nocere*" (first do no harm) or "to cure when possible, to relieve often, and to comfort always." The core values on which these maxims were grounded—beneficence and nomaleficence—were unquestionably formulated by physicians during the long reign of paternalism as the overarching paradigm for the professional–patient relationship. What constituted benefit and harm, and when the zealous pursuit of cure should yield to the provision of comfort, or more radically still, occur simultaneously, was for the physician, not the patient to determine. In the latter half of the 20th century, particularly but certainly not exclusively in the United States, the evolution of medical jurisprudence and the revolution in bioethics challenged the legitimacy of the paternalistic paradigm. This challenge was grounded upon an emerging principle of bioethics—respect for individual patient autonomy. Indeed, by the end of that century, paternalism had become almost completely discredited, replaced by a new paradigm grounded on the legal duty to obtain informed consent (and to accept an informed refusal) supported by and in turn operating in affirmation of the most recent bioethical principle.[2] The new paradigm for the professional–patient relationship became that of shared decision making.[3]

While beneficence and nonmaleficence were retained among the core principles of modern bioethics along with a fourth justice, the clinician was no longer considered the final arbiter of what constituted benefit and harm in the care of any particular patient. It is, after all, the patient who must endure the rigors of medical interventions and/or the burdens of disease. Thus, in the case of intractable disputes between clinician and patient, the patient has come to be recognized as the final arbiter. The dissenting clinician's option is to disengage from the relationship (but not precipitously so as to constitute abandonment) when and if respecting the patient's wishes compromises professional ethics or personal conscience.[4] The relief of pain and suffering, however, was not an integral part of this transformative process. Only quite recently have the legal, ethical, and public policy dimensions of pain management and palliative care begun to receive the attention they deserve, thereby properly placing them within the new bioethical, jurisprudential, and sociocultural framework. Providing the details of this process will be the task of this chapter, and the others in this section of the text.

The Duty to Relieve Pain and Suffering

When, over 2 decades ago, Eric Cassell began his seminal article on suffering and medicine in the *New England Journal of Medicine*, he did not think it necessary to build an extensive case for the proposition that physicians have a duty to relieve pain and suffering that dates back into antiquity. Nevertheless, his initial inquiries into the subject matter revealed a curious phenomenon: Contemporary patients and laypersons attached appreciably more significance to that duty than did his physician colleagues.[5] It is this disparity between lay persons and health care professionals in the prioritization of the need for and duty to provide pain relief that caused, or at least significantly contributed to, the jury verdicts in legal cases alleging undertreatment of pain, which we consider in Chapter 16. If, in the ethos of ancient medicine, the relief of pain and suffering was the essence of beneficence (doing good) and nonmaleficence (avoiding harm), then something transformative took place en route to modern medicine. Otherwise, the opening passage of the preface to Eric Cassell's book would be incomprehensible. That passage, a remarkably stinging indictment of his own profession, reads: "The test of a system of medicine should be its adequacy in the face of suffering . . . modern medicine fails that test."[6] Cassell analyzes in great depth important distinctions between pain and suffering, including notable instances in which a person can experience pain but not suffer, as well as suffer in the absence of pain. However, most pertinently to this chapter and text, he observes that pain is the most common cause of suffering and people in pain experience suffering when it is severe, uncontrolled, and seemingly without end.

Curative v. Palliative Paradigms of Patient Care

According to Cassell, the willful blindness that afflicts modern medicine with regard to pain and suffering relates to the complex nature of persons and the reductionistic tendencies of modern medical science. He cogently expresses the nub of the problem when he declares: "Bodies do not suffer; persons suffer." The implications of this proposition are clear but nonetheless potentially controversial: If a clinician cannot relate to the patient as a person, rather than as a body that is merely the locus of some disease process, then he or she cannot even recognize suffering, and certainly cannot begin to competently and compassionately respond to it. Unsurprisingly, many clinicians view this as a gross exaggeration, verging upon caricature. However, other credible sources bolster Cassel's point. Consider, for example, the assertions of Yale surgeon Sherwin Nuland in his book *How We Die*:

> . . . the challenge that motivates most persuasively; the challenge that makes each of us physicians continue ever trying to improve our skills; the challenge that results in the dogged pursuit of a diagnosis and a cure; the challenge that has resulted in the astounding progress of late-twentieth century clinical medicine—that foremost of challenges is not primarily the welfare of the individual human being, but rather, the solution of the The Riddle of his disease.[7]

Nuland is describing, with only a bit of grandiosity, one of the essential elements of the curative model cogently presented several years later by Ellen Fox.[8] For ease of analysis, her delineation of the essential features of the curative and palliative models of patient care is illustrated below.

Curative Model	Palliative Model
• analytic and rational	humanistic and personal
• clinical puzzle-solving	patient as person
• mind–body dualism	mind–body unity
• disvalues subjectivity	privileges subjectivity
• biomedical model	biocultural model
• discounts idiosyncrasy	respects idiosyncrasy
• death = failure	unnecessary suffering = failure

As illustrated above, point by point the essential features of the reigning curative model are the diametric opposite of the palliative model, the latter being the one that presumably must be followed in order to respond appropriately to the pain and suffering associated with both acute and chronic illness. The clinical puzzle-solving element is precisely what Nuland waxes so euphorically about in his discussion of the zealous pursuit of "the riddle," which he maintains is the primary motivator and the ultimate goal of the best clinicians.

As previously indicated, ethical issues in end-of-life care will be the special focus of Chapter 13 of this volume. Nevertheless, it is worth noting the stark contrast in the perspective on death and dying between the two models. The view of many clinicians in the full grip of the curative model that a patient's death is the ultimate medical failure has led, as Nuland himself admits, to situations in which medical specialists have "convinced patients to undergo diagnostic or therapeutic measures at a point in illness so far beyond reason that The Riddle might better have remained unsolved."[7] The type of clinical situations to which Nuland refers, particularly when patients are intentionally deceived or kept in the dark about the grimness of their prognosis or the dismal prospect that disease-directed interventions will produce any benefit, constitute a form of what might reasonably be characterized not only as "medical futility" but also as "therapeutic belligerence."[9]

THE PHENOMENON OF UNDERTREATED PAIN

The zealous, single-minded pursuit of a diagnosis and the relentless delivery of disease-directed interventions means, as a practical matter, that precious little professional time, energy, or attention is available for assessing and managing pain or suffering, even for patients in the intensive care unit who may be unlikely to leave the hospital alive. That is the bleak conclusion reached by the investigators in the formidable Study to Understand Prognoses, Preferences for Outcomes, and Risks of Treatment (SUPPORT) project in the mid-1990s.[10] The SUPPORT principal investigators sought to evaluate the quality of care in the intensive care unit of five premier academic medical centers across the country. The ICU, of course, is the locus of patient care in which the curative (disease-directed) paradigm of high technology patient care reigns supreme. The findings of the SUPPORT investigators are quite concerning with regard to such considerations as the relief of pain and suffering, the extent to which a patient's plan of care had been discussed with the patient or her proxy, or the likelihood that code status was consistent with what was known about the patient's wishes or values. For purposes of this discussion, at least three fundamental principles of bioethics were frequently violated in ICU care: respect for patient autonomy, beneficence, and nonmaleficence. More particularly, SUPPORT revealed that there was at best a 50–50 chance that the care provided to patients was consistent with their wishes, values, or written directives, and half of the patients studied were believed to be experiencing significant pain or distress in the last days of their lives.

Similar disappointing findings about pain and symptom management have been reported in the care of pediatric intensive care unit patients,[11] nursing home patients,[12] and in outpatient care of cancer patients.[13] The pervasiveness of deficiencies in pain and symptom management across the life span of patients, types of disease, and settings of care strongly suggests a problem that emanates from core issues in medicine and society to which we now must turn. Otherwise, we would be compelled to consider a highly implausible proposition; that is, that health care professionals are truly indifferent to the pain and suffering of their patients.

Identifying the Barriers to Pain Relief

In the last decade or two, an unprecedented amount of attention has been paid to the root causes of undertreated pain. A consistently cited set of barriers has been identified. At a basic level, these barriers exist with regard to all types of pain: acute, chronic noncancer, and pain associated with terminal illness. Certain barriers, as we shall duly note, are exacerbated in patients with chronic pain. The general categories into which these barriers are divided are professional, patient, and societal in nature and origin.

Professional Barriers

In one sense, as I will endeavor to make clear, the professional barriers to pain relief are the most ethically significant, given the fiduciary nature of the clinician–patient relationship. The key elements utilized in assessing professional competence are knowledge, skills, and attitudes. Deficiencies in any one of these elements can result in inadequate and hence substandard patient care. Deficiencies in more than one for any type of patient care will markedly increase the likelihood that substandard care will result. Marked deficiencies in each of these dimensions have been documented in physicians (of all specialties), nurses, and pharmacists.[14–16] Behavior, or more particularly, professional conduct, is the ultimate consideration. For it is when deficiencies in knowledge, skills, and attitudes concerning the assessment and management of pain coalesce to produce substandard care that their ethical implications become most significant. Given the pervasiveness of pain across the clinical spectrum, only rarely may any clinician legitimately claim that such deficiencies pose no threat of harm to patients. As we shall further consider shortly, however, even clinicians who possess the requisite knowledge, skills, and attitudes may be reluctant to translate them consistently into effective pain management, particularly when what is clinically indicated may be opioid analgesia, because of fears of regulatory scrutiny or other forms of potential legal liability.

None other than John Bonica himself pointed out many years ago that no medical school has been so bold and innovative as to establish and maintain a formal, required curriculum in assessing and treating the most common problem of patients who seek medical care—pain.[17] The glaring deficiency that he described nearly 20 years ago persists. In data ascribed to the Association of American Medical Colleges in 2003, only 3% of medical schools have a separate required course in pain management, and only 4% require students to take a course in end-of-life care.[18]

The absence of any solid evidence of a formal curriculum in the assessment and management of pain in most institutions warrants the conclusion that none actually exists. Some defenders of the status quo have argued that the requisite knowledge, skills, and attitudes are imparted in other, less formal but perfectly acceptable ways, such as in the care of actual patients in the clinical

years of medical education. What undermines these assertions is the strong evidence that health care professionals continue to graduate and obtain licensure with major deficits in knowledge, skills, and attitudes concerning pain management and its relevance to quality in patient care.

The ethical significance of this phenomenon is the aforementioned "culpability of cultivated ignorance." The absence of a pain curriculum in medical and other educational programs in the health professions may be an important reason why pain is often undertreated, but is not an excuse for it. Medical schools have been, and continue to be, major culprits in the epidemic of pain. It is not merely an absence of required course work on up-to-date pain assessment and management techniques, but also myths and misconceptions about the risks and purportedly unmanageable side effects of opioids that are deeply entrenched in the minds of clinical faculty and which are passed on from one generation of physicians to the next.[19] That is perhaps why, when the American Medical Association developed the Education for Physicians on End-of-Life Care Project (EPEC), it adopted a train-the-trainer approach in the hope of maximizing the dissemination of current thinking on palliative care to experienced practitioners rather than medical students or residents.[20] When one enters a profession, one assumes a moral responsibility to ensure that one possesses and consistently applies the knowledge and skills essential to minimal competence. That one may in some instances enter the profession with certain deficiencies does not provide a legitimate basis for cultivating the ignorance that may be originally attributable to curricular deficiencies. The medical school curriculum should reflect the current standard of care and anticipate future improvements to it, but it does not set that standard in any definitive sense.

In California, the continuing absence of a pain curriculum in medical schools, combined with increasing public awareness of and outrage over a national, indeed international, epidemic of undertreated pain, moved one crusading member of the California Assembly to introduce and successfully pursue a statute mandating two things: (1) that pain management and end-of-life care be part of the medical school curriculum for applicants seeking a license as a California physician after June 1, 2000; and (2) that inpatient health facilities include pain as a fifth vital sign assessed along with other vital signs and noted in the patient's medical record.[21] In yet another example of lawmakers interceding to address professional deficiencies, the California Assembly in 2001 enacted a statute requiring that all licensed physicians in the state (with the exception of radiologists and pathologists) receive a minimum of 12 hours of continuing medical education prior to January 1, 2007.[22]

These and the other legislative measures described hereinafter actually run counter to a well-established tradition in American government to leave the professions, particularly the health professions, virtually unfettered latitude and discretion to manage their affairs. Only when substantial evidence accumulates—and results in a high level of public concern—are lawmakers prompted to intercede. When morally troubling circumstances are allowed to persist by those who ostensibly have the power and authority to address them through nonlegal measures, the law has been invoked to address the problem. A graphic example was the Nuremberg Code that emerged from the Nuremberg Tribunal's prosecution of the Nazi doctors. The first principle of the Nuremberg Code was the right of human research subjects to informed consent. Twenty-five years later, when the public became aware that a number of clinical trials conducted by prominent medical researchers in the United States were openly and notoriously violating the Code, which was an ethical–professional, not necessarily a legal mandate, the federal government stepped in with the first of what became many regulations of federally funded research involving human subjects.[23]

Similarly, in the early 1980s a phenomenon known as "patient dumping" became the subject of significant public awareness and concern. When indigent or uninsured patients presented to emergency rooms, they were with increasing frequency shunted off to other (usually government operated) hospitals for care, often with deleterious consequences from the delay in properly addressing an unstable medical condition. When neither the health professions nor national hospital organizations demonstrated any inclination to address the problem, the Congress of the United States passed the Emergency Medical Treatment and Active Labor Act (EMTALA), which imposed a mandate on all emergency departments to provide a medical screening examination to patients upon arrival, and prohibiting transfer of any patient found to be in an unstable medical condition prior to stabilization except under certain carefully described situations.[24] Notably, EMTALA recognized pain as an indication of an unstable medical condition requiring prompt attention and effective remediation. These instances indicate that it is often the failure or refusal of health care institutions and/or professionals to put their own houses in order that prompts major governmental intervention in order to address an otherwise seemingly intractable problem.

One must ask whether there is a causal connection between the failure of health professional schools to recognize the need for a pain curriculum, and the failure of the health professions and the institutions in which health care is delivered to make the prompt, effective, and consistent assessment and management of pain a priority in patient care. We noted early in this chapter how Eric Cassell was perplexed by the seeming indifference to the phenomenon of suffering on the part of physicians given the traditional core values of medicine. The same is true for pain, since another professional barrier has been characterized as the failure of health care institutions and professionals to make pain relief a priority in patient care. One of the primary objectives of many of the policies discussed in Chapter 14 of this text, particularly the Federation of State Medical Boards (FSMB) Model Policy and the Joint Commission Accreditation Manual standards on pain management, was to disabuse their target audience of the persistent notion that effective pain management was not an essential feature of sound patient care.

The final professional barrier to effective pain management is fear of regulatory scrutiny and potential legal liability (civil or criminal). There is little question that the nidus of this concern is opioid analgesia. There is quite simply no discussion about such concerns arising out of nonpharmacological pain management strategies. When one looks at the record of disciplinary actions by state medical boards, those relating in any manner to pain management practices were invariably characterized as excessive prescribing of opioids. Such cases will be addressed in detail in Chapter 15 of this text. It is for this reason that the previously mentioned FSMB policy is of such potential significance, for it seeks to shift the focus of medical boards from "overprescribing" or "underprescribing" of opioids to inappropriate prescribing, since both extremes pose risks to patients.

From an ethical perspective, it is a troubling state of affairs when clinicians fear that they are at risk of disciplinary action by their professional licensing board if they follow current national clinical practice guidelines on the use of opioid analgesics. Their concerns have not been without foundation, for an initial survey of the knowledge and attitudes of state medical licensing board members regarding opioids and pain management revealed significant knowledge deficits and attitudes that were at best unsupportive and at worst hostile toward the use of opioids, especially for patients with chronic noncancer pain.[25] One analysis of the prevailing attitude among medical board members concerning opioid analgesia characterized it as an "ethic of underprescribing."[26] A follow-up study conducted after the promulgation of FSMB guidelines on prescribing opioids and a series of workshops across the country on pain management for medical board members revealed some improvement in areas that might be reassuring to those whom boards are charged with regulating, but also noted the need for further education and wider acceptance of the FSMB model guidelines/policy.[27]

When medical and other health professions' boards issue new and presumably more enlightened policies on pain management, one cannot presume that most affected clinicians will become aware of them. There is still less of a basis to expect that these policies will, in the short term, have a direct and immediate impact on clinical practice even among clinicians who become aware of them. In the event that these new or updated policies were to become part of a mandatory continuing professional education program, there is nevertheless reason for concern that they would in fact be likely to significantly improve the usual custom and practice of minimizing the clinical significance of pain that has been mentored, modeled, and followed by generations of professionals.[28] Concerted efforts must be made to reform practice patterns and the underlying clinical culture that sustains them by infusing more enlightened attitudes about the importance of pain relief to patient health and well-being.

The regulatory barriers also include the federal Controlled Substances Act, the policies and procedures of the Drug Enforcement Administration, and criminal prosecutions of physicians for drug diversion or trafficking when their prescribing practices are deemed far outside the ambit of mainstream medicine. These issues are dealt in depth in Chapters 14 and 15 of this volume. The ethics of public policy formulation and law enforcement strategies and tactics are somewhat beyond the scope of this chapter. Nevertheless, such practices are fraught with moral implications because they affect the lives of many people. Much of the impetus for the new emphasis on balance intended to moderate between seemingly competing considerations of preventing drug abuse and diversion, on the one hand, and ensuring that patients in pain receive the analgesics they require for effective relief, has been based on legitimate concerns that state and federal regulatory and law enforcement measures have been obsessively focused on the former and virtually indifferent to the latter. We will consider the moral dimensions of pain policy and law further from the perspective of the health care professional in a subsequent section of this chapter as well, when we take up the demands of professionalism to make the patient's needs and interests primary in a fiduciary relationship.

Patient Barriers

In one sense at least, it should not be surprising that if clinicians commonly labor under myths and misinformation about the clinical significance of pain and the risk and side effects of opioids, so too will patients. Traditionally clinicians were the primary source of patient information on medicine and health. If they did not themselves possess accurate and up-to-date information about the risks and benefits of pharmacological and nonpharmacological modalities of pain relief, they would not be able to educate their patients. Indeed, that is why pain management has historically been an area of clinical practice in which truly informed patient consent was virtually nonexistent. Now, however, in the Internet age, patients and family members may actually access up-to-date information on pain and its management as or more often than their physicians.

Without adequate information concerning the available range of pain management interventions and their risks and benefits, patients had no basis upon which to formulate reasonable expectations with regard to pain relief. A major public survey on pain in the United States conducted in 1997 revealed that not only is pain pervasive, but the most common reason why people avoid seeking medication to relieve their pain is fear of addiction or physical dependence.[29] Patients may also avoid seeking medical care when they experience pain because they fear it may be caused by some serious, perhaps even life-threatening, condition. Finally, patients experiencing pain that is associated with conditions for which they are currently receiving treatment may not complain about their pain and seek more effective pain relief because of a mistaken assumption that pain is an unavoidable concomitant of therapy or that their physician would certainly be providing as much pain relief as possible. It is these latter perspectives that help explain how, until the legal cases discussed in Chapter 15 arose, no malpractice claims based upon negligent pain management had been brought despite an epidemic of undertreated pain.[30]

Societal Barriers

Pain and suffering are not just immensely complex and highly individualized human experiences. They occur within familial and other interpersonal contexts, as well as social, organizational, and governmental configurations. Pain in particular may be a symptom of an underlying condition, but it may also, in the case of chronic noncancer pain, become a condition itself, hence the appropriateness of the term "chronic pain syndrome." These are by definition, as Arthur Kleinman has observed, "conditions in which the degree of pathology does not seem to explain the severity of perceived pain or the limitations in bodily functioning the pain produces."[31] This marked disparity between the patient's pathophysiology and reports (often interpreted as complaints) of pain and disability produces a strong element of skepticism, not only on the part of clinicians from whom the patient seeks care, but also from family and friends. These doubts about the veracity of the patient's experience of chronic pain can exacerbate the feelings of isolation and abandonment that characterize the chronic pain patient. At the end of this chapter we further consider the special challenges for the clinician posed by the chronic pain patient.

American culture in particular has precious little patience with or sympathy for the chronically ill. Indeed, much of the recent momentum within the disability rights movement has been an understandably strong reaction to the widespread perception among the healthy and able-bodied that certain profoundly disabling conditions are categorically incompatible with any quality of life whatsoever. In response to such pervasive attitudes, perhaps the most high-profile disability rights organization took the name "Not Dead Yet." Their message is clear to society in general and health professionals in particular: We do not seek your assistance in ending what *you* consider our miserable existence, but rather in enhancing what *we* consider to be our quality of life and our ability to be active and engaged members of our community.

ETHICAL IMPLICATIONS OF THE BARRIERS

There is a new emphasis in both undergraduate and graduate medical education on professionalism and communication.[32] In some small measure, such curricular reforms may begin to address the larger and more fundamental problem identified by previously cited commentators such as Cassel, Fox, Kleinman, and Morris that is posed by medicine's predilection for biological reductionism and obsession with diagnostic and disease-directed interventions. The none-too-subtle point is that one does not enter into a professional relationship with or provide care to a disease process. While a certain cadre of clinicians may romanticize the pursuit of "the riddle" of disease, the professional relationship (fiduciary in nature) and communication are necessarily with the personhood, not the disease of the patient. The assessment of pain, for example, is all about effective communication between patient and physician concerning the subjective experience of pain. If effective pain assessment is absolutely essential to providing effective pain relief, then the clinician must be able to understand and appreciate the patient's experience of illness in a manner and to an extent that may not be true for other aspects of patient care.

The concept of holding oneself out as a professional and the ethical demands of entering into a fiduciary relationship with another person entail the acquisition, utilization, and maintenance of the knowledge, skills, and attitudes necessary to ensure minimally sufficient competence. When a significant percentage of the practitioners of a profession such as medicine or nursing have been found to have major deficiencies in something as pervasive as pain and as integral to good patient care as are its assessment and management, invariably major ethical issues arise. It is in the recognition of these ethical issues that one demonstrates a grasp of the close relationship between ethics and professionalism. Yet there was a period in the early years of the movement to address the widespread phenomenon of undertreated pain when, as noted in the beginning of this chapter, there was little acknowledgment of, and hence attention to, the ethical dimensions of these professional deficiencies.

Turning from barriers associated with knowledge deficits and problematic attitudes toward the significance of pain and its relief to those associated with legal and regulatory concerns, we encounter a challenging ethical quandary. As described in detail in Chapter 14, the regulation of opioid analgesics has created a hostile environment toward their widespread use in pain management. Regulatory barriers, including a pattern of medical board disciplinary actions against physicians for so-called "overprescribing" of opioids, have, as previously noted, caused physicians to feel at risk even if they are scrupulously following state-of-the-art clinical practice guidelines.

A fundamental ethical question posed by this situation is: To what extent is it reasonable to expect, indeed to demand, that physicians routinely engage in acts of moral courage in order to ensure that their patients with pain receive the medications that they require for relief? The essence of the duty imposed upon a professional when entering into a fiduciary relationship is that the other person's interests become primary, and any potential conflict of interest shall be resolved in favor of the person to whom the professional duty is owed. Therefore, prescribing inadequate doses of analgesics or opioids from a lower schedule of the Controlled Substances Act (e.g., Schedule III–V) when those from a higher schedule (e.g., Schedule II) are medically indicated in order to avoid regulatory scrutiny would constitute a breach of fiduciary duty. It is also the case, however, that a public policy posture and regulatory regime that routinely demands acts of moral courage on the part of professionals is a fundamentally flawed system that is vulnerable to strong moral critique. Such a critique is at least implied in the Report Card on state and federal pain policies that has been issued by the Pain & Policy Studies Group and which is discussed in some detail in Chapter 14.

EMBRACING A NEW ETHIC OF PAIN RELIEF

While it is important to understand the historical context in which formerly prevailing attitudes toward pain and its relief with opioids developed and ultimately became so pervasive and persistent, we must continue the momentum that has followed from more enlightened attitudes in order to address emerging ethical concerns. The clinical specialty of pain medicine has played a major role in the progress that has been achieved in the last 2 decades. Ultimately, however, each of the health professions has a responsibility to cultivate within its practitioners the knowledge, skills, and attitudes that are essential to the provision of effective pain management. The need for highly trained physicians and nurses in pain and palliative care will continue to grow, but so too will the need for all physicians and nurses to possess certain minimal core competencies in the assessment and management of pain.

A chapter on the ethics of pain management would be woefully inadequate if it did not address some of the special issues and problems of chronic pain patients. It is in this patient population, for reasons we will consider, that the efforts to identify an appropriate balance between the long-standing War on Drugs and the newly-minted War on Pain are primarily focused. Having already noted Arthur Kleinman's seminal work on the plight of the patient with chronic pain, we now must turn to emerging policies, protocols, and guidelines on care of the chronic pain patient, and their sometimes overlooked ethical dimensions. One of the new shibboleths in pain medicine is "pharmacovigilence."[33] The implicit premise of this concept is that clinicians are not truly confronted with a genuine moral dilemma of providing effective pain relief for patients or preventing drug abuse and diversion. The basic presupposition appears to be that the parameters delineated by pharmacovigilance, as conceived by some of the thought leaders in pain medicine, enable a responsible prescribing professional to provide appropriate and effective pain relief to patients while at the same time significantly minimizing the known risk of addiction posed by opioids or their diversion to persons who have no legitimate need for them. In other words, pharmacovigilant pain management recognizes the need in clinical practice for a kind of balance that is similar to the balance sought in laws, regulations, and public policies affecting opioid analgesics as discussed in Chapter 14 of this text.

While in theory all opioid prescribing, indeed, all prescribing of medications of any type should reflect pharmacovigiliance, the term has most often been invoked in the context of chronic pain management. While the available data support the conclusion that all types of pain have been undertreated, the plight of chronic noncancer pain patients has been particularly bleak because it is not uncommon for their reports of pain to exceed the tangible clinical evidence that would appear to support their legitimacy. Furthermore, patients who have just undergone major surgical procedures, been the victims of traumatic injury, or who are facing terminal conditions, do not encounter the same credibility problems when they report high levels of pain and seek relief. The phenomenon of pseudoaddiction, in which patients with genuine pain that has been undertreated engage in behaviors that cause them to appear to be drug seeking (in some illegitimate sense), is most prevalent in the population of chronic noncancer pain patients.[34] While it was once thought that undertreatment of pain at the end of life was the driving force behind the movement to legalize the prescribing of lethal doses of medication at the request of patients with terminal illness, the data accumulated as a result of the Oregon Death With Dignity Act reveal that undertreated pain is actually not even among the five most frequently cited reasons why dying patients seek a lethal prescription.[35]

Some of the practices that have come to be advocated with increasing frequency under the rubric of "pharmacovigilance" or responsible opioid prescribing are opioid contracts and random urine drug screens. Both approaches raise critical questions of an ethical nature about the role of trust in the clinician–patient relationship, as well as questions about why patients with chronic pain are special cases that require such measures when other patients whose conditions necessitate treatment with potentially dangerous medications and strict adherence to clinician recommendations do not. We will focus here particularly on the contracts/agreements that are being so widely promoted, the form that they take, the benefits that are claimed by their proponents, and the risks they pose to the establishment and maintenance of trust in the clinician–patient relationship.

There is an ethically more and less benign way in which to view and characterize the nature and role of these documents. The more benign approach is to simply consider the contract or agreement under the traditional rubric of a written informed consent document. Informed consent is a foundational concept in both medical ethics and medical jurisprudence, and the primary mechanism by which respect for individual patient autonomy is

demonstrated.[36] The execution by patients of consent forms is a routine practice for any invasive medical procedure or other therapeutic measure. Thus, to the extent that an opioid contract were nothing more than a patient's written informed consent to undergo opioid therapy, acknowledging thereby both the risks and benefits associated with it, there would be nothing remarkable about it and certainly nothing that would raise serious ethical concerns.

The authors of one important article on the subject state: "The contract is ideally intended to enhance the therapeutic relationship by initiating and supporting an alliance between the patient and the physician. It may enable a patient to have an active role in treatment. . . ."[37] The key word in this passage may be "ideal," for there is growing concern among some that the primary reasons why opioid contracts are becoming routine among those physicians who are willing to consider opioid therapy for chronic noncancer pain patients relate to risk management and regulatory/law enforcement considerations rather than patient well being. For example, one review of opioid contracts that are currently in use revealed that over 90% had specific conditions warranting disciplinary termination of the agreement by the physician (e.g., for violating terms of the contract or missing appointments) and nearly 70% required submission to random drug screens, whereas only 5% stated the potential benefits of opioid therapy and just 3% provided general information regarding treatment.[37] Since the latter two elements are most typically found on consent forms, their absence seriously undermines the argument that these contracts are merely more elaborate or formal consent documents.

Such contract provisions emphasize the physician's power to impose conditions of treatment upon patients rather than the autonomy of the patient to participate meaningfully in the consideration of therapeutic options according to the paradigm of shared decision-making.[38] Interestingly, the American Academy of Pain Medicine (AAPM) features a "Sample Agreement" for "Long-term Controlled Substances Therapy for Chronic Pain" on its Web site, but the document also declares itself to be "a consent form." This agreement/consent form contains 19 provisions, including the more common ones, such as obtaining all opioid prescriptions from a single physician and filling them at a single pharmacy. The form advises that unannounced urine or serum toxicology screens may be "requested," to which the patient is "required" to submit. While, as previously noted, a typical consent form consists in large measure of a description of the proposed intervention, its anticipated benefits and risks, as well as the alternatives, the AAPM agreement/form states: "the risks and benefits of these therapies are explained elsewhere (and you acknowledge that you have received such explanation)."[39]

The absence of such detailed therapeutic agreements in most other clinical settings in which the modalities of treatment and the need for patient adherence to the therapeutic regimen are of equal importance to patient well-being (e.g., cancer chemotherapy) suggests that chronic noncancer pain patients who require opioid analgesia for effective relief warrant a heightened level of suspicion. Furthermore, the widespread and routine use of opioid contracts by many physicians for all of their chronic noncancer pain patients receiving opioid therapy, but not for acute pain or pain associated with terminal illness, implies that there is something intrinsically untrustworthy or suspicious about this category of patient.[40] Clearly, however, merely being a victim of chronic noncancer pain that happens to be refractory to nonopioid analgesics is not inherently suspicious. Such patients and syndromes exist, and a consensus of thought leaders in pain medicine has emerged in support of the position that opioid analgesia should generally be offered to these patients unless there are specific and significant contraindications.[41]

Recent acknowledgment that earlier estimations of the risk of addiction associated with opioid analgesia were much too low does not undercut this consensus view. The best current evidence is that the incidence of addictive disorders (of all types) in the general population ranges from 3% to 26%, while the rate for hospitalized patients is 19% to 25%, and for major trauma patients as high as 40% to 60%.[42] It is important to note that recently formulated model pain policies do not recommend the routine use of either opioid agreements or urine drug screens in all patients—even all chronic noncancer pain patients—but rather those patients who in the exercise of sound clinical judgment are deemed to pose a "high risk for medication abuse or have a history of substance abuse."[43] Approaches to screening for addiction prior to the initiation of chronic opioid therapy as well as assessing for addiction during therapy (exclusive of urine toxicology screening) have been identified and utilized.[44]

The imposition of random urine drug screening as one condition precedent to offering opioid therapy to a patient appears to have become a common practice among clinicians whose practice includes patients with persistent pain problems. As with opioid agreements themselves, random drug screens may be required of all patients who receive opioid analgesia for an extended period, not simply those whose histories raise questions or concerns about the likelihood that they will take the medications as directed. In this way it might be argued that all patients for whom opioid analgesia is indicated are treated the same, rather than certain patients being stigmatized by differential treatment that calls their capacity to adhere to the treatment protocol in question. Nonadherence to chronic opioid therapy may take a variety of forms, including consuming more (or less) than the amount of the prescribed drug directed by the prescribing clinician, using opioids obtained from other sources, and failing to take the drug prescribed, whether or not the drug is then sold or otherwise diverted from legitimate medical use.

Failure to comply with instructions concerning the taking of medication is not unique to chronic pain patients, and the risks of such behaviors by patients can have serious consequences in many different clinical settings, including diabetes, hypertension, epilepsy, and cancer therapy, to name only a few.[44] Nevertheless, it has not yet become routine to insist on prescription medication agreements and laboratory screening for those patients, even when studies suggest that in some patient populations nonadherence to therapeutic regimens may exceed 50%.[45,46]

One important distinction between nonadherence to opioid therapy and nonadherence to other pharmacological regimens that do not involved prescription medications that are subject to diversion and abuse is the risk posed to society. A patient who must take a prescription medication for a serious medical condition but who fails to do so as directed in most instances places only him or herself at risk of adverse consequences. However, when nonadherence to opioid therapy takes the form of selling or otherwise diverting these medications, there are significant adverse societal implications. There is no question that clinicians have responsibilities to their communities and the society at large and not only to their individual patients. Sometimes, as in the case of public health emergencies, there may be genuine conflicts between these two responsibilities. However, minimizing the risk of opioid addiction and diversion through the responsible use of treatment agreements and adherence monitoring enables the clinician to meet his or her obligations to both individual patient and society. As with the informed consent and information disclosure process itself, the manner in which such approaches are taken is every bit as important as the details of the approach itself. Moreover, it may well be the case that the wider use of measures to warn patients about the risks of nonadherence to prescription medication regimens and to monitor such adherence may be a necessary and appropriate response by the health professions to the data documenting the extent to which patients fail to take their medications as prescribed.

What is needed but presently does not exist are rigorous empirical studies evaluating the effects of patient agreements and drug screening on adherence to or the outcomes of treatment regimens.[38]

It would not be surprising to find that some of the high profile federal prosecutions of physicians with very liberal prescribing practices described in detail in Chapter 15 of this text have fueled the widespread adoption of rigorous opioid contract provisions. Those physicians were alleged to have, among other things, engaged in a form of willful blindness to a host of red flags that some of their patients either had no legitimate medical need for opioids or were flagrantly abusing or selling their medications. The recordkeeping and monitoring by the physicians was poor to nonexistent.

CONCLUSION

The ethics of pain management are in a profound state of flux. Neither the terms evolution nor revolution seem to be an apt characterization, for such terms suggest a gradual and organic development process on the one hand or a transformational paradigm shift on the other, neither of which can be supported by the existing evidence. Rather, the current state of affairs might well be characterized, without risk of serious exaggeration, as a battle for the soul of medicine. For as we noted at the very beginning of this chapter, seminal works on the place of pain and suffering in the context of the patient's experience of illness consistently remind us that their relief is a core value of medicine with roots running back to the very origins of the profession. In the modern era, when organized medicine has confronted phenomena such as physician-assisted suicide (aid in dying) or physician participation in lethal injection, prominent voices in opposition to the legitimacy of the physician's role in such practices have consistently invoked statements of principle such as the following: "Healing the sick and alleviating suffering is the primary role of physicians in U.S. society."[48] Yet those same voices have, for the most part, been silent in the midst of an epidemic of undertreated pain that afflicts chronic noncancer pain patients disproportionately. It has fallen to organizations such as the World Health Organization (WHO) and the International Association for the Study of Pain (IASP) to call for the recognition of pain relief as a human right.[49]

In no other aspect of patient care has the fundamental role of trust in the clinician–patient relationship become more of a pivotal issue than in the care of patients with chronic noncancer pain. With the proliferation of detailed opioid contracts including provisions for routine urine drug screens and rigidly specified grounds for terminating the relationship for nonaderence, we may be at risk of distrust becoming the reigning paradigm.[50] A shibboleth of the cold war era was "trust but verify." This approach may well have a place in patient care and the standard of care with which clinicians must comply. The challenge to the health professions posed by the current ambivalence toward patients requiring opioid analgesia for moderate to severe noncancer pain is formidable. On one hand are prominent voices such as the WHO and the IASP calling for recognition of a human right to pain relief for all patients. On the other hand are dire warnings to clinicians about deceptive, drug-seeking patients who must be engaged with extreme caution, a robust skepticism, rigorous scrutiny, as well as all of the other essential elements of pharmacovigilance. The establishment of a solid consensus among clinical and regulatory stakeholders as to where we ought to situate a healthy and reasonable balance between extreme, unrealistic naiveté and a rigid, pervasive cynicism about the role of trust in the care of patients with persistent pain should become a high priority for all conscientious and caring professionals.

References

1. Morris DM. *The Culture of Pain*. Berkeley: University of California Press; 1991:190–192.
2. Faden RR, Beauchamp TL, King NMP. *A History and Theory of Informed Consent*. New York: Oxford University Press; 1986.
3. Rothman DJ. *Strangers at the Bedside: A History of How Law and Bioethics Transformed Medical Decision Making*. New York: Basic Books; 1991.
4. Veatch RM. *The Patient-Physician Relationship: The Patient As Partner*. Bloomington, Ind: Indiana University Press; 1991.
5. Cassel EJ. The nature of suffering and the goals of medicine. *N Engl J Med* 1982;306:639–645.
6. Cassel EJ. *The Nature of Suffering and the Goals of Medicine*. New York: Oxford University Press;1991:vii.
7. Nuland SB. *How We Die: Reflections on Life's Final Chapter*. The lessons learned. New York: Alfred A. Knopf; 1994:248–249.
8. Fox E. Predominance of the curative model of medical care. A residual problem. *JAMA* 1997;278:761–763.
9. Pellegrino ED, Thomasma DM. *For the Patient's Good: The Restoration of Beneficence in Health Care*. New York: Oxford University Press; 1988:94.
10. The SUPPORT Principle Investigators. A controlled trial to improve care of seriously ill hospitalized patients. The study to understand prognoses and preferences for outcomes and risks of treatments (SUPPORT). *JAMA* 1995;274:1591–1598.
11. Wolfe J, Grier HE, Klar N, et al. Symptoms and suffering at the end of life in children with cancer. *N Engl J Med* 2000;342:326–333.
12. American Geriatrics Society. The management of persistent pain in older persons: AGS panel on persistent pain in older persons. *J Am Geriatr Soc* 1998;46:635–651.
13. Cleeland CS, Gonin R, Hatfield AK, et al. Pain and its treatment in outpatients with metastatic cancer. *N Engl J Med* 1994;330:592–596.
14. Von Roenn JH, Cleeland CS, Gonin R, et al. Physician attitudes and practices in cancer pain management. A survey from the Eastern Oncology Group. *Ann Intern Med* 1993;119:121–126.
15. Sanderson L. Review. Attitudes to and knowledge about pain and pain management of nurses working with children with cancer: a comparative study between UK, South Africa, and Sweden. *J Res Nurs* 2007;12:517–519.
16. Joranson DE, Gilson AM. Pharmacists' knowledge and attitudes about pain medication in relation to federal and state policies. *J Am Pharm Assoc (Wash)* 2001;41:213–220.
17. Weiner RS. An interview with John J. Bonica, MD. *Pain Practitioner* 1989;1:2.
18. Silverman J. Students need more pain management training: education effort underway. OB/GYN News. Available at: http://www.obgynnews.com/article/S0029-7434(03)70079-2/fulltext. Accessed October 15, 2003.
19. Hill CS Jr. When will adequate pain management be the norm? *JAMA* 1995;274:1881–1882.
20. The EPEC™ Project. Available at: http://www.epec.net/EPEC/Webpages/index.cfm. Accessed May 5, 2009.
21. Thomson H. A new law to improve pain management and end-of-life care. *West J Med* 2001;174:161–162.
22. CA Bus & Prof Code Act, 10 § 2190.5.
23. Frankel MS. *The Public Health Service Guidelines Governing Research Involving Human Subjects*. Washington, DC: George Washington University Program of Policy Studies in Science and Technology Monograph No. 10; 1972:20–21.
24. Emergency Medical Treatment and Active Labor Act, 42 USC §1395dd.
25. Joranson DE, Cleeland CS, Weissman DE, et al. Opioids for chronic cancer and non-cancer pain: a survey of State Medical Boards. *Fed Bull: J Med Licensure Discipline* 1992;79:15–49.
26. Martino AM. In search of a new ethic for treating patients with chronic pain: what can medical boards do? *J Law Med Ethics* 1998;26:332–349, 263.
27. Gilson AM, Joranson DE. Controlled substances and pain management: changes in knowledge and attitudes of state regulators. *J Pain Symptom Manage* 2001;21:227–237.
28. Max MB. Improving outcomes of analgesic treatment: is education enough? *Ann Intern Med* 1990;113:885–889.
29. Bostrom M. Summary of the Mayday Fund Survey: public attitudes about pain and analgesics. *J Pain Symptom Manage* 1997;13:166–168.
30. Dawson R, Spross JA, Jablonski ES, et al. Probing the paradox of patient's satisfaction with inadequate pain management. *J Pain Symptom Manage* 2002;23:211–220.
31. Kleinman A. *The Illness Narratives: Suffering, Healing & the Human Condition*. Vulnerability of Pain and the Pain of Vulnerability. New York: Basic Books;1988:59.
32. Whitcomb ME. Professionalism in medicine. *Acad Med* 2007;82:1009.
33. Fishman SM. *Responsible Opioid Prescribing: A Physician's Guide*. Washington, DC: Federation of State Medical Boards and Waterford Life Sciences; 2007:Appendix A.
34. Weissman DE, Haddox JD. Opioid pseudoaddiction. *Pain* 1989;36:363–366.
35. Oregon Death with Dignity Act Annual Report, March 2007. Available at: http://www.oregon.gov/DHS/ph/pas/ar-index.shtml. Accessed December 16, 2007.
36. Meisel A, Kuczewski M. Legal and ethical myths about informed consent. *Arch Intern Med* 1996;156:2521–2526.
37. Fishman SM, Bandman TB., Edwards A, et al. The opioid contract in the management of chronic pain. *J Pain Symptom Manage* 1999;18:27–37.
38. Arnold RM, Han PK, Seltzer D. Opioid contracts in chronic nonmalignant pain management: objectives and uncertainties. *Am J Med* 2006;119:292–296.
39. American Academy of Pain Medicine. Long-term controlled substances therapy for chronic pan – sample Agreement. Available at: http://www.painmed.org/pdf/controlled_substances_sample_agrmt.pdf. Accessed May 6, 2009.
40. Miller J. The other side of trust in health care: prescribing drugs with the potential for abuse. *Bioethics* 2007;21:51–60.
41. Savage SR. Assessment for addiction in pain-treatment settings. *Clin J Pain* 2002;18:S28–S38.
42. American Academy of Pain Medicine and American Pain Society. Consensus statement: the use of opioids for the treatment of chronic pain. Available at: http://www.painmed.org/pdf/opioids.pdf. Accessed May 6, 2009.
43. Federation of State Medical Boards of the United States. Model policy for the use of controlled substances for the treatment of pain (2004). Available at: http://www.fsmb.org/pdf/2004_grpol_Controlled_Substances.pdf. Accessed May 6, 2009.
44. Fishman SM, Wilsey B, Yang J, et al. Adherence monitoring and drug surveillance in chronic opioid therapy. *J Pain Symptom Manage* 2000;20:293–307.
45. Cramer JA, Mattson RH, Prevey ML, et al. How often is medication taken as prescribed? A novel technique. *JAMA* 1989;261:3273–3277.
46. Levine AM, Richardson JL, Marks G, et al. Compliance with oral drug therapy in patients with hematologic malignancy. *J Clin Oncol* 1987;5:1469–1476.
47. Beauchamp TL, Childress JF. *Principles of Biomedical Ethics*. 4th ed. New York, Oxford University Press; 1994:163–170.
48. Black L, Sade RM. Lethal injection and physicians: state law vs medical ethics. *JAMA* 2007;298:2779–2781.
49. World Health Organization. Pain relief a human right. Available at: http://www.who.int/mediacentre/news/releases/2004/pr70/en/. Accessed May 6, 2009.
50. Victor L, Richeimer SH. Trustworthiness as a clinical variable: the problem of trust in the management of chronic, nonmalignant pain. *Pain Med* 2005;6:385–391.

CHAPTER 13 ■ ETHICAL ISSUES IN THE CARE OF DYING PATIENTS

DAVID BARNARD

INTRODUCTION

The Quest for Moral Order Amid Existential Disorder

To the dying person his doctor, however much he is trusted and regarded as a source of treatment, is no longer one with the power to cure; to the doctor, the patient has become one whose death, despite every possible effort, he is impotent to prevent. This gives rise to problems in the special professional relationship which often develops between a patient and his doctor, and besides that they have the difficulties that face any two people trying to adjust to the fact that one of them is shortly going to die.[1]

This comment by John Hinton is a pointed reminder that the patient's nearness to death places the patient and the doctor in a challenging and disturbing place, both in their relationship with each other and in their sense of personal identity. The direct encounter with death—in the guise of the death of the patient—has the power to disrupt the doctor's relationship and communication with the dying person, throw ordinarily rational decision making into confusion, and capsize carefully wrought treatment plans.

Robert Burt has commented on the "inherent unruliness of death and the persistence of individual and social ambivalence about death" as features that limit our ability to fashion social policies and practice guidelines that are free of moral ambiguity or the possibility for evil and abuse. At the conclusion of his study of the conflict-ridden policies governing abortion, the death penalty, and physician-assisted death in the United States during the last half-century, Burt writes,

Here is the paradox that we must learn to live with in regulating death: that we must teach ourselves, through our rational intellectual capacities, that our rational intellect cannot adequately comprehend, much less adequately control, death. We are no more compassionate, honorable, or intelligent than our predecessors who embraced the pursuit of rational mastery over death and were led, without acknowledgment, into unreasoned evil. We would do better to admit, as W.H. Auden acknowledged, that "Death is not understood by Death; nor You, nor I."[2]

The Contributions and Limitations of Ethical Analysis in End-of-Life Care

Hinton and Burt suggest that the psychological and existential dimensions of the encounter with death destabilize the doctor–patient relationship and rational decision making. They also require acknowledgment of the limitations as well as the contributions of ethical analysis in end-of-life care. At the most general level, the discipline of ethics itself embodies the cacophony of voices, worldviews, cultural frameworks, and value systems characteristic of postmodernity. As philosophers such as Alasdair McIntyre[3] and H. Tristram Englehardt[4] argue, no single, overarching standpoint or scale of values commands universal allegiance in a secular, pluralist society that is committed to the peaceable resolution of differences. Yet without such a universally compelling standpoint, there is no means short of force to eliminate the contradictions between philosophical systems or the competing claims of multiple moral communities.

Two aspects of uncertainty more specifically related to clinical ethics near the end of life are worth particular note at the outset. Consider the commonly accepted public consensus on the ethics of end-of-life care. Its main points include the following:

1. Competent adults may refuse medical treatment.
2. Treatment refusals may include all forms of life-sustaining medical treatment, including artificially provided nutrition and hydration.
3. Complying with a competent adult's informed wishes to refuse or discontinue life-sustaining treatment should be considered neither homicide nor assisted suicide.
4. From a moral and legal point of view, there is no difference between withholding a treatment (not starting it) and withdrawing a treatment (stopping it after it has been started), if the treatment in question is inconsistent with a competent patient's informed preferences.
5. For a patient who is terminally ill and who values comfort over prolongation of life, symptom control that has as a side effect the shortening of life is morally permissible and is not the moral equivalent of active euthanasia.
6. Incompetent or otherwise nonautonomous people have the same rights as competent people in these matters, with their wishes expressed either in the form of an advance directive or by a person authorized to make health care decisions for them.

To call these points the "public consensus" means that they capture a broad agreement in the bioethics literature, policy statements of professional organizations, judicial decisions, and the actions of state legislatures on the matters in question.[5] It is probably safe to say that these points organize the notes of nearly every medical school and nursing school lecturer on the topic of "the ethics of end-of-life care," and that they are the guiding principles brought to bear on individual cases by the vast majority of clinical ethics consultants at large in the corridors of U.S. hospitals. And yet it must be admitted that the consensus, though undoubtedly broad-based intellectually and influential clinically, masks substantial differences and disagreements within the health professions and the larger society. These differences encompass matters such as the relative weight to be accorded to individual autonomy and the general welfare; the validity of the distinction between, say, "killing" and "allowing to die"; or the proper characterization of artificially provided nutrition and hydration as either "medical treatment" or "basic, humane care."

A second aspect of uncertainty stems from the potential disconnect between an individual health professional's espoused values and ethical commitments, and his or her ability to act according to those commitments in specific clinical situations. To take one of many examples, since the 1960s there has been an enormous shift in physicians' stated attitudes toward disclosing bad news to their patients. Whereas physicians have historically been reluctant to discuss bad diagnoses such as cancer directly with patients for fear of depressing them or eliminating hope,[6] by the late 1970s physicians who responded to surveys overwhelmingly favored full disclosure of a cancer diagnosis to the patient.[7] Patients themselves usually want to know the truth of their cancer diagnosis, and most also want a realistic estimate of how long they are likely to live. Yet when Baile and his colleagues surveyed more than 500 oncologists attending a meeting of the American Society of Clinical Oncology (ASCO), nearly one half rated their ability to break bad news as only fair or poor, and two thirds rated themselves as not very comfortable or uncomfortable dealing with their patients' resulting emotions. Only half had received any training in the subject.[8] These findings are consistent with the fact that, while many studies report general satisfaction on the part of patients and families with the information disclosure process,[9] other studies report significant dissatisfaction with the level of information or emotional support that patients receive from their doctors.[10,11]

With these considerations and qualifications in mind, this discussion of ethical issues in end-of-life care will attempt to bring to bear the public consensus mentioned above on four major themes:

1. The transition from curative to palliative and end-of-life care,
2. surrogate decision making,
3. responding to demands for nonbeneficial treatment, and
4. physician-assisted death.

Though, for the reasons noted, ethical analysis cannot pretend to eliminate moral doubt and disagreement—particularly on some of the most contested issues in these domains—some goals are quite realistic. These include: (1) providing a blueprint or template for careful and systematic ethical scrutiny of a clinical situation, thereby minimizing the risk that important, morally relevant considerations will be left out of account; (2) organizing the dialogue among the various parties to an ethical dispute, thereby assuring that the concerns and perceptions of everyone with a stake in the outcome of a clinical decision are taken seriously; (3) providing a method for isolating particular sources of ethical disagreement, thereby making possible either the marshalling of additional facts or arguments to produce agreement, or allowing people unable to agree to recognize their mutual good faith; (4) pointing to areas of agreement as the basis for creative problem solving that leads to decisions and actions consistent with people's most important values; and (5) encouraging educational efforts for health professionals—especially in the realm of patient-provider communication—to bring professionals' behavior more fully in line with their avowed values and beliefs.

THE TRANSITION FROM CURATIVE TO PALLIATIVE AND END-OF-LIFE CARE

Patients with serious disease and their physicians usually share three goals for the patient's care: cure or long-lasting remission, prolongation of survival, and comfort and quality of life. As prospects for the first and second goals dim with the progression of disease or the exhaustion of available curative therapies, physicians have the opportunity, and the challenge, of recommending that the third goal—now usually referred to generically as "palliative care"—become the main focus of the patient's continuing care. The World Health Organization defines palliative care as "the active total care of patients whose disease is not amenable to curative treatment. Control of pain, of other symptoms, and of psychological, social, and spiritual problems is paramount. The goal of palliative care is the achievement of the best possible quality of life for patients and their families."[12] J. Andrew Billings has suggested a more patient- and family-friendly definition:

Palliative care is a special service, a team approach to providing comfort and support for persons living with a life-threatening illness and for their families. We are a nurse, social worker, chaplain, and physicians who work with your current health-care team to assure that you and your family receive excellent pain control and other comfort measures, get the information you want to participate in decisions about your care, receive emotional and spiritual support and practical assistance, obtain expert help in planning for care outside the hospital, continue getting good services in the community, and overall enjoy life as best you can, given your condition. We try to coordinate and tailor a package of services that best suits your values, beliefs, wishes, and needs in whatever setting you are receiving care.[13]

For the doctor, arriving at the decision to focus primarily on palliative care rather than continuing active, disease-modifying therapy can be complicated. It usually combines scientific and technical skills related to prognosis and clinical judgment; communication skills, often involving bad news and the need to respond sensitively to the patient's emotions; and negotiation of treatment preferences. Billings' description of the doctor's role at this juncture is:

The patient and the family need a doctor who respects their expertise and can help them clarify and choose what they want, yet who is authoritative, helping to bring clarity and control by saying, "Let's keep trying" or "Let's face the music, it's time to stop."[14]

Billings' formulation strikes a balance between the two poles that have characterized ethical debates about the doctor–patient relationship for the past several decades: the doctor as neutral respecter of patient autonomy, and the doctor as authority figure under whose guidance patients suspend their own preferences in favor of the doctor's superior insight into their best interests. Despite the strong emphasis on patient autonomy and self-determination in the bioethics literature, when patients are faced with very serious disease and complicated choices, few want to be left completely on their own to make treatment decisions. Billings' formulation captures this reality by emphasizing both respect for the patient's ultimate decision making authority (consistent with the foundational value of informed consent) and the commitment not to abandon the patient by withholding the physician's best professional judgment.

Negotiating Treatment Preferences: The Ideal Decision-Making Process

From the standpoint of ethics, treatment decisions near the end of life, as at any other juncture in health care, ought to be structured by the notion of informed consent.[15] To be valid, the patient's consent should be informed and free of duress or coercion, and should reflect the patient's genuine values and preferences. An ideal decision-making process for medical care would include the following elements:

- *Joint participation* of doctor and patient, with additional participation of significant others of the patient's choice;
- *Clear and truthful communication* by the physician;
- *Clear and thoughtful deliberation* by the patient;
- *Consideration*, by both doctor and patient, of medical and nonmedical factors, including:
  - The patient's medical condition and options for treatment (including no treatment);
  - The reasonable probabilities that particular goals can be achieved;
  - The reasonably expected proportion of benefits of treatment to harmful or painful side effects;
  - The patient's values and life goals;
  - The patient's assessment of his or her quality of life, and the essential elements for a positive quality of life;
  - The patient's tolerance for risks and uncertainty;

- *So that*, the resulting decision:
  - Reflects a reasonable accommodation to the medical facts;
  - Is consistent with the patient's values and the physician's conscience.

Departures From the Ideal

In the end-of-life context, several factors are likely to complicate the ideal framework outlined above. They can be divided into two large groups: factors related to the uncertainty of prognosis and clinical judgment, and factors related to attitudes and values of both patients and physicians. After some discussion of each of these, this section will conclude with some suggestions for approaching conversations with patients that attempt to accommodate both prognostic uncertainties and emotional reactions.

Prognosis and Clinical Judgment

There are now a number of resources available for physicians to consult for prognostic information across a wide range of diseases and conditions, for example, in advanced cancer,[16] heart failure,[17] end-stage chronic obstructive pulmonary disease,[18] dementia,[19] cirrhosis,[20] and coma following cardiopulmonary resuscitation.[21] While the general outcomes and trajectories of diseases that are the major causes of death in the United States are known, and a typical patient's survival (assuming accurate diagnosis) can usually be estimated within a known range of probabilities, when any particular individual will die remains an inexact prediction. *Most people appreciate this, however, and the inability to give very precise predictions of a patient's remaining life expectancy should not be a barrier to physicians' participating in discussions with patients who want to have some realistic idea of their situation.* As will be described further below, the most important question for the physician is the level of information a patient desires to receive. The question, "Doctor, how long am I going to live?" cannot be answered helpfully without some initial exploration of the meaning the question has to the patient, what has motivated the question, and the patient's preferred level of detail.

A physician's prognostic accuracy seems to vary inversely with the length of time the physician has known the patient. The longer the relationship, the more likely it is that the physician will overestimate the patient's remaining time.[22] While the mechanism of this effect is not clearly established, the possibility of the physician's emotional attachment to the patient and investment in his or her survival cannot be ruled out. Lamont and Christakis comment in relation to this data that a palliative medicine specialist, or some other physician with relevant expertise but with no prior relationship to the patient, is likely to be a helpful resource to the treating physician in formulating prognostic information for individual patients.[23]

Another tendency of physicians that can diminish the usefulness of prognostic information is to provide it solely in terms of the quantity of remaining life (weeks, months, or years), without attempting to describe the quality of life the patient is likely to enjoy. Especially for people with chronic, degenerative conditions or conditions for which available disease-modifying therapies have significant side effects, their remaining quality of life is likely to be as important as a bare estimate of survival. Some issues that are likely to be of particular interest to the patient include the pace and timing of decreases in functional and/or cognitive status, pain and discomfort and the availability of the means to relieve them, loss of independence, and the expected burden on caregivers. It bears repeating that the physician's offer to go into detail on any of these matters should be contingent on a signal from the patient that he or she does in fact want to discuss them. Some people would prefer *not* to have such a clear image of impending decline to look forward to, though they may wish someone in the family to have this information so as to be better prepared.

Patients' Attitudes and Values

The physician's first responsibility in preparing for a conversation about treatment preferences in the setting of end-life care is to assess the patient's emotional and cognitive capacity to participate in the conversation. Among the emotional and attitudinal factors that may cause patients to depart from the ideal decision-making process outlined above are the patient's denial of the seriousness of the disease, or the presence of depression or other psychiatric disorders, as well as other forms of cognitive impairment that may be related either to the disease or its treatment. Appropriate treatment of the underlying causes of the cognitive impairment should be the first order of business. If this is not possible, the physician should consider the availability of a surrogate decision maker, as discussed in the next section.

Other emotional factors short of psychiatric impairment can diminish the patient's capacity to participate meaningfully in these discussions. For example, some patients may appear determined to *continue* pursuing active treatment for their disease because they believe other people want them to do this, not because it is their own preference. Some patients may worry about family members' ability to cope with the patient's worsening illness, or about their future security and well-being once the patient has died. Some patients may find it hard to reject treatments because they do not want to disappoint the doctor.

On the other hand, patients may *reject* further treatments not because they genuinely believe this is in their best interest but because treatment refusal is a language for expressing other concerns, such as fear (of being a burden to others, of the treatment, of the process of dying), anger, exhaustion, helplessness, mistrust, or unrelieved physical symptoms. A similar phenomenon can underlie patients' requests for physician-assisted death. In either context, sensitive exploration of the background and motivations underlying the patient's stated preferences is essential before the physician concludes that he or she has a clear understanding of the patient's perspective.

Physicians' Attitudes and Values

Several factors on the physician's side can also cause a dialogue about treatment preferences to deviate from the ideal. The physician's counterpart to the patient's denial is the tendency alluded to above for physicians to overestimate expected survival, especially for patients with whom they have had long-term relationships. It is often easier to perceive the deterioration in the patients of one's colleagues than in one's own patients.

A number of conceptual and philosophical commitments may also lead physicians to minimize or avoid open discussion with the patient about the transition from curative to palliative care. For example, medical training is primarily focused on providing the tools and skills necessary for the active investigation, diagnosis, and treatment of pathology. This instills an ideology of intervention, according to which any pathological state or process that is potentially reversible *should* be reversed. To stand back and look at the "big picture"—to accompany a patient into death without investigating or treating conditions for which (at least short term) remedies are available—requires a shift in perspective that many physicians find very difficult and contrary to their professional identity.

A closely related issue, especially in academic medical centers, is the imperative of research and therapeutic innovation. From this perspective, it is precisely the point in the patient's illness when all known effective remedies have been exhausted that presents the greatest opportunity for scientific progress. The research imperative demands that these opportunities be seized for trials of new and unproven treatments, to push back the boundaries of medical power. Many patients (especially if they are of a socioeconomic status that has entitled them to regular access to health care) are themselves caught up in the ideology of medical progress, having absorbed a lifetime of exhortations from doctors and hospitals to avail themselves of regular checkups and the very latest in medical technology to ensure a longer, happier life.

The power of medical technology to forestall the time of death, especially in the intensive care unit, gives rise, in Daniel Callahan's phrase, to an ideology of "technological brinkmanship."[24] This is the idea that we can and should employ our technology for its maximum life-extending benefit, and then back off just at the point—but no later—when its marginal benefits begin to be outweighed by its burdens and costs. The reality is that the point of diminishing return is almost always only discernible in retrospect, after the patient has been subjected to a period of intensive and invasive treatments to no positive end, and the family is left to wonder why the patient couldn't have enjoyed a more peaceful death.

The availability of technology to forestall death creates an additional psychological pressure. This derives from the apparently observable fact that the death of any individual patient (especially in the ICU) almost always results from a decision to withhold or withdraw medical treatment. In other words, while in principle we ought to be able to take comfort from the fact that death is natural and universal—as in the ancient syllogism, "Socrates is a man; all men are mortal, therefore Socrates is mortal"—death for *this* patient *now* seems to us always to be optional, and its psychological reality for the doctor is that the death occurred only because he or she brought it about when he or she recommended, or acquiesced when the patient or family requested, termination of treatment.

Finally, a very common concern for physicians faced with recommending the transition from curative to palliative care (identified by nearly 60% of the respondents to Baile and colleagues' ASCO survey as the most difficult part of breaking bad news) is "being honest without taking away hope." This is particularly the case when "hope" is uniquely identified with the prospects for cure or significantly extended life. In fact, there are many other objects of patients' and families' hope that physicians almost always can help them realize; for example, comfort and freedom from pain, companionship, completion of important tasks, security for those who will be left behind.[25] Indeed, as suggested by Billings' previously quoted definition, these concerns are precisely the focus of palliative care. Nevertheless, the strong association between the shift to palliation from active treatment and "giving up all hope" can lead physicians to dread serious discussion of a patient's end-of-life treatment preferences.

Communication With Patients About Treatment Preferences Near the End of Life

The physician has four primary goals in the dialogue with a patient in the context of end-of-life decision making:

1. To learn about the patient's preferences for receiving information, and to assess the patient's coping style when confronting threatening situations;
2. To provide the patient with sufficient information about his or her current and projected medical situation and corresponding therapeutic and supportive options to enable the patient to make choices that reflect his or her values and preferences;
3. To establish rapport and trust in order to enhance the physician's credibility as a source of reliable information and interpersonal support;
4. To so balance genuine appreciation of the clinical situation with realistic optimism as to empower the patient—by mobilizing his or her adaptive capacities and social supports—to maximize his or her quality of life for as long as possible.

The goal of effective information transfer, while obviously of cardinal importance, is only one of several goals. If the others are not also satisfied, information transfer itself may not successfully occur. For this reason, most expert opinion on communication with patients about bad news—which for the purposes of this chapter will embrace not only prognostic disclosures but also discussions of referral to palliative care or hospice, responding to requests for nonbeneficial treatment, and requests for physician-assisted death—recommends that the physician address the interpersonal and emotional dimensions of communication as well as the clear presentation of scientific facts.

In an extensive literature review Penelope Schofield and her colleagues[26] identified 10 major considerations for communication about the transition from curative cancer treatment to palliative care:

1. Preparation prior to the discussion.
2. Eliciting the person's understanding of the illness and preferences for information transfer.
3. Providing information.
4. Responding to emotional reactions.
5. Negotiating new goals of care.
6. Arranging for continuity of care.
7. Addressing family concerns.
8. Acknowledging cultural and linguistic diversity.
9. Concluding the discussion.
10. Documenting the discussion and appropriately informing other members of the treatment team.

Baile and colleagues[8] consolidate these dimensions in a six-step protocol with the mnemonic **SPIKES**. In their formulation the physician's communication with the patient proceeds as follows:

Step 1: SETTING UP the Interview
Mental rehearsal, arranging for a private setting, involvement of significant others, sitting down, making eye contact, and taking steps to avoid interruption.
Step 2: Assessing the Patient's PERCEPTION
Ask before telling: Ascertain what the patient knows, how they want to receive information; for example, "What have you been told about your medical condition so far?" or "What is your understanding of the reasons we did the MRI?"
Step 3: Obtaining the Patient's INVITATION
Ask before telling: Ascertain the patient's preference for receiving information, recognizing that shunning information is a valid psychological response for some people. Asking this at the time of test ordering can help set the stage; for example, "How would you like me to give you the test results? Would you like all of the information, or just the big picture, with more time for us to talk about a treatment plan? Is there anyone else with whom you would prefer us to discuss this information?" Lamont and Christakis[23] suggest: "Some people want to know everything possible about their illness and others prefer to know very little. How much about your illness do you want to know from me today?"
Step 4: Giving KNOWLEDGE and Information to the Patient
Give a "warning shot"; for example, "Unfortunately I've got some bad news to tell you. . ." Start at the patient's comprehension level, avoiding technical words (say "spread" rather than "metastasize"); give information in small chunks with pauses to check understanding; avoid phrases such as "there is nothing more we can do."
Step 5: Addressing the Patient's EMOTIONS with Empathic Responses
Another mnemonic, **NURSE**, is helpful here.
Name the emotion: You look (sound) as if this is a real shock to you.
Understand: I cannot imagine what it is like to be so sick.
Respect: I really appreciate how you have been coping with this.
Support: I want you to know that regardless of what happens I will be there for you.

Explore: Tell me more.

Step 6: STRATEGY and SUMMARY

Ask before telling: Determine whether the patient wants to discuss future treatment plans at the present time; check the patient's overall understanding of what has been said; present treatment options if appropriate in the moment; offer time for the patient to reflect; offer to be available for questions that may arise after the interview; schedule a follow-up appointment.

In summary, the physician–patient dialogue about the transition from active treatment to palliative care can help the physician fulfill several aspects of the ideal decision-making process. By acknowledging emotional aspects of the situation that are likely to be present on both sides, by offering patients the opportunity to receive information—or not—at their own pace, by examining one's professional biases and assumptions that may hinder an open discussion of the patient's circumstances and the realistic benefits of a palliative approach, and by attention to the interpersonal as well as factual aspects of information transfer, the physician is most likely to support treatment decisions by patients that reflect their genuine values, and also to strengthen the foundations for the physician's role as a supportive companion to the patient throughout the course of the illness.

SURROGATE DECISION MAKING

At the time end-of-life treatment decisions have to be made, patients may not be able to speak clearly for themselves. They may be too sick to speak, too confused to listen to medical information or to deliberate about preferences, or even completely unconscious and beyond any communication at all. Typical contexts when patients lack decisional capacity near the end of life include patients suffering from dementia or other long-term cognitive impairment; patients suffering from delirium as a consequence of their disease or side effects of its treatment (e.g., metabolic derangements, drug-induced delirium, "ICU psychosis,"), severely depressed patients, patients with waxing and waning mental capacity, or who give inconsistent, contradictory answers to treatment-related questions within a short period of time; postoperative patients under the influence of anesthetics or medications to promote ventilator compliance; patients suffering loss of consciousness due to stroke, cardiac arrest, or other traumatic event; and patients in coma or persistent vegetative state.

Surrogate decision-making is the process by which these patients may be brought as close as possible to the ideal decision-making process described above. It involves the following basic elements: (1) assessment of the patient's decisional capacity; (2) for patients deemed lacking in capacity, attempts to rule out or eliminate reversible causes; (3) identification of an appropriate surrogate; (4) clarifying the surrogate's roles and responsibilities; and (5) anticipating, where possible, future needs for surrogate decision making through a process of advance care planning.

Assessing Decisional Capacity

Decisional capacity is task specific. Someone may be properly judged capable of making some decisions—jello or custard for dessert, baseball or NASCAR on TV—and incapable of making other decisions—financial investments, whether or not to enter a nursing home, or, most relevant here, the choice of medical treatments in the setting of advanced disease. For the latter, the patient's capacity should be assessed in terms of:

- **Understanding:** Does the patient understand the meaning of the diagnostic or prognostic information provided to him or her? Can the patient restate the information in his or her own words in a way that demonstrates this understanding?

- **Appreciation:** Does the patient appreciate the implications of the information for himself or herself? Does he or she appreciate that decisions have to be made from among alternative treatment plans, and that his or her input is necessary for these decisions?

- **Deliberation:** Can the patient weigh the alternative treatments according to his or her personal goals and values?

- **Communication:** Can the patient communicate his or her treatment preferences in an understandable manner? Do the patient's stated preferences appear logically related to the patient's goals?

There is no rigid, quantifiable measure of the patient's abilities in these domains. In general, the more significant the decision that needs to be made—in terms of risks, benefits, and side effects—the more stringent our standards should be in satisfying ourselves that the patient has the requisite capacity.[27]

Contrary to common practice, especially in hospitals where psychiatric consultation is readily available, a formal psychiatric consultation is not required to assess a patient's decisional capacity. Nonpsychiatrist physicians ordinarily are capable of forming a reasonable judgment of the patient's abilities in these four domains. Moreover, even if a psychiatric consultant judges the patient to have capacity, it remains the attending physician's responsibility to satisfy himself or herself that the patient is in fact capable of giving informed consent before proceeding with treatment. Where psychiatric opinion is most relevant is when the physician suspects mental illness or delirium as the (possibly reversible) cause of the patient's lack of capacity, or where appointment of a legal guardian is anticipated, in which case the court will be interested in authoritative medical opinion.

Ruling Out or Eliminating Reversible Causes of Incapacity

Reversible causes of incapacity can be biological or situational. Biological causes include transient delirium, treatable depression, or the side effects of anesthetic or analgesic medications. Situational causes include anxiety or fear as an immediate consequence of receiving bad news, confusion or anxiety due to the effects of hospitalization, the sensory overload of the ICU, and/or separation from familiar people. Before deciding that a patient's lack of capacity warrants turning to a surrogate, realistically assess the importance of making particular decisions right away. If urgent decisions are not required, attempt to diagnose and eliminate the patient's incapacity. This could entail adjustments of medication, psychosocial intervention, or simply the passage of time.

Identifying a Surrogate

If the gold standard for ethical health care decision making is the thoughtful participation of an informed patient, the gold standard for surrogate decision making involves a surrogate who is:

- **authorized** by the patient, because the patient considers the surrogate to be trustworthy and in the best position to advocate for the patient's best interests;

- **willing** to accept the patient's trust and to fulfill the role of surrogate in good faith;

- **informed**, through prior acquaintance or explicit conversation with the patient, about the patient's values and preferences regarding medical care near the end of life;

- **capable** of understanding the physician's explanations of the patient's condition and weighing treatment options in light of the patient's preferences;

■ **available** to represent the patient's interests at the time decisions have to be made.

Since Congress passed the Patient Self-Determination Act in 1990 in the wake of the *Nancy Cruzan* decision of the U.S. Supreme Court, there have been many local and national efforts to encourage people to identify a surrogate in case of their own future incapacity. All 50 states have adopted legislation authorizing health care decision making by surrogates under various criteria and qualifications, for example, the state of the patient's health (usually the patient must be "terminally ill" as variously defined, permanently unconscious, or in an advanced stage of a serious, incurable condition), the process by which the surrogate has been designated, and the scope of the surrogate's authority. Despite these efforts, most people for whom end-of-life medical decisions must be made have not designated a surrogate in advance.[28]

A number of states have addressed this gap legislatively by prescribing, in lexical order, the persons who are empowered to act as the patient's surrogate. A typical ordering begins with the patient's spouse, and then moves in descending order through adult children, parents, adult siblings, adult grandchildren, and (only then) other adults who may be in a position to know the patient's beliefs about medical treatment. In states where this regime applies, physicians as well as patients may be faced with the situation where the prescribed surrogate does not fulfill the criteria noted above as well as someone lower on the list—or not on the list at all. Gay partners, for example, have legitimate reason to fear exclusion and disenfranchisement in decision making for each other under strict interpretations of these surrogacy laws.

From the point of view of ethics, the physician's primary responsibility as the patient's advocate is to identify the surrogate who meets those criteria to the greatest extent. In cases where that person is available and willing to serve in the role, but another, less qualified, person with lexical priority is expressing conflicting preferences for care, it is advisable for the physician to seek consultation from an ethics committee or from a hospital's legal counsel.

The Surrogate's Roles and Responsibilities

The surrogate's primary responsibility is to interpret the physician's recitation of the patient's medical condition and recommended treatment in light of what the surrogate has reason to believe are *the patient's* relevant values, preferences, and life goals. This is the "substituted judgment" standard for surrogate decision making. Unless the surrogate has been instructed differently by the patient, he or she ought to try to the best of his or her ability to express treatment preferences that reflect the patient's goals and values, and not the surrogate's, if there is a conflict between them. If the surrogate is not certain what the patient would prefer in a given situation, or if, despite a good faith effort on the part of all who are in a position to know, there is simply no evidence whatsoever of the patient's likely preference, the surrogate ought to make the decision that appears to be, from an objective point of view, in the patient's best interests. Ordinarily this is determined by weighing, in the most informed manner possible, the likely benefits (to the patient) of various proposed treatments—or no treatment—against their likely burdens (again to the patient). This is (not surprisingly) the "best interests" standard for surrogate decision making.

Physicians and other members of the health care team have potential roles to play in helping surrogates do their job. Their most obvious role is to provide clear and helpful prognostic information and descriptions of proposed treatments according to the protocols outlined in the previous section. But they may also be able to enhance the surrogate's ability to represent the patient's interests and preferences by engaging in dialogue with the surrogate about the patient. The content of that dialogue will be suggested by the discussion in the next section of the most useful elements of an advance directive for health care.

A Realistic Process of Advance Care Planning

Most commentators agree that policies to encourage people to use advance directives to prepare for future end-of-life decision making have been largely unsuccessful.[28,29] As noted above, only a minority (between 20%–30%) of American adults have filled out an advance directive. Evidence suggests that even for those who have them, advance directives do not influence decision making. Most particularly, if people expect that filling out an advance directive will ensure that the medical decisions made during their future incapacity will match the choices they themselves would have made had they been able to participate in those decisions themselves, they will almost certainly be disappointed.

Common difficulties are that the documents cannot be located when they are needed, they are too vague to give useful guidance in the patient's actual circumstances, or the patient's stated preferences are ignored in favor of a course of action that physicians and/or family members believe is more in accord with the patient's present best interests. Hickman et al.[29] have listed some of the main factors that may explain these difficulties. These include:

1. An overemphasis on the patient's legal rights to refuse medical care, as opposed to the more general objective of enhancing people's ability to influence their care according to their goals and values;
2. Insufficient efforts by health professionals to educate patients as to realistic outcomes of various medical interventions;
3. Overemphasis on patients' preferences for specific medical interventions, rather than the effort to ascertain the patient's views about goals and values, and about what constitutes an acceptable quality of life;
4. The assumption that the planning process is complete as soon as an advance directive has been filled out, rather than viewing the process as ongoing and subject to periodic reassessment and revision of the patient's goals in light of changing medical circumstances;
5. Failure to involve family members or other important people in the patient's life in discussions about preferences for medical care;
6. Absence of system-wide policies and procedures to ensure that patients' preferences for care are known and respected wherever the patient may be receiving care;
7. Low community awareness of issues related to end-of-life planning;
8. State advance directive laws that introduce barriers into the advance planning process.

Three Basic Problems

As significant as Hickman and colleagues' barriers are for explaining the lack of public enthusiasm for the advance care planning process, there are three basic problems with advance directives that frequently lead to frustration and disappointment even when patients have gone to the trouble of creating one. All three are related to the nature of medical care for the critically ill, and the existential predicament of the person facing death. Stated briefly, and somewhat too simply, they are:

(1) Unpredictability. Because of the probabilistic and uncertain nature of prognosis, it is extremely unlikely that the scenarios a healthy person imagines when filling out his or her advance directive—either sitting at the kitchen table or in the doctor's office—will match the actual circumstances the patient or surrogate will face in the future. The more general the terms of the advance directive, in order to capture a range of possibilities broad enough to fit an unknown and unknowable future, the less use they will be in providing specific guidance about treatment preferences. This is a structural problem that no preprinted advance directive form—no matter how elaborately or imaginatively it has been constructed—can solve.

(2) Uncertainty. Related to the unpredictability of the time and manner of death in general is a more specific uncertainty as to the potential benefit of any particular medical intervention or treatment that might be used near the end of the incapacitated person's life. Consider, for example, treatments such as antibiotics, oxygen therapy, blood transfusions, or even more invasive procedures such as kidney dialysis. All of these are typically among the items that, in advance directives, people indicate the desire *to refuse* in the case of terminal illness. Yet each of these, while not capable of reversing the dying process, may be very useful for more particular goals such as alleviating pain, clearing mental confusion, or simply keeping a person alive long enough for family or friends to gather at the bedside for a final farewell. The question, "If you were mentally incapacitated and terminally ill, would you want blood products or antibiotics?" (for example) is practically meaningless when asked far in advance.[30]

(3) Ambivalence. The desire for a gentle death, free of tubes and machines, coexists in most of us with the powerful desire to stay alive. It is very difficult to predict how, in the moment of truth, a particular patient will respond to even a tiny chance of success for a life-prolonging treatment, when the alternative to trying the treatment is likely to be imminent death. The difficulty of extrapolating a patient's real-time choices from previous discussions is compounded by the "framing effect," in which those choices will be strongly influenced by the way the alternatives are actually described.[31]

A Realistic Approach

It is a disservice to patients and families to represent advance care planning as a method of assuring the ability to exert control over the medical treatments they will receive at the end of life. Nevertheless, proponents of advance care planning frequently urge people to complete an advance directive, or a durable power of attorney for health care, precisely to "take charge" of their future medical care or, with respect to some dreadful twilight state between life and death in an Intensive Care Unit, to "make sure this can never happen to you." They encourage people to believe that if they are incapacitated, but have planned in advance and filled out the proper documents, the treatment decisions that will be made for them will match the decisions they themselves would make if, miraculously, they could be restored to full capacity, process all currently relevant medical information, and then decide which treatments should be applied. For all of the reasons mentioned above, this is misleading overstatement.

There are, however, some very realistic and meaningful goals that advance care planning *can* help people achieve. One goal is to promote honest and open communication about important values and life goals within families, and between patients, families, and health professionals, in the face of serious illness. This type of communication is often of great intrinsic value, whether or not it bears any relation to specific treatment choices. Another goal is to arrange for future medical decisions to be made, in case of future incapacity, by someone whose love and care the principal trusts—not on the assumption that this individual will infallibly make the "right" decision (if "right" means matching exactly the decision the principal would have made)—but because, since *any* surrogate is likely to be "wrong," it is often of great comfort to know that the decision maker is someone who really cares about you and is probably going to do his or her best to serve your best interests. Finally, advance planning is an

opportunity to reflect on those qualities of life that make life worth holding onto and, conversely, those qualities that might be worse than death, and to communicate those values to a surrogate, who can then compare the likely outcomes of real-time medical alternatives to those benchmarks, and make choices in their light.[32]

A reasonable and useful advance care planning document should probably contain information along the following lines. Beyond their value in suggesting what an advance directive should contain, these items are also intended to suggest some of the questions that physicians can ask—directly of patients in advance, or to help surrogates fulfill their roles in order to fashion a treatment plan more likely than not to respect patient values.

1. Identification of a preferred surrogate decision maker, and at least one back-up.

2. Statement of the extent of the surrogate's authority, and how much flexibility the surrogate has in responding to real-time circumstances in ways that might depart from any specific instructions.

3. Evidence that the surrogate is aware of his or her appointment and understands the scope of his or her authority.

4. A statement from the principal describing the qualities and aspects of life that the principal considers necessary for a minimally acceptable quality of life, accompanied by instructions to the surrogate to request the application or continuation of *any and all* medical treatments that have a reasonable likelihood—according to accepted medical judgment—of restoring to the principal that quality of life for a reasonable period of time. Similarly, the surrogate is instructed to decline or insist on the withdrawal of *any and all* medical treatments if those treatments do not have a reasonable chance—according to accepted medical judgment—of achieving or maintaining that quality of life for a reasonable period of time.

5. In general the document should *not* specify particular treatments that the principal does or does not want. The statement in (4) should provide sufficient guidance for the physician to make these specific treatment decisions in light of the principal's overall criteria for an acceptable quality of life, combined with the principal's preference for resolving medical uncertainties—see (7). However, there may be some special circumstances in which particular treatments should be mentioned; for example, a Jehovah's Witness may wish to decline blood or blood products; or a person who has previously been resuscitated and placed on a mechanical respirator may have become convinced by the experience that he or she would never want it to be repeated; or in states that require the administration of artificial nutrition and hydration unless they are explicitly included among treatments to be withheld. Otherwise, the broad statement of values (4) and preference for resolution of uncertainties (7) should suffice for most people.

6. A statement of the principal's willingness to undergo trial periods of medical treatments when physicians are uncertain of their likely benefit, as defined in (4), accompanied by a clear statement of the surrogate's authority to stop those treatments after the agreed-upon trial period has ended.

7. A statement of the principal's preference either that genuine medical uncertainties be resolved in favor of *more* aggressive treatment or *less* aggressive treatment, with a clear additional statement that the surrogate has the ultimate authority to resolve disagreements between conflicting medical opinions.

8. A statement by the principal that he or she wants all necessary measures to maintain comfort and to treat pain, and that when medical treatments are deemed incapable of achieving the goals defined in (4), pain and other symptoms should be treated aggressively even if adequate treatment carries the risk of hastening death. The statement should include the desire for treating physicians to consult with qualified specialists in

pain management and palliative care whenever they or the surrogate deems it appropriate.

It should be said in conclusion that many, many people experience end-of-life decision making that is smooth and uncomplicated, and for many, many survivors the death of a loved one, while sad, is neither chaotic nor traumatic. When things go awry, or people are anguished and bewildered by events that seem to be tumbling out of control, it is usually not the fault of a missing or poorly worded living will or durable power of attorney for health care. Recall the perspectives of Hinton and Burt in the introduction. Death carries enormous power to frighten us and to discombobulate the best laid plans. Despite our rhetoric of *management* of symptoms, or of *directing* our health care providers to do (or not to do) this or that, we do not control death. In its presence we bear witness, and do the best we can.

RESPONDING TO DEMANDS FOR NONBENEFICIAL TREATMENT

The ethical consensus respecting a competent adult's right to *refuse* medical treatment—even life-sustaining treatment when the refusal is contrary to the physician's professional judgment—does not extend to the patient's or family's right to *demand* medical treatments that, in the physician's professional judgment, offer no prospect of patient benefit. This difference in the moral and legal status of refusals and demands occasionally gives rise to conflicts that are among the most vexing and emotionally draining that can occur in end-of-life care. Taken to their limit these conflicts can be so destructive, not only of the physician–patient–family relationship but of the atmosphere and milieu of the patient's dying that loved ones will take with them in memory, that prevention is the physician's foremost ethical responsibility. Preventive measures are not always successful, but their chances can be improved through systematic analysis of the nature of a conflict in its early manifestations ("differential diagnosis"), and a range of communication and conflict resolution strategies.

The Ethical Basis of the Conflict

Ethically, the difference in physicians' obligations toward refusals of treatment and demands for treatment stems from the way ethics and law customarily interpret the concepts of autonomy and self-determination. In bioethics, respect for personal autonomy and self-determination is rooted in the ideas of privacy and bodily integrity. The idea is that—with very few exceptions, such as a potential public health emergency—a person ought to be able to control what is done to, with, or for his or her own body. This is the foundation for the requirement of informed consent, and for the patient's right to say "No" to the physician's recommendations for (even life-saving) treatment. Courts have tested the claim of patient self-determination, or the patient's right to say "No," against potentially competing claims such as the state's interest in preserving life, the interests of third parties (e.g., spouses or minor children), the integrity of the medical profession, and the prevention of suicide. In every case almost all courts have come down in favor of self-determination. The competing interests have been uniformly seen as too abstract, too remote, or too weak to override the individual's interests in preventing the violation of his or her bodily integrity and in limiting the power of others to enforce values or life goals that he or she does not share.[33]

The matter is quite different for the person who demands a particular treatment. (This distinction applies equally to the context of requests for physician-assisted death, which are discussed in the next section.) Here it is no longer a question of an individual protecting his or her bodily integrity by drawing a boundary and saying: "Do not cross." Respecting this essentially negative right (the right to be let alone) requires physicians and everyone else simply to do nothing. The person who demands a treatment, however, would compel the physician, and potentially many other people, to act affirmatively to supply the treatment. Many more public and professional interests and resources are implicated in the positive satisfaction of a demand than in the negative respect for a refusal. And, especially when the demand is for a treatment that, according to accepted medical opinion, will not benefit the patient, ethical opinion is far more deferential to competing societal and professional interests than in the case of patients who are asserting their negative right to be let alone.

It is worth noting in this last connection that only a very few courts have explicitly addressed the question of patients' demands for life-saving treatment against widely accepted medical opinion, and up to now no clear judicial trend has emerged.[34] Among the most likely reasons for the relative lack of such cases is hospitals' reluctance, despite their desire to support physicians' professional judgment, to bear the costs and potential damage to their public image of going to court to force the removal of life-sustaining treatment over a family's vehement protests. However, as noted above, there are other, better reasons to avoid recourse to the very public, adversarial forum of a court of law to resolve these conflicts. Preserving a therapeutic relationship and protecting the sacred personal environment of the deathbed are very worthy motivations for the physician's efforts to find a more constructive resolution.

The Clinical Context of the Conflict

Many clinical scenarios have the potential to bring doctors into conflict with patients or their families over the continuation of medical treatments of little or no likely patient benefit; for example, continuous blood transfusion for the patient with inoperable bleeding, full resuscitation efforts for the elderly patient with sepsis and multiorgan failure, additional courses of high toxicity anticancer treatment for the patient for whom both standard and experimental therapies have failed to slow the spread of the disease. The paradigm case, however, continues to be the noncommunicative, ventilator-dependent patient, kept alive by mechanical means while suffering inexorable bodily deterioration and discomfort with little prospect of improvement. This is the patient who, in K. Danner Clouser's words—as vividly applicable today as when he wrote them 30 years ago—"is on the borderline between treatment and torture, where therapeutic hope has vanished, and pain without point has taken over. The doctor's time-honored admonition to preserve life and lessen pain is at a stupefying impasse."[35]

Faced with a family's continuing insistence that "everything be done," including, if necessary, chest compressions and electric shocks to the heart in order to keep the patient alive, the medical team chafes in resentment at another "family that doesn't get it." Every evening, when the family arrives at the ICU the same routine plays out: a physician from the team recites the grim medical facts, points to the patient's deteriorating body, and urges the family to allow them to withdraw the ventilator so the patient can die peacefully. The family listens to the explanations—the descriptions of failing organs, alarming laboratory values, hopelessly long odds—and insists that everything be done. The team wonders why a supposedly loving family is being so selfish and cruel, and how it is possible for the obstinacy of one family to commandeer enormous medical resources that could and should be put to much better use. The family wonders why the doctors keep badgering them with their litany of doom and gloom when they should simply be about their business of keeping their loved one alive, and how it is possible that the hospital can be so indif-

TABLE 13.1

CONFLICTS OFTEN RESOLVABLE

- Lack of comprehension
- Emotional barriers to processing information
- Disagreement about the patient's preferences
- Narrow understanding of "hope" and "caring"
- Mistrust of health care team
- Team conflict and mixed messages

ferent to the value of the life which the family has entrusted to it.

Differential Diagnosis of the Conflict

The frustrated medical team's epithet, "The family doesn't get it," is often shorthand for a common diagnosis of the cause of the impasse; namely, that for all of the medical team's efforts to be clear about the patient's serious medical condition and grim prognosis, the family has yet to fully comprehend. With every passing day, with its presentation of facts, laboratory values, and statistics, the team's hypothesis appears to be confirmed by the family's implacable opposition to changing the patient's level of care. Perhaps, the team reflects, we are using too many big words. Perhaps this is not a very well educated family. Maybe English is not their native language. The team redoubles its efforts to educate the family about the seriousness of the situation, only to remain stuck with the same result.

In fact there are several possible explanations for the conflict between the doctor and the family, of which a lack of intellectual understanding is only one, and not the most common in any event. But if lack of understanding is *not* the principal source of the conflict, then repeated efforts to lecture the family about the medical facts are no more likely to resolve the impasse than a course of antibiotics is likely to succeed in treating a viral infection. From the outset, therefore, an ethics of prevention requires careful discrimination among the possibilities. Tables 13.1 and 13.2 suggest a differential diagnosis of physician–family conflicts surrounding medically nonbeneficial treatments.

The principal difference between the two tables is that, in principle at least, all of the issues in Table 13.1 are amenable to resolution through sensitive, therapeutic dialogue, whereas the issues in Table 13.2 represent potentially intractable clashes of values or worldviews. Therefore, a good first step for the team is to try to elicit as specifically and clearly as possible all apparent sources of disagreement, sorting them if possible into the two categories, and choosing strategies of mediation or conflict resolution accordingly.[36]

In Table 13.1, for example, even though problems of intellectual comprehension are infrequently at the bottom of profound disagreements about life-sustaining treatment, the team has the responsibility (always implicit in the ideal decision-making process outlined above) of communicating information about the

TABLE 13.2

CONFLICTS OFTEN INTRACTABLE

- Disagreement on legitimate goals of medical care
- Disagreement on acceptable probabilities of success, or trade-offs between potential benefits and burdens
- Disagreement on an acceptable quality of life
- Waiting for a miracle

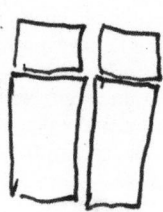

FIGURE 13.1 Physician's sketch of infant heart in apocryphal story of miscommunication.

patient's illness in a language and in a setting that are optimally conducive to patient/family comprehension. It is worthwhile cultivating the skill of inquiring, in a noncondescending way, whether a family can repeat back to the team the essence of the information the team has tried to convey. (An apocryphal story recounts the experience of a surgeon who hastily sketched the chambers of a baby's heart for a new mother, in an effort to explain the need for a valve repair, in a schematic diagram similar to what's shown in Figure 13.1, only to hear the mother report to the father that their baby's problem was that it had been born with a square heart.) Genuine misconceptions and misunderstanding usually can be corrected with appropriate educational strategies.

Other issues in Table 13.1, however may deserve more consideration. For example:

- What may appear to be lack of intellectual comprehension may be a manifestation of emotional barriers to taking in information. The information may be too threatening, too unexpected, or too evocative of a deepest dread to be absorbed without the protective shields of numbing or denial. Most situations permit periods of supportive accompaniment of the shell-shocked, grief-stricken family before pressing forward with the team's recommendations to change the focus of care. Communication strategies discussed above, particularly under the SPIKES and NURSE mnemonics, can be of great value in this setting.

- The team and family may have different understandings, or evidence, of the patient's likely preferences. The patient may have expressed one view to the doctor, and another to the family. Language in an advance directive may suggest one thing to the team, but something quite different to family members who were present when the document was filled out. A tension-lowering approach in this setting is for someone (perhaps an ethics consultant) to open a physician–family conference with the statement, "Everyone in this room is trying to do exactly the same thing, which is to give [your husband, father, brother] the care that he would want if he could speak with us now. Our challenge is to figure out what that is. Let's go over what each of us knows about his likely preferences at this point, and how we learned this information."

- Patients as well as physicians may equate "hope" exclusively with hope for cure or prolongation of life, and "care" with the provision of maximal medical treatment. Efforts to expand hope include achievable goals more consistent with the patient's condition, and suggestions to the family of ways to express love and care through their presence, voice, and

TABLE 13.3

CHECKLIST FOR THE TEAM

- Do team members agree on diagnosis and prognosis?
- Have team members and family compared sources of information about the patient's preferences?
- Is the team speaking to the family with one voice?
- Has the team identified a spokesperson with the greatest rapport and credibility in the eyes of the family?

touch, may offer the family emotional space to adjust their expectations of the medical team.

- Especially for families from marginalized, economically disadvantaged communities, the recommendation to limit intensive medical care can appear to repeat long-standing patterns of social injustice and deprivation. The medical team may represent one more agent of an oppressive power structure. In this setting, the family is unlikely to trust the team's recommendations, even when they are made in good faith on the basis of solid scientific evidence. If the team suspects this dynamic may be at work, explicitly naming the lack of trust and offering to call in more trusted individuals from the family's community may diffuse the conflict and promote eventual agreement on a treatment plan.
- Perhaps most common of all preventable or remediable sources of conflict, especially in the ICU, are mixed messages to the family about the patient's condition. The attending physician may prepare the family for the patient's inevitable death based on the overall combination of downward-trending prognostic indicators, only to have a specialist consultant come by later to tell the family that "the [lungs, kidneys, blood counts] look a bit better today." A team that repeatedly sends mixed signals to the family should not be surprised when the family holds fast to the most optimistic statements, and insists on staying the course. The most urgent task is for the team to arrive at its own internal consensus.

A brief checklist (see Table 13.3) can be part of a preventive ethics strategy to help the team first ascertain whether it is in fact dealing with a Table 13.1 type of conflict, and, second, maximize its chances of resolving it.

Table 13.2 conflicts are more difficult to resolve solely within the context of therapeutic dialogue. This is because the terms of the disagreement reflect value differences or worldviews that are not necessarily amenable to rational persuasion, or which supply disputants with individually convincing yet mutually incompatible interpretations of agreed upon facts. Institutional policies for mediation, which may include mandatory consultations with an ethics committee, and—if these efforts fail to break the impasse—offers to transfer the care of the patient either to another physician or to another institution, are options of almost last resort.[36] In the extreme case, none of these options is feasible. The institution may then be faced with the choice of going to court to obtain judicial authorization to stop the treatment—with no certainty of success but the virtual certainty of cementing the family's enduring resentment. Alternatively, it may recognize that there are (fortunately rare) instances where, for reasons of compassion, "professional medical judgment" and "the rational use of medical resources" may yield to a family's indomitable will. Though the team may view the patient's dying as needlessly prolonged and even horrible, in the circumstances of a family's passionate intransigence it may be the least poor outcome.

PHYSICIAN-ASSISTED DEATH

The vast attention paid to physician-assisted death in discussions of ethics at the end of life is far out of proportion to its actual significance in the experiences of most dying patients and their families. For most people, far more important issues are related to maintaining the energy and stamina to pursue valued activities and relationships amid the burdens of illness and obtaining timely, skilled help with pain, anxiety, and other symptoms. Even in Oregon, whose Death with Dignity Act legalizing physicians' prescriptions of lethal doses of medication for terminally ill patients spawned fears of a "suicide mecca" in the Northwest, the 46 deaths in 2006 that occurred under the law amounted to one-seventh of 1% of all deaths in the state that year.[37] Nevertheless, the issue commands attention, in part because of legitimate public concerns about the quality of care that our society makes available to the dying, and because requests for physician-assisted death confront physicians with troubling questions about the proper boundaries of medical practice and the nature of their duty to relieve suffering.

Terminology

As with many contested social practices, the language used to describe the various ways physicians can be involved in hastening the time of a patient's death has evolved through many phases and fashions, with people's preferred language often reflecting their prior moral evaluation of the practices in question. Thus, the literature abounds in discussions of the differences between "killing patients" and "allowing patients to die" or the differences between "passive euthanasia" and "active euthanasia,"[38] and—more recently—the preference of organizations such as the American Public Health Association[39] and the American Academy of Hospice and Palliative Medicine[40] for the term "physician-assisted death" rather than "physician-assisted suicide." What seems to be at issue in the debates about terminology is the recognition that *how we characterize* an action (or an omission) often predetermines judgments of its moral status.

Because "killing" is nearly universally condemned in all but very carefully circumscribed situations, proponents of physician actions (or omissions) that hasten a patient's death take pains to argue that those actions or omissions are not instances of "killing." Similarly, because "suicide" carries wide social stigma and is often associated with mental illness, patients who make use of physician-provided lethal prescriptions and the physicians who provide them prefer to characterize what they are doing in terms other than committing or aiding in "suicide." In fact, there is usually room for reasonable people to disagree about the most accurate characterization of many actions. This is one reason why, as mentioned at the beginning of this chapter, the public consensus on many aspects of end-of-life care (including, of most pertinence here, the idea that respecting patient wishes for aggressive symptom management that foreseeably hastens death is neither assisted suicide nor active euthanasia) masks considerable uncertainty and debate within society.

For convenience, the rest of this section will employ the term "physician-assisted death" to refer to a spectrum of actions and omissions by which physicians may have a more or less direct role in bringing about the death of an incurably ill patient sooner than the patient might have died without the physician's involvement. There is a fairly strong public and professional consensus (with the qualifications previously mentioned) about the moral status of many points along the spectrum.

Ethical Considerations Along the Clinical Spectrum

There are at least six reasonably distinct actions or roles that a physician might take in the care of a terminally ill patient that could advance the timing of the patient's death. Two lie at opposite ends of the ethical and legal spectrum. Respecting the competent patient's wishes to forego or remove life-sustaining treatment is universally accepted ethically and legally in the United States. Administering a lethal injection with the intent of immediately ending the patient's life ("active euthanasia") is universally rejected legally in the United States, and—though not universally condemned ethically—commands the least widespread support in the ethical literature. In between are four actions that remain somewhat controversial though in varying degrees, always allowing for the fact that characterizing an action as one of these four is itself often a morally significant choice.[41,42]

These four intermediate actions include:

- Aggressive symptom management, usually with opiates and sedatives, despite the risk of hastening the patient's death. The paradigm case is the use of large doses of morphine for pain relief that have the effect of causing fatal respiratory depression. In fact this is an extremely *unlikely* side effect of skillful opioid administration to a patient who has been receiving chronic opioid therapy for pain relief for a period of time. Nevertheless, the scenario is frequently brought up in discussion of the "rule of double effect." This is the notion, originating in Catholic moral theology, that an action with foreseeable but unintended bad effects (here the death of the patient) may under certain conditions be undertaken with the primary intent of bringing about its good effect (here, the relief of pain). The extensive debate over the philosophical coherence and clinical applicability of the rule of double effect is beyond the scope of this chapter.[43–45] For present purposes it is sufficient to note that the basic concept of treating patient suffering aggressively with appropriate medical therapies, even at the risk of the patient's earlier death as a side effect of the therapy, is well accepted clinical practice and appears also to have received the sanction of at least some justices of the U.S. Supreme Court.

- Sedating the consenting, terminally ill patient to the point of unconsciousness to protect the patient from otherwise intractable physical or emotional suffering, while also withholding artificially provided nutrition and hydration. This sits on the borderline between the previous action (and its common justification via the rule of double effect) in combination with the universally accepted practice of respecting patient refusals of medical treatment, on the one hand, and the far more controversial action of injecting patients with a lethal dose of medication. The argument against the practice is that, while the sedatives themselves are not administered in an intentionally lethal dose as in the case of "active euthanasia," in combination with the withholding of nutrition and hydration the patient's death is as inevitable as it would be at the higher dose. That it takes place more slowly, in this view, should not affect the characterization of the action as ("slow") active euthanasia.[46] To this comes the rejoinder that, unlike active euthanasia, with its clear intent for immediate death, "terminal sedation"—as the practice is commonly known—is in principle always reversible (sedatives can be lightened to give the patient the opportunity to interact and change course if desired), and remains focused on alleviation of discomfort, not on bringing about the patient's death.

- Counseling the patient about voluntarily stopping eating and drinking and, if the patient decides to do this, providing medication as needed to alleviate possible discomforts or anxiety over the ensuing period of the patient's death from dehydration. This is another borderline action. On the one hand, it has been advocated as a solution to the moral conundrum posed by physician-provided prescriptions for lethal injection because the patient is solely responsible for his or her lack of nutrition and hydration, and his or her death is simply the result of the patient's exercise of the well-accepted right to be free of bodily intrusion. It is further argued that the determination required on the patient's part to persist in refusal of eating or drinking until death is a safeguard against subtle manipulation or coercion of the patient. On the other hand, the physician clearly has played some significant role. Without the physician's education of the patient about the option, his or her assurances of providing comfort measures, and actually providing them, many people would probably never consider this option at all, much less pursue it to its conclusion.

- Providing a prescription for a lethal dose of medication at the patient's request, and counseling the patient about how to take the medication so as to ensure a painless death, after ensuring the patient's mental competence, providing information about palliative care as an alternative, and requiring both oral and written requests separated by a waiting period. This is the Oregon Death with Dignity Act. As with the previous action, the patient takes all of the decisive steps to bring about his or her death, and may decide at many points to change his or her mind (indeed, of the 65 patients who received prescriptions in Oregon in 2006, 35 took the medication, 19 died of their disease, and 11 were still alive at the end of the year).[37] By calculating the effective dose, writing the prescription, and counseling the patient on how to ingest the medication, however, the physician is complicit in the patient's death in a way that he or she would not be were the patient to end his or her life in a completely private act.

Two Levels of Response: Social Policy and Clinical Care

There are two important levels of response to the issue of physician-assisted death: the level of social policy (i.e., which actions along the clinical spectrum should be legally permitted or prohibited) and the level of clinical care (i.e., how individual physicians should respond to their patients who request help in advancing the time of their death).

Social Policy

At the level of social policy there are once again two positions at the ends of a spectrum, with ongoing, active debates about positions in between.[38] One end is occupied by advocates of a thoroughgoing libertarianism: the choice to end one's life at the time and in the manner of one's own choosing is so bound up with personal privacy and self-determination that no limits should be set on the actions of fully informed, mentally competent adults, and least of all of a physician to help a terminally ill, suffering patient achieve a swift and painless death. The other end views physicians' direct involvement in assisted death—at least in the forms of providing prescriptions or injecting lethal medication—as so contrary to the role and professional identity of the physician, and so destructive of important societal values, as to require universal and permanent legal prohibition.[47] Physicians, on this view, should abstain from the practice even where it is legally permitted.

The most active debate takes place between these extremes. The essential dispute is this: Given the improvement in the science and technique of palliative care and pain management over the last 20 years or so (much of which is documented elsewhere in this volume), is the number of people whose physical or existential anguish near the end of life is beyond the reach of effective palliation large enough to justify the societal risks that could accompany widespread legalization of physician-assisted death in its most direct and active forms? Those who say no—and at the state level that would include, as of now, all states in the U.S. except Oregon—worry that the possibilities for various types of abuse in a permissive legal system outweigh the benefits to the very small number of people who truly have no other options.

These abuses might include acts of desperation by people without reliable access to medical care of any sort, much less state-of-the-art palliative care; subtle coercion of people to take advantage of legal means to end their lives, playing on their common desire not to be a burden on others; or misguided compassion of caregivers who are ignorant of comfort measures and social supports that could have provided the patient with more options for maintaining dignity and comfort.[2]

Those who say yes would argue that these hypothetical, even if theoretically plausible, worries should not outweigh the actual suffering of identifiable people who are ravaged by disease and dying in uncontrolled misery or humiliation. Given what even most opponents concede, that there are indeed some patients (small though their number might be) whose suffering is not remediable with standard measures of palliative care, proponents of legalization believe the more active forms of physician assistance should be available—and socially permissible—as a last resort.[48] They contend that the Oregon experience itself should reassure skeptics that safeguards against abuse can work;[49] and that, even if legally prohibited, physician-assisted death in its active forms is and will be carried out, and that legalization will allow a more public, well-regulated practice to take the place of the "euthanasia underground."[50]

Clinical Care

Regardless of the resolution of these issues at the social and political level, individual physicians should be prepared to deal compassionately and therapeutically with patients who raise the possibility of physician-assisted death. Opponents and proponents of legalization of the more active forms of physician involvement usually agree that excellent palliative care—the full array of active management and support of physical, psychosocial, and spiritual distress—is the standard of care for the seriously ill patient near the end of life. Quill and Arnold[51] outline a set of responses within the physician–patient relationship and the therapeutic dialogue that can help assess and respond to patients, independent of the physician's personal moral beliefs or the legal environment of his or her practice. They recommend that the physician who receives a request from a patient to help hasten death:

- **CLARIFY** what the patient is communicating: General thoughts about the desirability of ending his or her life? Wondering about the future if his or her condition deteriorates? Asking for help right now?
- **SUPPORT** the patient by giving reassurance that whatever the patient feels or desires, the physician is prepared to work together to find a mutually acceptable solution.
- **EVALUATE** the patient's mental state and decision-making capacity; whether the request seems commensurate with the level of unrelieved suffering; whether there is evidence of treatable depression.
- **EXPLORE** the many possible sources of intolerable suffering; for example, poorly controlled physical symptoms, loneliness, sleep disturbances and exhaustion, psychological or spiritual anguish.
- **RESPOND** to the emotions associated with the patient's request. Take them seriously while also trying to separate your own emotions from those of the patient.
- **INTENSIFY TREATMENT**, with the help of a multidisciplinary team, of any potentially reversible elements of the patient's suffering.

Only when all of these steps have been completed, Quill and Arnold recommend, should the physician respond directly to a patient's persistent request for hastened death. Physicians who believe that affirmative assistance is justified beyond steps that fall within ethically or legally accepted practice have a genuine moral dilemma. Some may feel compelled to inform the patient that, despite their sympathy and solidarity, they cannot cross a particular legal or ethical boundary, but may be willing to refer the patient to another physician. Others may be willing to, in Quill's words—cited in a very valuable essay by John Arras[52]—"take small risks for people [they] really know and care about."

CONCLUSION: BEYOND THE PATIENT–PHYSICIAN DYAD

Good care for a dying patient depends on more than the skillful efforts of the most conscientious physician. Dying is both an intensely private and an inherently social process. The ramifications of the patient's illness spread throughout his or her social network, both in space—to family, intimate friends, workmates, and so on—and in time—lasting throughout the grief and bereavement of the survivors. Palliative care, which sets itself the task of ministering not only to the patient but also to the "family as the unit of care," necessarily raises ethical and policy questions beyond the patient–physician dyad.

Some of these issues are closely connected to some of the familiar topics of clinical ethics, such as protecting the confidentiality of medical information or weighing the preferences or needs of family members against potentially incompatible wishes of the patient (e.g., the patient who insists on remaining at home to die even as family members are pushed beyond their physical or emotional limits by the demands of home-based care). Issues such as these push against an individualistic ethic that places the physician's obligations to the best interests of his or her patient above all other moral considerations,[53] and they often call for skills of negotiation and mediation that are not typically included in the interviewing and communication skills training in medical schools.

Other issues touch on broader questions of public policy and the allocation of society's resources. Excellent palliative care requires *systems* of care that can match the particular needs of patients and their families to appropriate resources, across all the sites of care typical of the prolonged, chronic illnesses that precede most deaths in our society.[54,55] These include, at a minimum:

- Systems to elicit and document meaningful information from patients about their values, preferences, and goals for medical care, and to make sure the documentation accompanies the patient wherever they are in the health care system;
- Systems to assure quality standards for the provision of palliative care in health care institutions, including hospitals, nursing homes, and personal care facilities;
- Systems to train health professionals in the principles and practices of palliative care;
- Systems for family and caregiver support that help families participate meaningfully in the lives and care of their dying loved ones without sacrificing their own physical, mental, and financial well-being;
- Systems for financing care that reward professionals for the time-intensive nature of patient and family support and communication in palliative care.

As has been mentioned more than once in this chapter, the enormous disruptive power of death makes it impossible for even the best systems and most dedicated individuals to ensure that every person dies according to their ideals and hopes for meaning, dignity, and comfort. And the physician is only one actor—albeit a very significant one—in the universal human process of coming to terms with life's ending. Families, faith communities, neighborhoods, civic groups, employers, professional caregivers, and many others have the opportunity and responsibility to help people die in ways that affirm the values and qualities that make life itself worthwhile. The best social policies, laws, and regulations that address the care of the dying will be those that make the efforts of all of these people easier rather than harder.

References

1. Hinton J. The dying and the doctor. In: Toynbee A, ed. *Man's Concern with Death*. St. Louis: McGraw-Hill; 1969.
2. Burt RA. *Death Is That Man Taking Names: Intersections of American Medicine, Law, and Culture*. Berkeley: University of California Press; 2002.
3. McIntyre A. *After Virtue*. Notre Dame, Ind: Notre Dame University Press; 1981.
4. Engelhardt HT Jr. *The Foundations of Bioethics*. 2nd ed. New York: Oxford University Press; 1996.
5. Meisel A. The legal consensus about forgoing life-sustaining treatment: its status and its prospects. *Kennedy Inst Ethics J* 1993:2(4):309–345.
6. Oken D. What to tell cancer patients. A study of medical attitudes. *JAMA* 1961;175:1120–1128.
7. Novack DH, Plumer R, Smith RL, et al. Changes in physicians' attitudes toward telling the cancer patient. *JAMA* 1979;241:897–900.
8. Baile WF, Buckman R, Lenzi R, et al. SPIKES-A six-step protocol for delivering bad news: application to the patient with cancer. *Oncologist* 2000;5:302–311.
9. Benbassat J, Pilpel D, Tidhar M. Patients' preferences for participation in clinical decision-making: a review of published surveys. *Behav Med* 1998;24:81–88.
10. Ford S, Fallowfield L, Lewis S. Can oncologists detect distress in their outpatients and how satisfied are they with their performance during bad news consultations? *Br J of Cancer* 1994;70:767–770.
11. Ford S, Fallowfield L, Lewis S. Doctor-patient interactions in oncology. *Soc Sci Med* 1996;42:1511–1519.
12. World Health Organization. *Cancer Pain Relief and Palliative Care. Technical Report Series 804*. Geneva, Switzerland: World Health Organization; 1990;11.
13. Billings JA. What is palliative care? *J Palliat Med* 1998;1(1):73–81.
14. Billings JA. On being a reluctant physician—strains and rewards in caring for the dying at home. In: Billings, JA, ed. *Outpatient Management of Advanced Cancer*. Philadelphia: Lippincott & Co; 1985:309–318.
15. Berg JW, Appelbaum PS, Lidz CW, et al. *Informed Consent: Legal Theory and Clinical Practice*. 2nd ed. New York: Oxford University Press; 2001.
16. Hauser CA, Stockler MR, Tattersall MH. Prognostic factors in patients with recently diagnosed incurable cancer: a systematic review. *Support Care Cancer* 2006;14:999–1011.
17. Levy WC, Mozaffarian D, Linker DT, et al. The Seattle Heart Failure Model: prediction of survival in heart failure. *Circulation* 2006;113:1424–1433.
18. Childers JW, Arnold RM, Curtis JR. Prognosis in end-stage chronic obstructive pulmonary disease #141. *J Palliat Med* 2007;10(3):806–807.
19. Mitchell SL, Kiely DK, Hamel MB, et al. Estimating prognosis for nursing home residents with advanced dementia. *JAMA* 2004;291:2734–2740.
20. D'Amico G, Garcia-Tsao G, Pagliaro L, et al. Natural history and prognostic indicators of survival in cirrhosis: a systematic review of 188 studies. *J Hepatol* 2006;44:217–231.
21. Wijdicks EFM, Hijdra A, Young GB, et al. Practice parameters: Prediction of outcome in comatose survivors after cardiopulmonary resuscitation (an evidence-based review). Report of the Quality Standards Subcommittee of the American Academy of Neurology. *Neurology* 2006;67:203–210.
22. Christakis NA, Lamont EB. Extent and determinants of error in doctors' prognoses in terminally ill patients: prospective cohort study. *BMJ* 2000;320:469–472.
23. Lamont EB, Christakis NA. Complexities in prognostication in advanced cancer: "to help them live their lives the way they want to." *JAMA* 2003;290(1)98–104.
24. Callahan D. *The Troubled Dream of Life: Living with Mortality*. New York: Simon and Schuster; 1993.
25. Herth K. Fostering hope in terminally-ill people. *J Adv Nurs* 1990;15:1250–1259.
26. Schofield P, Carey M, Love A, et al. 'Would you like to talk about your future treatment options'? Discussing the transition from curative cancer treatment to palliative care. *Palliat Med* 2006;20:397–406.
27. Appelbaum PS, Grisso T. Assessing patients' capacities to consent to treatment. *N Engl J Med* 1988;319(25):1635–1638.
28. Fagerlin A, Schneider CE. Enough. The failure of the living will. *Hastings Cent Rep* 2004;34(2):30–42.
29. Hickman SE, Hammes BJ, Moss AH, et al. Hope for the future: achieving the original intent of advanced directives. *Hastings Cent Rep* 2005;Spec No: S26–S30.
30. Brett AS. Limitations of listing specific medical interventions in advanced directives. *JAMA* 1991;266(6):825–828.
31. Tversky A, Kahneman D. The framing of decisions and the psychology of choice. *Science* 1981;211:453–458.
32. Barnard D. Advance care planning is not about "getting it right." *J Palliat Med* 2002;5:475–481.
33. Meisel A. *The Right to Die*. 2nd ed. New York: Aspen; 1985.
34. Helft PR, Siegler M, Lantos J. The rise and fall of the futility movement. *N Engl J Med* 2000;343:293–296.
35. Clouser KD. Allowing or causing: another look. *Ann Intern Med* 1977;87:622–624.
36. Back AL, Arnold RM. Dealing with conflict in caring for the seriously ill: "it was just out of the question." *JAMA* 2005;293(11):1374–1381.
37. The Oregon Public Health Division [homepage on the Internet]. Summary of Oregon's death with Dignity Act- 2006. Available at: http://egove.oregon.gov/dhs/ph/pas/docs/year9.pdf. Accessed November, 2007.
38. Battin MP, Rhodes R, Silvers A, eds. *Physician-Assisted Suicide: Expanding the Debate*. New York: Routledge; 1998.
39. American Public Health Association. [homepage on the Internet]. Supporting appropriate language used to discuss end-of-life choices. Available at: http://www.apha.org/advocacy/policy/policysearch/default.htm?id = 1345. Accessed April 17, 2009.
40. American Academy of Hospice and Palliative Medicine. [homepage on the Internet]. Position statements. Physician-assisted death. Available at: http://www.aahpm.org/positions/suicide.html. Accessed April 17, 2009.
41. Quill TE, Lee BC, Nunn S. Palliative treatments of last resort: choosing the least harmful alternative. University of Pennsylvania Center for Bioethics Assisted Suicide Consensus Panel. *Ann Intern Med* 2000;132:488–493.
42. Quill TE, Lo B, Brock DW. Palliative options of last resort: a comparison of voluntarily stopping eating and drinking, terminal sedation, physician-assisted suicide, and voluntary active euthanasia. *JAMA* 1997;278(23):2099–2104.
43. Quill TE, Dresser R, Brock DW. The rule of double effect—a critique of its role in end-of-life decision making. *N Engl J Med* 1997;337:1768–1771.
44. Sulmasy DP, Pellegrino ED. The rule of double effect: clearing up the double talk. *Arch Intern Med* 1999;159:545–550.
45. Fohr SA. The double effect of pain medication: separating myth from reality. *J Palliat Med* 1998;1:315–328.
46. Billings JA, Block SD. Slow euthanasia. *J Palliat Care* 1996;12(4):21–30.
47. Pellegrino ED. Doctors must not kill. *J Clin Ethics* 1992;3:95–102.
48. Quill TE. Doctor, I want to die, Will you help me? *JAMA* 1993;270:870–873.
49. Okie S. Physician-assisted suicide—Oregon and beyond. *N Engl J Med* 2005;352(16):1627–1630.
50. Magnusson RS. *Angels of death: Exploring the euthanasia underground*. New Haven, Conn: Yale University Press; 2002.
51. End of Life/Palliative Education Resource Center. Medical College of Wisconsin. Quill Timothy E, Arnold Robert. Fast fact and concept #156: evaluating requests for hastened death. Available at: http://www.eperc.mcw.edu/fastFact/ff_156.htm. Accessed November 30, 2007.
52. Arras JD. Physician-assisted suicide: A tragic view. In: Battin MP, Rhodes R, Silvers A, eds. *Physician-Assisted Suicide: Expanding the Debate*. New York: Routledge; 1998:63–72.
53. Randall F, Downie RS. *Palliative Care Ethics: A Companion for All Specialties*. 2nd ed. Oxford, England: Oxford University Press; 1999.
54. The Robert Wood Johnson Foundation: Last Acts. Means to a better end: a report on dying in America today. Available at: http://www.rwjf.org/pr/product.jsp?id = 15788. Accessed April 17, 2009.
55. Field M, Cassel C, eds and the Institute of Medicine (US), Committee on Care at the End of Life. *Approaching Death: Improving Care at the End of Life. Institute of Medicine*. Washington, DC: The National Academy Press; 1997.

CHAPTER 14 ■ LAWS AND POLICIES AFFECTING PAIN MANAGEMENT

AARON M. GILSON

INTRODUCTION

Prevalence of Unrelieved Pain is a Public Health Problem

In *Illness as Metaphor*, author Susan Sontag wrote:

> Illness is the night-side of life, a more onerous citizenship. Everyone who is born holds dual citizenship, in the kingdom of the well and in the kingdom of the sick. Although we all prefer to use only the good passport, sooner or later each of us is obliged, at least for a spell, to identify ourselves as citizens of that other place.[1]

Of course, with sickness and disease often comes the experience of pain. In fact, pain is one of the most common physical complaints upon a person's admission into the health care system, and moderate to severe pain is frequently reported to be experienced throughout hospitalization, during treatment, and even after discharge. The National Institutes of Health (NIH) estimate that 100 million Americans suffer from chronic pain, including pain associated with the disease of cancer,[2] and recent research suggests that the prevalence of pain in people with cancer can range from 14% to 100%, depending on chronicity, severity, and site of the disease.[3] In addition, the prevalence of chronic noncancer pain in patients seen in the primary care setting shows an approximate range of 5% to 33%,[4] and a 2006 American Pain Foundation (APF) survey found that fewer than 40% of people with severe chronic noncancer pain reported that their pain was under control.[5] The costs of pain, both emotional and financial, can be enormous.[6] Untreated or undertreated severe pain at any stage of disease or condition can limit a person's functioning, productivity, and ability to interact socially; sometimes pain even destroys the will to live.[7] A 2003 study published in the *Journal of the American Medical Association* indicated that unrelieved pain annually exceeds $61 billion in lost productivity,[8] while a previous NIH estimation exceeded $100 billion per year in lost productivity and wages and in medical expenses.[9] The financial cost of chronic pain is considered similar to that of cancer or cardiovascular disease.[10] Increasingly, unrelieved pain is recognized as a significant public health problem in the United States.

Issues of public health demand a public health approach to develop informed and organized responses to these health problems.[11] A public health approach is intended to protect the community and enhance the health and quality of life of this population by making available effective and economical interventions.[12] Utilizing a social systems perspective, which incorporates input from various levels of the government (including administrative agencies), health care, education, and welfare systems, often is necessary to guide effective interventions.[13] As inadequate pain management becomes accepted as an important public health issue, efforts to rectify this situation will necessarily involve the systematic utilization of methods to measure outcomes of improved treatment. Some of the most frequent outcome measures, including reduction in pain scores and indicators of quality of life enhancement, must be considered alongside more long-term objectives that denote optimal levels of health status. Before such approaches and outcomes can be conceptualized and achieved, however, the numerous factors that can combine to result in unrelieved pain for patients with chronic diseases or conditions must be understood.

Barriers to the Effective Use of Opioid Analgesics for Pain Management

Unlike most countries in the world, the problem of unrelieved pain in the U.S. is not a function of needed medications being unavailable. However, patients who experience chronic severe pain often do not have access to prescription opioid analgesics, which are the only medications currently indicated for treating this level of pain. This situation relates directly to the equity of health care services. Access to effective pain management requiring prescription opioids remains inequitable, and the reasons for this represent a variety of issues.

Health care organizations and national experts suggest that a number of diverse factors can interfere with the medical use of opioid analgesics for the treatment of pain and can negatively impact patients' access to effective pain relief. Most studies have focused on issues in the patient or clinical domains, such as: (1) patient and family perceptions about the use of opioids for pain relief[7,14-20]; (2) patient characteristics such as race or ethnicity, substance abuse history, or the community in which they live[21-31]; and (3) knowledge and attitudes of health care professionals about the legitimate use of opioids.[28,32-45]

When treating pain with opioid analgesics, clinicians must determine how to maximize benefit and minimize harm, which they have generally not been trained to do. Health care practitioners' willingness to manage chronic pain with opioids often is impacted by unfamiliarity with pain management in general and with the relevant medications in particular, as well as by the perceived likelihood of iatrogenic harm to the patient and risk of regulatory or criminal sanctions resulting from prescribing the medications. As a result, there remains an urgent need to enhance the skills, awareness, and confidence of health care providers, and to explore the motivations and challenges to get both practitioners and patients involved in initiatives promoting pain management services.

Many of the clinical and patient factors previously mentioned can contribute to the high prevalence of unrelieved pain in the U.S., including characteristics of the health care system and health care professionals. Restrictive federal and state policies relating to drug control and health care practice (referred to as regulatory barriers) also are recognized as potential impediments to pain management, especially considering the extent that practitioners know of and adhere to such policies. Since the early 1990s, national health care organizations have frequently voiced concern about the possible detrimental effects of regulatory barriers. In 1994, the Agency for Health Care Policy and Research (now the Agency for Health Care Research and Quality) published clinical practice guidelines for cancer pain relief, which recognized the existence of regulatory barriers, and recommended that drug abuse prevention laws not hamper the appropriate use of opioids for cancer pain.[46] Around that time the American Cancer Society sponsored a workshop to define priorities in cancer pain-related research that included policy and regulatory issues.[47] The American Cancer Society (ACS) later convened a Cancer Pain Management Policy Review Group to discuss regulatory challenges facing cancer pain management, with an emphasis on ensuring access to appropriate treatment given the recent national attention on the nonmedical use of pain medications. The Review Group developed several policy statements about various aspects of cancer pain management,[48–50] including a description of regulatory barriers affecting quality pain treatment.[51] In the last few years, the ACS,[48] as well the Institute of Medicine (IOM)[52] and the NIH,[53] have called for studies to improve pain management and identify the legal and regulatory impediments to using opioids for pain relief. For the U.S., this involves an understanding and examination of both federal and state laws.

Policies Governing the Use of Opioid Analgesics for Pain Management

Governments, both federal and state, can create and change public policies that influence health. Laws reflect governmental decisions that are largely influenced by social values, but provide the legal basis for actions that affect public health, including pain management. For example, given the increasing recognition of pain relief as a basic human right,[54] health care facility licensing standards (e.g., for hospitals, nursing homes, residential care units, and hospices) recently are making the assessment and relief of pain a regulatory mandate and, therefore, a treatment expectation for the patients who require these services. The World Health Organization (WHO) embraces the incorporation of human rights principles, acknowledging the need to "balance effective responses to disease risks" with respect for fundamental individual freedoms.[55] However, a patient receiving effective pain relief currently is viewed more as a right in the moral sense, but generally is not supported by law.

Legislative bodies typically create laws (i.e., statutes) that are broad and general, and depend on the relevant regulatory agency to interpret and implement the laws. In fact, legislatures that avoid making considerably detailed law would likely require less frequent amendments to such laws, because the accompanying regulations contain the professional or technical details that would need to be revised periodically to keep pace with changing practice standards. For medicine, the legislature grants authority to the state medical board to define and implement its laws through regulation (or administrative rules); regulations must be consistent with legislative provisions. Even given this structured process, pain-related law has not kept pace with advances in medical and scientific understanding. Although professional boards generally have frequently revised their pain management policies in reaction to updated professional standards, legislation has been slow to change. This has particular implication for pain management issues related to opioid prescribing, where such legislation tends to have extensive detail and may not reflect current medical standards (see the section State Pain Policy Development: An Emerging Trend).

In 2007, the journal *Pain Medicine* published B. Todd Sitzman's President's Message to the American Academy of Pain Medicine readership, entitled "Guiding Principles for the Pain Medicine Physician—In a Not So Ideal World."[56] According to Dr. Sitzman, an ideal clinical world for practicing pain medicine physicians would be characterized by, among other things:

no governmental or third-party oversight; addiction to prescribed analgesics would not exist; . . . and for good measure, professional liability and attorneys would not exist.[56]

As Dr. Sitzman recognizes, health care professionals must practice in an environment of legal and regulatory influences, and where some patients with pain also have an addictive disease. Although practitioners generally do not receive training in legal and regulatory issues related to prescribing opioid analgesics, and are not familiar with the federal and state laws that govern their practice, there has been an increasing call for clinicians to acquire knowledge of the policies under which they practice.[57,58] This chapter attempts to create a resource to address this need by describing the three layers of laws creating the policy framework for both the diversion and legitimate medical use of opioid analgesics: (1) international treaties governing drug control; (2) federal statutes and regulations governing drug control, which includes the legal parameters for prescribing controlled substances; and (3) state statutes and regulations governing drug control and health care practice, including prescribing controlled substances. The chapter also discusses other legal and regulatory influences on prescribing practices, and provides recommendations to practitioners about what they can do in their state to improve pain management.

INTERNATIONAL TREATIES: ESTABLISHING BALANCE BETWEEN DRUG CONTROL AND MEDICAL USE

Treaties form the basic legal framework to control international and domestic production and distribution of drugs that have a recognized abuse liability. The drugs subject to these more rigorous controls are therefore referred to as "controlled substances," and include, but are not limited to, opioid analgesics. The principal treaty establishing controls for opioid analgesics used to treat severe pain is the Single Convention on Narcotic Drugs of 1961 (Single Convention).[59] It should be understood that the term "narcotic," which includes opioid analgesics, is now primarily used in legal contexts, such as in reference to the international drug control treaty or relevant laws; "narcotic," which generally is defined as an agent that produces stupor or insensibility, is no longer considered "useful in a pharmacological context" when describing opioid medications.[60] The Single Convention establishes a number of basic requirements for a country's laws and regulations to create effective measures against drug abuse and diversion. Many of these measures relate directly to the health care setting, including:

- A country's government must duly authorize everyone involved in the medical distribution of narcotic drugs,
- Medical prescriptions must be used to provide narcotic drugs to patients and may be issued only by health care professionals duly authorized under national law, and
- Authorized personnel are responsible for security, record-keeping, and reporting (Article 30: Trade and Distribution).[59]

Although established as international law aimed at preventing drug abuse, this treaty also recognizes that many controlled substances are indispensable to public health and that there is a need to ensure their availability for legitimate medical and scientific purposes.[59] Becoming a party to this treaty obligates a government to take steps to make controlled substances available in adequate amounts to effectively treat medical conditions. Most, but not all, of the world governments are parties to the Single Convention, including the U.S., which means that they formally accept the obligation to develop a legislative and administrative framework to implement the treaty's objectives.[61]

The long-standing dual obligation of country governments to (1) establish a system of controls to prevent abuse, trafficking, and diversion of controlled substances, and (2) simultaneously assure their medical availability is referred to as "balance." Balance maintains that opioid analgesics, although designated as controlled substances, also are essential drugs, are absolutely necessary for adequate pain relief, and must be accessible to patients who need them for medical purposes. Within this framework, the "controlled substances" status of these medications is not meant to diminish their medical usefulness or create the perception that practitioners should avoid their use. Moreover, the principle of balance does not sanction medication use outside an established system of control, recognizing that only properly licensed health care practitioners can use opioid analgesics for legitimate medical purposes in the course of professional practice. Governments that achieve and implement balanced policy continue to maintain an opioids supply sufficient to meet medical demand, and empower practitioners to prescribe, dispense, and administer opioids in the course of professional practice and in response to individual patient needs.

The International Narcotics Control Board (INCB), a United Nations-affiliated agency responsible for monitoring governments' implementation of the Single Convention, has historically observed, and continues to note, that the global medical need for opioid analgesics is not being fully met.[62–64] Opioids remain insufficiently available to meet medical needs throughout the world for many reasons, including severely restrictive (or unbalanced) drug control policies[65–67]; the overriding concern about drug abuse and addiction also has motivated the creation of laws that hamper the appropriate medical use of opioids, including for the treatment of cancer pain[65,68]:

> . . . the reaction of some legislators and administrators to the fear of drug abuse developing or spreading has led to the enactment of laws and regulations that may, in some cases, unduly impede the availability of opiates. The problem may also arise as a result of the manner in which drug control laws and regulations are interpreted or implemented.[62]

Recently, the Council of Europe,[69] WHO HIV/AIDS,[70] the INCB,[71] and the UN Economic and Social Council[72] have called for governments to identify and address regulatory barriers in their narcotics control policies.

For example, a common requirement found in international drug control policies has been and continues to be Multiple Copy Prescription Programs (MCPPs), which the Single Convention encourages when a country's government considers such a control measure necessary or desirable (Article 30(2)(b)(ii)).[59] MCPPs typically require physicians to issue prescriptions using a special form so that a designated regulatory or enforcement agency can monitor the prescribing and dispensing of certain drugs. MCPPs are designed and enacted primarily to prevent forgery of narcotic prescriptions and can vary in type, from the use of prescription pads with counterfoil or carbon pages, to an extreme where the physician must complete the same required prescription information repeatedly on a number of separate forms. These serialized prescription forms are government-issued, but they may be difficult to obtain and can increase the health care and social stigma associated with opioid medications.[73,74] As early as 1990, the WHO Expert Committee on Cancer Pain Relief and Active Supportive Care addressed how special government-issued prescription forms can impact prescribing:

> Record-keeping and authorization requirements should not be such that, for all practical purposes, they eliminate the availability of opioids for medical purposes. Multiple-copy prescription programmes are cited as means of reducing careless prescribing and 'multiple doctoring' (patients registering with several medical practitioners in order to obtain several prescriptions for the same, or similar drugs). There is some justification for (this), but the extent to which these programmes restrict or inhibit the prescribing of opioids to patients who need them should also be questioned.[75]

More recently, some governments have concluded that MCPPs create burdens to physicians' practice that can unduly limit access to covered medications, and have changed the requirements of these programs to respond to these problems—this has occurred recently in Austria,[76] Italy,[77] and in numerous states in the U.S.[73,78] These positive programmatic changes do not undermine MCPPs' drug control capacities, but rather make it less likely that they hinder patient care. Other ways that countries have established overly restrictive drug monitoring and control systems include establishing extremely short medication supply limits (e.g., 3 days)[79] and only allowing physicians with certain specialties to prescribe.[80]

It is apparent that the international narcotics control treaty is intended to maintain drug availability for medical purposes, which the World Health Assembly[54,81,82] recently reaffirmed. However, some countries have implemented the treaty too strictly, which makes the use of opioid drugs for pain management difficult if not impossible—such countries do not have balanced drug control or professional practice policies. Given this reality, it is important to understand the current status of U.S. statutes and regulations. The next section describes the extent that the U.S. is continuing to balance its obligation to prevent medication diversion and abuse against its responsibility to ensure the appropriate medical use of opioid analgesics.

FEDERAL LAW: PRESERVING BALANCE BETWEEN DRUG CONTROL AND MEDICAL USE

The Federal Food, Drug, and Cosmetic Act

Under the authority of the Federal Food, Drug, and Cosmetic Act of 1962 (FFDCA), the Food and Drug Administration (FDA), which is part of the Department of Health and Human Services, is responsible for promoting public health by ensuring that all new drugs, including opioids and other controlled substances, are safe and effective for marketing and for human use under medical supervision.[83] The FDA's approval decisions for marketing a particular drug always involve an assessment of the benefits and risks, including its abuse liability. The drug manufacturer must provide to the FDA all relevant data related to safety by the time a new drug application is submitted.[84] When the benefits of a drug are considered to outweigh its risks, and when the labeling instructions allow for safe and effective use, only then does the FDA consider the drug safe for approval and marketing.

When reviewing a new drug application, a determination can be made that the manufacturer also must submit plans for a risk evaluation and mitigation strategy (REMS). The REMS contains steps to address morbidity and mortality, and requires a timetable to assess the strategy at 18 months, 3 years, and 7 years after the strategy is approved.[85] Additional elements of the strategy can include a communications plan to health care practitioners about the drug, such as: (1) sending letters, (2) disseminating information about the REMS to explain certain safety protocols or to encourage implementation by health care practitioners of applicable components of the REMS, and (3) use professional societies to disseminate information about serious drug risks and protocols to enhance safety.[85]

The FDA also is responsible for reviewing product labeling, and for ensuring that post-marketing promotional materials are consistent with the approved labeling. Historically, the FDA's statutory authority applied primarily to pre-marketing testing and, after drug approval, the agency's role was limited. However, in September 2007, the FFDCA was expanded to comprise active post-market risk identification for approved drugs,[86] which includes ongoing analysis of drug safety data from disparate data sources as well as adverse event surveillance using electronic data from the Federal government and the private sector. Once enacted, this collaborative process is designed to improve the quality and efficiency of post-marketing drug safety risk-benefit analysis, and to allow for the public disclosure of safety and effectiveness data in a timely and systematic manner.

Once the FDA approves a medication, a physician can prescribe, and a pharmacist can dispense, that medication for "off-label" uses (i.e., uses not included in the approved labeling) if there is a recognized medical basis for those uses.[87,88]

> Once (an approved) new drug is in a local pharmacy after interstate shipment, the physician may, as part of the practice of medicine, lawfully prescribe a different dosage for his patient, or may otherwise vary the condition for use from those approved in the package insert, without informing or obtaining the approval of the Food and Drug Administration. This interpretation of the Act is consistent with the Congressional intent as indicated in the legislative history of the 1938 Act and the Drug Amendments of 1962. Throughout the debate leading to the enactment, there were repeated statements that Congress did not intend the Food and Drug Administration to interfere with medical practice and references to the understanding that the bill did not purport or regulate the practice of medicine as between the physician and the patient.[89]

The FDA again corroborated this statement in their FDA Consumer Magazine.

> New uses for drugs are often discovered, reported in medical journals and at medical meetings, and subsequently may be widely used by the medical profession. . . . When physicians go beyond the directions given in the package insert it does not mean they are acting illegally or unethically and Congress did not intend to empower the FDA to interfere with medical practice by limiting the ability of physicians to prescribe according to their best judgment.[90]

As this statement suggests, evidence supporting effective off-label use usually results from post-marketing studies or from an accumulation of case reports by independent investigators. The FFDCA does not restrict a physician's prescribing either to recommended doses or to labeled indications, which is a clear message contained in the forward to the *Physician's Desk Reference*.[91] Off-label uses simply reflect a physician's lawful ability to prescribe for a medical purpose and in the interest of the patient according to his or her best knowledge and judgment.[92]

Of course, prescribing decisions, including whether the medication is intended for a labeled or off-label indication, are part of medical practice. The FFDCA is intended neither to regulate medical practice[93] nor to interfere with the authority of a licensed health care practitioner to use controlled substances for a legitimate medical purpose.[94] It is the responsibility of the states, and not the federal government, to regulate professional health care practice. However, both the state and the federal governments share drug control responsibilities.

Federal Controlled Substances Law

Controlled substances laws provide an additional layer of control over the distribution of prescription drugs that have an abuse liability (i.e., use criteria related to the potential to produce psychological or physical dependence), establishing a closed distribution system to minimize their abuse, trafficking, and diversion. The federal Controlled Substances Act (CSA),[95] part of the Comprehensive Drug Abuse Prevention and Control Act of 1970,[96] is the principal drug control law in the U.S. and conforms to the international treaties—it establishes criminal penalties for the illicit possession, manufacture, and trafficking of controlled substances and prohibits their nonmedical use, while at the same time recognizing that they are necessary for public health and that their medical availability must be ensured. The CSA creates a comprehensive regulatory framework assuring that controlled substances are only produced and distributed through proper channels and for proper medical purposes. In fact, the CSA is a culmination of more than 50 pieces of federal legislation adopted since 1914 relating to drug control and diversion.[96]

The CSA specifies five classification schedules for controlled substances, each carrying different penalties for unlawful uses. A drug's medical usefulness and abuse liability form the basis for the decision to assign it to a particular schedule.[97] Schedule I drugs have no currently accepted medical use, no accepted safety for use under medical supervision, and a high potential for abuse (e.g., ecstasy, heroin, LSD, marijuana, methaqualone, and peyote), and are available only for scientific research. Drugs that have an FDA-approved medical use are placed in Schedules II through V according to potential for abuse in the following manner:

- Schedule II drugs have the highest potential for abuse, and include such opioids as codeine, fentanyl, hydromorphone, meperidine, methadone, morphine, and oxycodone, as well as nonopioids such as short-acting barbiturates (e.g., pentobarbital), amphetamines (e.g., methamphetamine, methylphenidate, and cocaine).
- Schedule III drugs have a lower abuse potential than Schedule II drugs, and include opioids such as hydrocodone- or codeine-combinations with aspirin or acetaminophen, as well as nonopioids such as buprenorphine, intermediate-acting barbiturates (e.g., butalbital), and the synthetic cannabinoid dronabinol.
- Schedule IV drugs have a lower abuse potential relative to drugs in Schedule III, and include opioids such as dextropropoxyphene, and pentazocine, as well as nonopioids such as benzodiazepines (e.g., alprazolam and diazepam), long-acting barbiturates (e.g., phenobarbital), and certain nonamphetamine stimulants (e.g., pemoline).
- Schedule V drugs have a lower abuse potential compared to drugs in Schedule IV and include compounds or preparations containing limited quantities of opioids such as codeine or opium, which may be used for over-the-counter preparations to treat cough or diarrhea, respectively, as well as antidiarrheals containing diphenoxylate and difenoxin.

Under federal law, the Drug Enforcement Administration (DEA) is the primary federal agency responsible for enforcing the CSA and, thus, has regulatory authority over controlled substances. The DEA is an agency of the federal Department of Justice, headed by the Attorney General of the United States.

To conduct research with, or manufacture, distribute, handle, dispense, administer, or prescribe, controlled substances, a person or business must be registered with the DEA (and, in some cases, also with the relevant state agencies).[98,99] Licensed and registered practitioners can prescribe, dispense, and administer controlled substances only for legitimate medical purposes and in the usual course of professional practice[100,101]; the DEA and federal courts have interpreted this to mean that prescriptions must be issued "in accordance with a standard of medical practice generally recognized and accepted in the United States."[102] Registrants' distribution of Schedule I and II controlled substances are made using a special order form (DEA Form 222) to monitor all transfers of these controlled substances within the "closed" system.[103,104] Prescriptions for Schedule II medications must be written and may not be refilled,[105,106] while five refills are permitted for drugs in Schedules III and IV.[107,108] Federal law allows oral or faxed (but not electronic) transmission of prescriptions for Schedule II controlled substances in medical emergencies under specific circumstances.[109] Federal law also allows for the partial dispensing and faxing (but not oral or electronic data transmission) of prescriptions under certain circumstances.[110] There are penalties, both criminal and civil, for violating federal requirements.

Although prescriptions for certain controlled substances must be in writing, and refills are limited, the fact that a drug has been approved for medical use does not change when it becomes a controlled substance. This principle is conveyed by the CSA statement that:

[M]any of the drugs included within this title have a useful and legitimate medical purpose and are necessary to maintain the health and general welfare of the American people.[111]

Overall, the legislative history, as well as language contained in the CSA itself (and its related regulations), makes it clear that efforts to prevent drug abuse and diversion are not to interfere with legitimate medical practice and appropriate patient care.[112]

The CSA Ensures Availability of Controlled Substances for Medical Purposes

The CSA authorizes the DEA to establish production quotas for a number of opioids and other controlled substances as a means to stem diversion resulting from excessive unused supplies.[113] Such quotas, however, must maintain sufficient supplies to accommodate all medical and scientific needs.[101] Despite this apparent standard, 20 years ago the DEA set a very low quota for methylphenidate to restrict its production in an effort to control diversion.[114] As a result, the methylphenidate supply was inadequate to treat patients with attention deficit disorder and narcolepsy, which are legitimate medical uses. An official statement was promulgated in response to this action, establishing the principle of an "undisputed proposition" of drug availability:

> The CSA requirement for a determination of legitimate medical need is based on the undisputed proposition that patients and pharmacies should be able to obtain sufficient quantities of methylphenidate, or of any Schedule II drug, to fill prescriptions. A therapeutic drug should be available to patients when they need it. To accomplish this, a smooth flow of distribution is required ... the harshest impact of actual or threatened shortages falls on the patients who must take methylphenidate, not on the manufacturers to whom the quotas directly apply. Actual drug shortages, or even threatened ones, can seriously interfere with patients' lives and those of their families.[114]

Following this statement, the DEA recalculated the methylphenidate quotas to accommodate its demand for medical purposes. The DEA has since expressed a willingness to grant additional quotas for opioids necessary to treat medical conditions including pain[115,116] and has not significantly reduced manufacturing quotas as a means to address the nonmedical use of prescription medications.

The CSA Does Not Regulate Medical Practice

Again, the federal government does not have the authority to regulate medical practice. This authority belongs to the states and is based on the police power in state constitutions, and underlies the medical practice acts that are designed to protect the public health and safety.[117] The CSA is not intended to supersede the authority of the FFDCA and provides no authority for the DEA to define or regulate medical practice,[95] including the treatment of pain in people with addictive disease and the indications for which a drug may be prescribed.

The DEA's enforcement authority is intended to relate to clinicians involved in unlawful distribution of controlled substances that is outside legitimate health care practice (i.e., behaviors that are clearly criminal in nature). To this end, a prescription for a controlled substance is only lawful when issued for a legitimate medical purpose and in the usual course of professional practice.[100] David Brushwood, a pharmacist and attorney and Professor in the College of Pharmacy at the University of Florida–Gainesville, interprets a useful distinction between the phrases "legitimate medical purpose" and "course of professional practice," which define the boundaries of practitioner investigations and prosecutions for the DEA:

> A practice that is not medical is neither legitimate nor legal under the DEA regulation. A practice that is medical is legitimate and is legal under the DEA regulation. DEA does not regulate within medical practice but simply discerns whether a practice is medical or nonmedical ... The DEA regulation has nothing to do with the credentials or qualifications of a health care provider. It has everything to do with the *activities* of the health care provider. If those activities are not professional health care activities, then they are illegal under the DEA regulations; if they are professional health care activities, they are legal. DEA has no authority to pass judgment on the merits of a professional practice. Its role is limited to determining whether a practice is a professional practice.[118]

Further evidence that the CSA was not intended to interfere with legitimate medical practice is found when Congress enacted a law in 1978 to implement another international treaty (i.e., the Convention of Psychotropic Substances of 1971).[119] Consequently, the control of psychotropic substances such as benzodiazepines became a responsibility within the CSA to:

> ... ensure that the availability of psychotropic substances to manufacturers, distributors, dispensers, and researchers for useful and legitimate medical and scientific purposes will not be unduly restricted ... and nothing in the Convention (on Psychotropic Substances) will interfere with ethical medical practice in this country as determined by the secretary of Health and Human Services on the basis of a consensus of the American medical and scientific community.[120]

The CSA Distinguishes Treatment of Addiction from Treatment of Pain

Under the CSA, it is not lawful to prescribe opioids for the purpose of treating addiction; this practice requires separate registration by the federal government as an Opioid Treatment Program (OTP), for the purpose of maintenance or detoxification of opioid addiction.[121] The use of medications approved for the purpose of addiction treatment, such as methadone and buprenorphine, must comply with federal and state regulations. Methadone, however, can be prescribed as an analgesic according to the same laws for prescribing any other Schedule II opioid.

The accurate application of terminology is central to shaping a balanced policy on drug control, especially in the U.S. where using opioids to maintain addiction (without a separate registration) is illegal. Addiction often is erroneously perceived as reflecting the development of physical dependence or tolerance, which are expected physiological consequences of using opioids for a prolonged period. Practitioners who consider these related, but separate, phenomena as synonymous can inappropriately label a pain patient as an "addict" and increase the risk of inadequate pain treatment. Given this situation, one must carefully differentiate between treating a patient's pain and maintaining or detoxifying a person with an addictive disease, and to understand and use terms correctly.

The CSA defines "addict" as:

> an individual who habitually uses any narcotic drug so as to endanger the public morals, health, safety, or who is so far addicted to the use of narcotic drugs as to have lost power of self-control with reference to his addiction.[122]

This definition is characterized by the use of circular, imprecise, and archaic language but, since the main component is loss of control and harm, it seems inapplicable to a patient with pain being treated with opioids. However, the CSA definition does not conform to the WHO's International Classification of Diseases concept of "dependence syndrome,"[123] the American Psychiatric Association's Diagnostic and Statistical Manual classification of "substance dependence,"[124] or the definition by the Liaison Committee on Pain and Addiction's (a consensus committee of the American Academy of Pain Medicine, the American Pain Society, and the American Society of Addiction Medicine).[125] Despite the CSA definition of "addict" not being considered a potential barrier to adequate pain relief, because it would not pertain to a legitimate patient, the language should be updated to conform more completely to current terminology and standards.

Although not contained in the CSA, in 1970 a definition of "drug dependent person" was added to the federal Public Health Service Act (now the Public Health and Welfare Act).[126] The Interstate and Foreign Commerce Committee of the House of Representatives[96] considered the adopted definition to be similar to the WHO's terminology of the time. "Drug dependent person" was defined as:

> a person who is using a controlled substance . . . and who is in a state of *psychic or physical dependence, or both,* arising from the use of that substance on a continuous basis. Drug dependence is characterized by behavioral and other responses which include a strong compulsion to take the substance on a continuous basis in order to experience its psychic effects or to avoid the discomfort caused by its absence [emphasis added].[126]

Although indeed similar, there is a critical interpretive distinction between the resulting U.S. legal term and the WHO term from which it was adopted. Unlike the U.S. definition, the WHO conceptualization did not provide the opportunity for physical dependence alone to characterize drug dependence. In 1998 the WHO reaffirmed this conceptualization when they replaced the term "drug dependence" with "dependence syndrome" and further emphasized the bio-psycho-social nature of compulsive drug seeking.[127] Even given the medical and scientific evolution of addiction-related terminology that has occurred in the last 30 years, the 1970 Public Health and Welfare definition continues to have the potential to legally codify as "drug dependent" a patient with pain who has been taking opioids for a prolonged period.

Despite the inconsistent and incorrect use of addiction-related terminology in federal law, it must be stressed that it remains lawful under federal laws to use opioids to treat pain in patients, even when they have a history of substance use or current addictive disease. For example, in 1993 the DEA initiated action to revoke an Ohio physician's prescribing authority because prescriptions were issued to patients who were "known" drug abusers and drug traffickers. A DEA administrative law judge ruled, however, that the physician's controlled substances prescriptions were lawful because they were issued for legitimate medical purposes (e.g., pain relief, muscle spasm, and anxiety).[128] This ruling represents the critical distinction between a practitioner's ability to prescribe controlled substances to treat pain, even though the patient has an addictive disease, and clearly criminal behavior in which controlled substances are distributed without regard to their purpose or ultimate use. Such a judgment upholds the fundamental principle that, when considering the legality of a particular prescribing practice, the determination must be based on the purpose of the prescribing and not solely on the type of patient being treated. A later section will address how this critical distinction relates to more recent criminal investigations and prosecutions of health care professionals for their prescribing practices.

Regulations Implementing the CSA Recognize Opioids as Appropriate to Treat Intractable Pain

Controlled substances regulations promulgated by the DEA in Chapter II of the Code of Federal Regulations (CFR) clearly state that practitioners who use opioids to treat intractable pain over an extended period are considered to be acting within the course of professional practice:

> This section is not intended to impose any limitations on a physician or authorized hospital staff to . . . administer or dispense (including prescribe) narcotic drugs to persons with intractable pain in which no relief or cure of is possible or none has been found after reasonable efforts.[129]

This CFR provision was adopted in 1974, during a time when the concept of intractable pain was beginning to be accepted into the medical lexicon. In the intervening years, however, it became apparent that the phrase "no relief . . . has been found after reasonable efforts" could be interpreted to mean that the medical use of controlled substances is not reasonable and therefore should be used *only* after attempting and failing other treatments.[78] Given this ambiguity, and its potential negative impact on patient care, the term "chronic pain" has been used with increasing frequency to denote pain that persists beyond the expected time of healing but can vary over time in relation to its severity or extent of associated disability.[130] Nevertheless, this statement from federal regulations provides further support for the need to recognize and maintain a clinical and legal acceptance of prescribing controlled substances for pain.

The CSA and Regulations Do Not Limit Prescription Amount or Duration

As stated previously, federal law establishes requirements for what constitutes a lawful controlled substance prescription. At this time neither the CSA nor the CFR sets limits on the amount or duration of medication for which a practitioner can prescribe, administer, or dispense at one time. This still seems to hold true even after December 19, 2007, when the DEA amended the CFR to allow practitioners to issue multiple prescriptions of a Schedule II controlled substance, each issued on the same date and filled sequentially (called a "prescription series").[131]

A prescription series is a method for a practitioner to provide a patient with a large enough amount of a Schedule II medication, for example for a 3-month supply, without using a single prescription. Rather, the practitioner can now issue several prescriptions, each for one-third of the total amount needed. These prescriptions, each issued on the same day and containing written instructions for the date on which they are to be dispensed, would be delivered to the pharmacist and then dispensed sequentially on the dates indicated on the prescriptions. This procedure allows patients access to the medications they need and results in fewer doses dispensed at a time, thereby reducing the potential for diversion. A practitioner's ability to specifically issue a prescription series for Schedule II controlled substances was not previously authorized within the CSA; the CSA, when adopted in 1970, did not address this practice because chronic pain was not a treatment priority at that time.[132]

The DEA said it wanted to reassure health care professionals and patients that it is legal for practitioners to provide a prescription series to individual patients during a single office visit,[132,133] and now authorizes multiple prescriptions for "a total of up to a 90-day supply of a Schedule II controlled substance."[131] The DEA has clarified that allowing a 90-day prescription series does not alter the fact that the CSA and the CFR do not limit the quantity or number of days for which a single prescription for a Schedule II controlled substance can be written.

> The (Final) rule in no way changes longstanding federal law governing the issuance of prescriptions for controlled substances . . . the CSA and DEA regulations contain no specific limit on the number of days worth of a schedule II controlled substance that a physician may authorize per prescription.[131]

In addition, the DEA has verified that the new prescription series rule does not establish additional practice standards to which health care professionals must conform, especially in relation to a practitioner's responsibility to minimize the potential for medication abuse and diversion.[134]

> Under this Final Rule, practitioners who prescribe controlled substances are subject to the same standard in preventing diversion as they always have been under the CSA and DEA regulations. Section 1306.12(b)(iii) of this Final Rule is intended to make clear that a practitioner may not simply comply with the other requirements of

this Final Rule while turning a blind eye to circumstances that might be indicative of diversion. Thus, section 1306.12(b)(iii) merely underscores that the longstanding requirement of providing effective controls against diversion remains in effect when issuing multiple schedule II prescriptions in accordance with this Final Rule.[131]

The intent of the CFR amendment is laudable, with the DEA wanting to reaffirm a practitioner's legal authority to issue a prescription series for Schedule II medications.[131,132,135] Multiple prescriptions for sequential dispensing permits health care professionals to better manage chronic pain in stable patients while exercising improved control over potential medication abuse and diversion, which is consistent with the principle of balance.[136] The DEA also recognizes the need to maintain balanced policy:

> ... DEA, through its enforcement of the CSA and its implementing regulations, must prevent the diversion and abuse of controlled substances while ensuring that there is an adequate supply for legitimate medical purposes. DEA supports the intent of this Final Rule to address patients' needs for schedule II controlled substances while preventing the diversion of those substances.[131]

Indeed, the prescription series regulation is an important recent federal step to improve the regulatory environment for both diversion control and pain management and palliative care.

STATE LAWS: NEEDING TO IMPROVE BALANCE BETWEEN DRUG CONTROL AND MEDICAL USE

Both federal and state laws govern the prescribing, dispensing, and administering of controlled substances. In addition, states are solely responsible for regulating health care practice, including medical, pharmacy, and nursing practice. State policies are generally not as balanced as international treaties and federal law.[137] For example, most state laws do not specifically recognize controlled medications as important to public health, which is a concept inherent in federal law.[111] Some state policies also place greater restrictions than do federal laws on the prescribing and dispensing of opioids, which can ultimately interfere with medical decision-making that should be based both on the expertise of the practitioner and the individual patient needs, rather than on governmental requirements. Policy impediments at the state level are known to contribute to inadequate pain management.[48,51,52,137-148] In response to this knowledge, both international organizations[65,75,149,150] and national organizations[51-53] have called for studies to improve pain management by identifying and addressing the legal and regulatory impediments to using opioids for pain relief. A number of governmental and national authorities, such as Congress,[95] the National Conference of Commissioners on Uniform State Laws,[144,145,151] and the Federation of State Medical Boards of the U.S., Inc. (the Federation)[138,139] have recommended controlled substances or medical practice policy that is balanced.

State Pain Policy Development: An Emerging Trend

Since the late 1980s, there has been an increasing number of state pain-specific policies, such as Intractable Pain Treatment Acts (IPTAs) and health care regulatory board regulations and guidelines or policy statements (Fig. 14.1). Such policy adoption typically promotes the safe and appropriate use of controlled substances and creates more balanced state policies, but in some cases has led to additional restrictions and requirements with the potential to create barriers to the effective treatment of pain. For example, IPTAs are statutes that create immunity from regulatory sanctions for physicians who prescribe opioids to patients with intractable pain, and thus are intended to improve access to pain management; however, many IPTAs impose additional requirements and restrictions on prescribing opioids to such patients.[137,152-154] IPTAs often imply that opioid use for "intractable pain" is outside of ordinary medical practice, which produces greater rather than less government regulation when treating pain with controlled substances. For physicians who prescribe to patients whose pain does not satisfy the definition of "intractable pain," there is question about whether an IPTA provides immunity. IPTAs also tend to not contain clear statements supporting enhanced pain management and access to care.

Some advocates have recently recognized the potential negative impact of these characteristics on patient care and have worked with the legislature to remove ambiguities and restrictions from their state's IPTA. Iowa and Michigan became the first states, in 2002, to delete the term "intractable pain" from law. More recently, Arizona, California, North Dakota, Oregon, Rhode Island, and Texas repealed a number of restrictive provisions from their IPTAs, including removing the term and definition of "intractable pain"; the resulting laws now govern treatment for all types of pain.

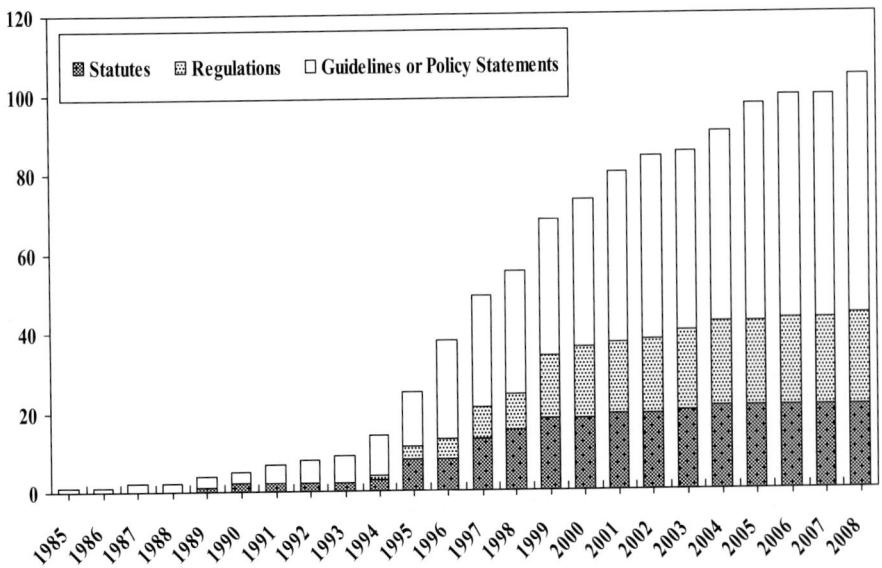

FIGURE 14.1 State pain policies, 1989-2008.

As an alternative approach to creating legislation, which often is difficult to modify to keep pace with evolutions in medical and scientific understanding, many states have instead chosen to develop health care regulatory board guidelines or regulations to encourage better pain management and to address physicians' fear of investigation and sanction.[137,155] Early reports have shown that concerns about regulatory scrutiny are prevalent and can hinder the availability of opioids for patient pain relief.[156–159] Since prescribing for pain management has become a more prominent part of professional practice, physicians have reported a reluctance to prescribe controlled substances out of a concern about regulatory oversight.[160–163] Fear of disciplinary action for opioid prescribing has been documented for a variety of other health care practitioners, including general practice physicians,[34,164–166] oncologists,[45] pain specialists,[167,168] medical residents,[44] pharmacists,[34,39] and nurses.[15,34,37,169] To directly address these concerns, for the past 20 years, health care regulatory boards have promulgated regulations, guidelines, and policy statements perpetuating the message that pain management and the appropriate use of controlled substances is an accepted part of professional practice; a typical goal of such policies is to reassure clinicians that they have nothing to fear from their licensing agency if reasonable professional practices are followed when using controlled substances for patient care.

Much of this recent policy activity was prompted by state medical board members' participation in pain management workshops sponsored periodically by the Pain and Policy Studies Group (PPSG) and the Federation since 1994.[36,170] The workshops emphasized the need for positive policy as a vehicle for providing guidance to licensees about using controlled substances for effective pain relief.

State medical boards' issuance of recommendations for pain management was aided considerably when, in 1998, the Federation adopted a policy template to promote consistency in state medical board policy, entitled *Model Guideline for the Use of Controlled Substances for the Treatment of Pain* (Model Guideline).[138] In May 2004, the Federation revised the Model Guideline as the *Model Policy for the Use of Controlled Substances for the Treatment of Pain* (Model Policy).[139] The Model Policy is substantially the same as the 1998 guideline, but encourages state boards to consider the failure to treat pain as worthy of disciplinary sanction; undertreated pain previously had been identified as an important clinical topic to address in state policy.[171] As of 2008, 32 states have adopted or adapted either the Model Guideline or Model Policy.

Evaluating the Quality of State Pain Policy

A criteria-based policy research methodology recently was developed to evaluate federal and state drug control and health care regulatory policies related to pain management, palliative care, and end-of-life care.[78,136,172–174] The basis for this policy evaluation was the aforementioned principle called balance, which is a fundamental and long-standing national and international principle of drug regulation and medical ethics. Balanced state policies do not establish barriers to appropriate health care practice and patient care, and will support pain management, including the use of controlled substances as an essential part of quality medical practice.[136] The principle of balance was used to derive 16 evaluation criteria. Each criterion relates to one of two categories: (1) positive provisions—policy language that can *enhance* pain relief, and (2) negative provisions—language that can *impede* pain relief (Table 14.1 contains each criterion). A complete description of the criteria, the evaluation methodology, and individual state policy profiles that contain the policy language from each state that satisfies each criterion, can be found in "Achieving Balance in Federal and State Pain Policy: A Guide to Evaluation" online at http://www.painpolicy.wisc.edu.

The most recent series of policy evaluations,[78,136,174] which were conducted in 2006, 2007, and 2008 and supported by grants

TABLE 14.1

CRITERIA USED TO EVALUATE STATE PAIN POLICIES

Positive provisions: Criteria that identify policy language with the potential to enhance pain management

1. Controlled substances are recognized as necessary for the public health
2. Pain management is recognized as part of general medical practice
3. Medical use of opioids is recognized as legitimate professional practice
4. Pain management is encouraged
5. Practitioners' concerns about regulatory scrutiny are addressed
6. Prescription amount alone is recognized as insufficient to determine the legitimacy of prescribing
7. Physical dependence or analgesic tolerance are *not* confused with "addiction"
8. Other provisions that may enhance pain management
   Category A: Issues related to health care professionals
   Category B: Issues related to patients
   Category C: Regulatory or policy issues

Negative provisions: Criteria that identify policy language with the potential to impede pain management

9. Opioids are considered a treatment of last resort
10. Medical use of opioids is implied to be outside legitimate professional practice
11. Physical dependence or analgesic tolerance are confused with "addiction"
12. Medical decisions are restricted
    Category A: Restrictions based on patient characteristics
    Category B: Mandated consultation
    Category C: Restrictions regarding quantity prescribed or dispensed
    Category D: Undue prescription limitations
13. Length of prescription validity is restricted
14. Practitioners are subject to additional prescription requirements
15. Other provisions that may impede pain management
16. Provisions that are ambiguous
    Category A: Arbitrary standards for legitimate prescribing
    Category B: Unclear intent leading to possible misinterpretation
    Category C: Conflicting (or inconsistent) policies or provisions

from the ACS and the Susan G. Komen for the Cure, as well as through a cooperative agreement with the Lance Armstrong Foundation, provide the findings described in this section.

Policy Evaluation Findings

Policy language was identified that promotes appropriate pain management and can enhance patient access to effective pain care; such language is common in the policies from state regulatory agencies, rather than from legislative statutes. The frequency with which states' policies contained such language in 2008[136] is as follows:

■ Recognizes medical use of opioid as legitimate professional practice (in all states)
■ Recognizes pain management as part of general medical practice (in 46 states)

- Addresses practitioners' concerns about regulatory scrutiny (in 40 states)
- Encourages pain management (in 39 states)
- Distinguishes addiction from physical dependence or analgesic tolerance (in 37 states)
- Recognizes that medication amount or duration are insufficient to determine legitimacy of a prescription (in 34 states)

Policy language that appears less frequently than the above concepts, but that also promotes effective pain control and patient care, was identified and relates to three broad domains: (1) health care practice issues (e.g., recognizes inadequate pain treatment as substandard medical practice that is subject to professional disciplinary action, recognizes that the goals of pain treatment should include improvements in patient functioning and quality of life, and recognizes the need for a multidisciplinary approach to pain management); (2) patient characteristics (e.g., recognizes that a patient's prior history or current status of drug abuse does not necessarily contraindicate appropriate pain management, and exempts certain patient populations from undue prescription requirements); and (3) regulatory or policy issues (e.g., establishes a legal responsibility for health care facilities to ensure that pain management is an essential part of patient care, and specifically acknowledges that drug control policies should not interfere with legitimate medical use of controlled substances). A state's drug control policy is considered unbalanced when it lacks these positive messages, because it focuses disproportionately on the abuse potential of opioids while failing to recognize their medical benefit when used appropriately.

In addition, some state policies, which were adopted to prevent drug abuse and substandard prescribing practices, can create unnecessary additional requirements that unduly restrict health care decision making and establish excessive burdens on caregivers and patients. In 2008, a number of state policy provisions did not conform to and even conflicted with current standards of professional practice, including language that:

- confuses physical dependence with addiction, thus suggesting that pain patients being treated with opioids may be "addicts" (in 16 states)
- prohibits prescribing to patients with addictive disease or a history of substance abuse, even if they have pain (in 8 states)
- requires a specialist consultation for every patient who is prescribed Schedule II controlled substances (in 8 states)
- places arbitrary limits on the amount of pain medications that can be prescribed and dispensed at one time (in 8 states) (see Table 14.2 for specific restrictions for each state)
- restricts opioids from being used unless other treatments have failed (in 6 states)
- places overly restrictive limits on the amount of time (less than 2 weeks) that a Schedule II prescription is valid (in 4 states) (see Table 14.3 for specific restrictions for each state)

These evaluations also consider laws that create and implement Prescription Monitoring Programs (PMP), which are primary diversion control mechanisms in the U.S., specifically at the state level. Until relatively recently, PMPs were characterized by the use of MCPPs, which are multiple-copy government-issued serialized prescription forms (usually required in triplicate or duplicate). The prescription forms were required for Schedule II medications only (i.e., the only medications indicated for severe pain) and the programs were administered by state law enforcement, such as the state Department of Justice. Their purpose was to provide law enforcement and prescribers and dispensers with information on "doctor shoppers," "scammers," and dishonest physicians. Unfortunately, prescription information collected by the programs was not real-time and often took months or even years to compile, which severely undermined their ability to actively monitor diversion or abuse activity. MCPPs focused exclusively on Schedule II medications, and used unique forms that practitioners had to order only from the government to prescribe those medications. As a result, the programs tended to stigmatize both the medications and the practitioners who prescribed them.[50] Research demonstrated that this stigmatization often motivated practitioners to prescribe lower-scheduled medications to avoid being monitored[74,175-179]; this phenomenon is called the "substitution effect."[74] Of course, lower-scheduled medications are not indicated to relieve severe pain, so the substitution effect usually meant a potential for undertreatment. On the other hand, law enforcement has tended to interpret decreased prescribing of Schedule II medications as evidence that the program was effective in reducing diversion.[180-182]

MCPPs largely have been replaced by Electronic Data Transfer (EDT) programs that collect prescription information about more than Schedule II controlled substances (usually Schedules II, III, and IV).[183-185] Monitoring multiple schedules minimizes a potential substitution effect because there are few other medications with which they could be replaced. EDT programs tend to be administered by state health agencies, such as the Pharmacy Board, and the policies that implement the programs generally emphasize that this effort to reduce abuse and diversion are not meant to interfere with appropriate patient care. The information from these programs is collected in a more timely fashion, although it is usually not real-time. However, there is still no generally available evidence to demonstrate the programs' effects either on practitioner prescribing or on incidents of medication abuse and diversion.

As of this writing, more than 38 states have legislation creating a PMP that is an EDT system for a variety of medication schedules. Over half of these programs were created in the last 3 years, as a result of federal funding under the Harold Rogers Prescription Drug Monitoring Program,[186] as well as the prospect of funding under the National All-Schedules Prescription Electronic Reporting Act (NASPER).[187] Both programs were designed to provide grants to states to develop PMPs. However, NASPER funds are contingent on the programs being EDT and applying to medications in Schedules II–IV; states can create programs with different characteristics, but they are not fundable under NASPER. Federal law mandates that the Secretary of Health and Human Services evaluate the safety and efficacy of the programs established through NASPER. In this context, "safety" refers to the extent that the programs avoid creating barriers to prescribing to patients for legitimate medical purposes, such as for pain management. "Efficacy" means the ability of the program to validly identify instances

TABLE 14.3

STATES WITH LAWS RESTRICTING SCHEDULE II PRESCRIPTION VALIDITY PERIOD

Delaware	7 days
Hawaii	3 days
Illinois	7 days
Vermont	10 days

TABLE 14.2

STATES WITH LAWS RESTRICTING SCHEDULE II PRESCRIPTION QUANTITY OR DURATION

Delaware	100 dosage units or 31-day supply
Massachusetts	30-day supply
New Hampshire	100 dosage units or 31-day supply
New Jersey	120 dosage units or 30-day supply
New York	30-day supply
Rhode Island	250 dosage units or 30-day supply
South Carolina	120 dosage units or 30-day supply
Utah	One-month's supply

of abuse and diversion. Although there seems to be less chance for EDTs to restrict patient care, especially when compared to MCPPs, there has yet to be documentation available to the general public detailing either the safety or efficacy of these programs.

In addition to the discrete occurrences of policy language that can either enhance or impede the adequate treatment of pain with opioid analgesics, some state policies contain requirements or concepts that are contradictory and can create ambiguous practice expectations. For example, as identified previously, policies in 37 states correctly define addiction as a psychological/behavioral disorder that is not synonymous with either physical dependence or tolerance. Laws in 16 states also have an archaic and incorrect definition, which could legally classify patients being treated chronically with opioids, only because they are physically dependent, as "addicts." As a result, 13 states have at least one policy that correctly defines addiction and another that defines the concept incorrectly. There is no clear guidance for practitioners in these states about how patients with pain who are being treated with opioids should be viewed, given the inconsistencies among the legal, regulatory, and health care classification. Achieving balanced policy often depends on potentially discrepant practice standards being identified and made consistent.

A Progress Report Card to Measure Changes in the Quality of State Pain Policies

The criteria-based evaluation of state pain policy also serves as the basis for a methodology to quantify a state's policy based on its quality, which can then be used to compare all states and track policy changes over time.[188–191] Using policy data from the state profiles, each state now has been assigned a grade for 2000, 2003, 2006, 2007, and 2008. The grades, and the methodology used to calculate the grades, are contained in the most recent report, entitled "Achieving Balance in State Pain Policy: A Progress Report Card", and is available online at http://www.painpolicy.wisc.edu.

Grades range from A to F, using mid-point grades (e.g., B+, C+, D+) to characterize more precisely each state's overall combination of positive and negative provisions. A high grade means a state had many positives and few negatives. An A is achieved only when a state has a high number of positive provisions and no instances of restrictive or ambiguous language, while an F would result if a state had many negative provisions and no positive language. Higher grades are associated with state policies that are more balanced and consistent with modern medicine. A lower grade means that a state's policies contain potential barriers to patient pain relief (i.e., provisions that contradict current medical knowledge, are not consistent with the policy guidance recommendations from authoritative sources, and fail to communicate the appropriate messages about pain management to professionals, patients, and the public).

Progress Report Card Findings

Results show that the quality of pain policies varies greatly across states but has continued to improve over time. Between 2003 and 2006, 35 states made changes to their policies, but 19 states had policy change sufficient to produce improvement in their grade.[188] Of these 19 states, Rhode Island made the greatest improvement, increasing from a D+ to a B in this 3-year period; this state also was unique because all the improvement resulted from legislative policy change. The Rhode Island legislature added positive language to its IPTA, and repealed a number of unduly restrictive requirements from its IPTA and CSA.

Between 2006 and 2007, the first time policy change was evaluated over a single year, 23 states showed some degree of policy change and, in 8 of those states, the change was sufficient to improve their grade.[190] Kansas and Wisconsin achieved an A. California and Wisconsin demonstrated the greatest improvement: California increased from a C to a B, while Wisconsin increased from a B to an A. As with Rhode Island in 2006, California realized its grade change primarily by repealing restrictive or ambiguous language from its IPTA. Alternatively, Wisconsin's grade improved because its medical board adopted a positive pain management policy statement. By 2007, 12% of states scored around the average (a grade of C), while 86% scored above the average, and only 2% fell below the average; no state received a grade of D or F. Alternatively, Georgia remained the only state with the lowest grade (D+) and the least balanced policies.

Between 2007 and 2008, seven states changed their policies enough to improve their overall grade.[191] Oregon achieved the highest grade (A), and joined Kansas, Michigan, Virginia, and Wisconsin as having the most balanced policies in the country. An A means that there is prevalent language in statutes or regulatory policies, or both, that promote safe and effective pain management, as well as there being no language that can restrict medical decision making or patient access to appropriate pain care. The five states achieving an A comprise approximately 10% of the U.S. population. Alternatively, states with a B or B+ make up around 50% of the U.S. population (owing to the large populations of California, Florida, and Ohio), while almost 40% live in states that have a grade of C or C+ (owing primarily to Illinois, New Jersey, New York, Pennsylvania, and Texas). Georgia demonstrated the largest improvement, increasing from a D+ to a B. This was accomplished primarily through the medical board repealing its 1991 pain policy (the oldest existing medical board pain policy) with a guideline that repealed three existing negative provisions and contributed seven positive provisions. By 2008, 88% of states scored above the average grade of C in 2008, while no state scored a D+, D, or F (see Table 14.4). This finding is quite an improvement over those obtained in 2000, the first year that this policy evaluation was conducted, when only 49% of states received above a C.

No states' grade decreased over the entire 8-year evaluation timeframe; for the most part, states have avoided adopting new policies that could impede pain management and the medical use of controlled substances. In fact, in 2008 and for the first time since the policy evaluations began in 2000, state legislatures and regulatory agencies have completely avoided adopting policy language that could create barriers to chronic opioid treatment for pain relief.

The Importance of Improving State Pain Policy

The messages and requirements contained in state policies that govern health care practice, including opioid analgesic prescribing, can influence medical decision making and, ultimately, patient pain relief. Health care licensing boards that create and implement policies recognizing pain management as part of quality medical practice and patient care can counter the concern professionals have about regulatory investigation or sanction for prescribing pain medications. Patients and patient advocates also can use the presence of such policy to support appropriate pain treatment and to justify activities to improve pain management practices. Conversely, restrictive and ambiguous health care board policies can create a regulatory environment that hampers adequate patient pain relief. Achieving more balanced pain policy, as evidenced by higher state policy grades, is a necessary part of an overall multifaceted plan to improve pain and symptom management while stemming prescription medication abuse and diversion.[136,191,192]

The last decade was a time of notable improvement in the quality of many states' drug control and professional practice policies. Generally, the substantial policy change witnessed in

TABLE 14.4

STATES' PAIN POLICY GRADES FOR 2008

Alabama	B+	Kentucky	B	North Dakota	B
Alaska	C+	Louisiana	C	Ohio	B
Arizona	B+	Maine	B+	Oklahoma	C+
Arkansas	B	Maryland	B	Oregon	A
California	B	Massachusetts	B+	Pennsylvania	C+
Colorado	B	Michigan	A	Rhode Island	B+
Connecticut	B	Minnesota	B+	South Carolina	C+
Delaware	C+	Mississippi	C+	South Dakota	B
District of Columbia	C+	Missouri	C+	Tennessee	C
Florida	B	Montana	C+	Texas	C
Georgia	B	Nebraska	B+	Utah	B+
Hawaii	B	Nevada	C	Vermont	B+
Idaho	B	New Hampshire	B	Virginia	A
Illinois	C	New Jersey	C+	Washington	B+
Indiana	C+	New Mexico	B+	West Virginia	B
Iowa	B	New York	C	Wisconsin	A
Kansas	A	North Carolina	B	Wyoming	C+

recent years has contributed to an abundance of positive messages about effective pain management, including statements to reduce licensees' concern about regulatory scrutiny with prescribing opioid analgesics. Much of this improvement results from individual health care regulatory boards taking advantage of the Federation's Model Guideline or Model Policy. In addition, health care regulatory boards (e.g., medical, osteopathic, pharmacy, and nursing) in some states have worked together to adopt joint guidelines for pain management, palliative care, and end-of-life care.[78,136,174] Such policies tend to emphasize the value of a multi-disciplinary approach to treating pain, recognize that the goal of pain treatment should include improvements in patient functioning and quality of life, and assure that a broader variety of health care practitioners should not fear disciplinary action from their licensing board. The trend of state medical boards to adopt policies about pain management (e.g., regulations, guidelines, or policy statements), either separately or collaboratively, has resulted in an overall substantial improvement in the quality of state pain policies.[192]

Activities by health care professionals, pain, cancer, and end-of-life care initiatives, state agencies, and patient groups also have led to state pain policy changing for the better.[137,141,193] Many of these initiatives have as one of their goals to positively affect pain management practices of clinicians in their state by removing policy barriers that can restrict patients' access to adequate pain relief.[158,194,195] Improving pain, palliative care, and end-of-life care policy also has been part of the activities of national organizations such as the Alliance of State Pain Initiatives (ASPI),[196] the ACS,[48,197] the American Society of Law, Medicine & Ethics,[198] the IOM,[52] the National Association of State Controlled Substances Authorities,[199] the National Association of Attorneys General,[200] and the NIH.[53,146]

For most states to achieve greater balance and consistency in their pain policies, more effort must focus on removing long-outdated restrictive or ambiguous language from state law, some of which has been present for 30 years or more. Repeal from law of archaic restrictive language seems to have received less attention compared to the work of professional licensing boards to adopt positive policy. For example, between 2000 and 2008 there was only a 27% reduction in restrictive or ambiguous language, whereas there was a 75% increase in positive language during the same period.[191] Although states can enact laws or other governmental policies that are stricter than federal law, and must be allowed to vary in their approaches to public policy, the creation of undue restrictions is not obligatory in laws designed to control drug diversion or regulate professional practice. It is clear that professional and regulatory organizations recognize the necessity of attaining balanced policies governing pain management practices, including prescribing opioid analgesics. Support for balanced policy also was recently reiterated by national law enforcement; when the DEA issued its new regulation regarding the prescription series, it recognized the dual purpose of the new rule to maintain an adequate supply of medications to patients with legitimate medical needs while improving the potential to control their abuse and diversion.[131] Maintaining such an approach will ensure that patient care decisions requiring medical judgment are not overly limited by governmental laws solely aimed at preventing drug abuse and diversion.

THE NEED TO IMPLEMENT AND COMMUNICATE POLICY

Changing state policy, like addressing any other single factor, is not usually sufficient in and of itself to guarantee patient access to effective pain relief and symptom control, but it should be considered a necessary activity when trying to attain a positive professional practice and regulatory environment for treating pain. Policy improvement is not the final objective, but rather the critical first step. Regulatory policy will have the greatest potential to impact practice when coupled with a sustained commitment by the health care licensing board to communicate and properly implement it. To be most effective, new state regulatory policy must be disseminated widely and repeatedly to licensees and the public, and implemented consistently by the relevant board members, and regulatory administrators, investigators, and attorneys, or it will have little practical value and no effect on patient pain care.

Health care regulatory boards (i.e., medical, osteopathic, pharmacy, and nursing) increasingly are recognizing the importance of communicating newly adopted policy and have developed efforts to educate practitioners about the boards' expectations for proper pain management with controlled substances, and that health care professionals who responsibly treat pain should not fear their licensing agency. A number of state regulatory boards have created ways to widely disseminate and communicate their positive policy messages to practitioners, including California, Kansas, Maryland, Minnesota, North Carolina, Ohio, and West Virginia. Educational methods include video presentations that are mandatory viewing for all new licensees, sections on the boards' websites dedicated to pain management and policy issues, and adopting laws that require health care regulatory agencies to periodically educate their licensees about the appropriate use of controlled substances to treat pain. Such methods suggest that many boards are serious about confronting unrelieved pain and understand that communication is an essential component of policy change.

THE NEED TO CONTINUALLY AVOID POTENTIALLY RESTRICTIVE STATE POLICY

Despite there being sustained improvements since 2000 in state statutes and regulatory policies addressing pain management and the use of controlled substances,[136,191] a recent multidisciplinary Guideline from Washington[201] could create a precedent for states to adopt potentially restrictive treatment policy for chronic non-cancer pain; although clinical practice guidelines do not meet the inclusion criteria for the PPSG policy evaluation methodology, this practice guideline warrants further dialogue and examination about its possible impact on patient care. The "Interagency Guideline on Opioid Dosing for Chronic Non-cancer Pain" was created by the Interagency Workgroup on Practice Guidelines (IWPG) representing the Departments of Corrections, Health, Labor and Industry, Social and Health Services, and Health Care Authority, and is not meant to apply to the treatment of cancer pain or pain at the end of life. After emphasizing the association between the "dramatic increase" in medical consumption of morphine and other opioids and rises in accidental deaths associated with opioid use, the practice guideline contains a purpose statement, which is to assist:

> . . . the practitioner in prescribing opioids in a safe and effective manner when instituting opioids for chronic non-cancer pain; when transitioning opioid treatment from acute to chronic non-cancer pain; and when weaning opioid if an opioid trial fails to yield improvements in function and pain [and] . . . managing opioid treatment for patients who are already above 120 mg morphine equivalents (MED) total daily opioid doses.[201]

Many recommendations are then provided to assist physicians in treating patients with chronic noncancer pain, including routine monitoring of treatment outcomes and consulting with other health care practitioners when needed. However, the guideline states that rarely, and only with a pain management consultation, should the total daily dose of opioid exceed 120 mg oral morphine equivalents for chronic noncancer pain. Such a condition has been perceived by many to establish a limit on the amount of medication that can be prescribed by practitioners who do not specialize in pain management.[202–205] Concern about this recommendation becoming a treatment standard largely relates to there being no scientific data to support 120 mg/day MED as a ceiling dose or as having sufficient treatment efficacy for patients with severe chronic pain, and the difficulty in identifying a practitioner who specializes in pain medicine, the reimbursement of these services[202–205]; in fact, experts commonly recognize that few patients with chronic pain have access to a pain specialist, given the dearth of such professionals.[206]

In addition, the Washington Interagency Guideline contains specific recommendations that, while similar, are more stringent than those contained in the Federation's Model Policy. For example, practitioners are suggested to consider prescribing opioids for any patient:

- only after other treatments have failed
- when treatment goals include improvements in both functioning *and* pain scores
- after establishing numerous risk management procedures, such as using single a prescriber/pharmacy, a signed opioid treatment agreement, and random urine drug screens

Although such clinical approaches can and should be used at a physician's discretion, based on individual patient circumstance,

seeming to require them for every patient runs counter to the approach of the national medical regulatory agency.[138,139,207] As a result, physicians and other health care providers in Washington could perceive this as unduly restrictive policy, and that failure to conform to the policy expectations when treating pain patients with opioids will prompt greater regulatory or legal oversight.

Perhaps the most disquieting aspect of this guideline is that it is promoted as an effective response to the abuse and diversion of prescription pain medications. It implies that health care professionals and misprescribing are the primary sources of illicitly used opioids, despite there being a question whether this causal attribution exists. In fact, there are few systematic studies identifying the mechanisms contributing to opioid diversion (e.g., prescribing practices, employee pilferage, pharmacy thefts, home and medicine cabinet burglaries, and Internet sales), or the extent to which such sources are each part of the overall problem. Initiatives to safely and successfully address diversion are essential, but only to the extent that they do not have the potential to undermine clinical decision making and their ability to adequately treat patients with legitimate medical conditions.

Soon after the Interagency Guideline was introduced, media coverage characterized the policy launch under the heading "Washington State weighs limiting narcotic doses,"[206] believing that the guideline "recommends a total maximum daily dose of 120 mg of morphine or its equivalent." An interviewed pharmacist echoed this belief, stating objection to the dose limit set by the guidelines and considering it inadequate for the types of patients he treats.[206] For the first year of its existence, the opioid guideline is considered "educational" only, which allows for an official process of obtaining feedback from Washington state health care professionals before it can be implemented. A primary goal of this "educational" process is "seeing research that demonstrates the safety and effectiveness of dosage above 120 mg morphine equivalents per day."[208,209] During this time, the IWPG also plans to assess the "adequacy of specialty consultation."[209] Ostensibly, these measures were put into place to support the laudable goal of

> [making] sure any interventions to prevent problematic use don't adversely affect the vast majority who are appropriately using their medications.[208]

Hopefully, to accurately meet this stated objective, additional evidence will be presented and considered about whether guideline implementation, and the perception of its contents, creates barriers for health care practitioners who provide pain management services using opioids. For any new policy considered for adoption, there has to be attention to new requirements that are placed on practice, and whether they could be restrictive. This is a concern that always needs to be kept in mind when trying to maintain balance: That in a state's continued efforts to improve pain management and drug control through policy adoption, unintentional limitations, or ambiguities are not created. It would be regrettable if a practice guideline designed to protect patient safety and prevent harm to public health from prescription opioid diversion instead contributed to the public health problem of unrelieved pain and inadequate patient care. Although this policy is the first of its kind, other states already have expressed interest in using it as a template.

HOW HEALTH CARE REGULATORY BOARDS AND LAW ENFORCEMENT CAN AFFECT PRACTITIONERS' USE OF CONTROLLED SUBSTANCES

Health care professionals who prescribe, dispense, or administer controlled substances are subject to: (1) federal and state laws governing their use of controlled substances, and (2) state laws and regulatory policies governing their professional practice, including their use of medications. Federal and state laws prohibit the nonmedical use of controlled substances, set potential penalties and sanctions for violations and are enforced by local, state, or federal law enforcement. State licensing boards establish minimum expectations (or standards) for health care practice and the use of controlled substances to treat pain, and can discipline practitioners for unprofessional conduct. Given this reality, not only is it important for practitioners to understand the legal and regulatory framework for opioid treatment of chronic pain, but it remains essential to realize what attitudes and beliefs the regulatory and law enforcement communities hold about the appropriateness of pain management and the use of opioid analgesics. How do regulators and law enforcement view practitioners who use opioids to treat pain, especially when the treatment involves chronic prescribing or patients with an addictive disease?

Pain Management and Medical Regulators: An Evolving Acceptance of This Health Care Practice

Since 1991, the Federation and the PPSG have cosponsored a series of national surveys of board members to assess across time changes in their knowledge and attitudes about issues related to the use of controlled substances for pain treatment. The surveys were initiated to determine the extent that physicians' reported concerns about regulatory discipline for their prescribing practices were warranted.[170,210] Many respondents to the earliest survey doubted that extended opioid prescribing for patients with chronic pain was legal and medically acceptable, especially when the patient had a history of substance abuse.[211] Medical regulators also tended to view "addiction" as synonymous with "physical dependence" or "tolerance," which could lead to the perception that any patient being treated with opioids is addicted. A second survey, conducted in 1997, showed encouraging improvements in beliefs and knowledge, but deficits remained in many regulators' concepts of what constitutes accepted prescribing practice and addiction.[35] The third survey, from 2004, was conducted to determine whether state board members' views about prolonged opioid use for pain have continued to improve over time, especially given the frequent policy adoption promoting appropriate and effective pain management.[36]

The 2004 survey contained 45 items, excluding the demographic variables, but only results for the most relevant items are discussed here. A number of survey items related to various aspects of clinical practice:

- 57% did not know that federal law imposes no limits on the amount of Schedule II controlled substances that can be prescribed at one time
- 9% did not believe, and 21% did not know, that physicians can lawfully prescribe methadone for pain
- 46% believed addiction was common when opioids are used for an extended period for pain relief
- 41% considered prescription amounts greater than those recommended in the *Physician's Desk Reference* or Product Package Insert as excessive and possibly inappropriate
- 35% did not know that federal law considered the medical use of controlled substances to treat intractable pain as acceptable practice
- 28% would doubt that a prescription order for more than one opioid for a single patient was legitimate

Interestingly, 37% of regulators reported that they were not familiar with the Federation's Model Guidelines, despite the fact that their own national organization actively disseminated the policy and even updated it in 2004 (before this survey was conducted).

Board members in 2004 were statistically more likely than those from the previous two surveys to correctly characterize addiction as compulsive use despite harm, and did not view it solely as "physical dependence." In addition, when asked to judge the legality of prescribing opioids for more than several months for several clinical scenarios, respondents in 2004 were more likely to view this practice as both lawful and medically acceptable for patients with cancer or noncancer pain, and even when the patient had a history of substance abuse. However, not surprisingly, when the patient scenario included a history of substance abuse, a much lower percentage of respondents considered this practice to be legal and acceptable. Only 21% of board members viewed prolonged opioid prescribing to a patient with chronic noncancer pain and a history of drug abuse as lawful, but this result compares favorably to the 1% of medical regulators considering it lawful in 1991.

Such findings suggest that, while most medical board members recognize the need for adequate pain relief, and maintain beliefs that are consistent with currently accepted medical practice standards, some continue to possess knowledge deficits and attitudes that do not conform to the Federation's promulgated standards. These deficits can have potentially profound implications for clinical practices involving opioid use, especially creating an environment of uncertainty for practitioners faced with treating pain in a patient with a history of substance abuse or an addictive disease. Regulators who hold these misconceptions can adversely influence disciplinary determinations.

Pain Management and Law Enforcement: Distinguishing Criminal Conduct from Unprofessional Practice

As stated previously, state licensing boards regulate professional practice and medical boards oversee physician practice, including controlled substances prescribing, to determine whether there are violations of statutes and regulations.[192] The CSA's legislative history demonstrates health care professionals' overriding concern that the drug control law ultimately would give law enforcement inappropriate authority over medical and scientific decisions[112]; abundant professional testimony resulted in Congress establishing a procedure in which the federal health agency (now the Department of Health and Human Services) makes medical determinations under the CSA. This history makes it clear that the federal government is obligated to create criteria for drug control, including the legal parameters for prescribing controlled substances, and to investigate intentional criminal conduct (e.g., issuing prescriptions *not* for a legitimate medical purpose and in the usual course of professional practice), while state administrative agencies regulate health care practice. Consequently, the responsibility to investigate physicians' clinical decisions to prescribe opioids belongs to the medical board.

However, the perception of increased law enforcement activity may be undermining a medical regulatory climate characterized by positive board policy that has developed in recent years. The 2004 national survey of medical board members described in the previous section showed that 11% of respondents believed that federal, state, or local law enforcement agencies, including the DEA, are more likely than their own boards to investigate a physician's improper prescribing practices.[36] Another 35% of board members viewed law enforcement as more involved in federal and state investigations and prosecutions of physicians due to their opioid prescribing practices.[36] This and other evidence[212] calls into question whether more prominent law enforcement involvement is superseding the generally more balanced health care regulatory environment that exists today. The DEA continually asserts that less than 1% of registered physicians have been criminally prosecuted for prescribing controlled substances,[213–215] and such prosecutions are related to conduct that is clearly criminal in nature (e.g., selling prescriptions, exchanging drug for sex, etc.). Despite these assurances, reports of law enforcement's unwarranted intrusions into legitimate health care persist.[215] Media coverage focusing on allegations, convictions, and acquittals of clinicians for manslaughter and murder, in relation to opioid prescribing and dispensing, perpetuates fear of possible criminal sanction.[216,217]

Cases involving questionable prescribing must be evaluated to determine whether the relevant practice is intentional criminal conduct or substandard professional practice.[58,218,219] Such a distinction remains critical to assure proper jurisdiction: good faith professional practice, even if poor, should insulate a practitioner from criminal prosecution[220]; both state and federal case law supports this distinction.[221] If a practitioner's conduct is intentionally outside legitimate professional practice, law enforcement interventions from federal, state, or local agencies seem warranted.[118] That is, a prescription issued or dispensed other than in good faith (i.e., the practitioner knew or intended that the prescription would not be used for a legitimate medical purpose) could form the basis for criminal sanctions.[118,213] It is likely that potentially unwarranted criminal charges against practitioners will become less frequent when investigations clearly and consistently consider criminal behavior as distinct from unprofessional conduct. Such a course of action ultimately can reduce the perception that pain management with opioids is at the periphery of legitimate professional practice, rather than being an integral treatment option.

PRACTITIONERS CAN IMPROVE PAIN MANAGEMENT POLICY IN THEIR STATE

Since the late 1990s especially, there seems to have been an evolution in the pain management field about how restrictive policy is viewed, from being a "condition" that is unavoidable and intractable to a "problem" about which something can be done.[221] Achieving balanced state policies governing pain management, through repealing restrictive or ambiguous language particularly in statutes and regulations and by adopting positive legislative or administrative policies, requires a strategic approach. Collaborating with members of the legislature or administrative agencies often is necessary for successful change. Increasingly, health care professionals have assumed a leadership role in helping shape state policy that avoids restrictive policy language and promotes effective pain care for patients.

With the objective of balanced state pain policy, the initial step is to recognize the potential impact that policy can have on pain management practice by understanding the policies' content; the types of policies determined to be in need of improvement can often dictate the path to take. Attempting to change statutory law requires legislature engagement, while improving regulatory policy involves collaborating with the relevant health care administrative agency such as the medical, pharmacy, or nursing board. A practitioner can begin this partnership either independently or as a member of an advisory committee. Also termed a task force or pain commission, an advisory committee is a legislatively mandated ad hoc group typically created to scan the legislative, regulatory, and health care environment to set an agenda to identify and remedy the particular issues in a state that create barriers to adequate pain treatment, which traditionally have included the development of educational programs for health care practitioners. Such barriers to patients' pain relief can vary considerably from state to state. Effective advisory committees usually comprise a multidisciplinary team of professionals (both governmental and nongovernmental), including members from a variety of health care professions and specialties.

The goals of advisory committees recently have included efforts to repeal restrictive or ambiguous provisions and to adopt positive policy as a means to enhance pain treatment. A diverse committee composition often is beneficial when wanting to enlist support from legislators, regulators, or other advocates willing to sponsor amendments to law to create more balanced state pain policies. Advisory committees also can function to educate policy makers about how certain provisions in current statutes and regulations have the potential to adversely impact patient care, which can serve to reduce the frequency of restrictive or ambiguous policy provisions in the future. As a result, successful collaborations between committee members and legislators can influence the legislative agenda within a state to diminish or avoid establishing barriers to the management of chronic pain for people with cancer or noncancer conditions.

Advisory committees are not the only forum in which practitioners can develop an understanding of, and effectively advocate for, balanced pain policy. Stakeholders have access to a variety of PPSG policy-related resources, including the policy evaluation reports that detail the content and quality of all states' statutes, regulations, and health care policies and that offer example language that can be incorporated into current policy to strengthen its messages regarding safe and effective pain relief. Also, national organizations such as APF or ASPI, the individual Pain Initiatives that are active in most states, or other unique state-level initiatives, can be valued resources for guidance. Such initiatives can be contacted to advise about resource mobilization, or to help identify state-level efforts currently underway to improve pain policy and to suggest a state legislator or regulator who can sponsor requests for policy reform.

Either alone, in conjunction with a state pain initiative, or as a member of a legislatively created advisory committee, practitioners now more than ever before are playing a successful role in improving statutes and regulations to optimize the appropriate medical use of opioid analgesics to treat chronic pain. Regardless of the forum used, however, any effort at policy change must avoid inadvertently creating additionally restrictive policy. Historically, as with IPTAs, some laws created to improve patient access to controlled substances ultimately impede medication use because they contain undue limits or treatment ambiguities. State-level stakeholders, including health care professionals, recently have recognized the reality that laws can create barriers to treating pain and have sought to repeal such limiting requirements, but such efforts are time-intensive and the first approach is not always successful and may require further windows of opportunity for action. Of course, it is expected that there will be less need to repeal language that can impede pain management when current or future policy development precludes potential barriers.

CONCLUSION

Controlled substances remain essential to maintain the quality of life for many patients experiencing severe chronic pain from cancer or noncancer origins. To navigate successfully through an environment characterized by heightened professional and societal concern about diversion and abuse of prescription controlled substances, we must remain cautious not to minimize or ignore the important role of opioid analgesics as an effective therapeutic modality, or to stigmatize patients with a chronic illness or condition who benefit from the prolonged use of opioid medications. We also must avoid stigmatizing those health care professionals who appropriately prescribe, dispense, or administer opioids. It is possible to contemporaneously address the dual public health problems of undertreated pain and prescription medication abuse/diversion without sacrificing either.

Given recent progress to reduce barriers in state policy, the principle of balance will likely continue to provide a useful framework for improving state policies governing health care practice and controlled substances prescribing. Practitioners, as well as members of regulatory and law enforcement agencies, have been working at an unprecedented level in recent years to achieve more balanced state pain policy and to systematically implement such policy. The medicolegal concept of balance also can be used to conceptualize the appropriate roles and responsibilities of health care professionals, members of regulatory agencies, and law enforcement officials when considering cases of pain treatment or stemming the potential for drug diversion. A practitioner's medical responsibility is pain relief, but he or she also plays an essential role in monitoring for the abuse and diversion of the medications that are prescribed and for identifying possible comorbidities that would inform treatment considerations. Conversely, drug control is chiefly a responsibility of law enforcement, and such efforts must not interfere in medication availability, health care practice, or patient care. From this national and international principle, it is clear that the actions of members of health care, regulation, and law enforcement often overlap in the areas of medication availability for pain relief and efforts to minimize abuse and diversion. Likewise, U.S. drug laws and regulations have a dual purpose: to provide ample authority to address diversion problems without impeding the use of controlled substances in the medical care of patients.

Pain policy that does not contain archaic medical concepts and restrictive provisions, but does recognize pain management as a part of quality medical practice and attempts to address concern about unwarranted investigation for appropriate prescribing, coupled with training for practitioners about prescribing to relieve chronic severe pain, will realize the greatest benefit to public health. Practitioners also would benefit from guidance about treating patients with pain who have a history of substance abuse or other comorbid conditions that create a more complex clinical situation. Such sustained activities have the potential to contribute substantially to enhanced treatment of patients suffering from chronic pain conditions.

Since the early 1990s, the Federation periodically has sponsored educational workshops for medical regulators, and medical boards in all but four states have issued at least one policy concerning the treatment of pain. These policies have communicated positive messages to physicians about prescribing opioids for pain relief. To capitalize on state medical boards' momentum to promote the appropriate use of controlled substances for pain management, in 2007 the Federation sponsored preparation of a handbook entitled "Responsible Opioid Prescribing: A Physician's Guide."[207] The Handbook is conceptualized as a companion document to the Federation's Model Policy, and provides a description for practitioners about how they can effectively accomplish in their everyday clinical practice the recommendations made for each of the outlined seven treatment steps: (1) evaluation of the patient, (2) treatment plan, (3) informed consent and agreement for treatment, (4) periodic review, (5) consultation, (6) medical records, and (7) compliance with controlled substances laws and regulations. The Federation plans to make a copy of this handbook eventually available to all physicians licensed in each state. It is anticipated that the handbook will become a valuable educational tool to inform practitioners about addressing the clinical, regulatory, and policy issues inherent in treating chronic pain with opioids.

Availability of the policy information and policy change tools described in this chapter can facilitate further improvement in statutes and regulations across the U.S., and engender greater practitioner knowledge about the requirements and restrictions contained in the policies under which they practice. Increased practitioner understanding of their states' statutes, regulations, and other health care policies, and the extent to which health care regulators officially recognize the legitimacy of effective pain management using controlled substances, has a great potential to reduce concerns about scrutiny for such practice. Notable progress in the policy environment was made in the last 8 years, and will likely continue given the increased interest and resources in this area. More than ever before, we are poised to enter an era when state drug control laws and regulations and health care

regulatory board policies create few significant barriers to appropriate and effective prescribing of controlled substances for pain relief.

References

1. Sontag S. *Illness as Metaphor.* New York, NY: Farrar, Straus and Giroux; 1977:3.
2. Gottlieb S. Speech before the American Pain Foundation. Remarks by the Deputy Commissioner for Medical and Scientific Affairs, Food and Drug Administration to the U.S. House of Representatives Committee on Energy and Commerce, Subcommittee on Health; December 8, 2005; Washington, DC.
3. Goudas LC, Bloch R, Gialeli-Goudas M, et al. The epidemiology of cancer pain. *Cancer Invest* 2005;23:182–190.
4. Reid MC, Engles-Horton LL, Weber MB, et al. Use of opioid medications for chronic noncancer pain syndromes in primary care. *J Gen Intern Med* 2002;17:173–179.
5. American Pain Foundation. *Voices of Chronic Pain.* New York, NY: David Michaelson & Company, LLC; 2006.
6. Cabe J, Springer S. *National Call to Action on Cancer Prevention and Survivorship.* Tucson, AZ: Excel Print Communications; 2008.
7. Institute of Medicine National Cancer Policy Board. *Improving Palliative Care for Cancer.* Washington, DC: National Academy Press; 2001.
8. Stewart WF, Ricci JA, Chee E, et al. Lost productive time and cost due to common pain conditions in the US workforce. *JAMA* 2003;290:2443–2454.
9. National Institutes of Health. *The NIH Guide: New Directions in Pain Research I.* Washington, DC, Government Printing Office; 1998.
10. International Association for the Study of Pain and European Federation of IASP Chapters. *Unrelieved Pain is a Major Global Health Care Problem.* November 16, 2006. Available at: http://www.iasp-pain.org.
11. Brownson RC, Baker EA, Leet TL, et al. *Evidence-Based Public Health.* New York, NY: Oxford University Press; 2003.
12. Stjernswärd J, Foley KM, Ferris FD. The public health strategy for palliative care. *J Pain Symptom Manage* 2007;33:486–493.
13. Turnock BJ. *Public Health: What It Is and How It Works.* Boston, Mass: Jones and Bartlett Publishers; 2004.
14. Breitbart W, Passik S, McDonald MV, et al. Patient-related barriers to pain management in ambulatory AIDS patients. *Pain* 1998;76:9–16.
15. Drayer RA, Henderson J, Reidenberg M. Barriers to better pain control in hospitalized patients. *J Pain Symptom Manage* 1999;17:434–440.
16. McCracken LM, Hoskins J, Eccleston C. Concerns about medication and medication use in chronic pain. *J Pain* 2006;7:726–734.
17. Schieffer BM, Pham Q, Labus J, et al. Pain medication beliefs and medication misuse in chronic pain. *J Pain* 2005;6:620–629.
18. Tolle SW, Tilden VP, Rosenfeld AG, et al. Family reports of barriers to optimal care of the dying. *Nurs Res* 2000;49:310–317.
19. Ward SE, Goldberg N, Miller-McCauley V, et al. Patient-related barriers to management of cancer pain. *Pain* 1993;52:319–324.
20. Weiss SC, Emanuel LL, Fairclough DL, et al. Understanding the experience of pain in terminally ill patients. *Lancet* 2001;357:1311–1315.
21. Cleeland CS, Gonin R, Baez L, et al. Pain and treatment of pain in minority patients with cancer. The Eastern Cooperative Oncology Group Minority Outpatient Pain Study. *Ann Intern Med* 1997;127:813–816.
22. Green CR, Baker TA, Sato Y, et al. Race and chronic pain: A comparative study of young black and white Americans presenting for management. *J Pain* 2003;4:176–183.
23. Green CR, Baker TA, Smith EM, et al. The effect of race in older adults presenting for chronic pain management: A comparative study of black and white Americans. *J Pain* 2003;4:82–90.
24. Green CR. Racial disparities in access to pain treatment. *Pain Clinical Updates* 2004;12(6):1–4.
25. Green CR, Ndao-Brumblay SK, West B, et al. Differences in prescription opioid analgesic availability: comparing minority and white pharmacies across Michigan. *J Pain* 2005;6:689–699.
26. Lusher J, Elander J, Bevan D, et al. Analgesic addiction and pseudoaddiction in painful chronic illness. *Clin J Pain* 2006;22:316–324.
27. Michna E, Ross EL, Hynes WL, et al. Predicting aberrant drug behavior in patients treated for chronic pain: Importance of abuse history. *J Pain Symptom Manage* 2004;28:250–258.
28. Morrison RS, Wallenstein S, Natale DK, et al. "We don't carry that"—Failure of pharmacies in predominantly nonwhite neighborhoods to stock opioid analgesics. *N Engl J Med* 2000;342:1023–1026.
29. Nicholson B, Passik SD. Management of chronic noncancer pain in the primary care setting. *South Med J* 2007;100:1028–1036.
30. Passik SD, Kirsh KL, McDonald MV, et al. A pilot survey of aberrant drug-taking attitudes and behaviors in samples of cancer and AIDS patients. *J Pain Symptom Manage* 2000;19:274–286.
31. Passik SD, Kirsh KL, Donaghy KB, et al. Pain and aberrant drug-related behaviors in medically ill patients with and without histories of substance abuse. *Clin J Pain* 2006;22:173–181.
32. Bonica JJ. Treatment of cancer pain: current status and future needs. In: Fields HL, Dubner R, Cerveo S, eds. *Advances in Pain Research and Therapy.* Vol 9. New York, NY: Raven Press; 1995:589–616.

33. Dobscha SK, Corson K, Flores JA, et al. Veterans Affairs primary care clinicians' attitudes toward chronic pain and correlates of opioid prescribing rates. *Pain Med* 2008;9:564–571.

34. Furstenberg CT, Ahles TA, Whedon MB, et al. Knowledge and attitudes of health-care providers toward cancer pain management: a comparison of physicians, nurses, and pharmacists in the State of New Hampshire. *J Pain Symptom Manage* 1998;15:335–349.

35. Gilson AM, Joranson DE. Controlled substances and pain management: Changes in knowledge and attitudes of state medical regulators. *J Pain Symptom Manage* 2001;21:227–237.

36. Gilson AM, Maurer MA, Joranson DE. State medical board members' beliefs about pain, addiction, and diversion and abuse: A changing regulatory environment. *J Pain* 2007;8:682–691.

37. Hollen CJ, Hollen CW, Stolte K. Hospice and hospital oncology unit nurses: a comparative survey of knowledge and attitudes about cancer pain. *Oncol Nurs Forum* 2000;27:1593–1599.

38. Jacobsen R, Sjøgren P, Møldrup C, et al. Physician-related barriers to cancer pain management with opioid analgesics: a systematic review. *J Opioid Manag* 2007;3:207–214.

39. Joranson DE, Gilson AM. Pharmacists' knowledge of and attitudes toward opioid pain medications in relation to federal and state policies. *J Am Pharm Assoc (Wash)* 2001;41:213–220.

40. Lin JJ, Alfandre D, Moore C. Physician attitudes toward opioid prescribing for patients with persistent noncancer pain. *Clin J Pain* 2007;23:799–803.

41. McMillan SC, Tittle M, Hagan S, et al. Knowledge and attitudes of nurses in veterans hospitals about pain management in patients with cancer. *Oncol Nurs Forum* 2000;27:1415–1423.

42. Passik SD, Byers K, Kirsh KL. Empathy and the failure to treat pain. *Palliat Support Care* 2007;5:167–172.

43. Portenoy RK, Sibirceva U, Smout R, et al. Opioid use and survival at the end of life: a survey of a hospice population. *J Pain Symptom Manage* 2006;32:532–540.

44. Roth CS, Burgess DJ, Mahowald ML. Medical residents' beliefs and concerns about using opioids to treat chronic cancer and noncancer pain: a pilot study. *J Rehabil Res Dev* 2007;44:263–270.

45. Von Roenn JH, Cleeland CS, Gonin R, et al. Physician attitudes and practice in cancer pain management: A survey from the Eastern Cooperative Oncology Group. *Ann Intern Med* 1993;119:121–126.

46. Jacox A, Carr DB, Payne R, et al. *Management of Cancer Pain. Clinical Practice Guideline Number 9*. Rockville, Md: Agency for Health Care Policy and Research, US Dept of Health and Human Services, Public Health Service; 1994. AHCPR publication 94–0592.

47. Advisory Group on Cancer Pain Relief. *American Cancer Society Advisory Group on Cancer Pain Relief: Agenda, Patient Services*. Atlanta, Ga: American Cancer Society; 1994.

48. Cancer Pain Management Policy Review Group. *American Cancer Society Policy Statement on Cancer Pain Management*. National Government Relations Department, American Cancer Society; 2001.

49. Cancer Pain Management Policy Review Group. *American Cancer Society Position Statement on Medicaid Prior Authorization for Pain Medications*. National Government Relations Department, American Cancer Society; 2001.

50. Cancer Pain Management Policy Review Group. *American Cancer Society Position Statement on Prescription Monitoring and Drug Utilization Review Programs*. National Government Relations Department, American Cancer Society; 2001.

51. Cancer Pain Management Policy Review Group. *American Cancer Society Position Statement on Regulatory Barriers to Quality Cancer Pain Management*. National Government Relations Department, American Cancer Society; 2001.

52. Field MJ, Cassel CK, eds. Institute of Medicine Committee on Care at the End of Life. *Approaching Death: Improving Care at the End of Life*. Washington, DC: National Academy Press; 1997.

53. National Institutes of Health Consensus Development Program. Symptom management in cancer: Pain, depression and fatigue. Statement prepared following a National Institutes of Health State-of-the-Science Conference on Symptom Management in Cancer; July 15–17, 2002; Bethesda, Md.

54. World Health Assembly. *Cancer Prevention and Control. WHA 58.22*. Geneva, Switzerland: World Health Organization; 2005.

55. World Health Organization. *WHO Policy Perspectives on Medicines. Equitable Access to Essential Medicines: A Framework for Collective Action*. Geneva, Switzerland: World Health Organization; 2004.

56. Stitzman BT. Guiding principles for the pain medicine physician—in a not so ideal world. *Pain Med* 2007;8:293–294.

57. Bolen J. Taking back your turf: Understanding the role of law in medical decision making in opioid management (Part I—overview). *J Opioid Manag* 2005;1:125–130.

58. Bolen J. Enough about barriers and fear already—the pain community needs to be proactive and take steps to stop the "roulette wheel." *Pain Med* 2007;8:438–440.

59. United Nations. *Single Convention on Narcotic Drugs, 1961, as Amended by the 1972 Protocol Amending the Single Convention on Narcotic Drugs, 1961*. New York, NY: United Nations; 1977.

60. Jaffe JH, Martin WR. Opioid analgesics and antagonists. In: Gilman AG, Rall TW, Nies AS, Taylor P, eds. *Goodman and Gilman's The Pharmacological Basis of Therapeutics*. 8th ed. New York, NY: Pergamon Press; 1990: 485–521.

61. International Narcotics Control Board. *Report of the International Narcotics Control Board for 2005*. New York, NY: United Nations; 2006.

62. International Narcotics Control Board. *Report of the International Narcotics Control Board for 1989: Demand for and Supply of Opiates for Medical and Scientific Needs*. Vienna, Austria: United Nations; 1989.

63. International Narcotics Control Board. *Report of the International Narcotics Control Board for 2002*. New York, NY: United Nations; 2003.

64. International Narcotics Control Board. *Report of the International Narcotics Control Board for 2006*. New York, NY: United Nations; 2007.

65. International Narcotics Control Board. *Report of the International Narcotics Control Board for 1995: Availability of Opiates for Medical Needs*. New York, NY: United Nations; 1996.

66. World Health Organization. Guiding principles for small national drug regulatory authorities. *World Health Organization Drug Info* 1989;3:43–50.

67. World Health Organization. *Cancer Pain Relief: With a Guide to Opioid Availability*. 2nd ed. Geneva, Switzerland: World Health Organization; 1996.

68. Forbes K. Opioids: Beliefs and myths. *J Pain Palliat Care Pharmacother* 2006; 20:33–35.

69. Council of Europe. Recommendation (2003) 24 of the Committee of Ministers to member states on the organisation of palliative care. Adopted by the Committee of Ministers at the 860th meeting of the Ministers' Deputies; November 12, 2003. Available at: http://www.coe.int/DefaultEN.asp.

70. World Health Organization HIV-AIDS. *Palliative Care*. Geneva, Switzerland: World Health Organization; 2004.

71. International Narcotics Control Board. *Report of the International Narcotics Control Board for 2004*. New York, NY: United Nations; 2005.

72. United Nations Economic and Social Council. *Demand for and Supply of Opiates Used to Meet Medical and Scientific Needs*. Report on the forty-eighth session of the Commission on Narcotic Drugs E/2005/28; 19 March 2004 and 7–11 March 2005; July 22, 2005. Resolution 2005–26.

73. Fishman SM, Papazian JS, Gonzalez S, Riches PS, Gilson AM. Regulating opioid prescribing through prescription monitoring programs: balancing drug diversion and treatment of pain. *Pain Med* 2004;5:309–324.

74. Wastila LJ, Bishop C. The influence of multiple copy prescription programs on analgesic utilization. *J Pharm Care Pain Symptom Control* 1996;4:3–19.

75. World Health Organization. *Cancer Pain Relief and Palliative Care: Report of the WHO Expert Committee on Cancer Pain Relief and Active Supportive Care (technical report series 804)*. Geneva, Switzerland: World Health Organization; 1990:39.

76. Beubler E, Eisenberg E, Castro-Lopes J, et al. Prescribing policies of opioids for chronic pain. *J Pain Palliat Care Pharmacother* 2007;21:53–55.

77. Blengini C, Joranson DE, Ryan KM. Italy reforms national policy for cancer pain relief and opioids. *Eur J Cancer Care (Engl)* 2003;12:28–34.

78. Pain & Policy Studies Group. *Achieving Balance in Federal and State Pain Policy: A Guide to Evaluation*. 4th ed. Madison, Wis: University of Wisconsin Paul P. Carbone Comprehensive Cancer Center; 2007.

79. Mosoiu D, Ryan KM, Joranson DE, et al. Reforming drug control policy for palliative care in Romania. *Lancet* 2006;367:2110–2117.

80. Green K, Kinh LN, Khue LN. *Palliative care in Viet Nam: Findings From a Rapid Situation Analysis in Five Provinces*. Hanoi, Vietnam: Ministry of Health; 2006.

81. World Health Assembly. *Ensuring Accessibility to Essential Medicines WHA 55.14*. Geneva, Switzerland: World Health Organization; 2002.

82. World Health Assembly. *Cancer Prevention and Control. Resolution EB114.R2*. Geneva, Switzerland: World Health Organization; 2004.

83. Federal Food Drug and Cosmetic Act, Title 21 USCS §393.

84. Federal Food Drug and Cosmetic Act, Title 21 USCS §355.

85. Federal Food Drug and Cosmetic Act, Title 21 USCS §355-1(e)(3).

86. Federal Food Drug and Cosmetic Act, Title 21 USCS §355(k)(3).

87. Federal Register, 48 FR 26733 (1983).

88. United States General Accounting Office. *Prescription Drugs: Implications of Drug Labeling and Off-label Use*. Washington, DC: United States General Accounting Office, GAO/T-HEHS-96-212; 1996.

89. Federal Register, 37 FR 16503 (1972):16503.

90. Food and Drug Administration. *FDA Consumer*. Rockville, Md: US Food and Drug Administration; 1975:7.

91. Thomson Health care. *Physicians' Desk Reference*. 58th ed. Montvale, NJ: Thomson PDR; 2004.

92. Federal Register, 40 FR 15394 (1975).

93. *United States v Evers*, 643 F2d 1043 5th Circuit (1981).

94. Federal Food Drug and Cosmetic Act, Title 21 USCS §396.

95. Controlled Substances Act. Pub L No. 91-513, 84 Stat 1242 (1970).

96. United States House of Representatives. *Comprehensive Drug Abuse Prevention and Control Act of 1970*. House Report No 91-1444 (September 10, 1970).

97. Controlled Substances Act, Title 21 USCS §812(c).

98. Controlled Substances Act, Title 21 USCS §823(e).

99. Controlled Substances Act, Title 21 USCS §823(f).

100. Code of Federal Regulations, Title 21 CFR §1306.04(a).

101. Controlled Substances Act, Title 21 USCS §826(a).

102. *United States v Moore*, 96 S. Ct. 335, 423 U.S. 122, 1975:139.

103. Code of Federal Regulations, Title 21 CFR §1305.03.

104. Controlled Substances Act, Title 21 USCS §828(a).

105. Code of Federal Regulations, Title 21 CFR §1306.12.

106. Controlled Substances Act, Title 21 USCS §829(a).

107. Code of Federal Regulations, Title 21 CFR §1306.22.

108. Controlled Substances Act, Title 21 USCS §829(b).
109. Code of Federal Regulations, Title 21 CFR §1306.11(d).
110. Code of Federal Regulations, Title 21 CFR §1306.13.
111. Controlled Substances Act, Title 21 USCS §801(1).
112. United States of America Congressional Record. *Proceedings and Debates of the 91st Congress Second Session.* Vol 116 - part 25. Washington, DC: United States Government Printing Office; 1970.
113. Controlled Substances Act, Title 21 USCS §826(c).
114. Federal Register, 53 FR 50593 (1988):50593–50594.
115. Federal Register, 59 FR 52991 (1994).
116. Federal Register, 72 FR 24608 (2007).
117. Annas GJ. Congress, controlled substances, and physician-assisted suicide: Elephants in mouseholes. *N Engl J Med* 2006;354:1079–1084.
118. Brushwood DB. Defining "legitimate medical purpose." *Amer J Health Syst Pharm* 2005;62:306–308.
119. United Nations. *Convention on Psychotropic Substances, 1971.* Geneva, Switzerland: United Nations; 1971.
120. Controlled Substances Act, Title 21 USCS §801a(3).
121. Controlled Substances Act, Title 21 USCS §823(g).
122. Controlled Substances Act, Title 21 USCS §802(1).
123. World Health Organization. *The ICD-10 Classification of Mental and Behavioral Disorders: Clinical Descriptions and Diagnostic Guidelines.* Geneva, Switzerland: World Health Organization; 1992.
124. American Psychiatric Association. *Diagnostic and Statistical Manual of Mental Disorders.* 4th ed. Washington, DC: American Psychiatric Association; 1994.
125. American Academy of Pain Medicine, American Pain Society, American Society of Addiction Medicine. *Definitions related to the use of opioids for the treatment of pain.* Glenview, Ill: AAPM, APS, ASAM; 2001.
126. Public Health and Welfare, Title 42 USC §201.
127. World Health Organization. *WHO Expert Committee on Drug Dependence: Thirtieth Report.* Geneva, Switzerland: World Health Organization; 1998.
128. Federal Register, 58 FR 37507 (1993).
129. Code of Federal Regulations, Title 21 CFR §1306.07(c).
130. Von Korff M, Miglioretti DL. A prognostic approach to defining chronic pain. *Pain* 2005;117:304–313.
131. Drug Enforcement Administration. *Issuance of Multiple Prescriptions for Schedule II Controlled Substances.* Arlington, Va: Drug Enforcement Administration. November 19, 2007:64921–64930. Docket No. DEA-287F.
132. Drug Enforcement Administration. *Issuance of Multiple Prescriptions for Schedule II Controlled Substances.* Arlington, Va: Drug Enforcement Administration. September 6, 2006:52715–52723. Docket No. DEA-286P.
133. Gilson AM, Joranson DE. The federal Drug Enforcement Administration "prescription series" proposal: continuing concerns. *J Pain Palliat Care Pharmacother* 2007;21:21–24.
134. Gilson AM, Joranson DE. Is the DEA's new "prescription series" regulation balanced? *J Pain Palliat Care Pharmacother* 2008;22(3):218–20.
135. Heit H. Health care professionals and the DEA: restoring the balance. *J Opioid Manag* 2006;2:310–311.
136. Pain & Policy Studies Group. *Achieving Balance in Federal and State Pain Policy: A Guide to Evaluation.* 5th ed. Madison, Wis: University of Wisconsin Paul P. Carbone Comprehensive Cancer Center; 2008.
137. Gilson AM, Maurer MA, Joranson DE. State policy affecting pain management: Recent improvements and the positive impact of regulatory health policies. *Health Policy* 2005;74:192–204.
138. Federation of State Medical Boards of the United States Inc. *Model Guidelines for the Use of Controlled Substances for the Treatment of Pain.* Euless, TX: Federation of State Medical Boards of the United States Inc; 1998.
139. Federation of State Medical Boards of the United States Inc. *Model Policy for the Use of Controlled Substances for the Treatment of Pain.* Dallas, TX: Federation of State Medical Boards of the United States Inc; 2004.
140. Fujimoto D. Regulatory issues in pain management. *Clin Geriatr Med* 2001; 17:537–551.
141. Gilson AM, Joranson DE, Maurer MA, et al. Progress to achieve balanced state policy relevant to pain management and palliative care: 2000–2003. *J Pain Palliat Care Pharmacother* 2005;19:13–26.
142. Merritt D, Fox-Grage W, Rothouse M, et al. *State Initiatives in End-of-life Care: Policy Guide for State Legislators.* Washington, DC: National Conference of States Legislatures; 1998.
143. Miaskowski C, Cleary J, Burney R, et al. *Guideline for the Management of Cancer Pain in Adults and Children. APS Clinical Practice Guidelines Series, No. 3.* Glenview, IL: American Pain Society; 2005.
144. National Conference of Commissioners on Uniform State Laws. *Uniform Controlled Substances Act.* Adopted at its Annual Conference Meeting in its Ninety-Ninth Year; July 13–20, 1990; Milwaukee, WI.
145. National Conference of Commissioners on Uniform State Laws. *Uniform Controlled Substances Act.* Adopted at its Annual Conference Meeting in its One-Hundred-and-Third-Year; July 29–August 5, 1994; Chicago, IL.
146. National Institutes of Health. State-of-the-Science Conference Statement: Improving End-of-Life Care. Draft statement prepared following a National Institutes of Health State-of-the-Science Conference on Improving End-of-Life Care; December 6–8, 2004; Bethesda, MD.
147. Rich BA. An ethical analysis of the barriers to effective pain management. *Camb Q Healthc Ethics* 2000;9:54–70.
148. Tucker KL. A new risk emerges: Provider accountability for inadequate treatment of pain. *Ann Long-Term Care* 2001;9:52–56.
149. World Health Organization. *Cancer Pain Relief and Palliative Care in Children.* Geneva, Switzerland: World Health Organization; 1998.
150. World Health Organization. *Achieving Balance in National Opioids Control Policy: Guidelines for Assessment.* Geneva, Switzerland: World Health Organization; 2000.
151. National Conference of Commissioners on Uniform State Laws. *Uniform Controlled Substances Act.* St. Louis, MO: NCCUSL; 1970.
152. American Alliance of Cancer Pain Initiatives. *Statement on Intractable Pain Treatment Acts (IPTA).* Madison, WI: AACPI; 2004.
153. Joranson DE. Intractable pain treatment laws and regulations. *Am Pain Soc Bull* 1995;5:1–3, 15–17.
154. Joranson DE, Gilson AM. State intractable pain policy: Current status. *Am Pain Soc Bull* 1997;7:7–9.
155. Gilson AM, Joranson DE. U.S. policies relevant to the prescribing of opioid analgesics for the treatment of pain in patients with addictive disease. *Clin J Pain* 2002;18:S91–S98.
156. Clark HW. Policy and medical-legal issues in the prescribing of controlled substances. *J Psychoactive Drugs* 1991;23:321–328.
157. Dahl JL, Joranson DE, Weissman DE. The Wisconsin cancer pain initiative: a progress report. *Am J Hospice Care* 1989;6:39–43.
158. New York State Public Health Council. *Breaking Down the Barriers to Effective Pain Management: Recommendations to Improve the Assessment and Treatment of Pain in New York State.* Albany, NY: New York State Department of Health; 1998.
159. Weissman DE, Joranson DE, Hopwood MB. Wisconsin physicians' knowledge and attitudes about opioid analgesic regulations. *Wis Med J* 1991; 671–675.
160. Johnson SH. Disciplinary actions and pain relief: Analysis of the Pain Relief Act. *J Law Med Ethics* 1996;24:319–327.
161. Martino AM. In search of a new ethic for treating patients with chronic pain: What can medical boards do? *J Law Med Ethics* 1998;26:332–349.
162. Hoffmann DE, Tarzian AJ. Achieving the right balance in oversight of physician opioid prescribing for pain: The role of state medical boards. *J Law Med Ethics* 2003;31:21–40.
163. Richard J, Reidenberg M. The risk of disciplinary action by state medical boards against physicians prescribing opioids. *J Pain Symptom Manage* 2005; 29:206–212.
164. Nowels D, Lee JT. Cancer pain management in home hospice settings: a comparison of primary care and oncologic physicians. *J Palliat Care* 1999; 15:5–9.
165. Weinstein SM, Laux LF, Thornby JI, et al. Physicians' attitudes toward pain and the use of opioid analgesics: results of a survey from the Texas Cancer Pain Initiative. *South Med J* 2000;93:479–487.
166. Zimbal M, Cleary J, Gilson AM, et al. Wisconsin physicians' beliefs and attitudes about the use of opioid analgesics. *J Pain* 2007;7(suppl 2):597.
167. Grahmann PH, Jackson KC 2nd, Lipman AG. Clinician beliefs about opioid use and barriers in chronic nonmalignant pain. *J Palliat Care Pharmacother* 2004;18:7–28.
168. Turk DC, Brody MC. What position do APS's physician members take on chronic opioid therapy? *Am Pain Soc Bull* 1992;2:1–5.
169. Hickman SE, Tolle SW, Tilden VP. Physicians' and nurses' perspectives on increased family reports of pain in dying hospitalized patients. *J Palliat Med* 2000;3:413–418.
170. Joranson DE, Gilson AM, Dahl JL, et al. Pain management, controlled substances, and state medical board policy: a decade of change. *J Pain Symptom Manage* 2002;23:138–147.
171. Tucker KL. Treatment of pain in dying patients. *N Engl J Med* 1998;338: 1231.
172. Joranson DE, Gilson AM, Ryan KM, et al. *Achieving Balance in Federal and State Pain Policy: A Guide to Evaluation.* University of Wisconsin Comprehensive Cancer Center, Madison, Wis: Pain & Policy Studies Group; 2000.
173. Pain & Policy Studies Group. *Achieving Balance in Federal and State Pain Policy: A Guide to Evaluation.* 2nd ed. Madison, WI: University of Wisconsin Comprehensive Cancer Center, 2003.
174. Pain & Policy Studies Group. *Achieving Balance in Federal and State Pain Policy: A Guide to Evaluation.* 3rd ed. Madison, WI: University of Wisconsin Paul P. Carbone Comprehensive Cancer Center; 2006.
175. Ross-Degnan D, Simoni-Wastila L, Brown JS, et al. A controlled study of the effects of state surveillance on indicators of problematic and non-problematic benzodiazepine use in a Medicaid population. *Int J Psychiatry Med* 2004;34: 103–123.
176. Simoni-Wastila L, Tompkins C. Balancing diversion control and medical necessity: The case of prescription drugs with abuse potential. *Subst Use Misuse* 2001;36:1275–1296.
177. Simoni-Wastila L, Ross-Degnan D, Mah C, et al. A retrospective data analysis of the impact of the New York triplicate prescription program on benzodiazepine use in Medicaid patients with chronic psychiatric and neurologic disorders. *Clin Ther* 2004;26:322–336.
178. Wagner AK, Soumerai SB, Zhang F, et al. Effects of state surveillance on new post-hospitalization benzodiazepine use. *Int J Qual Health Care* 2003;15: 423–431.
179. Wastila LJ, Bishop C. The influence of multiple copy prescription programs (MCPPs) on analgesic utilization. *J Pharm Care Pain Symp Contr* 1996;4(3): 3–19.
180. United States General Accounting Office. *Prescription Drug Monitoring: States Can Readily Identify Illegal Sales and Use of Controlled Substances.*

Washington, DC: United States General Accounting Office; 1992. GAO/HRD-92-115.

181. United States General Accounting Office. *Prescription Drugs: State Monitoring Programs Provide Useful Tool to Reduce Diversion.* Washington, DC: United States General Accounting Office; 2002. GAO-02-634.

182. American Society of Addiction Medicine. Pain and addiction medicine. 2003. Available at: http://www.asam. org/pain/pain_and_addiction_medicine.htm.

183. American Alliance of Cancer Pain Initiatives. *Statement on State Prescription Monitoring Programs.* Madison, WI: AACPI; 2002.

184. Brushwood DB. Maximizing the value of electronic prescription monitoring programs. *J Law Med Ethics* 2003;31:41–54.

185. Joranson DE, Carrow GM, Ryan KM, et al. Pain management and prescription monitoring. *J Pain Symptom Manage* 2002;23:231–238.

186. Alliance of States with Prescription Monitoring Programs. BJA announces 2009 PDMP grant solicitation. *The Alliance Monitor* 2009;1(1):1.

187. Public Health and Welfare, Title 42 USC §280g-3 (2005).

188. Pain & Policy Studies Group. *Achieving Balance in State Pain Policy: A Progress Report Card.* University of Wisconsin Comprehensive Cancer Center, Madison, WI; 2003.

189. Pain & Policy Studies Group. *Achieving Balance in State Pain Policy: A Progress Report Card.* 2nd ed. Madison, WI: University of Wisconsin Comprehensive Cancer Center; 2006.

190. Pain & Policy Studies Group. *Achieving Balance in State Pain Policy: A Progress Report Card.* 3rd ed. Madison, WI: University of Wisconsin Paul P. Carbone Comprehensive Cancer Center; 2007.

191. Pain & Policy Studies Group. *Achieving Balance in State Pain Policy: A Progress Report Card.* 4th ed. Madison, WI: University of Wisconsin Paul P. Carbone Comprehensive Cancer Center; 2008.

192. Gilson AM, Joranson DE, Maurer MA. Improving state pain policies: Recent progress and continuing opportunities. *CA Cancer J Clin* 2007;57:341–353.

193. Gilson AM, Joranson DE, Maurer MA. Improving state medical board policies: Influence of a model. *J Law Med Ethics* 2003;31:119–129.

194. Maryland State Advisory Council on Pain Management. *Final Report to the General Assembly.* Annapolis: Maryland State Advisory Council on Pain Management; 2004.

195. Michigan Department of Consumer & Industry Services. *Pain and Symptom Management Advisory Committee Report.* Lansing, MI: Michigan Department of Consumer and Industry Services; 2002.

196. Dahl JL, Bennett ME, Bromley MD, et al. Success of the State Pain Initiatives. *Cancer Pract* 2002;10:S9–S13.

197. Connecticut Cancer Pain Initiative, American Cancer Society New England Division. *Connecticut Pain Summit: Promoting Proper Use of Opioid Analgesics, Report and Recommendations.* Meriden, CT: American Cancer Society New England Division; 2003.

198. Johnson SH. Providing relief to those in pain: a retrospective on the scholarship and impact of the Mayday project. *J Law Med Ethics* 2003;31:15–20.

199. National Association of State Controlled Substances Authorities. NASCSA Resolution 99-01. *A resolution endorsing the model guidelines for the use of controlled substances for the treatment of pain.* Adopted at the NASCSA 15th Annual Educational Conference; October 29, 1999; Coeur d'Alene, Idaho.

200. National Association of Attorneys General. *Resolution calling for a balanced approach to promoting pain relief and preventing abuse of pain medications.* Adopted at the National Association of Attorneys General Spring Meeting; March 17–20, 2003; Washington, DC.

201. Agency Medical Director's Group. *Interagency guideline on opioid dosing for chronic non-cancer pain.* October 12, 2006. Available at: http://www.agencymeddirectors.wa.gov/Files/OpioidGdline.pdf.

202. American Pain Foundation. *APF position statement on Washington State Interagency Guideline on Opioid Dosing for Chronic Non-Cancer Pain: An educational pilot to improve care and safety with opioid treatment.* May 2007. Available at: http://www.painfoundation.org/PositionStatements/WAOpioidGuideline2007.pdf.

203. American Pain Society. *The Washington State Agency Medical Directors Group (AMDG) published guidelines on opioid dosing for chronic non-cancer pain.* July 19, 2007. Available at: http://www.doctordeluca.com/Library/WOD/WSG/APStoAMDGreWaGuidelines07.pdf.

204. Oregon Pain Management Commission. Oregon Pain Management Commission position on the Washington state Interagency Guideline on opioid dosing for chronic non-cancer pain. 2007.

205. Peppin J. Washington state develops guideline for opioid dosing of chronic noncancer pain. *Pain Medicine Network* 2008;23:3.

206. Brody JE. Many treatments can ease chronic pain. *New York Times.* November 22, 2007.

207. Fishman SM. *Responsible Opioid Prescribing: A Physician's Guide.* Washington, DC: Waterford Life Sciences; 2007.

208. Magill-Lewis J. Washington State weighs limiting narcotic doses. *Drug Topics.* January 8, 2007.

209. Agency Medical Director's Group. *Washington State's draft guidelines for opioids for chronic non-cancer pain: Frequently asked questions.* October 4, 2006. Available at: www.lni.wa.gov/news/files/2006-10-04%20FAQ_v8.pdf.

210. Joranson DE, Gilson AM. Improving pain management through policy making and education for medical regulators. *J Law Med Ethics* 1996;24:344–347.

211. Joranson DE, Cleeland CS, Weissman DE, et al. Opioids for chronic cancer and non-cancer pain: a survey of state medical board members. *Fed Bull: J Med Licsen & Disc* 1992;79:15–49.

212. Brushwood DB. Professional casualties in America's war on drugs. *Am J Health Syst Pharm* 2003;60:2004–2006.

213. Drug Enforcement Administration. *DEA Administrator Karen Tandy's Remarks on Hurwitz Sentencing.* News Release issued April 14, 2005. Available at: www.usdoj.gov/dea/pubs/pressrel/pr041405b.html.

214. Gallagher CA. *DEA Perspectives.* 7th International Conference on Pain and Chemical Dependency; June 24, 2007; New York, NY.

215. Gallagher CA. *Pain medicine through the eyes of the DEA.* Presented at: Opioid Therapy for Chronic Pain: Safe and Effective Prescribing—Clinical, Ethical, Legal, and Regulatory Concerns; November 10, 2007; Washington, DC.

216. Goldenbaum DM, Christopher M, Gallagher RM, et al. Physicians charged with opioid analgesic-prescribing offenses. *Pain Med* 2008;9:737–751.

217. Brushwood DB. Drug control policy out of balance. *Pain & The Law* September 4, 2003.

218. Jung B, Reidenberg MM. Physicians being deceived. *Pain Med* 2007;8:433–437.

219. Ziegler SJ. Pain, patients, and prosecution: Who is deceiving whom? *Pain Med* 2007;8:445–446.

220. Brushwood DB. The "general recognition and acceptance" standard of objectivity for good faith in prescribing: Legal and medical implications. *J Pain Palliat Care Pharmacother* 2007;21:35–38.

221. Edmondson WAD, Rowe GS, Goddard T, et al. Docket No. DEA61: *Comment on Dispensing of Controlled Substances for the Treatment of Pain.* Washington, DC: National Association of Attorneys General. March 21, 2005.

222. Kingdon JW. *Agendas, Alternatives, and Public Policies.* 2nd ed. New York: Addison-Wesley Educational Publishers, Inc; 2003.

CHAPTER 15 ■ LITIGATION INVOLVING PAIN MANAGEMENT

BEN A. RICH

INTRODUCTION

In recent years, issues arising in the context of pain management have increasingly been raised in the context of law and public policy. Indeed, one of the major professional journals, *Pain Medicine*, now has an entire section devoted to this area of activity (i.e.,

forensic pain medicine). While technically forensic pain medicine encompasses all instances in which pain medicine and the law converge, this chapter will focus on the area of convergence that is most often associated with the term forensic—litigation. The other aspects of law and public policy affecting pain management are covered in Chapter 14.

American jurisprudence is divided into two broad categories

of jurisdiction—state and federal—and four distinct domains within both categories: administrative, civil, criminal, and constitutional. Cases involving pain management have arisen in all four domains, and in this chapter we will consider the important cases in each and identify the important lessons for practitioners. We will begin with administrative proceedings, all of which involve disciplinary actions by state medical licensing boards against physicians. In reviewing these cases, it will become clear how the pendulum has been shifting in the last decade from concerns about so-called "over-prescribing" of opioid analgesics to cases in which physicians have been charged with unprofessional or substandard practice for their failure to demonstrate a minimally sufficient level of knowledge or skill in the assessment and management of pain. These proceedings reflect a policy trend among medical boards to emphasize the important role of pain management in patient care. That trend is more fully discussed in Chapter 14.

The aspect of civil litigation that most often involves health care professionals is medical malpractice. Such claims are a species of tort claim in which an injured party, the plaintiff, asserts that they have sustained damages as a result of the negligence of the other party, the defendant. Medical malpractice claimants, in order to be successful, must establish four essential elements. The first element is the existence of a duty owed by the defendant to the plaintiff. The generic characterization of such a duty is "due care."[1] In professional liability cases this translates to compliance with the prevailing standard of care. However, a health care professional–patient relationship must exist before such a duty may be deemed to have arisen.

The second element is breach of the duty owed, hence in medical malpractice litigation a material departure from the standard of care. A dispute as to what constitutes the relevant standard of care by which the defendant professional's conduct is to be evaluated is usually the critical issue in a medical malpractice case, and the outcome often depends on whose expert witness or witnesses are deemed by the jury to be most convincing. Consequently, medical malpractice cases have come to be characterized as little more than a "battle of the experts." Traditionally the usual custom and practice of physicians in the same or similar situations to the defendant has set the standard of care. Evidence of compliance by the defendant physician with the custom tended to create an irrebuttable presumption that the applicable standard of care had been met. Over the last several decades there has been a gradual trend by the courts toward a recognition of instances in which the custom and practice of clinicians has lagged noticeably far behind advances in medical science and technology, or physicians have failed to adopt safer or more effective clinical practices such as those advocated by national clinical guidelines. In such situations, the courts have acknowledged that rigid and unreflective adherence to the customary practice might demonstrate a failure to exercise appropriate clinical judgment. We will consider that issue further in the section of the chapter pertaining to civil litigation.

The third element of a tort claim is damage or injury. The breach of a duty of due care that fails to produce an injury or other harm is, from a strictly legal perspective, of no consequence. It is characterized in the law as *damnum absque injuria* (a wrong without injury). Such circumstances may be of interest to risk managers and quality improvement personnel, but they do not give rise to tort liability. The intriguing aspect of harm in the context of pain management is whether subjecting patients to unnecessary pain through substandard care would be deemed by juries as on the same level as medical errors that produce demonstrably physical injury or even death. The cases we will examine confirm that this is indeed the case, at least for patients who were at the end of life.

Finally, the plaintiff must establish that the breach of the duty of care by the defendant was the proximate (direct and immediate) cause of the damage or injury he or she sustained. In the cases we will be considering, the plaintiff must persuade the jury that pain management consistent with the standard of care would have, to a reasonable degree of medical probability, ensured that the patient did not suffer.

In the fourth section of the chapter we will review criminal prosecutions by both the state and federal governments that concern the prescribing of opioid analgesics for terminal or chronic noncancer pain patients. Finally, in section 5, we will consider three U.S. Supreme Court cases in which Constitutional issues are raised in the context of cases related to pain management and/or end-of-life care.

ADMINISTRATIVE PROCEEDINGS

Until recently, disciplinary actions by state medical licensing boards involving the prescribing of opioid analgesics targeted the phenomenon of "overprescribing," and it was the leading cause of both investigations and disciplinary actions.[2] Some of these actions were well-founded efforts to punish physicians who prescribed controlled substances inappropriately or without a legitimate medical purpose, thereby endangering their patients and/or society. Others, however, sought to punish physicians who were engaged in a good faith effort to manage chronic noncancer pain, and demonstrated either a dismissal by the boards of the plight of chronic pain patients or an ignorance of the risks, side effects, and benefits of opioid analgesia.[3] We will consider two cases from the second group in which the practices of the accused physicians were ultimately vindicated by state appellate court decisions.

In the Matter of DiLeo

Dr. Lucas DiLeo, a general practitioner, prescribed opioid analgesics for some of his patients with significant chronic nonmalignant pain. One of these patients, for example, was an iron worker who had fallen over 40 feet onto concrete and sustained 153 fractures, 93 in the face, as well as shattering his knees, ankles, and left femur. He underwent 10 operations, and continued thereafter to suffer with chronic pain. In 1992 the Louisiana Board of Medical Examiners filed an administrative complaint against Dr. DiLeo alleging that his prescribing of opioids to seven patients (an eighth patient was treated for obesity with a combination of Didrex and Xanax) was not for a legitimate medical purpose, demonstrated incompetence, and fell outside acceptable standards of medical practice.

The Board's expert witness, Dr. Linda Stuart, a board certified family practitioner and addiction specialist, did not question that the seven patients receiving opioids had serious pain problems nor did she challenge the doses prescribed as excessive. However, she did testify that in her opinion opioid analgesia was provided for too long a period of time, thereby posing an unacceptable risk of addiction and withdrawal symptoms. She acknowledged, however, that there were different schools of thought on this issue in the medical profession. As for the obesity patient, Dr. Stuart questioned the prescribing of Didrex and Xanax at the same time, since she considered the former to be a stimulant while the latter was a depressant.

Five of Dr. DiLeo's patients testified on his behalf, as did a physician whose specialty was internal medicine/endocrinology. The medical board ruled against Dr. DiLeo, and that ruling was affirmed by a trial court. The Louisiana Court of Appeals reversed and dismissed all charges against him after finding that no evidence had been presented by the Board to support Dr. Stuart's assertion that the duration of Dr. DiLeo's prescriptions was excessive. Indeed, the Court of Appeals held that the Board had failed to present any evidence as to what the relevant standard of medical practice was for prescribing opioids for chronic pain.

In the absence of such evidence, the unsupported assertions of Dr. Stuart were insufficient to justify the disciplinary measures imposed on Dr. DiLeo, and the charges against him were deemed by the court to be arbitrary, capricious, and an abuse of the Board's discretion.[4]

Hoover v. Agency for Health Care Administration

Katherine Hoover, MD was a board certified internist who had a number of chronic pain patients in her practice. For some of them she elected to prescribe opioid analgesics for an extended period of time. The state medical board took a dim view of this, and initiated disciplinary proceedings for "inappropriately and excessively" prescribing Schedule II drugs to seven patients. The board's case against Dr. Hoover consisted of two physicians who had reviewed pharmacy computer printouts documenting the prescriptions written for these patients by Dr. Hoover, and their opinions that the dosages she had prescribed were "excessive, perhaps lethal." None of these patients had, in fact, suffered any adverse effects from the prescriptions written by Dr. Hoover. Rather, they rallied to her support because she had diligently and successfully worked to manage their pain and restore their ability to function, whereas other physicians had either discounted their reports of pain or refused to prescribe opioids.

The board's experts did not review the medical records for any of these patients. Also, upon cross-examination, these "experts" acknowledged that they did not treat chronic pain patients in their practice. Indeed, under the more stringent standards for expert testimony that have developed in the last 10 years, one could reasonably argue that the medical board's experts were not really experts in pain management. The hearing officer in the case may have taken the same view, since she ultimately ruled that the evidence presented at the hearing supported a conclusion that Dr. Hoover's care of these patients was entirely appropriate. Nevertheless, the Board of Medicine took the remarkable step of disregarding the hearing officer's findings and conclusions, and imposed sanctions that included an administrative fine of $4000, CME on the prescribing of "abusable drugs," and 2 years of probation.

Dr. Hoover appealed, and in a scathing opinion by a three-judge panel of the Florida Court of Appeals, the ruling of the medical board was reversed. Noting a disturbing pattern and practice by the medical board, the opinion declared: "the board has once again engaged in the uniformly rejected practice of over-zealously supplanting a hearing officer's valid findings of fact regarding a doctor's prescription practices with its own opinion in a case founded on a woefully inadequate quantum of evidence."[5] Elsewhere in the opinion, the court referred to the board's "draconian policy of policing pain prescription practice." Similar to the decision by the Louisiana Court of Appeals in DiLeo, the Florida court noted that the medical board had failed to introduce competent, credible evidence of the standard of care by which Dr. Hoover's prescribing practices could be evaluated.

One very important implication of the DiLeo and Hoover cases is that the courts will not simply sit back and allow medical boards to declare what the standard of care is in any particular clinical situation. Rather, the board must present persuasive evidence in support of the prevailing standard of care. Moreover, such cases as these appear to represent an "ethic of underprescribing" on the part of state medical boards that persisted for decades.[6] It was the deeply engrained and pervasive nature of this ethic that prompted some state legislatures to adopt the intractable pain treatment acts (IPTA) that are discussed in Chapter 14. The thrust of such legislation was to send a message that the public policy of the state should not be to discourage physicians from providing effective pain management to patients with chronic nonmalignant pain, even if in some cases that would involve the extended use of opioid analgesics. The Hoover case suggests how difficult it was to surmount the prevailing ethic in some boards, since that case was brought shortly after the State of Florida had enacted an IPTA. The medical board rationalized its attempt to discipline Dr. Hoover by arguing that she had treated the patients in question prior to the effective date of the Florida law. The Florida Court of Appeals critiqued the cramped and legalistic way in which the Board attempted to flaunt the statute, noting that what the Board failed or refused to recognize was that the public policy of the state did not support its approach to punishing physicians who dared to prescribe opioids to patients with chronic noncancer pain.

Beginning in the mid-1990s, a few state medical boards adopted policies on pain management that were intended to reassure physicians that the board was not, in fact, hostile to good pain management practice, and sought to outline how physicians could care for such patients in a manner that was consistent with good medical practice. Then, in 1998, the Federation of State Medical Boards (FSMB) promulgated model guidelines for the use of controlled substances for the treatment of pain.[7]

The gradual dissemination of medical board policies promoting effective pain relief as an essential component of quality patient care signaled the beginning of a paradigm shift. Heretofore, the idea that if there could be such a thing as overprescribing of opioids, then as a matter of logic and consistency there must be an opposite side to the coin (i.e., underprescribing of opioids) seemed to be unintelligible to many medical boards. The inconsistency between perception and reality was truly remarkable. Whereas the medical literature in the 1980s and 1990s was replete with data indicating that pain was significantly undertreated in almost all patient care settings, no medical board had ever encountered a case in which underprescribing was deemed to constitute incompetent or unprofessional conduct.[8]

Oregon Board of Medical Examiners (OBME) v. Bilder

Paul A. Bilder is a pulmonary specialist who in the late 1990s was practicing in a small Oregon community. In 1999, the OBME initiated disciplinary action against Bilder following an investigation of complaints concerning his alleged failure to properly manage the pain and other distressing symptoms of six patients over a period of 5 years. The disciplinary action ultimately led to a Stipulated Order in which Bilder agreed to certain remedial measures.[9] Two of the six were elderly patients with metastatic cancer who were enrolled in hospice. In each instance the hospice nurse requested an increase in the dosage of pain medication in what turned out to be the last hours of the patient's life which Dr. Bilder refused to provide because he considered the amount requested excessive. In the other three cases, he refused to provide morphine or similar pain medication to a patient with CHF who was DNR and gasping for breath. The other three cases involved patients who were ventilator-dependent because of COPD or pneumonia. Dr. Bilder ordered paralytic agents but refused to order anti-anxiolytics or pain medication.

By the terms of the Stipulated Order, Dr. Bilder agreed to a 10-year probation, a formal reprimand, successful completion of the Board's Physician's Evaluation Education Renewal Program and an approved course in physician–patient communication, as well as continuing psychiatric treatment with regular reports from the treating psychiatrist to the Board. The Oregon Board once again found it necessary to take disciplinary action against Dr. Bilder 2 years later for similar instances of failure or refusal to appropriately respond to clear indications of patient suffering.[10]

Accusation of Eugene Whitney, MD

In 2003, California became the second state to take disciplinary action against a physician for failure to provide appropriate pain relief. The patient in question was an 85-year-old man with advanced mesothelioma. The care of Lester Tomlinson in the last weeks of his life was the subject of both civil litigation and medical board disciplinary action. The civil litigation will be discussed in the next section of this chapter.

Mr. Tomlinson spent 5 days in a local hospital receiving treatment for pneumonia and pleural effusion. He was then transferred to a skilled nursing facility (SNF) and came under the care of Eugene B. Whitney, MD, for the duration of his stay, which ended with his death approximately 3 weeks later.[11] The care of Mr. Tomlinson at the SNF generated a great deal of contention between the members of his family (wife and daughter) and the caregivers. Each administration of pain medication, which began on the fourth day following his transfer from the hospital, was precipitated by a complaint from the family that he was in pain. Medication orders progressed from Restoril to Vicodin to various strengths of Duragesic patch. Only after the family specifically requested morphine for Mr. Tomlinson's increasing pain did Dr. Whitney discontinue the Vicodin and ordered Roxanol 20 mg, 10 mg orally every 6 hours.

Dr. Whitney saw Mr. Tomlinson only once during that period of time, 2 days after the first administration of Roxanol. He found the patient to be in pain and ordered MS Contin oral solution 10 mg every 4 hours as needed. As noted in the medical board charges against Dr. Whitney, MS Contin comes in tablet form only, and should be provided on a regular schedule, not on an "as needed" basis. Dr. Whitney discontinued the prior order 2 days later and instead ordered MS Contin 5 mg every 2 hours for breakthrough pain. As further noted in the medical board accusation, halving the dose of an opioid analgesic and doubling the frequency of administration will not increase the analgesic potency. Nursing notes at the SNF in the subsequent 2 days until Mr. Tomlinson's death indicate uncontrolled pain and anxiety.

The Medical Board of California charged Dr. Whitney with unprofessional conduct and incompetence for his failure "to understand the unique properties of Roxanol solution and MS Contin tablets and to prescribe the medications properly."[11] The Board and Dr. Whitney entered into a Stipulation for Public Reprimand, the terms and conditions of which require that he obtain continuing medical education in pain management, the prescribing of opioid analgesics, and communication with patients and families.[12]

At this point it is still too early to conclude that the medical board actions against Drs. Bilder and Whitney represent any sort of paradigm shift in philosophy and practice of medical boards generally in regard to opioid prescribing by their licensees. Two cases do not constitute a trend. Nevertheless, the Federation of State Medical Boards Model Policy concerning controlled substances for pain relief, updated and expanded in 2004, contains language that is strongly suggestive of a new paradigm. The Model Policy makes the following assertions:

- the state medical board will consider inappropriate treatment, including the undertreatment of pain, a departure from an acceptable standard of practice;
- the state medical board views pain management to be important and integral to the practice of medicine;
- the inappropriate treatment of pain includes nontreatment, undertreatment, overtreatment, and the continued use of ineffective treatments.[13]

As of mid-2007, a majority of state medical boards had adopted the model policies or promulgated policies that emphasized the need to incorporate sound pain management practices into patient care.[14] To some extent the shift in attitudes about the role of pain management in patient care, and the influence of those new attitudes in the formulation of medical practice guidelines and policies, can be traced to a few dramatic legal cases. We turn now to these cases and their role in informing public attitudes and public policies about pain and its management.

CIVIL LITIGATION

Despite growing evidence in the clinical literature that pain is often undertreated, and a medical malpractice crisis purportedly arising out of a plethora of malpractice claims yielding significant monetary damage awards, prior to 1990 there had never been a malpractice suit seeking damages for failure to provide appropriate pain relief.

While somewhat speculative, there are several possible explanations of this curious state of affairs. First, the phenomenon of widespread undertreated pain was not well known outside of the health professions. It had yet to become a featured topic in the print or electronic media. Moreover, laypersons held the erroneous belief that pain was the inevitable result of traumatic injury, serious illness, or a major surgical procedure. Finally, the generally high repute in which health care professionals were held presupposed that they would most certainly not allow a patient to experience unnecessary pain or suffering. The pervasiveness of pain in the clinical setting must, on this view, result from the sheer intractability of the pain associated with major illness, and most certainly with the process of dying. From this perspective, the case we now consider is all that more remarkable in its outcome.

Estate of Henry James v. Hillhaven Corporation

Henry James was a 75-year-old man who carried the diagnosis of stage III adenocarcinoma of the prostate with metastasis to the lumbar sacral spine and left femur. In December of 1986 and January of 1987 he spent nearly 2 months in a local hospital receiving treatment for a pathological hip fracture. During that hospitalization, in addition to bone debridement and radiation therapy, Mr. James was evaluated by hospice and received Roxanol 150 mg every 3 to 4 hours around the clock for his pain. Progress notes indicate that his pain was well controlled on this regimen.

After a very short stay at home, he was admitted to a nursing home owned and operated by the Hillhaven Corporation. The continuing orders for pain medication included 150 mg per day of Roxanol, along with 2 tablets of Tylenol every 4 hours as needed and Darvocet-N 100 mg. His family had ensured that he received the medication when he was at home, and made certain that the nursing home staff was aware of it upon his admission.[15]

In preparation of the SNF admission documents, a nurse offered the opinion that Mr. James was addicted to morphine and on that basis declared her intent to significantly reduce the amount of opioid analgesia and replace it with a tranquilizing agent. Remarkably, she was able to effectuate this change in the pain management regimen without the review and approval of the patient's physician. His family learned about the change only after he had been discharged from the facility and was interviewed by investigators for the North Carolina Department of Human Resources, the licensing agency for the facility. Their investigation revealed that at no time during his 23-day stay did he receive pain medication as ordered.[15]

Thereafter, the family consulted an attorney and suit was filed against the nurse and the facility for failure to properly treat Mr. James' pain.[16] In order to prevail in such a case, the plaintiff (Mr. James' estate) had to establish by a preponderance of the evidence that (1) a recognized standard of care for the management of his pain existed, (2) the standard was violated by the defendants, and (3) the departure from the standard of care caused him to experience pain. If the jury answered each of those questions in the affirmative, then it must proceed to determine what several weeks of unnecessary pain should be worth in monetary damages. During the course of the trial expert witnesses called by the plaintiff challenged the position taken by the nurse at the Hillhaven facility that the dose of morphine prescribed for Mr. James was excessive and not necessary to control his pain.[17]

The jury answered each of the questions in the affirmative and awarded the plaintiff compensatory damages of $7.5 million. However, the jury did not stop with that award. In a civil action, when a defendant's conduct is sufficiently egregious to meet certain criteria, punitive damages may be awarded. The purpose of such damages, as the term suggests, is not to compensate the plaintiff, but rather to make a negative example of and punish the defendant. The jury in this case assessed another $7.5 million in punitive damages. Apparently, the jurors were convinced that there is or ought to be something like a right to effective pain relief, at least for patients in the circumstances of Mr. James, and that the defendant corporation and/or its agent consciously disregarded that right and in the process subjected an elderly, dying patient to unnecessary pain and suffering. In a subsequent section of this chapter we will consider two cases in which the U.S. Supreme Court appears to adopt a similar position as a matter of constitutional law.

Several years after the verdict and subsequent out-of-court (and confidential) settlement of the *James v. Hillhaven* case, North Carolina joined a number of other states in enacting tort reform legislation. Consequently, the same result could not be achieved today even in the same or a very similar case. Punitive damages are now capped at three times the amount of compensatory damages or $250,000, whichever is greater. Furthermore, punitive damages cannot even be sought unless the plaintiff can prove by clear and convincing evidence (a higher burden of proof than a preponderance of the evidence) one of the following aggravating factors: (1) the defendant acted out of malice, (2) fraudulently, or (3) in willful and wanton disregard of the rights or safety of the defendant. Punitive damages could not be recovered from a corporation (such as Hillhaven) unless the officers, managers, or directors participated in or condoned the conduct that constituted the aggravating factors.[18]

William Bergman v. Wing Chin, MD and Eden Medical Center

William Bergman was an 85-year-old man in severe pain when he arrived at the Emergency Department (ED) of Eden Medical Center. He had been taking the Vicodin prescribed by his physician, but without receiving adequate relief. He was given morphine by the ED physician, and experienced significant relief. In order to do a more extensive workup, he was admitted to the hospital and came under the care of a hospitalist, Wing Chin, MD. Out of concerns about the side effects of morphine, in particular respiratory depression, Dr. Chin discontinued it and wrote a standing order for Demerol, 25–50 mg every 4 hours "as needed." This order remained in place throughout the 5-day hospital stay, during which the nurses charted pain levels in the range of 7–10 on the standard 10-point scale. On the date of Mr. Bergman's discharge, his numerical pain score was noted to be a 10; nevertheless, Dr. Chin planned to send him home with a prescription for Vicodin. When Mr. Bergman's daughter protested, Dr. Chin ordered another administration of Demerol and a fentanyl patch.

During the hospitalization, the medical work up was strongly suggestive of lung cancer, although Mr. Bergman refused to consent to a lung biopsy that Dr. Chin believed was indicated in order to make a definitive diagnosis. Despite a diagnosis Dr. Chin deemed less than definitive, shortly following his discharge Mr. Bergman came under the care of a hospice nurse, who prevailed upon another physician in the community to write a prescription for morphine after she found the fentanyl patch to be inadequate to manage Mr. Bergman's pain. He died 3 days following discharge. No autopsy was performed. The cause of death was considered to be complications from lung cancer.[19]

The children of William Bergman became convinced that the last days of their father's life were severely compromised by a clinical failure to provide effective pain relief. Their conviction resulted in part from a review of his medical record by an expert secured through the assistance of the organization Compassion in Dying (now Compassion and Choices). The family initially filed a complaint against Dr. Chin with the Medical Board of California. In an interesting approach to the case, the Board's own investigation and independent expert review confirmed that the pain relief Dr. Chin provided to Mr. Bergman was inadequate. Nevertheless, the Board notified the family that it would not take any adverse disciplinary action against Dr. Chin based upon only one episode of inadequate patient care. Displeased by this response, and with continuing support from Compassion in Dying, the Bergman family secured legal counsel and filed a civil action against Dr. Chin and Eden Medical Center. The medical center settled with the plaintiffs prior to trial.

The complaint against Dr. Chin that was tried to a jury was unusual in that it was not a straightforward medical malpractice claim. Such a claim could not have any chance of success in California because, as a result of tort reform legislation, damages for pain and suffering resulting from medical malpractice can only be recovered by the patient; they are not deemed to "survive" such that they can be recovered following the patient's death by the personal representative. The only challenge to the medical care provided by Dr. Chin related to his alleged failure to properly manage Mr. Bergman's pain, hence the only damages that could be awarded would be for unnecessary pain and suffering. However, if the pain and suffering can be proven to have resulted from acts or omissions that constitute "elder abuse," under California law the personal representative of the "victim" of the abuse can recover damages. Consequently, the Bergman family's suit against Dr. Chin and the hospital alleged elder abuse.

Another complicating factor about an elder abuse claim in California is that it carries an elevated burden of proof. Rather than a mere preponderance of the evidence, the plaintiff must establish by "clear and convincing evidence" that the defendant was guilty of recklessness, fraud, or malice in perpetrating physical, financial, or fiduciary abuse or neglect.[20] Prior to this case, no physician had ever been accused of elder abuse, and the claim that failure of a health care professional to provide effective pain management might constitute a violation of the statute was an even further stretch. From all appearances, the trial of the case proceeded as would a typical medical malpractice claim. The plaintiffs offered the testimony of two physician expert witnesses, both of whom testified that there were serious problems with the type, dose, and schedule of administration of analgesia to Mr. Bergman while a patient at Eden Medical Center. In rebuttal, Dr. Chin called two physician expert witnesses who testified that in their opinion the measures he employed in an effort to manage Mr. Bergman's pain did not constitute a material departure from the custom and practice of similar physicians caring for patients like Mr. Bergman.[21]

During the course of the trial, despite Dr. Chin's contention that there was no conclusive evidence that Mr. Bergman had lung cancer, the judge allowed the plaintiffs to introduce into evidence the Agency for Health Care Policy and Research Clinical Practice Guideline *Managing Cancer Pain*. That evidence tended to bolster the testimony of the plaintiff's experts that Dr. Chin's pain management strategy was deficient in significant ways. The guideline provides, for example:

▪ Treatment of persistent or moderate to severe pain should be based on increasing the opioid potency or dose;

- Medications for persistent cancer-related pain should be administered on an around-the-clock basis with additional "as needed" doses, because regularly scheduled dosing maintains a constant level of drug in the body and helps prevent recurrence of the pain;
- Meperidine (Demerol) should not be used if continued opioid use is anticipated.[22]

Dr. Chin testified that he had no familiarity with these or with the Medical Board of California's 1994 guidelines and policy on pain management. He also stated that he did not take the nurses' notes on Mr. Bergman's pain levels into account because he did not have any confidence in that form of pain assessment.

The nurses involved in the care of Mr. Bergman testified on behalf of Dr. Chin that whenever Mr. Bergman reported pain in the moderate to severe range, they administered another 25 mg dose of Demerol consistent with the standing order. Interestingly, however, they testified that the reason the medical record did not reflect what they insisted to have been consistent achievement of pain relief in response to these administrations was that at Eden Medical Center pain was charted "by exception." In other words, pain was only noted when it was outside of normal limits. Such an approach begs the question of what constitutes an authoritative source for the "normal limits" of pain for any particular patient. This charting anomaly worked against the defendant, because the medical record was replete with pain levels in the moderate-to-severe range each day, but not in the mild to nonexistent range that would have supported their claim that the opioids administered to Mr. Bergman during his hospitalization were sufficient to meet his needs.

Ultimately, the jury reached a verdict in favor of the plaintiffs, and awarded $1.5 million in damages. They came within one vote of awarding an additional amount in punitive damages. The trial judge reduced the award to $250,000 on the theory that the statutory cap on monetary damage awards for medical malpractice claims applied even though this claim was filed pursuant to the elder abuse statute. The judge awarded nearly $1 million in attorney fees and litigation costs to the plaintiffs as well. Outstanding posttrial issues were resolved by confidential agreement between the parties; hence, no appeal was taken by either side.

News of the verdict in the Bergman v. Chin case shook the medical community. The stark contrast between the reaction of the Medical Board of California to the allegations in the case and that of the lay jury seemed to support an observation by the physician Eric Cassell nearly 20 years earlier: "The relief of suffering, it would appear, is considered one of the primary ends of medicine by patients and lay persons, but not by the medical profession."[23] Because the verdict came in the context of an elder abuse claim against Dr. Chin, it seemed particularly punitive in nature, and raised the issue of how to most appropriately and effectively "rehabilitate" physicians whose knowledge, skills, and/or attitudes were not conducive to the effective assessment and management of pain. We will revisit this issue after the discussion of the Tomlinson case that follows.

Tomlinson v. Bayberry Care Center, et al.

We have previously discussed the Tomlinson case in the context of the elder abuse claims filed against both the acute and long-term care facilities in which the patient received care in the last month of his life, as well as the physicians who were responsible for that care in both clinical settings. The claims in that case bore a striking resemblance to the claims in the Bergman v. Chin case.[24] Perhaps because of the jury verdict in the prior case, as noted, all of the defendants in Tomlinson settled prior to trial. Interestingly, as alluded to previously, the Medical Board of California took a much different position in dealing with the complaint by the Tomlinson family against Dr. Eugene Whitney, who was the responsible physician when Mr. Tomlinson was in the skilled nursing facility (Bayberry Care Center) than it did with regard to the complaint filed by the Bergman family against Dr. Chin. The Medical Board of California sanctioned Dr. Whitney for his failure "to understand the unique properties of Roxinol solution and MS Contin tablets and to prescribe the medications properly" pursuant to a stipulated disciplinary order he entered into with the Board. He was required to undergo an extensive evaluation of his professional knowledge and skills and work with the Board in developing a detailed remediation plan.[26] Also, the California Department of Health Services issued a Notice of Deficiency against Bayberry Care Center based upon the many problems with the care Mr. Tomlinson received at that facility.[25]

Just as one can speculate that the defendants in the elder abuse claims by the Tomlinson family were motivated to settle prior to trial because of the earlier jury verdict against Dr. Chin, it is also tempting to suggest that the decision of the Medical Board of California to take disciplinary action against Dr. Whitney in response to the complaint filed against him by the Tomlinson family was influenced by the highly negative public response to the Board's refusal to take similar action against Dr. Chin, particularly when a lay jury deemed the same conduct not just malpractice but elder abuse and the California legislature was motivated to pass a law mandating continuing medical education in pain management for California physicians. It is certainly possible that one influenced the other, but there is no way to authoritatively establish that proposition.

CRIMINAL LITIGATION

Criminal prosecutions of health care professionals for acts or omissions resulting in death or grave harm to patients are exceedingly rare.[26] By far the most common means of imposing sanctions on health professionals for negligent or even reckless patient care are those we have already considered—disciplinary action by state licensing boards or professional liability (malpractice) claims. The exceptional case that prompts a criminal prosecution is almost invariably one involving the death of the patient and conduct by the professional that is considered egregious in nature or in the extent to which it departs from a consensus view of what constitutes the parameters of responsible professional conduct.

Since our focus is necessarily on pain management and palliative care, we will consider several instances in which physicians have been prosecuted in either state or federal court. Some of the more high profile state prosecutions have involved the care of dying patients, whereas those in federal court have been pursuant to the Controlled Substances Act and involved prescribing opioids for chronic noncancer pain patients. We begin with a highly instructive state prosecution.

State v. Naramore

In 1994, the Attorney General of Kansas filed a two-count criminal complaint against L. Stanley Naramore, D.O. Both counts related to his care of patients almost 2 years before who were facing terminal conditions. Early in 1996 a jury returned guilty verdicts related to each count and the court sentenced Dr. Naramore to concurrent terms of 5 to 20 years. We will focus on the case that gave rise to the first count, and on the subsequent reversal of both convictions by the Kansas Court of Appeals.

The patient, Ruth Leach, was a 78-year-old woman suffering from advanced breast cancer that had metastasized to her bones, lungs, and brain. While a patient at St. Francis Hospital in the small Kansas town by the same name, her condition continued to deteriorate and the fentanyl patches no longer controlled her pain. She was restless and agitated, and the nurse on duty suggested to the family that Dr. Naramore be called and asked to prescribe stronger pain medication. Upon arriving at the hospital, he examined Ruth Leach and spoke with her two adult children. Together they reached a decision to increase her pain medication in an effort to control her pain. Naramore explained that there was a risk of depressed respiration. He then administered 4 mg of Versed and 100 micromilligrams of fentanyl. Thereafter, the nursing notes indicate that the patient's respiration slowed and grew irregular.

From this point on the accounts of what transpired take on a curious, disjointed quality. To the extent they are accurate, it is not difficult to understand why there was a failure to maintain a consensus among the family and caregivers concerning the goals of care and how each subsequent action would be consistent with the reasonable pursuit of those goals.

The patient's son, who had training as an emergency medical technician, is reported to have asked Dr. Naramore if his mother was dying, and Naramore was said to have observed that she was, but that the effects of the fentanyl could be reversed by the administration of Narcan. This statement suggested to the patient's son and the nurse on duty that an overdose of pain medication must have been given. Thereafter, when Dr. Naramore began to prepare for continuing IV infusion of analgesics, the son insisted that he not administer any more, and was quoted as saying: "I'd rather my mother lay there and suffer for 10 more days than you do anything to speed up her death." In an effort to dissuade the son, Dr. Naramore told him: "it just gets terrible from here on out . . . the next few days are going to be absolutely terrible."[27] When the son remained intransigent and assured Dr. Naramore that he would hold the doctor accountable for anything that happened, Dr. Naramore withdrew from the case. The next day Ruth Leach was transported to another hospital, where she was given morphine for her pain and died 3 days later of her underlying terminal illness.[28]

As a result of the events described above, Ruth Leach's family became convinced, and they in turn persuaded the Kansas Attorney General, that Dr. Naramore had intended to hasten her death through administration of excessive doses of analgesics. Dr. Naramore was charged with attempted first-degree murder of Ruth Leach. At the same time, he was charged with second-degree murder of another patient from about the same time period, Chris Willt.

In order to convict a defendant of attempted first-degree murder, the jury must find that the prosecution has proven beyond a reasonable doubt that the defendant: (1) performed an overt act toward the commission of the crime; (2) did so with the intent to commit the crime of first-degree murder; and (3) failed to complete the commission of that crime. The elements of murder in the first degree include intent to kill a person, the intentional performance of an overt act toward that end that is both deliberate and premeditated.[27]

The prosecution presented several medical experts whose testimony supported the charge that Dr. Naramore had attempted to murder Ruth Leach. The Director of Emergency Medicine at the University of Kansas Medical Center testified that in his opinion Ruth Leach was near death after the administration of Versed and fentanyl, and that she would have died if the morphine Dr. Naramore had ordered had in fact been administered. This view was similarly expressed by a specialist in anesthesiology and critical care medicine at the University of Vermont College of Medicine who had previously practiced in Kansas. He testified that a dose of Versed combined with that of the fentanyl were excessive and in short order would have caused the patient to stop breathing. An additional respiratory depressant such as morphine would simply have added to the certainty of her death.

In his defense, Dr. Naramore called several expert witnesses. One of these, a physician who had cared for Ruth Leach for 5 years prior to her death, noted that she had received a variety of medications for her pain, none of which had brought it under control. He found it to be "phenomenal" that anyone would

accuse Dr. Naramore of trying to kill her under these circumstances. A family physician from another small Kansas community said that if Dr. Naramore had actually intended to kill Ruth Leach he would have used 10 times the dosage administered. He characterized the care provided as "concerned and compassionate."

Another witness for Dr. Naramore was the president of the Kansas Association of Osteopathic Medicine and a family medicine practitioner. He believed that Dr. Naramore's efforts to control Ruth Leach's pain and distress at the end of her life were exemplary. Finally, another family physician who served on the peer review committee for Blue Cross/Blue Shield of Kansas testified that given her significant history of opioid analgesia and the extent of her distress at the time, the dosages of Versed and fentanyl were reasonable and in no sense an overdose.

The convictions of Dr. Naramore for the attempted murder of Ruth Leach and for the second-degree murder of the other patient were reviewed and reversed by the Kansas Court of Appeals. In its opinion, the Court of Appeals made numerous references not only to the expert witness testimony on his behalf at trial, but also to *amicus curiae* (friend of the court) briefs filed on behalf of Dr. Naramore by the Kansas Association of Osteopathic Medicine, the American Osteopathic Association, and the Kansas Medical Society. The court also noted that it had done its own substantial research on the subject of palliative care for terminally ill patients. Its review of the case law revealed "no criminal conviction of a physician for the attempted murder or murder of a patient which has ever been sustained on appeal based upon evidence of the kind presented here."[27]

In arriving at its decision that the criminal convictions must be reversed, the Court of Appeals noted and relied heavily upon the several expert witnesses who testified not only that Dr. Naramore's care of Mrs. Leach could not be reasonably characterized as indicative of an intent to kill her, but that in their professional judgment the care he provided was medically appropriate under the circumstances and hence within the applicable standard of care. The following language of the court is highly instructive and hence merits direct quotation:

> We have made a thorough review of the record [of the trial court proceedings], which contains a wealth of undisputed evidence and expert medical testimony. We find that no rational jury could find criminal intent and guilt beyond a reasonable doubt based on the record here. When the issue is whether there is reasonable doubt, a jury is not free to disbelieve undisputed facts. What occurred here is generally known. The jury was not free to disbelieve that there was substantial competent medical opinion in support of the proposition that Dr. Naramore's actions were not only noncriminal, but were medically appropriate.
> . . . When there is such strong evidence supporting a reasonable, noncriminal explanation for the doctor's actions, it cannot be said that there is no reasonable doubt of criminal guilt . . . All three *amicus* briefs . . . note that if criminal responsibility can be assessed based solely on opinions of a portion of the medical community which are strongly challenged by an opposing and authoritative medical consensus, we have criminalized malpractice, and even the possibility of malpractice. The instant case is a very good example of this.[27]

The above-quoted language of the court, and subsequent statements in the court's decision regarding the absence of any jury instructions "relating to the medical and moral responsibilities of care givers for the critically or terminally ill patient" are of considerable consequence because of their implications for a wide range of criminal prosecutions of physicians for care provided in an effort to manage the pain and adverse symptoms associated with terminal and serious chronic conditions.

Not only have state criminal prosecutions of health care professionals been relatively infrequent[28]; as illustrated by the Naramore charges, some of those have not been carefully screened by prosecutors prior to their initiation, so that even if they result in a conviction at trial, they do not survive the appellate review process. At the end of this chapter we will consider a set of recommendations for further insulating health care professionals from the risk of such prosecutions.

FEDERAL CRIMINAL PROSECUTIONS

Recent federal criminal prosecutions of physicians pursuant to the Federal Controlled Substances Act (CSA) for prescribing practices in the care of chronic noncancer pain patients are not entirely aberrational. They follow in the history and tradition of earlier cases, and the appellate courts reviewing these cases cite the earlier decisions profusely as correctly interpreting and applying the intent of the Congress when enacting the CSA. It therefore behooves us to review key elements of one such precedent-setting case before taking up the contemporary examples.

United States v. Rosen (1978)

Although Dr. Isadore Rosen was prosecuted under the CSA for prescribing controlled substances to patients for weight loss as part of an "obesity practice," and not for pain management, the language of the appellate court decision and its analysis of the CSA are often cited in later cases involving the prescribing of controlled substances for pain. Also, the prosecution of Dr. Rosen was based in large measure on the testimony of undercover law enforcement agents who came to him posing as patients seeking to lose weight. The use of such tactics generally gives rise to a claim of "entrapment" by the defendant; that is, that the government agents induced him to engage in one or more unlawful acts that he was not otherwise contemplating and in which he never would have engaged but for their inducement. As often happens, the court in *Rosen* easily disposed of this defense by noting "When a person is shown to be ready and willing to violate the law, the providing of an opportunity therefore by undercover agents or police officers is not entrapment."[29]

In order to convict Dr. Rosen of the 25 counts of distributing controlled substances in violation of the CSA with which he was charged, the government had to prove the following three elements of the offense beyond a reasonable doubt:

1. That he distributed or dispensed a controlled substance;
2. That he acted knowingly and intentionally; and
3. That he did so other than for a legitimate medical purpose and in the usual course of his professional practice.

Dr. Rosen conceded the first two elements, but asserted as to the third that each of the agents who came to him posing as patients presented symptoms for which the drugs he prescribed or dispensed were medically appropriate. It is important to note that while the prescribing of certain types of medications for the purpose of weight reduction is subject to some controversy, for purposes of this decision the court noted that all of the drugs prescribed by Dr. Rosen have legitimate therapeutic uses.

The crux of Dr. Rosen's argument on appeal of his criminal conviction was that the trial court relied on what it considered to be evidence of substandard medical practice as a basis for finding criminal intent. This point is critical as it will arise in the discussion of more recent prosecutions under the CSA. If the third element listed above is deemed to have been established beyond a reasonable doubt by the evidence, then the courts treat the physician not simply as a negligent, or even in some instances a reckless physician, but simply as a drug dealer. The court in Rosen reviewed a number of earlier convictions under the CSA and identified the following list of "red flags" suggesting that a physician may be acting illegitimately or outside the course of professional practice.

1. An inordinately large quantity of controlled substances was prescribed.
2. Large numbers of prescriptions were issued.
3. No physical exam was given.
4. The physician warned the patient to fill the prescriptions at different pharmacies.
5. The physician issued prescriptions to a patient known to be delivering the drugs to others.
6. The physician prescribed controlled substances at intervals inconsistent with legitimate medical treatment.
7. The physician used street slang rather than medical terminology for the drugs prescribed.
8. There was no logical relationship between the drugs prescribed and treatment of the condition allegedly existing.
9. The physician wrote more than one prescription on occasions in order to spread them out.[30]

The routine followed by Dr. Rosen's weight loss "clinic" included many of these red flag elements according to the testimony of the government agents who posed as patients seeking to lose weight. In particular, Dr. Rosen did not take a medical history or perform a physical exam other than to have the patients weighed and their blood pressure taken on the first visit by a staff member who was not a nurse. He provided no instructions on how to take the medications or warnings of risks or side effects to be concerned about, nor did he schedule follow-up appointments. Based upon this and other evidence at trial, the court of appeals ruled that the government had met its burden of proof that Dr. Rosen's prescribing or dispensing of controlled substances to the undercover agents was not in good faith for legitimate medical purposes in the course of his professional practice.

United States v. Hurwitz

Dr. William Hurwitz was a medical doctor who operated a pain medicine practice in McLean, Virginia. So widespread was his reputation as a liberal prescriber of opioids that many of his patients came from great distances—39 states—seeking medications from him that other physicians would not prescribe. In 1992, he was reprimanded by the District of Columbia medical board because of his "liberal" prescribing practices, and in 1996 the Virginia board revoked his license, and subsequently reinstated it with ongoing monitoring of his prescribing practices. Ostensibly that monitoring was still taking place when, in 2004, a federal grand jury indicted him on 62 counts, including drug trafficking resulting in death and serious bodily injuries, health care fraud, and criminal forfeiture. He was subsequently convicted on 50 of those counts and sentenced to 25 years in prison.[30] Throughout the criminal process, Dr. Hurwitz was portrayed by the federal prosecutor and officials of the Drug Enforcement Administration as "no different from a cocaine or heroin dealer peddling poison on the street corner."[30] At the trial, however, several nationally prominent experts in pain medicine testified on behalf of Dr. Hurwitz. During the trial, immediately following the testimony of the government's chief expert witness, six former presidents of the American Pain Society (APS) took the unprecedented step of sending a letter to the trial judge expressing their deep concerns about "serious misrepresentations" that had been made by the government's expert, who was also a past president of the APS.

When Dr. Hurwitz appealed his convictions to the Fourth Circuit Federal Court of Appeals, the American Academy of Pain Medicine, the American Pain Foundation, and a group of nationally prominent experts in pain management, among others, filed *amicus curiae* (friend of the court) briefs in support of his appeal. These briefs asserted, among other points, that "seriously erroneous rules of law and scientific theories [were] relied upon to convict [Dr. Hurwitz]."[32]

It is important to understand the significance one can reasonably attach to the willingness of these prominent organizations and individual members of the pain medicine community to go on record in this case. The government's position was that Dr. Hurwitz's prescribing of controlled substances had absolutely nothing to do with pain management. It was drug trafficking, pure and simple. The persons to whom he dispensed or prescribed these drugs were not patients, but rather drug seekers who sought either to feed their addiction or further disseminate them in the illicit market for prescription drugs.[32] The thrust of the argument on the other side was not that Dr. Hurwitz was practicing exemplary medicine, or in some instances even prescribing within the minimal standard of acceptable care for chronic pain patients, but rather that however far out of the mainstream his prescribing practices were, he was nevertheless a physician and not a drug dealer. The appropriate societal sanctions for physicians who practice negligently are medical malpractice liability claims or disciplinary action by licensing boards. In egregious circumstances, appropriate sanctions might include the permanent revocation of licensure. Nevertheless, physicians who practice substandard medicine are nonetheless physicians, and their patients remain patients in need of medical care, even if in some instances the care they require is for addiction.

The Fourth Circuit Court of Appeals reversed the Hurwitz conviction and remanded the case to the District Court for a new trial. In doing so, it sought to make clear where the trial judge had erred, and how the retrial should be conducted so as to provide Dr. Hurwitz with a fair trial. At the end of the new trial, he was convicted of 16 counts of drug trafficking and sentenced to 57 months in prison. Taking into consideration the amount of time he has already spent, it is likely that he will be released in late 2008 or early 2009.

United States of America v. McIver

Dr. Ronald McIver had approximately 1,000 patients in his South Carolina practice, most of whom saw him because of problems with chronic noncancer pain. In response to reports from the Columbia, South Carolina police department about Dr. McIver's prescribing practices, the DEA initiated an investigation of his practice in 2002. Based upon investigatory findings that among McIver's patients there were those who regularly received prescriptions for what were characterized as "massive quantities" of oxycodone, Dilaudid, OxyContin, methadone, and morphine, he was indicted on 15 counts of drug trafficking related to his treatment of 10 patients, 9 of whom testified for the government at his trial. The remaining patient was deceased, the cause of death having been characterized as an "oxycodone overdose."[33]

The major thrust of the prosecution's case at trial was based upon the expert testimony of a Dr. Steven Storick, an anesthesiologist who the court deemed to be duly qualified as an expert in pain management. After reviewing the medical records of the patients in question, he concluded that Dr. McIver's treatment of several of them fell outside the parameters of legitimate medical practice. For example, in the case of a patient with a history of substance abuse, Dr. Storick asserted that prescribing opioids to such a patient was "like pouring gasoline on a fire." A medicaid patient who sought treatment from Dr. McIver for fibromyalgia traveled almost 3 hours to see him, paid for his services in cash, and filled prescriptions for methadone, OxyContin, oxycodone, and morphine costing thousands of dollars. The patient testified that she sold the methadone and morphine, and was addicted to oxycodone. With regard to her treatment, Dr. Storick testified that Dr. McIver's conduct was "way outside the course of legitimate medical treatment."[33]

The jury convicted Dr. McIver of multiple counts of unlawful distribution of a controlled substance, and one that resulted in death. He was sentenced to 30 years in prison. On appeal to the Fourth Circuit Court of Appeals, the same court that granted Dr. Hurwitz a new trial, Dr. McIver's counsel attacked Dr. Storick's testimony as reflective of a hostile and suspicious approach to the care of chronic noncancer pain patients in that he insisted upon objective signs of tissue damage before prescribing opioids, and he refused to acknowledge that physicians could be deceived by some patients' reports of pain and yet still be legitimately prescribing opioids for them based upon a reasonable belief that they had significant pain.

The appeal also challenged the jury instructions, which Dr. McIver claimed suggested to the jury that he could be convicted if he "deviated drastically from accepted medical practice." The Court of Appeals, in affirming the conviction, disagreed, noting that the jury was instructed that the prosecution must prove not only that the defendant acted "outside the course of professional practice" but also that he acted "for other than a legitimate medical purpose."[34]

Before concluding the discussion of these federal prosecutions of physicians who were at the far liberal end of the prescribing continuum, it may be helpful to delineate the parameters of that entire continuum, and perhaps even to suggest where, as a matter of law and public policy, the line should be drawn between "the bounds of medicine" and the realm of drug dealing and trafficking by health care professionals. The thrust of the argument goes something like this: Just as we do not criminally prosecute clinicians whose failure or refusal to provide pain relief subjects some of their patients to physical and mental anguish, neither ought we to criminally prosecute clinicians whose excessive prescribing creates or exacerbates some of their patients' addiction disorders or propensity to engage in drug dealing under the guise of being a pain patient. In the most egregious instances at both ends of the continuum, the appropriate public policy stance is to suspend or permanently revoke their professional licensure.

Currently, however, at least clinicians at the far liberal end of the prescribing continuum, such as Hurwitz and McIver, prosecutors, and judges (through approved jury instructions) invite juries to act as though no real physician–patient relationship existed. As suggested by the Kansas Court of Appeals in the Naramore case, whenever the criminally charged clinician is able to present expert testimony that what he or she did was within the "bounds of medicine," the mere fact that the prosecution can offer expert testimony maintaining that it was not should never be sufficient for a conviction. Such a conflict of testimony should necessarily create the reasonable doubt that precludes a jury verdict against a criminal defendant.

CONSTITUTIONAL CASES

Several decisions by the Supreme Court of the United States in the last 10 years have addressed issues related to the treatment of pain. Each case also involved highly controversial ethical and political issues: physician-assisted suicide and medical marijuana. As is typical of the Supreme Court, the rulings in each case were not an effort to decide which side was correct on the ethics or the politics, but rather to determine what was consistent with the Constitution and a reasonable interpretation and application of federal statutes.

The first of these, the companion cases of *Washington v. Glucksberg*[36] and *Vacco v. Quill*[37] decided in 1997, directly involved the question of whether there was a constitutional right on the part of dying patients to be able to acquire lethal doses of medication from willing physicians for purposes of hastening their death. In the process of unanimously ruling that there was no such constitutional right, five of the nine justices joined in two concurring opinions that have been interpreted as a recognition by a majority of the court of a constitutional right on the part of terminal patients to receive palliative care.[37] The language from these companion cases most consistently cited for this proposition include the following passage from the concurring opinion by Justice O'Connor:

> The parties and amici agree that in these states [Washington and New York] a patient who is suffering from a terminal illness and who is experiencing great pain has no legal barriers to obtaining medication, from qualified physicians, to alleviate that suffering, even to the point of causing unconsciousness and hastening death.

combined with language from a separate opinion by Justice Breyer:

> Were the legal circumstances different [than in Washington and New York]—for example were state law to prevent the provision of palliative care, including the provision of drugs as needed to avoid pain at the end of life—then the law's impact upon serious and otherwise unavoidable physical pain (accompanying death) would be more directly at issue. And as Justice O'Connor suggests, the Court might have to revisit its conclusions in these cases.

The focus upon pain and suffering at the end of life by the concurring justices may simply be a consequence of the fact that a right to lethal medication was asserted by the plaintiffs in these cases only as to patients with terminal illness. However, a right to appropriately aggressive palliative care as opposed to a lethal prescription, especially if defined quite broadly as the relief of pain and suffering, might be of even greater significance for a patient with severe chronic noncancer pain than for a terminally ill patient, since it could persist for years or decades rather than merely weeks or months. Only future cases will illuminate whether there might be constitutional protection from unreasonable governmental barriers to pain relief for such patients.

The constitutionality of the Oregon Death With Dignity Act (ODWDA), pursuant to which the state of Oregon legalized and regulated physician-assisted suicide (referred to by its proponents as physician aid in dying) was not directly at issue in either *Glucksberg* or *Quill*. However, those decisions by implication upheld the ODWDA since they determined that there is neither a constitutional right to nor a constitutional prohibition of such a practice. Consequently, it is a matter for each individual state to determine as part of its authority to regulate the practice of health care professionals.

In 2001, Attorney General John Ashcroft issued an Interpretive Rule (IR) of the federal Controlled Substances Act (CSA), maintaining that prescribing a controlled substance for the purpose of assisting a patient in ending their life, even pursuant to a state statutory scheme such as the ODWDA, contravened the CSA and rendered the prescriber vulnerable to federal prosecution. Since all lethal prescriptions written pursuant to the ODWDA were federally controlled substances, the Ashcroft IR would essentially nullify the Oregon law. The State of Oregon immediately challenged the IR in federal court and obtained first a temporary restraining order and subsequently an injunction prohibiting enforcement of the IR pending resolution by the courts. When Ashcroft resigned as Attorney General, his successor Alberto Gonzales decided to continue the legislation. By then, review of adverse rulings by the federal district and Ninth Circuit Court of Appeals had been sought and the case was pending before the U.S. Supreme Court.

The central issue decided by the Supreme Court in Gonzales v. Oregon was: "who decides whether a particular activity is 'in the course of medical practice' or 'done for a 'legitimate medical purpose.' "[38] The Attorney General claimed authority under the CSA to define standards of medical practice at least insofar as the prescribing of scheduled drugs. Taking into consideration the legislative history of the CSA, the Supreme Court majority ruled that the intent of Congress was to combat a national problem of recreational drug abuse by ensuring that scheduled narcotics were secured within the health care setting through the prescribing by licensed practitioners for legitimate medical purposes. Nothing in the language or the legislative history of the CSA suggests that Congress intended to confer on the Attorney General, in his

capacity of law enforcement, to usurp the usual authority of the individual states in regulating the practice of medicine, which includes the writing of prescriptions. For this and other reasons discussed at length by the Court, the IR was held to exceed the authority of the Attorney General under the CSA.

The last case we will consider, which was decided before *Gonzales v. Oregon*, was *Gonzales v. Raich*. The plaintiffs in this case, Angel Raich and Diane Monson, were California residents suffering from a variety of serious medical conditions. Raich carries at least ten diagnoses, including an inoperable brain tumor, seizure disorder, and several chronic pain syndromes. Monson suffers from severe chronic back pain and muscle spasms related to a degenerative disease of the spine.

California is one of ten states that have enacted legislation insulating seriously ill patients or their physicians from prosecution under state law for cultivating or possessing cannabis for use by the patient pursuant to the physician's written recommendation or approval. The plaintiffs in this case argued that they were being treated by board-certified family practitioners who had determined after prescribing a wide variety of standard medications that marijuana is the only drug available that provides effective relief of their symptoms.[40] As a Schedule 1 drug, the CSA recognizes no legitimate basis for patients such as Raich and Monson to possess or use marijuana, even though their physicians authorized it pursuant to the California statute. The plaintiffs filed suit against Attorney General Ashcroft and the administrator of the DEA in federal district court seeking declaratory and injunctive relief preventing the federal government from prosecuting them under the CSA. The crux of their argument was that enforcement of the CSA against them required that interstate commerce be implicated in their acquisition and use of medical marijuana. The district court ruled against the plaintiffs, finding that the Commerce Clause of the Constitution applied to them despite the fact that the marijuana they used was grown in California.

The Ninth Circuit Court of Appeals reversed the district court, holding that the plaintiffs' intrastate, noncommercial cultivation, possession, and use of marijuana for personal medical purposes on the advice of a physician does not constitute drug trafficking. Much of the court's discussion involved arcane legal principles and Supreme Court precedents. Ultimately, it was these very principles and precedents that provided the basis for the Supreme Court's reversal of the Ninth Circuit. Simply stated, the Court held that "Congress' power to regulate interstate markets for medicinal substances encompasses the portions of those markets that are supplied with drugs produced and consumed locally. . . . The CSA is a valid exercise of federal power, even as applied to the troubling facts of this case."[39] Thus the Court's ruling in *Raich* cannot be understood as a pronouncement on the clinical question of whether the known risks and purported benefits of medical marijuana use ever justify a physician recommending it to patients when standard therapies are found to be inadequate.

LESSONS FROM THE LITIGATION

Generalizations that meet minimal criteria of accuracy and practicality concerning the lessons one should learn from the varieties of litigation surveyed in this chapter are both difficult and dangerous. They are difficult because of the wide variation in cases; for example, state and federal courts, some patients who were dying, others facing chronic noncancer pain, still others who were addicted to prescription drugs or simply "planted" as a part of ongoing investigations by law enforcement. They are dangerous when they constitute gross oversimplifications of complex phenomena that have only superficial similarities. Nevertheless, some attempt at synthesis is both necessary and appropriate.

■ Lesson 1: A new medical ethos has clearly emerged, grounded on the recognition that timely and effective assessment and management of all types of pain is essential to sound patient care. Nationally recognized clinical practice guidelines and organizational policies (such as the Joint Commission) affirm this basic proposition.

■ Lesson 2. Evidence- or consensus-based guidelines and policies reinforce the proposition that there are recognized standards of care for the management of acute, chronic noncancer, and pain associated with terminal illness. These standards apply to all clinicians who care for patients with pain, and not merely pain medicine or palliative care specialists.

■ Lesson 3. Material departures from these standards render clinicians vulnerable to a variety of adverse legal consequences. Egregiously conservative approaches to opioid analgesia may result in civil liability for undertreatment of pain or professional licensing board sanctions. Excessively liberal approaches to the prescribing of opioids, particularly when a reasonable clinician would have recognized red flags or other warning signs, may result in criminal prosecution at the state or federal level.

■ Lesson 4. Prudent practitioners should ensure that their knowledge, skills, and attitudes (at least insofar as they affect professional practice) are informed by the current authoritative clinical practice guidelines and policy statements. When that is the case, their approach to pain management will reflect a reasonable balance between effective pain management for their patients and due diligence to ensure that their prescribing practices are neither harming their patients nor contributing to the phenomena of prescription drug abuse and diversion.

■ Lesson 5. As with any other aspect of patient care, timely, accurate, and thorough documentation in the medical record that reflects not only what was done, but also what informed the decision on what to do and what alternatives were considered is absolutely essential. In every legal setting, incomplete, inaccurate, or untimely documentation of professional conduct is problematic, sometimes devastatingly so.

■ Lesson 6. Clinicians who heed lessons 1–5 above are not at any serious risk of adverse legal action arising out of their responsible efforts to relieve the pain of their patients.

References

1. Prosser WL, Keeton WP, Dobbs DB, et al. *Prosser and Keeton on Torts.* 5th ed. St. Paul, Minn: West Publishing Co; 1984.
2. Brookoff D. Commentary on state medical boards and pain management. *J Pain Symptom Manage* 1998;15;381–382.
3. Gilson AM, Joranson DE. Controlled substances and pain management: changes in knowledge and attitudes of state medical regulators. *J Pain Symptom Manage* 2001;21:227–237.
4. Matter of DiLeo, 661 So. 2d 162 (1995).
5. *Hoover v Agency for Health Care Administration*, 676 So. 2d 1380 (1996).
6. Martino AM. In search of a new ethic for treating patients with chronic pain: what can medical boards do? *J Law Med Ethics* 1998;26:332–349, 263.
7. Federation of State Medical Boards of the United States. Model Guidelines for the Use of Controlled Substances for the Treatment of Pain. Federation of State Medical Boards of the United States; 1998.
8. Hill, CS. The negative influence of licensing and disciplinary boards and drug enforcement agencies on pain treatment with opioid analgesics. *J Pharm Care Pain and Symptom Control* 1993;1:43–62.
9. Oregon Board of Medical Examiners. Stipulated Order In the Matter of Paul A. Bilder, M.D. September, 1999.
10. Oregon Board of Medical Examiners Actions Report. Available at: http://www.oregon.gov/BME/Actions/.BOARDACTIONS2003.pdf. Federation of State Medical Boards of the United States; accessed May 14, 2009.
11. Medical Board of California. In the Matter of the Accusation Against Eugene B. Whitney, M.D. March, 2003.
12. Medical Board of California. In the Matter of the Accusation Against Eugene B. Whitney, MD. Decision, December, 2003.
13. Federation of State Medical Boards of the United States, Inc. Model Policy for the Use of Controlled Subtances for the Treatment of Pain. Adopted May, 2004.
14. Federation of State Medical Boards. Pain management overview by state 2006. Available at: http://www.fsmb.org/pdf/copy of grpol pain management.pdf. Accessed May 14, 2009.
15. Cushing M. Pain management on trial. *Am J Nurs* 1992;92:21–23.
16. *Estate of Henry James v Hillhaven Corp*, No. 89 CVS 64 (N.C. Super. Ct. Jan. 15, 1991)
17. Shapiro RS. Liability issues in the management of pain. *J Pain Symptom Manage* 1994;9(3):146–52.
18. NC Gen Stat §§10–15(b), 1D-25 (2003).
19. Rich BA. Moral conundrums in the courtroom: reflections on a decade in the culture of pain. *Camb Q Healthc Ethics* 2002;11:180–190.
20. California Welfare and Institutions Code, §15610 (2006).
21. *Bergman v Chin*, No. H205732-1 (Superior Court of Alameda County, CA 1999).
22. Agency for Health Care Policy and Research. Clinical Practice Guideline No. 9 Management of Cancer Pain. Washington, DC: US Department of Health and Human Services; 1994.
23. Cassell EJ. The nature of suffering and the goals of medicine. *N Engl J Med* 1982;306:639–645.
24. *Tomlinson v Bayberry Care Center*, No. C 02-00120, (Contra Costa County Superior Court, 2002).
25. Annas GJ. Medicine, death, and the criminal law. *N Engl J Med* 1995;333:527–530.
26. Medical Board of California. In the Matter of the Accusation Against Eugene V. Whitney, M.D. No. 12 2002 133376. Stipulation for Public Reprimand. Filed January 14, 2004.
27. *State v Naramore*, 965 P. 2d 211 (Kan. Ct. App. 1998). cert. denied.
28. Alpers A. Criminal act or palliative care? Prosecutions involving the care of the dying. *J Law Med Ethics* 1998;26:308–331.
29. *United States v Rosen*, 582 F. 2d 1032, 1033 (1978).
30. United States Attorney Eastern District of Virginia. News Release. April 14, 2005.
31. DEA administrator Karen Tandy's remarks on Hurwitz sentencing. US Drug Enforcement Administration Web site. Available at: http://www.dea.gov/pubs/pressrel/pr041405b.html. Accessed April 14, 2005.
32. *United States v. Hurwitz*, 459 F.3d 463 (4th Cir. 2006).
33. *United States v. McIver*, 470F.3d 550 (4th Cir. 2006).
34. *McIver, DO v United States of America*, Petition for a Writ of Certiorari to the Supreme Court of the United States (2007).
35. *Washington v Glucksberg*, 521 US 702 (1997).
36. *Vacco v Quill*, 521 US 793 (1997).
37. Burt Robert A. The Supreme Court Speaks—not Assisted suicide but a constitutional right to palliative care. *N Engl J Med* 1997;337:1234–1236.
38. *Gonzales v. Oregon*, 546 v.s. 243 (2006).
39. *Gonzales v. Raich*, 545 v.s. 1 (2005).

CHAPTER 16 ■ OPIOID POLICY, AVAILABILITY, AND ACCESS IN DEVELOPING AND NONINDUSTRIALIZED COUNTRIES

DAVID E. JORANSON, KAREN M. RYAN, AND MARTHA A. MAURER

INTRODUCTION

More than two decades ago, an expert committee of the World Health Organization (WHO) concluded that most pain due to cancer could be relieved if health professionals would use a relatively simple analgesic method and if patients could have access to opioids such as oral morphine.[1] The WHO analgesic method also has been endorsed for relief of pain due to HIV/AIDS.[2]

United Nations (UN) health and regulatory agencies repeatedly have appealed to health professionals, their organizations, and governments to cooperate in order to implement the WHO analgesic method and remove barriers that block patient access to opioid pain medications.[3–7] Although drug regulations and opioid availability have improved in some countries, the vast majority of cancer and AIDS patients in the developing world, and many in developed countries, still lack access to these essential medications. This chapter focuses on opioids that are indicated for moderate to severe pain associated with cancer and AIDS, such as morphine, oxycodone, and fentanyl.

A further disparity exists in reported medical consumption of opioid analgesics between developed nations with a small proportion of the global population and the large and growing population of developing countries. With the shifting burden of cancer and AIDS to developing countries, the public health problem of inadequate availability of pain medications is deepening.[8,9]

Health professionals who manage pain must know about the regulation of opioid analgesics. Just as effective clinical management of pain rests on a body of knowledge, treatment methods, and communication between the clinician and patient, so the task of ensuring access to pain medications in any country depends on knowing the role and responsibilities of national governments and on communication between drug regulators and health professionals.

This chapter outlines the body of knowledge about government drug control policy and the methods that are being developed to assist health professionals and governments to improve opioid analgesic availability and access. "Opioid availability" refers to whether a country has stocks of opioid analgesics either at the manufacturer or retail level of the drug distribution system. The term may be used in referring to the presence of opioids within a country, or at any point throughout the drug distribution system, including in the health care facilities that provide medical care for patients. Alternatively, "opioid accessibility" refers to patients' ability to obtain the opioid pain medications they need for pain relief. Clearly, patient access is not possible unless opioids are available in a country. Therefore opioids may be legally available within a country or even a health care facility, but patients may not be able to access them for a variety of reasons. Cooperation of governments with pain and palliative care experts and their national and international organizations is emphasized.

PAIN RELIEF IS PART OF CANCER AND AIDS CONTROL

The global incidence and prevalence of cancer and HIV/AIDS is a public health problem of great concern. The WHO estimates that there are 22 million people with cancer in the world. Each year approximately 10 million individuals are diagnosed with cancer, and more than 6 million die from this noncommunicable disease. Experts predict that these numbers will double by 2020, with major impacts on developing countries where it is estimated that the majority of new cases and deaths from cancer, including children, will occur.[8,9] The global occurrence of HIV/AIDS is also a critical public health problem. The Joint United Nations Programme on HIV/AIDS (UNAIDS) indicated that in 2007, 33.2 million people were living with HIV/AIDS, a communicable disease, and 2.1 million people died from AIDS.[10]

During the course of their disease, people living with AIDS and cancer survivors experience pain as well as a variety of other symptoms that will negatively impact the quality of their lives.[11] Those nearing the end of life are likely to experience even more severe symptoms.[2,12–15] Common symptoms of cancer include pain, fatigue, anxiety, constipation, cough, depression, dyspnea, and nausea.[1] Patients with cancer or AIDS often have severe pain, particularly during the late stages of the disease.[13,15–19] In the developing world, most cancers are diagnosed in late stage.[16,17] Pain can be due to the disease itself, the treatment of the disease, or another concurrent disorder.

Pain and Palliative Care

Palliative care, including the critically important component of pain management, is a model of care aimed at relieving symptoms of disease and its treatment and improving the patient and family's quality of life throughout the course of the disease. The WHO has long recognized that relieving pain and other symptoms in cancer[1] and AIDS[2,20] is a necessary part of palliative care, including for children.[21]

Palliative care and pain relief medicines should be available and accessible to all individuals who have pain and other symptoms.[2,12] In 2002[22] and 2003,[9] the WHO emphasized that palliative care be part of any national program aimed at reducing the overall burden of cancer, and that it is the government's public health responsibility to develop a policy and program to address palliative care needs in the country. The WHO has expanded its recommendations to include HIV/AIDS control programs: "Palliative care is an essential component of a comprehensive package of care for people living with HIV/AIDS because of the variety of symptoms they can experience—such as pain . . ."[2]

There is a strong international imperative that palliative care, including pain management, should be included in national cancer and HIV/AIDS control efforts. The WHO has reaffirmed the necessity of including palliative care as a critical component of cancer or AIDS control efforts in a country.[23,24] At the country level, national policies should provide a policy framework for developing and expanding health care services to reach patients who need disease treatment as well as relief of pain and other symptoms.

In 2007, the WHO published a guide for developing effective national cancer control programs that include palliative care. This guide reiterated that national palliative care plans must include policy to provide for the medications necessary to manage symptoms associated with cancer, including opioid analgesics for pain.[25]

OPIOIDS ARE ESSENTIAL MEDICINES

There are many useful therapies for treating cancer pain, including pharmacological and nonpharmacological approaches. Opioid analgesics, and in particular orally administered morphine, are regarded by international health experts as the gold standard for relieving moderate to severe pain due to cancer or AIDS. The WHO Expert Committee on the Selection and Use of Essential Medicines has designated morphine and other opioid analgesics as *essential medicines*, which are those medicines that ". . . satisfy the priority health care needs of the population. They are selected with due regard to public health relevance, evidence on efficacy and safety, and comparative cost-effectiveness. Essential medicines are intended to be available within the context of functioning health systems at all times in adequate amounts, in the appropriate dosage forms, with assured quality and adequate information, and at a price the individual and the community can afford. The implementation of the concept of essential medicines is intended to be flexible and adaptable to many different situations; exactly which medicines are regarded as essential remains a national responsibility."[26]

The first WHO essential medicines list, issued in 1977, identified 208 essential medicines for treating the global disease burden, and included morphine to treat pain, thereby recognizing its benefit to public health.[27] In 2007, the 15th edition celebrated the 30th anniversary of the Model Essential Medicines List.[28] This list identified 340 essential medicines and included only morphine, immediate and sustained release, as an opioid analgesic appropriate for the treatment of moderate to severe pain. Currently, 156 of 193 WHO member states have official essential medicines lists.

In 2005, the WHO Cancer Control Program requested that the International Association for Hospice and Palliative Care (IAHPC) recommend a list of essential medicines specifically for palliative care. In 2006, a committee of the International Association for Hospice and Palliative Care Board members and external advisors from 29 pain and palliative care organizations guided the process of identifying the medications to treat the most prevalent symptoms in palliative care. The effort focused on efficacy and safety of medications, with the presumption that cost considerations will be made at the national level. The committee recommended 33 essential medicines (14 are also on the WHO list of essential medicines); the list can be online accessed at http://www.hospicecare.com/resources/pdf-docs/iahpc-list-em.pdf. The list includes four opioid analgesics to treat moderate to severe pain: transdermal fentanyl, methadone, morphine (both immediate and sustained release preparations), and oxycodone. If accepted, this list would expand WHO's list of essential medicines to treat moderate to severe pain, which presently includes only morphine (both immediate and extended release). The WHO will be conducting cost effectiveness analyses and evidence-based reviews of the recommended medications to determine whether it will adopt this list of essential medicines for inclusion in its list for palliative care. Meanwhile, the IAHPC encourages countries to use the list as a model when developing their own lists of essential medicines according to resources and needs.

OPIOID ANALGESICS ARE CONTROLLED DRUGS

Opioid analgesics, in addition to being medicines that are essential for relieving pain, have a potential for abuse and drug dependence. They are "controlled" by an international law called the Single Convention on Narcotic Drugs, 1961, as amended by the 1972 Protocol Amending the Single Convention on Narcotic Drugs, 1961 (Single Convention) (see Fig. 16.1)[29] as "narcotic drugs," a legal term that will be used where the context requires. This chapter addresses opioid analgesics that are agonists with no ceiling effect that can relieve moderate to severe pain, such as morphine, fentanyl, oxycodone, and hydromorphone. This chapter does not address codeine, which is not a pure agonist, or other partial or mixed agonists, such as buprenorphine and pentazocine, which are controlled under the Convention on Psychotropic Substances, 1971.[30]

Nearly every government, or party, in the world has formally acceded to the Single Convention. As of 2006, 181 countries were Parties to the Single Convention, representing 99.6% of the world's population. In so doing, each has agreed to adopt laws, regulations, and administrative procedures to carry out the aims of the Single Convention. The Single Convention establishes obligations to which national governments have acceded, to control opioids and also to make them available for medical purposes.

The premise of the Single Convention rests on the recognition that the consequences of addiction to narcotic drugs pose a threat to society that governments must address: ". . . addic-

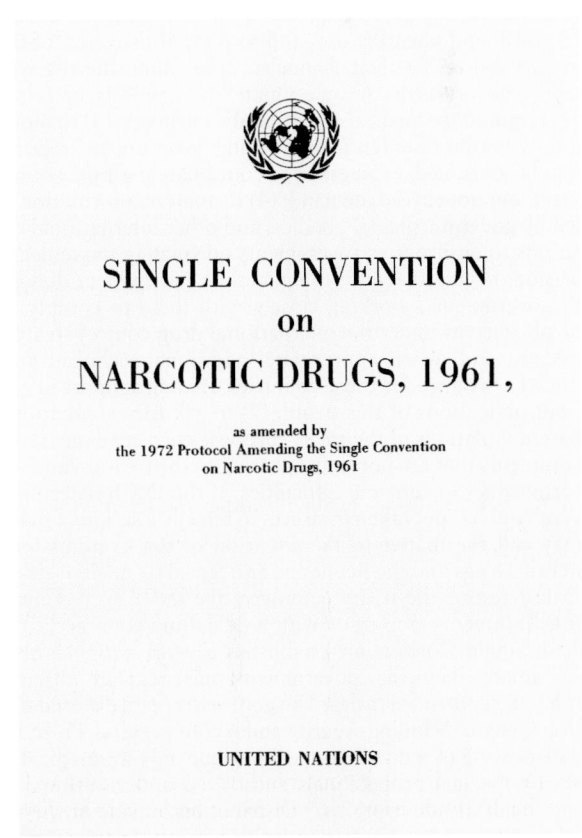

FIGURE 16.1 The United Nations Single Convention on Narcotic Drugs, 1961.

tion to narcotic drugs constitutes a serious evil for the individual and is fraught with social and economic danger to mankind."[28] The Single Convention establishes an international government framework of prohibitions and requirements concerning the legitimate production, manufacture, and distribution that is intended to prevent illicit trafficking, nonmedical use of narcotic drugs, and diversion, which is the illegal movement of controlled medications from the licit distribution system into the illicit market. The most restrictive category under the Single Convention is Schedule I, which includes narcotic drugs considered to be highly addictive and liable to abuse. Morphine and other opioids such as fentanyl, oxycodone, and pethidine are controlled in Schedule I.

According to the Single Convention, several UN organizations have roles in the procedure to schedule drugs. The WHO Expert Committee on Drug Dependence has the responsibility of providing recommendations to the Commission on Narcotic Drugs regarding scheduling drugs.[31] This role is critically important as scheduling decisions can have major implications for the availability of drugs for medical care.

The principal *international* requirement is that legitimate trade in narcotic drugs is regulated, including the cultivation of opium and manufacture of medicinal opioids such as codeine and morphine. To prevent diversion, an import-export system is established to limit trade to the amounts necessary for medical use; trade is regulated by the International Narcotics Control Board (INCB) in Vienna, Austria.

The INCB was established in 1968 as an independent and quasi-judicial monitoring body to implement UN international drug control conventions.[31] The 13 members of the INCB are elected by the Economic and Social Council of the UN and serve as individuals rather than representatives of their governments. The WHO nominates three members who have medical, pharmacological, or pharmaceutical experience. The INCB's responsibilities in regard to opioids include: (1) to ensure, in cooperation with governments, that adequate supplies of drugs are available for medical and scientific uses and to prevent diversion of drugs from licit sources to illicit channels; (2) to administer the system whereby governments must estimate the amounts of narcotic drugs required for medical and scientific purposes; (3) to monitor licit distribution of narcotic drugs using governments' reports of amounts consumed, in an effort to coordinate a supply sufficient to meet, but not exceed, demand; (4) to analyze information provided by governments, UN bodies, and other international organizations to ensure that governments adequately implement the provisions of the treaty; (5) to maintain a "permanent dialogue" with governments, working closely with them to comply with their obligations under the international drug control treaty; (6) to recommend, when appropriate, additional technical and/or financial assistance for those countries needing support in carrying out obligations of this treaty; (7) to ask for explanations of apparent violations of the treaty, propose corrective measures to governments that are not fully adhering to the treaties, and assist governments to overcome difficulties. If the INCB determines a government has not taken measures to remedy a serious situation, it may call the matter to the attention of the Commission on Narcotic Drugs and the Economic and Social Council of the UN. As a last resort, the treaty empowers the INCB to recommend that governments stop trade with a defaulting country.[31]

The Single Convention establishes several *national* obligations, among them that governments must regulate all entities that handle controlled drugs. The goal is to create a closed distribution system, including security and record keeping. Prescribing and dispensing to individuals must be done only for medical purposes by medical professionals authorized under national law, using "medical prescriptions." Distribution outside of the regulated system is prohibited in order to prevent diversion of controlled drugs from medical to nonmedical uses. There is little if any diversion of narcotic drugs from the licit international trade, despite the large number of transactions involved; most diversion of narcotic drugs occurs within domestic circuits.[32] Efforts to prevent diversion should be balanced so as not to interfere in medical practice and patient care.[33,34]

Examples of efforts to lessen the risks of abuse and diversion include risk management plans before marketing of new controlled drugs[35,36]; guidance for clinicians on how to safeguard controlled drugs[37]; education for clinicians about how to assess patients for abuse and drug dependence as well as for pain; and ethics guidelines for how pain medicine specialists can balance the benefits and risks of opioid treatment.[38]

CONTROLLED MEDICINES SHOULD BE AVAILABLE

In addition to controlling drugs to prevent their diversion and nonmedical use, the Single Convention stipulates a second obligation to ensure adequate availability of narcotic drugs for medical and scientific purposes. The Single Convention clearly recognizes the importance of narcotic drugs as analgesic medications, and asserts that medical access to opioids for relief of pain is to be assured by governments, since they are obligated to conform their laws to the Single Convention, ". . . the medical use of narcotic drugs continues to be indispensable for the relief of pain and suffering and that adequate provision must be made to ensure the availability of narcotic drugs for such purposes."[39]

The drug availability obligation is no less important than drug control, but it is poorly understood and implemented by health professionals and governments. There is no indication that the medical value of controlled drugs is lessened as a result of scheduling under the Single Convention. Scholars of international narcotic drug policy have concluded that the Single Convention, as amended, recognizes that the basic purpose of international drug control is to reduce the availability of drugs for nonmedical purposes, but "that this should not affect or limit their therapeutic use."[40]

Government Mechanisms to Ensure Adequate Drug Availability

The INCB recognizes *both* drug control and drug availability obligations of governments:

> One of the objectives of the Single Convention on Narcotic Drugs, 1961 . . . is to ensure the availability of opiates, such as codeine and morphine, that are indispensable for the relief of pain and suffering, while minimizing the possibility of their abuse or diversion.[3]

To accomplish this objective, the Single Convention requires that governments adopt laws, regulations, and administrative procedures to implement two specific mechanisms that are intended to ensure adequate availability of opioid analgesics in countries, while preventing nonmedical use. First, governments must annually establish an estimate of the amounts of opioids that will be required for all medical and scientific needs for the coming year. Licit trade in narcotic drugs can be lawfully conducted only within this amount. If imports exceed a country's estimated requirements, exporters are obligated to refrain from further trade with the country. Governments are encouraged to develop valid estimation methods, to establish estimates that take increasing demand into consideration, to cooperate with health professionals to obtain information about unmet needs, and to increase the estimate whenever necessary to always satisfy medical needs. Second, governments must report the amounts of each narcotic drug consumed (i.e., distributed to the retail level), to allow identification of consumption that either exceeds or falls short of the estimate.

Implementation of Drug Availability: The Competent National Authority

Each Party to the Single Convention is expected to establish a drug control program not only to prevent illicit trafficking and diversion, but also to ensure the adequate availability of narcotic drugs for medical and scientific purposes[5] and to designate an agency called the Competent National Authority (CNA) to implement the functions required by the Single Convention. This office is usually located in the pharmaceutical department of the Ministry of Health, the national drug control or public security agency, or the functions may be divided between agencies. The CNA is the principal national administrative authority for carrying out the estimation and statistical reporting procedures that are necessary for ensuring that opioid analgesics are adequately available for medical and scientific purposes. Guidelines for estimating the amounts of opioids required for medical and scientific use and for reporting consumption statistics are useful for those who want to understand the administrative procedures to be followed by CNAs.[41,42] The INCB provides guidelines for CNAs to comply with the Single Convention, including the administration of effective mechanisms to ensure opioid availability.[43]

DISPARITIES IN OPIOID CONSUMPTION

The Single Convention requirement that national governments report annual consumption statistics provides a unique source of data to describe global and national opioid consumption trends and to study disparities. Consumption means the amounts of opioid analgesics distributed for medical purposes to the "retail" level in a country (i.e., to those institutions and programs that are licensed to dispense to patients, such as hospitals, nursing homes, pharmacies, hospices, and palliative care programs). The INCB uses consumption statistics to: (1) monitor compliance of governments with the provisions of the Single Convention; (2) identify trade discrepancies between importing and exporting countries, (3) detect imbalances between quantities of medications available and disposed within a country; (4) identify trends in the worldwide availability of opioids and other drugs for medical needs; and (5) monitor and maintain a global balance of supply and demand of opioids for medical and scientific needs.[42]

Opioid consumption statistics have several useful applications for those who study and improve opioid availability to: (1) identify whether a country has available opioids that can relieve moderate to severe pain, (2) learn whether the amounts indicate any substantial current consumption or progress over time,[14] and (3) evaluate the outcome of efforts to improve opioid availability.

Consumption statistics provided in INCB reports have several limitations that should be considered when using them as an indicator of opioid availability:

1. Some governments report late, do not report for a particular year or period, or make inaccurate reports, which results in incomplete or invalid information for that year. Consequently, the amounts for the most recent year may be underreported; these deficiencies may be corrected in subsequent years.
2. The INCB's published reports do not provide data on small quantities; instead, the symbol "<<" signifies that a country reported between 0 and 0.499 kg, and also rounds up to 1 kg reported amounts that were reported between 0.5–0.999.[32] Although not available from the INCB's published reports, consumption of small amounts can nevertheless be important, especially in countries with small populations or in those which are just beginning to address their needs.
3. Consumption statistics do not distinguish between clinical

uses for opioids, as in methadone for treatment of pain or drug dependence, or fentanyl for analgesia or anesthesia.
4. Consumption statistics do not distinguish between programs that use opioid analgesics such as hospitals and hospices.
5. Consumption statistics do not indicate which products or dosage forms of an opioid are available within a country (i.e., whether an opioid is in oral, parenteral, or transdermal form).
6. Consumption statistics are not a valid clinical indicator of the quality of pain control in a country.

Morphine Equivalence Metric

The WHO has considered a country's annual consumption of morphine to be an indicator of the extent that opioids are used to treat severe cancer pain and an index to evaluate improvements in pain management.[13,14] The WHO and the INCB have long recognized that pain is inadequately treated owing to low consumption of morphine in most countries, and great disparities between countries.[44,45] Additional opioid analgesic medications and formulations such as fentanyl, hydromorphone, and oxycodone have been introduced in global and national markets over the past 20 years and should be taken into consideration when studying opioid consumption in a country, region, and globally. To what extent does consumption of morphine alone compared with other opioids adequately describe a country's medical use of opioids?

To address this question, the Pain & Policy Studies Group/ WHO Collaborating Center for Policy and Communications in Cancer Care (PPSG/WHOCC) developed a metric called morphine equivalence (ME) for each principal opioid used to treat moderate to severe pain that is expressed in terms of morphine equivalence and adjusted for population. The ME allows an equianalgesic comparison of the consumption of morphine with other opioid medications at the national, regional, and global levels.[45] A total ME statistic combines consumption of several principal opioid analgesics into one metric. The following study drugs were selected to calculate the total ME because they are the opioids that are indicated for severe pain: fentanyl, hydromorphone, methadone, morphine, oxycodone, and pethidine. We used conversion formulas established by the WHO Collaborating Centre for Drug Statistics Methodology in Oslo, Norway.[46] These data were obtained directly from the INCB, thereby eliminating the small quantity limitation; the other limitations of opioid consumption statistics apply to ME data.

Global Trends

The 30-year trend ending in 2005 in Figure 16.2 shows that prior to 1986, morphine ME was very low and stable throughout the world; it was paralleled by total ME. After WHO announced its cancer pain relief three-step analgesic ladder in 1986 and encouraged use of oral morphine, morphine ME began to increase; total ME increased more rapidly and diverged from morphine ME. With the emergence of additional opioids and dosage forms in the mid-1990s, total ME increased even more, so that morphine ME became less and less of a valid indicator of global opioid consumption. In 1986, global morphine ME was 50% of total ME, compared to 14% in 2005. In recent years, fentanyl, methadone, oxycodone, and hydromorphone, respectively, accounted for the greatest portion of opioid consumption, at least for the global aggregate data.

Of interest is the long-term decline in consumption of pethidine (meperidine), likely due to increasing recognition of the potential risks associated with accumulation of the toxic metabolite norpethidine. Pethidine has been used in many countries mainly by injection for postoperative pain because of a perception that its very short duration of action reduces the risk of dependence. Pethidine is no longer recommended by the WHO for the treat-

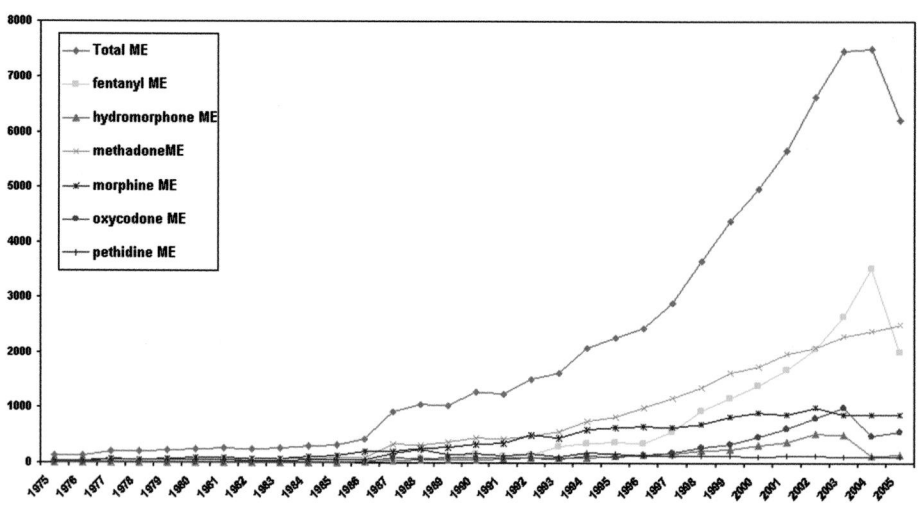

FIGURE 16.2 Global opioid consumption, ME by drug and total ME, mg/capita.

ment of pain[28] although it continues to be used. Programs that move away from pethidine should ensure that other suitable opioids are accessible; if pethidine is available, there should be no regulatory barrier to this transition, as pethidine and other opioids such as morphine are controlled in the same schedule and should be subject to the same international and national controls.

Disparities in Consumption Among High- and Low-Income Countries

At the national and regional level, there are great disparities in the amount of morphine consumed between high- and low-income countries. The INCB has consistently reported that a small number of high-income countries consume most of the morphine in the world, while the remaining countries, which have over 80% of the world's population, consume a small fraction.[47] Is this striking disparity unique to morphine consumption, or are there similar disparities for total ME?

Major disparities in ME are also evident when geographic regions are compared. Table 16.1 shows the milligram per capita total ME for six regions compared to the global total ME for 1975, 1986, and 2005. Global total ME increased fourfold between 1975 and 1986 and 14-fold from 1986 to 2005. Similarly, each of the regions experienced increases in total ME during the 30-year period; however, there were striking disparities between the regional total ME as a percentage of the global total ME. The total ME for Africa, a region with mostly low-income countries, was consistently the smallest percentage of total global ME and

experienced a slight decrease between 1986 and 2005. The regional total ME for Asia, Central and South America, and the Middle East, also regions with predominantly low-income countries, were similar to Africa, representing relatively small percentages of the global total ME and experiencing decreases in the percentage of total global ME between 1986 and 2005. In contrast, Europe, a region with a number of high-income countries, had the largest percentage of total global ME throughout the 30-year period, with a substantial increase in the last 20 years. In 2005, these data showed that Europe and the four high-income countries of Australia, Canada, New Zealand, and the United States represented over 85% of the global total ME.

Country Comparisons

In some countries, morphine alone continues to be a valid indicator of total ME but not in others. Two European countries are compared: the Russian Federation and Belgium. In the Russian Federation, the low and relatively stable consumption of morphine ME has paralleled that of total ME. In Belgium, fentanyl ME has always accounted for the increasing trend in total ME. These differences are interesting and no doubt related to social, cultural, or economic differences between the countries.

Additional studies using the ME statistic are needed to further examine the role of opioid consumption as an indicator of treating pain over the past 20 years. What other events in the pain management/palliative care field may have influenced the changes in the consumption of strong opioids? What are the countries

TABLE 16.1

GLOBAL AND REGIONAL TRENDS IN TOTAL ME (MG/CAPITA)

Year	Africa Total ME	Middle East Total ME	Central and South America Total ME	Asia Total ME	Australia, Canada, New Zealand, U.S. Total ME	Europe Total ME	Global Total ME
1975	3.21 (2%)	7.66 (6%)	8.29 (6%)	10.08 (8%)	41.58 (34%)	53.10 (43%)	123.92
1986	8.99 (2%)	23.05 (5%)	72.63 (16%)	50.16 (12%)	99.6 (23%)	175.38 (41%)	430.93
2005	31.46 (1%)	141.717 (2%)	97.41 (2%)	212.95 (3%)	1551.66 (25%)	4189.31 (67%)	6218.61

Values in parentheses indicate the region's percentage of the global total ME for that year.
Percentages added across rows may not total 100% due to rounding.

for which morphine consumption alone was the most and least accurate, and what might this signify? What are the strong opioids that account for most of the global and regional increase in consumption? The ME statistic may be a useful tool to examine these types of questions at the global, regional, and national levels.

Finally, we identified an important contribution for fentanyl and methadone in the total ME increase over time. Future studies should correct for these medications' other clinical indications to focus solely on their use for pain relief, especially methadone's use for addiction treatment. This procedure will ultimately provide a much more precise measure of national opioid consumption for pain treatment.

BARRIERS: HEALTH PROFESSIONALS AND GOVERNMENTS

A number of factors, or barriers, contribute to inadequate availability of opioid analgesics[49]; their presence and severity vary from country to country. Weakness of health care infrastructure and problems in access to basic services is a typical constraint to obtaining pain relief and palliative care that is found especially, but not only, in developing countries, and in countries with remote areas and challenging geography. This chapter concentrates on the opioid-related barriers involving health professionals, government drug regulatory policies, and drug distribution systems.

Since national laws control drug availability and access, it is useful to know how government drug regulators perceive the issues relating to opioid availability. The INCB surveyed government drug control authorities about barriers in their countries; Table 16.2 lists these barriers.[5] Although the survey was conducted in 1995, the barriers are similar to those of today. Approximately 10 years later, Help the Hospices surveyed health care professionals and hospice or palliative care staff from Asia, Africa, and Latin America about barriers to accessing pain relieving medications and, in particular, oral morphine.[50] Sixty-nine surveys were returned, representing 31 countries and all 3 regions. The barriers to accessing oral morphine can be summarized by the following: (1) excessively strict national laws and regulations; (2) fear of addiction, tolerance, and side effects; (3) poorly developed health care systems and supply; and (4) lack of knowledge on the part of health care professionals, the public, and policy makers.

TABLE 16.2

BARRIERS IDENTIFIED BY 1995 INCB SURVEY

- Fear of addiction to opioids
- Lack of training of health care professionals about the use of opioids
- Laws or regulations that restrict the manufacturing, distribution, prescribing, or dispensing of opioids
- Reluctance to prescribe or stock opioids stemming from fear of legal consequences
- Overly burdensome administrative requirements related to opioids
- Insufficient amount of opioids imported or manufactured in the country
- Fear of diversion
- Cost of opioids
- Inadequate health care resources, such as facilities and health care professionals
- Lack of national policy or guidelines related to opioids

It is important to identify the barriers in a country, distinguish between them, and choose intervention strategies that can be effective. For example, it would be ineffective to use professional education to change strict prescription regulations; changing strict regulations could be part of an effort to alleviate physicians' fears of addiction and of being investigated, but would not do much to change the low priority of pain management or address reimbursement issues. A survey has been developed to gather information about barriers.[51] Once identified, for example, using a convenience survey of participants at a conference, barriers can be studied, prioritized, and categorized: (1) knowledge and attitudes about pain, opioids, and addiction; (2) opioid regulatory policy; (3) the drug distribution system; and (4) cost of opioid analgesics.

Knowledge and Attitudes About Pain, Opioids, and Addiction

Incorrect knowledge about pain, opioids, and addiction often underlies attitudes and can result in medical and institutional practices that block access to opioid analgesics. If professionals who are responsible for regulating drugs are misinformed about addiction, now referred to as *dependence syndrome* in the WHO International Classification of Diseases–10,[52] or have outdated attitudes about the benefits and risks of opioids, they may not be able to accept that there is an unmet need for opioid analgesics and be reluctant to examine regulatory policies for barriers.[1] The International Association for Pain and Chemical Dependency (IAPCD) provides an international forum for considering the relationship between pain and addiction.[53] IAPCD is an international organization with the objective of fostering communication and cooperation among professionals in health care, law enforcement, policy, and regulation in an effort to improve pain management for all patients, including those with a history of, or current, addictive disorders.

Inadequate Education of Health Professionals

The governments who responded to the 1995 INCB survey frequently identified insufficient education of health professionals as a barrier to opioid availability.[5] If health care professionals do not understand the importance of pain management, or how to assess and treat pain, they may be reluctant to care for pain patients or lack the confidence to prescribe medications like morphine. Indeed, given the major advances in knowledge about pain, opioids, and addiction, it is likely that what health professionals and the public learned 20 years ago is inaccurate by today's standards.

Exaggerated Fears of Opioid Dependence Syndrome

The barrier identified most frequently by government narcotic regulators in the 1995 INCB survey was concern about addiction to opioids.[5] Overstated concerns about the risk of dependence syndrome and side effects preventing adequate treatment of pain or regulatory reform is a phenomenon that has been called "opiophobia."[54,55] Early definitions of dependence syndrome were developed by experts in addiction before opioid pain management became a priority. These experts believed that mere exposure to morphine produced dependence syndrome,[56] and that physical dependence, expected in extended use of opioids, was the principal characteristic of dependence syndrome and therefore to be prevented.[52] New knowledge about pain and dependence syndrome has led to official recognition that diagnosis of drug dependence depends on the principal characteristics of compulsive behavior and continued use despite harm, whether or not physical dependence or tolerance is present.[57] Despite evidence that addiction or dependence syndrome—when defined and applied correctly—is not inevitable or even common when opioids are used to relieve pain in patients without a history of substance abuse, fears of addiction continue to impact the treatment decisions of health care professionals resulting in suboptimal pain relief.[58] There is no question that some individuals are susceptible to addiction/dependence syndrome, so a competent assessment of the patient including substance abuse history is indicated, as well as monitoring for warning signs.

Misunderstanding of Side Effects

Patients and families sometimes fear that using opioids to manage pain will result in side effects that cannot be managed.[58] Several side effects are associated with the medical use of opioids, including constipation, fatigue, nausea, vomiting, itching, drowsiness, confusion, and sedation.[13] Health care professionals and patients should realize that side effects are predictable and should be anticipated and treated.[59] Most patients will experience a reduction in many of the side effects, such as sedation and nausea, within the first week of opioid therapy. Constipation does not diminish so clinicians should always advise patients to begin a bowel regimen with opioid therapy.[59] When side effects persist despite treatment, adjustment of the dose and trials of other opioids are indicated.

Fear That Opioids Will Hasten Death

Some fear that the use of opioids for pain at the end of life in terminally ill patients will hasten death owing to the side effect of respiratory depression. This has been shown to be more a myth than reality.[60] Respiratory depression can be a concern when opioids are administered by poorly trained physicians, when the patient has not used opioids previously and the starting dose is too high, when the dose exceeds what is necessary to relieve a patient's pain, when the dose is increased too rapidly, or when the patient does not adhere to the directions for use. However, studies have found that incremental dose increases to relieve pain are safe when pain is severe.[61] If respiratory depression occurs during treatment, it can be reversed by the administration of an opioid antagonist medication such as naloxone, which should be available. Rather than shortening patient survival, some studies suggest that adequate relief from pain can improve quality of life and possibly survival.[61,62]

Health Care Professionals Fear Legal Sanction

The INCB survey showed that governments realize that health care professionals fear legal sanctions. This is a significant barrier leading to reluctance to prescribe opioid analgesics. The WHO has also recognized that health care professionals may be reluctant to prescribe or stock opioid medications if they make a mistake or perceive a risk of losing their professional license, or even criminal prosecution based on misunderstanding of pain, opioids, and addiction.[13] Consequently, it is important that the WHO[13,63] and the INCB[5] have recognized that overly restrictive laws and regulations impede adequate opioid availability in some countries.

Government Regulatory Policy

Clearly, governments' main responsibility is to protect public health and safety; so it is reasonable and necessary for governments to take steps to prevent harm caused by diversion of opioid analgesics to nonmedical uses. But the relevant policies and activities should not interfere in medical practice and patient care. The Single Convention establishes a number of basic requirements for national laws and regulations to establish a "closed" distribution system to prevent diversion:

- everyone involved in the industrial production and medical distribution of narcotic drugs must be authorized to do so by the government;
- medical prescriptions, the format to be decided by governments, must be used to provide opioids to legitimate patients, and only for medical purposes;

- "counterfoil" prescription forms with several copies may be used but they are not required; and
- security, record keeping, and reporting requirements must be observed.[39]

A lack of understanding about how international law intends there to be a balance between controlling diversion and drug availability can lead to overly restrictive regulation of opioid medications. Pain and palliative care advocates should also avoid making opioids available *without* a control system; this would also be unbalanced and could lead to public health and safety consequences.

It should be noted that the systems established by governments to regulate prescription and distribution of opioids were designed before the value of the oral use of opioid drugs for cancer pain management was recognized. These systems were developed to prevent the diversion and abuse of opioids and not to prevent the use of opioids for pain relief.[1]

It is clear that some countries have gone beyond the minimum control measures required by the Single Convention and have established very stringent controls, especially in relation to drug prescription and distribution.[1] The INCB has recognized that some legislators and administrators have overreacted to drug abuse and have enacted laws, regulations, and administrative policies that impede the availability of opiates for medical purposes.[3] These include complex prescription forms and prescription books that must be obtained from the government with considerable difficulty, restrictions that limit the diagnoses of eligible patients, limitations on prescription amount to a few days, limitations on daily dose, and elaborate licensing requirements for palliative care programs. In countries with states, as in India and the U.S., some states have enacted restrictive laws and regulations that interfere with opioid distribution and patient access to opioid pain medications.[64,65]

The Single Convention clearly recognizes that governments have the right to regulate narcotic drugs more strictly than required by the Single Convention. The 34th WHO Expert Committee on Drug Dependence (ECDD) discussed the impact of unduly strict national laws on the medical availability of controlled medications, acknowledging there are countries where stricter measures are applied than are required by the Conventions. While recognizing that this is permissible, the ECDD said that governments should bear in mind that the aims of the Single Convention are to ensure availability for medical use as well as to prevent abuse. The ECDD called on national authorities to carefully consider whether ". . . .any such measure currently in force could be modified to permit access for patients in need."[66]

Drug Distribution Systems

In any country, opioid medications must first be approved and then procured by importation or domestic manufacture from narcotic raw materials or drugs seized by law enforcement. A system of government-regulated distributors then distributes to the retail level of pharmacies, hospitals, clinics, nursing homes, hospices, and palliative care programs, where registered health care professionals prescribe and dispense them to patients. The entire system of medication acquisition and disbursement is referred to as the drug distribution system. Figure 16.3 illustrates the key components of a drug distribution system and Table 16.3 presents examples of drug distribution system barriers.

Cost of Opioid Analgesics

The cost of opioid analgesic products has been identified by international organizations and researchers as a barrier to opioid availability and access.[67-69] Comparative studies have reported

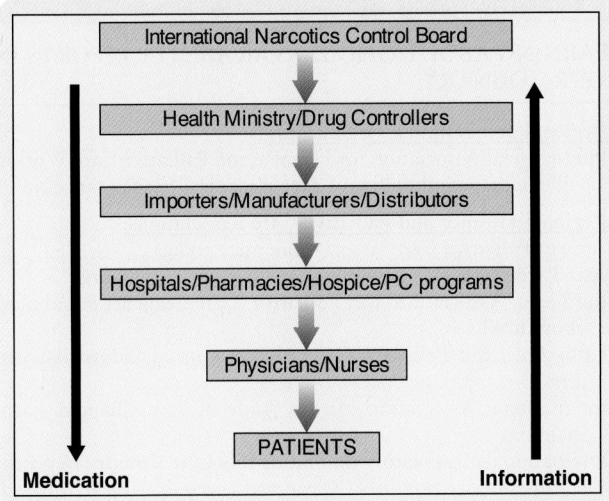

FIGURE 16.3 Drug distribution system.

wide variability in the cost of opioids analgesics throughout the world. One study of developed and developing countries found the cost of opioids relative to income was significantly higher in developing countries than in developed countries.[69] Another comparative study of codeine, fentanyl, morphine, and tramadol in nine developed Western European countries found great variability in the cost of opioids. The wholesale price of morphine was consistently the lowest of all the opioids in each of nine countries over the 3-year study period.[69] A recent survey of cancer pain treatment in Latin American countries revealed that a patient's inability to pay for opioid medications was one of the central reasons they are not prescribed.[68]

UNITED NATIONS' RECOMMENDATIONS

Although there have been efforts to inform health professionals and their organizations about the need to work with government,[50,70] this subject is not well understood among most health care professionals and their organizations because it is not ordi-

TABLE 16.3

EXAMPLES OF DRUG DISTRIBUTION SYSTEM BARRIERS

- Government has not made procurement arrangements for the importation or domestic manufacture of needed opioids.
- There are delays in government decision making about procurement.
- Government's official estimate of type and quantity of opioids required is insufficient.
- The government's method for estimating opioid requirements does not take into consideration the actual needs.
- Manufacturers and distributors do not distribute opioids in a timely way.
- The number of health professionals, pharmacies, and patient care facilities authorized to procure and dispense opioids to patients who need them is insufficient.
- Governments do not have the systems in place to guarantee a safe and effective transfer of medications from wholesalers to retailers.

narily included in medical education. A brief historical review of the recommendations of UN bodies shows they have made a number of useful observations and recommendations to governments and health professionals, including that they should cooperate with each other to ensure adequate availability of opioids for medical purposes including pain relief throughout the world. Indeed, representatives of national governments, acting through their membership in UN bodies such as the Economic and Social Council and its Commission on Narcotic Drugs, and the World Health Assembly, have for a number of years requested governments to evaluate their national drug control policies for impediments and to improve the availability of opioid analgesics for medical purposes.

Beginning in 1989, a consultation between the INCB and the WHO Cancer Unit, then led by Dr. Jan Stjernsward, produced an authoritative recognition of the opioid availability problem and a strong recommendation that governments should act to evaluate their national laws. The INCB requested governments throughout the world to "examine the extent to which their health-care systems and laws and regulations permit the use of opiates for medical purposes, identify possible impediments to such use and develop plans of action to facilitate the supply and availability of opiates for all appropriate indications."[3]

In 1990, the WHO Expert Committee on Cancer Pain Relief and Active Supportive Care made a recommendation similar to that of the INCB, requesting that national governments should conduct a "regular review [of legislation], with the aim of permitting importation, manufacture, prescribing, stocking, dispensing and administration of opioids for medical reasons, . . . [and] review of the controls governing opioid use, with a view to simplification, so that drugs are available in the necessary quantities for legitimate use."[4]

In 1995, the INCB returned to the subject of opioid availability for pain relief and conducted a survey to determine whether governments had responded to its 1989 recommendations. The responses of the 65 responding governments were analyzed and published along with several pointed conclusions and recommendations including that "governments that have not done so should determine whether there are undue restrictions in national narcotics laws, regulations or administrative policies that impede prescribing, dispensing or needed treatment of patients with narcotic drugs, or their availability and distribution for such purposes, and should make the necessary adjustments."[5] The INCB outlined its expectations for governments under the Single Convention: "A national drug control programme should have legislative authority reflecting the provisions of the 1961 Convention, delegation of responsibility for implementation, including administrative responsibility for managing import and export licenses, estimating medical requirements, reporting required statistics and supervising adequate controls over distribution. Controls over the professionals and medical facilities that distribute narcotic drugs should ensure accountability and prevent diversion while making narcotic drugs available to the patients who need them. Controls should not be such that for all practical purposes they eliminate the availability of narcotic drugs for medical purposes."[5]

The INCB called specific attention to the role of health professionals, recommending that their organizations, including the International Association for the Study of Pain (IASP), teach students and practitioners about the medical use of opioids, their adequate control, and the correct use of terms related to dependence.[5] The INCB further recommended that IASP and other nongovernment organizations establish ongoing communication about national requirements, unmet medical needs, and impediments to availability with the CNAs in their countries. Such recommendations are consistent with the ethical responsibilities of physicians to comply with all laws and regulations but also to work toward changing them if they interfere in the practice of medicine and patient care.[38]

The INCB requested and received a number of comments from

national chapters of the IASP including from Canada, Chile, Colombia, Hungary, Japan, Kenya, Malaysia, New Zealand, the Philippines, Republic of Korea, Russian Federation, Singapore, Slovakia, the United Kingdom, and the U.S. Summaries of these comments were included in the INCB's report (see http://www.incb.org/pdf/e/ar/1995/suppl1en.pdf)

One INCB recommendation in particular was to the WHO to develop "methods that can be used by government and nongovernment organizations to identify impediments to the appropriate medical availability of narcotic drugs."[5] Subsequently, the WHO revised its seminal publication *Cancer Pain Relief*[1] to include a Guide to Opioid Availabilty[13] and designated the Pain and Policy Studies Group (PPSG) at the University of Wisconsin to be a WHO Collaborating Center (WHOCC), with terms of reference to develop methods to improve opioid availability. The PPSG/WHOCC drafted international guidelines for evaluating national opioids control policy. In 2000, the WHO and the INCB approved them, emphasizing that governments should use the guidelines to examine their laws and regulations and health care systems to identify impediments and to ensure that opioid medications are always available to patients when they are needed.[73] The WHO also proposed that governments encourage health care workers to report to the appropriate authorities any instance in which oral opioids are not available for cancer patients.[1]

In 2005, the UN Economic and Social Council adopted a resolution about the treatment of pain using opioids,[6] found online at http://www.un.org/docs/ecosoc/documents/2005/resolutions/Resolution%202005-25.pdf. It recognizes that medical use of narcotic drugs is indispensable for the relief of pain and suffering, that low national consumption of opioids is a matter of great concern, and that opioids such as morphine should be available at all times in adequate amounts and appropriate dosage forms to relieve severe pain. A resolution by the World Health Assembly[7] in the same year called for the development of a funding mechanism to facilitate the actions necessary to improve the availability of opioids for the treatment of pain.[72] See online at http://www.who.int/gb/ebwha/pdf_files/WHA58-REC1/english/A58_2005_REC1-en.pdf and http://www.who.int/medicines/areas/quality_safety/Framework_ACMP_withcover.pdf

Taken together, these findings and resolutions form an unmistakable and uncontroversial imperative from the highest level of international and national government health and regulatory authorities in the world that governments and health professionals should work together to identify and remove impediments to the adequate availability of opioids for medical purposes.

METHODS AND EXAMPLES

There are several approaches to consider when implementing the United Nations' recommendations to review drug control policies and address identified barriers to opioid availability. The following section outlines approaches, methods, tools, and resources that national governments or palliative care advocates can use to develop and implement a national project to improve opioid availability.

The specific activities and the order in which they are carried out may not be the same in every country because of differing national situations. We discuss a general approach for a national project, but the activities outlined should be considered flexible and be adapted to a country's situation. Some of the activities may already have occurred, or may need to be repeated to garner broader support and new steps or stakeholders may emerge as the project develops. A national project usually begins as a result of leadership of one or more professionals in pain management, palliative care, or drug regulation.

TABLE 16.4

LEARNING ABOUT OPIOID AVAILABILITY EFFORTS IN YOUR COUNTRY

Regional and National Organizations:
International Association for Hospice and Palliative Care Worldwide hospice and palliative care directory: hospicecare.com/

Regional Hospice and Palliative Care Associations:
African Palliative Care Association: apca.co.ug/
Asia Pacific Hospice Palliative Care Network: aphn.org/
European Association for Palliative Care: eapcnet.org/about/about.html
Latin American Palliative Care Association: cuidadospaliativos.org/
International Association for the Study of Pain Chapters: iasp-pain.org
International Observatory on End-of-Life Care Country Reports:
The Observatory provides "Clear and accessible research-based information about hospice and palliative care provision in the international context. We present public health and policy data relating to hospice and palliative care services. This is complemented by material drawn from the social and cultural analysis of end of life issues, including ethnographic, historical and ethical perspectives. You will find data here for over 61 countries in Eastern Europe, Central Asia, Africa, South America and the Middle East in ways which facilitate cross-national and regional comparison and analysis." eolc-observatory.net/global_analysis/index.htm

---

Assessing the Country Opioid Availability Situation

An important initial step when beginning an effort to improve opioid availability is to collect and review available information about a country's pain and palliative care situation, such as how much opioid medication is currently being used, and if there are activities underway to improve opioid availability. There are a number of resources that can provide this type of information, such as the Country Profiles on the PPSG/WHOCC website, which will be discussed in greater depth in the next section. Sometimes a more formal needs assessment has been accomplished,[72] however, it is very important to assess those factors that relate directly to the unmet needs for opioid analgesics and how they are controlled and distributed. Table 16.4 offers suggestions for identifying the extent and nature of existing efforts by regional or national organizations toward improving palliative care or opioid availability in a particular country. With increasing interest in opioid availability in many parts of the world, it is important for the planners to identify those who are interested or already involved in order to exchange information and coordinate activities.

Identification of Barriers to Opioid Availability

After an assessment of the situation and stakeholders in a country, the next step in the process may be to identify the regulatory barriers to adequate opioid availability. The WHO Achieving Balance Guidelines is the central resource; it offers a framework for understanding and specific criteria for assessing regulatory barriers. The criteria are recommended by international authorities.[74] The Guidelines were approved by a group of international experts in pain management and drug regulation and were reviewed and endorsed by the INCB, so they constitute the highest level of international health and drug regulatory consensus.

The WHO Guidelines are based on the principle of "Balance" which is derived from the Single Convention. This principle asserts that governments' obligation to control narcotic drugs is not only to prevent drug abuse, but also to ensure the availability of opioid analgesics for medical purposes. Controls aimed at preventing drug abuse and diversion must not interfere with the adequate availability of opioid analgesics for patients' pain relief; drug abuse controls that interfere in opioid availability and patient access to effective pain care would be considered out of balance and should be identified and corrected.

Sixteen guidelines are recommended for use in assessing the adequacy of national drug control policy and administration, and encourage governments and health care professionals to cooperate in a study process using the guidelines. Each guideline or criteria is explained and documented; the guidelines should be used to evaluate the adequacy of: (1) policy language in laws and regulations, (2) administration of the estimates and statistics system, and (3) the functioning of the system that distributes opioid pain medications.

The Guidelines contain a Self Assessment Checklist (SAC) that can be used to familiarize the planners with the nature of the evaluation criteria, to guide an assessment activity within a group of interested parties, and to summarize findings.[74] Once barriers are identified, additional information and review may be necessary to refine the analysis so that it is specific enough to discuss with regulators and to guide strategic planning of interventions.

Other methods to identify barriers may be used as well, such as interviews with key informants or focus groups with those who are familiar with patient care, unmet needs, and the national regulatory framework (e.g., clinicians, pharmacists, and regulators).[45]

Mechanisms of Change

Making change in national policy usually requires a government mechanism to allow the needs and action plans to be discussed and agreed upon. A direct dialogue between health professionals and government regulators can result in modifications to regulatory policy. Sometimes a more formal mechanism such as a task force or commission is needed to convene the stakeholders and guide a strategic planning process. A task force or commission appointed by the government can be a powerful mechanism, since government willingness to examine policy is a necessary component of changing government policy. Less formal methods such as a committee or task force of a nongovernment organization may be a good place to begin to study the problem, review relevant literature, raise awareness, and formulate a preliminary analysis. In any case, thoughtful fair leadership is always needed from one or more individuals who have the time, energy, credibility, communication ability, and willingness to listen and guide a process. The relevant body should prepare a report of its deliberations, including information about the needs, barriers, results of the policy evaluation, and recommended changes. The recommendations do not need to be limited to government regulations, and may include other aspects of national policy and program that are relevant to meeting the needs of people with cancer and HIV/AIDS. Needs assessments, such as the WHO Achieving Balance Guidelines, can provide a structure for the deliberations. The report should reflect a consensus so that points of disagreement, which could block later progress, are resolved early in the process. The following examples illustrate successful mechanisms that guided the policy change process in Italy and Uganda.

Italian Ministerial Workgroup

In 1998, health care organizations publicly requested the Italian Ministry of Health and other nongovernment organizations to address barriers to opioid availability by amending the opioid prescribing laws.[75] The Drug Department of the Ministry of Health responded by appointing a multidisciplinary workgroup of physicians, pharmacists, and representatives of the Ministry of Health who had experience in cancer, pain management, palliative care, opioid legislation, and pharmacology. The objectives of the workgroup were: (1) to recommend changes to the Italian national opioid prescribing law, (2) to identify and make available the drugs necessary for pain relief, and (3) to develop educational information on cancer pain management to educate the public and health care professionals.[76] Leadership was provided by leading palliative care physicians who reached out to the PPSG/ WHOCC for technical assistance.

Ugandan Ministry of Health Study Group

In 1998, the Ugandan Ministry of Health invited staff from Hospice Africa Uganda, a nongovernment organization that had pioneered community-based palliative care in rural and urban Uganda, to be technical experts in a pilot study looking at the viability and safety of using morphine to treat chronic pain at the community level.[77] The study involved semi-structured interviews with key informants, direct observation of morphine distribution throughout the country, and audits of clinical care quality. The Ministry's leadership and involvement with the study enhanced the government's awareness of the need to make policy change.

The Strategic Plan

Developing a strategic plan to address barriers to opioid availability is a critical phase in a national project. The strategic planning process typically begins after the leaders have reviewed the literature, and used the BOAT and the SAC and/or other techniques to identify barriers.

In an effort to make a strategic plan realistic and achievable, the plan should focus on three to five of the most important opioid availability/access problems in a country which, if successfully addressed, would contribute to significant immediate and sustained improvements in patient access to pain medications. A strategic planning process requires some preparation, and can take place during a national event such as a workshop or commission, or in a regional workshop where country teams meet separately to develop and then share their strategic plans for comment.

Regional Workshops

Several workshops to improve opioid availability have been organized cooperatively between the WHO, PPSG/WHOCC, and national and/or regional nongovernment organizations that have an interest in relieving pain due to cancer and HIV/AIDS.[20,78–84] These 3-day regional workshops involved carefully selected teams of health care and regulatory professionals, including a representative of the CNA, from five or six countries in the same region. Drawing together countries in a particular region allows for participants to learn together about the methods to improve opioid availability, as well as common challenges and opportunities among the participating countries. These workshops culminate in a strategic planning process and specific action plans, and sometimes result in country teams working to implement a national project to address barriers to opioid availability. Leadership, availability of resources, and technical cooperation are critically important to successful follow-up implementation of strategic plans.

National or State Workshops

A national or state workshop involving the stakeholders (e.g., regulators, expert health care practitioners, and patient care programs) can be a useful mechanism to initiate or continue the dialogue that is needed to improve opioid availability for medical needs. A workshop can be an opportunity to increase awareness by reviewing relevant literature, exchanging information among the stakeholders about pain management, palliative care, laws and regulations, and need for opioids leading to a report. Workshop participants can develop an action plan to submit to the government for its approval and action. The following example highlights a recent national workshop in Colombia.

Colombia

The CNA in Colombia is the Fondo Nacional de Estupefacientes (FNE) of the Ministry of Health. In cooperation with the PPSG/WHOCC and the WHO, the Fondo convened a national workshop of drug regulators and palliative care physicians in November 2007 to examine the procurement and distribution systems for opioid analgesics throughout the country. The goal was to improve these systems so that patients have better access to these essential pain medications from a well-functioning distribution system. The workshop, hosted by the Universidad de la Sabana, included representatives from the Ministry of Health (MOH), the WHO, the Pan American Health Organization (PAHO), the PPSG/WHOCC, the Colombian National Cancer Institute (INC), the International Association for Hospice and Palliative Care (IAHPC), the Colombian Chapter of the International Association for the Study of Pain (ACED), and the Colombian Association for Palliative Care. This workshop yielded excellent communication between health care practitioners and regulators from the 32 states in 6 national regions. Six regional break-out sessions were used to identify problems and obstacles as well as solutions. The six groups reported on their findings in a plenary session, where a strategy session was held to discuss possible solutions and to decide on recommendations to be presented to the FNE.

Implementation of Policy Changes

Improving national policy by itself is not sufficient to improve opioid availability and patient access. It is critically important to work with relevant government and nongovernment organizations to implement policy changes: this may include communication of policy changes to the public via the media (e.g., newspaper articles, radio announcements); for example, education of health care professionals, drug regulators, and law enforcement, including how the policy changes will impact their professional responsibilities. The following example from Kerala, India, illustrates the importance of translating policy changes into practice to positively affect patient care.

Kerala, India

In 1999, a task force appointed by the Kerala Health Secretary was successful in simplifying the state morphine rules, and a national policy was changed which exempted palliative care programs from the requirement to have a "drug license" to dispense morphine (which requires employing a pharmacist, a substantial cost to the program).[64] The policy improvements enhanced the efforts of the Pain and Palliative Care Society, a nongovernment organization based in Kerala, to expand greatly the number of palliative care clinics throughout the state to reach patients in rural and remote areas. The number of palliative care clinics in Kerala increased from 21 in 2000 to 68 in 2006.[85]

Case Example–Romania

The following example summarizes a recent national policy project to improve opioid availability and accessibility in Romania. This example highlights a series of activities and tools that were used by the Romanian leaders to achieve policy change and embark on implementation.

Regional Workshop

In 2002, the PPSG/WHOCC, the WHO European regional office (EURO), and the Open Society Institute (OSI) sponsored a 3-day regional workshop in Budapest, Hungary,[45] entitled *Assuring Availability of Opioid Analgesics for Palliative Care*. The workshop was attended by teams of health are professionals and drug regulators from six Eastern European countries: Bulgaria, Croatia, Hungary, Lithuania, Poland, and Romania.

Strategic Planning

During the workshop, the six country teams used the WHO Guideline's SAC to identify barriers to opioid availability and develop an action plan for addressing those barriers. The team of Romanian health care professionals and drug regulators identified lack of morphine in most hospital pharmacies, severe restrictions on the out-patient use of opioids, and a complex regulatory system for prescribing opioids.[45]

Readiness for Policy Change

The workshop organizers had limited resources for follow-up and decided to choose one country on which to concentrate. Romania was identified as the country with the most potential for making policy changes because (1) it had many regulatory barriers that restricted patient access to opioids, (2) it had palliative care leaders who were highly motivated to work on making changes, and (3) the Ministry of Health, where the Competent Authority was located, was willing to establish a palliative care commission to evaluate national drug control policy and provide recommendations for change.[45]

Establishing a Mechanism: A Ministry of Health Commission

A Commission was a critical factor contributing to the successful policy change process in Romania. Following the regional workshop in 2002, the Romanian Ministry of Health appointed a Commission of Pain and Palliative Care specialists to study the narcotics control policies using the WHO Guidelines. The Commission requested assistance from the PPSG who assisted with the review and analysis of policies. A report of recommended policy changes was prepared and presented to the Minister of Health. This report became the basis for the changes in law and regulations that followed.[45]

Policy Change

The Minister of Health directed the Pharmaceutical Department to draft new legislation removing barriers that had been identified according to the Commission's recommendations. The proposed law was adopted by the Romanian Parliament in 2005. A team from the Ministry of Health CNA and the Commission came to the University of Wisconsin in 2004 to concentrate on drafting a regulation to implement the new law. The regulations, from which remaining barriers were removed, were approved in 2006 and became effective in 2007.[86]

Implementing Policy Changes

A process to implement the new law and regulations began with a meeting in Bucharest in 2006. All the major stakeholders, including representatives of palliative care, cancer, HIV/AIDS, the CNA, medical education, and the anti-drug law enforcement agency convened for a day to discuss how the new law and regulations would be successfully implemented. The meeting, titled "Implementing a modern and balanced opioid legislation in Romania," was attended by approximately 40 people, including the Vice Chair of the Parliament Commission for Health. The meeting provided an opportunity to educate all parties about opioids for treating pain under the new law and regulations. It was also an opportunity to clarify any questions and to clear any doubts so there would be a consensus.

Educational Program

The Palliative Care Commission also recognized that it was necessary to develop a national education program and a curriculum to re-educate health care practitioners about how to prescribe opioid analgesics under the new regulations so as to improve pain management. A new Curriculum Planning Committee, including experts in palliative care and pharmacy from the University of Wisconsin, was developed to prepare a training of trainers program to reach physicians and pharmacists throughout the country. It consists of 20 hours of classroom teaching on two consecutive weekends and 6 hours of clinical practice in each participant's own setting. The courses include interactive case studies, are recognized by the Ministry of Health, and are nationally accredited for continuing medical education by the College of Physicians and Pharmacists.[86] In the first year, approximately 2,200 physicians were trained (D. Mosoiu, personal communication, October 30, 2007).

NEW RESOURCES FOR NATIONAL POLICY PROJECTS

Several new resources are being developed to support policy reform activities and to accelerate the rate of change in the world.[87]

International Pain Policy Fellowship

The PPSG/WHOCC has learned that making policy and systems change in a country is more likely to be successful if three criteria are met:

1. A demonstrated unmet need for opioid analgesics for pain management due to regulatory barriers.
2. A committed pain or palliative care "champion" to work with the PPSG and also the government.
3. A demonstrated government commitment to address regulatory barriers.

In order to expand leadership for change in more countries, the PPSG/WHOCC developed an International Pain Policy Fellowship (IPPF), supported by a grant from the Open Society Institute's International Palliative Care Initiative. The IPPF seeks to provide candidates with the knowledge and skills necessary to develop and implement a project to improve the availability of pain medications for pain relief and palliative care in their respective countries. The 2-year Fellowship is intended for health professionals (for example pharmacists, oncologists, AIDS clinicians, pain and palliative care physicians), health care administrators, policy experts, or lawyers from low- or middle-income countries who have an interest in drug policy advocacy to improve availability of opioid analgesics for pain relief and palliative care.

The Fellowship consists of (1) education regarding the role of international drug control treaties, governments, health care professionals, and opioid analgesics in the treatment of pain; (2) a 1-week training session at the University of Wisconsin Paul P. Carbone Comprehensive Cancer Center in Madison, Wisconsin; and (3) follow-up technical assistance to the Fellows for the duration of the 2-year Fellowship. The training curriculum covers the relationships between disease, pain, palliative care, inadequate opioid availability; examines the international legal framework for drug control, national government responsibilities to ensure

drug availability, and examples of regulatory barriers; and provides resources for evaluating national policy as well as examples of their use. This specialized curriculum, based in large part on the WHO Guidelines, "Achieving Balance in National Opioids Control Policy," addresses the dual, often competing, characteristics of opioid analgesics: their necessity for pain relief but also their potential for abuse.

The application process is competitive, based on demonstrated national leadership to develop pain management and/or palliative care; the strength of commitment to improving opioid availability in their country; position in national cancer, AIDS, pain, or palliative care association(s); and potential ability to develop a working relationship with government officials. Those selected as finalists are invited to a telephone interview for more in-depth discussions and examination of the potential for a successful Fellowship.

The inaugural IPPF was held in October 2006 with eight Fellows from Argentina, Colombia, Nigeria, Panama, Serbia, Sierra Leone, Uganda, and Vietnam. Additional funding provided by the United States Cancer Pain Relief Committee allowed seven members of an International Expert Collaboration in palliative care and opioid availability to attend the training session to assist PPSG/WHOCC staff to present the curriculum, guide the discussions, assist with country Action Planning, and follow up. These global experts have maintained follow-up communication and mentoring, in conjunction with PPSG/WHOCC staff, during the remainder of the 2-year Fellowship.

At the end of the week, the Fellows prepared detailed national Action Plans that will guide their activities to improve patient access to opioid analgesics for the next 2 years, in collaboration with the PPSG/WHOCC.

In September 2007, the *New York Times* published a series about the global undertreatment of pain including in India[87] and Sierra Leone.[89] One article highlighted the situation in Sierra Leone, including the work of the International Pain Policy Fellow, who is the founder and Executive Director of Shepherd's Hospice in Freetown. He is implementing his action plan to improve patient access to pain medication. Working with the government, he is making progress to import oral morphine at the hospice to provide patients with appropriate pain management, he has trained his staff on the appropriate uses and handling of morphine, and he is taking part in a national Palliative Care Task Force.

These Action Plans are ambitious, each addressing unique and dynamic national environments characterized by political changes (such as national elections) and other unforeseen factors that impact national health care priorities. Consequently, the PPSG/WHOCC obtained funding from the Lance Armstrong Foundation to reconvene the 2006 class of fellows to discuss progress and challenges as they work toward the objectives outlined in their national Action Plan. The 3-day meeting allowed for (1) an update and discussion with each country on progress and barriers in the past 12 months; (2) break-out into small groups to revise the Action Plan, if necessary; (3) a report from each Fellow on their Action Plan revisions for the remainder of their Fellowship; and (4) preliminary exploration of the meaning of cancer survivorship in developing countries. This type of meeting can capitalize on the inevitable changes in national landscape that will occur during a 2-year period by providing a real-time forum to review and respond to both their achievements and challenges, and to utilize the collective experiences of the entire group that may allow Fellows to share methods for handling a particular obstacle that may be common among them.

IPPF Progress

Vietnam. On 27 March 2007, a national workshop, "Workshop on Supply, Management and Use of Opioids in Palliative Care" was held in Hanoi, Vietnam. The workshop, which included a broad range of stakeholders from throughout the country, was successful in accomplishing the following stated objectives: (1) to enhance understanding of the Principle of Balance in national narcotics control policies and the WHO- and INCB-supported narcotics policies, and (2) to agree on the action plan for 2007–2008 to ensure the availability of opioids used in palliative care. Participants divided into small working groups to discuss the action plan and to assign tasks. A consensus was reached that revisions and enhancements should be made to the current regulation on the supply, management, production, and use of opioids in palliative care. The following day, the Ministry of Health formally approved the new Action Plan. The Ministry of Health will now develop new prescribing regulations for opioids to improve availability which include the following policies aimed at improving availability as well as control:

1. The prescription length for opioids for terminal cancer and AIDS patients will be increased from 7 to 30 days.
2. The maximum dose of opioid prescriptions which was 30 mg will be eliminated.
3. The requirement for physicians and pharmacies to maintain opioid prescription records will be reduced from 5 to 2 years.
4. Opioids will be available in all districts throughout the country. If a district has no pharmacy that stocks opioids, the pharmacy of the district hospital will be required to stock opioids.
5. The Drug Administration of Vietnam (DAV) within the MoH revised its regulations on Procurement, Purchase, Distribution, Storage & Dispensing of Narcotic and Psychotropic Drugs following WHO, INCB guidelines.
6. The DAV will regulate conditions for production, importation, exportation, storage, distribution, and retailing of opioids and psychotropic drugs.
7. Any pharmacy that meets the standards of "Good Pharmacy Practice" (GPP) and "Good Store Practice" (GSP) will be able to sell opioids and psychotropic drugs. (In the past, only very few pharmacies could do this.)
8. Requirements for reporting of controlled medication supply and distribution and of estimated need will be revised in line with a newly designed, decentralized supply chain.
9. Templates for reporting, estimation, and bookkeeping will be revised to be in line with the improved management system.

Planning is underway for the second class of International Pain Policy Fellows in 2008.

Internet Course

Another way to accelerate change is to make the body of knowledge and experience more easily accessible to an international audience. Funded by the National Hospice and Palliative Care Organization (NHPCO), the PPSG/WHOCC developed a Web-based course about national drug control policies' impact on access to opioid analgesics for pain relief that will be available free of charge in 2008. The aim of the course is for learners to understand the body of knowledge encompassing the evaluation and improvement of national policies that govern the medical availability of opioid analgesics for cancer and AIDS patients. The course is intended for an international audience of health care professionals, local and national policy advocates, government drug regulatory personnel, national health policy advisors, and medical scholars. The course is accessible via the PPSG/WHOCC Web site (http://www.painpolicy.wisc.edu/on-line_course/welcome.htm).

Essential Elements of National Drug Control Policy

A question often encountered during the course of the PPSG/WHOCC's policy evaluation work in a number of countries is whether there exists a balanced model law that could be adopted or adapted to simplify drafting of new legislation. Although several model laws have been produced by UN agencies, PPSG/WHOCC has found none that address adequately the obligation to ensure drug availability. Further, our experience shows there is great variability among national laws. Each country has its own cultural history and health care systems. Their laws are so unique that wholesale replacement with a one-size-fits-all is not likely to be accepted. Consequently, the PPSG/WHOCC developed, in consultation with the WHO, the UN Office of Drugs and Crime, and the INCB, a report about the "essential elements" of a modern national opioids control policy that will present reasonable expectations for national policies, based on the obligations that were established in the Single Convention and the subsequent official interpretations of the drug control conventions and expert guidance from international health and regulatory bodies. See report at http://www.painpolicy.wisc.edu/internat/model_law_eval.pdf.

PPSG/WHOCC Web Site Resources

Some important parts of the body of knowledge regarding opioid availability are not easily accessible. The PPSG/WHOCC has established an international section of its website (http://www.painpolicy.wisc.edu) to provide worldwide public access to key resources and information. The international section contains most of PPSG/WHOCC's international publications and links to other important articles about opioid availability; monographs that present the opioid consumption trends globally, regionally, and nationally; as well as links to other relevant resources and organizations pertinent to specific countries. The 2000 WHO guidelines, "Achieving Balance in National Opioids Control Policy," in 23 languages, are readily accessible from the home page and from each country page.

Country Profiles

A new and useful place to begin learning about the status of opioid consumption in a country is the Country Profile on the PPSG website. These profiles include: (1) the country population and a map, (2) the country's status of adherence to the Single Convention and whether the country has reported consumption statistics and submitted estimates to the INCB, (3) the contact information for the Competent National Authority, (4) opioid consumption statistics, and (5) links to relevant national resources regarding pain, palliative care, and opioid availability.

CONCLUSION

Deepening disparities between high-, low-, and middle income countries in the extent of availability of opioid pain medicines means that pain and suffering in the world is an increasing public health problem. This is cause for alarm and should precipitate concerted action by health professionals, their organizations, and their governments. Actions should be guided by an understanding not only of the need for pain medicines, but also the barriers, the drug control policy framework, and how to work with government drug regulators.

However, health care professionals from any country are not likely to know about these topics because they have not generally been included in basic professional education or continuing education about pain and palliative care. The purpose of this chapter is to outline the body of knowledge, methods, and experience that is relevant to understanding and improving national opioid availability and patient access to pain medicines.

How can this information be applied? Pain and palliative care specialists often are involved in the planning and delivery of training and education for colleagues in other countries, where availability and access to opioid pain medicines is likely to be limited. Each of these occasions presents an opportunity, if not an ethical imperative, for the visiting professional to learn about the national opioid situation and to address availability and access issues knowledgeably and appropriately.

This approach might result in presentations that include a discussion of the pharmacology of analgesics with emphasis on the opioids that are necessary to relieve severe pain, discussion of the types of barriers that may interfere in pain relief, explanation of national governments' obligation to ensure *adequate* opioid availability and the role of the Competent National Authority, encouragement to address the barriers, and where to find resources that can be used to improve opioid availability and access.

Although the body of knowledge about the control and availability of opioid analgesics may not be well known, the process of working with individual countries to improve opioid availability borrows from a method with which health professionals are very familiar. The elements of the medical model can be applied to solving problems in opioid availability: evaluation, diagnosis, and a treatment plan. Indeed, health care professionals and governments in India, Romania, and Uganda have worked together to diagnose opioid availability barriers and implement action plans to remove the barriers. New efforts to diagnose and treat barriers are being led by International Pain Policy Fellows in other low- and middle income countries.

There are hopeful signs of progress in some countries, but it is not likely that this progress—which is still in an early developmental phase—is sufficient to gain on the deepening global disparities in access to pain relief medications. Greater leadership will be needed from international drug control bodies, national governments, and from individual health professionals and their organizations.

References

1. World Health Organization. *Cancer Pain Relief.* Geneva, Switzerland: World Health Organization; 1986.
2. World Health Organization HIV–AIDS. *Palliative Care.* Geneva, Switzerland: World Health Organization; 2004.
3. International Narcotics Control Board. *Report of the International Narcotics Control Board for 1989: Demand for and supply of opiates for medical and scientific needs.* Vienna, Austria: United Nations; 1989:E.89 XI.5.
4. World Health Organization. *Cancer pain relief and palliative care: Report of the WHO Expert Committee on Cancer Pain Relief and Active Supportive Care.* Geneva, Switzerland: World Health Organization; 1990: WHO Technical Report Series, No. 804.
5. International Narcotics Control Board. *Report of the International Narcotics Control Board for 1995: Availability of opiates for medical needs.* New York: United Nations; 1996.
6. United Nations Economic and Social Council. *Treatment of pain using opioid analgesics; Resolution 2005–25.* Report on the forty-eighth session of the Commission on Narcotic Drugs E/2005/28; 19 March 2004 and 7–11 March 2005; Issued 22 July 2005. Available at: http://www.un.org/docs/ecosoc/documents/2005/resolutions/Resolution%202005–25.pdf.
7. World Health Assembly. *Cancer Prevention and Control.* Geneva, Switzerland: World Health Organization; 2005:WHA 58.22
8. Boyle P. The globalisation of cancer. *Lancet* 2006;368:629–630.
9. World Health Organization. *World Cancer Report.* Lyon, France: IARC Press; 2003.
10. United Nations Programme on HIV/AIDS, World Health Organization. *AIDS Epidemic Update.* Geneva, Switzerland: UNAIDS Information Centre; 2007.
11. Burton AW, Fanciullo GJ, Beasley RD, et al. Chronic pain in the cancer survivor: A new frontier. *Pain Med* 2007;8(2):189–198.
12. World Health Organization. *Symptom Relief in Terminal Illness.* England: Scientific Publishing/Clays; 1998.
13. World Health Organization. *Cancer Pain Relief: With a Guide to Opioid Availability.* 2nd ed. Geneva, Switzerland: World Health Organization; 1996.
14. Foley KM, Wagner JL, Joranson DE, et al. Pain control for people with cancer and AIDS. In: Jamison DT, Breman JG, Measham AR, et al., eds. *Disease Control Priorities in Developing Countries.* New York: Oxford University Press; 2006:981–993.
15. Frich LM, Borgbjerg FM. Pain and pain treatment in AIDS patients: A longitudinal study. *J Pain Symptom Manage* 2000;19(5):339–347.
16. Goudas LC, Bloch R, Gialeli-Goudas M, et al. The epidemiology of cancer pain. *Cancer Invest* 2005;23:182–190.
17. Davis MP, Walsh D. Epidemiology of cancer pain and factors influencing poor pain control. *Am J Hosp Palliat Care* 2004;21(2):137–142.
18. Breitbart W, Rosenfeld BD, Passik SD, et al. The undertreatment of pain in ambulatory AIDS patients. *Pain* 1996;65:243–249.
19. Larue F, Fontaine A, Colleau SM. Underestimation and undertreatment of pain in HIV disease: Multicentre study. *BMJ* 1997;314:23–28.
20. World Health Organization. *A community health approach to palliative care for HIV/AIDS and cancer patients in sub-Saharan Africa.* Geneva, Switzerland: World Health Organization; 2004.
21. World Health Organization. *Cancer Pain Relief and Palliative Care in Children.* Geneva, Switzerland: World Health Organization in collaboration with the International Association for the Study of Pain; 1998.
22. World Health Organization. *National Cancer Control Programmes: Policies and Managerial Guidelines.* 2nd ed. Geneva, Switzerland: World Health Organization; 2002.
23. World Health Organization Programme on Cancer Control. *Strategies to improve and strengthen cancer control programmes in Europe.* WHO Consultation held in Geneva, Switzerland; 25–28 November 2003.
24. World Health Organization, International Union Against Cancer. *Global Action Against Cancer.* Geneva, Switzerland: World Health Organization; 2005.
25. World Health Organization. *Cancer Control: Knowledge into Action–Palliative Care.* Geneva, Switzerland: World Health Organization; 2007
26. World Health Organization. *Essential medicines* (website). Geneva, Switzerland: World Health Organization; 2005.
27. World Health Organization. *Essential Medicines – WHO Model List.* 1st ed. Geneva, Switzerland: World Health Organization; 1977.
28. World Health Organization. *Essential Medicines – WHO Model List.* 15th ed. Geneva, Switzerland: World Health Organization; 2007.
29. United Nations. *Single convention on narcotic drugs, 1961, as amended by the 1972 protocol amending the single convention on narcotic drugs, 1975.* New York: United Nations; 1977.
30. United Nations. *Convention on Psychotropic Substances.* Geneva, Switzerland: United Nations; 1971.
31. International Narcotics Control Board. *1961 Single Convention on Narcotic Drugs: Part 1: The International Control System for Narcotic Drugs.* Vienna, Austria: International Narcotics Control Board; 2005.
32. International Narcotics Control Board. *Report of the International Narcotics Control Board for 2006.* New York: United Nations; 2007.
33. Joranson DE. Why is a balanced policy important, and do we have it now? In: Wilford BB, ed. *Balancing the response to prescription drug abuse, report of a national symposium on medicine and public policy.* Chicago, Ill: American Medical Association, Department of Substance Abuse; 1990:1–6.
34. Joranson DE. Guiding principles of international and federal laws pertaining to medical use and diversion of controlled substances. In: Cooper JR, Czechowicz DJ, Molinari SP, et al., eds. *Impact of prescription drug diversion control systems on medical practice and patient care: monograph 131.* Rockville, MD: U.S. Department of Health and Human Services, Public Health Service, National Institutes of Health, National Institute on Drug Abuse; 1993:18–34.
35. Katz NP, Adams EH, Benneyan JC, et al. Foundations of opioid risk management. *Clin J Pain* 2007;23(2):103–118.
36. Cicero TJ, Dart RC, Inciardi JA, et al. The development of a comprehensive risk-management program for prescription opioid analgesics: Researched abuse, diversion and addiction-related surveillance (RADARS). *Pain Med* 2007; 8(2):157–170.
37. Department of Health, Medicines Pal. *Safer management of controlled drugs: A guide to good practice in secondary care* England; 2007.
38. American Academy of Pain Medicine Council on Ethics. *Ethics Charter.* Glenview, IL: American Academy of Pain Medicine; 2005.
39. United Nations. *Single Convention on Narcotic Drugs, 1961.* Geneva, Switzerland: United Nations; 1973.
40. Bayer I, Ghodse H. Evolution of international drug control, 1945–1995. *Bull Narc* 1999; 51(1–2):1–17.
41. International Narcotics Control Board. *1961 Single Convention on Narcotic Drugs: Part 2: The Estimates System for Narcotic Drugs.* Vienna, Austria: International Narcotics Control Board; 2005.
42. International Narcotics Control Board. *1961 Single Convention on Narcotic Drugs: Part 3: The Statistical Returns System for Narcotic Drugs.* Vienna, Austria: International Narcotics Control Board; 2005.
43. International Narcotics Control Board. *Guidelines for National Comptetent Authorities.* Vienna, Austria: International Narcotics Control Board; 2007.
44. International Narcotics Control Board. *Report of the International Narcotics Control Board for 2004.* New York: United Nations; 2005.
45. Mosoiu D, Ryan KM, Joranson DE, et al. Reform of drug control policy for palliative care in Romania. *Lancet* 2006;367(9528):2110–2117.
46. Ryan KM, Joranson DE, Gilson AM. Toward a more complete indicator of opioid consumption trends. Paper presented at: 7th International Conference on Pain & Chemical Dependency; New York; June 21–24 2007. Madison, WI, University of Wisconsin Pain & Policy Studies Group/WHO Collaborating Center for Policy and Communications in Cancer Care; 2007.
47. World Health Organization Collaborating Centre for Drug Statistics Methodology. *Anatomical Therapeutic Chemical/Defined Daily Dose.* Oslo, Norway: Norwegian Institute of Public Health; 2007.
48. International Narcotics Control Board. *Report of the International Narcotics Control Board for 2003.* New York: United Nations; 2004.
49. Rhymes JA. Barriers to effective palliative care of terminal patients. An international perspective. *Clin Geriatr Med* 1996;12(2):407–416.

50. Adams V. *Access to pain relief: An essential human right.* London: Help the Hospices for the Worldwide Palliative Care Alliance; 2007.
51. Joranson DE. Availability of opioids for cancer pain: Recent trends, assessment of system barriers, new World Health Organization guidelines, and the risk of diversion. *J Pain Symptom Manage* 1993;8(6):353–360.
52. World Health Organization. *The ICD-10 Classification of Mental and Behavioral Disorders: Clinical Descriptions and Diagnostic Guidelines.* Geneva, Switzerland: World Health Organization; 1992.
53. International Association of Pain and Chemical Dependency. International Association of Pain and Chemical Dependency website. Accessed January 29, 2008.
54. Morgan JP. American opiophobia: Customary underutilization of opioid analgesics. In: Hill CS, Fields WS, eds. *Advances in Pain Research and Therapy.* Vol 11. New York: Raven Press; 1989:181–189.
55. Bennett DS, Carr DB. Opiophobia as a barrier to the treatment of pain. *J Pain Palliat Care Pharmacother* 2002;16(1):105–109.
56. World Health Organization. *WHO expert committee on drugs liable to produce addiction: Third report.* Geneva, Switzerland: World Health Organization; 1952:technical report series 57.
57. World Health Organization. *The ICD-10 classification of mental and behavioural disorders: Clinical descriptions and diagnostic guidelines.* F1x.2 Dependence syndrome; Geneva, Switzerland; 2006 version.
58. Forbes K. Opioids: Beliefs and myths. *J Pain Palliat Care Pharmacother* 2006; 20(3):33–35.
59. Doyle D, Hanks GWC, Cherny N, et al. *Oxford Textbook of Palliative Medicine.* 3rd ed. New York: Oxford University Press; 2004.
60. Fohr SA. The double effect of pain medication: Separating myth from reality. *J Palliat Med* 1998;1(4):315–328.
61. Portenoy RK, Sibirceva U, Smout R, et al. Opioid use and survival at the end of life: A survey of a hospice population. *J Pain Symptom Manage* 2006;32(6): 532–540.
62. Bercovitch M, Adunsky A. Patterns of high-dose morphine use in a home-care hospice service. *Cancer* 2004;101:1473–1477.
63. World Health Organization. *Guiding principles for small national drug regulatory authorities.* World Health Organ Drug Info 1989;3(2):43–50.
64. Joranson DE, Rajagopal MR, Gilson AM. Improving access to opioid analgesics for palliative care in India. *J Pain Symptom Manage* 2002;24(2):152–159.
65. Gilson AM, Joranson DE, Maurer MA. Improving state pain policies: Recent progress and continuing opportunities. *CA Cancer J Clin* 2007;57(6):341–353.
66. World Health Organization. *WHO expert committee on drug dependence: thirty-fourth report.* Geneva, Switzerland: World Health Organization; 2006.
67. Mercadante S. Costs are a further barrier to cancer pain management. *J Pain Symptom Manage* 1999;18(1):3–4.
68. Moyano J, Ruiz F, Esser S, et al. Latin American survey on the treatment of cancer pain. *Eur J Palliat Care* 2006;13(6):236–240.
69. De Conno F, Ripamonti C, Brunelli C. Opioid purchases and expenditure in nine western European countries: 'Are we killing off morphine?' *Palliat Med* 2005;19:179–184.
70. De Lima L, Sweeney C, Palmer JL, et al. Potent analgesics are more expensive for patients in developing countries: A comparative study. *J Pain Palliat Care Pharmacother* 2004;18(1):59–70.
71. Colleau SM. Highlights of the INCB report. *Cancer Pain Release* 1996; 9(suppl):1–4.
72. World Health Organization. *Access to Controlled Medications Programme - Framework.* Geneva, Switzerland: World Health Organization; 2007.
73. Green K, Kinh LN, Khue LN. *Palliative Care in Vietnam: Findings from a Rapid Situation Analysis in Five Provinces.* Hanoi, Vietnam; 2006.
74. World Health Organization. *Achieving balance in national opioids control policy: Guidelines for assessment.* Geneva, Switzerland: World Health Organization; 2000.
75. Federazione Nazionale Ordini dei Medici Chirurghi e Odontoiatri, Associazione Europea per le Cure Palliative, Associazione Italiana di Oncologia Medica, et al. *Proposta di modifica della legge sugli stupefacenti.* S I M G Rivista di Politica Professionale della Medicina Generale 1998;8(Ottobre):10–12.
76. Blengini C, Joranson DE, Ryan KM. Italy reforms national policy for cancer pain relief and opioids. *Eur J Cancer Care (Engl)* 2003;12(1):28–34.
77. Logie DE, Harding R. An evaluation of a morphine public health programme for cancer and AIDS pain relief in Sub-Saharan Africa. *BMC Public Health* 2005;5(82):1–7.
78. Joranson DE, Nischik JA, Gilson AM, et al. *Consumo de analgésicos opioides en el mundo y la región andina. Preparado para: Taller de Reguladores: Asegurando Disponibilidad de Analgésicos Opioides para Cuidados Paliativos;* Quito, Ecuador; 3–5 Diciembre de 2000. Madison, WI: University of Wisconsin Pain & Policy Studies Group/WHO Collaborating Center for Policy and Communications in Cancer Care; 2000.
79. World Health Organization Regional Office for Europe. *Assuring availability of opioid analgesics for palliative care.* Meeting report of opioid availability workshop held in Budapest, Hungary; February 25–27, 2002. Copenhagen, Denmark, World Health Organization Regional Office for Europe; 2002.
80. Pain & Policy Studies Group. *Availability of opioid analgesics in Eastern Europe and the world.* Prepared for the Workshop on Assuring Availability of Opioid Analgesics for Palliative Care; Budapest, Hungary; February 25–27, 2002. Madison, WI: University of Wisconsin Pain & Policy Studies Group/WHO Collaborating Center for Policy and Communications in Cancer Care; 2002.
81. Pain & Policy Studies Group. *Availability of opioid analgesics in Africa and the world.* Prepared for the WHO meeting, "A Community Health Approach to Palliative Care for HIV/AIDS and Cancer Patients in Africa"; Gaborone, Botswana; July 9–12, 2002. Madison, WI: University of Wisconsin Pain & Policy Studies Group/WHO Collaborating Center for Policy and Communications in Cancer Care; 2002.
82. Pain & Policy Studies Group. *Availability of Morphine and Pethidine in the World and Africa, With a special focus on: Botswana, Ethiopia, Kenya, Malawi, Nigeria, Rwanda, Tanzania, Zambia.* Prepared for Advocacy for Palliative Care in Africa: A Focus on Essential Pain Medication Accessibility. Entebbe, Uganda; June 27–29, 2006. Madison, WI: University of Wisconsin Pain & Policy Studies Group/WHO Collaborating Center for Policy and Communications in Cancer Care; 2006.
83. African Palliative Care Association. *Advocacy workshop for palliative care in Africa.* Kampala, Uganda: African Palliative Care Association; 2007.
84. Pain & Policy Studies Group. *Availability of morphine and pethidine in the world and Africa with a special focus on: Cameroon, Cote d'Ivoire, Ghana, Nigeria, Sierra Leone, The Gambia.* Prepared for Advocacy for Palliative Care in Africa: A Focus on Essential Pain Medication Accessibility; May 9–11, 2007. Madison, WI: University of Wisconsin Pain & Policy Studies Group/WHO Collaborating Center for Policy and Communications in Cancer Care; 2007.
85. Kumar S. Kerala, India: A regional community-based palliative care model. *J Pain Symptom Manage* 2007;33(5):623–627.
86. Mosoiu D, Mungiu OC, Gigore B, et al. Romania: Changing the regulatory environment. *J Pain Symptom Manage* 2007;33(5):610–614.
87. Ryan KM. The Pain & Policy Studies Group. *J Pain Palliat Care Pharmacother* 2007;21(4):35–37.
88. McNeil DG. In India, a quest to ease the pain of the dying. *The New York Times.* September 11, 2007;D1–D5.
89. McNeil DG. Drugs banned, world's poor suffer in pain. *The New York Times.* September 10, 2007;A1–A12.

CHAPTER 17 ■ MEDICAL EVALUATION OF THE CHRONIC PAIN PATIENT

GORDON IRVING AND PAM SQUIRE

INTRODUCTION

Evaluation of a patient with acute pain is usually straightforward. A simple history of the presenting painful condition, physical evaluation, and appropriate investigation is standard and in most cases adequate. Persistent pain with a limited focus such as osteoarthritis of one or two joints without significant comorbidities can also be relatively straightforward and a limited pain assessment is appropriate. Chronic pain, however, is much more complex, with patients often developing anxiety and depression. They may also exhibit somatic preoccupation as well as a tendency to develop other life problems. The pathological cause of the pain (the pain generator) may be unknown (as in fibromyalgia). The intensity of the pain may seem to be out of proportion to any obvious pathology. Faced with a disease they do not understand and anxious about hurting themselves further, many patients will avoid activities that may exacerbate their pain, which eventually leads to feelings of unworthiness and poor self-esteem. Compounding these issues, the medications themselves may contribute to reduced functionality.

The effect of these complex interplays between pain and its comorbidities results in a life that spirals downward, often becoming pain-centered with life deterioration of such severity that many of these patients admit to suicidal ideation. Failure to identify and address all factors contributing to the patient's "total pain" will prevent the implementation of effective treatment strategies, often leading to mutual frustration between patient and physician. The objective of a pain assessment is to determine all of these relevant factors. The initiative on Methods, Measurement, and Pain Assessment in Clinical Trials (IMMPACT)[1,2] were published primarily to improve and standardize methodology in clinical trials but can be modified for practicing clinicians.[3] This chapter utilizes some of the IMMPACT recommendations and suggests a format to document the evaluation in a way that facilitates both sharing and transfer of information between health care professionals. Time efficient, validated tools designed to expedite an assessment done in either a multidisciplinary clinic or by a solo practitioner assessment have been included. Sourcing information for these tools is available at the end of the chapter.

PROCESS OF ASSESSMENT

A multidisciplinary team best evaluates complex chronic pain patients. However, in today's health care environment, the time to evaluate complex pain patients is often limited and assessments are commonly completed by a solo practitioner. In this chapter, interview techniques to reduce this burden and patient completed questionnaires have been included or Internet referenced. Pain assessments using electronic questionnaires that integrate into existing electronic medical records (EMRs) are becoming more common. Any Web-based questionnaire should allow drop down boxes if an answer is positive, enabling greater detail to be asked. Ideally, it should also allow integration with the practitioner's EMR and the patient's own personal electronic health record if they have one. The use of Web-based or paper questionnaires should save the practitioner time and enable more focused questioning.

Initial and follow-up assessments will be handled differently, depending on whether the practitioner is a primary health care giver or a pain specialist.

A detailed examination of the patient presenting with specific pain syndromes (e.g., low back pain, headaches, complex regional pain syndromes) will not be addressed in this chapter. These are described in the chapters allotted to those problems. Details of the psychological and psychiatric assessments will also be covered in other chapters. In this chapter, the authors present a general guide to the clinician.

General Guidelines

Assessment and treatment of a patient with complex pain begins with the recognition that a complete pain cure is unlikely. The best results are achieved by utilizing approaches that involve both the available community resources as well as the patient taking more responsibility in their own therapy. Involvement by the patient in decision-making and goal setting is important. Improving the patient's physical and mental functioning is the goal.

Time Allotment

This depends on the type of practice. A pain specialist may allot 30 to 90 minutes to assess a new patient; the busy primary care practitioner may only have 15 to 20 minutes. The use of a physician extender (either a self-completed questionnaire or another person who can document this information for the physician) can speed up the encounter by having the patient's history available before the practitioner enters the examination room. Alternatively, the assessment can be divided and information can be completed over several different visits.

An initial comprehensive questionnaire can be sent to the patient prior to the consultation (see Appendix), or a Web-based one developed. Asking the patient to arrive 20 to 30 minutes early prior to the initial appointment enables relevant paperwork and insurance verification to take place, and gives time for the patient to complete questionnaires if not already done. A companion, preferably a significant other, should accompany the patient when possible for the initial evaluation and when optimizing or initiating new therapies. By having this individual sit at the patient's side, much information can be gathered about the couple's relationship by body language as well as by visual and verbal expression. The companion may also contradict or confirm whether a therapy is working, either verbally or by gesture.

Successful evaluation of a patient with complex pain by a clinician is facilitated by the development of a mutually trusting relationship. Patients should have the feeling that they have been listened to, their fears have been acknowledged, and that the practitioner is "there for them." This latter statement does not imply the practitioner has to feel the suffering of the patient.

The practitioner should remain empathic, not sympathetic, to the patient's issues.

OUTLINE OF A MULTIDIMENSIONAL ASSESSMENT FOR PERSISTENT PAIN HISTORY

The following format for documentation of a multidimensional pain assessment is recommended for complex patients. It serves to ensure that all the various dimensions of pain have been assessed and serves, when dictated in this format, to facilitate communication with other treating clinicians.[4,5]

Pain History

- Details of pain history and associated symptoms
- Details of previous consults and investigations
- Previous treatments tried and details of the outcomes
- Current medications, including over-the-counter medications and other treatments.

History of Past Health Relevant to the Presenting Problem

- Those comorbidities that could influence the manifestation of the pain syndrome (dementia, diabetes)
- Those comorbidities that could influence treatment (renal failure, cardiovascular disease, sleep disturbance)

Psychiatric Comorbidity

- Anxiety, depression, bipolar disorder, posttraumatic stress disorder (PTSD), adult attention deficit hyperactivity disorder (ADHD)

Psychosocial Factors

- Individual personality features which impact pain (catastrophizing, health-related anxiety, pain-related fear and associated avoidance behaviors)
- Factors that may contribute to pain interruption of life (solicitous spouse, meaning of the pain)
- Other factors (specific family or cultural issues, employment history, litigation issues, financial situation, family and/or community support)
- Pain coping strategies
- Relevant family history, including sexual abuse and adverse childhood events

Risk of Addiction

- Screening—if opioids or cannabinoids are currently being used, requested, or will be considered; determine if the addiction risk is low, medium, or high[6]
- Smoking history[7,8]
- Previous drug and/or alcohol exposure and related outcomes (attendance at drug or alcohol detoxification or rehabilitation programs or legal or social problems)
- Family history of drug, alcohol, or psychological/psychiatric problems[9]

Assessment of Function

- To determine the impact of the pain on a person's life and provide a baseline for follow-up assessment
- It should cover all of the relevant areas and usually includes impact of pain on domains such as employment, social, recreational, family, or home responsibilities. It should assess self care, sleep, and ideally evaluate the overall quality of life

Goals

- Determine patient goals to direct treatment and evaluate effectiveness of therapeutic interventions

Physical Examination

- Mental status examination as appropriate
- General physical examination and, if appropriate, look for evidence of substance abuse/misuse and document its presence or absence
- Focused pain examination, paying attention to musculoskeletal and neurological examination
- Further investigations or consults as needed and consider:
  - urine drug testing
  - medication logs
  - diaries to assess pain, sleep, activity, or other relevant behaviors
  - informed consent documentation, opioid or behavioral contracts.

Follow-Up Visit

- To review goal achievement
- To review "homework" (pain diaries, medication logs)
- To interview a significant other
- Need to document (5As):
  - Analgesic response both to pain score and function
  - Activity response
  - Adverse events (to treatment)
  - Aberrant drug-related behavior if potentially addictive medications such as opioids and /or cannabinoids are prescribed
  - New Action plan of care

THE PAIN HISTORY

It is important to document medical etiologies of all contributing pain diagnoses. The pain may be categorized according to the taxonomy of the International Association for the Study of Pain (IASP).[10] The mechanism, if known, date of onset and overall severity, and factors that worsen or improve pain should be noted. Having a routine when evaluating a patient ensures capture of all the relevant data. It can be formally done during an interview by having the history form outlined with headings or captured by a questionnaire. For children or patients with cognitive impairment, a caregiver should be present to provide additional information.

The Short Form of the McGill Pain Questionnaire (SF-MPQ)[11] is a self-report measure of pain quality. The Brief Pain Inventory (BPI)[12] is another self-reporting tool that includes a pain diagram and several scales to assess pain severity and interference with function and is recommended by IMMPACT.

The acronym OPQRST has been suggested as a mnemonic for assessing each individual pain problem.

O = Onset
P = Provocative/Palliative
Q = Quality/Character (Does it have neuropathic features?)
R = Region/Radiation
S = Severity/Intensity
T = Timing of pain (Continuous or intermittent?)

O: Onset of Pain

How pain began is often informative.

In many cases the initial acute pain is well documented with an understandable etiology. In other cases, there does not appear to be an obvious organic cause. In these cases the physician has to be careful not to ascribe the pain to psychogenic causes but to accept the patient's description.[13]

P: Provocative/Palliative

Assessing what provokes or relieves the pain provides valuable clues to the diagnosis.

Leg and back pain due to spinal stenosis has a characteristic pattern of worsening with walking or standing, with the pain being totally relieved with sitting or lying. Neuropathic pain can present with spontaneous pain or pain provoked by different stimuli such as cold, light touch, or the brushing of sheets. It is usually improved with heat, often the opposite of inflammatory pain.

Q: Quality or Character

Neuropathic pain symptoms include numbness, tingling, pins and needles, electric shocks or shooting pain, and hot or burning pains. Questionnaires to identify neuropathic pain (and differentiate it from nociceptive pain) include the LAANS scale,[14,15] The Neuropathic Pain Questionnaire,[16,17] painDetect,[18] the DN4[19] and ID-Pain,[20] and the Neuropathic Pain Scale.[21] Associated symptoms are often important in formulating a diagnosis. A severe recurrent bilateral headache accompanied by photophobia, phonophobia, nausea, and vomiting in an otherwise healthy female suggests a migraine. In patients with suspected neuropathic pain it is important to ask about associated symptoms involving activation of the sympathetic nervous system. Inquire about changes in hair and nail growth, sweating, skin color and temperature, or swelling. The latter four may not be evident on the day of examination as they are often intermittent. They can sometimes be documented by photograph if the patient is able to provide this. Many patients with complex regional pain syndromes will have subtle motor abnormalities. They may volunteer weakness but not mention tremor, dystonia, or motor incoordination unless specifically asked. Patients with neuropathic pain may also experience altered and sometimes bizarre sensations and, since many pain patients struggle to have their pain believed, they may not volunteer certain information. For example, they may hesitate to describe formication (a sensation of bugs crawling under their skin), or a sudden feeling of cold water running down one leg, for fear of appearing "crazy." Asking directly about these types of symptoms is helpful.

R: Region/Radiation

The different sites of pain can be visually represented by having the patient draw their pain on a pain diagram. Neuropathic characteristics can be represented at the same time by using symbols

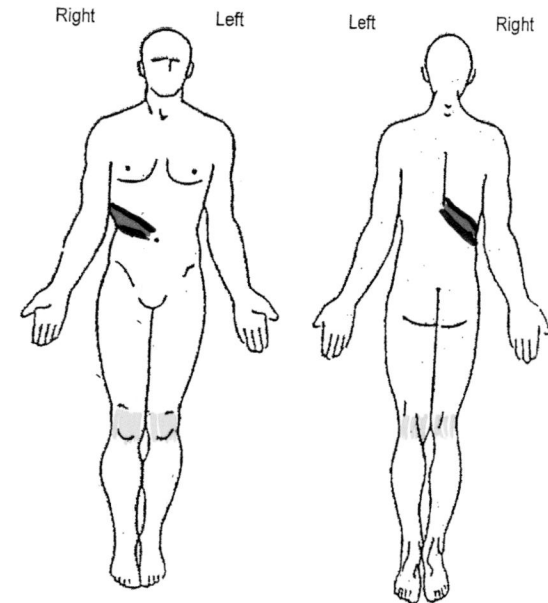

Name _____   Date _____

Please color the areas where you experience pain. Use one of these five coloring pens to shade the specific type of pain that you are experiencing. Then circle with a pen all areas of pain and starting with the worst, number the areas in order of severity.

Red   - burning   If you have other pain   Yellow - Aching
Green - tingling   sensations name them
Blue - numbness   here and color as black   Black - _____
                     or yellow

FIGURE 17.1 The pain diagram of a patient with postherpetic neuralgia and bilateral osteoarthritis of the knees.

or adding colors to the diagram (i.e., red for burning, green for tingling, blue for numbness) (Fig. 17.1).

S: Severity/Intensity

There are several different rating scales validated as measures of pain severity. The one chosen should be appropriate for the patient's abilities and preferences. The Numeric Rating Scale (NRS) is the most commonly used. A patient simply rates pain on a scale between 0 and 10 where "0" represents no pain and "10" represents the "worst pain imaginable." The visual analogue scale (VAS) consists of a 10-cm line anchored at the 0 end with the words "no pain" and at 10 with "the worst imaginable pain." The patient then makes a mark on the line consistent with their pain rating.

Many physicians have difficulty when patients rate their pain score with a number that seems to be at odds with their demeanor and functionality. Acknowledging to the patient that you believe they must have significant pain and then offering further anchors to the scale often results in a different rating that may be more meaningful in follow-up. The following script may be helpful in a patient who has rated their pain as 15/10:

"I believe you have pain that is severe and it is obviously very distressing to you but I am not quite sure how to interpret your rating because I do need a number between 0 and 10. If I say 0 means absolutely no pain and 10 out of 10 pain would be severe burns to most of your body or the pain you would feel if your hand was caught in a meat grinder, where would you rate your pain?" A patient who initially described their pain as 15/10 will often adjust their rating when belief, acknowledgment, and new anchors are provided.

Infants, children, the elderly, and others with cognitive impairment all require pain assessment scales designed to address their individual needs. Many different scales have been developed for these special populations and the reader is directed to separate chapters in this book for more detail.

T: Timing of Pain

The timing of pain can provide diagnostic clues to pain etiology. Neuropathic pain is often spontaneous. Patients report episodes of severe pain without any provocation while nociceptive pain, such as osteoarthritis of the hip, is usually not severe unless provoked by use. The typical timing of cluster headaches differentiates it from the ice pick headache and the intermittent nature of trigeminal neuralgia would differentiate it from herpes zoster pain of the fifth cranial nerve.

Previous Treatments Tried and Details of the Outcomes

The initial questionnaire should allow the patient to list all the therapeutic modalities they are currently using or have used in the past. These could include prescription medications, nonprescription or complementary formulations, as well as interventions such as biofeedback, physiotherapy, massage therapy, anesthetic pain blocks, or surgeries. It is important to determine which ones the patient feels are useful as well as which were ineffective or produced intolerable side effects.

Current Medications Including Over-the-Counter and Other Treatments

A complete list of the patient's present medication should be recorded and any changes documented at each follow up. This is especially important if the patient is seeing other specialists who are prescribing medications as this poses an increased risk for unsuspected drug interactions. Inquire about other alternative therapists treating and/or prescribing nonprescription medications, herbs, or supplements. Many of these interact with prescribed medications or create other side effects and should be documented (for specific information go to the Memorial Sloan-Kettering Cancer Center Web site at www.mskcc.org/aboutherbs)

HISTORY OF PAST HEALTH RELEVANT TO THE PRESENTING PROBLEM

Medical history relating to the possible etiology of the pain is important as it may predict other pain problems either currently or in the future (i.e., multiple sclerosis or Parkinson's). Document history of comorbidities that could influence either the manifestation of the pain (i.e., dementia) or treatment choices (i.e., liver or renal insufficiency).

Many comorbidities occur in patients suffering chronic pain. Common relevant comorbidities include:

- **Dementia:** This may alter the manifestation of pain. Simple tests such as the mini mental status should be available to give to patients who are suspected of being in the early stages of dementia. Pain and depression scales should be appropriate for the degree of cognitive impairment. It is important to have a caregiver present at the evaluation in these situations.

- **Renal or hepatic compromise:** These will obviously affect many metabolic functions and reactions to medications. Initial baseline laboratory tests should be considered before commencing or continuing to prescribe many medications.
- **Sleep disturbance:** The relationship between pain and sleep dysfunction can be complex and over 70% of patients with chronic pain report sleep disturbance.[22] Most patients report that sleep is interrupted due to pain and many develop unhealthy sleep patterns. A sleep history should always be asked with questions to identify sleep apnea, restless leg syndrome, and monoclonic leg movements. Patients with PTSD may have significant sleep disturbance from nightmares. Effective treatment of sleep disturbance will involve assessing and treating all of the contributing factors.

PSYCHIATRIC COMORBIDITIES

Anxiety and depression are common and may decrease the patient's tolerance to pain, in turn reducing their coping ability. There are many different assessment tools for depression. Ideally, a tool validated for chronic pain patients should be used. The IMMPACT committee[23] recommended using the Beck Depression Inventory (BDI). A change of ≥5 points on the BDI was recommended by IMMPACT to be considered a reasonable estimate of a clinically important change when assessing treatment efficacy in follow-up.

Other validated easy to use depression tools include the Hamilton Depression Scale, the Zung Self-Rating Depression Score, and the Hospital Anxiety and Depression Scale (HADS).

The HADS can also be used for anxiety as can the General Anxiety Disorder Scale (GAD7) and the Beck Anxiety Inventory.

Other psychiatric comorbidities that may affect pain management and should be assessed include bipolar disorder, PTSD, and ADHD.

PSYCHOSOCIAL ASSESSMENT

Psychosocial factors are important variables in the comprehensive assessment of chronic pain. Numerous relevant factors have been described and there are multiple assessment tools and measures to evaluate them. Unfortunately, at present there is no consensus in the literature to direct the clinician regarding choice of these measures. Using a "prototypical" pain assessment battery, Davidson et al.[24] determined that a 7-factor model could be extracted. The dimensions they determined should be measured included pain and disability, pain description, affective distress, support, positive coping strategies, negative coping strategies, and activity.

Two key individual personality features that impact pain include catastrophizing and health related anxiety. Persons who catastrophically misinterpret innocuous bodily sensations, including pain, are likely to become fearful of pain, which results in at least two processes. First, pain-related fear is associated with avoidance behaviors and the avoidance of movement and physical activity in particular. Avoidance also means withdrawal from rewarding activities such as work, leisure, and family. Second, pain-related fear is associated with increased bodily awareness and pain hypervigilance. Hypervigilance, depression, and disuse are associated with increased pain levels and, hence, would exacerbate the painful experience.

Validated tools to screen for these features include the Pain Catastrophizing Scale (PCS) and the Tampa Scale of Kinesophobia (TKS).[25] Patients with higher scores should have further assessment. Another simple option is to simply have the patient list their fears. There is evidence that identifying and modifying the patient's specific fears can improve outcomes.[26]

Other factors that may contribute to pain interruption of life include the influence of others (e.g., a spouse that is particularly solicitous), litigation issues, financial security, and status of health care coverage. If a patient has to pay a significant amount of money out of pocket for his or her medications, the prescription may not be filled. A brief employment history should focus on whether the patient is able to return to the previous employment, if they enjoyed their job, and if they are considering or actively retraining for other employment. Whether the patient is receiving wages while off work and whether or not a lawyer is involved may influence return to work. These factors have a major effect on successful pain management and should not be overlooked on the initial evaluation. The family or community support system of the patient is important in assessing the individual's social isolation.

The Multidimensional Pain Inventory Interference Scale (MPI)[27] is a 60-item self-reporting tool. It assesses pain patients' affective, cognitive, and behavioral responses to pain. IMMPACT suggests utilizing this tool.[1,2]

Coping strategies can be assessed by using the Chronic Pain Coping Index (CPCI),[28] a 65-item measure of cognitive and behavioral coping strategies.

If available, a referral to a clinical psychologist specializing in pain should be made if one or more of the following factors have been identified: pronounced emotional disturbance; pain behavior enabled by the family; possible secondary gain; failure to respond to several treatment modalities; reports of pain severity or functional impairment which seem inconsistent with disability; or excessive use of health care services.[29]

RISK OF ADDICTION SCREENING

The disease of addiction exists as a spectrum disorder and can complicate the management of a patient with persistent pain. Assessment of addiction risk is covered in this textbook in a separate chapter and the reader is referred there for further details. Standard assessment tools to define risk are listed in Table 17.1, as are other resources to assist with urine drug testing and follow-up documentation of high-risk individuals.

ASSESSMENT OF FUNCTION

Pain can affect functioning through its effect on physical, emotional, and cognitive functioning. Pain interrupts memory tasks, specifically ones that require attentional resourcing for controlled processing of information.[30] Simple tasks may therefore not be as impaired by pain as tasks that require more complex attention.

Assessment of loss of functionality can be assessed using different functionality questionnaires including the Pain Disability Index (PDI)[31] and the last 7 questions of the BPI. Disease-specific tools can also be used, such as the WOMAC scale for osteoarthritis, the Roland score for low back pain, or the Fibromyalgia Impact Score for fibromyalgia. These and others can be found in Wittink and Carr's source book.[32] Utilizing these self-reporting tools allows some objective documentation of functionality change, which is helpful in determining treatment efficacy and tracking outcome.

GOALS

Goal setting seeks to determine which specific social, recreational, or occupational tasks or roles are important to the patient. Examples of tasks in these categories include going out to see a movie (social), skiing (recreational), or being able to lift heavy objects (occupational). Roles in these domains could include active participation as a church committee member (social), soccer coach (recreational), or as a mother or lawyer (occupational). Determining appropriate goals is an important part of the pain assessment as it will help to direct treatment. People resist coercion, therefore

when getting the patient to identify achievable goals, it is important to influence and not control. Goals need to be measurable, for example "to walk 3 blocks" not "exercise more." They should reflect the patient's current abilities. Identifying up to three goals is a reasonable starting point.

If a patient cannot achieve his or her goals, the practitioner should reassess the goals made, find out what barriers prevented the patient from completing their goal, and assist in reframing the goal to something more achievable in the short term. The goal, however, should always be one that the patient identifies. Evaluation by a psychologist may provide some helpful insights when constructing or re-evaluating goals.

If treatment goals are not met and the PDI or BPI score does not improve, it may be reasonable to assume current treatment is not effective and should be changed. Documenting that a patient has achieved or exceeded goals and has achieved a drop in the PDI score over 6 months can corroborate treatment efficacy.

PHYSICAL EXAMINATION

The examination is usually a focused examination based on the patient's history. The goal is to determine the etiology of the pain (if possible) and to determine, if appropriate, the presence or absence of neuropathic pain and physical signs of substance abuse or misuse. The following evaluation outline for a physical examination is suggested.

General Exam: Observe, Identify, and Document

- Mental status—consider a mini mental status exam if there are concerns about cognitive impairment. Comment on mood, displays of emotion, or evidence of impairment (slurred speech, difficulty remaining alert) and any smell of substance of abuse on breath, body, or clothes
- General appearance (whether it matches photo ID may be appropriate to comment on depending on the specific situation)
- Blood pressure, heart rate, weight, and height
- Stance and gait
- Mobilization aids (what, how, and why they are used)
- Signs of substance abuse including needle marks on lower arm, leg, or bottom of feet; rhinorrhea; red palms; spider veins on chest; and pupil diameter
- Evidence of any tremors, muscle atrophy, trophic changes, or deformities

Site of Pain

Perform a focused examination of the musculoskeletal system.

LOOK for:

- Positional relief postures (i.e., avoids weight bearing on one buttock, turns body instead of neck, prefers to stand and lean)
- Pain distraction signs (i.e., permanent heating pad burn marks, excessive teeth wear from clenching or grinding, joint damage in hand from chronically exerting excessive pressure on a painful area)
- General posture (i.e., head forward posture, exaggerated lumbar lordosis)
- Alignment of spine, shoulders, pelvis, and legs
- Symmetry
- Deformities, visible muscle spasm, atrophy, hypertrophy, scars, and birthmarks
- Leg length asymmetry

TABLE 17.1

SELECTED ASSESSMENT TOOLS RELEVANT FOR PAIN ASSESSMENT

Tool	Web source of tool
1. Pain Assessment Documentation Tool (PADT)	The National Pain Education Council www.npecweb.org/default.asp
2. Brief Pain Inventory	The National Pain Education Council at www.npecweb.org/default.asp
3. Short Form McGill Pain Questionnaire	This website is a pdf that includes the SF-MPQ as well as a pain diagram. It is available for download with the authors permission. http://www.npcrc.org/usr_doc/adhoc/painsymptom/McGill%20Pain%20Inventory.pdf
4. The Neuropathic Pain Scale	PainEdu.org at www.painedu.org/tools.asp
5. The Beck Depression Inventory	This website is a resource center and provides comprehensive information on this tool as well as information regarding purchasing the tool. http://www.musc.edu/dfm/RCMAR/Beck.html
6. Mixed psychological and psychiatric assessment: Personality Assessment Inventory	This website provides information regarding this tool and purchasing it. http://www.sigmaassessmentsystems.com/assessments/pai.asp
7. Psychological assessment: The Minnesota Multiphasic Personality Inventory (MMPI)	This website provides information regarding this tool and purchasing it. http://www.pearsonassessments.com/tests/mmpi_2.htm
8. Psychological assessment: The Pain Catastrophizing Scale[34]	The scale: www.workcover.vic.gov.au/wps/wcm/resources/file/eb5cdc42c0d724e/pain_catastrophizing_scale.pdf Scoring it: www.workcover.vic.gov.au/wps/wcm/resources/file/eb5cdf42c0ec0c8/pain_catastrophizing_scale_scoring_information.pdf
9. Psychological Assessment to assess fear of movement. The Tampa Scale for Kinesiophobia	www.workcover.vic.gov.au/wps/wcm/resources/file/eb5c6742bb4ae48/tampa_scale_kinesiophobia.pdf
10. Tools to assess addiction risk. Review of 9 validated tools and downloadable selected tools	Emerging Solutions in Pain at www.emergingsolutionsinpain.com
11. To assess risk of opioid misuse in a patient already on opioids. The Current Opioid Misuse Measure (COMM)®	PainEdu.org at www.painedu.org/tools.asp
12. Urine Drug Testing	To view a recorded presentation on Urine Drug Testing: A Therapeutic Approach by Douglas L. Gourlay go to :http://aapm.confex.com/aapm/2007am/techprogram/P1671.HTM To download a free pdf copy of Urine Drug Testing in Clinical Practice (authors Doug Gourlay, Howard Heit and Yale Caplan) go to http://www.familydocs.org/files/UDTmonograph.pdf)
13. Functionality Assessment: 1. The Pain Disability Index Score 2. The Brief Pain Inventory	1. See Appendix 2. The National Pain Education Council website http://www.npecweb.org/clinicaltoolbox.asp?id=26&selMenu=15
14. Informed consent documentation, opioid or behavioral contracts	PainEdu.org at www.painedu.org/tools.asp The National Pain Education Council at www.npecweb.org/default.asp Emerging Solutions in Pain at www.emergingsolutionsinpain.com

FEEL for:

- Bony landmarks
- Tenderness, swelling, crepitus, contour or bogginess of joint, muscle, ligament, bursa, or bone
- Trigger points (some clinicians quantify these with a pressure algometer)
- Evidence of damage to the local myotomal segment which includes:
    - Denervation sensitivity of the local spinal segment resulting in:
- Trophedema. This can be documented by the matchstick test—trophedema is nonpitting to digital pressure, but if the end of a matchstick is pushed into the skin it will form a clear-cut indentation that persists for several minutes.
- Peau d'orange effect of the skin in the area affected

MOVE to assess:

- Individual joints for swelling, crepitus, redness, warmth, and range of motion (active/passive)

- Muscle tone
- Muscle weakness
- Specific maneuvers (i.e., the impingement test to assess the shoulder, the hip flexion adduction internal rotation (FAIR) test of the hip to assess the piriformis muscle)

Neurological Exam

LOOK for or ASK ABOUT:

- Signs of sensory avoidance (specific clothing to avoid clothes brushing, wearing dark glasses in the examination room, poor oral hygiene in patients with mouth pain)
- Skin lesions (i.e., scarring from varicella zoster, foot ulcers with diabetic neuropathy)
- Swelling of the painful area (neurogenic edema) (ask if this occurs if not present, as in many patients this can be an intermittent feature)
- Changes in skin color (again, ask if this occurs if not present as in many patients this can be an intermittent feature. A photo by the patient can also provide documentation of these signs)
- Altered sweating (ask about if not present)
- Trophic changes (loss of hair, thinning skin, cracked dry skin, altered nails)
- Secondary changes associated with chronic peripheral neuropathy (e.g., Charcot neuropathic foot destruction with necrotic arthropathy and chronic ulcers on the plantar surface)
- Evidence of autonomic dysfunction (especially with complex regional pain syndrome or peripheral diabetic polyneuropathy)

- Involuntary movements: tremors, myoclonus, tics, dystonia, fasciculations, or others
- Specific tests (i.e., Adson's test for thoracic outlet syndrome, straight leg raising for lumbar radiculopathy)

FEEL for:

- Temperature differences between affected and unaffected areas (some clinicians document this objectively with a temperature probe)
- Edema, swelling, tenderness

MOVE to assess:

- Cranial nerves
- Gait
- Balance and coordination; finger tapping, rapid alternating movements, finger nose and heel-shin testing, Romberg
- Tone:
    - Spasticity = eliciting the "clasp knife phenomenon," which predominates in the upper limb flexors and the lower limb extensors
    - Rigidity = uniform resistance that worsened during the range of movement; usually worsens with distraction
    - Paratonia = describes increased resistance because the patient has difficulty consciously relaxing the muscle. This usually improves with distraction.
    - Hypotonia = decreased tone
- Motor function (Table 17.2):
    - Pronator drift: With the patient standing with both arms extended and palms up (supinated) look for one arm to drift downward and begin to turn palm down (pronate). A positive test is a subtle indicator of upper motor neuron weakness (in which supination is weaker than pronation)

TABLE 17.2

SENSORIMOTOR NERVE DISTRIBUTION

Movement	Nerve root	Key sensory area	Peripheral nerve
Hip flexion	L2–L3	L2 = Medial midthigh L3 = medial knee	Femoral
Knee extension (deep knee bend)	L3–L4	L4 = medial calf (test just above medial malleolus) L5 = lateral calf and dorsum foot (test area above second toe)	Femoral
Ankle dorsiflexion (heel walk)	L4–L5	L4 = medial calf L5 = lateral calf and dorsum foot	Peroneal
Hip extension (compare buttock squeeze)	L4–L5	As above	Gluteal
Knee flexion	L5–S1	S1 = posterolateral foot and ankle (test base of 5th toe)	Sciatic
Ankle plantarflexion (toe walk)	S1–S2	S2–posterior thigh and popliteal fossa	Tibial
Anal sphincter weakness (finger squeeze during exam)	S2–S4	S3–S5–perianal area	
Shoulder abduction	C5	C5–lateral upper arm/lateral epicondyle	Axillary
Elbow flexion	C5–C6	C6–thumb	Musculocutaneous
Elbow extension	C6–C7	C7–middle finger	Radial
Wrist extension	C6–C7		Radial
Wrist flexion	C7–C8	C8—5th finger	Median
Finger flexion	C8		Median
Finger extension	C8		Radial
Finger abduction	T1	T1–ulnar forearm/medial epicondyle	Ulnar

■ In the arms, test resisted shoulder abduction C5, elbow flexion C5–C6, elbow extension C6–C7, wrist extension C6–C7, wrist flexion C7–C8, finger flexion C8, finger extension C8, and finger abduction T1. In the legs, test hip flexion L3–L4, hip extension L4–L5, knee flexion L5–S1, knee extension L3–L4, ankle dorsiflexion L4–L5, and ankle plantar flexion S1–S2.

Score power by
0 = No contraction
1 = Visible muscle twitch but no movement of the joint
2 = Weak contraction insufficient to overcome gravity
3 = Weak contraction able to overcome gravity but no additional resistance
4 = Weak contraction able to overcome some resistance but not full resistance
5 = Normal; able to overcome full resistance

■ Reflexes:
  ■ C5–C6 roots the biceps and brachioradialis reflexes:
  ■ C6–C7 roots (mainly C7) the triceps reflex
  ■ L3–L4 roots (mainly L4) the knee jerk
  ■ S1 roots the ankle jerk
  ■ Score reflexes by
    0 = No observable reflex
    1 = Trace reflex
    2 = Normal reflex
    3 = Brisk reflex
    4 = Nonsustained clonus (two or less beats of clonus)
    5 = Greater than three beats of clonus or sustained clonus
    Anal "wink" reflex in a patient with suspected cauda equina syndrome (scratch the perianal skin about 2 cm away from the anus and look for muscle contraction to cause an "anal wink")

Patients with peripheral neuropathy may have diminished or absent reflexes. If they do not, look carefully for evidence of upper motor neuron dysfunction.

Signs of Upper Motor Neuron Dysfunction

■ Hyperreactive reflexes
■ Spasticity
■ Positive Babinski sign
■ Positive pronator drift sign
■ Weakness that is predominant in the arm extensors and leg flexors

Signs of Lower Motor Neuron Dysfunction

■ Absent or hyporeactive reflexes
■ Tone normal or reduced
■ Negative Babinski sign
■ Atrophy and fasciculations
■ Weakness that is predominant in arm flexors and leg extensors

Mixed upper and lower motor neuron dysfunction can present with hyperreflexia and spasticity mixed with depressed reflexes and weakness in patients with cervical myeloradiculopathy.

Bedside Method for Quantitative Sensory Pain Testing

Many clinicians find it useful to have the patient complete a colored pain diagram as it helps to direct the sensory testing (see Fig. 17.1 or Appendix 4). Using the diagramed symptoms of neuropathic pain, determine if the area of pain, tingling, or numbness colored by the patient is associated with sensory changes.

Patients are examined for the following modalities:

Light Touch

Lightly brush the skin. This can be performed at the bedside with a cotton wisp, cotton-wool tip, Q-tip, foam brush, or paint brush. In cases of decreased light touch, testing begins in the area of reduced or absent sensation and is slowly advanced until the sensate area is reached. With areas of increased sensitivity, testing should start over the normal skin and move toward the sensitive area. Once the patient feels any change in sensation the point on the skin is marked.

Drawing the area of abnormality on the skin can help to determine the pattern of loss (single nerve territory, polyneuropathy, or nondermatomal). If light touch is normal it is still important to test for pinprick and temperature, as these tests evaluate different small fiber components of the nerve.

VIBRATION: TESTING

Vibration sense is often tested with a 128-Hz tuning fork. Test over the bony prominences moving from distal to proximal. In subjects with distal symmetric polyneuropathy, the tuning fork is placed over the interphalangeal joint of the big toe. If no vibration is noted, move to the medial malleolus and repeat the exam. If still unable to sense vibration, the test is repeated over the patella. For the hands, test over the second distal interphalangeal joint, and move proximally to the ulnar styloid and lateral epicondyle if no vibration is felt.

Punctate/Pinprick

This can be evaluated with a safety pin, unbent paper clip, or a more standardized device such as a Neuropen. The size and angle of the sharp tool can significantly affect the intensity of the stimulus and can produce differing clinical evaluation results. The Neuropen has a standardized probe tip and is designed to allow production of a consistent stimulus. Perform the testing in the area with the abnormal positive or negative sensations.

Warm and Noxious Heat Testing

For bedside testing, thermal evaluation can be done by heating the round end of a tuning fork in warm or hot water. There are no commercially available small devices for standard bedside testing of warmth or heat pain. It is difficult to get the tuning fork to the correct temperature for heat pain testing. This test is most useful to confirm the involvement of small fibers when evaluating for a possible small fiber neuropathy. This most often occurs in a patient whose pain drawing suggests a peripheral neuropathy but in whom sensation to vibration and light touch was normal.

Cool and Noxious Cold Testing

For cool testing a tuning fork is held under cool water and applied to the area of altered skin sensation. For cold pain the tuning fork is immersed in ice water. Comparison is made with the established control site. Have the patient report the sensation. (Does it actually feel cool? In some patients it feels paradoxically hot.)

REDUCED SENSATION: Have the patient express the degree of loss by utilizing a simple 1 to 100 scale of a dollar. Ask "If this is a dollar (stimulating the normal area), then how much is this worth? (now stimulating the area of sensory loss). Responses of 90 cents reflect a very different degree of loss than a reply of 10 cents.

INCREASED SENSATION: In the case of a sensation that should have been painful (pinprick, noxious heat or cold) have the patient grade the pain in the normal area first (0–100) and then grade the abnormal area which they should rate as higher than the normal area.

Record **dysesthesia** if the nonpainful stimulus was felt as increased but not painful and write a description of the sensation (e.g., numb, pins and needles).

Record **hyperalgesia** if the stimulus was a normally painful stimulus (pinprick, heat or cold pain) but it produced more pain than the unaffected normal test site. Grade intensity (0–100).

Record **allodynia** if the stimulus was nonpainful (brush, vibration, warm, cool) and either the threshold was normal or decreased (stimulus intensity reported as the same or more than the normal site) and the patient reported pain from the stimulus. Grade intensity (0–100).

Record **hyperpathia** if the stimulus threshold is increased (stimulus intensity reported as less than the normal site) and the patient reports it as painful. Grade intensity (0–100).

Further Investigations or Consults

Other investigations may include specific radiological or EMG testing, a sleep study, specific or baseline laboratory investigations, or urine toxicology screening. Referral to appropriate specialists for further assessments should be requested as needed.

FOLLOW-UP VISITS

Ideally the first follow-up visit should be within a few weeks to allow assessment of treatment efficacy and tolerability and review of any testing, consults, or "homework" requested. A follow-up form given to the patient to complete prior to being seen may be helpful. It should include questions about the goals achieved and efficacy of any therapy started (see Appendix).

The 5A's have been suggested as a useful acronym to document follow-up visits and evaluate the efficacy therapy. These are Adverse events (to treatment), Affect (mood), Activities (progress toward goals/functionality outcomes), Aberrant drug–related behavior if opioids are prescribed, and Action taken.[33]

CONCLUSION

Assessment and reassessment must be built into every treatment plan. Patients should leave each visit, whether an initial visit or a follow-up, with a definite and agreed plan. Patients should also be repeatedly reminded that it will take effort on their part to reach relevant goals (see Appendix).

Nonadherence, or questioning an agreed treatment plan, occurs in up to 50% of patients, but merely repeating the original reasoning will often be ineffective. Patients need to be involved in a discussion about any concerns or objections they may have to the treatment plan as it evolves. For any trial of treatment, a reasonable time to expected improvement must be defined early on (e.g., up to 3–4 weeks for an antidepressant to work, 2–3 weeks before improvement in pain may be felt with the same drug). With physical therapy it may take three to four sessions for ongoing improvement. If there are no recognizable improvements after the agreed upon trial time, that particular therapy should be changed or stopped.

Working with a chronic pain patient can be immensely satisfying, as the practitioner sees a patient begin to take more responsibility for their often disabling, all-encompassing pain, and improve their quality of life and function. Having an organized

way of getting the patient to give a comprehensive history and validating their pain but not being drawn into their "stories" is a skill that takes time to develop, but being prepared by using some of the suggestions outlined in this chapter and appendix should speed up the "learning curve." Equally important from the practitioner's point of view is to not do it alone, but involve the patient, their significant other, and other community resources. An integrative approach provides the best possible outcome for patients with chronic pain.

APPENDIX 1: INITIAL PAIN QUESTIONNAIRE

Name   Date
Age

Please list your main areas of pain, how long you have had pain in each area, and how severe the pain is on average (e.g., low back pain 10 years moderately painful).

Area	how long years	months	Mild pain/moderate pain/severe pain
1			
2			
3			
4			
5			

Briefly describe how each of the pain problems you listed above started (e.g., "after surgery to my knee," "after a car accident").
Area 1
Area 2
Area 3
Area 4
Area 5

Surgical History

Have you had any surgeries directly related to your pain problem(s):   Yes   No

If yes, complete the information.

Name and year of surgery (e.g., lumbar fusion, 1985; knee surgery, 1998):

1	Year
2	Year
3	Year
4	Year
5	Year

Have you had other surgeries NOT related to your pain problems?   Yes   No

If yes please complete the following information:

Name and year of surgery (e.g., appendectomy 1993, tonsillectomy 2001).

1	Year
2	Year
3	Year
4	Year
5	Year

Allergies

Are you allergic to any medication? (An allergy means a rash, swelling, difficulty in breathing. It does NOT mean causing a stomach upset or dizziness):   Yes   No

If yes, please list them:

Present Medication

How satisfied are you with your present pain medications? 5-point scale from extremely satisfied to extremely dissatisfied Please list all prescription medications you are taking that are NOT for pain (e.g., blood pressure, cholesterol, heart, blood thinners) and how many times a day:

Name   Dose   Times per day   Date started   Prescribing doctor

Please list all other nonprescription medications you are taking (e.g., Tylenol, Advil, Aleve, vitamins, herbal supplements, homeopathic remedies).

Pain Medication

What pain medications have you taken in the past? Your pharmacist may be able to help you with a list.

Opioid (Narcotic) Medication (Vicodin, Percocet, Darvocet, Morphine, Fentanyl, Demerol, Methadone

Have you been given opioid (narcotic) medication for your pain? Yes   No

If yes have they improved your activity or general level of function?
No   a little bit   somewhat   quite a bit   very much

Do you feel your doctor is reluctant to prescribe opioids? Yes   No

Are you concerned about addiction if you are prescribed opioids: Yes   No

Are any members of your family concerned about addiction if you are prescribed opioids?   Yes   No

Past Medical History

Have you had any of these conditions either now or in the past?

Heart and Blood Vessels

High blood pressure
Angina
A heart attack
Congestive cardiac failure

Lungs

Shortness of breath easily
Asthma

Liver/Kidneys

Hepatitis
Other liver problems
Kidney problems
Bladder problems

Metabolic/Intestinal Tract

Diabetes
Thyroid disease
Acid reflux
Stomach ulcer
Dark black stools
Blood in stools
Have you had an unexplained weight loss of more than 10 pounds in the last 6 months?

Nervous System

Loss of balance
Seizures
Stroke
Paralysis
Peripheral neuropathy

Muscles and Joints

Neck/back problems
Joint pains

Other

Cancer
HIV

Psychological

Anxiety
Panic disorder
PTSD
ADHD (Adult hyperactivity disorder)
Bipolar
Schizophrenia
Depression
Any history of addiction or substance abuse: Yes   No

Please note, if you answer yes to this or other similar questions it will NOT mean you don't receive the best treatment your provider can give you, nor will it necessarily mean you don't get strong pain medicine (narcotics) but it will help him or her to offer you the safest treatment plan the two of you together can determine.
If yes was it to:
Alcohol
Prescription drugs?
Other drugs?
Exposure to toxins such as asbestos, dyes, printing rubber, arsenic, etc.?

Are you pregnant now?   Yes   No

If all your pain was gone how healthy would you be (100% being full health)_____%
ER visits

In the PAST YEAR have you been treated in the Emergency Room for your pain problem   YES   NO
If yes 1   2–3   4–6   7–10   More than 10 times

Health care visits

In the past 3 months how many times have you been to your regular health care provider or specialist for your pain problem

(MD, ARNP, PA) 0 1 2–3 4–6 7–10 More than 10 times

In the past 3 months how many times have you been to your physical therapist for your pain problem 0 1 2–3 4–6 7–10 More than 10 times

In the past 3 months how many times have you seen an alternative health care provider for your pain problem (chiropractor, homeopath, naturopath, acupuncturist) 0 1 2–3 4–6 7–10 More than 10 times

Pain Score

Click the number that best describes your baseline or constant level of pain over the past few days when taking your pain medication:

0   1   2   3   4   5   6   7   8   9   10
No pain   worst possible pain

Click the number that best describes your worst level of pain over the past few days, when taking your pain medication:

0   1   2   3   4   5   6   7   8   9   10
No pain   worst possible pain

How many times on average over the past few days did your worst pain occur?
1–2   3–4   5–6   7–8   More than 8

Have you ever had the following types of treatment for your PRESENT pain problem(s) and what was the result?
No   Improved   No change   Worse

Occupational Therapy
Physical therapy
Passive (heat, gentle massage, ultrasound)
Mobilizations
Exercises
TENS
Chiropractic manipulations
Deep tissue massage
Psychological counseling for pain
Biofeedback
Trigger point injections
Joint injections
Epidural steroid injections
Facet joint injections
Nerve blocks
Other local anesthetic or steroid injections

Have you had any of the following tests for your pain:

Blood tests	No	Yes
X rays	No	Yes
MRI	No	Yes
Cat (CT)Scan	No	Yes
EMG	No	Yes
Bone Scan	No	Yes
Myelogram	No	Yes
Discogram	No	Yes
Ultrasound	No	Yes

Social History

This is important for physicians who treat your pain to know because HOW you grew up affected how your pain sensing system developed and your current environment and state of mind can affect both your pain and how easy it is to cope with it.

Did you have a happy childhood?   Yes   No

Have you ever been sexually and or physically abused?   Yes   No

If yes was it before you were an adult?   Yes   No

Do you currently feel threatened in your environment?   Yes   No

Have you ever seriously considered or attempted suicide?   Yes   No

Do you have a suicide plan at the moment?   Yes   No

Are you: married, divorced, widowed, single, living with someone?

Do you have any children?   Yes   No
If yes how old are they? _____

Do you smoke?   Yes   No

If yes
Less than half a pack a day
Half to one pack a day
One or more packs a day.

Is the best smoke of the day the first one in the morning?
Yes   No

If you are a former smoker when did you stop?

Do you drink alcohol?   Yes   No

If yes
Less than 6 drinks per week?
7–24 drinks per week?
Over 24 drinks per week?

Do you binge drink?

Do you drink to decrease your pain   Yes   No

Have you or your doctor ever thought you had a problem with pain medication?   Yes   No

In the past 10 years have you ever tried street drugs?   Yes   No

If yes
Marijuana
Cocaine
Heroin
Other

Are you using any of these drugs presently?

Family History

Do you have any members of your immediate family who suffer from
Chronic pain   Yes   No
Diabetes   Yes   No
Headaches/migraines   Yes   No
Severe arthritis   Yes   No
The same pain complaints as you have   Yes   No
Any family history of addiction or substance abuse   Yes   No

If yes was it to
Alcohol?
Prescription drugs?
Other drugs?

Work History

What is your occupation? Are you:
Employed full time
Employed part time
Unemployed because of pain
Unemployed because of other reasons

Retired because of pain

In school or retraining because of pain

Homemaker

How satisfied are you with your current job?
Very satisfied,   Neutral,   Very dissatisfied

Do you have problems getting along with your co-workers?
No   Yes

Do you have an attorney working on your injury claim?
No   Yes

If you are not working at present do you think you will be able to return to the same sort of job that you were doing before your pain?
No   Yes   Not applicable

Are you actively considering a change of employment or a retraining program?
No   Yes   Not applicable

Overall, on a scale of 0–10 how close are you to returning to work (10 means ready to work full time, 0 means you are not even close to work at any job)
0   1   2   3   4   5   6   7   8   9   10

Do you suffer from headaches? ☐ Yes   ☐ No

IF YES
   In the past two weeks did you suffer from headaches? (one possible answer)

      ☐ I had mild headaches which came infrequently
      ☐ I had moderate headaches which came infrequently
      ☐ I had moderate headaches which came frequently
      ☐ I had severe headaches which came infrequently
      ☐ I had headaches almost all the time

   Type of headaches (mark the ones that best describe your main headaches)

      ☐ Are your headaches one sided? Yes No
      ☐ Are they worsened by, or do they cause you to avoid physical activity? Yes No
      ☐ Do they cause you to feel sick or to vomit? Yes No
      ☐ Does bright light or any noise make the headache worse? Yes No

Constipation
Do you suffer from constipation (less than 3 bowel movements a week) Yes   No

Do you suffer from all over body pains or have you been told you suffer from fibromyalgia? ☐ Yes   ☐ No

Sleep History

Have you been told you snore a lot? Yes No

Have you been told you often gasp for breath or stop breathing during sleep? Yes   No

Have you been diagnosed with sleep apnea? Yes   No

Are you a restless sleeper? Yes   No

Do you often have problems with restlessness (creeping, crawling or other uncomfortable feelings) in the legs keeping you awake? Yes   No

Does your bed partner report that your legs jerk during sleep? Yes   No   Don't know

Do you feel rested when you wake up in the morning? Yes   No

Do you use any of these substances regularly in the four hours before going to bed?
Alcohol
Caffeine (coffee, tea, sodas)
Tobacco
Decongestants

Beta blockers (for blood pressure or heart problems, such as atenolol, propranolol)

Have you ever had a sleep study?   Yes   No

Physical Function and Quality of Life Questions

Mood Disorders

Has there ever been a period of time when you were not your usual self and (while not using drugs or alcohol). ☐ Yes ☐ No

...you felt so good or so hyper that other people thought you were not your normal self, or you were so hyper that you got into trouble? ☐ Yes   ☐ No

Has a health professional ever told you that you have manic-depressive illness or bipolar disorder?   Yes   No

Depression Questionnaire

During the past month have you often been bothered by feeling down, depressed, or hopeless?   Yes   No

During the past month have you often been bothered by having little interest or pleasure in doing things?   Yes   No

Anxiety

Over the last 2 weeks, how often have you been bothered by the following problems?

		Not at all	Several days	More than half of the days	Nearly every day
1	Feeling nervous, anxious or on edge	0	1	2	3
2	Not being able to stop or control worrying	0	1	2	3
3	Worrying too much about different things	0	1	2	3
4	Trouble relaxing	0	1	2	3
5	Being so restless that it is hard to sit still	0	1	2	3
6	Becoming easily annoyed or irritable	0	1	2	3
7	Feeling afraid as if something awful might happen	0	1	2	3

If you checked off any problems, how difficult have these problems made it for you to do your work, take care of things at home, or get along with other people?

Not difficult at all	Somewhat difficult	Very difficult	Extremely difficult
○	○	○	○

PTSD

In the past month have you:

Had repeated, disturbing *thoughts,* or *images* or flashbacks of a stressful experience?   Yes   No

Several times avoided *having feelings* related to a stressful experience? Yes No

ADHD

Check the box that best describes how you have felt and conducted yourself over the past six months.

Never   Rarely   Sometimes   Often   Very often

1. How often do you have trouble wrapping up the final details of a project once the challenging parts have been done?
2. How often do you have difficulty getting things in order when you have to do a task that requires organization?
3. How often do you have problems remembering appointments or obligations?
4. When you have a task that requires a lot of thought, how often do you avoid or delay getting started?
5. How often do you fidget or squirm with your hands or feet when you have to sit down for a long time?
6. How often do you feel overly active and compelled to do things, like you were driven by a motor?

Pain Disability Index [PDI]

The rating scales below are designed to measure the degree to which aspects of your life are disrupted by chronic pain. In other words, we would like to know how much your pain is preventing you from doing what you would normally do, or from doing it as well as you normally would. Respond to each category by indicating the *overall* impact of pain in your life, not just when the pain is at its worst.

For each of the 7 categories of life activity listed, please circle the number on the scale, which describes the level of disability you typically experience. A score of 0 *means no disability at all,* and a score of 10 *signifies that all of the activities in which you would normally be involved have been totally disrupted or prevented by your pain.*

Family / home responsibilities: This category refers to activities related to the home or family. It includes chores or duties performed around the house (e.g., yard work) and errands or favors for other family members (e.g., driving the children to school).

0   1   2   3   4   5   6   7   8   9   10
No disability   Worst disability

Recreation: This category includes hobbies, sports, and other similar leisure time activities.

0   1   2   3   4   5   6   7   8   9   10
No disability   Worst disability

Social Activity: This category refers to activities which involve participation with friends and acquaintances other than family members. It includes parties, theater, concerts, dining out, and other social functions.

0   1   2   3   4   5   6   7   8   9   10
No disability   Worst disability

Occupation: This category refers to activities that are a part of or directly related to one's job. This includes nonpaying jobs as well, such as that of a home maker or volunteer worker.

0 1 2 3 4 5 6 7 8 9 10
No disability   Worst disability

Sexual Behavior: This category refers to the frequency and quality of one's sex life.

0   1   2   3   4   5   6   7   8   9   10
No disability   Worst disability

Self-Care: This category includes activities which involve personal maintenance and independent daily living (e.g., taking a shower, driving, getting dressed, etc.).

0   1   2   3   4   5   6   7   8   9   10
No disability   Worst disability

Life-support Activity: This category refers to basic life-supporting behaviors such as eating, sleeping, and breathing.

0   1   2   3   4   5   6   7   8   9   10
No disability   Worst disability

Goals for Treatment

Please put down four things in your life which you can't do or have difficulty doing because of your pain, and which you would most DEARLY like to do if the treatments decrease your pain by 50%.

These four things can't be vague or general such as "to be free of pain" or "to be whole again." They have to be activities which can be measured and which someone else could see you doing. For instance if you have been very inactive and wish to change this write "walk 3 blocks" instead of "increase exercise."

1 _____
2 _____
3 _____
4 _____

APPENDIX 2: FOLLOW UP/ PROGRESS NOTE

What new medications (prescribed and over the counter) are you taking for your pain (how much and how often?)

_____
_____

How would you best describe your pain? (please check all that apply)

Dull, throbbing, aching   shock-like, numb, or tingling   burning

Has the sort of pain changed since your last visit? No Yes

Please rate your pain by circling the one number that best describes your pain on the average over the past few days (while taking your pain medication)

1   2   3   4   5   6   7   8   9   10

Please circle the number that best describes your pain at its worst in the last 24 hours

1   2   3   4   5   6   7   8   9   10

How many times did your pain get to its worst level during the last 24 hours?

1–2   3–4   5–6   7–8   More than 8

What makes your pain worse?

Standing   Walking   Sitting   Bending   Ice   Heat
Other _____

What makes your pain better?

Standing   Walking   Sitting   Bending   Ice   Heat
Other _____

Did the pain medicine cause a problem

	No	Mild	Moderate	Severe
Nausea				
Constipation				
Drowsiness				
Confusion				
Dry mouth				
Headache				
Weight gain				
Sexual problems				

(Brief Pain Inventory) To what degree has pain interfered with the following activities (1 = no interference, 10 = maximum interference

Your sleep	1....2....3....4....5....6....7....8....9....10
General activity	1....2....3....4....5....6....7....8....9....10
Mood	1....2....3....4....5....6....7....8....9....10
Walking ability	1....2....3....4....5....6....7....8....9....10
Normal work (at home and outside)	1....2....3....4....5....6....7....8....9....10
Relations with others	1....2....3....4....5....6....7....8....9....10
Enjoyment of life	1....2....3....4....5....6....7....8....9....10

Did you achieve your physical goals since your last visit? (These are activities that pain had stopped you doing?)
No Didn't try Almost achieved Achieved Achieved and more

What new goals are you setting yourself to be achieved by the next visit?

Do you need refills of your pain medications   Yes   No

Please list problems in order of importance you want to discuss with your health care practitioner.

APPENDIX 3: GOAL SETTING

A goal is something we would like to do in the next month to 6 months, such as walking, water exercise, visiting family, doing things with friends, or controlling your diabetes.

Goals are generally too big to work on all at once, so start one step at a time and with smaller goals. For example, your pain will have limited your physical activity so it is important to exercise, but doing too much all at once may make your pain worse temporarily. You might start with deciding what type of exercise to do, then where to go to exercise, how much time I will spend exercising when first starting, and maybe asking a friend or family member to exercise with you.

Decide what goals to make **this month** and how to do it.

Important points about goals, they should be something:

1. You want to do—not what your doctor, nurse, family, or anyone else thinks you should do.
2. Realistic—something you think you can REALLY do this month.
3. Specific—for example, doing more exercise is not specific, but walking 10 minutes twice a day IS.
    What? Walking more
    How much? 10 minutes
    How often? Twice a day: 4 times a week
4. How confident are you that you can succeed? This usually means a level of 7 or more on a confidence scale (0 = don't think I can do it to 10 = I definitely think I will complete the goal)

Goal Setting Worksheet

Date: _____

Use the following worksheet to assist you in identifying your goals.

1. **Choose one of the activities below:**
    To improve my pain I will:
    1. Choose one of the activities below:
        _____ Work on something that's bothering me.
        _____ Stay more physically active!
        _____ Take my medications as prescribed.
        _____ Improve my food choices.
        _____ Reduce my stress.
        _____ Cut down on smoking.
        _____ Other

2. **Choose your confidence level:**
    This is how sure I am that I will be able to meet my goal over the next month.

1	5	10
Not sure	Somewhat sure	Very sure

3. Chosen Goal one:
What: _____
How much/often: _____
Confidence level =

Chosen Goal Two:
What: _____
How much/often: _____
Confidence level =

APPENDIX 4: PAIN DIAGRAM

Name _____   Date _____

Please color the areas where you experience pain. Use one of these five coloring pens to shade the specific type of pain that you are experiencing. Then circle with a pen all areas of pain and, starting with the worst, number the areas in order of severity.

Red	— burning	If you have other	Yellow	— _____
Green	— tingling	pain sensations,		— _____
Blue	— numbness	name them here	Black	
		and color as		
		black or yellow		

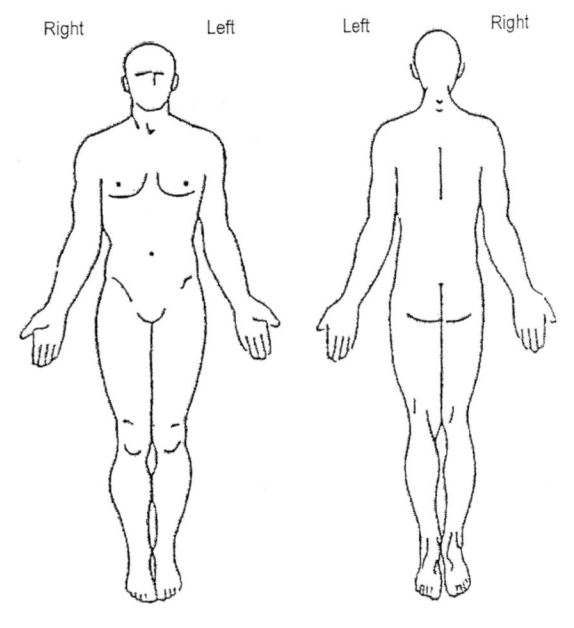

Right   Left   Left   Right

References

1. Dworkin RH, Turk DC, Farrar JT, et al. Core outcome measures for chronic pain clinical trials: IMMPACT recommendations. *J Pain* 2005;113:9–19.
2. Dworkin RH, Turk DC, Wyrwich KW, et al. Interpreting the clinical importance of treatment outcomes in chronic pain clinical trials: IMMPACT recommendations. *J Pain* 2008;9:105–121.
3. Breivik H, Borchgrevink PC, Allen M, et al. Assessment of pain. *Br J Anaesth* 2008;101:17–24.
4. Backonja MM, Argoff CE. Neuropathic pain: definition and implications for research and therapy. *J Neuropathic Pain Sympt Palliat* 2005;1:11–17.
5. Squire P. Does ineffective communication confound multidimensional pain assessment? *J Pain* 2007;8(12):903–905.
6. Gourlay DL, Heit HA, Almahrezi A. Universal precautions in pain medicine: a rational approach to the treatment of chronic pain. *Pain Med* March–April, 2005;6(2):107–112.
7. Jamison RN, Stetson BA, Parris WC. The relationship between cigarette smoking and chronic low back pain. *Addict Behav* 1991;16(3–4):103.

8. Webster LR, Webster RM. Predicting aberrant behaviors in opioid-treated patients: prelminary validation of the Opioid Risk Tool. *Pain Med* 2005;6(6): 432–442.
9. Michna E, Ross EL, Hynes WL, et al. Predicting aberrant drug behavior in patients treated for chronic pain: importance of abuse history. *J Pain Symptom Manage* 2004;28:250–258.
10. Mersky H, Bogduk N. Classification of chronic pain. Seattle, WA, IASP Press, 1994.
11. Melzac R. The short-form McGill Pain Questionnaire. *J Pain* 1987;30: 191–197.
12. Cleeland CS, Ryan KM. Pain assessment: global use of the Brief Pain Inventory. *Ann Acad Med* 1994;23:129–138.
13. Brokoff D. Chronic pain: 1. A new disease? *HospPract* September 22, 2005.
14. Bennett MI. The LANSS pain scale: the Leeds assessment of neuropathic symptoms and signs. *Pain* 2001;92(1–2):147–157.
15. Bennett MI, Smith BH, Torrance N, Potter J. The S-LANSS score identifying pain of predominantly neuropathic origin: validation for use in clinical and postal research. *Pain* 2005;6(3):149–158.
16. Krause SJ, Backonja MM. Development of a neuropathic pain questionnaire. *Clin J Pain* 2003;19:306–314.
17. Backonja MM, Krause SJ. Neuropathic pain questionnaire-short form. *Clin J Pain* 2003;19:315–316.
18. Freynhagen R, Baron R, Gockel U, Tolle T. painDETECT: a new screening questionnaire to detect neuropathic components in patients with back pain. *Curr Med Res Opin* 2006;22:1911–1920.
19. Bouhassira D, Attal N, Alchaar H, et al. Comparison of pain syndromes associated with nervous or somatic lesions and the development of a new neuropathic pain diagnostic questionnaire (DN4). *Pain* March, 2005;114 (1–2):29–36.
20. Portenoy R. Development and testing of a neuropathic pain screening questionnaire: ID pain. *Curr Med Res Opin* 2006;22:1555–1565.
21. Galer BS, Jensen MP. Development and preliminary validation of a pain measure specific to neuropathic pain: the Neuropathic Pain Scale. *Neurology* 1997; 48:332–338.
22. Argoff CE. The coexistence of neuropathic pain, sleep, and psychiatric disorders: a novel treatment approach. *Clin J of Pain* 2007;23:15–22.
23. Dworkin RH, Turk DC, Wyrwich KW, et al. Interpreting the clinical importance of treatment outcomes in chronic pain clinical trials: IMMPACT recommendations. *J Pain* February, 2008;9(2):105–121.
24. Davidson M, Tripp DA, Fabrigar LR, Davidson PR. Chronic pain assessment: a seven-factor model. *Pain Res Manage* 2008;13(4):299–308.
25. Swinkels-Meewisse EJ, Swinkles RA, Verbeek AL, Vlaeyen JW, Oostendorp RA. Psychometric properties of the Tampa Scale for kinesiophobia and the fear-avoidance beliefs questionnaire in acute low back pain. *Man Ther* 2003; 8:29–36.
26. Woods MP, Asmundson GJ. Evaluating the efficacy of graded in vivo exposure for the treatment of fear in patients with chronic back pain: a randomized controlled clinical trial. *Pain* June, 2008;136(3):271–280.
27. Kerns RD, Turk DC, Rudy TE. The West Haven-Yale Multidimensional Pain Inventory (WHYMPI). *Pain* 1985;23:345–356.
28. Jensen MP, Turner JA, Romano JM, Strom SE. The chronic pain coping inventory: development and preliminary validation. *Pain* 1995;60:203–216.
29. Marrero M. Psychological evaluation. In: Ramamurthy S, ed. *Decision Making in Pain Management.* Mosby 2006;15.
30. Morley S. Psychology of pain. *Br J Anaesth* 2008;101(1): 25–31.
31. Pollard CA. Preliminary validity study of the pain disability index. *Percept Mot Skills* 1984;59:974–981.
32. Wittink HM, Carr DB. *Pain Management: Evidence, Outcomes, and Quality of Life.* London: A Sourcebook. 2008:361–376.
33. Gourlay DL, Heit HA, Almahrezi A. Universal precautions in pain medicine: a rational approach to the treatment of chronic pain. *Pain Med* March–April, 2005;6(2):107–112.
34. Sullivan HJL, Bishop SR, Pivik J. The Pain Catastrophizing Scale: development and validation. *Psychol Assess* 1995;7:524–532.

CHAPTER 18 ■ ELECTRODIAGNOSTIC EVALUATION OF ACUTE AND CHRONIC PAIN SYNDROMES

DOUGLAS G. CHANG AND ELAINE S. DATE

INTRODUCTION

Before a clinician can treat pain effectively, the utmost must be done to identify what condition is being treated, and identify what may be causing pain. For this purpose, electrodiagnostic studies are important in the evaluation of acute and chronic pain syndromes. They give valuable, quantitative information on the physiologic health and functioning of nerve and muscle. They help localize injuries, quantify the extent of injury, suggest age of injury, and give valuable prognostic information that can change treatment protocols. They can monitor interval progression. All of this complements the static, anatomic structural information provided by radiological imaging studies. In other words, radiological imaging can identify anatomy that may or may not be the cause of symptoms. Electrodiagnostic studies can quantify symptoms (e.g., show evidence of spinal nerve root compression) but cannot identify the anatomic cause (e.g., infection, tumor, or disk herniation). Together, electrodiagnostic and radiologic studies are extensions of the physical exam and serve to refine the differential diagnosis suggested by a clinical presentation.

Common reasons for ordering electrodiagnostic studies include symptomatic complaints (weakness, pain, numbness and/ or tingling in an extremity) and physical examination findings (focal neurological deficits in deep tendon reflexes, strength or sensory losses). Typical clinical scenarios involve radiculopathies, entrapment syndromes, trauma, and metabolic pathology seen in diabetes and alcoholism. Other important scenarios include rheumatologic disease, neuromuscular disease, and various infectious and neoplastic neuropathies. Further details about these conditions can be found in several electrodiagnostic textbooks.[1,2,3,4,5,6]

Practically, electrodiagnostic studies should be thought of when the diagnosis is in doubt, either during the initial patient presentation or as the result of nonresponse to treatment. The studies can evaluate the possibility of additional lesions (e.g., concomitant nerve entrapment syndromes, peripheral neuropathies, and so-called "double crush syndromes"), be used to follow the interval progression of both operative and nonoperative treatments, and provide pre-operative baselines. The objectives of this chapter are to introduce basic principles of electrodiagnosis. Hopefully, this will provide information on when to order electrodiagnostic tests, and help interpret and utilize the resulting electrodiagnostic reports.

TERMINOLOGY

Electrodiagnostic studies involve two components: nerve conduction studies (NCS) and needle electromyography (EMG). Al-

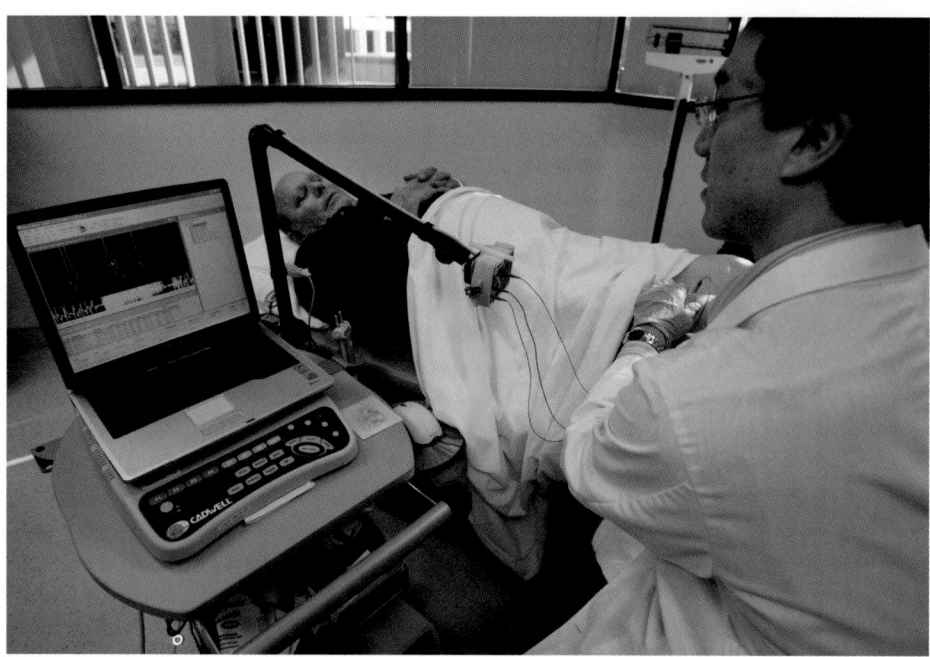

FIGURE 18.1 A typical configuration for an electrodiagnostic study. In this figure, a monopolar electrode (*orange*) is inserted into the right vastus medialis of a subject. On the computer monitor (*left*) appear the motor unit potentials from voluntary muscular contractions. The equipment for a nerve conduction study would vary slightly from this picture; instead of a needle electrode, there would be recording electrodes.

though the term EMG strictly refers to the direct needle examination of muscle, EMG is often used generically to refer to electrodiagnostic studies as a whole. A typical setup is depicted in Figure 18.1.

Nerve conduction studies involve electrical stimulation to evaluate peripheral nerve function. Electrical conduction abnormalities can suggest injury to myelin (from slowed conduction velocity or delayed response), axons (with diminished amplitude response or temporally dispersed waveforms), or the neuromuscular junction (diminished amplitude response with repetitive stimulation). The distribution of abnormalities distinguishes focal from diffuse global processes.

So-called "late responses" are variations of nerve conduction studies. Two common studies are the "H-reflex" and "F-wave." The H-reflex is an electrically measurable analog of the ankle deep tendon reflex. The H-reflex and ankle deep tendon reflex are specific for the S1 monosynaptic spinal reflex arc. In the H-reflex, an electrical stimulus is applied to the tibial nerve behind the knee, which elicits a wave of depolarization that travels proximally on Ia afferents. The wave traverses the spinal reflex arc, synapses on the anterior horn cell, and elicits an efferent volley, causing depolarization of the calf muscle. The H-wave may be delayed or lost bilaterally in large nerve fiber pathology, and unilaterally with unilateral S1 nerve root lesions that may have occurred in the indeterminate past. Therefore it cannot distinguish acute from chronic injury. It will be abnormal with advanced age, tibial or sciatic nerve injuries, and peripheral neuropathies.[7]

F-waves are late responses from the axons of motor neurons in a peripheral nerve as well as the spinal cord. The F-wave may be obtained from practically any muscle, but typically is used to evaluate cervical spinal nerve root function via the median nerve. The clinical utility is not agreed upon,[1] but it may be helpful with three scenarios. These are diabetic neuropathy, Guillain-Barré syndrome, and multifocal motor neuropathy with conduction block. F-waves are usually abnormal in radiculopathies only when significant disease is present. Many practitioners do not suggest routine F-wave studies in the workup of focal entrapment neuropathies such as carpal tunnel syndrome.[1]

Somatosensory evoked potentials (SSEP) measure conduction between a large peripheral nerve and the cerebral cortex or spinal cord. SSEP is sensitive to certain lesions in the central nerve system pathways, such as may occur in multiple sclerosis, spinal

cord injury or tumor, and compressive myelopathies. It has poor detection of radiculopathies and the CNS motor pathways.[7]

EMG OVERVIEW

EMG Procedure

Electromyography studies involve insertion of a needle electrode, typically about 23 gauge to 25 gauge in size, into muscle tissue and recording the resultant electrical activity (as seen on the computer monitor in Figure 18.1). The muscle is examined while at rest and during contraction. This provides information about muscle motor unit health and function. Various muscles are examined, and the pattern of pathology seen across all the muscles gives information about the overall disease process.[8] Each muscle is routinely examined in four stages (during initial needle insertion, at rest, and during minimal contraction and maximal contraction). Several findings are described. In the first stage there is insertional activity; in the second stage we look for abnormal spontaneous activity. The third stage evaluates the motor unit potentials (amplitude, configuration, and recruitment). In the fourth stage, the interference pattern is examined.

Stages of the EMG Examination and Typical Findings

Insertional activity is a volley of electrical potentials that is provoked by the initial mechanical irritation of needle insertion and movement. It lasts a few milliseconds. If muscle fibers have degenerated, there are fewer electrically excitable cells available. As a result, there is reduced insertional activity.

Secondly, the electrical activity of the muscle at rest is examined. Normally there should be electrical silence when needle movement ceases. Abnormal spontaneous activity arises from persistent electrical potentials that occur despite the lack of needle movement. It is a sign of unstable muscle membranes. The abnormal spontaneous activity can take the form of fibrillation potentials, positive sharp waves, and complex repetitive discharges

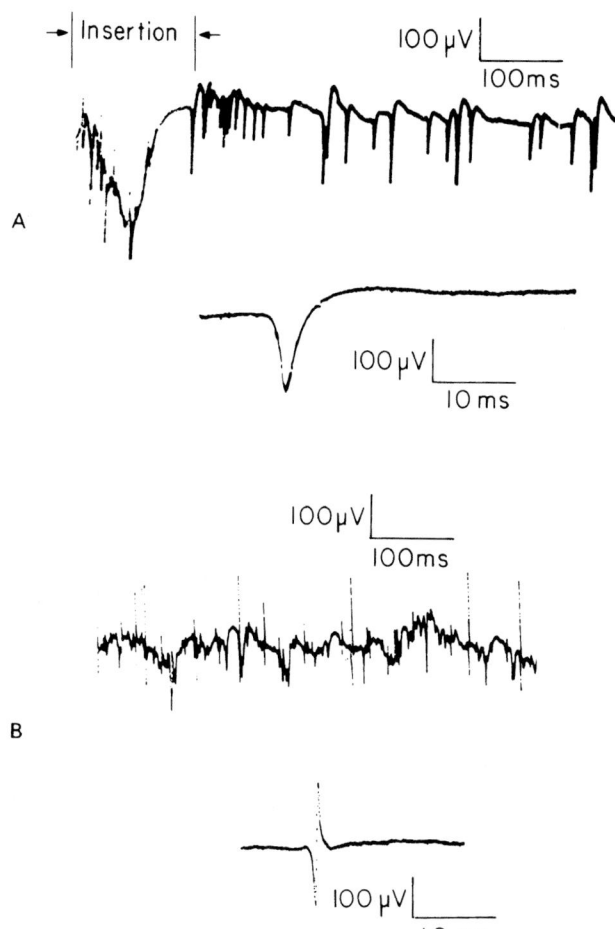

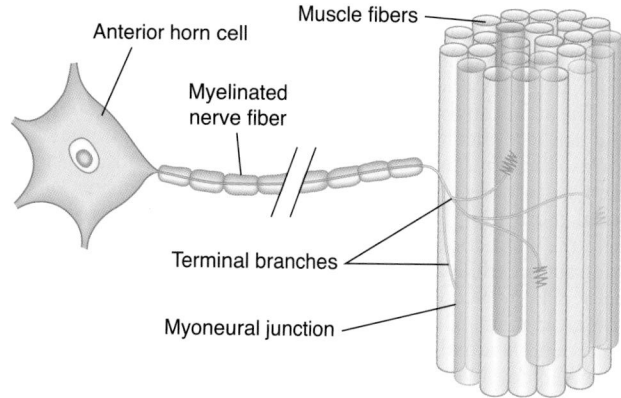

FIGURE 18.3 The components of a single motor unit. The muscle fibers of the unit (*shaded*) are interspersed among fibers of other units. The myoneural junctions are located approximately midway between the ends of the muscle fibers.

FIGURE 18.2 Involuntary needle electromyography action potentials at rest (negative values are above the baseline). (**A**) Insertion potentials are seen in the first 250 ms of this record. They were produced as the needle sliced through muscle fibers. The insertion potentials are followed by a train of positive sharp waves. A single positive sharp wave is also illustrated. (**B**) Fibrillation potentials. The sharp spikes are seen against a background of positive sharp waves. A single fibrillation potential is also illustrated.

(Fig. 18.2). Spontaneous and benign endplate spikes and endplate noise can also be observed occasionally.

In the third stage, the subject is asked to contract the muscle minimally to study the motor unit potentials (MUP). A muscle motor unit is defined as all the muscle fibers innervated by a single motor neuron (Fig. 18.3). The motor unit potential is the electrical discharge of the contracting motor unit. MUP amplitude, duration, shape, and discharge frequency is recorded (Fig. 18.4).

These parameters are usually commented upon in an electrodiagnostic report and carry clinical implications. The findings can be described as "normal," "myopathic," or "neuropathic." MUP amplitude can be decreased with loss of muscle fibers (e.g., myopathy), axonal neuropathy, or motor neuron disease. It can be increased because of reinnervation with spatially larger motor units (e.g., recovery from neuropathy). MUP duration can be decreased with atrophy of muscle fibers (seen in myopathy), or increased with reinnervation with spatially dispersed muscle fibers (seen in recovery from neuropathy or myopathy).

In the fourth stage, the subject is asked to gradually increase the force of muscular contraction up to maximal effort. The number and firing rates during recruitment are evaluated. With progressively forceful contraction in normal muscle, the recruitment

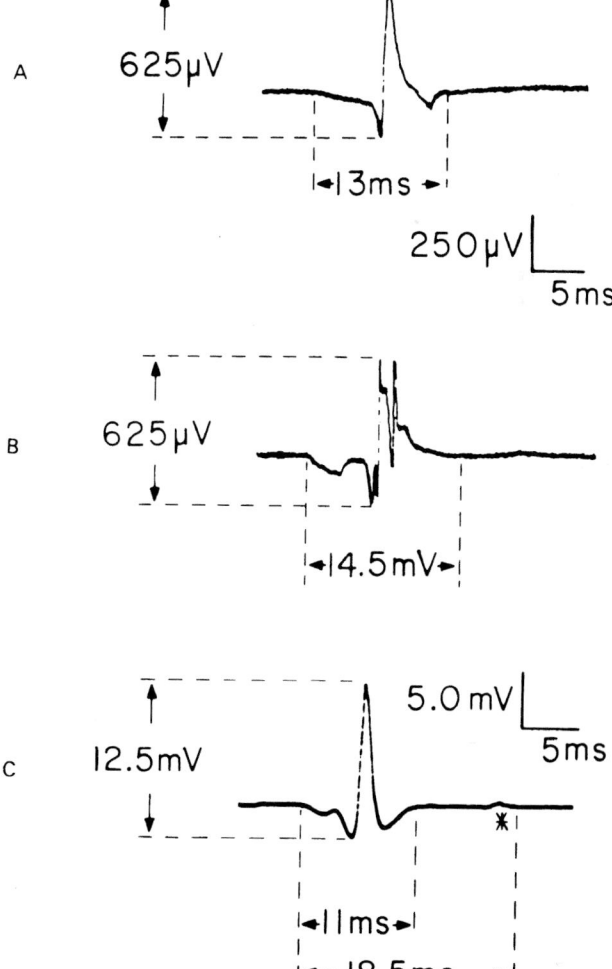

FIGURE 18.4 Samples of motor unit action potentials recorded by monopolar needle electrodes. (**A**) Normal triphasic wave. (**B**) Polyphasic (eight phases) wave of longer duration and of similar amplitude. (**C**) Large amplitude potential with a triphasic basic component and a small late component, a satellite potential (*). Note amplitude calibration in **C** compared with that in **A** and **B**.

of muscle fibers follows a pattern: An individual muscle fiber will fire and reach a frequency of 15 to 20 Hz, at which point a second fiber will be recruited. The second fiber will reach a frequency of 15 to 20 Hz and then a third fiber is recruited, and so on.

The actual analysis of recruitment patterns is rather subjective and can be difficult. Modern computerized analysis of the waveforms is helpful, but the whole process also depends on the patient's effort. Because of pain, language, comprehension, or personal motivation level, the patient may not be able to comply with the instructions to provide a slow and progressively forceful contraction while a needle electrode is embedded in the muscle belly. Maximal contraction in normal muscle reveals the discharge of many MUPs, which flood the screen. The interference pattern at maximal contraction is evaluated subjectively from the observed density of electrical spikes, along with their amplitude, frequency, and sound.

In disease states, there are characteristic patterns of firing, recruitment, and interference that suggest either muscle denervation (neuropathies) or muscle fiber destruction (myopathies). Neuropathic disease processes denervate the motor unit acutely. This is followed by re-innervation from collateral sprouting of nearby surviving motor units. As a result, the motor units become bigger because the fewer surviving neurons assume control over more and more of the muscle fibers. When the bigger motor units fire, there is an observable pattern of muscle fiber recruitment that is termed a "neurogenic" recruitment pattern. This is also called "decreased recruitment" or "reduced recruitment." There are decreased numbers of MUPs, firing later at increased rates, in order to meet the force demanded of the muscle.

On the other hand, the so-called myopathic recruitment pattern (also called "early" or "increased" recruitment) comes from the fact that insufficient force is generated by any given motor unit, and additional motor units are recruited earlier or more rapidly than expected. The observation is that there are too many motor units firing for the amount of contraction requested. There is an increased number of MUPs, firing faster, and earlier in the myopathic disease state.

Summary of EMG Findings

The EMG findings in upper and lower motor neuron disorders and myogenic lesions are summarized in Table 18.1, which was adapted from Kimura.[2] The exact findings seen in a given subject depend on the disease process itself, as well as the timing of the electrodiagnostic exam in relation to the disease process. In normal muscle, there is brief insertional activity, no spontaneous activity, motor unit potentials (MUPs) of 0.5 mV to 1.0 mV and 5 msec to 10 msec duration, and full interference pattern.

In neuropathic lesions, the EMG findings show normal to increased insertional activity, normal (silent) to abnormal spontaneous activity (with positive sharp waves and/or fibrillation potentials), MUPs that are normal to large amplitude with increased duration, complex configuration, and limited recruitment. During maximal contraction (stage 4) there is a reduced interference pattern.

In myopathic lesions, the EMG findings show normal to increased insertional activity and sometimes there are myotonic discharges. There can be normal (silent) to abnormal spontaneous activity (with positive sharp waves and/or fibrillation potentials). The MUPs have small amplitudes with early recruitment and myotonic discharges may be seen. The interference pattern is full but of low amplitude.

NERVE CONDUCTION STUDIES OVERVIEW

The intraneural anatomy of the nerve fiber gives our bodies a functional reserve that protects us against catastrophic loss with partial nerve injuries. The peripheral nerves are similar to insulated cables, and are composed of individual nerve fibers traveling together in bundles, called fascicles. However, the internal organization of the peripheral nervous system is unlike a cable, and does not have the somatotopic organization seen in the brain and spinal cord of the central nervous system. In the peripheral nervous system, the fascicles exchange nerve fibers in an interwoven course along the nerve (see Fig 18.5).[6] Therefore, a partial nerve injury in the peripheral nervous system does not result in a Brown-Sequard–like scenario that might result from a partial injury in the central nervous system spinal cord. In the peripheral nervous system, a partial nerve injury will often result in partial function of most muscles because of spared fascicles. Furthermore, each of the nerves distal to the injury will have at least some abnormality that will be detectable. It is the intraneural

---

TABLE 18.1

TYPICAL EMG FINDINGS SEEN IN NORMAL, NEUROGENIC, AND MYOGENIC LESIONS

EMG Stage	Normal	Neuropathic lesion	Myopathic lesion
1. Insertional activity	Normal (brief)	Normal–increased	Normal–increased Myotonic discharges
2. Spontaneous activity	Normal (silent)	Normal (silent) Fibrillation potentials Positive sharp waves	Normal (silent) Fibrillation potentials Positive sharp waves
3. Motor unit potentials	0.5–1.0 mV amplitude 5–10 msec duration Normal recruitment	Normal to large amplitude Normal to increased duration Normal to limited recruitment	Small amplitude Early recruitment Myotonic discharges
4. Interference pattern	Full	Reduced	Full Low amplitude

(Adapted from Kimura J. *Electrodiagnosis in Diseases of Nerve and Muscle: Principles and Practice.* 3rd edition. New York: Oxford University Press; 2001.)

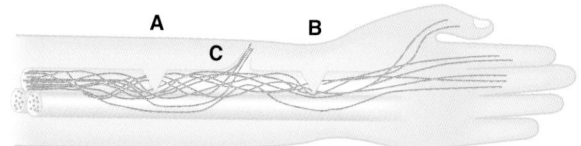

FIGURE 18.5 Typical mammalian nerve, involving the movement of axons from one fascicle to another during their course. Here lesions at A and B may be easily distinguished electromyographically by the fact that lesion A produces changes in the distribution of branch C, whereas the lesion at B does not. (Redrawn from Pease WS, Lew HL, Johnson EW. *Johnson's Practical Electromyography*. Philadelphia: Lippincott Williams & Wilkins; 2007.)

anatomy that permits partial function after a nerve injury and allows electrodiagnostic studies to pinpoint a lesion.

Nerve conduction studies test the integrity of the peripheral nervous system, both sensory and motor. The techniques are standardized, and there are banks of reference data.[8] Reference data are established in age-matched normals without neurological complaints. However, subjects at the extremes of age or limb size may not fall within these norms. In these cases, the sensitivity of NCS can be increased if a contralateral asymptomatic limb is used for the control.[6]

In motor nerve testing, the peripheral nerve is stimulated by passing electrical currents through the skin to produce synchronized muscle contraction "downstream," or distally. The motor response is recorded with surface recording electrodes (Fig. 18.6) placed over the muscle being studied. The recording is referred to as a compound motor action potential (CMAP), with the key parameters being onset latency and amplitude. Latency is the time between the stimulus and observed response. It measures conduction in the fastest nerve fibers. Amplitude (and area) is a result both of the total number of fibers conducting electrical signal and their degree of synchrony (see Fig. 18.7). Conduction velocity of a nerve is determined by measuring the distance between two stimulation sites along the course of a nerve, and com-

paring the latency measurements. Surface stimulators consist of two electrodes placed 1.5 to 3.0 cm apart (Fig. 18.8).

Sensory nerve testing involves techniques and analysis similar in concept to motor testing, although there are a few differences. The electrodes come in different shapes and forms (see Fig. 18.8). Sensory nerves may be tested in an antidromic fashion, stimulating the nerve proximally and recording a response distally (Fig. 18.9). They may also be tested in an orthodromic fashion, stimulating the nerve distally and recording the response proximally. The response from either technique is referred to as a sensory nerve action potential (SNAP).

Neural pathology may be identified by examining the CMAP and SNAP parameters (Fig. 18.10). In general, demyelinative neural pathology will lead to prolonged latency measurements and slowed conduction velocity. A long demyelinated nerve segment will have conduction velocities less than 20 m/second.[6] On the other hand, with axonal pathology there is no slowing of conduction in individual fibers. Instead there is loss of axons, which results in decrements of the CMAP amplitude. In actuality, many disease states, such as a compression neuropathy, will result in a combined demyelinative, axonal loss picture of varying proportions. Also, if the pathology is severe, absent responses can occur with either process.

Pathology of the myelinated neuron comes in three patterns: conduction slowing, segmental conduction block, and full-length conduction loss. Conduction slowing can be seen in demyelination, remyelination, and reinnervation. Conduction block occurs at a specific location along the nerve. It is frequently caused by local trauma, ischemia, autoimmune, metabolic, or vascular disease. Axons are spared, and the segments above and below the lesion will conduct signals normally.

Axon loss occurs in various disease states and injuries. Many diseases result in partial axon loss. Some examples include diabetic neuropathy, vitamin E deficiency, alcoholic neuropathy, chronic renal failure with uremia, and hereditary neuropathies such as Charcot-Marie-Tooth disease. Complete axon loss, following a stab wound, for example, results in a characteristic pic-

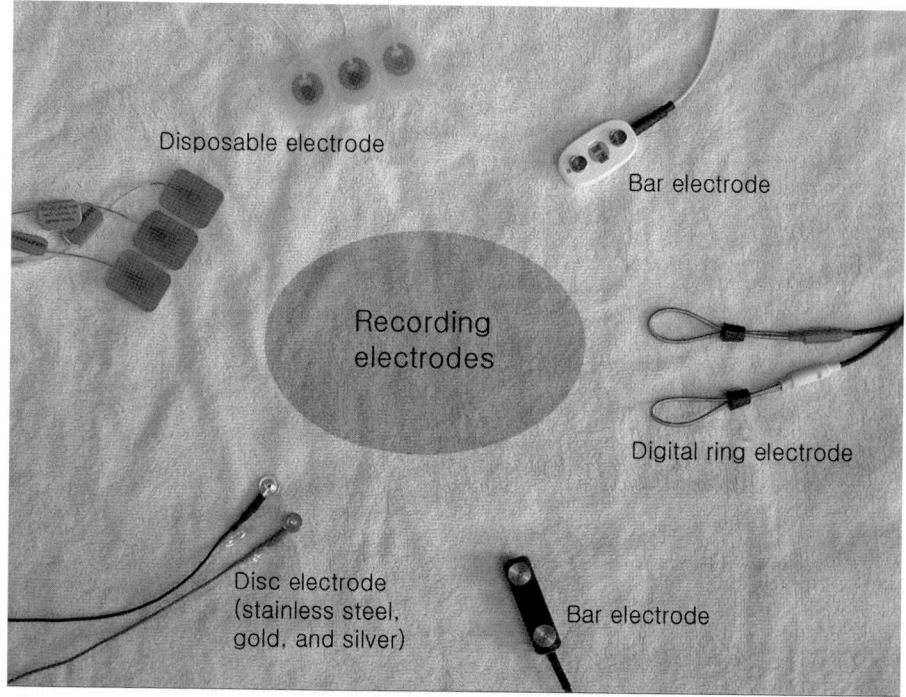

FIGURE 18.6 Different types of surface recording electrodes. (From Lee HJ, DeLisa JA. *Manual of Nerve Conduction Study and Surface Anatomy for Needle Electromyography*. Philadelphia: Lippincott Williams & Wilkins; 2005.)

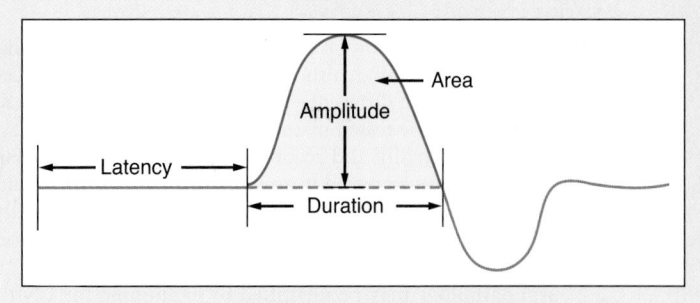

FIGURE 18.7 CMAP parameters. (Redrawn from Lee HJ, DeLisa JA. *Manual of Nerve Conduction Study and Surface Anatomy for Needle Electromyography*. Philadelphia: Lippincott Williams & Wilkins; 2005.)

ture. For 3 to 7 days after complete axonal injury, the distal nerve will continue to conduct because there are enough stored materials and energy sources for independent function.[6] After this period, the conduction of the distal nerve will fail completely because of neural dissolution, a process known as Wallerian degeneration.

Regeneration of the injured distal nerve segments can occur as long as the nerve cell body is intact. Additionally, there must be some connective tissue integrity about the nerve fiber to provide a permissive environment and conduit for regeneration. In a frankly severed nerve, surgical approximation is required to permit regeneration. After interruption of the axons, the cell body requires about a month before regeneration occurs. Thereafter, the regrowth occurs at a rate of an inch per month. Motor nerves may then require yet another month after the regenerating nerve establishes connection to the muscle in order to establish new myoneural junctions.

PATIENT PREPARATION

The patients should be placed in the most comfortable position possible on an exam table or chair, with pillows and blankets. To reduce anxiety and fear of pain, provide an opportunity to counsel and educate the patients about the procedure. Expose the area to be studied and clean the skin with an alcohol pad. It is helpful to inform patients not to use heavy lotions or creams on their skin. An important environmental factor is temperature, to the extent that every EMG report should report the skin temperature among the test data. The patients must be kept warm to avoid temperature artifacts in the study. Cool limbs will result in slowed nerve conduction and latency measurements, and increased amplitudes. This may have nothing to do with any neural pathology. A wrist temperature of 32° C and ankle temperature of 29° C is considered standard. Many laboratories have warmer requirements. Temperature regulation can be accomplished with

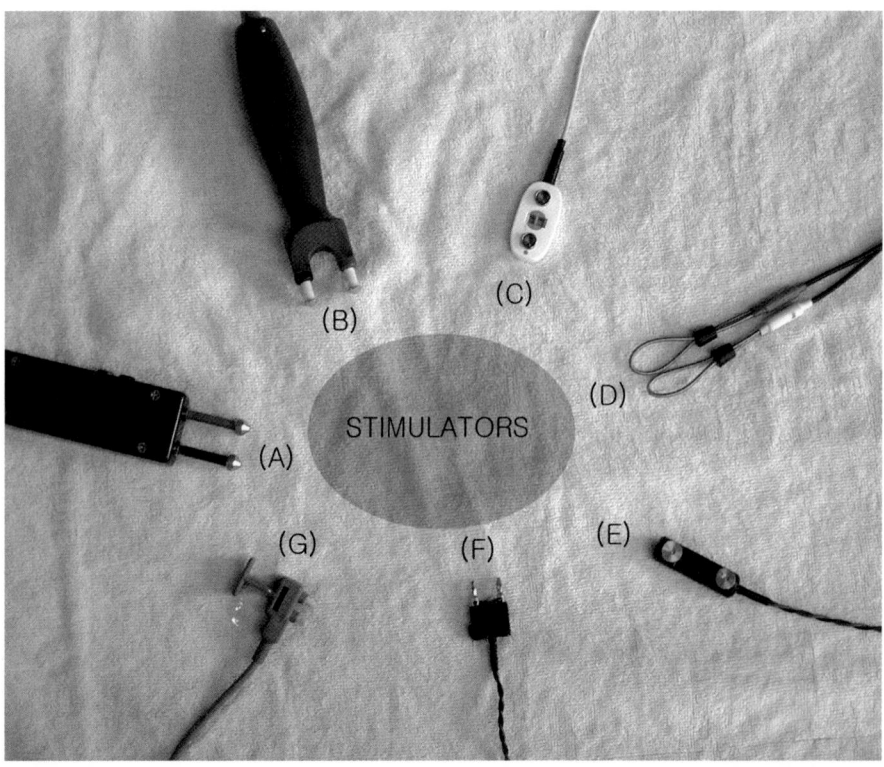

FIGURE 18.8 Different types of stimulators. (From Lee HJ, DeLisa JA. *Manual of Nerve Conduction Study and Surface Anatomy for Needle Electromyography*. Philadelphia: Lippincott Williams & Wilkins; 2005.)

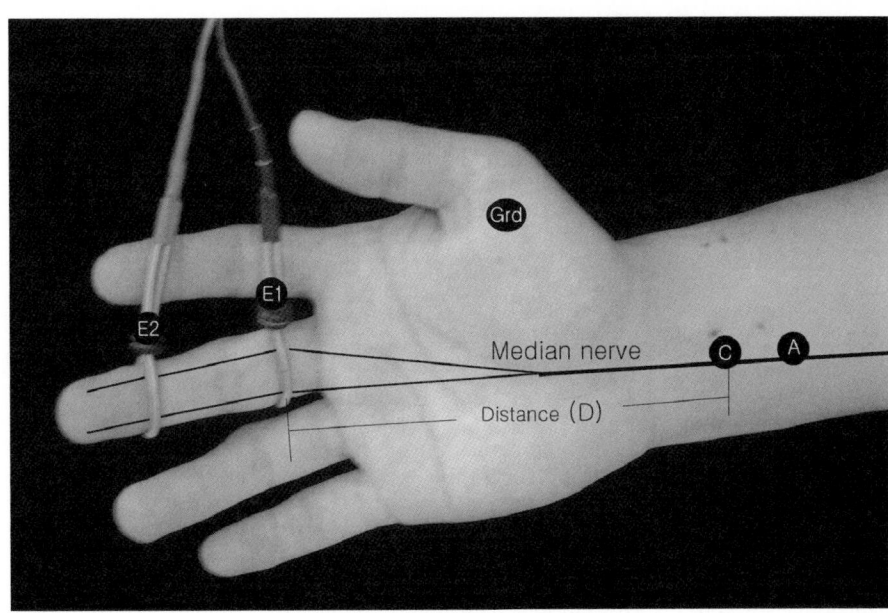

A

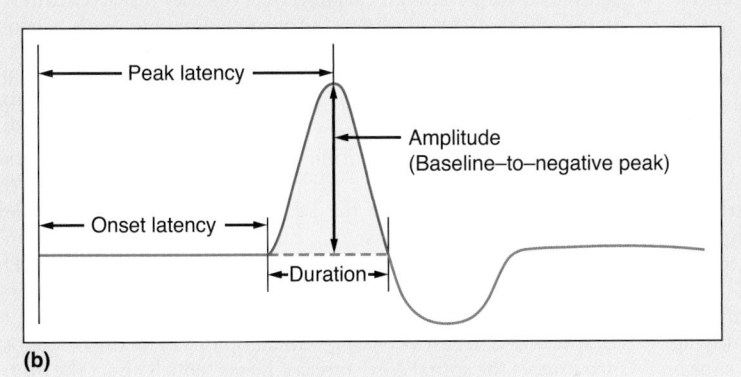

FIGURE 18.9 (**A**) Antidromic sensory conduction studies of the median nerve. (**B**) Sensory nerve action potential parameters from antidromic median nerve conduction studies. (From Lee HJ, DeLisa JA. *Manual of Nerve Conduction Study and Surface Anatomy for Needle Electromyography.* Philadelphia: Lippincott Williams & Wilkins; 2005.)

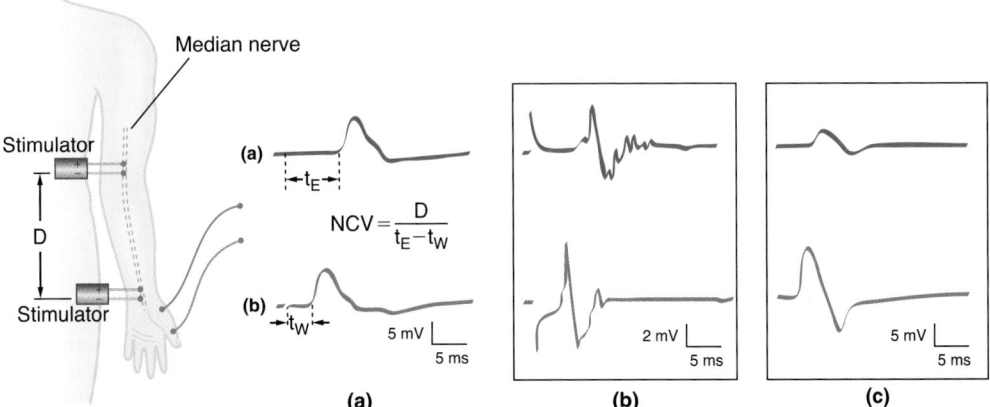

FIGURE 18.10 Schematic representation of the determination of median nerve motor conduction velocity (NCV) from the elbow to wrist, illustrating three different types of responses: t_E and t_W are the latencies from time of stimulation to time of onset of response of the muscle, from elbow and wrist stimulation, respectively. D is the distance between the two points of stimulation. (**A**) A normal response. Note that the amplitude of the response from the elbow and wrist stimulations are essentially equal, as are the wave shapes. (**B**) Temporal dispersion associated with segmental demyelination. Note the smaller amplitude of the response on elbow stimulation compared with stimulation at the wrist, as well as distortion of the wave when the elbow response is compared with the wrist response. (**C**) Partial neurapraxic block between the two points of stimulation. Note the much smaller response from elbow stimulation without distortion of wave form when compared with the response on wrist stimulation.

a combination of heating pads, blankets, and heat lamps. Sometimes a patient can be asked to exercise or drink hot beverages. Last, temperature correction factors exist to normalize the electrophysiologic data obtained from suboptimal studies.[1,8]

SPECIAL CONSIDERATIONS

For patients, the EMG experience is generally an uncomfortable one. Perception of pain is affected by various psychological factors (advice from friends, fear of needles, sound emanating from the medical instrumentation speaker, unfamiliarity with the test). Certainly, the puncture of skin by the electrode and movement through the tissue fascia contributes most of the pain. Some areas are more painful than others; the most painful are the cervical and lumbosacral paraspinal muscles and the hand intrinsics. Concentric needles, favored by electrodiagnosticians trained in neurology, are more painful than the monopolar, Teflon coated needles, favored by those trained in the field of physical medicine and rehabilitation. Rarely, a short-acting benzodiazepine may be required for anxious patients.

There are no absolute contraindications to a focused EMG exam, but the risk–benefit ratio should be weighed. Relative contraindications include bleeding risk in patients with mild thrombocytopenia, whose platelet counts are below 50,000/mm.[3] In patients with anticoagulation there are some special considerations. Coumadin should be stopped 3 days prior to the needle exam. A follow-up check of serum coagulation parameters is usually not necessary. Treatment dose, subcutaneous low molecular weight heparin should be stopped 12 hours prior to the study. Other strategies include gentle use of a small EMG needle (e.g., 30 gauge) and being selective about which muscles to test (avoiding deep muscles that are difficult to manually compress or muscles that are near vital blood vessels or nerves). No particular precaution is needed with patients on prophylactic heparin or other medications such as aspirin, clopidogrel, and nonsteroidal anti-inflammatory medications.[9]

Pneumothorax is a rare but potentially catastrophic complication of EMG studies. Some caution should be used when studying the muscles of the shoulder girdle (e.g., serratus anterior, supraspinatus, rhomboid) and paraspinals near the cervicothoracic junction.

With regard to NCS examinations, there are precautions advised in patients with implanted pacemakers and cardioverter-defibrillators. There are no known complications of nerve conduction studies in patients with regular, implanted pacemakers.[9] General guidelines suggest that NCS studies be performed more than 6 inches away from the pacemaker, using a stimulus duration of 0.2 ms or less, and a stimulus rate less than 1 Hz. For patients with an implantable automatic cardioverter-defibrillator, there is a greater theoretical risk and a consultation with a cardiologist is recommended. One option is to deactivate the device and provide cardiac monitoring during the study.[9]

The only other medication consideration is stopping the use of pyridostigmine in patients being tested for a neuromuscular junction disease such as myasthenia gravis or Lambert-Eaton syndrome.

Last, after the needle EMG examination, a patient's serum creatine phosphokinase (CPK) may be mildly elevated for up to 3 days. This may affect the workup for myopathy.

PATHOLOGICAL CONDITIONS

The EMG-NCS examination can provide diagnostic information to help clarify the diagnosis. It is useful in several situations, such as radiculopathy, focal nerve entrapment syndromes, trauma, and peripheral neuropathies due to such conditions as diabetes, hypothyroidism, or alcohol abuse. It is vital for the diagnosis of

other conditions such as neuromuscular junction disease (e.g., myasthenia gravis, Lambert-Eaton syndrome, botulism), neuropathies (e.g., Guillain-Barré syndrome, amyotrophic lateral sclerosis), and myopathies (e.g., the inheritable dystrophies and inflammatory myositis conditions). Although pain management clinicians need to be mindful of these important conditions, these diseases are not regularly encountered in a typical pain management practice. Therefore, for the sake of brevity, the ensuing discussion will not focus on these conditions. Only a brief summary will be presented at the end of the section. Further details are described in common neurology and electrodiagnostic medicine texts.[1,2,3,4,5,6]

Radiculopathies

With many patients suspected of having a radiculopathy, there is little practical value from electrodiagnostic testing. This is the case for a younger patient with a consistent history of radicular pain, a neurological exam with focal deficits, and advanced radiological images showing spinal stenosis at the appropriate neurological level. However, many patients do not have such a tidy presentation. With a more complex presentation, electrodiagnostic testing is extremely valuable. This is not an uncommon presentation: an older patient with confounding past medical (e.g., diabetes) and surgical (e.g., carpal tunnel release) history, scattered neurological exam findings, and spine imaging with various stages of degenerative change identifiable at several levels.

The electrodiagnostic nerve conduction findings in a radiculopathy are explainable with an anatomic discussion (see Fig. 18.11). Spinal radiculopathies usually involve stenosis of the spinal nerve roots at a location that lies proximal to the dorsal root ganglion (DRG). The peripheral nerve cell bodies of the sensory neurons reside in the DRG and send their nerve fibers distally. Usually in the case of a radiculopathy, there are normal sensory nerve conduction studies because of this anatomy. (The site of stenosis is proximal to the entirety of the sensory nerve cell bodies and tracts.) In contrast, motor nerve function can be compromised in cases of severe radiculopathy. The site of stenosis may impact the spinal cord anterior horns, which affect the motor nerve cell bodies and result in axon loss in the motor nerve fiber tracts. This loss can appear with amplitude loss in the motor nerve conduction studies. For example, a severe L5 radiculopathy could result in decreased CMAP amplitude in the deep peroneal nerve conduction studies to the extensor digitorum brevis. In general, however, radiculopathies do not result in observable abnormalities in the nerve conduction studies.

Needle EMG exam is a very specific investigation in cases of radiculopathy, with poor sensitivity. The EMG diagnosis of an acute or subacute radiculopathy depends on the observation of abnormal spontaneous activity, with positive sharp waves and fibrillation potentials. Such spontaneous activity should be seen in two peripheral muscles that share the same nerve root origin, but are innervated by different peripheral nerves. An example involves the abducens pollicis brevis (APB) and first dorsal interosseus (1st DI) muscles of the hand. Both of these muscles originate from the C8 and T1 nerve roots. However, the APB is innervated by the median nerve, whereas the 1st DI is innervated by the ulnar nerve. The diagnosis of acute radiculopathy can also be made with the observation of abnormal spontaneous activity in one peripheral muscle and one proximal trunk muscle, such as the paraspinal muscles. An example would be the APB and the lower cervical spine multifidus muscles. Nerve root innervation of the muscles has some degree of individual anatomical variation. Nevertheless, there are commonly accepted tables to guide the electromyographer (see Table 18.2). A reasonable radiculopathy screen should involve at least five muscles in an affected limb, with consideration for the proximal trunk musculature as well.[10]

The needle EMG examination does not have good sensitivity,

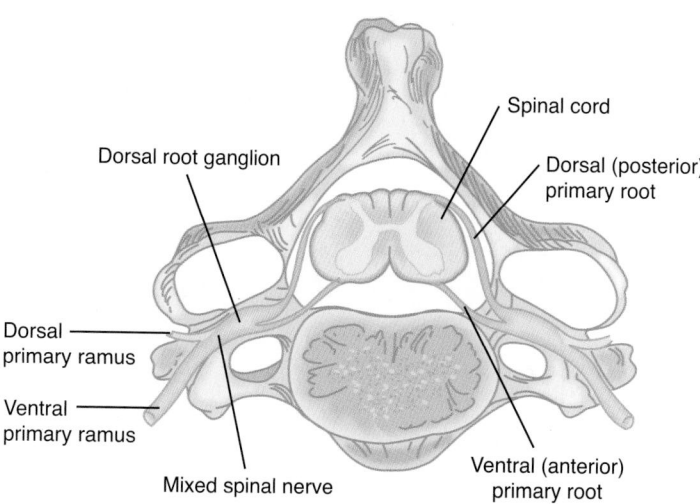

FIGURE 18.11 Relationship between the spinal cord, roots, and the ventral and dorsal rami. Note that the dorsal root ganglion is at the intervertebral foramen. (Redrawn from Pease WS, Lew HL, Johnson EW. *Johnson's Practical Electromyography*. Philadelphia: Lippincott Williams & Wilkins; 2007.)

and an exam that does not uncover abnormal spontaneous activity should not be taken as evidence that the patient is not suffering from a radiculopathy. There are several reasons why a needle EMG exam might not show muscle abnormalities in the presence of a true radiculopathy. A false negative result can arise from sampling errors. For example, there are several L5 innervated muscles to examine with a needle electrode. The electromyographer may choose to examine the peroneus longus (L5) and anterior tibialis (L4, L5) muscles, but the muscle abnormalities could be limited to the flexor digitorum longus and medial head of the gastrocnemius (L5, S1). There may not be representative muscle

groups to sample; for example, in a C3 radiculopathy. Furthermore, a given muscle should be sampled with a needle placed in four or five different locations within the muscle. The ability of the patient to cooperate (by keeping relaxed during an uncomfortable needle exam) can introduce muscle noise artifacts that make it difficult to see or hear subtle spontaneous muscle activity. The timing of the EMG needle exam can also affect results. Abnormal spontaneous activity disappears with time even though clinical symptoms persist. The likelihood of false negative exams increase with cervical spine radiculopathies lasting longer than 6 months, and with lumbosacral radiculopathies lasting longer than 12 to 18 months.[10,11] Proximal muscles heal faster than distal muscles, and false negative results are more likely in a high cervical or high lumbar radiculopathy than with a radiculopathy affecting a lower nerve root.

False-positive examinations are rare. The false-positive problem arises from the diagnosis of a radiculopathy, when there is actually a more systemic problem such as a polyradiculopathy, plexopathy, or motor neuron disease. The false-positive problem comes either from a deficient study (not sampling enough muscles during EMG or performing adequate NCS), or from testing too early in the disease process before widespread findings are apparent.

Entrapment Syndromes

Carpal Tunnel Syndrome (CTS)

A common nerve entrapment scenario is carpal tunnel syndrome, which results from compression of the median nerve under the transverse carpal ligament, which provides the "roof" of the carpal tunnel in the palmar wrist. This may result in a median nerve neuropathy. The clinical scenario is well described. Patients may complain of pain, numbness, and tingling of the entire hand or in a distribution limited to the median nerve dermatome. Radiation of symptoms into the forearm is not uncommon. Nocturnal exacerbation is typical, when it is presumed that the wrist is held in extreme flexion or extension during sleep. Predisposing factors include previous Colles' fracture, rheumatoid arthritis, diabetes, gout, pregnancy, thyroid conditions, multiple myeloma, and tuberculosis. However, most patients are otherwise healthy. On physical exam, the symptoms may be exacerbated by tapping on the carpal tunnel of the wrist (Tinel's sign) or by prolonged wrist flexion (Phalen's sign). Patients may also complain of neck pain. Clinical series do demonstrate some increased association between cervical spine degenerative disease, ulnar nerve pathology

TABLE 18.2

REPRESENTATIVE MUSCLE NERVE ROOT AND PERIPHERAL NERVE INNERVATION

Muscle	Spinal cord level	Peripheral nerve
Upper limb		
Supraspinatus	C5, C6	Suprascapular
Deltoid	C5, C6	Axillary
Biceps brachii	C5, C6	Musculocutaneous
Brachioradialis	C5, C6	Radial
Pronator teres	C6, C7	Median
Triceps brachii	C6, C7, C8	Radial
Extensor indicis proprius	C7, C8	Radial
Abductor pollicis brevis	C8, T1	Median
Dorsal interossei	C8, T1	Ulnar
Abductor digiti minimi	C8, T1	Ulnar
Lower limb		
Adductor longus	L2, L3, L4	Obturator
Vastus medialis	L2, L3, L4	Femoral
Anterior tibialis	L4, L5	Deep peroneal
Gluteus medius	L4, L5, S1	Superficial gluteal
Peroneus longus	L5, S1	Superficial peroneal
Flexor digitorum longus	L5, S1	Tibial
Biceps femoris short head	L5, S1	Sciatic (peroneal)
Gastrocnemius	S1	Tibial

at the cubital tunnel, and median nerve pathology at the carpal tunnel.[5] Thus, an electrodiagnostic examination is helpful to determine which factors may be contributing most to a patient's symptomatology.

Carpal tunnel syndrome is fundamentally a clinical diagnosis. In the syndrome, electrodiagnostic studies will demonstrate conduction abnormalities of the sensory and/or motor nerve branches of the median nerve only. In mild cases, abnormalities of the sensory nerve SNAPs will precede abnormalities of the motor nerve CMAPs, although the reverse may occur. If the SNAPs are recorded between the wrist and digits, an abnormality may not be localized to the wrist. The abnormal SNAPs could also be the result of proximal compression (e.g., pronator teres syndrome) or a diffuse neuropathy. Any of these conditions would produce distal abnormalities. A better localizing feature would be slowing of the CMAP distal latency, and normal forearm conduction velocity. In severe cases, slowing of the median motor nerve conduction velocity is seen in the forearm. This slowing, occurring proximal to the wrist, may be due to retrograde changes in the nerve. Severe cases of carpal tunnel syndrome may demonstrate axonal loss in the distal median nerve innervated muscles (i.e., abducens pollicis brevis [APB]).

For these reasons, CTS evaluation should include sensory and motor nerve conduction studies of both the ulnar and median nerves. The sensory exam of choice is *antidromic*, meaning the electrical stimulus is applied proximally on the median nerve and the recording is made distally. If this exam is "normal," a short segment *orthodromic* sensory exam is indicated because the orthodromic studies have less likelihood of false negative results with higher sensitivity.[12] With regard to the ulnar nerve, electrodiagnostic studies show that 15% to 40% of patients with CTS also have objective evidence of ulnar nerve dysfunction.[1] The likely explanation is that many CTS patients may have a predisposition to multiple entrapment neuropathies, or a more generalized peripheral neuropathy.

Last, the CTS evaluation should also include needle exam of the APB to determine the presence of axon loss. The needle EMG exam is less sensitive than NCS in the evaluation of CTS, because the pathology is mainly demyelination. (Demyelinative processes affect the sensory nerve responses with slowing and prolongation of the SNAP latency.) The needle exam is usually not too revealing in most CTS cases until late in the disease. If there is evidence of membrane instability in the APB, then it is important to sample another C8–T1 innervated muscle to evaluate for a cervical radiculopathy. The first dorsal interosseus muscle is a good muscle to sample because it is a C8–T1 muscle innervated by the ulnar nerve. Also, needle sampling of C6–C7 innervated muscles (e.g., pronator teres or flexor carpi radialis) can be helpful, because C6 and C7 radiculopathies commonly present with thumb and hand pain. Last, 11% of patients with CTS have a concomitant cervical radiculopathy,[1] a phenomenon termed "double crush syndrome."

Several schemes have been established to diagnose and rate the severity of carpal tunnel syndrome.[1] However, there are no universally accepted criteria or standards. The diagnosis is fundamentally a clinical decision. The severity can be rated with electrodiagnostic findings according to one scheme[1] as mild (median sensory nerve abnormalities), moderate (median sensory and motor nerve abnormalities), and severe (median sensory and motor nerve abnormalities, along with needle EMG abnormalities). A reasonable treatment approach could utilize splinting for mild cases, splinting and steroid injections for moderate cases, and surgery for severe cases.

Case example: A 56-year-old female with mild central canal stenosis at C3–C4 and C5–C6, with moderately severe right C5–C6 neuroforaminal stenosis (Fig. 18.12) was treated with three cervical epidural steroid injections during the course of a year. The shots were mildly helpful in treating her bilateral hand

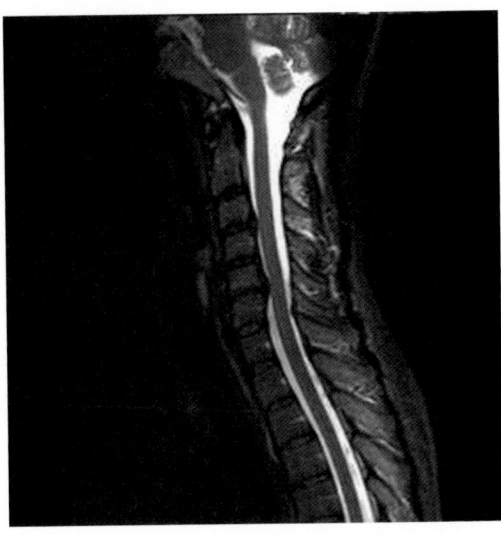

FIGURE 18.12 Sagittal T-2 image of the cervical spine, showing multilevel degenerative disk disease with mild central canal stenosis at C5–C6 and C3–C4. Axial images (not shown) demonstrate moderate to severe right neuroforaminal stenosis at C5–C6.

and forearm pain. Because of the muted benefit of epidural injections, an electrodiagnostic study was ordered.

Evaluation of the left median nerve compound motor action potential (CMAP) had normal amplitude with decreased latency and normal conduction velocity across the forearm. The right median nerve CMAP had decreased latency, amplitude, and conduction velocity. These results demonstrated a bilateral median nerve sensorimotor mononeuropathy. On the left there was evidence of demyelination, on the right there was evidence of demyelination with axon loss. Both sides are consistent with a diagnosis of moderate carpal tunnel syndrome. The EMG exam refocused the treatment plan.

Traumatic Syndromes

Trauma can cause a nerve injury in just about any part of the body. Some of the more common scenarios are presented in Table 18.3, adapted from Liveson.[5] Nerve resection can occur with fractures or penetrating injuries. Traction injuries are commonly seen with dislocations or vaginal and obstetrical procedures. Compression injuries may result from blunt trauma, hematomas, compartment syndromes, or positioning issues during surgery.

During the acute phase (within 4 weeks of injury), the electrodiagnostic exam is used to identify injury location, the possibility of muscle paralysis, and nerve continuity. It can be important in the acute phase to identify outright nerve injury, as opposed to pain inhibited function or cognitive impairment (e.g., an obtunded patient). If no volitional motor activity is observed with the needle EMG exam, then there is no nerve conduction to the muscle. This could be because of complete severance of the nerve, or temporary conduction block (neuropraxia). If some motor unit potentials are seen, then there is neural continuity to the muscle. Nerve conduction studies give information about neural transmission.

In the chronic phase, the needle EMG becomes very useful. If nerve transaction or axon death exists, then there will be observable membrane instability with abnormal spontaneous activity. The nerve interruption is complete if membrane instability is present and no voluntary motor unit potentials are present. The location of the injury can be identified by strategically examining muscles along the course of a particular nerve. In the chronic

TABLE 18.3

ANATOMIC SITES SUSCEPTIBLE TO TRAUMATIC NERVE INJURY

Traumatic event	Vulnerable nerve
Upper limb	
Penetrating neck wound, traction injury at birth	Brachial plexus
Shoulder dislocation, intramuscular injection	Axillary
Humerus (spiral groove) fracture, pressure	Radial
Elbow subluxation, fracture, dislocation	Ulnar
Humerus, elbow, radioulnar joint fractures	Median
Lower limb	
Regional anesthesia (femoral block)	Femoral
Hip, pelvic fracture	Sciatic (peroneal > tibial)
Knee injuries	Peroneal
Ankle fractures	Tibial, peroneal

phase, nerve conduction studies permit the distinction between temporary conduction block and complete axon interruption. Serial examinations over time can document interval progress and healing.

Peripheral Polyneuropathies

There are many different types of acquired peripheral polyneuropathies involving infectious, toxic, metabolic, pharmacologic, hereditary, auto-immune, nutritional, systemic illness–related, malignant, and endocrine disorders.[13] Most polyneuropathies cause distal, symmetrical weakness and/or sensory loss. The sensory deficit is frequently most severe in the distal extremities ("stocking-glove" distribution). Occasionally, a polyneuropathy will preferentially affect the proximal limbs. The disorder may present over a variable time course, and the predominant neurological deficit may involve motor, sensory, autonomic, or combinations thereof.

Leprosy

Leprosy (Hansen disease) is the most common cause of polyneuropathy worldwide. In this disease, *mycobacterium leprae* invades Schwann cells, endoneurium, and perineurium. Three manifestations of the disease are recognized: lepromatous, borderline, and tuberculoid. The host's immunologic status determines which form of the disease develops. Patients may develop generalized symmetric sensorimotor polyneuropathies, mononeuropathies, and mononeuropathy multiplex.[1]

Diabetic Neuropathy

The most common cause of neuropathy in the United States is diabetes.[6] The common etiology involves chronic hyperglycemia; however, there appear to be diverse causes. The precise mechanism is not known, but direct axonal injury due to hyperglycemia, autoimmune injury with antineural antibodies, and increased intraneural pressure and ischemia seem to be contributing factors.[14] Additionally, patients with renal failure independent of diabetes develop a sensorimotor neuropathy due to uremia. About half of the patients with diabetes have a distal symmetric polyneurop-

athy. It is most common in patients older than 50 years. Patients experience sensory complaints with dysesthesia, painful paresthesias, and sensory loss in the distal extremities. Early signs include decreased perception of vibration and pain. In progressed cases, proprioception is affected and there is weakness in the distal muscles. Painless injuries and loss of balance are common. Later, proximal weakness can occur.

Most asymptomatic, neurologically intact diabetic patients have conduction velocities that are mildly slow, around the lower limit of normal.[6] As the severity of the neuropathy advances, sensory amplitudes disappear in the lower extremities. Motor amplitudes become reduced. Abnormal temporal dispersion and partial conduction block are not common. Needle EMG findings will show abnormal spontaneous activity in the distal muscles.

A pure autonomic neuropathy is rare, but some degree of autonomic involvement is present in most patients. Autonomic symptoms may involve sudomotor (dry skin), papillary (poor dark adaptation), cardiovascular (orthostatic hypotension), urinary (incontinence, impotence), or gastrointestinal (constipation).

There are several other presentations of diabetic neuropathies. Some diabetic patients will have a polyneuropathy affecting mainly the small-diameter sensory fibers (A delta and C fibers) that manifests as painful paresthesias. Another presentation is diabetic neuropathic cachexia, which involves a precipitous and profound weight loss. It is rather uncommon. Mononeuropathies are more common in diabetics (refer to the previous entrapment neuropathy section). A diabetic femoral neuropathy may present with pain, weakness, and atrophy of muscles innervated by the femoral nerve. The presentation of a diabetic polyradiculopathy resembles a radiculopathy due to spinal degeneration (see the previous radiculopathy section).[15] The neuropathy usually begins with severe, unilateral pain in the low back, hip, and thigh. However, multiple spinal nerve roots are involved and there is weakness in the expected myotomal distributions. Coexisting symmetrical polyneuropathy often is present.

The presentation of a patient with diabetes can arise from a combination of degenerative musculoskeletal and nervous system etiologies. The electrodiagnostic exam helps to refine the diagnosis, direct treatments, and establish treatment expectations.

Disorders of Muscle

Myopathy refers to a problem in skeletal muscle. A myopathy usually presents with symmetrical proximal weakness. The sensory exam is normal. Deep tendon reflexes are depressed. Muscle atrophy and weakness is present. Occasionally, the lost muscle is replaced by fat and pseudohypertrophy (increase in the apparent muscle size) results. Myopathies are generally painless, but some cases are painful with muscle tenderness. Hereditary myopathies include the muscular dystrophies, dystrophic myotonias, congenital myopathies, metabolic myopathies, and mitochondrial myopathies. Acquired myopathies involve inflammatory, infectious, endocrine, electrolyte disturbances, malignancy, toxins, and systemic disease.[1]

Duchenne Muscular Dystrophy (DMD)

One devastating example of a hereditary muscle disorder is Duchenne muscular dystrophy (DMD). It is an X-linked disease affecting boys that usually results in death before the age of 20. A milder form is Becker muscular dystrophy. Both dystrophies involve a defect in the gene product dystrophin.

Myotonic Dystrophy

Another type of heritable myopathy is myotonic dystrophy. The molecular defect involves myotonin protein kinase. There is distal muscle weakness and atrophy, and a characteristic facial appearance involving additional atrophy of the temples and jaws. Cardiac abnormalities present in more than 50% of patients. Endocrine abnormalities, such as testicular atrophy and diabetes, are common. A key feature is *myotonia*, delayed relaxation of skeletal muscle after contraction (e.g., inability to relax grip after a handshake). Serum creatine kinase levels are usually normal. Motor and sensory nerve conduction studies are usually normal. Needle EMG will reveal a striking finding called the myotonic discharge, which involves waxing and waning of both the amplitude and frequency of motor units.

Disorders of Neuromuscular Junction

Myasthenia Gravis

Disorders of the neuromuscular junction are rare. In myasthenia gravis, the density of postsynaptic acetylcholine receptors is reduced at the neuromuscular junction. The geometry of the end plate is also disturbed. As a result, the amplitude of the endplate potential is reduced and may fail to reach the necessary threshold to produce a muscle action potential. The patient experiences easy fatigability and weakness. An initial effort may produce strong muscular contraction, but subsequent efforts get progressively weaker. In one variation, the disorder is ocular, affecting all eye muscles. The diagnosis rests on a form of nerve conduction testing called repetitive nerve stimulation. Treatment is directed at blocking acetylcholinesterase in order to prolong neurotransmitter function. Immunosuppressive therapies, including thymectomy, may be of benefit.

CONCLUSION

The basics of electrodiagnostic studies were outlined in this chapter. The technical aspects of nerve conduction studies and electromyographic needle exam were presented. Patient preparation factors were identified. Radiculopathies, entrapment syndromes, trauma, polyneuropathies, and a few myopathic conditions were discussed. The approach has been practical and applied, with the anesthesiology pain management audience (who may never have performed an EMG) in mind. Neurology and physical medicine and rehabilitation "purists" might find this review too brief.

Everyone, regardless of background, is directed to more comprehensive textbooks dedicated exclusively to the art and practice of electrodiagnosis.

There are limitations and subjective aspects to every electrodiagnostic exam. However, in the end, electrodiagnostic studies help to refine and clarify the diagnosis, set expectations, and can radically change treatment plans. The bottom line is that electrodiagnostic studies are an important tool that must not be overlooked by physicians who treat pain.

References

1. Dumitru D, Amato A, Zwarts M, eds. *Electrodiagnostic Medicine.* 2nd edition. Philadelphia: Hanley & Belfus; 2001.
2. Kimura J. *Electrodiagnosis in Diseases of Nerve and Muscle: Principles and Practice.* 3rd edition. New York: Oxford University Press; 2001.
3. Oh S. *Clinical Electromyography: Nerve Conduction Studies.* 3rd ed: Lippincott Williams & Wilkins; 2002.
4. Weiss L, Silver J, Weiss J, eds. *Easy EMG.* 1st ed: Butterworth-Heinemann; 2004.
5. Liveson J. *Peripheral Neurology: Case Studies.* New York: Oxford University Press; 2000.
6. Pease WS, Lew HL, Johnson EW, eds. *Johnson's Practical Electromyography.* 4th edition. Philadelphia: Lippincott Williams & Wilkins; 2007.
7. Carragee E. Electromyography, local blocks/injections, discograms. In: Bono C, Garfin S, eds. *Orthopaedic Surgery Essentials Spine.* Philadelphia: Lippincott Williams & Wilkins, 2004:28–34.
8. Lee H, DeLisa J. *Manual of Nerve Conduction Study and Surface Anatomy for Needle Electromyography.* 4th edition. Philadelphia: Lippincott Williams & Wilkins, 2005.
9. Al-Shekhlee A, Shapiro B, Preston D. Iatrogenic complications and risks of nerve conduction studies and needle electromyography. *Muscle Nerve* 2003; 27:517–526.
10. Wilbourn A, Aminoff M. AAEM minimonograph 32: the electrodiagnostic examination in patients with radiculopathies. *Muscle Nerve* 1998;21: 1612–1631.
11. Waylonis G. Electromyographic findings in chronic cervical radicular symptoms. *Arch Phys Med Rehabil* 1968;49:407–412.
12. Lew H, Date E, Pan S, et al. Sensitivity, specificity, and variability of nerve conduction velocity measurements in carpal tunnel syndrome. *Arch Phys Med Rehabil* 2005;86:12–16.
13. Donofrio P, Albers J. Polyneuropathy: classification by nerve conduction studies and electromyography. *Muscle Nerve* 1990;13:889–903.
14. Zochodne D. Diabetes mellitus and the peripheral nervous system: manifestations and mechanisms. *Muscle Nerve* 2007;36:144–166.
15. Dyck P, Windebank A. Diabetic and nondiabetic lumbosacral radiculoplexus neuropathy: new insights into pathophysiology and treatment. *Muscle Nerve* 2002;25:477–491.

CHAPTER 19 ■ DIAGNOSTIC IMAGING OF PAIN

ASAKO MIYAKOSHI AND KENNETH R. MARAVILLA

INTRODUCTION

Pain is a major indication for imaging examinations. Imaging protocols are tailored based on acuteness, character, and location of the pain and the presumed diagnosis. Since, most of the time, the differential diagnoses of acute pain are relatively limited based on history and physical examination but can be of surgical emergency, primary imaging study for the patient with acute pain will typically confirm or exclude the presumed diagnosis based on history and physical examination (acute fracture, intracranial hemorrhage, aortic dissection, pneumothorax, pneumoperito-

neum, etc). For patients with recurrent or persistent pain whose diagnosis remains obscure after routine imaging workup, the role of imaging could be expanded. Specialized imaging techniques can help detect subtle evidence of disease, direct therapy, and help identify patients for surgical or radiological intervention.

A comprehensive discussion of radiographs, computed tomography (CT), magnetic resonance imaging (MRI), ultrasound, and radionuclide examinations for evaluation of pain should include almost all radiological subspecialties. This is beyond the scope of this chapter and can be found in most general radiology textbooks. This chapter is dedicated to the evaluation of the pain in the nervous system and reviews the imaging approach to several regional pain syndromes as well as imaging techniques that can be used to select surgical candidates among patients with back pain, tic douloureux, and peripheral nerve entrapment syndromes. Techniques and indications for MRI of the cranial nerves and posterior fossa vasculature, discography for nonradicular back and neck pain, and high-resolution MRI of the brachial plexus and peripheral nerves are discussed.

HEADACHE

Headache is a common symptom. Choosing the patient who should have a cranial imaging study can be challenging (see Chapter 62). The diagnostic yield of neuroimaging examinations in patients with headache and a normal neurologic examination, or in patients with typical migraine, is low (Table 19.1).[1] Specific clinical features associated with significant intracranial abnormality, however, should prompt neuroimaging: Acute onset of an extremely severe headache, including thunderclap headache, worsening subacute headache, headache associated with focal neurologic signs or cognitive impairment (in patients without a history of migraine), new headache in patients older than age 50, and headache in immunocompromised patients or patients with known malignancy.[1-4] Patients over the age of 65 with new onset of pathologic headache have a 15% incidence of serious intracranial disease, including temporal arteritis, tumor, and infarct. In contrast, patients younger than age 65 have only a 1.5% incidence of detectable underlying pathology.[5]

Acute Headache

Severe, acute headache, especially if associated with neurologic abnormality or depressed sensorium, suggests possible subarachnoid hemorrhage (SAH). The devastating consequences of untreated ruptured aneurysm require prompt exclusion of SAH in this setting. Diagnosis is best made by CT demonstration of hyperdense blood in the subarachnoid space or detection of xanthochromic cerebrospinal fluid (CSF) on lumbar puncture in patients with a negative CT examination.[6] CT sensitivity for detection of SAH is reduced as the time interval from hemorrhage increases.[1] If SAH is present, subsequent imaging is directed at detecting an aneurysm (Fig. 19.1) or arteriovenous malformation (Fig. 19.2). Venous sinus thrombosis (Figs. 19.3 and 19.4),[7,8] benign perimesencephalic SAH,[9] arterial dissection[10,11] (Fig. 19.5), and migraine can also present as severe acute headache.

Imaging the patient with suspected SAH should begin with nonenhanced CT. Cisterns and sulci must be carefully examined for hyperdense acute blood, which can be subtle if the amount of hemorrhage is small, or if the study is performed more than 24 hours after the bleed occurred. Nonenhanced CT has a sensitivity of 98%[6] within 12 hours, or on a more recent study, 100% on emergency CTs.[12] In patients with high suspicion for SAH who have a negative CT, lumbar puncture should be performed

for the uncommon but possible false negative CT.[6,13] In the absence of SAH, nonenhanced CT can detect signs of other pathologies, including increased density within a thrombosed dural venous sinus, venous infarction, and edema associated with intracranial mass lesions. If subtle abnormalities are found on nonenhanced CT, further imaging evaluation includes contrast-enhanced CT or MRI. In the absence of SAH, MRI is a more sensitive technique to evaluate the patient for other causes of headache, including dural venous sinus occlusion, venous infarct, and intracranial infection. If SAH is detected, CTA or DSA is generally used to further evaluate the location and features of an aneurysm or arteriovenous malformation.

Magnetic resonance angiography (MRA) and CT angiography (CTA) are useful for rapid, noninvasive diagnosis of intracranial vascular lesions. CTA is a dynamic, CT-based angiographic technique in which thin slice images are obtained rapidly and continuously during the first pass of the arterial phase of an intravenous contrast infusion. Using state-of-the-art multidetector CT, axial images covering the entire cerebral vessels can be acquired in a few seconds. Using rapid computer processing, planar and three-dimensional (3D) reconstructions can be created to display the enhanced blood vessels in a manner analogous to the projection images from catheter angiography. CTA can be easily performed immediately following the initial noncontrast CT while the patient is still on the CT table. MRA is also possible to obtain, but it is more time consuming and may not be suitable when the patient is unable to hold still and requires close monitoring. The quality of CTA in detecting aneurysms is comparable to digital subtraction angiography (DSA). However, DSA is considered to be superior to CTA for detecting small aneurysms (<5mm), especially with 3D rotational angiography. 3D rotational angiography also allows for more precise evaluation and measurement of aneurysms.[14-19] CTA or MRA can assist in the rapid diagnosis or exclusion of aneurysms and arteriovenous malformations in the acutely ill patient. These images are also used to clarify subtle findings in patients with questionable abnormalities on noncontrast CT. Similarly, carotid dissection can be detected by imaging the upper cervical vasculature with the above-described imaging techniques (see Fig. 19.5).[20,21]

Chronic Headache

Image findings are unrevealing in most cases of isolated chronic headache. Intracranial lesions can present primarily with headache, but usually are associated with other neurologic signs or symptoms.[22] When headaches are caused by underlying pathologic disorders, the differential diagnosis is broad. Serious primary conditions include intraparenchymal, dural, or skull base tumors[23]; unruptured aneurysms[24]; abscesses; arterial dissection[25]; venous sinus thrombosis; and arteriovenous malformations. A normal CT or MRI without intravenous contrast excludes most intracranial masses, and can reassure the clinician and justify continued clinical observation and symptomatic treat-

---

TABLE 19-1

NEUROIMAGING YIELD IN HEADACHE

| Headache type | Percentage of patients with underlying condition | | | | | |
	Tumor	Arteriovenous malformation	Hydrocephalus	Aneurysm	Subdural hematoma	Infarct
Normal examination	0.8	0.2	0.3	0.1	0.2	1.2
Migraine	0.3	0.07	—	0.7	—	—

Adapted from Evans RW. Diagnostic testing for the evaluation of headaches. *Neurol Clin* 1996;14:1–26.

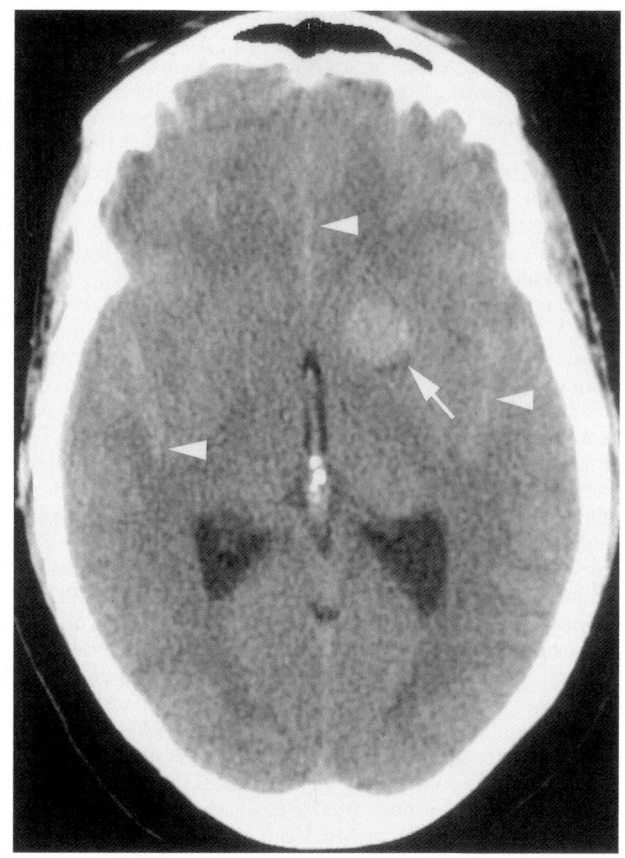

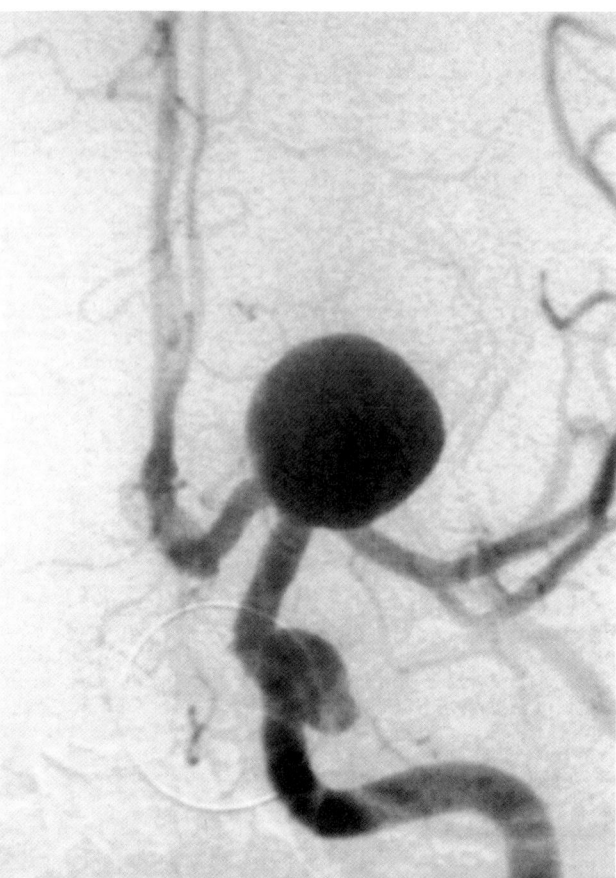

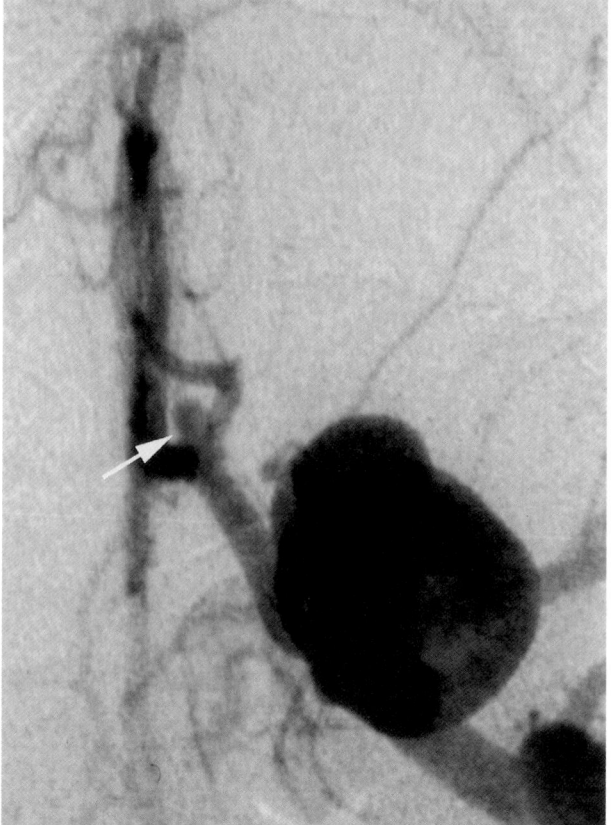

FIGURE 19.1 Subarachnoid hemorrhage caused by ruptured terminal internal carotid artery aneurysm. (**A**) Nonenhanced computed tomography shows hyperdense aneurysm (*arrow*) and blood within interhemispheric and sylvian fissures (*arrowheads*). The ventricles are mildly enlarged and clot is present within the third ventricle. (**B**) Left internal carotid artery arteriogram shows a 2-cm aneurysm arising from the termination of the internal carotid artery. (**C**) A second, unruptured aneurysm is seen at the junction of the left anterior cerebral artery and the anterior communicating artery (*arrow*).

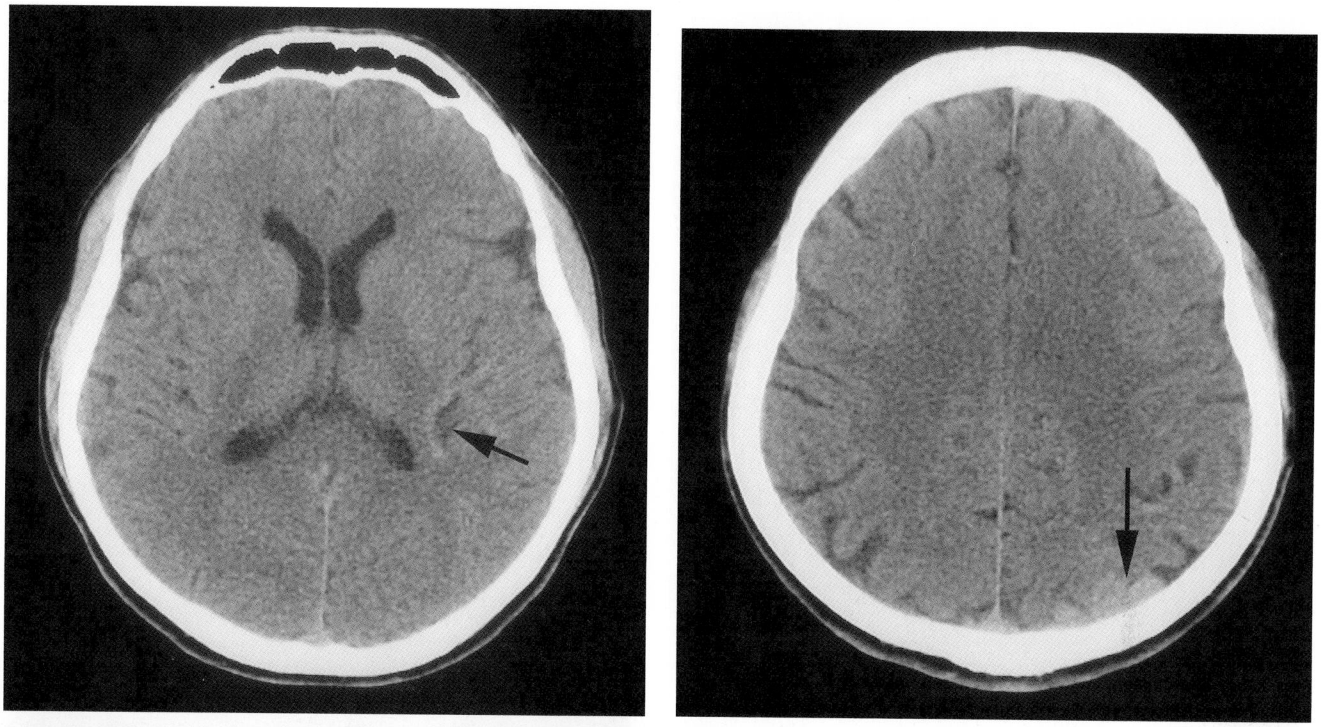

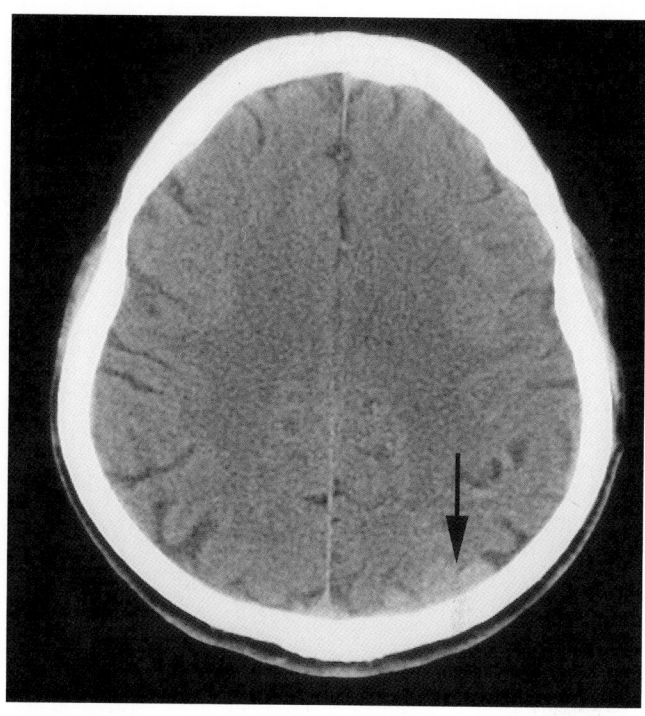

FIGURE 19.2 Arteriovenous malformation. A 39-year-old man with several days' headache. (**A**) Noncontrast computed tomography shows enlarged, slightly hyperdense vessels in the sylvian fissure (*arrow*). (**B**) Hyperdense, dilated veins at the varietal vertex (*arrow*). (**C**) Computed tomographic angiography shows the arteriovenous malformation nidus as well as dilated feeding arteries and peripheral draining veins.

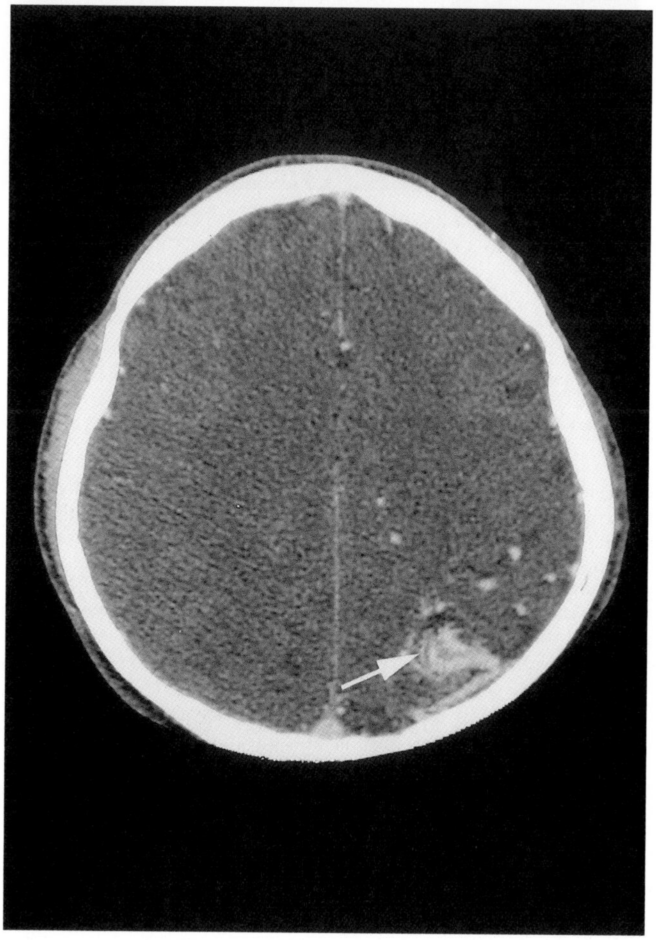

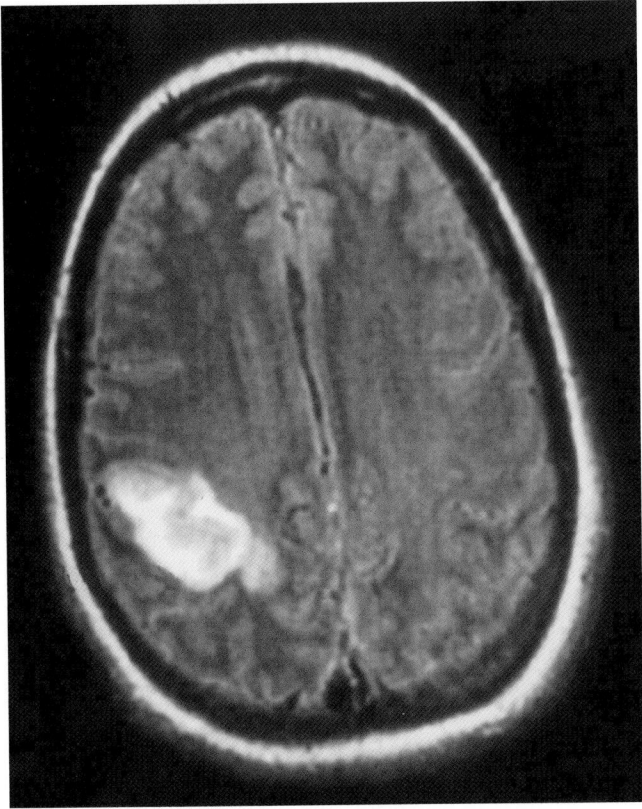

A

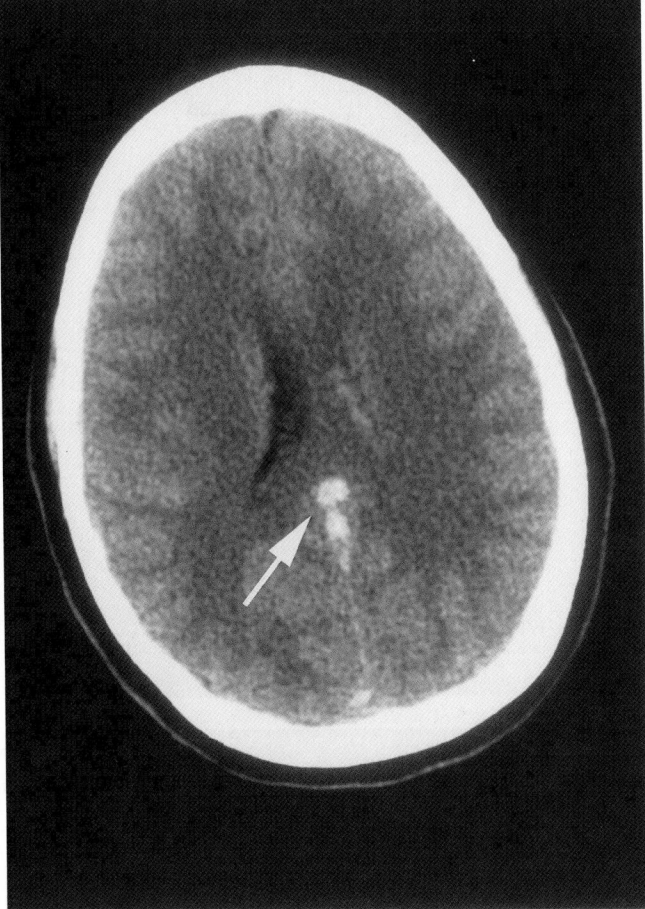

B

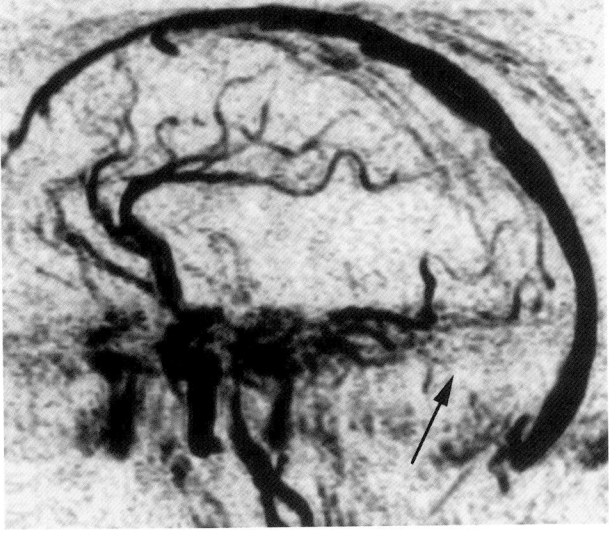

C

FIGURE 19.3 Venous sinus thrombosis with cortical infarct. A 26-year-old postpartum woman with headache and left hemiparesis. (A) Axial FLAIR image at level of centrum semiovale shows increased signal in precentral gyrus, indicating cortical infarct. (B) Nonenhanced computed tomography shows high attenuation in vein of Galen and straight sinus (*arrow*). (C) Magnetic resonance venogram shows absence of flow through straight sinus with patent sagittal and transverse sinuses.

ment. If the clinical evaluation points toward metastasis, abscess, or a vascular process, then contrast-enhanced CT or MRI is an appropriate study. Conventional plain-film radiography may be used as a screening method for various pathological conditions of the sinonasal cavities. However, CT scanning remains the study of choice for the imaging evaluation of acute and chronic inflammatory diseases of sinonasal cavities.

Acute Sinusitis

Acute sinusitis is a common cause of headache or facial pain. Conventional plain radiography may be used. It is specific but not sensitive in detecting sinus mucosal abnormalities.[26,27] Screening sinus CT is more sensitive than plain radiography and is now

used routinely at our center. Designed as a rapid, limited CT examination targeted only at the paranasal sinuses, this study can be performed at only a modestly increased cost compared with plain films. CT has the additional advantages of evaluating the middle ear and mastoid air cells, as well as the subtle bony and mucosal changes reflecting chronic sinusitis. In the patient with recurrent sinusitis, thin section, high resolution coronal CT assists in planning of endoscopic sinus surgery (Fig. 19.6).[28]

Intracranial Hypotension

The syndrome of CSF hypotension is characterized by positional headache and variable symptoms of nausea, vomiting, and visual, auditory, or vestibular disturbances. Normal CSF pressure in the

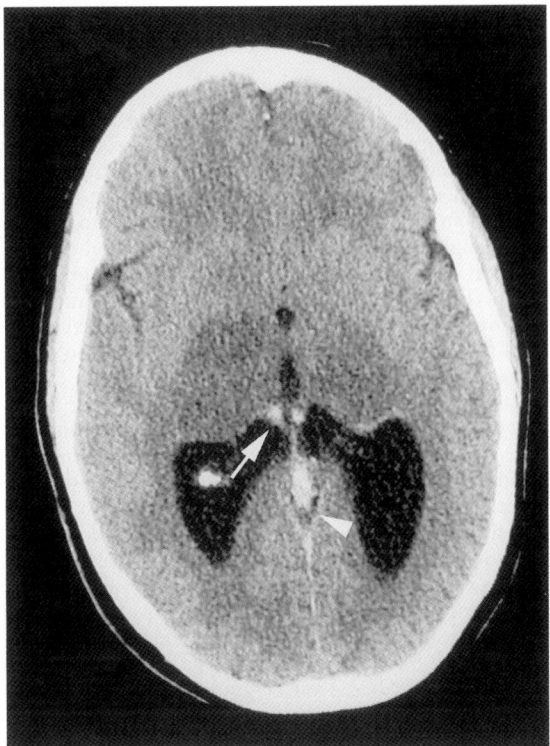

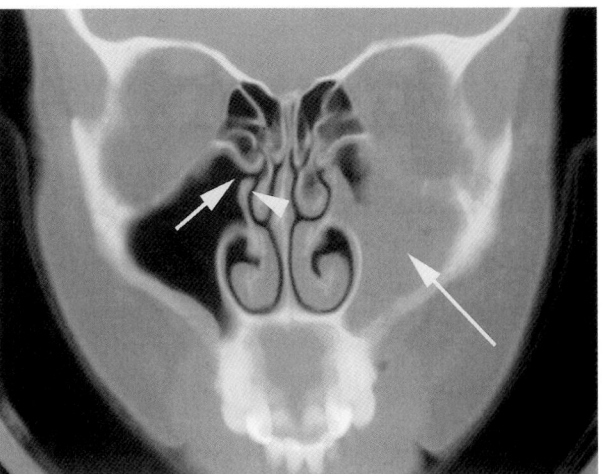

FIGURE 19.6 Chronic sinusitis. Coronal, nonenhanced screening sinus computed tomography through the face shows opacification of the left maxillary sinus caused by chronic inflammation (*long arrow*). The ostiomeatal unit (*short arrow*) and uncinate process (*arrowhead*) are clearly demonstrated on the opposite side.

FIGURE 19.4 Venous sinus thrombosis with bilateral thalamic infarcts in a 24-year-old woman with 4 days of headache followed by several hours of nausea and depressed consciousness. Nonenhanced computed tomography shows low attenuation changes in both thalami, with increased attenuation in the internal cerebral veins (*arrow*) and straight sinus (*arrowhead*).

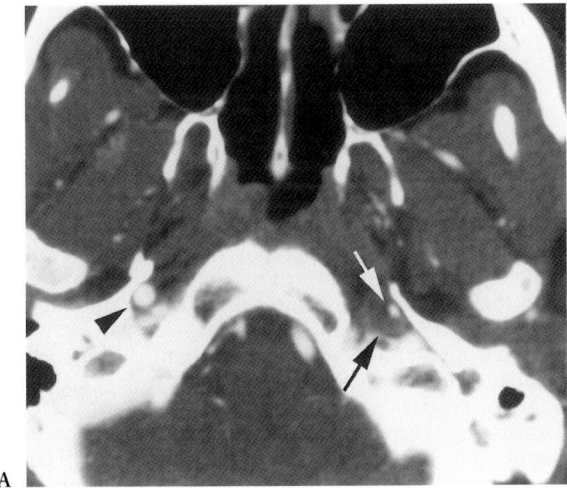

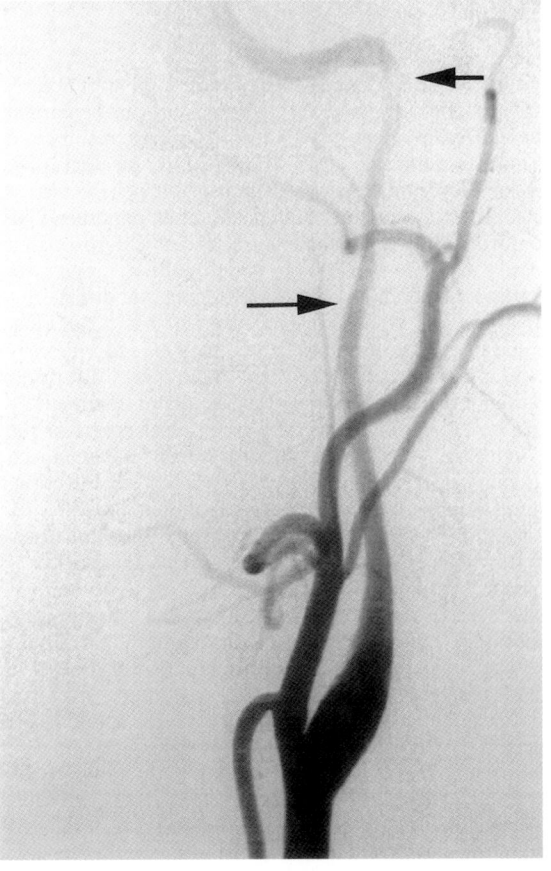

FIGURE 19.5 Internal carotid artery dissection in a 37-year-old man with headache and left pupillary constriction. (**A**) Computed tomographic angiography at skull base shows decreased caliber of left internal carotid artery (*white arrow*) at the skull base. Intramural hematoma surrounds the narrowed lumen (*black arrow*). Normal right internal carotid artery (*arrowhead*). (**B**) Left internal carotid arteriogram shows smooth narrowing of distal cervical internal carotid with near complete occlusion at the skull base (*arrows*).

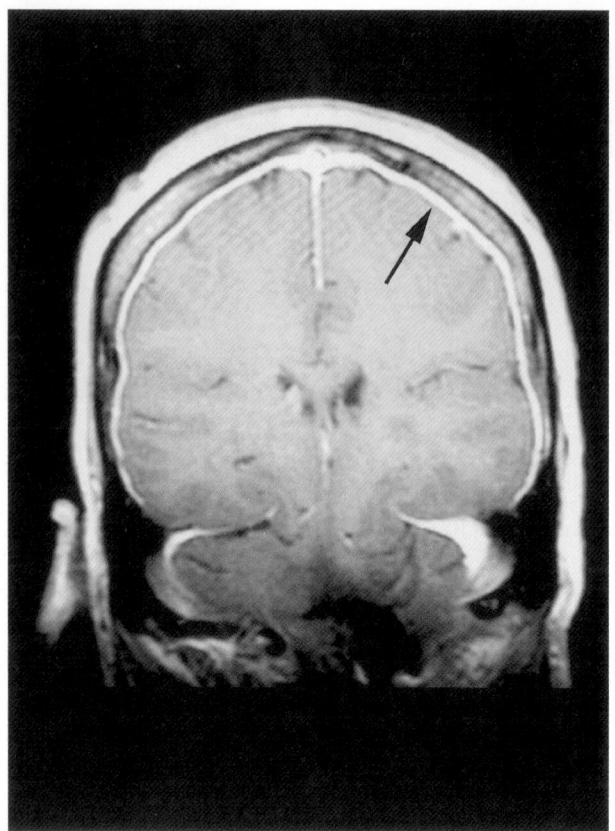

FIGURE 19.7 Cerebrospinal fluid hypotension caused by overshunting. A 54-year-old woman with ventriculoperitoneal shunt. Diffuse dural thickening and enhancement (*arrow*) caused by shunt valve with insufficient resistance. Similar findings may be seen in patients with postlumbar puncture, dural tears, or posttraumatic cerebrospinal fluid leaks.

recumbent position, and in the absence of prior lumbar puncture, is between 7 and 18 cm H_2O. CSF hypotension can be caused by spontaneous development of a CSF leak[29] or may result from diagnostic lumbar puncture, epidural anesthesia, myelography, head injury, or overdrainage of CSF shunts.[30]

Spontaneous, posttraumatic, and postlumbar puncture CSF hypotension probably reflects chronic leakage of CSF through a dural defect.[31] Cranial MRI with gadolinium demonstrates smooth, continuous enhanced dural thickening, subdural effusions, and downward vertical displacement of the brain (Fig. 19.7). In some cases, the dural thickening may extend inferiorly to involve the spinal canal as well. These findings may disappear with resolution of CSF hypotension after successful treatment by blood patch, epidural saline injection, or surgical repair of the defect.[32–34] Headache with MR findings of diffuse enhanced dural thickening, not explained by prior surgery or infection, should prompt a diligent search for occult spontaneous CSF leak. An occult, spontaneous leak may occur through the skull base, or, less frequently, via a spinal dural defect. Recently, MR myelography has been attempted and seems promising as a noninvasive test to detect the source of the leak in spontaneous intracranial hypotension.[35–38] On MR myelogram, epidural collection, engorgement of a venous plexus, and irregularity of the nerve sleeve at the leakage site can be seen.

FACIAL PAIN

Intractable trigeminal neuralgia (tic douloureux) can be related to irritation of the nerve from a branch of the superior, anterior,

or posterior inferior cerebellar artery that contacts the cisternal portion of the fifth cranial nerve near its exit from the pons[39] (see Chapter 67). Surgical intervention with placement of a prosthesis to separate the offending vessel from the root entry zone of the cranial nerve is often effective in relieving symptoms.[40] Diagnosis of vascular loops in the prepontine cistern and cerebellopontine angle was difficult before the development of MRI. Thin section balanced steady-state free precession gradient-echo techniques (BFFE, FIESTA, true FISP), MRA, and multiplanar or 3D reformatting can accurately demonstrate cisternal vessels and nerves in the posterior fossa and aid in identification of surgical candidates.[41–45]

The diagnosis of vascular loop syndrome is made by demonstration of a blood vessel contiguous with, or preferably distorting, a cranial nerve close to its origin from the brainstem at the root entry zone. This portion of the nerve is sensitive to irritation from pulsations in the contacting artery. The diagnosis is based on appropriate clinical symptoms as well as definitive MRI/MRA findings, because 49% asymptomatic patients show vascular loops contacting the cranial nerve origins.[44] Diffusion tensor imaging may be useful to support the diagnosis. Asymmetric decrease of fractional anisotropy in the affected nerve could be visualized[46] (Fig. 19.8). Image findings alone do not justify surgical treatment, which is based on symptom severity and failure of medical therapy. Other causes of trigeminal nerve dysfunction include mass lesions near the trigeminal nerve such as meningioma, schwannoma, arachnoid cyst, cholesteatoma, and epidermoid cyst.[47,48] These can be diagnosed by conventional cranial MRI and CT.

Vascular loops can compromise other cranial nerves in the basal cisterns. Chronic vertigo can be caused by posterior fossa vessels contacting the root entry zone of the eighth nerve (see Fig. 19.9) and compression of the intracisternal seventh nerve can result in hemifacial spasm. High-resolution MRI/MRA can be used to identify potential vascular loop syndromes causing these symptoms.

SPINAL PAIN

Overview

Technical advances in surgical fusion of lower lumbar vertebrae have resulted in safer, less invasive operations and have generated renewed interest in diagnostic tests that might predict a favorable surgical outcome for the back pain patient.[49–51] Conventional MRI, CT, and CT myelography can accurately evaluate spinal canal or neuroforaminal stenosis, lumbar disc protrusion, extrusion, or sequestration in the patient with pain and radiculopathy[52] (Fig. 19.10). Gadolinium-enhanced MRI can distinguish between postsurgical scar and recurrent disc herniation in the patient with prior back surgery and persistent or recurrent pain.[53] Scar tissues have a blood supply and demonstrate contrast enhancement, whereas herniated disc does not have a direct blood supply and only minimally enhances by diffusion of contrast. The difference of the enhancement is more conspicuous by using an ionic contrast medium.[54] Although CT and MRI are helpful to depict degenerative changes and disc pathology, because of the prevalence of degenerative changes, annular tears, and disc bulge and focal protrusion in asymptomatic patients, CT or MRI findings alone do not prove that a given disc is the cause of the individual patient's pain.[55] The less common findings of moderate or severe central stenosis, root compression, and extrusions are likely to be diagnostically and clinically relevant.[56]

Benign versus Malignant Compression Fracture

Water-fat in-phase and opposed-phase gradient recalled-echo sequences are promising in differentiating pathologic compression fractures from benign compression fractures.[57] In this method,

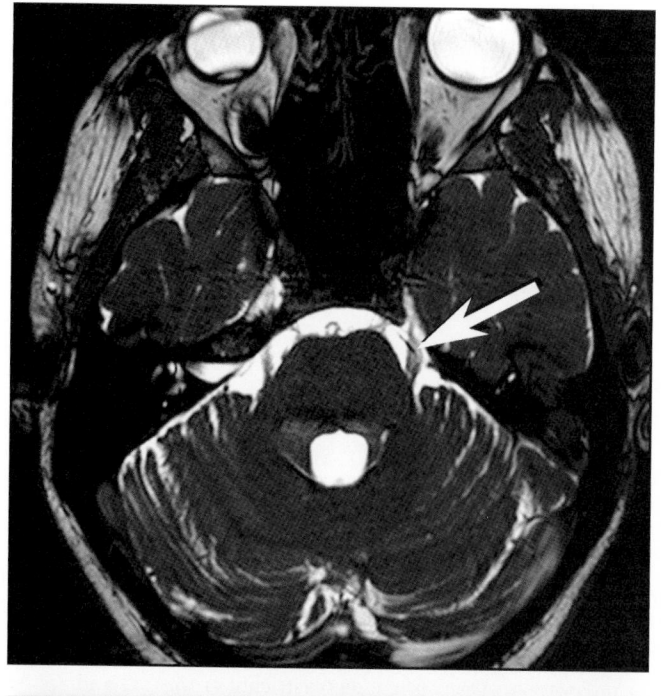

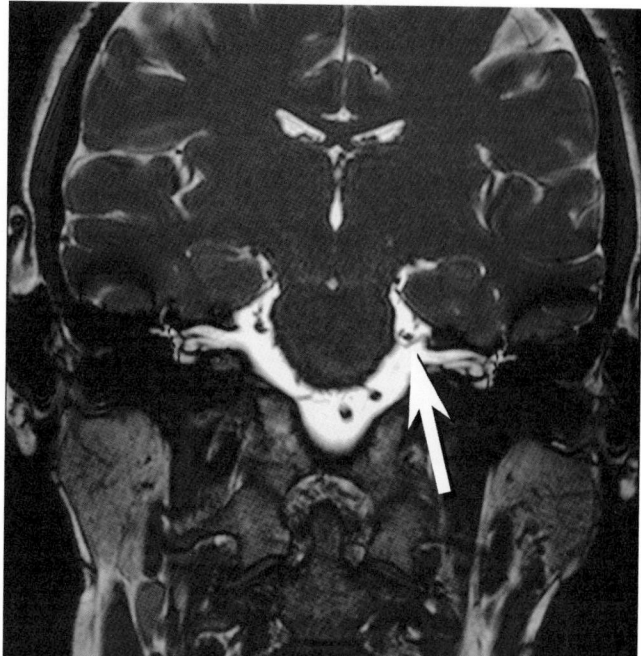

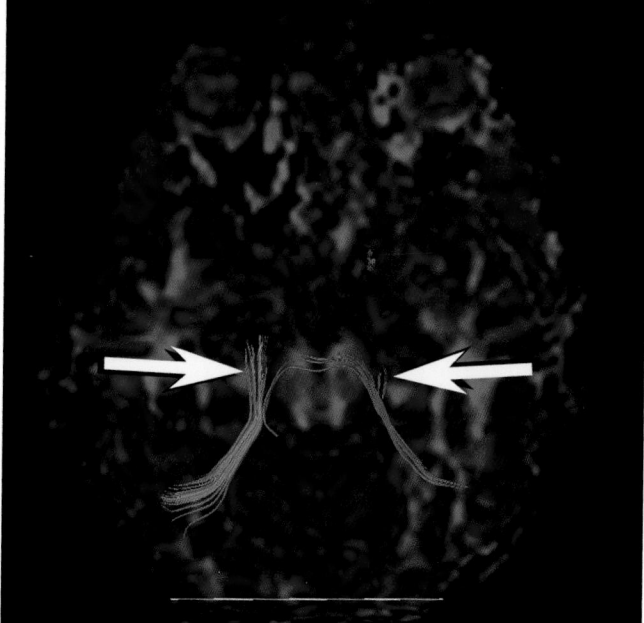

FIGURE 19.8 Vascular loop compression of the trigeminal nerve. **(A)** Axial balanced fast field echo (BFFE) image and **(B)** coronal BFFE image demonstrate the left superior cerebellar artery branch runs immediately inferior to the cisternal segment of the left trigeminal nerve (*arrows*) with possible compression. **(C)** Diffusion tensor imaging (DTI) clearly delineates the asymmetry of the trigeminal nerves (*arrows*) with decreased anisotropy on the left (*right arrow*), which is suggestive of vascular compression.

signal intensity ratio on opposed-phase images compared to in-phase images of >0.8 suggests malignancy since malignant processes replace normal fatty marrow.

Discogenic Pain

Before the advent of spinal CT and MRI, discography was the only radiologic technique for directly assessing the anatomy and integrity of the intervertebral disc. From this anatomic standpoint, CT and MRI have replaced discography.[58] The current role of discography is as a provocative test, with the aim of selecting patients with a greater likelihood of improvement after spinal fusion procedures. Discography involves injection of radiographic contrast material into an anatomically abnormal (sus-

pect) disc and one or two normal (control) discs, and recording the patient's reported pain sensations during injection (Fig. 19.11).[59] A positive test result is indicated by reproduction of the patient's symptoms during injection of a morphologically abnormal disc, without similar discomfort on injection of control disc levels.[60] Discography is a unique provocative test for discogenic pain, but patients' reporting symptoms during disc injection can be affected by psychological factors as well as the interview technique.[61,62] The discographic identification of a painful disc also does not guarantee that the patient will respond to surgical fusion at that level.[63,64] Concordant pain could be present in patients with mild low back pain who do not seek treatment.[65] Because ongoing controversy exists as to the accuracy and value of discography,[66–68] its utilization largely depends on each clinician. Discography is probably best indicated before proposed sur-

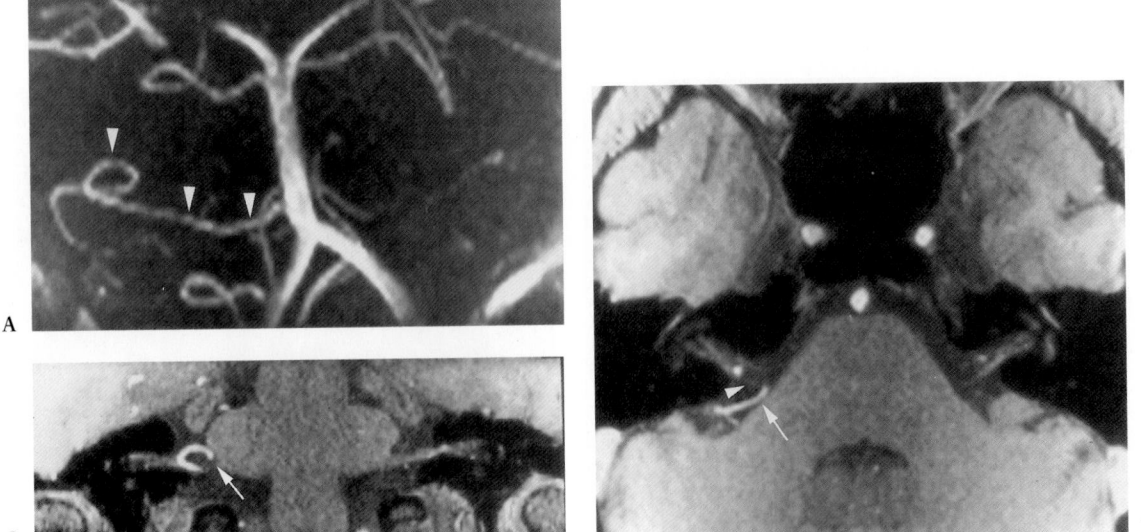

FIGURE 19.9 Vascular loop compression of the eighth nerve. (**A**) Anteroposterior projection of a MRA of the vertebral basilar arterial system shows a good demonstration of a prominent right anterior inferior cerebellar artery (*arrowheads*). However, this standard MRA display does not allow one to determine the relationship of the looping portion of the vessel to the underlying neural structures. (**B**) Axial source image of the MRA now shows a good demonstration of a vascular loop (*arrow*), which lies contiguous with the eighth nerve near its origin from the brainstem. (**C**) Coronal reformatted image from the MRA data set confirms the contiguous position of the vascular loop with the eighth nerve near its root entry zone (*arrow*).

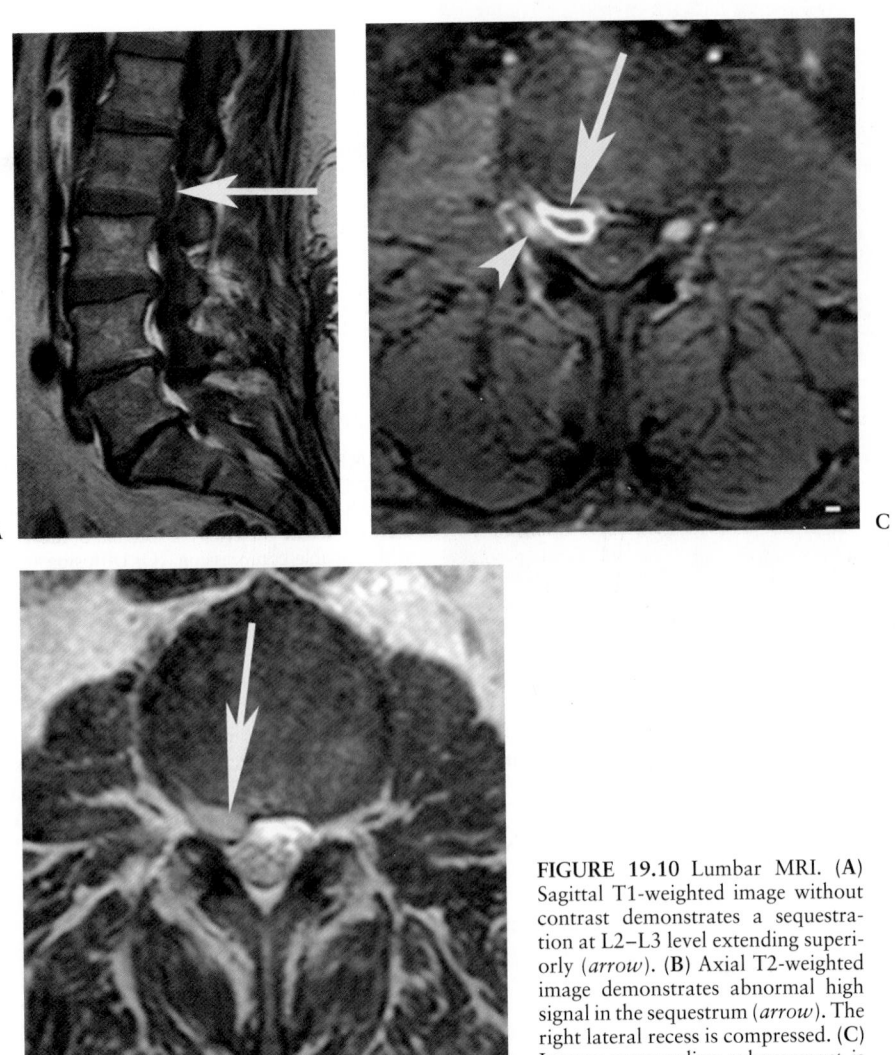

FIGURE 19.10 Lumbar MRI. (**A**) Sagittal T1-weighted image without contrast demonstrates a sequestration at L2–L3 level extending superiorly (*arrow*). (**B**) Axial T2-weighted image demonstrates abnormal high signal in the sequestrum (*arrow*). The right lateral recess is compressed. (**C**) Intense surrounding enhancement is present (*arrow*). The exiting right L2 nerve is compressed (*arrowhead*).

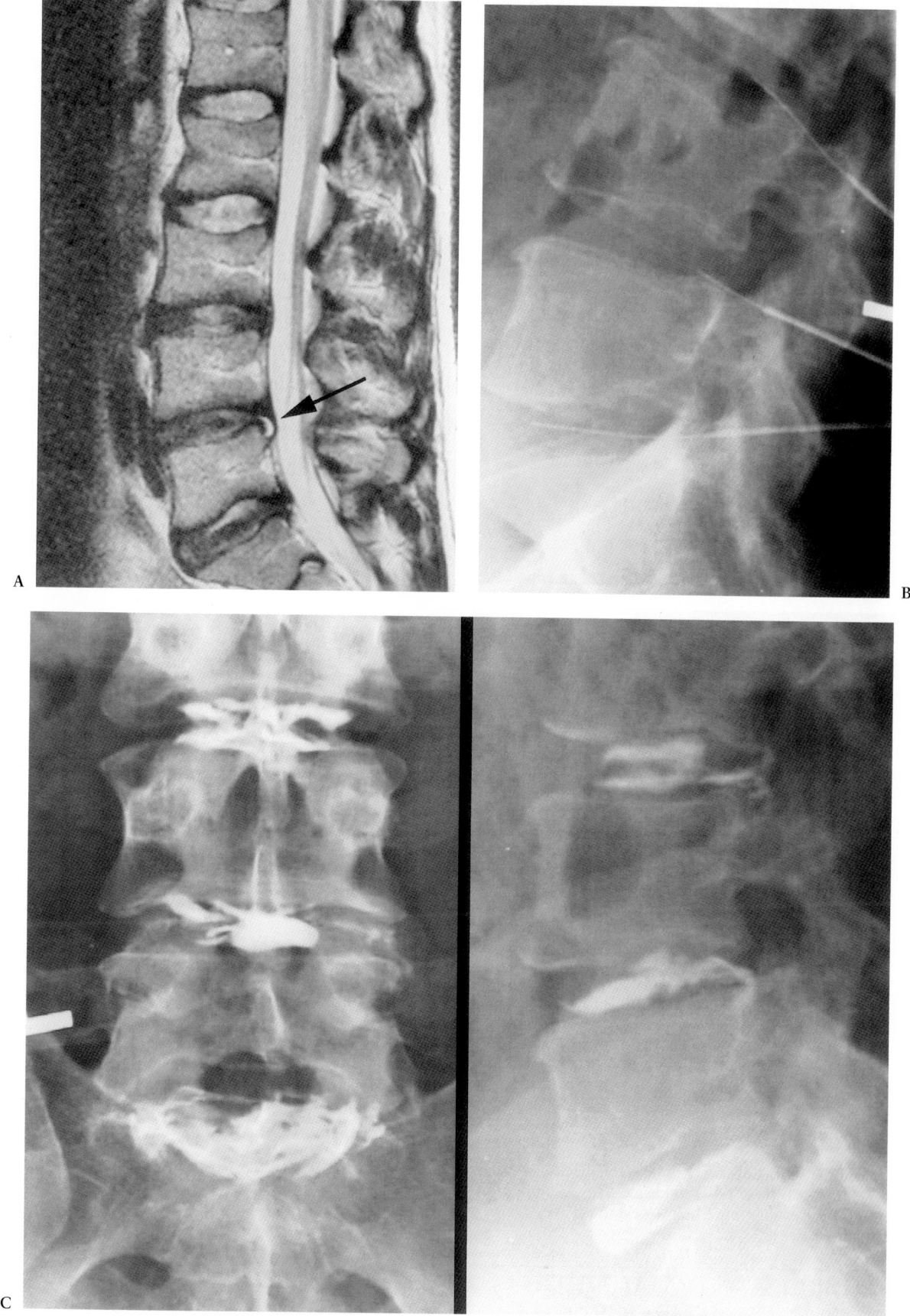

FIGURE 19.11 Discogram. A 34-year-old man with chronic lower back pain with radiation to left leg. (**A**) Sagittal T2-weighted lumbar magnetic resonance imaging examination demonstrates an annular tear at L-4–5 as well as mild disk desiccation at L-3–4 and L-5–S-1. (**B**) Lateral fluoroscopic spot film showing placement of 25-gauge Chiba needles within the intervertebral discs at L-3–4, L-4–5, and L-5-S-1. (**C**) Antero-posterior (*left*) and lateral (*right*) fluoroscopic images after injection of contrast material. During contrast injection, the patient reported no pain at L-3–4, mild (2/10) pain similar to clinical symptoms at L-4–5, and minimal (1/10) pain unlike clinical symptoms at L-5–S-1.

(continues)

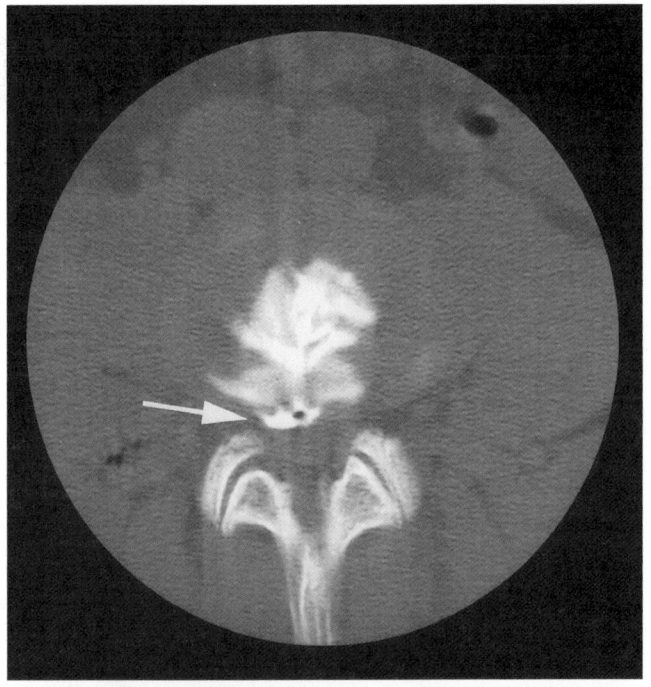

D

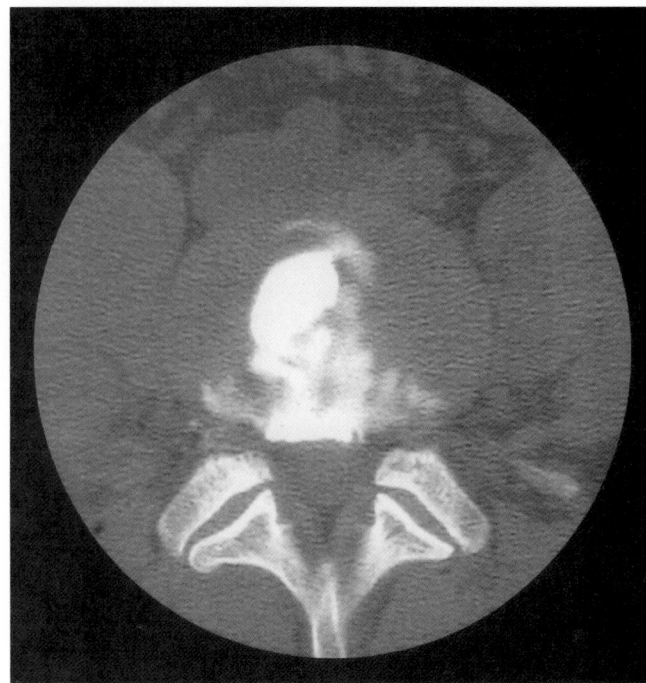

E

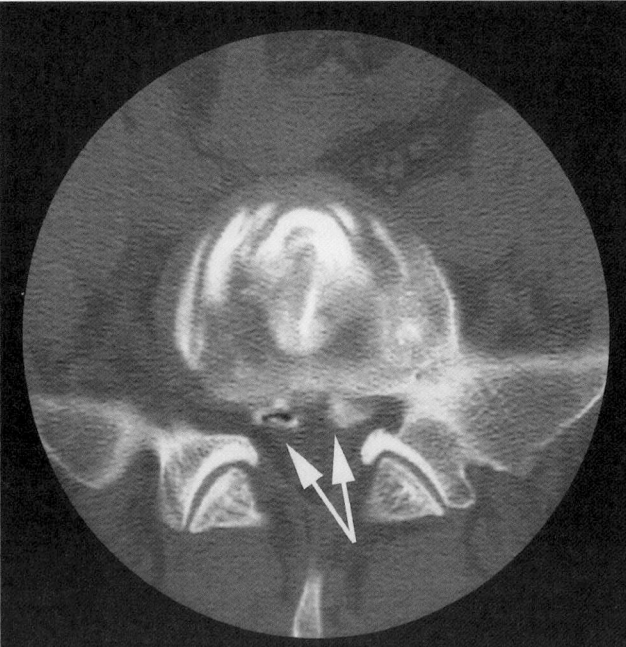

F

FIGURE 19.11 (*continued*) (**D**) Postdiscography axial CT through L-3–4. Internal fissures and small central annular tear (*arrow*). (**E**) Axial CT through L-4–5. Internal fissures. (**F**). Axial CT through L5–S1. Internal fissures and annular tear with focal herniation (*arrow*).

gical therapy in the setting of severe, intractable back pain without radiculopathy or CT or MRI evidence of disc herniation. In this setting, discography may help to establish the levels of symptomatic disc disease.

LIMB PAIN AND MAGNETIC RESONANCE NEUROGRAPHY

Magnetic Resonance Neurography

Magnetic resonance neurography (MRN) is targeted to the peripheral nervous structures using a high resolution matrix. Images are obtained along the courses of the nerves of interest. The pri-

mary purpose of MRN is to delineate any abnormality of the nerve and detect the cause. The current indications include mass, compressive neuropathy, nerve entrapment syndromes, unexplained neuropathy or plexopathy, traumatic nerve injury, and posttreatment nerve evaluation. With the advance of available surgical techniques, accurate presurgical evaluation of the nerve abnormality is becoming more and more important. MRI of the cervical or lumbar spine and MRN of the brachial or lumbosacral plexus and peripheral nerves permit direct visualization of the nervous structures and can confirm the presence of neural irritation, edema, or compression.[69–73] Pathologic states caused by variant anatomy, prior trauma, scar tissue or mass lesion, and musculoskeletal causes of pain can be excluded (Figs. 19.12 to 19.14). MRI of distal musculature can provide evidence of denervation in the distribution of a given peripheral nerve (Figs. 19.15

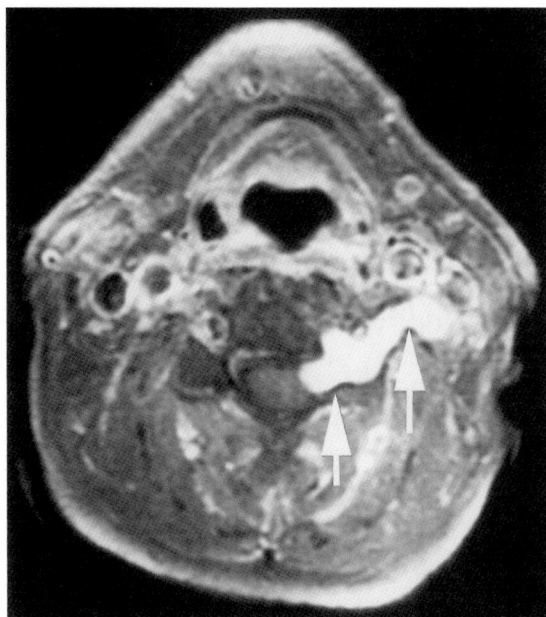

FIGURE 19.12 C-5 schwannoma. An 81-year-old man with 4 years of left upper extremity pain and dysesthesia. Axial and coronal short tau inversion recovery images reveal a dumbbell-shaped high signal intensity extradural mass involving the left C-4/5 neural foramen (*arrows*).

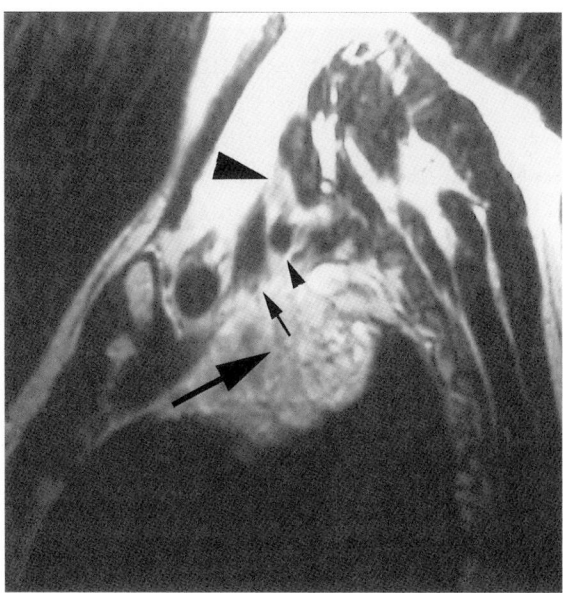

FIGURE 19.14 Pancoast's tumor. A 42-year-old man with mild cough. Posterior superior mediastinal mass was identified on plain radiograph. Sagittal T2 images demonstrate the pulmonary apex mass (*long arrow*) that abuts but does not surround the subclavian artery (*small arrowhead*). At surgery, the mass was found to be a lung cancer. Small arrow: anterior scalene muscle; large arrowhead; brachial plexus.

and 19.16).[74–76] In rat models, increased T2 signal is seen in the denervated muscles within 48 hours after a denervation event. This peaks at about 2 to 4 weeks. If there is nerve regeneration, the abnormal muscle signal resolves in 6 to 8 weeks. But without regeneration of the nerve, denervation changes of the muscle progresses and eventually causes muscle atrophy with fatty infiltration and resolution of high T2 signal several months later.[75,77–79]

Neurogenic pain involving the neck, shoulder, and the upper extremity can result from cervical nerve root compression, bra-

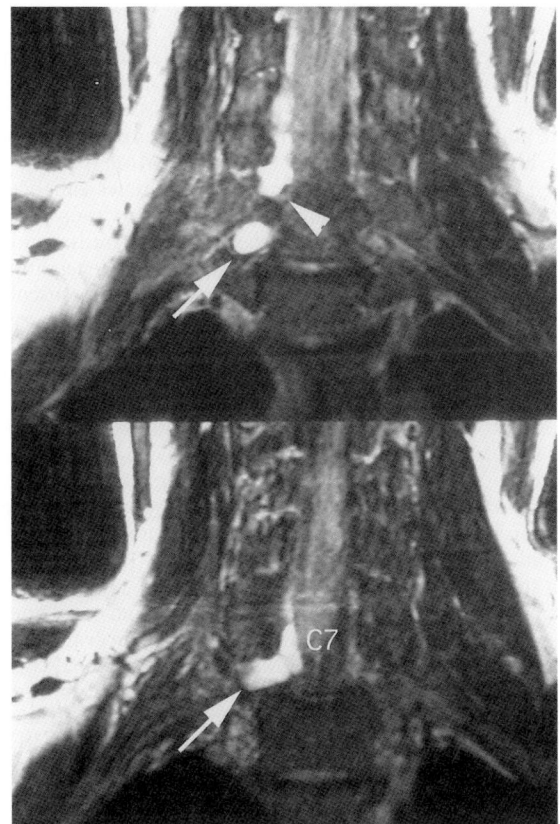

FIGURE 19.13 Nerve root avulsion. A 25-year-old man with traumatic injury to the right brachial plexus following a motorcycle accident that resulted in a flail upper extremity. After the accident he suffered from daily, intermittent, lancinating pain. Electromyography demonstrated absent cortical and brainstem response to stimulation of median and ulnar nerves and upper trunk of brachial plexus (C-6–8 roots). Coronal T1 and short tau inversion recovery images show proximal meningeal diverticuli at C-6, C-8, and T-1 (*arrow*) as well as abnormal signal in the right brachial plexus.

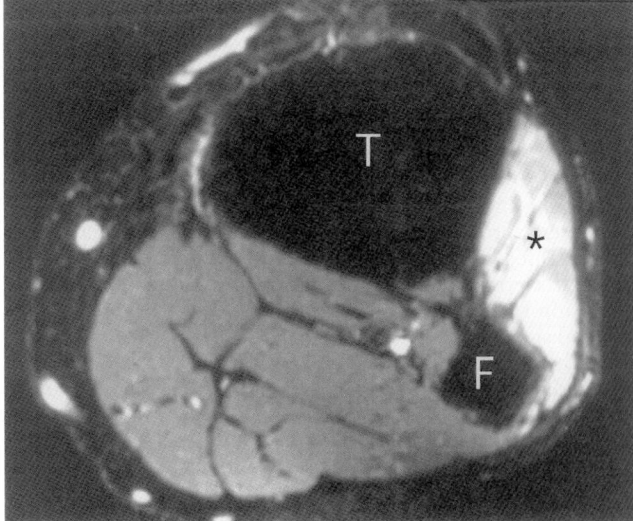

FIGURE 19.15 Subacute denervation in the distribution of the peroneal nerve. This axial short tau inversion recovery image of the proximal calf at the level of the fibular head (*F*) and the tibial metaphysis (*T*) demonstrates markedly hyperintense signal intensity within the anterior compartment muscles (*asterisk*). Note the muscles of the posterior calf for comparison, which show normal signal intensity. This illustrates the typical appearance of acute and subacute denervation that in this case followed severe injury to the left common perineal nerve.

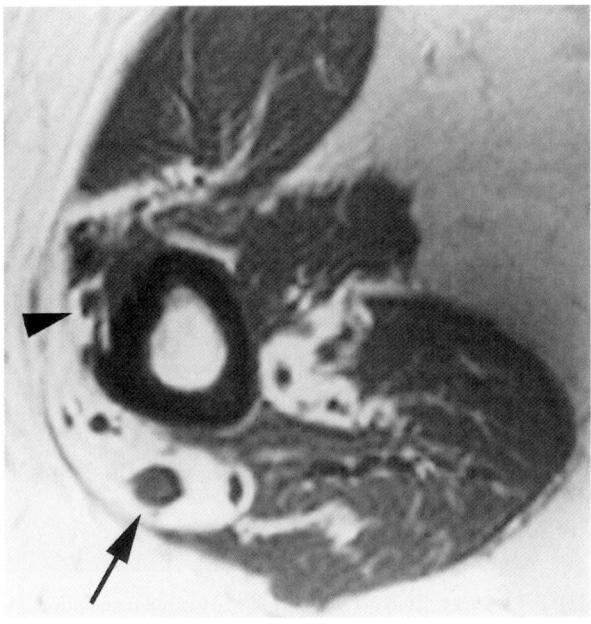
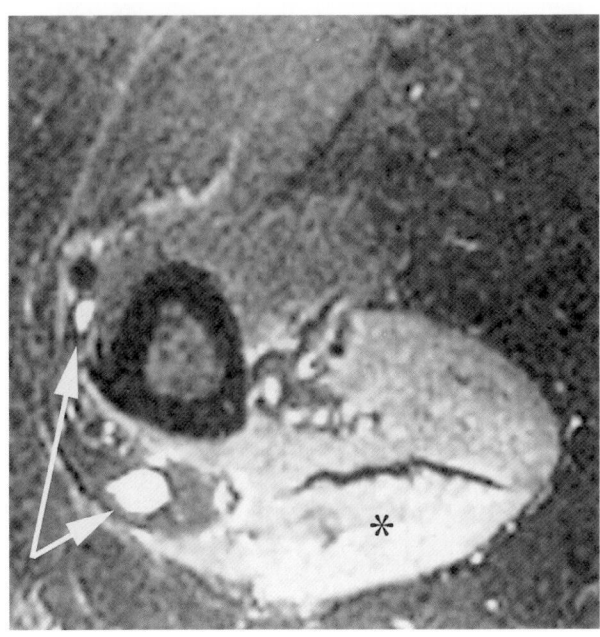

FIGURE 19.16 Ulnar and radial nerve injury. This patient suffered a severe left brachial plexus injury, with radial and ulnar neuropathy. (**A**) T1-weighted axial image through the left upper arm showing location of the radial (*arrow*) and ulnar (*arrowhead*) nerves. T1 sequences generally demonstrate anatomic relationships better than corresponding short tau inversion recovery sequences. (**B**) Short tau inversion recovery image showing increased signal in radial and ulnar nerves (*arrows*) as well as increased signal in triceps muscle (*asterisk*).

chial plexopathy, thoracic outlet syndrome (TOS), ulnar nerve entrapment at the elbow, or median nerve compression at the carpal tunnel.

Neurogenic pain involving the lower back, hips, and legs can result from lumbar nerve compromise, lumbosacral plexopathy, and an abnormality along the sciatic nerve (see Chapters 40, 69, and 71). MRN is particularly useful for patients with unexplained neuropathy, for whom surgical intervention is planned, or when the anatomic site of abnormality remains unclear after clinical examination and electrodiagnostic studies.[72,80] However, because only a relatively small field of view (FOV) can be imaged with high spatial resolution, it is necessary to clinically establish the site of a suspected neuropathic lesion as accurately as possible before using MRN. Imaging is then focused on the site of maximum clinical suspicion.

Brachial plexus, cervical root, or lumbosacral MRI is optimally performed using a phased-array RF coil and a large matrix size. These specialized receiver coils obtain detailed images by combining high signal-to-noise information from multiple coil elements to produce a very detailed image.[72] Coronal and sagittal T1-weighted images provide superb anatomic definition. Frequency selective fat saturation fast spin echo T2 and short tau inversion recovery (STIR) sequences are sensitive to changes in normal signal intensity within the roots, trunks, and cords of the brachial plexus and lumbosacral plexus. The former has better signal-to-noise ratio. STIR sequences suppress signal from fat more homogeneously, increasing the conspicuity of abnormal nerves. It is often helpful to image both sides of the patient simultaneously for comparison with the asymptomatic side.[81] Optimal MR neurography at the elbow, wrist, arm, thigh, knee, and ankle also requires high-resolution surface coils, a large matrix size, T1, fast spin echo T2, and STIR sequences. Imaging is conducted in the axial plane (perpendicular to the nerve) and either in the coronal or sagittal plane. Normal nerves demonstrate iso- or slightly high T2 signal compared to muscles. Fasciculated appearance can be seen especially within a large nerve such as the sciatic nerve due to interfascicular adipose tissues. Abnormal changes in peripheral nerves identified by MR neurography include focal or generalized enlargement of the nerve, increased signal on T2

and STIR sequences, loss of fascicular architecture, enhancement after administration of gadolinium, and displacement or compression of the nerve by soft tissue or osseous masses.[72,73,80] Acute and subacute denervation of musculature supplied by peripheral nerves is evident as increased signal on T2 and STIR sequences, loss of muscle volume, and sometimes enhancement after gadolinium administration. Chronic denervation results in marked loss of muscle mass together with fatty infiltration. The increased T2 changes seen in acute and subacute denervation are not seen. Axial T2 or STIR images of the abnormal musculature supplied by an injured peripheral nerve can identify denervation and are an indirect but effective means of determining the affected nerve and level of injury (see Figs. 19.15 and 19.16).[69] The 3D T1-weighted data set may also be used for better anatomical evaluation of the nerve.[82] Extremity pain, dysesthesia, and weakness can result from entrapment of nerve roots, compression, injury, or infiltration of the brachial, lumbar, or sacral plexi and compression of peripheral nerves at several sites.[83,84] Anatomical diagnosis is not always clear and may require imaging of the spine or trunk as well as the affected extremity.

In summary, cervical spine MRI, CT, or CT myelography can demonstrate intervertebral disc herniation, spinal canal and neuroforaminal stenoses, and degenerative changes in evaluating radiculopathy. Contrast-enhanced MR can identify spinal cord and vertebral tumors in addition to postoperative scars. Brachial plexus and pelvic MRI, using high-resolution phased array coils, can define the course of nerve roots, trunks, divisions, and cords in the patient with plexopathy, as well as detect masses, traumatic injuries, and inflammatory changes[81] (see Figs. 19.12 and 19.13). Direct imaging of peripheral nerves at common sites of entrapment can confirm the location of repetitive stress injury or tumor, and help clinicians select patients who might benefit from decompressive surgery (Fig. 19.17; see Fig. 19.16).[80]

Thoracic Outlet Syndrome

Thoracic outlet syndrome (TOS) is a group of disorders associated with the nervous and vascular structures from the base of

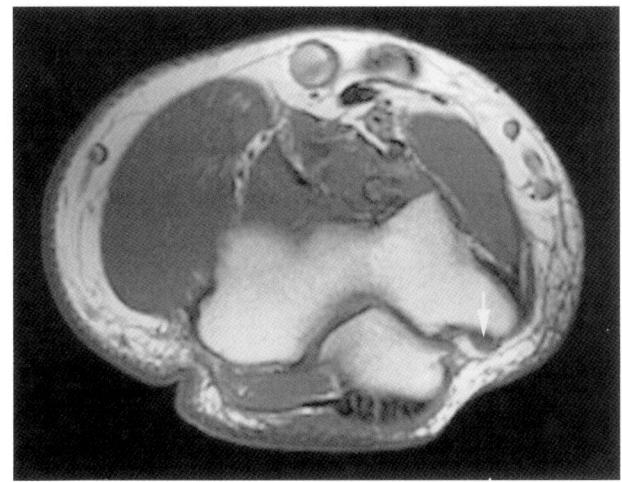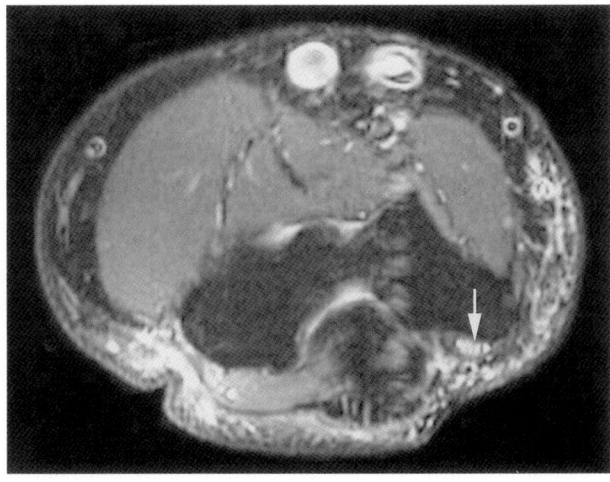

A   B

FIGURE 19.17 Ulnar entrapment. Axial T1 (**A**) and short tau inversion recovery (STIR) (**B**) images of the right elbow taken at the level in which the ulnar nerve passes through the cubital tunnel. (**A**) On this T1-weighted image, a normal sized right ulnar nerve is nicely demonstrated surrounded by perineural fat (*arrow*). (**B**) The STIR image, however, demonstrates abnormally increased hyperintensity within the nerve that is abnormal (*arrow*) and that, in the presence of appropriate symptoms, is an indication of ulnar nerve entrapment.

the neck to the axilla (see Chapter 40). Most patients have a controversial syndrome characterized by variable supraclavicular and upper extremity pain, dysesthesia, and weakness without the presence of an anomalous cervical rib or objective physical examination or electromyographic findings of nerve abnormality.[85] Because musculoskeletal inflammatory conditions, complex regional pain syndromes, and distal compressive neuropathies can have similar symptoms, the diagnosis of TOS can be extremely difficult. Although decompression of the inferior brachial plexus and subclavian vessels by transaxillary resection of the first rib has been successful in management of some patients with TOS, generally after a trial of physical therapy, the decision to operate is rarely straightforward. There are three forms of TOSs: arterial, venous, and neurogenic. Neurogenic TOS is considered to be most common, consisting of more than 90% of all TOS cases. But more than one form may coexist.[86] Neurogenic TOS is difficult to diagnose. Patient symptoms are subtle and confusing, but generally show chronic progression. It is usually considered to be associated with chronic compression and entrapment. Primary use of EMG is to exclude other peripheral neuropathies, rather than to rule in TOS. A minority of patients (less than 10%) have a predominately vascular form of TOS with symptoms resulting from subclavian artery compression or venous insufficiency and possible thrombosis.[87] Arterial TOS is due to compression of the subclavian artery or axillary artery and typically presents with upper extremity arterial insufficiency symptoms or embolic episodes, and ultrasound or arteriography demonstrates subclavian artery aneurysm, arterial thrombosis, or distal emboli. Venous TOS (Paget-Schroetter syndrome) is due to thrombosis caused by compression of the subclavian or axillary vein and typically presents with upper limb swelling, pain, and cyanosis. It is significant in that it can result in pulmonary embolism.

The role of imaging in suspected TOS is not clearly established at present and more investigation is required to evaluate the validity of imaging.[88]

If cervical radiographs visualize the cervical ribs, the diagnosis is easily made. And it is usually due to arterial compression. But most cases of neurogenic TOS are not associated with cervical ribs. Neurogenic TOS may be imaged with MR neurography of the brachial plexus which may show an angular deformity of the course of the brachial plexus trunks as they pass through the area of the scalene triangle with or without accompanying increase in T2 signal of the affected nerve(s).

Ultrasound is useful for vascular evaluation including dynamic evaluation of vascular systems in different arm positions and in a seated position and detects arterial stenoses even when the MRI is negative.[89] Significant (>70%) stenosis can also be seen in 19% of the normal population with abducted arm position. Ultrasound can demonstrate thrombosis in the subclavian-axillary venous system. Its sensitivity is over 90% with variable specificity.[90–92] However, ultrasound is largely operator dependent and the clavicle may limit the observation window.

CT is useful in evaluation of bony and vascular structures but inferior to MRI in regard to soft tissue evaluation. CT scanning in neutral and elevated arm position is useful to evaluate vascular compression especially with reformatted multidimensional or 3D reconstructions.[93, 94] However, this requires radiation to the patients and iodine contrast.

MRI is an emerging modality in evaluation of thoracic outlet syndrome.[95,96] It is noninvasive, does not require radiation, and demonstrates good soft tissue delineation. Panegyres and colleagues reported sensitivity of 79% and specificity of 87.5% for the detection of distortion or displacement of the brachial plexus or subclavian vessels.[95] Contrast enhanced MRA is also useful to evaluate vascular compression,[97] especially with abducted arm position.[98–100] However, arterial compression can be seen in the normal population (0% to 1.39%). Venous compression is seen more frequently in normal populations (41.7% to 47%). Therefore, clinical correlation is important. Scanning in two positions is also useful to evaluate neural compression. Nervous compression on the provocative position is only seen in patients but not in controls.[101,102] The costoclavicular distance also significantly decreases by the provocative position in patients.[101–104]

Piriformis Syndrome

Piriformis syndrome is nondisc origin leg pain caused by compression of the sciatic nerve by the asymmetrically enlarged piriformis muscle or by an associated fibrous band. On MR, abnormal T2 high signal can be present in the affected sciatic nerve.[105,106] Filler reported that piriformis muscle asymmetry and sciatic nerve hyperintensity at the sciatic notch exhibited a 93% specificity and 64% sensitivity on MR in distinguishing patients with piriformis syndrome from those without who had similar symptoms.

Peripheral Nerve Entrapment Syndromes

Carpal tunnel syndrome is the most common form of nerve entrapment and is the result of median nerve compression at the carpal tunnel (see Chapter 71). Clinical features, usually sufficient for diagnosis, include paresthesia and hyperesthesia in the median nerve distribution, radiation of pain along the volar aspect of the forearm, nocturnal pain, exacerbation with repetitive movements, and atrophy of the thenar muscles. Carpal tunnel syndrome is most often caused by repetitive injury of the median nerve within a compromised carpal tunnel volume, but can also be caused by focal space-occupying lesions, local inflammatory processes, or metabolic derangements related to systemic illness.[107,108] Proximal nerve entrapment in the cervical spine, thoracic outlet, and along the course of the median nerve can mimic carpal tunnel syndrome. The pronator syndrome and the anterior interosseous syndrome are distal median nerve compression syndromes in which the nerve is compressed by the two heads of the pronator teres, or after the branching of the anterior osseous nerve, along the interosseous membrane, respectively. Both of these syndromes can produce symptoms identical to carpal tunnel syndrome.[72]

Although ultrasound and CT have been used to evaluate anatomy of the carpal tunnel and visualize the median nerve,[109] MR is superior to these technologies in confirming the diagnosis of carpal tunnel syndrome, by virtue of its greater contrast sensitivity and its ability to detect abnormal signal intensity changes within a compressed median nerve. A coronal T1 scout image allows selection of axial scan levels through the wrist. Axial T1 and STIR (or T2) images should be obtained at the distal radiocarpal joint, proximal carpal tunnel, distal carpal tunnel, and metacarpal bases. Dedicated phased-array coils are valuable in increasing image quality to better demonstrate these small structures (Fig. 19.18).[69]

Findings in carpal tunnel syndrome include increased girth of the median nerve proximal to the carpal tunnel, flattening of the nerve within the tunnel, increased bowing of the flexor retinaculum, and increased signal intensity of the median nerve on T2 and STIR sequences. Ganglion cysts, lipomas, posttraumatic or degenerative bony deformities, and other soft tissue tumors are easily identified on MRI. Thickening or separation of tendons with increased signal changes on T2 or STIR sequences indicates tenosynovitis. Often idiopathic, it can also be caused by trauma, rheumatoid arthritis, and chronic infection. Amyloid, gout, acro-

megaly, hypothyroidism, and other systemic diseases associated with carpal tunnel syndrome are generally diagnosed on the basis of clinical, laboratory, and plain film findings.[110–113]

Additional entrapment syndromes are also found with the ulnar nerve in the cubital tunnel at the elbow and Guyon's canal in the wrist[114] with common symptoms being tingling sensation on the ring and little fingers. On MRN of the elbow, abnormal signal and enlargement of the nerve can be seen.[115] Common peroneal nerve entrapment around the fibular head can be seen as T2 high signal within the nerve.[76] High-resolution, surface coil MRI can be diagnostic, but its application requires careful attention to the anatomy of the particular nerve involved.[69]

IMAGING GUIDED INJECTION

Imaging studies play an important role in the facilitation of diagnostic and therapeutic nerve blocks, vertebroplasty, and kyphoplasty (see Chapters 99 to 103). Accurate placement of needles for the injection of local anesthetic or neurolytic substances can be confirmed by radiographs, fluoroscopy, or CT scanning. These imaging techniques can prove the localization of a needle at a specific anatomic site and confirm the actual nerve or nerve root that is being blocked. The injection of a contrast agent with a local anesthetic solution can reveal the distribution of the agent used and confirm which nerves have been exposed to the anesthetic solution. This is particularly important when a surgical decision is based on the responses to nerve blocks. These techniques are particularly useful in patients whose anatomy has been distorted by disease processes or prior surgical procedures. The development of open magnet MR scanning may lead to an increase in the use of this imaging technology in the performance of image guided nerve blocks.

Radiography is commonly used to confirm the placement of needles in the performance of facet joint blocks, paravertebral somatic nerve blocks, or transsacral blocks. Fluoroscopy is used in the placement of epidural electrodes or catheters. Surgical procedures such as gangliolysis of the trigeminal nerve or radiofrequency rhizolysis or spinal nerves are performed with fluoroscopy. CT scans are commonly used for celiac plexus block. Modern imaging techniques facilitate the use of nerve blocks by providing proof of the exact location of the needle or the spread of injectate.

For vertebroplasty, the role of imaging procedures includes

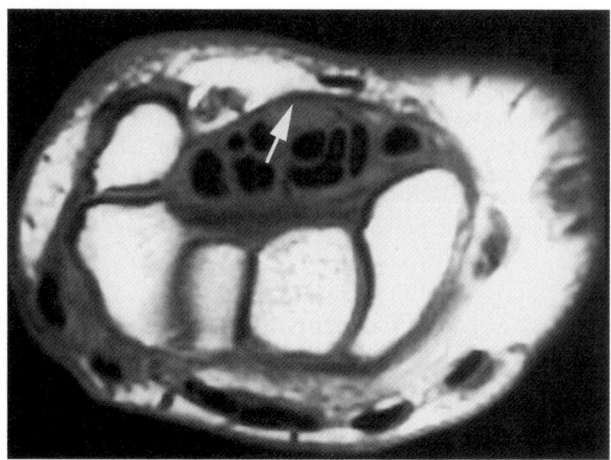
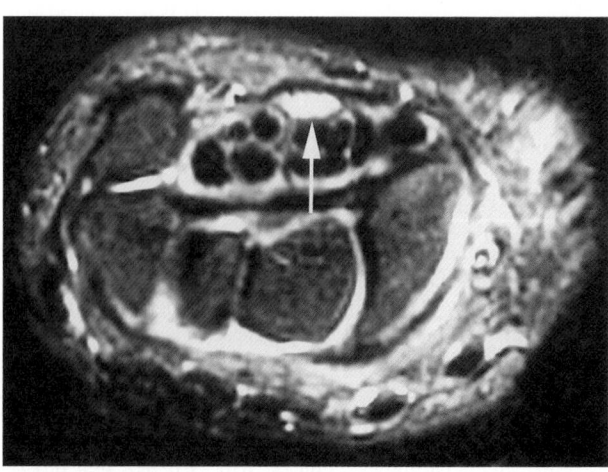

A

B

FIGURE 19.18 Carpal tunnel syndrome secondary to tenosynovitis. **(A)** Axial T1 image through the carpal tunnel shows increased girth of the median nerve and bowing of the flexor retinaculum (*arrow*). **(B)** Corresponding axial short tau inversion recovery image shows increased signal in the median nerve (*arrow*), as well as high signal fluid surrounding the tendon sheaths.

preprocedural evaluation to assess for the degree of the vertebral compression, exclude findings which contraindicate the procedure such as unstable fracture, neural foraminal involvement, and osteomyelitis of the target vertebra.

FUTURE APPLICATION OF PAIN IMAGING

Recent advances in functional brain imaging have started to reveal the complex process of the pain mechanism. Patterns of brain activation with various pain syndromes are being explored and the responses of individuals with chronic pain versus control subjects undergoing identical painful stimuli are beginning to reveal some interesting findings. How these will influence management of patients with chronic pain is yet to be defined.

CONCLUSION

Diagnostic imaging in patients with acute pain has a clearly defined role in establishing or confirming a pathologic diagnosis and directing medical, surgical, or radiologic intervention. Patients suffering from chronic, recurrent, or intractable pain from degenerative disease, anatomic variations, chronic inflammatory conditions, neoplasm, and postoperative or posttraumatic scarring may benefit from specialized imaging examinations for the determination of etiology, treatment planning, and prediction of the outcome of directed therapy.

References

1. Evans RW. Diagnostic testing for the evaluation of headaches. *Neurol Clin* 1996;14:1–26.
2. Perkins AT, Ondo W. When to worry about headache. Head pain as a clue to intracranial disease. *Postgrad Med* 1995;98:197–201, 204–208.
3. Silberstein SD. Evaluation and emergency treatment of headache. *Headache* 1992;32:396–407.
4. Detsky ME, McDonald DR, Baerlocher MO, et al. Does this patient with headache have a migraine or need neuroimaging? *JAMA* 2006;296(10): 1274–1283.
5. Pascual J, Berciano J. Experience in the diagnosis of headaches that start in elderly people. *J Neurol Neurosurg Psychiatry* 1994;57:1255–1257.
6. van der Wee N, Rinkel GJ, Hasan D, et al. Detection of subarachnoid haemorrhage on early CT: is lumbar puncture still needed after a negative scan? *J Neurol Neurosurg Psychiatry* 1995;58:357–359.
7. Pannke TS. Cerebral dural sinus thrombosis. *Ann Emerg Med* 1991;20: 813–816.
8. de Bruijn SF, Stam J, Kappelle LJ. Thunderclap headache as first symptom of cerebral venous sinus thrombosis. CVST Study Group. *Lancet* 1996;348: 1623–1625.
9. Wijdicks EF, Schievink WI, Miller GM. Pretruncal nonaneurysmal subarachnoid hemorrhage. *Mayo Clin Proc* 1998;73:745–752.
10. Guillon B, Biousse V, Massiou H, et al. Orbital pain as an isolated sign of internal carotid artery dissection. A diagnostic pitfall. *Cephalalgia* 1998;18: 222–224.
11. Guillon B, Brunereau L, Biousse V, et al. Long-term follow-up of aneurysms developed during extracranial internal carotid artery dissection. *Neurology* 1999;53(1):117–122.
12. Boesiger BM, Shiber JR. Subarachnoid hemorrhage diagnosis by computed tomography and lumbar puncture: are fifth generation CT scanners better at identifying subarachnoid hemorrhage? *J Emerg Med* 2005;29(1):23–27.
13. Sidman R, Connolly E, Lemke T. Subarachnoid hemorrhage diagnosis: lumbar puncture is still needed when the computed tomography scan is normal [see comments in *Acad Emerg Med* 1996;3(9):823]. *Acad Emerg Med* 1996; 3:827–831.
14. Hoh BL, Cheung AC, Rabinov JD, et al. Results of a prospective protocol of computed tomographic angiography in place of catheter angiography as the only diagnostic and pretreatment planning study for cerebral aneurysms by a combined neurovascular team. *Neurosurgery* 2004 Jun;54(6):1329–1340; discussion 1340–1342.
15. Chen W, Wang J, Xin W, et al. Accuracy of 16-row multislice computed tomographic angiography for assessment of small cerebral aneurysms. *Neurosurgery* 2008;62(1):113–121; discussion 121–122.
16. McKinney AM, Palmer CS, Truwit CL, et al. Detection of aneurysms by 64-section multidetector CT angiography in patients acutely suspected of having an intracranial aneurysm and comparison with digital subtraction and 3D rotational angiography. *AJNR Am J Neuroradiol* 2008;29(3):594–602.
17. Pedersen HK, Bakke SJ, Hald JK, et al. CTA in patients with acute subarachnoid haemorrhage. A comparative study with selective, digital angiography and blinded, independent review. *Acta Radiol* 2001;42(1):43–49.
18. Romijn M, Gratama van Andel HA, van Walderveen MA, et al. Diagnostic accuracy of CT angiography with matched mask bone elimination for detection of intracranial aneurysms: comparison with digital subtraction angiography and 3D rotational angiography. *AJNR Am J Neuroradiol* 2008;29(1): 134–139. Epub 2007 Oct 10.
19. Dammert S, Krings T, Moller–Hartmann W, et al. Detection of intracranial aneurysms with multislice CT: comparison with conventional angiography. *Neuroradiology* 2004;46(6):427–434.
20. Anderson GB, Findlay JM, Steinke DE, et al. Experience with computed tomographic angiography for the detection of intracranial aneurysms in the setting of acute subarachnoid hemorrhage. *Neurosurgery* 1997;41:522–527; discussion 527–528.
21. Hope JK, Wilson JL, Thomson FJ. Three-dimensional CT angiography in the detection and characterization of intracranial berry aneurysms [see comments in *AJNR Am J Neuroradiol* 1997;18(4):790–792]. *AJNR Am J Neuroradiol* 1996;17:439–445.
22. Weingarten S, Kleinman M, Elperin L, et al. The effectiveness of cerebral imaging in the diagnosis of chronic headache [see comments in *Arch Intern Med* 1993;153(13):1613–1614]. *Arch Intern Med* 1992;152:2457–2462.
23. Masson C, Lehericy S, Guillaume B, et al. Cluster-like headache in a patient with a trigeminal neurinoma. *Headache* 1995;35:48–49.
24. Smith WS, Messing RO. Cerebral aneurysm presenting as cough headache. *Headache* 1993;33:203–204.
25. Guillon B, Levy C, Bousser MG. Internal carotid artery dissection: an update. *J Neurol Sci* 1998;153:146–158.
26. Aaløkken TM, Hagtvedt T, Dalen I, et al. Conventional sinus radiography compared with CT in the diagnosis of acute sinusitis. *Dentomaxillofac Radiol* 2003;32(1):60–62.
27. Timmenga N, Stegenga B, Raghoebar G, et al. The value of Waters' projection for assessing maxillary sinus inflammatory disease. *Oral Surg Oral Med Oral Pathol Oral Radiol Endod* 2002;93(1):103–109.
28. Mafee MF. Modern imaging of paranasal sinuses and the role of limited sinus computerized tomography; considerations of time, cost and radiation. *Ear Nose Throat J* 1994;73:532–534, 536–538, 540–542.
29. Blank SC, Shakir RA, Bindoff LA, et al. Spontaneous intracranial hypotension: clinical and magnetic resonance imaging characteristics. *Clin Neurol Neurosurg* 1997;99:199–204.
30. Ferrante E, Riva M, Gatti A, et al. Intracranial hypotension syndrome: neuroimaging in five spontaneous cases and etiopathogenetic correlations. *Clin Neurol Neurosurg* 1998;100:33–39.
31. Khurana RK. Intracranial hypotension. *Semin Neurol* 1996;16:5–10.
32. Bourekas EC, Lewin JS, Lanzieri CF. Postcontrast meningeal MR enhancement secondary to intracranial hypotension caused by lumbar puncture. *J Comput Assist Tomogr* 1995;19:299–301.
33. Pannullo SC, Reich JB, Krol G, et al. MRI changes in intracranial hypotension. *Neurology* 1993;43:919–926.
34. Fishman RA, Dillon WP. Dural enhancement and cerebral displacement secondary to intracranial hypotension. *Neurology* 1993;43:609–611.
35. el Gammal TA, Crews CE. MR myelography of the cervical spine. *Radiographics* 1996;16(1):77–84.
36. Matsumura A, Anno I, Kimura H, et al. Diagnosis of spontaneous intracranial hypotension by using magnetic resonance myelography. Case report. *J Neurosurg* 2000;92(5):873–876.
37. Chiapparini L, Ciceri E, Nappini S, et al. Headache and intracranial hypotension: neuroradiological findings. *Neurol Sci* 2004;25(suppl 3):S138–141.
38. Tomoda Y, Korogi Y, Aoki T, et al. Detection of cerebrospinal fluid leakage: initial experience with three-dimensional fast spin-echo magnetic resonance myelography. *Acta Radiol* 2008;49(2):197–203.
39. Baldwin NG, Sahni KS, Jensen ME, et al. Association of vascular compression in trigeminal neuralgia versus other "facial pain syndromes" by magnetic resonance imaging. *Surg Neurol* 1991;36:447–452.
40. Brisman R. Surgical treatment of trigeminal neuralgia. *Semin Neurol* 1997; 17:367–372.
41. Kumon Y, Sakaki S, Kohno K, et al. Three-dimensional imaging for presentation of the causative vessels in patients with hemifacial spasm and trigeminal neuralgia. *Surg Neurol* 1997;47:178–184.
42. Majoie CB, Verbeeten B Jr, Dol JA, et al. Trigeminal neuropathy: evaluation with MR imaging. *Radiographics* 1995;15:795–811.
43. Majoie CB, Hulsmans FJ, Verbeeten B Jr, et al. Trigeminal neuralgia: comparison of two MR imaging techniques in the demonstration of neurovascular contact [see comments in *Radiology* 1998;208(2):550–552]. *Radiology* 1997; 204:455–460.
44. Kakizawa Y, Seguchi T, Kodama K, et al. Anatomical study of the trigeminal and facial cranial nerves with the aid of 3.0-tesla magnetic resonance imaging. *J Neurosurg* 2008;108(3):483–490.
45. Miller J, Acar F, Hamilton B, et al. Preoperative visualization of neurovascular anatomy in trigeminal neuralgia. *J Neurosurg* 2008 Mar;108(3):477–482.
46. Herweh C, Kress B, Rasche D, et al. Loss of anisotropy in trigeminal neuralgia revealed by diffusion tensor imaging. *Neurology* 2007;68(10):776–778.

47. Klieb HB, Freeman BV. Trigeminal neuralgia caused by intracranial epidermoid tumour: report of a case. *J Can Dent Assoc* 2008;74(1):63–65.
48. Ogütcen–Toller M, Uzun E, Incesu L. Clinical and magnetic resonance imaging evaluation of facial pain. *Oral Surg Oral Med Oral Pathol Oral Radiol Endod* 2004;97(5):652–658.
49. Hacker RJ. Comparison of interbody fusion approaches for disabling low back pain. *Spine* 1997;22:660–665; discussion 665–666.
50. Ray CD. Threaded fusion cages for lumbar interbody fusions. An economic comparison with 360 degree fusions. *Spine* 1997;22:681–685.
51. Ray CD. Threaded titanium cages for lumbar interbody fusions. *Spine* 1997; 22:667–679; discussion 679–680.
52. Bueff HU, Van der Reis W. Low back pain. *Prim Care* 1996;23:345–364.
53. Russo R, Cook P. Diagnosis of low back pain: role of imaging studies. *Occup Med* 1998;13:83–96.
54. Haughton V, Schreibman K, De Smet A. Contrast between scar and recurrent herniated disk on contrast-enhanced MR images [published correction appears in *AJNR Am J Neuroradiol* 2003;24(2):296]. *AJNR Am J Neuroradiol* 2002;23(10):1652–1656.
55. Stadnik TW, Lee RR, Coen HL, et al. Annular tears and disk herniation: prevalence and contrast enhancement on MR images in the absence of low back pain or sciatica. *Radiology* 1998;206:49–55.
56. Jarvik JJ, Hollingworth W, Heagerty P, et al. The Longitudinal Assessment of Imaging and Disability of the Back (LAIDBack) Study: baseline data. *Spine* 2001;26(10):1158–1166.
57. Erly WK, Oh ES, Outwater EK. The utility of in-phase/opposed-phase imaging in differentiating malignancy from acute benign compression fractures of the spine. *AJNR Am J Neuroradiol* 2006;27(6):1183–1188.
58. Schneiderman G, Flannigan B, Kingston S, et al. Magnetic resonance imaging in the diagnosis of disc degeneration: correlation with discography. *Spine* 1987;12:276–281.
59. Kinard RE. Diagnostic spinal injection procedures. *Neurosurg Clin N Am* 1996;7:151–165.
60. Tehranzadeh J. Discography 2000. *Radiol Clin North Am* 1998;36:463–495.
61. Block AR, Vanharanta H, Ohnmeiss DD, et al. Discographic pain report. Influence of psychological factors. *Spine* 1996;21:334–338.
62. Ohnmeiss DD, Vanharanta H, Guyer RD. The association between pain drawings and computed tomographic/discographic pain responses. *Spine* 1995;20: 729–733.
63. Parker LM, Murrell SE, Boden SD, et al. The outcome of posterolateral fusion in highly selected patients with discogenic low back pain [see comments in *Spine* 1997;22(12):1419–1420]. *Spine* 1996;21:1909–1916; discussion 1916–1917.
64. Carragee EJ, Lincoln T, Parmar VS, et al. A gold standard evaluation of the "discogenic pain" diagnosis as determined by provocative discography. *Spine* 2006;31(18):2115–2123.
65. Carragee EJ, Alamin TF, Miller J, et al. Provocative discography in volunteer subjects with mild persistent low back pain. *Spine J* 2002;2(1):25–34.
66. Bogduk N, Modic MT. Lumbar discography. *Spine* 1996;21:402–404.
67. Carragee EJ, Alamin TF, Carragee JM. Low-pressure positive discography in subjects asymptomatic of significant low back pain illness. *Spine* 2006;31(5): 505–509.
68. Carragee EJ, Barcohana B, Alamin T, et al. Prospective controlled study of the development of lower back pain in previously asymptomatic subjects undergoing experimental discography. *Spine* 2004;29(10):1112–1117.
69. Aagaard BD, Maravilla KR, Kliot M. MR neurography. MR imaging of peripheral nerves [published correction appears in *Magn Reson Imaging Clin N Am* 1998;6(2):x]. *Magn Reson Imaging Clin N Am* 1998;6:179–194.
70. Dailey AT, Tsuruda JS, Goodkin R, et al. Magnetic resonance neurography for cervical radiculopathy: a preliminary report. *Neurosurgery* 1996;38: 488–492; discussion 492.
71. Kuntz C 4th, Blake L, Britz G, et al. Magnetic resonance neurography of peripheral nerve lesions in the lower extremity. *Neurosurgery* 1996;39: 750–756; discussion 756–757.
72. Maravilla KR, Bowen BC. Imaging of the peripheral nervous system: evaluation of peripheral neuropathy and plexopathy [see comments in *AJNR Am J Neuroradiol* 1998;19(6):1001]. *AJNR Am J Neuroradiol* 1998;19:1011–1023.
73. Moore KR, Tsuruda JS, Dailey AT. The value of MR neurography for evaluating extraspinal neuropathic leg pain: a pictorial essay. *AJNR Am J Neuroradiol* 2001;22(4):786–794.
74. Polak JF, Jolesz FA, Adams DF. Magnetic resonance imaging of skeletal muscle. Prolongation of T1 and T2 subsequent to denervation. *Invest Radiol* 1988;23(5):365–369.
75. Wessig C, Koltzenburg M, Reiners K, et al. Muscle magnetic resonance imaging of denervation and reinnervation: correlation with electrophysiology and histology. *Exp Neurol* 2004;185(2):254–261.
76. Koltzenburg M, Bendszus M. Imaging of peripheral nerve lesions. *Curr Opin Neurol* 2004;17(5):621–626.
77. Aagaard BD, Lazar DA, Lankerovich L, et al. High-resolution magnetic resonance imaging is a noninvasive method of observing injury and recovery in the peripheral nervous system. *Neurosurgery* 2003;53(1):199–203; discussion 203–204.
78. Kikuchi Y, Nakamura T, Takayama S, et al. MR imaging in the diagnosis of denervated and reinnervated skeletal muscles: experimental study in rats [published correction appears in *Radiology* 2004;230(2):597]. *Radiology* 2003;229(3):861–867. Epub 2003 Oct 23.

79. Bendszus M, Koltzenburg M, Wessig C, et al. Sequential MR imaging of denervated muscle: experimental study. *AJNR Am J Neuroradiol* 2002;23(8): 1427–1431.
80. Filler AG, Kliot M, Howe FA, et al. Application of magnetic resonance neurography in the evaluation of patients with peripheral nerve pathology. *J Neurosurg* 1996;85:299–309.
81. Blake LC, Robertson WD, Hayes CE. Sacral plexus: optimal imaging planes for MR assessment. *Radiology* 1996;199:767–772.
82. Freund W, Brinkmann A, Wagner F, et al. MR neurography with multiplanar reconstruction of 3D MRI datasets: an anatomical study and clinical applications. *Neuroradiology* 2007;49(4):335–341. Epub 2007 Jan 5.
83. Rosenberg ZS, Beltran J, Cheung YY, et al. The elbow: MR features of nerve disorders. *Radiology* 1993;188:235–240.
84. Rosenberg ZS, Bencardino J, Beltran J. MR features of nerve disorders at the elbow. *Magn Reson Imaging Clin N Am* 1997;5:545–565.
85. McGough EC, Pearce MB, Byrne JP. Management of thoracic outlet syndrome. *J Thorac Cardiovasc Surg* 1979;77:169–174.
86. Degeorges R, Reynaud C, Becquemin JP. Thoracic outlet syndrome surgery: long-term functional results. *Ann Vasc Surg* 2004;18(5):558–565. Epub 2004 Aug 6.
87. Ohkawa Y, Isoda H, Hasegawa S, et al. MR angiography of thoracic outlet syndrome. *J Comput Assist Tomogr* 1992;16:475–477.
88. Estilaei SK, Byl NN. An evidence-based review of magnetic resonance angiography for diagnosing arterial thoracic outlet syndrome. *J Hand Ther* 2006; 19(4):410–419; quiz 420.
89. Demondion X, Vidal C, Herbinet P, et al. Ultrasonographic assessment of arterial cross-sectional area in the thoracic outlet on postural maneuvers measured with power Doppler ultrasonography in both asymptomatic and symptomatic populations. *J Ultrasound Med* 2006;25(2):217–224.
90. Baxter GM, Kincaid W, Jeffrey RF, et al. Comparison of colour Doppler ultrasound with venography in the diagnosis of axillary and subclavian vein thrombosis. *Br J Radiol* 199;64(765):777–781.
91. Köksoy C, Kuzu A, Kutlay J, et al. The diagnostic value of colour Doppler ultrasound in central venous catheter related thrombosis. *Clin Radiol* 1995; 50(10):687–689.
92. Longley DG, Yedlicka JW, Molina EJ, et al. Thoracic outlet syndrome: evaluation of the subclavian vessels by color duplex sonography. *AJR Am J Roentgenol* 1992;158(3):623–630.
93. Remy–Jardin M, Doyen J, Remy J, et al. Functional anatomy of the thoracic outlet: evaluation with spiral CT. *Radiology* 1997;205(3):843–851.
94. Remy–Jardin M, Remy J, Masson P, et al. CT angiography of thoracic outlet syndrome: evaluation of imaging protocols for the detection of arterial stenosis. *J Comput Assist Tomogr* 2000;24(3):349–361.
95. Panegyres PK, Moore N, Gibson R, et al. Thoracic outlet syndromes and magnetic resonance imaging [see comments in *Brain* 1995;118 (Pt 3): 819–821]. *Brain* 1993;116(Pt 4):823–841.
96. Demondion X, Boutry N, Drizenko A, et al. Thoracic outlet: anatomic correlation with MR imaging. *AJR Am J Roentgenol* 2000;175(2):417–422.
97. Cosottini M, Zampa V, Petruzzi P, et al. Contrast-enhanced three-dimensional MR angiography in the assessment of subclavian artery diseases. *Eur Radiol* 2000;10(11):1737–1744.
98. Dymarkowski S, Bosmans H, Marchal G, et al. Three-dimensional MR angiography in the evaluation of thoracic outlet syndrome. *AJR Am J Roentgenol* 1999;173:1005–1008.
99. Hagspiel KD, Spinosa DJ, Angle JF, et al. Diagnosis of vascular compression at the thoracic outlet using gadolinium-enhanced high-resolution ultrafast MR angiography in abduction and adduction. *Cardiovasc Intervent Radiol* 2000;23(2):152–154.
100. Charon JP, Milne W, Sheppard DG, et al. Evaluation of MR angiographic technique in the assessment of thoracic outlet syndrome. *Clin Radiol* 2004; 59(7):588–595.
101. Demondion X, Bacqueville E, Paul C, et al. Thoracic outlet: assessment with MR imaging in asymptomatic and symptomatic populations. *Radiology* 2003; 227:461–468.
102. Demirbag D, Unlu E, Ozdemir F, et al. The relationship between magnetic resonance imaging findings and postural maneuver and physical examination tests in patients with thoracic outlet syndrome: results of a double-blind, controlled study. *Arch Phys Med Rehabil* 2007;88(7):844–851.
103. Smedby O, Rostad H, Klaastad O, et al. Functional imaging of the thoracic outlet syndrome in an open MR scanner. *Eur Radiol* 2000;10(4):597–600.
104. Remy–Jardin M, Remy J, Masson P, et al. Helical CT angiography of thoracic outlet syndrome: functional anatomy. *AJR Am J Roentgenol* 2000;174(6): 1667–1674.
105. Lewis AM, Layzer R, Engstrom JW, et al. Magnetic resonance neurography in extraspinal sciatica. *Arch Neurol* 2006;63(10):1469–1472.
106. Filler AG, Haynes J, Jordan SE, et al. Sciatica of nondisc origin and piriformis syndrome: diagnosis by magnetic resonance neurography and interventional magnetic resonance imaging with outcome study of resulting treatment. *J Neurosurg Spine* 2005;2(2):99–115.
107. Cantatore FP, Dell'Accio F, Lapadula G. Carpal tunnel syndrome: a review. *Clin Rheumatol* 1997;16:596–603.
108. Mesgarzadeh M, Triolo J, Schneck CD. Carpal tunnel syndrome. MR imaging diagnosis. *Magn Reson Imaging Clin N Am* 1995;3:249–264.
109. Buchberger W, Schön G, Strasser K, et al. High-resolution ultrasonography of the carpal tunnel. *J Ultrasound Med* 1991;10:531–537.

110. Allmann KH, Horch R, Uhl M, et al. MR imaging of the carpal tunnel. *Eur J Radiol* 1997;25:141–145.
111. Radack DM, Schweitzer ME, Taras J. Carpal tunnel syndrome: are the MR findings a result of population selection bias? [see comments in *AJR Am J Roentgenol* 1998;171(1):268–269]. *AJR Am J Roentgenol* 1997;169:1649–1653.
112. Mesgarzadeh M, Schneck CD, Bonakdarpour A. Carpal tunnel: MR imaging. Part I. Normal anatomy. *Radiology* 1989;171:743–748.
113. Mesgarzadeh M, Schneck CD, Bonakdarpour A, et al. Carpal tunnel: MR imaging. Part II. Carpal tunnel syndrome. *Radiology* 1989;171:749–754.
114. Zeiss J, Jakab E, Khimji T, et al. The ulnar tunnel at the wrist (Guyon's canal): normal MR anatomy and variants. *AJR Am J Roentgenol* 1992;158:1081–1085.
115. Grant GA, Britz GW, Goodkin R, et al. The utility of magnetic resonance imaging in evaluating peripheral nerve disorders. *Muscle Nerve* 2002;25(3):314–331.

CHAPTER 20 ■ MEASUREMENT OF PAIN

MARK P. JENSEN

INTRODUCTION

Valid and reliable pain assessment is essential for successful pain care. Adequate assessment is also necessary to determine the efficacy of pain treatments in clinical trials, and for understanding the mechanisms of those effects. The clinician or researcher who wishes to use the most useful measures and strategies for pain assessment is faced with a large, and growing, number of options and decisions. The purpose of this chapter is to make those decisions easier.

The chapter begins with a brief discussion of several important issues that clinicians and researchers need to consider when choosing from among pain measures and designing pain assessment procedures, including: (1) evaluating the reliability, validity, and utility of pain measures; (2) determining the number of pain problems to assess; (3) choosing the pain domain(s) to assess; and (4) selecting the time period of assessment (e.g., current pain experience versus recall of pain over the last day, week, or longer). The bulk of the chapter then reviews the available psychometric information regarding measures of six pain domains: pain intensity, pain affect, pain quality, pain site, pain's temporal characteristics, and pain interference. Next, the chapter briefly discusses strategies for assessing pain in special populations (e.g., infants and young children, the demented geriatric patient, or other patients who might have difficulty expressing themselves verbally). It ends with a summary of recommendations.

Validity, Reliability, and Utility in the Context of Pain Assessment

No measure is perfect. No one measure assesses all pain domains, nor is any single measure useful in all settings and with all populations. Moreover, because of the imperfection of available instruments, it is theoretically possible to modify any existing measure to improve it further, or to develop new and better measures to replace existing ones. As a result, new pain assessment procedures and measures are constantly being developed and published. Thus, the clinician or researcher seeking to find the best measure for his or her needs should not only be aware of the existing pain assessment literature, but should also know how to evaluate new measures as they are published.[1] The following section seeks to facilitate this task by briefly summarizing the three key issues that should be considered when evaluating any pain measure: *validity, reliability,* and *utility*.

Validity

Validity refers to the appropriateness, meaningfulness, and usefulness of a measure for a specific purpose. It is generally seen as the most important consideration in the evaluation of a measure.[2] Validity always needs to be evaluated with respect to the specific purpose a measure or instrument will be used for; measures are not inherently "valid" or "invalid" in and of themselves. For example, a hammer is not inherently valid. It is valid (useful) for driving nails into wood, but invalid for washing dishes.

Rarely, if ever, can the validity of a measure be determined with a single study. Rather, support for the validity of a measure is usually established over time and with a series of studies. When evaluating the validity of a potential measure, the clinician or investigator should consider *content, construct,* and *criterion* validity.

Content Validity. Content validity concerns the degree to which the items of a measure represent a defined universe or domain of interest. For example, if a measure of a patient's *usual* pain or *average* pain over the last month is needed, then a single rating of current pain would not usually be considered to have content validity for assessing this construct, because pain can vary so much from one moment to another. Similarly, if a measure of the impact of pain on a patient's life is needed, and a measure includes items that ask only about pain's impact on sleep and mobility (but not other important daily activities), the measure would not generally be viewed as adequately representing the domain of pain interference. Thus, a critical question that every test user should ask is whether or not a potential measure assesses or represents all of the key components of the domain of interest. If the measure does not meet this standard, it does not have content validity.

Construct Validity. Construct validity refers to how well the items of a measure perform as measures of the domain or construct of interest. Two measures can have similar content validity—that is, both may contain items that assess the critical components of some pain construct—but have different construct validity. For example, if two measures ask about pain interference with the same set of activities, yet respondents are asked to indicate the extent of interference with each activity using different response levels (for example, yes/no response in one measure versus 0–10 scales in the second), the latter measure may evidence more precision than the former. The more precise measure may represent the construct better, and have more construct validity than the less precise one, despite the fact that the two measures have similar content validity. Similarly, if the language used in the items of one measure is clear and succinct and the other confusing and complex, the former measure would likely contain less error than the latter measure, and therefore better represent the construct of interest. Thus, factors other than content validity will impact how the scores obtained from different measures behave, especially with respect to their associations with other important pain-related measures and the precision with which they represent the domain of interest. Evidence for the construct validity of a measure generally comes from studies that demonstrate strong associations between a measure's score and other measures of the same construct, and weak to moderate associations with measures of other constructs.

Criterion Validity. Criterion validity refers to a measure's associations with one or more key outcome criteria. Usually, the most important criterion of a pain measure is the responsivity of the measure to the effects of a pain treatment, or to changes in pain over time, because pain measures are most often used for detecting these differences and changes. Pain measures that are proposed to be used as outcome measures in clinical trials should therefore have evidence that they are able to detect treatment effects or show expected changes in pain over time.

But not all pain measures are designed to assess treatment efficacy. A number of measures of pain quality, for example, and as described later in this chapter, were designed to distinguish from among different types of pain (e.g., neuropathic versus nociceptive). The validity of such measures should be determined by their ability to perform the task they were designed for or that they will be used for; their validity as measures of treatment efficacy need only be of concern when or if they are being considered for that specific purpose.

Reliability

Reliability refers to the extent to which the score from a test is free from errors of measurement. Many factors, other than a patient's experience of pain, could potentially influence his or her response to a pain measure or scale. Such factors could include the specific assessment setting (e.g., home versus clinic), assessment burden (e.g., single assessment versus a daily diary), the person administering the measure (e.g., research assistant, nurse, spouse, primary health care provider), other subjective experiences and feelings (e.g., being more or less fatigued or upset), motivational factors (e.g., desiring to appear stoic, wanting a prescription for a specific medication), ethnicity or culture, and previous learning experiences (e.g., the consequences of reporting of higher versus lower pain levels), among many others. The variability in a pain score (the "variance") that is associated with these other factors, and that is not associated with the specific domain of interest, is considered error variance. Although no measure is 100% reliable, the best measures demonstrate relatively little influence of these other factors and potential sources of error.

Higher error variance means lower reliability. Unlike validity, which is considered with respect to the proposed use of the measure, reliability is usually considered to exist within a measure. However, it is also possible for a measure to be more reliable in some settings or with some populations then in others. For example, as described in more detail later in this chapter, Visual Analogue Scales of pain intensity (where the respondent is asked to make a mark on a line that represents the perceived magnitude of pain) have been found to be more difficult for patients with cognitive deficits than with patients who do not exhibit cognitive deficits. These measures, then, might be considered to be inadequately reliable in populations at risk for cognitive deficits, although evidence indicates that they are adequately reliable in otherwise healthy adults. Thus, it is important that the reliability of any measure be established for the specific population with whom the measure will be used, or at least in samples of individuals who are similar to the population with whom the measure will be used.

Utility

Finally, issues of reliability and validity need to be considered in light of a measures' utility, given that there is often a trade-off among these. For example, to maximize the content validity of a measure of pain interference, one would want the measure to assess the pain interference of all, or nearly all, of the possible (100s? 1,000s?) activities a person could engage in. Such a measure, although it would have clear content validity, would not be practical; no one would use it. Similarly, to maximize the content validity of a measure of a patient's usual pain over the course of the last month, one might ask the patient to report on his or her current pain every hour for 30 days, and then average those responses into a single index of average pain. But few patients would be willing to perform this assessment task, and the costs of ensuring complete data for such a measure would be prohibitively expensive for most clinicians and many researchers. Deciding on which measure(s) to use for a particular application often comes down to selecting the measure that is both adequately valid and most practical.

How Many Pain Problems Should Be Assessed?

Patients often have more than one pain problem. For example, the majority of individuals with spinal cord have chronic pain, and the majority of these report pain at more than one site.[3] Clinicians and those researchers who do not limit their sample to the (few) patients with only one pain problem are faced with the difficult task of determining the number of pain problems to assess in any one patient or study participant. If only one "primary" pain problem is assessed at a clinic visit, but on the next visit a different "primary" pain problem emerges as the most distressing, then it would be very difficult to track the effects of pain treatment from one clinic visit to the next.

Similarly, researchers who limit the number of pain problems assessed to just one primary problem run the risk of underestimating the magnitude of pain and its impact in their research findings. On the other hand, it may not be practical to assess every pain problem in every patient seen in the clinic or in every participant of a research study. These considerations suggest that, in many situations, patients should have the opportunity to report on more than one pain problem, but not necessarily always be required or expected to report on every pain problem that they have at every assessment point.

But how many pain problems should be assessed? Two? Five? More? One approach to deal with this issue is to begin by assessing pain "in general"; for example, asking patients to consider all of their pain problems together when rating the overall average magnitude or intensity of their pain and the impact of pain on their lives. This is a practical solution, especially for assessing pain interference, since it may be very difficult for patients to identify the unique contribution of each different pain problem to interference with different activities. Moreover, assessing global pain intensity and interference allows the clinician or researcher to have a single primary measure of these two key pain domains, making analyses and tracking over time easier.

However, limiting assessment to only pain "in general" may oversimplify assessment, and also interfere with determining the true effects of pain treatment. For example, if a pain treatment reduces the pain associated with one pain problem (headache) but not another (low back pain), the specific effect of the treatment on headache pain might be less noticeable or even lost altogether if a measure of "general" pain intensity is used. So, in many situations, allowing for the assessment of more than one pain problem would be useful.

Unfortunately, however, there is not yet a clear consensus in the field concerning the best number of pain problems to assess. In the clinical setting, it probably makes sense to assess as many of the pain problems that are of concern to the patient. If the patient experiences eight unique pain problems, and views each as a significant problem that contributes to dysfunction, then perhaps each of these should be assessed, at least at the initial evaluation, and then tracked at subsequent clinic visits as appropriate.

When determining how many pain problems to assess in a research study, the number of problems that should be assessed would vary as a function of the research question(s) being asked and the specific population being studied. One reasonable option would be to select the number of pain problems to assess that would capture the majority of patients in the population. For example, in persons with spinal cord injury, it has been recommended that investigators should consider assessing basic information (such as pain location and intensity) for up to three presenting pain problems.[4] In this instance, three was chosen as a way to balance the need for a thorough assessment against the need to minimize assessment burden, keeping in mind that the majority of persons with spinal cord injury and pain report three or fewer pain problems.[3] Although it is unlikely that a single upper limit of pain problems can be identified that should be assessed in every research project and with every patient population, each investigator should at least consider this issue when developing assessment protocols.

Which Pain Domain(s) Should Be Assessed?

Clinicians and researchers have long recognized that pain is a multidimensional experience that includes a number of measurable qualities such as intensity, affect (global bothersomeness of the pain experience as well as the impact of pain on emotional functioning), sensory quality, spatial quality (location), temporal quality, and impact on or interference with daily activities.[5,6] Although the focus of pain assessment in clinical and research settings has often been, and continues to be, on pain intensity,[7] there has been an increased interest in the assessment of pain's other domains.[8]

It is important that clinicians and investigators consider assessing more than just pain intensity for a number of important reasons. First, limiting assessment to only pain intensity leaves clinicians and researchers in the difficult position of having limited information about the presenting pain problem(s). In a clinical situation, changes in a pain domain not assessed might end up being critical for understanding the effects of a pain treatment (for example, if pain qualities are not assessed, and a treatment reduces the "aching" and "deep" qualities of a pain problem, but perhaps not average pain intensity overall; or if a treatment produces a decrease in the impact of pain on sleep or other areas of functioning, even when there has been a minimal impact on pain intensity). For this reason, anyone interested in assessing pain should at least consider all of the pain domains when determining which ones to assess, and perhaps only avoid those domains they are certain will not be important to treatment (for clinicians) or understanding (for researchers).

One of the factors that might determine the selection of fewer domains and measures (e.g., perhaps choosing to assess just pain intensity and pain quality) over a more comprehensive assessment (e.g., including measures of pain site, pain interference, and the temporal qualities of pain, as well as perhaps more general measures of psychological and physical functioning) is whether the pain problem being assessed is more acute or chronic. Acute pain, which may be defined as pain resulting from current or very recent damage to tissue, includes pain from medical procedures

(e.g., injections, lumbar punctures, surgery) as well as both major and minor physical injuries. Because many acute pain problems tend to resolve quickly in most individuals, their impact tends to be transitory. In this situation, and if the focus of treatment is on just one or two pain domains (e.g., pain intensity, mood), then it may be appropriate to assess only one or two pain domains.

Chronic pain, on the other hand, tends to be more complex than acute pain. Patients' responses to chronic pain can vary a great deal, and its impact can be quite variable. For chronic pain, then, in both clinical and research settings, and in order to ensure a thorough understanding of the pain problem, more pain domains, and perhaps more measures that assess these domains, are often required.

Recall Ratings versus Summary Scores From Multiple Ratings Using Diaries

Often, the clinician or researcher wishes to have a measure of a patient's usual, least, or worst pain during a specific period of time. A single measure or rating of current pain is not likely going to be an adequate index of usual pain, given that pain can vary from one moment to another. So what is the best way to assess usual pain? Currently, the two viable options are: (1) ask the respondent to provide multiple ratings of current pain on pain diaries during the epoch of interest (e.g., four times/day for 7 days), and then compute the average, worst, and least pain levels from the ratings obtained, or (2) assess pain once, but ask the respondent to provide a *recall* rating of their average, worst, and least pain over the epoch of interest (e.g., asking respondents to rate their average, worst, and least pain intensity during the past week). Deciding between these two options has significant implications for the cost of a study and the reliability and validity of the obtained scores. However, each approach has strengths and weaknesses, and pain assessment experts have not yet reached a clear consensus on which option should be recommended.

Support for the first approach, using multiple assessment from diary data (most often obtained electronically using palm-top computers or automated telephone recordings) comes from studies that have demonstrated (1) a biasing impact of recent pain and worst pain (also known as "end" and "peak" effects) on recall ratings[9–11] and (2) the ability of electronic diaries (through the use of palm-top computers that can obtain ratings throughout the day, and download the ratings onto a server) or phone diaries to obtain multiple pain ratings over time, making it possible to average these ratings into a highly reliable measure of average pain.[12,13] These considerations provide a strong incentive to use diary assessments. In general, when diaries are required, electronic or phone diaries are preferred over paper-and-pencil ones, given the frequency with which patients use paper-and-pencil diaries inappropriately.[14,15] Because of the reported strengths of diary approaches, there has been a recent significant increase in the use of this approach to collect data in clinical trials.[16–19]

However, there are three findings from studies of diary pain assessment, and one practical issue, that make some investigators hesitant to embrace a diary approach to pain assessment, especially for use in clinical trials. First, as a practical issue, diary data are expensive. The financial cost of the hardware and software associated with data collection via electronic diaries may be beyond the means of some investigators. Related to this, there is also a cost in terms of patient assessment burden. It is not yet clear how many times per day a patient needs to report pain in order to adequately capture their usual pain experience. Some procedures require only one assessment per day[14,20–22] but it is more common to ask patients to provide three[22] or even more (four to six times[16,18,23]) ratings per day. This requires a significant effort on the part of patients. To the extent that much less costly recall ratings (that only require one assessment) may be adequately valid (and data suggest that they are, see later), investigators may save substantial resources and significantly decrease the patient assessment burden, if recall ratings are used instead of diary ratings.

A second problem with diary data is that using this approach will result in missing data. The reported percentages of missing data points from electronic diary studies range from 6%[15] to 17%.[24] The reported rates of study participants who provide incomplete data (that is, at least some missing data during the study period) range from 17%[14] to 46%.[20] The primary reason reported for missing electronic data is that the patient did not hear the alarm or cue asking for the assessment.[25] Other reasons given include: the alarm going off at an inconvenient time, the participant being too busy to respond, technical difficulties with the computer, emotional reasons, and pain being too severe at the time of assessment.[25] When data are missing, investigators need to either remove subjects from the analyses (which limits the generalizability of the findings and runs the risk of resulting in findings that overstate the impact of treatment) or use some approach to impute the missing data (that is, estimate what the missing ratings might have been, had all subjects provided complete data). A variety of data imputation procedures can be used for clinical trial data, such as "last observation carried forward," which involved taking the most recent rating obtained, and replacing all missing values with that rating.[16] A more conservative approach is to replace missing values with pretreatment ratings. Regardless of the approach used, however, data imputation adds error; imputed data are estimates only. And there is no evidence that the error added with data imputation is any less then the error that exists in recall ratings. In fact, the error added by the need to impute missing scores could potentially be greater than that associated with recall bias, so the use of diary data over recall ratings could potentially result in a more costly and effort-intensive assessment procedure that is ultimately also less reliable.

A third issue is that the use of electronic diaries limits the subjects who can participate in a study. For example, in one electronic diary study that approached 52 possible participants, 6 refused participation outright, one did not have the motor ability to hold the computer stylus, and 5 had visual problems that interfered with their ability to read the computer display.[20] By limiting the participants in clinical trials to those who are able and willing to use electronic diaries, their use in these trials limits the generalizability of the study findings.

Also, research supports the conclusion that recall ratings are adequately valid for most research purposes. Although research does indicate that there can be both peak and end effects that bias recall ratings, these effects tend to be small.[9] Moreover, research indicates that the correlations between recalled average pain (in the previous 7 days) and actual average pain during that same period (as assessed by diaries) are quite strong (correlation coefficients range from 0.68 to 0.99[26–32])—well within a range that indicate they carry valid variance as measures of average or usual pain. In short, recall ratings reflect actual average pain, and are therefore valid indicants of that pain.

Finally, and perhaps most critically, the research finding that provides the most support for the validity of recall ratings as outcome measures in pain clinical trials is indisputable: recall ratings are responsive to the effects of pain treatments known to impact pain. Hundreds, if not thousands, of clinical trials have shown that effective treatments for chronic pain result in reductions in recall ratings of average pain.

In summary, although data from pain diaries could potentially be more valid as measures of average pain than recall ratings are among those who provide complete data, scores from such data could also result in more measurement error (when data need to be imputed), create problems with generalizability (when subjects who cannot complete diaries or those who provide missing data are excluded), or both. Although some of the sources of error in recall ratings are now better known, those associated with peak (most pain) and end (most recent pain) effects tend to have only small effects on recall ratings. Most importantly, research consistently shows that the bulk of the variance of recall ratings is related to actual pain scores, and that recall ratings are responsive to treatment effects. Thus, recall ratings can be used as valid measures of usual pain in clinical trials.

MEASURING PAIN'S DOMAINS

Measuring Pain Intensity

The single pain domain assessed most often in clinical and research settings is pain intensity, or the magnitude of felt pain.[33] The three most commonly used scales to assess pain intensity are (1) the Visual Analogue Scale (VAS), (2) the Numerical Rating Scale (NRS), and (3) the Verbal Rating Scale (VRS) (Fig. 20.1). The results from research across many different pain populations yield fairly consistent findings concerning the psychometric properties of these measures[5,8] and may be summarized as follows:

1. Each of these measures is adequately valid and reliable as a measure of pain intensity in most settings.
2. For both VAS and 0–10 NRS scales, changes (decreases) between about 30% to 35% appear to indicate a meaningful change in pain to patients across patient populations.
3. For 0–10 NRS scales, the rating chosen has a specific meaning in terms of the impact of pain on functioning. In most samples, ratings in the 1–4 range have a minimal impact on pain, and can be viewed as representing "mild" pain. Once ratings reach 5 or 6, patients report that pain has a greater impact on functioning; these ratings can be viewed as "moderate" pain. Ratings ranging from 7–10 have the greatest impact on functioning, and can be viewed as representing "severe" pain.
4. When examined, single-item measures of pain intensity appear to have adequate test-retest stability (often, but not always, greater than 0.80) over short periods of time.
5. There are fairly consistent differences between available measures in terms of their failure rates. VASs usually show higher

Visual Analogue Scale

No pain   Pain as
                                        bad as it
                                        could be

Numerical Rating Scale

0   1   2   3   4   5   6   7   8   9   10
No pain   Pain as
                                            bad as it
                                            could be

Verbal (Categorical) Rating Scale

( ) No pain
( ) Mild pain
( ) Moderate pain
( ) Severe pain

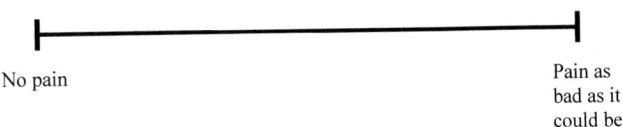

FIGURE 20.1 The Visual Analogue Scale (VAS), Numerical Rating Scale (NRS), and Verbal Rating Scale (VRS).

failure rates than NRSs and VRSs, and NRSs tend (when differences are found) to show slightly greater failure rates than VRSs, probably related to the increased complexity of matching a sensation to a line length versus a number or verbal descriptor.

6. In terms of preferences, patients tend to prefer VRSs and NRSs over VASs.

Recommendations for Assessing Pain Intensity

Given the empirical support for the validity and reliability of VASs, NRSs, and VRSs as measures of pain intensity, any of these could reasonably be employed in most clinical settings or as outcome measures in clinical trials. Primarily because of (1) differences in failure rates between these measures in some populations (supporting NRSs and VRSs over VASs),[34] (2) the evidence that some people can differentiate between more than just four or five levels of pain between from "no pain" and "extreme pain,"[35,36] and (3) the potential benefits of standardizing pain intensity assessment to allow for increased comparisons between studies, the field has recently moved toward recommending that clinicians and researchers consider first using the 0–10 NRS (see Fig. 20.1) over other pain intensity measures.[8]

Of course, there may be times when the 0–10 scale may not be appropriate. This scale requires the respondent to match his or her pain experience to a number, a task that may not be that easy for the very young, the extremely elderly, or individuals who are very ill. In these cases, and perhaps others, alternative pain intensity measures may be needed (see final section on assessing pain in special populations).

Measuring Pain Affect

The affective quality of pain includes both the general unpleasantness and/or bothersomeness of the pain sensation, as well as the many varieties of affect (fear, anger, sadness, frustration, feelings of hopelessness) that pain can produce—especially as it becomes chronic. The most common measures of general, global pain unpleasantness are single-item rating scales (VASs, NRSs, and VRSs) that use endpoints that reflect extreme levels of unpleasantness (e.g., for a 0–10 NRS or 100 mm VAS, "not bad at all" for the 0 rating or 0 mm mark, and "the most unpleasant feeling possible for me" for the 10 rating or 100 mm mark[37]). In general, these measures have proven useful in highly controlled laboratory studies that seek to differentiate intensity from affective components of pain.[37,38]

On the other hand, outside of the laboratory setting, patients appear to treat single-item VAS, NRS, and VRS measures of pain unpleasantness much like measures of pain intensity, so that the two are often indistinguishable from one another in clinical populations.[39,40] Moreover, one might question the content validity of single-item measures of affect, given the complex and multidimensional nature of emotional experience.

Pain affect can also be assessed using multiple-item scales, the most common of which are the affect subscale of the McGill Pain Questionnaire (MPQ[41]) and its associated short form, the MPQ-SF[42] (Fig. 20.2). The original MPQ contains 78 descriptors that are categorized into 20 subgroups, 5 of which assess the impact of pain on affect. The five affective domains are: tension (assessed using "tiring" and "exhausting" descriptors), autonomic (assessed using "sickening" and "suffocating" descriptors), fear (assessed using "fearful," "frightful," and "terrifying" descriptors), punishment (assessed using "punishing," "grueling," "cruel," "vicious," and "killing" descriptors), and affective miscellaneous (assessed using "wretched" and "blinding" descriptors).[41] Within each domain, when administered the MPQ, respondents are asked to circle or mark the single descriptor within each group that most accurately reflects or describes their pain. Descriptors are then ranked according to their position in the word set. The Pain Rating Index (PRI), which can be computed for each of the four primary MPQ subscales, including the affective subscale, is the sum of the rank values of these descriptors.

The short form of the MPQ (MPQ-SF) contains 15 descriptors, 4 of which come from the MPQ Affective subscale ("tiring-exhausting," "sickening," "fearful," and "punishing-cruel").[42] However, unlike the MPQ, which requires respondents to select a single descriptor from each category list that best describes their pain, respondents to the MPQ-SF are allowed to rate the severity of each item individually on a four-point Likert scale (0 = none to 3 = severe). A severity or intensity score can then be calculated for the Affective subscale (as well as for Sensory and Total scale scores, see next section on pain quality assessment). Research has shown that the correlations between the corresponding scales on the MPQ and MPQ-SF are high (rs range, 0.68 to 0.92).[42-44]

There is a substantial amount of data supporting the validity of the MPQ and MPQ-SF Affective subscales. First, like the other MPQ and MPQ-SF scales, the Affective subscale has been shown to be responsive to pain treatment.[45-47] Additional support for the validity of the MPQ-Affective scale as a measure of the affective component of pain, specifically, was reported by Ahles and colleagues, who found that this scale was more strongly associated with measures of psychological distress than with measures of pain intensity.[48] Also, Kremer and colleagues reported that patients with cancer report a greater affective component of their pain on the MPQ-Affective scale than patients with low back pain, consistent with the hypothesis that cancer pain may be associated with higher levels of affect (e.g., be more worrisome and cause more fear) than low back pain.[49] Given the strong associations between the original MPQ and SF-MPQ Affective scales, it is likely that the findings for the Affective MPQ scale would likely be similar for the SF-MPQ, although research confirming this has yet to be performed.

Recommendations for Assessing Pain Affect

Although single-item measures of pain affect or pain bothersomeness have demonstrated validity in highly controlled laboratory studies, supporting their use in this setting, they have shown less discrimination (from single-item measures of pain intensity) in clinical populations. Thus, with clinical populations, when an index of pain affect is needed, clinicians and researchers should strongly consider administering the MPQ or MPQ-SF Affective items. The MPQ Affective scale, having a longer history than the MPQ-SF, has more empirical support for its reliability and validity. However, given the strong associations between the MPQ and MPQ-SF scales, their high degree of item overlap, and the relative brevity and greater simplicity of the MPQ-SF for scoring, adequate evidence exists to support the use of the MPQ-SF as well.

Measuring Pain Quality

The experience of pain consists of much more than its magnitude or intensity and affective components. Pain is also often described using a number of different qualities, such as "burning," "aching," and "tender," among many others. Although historically clinicians and researchers have focused on pain intensity as the single most important pain domain to assess,[33] there has been a recent upsurge of interest in the assessment of pain qualities. The two primary purposes of such measures are: (1) to help diagnose the pain problem and (2) to more thoroughly describe the pain experience and determine the effects of pain treatments on that experience.

Using Pain Quality Measures as Diagnostic Aides

A growing body of research supports the conclusion that different pain qualities are associated with different causes, sources, or

Short-Form McGill Pain Questionnaire
(SF-MPQ)

A. PLEASE DESCRIBE YOUR PAIN DURING THE LAST WEEK. *(Check off one box per line.)*

	None	Mild	Moderate	Severe
1. Throbbing	0 ☐	1 ☐	2 ☐	3 ☐
2. Shooting	0 ☐	1 ☐	2 ☐	3 ☐
3. Stabbing	0 ☐	1 ☐	2 ☐	3 ☐
4. Sharp	0 ☐	1 ☐	2 ☐	3 ☐
5. Cramping	0 ☐	1 ☐	2 ☐	3 ☐
6. Gnawing	0 ☐	1 ☐	2 ☐	3 ☐
7. Hot-burning	0 ☐	1 ☐	2 ☐	3 ☐
8. Aching	0 ☐	1 ☐	2 ☐	3 ☐
9. Heavy (like a weight)	0 ☐	1 ☐	2 ☐	3 ☐
10. Tender	0 ☐	1 ☐	2 ☐	3 ☐
11. Splitting	0 ☐	1 ☐	2 ☐	3 ☐
12. Tiring-Exhausting	0 ☐	1 ☐	2 ☐	3 ☐
13. Sickening	0 ☐	1 ☐	2 ☐	3 ☐
14. Fear-causing	0 ☐	1 ☐	2 ☐	3 ☐
15. Punishing-Cruel	0 ☐	1 ☐	2 ☐	3 ☐

B. PLEASE RATE YOUR PAIN DURING THE LAST WEEK.

The following line represents pain of increasing intensity from "no pain" to "worst possible pain". Place a vertical mark (|) across the line in the position that best describes your pain **during the last week.**

No Pain ———————————————————————— **Worst Possible Pain**

☐☐☐
Score in mm
(Investigator's use only)

C. CURRENT PAIN INTENSITY
0 ☐ No pain
1 ☐ Mild
2 ☐ Discomforting
3 ☐ Distressing
4 ☐ Horrible
5 ☐ Excruciating

Questionnaire Developed by: Ronald Melzack

FIGURE 20.2 The Short-Form McGill Pain Questionnaire (SF-MPQ). (Copyright © R. Melzack, 1984, 1987. Reproduced with permission.)

types of pain. In one study supporting this conclusion, Chang and colleagues[50] induced skin pain and muscle pain in human subjects through the use of intracutaneous and intramuscular injection of capsaicin into the left forearm, respectively. Although ratings of global pain intensity were very similar for both the skin and muscle pain, capsaicin injection into skin and muscle produced distinctly different pain qualities, as described by the subjects. When capsaicin was injected into the skin, subjects described their pain as sharp, cutting, and burning; pain induced by intramuscular capsaicin injection was described as throbbing, pulsing, and tingling. The results of this study support the idea that different pain mechanisms or sources of pain produce different pain sensations, and that these differences can be reliably assessed through the assessment of specific pain qualities. Also, it is generally thought that different nociceptors and fibers underlie different pain sensations, with the myelinated A-delta fibers responsible for localized "sharp," "stinging," and "shooting" pain, and the unmyelinated C-fibers responsible for less localized dull pain sensations.[51–53]

To date, five measures of pain quality have been developed that are specifically designed to assist in the diagnosis or classification of pain. They include: (1) the Leeds Assessment of Neuropathic Symptoms and Signs,[54] (2) the Self-Report Leeds Assessment of Neuropathic Symptoms and Signs,[55] (3) the Neuropathic Pain Questionnaire,[56] (4) the Neuropathic Pain Questionnaire–Short Form,[57] and (5) the Neuropathic Pain Diagnostic Questionnaire (DN4).[58]

Leeds Assessment of Neuropathic Symptoms and Signs. The Leeds Assessment of Neuropathic Symptoms and Signs (LANSS)[54] was perhaps the first measure designed specifically to distinguish neuropathic from nociceptive pain. It has two components: a pain questionnaire and a sensory testing component. The pain questionnaire consists of five items that ask respondents to indicate, yes or no, if their pain could be described as: (1) "[consisting of] strange, unpleasant sensations . . . like pricking, tingling, pins and needles"; (2) "[making] . . . the skin in the painful area look different from normal . . . like mottled or looking more red . . ."; (3) "[making] . . . the affected skin abnormally sensitive to touch . . ."; (4) "[coming] . . . on suddenly and in bursts for no apparent reason . . . like electric shocks, jumping and bursting . . ."; (5) "[feeling] . . . as if the skin temperature in the painful area has changed abnormally . . . like hot and burning . . ." The sensory testing component asks a clinician to test for allodynia (by lightly stroking a nonpainful and the painful area with cotton wool) and to test for altered pin-prick threshold (by comparing the patient response to a 23-gauge needle mounted inside of a syringe barrel placed gently on the skin in a nonpainful and then in the pain area). Each response is weighted, and the weights of all positive responses are summed to create a total score, with a score of less than 12 indicating an unlikelihood that neuropathic mechanisms are contributing to the patient's pain, and a score of 12 or greater indicating that neuropathic mechanisms are likely to be contributing to the patient's pain.

The LANSS showed a high rate (85%) of accurate classification for neuropathic versus nonneuropathic pain in the original development sample that was replicated in a cross-validation sample (82% accuracy).[54] This high level of accuracy was subsequently replicated in additional samples of patients (one sample with cancer[59] and a second with mixed chronic pain conditions[60]). The internal consistency of LANSS is high (Cronbach's alpha = 0.74),[54] indicating adequate reliability, and the LANSS items have also demonstrated an ability to discriminate between patients with fibromyalgia and patients with rheumatoid arthritis.[61] Finally, although the LANSS was not designed to be a measure of treatment outcome, one study demonstrated significant beneficial effects for transcranial magnetic stimulation for central (poststroke) and peripheral (trigeminal neuralgia) pain using the LANSS as an outcome measure.[62]

However, the LANSS has also been criticized as being difficult to administer, and concerns have been raised about using a sharp needle for assessing pin-prick threshold differences.[63] Specifically (1) the allodynia item was viewed as ambiguous given that this item does not provide an option for scoring patients with both sensory deficits and no allodynia and (2) using a sharp needle for pin-prick detection may pierce the skin in patients with fragile skin. In response to these concerns, the LANSS developer clarified that (1) if the patient has sensory deficits in the painful area and does not report allodynia, the allodynia item should be scored as "0" and (2) clinicians need not use a sharpened needle to detect differences in pin-prick threshold if this is deemed as unsafe for a particular patient—dulled (but sterile) pins could be used instead. The important issue for this item is whether a difference in sensation or threshold exists between the painful and a nonpainful area when a pin-prick is applied to both. Also, of four studies that have provided cross-validation psychometric data concerning the LANSS, three did not report significant difficulties using this measure.[60–62] One study reported that 6 of 26 patients required assistance with the five pain quality items (but did not report any difficulties with the sensory items).[59] In this latter study, if the pain quality being assessed was not clearly present (i.e., if either the patient or clinician was unsure), it was scored as absent. The resulting accuracy for discrimination of the LANSS when scored in this way was still high (86%).[59]

Self-Report Leeds Assessment of Neuropathic Symptoms and Signs. One potential drawback to the LANSS, that could limit its use in some clinical and research settings, is that it requires a trained clinician to administer. To address this limitation, a self-report version of the LANSS (S-LANSS) has been developed.[55] The S-LANSS includes the same five pain quality items of the LANSS. However, the sensory items were modified to allow patients to self-administer them by: (1) gently rubbing the painful and a nonpainful area with their index finger for the allodynia item and (2) gently pressing the painful and a nonpainful area with a finger tip to assess static allodynia. The S-LANSS has demonstrated an ability to correctly classify 75% of 200 patients with mixed chronic pain problems as having neuropathic versus nociceptive pain.[55] When administered by a clinician, however, its accuracy rate increased to 80%.[55] Finally, the internal consistency of the S-LANSS (Cronbach's alpha = 0.76) supports its reliability as well as the conclusion that the S-LANSS items tap into the same underlying dimension.

Neuropathic Pain Questionnaire. The Neuropathic Pain Questionnaire (NPQ)[56] has 12 items that assess two global affective pain domains (unpleasant and overwhelming pain) and 10 specific pain descriptors (burning, sensitive, shooting, numb, electric, tingling, squeezing, freezing, increased pain due to touch, increased pain due to weather changes). The items were selected from a larger pool of items specifically because of their ability to discriminate between patients with neuropathic and nonneuropathic pain.

When completing the NPQ, respondents are asked to rate each item using a 0 to 100 severity scale. The ratings are then weighted based on their demonstrated ability to discriminate between pain types; items with better discriminative ability are given more weight. The weighted scores are then summed into a total, with total scores below 0 suggesting nociceptive pain, and scores of 0 or above suggesting neuropathic pain. The sensitivity and specificity of the NPQ for discriminating neuropathic from nociceptive pain were found to be 75% and 78% in the scale development sample, respectively. Cross-validation yielded a sensitivity of 67% and a specificity of 75%.[56]

Neuropathic Pain Questionnaire–Short Form. A short form of the NPQ has also been developed (NPQ-SF),[57] with the idea that this could be used in settings where subject assessment burden is a primary concern (e.g., survey research). A discriminant function analysis was used to select only those items from the pool of 12 NPQ items that contributed statistically significantly to the ability to classify patients with neuropathic versus nonneuropathic pain. Three items emerged from these analyses: numbness, tingling pain, and increased pain due to touch. In the scale development sample, these three items had a 73% classification accuracy rate, indicating that NPQ-SF was only slightly less accurate in its predictive power than the original NPQ, despite its brevity.[57]

Neuropathic Pain Diagnostic Questionnaire. The Neuropathic Pain Diagnostic Questionnaire (DN4)[58] is the most recently developed measure that was designed to discriminate between neuropathic and nonneuropathic pain. It is administered by a clinician, and begins by asking patients if they do or do not experience their pain as having burning, painful cold, or electric shock qualities. Patients are then asked to indicate if they do or do not experience tingling, pins and needles, numbness, or itching in the same area that they experience pain. Finally, and similar to the LANSS, the evaluating clinician determines if hypoesthesia (decreased sensitivity) to touch or to pinprick exists in the painful area, and whether lightly brushing the area elicits pain. In the initial study, the DN4 yielded a very high level of accuracy (86%; sensitivity, 83%; and specificity, 90%) for distinguishing patients with and without neuropathic pain.[58]

Pain Quality Scales as Descriptive and Outcome Measures

Pain quality measures may also be used to describe the pain associated with different pain conditions, as well as to identify the effects of pain treatments on various qualities of the pain experience. To the extent that different pain qualities are linked to different pain mechanisms, then understanding the effects of pain treatments on those qualities may be used to better understand the mechanisms of pain treatments. In addition, given the evidence (reported later) that different pain treatments have different effects on various pain qualities, pain clinicians could potentially use pain quality assessment for helping to select from among different treatment options. For example, clinicians may offer patients reporting their pain as primarily "aching" those treatments shown to impact "aching" pain most effectively, while providing patients who describe their pain as "electrical" with treatments that have been shown to reduce "electrical" pain sensations.

To date, five measures have been developed to assess pain quality, and have been used as outcome measures in clinical trials. They include (1) the McGill Pain Questionnaire (MPQ),[41] (2) the Short-Form McGill Pain Questionnaire (MPQ-SF),[42] (3) the Neuropathic Pain Symptom Inventory (NPSI),[64] (4) the Neuropathic Pain Scale (NPS),[65] and (5) the Pain Quality Assessment Scale (PQAS).[66]

McGill Pain Questionnaire. The MPQ was introduced previously in the context of assessing pain affect. In addition to assessing affective pain domain, the 78 MPQ descriptors can also be scored to assess sensory pain (10 sensory categories, such as temporal, punctuate pressure, and thermal pain, assessed using 42 descriptors), evaluative pain (one category, assessed using five descriptors), and miscellaneous pain (four categories that do not clearly fall into sensory or affective components, assessed using 17 descriptors).[41]

As described previously, respondents are asked to select the single descriptor from each of the 20 categories (the number of descriptors listed per category varies from 2 to 6) that best describes his or her pain, and the rank order of the descriptors in each category are summed to compute sensory, affective, evaluative, miscellaneous, and total scores.

Support for the usefulness of the MPQ comes from the fact that it has been used in hundreds of studies, and has been trans-

lated into at least 20 languages.[67] Moreover, a three factor (sensory, affective, and evaluative domains) structure of the MPQ has been confirmed in two studies,[68,69] although the high degree of association among these subscales suggests some limitations in discriminative validity of the primary MPQ scales.[68] Also, and of primary importance, the MPQ scales have demonstrated validity as outcome measures given their responsivity to changes produced by pain treatments.[47,75,76]

A number of studies have examined the reliability of the MPQ. In populations of patients with cancer pain, studies have found that responses to the MPQ are generally consistent over the time span of several days.[77–79] In a study with patients with low back pain, Love and colleagues[78] found adequate test-retest stability for the MPQ scale scores (total: r = 0.83; sensory: r = 0.76; affective: 0.78) over the course of several days.

Despite the many strengths of the MPQ, it also has some limitations. First, although it only takes about 5 minutes to complete by someone familiar with the measure, the MPQ includes a large number of descriptors that are rarely used by some individuals with pain; 78 descriptors suggests a very high degree of content validity, but this many descriptors may not be needed to adequately describe pain quality in many populations. Pain quality measures with fewer items may be adequately thorough, while also still providing adequate content validity. Indeed, this limitation may be one reason that the short-form version of the MPQ, described later, was developed.

A second limitation of the MPQ concerns the way it is scored. Although it probably makes sense to combine multiple affective responses into a composite Affective scale, there may be limitations in combining a large number of different sensory descriptors into a composite sensory scale. Primary among these is the possibility that such a procedure does not allow investigators to detect the impact of treatments on specific pain descriptors. A significant effect of a pain treatment on the MPQ sensory pain scale could have been due to its modest effects on many different pain qualities, or a large effect on just a few. One of the important reasons to assess pain quality in clinical trials is to determine the effects of treatment on specific pain qualities; scoring the MPQ descriptors into composite scales does not allow for this.

Also, because it is unlikely that pain treatments impact all pain qualities in the same way, the use of composite pain quality scores, based on many different items (recall that the MPQ sensory scale assesses 10 quality domains using 42 descriptors), runs the risk of reducing one's ability to detect significant effects. When using composite measures in clinical trials that include items that are not affected by treatment, or are affected only minimally, the effect size for the total scale is reduced. Indeed, when differences are found, the MPQ scale scores tend to be less responsive to treatment effects than single-item pain intensity ratings.[80–82]

Short-Form McGill Pain Questionnaire. The Short-Form McGill Pain Questionnaire (SF-MPQ) was developed as a measure that balances the need for pain quality data against the need to minimize assessment burden (see Fig. 20.2).[42] As previously mentioned in the Affect section, the SF-MPQ consists of 15 descriptors, each of which can be rated on a four-point severity scale from "none" to "severe." The 15 items were selected based on their frequency of endorsement by patients with a variety of pain disorders. Eleven of the descriptors assess sensory pain (throbbing, shooting, sharp, cramping, gnawing, hot-burning, aching, heavy, tender, and splitting), and, as described previously, four items assess affective pain.

Evidence supporting the validity of both SF-MPQ scales includes data showing a strong association between the sensory and affective scales scored from the SF-MPQ and the original MPQ sensory and affective subscales.[42–44] Also, a number of studies have demonstrated that the SF-MPQ is responsive to pain treatments, providing additional critical support for the validity of the SF-MPQ as an outcome measure.[83–85] Finally, because each SF-MPQ item is individually rated, SF-MPQ responses could theoretically be used in clinical trials to look at the specific effects of pain interventions on particular pain qualities, although this strength of the SF-MPQ has yet to be capitalized on.

Limitations of the SF-MPQ include the fact that some descriptors common to neuropathic pain (e.g., electrical, tingling) are not included in the measure, limiting its utility in individuals with neuropathic pain. An additional limitation of the SF-MPQ concerns scoring. As discussed previously with respect to the MPQ, if the items are combined into scale scores, these scores may be less sensitive to treatment effects than are individual ratings of pain intensity or individual descriptor ratings. This makes the SF-MPQ scale scores, perhaps, less useful than global pain intensity ratings or even the individual SF-MPQ items as outcome measures.

Neuropathic Pain Symptom Inventory. The Neuropathic Pain Symptom Inventory (NPSI)[64] includes 12 items that were selected to assess four global domains of neuropathic pain (spontaneous ongoing pain, spontaneous paroxysmal pain, evoked pain, and paresthesias/dysesthesia). Respondents rate the severity or intensity of each descriptor item on 0 to 10 numerical rating scales. Two additional items assess the temporal qualities of pain (number of hours of spontaneous pain in the past 24 hours, number of paroxysms during the last 24 hours).

As reported in the initial development study, short-term (3 hours) and long-term (1 month) test-retest stability of the NPSI items were shown to be very high, as measured by intra-class correlation coefficients (short-term: range 0.87–0.98; long-term: 0.78–0.98). Also, validity for the evoked pain items was evidenced through their significant associations (rs range 0.66–0.73) with related clinician scores of pain evoked by brushing, pressure, and cold stimuli. Changes in the NPSI total score were also found to be associated significantly with patient and provider ratings of global improvement over a one-month period. However, to date, no other studies using the NPSI have been reported.

Neuropathic Pain Scale. The Neuropathic Pain Scale (NPS) was developed as a measure of neuropathic pain to both (1) describe neuropathic pain qualities in different pain populations, and (2) document the impact of pain treatments on pain qualities in clinical trials.[64] The NPS includes 10 items, two that assess global pain intensity and unpleasantness, and eight that reflect specific pain domains (six pain qualities and two spatial characteristics) likely to be reported by patients with neuropathic pain syndromes:

Respondents rate each item on a scale from 0 to 10, with 0 being "no ____" or "not ____" and 10 corresponding to "the most ____ sensation imaginable." An eleventh item allows patients to report the temporal nature of their pain (constant with intermittent increases, intermittent, or constant with fluctuation). Rather than combining the individual item ratings into scale scores, the NPS items were intended primarily to be used for assessing distinct pain qualities, which could then be used to create a profile of a person's pain quality experience. A growing body of research supports the validity of the NPS for describing neuropathic pain conditions,[86–88] distinguishing between pain diagnoses,[55,64,86] predicting treatment outcome,[89] and other symptoms,[90] and detecting treatment effects.[64,71,91–97]

The NPS has also shown utility for identifying the pain qualities affected by different pain treatments.[65,71,93,97] For example, a recent study examined the effectiveness of the NPS for assessing changes in pain qualities in three groups (peripheral neuropathic pain, low back pain, and osteoarthritis) of patients treated with open label lidocaine patch 5%.[93] Although significant changes in almost all NPS pain qualities were found, significantly larger changes were seen for NPS items measuring sharp and deep pain than for items measuring cold, sensitive, or itching pain.[93] In

another study, controlled-release oxycodone was found to be associated with decreases in sharp, dull, deep, and surface pain, but had little impact on hot, cold, itchy, or sensitive pain in patients with painful diabetic neuropathy.[66] In a sample of patients with mixed neuropathic pain conditions, intravenous lidocaine and phentolamine were found to have similar effects on 8 of 10 NPS items, although lidocaine had a greater effect on global pain unpleasantness and deep pain.[65] Finally, one study showed that tizanidine for neuropathic pain impacted the hot, cold, and sensitive NPS items (as well as global intensity and unpleasantness) after 2 weeks of treatment, and then impacted sharp, dull, and deep pain NPS items after 8 weeks, indicating that the NPS may be used to show how treatments impact various pain qualities over time.[96]

Another strength of the NPS is its brevity, which makes it potentially useful in survey research and in settings where assessment burden may be a significant issue. Also, the NPS has been translated into 24 languages, and so may be useful for cross-cultural research comparing neuropathic pain conditions and treatments across cultures.

Although the NPS was originally designed to be scored to create a "profile" of sensation severity across different pain qualities, it is possible to combine the items into composite scores. Galer and colleagues,[91] for example, created four different NPS composite scores when examining the effects of a lidocaine patch 5% in a sample of patients with postherpetic neuralgia: an average of all 10 items (NPS10), an average of the eight specific descriptors excluding the global ratings of pain intensity and unpleasantness (NPS8), an average of the eight items that do not reflect allodynia (i.e., excluding the "sensitive" and "surface" items; NPS NA), and an average of four items thought to reflect nonperipheral pain mechanisms ("dull," "deep," "sharp," and "burning" items; NPS4). However, concerns about the use of composite scores from pain quality measures, raised above with respect to the MPQ, are also relevant here; use and interpretation of composite pain quality scores, regardless of the measure used for item selection, needs to proceed with caution.

The primary limitation of the NPS is associated with one of its strengths—its brevity. The NPS does not assess a number of pain qualities that are commonly reported by patients with some neuropathic pain conditions, such as shooting, electrical, and tingling pain. Also, the NPS does not assess some pain qualities experienced by individuals with nonneuropathic pain, limiting its utility in populations with musculoskeletal problems, such as individuals with low back pain or arthritis.

Pain Quality Assessment Scale. The Pain Quality Assessment Scale (PQAS; Fig. 20.3)[5,98] was developed to make available a measure that had the strengths of the NPS, but without its primary limitation. It uses the existing 10 NPS items as a starting point, but then also includes 10 additional items to create a measure capable of assessing the most common pain qualities seen across a variety of chronic pain conditions.[66] In addition to the original NPS items, the PQAS includes the following pain qualities to make it possible to assess additional common neuropathic and nociceptive pain qualities: tender, shooting, numb, electrical, tingling, cramping, radiating, throbbing, aching, and heavy. Like the NPS, the PQAS includes an additional item to differentiate between three primary temporal patterns of pain: intermittent (i.e., variable pain with some pain free periods), variable (variable pain without pain-free periods), and stable (i.e., constant pain with little variation). Thus, the final 21-item PQAS was intended to be comprehensive enough to capture the majority of a patient's pain experience, yet also be brief enough to minimize assessment burden.

All of the data that support the validity of the NPS also support the PQAS, since the NPS items are contained in the PQAS. In addition, in the first published report using the PQAS items, it was found that all 10 of the new PQAS items (i.e., the non-NPS

PAIN QUALITY ASSESSMENT SCALE (PQAS)

<u>Instructions:</u> There are different aspects and types of pain that patients experience and that we are interested in measuring. Pain can feel sharp, hot, cold, dull, and achy. Some pains may feel like they are very superficial (at skin-level), or they may feel like they are from deep inside your body. Pain can also be described as unpleasant.

The Pain Quality Assessment Scale helps us measure these and other different aspects of your pain. For one patient, a pain might feel extremely hot and burning, but not at all dull, while another patient may not experience any burning pain, but feel like their pain is very dull and achy. Therefore, we expect you to rate very high on some of the scales below and very low on others.

Please use the 19 rating scales below to rate how much of each different pain quality and type you may or may not have felt ***OVER THE PAST WEEK, ON AVERAGE.***

Place an "X" through the number that best describes your pain. For example:

| 0 | 1 | 2 | ☒ | 4 | 5 | 6 | 7 | 8 | 9 | 10 |

---

1. Please use the scale below to tell us how **intense** your pain has been over the past week, on average.

No pain | 0 | 1 | 2 | 3 | 4 | 5 | 6 | 7 | 8 | 9 | 10 | The most **intense** pain sensation imaginable

2. Please use the scale below to tell us how **sharp** your pain has felt over the past week. Words used to describe sharp feelings include "<u>like a knife</u>," "<u>like a spike</u>," or "<u>piercing</u>."

Not sharp | 0 | 1 | 2 | 3 | 4 | 5 | 6 | 7 | 8 | 9 | 10 | The most **sharp** sensation imaginable ("like a knife")

3. Please use the scale below to tell us how **hot** your pain has felt over the past week. Words used to describe very hot pain include "<u>burning</u>" and "<u>on fire</u>."

Not hot | 0 | 1 | 2 | 3 | 4 | 5 | 6 | 7 | 8 | 9 | 10 | The most **hot** sensation imaginable ("burning")

4. Please use the scale below to tell us how **dull** your pain has felt over the past week.

Not dull | 0 | 1 | 2 | 3 | 4 | 5 | 6 | 7 | 8 | 9 | 10 | The most **dull** sensation imaginable

5. Please use the scale below to tell us how **cold** your pain has felt over the past week. Words used to describe very cold pain include "<u>like ice</u>" and "<u>freezing</u>."

Not cold | 0 | 1 | 2 | 3 | 4 | 5 | 6 | 7 | 8 | 9 | 10 | The most **cold** sensation imaginable ("freezing")

6. Please use the scale below to tell us how **sensitive** your skin has been to light touch or clothing rubbing against it over the past week. Words used to describe sensitive skin include "<u>like sunburned skin</u>" and "<u>raw skin</u>."

Not sensitive | 0 | 1 | 2 | 3 | 4 | 5 | 6 | 7 | 8 | 9 | 10 | The most **sensitive** sensation imaginable ("raw skin")

FIGURE 20.3 The Pain Quality Assessment Scale (PQAS). (Copyright © Jensen, Galer, and Gammaitoni, 2006. Reproduced with permission.)   *(continues)*

7. Please use the scale below to tell us how **tender** your pain is when something has pressed against it over the past week. Another word used to describe tender pain is "like a bruise."

Not tender | 0 | 1 | 2 | 3 | 4 | 5 | 6 | 7 | 8 | 9 | 10 | The most **tender** sensation imaginable ("like a bruise")

8. Please use the scale below to tell us how **itchy** your pain has felt over the past week. Words used to describe itchy pain include "like poison ivy" and "like a mosquito bite."

Not itchy | 0 | 1 | 2 | 3 | 4 | 5 | 6 | 7 | 8 | 9 | 10 | The most **itchy** sensation imaginable ("like poison ivy")

9. Please use the scale below to tell us how much your pain has felt like it has been **shooting** over the past week. Another word used to describe shooting pain is "zapping."

Not shooting | 0 | 1 | 2 | 3 | 4 | 5 | 6 | 7 | 8 | 9 | 10 | The most **shooting** sensation imaginable ("zapping")

10. Please use the scale below to tell us how **numb** your pain has felt over the past week. A phrase that can be used to describe numb pain is "like it is asleep."

Not numb | 0 | 1 | 2 | 3 | 4 | 5 | 6 | 7 | 8 | 9 | 10 | The most **numb** sensation imaginable ("asleep")

11. Please use the scale below to tell us how much your pain sensations have felt **electrical** over the past week. Words used to describe electrical pain include "shocks," "lightning," and "sparking."

Not electrical | 0 | 1 | 2 | 3 | 4 | 5 | 6 | 7 | 8 | 9 | 10 | The most **electrical** sensation imaginable ("shocks")

12. Please use the scale below to tell us how **tingling** your pain has felt over the past week. Words used to describe tingling pain include "like pins and needles" and "prickling."

Not tingling | 0 | 1 | 2 | 3 | 4 | 5 | 6 | 7 | 8 | 9 | 10 | The most **tingling** sensation imaginable ("pins and needles")

13. Please use the scale below to tell us how **cramping** your pain has felt over the past week. Words used to describe cramping pain include "squeezing" and "tight."

Not cramping | 0 | 1 | 2 | 3 | 4 | 5 | 6 | 7 | 8 | 9 | 10 | The most **cramping** sensation imaginable ("squeezing")

14. Please use the scale below to tell us how **radiating** your pain has felt over the past week. Another word used to describe radiating pain is "spreading."

Not radiating | 0 | 1 | 2 | 3 | 4 | 5 | 6 | 7 | 8 | 9 | 10 | The most **radiating** sensation imaginable ("spreading")

15. Please use the scale below to tell us how **throbbing** your pain has felt over the past week. Another word used to describe throbbing pain is "pounding."

Not throbbing | 0 | 1 | 2 | 3 | 4 | 5 | 6 | 7 | 8 | 9 | 10 | The most **throbbing** sensation imaginable ("pounding")

FIGURE 20.3 (*continued*)

16. Please use the scale below to tell us how **aching** your pain has felt over the past week. Another word used to describe aching pain is "like a toothache."

Not aching | 0 | 1 | 2 | 3 | 4 | 5 | 6 | 7 | 8 | 9 | 10 | The most **aching** sensation imaginable ("like a toothache")

17. Please use the scale below to tell us how **heavy** your pain has felt over the past week. Other words used to describe heavy pain are "pressure" and "weighted down."

Not heavy | 0 | 1 | 2 | 3 | 4 | 5 | 6 | 7 | 8 | 9 | 10 | The most **heavy** sensation imaginable ("weighted down")

18. Now that you have told us the different types of pain sensations you have felt, we want you to tell us overall how **unpleasant** your pain has been to you over the past week. Words used to describe very unpleasant pain include "annoying," "bothersome," "miserable," and "intolerable." Remember, pain can have a low intensity but still feel extremely unpleasant, and some kinds of pain can have a high intensity but be very tolerable. With this scale, please tell us how **unpleasant** your pain feels.

Not unpleasant | 0 | 1 | 2 | 3 | 4 | 5 | 6 | 7 | 8 | 9 | 10 | The most **unpleasant** sensation imaginable ("intolerable")

19. Finally, we want you to give us an estimate of the severity of your <u>deep</u> versus <u>surface</u> pain over the past week. We want you to rate each location of pain separately. We realize that it can be difficult to make these estimates, and most likely it will be a "best guess," but please give us your best estimate.

HOW INTENSE IS YOUR *DEEP* PAIN?

No **deep** pain | 0 | 1 | 2 | 3 | 4 | 5 | 6 | 7 | 8 | 9 | 10 | The most **intense deep** pain sensation imaginable

HOW INTENSE IS YOUR *SURFACE* PAIN?

No **surface** pain | 0 | 1 | 2 | 3 | 4 | 5 | 6 | 7 | 8 | 9 | 10 | The most **intense surface** pain sensation imaginable

20. Pain can also have different time qualities. For some people, the pain comes and goes and so they have some moments that are completely without pain; in other words the pain "comes and goes". This is called **intermittent** pain. Others are never pain free, but their pain types and pain severity can vary from one moment to the next. This is called **variable** pain. For these people, the increases can be severe, so that they feel they have moments of very intense pain ("breakthrough" pain), but at other times they can feel lower levels of pain ("background" pain). Still, they are never pain free. Other people have pain that really does not change that much from one moment to another. This is called **stable** pain. Which of these best describes the time pattern of your pain (please select only one):

( ) I have **intermittent** pain (I feel pain sometimes but I am pain-free at other times).
( ) I have **variable** pain ("background"pain all the time, but also moments of more
       pain, or even severe "breakthrough pain or varying types of pain).
( ) I have **stable** pain (constant pain that does not change very much from one moment to
       another, and no pain-free periods).

PQAS Copyright © Jensen, Galer, and Gammaitoni 2006

FIGURE 20.3 (*continued*)

items) were responsive to the effects of both lidocaine patch 5% and a corticosteroid injection in a sample of patients with carpal tunnel syndrome.[98] These findings indicate that the PQAS may be even more useful than the NPS for identifying the specific effects of pain treatments on different qualities of neuropathic pain, although more research is needed to determine if the new items continue to evidence validity as outcome measures in other neuropathic pain populations, as well as in populations of persons with nonneuropathic pain.

Recommendations for Assessing Pain Quality

There is clearly a very large interest in the development, if not the use of, pain quality measures. A fair number of such measures now exist, and additional pain quality measures and modifications of pain quality measures seem to be developed and published on a regular basis. At this point, the LANSS (or S-LANSS in survey research) has the most evidence supporting its validity as a measure for distinguishing neuropathic from nonneuropathic pain, and the NPS has the most empirical evidence supporting its validity as a measure of the distinct pain qualities impacted by pain treatments.

However, both the LANSS and the NPS have limitations, and it is likely that each can be improved further. Concerning the LANSS or S-LANSS, improvements could potentially be made by adding items or pain quality domains to these measures that have been shown to discriminate neuropathic from nonneuropathic pain in other studies measures. These include, for example, "squeezing" (from the NPQ and DN4), "freezing" (from the NPQ) or "painful cold" (from the DN4), and "itching" (from the DN4). Indeed, even though the NPS was not specifically developed to discriminate between neuropathic and nonneuropathic pain, five NPS items have been shown to differ between patients with these types of pain, and four of these ("sharp," "cold," "itchy," and "surface" pain) are not included on the LANSS.[55,99] Inclusion of items that reflect these pain qualities, and possibly others, may enhance the accuracy of the LANSS and S-LANSS even further.

Similarly, although the NPS has been used more than any other pain quality measure for identifying the specific pain qualities impacted by pain treatments, it has limited content validity. This limitation was what inspired the development of the PQAS, which includes pain qualities common to patients with neuropathic and nonneuropathic pain conditions. Thus, it is likely that the PQAS will ultimately prove more useful than the NPS, and might be considered over the NPS when a measure of pain's effects on specific pain qualities is needed, especially given the fact that all of the NPS items are included in the PQAS.

Ultimately, it is possible that pain quality scales (or subscales of measures such as the MPQ or PQAS) may be developed that are specific for each pain problem or pain type. Once the pain qualities most closely associated with low back pain, for example, are identified, it may be most practical to administer measures that just assess those qualities in samples of patients with low back pain. In a sample of persons with carpal tunnel syndrome, the pain qualities assessed by the PQAS that were reported as most severe (as defined by average ratings of 4.00 or more on a 0–10 scale) included sharp, tender, shooting, numb, electrical, tingling, cramping, deep, and surface pain.[98] Numb (average rating, 7.13/10) and tingling (average rating, 6.98/10) were particularly high in this sample. Moreover, as might be expected, the pain qualities that were rated as most severe pretreatment were the qualities that tended to show the greatest improvement with pain treatment.[98] Based on these findings, a PQAS Carpal Tunnel subscale (PQAS-CT) could be envisioned that included just these nine items, and a composite score made up of such a scale might be shown to be more responsive to effective pain treatment than a composite made up of all of the PQAS sensory items. But replications of research using the PQAS and other pain quality measures are needed to ensure that no critical pain quality is left out when diagnosis-specific measures are developed.

Measuring Pain's Spatial Characteristics

Pain can occur both at different body locations (e.g., head, leg), or at different depths (e.g., "surface" or "deep" pain). The two most common strategies used for assessing the body location of pain are the pain drawing and the pain site checklist. A pain drawing consists of an outline of a human form, and respondents are simply asked to mark or shade in the areas on the drawing which correspond to pain they are currently experiencing. Pain drawings are included in a number of standard pain questionnaires, such as the MPQ,[41] the LANSS,[54] and the original (non-short form) BPI.[100] One published pain drawing allows the assessor to use a template to score the patient's response, both for the specific area that has been shaded, as well as for "pain extent" (which reflects the total number of areas that have been shaded).[101]

A site checklist is a simple list of possible sites for pain, and the respondent is asked to indicate which site(s) are currently painful.[102] Like pain drawings, site checklists can be scored for both the specific site(s) chosen, as well as for "pain extent" (total number of sites chosen). The presence and severity of "deep" and "surface" pain can be determined by asking respondents to rate each (see the PQAS reflecting these in Fig. 20.3).

Although research suggests that scores derived from measures of pain site (i.e., "pain extent" as represented by the number or percent of body area involved) predict, in some patients, disability, pain interference, medication use, return to work, and psychological functioning, this same body of research indicates that these associations are not consistent and not always strong.[32] This suggests that measures of pain's spatial characteristics should not be used as proxy measures of psychopathology or disability.

On the other hand, pain drawings, pain site checklists, and measures of the relative depth of pain are well suited for descriptive purposes. For example, research in patients with spinal cord injury has used pain drawings and pain site to describe the frequency of pain experienced at different body sites, as well as the relationship between pain location or number of pain sites and other related variables.[102,103]

Recommendations for Assessing Pain Site

Pain drawings, pain site checklists, and severity ratings of pain's perceived depth have all been used successfully to describe the pain in different populations, and measures of the latter domain, as items from the NPS and PQAS, have demonstrated responsiveness as outcome measures in clinical trials. Decisions about which to use in any one setting or with any one population will largely depend on the preference of the assessor, and practical issues concerning how the data will be used. Clinicians often prefer pain drawings, given that they provide a global overview of how patients experience the location(s) of their pain. However, when used in research, pain drawings require an additional step (usually with the aid of a template) to objectively determine the specific site(s) selected. Pain checklists may be more practical for the researcher, given that coding for the specific sites (e.g., legs, low back, head, etc.) is completed by the respondent once the checklist has been administered and completed.

Measuring Pain's Temporal Characteristics

The temporal aspects of pain, such as its variability, frequency, and duration, as well as its pattern across time (over minutes, hours, days, or months) can be assessed by asking patients to rate their pain on multiple occasions over time using pain diaries.

The specific temporal domains of interest can then be operationalized by computing scores from the diary ratings. Based on diary data, *pain variability* can be operationalized as the standard deviation of pain intensity ratings during a specific epoch, *frequency of "breakthrough" pain* as the number of times pain reached and exceeded a specific cutoff (e.g., 7 or more on a 0–10 scale for severe breakthrough pain, or 5 or more for moderate to severe breakthrough pain[104]), and *pain duration* as the number of hours that pain was rated as being above a specific cutoff, for example 5 or more on a 0 to 10 scale for duration of "moderate to severe" pain.[104]

Diary data can also be used to identify *temporal patterns*. Jamison and Brown,[105] for example, identified six different temporal pain pattern types (e.g., steady increase over the course of a day, steady decrease, curvilinear pattern, no consistent pattern) based on diary data. They found that the group of patients that showed no clear consistent pattern from one day to the next also reported the greatest emotional distress.[105] van Grootel and colleagues identified two primary patterns of pain intensity from diary data in a sample of patients with temporomandibular disorders: (1) those reporting higher levels of pain later in the day and (2) those reporting higher levels of pain in the morning; with the former group reporting higher overall levels of pain intensity, more difficulty falling asleep at bedtime, more widespread pain, and greater endorsement about the role of a physician in managing their pain problem.[106] These findings suggest the possibility that the time pattern of pain experience may play a role in how patients think about or manage their pain.

Another way to assess pain pattern is to describe different temporal patterns to patients, and allow them to select the description that best describes their pain. For example, an item from the PQAS (see Fig. 20.3) asks patients to indicate which of the following best describes their pain: (1) I have intermittent pain (I feel pain sometimes but I am pain-free at other times); (2) I have variable pain ("background" pain all the time, but also moments of more pain, or even severe "breakthrough" pain or varying types of pain); (3) I have stable pain (constant pain that does not change very much from one moment to another, and no pain-free periods). One study found that these temporal characteristics differed as a function of neuropathic versus nonneuropathic pain, with patients rated by physicians as having "possible" neuropathic pain being more likely to endorse having variable pain then patients rating as being "unlikely" to have neuropathic pain.[99]

Recommendations for Assessing Pain's Temporal Characteristics

Either diary-based measures or categorical scales may be used to assess pain's temporal characteristics. Categorical scales require less investigator effort than diary-based measures, but diary-based measures allow for greater flexibility in coding different temporal patterns then categorical scales. Both types of measures have some, albeit limited, support for their predictive validity. Neither has yet been used as outcome measures, so their utility for determining the impact of pain treatment has yet to be determined.

Overall, then, although the temporal dimension of pain can be assessed, there is not yet adequate empirical support for concluding that assessment of the temporal characteristics of pain provides information that is critical to understanding a patient's pain, or the impact of treatment on that pain. More research is needed to compare the utility and validity of measures of pain's temporal characteristics to draw conclusions about the clinical and research importance of this pain domain, and the best way(s) to assess it.

Measuring Pain Interference

Pain interference refers to the extent to which pain interferes with day-to-day functioning. The two most commonly used measures of pain interference are the Brief Pain Inventory Pain Interference (BPI) scale[100] (see Fig. 41.3) and the Interference scale of the West Haven-Yale Multidimensional Pain Inventory (WHYMPI).[107]

Brief Pain Inventory Pain Interference Scale

The BPI Interference scale includes seven items that assess the extent to which pain has interfered with: general activity, mood, walking ability, normal work (including both work outside the home and housework), relations with other people, sleep, and enjoyment of life. Respondents are asked to rate the degree of pain interference with each activity on 0 (does not interfere) to 10 (completely interferes) numerical scales. The responses to the seven items are then averaged to form the Pain Interference scale score.

Factor analyses of responses show that the seven interference items load together onto a single factor,[100,108–116] and that the scale has excellent internal consistency (with alphas ranging from .78 to .91).[104,109,110,113–115] One study used multidimensional scaling to determine the factors underlying the BPI Pain Interference items in a large sample of 1,843 persons with metastatic cancer.[117] These analyses yielded two underlying interference dimensions: interference with activity (walking, work, general activity, sleep) and affectivity-related interference (relations, mood, enjoyment of life), suggesting the possibility of alternate scoring and use of the BPI Pain Interference scale. However, this alternate scoring has yet to be used or tested in additional samples. The BPI Pain Interference scale is associated, as would be expected, with measures of pain intensity.[112,118,119] The BPI Interference scale has been increasingly used as an outcome measure in clinical trials, and evidence demonstrating changes in the BPI Interference scale score supports its validity for this purpose.[92,120–123]

Recently, the BPI Interference scale was slightly modified (with permission from the copyright holder of the BPI) so that it could be used in persons with physical disabilities.[124–126] Perhaps the most important modification was to change the wording of the interference with walking item to ask respondents to rate the degree of interference with "mobility (ability to get around)." This change makes it possible for individuals who have mobility restrictions unrelated to pain (i.e., who are wheelchair users) to rate the impact of pain on their mobility. Since many of these individuals would be unable to walk even if they had no pain, the original wording of this item would not be appropriate.

The other modification made was to increase the content validity of the scale by including items asking about pain interference with self-care, recreational activities, and social activities,[125] as well as items asking about interference with communication and learning new information or skills.[124,126] These five activity domains are important to many individuals with disabilities, and also reflect functioning domains defined as relevant and unique by the WHO's International Classification of Functioning, Disability, and Health.[127] Given the psychometric strength of the original BPI interference items, it is perhaps not surprising that the 10- and 12-item modified scales also have strong psychometric properties. First, the internal consistency of the modified scales are uniformly high (range, 0.89 to 0.96) in three samples of persons with disabilities, including individuals with cerebral palsy,[125] spinal cord injury,[126] and multiple sclerosis.[124] Second, like the original BPI Interference scale, the modified and expanded scales show strong associations with measures of pain intensity (correlation coefficients range, 0.61 to 0.66), consistent with what would be expected if they measured the extent to which pain interfered with functioning.[125,126] Finally, factor analyses of the modified and expanded items show that new items all load strongly on a pain interference factor that is related to, but also distinct from, a pain intensity factor.[124]

However, although the modification of the original walking BPI item makes it possible for individuals who have difficulties walking for reasons other than pain to respond to that item, and the addition of items increases the content validity of the BPI, it is not clear that these modifications substantially improve other psychometric properties of the scale. For example, the internal consistency of a scale made up of 10 items (αs = 0.95 to 0.96[124,126]) is not that much larger than the original seven-item scale (α = 0.92 to 0.93[124,126]) in these same samples, suggesting that if scale brevity is important, the original 7 BPI items may provide as good a measure of pain impact as the expanded 10- or 12-item version.

West Haven Yale Multidimensional Pain Inventory Pain Interference Scale

Another measure of pain interference is the Interference scale of the West Haven-Yale Multidimensional Pain Inventory (WHYMPI).[107] The entire WHYMPI consists of three parts. Part 1 contains 20 items that assess five key pain-related domains: interference, support, pain severity, self-control, and negative mood. Parts 2 and 3 assess spouse responses to patient pain behaviors and participation in various life activities, respectively. The Interference scale contains nine items that assess the perceived degree to which pain affects: (1) four daily activities (social activities, work, daily activities, and chores), (2) satisfaction with three activities (social activities, family activities, work), and (3) social relationships (friendships, marital, and family relationships).

Support for the reliability and validity of the WHYMPI Interference scale as a measure of pain interference comes from a number of sources. First, factor analyses show that the nine pain interference items loaded together on a single scale that is distinct from the other WHYMPI scales.[107,128] The items show an excellent internal consistency (α range = 0.90 to 0.91),[107,128] as well as a high degree of stability (r = 0.86)[107] over a 2-week period. The WHYMPI Interference scale also shows an expected strong association with pain severity (rs range = 0.49 to 0.70).[128,129] Importantly, the WHYMPI Interference scale has also shown responsivity to change associated with treatment.[129–133]

Recommendations for Assessing Pain Interference

Both the BPI and WHYMPI of pain interference scales were constructed using sound scale development strategies, and each has support for its reliability and validity as a measure of pain interference. Also, each measure is relatively brief and easy to administer, complete, and score. However, to date, the BPI Interference scale has the most empirical support for its reliability and validity. Moreover, it has been translated into many different languages, and has been adapted for and validated in disabled populations, making it possible to compare pain interference across different cultures and populations. Thus, unless there is a clear reason not to use the BPI, it appears to be an excellent first choice when a measure of pain interference is needed both in the clinic and in research settings.

MEASURING PAIN IN SPECIAL POPULATIONS

Although the measures described and recommended for use in this chapter so far can be used by many patients in most settings, there are special populations that may require different measures or approaches. These include patients that are at risk for cognitive deficits (e.g., patients with head injuries, the elderly, the very ill) or who may not yet have reached an adequate developmental stage to understand the measure or the tasks that the measure requires (e.g., infants and toddlers). A detailed review of the many measures and procedures for assessing pain in special populations is beyond the scope of this chapter, and the interested reader is referred to other more detailed reviews to obtain information

concerning the available options (for children[134,135]; for the elderly[136–138]; for individuals with limited communication abilities[137,139]; for individuals with cancer[140]). In general, when assessing pain in special populations who are unable to provide valid responses to standard measures, the clinician and researcher has two options: (1) to simplify the assessment strategy to a level that can be understood by the patient or (2) to depend on observation of behaviors known to reflect pain experience.

Simplified Measures of Pain

Simple Pain Measures to Consider

Of the two options to consider when selecting a pain assessment approach for special populations, the first option, using a simplified measure of pain, may be considered a better option to select whenever possible and practical given the facts that (1) only patients have direct access to their pain experience, and so are in the best position to describe this experience and (2) observational measures of pain behaviors show, at best, only moderate associations to patient reports of pain experience.[141]

Of the three primary pain intensity measures used most often in pain research and clinical settings, evidence indicates that VRSs tend to be easier for patients to understand and use than NRSs, and that NRSs are easier for patients to understand and use than VASs,[40,142–145] making simple VRSs (e.g., none, mild, moderate, severe) a natural choice to consider when a simple measure of pain is needed. Another measure to consider in this situation is a face scale. Face scales consist of line drawings of faces, each of which represent expressions that communicate different levels of pain and distress. Although a number of such scales have been developed, one that has many strengths is the Faces Pain Scale–Revised (FPS-R, Fig. 20.4). An earlier version of the FPS-R[146] as well as the FPS-R have been shown to be easier to comprehend by older patients and patients with dementia than either a VRS or a VAS,[147,148] suggesting that this measure may be useful when even simple VRSs are too complex for the patient or population being studied. Also, the instructions for the FPS-R are available in many languages (currently 34), and information about the FPS-R is readily available and kept updated on a website (www.painsourcebook.ca).

There is ample evidence supporting the reliability and validity of the FPS-R as a measure of pain intensity (see review[137]). For example, the FPS-R of pain intensity is strongly associated with other measures of pain intensity,[148,149] and shows adequate test-retest stability over a 2-week interval (r = 0.76).[148] Also, the FPS-R shows responsivity to treatments known to impact pain, including in a clinical trial involving children as young as 4 to 6 years old,[150] a trial involving children 5 to 12 years old,[149] and one that used the FPS-R in children aged 3 to 12 years old.[151] Interestingly, although the NRS tends to be preferred over other scales by older patients who are not cognitively impaired, the FPS-R is preferred over other pain measures by elderly patients who have cognitive impairments.[148] However, one study reported that over half of a sample of 6-year-olds had difficulty understanding and using the FPS-R,[152] suggesting that when designing a pain trial with very young children, either: (1) adequately large numbers of participants may be needed to overcome possible unreliability of the measure or (2) if limited numbers of possible participants are available, an alternative measure or procedure (such as a pain behavior observation procedure) may be needed.

A final option to consider in special populations is the "Box Scale," which is basically a Numerical Rating Scale presented with the numbers surrounded by boxes.[153] Respondents are asked to indicate on this scale the single number that represents their pain intensity level. Because of the way the measure is presented, respondents are given two cues to help them identify dif-

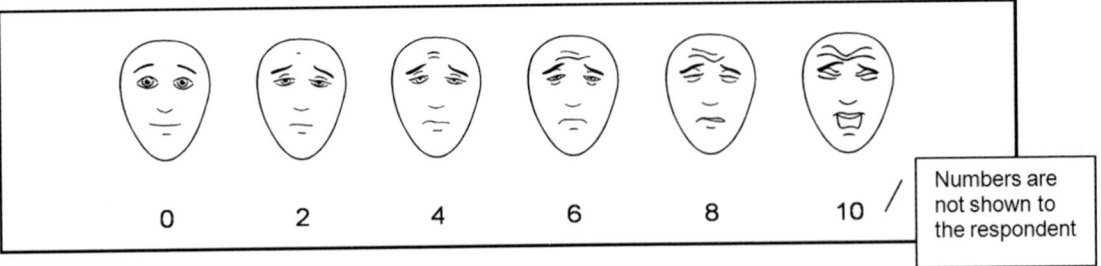

Numbers are not shown to the respondent

FIGURE 20.4 The Faces Pain Scale–Revised (FPS-R). Instructions to the respondent are: "These faces show how much something can hurt. This face [point to left-most face] shows no pain [or hurt]. The faces show more and more pain [point to each from left to right] up to this one [point to right-most face]—it shows very much pain. Point to the face that shows how much you hurt [right now]." Do not use words like "happy" or "sad." This scale is intended to measure how the respondents feel inside, not how their face looks. Numbers are not shown to the respondent; they are shown here only for reference. The instructions for administration are currently available in over 31 languages from www.painsourcebook.ca. (From Hicks CL, von Baeyer CL, Spafford PA, et al. The Faces Pain Scale – Revised. Toward a Common Metric in Pediatric Pain Measurement. *Pain* 2001;93:173–183. Used with permission from IASP®.)

ferent pain levels: both a number and a visual analogue. Although not a great deal of research has been performed using such measures, the research that has been performed suggests the possibility that box scales may be even easier for elderly individuals to comprehend and use than verbal categorical scales or faces scales.[153] More research is needed to explore this possibility, but until such research is performed, clinicians may wish to consider including box scales as an option when choosing a measure to use with a special client who has difficulties with other measures.

Selecting the Best Measure for a Patient or Population

One way to determine which measure to use in any one patient in the clinical setting is to begin by asking him or her to provide pain ratings using a number of different measures (for example, a NRS, a VRS, the FPS-R, and perhaps a box scale) for *six* domains of pain intensity: his or her own current pain, his or her own worst, least, and average pain during a specific period of time (e.g., the past 24 hours), the rating he or she would make on the scales that would represent mild pain, and the rating he or she would make on the scales that would represent severe pain. The patient's responses to the measures could then be examined to determine which scale(s) show(s) the most consistent response; that is, the scales for which his or her own least pain is rated lower than worst pain, ratings of his or her own current and average pain ratings fall within the least-worst range, and the ratings they selected as representative of "mild" and "severe" pain fall within an expected range (e.g., severe pain is rated higher than mild pain, and both are rated higher than the lowest possible response on the scale). Evidence indicates that even among individuals with severe dementia, the majority can provide a valid response to at least one type of scale, although the scale that is most useful for any one patient may differ between individuals.[147] Thus, by first trying different scales with patients who are at risk for having difficulties with standard measures, the clinician can determine for each patient that measure or scale that provides the most consistent response, and that the patient indicates is easiest for him or her to use. This is the scale that could then be used with that patient in future clinical encounters.

Selecting a measure to use in a clinical trial involving populations of patients who may have difficulty comprehending or using pain measures is more challenging, given that there is no single measure that is universally valid for every individual. In this situation, it probably makes the most sense to: (1) select the single measure that is most likely to be valid for the most study participants (for example, either a simple VRS or the FPS-R); (2) ensure that the measure is adequately explained to all study participants; (3) ensure adequate power (e.g., large sample sizes) to deal with

possible decreases in reliability of assessment due to possible difficulties with the measure in some study participants; and (4) consider using ability to comprehend and use the measure (as determined, for example, by an ability to provide a consistent response when asked to rate current, least, average, most, "mild" and "moderate" pains, see previous discussion) as an eligibility criterion for participation in the study. If the study population of interest is known to include at least some participants who will not be able to provide a valid response on a self-report pain measure, and adequate sample sizes are not available to address possible increased unreliability in assessment because of this potential problem (or there is a need to determine the effects of the treatment even among those who are unable to validly describe their pain), then the use of pain behavior observation scales or procedures may be indicated.

Behavior Observation Measures

A large number of pain behavior observation scales and measures have been developed for use as proxy measures of pain when self-report scales cannot be used, for example, in preverbal children or in nonverbal adults. The field has not yet come to a consensus regarding which one of the available measures is the most valid and reliable in most populations. The interested reader is referred to the published reviews for the most up-to-date summary of the state of the science concerning these measures.[135,137,138,154]

Briefly, all of the available measures contain a list of behaviors commonly thought to be associated with the experience of pain, such as moaning, crying, furrowing one's brow, grimacing, and rubbing a body part, among many others. The scales often score the behaviors as being present or absent, but they sometimes ask the observer to rate the behaviors along a continuum of frequency or intensity. Item responses are then summed to create total pain behavior scores or subscales for specific classes of behaviors, such as vocal, social, and activity pain behavior subscales. One review of pediatric measures[135] recommended two scales for assessing pain intensity associated with medical procedures (the Face, Legs, Activity, Cry, and Consolability, or FLACC scale[155]; and the Children's Hospital of Eastern Ontario Pain Scale, or CHEOPS[156]), one for assessing postoperative pain in the hospital (FLACC), one for assessing postoperative pain at home (Parents' Post-operative Pain Measure, or PPPM[157]), one for assessing pain in critical care (the COMFORT scale[158]), and two for assessing pain related fear or anxiety (the Procedure Behavior Check List, or PBCL[159]; and the Procedure Behavioral Rating Scale–

Revised[160]). A review of pain behavior measures in elderly individuals with dementia concluded that two scales appear most valid and useful in these populations: the Pain Assessment Checklist for Seniors with Limited Ability to Communicate (PAC-SLAC)[161]; and the DOLOPLUS 2.[162]

CONCLUSION

When considering which pain domains to assess for research or clinical purposes, investigators and clinicians must balance the need for a thorough assessment against the needs of the patient for minimal assessment burden. When determining this balance, all of the possible pain domains (intensity, affect, quality, temporal characteristics, and impact or interference) should at least be considered. Moreover, it is important to remember that many patients with pain often report more than one pain problem.

The ideal assessment, even when assessment needs to be brief, would probably involve assessing up to at least three "primary" or "most bothersome" pain problems, and include an evaluation of their intensities and locations. For assessing intensity of each pain problem or pain site, the data from a large number of studies in persons with chronic pain suggest that 0 to 10 scales of pain intensity (with 0 = no pain and 10 = pain as bad as you can imagine) have the most strengths and fewest weaknesses of the available measures.

To assess pain site, pain drawings have been used more often then site checklists in published research. However, pain site checklists are easier to score, given that pain drawings require a second step of scoring to determine the location(s) and extent of pain, and there is no evidence to suggest that patients' responses to site checklists are any less valid than their responses to pain drawings. For these reasons, a site checklist, providing that the sites listed are adequately comprehensive, may be more practical in many research situations, although clinicians may prefer pain drawings for the overall gestalt that such measures can provide concerning how the patient views pain in his or her own body.

Whether or not to assess the temporal pattern(s) of the different pain problems would be important (1) if altering the temporal pattern of pain is a goal of treatment or (2) if knowledge about the temporal pattern is needed to help diagnose the pain problem. The available data indicate that pain's continuous versus intermittent nature can predict important functional outcomes, with continuous pain associated with poorer outcomes, suggesting that some assessment of this aspect of pain may be useful. A simple categorical question (e.g., such as that included on the PQAS) appears to be adequate for assessing this characteristic of pain. More research is needed to determine the relative validity and utility of assessing other temporal characteristics of each pain problem.

Although pain does have an affective component, pain affect is not frequently measured in pain research. This may be due, in part, to the strong associations found between measures of pain intensity and pain affect; pain that is more severe usually bothers people more. There are, however, a number of situations in which it may be appropriate to assess pain affect in addition to pain intensity. For example, when evaluating the effects of treatments, such as cognitive-behavioral treatments, that might have a greater impact on the affective or suffering component of pain than on pain intensity. In these situations, because of its brevity and demonstrated validity, the pain affect scale of the short-form MPQ is probably the best choice.

Although more research is needed to identify the pain quality scales (and items) that best classify pain types (e.g., neuropathic vs. nonneuropathic), at this point, the LANSS has the most empirical support for this purpose. To assess pain qualities for describing pain or determining the effects of treatment on pain qualities, the NPS has the most empirical support. However, the NPS has limited content validity. Because the PQAS includes all of the

NPS items, it also has support for its validity as a measure of pain quality in treatment outcome studies. However, the additional items in the PQAS means that it has greater content validity then the NPS, and so may prove to be more useful for many populations of persons with pain.

Research has confirmed what many clinicians and patients with chronic pain already know: Pain can have a significant negative impact on important activities. Assessing the critical domain of pain interference should be strongly considered by both clinicians and researchers. Clinicians could use this information to help target treatments (e.g., substantial impacts on mood might suggest the need for treatments that could address mood disturbances, while substantial impact on sleep would suggest the need for treatments that could help the patient sleep better), as well as track the efficacy of different pain treatments that are provided. Researchers could, and in many cases probably should, assess pain interference as a secondary outcome in clinical trials in order to determine whether or not the treatment being examined has any benefits on the patient's life beyond its effects on pain. For assessing this domain, the seven BPI pain interference items (with the "walking" item modified in samples of patients with physical disabilities so these patients can rate the interference of pain on "mobility [ability to get around]") appear to have the most strengths of the available measures.

In populations of patients who might have limited ability to communicate or to use the measures recommended above, clinicians can select from among the simpler measures, such as simple categorical scales or the FPS-R. Among patients who demonstrate an inability to understand or use these measures, then a very simple dichotomous question ("Do you have bothersome pain?") or some of the validated pain behavior observation scales may be needed.

One final point can be made concerning the pain assessment: In any setting, it is critical to remember that we are ultimately assessing individuals—not pain. Many of the measures that we use have extensive support for their reliability and validity, and can provide numbers and ratings that can be used to help determine the efficacy of pain treatments, the need to continue or discontinue those treatments, and the possible need to provide additional treatments. But all of the numbers and ratings provided by patients and research subjects come from people, many of whom may be suffering a great deal. Measures, surveys, and questions can never replace the need to listen with compassion to the people we serve. The experience of a person reporting a pain level of "7" (out of 10) will rarely, if ever, be the same as the experience of another person reporting that same pain level. Much more important than obtaining a pain rating or score is an understanding of patients and their experience. We serve our patients best when we remember to take the time to listen.

References

1. Jensen MP. Questionnaire validation: a brief guide for readers of the research literature. *Clin J Pain* 2003;19:345–352.
2. American Educational Research Association, American Psychological Association, National Council on Measurement in Education. *Standards for Educational and Psychological Testing.* Washington, DC: American Educational Research Association;1999.
3. Turner JA, Cardenas DD. Chronic pain problems in individuals with spinal cord injuries. *Semin Clin Neuropsych* 1999;4:186–194.
4. Jensen MP, Stoelb BL, Molton IR. Measuring pain in persons with spinal cord injury. *Top Spinal Cord Inj Rehabil* 2007;13:20–34.
5. Jensen MP. Pain assessment in clinical trials. In: Wittink H, Carr D, eds. *Pain Management: Evidence, Outcomes, and Quality of Life in Pain Treatment.* Amsterdam: Elsevier. In press.
6. Melzack R, Torgerson WS. On the language of pain. *Anesthesiol* 1971;34:50–59.
7. Jensen MP. The validity and reliability of cancer pain measures. *J Pain* 2003;4:2–21.
8. Dworkin RH, Turk DC, Farrar JT, et al. Core outcome measures for chronic pain clinical trials: IMMPACT recommendations. *Pain* 2005;113:9–19.
9. Jensen, MP, Mardekian J, Lakshminarayanan M, et al. Validity of 24-hour

recall ratings of pain severity: biasing effects of "peak" and "end" pain. *Pain*. In press.

10. Redelmeier DA, Kahneman D. Patients' memories of painful medical treatments: real-time and retrospective evaluations of two minimally invasive procedures. *Pain* 1996;66:3–8.

11. Redelmeier DA, Katz J, Kahneman D. Memories of colonoscopy: a randomized trial. *Pain* 2003;104:187–194.

12. Jamison RN, Raymond SA, Levine JG, et al. Electronic diaries for monitoring chronic pain: 1-year validation study. *Pain* 2001;91:277–285.

13. Lewis B, Lewis D, Cumming G. Frequent measurement of chronic pain: an electronic diary and empirical findings. *Pain* 1995;60:341–347.

14. Palermo TM, Valenzuela D, Stork PP. A randomized trial of electronic versus paper pain diaries in children: impact on compliance, accuracy, and acceptability. *Pain* 2004;107:213–219.

15. Stone AA, Shiffman S, Schwartz JE, et al. Patient compliance with paper and electronic diaries. *Control Clin Trials* 2003;24:182–199.

16. Evans SR, Simpson DM, Kitch DW, et al. Neurologic AIDS Research Consortium; AIDS Clinical Trials Group. A randomized trial evaluating Prosaptide for HIV-associated sensory neuropathies: use of an electronic diary to record neuropathic pain. *PLoS ONE* 2007;25:551.

17. Han SH, de Klerk JM, Tan S, et al. The PLACORHEN study: a doubleblind, placebo-controlled, randomized radionuclide study with (186)Re-etidronate in hormone-resistant prostate cancer patients with painful bone metastases. Placebo Controlled Rhenium Study. *J Nucl Med* 2002;43:1150–1156.

18. Roelofs J, Peters ML, Patijn J, et al. An electronic diary assessment of the effects of distraction and attentional focusing on pain intensity in chronic low back pain patients. *Br J Health Psychol* 2006;11:595–606.

19. Turner JA, Mancl L, Aaron LA. Brief cognitive-behavioral therapy for temporomandibular disorder pain: effects on daily electronic outcome and process measures. *Pain* 2005;117:377–387.

20. Gaertner J, Elsner F, Pollmann-Dahmen K, et al. Electronic pain diary: a randomized crossover study. *J Pain Symptom Manage* 2004;28:259–267.

21. Heiberg T, Kvien TK, Dale Ø, et al. Daily health status registration (patient diary) in patients with rheumatoid arthritis: a comparison between personal digital assistant and paper-pencil format. *Arthritis Rheum* 2007;57:454–460.

22. Stinson JN, Stevens BJ, Feldman BM, et al. Construct validity of a multidimensional electronic pain diary for adolescents with arthritis. *Pain* 2007. Epub ahead of print.

23. Litcher-Kelly L, Kellerman Q, Hanauer SB, et al. Feasibility and utility of an electronic diary to assess self-report symptoms in patients with inflammatory bowel disease. *Ann Behav Med* 2007;33:207–212.

24. Peters ML, Sorbi MJ, Kruise DA, et al. Electronic diary assessment of pain, disability and psychological adaptation in patients differing in duration of pain. *Pain* 2000;84:181–192.

25. Aaron LA, Mancl L, Turner JA, et al. Reasons for missing interviews in the daily electronic assessment of pain, mood, and stress. *Pain* 2004;109:389–398.

26. Bolton JE. Accuracy of recall of usual pain intensity in back pain patients. *Pain* 1999;83:533–539.

27. Jamison RN, Sbrocco T, Parris WC. The influence of physical and psychosocial factors on accuracy of memory for pain in chronic pain patients. *Pain* 1989;37:289–294.

28. Jamison RN, Raymond SA, Slawsby EA, et al. Pain assessment in patients with low back pain: comparison of weekly recall and momentary electronic data. *J Pain* 2006;7:192–199.

29. Jensen MP, Turner LR, Turner JA, et al. The use of multiple-item scales for pain intensity measurement in chronic pain patients. *Pain* 1996;67:35–40.

30. Kikuchi H, Yoshiuchi K, Miyasaka N, et al. Reliability of recalled self-report on headache intensity: investigation using ecological momentary assessment technique. *Cephalalgia* 2006;26:1335–1343.

31. Stone AA, Broderick JE, Kaell AT, et al. Does the peak-end phenomenon observed in laboratory pain studies apply to real-world pain in rheumatoid arthritics? *J Pain* 2000;1:212–217.

32. Stone AA, Broderick JE, Shiffman SS, et al. Understanding recall of weekly pain from a momentary assessment perspective: absolute agreement, between- and within-person consistency, and judged change in weekly pain. *Pain* 2004; 107:61–69.

33. Litcher-Kelly L, Martino SA, Broderick JE, et al. A systematic review of measures used to assess chronic musculoskeletal pain in clinical and randomized controlled clinical trials. *J Pain* 2007. Epub ahead of print.

34. Jensen MP, Karoly P. Self-report scales and procedures for assessing pain in adults. In: Turk DC, Melzack R, eds. *Handbook of Pain Assessment*. 2nd ed. New York: Guilford Publications; 2001:15–34.

35. Hardy JD, Wolff HG, Goodell H. *Pain Sensations and Reactions*. Baltimore: Williams and Wilkins; 1952.

36. Jensen MP, Turner JA, Romano JM. What is the maximum number of levels needed in pain intensity measurement? *Pain* 1994;58:387–392.

37. Price DD, Barrell JJ, Gracely RH. A psychophysical analysis of experimental factors that selectively influence the affective dimension of pain. *Pain* 1980; 8:137–149.

38. Price DD, Harkins SW, Baker C. Sensory-affective relationships among different types of clinical and experimental pain. *Pain* 1987;28:297–307.

39. Gaston-Johansson F, Franco T, Zimmerman L. Pain and psychological distress in patients undergoing autologous bone marrow transplantation. *Oncol Nurs Forum* 1992;19:41–48.

40. Jensen MP, Karoly P, O'Riordan EF, et al. The subjective experience of acute pain: an assessment of the utility of 10 indices. *Clin J Pain* 1989;5:153–159.

41. Melzack R. The McGill Pain Questionnaire: major properties and scoring methods. *Pain* 1975;1:277–299.

42. Melzack R. The short-form McGill Pain Questionnaire. *Pain* 1987;30:191–197.

43. Dudgeon D, Raubertas RF, Rosenthal SN. The short-form McGill Pain Questionnaire in chronic cancer pain. *J Pain Symptom Manage* 1993;8:191–195.

44. Putzke JD, Richards JS, Hicken BL, et al. Pain classification following spinal cord injury: the utility of verbal descriptors. *Spinal Cord* 2002;40:118–127.

45. Georgoudis G, Oldham JA, Watson PJ. Reliability and sensitivity measures of the Greek version of the short form of the McGill Pain Questionnaire. *Eur J Pain* 2001;5:109–118.

46. Rowbotham M, Harden N, Stacey B, et al. Gabapentin for the treatment of postherpetic neuralgia: a randomized controlled trial. *JAMA* 1998;280:1837–1842.

47. Viola V, Newnham HH, Simpson RW. Treatment of intractable painful diabetic neuropathy with intravenous lignocaine. *J Diabetes Complications* 2006;20:34–39.

48. Ahles TA, Blanchard EB, Ruckdeschel JC. The multidimensional nature of cancer-related pain. *Pain* 1983;17:277–288.

49. Kremer EF, Atkinson JH Jr, Ignelzi RJ. Pain measurement: the affective dimensional measure of the McGill Pain Questionnaire with a cancer pain population. *Pain* 1982;12:153–163.

50. Chang PF, Arendt-Nielsen L, Graven-Nielsen T, et al. Comparative EEG activation to skin pain and muscle pain induced by capsaicin injection. *Int J Psychophysiol* 2004;51:117–126.

51. Ahlquist ML, Franzén OG. Encoding of the subjective intensity of sharp dental pain. *Endod Dental Traumatol* 1994;10:153–166.

52. Beise RD, Carstens E, Kohllöffel LU. Psychophysical study of stinging pain evoked by brief freezing of superficial skin and ensuing short-lasting changes in sensations of cool and cold pain. *Pain* 1998;74:275–286.

53. Ngassapa DN. Comparison of functional characteristics of intradental A- and C-nerve fibres in dental pain. *East Afr Med J* 1996;73:207–209.

54. Bennett M. The LANSS Pain Scale: the Leeds assessment of neuropathic symptoms and signs. *Pain* 2001;92:147–157.

55. Bennett MI, Smith BH, Torrance N,et al. The S-LANSS score for identifying pain of predominantly neuropathic origin: validation for use in clinical and postal research. *J Pain* 2005;6:149–158.

56. Krause SJ, Backonja M. Development of a neuropathic pain questionnaire. *Clin J Pain* 2003;19:306–314.

57. Backonja MM, Krause SJ. Neuropathic pain questionnaire—short form. *Clin J Pain* 2003;19:315–316.

58. Bouhassira D, Attal N, Alchaar H, et al. Comparison of pain syndromes associated with nervous or somatic lesions and development of a new neuropathic pain diagnostic questionnaire (DN4). *Pain* 2005;114:29–36.

59. Potter J, Higginson IJ, Scadding JW, et al. Identifying neuropathic pain in patients with head and neck cancer: use of the Leeds Assessment of Neuropathic Symptoms and Signs Scale. *J R Soc Med* 2003;96:379–383.

60. Yucel A, Senocak M, Kocasoy Orhan E, et al. Results of the Leeds Assessment of Neuropathic Symptoms and Signs Pain Scale in Turkey: a validation study. *J Pain* 2004;5:427–432.

61. Martínez-Lavin M, López S, Medina M, et al. Use of the Leeds assessment of neuropathic symptoms and signs questionnaire in patients with fibromyalgia. *Semin Arthritis Rheum* 2003;32:407–411.

62. Khedr EM, Kotb H, Kamel NF, et al. Long-lasting antalgic effects of daily sessions of repetitive transcranial magnetic stimulation in central and peripheral neuropathic pain. *J Neurol Neurosurg Psychiatry* 2005;76:833–838.

63. Backonja MM. Need for differential assessment tools of neuropathic pain and deficits of the LANSS pain scale. *Pain* 2002;97:229–230.

64. Bouhassira D, Attal N, Fermanian J, et al. Development and validation of the Neuropathic Pain Symptom Inventory. *Pain* 2004;108:248–257.

65. Galer BS, Jensen MP. Development and preliminary validation of a pain measure specific to neuropathic pain: the Neuropathic Pain Scale. *Neurology* 1997;48:332–338.

66. Jensen MP, Friedman M, Bonzo D, et al. The validity of the Neuropathic Pain Scale for assessing diabetic neuropathic pain in a clinical trial. *Clin J Pain* 2006;22:97–103.

67. Melzack R, Katz J. The McGill Pain Questionnaire: appraisal and current status. In: Turk DC, Melzack R, eds. *Handbook of Pain Assesment*. 2nd ed. New York: Guilford Press; 2001:35–52.

68. Lowe NK, Walker SN, MacCallum RC. Confirming the theoretical structure of the McGill Pain Questionnaire in acute clinical pain. *Pain* 1991;46:53–60.

69. Turk DC, Rudy TE, Salovey P. The McGill Pain Questionnaire reconsidered: confirming the factor structure and examining appropriate uses. *Pain* 1985; 21:385–397.

70. Burchiel KJ, Anderson VC, Brown FD, et al. Prospective, multicenter study of spinal cord stimulation for relief of chronic back and extremity pain. *Spine* 1996;21:2786–2794.

71. Kalso E, Tasmuth T, Neuvonen PJ. Amitriptyline effectively relieves neuropathic pain following treatment of breast cancer. *Pain* 1996;4:293–302.

72. Lynch ME, Clark, AJ, Sawynok J. Intravenous adenosine alleviates neuropathic pain: a double blind placebo controlled crossover trial using an enriched enrollment design. *Pain* 2003;103:111–117.

73. Nikolajsen L, Hansen CL, Nielsen J, et al. The effect of ketamine on phantom

pain: a central neuropathic disorder maintained by peripheral input. *Pain* 1996;67:69–77.

74. Shupak NM, McKay JC, Nielson WR, et al. Exposure to a specific pulsed low-frequency magnetic field: a double-blind placebo-controlled study of effects on pain ratings in rheumatoid arthritis and fibromyalgia patients. *Pain Res Manag* 2006;11:85–90.

75. Tannock I, Gospodarowicz M, Meakin W, et al. Treatment of metastatic prostatic cancer with low-dose prednisone: evaluation of pain and quality of life as pragmatic indices of response. *J Clin Oncol* 1989;7:590–597.

76. Tesfaye S, Watt J, Benbow SJ, et al. Electrical spinal-cord stimulation for painful diabetic peripheral neuropathy. *Lancet* 1996;348:1698–1701.

77. Graham C, Bond S, Gerkovich M. Use of the McGill Pain Questionnaire in the assessment of cancer pain: reliability and consistency. *Pain* 1980;8:377–387.

78. Love A, Leboeuf C, Crisp TC. Chiropractic chronic low back pain sufferers and self-report assessment methods. Part I. A reliability study of the Visual Analogue Scale, the Pain Drawing and the McGill Pain Questionnaire. *J Manipulative Physiol Ther* 1989;12:21–25.

79. Walsh TD, Leber B. Measurement of chronic pain: Visual Analogue Scale and McGill Pain Questionnaire compared. *Adv Pain Res Ther* 1983;5:897–899.

80. Jenkinson C, Carroll D, Egerton M, et al. Comparison of the sensitivity to change of long and short from pain measures. *Qual Life Res* 1995;4:353–357.

81. Bellamy N, Campbell J, Syrotuik J. Comparative study of self-rating pain scale in osteoarthritis patients. *Curr Med Res Opin* 1999;15:113–119.

82. Graff-Radford SB, Shaw LR, Naliboff BN. Amitriptyline and fluphenazine in the treatment of postherpetic neuralgia. *Clin J Pain* 2000;16:188–192.

83. Chandra K, Shafiq N, Pandhi P, et al. Gabapentin versus nortriptyline in post-herpetic neuralgia patients: a randomized, double-blind clinical trial—the GONIP Trial. *Int J Clin Pharmacol Ther* 2006;4:358–363.

84. Rosenstock J, Tuchman M, LaMoreaux L, et al. Pregabalin for the treatment of painful diabetic peripheral neuropathy: a double-blind, placebo-controlled trial. *Pain* 2004;110:628–638.

85. Siddall PJ, Cousins MJ, Otte A, et al. Pregabalin in central neuropathic pain associated with spinal cord injury: a placebo-controlled trial. *Neurology* 2006;67:1792–1800.

86. Carter GT, Jensen MP, Galer BS, et al. Neuropathic pain in Charcot-Marie-Tooth disease. *Arch Phys Med Rehabil* 1998;79:1560–1564.

87. Galer BS, Gianas A, Jensen MP. Painful diabetic polyneuropathy: epidemiology, pain description, and quality of life. *Diab Res Clin Prac* 2000;47:123–128.

88. Galer BS, Henderson J, Perander J, et al. Course of symptoms and quality of life measurement in complex regional pain syndrome: a pilot survey. *J Pain Symptom Manage* 2000;20:286–292.

89. Fishbain DA, Lewis J, Cole B, et al. Multidisciplinary pain facility treatment outcome for pain-associated fatigue. *Pain Med* 2005;6:299–304.

90. Fishbain DA, Lewis JE, Cole B, et al. Lidocaine 5% patch: an open-label naturalistic chronic pain treatment trial and prediction of response. *Pain Med* 2006;7:135–142.

91. Galer BS, Jensen MP, Ma T, et al. The lidocaine patch 5% effectively treats all neuropathic pain qualities: results of a randomized, double-blind, vehicle-controlled, 3-week efficacy study with use of the neuropathic pain scale. *Clin J Pain* 2002;18:297–301.

92. Gammaitoni AR, Galer BS, Lacouture P, et al. Effectiveness and safety of new oxycodone/acetaminophen formulations with reduced acetaminophen for the treatment of low back pain. *Pain Med* 2003;4:21–30.

93. Jensen MP, Dworkin RH, Gammaitoni AR, et al. Assessment of pain quality in chronic neuropathic and nociceptive pain clinical trials with the Neuropathic Pain Scale. *J Pain* 2005;6:98–106.

94. Levendoglu F, Ogün CO, Ozerbil O, et al. Gabapentin is a first line drug for the treatment of neuropathic pain in spinal cord injury. *Spine* 2004;28:743–751.

95. Moseley GL. Graded motor imagery is effective for long-standing complex regional pain syndrome: a randomised controlled trial. *Pain* 2004;108:192–198.

96. Semenchuk MR, Sherman S. Effectiveness of tizanidine in neuropathic pain: an open-label study. *J Pain.* 2000;1:285–292.

97. Tai Q, Kirshblum S, Chen B, et al. Gabapentin in the treatment of neuropathic pain after spinal cord injury: a prospective, randomized, double-blind, crossover trial. *J Spinal Cord Med.* 2002;25:100–105.

98. Jensen MP, Gammaitoni AR, Olaleye DO, et al. The Pain Quality Assessment Scale: assessment of pain quality in carpal tunnel syndrome. *J Pain* 2006;7:823–832.

99. Bennett MI, Smith BH, Torrance N, et al. Can pain can be more or less neuropathic? comparison of symptom assessment tools with ratings of certainty by clinicians. *Pain* 2006;122:289–294.

100. Cleeland CS, Ryan KM. Pain assessment: global use of the Brief Pain Inventory. *Ann Acad Med Singapore* 1994;23:129–138.

101. Margolis RB, Tait RC, Krause SJ. A rating system for use with patient pain drawings. *Pain* 1986;24:57–65.

102. Jensen MP, Hoffman AJ, Cardenas DD. Chronic pain in individuals with spinal cord injury: a survey and longitudinal study. *Spinal Cord* 2005;43:704–712.

103. Widerström-Noga EG, Duncan R, Turk DC. Psychosocial profiles of people with pain associated with spinal cord injury: identification and comparison with other chronic pain syndromes. *Clin J Pain* 2004;20:261–271.

104. Serlin RC, Mendoza TR, Nakamura Y, et al. When is cancer pain mild, moder-

ate or severe? grading pain severity by its interference with function. *Pain* 1995;61:277–284.

105. Jamison RN, Brown GK. Validation of hourly intensity profiles with chronic pain patients. *Pain* 1991;45:123–128.

106. van Grootel RJ, van der Glas HW, Buchner R, et al. Patterns of pain variation related to myogenous temporomandibular disorders. *Clin J Pain* 2005;21:154–165.

107. Kerns RD, Turk DC, Rudy TE. The West Haven-Yale Multidimensional Pain Inventory (WHYMPI). *Pain* 1985;23:345–356.

108. Cleeland CS, Ladinsky JL, Serlin RC, et al. Multidimensional measurement of cancer pain: comparisons of US and Vietnamese patients. *J Pain Sympt Manag* 1998;3:23–27.

109. Caraceni A, Mendoza TR, Mencaglia E, et al. A validation study of an Italian version of the Brief Pain Inventory (Breve Questionario per la Valutazione del Dolore). *Pain* 1996;65:87–92.

110. Wang XS, Mendoza TR, Gao SZ, et al. The Chinese version of the Brief Pain Inventory (BPI-C): its development and use in a study of cancer pain. *Pain* 1996;67:407–416.

111. Uki J, Mendoza T, Cleeland CS, et al. A brief cancer pain assessment tool in Japanese: The utility of the Japanese Brief Pain Inventory—BPI-J. *J Pain Symptom Manage* 1998;16:364–373.

112. Ger LP, Ho ST, Sun WZ, et al. Validation of the Brief Pain Inventory in a Taiwanese population. *J Pain Symptom Manage* 1999;18:316–322.

113. Radbruch L, Loick G, Kiencke P, et al. Validation of the German Version of the Brief Pain Inventory. *J Pain Symptom Manage* 1999;18:180–187.

114. Saxena A, Mendoza T, Cleeland CS. The Assessment of Cancer Pain in North India: the validation of the Hindi Brief Pain Inventory—BPI-H. *J Pain Symptom Manage* 1999;17:27–41.

115. Mystakidou K, Mendoza T, Tsilika E, et al. Greek brief pain inventory: validation and utility in cancer pain. *Oncol* 2001;60:35–42.

116. Zelman DC, Gore M, Dukes E, et al. Validation of a modified version of the brief pain inventory for painful diabetic peripheral neuropathy. *J Pain Symptom Manage* 2005;29:401–410.

117. Cleeland CS, Nakamura Y, Mendoza TR, et al. Dimensions of the impact of cancer pain in a four-country sample: new information from multidimensional scaling. *Pain* 1996;67:267–273.

118. Daut RL, Cleeland CS. The prevalence and severity of pain in cancer. *Cancer* 1982;50:1913–1918.

119. McMillan SC, Williams FA, Chatfield R, et al. A validity and reliability study of two tools for assessing and managing cancer pain. *Oncol Nurs Forum* 1988;5:735–741.

120. Armstrong DG, Chappell AS, Le TK, et al. Duloxetine for the management of diabetic peripheral neuropathic pain: evaluation of functional outcomes. *Pain Med* 2007;8:410–418.

121. Arnold LM, Goldenberg DL, Stanford SB, et al. Gabapentin in the treatment of fibromyalgia: a randomized, double-blind, placebo-controlled, multicenter trial. *Arthritis Rheum* 2007;56:1336–1344.

122. Wardley A, Davidson N, Barrett-Lee P, et al. Zoledronic acid significantly improves pain scores and quality of life in breast cancer patients with bone metastases: a randomised, crossover study of community vs hospital bisphosphonate administration. *Brit J Cancer* 2005;92:1869–1876.

123. White WT, Patel N, Drass M, Nalamachu S. Lidocaine patch 5% with systemic analgesics such as gabapentin: a rational polypharmacy approach for the treatment of chronic pain. *Pain Med* 2003;4:321–330.

124. Osborne TL, Raichle KA, Jensen MP, et al. The reliability and validity of pain interference measures in persons with multiple sclerosis. *J Pain Symptom Manage* 2006;32:217–229.

125. Tyler EJ, Jensen MP, Engel JM, et al. The reliability and validity of pain interference measures in persons with cerebral palsy. *Arch Phys Med Rehabil* 2002;83:236–239.

126. Raichle KA, Osborne TL, Jensen MP, et al. The reliability and validity of pain interference measures in persons with spinal cord injury. *J Pain* 2006;7:179–186.

127. World Health Organization. *International classification of functioning, disability and health.* Geneva, Switzerland: World Health Organization; 2001.

128. Bernstein IH, Jaremko ME, Hinkley BS. On the utility of the West Haven-Yale Multidimensional Inventory. *Spine* 1995;20:956–963.

129. Strong J, Westbury K, Smith G, et al. Treatment outcome in individuals with chronic pain: is the Pain Stages of Change Questionnaire (PSOCQ) a useful tool? *Pain* 2002;97:65–73.

130. Kjellby-Wendt G, Styf J, Carlsson SG. Early active rehabilitation after surgery for lumbar disc herniation: a prospective, randomized study of psychometric assessment in 50 patients. *Acta Orthop Scand* 2001;72:518–524.

131. Thieme K, Gromnica-Ihle E, Flor H. Operant behavioral treatment of fibromyalgia: a controlled study. *Arthritis Rheum* 2003;49:314–320.

132. Turner-Stokes L, Erkeller-Yuksel F, Miles A, et al. Outpatient cognitive behavioral pain management programs: a randomized comparison of a group-based multidisciplinary versus an individual therapy model. *Arch Phys Med Rehabil* 2003;84:781–788.

133. Worrel LM, Krahn LE, Sletten CD, et al. Treating fibromyalgia with a brief interdisciplinary program: initial outcomes and predictors of response. *Mayo Clin Proc* 2001;76:384–390.

134. McGrath PA, Gillespi J. Pain assessment in children and adolescents. In: Turk DC, Melzack R, eds. *Handbook of Pain Assessment.* 2nd ed. New York: The Guilford Press; 2001:97–118.

135. von Baeyer CL, Spagrud LJ. Systematic review of observational (behavioral)

measures of pain for children and adolescents aged 3 to 18 years. *Pain* 2007; 127:140–150.

136. Gagliese L. Assessment of pain in elderly people. In: Turk DC, Melzack R, eds., *Handbook of Pain Assessment.* 2nd ed. New York: The Guilford Press; 2001:119–133.

137. Hadjistavropoulos T, Herr K, Turk DC, et al. An interdisciplinary expert consensus statement on assessment of pain in older persons. *Clin J Pain* 2007; 23:S1–S43.

138. Zwakhalen SM, Hamers JP, Abu-Saad HH, et al. Pain in elderly people with severe dementia: a systematic review of behavioural pain assessment tools. *BMC Geriatr* 2006;6:3.

139. Hadjistavropoulos T, von Baeyer C, Craig KD. Pain assessment in persons with limited ability to communicate. In: Turk DC, Melzack R, eds. *Handbook of Pain Assessment.* 2nd ed. New York: The Guilford Press;2001:134–149.

140. Anderson KO, Syrjala KL, Cleeland CS. How to assess cancer pain. In: Turk DC, Melzack R, eds. *Handbook of Pain Assessment.* 2nd ed. New York: The Guilford Press; 2001:579–600.

141. Labus JS, Keefe FJ, Jensen MP. Pain intensity and pain behavior: when are they correlated? *Pain* 2003;102:109–124.

142. Ferrell BA, Ferrell BR, Rivera L. Pain in cognitively impaired nursing home patients. *J Pain Symptom Manage* 1995;10:591–598.

143. Jensen MP, Karoly P, Braver S. The measurement of clinical pain intensity: a comparison of six methods. *Pain* 1986;27:117–126.

144. Herr KA, Spratt K, Mobily PR, et al. Pain intensity assessment in older adults: use of experimental pain to compare psychometric properties and usability of selected pain scales with younger adults. *Clin J Pain* 2004;20:207–219.

145. Littman GS, Walker BR, Schneider BE. Reassessment of verbal and visual analog ratings in analgesic studies. *Clin Pharmacol Ther* 1985;38:16–23.

146. Bieri D, Reeve RA, Champion GD, et al. The Faces Pain Scale for the self-assessment of the severity of pain experienced by children: development, initial validation and preliminary investigation for ratio scale properties. *Pain* 1990; 41:139–150.

147. Pautex S, Michon A, Guedira M, et al. Pain in severe dementia: self-assessment or observational scales? *J Am Geriatr Soc* 2006;54:1040–1045.

148. Ware LJ, Epps CD, Herr K, et al. Evaluation of the Revised Faces Pain Scale, Verbal Descriptor Scale, Numeric Rating Scale, and Iowa Pain Thermometer in older minority adults. *Pain Manag Nurs* 2006;7:117–125.

149. Spafford PA, von Baeyer CL, Hicks CL. Expected and reported pain in chil-

dren undergoing ear piercing: a randomized trial of preparation by parents. *Behav Res Ther* 2002;4:253–266.

150. Wood C, von Baeyer CL, Bourrillon A, et al. Self-assessment of immediate post-vaccination pain after two different MMR vaccines administered as a second dose in 4- to 6-year-old children. *Vaccine* 2004;23:127–131.

151. Migdal M, Chudzynska-Pomianowska E, Vause E, et al. Rapid, needle-free delivery of lidocaine for reducing the pain of venipuncture among pediatric subjects. *Pediatrics* 2005;115:393–398.

152. Stanford EA, Chambers CT, Craig KD. The role of developmental factors in predicting young children's use of a self-report scale for pain. *Pain* 2006;120: 16–23.

153. Chibnall JT, Tait RC. Pain assessment in cognitively impaired and unimpaired older adults: a comparison of four scales. *Pain* 2001;92:173–186.

154. van Herk R, van Dijk M, Baar FP, et al. Observation scales for pain assessment in older adults with cognitive impairments or communication difficulties. *Nurs Res* 2007;56:34–43.

155. Merkel SI, Voepel-Lewis T, Shayevitz JR, et al. The FLACC: a behavioral scale for scoring postoperative pain in young children. *Pediatr Nurs* 1997; 23:293–297.

156. McGrath PJ, Johnson G, Goodman JT, et al. CHEOPS: a behavioral scale for rating postoperative pain in children. In: Fields HL, Dubner R, Cervero F, eds. *Advances in Pain Research and Therapy.* Vol 9. New York, Raven Press;1985:395–402.

157. Chambers CT, Reid GJ, McGrath PJ, et al. Development and preliminary validation of a postoperative pain measure for parents. *Pain* 1996;68: 307–313.

158. Ambuel B, Hamlett KW, Marx CM, Blumer JL. Assessing distress in pediatric intensive care environments: the COMFORT scale. *J Pediatr Psychol* 1992; 17:95–109.

159. LeBaron S, Zeltzer L. Assessment of acute pain and anxiety in children and adolescents by self-reports, observer reports, and a behavior checklist. *J Consult Clin Psychol* 1984;52:729–738.

160. Katz ER, Kellerman J, Siegel SE. Behavioral distress in children with cancer undergoing medical procedures: developmental considerations. *J Consult Clin Psychol* 1980;48:356–365.

161. Fuchs-Lacelle S, Hadjistavropoulos T. Development and preliminary validation of the pain assessment checklist for seniors with limited ability to communicate (PACSLAC). *Pain Manag Nurs* 2004;5:37–49.

162. Lefebre-Chapiro L, Doloplus group. The Doloplus-2 scale-evaluating pain in the elderly. *Euro J Palliative Care* 2001;8:191–194.

CHAPTER 21 ■ PSYCHOLOGICAL AND PSYCHOSOCIAL EVALUATION

TATIANA D. STARR, LAUREN J. ROGAK, KENNETH L. KIRSH, AND STEVEN D. PASSIK

INTRODUCTION

Over the past 30 years it has become increasingly evident that psychological factors have a significant impact on the overall experience of chronic pain.[1–3] Chronic pain is more than ongoing and recurrent physical pain; it involves a persons' psychological and social well-being. Research examining behavioral and psychosocial evaluation in the context of persistent pain has led to new developments in psychological assessments, including the advancement and incorporation of well-validated measures to round out the multidisciplinary process of pain management.[4] Clinicians and researchers have also developed approaches that have the potential to significantly enhance patient adjustment to pain as well as aid in prevention and management of psychological and behavioral issues that arise as a result of chronic pain.[5–9] This chapter reviews the various psychosocial concepts which may be related to pain and should be targeted for effective assessment. We seek to touch on the prevalence, association, assessment, evaluation, and treatment of each relationship.

PSYCHOPATHOLOGY

It is well established that patients with chronic pain frequently present with a number of comorbid psychiatric conditions including depression, anxiety, and personality disorders.[10] Research has also demonstrated a significantly higher incidence of these disorders among chronic pain patients in comparison to other medically ill populations as well as the general population.[11] Additionally, an estimated 50% of individuals with chronic pain have comorbid depression and/or anxiety,[10] and although these disorders are viewed conceptually as two distinct conditions, the high prevalence of comorbidity and overlapping symptoms have the potential to complicate assessment.[12–14] The majority of self-report measures of depression and anxiety are highly correlated with each other and the lack of discriminant validity among these measures creates additional barriers toward assessment.[12–16] Complications associated with measurement of mood disorders have additional consequences when assessing these conditions in the chronic pain population. An assessment method that distinguishes between symptoms common to these mood disorders is essential in accurately guiding specifically tailored interventions as misunderstanding these interactions can lead to unsuitable treatment approaches.

Depression

There has been a growing interest in the relationship between depression and chronic pain due to the high prevalence rates encountered coupled with general lack of standard assessment and treatment methods.[17] The research on this association is vast but remains inconclusive. One small certainty is that there is an extraordinary amount of suffering experienced by chronic pain patients who struggle with depression. Whether depression was pre-morbid or manifested as a result of the pain condition, the burdens of coexisting pain and depression should not be ignored. Although there is more work to be done, there has been enormous progress in understanding, assessing, evaluating, and treating these patients.[17,18]

The diagnostic definition of depression was developed from a psychiatric framework and has not been adapted appropriately to apply to the chronic pain population, adding to diagnostic difficulties.[19] The broad range of depression assessment tools (i.e., self-report, structured and unstructured interviews, projective tests), makes it difficult to compare studies of patients with chronic pain and those with depression.[17] Although many theories of pain have been established, the biopsychosocial model may be the most useful as it addresses the integration of biological mechanisms, psychological and social factors, and addresses each as an individual facet while determining a multifaceted approach to evaluate and treat a patient comprehensively.[20]

Epidemiological studies[18] show that major depressive disorder (MDD) is shown in 5% to 10% of primary care settings. This represents an underestimation of the prevalence seen in pain populations, as many individuals have depressive symptoms that do not meet the full criteria to be diagnosed as MDD as outlined by the *Diagnostic and Statistical Manual of Mental Disorders* (DSM-IV).[21] The implication is that these conditions are coexisting more commonly and have the potential to exacerbate one another. This also raises the issue that they may be treated together to maximize a healthy lifestyle.[22]

The overlap of pain and depression is seen in 30% to 60% of patients.[22] When the etiology for the pain is unknown, depression rates have been shown to be higher.[23] Additionally, those patients with chronic pain, defined as the presence of pain for most days within a month, are three times more likely to meet the diagnostic criteria outlined for depression as those without a diagnosis of chronic pain.[24] Research has also shown that the more severe, frequent, and enduring the painful condition, the more severe any corresponding depression will be.[25] Further, the extent of depressive symptoms has been correlated with level of acceptance of chronic pain as facilitated by a basic idea of the perception of what the future held, with poor acceptance leading to greater depth of depression.[26]

A close look at the association between prevalence rates of pain and depression raises the question as to why chronic pain patients are not all depressed.[27] The prevalence rates of pain and depression are high but not universal. Research comparing depressed, nondepressed, and mildly depressed pain patients proposes that difficulty in coping and negative perceptions of self-control are correlated with the advent of depression in pain patients.[28] Some research proposes two facets that may mediate the effects of pain and depression: a patient's perspective of the role of pain in their life and their ability to maintain control over the pain.[29,30] Thus, the more perceived control a person believes they have in life, and the smaller role they allow the pain to play, the less likely they will become depressed.[29,30]

Assessment and Evaluation

The body of literature on the diagnostic and treatment implications of comorbid depression and pain is growing rapidly. However, one issue always seems to emerge: due to the nature of each individual illness, pain can result from depression or depression can result from pain. This adds to diagnostic difficulties and complicates decisions regarding which illness might be considered primary and whether both issues need to be treated through medication trials. It is important to delineate the true diagnosis (or both if a comorbid diagnosis is appropriate) so that medications can be streamlined and given appropriately. For instance, the pain patient with increased agitation presenting with pseudodepressed mood might see remarkable mood improvement simply from treating the pain condition aggressively. If the patient responds to the pain medication alone, we have spared them another medication (or set of medications) for depression and anxiety which would have potentially added side effects for no appreciable gain in mood or function. In either case, we do need to be aware of the interrelationships between pain and mood and ultimately focus on helping the patient integrate into a healthy way of living.[22,31]

In many cases, chronic pain patients are only followed by a primary care physician due to the fact that there are simply not enough chronic pain specialists and they are often concentrated in metropolitan areas. The high rate of comorbidity between chronic pain and mental disorders, including depression, is not standard knowledge for primary care physicians. Therefore, it is not a guarantee that a physician will recognize the symptoms of such disorders. Primary care physicians are then left to assess, evaluate, and proceed to the best of their ability when faced with a patient with this comorbidity.[31] Recognition of depression in the chronic pain patient has caused difficulty in the primary care setting.

Few diagnostic tools and structured interviews for diagnosing depression take into account the presence of chronic pain. Therefore, patients in pain may not show the "common" depressive symptoms.[19,22] They may present with those that aren't the direct markers of an MDD. Consequently, it has been seen that patients with comorbid pain and depression do not commonly present symptoms of dysphoria, anhedonia, hopelessness, melancholy,[22] guilt, or self-vilification[19] but show more somatic symptoms, feelings of sadness,[22] negative cognitive biases, and a self-focused and health-oriented perspective.[19]

Initial psychosocial screenings in patients with depression should include the emotional impact pain has on daily activities, past and present pain treatments (successes and failures), and their goals and expectations for relief of pain. The answers to these questions, as well as clinical judgment, will lead to a need for a comprehensive interview. This interview should go into more depth than the initial questions and may include details regarding how daily activities are affected (e.g., impact on interpersonal relationships, coping with physical and emotional symptoms, substance abuse, and historical and current psychological symptoms and diagnosis, if relevant).[27]

Pain-Related Anxiety, Catastrophization, and Anxiety Sensitivity

Pain-related anxiety is a complex psychological construct surrounding a variety of cognitive, behavioral, and physiological responses to the pain experience.[32,33] Anxiety is an important factor in predicting patient outcomes, particularly regarding how well the patient will adapt to their pain.[34-37] Research has demonstrated that anxiety precipitates muscular contraction, vasoconstriction, and pain-inciting chemicals that increase pain severity.[3] Pain-related anxiety has also been associated with catastrophizing,[38] placing greater focus on bodily sensations[39] and avoidance of physical activities.[35]

Catastrophizing around pain refers to an appraisal process or an attempt to cognitively cope with pain.[47] A consistent finding in the past two decades is that catastrophizing during, and in anticipation of, pain may result in greater psychological distress and a more intense pain experience.[40–48] While positive coping attempts involve adaptive thoughts and behaviors to manage pain, catastrophizing involves negative or intrusive thoughts that exaggerate the severity of the pain and generates feelings of helplessness regarding how to control it.[45,47,49] Catastrophizing includes three components: magnification, rumination, and helplessness that lead to increased pain-related behaviors.[43] Such behaviors include higher rates of health care usage,[2] increased use of pain medications,[44] and prolonged hospitalization.[50] Patients who catastrophize report more intense pain, psychological distress, and disability compared to other patients.[43,44,47] The concept of pain catastrophizing has gained recognition as one of the most important predictors of pain, and it is estimated to account for approximately 7% to 31% of the variance among pain ratings.[51] It has also been found that catastrophizing is a stronger predictor of poor pain outcomes than depression.[20,48,52]

The term *anxiety sensitivity* refers to fear associated with symptoms related to anxiety that are based on the belief that these sensations have negative social, psychological, or somatic consequences.[53] This perspective represents a stable psychological construct that magnifies anxiety and fear in response to stimuli that is potentially anxiety-evoking.[54] Individuals with high anxiety sensitivity may be more susceptible to panic attacks. In the absence of effective emotional regulatory techniques, patients who perceive physiological sensations, such as an autonomic arousal, as a sign of danger or harm may experience heightened levels of anxiety.[55] Research assessing the relationship between chronic pain and anxiety sensitivity has shown evidence that individuals with chronic pain tend to experience higher levels of anxiety related to somatic symptoms.[56] In addition, those patients with heightened anxiety sensitivity have been found to report increased levels of persistent pain more frequently.[57] Heightened levels of anxiety sensitivity may also intensify pain sensations in patients when exposed to anxiety-producing stimuli.[58] Anxiety sensitivity has also been recently linked to the development of higher levels of pain-related fear, specifically fear of consequences associated with the experience of pain sensations. Elevated levels of anxiety sensitivity may then lead to avoidance of activities that may induce or increase pain.[59] Such avoidance over a long period of time may take a physical and emotional toll on the patient, leading to decreased socializing, diminished physical activity, and secondary behavioral problems (e.g., deconditioning and weight gain).[60] This response pattern tends to be cyclical, with emotional responsiveness and diminished physical capacity eliciting avoidance and reconfirming the patient's apprehension concerning their pain experience.[61]

lizing the PASS have indicated that patients with chronic pain exhibit higher levels of pain-related anxiety, tend toward overpredicting their pain intensity, cope poorly with painful sensations, and demonstrate greater somatic reactivity in expectation of pain-eliciting physical activities.[38] The primary function of the PASS is to facilitate the study of anxiety and fear associated with pain and to improve treatment outcomes. It may also have particular clinical utility in identifying empirical subtypes of chronic pain patients who may have different responses to treatment regimens. For example, patients found to manifest fear of pain primarily in the physiological response system may benefit more from an intervention such as relaxation training rather than cognitive restructuring.[35] The PASS[35] is also used to assess catastrophizing in chronic pain patients.[62] Although the PASS is generally not considered a catastrophizing measure, two of the subscales included are closely related. These scales (fear and cognitive anxiety) are also highly correlated with the six-item catastrophizing scale on the Coping Strategies Questionnaire.[62]

The Pain Catastrophizing Scale (PCS)[43] is used more frequently to assess pain catastrophizing. It was developed based on definitions of catastrophizing and measure it based on three dimensions including rumination, helplessness, and magnification.[62] The PCS can be useful in gaining a greater understanding of the psychological processes that lead to heightened physical and emotional distress in response to painful experiences. From a clinical perspective, the PCS could aid in identifying individuals who have greater susceptibility to aversive medical procedures such as surgery or chemotherapy.[63]

Anxiety sensitivity is frequently measured using the Anxiety Sensitivity Index (ASI).[64] Research has demonstrated that the ASI has utility in longitudinally predicting panic attacks[65] and heightened anxious responding.[66] The ASI is comprised of a hierarchical structure measuring three major factors including: (1) physical concerns (fears associated with adverse physical outcomes); (2) psychological concerns (fears associated with losing control cognitively); and (3) social concerns (fears associated with public display of anxious symptoms).[67–69]

It is common for chronic pain patients to experience anxiety about the meaning of their pain and how it will impact their daily lives now and in the future. The threat of severe pain can have such a profound effect that individuals may have difficulty disengaging from it, and such fears can lead to avoidance and inactivity, and ultimately greater disability.[70] The pain experience may instigate a set of increasingly negative thoughts and fears, and these processes, which are not driven solely by the actual sensory experience of pain, can have a tremendous influence on the patient's functioning and pain tolerance.[71–73] In fact, factors related to anxiety, including fear and avoidance, have been found to be stronger predictors of persistent pain than biomedical factors.[74] Clearly, pain-related anxiety, pain catastrophizing, and anxiety sensitivity all play important roles in amplifying the pain experience and such issues must be assessed and addressed in treatment.

Assessment and Evaluation

The emotional and cognitive responses to and in anticipation of pain are important factors in determining the extent of patients' distress and suffering. As such, self-report measures have been developed to gain a subjective assessment of the specific dimensions associated with pain-related anxiety, catastrophization, and anxiety sensitivity. These instruments help guide clinicians' understanding of the patient's emotional and cognitive responses to pain, and ultimately aid in developing a treatment plan to minimize distress and increase overall functioning.[35]

The Pain Anxiety Symptoms Scale (PASS) was developed to measure pain-related anxiety on four dimensions: (1) pain-specific appraisals; (2) cognitive symptoms; (3) physiological symptoms; and (4) escape and avoidance behavior.[35] Studies uti-

Posttraumatic Stress Disorder

Posttraumatic stress disorder (PTSD) develops after a person experiences a traumatic event wherein a person's well-being feels threatened. The DSM-IV[21] categorizes the symptoms into three constructs: (1) re-experiencing the event (e.g., intrusive thoughts and reminders), (2) avoidance and emotional numbing (e.g., restricted affect), and (3) hyperarousal (e.g., insomnia). Additionally, symptoms manifest with intense fear, helplessness, and avoidance of stimuli.[21] A major distinction between PTSD and other psychiatric disorders is that it is necessitated by an initial stressor.[21] In the past, PTSD was only conceptualized as a disorder that occurred in war veterans and rape victims.[75] However, definitions of this initial stressor have expanded to an unending range of events, some of which include serious medical illnesses, abuse, natural disasters, and violence.[21]

When looking at patients with PTSD, chronic pain has been seen as the most prevalent co-occurring physical problem.[76,77] There has been growing interest in the relationship between pain and PTSD, and the increased risk of chronic pain in PTSD patients.[76] A breakdown of the symptoms commonly associated with both these disorders demonstrates large overlap. For example, both are characterized with anxiety, avoidance, and increased somatic responses.[76] This symptom overlap is important to the understanding of the overall clinical picture of a patient who presents with both PTSD and chronic pain.

Assessment and Evaluation

PTSD is a disorder that is dependent on assessment and treatment since the debilitating symptoms do not recede on their own. People suffering with PTSD have been shown to be at an increased risk for suicide, social isolation, substance abuse, psychiatric disorders (depression, anxiety), insomnia, and medical illness (asthma, chronic pain).[78] Therefore, a comprehensive assessment and evaluation of each patient is essential in order to determine the frequency and severity of their symptoms which can aid in tailoring a treatment plan specific to their particular needs.

The Modified PTSD Symptom Checklist (MPSS) is a self-report scale used to measure general symptoms of PTSD.[79] The checklist is based on the diagnostic criteria of PTSD as outlined by the DSM-IV[21] and allows patients to rate the frequency and severity of their symptoms along either a four point scale (for frequency) or a five point scale (for severity).[80] A study employing this measure with a population of patients with comorbid PTSD and chronic pain found that chronic pain patients showed higher rates of frequency and severity in PTSD symptoms suggesting that these patients have a hyper-awareness and sensitivity to bodily sensations.[80] Findings such as this illustrate the need to further understand both disorders exclusively and mutually in order to provide the most effective treatment. Additionally, it is well-known that self-report measures, although beneficial, lack invaluable clinical judgment. Therefore, implementing a comprehensive psychosocial evaluation will give a clinician a more complete clinical picture and allow them to tailor treatments based on the more prevalent symptoms.

It is clear that negative moods play a significant role in influencing treatment motivation and compliance. For example, patients with pain-related anxiety may struggle with continuous fear of activities that they perceive as too dangerous or demanding, and patients with comorbid depression who feel hopeless may lack the motivation to seek treatment. An essential component of pain management requires clinicians to keep a watchful eye on patients' moods in order to provide optimal care.[81]

The frequent prevalence of PTSD and chronic pain, in conjunction with the negative impact they can have on each other by exacerbating symptoms and hindering treatment, shows the need for comprehensive assessment as well as further research. Hopefully, future research should include examination of a broader population. By assessing patients who suffer from comorbid PTSD and chronic pain in a multitude of settings (e.g., pain clinics, community settings, mental health clinics, outpatients, inpatients, and the general population), we will gain a greater understanding of each disorder, their relationship, and how to better treat them.

ADJUSTMENT TO CHRONIC PAIN

Individuals with chronic pain face numerous experiences in which their pain serves to elicit responses that have a significant impact on their everyday functioning. Chronic pain does not imply inca-

pacitation; although the effects of having a long-term painful condition can be disabling for some patients, others are able to live full, productive lives.[82,83] The primary goal of treatment for chronic pain is undoubtedly to eliminate or reduce the pain,[84] utilizing interventions that focus on prolonged analgesia of the physical symptoms.[85] However, total, lasting relief is uncommon and some patients show little to no improvement even in the short-term.[86] When patients are unable to achieve sufficient pain relief, their condition can become overwhelming and lead to decreased levels of functioning and greater disability. When this occurs, the treatment goals often shift focus from the physical aspect of the pain, and toward alternatives that take into account other influences that affect the patient's overall functioning.[87]

Responses to Pain: Coping and Acceptance

Recent evidence suggests that patients' overall level of functioning is strongly influenced by the way in which they respond to their pain.[82] Coping techniques in response to persistent pain have been a focal point of treatment over the past two decades.[88] These techniques have been found to yield positive outcomes,[89,90] and, as a result, have become widely accepted among the pain community, and have been utilized as the primary approach to pain adjustment.[91] Coping can be broadly defined as the deliberate effort to manage or alleviate the negative effect of stress.[92–94] In the context of chronic pain, coping has been referred to as a method to control either the level of pain, or the reaction to the pain.[91] Patients who view their pain as intolerable may make intense efforts to control the severity of their pain.[85] These efforts can be beneficial when they lead to sustained relief and improvement in functioning.[84] Conversely, they can also become problematic when they dominate other important aspects of the patient's life, creating additional undesirable side effects, or shifting the patient's priorities from valuable aspects of their life toward continuous efforts to reduce or eliminate their pain.[84] Problems associated with coping often stem from unsuccessful attempts to control or avoid the pain,[84] and repeated failures at achieving relief frequently leads to increased feelings of frustration and discouragement which only exacerbate the problem.[91]

Coping has also been conceptualized as a form of avoidance.[39,84,85] Previous research indicates a strong relationship between excessive avoidance of pain and increased discomfort and disability.[39,95,96] Patients who do not accept the fact that they have chronic pain are more likely to seek out any possible intervention to treat or reduce their pain. For these patients, this approach may not be in their best interest because they may exhaust all possible treatment options with a small chance of achieving lasting relief.[85]

Accumulating research is now supporting acceptance-based approaches to living with unrelieved chronic pain.[84] Acceptance is not a method of coping but, rather, a lifestyle that incorporates acknowledgment of pain, and a willingness to experience it.[82,85] Accepting pain means continuing to work toward living a satisfying and fulfilling life despite the pain and choosing to refrain from fruitless attempts to change, reduce, or eliminate the pain past what can be reasonably achieved.[82,85] This idea may be counterintuitive for many patients since our natural inclination is toward avoiding or controlling undesirable and distressing experiences. It is important, however, to note that acceptance neither means submitting to a life of suffering, nor is it a decision to give up all attempts to feel better. Rather, it promotes making a reasonable distinction between what can be controlled, and what can not.[82,84]

Research evaluating the impact of acceptance on patient functioning has demonstrated greater patient adaptation to pain beyond the effect of increased pain intensity or pain-related depression and anxiety.[85,97,98] Additionally, incorporating a perspective that focuses more on acceptance may lead the patient with chronic pain to generally have a greater sense of self-control.[99] A number of studies have shown evidence that patients who accept chronic pain function significantly better, reporting less pain, emotional distress, and disability.[84,85,87,91] They also report better work status and have less frequent medical visits.[97]

Assessment and Evaluation

The majority of studies that examine coping with chronic pain have utilized the Coping Strategies Questionnaire (CSQ), which assesses five strategies for coping with pain: (1) ignoring the pain; (2) distancing from the pain; (3) distraction; (4) coping self-statements; and (5) praying.[88,100] Patients use a rating scale to indicate how frequently they use each strategy to cope with their pain.[88] A major concern with the assessment of these strategies is the emphasis on cognitive processes. Some research has indicated that praying, distancing from the pain, and distraction were unhelpful coping strategies and associated with increased difficulty in patient functioning[88] and increased pain.[91] Coping, as a psychological framework for chronic pain patients, has received criticism surrounding the paucity of empirical data clarifying which behavioral strategies in response to pain are helpful.[91] The CSQ, as well as other coping inventories, rely heavily on reporting thoughts, or attempts to change thoughts, rather than behaviors. This emphasis can be problematic because it may distance the respondent further from the perspective of overt behavior where a great deal of daily activity occurs and can significantly limit assessment methods.[91]

The most widely used measure of acceptance of chronic pain is the Chronic Pain Acceptance Questionnaire (CPAQ).[82] The CPAQ is a 20-item self-report measure that assesses acceptance on two domains: (1) activity engagement (e.g., "I am getting on with the business of living no matter what my level of pain is") and (2) pain willingness (e.g., "I would gladly sacrifice important things in my life to control this pain better").[97] In a study comparing the utility of the CSQ and the CPAQ in guiding treatment, the CPAQ was found to offer greater utility because of its inclusion of items that fit an activity-related treatment approach, including such aspects as awareness of pain without wrestling with pain, mindfulness, and moving away from controlling or changing the pain.[88] The development of the CPAQ has led to innovative treatment approaches focused on cognitive, emotional, and behavioral change.[88]

Individuals diagnosed with persistent pain are often confronted with the reality of their chronicity, often being told they have to "learn to live with the pain."[91] It has recently been argued that limiting unsuccessful coping strategies should be the primary focus of treatment.[101] Interventions aimed at disengaging patients from the perceived struggle associated with controlling their condition have significant potential for development in this area.[91]

There is a large degree of overlap between coping strategies and adopting an acceptance perspective. Perhaps the most effective approach to treatment would include a cooperative effort between both models of adjustment to chronic pain. Some research supports the idea that there is more than one path to adopting an acceptance perspective. For example, using cognitive behavioral strategies that focus on obtaining control over painful experiences may actually make the pain become more acceptable.[102] The outcome of greater acceptance may be due to decreased avoidance and increased pain exposure, thus leading patients to experience less emotional reactions and recognize that different circumstances may be associated with variable pain levels, and the pain may not be as debilitating as they had once believed.[85] The decision to cope with or accept pain is not a solitary choice. Learning to live with chronic pain is a continuous experience that requires a balance between control strategies and acceptance.

LIFESTYLE HABITS AND MOTIVATION TO CHANGE

Living with chronic pain requires major lifestyle adjustments. To this end, when faced with a persistent chronic pain condition, a decision must be made to learn how to incorporate the necessary adjustments into daily life. In both the chronic pain population and the general population, maladaptive lifestyle habits are common. These can include smoking, overeating, not exercising, gambling etc. These lifestyle habits, in conjunction with chronic pain, create added obstacles which must be resolved to help make a smoother transition more feasible. Psychological interventions tailored to these individuals help manage the effects of living with chronic pain and achieving a balance between these new obstacles in life.

The chronic pain population is unique. These patients are facing new challenges and are adding an unseen variable to their current lifestyle. Not only does the chronic pain condition vary from patient to patient, but each person presents with a unique lifestyle comprised of both good and bad habits. This causes difficulties for the treating physicians. In order for their primary care physician to help, these patients have to be ready to adopt a self-management perspective.[103] A way to start the intervention process is by implementing a patient-centered therapeutic approach. This technique is based on the patients' perspective about their pain and their lifestyle in general. The foundation is built on patients' present feelings as well as their expectations and future goals.[104] Within a patient-centered treatment approach, the primary responsibility is given to the patient who, in turn, is encouraged to set goals and work toward achieving those goals. It is the responsibility of the clinician to help foster the global goals and to help formulate techniques to manage the day-to-day experiences. In effect, the clinician takes on the role of a mentor and consultant. Furthermore, this role must be set with boundaries and limits. Specifically regarding advice giving, it is not the responsibility of the clinician to tell the patient what the goals are and how to achieve them. Rather, they should approach the patient with empathy and compassion when offering advice and employ reflective listening techniques.[105,106] Types of reflective statements include repetition and rephrasing what a patient is saying, continuation of thoughts and reflecting on the feelings they express. The success of reflective listening relates back to the idea that the patient is in the center of the therapy which becomes a collaboration rather than traditional treatment.[103,106]

The Stages of Change

Similarly to how the degree of pain varies with each patient, they also differ in their readiness and confidence to self-manage the pain.[107] In addition, cognitive behavioral interventions will not succeed when there is any resistance from the patient. The Stages of Change were developed to benefit those individuals who were not ready to change their lifestyle and to move along those that were on the path.[108] This is the most innovative construct coming from the Transtheoretical Model (TTM), a comprehensive protocol of therapeutic interventions.[103,106]

The literature pertaining to the Stages of Change model within the framework of patients with chronic pain reveals that, beyond living with chronic pain, these patients suffer from secondary negative consequences which they have the power to control, including social isolation and decreased physical stamina.[109] Utilizing a behavioral model and framework will allow these patients to make the necessary changes by reducing these secondary consequences. The five original stages of change are: (1) precontemplation (individual is not considering change and further may not recognize the need for change); (2) contemplation (the idea of changing behaviors is considered but not yet implemented); (3)

preparation (plans are set in motion to make changes in behavior); (4) action (a plan has been set and techniques are being employed); and (5) maintenance (the goal has been met and behavior has been changed, however it must be continuously worked on to keep this stable).[109] These stages are fluid, meaning that a person can move back and forth through them as they reach goals, reassess goals, or falter and regress.[108] Additionally, even successfully reaching a goal does not allow a person to skip a stage. Actual success is achieved when the person moves through each stage.[109]

Assessment and Evaluation

Readiness to change is defined as a process of behavioral change, as opposed to one isolated event. People can alter their levels of motivation, confidence to change, desire to receive help, or choice to internalize. All of these varied emotions and stages became the basis for the distinct stages.[108] There seems to be a correlation between a person's readiness to change and the ability to successfully change a behavior.[110] The idea of the TTM and using motivation as an approach to self-management is tied very tightly with the readiness of a patient. There is a vast amount of literature following this idea and deconstructing the theories and assessments in order to formulate the most effective way to apply this to the chronic pain population.[107,110]

The first and most widely recognized assessment of the Stages of Change is the University of Rhode Island Change Assessment Questionnaire (URICA).[111] This was developed initially to assess psychiatric outpatients' level of motivation to adopt specific treatment. Kerns and colleagues[107] adapted this for the chronic pain population into the Pain Stages of Change Questionnaire (PSOCQ). Some of the content was altered, but the biggest change was to remove the third stage, preparation. When adapted for a pain population, the focus of each stage remains mostly the same. In precontemplation, a patient sees their pain as strictly medical, thereby requiring only those related interventions. In contemplation, a patient may recognize that they can intervene on their own behalf aside from using the medical techniques. In action, a patient takes on a self-management approach and implements a plan to change their lifestyle. In the last stage, maintenance, patients have acquired the necessary skills to manage their chronic pain and have a lifestyle plan in place to follow.[112]

The motivational strategies that have been employed to work along with the Stages of Change center around assessing what the patient wants to change, what they want to get out of the therapy, and generating a picture of their ideal lifestyle, which should help to foster authentic self-management. Assessing and evaluating these goals early on and continuously coming back to them is mutually beneficial and will help to establish and maintain rapport between patient and physician. This also will help a patient keep to the set agenda and opens the door for the physician to ask a patient for clarification when needed. Use of direct, open-ended questions in this dialogue will prevent confusion and even conflict later on.

There are a number of specific strategies which can be useful, including the employment of open-ended questions and reflective listening.[113] These help to bring the patient to a higher level of confidence and recognition of the importance of self-management. This will lead to the formulation of an agenda that is specific to the patient. Also, examining the pros and cons of behavior change will bring about the negatives and positives associated with self-management and aid in minimizing the ambivalence a patient may be feeling. Third, the physician can elicit concerns about the status quo if a behavior is not changed. Bringing these concerns to the surface will endorse the need for change and consequences if the behavioral change is not pursued. Last, the physician can help to brainstorm solutions and aid in coming up with a multitude of ideas that will help maintain or increase a patient's confidence in their ability to change.[103]

Reverting back to the idea of a patient-centered therapeutic approach, goals and treatments will differ for each patient. In addition, the simple idea of readiness to self-manage is going to vary along a continuum as well. The Stages of Change was formulated with this exact idea in mind, focusing on the idea that a patient should find their place with the stages organically.

Habits are deeply ingrained in our daily lives and we must remember that making the decision to change, implementing a plan, and maintaining that change for any length of time is a difficult feat for anyone. When the additional obstacle of experiencing chronic pain is present, the need to adapt lifestyles is that much more difficult and important. In the chronic pain population, the patient must reach a level where they no longer see medical treatment as the only way to ease suffering.[103] This helps them to take back control of their lives and not allow the pain to overshadow their chosen lifestyle. Further research is needed to understand how a person succeeds and fails in this feat, using such techniques as the Stages of Change. This can lead to the formulation of a standard program where patients have a framework to use as a baseline for comparison and to monitor progress.

CHEMICAL HEALTH

Chemical Coping

Chemical coping is a construct that stemmed from the recognition of the grey area between perfect compliance and aberrancy in medication usage.[114] This idea was cultivated by Bruera and colleagues[115] as a way to illustrate an archetype of maladaptive coping via substances. This construct was first applied to a sample of cancer patients with high rates of historical substance abuse, which was furthered by the distress associated with cancer.[115] More recently, this idea is being extended from cancer patients into chronic pain populations.[114]

There are distinctive traits associated with patients in the chronic pain population who might be considered chemical copers. Stress has been seen as a major catalyst in this population and chemical copers have a tendency to increase drug dose and deviate from the treatment path when stress seems unmanageable. Additionally, chemical copers do not tend to set psychosocial goals and are disinterested in nonpharmacological treatments.[114]

There are several associated features within the construct of chemical coping: (1) self-medication,[116] (2) sensation seeking, (3) alexithymia, and (4) somatization. The self-medication hypothesis purports that patients misuse substances in order to relieve feelings of physical or emotional distress and that they have an affinity toward specific pharmacological substances.[116] Sensation seeking is defined as an inclination toward a multitude of complicated and powerful experiences and a desire to go beyond the norm to obtain these feelings. Chemical coping is a strategy used to avoid feelings of distress, whereas the goal of sensation seeking is an alternative to everyday states of mind.[114] Alexithymia is present when a person has the inability to manage and comprehend their emotions and feelings. These patients present with somatic complaints and have little to no emotional connection thereby solely relying on physical feelings.[117] The last associated feature is that of somatization wherein physical complaints have no physiological basis. These patients are not always aware that they are misconstruing emotional distress as physical symptoms and are likely to be resistant to accepting this meassage.[118]

Impulsivity

Impulsivity is a complex behavioral construct that requires further examination within the chronic pain population.[119] Different aspects of impulsivity include decreased ability to delay gratification, tendency toward the present moment, risk-taking, poor planning, proneness to boredom, sensation-seeking, reward sensitivity, adventuresomeness, acting without predetermined thought, and hedonism.[120,121] Due to the multidimensional nature of impulsivity, these aspects may manifest in varying behavioral degrees depending on the context in which they are presented. Since it applies to a diverse range of contexts, impulsivity is a common diagnostic criterion for many disorders in the DSM-IV,[21] and has also been implicated as a risk factor for disorders such as alcoholism, eating disorders, and pathological gambling.[120] Longitudinal studies have shown evidence supporting the idea that impulsivity is a risk factor in children for later development of substance abuse issues,[122,123] and cross-sectional studies have demonstrated an association between impulsiveness and substance use in a sample of college students.[124] Impulsiveness may also be linked to other types of impulse-control related behaviors including criminal activity and repeated aggression.[125] The relationship between impulsivity and substance abuse has also been examined in patient populations, demonstrating that patients who are substance abusers score higher on personality measures of impulsivity relative to control groups.[126–133]

A proclivity toward impulsive behavior has important clinical implications in chronic pain patients. This can become problematic because pain patients taking potentially abusable medications such as opioids may be at greater risk for abuse. There are a number of risk factors that have been associated with substance abuse that relate to impulsive behavior. Women with a history of preadolescent sexual abuse are at greater risk for substance abuse and mental disorders.[134–136] Trauma experienced as a result of this abuse can also lead to other psychological disorders such as PTSD[137] and personality disorders.[11] Chronic pain patients who present with a comorbid personality disorder such as borderline personality disorder (BPD) may be at particular risk for substance abuse.[11] Patients with BPD tend to have more intermittent patterns of drug abuse as a result of their characteristic impulsivity and frantic efforts to self-regulate their emotional distress and feelings of emptiness and boredom. This self-medicating, impulsive behavior is often chaotic in nature and in line with their other desperate attempts to act out, such as pursuing the self-regulating effects of food or interpersonal contacts.[138] Impulsive substance abuse has also been found to be largely associated with other psychological disorders including attention-deficit hyperactivity disorder (ADHD), depression, anxiety, obsessive compulsive disorder (OCD), schizophrenia, and bipolar disorder.[139]

Assessment

Self-report measures have been developed to assess impulsivity such as the Barratt Impulsiveness Scale (BIS-10)[133,140] and the Eysenck Personality Questionnaire.[141] However, there are a number of limitations associated with these instruments. First, these measures were generally developed to assess impulsivity in healthy volunteers, not in medically ill populations.[142] Additionally, when respondents are asked to rate items on long-term personality traits such as "I act on impulse," there is a large potential for bias.[143]

Impulsivity can be a predictor and risk factor when viewed within the framework of aberrant drug-taking behaviors. Markers of impulsivity include criminal behavior, history of personal or family substance abuse, history of childhood sexual abuse, and psychological disorders.[137,139] The Opioid Risk Tool (ORT) is a five-item self-report measure that evaluates risk potential for opioid abuse. It was developed based on empirical research linking the aforementioned markers to the level of risk associated with opioid abuse.[137] This measure has clinical utility in evaluating patients prior to initiation of opioid therapy thus allowing clinicians to classify patients into one of three categories; low,

moderate, or high risk. The simplicity of the ORT allows the clinician to begin treatment while monitoring the underlying risk factors. Furthermore, the clinician is able to tailor treatment to meet the individual needs of each patient.[139]

In the pain population, chemical health should be part of the initial and ongoing assessment. The goal of psychotherapy in chronic pain syndromes needs to be focused on the differentiation between emotional and physical pain. This is especially true in individuals with tendencies toward chemical coping and impulsivity. This will allow the physician to combat repercussions faced as a result of pharmacological misuse as well as tend to the psychosocial components of living with chronic pain.[114]

CONCLUSION

Increasing attention on chronic pain has led to significant advances in assessment and treatment with greater understanding of the implications of psychological and psychosocial conditions within the chronic pain population. Although recent contributions have improved assessment and evaluation methods of these patients, further research is needed to determine a standard of care.

References

1. Compas BE, Haaga DA, Keefe FJ, et al. Sampling of empirically supported psychological treatments from health psychology: smoking, chronic pain, cancer, and bulimia nervosa. *J Consult Clin Psychol* 1998;66(1):89–112.
2. Gil KM, Abrams MR, Phillips GG, et al. Sickle cell disease pain: 2. Predicting health care use and activity level at 9-month follow-up. *J Consult Clin Psychol* 1992;60(2):267–273.
3. Turk DC, Okifuji A. Chronic pain. In: Christensen AJ, Antoni MH, eds. *Chronic Physical Disorders: Behavioral Medicine's Perspective: The Blackwell Series in Health Psychology and Behavioral Medicine.* Malden, MA: Blackwell Publishers; 2002:165–190.
4. Keefe FJ, Rumble ME, Scipio CD, et al. Psychological aspects of persistent pain: current state of the science. *J Pain* 2004;5(4):195–211.
5. Ehde DM, Jensen MP, Engel JM, et al. Chronic pain secondary to disability: a review. *Clin J Pain* 2003;19(1):3–17.
6. Linton SJ. Occupational psychological factors increase the risk for back pain: a systematic review. *J Occup Rehabil* 2001;11(1):53–66.
7. Linton SJ. Early identification and intervention in the prevention of musculoskeletal pain. *Am J Ind Med* 2002;41(5):433–442.
8. Linton SJ, van Tulder MW. Preventive interventions for back and neck pain problems: what is the evidence? *Spine* 2001;26(7):778–787.
9. Turner JA. Educational and behavioral interventions for back pain in primary care. *Spine* 1996;21(24):2851–2857; discussion 2858.
10. Weisberg JN, Boatwright BA. Mood, anxiety, and personality traits and states in chronic pain. *Pain* 2007;133(1–3):1–2.
11. Weisberg JN. Personality and personality disorders in chronic pain. *Curr Rev Pain* 2000;4(1):60–70.
12. Clark LA, Watson DD. Tripartite model of anxiety and depression: psychometric evidence and taxonomic implications. *J Abnorm Psychol* 1991;100(3):316–336.
13. Gotlib IH, Cane DB. Self-report assessment of depression and anxiety. In: Kendall PC, Watson D, eds. *Anxiety and Depression: Distinctive and Overlapping Features.* New York: Academic Press; 1989:131–169.
14. Mendels J, Weinstein N, Cochrane C. The relationship between depression and anxiety. *Arch Gen Psychiatry* 1972;27:649–653.
15. Reidy J, Keogh E. Testing the discriminant and convergent validity of the Mood and Anxiety Symptoms Questionnaire using a British sample. *Pers Indiv Differ* 1997;23:337–344.
16. Tanaka-Matsumi JJ, Kameoka VA. Reliabilities and concurrent validities of popular self-report measures of depression, anxiety, and social desirability. *J Consult Clin Psychol* 1986;54(3):328–333.
17. Dersh J, Polatin PB, Gatchel RJ. Chronic pain and psychopathology: research findings and theoretical considerations. *Psychosom Med* 2002;64(5):773–786.
18. Katon W, Schulberg H. Epidemiology of depression in primary care. *Gen Hosp Psychiatry* 1992;14(4):237–247.
19. Pincus T, Santos R, Morley S. Depressed cognitions in chronic pain patients are focused on health: evidence from a sentence completion task. *Pain* 2007;130(1–2):84–92.
20. Keefe FJ, France CR. Pain: biopsychosocial mechanisms and management. *Curr Dir Psychol Sci* 1999;8:137–141.
21. American Psychiatric Association. *Diagnostic and Statistical Manual of Mental Disorders.* 4th ed. Washington, DC: Author; 1994.

22. Bair MJ, Robinson RL, Katon W, et al. Depression and pain comorbidity: a literature review. *Arch Intern Med* 2003;163(20):2433–2445.

23. Magni G, Merskey H. A simple examination of the relationships between pain, organic lesions and psychiatric illness. *Pain* 1987;29(3):295–300.

24. Magni G, Marchetti M, Moreschi C, et al. Chronic musculoskeletal pain and depressive symptoms in the National Health and Nutrition Examination. I. Epidemiologic follow-up study. *Pain* 1993;53(2):163–168.

25. Fishbain DA, Cutler R, Rosomoff HL, et al. Chronic pain-associated depression: antecedent or consequence of chronic pain? A review. *Clin J Pain* 1997;13(2):116–137.

26. Morley S, Davies C, Barton S. Possible selves in chronic pain: self-pain enmeshment, adjustment and acceptance. *Pain* 2005;115(1–2):84–94.

27. Turk DC. Psychosocial factors in chronic pain patients. In: McCarberg BH, Passik SD, eds. *Expert Guide to Pain Management*. Philadelphia: American College of Physicians; 2005:271–290.

28. Kerns RD, Haythornthwaite JA. Depression among chronic pain patients: cognitive–behavioral analysis and effect on rehabilitation outcome. *J Consult Clin Psychol* 1988;56(6):870–876.

29. Rudy TE, Kerns RD, Turk DC. Chronic pain and depression: toward a cognitive–behavioral mediation model. *Pain* 1988;35(2):129–140.

30. Turk DC, Okifuji A, Scharff L. Chronic pain and depression: role of perceived impact and perceived control in different age cohorts. *Pain* 1995;61(1):93–101.

31. Twillman RK. Mental disorders in chronic pain patients. *J Pain Palliat Care Pharmacother* 2007;21(4):13–19.

32. McNeil DW, Turk CL, Ries BJ. Anxiety and fear. In: Ramachandran VS, ed. *Encyclopedia of Human Behavior*. Vol 1. San Diego: Academic Press; 1994:151–163.

33. Zinbarg RE. Concordance and synchrony in measures of anxiety and panic reconsidered: a hierarchical model of anxiety and panic. *Behav Ther* 1998;29(2):301–323.

34. Vlaeyen JW, Linton SJ. Fear-avoidance and its consequences in chronic musculoskeletal pain: a state of the art. *Pain* 2000;85(3):317–332.

35. McCracken LM, Zayfert CC, Gross RT. The Pain Anxiety Symptoms Scale: development and validation of a scale to measure fear of pain. *Pain* 1992;50(1):67–73.

36. Waddell G, Newton M, Henderson I, et al. A Fear-Avoidance Beliefs Questionnaire (FABQ) and the role of fear-avoidance beliefs in chronic low back pain and disability. *Pain* 1993;52(2):157–168.

37. Vlaeyen JW, Kole–Snijders AM, Boeren RG, et al. Fear of movement/(re)injury in chronic low back pain and its relation to behavioral performance. *Pain* 1995;62(3):363–372.

38. McCracken LM, Gross RT, Sorg PJ, Edmands TA. Prediction of pain in patients with chronic low back pain: effects of inaccurate prediction and pain-related anxiety. *Behav Res Ther* 1993;31(7):647–652.

39. McCracken LM, Gross RT, Aikens JJ, Carnrike CL. The assessment of anxiety and fear in persons with chronic pain: a comparison of instruments. *Behav Res Ther* 1996;34(11–12):927–933.

40. Keefe FJ, Kashikar–Zuck S, Robinson E, et al. Pain coping strategies that predict patients' and spouses' ratings of patients' self-efficacy. *Pain* 1997;73(2):191–199.

41. Keefe FJ, Brown GK, Wallston KA, et al. Coping with rheumatoid arthritis pain: catastrophizing as a maladaptive strategy. *Pain* 1989;37(1):51–56.

42. Sullivan MJ, D'Eon JL. Relation between catastrophizing and depression in chronic pain patients. *J Abnorm Psychol* 1990;99(3):260–263.

43. Sullivan MJ, Thorn B, Haythornthwaite JA, et al. Theoretical perspectives on the relation between catastrophizing and pain. *Clin J Pain* 2001;17(1):52–64.

44. Jacobsen PB, Butler RW. Relation of cognitive coping and catastrophizing to acute pain and analgesic use following breast cancer surgery. *J Behav Med* 1996;19(1):17–29.

45. Bishop SR, Warr D. Coping, catastrophizing and chronic pain in breast cancer. *J Behav Med* 2003;26(3):265–281.

46. Zaza C, Baine N. Cancer pain and psychosocial factors: a critical review of the literature. *J Pain Symptom Manage* 2002;24(5):526–542.

47. Thorn BE, Boothby JL, Sullivan MJL. Targeted treatment of catastrophizing for the management of chronic pain. *Cogn Behav Pract* 2002;9(2):127–138.

48. Geisser ME, Robinson ME, Keefe FJ, et al. Catastrophizing, depression and the sensory, affective and evaluative aspects of chronic pain. *Pain* 1994;59(1):79–83.

49. Sullivan M, Ferrell B. Ethical challenges in the management of chronic nonmalignant pain: negotiating through the cloud of doubt. *J Pain* 2005;6(1):2–9.

50. Gil KM, Thompson RJ, Keith BR, et al. Sickle cell disease pain in children and adolescents: change in pain frequency and coping strategies over time. *J Pediatr Psychol* 1993;18(5):621–637.

51. Sullivan MJ, Thorn B, Haythornthwaite JA, et al. Theoretical perspectives on the relation between catastrophizing and pain. *Clin J Pain* 2001;17(1):52–64.

52. Sullivan MJ, Stanish W, Waite H, et al. Catastrophizing, pain, and disability in patients with soft-tissue injuries. *Pain* 1998;77(3):253–260.

53. Reiss S, McNally RJ. Expectancy model of fear. In: Reiss S, Bootzin RR, eds. *Theoretical Issues in Behavior Therapy*. San Diego: Academic Press; 1985:107–121.

54. Taylor S, Cox BJ. Anxiety sensitivity: multiple dimensions and hierarchic structure. *Behav Res Ther* 1998;36(1):37–51.

55. Zvolensky MJ, Eifert GH, Lejuez CW, et al. The effects of offset control over 20% carbon dioxide-enriched air on anxious responding. *J Abnorm Psychol* 1999;108(4):624–632.

56. Craig KD. Emotional aspects of pain. In: Wall PD, Melzack R, eds. *The Textbook of Pain*. Edinburgh: Churchill Livingstone; 1994:261–274.

57. Schmidt NB, Telch MJ. Nonpsychiatric medical comorbidity, health perceptions, and treatment outcome in patients with panic disorder. *Health Psychol* 1997;16(2):114–122.

58. Schmidt NB, Cook JH. Effects of anxiety sensitivity on anxiety and pain during a cold pressor challenge in patients with panic disorder. *Behav Res Ther* 1999;37(4):313–323.

59. Asmundson GJG. Anxiety sensitivity and chronic pain: Empirical findings, clinical implications, and future directions. In: Taylor S, ed. *Anxiety Sensitivity: Theory, Research, and Treatment of the Fear of Anxiety*. Mahwah, NJ: Erlbaum; 1999:269–285.

60. McCracken LM. "Attention" to pain in persons with chronic pain: a behavioral approach. *Behav Ther* 1997;28:271–284.

61. Zvolensky MJ, Goodie JL, McNeil DW, et al. Anxiety sensitivity in the prediction of pain-related fear and anxiety in a heterogeneous chronic pain population. *Behav Res Ther* 2001;39(6):683–696.

62. Turner JA, Aaron LA. Pain-related catastrophizing: what is it? *Clin J Pain* 2001;17(1):65–71.

63. Sullivan MJ, Bishop SR, Pivik J. The pain catastrophizing scale: development and validation. *Psychol Assess* 1995;7(4):524–532.

64. Reiss S, Peterson RA, Gursky DM, et al. Anxiety sensitivity, anxiety frequency and the prediction of fearfulness. *Behav Res Ther* 1986;24(1):1–8.

65. Schmidt NB, Lerew DR, Jackson RJ. Prospective evaluation of anxiety sensitivity in the pathogenesis of panic: replication and extension. *J Abnorm Psychol* 1999;108(3):532–537.

66. Zvolensky MJ, Eifert GH. A review of psychological factors/processes affecting anxious responding during voluntary hyperventilation and inhalations of carbon dioxide-enriched air. *Clin Psychol Rev* 2001;21(3):375.

67. Zinbarg RE, Mohlman J, Hong NN. Dimensions of anxiety sensitivity. In: Taylor S. *Anxiety Sensitivity: Theory, Research, and Treatment of the Fear of Anxiety*. Mahwah, NJ: Erlbaum; 1999.

68. Stewart SH, Taylor S, Baker JM. Gender differences in dimensions of anxiety sensitivity. *J Anxiety Disord* 1997;11(2):179–200.

69. Zinbarg RE, Brown TA, Barlow DH. Hierarchical structure and general factor structure saturation of the Anxiety Sensitivity Index: evidence and implications. *Psychol Assess* 1997;9:277–284.

70. Boersma K, Linton SJ. Psychological processes underlying the development of a chronic pain problem: a prospective study of the relationship between profiles of psychological variables in the fear-avoidance model and disability. *Clin J Pain* 2006;22(2):160–166.

71. Feuerstein M, Beattie P. Biobehavioral factors affecting pain and disability in low back pain: mechanisms and assessment. *Phys Ther* 1995;75(4):267–280.

72. Vlaeyen JW, Crombez G. Fear of movement/(re)injury, avoidance and pain disability in chronic low back pain patients. *Man Ther* 1999;4(4):187–195.

73. Vlaeyen JW, Linton SJ. Fear-avoidance and its consequences in chronic musculoskeletal pain: a state of the art. *Pain* 2000;85(3):317–332.

74. Asmundson GJ. Anxiety and related factors in chronic pain. *Pain Res Manag* 2002;7(1):7–8.

75. March JS. What constitutes a stressor? The "Criterion A" issue. In: Davidson JRT, Foa E, eds. *Posttraumatic Stress Disorder: DSM-IV and Beyond*. Washington, DC: American Psychiatric Press Inc; 1993:37–54.

76. Asmundson GJ, Coons MJ, Taylor S, et al. PTSD and the experience of pain: research and clinical implications of shared vulnerability and mutual maintenance models. *Can J Psychiatry* 2002;47(10):930–937.

77. Shiperd JC, Keyes M, Jovanic T, et al. Veterans seeking treatment for posttraumatic stress disorder: what about comorbid chronic pain? *J Rehabil Res Dev* 2007;44(2):153–166.

78. Wilson JF. Posttraumatic stress disorder needs to be recognized in primary care. *Ann Intern Med* 2007;146(8):617–620.

79. Foa EB, Riggs DS, Dancu CV, et al. Reliability and validity in a brief instrument for assessing post-traumatic stress disorder. *J Trauma Stress* 1993;6:459–473.

80. Bonin M, Norton GR, Frombach I, et al. PTSD in different treatment settings: a preliminary investigation of PTSD symptomatology in substance abuse and chronic pain patients. *Depress Anxiety* 2000;11(3):131–133.

81. Gatchel RJ, Peng YB, Peters ML, et al. The biopsychosocial approach to chronic pain: scientific advances and future directions. *Psychol Bull* 2007;133(4):581–624.

82. McCracken LM, Vowles KE. Acceptance of chronic pain. *Curr Pain Headache Rep* 2006;10:90–94.

83. Jensen MP, Turner JA, Romano JM, et al. Coping with chronic pain: a critical review of the literature. *Pain* 1991;47(3):249–283.

84. McCracken LM, Carson JW, Eccleston CC, et al. Acceptance and change in the context of chronic pain. *Pain* 2004;109(1–2):4–7.

85. McCracken LM. Learning to live with the pain: acceptance of pain predicts adjustment in persons with chronic pain. *Pain* 1998;74(1):21–27.

86. Turk DC. Customizing treatment for chronic pain patients: who, what, and why. *Clin J Pain* 1990;6(4):255–270.

87. McCracken LM, Eccleston CC, Bell LL. Clinical assessment of behavioral coping responses: preliminary results from a brief inventory. *Eur J Pain* 2005;9(1):69–78.

88. McCracken LM, Eccleston CC. A comparison of the relative utility of coping and acceptance-based measures in a sample of chronic pain sufferers. *Eur J Pain* 2006;10(1):23–29.

89. Morley SS, Eccleston CC, Williams AA. Systematic review and meta-analysis

of randomized controlled trials of cognitive behaviour therapy and behaviour therapy for chronic pain in adults, excluding headache. *Pain* 1999;80(1–2): 1–13.

90. McCracken LM, Turk DC. Behavioral and cognitive–behavioral treatment for chronic pain: outcome, predictors of outcome, and treatment process. *Spine* 2002;27(22):2564–2573.

91. McCracken LM, Eccleston CC. Coping or acceptance: what to do about chronic pain? *Pain* 2003;105(1–2):197–204.

92. Burish TG, Bradley LA. Coping with chronic disease: definitions and issues. In: Burish TG, Bradley LA, eds. *Coping with Chronic Disease: Research and Applications*. New York: Academic Press; 1983:3–12.

93. Coyne JC, Holroyd K. Stress, coping and illness: a transactional perspective. In: Millon T, Green C, Meagher R, eds. *Handbook of Health Care Clinical Psychology*. New York: Plenum Press; 1982.

94. Lazarus RA, Folkman S. *Stress, appraisal, and coping*. New York: Springer; 1984.

95. Asmundson GJ, Norton PJ, Norton GR. Beyond pain: the role of fear and avoidance in chronicity. *Clin Psychol Rev* 1999;19(1):97–119.

96. Bortz WM. The disuse syndrome. *West J Med* 1984;141(5):691–694.

97. McCracken LM. Social context and acceptance of chronic pain: the role of solicitous and punishing responses. *Pain* 2005;113(1–2):155–159.

98. McCracken LM, Spertus IL, Janeck AS, et al. Behavioral dimensions of adjustment in persons with chronic pain: pain-related anxiety and acceptance. *Pain* 1999;80(1–2):283–289.

99. Jacob MC, Kerns RD, Rosenberg R, et al. Chronic pain: intrusion and accommodation. *Behav Res Ther* 1993;31(5):519–527.

100. Tan G, Jensen MP, Robinson–Whelen S, et al. Coping with chronic pain: a comparison of two measures. *Pain* 2001;90(1–2):127–133.

101. Geisser ME, Robinson ME, Riley JL. Pain beliefs, coping, and adjustment to chronic pain. *Pain Forum* 1999;8:161–168.

102. Geiser DS. A comparison of acceptance-focused and control-focused psychological treatments in a chronic pain treatment center. Unpublished doctoral dissertation: University of Nevada, Reno; 1992.

103. Douaihy AB, Jensen MP, RJ, J. Motivating behavior change in patients with chronic pain. In: McCarberg BH, Passik SD, eds. *Expert Guide to Pain Management*. Philadelphia: American College of Physicians; 2005:217–231.

104. Stewart MA, Brown JB, Weston WW, et al. *Patient-Centered Medicine: Transforming the Clinical Method*. Thousand Oaks, CA: Sage Publications; 1995.

105. Ashenden R, Silagy C, Weller D. A systematic review of the effectiveness of promoting lifestyle change in general practice. *Fam Pract* 1997;14(2): 160–176.

106. Miller WR, Rollnick S. *Motivational Interviewing: Preparing People to Change Addictive Behavior*. 2nd ed. New York: The Guilford Press; 2002.

107. Kerns RD, Rosenberg R, Jamison RN, et al. Readiness to adopt a self-management approach to chronic pain: the Pain Stages of Change Questionnaire (PSOCQ). *Pain* 1997;72(1–2):227–234.

108. Prochaska JO, DiClemente CC, Norcross JC. In search of how people change. Applications to addictive behaviors. *Am Psychol* 1992;47(9):1102–1114.

109. Dijkstra A. The validity of the stages of change model in the adoption of the self-management approach in chronic pain. *Clin J Pain* 2005;21(1):27–37; discussion 69–72.

110. Dijkstra A, Vlaeyen JW, Rijnen H, et al. Readiness to adopt the self-management approach to cope with chronic pain in fibromyalgic patients. *Pain* 2001; 90(1–2):37–45.

111. McConnaughy EA, Prochaska JO, Velicer W. Stages of change in psychotherapy: Measurement and sample profiles. *Psychotherapy* 1983;20:368–375.

112. Strong J, Westbury K, Smith G, et al. Treatment outcome in individuals with chronic pain: is the Pain Stages of Change Questionnaire (PSOCQ) a useful tool? *Pain* 2002;97(1–2):65–73.

113. Rollnick S, Mason P, Butler C. *Health Behavior Change: A Guide for Practitioners*. Edinburgh: Harcourt Publishers; 1999.

114. Kirsh KL, Jass C, Bennett DS, et al. Initial development of a survey tool to detect issues of chemical coping in chronic pain patients. *Palliat Support Care* 2007;5(3):219–226.

115. Bruera E, Moyano J, Seifert L, et al. The frequency of alcoholism among patients with pain due to terminal cancer. *J Pain Symptom Manage* 1995; 10(8):599–603.

116. Khantzian EJ. The self-medication hypothesis revisited: the dually diagnosed patient. *Primary Psychiatry* 2003;10:47–48, 53–54.

117. Sifneos PE. Alexithymia: past and present. *Am J Psychiatry* 1996;153(7 suppl):137–142.

118. Avila LA. Somatization or psychosomatic symptoms? *Psychosomatics* 2006; 47(2):163–166.

119. Gerbing DW, Ahadi SA, Patton JH. Toward a conceptualization of impulsivity: components across the behavioral and self-report domains. *Multivariate Behav Res* 1987;22:357–379.

120. Cyders MA, Smith GT, Spillane NS, et al. Integration of impulsivity and positive mood to predict risky behavior: development and validation of a measure of positive urgency. *Psychol Assess* 2007;19(1):107–118.

121. Vitaro F, Arseneault L, Tremblay RE. Impulsivity predicts problem gambling in low SES adolescent males. *Addiction* 1999;94(4):565–575.

122. Dawes MA, Tarter RE, Kirisci L. Behavioral self-regulation: correlates and 2 year follow-ups for boys at risk for substance abuse. *Drug Alcohol Depend* 1997;45(3):165–176.

123. White JL, Moffitt TE, Caspi A, et al. Measuring impulsivity and examining its relationship to delinquency. *J Abnorm Psychol* 1994;103(2):192–205.

124. Jaffe LT, Archer RP. The prediction of drug use among college students from MMPI, MCMI, and sensation seeking scales. *J Pers Assess* 1987;51(2): 243–253.

125. Stanford MS, Barratt ES. Impulsivity and the multi-impulsive personality disorder. *Pers Indiv Differ* 1992;7:831–834.

126. Allen TJ, Moeller FG, Rhoades HM, et al. Impulsivity and history of drug dependence. *Drug Alcohol Depend* 1998;50(2):137–145.

127. Chalmers D, Olenick NL, Stein W. Dispositional traits as risk in problem drinking. *J Subst Abuse* 1993;5(4):401–410.

128. McCormick RA, Taber J, Kruedelbach N, et al. Personality profiles of hospitalized pathological gamblers: the California Personality Inventory. *J Clin Psychol* 1987;43(5):521–527.

129. Rosenthal TL, Edwards NB, Ackerman BJ, et al. Substance abuse patterns reveal contrasting personal traits. *J Subst Abuse* 1990;2(2):255–263.

130. Sher KJ, Trull TJ. Personality and disinhibitory psychopathology: alcoholism and antisocial personality disorder. *J Abnorm Psychol* 1994;103(1):92–102.

131. Cookson H. Personality variables associated with alcohol use in young offenders. *Pers Indiv Differ* 1994 16:179–182.

132. Eisen SV, Youngman DJ, Grob MC, et al. Alcohol, drugs and psychiatric disorders: a current view of hospitalized adolescents. *J Adolesc Res* 1992; 7(2):250–265.

133. Patton JH, Stanford MS, Barratt ES. Factor structure of the Barratt impulsiveness scale. *J Clin Psychol* 1995;51(6):768–774.

134. Kendler KS, Bulik CM, Silberg J, et al. Childhood sexual abuse and adult psychiatric and substance use disorders in women: an epidemiological and cotwin control analysis. *Arch Gen Psychiatry* 2000;57(10):953–959.

135. Mullen PE, Martin JL, Anderson JC, et al. Childhood sexual abuse and mental health in adult life. *Br J Psychiatry* 1993;163:721–732.

136. Zickler P. Childhood sex abuse increases risk for drug dependence in adult women. *NIDA Notes* 2002;17(1).

137. Webster LR, Webster RM. Predicting aberrant behaviors in opioid-treated patients: preliminary validation of the Opioid Risk Tool. *Pain Med* 2005; 6(6):432–442.

138. Hay JL, Passik SD. The cancer patient with borderline personality disorder: suggestions for symptom-focused management in the medical setting. *Psycho-oncology* 2000;9(2):91–100.

139. Webster LR. Assessing abuse potential in pain patients. *Medscape Neurology and Neurosurgery* 2004;6(1).

140. Barratt ES. Factor analysis of some psychometric measures of impulsiveness and anxiety. *Psychol Rep* 1965;16:547–554.

141. Eysenck SB, Eysenck HJ. The place of impulsiveness in a dimensional system of personality description. *Br J Soc Clin Psychol* 1977;16(1):57–68.

142. Moeller FG, Barratt ES, Dougherty DM, et al. Psychiatric aspects of impulsivity. *Am J Psychiatry* 2001;158(11):1783–1793.

143. Kertzman S, Grinspan H, Birger M, et al. Computerized neuropsychological examination of impulsiveness: a selective review. *Isr J Psychiatry Relat Sci* 2006;43(2):74–80.

CHAPTER 22 ■ DISABILITY EVALUATION IN PAINFUL CONDITIONS

JAMES P. ROBINSON AND RAYMOND C. TAIT

INTRODUCTION

The third edition of *Bonica's Management of Pain* contains a chapter on disability assessment in patients with chronic pain written by one of the present authors (JPR).[1] It outlines fundamental conceptual dilemmas that must be faced by any individual or institution that grapples with the problem of how to compensate fairly people who report incapacitation from pain.

As discussed in the third edition, issues related to pain and disability are problematic at several levels. At a societal level, they challenge institutions charged with the responsibility of developing policies regarding disability benefits that bear on individuals who report incapacitating pain. At a much more concrete level, they confound clinicians who are faced with the challenge of whether or not to support requests by their patients for disability benefits and what metric they should apply if they decide to do so.

The present chapter builds on concepts discussed in the previous chapter on disability. In particular, we identify questions which bear on policies for determining pain-related disability and which are amenable to empirical study, and we review the small steps that have been taken to answer these questions. To some degree, these small steps begin to flesh out the concept of "disability science" described in the third edition chapter. The current chapter also summarizes the developments that have occurred in social policies relative to pain and disability during the 7 years since the latter chapter was written.

Finally, we briefly consider the types of decisions that treating physicians are required to make regarding their patients in order to comply with regulations established by disability agencies, and strategies that clinicians might follow when they make disability determinations for patients who they are treating. We note at the outset, however, that the challenges for clinicians are essentially identical to those that existed 7 years ago, secondary to a failure to address critical issues at the levels of policy formation and disability science.

The material contained in this chapter is most relevant to individuals with chronic pain who live in the United States, report incapacitation secondary to their pain, and seek disability benefits of some kind. The chapter focuses on disability programs in the United States for the simple reason that these are the ones with which the authors are most familiar. While the need to specify the jurisdictions considered in this chapter highlights the important fact that disability policies are extremely variable from one jurisdiction to another, the reader will also note that some of the issues raised in the following pages cut across jurisdictions and apply more broadly to the difficulties that clinicians and disability evaluators face when assessing a subjective phenomenon such as pain.

REVIEW OF KEY CONCEPTS

Impairment and Disability

Disability

Two concepts that are fundamental in the area of disability involve "impairment" and "disability." Unfortunately, these terms do not have unique definitions, because different disability agencies define them in slightly different ways. The two concepts are compared in Table 22.1.

In its broadest meaning, disability refers to an inability to carry out necessary tasks in any important domain of life because of a medical condition. For example, a C5 quadriplegic is disabled in the sense of being unable to carry out many basic activities of daily living (ADLs). This chapter focuses on the more restricted concept of work disability, which can be informally defined as the inability to carry out work-related tasks because of a medical condition.

It is important to distinguish between self-reported disability and disability as a social construct. In medical research, it is common for investigators to use self-reported disability as an outcome variable. For example, patients might be asked to complete the Roland-Morris scale, which assesses the extent to which they are limited in ADLs because of low back pain.[2] As a completely different matter, a patient with chronic pain might apply for work disability benefits from a workers' compensation carrier or some other agency that manages disability benefits. If the disability agency determines that the patient is eligible for benefits, he/she is granted the social status of being work disabled. As a consequence of this determination, he/she is exempted from selected customary societal obligations (i.e., working) and is likely to receive disability payments to compensate for lost income. This chapter focuses on the latter aspect of disability, work disability as a social construct.

Work disability can be subcategorized in several ways. The most important distinctions are between total and partial disability, and between temporary and permanent (or long-term) disability. Various disability agencies have programs tailored to these different categories of work disability. For example, the U.S. Social Security Administration (SSA) disability programs are designed for people who are permanently and totally disabled[3]; workers' compensation time loss benefits are paid to individuals who are totally, temporarily disabled; many private disability insurance policies provide benefits when an individual is disabled from performing his or her usual work, even if he or she is not totally disabled. In this chapter we will focus on permanent, pain-related disability.

Impairment

As with the term, disability, "impairment" does not have a unique definition. The American Medical Association's *Guides to the Evaluation of Permanent Impairment*, 5th edition (AMA Guides), provides one definition: "A loss, loss of use, or derangement of any body part, organ system, or organ function."[4] The World Health Organization (WHO) gives the following definition: "Impairments are problems in body function or structure as a significant deviation or loss."[5] The definition given in the 6th edition of the AMA Guides[6] is similar to the one used by WHO. Finally, the SSA offers the following definition: "Anatomical, physiological, or psychological abnormalities that can be shown by medically acceptable clinical and laboratory diagnostic

TABLE 22.1

IMPAIRMENT VERSUS DISABILITY

	Impairment	Disability
Typical Definition	A loss, loss of use, or derangement of any body part, organ system, or organ function†	The inability to engage in any substantial gainful activity by reason of any medically determinable physical or mental impairment(s) which can be expected to result in death or which has lasted or can be expected to last for a continuous period of not less than 12 months‡
Purpose	Determine the extent to which organs/body parts of an individual are compromised	Determine limitations in an individual's ability to perform various activities because of a medical condition
Level of analysis	Organs or body parts	The whole person
Subtypes	Irrelevant	Temporary vs. permanent Total vs. partial Work-related vs. other domains (e.g., inability to perform ADLs)

†Cocchiarella L, Andersson GBJ, eds. *Guides to the Evaluation of Permanent Impairment*. 5th ed. Chicago, Illinois: AMA Press, 2001.
‡Disability evaluation under Social Security. SSA Publication No. 64-039. Washington, D.C.: U.S. Government Printing Office, 2006.

techniques."[7] The present essay focuses on impairment as conceptualized by the AMA Guides, 5th and 6th editions.[4,6]

Although these definitions of impairment differ somewhat, they all emphasize that impairments are biomedical abnormalities that can be analyzed at the level of organs or body parts. In fact, a critical distinction between impairment and disability is that they address limitations at different levels of analysis—impairment refers to a limitation in the function or structure of an organ or body part, whereas disability refers to a limitation in the behavior of a person. This distinction is reflected in the syntax used to describe impairments and disabilities. For example, one would say "Ms. Smith's right leg is weak because of her polio" to describe her impairment, and "Ms. Smith is unable to walk up stairs" to describe her consequent disability.

While it is possible to distinguish conceptually between impairment (meaning dysfunction of an organ or body part) and disability (meaning an activity limitation secondary to an impairment), the distinction is often unclear in actual practice. For example, the notion of a measurably dysfunctional organ does not readily apply to psychiatric impairments. It is also difficult to make the distinction in conditions in which incapacitation is attributed to pain.

Associations Between Impairment and Disability

As many observers have noted, evaluations of impairment and evaluations of work disability can yield discrepant results. At one extreme (e.g., a violinist with amputation of the second and third digits of the left hand), an individual can have modest impairment, but severe work disability. At the opposite extreme (e.g., Stephen Hawking), an individual can have severe impairment but little or no work disability. But disability agencies typically assume a strong link between impairment and disability. First, they construe impairment as a necessary condition for disability. The logic underlying this requirement is simple. Disability programs are designed to assist individuals who are unable to compete in the workplace because of a medical condition. In essence, disability programs attempt to partition individuals who fail in the workplace into two large groups: those who fail because of a medical condition, and those who fail for nonmedical reasons. The distinction is necessary because there are many potential nonmedical reasons that may restrict employment, including a lack of demand for a job applicant's skills or an applicant's lack of motivation. Disability programs require evidence that an applicant has a medical problem underlying his/her workplace failure. Impairment provides the needed evidence, since it can be viewed as a marker that an individual has a medical problem which diminishes his/her capability. Conversely, if an individual has no identifiable impairment, this implies that employment limitations may not be due to a medical condition.

Second, disability agencies typically assume that the severity of a patient's impairment correlates with the degree and/or probability of his/her being disabled from work. Even when an agency compensates for work disability and not for impairment, it will often seek information about a patient's impairment to rationalize its decision about whether or not to award disability benefits. In this chapter, we will use the term "impairment" when the emphasis is on medical evaluation of the severity of an individual's derangement of organs or body parts, and "disability" when the emphasis is on evaluation of an individual's ability to work.

Institutions Involved With Disability

Communities frequently provide assistance to individuals who are incapacitated. This type of helping behavior can be seen not only in modern societies, but also in primitive ones. Indeed, evidence of such assistance even can be seen in communities of infra-human primates.[8] During the last 100 years, the informal understandings that have existed in communities regarding help for the infirm have been supplemented or replaced by formal disability programs. The development of such programs–for example, the Social Security Disability Insurance (SSDI) and the Supplemental Security Income (SSI) programs run by the SSA—has changed the dynamics of disability. In order to receive benefits, an individual having a medical problem that hinders activity must submit an application to an agency that administers a disability program. Adjudicators from the agency then determine whether the applicant meets eligibility criteria for benefits. In order to make this determination, the adjudicators typically request medical information from the applicant's treating physicians. Due to this need for pertinent medical information, physicians are routinely drawn into the disability determination process. This is true not only for SSI and SSDI, but also for other disability systems such as workers' compensation, the Veterans Administration, and private disability insurance programs.

When assessing impairment or disability, the physician must do so within the guidelines of the system within which the disability determination is to be made. In the present chapter, the term "disability agency" is used to refer to any insurance company or governmental organization that evaluates disability applications or dispenses disability benefits. A detailed discussion of different disability agencies can be found elsewhere.[9] In the United States, the disability agencies that physicians are most likely to encounter are the SSA, the Veterans Administration, the workers' compensation system, and various disability programs administered by private insurance companies. It is important to be aware that these agencies differ markedly with respect to their missions, their definitions of key concepts, and the demands they make on physicians. This chapter makes frequent references to the 5th and 6th editions of AMA Guides.[4,6] As the title indicates, that book describes procedures that can be used to determine the severity of impairment for claimants with a wide range of medical disorders. The book is important to any discussion of pain-related disability for two reasons. First, it is the most comprehensive work available on the evaluation of impairment. Second, many disability agencies require that applicants for disability be evaluated according to principles set out in the AMA Guides. Hence, it is imperative that physicians who provide disability evaluations become familiar with the principles described in the AMA Guides. At the time of this writing, most disability agencies rely on the 5th edition of the AMA Guides. However, the recently published 6th edition will almost certainly supersede the 5th edition in the near future.

The Administrative Imperative

As noted previously, disability programs are run by bureaucracies that can have distinct, and often unique, imperatives. For example, the SSA, which runs the two largest disability programs in the United States, strives for uniformity, objectivity, and cost containment in its disability evaluation procedures.[10] However sensible these goals are from a bureaucratic standpoint, they often are at odds with the clinical realities of patients with chronic pain.[11] In particular, the administrative imperative for objectivity leads agencies to assume that incapacitation associated with an injury or illness is (or should be) "transparent" to a physician (i.e., that the activity limitations described by patients should be highly correlated with evidence of tissue damage or organ dysfunction objectively assessed by a physician).

The administrative requirement that impairment/disability decisions be based on objective medical evidence of derangement in an organ or body part conflicts fundamentally with the evaluation of incapacitation secondary to pain. People with chronic pain typically attribute their pain and activity limitations to dysfunction of an organ or body part. But these subjective reports often are difficult to assess, primarily because examination of the involved organ or body part often does not reveal objective abnormalities that make the pain reports inevitable.[12] It often appears to an observer that the affected organ or body part is capable of functioning, but that the claimant *does not use it normally* because of pain.[13]

CONCEPTUAL PROBLEMS IN EVALUATING PAIN-RELATED DISABILITY

The Fundamental Dilemma

A key feature of pain is its subjectivity. Physicians and other observers can make inferences about a claimant's pain, but cannot directly experience it. To examine the significance of this feature of pain, it is useful to consider two conceptually distinct factors that might be considered in impairment ratings: objective factors such as atrophy of a limb or reduced ejection fraction and subjective factors such as pain. While objective medical factors can be assessed via methods (e.g., laboratory assays or imaging studies) that are independent of the subjective experiences and communications of a claimant, the assessment of subjective factors requires an examiner to interpret the behavior and communications of the claimant and to use these sources of information to infer the claimant's subjective experiences.

Disability agencies clearly and consistently attach great weight to objective factors in the determination of disability. The agencies, however, are inconsistent with respect to the weight (and legitimacy) that they attach to subjective factors. For example, the SSA specifically requires adjudicators to consider pain when they evaluate applicants for SSDI or SSI programs.[14] In sharp contrast, the Washington State Department of Labor and Industries specifically mandates that pain should not be considered in disability determinations regarding injured workers.[15]

It is worth noting that the challenge of assessing subjective factors is not limited to conditions in which chronic pain plays a major role. Very comparable assessment issues arise when impairment associated with mental illness is assessed. There are no established laboratory or imaging studies that identify an individual who suffers from depression or schizophrenia. In diagnosing these conditions and determining the extent of impairment associated with them, an examiner is forced to rely primarily on the verbal and nonverbal behaviors of a patient.

Pain versus Other Manifestations of Disorders: The Embeddedness Problem

One conceptual problem in any discussion of pain-related impairment is that pain is not completely distinct from organ/body part dysfunction. Rather, it is usually most appropriate to construe pain as a "component" of a medical disorder. From this perspective, it is arbitrary to examine the significance of pain in isolation from the medical condition underlying the pain, just as it would be arbitrary to evaluate shortness of breath in isolation from congestive heart failure. It would seem conceptually appropriate to evaluate a medical disorder as an entity with characteristic signs, symptoms, and pathophysiology. An impairment rating based on such an evaluation would take into account all manifestations of the disorder, including pain. Many disability agencies follow this logic: that is, they construe pain as one of many manifestations of injuries or diseases. This conceptualization involves the implicit assumption that impairment ratings based on objective evidence of derangement of organs or body parts capture the burden of illness borne by an individual, including the burden imposed by pain.

Unfortunately, this apparently plausible approach to the assessment of pain in the context of impairment ratings can run into either of two complications. First, pain severity may not (and often does not) correlate well with objective indicators of organ/body part dysfunction. In fact, empirical evidence has consistently demonstrated a low concordance between self-reports of pain and behavioral functioning (such as ADLs) or physiologic indices.[16,17] In such situations, impairment ratings based strictly on objective findings are likely to fail to capture the burden of illness of the disorder.

A second and even more difficult situation involves conditions that are associated with severe pain but are not amenable to conventional impairment ratings because they are not associated with unequivocal objective findings. In these conditions, it is not possible to make impairment ratings on the basis of such findings. Common examples include headache disorders and fibromyalgia.

TOWARD A SCIENTIFIC APPROACH TO PAIN-RELATED DISABILITY

Progress Since the Third Edition of *Bonica's Management of Pain*

The chapter on disability evaluation in the 3rd edition discussed conceptual dilemmas associated with the evaluation of pain-related disability and noted the paucity of scientific data that might help resolve these dilemmas. Unfortunately, the last 7 years have witnessed little progress in "disability science" that might inform a more rational approach to pain-related disability. Several problems have impeded progress.

Although some of the conundrums relevant to pain-related disability are amenable to empirical research (see later), there is a paucity of published studies that address relevant issues. Moreover, we are not aware of any attempt to synthesize empirical data that might be relevant to pain-related disability, much less attempt to consider the significance of such data for policy. As a result, the debate between those who consider pain an important element of disability determination and those who do not continues to rely on rhetoric rather than scientific data. Unfortunately, the rhetoric has only served to polarize the respective positions.

There is also a dearth of conceptual papers relevant to pain-related disability in the medical literature. For example, although there has been heated debate about the appropriate way to treat pain in the 6th edition of the AMA Guide,[18] we are not aware of any published paper in which proponents and opponents have presented their arguments relative to the place of pain assessment in impairment/disability evaluations. While relevant papers have been generated within disability agencies,[15] these are generally not available to the broad academic and/or disability determination community.

In particular, we are not aware of any published paper that weighs the relative importance of two key issues relevant to pain-related disability. One is that pain appears to be *relevant* to the incapacitation of many individuals (see later). The other is that incapacitation associated with pain is *difficult to assess*. Those who advocate giving great weight to pain in disability determinations emphasize the first point; opponents emphasize the second.

Agencies with different policies regarding pain-related disability have not published results of research on the effects of their policies and appear not to have tracked them carefully.[19] Also, it appears that there is little communication among disability agencies, perhaps because they often operate with different disability determination policies. As a result, the debate regarding pain-related disability has not been informed by the various experiments of nature represented by policies of different disability agencies. For example, as far as we know, the SSA and the Washington State Department of Labor and Industries have not compared the effects of their very different policies regarding the determination of pain-related disability.

Despite these caveats, a few contributions to the problem of pain-related disability have appeared in the last 7 years. In particular, the AMA Guides 5th edition[4] and the AMA Guides 6th edition[6] provide detailed discussions of problems in assessing impairment associated with pain. Also, the primary authors of the chapter on pain-related impairment in the 5th edition subsequently published a paper addressing conceptual issues regarding the evaluation of pain-related impairment.[13] Two law professors have published a detailed discussion of SSA regulations related to pain, along with crucial legal judgments regarding these regulations.[20] Finally, Waddell[21] has published a fascinating historical review of efforts by various jurisdictions in Canada to address pain-related disability. Although we note attention in these disparate venues to the problem of pain in the determination of disability, we also note the rather scattered nature of this attention. Clearly, the problem is sufficiently complex and of sufficient importance to merit a more integrated approach, such as that commissioned by the Institute of Medicine 20 years ago.[11]

Empirical Approaches to Pain-Related Disability

Several empirical issues bear on the feasibility of awarding disability benefits to individuals with incapacitating pain (Table 22.2). Specifically, the following questions are relevant and amenable to research: (1) What is the epidemiology of incapacitating chronic pain? (2) What is the relative contribution of objective factors and subjective factors to incapacitation in various medical conditions? (3) How accurate are physicians in assessing the burden of pain-related illness that individuals actually face? (4) Do the awards currently being provided by disability agencies match the future burden of illness/injury of claimants who report incapacitating pain? In the following sections, we discuss the rather limited data that bear on these questions.

Epidemiology of Pain-Related Disability

Analysis of the epidemiology of pain-related disability is compromised by the fact that it is difficult to get relevant data from disability agencies. There are several reasons for this difficulty. One is that there are multiple disability agencies that develop their own methods for recording and storing data about disability applicants and beneficiaries. There is no central repository for such data. Hence, access to such data, if it were to occur, would be piecemeal at best. Second, relevant data from private disability agencies are generally proprietary and not readily shared with

---

TABLE 22.2

EMPIRICAL ISSUES THAT BEAR ON THE FEASIBILITY OF EVALUATING PAIN-RELATED IMPAIRMENT AND DISABILITY

1. What is the epidemiology of incapacitating chronic pain?
2. What is the relative contribution of objective factors and subjective factors to incapacitation in various medical conditions?
3. How accurate are physicians in assessing the burden of pain-related illness that individuals actually face?
4. Do the awards currently being provided by disability agencies match the actual burden of illness/injury of claimants who report incapacitating pain?

the public. Third, medico-legal records related to disability claims have a limited shelf life; not only do most lawyers that represent disability claimants destroy records within 3 years of claim settlement, many agencies do so, as well.

Finally, disability agencies generally do not record information about claimants in ways that facilitate the study of pain in the incapacitation of beneficiaries. Although, as noted previously, disability agencies differ in the manner in which they code medical information regarding claimants, their general tendency is to rely on traditional diagnostic categories such as those given in ICD-9. The categories in ICD-9 do not provide direct information about the role of pain in incapacitation. While at least one agency, the SSA, has instructed adjudicators to gather such information, these data have not been gathered systematically enough to be useful.[19]

In the face of these limitations, the best available strategy for investigating the role of pain in claimants' reports of incapacitation is to look for proxies—conditions in which activity limitations are governed primarily by pain, and where the pain that patients report is not closely associated with objective findings of organ/body part derangement. Of course, the determination that a condition designated by an ICD-9 diagnosis is a pain syndrome involves judgment, and disagreements are inevitable. But in the absence of better data, we will consider sprains/strains and lumbar spine conditions to be representative conditions in which pain is the dominant reason for incapacitation, and objective findings of loss of function of the affected body area are minimal or inconclusive.

In identifying sprains/strains as proxies for pain syndromes, we recognize that these can be very specific diagnoses based on definable injuries to ligaments or muscles. For example, a tear of the anterior cruciate ligament would be coded as a sprain. However, informal observation suggests that the latter example is relatively rare. In most instances, a diagnosis of sprain/strain is made when an individual complains of pain, but there are no clear-cut findings of injury in the symptomatic area. Thus, when a patient complains of pain in his/her spine, upper extremity, or lower extremity, an examining physician typically considers the possibility that the patient's symptoms might be the result of a definable musculoskeletal abnormality (e.g., fracture) or neurologic abnormality (e.g., carpal tunnel syndrome). If such well defined conditions are ruled out, a diagnosis of sprain/strain is often the default option.

We consider most diagnoses of lumbar spine disorders to be proxies for pain syndromes because the incapacitation of individuals is generally not attributable to measurable mechanical failure of the spine, or to a loss of neurologic function in a lower extremity. Rather, the individuals are incapacitated by pain as they try to engage in various activities.[1,13]

Useful data about sprains/strains and low back disorders come from the Bureau of Labor Statistics (BLS).[22] For example, in 2003, there were 1,315,920 work injuries and occupational illnesses in the United States that required a worker to take time off work. Of these, 43% were coded as sprains/strains, and 18% as back injuries. (These two categories overlap, since most back injuries are coded as back strains/sprains.) BLS data on claims that require prolonged time away from work (more than 30 days) indicate similar trends: 43% of such claims were for sprains/strains, and 21.4% were for back injuries. Finally, unpublished data from the Washington State Department of Labor and Industries from 2003[23] provide information on work injuries that lead to more than 120 days off work. Twenty-one percent of these claims were for sprains/strains of the back. Although these data do not directly address permanent disability, there is strong evidence that the probability of indefinite work disability is high among workers who miss substantial periods of time from work shortly after their injuries.[24]

In summary, the previous data indicate that disorders characterized by pain that is at best loosely correlated with objective findings account for a very substantial proportion of protracted work disability claims. These data underline the importance of developing systems to evaluate claims of incapacitation secondary to pain.

Relative Contributions of Objective versus Subjective Factors in Disability

As described previously, pain is typically "embedded" in various medical disorders. Thus, it is often the case that when individuals complain of persistent pain, the pain can plausibly be attributed to a medical condition that is associated with objective indicators of organ/body part derangement. For example, a patient with significant coronary artery stenosis would have understandable reasons for his/her complaints of chest pain. In conditions where objective indicators of organ/body part derangement typically occur in conjunction with characteristic pain, the severity of an individual's incapacitation could in principle be assessed either by (1) evaluating the severity of the objective indicators, (2) by gathering subjective data from him/her about the burden of illness imposed by the condition because of pain, or (3) by some combination of the two strategies. Which of the approaches provides data that are most closely associated with the degree of incapacitation that the individual demonstrates?

Once some indicator of incapacitation has been defined (e.g., ability to work, or ability to perform ADLs), the previous question can be framed as a problem in prediction, and can be modeled by the following regression equation:

$$\text{Predicted } Y = f(X_1, X_2, \ldots\ldots X_n; x_1, x_2, \ldots\ldots\ldots x_m)$$

Where:

Predicted Y = a claimant's predicted ability to perform ADLs

$X_1, X_2, \ldots\ldots X_n$ = the claimant's "scores" on indices of organ or body part derangement

$x_1, x_2, \ldots\ldots\ldots x_m$ = the claimant's "scores" for self-reported pain severity, and severity of limitations imposed by pain

This conceptualization of the problem of assessing the role of subjective factors (pain) versus indicators of organ/body part derangement in incapacitation invites empirical exploration. Specifically, for a given medical condition, it would be possible to investigate correlations between: (1) organ or body part indices and self-report variables; (2) organ or body part indices and incapacitation; and (3) self-report variables and indices of incapacitation. Correlations among these classes of variables will, of course, depend on the medical condition under consideration and on the specific measures used to assess relevant variables. At one extreme, objective measures of organ dysfunction/derangement might accurately predict the degree of incapacitation of individuals with a given medical disorder, and subjective data might add nothing to the predictive equation. Alternatively, it is possible that subjective data are needed to maximize prediction of incapacitation.

It is beyond the scope of this chapter to review research in this complex area in any depth. However, in the specific case of noncatastrophic low back pain, self-report measures demonstrate the following statistical properties: (1) they are only modestly associated with objective indicators of spine dysfunction and (2) they are substantially correlated with functional outcome measures such as ability to perform ADLs.[25–36] Thus, a system to predict functional status among low back pain claimants is likely to be more accurate if it incorporates self-report data in addition to indices of spine function than if it relies solely on objective indices of spine function.

Judging Pain and Disability: Bias and Accuracy

As has been noted previously, the subjective nature of pain and the frequent failure of pain reports to correlate with available medical evidence greatly complicate disability determination. Patients can report severe pain in the absence of medical evidence[37,38] and they can describe little or no pain despite obvious lesions.[31] The inherent difficulties in evaluating patients' reports about their pain are magnified when the patients become claimants for benefits from disability agencies that require objective evidence of impairment.[39] A key question amenable to empirical research is whether examiners are capable of accurately judging the burden of illness borne by individuals who report incapacitating pain.

Historically, concerns regarding judgments of pain-related disability have been framed as a problem of inter-rater reliability.[40–42] Much of the focus of these concerns has centered on low back pain, secondary to its uncertain pathogenesis, its prevalence, and its associated costs, both medical and societal.[39,43–45] Unfortunately, systematic efforts to improve inter-rater reliability among disability examiners have met with somewhat mixed success.[46] Indeed, there is increasing evidence that variability in disability determination decisions may be a function of more than inter-rater error.[47,48] In particular, the variability may reflect uncertainty that is inherent in judging subjective phenomena such as pain.

Decisions made in the context of uncertainty have received considerable scrutiny in recent years,[49,50] although little directly involves decisions made regarding pain-related disability. That literature suggests that such decisions often are influenced by intuitive, rather than rational-deductive processes.[51] Moreover, when phenomena lack clear and specific evidence (as is common with chronic pain), judges tend to discount their importance.[52] Because pain is highly reliant upon self-report and often lacking objective evidentiary support, it is not surprising that observers (both lay and medical) tend to underestimate pain when patients report severe pain.[53,54] Although the precise mechanisms underlying this tendency are unclear, there is little doubt that the tendency to discount high levels of pain is consistent and widespread.

Negative stereotypes also exist for patients with symptoms of chronic pain and can influence assessment processes,[55,56] especially for those involved in compensation/litigation proceedings.[57] When observers are asked to make judgments of pain and pain-related disability for patients who fall into the latter category, those stereotypes have been shown to operate: judgments of symptom severity are significantly lower for patients involved in litigation proceedings than patients who are not.[58] Similarly, negative stereotypes exist for patients who describe severe pain without supporting medical evidence, as is often the case for patients with diagnoses of lumbar sprain/strain. Judgments of pain intensity and pain-related disability for patients without supporting medical evidence are reliably and substantially lower than those for patients with such evidence.[59,60] Not only does each of the above factors influence ratings of pain and disability independently, the factors have an additive effect when they are combined. Hence, litigating patients who report high levels of pain without supporting medical evidence present a very disadvantaged picture to examiners charged with making disability determinations.[61]

Aside from the situational factors described, several patient features also may systematically influence the disability determination process, potentially undermining its validity for pain-related conditions. For example, there is growing evidence that the race of an applicant can influence impairment[47] and disability ratings.[48] Further, socioeconomic status (SES) may influence ratings, such that lower SES applicants may receive lower ratings than do those from higher SES levels.[62] Finally, while less studied with regard to disability, gender also has been shown to influence observer estimates of pain: research has shown that women are seen as more emotional and more likely to over-report pain than men.[63] If the proclivity to discount pain reports from women extrapolates to a similar tendency in regard to their reports of pain-related dysfunction, women may be another group that is at risk of receiving lower ratings when disability is determined.

In addition to patient and situational factors, several characteristics of the rater may influence his/her disability ratings. One involves the rater's experience. Raters with more experience seem to underestimate pain to a greater degree than do those with less experience.[64–66] The precise mechanisms associated with this predisposition are unclear, but may have something to do with the fact that highly experienced clinicians draw upon increased levels of exposure to severe pain among patients that they have seen, such that the anchor points that describe "severe pain" differ from those of less experienced clinicians. Similarly, there is some evidence that a physician's specialty also may moderate his or her ratings; those whose specialties expose them to patients with catastrophic injuries and/or illnesses may rate pain and disability at lower levels than those whose practices comprise patients with more commonplace problems.[60] Each of these findings may have implications for disability determination: physicians who perform disability determinations usually are highly experienced and many also are surgeons. Thus, disability examiners may have characteristics that predispose them to underestimate levels of pain and pain-related disability in patients who present with a primary complaint of pain.

The Detection of Deception

The previous discussion focuses on general factors that influence evaluators when they rate disability in patients with chronic pain. However, it does not specifically address one key issue that bears on these ratings: the ability of evaluators to determine when patients are exaggerating their incapacitation or are deliberately feigning incapacitation.

Deception must be seen against the broader background of social influence. Throughout their lives, people develop strategies to meet their needs by influencing others.[67] The strategies they develop may be explicit and carefully planned, but they are often implicit and unplanned. When individuals develop medical problems, they frequently find that their needs can be met only if they can influence the physicians and other professionals with whom they interact. At a very basic level, patients want to be respected and thought of as "legitimate" by these professionals.[68] This is particularly true for patients with primary complaints of pain, many of whom may have been accused of malingering or having psychiatric problems.[56] Patients who are sensitive to such issues appear to present themselves clinically in a manner that lessens the likelihood of such accusations; they appear to downplay emotional aspects of pain and to emphasize its biological determinants.[69] Similarly, patients with pain problems may feel that they need certain kinds of treatment, such as chronic opioid therapy. They can satisfy this need only if they can convince their physicians that such therapy is appropriate. Patients who are applying for disability have an obvious need to convince disability evaluators of the legitimacy of their claims.

It stands to reason that pain patients will adapt interpersonal strategies they have developed in the past to the task of influencing health professionals so as to meet their needs. These strategies are subtle enough so that it is difficult to enumerate them or to decide which strategies deserve the appellation "deception". To put the matter differently, while it is possible to identify extremes of patient behavior—one anchored by complete forthrightness, and the other by deliberate, planned deception—many patients occupy a "gray zone" somewhere in the middle. They demonstrate "exaggerated" pain behavior or report "excessive" incapacitation from their pain, but do not appear to be deliberately falsifying information that they provide.[70-72] Terms like symptom magnification are often used to describe such presentations.

Outright deceit (malingering) by patients is a form of fraud.[73] There is a general consensus that patients who are malingering should not receive disability benefits. In practice, however, secondary to the subjective nature of pain and the uncertainties inherent in its evaluation, it is extremely difficult to discern outright deceit with confidence because that judgment ultimately resides in the eye of the beholder. Some physicians will find evidence of symptom magnification and suspect deliberate deception whenever a claimant reports symptoms or a degree of incapacitation that cannot be easily explained on the basis of objective findings. But as discussed, chronic pain poses a dilemma precisely because patients report incapacitation that cannot be fully explained on the basis of objective findings. To put the matter differently, pain patients almost always have symptom magnification relative to their objective findings, but this should not be automatically construed as evidence that they do not have valid claims.

There is an abundant literature on deception by patients with various medical complaints. Much of this comes from forensic settings. A few points deserve mention. First, frank malingering is a problem in patients with chronic pain, with prevalence estimates of up to 10%.[74] In particular, investigators have expressed concern that individuals with chemical dependency might present themselves as suffering from chronic pain in order to get opioids.[75] Second, evidence available from forensic research and other settings suggests that physicians are not particularly skilled at identifying deception on the part of pain patients.[75-78] Third, research on the ability of physicians to detect deception is hampered by conceptual ambiguity about what constitutes deception on the part of patients with chronic pain.

It is beyond the scope of this chapter to provide a detailed review of literature on the ability of disability evaluators to detect deception on the part of claimants with chronic pain. It is important to note, though, that a thorough analysis of the scientific basis for disability evaluation in the context of chronic pain would need to include a consideration of this literature.

Systemic Factors

While the research cited above raises concerns about the reliability and validity of disability determination examinations at the level of the individual claimant, those results do not obviate the need to examine disability determination processes at the systemic level. Indeed, the disability determination system is constructed in a manner that may mitigate the effects of a single examiner or examination. In fact, when substantive disagreement exists in regard to an applicant's level of disability, it is common for several medical opinions to be obtained, each of which is considered when an administrative law judge reaches a final determination.[79]

The issue of systemic fairness was examined for the State of California in a study commissioned through the RAND Institute for Civil Justice.[80] Because of the scale of the project, we will describe it in some detail. A crucial element of the study methodology involved the computation of actual earnings loss; this was derived from a comparison of the earnings of workers applying for workers' compensation benefits with a cohort of workers in similar occupations over the years of the study (January 1, 1991 to April 1, 1997). By comparing actual earnings loss with actual benefits, the study investigators were able to assess the equity of the system.

Study findings of most relevance to this chapter involved the "horizontal" and "vertical" equity of disability determinations for workers' compensation claims. Horizontal equity involved analysis of benefits relative to actual loss of earnings for workers who sustained injuries to different body parts (e.g., shoulder vs. low back). Horizontal equity would be demonstrated if the ratio between disability benefits and earning losses was the same for workers with different types of injuries. Vertical equity, on the other hand, involves the proportionality of benefits to different levels of actual earnings loss; vertical equity would be demonstrated if workers with a greater loss of earnings also received higher benefits than those with a lower loss of earnings.

Study findings relative to these metrics were mixed. In regard to horizontal equity, researchers found that injuries to some body parts (e.g., shoulders) were compensated at higher levels than injuries to other body parts (e.g., knee). For vertical equity, results appeared more encouraging: benefits correlated strongly with actual earnings loss. At a general level, therefore, the disability determinations seemed to reflect vertical equity in the California system.

The latter finding, however, masked significant inconsistencies in the data. Of particular note for this chapter, there was significant inconsistency in impairment ratings between physicians who were retained by applicants versus those retained by the defense. Further, those inconsistencies were greatest in conditions that required the subjective judgment of an examiner, typically involving multiple-impairment cases. While the report did not break out data specific to the issue of pain, its findings are of particular note relative to multiple impairments involving the back, for example, back and psychiatric disorders and back and lower extremity; both common among patients with chronic back pain. Among applicants with both back and lower extremity impairments, the average applicant rating exceeded the average defense rating by 86%. Among applicants with both back and psychiatric impairments, the difference averaged 94%. These data suggest that the factors described that operate at the level of the medico-legal encounter had systemic effects that apparently influenced final disability determination findings.

Related concerns are raised by other research more specific to disability applicants with low back pain. For example, a recent study followed these applicants approximately 2 years after claim settlement, collecting information regarding their functional status at that time.[62] The study found very little correlation between disability ratings and measures of functional status, including levels of pain severity, psychological distress, and disability/employment. Not only were the correlations between disability ratings and functional status weak, the correlations generally reflected an inverse relationship: claimants who had received higher disability ratings reported fewer functional problems. These data, although reflecting disability determination processes in only one state, nonetheless raise significant questions regarding the validity of current disability determination paradigms for applicants with pain as a primary cause of disablement.

Aside from the issues of equity and validity raised by the previous studies, other research suggests that systemic disparities may exist in the management of pain in workers with occupational injuries. Race/ethnicity and SES appear to be associated with levels of treatment, such that the rates of surgery and overall levels of medical care have been shown to be lower for African Americans and for lower SES applicants.[48,81] Moreover, because both surgery and level of medical care predict final disability ratings, the differences in treatment indirectly affected disability settlements for the latter groups. Further, race and SES also contributed directly to disability ratings, such that African American race was negatively associated with those ratings and SES positively associated with ratings. Finally, the clinical adjustment of African Americans and of poorer applicants was worse than that of their Caucasian and more affluent counterparts after their claims were settled.[82] Hence, the limited available data suggest that disability determination systems may disadvantage minority and lower SES applicants with low back pain in terms of treatment, claim settlement, and long-term outcomes.

Conclusion

While research that bears directly and indirectly on disability determination processes remains quite limited for patients with pain, it is sufficient to raise substantial questions about the validity and equity of those systems. At the level of the medico-legal encounter, there is reason to believe that situational, patient, and provider factors contribute to systematic variability in ratings. At the level of the disability system, there is reason to believe that significant inequities are meted out to applicants with a primary complaint of pain, and those inequities may impact applicants at multiple levels: in the delivery of care, in claim settlement, and in postsettlement outcomes.

The scientific evidence is limited in a number of ways beyond its relative scarcity. First, the research is limited geographically. Because it has occurred primarily at the state level (e.g., California, Missouri), there is a real need for a broader examination of disability systems at a multi-state or national level. Second, research has focused primarily on workers' compensation systems; there is a need to examine other systems for disability determination (SSA disability, Veterans' Affairs, etc.). Finally, much of the research has focused on low back pain. While low back pain constitutes a substantial dilemma for disability determination systems (especially in the absence of verifiable objective impairment), it certainly is not the only condition for which pain represents the primary source of dysfunction. For example, fibromyalgia and other forms of musculoskeletal pain also are widespread causes of disability.[83–86] As such, these conditions also merit specific empirical attention if a more valid and equitable approach to disability determination is to be undertaken.

PAIN-RELATED IMPAIRMENT/ DISABILITY: CHALLENGES FOR THE CLINICIAN

Physicians play a crucial role in the roughly 7 million disability evaluations that are done annually in the United States. Sometimes physicians are hired by insurance companies or disability agencies to perform independent medical examinations on patients whom they are not treating. In other instances, physicians are asked (or required) to make disability judgments about patients whom they are treating.

Treating physicians have good reason to feel discomfort when they make disability judgments about their patients. In a general way, the process of disability evaluation places a physician in the middle, between his/her patient and a variety of disability agencies. In the best of circumstances, this often has the feel of fitting a round peg into a square hole, since the administrative categories established by disability agencies often do not match the clinical realities of patients. In the worst case, clinicians end up feeling caught in the crossfire between warring adversaries. They may perceive employees of disability agencies as unenlightened bureaucrats who make excessive demands for documentation and seem to lose the forest for the trees. At the same time, they may perceive their patients as reporting extraordinary amounts of incapacitation, and trying to enlist physicians as allies in their battles with disability agencies. It is beyond the scope of this chapter to discuss the multiple challenges that clinicians face as they interface between their patients and disability agencies. Detailed discussions of these issues are available.[12,87–90] We will thus confine ourselves to a few salient comments.

1. Treating physicians usually prefer to avoid the task of rendering judgments about whether their patients are disabled from work. Unfortunately, this is typically not an option. Disability agencies generally will not grant disability benefits to an applicant unless his/her treating physician supports the application. Thus, if a physician fails to complete disability forms for his/her patient, the patient is penalized.
2. The types of data required by physicians and the manner in which physician information is processed vary widely from one disability agency to another. In order to address a patient's requests fairly, a physician must be familiar with the disability agency with which he or she is interacting.
3. Disability agencies routinely insist that treating physicians base their judgments about disability on objective findings. As noted previously, if this demand is followed, patients incapacitated by pain would never receive disability. As discussed by Robinson,[12] treating physicians often need to reject the administrative demand for objectivity.

CONCLUSION

This chapter has focused on problems associated with disability evaluation for chronic pain at a societal level. We have described some of the dilemmas and controversies in this area, have outlined research issues that bear on the question of whether pain-related disability can be reliably and validly assessed, and have briefly discussed research on these issues. Our goal has been to demonstrate the possibility (and need) of performing empirical research on pain-related disability rather than to exhaustively review the research that has been done thus far. The research that we have reviewed supports the following conclusions: (1) incapacitation secondary to pain occurs frequently in the workplace; (2) in at least some highly prevalent conditions, it is necessary to consider subjective information (especially pain) in order to predict how incapacitated patients are likely to be; (3) the ability of clinicians to "decode" the verbal messages that patients provide about their pain and their burden of illness is limited; and (4) current systems for awarding disability benefits probably underestimate the burden of illness created by chronic pain.

In our opinion, policies regarding pain-related disability are in disarray. Disability agencies vary widely in the way they approach this problem. For example, the SSA requires adjudicators to consider pain when they evaluate disability applications, while the Washington State Department of Labor and Industries requires adjudicators *not* to consider pain. There appears to be little communication between agencies about the pros and cons of various policies regarding pain-related disability, and the medical literature on the subject is virtually nonexistent.

In our view, several steps must occur if rational policies regarding pain-related disability are to emerge (Table 22.3). First, there needs to be a dialogue about the problems associated with assessing pain-related disability. This dialogue will be productive only if it addresses both horns of the dilemma of pain-related disability simultaneously—the relevance of pain to work incapacity and the difficulty of assessing the burden of pain. Second, further research is needed on the empirical issues described previously, and other researchable questions regarding pain-related disability policy should be identified. Third, disability agencies need to assess the effectiveness of policies they have developed regarding

TABLE 22.3

STEPS NEEDED TO DEVELOP RATIONAL POLICIES REGARDING PAIN-RELATED DISABILITY

1. Dialogue among professionals about the problems associated with assessing pain-related disability.
2. Simultaneous consideration of the relevance of pain to work incapacity and the difficulty of assessing the burden of pain.
3. Further research on empirical issues that bear on the feasibility of assessing pain-related disability.
4. Assessment by disability agencies of the effectiveness of their current policies for evaluating pain-related disability.
5. Better communication among disability agencies regarding policies for evaluating pain-related disability.

pain-related disability; it would be advantageous if they could establish channels of interagency communication in conducting these assessments. A related point is that it is important that questions related to the determination of pain-related disability be addressed on a wider stage than has been the case thus far. Most research has been constrained by geographic limitations; studies on a national scope are needed if a piecemeal approach to this issue is to be avoided.

In the absence of rational policies regarding pain-related disability, it is difficult to provide guidance to the clinician who addresses pain-related disability in patients he/she treats. We have outlined a few rules of thumb that we believe will help such clinicians, and have referred to publications in which one of us (JPR) has discussed the practical problems of disability management by clinicians in more detail. However, we are convinced that clinicians will not get any respite until disability agencies come to terms with the problems of pain-related impairment/disability, and develop empirically driven rules and assessment methods that are consistent and acceptable to treating physicians.

ACKNOWLEDGMENT

This work was supported in part by grant R01 HS014007 from the Agency for Healthcare Research and Quality.

References

1. Robinson JP. Evaluation of function and disability. In: Loeser JD, ed. *Bonica's Management of Pain*. 3rd ed. Philadelphia: Lippincott Williams & Wilkins; 2001.
2. Schiphorst Preuper HR, Reneman MF, Boonstra AM, et al. The relationship between psychosocial distress and disability assessed by the Symptom Checklist-90-Revised and Roland Morris Disability Questionnaire in patients with chronic low back pain. *Spine* 2007;7(5):525–530.
3. *Disability evaluation under Social Security*. Washington, DC: U.S. Government Printing Office; 2006. SSA Publication No. 64–039.
4. Cocchiarella L, Andersson GBJ, eds. *Guides to the Evaluation of Permanent Impairment*. 5th ed. Chicago, IL: AMA Press; 2001.
5. World Health Organization. *International Classification of Functioning, Disability and Health*. Geneva: World Health Organization; 2001.
6. Rondinelli RD, ed. *Guides to the Evaluation of Permanent Impairment*. 6th ed. Chicago: American Medical Association; 2008.
7. *Disability Evaluation Under Social Security*. Washington, DC: U.S. Government Printing Office; 1994. SSA Publication No. 64–039.
8. Fabrega H. *Evolution of Sickness and Healing*. Berkeley: University of California Press; 1997.
9. Demeter SL, Andersson GBJ, Smith GM. *Disability Evaluation*. Chicago: American Medical Association; 1996.
10. Derthick M. *Agency Under Stress*. Washington, DC: The Brookings Institution; 1990.
11. Osterweis M, Kleinman A, Mechanic D, eds. *Pain and Disability*. Washington, DC: National Academy Press; 1987.
12. Robinson, JP. Disability evaluation in painful conditions. In: Turk DC, Melzack R, eds. *Handbook of Pain Assessment*. 2nd ed. New York: The Guilford Press; 2001.
13. Robinson JP, Turk DC, Loeser JD. Pain, impairment, and disability in the AMA Guides. *J Law Med Ethics* 2004;32(2):315–326.
14. Dorf V. Disability evaluation in the Social Security Administration. In: RF Schmidt, WD Willis, eds. *Encyclopedic Reference of Pain*. Berlin: Springer–Verlag; 2007.
15. *Medical Examiner's Handbook: Impairment ratings and independent medical examinations in Washington State Workers' Compensation*. Olympia, Washington: Department of Labor and Industries; 2005. Publication F252-001 1-000.
16. Flores L, Gatchel R, Polatin PB. Objectification of functional improvement after nonoperative care. *Spine* 1997;22:1622–1633.
17. Gatchel RJ. Comorbidity of chronic mental and physical health disorders: the biopsychosocial perspective. *Am Psychol* 2004;59:792–805.
18. Rondinelli R. Personal communication, September, 2007.
19. Dorf V. Personal communication, October, 2007.
20. Schneider EK, Simeone JJ. Pain and disability under Social Security: time for a new standard. *J Health Law* 2001;34(3):459–485.
21. Waddell G. *Compensation for Chronic Pain*. London: The Stationery Office; 2004.
22. United States Department of Labor; Bureau of Labor Statistics. Cases and demographic characteristics of work-related injuries and illnesses involving days

23. away from work. Available online at http://www.bls.gov/iif/oshcdnew.htm. Accessed January 21, 2008.
23. Lisann Rolle, Department of Labor and Industries, personal communication, July, 2005.
24. Cheadle A, Franklin G, Wolfhagen C, et al. Factors influencing the duration of work-related disability: a population-based study of Washington State workers' compensation. *Am J Public Health* 1994;84(2):190–196.
25. Cox ME, Asselin S, Gracovetsky SA, et al. Relationship between functional evaluation measures and self-assessment in nonacute low back pain. *Spine* 2000;25:1817–1826.
26. Deyo RA, Andersson G, Bombardier C, et al. Outcome measures for studying patients with low back pain. *Spine* 1994;19:2032S–2036S.
27. Lee CE, Simmonds MJ, Novy DM, et al. Self-reports and clinician-measured physical function among patients with low back pain: a comparison. *Arch Phys Med Rehabil* 2001;82:227–231.
28. Severeijns R, Vlaeyen JWS, van den Hout MA, et al. Pain catastrophizing predicts pain intensity, disability, and psychological distress independent of the level of physical impairment. *Clin J Pain* 2001;17:165–172.
29. Waddell G. 1987 Volvo award in clinical sciences. A new clinical model for the treatment of low-back pain. *Spine* 1987;12:632–644.
30. Boden SD, Davis DO, Dina TS, et al. Abnormal magnetic-resonance scans of the lumbar spine in asymptomatic subjects. *J Bone Joint Surg Am* 1990;72: 403–408.
31. Jensen MC, Brant–Zawadski MN, Obuchowski N, et al. Magnetic resonance imaging of the lumbar spine in people with back pain. *New Engl J Med* 1994; 331:69–73.
32. Boos N, Semmer N, Elfering A, et al. Natural history of individuals with asymptomatic disc abnormalities in magnetic resonance imaging: predictors of low back pain-related medical consultation and work incapacity. *Spine* 2000;25: 1482–1492.
33. Borenstein DG, O'Mara JW Jr, Boden SD, et al. The value of magnetic resonance imaging of the lumbar spine to predict low-back pain in asymptomatic subjects: a seven-year follow-up study. *J Bone Joint Surg Am* 2001;83-A: 1306–1311.
34. Wiesel SW, Tsourmas N, Feffer H, et al. A study of computer-assisted tomography. 1. The incidence of positive CAT scans in an asymptomatic group of patients. *Spine* 1984;9:549–551.
35. Jarvik JJ, Hollingworth W, Heagerty P, et al. The Longitudinal Assessment of Imaging and Disability of the Back (LAIDBack) Study: baseline data. *Spine* 2001;26:1158–1166.
36. Carragee E, Alamin T, Cheng I, et al. Does minor trauma cause serious low back illness? *Spine* 2006;31(25):2942–2949.
37. Beattie PF, Meyers SP. Magnetic resonance imaging in low back pain: general principles and clinical issues. *Phys Ther* 1998;78:738–753.
38. Fraser RD, Sandhu A, Gogan WJ. Magnetic resonance imaging findings 10 years after treatment for lumbar disc herniation. *Spine* 1995;20:710–714.
39. Hadler NM. Work incapacity from low back pain: the international quest for redress. *Clin Orthop Relat Res* 1997;336:79–93.
40. Greenwood JG. Low-back impairment-rating practices of orthopaedic surgeons and neurosusrgeons in West Virginia. *Spine* 1985;10:773–776.
41. Osterweis M, Kleinman A, Mechanic D, eds. *Pain and Disability: Clinical, Behavioral, and Public Policy Perspectives*. Institute of Medicine Committee on Pain, Disability and Chronic Illness Behavior. Washington, DC: National Academy Press; 1987.
42. Rucker KS, Metzler HM. Predicting subsequent employment status of SSA disability applicants with chronic pain. *Clin J Pain* 1995;11:22–35.
43. Deyo RA, Cherkin D, Conrad D, et al. Cost, controversy, crisis: low back pain and the health of the public. *Annu Rev Public Health* 1995;12:141–156.
44. Fordyce WE. *Back Pain in the Workplace*. Seattle: IASP Press; 1995.
45. Waddell G. Low back pain: a twentieth century health care enigma. *Spine* 1996;21:2820–2825.
46. Clark W, Haldeman S. The development of guideline factors for the evaluation of disability in neck and back injuries. *Spine* 1993;18:1736–1745.
47. Tait RC, Chibnall JT. Work injury management of refractory low back pain: relations with ethnicity, legal representation, and diagnosis. *Pain* 2001;91: 47–56.
48. Tait RC, Chibnall JT, Andresen EM, et al. Management of occupational back injuries: differences among African Americans and Caucasians. *Pain* 2004;112: 389–396.
49. Kahneman D. A perspective on judgment and choice. *Am Psychol* 2003;58: 697–720.
50. Tversky A, Kahneman D. Availability: a heuristic for judging frequency and probability. *Cognit Psychol* 1973;5:207–232.
51. Burgess DJ, van Ryn M, Crowley–Matoka M, et al. Understanding the provider contribution to race/ethnicity disparities in pain treatment: insights from dual process models of stereotyping. *Pain Med* 2006;7:119–134.
52. Redelmeier DA, Koehlor DJ, Liberman V, et al. Probability judgment in medicine: discounting unspecified possibilities. *Med Decis Making* 1995;15: 227–230.
53. Grossman SA, Sheidler VR, Swedeen K, et al. Correlation of patient and caregiver ratings of cancer pain. *J Pain Symptom Manage* 1991;6:53–57.
54. Solomon P. Congruence between health professionals' and patients' pain ratings: a review of the literature. *Scand J Caring Sci* 2001;15:174–180.
55. Marbach JJ, Lennon MC, Link BG, et al. Losing face: sources of stigma perceived by chronic facial pain patients. *J Behav Med* 1990;13:583–604.

56. Merskey H, Teasell RW. The disparagement of pain: social influences on medical thinking. *Pain Res Manage* 2000;5:259–270.
57. Mendelson G. Compensation and chronic pain. *Pain* 1992;48:121–123.
58. Chibnall JT, Tait RC. Social and medical influences on attributions and evaluations of chronic pain. *Psychol Health* 1999;14:719–729.
59. Chibnall JT, Tait RC, Ross L. The effects of medical evidence and pain intensity on medical student judgments of chronic pain patients. *J Behav Med* 1997;20:257–271.
60. Chibnall JT, Tait RC, Merys S. Disability management of low back injuries by employer-retained physicians: ratings and costs. *Am J Ind Med* 2000;38:529–538.
61. Tait RC, Chibnall JT. Physician judgments of patients with intractable low back pain. *Soc Sci Med* 1997;45:1199–1205.
62. Tait RC, Chibnall JT, Andresen EM, et al. Disability determination: validity with occupational low back pain. *J Pain* 2006;7:951–957.
63. Martin R, Lemos K. From heart attacks to melanoma: do common sense models of somatization influence symptom interpretation for female victims? *Health Psychol* 2002;21:25–32.
64. Choiniere M, Melzack R, Girard N, et al. Comparisons between patients' and nurses' assessment of pain medication efficacy in severe burn injuries. *Pain* 1990;40:143–152.
65. Marquie L, Raufaste E, Lauque D, et al. Pain rating by patients and physicians: evidence of systematic pain miscalibration. *Pain* 2003;102:289–296.
66. Prkachin KM, Solomon P, Hwang T, et al. Does experience influence judgments of pain behaviour? Evidence from relatives of pain patients and therapists. *Pain Res Manag* 2001;6:105–112.
67. Goffman E. *The Presentation of Self in Everyday Life.* Garden City, New York: Doubleday; 1959.
68. Shorter E. *From Paralysis to Fatigue.* New York: The Free Press; 1992.
69. Deshields TL, Tait RC, Gfeller JD, et al. Relationship between social desirability and self-report in chronic pain patients. *Clin J Pain* 1995;11(3):189–193.
70. Sterling M, Jull G, Vicenzino B, et al. Sensory hypersensitivity occurs soon after whiplash injury and is associated with poor recovery. *Pain* 2003; 104:509–517.
71. Ferrari R. The clinical relevance of symptoms amplification. *Pain* 2004;107:276–277.
72. Greve KW, Bianchini KJ. More on the clinical and scientific relevance of 'symptom amplification' and psychological factors in pain. *Pain* 2004;110(1–2):499–500; author reply 500–502.
73. Mendelson G, Mendelson D. Malingering pain in the medicolegal context. *Clin J Pain* 2004;20(6):423–432.
74. Fishbain DA, Cutler R, Rosomoff HL, et al. Chronic pain disability exaggeration/malingering and submaximal effort research. *Clin J Pain* 1999; 15(4):244–274.
75. Jung B, Reidenberg MM. Physicians being deceived. *Pain Med* 2007;8(5):433–437.
76. Hall HV, Pritchard DA. *Detecting Malingering and Deception.* Delray Beach, Florida: St. Lucie Press; 1996.
77. Craig KD, Badali MA. Introduction to the special series on pain deception and malingering. *Clin J Pain* 2004;20(6):377–382.
78. Hill ML, Craig KD. Detecting deception in pain expressions: the structure of genuine and deceptive facial displays. *Pain* 2002;98(1–2):135–144.
79. Hinderer SR, Rjondinelli RD, Katz RT. Measurement issues in impairment rating and disability evaluation. In: Rondinelli RD, Katz RT, eds. *Impairment Rating and Disability Evaluation.* Philadelphia: WB Saunders; 2000:35–52.
80. Reville RT, Seabury SA, Neuhauser FW, et al. An Evaluation of California's Permanent Disability Rating System. Santa Monica, CA: RAND Corporation; 2005. MG-258.
81. Chibnall JT, Tait RC, Andresen EM, et al. Race differences in diagnosis and surgery for occupational low back injuries. *Spine* 2006;31:1272–1275.
82. Chibnall JT, Tait RC, Andresen EM, et al. Race and socioeconomic differences in post-settlement outcomes for African American and Caucasian workers' compensation claimants with low back injuries. *Pain* 2005;114:462–472.
83. Gervais RO, Russell AS, Green P, et al. Effort testing in patients with fibromyalgia and disability incentives. *J Rheumatol* 2001;28:1892–1899.
84. White KP, Speechley M, Harth M, et al. Comparing self-reported function and work disability in 100 community cases of fibromyalgia syndrome versus controls in London, Ontario: the London Fibromyalgia Epidemiology Study. *Arthritis Rheum* 1999;42:76–83.
85. Wolfe F. Disability and the dimensions of distress in fibromyalgia. *J Musculoskel Pain* 1993;1:65–88.
86. Wolfe F, Anderson J, Harkness D, et al. Work and disability status of persons with fibromyalgia. *J Rheumatol* 1997;24:1171–1178.
87. Robinson JP. Pain and disability. In: Jensen TS, Wilson PR, Rice A, eds. *Clinical Pain Management: Chronic Pain.* London: Edward Arnold Limited; 2002.
88. Robinson JP, Turk DC. Compensation, disability assessment, and pain in the workplace. In: Schmidt RF, Willis WD, eds. *Encyclopedic Reference of Pain.* Berlin: Springer–Verlag, 2007.
89. Robinson JP. Disability management in primary care. In: McCarberg B, Passik SD, eds. *Expert Guide to Pain Management.* American College of Physicians; 2005.
90. Robinson JP, Seroussi RE. Impairment rating and disability determination. In: Braddom RL, ed. *Physical Medicine and Rehabilitation.* 3rd ed. Philadelphia: Elsevier; 2007.

CHAPTER 23 ■ MULTIDISCIPLINARY ASSESSMENT OF PATIENTS WITH CHRONIC PAIN

DENNIS C. TURK AND JAMES P. ROBINSON

INTRODUCTION

This chapter deals with the multidisciplinary assessment of patients with chronic noncancer pain. In order to be specific, especially with regard to the medical evaluation of chronic pain patients, we organize the discussion around a typical and common chronic pain problem (e.g., persistent cervical spine pain). We note, though, that many of the concepts in the chapter are relevant to the assessment of virtually any chronic pain patient. In particular, concepts related to the assessment of psychological factors, social factors, and functional limitations have wide applicability.

A key premise in this chapter is that multiple factors influence the symptoms and functional limitations of patients with chronic pain. As a consequence, we believe that evaluation along multiple dimensions, performed by professionals with a variety of skills, provides important insights into the factors governing the complaints of these patients and assists in treatment planning.

CONCEPTUAL ISSUES

Conundrums in the Assessment of Pain

How we think about symptoms such as pain influences the way in which we go about evaluating patients. Physicians and the lay public alike tend to assume that some underlying pathology is both a necessary and a sufficient cause of the symptoms reported and experienced by patients. Consequently, medical assessment usually begins with taking a thorough history and performing a physical examination, followed by, when deemed appropriate, laboratory tests and diagnostic imaging procedures in an attempt to identify or confirm the presence of an underlying pathology that *causes* the symptom (see later). In the absence of identifiable organic pathology, the physician may assume that the report of symptoms stems from psychological factors (i.e., personality characteristics, psychopathology, malingering). A psychological evaluation may be requested to detect the underlying psychological factors that underlie the patient's reports. Thus, there is a duality where the report of symptoms is attributed to *either* somatic *or* psychogenic mechanisms. This dualistic perspective dates back at least to the 17th century and the philosopher René Descartes. The assumption that symptoms that cannot be explained by medical findings must originate from psychological distress is, albeit unfortunately common, overly simplistic and inconsistent with current scientific understanding. The dichotomous view is incomplete and, as described throughout this chapter, is not compatible with available research evidence or the current understanding of chronic pain.[1]

Over the years, research has revealed puzzling observations that challenge the presumed isomorphism between pain and organic pathology. For example, the exact pathophysiology underlying some of the most common and recurring acute (e.g., primary headache) and chronic (e.g., back pain, fibromyalgia [FM]) pain problems is largely unknown. Conversely, several studies using plain radiography, computed tomography (CT), and magnetic resonance imaging (MRI) reveal that more than 30% of *asymptomatic* individuals have structural abnormalities such as herniated discs and spinal stenosis that would be accepted as valid explanations of pain if the individuals had been symptomatic.[2-6] In the case of FM, although a number of endocrine, immunological, and neurochemical perturbations have been investigated, there is currently no consensus regarding the causal mechanisms for the symptoms reported.[7] Thus, we are confronted with a rather strange set of circumstances: people with no identified organic pathology who report severe pain and, conversely, others with significant pathology who are apparently pain free.

A Conceptual Model for Assessing Pain

The conundrums described suggest that multiple factors likely contribute to persistent pain and related disability. There is a growing consensus that these consist of (1) genetic composition,[8] (2) physical pathology associated with trauma or disease, (3) alterations in the peripheral and central nervous system attributable to initial insult (peripheral and central sensitization), (4) psychological contributors including prior learning history and available coping resources (e.g., emotional support, financial resources, acquired coping skills), and (5) environmental influences (e.g., response by significant others, disability compensation, features inherent in the workplace) that all likely interact. A comprehensive evaluation should provide information about each of these factors, although examination of unique genetic contributions is in its infancy at this time but will likely be gaining attention in the coming years. Thus, in this chapter we will describe a general strategy for assessing factors 2 to 5.

Pain Behavior

It is useful to begin a discussion of assessment of patients with chronic pain with the concept of pain behaviors. Pain is a subjective perception and there is currently no objective way to know about the experience of pain other than by patients' behavior. Pain behaviors include verbal behaviors (i.e., statements about pain). They also include nonverbal behaviors such as limping or wincing. These pain behaviors are sources of communication; they convey to others the presence and severity of pain.

The challenge for an examiner is how to interpret patients' pain behaviors. Although these behaviors are sometimes determined entirely by an abnormal biological process in the area of injury, they are typically also influenced by changes in nervous system encoding and processing of nociceptive signals, by a patient's beliefs and appraisals, emotional status, coping strategies, and by the social environment.

Classes of Variables Underlying Pain Behavior

We will return to more formal assessment of pain behaviors later in this chapter. For now, a useful way to conceptualize this challenge is to think of a prediction equation with multiple unknowns:

$$PB = f(Xa1, Xa2 \ldots Xan1; Xb1, Xb2 \ldots \ldots Xbn2; Xc1, Xc2 \ldots \ldots Xcn3; Xd1, Xd2 \ldots Xdn4)$$

Where PB = the pain behavior that a patient demonstrates, and predictor variables are organized into four categories, such that Xa1, Xa2. . .Xan1 refer to biomedical factors at the end organ where the patient reports pain; Xb1, Xb2 . . . . . . Xbn2 refer to alterations in nervous system function (especially central nervous system sensitization) that perpetuate pain after nociceptive impulses from the end organ have diminished or ceased; Xc1, Xc2 . . . . Xcn3 refer to psychological variables; and Xd1, Xd2 . . . Xdn4 refer to social or contextual variables that influence pain behavior.[9a]

The prediction equation emphasizes the multiplicity of factors that influence patients' expressions of pain and highlights the dilemma facing an evaluating physician. The dilemma is that it is extremely difficult to determine the weights that should be assigned to various factors for an individual patient. To make matters even worse, there is no consensus about what the possible variables within various categories are (e.g., to specify the types of psychological factors that may affect a patient's pain behavior).

In accordance with the model, the discussion is organized around the assessment of medical factors, central nervous system sensitization, psychological factors, and social factors in chronic pain patients. We also consider the assessment of the severity of functional incapacitation in these patients.

ASSESSMENT OF MEDICAL FACTORS

A careful medical evaluation is a basic element in a multidisciplinary evaluation of a patient with chronic pain. The general goals of such an evaluation are to: (1) make a medical diagnosis; (2) determine whether additional diagnostic testing is needed; (3) make a judgment about the extent to which medical data regarding a patient adequately explain his or her symptoms and the severity of his or her apparent incapacitation; (4) determine whether there is any medical or surgical treatment that has a reasonable chance of reversing the pathophysiologic processes underlying the patient's pain; (5) determine whether there are any symptomatic treatments that should be prescribed if a reversal of pathophysiology is not possible; and (6) establish the objectives of treatment.

The specific procedures that physicians perform and the differential diagnostic possibilities they entertain vary enormously with patients' symptoms and presumed medical disorders. For example, the medical evaluation of a patient with pelvic pain is entirely different from the evaluation of a patient with neck pain. Also, the medical evaluation of a pain patient depends on the chronicity of the patient's symptoms and the medical evaluations and diagnostic testing that the patient has already undergone.

In order to be reasonably specific, the discussion here focuses on the medical evaluation of patients with persistent neck pain following a "whiplash" injury. Although some of the procedures are specifically relevant to this patient population, many of them can be employed in the evaluation of virtually any chronic pain patient.

There is no uniformly accepted algorithm for evaluating neck pain patients. In fact, as will be discussed, physicians differ sharply about some aspects of such evaluations. The approach discussed later is summarized in Figure 23.1, which identifies key questions that should be asked in the evaluation of a patient with persistent neck pain.

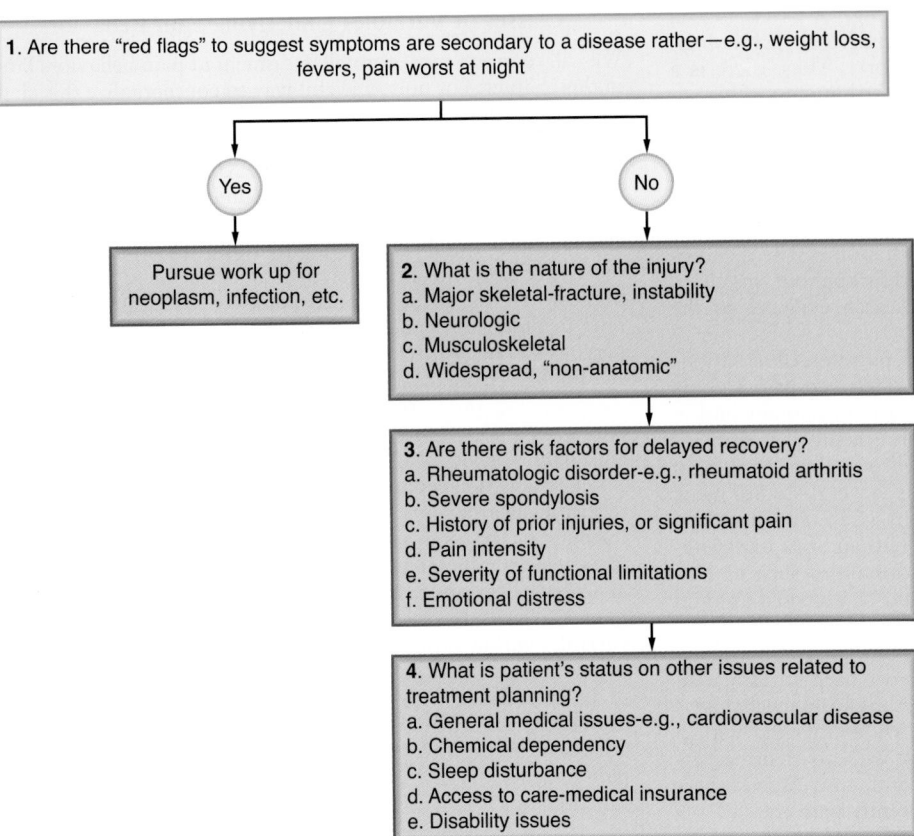

FIGURE 23.1 Key issues to address in the medical evaluation of chronic pain patients.

Are There Red Flags?

Although the assumption in this section is that the patient is undergoing evaluation for residuals of a neck injury, occasionally the physician will find that the patient has misattributed his or her symptoms, and is actually symptomatic because of a disease rather than because of any injury.

1. A general medical history that addresses issues such as weight loss or fevers should alert the physician to focus on the possibility of neoplasm or infection.[9]
2. If symptoms appear to be the result of injury, what is the nature of the injury?
   a. Neurologic disorders. The physician needs to be alert to clinical evidence of a cervical radiculopathy or a myelopathy. Evidence for these possibilities is obtained from the patient's history (e.g., pain and paresthesias into an extremity in a segmental distribution) and a careful neurologic examination.
   b. Major skeletal injuries. When a history of significant trauma is elicited, radiologic studies are needed to rule out the possibility that a patient has a spinal fracture, or a ligamentous injury severe enough to yield instability. X-rays that include flexion and extension views are usually sufficient.
   c. Widespread "nonanatomic" pain. Physicians who practice musculoskeletal medicine try to explain symptoms following an injury in terms of some structural lesion in joints, periarticular tissues, muscles, and nerves in the body region where the patient is symptomatic.[10] Although this approach often uncovers a potential cause, the symptoms of some patients with chronic pain do not fit a pattern that suggests some discrete injury to a musculoskeletal struc-

ture. For example, Figure 23.2 is a pain drawing provided by a chronic pain patient reporting initially lower back pain sustained when lifting a heavy box on her job. Although the patient reported that the only injuries she sustained were localized, the figure indicates that she was now experiencing widespread pain. In interpreting such figures, it is important to note that research has demonstrated that irritation of intervertebral discs and facet joints produce characteristic patterns of referred pain.[11,12] Thus, it is sometimes possible to explain widespread symptoms as indications of referred pain. However, the drawing shown in Figure 23.2 does not lend itself to such an interpretation, since it does not conform to any known pattern of referred pain from a spinal structure. The most plausible interpretation of such widespread pain is that it is a manifestation of altered perception based on central nervous system sensitization (CNSS, described later) or psychological factors.
   d. Musculoskeletal pain apparently emanating from joints of the spine. Patients who present with localized axial cervical spine pain or pain in a pattern suggesting referral from a joint in the cervical spine[11,12] are often very difficult to evaluate medically. In principle, such pain could be the product of irritation of several different structures in the cervical spine, including intervertebral discs, facet joints, and various ligaments. Since a physical examination typically does not identify the structural basis of axial cervical spinal pain, the examining physician is faced with the challenge of deciding whether to refer such a patient for advanced evaluation procedures as discussed later.

Are There Risk Factors for Delayed Recovery?

It is important to evaluate such risk factors in a patient with chronic neck pain. Unfortunately, research on the validity of

Chronic Pain Clinic Evaluation

Use the pictures below to show the origin of your pain (mark with a solid dot)

Does the pain travel or radiate anywhere? (mark with a broken line) *no*

Is the pain external (outside)? (Mark with an "E") or
Is the pain internal (inside)? (mark with an "I") or both

How much pain do you feel? (mark the area(s) with appropriate number below) *I can't answer*

1= Mild 2= Uncomfortable 3= Distressing (fairly severe) 4= Very Severe/horrible 5= unbearable

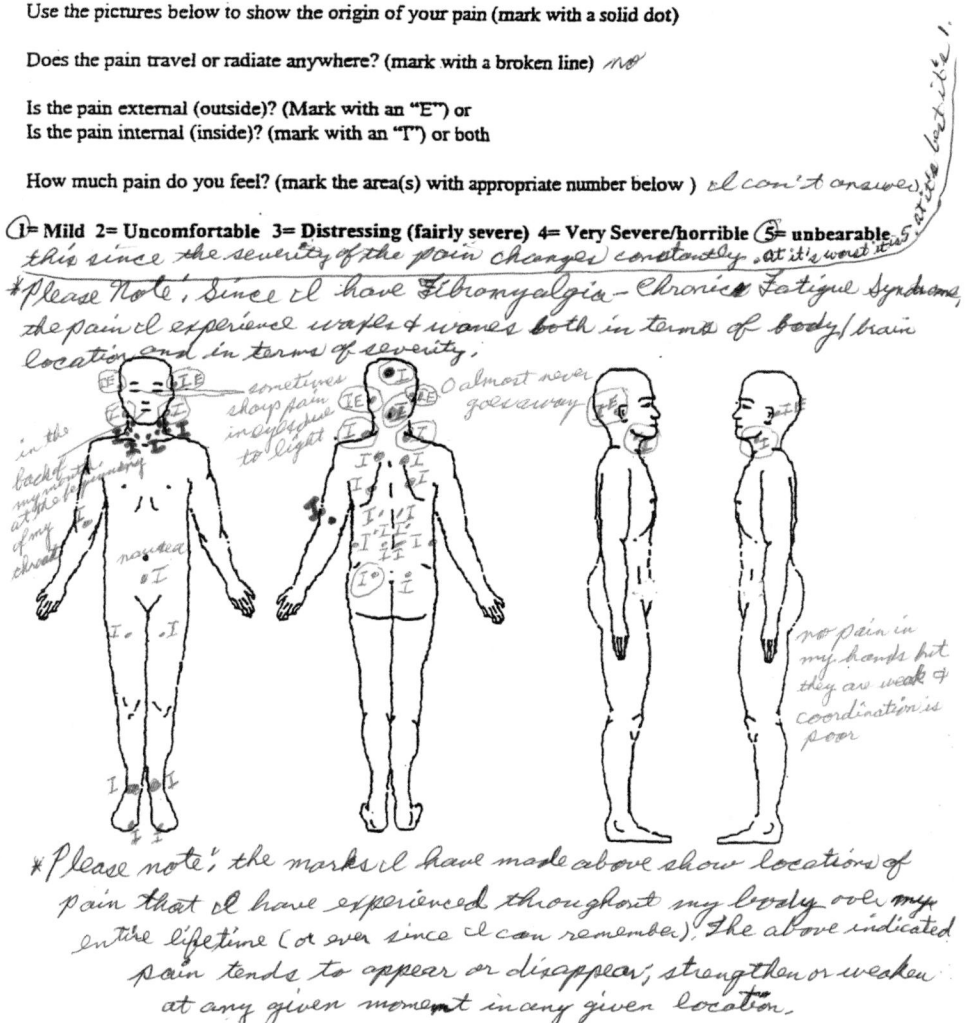

FIGURE 23.2 Patient indication of pain location.

many potential indicators is lacking. Thus, the following list of indicators should be viewed as *plausible* candidates for consideration during the medical evaluation of a chronic pain patient, rather than as proven predictors.

- Presence of a systemic disorder of the musculoskeletal system, such as rheumatoid arthritis or one of the muscular dystrophies.
- History of prior spinal injuries, or of significant prior symptoms in the absence of injury
- Evidence of severe spondylosis
- High pain intensity
- Severe functional limitations on examination
- Evidence of severe emotional distress

- Various general medical conditions. For example, if a patient has severe cardiovascular disease, this may have implications for his or her ability to function in a physical therapy program.
- Chemical dependency. The patient's history in this domain is important because it may bear on the appropriateness of prescribing opioids or sedatives.
- Sleep disturbance. Disturbed sleep is a common symptom reported by chronic pain patients, and most clinicians who treat these patients accept the premise that disordered sleep plays a role in perpetuating symptoms and disability. Thus, if a patient reports significantly disturbed sleep, a treatment plan for him or her should include interventions to promote normalization of sleep.
- Disability and litigation issues (discussed later).

Are There Other Issues That Bear on the Patient's Prognosis Or Have Implications for Treatment Planning?

An enormous number of issues have the potential to influence treatment planning for a chronic pain patient. Some of the most commonly encountered ones are:

Specific Evaluation Procedures

The physician should gather information on most or all of the questions outlined. Broadly speaking, this information will come from three sources: the patient's history, the physical examination, and ancillary studies.

History

It is beyond the scope of this chapter to discuss the elements of a thorough history. It is worth noting, though, that in evaluating a chronic pain patient, the physician should pay careful attention to certain historical items that are considered only cursorily in other clinical settings. In particular, the physician should be careful to assess the patient's history with respect to chemical dependency, his or her reported level of incapacitation, and his or her status with respect to litigation and compensation.

Physical Examination

A neurological and musculoskeletal examination should be performed on all patients with chronic cervical spine pain. In a patient with a normal neurological examination, a musculoskeletal evaluation of the neck (including assessment of soft tissue hypersensitivity and range of motion) is often not especially revealing.[13] In particular, it is virtually impossible to identify a distinct pain generator on the basis of a physical examination of such patients. But some useful information can be gleaned from a musculoskeletal examination. First, the physician can determined the severity of the patient's functional limitations, especially restricted motion of the spine and pain-inhibited weakness of neck and extremity muscles. Second, the physician can check for hyperalgesia over muscles of the neck and shoulder girdle, as well as more widespread hyperalgesia involving remote sites. Third, the physician can determine whether the patient demonstrates significant apprehension and "nonorganic signs."[14,15] Research indicates that patients with nonorganic signs usually have significant somatic anxiety. This emotional distress may impair their recoveries, and may be a focus of treatment.

One caution about physical examination concerns the reliability of the assessment of factors such as range of motion. Evidence suggests that the inter-rater reliability of commonly performed physical examination tests is limited[16,17] and thus it is important to determine whether findings on a single examination are consistent with a patient's history, previous examination findings, and diagnostic tests.

Ancillary Studies

Although laboratory studies and electrodiagnostic evaluations are occasionally helpful in the assessment of chronic pain patients, imaging modalities are the procedures that are done the most frequently. There is significant controversy about how and when imaging should be done on chronic pain patients. When judged against guidelines, one-third to two-thirds of spinal CT and MRI imaging may be inappropriate,[18–20] High imaging rates can be problematic because irrelevant but alarming findings, including herniated discs, are common in asymptomatic people.[2,3,21] Without attempting to resolve these controversies in any systematic way, we suggest the following: (1) for chronic pain involving a trauma, it is reasonable to check for the possibility of a fracture or significant spinal instability using plain x-rays of the spine; (2) additional imaging is generally not needed for such a patient, however, if there is some clinical evidence of a neurologic injury, an MRI scan is generally indicated; and (3) CT scans and bone scans usually have a limited role—they can be obtained to identify an occult fracture or an inflamed facet joint.

Many controversies regarding ancillary studies arise in relation to patients with localized axial cervical spinal pain and no evidence of major skeletal trauma. The basis for the controversies is that some physicians believe that such pain can be ascribed to well-defined injuries to structures in the cervical spine, whereas other physicians are much more skeptical. The following discussion addresses issues related to three types of structural lesions that have been proposed to explain persistent axial pain.

Ligamentous Injuries. Some investigators have reported that ligamentous injuries play a significant role in whiplash injuries[22,23]

and that the severity of self-reported disability among people with these injuries correlates with the severity of ligamentous injuries found on MRI scans. However, research on asymptomatic people[24,25] and ones with neck pain secondary to cervical spondylosis rather than injury[26] suggest that the MRI signals which some investigators have interpreted as indicators of ligamentous injuries should actually be considered normal variants or indicators of cervical degenerative disc disease.

Disc Pathology. Some investigators have advocated the use of cervical discography to identify painful intervertebral discs in the cervical spine.[27–29] The presence of an abnormal discogram, defined on the basis of some combination of the morphology of discs and the pain responses of a patient during the procedure, is viewed as an indication for a cervical spinal fusion.[30] However, the validity of using discography to determine that a disc is the pain generator for a patient with spinal pain has been questioned,[31] as have the results of spinal surgery based on abnormal discography.[32] See Chapter 100 for a detailed discussion of the utility of diagnostic discography.

Facet Joint Injury. Bogduk and colleagues[33–35] have asserted that facet joint injuries often underlie persistent cervical pain, and have pioneered techniques for identifying the structural basis of patients' reports of symptoms by careful application of injection procedures designed to provoke or palliate pain. Using these techniques, they have reported that approximately 70% of individuals with persistent neck pain following motor vehicle collisions have pain mediated by one or more of the cervical facet joints. Equally importantly, they have demonstrated that when patients diagnosed with facet-joint-mediated receive facet neurotomies designed to denervate the affected facet joint, approximately 70% experience prolonged symptom relief.[36,37] Although attempts to replicate these provocative results have met with only partial success,[38] the research by Bogduk and others strongly supports the conclusion that at least some individuals with persistent neck pain do have facet arthropathies.

It is beyond the scope of this chapter to review the controversies surrounding the value of discography, medial branch blocks, and ligament injuries diagnosed by MRI (see Chapter 97 for a detailed discussion). Instead, we will offer a few opinions that are consistent with those of leaders in the area of spine care. First, chronic pain patients with obvious concomitant psychological dysfunction or obvious markers of CNSS should not be referred for diagnostic procedures that rely on pain provocation and palliation.[32] Second, the interpretation of discography is so uncertain that we would not recommend it in any circumstance; however, leading experts continue to debate the utility of diagnostic discography. Third, there is research support for the use of medial branch blocks to detect facet arthropathies, combined with treatment of facet joint mediated pain by means of radiofrequency ablations of the appropriate medial branches.[36,37] We believe referral for medial branch blocks is appropriate for patients with chronic whiplash pain who continue to report symptoms despite conservative treatment and who have no evidence of either CNSS or significant psychological dysfunction. Finally, we do not recommend attempting to diagnose ligament injuries by means of MRI scans, in part because of questions about the validity of such diagnoses and in part because there is currently no widely accepted treatment for subtle ligament injuries diagnosed by MRI (as opposed to gross ligament injuries that cause instability).

Conclusion

The previous discussion addresses the medical evaluation of chronic pain within the context of patients with cervical spinal pain. Some of the examination steps and clinical decisions are broadly relevant to almost any patient with chronic pain. Others, however, are specific to patients with this kind of condition. We have gone into some detail in order to make the point that medical decision-making in relation to cervical spine pain is far from simple. It is our opinion that in order for pain patients to participate fully in evaluations of nonmedical factors contributing to their pain, they need to be confident that their problem has been evaluated thoroughly from a medical perspective. Thus, it is important for physicians participating in a multidisciplinary team either to have a lot of expertise in medical aspects of the problems that afflict their patients, or to consult with colleagues who have this expertise.

ASSESSMENT OF CENTRAL NERVOUS SYSTEM SENSITIZATION

During the past 20 years, CNSS has emerged as an important phenomenon in chronic pain.[39,40] Early research on nonhumans demonstrated that CNSS was associated with characteristic changes in the behavior of dorsal horn neurons in the spinal cord, including a lowered response threshold and an expansion of receptive fields.[41] Expansion of receptive fields was postulated to correlate with referral of pain, and lowered response threshold with hyperalgesia.[42,43] It is beyond the scope of this chapter to discuss the vast literature on central and peripheral nervous system sensitization.

Research indicates that people with chronic pain demonstrate reduced thresholds to multiple modalities of sensory stimulation, including pressure, thermal, and electrical stimuli.[44,45] These abnormalities occur when stimuli are applied to the specific location of the reported pain and even to body regions where patients do not experience clinical pain. Other research has shown that withdrawal reflexes can be elicited among chronic pain patients at lower stimulus intensities than the ones required to elicit the reflexes in healthy people. These findings have been interpreted by several researchers as evidence of CNSS among people with persistent pain[42] and as a central feature in the development of neuropathic pain.[40]

Although these proposals have not been conclusively proven, the widespread belief among many neuroscientists and pain specialists that CNSS is a major factor in chronic pain has implications for the evaluation and treatment of the condition. Practitioners who treat chronic pain patients need to be aware that CNSS may be playing a role in the reports of their patients. Also, they should be aware that many of the inferential rules followed by physicians when they interpret reports of pain are based on a simple model of an isomorphic correspondence between symptoms and dysfunction of tissues (nerves, joints, periarticular tissues, muscles) in the region where the patient indicates pain. The inferential rules are simply not valid when CNSS has occurred. For example, stocking glove numbness has long been considered a nonphysiologic complaint, but it can logically be interpreted as a result of CNSS.[46] Finally, to the extent that persistent chronic pain is mediated by altered nervous system responsivity rather than by ongoing nociceptive input from specific body locations, there is no reason to expect a one-to-one relation between symptoms and a definable structural lesion.

Given the potential importance of CNSS in the symptoms and functional limitations of pain patients, it would be highly desirable to have sensitive and specific tests to determine whether it is occurring in individual patients. Unfortunately, no such definitive assessment tools exist. In this regard, it is important to note that the original research demonstrating CNSS was performed on animals, and that the determination of whether CNSS had developed was made via microelectrode recordings from the dorsal horn of the spinal cord or other CNS structures. For obvious ethical reasons, these invasive procedures are not performed on humans. In the absence of data from direct monitoring of the CNS, investigators of pain in humans have, as noted previously, relied on analogies between clinical phenomena in patients and phenomena demonstrated in animal research. In particular, widespread soft tissue hyperalgesia is considered an indicator of CNSS.[47,48]

The existence of CNSS complicates our understanding of chronic pain, and the process of assessing individuals who report persistent symptoms. At a conceptual level, CNSS challenges the simple dichotomy between organic pain and psychogenic pain that held sway in the orthopedic literature of a generation ago.[10] At the level of clinical evaluation of an individual patient, the absence of definitive tests to determine the presence of CNSS makes it difficult for a clinician to rule in or out the hypothesis that it is affecting symptoms. The ambiguity introduced by CNSS is increased by the fact that although it is usually identified in the context of an examination by a physician, it is not a medical diagnosis in the usual sense. For example, the *International Classification of Disease*, 10th edition, does not include any codes that can be used to designate that a patient's pain is a reflection of CNSS. Also, no clear delineation has been drawn between CNSS versus psychological factors as a cause of persistent symptoms. The evaluation of CNSS is given a separate section in this chapter because of its ambiguous middle ground status between traditional medical processes and psychological processes.

ASSESSMENT OF PSYCHOLOGICAL FACTORS

A comprehensive psychological evaluation of a pain patient is a fundamental component of a multidisciplinary evaluation. It addresses the specific psychosocial, behavioral, and cognitive factors such as current mood (anxiety, depression, anger), interpretation of the symptoms, expectations about the meaning of symptoms, and the responses to the patient's symptoms by significant others (e.g., family members, coworkers), each of which contributes to the subjective experience of pain. This type of information should be included in the development of a comprehensive treatment plan.

Psychological Factors as Causes versus Consequences of Chronic Pain

Psychological Factors as Causal Agents in Development of Chronic Pain

Patients often resist psychological evaluations, because they intuitively sense that the outcome of such evaluations might be the conclusion that their pain is a result of psychological dysfunction rather than the injury to which they attribute their symptoms. Indeed, early reports suggested that pre-existing psychopathology or neurotic traits might be the underlying mechanisms for unremitting chronic pain.[49,50] As early as 1953, Gay and Abbot[49] mentioned "neurotic reactions" noting that particular psychological factors predisposed an individual to chronic problems after an injury. In 1982, Blumer and Heilbronn[51] postulated that patients with chronic symptoms had a distinct personality type that predisposed them to developing chronic pain—"pain-prone personality." They specifically suggested that persistent symptoms offered a solution for their pre-existing neurosis. There has been little empirical support indicating that the majority of chronic pain patients manifest character traits comprising a common and unique disposition.[52] However, some studies have noted the high lifetime prevalence of psychiatric diagnoses observed in chronic pain patients[53] and prospective studies that followed healthy individuals who subsequently develop back pain[21] and from acute injuries to the presence of disabling pain[54] have observed that premorbid psychological factors were the best predictor of persistent pain chronicity.

Psychological Consequences of Chronic Pain

Psychological symptoms following the onset of pain have also been thoroughly documented. Acute and long-lasting psychological symptoms following symptom onset are prevalent.[55,56] Disabling emotional symptoms have been observed in as many as 59% of people following initial pain onset.[53]

A number of studies have implicated the role of the patient's idiosyncratic appraisals of his or her symptoms, expectations regarding the cause of the symptoms, and the meaning of the symptoms, in addition to organic factors, as essential in understanding the individual's report of pain and subsequent disability.[21,57-59] Moreover, the patient's current mood, ways of coping with symptoms, and responses by significant others including physicians may modulate the experience of pain, particularly chronic or recurrent pain.[60,61] Failure to address these factors can result in poor response to treatments that focus exclusively on somatic causes.

The results of many studies implicate psychological symptoms as *concomitants* rather than *precursors* to chronic symptoms after chronic pain.[62] Initial reaction to an injury, rather than the pre-existing psychological status, has been shown to predict chronicity.[63,64] It seems reasonable that pre-existing psychological status may predispose *some* individuals to chronic emotional disturbances following an injury. For example, acute emotional distress has been shown to be related to pain severity one month following a motor vehicle collision.[65] The correct answer is probably somewhere in the middle where pre-existing psychological disturbances, immediate emotional reaction, coupled with medical complications contribute to chronicity of pain, at least for some people. In either case, these studies underscore the importance of evaluating psychological factors for all chronic pain patients.

Elements of the Psychological Evaluation

Table 23.1 contains a brief set of salient issues with the acronym ACT-UP (Activity, Coping, Think, Upset, People's responses) that can be used as a guide for interviewing patients who report persistent or recurring symptoms. Generally, a referral for evaluation may be indicated where disability greatly exceeds what would be expected based on physical findings alone, when patients make excessive demands on the health care system, when the patient persists in seeking medical tests and treatments when these are not indicated, when patients display significant emotional distress (e.g., depression or anxiety), or when the patient displays evidence of addictive behaviors or continual nonadherence to the prescribed regimen. Table 23.2 contains a detailed outline of the areas that should be addressed in a more extensive psychological interview for pain patients.

TABLE 23.1

BRIEF PSYCHOSOCIAL SCREENING: ACT-UP

Activities: How is your pain affecting your life (i.e., sleep, appetite, physical activities, relationships)?

Coping: How do you deal/cope with your pain (what makes it better/worse)?

Think: Do you think your pain will ever get better?

Upset: Have you been feeling worried (anxious)/depressed (down, blue)?

People: How do people respond when you have pain?

Interviews

A psychological interview with chronic pain patients is typically semi-structured. A structured format of psychiatric interview[66] can be incorporated as a tool to examine psychopathology. However, a psychological interview with pain patients needs to go beyond an assessment of psychopathology, since its main purpose is to assess a wide range of psychosocial factors (not just psychopathology) related to a patient's symptoms and disability.

When conducting an interview with chronic pain patients the health care professional should focus not only on gathering information provided by the patient, but also on observing patients' pain behaviors and the manner in which they convey information. We discuss some specific measures that have been proposed to systematically assess pain behaviors later.

Chronic pain patients' beliefs about the cause of symptoms, their trajectory, and beneficial treatments will have important influences on emotional adjustment and adherence to therapeutic interventions. A habitual pattern of maladaptive thoughts may contribute to a sense of hopelessness, dysphoria, and unwillingness to engage in activity. These reactions, in turn, deactivate the patient and severely limit his or her physical and emotional adaptation. The interviewer should also determine both the patient's and the significant others' expectancies and goals for treatment. An expectation that pain will be eliminated completely may be unrealistic and will have to be addressed to prevent discouragement when this outcome does not occur. Setting appropriate and realistic goals is an important process in pain rehabilitation as it requires the patient to attain better understanding of chronic pain and goes beyond the dualistic, traditional medical model.

In order to help chronic pain patients understand the psychosocial aspects of pain, attention should focus on the patients' reports of specific thoughts, behaviors, emotions, and physiological responses that precede, accompany, and follow pain episodes or exacerbation, as well as the environmental conditions and consequences associated with cognitive, emotional, and behavioral responses in these situations. During the interview, the clinician should attend to the temporal association of these cognitive, affective, and behavioral events; their specificity versus generality across situations; and the frequency of their occurrence, to establish salient features of the target situations, including the controlling variables. The interviewer seeks information that will assist in the development of potential alternate responses, appropriate goals for the patient, and possible reinforcers for these alternatives.

Patients with chronic pain problems often consume a variety of medications. It is important to discuss a patient's medications during the interview, as many pain medications (particularly opioids) are associated with side effects that may mimic emotional distress. A clinician, for example, should be familiar with side effects that result in fatigue, sleep difficulties, and mood changes to avoid misdiagnosis of depression. A general understanding of commonly used medications for chronic pain is important, as some patients also may use opioid analgesics to manage mood. During the interview potential psychological dependence and aberrant drug seeking behaviors on pain-relieving medications should be evaluated. In some states, a physician is able to obtain a record of prescriptions of controlled substances. When in doubt, a psychologist may recommend that such a record be obtained and request urine toxicology screening to rule out substance abuse problems (including diversion) and aberrant opioid taking behaviors.[67]

Self-Report Inventories

In addition to interviews, a number of assessment instruments designed to evaluate patients' attitudes, beliefs, and expectancies about themselves, their symptoms, and the health care system

TABLE 23.2

AREAS ADDRESSED IN PSYCHOLOGICAL INTERVIEWS

Experience of pain and related symptoms
- Location and description of pain (e.g., "sharp," "burning")
- Onset and progression
- Perception of cause (e.g., trauma, virus, stress)
- What has the patient been told about the symptoms and condition? Does the patient believe that this information is accurate?
- Exacerbating and relieving factors (e.g., exercise, relaxation, stress, massage)
- Pattern of symptoms (e.g., worse certain times of day or following activity or stress)
- Sleep habits (e.g., difficulty falling to sleep or maintaining sleep, sleep hygiene)
- Thoughts, feelings, and behaviors that precede, accompany, and follow fluctuations in symptoms

Treatments received and currently receiving
- Medication (prescribed and over-the-counter). How helpful have these been?
- Pattern of medication use (*prn*, time-contingent), changes in quantity or schedule
- Physical modalities (e.g., physical therapy). How helpful have these been?
- Exercise (e.g., Do they participate in a regular exercise routine? Is there evidence of deactivation and avoidance of activity due to fear of pain or exacerbation of injury?). Has the pattern changed (increased, decreased)?
- Complementary and alternative (e.g., chiropractic manipulation, relaxation training). How helpful have these been?
- Which treatments have they found the most helpful?
- Compliance (adherence) with recommendations of health care providers.
- Attitudes toward previous health care providers

Compensation and litigation
- Current disability status (e.g., receiving or seeking disability, amount, percent of former job income, expected duration of support)
- Current or planned litigation

Responses by patient and significant others
- Typical daily routine
- Changes in activities and responsibilities (both voluntary and obligatory) due to symptoms
- Changes in significant other's activities and responsibilities due to patient's symptoms
- Patient's behavior when pain increases or flares up
- Significant others' responses to behavioral expressions of pain
- What does the patient do when pain is not bothering him or her (uptime activities)?
- Significant other's response when patient is active
- Impact of symptoms on interpersonal, family, marital, and sexual relations (e.g., changes in desire, frequency, or enjoyment)
- Activities that patient avoids because of symptoms
- Activities continued despite symptoms
- Pattern of activity and pacing of activity (can use activity diaries that ask patients to record their pattern of daily activities [e.g., sitting, standing, walking] for several days or weeks)

Coping
- How does the patient try to cope with his or her symptoms? Does patient view himself or herself as having any role in symptom management? If so, what role?
- Current life stresses
- Pleasant activities

Educational and vocational history
- Level of education completed, including any special training
- Work history
- How long at most recent job?
- How satisfied with most recent job and supervisor?
- What like least about most recent job?
- Would the patient like to return to most recent job? If not what type of work would the patient like?
- Current work status, including homemaking activities
- Vocational and avocational plans

(continued)

TABLE 23.2

CONTINUED

Social history
- Relationships with family or origin
- History of pain or disability in family members
- History of substance abuse in family members
- History of or current, physical, emotional, and sexual abuse. Was the patient a witness to abuse of someone else?
- Marital history and current status
- Quality of current marital and family relations

Alcohol and substance use
- Current and history of alcohol use (quantity, frequency)
- History and current use of illicit psychoactive drugs
- History and current use of prescribed psychoactive medications
- Consider the CAGE questions as a quick screen for alcohol dependence (Mayfield, McLeod, & Hall, 1974). Depending on response consider other instruments for alcohol and substance abuse (Allen & Litten, 1998).

Psychological dysfunction
- Current psychological symptoms/diagnosis (depression including suicidal ideation, anxiety disorders, somatization, posttraumatic stress disorder). Depending on responses, consider conducting structured interview such as the Structured Clinical Interview for DSM-IV-TR (SCID) (American Psychiatric Association, 1997).
- Is the patient currently receiving treatment for psychological symptoms? If yes, what treatments (e.g., psychotherapy or psychiatric medications). How helpful are the treatments?
- History of psychiatric disorders and treatment including family counseling
- Family history of psychiatric disorders

Concerns and expectations
- Patient concerns/fears
- Explanatory models of pain held by the patient
- Expectations regarding the future and treatment (will get better, worse, never change)
- Attitude toward rehabilitation versus "cure"

Treatment goals

Adapted from Mayfield, McLeod, & Hall, 1974; Allen & Litten, 1998; and American Psychiatric Association, 1997.

have been developed and published. One survey[68] of clinicians who treated pain indicated that the five most frequently used instruments in the assessment of pain, in order of frequency, were: the McGill Pain Questionnaire,[69,69a] Beck Depression Inventory (BDI),[70,71] Multidimensional Pain Inventory,[72] Coping Strategies Questionnaire,[73] and the Oswestry Low Back Pain Questionnaire.[74]

Standardized instruments have advantages over semi-structured and unstructured interviews. They are easy to administer, require less time, assess a wide range of behaviors, obtain information about behaviors that may be private (sexual relations) or unobservable (thoughts, emotional arousal), and, most importantly, they can be submitted to analyses that permit determination of their reliability and validity. These instruments should not be viewed as alternatives to interviews; rather, they may suggest issues to be addressed in more depth during an interview or investigated with other measures.

There is an important caveat when interpreting the results of self-report inventories. Studies of the psychometric properties of self-report inventories typically involve data collection from a large number of patients. As reliability estimates are influenced by sample size, it follows that the measurement error of questionnaire data from one person should be expected to be much greater than that found in reports based on group data. One way to address concerns about reliability with some measures is to collect data at multiple points over time rather than simply comparing pretreatment and posttreatment data.

Problem Areas to Assess

Assessment of Emotional Distress

The results of numerous studies suggest that chronic pain is often associated with emotional distress, particularly depression, anxiety, anger, and irritability. The presence of emotional distress in people with chronic pain presents a challenge when assessing symptoms such as fatigue, reduced activity level, decreased libido, appetite change, sleep disturbance, weight gain or loss, and memory and concentration deficits. These symptoms are often associated with pain and have also been considered "vegetative" symptoms of depressive disorders. Improvements or deterioration in such symptoms, therefore, can be a result of changes in either pain or emotional distress.

Both the BDI and BDI-2[70,71] and the Profile of Mood States[75] have well-established reliability and validity in the assessment of symptoms of depression and emotional distress, and they have been used in numerous clinical trials in psychiatry and an increasing number of studies of patients with chronic pain.[76] In research in psychiatry and chronic pain, the BDI provides a well-accepted criterion of the level of psychological distress in a sample and its response to treatment. The Profile of Mood States (POMS)[75] assesses six mood states—tension-anxiety, depression-dejection, anger-hostility, vigor-activity, fatigue-inertia, and confusion-bewilderment—and also provides a summary measure of total mood disturbance. Although the discriminant validity of the POMS scales in patients with chronic pain has not been adequately documented, it has scales for the three most important dimensions of emotional functioning in chronic pain patients (depression, anxiety, and anger) and also assesses three other dimensions that are very relevant to chronic pain and its treatment, including a positive mood scale of vigor-activity. Moreover, the POMS has demonstrated beneficial effects of treatment in some (but not all) recent chronic pain trials.[77,78] For these reasons, administration of the BDI and the POMS are reasonable choices as brief measures of emotional distress.

As noted previously, various symptoms of depression—such as decreased libido, appetite or weight changes, fatigue, and memory and concentration deficits—are also commonly believed to be consequences of chronic pain and the medications used for its treatment.[79] It is unclear whether the presence of such symptoms in patients with chronic pain (and other medical disorders) should nevertheless be considered evidence of depressed mood, or whether the assessment of mood in these patients should emphasize symptoms that are less likely to be secondary to physical disorders.[80]

Assessment of Fear. Many patients with chronic pain, especially those who attribute their symptoms to trauma, are fearful of engaging in activities that they believe may either contribute to further injury or exacerbate their symptoms. Avoidance of activities may, in the short term, lead to symptom reduction. But over time restriction of activities is likely to lead to decreased functional capacities as a result of deconditioning. Also, avoidance of activity has the unfortunate consequence of preventing corrective feedback. Health care providers may inadvertently contribute to avoidance of activity by providing patients with cervical collars that restrict neck movements and advising them to avoid activities that hurt (i.e., hurt = harm). They may contribute to the patient's anxiety that something is seriously wrong with their bodies by continuing to order sophisticated diagnostic tests in search of occult physical pathology.

Assessment of Coping and Psychosocial Adaptation to Pain. Historically, psychological measures designed to evaluate psychopathology have been used to identify specific individual differences associated with reports of pain, even though these measures were usually not developed for or standardized on samples of medical patients. However, it is possible that responses by medical patients may be distorted as a function of the disease or the medications that they take. For example, common measures of depression ask patients about their appetites, sleep patterns, and fatigue. Because disease status and medication can affect responses to such items, patients' scores may be elevated, thereby distorting the meaning of their responses. As a result, a number of measures have been developed for use specifically with pain patients. Instruments have been developed to assess psychological distress, the impact of pain on patients' lives, feeling of control, coping behaviors, and attitudes about disease, pain, and health care providers and the patient's plight.[81]

Assessment of Pain

Although all members of a multidisciplinary assessment team ask questions about pain when they evaluate a patient, the psychologist typically delves into this area in more depth than physicians or other members of a multidisciplinary evaluation team. Psychologists typically rely on a variety of tools to assess the pain experiences of patients, and consider several dimensions of these experiences.

Pain Intensity. Self-report measures of pain often ask patients to quantify their pain by providing a single, general rating of pain: "Is your usual level of pain 'mild,' 'moderate,' or 'severe'?" or "Rate your typical pain on a scale from 0 to 10 where 0 equals no pain and 10 is the worst pain you can imagine." There are a number of simple methods that can be used to evaluate current pain intensity—numerical scale (NRS), verbal ratings scales (VRS), and visual analog scales (VAS).

Each of the commonly used methods of rating pain intensity, NRS, VRS, and VAS, appear sufficiently reliable and valid and no one method consistently demonstrates greater responsiveness in detecting improvements associated with pain treatment.[82] However, there are important differences among NRS, VRS, and VAS measures of pain intensity with respect to missing data stemming from failure to complete the measure, patient preference, ease of data recording, and ability to administer the measure by telephone or with electronic diaries. NRS and VRS measures tend to be preferred over VAS measures by patients, and VAS measures usually demonstrate more missing data than do NRS measures. Greater difficulty completing VAS measures is associated with increased age and greater opioid intake, and cognitive impairment has been shown to be associated with inability to complete NRS ratings of pain intensity.[82] Patients who are unable to complete NRS ratings may be able to complete VRS pain ratings (e.g., none, mild, moderate, severe). Other measures are available to assess pain in children and those who are unable to verbally communicate (e.g., stroke patients, mentally-impaired).[83]

There has been some concern expressed that retrospective reports may not be valid, as they may reflect current pain severity that serves as an anchor for recall of pain severity over some interval.[84,85] More valid information may be obtained by asking about current level of pain, pain over the past week, worst pain of the last week, and lowest level of severity over the last week. This has also led to the use of daily diaries that are believed to be more accurate as they are based on real-time rather than recall. For example, patients are asked to maintain regular diaries of pain intensity with ratings recorded several times each day (e.g., at meals and bedtime) for several days or weeks. One problem noted with the use of paper-and-pencil diaries is that patients may not follow the instruction to provide ratings at specified intervals. Rather, patients may complete diaries in advance ("fill forward") or shortly before seeing a clinician ("fill backward").[86] These two reporting approaches undermine the putative validity of diaries. As an alternative to the paper-and-pencil diaries, a number of commentators have advocated for the use of electronic devices that can prompt patients for ratings and "time stamp" the actual ratings, thus facilitating real-time data capture. Although there are numerous advantages to the use of advanced technology to improve the validity of patient ratings, they are not without potential problems, including hardware problems, software problems, and user problems.[87] These methods are also costly and, although they may be appropriate for research studies, their usefulness in clinical settings may be limited.

Pain Quality. Pain is known to have different sensory and affective qualities in addition to its intensity, and measures of these components of pain may be used to more fully describe an individual's pain experience.[88] It is possible that the efficacy of pain treatments varies for different pain qualities, and measures of pain quality may therefore identify treatments that are efficacious for certain types of pain but not for overall pain intensity. Assessment of specific pain qualities at baseline also makes it possible to determine whether certain patterns of pain quality moderate the effects of treatment. The Short-Form McGill Pain Questionnaire[69a] assesses 15 sensory and affective pain descriptors and its sensory and affective subscales have demonstrated responsivity to treatment in a number of clinical trials.[77,78]

Pain Modifiers. For the majority of people with chronic pain, pain severity varies. Thus, it is useful to inquire as to what the patient believes makes his or her pain worse. For example, are their specific activities that result in increase in symptoms? Are their certain circumstances that contribute to exacerbation of pain such as stress including interpersonal conflicts? Does pain vary with time of day? For example, does the patient notice that his or her pain is worse in the morning or later in the day? In the same way it is important to identify factors that magnify or initiate pain episodes, it is important to ask about what factors result in reductions of pain. For example, do medication, rest, heat or cold, distraction, or exercise result in reductions of pain severity or even elimination of symptoms for some period.

Assessment of Overt Expressions of Pain

As noted previously, patients display a broad range of responses that communicate to others that they are experiencing pain, distress, and suffering. Some of these pain behaviors may be controllable by the person, whereas others are not. Informally, a health care provider can observe patients' behaviors during their interviews and examinations. It is useful to observe patients in multiple contexts when possible. When patients know they are being observed and are presenting information to a healthcare provider they may use behavior to convey information in ways most likely to support the impact of their symptoms. They may feel a need to convince the health care provider of the severity of their symptoms, functional limitations, and distress. Thus, observation of the patient in the waiting room, when ambulating to the examination room, and when departing may allow the clinician to establish the stability and consistency of pain behaviors. We have also found it useful to observe patients in the presence of a significant other to note differences in behaviors when the significant other is present and absent and also how the significant other responds to the patient's pain behaviors.

A number of different observational procedures have been developed to identify and quantify pain behaviors. Structured methods that require patients to engage in a set of behaviors during which their behavior is observed and rated have been proposed by Keefe and colleagues.[89,90] Such structured approaches may be useful in research studies but can be cumbersome in clinical settings. Several investigators have developed observational Pain Behavior Checklists[91,92] that can be used in any setting. Although they have the advantage of efficiency, these methods may be less appropriate to compare among patients who are viewed in different contexts (e.g., during a physical examination or interview). The context may influence the behaviors observed. For example, the nature of pain behaviors observed might be quite different during a stressful physical examination compared to an interview. The number and nature of pain behaviors might be influenced by the presence of significant others during the observation period. At a minimum it is important to note the context in which the behaviors were observed. Studies using pain behavior checklists have found a significant association between these self-reports and behavioral observations. A variant of this observational procedure was developed by Kerns et al.[92a] who developed a self-report version in which patients endorsed specific behaviors that they engaged in when they were experiencing pain.

Uses of the health care system and analgesic medication are other ways to assess pain behaviors. Patients can record the times when they take medication over a specified interval such as a week. Diaries not only provide information about the frequency and quantity of medication but may also permit identification of the antecedent and consequent events of medication use. Antecedent events might include stress, boredom, or activity. Examination of antecedents is useful in identifying patterns of medication use that may be associated with factors other than pain per se. Similarly, patterns of response to the use of analgesic, may be

identified. Does the patient receive attention and sympathy whenever he or she is observed by significant others taking medication? That is, do significant others provide positive reinforcement for the taking of analgesic medication and thereby unwittingly increase medication use?

ASSESSMENT OF SOCIAL FACTORS

Social factors are construed as factors in the social environment that influence people independent of their individual psychological characteristics. A good example is the receipt of workers' compensation benefits. There is good evidence that injured workers respond less well to a variety of treatments than individuals with similar medical conditions who do not have workers' compensation claims.[93,94] Although participation in the workers' compensation system exerts its negative influence through effects on the perceptions, goals, and attitudes of injured workers, the influence appears to be robust and not dependent on any particular psychological characteristics of the affected individuals.

Social factors include demographic variables that influence the presentation and clinical course of people with painful conditions. In particular, research indicates that an individual's clinical presentation is associated with his or her age, gender, ethnicity,[95,96] and education level.[97,98]

The social factors that have attracted the most research attention in relation to chronic pain are participation in litigation and participation in a workers' compensation system.[94,99] A significant proportion of individuals involved in injuries file personal injury claims. Research on the relation between litigation and clinical course, however, has been contradictory. For example, whereas several recent studies have reported a negative effect of attorney involvement and litigation on recovery from whiplash disorders,[100,101] Scholten-Peeters et al.[102] concluded in a comprehensive review that "often mentioned factors like age, gender, and compensation do not seem to be of prognostic value" in relation to the clinical course. It is beyond the scope of this chapter to review the often contentious literature on the effect of litigation/attorney involvement on outcomes of chronic pain.[103–107] Our interpretation of this literature is that it does, on balance, support the hypothesis that attorney involvement and participation in litigation is a negative prognostic factor for individuals with pain associated with physical injury. There is also evidence that injured workers with workers' compensation claims respond poorly to a variety of treatments compared to individuals with the same medical conditions, but without workers' compensation claims.[94]

Important social factors also include influences from an individual's immediate social environment. For example, there is good evidence that pain patients generally demonstrate more dramatic pain behaviors when they are in the presence of solicitous spouses.[108]

In multidisciplinary evaluations, social factors are usually evaluated by a psychologist. The evaluation of some social factors is straightforward. These include demographic variables, compensation status, and litigation status. The assessment of influences in a patient's immediate social environment is more difficult, but psychologists typically attempt to determine how a patient communicates his or her pain to significant others, and how the significant others respond to these cues.

ASSESSING FUNCTIONAL IMPACT

A major focus of the discussion above has been on the identification of factors underlying the symptoms of a chronic pain patient. It is important to note, though, that the identification of factors that qualitatively play a role in a patient's symptoms is not the same as an explanation of the severity of these symptoms, or the extent to which the patient is disabled by them. Thus, we recommend that an evaluation of any chronic pain patient should include an assessment of the extent to which the patient is affected by his or her symptoms. When a multidisciplinary evaluation is done, physical therapists, vocational rehabilitation counselors, physicians, and psychologists may participate in the evaluation of function among pain patients.

Conceptually, the impact of chronic pain on function can be subdivided into: (1) the ability of patients to function in the sense of performing activities of daily living; (2) their physical capacities as demonstrated in a structured setting; and (3) their ability to function in adult roles such as work.

Self-Report Measures of Function

Self-report measures have been developed to assess people's reports of their abilities to engage in a range of functional activities such as the ability to walk up stairs, to sit for specific periods of time, the ability to lift specific weights, perform activities of daily living, as well as the severity of the pain experienced upon the performance of these activities.[109] There are a number of well-established, psychometrically supported generic (e.g., Short-Form 36[110]), pain-specific (e.g., Brief Pain Questionnaire Interference Scale[111]; Pain Disability Index[112]; MPI Interference Scale[72]), and back-pain specific (Oswestry Low Back Pain Disability Questionnaire[74]) measures of functional status.

The Oswestry Disability Index is a 10-item scale that asks patients about disability associated with back pain.[74] It has the advantage of being a disease-specific instrument. In general, disease-specific measures are designed to evaluate the specific effects of a disorder that may not be assessed by a generic measure.[113] In addition, responses on disease-specific measures will generally reflect the effects of comorbid conditions on physical functioning, which may confound the interpretation of change occurring over the course of a trial when generic measures are used. Disease-specific measures may be more sensitive to the effects of treatment on function, but generic measures provide information about physical functioning and treatment benefits that can be compared across different conditions and studies.[113,114] Each of these approaches has strengths. Decisions regarding whether to use a disease-specific or a generic measure, or some combination, will depend on the purpose of the assessment. For individual patients in clinical practice it would be most appropriate to use measures developed on samples with comparable characteristics. If the clinician wishes to compare across a group of patients, then one of the broader-based pain-specific measures should be considered. If the assessment is being performed as part of a research study, some combination might be appropriate to compare chronic pain samples with a larger population of people with diverse medical diseases (e.g., SF-36).

The physical capacities of pain patients are typically assessed by physical and occupational therapists. In some clinical settings, evaluation protocols are developed informally by individual therapists, sometimes in conjunction with a physician. In other settings, formal assessment protocols are used. Although the validity of such protocols has been questioned,[115,116] they are frequently used—particularly when injured workers are being evaluated. The purpose of such evaluations is to obtain objective information about the capabilities of patients. In clinical settings, this information is used in the planning of rehabilitative treatment. In more adversarial settings (e.g., workers' compensation), physical capacities data are used when adjudicative decisions about claims are made.

Ideally, a multidisciplinary evaluation would include having a vocational rehabilitation counselor perform a comprehensive evaluation of the work status of pain patients, and their potential for vocational rehabilitation. In many situations, though, the job of assessing vocational disability falls on the physician or psychol-ogist on the multidisciplinary team. We are not aware of standardized instruments to assess the vocational status of pain patients. In the absence of a standard instrument, we recommend that clinicians assessing these patients address the following issues: (1) Is the patient currently working? (2) If the patient is not working, is this related to his or her health? (3) How long has the patient been out of the workforce? (4) Is he or she receiving any kind of work disability benefits? Which ones?

ORGANIZATION OF MULTIDISCIPLINARY EVALUATIONS

As discussed previously, the professionals who might participate in multidisciplinary evaluations include physicians, psychologists, vocational rehabilitation counselors, physical and occupations therapists, and perhaps other professionals. An obvious question is: How do these professionals orchestrate their evaluations and communicate with each other?

The model that has received the most attention in research literature has been multidisciplinary intensive pain rehabilitation.[117] In the United States, the multidisciplinary pain centers and functional restoration programs that provided intensive pain rehabilitation began in the late 1960s, flourished during the 1980s and early 1990s, and more recently have been in decline.[118]

Given the decline in intensive pain rehabilitation programs, it will probably be necessary in the future for professionals involved in the evaluation of patients with chronic pain to develop a number of informal strategies for working together. There are almost certainly a variety of models that can succeed. The key issue is for professionals to work together in acquiring data on the multiple dimensions that affect chronic pain patients, and to communicate with each other so that the patients benefit from the data that are gathered.

CONCLUSION

Pain and associated symptoms are the results of a complex interplay of factors. Assessment and treatment of chronic pain can be complicated by the web of influential factors that modulate the overall pain experience and associated disability. Furthermore, traditional biomedical approaches with diagnostic tests are often not helpful because structural damage and persistent pain complaints do not necessarily coincide. Pain research in the last three decades has repeatedly shown that pain is not just a physiological phenomenon, and that a range of "person variables," such as psychosocial, environmental, and behavioral factors, play a significant role in determining the occurrence, severity, and quality of pain. Given the multifactorial nature of chronic pain, adequate assessment requires an interdisciplinary team approach. In this chapter, we discussed the assessment of medical factors, altered CNS processing, psychological factors, and social factors in patients with chronic pain. We introduced a number of self-report inventories that can be used in conjunction with interviews and medical examinations. As we have repeatedly stressed, an adequate assessment of patients with chronic pain means the evaluation of the person with the symptoms. We must not just focus on the pathology or symptom report, but must reach out to understand the person and his or her well-being. Although there is no shortcut in this, the delineation of relevant medical, psychosocial, and behavioral factors contributing to pain in a patient are critical in planning and executing a successful treatment plan.

ACKNOWLEDGMENT

Preparation of this chapter was supported by a grant from the National Institutes of Health/ National Institute of Arthritis and Musculoskeletal and Skin Disorders (R01AR044724).

References

1. Turk DC, Flor H. Chronic pain: a biobehavioral perspective. In: Gatchel RJ, Turk DC, eds. *Psychosocial Factors in Pain: Critical Perspectives*. New York: Guilford Press; 1999:18–34.
2. Boden SD, Davis DO, Dina TS, et al. Abnormal magnetic-resonance scans of the lumbar spine in asymptomatic subjects. A prospective investigation. *J Bone Joint Surg Am* 1990;72:403–408.
3. Jensen MC, Brant–Zawadski MN, Obuchowski N, et al. Magnetic resonance imaging of the lumbar spine in people with back pain. *N Engl J Med* 1994; 331:69–73.
4. Boos N, Semmer N, Elfering A, et al. Natural history of individuals with asymptomatic disc abnormalities in magnetic resonance imaging: predictors of low back pain-related medical consultation and work incapacity. *Spine* 2000;25:1482–1492.
5. Borenstein DG, O'Mara JW Jr, Boden SD, et al. The value of magnetic resonance imaging of the lumbar spine to predict low-back pain in asymptomatic subjects: a seven-year follow-up study. *J Bone Joint Surg Am* 2001;83-A: 1306–1311.
6. Jarvik JJ, Hollingworth W, Heagerty P, et al. The Longitudinal Assessment of Imaging and Disability of the Back (LAIDBack) Study: baseline data. *Spine* 2001;26:1158–1166.
7. Pillemer S, Bradley LA, Crofford LJ, et al. The neuroscience and endocrinology of fibromyalgia. *Arthritis Rheum* 1997;40:1928–1939.
8. Buskila D. Genetics of chronic pain states. *Best Pract Res Clin Rheumatol* 2007;21:535–547.
9. Chou R, Qassem A, Snow V, et al. Diagnosis and treatment of low bck pain: a joint clinical practice guideline from the American College of Physicians and the American Pain Society. *Ann Intern Med* 2007;147:478–491.
9a. Turk DC, Robinson JP. Assessment of patients with whiplash associated disorders: a comprehensive approach. In: Duckworth MP, Iezzi A, O'Donohue W, eds. *Motor Vehicle Collisions: Medical, Psychosocial, and Legal Consequences*. New York: Elsevier; 2008: 187–227.
10. Robinson JP, Ricketts D, Hanscom DA. Musculoskeletal pain. In: Merskey H, Loeser JD, Dubner R, eds. *The Paths of Pain*. Seattle: IASP Press; 2005: 1975–2005.
11. Dwyer A, Aprill C, Bogduk N. Cervical zygapophyseal joint pain patterns. I: A study in normal volunteers. *Spine* 1990;15:453–457.
12. Slipman CW, Plastaras C, Patel R, et al. Provocative cervical discography symptom mapping. *Spine J* 2005;5:381–388.
13. Bodguk N, McGurik B. *Management of Acute and Chronic Neck Pain: An Evidence-Based Approach*. New York: Elsevier; 2006.
14. Waddell G, McCulloch JA, Kummel E, et al. Nonorganic physical signs in low-back pain. *Spine* 1980;5:117–125.
15. Main CJ, Waddell G. Behavioral responses to examination. A reappraisal of the interpretation of "nonorganic signs." *Spine* 1998;23:2367–2371.
16. Hunt DG, Zuberbier OA, Kozolowski AJ, et al. Reliability of the lumbar flexion, lumbar extension, and passive straight leg raise test in normal populations embedded within a complete physical examination. *Spine* 2001;26: 2714–2718.
17. Nitschke JE, Nattrass CL, Disler PB, et al. Reliability of the American Medical Association guides' model for measuring spinal range of motion. Its implication for whole-person impairment rating. *Spine* 1999;24:262–268.
18. Rao JK, Kroenke K, Mihaliak KA, et al. Can guidelines impact the ordering of magnetic resonance imaging studies by primary care providers for low back pain? *Am J Manag Care* 2002;8:27–35.
19. Schroth WS, Schectman JM, Elinsky EG, Et al. Utilization of medical services for the treatment of acute low back pain: conformance with clinical guidelines. *J Gen Intern Med* 1992;7:486–491.
20. Weiner DK, Kim YS, Bonino P, et al. Low back pain in older adults: are we utilizing healthcare resources wisely? *Pain Med* 2006;7:143–150.
21. Jarvik JG, Hollingworth W, Heaqgerty PJ, et al. Three-year incidence of low back pain in an initially asymptomatic cohort: clinical and imaging risk factors. *Spine* 2005;30:1541–1548.
22. Stemper BD, Yoganandan N, Pintar FA, et al. Anterior longitudinal ligament injuries in whiplash may lead to cervical instability. *Med Eng Phys* 2006;28: 515–524.
23. Tominaga Y, Ndu AB, Coe MP, et al. Neck ligament strength is decreased following whiplash trauma. *BMC Musculoskelet Disord* 2006;7:103.
24. Roy S, Hol PK, Laerum LT, et al. Pitfalls of magnetic resonance imaging of alar ligament. *Neuroradiology* 2004;46:392–398.
25. Wilmink, JT, Patijn J. MR imaging of alar ligament in whiplash-associated disorders: an observer study. *Neuroradiology* 2001;43:859–863.
26. Saifuddin A, Green R, White J. Magnetic resonance imaging of the cervical ligaments in the absence of trauma. *Spine* 2003;28:1686–1691; discussion 1691–1692.
27. Cohen SP, Hurley RW. The ability of diagnostic spinal injections to predict surgical outcomes. *Anesth Analg* 2007;105:1756–1775.
28. Wieser ES, Wang JC. Surgery for neck pain. *Neurosurgery* 2007;60(1 supp11):S51–S56.
29. Zheng Y, Liew SM, Simmons ED. Value of magnetic resonance imaging and discography in determining the level of cervical discectomy and fusion. *Spine* 2004;29:2140–2145; discussion 2146.
30. Carragee EJ, Alamin TF, Carragee JM. Low-pressure positive discography in subjects asymptomatic of significant low back pain illness. *Spine* 2006;31: 505–509.
31. Carragee EJ, Alamin TF, Miller JL, et al. Discograhic, MRI and psychosocial determinants of low back pain disabilty and remission: a prospective study in subjects with benign persistent back pain. *Spine J* 2005;5:24–35.
32. Carragee EJ, Lincoln T, Parmar VKS, et al. A gold standard evaluation of the "discogneic pain" diagnosis as determined by provocative discography. *Spine* 2006;31:2115–2123.
33. Bogduk N. Diagnostic nerve blocks in chronic pain. *Best Pract Res Clin Anaesthesiol* 2002;16:565–578.
34. Gibson T, Bogduk N, Macpherson J, et al. Crash characteristics of whiplash associated chronic neck pain. *J Musculoskeletal Pain* 2000;8:87–95.
35. Lord S, Barnsley L, Wallis BJ, et al. Chronic cervical zygapophyseal joint pain after whiplash: a placebo-controlled prevalence study. *Spine* 1996;21: 1737–1745.
36. Lord SM, Barnsley L, Wallis BJ, et al. Percutaneous radio-frequency neurotomy for chronic zygapophysial-joint pain. *N Engl J Med* 1996;335: 1721–1726.
37. McDonald G, Lord SM, Bogduk N. Long-term follow-up of patients treated with cervical radiofrequency neurotomy for chronic neck pain. *Neurosurgery* 1999;45:61–68.
38. Manchikanti L, Singh V, Rivera J, et al. Prevalence of cervical facet joint pain in chronic neck pain. *Pain Physician* 2002;5:243–249.
39. Ji RR, Kohno T, Moore KA, et al. Central sensitization and LTP: do pain and memory share similar mechanisms? *Trends Neurosci* 2003;26:696–705.
40. Woolf CJ, Mannion RJ. Neuropathic pain: aetiology, symptoms, mechanisms, and management. *Lancet* 1999;353:1959–1964.
41. Hoheisel U, Mense S. Long-term changes in discharge behaviour of cat dorsal horn neurons following noxious stimulation of deep tissues. *Pain* 1989;36: 239–247.
42. Curatolo M, Arendt–Nielsen L, Petersen–Felix S. Evidence, mechanisms, and clinical implications of central hypersensitivity in chronic pain after whiplash injury. *Clin J Pain* 2004;20:469–476.
43. Robinson JP, Arendt–Nielsen L. Muscle pain syndromes. In: Braddom R. ed. *Physical Medicine and Rehabilitation*. 3rd ed. Edinburgh: Elsevier/Saunders; 2007:989–1020.
44. Kasch H, Qerama E, Bach FW, et al. Reduced cold pressor pain tolerance in non-recovered whiplash patients: a 1-year prospective study. *Eur J Pain* 2005; 9:561–569.
45. Sterling M, Jull G, Vicenzino B, et al. Characterization of acute whiplash-associated disorders. *Spine* 2004;29:182–188.
46. Gun RT, Osti OL, O'Riordan A, et al. Risk factors for prolonged disability after whiplash injury: a prospective study. *Spine* 2005;30;386–391.
47. Banic B, Petersen–Felix S, Andersen OK, et al. Evidence for spinal cord hypersensitivity in chronic pain after whiplash injury and in fibromyalgia. *Pain* 2004;107:7–15.
48. Curatolo M, Arendt–Nielsen L, Petersen–Felix S. Central hypersensitivity in chronic pain: mechanisms and clinical implications. *Phys Med Rehabil Clin N Am* 2006;17:287–302.
49. Gay J, Abbot K. Common whiplash injuries of the neck. *JAMA* 1953:152: 1698–1704.
50. Hodge JR. The whiplash neurosis. *Psychosomatics* 1971;12:245–249.
51. Blumer D, Heilbronn M. Chronic pain as a variant of depressive disease: the pain-prone disorder. *J Nerv Ment Dis* 1982;170:381–406.
52. Turk DC, Salovey P. "Chronic pain as a variant of depressive disease": a critical reappraisal. *J Nerv Ment Dis* 1984;172:398–404.
53. Kroenke K, Price RK. Symptoms in the community. Prevalence, classification, and psychiatric comorbidity. *Arch Intern Med* 1993;153:2474–2480.
54. Polatin PB, Kinney RK, Gatchel RJ, et al. Psychiatric illness and chronic low back pain. The mind and the spine—which goes first? *Spine* 1993;18:66–71.
55. Banks SM, Kerns RD. Explaining high rates of depression in chronic pain: a diathesis-stress framework. *Psychol Bull* 1996;119:95–110.
56. Von Korff M, Simon G. The relationship between pain and depression. *Br J Psychiat Suppl* 1996;168:101–108.
57. Jensen MP, Turner JA, Romano JM, et al. Relationship of pain-specific beliefs to chronic pain adjustment. *Pain* 1994;57:301–309.
58. Jensen MP, Romano JM, Turner JA, et al. Patient beliefs predict patient functioning: further support for a cognitive-behavioral model of chronic pain. *Pain* 1999;81:95–104.
59. Carragee EJ, Barcohana B, Alamin T, et al. Prospective controlled study of the development of lower back pain in previously asymptomatic subjects undergoing experimental discography. *Spine* 2004;29:1112–1117.
60. Fordyce WE. *Behavioral Methods for Chronic Pain and Illness*. St. Louis, CV Mosby; 1976.
61. Turk DC, Okifuji A, Scharff L. Chronic pain and depression: role of perceived impact and perceived control in different age cohorts. *Pain* 1995;61:93–101.
62. Rudy TE, Kerns RD, Turk DC. Chronic pain and depression: toward a cognitive–behavioral mediational model. *Pain* 1988;35:129–140.
63. Drottning M, Staff PH, Levin L, et al. Acute emotional response to common whiplash predicts subsequent pain complaints – a prospective study of 107 subjects sustaining whiplash injury. *Nordic J Psychiatry* 1995;49:293–300.
64. Gargan M, Bannister G, Main C, et al. The behavioral response to whiplash injury. *J Bone Joint Surg Br* 1997;79:523–526.
65. Mayou R, Bryant B, Duthie R. Psychiatric consequences of road traffic accidents. *BMJ* 1993;307:647–651.
66. American Psychiatric Association. *User's Guide for the Structured Clinical*

Interview for DSM-IV Axis I Disorders SCID-1: Clinician version. Washington, DC: American Psychiatric Press; 1997.

67. Turk DC, Swanson KS, Gatchel RJ. Predicting opioid misuse by chronic pain patients: a systematic review and literature synthesis. *Clin J Pain.* 2008;24:497–808.

68. Piotrowski C. Review of the psychological literature on assessment instruments used with pain patients. *N Am J Psychol* 2007;9:303–306.

69. Melzack R. The McGill Pain Questionnaire: major properties and scoring methods. *Pain* 1975;1:277–299.

69a. Melzack R. The short-form McGill Pain Questionnaire. *Pain* 1987;30:191–197.

70. Beck AT, Ward CH, Mendelson M, et al. An inventory for measuring depression. *Arch Gen Psychiatry* 1961;4:561–571.

71. Beck AT, Steer RA, Ball R, et al. Comparison of Beck Depression Inventories -IA and -II in psychiatric outpatients. *J Pers Assess* 1996;67:588–597.

72. Kerns RD, Turk DC, Rudy TE. The West Haven–Yale Multidimensional Pain Inventory (WHYMPI). *Pain* 1985;23:345–356.

73. Rosenstiel AK, Keefe FJ. The use of coping strategies in chronic low back pain patients. *Pain* 1983;17:33–44.

74. Fairbank JC, Couper J, Davies JB, et al. The Oswestry low back pain disability questionnaire. *Physiotherapy* 1980;66:271–273.

75. McNair DM, Lorr M, Droppleman LF. *Profile of Mood States.* San Diego: Educational and Industrial Testing Service; 1971.

76. Kerns RD. Assessment of emotional functioning in pain treatment outcome research. Presented at the second meeting of the Initiative on Methods, Measurement, and Pain Assessment in Clinical Trials (IMMPACT-II); April 2003. Available at http://www.immpact.org/meetings.html.

77. Dworkin RH, Corbin AE, Young JP, et al. Pregabalin for the treatment of postherpetic neuralgia: a randomized, placebo-controlled trial. *Neurology* 2003;60:1274–1283.

78. Rowbotham MC, Harden N, Stacey B, et al. Gabapentin Postherpetic Neuralgia Study Group. Gabapentin for the treatment postherpetic neuralgia: a randomized controlled trial. *JAMA* 1998;280:1837–1842.

79. Gallagher RM, Verma S. Mood and anxiety disorders in chronic pain. In: Dworkin RH, Breitbart WS, eds. *Psychosocial Aspects of Pain: A Handbook for Health Care Providers.* Seattle: IASP Press; 2004:589–606.

80. Wilson KG, Mikail SF, D'Eon JL, et al. Alternative diagnostic criteria for major depressive disorder in patients with chronic pain. *Pain* 2001;91:227–234.

81. Turk DC, Melzack R. eds. *Handbook of Pain Assessment.* 1st ed./2nd ed. New York, Guilford;1991/2001.

82. Jensen MP, Karoly P. Self-report scales and procedures for assessing pain in adults. In: Turk DC, Melzack R, eds. *Handbook of Pain Assessment.* 2nd ed. New York: Guilford Press; 2001:15–34.

83. Hadjistavropoulos T, von Baeyer C, Craig KD. Pain assessment in persons with limited ability to communicate. In: Turk DC, Melzack R, eds. *Handbook of Pain Assessment,* 2nd ed. New York: Guilford Press; 2001:134–152.

84. Gendreau M, Hufford MR, Stone AA. Measuring clinical pain in chronic widespread pain: selected methodological issues. *Best Pract Res Clin Rheumatol* 2003;17:575–592.

85. Stone AA, Shiffman, S. Capturing momentary, self-report data: a proposal for reporting guidelines. *Ann Behav Med* 2002;24:236–243.

86. Stone AA, Shiffman S, Schwartz JE, et al. Patient compliance with paper and electronic diaries. *Control Clin Trials* 2003;24:182–199.

87. Turk DC, Burwinkle T, Showlund M. Assessing the impact of chronic pain in real-time. In: Stone A, Shiffman S, Atienza A, et al, eds. *The Science of Real-time Data Capture: Self-reports in Health Research.* New York: Oxford University Press; 2007:204–228.

88. Price DD, Harkins SW, Baker C. Sensory-affective relationships among different types of clinical and experimental pain. *Pain* 1987;28:297–307.

89. Keefe FJ, Block AR. Development of an observation method for assessing pain behavior in chronic low back pain. *Behav Ther* 1982;12:363–375.

90. Keefe FJ, Williams DA, Smith SJ. Assessment of pain behaviors. In: Turk DC, Melzack RJ, eds. *Handbook of Pain Assessment.* 2nd ed. New York: Guilford Press; 2001:170–190.

91. Richards JS, Nepomunceno C, Riles M, et al. Assessing pain behavior: the UAB Pain Behavior Scale. *Pain* 1992;14:313–338.

92. Turk DC, Wack JT, Kerns RD. An empirical examination of the "pain behavior" construct. *J Behav Med* 1985;9:119–130.

92a. Kerns RD, Haythornthwaite J, Rosenberg R, et al. The Pain Behavior Checklist (PBCL): factor structure and psychometric properties. *J Behav Med* 1991;14:155–167.

93. Atlas SJ, Tosteson TD, Hanscom B, et al. What is different about worker's compensation patients? Socioeconomic predictors of baseline disability status among patients with lumbar radiculopathy. *Spine* 2007;32:2019–2026.

94. Harris I, Mulford J, Solomon M, et al.. Association between compensation status and outcome after surgery: a meta-analysis. *JAMA* 2005;293:1644–1652.

95. Hernandez A, Sachs–Ericsson N. Ethnic differences in pain reports and the moderating role of depression in a community sample of Hispanic and Caucasian participants with serious health problems. *Psychosom Med* 2006;68:121–128.

96. Watson PJ, Latif RK, Rowbotham DJ. Ethnic differences in thermal pain responses: a comparison of South Asian and White British healthy males. *Pain* 2005;118:194–200.

97. Berglund A, Bodin L, Jensen I, et al. The influence of prognostic factors on neck pain intensity, disability, anxiety and depression over a 2-year period in subjects with acute whiplash injury. *Pain* 2006;125:244–256.

98. Holm LW, Carroll LJ, Cassidy JD, et al. Factors influencing neck pain intensity in whiplash-associated disorders. *Spine* 2006;31:E98–104.

99. Mendelson G, Mendelson D. Legal aspects of the management of chronic pain. *Med J Aust* 1991;155:640–642.

100. Dufton JA, Kopec JA, Wong H, et al. Prognostic factors associated with minimal improvement following acute whiplash-associated disorders. *Spine* 2006;31:E759–765; discussion E766.

101. Gun RT, Osti OL, O'Riordan A, et al. Risk factors for prolonged disability after whiplash injury: a prospective study. *Spine* 2005;30:386–391.

102. Scholten–Peeters GM, Verhagen AP, Bekkering GE, et al. Prognostic factors of whiplash associated disorders: a systematic review of prospective cohort studies. *Pain* 2003;104:303–322.

103. Cassidy JD, Carroll LJ, Cote P, et al. Effect of eliminating compensation for pain and suffering on the outcome of insurance claims for whiplash injury. *N Engl J Med* 2000;342:1179–1186.

104. Clionsky M. Effect of eliminating compensation for pain and suffering on the outcome of insurance claims. *N Engl J Med* 200;343:1119.

105. Freeman MD, Rossignol AM. Effect of eliminating compensation for pain and suffering on the outcome of insurance claims. *N Engl J Med* 2000;343:1118–1119.

106. Merskey H, Teasell RW. Effect of eliminating compensation for pain and suffering on the outcome of insurance claims. *N Engl J Med* 2000;343:1119.

107. Russell RS. Effect of eliminating compensation for pain and suffering on the outcome of insurance claims. *N Engl J Med* 2000;343:1119–1120.

108. Thieme K, Spies C, Sinha P, et al. Predictors of pain behaviors in fibromyalgia syndrome patients. *Arthritis Care Res* 2005;53:343–350.

109. Wind H, Gouttebarge V, Kuijer PP, et al. Assessment of functional capacity of the musculoskeletal system in the context of work, daily living, and sport: a systematic review. *J Occup Rehabil* 2005;15(2):253–272.

110. Ware JE Jr, Sherbourne CD. The MOS 36-item short-form health survey (SF-36). *Med Care* 1992;30:473–483.

111. Cleeland CS, Ryan KM. Pain assessment: global use of the Brief Pain Inventory. *Ann Acad Med Singapore* 1994;23:129–138.

112. Pollard CA. Preliminary validity study of the Pain Disability Index. *Percept Mot Skills* 1984;59:974.

113. Dworkin RH, Nagasako EM, Hetzel RD, et al. Assessment of pain and pain-related quality of life in clinical trials. In: Turk DC, Melzack R, eds. *Handbook of Pain Assessment.* 2nd ed. New York: Guilford; 2001:659–692.

114. Guyatt GH, Feeney DH, Patrick DL. Measuring health-related quality of life. *Ann Intern Med* 1993;118:622–629.

115. King PM, Tuckwell N, Barrett TE. A critical review of functional capacity evaluations. *Phys Ther* 1998;78:852–866.

116. Gouttebarge V, Wind H, Kuijer PP, et al. Reliability and validity of Functional Capacity Evaluation methods: a systematic review with reference to Blankenship system, Ergos work simulator, Ergo-Kit and Isernhagen work system. *Int Arch Occup Environ Health* 2004;77:527–537.

117. Loeser JD, Turk DC. Multidisciplinary pain management. In: Loeser JD, Butler SH, Chapman CR, et al., eds., *Bonica's Management of Pain.* 3rd ed. Baltimore: Lippincott, Williams & Wilkins; 2001;2069–2080.

118. Schatman ME. The demise of multidisciplinary pain management clinics? *Practical Pain Manage* 2006;6:30–41.

CHAPTER 24 ■ PAINFUL NEUROPATHIES

DAVID WALK AND MISHA-MIROSLAV BACKONJA

PAIN AS A SYMPTOM OF NEUROPATHY

Neuropathy is a common clinical problem. Pain merits attention in any discussion of neuropathy for several reasons. First, insofar as pain varies among neuropathy etiologies, the presence, absence, and type of pain when present can contribute to the diagnostic process. Second, for many people with neuropathy, pain is the chief complaint and the only cause of disability. The traditional neurological focus on deficits rather than positive sensory phenomena does not serve these patients well. Finally, and perhaps most importantly, pain is a neurological symptom. The study of pain due to nerve dysfunction is providing important insights into the function of the nervous system, as has the study of other neurologic symptoms in the past.

THE EVALUATION AND DIAGNOSIS OF NEUROPATHY

Neuropathy Classification

The approach to the diagnosis of neuropathy is fully covered in textbooks devoted to this topic.[1,2] The present section is a conceptual overview to allow readers unfamiliar with neuromuscular practice to better understand the balance of this chapter. Throughout this section, specific neuropathies will be named for the purpose of illustration only. More comprehensive and detailed information about specific types of neuropathy can be can be found later in this chapter under "Painful Neuropathies."

The four principal questions to address in the etiologic classification of neuropathy are the *time course* of symptoms, the *distribution* of neuropathy symptoms and signs, the *modalities* affected (motor, small fiber sensory, large fiber sensory, and autonomic), and the primary *locus of pathology* (axon or myelin). Answers to these four questions will narrow the differential diagnosis substantially.

Time course is self-explanatory. Many common neuropathies, particularly those due to metabolic or genetic conditions, progress insidiously and at a regular pace over years. Some, such as chronic inflammatory demyelinating polyradiculoneuropathy (CIDP), can progress over a period of weeks to months, and often with unpredictable relapses or remissions. Relatively few neuropathies present with florid findings over a matter of days to weeks; among these are Guillain-Barre syndrome (which progresses rapidly in a predictable fashion to a nadir within 2 to 4 weeks), toxic neuropathies (which can present rapidly upon neurotoxin exposure and commonly progress in a predictable fashion until days, weeks, or even months after removal of the cause), and necrotizing peripheral nerve vasculitis (which usually progresses in a stepwise fashion over days to weeks until effective therapy is instituted).

The *distribution of neuropathy symptoms and signs* can be identified by the history and confirmed by the examination and electrophysiological studies. Most neuropathies conform to one of three patterns: symmetric, length dependent; asymmetric, nonlength dependent; and multifocal. The symmetric, length dependent pattern begins with symptoms in both feet and progresses rostrally in a symmetric fashion. The pattern and rate of change are uniform. Symptoms usually do not appear in the hands until lower limb symptoms have progressed to the proximal calves or thighs. Symptoms appear last in the trunk and face. The term *length dependent* refers to the fact that nerve dysfunction in these patients begins in the longest axons and progresses rostrally. The implication vis-à-vis pathophysiology is that all nerves are exposed in equal measure to a systemic stressor, and that the effect of this stressor on nerve function is closely correlated to the distance of the nerve terminal from the cell body. Many metabolic, toxic, and genetic disorders of nerve present in a symmetric, length-dependent pattern. Asymmetric, nonlength-dependent neuropathies are widespread but can affect proximal and distal nerve segments concomitantly and do not present in a symmetric fashion. CIDP typically demonstrates this distribution. Multifocal neuropathies affect individual named nerves or nerve trunks, often with a stepwise progression. Necrotizing vasculitis, granulomatous disorders, hereditary neuropathy with liability to pressure palsies (HNPP), and lymphomatous infiltration are examples of conditions that can present in this fashion. When a sufficient number of nerves are affected, multifocal neuropathies become confluent and are thereby transformed into the asymmetric, nonlength dependent pattern.

The *modalities affected* refers to motor axons, large fiber (Aβ myelinated) sensory axons, small fiber (A∂ and C) sensory axons, and autonomic (cardiorespiratory, vasomotor, and visceromotor) axons. As with *distribution*, the involvement of these fiber classes can be identified by the history and confirmed by the neurological examination and electrophysiological studies; in addition, numerous clinical tools have been developed in recent decades to assist in the confirmation of small fiber sensory and autonomic involvement. Virtually all neuropathies demonstrate prominent involvement of sensory axons, and most symmetric, length-dependent neuropathies with metabolic or toxic etiologies are clinically sensory-predominant or pure sensory neuropathies until they are relatively advanced. The relative involvement of large and small sensory axons varies among, and in some cases within, etiologies. Patients with clinical findings isolated to small-fiber modalities are often referred to as having small-fiber neuropathy (SFN), although there is evidence that this progresses over time to involve both small- and large-fiber types. SFN can be seen in diabetes or HIV infection but is also often idiopathic. Not surprisingly, large-fiber sensory symptoms predominate in those neuropathies in which the primary pathology is a disorder of myelin, such as Charcot-Marie-Tooth (CMT) type I or CIDP. Necrotizing vasculitis, CMT, and CIDP are among the relatively common neuropathies that usually demonstrate prominent motor and sensory involvement. Motor neuropathies without discernible sensory or autonomic involvement are so uncommon in general clinical practice that patients presenting with isolated weakness in a pattern suggesting neuromuscular disease should be considered to have a disorder of motor neurons, neuromuscular transmission, or muscle until proven otherwise. The few neuropathies that can present as pure motor disorders include multifocal motor neuropathy (MMN) and the neuropathy of acute lead intoxication, and both are rare conditions. Few neuropathies, including those associated with amyloidosis and type I diabetes mellitus, have clinically significant autonomic involvement.

The *primary locus of pathology (axon or myelin)* is most reliably determined by nerve conduction studies and by nerve biopsy, although the neurological examination can be used to draw inferences about this. For example, muscle stretch reflexes are lost early in CIDP, and sometimes in the absence of substantial weakness of the muscle in question. By contrast, because demyelination alone does not result in denervation, denervation atrophy does not develop unless or until there is secondary axonal injury from longstanding demyelination. Thus, CIDP is often associated with early loss of reflexes and relative preservation of muscle bulk in the face of significant weakness. By contrast, axonal neuropathies result in relative preservation of reflexes and early atrophy of clinically affected muscles. Nonetheless, these clinical clues require confirmation by nerve conduction studies which, if interpreted correctly, provide reliable information about the primary pathologic substrate. For this reason, nerve biopsy is rarely needed to determine whether the primary pathology is of the axon or myelin, though it is occasionally useful in demonstrating the nature of the pathologic process. The only common disorders of peripheral myelin are Guillain-Barré syndrome, CIDP, and CMT type I.

Pain is common in some neuropathies and uncommon in others. There are pain descriptors that are common in painful neuropathies and less common in other painful conditions. This clinical observation has led to the development of several neuropathic pain questionnaires.[3–6] The process of validating such questionnaires has resulted in the identification of several symptoms that correlate well with the presence of neurologic dysfunction. These include paresthesias, spontaneous burning, numbness, shooting pains, and tactile allodynia.[7]

The presence, absence, and character of neuropathic pain can help the clinician identify the most likely type and etiology of a patient's neuropathy. For example, neuropathic pain is one of the defining characteristics of small fiber neuropathy. Allodynia is almost universally present in postherpetic neuralgia and is common in other sensory neuronopathy syndromes. Severe, aching, boring pain is an essential feature of neuralgic amyotrophy and a common complaint in necrotizing vasculitis. By contrast, CMT may be associated with musculoskeletal pain but the presence of prominent neuropathic pain would put this diagnosis in doubt. A neuropathic pain symptom questionnaire should be included in every diagnostic evaluation for neuropathy.

History, Examination, and Diagnostic Studies

The medical history of a patient with neuropathy should include a systematic assessment of positive and negative sensory symptoms, motor symptoms, and autonomic symptoms. The neuropathy symptom profile instrument includes all of these.[8] As noted previously, neuropathic pain questionnaires allow systematic and comprehensive assessment of spontaneous and stimulus-evoked positive sensory symptoms, as well as pain descriptors, in patients with neuropathic pain.

The examination of the patient with neuropathy must include

bedside assessments of both large and small fiber sensory modalities.

In addition to the standard neurological examination, several laboratory investigations have proven valuable in the assessment of neuropathy in general and painful neuropathy in particular. These include psychophysical, neurophysiological, and anatomic investigations.

Psychophysical tests investigate the relationship between physical stimulus properties and corresponding perceptions of the stimulus.[9] The sensory component of the standard neurological examination is a series of psychophysical tests. The term "quantitative sensory testing" (QST) is often used to describe one of several psychophysical testing paradigms for quantitative determination of thermal or mechanical perception thresholds. In addition to threshold testing, QST can be used to obtain a subjective intensity rating in response to a fixed stimulus. For example, QST can be used to establish either a thermal pain threshold or the perceived intensity of pain evoked by a thermal stimulus of fixed intensity. Like the neurologic examination, QST can be used to determine whether a subject's sensory perception is normal and as a monitoring tool.[10,11]

There is growing interest in developing a standardized assessment protocol for neuropathic pain to include tests of thermal, mechanical, and even chemical allodynia and hyperalgesia. It is hoped that comprehensive assessments of neuropathic pain features such as these will allow clinicians to identify patterns of pain phenotypes that reveal clues to the unique causes and treatments of neuropathic pain in individual patient groups, much as the development of the now-standard neurologic examination has proved useful in lesion localization and disease pattern recognition. Thermal allodynia and hyperalgesia can be tested along with thermal sensory threshold testing, using commercially available devices. A comprehensive test of sensory thresholds, allodynia, and hyperalgesia has been designed and implemented by the German Neuropathic Pain study group.[12] A simpler test which combines mapping of areas of allodynia or hyperalgesia with fixed stimulus intensity rating and multimodality neuropathic pain assessment has been proposed by the Neuropathic Pain Research Consortium (NPRC) in the United States.[13] These efforts are still in their infancy and await further validation and large-scale implementation.

Neurophysiologic studies investigate the activity of electrically excitable tissues (nerve or muscle cells) either at rest, during normal activity, or in response to externally applied stimuli. In the context of peripheral nerve disease, the most commonly used neurophysiologic studies are nerve conduction studies and electromyography (NCS/EMG). As noted in the previous section, NCS/EMG can provide objective evidence of dysfunction of large myelinated (Aβ) nerves, valuable evidence of whether the primary pathology is in the myelin or axon, and information about the distribution of disease.

One of the major limitations of NCS/EMG is that it provides no information about the function of small myelinated (Aδ) or unmyelinated (C) fibers. Because NCS/EMG has been the principal confirmatory and investigational tool in the neuromuscular field since its inception, there has therefore been little or no recognition of the existence of neuropathy preferentially affecting small axons until very recently. The advent of immunohistochemical staining of skin biopsy tissue for evaluation of epidermal nerve fibers (ENFs) has allowed the identification of patients with normal nerve conduction studies but loss of cutaneous nerves.[14,15] In most cases there are corresponding signs of abnormal nociception, consisting of both sensory loss and spontaneous or stimulus-evoked neuropathic pain,[16,17] although such patients likely lose large (Aβ) fibers over time as well.[18] The syndrome of neuropathic pain with impaired thermal and nociceptive sensation, loss of ENFs, and relatively normal nerve conduction studies is often referred to as "small fiber neuropathy" in recognition of the fact that the clinical and laboratory features of this condition are largely referable to loss or dysfunction of the small caliber Aδ and C fibers. The ability to diagnose small fiber neuropathy with ENF density evaluation has spurred tremendous interest in this syndrome.

Pathologic examination of peripheral nerve trunks also plays an important role in neuropathy diagnosis in selected cases. While NCS/EMG are usually adequate to confirm a diagnosis of neuropathy, define the geographic distribution, and identify whether the primary pathology is demyelination or axon loss, nerve biopsy is occasionally needed to identify those etiologies, such as vasculitis or amyloidosis, that are primarily pathologic diagnoses. Nerve biopsy can also be used to support a diagnosis of CIDP or other chronic demyelinating neuropathies.[19]

PAINFUL NEUROPATHIES

There is a higher incidence of pain among some etiologic categories of neuropathy than others. In this section we describe those common neuropathies that are often painful.

Distal Symmetric Polyneuropathies

Metabolic Causes

Diabetic Neuropathy. The most common cause of distal symmetric polyneuropathy in the developed world is diabetes. Diabetic neuropathy is often but not always painful. The prevalence of painful neuropathy symptoms in one community study of diabetics was 16%.[20] All features of neuropathic pain, including mechanical or thermal allodynia, hyperalgesia, spontaneous shooting pains, and spontaneous burning, may occur. Like the sensory deficits of diabetic neuropathy, diabetic neuropathy pain presents in a length-dependent, symmetric pattern. Therefore, focal neuropathic pain in a diabetic should prompt consideration of an alternative etiology for the pain. Mononeuropathies in diabetes are discussed later under the heading "painful mononeuropathy multiplex and focal neuropathic syndromes."

There is no established metabolic or genetic distinction between diabetics whose neuropathy is or is not associated with neuropathic pain, although it has been suggested that neuropathic pain often develops early in the course of nerve injury and recedes when neuropathy becomes more severe. There is no firm evidence that any one of the several proposed mechanisms of diabetic neuropathy is responsible for diabetic polyneuropathy pain.

Experimental models of diabetic neuropathy have provided evidence that pain in diabetic neuropathy may be due to pathology at multiple sites in the nervous system. Work in the streptozotocin model has demonstrated altered expression of sodium channels in primary afferent neurons,[21] COX-2 release from oligodendrocytes and dysregulation of inhibitory interneurons in the spinal cord,[22,23] and altered descending inhibition of pain.[24] It remains to be determined whether these mechanisms apply in people with diabetic neuropathy.

Investigation of the syndrome of small fiber neuropathy has revealed a disproportionate number of patients with impaired glucose tolerance (IGT), suggesting that the etiology of neuropathy in such cases is incipient diabetes and the mechanism is the same as that of diabetic neuropathy. Although appealing, this remains a hypothesis only. Many such patients also have the metabolic syndrome, presently defined as at least three of the following: central obesity, elevated serum triglycerides, reduced serum HDL, elevated blood pressure, and elevated fasting plasma glucose.[25] Among disorders of lipids, hypertriglyceridemia in particular has been found to be prevalent in this syndrome.[26,27] Conversely, there is some evidence that, among diabetics, the prevalence or severity of neuropathy is greater if other components of the metabolic syndrome are present.[28,29] These observa-

tions suggest that microvascular disease exacerbates the nerve injury associated with hyperglycemia.

Infectious Causes

Both HIV infection and several of the commonly used highly active antiretroviral therapies (HAART) for HIV infection are associated with distal symmetric polyneuropathy.[30–32] The two etiologies may coexist and the neuropathies associated with them are clinically indistinguishable; therefore, initial management for DSP in a patient on HAART usually consists of a therapeutic trial of medication change or discontinuation. DSP is most closely associated with the use of dideoxynucleoside analogues stavudine (D4T), zalcitabine (ddC), and didanosine (ddI). The mechanism of this effect is believed to be the inhibition of mitochondrial DNA polymerization, leading to mitochondrial dysfunction and, in turn, reduced energy availability. DSP in HIV infection commonly presents with symptoms of small-fiber involvement, with prominent pain and paresthesias. The mechanism of HIV neuropathy is unknown, although there is some experimental evidence implicating inflammatory mechanisms triggered by infection of periaxonal Schwann cells.[30]

Chronic hepatitis C virus (HCV) infection is a well-recognized cause of polyneuropathy. Distal symmetric polyneuropathy, mononeuropathy multiplex, and cranial neuropathy can all be seen in this context. Polyneuropathy due to HCV infection is usually, but not always, associated with secondary cryoglobulinemia, and nerve biopsy often demonstrates features suggestive or diagnostic of vasculitis.[33] Depending on the severity and time course of the condition, as well as the pathologic findings, treatment can be supportive or may include antiviral therapy, immunomodulating therapy, or both.[33,34]

Lyme disease is a well-recognized cause of cranial neuropathy and polyradiculopathy. Less commonly, polyneuropathy and mononeuropathy multiplex have been described in the context of Lyme disease. While direct infection is difficult to demonstrate, a diagnosis of peripheral nervous system Lyme disease can be inferred in the context of a subacute progressive neuropathy with clinical and serologic evidence of Lyme and clinical improvement with antibiotic therapy. Lyme radiculopathy, polyneuropathy, and mononeuropathy multiplex can all be associated with pain.[35,36]

Toxic Neuropathies

Neurotoxic substances impair a number of neural processes such as protein synthesis, axonal transport, and myelin maintenance. Exposure to several industrial toxins is well known to lead to polyneuropathy. These usually cause motor symptoms and signs, although painful and dysesthetic symptoms may ensue in a minority of patients. Very few pathological studies have been conducted in humans. N-hexane, a common ingredient in household glue, and methyl-n-butyl ketone, an industrial solvent, are known to cause focal swelling of axons to two to three times their normal diameter and can result in painful neuropathy.[37,38]

Several pharmaceutical agents may cause painful polyneuropathy. Vincristine, taxol, paclitaxel, and docetaxel all cause polyneuropathy with pain and dysesthesias. Recent evidence implicates mitochondrial dysfunction and changes in calcium-channel expression in chemotherapy-induced neuropathy, which will probably dictate treatment strategies for this type of painful polyneuropathy.[39,40]

Many other drugs are known to cause polyneuropathies which are not always painful. Among these are isoniazid, gold, disulfiram, nitrofurantoin, amiodarone, and benzafibrate.

Nutritional Neuropathies

Pyridoxine Deficiency From Isoniazid Use. Isoniazid is an effective and inexpensive antituberculosis drug but it is associated with distal neuropathy when administered in high doses. Patients with a genetic predisposition for slow metabolism of isoniazid are more susceptible to this adverse effect. Isoniazid interferes with essential metabolic functions of pyridoxine, leading to axonal damage. This axonopathy affects small and large fibers, causing motor deficits, sensory deficits, and pain. Pain is described as deep aching pain in calf muscles and burning paresthesiae in upper and lower extremities. Oral pyridoxine in doses of 30–100 mg per day can prevent or reverse isoniazid neuropathy. Excessive doses should be avoided since pyridoxine itself can cause neuropathy if given in excess.

Beriberi. Beriberi is the most widely recognized nutritional neuropathy and is a disease of the peripheral nerves and heart[41] caused by thiamine deficiency. If the heart is affected it presents with heart failure (wet beriberi) but the majority of patients present with neuropathy alone (dry beriberi). Presenting symptoms are slowly progressive distal weakness, paresthesiae, and pain. Rarely beriberi develops acutely. There are multiple presentations of pain symptoms, including dull, constant ache, lancinating brief pain similar to tabes dorsalis, tightness, and burning. Unlike idiopathic distal symmetric small fiber neuropathy, in beriberi burning usually involves the hands as well as the feet shortly after onset. Physical examination reveals symmetric sensory loss across all modalities as well as positive phenomena such as allodynia, hyperalgesia, and hyperpathia, as well as distal weakness and areflexia. Large-fiber involvement is demonstrated by nerve conduction studies.[42] Nutritional supplementation with thiamine is essential. With treatment, beriberi neuropathy improves slowly.

Pellagra Neuropathy. Pellagra is a nutritional disorder which when fully developed affects the skin, gastrointestinal, hematopoietic, and nervous systems. Nervous system manifestations include encephalopathy, myelopathy, and neuropathy. Neuropathy is infrequent but can be quite disabling.

Alcohol Neuropathy. It is well established that excessive and prolonged intake of alcohol is associated with a distal symmetric polyneuropathy which is often characterized by distal paresthesias, burning, and other features of neuropathic pain. The precise cause of alcohol polyneuropathy is unknown. For decades, the principal question has been whether alcohol polyneuropathy is due solely to deficiency of thiamine and, perhaps, other B vitamins, or is due to a direct toxic effect of alcohol, its metabolites, or even other neurotoxins in alcoholic beverages. Support for a neurotoxic role of alcohol comes from an animal model of alcoholic neuropathy in which rats that are provided adequate nutritional supplementation along with alcohol develop polyneuropathy.[43] Some interesting clinical observations support this as well. For example, alcohol polyneuropathy is prevalent among Danish alcoholics despite the fact that beer, which is the alcoholic beverage of choice in that country, is supplemented with B vitamins.[44] In addition, an elegant series of studies of Japanese alcoholics has demonstrated that neuropathy is prevalent among alcoholics with normal serum thiamine levels, and that sural nerve pathology differs between alcoholics with and without thiamine deficiency.[45]

Neuromuscular Manifestations of Intestinal Malabsorption After Bariatric Surgery and Other Gastrointestinal Surgical Procedures. The growing use of bariatric surgery has led to resurgence in awareness of neurological disorders associated with malabsorption, some of which can be associated with neuropathic pain. Wernicke's encephalopathy, beriberi, and subacute combined degeneration due to vitamin B12 or copper deficiency are among the neurologic disorders attributable to known deficiency states that have been described after bariatric surgery. In some cases a presumed nutritional myeloneuropathy has been ascribed to multiple nutritional deficiencies or deficiency of an

unknown nutrient in such patients. Neuropathic pain can occur in beriberi and in subacute combined degeneration, the latter most likely as a result of an associated sensory neuropathy.

Hereditary Neuropathies

Charcot-Marie-Tooth (CMT) is the most common hereditary neuropathy, with an estimated prevalence of 40 per 100,000.[46] The clinical syndrome is a progressive symmetric length-dependent motor and sensory neuropathy. CMT differs from the length-dependent polyneuropathy seen in diabetes and most other metabolic, nutritional, and toxic disorders because, in CMT, weakness and atrophy are prominent early signs and both upper and lower extremities are typically affected. Most forms of CMT are inherited in an autosomal-dominant fashion, the exception being the X-linked form (CMTX). Neuropathic pain is uncommon in CMT, and when it occurs it is usually not the most prominent symptom. Fatigue, neuromuscular discomfort, and aching pain from foot deformities and overuse syndromes do occur. Acute intermittent porphyria is an autosomal dominant disorder with neuropathy which may have pain as one of the presenting symptoms, but pain is always overshadowed by weakness.

Fabry's Disease. Fabry's disease is perhaps the sole hereditary neuropathy in which neuropathic pain is the cardinal symptom. Fabry's disease is a multisystem disorder affecting peripheral nerves, kidneys, heart, and skin. It is inherited in X-linked recessive fashion and its symptoms start in childhood or adolescence. The biochemical abnormality is a deficiency of alpha-galactosidase, a lysosomal enzyme. The estimated prevalence is about 2 per 100,000 males.[47]

The clinical features include red punctate skin lesions in the lower body and thighs, corneal opacifications, cardiac and renal failure, and polyneuropathy. Cardiac and renal failure are terminal events for these patients. The neuropathy of Fabry's disease is characterized by continuous burning pain in the hands and feet, with spontaneous paroxysms of more severe pain. On examination there are surprisingly modest sensory deficits, and muscle stretch reflexes are preserved. Nerve conduction studies are usually normal. In addition to pain, patients with Fabry's disease have marked autonomic dysfunction manifesting with episodic diarrhea, vomiting, urinary retention, and diminished sweating. Gastrointestinal symptoms can be relieved with metoclopramide.[48,49]

While idiopathic SFN preferentially affects small fibers, Fabry's disease may be unique in that it appears to exclusively affect small myelinated and unmyelinated axons, at least until such time as renal insufficiency occurs and causes a superimposed mixed polyneuropathy. This has been demonstrated pathologically by comparison of epidermal nerve fiber density with sural nerve morphometry in the same patients. Interestingly, the same study demonstrated a loss of epidermal nerve fibers immediately after an episode of pain in two subjects, suggesting that painful episodes in Fabry's disease reflect acute nerve injury. Enzyme replacement therapy has been shown to have multiple benefits, including an improvement in the Brief Pain Inventory, but not in ENF density or thermal thresholds. Clearly, more needs to be learned about the effect of enzyme replacement therapy on the neuropathy of Fabry's disease.[48,49]

Amyloid Neuropathy. Neuropathy is a common, early, and often prominent manifestation of amyloidosis.[50] Neuropathy can occur in both familial and acquired amyloidosis. There are several distinct clinical groups of familial (transthyretin) amyloidosis but all of them have an autosomal dominant inheritance pattern. The prevalence varies greatly among ethnic groups. The initial symptoms are numbness, paresthesiae, and pain in the feet and lower legs. Autonomic involvement is also common, manifesting with abnormal pupillary reflexes, miosis, anhidrosis, orthostatic hypotension, diarrhea alternating with constipation, and impotence. Cranial nerve involvement manifests late in the disease. About half of the patients have neuropathic symptoms at onset, while half present with cardiac, hematologic, or renal dysfunction. Patients with familial amyloid polyneuropathy can benefit from liver transplantation.[51] The prognosis of primary (nonfamilial) amyloidosis is very poor.[52]

Other Widespread but Nonlength-Dependent Neuropathies

Neuropathy with Paraproteinemia

Monoclonal gammopathy, defined as the presence of a single clone of immunoglobulin identified via serum protein electrophoresis or immunofixation, is common in the elderly. While sometimes due to myeloma or lymphoma, monoclonal gammopathy can present in the absence of a malignant lymphoproliferative disorder and, in such cases, is referred to as monoclonal gammopathy of undetermined significance (MGUS). There is an increased prevalence of neuropathy among individuals with MGUS, and an increased prevalence of MGUS among individuals with otherwise unexplained neuropathy.[52] Despite this, with the exception of a few well-characterized specific antibody-mediated syndromes, such as the syndromes associated with IgM antibodies to the sulfated glucuronyl paragloboside epitope of myelin-associated glycoprotein (MAG-SGPG)[53] and disialosyl antibodies, there is no compelling evidence of a causal relationship between MGUS and neuropathy. Nonetheless, the association is sufficiently common that it is prudent to obtain a serum protein immunofixation as part of the evaluation of idiopathic neuropathy, particularly in patients over the age of 60, and to consider that MGUS in a patient with neuropathy may represent more than a chance association.

Several clinical phenotypes, both axonal and demyelinative, have been described in neuropathy with MGUS. CIDP, a chronic acquired demyelinating neuropathy that usually responds to immune manipulation, is occasionally associated with MGUS. Distal acquired demyelinating syndrome (DADS) is an indolent syndrome of sensory ataxia, often with distal weakness, with electrophysiologic evidence of distal-predominant demyelination. DADS is usually associated with an IgM monoclonal gammopathy which, in about two-thirds of cases, is directed against MAG-SGPG.[54]

Axonal pathology is also common in MGUS-neuropathy, particularly among patients with IgG and IgA monoclonal proteins. Axonal MGUS-neuropathy is usually an indolent condition with prominent negative and positive sensory symptoms.

Neuropathy can be associated with lymphoproliferative malignancies as well. Perhaps most notably, polyneuropathy is part of the POEMS syndrome, an acronym which refers to polyneuropathy, organomegaly, endocrinopathy, M-spike, and skin changes. POEMS syndrome most often occurs in the setting of osteosclerotic myeloma, multiple myeloma, or angiofollicular lymph node hyperplasia (Castleman's syndrome). The polyneuropathy in POEMS syndrome, unlike most polyneuropathies associated with MGUS, is usually progressive and disabling but does often respond to appropriate treatment of the associated lymphoproliferative syndrome. Electrophysiologic studies usually reveal a primary demyelinative pattern.[55]

Neuropathic pain can occur with all paraproteinemic polyneuropathies. While negative sensory symptoms usually predominate in acquired demyelinating neuropathies, pain and paresthesias can occur and are occasionally severe. While speculative, it is possible that this reflects dysfunction or ectopic discharge of small myelinated nociceptors, loss of collateral inhibition of afferent input from small myelinated and unmyelinated axons, or sensitization due to the expression of inflammatory cytokines in nerve.

Autoimmune Demyelinating Neuropathies

Guillain-Barré Syndrome. Guillain-Barré syndrome (GBS) is an inflammatory polyneuropathy with an estimated annual incidence rate of 1.2–1.9 per 100,000.[56] The syndrome is characterized by rapidly progressive, widespread, and often severe weakness of the limbs and cranial musculature with areflexia. Approximately 10% of patients require ventilatory support. Weakness reaches a nadir within 4 weeks, with substantial spontaneous recovery in the majority of patients. Nonetheless, despite a generally good prognosis for recovery of strength, many patients are left with considerable fatigue, and some with distal weakness and paresthesias.

Electrophysiologic investigations demonstrate features of demyelination, including focal motor conduction block, in most patients with GBS. This is concordant with pathologic investigations which demonstrate lymphocytic infiltration and macrophage-mediated demyelination of nerve roots and peripheral nerves.[57] Thus, until recently the descriptive term acute inflammatory demyelinating polyradiculoneuropathy (AIDP) was considered synonymous with GBS. Occasional patients with evidence of axon loss were felt to have suffered secondary axonal injury in a fulminant demyelinating disease. In 1995, a seminal description of Chinese patients with a epidemic form of GBS without electrophysiologic or pathologic features of demyelination led to the elucidation of GBS subtypes, now referred to as acute motor axonal neuropathy (AMAN) and acute motor axonal sensory-motor neuropathy (AMSAN),[58] which appear to reflect immunologically mediated disruption of paranodal sodium channels, leading to reversible conduction failure without myelin disruption.[59] Whether they are AIDP, AMAN, or AMSAN, all forms of GBS often develop several weeks following a systemic infection, suggesting molecular mimicry as a triggering event, but AMAN in particular is strongly associated with preceding gastrointestinal infection with *Campylobacter jejuni* and the subsequent development of serum IgG antibodies directed against ganglioside GM1, which are probably pathogenic.[59] Pain has been reported to be one of the presenting symptoms in more than three quarters of patients with GBS, and in many it precedes weakness. Pain is present throughout the course of GBS and in half of those patients it is rated as severe. Pain intensity upon admission does not correlate with neurological disability.[60] The major pain syndromes observed in GBS are back and leg pain, dysesthetic extremity pain, and myalgic extremity pain.[61]

About two-thirds of patients experience back and leg pain at some time during the course of GBS. This pain is usually described as a deep, aching, or throbbing pain in the low back frequently radiating to the buttocks, thighs, and occasionally to the calves. This pain may reflect root inflammation or endoneurial edema. Dysesthetic extremity pain, described as burning, tingling, or shock-like, involves the legs more frequently than the arms, and is also common in GBS. This type of pain is present in a minority of patients upon admission, although about half experience dysesthetic pain sometime during the course of the illness. It may persist indefinitely in 5% to 10%.[60] It is postulated that neuropathic pain of this type is due to ectopic impulse formation at sites of demyelination and axonal degeneration or regeneration.[62] Myalgic extremity pain, described as aching or cramping pain, often with joint stiffness, is less frequent than radicular low back pain. This pain is most notable during the passive and active assisted exercises associated with physical therapy.[61]

A recent review of pain symptoms in GBS demonstrated that backache, interscapular pain, and myalgias are most common early in the course of the disease and generally resolve during the recovery phase, while dysesthesias and paresthesias are more likely to persist, sometimes for months or longer.[61] This is compatible with the theorized etiologies noted previously.

Pain Management in Guillain-Barre Syndrome. In a prospective study, 75% of patients required oral or parenteral opioids to provide adequate pain relief.[60] Epidural morphine has been used as an alternative to systemic opioids in ventilated patients with primarily low back and leg pain.[63] In nonventilated patients in the acute stage of illness, opioid analgesics must be titrated carefully because of increased risk of respiratory depression. During the recovery phase, when muscle and joint pain is routinely precipitated by passive and active exercises, immediate-release codeine or morphine can be given an hour or two prior to treatment to facilitate compliance with physical therapy. Most patients do not require opioid analgesics beyond the first 8 weeks of illness.

A wide variety of medications used to manage neuropathic pain in other settings can be used in GBS, although caution should be taken with medications that can exacerbate hypotension or precipitate cardiac arrhythmias because of the autonomic instability which is common in GBS.

There are no controlled studies on the efficacy of any treatment of pain associated with GBS.

Chronic Inflammatory Demyelinating Polyradiculoneuropathy. Chronic inflammatory demyelinating polyradiculoneuropathy (CIDP) is a chronic peripheral nervous system disorder which can have progressive, relapsing-remitting, and monophasic courses. The prevalence of CIDP has been estimated at 0.8 to 1.9 per 100,000. In contrast to GBS, association with preceding viral illnesses is uncommon. Some autoimmune and infectious disorders, such as MGUS, lupus, and HIV infection, have been associated with CIDP, but most cases are unrelated to systemic illness. The presenting symptoms are numbness and/or weakness with hyporeflexia progressing over at least 8 weeks' time. Pain may or may not occur but, when it does, it can have any of the features of neuropathic pain. Therapy is aimed at treating the underlying disease process with immunotherapy, usually steroids or IVIg.[64,65] Pain management should follow the basic principles of neuropathic pain pharmacological therapy.

Painful Mononeuropathy Multiplex and Focal Neuropathic Syndromes

The conditions discussed next are commonly associated with substantial pain. About 50% of vasculitic neuropathies are painful and, when present, the pain is usually severe, requiring treatment with multiple medications including narcotic analgesics. In addition to characteristic features of neuropathic pain, a deep, aching, boring pain is often present in peripheral nerve vasculitis. This has been attributed to infarction of vasa nervorum. Immunohistological studies have demonstrated a correlation between neuropathic pain and the presence of cytokines in nerve biopsy specimens, and it is a common observation that the pain of vasculitic neuropathy is alleviated promptly by steroid therapy.

Like vasculitic neuropathy, the pain of neuralgic amyotrophy and diabetic amyotrophy also often has a deep, aching quality and, if treated promptly, often improves with immunomodulating therapy.

Vasculitic Neuropathy

Vasculitis is an autoimmune disorder characterized by inflammation and necrosis of blood vessel walls. The principal primary systemic vasculitides affecting peripheral nerve include polyarteritis nodosa, Churg-Strauss syndrome, and Wegener's granulomatosis. Peripheral nerve vasculitis also occurs as a complication of systemic inflammatory and infectious disorders, including lupus, rheumatoid arthritis, Sjogren's syndrome, progressive sys-

temic sclerosis, chronic hepatitis C infection, and HIV infection. Peripheral nerve vasculitis can also occur in isolation. While immunomodulation is almost always indicated, important differences exist in therapy and prognosis between the types of vasculitis, making classification important.[66] Thus, a comprehensive general medical evaluation and serologic studies relevant to the aforementioned disorders are indicated if vasculitis is suspected. The diagnosis can only be confirmed by tissue biopsy; in cases of peripheral nerve involvement, the sural, superficial peroneal, and superficial radial nerves are most commonly studied. Ideally a biopsy should be taken from a nerve that is affected, based upon clinical and electrophysiologic criteria, but not one that has undergone severe and longstanding injury. The diagnostic histological finding is transmural lymphocytic infiltration and fibrinoid degeneration of the medium size arteries in the epineurium and axonal degeneration that is nonuniform both within and between nerve fascicles.[19]

Most patients with neuropathy due to vasculitis experience sensory loss and weakness in a multifocal pattern, although in longstanding vasculitis the deficits can become confluent and mimic a symmetric process. In about 20% of cases of peripheral nerve vasculitis, the presentation is of a distal symmetric polyneuropathy at onset. When present, as it is in about 50% of cases, pain has characteristics of acute neuropathic pain as well as a continuous deep, aching pain.

The primary treatment goal in vasculitic neuropathy is control of the underlying disease process. This usually requires prompt and aggressive immunotherapy with corticosteroids and, in some circumstances, other immonomodulatory agents such as cyclophosphamide. The pain associated with necrotizing vasculitis is different in character and pathogenesis than the neuropathic pain associated with nonvasculitic neuropathy. A combination of opioids and other medications indicated specifically for neuropathic pain is usually required in this setting.

Neuralgic Amyotrophy

Neuralgic amyotrophy (NA) usually manifests as sudden, severe, deep aching pain in the shoulder girdle and proximal upper limb, followed within days to weeks by marked atrophy and weakness and relatively modest sensory loss. Weakness can be isolated to the distribution of one or two nerve trunks only, and can include nerves, such as the phrenic nerve, which involve the upper body but not the upper limb per se. Commonly affected nerves include the long thoracic, suprascapular, phrenic, musculocutanoues, and anterior interosseous. NA occurs primarily in patients between 20 and 40 years of age and is more common in men than women. It is also known as idiopathic brachial neuritis and as Parsonage-Turner syndrome. The etiology of this syndrome is not established, although the following clinical observations suggest that it may be dysimmune. First, NA often follows a viral infection, as is the case in GBS. Second, NA often begins with severe focal pain followed by atrophy and weakness, as is often the case in vasculitic neuropathy. Third, NA is a mononeuropathy multiplex, which is the most common pattern seen in peripheral nerve vasculitis. Careful clinical and electrodiagnostic examination often reveals differential fascicular involvement within a nerve trunk. The natural history of neuralgic amyotrophy is of very gradual improvement over the course of 1 to 2 years, as axonal regeneration occurs. Empiric immunotherapy is occasionally used. It is our impression that steroid therapy accelerates recovery and pain relief, but this has not been evaluated systematically.[67,68]

Pain in NA is usually described as deep, aching, and severe. It is made worse with movements of the affected limb and, as a result, patients often avoid movement at the shoulder joint, resulting at times in a secondary adhesive capsulitis (frozen shoulder). Deep aching pain generally improves over a matter of weeks, but can persist and can be followed by painful paresthesias and dysesthesias. Residual weakness and pain can occur. A hereditary form, known as hereditary neuralgic amyotrophy (HNA), has been identified and may represent a substantial proportion of cases.[69] HNA is inherited in an autosomal dominant fashion and has been linked to a mutation in the SEP9 gene, which is responsible for the formation of a possible cytoskeletal protein.[70]

Diabetic Amyotrophy

Like neuralgic amyotrophy, diabetic amyotrophy is a well-recognized syndrome characterized by sudden, severe pain, usually in the proximal segment of the limb, followed shortly thereafter by striking atrophy and weakness. Unlike neuralgic amyotrophy, diabetic amyotrophy usually affects the lower limb, although similar presentations involving the upper limb have been described. Also unlike neuralgic amyotrophy, and as indicated by the name, diabetic amyotrophy occurs almost exclusively in diabetics, although an identical syndrome has been described in patients with impaired glucose tolerance. This syndrome is also known as the Bruns-Garland syndrome and as diabetic lumbosacral radiculoplexus neuropathy, which describes the postulated localization of the pathology. Biopsy of proximal cutaneous nerves has demonstrated features of microvasculitis.[71] In keeping with this, there is extensive anecdotal evidence of prompt resolution of pain, and possible acceleration of recovery, after immune manipulation with steroids or intravenous immunoglobulin.

Other Diabetic Mononeuropathies

All healthcare providers should also be familiar with diabetic mononeuropathies, because of their clinical management implications as well as the striking pain associated with these conditions. In addition to inducing a predisposition to entrapment neuropathies, diabetes is associated with several acute, painful mononeuropathies or focal neuropathic syndromes affecting cranial nerves (third, fourth, sixth, seventh), roots (thoracic radiculopathy), and root/plexus (diabetic amyotrophy). In addition, a multifocal polyneuropathy ("diabetic mononeuropathy multiplex") can occur in the setting of diabetes. There is published evidence, supported by biopsy material, that several of these diabetic mononeuropathy syndromes are vasculitic.[72]

Recognizing clear risks associated with both treatments in this population, there is also anecdotal evidence that immunotherapy with steroids or immunoglobulin infusions may accelerate pain relief and possibly recovery of function in diabetic focal neuropathies.[73] A sudden, focal, painful neuropathy in diabetes is not due to "diabetic neuropathy" as the term is usually meant, and should be investigated promptly to determine whether it represents another condition or a recognized diabetic mononeuropathy.

Sensory Neuronopathies

The following conditions are believed to reflect pathology in the cell bodies of sensory neurons. Postherpetic neuralgia follows reactivation of a viral infection, while the others are believed to represent primary dysimmune processes. In all cases, neuropathic pain is often the principal symptom. The high prevalence of neuropathic pain in sensory neuronopathies may be attributable to the presence of an inflammatory process in relative proximity to the dorsal horn of the spinal cord.

Postherpetic Neuralgia

Postherpetic neuralgia (PHN) is one of the most common and disabling neuropathic pain states. A recent epidemiologic survey estimated the incidence of herpes zoster at 4.1 per 1,000 person-years, with PHN developing in 18% of cases.[74] Herpes zoster is due to a reactivation of varicella-zoster virus (VZV), which remains sequestered and clinically dormant in cells of sensory ganglia after an initial infection but becomes reactivated in the context of age-related or disease-related reduction in cell-mediated immunity to the virus. There is some evidence of persistent active infection in patients with PHN. PHN is presumed to be due to sensitization of nociceptors and central sensitization after herpes zoster. PHN is more likely to occur in patients with pain associated with acute zoster and patients with zoster affecting multiple dermatomes. There is a positive correlation between age at the time of developing herpes zoster and the likelihood of developing PHN.[75,76] Several studies have demonstrated that antiviral treatment of herpes zoster substantially reduces the risk of developing PHN and the duration of PHN if it develops.[77–79] PHN is described in greater detail in Chapter 27.

Sjogren's Syndrome

Sjogren's syndrome (SS) is a systemic autoimmune disorder. The cardinal features are sicca syndrome, supported by objective evidence of diminished tear production, salivary gland inflammation, and serologic evidence of antibodies highly correlated with this disorder.[80] SS is commonly associated with disease of both the peripheral and central nervous systems. The range of neurologic disorders that have been associated with SS is remarkably broad, including multiple sclerosis-like cerebral disorders, myelopathy, polyradiculoneuropathy, sensory neuronopathy, vasculitic mononeuropathy multiplex, and myositis.[81] The peripheral nervous system disorders for which the association with SS is clearest are sensory neuronopathy and vasculitic neuropathy. In patients with SS, sensory neuronopathy can present with sensory ataxia, neuropathic pain, or both, presumably reflecting the relative involvement of large and small sensory neurons. Sensory neuronopathy from SS is usually an indolent, progressive condition.[81–83] Evidence of response to immunotherapy is anecdotal. Dysimmune sensory neuronopathy can occur as an idiopathic phenomenon as well.

As with other systemic autoimmune conditions, necrotizing peripheral nerve vasculitis from SS is a rapidly progressive, disabling, and commonly painful condition which nonetheless does respond to immunotherapy.

Paraneoplastic Sensory Neuronopathy

Paraneoplastic sensory neuronopathy is one of several paraneoplastic syndromes associated with the presence of anti-Hu antibodies which is encompassed under the rubric of paraneoplastic encephalomyelitis. The predominant clinical syndrome is a sensory ataxia rather than neuropathic pain. Paraneoplastic sensory neuronopathy may respond to treatment of the tumor and, occasionally, immunomodulating therapy, but the prognosis is nonetheless poor.[84]

Toxic Neuronopathy

Cisplatin is an antineoplastic agent known to cause sensory loss and neuropathic pain. The pathophysiology is felt to be disruption of mitochondrial DNA synthesis resulting in a sensory neuronopathy.[85–87]

TREATMENT OF PAINFUL NEUROPATHIES

General Principles of Therapy

Treatment of neuropathy and neuropathic pain are complementary. Treatment of neuropathy is targeted at the underlying disease process. Such therapy should be administered as soon as possible to control or even reverse the process responsible for neuropathy and neuropathic pain. Nevertheless in the authors' experience patients commonly report persistent neuropathic pain even after stabilization or reversal of neuropathy. This is particularly true in vasculitic neuropathy, where progressive weakness and sensory loss can be aborted with steroid therapy but pain often persists even years after resolution of necrotizing vasculitis. Assuming that inflammation and injury in peripheral nerve terminals has stabilized or receded in these cases, this observation might be attributable to central sensitization.

Analgesia Therapy: Guidelines for Pharmacotherapy

Treatment of neuropathic pain should begin as soon as possible and in tandem with treatment of neuropathy. Postulated mechanisms of neuropathic pain and neuropathic pain pharmacotherapy are addressed in other chapters. Here we will address treatment of painful neuropathy in particular.

Diabetic neuropathy is the most prevalent painful neuropathy in developed countries and has therefore been most widely studied as a target for treatment of neuropathic pain from neuropathy. It follows, therefore, that most clinical trial data regarding efficacy of analgesic treatments in painful neuropathy were obtained in patients with diabetic neuropathy pain and that there is little formal evidence that these data apply to other etiologies.

Primary outcome measures of most large clinical trials are overall change in pain severity and improvement in quality of life indicators. There is a growing recognition that clinical trial design in neuropathic pain should also include systematic evaluation of individual neuropathic pain symptoms and signs.[88] Thus, there is potential utility in the systematic evaluation of the effect of treatments on specific neuropathic pain symptoms, such as paresthesias, dysesthesias, and burning; neuropathic pain descriptors, such as sharp, dull, stabbing, or exhausting; and neuropathic pain signs, such as dynamic mechanical allodynia, punctate hyeralgesia, thermal allodynia, and thermal hyperalgesia. It is not clear at present whether it is better to ask the question "which treatment is best for neuropathic pain from this disease?" or, rather, "which treatment is best for this neuropathic pain symptom/sign complex?" Implied in the latter is the hypothesis that pain symptoms and signs inform us about the principal mechanisms of pain in a given individual, which in turn may match the mechanism of action of a particular treatment.

For now, however, evidence-based treatment of neuropathic pain from neuropathy is based largely on evidence of reduction in overall pain severity in diabetic neuropathy and few other conditions, and practitioners are obliged to extrapolate from these data. Most large clinical trials in this arena are industry-supported pivotal trials of the agent in question against placebo. There is very little evidence comparing treatments against each other. One way to try to make such a comparison is by comparing the number needed to treat (NNT), defined as the average number of individuals that must be treated with a medication to obtain a defined degree of pain relief in one subject.[89] NNT takes into consideration treatment failures for any reason, both lack of efficacy and lack of tolerability. While NNT is usually based upon 50% improvement, it has been shown that 30% improvement in pain severity or a reduction in pain severity by at least 2 points on a 0 to 10 Likert scale is clinically meaningful.[90,91]

The medication classes with the best evidence for efficacy in the management of neuropathic pain are tricyclic antidepressants (TCAs), $\alpha_2\delta$ ligands, serotonin and norepinephrine reuptake inhibitors (SNRIs), and opioids.[92] Tramadol, which is believed to both inhibit serotonin and norepinephrine reuptake and act as a mu-opioid agonist, has demonstrated efficacy as well.

Tricyclic Antidepressants

Tricyclic antidepressants are believed to derive their analgesic effect from serotonin and norepinephrine reuptake inhibition as well as sodium channel blockade. The benefit is independent of an antidepressant effect. Most undesirable effects from this class derive from its anticholinergic properties. TCAs have been demonstrated to be beneficial in relieving neuropathic pain from diabetic neuropathy in several small series. A recent Cochrane review found an overall class NNT of 3.6 for moderate pain relief among 17 studies of TCAs for neuropathic pain.[93] TCAs should be used with caution in patients at risk for cardiac arrhythmias because they can prolong the QT_c interval. The most common side effects of the tricyclics are due to their anticholinergic activity and include constipation, dry mouth, blurred vision, cognitive changes, tachycardia, and urinary hesitancy. Sedation and weight gain may occur from antihistaminergic activity. Alpha-adrenergic receptor blockade may result in orthostatic hypotension. All of these potential side effects can be minimized by slow titration. Nortriptyline and desipramine are better tolerated than their parent drugs, amitriptyline and imipramine. Contraindications to the tricyclics include closed-angle glaucoma, benign prostatic hypertrophy, and acute myocardial infarction.

Treatment with a tricyclic should be initiated with a dose of 10 mg or 25 mg a few hours before bedtime to minimize daytime sedation. The lower 10 mg dose should be prescribed for the elderly, frail, or side effect-prone patient. The dose is titrated by one tablet, 10 or 25 mg, every 7 days if the patient has poor pain relief and does not complain of intolerable side-effects. The majority of patients will report significant pain relief or intolerable side effects within the dose range of 30 to 150 mg. The mean dose of amitriptyline that often results in pain reduction is 75 to 150 mg/day. Onset of the analgesic effect occurs within 1 to 2 weeks and peaks around 4 to 6 weeks.[94,95] Improvement in sleep, mood, and anxiety can augment the benefit of pain control.

$\alpha_2\delta$ Ligands

Mechanical allodynia in neuropathic pain is believed to be mediated in part by increased expression of N-type calcium channels in the central terminals of primary afferent neurons, resulting in pathologically enhanced neurotransmission in the dorsal horn. Gabapentin and pregabalin are chemically related compounds that have been shown to have a modulatory effect via binding to the $\alpha_2\delta$ subunit of the calcium channel. Several studies have demonstrated that gabapentin alleviates diabetic neuropathy pain at doses ranging from 900 to 3600 mg per day, with a combined NNT for 50% pain relief of 2.9. Two small series comparing gabapentin with amitriptyline demonstrated improvement in pain ratings with both drugs and no statistically significant difference in benefit between them.[96,97] It should be noted, however, that serious adverse events can occur with amitriptyline and are virtually unknown with gabapentin. Gabapentin can cause weight gain, reversible cognitive symptoms, and peripheral edema.

Gabapentin bioavailability is limited because absorption from the gastrointestinal tract is dependent on a single saturable active transport mechanism. Pregabalin shares gabapentin's presumed mechanism of action but demonstrates more linear kinetics than gabapentin. Presumably for this reason pregabalin is absorbed more quickly and demonstrates more linear kinetics than gabapentin. Pregabalin has been shown to be effective in relieving the pain of diabetic neuropathy, with NNTs for 50% pain relief of 3.4 and 3.3 for the 300 mg/day and 600 mg/day doses, respectively.[98,99] Like gabapentin, pregabalin can cause cognitive side effects which are usually mild to moderate in severity, as well as weight gain and peripheral edema.

Serotonin and Norepinephrine Reuptake Inhibitors

Serotonin and norepinephrine reuptake inhibition is believed to alleviate neuropathic pain by facilitating descending inhibition of afferent pain signaling. This descending inhibition is mediated by neurons of the rostroventral medulla. It is believed that both neurotransmitters are important in this pathway, which may explain the observation that selective serotonin reuptake inhibitors (SSRIs) alone are of little benefit in alleviating pain from neuropathy.[93] Duloxetine, an SNRI with relative balance between serotonergic and noradrenergic effects, has demonstrated efficacy in relieving pain from diabetic neuropathy, with an NNT for 50% pain relief of 4.3 at a dose of 60 mg/day and 3.8 at a dose of 120 mg/day.[100] Venlafaxine, an SNRI with balanced pharmacology at high doses, has also been shown to be beneficial, with an NNT of 4.5 for 50% pain relief in the 150 to 225 mg dose range.[101] SNRIs can cause nausea, hyperhidrosis, and sexual side effects in some patients. While they do not have substantial anticholinergic properties, they can cause some symptoms of dry mouth and dizziness, possibly on a noradrenergic basis; however, these effects are probably less frequent or severe than with tricyclic medications. Combining SNRIs with other serotonergic agents, including other antidepressants, triptans, and tramadol, should be done with caution because of the risk of serotonin syndrome. SNRIs are also known to inhibit the metabolism of other antidepressants, thus substantially increasing blood levels of such drugs when they are used in combination. For these reasons, it is usually best to avoid the use of SNRIs with other antidepressants, and to consider using one SNRI or tricyclic agent alone to treat both pain and depression if treatment of both conditions is indicated.

Opioids

Opioids strongly inhibit central nociceptive neurons mainly through interaction with μ-opioid receptors, producing neuronal membrane hyperpolarization. Controlled-release oxycodone has been shown to reduce pain from diabetic neuropathy in two small randomized controlled trials, with an NNT for moderate pain relief of 2.6 in one.[102,103] Administration of opioids requires specific treatment programs for patients with a history of chemical dependence and caution in patients with pulmonary disease. Opioid-induced dependence, tolerance, and hyperalgesia are risks of opioid use, although these may be less common in patients with chronic, stable neuropathy than some other chronic pain states. Prophylactic treatment of common side-effects such as nausea or constipation can improve patient compliance.

Tramadol

Tramadol is both an inhibitor of serotonin and norepinephrine reuptake and a μ-opioid agonist. Tramadol has been shown to effectively alleviate pain in diabetic neuropathy as well as a mixed group of neuropathy patients among whom many had diabetic neuropathy.[104,105] Tramadol has a short duration of action and therefore is given every four to six hours or is used on an as-needed basis as an adjuvant medication. It is now also available in an extended release formulation.

Other Pharmacological Agents

Several other agents approved for the treatment of epilepsy have demonstrated limited evidence of efficacy in the management of pain from neuropathy. These include oxcarbazepine, which has demonstrated benefit in one randomized controlled study in diabetic neuropathy pain, lamotrigine, and topiramate, both agents which have demonstrated conflicting results in randomized controlled trials for pain from diabetic neuropathy.[106–110] Despite limited evidence of efficacy, these have all been used on occasion as second- or third-line agents for patients who have not responded to or tolerated other treatments. Carbamazepine, which is approved for pain from trigeminal neuralgia, has been found to be effective in two double-blind placebo-controlled studies for control of pain in diabetic neuropathy.[111,112] Prior to the availability of many of the aforementioned agents for neuropathic pain management, phenytoin was shown to be effective in controlled trials of pain from diabetic polyneuropathy[113] and pain in Fabry's disease.[114] Phenytoin is no longer commonly used to treat pain due to neuropathy.

Bupropion, a unique agent which inhibits norepinephrine and dopamine uptake, has shown benefit in one study involving pain from a variety of neuropathy etiologies.[115]

Acetyl-L-carnitine (ACL) is believed to have several potentially neuroprotective properties that have led to extensive study of this agent as a treatment for diabetic, HIV, and chemotherapy-induced neuropathy.[116–118] It also has analgesic properties. ACL has been administered at doses between 1 and 3 g per day. Alpha-lipoic acid, a potent antioxidant, has also been studied as a potential treatment of both diabetic neuropathy and diabetic neuropathy pain. The recently-completed SYDNEY 2 trial showed that daily oral therapy at a dose of 600 mg/day, the lowest dose yet studied, reduced the neuropathy total symptom score by 50% or greater with an NNT of 2.8.[119,120]

Topical Agents

Capsaicin stimulates the release of substance P from small caliber primary afferent neurons and is believed to alleviate neuropathic pain with regular use by exhausting stores of substance P. Capsaicin also causes prompt epidermal denervation so reliably that capsaicin denervation has become an important human model of neuropathy. While capsaicin can alleviate neuropathic pain with sustained use, it also causes considerable burning discomfort which limits its use. A high-potency capsaicin patch is presently undergoing clinical trials.

Topical lidocaine, a local anesthetic which acts via sodium channel blockade, has been approved for the treatment of postherpetic neuralgia. It is used on occasion to treat cutaneous pain from other neuropathic conditions as well. Systemically administered lidocaine, mexiletine, and tocainide have also been demonstrated to have analgesic effects for control of diabetic neuropathic pain and in postherpetic neuralgia.[121–123] Systemically administered local anesthetics block ectopic discharges due to experimental peripheral nerve injury and in axotomized dorsal root ganglion cells of the peripheral nerves,[124] probably by blocking sodium channels.[125] In addition, there is evidence that lidocaine and similar local anesthetics have actions on G protein-coupled receptors that can result in long-lasting modulation of pain via effects both on sensitization and on the immune response to nerve injury.[126]

Principles of Pharmacotherapy for Pain from Neuropathy

Polypharmacy is common in the treatment of pain from neuropathy for several reasons. First, neuropathy pain can be treated with several classes of agents, with different postulated mechanisms of action. Second, on a more practical level, there is (fortuitously) relative compatibility among these medication classes. And, finally, despite evidence that these treatments are generally efficacious, it is uncommon to achieve complete or even adequate pain relief with a single agent, while it is common to encounter significant adverse effects. Therefore, one usually begins with slow upward titration of one of the first-line drugs (SNRIs, α₂δ ligands, or tricyclics), followed by the addition of another first-line agent (but generally *not* an SNRI *with* a tricyclic) if pain relief is inadequate at the highest tolerated dose of the first drug. Because these are generally chronic conditions, there is no need to titrate faster than tolerability will permit. Opioids or tramadol are often used as second-line agents or as rescue drugs and are particularly helpful for patients who can predict an increase in pain after a physically active day. Topical and nonpharmacological treatments are particularly valuable as add-on therapy for patients who do not tolerate medication well. Cognitive-behavioral therapy, discussed in Chapter 82, can be very helpful because it is often the distress associated with pain, perhaps more than the pain itself, that causes pain-related disability.

UNRESOLVED QUESTIONS

There have been no attempts to evaluate whether successful treatment with an analgesic medication alters the natural history of pain. There is also insufficient evidence to guide duration of therapy. For example, do patients who report significant pain relief with a certain medication need to be treated with that particular medication at that dose indefinitely? Most pivotal clinical trials in this field run for about 12 weeks' duration, which is woefully inadequate in the context of conditions that usually persist for years.

The mechanisms of neuropathic pain in people with neuropathy also require considerably more study. Much of our understanding of mechanisms, such as ectopic and ephaptic transmission, neurogenic inflammation, descending modulation, and peripheral and central sensitization, comes from animal models that do not mimic human neuropathies. A better understanding of mechanism will likely require better investigation of people with neuropathy. Just as the diagnosis and management of conditions causing neurologic deficit rely upon an ever-more sophisticated clinical/laboratory/radiographic correlation, so too must the management of pain from neuropathy advance with the help of evidence gleaned in a systematic fashion from neuropathic pain questionnaires, neuropathic pain examinations, and relevant imaging, pathologic, and laboratory tools.

References

1. Dyck PJ, Thomas PK, eds. *Peripheral Neuropathy*. 4th ed. Philadelphia: Elsevier Saunders; 2005.
2. Schaumberg HH, Berger AR, Thomas PK, eds. *Disorders of Peripheral Nerves*. Philadelphia: F.A. Davis; 1992.
3. Bennett M. The LANSS pain scale: the Leeds assessment of neuropathic symptoms and signs. *Pain* 2001;92:147–157.
4. Galer BS, Jensen MP. Development and preliminary validation of a pain measure specific to neuropathic pain: the neuropathic pain scale. *Neurology* 1997; 48:332–338.
5. Bouhassira D, Attal N, Fermanian J, et al. Development and validation of the neuropathic pain symptom inventory. *Pain* 2004;108:248–257.
6. Krause SJ, Backonja MM. Development of a neuropathic pain questionnaire. *Clin J Pain* 2003;19:306–314.
7. Bennett MI, Attal N, Backonja MM, et al. Using screening tools to identify neuropathic pain. *Pain* 2007;127:199–203.
8. Dyck PJ, Karnes J, O'Brien PC, et al. Neuropathy symptom profile in health, motor neuron disease, diabetic neuropathy, and amyloidosis. *Neurology* 1986;36:1300–1308.
9. Savage CW. The Measurement of Sensation. Berkeley: University of California Press; 1970.
10. Hansson P, Backonja M, Bouhassira D. Usefulness and limitations of quantitative sensory testing: clinical and research application in neuropathic pain states. *Pain* 2007 6;129(3):256–259.
11. Greenspan JD. Quantitative assessment of neuropathic pain. *Curr Pain Headache Rev* 2001;5:107–113.
12. Rolke R, Magerl W, Campbell KA, et al. Quantitative sensory testing: a comprehensive protocol for clinical trials. *Eur J Pain* 2006;10:77–88.
13. Walk D, Sehgal N, Moeller-Bertram T, et al. Quantitative sensory testing and mapping: a review of non-automated quantitative methods for examination of the patient with neuropathic pain. *Clin J Pain* 2009;25:632–640.
14. Hoitsma E, Reulen JP, de Baets M, et al. Small fiber neuropathy: a common and important clinical disorder. *J Neurol Sci* 2004;227:119–130.
15. Periquet MI, Novak V, Collins, MP, et al. Painful sensory neuropathy: prospective evaluation using skin biopsy. *Neurology* 1999;53:1641–1647.
16. Lacomis D. Small-fiber neuropathy. *Muscle Nerve* 2002;26:173–188.
17. Walk D, Wendelschafer-Crabb G, Davey C, et al. Concordance between epidermal nerve fiber density and sensory examination in patients with symptoms of idiopathic small fiber neuropathy. *J Neurol Sci* 2007;255:23–26.
18. Walk D, Zaretskaya M, Parry GJ. Symptom duration and clinical features in painful sensory neuropathy with and without nerve conduction abnormalities. *J Neurol Sci* 2003;214:3–6.
19. Said G. Indications and usefulness of nerve biopsy. *Arch Neurol* 2002;59: 1532–1535.
20. Daousi C, MacFarlane IA, Woodward A, et al. Chronic painful peripheral neuropathy in an urban community: a controlled comparison of people with and without diabetes. *Diabet Med* 2004;21:976–982.
21. Hong S, Morrow TJ, Paulson PE, et al. Early painful diabetic neuropathy is associated with differential changes in the tetrodotoxin-sensitive and -resistant sodium channels in dorsal root ganglion neurons in the rat. *J Biol Chem* 2004; 279:29341–29350.
22. Calcutt NA, Backonja MM: Pathogenesis of pain in peripheral diabetic neuropathy. *Curr Diab Rep* 2007;7:429–434.
23. Ramos KM, Jiang Y, Svensson CI, et al. Pathogenesis of spinally mediated hyperalgesia in diabetes. *Diabetes* 2007;56:1569–1576.
24. Paulson PE, Wiley JW, Morrow TJ. Concurrent activation of the somatosensory forebrain and deactivation of periaqueductal gray with diabetes-induced neuropathic pain. *Exp Neurol* 2007;208:305–313.
25. Grundy SM, Cleeman JI, Daniels SR, et al. Diagnosis and management of the metabolic syndrome. *Circulation* 2005;112:2735–2752.
26. Hughes RA, Umapathi T, Gray IA, et al. A controlled investigation of the cause of chronic acquired idiopathic axonal polyneuropathy. *Brain* 2004;127: 1723–1730.
27. McManis PG, Windebank AJ, Kiziltan M. Neuropathy associated with hyperlipidemia. *Neurology* 1994;44:2185–2186.
28. Isomaa B, Henricsson M, Almgren P, et al. The metabolic syndrome influences the risk of chronic complications in patients with type II diabetes. *Diabetologia* 2001;44:1148–1154.
29. Tesfaye S, Chaturvedi N, Eaton SE, et al. Vascular risk factors and diabetic neuropathy. *N Engl J Med* 2005;352:341–350.
30. Cornblath DR, Hoke A. Recent advances in HIV neuropathy. *Curr Opin Neurol* 2006;19:446–450.
31. Wulff EA, Wang AK, Simpson DM. HIV-associated peripheral neuropathy: epidemiology, pathophysiology and treatment. *Drugs* 2000;59(6): 1251–1260.
32. Morgello S, Estanislao L, Simpson D, et al. HIV-associated distal sensory polyneuropathy in the era of highly active antiretroviral therapy. *Arch Neurol* 2004;61:546–551.
33. Nemni R, Sanvito L, Quattrini A, et al. Peripheral neuropathy in hepatitis C virus infection with and without cryoglobulinaemia. *J Neurol Neurosurg Psychiatry* 2003;74(9):1267–1271.
34. Nemni R, de Freitas MR. Infectious neuropathy. *Curr Opin Neurol* 2007; 20(5):548–552.
35. Halperin JJ. Lyme disease and the peripheral nervous system. *Muscle Nerve* 2003;28:133–143.
36. Said G. Infectious neuropathies. *Neurol Clin* 2007;25:115–137.
37. London Z, Albers JW. Toxic neuropathies associated with pharmaceutic and industrial agents. *Neurol Clin* 2007;25:257–276.
38. Umapathi T, Chaudhry V. Toxic neuropathy. *Curr Opin Neurol* 2005;18: 574–580.
39. Flatters SJ, Bennett GJ. Studies of peripheral sensory nerves in paclitaxel-induced painful peripheral neuropathy: evidence for mitochondrial dysfunction. *Pain* 2006 Jun;122(3):245–257.
40. Xiao W, Boroujerdi A, Bennett GJ, et al. Chemotherapy-evoked painful peripheral neuropathy: analgesic effects of gabapentin and effects on expression of the alpha-2-delta type-1 calcium channel subunit. *Neuroscience*. 2007 Jan 19;144(2):714–720.
41. Kril JJ. Neuropathology of thiamine deficiency disorders. *Metab Brain Dis* 1996;11(1):9–17.
42. Djoenaddi W, Notermans SL, Lilisantoso AH. Electrophysiologic examination of subclinical beriberi polyneuropathy. *Electromyogr Clin Neurophysiol* 1995;35:439–442.
43. Bosch EP, Pelham RW, Rasool CG, et al. Animal models of alcoholic neuropathy: morphologic, electrophysiologic, and biochemical findings. *Muscle Nerve* 1979;2(2):133–144.
44. Behse F, Buchtal F. Alcoholic neuropathy: clinical, electrophysiological, and biopsy findings. *Ann Neurol* 1977;2:95–110.
45. Koike H, Sobue G. Alcoholic neuropathy. *Curr Opin Neurobiol* 2006;19: 481–486.
46. Laski JR, Garcia A. Charcot-Marie-Tooth peripheral neuropathies and related disorders. In: Scriver CR, Beaudet AL, Sly WS et al., eds. *The Metabolic and Molecular Bases of Inherited Diseases*. New York: McGraw-Hill; 2001: 5759–5788.
47. Desnick RJ, Ioannou YA, Eng CM. Alpha-galactosidase A deficiency: Fabry disease. In: Scriver CR, Beaudet AL, Sly WS, et al., eds. *The Metabolic and Molecular Bases of Inherited Diseases*. 8th ed. New York: McGraw-Hill; 2001:3733–3774.
48. Beck M, Ricci R, Widmer U, et al. Fabry disease: overall effects of agalsidase alfa treatment. *Eur J Clin Invest* 2004;34:838–844.
49. Schiffmann R, Hauer P, Freeman B, et al. Enzyme replacement therapy and intraepidermal innervation density in Fabry disease. *Muscle Nerve* 2006;34: 53–56.
50. Adams RD, Victor M. *Principles of Neurology*. New York: McGraw-Hill; 1993.
51. Bergethon PR, Sabin TD, Lewis D, Simms RW, Cohen AS, Skinner M. Improvement in the polyneuropathy associated with familial amyloid polyneuropathy after liver transplantation. *Neurology* 1996;47:944–951.
52. Kwan JY. Paraproteinemic neuropathy. *Neurol Clin* 2007;25:47–69.
53. Steck AJ, Stalder AK, Renaud S. Anti-myelin-associated glycoprotein neuropathy. *Curr Opin Neurol* 2006;19:458–463.
54. Katz JS, Saperstein DS, Gronseth G, et al. Distal acquired demyelinating symmetric neuropathy. *Neurology* 2000;54:615–620.
55. Sung JY, Kuwabara S, Ogawara K, et al. Patterns of nerve conduction abnormalities in POEMS syndrome. *Muscle Nerve* 2002;26:189–193.
56. Hughes RA, Cornblath DR. Guillain-Barre Syndrome. *Lancet* 2005;366: 1653–1666.
57. Richardson EP Jr, De Girolami U. *Pathology of the Peripheral Nerve*. Philadelphia: W.B. Saunders; 1995.
58. Griffin JW, Li CY, Ho TW, et al. Guillain-Barre syndrome in northern China. The spectrum of neuropathological changes in clinically defined cases. *Brain* 1995;118:577–595.

59. Yuki N, Kuwabara S. Axonal Guillain-Barré syndrome: carbohydrate mimicry and pathophysiology. *J Peripher Nerv Syst* 2007;12:238–249.

60. Moulin DE, Hagen N, Feasby TE, et al. Pain in Guillain-Barre syndrome. *Neurology* 1997;48:328–331.

61. Ruts L, van Koningsveld R, Jacobs BC, et al. Determination of pain and response to methylprednisolone in Guillain-Barré syndrome. *J Neurol* 2007; 254:1318–1322.

62. Devor M. The pathophysiology of damaged peripheral nerves. In: Wall PD, ed. *Texbook of Pain*. New York: Churchill Livingston; 1989:63–81.

63. Genis D, Busquets C, Manubens E, et al. Epidural morphine analgesia in Guillain-Barré syndrome. *J Neurol Neurosurg Psych* 1989;52:999–1001.

64. Hughes RA, Bouche P, Cornblath DR, et al. European Federation of Neurological Societies/Peripheral Nerve Society guideline on management of chronic inflammatory demyelinating polyradiculoneuropathy: report of a joint task force of the European Federation of Neurological Societies and the Peripheral Nerve Society. *Eur J Neurol* 2006;13(4):326–332.

65. Lewis RA. Chronic inflammatory demyelinating polyneuropathy. *Neurol Clin* 2007;25:71–87.

66. Kissel JT Mendel JR. Vasculitic neuropathy. In: Johnson RT, ed. *Current Therapy in Neurology Disease*. 4th ed. B.C. Decker; 1993:365–368.

67. van Alfen N, van Engelen BG. The clinical spectrum of neuralgic amyotrophy in 246 cases. *Brain* 2006;129:438–450.

68. Nakajima M, Fujioka S, Ohno H, et al. Partial but rapid recovery from paralysis after immunomodulation during early stage of neuralgic amyotrophy. *Eur Neurol* 2006;55:227–229.

69. van Alfen N, Gabreëls-Festen AA, Ter Laak HJ, et al. Histology of hereditary neuralgic amyotrophy. *J Neurol Neurosurg Psychiatry* 2005;76:445–447.

70. Kuhlenbäumer G, Hannibal MC, Nelis E, et al. Mutations in SEPT9 cause hereditary neuralgic amyotrophy. *Nat Genet* 2005;37(10):1044–1046.

71. Kelkar P, Masood M, Parry GJ. Distinctive pathologic findings in proximal diabetic neuropathy (diabetic amyotrophy). *Neurology* 2000;12;55(1): 83–88.

72. Kelkar P, Parry GJ. Mononeuritis multiplex in diabetes mellitus: evidence for underlying immune pathogenesis. *J Neurol Neurosurg Psychiatry* 2003;74: 803–806.

73. Tracy JA, Dyck PJ. The spectrum of diabetic neuropathies. *Phys Med Rehabil Clin N Am* 2008;19:1–26.

74. Yawn BP, Saddier P, Wollan PC, et al. A population-based study of the incidence and complication rates of herpes zoster before zoster vaccine introduction. *Mayo Clin Proc* 2007;82(11):1341–1349.

75. Niv D, Maltsman-Tseikhin A. Postherpetic neuralgia: the never-ending challenge. *Pain Pract* 2005;5(4):327–340.

76. Weinberg JM. Herpes zoster: epidemiology, natural history, and common complications. *J Am Acad Dermatol* 2007;57:S130–S135.

77. Tyring S, Barbarash RA, Nahlik JE, et al. Famciclovir for the treatment of acute herpes zoster: effects on acute disease and postherpetic neuralgia. A randomized, double-blind, placebo-controlled trial. *Ann Intern Med* 1995; 123:89–96.

78. Quan D, Hammack BN, Kittelson J, et al. Improvement of postherpetic neuralgia after treatment with intravenous acyclovir followed by oral valacyclovir. *Arch Neurol* 2006;63:940–942.

79. Jackson JL, Gibbons R, Meyer G, Inouye L. The effect of treating herpes zoster with oral acyclovir in preventing postherpetic neuralgia. A meta-analysis. *Arch Intern Med* 1997;157(8):909–912.

80. Vitali C, Bombardieri S, Jonsson R, et al. Classification criteria for Sjögren syndrome: a revised version of the European criteria proposed by the American-European Consensus Group. *Ann Rheum Dis* 2002;61:554–558.

81. Delalande S, de Seze J, Fauchais AL, et al. Neurologic manifestations in primary Sjögren syndrome: a study of 82 patients. *Medicine(Baltimore)* 2004; 1583(5):280–291.

82. Mori K, Iijima M, Koike H, et al. The wide spectrum of clinical manifestations in Sjögren's syndrome-associated neuropathy. *Brain* 2005;128:2518–2534.

83. Gorson KC, Herrmann DN, Thiagarajan R, et al. Non-length dependent small fibre neuropathy/ganglionopathy. *J Neurol Neurosurg Psychiatry* 2008;79(2): 163–169.

84. Vedeler CA, Antoine JC, Giometto B. Management of paraneoplastic neurological syndromes: report of an EFNS task force. *Eur J Neurol* 2006;13: 682–690.

85. London Z, Albers JW. Toxic neuropathies associated with pharmaceutic and industrial agents. *Neurol Clin* 2007;25:257–276.

86. Umapathi T, Chaudhry V. Toxic neuropathy. *Curr Opin Neurol* 2005;18: 574–580.

87. Krarup-Hansen A, Helweg-Larsen S, Schmalbruch H, et al. Neuronal involvement in cisplatin neuropathy: prospective clinical and neurophysiological studies. *Brain* 2007;130:1076–1088.

88. Dworkin RH, Turk DC, Wyrwich KW, et al. Interpreting the clinical importance of treatment outcomes in chronic pain clinical trials: IMMPACT recommendations. *J Pain* 2008;9(2):105–121.

89. Cook RJ, Sackett DL. The number needed to treat: a clinically useful measure of treatment effect. *BMJ* 1995;310:452–454.

90. Farrar JT, Portenoy RK, Berlin JA, et al. Defining the clinically important difference in pain outcome measures. *Pain* 2000;88:287–294.

91. Farrar JT, Berlin JA, Strom BL. Clinically important changes in acute pain outcome measures: a validation study. *J Pain Symptom Manage* 2003;25(5): 406–411.

92. Dworkin RH, O'Connor AB, Backonja M, et al. Pharmacologic management of neuropathic pain: evidence-based recommendations. *Pain* 2007;132(3): 237–251.

93. Saarto T, Wiffen PJ. Antidepressants for neuropathic pain. *Cochrane Database Syst Rev* 2007;(4):CD005454.

94. Max MB, Culnane M, Schafer SC, et al. Amitriptyline relieves diabetic neuropathy pain in patients with normal or depressed mood. *Neurology* 1987; 37:589–596.

95. Max MB, Schafer SC, Culnane M, et al. Amitriptyline, but not lorazepam, relieves postherpetic neuralgia. *Neurology* 1988;38:1427–1432.

96. Rao RD, Michalak JC, Sloan JA, et al. Efficacy of gabapentin in the management of chemotherapy-induced peripheral neuropathy: a phase 3 randomized, double-blind, placebo-controlled, crossover trial (N00C3). *Cancer* 2007; 110(9):2110–2118.

97. Wiffen PJ, McQuay HJ, Edwards JE, et al. Gabapentin for acute and chronic pain. *Cochrane Database Syst Rev* 2005 Jul 20;(3):CD005452.

98. Rosenstock J, Tuchman M, LaMoreaux L, et al. Pregabalin for the treatment of painful diabetic peripheral neuropathy: a double-blind, placebo-controlled trial. *Pain* 2004;110:628–638.

99. Lesser H, Sharma U, LaMoreaux L, et al. Pregabalin relieves symptoms of painful diabetic neuropathy: a randomized controlled trial. *Neurology* 2004; 63:2104–2110.

100. Goldstein DJ, Lu Y, Detke MJ,et al. Duloxetine vs. placebo in patients with painful diabetic neuropathy. *Pain* 2005;116:109–118.

101. Rowbotham MC, Goli V, Kunz NR, et al.. Venlafaxine extended release in the treatment of painful diabetic neuropathy: a double-blind, placebo-controlled study. *Pain* 2004;110:697–706.

102. Watson CP, Moulin D, Watt-Watson J, et al. Controlled-release oxycodone relieves neuropathic pain: a randomized controlled trial in painful diabetic neuropathy. *Pain* 2003;105:71–78.

103. Gimbel JS, Richards P, Portenoy RK. Controlled-release oxycodone for pain in diabetic neuropathy: a randomized controlled trial. *Neurology* 2003;60: 927–934.

104. Harati Y, Gooch C, Swenson M, et al. Double-blind randomized trial of tramadol for the treatment of the pain of diabetic neuropathy. *Neurology* 1998;50:1842–1846.

105. Sindrup SH, Andersen G, Madsen C, et al. Tramadol relieves pain and allodynia in polyneuropathy: a randomized, double-blind, controlled trial. *Pain* 1999;83:85–90.

106. Beydoun A, Kobetz SA, Carrazana EJ. Efficacy of oxcarbazepine in the treatment of painful diabetic neuropathy. *Clin J Pain* 2004;20:174–178.

107. Eisenberg E, Lurie Y, Braker C, et al. Lamotrigine reduces painful diabetic neuropathy: a randomized, controlled study. *Neurology* 2001;57:505–509.

108. Vinik AI, Tuchman M, Safirstein B, et al. Lamotrigine for treatment of pain associated with diabetic neuropathy: results of two randomized, double-blind, placebo-controlled studies. *Pain* 2007;128:169–179.

109. Thienel U, Neto W, Schwabe SK, et al. Topiramate in painful diabetic polyneuropathy: findings from three double-blind placebo-controlled trials. *Acta Neurol Scand* 2004;110:221–231.

110. Raskin P, Donofrio PD, Rosenthal NR, et al. Topiramate vs. placebo in painful diabetic neuropathy: analgesic and metabolic effects. *Neurology* 2004;63: 865–873.

111. Rull JA, Quibrera R, González-Millán H, et al. Symptomatic treatment of peripheral diabetic neuropathy with carbamazepine (Tegretol): double-blind crossover trial. *Diabetologia* 1969;5:215–218.

112. Wilton TD. Tegretol in the treatment of diabetic neuropathy. *S Afr Med J* 1974;48:869–872.

113. Chadda VS, Mathur MS. Double blind study of the effects of diphenylhydantoin sodium diabetic neuropathy. *J Assoc Physicians India* 1978;26:403–406.

114. Lockman LA, Hunninghake DB, Krivit W, et al. Relief of pain of Fabry's disease by diphenylhydantoin. *Neurology* 1973;23:871–875.

115. Semenchuk MR, Sherman S, Davis B. Double-blind, randomized trial of bupropion SR for the treatment of neuropathic pain. *Neurology* 2001;57: 1583–1588.

116. De Grandis D. Acetyl-L-carnitine for the treatment of chemotherapy-induced peripheral neuropathy. *CNS Drugs* 2007;1(suppl 21):39–43.

117. Sima AA. Acetyl-L-carnitine in diabetic polyneuropathy: experimental and clinical data. *CNS Drugs* 2007;1(suppl 21):13–23.

118. Youle M. Acetyl-L-carnitine in HIV-associated antiretroviral toxic neuropathy. *CNS Drugs* 2007;1(suppl 1):25–30.

119. Foster TS. Efficacy and safety of alpha-lipoic acid supplementation in the treatment of symptomatic diabetic neuropathy. *Diabetes Educ* 2007;33(1): 111–117.

120. Ziegler D, Ametov A, Barinov A, et al. Oral treatment with alpha-lipoic acid improves symptomatic diabetic polyneuropathy: the SYDNEY 2 trial. *Diabetes Care* 2006;29:2365–2370.

121. Rowbotham MC, Reisner-Keller LA, Fields HL. Both intravenous lidocaine and morphine reduce the pain of postherpetic neuralgia. *Neurology* 1991;41: 1024–1028.

122. Kastrup J, Petersen P, Dejgård A, et al. Intravenous lidocaine infusion—a new treatment of chronic painful diabetic neuropathy? *Pain* 1987;28:69–75.

123. Bach FW, Jensen TS, Kastrup J, at al. The effect of intravenous lidocaine on nociceptive processing in diabetic neuropathy [see comments]. *Pain* 1990;40: 29–34.

124. Devor M, Wall PD, Catalan N. Systemic lidocaine silences ectopic neuroma and DRG discharge without blocking nerve conduction. *Pain* 1992;48: 261–268.

125. Devor M LP, Matzner O. Sodium channel accumulation in the injured axons as a substrate for neuropathic pain. In: Boivie J, Hansson P, Lindblom U, eds. *Touch, Temperature, and Pain in Health and Disease: Mechanisms and Assessments*. Seattle, WA: IASP Press; 1994:207–230.

126. Amir R, Argoff CE, Bennett GJ, et al. The role of sodium channels in chronic inflammatory and neuropathic pain. *J Pain* 2006;7(suppl 3):S1–S29.

CHAPTER 25 ■ COMPLEX REGIONAL PAIN SYNDROME

R. NORMAN HARDEN AND STEPHEN P. BRUEHL

INTRODUCTION

Complex regional pain syndrome (CRPS) is the current diagnostic label for the syndrome previously known by various names, including reflex sympathetic dystrophy (RSD), causalgia, Sudeck's atrophy, shoulder–hand syndrome, neuroalgodystrophy, and reflex neurovascular dystrophy. It was originally recognized as a distinct pain syndrome seen among Union veterans of the Civil War following traumatic nerve injury (causalgia).[1] It is an inflammatory and neuropathic pain disorder principally characterized by involvement of the autonomic nervous system. It is often a chronic disease that involves a full measure of biopsychosocial features, and it can become significantly disabling in some cases.

EPIDEMIOLOGY

Epidemiological data regarding CRPS in the general population are limited, although two large-scale studies are available. Sandroni reported an incidence of 5.46 new cases of CRPS-I per 100,000 annually[2] (Table 25-1 gives the distinction between types I and II). A larger more recent study using current International Association for the Study of Pain (IASP) diagnostic criteria reported an incidence as high as 25.2 new cases per 100,000 annually.[3] Based on this reported incidence, over 50,000 new cases of CRPS-I could be anticipated annually in the United States alone.[4] For physicians making pain diagnoses, the incidence of CRPS in relevant at-risk populations (e.g., postfracture) may be more clinically relevant. Large scale well-designed studies studying this issue are lacking. Several smaller prospective studies suggest that acute CRPS-I may develop in up to 11% to 18% of patients following fracture or total knee arthroplasty, although in some cases the condition may resolve relatively quickly with conservative care.[5–7]

TABLE 25.1

IASP DIAGNOSTIC CRITERIA FOR COMPLEX REGIONAL PAIN SYNDROME*

1) The presence of an initiating noxious event or a cause of immobilization.
2) Continuing pain, allodynia, or hyperalgesia with which the pain is disproportionate to any inciting event.
3) Evidence at some time of edema, changes in skin blood flow, or abnormal sudomotor activity in the region of pain.
4) This diagnosis is excluded by the existence of conditions that would otherwise account for the degree of pain and dysfunction.

Type I: Without obvious nerve damage (aka RSD)
Type II: With obvious nerve damage (aka Causalgia)

*Modified from Mersky and Bogduk[107]

Based on available epidemiological data, fractures and sprains appear to be the most common events triggering CRPS. CRPS appears to be more common in the upper extremities, is more common in females, and is most likely to occur in the 50–70 year age range.[2,3]

PATHOPHYSIOLOGY

CRPS remains one of the most enigmatic and difficult to treat of all pain conditions. Although excellent clinical characterizations started to appear in the literature in the late 1800s,[1] a definitive pathophysiology remains to be determined. This fact, to a great extent, explains the relative lack of clinical progress to date. In the following section, animal and human models that have relevance to understanding CRPS will be described, and then several pathophysiological mechanisms that may contribute will be reviewed. There is increasing consensus that CRPS is unlikely to be caused by a single pathophysiological mechanism.[8] Rather, it is likely to be the result of multiple interacting mechanisms, with varying relative contributions of these mechanisms across different patients.

Animal Models

There are several animal models that may shed light on the mechanisms of CRPS, albeit indirectly. However, as always, one must be cautious in extrapolating from animal models to human syndromes. The most useful animal model, best paralleling CRPS-II (causalgia) in which major nerve injury is a key feature, is the chronic constriction injury model in rat that was first described by Bennett and colleagues.[9] This model produces some behavioral features (e.g., guarding, disuse) that mimic some of the features of human CRPS (e.g., allodynia, hyperpathia, spontaneous pain) as well as some of the sympathetic abnormalities.[9] This model has been utilized in the preclinical screening of pharmacological interventions for CRPS. Another model that may be useful is the spinal nerve injury model,[10] although there is some controversy as to whether this model produces sympathetically maintained pain (SMP) and how similar the resulting pain syndrome is to human CRPS.[8,11] A third model, involving partial ligation of the sciatic nerve, may also have some relevance to human CRPS-II.[12] All three models likely generate ectopic activity at the site of injury and/or the dorsal root ganglion which may (or may not) be responsive to sympathetic outflow and which may cause/maintain central sensitization.[13] These models also result in various other phenomena putatively related to CRPS, such as sprouting of fibers in lamina II of the dorsal horn.[14,15] All of the models above appear most relevant to understanding CRPS-II, although two less widely-used models may be relevant to understanding CRPS-I (no major nerve injury evident). Models using tetanic electrical stimulation[16] and an ischemic reperfusion injury[17] appear to produce a syndrome that mimics some of the features of CRPS-I in the absence of signs of nerve injury.[16] These animal models may help somewhat in understanding mechanisms of CRPS, but their ultimate value may be in screening pharmaceutical interventions.

Human Models

Intracutaneous injection of capsaicin in humans induces burning pain and cutaneous mechanical hypersensitivity (allodynia) and as such may represent a useful model to study certain features of CRPS. The capsaicin model demonstrates the impact of intense nociceptive stimulation of normal skin with the rapid development of areas of primary and secondary hyperalgesia, allodynia, wheal, and flare.[18–20] This model results in hyperalgesia to suprathreshold heat within the capsaicin-induced secondary hyperalgesic skin, despite the absence of changes in heat pain threshold.[21] Another interesting human model of CRPS-like pain is the controlled heat injury model, which also leads to a zone of secondary hyperalgesia to suprathreshold heat.[22] These models and other lines of evidence suggest a primary role of central sensitization in CRPS[23–25]; however, overlapping regions of flare/vasodilatation and hyperalgesia may also suggest peripheral sensitization.[26] Polymodal C receptors likely mediate the temperature allodynia,[21,27] polymodal A receptors the pinprick hyperalgesia,[28] and A-beta receptors the mechanical allodynia[20] in these models. Whole-body cooling (to induce sympathetic activation) and sympathetic block have shown no effects on features of either the capsaicin or heat injury models,[22,29] although phentolamine (an adrenergic antagonist) reduces the area of allodynia in the capsaicin model.[30] Given these mixed findings, the value of these models in understanding interactions between sympathetic nervous system activity and pain in CRPS remains uncertain. While some features of these models are concordant with signs and symptoms of CRPS, the usefulness of these normal nociception models in unraveling disease specific mechanisms in CRPS is limited to date. As with animal models, a primary use of these human models may be in the testing of interventions for CRPS.[21,31]

Inflammation

Clinical evidence indicates that some features of acute/early CRPS often attributed exclusively to sympathetic hypofunction (i.e., vasodilatation, swelling, and edema) could perhaps be better explained by an exaggerated localized inflammatory process.[32] Sudeck was the first to propose this, along with a "patchy inflammatory osteoporosis,"[33] and Goris revitalized this idea more recently.[34] Consistent with inflammatory mechanisms, one experimental study demonstrated that 82% of acute CRPS patients exhibited a progressive accumulation of immunoglobulin in the affected extremity relative to the unaffected extremity, compared to only 17% of chronic CRPS patients[35] (In this study Oyen et al.[35] arbitrarily defined chronic as 5 months or more since onset. It is more common to label the syndrome chronic after 6 months.) Analyses of joint fluid and synovial biopsies in CRPS patients have shown an increase in protein concentration, synovial hypervascularity, and neutrophil infiltration.[36–38] Free radicals, suspected to play a prominent role in inflammation and ischemic damage, recreate acute CRPS symptomatology in a rat model (vasomotor abnormalities, edema, and pain behavior), and this is the partial rationale for some investigators recommending free radical scavengers in acute CRPS patients.[39] From these lines of evidence, it is logical to conclude that an inflammatory component is likely in CRPS-I, particularly in the early phase.[39,40]

A shift toward a proinflammatory cytokine profile in patients with CRPS suggests a potential pathogenic role for these compounds in the generation of pain.[41] In plasma, no alterations in inflammatory mediators were observed in CRPS patients. However, in blister fluid obtained in the region of CRPS pain, signifi-

cantly higher levels of interleukin 6 (IL-6) and tumor necrosis factor (TNF)-α were observed in the involved extremity relative to the uninvolved extremity.[42] In addition, significantly elevated cerebrospinal fluid levels of proinflammatory cytokines (interleukin 1b [IL-1b], IL-6) have been shown in CRPS patients compared to healthy controls and those with other types of pain.[41] Results to date do not support genetic factors as determinants of the cytokine profile that may contribute to CRPS.[43] Mast cells also appear to be involved in inflammatory reactions observed in CRPS-I and probably play a role in the production of proinflammatory cytokines such as TNF-α.[42]

Animal studies demonstrate that the sympathetic nervous system can influence the intensity of an inflammatory process.[44–47] In human pain models, sympatholytic procedures can reduce pain, inflammation, and edema.[48,49] A possible autoimmune etiology of CRPS in some cases has also been proposed, and autoantibodies against nervous system structures have been described in some patients.[50] Some evidence suggests that "neurogenic inflammation" is facilitated in CRPS patients. Transcutaneous electrical stimulation caused increased axon reflex vasodilatation and provoked protein extravasation only in CRPS patients, whereas it resulted in decreased axon reflex vasodilatation in healthy controls.[51]

Afferent Dysfunction

CRPS is characterized by "disproportionate" spontaneous and evoked pain (e.g., hyperalgesia, thermal, and mechanical allodynia). Whether these sensory symptoms are due to peripheral and/or central sensitization is the subject of considerable debate and investigation. Sensory impairment occurs in more than 70% of CRPS patients.[52,53] Although traditionally these sensory changes were thought to occur in a distal, regional distribution along with characteristic autonomic disturbances, some early data suggest that the afferent disturbances may be hemilateral or quadrantic.[54] Recent observations corroborate that CRPS may be associated with more generalized sensory impairments.[55,56] The types of remote sensory abnormalities described include the allodynia and hyperalgesia typical of CRPS, but also hypoesthesia and other dysesthesias. Psychophysical technologies, such as temperature quantitative sensory testing, reveal that ipsilateral hypoalgesia is common and contralateral hypoesthesia may occur in some cases.[56] Patients found to have generalized sensory impairment were also found to have ipsilateral weakness.[55] Another study showed that patients with generalized sensory impairment had ipsilateral hemibody increases in thresholds for touch, thermal sensation, and heat pain, whereas those with sensory deficits limited to the distal affected limb showed touch threshold elevations only in the affected limb.[56] In this trial, 46% of patients showed abnormalities in nerve conduction testing and 24% abnormalities in somatosensory evoked potentials, although these abnormalities did not correspond to the extent of sensory impairments observed on quantitative sensory testing.[56] These studies and others suggest that the sensory impairments in CRPS often extend beyond the area affected by pain, and up to 50% of subjects show hypoesthesia and hypoalgesia in a quadrantic or hemibody distribution ipsilateral to the pain. These effects are more likely to occur with greater CRPS chronicity, suggesting centralization of the pathology over time.

Skin biopsies have revealed decreased C-fiber and A-delta fiber axonal densities in the affected limb of CRPS-I patients compared to the unaffected side.[57] It is not known whether such changes are primary to the disease or a consequence of nutritional changes and ischemia caused by chronic vasoconstriction and inflammation.[33] These changes could help account for some of the sensory alterations described above that may occur in CRPS-I (as well as CRPS-II).[58,59]

Central Dysfunction

There is considerable evidence supporting centralization of the pathology in chronic CRPS.[54,60–62] Further support comes from evidence suggesting presence of sympathetic and motor dysfunction in the region of pain (see discussion below). An acute nociceptive barrage from an inciting trauma or due to peripheral sensitization and/or neurogenic inflammation can cause rapid changes in the central nervous system (brain and spinal cord), a process commonly referred to as central sensitization.[63] As a corollary, it has been hypothesized that normalization of afferent activity will reset and/or dampen this sensitization (e.g., increased functional input on large fiber tracts may modulate or normalize activity of small fiber tracts or "shut the pain gate").[64]

Evidence for supraspinal central mechanisms in CRPS also derives from studies using neuroimaging techniques that permit exploration of changes in information processing in the brains of CRPS patients. Studies using magnetoencephalography (MEG), quantitative electroencephalogram, functional MRI (fMRI), and positron emission tomography (PET) techniques all indicate that alterations of afferent input lead to cortical and thalamic plasticity and reorganization of sensory representations in patients with CRPS-I.[65–69] Increased brain responsiveness among CRPS patients in some imaging studies also supports the presence of central sensitization.[68] Some studies suggest a reduced size of the motor cortex devoted to the affected limb in unilateral CRPS-I patients compared to the unaffected side,[68] and the relevance of such brain changes to clinical symptoms is supported by the fact that degree of this shrinkage correlates with the degree of hyperalgesia to pinprick.[70] Functional MRI studies indicate different patterns of cortical activation to pinprick in the CRPS affected side (S1, S2, insula, frontal, anterior cingulate cortex) compared to the unaffected side (S1, S2, insula only).[71] Moreover, prospective research using MEG indicates that stimulation of early, unilateral CRPS-I subjects leads initially only to contralateral activation, whereas after 3 years of CRPS, the same stimulation leads to bilateral activation.[68] Such results suggest one possible brain mechanism by which reported contralateral spreading of CRPS symptoms may occur. Imaging studies suggest that CRPS-related brain changes like those described above may reverse after successful treatment; thus, a reduction or resolution of CRPS pain may correlate with resetting of the cortical reorganization associated with the disorder.[70,72]

Sympathetic Dysfunction

Although autonomic dysfunction has long been implicated as a key mechanism involved with CRPS pathology, the actual role of the sympathetic nervous system (SNS) is incompletely characterized.[73] A seminal role of the SNS in CRPS is pivotal in most diagnostic criteria, emphasizing signs and symptoms of autonomic disturbance (e.g., vasomotor, sudomotor, and fluid regulation changes).[52,74,75] The crucial role of the SNS in at least some cases of CRPS is also suggested by the fact that sympatholytic blocks cause substantial pain relief in a subset of patients (those with sympathetically-maintained pain; e.g., Wasner et al.[76] and see below). Because of the frequent beneficial response empirically seen to sympathetic blocks in chronic, cold, blue, sweaty CRPS, logically, sympathetic hyperactivity was originally thought to be a primary pathophysiological mechanism.[77] However, an analysis of the current available data provides evidence that sympathetic vasoconstrictor activity is inhibited rather than enhanced, at least in early CRPS.[78,79] The clinical presentation of CRPS appears to take two distinct forms, which may be sequential. Acutely, vasodilatation and sudomotor dysfunction (hot, red, occasionally dry) is characteristically observed; in contrast, patients with chronic CRPS often exhibit signs of vasocon-

striction and hyperhydrosis (cold, blue, sweaty).[80] This apparent temporal progression of vasomotor dysfunction from hypoactive to hyperactive is in accord with the sequential changes in rat paw temperature observed in the chronic constriction injury animal model of CRPS.[81] In a series of human studies examining thermoregulation and sympathetic reflexes in response to whole-body warming or cooling using a thermal suit, Wasner and colleagues[76,78] have corroborated the temporal progression from acute, relative sympathetic hypofunction, through an intermediate stage, to a chronic state of relative hyperfunction. Whole-body cooling, a very effective stimulus to tonically activate cutaneous vasoconstrictor pathways, induced a much lower level of vasoconstriction in the affected side as compared with the healthy side in acute CRPS patients.[76] Wasner[78] also reported a significant negative correlation ($p < 0.001$) between the duration of the disease and the maximal temperature difference between the affected and unaffected sides achieved during this thermoregulatory testing. The cold symptom pattern often seen in chronic CRPS is most likely related to adrenergic receptor supersensitivity, perhaps resulting from early sympathetic hypofunction due to local sympathetic nerve damage,[82] decreased central drive, or both. This hypothesis is supported by studies examining plasma catecholamines in CRPS and studies using PET scanning techniques.[83–85] These mechanisms do not exclude processes at the capillary and venular site of the vascular bed that may involve the sympathetic and unmyelinated afferent neurons[86] that could contribute to neurogenic inflammation and edema.[49]

Results of thermoregulatory sweat tests and quantitative sudomotor axon tests often reveal increased sudomotor activity in acute CRPS; however, only results of the former are increased in chronic CRPS.[76,87] While these sudomotor changes are not entirely in line with the pattern of reported vasomotor changes in CRPS, they do support a central sympathetic dysregulation in this acute period that is in accord with known thermoregulatory mechanisms.[76,87] The dysfunctional effectors of the SNS that are most prominent in CRPS (vasomotor and sudomotor) are thermoregulatory and are thought to be primarily under hypothalamic control.[73,88] It is important to note that these sympathetic signs and symptoms are highly variable between patients and even within patients over time.[89,90]

During the 1980s and early 1990s, many clinicians and researchers considered the presence of SMP to be a central feature of CRPS. SMP was corroborated by reports of significant analgesia when the efferent sympathetic nerve supply to the affected area was blocked.[91–93] The concept of SMP remains potentially useful clinically, as it suggests an intervention that may provide a relatively pain-free window of opportunity so that responsive patients might begin a functional restoration course. Physiologically, it is well established that nociceptive afferents are not influenced by sympathetic fibers under normal conditions,[94,95] and the specific role of the SNS in perpetuating pain in pathological states such as CRPS is not clear.[96] However, evidence from several studies suggests potential direct interactions between SNS activity and CRPS pain. Drummond[97] introduced a small dose of norepinephrine into capsaicin-treated skin by iontophoresis and showed markedly increased thermal hyperalgesia. Moreover, injection of adrenergic agonists into the symptomatic limb of CRPS patients often provokes or enhances pain, even if the limb has been sympathectomized.[92,98,99] These findings are consistent with the clinical observation that CRPS pain often increases in cold weather or in response to psychological stress, when catecholamine secretion would be expected to increase.[76] Experimentally evoking the startle response also causes increased pain intensity in CRPS-I patients, presumably via sympathetic activation, and these pain changes are paralleled by significantly greater vasoconstriction on the affected side versus the unaffected side.[100] Many of the motor abnormalities of CRPS have also been reported to improve with sympatholytic blocks, implying that some of these motor symptoms may also be sympathetically maintained.[101] Despite the hyperalgesic impact of increased SNS activity on CRPS pain in experimental studies and the common clinical assumption that SNS hyperactivity contributes directly to CRPS pain, unilateral fracture patients who later developed CRPS showed impaired SNS shortly after injury (recorded with laser Doppler fluxmetry).[102] In addition, presence of impaired SNS function shortly after facture prospectively predicted who later developed acute CRPS-I.[102]

A theoretical synthesis of this SNS data: there is acute damage to small efferent sympathetic fibers with the original trauma (such as a fracture or crush injury) resulting in relative sympathetic hypofunction (hot, red, dry). Soon thereafter, cholinergic receptor upregulation occurs in the target tissues (vessels, sweat glands) and importantly, adrenergic receptors may become activated/sensitized on afferent pain fibers as well. Ultimately, there may be regeneration of sympathetic fibers into this pathologically altered region (or restitution/upregulation of central sympathetic drive), giving the clinical appearance of sympathetic hyperfunction (cold, blue, sweaty), and providing direct stimulation of noradrenergically sensitized nociceptors.[78,80,82,83]

Trophic, Dystrophic, and Nutritional Abnormalities

Tropic/dystrophic changes to skin (thin and glossy or thickened), nails (thickened, striated), and hair growth (increased or decreased) are ubiquitous in reports of chronic CRPS symptomatology, but are of unknown etiology. These changes may simply be due to relative hypoxia with chronic vasoconstriction,[58,103,104] and a similar process could also lead to the observed nerve drop out[57] and osteopenia[33] reported in CRPS. There is evidence of cellular hypoxia or impaired oxygen utilization in the CRPS affected side compared to the unaffected side based on magnetic resonance spectroscopy.[105] Skin capillary hemoglobin oxygenation has also been shown to be decreased on the affected side in CRPS patients as determined by microlight guide spectrophotometry.[104] Skin, but not venous lactate, was also reported to be increased on the affected side as measured by dermal microdialysis, suggesting decreased oxygenation.[103] The decreased range of motion often seen in CRPS could be due in part to trophic changes of joints, tendons, or ligaments. It is also possible that many of these changes could be caused by inflammation as originally suggested by Sudeck[33] or by hormonal changes.[106]

Motor and Movement Disorders

Although older diagnostic criteria do not mention motor or movement disorders,[107] newer empirically derived criteria and clinical experience feature motor system abnormalities prominently.[75,108] Most CRPS patients show weakness, spasm, tremor, bradykinesia, and range of motion abnormalities,[109] while a minority (~10%) may show more dramatic aberrations such as dystonia.[110] Weakness of skeletal muscles of the affected distal extremity is common.[110] Tremor may occur in as many as 70% of patients with upper extremity CRPS, with most represented by an apparent increase in physiologic tremor.[108,109] This tremor may decrease with sympathetic block or sympathectomy, suggesting that some motor features of CRPS may be sympathetically maintained.[109] Muscle spindles have extensive adrenergic innervation[111] and may become sensitized as the vasomotor system does. Inflammatory mediators, especially cytokines, may also sensitize muscle spindles.[112] Bradykinesia is a common abnormality in CRPS and is likely a central abnormality at a spinal and/or cortical level.[108,109] Cerebral motor processing abnormalities have been shown in CRPS with kinematic and grip force analysis.[113] Increased reactivity of the motor cortex has been shown

by MEG[68] and transcranial magnetic stimulation studies.[114] In sum, numerous findings suggest clinically-important motor abnormalities in CRPS that may be of central origin. There is some evidence that there may be an incongruity between sensory input and motor output, and this hypothesis has been used as the rationale for a treatment that involves "normalizing" the sensory input with mirror therapy.[115] An apparent motor neglect syndrome could also contribute to significant motor dysfunction in some patients, further suggesting a central etiology of the motor dysfunction of CRPS.[116] CRPS-related motor dysfunction may worsen problems with disuse (see below). An area of interest in motor dysfunction is the basal ganglia, as this is an area of somatosensory and motor processing ideally positioned to explain motor aberrations in CRPS.[117] Chronic nociceptive input to the basal ganglia may lead to abnormal programming of motor tasks in CRPS patients.

Immobilization and Disuse

Patients with prolonged casting/immobilization of a limb present with many signs and symptoms considered characteristic of CRPS (e.g., sensory disturbances, vasomotor and sudomotor asymmetry, atrophic and dystrophic changes including osteopenia[118]). In rats, casting of hind paw for 4 weeks led to warmer limbs, edema, enhanced cellular extravasation, allodynia, and periarticular osteopenia that reversed after removing the casts, and rats casted after tibial fracture showed vasomotor and nociceptive abnormalities that persisted for several months longer than casting alone.[119] The potential contribution of disuse to CRPS symptomatology provides a primary rationale for functional restoration as treatment.[120,121]

Genetics

One of the unsolved questions in human pain is why only a minority of patients develop chronic pain after identical inciting events (e.g., nerve lesions).[122,123] In contrast, in animal models of nerve lesion, almost all animals develop neuropathic pain behavior.[9,10,12,124,125] In CRPS specifically, it is interesting to consider why some individuals who have frequent, sometimes severe injuries never develop CRPS (e.g., soccer players, American football players); yet in others, trivial injuries may lead to full blown CRPS (e.g., intravenous starts, minor sprains).[122] As always, there may be environmental considerations that predispose, but genetic factors will ultimately prove to be important. The human leucocyte antigen (HLA) molecules encoded by genes of the major histocompatibility complex (MHC) may contribute to several neurologic disorders including CRPS.[126] An early report described three families with two or more members in each affected by CRPS, suggesting the possibility that CRPS risk was heritable.[127] In small studies, the HLA loci A3, B7, DQ1(06), DR2(15) and DR13 are specifically implicated.[128–130] One Japanese study suggests an association between CRPS and the angiotensin-converting enzyme gene (non-MHC axis) and notes elevated angiotensin II in CRPS patients.[131] At present, data regarding possible genetic contributions to CRPS are rather limited, but are sufficient to justify further exploration of this very plausible contribution to pathophysiology.

A Convergent Pathophysiologic Theory

These seemingly divergent factors that are proven, theorized, or hypothesized to be involved in the pathophysiology of CRPS can be synthesized.[8] The peripheral factors such as nerve and tissue damage and inflammation (regional and neurogenic) cause an afferent barrage that begins the process of peripheral and central sensitization. Central effects such as changes in the dorsal horn, brainstem, limbic areas, and cortex acutely and chronically occur. An efferent response evolves as feedback from all these areas

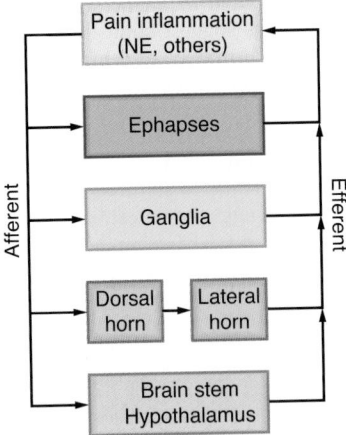

FIGURE 25.1 CRPS maintained and reinforced by nested, reverberating, feed forward (afferent) and feedback (efferent) loops. Overlaying this are the vectors of genetics (endogenous) and sociologic operant paradigms (exogenous).

along the motor (cortico-spinal) and sympathetic (limbic-hypothalamic-brainstem) systems. This efferent outflow may then substantially impact the peripheral dynamic by affecting the nutritional and inflammatory stasis in the damaged region. All of these sites interconnect, for instance by ephapses and short loops in the CNS (e.g., the sensory to sympathetic ganglion, dorsal to lateral horn, brainstem, etc.). Overlying all of this is variance in response on the basis of genetics (nature) and psychosocial factors (nurture). Thus, nested feedback and feed forward loops and cascades within the neuroaxis develop. Importantly, these feedback and feed forward loops can be self maintaining and can spread (come to involve more and more elements of the central nervous) (Fig. 25.1).

DIAGNOSIS

In the past, CRPS was diagnosed using a variety of nonstandardized and idiosyncratic diagnostic systems,[74,132–134] each of which was derived from the authors' clinical experiences and none of which achieved wide acceptance. This lack of a common diagnostic criteria hindered clinical progress for decades.

The International Association for the Study of Pain Criteria

After much debate, the name for the syndrome was ultimately changed to CRPS at a consensus workshop in Orlando, Florida, in 1994,[45,135] with the new name and diagnostic criteria codified by the IASP taskforce on taxonomy (see Table 25-1).[107] This new diagnostic entity was meant to be descriptive, general, and not to imply any pathophysiology (including any direct role for the sympathetic nervous system). According to these criteria, CRPS can be diagnosed regardless of whether the pain is sympathetically-maintained (SNS block responsive) or sympathetically-independent. These IASP-endorsed criteria had the potential to lead to improved clinical communication and greater generalizability across research samples.[45] However, realization of this potential has been somewhat limited by the fact that these criteria were derived solely by consensus. Also, since publication in 1994, utilization of the criteria has been sporadic (although increasing) in the literature,[136] and certain groups have resisted the change (especially certain advocacy groups and payors). As a consequence, the full benefits of common, clearly-defined criteria have not been completely realized.

Experience gained in developing diagnostic criteria in headache and psychiatric disorders indicates that consensus-based criteria can be significantly improved by systematic empirical validation[137] and consensus-derived criteria that are not subsequently validated may lead to over- or underdiagnosis, thus reducing the ability to provide timely, optimal treatment. Results of validation studies to date suggest that the IASP criteria are adequately sensitive (i.e., rarely miss a case of actual CRPS); however, both internal and external validation research suggest potential problems with specificity (overdiagnosis).[75,138,139] The current IASP criteria implicitly assume that signs and symptoms of vasomotor, sudomotor, and edema-related changes provide redundant diagnostic information; that is, presence of any one of these is sufficient to meet criterion 3 (see Table 25-1). This combination of multiple distinct elements of the syndrome into the same diagnostic criterion and allowing patient-reported symptoms are likely elements contributing to overdiagnosis in the IASP scheme.[75,140] An additional weakness of these criteria is the failure to include motor/trophic signs and symptoms, which could lead to important information being ignored that may help discriminate CRPS from other syndromes.

These conclusions are supported by the results of factor analysis (a statistical pattern recognition technique) that was conducted in a series of 123 CRPS patients. These results indicated that signs and symptoms of CRPS clustered into four statistically-distinct subgroups.[75] The first of these subgroups was a set of signs and symptoms indicating abnormalities in pain processing (e.g., allodynia, hyperalgesia). Skin color and temperature changes characterized the second subgroup, indicative of vasomotor dysfunction. Edema and sudomotor dysfunction (e.g., sweating changes) combined to form a third unique subgroup. The finding that vasomotor signs and symptoms were statistically-distinct from those reflecting sudomotor changes/edema is in contrast to the IASP criteria, which treats all three of these as diagnostically equivalent. A fourth and final subgroup was identified that included motor and trophic signs and symptoms. Numerous studies have described various signs of motor dysfunction (e.g., dystonia, tremor) as important characteristics of this disorder,[116,134,141] and trophic changes have frequently been mentioned in historical clinical descriptions. The absence of both of these features from current IASP criteria is therefore notable, especially given factor analytic findings that this subgroup of signs and symptoms does not overlap significantly with other characteristics of CRPS currently used in diagnosis.

External validity, which addresses the ability of the diagnostic criteria to distinguish CRPS patients from those with other types of pain conditions, is also an important issue. In the absence of a definitive pathophysiology of CRPS and thus the absence of a definitive objective test to serve as a criterion standard, providing evidence for the external validity of diagnostic criteria is challenging.[142] However, the upper limit of external validity can be evaluated by using the original criteria themselves as a reference point.[75,138,142] In this methodology, a CRPS patient group is identified using a strict application of the IASP/CRPS criteria with a comparison group of non-CRPS neuropathic pain patients defined by independent diagnostic information (e.g., diabetic neuropathy diagnosed by presence of chronic diabetes with ascending symmetrical pain and corroborated by electrodiagnostic studies). Existing criteria and modifications to these criteria can then be evaluated with regard to their ability to distinguish between these two groups based on patterns of signs and symptoms. This model was used to test the utility of the IASP/CRPS criteria for discriminating between 117 patients meeting IASP criteria and 43 neuropathic pain patients with established non-CRPS etiology. The IASP/CRPS criteria and decision rules (e.g., "evidence at some time" of edema *or* color changes *or* sweating changes satisfy criterion 3) did discriminate significantly between the CRPS and non-

CRPS groups. However, closer examination of the results indicated that while diagnostic sensitivity (i.e., being able to detect the disorder when it is present) was quite high (0.98), specificity (i.e., minimizing false positive diagnoses) was poor (0.36), and a positive diagnosis of CRPS was likely to be correct in as few as 40% of cases.[75,139]

For clinical purposes, sensitivity is extremely important. On the other hand, the issue of specificity is quite important for selection of research samples, as well as for minimizing unnecessary, potentially invasive treatments. The clinical implication of high sensitivity at the expense of specificity is that CRPS may be overdiagnosed and, ultimately, overtreated. It also has the very significant downside of identifying pathophysiologically heterogeneous groups for research, contributing potentially to negative results in clinical trials.[75]

The "Budapest" Criteria

A meeting of international researchers and clinicians with expertise in CRPS (the "Budapest Group") was held in Budapest, Hungary, in 2003 to make consensus recommendations on proposed revisions to the current IASP diagnostic criteria. The criteria ultimately proposed by the Budapest Group were consensus-based modifications of the criteria that were statistically derived from the validation studies, as above.[75,139] These modified criteria assessed CRPS characteristics within each of the four statistically-derived factors described above. Given evidence that objective signs on examination and patient-reported symptoms both provide useful, but nonidentical information, the modified criteria required the presence of signs and symptoms of CRPS for diagnosis.[75,138,143] A test of these modified criteria regarding their ability to discriminate between the CRPS and non-CRPS neuropathic pain groups indicated that they could increase diagnostic accuracy.[75,142] Results indicated that a decision rule requiring that two of four sign categories and three of four symptom categories be positive for a diagnosis to be made resulted in a sensitivity of 0.85 and a specificity of 0.69. This decision rule represented a good compromise between identifying as many patients as possible in the clinical context while substantially reducing the high level of false positive diagnoses associated with current IASP criteria. This decision rule was therefore adopted in a set of proposed clinical diagnostic criteria endorsed by the Budapest Group (summarized in Table 25-2).[75,143]

The proposed clinical diagnostic criteria described reflected an improvement over current IASP criteria for clinical purposes, but still suffered from less than optimal specificity for use in the research context.[143] Tests of the modified CRPS criteria above indicated that modifying the decision rules to require that two of four sign categories and four of four symptom categories be positive for diagnosis to be made resulted in a sensitivity of 0.70 and a specificity of 0.94. Of all the permutations tested, this decision rule resulted in the greatest probability of accurate diagnosis for both CRPS and non-CRPS patients (approximately 80% and 90% accuracy, respectively).[75,139,140,143] This high level of specificity was considered desirable in the research context by the Budapest Group, and therefore was adopted as part of a set of proposed research diagnostic criteria.[140,143] Current distinctions between CRPS-I and CRPS-II subtypes, reflecting respectively the absence and presence of evidence of peripheral nerve injury, were ultimately retained despite ongoing questions by the consensus group as to whether such distinctions have clinical utility.[143]

Thus, CRPS is a clinical diagnosis, made with simple bedside testing techniques known by all physicians. Technical testing procedures are sometimes used to corroborate or objectively document clinical impressions (e.g., thermography, bone scans).[40] To date none of these have been formally validated.

TABLE 25.2

"BUDAPEST" DIAGNOSTIC CRITERIA FOR CRPS

General Definition of the Syndrome

CRPS describes an array of painful conditions that are characterized by a continuing (spontaneous and/or evoked) regional pain that is seemingly disproportionate in time or degree to the usual course of any known trauma or other lesion. The pain is regional (not in a specific nerve territory or dermatome), but may spread, and usually has a distal predominance of abnormal sensory, motor, sudomotor, vasomotor, and/or trophic findings. The syndrome shows variable progression over time.

To make a clinical* diagnosis, the following criteria must be met:
1) Continuing pain, which is disproportionate to any inciting event.
2) Must report at least one symptom in **three of the four** following categories:
   —**Sensory:** Reports of hyperesthesia and/or allodynia.
   —**Vasomotor:** Reports of temperature asymmetry and/or skin color changes and/or skin color asymmetry.
   —**Sudomotor/Edema:** Reports of edema and/or sweating changes and/or sweating asymmetry.
   —**Motor/Trophic:** Reports of decreased range of motion and/or motor dysfunction (weakness, tremor, dystonia) and/or trophic changes (hair, nail, skin).
3) Must display at least one sign **at time of evaluation** in **two or more** of the following categories:
   —**Sensory:** Evidence of hyperalgesia (to pinprick) and/or allodynia (to light touch and/or deep somatic pressure and/or joint movement).
   —**Vasomotor:** Evidence of temperature asymmetry and/or skin color changes and/or asymmetry.
   —**Sudomotor/Edema:** Evidence of edema and/or sweating changes and/or sweating asymmetry
   —**Motor/Trophic:** Evidence of decreased range of motion and/or motor dysfunction (weakness, tremor, dystonia) and/or trophic changes (hair, nail, skin).
4) There is no other diagnosis that better explains the signs and symptoms.

*For research purposes, diagnostic decision rule should be at least one symptom **in all four** symptom categories and at least one sign observed at evaluation in two or more sign categories (modified from Harden[143]).

Sequential Stages of Complex Regional Pain Syndrome?

Although not part of clinical diagnosis per se, it is lore among clinicians that CRPS entails three sequential stages that differ in patterns of signs and symptoms. This traditional staging model is summarized by Bonica.[132] The early, acute stage of CRPS (Stage I) was characterized by pain/sensory abnormalities (e.g., hyperalgesia, allodynia), vasomotor and sudomotor dysfunction, and prominent edema. Stage II (Dystrophic Stage) was proposed to occur 3–6 months after onset, and to be characterized by more marked pain/sensory dysfunction, with continued evidence of vasomotor dysfunction and development of significant motor/trophic changes. Stage III (Atrophic Stage) was characterized by decreased pain/sensory disturbance, continued vasomotor disturbance, and markedly increased motor/trophic changes. Although until recently, there had been only limited empirical tests of this hypothesized staging of CRPS, the concept has frequently been accepted as fact in the CRPS literature.[132,144,145]

The limited available prospective research that followed patients who develop CRPS-like symptoms after surgery, fracture, or severe hand injury suggests that in many cases the condition does not progress through increasingly problematic stages like those described above.[6,52,146,147] Retrospective surveys completed by CRPS patients with an average pain duration of over 3 years similarly indicate that CRPS symptoms often tend to remain stable or improve, rather than progressively deteriorate.[138] More recently, the statistical technique of cluster analysis was used to test for evidence of sequential stages.[148] Specifically, three unique subgroups were identified, with patients in each subgroup displaying statistically similar patterns of symptoms but that there were no significant pain duration differences between the three subgroups; in contrast to the traditional staging model, the group with the most motor/trophic signs and symptoms had a slightly shorter mean pain duration.[148] Findings such as these suggest the possibility that the presumed sequential stages often reported by clinicians may reflect CRPS subtypes, rather than an actual staging that follows a progressive, deteriorating course. There is some evidence that "temperature staging" may occur; early CRPS may tend to present with increased temperature ("hot CRPS") and longer duration CRPS to present with decreased temperature ("cold CRPS").[79,149] Data are not yet sufficient to conclude whether such temperature staging occurs in all patients.

Psychological Factors in Complex Regional Pain Syndrome

It is critical to properly deem CRPS (as all chronic pain conditions) as a biopsychosocial disease; as such, it is crucial to clinical success that psychologic and sociologic diagnoses be identified and targeted for intervention. Psychologic factors could theoretically influence onset or maintenance of CRPS via adrenergic mechanisms believed to contribute to CRPS pathophysiology as described above.[82,83,86,93,149,150] The impact of catecholamine release in the pathophysiologic mechanisms described above may be important to recognize given that psychologic factors such as life stress and dysphoric emotional states (e.g., anxiety, anger, depression) can be associated with increased catecholaminergic activity.[151,152] For example, levels of plasma epinephrine were found to correlate significantly with depressive symptoms in a sample of 16 CRPS patients.[153] Similarly, plasma norepinephrine levels were significantly higher in a sample of 15 CRPS patients than in age- and gender-matched healthy controls, and these elevations were associated significantly with higher scores on a measure of posttraumatic stress symptoms.[154] It is plausible that stress and emotional distress could, through their impact on catecholamine release, interact with adrenergically-mediated pathophysiologic mechanisms to contribute to onset or maintenance of CRPS. Interestingly, recent evidence suggests that elevated stress levels in CRPS patients may also be associated with altered immune response, which could potentially impact CRPS as well.[154]

Examination of the historical CRPS literature frequently reveals the implicit assumption that psychologic dysfunction (usually emotional disorders) contributes to CRPS in at least some patients. This assumption probably colored physicians' conceptualization of CRPS patients, despite the absence until 10 years ago of a significant body of controlled studies examining this issue. In the existing research literature, most studies assessing the role of psychologic factors in CRPS have been limited to case series descriptions or cross-sectional psychologic comparisons between CRPS patients and non-CRPS chronic pain patients.[155]

The ability to make conclusions about psychologic factors contributing to onset of CRPS depends on prospective research designs, which are rare in the CRPS literature. One prospective study indicated that higher levels of anxiety symptoms prior to total knee arthroplasty were associated with greater likelihood of displaying CRPS-like symptoms at 1 month post surgery.[6] These latter findings would be consistent with the psychophysiologic

model proposed above. However, it is notable that neither anxiety nor depression predicted occurrence of CRPS-like symptoms at 6 months, so the long-term impact of psychologic factors on development of chronic CRPS remains unclear. Even if the psychophysiologic model is accurate, this should not be taken to imply that the presence of psychological risk factors alone would be either necessary or sufficient to cause CRPS. For example, one prospective study indicated that among 88 consecutive patients assessed shortly after acute distal radius fracture, 14 had significantly elevated life stress but did not develop CRPS, and the one patient who did develop CRPS had no apparent psychologic risk factors (i.e., no major life stressors, average emotional distress levels).[156]

In the absence of other prospective studies, the question of whether psychologic factors affect the development and maintenance of CRPS must be addressed solely on the basis of case reports and retrospective or cross-sectional research designs which do not allow causation to be inferred. Two uncontrolled retrospective case series reported a relationship between onset of CRPS and contemporaneous emotional loss or major life stressors,[157,158] although these can at best be considered anecdotal. The only controlled study regarding the role of life stress in CRPS onset found that 80% of patients in a CRPS sample recalled a stressful life event temporally concurrent with the initiating physical trauma, in contrast to only 20% of non-CRPS controls.[159] Although this suggests that stressful life events occurring concurrently with a physical trauma may contribute to development of CRPS, this study's findings still must be viewed with caution due to its retrospective design.

If psychologic dysfunction is somehow uniquely involved in onset or maintenance of CRPS, one might expect an increased prevalence of psychiatric disorders or elevated levels of emotional distress in this population. Based on structured interviews, estimates for prevalence of Axis I psychiatric disorders (e.g., anxiety and depressive disorders) in CRPS patients indicate a prevalence ranging from 24% to as high as 65%.[56,160,161] It should be noted that only Monti et al.[160] included a non-CRPS chronic pain control group, and these authors reported that prevalence of Axis I disorders was not significantly higher in CRPS compared to non-CRPS pain patients. None of the studies above documented psychiatric status prior to CRPS onset and therefore cannot address the issue of causality. At present, there is no evidence that CRPS patients suffer from diagnosable psychiatric disorders at a higher rate than do other chronic pain patients.

Controlled studies have also addressed the issue of whether CRPS patients are more emotionally distressed than other types of chronic pain patients. Several cross-sectional studies have found that CRPS patients report being more emotionally distressed than non-CRPS pain patients, in terms of greater depression and/or anxiety levels.[159,162–165] These findings for depressed mood may be relevant when one considers that in a study using time series diary methodology, depression levels on a given day were a significant predictor of CRPS pain intensity on the following day.[166]

More recently, results of a prospective study indicated that patients displaying signs and symptoms of CRPS 6 months following total knee replacement reported significantly higher levels of anxiety than did patients not displaying CRPS, despite the fact that both groups were continuing to experience at least some degree of pain.[6] However, baseline anxiety and depression did not predict CRPS status at 6 months, suggesting that the observed elevations in psychologic distress were a result of CRPS pain rather than a cause. In light of these findings, one possible explanation for elevated distress often reported in CRPS patients relative to non-CRPS chronic pain patients might be that the unusual and sometimes dramatic symptomatology of CRPS (e.g., allodynia, hyperalgesia, vasomotor changes, significant edema, motor changes) is more distressing than experiencing more common forms of chronic pain. Moreover, the validity of these symptoms are often questioned by health care providers, potentially adding to patient distress.

Some studies suggest CRPS patients are more distressed than comparable non-CRPS chronic pain patients, yet other studies have reported no such differences. For example, work by Ciccone and colleagues[165] provided only partial support for this hypothesis, finding that CRPS patients reported more somatic symptoms of depression than non-CRPS patients with local neuropathy, yet displayed no emotional differences relative to low back pain patients. Other studies have found no evidence of elevated distress among CRPS patients compared to low back pain patients[167,168] or headache patients.[167] In the absence of additional well-controlled studies, it remains unclear whether the findings suggesting uniquely elevated distress in CRPS patients are an artifact of sample selection.

Two studies report that emotional distress, when present, may have a greater impact on pain intensity in CRPS than in other types of chronic pain.[164,169] For example, correlations between pain intensity and both anxiety and anger expressiveness are significantly stronger in CRPS patients than in non-CRPS chronic pain patients.[164,169] These results suggest that even if CRPS patients are not uniquely distressed, the impact of that distress may be unique, possibly due to the hypothesized adrenergic interactions described above. These findings could have significant treatment implications, as psychologic interventions that reduce distress may directly contribute to reductions in CRPS symptoms (e.g., pain, vasomotor changes).

Another important operant mechanism that may contribute to CRPS is the sometimes dramatic disuse that patients develop in an effort to avoid stimuli that may trigger. Even in healthy individuals, prolonged disuse leads to temperature/color changes and hyperalgesia similar to those observed in CRPS.[118] Significant inverse correlations between CRPS pain intensity and ability to carry out activities of daily living suggest that pain avoidance is likely one of the common reasons for CRPS-related activity impairments.[159] Learned disuse, reinforced by either avoidance of actual pain or reduced anxiety subsequent to avoiding anticipated pain exacerbations (kinesophobia), may prevent desensitization and eliminate the normal tactile and proprioceptive input from the extremity that may be necessary to restore normal central signal processing.[170,171] Learned disuse may also inhibit the natural movement-related pumping action that helps prevent accumulation of catecholamines, tachykinins, and other nociceptive and inflammatory mediators in the affected extremity, which may impact negatively on CRPS signs and symptoms.[51] Pain-related learned disuse might therefore interact with other pathophysiological mechanisms to help maintain and exacerbate both the pain-related and autonomic features of CRPS (see below).[155]

In summary, while the contribution of psychologic factors to the development and maintenance of CRPS is largely speculative, it is theoretically consistent and highlights the importance of addressing psychologic factors in the clinical management of CRPS.

TREATMENT

The Rationale for Functional Restoration

CRPS can be a very challenging condition to successfully manage. It is biomedically multifaceted and should be treated as such.[172] The patient presentation often changes over time, and the natural history is variable and poorly understood. Evidence for efficacy of various treatment modalities is scarce and has developed slowly,[120] due in large part to the vagaries of diagnosis. The only treatment methodology that can have a reasonable chance of successfully bridging the varied presentation and mechanisms of disease and the profound gaps in treatment evidence is a systematic and orderly interdisciplinary approach.[173] Interdisciplinary treatment is defined as a dedicated, coherent, coordinated, specially trained group of relevant professionals that meet regularly to plan, coordinate care, and adapt to treatment eventualities.[143] It is critical to identify and aggressively treat all spheres of the pain experience in CRPS; obsessing with the biomedical alone dooms the clinician and patient to failure, especially in CRPS in which pathophysiology is incompletely characterized. Psychosocial targets that may impact pain and dysfunction are often readily and effectively treatable, and should be embraced as important avenues of help.

Pain is a central component of CRPS diagnosis and must figure prominently in any treatment regimen. However, its subjective nature makes this symptom a moving target that can only be effectively addressed by addressing not only subjective pain but also learned pain behavior and dysfunction. Thus, it is critical to target both subjective and objective clinical benchmarks and outcomes. Ideally, the treatment of CRPS should rely upon an intuitive, measurable, and stepwise functional restoration algorithm as the pivotal feature of treatment.[148,171,174] This line of reasoning has been codified by two large international consensus-building conferences.[171,175] The Initiative on Methods, Measurement, and Pain Assessment in Clinical Trials has concluded that physical functioning is a "core domain" in the assessment of pain treatment efficacy, second only to pain assessment.[176,177] Functional restoration emphasizes physical activity ("reanimation"), desensitization and normalization of sympathetic tone in the affected limb, and involves a steady progression from the most gentle, least invasive interventions to the ideal of complete rehabilitation in all aspects of the patient's life (Fig. 25.2).[143,171,175] Although the benefits of functional restoration are intuitive (and are becoming dogma), the evidence as to which modalities are optimal, when to use what and for how long, is currently unavailable.[143,175,178] In a early pivotal paper, Davidoff et al.[174] conducted a prospective uncontrolled study in RSD that supported the functional restoration approach with three key findings: (1) that objective functional components and biometric data could be quantified longitudinally; (2) that these components were reactive enough to display change over time (e.g., in response to a functional restoration-based interdisciplinary program); and (3) that they were associated with improvements in subjective outcomes (e.g., decreased pain). This study supplied a primary rationale for a reliance on functional measures as the basis for assessing success in the treatment of CRPS. Various uncontrolled studies suggest that CRPS patients benefited from certain physiotherapeutic modalities, including stress loading and isometric techniques.[170] Oerlemans et al.[178,179] conducted a prospective controlled study of 135 CRPS patients with pain located in an upper extremity and reported that both physical therapy (PT) and occupational therapy (OT) proved valuable in managing pain, restoring mobility, and reducing impairment. Birklein et al.[87] similarly found that pain reports were notably lower for patients undergoing PT.

Immobilization is recognized as a possible cause and/or perpetuating factor in the syndrome.[107] Patients (and animals) with prolonged casting of a limb often have many signs and symptoms considered part of the CRPS syndrome: vasomotor and sudomotor asymmetry, trophic/dystrophic changes including osteopenia, and occasionally sensory disturbances.[180] Diminished active range of motion is common in early CRPS,[181] and CRPS is associated with significantly reduced mobility and impaired ability to use the affected area normally.[182] Thus, normalized movement is a key objective in treating central changes linked with the syndrome, loosely categorized under the rubric of "altered central processing" and salient to this argument, "neglect."[183] "Pain-related fear is more disabling than pain itself," and this fear appears to be a dynamic clinical factor in CRPS.[184,185] The ability to impact this kinesophobia seen in most CRPS patients clinically provides a persuasive argument for functional restoration as fundamental. Meta-analyses have shown that an interdisciplinary

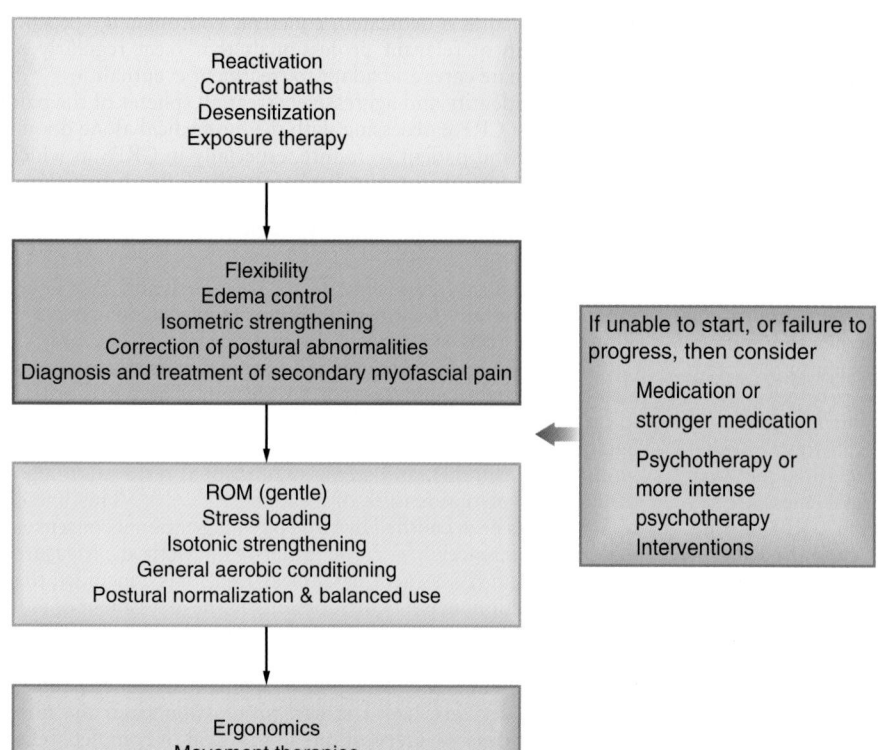

Reactivation
Contrast baths
Desensitization
Exposure therapy

Flexibility
Edema control
Isometric strengthening
Correction of postural abnormalities
Diagnosis and treatment of secondary myofascial pain

If unable to start, or failure to progress, then consider

Medication or stronger medication

Psychotherapy or more intense psychotherapy
Interventions

ROM (gentle)
Stress loading
Isotonic strengthening
General aerobic conditioning
Postural normalization & balanced use

Ergonomics
Movement therapies
Normalization of use
Vocational/functional rehabilitation

FIGURE 25.2 Functional restoration algorithm. From the outset, in appropriate cases, the patient should have access to medications and/or psychotherapy and/or injections. If the patient cannot begin, or fails to progress, at any step or in any regard, the clinical team should consider starting (or adding) more or stronger medications and/or more intensive psychotherapies and/or interventions (modified with permission from Harden[172]).

approach like that used in comprehensive functional restoration programs for CRPS improves symptoms in patients with chronic pain.[186,187]

Rehabilitation-Based Treatment Modalities

Occupational therapists are the ideal therapeutic leaders in the functional restoration process, as they are trained in the biopsychosocial principles of disease and are primary in functional assessment and treatment.[188] OT begins with an assessment of the patient's status and current function (e.g., range of motion, activities of daily living, edema). OT treatment should aim to normalize sensation and posture, decrease muscle guarding, minimize edema, and increase normal use.[189,190] Specialized garments, bandaging, and manual edema mobilization techniques can help manage edema.[191] Regular use of the affected limb during everyday tasks is promoted and strongly reinforced throughout the rehabilitation process. A stress loading ("scrubbing" and carrying) program should be implemented as soon as possible.[170,192] Later, treatments emphasizing active range of motion, coordination/dexterity, strengthening, and proprioceptive neuromuscular facilitation can be applied (see Fig. 25.2).[193] In extreme CRPS cases, functional splinting may be required to encourage improved circulation/nutrition to the affected area as well as to promote more normal tissue length/positioning during rehabilitation.

PT plays an equally critical role in functional restoration.[194,195] PT emphasizes range of motion, flexibility, posture, and later, weight-bearing and strength through the use of gentle progressive exercise. PT must be executed within the bounds of the patient's tolerance,[196] and never when the affected limb is insensate (such as immediately after a block).[197] Inappropriately aggressive PT can trigger extreme pain, edema, distress, and fatigue, and may in turn exacerbate the inflammation and sympa-

thetic symptoms of CRPS. Oerleman's group has shown that PT (and to a lesser extent OT) improves pain scores and "active mobility" versus controls.[178,179,198] In children with CRPS, a single-blind, randomized trial of PT combined with cognitive–behavioral therapy demonstrated significant improvement on five measures of pain and function[199] and in a prospective review of 103 children with CRPS, intensive PT (aerobic, hydrotherapy, and desensitization) supplemented by psychologic counseling was effective.[190] The therapy program should be primarily based on functional goals and achieved through active or active-assisted means or the use of low-tech devices (e.g., swiss balls, foam rolls, etc.). PT should encourage pacing and include rest breaks and relaxation techniques as well. Mat exercises provide strengthening of both the extremity and the postural muscles in a non–weight-bearing approach and may include movement therapies such as Feldenkrais or Pilates. Virtually all patients with advanced CRPS will present with myofascial pain syndrome of the supporting joint, and effective treatment of this is critical to optimize outcomes. Aquatic therapy can be quite valuable to CRPS patients because of its hydrostatic/compressive principles and its buoyancy effect.[190] Massage, electrostimulation, ultrasound, and contrast baths are empirical modalities administered by PT (see Fig. 25.2).[195]

The recreational therapist is often the first clinician to succeed in getting the CRPS patient to initiate increased movement. The incentive of returning to a favorite pastime is often the appropriate reinforcer to modify kinesophobia and bracing.[200] Through the use of modifications, adaptive equipment, and creative problem solving (e.g., large handled gardening equipment, bowling with the nondominant hand, etc.), a patient can enhance self efficacy and develop confidence through previously lost recreational activities (see Fig. 25.2).[195]

The vocational rehabilitation (VR) counselor helps prepare the appropriate CRPS patient for the ultimate functional restoration: return to work. Consultation with employer, supervisor, employee health nurse and work site visits are potential interactions initiated by VR. The VR counselor uses information from medical, occupational, educational, financial, and labor markets interfaced with the client's job description/analysis to attempt to reset negative operant paradigms and operationalize the benefits of work.[195] The VR counselor should participate in the work capacity evaluation, transferable skills analysis, job-specific reconditioning, work hardening, and functional capacities evaluation, and be central in the development and documentation of modifications, restrictions, return-to-work assessments, and work release documents.[195,201,202] VR counselor, occupational therapist, and responsible physician work closely together in these tasks, with an ideal goal of return to the original job with the original employer (see Fig. 25.2). The sociologic issues surrounding CRPS are pervasive, but very poorly characterized. The best approach to managing these is to compassionately and firmly pursue the goals of optimal functional restoration while proactively providing tools for closure in the forensic and compensation arenas.

Because the symptoms of CRPS patients encompass all the biopsychosocial complexities of chronic pain, the best hope of helping patients is the adoption of a systematic, stable, empathetic, and, above all, interdisciplinary approach that addresses those symptoms.[195] Pharmacotherapy, psychotherapy, and interventional techniques should be efficiently deployed for patients who either cannot begin or fail to progress using the interdisciplinary functional restoration approach outlined above. Many patients will require medication and psychotherapy from the beginning to be successful in the pivotal functional restoration algorithm (see Fig. 25-2).[195,203] That functional restoration can and should be the central intervention and outcome standard in CRPS is a theory that must be tested. Until then, the interdisciplinary approach for treating patients with CRPS clearly remains the most pragmatic, helpful, and cost-effective therapeutic approach available today.

Pharmacotherapy

In the 130 years since Weir-Mitchell recommended laudanum (tincture of opium) and the use of a new invention, the hypodermic syringe, to perform cocaine nerve blocks,[1] multiple pharmacotherapeutic interventions for CRPS have been described.[57,121,203] Unfortunately, there are very few randomized controlled trials (RCTs) in CRPS.[120] The best empirical approach must therefore employ the limited data available, extrapolate from better evidence that is available in related conditions (e.g., neuropathic pain),[204] and pragmatically utilize sequential drug trials in each unique case based on putative mechanisms, driven by close monitoring of outcome and risk (Table 25-3). Pharmacotherapy in CRPS, as with most chronic pain syndromes, achieves the greatest benefit when used in conjunction with an interdisciplinary approach to treatment. In CRPS patients, the initial pain intensity is often sufficient that pharmacotherapy may be necessary to begin available nonpharmacologic treatments, and rational polypharmacy is usually required to optimize analgesia.[121,203] In treating CRPS, the clinician must construct a drug regimen that draws from two basic classes of medications: prophylactic drugs (for maintenance, drugs used on a scheduled basis) to obtain base line analgesia and abortive drugs (rescue agents, pro re nata) for breakthrough pain or symptom flares. Although analgesia for its own sake has obvious value, a unifocal palliative strategy without concurrent functional restoration is useless in CRPS.[143,171,203]

Nonsteroidal anti-inflammatory drugs (NSAIDs), corticosteroids, Cox-2 inhibitors, and free-radical scavengers are generally used to treat CRPS pain in the context of discernible inflammation. As described previously, there is evidence that inflammatory

TABLE 25.3

PHARMACOTHERAPY CONSIDERATIONS

Condition/Presentation	Suggested Response
Mild to moderate pain	Simple analgesics and/or blocks
Excruciating, intractable pain	Opioids and/or blocks or later, more experimental interventions
Inflammation/swelling and edema	Steroids, systemic or targeted (acutely) or NSAIDs (chronically); immunemodulators
Depression, anxiety, insomnia	Sedative, analgesic antidepressant/anxiolytics (and/or psychotherapy)
Significant allodynia/hyperalgesia	Anticonvulsants and/or other sodium channel blockers and/or N-methyl-D-aspartate-receptor antagonists
Significant osteopenia, immobility, and trophic changes	Calcitonin or bisphosphonates
Profound vasomotor disturbance	Calcium channel blockers, sympatholytics and/or blocks

These very general guidelines are overruled by individual patient presentation. It is also important to note that certain drugs, such as bisphosphonates, may be associated with analgesia as well as the more primary action (modified with permission from Harden[172]).

components are critical to the development or perpetuation of CRPS, especially early in the course.[42,205] Anti-inflammatory medications can be used for both rescue and prophylaxis. NSAIDs have shown mixed results in several clinical trials of neuropathic pain, including one trial that showed that NSAIDs had no value in treating CRPS-I.[206] Even though Cox-2 selective inhibitors have not been properly assessed in CRPS, they have been used anecdotally.[207]

Oral corticosteroids are the only anti-inflammatory drugs with strong evidence in CRPS,[120,208] and there are two RCTs supporting their efficacy, at least in acute CRPS.[209,210] Given the data, a short course of steroids in acute CRPS with inflammatory features is indicated, but longer courses have a questionable risk benefit ratio[120] as there are numerous obvious contraindications to chronic steroid use. Free radical oxygen species are known to have a role in inflammatory processes and may be involved in CRPS; thus specific antioxidants in theory might have a role in CRPS treatment.[34] One RCT of the antioxidant vitamin C was found to reduce the incidence of RSD in patients with wrist fractures.[211] Neuroimmune modulators affecting inflammation, such as thalidomide,[212,213] lenalidomide,[214] etanercept, and infliximab,[215] all have some open label support in CRPS, and RCTs of some of these are ongoing.

There is anecdotal support for anticonvulsant drugs in CRPS, but no RCTs. There are meta-analytic and systematic reviews compiling evidence for the efficacy of certain anticonvulsant compounds as prophylactic agents in other forms of neuropathic pain,[216–219] and the diverse mechanisms of action of some anticonvulsants theoretically should be useful in addressing some of the putative pathophysiologic mechanisms underlying CRPS.[121,221] Gabapentin, Pregabalin, and Carbamezepine have strong evidence supporting their use in neuropathic pain conditions and anecdotal support in CRPS.[221–227]

There are also several meta-analyses of the analgesic efficacy of antidepressant/anxiolytics (ADs) in neuropathic conditions,[216,217,228,229] with some low-quality evidence supporting the use of ADs in CRPS.[120,230] These drugs have obvious use in managing some of the comorbidities in CRPS, such as major depression and anxiety.[121,229] Second generation ADs have not been studied in CRPS, but the so-called serotonin/ norepinephrine reuptake blockers show some promise.

The use of opioids for general chronic pain management is still the subject of some controversy,[120,231] but this class has anecdotal support for both abortive and prophylactic treatment in CRPS.[232] Only one RCT has been conducted specifically in CRPS, with negative results.[227] In general, neuropathic pain does not respond to opioids as well as nociceptive pain[233–236]; consequently, neuropathic pain may require higher doses (with an increase in the risk of side effects). Moreover, some animal data suggest that long-term opioid use may actually evoke symptoms characteristic of CRPS, such as allodynia and hyperpathia.[237] N-methyl-D-aspartate receptor antagonists (e.g., MK-801, ketamine, amantadine, and dextromethorphan), which theoretically should reduce central sensitization, have been considered for the treatment of neuropathic pain, but some of these have proven too toxic for regular clinical use in oral formulations.[238–242] Ketamine has shown favorable results in case reports of patients with CRPS.[243–245] There is some ongoing interest in high dose anesthetic ketamine protocols,[246] although there are no well-controlled studies supporting this approach. Amantadine has shown some benefit in neuropathic pain.[247,248] Dextromethorphan may augment the effect of other medications, especially opioids.[249]

Clonidine has been considered for the treatment of CRPS,[250] but most often by the epidural route.[251] A case series showed that transdermal clonidine could reduce local CRPS-induced hyperalgesia and allodynia,[252] but results of a systematic review failed to support the efficacy of this treatment approach.[120] Nifedipine has demonstrated some benefit in uncontrolled trials, particularly for the management of vasoconstriction.[253,254] Phenoxybenzamine and phentolamine have some low-quality evidence supporting their use in CRPS.[91,253–256] Calcitonin is one of the best-studied drugs in the treatment of CRPS.[257–260] A meta-analysis of a limited number of controlled calcitonin studies supported the therapeutic value of intranasal doses of 100–300 U per day for the management of CRPS.[259,261] However, one study reported no improvement after administration of 200 IU twice daily for 4 weeks.[257]

There are two positive randomized studies of bisphosphonates for the treatment of CRPS.[262,263] Two smaller RCTs and one case series of oral pamidronate have also suggested some benefit.[264,265] The impact of these drugs on the osteopenia (Sudeck's atrophy) that is often prominent in chronic CRPS is unknown.

Topical medications may also be of some use in management of CRPS. There is limited research endorsing the use of local anesthetic creams in neuropathic pain,[266] but RCTs have not been performed. A patch containing 5% lidocaine is FDA-approved for the management of postherpetic neuralgia, and is used anecdotally for CRPS.[267,268] A study of high-dose topical capsaicin with pretreatment with regional anesthesia demonstrated partial efficacy.[269] In one high-quality study, the topical free radical scavenger dimethyl sulfoxide (50% cream for 2 months) showed significant pain reduction when compared with placebo.[270] Topical clonidine has been mentioned, as above.[252]

In most cases, no single drug will provide sufficient analgesia long-term, nor will it completely prevent the need for abortive/ rescue agents. This clinical reality usually requires multiple medications to adequately manage the pain (see Table 25-3). There are numerous other medications that have been anecdotally mentioned as treatments for CRPS (e.g., case reports), but there is insufficient evidence to justify their inclusion in this chapter.

Psychologic Interventions

As psychologic and sociologic factors often contribute to CRPS pain and dysfunction and given the relative effectiveness of psychotherapeutic interventions, it is clear psychologic and behavioral treatments must play an important role in CRPS management.[172,173,272] Such interventions are likely to be maximally effective if provided in the context of multidisciplinary care. Psychologic interventions for CRPS, typically based on cognitive–behavioral therapy principles, should target learned disuse, fear of pain, cognitive responses to CRPS (e.g., catastrophizing), life stress, and emotional distress that may contribute to maintenance or exacerbation of the disorder.[172,173] Training in relaxation techniques (progressive muscle relaxation, breathing relaxation, autogenics, imagery) is of anecdotal use in giving patients some degree of control over their symptoms, particularly if complemented with biofeedback (especially thermal and myogenic). Moreover, as in all types of chronic pain, better pain coping skills may lead to improved functioning and quality of life and increased ability to self-manage pain.[172] At minimum, such treatments are likely to enhance patients' sense of control over the condition, and thereby reduce fears that may be a barrier to achieving success in functional therapies. Interventions that target a family's reinforcing responses to the patient's pain may also be helpful in addressing problems with learned disuse and dysfunction. It should be noted that the psychologic interventions above will only be successful to the extent that patients are willing to accept some responsibility for managing their condition, as opposed to an exclusive focus on achieving a medical "cure." Facilitating this cognitive shift to a self-management approach is often the first step necessary to achieve successful outcomes in both functional and psychologic therapies.[172]

A number of studies have addressed efficacy of psychologic interventions for CRPS, although nearly all of these reflect uncontrolled designs that permit only limited conclusions to be drawn. An additional caveat regarding these studies is that the criteria used to diagnose CRPS were often not adequately described and in all likelihood varied substantially across studies. This lack of consistent or specified diagnostic criteria limits the ability to generalize these results to patients diagnosed according to current IASP criteria.

Only one randomized trial specifically testing psychologic interventions in CRPS patients has been published to date. In this pilot study, Fialka et al.[272] randomized treatment for 18 CRPS patients to receive either home PT or home PT plus once-weekly autogenic relaxation training for 10 weeks. In this small trial, both groups showed similar improvements in pain, range of motion, and edema, although patients in the PT + Autogenics group could demonstrate significantly greater improvements in limb temperature.[272] The impact of this learned control over vasomotor tone and the probable improvement is self efficacy are unknown.

Results of several published case studies and small case series in adult CRPS patients further support the potential utility of a variety of psychologic techniques, including relaxation training, imagery, and thermal and muscular biofeedback. In all of these studies, 75% to 100% pain relief was reported, despite the fact that these patients had chronic CRPS that had failed to improve with previous medical treatments.[271,273–276] It should be noted that the complete resolution of symptoms described in some of these cases using only psychologic interventions may be atypical. While the uncontrolled designs used in these studies prevent definitive conclusions from being drawn regarding the efficacy of psychologic techniques for CRPS, they clearly support the recommendation that such techniques should play an important role in effective interdisciplinary treatment. Key to this analysis is the very favorable risk-benefit ratio.[172]

Other research has addressed psychotherapy in the context of multidisciplinary treatment, suggesting that integration of psychologic methods with medical and PT may be helpful in managing CRPS.[179,190,199,277] Two RCTs examining efficacy of physical therapy for CRPS have included components of psychologic treatment in the therapy package. Oerlemans et al.[179,277] tested a PT protocol that included relaxation exercises and cognitive interventions (designed to increase perceived control over pain). This combined intervention was found to produce significantly greater improvements in pain, active range of motion, and impairment levels than were observed in the social work control group.[179,277] In another RCT of physical therapy, Lee et al.[199] examined two different frequencies of PT treatment (once per week versus three times per week) for child and adolescent CRPS patients, with both groups additionally receiving six sessions of cognitive–behavioral treatment. Although no attentional control group was available for comparison, both groups were found to improve significantly in terms of pain and function when compared to their pretreatment baselines.[199] While the multicomponent interventions in both of these studies do not indicate the unique efficacy of psychologic interventions, they do suggest that psychologic treatment in combination with PT may prove effective in a rehabilitation-focused approach to management of CRPS.[172] The efficacy of psychologic interventions for CRPS would not be surprising, given the strong evidence of their utility in other types of chronic pain.[278–285]

Interventional Therapies

Multiple interventional therapies, including a variety of nerve blocks, infusions, stimulators, and implants have been used over the years for management of CRPS.[175,286] Because the sympathetic nervous system is traditionally implicated in the symptomatology and perhaps the pathogenesis of the syndrome, it is logical (but unfortunately not evidence-based) that sympathetic nerve blocks (SNBs) and surgical sympathectomies have played a prominent role in the treatment (and diagnosis) of CRPS.[132,287] In fact, CRPS diagnosis at one time was determined primarily based on a positive response to a sympathetic block.[74] However, at present, analgesia to SNBs merely indicates the presence of SMP. SMP is a subset of CRPS, whereas some CRPS patients display sympathetically-independent pain.[288] The presence of SMP provides a rationale for using SNBs to relive pain and to provide a therapeutic window to allow initiation of, or continued participation in, functional restoration.

Ideally, the pain relief following SNB should outlast the somatic effect of the local anesthetic and may be very long-lasting in some cases.[289,290] A systematic review of local anesthetic blocks included 19 retrospective reports, 5 prospective case series, 2 nonrandomized controlled studies, and 3 RCTS; unfortunately, due to the wide range of methodology in the studies, the results were inconclusive.[291] In the absence of better evidence, if a SNB provides good analgesia in a specific patient, then a short series of empiric blocks in conjunction with active reactivation-focused therapy is advocated based on consensus recommendations.[175,286]

The brachial plexus is anatomically well suited for continuous regional anesthesia in upper extremity CRPS because of its well-defined perivascular compartment and the close proximity to nerves supplying the upper extremity.[286,292,293] Axillary blocks and catheters have their advocates.[294] Epidural infusions of local anesthetics and sympatholytics (single or continuous infusions) are used empirically and have some research support.[251,295,296] Intrathecal analgesia has less support[297] with the exception of research using baclofen.[297,298] The complications of these interventions must be weighed versus the putative benefits and include bleeding, infection, intravascular injection, intrathecal injection, epidural abscess, pneumothorax, and others.[251,286,299]

Use of systemic infusions, especially of sympatholytics such as phentolamine, has been proposed for both treatment and diagnosis of CRPS. One early study showed positive results with guanethidine regional infusion.[302] A later study suggested that neither placebo, phentolamine, nor phenylephrine infusions conferred any benefit.[301] Phentolamine infusion is now seldom used therapeutically and principally used as a putative diagnostic tool to differentiate sympathetically independent pain from SMP.

Intravenous regional anesthesia (IVRA) is a procedure that allows infusion of medications directly into the affected region, usually using a variety of sympatholytic agents.[302] IVRA with guanethidine, lidocaine, bretylium, clonidine, droperidol, ketanserin, or reserpine have been described.[120,207,261] Although three IVRA studies with active controls have shown positive results,[303–305] the majority of studies and results of meta-analysis suggest no significant benefits.[120,207,261,306,307] Some authors advocate combination drug IVRA therapy,[308,309] and the use of new agents with this technology may eventually establish the worth of this technique (e.g., anticytokine agents).

As surgery is often mentioned as a cause of CRPS, it is somewhat illogical to consider surgery as an effective treatment. Nonetheless, surgical sympathectomy has a long anecdotal history in the treatment of RSD,[287,310] and more recently, endoscopic and radiofrequency sympathectomy have been tried.[311,312] There are no RCTs available and the risks are significant.[310,313] There is also no strong evidence and specifically no RCTs, supporting the efficacy of neurolytic procedures, either chemical or radiofrequency.[286]

There is one prospective RCT comparing spinal cord stimulation versus conservative therapy for upper extremity CRPS.[314] This trial showed a significant reduction in pain and a positive global perceived effect at 6 months, without functional improvement. Marginal improvement in these features, as well as in health-related quality of life, were maintained at 2 years.[315] A definitive trial has never been performed. There are several case reports predictably supportive of the procedure.[316,317] There are a variety of other interventions that have been mentioned, such as peripheral nerve stimulation or cortical stimulation, but there is no compelling evidence supporting such interventions to date.[318,319]

In the face of this lack of evidence for most interventions in CRPS, it is incumbent on the clinician to carefully consider and fully educate patients as to the risks and cost of any intervention entertained, and not overplay anecdotal benefits. One recommended strategy is to use interventional treatments for CRPS only in patients who are having difficulty either starting or progressing in a functional restoration/interdisciplinary program, starting with less invasive blocks, then infusions, and finally, if necessary, progressing to the more experimental neurostimulation techniques.[286]

Other Therapeutic Modalities

Hyperbaric oxygen therapy has been assessed in one RCT and produced a significant decrease in pain and edema versus "normal air."[320] These results need replication, but cost–benefit considerations will also be important. Although acupuncture is mentioned in many treatment reviews, there is only one small RCT in CRPS, and this trial failed to show significance. The authors noted that a definitive trial was planned, but this has been pending since 1999.[321] There is no evidence supporting the use of chiropractic manipulation in CRPS.[322] There are many, many other interventions that have been mentioned in the literature, but without experimental support. Discussion of the myriad anecdotes extant is far beyond the scope of this effort. Obviously, there is a critical need for well-designed, well-executed, randomized, and if possible placebo-controlled trials in CRPS.

In summary, because the symptoms of CRPS patients encompass all the biopsychosocial complexities of chronic pain, the best hope of helping our patients is the adoption of a systematic, stable, empathetic, and, above all, interdisciplinary approach that addresses those symptoms. Drugs, psychotherapy, and interventions should be efficiently deployed for patients who either cannot begin or fail to progress using the interdisciplinary approach outlined here. Many patients will require medication and psychotherapy from the beginning to be successful in the pivotal functional restoration algorithm. Treatment guidelines that center on progressive functional restoration delivered by an interdisciplinary team are traditional, have substantial empiric and anecdotal support, and have been assessed and ultimately codified by three large, expert, consensus-building conferences. Although high-level evidence supporting the rationale for interdisciplinary treatment of CRPS is fairly sparse (as it is for any treatment of CRPS), much stronger evidence exists for the efficacy of the interdisciplinary approach in other pain conditions, such as chronic low back pain. That functional restoration can and should be the central intervention and outcome standard in CRPS is a theory that must be tested (see Fig. 25.2). Until then, the interdisciplinary approach for treating patients with CRPS remains the most pragmatic, helpful and cost-effective therapeutic approach available today.[172]

References

1. Mitchell SW. *Injuries of Nerves and Their Consequences*. Philadelphia: JB Lippincott; 1872.
2. Sandroni P, Benrud-Larson LM, McClelland RL, et al. Complex regional pain syndrome type I: incidence and prevalence in Olmsted county, a population-based study. *Pain* 2003;103(1–2):199–207.
3. de Mos M, de Bruijn AG, Huygen FJ, et al. The incidence of complex regional pain syndrome: a population-based study. *Pain* 2007;129(1–2):12–20.
4. Bruehl S, Chung OY. How common is complex regional pain syndrome-Type I? *Pain* 2007;129(1–2):1–2.
5. Gradl G, Gierer P, Ewert A, et al. Radio-radial external fixation in the treatment of distal radius fractures allows for free wrist motion [in German]. *Zentralbl Chir* 2003;128(12):1014–1019.
6. Harden RN, Bruehl S, Stanos S, et al. Prospective examination of pain-related and psychological predictors of CRPS-like phenomena following total knee arthroplasty: a preliminary study. *Pain* 2003;106(3):393–400.
7. Puchalski P, Zyluk A. Complex regional pain syndrome type 1 after fractures of the distal radius: a prospective study of the role of psychological factors. *J Hand Surg Br* 2005;30(6):574–580.
8. Harden R, Baron R, Janig W. Preface. In: Harden R, Baron R, Janig W, eds. *Complex Regional Pain Syndrome*. Seattle: IASP Press; 2001:xi–xiii.
9. Bennett GJ, Xie YK. A peripheral mononeuropathy in rat that produces disorders of pain sensation like those seen in man. *Pain* 1988;33:87–107.
10. Kim SH, Chung JM. An experimental model for peripheral neuropathy produced by segmental spinal nerve ligation in the rat. *Pain* 1992;50(3):355–363.
11. Jänig W. CRPS-I and CRPS-II: a strategic view. In: Harden RN, Baron R, Jänig W, eds. *Complex Regional Pain Syndrome*. Seattle: IASP Press; 2001: 3–19.
12. Seltzer Z, Dubner R, Shir Y. A novel behavioral model of neuropathic pain disorders produced in rats by partial sciatic nerve injury. *Pain* 1990;43(2): 205–218.
13. Yoon YW, Na HS, Chung JM. Contributions of injured and intact afferents to neuropathic pain in an experimental rat model. *Pain* 1996;64(1):27–36.
14. Noguchi K, Kawai Y, Fukuoka T, et al. Substance P induced by peripheral nerve injury in primary afferent sensory neurons and its effect on dorsal column nucleus neurons. *J Neurosci* 1995;15(11):7633–7643.
15. Kohama I, Ishikawa K, Kocsis JD. Synaptic reorganization in the substantia gelatinosa after peripheral nerve neuroma formation: aberrant innervation of lamina II neurons by Abeta afferents. *J Neurosci* 2000;20(4):1538–1549.
16. Vatine JJ, Argov R, Seltzer Z. Brief electrical stimulation of c-fibers in rats produces thermal hyperalgesia lasting weeks. *Neuroscience Lett* 1998;246(3): 125–128.
17. Coderre TJ, Xanthos DN, Francis L, et al. Chronic post-ischemia pain (CPIP): a novel animal model of complex regional pain syndrome-type I (CRPS-I; reflex sympathetic dystrophy) produced by prolonged hindpaw ischemia and reperfusion in the rat. *Pain* 2004;112(1–2):94–105.
18. Culp WJ, Ochoa J, Cline M, et al. Heat and mechanical hyperalgesia induced by capsaicin. Cross modality threshold modulation in human C nociceptors. *Brain* 1989;112(pt 5):1317–1331.
19. Simone DA, Baumann TK, LaMotte RH. Dose-dependent pain and mechanical hyperalgesia in humans after intradermal injection of capsaicin. *Pain* 1989; 38(1):99–107.
20. Gracely RH, Lynch SA, Bennett GJ. Painful neuropathy: altered central processing maintained dynamically by peripheral input. *Pain* 1992;51(2): 175–194.
21. Andersen OK, Yucel A, Arendt-Nielsen L. Human models of hyperalgesia induced by capsaicin—a discussion of secondary hyperalgesia to heat. In: Harden R, Baron R, Jänig W, eds. *Complex Regional Pain Syndrome Progress in Pain Research and Management*. Seattle: IASP Press; 2001:165–181.
22. Pedersen JL, Kehlet H. Secondary hyperalgesia to heat stimuli after burn injury in man. *Pain* 1998;76(3):377–384.
23. LaMotte RH, Shain CN, Simone DA, et al. Neurogenic hyperalgesia: psycho-physical studies of underlying mechanisms. *J Neurophysiol* 1991;66(1): 190–211.
24. Torebjörk HE, Lundberg LE, LaMotte RH. Central changes in processing of mechanoreceptive input in capsaicin-induced secondary hyperalgesia in humans. *J Physiol* 1992;448:765–780.
25. Sang CN, Gracely RH, Max MB, et al. Capsaicin-evoked mechanical allodynia and hyperalgesia cross nerve territories. Evidence for a central mechanism. *Anesthesiology* 1996;85(3):491–496.
26. Serra J, Campero M, Ochoa J. Flare and hyperalgesia after intradermal capsaicin injection in human skin. *J Neurophysiol* 1998;80(6):2801–2810.
27. LaMotte R. Neurophysiological mechanisms of cutaneous sensory hyperalgesia in the primate. In: Willis WD, ed. *Hyperalgesia and Allodynia*. New York: Raven Press; 1992:175–185.
28. Ziegler EA, Magerl W, Meyer RA, et al. Secondary hyperalgesia to punctate mechanical stimuli. Central sensitization to A-fibre nociceptor input. *Brain* 1999;122 (pt 12):2245–2257.
29. Baron R, Wasner G, Borgstedt R, et al. Effect of sympathetic activity on capsaicin-evoked pain, hyperalgesia, and vasodilatation. *Neurology* 1999; 52(5):923–932.
30. Liu M, Max MB, Parada S, et al. The sympathetic nervous system contributes to capsaicin-evoked mechanical allodynia but not pinprick hyperalgesia in humans. *J Neurosci* 1996;16(22):7331–7335.
31. Petersen KL, Rowbotham MC. A new human experimental pain model: the heat/capsaicin sensitization model. *Neuroreport* 1999;10(7):1511–1516.
32. van der Laan L, Goris R. The role of an exaggerated regional inflammatory response in the pathophysiology of CRPS. In: Harden R, Baron R, Jänig W, eds. *Complex Regional Pain Syndrome Progress in Pain Research and Management*. Seattle: ISAP Press; 2001:183–191.
33. Sudeck P. Die sogen akute Knochenatrophie als ntzudndengsvorgang. *Der Chirurg* 1942;15:449–458.
34. Goris RJ. Treatment of reflex sympathetic dystrophy with hydroxyl radical scavengers. *Unfallchirurg* 1985;88(7):330–332.
35. Oyen WJ, Arntz IE, Claessens RM, et al. Reflex sympathetic dystrophy of the hand: an excessive inflammatory response? *Pain* 1993;55(2):151–157.
36. Kozin F, McCarty DJ, Sims J, et al. The reflex sympathetic dystrophy syndrome. I. Clinical and histologic studies: evidence for bilaterality, response to corticosteroids and articular involvement. *Am J Med* 1976;60:321–331.
37. Hannington-Kiff JG. Relief of Sudeck's atrophy by regional intravenous guanethidine. *Lancet* 1977;1(8022):1132–1133.
38. Renier JC, Arlet J, Bregeon C, et al. The joint in algodystrophy. Joint fluid, synovium, cartilage [in French]. *Rev Rhum Mal Osteoartic* 1983;50(4): 255–260.
39. van der Laan L, Goris RJ. Reflex sympathetic dystrophy. An exaggerated regional inflammatory response? *Hand Clin* 1997;13(3):373–385.
40. Leitha T, Korpan M, Staudenherz A, et al. Five phase bone scintigraphy supports the pathophysiological concept of a subclinical inflammatory process in reflex sympathetic dystrophy. *Q J Nucl Med* 1996;40(2):188–193.
41. Uçeyler N, Eberle T, Rolke R, et al. Differential expression patterns of cytokines in complex regional pain syndrome. *Pain* 2007;132(1–2):195–205.
42. Huygen FJ, De Bruijn AG, De Bruin MT, et al. Evidence for local inflammation in complex regional pain syndrome type 1. *Mediators Inflamm* 2002; 11(1):47–51.
43. van de Beek WJ, Remarque EJ, Westendorp RG, et al. Innate cytokine profile in patients with complex regional pain syndrome is normal. *Pain* 2001;91(3): 259–261.
44. Levine JD, Taiwo YO, Collins SD, et al. Noradrenaline hyperalgesia is mediated through interaction with sympathetic postganglionic neurone terminals rather than activation of primary afferent nociceptors. *Nature* 1986; 323(6084):158–160.
45. Jänig W, Stanton-Hicks M. *Reflex Sympathetic Dystrophy: A Reappraisal*. Seattle: IASP Press; 1996.
46. Perl ER. Cutaneous polymodal receptors: characteristics and plasticity. *Prog Brain Res* 1996;113:21–37.
47. Green PG, Luo J, Heller PH, et al. Further substantiation of a significant role for the sympathetic nervous system in inflammation. *Neuroscience* 1993; 55(4):1037–1043.
48. Levine JD, Fye K, Heller P, et al. Clinical response to regional intravenous guanethidine in patients with rheumatoid arthritis. *J Rheumatol* 1986;13(6): 1040–1043.
49. Blumberg H, Hoffmann U, Mohadjer M, et al Clinical phenomenology and mechanisms of reflex sympathetic dystrophy: emphasis on edema. In: Gebhart GF, Hammond DL, Jensen TS, eds. *Proceedings of the 7th World Congress on Pain*. Seattle: IASP Press; 1994:455–481.
50. Blaes F, Tschernatsch M, Braeu ME, et al. Autoimmunity in complex-regional pain syndrome. *Ann NY Acad Sci* 2007;1107:168–173.
51. Weber M, Birklein F, Neundörfer B, et al. Facilitated neurogenic inflammation in complex regional pain syndrome. *Pain* 2001;91(3):251–257.
52. Veldman PH, Reynen HM, Arntz IE, et al. Signs and symptoms of reflex sympathetic dystrophy: prospective study of 829 patients. *Lancet* 1993;342: 1012–1016.
53. Boas RA. Sympathetic nerve blocks: in search of a role. *Reg Anesth Pain Med* 1998;23(3):292–305.
54. Leriche R, Fontaine R. Sur la sensibilite de la chaine sympathique cervicale et des rameaux communicants chez l'homme. *Gaz Hop Civ Milit* 1925;36: 581–583.
55. Thimineur M, Sood P, Kravitz E, et al. Central nervous system abnormalities

in complex regional pain syndrome (CRPS): clinical and quantitative evidence of medullary dysfunction. *Clin J Pain* 1998;14(3):256–267.

56. Rommel O, Malin JP, Zenz M, et al. Quantitative sensory testing, neurophysiological and psychological examination in patients with complex regional pain syndrome and hemisensory deficits. *Pain* 2001;93(3):279–293.

57. Oaklander AL, Rissmiller JG, Gelman LB, et al. Evidence of focal small-fiber axonal degeneration in complex regional pain syndrome-I (reflex sympathetic dystrophy). *Pain* 2006;120(3):235–243.

58. Birklein F, Weber M, Ernst M, et al. Experimental tissue acidosis leads to increased pain in complex regional pain syndrome (CRPS). *Pain* 2000;87(2):227–234.

59. Harden R. Interdisciplinary management/functional restoration. *J Neuropathic Pain Symptom Palliation* 2006;2:57–67.

60. Rommel O, Gehling M, Dertwinkel R, et al. Hemisensory impairment in patients with complex regional pain syndrome. *Pain* 1999;80(1–2):95–101.

61. Rommel O, Thimineur M. Clinical evidence of central sensory disturbances in CRPS. In: Harden RN, Baron R, Jänig W, eds. *Complex Regional Pain Syndrome Progress in Pain Research and Management.* Seattle: IASP Press; 2001:193–208.

62. Sieweke N, Birklein F, Riedl B, et al. Patterns of hyperalgesia in complex regional pain syndrome. *Pain* 1999;80(1–2):171–177.

63. Ji RR, Kohno T, Moore KA, et al. Central sensitization and LTP: do pain and memory share similar mechanisms? *Trends Neurosci* 2003;26(12):696–705.

64. Melzack R, Wall PD. Pain mechanisms: a new theory. *Science* 1965;150:971–979.

65. Maihöfner C, Handwerker HO, Neundörfer B, et al. Patterns of cortical reorganization in complex regional pain syndrome. *Neurology* 2003;61(12):1707–1715.

66. Pleger B, Tegenthoff M, Schwenkreis P, et al. Mean sustained pain levels are linked to hemispherical side-to-side differences of primary somatosensory cortex in the complex regional pain syndrome I. *Exp Brain Res* 2004;155(1):115–119.

67. Maleki J, LeBel AA, Bennett GJ, et al. Patterns of spread in complex regional pain syndrome, type I (reflex sympathetic dystrophy). *Pain* 2000;88(3):259–266.

68. Juottonen K, Gockel M, Silén T, et al. Altered central sensorimotor processing in patients with complex regional pain syndrome. *Pain* 2002;98(3):315–323.

69. Fukumoto M, Ushida T, Zinchuk VS, et al. Contralateral thalamic perfusion in patients with reflex sympathetic dystrophy syndrome. *Lancet* 1999;354(9192):1790–1791.

70. Maihöfner C, Handwerker HO, Neundörfer B, et al. Cortical reorganization during recovery from complex regional pain syndrome. *Neurology* 2004;63(4):693–701.

71. Maihöfner C, Forster C, Birklein F, et al. Brain processing during mechanical hyperalgesia in complex regional pain syndrome: a functional MRI study. *Pain* 2005;114(1–2):93–103.

72. Pleger B, Tegenthoff M, Ragert P, et al. Sensorimotor retuning [corrected] in complex regional pain syndrome parallels pain reduction. *Ann Neurol* 2005;57(3):425–429.

73. Jänig W, Häbler HJ. Organization of the autonomic nervous system: structure and function. In: Vinken PJ, Bruyn GW, eds. *The Autonomic Nervous System, Part I: Normal Functions, Handbook of Clinical Neurology.* Amsterdam: Elsevier Science; 1999:1–52.

74. Gibbons JJ, Wilson PR. RSD score: criteria for the diagnosis of reflex sympathetic dystrophy and causalgia. *Clin J Pain* 1992;8:260–263.

75. Harden RN, Bruehl S, Galer BS, et al. Complex regional pain syndrome: are the IASP diagnostic criteria valid and sufficiently comprehensive? *Pain* 1999;83:211–219.

76. Wasner G, Drummond PD, Birklein F, et al. The role of the sympathetic nervous system in autonomic distrubances and "sympathetically maintained pain" in CRPS. In: Harden RN, Baron R, Jänig W, ed. *Complex Regional Pain Syndrome.* Seattle: IASP Press; 2001:89–118.

77. Bonica JJ. Causalgia and other reflex sympathetic dystrophies. In: Bonica JJ, Liebeskind JC, Albé-Fessard DG, eds. *Proceedings of the Second World Congress on Pain, Advances in Pain Research and Therapy.* New York: Raven Press; 1979:141–166.

78. Wasner G, Heckmann K, Maier C, et al. Vascular abnormalities in acute reflex sympathetic dystrophy (CRPS I): complete inhibition of sympathetic nerve activity with recovery. *Arch Neurol* 1999;56(5):613–620.

79. Wasner G, Schattschneider J, Heckmann K, et al. Vascular abnormalities in reflex sympathetic dystrophy (CRPS I): mechanisms and diagnostic value. *Brain* 2001;124(Pt 3):587–599.

80. Birklein F, Riedl B, Claus D, et al. Pattern of autonomic dysfunction in time course of complex regional pain syndrome. *Clin Auton Res* 1998;8(2):79–85.

81. Wakisaka S, Kajander KC, Bennett GJ. Abnormal skin temperature and abnormal sympathetic vasomotor innervation in an experimental painful peripheral neuropathy. *Pain* 1991;46(3):299–313.

82. Kurvers H, Daemen M, Slaaf D, et al. Partial peripheral neuropathy and denervation induced adrenoceptor supersensitivity: functional studies in an experimental model. *Acta Orthop Belg* 1998;64(1):64–70.

83. Harden RN, Duc TA, Williams TR, et al. Norepinephrine and epinephrine levels in affected versus unaffected limbs in sympathetically maintained pain. *Clin J Pain* 1994;10(4):324–330.

84. Goldstein DS, Tack C, Li ST. Sympathetic innervation and function in reflex sympathetic dystrophy. *Ann Neurol* 2000;48(1):49–59.

85. Drummond PD, Finch PM, Smythe GA. Reflex sympathetic dystrophy: the

significance of differing plasma catecholamine concentrations in affected and unaffected limbs. *Brain* 1991;114(Pt 5):2025–2036.

86. Arnold JM, Teasell RW, MacLeod AP, et al. Increased venous alpha-adrenoceptor responsiveness in patients with reflex sympathetic dystrophy. *Ann Intern Med* 1993;118(8):619–621.

87. Birklein F, Riedl B, Sieweke N, et al. Neurological findings in complex regional pain syndromes—analysis of 145 cases. *Acta Neurol Scand* 2000;101(4):262–269.

88. Janig W, McLachlan EM. Neurobiology of the autonomic nervous system. In: Mathias CJ, Bannister R, eds. *Autonomic Failure.* 4th Ed. Oxford: Oxford University Press; 1999:3–15.

89. Sherman RA, Karstetter KW, Damiano M, et al. Stability of temperature asymmetries in reflex sympathetic dystrophy over time and changes in pain. *Clin J Pain* 1994;10(1):71–77.

90. Tahmoush AJ, Malley J, Jennings JR. Skin conductance, temperature, and blood flow in causalgia. *Neurology* 1983;33(11):1483–1486.

91. Raja SN, Treede RD, Davis KD, et al. Systemic alpha-adrenergic blockage with phentolamine: a diagnostic test for sympathetically maintained pain. *Anesthesiology* 1991;74:691–698.

92. Torebjörk E, Wahren L, Wallin G, et al. Noradrenaline-evoked pain in neuralgia. *Pain* 1995;63(1):11–20.

93. Baron R, Maier C. Reflex sympathetic dystrophy: skin blood flow, sympathetic vasoconstrictor reflexes and pain before and after surgical sympatectomy. *Pain* 1996;67:317–326.

94. Jänig W, Koltzenburg M. What is the interaction between the sympathetic terminal and the primary afferent fiber? In: Basbaum AI, Besson JM, eds. *Towards a New Pharmacotherapy of Pain.* Chichester: John Wiley & Sons; 1991:331–352.

95. Jänig W, Koltzenburg M. Possible ways of sympathetic afferent interaction. In: Jänig W, Schmidt RF, eds. *Reflex Sympathetic Dystrophy: Pathophysiological Mechanisms and Clinical Implications.* New York: VCH Verlagsgesellschaft; 1992:213–243.

96. Verdugo RJ, Campero M, Ochoa JL. Phentolamine sympathetic block in painful polyneuropathies. II. Further questioning of the concept of "sympathetically maintained pain." *Neurology* 1994;44:1010–1014.

97. Drummond PD. Noradrenaline increases hyperalgesia to heat in skin sensitized by capsaicin. *Pain* 1995;60(3):311–315.

98. Wallin BG, Torebjörk E, Hallin RG. Preliminary observations on the pathophysiology of hyperalgesia in the causalgic pain syndrome. In: Zotterman Y, ed. *Sensory Functions of the Skin in Primates.* Oxford: Pergamon Press; 1976:489–502.

99. Ali Z, Raja SN, Wesselmann U, et al. Intradermal injection of norepinephrine evokes pain in patients with sympathetically maintained pain. *Pain* 2000;88(2):161–168.

100. Drummond PD, Finch PM, Skipworth S, et al. Pain increases during sympathetic arousal in patients with complex regional pain syndrome. *Neurology* 2001;57(7):1296–1303.

101. Deuschl G, Blumberg H, Lücking CH. Tremor in reflex sympathetic dystrophy. *Arch Neurol* 1991;48(12):1247–1252.

102. Schürmann M, Gradl G, Zaspel J, et al. Peripheral sympathetic function as a predictor of complex regional pain syndrome type I (CRPS I) in patients with radial fracture. *Auton Neurosci* 2000;86(1–2):127–134.

103. Birklein F, Weber M, Neundörfer B. Increased skin lactate in complex regional pain syndrome: evidence for tissue hypoxia? *Neurology* 2000;55(8):1213–1215.

104. Koban M, Leis S, Schultze-Mosgau S, et al. Tissue hypoxia in complex regional pain syndrome. *Pain* 2003;104(1–2):149–157.

105. Heerschap A, den Hollander JA, Reynen H, et al. Metabolic changes in reflex sympathetic dystrophy: a 31P NMR spectroscopy study. *Muscle Nerve* 1993;16(4):367–373.

106. Sternberg WF, Mogil J. Genetic and hormonal basis of pain states. *Clin Anesthesiol* 2001;15(2):229–245.

107. Merskey H, Bogduk N. *Classification of Chronic Pain: Descriptions of Chronic Pain Syndromes and Definitions of Pain Terms.* 2nd ed. Seattle: IASP Press; 1994.

108. Schwartzman RJ, Popescu A. Reflex sympathetic dystrophy. *Curr Rheumatol Rep* 2002;4(2):165–169.

109. Deuschl G, Blumberg H, Lücking CH. Tremor in reflex sympathetic dystrophy. *Arch Neurol* 1991;48:1247–1252.

110. Baron R, Jänig W. Human experimentation. In: Harden RN, Baron R, Jänig W, eds. *Complex Regional Pain Syndrome.* Seattle: IASP Press; 2001:239–246.

111. Marsden CD, Meadows JC, Lange GW. Effect of speed of muscle contraction on physiological tremor in normal subjects and in patients with thyrotoxicosis and myxoedema. *J Neurol Neurosurg Psychiatry* 1970;33(6):776–782.

112. Gazda LS, Milligan ED, Hansen MK, et al. Sciatic inflammatory neuritis (SIN): behavioral allodynia is paralleled by peri-sciatic proinflammatory cytokine and superoxide production. *J Peripher Nerv Syst* 2001;6(3):111–129.

113. Schattschneider P, Hébert C, Jouffrey B. Orientation dependence of ionization edges in EELS. *Ultramicroscopy* 2001;86(3–4):343–353.

114. Schwenkreis P, Janssen F, Rommel O, et al. Bilateral motor cortex disinhibition in complex regional pain syndrome (CRPS) type I of the hand. *Neurology* 2003;61(4):515–519.

115. McCabe CS, Haigh RC, Ring EF, et al. A controlled pilot study of the utility of mirror visual feedback in the treatment of complex regional pain syndrome (type 1). *Rheumatology (Oxford)* 2003;42(1):97–101.

116. Galer BS, Butler S, Jensen MP. Case report and hypothesis: a neglect-like syndrome may be responsible for the motor disturbance in reflex sympathetic dystrophy (Complex Regional Pain Syndrome-1). *J Pain Sym Manage* 1995; 10:385–391.

117. Jääskeläinen SK, Rinne JO, Forssell H, et al. Role of the dopaminergic system in chronic pain—a fluorodopa-PET study. *Pain* 2001;90(3):257–260.

118. Butler S. Disuse and CRPS. In: Harden RN, Baron R, Jänig W, eds. *Complex Regional Pain Syndrome*. Seattle: IASP Press; 2001:141–150.

119. Guo TZ, Offley SC, Boyd EA, et al. Substance P signaling contributes to the vascular and nociceptive abnormalities observed in a tibial fracture and rat model of complex regional pain syndrome type I. *Pain* 2004;108(1–2): 95–107.

120. Kingery WS. A critical review of controlled clinical trials for peripheral neuropathic pain and complex regional pain syndromes. *Pain* 1997;73:123–139.

121. Harden RN. Pharmacotherapy. In: Harden RN, ed. *Complex Regional Pain Syndrome: Treatment Guidelines*. Milford: RSDSA Press; 2006:25–36.

122. Richards RL. Causalgia. A centennial review. *Arch Neurol* 1967;16:339–350.

123. Sunderland S. *Nerve Injuries and Their Repair*. Edinburgh: Churchill Livingstone; 1991.

124. Blenk KH, Häbler HJ, Jänig W. Neomycin and gadolinium applied to an L5 spinal nerve lesion prevent mechanical allodynia-like behaviour in rats. *Pain* 1997;70(2–3):155–165.

125. Decosterd I, Woolf CJ. Spared nerve injury: an animal model of persistent peripheral neuropathic pain. *Pain* 2000;87(2):149–158.

126. Mailis A, Wade JA. Genetic considerations in CRPS. In: Harden RN, Baron R, Jänig W, eds. *Complex Regional Pain Syndrome*. Seattle: IASP Press; 2001: 227–237.

127. Greipp ME, Thomas AF. Familial occurence of reflex sympathetic dystrophy. *Clin J Pain* 1991;7(1):48.

128. Mailis A, Wade J. Profile of Caucasian women with possible genetic predisposition to reflex sympathetic dystrophy: a pilot study. *Clin J Pain* 1994;10(3): 210–217.

129. van de Beek WJ, Roep BO, van der Slik AR, et al. Susceptibility loci for complex regional pain syndrome. *Pain* 2003;103(1–2):93–97.

130. Kemler MA, van de Vusse AC, van den Berg-Loonen EM, et al. HLA-DQ1 associated with reflex sympathetic dystrophy. *Neurology* 1999;53(6): 1350–1351.

131. Kimura T, Komatsu T, Hosoda R, et al. Angiotensin-converting enzyme gene polymorphism in patients with neuropathic pain. In: Devor M, Rowbotham MC, Wiesenfeld-Hallin D, eds. *Proceedings of the 9th World Congress on Pain, Progress in Pain Research and Management*. Seattle: IASP Press; 2000: 471–476.

132. Bonica JJ. *The Management of Pain*. Philadelphia: Lea and Febiger, 1953.

133. Kozin F, Ryan LM, Carerra GF, et al. The reflex sympathetic dystrophy syndrome III: Scintigraphic studies, further evidence for the therapeutic efficacy of systemic corticosteroids, and proposed diagnostic criteria. *Am J Med* 1981; 70:23–30.

134. Wilson PR, Low PA, Bedder MD, et al. Diagnostic algorithm for complex regional pain syndromes. In: Jänig W, Stanton-Hicks M, eds. *Progress in Pain Research and Management*, vol. 6. Seattle: IASP Press; 1996:93–106.

135. Stanton-Hicks M, Jänig W, Hassenbusch S, et al. Reflex sympathetic dystrophy: changing concepts and taxonomy. *Pain* 1995;63:127–133.

136. Reinders MF, Geertzen JH, Dijkstra PU. Complex regional pain syndrome type I: use of the International Association for the Study of Pain diagnostic criteria defined in 1994. *Clin J Pain* 2002;18(4):207–215.

137. Merikangas KR, Frances A. Development of diagnostic criteria for headache syndromes: lessons from psychiatry. *Cephalalgia* 1993;13(suppl 12):34–38.

138. Galer BS, Bruehl S, Harden RN. IASP diagnostic criteria for complex regional pain syndrome: a preliminary empirical validation study. *Clin J Pain* 1998; 14:48–54.

139. Bruehl S, Lofland KR, Semenchuk EM, et al. Use of cluster analysis to validate IHS diagnostic criteria for migraine and tension-type headache. *Headache* 1999;39:181–189.

140. Harden R, Bruehl S. Diagnostic criteria: the statistical derivation of the four criterion factors. In: Wilson PR, Stanton-Hicks M, Harden RN, eds. *CRPS: Current Diagnosis and Therapy*. Seattle: IASP Press; 2005:45–58.

141. Schwartzman RJ, Kerrigan J. The movement disorder of reflex sympathetic dystrophy. *Neurology* 1990;40:57–61.

142. Bruehl S, Harden RN, Galer BS, et al. External validation of IASP diagnositic criteria for complex regional pain syndrome and proposed research diagnostic criteria. *Pain* 1999;81:147–154.

143. Harden RN, Bruehl S, Stanton-Hicks M, et al. Proposed new diagnostic criteria for complex regional pain syndrome. *Pain Med* 2007;8(4):326–331.

144. DeTakats G. Reflex dystrophy of the extremities. *Arch Surg* 1937;34:939.

145. Schwartzman RJ, McLellan TL. Reflex sympathetic dystrophy: a review. *Arch Neurol* 1987;44:555–561.

146. Bickerstaff DR, Kanis JA. Algodystrophy: an under-recognized complication of minor trauma. *Br J Rheumatol* 1994;33(3):240–248.

147. Zyluk A. The natural history of post-traumatic reflex sympathetic dystrophy. *J Hand Surg (Br)* 1998;23(1):20–23.

148. Bruehl S, Harden RN, Galer BS, et al. Complex regional pain syndrome: are there distinct subtypes and sequential stages of this syndrome? *Pain* 2002;95: 119–124.

149. Birklein F, Riedl B, Neundörfer B, et al. Sympathetic vasoconstrictor reflex pattern in patients with complex regional pain syndrome. *Pain* 1998;75(1): 93–100.

150. Jänig W, Baron R. The role of the sympathetic nervous system in neuropathic pain: Clinical observations and animal models. In: Hansson PT, Fields HL, Hill RG, et al., eds. *Neuropathic Pain: Pathophysiology and Treatment*. Seattle: IASP Press; 2001:125–149.

151. Charney DS, Woods SW, Nagy LM, et al. Noradrenergic function in panic disorder. *J Clin Psychiatry* 1990;51(suppl A):5–11.

152. Light KC, Kothandapani RV, Allen MT. Enhanced cardiovascular and catecholamine responses in women with depressive symptoms. *Int J Psychophysiol* 1998;28(2):157–166.

153. Harden RN, Rudin NJ, Bruehl S, et al. Increased systemic catecholamines in complex regional pain syndrome and relationship to psychological factors: a pilot study. *Anesth Analg* 2004;99(5):1478–1485, table of contents.

154. Kaufmann I, Eisner C, Richter P, et al. Psychoneuroendocrine stress response may impair neutrophil function in complex regional pain syndrome. *Clin Immunol* 2007;125(1):103–111.

155. Bruehl S. Do psychological factors play a role in the onset and maintenance of CRPS? In: Harden R, Baron R, Jänig W, eds. *Complex Regional Pain Syndrome*. Seattle: IASP Press; 2001:279–290.

156. Dijkstra PU, Groothoff JW, ten Duis HJ, et al. Incidence of complex regional pain syndrome type I after fractures of the distal radius. *Eur J Pain* 2003; 7(5):457–462.

157. Van Houdenhove B. Prevalence and psychodynamic interpretation of premorbid hyperactivity in patients with chronic pain. *Psychother Psychosom* 1986; 45(4):195–200.

158. Egle UT, Hoffmann SO. Psychosomatic correlations of sympathetic reflex dystrophy (Sudeck's disease). Review of the literature and initial clinical results [in German]. *Psychother Psychosom Med Psychol* 1990;40(3–4): 123–135.

159. Geertzen JH, de Bruijn-Kofman AT, de Bruijn HP, et al. Stressful life events and psychological dysfunction in Complex Regional Pain Syndrome type I. *Clin J Pain* 1998;14(2):143–147.

160. Monti DA, Herring CL, Schwartzman RJ, et al. Personality assessment of patients with complex regional pain syndrome type I. *Clin J Pain* 1998;14(4): 295–302.

161. Rommel O, Willweber-Strumpf A, Wagner P, et al. Psychological abnormalities in patients with complex regional pain syndrome (CRPS) [in German]. *Schmerz* 2005;19(4):272–284.

162. Hardy M, Merritt W. Psychological evaluation and pain assessment in patients with reflex sympathetic dystrophy. *J Hand Ther* 1988;1:155–164.

163. Geertzen JHB, de Bruijn H, de Bruijn-Kofman AT, et al. Reflex sympathetic dystropohy: early treatment and psychological aspects. *Arch Phys Med Rehabil* 1994;75:442–446.

164. Bruehl S, Husfeldt B, Lubenow TR, et al. Psychological differences between reflex sympathetic dystrophy and non-RSD chronic pain patients. *Pain* 1996; 67:107–114.

165. Ciccone DS, Bandilla EB, Wu W. Psychological dysfunction in patients with reflex sympathetic dystrophy. *Pain* 1997;71(3):323–333.

166. Feldman SI, Downey G, Schaffer-Neitz R. Pain, negative mood, and perceived support in chronic pain patients: a daily diary study of people with reflex sympathetic dystrophy syndrome. *J Consult Clin Psychol* 1999;67(5): 776–785.

167. Haddox JD, Abram SE, Hopwood MH. Comparison of psychometric data in RSD and radiculopathy. *Reg Anesth* 1988;13:27.

168. DeGood DE, Cundiff GW, Adams LE, et al. A psychosocial and behavioral comparison of reflex sympathetic dystrophy, low back pain, and headache patients. *Pain* 1993;54(3):317–322.

169. Bruehl S, Chung OY, Burns JW. Differential effects of expressive anger regulation on chronic pain intensity in CRPS and non-CRPS limb pain patients. *Pain* 2003;104(3):647–654.

170. Carlson LK, Watson HK. Treatment of reflex sympathetic dystrophy using the stress-loading program. *J Hand Ther* 1988;1:149–154.

171. Stanton-Hicks M, Baron R, Boas R, et al. Complex regional pain syndromes: guidelines for therapy. *Clin J Pain* 1998;14:155–166.

172. Harden R. *Complex Regional Pain Syndrome: Treatment Guidelines*. Milford: RSDSA Press; 2006.

173. Harden R. The rationale for integrated functional restoration. In: Wilson P, Stanton-Hicks M, Harden R, eds. *CRPS: Current Diagnosis and Therapy*. Seattle: IASP Press; 2005:163–172.

174. Davidoff G, Morey K, Amann M, et al. Pain measurement in reflex sympathetic dystrophy syndrome. *Pain* 1988;32(1):27–34.

175. Stanton-Hicks MD, Burton AW, Bruehl SP, et al. An updated interdisciplinary clinical pathway for CRPS: report of an expert panel. *Pain Pract* 2002;2(1): 1–16.

176. Turk DC, Dworkin RH, Allen RR, et al. Core outcome domains for chronic pain clinical trials: IMMPACT recommendations. *Pain* 2003;106(3): 337–345.

177. Revicki DA, Ehreth JL. Health-related quality of life assessment and planning for the pharmaceutical industry. *Clin Ther* 1997;19(5):1101–1115.

178. Oerlemans HM, Oostendorp RA, de Boo T, et al. Pain and reduced mobility in complex regional pain syndrome I: outcome of a prospective randomised controlled clinical trial of adjuvant physical therapy versus occupational therapy. *Pain* 1999;83(1):77–83.

179. Oerlemans HM, Goris JA, de Boo T, et al. Do physical therapy and occupational therapy reduce the impairment percentage in reflex sympathetic dystrophy? *Am J Phys Med Rehabil* 1999;78(6):533–539.

180. Butler SH, Nyman M, Gordth T. Immobility in volunteers produces signs and

symptoms of CRPS I and a neglect-like state. *Abstracts: 9th World Congress on Pain.* Seattle: IASP Press; 1999.

181. Schürmann M, Gradl G, Andress HJ, et al. Assessment of peripheral sympathetic nervous function for diagnosing early post-traumatic complex regional pain syndrome type I. *Pain* 1999;80(1–2):149–159.

182. Kemler MA, de Vet HC. Health-related quality of life in chronic refractory reflex sympathetic dystrophy (complex regional pain syndrome type I). *J Pain Symptom Manage* 2000;20(1):68–76.

183. Galer BS, Jensen M. Neglect-like symptoms in complex regional pain syndrome: results of a self-administered survey. *J Pain Symptom Manage* 1999; 18(3):213–217.

184. Crombez G, Vlaeyen JW, Heuts PH, et al. Pain-related fear is more disabling than pain itself: evidence on the role of pain-related fear in chronic back pain disability. *Pain* 1999;80:329–339.

185. Boersma K, Linton S, Overmeer T, et al. Lowering fear-avoidance and enhancing function through exposure in vivo: a multiple baseline study across six patients with back pain. *Pain* 2004;108(1–2):8–16.

186. Flor H, Fydrich T, Turk DC. Efficacy of multidisciplinary pain treatment centers: a meta-analytic review. *Pain* 1992;49:221–230.

187. Guzmán J, Esmail R, Karjalainen K, et al. Multidisciplinary rehabilitation for chronic low back pain: systematic review. *BMJ* 2001;322(7301):1511–1516.

188. Severens JL, Oerlemans HM, Weegels AJ, et al. Cost-effectiveness analysis of adjuvant physical or occupational therapy for patients with reflex sympathetic dystrophy. *Arch Phys Med Rehabil* 1999;80:1038–1043.

189. Swan M. *Treating CRPS: A Guide for Therapy.* Milford, CT: RSDSA Press; 2004.

190. Sherry DD, Wallace CA, Kelley C, et al. Short- and long-term outcomes of children with complex regional pain syndrome type I treated with exercise therapy. *Clin J Pain* 1999;15(3):218–223.

191. Uher EM, Vacariu G, Schneider B, et al. Comparison of manual lymph drainage with physical therapy in complex regional pain syndrome, type I. A comparative randomized controlled therapy study [in German]. *Wien Klin Wochenschr* 2000;112(3):133–137.

192. Watson HK, Carlson L. Treatment of reflex sympathetic dystrophy of the hand with an active "stress loading" program. *J Hand Surg [Am]* 1987; 12(suppl 5, pt 1):779–785.

193. Voss D, Ionta M, Myers B. Proprioceptive neuromuscular facilitation. In: Voss D, Ionta M, Myers B, eds. *Patterns and Techniques.* 3rd ed. New York: Harper & Row, 1985:xvii.

194. Rho RH, Brewer RP, Lamer TJ, et al. Complex regional pain syndrome. *Mayo Clin Proc* 2002;77(2):174–180.

195. Harden RN, Swan M, King A, et al. Treatment of complex regional pain syndrome: functional restoration. *Clin J Pain* 2006;22(5):420–424.

196. Birklein F, Handwerker HO. Complex regional pain syndrome: how to resolve the complexity? *Pain* 2001;94(1):1–6.

197. Phillips ME, Katz JA, Harden RN. The use of nerve block in conjunction with occupational therapy for complex regional pain syndrome type I. *Am J Occupat Ther* 2000;54:544–549.

198. Oerlemans HM, Oostendorp RA, de Boo T, et al. Pain and reduced mobility in complex regional pain syndrome I: outcome of a prospective randomised controlled clinical trial of adjuvant physical therapy versus occupational therapy. *Pain* 1999;83(1):77–83.

199. Lee BH, Scharff L, Sethna NF, et al. Physical therapy and cognitive-behavioral treatment for complex regional pain syndromes. *J Pediatr* 2002;141(1): 135–140.

200. Russ R. Pain, the disease. Available at: http://www.acofp.org/member%5Fpublications/canov_02.html. Accessed August 14, 2005.

201. Sanders S, Harden R, Benson S, et al. Clinical practice guidelines for chronic non-malignant pain syndrome patients II: An evidence-based approach. *J Back Musculoskel Rehabil* 1999;13:47–58.

202. State of Colorado DoLaE. Reflex sympathetic dystrophy/complex regional pain syndrome medical treatment guidelines; 1998. Available at: http://www.state.co.us/gov.

203. Harden RN. Pharmacotherapy of complex regional pain syndrome. *Am J Phys Med Rehabil* 2005;84(3 suppl):S17–S28.

204. Beydoun A. Neuropathic pain: from mechanisms to treatment strategies. *J Pain Symptom Manage* 2003 May;25(5 suppl):S1–S3.

205. van der Laan L, Veldman PH, Goris RJ. Severe complications of reflex sympathetic dystrophy: infection, ulcers, chronic edema, dystonia, myoclonus. *Arch Phys Med Rehabil* 1998;79:424–429.

206. Rico H, Merono E, Gomez-Castresana F, et al. Scintigraphic evaluation of reflex sympathetic dystrophy: comparative study of the course of the disease under two therapeutic regimens. *Clin Rheumatol* 1987;6(2):233–237.

207. Pappagallo M, Rosenberg A. Epidemiology, pathophysiology, and management of complex regional pain syndrome. *Pain Pract* 2001;1(1):11–20.

208. Forouzanfar T, Köke AJ, van Kleef M, et al. Treatment of complex regional pain syndrome type 1. *Eur J Pain* 2002;6:105–122.

209. Christensen K, Jensen EM, Noer I. The reflex dystrophy syndrome response to treatment with systemic corticosteroids. *Acta Chir Scand* 1982;148(8): 653–655.

210. Braus DF, Krauss JK, Strobel J. The shoulder-hand syndrome after stroke: a prospective clinical trial. *Ann Neurol* 1994;36(5):728–733.

211. Zollinger PE, Tuinebreijer WE, Kreis RW, et al. Effect of vitamin C on frequency of reflex sympathetic dystrophy in wrist fractures: a randomized trial. *Lancet* 1999;354(9195):2025–2028.

212. Schwartzman RJ, Chevlen E, Bengtson K. Thalidomide has activity in treating complex regional pain syndrome. *Arch Intern Med* 2003;163(12):1487–1488; author reply 1488.

213. Prager J, Fleischman J, Lingua G. *Open label clinical experience of thalidomide in the treatment of complex regional pain syndrome type I.* Los Angeles: California Pain Medicine Centers and Reflex Sympathetic Dystrophy Institute; 2003:Poster 868.

214. Schwartzman RJ, Irving G, Wallace M, et al. A multicenter, open-label 12-week study with extension to evaluate the safety and efficacy of lenalidomide (CC-5013) in the treatment of complex regional pain syndrome type 1. 2005. Abstract. 11th World Congress on Pain. Seattle. IASP Press, p. 586.

215. Breu G, Harrington M. Paula's secret struggle. *People* 2005;63(17):68–72.

216. Sindrup SH, Jensen TS. Efficacy of pharmacological treatments of neuropathic pain: an update and effect related to mechanism of drug action. *Pain* 1999; 83(3):389–400.

217. Collins SL, Moore RA, McQuay HJ, et al. Antidepressants and anticonvulsants for diabetic neuropathy and postherpetic neuralgia: a quantitative systematic review. *J Pain Symptom Manage* 2000;20(6):449–458.

218. McQuay H, Carroll D, Jadad AR, et al. Anticonvulsant drugs for management of pain: a systematic review. *BMJ* 1995;311(7012):1047–1052.

219. Wiffen P, Collins S, McQuay H, et al. Anticonvulsant drugs for acute and chronic pain. *Cochrane Database Syst Rev* 2000;3:CD001133.

220. Hord ED, Oaklander AL. Complex regional pain syndrome: a review of evidence-supported treatment options. *Curr Pain Headache Rep* 2003;7(3): 188–196.

221. Rowbotham M, Harden N, Stacey B, et al. Gabapentin for the treatment of postherpetic neuralgia: a randomized controlled trial. *JAMA* 1998;280(21): 1837–1842.

222. Backonja M, Beydoun A, Edwards KR, et al. Gabapentin for the symptomatic treatment of painful neuropathy in patients with diabetes mellitus: a randomized controlled trial. *JAMA* 1998;280(21):1831–1836.

223. Mellick GA, Mellick LB. Reflex sympathetic dystrophy treated with gabapentin. *Arch Phys Med Rehabil* 1997;78(1):98–105.

224. Wheeler DS, Vaux KK, Tam DA. Use of gabapentin in the treatment of childhood reflex sympathetic dystrophy. *Pediatr Neurol* 2000;22(3):220–221.

225. Burchiel KJ. Carbamazepine inhibits spontaneous activity in experimental neuromas. *Exp Neurol* 1988;102:249–253.

226. Rull J, Quibrera R, Gonzalez-Millan H, et al. Symptomatic treatment of peripheral diabetic neuropathy with carbamizepine: double-blind crossover study. *Diabetologia* 1969;5:215–220.

227. Harke H, Gretenkort P, Ladleif HU, et al. The response of neuropathic pain and pain in complex regional pain syndrome I to carbamazepine and sustained-release morphine in patients pretreated with spinal cord stimulation: a double-blinded randomized study. *Anesth Analg* 2001;92(2):488–495.

228. McQuay HJ, Tramèr M, Nye BA, et al. A systematic review of antidepressants in neuropathic pain. *Pain* 1996;68:217–227.

229. Sindrup SH, Jensen TS. Pharmacologic treatment of pain in polyneuropathy. *Neurology* 2000;55(7):915–920.

230. Watson CP, Vernich L, Chipman M, et al. Nortriptyline versus amitriptyline in postherpetic neuralgia: a randomized trial. *Neurology* 1998;51(4): 1166–1171.

231. Harden RN. Chronic opioid therapy: another reappraisal. *American Pain Society Bulletin* 2002;12(1):1,8–12.

232. Eisenberg E, McNicol ED, Carr DB. Efficacy and safety of opioid agonists in the treatment of neuropathic pain of nonmalignant origin: systematic review and meta-analysis of randomized controlled trials. *JAMA* 2005;293(24): 3043–3052.

233. Dellemijn PL, van Duijn H, Vanneste JA. Prolonged treatment with transdermal fentanyl in neuropathic pain. *J Pain Symptom Manage* 1998;16(4): 220–229.

234. Cherny NI, Thaler HT, Friedlander-Klar H, et al. Opioid responsiveness of cancer pain syndromes caused by neuropathic or nociceptive mechanisms: a combined analysis of controlled, single-dose studies. *Neurology* 1994;44(5): 857–861.

235. Portenoy RK, Foley KM, Inturrisi CE. The nature of opioid responsiveness and its implications for neuropathic pain: new hypotheses derived from studies for opioid infusions. *Pain* 1990;43:273–286.

236. Dellemijn P. Are opioids effective in relieving neuropathic pain? *Pain* 1999; 80(3):453–462.

237. Mao J, Price DD, Caruso FS, et al. Oral administration of dexromethorphan prevents the development of morphine tolerance and dependence in rats. *Pain* 1996;67:361–368.

238. Eide PK, Jørum E, Stubhaub A, et al. Relief of post-herpetic neuralgia with the N-methyl-D-aspartic acid receptor antagonist ketamine: a double-blind, cross-over comparison with morphine and placebo. *Pain* 1994;58:347–354.

239. Mao J, Price DD, Mayer DJ, et al. Intrathecal MK-801 and local nerve anesthesia synergistically reduce nociceptive behaviors in rats with experimental peripheral mononeuropathy. *Brain Res* 1992;576:254–262.

240. Nelson KA, Park KM, Robinovitz E, et al. High dose oral dextromethorphan versus placebo in painful diabetic neuropathy and postherpetic neuralgia. *Neurology* 1997;48:1212–1218.

241. Qian J, Brown SD, Carlton SM. Systemic ketamine attenuates nociceptive behaviors in a rat model of peripheral neuropthy. *Brain Res* 1996;715:51–62.

242. Tal M, Bennett GJ. Dextromorphan relieves neuropathic heat-evoked hyperalgesia in the rat. *Neurosci Lett* 1993;151:107–110.

243. Takahashi H, Miyazaki M, Nanbu T, et al. The NMDA-receptor antagonist ketamine abolishes neuropathic pain after epidural administration in a clinical case. *Pain* 1998;75(2–3):391–394.

244. Harbut RE, Correll GE. Successful treatment of a nine-year case of complex regional pain syndrome type-I (reflex sympathetic dystrophy) with intravenous ketamine-infusion therapy in a warfarin-anticoagulated adult female patient. *Pain Med* 2002;3(2):147–155.

245. Gammaitoni A, Gallagher R, Welz-Bosna M. Topical ketamine gel: possible role in treating neuropathic pain. *Pain Med* 2000;1(1):97–100.

246. Kiefer R, Rohr P, Unertl K, et al. Recovery from intractable complex regional pain syndrome type I (RSD) under high-dose intravenous ketamine-midazolame sedation. *Neurology* 2002;suppl 3:A474.

247. Pud D, Eisenberg E, Spitzer A, et al. The NMDA receptor antagonist amantadine reduces surgical neuropathic pain in cancer patients: a double blind, randomized, placebo controlled trial. *Pain* 1998;75(2–3):349–354.

248. Eisenberg E, Pud D. Can patients with chronic neuropathic pain be cured by acute administration of the NMDA receptor antagonist amantadine? *Pain* 1998;74(2–3):337–339.

249. Sang CN. NMDA-receptor antagonists in neuropathic pain: experimental methods to clinical trials. *J Pain Symptom Manage* 2000;19(1 suppl): S21–S25.

250. Tracey DJ, Cunningham JE, Romm MA. Peripheral hyperalgesia in experimental neuropathy: Mediation by alpha-2 and renoreceptors on post-ganglionic sympthetic terminals. *Pain* 1995;60:217–327.

251. Rauck RL, Eisenach JC, Jackson K, et al. Epidural clonidine for refractory reflex sympathetic dystrophy. *Anesthesiology* 1993;79:1163–1169.

252. Davis KD, Treede RD, Raja SN, et al. Topical application of clonidine relieves hyperalgesia in patients with sympathetically maintained pain. *Pain* 1991; 47(3):309–317.

253. Muizelaar JP, Kleyer M, Hertogs IA, et al. Complex regional pain syndrome (reflex sympathetic dystrophy and causalgia): management with the calcium channel blocker nifedipine and/or the alpha-sympathetic blocker phenoxybenzamine in 59 patients. *Clin Neurol Neurosurg* 1997;99(1):26–30.

254. Prough DS, McLeskey CH, Poehling GG, et al. Efficacy of oral nifedipine in the treatment of reflex sympathetic dystrophy. *Anesthesiology* 1985;62(6): 796–799.

255. Ghostine SY, Comair YG, Turner DM, et al. Phenoxybenzamine in the treatment of causalgia. Report of 40 cases. *J Neurosurg* 1984;60(6):1263–1268.

256. Dellemijn PL, Fields HL, Allen RR, et al. The interpretation of pain relief and sensory changes following sympathetic blockade. *Brain* 1994;117(pt 6): 1475–1487.

257. Bickerstaff DR, Kanis JA. The use of nasal calcitonin in the treatment of posttraumatic algodystrophy. *Br J Rheum* 1991;30:291–294.

258. Gobelet C, Meier JL, Schaffner W, et al. Calcitonin and reflex sympathetic dystrophy syndrome. *Clin Rheum* 1986;5:382–388.

259. Gobelet C, Waldburger M, Meier JL. The effect of adding calcitonin to physical treatment on reflex sympathetic dystrophy. *Pain* 1992;48:171–175.

260. Braga PC. Calcitonin and its antinociceptive activity: animal and human investigations 1975–1992. *Agents Actions* 1994;41(3–4):121–131.

261. Perez RS, Kwakkel G, Zuurmond WW, et al. Treatment of reflex sympathetic dystrophy (CRPS type I): a research synthesis of 21 randomized clinical trials. *J Pain Symptom Manage* 2001;21(6):511–526.

262. Varenna M, Zucchi F, Ghiringhelli D, et al. Intravenous clodronate in the treatment of reflex sympathetic dystrophy syndrome. A randomized, double blind, placebo controlled study. *J Rheumatol* 2000;27(6):1477–1483.

263. Adami S, Fossaluzza V, Gatti D, et al. Bisphosphonate therapy of reflex sympathetic dystrophy syndrome. *Ann Rheum Dis* 1997;56(3):201–204.

264. Robinson JN, Sandom J, Chapman PT. Efficacy of pamidronate in complex regional pain syndrome type I. *Pain Med* 2004;5(3):276–280.

265. Kubalek I, Fain O, Paries J, et al. Treatment of reflex sympathetic dystrophy with pamidronate: 29 cases. *Rheumatology (Oxford)* 2001;40(12): 1394–1397.

266. Attal N, Brasseur L, Chauvin M, et al. Effects of single and repeated applications of a eutectic mixture of local anaesthetics (EMLA) cream on spontaneous and evoked pain in post-herpetic neuralgia. *Pain* 1999;81(1–2):203–209.

267. Galer BS, Rowbotham MC, Perander J, et al. Topical lidocaine patch relieves postherpetic neuralgia more effectively than a vehicle topical patch: results of an enriched enrollment study. *Pain* 1999;80(3):533–538.

268. Devers A, Galer BS. Topical lidocaine patch relieves a variety of neuropathic pain conditions: an open-label study. *Clin J Pain* 2000;16(3):205–208.

269. Robbins WR, Staats PS, Levine J, et al. Treatment of intractable pain with topical large-dose capsaicin: preliminary report. *Anesth Analg* 1998;86(3): 579–583.

270. Zuurmond WW, Langendijk PN, Bezemer PD, et al. Treatment of acute reflex sympathetic dystrophy with DMSO 50% in a fatty cream. *Acta Anaesthesiol Scand* 1996;40(3):364–367.

271. Alioto JT. Behavioral treatment of reflex sympathetic dystrophy. *Psychosomatics* 1981;22(6):539–540.

272. Fialka V, Korpan M, Saradeth T, et al. Autogenic training for reflex sympathetic dystrophy: a pilot study. *Complement Ther Med* 1996;4:103–105.

273. Barowsky EI, Zweig JB, Moskowitz J. Thermal biofeedback in the treatment of symptoms associated with reflex sympathetic dystrophy. *J Child Neurol* 1987;2(3):229–232.

274. Blanchard EB. The use of temperature biofeedback in the treatment of chronic pain due to causalgia. *Biofeedback Self Regul* 1979;4(2):183–188.

275. Kawano M, Matsuoka M, Kurokawa T, et al. Autogenic training as an effective treatment for reflex neurovascular dystrophy: a case report. *Acta Paediatr Jpn* 1989;31(4):500–503.

276. Gainer MJ. Hypnotherapy for reflex sympathetic dystrophy. *Am J Clin Hypn* 1992;34(4):227–232.

277. Oerlemans HM, Oostendorp RA, de Boo T, et al. Adjuvant physical therapy versus occupational therapy in patients with reflex sympathetic dystrophy/complex regional pain syndrome type I. *Arch Phys Med Rehabil* 2000;81(1): 49–56.

278. Carlson CR, Hoyle RH. Efficacy of abbreviated progressive muscle relaxation training: A quantitative review of behavioral medicine research. *J Consult Clin Psychol* 1993;61:1059–1067.

279. Stetter F, Kupper S. Autogenic training: a meta-analysis of clinical outcome studies. *Appl Psychophysiol Biofeedback* 2002;27(1):45–98.

280. Eccleston C, Morley S, Williams A, et al. Systematic review of randomized controlled trials of psychological therapy for chronic pain in children and adolescents, with a subset meta-analysis of pain relief. *Pain* 2002;99(1–2): 157–165.

281. Holroyd KA, Penzien DB. Pharmacological versus non-pharmacological prophylaxis of recurrent migraine headache: a meta-analytic review of clinical trials. *Pain* 1990;42(1):1–13.

282. Crider AB, Glaros AG. A meta-analysis of EMG biofeedback treatment of temporomandibular disorders. *J Orofac Pain* 1999;13(1):29–37.

283. Astin JA, Beckner W, Soeken K, et al. Psychological interventions for rheumatoid arthritis: a meta-analysis of randomized controlled trials. *Arthritis Rheum* 2002;47(3):291–302.

284. Sim J, Adams N. Systematic review of randomized controlled trials of non-pharmacological interventions for fibromyalgia. *Clin J Pain* 2002;18(5): 324–336.

285. Devine EC. Meta-analysis of the effect of psychoeducational interventions on pain in adults with cancer. *Oncol Nurs Forum* 2003;30(1):75–89.

286. Burton AW. Interventional therapies. In: R. HN, ed. *Complex Regional Pain Syndrome: Treatment Guidelines*. Milford: RSDSA Press; 2006:51–61.

287. Evans J. Sympathectomy for reflex sympathetic dystrophy: report of 29 cases. *JAMA* 1946;132:620–623.

288. Jänig W, Häbler HJ. Sympathetic nervous system: contribution to chronic pain. *Prog Brain Res* 2000;129:451–468.

289. Price DD, Long S, Wilsey B, et al. Analysis of peak magnitude and duration of analgesia produced by local anesthetics injected into sympathetic ganglia of complex regional pain syndrome patients. *Clin J Pain* 1998;14:216–226.

290. Burton AW, Conroy BP, Sims S, et al. Complex regional pain syndrome type II as a complication of subclavian line insertion (letter). *Anesthesiology* 1998; 89:804.

291. Cepeda MS, Lau J, Carr DB. Defining the therapeutic role of local anesthetic sympathetic blockade in complex regional pain syndrome: a narrative and systematic review. *Clin J Pain* 2002;18:216–233.

292. Raj PP, Montgomery SJ, Nettles D, et al. Infraclavicular brachial plexus block—a new approach. *Anesth Analg* 1973;52(6):897–904.

293. Raj P. Nerve blocks: Continuous regional analgesia. In: Raj P, ed. *Practical Management of Pain*. 3rd ed. St Louis: Mosby; 2000:710–722.

294. Wang LK, Chen HP, Chang PJ, et al. Axillary brachial plexus block with patient controlled analgesia for complex regional pain syndrome type I: a case report. *Reg Anesth Pain Med* 2001;26(1):68–71.

295. Cooper DE, DeLee JC, Ramamurthy S. Reflex sympathetic dystrophy of the knee. Treatment using continuous epidural anesthesia. *J Bone Joint Surg Am* 1989;71(3):365–369.

296. Koning H, Christiaans C, Overdijk G, et al. Cervical epidural blockade and reflex sympathetic dystrophy. *Pain Clinic* 1995;8:239–244.

297. Lundborg C, Dahm P, Nitescu P, et al. Clinical experience using intrathecal (IT) bupivacaine infusion in three patients with complex regional pain syndrome type I (CRPS-I). *Acta Anaesthesiol Scand* 1999;43(6):667–678.

298. van Hilten BJ, van de Beek WJ, Hoff JI, et al. Intrathecal baclofen for the treatment of dystonia in patients with reflex sympathetic dystrophy. *N Engl J Med* 2000;343:625–630.

299. Du Pen SL, Peterson DG, Williams A, et al. Infection during chronic catheter epidural catheterization: diagnosis and treatment. *Anesthesiology* 1990;73: 905–909.

300. Arnér S. Intravenous phentolamine test: diagnostic and prognostic use in reflex sympathetic dystrophy. *Pain* 1991;46:17–22.

301. Verdugo RJ, Ochoa JL. Sympthetically maintained pain I. Phentolamine block questions the concept. *Neurology* 1994;44:1003–1010.

302. Hannington-Kiff JG. Intravenous regional sympathetic block with guanethidine. *Lancet* 1974;1(7865):1019–1020.

303. Hord AH, Rooks MD, Stephens BO, et al. Intravenous regional bretylium and lidocaine for treatment of reflex sympathetic dystrophy: a randomized, double-blind study. *Anesth Analg* 1992;74(6):818–821.

304. Bonelli S, Conoscente F, Movilia P, et al. Regional intravenous guanethidine versus stellate ganglion blocks in reflex sympathetic dystrophy: a randomized trial. *Pain* 1983;16(3):297–307.

305. Reuben S, Sklar J. Intravenous regional analgesia with clonidine in the management of complex regional pain syndrome of the knee. *J Clin Anesth* 2002; 14:87–91.

306. Ramamurthy S, Hoffman J. Intravenous regional guanethidine in the treatment of reflex sympathetic dystrophy/causalgia: a randomized double-blind study. *Anesth Analg* 1995;81:718–723.

307. Jadad AR, Carroll D, Glynn CJ, et al. Intravenous regional sympathetic dys-

trophy: A systemic review and a randomized, double-blind crossover study. *J Pain Symptom Manage* 1995;10:13–20.

308. Lubenow T, Dragisic B, Breuhl S, et al. Bretylium, lidocaine, phentolamine, and hydrocortisone in combination for IV regional sympathetic blocks in the treatment of reflex sympathetic dystrophy. Paper presented at: Annual Meeting of the American Academy of Pain Management; 1996; p. A121.

309. Suresh S, Wheeler M, Patel A. Case series: IV regional anesthesia with ketorolac and lidocaine: is it effective for the management of complex regional pain syndrome 1 in children and adolescents? *Anesth Analg* 2003;96:694–695.

310. Kim K, DeSalles A, Johnson J, et al. Sympathectomy: open and thoracoscopic. In: Burchiel K, ed. *Surgical Management of Pain*. New York: Thieme Publishers; 2002:688–700.

311. Robertson DP, Simpson RK, Rose JE. Video-assisted endoscopic thoracic ganglionectomy. *J Neurosurg* 1993;79:238–240.

312. Wilkinson H. Percutaneous radiofrequency upper thoracic sympathectomy. *Neurosurgery* 1996;38:715–725.

313. Mockus MB, Rutherford RB, Rosales C, et al. Sympathectomy for causalgia. Patient selection and long-term results. *Arch Surg* 1987;122(6):668–672.

314. Kemler MA, Barendse GA, van Kleef M, et al. Spinal cord stimulation in patients with chronic reflex sympathetic dystrophy. *N Engl J Med* 2000;343:618–624.

315. Kemler MA, De Vet HC, Barendse GA, et al. The effect of spinal cord stimulation in patients with chronic reflex sympathetic dystrophy: two years' follow-up of the randomized controlled trial. *Ann Neurol* 2004;55(1):13–18.

316. Grabow TS, Tella PK, Raja SN. Spinal cord stimulation for complex regional pain syndrome: an evidence-based review of the literature. *Clin J Pain* 2003; 19(6):371–383.

317. Turner JA, Loeser JD, Deyo RA, et al. Spinal cord stimulation for patients with failed back surgery syndrome or complex regional pain syndrome: a systematic review of effectiveness and complications. *Pain* 2004;108(1–2):137–147.

318. Burton AW, Hassenbusch SJ III, Warneke C, et al. Complex regional pain syndrome (CRPS): survey of current practices. *Pain Pract* 2004;4(2):74–83.

319. North RB, Levy RM. Consensus conference on the neurosurgical management of pain. *Neurosurgery* 1994;34(4):756–760,discussion 760–761.

320. Kiralp MZ, Yildiz S, Vural D, et al. Effectiveness of hyperbaric oxygen therapy in the treatment of complex regional pain syndrome. *J Int Med Res* 2004; 32(3):258–262.

321. Korpan MI, Dezu Y, Schneider B, et al. Acupuncture in the treatment of posttraumatic pain syndrome. *Acta Orthop Belg* 1999;65(2):197–201.

322. Muir JM, Vernon H. Complex regional pain syndrome and chiropractic. *J Manipulative Physiol Ther* 2000;23(7):490–497.

CHAPTER 26 ■ PHANTOM PAIN

HOWARD S. SMITH, IRFAN LALANI, AND CHARLES E. ARGOFF

INTRODUCTION

In 1871, Civil War surgeon Silas Weir Mitchell[1] popularized the concept of phantom limb pain (PLP) and coined the term *phantom limb* with publication of a long-term study on the fate of Civil War amputees. Phantom limb sensations may occur in roughly 85% of amputees and tend to be seen in the first 3 weeks after amputation,[2] although less commonly may develop 1 to 12 months following amputation.[3] Most phantom sensations generally resolve without treatment after 2 to 3 years.

Phantom pain refers to pain perceived in a missing body part and may occur in about 50% to 80% of all amputees.[4] Pain may be related to certain positions or movements of the phantom and may be elicited or exacerbated by a range of physical factors (e.g., changes in weather or pressure on the residual limb) and psychological factors (e.g., emotional stress). It seems to be more intense in the distal portions of the phantom and can have several different qualities, such as stabbing, throbbing, burning, or cramping.[5]

Residual limb pain—previously referred to in the literature as stump pain—refers to a regional pain restricted to the distal residual part. Unlike phantom pain, it occurs in the area of the body that actually exists. Patients may also experience feelings of tingling, itching, cramping, or involuntary movements in the residuum.

Commonly, the phantom is exactly the same size and shape as the missing limb immediately after the amputation.[6] Over time, the phantom may gradually reduce in size and shorten into the residual limb (telescope) so that eventually only the foot, hand, or digits are left on the stump.[7–10] Hill proposed that telescoping occurred in one-third of amputees.[11]

The exteroceptive component describes the feelings within the phantom. Examples are "pins and needles," "tingling," "tickling," "itching," "numbness," and "like it is asleep."[7,11–16] Super-added sensations are the sensation of an object such as a ring, wristwatch, or shoe still being present on the phantom[17,18]
or the return of a painful condition such as an ingrown toenail that existed some time before the amputation.[9,19] Super-added sensations were identified by 5 of 68 amputees (7%) in one study.[10,20] Exteroceptive sensations included pins and needles (50%) and itching (42.9%).[10] The high report of itching is interesting in terms of the mechanism of both PLP and itch. It has been found that similar areas of the brain, including the premotor areas, are involved in both sensations.[21,22]

EPIDEMIOLOGY

In 1983 Sherman et al. published a survey of 590 war veteran amputees in which 85% reported phantom pain.[23] A study with 2,694 amputees showed that 51% experienced PLP severe enough to hinder lifestyle on more than 6 days per month, 21% reported daily pain over a 10- to 14-hour period and 27% for more than 15 hours per day.[24] The incidence of PLP increases with more proximal amputation. Residual limb pain is reported in up to 50% of amputees.[25–31]

PLP has been reported to occur as early as 1 week after amputation and as late as 40 years after amputation.[32,33] Phantom pain may diminish with time and eventually fade away. However, some prospective studies indicate that even 2 years after amputation, the incidence is not greatly diminished from that at onset.[31,34]

MODULATION OF PHANTOM PAIN

The development of PLP can best be described as multifactorial. It is becoming appreciated that preamputation pain is a risk factor for the development of significant PLP.[14,35–37] Phantom pain may mimic preamputation pain.[17,38]

Phantom pain may be modulated by multiple factors, both internal as well as external. Exacerbations of pain may be produced by trivial, physical, or emotion stimuli. Anxiety, depression, urination, cough, defecation, sexual activity, cold environment, or changes in the weather may worsen PLP.[23,34,39–44] It also has been reported that general, spinal, or regional anesthesia in amputees may cause appearance of phantom pain in otherwise pain free subjects.[45–50]

PATHOPHYSIOLOGY OF PHANTOM PAIN

The mechanisms underlying phantom pain are complex and incompletely understood. It is highly likely that phantom pain is mediated by a complex interaction between the brain, spinal cord, and periphery.

Postamputation, damaged C-fiber and A-fiber axons generally undergo ineffective regeneration to form neuromas (e.g., enlarged and disorganized endings of C fibers and demyelinated A fibers that show an increased rate of spontaneous activity[5]) in the residual limb. About 30% of the time these neuromas may act as "pain generators" of PAP.[5] Mechanical (e.g., pressure [Tinel's sign]) and chemical (e.g., norepinephrine) stimulation may further increase the rate of discharge, which seems to be mainly related to spontaneous ectopia (neuronal discharge that is generated along the axon or in the soma), as a consequence of nerve injury and seems to be a result of the upregulation or novel expression of sodium channels.[51,52] These neuromas have aberrant sodium channel expression resulting in increased spontaneous and evoked discharges. These discharges can be provoked by innocuous stimuli such as pressure, light touch, and change in temperature and may be perceived as painful. Clinically, this mechanism appears to be corroborated by the observation that stump and phantom pain can be temporarily reduced in some (but not all) patients by injection of local anesthetics into stump neuromas. Ectopic discharges can also occur at the level of the dorsal root ganglion (DRG), independently of stump neuromas. This can result in amplification of peripheral signals and recruitment of neighboring neurons.

The sympathetic nervous system may play a role in potentiating phantom pain. Sympathetic nerve blocks can temporarily relieve phantom pain in some patients whereas injection of norepinephrine can exacerbate pain. Catecholamines can promote firing of peripheral mechanoreceptors, which in turn may activate sensitized dorsal horn neurons. Increased sympathetic tone can also promote ephaptic neuronal transmission in the periphery. Sympathetic tone is inversely related to skin temperature at the amputated stump.[5] Investigators have also shown an inverse relationship between phantom pain and skin temperature, suggesting that sympathetic tone promotes pain sensation.[5]

Peripheral nerve injury is also accompanied by reorganization of signal processing at the spinal cord level. Selective degeneration of unmyelinated C fibers results in functional denervation of lamina II neurons in the dorsal horn. A compensatory arborization of Aδ and Aβ fibers "sprouting" into lamina II can occur.[53,54] This change in innervation is accompanied by phenotypic switching, whereby Aβ fiber terminals release substance P, a nociceptive peptide. These changes may form the anatomic and neurochemical substrate for the clinical phenomenon of allodynia, where a non-noxious mechanical stimulus is perceived as painful.

Increased excitatory input at the dorsal horn following nerve injury can cause apoptosis of inhibitory interneurons expressing GABA and glycine. Activation of migroglia after neural injury can result in release of BDNF (brain derived neurotrophic factor), which promotes phenotypic switching of inhibitory interneurons, may lead to release excitatory neurotransmitters (e.g., glutamate). Opioid receptors are also downregulated along with upregulation of cholecystokinin, which is an endogenous opioid receptor antagonist.

Nikolajsen and Jensen[55] explained that the pharmacology of spinal sensitization involves increased activity in N-methyl-D-aspartate (NMDA) receptor-complex,[56] and many aspects of the central sensitization can be reduced by NMDA receptor antagonists. This was supported in human amputees where the evoked stump or phantom pain produced by repetitive stimulation of the stump by non-noxious pinprick was reduced by the NMDA receptor antagonist ketamine.[55]

Waxman and Hains proposed that abnormal expression of Nav 1.3 sodium channels in the 2nd and 3rd order neurons along nociceptive pathways after spinal cord injury may make these neurons hyperexcitable.[52] These neurons may then function as pain amplifiers/generators and conceivably contribute to phantom phenomena.

Peripheral injury after amputation is also accompanied by remapping of supraspinal synaptic networks, including those in the primary somatosensory cortex. Some patients with PLP exhibit "topographical remapping," where stimulation of an unaffected site (e.g., face) will result in a sensation perceived in the phantom limb. Functional imaging studies have shown activation of areas in the primary somatosensory cortex and are both adjacent and distant from the area normally subserving the affected limb. Topographical remapping appears to correlate with persistence of phantom pain, with data showing that upper extremity amputees with phantom pain have expansion of the mouth area into the hand area in the sensory homunculus (primary somatosensory cortex). These findings have also been described in the primary motor cortex of amputees, with good correlation between reorganization and presence of phantom pain symptoms.

Melzack observed that a substantial number of children who are born without a limb feel a phantom of the missing part and suggested the existence of a neural network, or *neuromatrix*, that subserves body sensation and has a genetically determined substrate that is modified by sensory experience.[59] Lotze et al. revealed that functional magnetic resonance imaging (MRI) data from amputees with pain and healthy volunteers during a lip pursing task were similar. In amputees with PLP, however, the cortical representation of the mouth extends into the region of the hand and arm. Giummarra et al. proposed that phantom pain may reflect a maladaptive failure of the neuromatrix to maintain global bodily constructs.[60] Cortical map reorganization may be facilitated via selective loss of C fibers, which occurs after amputations. C fibers appear to have an important role in the maintenance of cortical maps.

Psychological factors can also play a role in the pathogenesis of phantom pain. Though these factors may not play a causative role, they may certainly modulate the pain experience.

Longitudinal diary studies showed that there is a significant relation between stress and the onset and exacerbation of episodes of phantom-limb pain, probably mediated by activity in the sympathetic nervous system and increases in muscle tension.[61] Patients who received less support before the amputation tend to report more phantom-limb pain.[62]

Animal work on stimulation-induced plasticity suggests that extensive behaviorally relevant (but not passive) stimulation of a body part leads to an expansion of its representation zone.[63] Intensive use of a myoelectric prosthesis is positively correlated with reduced cortical reorganization and analgesic effects.[64] These effects could not be achieved with standard medical treatment and general psychological counseling because it is felt that in order to achieve analgesia, input into the amputation zone of the cortex is needed in order to "undo" the reorganizational changes induced by amputation. Similar beneficial effects on phantom pain and cortical activation were reported for imagined movement of the phantom, and may also occur to some degree with mirror treatment (where a mirror is used to trick the brain into perceiving movement of the phantom when the intact limb is moved).[65]

PREVENTION OF PHANTOM PAIN

PLP cannot currently be completely prevented; however, perioperative epidural techniques, peripheral nerve catheter techniques, or other analgesic strategies utilized preoperatively, intraoperatively, and postoperatively may at least address postoperative pain control better than not employing any specific perioperative analgesic techniques.[66–72]

Madabhushi and colleagues reported on a patient with a history of PLP from a below-knee amputation who then came for an above-knee amputation in the same extremity.[71] Before transection, the sciatic nerve was infiltrated with 0.25% bupivacaine 5 mL and clonidine 50 mcg. After the nerve was severed, a 20-gauge epidural catheter was inserted into the nerve sheath and externalized laterally through a separate skin incision. Before closure, 0.25% bupivacaine 10 ml and clonidine 50 mcg was injected, and then 0.1% bupivacaine and clonidine 2 mcg/mL was infused perineurally for the first 96 hours postoperatively. The mean postoperative pain score (from 0 to 10) for 96 hours was 1.2 ± 0.7.[71] The patient required a total of 10 mg of oxycodone postoperatively. Over a 1-year follow-up period the patient never reported stump or phantom pain.[71]

TREATMENT OF PHANTOM PAIN

Phantom pain often requires a multimodal approach to treatment. Treatment options include behavioral techniques, antidepressants, anticonvulsants, opioid and nonopioid analgesics, transcutaneous electrical nerve stimulators (TENS), neural blockade, spinal cord stimulation, and motor cortex stimulation. There remains a paucity of data from large randomized controlled trials to guide treatment options. As a general rule, initial treatments should be low risk, low cost, and noninvasive, with more expensive and invasive treatments reserved for patients who fail conservative care.

PHARMACOLOGIC INTERVENTIONS

Antidepressants

Antidepressants are commonly used for many painful conditions but especially for neuropathic pain. Although, antidepressants are utilized for the treatment of PAP conditions, they have not been well studied for PAP. Wilder-Smith et al. studied 94 treatment-naïve posttraumatic limb amputees with phantom pain (intensity: mean visual analog scale score [0–100, 40 [95% confidence interval, 38–41]) who were randomly assigned to receive individually titrated doses of tramadol, placebo (double-blind comparison), or amitriptyline (open comparison) for 1 month. Wilder-Smith and colleagues concluded that in treatment-naïve patients, both amitriptyline and tramadol provided excellent and stable phantom limb and stump pain control with no major adverse events.[73] Alternatively, Robinson et al. studied 39 persons with amputation-related pain lasting more than 6 months in a 6-week randomized controlled trial of amitriptyline (titrated up to 125 mg/day) or an active placebo (benztropine mesylate).[74] No significant differences were found between the treatment groups in outcome variables when controlled for initial pain scores, thus not supporting the use of amitriptyline in the treatment of postamputation pain.[74]

Kuiken et al. studied four individuals with PLP for at least 3 months after amputation.[75] All subjects received oral mirtazapine between 7.5 and 30 mg/day.[75] An 11-point numeric rating scale (0 to 10) measured pain intensity and relief during monitored outpatient follow-up visits. Mirtazapine use improved the PLP experienced by these subjects by at least 50%, measured by a numerical rating scale-11 (NRS-11).[75] Subjects with PLP-related sleeping difficulties reported the greatest pain relief concomitant with improved sleep quality.[75]

Antiepileptic Drugs

Carbamazepine, an anticonvulsant (and heterocyclic), has also been well documented for use in neuropathic pain syndromes and serves as a potent sodium channel blocker. Historically, it has also been the most commonly prescribed anticonvulsant for pain. Despite this, the results of its efficacy on PLP have been mixed. Patterson reported cases of phantom pain that were alleviated with the use of oral carbamazepine.[76,77] However, only brief, shock-like pain was assessed.[76] There are no studies that have shown its effectiveness in treating any of the other qualities of pain.

The effectiveness of gabapentin in postamputation PLP was studied in a randomized, double-blind, placebo-controlled, crossover study by Bone et al.[78] They evaluated analgesic efficacy of gabapentin in PLP in patients attending a multidisciplinary pain clinic. The daily dose of gabapentin was titrated in increments of 300–2400 mg or the maximum tolerated dose. Nineteen eligible patients were randomized, of whom 14 completed both arms of the study. Both placebo and gabapentin treatments resulted in reduced VAS scores compared with baseline. However, the pain intensity difference was significantly greater than placebo for gabapentin therapy at the end of the treatment. They concluded that after 6 weeks, gabapentin monotherapy was better than placebo in relieving postamputation PLP.

Nikolajsen et al. examined whether postoperative treatment with gabapentin could reduce postamputation residual limb and phantom pain and concluded that gabapentin administered in the first 30 postoperative days after amputation does not reduce the incidence or intensity of postamputation pain.[79] Pregabalin may exhibit analgesic effects on postamputation pain states but has not yet been evaluated.

Four PLP subjects[80] were treated during a larger prospective, double-blind, randomized, placebo-controlled pilot study conducted to test the efficacy of topiramate in managing various neuropathic pain conditions associated with rehabilitation.[80]

Three of the four subjects who had experienced over 2 years of refractory PLP experienced significantly reduced pain after treatment with topiramate.[80]

Opioids

Mishra et al. reported a case of intractable PLP whose pain did not respond to usual treatment and only a high dose of morphine made the patient totally pain free.[81]

Wilder-Smith et al. evaluated a recent study, 94 treatment-naive posttraumatic limb amputees with phantom pain who were randomly assigned to receive individually titrated doses of tramadol (mean dose 448mg) or placebo (double-blind comparison) for 1 month. It was found that tramadol provided excellent and stable phantom limb and residual limb pain control with no major adverse events.[73] A review found a 50% to 90% reduction in pain at 12 to 26 months with methadone 10–20 mg per day.[82]

Huse and colleagues studied the efficacy of oral long-acting morphine sulfate (MS) against placebo in a double-blind crossover design in 12 patients with PLP after unilateral leg or arm amputation.[83] The dose of MS was titrated to at least 70 mg/day and at highest 300 mg/day.[83] Pain, reorganization of somatosensory cortex, and pain thresholds were assessed pre- and posttreatment.[83] A significant pain reduction was found during MS therapy but not during placebo. A clinically relevant response to MS (pain reduction of more than 50%) was evident in 42%, with a partial response (pain reduction of 25% to 50%) in 8% of the patients.[83] Neuromagnetic imaging utilizing magnetoencephalographic recordings of three patients showed initial evidence for reduced cortical reorganization with MS treatment concurrent with the reduction in pain intensity.[83] Huse et al. concluded that opioids show efficacy in the treatment of PLP and may also potentially influence cortical reorganization.[83]

Intravenous lidocaine and morphine have also been evaluated for their therapeutic use in postamputation pain. Wu et al. conducted a randomized double-blind trial to compare the analgesic effects of intravenous morphine and lidocaine on postamputation stump and phantom pains.[84] A bolus of morphine, lidocaine, and an active placebo (diphenhydramine) were used over a span of 3 consecutive days. The results showed that 31 of 32 subjects enrolled completed the study. Eleven subjects had both stump and phantom pains, 11 and 9 subjects had stump and phantom pain alone, respectively. Compared with placebo, morphine reduced both residual limb and phantom pains significantly. In contrast, lidocaine decreased residual limb pain but not phantom pain. The authors concluded that the mechanisms of residual limb pain and phantom pain are different.[84]

NMDA Receptor Antagonists

Stannard and Porter described three cases in which PLP was successfully treated with ketamine hydrochloride.[85] Nikolajsen et al. administered ketamine intravenously to a patient with established stump pain in a double-blind saline-controlled fashion.[86] Following infusion, stump pain was alleviated for 31 hours.[86] Ketamine reduced the allodynic area and wind-up like pain and increased pressure-pain thresholds.[86] Treatment was started with ketamine 50 mg × 4 per day dissolved in juice.[104] No side effects or development of tolerance were observed during a 3-month treatment period.[86]

Nikolajsen et al. administered ketamine (bolus at 0.1 mg/kg/ 5 min followed by an infusion of 7 micrograms/kg/min) intravenously to 11 patients with established stump and PLP in a double-blind saline-controlled study.[57] All 11 patients responded with a decrease in the rating of stump and PLP assessed by visual analogue scale (VAS) and McGill Pain Questionnaire (MPQ).[57] Ketamine increased pressure-pain thresholds significantly. Wind-up like pain (pain evoked by repeatedly tapping the dysaethetic skin area) was reduced significantly by ketamine.[57] In contrast, no effect was seen on pain evoked by repeated thermal stimuli. Side effects were observed in nine patients.[57]

Although calcitonin may have analgesic effects for PAP postoperatively,[87] it does not appear to be effective for chronic PAP conditions.[88] Eichenberger et al. conducted a randomized, double-blind, crossover study in which 20 patients received four IV infusions of 200 IE calcitonin; ketamine 0.4 mg/kg (only 10 patients); 200 IE of calcitonin combined with ketamine 0.4 mg/ kg; placebo; and 0.9% saline. Intensity of phantom pain (visual analog scale) was recorded before, during, at the end, and the 48 hours after each infusion.[88] Ketamine, but not calcitonin, reduced PLP.[88] The combination was not superior to ketamine alone.[88]

TRPV1 Modulators

Topical capsaicin was also utilized for the treatment of PLP. In a study performed in a double-blind fashion with 24 patients, the authors concluded that capsaicin may be used as an alternative treatment for PLP.[89] Future developments may produce higher strength capsaicin products, more potent capsaicin analogues, TRPV1 antagonoists, and intravenous capsaicin formulations.

Interventional Therapy

A wide variety of types of neural blockade have been utilized in the treatment of PLP, including trigger point injections, sympa

thetic blocks, stump injections, peripheral nerve blocks, epidural, and subarachnoid blocks.[23] Despite this, studies have shown that only 14% of patients report a significant temporary change and 5% report a prolonged change with these blocks.[23]

The use of neural blockade in the treatment of PLP is largely based on anecdotal reports in the literature.[90–92] Blankenbaker[90] reported that sympathetic blocks are successful if amputees are treated soon after the onset of PLP. However, Halbert et al.,[93] in a systematic review to evaluate evidence for the optimal management of acute and chronic phantom pain, were unable to find any trials that met criteria for inclusion.

The use of botulinum-toxin A injections in PLP patients has also been utilized for residual limb pain control. It is conceivable that muscle tension, perhaps resulting from cortical reorganization, may contribute to phantom pain as a trigger of spinal reflexes and botulinum toxin by muscle relaxation in the stump or via inhibition of the release of various neurotransmitters may lead to analgesia. In a small pilot trial, researchers injected 100 IU botulinum-toxin A in four muscle-trigger points of an amputation stump. It was found that the use of botulinum toxin A reduced phantom pain about 60% to 80%.[94]

Kern et al. administered a total dose of 2500 IU of botulinum toxin type B (Neurobloc, Elan Pharma, Munich, Germany) to the arm amputation stumps, 5000 IU for one amputation of the lower leg, and 2500 IU to the other lower leg amputation of a patient with a very low baseline body weight.[95] Two patients reported that the injection was very painful. All patients experienced a reduction in stump pain, which lasted for many weeks.[95] Other reports included a reduction in the frequency of pain attacks, cessation of "balloon feelings," improvement in stump allodynia, and decreased occurrence of involuntary stump movements. In addition, quality of sleep at night significantly improved in one patient.[95]

Multiple other cases have been reported of botulinum toxin injections into the stump for PLP.[95,96]

Furthermore, Kern and colleagues suggested that by diminishing muscle tone, pain, and hyperhidroses, botulinum toxin may facilitate prosthesis use.[96] Four postamputation patients (one with phantom pain, three with stump pain) were each treated with 100 IU botulinum toxin A, divided between several trigger points in the distal stump musculature. In one female patient (along with a pronounced reduction in phantom pain) hyperhidrosis of the stump ceased completely, probably after diffusion of the drug into the dermal sweat glands, leading to longer and safer use of the prosthesis. Intentional intradermal injection for this purpose therefore could be potentially valuable. Another patient was able to use her prosthesis for the whole day again after botulinum toxin A treatment for substantial stump pain, compared with only 4 hours a day before treatment. In two male patients, residual limb pain while wearing the prosthesis subsided to a considerable extent, and one of the two reported an improvement in steadiness of gait. They suggested that stump treatment with botulinum toxin in rehabilitative medicine should be investigated in more detail.[96]

Dahl and Cohen treated six soldiers with residual limb and phantom pain with a series of perineural etanercept injections.[97] Five of the six patients reported significant improvements in residual limb pain at rest and with activity, PLP, functional capacity, and psychologic well-being 3 months after injections.[97] The one soldier who failed therapy was the only patient who presented with pain greater than 1 year in duration. At the reduced doses administered, no adverse effects were observed. These results seem to warrant further large well-designed studies.[97]

Neuromodulation

Transcutaneous electrical nerve stimulation has been used with some success in the treatment of phantom pain. Katz and Melzack reported that 10 minutes after receiving low frequency (4 Hz) high intensity (10–30 V) auricular TENS, phantom pain patients demonstrated a modest, yet statistically significant decrease in pain as measured by the McGill Pain Questionnaire.[98] Investigators have reported good to excellent results in roughly 25% of patients treated with TENS.[98,99]

Spinal cord stimulation (SCS) has also been used for PLP. Seigfried et al. reported that 51% of patients with SCS had a 50% or more decrease in pain, but without long term follow-up.[100]

Bittar and colleagues concluded that deep brain stimulation (DBS) has been utilized successfully for the treatment of phantom limp pain with a resultant decreased pain, decreased opiate intake, and improved quality of life.[101] Bittar et al. published a meta-analysis supporting this pain improvement as well, especially in the burning component—perhaps via a reorganization in the central nervous system.[102]

Sol et al. used chronic motor cortex stimulation (CMCS) in 3 patients with intractable PLP after upper limb amputation.[103] Functional magnetic resonance imaging (fMRI) correlated to anatomical MRI permitted frameless image guidance for electrode placement. Pain control was obtained for all the patients initially and the relief was stable in 2 of the 3 patients at 2 year follow-up. FMRI data may be useful in assisting the neurosurgeon in electrode placement for this indication.[103]

Surgical Interventions

PLP has generally been difficult to treat with surgical interventions. Part of the difficulty in addressing PLP/stump surgically lies in the postsurgical restriction or growth retardation of stump neuromas. Residual limb neuromas develop at the site of the severed end of peripheral nerves. Surgical management may involve implanting the end of severed nerves into a nearby/adjacent large muscle belly, which may alleviate stump pain somewhat, although it does not permanently cure patients.[104]

Sakai et al. theorized that preventing neuroma formation might also significantly decrease the incidence of postamputation stump pain. Techniques to prevent neuroma formation include nerve transposition of ligation, embedding the nerve end in bone or muscle, and capping the nerve stump with a nerve graft, epineurium, or atelocollagen.[105,106]

Sehirlioglu et al. retrospectively studied 75 patients who were treated for painful neuroma after lower limb amputation following landmine explosions between the years 2000 and 2006.[107] The average time period from use of prosthesis to start of symptoms suggesting neuroma was 9.6 months. The average time period from start of pain symptoms to neuroma surgery was 7.8 months. All clinically proven neuromas were surgically resected.[107] In the mean follow-up of 2.8 years, all patients were satisfied with the end results and all were free of any pain symptoms.[107] In a painful residual with clinical diagnostic findings of neuroma if conservative measures fail, surgery may be considered as a therapeutic option.[107]

Aggressive surgical techniques, such as anterolateral cordotomy and dorsal root entry zone (DREZ) lesions, have been attempted in PLP but do not have large multicenter studies supporting their use at all and have significant morbidity and some mortality.

Behavioral Medicine Interventions

Many psychological modalities have been attempted to manage those with PLP, including cognitive behavioral therapy, biofeedback, and muscular training.[108]

Biofeedback treatments resulting in vasodilatation or decreased muscle tension in the residual limb may help to reduce PLP and seem promising in patients in whom peripheral factors contribute to the pain.[109] Harden et al. conducted a pilot study that examined the effectiveness of biofeedback in the treatment of nine individuals with PLP who received up to seven thermal/autogenic biofeedback sessions over the course of 4–6 weeks.[110] Pain was assessed daily using the visual analog scale (VAS), the sum of the sensory descriptors, and the sum of the affective descriptors of the McGill short form. Interrupted time-series analytical models were created for each of the participants, allowing biofeedback sessions to be modeled as discrete interventions.[110] Analyses of the VAS revealed that a 20% pain reduction was seen in five of the nine patients in the weeks after session four, and that at least a 30% pain reduction (range: 25% to 66%) was seen in six of the seven patients in the weeks following session six.[110]

Relaxation training has also been shown to provide significant benefit in many patients. One report noted that 12 of 14 patients with chronic PLP improved with muscular relaxation training.[108] Hypnotic imagery has been used alone and with relaxation training; however, further studies need to be done before any conclusions regarding this therapy can be made.[111]

Ramachandran and Rogers-Ramachandran[112] described another behaviorally oriented approach: a mirror was placed in a box, and the patient inserted his or her intact arm and the residual limb. He or she was then asked to look at the mirror image of the intact arm, which is perceived as an intact hand where the phantom used to be, and to make symmetrical movements with both hands, thus suggesting real movement from the lost arm to the brain. This procedure may re-establish control over the phantom limb and alleviate pain in some patients, although controlled data are lacking.

Graded motor imagery is a promising, nonpharmacological means of treating PLP. A randomized controlled trial using graded motor imagery to treat CRPS I and PLP showed NNT of 3 at 6 months for a composite end point of 50% pain reduction and improvement in function.[113] Patients in the placebo arm of this study received standard physical therapy and usual medical care. Graded motor imagery involves training patients to improve right/left discrimination and imagine pain free movements of affected and normal limbs followed by practicing pain free movements with the aid of a mirror box.[113]

Murray et al. reported three participants who experienced PLP (two with an upper-limb amputation, and one with a lower-limb amputation) that took part in between two and five immersive virtual reality (IVR) sessions over a 3-week period.[114] The movements of participants' anatomical limbs were transposed into the movements of a virtual limb.[114] All participants reported the transferal of sensations into the muscles and joints of the phantom limb, and all participants reported a decrease in phantom pain during at least one of the sessions.[114] The authors suggested the need for further research studying IVR for PLP using controlled trials.

Schneider et al. evaluated eye movement desensitization and reprocessing (EMDR) treatment with extensive follow-up.[115] Five patients with PLP ranging from 1 to 16 years who were on extensive medication regimens underwent 3 to 15 sessions of EMDR, which was used to treat the pain and the psychological ramifications.[115] EMDR resulted in a significant decrease or elimination of phantom pain, reduction in depression and posttraumatic stress disorder (PTSD) symptoms to subclinical levels, and significant reduction or elimination of medications related to the phantom pain and nociceptive pain at long-term follow-up.[115] Further research is needed to explore the theoretical and treatment implications of this information-processing approach.[115]

Miscellaneous Treatments for Residual Limb Pain

Chronic residual limb pain may occur as a result of skin pathology, vascular insufficiency, infection, bone spurs, or neuromas.[11,106,34,39]

Fitting of a prosthetic socket is a critical stage in the process of rehabilitation of a trans-tibial amputation (TTA) patient, because a misfit may cause pressure ulcers or a deep tissue injury (DTI; necrosis of the muscle flap under intact skin) in the residual limb.[116] To date, prosthetic fitting topically depends on the subjective skills of the prosthetist, and is not supported by biomedical instrumentation that allows evaluation of the quality of fitting.[116] Portnoy et al. concluded that real-time patient-specific finite element (FE) analysis of internal stresses in deep soft tissues of the residual limb in TTA patients is feasible.[116] This method may be improving the fitting of prostheses in the clinical setting and protecting the residual limb from pressure ulcers and DTI.[116]

The use of a myoelectric prosthesis might be one way to influence phantom-limb pain. Intensive use of a myoelectric prosthesis was positively associated with both less phantom-limb pain and less cortical reorganization.[117]

Topical clonidine patches (and other topical therapies) have been utilized on the residuum, but have not been studied. For relatively superficial neuromas, lidocaine via iontophoresis (e.g., LidoSite® patch [developed and manufactured by Vyteris, Inc. of Fair Lawn, NJ]), theoretically may be useful.

Gruber et al. prospectively evaluated "neurosclerosis" of residual limb neuromars, present after amputation,[118] on 82 patients by means of high-resolution sonographically guided injection with up to 0.8 mL of 80% phenol solution. During treatment, all patients had marked improvement in terms of reduction of pain measured with a visual analog scale.[118] Twelve (15%) of the subjects were pain free after one to three treatments, with 9 of the 12 achieving relief with the initial instillation.[118] After 6 months, patients had an overall decrease in median VAS score from 10.0 ± 1.5 (SD) (range, 2–10) to 3.0 ± 2.6 (range, 1–10) after one (25 patients), two (12 patients), and three treatment sessions (15 patients). At the 6-month follow-up evaluation, 20 (38%) of the 52 patients reported almost unnoticeable pain, and 33 (64%) reported pain equal to the minimum pain they had reached during phenol injection therapy. In 18 (35%) of the 52 patients, the incidence of painful periods had markedly decreased.[118] The "neurosclerosis" procedure had a low complication rate (5% rate of minor complications, 1.3% rate of major complications).[118]

Pulsed radiofrequency (PRF) treatment of the dorsal root ganglion (DRG) at the L4 and L5 nerve root level was utilized as a therapeutic option for two patients with peripherally mediated intractable stump pain. A decrease in pain intensity and improved toleration of the limb prosthesis was appreciated in both patients.[106]

Anecdotes of other analgesic strategies such as acupuncture[119] and electroconvulsive therapy (ECT)[120] for PAP conditions exist.

SUMMARY

Phantom pain remains an incompletely understood, difficult to treat pain condition. It is present in a majority of postamputation patients. It is one of the painful conditions in which an obvious loss of sensory information coupled with a disruption of the nervous system leads to pain. Phantom pain also appears to be a painful condition in which the involvement of supraspinal mechanisms may be more intuitive than other painful conditions. Optimal treatment approaches involve the coordination of an interdisciplinary pain medicine team familiar with the therapy of postamputation pain syndromes. Pharmacologic treatment approaches, physical medicine and rehabilitation treatment approaches, behavioral medicine treatment approaches, neuromodulation treatment approaches, and interventional treatment approaches may all be needed in combinations to achieve optimal outcomes. Much basic and clinical research is still required to get a better handle of pathophysiologic mechanisms, prevention strategies, and optimal treatment approaches/situations for a variety of patient and phantom pains.

References

1. Mitchell SW. *Injuries of Nerves and Their Consequences.* London: Smith Elder; 1872.
2. Parkes CM. Factors determining the persistence of phantom pain in the amputee. *J Psychosom Res* 1973;17:97–108.
3. Gillis L. The management of the painful amputation stump: a new theory for the phantom phenomena. *Br J Surg* 1964;51:87–95.
4. Jensen TS, Nikolajsen L. Phantom pain and other phenomena after amputation. In: Wall P, Melzack R, eds. *Textbook of Pain.* 4th ed. Edinburgh: Churchill Livingstone; 1999:799–814.
5. Flor H. Phantom-limb pain: characteristics, causes, and treatment. *Lancet Neurology* 2002;1:182–189.
6. Melzack R, Wall P. *The Challenge of Pain.* London: Penguin; 1984.
7. Montoya P, Larbig W, Grulke N, et al. The relationship of phantom limb pain to other phantom limb phenomena in upper extremity amputees. *Pain* 1997;72:87–93.
8. Jensen TS, Rasmussen P. Phantom pain and related phenomena after amputation. In: Melzack R, Wall P, eds. *Textbook of Pain.* London: Churchill Livingstone; 1989.
9. Katz J. Psychophysical correlates of phantom limb experience. *J Neurol Neurosurg Psychiatry* 1992;55:811–821.
10. Richardson C, Glenn S, Nurmikko T, et al. Incidence of phantom phenomena including phantom limb pain 6 months after major lower limb amputation in patients with peripheral vascular disease. *Clin J of Pain* 2006;22:353–358.
11. Hill A. Phantom limb pain: a review of the literature on attributes and potential mechanisms. *J Pain Symptom Manage* 1999;17:125–142.
12. Vaida G, Friedmann LW. Postamputation phantoms: a review. *Phys Med Rehabil Clin North Am* 1991;2:325–353.
13. Wilkins KL, McGrath PJ, Finley GA, et al. Phantom limb sensations and phantom limb pain in child and adolescent amputees. *Pain* 1998;78:7–12.
14. Krane EJ, Heller LB. The prevalence of phantom sensation and pain in pediatric amputees. *J Pain Symptom Manage* 1995;10:21–29.
15. Ramachandran VS, Rogers-Ramachandran D. Synaesthesia in phantom limbs induced with mirrors. *Proc Biol Sci* 1996;263:377–386.
16. McGrath PA, Hillier LM. Phantom limb sensations in adolescents: a case study to illustrate the utility of sensation and pain logs in pediatric clinical practice. *J Pain Symptom Manage* 1992;7:46–53.
17. Katz J, Melzack R. Pain memories in phantom limbs: review and clinical observations. *Pain.* 1990;43:319–336.
18. Wesolowski JA, Lema MJ. Phantom limb pain. *Reg Anaesth* 1993;18:121–127.
19. Melzack R. Phantom limbs. *Sci Am* 1992;266:120–126.
20. Pohjolainen T. A clinical evaluation of stumps in lower limb amputees. *Prosthet Orthot Int* 1991;15:178–184.
21. Hsieh JC, Hagermark O, Stahle-Backdahl M, et al. Urge to scratch represented in the human cerebral cortex during itch. *J Neurophysiol* 1994; 72: 3004–3008.
22. Drzezga A, Darsow U, Treede RD, et al. Central activation by histamine-induced itch: analogies to pain processing: a correlational analysis of O-15 H2O positron emission tomography studies. *Pain* 2001; 92: 295–305.
23. Sherman RA, Sherman CJ. Prevalence and characteristics of chronic phantom limb pain among American veterans: results of a trial survey. *Am J Phys Med* 1983;62:227–238.
24. Sherman RA, Sherman CJ, Parker L. Chronic phantom and stump pain among American veterans: results of a survey. *Pain* 1984;18:83–95.
25. Alamo Tomillero F, Rodriguez de la Torre R, Caba Barrientos F, et al. Prospective study of prevalence and risk factors for painful phantom limb in the immediate postoperative period of patients undergoing amputation for chronic arterial ischemia. *Rev Esp Anestesiol Reanim* 2002;49:295–301.
26. Gallagher P, Allen D, Maclachlan M. Phantom limb pain and residual limb pain following lower limb amputation: a descriptive analysis. *Disabil Rehabil* 2001;23:522–530.
27. Ehde DM, Czerniecki JM, Smith DG, et al. Chronic phantom sensations, phantom pain, residual limb pain, and other regional pain after lower limb amputation. *Arch Phys Med Rehabil* 2000;81:1039–1044.
28. Wilkins KL, McGrath PJ, Finley GA, et al. Phantom limb sensations and phantom limb pain in child and adolescent amputees. *Pain* 1998;78:7–12.
29. Sherman RA, Sherman CJ. A comparison of phantom sensations among amputees whose amputations were of civilian and military origins. *Pain* 1985;21:91–97.
30. Helm P, Engel T, Holm A, et al. Function after lower limb amputation. *Acta Orthop Scand* 1986;57:154–157.
31. Nikolajsen L, Illkjaer S, Kroner K, et al. The influence of preamputation pain on post amputation stump and phantom pain. *Pain* 1997;72:393–405.
32. Ribera H, Cano P, Dora A, et al. Phantom limb pain secondary to post-traumatic stump hematoma 40 years after amputation: description of one case. *Revista de la Sociedad Espanola del Dolor* 2001;8:217–220.

33. Rajbhandari SM, Jarett JA, Griffiths PD, et al. Diabetic neuropathic pain in a leg amputated 44 years previously. Pain 1999;83:627–629.
34. Jensen TS, Krebs B, Nielsen J, et al. Immediate and long-term phantom limb pain in amputees: incidence, clinical characteristics and relationship to pre-amputation limb pain. Pain 1985;21:267–278.
35. Hagberg K, Brånemark R. Consequences of non-vascular trans-femoral amputation: a survey of quality of life, prosthetic use and problems. Prosthet Orthot Int 2001;25:186–194.
36. Devor M, Govrin-Lippman R, Angelides K. Na+ channels immunolocalization in peripheral mammalian axons and changes following nerve injury and neuroma formation. J Neurosci 1993;135:1976–1992.
37. Houghton AD, Nicolls G, Houghton AL, et al. Phantom pain: natural history and association with rehabilitation. Ann R Coll Surg Engl 1994;76:22–25.
38. Sherman RA. Phantom limb pain. Mechanism-based management. Clin Podiatr Med Surg 1994;11:85–106.
39. Jensen TS, Krebs B, Nielsen J, et al. Phantom limb, phantom pain and stump pain in amputees during the first 6 months following limb amputation. Pain 1983;17:243–256.
40. Bailey AA, Moersch FP. Phantom limb. Can Med Assoc J 1941;45:37–42.
41. Wall R, Novotny-Joseph P, MacNamara TE. Does preamputation pain influence phantom limb pain in cancer patients? South Med J 1985;78:34–36.
42. Frazier SH. Psychiatric aspects of causalgia, the phantom limb, and phantom pain. Dis Nerv Syst 1966;27:441–451.
43. Saris SC, Iacono RP, Nashold BS. Dorsal entry zone lesions for post amputation pain. J Neurosurg 1985;62:72–76.
44. Sherman RA, Barja RH, Bruno GM. Thermographic correlates of chronic pain: analysis of 125 patients incorporating evaluations by a blind panel. Arch Phys Med Rehabil 1987;68:273–279.
45. Miles JE. Phantom limb syndrome occurring during spinal anesthesia: relationship to etiology. J Nerv Ment Dis 1956;123:365–368.
46. Mackenzie N. Phantom limb pain during spinal anaesthesia. Recurrence in amputees. Anaesthesia 1983;38:886–887.
47. Martin G, Grant SA, MacLeod DB, et al. Severe phantom leg pain in an amputee after lumbar plexus block. Reg Anesth Pain Med 2003;28:475–478.
48. Murphy JP, Anandaciva SP. Phantom limb pain and spinal anaesthesia. Anaesthesia 1984;39:188.
49. Sellick BC. Phantom limb pain and spinal anaesthesia. Anesthesiology 1985;62:801–802.
50. Lee ED, Donovan K. Reactivation of phantom limb pain after combined interscalene brachial plexus block and general anesthesia: successful treatment with intravenous lidocaine. Anesthesiology 1995;82:295–298.
51. Devor M, Govrin-Lippman R, Angelides K. Na+ channels immunolocalization in peripheral mammalian axons and changes following nerve injury and neuroma formation. J Neurosci 1993;135:1976–1992.
52. Devor M, Jänig W, Michaelis M. Modulation of activity in dorsal root ganglion neurones by sympathetic activation in nerve-injured rats. J Neurophysiol 1994;71:38–47.
53. Mannion RJ, Doubell TP, Gill H, et al. Deafferentation is insufficient to induce sprouting of A-fibre central terminals in the rat dorsal horn. J Comp Neurol 1998;393:135–144.
54. Ma QP, Tian L, Wollf CJ. Resection of sciatic nerve retriggers central sprouting of A-fibre primary afferents in the rat. Neurosci Lett 2000;288:215–218.
55. Nikolajsen L, Jensen TS. Postamputation pain. In: Melzack R, Wall PD, eds. Handbook of Pain Management. Edinburgh: Churchill Livingstone. 2003;247–257.
56. Doubell TP, Mannion RJ, Woolf CJ. The dorsal horn: state-dependent sensory processing, plasticity and the generation of pain. In: Wall PD, Melzack R, eds. Textbook of Pain. 4th ed. Edinburgh, New York: Churchill Livingstone. 1999;165–181.
57. Nikolajsen L, Hansen CL, Nielsen J, et al. The effect of ketamine on phantom limb pain: a central neuropathic disorder maintained by peripheral input. Pain 1996;67:69–77.
58. Waxman SG, Hains BC. Fire and phantoms after spinal cord injury: Na+ channels and central pain. Trends Neurosci 2006;29:207–215.
59. Melzack R. Phantom limbs and the concept of a neuromatrix. Trends Neurosci 1990;13:88–92.
60. Giummarra MJ, Gibson SJ, Georgiou-Karistianus N, et al. Central mechanisms in phantom limb perception: the past, present and future. Brain Res Rev 2007;54:219–232.
61. Arena JG, Sherman RA, Bruno GM, et al. The relationship between situational stress and phantom limb pain: cross-lagged correlational data from six-month pain logs. J Psychosom Med 1990;34:71–77.
62. Gallagher P, Allen D, Maclachlan M. Phantom limb pain and residual limb pain following lower limb amputation: a descriptive analysis. Disabil Rehabil 2001;23:522–530.
63. Jenkins WM, Merzenich MM, Ochs MT, et al. Functional reorganization of primary somatosensory cortex in adult owl monkeys after behaviorally controlled tactile stimulation. J Neurophysiol 1990;63:82–104.
64. Lotze M, Grodd W, Birbaumer N, et al. Does use of a myoelectric prosthetis prevent cortical reorganization and phantom limb pain? Nature Neurosci 1999;2:501–502.
65. Chan BL, Witt R, Charrow AP, et al. Mirror therapy for phantom pain. N Engl J Med 2007;357:2206–2207.
66. Gehling M, Tryba M. Prophylaxis of phantom pain: is regional analgesia ineffective? Schmerz 2003;17:11–19.
67. Jahangiri M, Jayatunga AP, Bradley JWP, et al. Prevention of phantom pain after major lower limb amputation by epidural infusion of diamorphine, clonidine, and bupivicaine. Ann R Coll Surg Engl 1994;76:324–326.
68. Wilson JA, Nimmo AF, Fleetwood-Walker SM, et al. A randomized double blind trial of the effect of pre-emptive epidural ketamine on persistent pain after lower limb amputation. Pain 2008;135:108–118.
69. Malawer MM, Buch R, Khurana JS, et al. Postoperative infusion continuous regional analgesia. A technique for relief of postoperative pain following major extremity surgery. Clin Orthop 1991;266:227–237.
70. Pinzur MS, Garla PGN, Pluth T, Vrbos L. Continuous postoperative infusion of a regional anesthetic after an amputation of the lower extremity: a randomized clinical trial. J Bone Joint Surg Am 1996;78:1501–1505.
71. Madabhushi L, Reuben SS, Steinberg RB, et al. The efficacy of postoperative perineural infusion of bupivacaine and clonidine after lower extremity amputation in preventing phantom limb and stump pain. J Clin Anesth 2007;19:226–229.
72. Grant AJ, Wood C. The effect of intra-neural local anaesthetic infusion on pain following major limb amputation. Scott Med J 2008;53:4–6.
73. Wilder-Smith CH, Hill LT, Laurent S. Postamputation pain and sensory changes in treatment-naive patients: characteristics and responses to treatment with tramadol, amitriptyline, and placebo. Anesthesiology 2005;103:6189–6128.
74. Robinson LR, Czernicki JM, Ehde DM, et al. Trial of amitriptyline for relief of pain in amputees: results of a randomized controlled study. Arch Phys Med Rehabil 2004;85:1–6.
75. Kuiken TA, Schechtman L, Harden RN. Phantom limb pain treatment with mirtazapine: a case series. Pain Pract 2005;5:356–360.
76. Patterson JF. Carbamazepine in the treatment of phantom limb pain. South Med J 1988;81:1100–1102.
77. Elliott F, Little A, Milbrandt W. Carbamazepine for phantom-limb phenomena. N Eng J Med 1976;295:678.
78. Bone M, Critchley P, Buggy DJ. Gabapentin in postamputation phantom limb pain: a randomized, double-blind, placebo-controlled, cross-over study. Reg Anesth Pain Med 2002;27:481–486.
79. Nikolajsen L, Finnerup NB, Kramp S, et al. A randomized study of the effects of gabapentin on postamputation pain. Anesthesiology 2006;105:1008–1015.
80. Harden RN, Houle TT, Remble TA, et al. Topiramate for phantom limb pain: a time-series analysis. Pain Medicine 2005;6:375–378.
81. Mishra S, Bhatnagar S, Singhal AK. High-dose morphine for intractable phantom limb pain. Clin J Pain 2007;23:99–101.
82. Bergmans S, Snijdelaar DG, Katz J, et al. Methadone for phantom limb pain. Clin J Pain 2002;18:203–205.
83. Huse E, Larbig W, Flo H, et al. The effect of opioids on phantom limb pain and cortical reorganization. Pain 2001;90:47–55.
84. Wu CL, Tella P, et al. Analgesic effects of intravenous lidocaine and morphine on post amputation pain: a randomized double blind, active placebo controlled, crossover trial. Anesthesiology 2002;96:841–848.
85. Stannard CF, Porter GE. Ketamine hydrochloride in the treatment of phantom limb pain. Pain 1993;54:227–230.
86. Nikolajsen L, Hansen PO, Jensen TS. Oral ketamine therapy in the treatment of postamputation stump pain. Acta Anaesthesiol Scand 1997;41:427–429.
87. Jaeger H, Maier C, Wawersik J. Postpoerative treatment of phantom pain and causalgias with calcitonin. Anaesthesist 1988;37:71–76.
88. Eichenberger U, Neff F, Sveticic G, et al. Chronic phantom limb pain: the effects of calcitonin, ketmaine, and their combination on pain and sensory thresholds. Anesth Anal 2008;106:1265–1273.
89. Atesalp AS, Ozkan Y, Komurcu M, et al. The effects of capsaicin in phantom limb pain. Agri 2000;12:30–33.
90. Blankenbaker WL. The care of patients with phantom limb pain in a pain clinic. Anesth Analg 1977;56:842–846.
91. Wassef MR. Phantom pain with probable reflex sympathetic dystrophy: efficacy of fentanyl infiltration of the stellate ganglion. Reg Anesth 1997;22:287–290.
92. Lierz P, Schroegendorfer K, Choi S, et al. Continuous blockade of both brachial plexus with ropivacaine in phantom pain: a case report. Pain 1998;78:135–137.
93. Halbert J, Crotty M, Cameron ID. Evidence for the optimal management of acute and chronic phantom pain: a systematic review. Clin J Pain 2002;18:84–92.
94. Kern U, Martin C, Scheicher S, et al. Treatment of phantom pain with botulinum-toxin A. A pilot study. Schmerz 2003;17:117–124.
95. Kern U, Martin C, Scheicher S, et al. Effects of botulinum toxin type B on stump pain and involuntary movements of the stump. Am Jo Phys Med Rehabil 2004;83:396–399.
96. Kern U, Martin C, Scheicher S, et al. Does botulinum toxin A make prosthesis use easier for amputees? J Rehabil Med 2004;36:238–239.
97. Dahl E, Cohen SP. Perineural injection of etanercept as a treatment for postamputation pain. Clin J Pain 2008;24:172–175.
98. Katz J, Melzack R. Auricular transcutaneous electrical nerve stimulation (TENS) reduces phantom limb pain. J Pain Symptom Manage 1991;6:73–83.
99. Katz J, France C, Melzack R. An association between phantom limb sensations and stump skin conductance during transcutaneous electrical nerve stimulation (TENS) applied to the contralateral leg; a case study. Pain 1989;36:367–377.
100. Seigfried J, Zimmerman M. Phantom and stump pain. Berlin: Springer Verlag; 1981:148–155.

101. Bittar RG, Otereo S, Carter H, et al. Deep brain stimulation for phantom limb pain. *J Clin Neuerosci* 2005;12:399–404.
102. Bittar RG, Kar-Purkayastha I, Owen SL, et al. Deep brain stimulation for pain relief: a meta-analysis. *J Clin Neurosci* 2005;12:515–519.
103. Sol JC, Casaux J, Roux FE, et al. Chronic motor cortex stimulation for phantom limb pain: correlation between pain relief and functional imaging studies. *Stereotact Funct Neurosurg* 2001;77:172–176.
104. Prantl L, Schremi S, Heine N, et al. Surgical treatment of chronic phantom limb sensation and limb pain after lower limb amputatino. *Plast Reconstr Surg* 2006;118:1562–1572.
105. Sakai Y, Ochi M, Uchio Y, et al. Prevention and treatment of amputation neuroma by an atelocollagen tube in rat sciatic nerves. *J Biomed Mater Res B Appl Biomater* 2005;73:355–360.
106. Ramanavarapu V, Simopoulos TT. Pulsed radiofrequency of lumbar dorsal root ganglia for chronic post-amputation stump pain. *Pain Physician* 2008; 11:561–566.
107. Sehirlioglu A, Ozturk C, Yazicioglu K, et al. Painful neuroma requiring surgical excision after lower lomb amputation caused by landmine explosions. *Int Orthop* 2007. In Press.
108. Sherman RA, Gall N, Gormley J. Treatment of phantom limb pain with muscular relaxation training to disrupt the pain-anxiety-tension cycle. *Pain* 1979; 6:47–55.
109. Sherman RA. Stump and phantom limb pain. *Neurol Clin* 1989;7:249–264.
110. Harden RN, Houle TT, Green S, et al. Biofeedback in the treatment of phantom limb pain: a time-series analysis. *Applied Psycho Biofeed* 2005:30:83–93.
111. Oakley DA, Whitman LG, Halligan PW. Hypnotic imagery as a treatment for phantom limb pain: two case reports and a review. *Clin Rehabil* 2002; 16:368–377.
112. Ramachandran VS, Rogers-Ramachandran D. Synaesthesia in phantom limbs induced with mirrors. *Proc R Soc Lond B Biol Sci* 1996;263:377–386.
113. Moseley GL. Graded motor imagery for pathologic pain: a randomized controlled trial. *Neurology* 2006;67:2129–2134.
114. Murray CD, Pettifer S, Howard T, et al. The treatment of phantom limb pain using immersive virtual reality: three case studies. *Disabil Rehabil* 2007;29: 1465–1469.
115. Schneider J, Hoffman A, Rost C, et al. EMDR in the treatment of chronic phantom limb pain. *Pain Med* 2008;9:76–82.
116. Portnoy S, Yarnitzky G, Yizhar Z, et al. Real-time patient-specific finite element analysis of internal stresses in the soft tissues of a residual limb: a new tool for prosthetic fitting. *Ann Biomed Eng* 2007;35:120–135.
117. Lotze M, Flor H, Grodd W, et al. Phantom movements and pain: an fMRI study in upper limb amputees. *Brain* 2001;124:2268–2277.
118. Gruber H, Glodny B, Bodner G, et al. Practical experience with sonographically guided phenol instillation of stump neuroma: predictors of effects, success, and outcome. *AJR Am J Roentgenol* 2008;190:1263–1269.
119. Bradbrook D. Acupuncture treatment of phantom limb pain and phantom limb sensation in amputees. *Acupunct Med* 2004;22:93–97.
120. Rasmussen KG, Rummans TA. Electroconvulsive therapy for phantom limb pain. *Pain* 2000;85:297–299.

CHAPTER 27 ■ HERPES ZOSTER AND POSTHERPETIC NEURALGIA

RAJBALA THAKUR, JOEL L. KENT, AND ROBERT H. DWORKIN

INTRODUCTION

The objective of this chapter is to provide an overview of the clinical presentation and management of herpes zoster and its most common complication, postherpetic neuralgia (PHN). Herpes zoster is a viral infection caused by the reactivation of the varicella-zoster virus (VZV). The primary varicella infection occurs when the patient contracts chicken pox. Following the resolution of chicken pox, the virus then remains dormant in dorsal sensory ganglia and cranial nerve ganglia for years to decades. Individuals are asymptomatic while the virus is dormant, and reactivation of VZV results in a characteristic vesicular dermatomal rash. Some patients with herpes zoster develop PHN, and this persisting neuropathic pain can last for years.

Herpes zoster afflicts millions of older adults worldwide each year and causes significant suffering and disability because of both the acute pain that occurs in association with the rash and the chronic pain that is present in those patients who develop PHN. VZV-induced neuronal destruction and inflammation causes pain that interferes with activities of daily living and reduces quality of life. Recent advances have improved our ability to both diminish the incidence of these conditions as well as manage the remaining cases more effectively. These advances include the development of a herpes zoster vaccine, consensus that antiviral therapy and aggressive pain management can reduce the burden of this disease, the identification of efficacious treatments for PHN, and the recognition of PHN as a study model for neuropathic pain research.

CLINICAL PICTURE AND NATURAL HISTORY OF HERPES ZOSTER

Herpes zoster is a neurodermatomal illness that does not cross the midline. Typically, a single dermatome is affected in immunocompetent patients, although in some cases, involvement of adjacent dermatomes can be seen due to normal variation of cutaneous innervation. In immunocompromised patients there can be cutaneous dissemination and, rarely, visceral dissemination. The sequence of events described in the following sections is typically observed.

Prodrome

Herpes zoster may begin with fatigue, headache, or flulike symptoms, including fever, neck stiffness, malaise, and nausea. This may be accompanied by unilateral dermatomal pain and abnormal sensations, including pruritis. The prodromal symptoms usually precede the appearance of a rash by 3 to 7 days, although longer periods have been reported. The prodrome probably occurs in association with the initiation of viral replication and the accompanying inflammatory response. This process results in ganglionitis, as well as the destruction of neurons and supporting cells in the dorsal root ganglion and accompanying dermatome.[1,2] In cases where patients experience a prolonged course of prodromal symptoms, diagnostic investigations are frequently undertaken to identify other medical conditions that may cause pain in the affected anatomical distribution. Common examples of this include pursuing the diagnosis of glaucoma in cases of herpes zoster ophthalmicus, sciatica in cases of sacral dermatomal involvement, and angina, renal colic, or cholecystitis in cases of truncal involvement. Diffuse or regional adenopathy is seen in a minority of cases and has not been correlated with any residual or long-term complications.

Rash

The reactivated virus replicates in the sensory ganglion and travels antidromically via the cutaneous nerves to the nerve endings at the dermoepidermal junction. Further replication in the skin results in tissue inflammation and necrosis which ultimately leads to the appearance of a rash in the same distribution as the prodrome. The rash is initially maculopapular and evolves into the classic appearance of grouped vesicle formations on an erythematous base. Regional lymphadenopathy may appear at this stage. Over the next 7 to 10 days the lesions progress to a pustular rash. Open lesions will develop superficial crusting. Scabs are cleared within 2 to 3 weeks. Skin in the affected region may be left completely normal or may develop a patchwork of either hypo- or hyperpigmented scarring (Fig. 27.1).

Pain

Pain often precedes or accompanies the herpes zoster rash.[3-5] Pain may be accompanied by other sensations such as itching, paraesthesias, and dysaesthesias. The timing of the pain may be constant or intermittent, and the quality of the pain is variously described as burning, throbbing, stabbing, electric shock-like, or various combinations of these. It is frequently associated with increased tactile sensitivity and allodynia (i.e., pain in response to a normally nonpainful stimulus). The pain may interfere with the patient's sleep and other aspects of physical and emotional functioning. The acute pain associated with herpes zoster gradu-

ally resolves in most patients around the time that the rash resolves. Pain that persists beyond the acute phase of the rash is considered subacute herpetic neuralgia or PHN, depending on its duration. A distinction between these three phases of pain associated with herpes zoster has been identified and is useful in both clinical and research settings. Acute herpetic neuralgia has been defined as pain that occurs within 30 days of rash onset, subacute herpetic neuralgia as pain that persists beyond 30 days from rash onset but that resolves before the diagnosis of PHN can be made, and PHN as pain that persists for 120 days or more after rash onset (Fig. 27.2).

Distribution of Herpes Zoster

Thoracic dermatomes are the most commonly affected sites. These are followed, in order of incidence, by the ophthalmic division of the trigeminal nerve, other cranial nerves, and cervical, lumbar, and sacral dermatomes (Table 27.1). The reason for this pattern is not understood, but it has been speculated that this may reflect the characteristic distribution of the chicken pox rash. The pattern of rash seen in herpes zoster follows the same centripetal distribution observed with the primary varicella infection. Patients can develop lesions in the adjoining dermatomes, and much less commonly, a diffuse cutaneous or even visceral dissemination can occur, most often in immunocompromised individuals.

Clinical Variants

Herpes Zoster Ophthalmicus (HZO)

HZO occurs in approximately 10% to 20% of herpes zoster cases. For unknown reasons, involvement of the ophthalmic branch of the fifth cranial nerve is five times as common compared with cases involving the maxillary or mandibular branches.

Order of Rash Progression

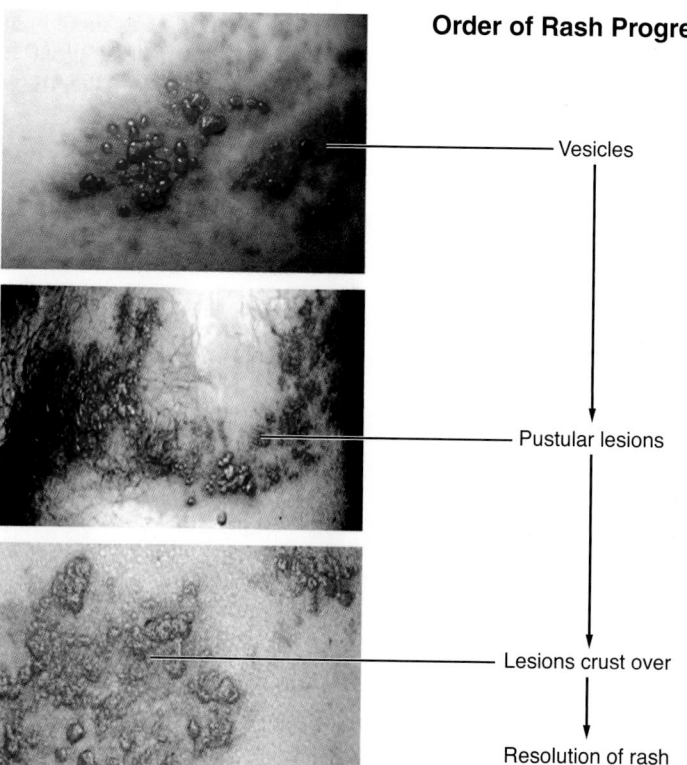

Vesicles

Pustular lesions

Lesions crust over

Resolution of rash

FIGURE 27.1 Herpes zoster rash progression. (From Weinberg M. Herpes zoster: epidemiology, natural history, and common complications. *J AM Acad Dermatol* 2007;57:S130–S135, with permission.)

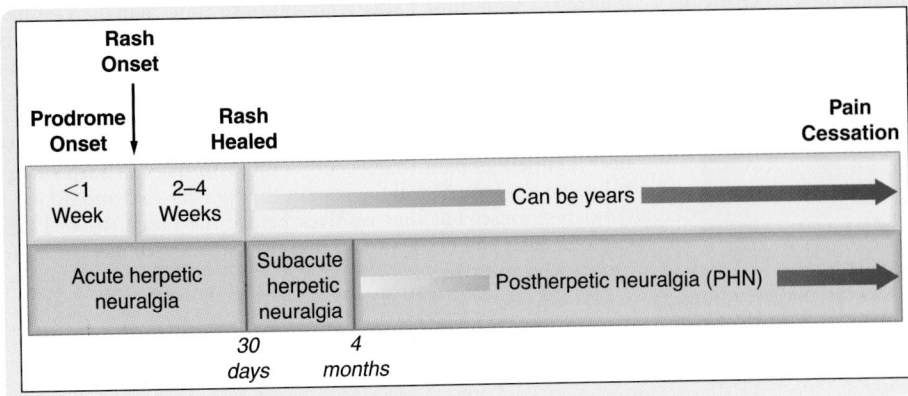

FIGURE 27.2 Natural history of herpes zoster and postherpetic neuralgia.

It is easily recognized by the presence of vesicles and erythema of the ipsilateral forehead and upper eyelid. HZO requires particularly prompt treatment and careful follow-up monitoring because of the possibility of ocular involvement, which occurs in approximately one-half of patients with HZO (Fig. 27.3).

Herpes Zoster Oticus (Ramsay-Hunt Syndrome)

This presentation of herpes zoster is relatively rare but this may reflect, at least in part, a failure to properly recognize and diagnose cases. Classically, herpes zoster oticus begins with otalgia and the formation of herpetiform vesicles within the external ear canal. Associated findings that may be present include facial paralysis resulting from facial nerve (cranial nerve VII) involvement, auditory symptoms including unilateral deafness, and/or vestibular symptoms. This condition may also result from zoster of the ninth or tenth cranial nerves because the external ear has complex innervation by branches of several cranial nerves (V, VII, IX, and X), as well as vertebral nerves C2 and possibly C3.

Zoster Sine Herpete

Herpes zoster infections presenting with only dermatomal pain in the absence of rash have been described in the literature for many years.[6,7] The actual prevalence of this condition is unknown. Positive serology in the acute or convalescent phase is the only definitive way to establish the diagnosis in such patients. Given that it would be rare to perform the required serological studies early in the disease course in most clinical settings, this diagnosis is rarely established in a definitive manner.

DIAGNOSIS OF HERPES ZOSTER

The diagnosis of herpes zoster is usually established based upon the clinical findings of a characteristic dermatomal rash (Fig.

TABLE 27.1

DERMATOMAL DISTRIBUTION OF HERPES ZOSTER IN IMMUNOCOMPETENT PATIENTS

Thoracic: up to 50% of all cases
Cranial: 10% to 20%
Cervical: 10% to 20%
Lumbar: 10% to 20%
Sacral: 2% to 8%
Generalized: <1%

27.4) and the presence of associated pain. The differential diagnosis frequently includes contact dermatitis. Herpes simplex virus (HSV) infection must also be considered, particularly if sacral dermatomes are involved. The main differentiating features of an HSV infection are that it tends to occur predominantly around the mouth or genitalia, there is a higher prevalence in younger patients verses the predilection for herpes zoster to afflict more elderly patients, and HSV has a propensity for recurrent outbreaks which are rare in herpes zoster. In cases of atypical presentations or when there is confusion as to whether VZV or HSV is the pathogen, diagnosis can be confirmed by laboratory testing.

Laboratory Testing

Viral Culture

Isolation of the virus in cell cultures can be done but takes 1 to 2 weeks to complete. The virus is also quite labile and may be difficult to recover from lesion swabs. This test has low sensitivity but high specificity. Treatment of presumed cases should not be delayed to await culture results given the prolonged turnaround time and low sensitivity (and thus high false negative rate) of the test.

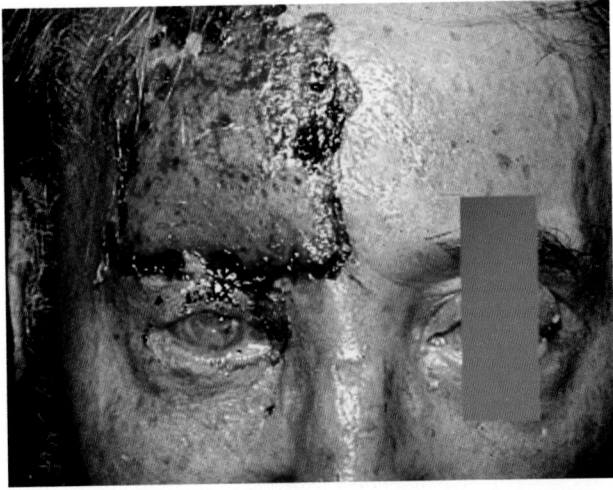

FIGURE 27.3 Ophthalmic zoster. (Reproduced from Dworkin RH, Johnson RW, Breuer J, et al. Recommendations for the management of herpes zoster. *Clin Infect Dis* 2007;44(1):S1–S26, with permission.)

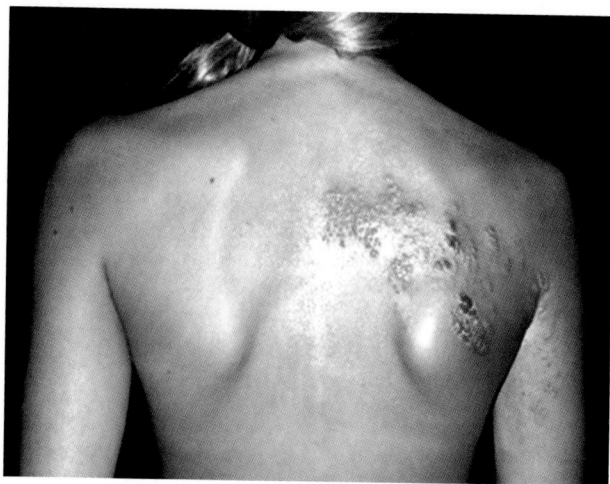

FIGURE 27.4 Herpes zoster rash in the T2 dermatomal distribution. (Reproduced from Dworkin RH, Johnson RW, Breuer J, et al. Recommendations for the management of herpes zoster. *Clin Infect Dis* 2007; 44(1):S1–26, with permission.)

Direct Immunofluorescence Assay

Direct immunofluorescence assay is often preferable to viral culture due to its low cost and rapid turnaround time, which can be within 3 hours. Sensitivity is approximately 90% but decreases if the lesions are beyond the vesicular stage.

Viral DNA Testing

Viral DNA can be detected in the vesicle fluid and cutaneous tissue by polymerase chain reaction (PCR) technology. It has the advantage that it can be effective even on old and crusted lesions. It has a turnaround time of 1 day but is generally more expensive than other approaches. This test has exceptional sensitivity and specificity of almost 100%.

Biopsy

A biopsy is not typically needed in clinical practice and should be reserved for difficult to diagnose cases. Histological findings of ballooning degeneration and acantholysis of keratinocytes resulting in intraepidermal vesicles are common to all herpes infections. Multinucleated giant cells with accentuation of nuclear material at the periphery of the nuclei are present. Underlying leukocytoclastic vasculitis is often a prominent finding and helps differentiate zoster from other herpesvirus infections.

Testing for Underlying Disorders

If clinically indicated, testing for HIV or occult malignancy may be advisable, but this is typically not necessary and is not recommended on a routine basis.

EPIDEMIOLOGY OF HERPES ZOSTER

The epidemiology of herpes zoster is primarily affected by a combination of the incidence of primary varicella infections in the population as well as age and level of immunosuppression in the population. At the present time, the lifetime incidence of herpes zoster is 20% to 30%. This incidence is likely to change in the future as a result of implementation of childhood varicella vaccination. At the present time herpes zoster is among the most common of neurological illnesses, affecting about 1 million people in

the United States,[8] 1.7 million in the European Union, 100,000 in Canada, and 80,000 in New Zealand and Australia annually. Primary varicella infection typically affects children in temperate climates and adolescents and young adults in tropical climates.[9] The incidence of herpes zoster in Asia and South America is not well studied, but is thought to follow the same pattern as in the U.S. and Europe despite regional differences in patient demographics for primary varicella infection.[10]

Increasing age is the most potent risk factor for herpes zoster in both immunocompetent and immunocompromised individuals (Table 27.2). The incidence of herpes zoster in all age groups is 1.2 to 4.8 cases per 1000 persons per year and increases to 7.2 to 11.8 cases per 1000 persons per year in persons older than 60.[11] The prevalence reaches approximately 50% in individuals living to be 85 years of age.[12,13]

Immunocompromised individuals have a relatively high risk for developing herpes zoster.[14] Patients with a history of HIV infection, solid organ and bone marrow transplantation, immunosuppressive chemotherapy, or systemic lupus erythematosus are 20 to 100 times more likely to develop herpes zoster compared to immunocompetent individuals. Immunocompromised individuals also experience higher recurrence rates of zoster compared to those who are immunocompetent.

Other factors that appear to increase the risk for herpes zoster that are less well replicated include Caucasian versus African-American racial group, presence of elevated psychological stress and/or physical trauma,[15,16] and being female.[17] Exposure to varicella antigen, either through contact with chicken pox or by vaccination, has a protective effect and reduces the incidence of herpes zoster.[8,18]

The epidemiology of varicella and herpes zoster is likely to change as childhood vaccination against the primary infection alters the long established relationships between humans and this viral infection. The incidence of primary varicella infections has declined dramatically in the United States since the implementation of routine childhood vaccination.[19] It has been hypothesized that there will be an initial increased incidence of herpes zoster in the coming decades as the opportunities for subclinical immune boosting in aging adults, which result from exposure to VZV, will decline due to the decreased incidence of chicken pox.[20–22] Adults living in regions where there is widespread varicella vaccination may therefore experience a higher incidence of herpes zoster compared with past generations unless herpes zoster immunization becomes widespread. Such vaccination would confer the immunological boost that past generations obtained through episodic exposure to children with chicken pox. In a similar manner, a single episode of herpes zoster boosts immunity to VZV and thereby appears to prevent recurrent bouts of zoster. This likely

TABLE 27.2

FACTORS ASSOCIATED WITH AN INCREASED INCIDENCE OF HERPES ZOSTER

1. Increasing age
2. Disease states
   HIV
   Lymphoproliferative disorders
3. Immunosuppressive therapy
   After organ transplant
   Chemotherapy
   Steroid treatment
4. Possible association with
   Caucasian vs. African-American racial group
   Psychological stress
   Physical trauma

explains why recurrent zoster is rare,[8,12,23,24] with an incidence generally estimated as less than 5%.[12,25–28] Eventually, as children immunized against VZV grow into adulthood, the number of adults infected with latent wild-type virus will decrease and the incidence of herpes zoster is expected to decline because the live attenuated virus used in the varicella vaccine appears to be less likely to reactivate and cause herpes zoster.

PATHOPHYSIOLOGY OF HERPES ZOSTER AND MECHANISMS OF ACUTE PAIN

As noted above, herpes zoster most commonly manifests in the distribution of a single dorsal sensory or cranial nerve ganglion. Why the reactivation occurs in one ganglion when latent virus is present throughout the patient's sensory ganglia is not clear. Declining cellular immunity is a major risk factor for reactivation of the virus, which is thought to occur when cell-mediated immunity falls below a critical level.[12] This impression is supported by evidence that even individuals with adequate levels of serum antibodies to VZV antigen can, over time, exhibit T cells with reduced ability to proliferate and defend against VZV infections.[23] Hence, cell-mediated immunity appears to play a crucial role in preventing reactivation of latent VZV (Fig. 27.5). Common causes of decreased cellular immunity include increasing age, various diseases, and immune-suppressing medical interventions, all of which are risk factors for herpes zoster.

During reactivation of the virus, newly synthesized viral particles are transported in a retrograde and anterograde fashion to the central and distal axons of the involved spinal or cranial sensory ganglion. Viral replication causes inflammatory and neural tissue injury in the affected dermatome,[1] which can ultimately result in infectious hemorrhagic necrosis and subsequent neuronal loss and scarring centered in the sensory ganglion of affected cranial and peripheral nerves.[1,29] Microscopic examination of the zoster affected ganglion shows significant hypocellularity and collagen scarring. The corresponding peripheral nerves may exhibit a long-lasting reduction in myelinated axons and increased numbers of small unmyelinated axons. These structural changes contribute to the pain and other characteristic sensory findings along the corresponding sensory dermatomes of the involved ganglion. Excessive electrical activity in the damaged peripheral nociceptors is the major cause of pain in the acute herpes zoster infection. Although VZV is a sensory-specific virus, involvement of anterior horn cells, autonomic neurons, and leptomeninges can be observed as a result of a bystander effect,[30] with consequent muscle weakness, palsy, and/or pleocytosis of spinal fluid.

COMPLICATIONS ASSOCIATED WITH HERPES ZOSTER

In general, the frequency and severity of complications are greater in older and immunocompromised individuals. The most common morbidity of herpes zoster in immunocompetent individuals is the development of PHN; this often severe pain can persist well beyond the resolution of herpes zoster. This complication will be discussed in detail in the second half of this chapter.

Ophthalmic Complications

The incidence of complications associated with HZO has been reported to be 2% to 6% of cases. A variety of complications have been described,[31] including retinitis, keratitis, iritis, scleritis, secondary glaucoma, and ptosis. These are obviously serious problems that can result in temporary or permanent deterioration in visual acuity or complete blindness. For these reasons, patients with ophthalmic zoster should be evaluated by an ophthalmologist as promptly as possible following diagnosis.

Motor Neuropathy

Motor nerve involvement is present in 5% to 15% of patients presenting with herpes zoster. Paresis in extraocular nerves, facial nerves, and a variety of other motor nerves has been described. Diaphragmatic paresis is not an uncommon occurrence with the involvement of the phrenic nerve, and intercostal nerve involvement may lead to paresis of intercostal muscles (Fig. 27.6). Involvement of cervical motor nerve roots may present as shoulder and arm weakness, and lower extremity weakness can occur when lumbosacral nerve roots are affected. In some cases, significant motor weakness may be the presenting symptom, and this can delay accurate diagnosis. In general, paresis improves with time and physical rehabilitation; however, the likelihood and completeness of muscle function recovery appears to decrease with older age and greater initial severity of the paralysis.

Rare Neurological Complications

VZV is a common cause of aseptic meningitis. Most patients with VZV meningitis experience a complete resolution of the symptoms in 1–2 weeks,[32] although meningeal involvement can result in long-term sequelae from subsequent scarring of the involved neural structures. Myelitis and encephalitis are other rare central manifestations of reactivated VZV. VZV encephalitis can present as an acute delirium accompanied by few focal neurologi-

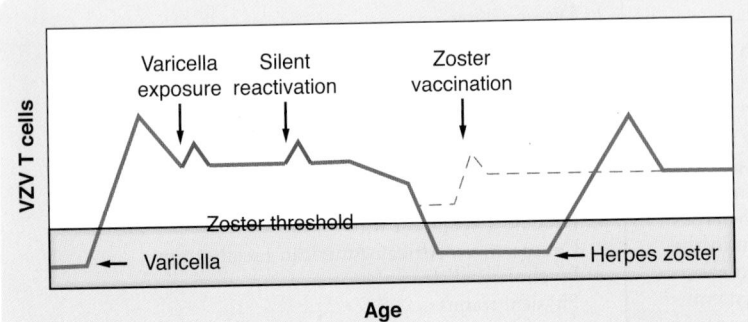

FIGURE 27.5 Host factors in VZV latency and reactivation. Varicella is the primary infection caused by VZV, and its resolution is associated with the induction of VZV-specific memory T cells (blue line). Memory immunity to VZV may be boosted periodically by exposure to varicella or silent reactivation from latency (red peaks). VZV-specific memory T cells decline with age. The decline below a threshold (black line below zoster threshold) correlates with an increased risk of zoster. The occurrence of zoster, in turn, is associated with an increase in VZV-specific T cells. The administration of zoster vaccine to older persons may prevent VZV-specific T cells from dropping below the threshold for zoster occurrence (dashed blue line). (Redrawn after Arvin A. Aging, immunity, and the varicella-zoster virus. *N Engl J Med* 2005;352:2266–2267, with permission.)

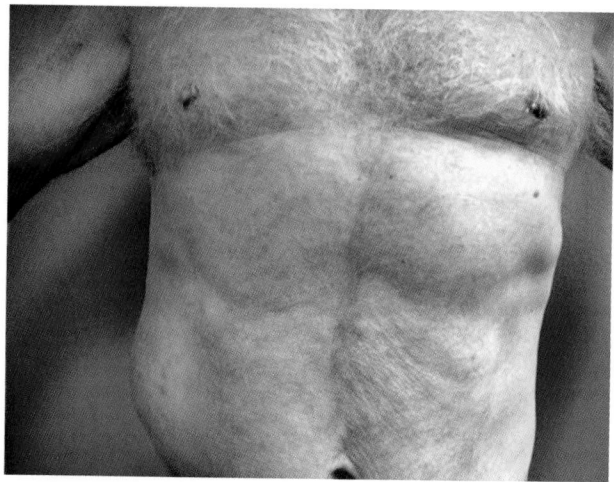

FIGURE 27.6 T8 motor neuropathy in an otherwise healthy 59-year-old man who presented with vesicles in the T8 distribution 4 weeks before this photo was taken. The patient was treated with an antiviral agent for 7 days and with analgesics as needed. As the rash resolved, this bulge became apparent; it is consistent with motor damage by varicella zoster virus to the muscles of the abdomen. (Reproduced from Dworkin RH, Johnson RW, Breuer J, et al. Recommendations for the management of herpes zoster. *Clin Infect Dis* 2007;44(1):S1–26, with permission.)

cal signs.[33] Factors that elevate the risk of central nervous system (CNS) involvement include the presence of altered immune function, cranial nerve or ophthalmic involvement, and evidence of cutaneous dissemination. Although more common in immunocompromised patients, CNS involvement has been reported in both immunocompetent and immunocompromised individuals[34] and in both children and adults.[35]

Visceral Complications

Visceral involvement in herpes zoster is rare but may result in organ dysfunction as a consequence of scar formation around the involved structures. In such cases, the associated signs and symptoms would be related to the specific structures mechanically affected by scarring.

Decreased Quality of Life

The acute pain associated with herpes zoster can cause significant suffering and is often accompanied by interference in the patient's ability to carry out normal activities of daily living. In addition, acute pain is associated with the greater use of analgesic medications and their attendant side effects, most notably sedation and constipation.[36–40] The resultant impact of herpes zoster on health-related quality of life is at least as great as what has been found with other chronic diseases such as diabetes or congestive heart failure.[39]

TREATMENT OF HERPES ZOSTER

All patients should have a thorough medical evaluation with added attention to factors related to the individual's immunocompetence. Patient education, reassurance, and supportive therapy are essential to allay fears and promote compliance with pharmacological therapy. The primary goals of pharmacological therapy are to reduce pain and prevent ongoing viral replication. Limiting viral replication has been shown to reduce the incidence

and severity of acute pain associated with herpes zoster. The primary pharmacological approaches include the use of antiviral therapy in conjunction with analgesic agents. Steroids have also been used, but their role is more controversial. The potential roles of neural blockade and neuroaugmentation strategies are also controversial.

Patient Education

It is important to educate patients and their family members about their disease. Patients and caretakers can be reassured that herpes zoster does not cause any illness in seropositive individuals who have contact with the patient. Herpes zoster does, however, pose a risk of viral transmission to individuals who do not have preexisting immunity to VZV. Given this, it is important for patients with herpes zoster to avoid contact with individuals who are known to be seronegative for VZV or have known or suspected immune system impairment, especially if it is unclear whether they have a history of chicken pox. Patients should be counseled regarding maintaining appropriate nutrition and optimal levels of social and physical activities. In addition, patients should be told to keep the rash area clean and to avoid application of ointments or adhesive dressings because these can cause skin irritation and secondary infections. Patients should inform their physician if fever, confusion, or other significant constitutional symptoms develop, and should return for further evaluation if rash healing appears delayed.

Antiviral Therapy

Antiviral therapy has been shown to be efficacious in suppressing viral replication and also has beneficial effects on both acute and chronic pain (Table 27.3).[41–43] Antiviral medication is recommended for all herpes zoster patients who are older, have a moderate to severe rash, have ophthalmic involvement, or are immunocompromised.[44] In current clinical practice, most physicians prescribe antiviral therapy to all patients with herpes zoster because of the very favorable risk benefit ratio of these medications. Antiviral treatment should be started as soon as possible; this should ideally be within 72 hours of the onset of rash, the inclusion criterion for initiating treatment in the clinical trials of antiviral agents in herpes zoster patients. The early initiation of antiviral therapy is intuitively logical and an important treatment objective. However, viral replication may continue beyond the third day after rash onset, suggesting that even delayed antiviral therapy may provide some benefit. Unfortunately, there are no well-designed clinical trials examining the efficacy of initiating antiviral therapy beyond 72 hours of rash onset. Two uncontrolled trials examined the effectiveness of antiviral treatment initiated at a later time and the results suggested that such treatment may have beneficial effects.[45,46] In clinical practice, the diagnosis of herpes zoster is often not made within 72 hours of the onset of symptoms; nevertheless, it is important to identify pa-

TABLE 27.3
BENEFITS OF ANTIVIRAL THERAPY[41,42,46,48,49,51,52,53]
• Inhibition of viral replication • Reduces duration of viral shedding • Hastens rash healing • Decrease in degree of neural damage • Decreases severity and duration of acute pain • Decreases duration of postherpetic neuralgia • Decreases incidence of postherpetic neuralgia

tients who could still benefit from antiviral medication even when it is initiated relatively late in the disease course. One example of patients who warrant such later initiation of treatment is those with ophthalmic zoster. The duration of viral shedding from the ocular surface is highly variable[47] and may continue for a longer period of time. Immunocompromised patients, those with disseminated zoster, and patients with neurological complications should also be started on antiviral medication irrespective of whether they are beyond 72 hours of rash onset.

There are two main classes of antiviral medication and these are differentiated by their reliance on viral phosphorylation to be activated. The first class of drugs requires phosphorylation by viral thymidine kinase and includes acyclovir, brivudin, famciclovir, and valacyclovir (Table 27.4). These drugs are phosphorylated to a triphosphate form that impairs viral replication by inhibiting viral DNA polymerase. Acyclovir, famciclovir, and valacyclovir are all available in the United States and are approved by the FDA for the treatment of herpes zoster. These medications are excreted renally, and dosages should therefore be adjusted in patients with renal insufficiency. Special dosing regimens are also needed in patients on dialysis. Acyclovir must be taken five times daily for 7 days, whereas famciclovir and valacyclovir are taken three times daily. Thus, patient compliance with famciclovir and valacyclovir is likely to be considerably greater than with acyclovir, and this may translate to somewhat greater efficacy. Famciclovir and valacyclovir may also be somewhat better than acyclovir in reducing the incidence of prolonged pain.[48-50] Although brivudin is currently not available in the United States, it has been approved for the treatment of herpes zoster in several other countries; it is dosed once daily for 7 days.

The second class of antiviral medications is not dependent on viral phosphorylation. These agents noncompetitively inhibit viral DNA polymerase, and include vidarabine, foscarnet, and cidofovir. Foscarnet is useful in patients with known resistance to acyclovir due to lack of viral thymidine kinase, which can be seen in patients with AIDS or prolonged exposure to acyclovir (as in transplant patients). Hence, this agent plays an important role in treating infections in individuals with known resistance to acyclovir.

Analgesic Treatment

Antiviral therapy does not completely abolish the acute pain associated with herpes zoster (nor does it completely prevent PHN), and supplemental analgesic medications are required in most pa-

TABLE 27.4

ANTIVIRAL MEDICATIONS FOR HERPES ZOSTER

All antivirals are renally excreted, hence dosage needs to be adjusted in patients with renal insufficiency, including patients on dialysis. Nausea and headache are common side effects.

Medication	Oral bioavailability	Dosage	Duration of treatment (Days)	Uncommon side effects	Special considerations
Acyclovir	15% to 30%	800 mg 5 times daily (every 4–5 h)	7–10	Neurotoxicity and nephrotoxicity	Additive nephrotoxic effects with cyclosporine
Famciclovir	77%	500 mg 3 times daily (approved dosage in United States; in some other countries, 250 mg 3 times daily is approved	7		Probenecid, theophylline increase levels of famciclovir. Digoxin levels increased
Valacyclovir	55%	1000 mg 3 times daily	7		Thrombotic thrombocytopenic purpura/hemolytic uremic syndrome reported at dosages of 8000 mg daily in immunocompromised patients
Foscarnet	NA	40–90 mg/kg I/V for induction and 120 mg/kg/day for maintenance therapy	10–14 days for induction and variable duration for maintenance	Nephrotoxicity, neurotoxicity, neutropenia, anemia	Increased risk of nephrotoxicity with cyclosporine. Increased risk of seizures with ciprofloxacin
*Brivudin		125 mg once daily	7		Contraindicated for patients treated with 5-fluorouracil or other 5-fluoropyrimidines because of drug interaction associated with severe and potentially fatal bone marrow suppression

*Not available in the United States

tients. Effective analgesia improves patient comfort and may also reduce the risk of PHN beyond what is achieved by antiviral therapy alone.[54,55] These considerations argue for aggressive management of the acute pain associated with herpes zoster. A multimodal analgesic strategy should be used to balance efficacy, safety, and tolerability of the medication regimen. Unfortunately, well-designed studies to delineate which combinations of therapies are optimal have not been conducted. In lieu of focused studies, clinicians must use the available data, extrapolate available information, and individualize therapy based on patient-specific factors. The World Health Organization analgesic ladder can be applied as one useful analgesic strategy with well-proven efficacy and ease of application. Patients with mild pain can be started on acetaminophen alone or in combination with a mild opioid analgesic such as tramadol. Nonsteroidal anti-inflammatory drugs (NSAID)s can also be used provided there are no contraindications to their use. Patients with moderate pain can be started on short-acting opioid medications and, if tolerated, can be converted to a timed-release preparation if clinically warranted. Opioids have not been well-studied in patients with herpes zoster, but one recent clinical trial did show that controlled-release oxycodone was superior to placebo in relieving acute pain within the first 2–3 weeks of rash onset, although the small sample size precluded an evaluation of the effect of this treatment on the development of PHN.[56]

If acute pain in herpes zoster patients is not adequately controlled with the analgesics mentioned above, other medications that have demonstrated efficacy in the treatment of chronic neuropathic pain can also be used in combination with antiviral therapy.[44] Gabapentin, pregabalin, and tricyclic antidepressants such as nortriptyline and desipramine can be considered in patients when conventional analgesic medications are not adequate in managing acute pain. Studies are limited, but a single-dose trial of 900 mg of gabapentin vs. placebo did demonstrate a reduction in acute pain over 6 hours in patients with herpes zoster.[57] Both gabapentin and pregabalin would seem like reasonable alternatives because they not only have efficacy in the treatment of PHN but have also demonstrated efficacy in reducing pain and analgesic requirements in some acute pain conditions.[58,59]

Although tricyclic antidepressants have not been well-studied in patients with herpes zoster, they have proven efficacy in chronic neuropathic pain and are additional rational choices for treating acute pain associated with herpes zoster. Dual reuptake inhibitors (selective serotonin and norepinephrine reuptake inhibitors) can be considered in lieu of tricyclic antidepressants given their more favorable side effect profiles. Both duloxetine and venlafaxine have demonstrated efficacy in painful diabetic peripheral neuropathy[60,61] and could thus be considered a potential therapy for the treatment of acute pain in patients with herpes zoster.

A pragmatic approach is to start with a short-acting opioid in combination with acetaminophen or an NSAID. Gabapentin or pregabalin can then be added if conventional analgesics are not entirely effective. Many clinicians would use one of these medications rather than a tricyclic antidepressant because of their generally safer side effect profile. The analgesic regimen should be tailored based on the individual patient's needs and tolerances (Table 27.5). Frequent follow up and reassessment are vital to assess efficacy and tolerability while titrating analgesic therapy.

Corticosteroids

The use of corticosteroids in the treatment of herpes zoster has been controversial.[62,63] One placebo-controlled trial demonstrated a benefit in terms of significantly accelerated return of uninterrupted sleep, cessation of analgesic therapy, and return to normal activity in patients treated with the combination of a corticosteroid and acyclovir as compared to those treated with

acyclovir alone.[63] The patients in this trial were 60 years of age on average and possessed no contraindications to corticosteroid treatment. Based on these results, the addition of oral corticosteroids can be considered in healthy older adults with moderate-to-severe pain unrelieved by antiviral therapy and analgesics, provided there are no contraindications to steroid use. Oral steroids are empirically used in VZV-induced facial nerve palsy or other cases of cranial neuritis, although there is limited evidence supporting the effectiveness of such treatment. It must be emphasized that corticosteroids should not be used alone in herpes zoster and must be initiated in combination with antiviral therapy.

Neural Blockade

If pain is not controlled with medical management, referral to a pain specialist should be considered for possible invasive interventions. Sympathetic blockade or neuraxial local anesthetic infusion can be considered. Additionally, perilesional infiltration of local anesthetics and steroids is advocated by some clinicians. All these interventions have been used for years in clinical practice but few controlled studies have been conducted to systematically examine their effects on herpes zoster acute pain or the development of PHN.[64,65] A recent randomized trial demonstrated significant reduction in acute pain following a single epidural injection of steroid and local anesthetic within the first month after rash onset as compared to standard therapy alone. The incidence of developing PHN, however, was not altered in this study.[66] In another study, continuous epidural infusion of local anesthetic with intermittent boluses was found to be superior to continuous infusion of saline and intermittent boluses of local anesthetic in reducing the time to complete resolution of pain in herpes zoster patients who were concomitantly treated with oral acyclovir.[67] This type of treatment requires home nursing care and careful coordination of care under the supervision of a pain physician and should only be considered in the small subset of patients who have relatively severe pain that is not adequately controlled by simpler measures.

There are also some data supporting the use of sympathetic blockade in the treatment of pain associated with herpes zoster.[64] These nerve blocks are used by some clinicians in cases where acute pain has been refractory to more conventional therapy. However, it is also hypothesized that sympathetic blockade may favorably affect the progression of herpes zoster acute pain to PHN because the effective treatment of acute pain may prevent the development of PHN, or at least decrease the severity of subsequent PHN. Unfortunately, randomized clinical trials evaluating this hypothesis are lacking.

Spinal Cord Stimulation

Spinal cord stimulation has been tried in a case series of four patients with herpes zoster and reported to be effective.[68] It is difficult to extrapolate these results to routine clinical practice as the majority of patients with herpes zoster have resolution of their symptoms as part of the natural history of the disease.

PREVENTION OF HERPES ZOSTER

Childhood Vaccination

The propensity to develop herpes zoster and PHN can ultimately be traced back to an individual's primary varicella infection. Thus, one obvious prevention strategy would include the prevention of the primary VZV infection through the use of varicella vaccination in childhood. Two types of vaccines are approved by

TABLE 27.5

PHARMACOLOGICAL OPTIONS THAT CAN BE CONSIDERED FOR TREATMENT OF ACUTE PAIN IN HERPES ZOSTER

Medication	Initial dose	Titration	Maximum daily dose	Side effects
Acetaminophen	500–1000 mg every 6 hrs as needed	Not needed	2.6 g in elderly; 4 g in younger patients	Liver toxicity with prolonged use; avoid alcohol use
NSAIDs (dosages given are for ibuprofen)	400 mg every 6 hrs as needed	Not needed	2400 mg	Gastrointestinal side effects, CV and renal toxicity and increased bleeding tendency
With Opioid analgesics (dosages given are for oxycodone)	5 mg every 4 h as needed	Increase by 5 mg 4 times daily every 2 days as tolerated; dosage can be converted to extended release opioid analgesic combined with short-acting medication as needed	No maximum dosage with careful titration	Nausea/vomiting, constipation, sedation, dizziness
Or Tramadol	50 mg once or twice daily	Increase by 50–100 mg daily in divided doses every 2 days as tolerated; dosage can be converted to extended release preparation combined with immediate release one as needed	400 mg daily (100 mg 4 times daily); for patients >75 years of age, 300 mg daily in divided doses	Nausea/vomiting, constipation, sedation, dizziness, seizures, postural hypotension
Gabapentin	300 mg at bedtime or 100–300 mg 3 times daily	Increase by 100–300 mg 3 times daily every 2 days as tolerated	3600 mg daily (1200 mg 3 times daily; reduce if renal function is impaired)	Sedation, dizziness, peripheral edema
Or Pregabalin	75 mg at bedtime or 75 mg twice daily	Increase by 75 twice daily every 3 days as tolerated	600 mg daily (300 mg twice daily; reduce if renal function is impaired)	Sedation, dizziness, peripheral edema
Tricyclic antidepressants, especially nortriptyline	25 mg at bedtime	Increase by 25 mg daily every 2–3 days as tolerated	150 mg daily	Sedation, dry mouth, blurred vision, weight gain, urinary retention
Oral corticosteroid (dosages given for prednisone)	60 mg daily for 7 days	After 60 mg daily for 7 days, decrease to 30 mg daily for 7 days, then decrease to 15 mg daily for 7 days, and then discontinue	60 mg daily	Gastrointestinal distress, nausea, changes in mood, edema

Note: Dose of opioids, pregabalin, and TCAs can be reduced in frail elderly individuals. Consider a screening electrocardiogram for patients with preexisting cardiac disease.
CV, Cardiovascular; NSAID, Non-steroidal anti-inflammatory drugs.
Adapted with permission from Dworkin RH, Johnson RW, Breuer J, et al. Recommendations for the management of herpes zoster. Clin Infect Dis 2007;44: S1–S26.

the FDA for vaccination in children from 12 months to 12 years of age; both are based on the Oka virus. The first agent is a single antigen vaccine, and the more recent vaccine is a combination product and protects against multiple childhood infections (i.e., measles, mumps, rubella, and varicella). The live attenuated Oka vaccine virus establishes latency in sensory ganglia, like wild-type VZV, but it appears to cause herpes zoster much less frequently. Hence, childhood varicella vaccination should eventually result in an overall decrease in the incidence of herpes zoster and PHN.

Varicella-Zoster Immunoglobulin

Temporary passive immunization may be required in specific circumstances. The United States Centers for Disease Control and Prevention currently recommends administration of varicella-zoster immune globulin (VZIG) to prevent or modify clinical illness in immunocompromised seronegative persons with recent exposure to patients with chicken pox or zoster. VZIG provides maximum benefit when administered as soon as possible after the presumed exposure, but VZIG may be effective if administered as late as 96 hours after exposure. Protection after VZIG administration lasts for an average of approximately 3 weeks. Treatment with VZIG should be followed by vaccination if possible.

Herpes Zoster Vaccination for Adults

Herpes zoster is caused by reactivation of VZV from a single sensory ganglion. It appears likely that seropositive adults derive a degree of protection from this viral reactivation by episodic exposure to children with chicken pox and a resulting boost in VZV-specific cellular immunity. With implementation of childhood vaccination programs and the decreased incidence of primary varicella infection in the general population, the majority of adults will not have such exposure and thus could have less protection against reactivation of VZV. Adult vaccination can confer the immunological boost to our current adult population that past generations had obtained through episodic exposure to children with chicken pox infections.

The Shingles Prevention Study—a large, multicenter, randomized, placebo-controlled trial—was conducted to evaluate the efficacy and safety of herpes zoster vaccination.[8] The results of the trial indicated that the herpes zoster vaccine reduces the likelihood of developing herpes zoster in immunocompetent individuals 60 years of age or older. Important results of this study included a decrease in the incidence of herpes zoster by 51.3%, a reduction in the overall burden of illness (BOI) by 61.1%, and a decrease in the incidence of PHN by 66.5%.[69] The effect on decreasing the incidence of herpes zoster was less in older subjects but the effect on reducing the severity of illness was greater in older subjects. Hence the overall reduction in BOI, the primary endpoint of the study, was maintained across all age groups. Based on these data, the FDA approved the use of the herpes zoster vaccine in individuals 60 years and older. This live, attenuated vaccine is contraindicated in children, pregnant women, and immunocompromised individuals. The vaccine has minor side effects, including local skin irritation. No clinically meaningful systemic side effects were observed. This vaccine is not interchangeable with the varicella vaccines used for the primary prevention of chicken pox; although all these vaccines contain the same attenuated strain of VZV, they vary in concentration of plaque forming units.

CLINICAL PICTURE OF PHN

PHN is the most common complication of herpes zoster in the immunocompetent patient. This condition results in significant patient suffering and causes a large economic burden to society. Our ability to diagnose and treat PHN has benefited from recent consensus among researchers as to its definitions and guidelines for treatment of chronic neuropathic pain conditions. Currently, the term PHN is used to describe dermatomal pain that persists for more than 120 days after the onset of the herpes zoster rash.[70] Pain persisting for more than 180 days after the rash onset is less likely to resolve and hence can be considered "well established PHN" to reflect its recalcitrant nature.[71]

A variety of signs and symptoms are characteristic of patients with PHN, although none are pathognomonic. These include various types of stimulus-independent pain, for example, intermittent sharp, shooting, or electric shock-like pain and continuous burning or throbbing pain. Stimulus-evoked pain is also very common in patients with PHN and includes tactile allodynia, one of the most debilitating symptoms associated with this condition. Tactile allodynia can be so severe that patients with truncal PHN may not be able to tolerate the sensation of clothing against their skin and those with craniofacial PHN may not be able to wear hats, glasses, or tolerate even breezes or air conditioning on the affected site. Hyperalgesia, which is an abnormally increased perception of pain in response to a painful stimulus, can occur with application of painful thermal or mechanical stimuli. These types of stimulus-independent and stimulus-evoked pain are caused by nerve damage (i.e., neuropathic pain), but musculoskeletal pain can also occur in patients with PHN as a result of excessive guarding of the affected area. Myofascial trigger points, atrophy, and reduced joint range of motion may be seen in severe cases where pain has resulted in excessive guarding.

Additional sensory abnormalities are also common in PHN. Involved areas may be hypoesthetic, which can occur even in regions that exhibit tactile allodynia. The areas of altered tactile sensitivity may become larger than the sites originally affected by the zoster rash. Alterations in temperature sensation have also been demonstrated. Various paresthesias and dysesthesias (abnormal or unpleasant but not painful sensations) can also occur. Chronic pruritis can persist or develop following herpes zoster and is particularly problematic for some individuals; it may be present with or without comorbid pain.

Areas of hyperpigmentation, hypopigmentation, or scarring may be present in the affected dermatomes following rash healing, and affected areas may also exhibit a persistent reddish or brownish hue. These cosmetic changes do not occur in all patients and the skin in the affected dermatome is normal in appearance in many patients with PHN.

Although less well-studied and generally less disabling than pain, altered motor function occurs in herpes zoster and can persist after rash healing. Facial paralysis may be evident in the form of ptosis or loss of the nasolabial fold in cases of facial nerve involvement. In cases of thoracic involvement, a truncal bulge resulting from intercostal muscle weakness may be present (Fig. 27.6).

Diagnosis and Assessment of PHN

PHN is diagnosed primarily based upon clinical findings. A history of herpes zoster rash, followed by persistent pain in the same distribution, usually establishes the diagnosis. Occasionally, patients report having a quiescent period between the resolution of the initial herpes zoster-associated pain and the onset of the pain associated with PHN. In a study of 156 patients with PHN, Watson et al.[76] noted that 25% of patients with a poor outcome said that they could recall a time after the rash when they had little or no pain. This pain free hiatus has been observed to last for a period of weeks to as much as 12 months. The recurrence of dermatomal pain is not associated with a recurrent episode of herpes zoster but may coincide with changes in the patient's emotional or physical status. As mentioned above, a clear history of rash may not be present in all patients. In these cases, a definitive diagnosis of VZV-related pain would require serial serologic assessments that are unlikely to be obtained in most clinical settings.

In addition to assessing the location, intensity, and characteristics of the pain, it is important to evaluate the overall impact that the pain has had on the patient. PHN can cause significant deleterious impacts on physical, emotional, and social functioning and therefore can have a widespread adverse effect on health-related quality of life.[72,74,77,78] PHN can result in fatigue, insomnia, anxiety, depression, and suicidal ideation, and careful screening for the presence of any psychiatric comorbidities or any escalation of pre-existing psychiatric symptoms should be performed.

Laboratory Diagnosis

Diagnostic tests have limited application in the clinical management of PHN patients. A variety of studies may be used but are predominately limited to clinical research settings. These include quantitative sensory testing (QST), skin biopsy, and nerve conduction studies. QST has been used to identify different phenotypic subtypes of PHN patients with distinct constellations of signs and symptoms, which are thought to reflect different pathophysiologic mechanisms. This is an especially interesting area of future research, and the hope is that such phenotypic subtypes will ultimately be used to guide mechanism-based treatment.

EPIDEMIOLOGY AND NATURAL HISTORY OF PHN

Systematic studies of the epidemiology of specific chronic pain conditions are very rare, and limited information is available regarding the incidence and prevalence of PHN. The lack of consistency in defining PHN hampers efforts to study its epidemiology, and estimates of the incidence and prevalence of PHN will vary depending on which definition is used. Estimates of the prevalence of PHN have ranged from 500,000 to 1 million in the United States,[79,80] but could decrease if herpes zoster vaccination becomes widespread. If PHN is defined as pain persisting beyond 120 days from rash onset,[70,81–83] available data indicate that 10% to 25% of herpes zoster patients will develop PHN[12,76,84–86]; however, the precise figures differ greatly depending on whether patients in the community or in clinical trials are studied.

PHN is a chronic pain syndrome that can last for years. There is a relative paucity of data on its natural history due to the lack of population-based studies of zoster-related pain. Multiple studies consistently indicate that the majority of patients experience resolution of pain over weeks to months following rash onset.[41,72,76,87] The presence of persistent pain 1 year after the initial diagnosis of PHN has been described to be present in 20% of patients over the age of 60.[25,88,51] There are few prospective studies that have followed patients for more than 6 months following the diagnosis of PHN. Hence, the exact number of patients who enjoy a complete resolution of PHN is unknown.

Risk Factors for PHN

The most well-established risk factors for PHN in patients with herpes zoster include older age, presence of a painful prodrome, greater severity of acute pain, and greater rash severity.[72,73] Increasing age is a particularly potent risk factor for the development of PHN. Approximately 20% of patients older than 50 years of age continue to have pain at 6 months after the onset of rash despite starting antiviral agents in a timely fashion.[41,49,73,74] Using a shorter duration of pain, patients 50 years of age or older were shown to have a 14.7-fold higher prevalence (95% CI, 6.8–32.0) of pain 30 days after rash onset compared with

TABLE 27.6

RISK FACTORS FOR PHN[17,25,83,88,89,90,91]

Well replicated
- Older age
- Severity of rash
- Severity of acute pain
- Prodromal pain

Less well replicated
- Female gender
- Greater sensory abnormalities in the affected dermatomes
- Polyneuropathy
- Psychosocial variables
- Ophthalmic distribution

patients younger than 50 years.[75] Elderly patients also seem to be predisposed to developing particularly refractory cases of PHN that do not respond to currently available treatments.[76] Other risk factors for PHN are listed in Table 27.6.

PATHOPHYSIOLOGY OF PHN

Viral replication is thought to result in a combination of neural and inflammatory damage, leading to sensitization of the peripheral and central sensory neural elements. There is evidence that various risk factors identified for the development of PHN make independent contributions to the likelihood of developing this chronic pain condition,[72,83] and these risk factors may reflect distinct underlying pathophysiological mechanisms. For instance, elderly patients who are at high risk for PHN are more likely to have a subclinical polyneuropathy, which may reduce the amount of viral damage needed to cause PHN.[92,93] Other examples of the possible relationships between risk factors for PHN and underlying mechanisms include the presence of a prodrome, reflecting earlier and more extensive viral damage in the affected sensory ganglion;[94] greater rash severity, reflecting greater damage to and loss of epidermal nerve fibers;[95–97] and severe acute pain, reflecting the initiation of processes that ultimately result in central and peripheral sensitization.[98,99] These relatively independent processes may combine to cause more severe cases of PHN.

More severe zoster infections are accompanied by greater neural damage, and it has been proposed that this neural damage contributes prominently to the development of PHN.[98] However, knowledge of the pathophysiological mechanisms of PHN is quite limited. It is mainly derived from autopsy and skin biopsy neuroanatomical studies and research on patterns of sensory dysfunction and pharmacologic response. A variety of pathophysiological mechanisms have been described and are hypothesized to be causally related to the qualitatively different types of pain associated with PHN. Different mechanisms may coexist in an individual patient, and there may be pathophysiologically distinct subgroups of patients.[100,101]

Modern anatomical understanding is based on data limited by the small number of patients studied to date. Watson[94] and colleagues compared autopsy tissue from patients with and without PHN following herpes zoster. They found that patients with PHN showed marked atrophy of the spinal cord dorsal horn on the ipsilateral versus contralateral side, a difference that was not present in the patients with a history of zoster but not PHN. Punch skin biopsy permits quantitative measurement of epidermal sensory nerve endings. Such studies have shown that PHN patients have reduced innervation density in the affected dermatome compared

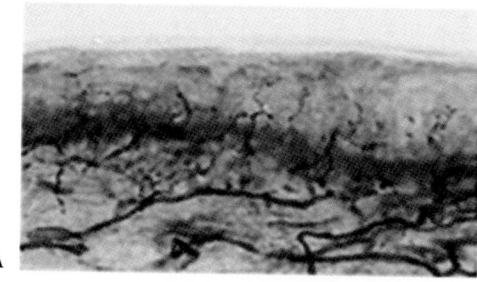

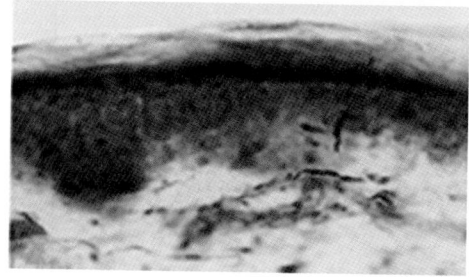

FIGURE 27.7 Representative, immunolabeled, dermal sensory nerve endings from skin biopsies of previously shingles-affected skin, with and without postherpetic neuralgia (PHN). (**A**) Biopsy from the previously affected shingles site on the back of a 75-year-old woman without PHN (1672 epidermal neuritis/mm^2). (**B**) Biopsy from the previous affected shingles site of a 72-year-old woman with PHN (145 neurites/mm^2). The epidermis is at the top of the image and the dermis is at the bottom. Individual neurites and neurite bundles are visible in the superficial dermis. (Reproduced from Oaklander AL. The density of remaining nerve endings in human skin with and without postherpetic neuralgia after shingles. *Pain* 2001;92:139–145, with permission.)

to the contralateral side (Fig. 27.7). Notably, in both the postmortem and skin biopsy studies, pathological features were only identified in PHN patients and were not found in patients with a history of zoster who did not go on to develop PHN.

Sensory testing can be used to investigate the function of small afferent fibers including nociceptors. This type of testing helps create a detailed sensory profile of the affected area. Rowbotham and Fields[100,101] have conducted an important series of studies of sensory dysfunction and pharmacologic response in an attempt to address the pathophysiology of PHN. The results of this research, along with that of others, have emphasized the role of central processes in interpreting sensory dysfunction and its relationship to pain in patients with PHN,[102–104] and have suggested that two different pathophysiological mechanisms contribute to the development of PHN—sensitization and deafferentation.

Both peripheral and central sensitization appear to contribute to PHN. Peripheral sensitization occurs predominately in small unmyelinated C fiber nociceptors. Clinically, there can be minimal sensory loss in areas of marked allodynia.[97,100,103] However, thermal sensory thresholds can be decreased (heat hyperalgesia) by up to 2° to 4° C[95,105] in allodynic regions. Heat hyperalgesia is a well-known consequence of peripheral nociceptor sensitization.[95] These observations all suggest that sensitization of C nociceptors can be responsible for the spontaneous burning pain and heat hyperalgesia seen in some patients. In many PHN patients, the area of mechanical or tactile allodynia is much larger than the area originally affected during herpes zoster and the painful area may continue to change with time. Allodynia in a subset of PHN patients may be caused by ectopic discharges from damaged C nociceptors maintaining a state of central sensitization.[100,106] The major excitatory neurotransmitter involved in spinal cord pain processing is glutamate, and binding at the NMDA receptor has been thought to play a key role in central sensitization.

Dynamic and tactile allodynia may also result from sprouting of A beta fibers into the superficial layers of the dorsal horn in response to partial loss of C fiber input. This sprouting may lead to connections between these fibers, which normally do not transmit pain, and the ascending pain pathways that were formerly responsive to C fiber input. This process would explain why non-painful stimuli such as light touch or pressure can become painful in patient with PHN.

Deafferentation may also be playing a significant role in the maintenance of PHN. In a subset of patients, there is a loss of both large and small diameter sensory afferent fibers. This loss of peripheral input can result in the development of spontaneous discharge in deafferented central neurons. This may produce constant pain in the area of sensory loss.[100] Interestingly, these patients may still suffer from severe mechanical allodynia.[107] Assuming that the dorsal root ganglion and central connections are lost in such patients, the pain may be due to intrinsic CNS changes.

The data above suggest that there may be subsets of patients within the PHN population who have different underlying mechanisms responsible for the generation and maintenance of their chronic pain. These different mechanisms may account for the varied presentations of pain in patients with PHN. Unfortunately, these observations have not yet been able to provide the foundation for a mechanism-based approach for selecting specific pharmacological treatment options in clinical practice. This, of course, would be an extremely desirable goal to improve the therapeutic effects of existing treatments.

TREATMENT OF PHN

Tricyclic antidepressants, various anticonvulsants, opioid analgesics, and topical lidocaine are efficacious in the management of PHN (Table 27.7). There is a limited role of invasive interventions and alternative modalities, but these are utilized for patients who are refractory to conservative modalities. The choice of which therapy is used is often individualized based upon the patient's comorbidities, concomitant medication use, and associated symptoms. Recent studies have evaluated the relative efficacy of these treatments.[108,109] Additionally, consensus recommendation and guidelines for the pharmacotherapeutic treatment of neuropathic pain, including PHN, have been published and serve as useful guides in selecting between the growing list of treatment options.[110–112] In clinical practice, certain anticonvulsants, topical lidocaine, and tramadol are often used as first-line medications, followed by tricyclic antidepressants and opioids. This is largely because the former agents are better tolerated in elderly patients. Needless to say, all patients should have a thorough assessment and treatment should be tailored to address their individual needs.

Anticonvulsants: Gabapentin and Pregabalin

Although a number of anticonvulsants have been used for many years for the treatment of PHN and other neuropathic pain conditions, the greatest evidence of efficacy exists for gabapentin and pregabalin. Both are well-tolerated and much less toxic than the first-generation anticonvulsants previously used to treat neuropathic pain. There is good evidence to support the use of gabapentin in PHN. Its use was associated with a statistically significant reduction in daily pain ratings as well as improvements in sleep, mood, and quality of life at daily dosages of 1800–3600 mg in two large clinical trials.[113,114] A meta-analysis of these trials indicated that the pooled NNT for gabapentin in the treatment of PHN is approximately 4.4 (95% CI, 3.3–6.1).[58] The precise mechanism of its analgesic action is not known, but evidence derived from rodent models suggests that gabapentin acts at the alpha-2 delta subunit of voltage dependent calcium channels to decrease calcium influx. This effect inhibits the release of the

TABLE 27.7

PHARMACOLOGICAL OPTIONS FOR THE TREATMENT OF PHN

Medication	Starting Dose	Dose-Escalation Scheme	Common Side Effects	Contraindications/Caution	Comments
Gabapentin	100–300 mg	Start qhs and increase to tid dosing; increase by 100–300 mg every 3 days to total dose of 1800–3600 mg	Somnolence, dizziness, fatigue, ataxia, peripheral edema, and weight gain	Decrease dose in patients with renal impairment. QOD dosing in dialysis patients	No clinically significant drug interactions, improved sleep Avoid sudden discontinuation
Pregabalin	50 mg tid or 75 mg bid	300–600 mg/day in 1 wk	Somnolence, fatigue, dizziness, peripheral edema and weight gain, blurred vision, and euphoria	Decrease dose in patients with renal impairment by 50% or more based on CL creatinine	Caution with concomitant use of ACE inhibitors-angioedema; Increased risk for weight gain and peripheral edema in patients on thiazolidinedione antidiabetic agents
Topical Lidocaine	5%, 1–2 patches	Can use up to 3 patches 12 h/d	Local erythema, rash, blisters	Known hypersensitivity to amide local anesthetics Caution in patients receiving class 1 antiarrhythmic drugs (e.g., tocainide and mexiletine)	No significant systemic side effects
Tramadol	50 mg every 6 hours prn	Can titrate up to 100mg q 6 hrs.; max daily dose: 400 mg Extended-release dosing once a day	Nausea/vomiting, constipation, drowsiness, and dizziness	Seizure disorder, concomitant use of SSRI, SSNRI, TCA medications. Decrease dose in patients with hepatic or renal disease	Available as combination products with ibuprofen/acetaminophen Extended release dose max is 300 mg/day
TCAs Nortriptyline Desipramine Amitryptiline	10–25 mg qhs	Increase by 10–25 mg weekly with a target dose of 75–150 mg	Sedation, dry mouth, blurred vision, weight gain, urinary retention, constipation, sexual dysfunction	Cardiac arrhythmic disease, glaucoma, suicide risk, seizure disorder. Concomitant use of tramadol, SSRI, or SSNRIs	The lower starting dose may be more appropriate in the elderly Amitryptyline has the most anticholinergic effects and hence less well tolerated by the elderly Obtain baseline ECG in patients with hx of cardiac disease
Opioids Morphine Oxycodone Methadone *Fentanyl patch	15 mg q 6 hrs prn 5 mg q 6 hrs prn 2.5 mg tid 12 mcg/hr	Titrate at weekly intervals balancing analgesia and side effects. If patient tolerating the medications can titrate faster	Nausea/vomiting, constipation, drowsiness and itching	Driving impairment and cognitive dysfunction during treatment initiation. Be careful in patients with sleep apnea. Additive effects of sedation with neuromodulators	Gradual titration monitoring GI and CNS side effects

ACE, Angiotensin-Converting Enzyme; CL, Clearance; CNS, Central Nervous System; GI, Gastro-intestinal; qhs, Every Night or At Every Bedtime; QOD, Every Other Day; SSNRI, Selective Serotonin-Norepinephrine Reuptake Inhibitor; SSRI, Selective Serotonin Reuptake Inhibitor; TCA, Tricyclic Antidepressant.
*May need to start a patient on short-acting opioid medications before changing over to a fentanyl patch.
Differences in recommended dosages of medications between tables 27.5 and 27.7 are in part because of the acuity of pain in herpetic neuralgia versus PHN.
Adapted with permission from Wu C and Raja S. An update on the treatment of postherpetic neuralgia. J Pain 2008;9:S19–S30

excitatory neurotransmitters, including glutamate.[115,116] As noted above, glutamate, via its effect at the NMDA receptor, is the primary neurotransmitter responsible for maintaining central sensitization.

Gabapentin is rapidly absorbed after oral administration. However, its absorption is mediated, at least in part, by a transport mechanism that becomes saturated at higher doses. This phenomenon reduces the bioavailability of gabapentin as the dose is increased. For example, the bioavailability of gabapentin at a dose of 300 mg is about 60%, but the bioavailability falls to 40% with a 600 mg dose. Peak serum concentrations are achieved approximately 3 hours after oral administration. Gabapentin does not exhibit significant protein binding, is eliminated unchanged via the kidneys, and is not metabolized by the liver.

The optimal dosing schedule for gabapentin has not been well characterized. A recent review suggested that dosing should be initiated at 300 mg on the first day, followed by 300 mg twice daily on the second day, and then increased to 300 mg three times daily on the third day.[117] At that point, the titration should be slowed down with a goal of reaching 600 mg three times daily over the ensuing 2 weeks. Daily dosages up to 3600 mg have been studied and shown efficacious.[113] The daily dosage should be divided into 3 or 4 doses per day as this drug has a relatively short half life. In elderly patients, dosages should be reduced and titration should be executed more slowly. In frail patients, it is typical to start with 100 mg/day, increasing by 100 mg every 3 to 4 days. Once patients are tolerating a daily dose of 600 mg, the titration rate may be increased by 300 mg/day every 3–4 days to a target of 1800–2400 mg/day. The titration schedule may need to be modified if efficacy is achieved at lower dosages or unmanageable side effects are encountered. Because gabapentin is excreted renally, dosages need to be adjusted in patients with renal insufficiency. Patients on dialysis should be started on a single dose of 100 mg given 1 hour after dialysis treatment on alternate days. This dose then can be titrated slowly and cautiously.

Side effects associated with gabapentin include somnolence, dizziness, peripheral edema, and gait or balance problems. In general these side effects are short lived, but they can require monitoring and, occasionally, dosage adjustment.

Pregabalin appears to have the same mechanism of action as gabapentin, and several large randomized clinical trials have demonstrated its efficacy in the treatment of PHN and other neuropathic pain conditions. Three double-blind trials comprising a total of 776 patients with PHN showed that pregabalin resulted in superior pain relief and improved pain-related sleep interference compared to placebo. Dosages in these studies ranged between 150–600 mg/day,[118] and both fixed as well as flexible dosing schedules have been efficacious in clinical trials.[119,120] Pregabalin can be given in two divided doses each day. Frequently reported side effects are the same as with gabapentin: somnolence, dizziness, peripheral edema, and balance problems.

Pregabalin has also been demonstrated to possess an anxiolytic effect[121,122] in patients with generalized anxiety disorder. Because patients with chronic pain often have comorbid anxiety disorders, it is possible that this anxiolytic effect may provide additional benefit in PHN patients. The analgesic efficacy and side effect profiles of gabapentin and pregabalin appear to be comparable. Pregabalin has greater convenience than gabapentin because of its twice daily dosing and simpler titration, however, and an effective analgesic dosage can be reached more rapidly with pregabalin.

Antidepressant Medications

Tricyclic Antidepressants

Tricyclic antidepressant medications have a number of proposed mechanisms that might explain their efficacy in the treatment of PHN. These include inhibition of the reuptake of norepinephrine and serotonin and sodium channel blockade.[123,124,125] There have been several clinical trials and meta-analyses of these agents demonstrating efficacy in the treatment of pain associated with PHN, with pooled data showing NNTs of 2.1–2.6.[58,126,127]

Amitriptyline has been the most widely studied antidepressant for PHN. Available evidence and clinical experience suggest that nortriptyline and desipramine[128] are equally effective[58,129] but are better tolerated than relatively more side effect prone amitriptyline. Thus, these secondary amine tricyclics are generally preferred, especially in elderly and frail patients. Both amitriptyline and nortriptyline are often helpful in patients with insomnia because of their sedating properties. Desipramine has significantly less sedation than these two medications and is thus preferred in patients who may be intolerant to the sedative effects of this class of medication.

Both significant side effects and toxicities must be considered when using tricyclic antidepressants. Major side effects include tachyarrhythmias, prolongation of QT intervals with the potential for the precipitation of life threatening arrhythmias, and the worsening of acute angle glaucoma. It would be prudent to review a baseline EKG before starting these medications in elderly patients or those who possess other risk factors for increased cardiac toxicity.[130,131] Minor side effects include dryness of mouth, dizziness, weight gain, sedation, constipation, urinary retention, and orthostatic hypotension. These medications should be started at a low dose, typically 25 mg at night, and titrated slowly to a target dose of 75–100 mg/day in a single evening dose. In elderly or frail individuals, these agents can be started using a 10 mg evening dose. Concomitant use with selective serotonin reuptake inhibitor antidepressants should be monitored carefully as there is a risk of developing toxic tricyclic serum levels and serotonin syndrome with such combinations.

Selective Serotonin and Norepinephrine Reuptake Inhibitors (Dual Reuptake Inhibitors)

Two antidepressant medications that are selective serotonin and norepinephrine reuptake inhibitors have shown efficacy in patients with painful diabetic and other peripheral neuropathies but have not been studied in PNH. Duloxetine is approved by the FDA for the treatment of painful diabetic peripheral neuropathy. Clinically, this medication seems to be better tolerated compared with tricyclic antidepressants and hence is being used in clinical practice for PHN. Two randomized clinical trials have shown that venlafaxine at higher dosages is also efficacious in painful diabetic and other peripheral neuropathies, but it has also not been studied in PHN.[111]

Opioid Analgesics

Historically, the role of opioid analgesics in the treatment of chronic nonmalignant pain, and particularly neuropathic pain, has been controversial. Recent evidence, however, has shown that this class of drugs is efficacious in neuropathic pain conditions, including PHN. They are now recommended as second or third line analgesics by several respected sources.[110,111,112] These sources reserve them as second and third line agents based upon concerns regarding their side effects, the potential for the development of tolerance, and concerns regarding misuse and abuse. The efficacy of these agents appears to be comparable to that of antidepressant and anticonvulsant medications.[132] The analgesic efficacy of oral oxycodone was evaluated in a double-blind, crossover trial in which treatment resulted in significant reductions in allodynia, steady pain, and spontaneous paroxysmal pain.[133] Oxycodone treatment also resulted in superior scores for global effectiveness, disability reduction, and patient preference compared to placebo. In another randomized crossover study, treatment with morphine (mean dose 91 mg/day) or methadone (mean dose 15 mg/day) was compared with placebo, and the opioids were associated with superior pain relief.[132] This study also made a direct comparison between opioids and tricyclic antidepressants. The NNT for opioids was 2.79 (2.01–4.6) compared to 3.73 (2.43–7.99) for the antidepressants.[132]

A quantitative review of pooled results for opioid therapy yielded an NNT of 2.67 (2.07–3.77).[58] It is noteworthy, however, that more frequent side effects were associated with the opioid therapy as compared to both tricyclics[132,134] and gabapentin[135] in head-to-head comparisons. If opioids are prescribed, the patients should be carefully counseled regarding common side effects such as nausea, sedation, urinary retention, pruritis, and constipation. Monitoring for immune suppression and hypogonadism is needed if opioid use is required chronically. Other adverse effects associated with chronic opioid use include tolerance, physical dependence, and opioid-induced hyperalgesia, which also require appropriate patient counseling and monitoring. Lastly, opioids cannot be prescribed without some risk of developing misuse, abuse, or addiction, but this appears to be relatively rare in elderly patients with no prior history of addictive disorders.

Clinical recommendations for the use of opioid analgesics in the treatment of PHN include the following: (1) use the lowest effective dose; (2) treatment can be initiated with short-acting opioids, for example, 5–10 mg oxycodone or 10–15 mg morphine every 4 hours as needed; (3) once a patient demonstrates tolerability to the initial opioid therapy, conversion can be made to a long-acting opioid preparation (controlled-release oxycodone or morphine, transdermal fentanyl patch, methadone, oxymorphone, or levorphanol), which can be further titrated up to an effective and well tolerated dose; (4) proactive effort should be made to anticipate and manage common side effects of nausea and constipation (with antiemetics and laxatives); and (5) regular assessment for efficacy and tolerability should be made. If the treatment is not effective, these medications should be tapered gradually to prevent the development of withdrawal symptoms.

Tramadol

Tramadol is an analgesic medication with a unique mechanism of action. It has a mu-agonist effect like opioids, but in addition it inhibits the reuptake of serotonin and norepinephrine like the antidepressants that are efficacious in neuropathic pain. It has been shown to possess efficacy in the treatment of PHN in a randomized, controlled trial in which a sustained release preparation was compared to placebo. Superior pain relief and improved quality of life was seen with tramadol,[136] and the NNT was 4.8 (CI 95%, 3.5–6.0). Tramadol can be dosed 50–100 mg every 4 hours on an as-needed basis. The daily dose should not exceed 400 mg. Lower doses should be used in the elderly and in patients with impaired renal function.

Adverse effects include nausea, vomiting, dizziness, constipation, urinary retention, somnolence, and headache. Concomitant use with medications that are inhibitors of CYP2D6, such as antidepressant medications, can lead to serotonin syndrome. Abuse of tramadol is thought to be rare but has been observed. Tramadol is associated with an increased risk of precipitating seizures in patients who have a history of seizures or who are also receiving drugs that can reduce the seizure threshold. These considerations usually result in clinicians avoiding tramadol in patients receiving CYP2D6 inhibitors or those patients at increased risk for seizures.

Topical Therapies

An inherent advantage of topical therapies is that they are associated with few systemic effects due to minimal systemic absorption of the medication. 5% lidocaine patches are the most commonly used topical modality for PHN in clinical practice and is the only one approved by FDA for this indication. Capsaicin cream and other compounded mixtures are used less commonly.

Topical Lidocaine

Five percent lidocaine patches result in a local analgesic effect. Clinical trials have shown greater efficacy with the use of lidocaine patches as compared to vehicle-controlled patches in PHN patients presenting with allodynia.[137,138] There was no significant difference in the side effects between patients receiving lidocaine versus the control patches. The suggested NNT is 4.4.[139] It is interesting to note that patients may respond well to topical lidocaine even if the skin at the targeted site appears to be completely devoid of nociceptors.[140] Lidocaine patches possess both excellent safety and tolerability profiles. Efficacy can be ascertained within 2 to 3 weeks of initiation of treatment, hence there is no need for a prolonged trial period. The side effects are minimal because of the minimal systemic absorption of the lidocaine. Lidocaine patches are not approved for use in herpes zoster and should not be used in patients with active zoster lesions.

Clinical recommendations for use of lidocaine patches in the treatment of PHN include the following: (1) the patches can be cut to fit the affected area (unlike fentanyl patches); (2) three patches can be applied with no additional risk of systemic side effects; (3) the recommendations are to keep the patches on for 12 hours and off for 12 hours but the patches can be left on for 18 hours at a time to improve effectiveness; (4) patches should be applied only on intact skin and directly over the area of maximum pain; (5) lidocaine gel has also been shown to be efficacious in patients with PHN and allodynia,[141] and its use can therefore be considered if lidocaine patches are not available, affordable, or their application is problematic.

Topical Capsaicin

Capsaicin is an extract of hot chili peppers and an agonist for the vanilloid receptor (TRPV1), which is present on afferent nociceptor terminals. There are no systemic effects with a local application. It is commercially available in two concentrations, 0.025% and 0.075%. Pooled data from two placebo-controlled studies demonstrated superior pain relief following 3–4 times/day application of 0.075% capsaicin to the painful areas compared to an inert topical agent. The NNT was 3.3.[142,143] Blinding in these studies was problematic given that capsaicin produces a distinct burning sensation on initial application. In clinical practice, it is difficult to use, especially in patients who are experiencing significant allodynia. Ironically, these are the very patients who would be expected to be most likely to benefit from this therapy. Recent large clinical trials have evaluated a single application of high concentration (8%) capsaicin following a local anesthetic application. The results of these studies indicate that this approach can produce prolonged relief of pain in some PHN patients.[144]

Low concentration capsaicin is rarely used as a first-line agent in patients with PHN. Patients should be warned about the unpleasant burning sensation it causes with initial application and to avoid contact with their eyes.

Other Topical Treatments

Topical anti-inflammatory preparations have been studied in a few randomized, placebo-controlled trials.[145] There was significant heterogeneity in these studies and definitive recommendations cannot be drawn from this literature. There have also been a few reports of other topical agents including tricyclic antidepressants and vincristine, as well as descriptions of novel delivery mechanisms, such as iontophoresis. The evidence for all these therapies is weak and they are generally not used in clinical practice.

Combination Therapy

Although the use of combination therapy is common in clinical practice, few clinical trials have provided an evidence base for this approach. One recent study has demonstrated that the combination of gabapentin and morphine was superior to either of these medications used alone in relieving pain in patients with either painful diabetic neuropathy or PHN.[135] The goal of combination therapy is to arrive at a balanced, multimodal approach that improves the efficacy and tolerability of treatment while minimizing side effects of the individual medications. Disadvantages of combination therapy include an increased risk of side effects as the number of medications is increased. It may also be difficult to determine which medication is responsible for side effects. Ideally, medications that can cause similar side effects (e.g., sedation) should not be started simultaneously. There should be a judicious interval of time (e.g., at least a week or more) before a new medication is introduced to the regimen.

Other Pharmacologic Therapies

A variety of other agents have been evaluated in the treatment of PHN and other neuropathic pain conditions. Several anticonvulsant and antidepressant medications besides those discussed above have shown evidence of efficacy in other neuropathic pain conditions in single clinical trials but lack convincing evidence of efficacy.[111] NMDA antagonists, including ketamine, dextromethorphan, and memantine, have been studied but no evidence is available for their efficacy in PHN. Similarly, the sodium channel blocker mexiletine has not demonstrated benefit in PHN, although there is some evidence of efficacy in painful diabetic peripheral neuropathy. However, this agent is usually avoided given its high toxicity profile. The use of all these medications can be considered in select circumstances, such as in cases where more conventional treatments have failed.

Invasive Treatments for PHN

A considerable percentage of PHN patients will not respond to currently available pharmacologic treatments. In these cases, a referral to a pain management center should be considered sooner rather than later. Invasive treatments may be considered for patients with refractory pain. A variety of interventional strategies have been described and examined as treatment options for PHN. Unfortunately, the studies conducted to date have either been relatively poorly controlled or have not been replicated by independent investigators (e.g., use of intrathecal methyl prednisone). Given the lack of objective evidence available to compare the efficacy of the various interventions available, the choice of specific therapy has been dependent on the treating physician's clinical experience. The lack of evidence demonstrating the efficacy of interventional treatments points more toward the lack of adequate research as opposed to the conclusion that these interventions are inherently ineffective.

Sympathetic Nerve Blocks

The sympathetic nervous system is considered to be important in mediating pain in some neuropathic pain conditions. It has been hypothesized that in the acute phase of herpes zoster, inflammation induces intense stimulation of the sympathetic nervous system leading to reduced intraneural blood flow with resultant neuronal hypoxia and endoneural edema. Other putative mechanisms of sympathetic nervous system involvement include the formation of ephaptic connections between the sensory system and the sympathetic system as well as the upregulation of adreno-

receptors. These phenomena could result in inappropriate activation of primary nociceptive fibers in response to sympathetic nervous system activation. Blockade of sympathetic nerves with local anesthetics may reverse these effects. Sympathetic nerve blocks have been used for the treatment of both the acute pain of herpes zoster and the chronic pain associated with PHN. Unfortunately, there is little high-quality evidence supporting the use of this treatment in patients with PHN. Retrospective data indicate that these blocks may provide temporary pain relief. These studies reported that 41% to 50% of patients with PHN noted short-term relief following the injection, but the effectiveness waned over time based on long-term follow up.[65] In clinical practice, sympathetic blocks are usually reserved as a second- or third-line treatment option in cases where more conservative treatments have been exhausted.

Neuraxial Blocks

Similar to the literature regarding sympathetic blockade, there is inadequate data to convincingly demonstrate that neuraxial therapy is both safe and effective for the routine treatment of PHN. One study has yielded encouraging results with the use of subarachnoid methylprednisolone,[146] but concerns regarding the association between this therapy and the development of adhesive arachnoiditis have precluded its routine use.

In clinical practice, epidural injections of both local anesthetic and steroids are used in patients with pain that has been refractory to conservative treatment. The authors will occasionally use continuous thoracic epidural analgesia with a home infusion pump for a period of 1–2 weeks in patients with intractable PHN pain for symptom palliation. We have observed this approach to be helpful for severe cases, but objective evidence for this therapy is lacking. It does require home nursing care and significant coordination of care by the treating physician. In general, it is reserved for the most severe cases.

Peripheral Nerve Blocks

Intercostal nerve blocks have been reported to provide long lasting relief in PHN patients.[147] The quality of the evidence is limited, much as it is for the other neural blockade techniques described above. Another intervention that is infrequently used is the injection of steroid into the involved dorsal root ganglion. This approach is performed in a nearly identical manner as that used for performing a transforaminal epidural steroid injection. If an inflammatory process at the level of the dorsal root ganglion is considered to play a role in the pathophysiology of PHN, then this treatment would seem rational. There is, however, no convincing evidence to support the routine use of this treatment.

Spinal Cord Stimulation

There has been an increasing role for neuromodulatory strategies in the management of chronic neuropathic pain conditions. Some encouraging data have been reported regarding the effects of spinal cord stimulation in patients suffering from PHN. In a case series of 28 patients (4 patients had herpes zoster and 24 patients had PHN), the effect of spinal cord stimulation was studied prospectively. Long-term relief was obtained in 82% of the patients with PHN.[68] Patients served as their own controls by intermittently switching their spinal cord stimulator off and then monitoring themselves for the reappearance of pain. This is an interesting case series, but confirmation of the benefit of spinal cord stimulation in PHN patients will require further studies with the inclusion of a formal control group.

Psychological Interventions

PHN has been demonstrated to adversely affect overall quality of life by impairing physical and emotional functioning. Studies have shown that the degree of catastrophizing predicts the level of pain in elderly patients with PHN,[148] and this has been shown to be independent of depressive symptoms. Although the effects of cognitive-behavioral therapy and other psychosocial treatments have not been specifically studied in patients with PHN, it would seem logical and prudent to utilize these treatments on an individualized patient basis. There is ample data to support the use of these therapies in other chronic pain conditions and it is reasonable to extrapolate this evidence of efficacy to the treatment of patients with PHN.

Transcutaneous Electrical Nerve Stimulation (TENS)

There have been conflicting responses reported to TENS therapy in patients with PHN. There are a few small case series[149,150] that showed beneficial effects with use of this treatment, but other similar reports failed to demonstrate any benefit. TENS is still clinically offered to many patients on a trial basis given its safety profile. Those patients who have a favorable response to the trial therapy can procure a TENS device for more long-term use.

SURGICAL APPROACHES

Multiple surgical approaches are described in the literature for the treatment of PHN. In general these are quite drastic procedures with no proven long-term benefit. Surgical treatments are largely avoided given the limited literature to support their use, their potential for serious sequelae, and the expanding list of safer and more efficacious options.

PREVENTION OF PHN

The prevention of PHN is obviously closely tied to the prevention of herpes zoster. Thus, the salutary effects of vaccines in preventing herpes zoster described earlier in this chapter, apply to the prevention of PHN as well. The beneficial effects of antiviral medication in decreasing the incidence and severity of PHN have also been reviewed above. These approaches are the mainstays in our arsenal to prevent PHN. There are only scant data to suggest any other therapies are genuinely helpful in preventing PHN.

A small, placebo-controlled, randomized trial evaluated the effect of 25 mg daily of amitriptyline initiated within 48 hours of rash onset in herpes zoster patients over 60 years of age.[151] Treatment with amitriptyline was associated with a 50% decrease in pain prevalence 6 months after rash onset. These results should be confirmed in a trial that controls for the presence of antiviral therapy. Although treatment with amitriptyline may have a beneficial effect in reducing the incidence of PHN, its use should be weighed carefully against potential side effects in elderly or otherwise frail patients.

Use of other medications that are efficacious in PHN, such as gabapentin and pregabalin, may decrease the severity of acute pain in herpes zoster and possibly reduce the incidence of PHN beyond what can be achieved by antiviral therapy alone. There are promising data in animal experiments to support this hypothesis, and results of a single-dose trial of gabapentin vs. placebo demonstrated a reduction in acute pain in patients with herpes zoster.[57]

Two double-blind, randomized, controlled trials of corticosteroids given for a 21-day duration in herpes zoster did not show any effect on the incidence or duration of PHN.[62,63] The data currently available do not support the routine use of corticosteroids as a strategy to prevent PHN.

The use of sympathetic blocks has been used for acute pain in herpes zoster and uncontrolled studies have claimed a reduction in the development of PHN.[152,153] Other studies, however, failed to replicate this effect.[154] Since the pain of herpes zoster and PHN improve over time as part of their natural history, a control group is critically important in any study of the effects of these and other treatments intended to reduce the incidence and duration of pain. Thus, currently available uncontrolled studies are inadequate to definitively support the routine use of sympathetic blocks as a strategy for preventing PHN. In clinical practice, injections are still used for pain management in patients who are refractory to conservative therapy. This is empirically recommended by some authors with the rationale that better pain control in the acute phase of herpes zoster is an important clinical objective in its own right and may also favorably affect the likelihood of developing PHN.

CONCLUSIONS

Herpes zoster and its most common complication, PHN, affect millions of people annually. Their epidemiology is expected to change in complex and potentially unpredictable ways as a result of the implementation of varicella and zoster vaccination programs. Nevertheless, it is difficult to imagine a complete disappearance of these challenging conditions in the near future. Hence, there is a need to develop improved strategies for the treatment of both herpes zoster and PHN. Ongoing research into the underlying mechanisms of these conditions will shape the direction of future treatments. For instance, a better understanding of the biological factors that contribute to the transition from acute to chronic pain may guide us toward therapies that will facilitate a more rapid and complete recovery of infected neurons. Genomic research also has the potential to guide us to new therapies.[155]

For now, clinicians should treat herpes zoster with antiviral therapy and analgesic medications. Corticosteroids should not be routinely prescribed, but can be considered in special circumstances, such as patients with ophthalmic involvement, associated motor deficits, or severe acute pain. Supplemental therapy with tricyclic antidepressants, gabapentin or pregabalin, and neural blockade can be considered in refractory cases where more conservatory therapy has failed, although the evidence base for these treatments is weak.[44] The treatment of PHN is likely to be an ongoing challenge, at least into the near future. At the present time, there is good evidence to support the use of some pharmacologic therapies, including tricyclic antidepressants, gabapentin and pregabalin, and topical lidocaine patches as well as opioid analgesics. The potential merits of each of these agents needs to be carefully balanced against each patient's ability to tolerate their side effects. This is a particularly salient consideration given that many patients with PHN are older or otherwise frail. Invasive modalities such as spinal cord stimulation may play an important role in the future, especially in patients with intractable pain. Further controlled clinical trials will be needed before this treatment approach can be recommended for widespread use. Finally, the role of patient and family education and psychological support cannot be overemphasized, given that the currently available treatments will not be effective for all patients.

Our major treatment recommendations may be summarized as follows:

1. Primary varicella vaccine in children is recommended to prevent chicken pox, and this is also expected to ultimately decrease the incidence of herpes zoster and PHN as vaccinated children become adults and replace those with wild-type virus in the population.
2. Herpes zoster vaccination is recommended for older immunocompetent adults to decrease the incidence of herpes zoster and PHN and to reduce the overall burden of illness.
3. Patients with herpes zoster should be treated with antiviral therapy as rapidly as possible to hasten the rate of healing,

minimize neural damage, decrease the pain caused by the acute infection, and decrease the incidence and duration of PHN.

4. Opioid analgesics, tricyclic antidepressants, gabapentin, and pregabalin can be used in patients with herpes zoster to treat acute pain, although it is important to recognize that few studies have investigated the efficacy of such treatments.

5. Tricyclic antidepressants, gabapentin, pregabalin, topical lidocaine patches, opioid analgesics, and tramadol should be used for the treatment of PHN given their well-established efficacy in this and other chronic neuropathic pain conditions.

6. Referral to a pain specialist should be made if pain control is inadequate despite the above measures

References

1. Head H, Campbell AW. The pathology of herpes zoster and its bearing on sensory localization. *Rev Med Virol* 1997;7(3):131–143.
2. Denny-Brown D, Adams RD, Fitzgerald PJ. Pathologic features of herpes zoster: a note on geniculate herpes. *Arch Neurol Psychiatry* 1944;51:216–231.
3. Dworkin RH, Nagasako EM, Johnson RW, et al. Acute pain in herpes zoster: the famciclovir database project. *Pain* 2001;94:113–119.
4. Haanpää M, Laippala P, Nurmikka T. Pain and somato-sensory dysfunction in acute herpes zoster. *Clin J Pain* 1999;15:78–84.
5. Haanpää M, Laippala P, Nurmikka T. Allodynia and pinprick hypesthesia in acute herpes zoster, and the development of postherpetic neuralgia. *J Pain* 2000;20:50–58.
6. Gilden DH, Dueland AN, Devlin ME, et al. Varicella-zoster virus reactivation without rash. *J Infect Dis* 1992;166(Suppl 1):S30–S34.
7. Lewis GW. Zoster sine herpete. *Br Med J* 1958;2:418–421.
8. Oxman MN, Levin MJ, Johnson GR, et al. for the Shingles Prevention Study Group. A vaccine to prevent herpes zoster and postherpetic neuralgia in older adults. *N Engl J Med* 2005;352:2271–2284.
9. Seward J. Epidemiology of Varicella. In: Arvin AM, Gershon AA, eds. *Varicella-zoster virus: Virology and clinical management.* Cambridge: Cambridge University Press; 2000:187–205.
10. Araújo LQ, MacIntyre CR, Vujacich C. Epidemiology and burden of herpes zoster and post-herpetic neuralgia in Australia, Asia, and South America. *Herpes* 2007;14(Suppl 2):2:40–44.
11. Schmader KE, Watson CP, Gnann JW. Epidemiological and clinical rationale for the herpes zoster vaccine. *J Infect Dis* 2008;19:Suppl 2:S207–S215.
12. Hope-Simpson RE. The nature of herpes zoster: a long-term study and a new hypothesis. *Proc R Soc Med* 1965;58:9–20.
13. Kurtzke JF. Neuroepidemiology. *Ann Neurol* 1984;16:265–277.
14. Gnann JW Jr, Whitley RJ. Clinical practice: herpes zoster. *N Engl J Med* 2002;347:340–346.
15. Schmader KE, George LK, Burchett BM, et al. Racial differences in the occurrence of herpes zoster. *J Infect Dis* 1995;171:701–704.
16. Thomas SL, Hall AJ. What does epidemiology tell us about risk factors for herpes zoster? *The Lancet Infect Dis* 2004;4:26–33.
17. Opstelten W, Van Essen GA, Schellevis F, et al. Gender as an independent risk factor for herpes zoster: a population-based prospective study. *Ann Epidemiol* 2006;16(9):692–695.
18. Thomas SL, Wheeler JG, Hall AJ. Contacts with varicella or with children and protection against herpes zoster in adults: a case-control study. *Lancet* 2002;360:678–682.
19. Goldman GS. Universal varicella vaccination: efficacy trends and effects on herpes zoster. *Int J Toxicol* 2005;24:205–213.
20. Brisson M, Gay NJ, Edmunds WJ, et al. Exposure to varicella boosts immunity to herpes-zoster: implications for mass vaccination against chickenpox. *Vaccine* 2002;20:2500–2507.
21. Schuette MC, Hethcote HW. Modeling the effects of varicella vaccination programs on the incidence of chickenpox and shingles. *Bull Math Biol* 1999;61(6):1031–1064.
22. Edmunds WJ, Brisson M. The effect of vaccination on the epidemiology of varicella zoster virus. *J. Infect* 2002;44:211–219.
23. Arvin A. Aging, immunity, and the varicella-zoster virus. *N Engl J Med* 2005;352:2266–2267.
24. Weller TH. Varicella and herpes zoster: changing concepts of the natural history, control, and importance of a not-so-benign virus. *N Engl J Med* 1983;309:1362–1368.
25. Ragozzino MW, Melton LJ III, Kurland LT, et al. Population-based study of herpes zoster and its sequelae. *Medicine (Baltimore)* 1982;61(5):310–316.
26. Donahue JG, Choo PW, Manson JE, et al. The incidence of herpes zoster. *Arch Intern Med* 1995;155(15):1605–1609.
27. Bowsher D. The lifetime occurrence of herpes zoster and prevalence of postherpetic neuralgia: a retrospective survey in an elderly population. *Eur J Pain* 1999;3(4):335–342.
28. Helgason S, Sigurdsson J, Gudmundsson S. The clinical course of herpes zoster: a prospective study in primary care. *Eur J Gen Pract* 1996;2:12–16.
29. Oaklander AL. The pathology of shingles: Head and Campbell's 1900 monograph. *Arch Neurol* 1999;56:1292–1294.
30. Haanpää M, Häkkinen V, Nurmikko T. Motor involvement in acute herpes zoster. *Muscle Nerve* 1997;20:1433–1438
31. Liesegang TJ. Varicella-zoster virus eye disease. *Cornea* 1999;18:511–531.
32. Echevarría JM, Casas I, Martinez-Martin P. Infections of the nervous system caused by varicella-zoster virus: a review. *Intervirology* 1997;40:72–84.
33. Jemsek J, Greenberg SB, Taber L, et al. Herpes zoster- associated encephalitis: clinicopathologic report of 12 cases and review of the literature. *Medicine (Baltimore)* 1983;62:81–97.
34. Verghese A, Sugar AM. Herpes zoster ophthalmicus and granulomatous angiitis: An ill- appreciated cause of stroke. *J Am Geriatr Soc* 1986;34:309–312.
35. Moriuchi H, Rodriguez W. Role of varicella-zoster virus in stroke syndromes. *Pediatr Infect Dis J* 2000;19:648–653.
36. Chidiac C, Bruxelle J, Daures JP, et al. Characteristics of patients with herpes zoster on presentation to practitioners in France. *Clin Infect Dis* 2001;33:62–69.
37. Coplan PM, Schmader K, Nikas A, et al. Development of a measure of the burden of pain due to herpes zoster and postherpetic neuralgia for prevention trials: adaptation of the brief pain inventory. *J Pain* 2004;5:344–356.
38. Katz J, Cooper EM, Walther RR, et al. Acute pain in herpes zoster and its impact on health-related quality of life. *Clin Infect Dis* 2004;39:342–348.
39. Lydick E, Epstein RS, Himmelberger D, et al. Herpes zoster and quality of life: a self-limited disease with severe impact. *Neurology* 1995;45:S52–S53.
40. Mauskopf J, Austin R, Dix L, et al. The Nottingham Health Profile as a measure of quality of life in zoster patients: convergent and discriminant validity. *Qual Life Res* 1994;3:431–435.
41. Wood MJ, Kay R, Dworkin RH, et al. Oral acyclovir therapy accelerates pain resolution in patients with herpes zoster: a meta-analysis of placebo-controlled trials. *Clin Infect Dis* 1996;22:341–347.
42. Jackson JL, Gibbons R, Meyer G, et al. The effect of treating herpes zoster with oral acyclovir in preventing postherpetic neuralgia: a meta-analysis. *Arch Intern Med* 1997;157:909–912.
43. Crooks RJ, Jones DA, Fiddian AP. Zoster-associated chronic pain: an overview of clinical trials with acyclovir. *Scand J Infect Dis* 1991;80:62–68.
44. Dworkin RH, Johnson RW, Breuer J, et al. Recommendations for the management of herpes zoster. *Clin Infect Dis* 2007;44(Suppl 1):S1–S26.
45. Decroix J, Partsch H, Gonzalez R, et al. on behalf of the Valacyclovir International Zoster Assessment Group (VIZA). Factors influencing pain outcome in herpes zoster: an observational study with valacyclovir. *J Eur Acad Dermatol Venereol* 2000;14:23–33.
46. Kurokawa I, Kumano K, Murakawa K. Clinical correlates of prolonged pain in Japanese patients with acute herpes zoster. *J Int Med Res* 2002;30:56–65.
47. Zaal MJ, Völker-Dieben HJ, Wienesen M, et al. Longitudinal analysis of varicella-zoster virus DNA on the ocular surface associated with herpes zoster ophthalmicus. *Am J Ophthalmol* 2001;131:25–29.
48. Degreef H. Famciclovir herpes zoster Clinical Study Group: famciclovir, a new oral antiherpes drug: results of the first controlled clinical study demonstrating its efficacy and safety in the treatment of uncomplicated herpes zoster in immunocompetent patients. *Int J Antimicrob Agents* 1994;4:241–246.
49. Beutner KR, Friedman DJ, Forszpaniak C, et al. Valaciclovir compared with acyclovir for improved therapy for herpes zoster in immunocompetent adults. *Antimicrob Agents Chemother* 1995;39:1546–1553.
50. Wassilew SW, Wutzler P. Oral brivudin in comparison with acyclovir for herpes zoster: a survey study on postherpetic neuralgia. *Antiviral Res* 2003;59:57–60.
51. Kost RG, Straus SE. Postherpetic neuralgia: pathogenesis, treatment, and prevention. *N Engl J Med* 1996;335:32–42.
52. Tyring S, Barbarash RA, Nahlik JE, et al. Collaborative Famciclovir Herpes Zoster Study Group: famciclovir for the treatment of acute herpes zoster: effects on acute disease and postherpetic neuralgia: a randomized, double-blind, placebo controlled trial. *Ann Intern Med* 1995;123:89–96.
53. Tyring SK, Beutner KR, Tucker BA, et al. Antiviral therapy for herpes zoster: randomized, controlled clinical trial of valacyclovir and famciclovir therapy in immunocompetent patients 50 years and older. *Arch Fam Med* 2000;9:863–869.
54. Dworkin RH, Perkins FM, Nagasako EM. Prospects for the prevention of postherpetic neuralgia in herpes zoster patients. *Clin J Pain* 2000;16(Suppl 2):S90–S100.
55. Dworkin RH, Schmader KE. Treatment and prevention of postherpetic neuralgia. *Clin Infect Dis* 2003;36:877–882.
56. Dworkin RH. Strategies for the prevention of neuropathic pain. In: Program and abstracts of expanding vistas in neuropathic pain, an official satellite of the 11th World Congress on Pain (Uluru, Australia). Seattle: International Association for the Study of Pain. Neuropathic Pain Special Interest Group; 2005:39.
57. Berry JD, Petersen KL. A single dose of gabapentin reduces acute pain and allodynia in patients with herpes zoster. *Neurology* 2005;65:444–447.
58. Hempenstall K, Nurmikko TJ, Johnson RW, et al. Analgesic therapy in postherpetic neuralgia: a quantitative systematic review. *PLoS Med* 2005;2:e164.
59. Dahl JB, Mathiesen O, Møniche S. Protective premedication: an option with gabapentin and related drugs? A review of gabapentin and pregabalin in the treatment of post-operative pain. *Acta Anaesthesiol Scand* 2004;48:1130–1136.
60. Rowbotham MC, Goli V, Kunz NR, et al. Venlafaxine extended release in the

treatment of painful diabetic neuropathy: a double-blind, placebo-controlled study. *Pain* 2004;110:697–706.

61. Goldstein DJ, Lu Y, Detke MJ, et al. Duloxetine vs. placebo in patients with painful diabetic neuropathy. *Pain* 2005;116:109–118.

62. Wood MJ, Johnson RW, McKendrick MW, et al. A randomized trial of acyclovir for 7 days or 21 days with and without prednisolone for treatment of acute herpes zoster. *N Engl J Med* 1994;330:896–900.

63. Whitley RJ, Weiss H, Gnann JW Jr., et al. Acyclovir with and without prednisone for the treatment of herpes zoster: a randomized placebo-controlled trial. *Ann Intern Med* 1996;125:376–383.

64. Wu CL, Marsh A, Dworkin RH. The role of sympathetic blocks in herpes zoster and postherpetic neuralgia. *Pain* 2000;87:121–129.

65. Kumar V, Krone K, Mathieu A. Neuraxial and sympathetic blocks in herpes zoster and postherpetic neuralgia: an appraisal of current evidence. *Reg Anesth Pain Med* 2004;29:454–461.

66. van Wijck AJ, Opstelten W, Moons KG, et al. The PINE study of epidural steroids and local anesthetics to prevent postherpetic neuralgia: a randomized controlled trial. *Lancet* 2006 367:219–224.

67. Manabe H, Dan K, Hirata K, et al. Optimum pain relief with continuous epidural infusion of local anesthetics shortens the duration of zoster-associated pain. *Clin J Pain* 2004;20:302–308.

68. Harke H, Gretenkort P, Ladleif HU, et al. Spinal cord stimulation in postherpetic neuralgia and in acute herpes zoster pain. *Anesth Analg* 2002;94(3):694–700.

69. Gnann JW Jr. Vaccination to prevent herpes zoster in older adults. *J Pain* 2008;9(Suppl 1):S31–S36.

70. Arani RB, Soong SJ, Weiss HL, et al. Phase-specific analysis of herpes zoster associated pain data: a new statistical approach. *Stat Med* 2001;20:2429–2439.

71. Dworkin RH, Gnann JW, Oaklander AL, et al. Diagnosis and assessment of pain associated with herpes zoster and postherpetic neuralgia. *J Pain* 2008;9(Suppl 1):S37–S44.

72. Dworkin RH, Schmader KE. The epidemiology and natural history of herpes zoster and postherpetic neuralgia. In: Watson CP, Gershon AA, eds. *Herpes zoster and postherpetic neuralgia.* 2nd revised and enlarged edition. New York: Elsevier; 2001:39–64.

73. Dworkin RH, Boon RJ, Griffin DR, et al. Postherpetic neuralgia: impact of famciclovir, age, rash severity, and acute pain in herpes zoster patients. *J Infect Dis* 1998;178(Suppl 1):S76–S80.

74. Dworkin RH, Portenoy RK. Pain and its persistence in herpes zoster. *Pain* 1996;67:241–151.

75. Choo PW, Galil K, Donahue JG, et al. Risk factors for postherpetic neuralgia. *Arch Intern Med* 1997;157:1217–1224.

76. Watson CP, Watt VR, Chipman M, et al. The prognosis with postherpetic neuralgia. *Pain* 1991;46:195–199.

77. Schmader K. Postherpetic neuralgia in immunocompetent elderly people. *Vaccine* 1998;16:1768–1770.

78. Schmader K. Herpes zoster in older adults. *Clin Infect Dis* 2001;32:1481–1486.

79. Bennett GJ. Neuropathic pain: An overview. In: Borsook D, ed. *Molecular Neurobiology of Pain.* IASP Press; 1997:109–113.

80. Bowsher D. The lifetime occurrence of herpes zoster and prevalence of postherpetic neuralgia: a retrospective survey in an elderly population. *Eur J Pain* 1999;3:335–342.

81. Dworkin RH, Portenoy RK. Proposed classification of herpes zoster pain. *Lancet* 1994;343:1648.

82. Desmond RA, Weiss HL, Arani RB, et al. Clinical applications for change-point analysis of herpes zoster pain. *J Pain Symptom Manage* 2002;23:510–516.

83. Jung BF, Johnson RW, Griffin DR, et al. Risk factors for postherpetic neuralgia in patients with herpes zoster. *Neurology* 2004;62:1545–1551.

84. Opstelten W, Mauritz WJ, de Wit NJ, et al. Herpes zoster and postherpetic neuralgia: incidence and risk indicators using a general practice research database. *Fam Pract* 2002;19(5):471–475.

85. di Luzio Paparatti U, Arpinelli F, Visonà G. Herpes zoster and its complications in Italy: an observational survey. *J Infect* 1990;38(2):116–120.

86. Czernichow S, Dupuy A, Flahault A, et al. Herpes zoster: incidence study among "sentinel" general practitioners. *Ann Dermatol Venereol* 2001;128(4):497–501.

87. Helgason S, Petursson G, Gudmundsson S, et al. Prevalence of postherpetic neuralgia after a first episode of herpes zoster: prospective study with long term follow up. *BMJ* 2000;321:794–796.

88. De Moragas JM, Kierland RR. The outcome of patients with herpes zoster. *AMA Arch Derm* 1957;75:193–196.

89. Hope-Simpson RE. Postherpetic neuralgia. *J R Coll Gen Pract* 1975;25(157):571–575.

90. Nagasako EM, Johnson RW, Griffin DR, et al. Rash severity in herpes zoster: correlates and relationship to postherpetic neuralgia. *J Am Acad Dermatol* 2002;46(6):834–839.

91. Higa K. Acute herpetic pain and post-herpetic neuralgia. *Eur J Pain* 1993;14(4):79–90.

92. Baron R, Haendler G, Schulte H. Afferent large fiber polyneuropathy predicts development of postherpetic neuralgia. *Pain* 1997;73:231–238.

93. McCulloch DK, Fraser DM, Duncan LP. Shingles in diabetes mellitus. *Practitioner* 1982;226:531–532.

94. Watson CP, Deck JH, Morshead C, et al. Post-herpetic neuralgia: further post-mortem studies of cases with and without pain. *Pain* 1991;44:105–117.

95. Rowbotham MC, Yosipovitch G, Connolly MK, et al. Cutaneous innervation density in the allodynic form of postherpetic neuralgia. *Neurobiol Dis* 1996;3(3):205–214.

96. Oaklander AL, Romans K, Horasek S, et al. Unilateral postherpetic neuralgia is associated with bilateral sensory neuron damage. *Ann Neurol* 1998;44:789–795.

97. Oaklander AL. The density of remaining nerve endings in human skin with and without postherpetic neuralgia after shingles. *Pain* 2001;92:139–145.

98. Bennett GJ. Hypothesis on the pathogenesis of herpes zoster-associated pain. *Ann Neurol* 1994;35(Suppl):S38–S41.

99. Scholz J, Broom DC, Kohno T, et al. Animal models of neuropathic pain induce apoptosis and a loss of GABAergic inhibition in the spinal dorsal horn. In: Dostrovsky JO, Carr DB, Koltzenburg M, eds. *Proceedings of the 10th World Congress on Pain.* Seattle: IASP; 2003; 387–395.

100. Fields HL, Rowbotham M, Baron R. Postherpetic neuralgia: irritable nociceptors and deafferentation. *Neurobiol Dis* 1998;5:209–227.

101. Rowbotham MC, Peterson KL, Fields HL. Is postherpetic neuralgia more than one disorder? *Pain Forum* 1998;7:231–237.

102. Bowsher D. Sensory change in postherpetic neuralgia. In: Watson CPN, ed. *Herpes Zoster and Postherpetic Neuralgia.* Amsterdam: Elsevier; 1993:97–103.

103. Baron R, Saguer M. Postherpetic neuralgia. Are C-nociceptors involved in signaling and maintenance of tactile allodynia? *Brain* 1993:116:1477–1496.

104. Baron R, Saguer M. Mechanical allodynia in postherpetic neuralgia: evidence for central mechanisms depending on nociceptive C-finer degeneration. *Neurology* 1995;45(Suppl 8):S63–S65.

105. Pappagallo M, Oaklander AL, Auatrano-Piacentini AL, et al. Heterogeneous patterns of sensory dysfunction in postherpetic neuralgia suggests multiple pathophysiologic mechanisms. *Anesthesiology* 2000;92(3):691–698.

106. Peterson KL, Fields HL, Brennum J, et al. Capsaicin-evoked pain and allodynia in post-herpetic neuralgia. *Pain* 2000;88(2):125–133.

107. Wasner G, Kleinert A, Binder A, et al. Postherpetic neuralgia: topical lidocaine is effective in nociceptor-deprived skin. *J Neurol* 2005;252(6):677–686.

108. Finnerup NB, Otto M, McQuay HJ, et al. Algorithm for neuropathic pain treatment: an evidence based proposal. *Pain* 2005;118:289–305.

109. Dworkin RH, Backonja M, Rowbotham MC, et al. Advances in neuropathic pain: diagnosis, mechanisms, and treatment recommendations. *Arch Neurol* 2003;60:1524–1534.

110. Attal N, Cruccu G, Haanpää M, et al. EFNS guidelines on pharmacological treatment of neuropathic pain. *Eur J Neurology* 2006;13:1153–1169.

111. Dworkin RH, O'Connor AB, Backonja M, et al. Pharmacological management of neuropathic pain: evidence-based recommendations. *Pain* 2007;132:237–251.

112. Moulin DE, Clark AJ, Gilron I, et al. Pharmacological management of chronic neuropathic pain: consensus statement and guidelines from the Canadian Pain Society. *Pain Res Manag* 2007;12:13–21.

113. Rowbotham MC, Harden N, Stacey B, et al. Gabapentin for the treatment of postherpetic neuralgia: a randomized controlled trial. *JAMA* 1998;280:1837–1842.

114. Rice ASC, Maton S, Postherpetic Neuralgia Study Group. Gabapentin in postherpetic neuralgia: a randomized, double-blind, placebo-controlled study. *Pain* 2001;94:215–224.

115. Bennett MI, Simpson KH. Gabapentin in the treatment of neuropathic pain. *Palliat Med* 2004;18:5–11.

116. Maneuf YP, Gonzalez MI, Sutton KS, et al. Cellular and molecular action of the putative GABA-mimetic, gabapentin. *Cell Mol Life Sci* 2003;60:742–750.

117. Backonja M, Glanzman RL. Gabapentin dosing for neuropathic pain: evidence from randomized, placebo-controlled clinical trials. *Clin Ther* 2003;25:81–104.

118. Frampton JE, Foster RH. Pregabalin in the treatment of postherpetic neuralgia. *Drugs* 2005;65:111–118.

119. Dworkin RH, Corbin AE, Young JP Jr, et al. Pregabalin for the treatment of postherpetic neuralgia: a randomized, placebo-controlled trial. *Neurology* 2003;60:1274–1283.

120. Freynhagen R, Strojek K, Griesing T, et al. Efficacy of pregabalin in neuropathic pain evaluated in a 12-week, randomized, double-blind, multicentre, placebo-controlled trial of flexible- and fixed-dose regimens. *Pain* 2005;115:254–263.

121. Montgomery SA, Tobias K, Zornberg GL, et al. Efficacy and safety of pregabalin in the treatment of generalized anxiety disorder: a 6-week, multicenter, randomized, double-blind, placebo-controlled comparison of pregabalin and venlafaxine. *J Clin Psychiatry* 2006;67:771–782.

122. Rickels K, Pollack MH, Feltner DE, et al. Pregabalin for treatment of generalized anxiety disorder: a 4-week, multicenter, double-blind, placebo-controlled trial of pregabalin and alprazolam. *Arch Gen Psychiatry* 2005;62:1022–1030.

123. Dick IE, Brochu RM, Purohit Y, et al. Sodium channel blockade may contribute to the analgesic efficacy of antidepressants. *J Pain* 2007;8:315–324.

124. Offenbaecher M, Ackenheil M. Current trends in neuropathic pain treatments with special reference to fibromyalgia. *CNS Spectr* 2005;10:285–297.

125. Guay DR. Adjunctive agents in the management of chronic pain. *Pharmacotherapy.* 2001;21:1070–1081.

126. Collins SL, Moore RA, McQuay HJ, et al. Antidepressants and anticonvul-

sants for diabetic neuropathy and postherpetic neuralgia: a quantitative systematic review. *J Pain* 2000;20:449–458.

127. Sindrup SH, Jensen TS. Efficacy of pharmacological treatments of neuropathic pain: an update and effect related to mechanism of drug action. *Pain* 1999; 83:389–400.

128. Rowbotham MC, Reisner LA, Davies PS, et al. Treatment response in antidepressant-naïve postherpetic neuralgia patients: double-blind, randomized trial. *J Pain* 2005;6:741–746.

129. Watson CP, Vernich L, Chipman M, et al. Nortryptiline vs. amitriptyline in postherpetic neuralgia: a randomized controlled trial. *Neurology* 1998;51: 1161–1171.

130. Sansone RA, Todd T, Meier BP. Pretreatment ECGs and the prescription of amitryptiline in an internal medicine clinic. *Psychosomatics* 2002;43: 250–251.

131. Vieweg WV, Wood MA. Tricyclic antidepressants, QT interval prolongation, and torsade de pointes. *Psychosomatics* 2004;45:371–377.

132. Raja SN, Haythornthwaite JA, Pappagallo M, et al. Opioids versus antidepressants in postherpetic neuralgia: a randomized, placebo-controlled trial. *Neurology* 2002;59:1015–1021.

133. Watson CP, Babul N. Efficacy of oxycodone in neuropathic pain: a randomized trial in postherpetic neuralgia. *Neurology* 1998;50:1837–1841.

134. Khoromi S, Cui L, Nackers L, et al. Morphine, nortriptyline and their combination vs. placebo in patients with chronic lumbar root pain. *Pain* 2007;130: 65–75.

135. Gilron I, Bailey JM, Tu D, et al. Morphine, gabapentin, or their combination for neuropathic pain. *N Engl J Med* 2005;352:1324–1334.

136. Boureau F, Legallicier P, Kabir–Ahmadi M, Tramadol in postherpetic neuralgia: A randomized, double blind, placebo-controlled trial. *Pain* 2003;104: 323–331.

137. Galer BS, Rowbotham MC, Perander J, et al. Topical lidocaine patch relieves postherpetic neuralgia more effectively than a vehicle topical patch: results of an enriched enrollment study. *Pain* 1999;80:533–558.

138. Rowbotham MC, Davies PS, Verkempinck, et al. Lidocaine patch: double-blind controlled study of a new treatment method for postherpetic neuralgia. *Pain* 1996;65:39–44.

139. Meier T, Wasner G, Faust M, et al. Efficacy of lidocaine patch 5% in the treatment of focal peripheral neuropathic pain syndromes: a randomized, double-blind, placebo-controlled study. *Pain* 2003;106:151–158.

140. Wasner G, Kleinert A, Binder A, et al. Postherpetic neuralgia: topical lidocaine is effective in nociceptor-deprived skin. *J Neurol* 2005;252:677–686.

141. Rowbotham MC, Davies PS, Fields HL. Topical lidocaine gel relieves postherpetic neuralgia. *Ann Neurol* 1995;37:246–253.

142. Bernstein JE, Korman NJ, Bickers DR, et al. Topical capsaicin treatment of chronic postherpetic neuralgia. *J Am Acad Dermatol* 1989;21:265–270.

143. Watson CP, Tyler KL, Bickers DR, et al. A randomized vehicle-controlled trial of topical capsaicin in the treatment of postherpetic neuralgia. *Clin Ther* 1993;15(3):510–526.

144. Backonja M. High-concentration capsaicin for treatment of PHN and HIV neuropathy pain. *Eur J Pain* 2007;11(1):S40.

145. De Benedittis G, Lorenzetti A. Topical aspirin/diethyl ether mixture versus indomethacin and diclofenac/diethyl ether mixtures for acute herpetic neuralgia and postherpetic neuralgia: A double-blind crossover placebo-controlled study. *Pain* 1996;65:45–52.

146. Kotani N, Kushikata T, Hashimoto H, et al. Intrathecal methylprednisolone for intractable postherpetic neuralgia. *N Engl J Med* 2000;343:1514–1519.

147. Doi K, Nikai T, Sakura S, et al. Intercostal nerve block with 5% tetracaine for chronic pain syndromes. *J Clin Anesth* 2002;14:39–41.

148. Haythornthwaite JA, Clark MR, Pappagallo M, et al. Pain coping strategies play a role in the persistence of pain in post-herpetic neuralgia. *Pain* 2003; 106:453–460.

149. Nathan PW, Wall PD. Treatment of postherpetic neuralgia by prolonged electrical stimulation. *Br Med J* 1974;3:645–647.

150. Haas LF. Postherpetic neuralgia. *Trans Opthalmol Soc NZ* 1977;29:133–136.

151. Bowsher D. The effects of pre-emptive treatment of postherpetic neuralgia with amitryptiline: A randomized, double-blind, placebo-controlled trial. *J Pain Symptom Manage* 1997;13:327–331.

152. Colding A. The effect of sympathetic blocks on herpes zoster. *Acta Anaesthesiol Scand* 1969;13:113–141.

153. Dan K, Higa K, Noda B. Nerve block for herpetic pain. In: Fields HL, Dubner R, Cervero F, eds. *Advances in Pain Research and Therapy.* New York: Raven; 1985;9:831–838.

154. Yanagida H, Suwa K, Corssen G. No prophylactic effect of early sympathetic blockade of postherpetic neuralgia. *Anesthesiology* 1987;66:73–79.

155. Shir Y, Zelster R, Vatine JJ, et al. Correlation of intact sensibility and neuropathic pain-related behaviors in eight inbred and out-bred rat strains and selection lines. *Pain* 2001;90:75–82.

CHAPTER 28 ■ CENTRAL PAIN STATES

JOEL D. GREENSPAN, ROLF-DETLEF TREEDE, RONALD R. TASKER, AND FREDERICK A. LENZ

Central pain is defined[1] as "pain associated with lesions of the central nervous system (CNS)" and is among the most intriguing, distressing, and intractable of chronic pain syndromes. For example, transection of the spinal cord can result in chronic pain below the level of the transection (spinal cord injury/SCI central pain), or a stroke can result in central pain on the opposite side of the body (central poststroke pain, CPSP). In both cases, the diagnosis of central pain is based on clear evidence of a CNS injury, evidence of pain and temperature sensory alterations, and the exclusion of other mechanisms of pain. The evidence of CNS injury rests on neurologic signs, radiologic, and electrical studies (see Chapters 18 and 19). Central pain belongs to the group of neuropathic pain syndromes and shares many features with these pain syndromes.[1–3] This chapter is divided into two sections, the first deals with SCI central pain and the second with CPSP. Each section deals both with basic and clinical considerations. A more general discussion of the different types of pain seen after injury to the spine and spinal cord may be found in Chapter 40.

SPINAL CORD INJURY CENTRAL PAIN

Incidence and Etiology

The diagnosis of SCI central pain may be obvious but is conservatively considered to be a diagnosis of exclusion. The patient presents for treatment of pain after therapy after completion of the causative event, such as trauma or transverse myelitis in multiple sclerosis (MS). In the case of trauma there may be pain from direct injury to the spine or the limbs which may confuse the issue. A recent study demonstrated that patients with SCI central pain (n = 20) could be identified by clinical criteria among a group of patients with SCI (n = 40).[4] These criteria included the presence of pain at least two spinal dermatomal levels below the level of SCI after exclusion of pain secondary to nociceptive, peripheral neuropathic, and psychogenic mechanisms. Only pa-

(Data from Tasker RR, DeCarvalho GT, Dolan EJ. Intractable pain of spinal cord origin: clinical features and implications for surgery. *Neurosurgery* 1992;77(3):373–378.)

TABLE 28.1

ETIOLOGY OF 127 CASES OF SCI CENTRAL PAIN

Diagnosis	% of Patients
Trauma	65
Iatrogenic	12
Inflammatory	9
Neoplasm	6
Skeletal pathology	2
Vascular pathology	2
Congenital lesions	4

tients with an injury above the conus medullaris were included because of the presence of combined injury to the central and peripheral nervous systems for lesions of the conus, that is, skeletal level above T10.

Trauma is the most common cause of spinal cord central pain, as shown in Table 28.1, which lists the etiology of pain in a series of 127 patients with SCI central pain.[5] In this series, 76.4% were men, and 57.4% were younger than 40 years at the time of the injury. Forty-two percent of the patients had lesions in the cervical area, 21% in the T1-9, and 37% in the T-10–L-2 areas; 32% of lesions were clinically complete, 64% incomplete, and 4% of patients had no clinically detectable sensory loss. There appeared to be no correlation between patterns of pain and etiology, level of injury, and completeness of spinal cord transaction. A retrospective study of 380 patients (questionnaire response rate 38%) who suffered from SCI revealed that 65.5% experienced pain, of which the steady, burning, dysesthetic component was the most common.[6]

Patients with traumatic SCI and central pain (n = 20) were compared with those with SCI but without central pain (n = 20) in a Danish prospective series.[4] There were no significant differences between these two groups by demographics, interval since injury, level of injury, posttraumatic interval, degree of disability, degree of spasticity, or sensory diminution.

The time of onset of SCI central pain after the causative event could be correlated with the mechanism of pain.[6] When onset was delayed beyond 1 year, 56% of these patients were found to suffer from a syrinx; 37% of those with onset before 1 year did so too. Although the pain rarely, if ever, subsides on its own, it may change slowly but significantly over time. The presence of facial pain or late onset of pain should alert the physician to the possibility of posttraumatic syringomyelia.[7]

A large series of patients with syringomyelia correlated MRI findings with clinical features.[8] This study identified segmental burning pain, hypersensitivity, and dysesthesias and trophic phenomena in patients with syringomyelia (51/137, 37%) at the time of presentation. Forty-three of these 51 (84%) had extension of the syrinx into the dorsolateral quadrant of the cord ipsilateral to the pain at the appropriate level.

Clinical Features

The clinical features and types of pain have been reported in 127 patients with SCI central pain.[7] The temporal course of the pain was characterized as: steady in 95% of cases, intermittent (usually shooting) in 31%, and evoked (allodynia, hyperpathia, or hyperesthesia) in 45%. Steady pain was usually causalgic (75%) or dysesthetic (28%). The dysesthetic element was variably described as tingling in 20%, numb in 6%, crawling in 2%, and pricking in 1%. The quality of pain sometimes included a mechanical component described as aching in 13%, had a sense of compression or distraction in 18% (crush, 3%; tight, 2%; squeeze, 2%; pull, 2%; pinch, 2%), whereas it was rhythmic in 9% (throb, 5%; cramp, 3%; pound, 1%; pump, 1%), cold in 4%, and had the feeling of a cut in 2%. These results are generally consistent with a smaller detailed study of 19 patients in which the following sensations commonly occurred: (30% to 70%): cutting, burning, piercing, radiating, and tight.[9] A steady, burning, dysesthetic component was the most common in a study of 102 SCI central pain patients.[7] The only obvious clinical correlation with pain type was the association of intermittent pain with lesions at the T10–L2 vertebral level.[7]

Patients with traumatic SCI and central pain are similar to those without central pain in terms of sensory alteration as measured by mechanical, thermal, and pain thresholds.[4] However, the populations of SCI with central pain were distinguished from those without by increased sensitivity to painful or nonpainful mechanical or temperature stimuli. This is consistent with another report of 16 patients with SCI and dysesthetic pain, comparing the somatosensory function in normal, painful, and nonpainful denervated skin.[10] No difference existed between the degree of deficit in dorsal column and spinothalamic tract function, but allodynia and wind-up were more common in painful than nonpainful denervated cutaneous areas in both studies.

The prevalence of a band of steady pain at the upper margin of sensory loss and diffuse pain below the level of injury is more characteristic of an incomplete lesion.[5] Visceral, perineal, and anal pain were more common in complete lesions. Pain may resemble that of musculoskeletal disease or muscle tension (see previous discussion, quality of pain). When this type of pain occurs in an innervated area above the level of injury, it may be associated with mechanical problems in traumatic SCI patients. However, such pain may occur below the level of a complete injury, and so may be neuropathic in origin. Alternately, there may be a painful or nonpainful phantom below the level of a complete lesion. In this series, facial pain was pathognomonic of a syrinx in the cervical area interfering with the descending tract of the trigeminal nerve.

Forty-seven percent of patients experienced allodynia or hyperalgesia or both, but only in areas of preserved sensation.[5,7] This was usually associated with spontaneous pain, although in 4% of patients, evoked pain occurred in isolation. It affected 39% of patients with complete lesions where it usually occurred as a band at the upper level of the sensory loss, and 51% of patients with incomplete lesions. In these latter it was found diffusely in 67%, and as a band at the upper level of the sensory deficit in 18%. Taking complete and incomplete lesions together, in 21% it occurred in a band at the upper level of the sensory loss, in 29% diffusely, and in 50% patchily below the patient's level. This was similar to the findings of a more recent Danish study in which 40% (8/20) of patients had allodynia to touch and one patient also had cold allodynia.[4] Seven of the eight had allodynia in the border of anesthetic area. One patient had pain below the lesion level and one had widespread allodynia, including face, when the spontaneous pain was severe. It could also occur in radicular distribution from damage to a root near the level of spine injury.

Patients with lesions of the cauda equina and conus pain often had a neuralgic intermittent component shooting down the legs.[5,7] This type of pain may well be the result of injury to both central and peripheral nervous systems, and affected 31% of patients. It was present in 82% of patients with complete T10–L2 lesions, and 64% of incomplete lesions at this level. Pain resembling abdominal or pelvic disease usually occurred below a level of complete sensory loss and often led to extensive investigation of the viscera, and even to abdominal surgery. These types of pain were not apparently observed in the more recent study which excluded patients with lesions of the conus.[4] These results suggest that injury to the central and peripheral nervous systems are responsible for these pain types.

These findings demonstrate that patients with SCI central pain, have diminution of STT mediated thermal sensation or pain sensation or both on quantitative sensory testing.[4,10,11] However, this characteristic does not identify the subset of patients with SCI central pain among those patients with SCI.[4] Therefore diminution of STT-mediated sensations is a necessary but not sufficient condition for the development of SCI central pain. All patients with SCI central pain have diminished thermal or pain sensation or both on quantitative sensory testing.[4,10,11] However, the presence of SCI central pain is correlated with the presence of hypersensitivity to cold or tactile stimuli. When compared to SCI patients without central pain, those with central pain more frequently had hypersensitivity to mechanical and cold stimulation at dermatomes corresponding to the lesion level. The intensity of brush-evoked pain at the lesion level is correlated with spontaneous pain below the level of the injury.[4] These results point to the role of brainstem, thalamic, and cortical neurons in somatic sensory pathways in the mechanism of central pain (see later discussion).

Animal Models

The best model of SCI lesions leading to central pain is the hypersensitivity of nonhuman primates with lesions of the anterolateral quadrant of the spinal cord.[12,13] The response of these monkeys with these lesions could be divided into those which recovered their prelesion purposive escape response and those which did not. The animals which did recover were those which had lesions extending medially into the grey matter of the spinal cord. The reflexive response to electrocutaneous stimuli was initially reduced contralaterally, but to some extent ipsilaterally. The recovery tended to be bilateral, leading to a greater reflexive response ipsilaterally. This pattern distinguished itself from the purposive/escape behavior, in which the changes tended to be contralateral.[13,14]

Anatomic studies of the thalamus have been carried out in monkeys with thoracic spinal cord lesions both of the ipsilateral anterolateral quadrant of the spinal cord and of the contralateral dorsal quadrant. Compared with controls these lesioned animals show decreased GABA immunoreactive elements in the thalamic ventrobasal nucleus.[15] Electron microscopic analysis demonstrates the presence of two types of GABAergic elements, including F elements which are mostly axonal terminals of the neurons in the thalamic reticular nucleus. The second type of terminal is a presynaptic dendrite of local interneurons (PSD). Results in three monkeys demonstrated significant decreases in both types of GABA immunoreactive elements in the ventral basal complex.

Detection of electrocutaneous stimuli was not impaired in these animals, suggesting that other spinal pathways, perhaps the ipsilateral STT, can transmit activity evoked by this electrocutaneous stimulus. Thalamic recordings in the hind limb representation of the ventral basal complex were carried out in these animals and demonstrated absent responses to thermal and mechanical somatic sensory stimuli, graded into the painful range. In the forelimb representation evoked responses were increased for thalamic multi-receptive cells (MR) which responded to both cutaneous brushing and compressive stimuli with activity that was not graded into the noxious range. In the forelimb representation low threshold spike (LTS) bursts were increased during spontaneous activity. In the hind limb representation there were no responses to somatic stimulation. Burst rates were increased, and firing rates between bursts were decreased, consistent with studies in humans.[16]

Thalamic recordings were also carried out in monkeys with thoracic anterolateral cordotomies.[17] Some of these animals showed increased responsiveness to electrocutaneous stimuli and thus may represent a model of central pain.[18] In comparisons with normal controls, MR cells in the monkeys with anterolateral cordotomies showed significant increases in the number of low threshold bursts occurring spontaneously or in response to brushing or compressive stimuli. Thalamic low threshold bursts were those associated with a low threshold calcium spike deinactivated by a prolonged hyperpolarization of the neuron membrane (approximately 100 ms). The changes in bursting behavior were widespread, occurring in the thalamic representation of upper and lower extremities, both ipsilateral and contralateral to the cordotomy.

The location of this bursting activity in the forelimb representation ipsilateral to the spinal injury suggests that bursting is not sufficient for pain which is contralateral in this syndrome.[19] However, such bursting could cause pain if activation of the bursting cell produced the sensation of pain consistent with the increased frequency of pain evoked by thalamic stimulation with a grouped/bursting pattern of pulses in patients with central pain.[20-22]

Some monkey species with anterolateral cordotomy display autotomy behavior (self-inflicted destruction of denervated parts of the body).[23] This behavior is often interpreted to indicate the presence of dysesthesias, and perhaps central pain.[24,25] The presence of autotomy in patients with congenital analgesia, and without the sensation of pain, has been taken to indicate that autotomy is not necessarily an indicator of chronic pain.[26]

Autotomy reactions have been studied following lesions of rodent spinal cord pathways.[27-29] Autotomy was not present after posterior quadrant sections, simultaneous section of ipsilateral, lateral, or anterolateral quadrants in addition to anterolateral quadrant section or hemisection on the other side of the spinal cord. The conclusion of these studies is that autotomy occurs only in cases where section of the anterolateral quadrant or one half of the spinal cord allows for sensory transmission through ipsilateral nociceptive pathways.

A number of studies of spinal cord injury in rats have led to models of the mechanism of spinal cord injury. Behavioral evidence of hyperalgesia and abnormal hypersensitivity of dorsal horn neurons has also been reported in rats after cavitary lesions of the spinal cord central gray. These cavitary lesions were created by injection of quisqualic acid, an excitotoxin acting at non-NMDA glutamate receptors.[30,31] This excitatotoxic SCI injury leads to a cascade of chemical and inflammatory events resulting in increased extracellular excitatory amino acid (EAA) concentrations, which may be important mediators of the delayed injury which occurs in this model. Studies by Hulsebosch have highlighted the role of the metabotropic EAA receptor (mGluR) class in the release of EAA.[32] Some receptors of this class (mGLuR) group I (mGluR1 and mGluR5), seem to activate several intracellular pathways that lead to increased extracellular EAA concentrations. The results demonstrate that this pathway can initiate a number of intracellular cascades which lead to increased extracellular EAA concentrations, possible mediators of the delayed injury and central neuropathic pain behaviors observed in this model.

A role for sodium channels in SCI central pain is suggested by studies carried out in rats with a spinal cord contusion injury.[33,34] In these animals the expression of non-tetrodotoxin (TTX) dependent sodium channels in dorsal horn and thalamic neurons may correlate with the presence of thalamic bursting behavior similar to that found in humans with SCI central pain. These animals also displayed spontaneous behaviors and responses to sensory stimulation consistent with those observed in central pain. Administration of anti-sense in these animals reversed thalamic bursting and the behaviors which are related to pain.[33] These studies suggest that the presence of non-TTX dependent sodium channels of this type may be the factor which leads to central pain, in response to or in addition to STT-mediated sensory attenuation, or both. It is unclear how these studies in rodents relate to the clinical features and treatment of human SCI central pain after complete or partial SCI.

Treatment of Spinal Cord Injury Central Pain: Medical Treatment

SCI central pain is a particularly refractory chronic pain syndrome. One-third to one-half of patients who experience SCI central pain have severe pain.[7] Chronic pain syndromes can almost never be eradicated and, even after successful treatment, the chronic pain of SCI tends to recur with time, regardless of the treatment modality. Therefore, initial treatment should be conservative and carry low risk. First, musculoskeletal and visceral causes of pain from spinal cord injury should be assessed and if identified, treatments directed at these causes can effectively relieve the pain. It is also important to evaluate and treat motor spasticity as treatment of spasticity may result in a significant reduction in pain. Treatments discussed in this chapter will focus on neuropathic pain since treatment of neuropathic pain is usually more difficult. Pharmacological treatment of SCI pain is the standard for most patients although there are a limited number of trials that can guide drug selection. A summary of controlled trials on the pharmacological treatment of SCI pain is presented in a paper by Basastrup and Finnerup.[35]

The anticonvulsant drugs have been studied the most of all antineuropathic agents and currently gabapentin and pregabalin are considered first-line drugs even though there are both positive and negative studies. The most comprehensive study was by Siddall et al. who used a flexible dosing schedule of pregabalin and found doses ranging from 150–600 mg (mean dose of 460 mg) were better than placebo.[36] Another recent trial supported these findings with pregabalin doses of up to 600 mg day being better than placebo.[37] Two trials with gabapentin using doses up to 3600 mg/day showed mixed results with one showing gabapentin better than placebo[38] and a second trial showing no difference from placebo.[39] A third study showed gabapentin no more effective than placebo; however, this study used doses up to only 1800 mg/day and only included seven subjects.[40] Trials with other anticonvulsant drugs lamotrigine and valproic acid have not been effective in the treatment of SCI pain.[41,42]

There is an extensive literature supporting the use of antidepressants for the treatment of neuropathic pain and therefore it is reasonable to believe that they have a place in the treatment of SCI pain. Only amitriptyline and trazodone have been subjected to randomized, placebo-controlled trials and the results have been mixed. One study at doses up to 150 mg/day of amitriptyline resulted in better pain relief than plabebo[39] whereas a second study using doses ranging from 10–125 mg/day showed no effect over placebo.[43] A study of trazodone at doses ranging from 50–150 mg/day showed no effect.[44] The selective serotonin reuptake inhibitors (SSRIs) and the selective norepinephrine reuptake inhibitors (SNRIs) have not been studied for SCI pain. These agents have a better side effect profile than the tricyclic antidepressants; however, the SSRI have demonstrated inconsistent effects in the treatment of neuropathic pain. Clinical trials with the SNRIs have consistently demonstrated efficacy and therefore are reasonable alternatives for SCI pain.

Sodium channel antagonists may have a role in the treatment of SCI pain. Galer and colleagues found intravenous (IV) lidocaine infusion was useful in patients with central pain in a population of mixed SCI and post-stroke central pain, although the effect in central pain was less than that in peripheral neuropathic pain.[45] A randomized control trial by Finnerup also showed a positive effect of IV lidocaine on SCI pain.[46] Mexiletine, an oral analogue of lidocaine, did not have any significant effect on SCI pain at a dose of 450 mg three times per day. There were severe side effects at this dose which is a limitation of mexiletine.[47]

The systemic opioids have been shown to be effective in the treatment of a variety of neuropathic pain syndromes; however, there are few studies in SCI pain. Only one study has looked at the effects of a systemic opioid on SCI pain. Attal et al. showed studied the effects of IV morphine on spontaneous and evoked pain of CPSP and SCI pain and found no difference from placebo.[48] A randomized double-blind crossover study compared the putative N-methyl-d-aspartate receptor antagonist ketamine and the opioid receptor agonist alfentanil.[49] Both agents reduced both spontaneous and evoked pain. Ketamine did not affect windup pain and was associated with significant side effects, although it did diminish allodynia. The recently published neuropathic treatment guidelines recommend the opioids as second-line therapy which is a reasonable approach for SCI pain.[50]

GABA receptors are widely distributed throughout the CNS and thought to control pain transmission.[229] A controlled trial of propofol (Diprivan 1% in an oil and water emulsion containing 10% soy bean oil, AstraZeneca) a putative $GABA_A$ agonist has found that propofol decreased spontaneous and evoked pain in a population of patients with SCI central pain and CPSP (see later discussion, Treatment of CPSP: Medical). Balofen, a $GABA_B$ agonist, is widely used to treat spasticity in SCI patients. There have been reports emerging in the literature on the effects of intrathecal baclofen on neuropathic pain. A small study in seven patients showed that a single dose of baclofen (50 mcg) decreased dysesthetic pain and spasm related pain in SCI patients.[52]

Studies have shown that intrathecal lidocaine reduces the pain of SCI suggesting that pain generators exist in the spinal cord of such patients.[53] A number of intrathecally delivered agents have been shown be effective in the treatment of SCI including the opioids, clonidine, baclofen, and the calcium channel antagonist ziconotide. In SCI central pain syndromes intraspinal delivery of opioids (alfentanil) was found to be effective for the treatment of spontaneous and evoked pain[49] while morphine was reported to be ineffective except in combination with clonidine.[54] Both epidural and intrathecal clonidine has been reported to relieve SCI pain.[55] Although the role of $GABA_B$ agonists on the treatment of SCI related spasticity is clear, the effects of these agents on SCI pain is less clear. A study by Herman et al. found that intrathecal baclofen reduced pain in a SCI central pain syndrome patients.[56] A study by Loubser and Akman showed no effect of intrathecal baclofen on SCI neuropathic pain.[57] There is one case report of two patients with SCI pain and spasticity that responded to the calcium channel blocker ziconotide.[58]

Treatment of Spinal Cord Injury Central Pain: Surgical Procedures

As discussed previously, there are a number of conservative options available for the treatment of SCI pain. Given the risks associated with surgical procedures, conservative therapies should be exhausted before using the more invasive therapies. If the patient fails systemic therapies, they should be first evaluated for spinal drug delivery since this therapy is reversible. The discussion of surgical procedures for SCI central pain must balance the limited success and incidence of complications, against the severity and impact of pain. Nondestructive procedures should be considered first. If destructive procedures are to be used, spinal procedures should be considered first. Aggressive medical therapy, psychological evaluation, and assessment of narcotic intake must be considered before commencing surgical treatment.[7]

Imaging studies help in the planning of operations which address the pain directly such as the dorsal root entry zone (DREZ) procedure and spinal cord stimulation (SCS). Imaging will also identify structural abnormalities such as a syrinx that, if progressive, must be dealt with first. If the preliminary investigation discloses the presence of a syrinx, it should first be treated by a procedure to shunt cyst fluid to the subarachnoid space or the pleural space.[8] Syringomyelia should be suspected in long-delayed onset of SCI central pain and in patients who show delayed changes in their neurologic status or who have facial pain.[7] Drainage of a syrinx relieved pain in the majority of patients (22/37, 59%), partially in 40%, and completely in 19% at 6 weeks after surgery. Any improvement was maintained for a year in only 24% of patients, all of whom retained unpleasant symptoms. In summary, the syrinx must be treated to prevent additional neurologic deficits; pain, when present, is not usually alleviated by treatment of the syrinx. Success after pain surgery is measured by the patient's pain ratings, quality of life scales, the patient's overall satisfaction with the procedure, and subsequent treatment, particularly consumption of analgesics.

One of the first procedures to be considered is spinal cord stimulation (SCS), because of its simplicity and low risk (see Chapter 95). It is indicated in SCI central pain patients in whom sufficient dorsal columns survive above the lesion so that stimulation produces paresthesiae in the patient's area of pain, although some consider that the success rate is too low to justify a trial.[5,60] The inability to produce adequate paresthesiae with SCS is the probable cause of the low success rate in treating SCI central pain.[7] Another problem is that spinal cord injury itself or the primary surgical treatment of the pain-causing lesion may have so disturbed the local anatomy that SCS carries a significant surgical risk.

Deep brain stimulation (DBS) of the thalamus, periventricular grey, or medial lemniscus bilaterally is sometimes considered for treatment of the steady component of SCI central pain when SCS fails.[7] Large retrospective series of DBS have reported mixed results in SCI central pain. An early report found that success (50% pain relief) occurred in the short term in 3/8 patients and 2/8 long term.[61] Another study found pain relief of 0% to 25% in 2/12 patients, and 25% to 50% in 1/12.[62,63] If SCS produces adequate paresthesiae and fails to relieve the pain, paresthesia-producing DBS also fails. Paresthesiae-producing DBS is preferable to periventricular DBS for the steady neuropathic pain, the latter being preferable for nociceptive pain.[61–64]

Local anesthetic diagnostic blocks performed proximal or distal to the causative lesion, are used to determine if pain relief is obtained after blocking a specific nerve or nerve group. If so, an ablative procedure of the same nerve or nerve group might be helpful.[65,66] Permanent section of the same neural structure affected by the block does not lead to long-term pain relief.[3] Nerve blocks may be useful in monoradicular syndromes by allowing confirmation of the fact that division of a particular root can stop the allodynia or hyperpathia. They also allow an assessment of the degree of sensory attenuation, particularly position sense, to be expected should that root be divided in an attempt to relieve the pain. Sympathectomy may be useful for complex regional pain syndrome type I that is superimposed on spinal cord injury (see Chapter 102).

The differential response of SCI central pain to stimulation or augmentative versus destructive procedures is a basic organizing principle of the surgical approaches to this type pain. Chronic stimulation that produces paresthesiae in the area of pain has limited efficacy for the relief of spontaneous, steady pain while destructive procedures such as cordotomy, cordectomy, and the DREZ operation are useful treatment for intermittent spontaneous pain or allodynia/hyperalgesia.[7]

Hypersensitivity following peripheral lesions may result from altered processing of peripheral stimuli in the dorsal horn, which is transmitted to the brain through the STT, resulting in pain.[59,67] It seems likely that hyperalgesia secondary to peripheral lesions would be relieved by medical or surgical strategies that block transmission in the STT either by destructive or augmentative procedures. The mechanism of hyperalgesia caused by spinal cord lesions is more difficult to understand because the causative lesion in these cases is proximal to the dorsal horn. Nevertheless, SCI

central pain can be relieved by transection of the STT, the DREZ procedure, and cordectomy (see Chapter 104).

There is a selective differential benefit of cordotomy on the neuralgic compared with the steady element of the patient's pain.[7,24,60] In a recent series (n = 39) undergoing cordotomy, mostly by the percutaneous technique, 54% enjoyed good relief and 32% fair relief of the neuralgic pain, 50% good relief and 25% fair relief of the evoked pain, and 6% good relief and 21% fair relief of the steady elements of SCI central pain.[5] However, percutaneous cordotomy carries a small risk of producing ipsilateral limb paresis, or impaired automatic respiration, and of aggravated bladder dysfunction, crucial matters for the spinal cord–injured patient with an incomplete lesion. Furthermore, the pain of many etiologies, perhaps including SCI central pain, tends to recur after cordotomy.[68,69] Long-term follow-up of Rosomoff series revealed that cordotomy initially relieved pain in 90% of patients, but that after 3 months relief had fallen to 84%, after 1 year to 61%, after 1 to 5 years to 43%, and after 5 to 10 years to 37%.

The DREZ operation has proved as successful as cordotomy and cordotomy in the relief of the neuralgic and evoked elements of spinal cord central pain. Like cordotomy, it results in an elevation of the patient's sensory level and requires a laminectomy. Conus DREZ may interfere with surviving bladder function. The DREZ procedure has been found to be most useful for the relief of end-zone pain (i.e., pain starting at the level of injury and extending distally), and not so effective for the diffuse, often sacrally distributed pain.[70] This procedure is most effective for pain in the dermatomes immediately caudal to the level of injury. Pain extending into areas remote from the injury site described as phantom, body, or diffuse burning pain is not very responsive.[71]

Destructive stereotactic procedures such as medial thalamotomy or mesencephalic pain tract section yield such poor relief of SCI central pain that they are contraindicated.[60,72,73]

The spontaneous, intermittent neuralgic component of SCI central pain has been recognized by many authors to be associated with conus and cauda lesions.[74] Such pain may be the result of root damage. Like hyperalgesia, it is relieved by interrupting the STT or inputs to the STT, by the DREZ operation, or by transection of the spinal cord.[7,75] In the literature concerning DREZ operation,[76,77] it is recognized that this procedure, like cordectomy,[7] is ineffective for the relief of the spontaneous, steady pain. However, it can relieve pain starting at the level of the lesion and extending caudally for a variable number of dermatomes as well as radicular pain.

The most common aspect of SCI central pain, the spontaneous, steady, causalgic, or dysesthetic element, is similar to that seen in all types of neuropathic pain. In spinal cord central pain, this is more characteristic of lesions above the level of the conus and can also occur in radicular distribution. This is the type of pain that is most difficult to relieve. It is not stopped by spinal cord transection above the level of the injury,[7] but responds best to chronic stimulation that produces paresthesiae in the area of the patient's pain.[78]

The relative merit of these destructive and augmentative procedures was assessed in a series of 127 patients with SCI central pain refractory to medical treatment.[7] The surgical procedures consisted of percutaneous cordotomy in 39 cases, cordectomy in 12, dorsal root entry zone (DREZ) surgery in 4, dorsal cord stimulation in 35, and brain stimulation in 13. Destructive surgery (cordotomy, DREZ surgery, or cordectomy) affected the three chief types of pain differently from treatment with SCS or brain stimulation. Destructive surgery resulted in reduction of steady pain in 26% of affected cases, of intermittent pain in 89%, and of evoked pain in 84%. Stimulation resulted in pain reductions in 36%, 0%, and 16% of cases, respectively. The differential effect of destructive surgery on steady and intermittent pain is consistent with published experience. These observations suggest differing mechanisms for the three types of pain.

In the patient with a conus/cauda lesion with significant neuralgic pain shooting up or down the legs below this level, relief is unlikely with SCS, although a trial may be attempted.[7] The next simplest step is a destructive procedure to interrupt the pain pathways such as cordotomy, cordectomy, or DREZ lesion. Transection of the spinal cord just above the level of the patient's injury is referred to as cordectomy. It is carried out at the expense of elevating the sensory level one or a few segments and of denervating the lower abdominal muscles.[7] However, the promise of therapies which may allow the spinal cord to heal makes this last approach unacceptable at present.

BRAIN CENTRAL PAIN

Central pain caused by lesions of the brain is as intractable as that arising from lesions of the spinal cord. It can arise from lesions of any etiology above of the spinal-medullary junction. Most cases of brain central pain are caused by strokes as shown in Table 28.2, which lists the etiology in 73 cases reported in Tasker's series.[5] This included hematomas which occurred in 17% of patients in the series. These lesions can be minimal or massive or associated with minor or major neurologic deficit. Like other types of neuropathic pain, it is idiosyncratic, often has a delayed onset, may occur in the absence of clinically detectable sensory loss, and commonly has three features: spontaneous steady pain, neuralgic pain, and evoked pain (allodynia and hyperpathia).[5] Papers by Head and Holmes and by Dejerine and Roussy[79] are pioneering studies of the clinical description of CPSP.[80,81]

TABLE 28.2

ETIOLOGY IN 73 CASES OF BRAIN CENTRAL PAIN (EXPRESSED AS PERCENTAGES)

Vascular	90.6%
Supratentorial	78.1
Thrombotic stroke	67.1
Spontaneous	57.5
Subarachnoid hemorrhage	2.7
Iatrogenic	
Artery ligation	2.7
Angiography	1.4
Postoperative	1.4
Trauma	1.4
Hematoma	11.0
Spontaneous	9.6
Thalamotomy lesion	1.4
Infratentorial	
Thrombotic stroke	6.9
Lateral medullary syndrome	5.5
Other	1.4
Hematoma	4.2
Hematobilia	1.4
Infection: Abscess	2.7
Vaccinia encephalitis	1.4
Other: Trigeminal tractotomy	1.4
Syringobulbia	1.4
Thalamic astrocytoma	1.4
Degenerative, not yet diagnosed	1.4

(From Tasker RR. *Central pain states.* In: Loeser JD, Butler SH, Chapman CR, Turk DC, eds. *Bonica's Management of Pain.* Philadelphia: Lippincott Williams & Wilkins; 2002.)

Clinical Features

Most cases of CPSP are caused by strokes. Brain central pain has been reported to be uncommon, occurring in only 1% to 2% of all strokes.[1,82] A more accurate estimate of the incidence may be that of Andersen and colleagues who studied 267 consecutive stroke patients at one institution over a 1-year post-stroke interval.[83] Two hundred seven survived more than 6 months, and were cognitively intact so that they could participate in sensory testing. Among this group, 47% had sensory abnormalities, while central pain developed in 8%, and a central nonpainful dysesthesia syndrome developed in 1 patient. All but one patient with CPSP also developed allodynia to heat or cold (9 patients each) or both. Central pain began by 1 month in 10 patients and after greater than 6 months in 3. Pain was mild in 6 (3%), and moderate to severe in 10 patients (5%).[83] Therefore, CPSP is not uncommon among patients with stroke and, when present, spontaneous and evoked pain are frequently severe.

Dejerine and Roussy have stated that stroke-induced pain depended on thalamic lesions. They coined the term "thalamic pain syndrome."[80] This statement and term was disputed by Biemond.[84] Modern imaging has confirmed that pain can arise from lesions in brainstem, thalamus, subcortical white matter, and cerebral cortex.[85-88] The location of nuclear thalamic lesions in these studies is unclear since they employed routine interpretation of CT and MRI scans.

There are three series of CPSP in which quantitative sensory testing was carried out along with descriptions of central pain qualities (Table 28.3). In one recent series, the patients' ongoing pain was characterized by temperature descriptors in eight (62%) cases, while mechanical descriptors were endorsed by nine (69%) patients.[89] These results are similar to those reported in the two comparable studies of CPSP.[86,90] Patients in the more recent study had higher pain ratings than did patients in the other two series, suggesting that there may be differences in the populations included in these studies.

The recent results are compared with previous studies of quantitative sensory testing reported as individual patients with CPSP.[86,90,91] Tactile hypoesthesia was documented in 50% of the patients tested, similar to the proportion reported in previous studies.[89] These previous studies documented hyperalgesia, by using a rotating von Frey hair[83] or a pin prick.[90] The sensations normally evoked by the rotating von Frey were not described; thus, it may not be appropriate to compare their results with the recent study.

All studies reported a large proportion of patients with cool hypoesthesia, while no more than 23% showed cold allodynia (Table 28.3). All studies described a small number of patients with bilateral cool hypoesthesia. All studies reported a large proportion of patients with warm hypoesthesia, but very few cases of heat allodynia. Thus, these studies demonstrated no clear relationship between compromise of painful sensation and allodynia within any particular submodality.

The most consistent characteristic of patients with CPSP is abnormal sensibility to some aspect of the STT-mediated sensations, particularly the innocuous thermal sensations of warmth (85%, 11/13), and cool (85%, 11/13) in patients with either CPSP[86,90] or SCI.[11] The patients show less consistent abnormalities of painful than nonpainful sensibility. Abnormal cold pain thresholds were observed in 9/13 patients, abnormal heat pain thresholds in only 1/13, and brush allodynia in 7/13. The other two series of patients with CPSP had higher proportions of abnormalities in cold, heat, and tactile pain sensibility than did the present series.[86,91]

A descriptive report of 73 patients with CPSP found that the onset of pain was often delayed, consistent with previous studies.[5,90] Pain in CPSP pain was commonly characterized by steady (usually burning 64.4%), dysesthetic (31.6%), intermittent pain

TABLE 28.3

COMPARISON OF SERIES OF PATIENTS WITH CPSP WHO WERE STUDIED CLINICALLY AND BY QUANTITATIVE SENSORY TESTING

Reference	89	85, 90	Descriptors, 86; sensory testing, 83
Burning cold/cold pain	53% overall; 38%, burning and cold; 15%, hot and cold	59%, 16/27	38%, 6/16 (freezing 3/16)
Mechanical pain	77% overall; 33%, sharp/stab; 23%, pressure heavy; tight/squeezing, 7% each	Aching 30%, pricking 30%, lacerating 26%	86%, 23/27
Pain rating	7.1 mean, 2.0 SD	2.5–7.9 mean by stroke location	3.3 median (0–7)
Touch—method	Von Frey for threshold; brushes for allodynia	V Frey for threshold, Pin prick for hyperalgesia	V Frey hair, V Frey rotating for hyperalgesia
Normal threshold	50%, 5/10	48%, 13/27	54%, 6/11
Hypoesthesia	50%, 5/10	52%, 14/27	27%, 3/11
Allodynia/Hyperalgesia	54% 7/13	16/27, 59% hyperalgesia	1/11 hyperalgesia
Cool—method	Peltier Medoc	Peltier Somedic, warm minus cool threshold	Peltier Somedic
Normal threshold	15%, 2/13	0/27	9%, 1/11
Hypoesthesia	85%, 11/13, 3 with equal bilateral hypoesthesia	Diff in cool-warm thresholds 17/27; larger change in cool 2/27	91%, 10/11
Cold pain—method	As above	As above	As above
Normal threshold	31%, 4/13	7% normal difference between cold & heat pain threshold	18%, 2/11-unaffected side lower
Hypoalgesia	46%, 6/13 (2 indeterminate)	93% abnormal difference between cold and heat pain threshold	45%, 5/11 (4/11-bilateral hypoalgesia)
Allodynia	23%, 3/13	No abnormally sensitive thresholds, but 5/22 (23%) reported discomfort to metal at room temperature	0/11
Warm—method	As above	As above	As above
Normal threshold	15%, 2/13	–	–
Hypoesthesia	85%, 11/13	Diff in cool-warm thresholds, 17/27; larger change in warm threshold, 8/27	11/11
Heat pain – method	As above	As above	As above
Normal	93%, 12/13	7% normal difference between cold and heat pain threshold	9%, 1/11
Hypoalgesia	7%, 1/13 (2 indeterminate)	93% abnormal difference between cold and heat pain threshold	91%, 10/11
Allodynia	0/13 (2 borderline)	No abnormally sensitive thresholds	0/11

The fourth column includes both clinical findings (n = 16)[86] and quantitative sensory testing (n = 11).[83] Similarly, the third column includes both clinical[85] and sensory testing results (both n = 27).[90] Another very large series could not be included because of quantitative sensory testing population statistics.[91] (From Greenspan JD, Ohara S, Sarlani E, Lenz FA. Allodynia in patients with post-stroke central pain (CPSP) studied by statistical quantitative sensory testing within individuals. *Pain* 2004;109:359–366, with permission.)

(16.4%), and allodynia or hyperalgesia (64.9%).[5] Distribution of intermittent pain was similar to that of spontaneous pain overall and to that of sensory diminution. Onset is often delayed between 1 and 4 weeks in 47% to 63% and greater than 4 weeks in approximately 20%.[5,83,92] Distribution of pain varied and bore no relation to any clinical features. Size, side, or location of the lesion; degree of sensory diminution; age; and sex all had no apparent relationship to the quality or severity of the pain.

The original description of the Dejerine-Roussy syndrome included abnormal movements and dystonia on the same side of the body as the pain.[80] Dystonia affected 8.2% of Tasker's series, all in patients with thalamic lesions,[5] although stroke-induced dystonia occurs regularly in the absence of central pain.[93] In the same series of patients with CPSP, 6.8% had tremor in addition to central pain, especially in the case of brainstem lesions, and so could be classified as midbrain or Holmes tremor.[94]

Lesions Resulting in Central Poststroke Pain

The recent version of the disinhibition hypothesis proposes that central pain results from a lesion involving a lateral, cold-signaling, STT pathway which projects to the insula through nucleus ventral medial posterior (VMpo; see later discussion).[95] According to this hypothesis, lesions of VMpo or posterior insula lead to cold hypoesthesia, which results in the burning pain of CPSP. Therefore, the location of thalamic and cortical strokes in CPSP provides a critical test of this hypothesis.

Lateral (Vc, Vcpc) and posterior thalamus (Vcpor, Vmpo, Po) and perisylvian or primary sensory cortex are most clearly linked to the sensory-discriminative aspect of pain. Injections of lidocaine into monkey VP, corresponding to human Vc, are associated with a decreased ability to detect small changes in temperature in both the innocuous and noxious range.[96] A study in patients with pure somatic sensory stroke (n = 21) identified 11 thalamic strokes, 9 lacunes, and 2 hemorrhagic strokes. The lacunes were confined to "posterior lateral thalamus probably involving the Vc." Five involved both tactile and thermal/pain sensations, six were lacunes which involved either tactile or thermal/pain sensations, and nine were located in the ventral posterior lateral thalamus of corresponding to Vc.[88,97,98] Six of these were small lacunes which were associated with diminution of some and sparing of other somatic sensory modalities. Although central pain was not explicitly assessed, most patients reported unpleasant sensations in areas of sensory deficits.

Four patients with CPSP secondary to small thalamic lesions were studied with quantitative sensory testing.[99] All had alterations of cold pain sensation (either allodynia or hypoalgesia), while three patients had cool hypoesthesia. The patient with the least involvement of Vc had normal cool detection thresholds, suggesting that a lesion involving a critical volume of Vc is required to impair this modality. Perception of warm was impaired only in lesions involving nuclei posterior to Vc, consistent with the effect of injection of local anesthetic into monkey ventral posterior thalamus (corresponding to human Vc).[88,96] Heat pain threshold was not abnormal in any of these cases. Tactile perception was always impaired on the involved side. In a subject with cold allodynia, a single subject protocol positron emission tomography (PET) study measured the responses to immersion of either hand in a 20°C waterbath. The scan during stimulation of the affected hand (evoking allodynic pain) was characterized by intense activation of contralateral sensorimotor cortex. Therefore, there appear to be modality-specific elements in the human posterior thalamus, but lesions of Vc are sufficient to impair cold sensibility and to produce CPSP.

Lesions of the thalamus and cortex have also been studied in imaging studies of patients with CPSP. Previous studies have used computed tomography (CT) to localize lesions in thalamus in patients with central pain (n = 12). In four cases the lesions involved the thalamus, all of which involved other structures in addition to the thalamus.[83] In a similar study of 27 patients with CPSP, 9 out of 27 had thalamic lesions that could not be further specified, of which 2 were limited to the thalamus.[100] In a study of magnetic resonance imaging (MRI) scans in patients with central pain, 49/70 patients had lesions including the "ventral posterior nucleus" (corresponding to Vc).[101] Finally, MRI- and atlas-based methods have been used to demonstrate that thalamic lacunes leading to CPSP were located in Vc and do not involve VMpo,[99,102] contrary to the hypothesis that VMpo involvement is critical for thalamic lesion induced central pain, cool hypoesthesia, and cold allodynia.[95]

Similar techniques have been used in studies of sensory function following cortical lesions. Lesions of cortical elements of the STT-thalamocortical system in patients with central pain involve the somatic sensory structures. Imaging analysis of patients with CPSP have identified lesions in the parietal lobe in 4/5 patients with cortical lesions leading to central pain[86]; precise anatomy of capsular lesions (2 patients) could not be further specified. In another study, patients with central pain had parietal lesions in all extrathalamic cases.[85] A prior study of MRI scans in patients with CPSP had cortical lesions localized to insula or parietal cortex.[101] A patient with compression of the retro-insula and the parietal operculum posterior to the central sulcus had elevated pain thresholds to mechanical, heat, and cold stimuli.[103] Decreased unpleasantness associated with experimental pain was reported in a series of insular strokes identified by CT scan.[104] A study employing comprehensive quantitative somatic sensory testing revealed that lesions of the parietal operculum decreased the discrimination of pain while lesions of the insula increased the tolerance for pain.[105] Lesions of SI reduce the ability to discriminate painful stimuli[106,107] and reduce chronic pain.[108] A case study of an isolated stroke in the arm area of S1 decreased pain discrimination but did not decrease the unpleasantness of pain.[79] Therefore, the precise insular and parietal lesions associated with CPSP are unclear.

Mechanisms of Central Pain: Imaging Studies of Spontaneous Pain

Functional imaging studies have reported both hypo- and hyperactivity of the thalamus in central pain patients. Multiple PET studies reported decreased cerebral blood flow (CBF) in the ipsilesional thalamus in central pain patients during rest.[109–112] Due to poor spatial resolution of these PET studies, the exact thalamic nuclei could not be specified. This relative thalamic hypoactivity could be reversed by motor cortex stimulation[113] or by repeated cycles of daily IV lidocaine infusion.[110] At the same time, motor cortex stimulation and lidocaine treatment reduced pain compared to the resting state. Similar decreases in thalamic perfusion have been found in chronic peripheral neuropathic pain, such that the thalamus contralateral to the affected body region exhibited substantially lower CBF than the ipsilateral thalamus.[114–116]

Hyperactivity of the thalamus has also been described, typically under conditions of increased pain. A single photon emission computed tomography (SPECT) study reported bilateral regional metabolic increases in the thalamus in a case of SCI central pain during the experience of spontaneous high intensity paroxysmal central pain. However, reduced thalamic blood flow was observed when the spontaneous pain was at a low intensity compared to resting values of healthy subjects.[117] However, these data are descriptive in nature; no statistical analyses were done. Other SPECT and PET studies of CPSP patients demonstrated hyperactivity in the thalamic area after stimulating the allodynic side compared to stimulating the nonallodynic side and/or to patients without allodynia.[109,118–120]

An interesting SPECT study in patients with CRPS demonstrated hyperperfusion of the thalamus contralateral to the painful limb compared to the ipsilateral thalamus in patients with symptoms for only 3–7 months, but hypoperfusion of the contralateral compared to the ipsilateral thalamic in patients with long-term symptoms (24–36 months).[121] In contrast, symmetric perfusion of bilateral thalami was found in controls. No differences between controls and patients were seen with symptoms of the disease for 10–13 months. It remains to be determined if the same holds for central pain. Therefore, thalamic spontaneous blood flow may be increased or decreased in central pain syndromes, perhaps related the duration of the syndrome. Blood flow activations evoked by allodynic stimuli in central pain are considered in later discussions.

Neurochemical Studies

The most basic study of neurochemistry in central pain reported changes in magnetic resonance spectroscopic (MRS) signals consistent with different classes of thalamic cells. An MRS study found that thalamic concentrations of the neuronal marker N-acetyl-aspartate (NA) and the glial cell marker *myo*-inositol (Ins) differed between patients with or without central pain after SCI.[122] Mean NA concentrations and the NA/Ins ratio were significantly lower for pain patients compared to pain-free patients. Mean Ins concentrations were higher for pain patients versus pain-free patients, and the difference approached significance. Further, NA concentrations were negatively correlated with pain intensity and Ins were positively correlated with pain intensity in the pain group. No significant differences were found between the right and left thalamus, but it is unclear if pain was localized unilaterally. These results reflect dysfunction or loss of neurons in the thalamus in patients with central pain secondary to spinal cord injury.

It has been suggested that up or down regulation of receptors may be involved in the development of central pain, which could also explain the delayed time course of the development of central pain.[101] Recent PET studies of opioid receptor binding in both healthy subjects and central pain patients can be interpreted in the light of a recent study of healthy volunteers.[123] This study demonstrated that many areas traditionally thought to be involved in pain processing have a high binding potential for opioids. Highest binding potentials were found in the thalamus (nuclei not identified), basal ganglia (putamen and caudate), amygdala, anterior cingulate cortex (ACC), midsagittal corpus callosum (MCC), and operculo-insular region. SI and MI have significantly less binding potential. No hemispheric differences were found.

Recent PET receptor binding studies demonstrate reduced nonspecific opioid-receptor binding in many of these areas in CPSP patients versus healthy controls.[124–126] Significant reduced regional binding was found independent of lesion site, mainly involving the thalamus, SII, insula, prefrontal cortex, ACC, and inferior parietal cortex (BA 40). Reduced radio-labeled opioid binding may reflect decreased binding of the exogenous ligand resulting from increased receptor occupancy by endogenous opioid peptides. However, the observation that two patients who received naloxone infusions did not develop increased pain contradicts this explanation.[126] Other explanations are loss of receptors due to the lesion, transneuronal degeneration, or receptor mechanisms such as receptor internalization or down-regulation.[125] Reduced opioid receptor binding in central pain patients may explain the poor response of these patients to opioid treatment.[127,128]

Up-regulation of receptors is also possible following lesion-induced denervation. SCI can also dysregulate sodium channel expression, specifically in neurons of the dorsal horn of the spinal cord and thalamus.[34] An imbalance of central excitatory and inhibitory mechanisms has been proposed to contribute to central pain. Pharmacological studies support the importance of neuronal hyperexcitability as a mechanism of central pain. Agents that inhibit hyperexcitability such as lidocaine (by blocking voltage-sensitive sodium channels), ketamine (by blocking NMDA receptors and thereby glutamatergic excitation), and lamotrigine (blocking both sodium channels and glutamate receptors) have been shown to be effective in relieving central pain.[129,130] Also increasing GABAergic inhibition with either baclofen or propofol has been shown to be effective.[129,130] However, it is not possible to identify the site of action of the agents in these clinical studies.

Motor Cortex and Central Pain

Motor cortex stimulation has been used for the treatment of central pain with success rates reported between 50% and 75%,[131,132] perhaps by modulation of activity in the spinal dorsal horn. Electrical stimulation of the motor cortex inhibited spinal neuronal responses to noxious pressure and pinch stimuli in a graded fashion, so that higher voltage of electrical stimulation reduced neuronal activity.[133] Motor cortex stimulation had no effect on the response to innocuous brush as recorded from wide dynamic neurons in lumbar spinal dorsal horn in rats. However, mixed results from motor cortex stimulation have been reported in monkeys so that motor cortex stimulation resulted in excitation or excitation followed by inhibition of STT cells.[133]

A recent imaging study shed new light on the possible underlying mechanism of motor cortex stimulation in relieving central pain. This recent PET blood flow study demonstrated that motor cortex stimulation in chronic neuropathic pain patients induced activation, partly during the stimulation period but mainly in the post-stimulation period, in the posterior mid-cingulate cortex (MCC), pregenual ACC, orbitofrontal cortex, putamen, thalamus, and brainstem (PAG and pons).[134] Regional CBF changes during this post-stimulation period correlated with pain relief. A functional connectivity analysis showed that these areas are all connected and provide a network that is influenced by motor cortex activation. Lack of efficacy of motor cortex stimulation in a subset of patients may be due to damaged corticospinal tracts or intracortical connections.

A recent study examined the effect of repeated sessions of repetitive transcranial magnetic stimulation (rTMS) at 20 Hz for 10 minutes each day on 5 successive days over the motor cortex. This pattern of stimulation reduced pain by about 40% compared to baseline and sham rTMS in patients with CPSP for at least 2 weeks after the end of the treatment.[135] Therefore, epidural or transcranial magnetic stimulation of motor cortex can have a substantial analgesic effect upon CPSP.

Involvement of the Spinothalamic Tract in the Mechanism of Central Pain

Many studies suggest that impairment of temperature and pain sensation are associated with the development of central pain.[136] A broad range of evidence links pain and temperature sensibility to the human STT, the principle somatic sensory nucleus (ventral caudal, Vc), and the nuclei below and behind. This thalamic area is involved in pain mechanisms based on the presence of a dense termination of the STT.[137,138] Stimulation of the STT produces thermal and pain sensations[139] and lesioning of the STT by cordotomy causes thermal and pain sensory loss.[140] In Vc or posterior/inferior to Vc, neurons respond to cold or painful stimulation[141–143] and stimulation may evoke painful or nonpainful heat and cold sensations.[142–144]

Temperature and pain sensation are signaled by the STT and surgical lesions leading to central pain often involve STT.[2] Therefore, it is reasonable to suppose that lesions of pain- and temperature-signaling pathways are common to all central pain syndromes. In fact, imaging studies (see previous discussion) outline anatomic evidence that lesions of STT-thalamocortical pathways are associated with CPSP.

These lesions also lead to sensitization of the STT-thalamocortical pathway in patients with CPSP. In such patients, electrical stimulation at micro-ampere current levels (microstimulation) in Vc and in the region inferior and posterior to Vc evokes pain sensations more commonly and nonpainful cold less commonly than in patients without central pain.[145,146] Stimulation of this region evoked pain more commonly in patients with hyperalgesia in the setting of central pain than in those without hyperalgesia.[21,137,142,144] Therefore, sensitization of this pathway may lead to the ongoing pain and hyperalgesia of central pain syndromes.

A broad range of evidence suggests that the cortical targets of these thalamic nuclei are involved in cold allodynia. The largest PET study of cold allodynia involved patients with a lateral medullary stroke (Wallenberg syndrome).[119] The allodynic test stimulus was a cold/mechanical stimulus described as "a cold non-noxious stimulus (ice in a flat plastic container) moved slowly" over the skin. When this stimulus was used on the affected side it produced activation of structures very similar to those activated in response to 20°C waterbath stimulation of the affected hand in a patient with CPSP secondary to a small stroke of the thalamic nucleus Vc.[99] These studies showed absence of ACC activation and the presence of sensorimotor activation. The sensorimotor responses were similar to those in another study in which healthy controls were stimulated with a 20°C waterbath, although ACC was activated in this study.[148]

This increased blood flow activation of sensorimotor cortex is consistent with hypersensitivity to electrical stimulation of Vc and primary somatic sensory cortex. Such stimulation produces pain more commonly in patients with central pain than those without.[20,21,142–144] Lesions of the sensorimotor cortex can dramatically relieve pain in patients with thalamic central pain.[151–153] Therefore, the evidence of blood flow, stimulation, and lesion studies forcefully makes the case that Vc and sensorimotor cortex are involved in the development of CPSP.

There is also evidence of sensitization of medial and intralaminar nuclei which receive nociceptive input, including medial dorsal nucleus. Electrical stimulation of the medial and intralaminar thalamus has evoked a range of effects and sensations which are usually unpleasant.[154] These sensations include dyspnea and dizziness,[154,155] pain and heat,[156] pupillary dilation and contraversive eye movements,[157] and nonspecific painful sensations.[158–160]

In Tasker's series of operative cases, burning and pain were evoked much more commonly by stimulation in medial and intralaminar thalamus than at other thalamic sites. Macrostimulation-induced burning was nearly always on the contralateral side of the body.[139] Forty-three percent of the sites where burning was evoked occurred in the 89% of patients with movement disorders, usually sporadically, in isolation from other pain sites, and 57% occurred in the 13% of patients operated on for chronic pain.[139] In the latter group, the pain sites were usually clustered. Burning was induced contralaterally without somatotopographic organization. Eighty percent of the sites at which stimulation induced burning occurred in the 41% of pain patients who experienced neuropathic pain; but only 20% occurred in the 59% with cancer pain. Similar results were obtained for the 67 points at which painful, nonburning responses were recorded.

The most detailed description of the pain evoked by stimulating these nuclei reported two types of sensation.[158,161] The first type was a diffuse, burning pain referred to the contralateral half of the body, or occasionally to the whole body. The sites at which these sensations were produced were usually concentrated near the posterior half of the internal medullary lamina, corresponding to the parvocellular regions of central medial, plus parafascicularis and limitans. The first response to stimulation was exacerbation of the patient's spontaneous pain. The other type of sensation was a generalized "unpleasant" sensation, not localized to a particular body part. The sites at which these sensations were produced were concentrated in the very medial and anterior regions, possibly the medial dorsal and periventricular nuclei. Rinaldi and coworkers have also produced sensations by microstimulation in the medial thalamus, but these were not considered painful.[162] Instead a sensation of "pulling" was produced by stimulation in parafascicularis, while throbbing was produced by stimulation in the central medial nucleus.[139,163,164]

The Disinhibition Hypothesis of Central Pain

The sensory abnormalities in patients with central pain speak to the hypothesis that central pain/dysesthesia syndromes are associated with lesions of a cool-signaling STT pathway which disinhibits a nociceptive STT pathway.[95] This hypothesis proposes that a cool-signaling STT pathway passing from spinal lamina 1 through a lateral thalamic nucleus VMpo to the insula normally inhibits a heat-pinch-cold (HPC) nociceptive STT pathway passing from spinal lamina 1 through a medial thalamic nucleus (medial, dorsal, ventral caudal part to the ACC).[95] In patients with central pain, it is proposed that a lesion of the lateral cool pathway disinhibits the medial pain pathway, so that cold allodynia and the burning, cold, ongoing pain of CPSP occur in the absence of cold sensibility.[95]

Several lines of evidence help to evaluate this hypothesis. A study of small thalamic lesions leading to central pain uniformly involved the human principal sensory nucleus (Vc) but did not involve the VMpo (see previous discussion).[99] Approximately 50% of patients with central pain described their pain with temperature descriptors, while only about 25% demonstrated cold allodynia.[89] In the same study, strong cold allodynia was associated with normal cool detection thresholds in one case. Cool hypoesthesia, while frequently present, was not significantly associated with cold allodynia, however, it may be related to burning and/or cold ongoing pain.[89] These studies do not support the disinhibition theory of central pain.

There is contrary evidence that CPSP is mediated through sensory pathways including the dorsal columns. Patients with SCI central pain uniformly have diminution or loss of pain and/or temperature sensation.[4,10,11] However, the degree of sensory diminution for thermal or pain sensations is not a predictor of central pain in the population of patients with SCI.[4,10] Therefore, compromise of STT function is a necessary but not sufficient condition for the development of central pain in patients with SCI. Abnormal sensitivity to tactile and thermal stimuli is more common in SCI patients with central pain than in those without. The intensity of tactile allodynia at the border of sensory loss is a significant predictor of the intensity of spontaneous pain in the levels below the lesion.[4] These results suggest that SCI central pain is associated with hyperactivity in neurons higher along the somatic sensory pathways including structures receiving input from the dorsal columns.[22] This is consistent with a range of anatomic and physiologic studies of CPSP as reviewed next.

Involvement of the Dorsal Column Pathway in the Mechanism of Central Pain

A study of quantitative sensory testing in CPSP described previously has also demonstrated that tactile allodynia is more often associated with normal tactile sensibility than tactile hypoesthesia.[89] Tactile sensibility measured by von Frey hairs and a moving brush are mediated through the dorsal column pathway,[165–167] more than the STT pathway.[167–170] Sensory testing in patients with lesions of the dorsal columns revealed mild deficits in tactile sensation, while lesions of the STT (sparing the dorsal columns) were associated with no deficit in tactile sensation.[171] Therefore, the reduced tactile thresholds in the recent study are likely due to decreased transmission of stimuli through the dorsal column-thalamic-cortical pathway.[89] In those patients with CPSP, brush allodynia occurred in the presence of normal tactile thresholds, implying no lesion of the dorsal column-thalamic-cortical pathway in those patients.[171]

These results support a model in which brush-evoked allodynia involves input to the forebrain through an intact pathway dorsal column–thalamic Vc–post central gyrus and parietal operculum.[166,172,173] Activation of afferents known to project through the dorsal columns was associated with unpleasant dysesthesias only in stroke patients with post-stroke dysesthesias, a variant of CPSP.[174] This suggests that post-stroke dysesthesias result from transmission of activity through the dorsal columns.

The involvement of the dorsal column pathway in central pain is supported by electrophysiologic studies of the forebrain. Microstimulation in Vc evokes painful sensations more commonly in patients with CPSP than in controls operated for treatment of either movement disorders or non-CPSP pain syndromes.[20,21] In patients with CPSP and hyperalgesia, microstimulation in Vc evoked pain more frequently than in patients without hyperalgesia.[21] Stimulation in Vc evoked pain more frequently in the representation of the part of the body where the patient experienced hyperalgesia than did stimulation in the representation of other parts of the body.[21] The pain-related function of Vc is demonstrated by the presence of STT terminals,[138] sites where stimulation evokes pain,[143] and recording studies which demonstrate that some cells in Vc respond differentially or selectively to painful stimuli.[167] In combination with the present results, these studies are strong evidence of a role for the dorsal column–thalamic Vc-somatic sensory cortical pathway (SI) in tactile allodynia.

A few imaging studies examined cortical activation after tactile-evoked allodynia. A PET study using the capsaicin experimental pain model reported similar activation patterns during nonpainful light brush stimulation and capsaicin induced experimental tactile allodynia mainly in SI, bilateral parietal lobule/SII, ACC, ipsilateral insula, and ipsilateral putamen.[175] Activation specific to allodynia was mainly observed in bilateral superior frontal gyrus, ipsilateral posterior insula, and ipsilateral inferior parietal lobule/SII. In a functional MRI (fMRI) study using this same capsaicin model,[176] SI and SII activation were only found during nonpainful mechanical stimulation using von Frey filaments. When stimulating the area that provoked secondary mechanical hyperalgesia, significant activation was found in the prefrontal cortex, and middle and inferior frontal gyrus. No activation in the ACC was found.

The only imaging study of clinical tactile allodynia was carried out in SCI central pain patients with STT injuries. Tactile allodynia in these patients produced a pattern of brain activation distinct from that of cold allodynia in patients with CI.[120] Tactile stimuli consisted of repetitive stroking with a soft brush applied in the allodynic area of patients with and without central pain and normal controls. The pattern of activation for tactile allodynia was very similar to nonpainful brushing in normal volunteers and patients without pain. In all groups, activation was observed in the contralateral SI, contralateral SII, inferior, and superior parietal areas. Activation specific to allodynia was elicited in the contralateral thalamus, bilateral middle frontal gyrus, caudate nucleus, and supplementary motor areas. Tactile allodynia was not associated with activation in the insula or anterior cingulate. The most striking activation shared by tactile and cold allodynia was activation of S1 cortex, although prefrontal cortex was activated most reliably.

Thalamic Low-Threshold Spike Bursting Activity in Central Pain

Thalamic low-threshold spike (LTS) bursting occurs at rates above those found in patients with movement disorders.[16] In patients with spinal transection, the highest rate of bursting occurs in cells that do not have peripheral receptive fields and that are located in the representation of the anesthetic part of the body. These cells also have the lowest firing rates in the interval between bursts (principal event rate).[16] The low firing rates suggest that these cells have decreased tonic excitatory drive and are hyperpolarized, perhaps due to loss of excitatory input from the STT.[177–180] Therefore the available evidence suggests that affected thalamic cells in patients with spinal transection were dominated by spike-bursting consistent with membrane hyperpolarization.[21,181–184]

Spike-bursting activity is maximal in the region posterior and inferior to the core nucleus of Vc.[16] Stimulation in this area evokes the sensation of pain more frequently than does stimulation in the core of Vc.[145,185–187] Thus, increased spike-bursting activity may be correlated with some aspects of the abnormal sensation (e.g. dysesthesia or pain) that these patients experience.

However, in patients with spinal transaction, the painful area and the area of sensory loss overlap.[16] Thus, the bursting activity might be related to sensory loss, rather than to pain.

These findings about spike-bursting activity in spinal patients have been called into question by a recent study in patients with chronic pain.[146] It has been reported that the number of bursting cells per trajectory in patients with movement disorders (controls) is not different from that in patients with chronic pain. However, there are significant differences between the two studies[16,146] in terms of patient population (spinal cord injury vs. mixed chronic pain), location of cells studied (Vc vs. anterior and posterior to Vc), and analysis methods (incidence of bursting cells vs. bursting parameters). The increase in bursting activity demonstrated in the earlier study is more applicable to SCI central pain.[16]

Further support for increased spike-bursts occurring in spinal cord transected patients is found in thalamic recordings from monkeys with unilateral thoracic anterolateral cordotomies.[17] Some of these animals showed increased responsiveness to electrocutaneous stimuli and thus may represent a model of central pain[18] (see previous discussion). The most pronounced changes in firing pattern were found in thalamic MR cells. In comparison with normal controls, MR cells in the monkeys with cordotomies showed significant increases in the number of bursts occurring spontaneously or when evoked by brushing or compressive stimuli. The changes in bursting behavior occurred in the thalamic representation bilaterally in upper and lower extremities.

The relationship between spike-burst firing and pain does not appear to be direct. Increased bursting is found in the thalamic representation of the monkey upper extremity and of the representation of the arm and leg ipsilateral to the cordotomy. Pain is not typically experienced in these parts of the body in patients with thoracic spinal cord transection or cordotomy.[11] Spike-bursts are increased in frequency during slow wave sleep in all mammals studied[181] including man.[188] However, such bursting could cause pain if grouped, or bursting stimulation pulses, which activate bursting cells can produce the sensation of pain, as previously reported.[20–22]

Evidence for Ipsilateral Mechanisms of Stroke Pain

Projected fields (PF) refer to the perceived location of sensations evoked by stimulation of the nervous system. We compared PFs with receptive fields (RFs) which refers to the part of the body where stimulation evokes a response in the nervous system. In patients with spinal transection thalamic stimulation produced pain referred to the part of the body which was anesthetic, although no RFs were found in thalamic neurons by stimulation of that part of the body. Therefore, the anesthetic part of the body retained intact PFs, demonstrating the following, that thalamic neurons and thalamocortical connections can be left intact and apparently isolated after a stroke, yet still capable of generating conscious effects, and presumably capable of activation by alternate somatosensory input, possibly to generate pain.

A CPSP patient had a massive right-sided thrombotic stroke causing left homonymous hemianopsia, spastic hemiplegia, and multimodality hemisensory hypoesthesia with allodynia and hyperpathia. Stereotactic exploration with microelectrode presence before DBS was carried out.[5] An extensive exploration of the region of Vc thalamus revealed no neuronal activity.

A hemispherectomized patient has been reported who complained of touch-evoked pricking and burning pain in her paretic hand, especially when the hand was cold.[189] QST demonstrated confused cool and warm temperatures on the paretic side, and confirmed that she had a robust allodynia to brush stroking that was enhanced at a cold ambient temperature. fMRI showed that during brush-evoked allodynia, brain structures implicated in normal pain processing, such as the posterior part of the anterior cingulate cortex, secondary somatosensory cortex, and prefrontal cortices, were activated. The fMRI findings thus indicate that the central pain in this patient was served by brain structures implicated in normal pain processing.

QST studies in patients undergoing cingulotomy for psychiatric disease suggest that hyperalgesia for thermal sensations is found postoperatively.[190,191] Single subject PET studies in one patient demonstrated preoperative contact heat pain-evoked activation of the bilateral MCC/SMA (supplementary motor area) and the left (contralateral) frontoparietal operculum.[191] Postoperative pain-evoked activation was demonstrated in the right (ipsilateral) perisylvian cortex but not of the MCC/SMA. This pattern would be unusual in a population study protocol of healthy controls,[192] although the ipsilateral activations occur commonly in an fMRI study of healthy single subjects.[193] Ipsilateral perisylvian activation has also been observed during the increased (allodynic) responses to thermal stimuli in patients with central pain related to lesions of the brain or spinal cord.[109,120,194]

A similar pattern has been found in neurogenic allodynia secondary to injection of capsaicin.[175] Experimental tactile allodynia following cutaneous injection of capsaicin led to activation of superior frontal gyrus (BA 10) bilaterally, insula bilaterally, portions of the inferior frontal gyrus (BA 47 contralaterally), putamen/globus pallidus ipsilaterally, SII/inferior, parietal lobule (BA 40) bilaterally, middle frontal gyrus (BA 6, 8, and 10), and cingulate gyrus (BA 24, midline/ipsilateral), and contralateral SI. These and the previously reviewed results suggest that ipsilateral activations are a common factor in increased ratings of pain following brain lesions, whether clinically significant or not.

The mechanism of the increased activation of ipsilateral perisylvian structures postoperatively may be disinhibition of pain-related inputs to these structures by the cingulotomy.[191,195-197] This disinhibition could lead to pain-related increased synaptic activity and blood flow. In addition, postoperative pain-related activation of the right (ipsilateral) parietal and insular cortex after cingulotomy might be consistent with reports of activation of right inferior parietal cortex following stimulation of either side.[198] In that study, pain intensity–dependent activation was not entirely lateralized, but was localized to contralateral regions of the primary somatosensory cortex, secondary somatosensory cortex, insular cortex, and bilateral regions of the cerebellum, putamen, thalamus, anterior cingulate cortex, and frontal operculum. In contrast, right sided activation was found in thalamus, inferior parietal cortex (BA 40), dorsolateral prefrontal cortex (BA 9/46), and dorsal frontal cortex (BA 6) in response to painful (and nonpainful) stimulation, regardless of the side of stimulation.

These observations implicate ipsilateral pathways in the generation of the steady pain and allodynia and hyperpathia that plague such patients. Whatever the ipsilateral paths responsible for the pain, they must be somatotopically organized to preserve the somatotopic features of the pain and capable of inducing steady pain and allodynia, incriminating the ipsilateral STT.

Treatment of Central Poststroke Pain: Medical Treatment

As with SCI pain, the number of studies on the treatment of CPSP is remarkably small. It is reasonable to postulate that therapies that work for SCI pain should also be effective for CPSP. Frese et al. provide a good summary of the pharmacologic treatments for CPSP.[199] There are several studies in the literature that specifically look at drug therapy for CPSP. The first randomized, placebo-controlled, crossover trial of chronic oral medication compared amitriptyline versus carbamazepine versus control and the results demonstrated statistically significant pain relief from the second week of the trial onward for amitriptyline but no pain

relief from carbamazepine at any time point.[85] Two thirds of patients were responders and there was a positive correlation between pain relief and plasma amitriptyline levels >300 ngmol/L. The majority of responders stayed on amitriptyline following the trial suggesting that this agent provided durable analgesia.

There are several studies evaluating the efficacy of the anticonvulsants in CPSP. A randomized, placebo-controlled crossover trial of the anti-epileptic agent lamotrigine showed a significant decrease in pain ratings for the last week of the trial (30%), at doses of 200 mg/day. No significant effect was found at lower doses (25 or 50mg/day); 44% of patients were identified as responders.[200] The hypothesis that amitriptyline is effective for the prevention of CPSP was examined in a randomized, double-blind, placebo-controlled trial of amitriptyline with 1-year follow-up.[201] At the termination of the trial (1 year follow-up), no statistically significant benefit was found.[201] Other open label studies on the efficacy of the anticonvulsants phenytoin, gabapentin, and zonisamide for CPSP are too small to draw conclusions.[202-204]

There have also been a number of trials of local anesthetic agents for the treatment of CPSP. In a double-blind, placebo-controlled study in 6 patients with CPSP and 10 with SCI pain, IV lidocaine resulted in a significant short term relief of spontaneous pain, mechanical allodynia, and mechanical hyperalgesia.[205] After completing this study, 12 subjects were started on oral mexiletine (400–800 mg/day) with no effect on pain.[206] Edmondson and colleagues also found an analgesic effect in response to IV lidocaine infusion analgesic in 4/4 CPSP patients. Mexiletine, an oral congener of lidocaine, produced durable analgesia (1 year) in two of these four patients, while intolerable side effects developed in the other two patients.[207] IV lidocaine led to significant decreases in ongoing pain, allodynia to static and dynamic (brush) stimuli in a study of three patients.[208] Lidocaine-induced spinal block successfully relieved CPSP with allodynia in two of three patients; one of the successes and the failure had thalamic lesions.[209]

Studies on systemic opioids have shown no effect or limited effects in CPSP. A double-blind, randomized trial of levorphanol on neuropathic pain showed almost no effect in a subset of five patients with CPSP.[127] A randomized, double-blind placebo-controlled proof of principle trial of methadone showed no change in the pain rating in one patient, and a 50% reduction in the other.[210] In a randomized, double-blind study of opioids for treatment of all categories of neuropathic pain most of the patients with CPSP did not complete the study.[127] Those who did complete the study had approximately a 25% decrease in pain. IV morphine and IV fentanyl had no effect on CPSP[211-216] and on the pain of MS[217]; however, IV alfentanil led to a significant decrease in spontaneous and evoked pain.[49] In another study, intrathecal morphine with clonazepam led to significant pain relief, although neither agent was effective alone.[218] A double-blind, placebo-controlled trial of IV naloxone did not produce analgesia in patients with CPSP.[219] However, an open label trial of intravenous naloxone reported that "pain and hyperpathia were completely obtunded" in 7 out of 13 CPSP patients studied, and "partially obtunded" in one patient.[220]

In a mixed population of patients with SCI central pain and CPSP, the injection of putative GABA agonist propofol produced significant relief of both spontaneous and evoked pain.[221] This double-blind, placebo crossover trial employed a subhypnotic bolus dose of propofol. Decreases in spontaneous pain and allodynia (both cold and tactile) were significantly greater following injections of propofol than placebo. Differences between SCI central pain and CPSP were not significant. Four patients, with pain secondary to SCI or thalamic hemorrhage, had worse pain after propofol but not after placebo.[222] Overall, the injections were well tolerated without hemodynamic side effects. Burning at the site of injection was observed for a few patients, and a few patients complained of short-lasting lightheadedness in both the propofol and placebo groups. In an uncontrolled study, IV thiopental, a GABA-a agonist, resulted in pain relief in 22 of 39 patients with CPSP. However, oral amobarbital did not result in any pain relief even at plasma levels equivalent to the thiopental infusions.[223] An early study reported intravenous infusions of 50 to 225 mg of sodium pentothal reduced CPSP in 73% of CPSP patients.[215] One study reported positive effects of intrathecal baclofen, a GABA-b agonist, in 6 of 8 patients with CPSP.[56]

Other trials examined the role of a noncompetitive NMDA blockers, dextromethorphan and ketamine, on CPSP. The first of these was also a randomized, double-blind, placebo-controlled, crossover trial which found that dextromethorphan was ineffective for the treatment of CPSP.[224] A similar trial of dextromethorphan in a group of patients with neuropathic pain of mixed etiology also found no benefit.[225] Studies of ketamine given intravenously in patients with CPSP led to transient analgesia which lasted for less than 3 hours in two out of three patients.[218]

There are few studies on cannabinoid receptor agonists in the treatment of neuropathic pain. One randomized controlled trial of cannabinoids in multiple sclerosis patients produced significant decreases in pain.[226] A similar study did not find an analgesic effect but found significant improvements in symptom control, particularly in the case of insomnia.[227]

On the basis of the effectiveness of amitriptyline and the proof of principle trial of mexiletine,[201] Bowsher suggested that CPSP should be treated first with a trial of adrenergic antidepressants, then mexilitine.[87] In the German literature, opioids have been proposed to have had a major role in the long-term treatment of central pain.[228] Two recent consensus conferences evaluating database searches regarding pharmacologic approaches to the treatment of neuropathic pain of all types recommended tricyclics and calcium channel ligands (gabapentin) as the first line of treatment and antiepileptic drugs plus opioids as the second line.[50,229] The data reviewed here are consistent with these recommendations and it is reasonable to apply these recommendations to the treatment of CPSP.

Treatment of Central Poststroke Pain: Surgical Procedures

As with SCI pain, all conservative therapies should be exhausted before resorting to surgical interventions. Reversible treatments such as stimulation should be considered before resorting to neuroablative procedures. Of the stimulation procedures, motor cortex stimulation has been the most studied.

Tsubokawa and colleagues described motor cortex stimulation for the treatment of CPSP, placing paddle-type electrodes designed for SCS extradurally parallel to the central sulcus 3 to 4 cm from the midline for upper limb, and 1 cm from midline for lower limb pain.[230] These authors applied stimulation below the threshold for motor events, at which level it usually caused tingling or mild vibration in the area of pain. Pain typically diminished after 5 to 10 minutes of stimulation, and pain relief outlasted a 10-minute period of stimulation by 2 to 6 hours. Thus, patients would typically use five to seven bouts of stimulation daily. They believed that to relieve neural injury pain, it was necessary to stimulate rostral to the *causative* lesion, hypothetically activating the fourth-order sensory neurons whose nonnociceptive impulses induced by cortex stimulation inhibited nociceptive neurons.

Yamamoto and colleagues[224] tried to correlate certain pharmacologic tests with the success of motor cortex stimulation. They concluded in 25 cases of CPSP with thalamic lesions and 14 with suprathalamic lesions that those patients whose pain was diminished by thiamylal and ketamine administration but not by morphine responded best to motor cortex stimulation. Ninety percent of 10 cases of CPSP so treated did well after 1 year of follow-up.[230] Eleven patients were described with CPSP, 73% of whom enjoyed initial pain relief, with 45% long-term pain relief at 2 years' follow-up.[231] A small series reported that 50% of six patients were effectively controlled by motor cortex stimulation.[232] More recent studies suggest that motor cortex stimulation provides moderate success rates varying approximately between 50% and 75% of patients with CPSP.[131,132]

The overall level of evidence supporting the use of motor cortical stimulation for the treatment of pain has been assessed in detail. A database study of the European Association of Neurology Panel on Neurostimulation for the Treatment of Pain concluded that the use of motor cortical stimulation was supported by multiple retrospective studies without validated measures of outcome in the case of upper extremity, amputation pain, (phantom and stump), CPSP, facial pain, and headache.[233,234] They concluded that there is convincing evidence that motor cortex stimulation (MCS) is useful in 50% to 60% of patients with CPSP and trigeminal neuropathic pain.

A number of different stimulation approaches have been adopted for treatment of CPSP. Seven patients treated with trigeminal stimulation for the relief of chronic neuropathic facial pain suffered from CPSP, three with lateral medullary syndrome, one with a middle cerebral artery area infarct, one with a massive thalamic and suprathalamic infarct, one with an infarct after internal carotid artery ligation, and one with neuropathic pain after a medullary trigeminal tractotomy.[215] Five of these seven patients reported relief during trial stimulation and went on to enjoy more than 50% ongoing pain relief after implantation of a permanent device, a good result. The chief complication of this procedure was superficial infection at hardware sites.

SCS was of no benefit in CPSP among twelve cases in Tasker's series.[7] In this series, six reported pain relief during trial stimulation and received a permanent stimulator, but only 17% of the original group experienced ongoing relief. In four patients, all with allodynia, hyperpathia, or both, SCS was unsuccessful because stimulation was perceived as painful. This observation recalls the experience described previously in which microstimulation of the tactile relay of thalamus is often painful in patients experiencing stroke-induced pain with allodynia, hyperpathia, or both.[20,21]

The dichotomy between paresthesia-producing thalamic stimulation versus PVG/periaqueductal grey DBS in nociceptive versus neuropathic pain is a basic principle which may be used in planning DBS.[8,62] Thus, paresthesia-producing DBS may be more appropriate for CPSP than PVG/periaqueductal grey DBS. Anecdotal evidence suggests that stimulating in the internal capsule is preferable to other sites,[235] but until larger numbers of patients have been reported it is difficult to draw conclusions (see Chapter 96).

Two large retrospective series of DBS have reported mixed results in CPSP. An early report found success (50% pain relief) occurred in the short term in 8/13 patients and 6/13 long-term (2–14 years).[61] In another retrospective series including 12 patients with CPSP, pain relief was rated at 0% to 25% (2/12), 25% to 50% in 1/12, and 50% to 75% in 1/12.[62] In Tasker's series, six patients, all of whom suffered from allodynia, hyperpathia, or both, found stimulating in the Vc painful, preventing use of that treatment modality. On the other hand, patients with neuropathic pain not caused by cerebral lesions who had allodynia or hyperpathia seldom found such stimulation painful.[237] In three patients with stroke-induced allodynia, hyperpathia, or both, PVG stimulation relieved the allodynia and hyperpathia. Microelectrode recordings and stimulation in patients with central pain demonstrated that stimulation in the region of nucleus Vc was painful more frequently in this group than in controls, and in patients with allodynia or hyperalgesia than in those without.[20,21]

A database search identified three recent studies using current standards of MRI target localization in thalamus or PAG/PVG.[233] The first described results in 15 patients with CPSP who identified success (pain relief >30%) in 67% of patients at long-term follow-up. The other reported on 21 patients with mixed neuropathic pain syndromes, and concluded that only 24% of patients had durable pain relief as defined by use of DBS for over 5 years. Another study compared the benefit of SCS, thalamic DBS, and MCS in 45 patients with CPSP, reported success with DBS in only 25% of patients. Overall, they considered that there was weak positive evidence for use of DBS peripheral neuropathic pain.[233] In CPSP, further trials were suggested because DBS results were equivocal and required further comparative trials.

Trigeminal subnucleus caudalis DREZ lesions have been reported to relieve facial pain of CPSP in one patient with CPSP caused by a pontine infarct and another with an arteriovenous malformation of the tectum of the mesencephalon.[237] Both patients suffered from facial pain that was relieved by a DREZ procedure on the trigeminal nucleus caudalis. The first patient had allodynia and some steady pain; the second had steady pain. In both cases, the DREZ procedure induced mild ipsilateral upper limb dysmetria.

Retrospective studies point to the effectiveness of lesions of the mesencephalic reticular formation and mesencephalic STT in the treatment of central pain.[238,239] There are also a number of anecdotal case reports of different procedures for the treatment of CPSP. Relief of evoked pain has been reported following lesions of the STT by cordotomy[2] and mesencephalic tractotomy.[240]

Medial thalamotomy has been reported to be effective in 25% to 89% of patients[161,162,241] although the durability of this effect is limited.[242] Success of this procedure was also reported as percent pain relief in a population of patients with mixed etiology, either central (33% pain relief, n = 20 patients), peripheral (55%, n = 53), or mixed central and peripheral pain (33%, n = 23).[242] In this, the largest study (n = 96 patients including central or peripheral neuropathic pain or both), significant complications were reported including three bleeds (two thalamic, one intraventricular) and two cases of thalamic vascular compromise or edema.

CONCLUSION

This review demonstrates that there are substantial clinical similarities between SCI central pain and CPSP. There is evidence that sensory compromise in modalities mediated through the STT is a necessary but not sufficient condition for the development of these syndromes. Other factors which may lead to the development of central pain may include the presence of blood products at the site of spinal cord injury, the expression of particular non-TTX dependent sodium channels, or the balance of neuromodulator inputs to the spinal cord, thalamusm or cortex. Agents that are proven effective in the clinic are noradrenergic antidepressants, and with the antiepileptic drug lamotrigine at relatively high doses. Destructive procedures targeting the spinal cord, thalamus, and midbrain may be effective for the intermittent, shooting pains or the evoked pain of these syndromes, at some risk. Motor cortex or thalamic stimulation may be effective for the treatment of the spontaneous pain of CPSP. Therefore, central pain remains a mysterious syndrome which has yielded grudgingly to medical and surgical treatment.[242]

Acknowledgment

The work involved in this paper was supported by the National Institutes of Health–National Institute of Neurological Disorders and Stroke (NS38493 and NS40059 to F.A.L. NS-39337 to JDG), and Deutsche Forschungsgemeinschaft Tr236/13-2 to RDT.

References

1. Casey KL. Pain and central nervous system disease: a summary and overview. In: Casey, ed. *Pain and Central Nervous System disease: The Central Pain Syndromes*. New York: Raven Press; 1991:1–11.
2. Cassinari V, Pagni CA. *Central Pain*. Cambridge, MA: Harvard University Press; 1969.
3. Tasker RR, Dostrovsky JO. Deafferentation and central pain. In: Wall PD, Melzack R, eds. *Textbook of Pain*. Edinburgh: Churchill Livingston; 1989:154–180.
4. Finnerup NB, Johannesen IL, Fuglsang-Frederiksen A, et al. Sensory function in spinal cord injury patients with and without central pain. *Brain* 2003;126(pt 1):57–70.
5. Tasker RR. Central pain states. In: Loeser JD, ed. *Bonica's Management of Pain*. Philadelphia: Lippincott Williams & Wilkins; 2002.
6. Fenollosa P, Pallares J, Cervera J, et al. Chronic pain in the spinal cord injured: statistical approach and pharmacological treatment. *Paraplegia* 1993;31(11):722–729.
7. Tasker RR, DeCarvalho GT, Dolan EJ. Intractable pain of spinal cord origin: clinical features and implications for surgery. *J Neurosurgery* 1992;77(3):373–378.
8. Milhorat TH, Kotzen RM, Mu HT, et al. Dysesthetic pain in patients with syringomyelia. *Neurosurgery* 1996;38(5):940–946.
9. Davidoff, G. and E. Roth, Clinical characteristics of central (dysesthetic) pain syndrome in spinal cord injury patients. In: Casey KL, ed. *Pain and Central Nervous System disease: The Central Pain Syndromes*. New York: Raven Press; 1991:77–83.
10. Eide PK. Pathophysiological mechanisms of the central neuropathic pain after spinal cord injury. *Spinal Cord* 1998;36:601–612.
11. Berić A, Dimitrijević MR, Linblom U. Central dysesthesia syndrome in spinal cord injury patients. *Pain* 1988;34(2):109–116.
12. Vierck CJ, Luck MM. Loss and recovery of reactivity to noxious stimuli in monkeys with primary spinothalamic cordotomies, followed by secondary and tertiary lesions of other cord sectors. *Brain* 1979;102(2):233–248.
13. Vierck CJ, Greenspan JD, and Ritz LA. Long-term changes in purposive and reflexive responses to nociceptive stimulatin following anterolateral chordotomy. *J Neurosci* 1990;10:2077–2095.
14. Boivie J. Central pain. In: Wall PD, Melzack R, eds. *Textbook of Pain*. Edinburgh: Churchill Livingstone; 1999.
15. Ralston DD, Doughterty PM, Lenz FA, et al. Plasticity of the inhibitory circuitry and neuronal responses in the primate somatosenory thalamus following lesions of the dorsal column and spinothalamic pathways. *Prog Pain Res Manag* 2000;16:427–434.
16. Lenz FA, Kwan HC, Martin R, et al., Characteristics of somatotopic organizations and spontaneous neuronal activity in the region of the thalamic principal sensory nucleus in patients with spinal cord transection. *J Neurophysiol* 1994;72(4):1570–1587.
17. Weng HR, Lee JI, Lenz FA, et al. Functional plasticity in primate somatosensory thalamus following chronic lesion of the ventral lateral spinal cord. *Neuroscience* 2000;101:393–401.
18. Vierck CJ. Can mechanisms of central pain syndromes be investigated in animal models? In: Casey KL, ed. *Pain and Central Nervous System disease: The Central Pain Syndromes*. New York: Raven Press; 1991:129–141.
19. Tasker RR, DeCarvallo G, Dostrovsky JO. The history of central pain syndromes, with observations concering pathophysiology and treatment. In: Casey KL, ed. *Pain and Central Nervous System disease: The Central Pain Syndromes*. New York: Raven Press; 1991:31–58.
20. Davis KD, Kiss ZH, Tasker RR, et al. Thalamic stimulation-evoked sensations in chronic pain patients and nonpain (movement disorder) patients. *J Neurophysiol* 1996;75:1026–1037.
21. Lenz FA, Gracely RH, Baker FH, et al. Reorganization of sensory modalities evoked by microstimulation in region of the thalamic principal sensory nucleus in patients with pain due to nervous system injury. *J Comp Neurol* 1998;399(1):125–138.
22. Lenz FA, Ohara S, Gracely RH, et al. Pain encoding in the human forebrain: binary and analog exteroceptive channels. *J Neurosci* 2004;24(29):6540–6544.
23. Levitt M. Postcordomoty spontaneous dysesthesia in macaques: recurrence after spinal cord transection. *Brain Res* 1989481:47–56.
24. Levitt M, Levitt JH. The deafferentation syndrome in monkeys: dysesthesias of spinal origin. *Pain* 1981;10:129–147.
25. Levitt M, The bilaterally symmetrical deafferentation syndrome in macaques after bilateral spinal lesions: evidence for dysesthesias resulting from brain foci and considerations of spinal pain pathways. *Pain* 1983;16:167–184.
26. Sweet WH. Animal models of chronic pain: their possible validation from human experience with posterior rhizotomy and congenital analgesia. *Pain* 1981;10:275–295.
27. Albe–Fessard DG, Rampin O. Neurophysiological studies in rats deafferented by dorsal root sections. In: Nashold BS, Ovelmen–Levitt J, eds. *Deafferentational Pain Syndromes: Pathophysiology and Treatment*. New York: Raven Press; 1991:125–139.
28. Ovelmen–Levitt J, Gorecki J, Nguyen KT, et al. Spontaneous and evoked dysesthesias observed in the rat after spinal cordotomies. *Stereotact Funct Neurosurg* 1995;65:157–160.

29. Ovelmen–Levitt J. The neurophysiology of deafferentation syndromes. In: Nashold BS, Ovelmen–Levitt J, eds. *Deafferentation Pain Syndromes: Pathophysiology and Treatment.* New York: Raven Press; 1991:103–123.

30. Yezierski RP, Park SH. The mechanosensitivity of spinal sensory neurons following intraspinal injections of quisqualic acid in the rat. *Neurosci Lett* 1993;157(1):115–119.

31. Yezierski RP, Santana M, Park SH, et al. Neuronal degeneration and spinal cavitation following intraspinal injections of quisqualic acid in the rat. *J Neurotrauma* 1993;10(4):445–56

32. Mills CD, Johnson KM, Hulsebosch CE. Group I metabotropic glutamate receptors in spinal cord injury: roles in neuroprotection and the development of chronic central pain. *J Neurotrama* 2002;19(1):23–42.

33. Hains BC, Saab CY, Waxman SG. Alterations in burst firing of thalamic VPL neurons and reversal by Na(v) 1.3 antisense after spinal cord injury. *J Neurophysiol* 2006;95(6):3343–3352.

34. Waxman SG, Hains BC. Fire and phantoms after spinal cord injury: Na+ channels and central pain. *Trends Neurosci* 2006;29(4):207–215.

35. Baastrup C, Finnerup NB. Pharmacological management of neuropathic pain following spinal cord injury. *CNS Drugs* 2008;22(6):455–475.

36. Siddall PJ, Cousins MJ, Otte A, et al. Pregabalin in central neuropathic pain associated with spinal cord injury: a placebo-controlled trial. *Neurology* 2006; 67(10):1792–1800.

37. Vranken JH, Dijkgraaf MG, Kruis MR, et al. Pregablin in patients with central neuropathic pain: a randomized, double-blind, placebo controlled trial of a flexible-dose regimen. *Pain* 2008;136(1–2):150–157.

38. Levendoglu F, Ögün CO, Ozerbil O, et al. Gabapentin is a first line drug for the treatment of neuropathic pain in spinal cord injury. *Spine* 2004;29(7): 743–751.

39. Rintala DH, Holmes SA, Courtade D, et al. Comparison of the effectiveness of amitriptyline and gabapentin on chronic neuropathic pain in persons with spinal cord injury. *Arch Phys Med Rehabil* 2007;88(12):1547–1560.

40. Tai, Q., et al., Gabapentin in the treatment of neuropathic pain after spinal cord injury: a prospective, randomized, double-blind, crossover trial. *J Spinal Cord Med* 2002;25(2):100–105.

41. Finnerup NB, Sindrup SH, Bach FW, et al. Lamotrigine in spinal cord injury pain: a randomized controlled trial. *Pain* 2002;96(3):375–383.

42. Drewes AM, Andreasen A, Poulsen LH. Valproate for treatment of chronic central pain after spinal cord injury. A double-blind cross-over study. *Paraplegia* 1994;32(8):565–569.

43. Cardenas DD, Warms CA, Turner JA, et al. Efficacy of amitriptyline for relief of pain in spinal cord injury: results of a randomized controlled trial. *Pain* 2002;96:365–373.

44. Davidoff G, Guarracini M, Roth E, et al. Trazodone hydrochloride in the treatment of dysesthetic pain in traumatic myelopathy: a randomized, double blind, placebo-controlled study. *Pain* 1987;29:151–161.

45. Galer BS, Miller KV, Rowbotham MC. Response to intravenous lidocaine infusion differs based on clinical diagnosis and site of nervous system injury. *Neurology* 1993;43:1233–1235.

46. Finnerup NB, Biering-Sørensen F, Johannesen IL, et al. Intravenous lidocaine relieves spinal cord injury pain: a randomized controlled trial. *Anesthesiology* 2005:102(5):1023–1030.

47. Chiou–Tan FY, Tuel SM, Johnson JC, et al. Effect of mexiletine on spinal cord injury dysesthetic pain. *Am J Phys Med Rehabil* 1996;75(2):84–87.

48. Attal N, Guirimand F, Brasseur L, et al. Effects of IV morphine in central pain: a randomized placebo-controlled study. *Neurology* 2002;58:554–563.

49. Eide PK, Stubhaug A, Stenehjem AE. Central dysesthesia pain after traumatic spinal cord injury is dependent on N-methyl-D-aspirate receptor activation. *Neurosurgery* 1995;37(6):1080–1087.

50. Dworkin R, O'Connor AB, Backonja M, et al. Pharmacologic management of neuropathic pain: evidence-based recommendations. *Pain* 2007;132(3): 237–251.

51. Kontinen VK, Dickenson AH. Effects of midazolam in the spinal nerve ligation model of neuropathic pain in rats. *Pain* 2000;85:425–431.

52. Herman RM, D'Luzansky SC, Ippolito R. Intrathecal baclofen suppresses central pain in patients with spinal lesions: a pilot study. *Clin J Pain* 1992; 8:338–345.

53. Loubser PG, Donovan WH. Evaluation of central spinal cord injury pain with diagnostic spinal anesthesia. *Anesthesiology* 1993;79:376–378.

54. Siddall PJ, Molloy AR, Walker S, et al. The efficacy of intrathecal morphine and clonidine in the treatment of pain after spinal cord injury. *Anesth Analg* 2000;91(6):1493–1498.

55. Glynn CJ, Jamous MA, Teddy PJ, et al. Role of spinal noradrenergic system in transmission of pain in patients with spinal cord injury. *Lancet* 1986;1986: 1249–1250.

56. Taira T, Tanikawa T, Kawamura H, et al. Spinal inthrathecal baclofen suppresses central pain after a stroke. *J Neurol Neurosurg Psychiatry* 1994;57(3): 381–382.

57. Loubser PG, Akman NM. Effects of intrathecal baclofen on chronic spinal cord injury pain. *J Pain Symptom Manage* 1996;12:241–247.

58. Ridgeway B, Wallace M, Gerayli A. Ziconotide for the treatment of severe spasticity after spinal cord injury. *Pain* 2000;85(1–2):287–289.

59. Simone DA, et al. Neurogenic hyperalgesia: a central neural correlates in responses of spinothalamic tract neurons. *J Neurophysiol* 1991;66:228–246.

60. Gybels JM, Sweet WH. *Neurosurgical Treatment of Persistent Pain.* Basel: Karger; 1989.

61. Hosobuchi Y. Subcortical electrical stimulation for control of intractable pain in humans. Report of 122 cases (1970–1984). *J Neurosurg* 1986;64(4): 543–553.

62. Rasche D, Rinaldi PC, Young RF, et al. Deep brain stimulation for the treatment of various chronic pain syndromes. *Neurosurg Focus* 2006;21(6):E8.

63. Richardson DE. Deep brain stimulation for pain relief. In: Wilkins RH, Rengachary SS, eds. *Neurosurgery.* New York: McGraw–Hill Book Company; 1985:2421–2426.

64. Bendok B, Levy RM. Brain stimulation for persistent pain management. In: Gildenberg PL, Tasker RR, eds. *Textbook of Stereotactic and Functional Neurosurgery.* New York: McGraw–Hill; 1998:1539–1546.

65. Kibler RF, Nathan PW. Relief of pain and paraesthesiae by nerve block distal to a lesion. *J Neurol Neurosurg Psychiatry* 1960;23:91–98.

66. North RB, Kidd DH, Zahurak M, et al. Specificity of diagnostic nerve blocks: a prospective, a randomized study of sciatica due to lumbosacral spine disease. *Pain* 1996;65(1):77–85.

67. Willis WD. Electrophysiological evidence for a role of altered dicharges of spinothalamic tract neurons in hyperalgesia. In: Dimitrijevic MR, ed. *Altered Sensations and Pain: Recent Achievements in Restorative Neurology III.* New York: Karger, Basel; 1990:153–164.

68. Rosomoff HL. Neurosurgical control of pain. *Ann Rev Med* 1969;20: 189–200.

69. Tasker RR. Percutaneous cordotomy: the lateral high cervical technique. In: Schmidek HH, Sweet WH, eds. *Operative Neurosurgical Techniques, Indications, Methods, and Results.* Philadelphia: WB Saunders; 1988:1191–1205.

70. Bullitt E, Friedman AH. DREZ lesions in the treatment of pain following spinal cord injury. In: Nashold BS, et al, eds. *The DREZ operation.* Park Ridge, IL: The American Association of Neurological Surgeons; 1996: 125–135.

71. Edgar RE, Best LG, Quail PA, et al. Computer-assisted DREZ microcoagultaion: posttraumatic spinal deafferentation pain. *J Spinal Disord* 1993;6(1): 48–56.

72. Tasker RR. Stereotaxic surgery. In: Wall PD, Melzack R, eds. *Textbook of Pain.* Edinburgh: Churchill Livingston; 1984:639–655.

73. Pagni CA. Central pain due to spinal cord and brain stem damage. In: Mezlack R, Wall PD, eds. *Textbook of Pain.* New York: Churchill Livingstone; 1994: 634–654.

74. Tasker RR, Tsudat T, Hawrylyshyn P. Clinical neurophysiological investigation of deafferentation pain. *Adv Pain Res Ther* 1983;5:713–738.

75. Sindou M, Mertens P, Wael M. Microsurgical DREZotomy for pain due to spinal cord and/or cauda equina injuries: long-term results in a series of 44 patients. *Pain* 2001;92(1–2):159–171.

76. Gorecki JP, Nashold BS Jr, Rubin L, et al. The Duke experience with nucleus caudalis DREZ coagulation. *Stereotact Funct Neurosurg* 1995;65(1–4): 111–116.

77. Friedman AH, Nashold BS. DREZ lesions for relief of pain related to spinal cord injury. *J Neurosurg* 1986;65(4):465–469.

78. Yezierski RP. Pain following spinal cord injury: the clinical problem and experimental studies. *Pain* 1996;68(2–3):185–194.

79. Ploner M, Freund HJ, Schnitzler A. Pain affect without pain sensation in a patient with a postcentral lesion. *Pain* 1999;81:211–214.

80. Dejerine J, Roussy G. La syndrome thalamique. *Rev Neurol* 1906;14: 521–532.

81. Head H, Holmes G. Sensory disturbance from cerebral lesions. *Brain* 1912; 34:102–254.

82. Bonica JJ. Introduction: semantic, epidemiologic and educational issues. In: Casey KL, ed. *Pain and Central Nervous System Disease: The Central Pain Syndromes.* New York: Raven Press; 1991:13–29.

83. Andersen G, Vestergaard K, Ingeman–Nielsen M, et al. Incidence of central post-stroke pain. *Pain* 1995;61(2):187–193.

84. Biemond A. The conduction of pain above the level of the thalamus opticus. *AMA Arch Neurol Psychiatry* 1956;75:231–244.

85. Leijon G., Boivie J. Central post-stroke pain-a controlled trial of amitriptyline and carbamazepine. *Pain* 1989;36:27–36.

86. Vestergaard K, Nielsen J, Andersen G, et al. Sensory abnormalities in consecutive unselected patients with central post-stroke pain. *Pain* 1995;61:177–186.

87. Bowsher D. The management of central post-stroke pain. *Postgrad Med J* 1995;71(840):598–604.

88. Hirai T, Jones EG. A new parcellation of the human thalamus on the basis of histochemical staining. *Brain Res Rev* 1989;14:1–34.

89. Greenspan JD, Ohara S, Sarlani E, et al. Allodynia in patients with post-stroke central pain (CPSP) studied by statistical quantitative sensory testing within individuals. *Pain* 2004;109(3):357–366.

90. Boivie J, Leijon G, Johansson I. Central post-stroke pain: a study of the mechanisms through analyses of the sensory abnormalities. *Pain* 1989;37(2): 173–185.

91. Bowsher D. Central pain: clinical and physiological characteristics. *J Neurol Neurosurg Psychiatry* 1997;61:62–69.

92. Boivie J, Leijon G. Clinical findings in patients with central post-stroke pain. In: Casey KL, ed. *Pain and Central Nervous System Disease.* New York: Raven Press; 1991:65–75.

93. Dooling EC, Adams RD. The pathological anatomy of posthemiplegic athetosis. *Brain* 1975;98:29–48.

94. Deuschl G, Bain P, Brin M. Consensus statement of the Movement Disorder Society on Tremor. Ad Hoc Scientific Committee. *Mov Disord* 1998;13(suppl 3):2–23.

95. Craig AD, Reiman EM, Evans A, et al. Functional imaging of an illusion of pain. *Nature* 1996;384(6606):258–260.

96. Duncan GH, et al., Thalamic VPM nucleus in the behaving monkeys. III Effects of reversible inactivation by lidocaine on thermal and mechanical discrimination. *J Neurophysiol* 1993;70:2086–2096.

97. Kim JS. Pure sensory stroke. Clinical–radiological correlates of 21 cases. *Stroke* 1992;23(7):983–987.

98. Schaltenbrand G, Walker AE. *Stereotaxy of the Human Brain*. New York: Thieme–Stratton; 1982.

99. Kim JH, et al. Lesions limited to the human thalamic principal somatosensory nucleus (ventral caudal) are associated with loss of cold sensations and central pain. *J Neurosci* 2007;27(18):4995–5004.

100. Leijon G, Boivie J, Johansson I. Central post-stroke pain-neurological symptoms and pain characteristics. *Pain* 1989;36:13–25.

101. Bowsher D, Leijon G, Thuomas KA. Central post-stroke pain: correlation of MRI with clinical pain characteristics and sensory abnormalities. *Neurology* 1998;51(5):1352–1358.

102. Montes C, Magnin M, Maarrawi J, et al., Thalamic thermo-algesic transmission: ventral posterior (VP) complex versus VMpo in the light of a thalamic infarct with central pain. *Pain* 2005;113(1–2):223–232.

103. Greenspan JD, Winfield JA. Reversible pain and tactile deficts associated with a cerebral tumor compressing the posterior insula and partiel operculum. *Pain* 1992;50(1):29–39.

104. Berthier M, Starkstein S, Leiguarda R. Asymbolia for pain: a sensory–limbic disconnection syndrome. *Ann Neurol* 1988;24(1):41–49.

105. Greenspan JD, Lee RR, Lenz FA. Pain sensitivity alterations as a function of lesion locations in the parasylvian cortex. *Pain* 1999;81(3):273–282.

106. Kenshalo DR, Anton R, Dubner R. The detection and perceived intensity of noxious thermal stimuli in monkey and man. *J Neurophysiol* 1989;62:429–436.

107. Russel CK, Horsley V. Note on the re-representation in the cebral cortex of the type of representation as it exsist in the spinal cord. *Brain* 1906;29:137–152.

108. White JC, Sweet WH. Its Mechanisms and Neurosurgical Control. Springfield, IL: Charles C. Thomas; 1955.

109. Peyron R, Garcia–Larrea L, Gregoire MC, et al. Parietal and cingulate processes in central pain. A combined positron emission tomography (PET) and functional magnetic resonance imaging (fMRI) study of an unusual case. *Pain* 2000;84(1):77–87.

110. Cahana A, Carota A, Montadon ML, et al. The long-term effect of repeated intravenous lidocaine on central pain and possible correlation in positron emission tomography measurements. *Anesth Analg* 2004;98(6):1581–1584.

111. Hirato M, Horikoshi S, Kawashima Y, et al. The possible role of the cerebral cortex adjacent to the central sulcus for the genesis of central (thalamic) pain—a metabolic study. *Acta Neurochir Suppl (Wien)* 1993;58:141–144.

112. Canavero S, Bonicalzi V. The neurochemistry of central pain: evidence from clinical studies, hypothesis and therapeutic implications. *Pain* 1998;74(2–3):109–114.

113. Peyron R, et al. Electrical stimulation of precentral cortical area in the treatment of central pain: electrophysiological and PET study. *Pain* 1995;62(3):275–286.

114. DiPero V, Jones AK, Iannotti F, et al. Chronic Pain: a PET study of the central effects of percutaneous high cervical cordotomy. *Pain* 1991(46):9–12.

115. Hsieh JC, Belfrage M, Stone–Elander S, et al. Central representation of chronic ongoing neuropathic pain studied by positron emission tomography. *Pain* 1995;63(2):225–236.

116. Iadarola MJ, Max MB, Berman KF, et al. Unilateral decrease in thalamic activity observed with PET in patients with chronic neuropathic pain. *Pain* 1995;63:55–64.

117. Ness TJ, San Pedro EC, Richards JS, et al. A case of spinal cord injury-related pain with baseline rCBF brain SPECT imaging and beneficial response to gabapentin. *Pain* 1998;78(2):139–143.

118. Cesaro P, Mann MW, Moretti JL, et al. Central pain and thalamic hyperactivity: a single photon emission computerized tomographic study. *Pain* 1991;47(3):329–336.

119. Peyron R, García–Larrea L, Grégoire MC, et al. Allodynia after lateral-medullary (Wallenberg) infarct: a PET study. *Brain* 1998;121:345–356.

120. Ducreux D, Attal N, Parker F, et al. Mechanisms of central neuropathic pain: a combined psychophysical and fMRI study in syringomyelia. *Brain* 2006;129(pt 4):963–976.

121. Fukumoto M, Ushida T, Zinchuk VS, et al. Contralateral thalamic perfusion in patients with reflex sympathetic dystrophy syndrome. *Lancet* 1999;354(9192):1790–1791.

122. Pattany PM, Yezierski RP, Widerström-Noga EG, et al. Proton magnetic resonance spectroscopy of the thalamus in patients with chronic neuropathic pain after spinal cord injury. *AJNR Am J Neuroradiol* 2002;23(6):901–905.

123. Baumgärtner U, Buchholz HG, Bellosevich A, et al. High opiate receptor binding potential in the human lateral pain system. *NeuroImage* 2006;30(3):692–699.

124. Willoch F, Tölle TR, Wester HJ, et al, Central pain after pontine infarction is associated with changes in opiod receptor binding: a PET study with 11C-diprenophine. *AJNR Am J Neuroradiol* 1999;20(4):686–690.

125. Willoch F, Schindler F, Wester HJ, et al. Central post-stroke pain and reduced opiod receptor binding within pain processing circuitries: a [11C]diprenorphine PET study. *Pain* 2004;108(3):213–220.

126. Jones AK, Watabe H, Cunningham VJ, et al. Cerebral decrease in opioid

127. receptor binding in patients with central neuropathic pain measured by [11C]diprenorphine binding and PET study. *Eur J Pain* 2004;8(5):479–485.

127. Rowbotham MC, Twilling L, Davies PS, et al. Oral opioid therapy for chronic peripheral and central neuropathic pain. *N Engl J Med* 2003;348(13):1223–1232.

128. Katz N, Benoit C. Opioids for neuropathic pain. *Curr Pain Headache Rep* 2005;9(3):153–160.

129. Nicholson BD. Evaluations and treatment of central pain syndromes. *Neurology* 2004;62(5 suppl 2):S30–S36.

130. Cohen S, Abdi S. Central pain. *Curr Opin Anesthesiol* 2002;15(5):575–581.

131. Rasche D, Ruppolt M, Stippich C, et al. Motor cortex stimulation for long-term relief of chronic neuropathic pain: a 10 year experience. *Pain* 2006;121(1–2):43–52.

132. Nguyen JP, Lefaucher JP, Le Guerinel C, et al. Motor cortex stimulation in the treatment of central and neuropathic pain. *Arch Med Res* 2000;31(3):263–265.

133. Yezierski RP, Gerhart KD, Schrock BJ, et al. A further examination of effects of cortical stimulation on primate spinothalamic tract cells. *J Neurophysiol* 1983;49(2):424–441.

134. Peyron R, Faillenot I, Mertens P, et al. Motor cortex stimulation in neuropathic pain. Correlations between analgesic effects and hemodynamic changes in the brain. A PET study. *Neuroimage* 2007;34(1):310–321.

135. Khedr EM, Kotb H, Kamel NF, et al. Longlasting antalgic effects of daily sessions of repetitive transcranial magnetic stimulation in central and peripheral neuropathic pain. *J Neurol Neurosurg Psychiatry* 2005;76(6):833–838.

136. Boive J. Central pain. In: Wall PD, Melzack R, eds. *Textbook of Pain*. Edinburgh: Churchill Livingston; 1994:871–902.

137. Blomquist A, Zhang ET, Craig AD. Cytoarchitectonic and immunohistochemical characterization of a specific pain and temperature relay, the posterior portion of the ventral medical nucleus, in the human thalamus. *Brain* 2000;123(pt 3):601–619.

138. Mehler WR. Some observations on secondary ascending afferent systems in the CNS. In: Knighton RS, Dumke PR, eds. *Pain*. Boston: Brown and Little; 1966:11–32.

139. Tasker RR, Organ LW, Hawrylyshyn P. *The Thalamus and Midbrain in Man: A Physiologic Atlas Using Electrical Stimulation*. Springfield, IL: Thomas; 1982.

140. Nathan PW, Smith MC. Some tracts of the anterior and lateral columns of the spinal cord. In: Knighton RS, Dumke PR, eds. *Pain*. Philadelphia: Lippincott, Williams, and Wilkins; 1996:47–58.

141. Lenz FA, et al. Neurons in the area of human thalamic nucleus caudalis respond to painful heat stimuli. *Brain Res* 1993;623(2):235–240.

142. Davis KD, Lozano RM, Manduch M, et al. Thalamic relay site for cold perception in humans. *J Neurophysiol* 1999;81(4):1970–1973.

143. Ohara S, Lenz FA. Medial lateral extent of thermal and pain sensations evoked by microstimulation in somatic sensory nuclei of human thalamus. *J Neurophysiol* 2003;90(4):2367–2377.

144. Lenz FA, Seike M, Richardson RT, et al. Thermal and pain sensations evoked by microstimulation in the area of human ventrocaudal nucleus. *J Neurophysiol* 1993;70(1):200–212.

145. Lenz FA, Byl NN. Reorganization in the cutaneous core of the human thalamic principal somatic sensory nucleus (Ventral caudal) in patients with dystonia. *J Neurophysiol* 1999;82(6):3204–3212.

146. Radahkrishnan V, Tsoukatos J, Davis KD, et al. A comparison of the burst activity of lateral thalamic neurons in chronic pain and nonpain patients. *Pain* 1999;80:567–575.

147. Hirato M, Watanabe K, Takahashi A, et al. Pathophysiology of central (thalamic) pain: combined change of sensory thalamus with cerebral cortex and central sulcus. *Stereotact Funct Neurosurg* 1994;62(1–4):300–303.

148. Casey KL, Minoshima S, Morrow TJ, et al. Comparison of human cerebral activation pattern during cutaneous warmth, heat pain, and deep cold pain. *J Neurophysiol* 1996;76(1):571–581.

149. Katayama Y, Tsubokawa T, Yamamoto T. Chronic motor cortex stimulation for central deafferentation pain: experience with bulbar pain secondary to Wallenberg syndrome. *Stereotact Funct Neurosurg* 1994;62(1–4):295–299.

150. Brown JA, Barbaro NM. Motor cortex stimulation for central and neuropathic pain: current status. *Pain* 2003;104(3):431–435.

151. White JC, Sweet WH. *Pain and the Neurosurgeon. A Forty Year Experience*. Springfield IL: Charles C. Thomas; 1969.

152. Soria ED, Fine EJ. Disappearance of the thalamic pain after parietal subcortical stroke. *Pain* 1991;44:285–288.

153. Canavero S, Bonicalzi V. *Central Pain Syndrome: Pathophysiology, Diagnosis, and Management*. New York: Cambridge Press; 2007.

154. Richardson DE. Thalamotomy for intractable pain. *Confin Neurol* 1967;29:139–145.

155. Richardson DE. Thalamotomy for control of chronic pain. *Acta Neurochir (Wien)* 1974;(suppl 21):77–88.

156. Sugita K, Doi T. The effects of electrical stimulation on the motor and sensory system during stereotaxic operations. *Confin Neurol* 1967;29:224–229.

157. Hassler R,Reichert T. Klinische und anatomische Befunde bei stereotakischen Schmerzoperationen im Thalamus. *Arch Psychiatr Nerverkr* 1959;200:93–122.

158. Sano K. Intralaminar thalamotomy (thalamolaminotomy) and posteromedial hypothalamotomy of the treatment of intractable pain. In: Krayenbuhl H, Maspes PE, Sweet WH, eds. *Progress in Neurosurgical Surgery*. Basel: Karger; 1977:50–103.

159. Fairman D, Llavallol MA. Thalamic tractotomy for the alleviation of intractable pain in cancer. *Cancer* 1973;31:700–707.

160. Fairman D. Evaluations of results in stereotactic thalamotomy for the treatment of intactable pain. *Confin Neurol* 1966;27:67–70.

161. Sano K. Stereotaxic thalamolaminotomy and posteromedial hypothalamotomy for the relief of intractable pain. In: Bonica JJ, Ventrafridda V, eds. *Advances in Pain Research and Therapy*. New York: Raven Press; 1979: 475–485.

162. Rinaldi PC, Young RF, Albe-Fessard D, et al. Spontaneous neuronal hyperactivity in the medial and intralaminar thalamic nuclei in patients with deafferentation pain. *J Neurosurg* 1991;74:415–421.

163. Hecaen H, et al. Coagulations limitees du thalamus dans les algies du syndrome thalamique. resultatsctherapeutiques et physiologiqes. *Rev Neurol* 1949;81:68–93.

164. Urabe SA, Tsubokawa T. Stereotaxic thalamotomy for the relief of intractable Tohoku pain. *J Exp Med* 1965;85:286–298.

165. Mountcastle VB. Central nervous mechanisms in mechanoreceptive sensibility. In: Brookhart JM, Mountcastle VB, eds. *Handbook of Physiology: The Nervous System Sensory Processes*. Bethesda, MD: American Physiological Society; 1984:789–878.

166. Lenz FA, Tasker RR, Kwan HC, et al. Single-unit analysis of the human ventral thalamic nuclear group: somatosensory responses. *J Neurophysiol* 1988;59(2):299–316.

167. Lee J, Dougherty PM, Antezana D, et al. Responses of neurons in the region of human thalamic principal somatic sensory nucleus to mechanical and thermal stimuli graded into the painful range. *J Comp Neurol* 1999;410(4):541–555.

168. Willis WD, Trevino DL, Coulter JD, et al. Responses of primate spinothalamic tract neurons to natural stimulation of hindlimb. *J Neurophysiol* 1974;37: 358–372.

169. Willis WD, Coggeshall RE. *Sensory Mechanisms of the Spinal Cord*. New York: Plenum Press; 1991.

170. Lenz FA, Gracely RH, Rowland LH, et al. A population of cells in the human thalamic principal sensory nucleus respond to painful mechanical stimuli. *Neurosci Lett* 1994;180(1):46–50.

171. Nathan PW, Smith MC, Cook AW. Sensory effects in man of lesion of the posterior columns and of some other afferent pathways. *Brain* 1986;109(pt 5):1003–1041.

172. Jones EG. *The Thalamus*. New York: Plenum Press; 1985.

173. Van Buren JM, Borke RC. *Variations and Connections of the Human Thalamus*. Berlin: Springer Verlag; 1972.

174. Triggs WJ, Berie A. Dysaesthesiae induced by physiological and electrical activation of posterior column afferents after stroke. *J Neurol Neurosurg Psychiatry* 1994;57(9):1077–1080.

175. Iadarola MJ, Berman KF, Zeffiro TA, et al. Neural activation during acute capsaicin-evoked pain and allodynia assessed with PET. *Brain* 1998;121: 931–947.

176. Kilgard MP, Merzenich MM. Cortical map reorganization enabled by nucleus basalis activity. *Science* 1998;279(5357):1714–1718.

177. Eaton SA, Salt TE. Thalamic NMDA receptors and nonciceptive sensory synaptic transmission. *Neurosci Lett* 1990;110(3):297–302.

178. Blomqvist A, Ericson AC, Craig AD, et al. Evidence for glutamate as a neurotransmitter in spinothalamic tract terminals in the posterior region of owl monkeys. *Exp Brain Res* 1996;108(1):33–44.

179. Ericson AC, Blomqvist A, Craig AD, et al. Evidence for glutamate as neurotransmitter in trigemino- and spinothalamic tract terminals in the nucleus submediius of cats. *Eur J Neurosci* 1995;7(2):305–317.

180. Dougherty PM, Li YJ, Lenz FA, et al. Evidence that excitatory amino acids mediate afferent input to the primate somatosenory thalamus. *Brain Res* 1996; 278(2):267–273.

181. Steriade M, Jones EG, Llinas RR. *Thalamic Oscillations and Signaling*. New York: Wiley, John & Sons; 1990.

182. Steriade M, Llinás RR. The functional states of the thalamus and the associated neuronal interplay. *Physiol Rev* 1988;68:649–742.

183. Steriade M, Deschenes M. The thalamus as a neuronal oscillator. *Brain Res Rev* 1984;8:1–63.

184. Davis KD, Kiss ZH, Luo L, et al. Phantom sensations generated by thalamic microstimulation. *Nature* 1998;391(6665):385–387.

185. Dostrovsky JO, Wells FEB, Tasker RR. Pain evoked by stimulation in human thalamus. In: Sjigenaga Y, ed. *International Symposium on Processing Nociceptive Information*. Amsterdam: Elsevier; 1991:115–120.

186. Halliday AM, Logue V. Painful sensations evoked by electrical stimulation in the thalamus. In: Somjen GG, ed. *Neurophysiology Studied in Man*. Amsterdam: Excerpta Medica; 1972:221–230.

187. Hassler R. Dichotomy of facial pain conduction in the diencephalon. In: Walker AE, ed. *Trigeminal Neuralgia*. Philadelphia: Saunders; 1970: 123–138.

188. Zirh AT, Lenz FA, Reich SG, et al. Patterns of bursting occuring in thalamic cells during parkinsonian tremor. *Neurosci Lett* 1997;83:107–121.

189. Olausson H, Marchand S, Bittar RG, et al. Central pain in a hemispherectomized patient. *Eur J Pain* 2001;5(2):209–217.

190. Davis KD, Hutchison WD, Lozano AM, et al. Altered pain and temperature perception following cingulotomy and capsulotomy in a patient with schizoaffective disorder. *Pain* 1994;59(2):189–199.

191. Greenspan JD, Coghill RC, Gilron I, et al. Quantitative somatic sensory testing and functional imaging of the response to painful stimuli before and after

192. cingulotomy for obsessive compulsive disorder (OCD). *Eur J Pain* 2008;12(8): 990–999.

192. Apkarian AV, Bushnell MC, Treede RD, et al. Human brain mechanisms of pain perception and regulation in health and disease. *Eur J Pain* 2005;9: 463–484.

193. Davis KD, Kwan CL, Crawley AP, et al. Functional MRI study of thalamic and cortical activations evoked by cutaneous heat, cold, and tactile stimuli. *J Neurophysiol* 1998;80(3):1533–1546.

194. Peyron R, Schneider F, Faillenot I, et al. An fMRI study of cortical representation of mechanical allodynia in patients with neuropathic pain: a combined psychophysical and fMRI study in syringomyelia. *Brain* 2004;129(pt 4): 963–976.

195. Lenz FA, Rios M, Chau D, et al. Painful stimuli evoke potentials recorded from the perisylvian cortex in humans. *J Neurophysiol* 1998;80(4):2077–2088.

196. Van Hoessen GW, Morecraft RJ, Vogt BA. Connections of the monkey cingulate cortex. In: Vogt BA, Gabriel M, eds. *Neurobiology of Cingulate Cortex and Limbic Thalamus: A Comprehensive Handbook*. Birkhauser: Boston, MA; 1993:249–284.

197. Vogt BA. Pain and emotion interactions in subregions of the cingulate gyrus. *Nat Rev Neurosci* 2005;6(7):533–544.

198. Coghill RC, Gilron I, Iadarola MJ. Hemispheric lateralization of somatosensory processing. *J Neurophysiol* 2001;85(6):2602–2612.

199. Frese A, Husstedt IW, Ringelstein EB, et al. Pharmacologic treatment of central post-stroke pain. *Clin J Pain* 2006;22:252–260.

200. Vestergaard K, Andersen G, Gottrup H, et al. Lamotrigine for central post-stroke pain: a randomised controlled trial. *Neurology* 2001;56(2):184–190.

201. Lampl C, Yazdi K, Röper C. Amitriptyline in the prophylaxis of central post-stroke pain. Preliminary results of 39 patients in a placebo-controlled, long-term study. *Stroke* 2002;33(12):3030–3032.

202. Agnew DC, Goldberg VD. A brief trial of phenytoin therapy for thalamic pain. *Bull Los Angeles Neurol Soc* 1976;41:9–12.

203. Attal N, Brasseur L, Parker F, et al. Effects of gabapentin on different components of neuropathic pain syndromes: a pilot study. *Eur J Neurol* 1998;40: 191–200.

204. Takahashi Y, Hashimoto K, Tsuji S. Successful use of zonisamide for central poststroke pain. *J Pain* 2004;5:192–194.

205. Attal N, Gaudé V, Brasseur L, et al. Intravenous lidocaine in central pain: a double-blind, placebo-controlled, psychophysical study. *Neurology* 2000; 54(3):564–574.

206. Awerbuch G, Sandyk R. Mexiletine for thalamic pain syndrome. *Int J Neurosci* 1990;55:129–33.

207. Edmonson EA, Simpson RK Jr, Stubler DK, et al. Systemic lidocaine therapy poststroke pain. *South Med J* 1993;86(10):1093–1096.

208. Kvarnström A, Karlsten R, Quiding H, et al. The analgesic effect of intravenous ketamine and lidocaine on pain after spinal cord injury. *Acta Anaesthesiol Scand* 2004;48(4):498–506.

209. Crisologo PA, Neal B, Brown R, et al. Lidocaine-induced spinal block can relieve central post-stroke pain: role of the block in chronic pain diagnosis. *Anesthesiology* 1991;74(1):184–185.

210. Morley JS, Bridson J, Nash TP, et al. Low-dose methadone has an analgesic effect in neuropathic pain: a double-blind randomized controlled crossover trial. *Palliat Med* 2003;17(7):576–587.

211. Mailis A, Amani N, Umana M, et al. Effect of intravenous sodium amytal on cutaneous sensory abnormalities, spontaneous pain and algometric pain pressure thresholds in neuropathic pain patients: a placebo-controlled study. *Pain* 1997;70(1):69–81.

212. Arner S, Meyerson BA. Lack of analgesic effect of opioids on neuropathic and idiopathic forms of pain. *Pain* 1988;33(1):11–23.

213. Portenoy RK, Foley KM, Inturrisi CE. The nature of opioid responsiveness and its implications for neuropathic pain: new hypothesis derived from studies of opioid infusions. *Pain* 1990;43(3):273–286.

214. Kupers R, Gybels JM. Responsiveness of chronic pain to morphine. *Lancet* 1992;340(8814):310–311.

215. Tasker RR. Deafferentation. In: Wall PD, Melzack R, eds. *Textbook of Pain*. Edinburgh: Churchill Livingston; 1984:119–132.

216. Dellemijin PL, Vanneste JA. Randomised double-blind active-placebo-controlled crossover trial of intravenous fentanyl in neuropathic pain. *Lancet* 1997;349(9054):753–758.

217. Kalman S, Osterberg A, Sörensen J, et al. Morphine responsiveness in a group of well-defined multiple sclerosis patients: a study with i.v. morphine. *Eur J Pain* 2002;6(1):69–80.

218. Backonja M, Arndt G, Gombar KA, et al. Response of chronic neuropathic pain syndromes to ketamine: a preliminary study. *Pain* 1994;56(1):51–57.

219. Bainton T, Fox M, Bowsher D, et al. A double-blind trial of naloxone in central post-stroke pain. *Pain* 1992;48(2):159–162.

220. Budd K. The use of opiate antagonist, naloxone, in the treatment of intractable pain. *Neuropeptides* 1985;5(4–6):419–422.

221. Canavero S, Bonicalzi V, Pagni CA, et al. Propofol analgesia in central pain: preliminary clinical observations. *J Neurol* 1995;242(9):561–567.

222. Canavero S, Bonicalzi V. Intraveneous subhyptonic propofol in central pain: a double blind, placebo-controlled, crossover study. *Clin Neuropharmacol* 2004;27(4):182–186.

223. Koyama T. Arakawa Y, Shibata M, et al. Effect of barbituate on central pain: difference between intravenous administration and oral administration. *Clin J Pain* 1998;14:86–88.

224. McQuay HJ, Carroll D, Jadad AR, et al. Dextromethorphan for the treatment of neuropathic pain: a double-blind randomised controlled crossover trial with integral n-of-1 design. *Pain* 1994;59(1):127–133.
225. Heiskanen T, Härtel B, Dahl ML, et al. Analgesic effects of dextromethorphan and morphine in patiets with chronic pain. *Pain* 2002;96:261–267.
226. Wade DT, Robson P, House H, et al. A preliminary controlled study to determine whether whole-plant cannabis extracts can improve intractable neurgenic symptoms. *Clin Rehabil* 2003;17(1):21–29.
227. Notcutt W, Price M, Miller R, et al. Initial experiences with medicinal extracts from cannabis for chronic pain: results from 34 'N of 1" studies. *Anesthesia* 2004;59(5): 440–452.
228. Strumpf M, Zenz M. Opioid therapy of central pain conditions-long-term therapy? An expanded indication for opiod drugs [In German]. *Fortschr Med* 1994;112(16):227–228.
229. Finnerup NB, Otto M, McQuay HJ, et al. Algorithm for neuropathic pain treatment: an evidence based proposal. *Pain* 2005;118(3):289–305.
230. Tsubokawa T, Katayama Y, Yamamoto T, et al. Chronic motor cortex stimulation for the treatment of centra pain. *Acta Neurochir Suppl (Wien)* 1991; 52:137–139.
231. Tsubokawa T, Katayama Y, Yamamoto T, et al. Chronic motor cortex stimulation in patients with thalamic pain. *J Neurourg* 1993;78(3):393–401.
232. Hosobuchi Y, Motor cortex stimulation for treatment of central pain. In: Devinsky O, ed. *Electrical and Magnetic Stimulation of the Brain and Spinal Cord*. Philadelphia: Saunders; 1993:115–117.
233. Cruccu G, Aziz TZ, Garcia-Larrea L, et al. EFNS guidelines on neurostimulation therapy for neuropathic pain. *Eur J Neurol* 2007;14(9):952–9790.
234. Coffey RJ, Lozano AM. Neurostimulation for chronic noncancer pain: an evaluation of the clinical evidence and recommendations for future trial designs. *J Neurosurg* 2006;105(2):175–189.
235. Adams JE, Hosobuchi Y, Fields HL. Stimulation of internal capsule for relief of chronic pain. *J Neurosurg* 1974;41(6):740–744.
236. Tasker RR, Viela–Filho, Deep brain stimulation for treatment of intractable pain. In: Youmans JR, ed. *Neurological Surgery*. Philadelphia: Saunders; 1996:3512–3525.
237. Sampson JH, Nashold BS. Facial pain due to vacular lesions of the brain stem relieved by dorsal root entry zone lesions in the nucleus caudalis. Report of two cases. *J Neurosurg* 1992;77:473–475.
238. Amano K, Iseki H, Notani M, et al. Rostral mesencephalic reticulotomy for pain relief. Report of 15 cases. *Acta Neurochir Suppl (Wien)* 1980;30:391–393.
239. Shieff C, Nashold BS. Stereotactic mesncephalic tractotomy for thalamic pain. *Neurol Res* 1987;99:101–104.
240. Nashold BS, Wilson WP, Slaughter DG. Stereotactic midbrain lesions for central dysesthesia and central pain. *J Neurosurg* 1969;30:116–126.
241. Niizuma H, Kwak R, Ikeda S, et al. Follow-up results of centromedian thalamotomy for central pain. *Appl Neurophysiol* 1982;45(3):324–325.
242. Jeanmonod D, Magnin M, Morel A, et al. Surgical control of the human thalamocortical dysrhythmia: I. Central lateral thalamotomy in neurogenic pain. *Thalamus and Related Systems* 2001;1(1):71–79.

CHAPTER 29 ■ THE PSYCHOPHYSIOLOGY OF PAIN

C. RICHARD CHAPMAN

INTRODUCTION

Psychophysiology is a field of study that seeks to relate subjective awareness and behavior to physiological events.[1–3] As a field of scientific inquiry, it concerns itself with central mechanisms of perception, cognition, and behavior, including learning, the emotions, and the relationship of brain activity to consciousness. As a clinical area, psychophysiology has classically addressed somatoform disorders, stress (most recently posttraumatic stress disorders), and affective disorders in general. As a field, psychophysiology is an important resource for the pain field for two primary reasons. On one hand, it offers a framework for understanding how stress contributes to pain, including the persistence of chronic pain. On the other hand, it uncovers links between cognitive processes (attention, expectancy, meaning, belief) and pain, as well as pain relief through psychological intervention.

Most physicians think of pain as an unpleasant sensation that originates in traumatized or inflamed tissues; however, pain is more than sensory information about the condition of the body. Strong emotion is an intrinsic part of pain. Any reasonable and unbiased observer studying mammals, particularly humans, would have to conclude that pain's affective features rather than its sensory properties govern behavioral responses to injury. People who experience pain do not quietly report the fact; they express negative emotions.

Is the affective dimension of pain as important as its sensory aspect? A lay writer described pain's qualities as comprising extreme aversiveness, an ability to annihilate complex thoughts and other feelings, an ability to destroy language, and a strong resistance to objectification.[4] Her perspective resonates with the lessons of everyday life: While pain has sensory features and lends itself to sensory description, it is above all else a powerful negative feeling state. One cannot evaluate and address the suffering of a person in pain without an appreciation of its emotional nature.

The International Association for the Study of Pain (IASP) acknowledged the central role of emotion in its keystone definition: "Pain [is] an unpleasant sensory and *emotional* experience associated with actual or potential tissue damage, or described in terms of such damage"[5] (emphasis added). This definition clearly emphasizes the role of affect as an intrinsic component of pain. Emotion is not a consequence of pain sensation that occurs after a noxious sensory message arrives at somatosensory cortex. Rather, it is a fundamental part of the pain experience.

Psychophysiology has revealed that emotion and cognition are interdependent. Strong emotions can alter thought processes, perceptions, beliefs, attitudes, and expectancies. Conversely, thoughts can generate negative or positive emotional states, and the physiological changes associated with such states can interact with tissue injury or inflammation and alter both the sensory and affective aspects of pain.

Because pain states never exist in isolation, it is important to consider the psychophysiological context of a pain problem. The cognitive, emotional, and physiological state of the patient presenting with pain is potentially very important for both assessment and intervention. I propose here that the best framework for characterizing this state is stress theory. Stress involves physiological arousal related to defense, derives in part from cognition, and generates physiological processes that feed emotions and feelings.

The purposes of this chapter are to describe the psychophysiology of pain and to explore the importance of psychophysiological mechanisms for the assessment and care of patients with pain. The psychophysiology of pain requires an incursion into mind–body issues, consideration of the nature of emotion and its interdependence with cognition, and the overarching influence of stress. In this chapter I show that:

> Pain (awareness of tissue trauma) has intrinsic emotional properties, including negative emotional arousal.
>
> The brain creates bodily states of arousal (negative emotions) in response to threat to biological and psychological integrity.
>
> The affective dimension of pain is intrinsically linked to the related processes of defense and stress, and the physiological mechanisms of these processes shapes the affective dimension of pain.

HISTORICAL PERSPECTIVE: MIND–BODY ISSUES

Through most of the 20th century, our understanding of the relationship between mental processes and the body stemmed directly from Cartesian notions of mind–body dualism. For Descartes, a 17th century philosopher and mathematician, human beings are dualistic: the mind and body are separate entities. Descartes described the life processes of the body as though they were clockwork mechanisms. The actions of the mind were, in his thinking, the workings of the soul.

Descartes believed that the awareness of pain, like awareness of other bodily sensations, must take place in a specific location where the mind observes the body. Dennett[6] termed this hypothetical seat of the mind the *Cartesian theater*. In this theater, the mind observes and interprets the array of multimodality signals that the body produces. The body is a passive environment; the mind is the nonphysical activity of the soul.

Today, most people will agree that such a theater of the mind cannot exist. Scientifically, the activity of the brain and the mind are inseparable; yet, Cartesian dualism is endemic in Western thought and culture. Classical approaches to psychophysiology stemmed from Cartesian thinking, as did psychophysics. Early work on psychosomatic disorders focused on mind–body relationships. Today, much of the popular movement favoring alternative medicine emphasizes the "mind–body connection," keeping one's self healthy through right thinking, and the power of the mind to control the immune system. It is hard to avoid Cartesian thinking when the very fabric of our language carries it along as we reason and speak.

Cartesian assumptions are a subtle but powerful barrier for someone seeking to understand the affective dimension of pain. Relegating emotions to the realm of the mind and their physiological consequences for the body is classical Descartes. It prevents us from appreciating the intricate interdependence of subjective feelings and physiology, and it detracts from our ability to comprehend how the efferent properties of autonomic nervous function can contribute causally to the realization of an emotional state. This chapter emphasizes the interdependence of mental processes and physiology. What we call the mind is consciousness, and consciousness is an emergent property of the activity of the brain. In a feedback-dependent manner, the brain regulates the physiological arousal of the body, and emotion is a part of this process.

EMOTIONS: DEFINITION AND MECHANISMS

What Are Emotions?

The first step in understanding pain as an emotion is appreciating the origins and purposes of emotion. Many physicians regard emotions as epiphenomenal feeling states associated with mental activity, subjective in character, and largely irrelevant to the state of a patient's physical health. In fact, emotions are primarily physiological and only secondarily subjective. Because they can strongly affect cardiovascular function, visceral motility, genitourinary function, and immune competence, patient emotions can have an important role in health overall and especially in pain management. Simple negative emotional arousal can exacerbate certain pain states such as sympathetically maintained pain, angina, headache, and fibromyalgia. It contributes significantly to musculoskeletal pain, pelvic pain, and other pain problems in some patients.

Emotions are complex states of physiological arousal and awareness that impute positive or negative hedonic qualities to a stimulus (event) in the internal or external environment. The objective aspect of emotion is autonomically and hormonally mediated physiological arousal. The subjective aspects of emotion, *feelings*, are phenomena of consciousness. Emotion represents in consciousness the biological importance or meaning of an event to the perceiver.

Emotion as a whole has two defining features: valence and arousal. Valence refers to the hedonic quality associated with an emotion—the positive or negative feeling attached to perception. Arousal refers to the degree of heightened activity in the central nervous system and autonomic nervous system associated with perception.

Although emotions as a whole can be either positive or negative in valence, pain research addresses only negative emotion. Viewed as an emotion, pain represents a threat to the biological, psychological, or social integrity of the person. In this respect, the emotional aspect of pain is a protective response that normally contributes to adaptation and survival. If uncontrolled or poorly managed in patients with severe or prolonged pain, it produces suffering.

Emotion in a Sociobiological Perspective

Psychologists have many frameworks for studying the psychology of emotion. I favor a sociobiological (evolutionary) framework because this way of thinking construes feeling states, related physiology, and behavior as mechanisms of adaptation and survival. Nature has equipped us with the capability of negative emotion for a purpose; bad feelings are not simply accidents of human consciousness. They are protective mechanisms that normally serve us well but, like uncontrolled pain, sustained and uncontrolled negative emotions can become pathological states that can produce both maladaptive behavior and physiological pathology.

By exploring the emotional dimension of pain from the sociobiological perspective, the reader may gain some insight about how to prevent or control the negative affective aspect of pain, which fosters suffering. Unfortunately, implementing this perspective requires that we change conventional language habits that involve describing pain as a transient sensory event. *Pain is a compelling and emotionally negative state of the individual that has as its primary defining feature awareness of, and adaptive adjustment to, tissue trauma.*

Adaptive Functions of Emotion

Emotions, including the emotional dimension of pain, characterize mammals exclusively, and they foster mammalian adaptation by making possible complex behaviors and adaptations. Importantly, they play a strong role in consciousness, producing and summarizing information that is important for selection among alternative behaviors. According to MacLean, emotions "impart subjective information that is instrumental in guiding behavior required for self-preservation and preservation of the species. The subjective awareness that is an affect consists of a sense of bodily pervasiveness or by *feelings localized to certain parts of the body*"[7] (emphasis added). Because negative emotions, such as fear, evolved to facilitate adaptation and survival, emotion plays an important defensive role. The ability to experience threat when encountering injurious events protects against life-threatening injury.

The strength of emotional arousal associated with an injury indicates and expresses the magnitude of perceived threat to the biological integrity of the person. Within the contents of consciousness, threat is a strong negative feeling state and not a pure informational appraisal. In humans, threatening events, such as injury, that are not immediately present can exist as emotionally-colored somatosensory images.

Phenomenal awareness consists largely of the production of images. Visual images are familiar to everyone: we can readily imagine seeing things. We can also produce auditory images by imaging a familiar tune, a bird song, or the sound of a friend's voice. Similarly, we can generate somatosensory images. We can, for example, imagine the feeling of a full bladder, the sensation of a particular shoe on a foot, or a familiar muscle tension or ache. Cognition operates largely on images and plays a strong role in the experience of symptoms.

Patients can react emotionally to the mental image of a painful event before it happens (e.g., venipuncture), or for that matter they can respond emotionally to the sight of another person's injury. The emotional intensity of such a feeling marks the adaptive significance of the event that produced the experience for the perceiver. In general, the threat of a minor injury normally provokes less feeling than one that incurs a risk of death. *The emotional magnitude of a pain is the internal representation of the threat associated with the event that produced the pain.*

Emotions and Behavior

Negative emotions compel action, such as fight or flight, along with expression through vocalization, posture, variations in facial musculature patterns, and alterations of activity. This represents communication and often elicits social support, thus contributing to survival. Darwin,[8] observing animals, noted that emotions enable communication through vocalization, startle, posture, facial expression, and specific behaviors. He held that emotions must be inborn rather than learned tendencies. Darwin pursued this issue by comparing the facial and other emotional expressions of children born blind with those of other children, reasoning that blind children would express emotion differently if emotion is primarily a learned behavior. As others have since confirmed,[9] Darwin learned that the basic blueprints for human emotional expression are innate.

Contemporary investigators who study emotions and human or animal social behavior emphasize that communication is a fundamental adaptive function of emotional expression.[10,11] Social mammals, including humans, depend upon one another or their social group as resources for adaptation and survival. The emotional expression of pain in the presence of supportive persons is socially powerful; it draws upon a fundamental sociobiological imperative: communicating threat and summoning assistance.

The Central Neuroanatomy of Emotion: Limbic Structures

The limbic brain represents an anatomical common denominator across mammalian species,[7] and emotion is a common feature of mammals. Consequently, investigators can learn much about human emotion by studying mammalian laboratory animals. Humans and animals differ in that the limbic brain is more developed in humans, the frontal lobes are unique to our species, and the interdependence of cognition and emotion is greatest in humans.

Early investigators focused on the role of olfaction in limbic function and this led them to link the limbic brain to emotion. Emotion may have evolutionary roots in olfactory perception. MacLean introduced the somewhat controversial term "limbic system" and characterized its functions.[12] He identified three main subdivisions of the limbic brain: amygdala, septum, and thalamocingulate[7] that represent sources of afferents to parts of the limbic cortex. He also postulated that the limbic brain responds to two basic types of input: interoceptive and exteroceptive. These refer to sensory information from internal and external environments, respectively. Figure 29.1 summarizes and extends this concept. Noxious signaling can arise from an injurious event in the external environment or from a pathological condition in the internal environment.

Over the last decade, numerous studies have employed functional brain imaging to investigate how the human brain responds to painful laboratory stimulation as well as how it behaves in chronic pain conditions. These studies reveal unequivocally that limbic structures involved in emotion and cognition are active during pain. In addition, related studies show that cognitive processes such as threat appraisal and perceived control are related to pain modulation. Apkarian et al.[13] performed a meta-analysis of the literature and extracted consensus that the following brain structures are consistently active during states of pain: thalamus, primary, and secondary somatosensory cortices, insular cortex, anterior cingulate, and the prefrontal cortices. Thalamus and the somatosensory cortices played a prominent role in early neurophysiological models of pain. Insular cortex may play a role in the somatosensory representation of the body, and it appears to integrate multimodal sensory information.[14] Craig[15] holds that anterior insula integrates emotional and motivational processes while anterior cingulate cortex activates in numerous pain-related and other studies involving emotion and cognition. Prefrontal cortices control the executive functions of the brain and the sense of self. They are involved in threat appraisal, meaning, and the integration of information from the internal and external environment.

Peripheral Neuroanatomy of Emotion: The Autonomic Nervous System

The autonomic nervous system (ANS) plays an major role in regulating the constancy of the internal environment, and it does so in a feedback regulated fashion under the direction of the hypothalamus, the solitary nucleus (nucleus tractus solitarius) and ventral lateral medulla, the amygdala, and other brain structures.[16,17] In general, it regulates activities that are not normally under voluntary control. The hypothalamus is the principal integrator of autonomic activity. Stimulation of the hypothalamus elicits highly integrated patterns of response that involve the limbic system and other structures.[18]

Many researchers hold that the ANS has three divisions: the sympathetic, the parasympathetic, and the enteric.[19,20] Others subsume the enteric under the other two divisions. Broadly, the sympathetic nervous system makes possible the arousal needed for fight and flight reactions, while the parasympathetic system governs basal heart rate, metabolism, and respiration. The enteric nervous system innervates the viscera via a complex network of interconnected plexuses.

The sympathetic and parasympathetic systems are largely mutual physiological antagonists—if one system inhibits a function, the other typically augments it. There are, however, important exceptions to this rule that demonstrate complementary or integratory relationships. The mechanism most heavily involved in the affective response to tissue trauma is the sympathetic nervous system.

During emergency or injury to the body, the hypothalamus uses the sympathetic nervous system to increase cardiac output, respiration rate, and blood glucose. It also regulates body temperature, causes piloerection, alters muscle tone, provides compensatory responses to hemorrhage, and dilates pupils. These responses are part of a coordinated, well-orchestrated response pattern called the defense response.[21–23] It resembles the better known orienting response in some respects, but it can only occur following a strong stimulus that is noxious or frankly painful. It sets the stage for escape or confrontation, thus serving to protect the organism from danger. In an awake cat both electrical stimulation of the hypothalamus and infusion of norepinephrine into the hypothalamus elicit a rage reaction with hissing, snarling, attack posture with claw exposure, and a pattern of sympathetic nervous system arousal accompanies this.[24–26] Circulating epinephrine and norepinephrine produced by the adrenal medulla during activation of the sympa-

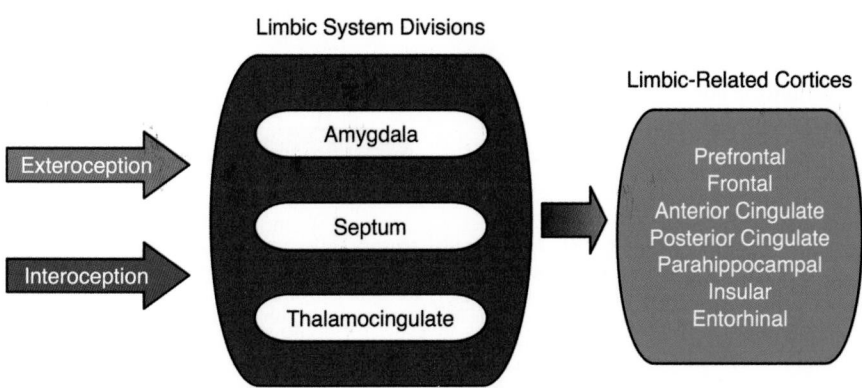

Limbic System Divisions

Exteroception

Interoception

Amygdala

Septum

Thalamocingulate

Limbic-Related Cortices

Prefrontal
Frontal
Anterior Cingulate
Posterior Cingulate
Parahippocampal
Insular
Entorhinal

FIGURE 29.1 Three subdivisions of the limbic brain and their relationship to limbic cortices. MacLean[7] proposed a three-part grouping of limbic structures and functions: amygdalar, septal, and thalamocingulate subdivisions. These divisions receive information, including noxious signaling, from the external environment (exteroceptors) and the internal environment (interoceptors). Cortical areas related to limbic function include the prefrontal and frontal cortices (related to executive function and sense of self), the cingulate cortices (the anterior cingulate cortex is related to attentional states), the parahippocampal and entorhinal cortices, which are important in memory, and the insular cortex (emotional–motivational integration).

thoadrenomedullary axis accentuate the defense response, fear responses, and aversive emotional arousal in general.

Autonomic Arousal and Subjective Experience

Because the defense response and related changes are involuntary in nature, we generally perceive them as something that the environment does to us. We typically describe such physiological changes, not as the bodily responses that they are, but rather as feelings. We might describe a threatening and physiologically arousing event by saying that "It scared me" or that "It made me really mad."

Phenomenologically, feelings seem to happen to us; we do not "do" them in the sense that we think thoughts or choose actions. Emotions are who we are in a given circumstance rather than choices we make, and we commonly interpret events and circumstances in terms of the emotions that they elicit. ANS arousal, therefore, plays a major role in the complex psychological experience of injury and is a part of that experience.

Early views of the ANS followed the lead of Cannon[21] and held that emergency responses and all forms of intense aversive arousal are undifferentiated, diffuse patterns of sympathetic activation. While this is broadly true, research has shown that definable patterns characterize emotional arousal, and that these are related to the emotion involved, the motor activity required, and perhaps the context.[16,17] An investigator attempting to understand how humans experience emotions must remember that the brain not only recognizes patterns of arousal; it also creates them.

The Role of Feedback

One of the primary mechanisms in the creation and management of emotion is feedback. Feedback means that information about the output of a system passes back to the input and thereby dynamically controls the level of the output. System self-regulation and self-organization depend upon feedback, as does self-direction. Feedback loops can be negative or positive. Negative feedback permits stability while positive feedback allows the organism to mount emergency responses. The regulatory processes of homeostasis and allostasis are negative feedback dependent. Negative feedback ensures system stability and maintains homeostasis. Feedback is positive when a variable changes and the system responds by changing that variable even more in the same direction, generating escalation and rapid acceleration.[27] This process abandons stability for instability. From an adaptation point of view, positive feedback loop capability is essential for meeting acute threat with defensive arousal. Each mode of operation has adaptive value as a short-range response in certain types of injurious events.

In general, defensive reactions involve a pattern of rapid arousal created through positive feedback that prepares the body and brain for emergency response, followed by a negative feedback-controlled transition to recovery and return to normalcy. Because smaller physiological systems are nested within larger physiological systems, higher order systems typically limit positive feedback processes in smaller systems. In some cases, top down regulation of positive feedback fails; for example, in a panic attack. In other cases, the event that triggered the emotion terminates and the positive feedback process then stops. Sustained periods of positive feedback have the potential for destructive consequences.

Feedback is the basis of neuroendocrine regulation, as I describe it below. Neuroendocrine feedback depends on bloodborne messengers that are typically hormones or peptides. The ANS uses feedback for afferent and efferent functions. The afferent mechanisms signal changes in the viscera and other organs while efferent activity conveys commands to those organs. Consequently, the ANS can maintain feedback loops related to viscera, muscle, blood flow, and other responses. The visceral feedback system exemplifies this process.

The feedback concept is central to the field of psychophysiology: Awareness of physiological changes elicited by a stimulus is a primary mechanism of emotion. The psychiatric patient presenting with panic attack, phobia, or anxiety is reporting a subjective state based on patterns of physiological signals and not an existential crisis that exists somewhere in the domain of the mind, somehow apart from the body. Similarly, the medical patient expressing emotional distress during a painful procedure, or during uncontrolled postoperative pain, is experiencing the sensory features of that pain against the background of a cacophony of sympathetic arousal and neuroendocrine stress response.

Relationship of Central and Peripheral Mechanisms

Figure 29.2 illustrates that noxious signaling undergoes parallel processing at the cognitive, affective, and sensory levels. An event representing a threat to biological integrity elicits strong patterns of sympathetic and neuroendocrine response. These, in turn, contribute to the awareness of the perceiver. Sensory processing provides information about the environment, but this information exists in awareness against a background of emotional arousal, either positive or negative, and that arousal may vary from mild to extreme.

The transition from acute to chronic pain may involve complex changes in these pathways. The HPA and SAM axes are vulnerable to dysregulation with prolonged exposure to a stressor or series of stressors. This can include prolonged noxious signal-

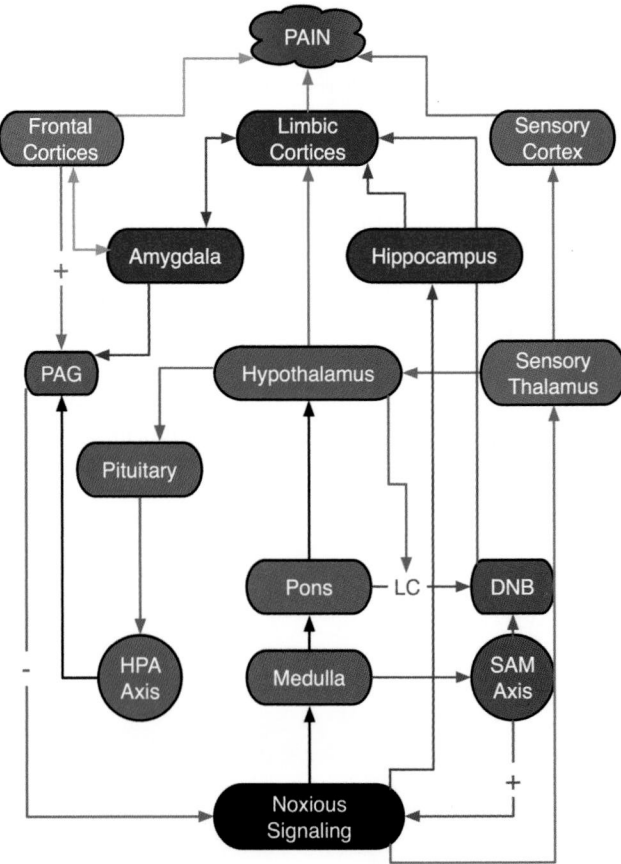

FIGURE 29.2 Parallel sensory, affective, and cognitive processing of noxious signaling arising from nociceptive or neuropathic sources. Parallel activation of sensory transmission and noradrenergic/limbic pathways leads to processing in somatosensory, limbic, and prefrontal/frontal cortical areas. In addition, noxious signaling triggers activity in the sympathoadrenomedullary (SAM) and the hypothalamo–pituitary–adrenocortical (HPA) axes. LC = locus coeruleus.

ing, as might occur with degenerative disease, or unrelenting noxious neuropathic signaling. Dysregulation in these systems may cause sensitization or impair normal inhibitory modulation. Moreover, neural networks associated with threat, dysphoria, or other negative emotions such as the frontal-amygdalar system may strengthen and become self-sustaining so that they can persist even in the absence of noxious signaling. Duric and McCarson[28] demonstrated that prolonged noxious signaling can produce stress-like damaging effects on the hippocampus, which is involved in the pathogenesis of depressive symptoms.

Noxious Signaling and Central Limbic Processing

Central sensory and affective pain processes share common sensory mechanisms in the periphery. As other chapters in this book describe, A-delta and C fibers serve as tissue trauma transducers (nociceptors) for both, the chemical products of inflammation sensitize these nociceptors, and peripheral neuropathic mechanisms such as ectopic firing excite both processes. In some cases neuropathic mechanisms may substitute for transduction as we classically define it, producing afferent signal volleys that appear, to the central nervous system, like signals originating in nociceptors. Differentiation of sensory and affective processing begins at the dorsal horn of the spinal cord. Sensory transmission follows spinothalamic pathways and transmission destined for affective processing takes place in spinoreticular pathways.

Noxious centripetal transmission engages multiple pathways: spinoreticular, spinomesencephalic, spinolimbic, spinocervical, and spinothalamic tracts,[29,30] as Figure 29.3 indicates. The spinoreticular tract contains somatosensory and viscerosensory afferent pathways that arrive at different levels of the brain stem. Spinoreticular axons possess receptive fields that resemble those of spinothalamic tract neurons projecting to medial thalamus, and, like their spinothalamic counterparts, they transmit tissue injury information.[31,32] Most spinoreticular neurons carry noxious signals and many of them respond preferentially to noxious activity.[33,34] The spinomesencephalic tract comprises several projections that terminate in multiple midbrain nuclei, including the periaqueductal gray, the red nucleus, nucleus cuniformis, and the Edinger-Westphal nucleus.[30] Spinolimbic tracts include the spinohypothalamic tract, which reaches both lateral and medial hypothalamus[35,36] and the spinoamygdalar tract that extends to the central nucleus of the amygdala.[37] The spinocervical tract, like the spinothalamic tract, conveys signals to the thalamus. All of these tracts transmit tissue trauma signals rostrally.

Central Neurotransmitter Systems

Central processing of noxious signals to produce affect undoubtedly involves multiple neurotransmitter systems. Four extrathalamic afferent pathways project to neocortex: the dorsal noradrenergic bundle (DNB) originating in the locus coeruleus (LC); the serotonergic fibers that arise in the dorsal and median raphe nuclei; the dopaminergic pathways of the ventral tegmental tract that arise from substantia nigra; and the acetylcholinergic neurons that arise principally from the nucleus basalis of the substantia innominata.[38] Of these, the noradrenergic and serotonergic pathways link most closely to negative emotional states.[39–41] The set of structures receiving projections from this complex and extensive network corresponds to classic definition of the limbic brain.[7,41–43]

Although other processes governed predominantly by other neurotransmitters almost certainly play important roles in the complex experience of emotion during pain, I emphasize the role of central noradrenergic processing here. This limited perspective offers the advantage of simplicity, and the literature on the role of central noradrenergic pathways in anxiety, panic, stress, and posttraumatic stress disorder provides a strong basis.[39,44] This processing involves two central noradrenergic pathways: the dorsal and ventral noradrenergic bundles (see Fig. 29.4).

Locus Coeruleus and the Dorsal Noradrenergic Bundle

Substantial evidence supports the hypothesis that noradrenergic brain pathways are major mechanisms of anxiety and stress.[39] The majority of noradrenergic neurons originate in the locus coeruleus (LC). This pontine nucleus resides bilaterally near the wall of the fourth ventricle. The locus has three major projections: ascending, descending and cerebellar. The ascending projection, the dorsal noradrenergic bundle (DNB), is the most extensive and important pathway for our purposes.[45] Projecting from the LC throughout limbic brain and to all of neocortex, the DNB accounts for about 70% of all brain norepinephrine.[46] The LC gives rise to most central noradrenergic fibers in spinal cord, hypothalamus, thalamus, hippocampus,[47] and, in addition, it projects to limbic cortex and neocortex. Consequently the LC exerts a powerful influence on higher-level brain activity.

The *noradrenergic stress response hypothesis* holds that any stimulus that threatens the biological, psychological or psychosocial integrity of the individual increases the firing rate of the LC, and this in turn results in increased release and turnover of norepinephrine in the brain areas involved in noradrenergic innervation. Studies show that the LC reacts to signaling from sensory stimuli that potentially threaten the biological integrity of the individual or signal damage to that integrity.[46] Spinal cord lamina one cells terminate in the LC.[31] The major sources of LC afferent input are the paragigantocellularis and prepositus hypoglossi nuclei in the medulla, but destruction of these nuclei does not block LC response to somatosensory stimuli.[48,49] Other sources of afferent input to the locus include the lateral hypothalamus, the amygdala and the solitary nucleus. Whether noxious signaling stimulates the LC directly or indirectly is still uncertain.

It is quite clear that noxious signaling inevitably and reliably increases activity in neurons of the LC, and LC excitation appears to be a consistent response to noxious signaling.[46,50–52] Notably,

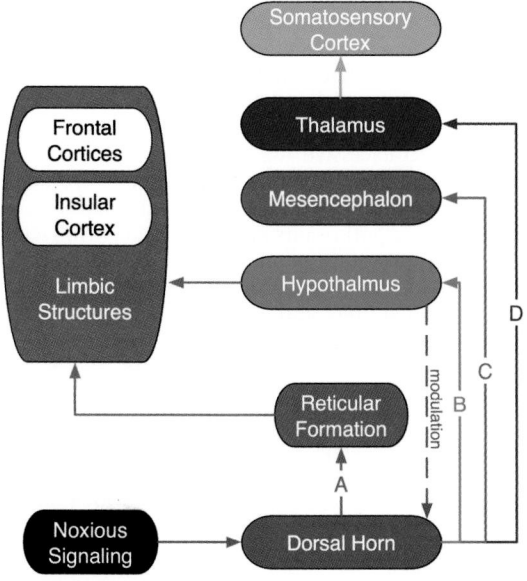

FIGURE 29.3 Multiple pathways of corticopetal noxious signal transmission. (**A**) Spinoreticular, (**B**) spinohypothalamic, (**C**) spinomesencephalic, and (**D**) spinothalamic.

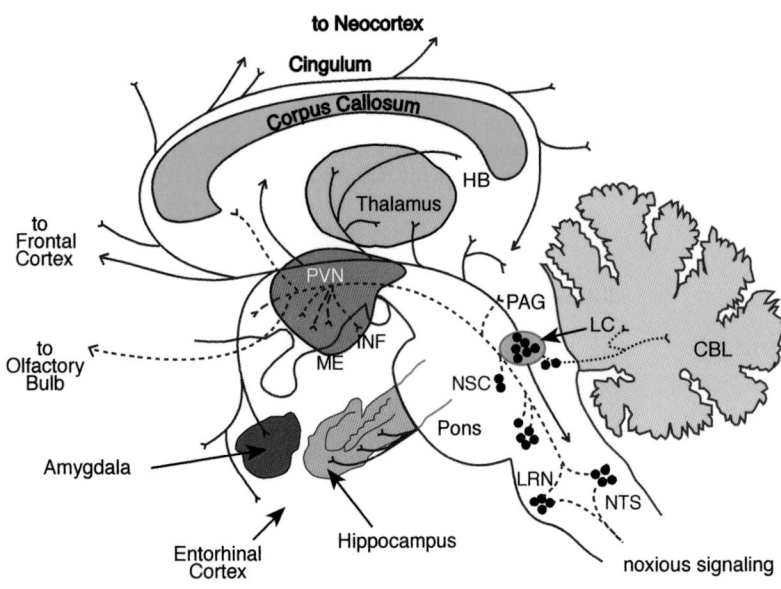

FIGURE 29.4 Central noradrenergic transmission. This parasagittal view identifies cell bodies of neurons that produce norepinephrine as black circles. The major projections of these cell bodies are the dorsal noradrenergic bundle (DNB) and the ventral noradrenergic bundle (VNB). The solid blue lines are DNB projections while the broken blue lines are VNB. The projection from the locus coeruleus (LC) to the cerebellum appears as a dotted line. Hypothalamus is orange. Noxious signaling from spinoreticular pathways excites the primarily noradrenergic LC, activating the DNB, which extends throughout the limbic brain and to neocortex. ME, median eminence; PAG, periaqueductal gray; HB, habenula; NSC, nucleus subcoeruleus; LRN, lateral reticular nucleus; NTS, nucleus tractus solitarius; INF, infundibulum; PVN, paraventricular nucleus of the hypothalamus; CBL, cerebellum.

this does not require cognitively-mediated attentional control since it occurs in anesthetized animals. Foote, Bloom, and Aston-Jones[53] reported that slow, tonic spontaneous activity at the locus in rats changed under anesthesia in response to noxious stimulation. Experimentally induced phasic LC activation produces alarm and apparent fear in primates,[54,55] and lesions of the LC eliminate normal heart rate increases to threatening stimuli.[56] In a resting animal, LC neurons discharge in a slow, phasic manner.[57]

The LC reacts consistently, but not exclusively, to noxious signaling. LC firing rates increase following non-noxious but threatening events, such as strong cardiovascular stimulation,[51,58] and certain visceral events, such as distention of the bladder, stomach, colon, or rectum.[46,59] Highly novel and sudden stimuli that could represent potential threat, such as loud clicks or light flashes, can also excite the LC in experimental animals.[57] Thus, the LC responds to biologically threatening or potentially threatening events, of which tissue injury is a significant subset. Amaral and Sinnamon[60] described the LC as a central analog of the sympathetic ganglia. Viewed in this way, it is an extension of the autonomic protective mechanism described above.

Invasive studies confirm the linkage between LC activity and threat. Direct activation of the DNB and associated limbic structures in laboratory animals produces sympathetic nervous system response and elicits emotional behaviors such as defensive threat, fright, enhanced startle, freezing and vocalization.[61] This indicates that enhanced activity in these pathways corresponds to negative emotional arousal and behaviors appropriate to perceived threat. LC firing rates increase two to threefold during the defense response elicited in a cat that has perceived a dog.[24] Moreover, infusion of norepinephrine into the hypothalamus of an awake cat elicits a defensive rage reaction that includes activation of the LC noradrenergic system. In general, the mammalian defense response involves increased regional turnover and release of norepinephrine in the brain regions that the LC innervates. The LC response to threat, therefore, may be a component of the partly "prewired" patterns associated with the defense response.

Increased alertness is a key element in early stages of the defense response. Normally, activity in the LC increases alertness. Tonically enhanced LC and DNB discharge corresponds to hypervigilance and emotionality.[39,53,62] The DNB is the mechanism for vigilance and defensive orientation to affectively relevant and novel stimuli. It also regulates attentional processes and facilitates motor responses.[38,41,46,63] In this sense, the LC influences the stream of consciousness on an ongoing basis and readies the individual to respond quickly and effectively to threat when it occurs.

LC and DNB support biological survival by making possible global vigilance for threatening and harmful stimuli. Siegel and Rogawski[64] hypothesized a link between the LC noradrenergic system and vigilance, focusing on rapid eye movement (REM) sleep. They noted that LC noradrenergic neurons maintain continuous activity in both normal waking state and non-REM sleep, but during REM sleep these neurons virtually cease discharge activity. Moreover, an increase in REM sleep ensues after either lesion of the DNB or following administration of clonidine, an alpha-2 adrenoceptor agonist. Because LC inactivation during REM sleep permits rebuilding of noradrenergic stores, REM sleep may be necessary preparation for sustained periods of high alertness during subsequent waking. Siegel and Rogawski contended that "a principal function of NE in the CNS is to facilitate the excitability of target neurons to specific high priority signals"[64(p226)]. Conversely, reduced LC activity periods (REM sleep) allow time for a suppression of sympathetic tone.

Both adaptation and sensitization can alter the LC response to threat. Abercrombie and Jacobs[65,66] demonstrated a noradrenergically mediated increase in heart rate in cats exposed to white noise. Elevated heart rate decreased with repeated exposure as did LC activation and circulating levels of norepinephrine. Libet and Gleason[67] found that stimulation via permanently implanted LC electrodes did not elicit indefinite anxiety. This indicates that the brain either adapts to locus excitation or engages a compensatory response to excessive LC activation under some circumstances. In addition, central noradrenergic responsiveness changes as a function of learning. In the cat, pairing a stimulus with a noxious air puff results in increased LC firing with subsequent presentations of the stimulus, but previous pairing of that stimulus with a food reward produces no alteration in LC firing rates with repeated presentation.[57] These studies show that, despite its apparently "prewired" behavioral subroutines, the noradrenergic brain shows substantial neuroplasticity. The emotional response of animals and people to a painful stimulus can adapt, and it can change as a function of experience.

From a different perspective, Bremner et al.[39] postulated that chronic stress can affect regional norepinephrine turnover and thus contribute to the *response sensitization* evident in panic disorder and posttraumatic stress disorder. Chronic exposure to a stressor (including perseverating noxious signaling) could create a situation in which noradrenergic synthesis cannot keep up with demand, thus depleting brain norepinephrine levels. Animals exposed to inescapable shock demonstrate greater LC responsiveness to an excitatory stimulus than animals who have experienced escapable shock.[68] In addition, such animals display "learned helplessness" behaviors—they cease trying to adapt to, or cope with, the source of shock.[69] From an evolutionary perspective, this is a failure of the defense response as adaptation; it represents surrender to suffering. Extrapolating this and related observations to patients, Bremner and colleagues[39] suggested that persons who have once encountered overwhelming stress and suffered exhaustion of central noradrenergic resources may respond excessively to similar stressors that they encounter at a later time.

The Ventral Noradrenergic Bundle and the Hypothalamo-Pituitary-Adrenocortical (HPA) Axis

The ventral noradrenergic bundle (VNB) originates in the LC and enters the medial forebrain bundle. Neurons in the medullary reticular formation project to the hypothalamus via the VNB.[70] Sawchenko and Swanson[71] identified two VNB-linked noradrenergic and adrenergic pathways to paraventricular hypothalamus in the rat: the A1 region of the ventral medulla (lateral reticular nucleus, LRN), and the A2 region of the dorsal vagal complex (the nucleus tractus solitarius, or solitary nucleus) which receives visceral afferents. These medullary neuronal complexes supply 90% of catecholaminergic innervation to the paraventricular hypothalamus via the VNB.[72] Regions A5 and A7 contribute in a comparatively minor way to the VNB.

The noradrenergic axons in the VNB respond to noxious stimulation[46] as does the hypothalamus itself.[73] Moreover, noxious-signaling neurons at all segmental levels of the spinal cord project to medial and lateral hypothalamus and several telencephalic regions.[30,35,36] These projections link tissue injury and the hypothalamic response, as do hormonal messengers in some circumstances.

The hypothalamic paraventricular nucleus (PVN) coordinates the HPA axis. Neurons of the PVN receive afferent information from several reticular areas including ventrolateral medulla, dorsal raphe nucleus, nucleus raphe magnus, LC, dorsomedial nucleus, and the nucleus tractus solitarius.[71,74,75] Still other afferents project to the PVN from the hippocampus, septum amygdala.[76] Nearly all hypothalamic and preoptic nuclei send projections to the PVN. This suggests that limbic connections mediate endocrine responses during stress. Feldman et al. note that limbic stimulation always increases adrenocortical activity in rats.

In responding to potentially or frankly injurious stimuli, the PVN initiates a complex series of events regulated by negative feedback mechanisms, as Figure 29.5 indicates. These processes ready the organism for extraordinary behaviors that will maximize its chances to cope with the threat at hand,[77] but they must limit overshooting and return to recover when the stressor has passed. While laboratory studies often involve highly controlled and specific noxious stimulation, real life tissue trauma usually involves a spectrum of afferent activity, and the pattern of activity may be a greater determinant of the stress response than the specific receptor system involved.[78] Traumatic injury, for example, might involve complex signaling from the site of injury, including inflammatory mediators, baroreceptor signals from blood volume changes, and hypercapnea. Tissue trauma normally initiates much more than noxious signaling.

Diminished noxious signal transmission during stress or injury helps people and animals to cope with threat without the distraction of pain. The medullary mechanisms involved in this are complex and include the response of the solitary nucleus to baroreceptor stimulation.[79] Laboratory studies with rodents indicate that animals placed in restraint or subjected to cold water develop analgesia.[80–82] Lesioning the PVN attenuates such stress induced analgesia.[83]

Some investigators[84,85] emphasize that neuroendocrine arousal mechanisms are not limited to emergency situations, even though most research emphasizes that such situations elicit them. In complex social contexts, submission, dominance, and other transactions can elicit neuroendocrine and autonomic responses, modified perhaps by learning and memory. This suggests that neuroendocrine processes accompany all sorts of emotion-eliciting situations.

The hypothalamic PVN supports stress-related autonomic arousal through neural as well as hormonal pathways. It sends direct projections to the sympathetic intermediolateral cell column in the thoracolumbar spinal cord and the parasympathetic vagal complex, both sources of preganglionic autonomic out-

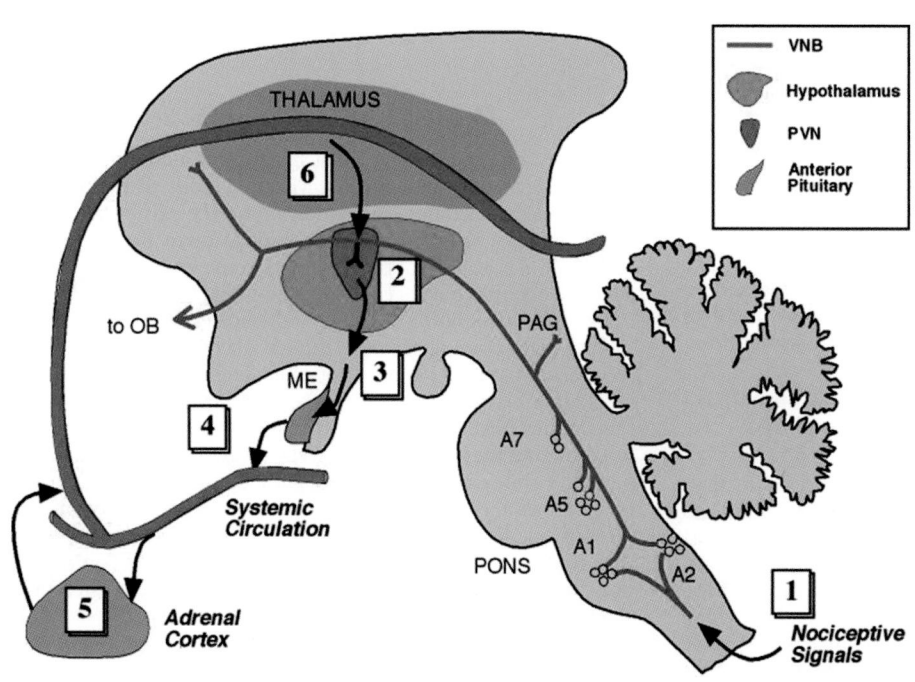

FIGURE 29.5 Response of the hypothalamo–pituitary–adrenocortical axis (HPA) to noxious signaling. The feedback modulated response involves six steps. In the first, noxious signaling excites the ventral noradrenergic bundle (VNB), including several medullary and pontine nuclei (designated A1, A2, A5, and A7). When such signals reach hypothalamus, they stimulate the paraventricular nucleus (PVN); this is Step 2. The PVN produces corticotropin releasing hormone (CRH). CRH-producing neurons extend from the PVN to the median eminence (ME) where they release CRH into the portal circulation, Step 3. At this point the response becomes neurohumoral rather than neuronal. The anterior pituitary responds to CRH by releasing adrenocorticotropin (ACTH) into the systemic circulation (Step 4). ACTH causes the adrenocortex to release corticosteroids into systemic circulation (Step 5). In addition to their extensive metabolic effects, the corticosteroids bind to receptors at the PVN (Step 6), thus closing the negative feedback loop.

flow.[86] In addition, it signals release of epinephrine and norepinephrine from the adrenal medulla. ACTH (adrenocorticotrophic hormone) release, while not instantaneous, is quite rapid: it occurs within about 15 seconds.[87] These considerations implicate the HPA axis in the neuroendocrinologic and autonomic manifestations of emotion associated with tissue trauma.

In addition to controlling neuroendocrine and autonomic nervous system reactivity, the HPA axis coordinates emotional arousal with behavior.[88] As noted above, stimulation of the hypothalamus in animals can elicit well-organized action patterns, including defensive threat behaviors and autonomic arousal.[89] The existence of demonstrable behavioral subroutines in animals suggests that the hypothalamus plays a key role in matching behavioral reactions and bodily adjustments to challenging circumstances or biologically relevant stimuli. Moreover, stress hormones at high levels may affect central emotional arousal, lowering startle thresholds and influencing cognition.[87] Saphier[90] observed that cortisol altered the firing rate of neurons in limbic forebrain. Clearly, stress regulation is a complex, feedback dependent, and coordinated process. The hypothalamus appears to coordinate behavioral readiness with physiological capability, awareness, and cognitive function.

Primary and Secondary Features of the Affective Dimension of Pain

The physiology of emotion suggests that the affective dimension of pain involves a two-stage mechanism. The primary mechanism generates an immediate experience akin to hypervigilance or fear. In nature, this rapid response to injury serves to disrupt ongoing attentional and behavioral patterns. At the same time, efferent messages from the hypothalamus, amygdala, and other limbic structures excite the autonomic nervous system, and this in turn alters bodily states. Cardiac function, muscle tension, altered visceral function, respiration rate, and trembling all occur, and awareness of these reactions creates a strong negative subjective experience. This body state awareness is the second mechanism of the affective dimension of pain.

Damasio[91] contended that visceral and other event-related, autonomically-mediated body state changes constitute "somatic markers." That is, they serve as messengers, delivering affective evaluations of perceptual experiences that either confirm or deny the potential threat inherent in an event. A somatic marker is essentially a somatic image. Perceptually, the brain operates on images that are symbolic representations of external and internal objects or events. Just as it is more efficient for a listener to work with words in language as opposed to phonemes, cognition is more efficient when it uses images rather than simple sensations. The somatic marker images associated with tissue trauma are often complex patterns of physiological arousal. They serve as symbolic representations of threat to the biological (and sometimes the psychological or social) integrity of the person. Like other images, they can enter into complex patterns of association. Because the secondary stage of the affective response involves images and symbols, it represents cognition as well as emotion.

EMOTION AND COGNITION

Negative emotions and somatic markers are much more than reactions to undesirable events; in nature they help an organism determine which things benefit and which things threaten survival, and they compel behavior consistent with such evaluations. Moreover, emotional expression communicates this judgment to others and thus sets up group approach or avoidance behaviors. MacLean[7] described emotion as a process that imparts subjective information. In these respects, our feelings approximate crude

intelligence. How we feel about something is often as important, or more important, than what we know about it. If emotion is a proto-intelligence, then evolutionarily newer structures, namely the later stages of cortical development, should have demonstrable links with limbic structures and functions.

Such interconnections exist. Parts of the frontal lobe (the dorsal trend) appear to have developed from rudimentary hippocampal formation while other parts (the paleocortical trend) originated in olfactory cortex. While these two areas interconnect anatomically, the former analyzes sensory information while the latter contributes emotional tone to that sensory information.[92(66–67)] Pribram,[93] noting that limbic function involves frontal and temporal cortex, offered a bottom-up concept for how cognition relates to feelings; that is, emotion determines cognition. However, the multimodal neocortical association areas project corticofugally to limbic structures,[94] which suggests that cognitions may drive emotions.

The debate on whether emotion or cognition is primary may never resolve. For immediate purposes, it seems best to conclude that knowing and feeling are closely interrelated. Still, these processes are not identical. We can know something about our feelings, and we can have emotional responses to what we know. The brain is a complex, dynamic organ, constantly constructing its internal model of reality from sensory input and memory storage. Feeling and thinking are major processes in this construction.

THE SENSE OF SELF

Cognitive Perspective

Pain informs the brain of injury to bodily integrity and its emotional aspect reflects the importance of that injury to the individual. An injury does not just cause objective harm, it harms "me." That is, it harms what I consider myself. Similarly, a social affront harms what I consider myself, and I might metaphorically describe the incident as something that "hurt" me. What constitutes the self? What would happen if an injured person had an altered or poorly developed sense of self? Clinical observations of schizophrenic patients and other psychiatric patients indicate that they sometimes mutilate themselves horribly and apparently with little or no pain.[95] This suggests that the sense of self may be an intrinsic part of the complex experience of pain because it is the focal point around which perceptions form and from which cognitions arise.

Multiple Perspectives on the Self

The *self* is a hierarchical construct that has different meanings at different levels of the neuraxis. Multiple levels of the self exist, and each level becomes a precondition for the existence of higher levels. At least two biological definitions merit inclusion in the construct. At the level of the human genome, the self is the unique genetic code that makes each of us an individual. It sets the basic rules of life by defining sex, size and features, and basic abilities.

At a higher biological level, the self is what the immune system recognizes as "me" versus "not me." The immunological self is an enigma because "me" and my genetic code are not identical. Our bodies host elaborate microbial ecosystems, and disturbing or damaging these systems (e.g., via antibiotic use) compromises health. Various microorganisms in our digestive tracts, oropharyngeal passages, and on our skin qualify as self to our immune systems; we live comfortably with them in a symbiotic relationship. Our microbial floras are clearly us, even though they do not carry our genetic code. For the immune system, there is no single chemical marker that defines individuality, nor is the self limited to certain biological structures. Thus, even at this basic level, the boundaries of the self are fuzzy.

At a neurological level, the self exists as a central representation of the body. Melzack[96–98] termed this the body neuromatrix. The brain maintains a detailed map of the body at several levels of the neuraxis. Study of phantom limb patients and patients born without limbs reveals that the brain has an elaborate internal representation of the body. If a person loses a leg, the brain maintains its representation of the leg and the person experiences a phantom limb. Even patients born without limbs have an internal sense or representation of the absent body parts. Thus, humans and almost certainly higher order animals carry within them a phenomenal representation of a body self.

These biological selves exist below the level of consciousness. They are very much a part of every person, but they normally play little or no part in what we think of as "me." Humans and animals do not differ with regard to self at this level.

Multiple psychological dimensions of the self also exist. At the most fundamental level there is the self-as-agent, which engages in biological adaptation and survival. From an evolutionary perspective, it is the agent that struggles to survive. The self-as-agent sets goals, chooses among alternatives, and engages in behaviors. Animals and humans share self-as-agent, and this self is, in part, social. That is, it exists not alone but in relation to others of its kind. Animals, including humans, engage in social dominance and submission. In this respect each organism defines its relationship to others, often via struggle or conflict. The defined relationship often determines the extent of one's opportunity to reproduce or one's access to the resources necessary for survival. The self-as-agent is primitive and does not require cognition. It is something that the individual does; not something that the individual experiences as a phenomenal reality. In other words, this is a self of behavior. It does not entail subjective awareness.

At a higher, and perhaps uniquely human, level the psychological self is also a point of view (self-as-perspective). It is the center of experiential gravity about which the brain organizes present circumstances, past history, future goals, and expectations. This is an inevitable outcome of the higher order self-organizing processes of the brain. This aspect of the self stems from recognition of one's physical being as an entity in the environment, and it becomes a frame of reference for all that happens to the person.

On still another level, the self represents the individual's complex sense of identity, to which I have referred above as "me," *vide supra*. This self-as-identity resembles the self-as-agent in some respects, but it is an age-dependent, autobiographically based narrative and interpretation, modified by the immediate circumstances and surroundings. Unlike the self-as-agent, the self-as-identity is the product of a developmental process and it changes over time.

Finally, every human has a sociological self. That is, we have an identity defined by our relationships to social groups and to society and culture as a whole. Gender roles, social class, education level, age roles, and our culture constrain who we are. To some degree, we are the roles that we play in our families, vocational settings, recreational pursuits, and elsewhere.

An injury to the body or a painful disease condition often has important social effects. A chronic pain syndrome might serve as a badge of honor for a former police officer wounded in the line of duty, and this would impact the extent to which he suffers. The pain of a patient dying of AIDS, who feels intense guilt toward his nuclear family for his homosexuality or drug abuse habits, takes on the opposite meaning. All pain occurs in the context of, and modifies, the sociological self. Consider the following examples: the fakir piercing himself in the public square of a European town, apparently without pain; the religious martyr dying a horrible death but apparently without pain; and the adolescent piercing her eyebrow and tongue with conspicuous pins for the social status that this brings. These cases all illustrate situations in which the sociological self gains from socially visible tissue trauma. These observations suggest that this aspect of the self can affect

pain behavior and possibly the experience of pain itself. The sociological self is uniquely human.

The role of sense of self in pain merits study, but as yet it has gained little or no attention from pain researchers. The constructs of self may prove important in defining the relationship of pain to suffering. The role of the sense of self in the initiation and organization of defense and stress responses merits inquiry.

STRESS, SICKNESS, AND PAIN

Basic Definitions: Stress, Homeostasis, and Allostasis

Human life entails repeated adverse physical and psychosocial events, and these challenges require an adaptive response. The brain mounts a coordinated, adaptive reaction characterized by physiological arousal. This response is often associated psychologically with the experience of threat or other negative affect. The term for this arousal reaction is the *stress response*, and any event that triggers such a response is a *stressor*. Some stressors are singular events, such as traffic accidents or surgery. Other stressors are constellations of vexing problems that never end. Examples include dysfunctional family relationships and vocational disorders. Stress and negative emotion feed one another, and the processes involved affect pain.

I have discussed the defense response above. It resembles the stress response and shares common mechanisms. The defense response and stress have historically different origins in science but seem to be different perspectives on a common adaptive mechanism. In order to integrate relevant information in these two fields, I consider the stress response to be a subset of the more general defense response. This position has the shortcoming of potentially obscuring an important distinction. Classically, the defense response pertained to threats appearing in the external environment and not the internal environment. However, the concept applies equally well to threatening internal events. The pain of a kidney stone, angina, or a migraine headache is threatening and can function as a stressor and elicit the physiological changes common to the defense response and the stress response.

In everyday life, stress is the resource-intensive process of mounting adaptive coping responses to challenges that occur in the external or internal environment. A stressor may be a physical or social event, an invading microorganism, or, in the case of a chronic pain, patient pain itself. Selye[77] first described this response as a syndrome produced by "diverse nocuous agents." He eventually characterized the stress response as having three stages: alarm reaction, resistance, and, if the stressor does not relent, exhaustion. The normal stress responses of daily living consist of the alarm reaction, resistance, and recovery. Stressors have as their primary features intensity, duration, and frequency. The impact of a stressor is the magnitude of the response it elicits. This impact involves cognitive mediation (thought processes) because it is a function of both the predictability and the controllability of the stressor.

A stressor can threaten homeostasis,[99] which strictly means a limited set of systems concerned with maintaining the essentials of the internal milieu. Homeostasis represents the control of internal processes truly necessary for life, such as thermoregulation, blood gases, acid base balance, fluid levels, metabolite levels, and blood pressure. Generic threats to homeostasis include environmental extremes, extreme exercise, depletion of essential resources, abnormal feedback processes, aging, and disease. Of course, various defensive processes must exist to protect homeostasis.

The term for the general adaptive process that protects against threats to homeostasis is *allostasis*. Allostatic processes dynamically adapt multiple internal systems to changes in the environment and coordinate their responses.[99,100] Allostasis exists when changes in the external or internal environment trigger physiological coping mechanisms such as autonomic arousal. These mechanisms ensure that the processes sustaining homeostasis stay within normal range. Allostasis is the essence of the stress response because it mobilizes internal resources to meet the challenge that a stressor represents. When a stressor, such as neuropathic signaling, persists for a long period of time, or when repeated stressors occur in rapid succession, allostasis may burn resources faster than the body can replenish them. The cost to the body of allostatic adjustment, whether in response to extreme acute challenges or to lesser challenges over an extended period of time, is called *allostatic load*.

Physiological Mechanisms of Stress

The major mechanisms of the stress response are the hypothalamo–pituitary–adrenocortical (HPA) axis based in the hypothalamic periventricular nucleus (PVN),[101] and the sympathoadrenomedullary (SAM) axis,[102] which includes the LC noradrenergic system (see Figure 29.1). The peripheral effectors of these mechanisms are the autonomic nervous system, the SAM circulating hormones, principally the catecholamines epinephrine (E) and norepinephrine (NE) together with the sympathetic cotransmitter neuropeptide Y (NPY),[103] all of which originate in the chromaffin cells of the adrenal medulla. Circulating catecholamines increase blood pressure and heart rate, dilate pupils, and increase skin conductance, thereby initiating arousal for the fight or flight response. The stress response involves hypothalamically-induced release of peptides derived from pro-opiomelanocortin (POMC) at the anterior pituitary. The POMC-related family of anterior pituitary hormones includes ACTH, β-lipotropin, β-melanocyte stimulating hormone, and β-endorphin.

The hypothalamic PVN initiates the HPA stress response and controls it through negative feedback mechanisms. Corticotropin-releasing hormone (CRH) produced at the PVN initiates the stress response. CRH initializes and coordinates the stress response at many levels,[104] including the LC.[105] It is the key excitatory central neurotransmitter and regulator in the endocrine response to injury.

The PVN triggers another aspect of the stress response in the SAM axis by recruiting catecholaminergic cells in the rostral ventrolateral medulla. This structure is a cardiovascular regulatory area involved, along with the solitary nucleus, in the control of blood pressure. The rostral ventrolateral medulla activates the solitary nucleus and, together with it, provides tonic excitatory drive to sympathetic vasoconstrictor nerves that maintain resting blood pressure levels. A normal stress response involves a complex pattern of autonomic arousal that includes increased blood pressure followed by a period of recovery when blood pressure and other aspects of arousal return to normal.

Neural Substrates

Viewing stress as a mechanism of defense brings additional neural substrates into focus. Chief among them are the medial hypothalamus, amygdala, and dorsal periaqueductal gray (PAG). These structures respond reliably but not exclusively to noxious signaling, interact with one another, and actively integrate cognitive, sensory, and emotional processes. Some pain researchers have begun to address the issue of integration. Tracey et al.,[106] for example, employed functional brain imaging to study subjects attending to or distracting themselves from painful stimuli cued with colored lights. Distraction and pain reduction occurred in conjunction with activation of the PAG, linking cortical control and the PAG.

Frontal-amygdalar circuits are a well-studied aspect of the defense response.[107–109] Cognitive variables such as interpretation, attention, and anticipation can influence amygdalar response through the frontal-amygdalar circuit. The amygdala, in turn, can influence the HPA axis.[110–112] Frontal influences also affect patterns of activity at the LC, which is a part of the SAM axis.

An important implication of viewing stress within the defense response framework is that endogenous cognitive activity (thoughts) generated during anticipation or memory reconstruction can activate complex neural circuits that mobilize the stress response in the absence of tissue trauma. In other words, mental activity has direct and deleterious physiological consequences. Chronic pain patients can stress themselves through negative thought processes, termed catastrophizing, and in so doing exacerbate and perpetuate their pain.[113]

The central nucleus of the amygdala projects to the PAG, which coordinates defensive behaviors.[114] In general, the amygdala is proving to be a key mechanism of conditioned fear.[115,116] It communicates with the hypothalamus via neural circuitry,[117,118] as well as the frontal cortices.

A second, and underestimated, aspect of the defense response depends predominantly upon the immune system. The brain controls the immune system via the actions of the sympathetic nervous system and the hypothalamic secretion of releasing factors into the bloodstream. These messenger substances activate the anterior pituitary via the HPA axis.[119] The pituitary body releases peptides related to pro-opiomelanocortin, such as ACTH and beta-endorphin, and these in turn trigger the release of glucocorticoids. Because the cells and organs of the immune system express receptors for these hormones, they can respond to humoral messenger molecules of central origin. In this way, the brain enlists the immune system in the defense response.

Immune Mechanisms

Just as the nervous system is the primary agent for detecting and defending against threat arising in the external environment, the immune system is the primary agent of defense for the internal environment. Kohl[120] described the immune system as "a network of complex danger sensors and transmitters." This interactive network of lymphoid organs, cells, humoral factors, and cytokines works interdependently with the nervous and endocrine systems to protect homeostasis.

Physical trauma produces specific tissue breakdown, triggering release of nitric oxide (NO), bradykinin, histamine, and peptides, some of which are immunostimulatory. The neuropeptides SP and NKA activate T cells and cause them to increase production of the pro-inflammatory cytokine IFN-g.[121] In addition, another pro-inflammatory cytokine, IL1-β, stimulates the release of SP from primary afferent neurons.[122] Thus, the neurogenic inflammatory response contributes to the immune defense response and at the same time is in part a product of that response.[123]

The immune system detects an injury event in at least three ways: (1) through bloodborne immune messengers originating at the site of injury; (2) through nociceptor-induced sympathetic activation and subsequent stimulation of immune tissues, and (3) through SAM endocrine signaling. Immune messaging begins with the acute phase reaction in the injured tissues.[124] Local macrophages, neutrophils, and granulocytes produce and release into intracellular space and circulation the pro-inflammatory cytokines Il-1, Il-6, IL-8, and TNF-α. This alerts and activates other immune tissues and cells that have a complex systemic impact.

The acute phase reaction to tissue trauma is the immune counterpart to noxious signaling in the nervous system in that it encompasses transduction, transmission, and effector responses. This is a feedback-dependent process. Sympathetic outflow following tissue injury can directly modulate many aspects of immune activity and provide feedback. This can occur because all lymphoid organs have sympathetic nervous system innervation[125] and because many immune cells express adrenoceptors.[126–128]

In addition to the familiar acute phase reaction, the immune system manifests several complex response patterns to tissue injury. In a primitive world, microbial invasion normally accompanies any breach of the skin, and when the microorganisms reach the bloodstream, sepsis occurs. Resultant inflammation therefore assists the immune system in defense. Redness, pain, heat, and swelling are its cardinal signs. The inflammatory process creates a barrier against the invading microorganisms and activates a variety of cells, including macrophages and lymphocytes, that find and destroy invaders. It also sensitizes the injured tissue and thereby minimizes the risk of further injury. Inflammation reduces function and increases pain by sensitizing nociceptors. Tracey[129] described the "inflammatory reflex" as an Ach-mediated process by which the nervous system recognizes the presence of, and exerts influence upon, peripheral inflammation. Through vagal and glossopharyngeal bidirectional processes, the nervous system modulates circulating cytokine levels.[130] Put another way, the nervous system can sense the activities of the immune system.

The Sickness Response

The immune system can mount a system-wide defense response characterized by fatigue, fever, and sickness with associated pain.[131–136] This is the "sickness response," and although it is cytokine mediated, it depends on the central nervous system. Macrophages and other cells release pro-inflammatory cytokines including IL1-β, IL-6, IL-8, IL-12, IFN-γ, and TNF-α in response to tissue trauma. These substances act on the vagus nerve, the glossopharyngeal nerve, the hypothalamus, and elsewhere to trigger a cascade of unpleasant, activity-limiting symptoms.[133,137]

Subjectively, the sickness response is a vivid and dysphoric experience characterized by fever, malaise, fatigue, difficulty concentrating, excessive sleep, decreased appetite and libido, stimulation of the HPA axis, and hyperalgesia. The sickness-related hyperalgesia may reflect the contributions of spinal cord microglia and astrocytes.[135] Functionally, this state is adaptive; it minimizes risk by limiting normal behavior and social interactions and forces recuperation. Curiously, this response does not always resolve with physical healing.

The Sickness Response and Depression

Mounting evidence supports the hypothesis that the sickness response and depression are related immune response patterns. This hypothesis derives from evidence that pro-inflammatory cytokines are agents of depression. The specific mechanisms are still at issue,[138] but pro-inflammatory cytokines instigate the behavioral, neuroendocrine, and neurochemical features of depressive disorders.[139–142] The therapeutic use of pro-inflammatory cytokines INF-α and IL-2 for cancer treatment produces depression,[143,144] and their administration generates hyperactivity and dysregulation in the HPA axis. These are common features of severe depression. The sickness response and depression overlap in that many of the behavioral manifestations of sickness are also manifestations of a depressive disorder. Whether sickness and depression constitute separate states of the system is still uncertain. It is becoming clear, however, that the immune defense responses associated with tissue damage contribute to bodily awareness and the complex, multidimensional experience of pain.

Summary

This review of mechanisms reveals that the emotional aspects of pain are the product of the defensive and stress responses that tissue trauma, a related stressor, or a constellation of stressors evokes. These responses comprise two forms of allostasis. At the neuroendocrine level, the defense response is an adaptive reaction characterized by sympathetic arousal, hypervigilance, and a sense of threat. However, a coordinated immune system adaptive defense response also occurs at the immune level. Mediated by pro-inflammatory cytokines, it produces a sense of sickness and curtails normal activity. The sickness response produces fatigue, general malaise, fever, and hyperalgesia typically experienced as musculoskeletal pain. Depression is apparently related to the sickness response in that both are the product of pro-inflammatory cytokines. Thus, the defensive responses generate negative emotions in the general domains of anxiety/threat, depression, and fatigue and sickness.

Stress and Chronic Pain

Stress and related defensive responses can promote chronic pain and related disability in at least three ways. First, noxious somatic or neuropathic signaling or central mechanism generating the perception of pain can function as stressors, thereby triggering a defense response and stress. As the mechanism discussion indicates, this can lead to negative emotional states, depressed mood, general sickness, and fatigue. If this is prolonged, patients typically undergo physical deconditioning that makes the pain worse. Second, psychosocial stressors such as dysfunctional family relationships or poor vocational adjustment can trigger the stress response and lead to all of the consequences noted above. Third, comorbid disorders and associated interventions are stressors and can contribute to pain by producing negative affective states, the sickness response, and, ultimately, physical deconditioning. Immunological diseases, cancer, diabetes, neurological disorders, and other disease states can increase patient vulnerability to chronic pain through these mechanisms.

The three mechanisms are not mutually exclusive: they can exist in any combination. The normal course of a stress response or defense response is immediate arousal with subsequent slow recovery to normalcy. When stressors confront a patient as a chain of events, the recovery process to the first may not finish before the second sets off another arousal pattern. A chain of stressors can dysregulate one or another feedback dependent aspect of the stress response system, such as the HPA axis. Hypercortisolemia, for example, characterizes almost half of severely depressed patients. Stress-induced chronobiological dysregulation is perhaps more common. Patients with chronic pain often complain of disturbed sleep patterns.

FUTURE DIRECTIONS

Psychophysiology is a rapidly expanding domain of inquiry. I have been able to cover only a small fraction of the field in this review. Other relevant areas include sleep and sleep disorders, chronobiology, physiological mechanisms of learning and memory, somatic representation, and psychoneuroimmunology. Painful conditions influence these various domains and in turn change in response to changes within these domains. Furthermore, functional brain imaging has opened new opportunities for pursing the relationship of brain activity to physical and psychological manipulations and also subjective experience. Building an interdisciplinary scientific evidence base in the domain of psychophysiology should be a priority in pain research because this field bridges psychological states and physiological health.

Multisymptom syndromes such as fibromyalgia syndrome, irritable bowel syndrome, and tempormandibular disorder pose major challenges in pain medicine and other medical areas. It is clear that these problems are related to stress, but the causal mechanisms of such disorders and their resistance to treatment remain ill-defined. These disorders are mind–body problems that refuse to yield to either purely physiological or purely psychological intervention. Psychophysiology is the only approach formally organized to pursue such mechanisms from an integrated body–mind perspective. Future research on the nature of multisymptom disorders and the development of management strategies or curative interventions can benefit from a psychophysiological approach.

Finally, psychophysiology as a field offers unique tools and methods for research that can address the mechanisms and benefits of interdisciplinary pain management. It is no surprise to experienced pain clinicians that psychological interventions and events have physiological consequences and, conversely, physiological events and interventions have psychological consequences. Psychophysiology as a field is well-positioned to characterize such phenomena and also to optimize interdisciplinary intervention through the coordinated examination of subjective and objective outcomes.

References

1. Andreassi JL. *Psychophysiology: Human Behavior and Physiological Response.* 2nd ed. Hillsdale, NJ: Lawrence Erlbaum Associates; 1989.
2. Cacioppo JT, Tassinary LG. Psychophysiology and psychophysiolociacal inference. In: Cacioppo JT, Tassinary LG, eds. *Principles of Psychophysiology: Physical, Social, and Inferential Elements.* New York: Cambridge University Press; 1990:3–33.
3. Hugdahl K. *Psychophysiology: The Mind-Body Perspective.* Cambridge: Harvard University Press; 1995.
4. Scarry E. *The Body in Pain: The Making and Unmaking of the World.* New York: Oxford University Press; 1985.
5. Merskey H. Pain terms: a list with definitions and a note on usage. Recommended by the International Association for the Study of Pain (IASP) Subcommittee on Taxonomy. *Pain* 1979;6:249–252.
6. Dennett D. *Consciousness Explained.* Boston: Little Brown; 1991.
7. MacLean PD. *The Triune Brain in Evolution: Role in Paleocerebral Functions.* New York: Plenum Press; 1990:425.
8. Darwin C. *The Expression of the Emotions in Man and Animals.* London: John Murray; 1872.
9. Thompson J. Development of facial expression of emotion in blind and seeing children. *Arch Psychol* 1941;37:264.
10. Ploog D. Biological foundations of the vocal expressions of emotions. In: Plutchik R, Kellerman H, eds. *Emotion: Theory, Research, and Experience.* New York: Academic Press; 1986:173–198.
11. Ploog D. Human neuroethology of emotion. *Prog Neuropsychopharmacol Biol Psychiatry* 1989;13(suppl):S15–S22.
12. MacLean PD. Some psychiatric implications of physiological studies on frontotemporal portion of limbic system (visceral brain). *Electroencehalogr Clin Neurophysiol* 1952;4:407–418.
13. Apkarian AV, Bushnell MC, Treede RD, et al. Human brain mechanisms of pain perception and regulation in health and disease. *Eur J Pain* 2005;9(4):463–484.
14. Nagai M, Kishi K, Kato S. Insular cortex and neuropsychiatric disorders: a review of recent literature. *Eur Psychiatry* 2007;22(6):387–394.
15. Craig AD. Interoception and emotion: a neuroanatomical perspective. In: Lewis, Haviland-Jones, Barrett, eds. *Handbook of Emotion.* 3rd ed. In Press.
16. Ledoux JE. The neurobiology of emotion. In: Ledoux JE, Hirst W, eds. *Mind and Brain: Dialogs in Cognitive Neuroscience.* Cambridge, MA: Cambridge University Press; 1986:301–354.
17. Ledoux JE. *The Emotional Brain: The Mysterious Underpinnings of Emotional Life.* New York: Simon and Shuster; 1996.
18. Morgane PJ. Historical and modern concepts of hypothalamic organization and function. In: Morgan PJ, Panksepp J, eds. *Handbook of the Hypothalamus.* New York: Marcel Dekker, Inc.; 1981:1–64.
19. Burnstock G, Hoyle CHV, eds. *Autonomic Neuroeffector Mechanisms.* Philadelphia: Harwood Academic Publishers; 1992.
20. Dodd J, Role LW. The anatomic nervous system. In: Kandel ER, Schwartz JH, Jessell TM, eds. *Principles of Neural Science.* 3rd ed. New York: Elsevier; 1991:761–775.
21. Cannon WB. *Bodily Changes in Pain, Hunger, Fear, and Rage.* New York: Appleton; 1929.
22. Sokolov EN. *Perception and The Conditioned Reflex.* Oxford: Pergamon Press; 1963.
23. Sokolov EN. The orienting response, and future directions of its development. *Pavlov J Biol Sci* 1990;25(3):142–150.
24. Barrett JA, Shaikh MB, Edinger H, et al. The effects of intrahypothalamic injections of norepinephrine upon affective defense behavior in the cat. *Brain Res* 1987;426(2):381–384.
25. Hess WR. Hypothalamus und die zantren des autonomen nervensystems: physiologie. *Archiv Psychiatr Nervenkr* 1936;104(548–557).
26. Hilton SM. Hypothalamic regulation of the cardiovascular system. *Br Med Bull* 1966;22:243–248.
27. Ferrell JE Jr. Self-perpetuating states in signal transduction: positive feedback, double-negative feedback and bistability. *Curr Opin Cell Biol* 2002;14(2):140–148.
28. Duric V, McCarson KE. Persistent pain produces stress-like alterations in hippocampal neurogenesis and gene expression. *J Pain* 2006;7(8):544–555.
29. Villanueva L, Bing Z, Bouhassira D, et al. Encoding of electrical, thermal, and mechanical noxious stimuli by subnucleus reticularis dorsalis neurons in the rat medulla. *J Neurophysiol* 1989;61:391–402.
30. Willis WD, Westlund KN. Neuroanatomy of the pain system and of the pathways that modulate pain. *J Clin Neurophysiol* 1997;14(1):2–31.
31. Craig AD. Spinal and trigeminal lamina I input to the locus coeruleus anterogradely labeled with Phaseolus vulgaris leucoagglutinin (PHA-L) in the cat and the monkey. *Brain Res* 1992;584(1–2):325–328.
32. Villanueva L, Cliffer KD, Sorkin LS, et al. Convergence of heterotopic nociceptive information onto neurons of caudal medullary reticular formation in monkey (Macaca fascicularis). *J Neurophysiol* 1990;63:1118–1127.
33. Bing Z, Villanueva L, Le Bars D. Ascending pathways in the spinal cord involved in the activation of subnucleus reticularis dorsalis neurons in the medulla of the rat. *J Neurophysiol* 1990;63:424–438.
34. Bowsher D. Role of the reticular formation in responses to noxious stimulation. *Pain* 1976;2:361–378.
35. Burstein R, Cliffer KD, Giesler GJ, eds. *The spinohypothalamic and spinotelecephalic tracts: direct nociceptive projections from the spinal cord to the hypothalamus and telencephalon.* New York: Elsevier; 1988.
36. Burstein R, Dado RJ, Cliffer KD, et al. Physiological characterization of spinohypothalamic tract neurons in the lumbar enlargement of rats. *J Neurophysiol* 1991;66(1):261–284.
37. Bernard JF, Besson JM. The spino(trigemino)pontoamygdaloid pathway: electrophysiological evidence for an involvement in pain processes. *J Neurophysiol* 1990;63(3):473–490.
38. Foote SL, Morrison JH. Extrathalamic modulation of corticofunction. *Annu Rev Neurosci* 1987;10:67–95.
39. Bremner JD, Krystal JH, Southwick SM, et al. *Noradrenergic Mechanisms in Stress and Anxiety: I. Preclinical Studies.* New York: Synapse; 1996:23(1):28–38.
40. Gray JA. *The Neuropsychology of Anxiety: An Enquiry into the Functions of the Septo-Hippocampal System.* New York: Oxford University Press; 1982.
41. Gray JA. *The Psychology of Fear and Stress.* 2nd ed. Cambridge: Cambridge University Press; 1987.
42. Isaacson RL. *The Limbic System.* 2nd ed. New York: Plenum Press; 1982.
43. Papez JW. A proposed mechanism of emotion. *Arch Neurol Psych* 1937;38:725–743.
44. Charney DS, Deutch A. A functional neuroanatomy of anxiety and fear: implications for the pathophysiology and treatment of anxiety disorders. *Crit Rev Neurobiol* 1996;10(3–4):419–446.
45. Fillenz M. *Noradrenergic Neurons.* Cambridge: Cambridge University Press; 1990.
46. Svensson TH. Peripheral, autonomic regulation of locus coeruleus noradrenergic neurons in brain: putative implications for psychiatry and psychopharmacology. *Psychopharmacology (Berl)* 1987;92:1–7.
47. Aston–Jones G, Foote SL, Segal M. Impulse conduction properties of noradrenergic locus coeruleus axons projecting to monkey cerebrocortex. *Neuroscience* 1985;15:765–777.
48. Rasmussen K, Aghajanian GK. Withdrawal-induced activation of locus coeruleus neurons in opiate-dependent rats: attenuation by lesions of the nucleus paragigantocellularis. *Brain Res* 1989;505(2):346–350.
49. Rasmussen K, Aghajanian GK. *Failure to Block Responses of Locus Coeruleus Neurons to Somatosensory Stimuli by Destruction of Two Major Afferent Nuclei.* New York: Synapse; 1989;4(2):162–164.
50. Korf J, Bunney BS, Aghajanian GK. Noradrenergic neurons: morphine inhibition of spontaneous activity. *Eur J Pharmacol* 1974;25:165–169.
51. Morilak DA, Fornal CA, Jacobs BL. Effects of physiological manipulations on locus coeruleus neuronal activity in freely moving cats. II. Cardiovascular challenge. *Brain Res* 1987;422:24–31.
52. Stone EA. Stress and catecholamines. In: Friedhoff AJ, ed. *Catecholamines and Behavior.* New York: Plenum Press; 1975:31–72.
53. Foote SL, Bloom FE, Aston–Jones G. Nucleus locus ceruleus: new evidence of anatomical and physiological specificity. *Physiol Rev* 1983;63:844–914.
54. Redmond DEJ, Huang YG. Current concepts. II. New evidence for a locus coeruleus–norepinephrine connection with anxiety. *Life Sci* 1979;25:2149–2162.
55. Grant SJ, Aston–Jones G, Redmond DE Jr. Responses of primate locus coeruleus neurons to simple and complex sensory stimuli. *Brain Res Bull* 1988;21(3):401–410.
56. Redmond DEJ. Alteration in the functions of the nucleus locus coeruleus: a possible model for studies of anxiety. In: Hannin I, Usdin E, eds. *Animal Models in Psychiatry and Neurology.* New York: Pergamon Press; 1977:293–306.
57. Rasmussen K, Morilak DA, Jacobs BL. Single unit activity of locus coeruleus neurons in the freely moving cat. I. During naturalistic behaviors and in response to simple and complex stimuli. *Brain Res* 1986;371(2):324–334.
58. Elam M, Svensson TH, Thoren P. Differentiated cardiovascular afferent regulation of locus coeruleus neurons and sympathetic nerves. *Brain Res* 1985;358:77–84.
59. Elam M, Svensson TH, Thoren P. Locus coeruleus neurons and sympathetic nerves: activation by visceral afferents. *Brain Res* 1986b;375:117–125.

60. Amaral DB, Sinnamon HM. The locus coeruleus: neurobiology of a central noradrenergic nucleus. *Prog Neurobiol* 1977;9:147–196.
61. McNaughton N, Mason ST. The neuropsychology and neuropharmacology of the dorsal ascending noradrenergic bundle—a review. *Prog Neurobiol* 1980;14:157–219.
62. Butler PD, Weiss JM, Stout JC, et al. Corticotropin-releasing factor produces fear-enhancing and behavioral activating effects following infusion into the locus coeruleus. *J Neurosci* 1990;10:176–183.
63. Elam M, Svensson TH, Thoren P. Locus coeruleus neurons and sympathetic nerves: activation by cutaneous sensory afferents. *Brain Res* 1986a;366: 254–261.
64. Siegel JM, Rogawski MA. A function for REM sleep: regulation of noradrenergic receptor sensitivity. *Brain Res Rev* 1988;13:213–233.
65. Abercrombie ED, Jacobs BL. Single-unit response of noradrenergic neurons in the locus coeruleus of freely moving cats. I. Acutely presented stressful and nonstressful stimuli. *J Neurosci* 1987a;7(9):2837–2843.
66. Abercrombie ED, Jacobs BL. Single-unit response of noradrenergic neurons in the locus coeruleus of freely moving cats. II. Adaptation to chronically presented stressful stimuli. *J Neurosci* 1987b;7(9):2844–2848.
67. Libet B, Gleason CA. The human locus coeruleus and anxiogenesis. *Brain Res* 1994;634(1):178–180.
68. Weiss JM, Simson PG. Depression in an animal model: focus on the locus ceruleus. *Ciba Found Symp* 1986;123:191–215.
69. Seligman ME, Weiss J, Weinraub M, et al. Coping behavior: learned helplessness, physiological change and learned inactivity. *Behav Res Ther* 1980;18(5): 459–512.
70. Sumal KK, Blessing WW, Joh TH, et al. Synaptic interaction of vagal afference and catecholaminergic neurons in the rat nucleus tractus solitarius. *J Brain Res* 1983;277:31–40.
71. Sawchenko PE, Swanson LW. The organization of noradrenergic pathways from the brain stem to the paraventricular and supraoptic neuclei in the rat. *Brain Res* 1982;257(3):275–325.
72. Assenmacher I, Szafarczyk A, Alonso G, et al. Physiology of neuropathways affecting CRH secretion. In: Ganong WF, Dallman MF, Roberts JL, eds. *The Hypothalamic–pituitary–adrenal Axis Revisited* 1987:149–161.
73. Kanosue K, Nakayama T, Ishikawa Y, et al. Responses of hypothalamic and thalamic neurons to noxious and scrotal thermal stimulation in rats. *J Thermobiol* 1984;9:11–13.
74. Peschanski M, Weil-Fugacza J. Aminergic and cholinergic afferents to the thalamus: experimental data with reference to pain pathways. In: Besson JM, Guilbaud G, Paschanski M, eds. *Thalamus and Pain*. Amsterdam: Excerpta Medica; 1987:127–154.
75. Lopez JF, Young EA, Herman JP, et al. Regulatory biology of the HPA axis: an integrative approach. In: Risch SC, ed. *Central Nervous System Peptide Mechanisms in Stress and Depression*. Washington, DC: American Psychiatric Press; 1991:1–52.
76. Feldman S, Conforti N, Weidenfeld J. Limbic pathways and hypothalamic neurotransmitters mediating adrenocortical responses to neural stimuli. *Neurosci Biobehav Rev* 1995;19(2):235–240.
77. Selye H. *The Stress of Life*. New York: McGraw–Hill; 1978.
78. Lilly MP, Gann DS. The hypothalamic–pituitary–adrenal-immune axis. A critical assessment. *Arch Surg* 1992;127(12):1463–1474.
79. Ghione S. Hypertension-associated hypalgesia. Evidence in experimental animals and humans, pathophysiological mechanisms, and potential clinical consequences. *Hypertension* 1996;28(3):494–504.
80. Amir S, Amit Z. The pituitary gland mediates acute and chornic pain responsiveness in stressed and non-stressed rats. *Life Sci* 1979;24:439–448.
81. Kelly DD, Silverman AJ, Glusman M, et al. Characterization of pituitary mediation of stress-induced antinociception in rats. *Physiol Behav* 1993;53: 769–775.
82. Bodnar RJ, Glusman M, Brutus M, et al. Analgesia induced by cold-water stress: Attenuation following hypophysectomy. *Physiol Behav* 1979;23: 53–62.
83. Truesdell LS, Bodner RJ. Reduction in cold-water swim analgesia following hypothalamic paraventricular nucleus lesions. *Physiol Behav* 1987;39: 727–731.
84. Henry JP. Neuroendocrine patterns of emotional response. In: Plutchik R, Kellerman H, eds. *Emotion: Theory, Research and Practice*. Orlando: Academic Press; 1986:37–60.
85. LeDoux JE, Iwata J, Cicchetti P, et al. Different projections of the central amygdaloid nucleus mediate autonomic and behavioral correlates of conditioned fear. *J Neurosci* 1988;8:2517–2529.
86. Krukoff TL. Neuropeptide regulation of autonomic outflow at the sympathetic preganglionic neuron: anatomical and neurochemical specificity. *Ann N Y Acad Sci* 1990;579:162–167.
87. Sapolsky RM. *Stress, the Aging Brain, and the Mechanisms of Neuron Death*. Cambridge: The MIT Press; 1992.
88. Panksepp J. The anatomy of emotions. In: Plutchik R, Kellerman H, eds. *Emotion: Theory, Research and Experience*. Orlando: Academic Press; 1986: 91–124.
89. Jänig W. Systemic and specific autonomic reactions in pain: efferent, afferent and endocrine components. *Eur J Anaesthesiol* 1985;2:319–346.
90. Saphier D. Cortisol alters firing rate and synaptic responses of limbic forebrain units. *Brain Res Bull* 1987;19:519–524.
91. Damasio AR. *Descartes' Error: Emotion and Reason in the Human Brain*. New York: Grosset/Putnam; 1994.
92. Pandya DN, Barnes CL, Panksepp J. Architecture and connections of the frontal lobe. In: Perecman E, ed. *The Frontal Lobes Revisited*. Hillsdale, NJ: Lawrence Erlbaum Associates; 1987:41–72.
93. Pribram KH. The biology of emotions and other feelings. In: Plutchik R, Kellerman H, eds. *Emotion: Theory, Research, and Experience*. New York: Academic Press; 1980:245–269.
94. Turner BH, Mishkin M, Knapp M. Organization of the amygdalopedal projections from modality-specific cortical association areas in the monkey. *J Comp Neurol* 1980;19:515–543.
95. Dworkin RH. Pain insensitivity in schizophrenia: a neglected phenomenon and some implications. *Schizophr Bull* 1994;20(2):235–248.
96. Melzack R. Phantom limbs and the concept of a neuromatrix. *Trends Neurosci* 1990;13:88–92.
97. Melzack R. Phantom limbs. *Sci Am* 1992;266(4):120–126.
98. Melzack R, Israel R, Lacroix R, et al. Phantom limbs in people with congenital limb deficiency or amputation in early childhood. *Brain* 1997;120(Pt 9): 1603–1620.
99. McEwen BS. The neurobiology of stress: from serendipity to clinical relevance. *Brain Res* 2000;886(1–2):172–189.
100. Korte SM, Koolhaas JM, Wingfield JC, et al. The Darwinian concept of stress: benefits of allostasis and costs of allostatic load and the trade-offs in health and disease. *Neurosci Biobehav Rev* 2005;29(1):3–38.
101. Tsigos C, Chrousos GP. Hypothalamic–pituitary–adrenal axis, neuroendocrine factors and stress. *J Psychosom Res* 2002;53(4):865–871.
102. Padgett DA, Glaser R. How stress influences the immune response. *Trends Immunol* 2003;24(8):444–448.
103. Zukowska Z, Pons J, Lee EW, et al. Neuropeptide Y: a new mediator linking sympathetic nerves, blood vessels and immune system? *Can J Physiol Pharmacol* 2003;81(2):89–94.
104. Elenkov IJ. Glucocorticoids and the Th1/Th2 balance. *Ann N Y Acad Sci* 2004;1024:138–146.
105. Rassnick S, Sved AF, Rabin BS. Locus coeruleus stimulation by corticotropin-releasing hormone suppresses in vitro cellular immune responses. *J Neurosci* 1994;14(10):6033–6040.
106. Tracey I, Ploghaus A, Gati JS, et al. Imaging attentional modulation of pain in the periaqueductal gray in humans. *J Neurosci* 2002;22(7):2748–2752.
107. Davidson RJ, Irwin W. The functional neuroanatomy of emotion and affective style. *Trends Cogn Sci* 1999;3(1):11–21.
108. Hariri AR, Mattay VS, Tessitore A, et al. Neocortical modulation of the amygdala response to fearful stimuli. *Biol Psychiatry* 2003;53(6):494–501.
109. Likhtik E, Pelletier JG, Paz R, et al. Prefrontal control of the amygdala. *J Neurosci* 2005;25(32):7429–7437.
110. Merali Z, Michaud D, McIntosh J, et al. Differential involvement of amygdaloid CRH system(s) in the salience and valence of the stimuli. *Prog Neuropsychopharmacol Biol Psychiatry* 2003;27(8):1201–1212.
111. Herman JP, Figueiredo H, Mueller NK, et al. Central mechanisms of stress integration: hierarchical circuitry controlling hypothalamo-pituitary–adrenocortical responsiveness. *Front Neuroendocrinol* 2003;24(3):151–180.
112. Pessoa L, Padmala S, Morland T. Fate of unattended fearful faces in the amygdala is determined by both attentional resources and cognitive modulation. *Neuroimage* 200528(1):249–255.
113. Keefe FJ, Rumble ME, Scipio CD, et al. Psychological aspects of persistent pain: current state of the science. *J Pain* 2004;5(4):195–211.
114. Misslin R. The defense system of fear: behavior and neurocircuitry. *Neurophysiol Clin* 2003;33(2):55–66.
115. Rosen JB. The neurobiology of conditioned and unconditioned fear: a neurobehavioral system analysis of the amygdala. *Behav Cogn Neurosci Rev* 2004; 3(1):23–41.
116. Pare D, Quirk GJ, Ledoux JE. New vistas on amygdala networks in conditioned fear. *J Neurophysiol* 2004;92(1):1–9.
117. Forray MI, Gysling K. Role of noradrenergic projections to the bed nucleus of the stria terminalis in the regulation of the hypothalamic–pituitary–adrenal axis. *Brain Res Rev* 2004;47(1–3):145–160.
118. Xu Y, Day TA, Buller KM. The central amygdala modulates hypothalamic–pituitary–adrenal axis responses to systemic interleukin-1beta administration. *Neuroscience* 1999;94(1):175–183.
119. Sternberg EM. Neuroendocrine factors in susceptibility to inflammatory disease: focus on the hypothalamic–pituitary–adrenal axis. *Horm Res* 1995; 43(4):159–161.
120. Kohl J. The role of complement in danger sensing and transmission. *Immunol Res* 2006;34(2):157–176.
121. Lambrecht BN. Immunologists getting nervous: neuropeptides, dendritic cells and T cell activation. *Respir Res* 2001;2(3):133–138.
122. Inoue A, Ikoma K, Morioka N, et al. Interleukin-1beta induces substance P release from primary afferent neurons through the cyclooxygenase-2 system. *J Neurochem* 1999;73(5):2206–2213.
123. Eskandari F, Webster JI, Sternberg EM. Neural immune pathways and their connection to inflammatory diseases. *Arthritis Res Ther* 2003;5(6):251–265.
124. Gruys E, Toussaint M, Niewold T, et al. Acute phase reaction and acute phase proteins. *J Zhejiang Univ SCI* 2005 2005;6B(11):1045–1056.
125. Elenkov IJ, Wilder RL, Chrousos GP, et al. The sympathetic nerve—an integrative interface between two supersystems: the brain and the immune system. *Pharmacol Rev* 2000;52(4):595–638.
126. Vizi ES, Elenkov IJ. Nonsynaptic noradrenaline release in neuro-immune responses. *Acta Biol Hung* 2002;53(1–2):229–244.

127. Kin NW, Sanders VM. It takes nerve to tell T and B cells what to do. *J Leukoc Biol* 2006;79(6):1093–1104.
128. Oberbeck R. Catecholamines: physiological immunomodulators during health and illness. *Curr Med Chem* 2006;13(17):1979–1989.
129. Tracey KJ. The inflammatory reflex. *Nature* 2002;420(6917):853–859.
130. Maier SF, Goehler LE, Fleshner M, et al. The role of the vagus nerve in cytokine-to-brain communication. *Ann N Y Acad Sci* 1998;840:289–300.
131. Dantzer R. Cytokine-induced sickness behavior: mechanisms and implications. *Ann N Y Acad Sci* 2001;933:222–234.
132. Elenkov IJ, Iezzoni DG, Daly A, et al. Cytokine dysregulation, inflammation and well-being. *Neuroimmunomodulation* 2005;12(5):255–269.
133. Watkins LR, Maier SF. Immune regulation of central nervous system functions: from sickness responses to pathological pain. *J Intern Med* 2005;257(2):139–155.
134. Watkins LR, Maier SF. Implications of immune-to-brain communication for sickness and pain. *Proc Natl Acad Sci U S A* 1996;96(14):7710–7713.
135. Wieseler–Frank J, Maier SF, Watkins LR. Immune-to-brain communication dynamically modulates pain: physiological and pathological consequences. *Brain Behav Immun* 2005;19(2):104–111.
136. Steinman L. Elaborate interactions between the immune and nervous systems. *Nat Immunol* 2004;5(6):575–581.
137. Romeo HE, Tio DL, Rahman SU, et al. The glossopharyngeal nerve as a novel pathway in immune-to-brain communication: relevance to neuroimmune surveillance of the oral cavity. *J Neuroimmunol* 2001;115(1–2):91–100.
138. Reiche EM, Morimoto HK, Nunes SM. Stress and depression-induced immune dysfunction: implications for the development and progression of cancer. *Int Rev Psychiatry* 2005;17(6):515–527.
139. Wichers M, Maes M. The psychoneuroimmuno-pathophysiology of cytokine-induced depression in humans. *Int J Neuropsychopharmacol* 2002;5(4):375–388.
140. Anisman H, Merali Z. Cytokines, stress and depressive illness: brain-immune interactions. *Ann Med* 2003;35(1):2–11.
141. Pucak ML, Kaplin AI. Unkind cytokines: current evidence for the potential role of cytokines in immune-mediated depression. *Int Rev Psychiatry* 2005;17(6):477–483.
142. Schiepers OJ, Wichers MC, Maes M. Cytokines and major depression. *Prog Neuropsychopharmacol Biol Psychiatry* 2005;29(2):201–217.
143. Wood LJ, Nail LM, Gilster A, et al. Cancer chemotherapy-related symptoms: evidence to suggest a role for proinflammatory cytokines. *Oncol Nurs Forum* 2006;33(3):535–542.
144. Raison CL, Capuron L, Miller AH. Cytokines sing the blues: inflammation and the pathogenesis of depression. *Trends Immunol* 2006;27(1):24–31.

CHAPTER 30 ■ PAIN AND LEARNING

ROBERT J. GATCHEL, BRIAN R. THEODORE, NANCY D. KISHINO, AND CARL NOE

INTRODUCTION TO PAIN AND LEARNING

One of the major contributions of the behavioral sciences to the area of medicine has been the application of learning principles to the development of effective illness management techniques. This has been especially true in the area of pain management. Before discussing these learning-based management techniques, an overview of the three major principles of learning will be provided.

OVERVIEW OF THE THREE MAJOR PRINCIPLES OF LEARNING

Classical Conditioning

Classical conditioning is one of the most basic forms of learning in which a learned association or connection develops between two stimuli or objects. As noted by Baum, Gatchel, and Krantz,[1] the eminent Russian physiologist Ivan Pavlov (1849–1936) was the first to describe the process of classical conditioning with his work on the conditioned reflex. Reflexes are specific, automatic, unlearned reactions elicited by a specific stimulus. For example, if you have ever touched a surface that you did not know was hot (such as a hot stove), you showed a reflexive behavior—the immediate withdrawal of your hand from the stove. Similarly, if a piece of dust suddenly enters your eye, your eye will automatically blink and begin to secrete tears. These **unconditioned reflexes** are automatic and have a great deal of survival value for the organism. Pavlov demonstrated that such unconditioned reflexes could be **conditioned**, or learned. While studying dogs in order to understand more fully the digestive process, he began to notice that many of the dogs secreted saliva (an unconditioned reflex to the sight or smell of food) before food was delivered to them. He observed that this phenomenon occurred whenever the dogs either heard the approaching footsteps of the laboratory assistant who fed them or had a preliminary glimpse of the food. In order to investigate this phenomenon more systematically, Pavlov developed a procedure for producing a conditioned reflex. This procedure came to be called **classical conditioning**. It is one of the most basic forms of learning.

Pavlov conducted a series of well-known studies on the process of classical conditioning using dogs as experimental subjects (Fig. 30.1). In these studies, Pavlov studied situations in which a neutral stimulus or event (such as a bell) was presented to a dog just prior to the presentation of food (an unconditioned stimulus that normally elicits an automatic unconditioned reflex of salivation). After a number of such presentations, the bell (now a conditioned stimulus) would elicit a conditioned or learned salivation re-

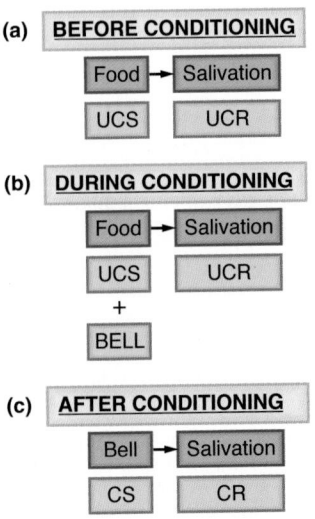

FIGURE 30.1 Pavlov's procedure of classical conditioning.

sponse when presented by itself in the absence of food. The conditioned reflex of salivation occurred to the bell alone. This represents the process of classical conditioning, and it is based on the learned association or connection between two stimuli, such that the bell is associated with food, that have occurred together at approximately the same point in time. An association is learned between a weak stimulus (such as the bell) and a strong stimulus (such as the sight of food) so that the weak stimulus comes to elicit the response originally controlled only by the stronger one (i.e., salivation).

Pavlov also subsequently demonstrated what would happen if the neutral stimulus, such as a bell, was presented just prior to the presentation of an aversive stimulus such as an electric shock or a pin prick. Normally, such aversive stimuli presented alone will produce a variety of negative responses such as whining/whimpering and fear-type reactions such as urination. When the bell preceded such an aversive stimulus, eventually the formerly neutral bell stimulus would automatically produce the negative emotional responses.

In another variety of this design, Pavlov then evaluated what would happen if, instead of preceding food with the sound of the bell, it was preceded by the aversive stimulus such as electric shock. What Pavlov found in this situation was that, after this conditioning, the dogs subsequently failed to demonstrate any negative emotional responses to the aversive stimulus. Instead, these dogs began perceiving these painful stimuli as signals that food was on the way. The electric shock now actually elicited salivation and approach behaviors!

Operant Conditioning

Operant conditioning (also referred to as instrumental conditioning) is a different form of learning that was originally formulated by Edward Thorndike (1874–1949), and then more comprehensively developed by B. F. Skinner (1904–1990). Unlike classical conditioning, operant conditioning develops new behaviors that bring about positive consequences or remove negative events. In classical conditioning, a new stimulus (such as a bell) is conditioned to elicit the same responses that had previously occurred to the unconditioned stimulus, whereas in operant conditioning, a new response is learned. For example, new behaviors that produce food, social approval, or other positive consequences, or that reduce damaging or aversive events, illustrate operant behavior. The behavior "operates" on the environment to bring about changes in it. Thus, animal training, such as that involved in the learned performance of circus animals, involves basic principles of operant conditioning. Although operant training has existed for centuries, the behaviorist revolution in psychology provided the first carefully delineated methods and procedures of operant conditioning so that such training could be accomplished most efficiently.[1] The key stimulus is **reinforcement**. Reinforcement refers to any consequence that increases the likelihood that a particular behavior will be repeated or that strengthens that behavior. **Extinction** involves the gradual decrease in the strength or tendency to perform a response due to the elimination of reinforcement. Based upon these principles, what came to be known as the "Skinner box" was devised as an enclosed plexiglas box in which there was a light above a lever. The lever could be pressed down by the animal with its paws (rats were used in these early studies). Below the lever was a food tray into which food pellets could be dispensed. The task of the animal was to learn that pressing the lever (a certain number of times or at a certain rate, predetermined by the experimenter) resulted in food pellets being dispensed in the food tray. Thus, the animal learned to operate on the environment (the lever in the box) in order to receive reinforcement (food pellets).

Once the above response was learned, one could then introduce different **reinforcement schedules** in order to produce different patterns of responding. Reinforcement could now require variable numbers of bar presses or could be available every so often. Also, a *discriminative stimulus* could be introduced, so that the rat received reinforcement for pressing the bar only when the light was on in the box. The animal would soon learn not to respond when the light was off. In this manner, the rat's bar-pressing behavior came under **stimulus** (e.g., light) **control**.

This same shaping procedure is used in training circus and other animals to perform complicated acts. Dolphins can be shaped to leap out of the water and lions can be taught to jump through flaming hoops in order to receive some reinforcement. These techniques are used in virtually every zoo and marine animal show.

Observational Learning

Finally, the third major form of learning is called observational learning. There has been a great deal of research indicating that learning can occur through simple observation without the presence of any form of tangible direct reinforcement. Such learning, besides being called *observational learning*, is sometimes called imitation learning, cognitive learning, vicarious learning, or modeling. Observational learning is defined simply as that learning which occurs without any apparent direct reinforcement.[2] Many behaviors can be acquired if an individual sees the particular behavior performed or modeled by another person. In addition, behavior is often strongly guided by social norms, resulting in a given individual being motivated to adopt a set of behaviors that are consistent with these norms.[3,4] Observational learning is one such mechanism that transmits knowledge of these norms to the individual. These norms can be either explicit or implicit, and they can operate at the level of specific groups an individual may identify with, in addition to norms dictated at the larger societal level.

One of the earliest laboratory studies of observational learning[5] involved nursery school children. One group of children observed an adult perform a series of aggressive acts, both verbal and physical, toward a large toy Bobo doll. Another group watched a nonaggressive adult, who simply sat quietly and paid no attention to the doll. A third group of children was not exposed to a model. Later, after being mildly frustrated, all children were placed in a room alone with the Bobo doll and their behavior was observed. It was found that the behavior of the two model groups tended to be similar to that of their adult model. That is, children who had viewed the aggressive adult performed more aggressive acts toward the doll in the free-play situation than the other groups and also made more responses that were exact imitations of the model's aggressive behavior. Those children who had observed a nonaggressive adult model performed significantly fewer aggressive responses than the aggressive model group.

OPERANT CONDITIONING AND PAIN

The Hallmark Work of Wilbert Fordyce

As discussed earlier, and as reviewed by Gatchel,[6] operant conditioning refers to the strengthening of a response and behavior through reward or reinforcement. That is to say, the probability that a behavior will be performed again is increased if it is followed by some form of reinforcement. Behavior is controlled by its consequences. If a behavior is followed by a reward, it has a high probability of recurring; if it is ignored or punished, it has a low probability of recurring. Obviously, a great deal of our everyday behavior is learned and maintained through operant conditioning. For example, most of us work because of the rewards (both tangible, such as money, and intangible, such as a pleasant work environment) that it produces.

In terms of pain, many times a person in pain will elicit a great deal of sympathy and attention (both of which are rewarding). In addition, suggestions are usually made by others to rest and stay inactive, pain-relieving medications are usually administered, and often financial compensation is provided. The longer these reinforcing consequences continue, the longer the patient is likely to display the maladaptive pain behaviors such as inactivity and avoidance of work. Thus, this type of learning or conditioning can significantly contribute to the maintenance of pain behavior.

As pointed out by Baum, Gatchel, and Krantz,[1] this operant conditioning conceptualization of pain was systematically employed in the operant pain treatment program originally developed at the University of Washington's Department of Rehabilitation Medicine by Fordyce and colleagues.[7] This program involved a 4 to 8 week inpatient period, designed to gradually increase the general activity level of the patient, and to decrease medication usage. The program was based on the assumption that, although pain may initially result from some underlying organic pathologic condition, environmental reinforcement consequences (such as attention of the patient's family and the rehabilitation staff) can modify and further maintain various aspects of "pain behavior," such as complaining, grimacing, slow and cautious body movements, requesting pain medication, and so on. Viewing pain as an operantly conditioned behavior, Fordyce assumed that the potentially reinforcing consequences, such as the concern and attention from others, rest, medication, avoiding unpleasant responsibilities and duties, as well as other events, frequently follow and reinforce the maladaptive pain behavior and, as a consequence, hinder the patient's progress in treatment.

In their treatment program, Fordyce and colleagues[7] systematically controlled environmental events (e.g., attention, rest, medication) and made them occur contingent on adaptive behaviors. A major goal of the program was to increase positive behaviors, such as participation in therapy and activity level, while simultaneously decreasing or eliminating negative pain behaviors. It should also be noted that members of the patient's family were actively involved in the treatment program and worked closely with the rehabilitation staff. They were taught how to react to the patient's behavior in a manner that would reduce pain and to maximize the patient's compliance with, and performance in, the rehabilitation program. Using this operant approach, the patient was basically taught to reinterpret the sensation of pain and tolerate it, while performing more adaptive behaviors that would gain the attention and approval of others. Such a program was initially conducted in the hospital, and would later be continued on an outpatient basis. These programs proved to be very successful at decreasing pain behaviors while increasing the levels of activities of daily living.

Of course, such examples do not imply that all pain is learned. The point being made is that our pain perceptions and responses often have a significant psychologic learning component that directly and significantly contributes to these experiences of pain. Thus, psychologic variables play a direct role in the pain experience. How one reacts to pain sensations is as important an issue as the specific physiologic mechanisms involved in transmitting and generating pain experiences. Pain is a complex behavior and not simply a sensory effect.

With the above view in mind, it is clear that one must conceptualize pain like any other form of complex behavior, consisting of multiple behavioral components. As Fordyce and Steger[8] have indicated, in order to describe pain, "there must be some form of pain behavior by which diagnostic inferences and treatment judgments can be made. A patient will signal the type of pain he or she is experiencing by describing the intensity, frequency, location, and type of pain experienced. In addition to these verbal cues available to the patient's environment as an indication of his or her pain, there is a myriad of nonverbal signs used to communicate pain experiences. These include grimaces, sighs, moans, limps, awkward or strained body positions, the use of a cane or crutch, and many other symbols associated in our society with discomfort or physical problems.

Traditionally, in attempts to describe pain, the focus was only on the physiologic or structural mechanisms underlying the report of pain and not on other components such as behavioral indices and self-report. The reliance on strictly one component, such as structural measures, does not yield a valid or precise measure of an individual's pain. Again, pain is a complex behavior and not purely a sensory event. One needs to consider multiple behavioral components in the assessment and treatment of this behavior.

Operant Conditioning and Chronic Pain: The Basics

Sanders[9] has provided an excellent overview of the key ingredients involved in the use of operant conditioning methods when managing chronic pain. Of course, as he appropriately points out, operant conditioning methods should not be viewed as the only technique to use in managing chronic pain. Rather, it is just one of a number of behavioral science methodologies that can be used in combination/unison with other methodologies. Operant techniques can be used to help significantly decrease many common overt pain behaviors, such as the following:

- Verbal pain behaviors, such as overt expressions of hurting (e.g., moaning, sighing, complaining, etc.)
- Nonverbal pain behaviors, such as limping, grimacing, over-reliance on a cane or brace, rubbing the affected area, etc.
- Overly sedentary activities, such as decreased activity level, sitting, and lying down.
- Overconsumption of medications and the sole reliance on other therapeutic devices to control pain.

Rather than engagement in the above maladaptive pain behaviors, the patient is encouraged and reinforced to engage in "well behaviors" that involve more positive activity and alteration away from the overfocusing on pain. Through a comprehensive approach, health care professionals, family members, and others reinforce and encourage these well behaviors while other effective pain management techniques are learned by the patient, such as biofeedback, stress management, coping skills, and appropriate pharmacotherapy, which is closely maintained. The overall goal is to increase function which will then be accompanied by a decrease in pain.[6]

CLASSICAL CONDITIONING AND PAIN

Aversive Classical Conditioning and Pain

As discussed earlier in this chapter, Pavlov conducted studies demonstrating that when an initially neutral stimulus (such as a bell) was presented just prior to the presentation of an aversive, painful stimulus (such as electric shock) which will, in turn, produce negative emotional responses (such as whimpering, fear, avoidance, etc.), then the bell itself will produce the negative emotional response when presented by itself. We then may generalize this to a patient who developed a sudden painful back problem at work, which does not go away after several days, after which just the act of going to work and anticipating lifting a heavy object may produce a negative emotional response such as fear of lifting and possible avoidance of the workplace because of pain.

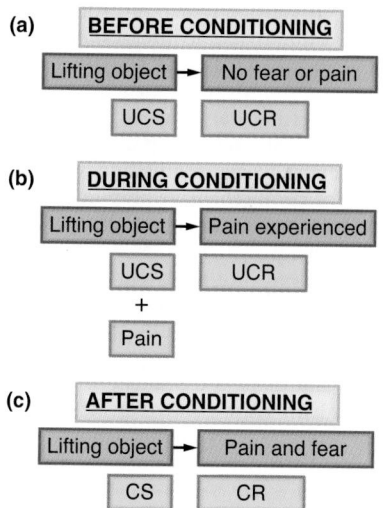

FIGURE 30.2 Classically conditioned fear and pain during a work task (lifting an object).

Classically Conditioned Fear/Avoidance and Pain

Figure 30.2 presents the conditioning sequence that a person may go through in the situation described above. (a) At first, before conditioning, there is no association between lifting an object at work and any avoidance of lifting because of fear of pain. (b) During conditioning, the individual now begins to experience some back pain while lifting objects at work. This pain becomes progressively worse over time, to the point that this person hesitates to lift anything because of fear of exacerbating the back pain he/she is already experiencing. (c) After conditioning, any prompting or requirement to lift an object automatically produces a fear response and active avoidance of any lifting to avoid pain. There is now a classically conditioned negative emotional response of lifting objects at work because of the fear of pain.

How can the above classically conditioned association between lifting and a fear of pain response be broken? As Pavlov's experiments have shown, just as a conditioned association can be learned, it can also be subsequently extinguished or broken under the right situations. One such method would be to initially teach patients how to correctly lift, while keeping their back muscles relaxed. The weight they are then asked to lift is kept relatively light and then progressively made heavier as the individual is able to lift a certain weight while relaxed and not experiencing any pain. The person is also taught appropriate pacing skills so that enough time is given between lifts for his or her back muscles to recuperate before performing the next lift. Thus, fear of lifting becomes "deconditioned" or extinguished in this work situation.

OBSERVATIONAL LEARNING AND PAIN

Observational learning is defined simply as that learning which occurs without any apparent direct reinforcement.[2] Many behaviors can be acquired if an individual merely sees the particular behavior displayed or modeled by another person. Examples of behaviors acquired by observational learning abound. For example, investigations of dental fears in children have revealed that the attitudes and feelings of a child's family toward dental treatment are important in determining that child's own anxiety toward dental treatment. In one such study, it was found that

children with anxious mothers showed significantly more emotionally negative behaviors during a tooth extraction than did children of mothers with low anxiety.[10]

In our society, there is a great deal of potential observational learning that can negatively influence comprehensive pain management effects. We are constantly being bombarded by advertisements that certain medications or pills will make us feel better. This, in turn, produces an unfortunate iatrogenic effect on patients who assume that there is some magic "silver bullet" pill or procedure that will automatically make them feel better and take away their pain. Unfortunately, such expectations are often not realized. Thus, patient education is often initially needed to dissuade patients of the notion that there is an immediate magical cure for their pain, especially as it becomes more chronic in nature.

Social norms can also influence an individual's response to pain, often through the mechanisms of observational learning. These normative influences play a role in behaviors associated with the reporting of pain, seeking treatment for pain, and level of pain tolerance. A study by Sternbach and Tursky[11] was among the earliest investigations that illuminated our further understanding of how normative factors influence responses to pain. In this study, the results implied that cultural differences associated with ethnicity played a role in an individual's tolerance of painful electrical stimulation. Parallel results in terms of ethnic differences were also demonstrated when physiological indices (such as heart rate and palmar skin resistance levels) were measured in response to painful electrical stimulation, despite relatively large intraethnic group variation.[12]

Recent studies have also demonstrated the role played by ethnic differences. For example, ethnicity has been reported to account for differences in self-reported levels of pain, as well as for tolerance of induced ischemic pain, during a study on a sample of chronic pain patients.[13,14] Cultural differences are also apparent in treatment preference and levels of health care utilization. A large population-based survey in the United States indicated that Caucasians had greater number of visits on average compared to African-Americans and Hispanics and were more likely to have received complementary or alternative therapies for chronic pain.[15]

Early research on the association between gender and responses to pain also indicated that females had a lower tolerance level for experimentally induced pain,[16] and were also more likely to report pain within clinical settings.[17] However, recent research has indicated that the extent of an individual's identification with their own gender group norms moderate their tolerance of pain. Gender differences in the tolerance of experimentally-induced pain are present only among individuals strongly identifying with social norms that dictate that men should tolerate more pain than women.[18] While it remains to be seen whether social norms also dictate gender differences in the probability of seeking treatment for pain, there is a demonstrable gender difference in health care utilization among chronic pain patients, with females being more likely to seek treatment for pain.[19]

INTEGRATING LEARNING PRINCIPLES IN THE TREATMENT OF PAIN

Cognitive–Behavioral Therapy and Pain

As Turk[20] has highlighted in his discussion of the cognitive-behavioral treatment (CBT) approach to pain, there are important behavioral learning theory principles that are part of this overall therapeutic perspective. Certainly, classical conditioning (a focus on eliminating conditioned fear avoidance), operant conditioning (such as not reinforcing pain behavior), and observational learning (such as education about the negative iatrogenic expectation of immediate pain relief) are all important components. However, in addition, Turk[20] appropriately points out the fact that cognitive factors, in addition to behavioral factors, need to be considered: "The critical factor for the C–B model, therefore, is not that events occur together in time or are operantly reinforced but that people learn to predict them based on experiences and information processing. They filter information through their preexisting knowledge and organized representations of knowledge (e.g., cognitive scheme) . . . and react accordingly . . . Because interaction with the environment is not a static process, attention is given to the ongoing reciprocal relationships among physical, cognitive, affective, social, and behavioral factors" (p. 140). This perspective is in keeping with the biopsychosocial approach to pain,[6] to be discussed later.

With this above perspective in mind, there is no doubt that CBT is an effective treatment modality for the management of pain. Morley, Ecclestan, and Williams,[21] on the basis of their systematic review of the scientific literature and a meta-analysis of randomized controlled trials, found that CBT produced significantly greater changes in self-reported pain and cognitive coping, as well as reduced behavioral expressions of pain, relative to waiting list control patients and alternative treatment control conditions. In a more recent comprehensive review, Gatchel and Okifuji[22] found comparable results. Table 30.1 provides a summary of some of the components of CBT, as delineated by Gatchel.[6]

Cognitive–Behavioral Therapy as an Essential Component of a Comprehensive Interdisciplinary Approach to Pain Management

The biopsychosocial perspective of pain is now accepted as the most heuristic approach to the understanding and treatment of pain disorders.[6,23] It views physical disorders, such as pain, as a result of a complex and dynamic interaction among physiologic, psychologic, and social factors that perpetuate and may worsen the clinical presentation. Moreover, each individual experiences pain uniquely. Therefore, the range of psychologic, social, and economic factors can interact with physical pathology to modulate a patient's report of symptoms and subsequent disability. As a consequence, a comprehensive biopsychosocial approach to assessment and treatment must be employed with each patient because of the unique interactions, as well as to tailor the treatment to the specific needs of the patient. This is why comprehensive interdisciplinary pain management programs have proven to be more therapeutic and cost-effective than traditional unimodal treatment approaches.[22]

Within an interdisciplinary treatment program, there is a comprehensive treatment team that consists of the following: physician/nurse team to deal with medical issues, psychologist or psychiatrist to deal with the psychosocial issues of patients, a physical therapist to address any issues related to physiologic bases of pain, as well as any issues related to physical progression toward recovery, and an occupational therapist who is involved in both physical and vocational aspects of the patient's treatment. For such a program to be effective, constant and efficient communication among all treatment personnel is imperative, during which patient progress can be discussed and evaluated. This is important so that patients hear the same treatment philosophy and message from each of the treatment team members. The overall goal is to produce an increase of functioning and the ability to manage pain and disability.

It is a major goal of the psychologist or psychiatrist to increase the patient's understanding of pain, as well as their coping skills required to manage the pain. This is where CBT plays a major role. Of course, in keeping with the biopsychosocial perspective, it is not a stand alone treatment, but must be integrated with the other components of therapy in order to yield the best long-term outcomes.[6]

CONCLUSION

Pain is a complex behavior and is, therefore, subject to the general principles of learning and behavior change. The three major principles of learning include classical conditioning, operant conditioning, and observational learning. These principles play an important role in the development of pain behavior (e.g., social or environmental factors that can reinforce maladaptive pain behavior). However, these learning principles can also be effectively utilized in the treatment and management of pain. The biopsychosocial approach to the treatment and management of pain emphasizes interdisciplinary treatment modalities and eschews a "one-size-fits-all" approach in dealing with pain. Learning principles are therefore an important component in this approach due to its flexibility in addressing complex behavioral history at the individual level. CBT incorporates these learning principles and has been documented as an effective component of interdisciplinary pain management.

TABLE 30.1

SUMMARY OF SOME OF THE MAJOR COMPONENTS OF COGNITIVE–BEHAVORIAL THERAPY

- Education of patients about pain and their particular syndrome.
- Engender in patients a self-management and coping skills perspective to pain.
- Help patients focus on increasing physical functioning and management of their pain, rather than expecting a sudden cure.
- Teaching biofeedback, relaxation, and stress management techniques.
- Providing patients with coping skills in other areas, such as with interpersonal problems, work-related problems, marital problems, etc.
- Emphasize to patients the importance of identifying, and then eliminating, maladaptive thoughts about pain.
- Provide patients with guidance about increasing activities of daily living (in order to distract them from pain), with appropriate pacing activities.
- Provide help to improve sleep.
- Review the appropriate use of potential adjunctive modalities, such as medications, exercise, and physical methods (e.g., cold and heat packs).
- Assist patients with appropriate goal setting for the future (e.g., when to return to work or other activities).
- Provide relapse prevention strategies in order to help cope with potential future relapses.

(Adapted from Gatchel RJ. Clinical Essentials of Pain Management. Washington, DC: American Psychological Association; 2005.)

References

1. Baum A, Gatchel RJ, Krantz DS, eds. An Introduction to Health Psychology. 3rd ed. New York: McGraw-Hill; 1997.
2. Bandura A. Principles of Behavior Modification. New York: Holt, Rinehart & Winston; 1969.
3. Turner JC. Social Influence. New York: Brooks/Cole; 1991.
4. Cialdini RB, Trost MR. Social influence: Social norms, conformity, and compliance. In: Gilbert D, Fiske S, Lindsey G, eds. The Handbook of Social Psychology. New York: McGraw-Hill; 1998:151–192.
5. Bandura A, Ross D, Ross SA. Imitation of film-mediated agressive models. J Abnorm Soc Psychol 1963;66:3–11.

6. Gatchel RJ. *Clinical Essentials of Pain Management*. Washington, DC: American Psychological Association; 2005.
7. Fordyce WE, Fowler RS Jr, Lehmann JF, et al. Some implications of learning in problems of chronic pain. *J Chronic Dis* 1968;21:179–190.
8. Fordyce WE, Steger JC. Chronic Pain. In: Pomerleau OF, Brady JP, eds. *Behavioral Medicine: Theory and Practice*. Baltimore: Williams & Wilkins; 1979:125–154.
9. Sanders SH. Operant conditioning with chronic pain: back to basics. In: Turk DC, Gatchel RJ, eds. *Psychological Approaches to Pain Management: A Practitioner's Handbook*. New York: Guilford Press; 2002:128–137.
10. Weisenberg M. Cultural and racial reactions to pain. In: Weisenberg M, ed. *The Control of Pain*. New York: Psychological Dimensions; 1977:201–232.
11. Sternbach RA, Tursky B. Ethnic differences among housewives in psychophysical and skin potential responses to electric shock. *Psychophysiology* 1965;1(3):241–246.
12. Tursky B, Sternbach RA. Further physiological correlates of ethnic differences in responses to shock. *Psychophysiology* 1967;4:67–74.
13. Campbell CM, Edwards RR, Fillingim RB. Ethnic differences in responses to multiple experimental pain stimuli. *Pain* 2005;113(1–2):20–26.
14. Edwards RR, Doleys DM, Fillingim RB, et al. Ethnic differences in pain tolerance: clinical implications in a chronic pain population. *Psychosom Med* 2001;63(2):316–323.
15. Portenoy RK, Ugarte C, Fuller I, et al. Population-based survey of pain in the United States: differences among white, African American, and Hispanic subjects. *J Pain* 2004;5(6):317–328.
16. Riley JL III, Robinson ME, Wise EA, et al. Sex differences in the perception of noxious experimental stimuli: a meta-analysis. *Pain* 1998;74(2–3):181–187.
17. Unruh AM. Gender variations in clinical pain experience. *Pain* 1996;65(2–3):123–167.
18. Pool GJ, Schwegler AF, Theodore BR, et al. Role of gender norms and group identification on hypothetical and experimental pain tolerance. *Pain* 2007;129:122–129.
19. McGeary DD, Mayer TG, Gatchel RJ, et al. Gender-related differences in treatment outcomes for patients with musculoskeletal disorders. *Spine J* 2003;3:197–203.
20. Turk DC. A cognitive-behavioral perspective on treatment of chronic pain patients. In: Turk DC, Gatchel RJ, eds. *Psychological Approaches to Pain Management: A Practitioner's Handbook*. 2nd ed. New York: Guilford Press; 2002:138–158.
21. Morley S, Eccleston C, Williams A. Systematic review and meta-analysis of randomized controlled trials of cognitive behaviour therapy and behaviour therapy for chronic pain in adults, excluding headache. *Pain* 1999;80:1–13.
22. Gatchel RJ, Okifuji A. Evidence-based scientific data documenting the treatment and cost-effectiveness of comprehensive pain programs for chronic nonmalignant pain. *J Pain* 2006; Nov;7(11):779–793.
23. Turk DC, Monarch ES. Biopsychosocial perspective on chronic pain. In: Turk DC, Gatchel RJ, eds. *Psychological approaches to pain management: a practitioner's handbook*. 2nd ed. New York: Guilford; 2002:5–29.

CHAPTER 31 ■ PSYCHIATRIC ILLNESS, DEPRESSION, ANXIETY, AND SOMATOFORM PAIN DISORDERS

AJAY D. WASAN, MARK D. SULLIVAN, AND MICHAEL R. CLARK

INTRODUCTION

Chronic pain and psychiatric illness are fundamentally linked in prevalence, pathophysiology, and patient outcomes.[1] Yet, the high rates of psychiatric illness in patients with chronic cancer and noncancer pain are still poorly understood. Diagnostic hierarchies taught to physicians in medical school and residency, impairment rating strategies used by compensation systems, and the natural scientific method used by medicine that looks for objective causes for clinical phenomena force us into a mind–body dualism. Engel did much of the early research to codify this Cartesian concept into the notion of psychogenic pain.[2] *Psychogenic pain* is defined as pain due to psychological factors in the absence of an organic basis for pain.[3] Subsequently, Merskey and others extended this concept into our lexicon of pain taxonomy.[4] If we cannot explain pain in terms of objective tissue pathology, Western biomedicine lures us to explain it in terms of patients' psychopathology.[5,6] Although this dichotomy has been popular in clinical settings historically, current scientific evidence for it is lacking.[7]

Evidence indicates that the majority of patients with chronic pain and psychiatric illness have a physical basis for pain in the body, whose perception is made worse by overlying psychiatric illness.[8] Epidemiologic evidence supports the use of inclusive rather than exclusive models of psychiatric diagnoses in medical settings that allows for the presence of both medical disease and mental disorders (i.e., a comorbidity model). Medical illness in no way excludes the possibility of a clinically important psychiatric illness. Medically ill patients are much more likely to have psychiatric illness than patients without medical illness. Psychiatric illness in no way precludes the possibility of a clinically important medical illness. Psychiatric illness is, in fact, associated with health behaviors and psychophysiologic changes known to promote medical illness. Even disorders seeming purely of the mind, such as conversion disorder, have been correlated to alterations in brain structure and function,[9] illustrating the interplay between mind and brain.

The structure of our clinical settings makes the integrated delivery of mental and physical health care difficult. Nowhere is this more important than in the care of the patient with chronic pain. Psychotherapeutic and psychopharmacologic interventions for chronic pain are rarely effective in isolation from somatic treatments, and the success of somatic treatments is diminished by co-occurring mental illness. Distress, disuse, and disability are important facets of a chronic pain problem, and all require clinical attention by the pain practitioner. Neglect of one of these components can result in treatment failure even in the presence of excellent care for the other components. Research has indicated that psychiatric comorbidity has an adverse impact on treatments for chronic pain, such as rehabilitation, spinal cord stimulation, or opioid therapy.[3,10] While the details of these interactions are quite relevant to understand, this chapter concentrates on the recognition and diagnosis of psychiatric illness in patients with chronic pain, a sizable task in itself. Similarly, psychiatric comorbidity has been shown to be particularly prevalent in and salient to the outcomes of a range of noncancer pain disorders (e.g., chronic low back pain,[11] fibromyalgia,[12] temporomandibular joint disorders,[13] chronic daily headache,[14] and chronic pelvic pain[15]). However, the specific role comorbid psychopathology plays in each of these disorders is beyond the scope of this chapter.

This chapter will first outline an approach to psychiatric diagnosis and to categorizing psychiatric symptoms in patients with chronic pain. Because of the breadth of psychiatric symptoms in pain patients, this section is substantial in order to provide a framework for organizing symptoms into diagnostic and treatment categories. Then the chapter will discuss the main illness categories of depression, anxiety, personality, and somatoform disorders. It is beyond this chapter to discuss to what extent a pain practitioner should evaluate and treat psychiatric problems and when to refer to a psychologist or psychiatrist.

PSYCHIATRIC NOSOLOGY AND DIAGNOSTIC AND TREATMENT APPROACHES

As noted, any discussion of psychiatric disorders in patients with chronic pain is haunted by the concept of psychogenic pain. We are drawn to the concept of psychogenic pain because it fills the gaps left when our attempts fail to explain clinical pain exclusively in terms of tissue pathology. Psychogenic pain, however, is an outdated concept that should be vanquished from our vocabulary of pain. Positive criterion for the identification of psychogenic pain, mechanisms for the production of psychogenic pain, and specific therapies for psychogenic pain are lacking. Furthermore, neuroimaging studies indicate that anticipated pain, imagined pain, or empathizing with the pain of another are associated with activations of the same brain areas involved in processing a painful stimulus, such as applied noxious heat (the lateral and medial pain systems).[16,17] Thus, there is a dynamic interaction between our mental states (mind) and brain function. The dichotomy between mind and body (including brain) underlying the concept of psychogenic pain is hollow. As will be discussed later in this chapter, it may be more useful to frame the contributions of the mind to pain perception in terms of a process of somatization.

Psychiatric diagnosis of many disorders, such as depression, can be helpful to the clinician and patient by pointing to specific effective therapies. The *Diagnostic and Statistical Manual of Mental Disorders* (DSM) lists the current diagnoses treated by psychiatrists and the specific symptoms that serve as descriptive criteria for each condition.[18] However, the DSM offers only consistency and reliability and does not differentiate the disorders according to the basic natures from which the phenomenology emerges, demonstrate any interrelationships among disorders, or prove that there is a criterion on which the validity of the diagnosis rests.[19] This is particularly true of psychiatric disorders in those with medical illness. Most psychiatrists tend to use the DSM as a guide to or an outline of the major diagnoses, not as a definitive diagnostic method. As a descriptive tool, many of the symptom lists for DSM diagnoses are quite complete and will be referred to throughout this chapter. However, when patients with chronic pain are in need of psychiatric care, they want to know the generative nature of their conditions and how to differentiate them for the sake of receiving prognoses and treatments.[20] The DSM and its descriptive companion, the biopsychosocial approach, offer only the ingredients and end products but not the recipes and processes for validation. Multidisciplinary pain treatment functions with the same limitations.[21,22] Without the method to determine a set of unique causes and direct specific treatments, the patient receives symptomatic treatments with the expected "partial" response. Despite the involvement of more disciplines, the message is clear cures for "organic" problems and management for "functional" problems. Cartesian dualism lives.

Patients with chronic pain come to or are referred to a psychiatrist because they are ill. In some way, they are considered a diagnostic dilemma.[23,24] Despite the utilization of extensive health care resources to perform an exhaustive evaluation, the patients remain ill. A temptation emerges to diagnose them with a psychogenic problem because no "good" cause can be found for their persistent pain and the accompanying disability and suffering.[25] The cause for their illness cannot be found until the investigation expands to include the domain of personal consciousness.[26] This realm contains not only the diseases of the brain (cerebral faculties) but also the disruptions of the motivational rhythms of behavior, the psychological constitution of the individual, and the personal chronicle of desire and encounters. All mental disorders are expressions of life under altered circumstances that affect characteristic mental capacities and generate particular expressions.[27,28] These distinctions allow for independently informed perspectives about the nature of mental disorders and what may have happened to generate the disorder. Four perspectives (diseases, behaviors, dimensions, and life stories) represent classes of disorders that each have a common essence and logical implications for causation and treatment.[29,30] In this approach to patient care, diseases are what people *have*; behaviors are what people *do*; dimensions are what people *are*; and life stories are what people *encounter*. The formulation of a patient with chronic pain should address the contributions from each perspective to the overall presentation and inform the design of a treatment plan that can address each component of the patient's illness. While the basis for a mental illness may be dominated by one perspective (i.e., the disease perspective in schizophrenia), generally each psychiatric diagnosis has contributions from each perspective that are responsible for the onset and maintenance of the disorder.

Diseases of the brain manifest psychologically. The psychological faculties of the brain include but are not limited to consciousness, cognition, memory, language, affect, and executive functions. Abnormalities in the structures or their associated functions of these faculties are expressed in the criteria that describe the common diagnoses such as delirium, dementia, panic disorder, and major depression. However, the patient may describe deficits in these faculties with difficulty and rely on somatic symptoms (e.g., pain) as incomplete proxies for these criteria. The physical symptoms occur because the brain is malfunctioning and suggesting pathology in the body. The unifying feature of diseases is a broken part within the individual that is causing pathology.[30] The pathology causes the characteristic signs and symptoms typically manifested by the affliction.[28] For the patient, there is no meaningful interpretation to be understood, no individual deficiency to be addressed, and no goal that is trying to be achieved. Finding a cure may repair the broken part, prevent the initial damage from progressing, or compensate for the pathology through secondary compensatory measures.

The perspective of *behavior* encompasses a wide range of actions and activities. The complex behaviors of human beings are designed with the purpose of achieving goals. Human consciousness is characterized by the regular, rhythmic alterations of attention and perception produced by internal drives that increase a person's motivation toward a particular activity.[30,31] The drive pushes the individual into action. Then, after the actions, the drive is satisfied and a state of satiety emerges. Over time, drives re-emerge with subsequent effects on the individual's perceptual attitude toward his setting. In addition, personal assumptions or external opportunities increase the likelihood of certain behaviors. These present a choice to the person, who must decide what action to take. After the choice is made and the behavior completed, external consequences emerge from the outcome and influence future actions. The person learns which choices are most effective. When aspects of choice and control over behavior become disrupted, physicians will be asked to address the distorted goals, excessive demands, damaging consequences, and a lack of responsiveness to negative feedback.[32,33] Eating disorders are but one example. Treatment of behavioral disorders begins with regaining temporary control of the situation by stopping the behavior.[34] Restricting the patient's actions and preventing these problematic behaviors eventually limits the chaos of destructive actions. This stable foundation is required for the patient to gain insight about and motivation toward appropriate choices that will result in less distress and more satisfaction.[35] This basis for the effectiveness of behavioral approaches to chronic pain management is outlined in other chapters.

In contrast, many mental disorders emerge not from a disease of the brain or some form of abnormal illness behavior but a patient's personal affective or cognitive constitution.[30,31] Each individual possesses a set of personal *dimensions*, such as intelligence, extraversion, and neuroticism. These traits describe who a person is, and they are carried into the world as a set of innate capabilities of their psychological makeup. Which traits are relied upon and how much of them a person possesses will determine his potential to cope with different situations. Some circumstances are overwhelming and provoke a person's vulnerability to distress. The patient cannot manage the situation and what is required because of who he is. Borderline personality disorder is an example. It is probably the most severe personality disorder and generally is evident prior to the onset of pain. Assessment of personality traits are discussed at greater length below. Treatment for disorders of the dimensional type focuses on remediation of specific deficiencies and guidance about overcoming potential vulnerabilities through adaptations such as education about, assistance with, or modification of the particular stressors.[22,34]

The *life story* perspective utilizes a narrative composed of a series of events that a person encounters and determines to be personally meaningful.[30,31] These self-reflections are the means by which a person judges the value of his life as a whole. They impart a sense of self as the agent of a life plan unfolding in a social setting as well as the reflective subject experiencing and interpreting the outcome of such plans and commitments. If events occur as planned, then the person feels on track and successful. However, if the sequence of events results in an unexpected or disappointing outcome, the person will feel a sense of distress about this failure. Life story disorders are interpretive responses to life encounters such as grief from loss or anxiety due to expected threats.[32,36,37] In patients with chronic pain, the demoralization resulting from the inability to work or perform normal duties is a good example. Treatment begins with the expectation to forge a narrative of setting and sequence that suggests some role of the patient in his life and that illuminates the troubled state of mind as the outcome of that role and course of events.[22,34] The effective treatment of life story disorders requires reframing and reinterpretation to remoralize the patient by transforming the story into one with the potential for success and fulfillment.

The four perspectives provide a comprehensive yet flexible approach to the evaluation of a patient in distress with chronic pain and other somatic symptoms.[30,38] The treatments prescribed are now designed from the individual formulation and relevant perspectives. If a patient's symptoms and distress continue, the physician must consider other factors that may have been overlooked. Usually these factors are within one of the perspectives initially thought to be less important. A new combination of therapies is then required to treat the patient successfully. In the discussion that follows, categories of psychiatric disorders as defined in the *Diagnostic and Statistical Manual*, fourth edition, of the American Psychiatric Association (*DSM-IV*, 1994) are used as an organizing strategy. Understanding the relevant contributions from each perspective is important to formulating treatment.

FRAMEWORK FOR DESCRIBING PSYCHIATRIC SYMPTOMS

Figure 31.1 illustrates common psychiatric symptoms in patients with chronic pain. However, Figure 31.1 does omit substance use disorders, which are beyond the scope of this chapter. It is important to note that approximately 15% of all patients with chronic pain have a comorbid substance use disorder, whether it is alcoholism or prescription opioid abuse, etc.[39] Psychiatry-based research and health psychology–based research have contributed important insights into characterizing the mental life of patients with chronic pain. The findings from these epistemologies overlap significantly, but, unfortunately, there is no agreed-upon model for integrating these results.[40] Common terms to describe the psychological condition in pain patients are heightened emotional distress, high negative affect, and elevated pain-related psychological symptoms (i.e., those that are a direct result of chronic pain, and when the pain is eliminated, the symptoms disappear). These can all be considered forms of psychopathology and psychiatric comorbidity, since they represent impairments in mental health and involve maladaptive psychological responses to medical illness. This approach melds methods of classification from psychiatry and behavioral medicine to describe the scope of psychiatric disturbances in patients with chronic pain. *Psychiatry* is the field of medicine that is concerned with someone's mental life, such as their emotions, experiences, thoughts, and behav-

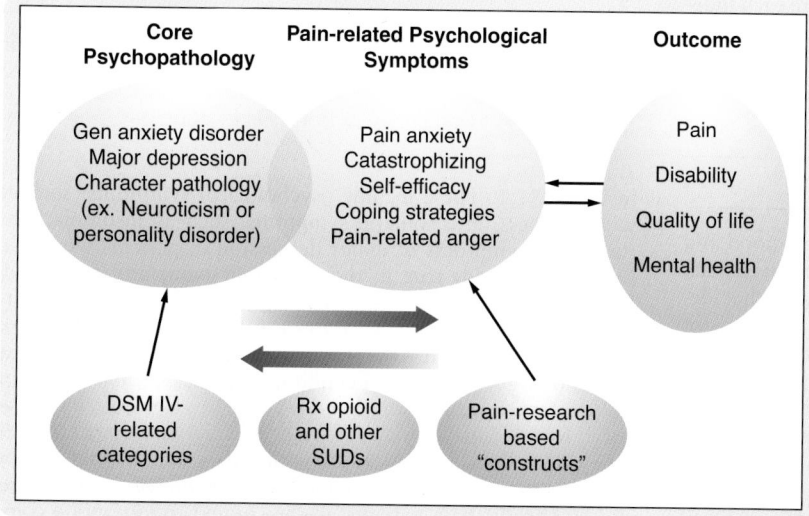

FIGURE 31.1 Common psychiatric symptoms in patients with chronic pain.

iors. It is focused particularly on disruptive, disordered, or pathological psychological states. Thus the constructs from pain-psychology are situated in Figure 31.1 as psychiatric symptoms, which in themselves can be at pathological levels, just as depression symptoms can rise to a level considered abnormal.

In pain patients the most common manifestations of psychiatric comorbidity involve one or more core psychopathologies in combination with pain-related psychological symptoms. For instance, poor pain self-efficacy or high levels of pain catastrophizing are most often found in conjunction with high levels of depression or anxiety symptoms.[41] These categories interact and some component of each are part and parcel of other psychopathologies. In other words, "lumping" (a diagnostic approach) and "splitting" (a construct-based approach) are both valid approaches to psychiatric phenomenology. As described in the previous section, not all patients and their psychiatric symptoms fit neatly into *DSM* categories of illness. This is true not just of those with chronic pain, and hence looking beyond *DSM* to broader and more specific methods of illness description and diagnosis is more prudent.

The pain-related psychological symptoms are described at length in other chapters, but it is important to understand how they interact with other psychiatric diagnoses. For example, pain-related anxiety (which includes state and trait anxiety related to pain) is the form of anxiety most germane to pain.[42] Elevated levels of pain-related anxiety (such as fear of pain) also meet *DSM-IV* criteria for an anxiety disorder due to a general medical condition. Since anxiety straddles both domains of core psychopathology and pain-related psychological symptoms, the assessment of anxiety in a patient with chronic pain (as detailed below) must include a review of manifestations of generalized anxiety as well as pain-specific anxiety symptoms (e.g., physiological changes associated with the anticipation of pain).

As indicated in Figure 31.1, elevated pain-related psychological symptoms have a clear, negative predictive relationship to many outcome areas. Poor coping skills often involve passive responses to chronic pain; for example, remaining bed-bound and mistakenly assuming that chronic pain is indicative of ongoing tissue damage as a reason for inactivity. Poor copers employ few self-management strategies (such as using ice, heat, or relaxation strategies for 10 to 20 minutes before resuming activities). Pain catastrophizing (cognitive distortions that are centered around pain), and low self-efficacy (a low estimate by the patient of what he/she is capable of doing) are linked with higher levels of pain and disability and worse quality of life.[40] A tendency to catastrophize often predicts poor outcome and disability, independent of other psychopathology such as major depression. Duration of chronic pain and psychiatric comorbidity are each independent predictors of pain intensity and disability. High levels of anger (which occur more often in men) can also explain a significant variance in pain severity.[43]

DEPRESSION

One must begin by distinguishing between depressed mood and the clinical syndrome of major depression. It is important to note, especially when working with chronic pain patients, that depressed mood or dysphoria is not necessary for the diagnosis of major depression. Anhedonia, the inability to enjoy activities or experience pleasure, is an adequate substitute. It is common for patients with chronic pain to deny dysphoria but to acknowledge that enjoyment of all activities has ceased, even those without obvious relation to their pain problem (e.g., watching television for a patient with low back pain).

The *DSM-IV* criteria for major depressive episodes are listed

---

TABLE 31.1

***DIAGNOSTIC AND STATISTICAL MANUAL*, FOURTH EDITION, CRITERIA FOR MAJOR DEPRESSIVE EPISODE**

A. Five (or more) of the following symptoms have been present during the same 2-week period and represent a change from previous functioning; at least one of the symptoms is either (1) depressed mood or (2) loss of interest or pleasure.
  1. Depressed mood most of the day, nearly every day, as indicated by either subjective report (e.g., feels sad or empty) or observation made by others (e.g., appears tearful). Note: In children and adolescents, can be irritable mood.
  2. Markedly diminished interest or pleasure in all, or almost all, activities most of the day, nearly every day (as indicated by either subjective account or observation made by others).
  3. Significant weight loss when not dieting or weight gain (e.g., a change of more than 5% of body weight in a month), or a decrease or increase in appetite nearly every day. Note: In children, consider failure to make expected weight gains.
  4. Insomnia or hypersomnia nearly every day.
  5. Psychomotor agitation or retardation nearly every day (observable by others, not merely subjective feelings of restlessness or being slowed down).
  6. Fatigue or loss of energy nearly every day.
  7. Feelings of worthlessness or excessive or inappropriate guilt (which may be delusional) nearly every day (not merely self-reproach or guilt about being sick).
  8. Diminished ability to think or concentrate, or indecisiveness, nearly every day (either by subjective account or as observed by others).
  9. Recurrent thoughts of death (not just fear of dying), recurrent suicidal ideation without a specific plan, or a suicide attempt or a specific plan for committing suicide.

B. The symptoms cause clinically significant distress or impairment in social, occupational, or other important areas of functioning.

C. The symptoms are not caused by the direct physiologic effects of a substance (e.g., a drug of abuse, a medication) or a general medical condition (e.g., hypothyroidism).

D. The symptoms are not better accounted for by bereavement (i.e., after the loss of a loved one) or the symptoms persist for longer than 2 months or are characterized by marked functional impairment, morbid preoccupation with worthlessness, suicidal ideation, psychotic symptoms, or psychomotor retardation.

From *Diagnostic and Statistical Manual*, 4th ed. Washington, DC: American Psychiatric Association, 1994:395, with permission.

---

in Table 31.1. These include psychological symptoms, such as worthlessness, and somatic symptoms, such as insomnia. The three core symptoms of major depression in patients with pain (which also holds true in those without pain) are low mood, impaired self-attitude, and neurovegetative signs.[44] It is important to note that somatic symptoms count toward a diagnosis of major depression unless they are caused by "the direct physiologic effects of a general medical condition" or medication. The poor sleep, poor concentration, and lack of enjoyment often experienced by patients with chronic pain are frequently attributed to pain rather than depression. However, they may or may not be a direct physiologic effect of pain. Given the high rates of depression in chronic pain patients, in the context of low mood complaints it is best to attribute these symptoms to a diagnosis of depression. Indeed, studies of depression in medically ill populations have generally found greater sensitivity and reliability with "inclusive models" of depression diagnosis than with models that try to identify the cause of each symptom.[45] Similarly, just as in those without pain, those with depression and pain are very likely to also have high levels of anxiety.[46,47]

Suicidal Ideation and Behavior

Suicide accounts for 1.8% of all deaths in the world.[48] In the United States, 4.6% of the population surveyed had made a suicide attempt and 13.5% reported a history of suicidal ideation.[49] The majority of suicide attempts occur within a year of the onset of suicidal ideation. The risk of suicidality is greatest in patients with affective disorders (e.g., depression and anxiety), personality disorders, substance use disorders, and chronic debilitating physical illnesses.[50,51] Depression is the most consistent and strongest predictor of suicidal ideation.[52] In one study of patients with major depressive disorder, 58% reported suicidal ideation during a current episode of illness.[53] Suicide was attempted by 15% of these patients with 95% preceded by suicidal ideation. Hopelessness, low levels of function, perceptions of poor social support, and disorders of alcohol use predicted suicidal ideation.

Medical illnesses and chronic pain in particular, increase the risk of suicide. In a study of suicide in the elderly, medical conditions such as congestive heart failure, chronic obstructive lung disease, seizure disorder and urinary incontinence were significantly associated with suicide with treatment for multiple illnesses increasing the risk.[54] Yet, except for bipolar disorder, the highest risk of suicide was found in patients with severe pain (OR = 7.52). Pain has been studied as a contributory factor in episodes of deliberate self harm involving patients with medical problems admitted to a general hospital.[55] Multiple studies have shown that patients with chronic pain are at greater risk for suicidal ideation, suicide attempts, and suicide completions.[56]

A recent comprehensive review notes that the likelihood of death by suicide in patients with chronic pain is 2 to 3 times the rate described in the general population.[51] The lifetime prevalence of suicide attempts in patients with chronic pain ranged from 5% to 14% and the rate of suicide attempts is double that found in the general population. The lifetime prevalence of suicidal ideation associated with chronic pain is approximately 20%. The rate of suicidal ideation in patients with chronic pain is estimated to be between 5% and 24%. While a number of methods are used to commit suicide, overdoses with medications are the most common. The relationship between chronic pain and suicidality is complex. While the associations are consistent, the cause and effect pathways of transition from suicidal ideation to suicide attempt to suicide completion are more difficult to describe. At this time, no successful algorithm exists and only an in-depth and longitudinal evaluation of the patient with chronic pain offers the best strategy for detecting who is considering suicide as a personal option. While understandable, it is not the norm to be suicidal even in those with severe pain. Most commonly, suicidality in a patient with chronic pain is indicative of an underlying psychiatric disorder. Thinking one is better off dead (a passive death wish) is not the same as actively trying or wanting to kill oneself (suicidality). It is important to bear this distinction in mind in evaluating any patient with thoughts about death.

Part of the concern regarding the association between chronic pain and suicidality lies in whether chronic pain is an independent risk factor for suicidal behavior or the presence of depression completely explains this association. A thorough review described the evidence for eight pain-specific risk factors of suicidality, which is defined as suicidal ideation, suicide attempt, or suicide completion.[51] The studies available suffer from significant limitations including inadequate assessments, retrospective designs, limited control groups, and the failure to distinguish between the potential risk factors of pain versus pain-related disability. However, the existing pain literature coupled with the general knowledge of suicide supports the following as the strongest predictors of suicidality: family history of suicide, previous suicide attempts, and presence of comorbid depression. Evidence exists for other risk factors including pain characteristics (intensity, location, type, duration), female gender, comorbid insomnia, catastrophizing and avoidance, desire for escape, helplessness and hopelessness, and problem-solving deficits.[57-59] The prevention of suicide should remain a priority for the care of patients with chronic pain.

Which Came First, Depression or Pain?

Patients with chronic pain often dismiss a depression diagnosis, stating that their depression is a direct reaction to their pain problem. Psychiatry has long debated the value of distinguishing a *reactive* form of depression caused by adverse life events from an *endogenous* form of depression caused by biological and genetic factors.[60] Life events are important in many depressive episodes, although they play a less important role in recurrent and severe or melancholic or psychotic depressions.[61] Only bereavement excludes someone from a depression diagnosis who qualifies on the basis of symptoms. Determining whether a depression is a *reasonable response* to life's stress may be important to patients seeking to decrease the stigma of a depression diagnosis and has been of interest to pain investigators (for a review, see Fishbain and colleagues).[8] It is not, however, important in deciding that treatment is necessary and appropriate. Indeed, no clinical benefit is gained from debating whether the depression caused the pain or the pain caused the depression, although such information may be useful in psychotherapy. If patients meet the diagnostic criteria outlined previously, it is likely that they can benefit from appropriate treatment. There is evidence that subsyndromal depression—depression symptoms not quite satisfying the threshold for major depression but debilitating nonetheless—also benefits from treatment, and should be treated.[62-64]

Prospective studies of patients with chronic musculoskeletal pain have suggested that chronic pain can cause depression,[65] that depression can cause chronic pain,[66] and that they exist in a mutually reinforcing relationship.[67] One fact raised to support the idea that pain causes depression is that the current depressive episode often began after the onset of the pain problem. The majority of studies appears to support this contention.[68] However, it has been documented that many patients with chronic pain (especially those disabled patients seen in pain clinics) have often had episodes of depression that predated their pain problem by years.[69] This has led some investigators to propose that there may exist a common trait of susceptibility to dysphoric physical symptoms (including pain) and to negative psychological symptoms (including anxiety and depression).[70,71] They conclude that "pain and psychological illness should be viewed as having reciprocal psychological and behavioral effects involving both processes of illness expression and adaptation."

It may be useful when initiating depression treatment to accept that the pain caused the depression because it builds rapport and is consistent with epidemiologic evidence about the current depressive episode. And most frequently, depression follows the onset of chronic pain and is not preceded by it.[72]

Differential Diagnosis

When considering the diagnosis of depression in the patient with chronic pain, important alternatives include bipolar disorder, substance-induced mood disorder, and dysthymic disorder (particularly if accompanied by a severe personality disorder, such as borderline personality disorder). Patients with bipolar disorder have extended periods of abnormally elevated as well as abnormally depressed mood. These periods of elevated mood need to last more than 1 continuous day and include features such as inflated self-esteem, decreased need for sleep, and racing thoughts. A history of manic or hypomanic episodes predicts an atypical response to antidepressant medication and increases the risk of antidepressant-induced mania. Substance-induced mood disorders can also occur in those with pain. Patients with chronic pain may be taking medications such as opioids, corticosteroids, dopamine-blocking agents (including antiemetics), or sedatives (including muscle relaxants) that produce a depressive syndrome. Current medication lists should be scrutinized before additional medications are prescribed for any patient.

Biological Tests for Depression

A variety of biological tests for depression have been investigated.[73] These tests have included the dexamethasone-suppression test, thyrotropin-releasing hormone stimulation test, clonidine-induced growth hormone secretion, and rates of imipramine binding to platelet membrane serotonin transporters. Of patients with major depression, 40% to 50% do not show normal suppression of morning plasma cortisol after receiving dexamethasone the night before. However, high false-positive rates for this dexamethasone-suppression test exist in patients who are pregnant; patients with dementia, alcoholism, anorexia nervosa, and other chronic debilitating diseases; and patients who are taking medications that induce microsomal enzymes, including barbiturates and opioids. This has limited the clinical value of this test.[74] The serotonin transport mechanism on platelet membranes is similar to that on serotonergic neurons. ^{3}H-imipramine binding to this platelet receptor is reduced in patients with major depression. It appears to be further reduced in patients who have both pain and depression.[75] Lower level of serotonin in the cerebral spinal fluid have been found in depressed patients and have been linked to suicidal ideation.[76] Although patients show significant differences on these tests, when considered as a group, substantial variation between individual patients limits the usefulness of these tests in the clinical setting. In the future, they may be able to provide a better understanding of the biochemical links between pain and depression.

Dysthymic Disorder

Dysthymic disorder is a chronic form of depression lasting 2 years or longer. The symptoms are generally less severe than those during an episode of major depression. Individuals with dysthymia can develop major depression as well. This combined syndrome has often been called *double depression*.[77] It is important to note dysthymia, because it is frequently invisible in medical settings, often being dismissed as "just the way that patient is." Dysthymia has been shown to respond to many antidepressants, including the selective serotonin reuptake inhibitors (SSRIs).[78] Treatment of double depression can be particularly challenging because of treatment resistance and concurrent personality disorders.[79] Psychiatric consultation should be considered when dysthymia or double depression is suspected.

Epidemiology of Depression

The prevalence of depression is much higher in medical settings and in patients with chronic illnesses than in the general population. It has been shown in studies using structured psychiatric interviews that a linear increase occurs in the prevalence of major depressive disorder when comparing community, primary care, and inpatient medical populations. Although 2% to 4% have major depression in the community, 5% to 9% of ambulatory medical patients and 15% to 20% of medical inpatients meet diagnostic criteria.[80] Primary care patients with major depression have been found to have more severe medical illness than those who are not depressed.[81] Even among community samples, the risk for depression appears to increase with worse perceived health status, number of chronic medical conditions, and number of medications taken.[82]

Prevalence rates of depression among patients in pain clinics have varied widely depending on the method of assessment and the population assessed. Rates as low as 10% and as high as 100% have been reported.[83] The reason for the wide variability may be attributable to a number of factors, including the methods used to diagnose depression (e.g., interview, self-report instruments), the criteria used (e.g., *DSM-IV*, cut-off scores on self-report instruments), the set of disorders included in the diagnosis of depression (e.g., presence of depressive symptoms, major depression), and referral bias (e.g., higher reported prevalence of depression in studies conducted in psychiatry clinics compared with rehabilitation clinics). The majority of studies report depression in more than 50% of chronic pain patients sampled.[84,85] There is a direct relationship between the duration of pain and the incidence of major depression. Certain chronic painful conditions are associated with higher rates of depression than others. For example, fibromyalgia, chronic daily headache, and chronic pelvic pain each are associated with higher rates than arthritis.[46,86]

Studies of primary care populations (in which generalization is less problematic) have revealed a number of other factors that appear to increase the likelihood of depression in patients with chronic pain. Dworkin and colleagues[87] reported that patients with two or more pain complaints were much more likely to be depressed than those with a single pain complaint. Number of pain conditions reported was a better predictor of major depression than pain severity or pain persistence.[87] Von Korff and colleagues developed a four-level scale for grading chronic pain severity based on pain disability and pain intensity: (a) low disability and low intensity; (b) low disability and high intensity; (c) high disability, moderately limiting; and (d) high disability, severely limiting. Depression, use of opioid analgesics, and doctor visits all increased as chronic pain grade increased.[88] Engel and colleagues showed that depression was associated with high total health care costs, but not high back pain costs among health maintenance organization patients with back pain.[89] When dysfunctional primary care back pain patients are studied for a year, those whose back pain improves also show improvement of depressive symptoms to normal levels.[90]

These epidemiologic studies provide solid evidence for a strong association between chronic pain and depression, but do not address whether chronic pain causes depression or depression causes chronic pain. As indicated previously, this question has more importance in medicolegal contexts than clinical contexts. Overall, in most instances depression follows the onset of pain.[72]

Pain and Depression: Mechanisms of Association

Beyond documenting the association of chronic pain and depression lies the question concerning mechanisms by which they may interact. Biological, psychological, and social mechanisms have been proposed to explain the high co-occurrence of chronic pain and depression. There is also substantial evidence (beyond the scope of this chapter to recount) that the following mechanisms underlie the other psychiatric comorbidities of pain, such as anxiety disorders.

Biological Theories

Pain Sensitivity. It is well documented that patients with major depression, or even depressive symptoms, have more pain complaints that those without depression. Studies have shown that 30% to 60% of depressed patients complain of pain.[91] These findings raise the possibility that depressed patients may have a greater sensitivity to noxious stimuli. In other words, depressed patients may have a reduced pain threshold. This has not been true in depressed patients without pain.[92,93] In patients with depression, anxiety, and pain, they appear more pain sensitive than those with chronic pain alone. Widerstrom-Noga and colleagues have demonstrated that patients with temporomandibular disorder and depression and anxiety symptoms were more sensitive to noxious stimuli and had lower pain thresholds.[94,95]

Biogenic Amines, Cytokines, and Neural Pathways. The highly variable relationship between injury severity and pain severity has been known since Beecher's studies of the soldiers at Anzio beach in World War II. Since the 1970s, great strides have been made in identifying the central nervous system mechanisms of endogenous pain modulation. Opioid and nonopioid branches to this system have been identified. Stimulation of the rostral ventromedial medulla or the dorsolateral pontine tegmentum produces behavioral analgesia in animals and inhibition of spinal pain transmission. The rostral ventromedial medulla is the principal source of serotonergic neurons that project to the spinal dorsal horn. The dorsolateral pontine tegmentum is the major source of noradrenergic neurons that project to the dorsal horn. Both neurotransmitters serotonin and norepinephrine inhibit nociceptive dorsal horn neurons when locally applied.[96] The descending inhibitory system is modulated by serotonin and norepinephrine, which are also thought to modulate mood. This is perhaps best illustrated by the effects of selective serotonin norepinephrine reuptake inhibitors (SNRIs) on depression and pain. The two drugs approved for use in this class are duloxetine and venlafaxine. Both are FDA approved antidepressants that have analgesic properties independent of their effects on mood.[97,98] These medications enhance serotonergic and noradrenergic neurotransmission. Additional studies indicate that opioid analgesia is enhanced in the presence of antidepressant treatment[99] and decreased after serotonin and norepinephrine depletion.[100] Therefore, it appears that biogenic amines play a critical role in endogenous pain modulation. To the extent that depletion or impaired function of amines such as serotonin and norepinephrine occurs in depression, this may contribute to the pain experienced and reported by those with major depression. Family history studies of depressed patients without pain illustrate that there is a heritable susceptibility to developing major depression.[101] It is thought that this genetic predisposition influences the vulnerability of biogenic amine systems.[102] Similarly, it has also been shown that those with major depression (without pain) have a diminished endogenous opioid response than healthy normals.[103]

Just as cytokine responses are important to the initiation and maintenance of chronic pain,[104] they have also been implicated in the pathogenesis of depression.[105] Depressed patients without pain have been found to have higher levels of proinflammatory cytokines and acute phase proteins. Administration of the cytokine interferon-alpha leads to depression in up to 50% of patients. Proinflammatory cytokines affect neurotransmitter metabolism, neuroendocrine function (particularly the hypothalamic-pituitary-adrenal axis), and synaptic plasticity.

Cortical Substrates for Pain and Affect. Advances in neuroimaging have linked the function of multiple areas in the brain which

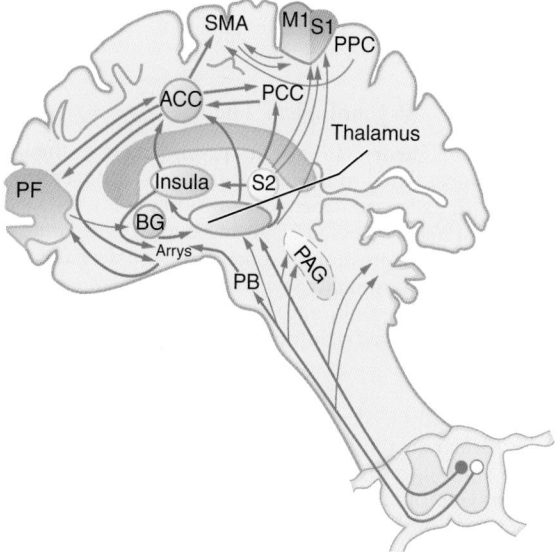

FIGURE 31.2 Supraspinal pathways of pain perception.

process pain and mood simultaneously, described at length in a previous chapter. This system is often termed the medial pain system or spinolimbic pain system.[106] These cortical areas (e.g., the anterior cingulate cortex [ACC], the insula, amygdala, and the dorsolateral prefrontal cortex [DLPFC]) form functional units through which psychiatric comorbidity may amplify pain and disability (Fig. 31.2). They are also laden with opioid receptors.[107] The ACC, insula, and DLPFC are less responsive to endogenous opioids in pain-free subjects with high negative affect (e.g., depression, anxiety, and anger symptoms).[108] Thus, high negative affect may diminish the effectiveness of endogenous and exogenous opioids through direct effects on supraspinal opioid binding. The medial pain system runs parallel to the spinothalamic tract and receives direct input from the dorsal horn of the spinal cord. The interactions among the function of these areas, pain perception, and psychiatric illness are still being investigated. But the spinolimbic pathway is involved in descending pain inhibition, whose function may be negatively affected by the presence of psychopathology. This, in turn, could lead to heightened pain perception. Coghill and colleagues have shown that differences in pain sensitivity between patients can be correlated with differences in activation patterns in the ACC, the insula, and the DLPFC.[109] The anticipation of pain—a form of anxiety for pain—is also modulated by these areas, suggesting a mechanism by which anxiety about pain can amplify pain perception. Ploghaus and colleagues have demonstrated that anticipation for an acute painful stimulus in healthy volunteers is marked by brain activation patterns throughout the medial pain system.[16]

Sleep Disturbance. Depression produces well-documented disturbances to sleep architecture. Polysomnographic recordings have documented reduced slow wave sleep, early onset of the first period of rapid eye movement (REM) sleep, and increased phasic REM sleep in patients with major depression.[110] Sleep continuity disturbances and increased phasic REM sleep tend to normalize with depression remission, even with psychotherapeutic treatment. However, reduction of REM latency and decreased slow wave sleep tend to persist despite clinical recovery. In sum, there appear to be *state* and *trait* elements to the sleep disturbance associated with depression. Studies have also demonstrated that sleep disturbance may be a result of chronic pain, which in turn can make it worse.[111] Fibromyalgia patients who were sleep deprived reported worsening pain and were found to be hyperalgesic (beyond their baseline pain) on pressure sensitivity testing.[112]

Thus, whether depression or pain precipitated or worsened a sleep disturbance, its presence makes pain worse and is an important link between the two conditions.

Psychological Theories

Psychodynamic Theory. In classic psychoanalytic theory,[113] depression is postulated to be derived from anger unconsciously turned inward, excessive dependence on others for self-esteem, and feelings of helplessness in achieving one's goals. Some have suggested that the depression in some chronic pain patients is a manifestation of a personality style that draws from early developmental conflicts of guilt, anger, and masochism.[114,115] From this perspective, chronic pain may be a symptom of depressive disorder.[116]

Psychoanalytic theory stresses the fundamental parallelism between mental and physical pain and the possible displacement from the former to the latter. Intrapsychic links between pain and depression suggest that pain may function as a *hysterical* or conversion symptom that may prevent the breakthrough of more severe depression. These intrapsychic links largely correspond with the dynamics of *pain proneness* that were originally described by Engel[117] and, in a further elaboration, connected with the concept of *masked depression* by Blumer and Heilbronn.

Blumer and Heilbronn[114] proposed a new psychological disorder, the "pain-prone" disorder, building on Engel's[117] notion of the pain-prone patient. In this view, pain should be considered as a variant of depressive disease. The central explanation is unconscious core conflicts. Core issues include "strong needs to be accepted and to depend on others, as well as marked needs to receive affection and to be cared for."

Pain in the absence of organic pathology is considered by Blumer and Heilbronn[114] to be a *depressive spectrum disorder*. According to this model, pain and depression are viewed as manifestations of a single, common disease process. Specifically, the pain-prone disorder is viewed as a masked "depressive equivalent . . . the prime expression of a muted depressive state." No empiric research has supported the psychoanalytic formulation as presented by Blumer and Heilbronn.[118,119]

Behavioral (Operant Conditioning) Theory. The behavioral model of depression concentrates on the most obvious symptom of depression, the motivational deficit characterized by a reduction in active behavior. A central feature of the behavioral model is response-contingent reinforcement (i.e., the responses from significant others to the individual's behavior). From this perspective, depressive behavior and depression are associated with low rates of positive reinforcement from the environment. Lack of positive reinforcement leads to a decrease in the frequency of the individual engaging in these behaviors and ultimately, they may be extinguished completely. These low rates of reinforcement may occur because (a) positive reinforcers in the environment may become less available, or aversive events in the environment may have become more prevalent; (b) the positive effect of previous reinforcers may have declined, or the negative impact of aversive events may have increased; or (c) the individual may lack the skills either to attain the available positive reinforcers or to cope with aversive aspects of the environment. When individuals experience low rates of positive reinforcement, they reduce the performance of those behaviors, unless they are self-reinforcing. The reduction of behavior decreases further opportunities to receive positive reinforcement.

In the case of chronic pain, the individual may reduce his or her behavior because of physical impairments or because of fear of additional pain or further injury. Thus, by the restriction in behavior and social contacts, chronic pain patients may reduce the opportunity to achieve positive reinforcement and to engage in previously rewarding activities and consequently become depressed. The family can also reinforce maladaptive behavior.

While many families of patients with chronic pain are supportive with the best of intentions, excessive catering to the patient at the expense of maintaining function can perpetuate illness behavior, leading to depression. In other words, patients can occupy the sick role for reasons other than causal disease.

Cognitive Theory. According to Beck,[120] people may be vulnerable to depression because, from an early age, they have possessed negatively biased conceptualizations (schemas) of themselves and their experiences. When they are challenged by stressful life events, these schema become activated, which in turn elicits negative thoughts about themselves, the world, and the future (the *negative cognitive triad*). These patients view themselves as hopeless, hapless, and helpless (i.e., "my life is not going to get better, no one can help me, and I can't help myself"). The latter can also be termed poor self-efficacy, or the belief that one is incapable of doing things to improve their life. Poor pain self-efficacy is the related belief that a patient cannot do anything to improve their pain or function.

In depressed patients, Beck suggests that the cognitive triad serves as a filter for incoming information. This filter creates a negative bias that serves to put a pessimistic light on information and reinforces the depressed state. It also creates low expectations about their ability and thus may lead to lack of effort. Moreover, these people tend to discount their performance, underestimating their accomplishments.

Beck's[120] cognitive theory of depression emphasizes the importance of peoples' appraisal processes. In particular, it is believed that depressed persons show faulty information processing reflected by errors of logic. Through these cognitive errors (collectively referred to as *cognitive distortions*), depressed persons systematically misinterpret or distort the meaning of events so as to consistently construe themselves, their world, and their experiences in a negative way (the negative cognitive triad). According to this perspective, differences in cognitive errors and cognitive distortions, in general, should differentiate depressed and nondepressed patients. One of the most common cognitive distortions is *catastrophizing*, a tendency to view the most negative possible outcome as the only likely outcome. Pain catastrophizing (discussed at length in previous chapters) is the extension of this concept to patients viewing their pain as unbearable, uncontrollable and leading to tissue damage. It has a significant co-occurrence and conceptual overlap with other depression and anxiety symptoms in pain patients. In other words, when pain patients with depression or anxiety catastrophize, they most often catastrophize over their pain.

Cognitive-Behavioral Perspective. The cognitive-behavioral perspective is based on five central assumptions: (a) People are active processors of information and not passive reactors. They attempt to make sense of information and determine what constitutes positive reinforcers. (b) Thoughts (e.g., appraisals, expectancies, beliefs) can elicit and influence mood, affect physiologic processes, have social consequences, and serve as impetuses for behavior; conversely, mood, physiology, environmental factors, and behavior can influence the nature and content of thought processes. (c) Behavior is reciprocally determined by both the individual and environmental factors. (d) People can learn more adaptive ways of thinking, feeling, and behaving. (e) Individuals should be active collaborative agents in changing their maladaptive thoughts, feelings, and behaviors.[121] From the cognitive-behavioral model, the way in which one thinks about pain and behaves in response to pain affects the extent of depression experienced. Like Beck's cognitive theory, its essential difference from the purely behavioral model is its view of patients as active interpreters of their environment.

Depression in chronic pain patients is postulated to result from patients' interpretations of the meaning and effect of their symptoms and their inability to exert any control over their symptoms.

It is only when patients interpret their pain as interfering with important life activities and believe that they (or anyone) can do little to control the symptoms that they become depressed (i.e., they become depressed when they feel helpless and hopeless to exert any control, overwhelmed by the disruption of their lives, and unable to attain significant positive reinforcement from previous activities).[67] Thus, the cognitive-behavioral approach integrates the principles of operant conditioning and behavioral techniques with the emphasis of cognitive theory on the patients' appraisals, beliefs, and attributions.[122]

Diathesis-Stress Model. This is discussed at length in other chapters, but should be restated here because it is the dominant model for understanding the interactions between pain and comorbid psychopathology, including depression.[3,123] This model frames the biological and psychological mechanisms discussed above as diatheses, or vulnerabilities. Under a condition of mental or physical stress, such as pain, the diatheses interact to produce the conditions of chronic pain and depression.[124,125] One can rephrase this notion such that in any given person genetic susceptibilities to chronic pain and/or mental illness interact with the environment (e.g., physical experience of acute pain, reinforcement from the family, inability to work) leading to changes in the functioning of mental processes (mind, such as negative cognitive schema) and brain (such as neurotransmitter systems and endogenous opioid response), resulting in chronic pain and psychiatric comorbidity.[126]

Anthropological Theories

Traditional and industrial societies appear to hold individuals less responsible for somatic symptoms than psychological symptoms. This difference may be especially prominent in modern Western biomedicine, in which symptom complexes are validated or invalidated through their correspondence with objective disease criteria.[127] A somatic "idiom of distress" may become the favored means for communicating distress of any origin that is overwhelming or disabling.[6,128] In other words, complaints about pain may be indicative of depression rather than a pain syndrome of a somatic origin. In many cultures including Western nations, pain is a more acceptable reason for disability than depression. Therefore, cultural incentives exist for translation of depression into pain. Because depressed patients have many physical symptoms, these can become the focus of clinical communication and concern. Giving patients with chronic pain permission to talk of distress in the clinical setting, using nonsomatic terms, can facilitate treatment as long as they do not feel that the somatic elements of their problem are being neglected or discounted.

This is one of the bedrock principles of narrative medicine,[129,130] which through the patient's description of their illness experience helps them to articulate the inter-relationships between their physical symptoms, psychological states, and their roles amongst family, coworkers, and within society. The physical symptoms of chronic pain and the pathophysiology underlying them can be thought of as the *disease* of chronic pain. The constellation of disease, a patient's psychological state, and their experience of suffering can be termed the *illness* of chronic pain.[129] Questions from the practitioner, such as "what have you lost as a result of your pain," "how do you manage with your pain," and "is it a lot of work to stay well despite having pain?" are important to evoking an illness narrative and describing these inter-relationships.[131]

Depression Treatment

Just as in the treatment of major depression in patients without chronic pain, the best quality treatment of depression in pain patients is to combine psychotherapy with medication management.[132,133] One of the most effective psychotherapy modalities in chronic pain patients is cognitive behavioral therapy (CBT), discussed below and in further detail in other chapters.

Pharmacologic Agents

In choosing an antidepressant agent in a patient with chronic pain, an important principle is that the medication should have independent analgesic properties. This means that the medication can be helpful for pain independent of its effect on mood (i.e., it works as an analgesic in those with and without depression). The two main classes with this property are the tricyclic antidepressants (TCAs) and the selective serotonin norepinephrine reuptake inhibitors (SNRIs). In the United States duloxetine and venlafaxine are the SNRIs currently available. The monoamine oxidase inhibitors (MAOIs, such as selegiline or tranylcypromine) are excellent antidepressants which do also have analgesic properties. But they are rarely used anymore except by psychiatrists (due to their side effect profile and medication interactions), and their use is confined to a third or fourth line agent in treatment resistant depression. Antidepressant medication can effectively treat depression in the presence of chronic pain, but there is some evidence that depression with comorbid pain is more resistant to treatment.[134] When depression accompanies chronic pain, as when it accompanies other chronic medical disorders, there may be some extra hurdles for depression treatment to overcome. These include aversive physical symptoms, severe deactivation, vocational dysfunction, marital conflict, social isolation, and concurrent medications. Comprehensive assessment of these issues and formulation of a treatment plan that takes them into account increase the likelihood of successful depression treatment in the chronic pain patient. If depression can be relieved, many other aspects of rehabilitation, such as physical therapy, are often much more easily accomplished. Pain often subsides with improvement in depressive symptoms.[135] Patients will typically report that they may still have pain but that, "it doesn't bother me anymore." This statement is very telling that the affective component of pain has significantly improved.

All currently marketed antidepressants are equally effective for the initial treatment of depression. However, there is some evidence that medications with effects on dual neurotransmitter systems, such as serotonin and norepinephrine (the SNRIs), are associated with a faster rate of improvement and lower rates of depression relapse.[136] Overall, whatever differences may exist among antidepressants in efficacy for neuropathic pain do not appear to affect their ability to treat depression.

The clinical art of depression treatment for those with chronic pain consists of establishing a solid therapeutic alliance around the problem of depression and finding a medication regimen with independent analgesic properties and a side-effect profile that the patient can tolerate. Because patients with chronic pain can be vigilant and catastrophic in thinking about somatic symptoms, care must be taken to educate them about antidepressant side effects. Sometimes it becomes necessary to initiate an antidepressant regimen at the lower doses used for geriatric patients to ease habituation to side effects. Because of their analgesic properties, the SNRIs and TCAs are the treatments of choice for patients with chronic pain and depression.

While the TCAs are considered first-line, their side effect profiles and the slower rate of titration needed to reach a therapeutic dose limit their usefulness compared to SNRIs. However, since the TCAs are used frequently in the management of neuropathic pain, it is very common to encounter a patient on lower doses of TCAs (10–75 mgs). Typically, these patients have acclimated too many of the side effects and gradual escalation of the dose to antidepressant ranges (approximately 100–300 mgs, depending on the compound) can easily be performed in the pain management setting. In monitoring their use for depression, it is important to obtain serum blood levels of TCAs to make sure that they are in the therapeutic range. Disadvantages of TCAs include a wide range of adverse effects, including anticholinergic effects, orthostatic hypotension, effects on the cardiac conduction system, weight gain, sedation, sexual dysfunction, restlessness, "jitteriness," heightened anxiety on initial dosing, and cardiotoxicity in overdose. Before starting a TCA, in those over 45 years or in any patient with a history of cardiac disease, the QTc interval on an EKG should be checked to see if it is <450 ms. Using TCAs in patients with QTc intervals >450 ms places them at a greater risk of developing torsades de pointes arrhythmia, even when lower doses of TCAs are used (10–75 mgs), as is common in pain medicine. Of the TCAs, nortriptyline has the lowest incidence of side effects, and thus is the preferred TCA for use in chronic pain patients, either for treatment of pain or depression. While nortriptyline is more sedating than desipramine, it has a lower incidence of orthostatic hypotension and dizziness. Nortriptyline also has a comparable rate of analgesia to amitriptyline, despite the latter perhaps having broader effects on multiple analgesic mechanisms, such as sodium channel blockade.

The selective serotonin reuptake inhibitors (SSRIs, those available in the United States include citalopram, escitalopram, fluoxetine, fluvoxamine, sertraline, and paroxetine) have become the most popular antidepressants because of their favorable side-effect profiles, but are more useful as second line agents in a pain population because they do not have significant independent analgesic properties. Nefazodone is a useful alternative for patients who have problems with agitation or insomnia on the SSRIs, but care must be taken to monitor liver enzymes. Bupropion has effects on dopamine and norepinephrine reuptake systems (DNRIs). Because of its energizing effects it is very useful in those with chronic pain, since many experience fatigue and poor concentration, either due to the pain itself or as side effects from pain medications. One study has shown that bupropion has analgesic properties in neuropathic pain.[137] More detailed information on prescribing antidepressants is available in one of the standard psychopharmacology manuals.[138–140] In situations of treatment resistant depression, studies have indicated that electroconvulsive therapy can be useful for treatment of depression and pain, across a variety of painful disorders.[141,142] However, no carefully controlled studies demonstrate the effectiveness of electroconvulsive therapy for treatment of chronic pain.

Chronic pain is frequently associated with insomnia and anxiety. It is, therefore, common that patients are treated with benzodiazepines or other sedatives (e.g., the muscle relaxers). Some patients begin taking these medications during the acute phase of the pain problem and then continue to take them for many months or years. Assessing chronic pain patients who take benzodiazepines for depression is important. These medications mask some symptoms of depression (e.g., initial insomnia, agitation), but they are not adequate treatments for depression. Indeed, dangerous levels of depression can develop under the cover of benzodiazepines. It has been suggested that benzodiazepines can induce depression with chronic use, but the evidence for this is not strong.[143] More important is the masking of depression by benzodiazepines.

Few conditions exist for which chronic benzodiazepines are the treatment of choice.[144] The treatment of choice for chronic anxiety disorders, which are almost always accompanied by depressive symptoms, is antidepressant medication.[145] Buspirone (a 5-HT$_{1a}$ partial agonist) is marketed as an anxiolytic, but is more similar to the antidepressants in its pharmacology and side-effect profile. It is a reasonable alternative to the benzodiazepines for the treatment of breakthrough anxiety, particularly for those who experience agitation on the antidepressants.

Psychotherapy

Psychodynamic Psychotherapy

In general, psychodynamic theory emphasizes the long-term predisposition to depression, rather than the losses that occur in the short term. Treatment of depression from the classical psychoanalytic perspective tries to help the patient achieve insights into the repressed conflict and often encourages outward release of hostility turned inward. In the most general terms, the goal of therapy is to uncover latent motivations for the patient's depression. The psychodynamic approach to the depressed individual with chronic pain emphasizes the importance of individual differences in patients based on their developmental history, intrapsychic conflicts, interpersonal difficulties, and the subsequent failure to adapt to chronic illness. Patients' premorbid characteristics are hypothesized to color their adaptation to their current situation and affect their vulnerability to depression.

Psychodynamic therapy emphasizes the need for patients to address unconscious conflicts that may contribute to and maintain the depression and makes use of the therapeutic relationship, assuming that the patient will transfer or project his or her feelings onto the therapist.[146] This approach can be contrasted with treatment based on operant conditioning, in which it is assumed that the basic principles of learning apply to all individuals and the environmental contingencies of reinforcement can influence the reports of pain, distress, and suffering . As a treatment for depression, there is no good standardization of psychodynamic therapy and thus it is difficult to evaluate the studies of its effectiveness.

Behavioral Model

As noted, the behavioral model of depression concentrates on the reduction in active behavior that is a central feature of depression. The focus of treatment for depression is on the shaping of behavior through the use of graded task assignments and response-contingent reinforcement. Depressed individuals are encouraged to engage in more activities and to behave in ways that are likely to be regarded more positively by others. In some instances, it is believed that depressed patients are deficient in certain skills necessary to achieve positive reinforcement. Social skills training may also be included when the therapist determines that the patient is deficient in specific skills (e.g., communication skills). Attention may also be given to assisting the patient in planning pleasant events that the patient will find reinforcing.

Cognitive Model

From the cognitive perspective, therapy is based on the rationale that an individual's affect and behavior are largely determined by the ways in which he or she construes the world and the therapeutic techniques were designed to identify, test, and correct distorted conceptualizations and the dysfunctional beliefs (schemas) underlying these cognitions. Beck's[120] therapy for depression is based on the assumption that the affected people engage in faulty information processing and reasoning and subscribe to a schema that is self-defeating. In particular, depressed people are subject to the negative cognitive triad, in which they have feelings of pessimistic helplessness about themselves, the world, and their future. The aim of the cognitive therapist is to identify and then help patients to correct these distorted ideas and also to improve their information processing and reasoning. In contrast to psychodynamic therapy, the focus is on the here and now. Thus, attention to the origin of dysfunctional schemas in the cognitive model is limited.

The therapeutic procedures are highly structured, time limited, and begin with the recognition of the connections between cognitions and affect, careful recording of these connections, collection of evidence for and against the ideas, followed by substitution of more adaptive and realistic interpretations. The cognitive approach is most frequently combined with behavioral techniques to treat patients with chronic pain, even though some debate exists about the compatibility of these approaches.[120,121]

Cognitive-Behavioral Model

No one cognitive-behavioral model exists, but rather sets of models that share a perspective and incorporate some common features, namely: (a) an interest in the nature and modification of patients' thoughts, feelings, and beliefs, as well as behaviors; and (b) some commitment to behavior therapy procedures in promoting change (e.g., graded practice, use of homework, training in relaxation, coping skills training, problem solving, and relapse prevention).[122]

Depressed people may focus attention selectively on and become preoccupied with somatic symptoms and their potentially ominous significance for their health and future. They may view themselves as helpless and their situation as hopeless and beyond their control. In depressed patients with chronic pain, the cognitive distortions often center around their pain, such as excessive fear of pain or fear of movement. To break this vicious circle, the cognitive-behavioral therapist applies a comprehensive approach to treatment that combines physical, psychological, behavioral, and social interventions. Coping skills training, problem-solving strategies, communications skills training, and directing patients to attend to their appraisals, interpretations, and beliefs surrounding pain are commonly used techniques. One of the most effective CBT methods in pain patients is to combine coping skills training focusing on fear of pain, re-injury, and movement with gradual activity and movement-based physical therapy.[147]

The cognitive-behavioral therapist attempts to assist patients to try new behaviors and to adopt more adaptive modes of thinking. Alterations in behavior become information that the patients are encouraged to use as the basis for changing their views of their situation and themselves from being helpless, hopeless, and out of their control to being resourceful and capable of exerting at least some control over their plights. Changing the cognitive schema by cognitive and behavioral means is designed to result in different interpretations of information about themselves and their futures. Thus, changing behaviors and thoughts may be reciprocally related and mutually reinforcing. Neither attending exclusively to behavior, as in the behavioral model, nor only attending to patients' thinking, as in the cognitive model, is adequate to alleviate depression.[121] The cognitive-behavioral approach has become a central component for treating depression in many multidisciplinary pain rehabilitation and functional restoration programs.

All of the psychological therapies emphasize patients' active role in alleviating depression. In contrast to the psychodynamic model, in which the therapist plays a relatively passive role, in behavioral, cognitive, and cognitive-behavioral therapies, the therapist takes an active, directive role, attempting to guide patients into changing their behavior and reorganizing their thinking and actions. The behavioral, cognitive, and cognitive-behavioral therapies are all centered in the present, compared with psychodynamic therapy, which focuses on the past.

ANXIETY DISORDERS

It is not unusual for patients with symptoms of pain to be anxious and worried. This is especially true when the symptoms are unexplained, as is often the case for chronic pain syndromes. For example, in a large-scale, multicenter study of fibromyalgia patients, between 44% and 51% of patients indicated that they were anxious.[148] In other clinic samples, rates of an anxiety disorder ranged from 16% to 29% among pain patients.[149,150] Most re-

searchers agree that the prevalence of anxiety disorders in patients with chronic pain is underestimated by these data.[1,56]

Anxiety and concern about symptoms are not synonymous with a psychiatric diagnosis of an anxiety disorder, necessarily. When anxiety is debilitating, it may meet criteria for an anxiety disorder. Anxiety disorders are a broad spectrum of disorders which include generalized anxiety disorder, posttraumatic stress disorder, obsessive-compulsive disorder and panic disorder. As noted earlier in this chapter, pain anxiety is the most prevalent and salient form of anxiety in pain patients.[151] Though distinct in some respects, there is significant overlap of pain anxiety symptoms with the constructs of fear of pain, fear of movement, and pain catastrophizing.[152] High levels of pain anxiety (which are impairing, maladaptive, and predictive of higher pain levels[153]) also meet *DSM-IV* criteria for anxiety due to a general medical condition.[154] While this diagnosis was intended originally for anxiety secondary to chronic hypoxemia or steroid use, for example, chronic pain is a medical condition primarily, and falls within the scope of this diagnostic category. Fears, worries, and preoccupations about pain are all secondary to having pain and if the pain resolves, so do these psychological symptoms.

Anxiety disorders frequently accompany other affective disorders, such as major depression, so clinicians should remain alert to the possibility of a mood disorder when patients complain of severe anxiety.[1] In general, the approach is to diagnose and treat initially the most prominent mood disorder in a patient, whether it be depression or anxiety. For instance, in a patient with significant depression and anxiety symptoms, if the depression symptoms seem to be greater or more debilitating than the anxiety symptoms, the diagnosis is major depression with anxious features. In these situations, addressing the depression will also improve the anxiety symptoms. In a major depression with significant overlying anxiety, clinicians will often choose an antidepressant with significant anti-anxiety properties, such as the SNRIs or SSRIs.

Generalized Anxiety Disorder

Table 31.2 outlines the criteria for generalized anxiety disorder (GAD). Generalized anxiety disorder is characterized by excessive nxiety and worry (apprehensive expectation) and difficulty controlling the worry for at least six months, accompanied by at least three of the following symptoms: restlessness or feeling keyed up, being easily fatigued, difficulty concentrating, irritability, muscle tension, or sleep disturbance.[1] There is significant debate whether a six month duration of symptoms is necessary to make the diagnosis, and many psychiatrists contend that this is unnecessarily lengthy.[155] Often there are significant associated depression symptoms, but they do not rise to the level of a major depressive disorder. It is very common for patients with GAD to also have panic attack symptoms or post-traumatic stress symptoms. There are trait and state (situational) components to anxiety disorder presentations in patients with pain. The trait components include excessive worry and concern, often about routine matters. The amount of worry and anxiety is out of proportion to the likelihood of the negative consequences occurring, and the patient has great difficulty controlling worry. In making a diagnosis of GAD, trait anxiety in this context does not imply that the symptoms or the tendency toward these symptoms have been present since the beginning of adulthood.

The situational (state) anxiety is often centered on the pain itself and its negative consequences (pain anxiety). Patients may have conditioned fear, believing that activities will cause uncontrollable pain, causing avoidance of those activities. Pain may also activate thoughts that a person is seriously ill.[42] Questions such as the following can be helpful: "Does the pain make you panic? If you think about your pain, do you feel your heart beat-

TABLE 31.2

DIAGNOSTIC AND STATISTICAL MANUAL, FOURTH EDITION, CRITERIA FOR GENERALIZED ANXIETY DISORDER

A. Excessive anxiety and worry (apprehensive expectation), occurring more days than not for at least 6 months, about a number of events or activities (such as work or school performance).

B. The person finds it difficult to control the worry.

C. The anxiety and worry are associated with three (or more) of the following six symptoms (with at least some symptoms present for more days than not for the past 6 months). Note: Only one item is required in children.
  1. Restlessness or feeling keyed up or on edge
  2. Being easily fatigued
  3. Difficulty concentrating or mind going blank
  4. Irritability
  5. Muscle tension
  6. Sleep disturbance (difficulty falling or staying asleep, or restless unsatisfying sleep)

D. The focus of the anxiety and worry is not confined to features of an Axis I disorder; the anxiety or worry is not about having a panic attack (as in a panic disorder), being embarrassed in public (as in social phobia), being contaminated (as in obsessive-compulsive disorder), being away from home or close relatives (as in separation anxiety disorder), gaining weight (as in anorexia nervosa), having multiple physical complaints (as in somatization disorder), or having a serious illness (as in hypochondriasis), and the anxiety and worry do not occur exclusively during posttraumatic stress disorder.

E. The anxiety, worry, or physical symptoms cause clinically significant distress or impairment in social, occupational, or other important areas of functioning.

F. The disturbance is not due to the direct physiological effects of a substance (e.g., a drug of abuse, a medication) or a general medical condition (e.g., hyperthyroidism) and does not occur exclusively during a mood disorder, a psychotic disorder, or a pervasive developmental disorder.

From *Diagnostic and Statistical Manual*, 4th ed. Washington, DC: American Psychiatric Association, 1994:395, with permission.

TABLE 31.3

DIAGNOSTIC AND STATISTICAL MANUAL, FOURTH EDITION, CRITERIA FOR PANIC ATTACK

A discrete period of intense fear or discomfort, in which four (or more) of the following symptoms developed abruptly and reached a peak within 10 minutes:

  1. Palpitations, pounding heart, or accelerated heart rate
  2. Sweating
  3. Trembling or shaking
  4. Sensations of shortness of breath or smothering
  5. Feeling of choking
  6. Chest pain or discomfort
  7. Nausea or abdominal distress
  8. Feeling dizzy, unsteady, lightheaded, or faint
  9. Depersonalization (feelings of unreality) or depersonalization (being detached from oneself)
  10. Fear of losing control or going crazy
  11. Fear of dying
  12. Paresthesias (numbness or tingling sensations)
  13. Chills or hot flushes
  14. Persistent concern about having additional attacks
  15. Worry about the implications of the attack or its consequences (e.g., losing control, having a heart attack, "going crazy")
  16. A significant change in behavior related to attacks

From *Diagnostic and Statistical Manual*, 4th ed. Washington, DC: American Psychiatric Association, 1994:395, with permission.

Panic Disorder

Panic disorder is a common, disabling psychiatric illness associated with high medical service use and multiple medically unexplained symptoms. The diagnosis of panic disorder requires recurrent, unexpected panic attacks (Table 31.3) followed by at least 1 month of worry about having another panic attack, the implications or consequences of the panic attacks, or behavioral changes related to the attacks. These attacks should not be the direct physiologic consequence of a substance or other medical condition. The panic attacks should not be better accounted for by another mental disorder, such as posttraumatic stress disorder (PTSD; see following discussion) or obsessive-compulsive disorder. At least two unexpected attacks are required for the diagnosis, although most patients have many more.

One of the most common problems with panic disorder is the fear of an undiagnosed, life-threatening illness. Patients with panic disorder can receive extensive medical testing and treatment for their somatic symptoms before the diagnosis of panic disorder is made and appropriate treatment initiated.

Epidemiology

Lifetime prevalence of panic disorder throughout the world is estimated to be 1.5% to 3.5%. One-year prevalence rates are from 1% to 2%. Panic disorder is two to three times more common in women than in men. Age of onset is variable, but most patients typically start between late adolescence and the mid-30s. Of all common mental disorders in the primary care setting, panic disorder is most likely to produce moderate to severe occupational dysfunction and physical disability.[158] It was also associated with the greatest number of disability days in the past month. In some studies, in pain patients it has a prevalence of 5% to 8%, significantly higher than the general population.[1,159]

ing fast? Do you have an overwhelming feeling of dread or doom? Do you experience a sense of sudden anxiety that overwhelms you when you feel more pain?"

The best quality of treatment for GAD is CBT plus medications. The CBT is pain-based as in major depression treatment. Psychotherapy alone is highly effective for anxiety disorders.[156] Successful CBT in patients with obsessive-compulsive disorder has been shown on neuroimaging studies to correlate to changes in the functioning of frontal lobe limbic areas.[157] As discussed, the most frequently chosen medication classes are the SNRIs or SSRIs. Unlike depression treatment and despite their lack of analgesic properties, in anxiety disorders the SSRIs are considered first line because of their efficacy over most other antidepressant classes. The TCAs can be effective, but higher doses are often needed which are difficult for patients to tolerate. Benzodiazepines should almost always be avoided, as discussed previously. Breakthrough anxiety can be addressed with buspirone, hydroxyzine, or low dose antipsychotics (which is beyond the scope of this discussion).

The most common complication of panic disorder is agoraphobia, or fear of public places. Patients with panic disorder learn to fear places where escape might be difficult or help not available in case they have an attack. One-half to two-thirds of patients with panic disorder also suffer from major depression. These patients are the most disabled panic disorder patients. The differential diagnosis of patients presenting with panic symptoms in the medical setting includes thyroid, parathyroid, adrenal, and vestibular dysfunction, seizure disorders, cardiac arrhythmias, and drug intoxication or withdrawal. Patients with panic disorder typically present in the medical setting with cardiologic, gastrointestinal, or neurologic complaints. These include chest pain, abdominal pain, and headaches.[160]

Chest pain is one of the most common complaints presented to primary care physicians, but a specific medical etiology is identified in only 10% to 20% of cases. From 43% to 61% of patients who have normal coronary arteries at angiography and 16% to 25% of patients presenting to emergency rooms with chest pain have panic disorder. A number of these patients eventually receive the diagnoses of vasospastic angina, costochondritis, esophageal dysmotility, or mitral valve prolapse. High rates of psychiatric disorders have been found in some of these groups as well.[161] Many of these patients remain symptomatic and disabled 1 year later despite reassurance concerning coronary artery disease.[162]

Patients with documented coronary disease also have elevated rates of panic disorder. A number of studies have found nearly identical rates of panic disorder in chest pain patients with and without coronary disease. Increased mortality has been noted in those with anxiety and coronary disease. These data point to the importance of remaining alert to both medical and psychiatric diagnoses in those presenting with chest pain. Patients with unexplained chest pain who were given low-dose imipramine (50 mg per day) reported significant reductions in pain regardless of whether they had increased anxiety symptoms or another psychiatric disorder. This has been postulated to be caused by a *visceral analgesic effect* of imipramine.[163] It is possible, however, that imipramine was treating subthreshold anxiety and depressive symptoms, because 63% of the sample had a history of these disorders at some point in their lives.

Approximately 11% of primary care patients present the problem of abdominal pain to their physician each year. Less than one-quarter of these complaints are associated with a definite physical diagnosis in the following year. Among the most common reasons for abdominal pain is irritable bowel syndrome. It is estimated that irritable bowel syndrome accounts for 20% to 52% of all referrals to gastroenterologists. Various studies have found that 54% to 74% of these patients with irritable bowel syndrome have associated psychiatric disorders. Walker and colleagues determined that patients with irritable bowel syndrome have much higher current (28% versus 3%) and lifetime (41% versus 25%) rates of panic disorder than a comparison group with inflammatory bowel disease.[164] This suggests that the psychiatric disorder was not simply a reaction to the abdominal distress.

Among 10,000 persons assessed in a community survey who consulted their physicians for headache, 15% of female and 13% of male subjects had a history of panic disorder. Further studies have suggested that migraine headache is most strongly associated with panic attacks.[165] Often, anxiety symptoms precede the onset of the headaches, whereas depressive symptoms often have their onset after the headaches. Some authors have suggested that a common predisposition exists with headaches (especially migraines and chronic daily headache), anxiety disorders, and major depression.

Treatment

Psychopharmacologic and psychotherapeutic treatments for panic disorder have been proven effective. The American Psychiatric Association has released a *Practice Guideline for the Treatment of Patients with Panic Disorder*.[166] Panic-focused cognitive-behavioral therapy and four classes of medications (SSRIs, tricyclic antidepressants, monoamine oxidase inhibitors, and benzodiazepines) have demonstrated effectiveness. These drugs may be used in combination with cognitive-behavioral therapy. Panic-specific cognitive-behavioral therapy includes psychoeducation, continuous panic monitoring, development of anxiety management skills, cognitive restructuring, and *in vivo* exposure. As discussed previously with depression, the SSRIs likely are the easiest antidepressants to use for panic disorder. However, starting doses should be halved to avoid any initial exacerbation of agitation or anxiety. Tricyclic antidepressants and monoamine oxidase inhibitors are now reserved for those patients who do not respond to the SSRIs. Benzodiazepines should only be used for early symptom control in conjunction with one of the other classes of effective medication.

POSTTRAUMATIC STRESS DISORDER

Diagnosis

At the time of initial physical trauma, patients who develop chronic pain may also experience overwhelming psychological trauma. George Crile, a surgeon and experimental physiologist, laid the foundation for our modern concept of psychological trauma. He suggested that fear is the memory of pain. This fear holds an adaptive advantage in directing individuals to anticipate and avoid injury. Freud added anxiety to our modern conceptualization. Anxiety is the capacity to imagine pain and not merely to remember it. In other words, anxiety is memory of pain set loose.[167]

After direct personal exposure to an extreme traumatic event, some individuals develop a syndrome that includes reexperiencing the event, avoidance of stimuli associated with the event, and persistent heightened arousal. PTSD was originally described after exposure to military combat, but is now recognized to occur after sexual or physical assault, natural disasters, accidents, life-threatening illnesses, and other events that induce feelings of intense fear, hopelessness, or horror. Persons may develop the disorder after experiencing or just witnessing these events. *DSM-IV* diagnostic criteria are shown in Table 31.4.

Epidemiology of PTSD in Chronic Pain Patients

Approximately 13% of all veterans returning from service in Iraq and Afghanistan receive diagnoses of PTSD. These constitute about half of all mental health diagnoses received.[168] Up to 80% of Vietnam veterans with PTSD report chronic pain in limbs, back, torso, or head.[169] Increased physical symptoms, including muscle aches and back pain, are also more common in Gulf War veterans with PTSD than in those without PTSD.[170] The prevalence of PTSD in medical populations has been shown to be quite high. For example, a number of patients presenting at medical clinics with myocardial infarctions[171] and cancer[172,173] often meet the criteria for PTSD. Averaging the prevalence rates of PTSD across a number of studies reveals that after motor vehicle accidents sufficient to require medical attention, 29.5% of patients meet the criteria for PTSD.[174] For more than one-half of these patients, the symptoms resolve within 6 months. In one study, 15% of idiopathic facial pain patients seeking treatment were found to have PTSD.[175] In another study, 21% of fibromyalgia patients were found to have PTSD.[176] Case reports have associated reflex sympathetic dystrophy (complex regional pain

TABLE 31.4

DIAGNOSTIC AND STATISTICAL MANUAL, **FOURTH EDITION, DIAGNOSTIC CRITERIA FOR POSTTRAUMATIC STRESS DISORDER**

A. The person has been exposed to a traumatic event in which both of the following were present:
  1. The person experienced, witnessed, or was confronted with an event or events that involved actual or threatened death or serious injury, or a threat to the physical integrity of self or others.
  2. The person's response involved intense fear, helplessness, or horror. Note: In children, this may be expressed instead by disorganized or agitated behavior.

B. The traumatic event is persistently reexperienced in one (or more) of the following ways:
  1. Recurrent and intrusive distressing recollections of the event, including images, thoughts, or perceptions. Note: In young children, repetitive play may occur in which themes or aspects of the trauma are expressed.
  2. Recurrent distressing dreams of the event. Note: In children, there may be frightening dreams without recognizable content.
  3. Acting or feeling as if the traumatic event were recurring (includes a sense of reliving the experience, illusions, hallucinations, and dissociative flashback episodes, including those that occur on awakening or when intoxicated). Note: In young children, trauma-specific reenactment may occur.
  4. Intense psychological distress at exposure to internal or external cues that symbolize or resemble an aspect of the traumatic event.
  5. Physiologic reactivity on exposure to internal or external cues that symbolize or resemble an aspect of the traumatic event.

C. Persistent avoidance of stimuli associated with the trauma and numbing of general responsiveness (not present before the trauma), as indicated by three (or more) of the following:
  1. Efforts to avoid thoughts, feelings, or conversations associated with the trauma.
  2. Efforts to avoid activities, places, or people that arouse recollections of the trauma.
  3. Inability to recall an important aspect of the trauma.
  4. Markedly diminished interest or participation in significant activities.
  5. Feeling of detachment or estrangement from others.
  6. Restricted range of affect (e.g., unable to have loving feelings).
  7. Sense of foreshortened future (e.g., does not expect to have a career, marriage, children, or normal life span).

D. Persistent symptoms of increased arousal (not present before the trauma), as indicated by two (or more) of the following:
  1. Difficulty falling or staying asleep.
  2. Irritability or outbursts of anger.
  3. Difficulty concentrating.
  4. Hypervigilance.
  5. Exaggerated startle response.

E. Duration of the disturbance (symptoms in criteria B, C, and D) is more than 1 month.

F. The disturbance causes clinically significant distress or impairment in social, occupational, or other important areas of functioning.

From *Diagnostic and Statistical Manual,* 4th ed. Washington, DC: American Psychiatric Association, 1994:427–429, with permission.

syndrome) with PTSD. Other studies suggest that 50% to 100% of patients presenting at pain treatment centers meet the diagnostic criteria for PTSD.[176,177] Among adult urban primary care patients, 23% had PTSD, of whom 11% had it noted in the medical record. The prevalence of PTSD, adjusted for demographic factors, was higher in participants with chronic pain, major depression, and anxiety disorders.[178]

Pain patients with PTSD have been shown to have more pain and affective distress than those without PTSD,[179] so it is not surprising that PTSD rates among pain patients increase as treatment settings become more specialized.

PTSD and Associations with Pain

The relationship between pain and PTSD is multifaceted, as suggested by the early thinking by Crile and Freud discussed previously. Pain and PTSD may result from a traumatic event. Sometimes acute pain can constitute the traumatic event, as described in a case of traumatic eye enucleation.[180] In a nationwide survey of patients admitted after trauma, 23% of injury survivors had symptoms consistent with a diagnosis of PTSD 12 months after their hospitalization.[181] Greater levels of early post-injury emotional distress and physical pain were associated with an increased risk of symptoms consistent with a PTSD diagnosis. Pain may also be a consequence of PTSD or a manifestation of it. In a sample of patients admitted to an orthopedic hospital, back pain after major trauma was not associated with measures of injury severity or demographic factors, but was significantly associated with the presence of posttraumatic stress disorder, the use of a lawyer, the presence of chronic illnesses, and lower education levels.[182] Functional brain imaging studies suggest altered processing of noxious signaling in the brain of patients with PTSD. In one study, patients with PTSD revealed increased activation in the left hippocampus and decreased activation in the bilateral ventrolateral prefrontal cortex and the right amygdala.[183] Much research remains to be done on the relative contributions of physical trauma and psychological trauma to chronic pain problems.

Treatment

It is best to institute treatment for PTSD as close in time to the trauma as possible. Acute crisis intervention may reduce the development of chronic PTSD and other complications, including, possibly, chronic pain. This treatment should establish support, promote acceptance of what happened, provide education and information about symptoms, and attend to general health needs. Beyond the acute phase, the cognitive-behavioral therapy treatment described for panic disorder earlier has been shown to be effective with PTSD as well. Stress-inoculation training, implosive therapy, and systematic desensitization have also been reported to have some efficacy.[175,184] Medications are rarely adequate as the sole treatment for PTSD. Controlled trials of tricyclic antidepressants, SSRIs, and monoamine oxidase inhibitors have demonstrated some benefit by 8 weeks at reducing core intrusive features. These benefits appear to be in addition to the antidepressant and antianxiety effects of these medications.[185] Recent PTSD treatment trials have demonstrated effectiveness of venlafaxine ER[186] and prazosin[187] but these trials have not specifically monitored the effects on pain.

PERSONALITY DISORDERS

Epidemiology

Several studies have reviewed the personality characteristics and disorders of patients with chronic pain.[149,150,188–190] The prevalence of personality disorders among clinic populations ranges from 31% to 81% and is greater than in the general population or in populations with either medical or psychiatric illnesses. The Minnesota Multiphasic Personality Inventory (MMPI) is the most widely used personality assessment tool of patients with chronic pain but is probably not purely a personality trait measure.[191–193] Previous studies have identified profiles defined by Minnesota Multiphasic Personality Inventory (MMPI) scale elevations that are proposed to be characteristic of chronic somatic symptoms such as pain.[194] The hypochondriacal reaction, conversion 'V' and neurotic triad profiles exhibit different multivariate relationships between other constructs such as somatization, coping strategies, depression, pain severity, and activity level.[195] However, while patients with chronic pain differ from nonchronic pain controls in their scale profiles on the MMPI, there is no single personality trait or disorder associated with medically unexplained chronic pain or chronic pain from "organic" diseases.

Overview of Personality Disorders

Personality pathology is best thought of along a continuum of traits present to greater or lesser degrees. Personality disorders described in the *DSM* represent the pathological extreme of personality traits. Patients with personality disorders are one type of "difficult patient" characterized by an inflexible, pervasive, and maladaptive inner experience and set of behaviors.[18,131] Traits have been conceptualized as dimensional aspects of individual variation while personality disorders are represented as categorical aberrations within the realm of psychopathology. This section will present an overview of personality pathology and not a discussion of the criteria for each specific personality disorder.

Analytic approaches undertaken to understand the features of temperament have described several core factors. The five-factor model is one of the most popular and characterized by the trait dimensions of neuroticism, extraversion, openness, agreeableness, and conscientiousness as described by the revised NEO Personality Inventory.[196–198] In contrast, the Temperament and Character Inventory (TCI) is comprised of four heritable and stable dimensions of temperament (Harm Avoidance, Novelty Seeking, Reward Dependence, Persistence) that represent individual differences in associative learning and three dimensions of character (Self-Directedness, Cooperativeness, Self-Transcendence) that develop over time as a function of social learning and maturation of interpersonal behavior.[199] This psychobiologic model defines personality as the interaction of temperament and character. Studies have described three dimensions (HA, SD, C) as a core feature of all personality disorders.[200] However, this profile has also been associated with other constructs such as depressive and anxiety disorders.[201,202]

Only a portion of the variance in the factors or dimensions characterizing personality disorders is explained by core personality traits.[203] Personality traits are generally considered to be enduring features of an individual. The stability of personality after age 30 has been consistently documented with long term follow-up studies.[204] Longitudinal studies also demonstrate that dimensional models of personality disorders may represent a manifestation of personality traits interacting with life events or illness consistent with the diathesis-stress model.[205,206] Caution should be exercised in making the diagnosis of a personality disorder in the presence of any illness. Personality traits should be appreciated as sustaining or modifying factors that have the potential to complicate the treatment process rather than as causes of or the sole explanation for illnesses such as chronic pain.[188] Personality vulnerabilities contribute to the degree of potential disability that individuals experience by modifying their response to pain. While these patients are more likely to be "difficult"

because of their complexity, their prognosis should not be viewed as hopeless or unresponsive to treatment.

The diathesis-stress model may partly explain the high rates of personality pathology but also, the decreases in these rates that have been observed with chronic pain treatment.[189,190] A comprehensive review of the effect of pain on the measurement of personality characteristics found substantial evidence that trait inventories are not pain state independent.[207] Pain treatment resulted in improvement in trait scores across the majority of studies that utilized the MMPI and measures of trait anxiety, coping/self-efficacy, and somatization/illness behavior. In a significant number of the studies reviewed, the trait changes could be attributed to improvements in pain. This state-trait interaction contradicts the notion that personality inventories catalog only enduring aspects of the individual. Instead, there is increasing evidence that a state disorder (psychiatric, medical, stress-related, pain) may distort the measurement of traits and that treatment of that condition will decrease the presumed trait disorder.[208–211] Just as personality pathology may improve with adequate pain treatment, personality disorders may emerge in the context of chronic pain, even if prior to pain there was no evidence of maladaptive personality traits. The explanation for this change may include several mechanisms or confounders including that trait measurements are being contaminated by state-specific questions, pain treatments (medications, cognitive-behavioral therapy) directly alter traits, pain treatments improve state disorders which were previously affecting trait measurement, test-retest related problems, and that standardized tests are actually measuring both states and traits.

Personality and Pain Treatment Outcome

Current research has focused on how personality relates to treatment outcome, the transition from acute to chronic pain, and the persistence of pain-related disability. However, results have been inconsistent and more likely to detect emotional distress and psychopathology. Recently, a Disability Profile based on elevations of 4 or more clinical scales of the MMPI-II has been proposed as more common than those described above.[1] In a prospective investigation of almost 1500 patients with chronic occupational spinal disorders, this Disability Profile was associated with 5 times the likelihood of having a personality disorder and 14 times the likelihood of having an Axis I disorder. While associated with high levels of psychopathology, patients with the Disability Profile compared to those with neurotic triad, conversion V, and normal profiles showed no significant differences in response to treatment with an interdisciplinary rehabilitation program. In a 30-year longitudinal study of healthy college students, elevations on MMPI scales 1 and 3 were associated with increased reports of chronic pain conditions at mid-life.[212] However, the magnitude of this association was small and the clinical significance was unclear.

In a similar study, patients with chronic pain due to nonspecific musculoskeletal disorders exhibited higher levels of harm avoidance (HA) and lower levels of self-directedness (SD) on the TCI.[213] This trait profile would characterize patients as cautious, insecure, pessimistic, lacking self-esteem and long term goals, failing to accept responsibility, and struggling with their identity. Another study of patients with chronic pain of all types identified the same profile plus low levels of cooperativeness (C).[150] Low levels of self-directedness have been associated with learned helplessness, poor self-efficacy, and an external locus of control. High levels of harm avoidance overlap with the construct of fear-avoidance behavior, fearful cluster C personality disorders, and the development of pain-related disability. The fear-avoidance model and expectancy model of fear provide explanations for the initiation and maintenance of chronic pain disability, proposing that anxiety sensitivity amplifies reactions such as avoidance of specific activities.[214–217] Anxiety sensitivity is a significant predictor of fear of, and anxiety about, pain.[218] Fear of pain, movement, reinjury, and other negative consequences that result in the avoidance of activities promote the transition to and sustaining of chronic pain and its associated disabilities such as muscular reactivity, deconditioning, and guarded movement.[219]

Fear-avoidance beliefs have been found to be one of the most significant predictors of failure to return to work in patients with chronic low back pain.[220] Operant conditioning reinforces disability if the avoidance provides any short-term benefits such as reducing anticipatory anxiety or relieving the patient of unwanted responsibilities. In a study of patients with chronic low back pain, improvements in disability following physical therapy were associated with decreases in pain, psychological distress, and fear-avoidance beliefs but not specific physical deficits.[221,222] Decreasing work-specific fears was a more important outcome than addressing general fears of physical activity in predicting improved physical capability for work among patients participating in an interdisciplinary treatment program.[223] These studies suggest that certain personality traits or profiles should alert the clinician to the presence of psychological problems and psychiatric disorders that would benefit from more specific treatments as opposed to defining a group of patients with chronic pain who should be condemned to no treatment because of an expected poor outcome.

SOMATOFORM DISORDERS, ILLNESS BEHAVIOR, AND SICK ROLE

Definitions

Sickness is a complicated psychological and social state that has been understood from a variety of perspectives over the years. We consider those of sick role, illness behavior, and somatoform disorder.

The concept of the *sick role* was first introduced by Talcott Parsons in 1951[224] and was formulated more concretely 12 years later.[225] The sick role is granted to an individual provided that he or she regards his or her condition as undesirable, and is not held responsible for it (i.e., under his or her control and able to be reversed voluntarily). If granted, the individual is allowed exemption from his or her usual obligations to a greater or lesser extent and is considered to be deserving of care and attention. Associated with the sick role are the obligations of seeking the advice and assistance of a person regarded as competent to diagnose and treat the condition and of cooperating with that person.

The basic concept of *illness behavior* was introduced by Mechanic and Volkart[226] and later fully formulated by Mechanic.[227] Mechanic's concept of illness behavior complements the sick role, because it delineates the contribution of the patient to the role-granting process. Illness behavior was originally defined as the ways in which individuals differentially perceive, evaluate, and respond to their symptoms. This concept proved to be an extremely useful one, because it has facilitated the empiric study of behaviors that are of considerable importance to clinicians and other health care providers, as well as to the individual's family and society.

Although useful as it stands, health care providers find Mechanic's definition restrictive because it refers to *symptoms* as the focus of behavior, and consequently deemphasizes actions directed toward avoidance of the illness. A slightly modified definition describes illness behavior as "the ways in which individuals experience, perceive, evaluate, and respond to their own health status." This definition recognizes the possibility that a person may be concerned about illness in the absence of symptoms.

Illness behavior is a concept more easily applied to individual patients than sick role and has therefore seen more use in clinical settings. However, it is dependent on social definitions of what constitutes legitimate illness. Although medical science determines what qualifies as *disease* based on objective changes in anatomy and physiology, society determines what qualifies as illness. These often follow each other quite closely, but there can be interesting discrepancies. Essential hypertension is a disease usually without symptoms. It has taken a concerted educational effort on the part of the medical profession to convince the public that it is an illness that should be monitored and treated. Chronic fatigue syndrome and fibromyalgia are illnesses increasingly recognized and accepted by the public. Because the medical profession has not been able to identify objective changes in physiology with these illnesses, many physicians question whether they qualify as legitimate diseases. Physicians, insurance companies, and compensation systems can find themselves in disagreement with patients experiencing chronic pain about whether a legitimate disease or illness is causing the pain.

Pilowsky introduced the concept of *abnormal illness behavior* for those situations in which physician and patient disagree about the applicability of the sick role to the patient's condition.[228] He contends that patients with truly abnormal illness behavior have extreme difficulty accepting the advice of any physician if it does not agree with their own appraisal of their health status. He cautions that misdiagnoses of abnormal illness behavior can occur when physician and patient do not share a common culture. We might add that it is also important to keep in mind the limitations of current diagnostic tests and disease criteria when diagnosing the patient's disagreement with his or her physician as pathologic.

Overview of Somatoform Disorders

Current psychiatric thinking frames the diagnoses of abnormal illness behavior or misuse of the sick role as somatoform disorders. The essential feature of the somatoform disorders is the presence of physical symptoms that suggest a general medical condition but are not fully explained by a general medical condition. These symptoms must cause impairment in social and occupational functioning. The somatoform disorders are distinguished from factitious disorders and malingering in that the symptoms are not intentionally or voluntarily produced in the somatoform disorders. Malingering is the deliberate feigning of symptoms for a clear gain, often financial. In factitious disorder, while there is a feigning of symptoms, the patient is only partially aware that they are doing so and their gain or benefit is much less clear. In factitious disorder, the maintenance of symptoms is for the psychological benefits of the sick role, similar to the gain in somatoform disorders.

In the majority of patients with pain and somatoform illness there is a physical basis (including functional or structural pathology, such as neuropathic pain) for at least a portion of the pain complaints, in which symptom-reporting is magnified by somatizing. Somatization is best thought of as a process (versus somatization disorder, discussed below). The spectrum of somatization includes amplification of symptoms, which entails "focusing upon the symptoms, racking with intense alarm and worry, extreme disability, and a reluctance to relinquish them."[229] Pain-related psychological symptoms amplify pain perception and disability. Hence, there is a tremendous overlap between the somatoform component of a chronic pain syndrome and other psychiatric comorbidities. In other words, in a patient with pain and any psychiatric comorbidity, somatization is a ubiquitous, mediating process by which pain and disability are worsened. It has psychological and physiological bases, which are still being elucidated. Similarly, pain complaints may become an "idiom of distress"[128] in which psychological distress or needs are communicated through the proxy of pain reporting. Four somatoform disorders may involve pain: somatization disorder, conversion disorder, hypochondriasis, and pain disorder (with or without a physical basis for pain). Somatoform disorders without any physical basis for pain are estimated to occur in 5% to 15% of patients with chronic pain who receive pain treatment.[230]

Somatization Disorder

Somatization disorder is a chronic condition characterized by a pattern of multiple and recurrent somatic complaints resulting in medical treatment and impairment in role functioning, but not explained by a general medical condition. For this particular somatoform diagnosis, the somatic symptoms must be persistent and pervasive. These complaints must begin before 30 years of age and last for a period of years. Diagnostic criteria are displayed in Table 31.5.

TABLE 31.5

DIAGNOSTIC AND STATISTICAL MANUAL, FOURTH EDITION, DIAGNOSTIC CRITERIA FOR SOMATIZATION DISORDER

A. A history of many physical complaints beginning before age 30 years that occur over a period of several years and result in treatment being sought or significant impairment in social, occupational, or other important areas of functioning.

B. Each of the following criteria must have been met, with individual symptoms occurring at any time during the course of the disturbance:
  1. Four pain symptoms: a history of pain related to at least four different sites or functions (e.g., head, abdomen, back, joints, extremities, chest, rectum, during menstruation, during sexual intercourse, or during urination).
  2. Two gastrointestinal symptoms: a history of at least two gastrointestinal symptoms other than pain (e.g., nausea, bloating, vomiting other than during pregnancy, diarrhea, or intolerance of several different foods).
  3. One sexual symptom: a history of at least one sexual or reproductive symptom other than pain (e.g., sexual indifference, erectile or ejaculatory dysfunction, irregular menses, excessive menstrual bleeding, vomiting throughout pregnancy).
  4. One pseudoneurological symptom: a history of at least one symptom or deficit suggesting a neurologic condition not limited to pain (conversion symptoms such as impaired coordination or balance, paralysis or localized weakness, difficulty swallowing or lump in throat, aphonia, urinary retention, hallucinations, loss of touch or pain sensation, double vision, blindness, deafness, seizures; dissociative symptoms such as amnesia; or loss of consciousness other than fainting).

C. Either 1 or 2:
  1. After appropriate investigation, each of the symptoms in criterion B cannot be fully explained by a known general medical condition or the direct effects of a substance (e.g., a drug of abuse or medication).
  2. When there is a related general medical condition, the physical complaints or resulting social or occupational impairment are in excess of what would be expected from the history, physical examination, or laboratory findings.

D. The symptoms are not intentionally produced or feigned (as in factitious disorder or malingering).

From *Diagnostic and Statistical Manual*, 4th ed. Washington, DC: American Psychiatric Association, 1994:449–450, with permission.

Many of the somatoform diagnoses, including somatization disorder, have their historic roots in the diagnosis of hysteria.[231] The Egyptians first ascribed multiple unexplained somatic symptoms to the displacement of other organs by a wandering uterus. In the seventeenth century, Thomas Sydenham dissociated hysteria from the uterus and associated it with psychological disturbances. In 1859, Briquet described the multisymptomatic and protracted course of the illness in 430 Parisian patients. This description was taken up in the 1950s by investigators at Washington University in St. Louis.[231] They described *Briquet's syndrome* as a multisymptomatic form of hysteria with 25 symptoms from 10 different symptom groups. By the publication in 1980 of *DSM-III*, the diagnosis had been streamlined to require 14 of 37 potential symptoms, and the name had been changed to *somatization disorder*. Through these changes, the essential feature of somatization disorder has remained multiple unexplained somatic symptoms producing disability and health care use. Somatization disorder must be distinguished from medical disorders producing multiple and scattered symptoms, such as multiple sclerosis or systemic lupus erythematosus. It must also be distinguished from panic disorder that also produces multiple somatic symptoms but is a more acute and treatable psychiatric disorder.

Epidemiology. The prevalence of somatization disorder in the community has been reported to be between 0.13% and 0.4%, with the vast majority of cases occurring in women.[232] Prevalence estimates in the primary care setting have ranged from 0.2% to 5.0%. Studies of patients referred to pain clinics have produced estimates from 8% to 12%. Although prevalence rates clearly increase when moving from community to primary care to tertiary care settings, somatization disorder patients remain in the clear minority in all settings. Unexplained somatic symptoms are a common problem in medical settings that extend far beyond the bounds of somatization disorder. Various attempts have been made to assess the prevalence of an abridged version of somatization disorder in primary care, requiring four to six unexplained symptoms (4.4% of patients) or three symptoms persistent over a 2-year period (8.2% of patients).[233] Even these abridged forms of somatization disorder are associated with increased rates of disability, health care use, and mood and anxiety disorders. Although the initial emphasis with Briquet's syndrome and somatization disorder was on a discrete, familial, even genetic, disorder, evidence suggests that somatization is a process that exists along a spectrum of severity.[234] A large international study confirms that medically unexplained somatic symptoms are common, whereas full somatization disorder is quite rare.[235] A great deal of confusion exists between somatization as a process and somatization as a disorder. Somatization as a process, meaning the somatic experience of distress, is ubiquitous.[236] It accounts for the majority of symptoms presented to primary care physicians. It is most frequently associated with transient stressors (therefore time limited) or acute psychiatric disorders (which are treatable). Somatization disorder is a rare, chronic, and treatment-resistant condition that characterizes the most severely and chronically distressed individuals. When clinicians use the term *somatizer* to refer to a patient with unexplained symptoms, it is unclear whether they are implying the process or the disorder.

Although somatization disorder frequently occurs within families and has a genetic component, it also appears to have a strong association with childhood physical and sexual abuse.[237] A significant percentage of patients who meet criteria for somatization disorder also meet criteria for borderline personality disorder.[238] This has led some investigators to question the independence of these diagnoses and others to stress their common origin in severe childhood abuse. Borderline personality disorder is a severe, chronic pattern of chaotic and dysfunctional interpersonal relationships. Diagnostic criteria are presented in Table 31.6.

In a study of 200 patients with back pain attending a pain clinic, 51% of patients had some personality disorder and 15%

TABLE 31.6

DIAGNOSTIC AND STATISTICAL MANUAL, FOURTH EDITION, DIAGNOSTIC CRITERIA FOR BORDERLINE PERSONALITY DISORDER

A pervasive pattern of instability of interpersonal relationships, self-image, and affects and marked impulsivity beginning by early adulthood and present in a variety of contexts, as indicated by five (or more) of the following:

1. Frantic efforts to avoid real or imagined abandonment. Note: Do not include suicidal or self-mutilating behavior covered in criterion 5.
2. A pattern of unstable and intense interpersonal relationships characterized by alternating between extremes of idealization and devaluation.
3. Identity disturbance: markedly and persistently unstable self-image or sense of self.
4. Impulsivity in at least two areas that are potentially self-damaging (e.g., spending, sex, substance abuse, reckless driving, binge eating). Note: Do not include suicidal or self-mutilating behavior covered in criterion 5.
5. Recurrent suicidal behavior, gestures, or threats, or self-mutilating behavior.
6. Affective instability caused by a marked reactivity of mood (e.g., intense episodic dysphoria, irritability, or anxiety usually lasting a few hours and only rarely more than a few days).
7. Chronic feelings of emptiness.
8. Inappropriate, intense anger or difficulty controlling anger (e.g., frequent displays of temper, constant anger, recurrent physical fights).
9. Transient, stress-related paranoid ideation or severe dissociative symptoms.

From *Diagnostic and Statistical Manual,* 4th ed. Washington, DC: American Psychiatric Association, 1994:654, with permission.

had borderline personality disorder determined by structured psychiatric interview.[239] This is a strikingly high prevalence of these disorders compared with other clinical populations. As discussed above, some controversy exists about the validity of these diagnoses, especially as to whether they constitute a cause or effect of the chronic pain problem.[240]

Treatment. Recognizing patients with somatization disorder is important, because they are among the most difficult patients to treat in the entire health care system. Above all, it is important to prevent iatrogenic damage to these patients through overly focused and invasive attempts to treat pain complaints. These patients are typically resistant to standard cognitive-behavioral treatment strategies used in chronic pain. They have extreme problems with trust and do not form therapeutic relationships easily. Any attempt to reframe somatic distress in emotional terms is likely to be experienced as an invalidation until a therapeutic alliance is well established. An adaptation of cognitive-behavioral therapy called *dialectical-behavioral therapy* has been shown effective for patients with borderline personality disorder, but has not been tested in patients with somatization disorder.[241]

Psychotropic medications have highly unpredictable effects in this group.[242] Any medications associated with tolerance and dependence, such as opioids and benzodiazepines, should be avoided, because they are often associated with clinical deterioration. Antidepressant medications also have unpredictable effects and should be prescribed only in collaboration with a psychiatrist. For patients with soft psychotic symptoms, such as depersonalization and derealization, low-dose antipsychotic medication may be of some benefit.

PAIN DISORDER

Diagnosis

In many prevalent pain syndromes (e.g., low back pain, headache, fibromyalgia), it is difficult to identify the tissue pathology giving rise to symptoms. When a somatic cause for pain cannot be identified, many clinicians begin to seek psychological causes. The identification of psychogenic pain is a difficult and perhaps impossible task. *Pain disorder* is the current psychiatric diagnosis that most closely corresponds to the diagnosis of psychogenic pain.

Because pain disorder is an important but problematic concept at the interface of pain medicine and psychiatry, it is important to understand some of the history of the concept. In *DSM-II* (published in 1968), no specific diagnoses existed that pertained to pain. Painful conditions caused by emotional factors were considered part of the psychophysiologic disorders. In 1980, *DSM-III* introduced a new diagnostic category for pain problems, *psychogenic pain disorder.*[243] To qualify, a patient needed to have severe and prolonged pain inconsistent with neuroanatomic distribution of nociceptors or without detectable organic etiology or pathophysiologic mechanism. Related organic pathology was allowed, but the pain had to be "grossly in excess" of what was expected on the basis of physical examination. Accepted evidence that psychological factors were involved in the production of the pain were (a) a temporal relationship between pain onset and an environmental event producing psychological conflict, (b) pain appearing to allow avoidance of some noxious event or responsibility, and (c) pain promoting emotional support or attention the individual would not have otherwise received. It is important to note that this kind of evidence never proves that psychological factors have caused a pain complaint.

Difficulties in establishing that pain was psychogenic led to changes in the diagnosis for *DSM-III-R,* which was published in 1987.[244] In *DSM-III-R,* the diagnosis was renamed *somatoform pain disorder,* and three major changes were made in the diagnostic criteria. The requirements for etiologic psychological factors and lack of other contributing mental disorders were eliminated, and a requirement for "preoccupation with pain for at least six months" was added. The diagnostic criteria were thus reduced to the following:

1. Preoccupation with pain for at least 6 months
2. Either a or b:
   a. Appropriate evaluation uncovers no organic pathology or pathophysiologic mechanism to account for the pain.
   b. When there is related organic pathology, the complaint of pain or resulting social or occupational impairment is grossly in excess of what would be expected from the findings.[245]

In *DSM-III-R,* therefore, somatoform pain disorder becomes purely a diagnosis of exclusion. The diagnosis is made when medical disorders are excluded in a patient *preoccupied* with pain.

The *DSM-IV* subcommittee on pain disorders found that, despite these changes, *somatoform pain disorder* was rarely used in research projects or clinical practice. They identified a number of reasons for this: (a) the meaning of "preoccupation with pain" is unclear, (b) whether pain exceeds that expected is difficult to determine, (c) the diagnosis does not apply to many patients disabled by pain in which a medical condition is contributory, (d) the term *somatoform pain disorder* implies that this pain is somehow different from organic pain, and (e) acute pain of less than 6 months' duration was excluded.[246] They therefore proposed the *DSM-IV* category of pain disorder described in Table 31.7.

The *DSM-IV* subcommittee has tried to devise a broader diagnostic grouping encompassing both acute and chronic pain prob-

TABLE 31.7

DIAGNOSTIC AND STATISTICAL MANUAL, FOURTH EDITION, DIAGNOSTIC CRITERIA FOR PAIN DISORDER

A. Pain in one or more anatomic sites is the predominant focus of the clinical presentation and is of sufficient severity to warrant clinical attention.

B. The pain causes clinically significant distress or impairment in social, occupational, or other important areas of functioning.

C. Psychological factors are judged to have an important role in the onset, severity, exacerbation, or maintenance of the pain.

D. The symptom of deficit is not intentionally produced or feigned (as in factitious disorder or malingering).

E. The pain is not better accounted for by a mood, anxiety, or psychotic disorder and does not meet criteria for dyspareunia.

Code as follows:

307.80, Pain disorder associated with psychological factors: Psychological factors are judged to have the major role in the onset, severity, exacerbation, or maintenance of the pain. (If a general medical condition is present, it does not have a major role in the onset, severity, exacerbation, or maintenance of the pain.) This type of pain disorder is not diagnosed if criteria are also met for somatization disorder.

Specify if:

Acute: duration of less than 6 months

Chronic: duration of 6 months or longer

307.89, Pain disorder associated with both psychological factors and a general medical condition: Both psychological factors and a medical condition are judged to have important roles in the onset, severity, exacerbation, or maintenance of the pain. The associated general medical condition or anatomic site of the pain (see following) is coded on axis III.

Specify if:

Acute: duration of less than 6 months

Chronic: duration of 6 months or longer

Note: The following is not considered to be a mental disorder and is included here to facilitate differential diagnosis.

Pain disorder associated with a general medical condition: A general medical condition has a major role in the onset, severity, exacerbation, or maintenance of the pain. (If psychological factors are present, they are not judged to have a major role in the onset, severity, exacerbation, or maintenance of the pain.) The diagnostic code for the pain is selected based on the associated general medical condition if one has been established (see Appendix G) or on the anatomic location of the pain if the underlying general medical condition is not yet clearly established—for example, low back (724.2), sciatic (724.3), pelvic (625.9), headache (784.0), facial (784.0), chest (786.50), joint (719.4), bone (733.90), abdominal (789.0), breast (611.71), renal (788.0), ear (388.70), eye (379.91), throat (784.1), tooth (525.9), and urinary (788.0).

From *Diagnostic and Statistical Manual*, 4th ed. Washington, DC: American Psychiatric Association, 1994:461–462, with permission.

lems. They wanted to have all the factors relevant to the onset or maintenance of the pain delineated and also to have a diagnostic category that does not require more training than the majority of *DSM-IV* users would be expected to have. These two requirements may not be compatible. Furthermore, no guidance is given in determining when psychological factors have a major role in pain or are considered important enough in the presence of a painful medical disorder to be coded as a separate mental disorder. Given the high rates of mood and anxiety disorders among disabled chronic pain patients, many patients most appropriate for the diagnosis would be excluded. Although depression and anxiety diagnoses point toward specific proven therapies, this is not true for pain disorder. The diagnosis thus continues covertly as a diagnosis of exclusion with neither clear inclusion criteria nor implications for therapy. However, these revised criteria are more useful in thinking about somatization as a psychiatric amplification process applied to pain.

Epidemiology

Because pain disorder has poor interrater reliability[247] and (as suggested previously) poor validity, there have been few epidemiologic studies of the *DSM* pain disorders. There have, however, been good studies of pain complaints and unexplained medical symptoms. In a study of adult health maintenance organization members, Von Korff and colleagues found the prevalence of pain over a 6-month period was 41% for back pain, 26% for headache, 17% for abdominal pain, 12% for chest pain, and 12% for facial pain.[248] These pain complaints were typically longstanding but nondisabling. However, 9% to 40% reported 1 or more days of disability in the past 6 months. Persons with a pain condition had higher levels of anxiety, depression, and nonpain somatic complaints.

Multiple studies have also demonstrated the association between medically unexplained symptoms (pain and nonpain) and psychiatric disorders. A linear relationship has been demonstrated between the lifetime number of medically unexplained physical symptoms and the lifetime number of depressive and anxiety disorders or the degree of neuroticism or harm avoidance the patient demonstrates on psychological testing.[249] Increased psychiatric morbidity has been repeatedly demonstrated for levels of unexplained medical symptoms far below the number required for a *DSM* diagnosis of somatization disorder.[250] This suggests that the somatoform disorders may be less distinct than implied by their separate *DSM* categories and that they have a strong kinship with the depressive and anxiety disorders. It may be more accurate and productive to think of somatization as a process present in varying degrees throughout the population rather than a set of disorders affecting a small subset of the population.[236]

Treatment

Because chronic pain often has multiple causes or contributing factors, it often does not respond to purely somatic or purely psychological modes of treatment. Persistent pain can set a vicious cycle of reinforcing features into motion that then becomes a self-perpetuating problem independent of the initiating illness or injury. Deactivation, depression, disuse, medication misuse, and vocational dysfunction are all common contributing factors to the suffering and disability associated with chronic pain. Although simpler cases of chronic pain may respond to an approach based on the biomedical model, this is not true for the extremely disabled or prolonged cases likely to be referred to psychiatrists or psychologists.

Patients with disabling chronic pain are prone to *doctor shopping*, in which they obtain medications and procedures from a number of physicians unknown to each other. It is not possible to successfully treat a patient with chronic pain who has not formed a solid and honest therapeutic alliance with his or her treating physician. When evidence of doctor shopping becomes apparent, the patient should be confronted immediately and a conversation opened about the doctor–patient relationship. If the patient does not agree to stop unannounced visits to other physicians, he or she should be dismissed from care, as it is impossible to provide appropriate service in this situation.

The needs of patients with disabling chronic pain often outstrip the resources of the most enlightened and eager primary care physician. These patients are most appropriately treated by a multidisciplinary team experienced in the treatment of chronic pain. Members of this team may include a psychiatrist, psychologist, neurologist, neurosurgeon, physical therapist, occupational therapist, nurse, and vocational counselor. Although each case does not require the expertise of each of these disciplines, all of these disciplines have expertise relevant to the management of chronic pain.

The treatment of chronic pain is in many ways counterintuitive to the clinician and the patient. Many medications used for acute pain are contraindicated. Relief from pain must often be secondary to reduction in disability and deactivation. Clinical phenomena that seem clearly caused by the pain (e.g., depression must be addressed before pain relief is possible).

Most important, pain is not itself a psychiatric disorder. Chronic pain is frequently complicated by psychiatric disorders, however. The most common of these is depression. Psychiatric treatment of these disorders has an important role to play in the rehabilitation of the chronic pain patient.

CONVERSION DISORDER

The essential feature of conversion disorder is an alteration in voluntary motor or sensory function that suggests a neurologic or general medical disorder. Classic examples include hysterical paralysis, blindness, or mutism. Psychological factors must be associated with the initiation or exacerbation of this deficit. Diagnostic criteria are displayed in Table 31.8.

TABLE 31.8

DIAGNOSTIC AND STATISTICAL MANUAL, FOURTH EDITION, DIAGNOSTIC CRITERIA FOR CONVERSION DISORDER

A. One or more symptoms or deficits affecting voluntary motor or sensory function that suggest a neurologic or other general medical condition.

B. Psychological factors are judged to be associated with the symptom or deficit because the initiation or exacerbation of the symptom or deficit is preceded by conflicts or other stressors.

C. The symptom or deficit is not intentionally produced or feigned (as in factitious disorder or malingering).

D. The symptom or deficit cannot, after appropriate investigation, be fully explained by a general medical condition, or by the direct effects of a substance, or as a culturally sanctioned behavior or experience.

E. The symptom or deficit causes clinically significant distress or impairment in social, occupational, or other important areas of functioning or warrants medical evaluation.

F. The symptom or deficit is not limited to pain or sexual dysfunction, does not occur exclusively during the course of somatization disorder, and is not better accounted for by another mental disorder.

Specify type of symptom or deficit:
  With motor symptom or deficit
  With sensory symptom or deficit
  With seizures or convulsions
  With mixed presentation

From *Diagnostic and Statistical Manual*, 4th ed. Washington, DC: American Psychiatric Association, 1994:457, with permission.

Great caution must be exercised in making the diagnosis of conversion disorder, because the presence of relevant psychological factors does not exclude the possibility of a concurrent organically caused condition.

In "Psychogenic Pain and the Pain-Prone Patient," George Engel proposed that psychogenic pain arose from guilt and an intolerance of success.[117] He indicated that it functioned as a substitute for loss or a replacement for aggression. He furthermore stated that "... patients with conversion hysteria constitute the largest percentage of the pain-prone population." Others have also contended that pain is probably the most common conversion symptom encountered clinically.[251] However, only case reports exist to support this contention. Pain is not a classic conversion disorder symptom, and it is controversial whether chronic pain can ever qualify as a conversion disorder by itself. Some, for example, have contended that reflex sympathetic dystrophy (complex regional pain syndrome) can be understood as a conversion reaction; however, this is highly controversial.[252] Some elements of conversion disorders appear to be present in reflex sympathetic dystrophy/complex regional pain syndrome patients (e.g., indifference or neglect toward the affected body part), although it is highly unlikely that the condition is entirely psychogenic.

Rather than labeling some chronic pain problems as conversion reactions and others as not, it may be more useful to understand what components of conversion reaction may be present in chronic pain problems. Again, the emphasis should be on thinking about somatoform illnesses as a process. Being ill surely creates problems in living for those affected, but it can also solve problems in living. For example, being ill provides an excuse for not being at school or not meeting a deadline at work. These interpersonal advantages of illness were originally recognized by Freud and termed *secondary gain*.

The term *secondary gain* has been distorted and misunderstood in the care of chronic pain, probably because of medicolegal pressures. A number of corrections are in order. First, all illnesses are characterized by some secondary gain, not just illnesses considered to be psychogenic. Being sick always has advantages as well as disadvantages. Second, secondary gain includes all potential interpersonal benefits of illness, not just monetary advantages. Many of the advantages of illness are quite subtle and individualized. Third, secondary gain must be understood in the context of *primary gain*, the intrapersonal advantages of illness. For example, focusing on pain rather than depression may allow patients to avoid self-blame and thereby achieve primary gain. This is a common phenomenon in chronic pain. Indeed, blame avoidance has been hypothesized by some to be one of the main functions of somatization.[253] Thus, traditional elements of conversion disorder may be present in many chronic pain problems without many pain problems qualifying as conversion disorders *per se*.

Purely psychogenic or conversion models of chronic pain have some questionable implications for diagnosis and therapy of chronic pain disorders. Interview of the patient with a suspected conversion disorder with the aid of a sodium amobarbital (Amytal) infusion has been a standard tool in psychiatric diagnosis.[254] More recently, lorazepam interviews have been substituted. It is more common that motor and sensory deficits than pain resolve under Amytal or benzodiazepine sedation. Furthermore, some patients have had violent or suicidal reactions to abrupt resolution of their somatic symptoms under Amytal, possibly caused by loss of face-saving primary gain aspects of the illness. Psychodynamic theories of the origin of conversion symptoms imply that psychological treatments alone will be effective.

Psychodynamic treatments for chronic pain, however, have little documented success. The most effective psychological treatments, such as cognitive-behavioral therapy, include a reactivation component that addresses the profound disuse and deconditioning found in many patients with chronic pain.

HYPOCHONDRIASIS

Many patients with chronic pain resist their physician's reassurance that "nothing is wrong" or that the "tests reveal nothing." These patients know that they hurt and cannot accept that a bodily cause cannot be identified for their pain. This has been described as *disease conviction* in the chronic pain literature. Disease conviction has been measured with the Illness Behavior Questionnaire, and Hypochondriasis is assessed with the Minnesota Multiphasic Personality Inventory. In *DSM-IV* there also exists a disorder called *hypochondriasis*. Diagnostic criteria are list in Table 31.9.

The prevalence of hypochondriasis in primary care has been reported to be 4% to 9%.[255] The prevalence of hypochondriasis in pain clinic populations is difficult to determine, but is likely to be high if patients are not excluded by qualifying for pain disorder, because of the likelihood of disagreement between patient and physician about the cause of the pain problem.

Treatments of hypochondriasis have attempted to shift patient focus from cure of the disease causing the symptoms to strategies of symptom management.[256] These strategies are common components of multidisciplinary pain treatment programs as well. It is indeed critical to achieve early in treatment some agreement with the patient about the cause of the pain that acknowledges the reality of the pain and yet points away from invasive attempts to cure disease or repair broken parts. The task is not to convince the patient that "nothing serious is wrong," because his or her pain may be severe and persistent. The task is to convince the patient that the appropriate treatment is different than the treatment he or she thought necessary.

TABLE 31.9

DIAGNOSTIC AND STATISTICAL MANUAL, FOURTH EDITION, DIAGNOSTIC CRITERIA FOR HYPOCHONDRIASIS

A. Preoccupation with fears of having, or the idea that one has, a serious disease based on the person's misinterpretation of bodily symptoms.

B. The preoccupation persists despite appropriate medical evaluation and reassurance.

C. The belief in criterion A is not of delusional intensity (as in delusional disorder, somatic type) and is not restricted to a circumscribed concern about appearance (as in body dysmorphic disorder).

D. The preoccupation causes clinically significant distress or impairment in social, occupational, or other important areas of functioning.

E. The duration of the disturbance is at least 6 months.

F. The preoccupation is not better accounted for by generalized anxiety disorder, obsessive-compulsive disorder, panic disorder, a major depressive episode, separation anxiety, or another somatoform disorder.

Specify if:

With poor insight: If, for most of the time during the current episode, the person does not recognize that the concern about having a serious illness is excessive or unreasonable.

From *Diagnostic and Statistical Manual,* 4th ed. Washington, DC: American Psychiatric Association, 1994:465, with permission.

CONCLUSION: PAIN AND SUFFERING AND PSYCHIATRY

Psychiatric diagnosis and treatment can add an essential and often neglected component to the conceptualization and treatment of chronic pain problems. The high rates of psychiatric comorbidity and the negative impact they have on chronic pain necessitate that a psychiatric assessment be part of any comprehensive pain evaluation. The expanse of psychiatric symptoms in patients with pain is broad and deep, and thus a comprehensive framework for describing psychiatric symptoms and the relationships between them is essential to thorough diagnosis and treatment. Advances in neuroimaging have elucidated some of the interrelationships between pain perception and psychological states, underscoring that most painful conditions have an affective component to the pain experience.

It is this disordered affective experience of pain and consequently, suffering, that form a key interaction between pain and overlying psychiatric disorders. It is absolutely critical to avoid a dualistic model that postulates that pain is either physical or mental in origin. This model alienates patients who feel blamed for their pain. It also is inconsistent with modern models of pain causation. Since the gate control theory of pain, multiple lines of evidence suggest that pain is a product of efferent as well as afferent activity in the nervous system. Tissue damage and nociception are neither necessary nor sufficient for pain. Indeed, it is now widely recognized that the relationship between pain and nociception is highly complex and must be understood in terms of the situation of the organism as a whole.

We are only beginning to understand the complexities of the relationship between pain and suffering. Pain usually, but not always, produces suffering. Suffering can, through somatization, produce pain. We have traditionally understood this suffering, as we have understood nociception, as arising from a form of pathology intrinsic to the sufferer. Hence, the traditional view that pain is caused by either tissue pathology (nociception) or psychological states (suffering). Psychiatric comorbidity represents an additional layer of suffering, which also magnifies the perception on pain. Yet this is still somewhat dualistic; an alternative model is to think of pain as a *transdermal process* with causes outside as well as inside the body. For humans, social pathology can be as painful as tissue pathology. We can investigate the physiology and the psychology of this *sociogenic* pain without losing sight of its origins in relations *between* people.

Psychiatric care for patients with chronic pain should occur within the medical treatment setting whenever possible. This is the most effective way to reassure patients that the somatic elements of their problems are not neglected. It also allows integration of somatic and psychological treatments in the most effective manner.[1] The success of multidisciplinary approaches to pain underscores the value of psychiatric assessment and treatment by the pain medicine provider.

References

1. Dersh J, Gatchel RJ, Mayer DJ, et al. Prevalence of psychiatric disorders in patients with chronic disabling occupational spinal disorders. *Spine* 2006; 31(10):1156–1162.
2. Engel GL. Psychogenic pain and the pain-prone patient. *Am J Med* 1959;26:899–918.
3. Dersh J, Polatin PB, Gatchel RJ. Chronic pain and psychopathology: research findings and theoretical considerations. *Psychosom Med* 2002;64:773–786.
4. Merskey H, Spear FG. Pain: *Psychological and Psychiatric Aspects,* ed. Balliere T, Cassell. 1967, London.
5. Sternbach R. Psychological aspects of chronic pain. *Clin Orthop Relat Res* 1977;129:150–155.
6. Good MJ, Pain as human experience: an anthropological perspective. Berkeley: University of California Press, 1992.

7. Birket-Smith M, Mortensen EL. Pain in somatoform disorders: is somatoform pain disorder a valid diagnosis? *ACTA Psychiatr Scand* 2002;106:103–108.

8. Fishbain D, Cutler R, Rosomoff H. Chronic pain associated depression: antecedent or consequence of chronic pain? A review. *Clin J Pain* 1997;13(2):116–137.

9. Aybek S, Kanaan RA, David AS. The neuropsychiatry of conversion disorder. *Curr Opin Psychiatry* 2008;21(3):275–280.

10. Wasan AD, Fernandez E, Pham LD, et al. The association between anxiety, depression, and reported disease severity in chronic rhinosinusitis. *Ann Otol Rhinol Laryngol* 2007;116(7):491–497.

11. Kinney RK, Gatchel R, Polatin P, et al. Prevalence of psychopathology in acute and chronic low back pain patients. *J Occup Rehabil* 1993;3:95–103.

12. Epstein S, Kay G, Clauw D, et al. Psychiatric disorders in patients with fibromyalgia: a multicenter investigation. *Psychosomatics* 1999;40:57–63.

13. Kight M, Gatchel RJ, Wesley L. Temporomandibular disorders: evidence for significant overlap with psychopathology. *Health Psychol* 1999;18:177–182.

14. Okasha A, Ismail MK, Khalil AH, et al. A psychiatric study of nonorganic chronic headache patients. *Psychosomatics* 1999;40:233–238.

15. Savidge C, Slade P. Psychological aspects of chronic pelvic pain. *J Psychosom Res* 1997;42:443–444.

16. Ploghaus A, Tracey I, Gati JS, et al. Dissociating pain from its anticipation in the human brain. *Science* 1999;284(5422):1979–1981.

17. Loggia ML, Mogil JS, Bushnell MC. Empathy hurts: compassion for another increases both sensory and affective components of pain perception. *Pain* 2008;136:168–176.

18. American Psychiatric Association. *Diagnostic and Statistical Manual of Mental Disorders*. 4th ed. Washington, DC: American Psychiatric Press Inc, 1994.

19. Mayou R, Kirmayer LJ, Simon G, et al. Somatoform disorders: time for a new approach in DSM-V. *Am J Psychiatry* 2005;162:847–855.

20. McHugh PR, Slavney PR. Methods of reasoning in psychopathology: conflict and resolution. *Compr Psychiatry* 1982;23:197–215.

21. Clark MR, Chodynicki MP. Pain management. In: Levenson JL, ed. *Textbook of Psychosomatic Medicine*. Arlington: American Psychiatric Publishing, Inc.; 2005:827–867.

22. Clark M, Cox T. Refractory chronic pain. *Psych Clin North Am* 2002;25(1):71–88.

23. Barsky AJ. A comprehensive approach to the chronically somatizing patient. *J Psychosom Res* 1998;45:301–306.

24. McHugh PR, Clark MR. Diagnostic and classificatory dilemmas. In: Blumenfield M, Strain JJ, eds. *Psychosomatic Medicine in the 21st Century*. Baltimore: Lippincott Williams & Wilkins, 2006:39–45.

25. Clark MR. Psychiatric conditions presenting as neurologic disease. Conversion disorder and hysteria. In: Johnson RT, Griffin JW, McArthur JC, eds. *Current Therapy in Neurological Diseases*. St. Louis: Mosby, 2002:428–431.

26. Kirmayer LJ, Groleau D, Looper KJ, et al. Explaining medically unexplained symptoms. *Can J Psychiatry* 2004;49:663–672.

27. Brown RJ. Psychological mechanisms of medically unexplained symptoms: an integrative conceptual model. *Psychol Bull* 2004;130:793–812.

28. Rief W, Barsky AJ. Psychobiological perspectives on somatoform disorders. *Psychoneuroendocrinology* 2005;30:996–1002.

29. McHugh PR. A structure for psychiatry at the century's turn the view from Johns Hopkins. *J Roy Soc Med* 1992;85:483–487.

30. McHugh PR, Slavney PR. *Perspectives of Psychiatry*. 2nd ed. Baltimore, MD: The Johns Hopkins University Press, 1998.

31. Slavney PR. *Perspectives on "Hysteria."* Baltimore, MD: The Johns Hopkins University Press, 1990.

32. Ford CV. Somatization and fashionable diagnoses: illness as a way of life. *Scand J Work Environ Health* 1997;23(Suppl 3):7–16.

33. Reuber M, Mitchell AJ, Howlett SJ, et al. Functional symptoms in neurology: questions and answers. *J Neurol Neurosurg Psychiatry* 2005;76:307–314.

34. Clark MR, Treisman GJ. Perspectives on pain and depression. *Adv Psychosom Med* 2004;25:1–27.

35. Stone J, Carson A, Sharpe M. Functional symptoms and signs in neurology: management. *Neurol Neurosurg Psychiatry* 2005;76(Suppl 1):i13–i21.

36. Kirmayer LJ, Robbins JM. Three forms of somatization in primary care: prevalence, co-occurrence, and sociodemographic characteristics. *J Nerv Ment Dis* 1991;179:647–655.

37. Rief W; Nanke A. Somatoform disorders in primary care and inpatient settings. *Adv Psychosom Med* 2004;26:144–158.

38. Clark MR, Swartz KL. A conceptual structure and methodology for the systematic approach to the evaluation and treatment of patients with chronic dizziness. *J Anxiety Disord* 2001;15:95–106.

39. Strain EC. Assessment and treatment of comorbid psychiatric disorders in opioid-dependent patients. *Clin J Pain* 2002;18(4 Suppl):S14–S27.

40. Keefe FJ, Rumble ME, Scipio CD, et al. Psychological aspects of persistent pain: current state of the science. *J Pain* 2004;5(4):195–211.

41. Wasan AD, Davar G, Jamison RN. The association between negative affect and opioid analgesia in patients with discogenic low back pain. *Pain* 2005;117:450–461.

42. McCracken L, Gross R, Aikens J, et al. The assessment of anxiety and fear in persons with chronic pain: a comparison of instruments. *Behav Res Ther* 1996;34(11):927–933.

43. Turk DC, Monarch ES. Biopsychosocial perspective on chronic pain. In: Turk DC, Gatchel R, eds. *Psychological Approaches to Pain Management*. Guilford Press: New York, 2002:3–29.

44. Novy DM, Nelson DV, Berry LA, et al. What does the Beck Depression Inventory measure in chronic pain?: a reappraisal of pain. 1995;61:261–270.

45. Koenig HG, George LK, Peterson BL, et al. Depression in medically ill hospitalized older adults: prevalence, characteristics, and course of symptoms according to six diagnostic schemes. *Am J Psychiatry* 1997;154:1376–1383.

46. White K, Nielson W, Harth M, et al. Chronic widespread musculoskeletal pain with or without fibromyalgia: psychological distress in a representative community adult sample. *J Rheum* 2002;29(3):588–594.

47. BenDebba M, Torgerson W, Long D. Personality traits, pain duration and severity, functional impairment, and psychological distress in patients with persistent low back pain. *Pain* 1997;72:115–125.

48. WHO. *The World Health Report 2004*. Geneva: World Health Organization, 2004.

49. Kessler RC, Borges G, Walters EE. Prevalence of and risk factors for lifetime suicide attempts in the National Comorbidity Survey. *Arch Gen Psychiatr* 1999;56:617–626.

50. Bernal M, Haro JM, Bernert S, et al. Risk factors for suicidality in Europe: results from the ESEMED study. *J Affect Disord* 2007;101:27–34.

51. Tang NK, Crane C. Suicidality in chronic pain: a review of the prevalence, risk factors and psychological links. *Psychol Med* 2006;36:575–586.

52. Moller HJ. Suicide, suicidality and suicide prevention in affective disorders. *Acta Psychiatr Scand Suppl* 2003(418):73–80.

53. Sokero TP, Melartin TK, Rytsala HJ, et al. Suicidal ideation and attempts among psychiatric patients with major depressive disorder. *J Clin Psychiatry* 2003;64:1094–1100.

54. Juurlink DN, Herrmann N, Szalai JP, et al. Medical illness and the risk of suicide in the elderly. *Arch Intern Med* 2004;164:1179–1184.

55. Theodoulou M, Harriss L, Hawton K, et al. Pain and deliberate self-harm: an important association. *J Psychosom Res* 2005;28:317–320.

56. Fishbain D. Approaches to treatment decisions for psychiatric comorbidity in the management of the chronic pain patient. *Med Clin North Am* 1999;83(3):737–759.

57. Edwards RR, Smith MT, Kudel I, et al. Pain-related catastrophizing as a risk factor for suicidal ideation in chronic pain. *Pain* 2006;126:272–279.

58. Smith MT, Edwards RR, Robinson RC, et al. Suicidal ideation, plans, attempts in chronic pain patients: factors associated with increased risk. *Pain* 2004a;111:201–208.

59. Smith MT, Perlis ML, Haythornthwaite JA. Suicidal ideation in outpatients with chronic musculoskeletal pain: an exploratory study of the role of sleep onset insomnia and pain intensity. *Clin J Pain* 2004b;20:111–118.

60. Frank E, Anderson B, Reynolds CF, et al. Life events and the research diagnostic criteria endogenous subtype. *Arch Gen Psychiatry* 1994;51:519–524.

61. Brown GW, Harris TO, Hepworth C. Life events and endogenous depression. *Arch Gen Psychiatry* 1994;51:525–534.

62. Mossey J, Gallagher RM, Tirumalasetti F. The effects of pain and depression on physical functioning in elderly residents of a continuing care retirement community. *Pain Med* 2000;1:340–350.

63. Ackermann RT, Williams JW. Rational treatment choices for non-major depressions in primary care: an evidence-based review. *J Gen Intern Med* 2002;17(4):293–301.

64. Lyness JM, Heo M, Datto CJ, et al. Outcomes of minor and subsyndromal depression among elderly patients in primary care settings. *Ann Intern Med* 2006;144(7):495–504.

65. Atkinson JH, Hampton J, Slater MA, et al. Prevalence, onset, and risk of psychiatric disorders in men with chronic low back pain: a controlled study. *Pain* 1991;45(2):111–121.

66. Magni G, Moreschi C, Rigatti Luchini S, et al. Prospective study on the relationship between depressive symptoms and chronic musculoskeletal pain. *Pain* 1994;56(3):289–297.

67. Rudy TE, Kerns RD, Turk DC. Chronic pain and depression: toward a cognitive behavioral mediation model. *Pain* 1988;35(2):129–140.

68. Brown GK. A causal analysis of chronic pain and depression. *J Abn Psychol* 1990;99(2):127–137.

69. Katon W, Egan K, Miller D. Chronic pain: lifetime psychiatric diagnosis and family history. *Am J Psych* 1985;142(10):1156–1160.

70. Blackburn-Munro G, Blackburn-Munro RE. Chronic pain, chronic stress, and depression: coincidence or consequence? *J Neuroendocrinol* 2001;13:1009–1023.

71. Von Korff M, Simon G. The relationship between pain and depression. *Br J Psychiatry* 1996;168(Suppl 30):101–108.

72. Dersh J, Mayer T, Theodore BR, et al. Do psychiatric disorders first appear preinjury or postinjury in chronic disabling occupational spinal disorders? *Spine* 2007;32:1045–1051.

73. Nemeroff CB, Krishnan KRR. Neuroendocrine alterations in psychiatric disorders. In: Nemeroff C, ed. *Neuroendocrinology*. Ann Arbor, MI: CRC, 1992.

74. American Psychiatric Association Taskforce on Laboratory Tests in Psychiatry. The dexamethasone suppression test: an overview of its current status in psychiatry. *Am J Psychiatry* 1987;144(10):1253–1262.

75. Mellerup ET, Dam H, Kim MY, et al. Imipramine binding in depressed patients with psychogenic pain. *Psychiatry Res* 1990;32(1):29–34.

76. Sullivan GM, Mann JJ, Oquendo MA, et al. Low cerebrospinal fluid transthyretin levels in depression: correlations with suicidal ideation and low serotonin function. *Biol Psychiatr* 2006;60:500–506.

77. Keller MB, Hirschfeld RM, Hanks D. Double depression: a distinctive subtype of unipolar depression. *J Affect Disord* 1997;45(1):65–73.

78. Thase ME, Fava M, Halbreich U, et al. A placebo-controlled, randomized clinical trial comparing sertraline and imipramine for the treatment of dysthymia. *Arch Gen Psychiatry* 1996;53(9):777–784.

79. Rush AJ, Thase ME. Strategies and tactics in the treatment of chronic depression. *J Clin Psychiatry* 1997;58(Suppl 13):14–22.

80. Katon WJ, Sullivan MD. Depression and chronic medical illness. *J Clin Psychiatry* 1990;51(Suppl):3–11.

81. Coulehan JL, Schulberg HC, Block MR, et al. Medical comorbidity of major depressive disorder in a primary medical practice. *Arch Intern Med* 1990; 150:2363–2367.

82. Palinkas LA, Wingard DL, Barrett-Connor E. Chronic illness and depressive symptoms in the elderly: a population-based study. *J Clin Epidemiol* 1990; 43(11):1131–1141.

83. Romano JM, Turner JA. Chronic pain and depression: does the evidence support a relationship? *Psychol Bull* 1985;97(1):18–34.

84. Fishbain D, Goldberg M, Meagher BR, et al. Male and female chronic pain patients characterized by DSM-III psychiatric diagnostic criteria. *Pain* 1986; 26:181–197.

85. Bair M, Robinson R, Katon W, et al. Depression and pain comorbidity: a literature review. *Arch Int Med* 2003;163:2433–2445.

86. McWilliams LA, Clara IP, Murphy PD, et al. Associations between arthritis and a broad range of psychiatric disorders: findings from a nationally representative sample. *J Pain* 2008;9(11):37–44.

87. Dworkin SF, Von Korff M, LeResche L. Multiple pains and psychiatric disturbance. An epidemiologic investigation. *Arch Gen Psychiatry* 1990;47(3): 239–244.

88. Von Korff M, Ormel J, Keefe FJ, et al. Grading the severity of chronic pain. *Pain* 1992;50(2):133–149.

89. Engel CC, Von Korff M, Katon WJ. Back pain in primary care: predictors of high health-care costs. *Pain* 1996;65(2–3):197–204.

90. Von Korff M, Deyo RA, Cherkin D, et al. Back pain in primary care. Outcomes at 1 year. *Spine* 1993;18:855–862.

91. Kroenke K, Price RK. Symptoms in the community. Prevalence, classification, and psychiatric comorbidity. *Arch Intern Med* 1993;153(21):2474–2480.

92. Adler G, Gattaz WF. Pain perception threshold in major depression. *Biol Psychiatry* 1993;34(10):687–689.

93. Dworkin RH, Clark WC, Lipsitz JD. Pain responsivity in major depression and bipolar disorder. *Psychiatry Res* 1995;56(2):173–181.

94. Widerstrom EG, Aslund PG, Gustafsson LE, et al. Relations between experimentally induced tooth pain threshold changes, psychometrics and clinical pain relief following TENS. A retrospective study in patients with long-lasting pain. *Pain* 1992;51(3):281–287.

95. Widerstrom-Noga E, Dyrehag LE, Borglum-Jensen L, et al. Pain threshold responses to two different modes of sensory stimulation in patients with orofacial muscular pain: psychologic considerations. *J Orofac Pain* 1998;12(1): 27–34.

96. Fields HL. *Pain.* New York: McGraw-Hill, 1987.

97. Sindrup SH, Bach FW, Masdsen C, et al. Venlafaxine versus imipramine in painful neuropathy: a randomized, controlled trial. *Neurology* 2003;60: 1284–1289.

98. Raskin J, Pritchett YL, Wang F, et al. A double-blind, randomized multicenter trial comparing duloxetine with placebo in the management of diabetic peripheral neuropathic pain. *Pain* 2005;6:346–356.

99. Gordon NC, Heller PH, Gear RW, et al. Temporal factors in the enhancement of morphine analgesia by desipramine. *Pain* 1993;53(3):273–276.

100. Carruba MO, Nisoli E, Garosi V, et al. Catecholamine and serotonin depletion from rat spinal cord: effects on morphine and footshock induced analgesia. *Pharmacol Res* 1992;25(2):187–194.

101. Hamet P, Tremblay J. Genetics and genomics of depression. *Metab Clin Exper* 2005;54(Supp 1):10–15.

102. Kato T. Molecular genetics of bipolar disorder and depression. *Psych Clin Neurosci* 2007;61:3–19.

103. Kennedy SE, Koeppe RA, Young EA, et al. Dysregulation of endogenous opioid emotion regulation circuitry in major depression in women. *Arch Gen Psychiatry* 2006;63:1199–1208.

104. Woolf CJ. Pain: moving from symptom control toward mechanism-specific pharmacologic management. *Ann Intern Med* 2004;140:441–451.

105. Raison CL, Capuron L, Miller AH. Cytokines sing the blues: inflammation and the pathogenesis of depression. *Trends Immunol* 2006;27(1):24–31.

106. Sprenger T, Valet M, Boecker H, et al. Opioidergic activation in the medial pain system after heat pain. *Pain* 2006;122:63–67.

107. Peyron R, Laurent B, Garcia-Larrea L. Functional imaging of brain responses to pain. A review and meta-analysis. *Neurophysiol Clin* 2000;30:263–288.

108. Zubieta JK, Ketter TA, Bueller JA, et al. Regulation of human affective responses by anterior cingulate and limbic mu-opioid neurotransmission arch. *Gen Psych* 2003;60(11):1145–1153.

109. Coghill RC, McHaffie JG, Yen YF. Neural correlates of interindividual differences in the subjective experience of pain. *Proc Natl Acad Sci U S A* 2003; 100(14):8538–8542.

110. Thase ME. Depression, sleep, and antidepressants. *J Clin Psychiatry* 1998; 59(Suppl 4):55–65.

111. Lautenbacher S, Kundermann B, Krieg J. Sleep deprivation and pain perception. *Sleep Med Rev* 2006;10:357–369.

112. Lentz MJ, Landis CA, Rothermel J, et al. Effects of selective slow wave sleep disruption on muscoskeletal pain and fatigue in middle aged women. *J Rheumatol* 1999;26:1586–1592.

113. Freud S. Mourning and melancholia. In: *Collected Papers.* London: Hogarth Press and the Institute of Psychoanalysis, 1917.

114. Blumer D, Heilbronn M. Chronic pain as a variant of depressive disease: the pain-prone disorder. *J Nerv Ment Dis* 1982;170(7):381–406.

115. Tinling DC, Klein RF. Psychogenic pain and aggression: the syndrome of the solitary hunger. *Psychosom Med* 1966;28:738–748.

116. von Knorring L, Perris C, Eisemann M, et al. Pain as a symptom in depressive disorders. II. Relationship to personality traits as assessed by means of KSP. *Pain* 1983;17(4):377–384.

117. Engel GL. Psychogenic pain and the pain-prone patient. *Am J Med* 1959; 26(6):899–918.

118. Bouchoms AJ, Litman RE, Baer L. Denial in the depressive and pain-prone disorders of chronic pain. *Clin J Pain* 1985;1:165–169.

119. Gupta MA. Is chronic pain a variant of depressive illness? A critical review. *Can J Psychiatry* 1986;31(3):241–248.

120. Beck AT. *Depression: Causes and Treatment.* Philadelphia: University of Pennsylvania Press, 1967.

121. Turk DC, Meichenbaum D. A cognitive-behavioral approach to pain management. In: Wall PD, Melzack R, eds. *Textbook of Pain.* London: Churchill Livingstone, 1994:1337–1348.

122. Turk DC, Meichenbaum D, Genest M. *Pain and Behavioral Medicine: A Cognitive-Behavioral Perspective.* New York: Guilford, 1983.

123. Turk DC. Anxiety and related factors in chronic pain: a diathesis-stress model of chronic pain and disability following traumatic injury. *Pain Res Manag* 2002;7(1):9–19.

124. Gatchel RJ. Psychological disorders and chronic pain: cause and effect relationships. In: Gatchel RJ, Turk DC, eds. *Psychological Approaches to Pain Management: A Practitioner's Handbook.* New York: Guilford Pub, 1996: 33–54.

125. Banks SM, Kern RD. Explaining high rates of depression in chronic pain: a diathesis-stress framework. *Psychol Bull* 1996,119:95–110.

126. Caspi A, Mofitt TE. Gene-environment interactions in psychiatry: joining forces with neuroscience. *Nat Rev Neurosci* 2006;7:583–590.

127. Fabrega H. The concept of somatization as a cultural and historical product of western medicine. *Psychosom Med* 1990;52(6):653–672.

128. Nichter M. Idioms of distress: alternatives in the expression of psychosocial distress: a case study from South India. *Cult Med Psychiatry* 1981;5(4): 379–408.

129. Kleinman A. *The Illness Narratives: Suffering, Healing, and the Human Condition.* New York: Basic Books, 1988.

130. Carr DB, Loeser JD, Morris DB. Why narrative? In: Carr DB, Loeser JD, Morris DB, eds. *Narrative, Pain, and Suffering.* Seattle: IASP Press, 2005: 3–13.

131. Wasan AD, Wootton J, Jamison RN. Dealing with difficult patients in your pain practice. *Reg Anesth Pain Med* 2005;30:184–192.

132. Wasan AD, Alpay M. Chapter 78: pain and the psychiatric co-morbidities of pain. In: Stern T, ed. *Comprehensive Clinical Psychiatry.* Philadelphia, PA: Elsevier, 2008.

133. Gilbody S, Bower P, Fletcher J, et al. Collaborative care for depression: a cumulative meta-analysis and review of longer-term outcomes. *Arch Intern Med* 2006;166(21):2314–2321.

134. Kroenke K, Shen J, Oxman TE, et al. Impact of pain on the outcomes of depression treatment: results from the RESPECT trial. *Pain* 2008;134: 209–215.

135. Salerno SM, Browning R, Jackson JL. The effect of antidepressant treatment on chronic back pain: a meta-analysis. *Arch Int Med* 2002;162(1):19–24.

136. Rosenzweig-Lipson S, Beyer CE, Hughes ZA, et al. Differentiating antidepressants of the future: efficacy and safety. *Pharmacol Therapeutics* 2007;113: 134–153.

137. Semenchuk MR, Sherman S, Davis B. Double-blind, randomized trial of bupropion SR for the treatment of neuropathic pain. *Neurol* 2001;57(9).

138. Janicak PG, Davis JM, Preskorn SH, et al. Indications for antidepressants. In: Janicak PG, Davis JM, Preskorn SH, et al. eds. *Principles and Practice of Psychopharmacotherapy.* Philadelphia, PA: Lippincott-Williams, 2001:193–214.

139. Maxmen JS, Ward NG. *Psychotropic Drugs: Fast Facts.* 2nd ed. New York: Norton, 1995.

140. Hyman SE, Arana GW, Rosenbaum JF. *Handbook of Psychiatric Drug Therapy.* 3rd ed. Boston, MA: Little, Brown and Company, 1995.

141. Wasan AD, Artin K, Clark MR. A case-matching study of the analgesic properties of electroconvulsive therapy. *Pain Med* 2004;5(1):50–58.

142. Bloomstein JR, Rummans TA, Maruta T, et al. The use of electroconvulsive therapy in pain patients. *Psychosomatics* 1996;37:374–749.

143. Dellemijn PL, Fields HL. Do benzodiazepines have a role in chronic pain management? *Pain* 1994;57(2):137–152.

144. Salzman C. The APA task force report on benzodiazepine dependence, toxicity, and abuse. *Am J Psychiatry* 1991;148(2):151–152.

145. Rickels K, Schweizer E. The treatment of generalized anxiety disorder in patients with depressive symptomatology. *J Clin Psychiatry* 1993;54(Suppl): 20–23.

146. Grzesiak RC, Ury GM, Dworkin RH. Psychodynamic psychotherapy with chronic pain patients. In: Gatchel RJ, Turk DC, eds. *Psychological Approaches to Pain Management: A Practitioner's Handbook*. New York: Guilford Press, 1996.

147. Brox JI, Reikeras O, Nygaard O, et al. Lumbar instrumented fusion compared with cognitive intervention and exercises in patients with chronic back pain after previous surgery for disc herniation: a prospective randomized controlled study. *Pain* 2006;122:145–155.

148. Wolfe F, Smythe HA, Yunnus MB, et al. The American College of Rheumatology 1990 criteria for the classification of fibromyalgia. Report of the multicenter criteria committee. *Arthritis Rheum* 1990;33(2):160–172.

149. Dersh J, Gatchel R, Polatin P, et al. Prevalence of psychiatric disorders in patients with chronic work-related musculoskeletal pain and disability. *J Occ Envir Med* 2002;44(5):459–468.

150. Conrad R, Schilling G, Bausch C, et al. Temperament and character personality profiles and personality disorders in chronic pain patients. *Pain* 2007;133: 197–209.

151. McCracken L, Zayfert C, Gross R. The pain anxiety symptoms scale: development and validation of a scale to measure fear of pain. *Pain* 1992;50:67–73.

152. Vancleef LM, Peters ML, Roelofs J, et al. Do fundamental fears differentially contribute to pain-related fear and pain catastrophizing? An evaluation of the sensitivity index. *Eur J Pain* 2006;10:527–536.

153. McCracken L, Gross R, Sorg P, et al. Prediction of pain in patients with chronic low back pain: effects of inaccurate prediction and pain-related anxiety. *Behav Res Ther* 1993;31(7):647–652.

154. Association AP. *Diagnostic and Statistical Manual of Mental Disorders*. 4th ed. Washington, DC: American Psychiatric Association, 1994.

155. Von Korff M, Crane P, Lane M, et al. Chronic spinal pain and physical-mental comorbidity in the United States: results from the National Comorbidity Survey Replication. *Pain* 2005;113(3):331–339.

156. Hunot V, Churchill R, Silva de Lima M, et al. Psychological therapies for generalized anxiety disorder. *Cochrane Database Syst Rev* 2007;24(1).

157. Linden DE. How psychotherapy changes the brain—the contribution of functional neuroimaging. *Molecular Psychiatry* 2006;11:528–538.

158. Ormel J, Von Korff M, Ustun TB, et al. Common mental disorders and disability across cultures. *JAMA* 1994;272(22):1741–1748.

159. Demyttenaere K, Bruffaerts R, Lee S, et al. Mental disorders among persons with chronic back or neck pain: results from the world mental health surveys. *Pain* 2007;129:332–342.

160. Zaubler TS, Katon W. Panic disorder and medical comorbidity: a review of the medical and psychiatric literature. *Bull Menninger Clin* 1996;60(2 Suppl A):A12–A38.

161. Carney RM, Freedland KE, Ludbrook PA, et al. Major depression, panic disorder, and mitral valve prolapse in patients who complain of chest pain. *Am J Med* 1990;89(6):757–760.

162. Beitman BD, Kushner MG, Basha I, et al. Follow-up status of patients with angiographically normal coronary arteries and panic disorder. *JAMA* 1991; 265(12):1545–1549.

163. Cannon RO, Quyyumi AA, Mincemoyer R, et al. Imipramine in patients with chest pain despite normal coronary angiograms. *N Engl J Med* 1994;330: 1411–1417.

164. Walker EA, Gelfand AN, Gelfand MD, et al. Psychiatric diagnoses, sexual and physical victimization, and disability in patients with irritable bowel syndrome or inflammatory bowel disease. *Psychol Med* 1995;25(6):1259–1267.

165. Stewart W, Breslau N, Keck PEJ. Comorbidity of migraine and panic disorder. *Neurology* 1994;44(Suppl 7):S23–S27.

166. American Psychiatric Association. Practice guideline for treatment of patients with panic disorder. *Am J Psychiatry* 1998;155(May 1998 suppl).

167. Kirmayer LJ, Young A, Hayton BC. The cultural context of anxiety disorders. *Psychiatry Clin North Am* 1995;18(3):503–521.

168. Eal KH, Bertenthal D, Miner CR, et al. Bringing the war back home: mental health disorders among 103,788 US veterans returning from Iraq and Afghanistan seen at Department of Veterans Affairs facilities. *Arch Intern Med* 2007; 167(5):476–482.

169. Beckham JC, Crawford AL, Feldman ME, et al. Chronic posttraumatic stress disorder and chronic pain in Vietnam combat veterans. *J Psychosom Res* 1997;43(11):379–389.

170. Baker DG, Mendenhall CL, Simbartl LA, et al. Relationship between posttraumatic stress disorder and self-reported physical symptoms in Persian Gulf War veterans. *Arch Intern Med* 1997;157(18):2076–2078.

171. Doerfler LA, Pbert L, DeCosimo D. Symptoms of posttraumatic stress disorder following myocardial infarction and coronary artery bypass surgery. *Gen Hosp Psychiatry* 1997;16(3):193–199.

172. Alter CL, Pelcovitz D, Axelrod A, et al. Identification of PTSD in cancer survivors. *Psychosomatics* 1996;37:137–143.

173. Cordova MJ, Andrykowski MA, Kenady DE, et al. Frequency and correlates of posttraumatic-stress-disorder-like symptoms after treatment for breast cancer. *J Consult Clin Psychol* 1995;63(6):981–986.

174. Blanchard EB, Hickling EJ. *After the Crash. Assessment and Treatment of Motor Vehicle Accident Survivors*. Washington, DC: American Psychological Association, 1997.

175. Aghabeigi B, Feinmann C, Harris M. Prevalence of post-traumatic stress disorder in patients with chronic idiopathic facial pain. *Br J Oral Maxillofac Surg* 1992;30(6):360–364.

176. Amir M, Kaplan Z, Neumann L, et al. Posttraumatic stress disorder, tenderness and fibromyalgia. *J Psychosom Res* 1997;42(6):607–613.

177. Muse M. Stress-related, post-traumatic chronic pain syndrome: behavioral treatment approach. *Pain* 1986;25(3):389–394.

178. Liebschutz J, Saitz R, Browner V, et al. PTSD in urban primary care: high prevalence and low physician recognition. *J Gen Intern Med* 2007;22(6): 719–726.

179. Geisser ME, Roth RS, Bachman JE, et al. The relationship between symptoms of post-traumatic stress disorder and pain, affective disturbance and disability among patients with accident and non-accident related pain. *Pain* 1996;66(2): 207–214.

180. Schreiber S, Galai-Gat T. Uncontrolled pain following physical injury as the core-trauma in post-traumatic stress disorder. *Pain* 1993;54(1):107–110.

181. Zatick DF, Rivara FP, Nathens AB, et al. A nationwide US study of post-traumatic stress after hospitalization for physical injury. *Psychol Med* 2007; 37(10):1469–1480.

182. Harris IA, Young JM, Rae H, et al. Factors associated with back pain after physical injury: a survey of consecutive major trauma patients. *Spine* 2007; 32(14):1561–1565.

183. Geuze E, Westenberg HG, Jochims A, et al. Altered pain processing in veterans with posttraumatic stress disorder. *Arch Gen Psych* 2007;64(1):76–85.

184. Solomon SD, Gerrity ET, Muff AM. Efficacy of treatment for posttraumatic stress disorder: an empirical review. *JAMA* 1992;268(2):633–636.

185. Davidson JR. Biological therapies for posttraumatic stress disorder: an overview. *J Clin Psychiatry* 1997;58(Suppl 9):29–32.

186. Davidson J, Baldwin D, Stein DJ, et al. Treatment of posttraumatic stress disorder with venlafaxine extended release: a 6-month randomized controlled trial. *Arch Gen Psych* 2006;63(10):1158–1165.

187. Raskind MA, Peskind ER, Hoff DJ, et al. A parallel group placebo controlled study of prazosin for trauma nightmares and sleep disturbance in combat veterans with post-traumatic stress disorder. *Biol Psych* 2007;61(8):928–934.

188. Vendrig AA. The Minnesota Multiphasic Personality Inventory and chronic pain: a conceptual analysis of a long-standing but complicated relationship. *Clin Psychol Rev* 2000;20:533–559.

189. Weisberg JN. Personality and personality disorders in chronic pain. *Curr Rev Pain* 2000;4:60–70.

190. Weisberg JN, Vaillancourt PD. Personality factors and disorders in chronic pain. *Semin Clin Neuropsychiatry* 1999;4:155–166.

191. Hathaway SR, McKinley JC. *Minnesota Multiphasic Personality Inventory Manual*. (rev ed). New York: Psychological Corporation, 1967.

192. Turk DC, Fernandez E. Personality assessment and the Minnesota Multiphasic Personality Inventory in chronic pain: underdeveloped and overexposed. *Pain Forum* 1995;5:104–107.

193. Vendrig AA, Derksen JJ, de Mey HR. MMPI-2 Personality Psychopathology Five (PSY-5) and prediction of treatment outcome for patients with chronic back pain. *J Pers Assess* 2000;74:423–438.

194. Sternbach RA. Psychological aspects of pain and the selection of patients. *Clin Neurosurg* 1974(21):223–233.

195. Riley JL, Robinson ME. Validity of MMPI-2 profiles in chronic back pain patients: differences in path models of coping and somatization. *Clin J Pain* 1998;14:324–335.

196. Norman WT. Toward an adequate taxonomy of personality attributes: replicated factors structure in peer nomination personality settings. *J Abnorm Soc Psychol* 1963;66:574–583.

197. Costa PT, McCrae RR. *The NEO Personality Inventory Manual*. Orlando: Psychological Assessment Resources, 1985.

198. Widiger TA, Lowe JR. Five-factor model assessment of personality disorder. *J Pers Assess* 2007;89:16–29.

199. Cloninger CR, Svrakic DM, Przybeck TR. A psychobiological model of temperament and character. *Arch Gen Psychiatry* 1993;50:975–990.

200. Svrakic DM, Whitehead C, Przybeck TR, et al. Differential diagnosis of personality disorders by the seven-factor model of temperament and character. *Arch Gen Psychiatry* 1993;50:991–999.

201. Hirano S, Sato T, Narita T, et al. Evaluating the state dependency of the temperament and character inventory dimensions in patients with a major depression: a methodological contribution. *J Affect Disord* 2002;69:31–38.

202. Grucza RA, Przybeck TR, Spitznagel EL, et al. Personality and depressive symptoms: a multi-dimensional analysis. *J Affective Disord* 2003;74: 123–130.

203. Nestadt G, Costa PT, Hsu FC, et al. The relationship between the five-factor model and latent Diagnostic and Statistical Manual of Mental Disorders, Fourth Edition personality disorder dimensions. *Compr Psychiatry* 2008;49: 98–105.

204. Terracciano A, Costa PT, McCrae RR. Personality plasticity after age 30. *Pers Soc Psychol Bull* 2006;32:999–1009.

205. Skodol AE, Gunderson JG, Shea MT, et al. The Collaborative Longitudinal

Personality Disorders Study (CLPS): overview and implications. *J Personal Disord* 2005;19:487–504.

206. Costa PT, Patriciu NS, McCrae RR. Lessons from longitudinal studies for new approaches to the DSM-V: the FFM and FFT. *J Personal Disord* 2005; 19:533–539.

207. Fishbain DA, Cole B, Cutler RB, et al. Chronic pain and the measurement of personality: do states influence traits? *Pain Med* 2006;7:509–529.

208. Loranger AW, Lenzenweger MF, Gartner AF, et al. Trait-state artifacts and the diagnosis of personality disorders. *Arch Gen Psychiatry* 1991;48: 720–728.

209. Bronisch T, Klerman G. Personality functioning: change and stability in relationship to symptoms and psychopathology. *J Personal Disord* 1991;5: 307–317.

210. Stuart S. Are personality assessments valid in acute major depression? *J Affect Disord* 1992;24:281–290.

211. Hellerstein DJ, Kocsis JH, Chapman D, et al. Double-blind comparison of sertraline, imipramine, and placebo in the treatment of dysthymia: effects on personality. *Am J Psychiatry* 2000;157:1436–1444.

212. Applegate KL, Keefe FJ, Siegler IC, et al. Does personality at college entry predict number of reported pain conditions at mid-life? A longitudinal study. *J Pain* 2005;6:92–97.

213. Malmgren-Olsson EB, Bergdahl J. Temperament and character personality dimensions in patients with nonspecific musculoskeletal disorders. *Clin J Pain* 2006;22:625–631.

214. Greenberg J, Burns JW. Pain anxiety among chronic pain patients: specific phobia or manifestation of anxiety sensitivity? *Behav Res Ther* 2003;41: 223–240.

215. Lethem J, Slade PD, Troup JDG, et al. Outline of fear-avoidance model of exaggerated pain perceptions. *Behav Res Ther* 1983;21:401–408.

216. Reis S. Expectancy theory of fear, anxiety, and panic. *Clin Psychol Rev* 1991; 11:141–153.

217. Vlaeyen JW, Linton SJ. Fear-avoidance and its consequences in chronic musculoskeletal pain: a state of the art. *Pain* 2000;85:317–332.

218. Zvolensky MJ, Goodie JL, McNeil DW, et al. Anxiety sensitivity in the prediction of pain-related fear and anxiety in a heterogeneous chronic pain population. *Behav Res Ther* 2001;39:683–696.

219. Asmundson GJG, Norton PJ, Norton GR. Beyond pain: the role of fear and avoidance in chronicity. *Clin Psychol Rev* 1999;19:97–119.

220. Waddell G, Newton M, Henderson I, et al. A fear-avoidance beliefs questionnaire (FABQ) and the role of fear-avoidance beliefs in chronic low back pain and disability. *Pain* 1993;52:157–168.

221. Mannion AF, Muntener M, Taimela S, et al. A randomized clinical trial of three active therapies for chronic low back pain. *Spine* 1999;24:2435–2448.

222. Mannion AF, Junge A, Taimela S, et al. Active therapy for chronic low back pain: part 3. Factors influencing self-rated disability and its change following therapy. *Spine* 2001;26:920–929.

223. Vowles KE, Gross RT. Work-related beliefs about injury and physical capability for work in individuals with chronic pain. *Pain* 2003;101:291–298.

224. Parsons T. *Social Systems.* London: Routledge and Kegan Paul, 1951.

225. Parsons T. *Social Structure and Personality.* New York: Free Press, 1964.

226. Mechanic D, Volkart EH. Stress, illness behavior, and the sick role. *Ann Soc Rev* 1961;26(1):51–58.

227. Mechanic D. The concept of illness behavior. *J Chron Dis* 196215:189–194.

228. Pilowsky I. The diagnosis of abnormal illness behavior. *NZ J Psychiatry* 1971; 5:136–141.

229. Barsky AJ. Patients who amplify bodily sensations. *Ann Intern Med* 1979; 91(1):63–70.

230. Sigvardsson S, von Knorring A, Bohman M. An adoption study of somatoform disorders. *Arch Gen Psychiatry* 1984;41(9):853–859.

231. van der Kolk BA, Herron N, Hostetler A. The history of trauma in psychiatry. *Psychiatry Clin North Am* 1994;17:583–600.

232. Smith GR. *Somatization Disorder in the Medical Setting.* Washington, DC: American Psychiatry Press, 1991.

233. Kroenke K, Spitzer RL, deGruy FVr, et al. Multisomatoform disorder. An alternative to undifferentiated somatoform disorder for the somatizing patient in primary care. *Arch Gen Psychiatry* 1997;54(4):352–358.

234. Liu G, Clark MR, Eaton WW. Structural factor analyses for medically unexplained somatic symptoms of somatization disorder in the Epidemiologic Catchment Area study. *Psychol Med* 1997;27(3):617–626.

235. Gureje O, Simon GE, Ustun TB, Goldberg DP. Somatization in a cross-cultural perspective: a WHO study in primary care. *Am J Psychiatry* 1997;154(7): 989–995.

236. Sullivan MD, Katon WJ. Somatization: the path from distress to somatic symptoms. *APS J* 1993;2:141–149.

237. Pribor EF, Yutzy SH, Dean JT, et al. Briquet's syndrome, dissociation, and abuse. *Am J Psychiatry* 1993;150:1507–1511.

238. Hudziak JJ, Bofffeli TJ, Kreisman JJ, et al. Clinical study of the relation of borderline personality disorder to Briquet's syndrome (hysteria), somatization disorder, antisocial personality disorder, and substance abuse disorders. *Am J Psychiatry* 1996;153(12):1598–1606.

239. Polatin PB, Gatchel RJ. Psychiatric illness and chronic low back pain. *Spine* 1993;18:66–71.

240. Weisberg JN, Keefe FJ. Personality disorders in the chronic pain population. *Pain Forum* 1997;6:1–9.

241. Binks CA, Fenton M, McCarthy L, et al. Psychological therapies for people with borderline personality disorder. *Cochrane Database Syst Rev* 2006; 25(1).

242. Hirschfeld RM. Pharmacotherapy of borderline personality disorder. *J Clin Psychiatry* 1997;58(Suppl 14):48–52.

243. American Psychiatric Association. *Diagnostic and Statistical Manual of Mental Disorders.* 3rd ed. Washington, DC: American Psychiatric Association Press, 1980.

244. Stoudemire A SJ. Psychogenic/idiopathic pain syndromes. *Gen Hosp Psychiatry* 1987;9:79–86.

245. American Psychiatric Association. *Diagnostic and Statistical Manual of Mental Disorders.* 3rd Revised ed. Washington, DC: American Psychiatric Association Press, 1987.

246. King SA, Strain JJ. Revising the category of somatoform pain disorder. *Hosp Comm Psychiatry* 1992;43:217–219.

247. Jantschek G, Rodewig K, von Wietersheim J, et al. Concepts of the psychosomatic disorders in the ICD-10: results of the Research Criteria Study. *Psychother Psychosom* 1995;63(2):112–123.

248. Von Korff M, Dworkin SF, LeResche L, et al. An epidemiologic comparison of pain complaints. *Pain* 1988;32(2):173–183.

249. Russo J, Katon W, Sullivan M, et al. Severity of somatization and its relationship to psychiatric disorders and personality. *Psychosomatics* 1994;35: 546–556.

250. Escobar JI, Burnham MA, Karno M, et al. Somatization in the community. *Arch Gen Psychiatry* 1987;44(8):713–718.

251. Ziegler FJ, Imboden JB, Meyer E. Contemporary conversion reaction: a clinical study. *Am J Psychiatry* 1960;116:901–910.

252. Ochoa JL, Verdugo RJ. Reflex sympathetic dystrophy: a common clinical avenue for somatoform expression. *Neurol Clin North Am* 1995;13(2): 351–363.

253. Bridges K, Goldberg D, Evans B, et al. Determinants of somatization in primary care. *Psychol Med* 1991;21(2):473–483.

254. Fackler SM, Anfinson TJ, Rand JA. Serial sodium amytal interviews in the clinical setting. *Psychosomatics* 1997;38:558–564.

255. Barsky AJ, Wyshak G, Klerman GL, et al. The prevalence of hypochondriasis in medical outpatients. *Soc Psychiatry Psychiatr Epidemiol* 1990;25:89–94.

256. Barsky AJ. Hypochondriasis. Medical management and psychiatric treatment. *Psychosomatics* 1996;37:48–56.

257. Apkarian AV, Bushnell MC, Treede RD, et al. Human brain mechanisms of pain perception and regulation in health and disease. *Eur J Pain* 2005;9: 463–484.

258. Price DD. Psychological and neural mechanisms of the affective dimension of pain. *Science* 2000;288:1769–1772.

CHAPTER 32 ■ THE PSYCHOLOGY OF ADDICTION

LAUREN J. ROGAK, TATIANA D. STARR, KENNETH L. KIRSH, AND STEVEN D. PASSIK

INTRODUCTION

Within the past several decades, the treatment of pain has made remarkable progress.[1,2] Pain assessment and treatment have became priorities of medical care ranks and are focused on attempting to bring relief to the overwhelming population of chronic pain patients.[3,4] Among these many efforts is the use of opioid therapy for the treatment of nonmalignant pain. Even with the potential benefits seen in association with opioid treatment, the pain community's rhetoric tended to trivialize addictions and the intricacy of risk stratification now seen as inherent to the proper delivery of opioid treatment.[5]

The integration of pain management and addiction medicine has been slow in coming. A fundamental inconsistency exists in specialists in addiction, who have a tendency to pinpoint the role of these drugs as a major cause of abuse, and pain specialists, who perceive them as essential medications for pain and suffering. These philosophical differences in these camps emphasizes the historical lack of communication between them.[6]

The gap in communication must be closed, given the significant prevalence and interactions between pain and chemical dependency. A multitude of surveys, both national and international, have shown a prevalence rate for chronic pain as high as 40%.[4] Domestic surveys of substance abuse have reported a prevalence of 6% to 10% of the population who use illicit drugs habitually and one-third have sampled one of these drugs at least once.[7–9] These prevalence rates suggest that clinicians will commonly encounter patients with comorbid pain and drug abuse.[6]

The growth of opioid therapy demands an ongoing evaluation of the associated benefits and risks. The populations are often merged as chronic pain patients are obviously not "immune" to problems of misuse, abuse, addiction, or diversion.[10]

Prevalence of Substance Abuse

It is estimated that 6% to 15% of the United States' population have some type of substance use disorder with approximately one-third having used illicit drugs.[7–9] Additionally, there has been a significant increase in prescription drug abuse over the past decade, with rates rising nearly 94%, from 7.8 million in 1992 to approximately 15.1 million in 2003.[11] The growing rates and high prevalence of prescription drug abuse raises concerns surrounding the use of such medications in the medical setting. When not used properly, opioids and central nervous system stimulants and depressants can be fatal.[12] In 2002, controlled substances were implicated in 30% of drug-related emergency room deaths and 23% of emergency room admissions.[11] According to the National Center on Addiction and Substance Abuse, approximately one-third of prescription drug abusers in 2000 were new users. Between 1992 and 2003, there was a 225% increase in new opioid abusers, 150% increase in new tranquilizer abusers, 127% increase in new sedative abusers, and a 171% increase in new stimulant abusers.[11]

The high prevalence of drug use, generally along with the overwhelming increase in prescription drug abuse, raises concerns regarding the manner in which pain is treated. Chronic pain pa-

tients who have current or remote histories of drug abuse face a number of physical and psychosocial concerns that could potentially affect their medical treatment and pain management. Even when patients do not have a history of abuse, questionable, problematic behaviors may manifest during pain treatment. It is evident that the interface between medical usage of potentially abusable prescription medications and the misuse and abuse of these drugs is complex and must be understood in order to provide optimal patient care.[12]

Definitions

Among the most significant challenges associated with management of substance abuse in chronic pain patients is the lack of clear, consistent terminology.[13] Defining abuse and addiction in medically ill populations can be highly problematic due to the current use of definitions that were originally developed to assess addicted populations without medical illness. The utilization of this terminology can create confusion in the clinical setting for a number of reasons. Many pain patients will be prescribed potentially abusable drugs such as opioids for legitimate medical purposes and subsequently experience the pharmacological phenomena of tolerance and physical dependence after long-term use.[13] This is further complicated by the fact that many clinicians do not specialize in treating cooccurring substance abuse, and often confuse behaviors associated with tolerance and dependance with abuse and addiction.[13] Therefore, it is inappropriate to apply this terminology to chronic pain patients as it further hinders the ability to distinguish between aberrant and appropriate drug-taking behaviors. Improper use of these terms also creates confusion and impedes the communication between the patient and clinician, which is a necessary component of adequate pain management.[12,14] Clarification of this terminology is a critical step in improving pain management and overall patient care.

Tolerance

Tolerance is defined as a pharmacological experience in which an increase in dosage is necessary to maintain the effects of the medication.[15,16] This phenomenon is not necessarily an indication of abuse or addiction, and the experience of tolerance is frequently associated with escalating pain or disease progression.[17–25] Tolerance to nonanalgesic effects (i.e., respiratory depression and cognitive impairment) are often seen in the clinical setting.[26] Tolerance to the analgesic effects of opioids has been reliably observed in animal models; however, analgesic tolerance rarely interferes with the clinical efficacy of opioids.[27] The need to increase the dosage is often indicative of progressing pain.[17,20,23,25,28–30] Clinically relevant analgesic tolerance, the need to increase the dosage without disease progression, seems to be a rare occurrence. There is also little evidence supporting the conclusion that tolerance significantly contributes to the development of addiction.[12]

Physical Dependence

There is considerable confusion among the medical community regarding the differences between physical dependence and addiction. Physical dependence is defined exclusively by the occurrence of a withdrawal syndrome after there is a sudden decrease in dosage or following the administration of an antagonist.[15,16,31] This phenomenon is likely to occur as a result of prolonged use of opioids when the prescribed dosage no longer offers sufficient pain relief. Physical dependence, much like tolerance, has also been conceptualized as a component of addiction[32,33] in that avoidance of withdrawal symptoms potentially lead to behavioral contingencies that reinforce drug-seeking behavior.[34] It is important to note, however, that the experience of physical dependence does not inevitably lead to complications during discontinuation of opioids in patients with nonmalignant pain[35] and cessation of opioid therapy frequently occurs without difficulty in cancer patients whose pain is diminished after completion of antineoplastic therapy. Animal models of opioid self-administration have also provided evidence demonstrating a fundamental distinction between physical dependence and addiction; these models have indirectly shown that persistent drug-taking behavior can continue despite the absence of physical dependence.[36]

Addiction

There are a number of issues surrounding the terms "addiction" and "addict." The confusion caused by using these labels to describe all patients who exhibit questionable drug-taking behaviors can be highly problematic. This is due to the lack of a discernible categorization between individuals who are engaging in aberrant drug-taking behaviors and those that are experiencing tolerance and physical dependence, thus needing to increase their dosage in order to achieve sufficient pain relief.[37] Clinicians and other medical professionals must be mindful in their application of these labels in order to avoid additional confusion. The terms "addict" and "addiction" should never be used in reference to a patient only believed to have the capacity for an abstinence syndrome. The term "physically dependent" is more appropriate in describing such patients. Medical staff should also be careful about using the word "dependent" without specifications toward physical or psychological dependence, which are both elements of addiction. With this in mind, use of the word "habituation" is also discouraged.[12]

Definitions of the terms "addict" and "addiction" should be based on the ability to identify questionable drug-related behaviors that fall outside cultural and societal norms. However, in categorizing aberrant drug-taking behaviors (e.g., escalating dosage or using medication for purposes other than prescribed) as unacceptable according to societal norms, it is not without the assumption that there is a universal understanding of the boundaries of normative behavior. If a significant proportion of patients demonstrate a specific type of behavior it could be considered normative and assessments regarding deviation from this norm would be influenced accordingly. However, in the context of prescription drug use, no empirical data exist that define the parameters of normative behavior. This issue was recently addressed in a pilot study performed at Memorial Sloan-Kettering Cancer Center (MSKCC). Findings indicated evidence concerning patients' attitudes supporting the misuse of drugs in response to symptom management issues. Additionally, women with HIV treated at MSKCC for palliative care were found to engage in aberrant drug-taking behaviors more commonly.[38]

Definition of Addiction in Medically Ill Populations

The prevalence of questionable drug-related behaviors among medically ill populations raises the issue of their predictive validity as an indication of any diagnosis related to substance abuse. Empirical data evaluating patients' drug-taking attitudes are needed to shed light on the prevalence of such behaviors across different medically ill populations.[12] Defining addiction is also complicated by changes that occur as a result of disease progression. It becomes increasingly difficult to establish clear distinctions between deterioration in physical and psychosocial functioning caused by the disease and treatments and the morbid effects of drug use.[12] This could potentially complicate efforts to assess the concept of "use despite harm," which is crucial to the diagnosis of addiction. For example, if a patient develops social withdrawal or changes in cognition following brain irradiation for metastases, it may be difficult to identify the nature of questionable drug-related behavior. Even if the cognitive deficits are associated with the medication used to treat the symptoms, this result might only reflect a small therapeutic window rather than the desire for these psychic effects on the patient's part.[12,14]

As previously mentioned, terminology that fails to distinguish the pharmacologic phenomena of tolerance and physical dependence frequently encountered in chronic pain patients creates additional barriers in identifying and treating addiction. A more suitable definition of addiction should focus on the chronicity of the disorder, characterized by "the compulsive use of a substance resulting in physical, psychological, or social harm to the user and continued use despite that harm."[39] Although this definition was taken from evaluation of addicted populations without medical illness, it addresses that addiction is, in essence, a psychological and behavior syndrome which allows it to flexibly apply to medically ill populations.[12] Concepts such as loss of control and compulsive drug use, as well as continued drug use despite harm, are essential components of an appropriate definition of addiction and should be included.[12] However, even with these ideas incorporated, these definitions still fall short in describing the broad scope of aberrant drug-taking behaviors that arise in the clinical setting.[12]

Pseudoaddiction

Assessing and interpreting drug-taking behaviors in the medical setting can be challenging. Even when there is an appropriate medical indication for drug use, the occurrence of questionable drug-related behavior is at the least an important sign that reevaluation of the patient's drug-taking regimen is necessary. When a drug-related behavior is classified as aberrant, it is important to further evaluate the behavior for a "differential diagnosis." Pseudoaddiction refers to the escalation of dosages in response to insufficient analgesia but with the behavior resolving once adequate pain relief is achieved.[40] Pseudoaddiction may be an appropriate consideration when a patient reports discomfort and distress associated with unremitting symptoms. Continuous requests for higher doses of medication, or sporadic unilateral dose escalation, may initially be perceived as addiction; however, it is likely such behaviors are indicative of desperation resulting from unrelieved pain and will cease once the patient experiences relief.

Pain specialists and addiction specialists have recently combined their efforts to develop a definition of a more universal and acceptable definition of addiction.[6] The following definition is currently endorsed by the American Society of Addiction Medicine, the American Pain Society, and the American Academy of Pain Medicine:

> Addiction is a primary, chronic, neurobiologic disease, with genetic, psychosocial, and environmental factors . . . It is characterized by behaviors that include one or more of the following: impaired control over drug use, compulsive use, continued use despite harm, and craving.[41]

Although this definition can be a helpful reference for clinicians and investigators, further research is necessary in order to empirically differentiate each of the criteria and to demonstrate the predictive validity of the numerous behaviors included in each.[6]

Aberrant Drug-Related Behaviors: Assessment and Differential Diagnosis

The concept of aberrant behavior was first put forward by Portenoy and then expanded on by Passik and Portenoy.[12,42,43] This concept suggests that pain clinicians who prescribe opioids are expected to see varieties of noncompliance behaviors, ranging on scales of commonality and aberrancy. A broad scope of aberrant drug-related behaviors is seen in the clinical setting because opioids and other potentially abusable drugs are prescribed for legitimate medical purposes. These behaviors range from those that are considered mild or limited (e.g., use of a prescribed dose to self-medicate a problem not intended by the clinician, such as insomnia) to severe or overwhelming behaviors (e.g., injection of an oral formulation) and have the potential to predict addiction[6] (Table 32.1). Noncompliance must be spoken about clearly and at length between patients and doctors, because typical signs of addictions are not applicable and may be misleading.[12]

Differential Diagnosis

Once the behaviors are detected, within the spectrum of aberrant drug-related behaviors, a differential diagnosis needs to be formulated so that a response can be made to bring the behavior under control.[6] A differential diagnosis should be explored if questionable behaviors occur during pain treatment (Table 32.2). These potential disorders will benefit from continuous and meticulous evaluation. The major goal of these assessments is to establish the nature of the problem for the overall purpose of developing a therapeutic intervention.[44,45]

Incorporated in the differential diagnosis of aberrant drug-related behaviors is the notion of "pseudoaddiction." An added challenge surfaces when patients have both pain and comorbid

---

TABLE 32.1

ABERRANT DRUG-RELATED BEHAVIORS

Behaviors more suggestive of an addiction disorder
Selling prescription drugs
Prescription forgery
Stealing or "borrowing" drugs from others
Injecting oral formulations
Obtaining prescription drugs from nonmedical sources
Obtaining drugs from multiple medical sources without informing or despite prohibition
Concurrent abuse of alcohol or illicit drugs
Multiple episodes of self-escalation of dose, despite warnings not to do so
Multiple episodes of prescription "loss"
Evidence of functional deterioration unexplained by the pain or other comorbidity
Repeated resistance to changes in therapy despite clear evidence of adverse effects

Behaviors less suggestive of an addiction disorder
Aggressive complaining about the need for more drug
Drug hoarding during periods of reduced symptoms
Requesting specific drugs
Openly acquiring similar drugs from other medical sources
Occasional unsanctioned dose escalation
Unapproved use of the drug to treat another symptom
Reporting psychic effects not intended by the clinician
Resistance to a change in therapy associated with "tolerable" adverse effects
Expression of family concerns

TABLE 32.2

DIFFERENTIAL DIAGNOSIS OF ABERRANT DRUG-RELATED BEHAVIOR

Addiction

Pseudoaddiction

Psychiatric disorders
    Axis 1 disorders (e.g., depression, anxiety, somatoform disorder)
    Axis 2 disorders (e.g., borderline personality, sociopath personality)

Encephalopathy (confusion in dose and interval of prescription)

Criminal intent

---

substance use disorders. An increase in self-reported distress for the lack of pain relief should be considered a marker of pseudoaddiction. An increase in drug-seeking behaviors may occur in those patients with addiction disorders as a result of experiences of uncontrolled pain. This can reflect both addiction and pseudoaddiction. This distinction is one of the most confounding differential diagnoses.[40]

Impulsive drug use may also be unrelated to both addiction and pseudoaddiction. Rather, it may be indicative of the presence of another psychiatric disorder. An example of this is seen in patients with borderline personality disorder who make use of prescription drugs to convey fear, anger, or other expressive emotions and may present with aberrant behaviors. Likewise, patients may self-medicate with opioids to suppress symptoms of anxiety, depression, or insomnia.[6]

In addition to the previously mentioned causes of problematic drug-related behaviors occurring in the clinical setting, there is a litany of more uncommon, yet probable sources seen. One example is that drugs are misused because of a state of confusion. Infrequently, patients will exhibit criminal behavior by selling controlled prescription drugs.[14,44]

The Four A's for Ongoing Monitoring

Recognizing potentially dangerous drug-taking behaviors is an important step toward providing optimal treatment and ongoing pain management. Extensive clinical experience has led to the development of a useful guideline for monitoring chronic pain patients receiving opioid treatment known as the "4 A's." This guideline incorporates the domains of pain relief, side effects, physical and psychosocial functioning, and the presence of any questionably aberrant or nonadherent drug-taking behaviors.[46] These domains are summarized as: (1) analgesia; (2) activities of daily living; (3) adverse side effects; and (4) aberrant drug-taking behaviors.[47] Ongoing monitoring of these domains throughout pain treatment provide clinicians with a framework that informs decision making and fosters adherence to therapeutic use of these controlled substances.[48]

Developing a Therapeutic Approach

As in any therapeutic approach, a comprehensive assessment and strategy must be based on a solid diagnostic foundation. When a clinician chooses to utilize opioid therapy for pain management, the clinician needs to be able to employ the current tenets for prescribing these medications. Additionally, these clinicians must assess each patient for the risks associated with misuse, abuse, addiction, and diversion, with the added responsibility of managing these risks over time. Those people within the chronic pain population who have a history of substance abuse require the prescribing clinician to be proficient in these aspects of treatment.[49]

Chronic pain can be described as nothing less than a multifaceted phenomenon that is often correlated with other symptoms and functional disturbances. Chronic pain is true to its name in its unceasing and unremitting nature. Therefore a cure is not a regular treatment result, but management is. As a result, the goals of therapy center about comfort, functional restoration, and improved quality of life.[6]

Assessment

A multidimensional syndrome, like chronic pain, requires a comprehensive assessment including compiling a history that focuses on the pain complaint, its consequences, prior treatments (e.g., prescribed and nonprescribed), relevant comorbidities, and other elements in a routine history. In regard to the pain itself, intensity, temporal features (e.g., onset, course), location, quality, and provoking or relieving factors should all be taken into account. The impact the pain has on a person's quality of life as well as the physical and psychosocial functioning needs to be accounted for.[6]

In addition to the comprehensive pain assessment, a detailed history of any drug abuse, including duration and frequency, is vital. In patients with a known history of substance abuse, the interview must gather detailed information on the specific pattern of addictive behaviors (e.g., drugs, routes, frequency of administration, means of acquisition, and means of financing). The perceived relationship between these behaviors and the pain should be clarified.[6] Adopting a nonjudgmental stance and using empathic and truthful communication is the best strategy to obtain a complete and honest history.[14,37,44] It is important to note that patients may have a history of misrepresenting their drug use for a variety of logical reasons, such as stigmatization, mistrust of the interviewer, or concerns regarding fears of undertreatment. Thus, there is a need to explain to a patient that the necessity of an accurate account of drug use is to concurrently prevent withdrawal states.[21,44,50]

Barriers to Treatment

Patients may become immersed in a routine where pain functions as a barrier to seeking treatment for addiction, with addiction potentially complicating treatment for chronic pain.[51] Also, as pain is undertreated, a patient's risk of escalating use and being perceived as abusing prescription medications and or other substances increases.[52]

The motivation behind substance abuse in the medical setting differs significantly from the seemingly pleasurable experience associated with social alcohol and even illicit drug use. In the clinical setting, patients' behavior is frequently motivated by avoidance of unpleasant physical experiences (i.e., pain) and the associated emotional consequences. Even though clinical observation demonstrates that addiction is a negative and unpleasant experience, clinicians may still perceive the motivation behind patient drug abuse as a desire to feel "high." The central premise of substance abuse and dependence is the out-of-control use despite the fact that there are substantial health, legal, and social consequences. This form of abuse is a struggle, and not motivated by an attempt to experience pleasure but rather an attempt to avoid experiencing discomfort.[53]

Chemically dependent patients spend a minimal amount of their time experiencing a "high." On the contrary, the majority of the time they feel depressed, isolated, and withdrawn and are often preoccupied with thoughts surrounding their drug use. It is important to recognize that substance abuse still persists despite the fact that there seems to be little reward associated with continued drug use. In addition, many addicts do not abuse drugs that produce feelings of euphoria, and these drugs frequently have unpleasant side effects.[53]

Guidelines for Treatment

There are several principles that can aid the clinician in ascertaining structure control and monitoring of addiction-related behaviors, whether the patients' substance abuse is current or historical.[50] An overarching guideline is to utilize outside consultants, such as pain and palliative care experts, social workers, and mental health professionals for an effective collaboration, or rather a multidisciplinary approach.[14,50]

Employing the widely accepted guidelines for cancer pain management will optimize long-term opioid therapy.[54,55] These stress patient self-report as the foundation for dosing, consistent monitoring, and the individualization of therapy in order to identify a complementary balance between efficacy and side effects,[50] and are valid for the concurrent treatment of side effects as the basis for enhancing the balance between both palliative and adverse effects.[21]

In response to unrelieved pain, aberrant drug-related behaviors may develop if the pain is undertreated. Despite understanding these behaviors as pseudoaddiction, their presence should be taken into serious consideration when prescribing medication.[50] Based on clinical experience, pseudoaddiction can lead patients with a history of substance abuse to genuinely becoming out of control.[56]

Maintaining open lines of communication will uphold a therapeutic environment with constant dialogue, which monitors the development of aberrant drug-taking behaviors. Regular evaluations are necessary for patients who are prescribed drugs with the potential for abuse, in addition to monitoring their behaviors regularly.[44] This is particularly true for those patients with a remote or current history of drug abuse, including alcohol abuse.

All patients with a history of abuse and addiction should be monitored especially closely. Patients who are actively abusing substances should be seen on a more regular basis than those patients who are not.[44,50]

Written agreements are helpful tools in structuring outpatient treatment. These agreements should clearly state the roles of each member of the team and the rules and expectations for the patient. Patients' behaviors should be used as the basis for the level of restrictions, and graded agreements that clearly state the consequences of aberrant drug use should be enforced.[44,50,57]

Within the context of outpatient management, a clinician may choose to refer patients to a 12-step program. This referral must stipulate that documented attendance is a condition for ongoing drug prescriptions.[44,50] Twelve-step programs pose a risk, because the liberal use of opioids may not be supported and the side effects misunderstood despite the patient's terminal status.

In order to endorse compliance and reveal any concurrent use of illicit substances or unprescribed licit drugs, patients with a history of aberrant drug use should be asked to submit to periodic urine toxicology screens. This will determine the early recognition of any aberrant drug-related behaviors. Patients should be provided with a detailed explanation that this is a method of monitoring, which can both reassure the clinician and provide a foundation for aggressive symptom-oriented treatment, thereby enhancing the therapeutic alliance.[44,58]

CONCLUSION

The emergent abuse of prescription drugs has mandated the field to take a new look at opioid prescribing and to seek balance in its risks and benefits. Today, all practitioners involved in pain management have the dual mission of relieving suffering while avoiding contributing to drug abuse and diversion. If all practitioners can become better acquainted with the principles of addiction medicine as they apply to the world of pain management, pain management can be kept safe and available for all who need it. The assessment of aberrant behaviors in patients with chronic pain is one key aspect of mastering these principles.[49]

The problem of prescription drug abuse has been amplified over the past decades. The initial reports that focused on the increasing production and use of opioids was not accompanied by a growth in the abuse and diversion of these drugs had an optimistic tone[59]; however, over time, magnitude of the problem has become more blatant.[49] As a result, it is up to the prescribers to acknowledge that there is a deteriorating environment around opioid use prompted by a significant level of public concern and to therefore follow guidelines meticulously. The problem of prescription drug abuse nationally is only part of the issue however.[49]

It has become well known[60,61] that, at least in the case of cancer patients, those with pain tolerate low levels of pain relief. Understanding the foundation of this level of satisfaction has been qualified by a complex combination of expectations, relationship issues (i.e., not wanting to distract the physician from treating their disease), past experiences with relief of pain, and goals of care.[48] This satisfaction with low levels of pain relief can be traced to the realistic fears of addiction and abuse.[48,49] In general, successful pain management is dependent on a mutual relationship and open communication between doctor and patient. The goal of chronic pain management is to enable people with pain to live a full and rewarding life in the face of chronic illness. As stated previously, however, this is complicated by the problems of drug abuse, addiction, and diversion.

References

1. Berry PH, Dahl JL. The new JCAHO pain standards: implications for pain management nurses. *Pain Manag Nurs* 2000;1(1):3–12.
2. SUPPORT Study Principal Investigators. A controlled trial to improve care for seriously ill hospitalized patients. The study to understand prognoses and preferences for outcomes and risks of treatments (SUPPORT). The SUPPORT Principal Investigators. *JAMA* 1995;274(20):1591–1598.
3. Osterweis M, Kleinman A, Mechanic D, eds. *Pain and Disability: Clinical, Behavioral, and Public Policy Perspectives*. Washington, DC: National Academy Press (Report of the Committee on Pain Disability and Chronic Illness Behavior. Institute of Medicine, National Academy of Sciences); 1987.
4. Verhaak PF, Kerssens JJ, Dekker J, et al. Prevalence of chronic benign pain disorder among adults: a review of the literature. *Pain* 1998;77(3):231–239.
5. Porter J, Jick H. Addiction rare in patients treated with narcotics. *N Engl J Med* 1980;302(2):123.
6. Portenoy RK, Lussier D, Kirsh KL, et al. In: Frances RJ, Miller SI, Mack AH, eds. *Clinical Textbook of Addictive Disorders*. 3rd ed. New York: Guilford Press; 2005:367–395.
7. Colliver JD, Kopstein AN. Trends in cocaine abuse reflected in emergency room episodes reported to DAWN. Drug Abuse Warning Network. *Public Health Rep* 1991;106(1):59–68.
8. Gfroerer J, Brodsky M. The incidence of illicit drug use in the United States, 1962–1989. *Br J Addict* 1992;87(9):1345–1351.
9. Regier DA, Farmer ME, Rae DS, et al. Comorbidity of mental disorders with alcohol and other drug abuse. Results from the Epidemiologic Catchment Area (ECA) Study. *JAMA* 1990;264(19):2511–2518.
10. Friedman DP. Perspectives on the medical use of drugs of abuse. *J Pain Symptom Manage* 1990;5(suppl 1):S2–5.
11. National Center on Addiction and Substance Abuse at Columbia University. *Under the counter: The Diversion and Abuse of Controlled Prescription Drugs in the US*. National Center on Addiction and Substance Abuse at Columbia University; 2005.
12. Passik SD, Olden M, Kirsh KL, et al. Substance abuse issues in palliative care. In: Berger A, Portenoy RK, Weissman DE, eds. *Principles and Practice of Palliative Care and Supportive Oncology*. 3rd ed. Philadelphia: Lippincott Williams & Wilkins; 2007:593–603.
13. Kirsh KL, Whitcomb LA, Donaghy L, et al. Abuse and addiction issues in medically ill patients with pain: attempts at clarification of terms and empirical study. *Clin J Pain* 2002;18:S52–S60.
14. Passik SD, Portenoy RK, Ricketts PL. Substance abuse issues in cancer patients. Part 1: prevalence and diagnosis. *Oncology (Williston Park)* 1998;12(4):517–521, 524.

15. Dole VP. Narcotic addiction, physical dependence and relapse. *N Engl J Med* 1972;286(18):988–992.
16. Martin WR, Jasinski DR. Physiological parameters of morphine dependence in man—tolerance, early abstinence, protracted abstinence. *J Psychiatr Res* 1969;7(1):9–17.
17. Chapman CR, Hill HF. Prolonged morphine self administration and addiction liability: evaluation of two theories in a bone marrow transplant unit. *Cancer* 1989;63:1636–1644.
18. Foley KM. Clinical tolerance to opioids. In: Basbaum AU, Besson JM, eds. *Towards a New Pharmacotherapy of Pain*. Chichester, UK: John Wiley and Sons; 1991:181.
19. France RD, Urban BJ, Keefe FJ. Long-term use of narcotic analgesics in chronic pain. *Soc Sci Med* 1984;19:1379–1382.
20. Kanner RM, Foley KM. Patterns of narcotic drug use in a pacer pain clinic. *Ann N Y Acad Sci* 1981;362:161–172.
21. Portenoy RK. Management of common opioid side effects during long-term therapy of cancer pain. *Ann Acad Med Singapore* 1994;23(2):160–170.
22. Portenoy RK, Foley KM. Chronic use of opioid analgesics in non-malignant pain: report of 38 cases. *Pain* 1986;25:171–186.
23. Twycross RG. Clinical experience with diamorphine in advanced malignant disease. *Int J Clin Pharmacol* 1974;7:187–198.
24. Urban BJ, France RD, Steinberger DL, et al. Long-term use of narcotic/antidepressant medication in the management of phantom limb pain. *Pain* 1986;24:191–196.
25. Zenz M, Strumpf M, Tryba M. Long-term opioid therapy in patients with chronic nonmalignant pain. *J Pain Symptom Manage* 1992;7:69–77.
26. Bruera E, Macmillan K, Hanson J, et al. The cognitive effects of the administration of narcotic analgesics in patients with cancer pain. *Pain* 1989;39(1):13–16.
27. Ling GS, Paul D, Simantov R, et al. Differential development of acute tolerance to analgesia, respiratory depression, gastrointestinal transit and hormone release in a morphine infusion model. *Life Sci* 1989;45(18):1627–1636.
28. Meuser T, Pietruck C, Radbruch L, et al. Symptoms during cancer pain treatment following WHO guidelines: a longitudinal follow-up study of symptom prevalence, severity and etiology. *Pain* 2001;93(3):247–257.
29. McCarberg BH, Barkin RL. Long-acting opioids for chronic pain: pharmacotherapeutic opportunities to enhance compliance, quality of life, and analgesia. *Am J Ther* 2001;8(3):181–186.
30. Aronoff GM. Opioids in chronic pain management: is there a significant risk of addiction? *Curr Rev Pain* 2000;4(2):112–121.
31. Redmond DE Jr, Krystal JH. Multiple mechanisms of withdrawal from opioid drugs. *Annu Rev Neurosci* 1984;7:443–478.
32. Technical report no. 516, youth and drugs. *World Health Organization*. Geneva; 1973.
33. American Psychiatric Association. *Diagnostic and Statistical Manual for Mental Disorders IV*. Washington, DC: Author; 1994.
34. Wikler A. *Opioid Dependence: Mechanisms and Treatment*. New York: Plenum Press; 1980.
35. Halpern LM, Robinson J. Prescribing practices for pain in drug dependence: a lesson in ignorance. *Adv Alcohol Subst Abuse* 1985;5(1–2):135–162.
36. Dai S, Corrigall WA, Coen KM, et al. Heroin self-administration by rats: influence of dose and physical dependence. *Pharmacol Biochem Behav* 1989;32(4):1009–1015.
37. Passik SD, Portenoy RK, Substance abuse issues in palliative care. In: Berger A, Portenoy R, D W, eds. *Principles and Practice of Supportive Oncology*. Philadelphia: Lippincott-Raven Publishers; 1998a.
38. Passik SD, Kirsh KL, McDonald MV, et al. A pilot survey of aberrant drug-taking attitudes and behaviors in samples of cancer and AIDS patients. *J Pain Symptom Manage* 2000;19(4):274–286.
39. Rinaldi RC, Steindler EM, Wilford BB, et al. Clarification and standardization of substance terminology. *JAMA* 1988;259(4):555–557.
40. Weissman DE, Haddox JD. Opioid pseudoaddiction—an iatrogenic syndrome. *Pain* 1989;36(3):363–366.
41. Savage SR, Joranson DE, Covington EC, et al. Definitions related to the medical use of opioids: evolution towards universal agreement. *J Pain Symptom Manage* 2003;26(1):655–667.
42. Portenoy RK. Chronic opioid therapy in nonmalignant pain. *J Pain Symptom Manage* 1990;5(suppl 1):S46–62.
43. Portenoy RK. Opioid therapy for chronic nonmalignant pain: current status. In: Fields HL, Liebeskind JC, eds. *Progress in Pain Research and Management. Vol 1. Pharmacological Approaches to the Treatment of Chronic Pain: New Concepts and Critical Issues*. Seattle: IASP Publicaitons; 1994.
44. Passik SD, Portenoy RK. Substance abuse disorders. In: Holland, JC, ed. *Psycho-oncology*. New York: Oxford University Press; 1998:576–586.
45. Passik SD, Kirsh KL, Whitcomb L, et al. Pain clinicians' rankings of aberrant drug-taking behaviors. *J Pain Palliat Care Pharmacother* 2002;16(4):39–49.
46. Passik SD, Kirsh KL, Whitcomb L, et al. A new tool to assess and document pain outcomes in chronic pain patients receiving opioid therapy. *Clin Ther* 2004;26(4):552–561.
47. Passik SD, Weinreb HJ. Managing chronic nonmalignant pain: overcoming obstacles to the use of opioids. *Adv Ther* 2000;17(2):70–83.
48. Kirsh KL, Passik SD. Managing drug abuse, addiction, and diversion in chronic pain. *Medscape Neurology & Neurosurgery* 2005;7(2).
49. Passik SD, Kirsh KL. Assessing aberrant drug-taking behaviors in the patient with chronic pain. *Curr Pain Headache Rep* 2004;8(4):289–294.

50. Passik SD, Portenoy RK, Ricketts PL. Substance abuse issues in cancer patients. Part 2: evaluation and treatment. *Oncology (Williston Park)* 1998;12(5):729–734; discussion 736, 741–742.
51. Savage SR. Addiction in the treatment of pain: significance, recognition, and management. *J Pain Symptom Manage* 1993;8(5):265–278.
52. Kemp C. Managing chronic pain in patients with advanced disease and substance-related disorders. *Home Healthc Nurse* 1996;14(4):255–261; quiz 262–263.
53. Passik SD, Theobald DE. Managing addiction in advanced cancer patients: why bother? *J Pain Symptom Manage* 2000;19(3):229–234.
54. American Pain Society, ed. *Principles of Analgesic Use in the Treatment of Acute Pain and Cancer Pain.* 5th ed. Glenview, IL: American Pain Society; 2003.
55. US Department of Health and Human Services. Clinical Practice Guideline No. 9. In: Washington DC: US Department of Health and Human Services, ed. *Vol Clinical Practice Guideline No. 9.* Agency for Health Care Policy and Research and Management of Cancer Pain; 1994.
56. Kirsh KL, Passik SD. Palliative care of the terminally ill drug addict. *Cancer Invest* 2006;24:425–431.
57. Fishman SM, Kreis PG. The opioid contract. *Clin J Pain* 2002;18(suppl 4):S70–75.
58. Weaver MF, Schnoll SH. Opioid treatment of chronic pain in patients with addiction. *J Pain Palliat Care Pharmacother* 2002;16(3):5–26.
59. Joranson DE, Ryan KM, Gilson AM, et al. Trends in medical use and abuse of opioid analgesics. *JAMA* 2000;283(13):1710–1714.
60. Dawson R, Spross JA, Jablonski ES, et al. Probing the paradox of patients' satisfaction with inadequate pain management. *J Pain Symptom Manage* 2002;23(3):211–220.
61. Passik SD, Kirsh KL. Re. Probing the paradox of patients' satisfaction with inadequate pain management. *J Pain Symptom Manage* 2002;24(4):361–363.

CHAPTER 33 ■ THE DOCTOR–PATIENT RELATIONSHIP IN PAIN MANAGEMENT: DEALING WITH DIFFICULT CLINICIAN–PATIENT INTERACTIONS

ROBERT N. JAMISON

Pain management physicians commonly have to deal with doctor–patient conflicts because of the nature of persons with chronic pain, the personalities of the pain practitioners who treat them, and added pressures stemming from the health care system. Persons with chronic pain frequently present with psychosocial stressors including sleep disturbances, loss of function, disability issues, and depression, which affect their ability to cope.[1] Medical conditions such as diabetes, hypertension, asthma, gastrointestinal distress, and other comorbidities such as substance abuse and psychiatric disorders make these patients challenging to manage. Chronic pain patients can be time-consuming when doctors are under increasing pressure to see more patients in a shorter amount of time. The need to provide detailed documentation and written justification of each treatment decision and to remain current with the latest treatments adds further time pressure for the pain practitioner. All of these conditions can add to difficulties that set up doctor–patient conflicts.[2]

Between 10% and 60% of patients treated in health care settings exhibit "difficult behavior,"[3–6] which can include extreme aggression, threats of homicide and suicide, and behavior related to substance abuse. Pain patients can be especially difficult since they have a tendency to be angry, mistrustful, anxious, and depressed.[7,8] Depression and anxiety disorders are two to three times more prevalent among chronic pain patients than in the general population,[9,10] and pain patients can frequently present with added behavioral symptoms of inflexibility, negativity, or entitled behavior.

The aim of this chapter is to describe difficult doctor–patient relationships in a pain center or primary care setting and focus on communication issues that may be useful in avoiding treatment dissatisfaction and possible legal reprisals. In this chapter I first review the reasons that patients can be difficult and identify those patients who are prone to exhibit problems. Next, I discuss some of the major issues that lead to doctor–patient conflicts and review possible communication strategies to help the pain specialist successfully manage these patients. Finally, I outline common clinical scenarios leading to potential doctor–patient conflicts and give appropriate responses that may be beneficial in dealing with difficult patients. As implied in the title, this chapter focuses on the doctor–patient relationship, although it should be noted that this same information could easily be applied to any clinician and any person receiving treatment.

DIFFICULT PATIENTS AND DIFFICULT DOCTOR–PATIENT RELATIONSHIPS

In a study of over 500 adults presenting to a primary care clinic, Jackson and Kroenke[6] found that treating physicians rated over 15% of their patients to be difficult. These difficult patients tended to have a depression or anxiety disorder, poor functional status, unmet expectations, reduced satisfaction, and a greater use of health care services. The study also showed that physicians who were less empathic were more likely to experience encounters with these patients as difficult. In a subsequent study, Jackson and Kroenke[11] found that patients' unmet expectations were common in those individuals experienced as difficult by the clinicians. These patients were also likely to have a mental disorder, with somatic symptoms, poorer function status, greater expectations for care, less satisfaction, and higher use of health services than patients who were not difficult ($p<.001$). Every clinician will encounter at least one extremely difficult patient who may require behavioral limit-setting and possible hospitalization and/or psychotropic medication.[12]

Vegni and colleagues,[13] after analyzing difficult doctor-patient relationships, concluded that the doctor's personal and professional issues as well as changes in the health care system are the chief contributors to conflicts. Likewise, Haas and others[2] identified the fact that difficult doctor-patient relationships can be based on (1) patient factors—medical, psychiatric, personality, and substance abuse risk, (2) physician factors—workload, communication skills, personality, level of experience, and practice setting, and (3) the health care system—financial and productivity pressures, fragmentation of care, availability of outside resources, and documentation and treatment guidelines. In a survey of 750 patients and 200 physicians performed by Roper Starch Worldwide Inc.,[14] the qualities of physicians that were most frustrating to patients were being too rushed (30%), hard to reach (19%), and not down to earth (11%). The qualities that described the most difficult patients were hostility or anger (49%), noncompliance (19%), and being too demanding or needy (19%).

Hahn and others[4] developed the Difficult Doctor-Patient Relationship Questionnaire (DDPRQ) and established its reliability and validity. The results of the DDPRQ, completed by physicians who had just concluded a patient encounter, showed that 10% to 21% of patient encounters were labeled as difficult. Most of these patients showed signs of psychosomatic symptoms and psychopathology. In subsequent studies by this same group[5,15] conducted in four primary care clinics, physicians rated 96 patients (15%) out of 627 to be difficult. Compared with patients who were described as not difficult, difficult patients had more functional impairment, higher health care utilization, lower satisfaction with care, and more psychiatric disorders of somatization, panic, dysthymia, anxiety, depression, and alcohol abuse or dependence.

Psychiatric and Personality Issues

Difficult pain patients can display destructive psychiatric behaviors such as suicidal ideation, self-mutilation, extreme noncompliance with treatment, or opioid misuse, and most pain specialists have little training in psychiatric assessment and treatment. Many clinicians avoid pain medicine practice altogether because of the emotional challenge of working each day with demanding and draining patients. Patients with pain can be fearful of flare-ups and worry that their clinic will be unresponsive to the urgency of their condition. Their heightened anxiety adds to a need for frequent contact with their doctors, resulting in endless emails and phone messages. Patient-relations departments of hospitals and the state boards of registration and medical examiners are notified most often by patients who complain that their doctor is unresponsive to their care. As a result, physicians should be watchful about the perception of inadequately treating or abandoning their patients.[16]

Epidemiological studies indicate that 35% of chronic back and neck pain sufferers in the United States have a comorbid depression or anxiety disorder[17] and up to half of all patients with chronic pain can have a comorbid psychiatric condition.[18,19] Further studies also report that patients who are most difficult frequently have a personality disorder, which includes psychotic episodes, impulsivity, superficiality, problems with interpersonal relations, and affective disorders.[20,21] Surveys of chronic pain clinic populations as a whole indicate that 50% to 80% of chronic pain patients have some signs of psychopathology, making this the most prevalent comorbidity in these patients.[10,19] Major depression alone is thought to affect 30% to 50% of patients,[7] with anxiety disorders being next most prevalent.[10,22] Outcome studies highlight the poor response of patients with psychiatric comorbidity to many different treatments for chronic pain,[23] especially those patients with chronic low back pain.[24,25] Boersma and Linton have shown that patients with chronic pain

with a combination of anxiety and depression have a 62% worse return to work rate at 1 year than those with no psychopathology.[26]

Opioid Therapy

Chronic pain patients with a mood disorder are likely to be prescribed opioids more often than those without a mood disorder, which can lead to doctor-patient conflicts. In a study of 50 Veterans Administration (VA) patients and 50 patients treated in outside primary care practices with opioids for noncancer pain, Carrington-Reid and colleagues found a 50% prevalence of major depression and a 20% prevalence of an anxiety disorder.[27] In a similar study, Breckenridge and Clark determined a high prevalence of mood disorder among pain patients who were prescribed opioids.[28] In a study of 191 patients examining factors that led pain physicians to prescribe opioids for noncancer pain, Turk and Okifuji concluded that neither pain severity nor objective physical pathology influenced the decision to prescribe.[29] Rather, greater affective distress and pain behaviors drove the decisions. Thus, patients with chronic pain and psychopathology are likely to be prescribed opioids, and these patients report greater pain intensity, more pain-related disability, and a larger affective component to their pain than those without psychopathology.[30] Patients with borderline and antisocial personality disorders can be commonly found in a pain management clinic. These patients often trigger the strongest negative reaction among their providers.

In terms of the impact of mood disorders on opioid response, a recent study examined the effects of intravenous (IV) opioid analgesia in chronic pain patients with high and low levels of psychiatric comorbidity.[31] Sixty patients with low back pain stratified into three groups of severity of psychological symptoms (low, moderate, and high) were given intravenous morphine and placebo in random order on separate visits and completed pain ratings over 3 hours at each session. The low-psychopathology group had a 40% greater reduction in pain with IV morphine than the high-psychopathology group ($p < .01$). This study found that patients with chronic pain who had a high degree of negative affect benefited less from opioids in controlling their pain than those with a low degree of negative affect.

Difficult "Normal" Patients

Not all patients with difficult behavior exhibit significant psychopathology, such as major depression or anxiety or a personality disorder. Patients who are otherwise "normal" can be perceived as difficult, for example, when they arrive at a pain center for treatment with unrealistic expectations about what should happen. They may have had problems with previous health care settings in which they were accused of exaggerating their pain. Lack of sleep, extreme fatigue, poor eating habits, and long travel to their appointments can also contribute to volatile and unstable behavior. They may experience their physicians as dismissive or skeptical of their pain, rather than being understanding and sympathetic. Even comparatively well-adjusted patients can sometimes develop the idea that their pain physician should be able to eliminate all of their pain and that failure to do so is tantamount to withholding treatment. This becomes critical when medication regimens involving opioids are concerned. Patients may worry about being prescribed adequate amounts of medication or undergoing withdrawal if they are to be tapered off opioids.

Some pain patients are entitled consumers who are no longer willing to be passive in their treatment but rather prefer to take control of their medical care. Medical information through the

Internet is more accessible than ever, and patients frequently come to their appointments armed with information about a particular therapy. Patients are increasingly opinionated about their care. They look to have a mutually respectful relationship with their health care providers and want to take an active role in the decision-making process. They become dissatisfied with their treatment when their provider is unresponsive to their suggestions and not willing to hear their own ideas. Cultural and ethnic differences can also act as barriers to an effective doctor–patient relationship.[32]

Comorbid Medical Conditions

Most persons with chronic pain also have significant medical conditions that impact treatment decisions. Some are medically challenging as well as being interpersonally difficult. Pain patients may report asthma, COPD, diabetes, coronary artery disease, hypertension, ulcers, kidney, bladder and liver problems, and history of cancer. Persons with chronic pain often smoke cigarettes, have gained weight, and have lost bone density. Multiple providers can prescribe multiple medications including blood thinners, blood pressure and heart disease medications, inhalers, and antidepressants. These patients are also noted for allergies and reactions to certain medications. Occasionally they have implanted medical devices (e.g., pacemakers, rods, stimulators) or wear prostheses. Some of the most challenging patients tend to be older, take many medications, have multiple psychosocial problems, have poor social support, limited education, and come from disadvantaged backgrounds.[33,34]

Kenny[35] points out in a survey study of 20 chronic pain patients and 22 pain specialists that differences in communication interactions—especially when patients embrace a medical model to explain their pain and physicians perceive a psychogenic etiology of pain—can significantly negatively affect the doctor–patient relationship. In a study of how and why physicians dismiss patients from their practice, 25 general practitioners identified two types of patients who tend to be dismissed over others: (1) patients who break the rules of the doctor–patient relationship or clinic practice, and (2) patients whose difficult personality makes it hard to care for them.[36]

Substance Use Disorders

There are notable links between chronic pain and substance abuse.[37,38] Studies show that 10% to 16% of patients treated in a general practice and 25% to 40% of hospitalized patients have problems related to drug or alcohol addiction.[39,40] Other studies indicate that patients with pain and high rates of mood disorders are at high risk for alcohol or opioid abuse.[41]

With the growing support of the use of opioid analgesics in the treatment of chronic pain, the United States Government General Accounting Office (GAO) recently recommended efforts to improve identification of abuse and diversion of controlled substances by health care providers.[42] Physicians are now in the difficult position of providing appropriate pain relief while minimizing the inappropriate use of pain medications by being ever watchful of substance use disorders.[43] Inappropriate use can include the following: selling and diverting prescription drugs; seeking additional prescriptions from multiple providers; concurrently using other illicit drugs; and manipulating the formulation to snort or inject the medications or use them in a manner in which they were not intended. It is important for the successful treatment of chronic noncancer pain to be able to frequently monitor patients on opioid regimens and to identify those patients who exhibit ongoing abuse behaviors, which can be an added burden to providers.[44,45]

Unfortunately, physicians can be deceived,[40] which is all the more reason that steps are needed to perform a thorough evaluation for risk factors and to closely monitor patients on opioid therapy. History of substance abuse further complicates treatment because it increases the potential for inadequate treatment of pain.[46] Thus, encounters with patients can be made difficult by underlying issues of substance abuse and addiction.

PHYSICIAN FACTORS

Difficult doctor–patient relationships are not completely due to the patient. The attitudes and behavior of the physicians play an important role as well. Some doctors take patient behavior personally instead of realizing that this is how the patient responds and behaves in other situations as well. An understanding of the patient's situation helps in depersonalizing any reactions that they may experience. Doctors who show disrespect or have inward anger toward their patients transmit negative emotions that lead to distrust. Some physicians have hidden feelings of inadequacy or poor self-esteem and others have an inability to listen to what the patient is saying.[47] Those personality and behavior qualities of doctors can lead to difficult relationships, including inward anger, impatience, lack of empathy, depression, poor self-esteem, and feelings of vulnerability.[48]

For health care providers, treating chronic pain patients can also lead to reactive feelings of being manipulated, which, in turn, can lead to extreme dislike for certain patients.[49] Because physicians are frequently under pressure to see patients within a short period of time, pain patients who show vague symptoms and who are unresponsive to many different interventions can be particularly frustrating, especially when the burden of providing treatment is shouldered alone instead of being shared by an interdisciplinary team. More problematic patient issues, including verbal abuse or physical threats to the clinician and staff, stalking, criminal behavior, and gross noncompliance, can trigger negative reactive emotions in the provider.

Krebs et al.[50] interviewed 1,391 physicians to assess personal and practice characteristics associated with greater frustration with patients. Physicians who were younger, worked more hours, had symptoms of depression and anxiety, were under higher stress, and had more patients with psychosocial and substance abuse problems reported increased frustration with their jobs. Tam[51] points out that pain clinicians may have extensive training in their area of expertise, but have had little instruction in communication skills.

HEALTH CARE SYSTEM FACTORS

Health care system factors also indirectly contribute to doctor–patient conflicts. Physicians frequently report being overworked and under constant pressure to be productive. The demands of the job include reading reports and meticulously documenting treatments. Many have also witnessed changes in health care financing and fragmentation of care. Commercial insurance carriers and the Joint Commission Centers for Medicare and Medicaid Services frequently revise regulations in medical record documentation. Physicians are more than ever being asked to expand their role in the identification and management of psychiatric conditions and addictive disorders.[52] Keeping abreast of the latest pharmacological therapies and screening devices can also be daunting.[53–56] Advances in information technology can radically transform decision-making and treatment processes, although there is no indication of whether they decrease the physician workload.[57,58] It has been suggested that the use of the Internet can have a negative effect on doctor–patient relationships by discrediting conventional therapies, misleading patients, and adding to consultation times.[57] Thus, productivity pressures from hospitals and medical centers, changes in health care financing, threats of legal repercussions related to treatment decisions, fragmentation of care, and the rising use of information technology can place burdens on the provider and add to additional external stress.

PATIENT INTERACTION STRATEGIES

It is surprising to some outsiders when patients cherish their pain provider even though their treatment outcomes are not successful. These patients may openly admit that their pain was made worse by a particular surgery or procedure, but still feel that their doctor did all that could have been done without placing fault or blame on him or her. Conversely, other patients may hold their physician directly at fault for a negative outcome in what they perceive was inadequate or faulty treatment, even though the treatment technique was appropriate without evidence of complications. The differences may lie in the interpersonal skills that the physician used to help deal with the poor outcome, diffusing conflicts and building patient rapport. These same skills may have been lacking in another provider who was accused of causing further problems. Thus, the medical expertise and competence of the clinician is not the only quality needed for acceptance and satisfaction of treatment, regardless of the outcome, but rather the nonspecific effects of the doctor–patient relationship play an important role. Here we review the components of positive doctor–patient relations, especially when dealing with challenging, difficult patients.

Much has been written on useful strategies in dealing with difficult patients, and an exhaustive review of the literature is beyond the scope of this chapter; however, a brief review of some studies will be useful. Elder and colleagues[59] interviewed 102 physicians who were identified as having excellent skills in interacting with difficult patients about how they identified, managed, and coped with these patients. The authors concluded that the key ingredients of changing a difficult encounter into a successful one included the use of empathy, appropriate use of power, and an understanding of the need for doctor–patient collaboration. Lown[60] also proposed strategies to deal with anger in the clinician–patient relationship, suggesting that clinicians who cultivate personal awareness, practice self-monitoring, understand the reasons for patient anger, demonstrate specific communication skills, set clear boundaries, and seek personal support are best at managing difficult patient encounters.

Halpern[49] also describes ways for physicians to manage difficult patients: recognize one's own emotions, attend to negative emotions, attune to patients' verbal and nonverbal emotional messages, and become receptive to negative feedback. These steps allow clinicians to reduce anger through increased empathy and ultimately increase therapeutic impact. Finally, Nasselle[61] felt that, by considering the difficulties in the relationship, doctors would be less prone to labeling patients as difficult. Strategies in managing difficult patients included acknowledging the problem, setting boundaries, using communication skills, and including external resources when necessary.

Patient-Focused Care

In a study on physicians' communication style and perceptions of patients, Street et al.[62] audio-taped and coded interactions among 29 physicians and 207 patients. They concluded that more positive communication from one participant led to similar responses from the other and that reciprocity and mutual influence had a strong effect on quality of care. Klitzman[63] interviewed 50 doctors who had experienced a serious illness in which they were required to be hospitalized as patients. Because of their own experiences as a patient, these physicians acknowledged increased sensitivity to patients' experiences and the importance of empathy in the doctor–patient relationship. They included hospital practice recommendations of charting with the patient present, acknowledging whenever they keep a patient waiting, and being sensitive to nonverbal aspects of care. Their conclusions are in keeping with the differences described by Irwin and Richardson[64] between patient-focused care and a disease-centered model of care. They loosely define patient-focused care as care we would like those we care most about to receive. Having a disease-focused management approach does not exclude having a good bedside manner; however, patient-focused care takes in the whole person's experience in a way that suggests understanding and caring. This point is well illustrated in a study of 316 cancer patients among whom satisfaction with pain management was strongly related to the doctor–patient relationship, and not related to the severity of the pain.[65] Likewise, studies of postoperative satisfaction with pain have been found to be more related to perception of care than actual report of pain.[66,67]

It has been suggested that poor communication style is the underlying problem in most medical–legal cases.[68] In a sample of 45 physician-related plaintiff dispositions, relationship issues appeared to be central to 71% of the lawsuits.[69] In fact, it has been suggested that the majority of negligence cases are not related to quality of care, but are brought on by inadequate doctor–patient communication—often occurring before the incident that leads to a claim.[70] By concentrating more on the medical than the human needs of the patient, there is an increased chance of breakdown in communication and a greater perception of inadequate care. Those physicians who are less prone to legal action demonstrate skills in listening, empathy, and expressing understanding.[68] Gafaranga and Britten[71] believe that the opening statement made by the physician during the first patient encounter may have a lasting impression on the relationship. Roy and others[72,73] have also shown that doctors who inform their patients of changes that impact their care in person rather than by mail have greater patient satisfaction. Back et al.[74] identified some common pitfalls of doctor–patient communication that they label as blocking, lecturing, depending on a routine, collusion, and premature reassurance. They encourage instead employing open-ended communication skills they label as "ask-tell-ask" and "tell me more." Caregivers who show good patient communication skills are ones who speak in a caring way with an open body posture and do not transmit the impression of defensiveness or indifference when they engage in conversation with their patients. Thus, as pointed out in some training programs, the secret of caring for patients is really caring for patients.

Pomm, Shahady, and Pomm[47] suggest that clinicians also need to understand the patient's perspective, attempt to actively listen to their patients, recognize what they can or cannot change, and get help from colleagues and friends for support if problems occur. They describe this as the CALMER approach to dealing with difficult patients (Catalyst for change, Alter thoughts to change feelings, Listen and then make a diagnosis, Make an agreement, Education and follow-up, Reach out and discuss feelings).[46] The literature on stages of change[75,76] also indicate that patients go through stages in which they are more prone to make positive behavioral changes than at other times. Physicians who recognize when a patient is not ready to change, despite the patient's giving lip service to what needs to be done, are less inclined to transmit disappointment when no changes are made.

COMMUNICATION FRAMEWORK: WIPS AND E'S

Different models have been promoted to improve doctor–patient communication. Kathleen Gordon (Connecting with Care, un-

TABLE 33.1

FOUR EXPECTATIONS FOR CLINICAL ENCOUNTERS (WIPS)

All patients want to:
1. Feel **W**elcome
2. Feel **I**mportant and informed
3. Believe their **P**erspective was understood
4. Feel **S**ecure that their needs will be met

TABLE 33.2

COMPONENTS OF EVERY PATIENT ENCOUNTER

1. **Engage** (Build rapport)
   a. Build rapport and professional partnership
   b. Greeting that is pleasant, warm, consistent
   c. Eye contact
   d. Consider barriers
   e. Nonverbal show of interest
   f. Be curious of how patient is doing
   g. Get patient's story with expectations and concerns

2. **Empathize** (Patient feels seen, heard, accepted)
   a. Listen and feed back what you hear
   b. Be aware of feelings, values, and thoughts
   c. Note body language and demeanor
   d. Reflect understanding
   e. Acknowledge and legitimize feelings
   f. Employ humor when appropriate

3. **Educate** (Inform and answer questions)
   a. Assess what the patient understands
   b. Address key concerns–let them know you reviewed their medical record
   c. Answer with compassion–what will happen; who will be there; what are the risks; what are some realistic expectations

4. **Enlist** (Invite the patient's involvement)
   a. Seek the patient's input on the treatment plan
   b. Ask for patient's agreement and active participation
   c. Provide options
   d. Negotiate priorities
   e. Explain what will happen if a problem arises

5. **End**
   a. Anticipate and forecast close of visit
   b. Summarize the encounter
   c. Review the plan and next steps
   d. Express personal confidence, caring, and hope
   e. Follow through

(Modified from Bayer Institute of Health Care Communication, 2001.)

published manual, 2006) identified what she believes are needs and expectations of all pain patients and used the letters WIPS (welcome, important and informed, perspective, and secure) to help remember what all patients expect during each doctor–patient encounter (Table 33.1. First, patients want to feel welcome. They like to believe that their provider is happy to see them and is concerned about their condition. Second, patients want to feel important and to be informed about what is going on and what will take place. The impression that there is mutual respect and collaboration is key to meeting these needs. Third, patients need to believe that their perspective is understood, which necessitates listening skills and body posture that convey a sense of caring. Fourth, the patient wants to feel secure that his or her doctor is competent and knows what needs to be done. To this end, patients like to have the expectation that their needs will be met as well as possible.

The Bayer Institute for Health Care Communication adopted a consensus model for essential elements of physician–patient communication.[77,78] Even if the encounter is brief, those clinicians who follow particular interaction strategies are able to improve patient rapport. These strategies are remembered as the 4 E's: (1) Engage, (2) Empathize, (3) Educate, and (4) Enlist. A revised version is presented in Table 33.2. First the clinician connects with the patient and builds rapport by greeting the patient warmly, having good eye contact, showing interest, and addressing any physical barriers by using nonverbal posturing that improves options for engagement (Engage). Second, the clinician listens to the patient and shows attentiveness by repeating the information back to the patient. The clinician acknowledges feelings and shows understanding. When appropriate, humor is also used (Empathize). Third, the clinician assesses the patient's understanding and informs the patient and answers any questions that might arise in order to address concerns and to alleviate anxiety (Educate). Fourth, the clinician seeks the patient's input about the treatment plan. Priorities are negotiated and different scenarios are discussed in order to address realistic expectations (Enlist). Finally, the clinician ends the encounter by summarizing the plan and outlining the next steps. Reassuring comments as well as positive concerns are expressed. The effective clinician will also be sure to follow through with what was discussed.

CLINICAL SCENARIOS

The following are some common scenarios encountered in a pain management clinic. How the clinician responds to these situations is important in preventing escalating problems and potential litigation. Although at times patients present with a borderline personality disorder or have an underlying substance use disorder, employment of communication techniques can make clinicians more adept at managing these situations and improving outcomes. The following brief scenarios were chosen to address some of the points raised above. As you read them, try and picture what you might do in these situations.

Scenario No. 1

You are seeing a patient for the first time. You begin to ask questions about the patient's medical history. The patient becomes very angry.

PATIENT: "*I sent you all of my records and medical notes. Didn't you even bother to read them? I keep having to repeat myself over and over again.*"
CLINICIAN: "*I am sorry that I have to ask you the same questions as everyone else, but I want to make sure that we do not miss anything. It is also important that I get a fresh look at how you are doing and what the main issues are. The goal is to improve your quality of life as best as possible and your patience and cooperation are important.*"

Main issues: This interaction might happen with a patient who has had many previous problematic contacts with health care providers. The clinician's appearing impatient and demanding will not help the situation. Rather, maintaining an open empathic stance, acknowledging the patient's frustration that the first session may be repetitive and tedious, and showing caring will encourage the patient to cooperate.

As with any initial interview, listening and understanding are vital. It is important to summarize the major concerns and to help reconcile the issues. Many physicians choose to ignore anger for fear that addressing it will bring out more anger or for worry that it will lead to greater time involvement. However, addressing the situation early will pay dividends later on. Appearing impatient or demanding cooperation is an invitation for patient dissatisfaction and increased difficulties later on.

Scenario No. 2

It is late afternoon and you have had several patients in the clinic with time-consuming complications. You are running 1 1/2 hours late. You enter the room to see your next patient and you can tell this patient is very upset about having to wait so long.

CLINICIAN: *"Hello Mrs. Black."*
PATIENT: (noticeably upset) *"I have been waiting a long time and I have to get back home. Can we hurry this up?"*
CLINICIAN: *"I recognize that you have been waiting a long time and I am sorry that you have had to wait so long. I hate it when anyone has to be kept waiting. As with all my patients, I want to spend as much time with you as you need."*

Main points: Apologizing ahead of time for any delay, even if it is for a short period, will acknowledge that you recognize that this person's time is valuable and he or she may be legitimately irritated. Validating the feelings of the patient first helps to defuse the situation. When running late, some clinicians make a point to quickly acknowledge that the patient is there and waiting and to let them know that they will be with them shortly.

Scenario No. 3

A patient is expecting to have a procedure, but the scheduler failed to put it in the schedule. You are running behind, and you can tell that this patient is very upset about the scheduling error.

CLINICIAN: *(Sits down facing the patient with good eye contact and caring body posture).* *"I need to apologize that there has been a mix-up about the schedule. I am afraid that we will not be able to do your procedure today."*
PATIENT: *"What? I have had this appointment for weeks and I brought a friend with me to drive me home. Why can't you just do it?"*
CLINICIAN: *"I can appreciate how upsetting this is especially when you have someone along with you. We simply can't do this today. Mistakes like this don't happen very often, and I am sorry that this happened to you. We will try and sort this out as best we can. I will have the scheduler set up another time as soon as possible."*

Main issues: It is important to reflect the patient's perspective. If a mistake was made, it is always best to admit it and apologize without making excuses or directing the blame at others. Coming up with excuses or reasons for the problem right away without listening would not help to defuse the situation. It is important to use active-listening techniques when patients are angry, including repetition, summary, validation, and empathy. Acknowledging that something will be done to help resolve the situation is important.

Scenario No. 4

A patient who calls and pages you often is pleasant when with you but is extremely disruptive while in the clinic. This patient is known to yell at the schedulers and the receptionist. Your receptionist insists that you speak to this patient.

CLINICIAN: *"Mrs. Smith, I need to speak to you about your behavior in the clinic. I am aware that you get angry and raise your voice with staff at the front desk. We need to follow a protocol in our clinic, which means that everyone must respect each other. We cannot permit shouting or swearing in the waiting room."*
PATIENT: *"But your receptionist has been rude to me and has accused me of coming just to get drugs. I don't put up with that from anybody."*
CLINICIAN: *"The staff here have difficult jobs to do, but we try and treat others with respect by not raising our voice or causing a scene. We expect the same from everyone who is being served here, including you. I am afraid that if you persist in this behavior we will not be able to continue to see you."*
PATIENT: *"I don't have a problem with you, doctor. But I can't stand some members of your staff."*
CLINICIAN: *"Whether you like them or not, you cannot be disruptive while you are here."*

Main issues: Some providers have difficulty in setting limits with difficult patients, but this is a case when firm limit-setting is needed. Stating that it is difficult to work with anyone who is disruptive in the clinic and identifying the expected behaviors without showing anger or being demanding or blaming is best. For patients who are very disruptive in the waiting room, inviting them to come to a clinic room and to meet to discuss the issues privately would help to prevent further escalation of behavior.

Scenario No. 5

An elderly patient becomes combative and delusional following a procedure. This patient requires sedation and restraints. Family members see this patient in restraints and are very angry.

FAMILY MEMBER: *"What are you doing to my mother? Is this a hospital or a prison? You should have notified us first. I want to transfer care to another facility."*
CLINICIAN: *"I can see why you would be upset seeing your mother in restraints. I want to reassure you that she is being cared for with her safety in mind."*
FAMILY MEMBER: *"But this can't be the way you are supposed to handle patients."*
CLINICIAN: *"I am sorry that you are upset, but we are doing this for her own safety. We try and take the greatest care with all our patients. Although your mother has been experiencing some of the effects of the medication, she will be fine."*

Main issues: It is important to be reassuring and matter of fact without reacting in a negative way. By acknowledging how the person may be feeling and checking to see if this is accurate, you allow the person to share his or her feelings. Helping the person to get some understanding of what is happening and why things are done according to protocol can also be valuable.

Scenario No. 6

A middle-aged man develops an infection following the implantation of a device. His goal was to decrease his opioid medication. Now he has more pain, is taking more opioids, and is very angry at the outcome. He returns with his wife and demands to know what will be done for his pain.

PATIENT: *[Noticeably angry and upset]* *"I am a lot worse off now since that failed procedure. What are you going to do about my pain?"*
CLINICIAN: *"I know that you had hope that this would help your pain, and it must be frustrating that you are experiencing more pain. Having a set-back like this is difficult for all of us. We need to work together to get you back to a better state."*

PATIENT: *"But things are even worse now than ever."*
CLINICIAN: *"I wish we could be 100% successful every time, but unfortunately that is not the case. I am afraid that this did not work out as we expected, but we will keep working on this and hopefully we will be able to turn this around soon."*

Main issues: In this case, underneath the anger, the patient is worried that he will be abandoned, and acknowledging this fear and worry as well as offering some reassurance is important. At first, allowing the patient to vent and express anger without becoming defensive or being angry in return can set the stage for greater partnership in the treatment process. It is important to speak slowly and calmly and to clarify expectations of treatment and limitations in the treatment process. Spending time with an angry patient despite levels of discomfort and helping to get the patient to commit to maintaining a mutual relationship in the treatment process are also important.

Scenario No. 7

A 42-year-old man was referred for treatment of his chronic back pain. He had two back surgeries following a work-related injury and has been taking opioids for his pain. His primary care provider has been prescribing his medication, and he was referred because he had been running out of his medication early and had an abnormal urine toxicology screen. This patient was seen on follow-up after having completed a comprehensive set of screening questionnaires, a structured interview with a psychologist, and a toxicology screen.

PATIENT: *"My doctor referred me to you because she no longer wants to write for my pain medication. She thinks that you should take over writing for my pain medication since you are at a pain center."*
CLINICIAN: *"Your interview and questionnaire information suggest that you are at high risk for having problems with opioids. This means that we will need to be very cautious. So, if I manage your medication I am going to have to require that you see me every 2 weeks, sign an opioid contract, give a urine screen once a month, and participate in substance compliance counseling. We may also find in the end that you are not a good candidate for opioids to treat your pain."*
PATIENT: *"You are just punishing me for being truthful about my drug history. Don't you realize that I have real pain and I need pain medication?"*
CLINICIAN: *"If you have heart problems I would not be giving you treatments that would cause problems for your heart. Your test results suggest that these medications can be a problem for you, and as a result we need to be very careful—for your sake and ours."*

Main issues: The physician does not talk down to the patient or accuse him of being a drug abuser, but instead educates him about the best course of treatment for someone with his risk factors. The suggestion is that there must be an up-front doctor–patient agreement and that cooperation will be needed. Ultimately the physician is expressing the final authority to decide what will be the best course of treatment.

SUMMARY AND CONCLUSIONS

Many things can contribute to patient conflicts when treating chronic pain: personality disordered patients, a busy work schedule, and ever-demanding regulations all can create problematic encounters. Despite the many patient factors that contribute to doctor–patient conflicts, some clinicians know how to recover from difficult patient interactions without long-term repercussions. Much is due to their skills in interpersonal relations and the

effects these skills have on patients' perception of their caregiver. Certain patients are difficult because of issues of psychiatric comorbidity and a substance use disorder, but the doctor's use of tested interpersonal communication skills can help to prevent the escalation of conflicts. It is important to have access to mental health professionals who can assist in working with the most difficult patients. Increased coordination and adequate communication among the other providers is also important. Ultimately, the employment of positive communication strategies can improve doctor–patient relations and minimize conflicts within a pain management practice.

ACKNOWLEDGMENT

Special thanks are extended to Kathleen Gordon and Edith Mariano from the Patient Family Relations Triaging Program, Brigham and Women's Hospital, for their invaluable assistance, and to the patients and staff of the Pain Management Center, BWH, Boston for their inspiration and support. Thanks also to Jaylyn Olivo for reviewing an earlier draft of this chapter.

References

1. Wasan AD, Wootton J, Jamison RN. Dealing with difficult patients in your pain practice. *Reg Anesth Pain Med* 2005;30:184–192.
2. Haas LJ, Leiser JP, Magill MK, et al. Management of the difficult patient. *Am Fam Physician* 2005;72:2063–2068.
3. Erb J. Assessment and management of the violent patient. In: Jacobson JL, Jacobson AM, eds. *Psychiatric Secrets*. 2nd ed. Philadelphia: Hanley & Belfus, Inc; 2001:440–447.
4. Hahn SR, Thompson KS, Wills TA, et al. The difficult doctor-patient relationship: somatization, personality and psychopathology. *J Clin Epidemiol* 1994; 47:647–657.
5. Hahn SR. Physical symptoms and physician-experienced difficulty in the physician-patient relationship. *Ann Intern Med* 2001;134:897–904.
6. Jackson JL, Kroenke K. Difficult patients encounters in the ambulatory clinic: clinical predictors and outcomes. *Arch Intern Med* 1999;159:1069–1075.
7. Fishbain DA, Cutler RB, Rosomoff HL, et al. Chronic pain-associated depression: antecedent or consequence of chronic pain? A review. *Clin J Pain* 1997; 13:116–137.
8. Sansone RA, Whitecar P, Meier BP, et al. The prevalence of borderline personality among primary care patients with chronic pain. *Gen Hosp Psychiatry* 2001; 23:193–197.
9. Holroyd KA. Recurrent headache disorders. In: Dworkin RH, Breitbart WS, eds. *Psychosocial Aspects of Pain: A Handbook for Health Care Providers.* Seattle, Wash: IASP Press; 2004:370–403.
10. Fishbain DA. Approaches to treatment decisions for psychiatric comorbidity in the management of the chronic pain patients. *Med Clin North Am* 1999; 83:737–760.
11. Jackson JL, Kroenke K. The effect of unmet expectations among adults presenting with physical symptoms. *Ann Intern Med* 2001;134:889–897.
12. Ward RK. Assessment and management of personality disorders. *Am Fam Physician* 2004;70:1505–1512.
13. Vegni E, Visioli S, Moja EA. When talking to the patient is difficult: the physician's perspective. *Commun Med* 2005;2:69–76.
14. What Americans really want from their doctor: Roper Starch survey results reveals what patients want and how they feel about whey they're getting. *Business Wire.* July 19,1996. Available at: http://findarticles.com. Accessed January 24, 2008.
15. Hahn SR, Kroenke K, Spitzer RL, et al. The difficult patient: prevalence, psychopathology, and functional impairment. *J Gen Intern Med* 1996;11:1–8.
16. Hoffmann DE, Tarzian AJ. Achieving the right balance in oversight of physician opioid prescribing for pain: the role of state medical boards. *J Law Med Ethics* 2003;31:21–40.
17. Von Korff M, Crane P, Lane M, et al. Chronic spinal pain and physical-mental comorbidity in the United States: results from the National Comorbidity Survey Replication. *Pain* 2005;113:331–339.
18. Dersh J, Gatchel R, Polatin P, et al. Prevalence of psychiatric disorders in patients with chronic work-related musculoskeletal pain and disability. *J Occup Environ Med* 2002;44:459–468.
19. Katon W, Egan K, Miller D. Chronic pain: lifetime psychiatric diagnoses and family history. *Am J Psychiatry* 1985;142:1156–1160.
20. Sansone RA, Sansone LA. Borderline personality disorder. Interpersonal and behavioral problems that sabotage treatment success. *Postgrad Med* 1995;97: 169–171, 175–176, 179.
21. Koekkoek B, van Meijel B, Hutschemaekers G. "Difficult patients" in mental health care: a review. *Psychiatr Serv* 2006;57:795–802.

22. Koenig TW, Clark MR. Advances in comprehensive pain management. *Psychiatr Clin North Am* 1996;19:589–611.
23. Nelson DV, Novy DM. Self-report differentiation of anxiety and depression in chronic pain. *J Pers Assess* 1997;69:392–407.
24. Evers AW, Kraaimaat FW, van Reil PL, et al. Cognitive, behavioral and physiological reactivity to pain as a predictor of long-term pain in rheumatoid arthritis patients. *Pain* 2001;9:139–146.
25. Harkins SW, Price DD, Braith J. Effects of extraversion and neuroticism on experimental pain, clinical pain, and illness behavior. *Pain* 1989;36:209–218.
26. Boersma K, Linton SJ. Screening to identify patients at risk: profiles of psychological risk factors for early intervention. *Clin J Pain* 2005;21:38–43.
27. Carrington-Reid M, Engles-Horton LL, Weber MB, et al. Use of opioid medications for chronic noncancer pain syndromes in primary care. *J Gen Intern Med* 2002;17:173–179.
28. Breckenridge J, Clark JD. Patient characteristics associated with opioid versus nonsteroidal anti-inflammatory drug management of chronic low back pain. *J Pain* 2003;4:344–350.
29. Turk DC, Okifuji A. What factors affect physicians' decisions to prescribe opioids for chronic noncancer pain? *Clin J Pain* 1997;13:330–336.
30. Passik SD, Kirsch KL, Whitcomb RK, et al. A new tool to assess and document pain outcomes in chronic pain patients receiving opioid therapy. *Clin Ther* 2004;26:552–561.
31. Wasan AD, Davar G, Jamison RN. The association between negative affect and opioid analgesia in patients with discogenic low back pain. *Pain* 2005;117:450–461.
32. Schouten BC, Meeuwesen L. Cultural differences in medical communication: a review of the literature. *Patient Educ Couns* 2006;64:21–34.
33. Schwenk TL. Caring about and caring for the psychosocial needs of patients. *J Fam Pract* 1987;24:461–463.
34. Crutcher JE, Bass MJ. The difficult patient and the troubled physician. *J Fam Pract* 1980;11:933–938.
35. Kenny DT. Constructions of chronic pain in doctor-patient relationships: bridging the communication chasm. *Patient Educ Couns* 2004;52:297–305.
36. Stokes T, Dixon-Woods M, McKinley RK. Breaking up is never easy: GPs' accounts of removing patients from their lists. *Fam Pract* 2003;20:628–634.
37. Ballantyne JC, LaForge KS. Opioid dependence and addiction during opioid treatment of chronic pain. *Pain* 2007;129:235–255.
38. American Psychiatric Association. *Diagnostic and Statistical Manual of Mental Disorders.* Washington, DC: American Psychiatric Association; 1994.
39. Kissen B. Medical management of alcoholic patients. In: Kissen B, Begleiter H, eds. *Treatment and Rehabilitation of the Chronic Alcoholic.* New York: Plenum Publishing; 1997.
40. Brown RL, Leonard T, Saunders LA, et al. The prevalence and detection of substance use disorders among inpatients ages 18–49: an opportunity for prevention. *Prev Med* 1998;27:101–110.
41. Jamison RN, Kauffman J, Katz NP. Characteristics of methadone maintenance patients with chronic pain. *J Pain Symptom Manage* 2000;19:53–62.
42. Office of Applied Studies. *Results from the 2003 National Survey on Drug Use and Health: National Findings.* Substance Abuse and Mental Health Services Administration; 2004.
43. Hampton T. Physicians advised on how to offer pain relief while preventing opioid abuse. *JAMA* 2004;292:1164–1166.
44. Savage SR. Assessment for addiction in pain treatment settings. Clin *J Pain* 2002;18:S28–S38.
45. Michna E, Ross EL, Hynes WL, et al. Predicting aberrant drug behavior in patients treated for chronic pain: importance of abuse history. *J Pain Symptom Manage* 2004;28:250–258.
46. Webster LR, Webster RM. Predicting aberrant behaviors in opioid-treated patients: preliminary validation of the Opioid Risk Tool. *Pain Med* 2005;6:432–442.
47. Pomm HA, Shahady E, Pomm RM. The CALMER approach: teaching learners six steps to serenity when dealing with difficult patients. *Fam Med* 2004;36:467–469.
48. O'Boyle M. Reactions to difficult patients. *Psychosomatics* 1998;29:368.
49. Halpern J. Empathy and patient-physician conflicts. *J Gen Intern Med* 2007;22:696–700.
50. Krebs EE, Garrett JM, Konrad TR. The difficult doctor? Characteristics of physicians who report frustration with patients: an analysis of survey data. *BMC Health Serv Res* 2006;6:128.
51. Tam M, Su M. How to manage difficult patients. 2006. Available at: http:/vitualis.workpress.com. Accessed November 19, 2007.
52. Hogan MF. The President's New Freedom Commission: recommendations to transform mental health care in America. *Psychiatr Serv* 2003;54:1467–1474.
53. Fiellin DA, O'Connor PG. Clinical practice. Office-based treatment of opioid-dependent patients. *N Engl J Med* 2002;347:817–823.
54. Willenbring ML, Olson DH. A randomized trial of integrated outpatient treatment for medically ill alcoholic men. *Arch Intern Med* 1999;159:1946–1952.
55. Weisner C, Mertens J, Tam T, et al. Factors affecting the initiation of substance abuse treatment in managed care. *Addiction* 2001;96:705–716.
56. Friedmann PD, Zhang Z, Hendrickson J, et al. Effect of primary medical care on addiction and medical severity in substance abuse treatment programs. *J Gen Intern Med* 2003;18:1–8.
57. Broom AF. The influence of the internet on patients' expectations. *Nature Clin Pract Urol* 2006;3:117.
58. Jamison RN, Fanciullo GJ, Baird JC. Computer and information technology in the assessment and management of patients with pain. *Pain Med* 2007;8:S83–S84.
59. Elder N, Ricer R, Tobias B. How respected family physicians manage difficult patient encounters. *J Am Board Fam Med* 2006;19:533–541.
60. Lown BA. Difficult conversations: anger in the clinician-patient/family relationship. *South Med J* 2007;100:40–42, 62.
61. Nisselle P. Difficult doctor-patient relationships. *Aust Fam Physician* 2000;29:47–49.
62. Street RL Jr, Gordon H, Haidet P. Physicians' communication and perceptions of patients: is it how they look, how they talk, or is it just the doctor? *Soc Sci Med* 2007;65:586–598.
63. Klitzman R. Improving education on doctor-patient relationships and communication: lessons from doctors who become patients. *Acad Med* 2006;81:447–453.
64. Irwin RS, Richardson ND. Patient-focused care: using the right tools. *Chest* 2006;130:73S–82S.
65. Dawson R, Spross JA, Jablonski ES, et al. Probing the paradox of patients' satisfaction with inadequate pain management. *J Pain Symptom Manage* 2002;23:211–220.
66. Jamison RN, Ross MJ, Hoopman P, et al. Assessment of postoperative pain management: patient satisfaction and perceived helpfulness. *Clin J Pain* 1997;13:229–236.
67. Kannan S, Jamison RN, Datta S. Maternal satisfaction and pain control in women electing natural childbirth. *Reg Anesth Pain Med* 2001;26:468–472.
68. Hegan T. The importance of effective communication in preventing litigation. *Med J Malaysia* 2003;58(Suppl A):78–82.
69. Piasecki M. *Clinical Communication Handbook.* New York: Blackwell Publishing; 2002.
70. Levinson W, Roter DL, Mullooly JP, et al. Physician-patient communication. The relationship with malpractice claims among primary care physicians and surgeons. *JAMA* 1997;277:553–559.
71. Gafaranga J, Britten N. "Fire away": the opening sequence in general practice consultations. *Fam Pract* 2003;20:242–247.
72. Roy MJ, Kroenke K, Herbers JE Jr. When the physician leaves the patient: predictors of satisfaction with the transfer of care in a primary care clinic. *J Gen Intern Med* 1995;10:206–210.
73. Roy MJ, Herbers JE, Seidman A, et al. Improving patient satisfaction with the transfer of care. A randomized controlled trial. *J Gen Intern Med* 2003;18:364–369.
74. Back AL, Arnold RM, Baile WF, et al. Approaching difficult communication tasks in oncology. *CA Cancer J Clin* 2005;55:164–177.
75. Prochaska JO, DiClemente CC. *The Transtheoretical Approach: Towards a Systematic Eclectic Framework.* Homewood, Ill: Dow Jones Irwin; 1984.
76. Kerns RD, Rosenberg R, Jamison RN, et al. Readiness to adopt a self-management approach to chronic pain: the Pain Stages of Change Questionnaire (PSOCQ). *Pain* 1997;72:227–234.
77. Keller VF, Carroll JG. A new model for physician-patient communication. *Patient Educ Couns* 1994;23:131–140.
78. Makoul G. Essential elements of communication in medical encounters: the Kalamazoo consensus statement. *Acad Med* 2001;76:390–393.

CHAPTER 34 ■ JOINT PAIN

GREGORY C. GARDNER

This chapter contains a discussion of the common causes of joint pain encountered in clinical practice. These are osteoarthritis (OA), rheumatoid arthritis, the spondyloarthropathies (ankylosing spondylitis, psoriatic arthritis, and reactive arthritis), and crystalline forms of arthritis (gout, pseudogout). In addition, there will be a brief discussion of two other types of rheumatologic disorders that present as joint pain: septic arthritis and polymyalgia rheumatica.

BASIC CONSIDERATIONS

Problem in Perspective

Data from the Centers for Disease Control and Prevention (CDC) indicate that, as of 2003, 43 million U.S. adults were affected by some form of arthritis (21% of the population) and it was the leading cause of disability in the U.S.[1] Self-reported arthritis is least common in Hawaii (17.9% of the survey sample) and highest in West Virginia (37.2%). By 2030, 67 million adults in the United States will be affected representing 20% of the projected population.[2] Women are more likely to report a musculoskeletal problem and are more often limited by its presence. The overall cost of musculoskeletal disease to the U.S. economy was estimated to be $86 billion in 2003 but numbers as high as $254 billion have been used as well.

Musculoskeletal disease is a worldwide phenomenon. In recognition of this, the Bone and Joint Decade was proposed by the United Nations in 1999 and formally launched on January 13, 2000, in Geneva, Switzerland, at the headquarters of the World Health Organization. The aim of the initiative is to raise the awareness of the increasing societal impact of musculoskeletal injuries and disorders; empower patients to participate in decisions about their care; increase funding for prevention activities and research; and promote cost-effective prevention and treatment of musculoskeletal injuries and disorders worldwide.[3] The official Bone and Joint Decade in the United States is from 2002 to 2011.

Joint Anatomy

Joints in the extremities are synovial (diarthrodial) joints that permit movement over a wide range[4] (Fig. 34.1). The joint is held together by a capsule of dense fibrous tissue and ligaments, and gains further support from overlying muscle and tendons. The inner surface of the joint capsule is covered by synovium, which consists of an intimal layer of specialized cells called *synoviocytes*, and an outer layer of highly vascularized connective tissue. Synoviocytes comprise one to three cell layers and are of two basic types, A and B. Type A synoviocytes are active in phagocytosis and type B cells synthesize hyaluronate, which is responsible in large part for the high viscosity of normal synovial fluid. Synovial fluid in a normal joint lubricates the surfaces of synovium and cartilage. The synovium is folded along the inside of the joint capsule and does not cover the load-bearing surface of articular cartilage. The connective tissue layer of synovium blends with periosteum, which does not cover the bone within the joint. The synovium has a rich network of capillaries, venules, and lymphatics and it is innervated by sympathetic nerve fibers. The knee and the sternoclavicular and radiocarpal joints contain discs of fibrocartilage that help to stabilize these joints when they rotate. The intervertebral facet joints are diarthrodial joints and are covered by synovium.

Amphiarthrodial joints are only slightly movable and include the symphysis pubis and the joints between vertebral bodies. The joint surfaces are separated by intervertebral discs. The sacroiliac joint has elements of both a diarthrodial and an amphiarthrodial joint.

Articular cartilage is composed of type 2 collagen and proteoglycans. Type 2 collagen is unique to joints and provides cartilage with form and tensile strength. Proteoglycan molecules are linked noncovalently to a long chain of hyaluronic acid and are interwoven within the network of collagen fibers. Proteoglycan molecules bind most of the water present in cartilage, which represents approximately 70% of the total weight of articular cartilage. The proteoglycan molecules are constrained within the meshwork of collagen fibers and are responsible for the resiliency of cartilage. Chondrocytes secrete collagen, proteoglycans, and enzymes that degrade the cartilaginous matrix. The process of remodeling and degradation is kept in balance unless the microenvironment of these cells is altered. Joints normally contain a small amount of synovial fluid, which is viscous, clear, and does not clot spontaneously. Normal synovial fluid contains fewer than 200 cells per cubic millimeter; most of these cells are mononuclear.

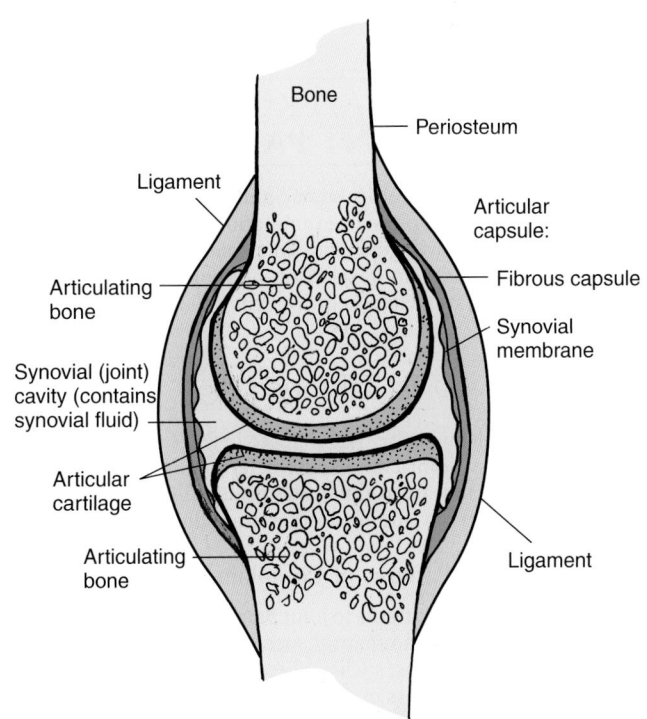

FIGURE 34.1 Schematic diagram of the anatomic features of a typical synovial joint seen in a section cut across the middle of the joint. (From Oatis CA. Kinesiology. *The Mechanics and Pathomechanics of Human Movement.* Baltimore: Lippincott Williams & Wilkins, 2003.)

Nerve and Blood Supply

Joints are supplied partly by articular nerves, which are branches of major peripheral nerves, and partly by branches of nerves supplying adjacent muscles as well as vasomotor sympathetic fibers. Nerve endings are distributed in the interstitial and perivascular tissue located in the subsynovium fibrous capsule, articular fat pads, and in the adventitial sheaths of arteries and arterioles supplying the joints. The periosteum is innervated, but articular cartilage and subchondral bone are not and, thus, not a direct source of pain in arthritis.

There are four types of receptors that supply joints.[5] Type I receptors are ovoid corpuscles with a thin connective tissue capsule and each is supplied by a small myelinated nerve fiber (5–8 mm in diameter) that arborizes within the capsule. The type I receptor occurs almost exclusively in the fibrous joint capsule, acts as a slowly adapting mechanoreceptor (stretch receptor), and resembles both structurally and functionally the Ruffini endings in the dermis. The type II receptor is approximately twice as large as the type I receptor and is supplied by a somewhat thicker myelinated fiber (8–12 mm in diameter) that usually ends as a single terminal within a rather thick laminated capsule. These receptors, which resemble the pacinian corpuscles, occur only in the fibrous joint capsule and have been shown to be rapidly adapting mechanoreceptors (acceleration receptors) that are sensitive to rapid movements. Type III receptors, which are the largest, are supplied by thick myelinated fibers that branch profusely. These receptors, which resemble the Golgi organs, are present in extrinsic and intrinsic ligaments (and not in the joint capsule) and adapt slowly and at high thresholds. Type IV receptors are represented by plexuses of fine unmyelinated fibers that occur in the fibrous joint capsules, ligaments, and subsynovial capsules and fat pads; they are considered to be the joint nociceptors.

An anastomotic plexus of blood vessels called the *periarticular anastomosis*, together with these nerves, surrounds the capsule and its branches penetrate the capsule. The periarticular anastomosis is fed by branches of arteries passing the joint and is the source of blood to the capillary bed in the synovial membrane and also to the epiphysis.

CLINICAL APPROACH TO JOINT PAIN

A variety of disorders, both systemic and local, cause joint pain. A history and a careful physical examination should be performed on each patient that will guide the clinician in developing a differential diagnosis and help in selection of appropriate laboratory and radiographic studies to help confirm a diagnosis.

History

The musculoskeletal history is composed of three parts: determining the pattern of joint complaints, determining the number of joints involved, and ascertaining the presence of other features that might help in developing a differential diagnosis.

Patterns of Complaints

There are three basic patterns to joint pain common to the rheumatologist. These are inflammatory, mechanical, and fibromyalgic. Inflammatory conditions, such as rheumatoid arthritis, are characterized by joint stiffness in the morning lasting at least 30 minutes but often several hours. Patients generally feel better after activity as the fluid accumulated during inactivity is pumped out of a swollen, stiff joint by the lymphatics, thus reducing the sensation of stiffness. The presence of inflammatory cytokines such as interleukin-1 (IL-1) or tumor necrosis factor (TNF) may cause fatigue, anorexia, or a loss of the sense of well-being. Joints may initially be stiff and painful but invariably become swollen. There is a subtype of inflammatory pain caused by the presence of bacteria, blood, or crystals. These conditions have an acute or subacute onset and cause severe pain. The affected person keeps the joint at 30 to 40 degrees of flexion and resists movement. This is the position of maximum joint volume and attempts to flex or extend the joint leads to decreased joint volume and, thus, increased joint fluid pressure. Pain is typically severe in these forms of arthritis.

Mechanical joint pain, typified by osteoarthritis, generally causes only 5 to 10 minutes of morning stiffness but affected joints become progressively more painful with activity. There may be discomfort for some period of time following use. Swelling may or may not be present or only present following stress. There are no systemic symptoms in patients with mechanical forms of arthritis.

Fibromyalgic pain is characterized by all over morning stiffness or pain, a period of loosening up late morning or early afternoon, followed by fatigue and increased pain as the afternoon progresses. Sleep is poor, memory may be reported to be poor, and activity and exercise are poorly tolerated and in fact patients will report being in bed for 1 or 2 days following a strenuous physical or even emotional event. Doing household chores may exacerbate the discomfort. Patients often describe their pain in dramatic terms such as hot pokers or ice picks being driven into a particularly painful area.

With experience, the clinician can with some ease categorize a patient's joint complaints into one of these three major types.

Number of Joints Affected

The next step in developing a differential diagnosis is determining the number of joints involved. There are three categories in joint number as well and include monoarthritis, pauciarthritis (2–5 joints affected), and polyarthritis (6 or more joints). Tables 34.1 to 34.3 give a general differential diagnosis based on inflammatory or mechanical joint pain pattern and number of joints involved. It is important to recognize that these are general guidelines because a polyarticular condition such as rheumatoid arthritis might initially present with less than six affected joints but progress over time to be polyarticular in character. Once a disease has been established for several weeks/months, these patterns tend to be more fixed.

TABLE 34.1

IMPORTANT CAUSES OF MONOARTHRITIS

Inflammatory	Mechanical
Infection	Osteoarthritis
Neisseria gonorrhoeae	Osteonecrosis
Other bacteria (especially Staphylococcus)	Trauma
Tuberculosis	Tumor
Fungi	
Lyme disease	
Crystals	
Monosodium urate	
Calcium pyrophosphate	
Hydroxyapatite	
Hemarthrosis	
Clotting disorder	
Anticoagulation therapy	
Trauma (ACL tear)	

TABLE 34.2

IMPORTANT CAUSES OF PAUCIARTHRITIS

Inflammatory	Mechanical
Infection *Neisseria gonorrhoeae* Other bacteria	Osteoarthritis
Crystals Monosodium urate	
Spondyloarthropathies Ankylosing spondylitis Psoriatic arthritis Reactive arthritis	
Miscellaneous Sarcoidosis Polymyalgia rheumatica	

TABLE 34.3

IMPORTANT CAUSES OF POLYARTHRITIS

Inflammatory	Mechanical
Infection Parvovirus Rubella Hepatitis C Hepatitis B Post-streptococcal arthritis	Osteoarthritis Hemochromatosis Acromegaly Ochromosis
Autoimmune diseases Rheumatoid arthritis Systemic lupus erythematosus Sjögren's syndrome Other autoimmune diseases (i.e., scleroderma)	
Miscellaneous Serum sickness	

Systemic Features of Arthritis

A variety of systemic or demographic features of illness also provide clues to the underlying diagnosis and will be discussed with the individual conditions.

Physical Examination

When evaluating a patient with musculoskeletal complaints, it is important to determine whether the joint complaint is articular, periarticular, or radiating from elsewhere. Joints should be examined for evidence of synovial proliferation, fluid, and bony enlargement. Tenderness, warmth, and any limitation of range of motion should be noted. Pain on passive motion of a joint suggests the possibility of inflammation in the joint or periarticular structures. Even though a patient may complain of a particular joint or joints, make sure to examine all joints. Milder abnormalities that may be present could provide useful information to make a diagnosis. Comparing an affected to a nonaffected joint often confirms the presence of swelling or deformity. Remember that "joint pain" may be the result of tendon, ligament, muscle, bone, or nerve abnormalities.

Examination of Synovial Fluid

Examination of the joint fluid is helpful in patients who have undiagnosed arthritis. Diagnosis of infectious or crystal-induced arthritis is established only by examination of joint fluid. Characteristics of the joint fluid in various rheumatic conditions are shown in Table 34.4. In inflammatory effusions, the cell count is usually elevated, with predominantly neutrophils. The fluid is cloudy, has reduced viscosity, and forms a fibrin clot. Normal joint fluid does not spontaneously clot because it contains no fibrinogen. Viscosity is reduced in inflammatory arthritis because of the breakdown of hyaluronate. A rough assessment of viscosity

TABLE 34.4

JOINT FLUID CHARACTERISTICS IN VARIOUS FORMS OF ARTHRITIS

Diagnosis	Appearance	Mucin clot[a]	White blood count (per mm³) leukocytes	% Neutrophils
Normal	Clear, straw colored	Good; firm	<200	<25
Osteoarthritis	Straw colored	Good; firm	<2000	<25
Rheumatoid arthritis	Yellow	Fair to poor; friable	5000–25,000 or greater	>65
Gout or pseudogout	Yellow, slightly cloudy	Fair to poor; friable	2000–75,000	>70
Spondylo-arthropathies	Yellow, slightly cloudy	Fair to poor; friable	2000–75,000	>50
Bacterial arthritis	Cloudy to purulent	Poor; friable	10,000, often >100,000	>75

[a]Mucin clot correlates with viscosity except with grossly purulent fluid.

can be made by forcing a drop of fluid through the end of the syringe. Fluid with poor viscosity drops like water. In normal joint fluid or noninflammatory conditions, a string trails the drop; the longer the string, the higher the viscosity.

Normal joint fluid usually contains fewer than 200 white cells per cubic millimeter and these cells are predominantly mononuclear. Cell counts greater than 75,000 per cubic millimeter and in which the cells are predominantly neutrophils suggest an infectious arthritis, but cell counts of this magnitude are also seen in noninfectious inflammatory joint diseases such as reactive arthritis or urate gout.

CLINICAL CONSIDERATIONS

Osteoarthritis

Osteoarthritis (OA) is characterized by progressive loss of articular cartilage leading to joint pain and limitation of movement. Weight-bearing and frequently used joints are most often affected. The disease is divided into a primary (idiopathic) form in which no predisposing factors are apparent and a secondary form that is associated with trauma, a metabolic disorder, or a congenital abnormality. Primary OA is the more common form but pathologically, the two forms are indistinguishable.

Epidemiology and Pathophysiology

OA is the most common form of arthritis worldwide and is the leading cause of disability in seniors.[6] The disease occurs in all races and geographic areas. Prevalence and severity increase with age. Under age 55 years, the frequency and joint distribution of OA in men and women are approximately the same. After age 55 years, OA of the knee is more common in women and OA of the hip in men.[7] OA can be demonstrated radiographically in almost all persons over the age of 75.[8] Weight-bearing joints such as the hips, knees, feet, and cervical and lumbosacral joints are most often affected. The distal and proximal interphalangeal (PIP) joints of the hands are also commonly involved. Certain occupations have been shown to predispose a person to OA. In coal miners, for example, OA of the shoulders and knees is more frequent, presumably because of the forces placed on these joints during work. Prize fighters are more likely to develop OA of their metatarsophalangeal joints, football players of their knees, and ballet dancers of their ankles. Hereditary factors also exist: Heberden's nodes (osteophytic deformity of the distal interphalangeal joints) are twice as frequent in mothers of affected persons and three times more frequent in sisters.[9] A single point mutation in the cDNA coding for type II collagen was found in family members with an inherited form of OA associated with a mild chondrodysplasia.[10,11] Previous major trauma and repetitive use of a joint increase the risk of developing OA. Age alone is a risk factor, with the prevalence of OA increasing after age 45 years. Obesity has been shown to be a definite risk factor for developing OA of the knees.[12,13]

The process of OA in the joint is well known. The cartilage initially shows fissuring and pitting, which eventually progress to erosions and denuded areas. The proteoglycan content of cartilage and the number of chondrocytes decrease in proportion to the degree of disease. Subchondral bone becomes thickened and has an eburnated, or ivory-like, appearance. Cysts appear in the subchondral bone, and the formation of new bone at the joint margins produces osteophytes or spurs. The synovium is thickened and contains a modest infiltration of lymphocytes, plasma cells, and an occasional multinucleated giant cell. The joint capsule and ligaments are hypertrophied. Figure 34.2 shows the progressive nature of OA in the knee via arthroscopy.

For many years treatment approaches to OA have focused on cartilage. To date no chondroprotective agent has been approved by the U.S. Food and Drug Administration even though several, such as doxycycline, have shown promise in animal studies. There is no data in human trials that they make an impact on the disease course. As one can imagine, such trials are difficult to do from a time perspective given the slowly progressive nature of the disease. Recently it has been argued by Felson and Kim that what is needed is a shift in our thinking about the approach to OA in general.[14] To successfully solve the problem of OA, a more global approach will be needed; that is, focus on intra- as well as extraarticular processes such as joint alignment, muscle strength, and other issues that influence loading forces across the joint.

Symptoms and Signs

OA may be limited to one or two joints or may occur in a generalized form involving many joints. Involved joints are stiff for 30 minutes or less in the morning and after periods of inactivity and pain develops with use. The involved joints often ache at night, and the ache can keep the patient awake. Night pain is caused in part by increased intraosseous venous pressure. As the disease progresses, pain becomes a constant feature of physical activity and can persist for several hours afterward. Eventually, restricted motion and joint deformities develop.

Primary OA most frequently affects the distal interphalangeal joints, the first carpometacarpal (CMC) joint, the scaphotrapezoid joint, the hips, knees, and first metatarsophalangeal (MTP) joint. The spine may also be affected, particularly the cervical and lumbar areas. *Heberden's nodes* usually develop after age 40 and are associated with OA of the distal interphalangeal joints. Similar nodes, called *Bouchard's nodes*, appear at the PIP joints (Fig. 34.3). At times, these nodes become red and painful to touch. Bony enlargement, small effusions, restricted motion, and angulation can be seen on physical examination. Radial subluxation of the first CMC joint gives a square appearance to this joint (shelf sign). A form of OA, referred to as *primary generalized OA*, appears most often in middle-aged women and affects the distal interphalangeal and proximal interphalangeal joints of the hand, the first CMC joint, knees, hips, and the first MTP joint. Episodes of inflammation are characterized by warmth, pain, and swelling of these joints.

OA of the hip is usually unilateral, but the opposite side is also affected in approximately 20% of patients.[15,16] Congenital or developmental abnormalities such as slipped capital femoral epiphysis, Legg-Calvé-Perthes syndrome, or hip dysplasia underlie many of the cases. OA follows avascular necrosis, which can be related to deep-water diving, glucocorticosteroid therapy, alcohol, or sickle cell disease. Hip pain is experienced in the groin, over the greater trochanter, in the buttock, or down the anterior and inner thigh. Pain might be referred to the distal thigh and upper knee because the obturator nerve and its branches supply both hip and knee. Hip disease can be mistaken for knee arthritis or trochanteric bursitis because hip pain can be referred to those locations. The pain of hip disease is often described as dull and aching and is initially experienced with physical activity. Later, night pain is also experienced. Patients might limp and have difficulty rising from a sitting position. Functional shortening of the leg caused by adduction and flexion contractures causes the patient to walk with a shuffling gait. Examination of the hip shows initially decreased internal rotation that is followed later by decreased extension, abduction, and flexion, as well as a flexion contracture.

The cause of OA of the knee is not known in most patients. Previous injury such as a torn meniscus or ligament predisposes the knee to secondary OA. The presence of an alignment abnormality such as genu varum (bow legs) or genu valgum (knock

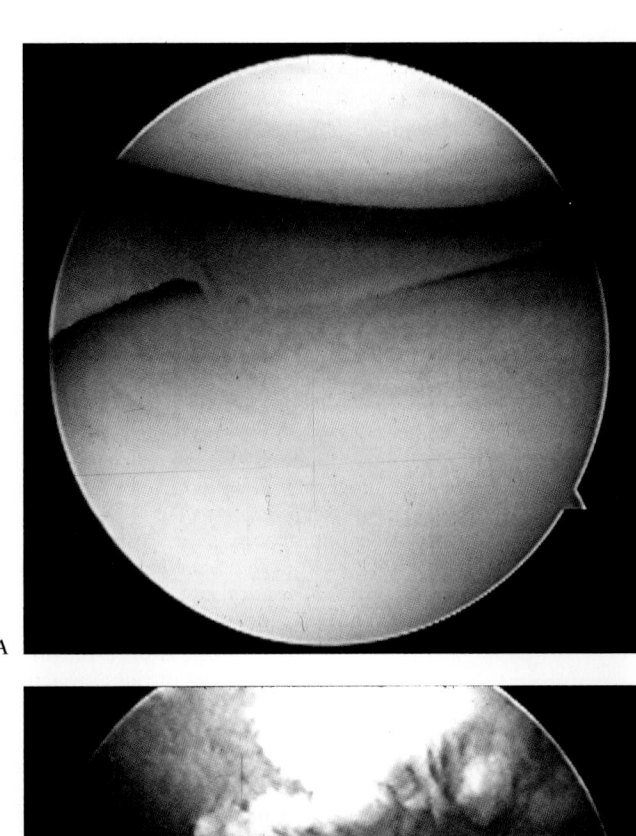

A

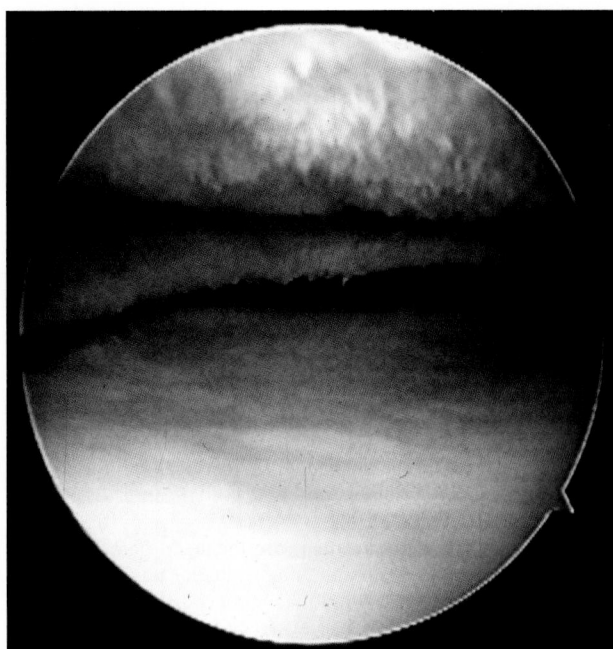

B

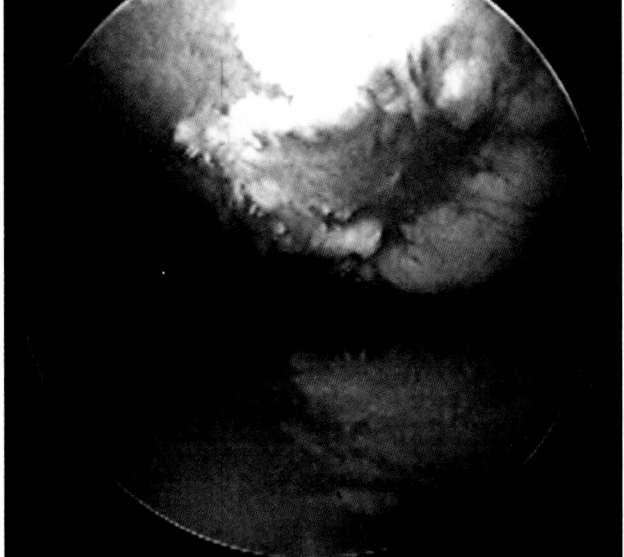

C

FIGURE 34.2 Progression of OA of the knee via arthroscopy. (**A**) Normal appearing knee. Note the smoothness of the articular cartilage of the femur as well as the meniscus. (**B**) Thickening and fissuring of the cartilage and meniscus. (**C**) Advanced OA of the knee with bare areas devoid of cartilage and loss of meniscal tissue.

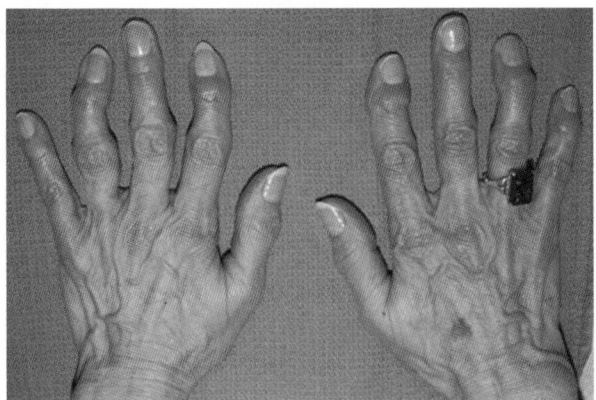

FIGURE 34.3 Osteoarthritis of the hands. Note Heberden's nodes (DIP joints) and Bouchard's nodes (PIP joints) in this patient with classic hand OA.

knees) increases the force directed through either the medial or lateral side of the knee and can lead to OA. These deformities are also acquired in OA as a result of destruction of either the medial or lateral articular cartilage. Obesity predisposes the knees to OA by the additional weight and by the thigh thickness, which places the legs in a genu varus position and increases the pressure on the medial compartment. Pain also can be localized to either the medial or lateral aspect of the joint depending on which compartment is primarily involved. Stiffness lasting less than 30 minutes is present in the morning or after prolonged rest during the day. Stiffness improves with activity but might return later in the day. Atrophy and weakness of the quadriceps muscle develop with progression of the arthritis. Crepitus might be noted with bending of the knee as well as an effusion. With more severe disease, a contracture may be present which increases the energy required to stand upright. With loss of ligamentous and muscle support, the knee becomes unstable, and the patient may be hesitant to walk on uneven surfaces. The knee might suddenly give way because of a pain reflex. A loose cartilaginous fragment, sometimes referred to as a *loose body*, can prevent the joint from being fully extended.

Patellofemoral arthritis occurs alone or in conjunction with arthritis of the other knee compartments, especially in older patients. The term *chondromalacia patellae* is often used interchangeably with patellofemoral arthritis, although some restrict this term to a self-limiting disorder occurring in adolescents and young adults. Patellofemoral arthritis is caused in some patients by improper tracking of the patella through the patellofemoral groove (trochlea). The patella is pulled to the lateral margin of the groove by a tight lateral patellar retinaculum or a relative weakness of the vastus medialis compared with the vastus lateralis of the quadriceps muscle. Lateral subluxation of the patella can also be caused by rotational malalignment of the femur and tibia.

In the spine, intervertebral discs and apophyseal (facet) joints are sites for OA. Involvement of intervertebral discs is referred to as *spondylosis*, whereas disease in the apophyseal joints is considered true OA. OA also affects the joints of Luschka (uncovertebral joints), which are located in the cervical spine between the superior process of one vertebral body and the inferior process of the vertebral body above it.

Symptoms of spine involvement are localized pain and stiffness, referred or dermatomal pain, and radicular pain from nerve root compression. Nerve root involvement produces paresthesias, decreased sensation, loss of muscle strength, and diminished or absent deep tendon reflexes. OA of the cervical spine causes either localized pain or pain referred to the occiput, shoulder, interscapular area, or arm, depending on the level affected. With upper cervical disease the pain tends to be referred to the occiput, and with lower cervical involvement it is referred to the shoulder, upper arm, or interscapular area. Neurologic manifestations are also caused by compression of the spinal cord by posteriorly directed osteophytes and by occlusion of the anterior spinal artery by a herniated disc. Cervical spine diseases are discussed in Chapter 67; lumbar spine in Chapters 71 through 75.

Secondary Osteoarthritis

OA can develop in joints that have been damaged. A torn knee meniscus or ligament can lead to incongruity of the joint surfaces resulting in OA. In addition, ligaments contribute to proprioceptive input and injury to these structures may increase the risk of developing OA.[17] OA may follow joint damage produced by infectious arthritis or an inflammatory arthritis such as rheumatoid arthritis. Neuropathic joint disease is a severe form of OA resulting from the loss of pain sensation, proprioception, or both.[17,18] Without these protective mechanisms, joints are subjected to repeated trauma, leading to progressive cartilage damage. Diabetes is the most common cause of neuropathic joint disease. Other causes include tabes dorsalis, syringomyelia, amyloidosis, meningomyelocele in children, and leprosy.

OA occurs in patients with excessively hypermobile joints. Patients with Ehler-Danlos syndrome, a hereditary disorder of connective tissue, develop OA of their hands, shoulders, knees, and ankles usually before age 40 years.[19] Debate exists regarding whether patients with idiopathic joint hypermobility are at risk of developing premature OA.[17]

Several metabolic disorders are associated with the development of OA. These include hemochromatosis, ochronosis, and acromegaly. Arthritis occurs in 20% to 50% of patients with hemochromatosis and may appear before other overt clinical manifestations.[20,21] Hands, knees, and hips are most commonly affected. A particularly characteristic finding is involvement of the second and third metacarpophalangeal (MCP) joints, which are rarely affected in primary OA. Ochronosis is a rare disorder caused by a hereditary deficiency of homogentisic acid oxidase, leading to accumulation of homogentisic acid in connective tissue. Deposits of homogentisic acid impart a blue-black hue to the sclerae and external cartilage of the ears. Arthritis appears in

middle age and involves most often the knees, shoulders, hips, and spine.[22] Approximately 60% of patients with acromegaly develop OA, which most often involves the spine, knees, hips, shoulders, and, occasionally, ankles.[23] The increased growth of articular cartilage causes joint surface incongruity and abnormal wear.

Laboratory Findings

Routine laboratory work is normal in patients with primary OA. If OA is found in unusual locations (MCP joints) or unusually early, unusual metabolic diseases or trauma may well be the case. In particular check for parathyroid hormone abnormalities with a PTH level and for hemochromatosis with iron studies (TIBC and FE with saturation level). The synovial fluid in OA is straw colored and has good viscosity. The cell count is usually less than 2000 white cells per cubic millimeter and the cells are predominantly mononuclear. Radiographs in early OA are usually normal, but as the disease progresses joint space narrowing, subchondral bone sclerosis, subchondral cysts, and osteophytes are observed (Fig. 34.4). Erosive OA is characterized by erosions on the joint surface, sclerosis of subchondral bone, and later by bony ankylosis. Radiographic abnormalities do not always correlate with clinical symptoms.

Treatment

Think about the treatment of OA as a program especially when the weight-bearing joints are involved. Basically the program consists of three parts: physical modalities, medications, and surgery. The goal in OA should not necessarily be 100% pain relief as no pain in a biomechanically abnormal joint may not be a good thing. The goal should be to reduce pain to a level that promotes quality of life and activity.

Physical modalities include education, weight loss if needed, joint protective aerobic exercises, range of motion exercises especially focusing on reduction of contractures, muscle strengthening exercises, assistive devices such as a cane, and attempts to affect alignment with off-loading knee braces or patellar taping if needed. The Arthritis, Diet, and Activity Promotion Trial demonstrated the benefit of promoting both exercise and weight loss in an 18-month program that examined both together versus either one alone.[24] The control group was healthy lifestyle. The combination group lost more weight than the weight loss group alone (5.7% of body weight vs. 4.9%) and the combination group had a 24% improvement in physical functioning and a 30% decrease in knee pain over the study period. The exercise group only showed improvement in walk time while the weight loss group showed no significant improvement in any of the variables related

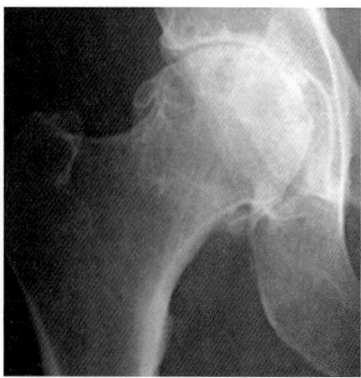

FIGURE 34.4 Osteoarthritis of the hip. The features of OA are well illustrated in this x-ray including joint space narrowing, subchondral cysts, osteophytes, and subchondral sclerosis (thickening of the bone where cartilage has been lost)

to the arthritis. Correct use of a cane can off-load a joint by up to 24% and has been shown to reduce pain in OA of the hip or knee. There is evidence for a modest benefit with the use of an off-loading knee brace designed to realign either a varus or valgus knee disalignment.[25]

The first-line pharmacologic therapy for OA is over-the-counter analgesics (e.g., acetaminophen, 1000 mg four times a day, or even less if it is effective). If the patient remains symptomatic after 2 to 4 weeks, low-dose ibuprofen or nonacetylated salicylates are indicated. If the response is still inadequate after 2 to 4 weeks, the patient should be placed on a full dose of a nonsteroidal drug. In the patient with risk factors for upper gastrointestinal (GI) bleeding or ulcer disease, a proton pump inhibitor should also be provided. There is one COX-2 inhibitor currently marketed in the United States (celecoxib) that could be used for patients at significant risk of GI bleeding if other options do not work. Because of a concern for cardiac toxicity from the COX-2 agents, use the recommend dose of no more than 200 mg per day. There was for a time some excitement about glucosamine based on a European trial published in *the Lancet* in 2001.[26] The data suggested not only a clinical benefit over placebo but also a possible disease modification of OA. A more recent U.S. five arm trial (glucosamine, chondroitin, combination, NSAID, and placebo) did not demonstrate an impressive effect of either nutraceutical in OA although the placebo response was impressive.[27]

Intra-articular corticosteroid injections are effective in OA and can be used as part of the overall program. How often can injections be given? For many years these were limited due to the concern about the development of Charcot joints. Again, the comments about not being too effective in controlling pain completely should be remembered. Data suggested that corticosteroid injections can be given every 3 months for at least 2 years with clinic benefit but no structural change. In the absence of data, injections should probably not be given more frequently than this.[28] Injectable hyaluronic acid is approved for use in OA of the knee. A recent meta-analysis of data on hyaluronic acid injections in knee OA suggests a small benefit especially for the higher molecular weight compounds.[29] Treatment with hyaluronic acid requires 3 to 5 injections and can be used in patients who fail more conservative therapy.

When a joint is severely damaged and painful, joint replacement should be considered. Total hip replacement has provided dramatic relief of pain and improvement of function. Placement of a knee or shoulder can also be quite helpful. Correction of a valgus or varus deformity by osteotomy of the knee improves weight distribution and extends the functional life of the joint. Rebuilding the first CMC joint and replacement of the PIP joint with a prothesis are now possible. Surgery is generally suggested for patients with a level of pain that is not controlled with physical modalities or medications and the patient is willing to endure a period of hospitalization and physical therapy.

Rheumatoid Arthritis

Rheumatoid arthritis is an inflammatory polyarthritis of unknown etiology and typically involves peripheral joints in a symmetric distribution. The worldwide prevalence varies from 0.097 to 2.900 per 1000.[30] In the United States, the prevalence is 1% to 2%.[31] Women are more commonly affected; the average ratio is 3:1. An association also exists with HLA-DR4, the prevalence being 48% to 59% in persons with this genetically determined antigen compared with 8% to 16% in the general Caucasian population.[32,33] Even though there is a genetic association, only 15% of the disease process is placed on genes as opposed to factors from the environment.

Etiology and Pathophysiology

Even though the etiology of rheumatoid arthritis remains unknown, significant advancements have been made in the understanding of the inflammatory events leading to joint injury and extraarticular manifestations. The hallmark of rheumatoid arthritis is the proliferation of synovium, which spreads over the articular surface as a pannus and damages cartilage, bone, and joint capsule. Harris has classified the pathophysiology of rheumatoid arthritis into four phases.[34] Stage I is characterized by the presentation of an as yet unknown antigen or antigens to T cells. In stage II, proliferation of T and B cells, as well as synovial angiogenesis, occurs. In stage III, synovial hypertrophy begins and neutrophils accumulate within the joint in response to chemotactic factors produced by the fixing of complement and the production of cytokines by macrophages and synoviocytes such as tissue necrosis factor-α, interleukin-1 (IL-1) and -6, and granulocyte macrophage cell-stimulating factor. Of interest, cytokines from macrophages and synoviocytes are present in abundance in the rheumatoid joint but typical T-cell cytokines such as IL-2 and interferon-γ are notably absent in established disease. Finally, stage IV is characterized by pannus formation and joint destruction.

B cells in the synovium have been shown to synthesize immunoglobulins, some of which have anti-IgG (rheumatoid factor) activity. Immune complexes consisting of IgG and anti-IgG form in the joint fluid and activate the complement system, which results in the formation of vasoactive and chemotactic factors. Polymorphonuclear white cells attracted to the joint by chemotactic factors phagocytize these immune complexes and secrete proteolytic enzymes within the synovial fluid. The most common form of rheumatoid factor is an IgM molecule directed against the *Fc* portion of IgG. IgG and IgA rheumatoid factors can also be found in patients with rheumatoid arthritis, and IgA rheumatoid factors in particular have been noted to be associated with more severe disease.[35]

The etiology of rheumatoid arthritis is uncertain, but research for many years has focused on the possibility of an arthrotropic infectious disease either triggering the inflammatory cascade or persisting in some form in the joint. An interesting piece of evidence is that rheumatoid arthritis was rare in the Old World before European exploration of the New World and seems to have appeared in Europe after this period.[36] Rheumatoid arthritis has been diagnosed via skeletal remains in certain Native American populations antedating the age of exploration, leading some to speculate that the disease is a New World phenomenon that was transmitted back to the Old World.

Symptoms and Signs

The typical patient with rheumatoid arthritis is a young to middle-aged woman who presents to her physician with a history of 2 to 3 months of joint pain and stiffness in her hands. Constitutional symptoms of fatigue, weight loss, and low-grade fever might also be present. The hands and other involved joints are stiff on arising in the morning. Stiffness might last from 30 minutes to 2 hours or longer. In severe disease, the patient might remain stiff most of the day.

Patients with involvement of the hands and wrists might have difficulty performing tasks such as lifting pots, washing their hair, and opening jars or doors. A firm handshake can be quite painful. Tingling and numbness of the thumb and index and middle fingers, which often occur at night, indicate compression of the median nerve by synovial tissue in the carpal tunnel (carpal tunnel syndrome). At times, the carpal tunnel syndrome produces pain radiating up the forearm and down into the hand. Rheumatoid arthritis can begin in the feet in the MTP joints. It is not unusual for a patient to attribute metatarsalgia to improperly fitting shoes before seeking medical attention.

On physical examination, the joints are swollen, tender to palpation, and warm but not hot. The combination of synovial proliferation and fluid gives the joint a boggy sensation on palpa-

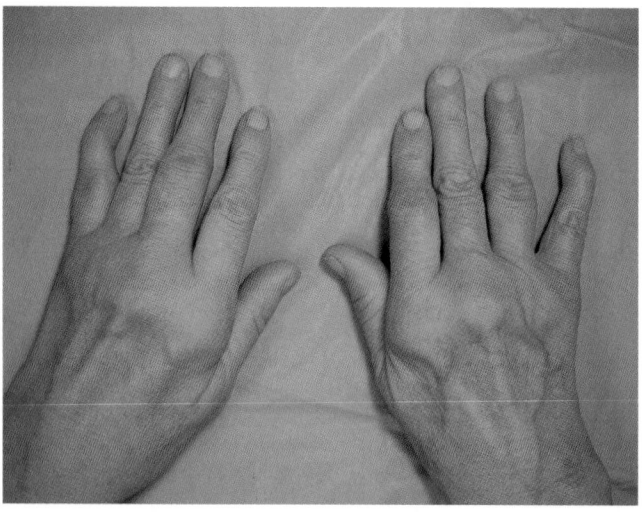

FIGURE 34.5 Example of rheumatoid arthritis of the hands. DIP joints are spared while the MCP and PIP joints are swollen. There is beginning to be some early ulnar deviation on the left hand.

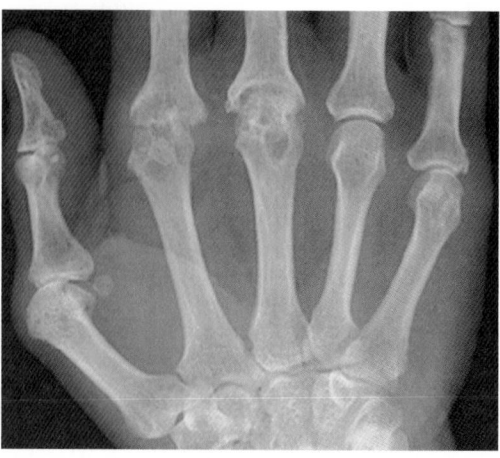

FIGURE 34.6 X-ray of rheumatoid arthritis of the right hand. Note the erosions and joint space narrowing at the second and third MCP joints.

tion (Fig. 34.5). Synovial proliferation in the flexor tendons of the fingers fills in the palm, giving it a flat appearance. The skin over the small joints often has a bluish discoloration resulting from venous engorgement. The hands may be cool and clammy. The range of joint motion is initially limited by pain and later by contractures. Ulnar deviation of the fingers at the metacarpal phalangeal joint is a common deformity in established disease and results from radial deviation of the wrist and slippage of the extensor tendons to the ulnar side of the MCP joints. Another common deformity of the hand that develops in chronic disease is the swan-neck deformity. This appearance results from flexion of the distal interphalangeal joint and MCP joint with hyperextension of the PIP joint. The boutonniere deformity is caused by avulsion of the extensor hood over the PIP joint, leading to a flexion deformity of this joint and hyperextension of the distal interphalangeal joint. In advanced disease, subluxation and flexion deformities are common and involve the knees, ankles, elbows, wrists, shoulders, hands, and feet.

The course of rheumatoid arthritis is highly variable. Fifteen percent of patients have complete remission, whereas 10% or less go on to destructive disease that responds poorly to all forms of therapy. Most patients fall between these two groups with variable periods of remission and relapse. Some patients experience significant disability, whereas others respond to treatment and function quite well throughout their lifetimes. Prognostic factors for more severe disease include the presence of high titers of rheumatoid factor, elevated cyclic citrullinated peptide (CCP) (see next section), presence of HLA-DR4, and more joints initially involved.

Laboratory Findings

Patients often have a normocytic normochromic anemia and an elevated erythrocyte sedimentation rate (ESR). Approximately 80% of patients have a positive rheumatoid factor test result. In the last several years, the CCP has emerged as an important diagnostic and prognostic test. It detects the presence of antibodies to citrullinated peptides and is 75% sensitive and 96% specific for rheumatoid arthritis. The higher levels are correlated with more erosive disease and may appear before overt arthritis has appeared.[37] Radiography in early disease reveals only juxta-articular osteopenia and soft tissue swelling. In more advanced disease one finds narrowing of joint spaces, erosions at the mar-

gins of the joint, and eventually subluxation (Fig. 34.6). The synovial fluid usually has a white blood cell count that varies from 5000 to 25,000 cells per cubic millimeter (most of the cells are neutrophils), decreased viscosity, and a low glucose level although this is rarely measured anymore (see Table 34.4).

Treatment

The treatment of rheumatoid arthritis has undergone considerable rethinking over the years. The time-honored approach to the treatment of rheumatoid arthritis has been based on the *pyramid*, in large part because of the philosophy that rheumatoid arthritis was a disabling but otherwise benign disease. Via the treatment pyramid, patients would receive nonsteroidal anti-inflammatory drugs (NSAIDs) or salicylates along with education and physical and occupational therapy and, as the disease progressed, more aggressive therapy with immunomodulating drugs known as DMARDs (disease modifying antirheumatic drugs) of increasing toxicity would be used. In 1965, up to 120 months would pass before a DMARD would be started.[40] A majority of patients with rheumatoid arthritis develop erosions after 2 years of disease and it has been found not to be the benign disease it was once thought to be. It has been suggested that we invert the pyramid; that is, begin with aggressive therapy up front to prevent erosive changes to joints that are generally not reversible and thus prevent the disability and potentially the mortality caused by unchecked rheumatoid arthritis.[39–41] Currently, most rheumatologists start a DMARD as soon as the diagnosis of rheumatoid arthritis is made and medication-induced remission rates in rheumatoid arthritis are now approaching 50% with the combination of methotrexate and anti-TNF biologics that will be discussed later.

Current Management of Rheumatoid Arthritis

Disease-Modifying Agents. Current therapy of rheumatoid arthritis is early diagnosis and early aggressive therapy especially for patients that have factors indicative of a poor prognosis—namely, high titer rheumatoid factor (or CCP) and a high number of joints involved at presentation. Patients with features that suggest more severe disease are typically started on methotrexate while patients without such features may be started on less potent DMARDs such as hydroxychloroquine or sulfasalazine. If after 3 to 6 months of therapy there is incomplete control of the disease, other agents are added to the regimen in particular the antitumor necrosis factor-α (anti-TNF) biologics.

Patients with early mild synovitis could be started on hydroxychloroquine.[42] This agent takes 8 to 12 weeks before it begins to affect the synovitis. Its mechanism of action is thought to be on the basis of increasing the pH of the vacuoles in antigen-presenting cells and gently disrupting the interaction of the major histocompatibility complex, with antigen thus affecting the way antigen is presented to T cells.[43]

Hydroxychloroquine is dosed by weight at 6.5 mg per kg per day in divided doses. Doses higher than this increase the risk for ocular toxicity. Common side effects include diarrhea, GI upset, and rash. Serious side effects are listed in Table 34.5 as well as a monitoring schedule. Improvement in morning stiffness and pain, as well as a decrease in the number of tender and swollen joints, and a reduction in acute-phase reactants (i.e., ESR or C-reactive protein [CRP]) are measures of success. Patients with more significant synovitis may be candidates for either sulfasalazine or methotrexate as single agents.

Sulfasalazine is another DMARD used for less severe disease. It is a combination of sulfapyridine and 5-aminosalicylic acid, which is cleaved by gut bacteria into two compounds. It is thought that the sulfapyridine moiety is the active one in rheumatoid arthritis.[42] It is dosed generally at 2000 mg in two divided doses and monitored as noted in Table 34.5. It takes 4 to 8 weeks for an effect to be apparent in most patients, and in some may be up to 12 weeks. Common side effects include GI upset, diarrhea, and rash. Severe agranulocytosis can occur and is idiosyncratic. Drug cessation resolves the cytopenias in most cases, but there have been a few cases requiring granulocyte colony-stimulating factor therapy. G6PD deficiency may lead to severe anemia in affected patients and should be checked before starting therapy if suspected.

Methotrexate is the current "workhorse" drug for rheumatoid arthritis. It is used by itself or, more and more frequently, in combination with other agents. In rheumatoid arthritis in particular, methotrexate plus something else seems to work better than either agent alone. The dose range and other characteristics are presented in Table 34.5. Methotrexate is a dihydrofolate reductase inhibitor. Its mode of action is uncertain but may be caused by an increase in adenosine, an anti-inflammatory compound.[44] Methotrexate has the advantage of being given once a week and can be given both orally and intramuscularly. Methotrexate begins to be effective generally in 3 to 8 weeks after initiation of therapy. Common side effects include stomatitis, nausea, GI upset, and mild hair thinning. Stomatitis in particular might respond to the addition of 1 mg of folic acid daily without affecting its activity in rheumatoid arthritis.

Leflunomide is a relatively new DMARD. The usual dose is 20 mg per day. Data indicate that it is similar to methotrexate in efficacy as well as toxicity. It has had, if you would, the misfortune to come to market at the same time as the anti-TNF biologic agents and thus has been somewhat overshadowed by the impressive results of these agents.

Biologic DMARDs. There are currently three anti-TNF DMARDs on the market with more on there way. Etanercept, infliximab, and adalimumab are anti-TNF agents that have been shown to be quite effective in not only controlling inflammation in rheumatoid arthritis but also preventing joint damage. In fact, data from the TEMPO study (Trial of Etanercept and Methotrexate with Radiographic and Patient Outcomes) indicates that the combination of methotrexate plus etanercept can prevent new erosion in 76% of patients over 3 years and even lead to filling in of previous erosions.[45] The other anti-TNF agents have similar numbers. Etanercept is administered subcutaneously once or twice a week; infliximab is given intravenously at 0, 2, and 6 weeks, and then every 8 weeks thereafter; and adalimumab is given subcutaneously every 2 weeks. Side effects can include leukopenia, reactivation of latent tuberculosis (TB), multiple sclerosis–like disease, and there is a concern for an increased prevalence of lymphomas in patients who use these drugs. The latter issue is difficult to

TABLE 34.5

DISEASE-MODIFYING ANTIRHEUMATIC DRUGS

Drug	Dose range	Route	Serious side effects	Monitoring
Hydroxy-chloroquine	200–600 mg/day	PO	Retinal toxicity, neuromyopathy	q 6–12 mo funduscopic and visual fields examination
Sulfasalazine	1000–3000 mg/day	PO	Leukopenia, sulfa hypersensitivity	CBC and platelets q 2–4 wk ∞ 3 mo, then CBC q 3 mo
Methotrexate	7.5–25.0 mg/wk	PO, IM, SQ	Bone marrow suppression, pneumonitis, hepatotoxicity	CBC, platelets, aspartate aminotransferase, albumin, and albumin q 4–8 wk
Leflunomide	10–20 mg/day after 100 mg/day for 3 days loading dose	PO	Hepatotoxicity, gastrointestinal distress, diarrhea, alopecia	LFTs q mo ∞ 6 mo, then every 3 mo. CBC would be reasonable early in course as well.
Etanercept	25 mg twice a week to 50 mg once a week	IM, SQ	Local injection site reaction, increased risk of infections, leukopenia, severe hepatitis in hepatitis B carriers, multiple sclerosis-like illness	Baseline CBC, LFT, hepatitis B, PPD; CBC, LFTs every 3–6 months
Infliximab	Initial dose: 3 mg/kg 2 wk: 5 mg/kg 6 wk: 5 mg/kg q 4–8 wk: 5–10 mg/kg	IV	Reactivation of TB, leukopenia, increased risk of infection, SLE-like disease, tumor risk uncertain, infusion reactions	Baseline CBC, LFT, hepatitis B, PPD; CBC, LFTs every 3–6 months
Adalimumab	40 mg	SQ	Similar to infliximab	Baseline CBC, LFT, hepatitis B, PPD; CBC, LFTs every 3–6 months

CBC, complete blood count; LFT, liver function test, PPD purified protein derivative.

ascertain as rheumatoid arthritis itself increases the risk of lymphomas. In addition to the anti-TNF biologics, two other biologic agents are now approved for rheumatoid arthritis. Rituximab, long used for treatment of lymphoma, is an anti-B cell agent, and abatacept is a molecule that inhibits T cell activation. These are currently used in patients who fail methotrexate plus an anti-TNF agent. In the next few years, there will be additional biologic agents for the treatment of rheumatoid arthritis.

Glucocorticoids. The anti-inflammatory mechanisms of glucocorticoids include altering leukocyte traffic and function, stabilizing lysosomal membranes of neutrophils and monocytes, and inhibiting the secretion of destructive enzymes including collagenase and elastase.[46] They also inhibit the products of arachidonic acid metabolism including prostaglandins and leukotrienes.

Studies have shown that low-dose glucocorticoids (defined as 7.5 mg or less of prednisone or the equivalent of another short-acting glucocorticoid) given in the morning by 10 AM reduces the progression of joint damage.[52] Also, the hypothalamic-pituitary-adrenal axis remains intact when low doses of prednisone are used. Low-dose prednisone treatment can be especially beneficial during initiation of treatment with a DMARD. Glucocorticoids are often used as bridge agents for patients diagnosed with rheumatoid arthritis; that is, 5 to 10 mg per day until the DMARD begins to work. In patients on corticosteroids, it is important to give calcium in the range of 1000 to 1500 mg per day and 400 units of vitamin D a day. Patients should be monitored closely for evidence of hypercalcemia and hypercalcinuria. A bisphosphonate (e.g., alendronate) may also reduce the bone loss of calcium in patients on corticosteroids.

Judicious intra-articular administration of corticosteroids can be quite useful in the treatment of rheumatoid arthritis. It is recommended that an individual joint be injected no more than three times at intervals of 6 months or longer. In a badly damaged joint or one that is soon to be replaced by a prosthetic joint, corticosteroids may be injected more frequently.

Surgery. Indications for orthopedic surgery in rheumatoid arthritis are twofold: pain unresponsive to medical management and loss of function. Synovectomy of selected joints provides alleviation of symptoms and improvement of function in the first year after operation, but may not provide a long-term effect. Removal of synovial tissue from the wrist and dorsal tendon sheath and resection of the ulnar head might prevent rupture of the extensor tendon. Patients with severely deformed hands can benefit from MCP arthroplasty. Patients with severe pain and loss of function can benefit from total joint replacement, especially the knee or hip. Metatarsal head resection can be of tremendous help in patients with painful metatarsal heads. Intermittent splinting of selected joints is beneficial.

Important Complications of Rheumatoid Arthritis Presenting with Pain

Carpal Tunnel Syndrome. Carpal tunnel syndrome is a common problem in rheumatoid arthritis caused by wrist synovitis that can lead to median nerve compression. Therapy is generally directed at the rheumatoid synovitis with DMARDs and anti-inflammatory agents. A wrist injection with corticosteroids may be helpful in many cases. Carpal tunnel release may be necessary in some cases.

Rheumatoid Vasculitis. This is a potentially life-threatening complication. Patients with long-standing, seropositive, erosive rheumatoid arthritis are generally at risk for this small to medium vessel vasculitis similar to polyarteritis nodosa. Patients may present with digital gangrene or symptoms of mononeuritis multiplex (i.e., footdrop). More serious complications include intestinal perforation or cardiac involvement. Kidneys are less commonly

involved than in polyarteritis nodosa. Treatment is with cyclophosphamide and high-dose prednisone.

Cervical Spine Disease. The synovial portions of the cervical spine can be involved in rheumatoid arthritis. This can lead to C1–2 instability or subaxial instability. Symptoms may be caused by cord or vascular compression and may include neck pain, shocklike sensation up or down the spine, and intermittent loss of consciousness when vertebral artery compression occurs. Before surgery, all patients with long-standing rheumatoid arthritis should have a set of lateral flexion and extension views of the cervical spine taken to evaluate the cervical spine for C1–2 subluxation.

Septic Arthritis. Patients with rheumatoid arthritis are at increased risk of septic arthritis caused by abnormal joint architecture, use of immunosuppressive drugs, and skin breakdown over high-pressure, biomechanically abnormal sites such as the feet. Patients often present with one joint out of proportion to the others in terms of pain or swelling and may have a paucity of systemic symptoms typical in nonrheumatoid patients. Detection is imperative because of the high mortality in such patients (i.e., 20% mortality if a single joint is infected and over 50% in patients with multiple joints involved).[48]

The Spondyloarthropathies

Ankylosing Spondylitis

Ankylosing spondylitis is an inflammatory arthritis involving sacroiliac joints and the spine. Inflammation also occurs at sites of tendon and ligament insertions (enthesitis). Hips and shoulders can also be affected. Peripheral arthritis is less common. Onset of disease is usually in the second or third decade, and men are predominantly affected. The histocompatibility antigen HLA-B27 is found in 90% or more of patients, fulfilling clinical criteria for ankylosing spondylitis.[49] The normal frequency of HLA-B27 in the Caucasian population is approximately 7%.

Pathophysiology. Synovitis in the apophyseal and costovertebral joints of the spine and peripheral joints is characterized by synovial hyperplasia with focal accumulation of lymphoid and plasma cells. Inflammation also involves cartilaginous joints, which include the intervertebral discs, manubriosternal joint, and symphysis pubis. Ossification of the outer layers of annulus fibrosus of the disc and the inner layers of the longitudinal ligaments forms syndesmophytes that eventually interconnect to give the spine the appearance of bamboo.

In recent years the enthesis (insertion of tendons, ligaments, and joint capsule to bone) has become an important tissue in understanding the pathophysiology of spondyloarthropathies.[50] These are common sites of inflammation and it appears that inflammation may begin on the bone side at areas rich in fibrocartilage such as enthesis and extend to surrounding tissues. The knee has some 32 enthesis alone and the concept of enthesitis explains the clinic finding of dactylitis or sausage digits in the spondyloarthropathies (Fig. 34.7).

Symptoms and Signs. The onset of the disease is usually in the second and third decades. The patient initially notes low back pain and stiffness, especially on arising in the morning. The stiffness of the back lasts for several hours in the morning and occurs after periods of activity during the day. The pain might radiate into either buttock, extend down the back of the leg to the knee, and can be mistaken for the pain caused by herniated disc. The pain might alternate from side to side. Involvement of the hips and shoulders causes pain, stiffness, and decreased motion. Peripheral joints other than the hips or shoulders are affected

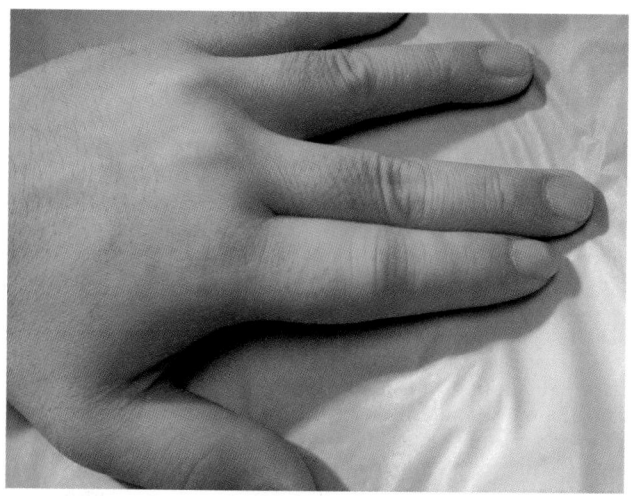

FIGURE 34.7 Classic example of dactylitis AKA "sausage digit" in a patient with a spondyloarthropathy (psoriatic arthritis in this case).

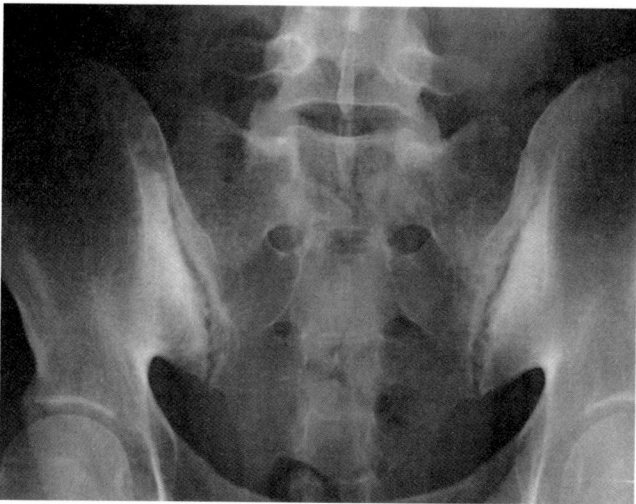

FIGURE 34.8 Ferguson view of the pelvis showing reactive bone changes around the SI joints as well as an indistinctness to the joints caused by erosions.

relatively infrequently. Costovertebral joint arthritis can cause chest pain similar to that of angina pectoris or pleurisy. The entire spine can become ankylosed. Ankylosis develops over several years, usually 10 years or more. The extent of involvement varies among patients and ranges from bilateral sacroiliitis to complete ankylosis of the spine. The spondylitis sometimes skips segments of the back. Atlantoaxial subluxation (with the potential danger of spinal cord compression) can occur, but this is observed less often in ankylosing spondylitis than in rheumatoid arthritis. The fused spine, especially the neck, is susceptible to fractures with trauma.

Acute iritis occurs in approximately one-third of the patients. A rare manifestation of ankylosing spondylitis is fibrosis of the upper lobes of the lung, which occurs late in the course of the disease. Also with long-standing disease dilatation of the proximal aorta may lead to insufficiency of the aortic valve and inflammation of the atrioventricular bundle can produce cardiac conduction abnormalities. Patients occasionally have significant constitutional symptoms of fever and weight loss.

On physical examination, sacroiliac tenderness is elicited by direct palpation or by maneuvers that stress the joint. A loss of normal lumbar lordosis occurs, giving the lumbar area an ironed-out appearance. Flexion is limited. Tenderness can be present over costovertebral joints, iliac crests, greater trochanter, and heels. Chest expansion is limited. In advanced disease the spine becomes rigid, fusing in varying degrees of flexion.

Laboratory Findings. The sedimentation rate or CRP can be elevated, and a mild hypoproliferative anemia can occur. The rheumatoid factor test result is negative and one would rarely mistake rheumatoid arthritis and ankylosing spondylitis. The synovial fluid is inflammatory (see Table 34.4). Radiography of the sacroiliac joints in early disease shows blurring and irregularity of the joint margins, followed later by subchondral erosions, sclerosis, and eventually fusion (Fig. 34.8). Bony spurs appear at tendinous insertions such as the sites of attachment of the Achilles tendon and plantar fascia. Radiography shows a straight lumbar spine, squared vertebrae, and syndesmophytes. Syndesmophytes extend along the outer aspect of the intervertebral disc and eventually form a bridge between adjacent vertebrae (bamboo spine).

Treatment. With the advent of the anti-TNF agents, the treatment philosophy has changed. There is now the hope of disease slowing or even remission similar to that seen with rheumatoid arthritis although it still remains to be seen whether that is indeed true. Most patients would still receive an NSAID initially but with partial response or evidence of radiographic progression most patients would now be put on an anti-TNF agent early in the course of the disease.

Nonsteroidal Anti-inflammatory Drugs. NSAIDs are especially useful in reducing inflammation and relieving pain, but they may not change the course of the disease. It is speculated, but not proven, that NSAIDs may encourage the patient to be more mobile and possibly lessen the chance of spine fusion. Preferred agents include indomethacin or a once-a-day agent such as piroxicam because of their anti-inflammatory activity. Any anti-inflammatory agent chosen usually needs to be dosed at an anti-inflammatory level (i.e., upper limit of dosing range) for benefit.

Disease-Modifying Antirheumatic Drugs. Sulfasalazine has been shown to be beneficial for the peripheral joint in ankylosing spondylitis, but not the spine.[51] Methotrexate has also been used for ankylosing spondylitis, but controlled trails are lacking. The anti-TNF agents have a significant impact on disease symptoms and also diminish both bone edema and enthesitis by serial MRI scan.[52,53] It has not been shown yet that they are definitive disease remitting agents yet but these medications have become important tools in the treatment of ankylosing spondylitis.

Physical Therapy. Physical therapy is directed at maintaining the erect posture of the patient. Patients should be encouraged to sleep in the prone position and to avoid using a pillow when sleeping on their backs. Anterior uveitis or iritis can be treated with topical or intraocular corticosteroids and in severe cases, methotrexate of the monoclonal anti-TNF agents such as adalimumab or infliximab can be used. Etanercept, a fusion protein, is not effective for uveitis. Patients with severe hip or shoulder disease can benefit from total shoulder replacement.

Important Complications of Ankylosing Spondylitis Presenting with Pain
Cauda Equina Syndrome. Patients with cauda equina syndrome generally have long-standing ankylosing spondylitis. The patient generally presents with progressive lower extremity weakness, pain, and loss of sensation in the lower extremities and perineum. Impotence and overflow incontinence are also frequently occurring problems. Radiographically, large dorsal arachnoid diverticula are seen on myelography or magnetic resonance imaging.[54]

Electromyography demonstrates multi-root involvement. Therapy with high-dose corticosteroids and surgery both have been disappointing.

Spondylodiskitis

Spondylodiskitis is a rare complication of long-standing ankylosing spondylitis. Patients have persistent mechanical-type back pain (pain with activity) rather than inflammatory low back pain (pain in the morning or with rest). It is caused by a mobile vertebral segment surrounded by fused segments. The focus of activity at the one segment may lead to significant inflammation and damage to the adjacent vertebral bodies, simulating infection. Infection generally needs to be ruled out and treatment is directed to immobilizing the segment either via brace and allowing it to fuse or refuse; occasionally it may need to be surgically fused.[55]

Vertebral Fracture. Vertebral segments connected by syndesmophytes are subject to fracture with even minor trauma.[55] The usual location for such fractures are the C5–7 vertebral segments; the fractures are typically caused by a hyperextension injury. Patients suspected of fracture should be evaluated by computed tomographic scan or bone scan to try to identify a potential fracture site, as plain radiography may not be able to demonstrate the fracture. Patients with such fractures have a relatively high morbidity and mortality even if identified, because of surgery or prolonged immobilization usually required for treatment. Only 40% of such patients return to their former level of activity.

Chronic Enthesitis. Enthesitis of Achilles tendon, plantar fascia, and occasionally the ribs can be a chronic source of pain and may be more resistant than spondylitis to usual therapies.[61] In such cases, indomethacin at maximum dose, use of a DMARD such as methotrexate, sulfasalazine, or an anti-TNF agent may be warranted. Refractory patients may benefit from low-dose radiation to the heel.[56]

Reactive Arthritis

Reactive arthritis (formally Reiter's syndrome) is defined as an asymmetric arthropathy involving predominantly joints of the lower extremities plus one or more of the following: urethritis or cervicitis, dysentery, mucocutaneous lesions, and inflammatory eye disease. It is also defined as an episode of arthritis lasting longer than 1 month that is associated with urethritis or cervicitis. The histocompatibility antigen HLA-B27 is present in approximately 80% of patients.[57] The reasons of the change in nomenclature for Reiter's to reactive arthritis is due to the involvement of Hans Reiter with the Nazi regime and the fact that the same syndrome had been described previously by others.

There appears to be a relationship between certain infections and a specific genetic background. Reactive arthritis can follow infections with *Shigella*, *Salmonella*, *Campylobacter*, or *Yersinia*.[58] An association also exists with urethritis associated with *Chlamydia* or *Mycoplasma* infections. In addition, reactive arthritis has been associated with human immunodeficiency virus (HIV) infection. Reactive arthritis develops in patients without these infections, however, and most patients with nonspecific urethritis do not develop this syndrome. The risk of an individual who has a positive result for HLA-B27 with nonspecific urethritis developing reactive arthritis is in the range of 20%. Up to 3% of individuals with nonspecific urethritis have been shown to develop a reactive arthritis. Reactive arthritis has a worldwide distribution and occurs more often in men. In postdysenteric reactive arthritis, the gender distribution is equal.

Symptoms and Signs

Arthritis affects several joints in an asymmetric fashion; knees and ankles are most often involved. Patients also experience pain in the feet and ankles secondary to inflammation at the insertion of the Achilles tendon and plantar fascia. Joints can remain swollen for several months. Swelling of two adjacent interphalangeal joints and adjoining tendon sheath results in a sausage digit or dactylitis. In approximately 20% of patients, spinal involvement occurs. Sacroiliitis is usually unilateral and spine involvement mild. Patients can also experience chest pain caused by inflammation at the tendinous insertions of the intercostal muscles.

The mucocutaneous lesions of reactive arthritis include oral ulcers, balanitis, and keratoderma blennorrhagica. The oral ulcers are shallow and irregular, and have a slightly erythematous base. These lesions are only present for several days. Balanitis usually begins as small painless vesicles that become hyperkeratotic. These lesions are painless and remain crusted in the circumcised patient. In the uncircumcised patient, lesions are moist and can become secondarily infected. Keratoderma blennorrhagica, a hyperkeratotic skin lesion similar to psoriasis, most commonly involves the feet. Sometimes it involves the hands, but it can be present almost any place on the body.

Conjunctivitis involves one or both eyes. Uveitis also occurs. Urethritis can precede or accompany the arthritis. Prostatitis is present in approximately 80% of patients.

As with ankylosing spondylitis, some patients may develop dilatation of the proximal aorta leading to aortic valve insufficiency.

The course of reactive arthritis is recurrent or persistent, with only an occasional patient experiencing transient, self-limited disease. In some patients, sexual intercourse with a certain partner appears to lead to an exacerbation of reactive arthritis. These patients should be advised to use a condom even though the benefit of this practice is questioned by some. No evidence exists that the use of an antibiotic prevents or alters the course of reactive arthritis.

Laboratory Findings

Routine laboratory test results are usually normal. The sedimentation rate is quite variable and does not correlate with disease activity. Synovial fluid shows an elevated white cell count ranging from 5000 to 50,000 cells per cubic millimeter, predominantly neutrophils. Radiography shows juxta-articular osteopenia, joint space narrowing, and bone erosions. Periostitis is present adjacent to the involved joints and at the insertion of tendons and fasciae. Erosions, sclerosis, and irregularity of the sacroiliac joint can be present and are usually unilateral. Changes of spondylitis are usually asymmetric, occur at various levels of the spine, and are similar to those seen in psoriatic arthritis. Testing for HLA-B27 is not necessary for diagnosis. This test should be reserved for patients who have asymmetric arthritis without other evidence of reactive arthritis.

Treatment

Treatment of reactive arthritis is similar to that of ankylosing spondylitis. NSAIDs are first-line therapy followed by sulfasalazine in refractory cases. Methotrexate or azathioprine can be used in more severe disease. Intra-articular corticosteroid can also be useful. The anti-TNF agents are less well studied in this condition but there is no reason to doubt their efficacy.

Complications of Reactive Arthritis Associated with Chronic Pain

Rare patients may have more persistent inflammatory eye disease requiring continuous ophthalmology care. Enthesitis can be severe in some cases of reactive arthritis. Chronic foot involvement can lead to erosive disease at the MTP.

Psoriatic Arthritis

Arthritis appears in 6% to 39% of outpatients with psoriasis depending on the population studied.[59] Hereditary factors play a role. An increased prevalence of psoriatic arthritis occurs in first-degree relatives with psoriasis. An association with HLA-B27 is seen in psoriatic arthritis with spondylitis, but not in patients with peripheral arthritis. Onset of psoriatic arthritis is usually in the third or fourth decade, and the gender ratio is approximately equal. In most patients, psoriasis precedes the arthritis by several years. Most patients with psoriatic arthritis have only a few joints that are involved, and, overall, the prognosis tends to be better than in rheumatoid arthritis. Psoriatic arthritis has been noted in patients with HIV infection.

Symptoms and Signs

Several patterns of arthritis are observed in patients with psoriasis. The majority of patients have an asymmetric oligoarthritis involving the proximal joints of the hands and feet. In approximately 10% of patients, arthritis affects predominantly the distal interphalangeal joints and is usually accompanied by psoriasis of the adjacent nail. Other patients have a symmetric polyarthritis similar to that seen in rheumatoid arthritis. These patients usually have negative results for rheumatoid factor. If the rheumatoid factor test or the CCP result is positive, the patient may have both rheumatoid arthritis and psoriasis. Patients can also manifest sacroiliitis, and variable degrees of spondylitis. In some patients the spine becomes ankylosed. A few patients have a severe, destructive, and deforming polyarthritis referred to as *arthritis mutilans*.

Joints are swollen, warm, and tender, and a digit may have the appearance of a sausage (see ankylosing spondylitis). Contractures and ankylosis of joints occur with long periods of persistent joint inflammation. In most cases there appears to be no definite correlation between the degree of skin involvement and joint disease.

Laboratory Findings

Laboratory findings include an elevated sedimentation rate and a hypoproliferative anemia. The rheumatoid factor test result is negative. The synovial fluid shows evidence of inflammation with elevated white cell counts; the cells are predominantly polymorphonuclear. A somewhat characteristic radiographic finding is that of the pencil-in-cup deformity caused by osteolysis, or whittling of the distal end of the middle phalanx, which produces a pencil point that projects into a widened cup-like erosion in the adjacent surface of the distal phalanx (Fig. 34.9). Radiography shows joint space narrowing, erosions, osteolysis, and ankylosis,

depending on the degree of clinical severity. The radiographic findings of the spine are similar to those found in patients with reactive arthritis.

Treatment

Initial treatment of psoriatic arthritis is aspirin or other NSAIDs. In patients with progressive disease, methotrexate, cyclosporine, sulfasalazine, and even hydroxychloroquine have been used successfully.[69] Low-dose oral corticosteroids as well as intra-articular corticosteroids can also be used. The tapering of corticosteroids in patients who have been on moderate to large doses may exacerbate the skin disease. The anti-TNF agents have an impressive effect on both skin and joints in many patients and are generally used with failure of methotrexate.[60]

Important Complications of Psoriatic Arthritis Presenting with Pain

See Ankylosing Spondylitis for a discussion of chronic enthesitis. For a discussion of carpal tunnel syndrome, see Rheumatoid Arthritis.

Arthritis Associated with Inflammatory Gastrointestinal Disease

Both ulcerative colitis and regional enteritis (Crohn's disease) are associated with peripheral arthritis and spondylitis.[61] Peripheral arthritis occurs in approximately 10% to 20% of patients with inflammatory bowel disease. Onset of peripheral arthritis is usually in the third or fourth decades. Both genders are equally affected. The arthritis usually follows the onset of colitis by months to years and involves only one or two joints. Arthritis is acute, lasts several days to several weeks, and leaves no residual damage. The knees and ankles are most frequently affected.

Ankylosing spondylitis is also associated with inflammatory bowel disease. The gender distribution is equal, in contrast to the male predominance observed in primary ankylosing spondylitis. The majority (70%) of patients with spondylitis associated with inflammatory bowel disease has positive results for HLA-B27. Asymptomatic bilateral sacroiliitis can be found in up to 15% of patients with inflammatory bowel disease. Frequency of HLA-B27 is not increased in patients with only peripheral arthritis. Synovial fluid analysis shows an inflammatory effusion.

Treatment

Peripheral joint symptoms are managed with salicylates or other NSAIDs. NSAIDs, however, may lead to an exacerbation of the inflammatory bowel disease. Peripheral arthritis often disappears after colectomy. Treatment of the spondylitis is similar to that described for ankylosing spondylitis.

Arthritis Caused by Deposition of Calcium Pyrophosphate

Deposition of calcium pyrophosphate dihydrate in the joint produces both an acute and chronic form of joint disease. The acute or subacute form is referred to as *pseudogout* because of its similarity to gout. *Chondrocalcinosis* refers to calcium pyrophosphate deposits in articular tissue that are detectable radiographically and occur in the absence of inflammatory arthritis. Pseudogout affects persons over the age of 40, men predominately. The knee is the most frequent site of acute arthritis, but the hip, shoulder, ankle, wrists, and bursae can be affected. Approximately 3% to 5% of the adult population has calcium pyrophosphate deposits in knee joints at the time of death. This disorder is associated with OA.

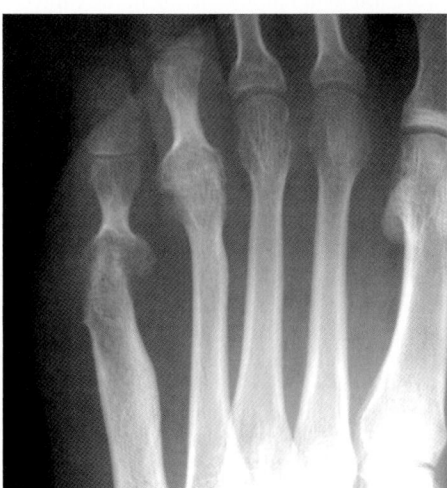

FIGURE 34.9 X-ray of the left foot in psoriatic arthritis demonstrating fusion of the fourth MTP and a developing pencil in a cup deformity of the fifth MTP.

Three forms of calcium pyrophosphate deposition disease (CPDD) are recognized: a hereditary form, CPDD associated with metabolic and other diseases, and an idiopathic form. The frequency of OA in CPDD varies from 40% to 70%. CPDD occurs in 41% of patients with hemochromatosis and in 5% to 15% with hyperparathyroidism.[62] An association is suspected in patients with diabetes mellitus, hypophosphatemia, Wilson's disease, ochronosis, and hypothyroidism.

Pathophysiology

The initial site of crystal formation is in articular cartilage. In idiopathic CPDD it is not clear whether the primary event is deposition of crystals in cartilage or whether the crystals develop as a consequence of disturbed cartilage metabolism. Increased inorganic pyrophosphate is found in the synovial fluid and probably reflects a local disorder of pyrophosphate metabolism leading to deposition of calcium pyrophosphate crystals in the joint.[63,64] Elevated levels are also found in patients with OA. Acute arthritis is brought on by shedding of crystals into the joint space. The mechanism for crystal shedding is the lowering of either calcium or pyrophosphate ions in synovial fluid.[65,66] The decreased concentration of ionized calcium results in movement of crystals from cartilage into synovial fluid. Crystals can also be shed into the synovial fluid as a consequence of mechanical disruption of cartilage. Attacks can follow trauma. In addition, crystals can be released as a result of degradation of cartilage by enzymes from polymorphonuclear white cells during episodes of bacterial arthritis or other forms of inflammatory arthritis. Increased enzyme activity is also present in OA.

Symptoms and Signs

Several patterns of joint disease are recognized.[62] In approximately 25% of patients, CPDD presents as an acute arthritis involving a single joint or a few joints at any given time. The clinical picture mimics that of acute gout, which accounts for the term *pseudogout*. The onset of joint swelling and pain is abrupt and severe and usually reaches a peak within 24 to 36 hours. An attack can last up to 14 days. The joint is swollen, red, and tender. The most common site of involvement is the knee, but attacks can involve other large joints such as the ankles, wrists, elbows, or hips. Also, the lumbar and cervical spine can be involved. Trauma, surgery, or severe medical illness can precipitate an attack. The same joint is often involved in subsequent attacks. Radiographic evidence of chondrocalcinosis may be present in affected joints.

Approximately 5% of patients with CPDD have a form of disease that mimics rheumatoid arthritis (*pseudorheumatoid disease*). Involvement of multiple joints, synovial proliferation, limitation of joint motion, and joint deformity can develop. Patients experience fatigue and morning stiffness. To further confuse the issue, calcium pyrophosphate deposition can occur in rheumatoid arthritis.

CPDD also occurs in a chronic form that is similar to OA. Multiple joints are involved and include the knees, wrists, MCP joints, hips, shoulders, elbows, and ankles. The disease involves middle-aged to elderly patients, predominantly women. CPDD can mimic neuropathic arthropathy and can also occur in patients with neuropathic joint disease.

The diagnosis of calcium pyrophosphate disease is established by identification of calcium pyrophosphate crystals in synovial fluid, both free and in polymorphonuclear white cells. The crystals appear as short rods, rhomboids, and cuboids and they have a sign of weakly positive birefringence under compensated polarized light. Radiography shows calcification in articular hyaline cartilage that is parallel to and separated from the subchondral bone. Calcifications in fibrocartilage are thick and irregular densities and are found in the menisci of the knee, symphysis pubis, annulus fibrosus, and the triangular cartilage of the wrist. Calcifications also occur in the Achilles, supraspinatus, and triceps tendons, but can involve any tendon. Changes in the joint are similar to those seen in OA with sclerosis of subchondral bone, joint space narrowing, and large subchondral cysts.

Treatment

The NSAIDs are effective in the treatment of acute and chronic joint disease. An NSAID is given for 10 to 14 days in patients with acute pseudogout. The drug can be continued indefinitely in patients with CCPD associated with OA. When an NSAID is contraindicated, another method of treatment for an acute attack is prednisone, starting with 40 mg the first day and gradually tapering over a 7-day period. Colchicine, 0.6 mg twice a day, is started on day 3 or 4 and continued for several weeks to avoid a flare of arthritis after prednisone is discontinued. Colchicine, 0.6 mg twice a day, can also be given prophylactically to reduce the number and length of attacks (see colchicine in section on gout). Aspiration of the involved joint followed by an injection of glucocorticoids reduces pain and swelling.

Urate Gout

Urate gout (as opposed to pyrophosphate gout or pseudogout) is characterized by elevated serum urate levels, recurrent attacks of acute arthritis involving a single joint or a few joints at any given time, and deposition of monosodium urate dihydrate (tophi) in and around joints, leading in some patients to a deforming and crippling arthritis. Renal stones also may form. These features are present in varying combinations.[67]

Recognized since ancient times, gout has been depicted in caricatures as affecting well-fed aristocrats overindulging in rich foods and wines. The disease has been referred to as the *king of diseases* and the *disease of kings*.[68]

The normal serum urate concentration is 5.1 ± 1.0 mg per dL in men and 4.0 ± 1.0 mg per dL in premenopausal women. After menopause, the level in women approximates that of men. The level in young boys is 3 to 4 mg per dL and increases to adult levels at puberty. Serum urate levels show a positive correlation with weight and surface area in various racial groups.[82] The prevalence of gout varies from 0.20 to 0.35 per 1,000.[69-71] The prevalence of gout increases with age and increasing levels of serum urate. In one study of men whose ages ranged from 35 to 44 years old, the prevalence was 15 per 1,000 men.[72]

Both genetic and environmental factors play a role in the expression of hyperuricemia and gout. For example, higher serum urate levels are found in Filipinos living in the United States compared with racially identical persons living in the Philippines. These persons are unable to excrete the greater uric acid load resulting from the higher purine content of the diet eaten in the United States.[73]

Etiology and Pathophysiology

Uric acid is a product of purine metabolism.[67] The serum urate concentration depends on the rate of uric acid production and excretion. Approximately two-thirds of uric acid is excreted in the urine and one-third into the gastrointestinal tract. Normally, uric acid is completely filtered through the glomeruli and completely reabsorbed in the proximal tubule. Secretion of uric acid occurs in the proximal tubule, followed by a second reabsorption in the proximal tubule.

Primary gout is defined by the absence of other diseases or conditions such as drugs that lead to hyperuricemia and gout. Approximately 90% of patients with primary gout have decreased renal clearance of uric acid resulting from reduced glomerular filtration, increased tubular reabsorption, reduced tubular secretion, or combinations of these factors. Evidence for a molecular renal defect is still lacking in the majority of patients.

Approximately 10% of patients are overproducers of uric acid. Overproduction is defined as the urinary excretion of more than 800 to 1,000 mg of uric acid in 24 hours while the patient is on a regular purine diet.

Two inborn errors of purine metabolism make up a small number of primary gout patients who are overproducers of uric acid. The first disorder is caused by a partial deficiency of the enzyme hypoxanthine-guanine phosphoribosyltransferase, which catalyzes conversion of hypoxanthine to inosinic acid and guanine to guanylic acid.[67] The second disorder is caused by increased 5-phosphoribosyl-1-pyrophosphate synthetase activity leading to elevated levels of intracellular 5-phosphoribosyl-1-pyrophosphate and overproduction of uric acid. These patients usually experience the onset of gouty arthritis in the second or third decade and have a high frequency of uric acid stones. Both diseases are inherited as an X-linked disorder, therefore affecting male subjects, with women as carriers. Some of these patients also have dysarthria, hyperreflexia, lack of coordination, and mental retardation. A severe form of the first disorder with almost a complete deficiency of this enzyme, referred to as the Lesch-Nyhan syndrome, is characterized by self-mutilation, choreoathetosis, and mental retardation.[74] This disorder is classified under secondary hyperuricemia or gout because the neurologic disorder is predominant.

Secondary gout is defined as gout or hyperuricemia occurring in patients with other disorders. Overproduction of uric acid results in hyperuricemia in patients with disorders associated with increased cell proliferation and turnover of nucleic acids. These disorders include myeloproliferative and lymphoproliferative diseases, multiple myeloma, polycythemia, pernicious anemia, hemoglobinopathies, and some carcinomas. The hereditary disorder glucose 6-phosphatase deficiency (von Gierke's glycogen storage disease) is also manifested by overproduction of uric acid. Secondary hyperuricemia can also result from renal failure or the effects of drugs or toxins on renal clearance of uric acid. Diuretic agents, low doses of aspirin (less than 2 g per day), alcohol, ethambutol, cyclosporine, and lead are some of the agents that decrease the clearance of uric acid and thereby raise the serum urate level.

Pathophysiology of Acute Gouty Arthritis

Acute gouty arthritis results from the inflammatory reaction to urate crystals that form in the joint space or are released into the joint from synovium or articular cartilage. Plasma becomes supersaturated with urate at concentrations of approximately 7 mg per dL.[67] This point has to be remembered when a laboratory "normal" level of uric acid is indicated to be 3 to 8 mg per dL. Factors in addition to supersaturation of plasma urate are necessary for crystal precipitation because most patients with hyperuricemia do not develop gout. The lower temperatures found in peripheral joints or tissues might contribute to urate precipitation at these sites. Urate is less soluble at 32°C, which is the temperature observed in a normal knee, compared with the core body temperature of 37°C.[75] Another mechanism for urate precipitation might be the faster reabsorption of extracellular fluid than urate from the joint space, resulting in a transient increased urate concentration and crystal formation.[76] Trauma or impact loading of a joint that breaks crystals loose from the joint surface is yet another possible mechanism and might explain the high frequency of gout at the base of the great toe, which is a joint subjected to great stress.

Urate crystals induce inflammation by several mechanisms.[67] Urate crystals activate Hageman's factor in joint fluid, leading to the formation of kinins that induce vasodilatation and increased vascular permeability. Urate crystals activate the complement system with the generation of leukocyte chemotactic factors and also stimulate the formation of leukotrienes from arachidonic acid. Furthermore, urate crystals can activate platelets, which secrete

several inflammatory mediators including prostaglandins. Urate crystals can also stimulate synovial lining cells and macrophages that secrete prostaglandins and collagenase.

The key to urate-induced inflammation is the polymorphonuclear white cell. Urate crystals activate toll-like receptors on the surface of cells that lead to the release of inflammatory mediators such as IL-1.[77] Crystals also bind IgG, leading to their attachment to and phagocytosis by polymorphonuclear white cells.[67] This process mediates the production of superoxide anions, which damage tissue. In addition, ingestion of crystals results in the release of chemotactic factors from the polymorphonuclear white cells, thus attracting more polymorphonuclear white cells. On ingestion by polymorphonuclear white cells, crystals are incorporated into phagosomes, which fuse with lysosomes. The rupture of phagolysosomes inside polymorphonuclear white cells damages these cells. Lysosomal and cytoplasmic enzymes are released into the joint space, resulting in tissue inflammation and injury.

Gouty arthritis often develops with fluctuation of serum urate levels. A rapid increase in serum uric acid results in precipitation of crystals in tissue or fluid. A rapid decrease in serum urate brings about release of urate from the joint surface into the joint space.

Drinking of alcohol is also associated with the precipitation of gouty attacks. Metabolism of ethanol results in an increased concentration of blood lactate, which blocks the renal excretion of uric acid by inhibiting tubular secretion and raising the serum urate level. Alcohol consumption also leads to accelerated degradation of adenosine triphosphate to adenosine monophosphate with accumulation of adenine nucleotides that are degraded to uric acid and other purine metabolites.[78] Beers and ales in particular increase the risk of gout due to the amount of purines these contain. The drinking of moonshine whiskey is associated with gouty arthritis and is referred to as *saturnine gout*.[79] Moonshine whiskey is often distilled in automobile radiators containing a lead core. Lead reduces the excretion of urate and decreases its solubility. In addition, lead may affect renal mechanisms for handling urate, leading to elevated levels.

Gout follows periods of fasting. During fasting the increased plasma level of acetoacetate and β-hydroxybutyrate interferes with renal excretion of urate.[80] Overindulgence of food and wine has often been associated with gout. When a large protein- and purine-rich diet is ingested along with copious amounts of wine or other liquor, the uric acid serum concentration rises because of increased formation and decreased excretion of sodium urate. Acute gouty arthritis attacks occur when drugs increase or lower the serum uric acid level. Attacks are precipitated by allopurinol, which lowers the uric acid concentrations, and thiazides or low doses of aspirin, which raise the level. Cyclosporine interferes with the renal excretion of uric acid and induces hyperuricemia and gout.[81] An increased frequency of gout is seen in transplant recipients receiving cyclosporine and may affect atypical joints such as the hips, sacroiliac joints, or shoulders.

Symptoms and Signs

Gouty arthritis occurs mainly in middle-aged and older men and after menopause in women. Approximately one-fourth of the patients have a family history of gout. Nephrolithiasis precedes the first attack of arthritis in approximately 10% of patients. The first attack occurs most often in the MTP joint of the great toe (podagra). Subsequent attacks might be separated by several months or even years. The involved joint usually returns to normal between attacks. In untreated cases, the attacks become more frequent and involve other joints, such as wrists, elbows, olecranon bursae, and the small joints of the hand. Gouty arthritis can occur in distal interphalangeal joints already involved with OA

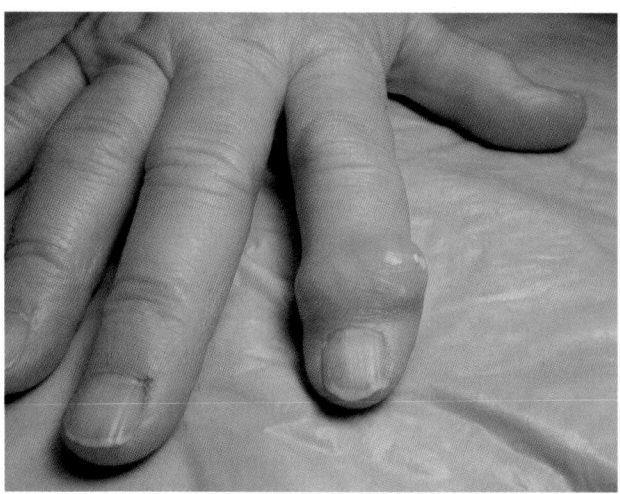

FIGURE 34.10 Tophaceous gout affecting the DIP joint.

and Heberden's nodes[82] (Figs. 34.10 and 34.11). Gout can be overlooked in these joints because acute inflammation can also occur with Heberden's nodes. Gouty arthritis of intervertebral joints, sacroiliac joints, and shoulders and hips is uncommon.

The typical attack of gout comes on acutely, often during the early hours of morning. Attacks also occur after surgery. Pain and swelling reach a peak within 24 hours. The joint is exquisitely tender, and overlying soft tissue is swollen and erythematous even to the degree that it could be mistaken for cellulitis. Pain is intense and throbbing. Patients are unable to tolerate even a light sheet touching the involved great toe. Jarring of the bed can make the patient wince with pain. The patient might even dread the landing of a fly on the involved toe. Both a low-grade fever and leukocytosis can accompany the attack, especially in polyarticular gout. An untreated attack of gout usually lasts for 1 to 2 weeks. Less severe attacks also occur that last only a few days.

Chronic tophaceous gout develops in some patients. Before the effective control of hyperuricemia, approximately one-half of the patients with episodes of gouty arthritis eventually developed deposits of monosodium urate dihydrate in and around joints as well as in other tissues. These deposits, referred to as *tophi*, usually become apparent at least 10 years after the onset of gouty arthritis. They develop in the olecranon, infrapatellar and prepa-

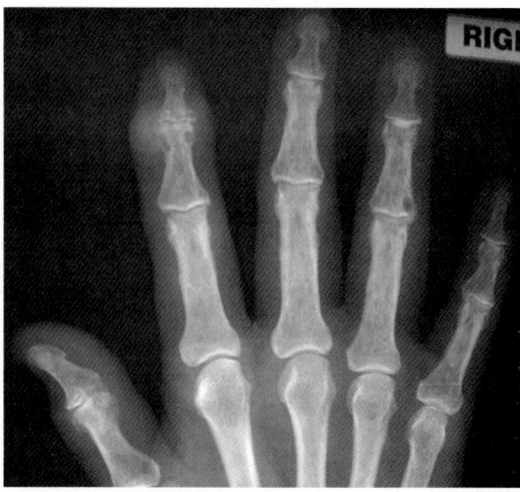

FIGURE 34.11 X-ray of same patient with tophaceous gout. Note erosions in the middle phalanx of the index finger caused by gout.

tellar bursae, Achilles tendons, synovium, subchondral bone, and, infrequently, in the cartilage of the ear. Tophi can ulcerate and drain material that contains microscopic needle-shaped crystals of monosodium urate. Patients with tophaceous gout have frequent episodes of acute gouty arthritis. Joint deformity and disability can be quite severe in the untreated patient.

Significant renal disease secondary to gouty nephropathy is rare. Proteinuria, decreased concentrating capacity, and a decrease in creatinine clearance might be present. Small deposits of urate are observed in the interstitium of the renal medulla. Nephrosclerosis and hypertension are frequently associated with gout.

Treatment of patients with underlying myeloproliferative or lymphoproliferative disorders results in extremely high levels of serum urate that can precipitate in the renal tubules, producing obstruction and oliguria. Patients should be treated with allopurinol and colchicine before treatment of the blood dyscrasia.

Renal calculi develop in approximately 20% of patients with gout. Hypertension, diabetes mellitus, and hypertriglyceridemia occur more frequently in patients with gout.

Laboratory Findings

Radiography of the affected joint in acute gouty arthritis is usually normal. When the first MTP joint is involved, radiography might show underlying changes of OA. The typical erosion caused by urate deposition is sharply defined and has a thin shell-like overhanging edge at the margins of the erosion. The diagnosis of gout is established by demonstration of the characteristic crystal of monosodium urate monohydrate in the synovial fluid or from tissue deposits. Crystals are found both in the polymorphonuclear white cells and free in fluid. The crystals in joint fluid are usually rod shaped and 7 to 10 μm in length. They are identified by use of polarized microscopy. With use of a first-order red compensator, crystals have a sign of strongly negative birefringence.[83] Crystals from tophi are long and needle-shaped and are not usually found in white cells.

Treatment

Treatment of a patient with gout has two components: treatment of the acute gouty arthritis and treatment of hyperuricemia. Each is treated independently. Even though they are closely interrelated, the drugs used for each are different. In fact, the indiscriminate use of a drug to lower the uric acid can exacerbate or prolong an attack of gouty arthritis.

Anti-inflammatory Drugs. For the acute attack of gouty arthritis, the patient is given indomethacin, 200 mg in four divided doses (50 mg every 6 hours) the first 24 hours, followed by 150 mg every day for 7 to 10 days. Other NSAIDs can also be used. NSAIDs for the treatment of acute gout should be avoided or used with caution in patients with symptomatic heart failure, renal failure, oliguria, or peptic ulcer disease. Glucocorticoids are also quite effective in treatment of acute gout. Prednisone is given over a 7-day period with an initial dose of 40 mg as a single dose and then gradually tapered over a 7-day period. To avoid a flare of arthritis when prednisone is discontinued, the patient is started on 0.6 mg of colchicine or an NSAID beginning on day 3 or 4 of prednisone therapy and continuing for several weeks. Methylprednisolone can be given intravenously to patients unable to take oral medications. The dose schedule for oral prednisone is followed. Intra-articular corticosteroids can also be used to treat gout in a large joint such as the knee.

In patients who experience frequent attacks of acute gouty arthritis, 0.6 mg colchicine once or twice a day is quite effective in preventing attacks. Patients on this prophylactic regimen can abort an acute attack by taking colchicine, 0.6 mg every hour for four to six doses, when they experience the first twinge of joint pain.

Myopathy and polyneuropathy may occur on maintenance doses of colchicine in patients who have renal insufficiency.[84] Myositis manifests as proximal muscle weakness and serum creatine kinase becomes elevated. These abnormalities return to normal 3 to 4 weeks after stopping the drug. Polyneuropathy also disappears on discontinuing colchicine. In addition, agranulocytosis or aplastic anemia can occur in patients with renal insufficiency who are on regular doses of colchicine because the plasma drug levels in these patients greatly increase.

Antihyperuricemic Drugs. Treatment of hyperuricemia in patients with gout is directed at preventing the formation of tophaceous deposits. It is not uniformly agreed that all patients with elevated uric acids and gouty arthritis require medications to lower their uric acid. If the patient already has tophaceous deposits in joints or subcutaneous tissue, then the uric acid should be lowered. On the other hand, an elevated uric acid of less than 10 mg per dL in a patient without tophi or frequent gouty attacks might not require treatment. Whether they have gout or not, persons with uric acid levels above 10 mg per dL are usually treated because of their higher risk of developing gout.

The uric acid concentration can be lowered by probenecid, which is a uricosuric agent.[85] In patients with normal renal function and no renal stones, probenecid is an effective agent. The dose of probenecid is 1 to 3 g per day given twice a day. The urine should be alkalinized to prevent precipitation of urate in the urinary tract. Sulfinpyrazone is another uricosuric drug. The usual daily dose is 300 to 400 mg per day, administered in three or four divided doses.

Serum uric acid level is effectively reduced by allopurinol, which is a potent inhibitor of xanthine oxidase.[85] This drug blocks the conversion of hypoxanthine to xanthine and xanthine to uric acid. This leads to the accumulation of other oxypurines in the blood. The daily dose of allopurinol is 300 to 800 mg per day, which is regulated to reduce uric acid to a concentration below 6 mg per dL. Allopurinol administration can precipitate an acute attack of gout, presumably because of fluctuation of sodium urate between tissue and blood. To prevent an acute gouty attack, allopurinol is started in a low dose and gradually increased. Colchicine, 0.6 mg once or twice a day, is given along with the allopurinol to prevent an acute attack.

The most significant side effect of allopurinol is a rash that occasionally progresses to a severe life-threatening exfoliative dermatitis. Transient leukopenia and abnormalities of liver function are observed in some patients. In patients treated for many years, xanthine stones may occur. These tend to occur in patients who are overproducers and hyperexcretors of uric acid.

Allopurinol is the drug of choice in patients with renal insufficiency who are unable to excrete a uric acid load. This drug is also indicated in patients with uric acid renal calculi. Allopurinol is more effective than probenecid in reducing tophi in patients with severe tophaceous gout. The addition of probenecid, however, further enhances the lowering of serum acid level.

Allopurinol is also indicated in patients with gout who are overproducers and hyperexcretors of urate (urine acid excretion greater than 1000 mg for 24 hours) because these patients are at greater risk for developing renal stones. No clear evidence exists that treatment of asymptomatic hyperuricemia in a person who is not a hyperexcretor is beneficial.

Allopurinol potentiates the action of 6-mercaptopurine and azathioprine. The dose of the cytotoxic agent is usually reduced by at least one-third in patients on allopurinol.

Infectious Arthritis

Nongonococcal Bacterial Arthritis

Acute bacterial or septic arthritis is a serious problem that requires prompt treatment to avoid joint damage.[86,87] Bacteria usually reach the joint by hematogenous spread from a primary infection elsewhere. Often, however, no primary source of infection is found. An infection in the adjacent bone or soft tissue can extend directly into the joint. Acute bacterial arthritis is most often caused by *Neisseria gonorrhea, Staphylococcus aureus, Streptococcus pneumoniae, Staphylococcus pyogenes,* or *Haemophilus influenzae,* with *Staphylococcus* spp. being the most common causative organisms. Gram-negative organisms include *Escherichia coli, Salmonella,* and *Pseudomonas* and are usually seen in patients who are immunosuppressed or use intravenous drugs.

Patients with diabetes mellitus or blood dyscrasias or those receiving glucocorticoids or immunosuppressive drugs are more susceptible to joint infection. Septic arthritis is more likely to occur in joints previously damaged by trauma or inflammatory arthritis. Patients with rheumatoid arthritis in particular have an increased risk of septic arthritis and an increased mortality rate.[88]

Pathophysiology. The synovium is edematous and infiltrated by neutrophils. As the disease progresses, small abscesses are present in the synovium and subchondral bone. Proteolytic enzymes from neutrophils damage the cartilage, bone, and joint capsule. Healing is manifested by proliferation of fibroblasts, which can lead to ankylosis.

Symptoms and Signs. The onset of bacterial arthritis is usually abrupt and associated with severe pain and fever. A shaking chill occasionally accompanies the onset. Any motion of the joint causes excruciating pain. The overlying skin is usually erythematous. In elderly patients and those who are on glucocorticoids, the symptoms can be less severe.

The joint affected most frequently by septic arthritis is the knee, which is involved in at least one-half of the cases. Other commonly involved joints are hips, shoulders, wrists, ankles, elbows, and sternoclavicular and sacroiliac joints. Involvement of the latter two joints has been noted in intravenous drug abusers. In the spine, the intervertebral disc space and adjacent vertebral bodies are infected. Infection in the hip is more difficult to recognize because swelling is less evident. Patients with hip infection might hold the thigh in adduction, flexion, and internal rotation. Pain is felt in the groin or thigh and is also referred to the anterior surface of the knee.

An overlying infected bursa or cellulitis can be mistaken for septic arthritis. It is important in aspirating a joint not to insert the needle through an infected bursa or cellulitis and possibly infect a normal joint.

Laboratory Findings. Joint fluid usually shows increased numbers of neutrophils ranging from 10,000 to greater than 100,000 per cubic millimeter. The white cell count in infected bursa fluid is not as high as observed in the joint. A peripheral blood leukocytosis might also be present. The synovial fluid glucose is usually less than 20% of a simultaneously drawn blood glucose when these two compartments are in equilibrium. Equilibrium is usually reached 6 hours after a meal. In gonococcal arthritis, however, the synovial fluid glucose is not significantly reduced. Gram stain performed on synovial fluid often shows bacteria except in gonococcal infections. Culture results of synovial fluid as well as blood are also often positive.

Radiography of the joint initially shows soft tissue swelling and distension of the joint capsule, followed later by juxta-articular osteoporosis and periosteal elevation. As the process continues, destruction of articular cartilage leads to joint space narrowing followed by bony erosions. Juxta-articular bone destruction might indicate osteomyelitis. In the spine, the initial change consists of narrowing of the disc space and proliferation of bone at vertebral margins. Osteolytic lesions in adjacent vertebrae are seen later. Radioisotope scans can be helpful in identifying infection in certain joints such as the hip, shoulder, spine, and sacroiliac joints, but inflammatory arthritides and degenerative joint disease also give a positive scan result.

Treatment. An infected joint requires immediate aspiration and rapid initiation of parenteral antibiotic therapy. It has been reported that joint outcome is best when patients are seen within 7 days of initial symptoms.[89] Joint fluid should be immediately cultured and a Gram stain performed. Vancomycin is the current suggested antibiotic for gram-positive infections (especially where methicillin-resistant *Staphylococcus aureus* [MRSA] infection is common) and generally a third-generation cephalosporin for gram-negative organisms. (The details of antibiotic therapy are beyond the scope of this text.) Antibiotics should be given intravenously for at least the first 2 weeks. A total of 6 weeks of antibiotic therapy is generally indicated but there is little evidenced based data with regard to length of therapy.[90] Antibiotics do not need to be infused into the joint. The joint should be adequately drained to prevent damage. Usually drainage can be accomplished with a large-gauge needle. Drainage reduces intra-articular pressure and removes pus, which is a source of proteolytic enzymes. Repeated aspirations are only necessary during the first few days of treatment. Surgical drainage is required when the joint cannot be adequately aspirated and irrigated by needle or when the cell count in the synovial fluid does not decline in spite of what appears to be adequate drainage. Surgical drainage via arthroscopy should also be considered in patients with underlying arthritis and those with prolonged symptoms (i.e., longer than 7 days).[88] During the first few days of treatment, splinting of the involved joint in extension makes the patient more comfortable and reduces the possibility of a flexion contracture. Daily physical therapy, once the acute process has resolved, improves the range of motion. In a severely damaged joint, bony fusion might be required.

Gonococcal Arthritis

Gonococcal arthritis is a frequent cause of bacterial arthritis in young adults. Women are more susceptible to gonococcal arthritis during menses and pregnancy. Persons who have a homozygous deficiency of complement component C5, C6, C7, or C8 are also susceptible to disseminated neisserial infections.[90] Patients with low complement levels caused by consumption of complement might also be more susceptible to disseminated neisserial infections.

Symptoms and Signs. Patients typically present with fever and migratory arthritis or arthralgias that evolve in several days into monoarticular arthritis. Patients also directly present with monoarticular arthritis. Wrists and knees are common sites of involvement, but any joint can be affected. Arthritis is manifested by swelling, erythema, and severe pain as in other bacterial arthritides. Skin lesions can accompany gonococcal arthritis. These lesions can be pustular, vesicular, or hemorrhagic and can ulcerate.

Laboratory Findings. Joint fluid shows increased numbers of polymorphonuclear white cells, but the white cell count might not be as high as in other bacterial infections. The joint fluid glucose is also not decreased to the low levels found in other bacterial joint infections.

Diagnosis. Gonococcal arthritis is suspected in a patient presenting with fever, typical skin lesions, and polyarthralgias or arthritis that evolves into monoarticular arthritis. Diagnosis is confirmed by positive culture results from synovial fluid or from blood, but culture results from these sites are positive in fewer than 50% of cases. Cultures from skin lesions are also usually negative. Gram stain or culture results from cervix, urethra, or rectum might be positive when joint, skin, and blood culture results are negative.

Treatment. The patient should be admitted to the hospital and receive parenteral antibiotics. Currently, the recommendation is to start a third-generation cephalosporin such as ceftriaxone since penicillin resistant strains are now widespread. The dose of ceftriaxone is 1 gram IV every 24 hours for 3 to 7 days. Most patients can be converted to oral antibiotic therapy in 48 hours. The patient is placed at bed rest for the first 2 days. Splinting of the affected joint provides pain relief. The infected joint should be immediately aspirated. The frequency of aspirations depends on the degree of inflammation. In most patients residual joint damage does not occur.

Polymyalgia Rheumatica

Polymyalgia rheumatica (PMR) is an inflammatory disease affecting people over the age of 50 years and typically those of Northern European ethnic background. Patients can generally remember the day or the week the symptoms began and the symptoms include marked stiffness of the shoulders and hip girdle regions, fatigue, and low-grade fever.[91] About 15% to 20% of patients may have joint swelling involving the wrists, finger joints, or the knees. Another feature that might be clue to PMR is a senior patient with bilateral "rotator cuff tendonitis." Patients my have rotator cuff signs and symptoms but it is unusual to have bilateral rotator cuff tendonitis. PMR is a synovitis and the tenosynovitis around the shoulder may lead to rotator cuff symptoms and signs. The general stiffness is often profound and a patient will describe significant difficulty getting out of bed. Patients will relate that they had to roll out of bed in order to get up. A related illness, giant cell arteritis (GCA), can present with manifestations of PMR but also includes headache and may include visual changes, jaw pain with chewing, and more pronounced systemic symptoms. It is important to recognize the difference between isolated PMR versus PMR plus GCA. If GCA is untreated it may lead to permanent visual loss in up to 50% or stroke in up to 10% of patients.

The laboratory hallmark of PMR is a markedly elevated ESR or CRP. A few patients (10% to 15%) may have normal levels and still have PMR, so the history is the key as well and the response to prednisone. Patients can also have mild anemia typical of other inflammatory diseases.

Treatment is, and has been for almost 50 years, prednisone. If suspected, an initial dose of 15 to 20 mg is sufficient in most patients with PMR, especially if a small portion is given in the evening. The initial dose is maintained for 4 to 6 weeks then slowly tapered. One taper regimen is to reduce the prednisone by 1 mg a week to 10 mg, 1 mg every 2 weeks to 5 mg, then 1 mg every month to 0 but there may be many small ups and downs on the prednisone dose. It must be recognized that the average length of disease duration is 24 months. If GCA is suspected, start the patients on high dose prednisone (40–60 mg per day) and refer to a rheumatologist. The patient will need to have temporal artery biopsy scheduled as soon as possible and may need additional therapy.

References

1. CDC. State Prevalence of Self-Reported Doctor-Diagnosed Arthritis and Arthritis-Attributable Activity Limitation—United States, 2003. *MMWR* 2006;55: 477–481.
2. Hootman JM, Helmick CG. Projections of US prevalence of arthritis and associated activity limitations. *Arthritis Rheum* 2006;54:226–229.
3. Bone and Joint Decade Website. Available online at http://www.usbjd.org/index.cfm.
4. Simkin PS, Gardner GC. Musculoskeletal system and joint physiology. In: Hochberg MC, Silman AJ, Smolen JS, et al, eds. *Textbook of Rheumatology*. Philadelphia: Mosby, 2003.
5. Brodal A. *Neurological Anatomy in Relation to Clinical Medicine*, 3rd ed. New York: Oxford University Press, 1981.

6. Prevalence of disabilities and associated health conditions among adults—United States, 1999. *MMWR Morb Mortal Wkly Rep* 2001;50:120–125.

7. Acheson RM, Collart AB. New Haven survey of joint diseases. *Ann Rheum Dis* 1975;34:379–387.

8. Lawrence JS, Bremner JM, Bier F. Osteoarthrosis. Prevalence in the population and relationship between symptoms and xray changes. *Ann Rheum Dis* 1966;25:1–24.

9. Stecher RM. Heberden's nodes. Heredity in hypertrophic arthritis of the finger joints. *Am J Med Sci* 1941;201:801–809.

10. Knowlton RG, Katzenstein PL, Moskowitz RW, et al. Genetic linkage of a polymorphism in the type II procollagen gene (COL2A1) to primary osteoarthritis associated with mild chondrodysplasia. *N Engl J Med* 1990;322:526–530.

11. Eyre DR, Weis MA, Moskowitz RW. Cartilage expression of a type II collagen mutation in an inherited form of osteoarthritis associated with a mild chondrodysplasia. *J Clin Invest* 1991;87:357–361.

12. Felson DT, Anderson JJ, Naimark A, et al. Obesity and knee osteoarthritis: the Framingham Study. *Ann Intern Med* 1988;109:18–24.

13. Felson DT, Zhang Y. An update on the epidemiology of knee and hip osteoarthritis with a view to prevention. *Arthritis Rheum* 1998;41:1343–1355.

14. Felson DT, Kim YJ. The futility of the current approaches to chondroprotection. *Arthritis Rheum* 2007;56:1378–1383.

15. Evarts CM. Challenge of the aging hip. *Geriatrics* 1969;24:112–119.

16. Lane NE. Osteoarthritis of the hip. *N Engl J Med* 2007;3587:1413–1421.

17. Sharma L, Pai YC. Impaired proprioception and osteoarthritis. *Curr Opin Rheumatol* 1997;9:253–258.

18. Bruckner FE, Howell A. Neuropathic joints. *Semin Arthritis Rheum* 1972;2:47–49.

19. Beighton P. Articular manifestations of the Ehlers-Danlos syndrome. *Semin Arthritis Rheum* 1972;1:246–261.

20. Askari AD, Muir WA, Rosner IA, et al. Arthritis of hemochromatosis. Clinical spectrum, relation to histocompatibility antigens, and effectiveness of early phlebotomy. *Am J Med* 1983;75:957–965.

21. Faraawi R, Harth M, Kertesz A, Bell D. Arthritis in haemochromatosis. *J Rheumatol* 1993;20:448.

22. Schumacher HR, Holdsworth DE. Ochronotic arthropathy. I. Clinicopathologic studies. *Semin Arthritis Rheum* 1977;6:207–246.

23. Bluestone R, Bywaters EG, Hartog M, et al. Acromegalic anthropathy. *Ann Rheum Dis* 1971;30:243–258.

24. Messier SP, Loeser RF, Miller GD, et al. Exercise and dietary weight loss in overweight and obese older adults with knee osteoarthritis: the Arthritis, Diet, and Activity Promotion Trial. *Arthritis Rheum* 2004;50:1501–1510.

25. Brouwer RW, van Raaij TM, Verhaar JA, et al. Brace treatment for osteoarthritis of the knee: a prospective randomized multi-centre trial. *Osteoarthritis Cartilage* 2006;14(8):777–783.

26. Reginster JY, Deroisy R, Rovati LC, et al. Long-term effects of glucosamine sulphate on osteoarthritis progression: a randomised, placebo-controlled clinical trial. *Lancet* 2001;357(9252):251–256.

27. Clegg DO, Reda DJ, Harris CL, et al. Glucosamine, chondroitin sulfate, and the two in combination for painful knee osteoarthritis. *N Engl J Med* 2006;354:795–808.

28. Raynauld JP, Buckland-Wright C, Ward R, et al. Safety and efficacy of long-term intraarticular steroid injections in osteoarthritis of the knee: a randomized, double-blind, placebo-controlled trial. *Arthritis Rheum* 2003;48(2):370–377.

29. Lo GH, LaValley M, McAlindon T, Felson DT. Intra-articular hyaluronic acid in treatment of knee osteoarthritis. *JAMA* 2003;290:3115–3121.

30. Mitchell D. Epidemiology. In: Utsinger PD, Zvaifler NJ, Ehrlich GE, eds. *Rheumatoid Arthritis*. Philadelphia: Lippincott, 1985:133–150.

31. Linos A, Worthington JW, O'Fallon WM, et al. The epidemiology of rheumatoid arthritis in Rochester, Minnesota: a study of incidence, prevalence and mortality. *Am J Epidemiol* 1980;111:87–98.

32. Stastny P. Association of the B-cell alloantigen DRw4 with rheumatoid arthritis. *N Engl J Med* 1978;298:869–871.

33. Weyland CM. New insights into the pathogenesis of rheumatoid arthritis. *Rheumatology* 2000;39(suppl. 1):3–8.

34. Harris ED. Rheumatoid arthritis. Pathophysiology and implications for therapy. *N Engl J Med* 1990;322:1277–1289.

35. van Zeben D, Hazes JMW, Zwinderman AH, et al. Clinical significance of rheumatoid factors in early rheumatoid arthritis: results of a follow up study. *Ann Rheum Dis* 1992;51:1029–1035.

36. Rothschild BM, Woods RJ, Rothschild C, et al. Geographic distribution of rheumatoid arthritis in ancient North America: implications for pathogenesis. *Semin Arthritis Rheum* 1992;22:181–187.

37. Avouac J, Gossec L, Dougados M. Diagnostic and predictive value of anti-citrullinated protein antibodies in rheumatoid arthritis: a systematic literature review. *Ann Rheum Dis* 2006;65;845–851.

38. Furst DE. Rheumatoid arthritis. Practical use of medications. *Postgrad Med* 1990;87:79–92.

39. Fuchs HA, Kaye JJ, Callahan LF, et al. Evidence of significant radiographic damage in rheumatoid arthritis within the first 2 years of disease. *J Rheumatol* 1989;16:585–591.

40. Scott DL, Symmons DPM, Coulton BL, et al. Long-term outcome of treating rheumatoid arthritis: results after 20 years. *Lancet* 1987;1:1108–1111.

41. Wilske KR, Healey LA. Remodeling the pyramid—a concept whose time has come. *J Rheumatol* 1989;16:565–567.

42. Gardner GC, Furst DA. Newer therapies for older adults with rheumatoid arthritis. *Drugs* 1995;7:420–437.

43. Fox RI. Mechanism of action of hydroxychloroquine as an antirheumatic drug. *Semin Arthritis Rheum* 1993;23(Suppl 1):82–91.

44. Cronstein BN. Low-dose methotrexate: a mainstay in the treatment of rheumatoid arthritis. *Pharmacol Rev* 2005;57:163–172.

45. van der Heijde D, Klareskog L, Landewé R, et al. Disease remission and sustained halting of radiographic progression with combination etanercept and methotrexate in patients with rheumatoid arthritis. *Arthritis Rheum* 2007;56:3928–3939.

46. Rhen T, Cidlowski JA. Anti-inflammatory actions of glucocorticoids: new mechanism for old drugs. *N Engl J Med* 2005;353:1711–1723.

47. Harris ED, Emkey RD, Nichols JE, et al. Low dose prednisone therapy in rheumatoid arthritis: a double blind study. *J Rheumatol* 1983;10:713–721.

48. Gardner GC, Weisman MH. Pyarthrosis in patients with rheumatoid arthritis: a report of 13 cases and a review of the literature from the past 40 years. *Am J Med* 1990;88:503–511.

49. Brewerton DA, Hart FD, Nicholls A, et al. Ankylosing spondylitis and HLA27. *Lancet* 1973;1:904–907.

50. Benjamin M, McGonagle D. The anatomical basis for disease localisation in seronegative spondyloarthropathy at entheses and related sites. *J Anat* 2001;199:503–526.

51. Dougados M, van der Linden S, Leirisalo-Repo M, et al. Sulfasalazine in the treatment of spondyloarthropathy. *Arthritis Rheum* 1995;5:618–627.

52. Calin A, Dijkmans BAC, Emery P, et al. Outcomes of a multicentre randomized clinical trial of etanercept to treat ankylosing spondylitis. *Ann Rheum Dis* 2004;63:1594–1600.

53. Marzo-Ortega H, McGonagle D, O'Connor P, Emery P. Efficacy of etanercept in the treatment of the entheseal pathology in resistant spondylarthropathy; a clinical and magnetic resonance imaging study. *Arthritis Rheum* 2001;44:2112–2117.

54. Mitchell MJ, Sartoris DJ, Moody D, et al. Cauda equina syndrome complicating ankylosing spondylitis. *Radiology* 1990;175:521–525.

55. Hunter T. The spinal complications of ankylosing spondylitis. *Semin Arthritis Rheum* 1989;19:172–182.

56. Grill V, Smith M, Ahern M, et al. Local radiotherapy for pedal manifestations of HLA-B27 related arthropathy. *Br J Rheumatol* 1988;27:390–392.

57. Brewerton DA, Caffrey M, Nicholls A, et al. Reiter's disease and HLA 27. *Lancet* 1973;2:996–998.

58. Calin A, Fries JF. An "experimental" epidemic of Reiter's syndrome, revisited: follow-up evidence on genetic and environmental factors. *Ann Intern Med* 1976;84:564–566.

59. Ritchlin C. Psoriatic disease: from skin to bone. *Nat Clin Pract Rheumatol* 2007;3:698–706.

60. Punzi L, Podswiadek M, Sfriso P, et al. Pathogenetic and clinical rationale for TNF-blocking therapy in psoriatic arthritis. *Autoimmun Rev* 2007;6:524–528.

61. Wollheim FA. Enteropathic arthritis. In: Kelley WN, Harris ED, Ruddy S, et al, eds. *Textbook of Rheumatology*, 5th ed. Philadelphia: Saunders, 1997:1006–1014.

62. Hamilton EBD. Disease associated with CPPD deposition disease. *Arthritis Rheum* 1976;19:353–357.

63. Russell RGG. Metabolism of inorganic pyrophosphate (PPi). *Arthritis Rheum* 1976;19:465–478.

64. Altman RD, Muniz OE, Pita JC, et al. Microanalysis of inorganic pyrophosphate (PPi) in synovial fluid and plasma. *Arthritis Rheum* 1973;16:171–178.

65. O'Duffy JD. Clinical studies of acute pseudogout attacks. Comments on prevalence, predispositions, and treatment. *Arthritis Rheum* 1976;19:349–352.

66. Bennett RM, Lehr JR, McCarty DJ. Factors affecting the solubility of calcium pyrophosphate dihydrate crystals. *J Clin Invest* 1975;56:1571–1579.

67. Choi HK, Mount DB, Reginato AM. Pathogenesis of gout. *Ann Intern Med* 2005;143:499–516.

68. Bywaters EGL. Gout in the time and person of George IV: a case history. *Ann Rheum Dis* 1962;21:325–338.

69. Evans JG, Prior IAM, Harvey HB. Relation of serum uric acid to body bulk, haemoglobin and alcohol intake in two South Pacific Polynesian populations. *Ann Rheum Dis* 1968;27:319–325.

70. Nishioka K, Mikanagi K. Hereditary and environmental factors influencing on the serum uric acid throughout ten years population study in Japan. *Adv Exp Med Biol* 1980;122A:155–159.

71. Currie WJC. Prevalence and incidence of the diagnosis of gout in Great Britain. *Ann Rheum Dis* 1979;38:101–106.

72. Zalokar J, Lellouch J, Claude JR. Serum urate and gout in 4663 young male workers. *Semin Hop Paris* 1981;57:664–670.

73. Healey LA, Bayani-Sioson PS. A defect in the renal excretion of uric acid in Filipinos. *Arthritis Rheum* 1971;14:721–726.

74. Lesch M, Nyhan WL. A familial disorder of uric acid metabolism and central nervous system function. *Am J Med* 1964;36:561–570.

75. Hollander JL, Stoner EK, Brown EM, et al. Joint temperature measurements in the evaluation of antiarthritic agents. *J Clin Invest* 1951;30:701–706.

76. Simkin PA. Concentration of urate by differential diffusion: a hypothesis for initial urate deposition. In: Sperling O, DeVries A, Wyngaarden JB, eds. *Purine Metabolism in Man*. New York: Plenum, 1974:547–550.

77. Akahoshi T, Murakami Y, Kitasato H. Recent advances in crystal-induced acute inflammation. *Curr Opin Rheumatol* 2007;19:146–150.

78. Faller J, Fox IH. Ethanol-induced hyperuricemia: evidence for increased urate

production by activation of adenine nucleotide turnover. *N Engl J Med* 1982; 307:1598–1602.

79. Halla JT, Ball GV. Saturnine gout: a review of 42 patients. *Semin Arthritis Rheum* 1982;11:307–314.
80. Maclachlan MJ, Rodnan GP. Effects of food, fast, and alcohol on serum uric acid and acute attacks of gout. *Am J Med* 1967;42:38–57.
81. Lin HY, Rocher LL, McQuillan MA, et al. Cyclosporine-induced hyperuricemia and gout. *N Engl J Med* 1989;321:287–292.
82. Simkin PA, Campbell PM, Larson EB. Gout in Heberden's nodes. *Arthritis Rheum* 1983;26:94–97.
83. Gatter RA. The compensated polarized light microscope in clinical rheumatology [editorial]. *Arthritis Rheum* 1974;17:253–255.
84. Kuncl RW, Duncan G, Watson D, et al. Colchicine myopathy and neuropathy. *N Engl J Med* 1987;316:1562–1568.
85. Terkeltaub RA. Gout. *N Engl J Med* 2003;349:1647–1655.

86. Goldenberg DL, Reed JI. Bacterial arthritis. *N Engl J Med* 1985;312:764–771.
87. Goldenberg DL. Bacterial arthritis. In: Kelley WN, Harris ED, Ruddy S, et al, eds. *Textbook of Rheumatology*, 5th ed. Philadelphia: Saunders, 1997: 1435–1449.
88. Gardner GC, Weisman MH. Pyarthrosis in patients with rheumatoid arthritis: a report of 13 cases and a review of the literature from the past 40 years. *Am J Med* 1990;88:503–511.
89. Ho G, Su EY. Therapy for septic arthritis. *JAMA* 1982;247:797–800.
90. Mathews CJ, Kingsley G, Field M, et al. Management of septic arthritis: a systematic review. *Ann Rheum Dis* 2007;66:440–445.
91. Petersen BH, Lee TJ, Snyderman R, et al. *Neisseria meningitidis* and *Neisseria gonorrhoea* bacteremia associated with C6, C7, or C8 deficiency. *Ann Intern Med* 1979;90:917–920.
92. Gardner GC. Polymyalgia rheumatica and giant cell arteritis. In: Rankel R, ed. *Conn's Current Therapy*. Philadelphia: WB Saunders, 2000:970–971.

CHAPTER 35 ■ MYOFASCIAL PAIN SYNDROME

JAN DOMMERHOLT AND JAY P. SHAH

INTRODUCTION TO MYOFASCIAL PAIN SYNDROME

Muscle pain is a common manifestation of many chronic pain conditions and is described as a diffuse, difficult to pinpoint, aching pain that may refer to deep somatic structures.[1,2] Muscle pain is common in all age groups, but chronic muscle pain is more frequent in the elderly than in younger populations.[3,4] Kellgren[5] was one of the first researchers to explore the diffuse nature of muscle pain and particular-referred pain patterns. Muscle-referred pain involves nociceptive specific neurons in the spinal cord and in the brainstem.[6,7] Wall and Woolf[8] have shown that muscle nociceptive afferents are especially effective in inducing neuroplastic changes in the spinal dorsal horn. Muscle pain activates specific cortical structures, such as the anterior cingulate gyrus, which is also involved in the emotional, affective component of pain.[9–11] Muscle pain is inhibited strongly by descending pain-modulating pathways, and, under normal circumstances, there is a dynamic balance between the degree of activation of dorsal horn neurons and the descending inhibitory systems.[12] Prolonged input from muscle nociceptors can be misinterpreted in the central nervous system and eventually can lead to allodynia and hyperalgesia and an expansion of receptive fields.[13]

Although muscle pain is very common, there is considerable controversy regarding the nature and relevance of muscle pain. Some clinicians consider muscle pain to be a secondary phenomenon to other diagnoses, such as tendonitis, muscle strain, inflammation, degeneration, or injuries to joints and nerves.[14] Gunn has proposed that all muscle pain (or more precisely, all myofascial pain) is the result of peripheral neuropathy, defined by Gunn as "a condition that causes disordered function in the peripheral nerve."[15] Gunn's model is based on Cannon and Rosenblueth's Law of Denervation, which states that the function and integrity of innervated structures is dependent on the free flow of nerve impulses.[16] When the flow of impulses is restricted, all innervated structures, including muscles, would become atrophic, highly irritable, and supersensitive.[15] In spite of a few early scientific outcome studies and numerous case reports, there are no studies that support the notion that myofascial pain is indeed always indicative of neuropathic pain. Gunn's model was never devel-

oped beyond the hypothetical stage, although he has denied that his approach is even based on a hypothetical model.[17] According to Gunn, his model is a "description of clinical findings that can be found by anyone who examines a patient for radiculopathy."[17]

Another example of muscle pain is the delayed onset of muscle soreness after eccentric exercise[18] which typically resolves in a few days and is generally of little concern to clinicians. Others view persistent muscle pain primarily as a manifestation of a presumed somatoform disorder.[19] With the development of orthopedic and manual medicine, physicians, chiropractors, and physical therapists directed their attention mostly to articular dysfunction, although early manual medicine pioneers Drs. James Cyriax and John Mennell did include muscle dysfunction in their thinking.[20–22] In this context, it is noteworthy that, although skeletal muscle comprises nearly half of the body's weight, it is the only organ in the human body that is not linked to a particular medical specialty. This has led Simons to suggest that muscle is an orphan organ, as further evidenced by the fact that muscle research and the development of a knowledge base of muscle-specific ailments, pathophysiology, and diagnostic and treatment options have not evolved until fairly recently.[23] The literature on myofascial pain is scattered among the literature of many different disciplines. One could wonder why persistent muscle pain and dysfunction have largely been ignored by the medical professions, but such contemplations are outside the scope of this chapter.

BRIEF HISTORICAL OVERVIEW

Over the past centuries, several articles and books have been published about muscle pain and dysfunction.[24,25] For example, in the 16th century, French physician Guillaume de Baillou (1538–1616) described specific muscle pain syndromes. In 1816, British physician Balfour reported observing muscles with "nodular tumors and thickenings which were painful to the touch, and from which pains shot to neighboring parts."[26] Muscle pain has been described by many different terms, including fibrositis, interstitial myofibrositis, myogeloses, nonarticular rheumatism, myofascial pain, idiopathic myalgia, myofasciitis, perineuritis, myodysneuria, and fibromyalgia. The publications by Kellgren, describing referred pain patterns from muscles and other soft tissues, strongly influenced physicians James Cyriax in England and Janet Travell in the United States. In 1942, Cyriax published his book *Massage, Manipulation and Local Anaesthesia* in which he devoted much attention to referred pain phenomena. Cyriax advocated treating nodules and taut bands of abnormal muscle tissue with deep friction massage.[27] Cyriax was very influential, and his work became a major aspect of modern manual medicine and manual therapy practice.[28]

At the time of Kellgren's first publications, Travell was a cardiologist and researcher. Initially, she was mostly interested in the applicability of Kellgren's findings to cardiac pain, but she quickly became interested in musculoskeletal medicine.[29] In 1942, she coauthored the first of many articles about the diagnosis and treatment of muscle pain.[30] In 1952, Travell and Rinzler published an article of observed pain referral patterns of 32 muscles (Fig. 35.1).[31]

At that time, there was virtually no research on muscle pain, and many of Travell's writings were based on her empirical observations and ability to establish clinical correlations. For example, Travell and Rinzler observed that the fascia generated similar referred pain patterns as the contractile elements of the muscle; she subsequently modified her terminology to "myofascial pain" to encompass both the fibrous and contractile aspects.[31] Interestingly, the similarities between referred pain patterns of fascia and muscle and the mechanical relationships between fascia and muscle were not further investigated until only a few years ago.[32]

Travell's work eventually culminated in the publication of a two-volume textbook on myofascial pain, which she coauthored with Dr. David Simons.[33,34] These books became known as the Trigger Point Manuals and they have been translated in multiple languages. The term "trigger point" was introduced by Steindler in 1940 in a paper on muscle pain.[35] Travell and Rinzler introduced the terms "myofascial trigger point" and "myofascial pain syndrome,"[31] which are now intricately linked to a particular theoretical model, referred to as the "integrated trigger point hypothesis."[36] The terms "muscle pain" and "myofascial pain" are sometimes used interchangeably; however, "muscle pain" is really a descriptive term while "myofascial pain," as introduced by Travell, is much more specific.[37]

Travell's concepts of myofascial pain did not gain wide acceptance in the manual medicine world and are not uniformly accepted even today. She is rarely mentioned in the manual medicine literature and is mostly remembered for blocking the profession of physical therapy from membership into the North American Academy of Manipulative Medicine, an organization she founded in 1966 with Mennell.[28] Travell did gain some recognition in the pain management world, however. A growing number of pain management clinicians and researchers are integrating Travell's model in their practices and laboratories. A survey of physician members of the American Pain Society showed overwhelming agreement that myofascial pain is a distinct clinical entity.[38] A second edition of Volume 1 of the Trigger Point Manual was published in 1999.[39]

In 1981, Simons and Travell developed a hypothetical model explaining the phenomena they observed. This model became known as the "energy crisis hypothesis."[40] The energy crisis hypothesis postulates that direct trauma and subsequent damage to the sarcoplasmic reticulum or the muscle cell membrane leads to an increase in calcium (Ca^{2+}) concentration, increased activation of actin and myosin, a relative shortage of adenosine triphosphate (ATP), and an impaired calcium pump, which in turn would increase the intracellular calcium concentration even more, completing the cycle.[40] Under normal physiological conditions, the calcium pump is responsible for returning intracellular Ca^{2+} to the sarcoplasmic reticulum against a concentration gradient, which requires a functional energy supply. In 1999, the energy crisis hypothesis was integrated into the integrated trigger point hypothesis.[39] In turn, several recent publications have expanded the integrated trigger point hypothesis based on electrodiagnos-

tic, histopathological studies, and other related fields.[36,41–44] This chapter provides an updated review of the etiology, mechanisms, pathophysiology, and clinical implications of myofascial trigger points, including the integrated trigger point hypothesis.

BASIC MYOFASCIAL PAIN CONCEPTS

During the past decade, research in the etiology, epidemiology, pathophysiology, diagnosis, and clinical management of myofascial pain has grown exponentially. Although the integrated trigger point hypothesis is not a perfect theoretical concept, it is the most comprehensive evidence-informed model currently available to explain the role of muscle tissue in acute and persistent pain conditions.[36] Researchers around the world are conducting basic trigger point research, prevalence studies, and clinical outcome studies. Their findings show that trigger points are associated with virtually all painful musculoskeletal problems, including migraines, tension-type headaches, craniomandibular dysfunction, epicondylalgia, low back pain, postlaminectomy syndrome, neck pain, disc pathology, carpal tunnel syndrome, osteoarthritis, radiculopathies, whiplash-associated disorders, fibromyalgia, postherpetic neuralgia, complex regional pain syndrome, etc.[41] Trigger points have also been associated with visceral dysfunction, including endometriosis, interstitial cystitis, irritable bowel syndrome, urinary/renal and gallbladder calculosis, dysmenorrhea, and prostadynia.[45–51] Although trigger points are reportedly the most common diagnosis responsible for chronic pain and disability, they are frequently overlooked in the clinic.[52] Trigger points have been reported in all age groups except infants.[3,39,53–56]

A trigger point is described as "a hyperirritable spot in skeletal muscle that is associated with a hypersensitive palpable nodule in a taut band."[39] By definition, trigger points are located within a taut band of contractured muscle fibers. Palpating for trigger points begins with identifying this taut band by palpating perpendicular to the fiber direction (Fig. 35.2).

Two recent studies confirmed the existence of taut bands using magnetic resonance elastography (MRE).[57,58] Taut bands are stiffer than relaxed muscle fibers, and the degree of stiffness can be assessed by phase-contrast analysis of vibration-induced cyclic shear waves.[57–60] Sikdar et al.[61] demonstrated that myofascial trigger points can be visualized using diagnostic ultrasound and sonoelastography. Myofascial trigger points are hypoechoic on two-dimensional ultrasound and appear stiffer than the surrounding muscle on vibration sonoelastography. An active trigger point produces symptoms, including local tenderness and pain, referral of pain or other paresthesia to a distant site, and peripheral and central sensitization. A latent trigger point is only painful when stimulated. Trigger points have characteristic motor, sensory, and autonomic features. Motor phenomena associated with trigger points include disturbed motor function, muscle weakness as a result of motor inhibition, muscle stiffness, and restricted range of motion. Nociceptive input can perpetuate altered motor control strategies and lead to muscle overload or disuse.[62,63] Lucas et al.[64] demonstrated that subjects with latent trigger points in several shoulder muscles featured altered shoulder abduction patterns when compared to healthy subjects. Autonomic aspects may include, among others, vasoconstriction, vasodilatation, lacrimation, and piloerection.[65]

To discuss the current research and the clinical implications of myofascial trigger points and the integrated trigger point hypothesis, a brief review of muscle physiology, the role of the motor endplate, muscle pain, dorsal horn, and central sensitization will be provided in the context of myofascial trigger points. The motor phenomena of trigger points are best explained by

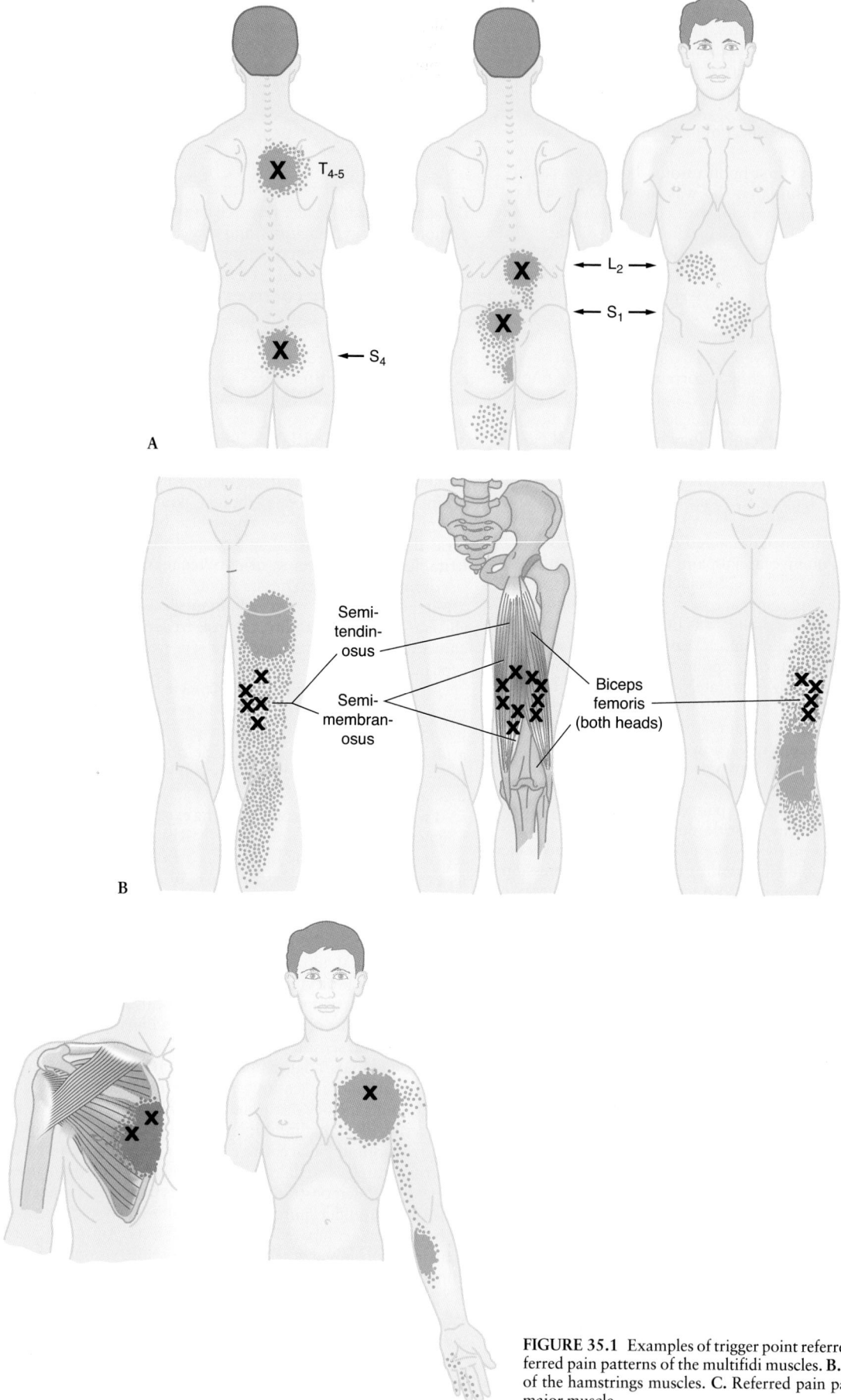

FIGURE 35.1 Examples of trigger point referred pain patterns. **A.** Referred pain patterns of the multifidi muscles. **B.** Referred pain patterns of the hamstrings muscles. **C.** Referred pain pattern of the pectoralis major muscle.

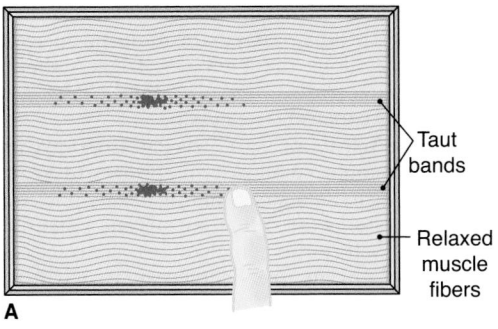

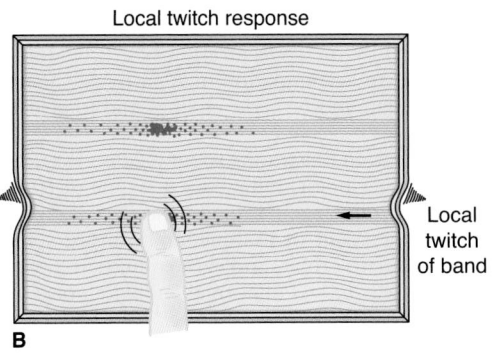

Local twitch response

Taut bands

Relaxed muscle fibers

Local twitch of band

A

B

FIGURE 35.2 Palpation of trigger points. As the palpating finger of the examiner moves from normal areas of muscle (**A**) and encounters a painful trigger point (**B**), a local twitch response often occurs within the muscle surrounding the trigger point. (Redrawn after Simons DG, Travell JG, Simons LS. *Travell and Simons' Myofascial Pain and Dysfunction; The Trigger Point Manual*. 2nd ed. Baltimore: Lippincott Williams & Wilkins; 1999.)

understanding the functions and structure of the motor endplate and the sarcomere assembly.

MUSCLE PHYSIOLOGY

Skeletal muscles consist of groups of fascicles, which are made of muscle fibers and myofibrils, accountable for contraction and relaxation of the fiber. The myofibril is approximately 1 to 2 μm in diameter and is separated from surrounding myofibrils by the

mitochondria, the sarcoplasmic reticulum, and the transverse tubular systems (T-tubules).

The T-tubules lie perpendicular to the long axis of the muscle fiber with two zones of transverse tubules to each sarcomere via the so-called dihydropyridine and ryanodine receptors. The main function of the T-tubules is to conduct impulses from the exterior to the interior of the muscle fiber with the release of Ca^{2+} from the sarcoplasmic reticulum, which is a store for the release and uptake of Ca^{2+}. Calcium is a prerequisite for muscle contractions. Muscle contractions occur after actin and troponin are activated by Ca^{2+}, allowing tropomyosin to shift its position and expose myosin-binding sites on actin, thus regulating the cross-bridge interactions between actin and myosin.[66] Myofibrils show a striated patterning when viewed under longitudinal electron micrograph scanning, which reflects the organization of thin actin and thicker myosin filaments. In addition to actin and myosin, there are several other important proteins, such as titin, nebulin, desmin, tropomyosin, troponin, and tropomodulin, among others, which together maintain the architecture and stability of the sarcomere (Fig. 35.3).[67–69]

Titin is the largest known vertebrate protein; it connects the Z-line with myosin filaments with cross-links from titin molecules of adjacent sarcomeres. Titin positions the myosin filaments at the center of the sarcomere as a spring.[70,71] One particular section of titin, the so-called PEVK domain or segment, is able to interact with actin filaments in close proximity to the Z-line, which may limit the degree of sarcomere contraction as the tip of the myosin filament may literally bounce back against a "viscous bumper" of the actin-titin interaction, similar to a dragnet.[72,73] Titin filaments are responsible for passive tension generation when sarcomeres are stretched, and provide muscle stiffness by virtue of its spring mechanism in the I-band. During sarcomere contractions, titin filaments are folded into a sticky gel-like structure at the Z-line.[68,70,71,74] Myofascial trigger points are thought to have a damaged sarcomere assembly; myosin filaments may have broken the actin-titin barrier and have literally gotten stuck in the sticky titin substance at the Z-line.[75]

Single molecules of nebulin span the full length of the actin filaments, and it is thought that nebulin actually dictates the architecture of actin with direct involvement of titin and the Z-line protein myopalladin.[76] Titin and nebulin interact at many levels, especially during myofibrillogenesis.[77] Nebulin connects to the proteins myopalladin and desmin in the Z-line.[78] Myopalladin binds to α-actinin, which in turn connects to actin and to titin.[78] Desmin filaments link adjacent Z-lines and interconnect the myofibrils with the sarcolemma, the nuclei, the T-tubules, the mito-

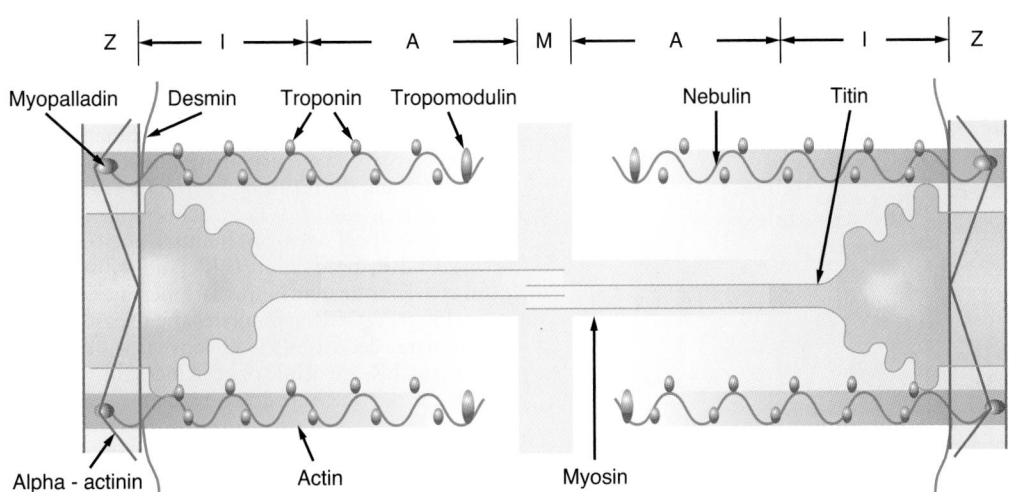

Z | I | A | M | A | I | Z

Myopalladin   Desmin   Troponin   Tropomodulin   Nebulin   Titin

Alpha-actinin   Actin   Myosin

FIGURE 35.3 Sarcomere.

chondria, and possibly the microtubules.[66,79] Nebulin acts as a stabilizing structure through its specific binding sites at different places at actin, but also at tropomyosin, troponin, and tropomodulin.[66,77,80,81] Nebulin regulates muscle contractions by inhibiting the cross-bridge formation until actin is activated by Ca^{2+}.[77]

A key feature of the integrated trigger point hypothesis is the presence of excessive acetylcholine (ACh) at the neuromuscular junction, which stimulates voltage-gated sodium channels of the sarcoplasmic reticulum and continuously increases intracellular Ca^{2+} levels. This results in ongoing activation of nebulin, troponin, and tropomyosin, and causes persistent muscle contractures consistent with myofascial trigger points. The role of the neuromuscular junction or motor endplate will be reviewed in the next section.

THE MOTOR ENDPLATE

The terms neuromuscular junction and motor endplate are used interchangeably, although technically, the neuromuscular junction refers to function, while the motor endplate refers to structure.[43] A motor endplate is the synapse between the terminal ends of motor neurons and skeletal muscle. The terminal branches of a single motor neuron terminate in multiple presynaptic boutons, which each contain many ACh vesicles.[82]

When nerve impulses from an α-motor neuron reach the motor nerve terminal, voltage-gated sodium (Na^+) channels are opened, which trigger a Na^+ influx that depolarizes the terminal membrane. Voltage-gated Ca^{2+} channels are opened, which causes an influx of Ca^{2+} and a quantal release of ACh and other molecules, such as ATP, from the nerve terminal into the synaptic cleft (Fig. 35.4). When two ACh molecules bind to a nicotinic ACh receptor (nAChR) across the synaptic cleft, the nAChR opens a cation-specific pore, which facilitates a Na^+ influx and a potassium (K^+) efflux across the muscle cell membrane. Each single quantum of ACh will depolarize the postsynaptic cell and trigger a miniature endplate potential (MEPP). A sufficient number of MEPP's will produce a depolarization and an action potential, which travels along the T-tubules, triggers the ryanodine receptor in the sarcoplasmic reticulum, and causes a release of Ca^{2+} from the sarcoplasmic reticulum.

As stated, the release of Ca^{2+} triggers tropomyosin to shift its position and nebulin to allow cross-bridges to form between the actin and myosin filaments, resulting in a muscle contraction. The K^+ efflux restores the resting membrane potential. During the brief period before the actual muscle contraction, ACh is hydrolyzed by the enzyme acetylcholinesterase (AChE) into acetate and choline. Choline is reabsorbed into the nerve terminal, where it is synthesized into ACh by acetyltransferase by combining choline and acetyl coenzyme A from the mitochondria. ACh release is not only activated by motor nerve stimulation, but it is also modulated by the concentration of AChE. Inhibition of AChE will cause an accumulation of ACh in the synaptic cleft, which may stimulate motor nerve endings and tonically activate nAChRs.

A 1993 publication illustrating spontaneous electrical activity in myofascial trigger points initiated a new line of research into the role of motor endplates.[83] Initially, the electrical activity was assumed to be the result of dysfunctional muscle spindles, but soon multiple human, rabbit, and even equine studies confirmed that the activity was in fact abnormal endplate noise, related to an excess of ACh at the motor endplate.[36,84-91] Wang and Yu[75] postulated that in myofascial trigger points, the contractures resulting from excessive ACh may cause myosin filaments to get stuck in sticky titin gel at the Z-line, thereby damaging the sarcomere assembly. The persistent contractures will compromise local blood vessels, reducing the local oxygen supply, which will result in hypoxia, a lowered pH, and hypoperfusion, which all contribute to muscle pain and dysfunction.[92] There is evidence that the oxygen saturation in myofascial trigger points is far below normal values.[93]

The reduced oxygen levels in myofascial trigger points and an increased metabolic demand result in a local energy shortage and a local shortage of ATP.[44] Under normal physiologic circumstances, presynaptic ATP inhibits the release of ACh. Inversely, a decrease in ATP leads to an increased ACh release. Insufficient postsynaptic ATP results in a failure of the calcium pump, increased levels of Ca^{2+}, and a Ca^{2+}-induced Ca^{2+} release. An increase in the Ca^{2+} concentration will reinforce muscle contractures. The local energy crisis is likely related to the finding of abnormal mitochondria in the nerve terminal and ragged red fibers, which are an indication of structural damage to the cell membrane and the mitochondria.[94]

The presence of excessive ACh can be the result of AChE insufficiency, an acidic pH, hypoxia, a lack of ATP, certain genetic mutations, drugs and particular chemicals, such as calcitonin-gene related peptide (CGRP), di-isopropylfluorophosphate, or organophosphate pesticides, and increased sensitivity of the nAChRs.[42,44,95] Myofascial tension or muscle hypertonicity, as seen in trigger points, may also enhance the excessive release of ACh.[96,97] There are many possible vicious cycles capable of maintaining the resulting contractures and trigger points. For example, hypoxia leads to an acidic milieu, muscle damage, and an excessive local release of multiple nociceptive substances, including CGRP, bradykinin (BK), and substance P (SP).[98] Hypoxia may even trigger an immediate increased ACh release at the motor endplate.[95] CGRP stimulates the release of ACh from the motor endplate, decreases the effectiveness of AChE, and upregulates the nAChR. An acidic pH enhances the release of calcitonin gene-related peptide and down-regulates AChE and causes hyperalgesia.[42,99,100]

There are many similarities between the mechanisms and consequences of myofascial trigger points and eccentric loading or eccentric exercise. Eccentric training or exposure is frequently characterized by a certain degree of cytoskeletal muscle damage.

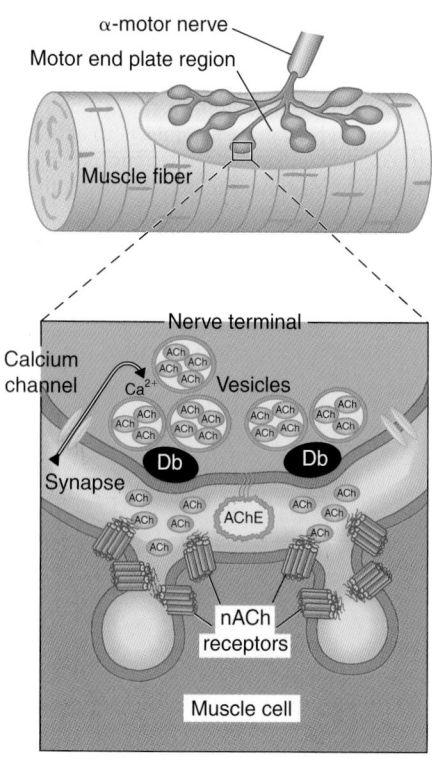

α-motor nerve

Motor end plate region

Muscle fiber

Nerve terminal

Calcium channel

Ca^{2+}

Vesicles

Db   Db

Synapse

AChE

nACh receptors

Muscle cell

FIGURE 35.4 The motor endplate.

Even very short bouts of eccentric exercise can result in a disorganization of the A-band, streaming of the Z-line, and a disruption of several cytoskeletal proteins, including titin, nebulin, vimentin, fibronectin, and desmin.[101–106] By comparison, postmortem histological studies of myofascial trigger points showed pathologic alterations of the mitochondria, as well as an increased width of A-bands and decreased width of I-bands in muscle sarcomeres of trigger points in 102 biopsies of the trapezius, gluteus medius, and gluteus maximus muscles. The samples were taken in a time period of 4–48 hours following death.[107,108] A biopsy study of trigger points in a dog gracilis muscle revealed a similar pattern of severely shortened sarcomeres in the center and lengthened sarcomeres outside the immediate trigger point region.[109] The diagnosis of trigger points in animals is basically the same as in human subjects. While an animal cannot verbalize recognition of pain, skilled palpation combined with an analysis of dysfunctional movement patterns will direct the investigator or clinician to clinically relevant trigger points.

There are other similarities between eccentric loading and myofascial trigger points, such as hypoxia, an impaired local circulation, and local and referred pain. Gerwin, Dommerholt, and Shah[42] suggested that eccentric contractions in unconditioned muscle or unaccustomed eccentric contractions are likely sources of myofascial trigger point development, which was confirmed by Itoh et al.[110] who demonstrated that eccentric exercise facilitated the formation of taut bands and myofascial trigger points in exercised muscle.

Yet, there are other possible causes of trigger points. Patients commonly report an onset of pain associated with trigger points following either acute, repetitive, prolonged, or chronic muscle overload. Piano students developed significantly decreased pressure thresholds over latent trigger points after only 20 minutes of continuous piano playing.[111] Computer operators developed trigger points after as little as 30 minutes of continuous typing.[112] In other words, low-level muscle contractions can contribute to the development of trigger points, which is best explained by the so-called Cinderella hypothesis.[113] According to the Cinderella hypothesis, low-level muscle contractions follow stereotypical patterns, where smaller motor units are recruited before and derecruited after larger motor units, which means that smaller type 1 fibers may be continuously activated during prolonged low-level contractions.[114,115] Low-level contractions have been shown to lead to muscle fiber degeneration, an increase in Ca^{2+} release, energy depletion, and the release of various cytokines, which all have been associated with the formation of trigger points.[116–119] During low-level contractions, the intramuscular pressure increases considerably especially near the muscle insertions, which may impair the local circulation, cause hypoxia, and eventually lead to trigger point formation.[41,120] As noted, motor phenomena associated with trigger points include disturbed motor function, muscle weakness as a result of motor inhibition, muscle stiffness, and restricted range of motion.

SENSITIZATION AND ACTIVATION OF MUSCLE NOCICEPTORS

To better understand the sensory aspects of myofascial trigger points, including local and referred tenderness, pain, and other paresthesia, as well as peripheral and central sensitization, a brief review of the current understanding of muscle nociceptors, spinal cord mechanisms, and sensitization is indicated.

Muscle nociceptors are dynamic structures that can be activated mechanically by deforming the axonal membrane of the nerve ending, as for example, following a blow to a muscle. They are also very susceptible to chemical activation by pain producing substances released from the surrounding tissues and immune cells.[121] Matched receptors at the nociceptor exist for a variety of substances including BK, prostaglandins (PG), serotonin (5-HT), protons (H^+), ATP, glutamate, and others, including the so-called purinergic and vanilloid receptors. Purinergic receptors bind ATP and stimulate nociceptors accordingly. Vanilloid receptors are especially sensitive under conditions of lowered tissue pH and muscle ischemia. Pain during tension-type headaches, tooth clenching, and bruxism is mediated by the vanilloid receptor molecule.[121] BK, 5-HT, and PG interact at many levels at the vanilloid receptors.[122] A combination of substances may have a synergistic effect in terms of local muscle pain production. For example, when injected together into the temporalis muscle of normal volunteers, BK, and 5-HT produce more pain than when each stimulant is injected alone.[123]

Moreover, the mechanism of chemical activation is of clinically greater interest, especially in evaluating chronic pain states where there often is little gross swelling evident. Endogenous substances such as BK, PG, and 5-HT are not only very effective at sensitizing or activating muscle nociceptors, but also cause local vasodilation. Therefore, the release of these substances can also lead to mechanoreceptor activation by distorting the normal tissue relationships. A sensitized muscle nociceptor has a lowered stimulation threshold into the innocuous range, such that it will respond to harmless stimuli like light pressure and muscle movement.[124]

The nociceptor terminals contain neuropeptides, such as SP and CGRP. When these substances are released, they stimulate local vasodilation, plasma extravasation, and liberation of sensitizing substances from the surrounding tissue. The effects of these neuropeptides are integral to the nociceptive response. Upon activation by a noxious stimulus, the nociceptor releases the stored neuropeptides, which directly influence the local microcirculation by stimulating vasodilation and increasing the permeability of the microvasculature.[125,126] More importantly, the secretion of the neuropeptides in sufficient quantity leads to a cascade of events, including the release of histamine from mast cells, BK from kallidin, 5-HT from platelets, and PGs from endothelial cells.[127] The cumulative effect is the increased production and release of sensitized substances in a localized region of edema in the muscle tissue. Therefore, the muscle nociceptor is not merely a passive structure designed to record potentially noxious stimuli. Rather, muscle nociceptors play an active role in the maintenance of normal tissue homeostasis by sensing the peripheral biochemical milieu and by mediating the vascular supply to peripheral tissue. With tissue injury, the secretion of SP and CGRP increases, leading to the response outlined above that can alter the responsiveness of the nociceptor. Muscle tenderness is mainly due to the sensitization of muscle nociceptors by BK, PG, and 5-HT, which may account for the exquisite tenderness found when firm pressure is applied over an active trigger point.[128]

As noted before, the activation of a nociceptive terminal is not primarily due to a nonspecific damage of the nerve ending by a strong stimulus. Rather, the binding of specific substances, including BK, PG, and 5-HT to their paired receptors on muscle nociceptors, is more often responsible.[124] Receptor responsiveness is dynamic. For example, inflammation alters the population of BK receptors at the nociceptive terminal. In normal muscle tissue, the B2 receptor is more prevalent. With tissue inflammation, an additional BK receptor (B1) is synthesized in the cell body of the ending in the dorsal root ganglion and inserted into the nociceptor terminal membrane. Unlike the B2 receptor, which is constitutively expressed, the B1 receptor is inducible and is involved in sensitization of the peripheral nociceptor. Induction and binding of the B1 receptor can also lead to the production of proinflammatory mediators, including tumor necrosis factor-α (TNF-α) and interleukin-1 β (IL-1β). Stimulation of B2 receptors leads to only transient increases in the intracellular calcium concentration and, for this reason, sensitization of the nociceptor is less likely. Conversely, stimulation of the B1 receptor results in prolonged elevation of intracellular Ca^{2+} concentration, which can lead to sustained peripheral sensitization.[129,130] If the conformational change of the BK receptor persists, even after the inflammation subsides, this maladaptive change may herald the transition from acute to chronic pain. Therefore, the degree to which muscle nociceptors in a trigger point become sensitized or activated will vary according to the balance of sensitizing substances in the muscle tissue and the threshold of their respective receptors. There may be a spectrum of nociceptor irritability based on this balance that distinguishes a normal muscle from a muscle with a latent or active trigger point.

CENTRAL SENSITIZATION

In addition to sensitization of the peripheral nociceptors, the pain and dysfunction induced by trigger points may also be due to alterations in the responsiveness of the dorsal horn. A chronic active trigger point may be the source of ongoing noxious input that sensitizes dorsal horn neurons and generates increased or referred pain to other spinal cord segments via central sensitization.[131,132] Conversely, a sensitized central nervous system may lead to a lowering of the activation threshold of the peripheral nociceptors in a trigger point, inducing the transition from a latent to an active trigger point. The latter may occur when trigger points develop secondary to referred pain from viscera, joints, or as a result of psychological stress. Giamberdino et al.[133] have established that visceral referred pain with hyperalgesia is usually associated with cutaneous hyperalgesia and with trigger points. Vecchiet et al.[134,135] measured significantly lower pain thresholds with electrical stimulation over active trigger points in the muscles, but also in the overlying cutaneous and subcutaneous tissues. With latent trigger points, the sensory changes did not involve the cutaneous and subcutaneous tissues.[134,135] Nociceptive input from the viscera may sensitize the central nervous system and indirectly lower the threshold for peripheral trigger point nociceptors. Because of this phenomenon, trigger points in the abdominal wall can be used for diagnostic purposes. Jarrell[51] found that the presence or absence of a trigger point in the abdominal wall helps to determine whether there is evidence of current or previously treated visceral disease. The presence of an abdominal wall trigger point predicted evidence of visceral disease in 90% of subjects. However, the absence of a trigger point was associated with no visceral disease in 64% of the subjects.[51,136] A recent cohort study of men with chronic pelvic pain syndrome found that abdominal pain or tenderness was present in 51% of patients, compared to only 7% of healthy controls.[137] Trigger points may be associated with joint dysfunction. Trigger points in the upper trapezius were found to correlate with cervical spine dysfunction at the C3 and C4 segmental levels, although a cause-and-effect relationship was not established.[138] A single spinal manipulation did induce changes in pressure pain sensitivity in latent trigger points in the upper trapezius muscle.[139] A brief review of basic muscle pain neurophysiology is useful to understand how central sensitization develops.

The primary peripheral sensing apparatus in muscle involves group III (thinly myelinated, low-threshold fibers) and group IV (unmyelinated, high-threshold fibers) afferent nerve fibers. These fibers cause aching, cramping pain when stimulated with microneural techniques. The central projections of these fibers share several important characteristics especially when compared to cutaneous nociception. First, a reduced spatial resolution because of a lower innervation density of muscle tissue will make it harder to localize muscle pain. Second, convergence of sensory input from skin, muscle, periosteum, bone, and viscera into lamina IV and V of the dorsal horn onto the wide dynamic range neuron can blur the identification of the origin of the pain. Third, divergence of sensory input into the dorsal horn-sustained noxious stimulation as demonstrated for example in group IV fibers in animal models can open previously ineffective synaptic connections in the dorsal horn, such that these fibers begin to respond to lower levels of stimulation, leading to mechanical allodynia and hyperalgesia.[124]

Compared to normal muscle and muscle with latent trigger points, a muscle with active trigger points is more tender and mechanically sensitive, suggesting that peripheral nociceptors are already sensitized. Once sensitized, the group IV afferent nerve fibers will fire at lower thresholds, even though they are normally high-threshold nociceptors. For example, in animal models, injection of BK into muscle will cause the group IV afferents to respond to much lower levels of stimulation, suggesting they have become sensitized.[140] Since muscle tenderness is mainly due to the sensitization of muscle nociceptors by BK, PGs, and 5-HT, peripheral sensitization by these substances presumably contributes to the tenderness seen in active trigger points and may contribute to the pain that individuals with active trigger points describe. Recent studies on the biochemical milieu of active trigger points in the upper trapezius muscle support this hypothesis.[141,142] Therefore, if an active trigger point in a muscle has elevated levels of these and other sensitizing biochemicals, any local muscle contraction that occurs with daily functional activities and postures may be sufficient to cause pain by activating the normally high-threshold nociceptors, which ordinarily do not respond to this type of mechanical activation.

Central sensitization is more readily induced as the activation threshold is lowered for peripheral muscle nociceptors. In animal models of pain, a nociceptive input from skeletal muscle is much more effective at inducing neuroplastic changes in the spinal cord than is input from the skin.[8] Experimentally induced myositis in animal models causes a marked expansion of the response of second order neurons beyond the muscle's target area of the dorsal horn. Hoheisel et al.[143] found that after a localized inflammatory reaction was created, noxious input from the gastrocsoleus (L5) muscle also activated second order neurons in the L3 segment. This segment would not ordinarily be activated by noxious stimulation of the gastrocsoleus in noninflamed muscle.[143] This study demonstrated an expansion of the receptive field in the dorsal horn as a result of a central sensitization. The L3 dorsal horn neurons became hyperexcitable after continuous nociceptive input from the inflamed L5 muscle. The sensitized surrounding segments caused the L3 segment to respond to previously ineffective afferent input.[143] This model of referred pain combines peripheral input and central processing and is known as the central hyperexcitability theory.[144] Supraspinal mechanisms contributing to referred pain have been explored by Niddam et al.,[9,10] who demonstrated that pain from myofascial trigger points involves enhanced activity in the somatosensory and limbic regions and suppressed hippocampal activity.

Expansion of the receptive field in the spinal cord with myositis-induced excitation is clinically relevant, helping to explain the unusual referral patterns seen in myofascial pain. For example, trigger points in the suboccipital muscles may refer to the frontal region of the head, and trigger points in the piriformis may cause pseudosciatica. In addition, central sensitization in animal models may explain the spread of muscle pain to other segments which become painful over time in patients with chronic myofascial pain. It may also explain the symptomatic hyperalgesia reported by many patients, as many of these neurons become hyperexcitable. It is likely that these myositis-induced changes in the spinal cord occur due to a rewiring of dorsal horn neurons in response to sustained peripheral drive from an irritable, sensitized muscle nociceptor, such as that found in an active trigger point.[132]

It is important to add that referred pain is not unique to muscle tissue or myofascial trigger points. All tissues, including fascia, intervertebral discs, internal organs, ligaments, and zygapophyseal joints are capable of referring pain.[5,14,133,144–148] Referred pain patterns from cervical zygapophyseal joints are very similar to those of trigger points in cervical muscles.[149] Clinically referred pain phenomena can be rather confusing, as patients frequently complain of pain in an area of the body where the pain did not originate. For instance, pain in the elbow region, often considered a local problem (e.g., epicondylitis), may in fact be referred pain from shoulder muscles.[150] Another example may be upper arm or shoulder pain originating in the distant infraspinatus muscle. Hsieh et al.[151] demonstrated that inactivating trigger points in the infraspinatus muscle inactivated trigger points in the anterior deltoid muscle. Similarly, pain in the region of the masseter muscle can be resolved by treating trigger points in the trapezius muscle.[152] Headley[153] has suggested that trigger points in one muscle may inhibit other muscles, especially in the area of referred pain. In other cases, muscle pain and trigger points may be secondary to other, nonmuscular disorders, such as internal organ, joint, or disc pathology. This finding underscores the necessity of an excellent and comprehensive differential diagnostic process to uncover the nuances of referred pain. Patients with osteoarthritis of the hip or knee joint were found to have significantly higher numbers of trigger points in muscles crossing these joints than healthy controls.[154] The correlations between pathological conditions and an increased number of trigger points may partially explain why localized painful conditions can become more widespread.[37]

SYNAPTIC CONNECTIONS IN THE DORSAL HORN

There are at least two functional types of synaptic connections in the dorsal horn. One is an "effective" synapse, where action potentials arriving at the presynaptic portion of the synapse exert a strong influence on the postsynaptic or second order neuron. There are a much larger number of "ineffective" synapses between primary afferents and second order neurons. They are considered ineffective because under normal circumstances they do not influence the postsynaptic neuron in a way that will propagate the action potential. These ineffective synapses are multisegmental, and there is anatomical evidence that deep somatic afferents can ramify and enter the dorsal horn of up to 6–7 segments.

The excitatory amino acid glutamate is the presynaptic transmitter for nociceptive information in dorsal horn neurons and can act on N-methyl-D-aspartate (NMDA) and the alpha-amino-3-hydroxy-5-methyl-4-isoxazolepropionic acid (AMPA) receptors at the postsynaptic site. Under normal conditions, only the AMPA receptor is active. Thus, when one sustains a blow to a muscle, a short train of nociceptive impulses from the injured muscle causes the presynaptic site in the dorsal horn to release glutamate. This glutamate release causes a brief activation of the AMPA receptor and postsynaptic neuron. Ineffective synapses limit sensation to specific areas. Though the train of impulses may reach segments of the dorsal horn normally thought to be outside the myotome of the injured muscle, ineffective synapses do not have AMPA receptors and the second order neurons will not fire at these levels. However, with an intense or sustained noxious input, SP is coreleased with glutamate. If this noxious barrage continues and sufficient quantities of SP are released, the NMDA receptor will release its magnesium plug and become responsive to glutamate. This allows the entry of Ca^{2+} ions into the cell of the second order neuron, leading to a cascade that results in the de novo synthesis of AMPA receptors at what were previously ineffective synapses. In this way, the release of SP in the dorsal horn in sufficient quantities will increase the efficacy of synaptic connections in the spinal cord, allowing the multisegmental spread of noxious input. This process explains how action potentials emanating from nociceptors in an L5 muscle can then excite neurons in the L3 segment.[124]

THE BIOCHEMICAL MILIEU OF MYOFASCIAL TRIGGER POINTS

Investigators at the U.S. National Institutes of Health (NIH) developed a clinical protocol to assess the local biochemical milieu of myofascial trigger points.[142] They designed, fabricated, and tested a novel 30-gauge microdialysis needle capable of the in vivo collection of small volumes (~0.5 μL) and subnanogram sizes (<75 kDa) of solutes from muscle tissue. The needle has the same size, shape, and handling characteristics of an acupuncture needle. Its features permit simultaneous sampling of the local biochemical milieu of muscle before, during, and after a local twitch response is elicited with the same needle (Fig. 35.5).

A local twitch response is an involuntary spinal cord reflex contraction of muscle fibers within a taut band, which can be elicited by manually strumming or needling of a taut band. Local twitch responses can be observed visually, recorded electromyographically, or visualized with diagnostic ultrasound.[155] When a trigger point is needled with a monopolar Teflon-coated electromyography needle, local twitch responses appear as high amplitude polyphasic discharges.[156,157] Eliciting local twitch responses is essential when using deep dry needling in clinical practice not only to accomplish optimal treatment results, but also to confirm that the needle is placed into a taut band, which is critically important when needling close to peripheral nerves or internal organs, such as the lungs.[158–160]

The microanalytical system allowed investigators to safely explore and measure the local biochemical milieu of muscle in subjects with and without pain and with and without trigger points at a standardized location in the upper trapezius muscle. In one study, 9 subjects were selected, and based on history and physical examination, classified into 3 groups:

- Group 1—*Normal* (no neck pain, no myofascial trigger point)
- Group 2—*Latent* (no neck pain, myofascial trigger point present)
- Group 3—*Active* (neck pain, myofascial trigger point present)

Samples were obtained continuously with the microdialysis needle at regular intervals, including at the time of needle insertion, elicitation of a local twitch response, and posttwitch.[142] The main outcome measures were pH and concentration levels of protons, SP, CGRP, BK, 5-HT, norepinephrine, TNF-α, and IL-

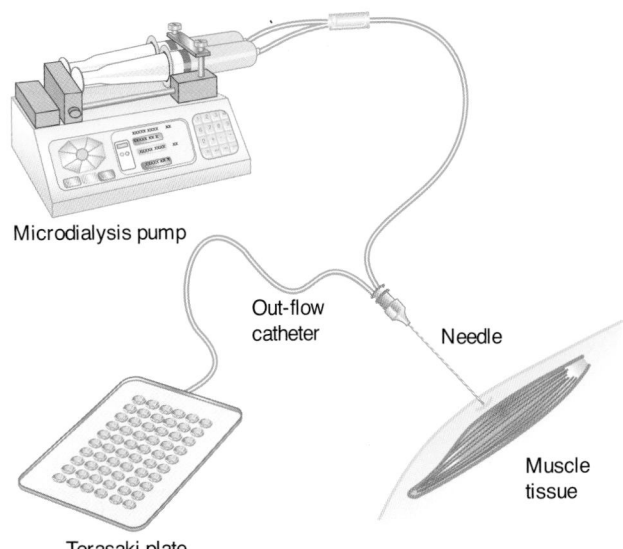

FIGURE 35.5 Schematic of perfusion pump and collection plate.

1β, determined by analysis of samples. Overall the amounts of SP, CGRP, BK, 5-HT, norepinephrine, TNF-α, and IL-1β were significantly higher in the *Active* group than either of the other two groups (p <0.01). The pH was also significantly lower in the *Active* group than the other two groups (p <0.03). In the *Active* group, the amounts of SP and CGRP were significantly lower at the end of sampling (posttwitch) than at baseline (p <0.02) (Fig. 35.6).

In a second study, the previous findings were confirmed, demonstrating that biochemicals associated with pain and inflammation are elevated in soft tissue in the vicinity of active trigger points.[141] The concentrations of these biochemicals, including protons, BK, SP, CGRP, TNF-α, IL-1β, 5-HT, and norepinephrine differentiate the *Active* group from the *Latent* and *Normal* groups. Two additional analytes sampled, IL-6 and IL-8, were likewise significantly higher in the *Active* group.[141]

The second study also included sampling of analyte levels from the biochemical milieu of a remote uninvolved site in the upper medial gastrocnemius muscle. Like the previous study, subjects were classified into groups based on physical findings of active, latent, or no upper trapezius trigger points. The upper medial gastrocnemius was examined and selected as a remote uninvolved site, and none of the participants had active or latent trigger points at this site. Analyte levels from this remote site were compared to levels in the upper trapezius with active, latent, and no

trigger points. In the *Active* group at needle insertion, analyte concentrations of the tested biochemical substances in the gastrocnemius were almost always lower than concentrations in the trapezius. The only exception was pH, which was the same in both muscles at needle insertion. Therefore, the biochemical milieu of an active trigger point in the upper trapezius differs quantitatively from a remote, uninvolved site in the gastrocnemius muscle.[141] They also found that subjects with an active trigger point in the upper trapezius have relatively elevated levels of these analytes in a remote, uninvolved muscle (the upper medial gastrocnemius) compared to gastrocnemius levels in latent and normal subjects (Fig. 35.7). This suggests that substances associated with pain and inflammation are not limited to local areas of trigger points or a single anatomical locus.[141] However, the elevated gastrocnemius concentrations in the *Active* group were lower than most analyte concentrations in the upper trapezius of the *Active* group.

Although there were no trigger points in the upper medial gastrocnemius for all subjects, analyte levels in this muscle were always significantly higher in the *Active* group than the *Normal* group and generally higher than analyte levels in the *Latent* group. This suggests that analyte abnormalities may not be limited to local areas of active (painful) trigger points in the upper trapezius, but are present in unaffected muscle remote from the active trigger points, albeit lower in concentration than in the

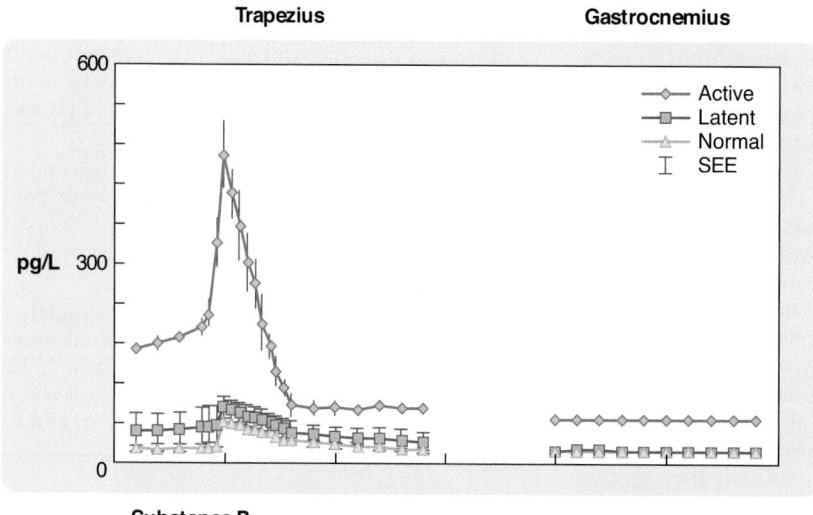

Substance P

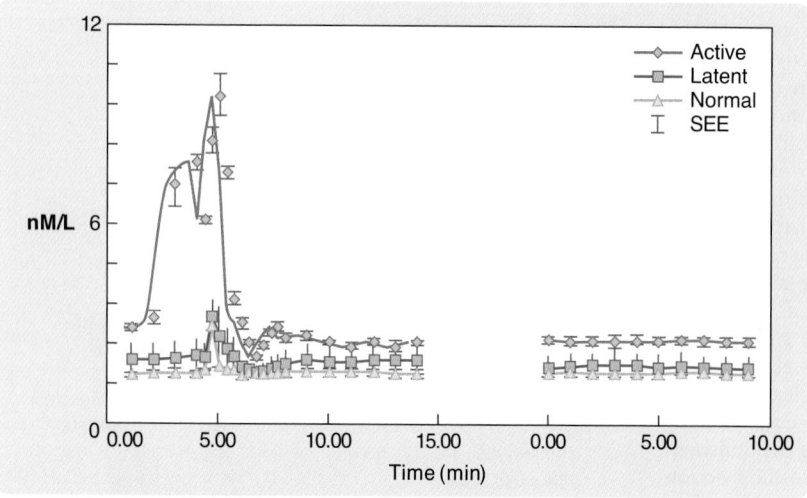

Norepinephrine

FIGURE 35.6 Analyte concentrations in trapezius compared to gastrocnemius, substance P, norepinephrine.

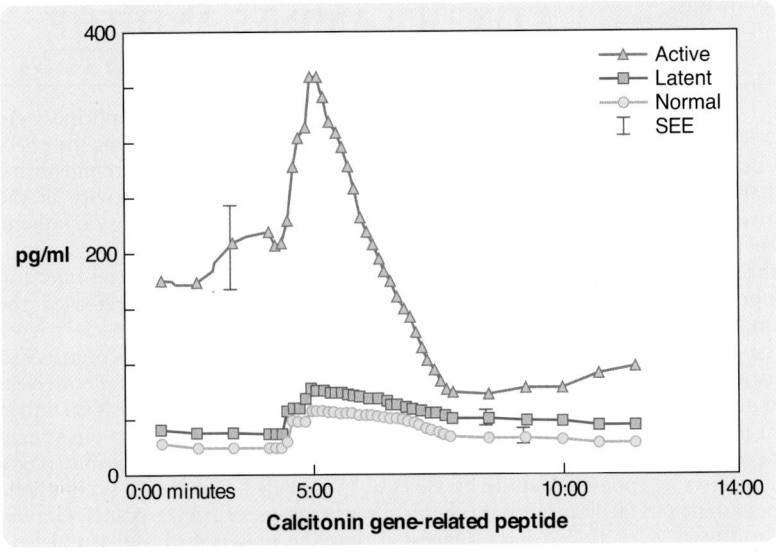

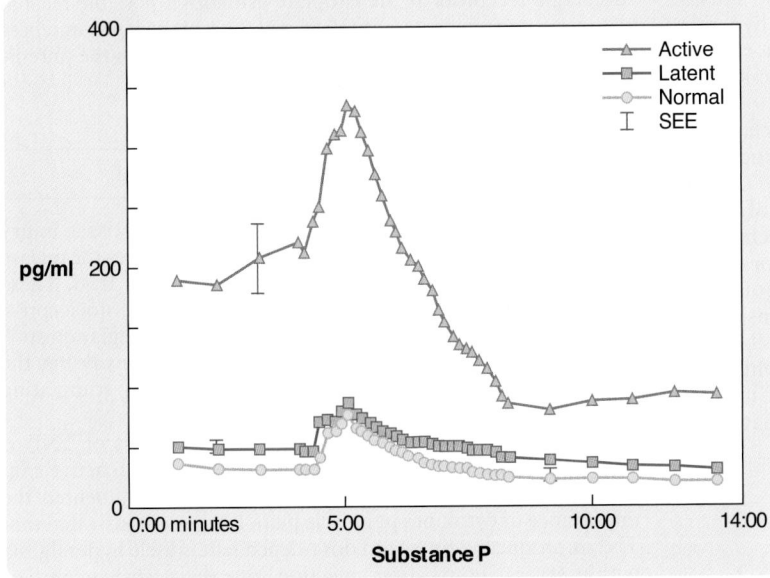

FIGURE 35.7 Concentrations of CGRP and SP across time. A local twitch response was elicited at 5 minutes.

trapezius. The slightly elevated analyte levels in the gastrocnemius may be a widespread phenomenon, possibly related to central sensitization in the *Active* group. There is a possibility that widespread elevation of analytes is a precursor to development of active (painful) trigger points. Conversely, individuals who are susceptible to developing active trigger points may have pre-existing elevated baseline levels of these analytes in muscles throughout their bodies. Further study of the natural history of this condition may elucidate whether the relatively elevated analyte levels in the gastrocnemius in the *Active* group follows the development of an active myofascial trigger point or if there is a baseline low-level elevation of these analytes that precedes the development of an active trigger point.

The NIH investigators demonstrated that it is possible to collect near real-time samples from soft tissue with minimal system perturbation and without harmful effects on subjects. They also showed proof-of-principle of the system's ability to distinguish among subjects who have clinically distinct soft tissue findings. In both studies, the microdialysis needle was used to elicit a local twitch response in the trapezius muscle of the *Active* and *Latent* groups. This caused dramatic changes in temporal sequencing of analyte levels with distinct curves observed among the three groups of subjects.[141,142] In clinical practice, eliciting local twitch

responses while needling active trigger points is believed to be therapeutic.[158–160] Audette et al.[161] found that in 61.5% of active trigger points in the trapezius and levator scapulae muscles, dry needling an active trigger point elicited a local twitch response in the same muscle, but on the opposite side of the body. Needling of latent trigger points resulted in unilateral local twitch responses only.[161] The authors suggested that this phenomenon may be another indication that active trigger points represent a greater degree of central sensitization.[161]

Until recently, myofascial pain was characterized primarily by a physical finding and symptom cluster without demonstrable pathology. Microdialysis sampling revealed that a unique biochemical milieu of substances associated with pain and inflammation exists in the vicinity of active trigger points in the upper trapezius and includes elevated concentrations of protons, SP, CGRP, BK, TNF-α, IL-1β, IL-6, IL-8, 5-HT, and norepinephrine. Further sampling of these and other substances, such as anti-inflammatory cytokines or peripheral opioids, may lead to an improved biochemical characterization of trigger points and identify those who are at risk for developing persistent symptoms. Furthermore, discovering if and which measurable substances are predictive of pain could lead to focused therapies in the future. The relevance of the research by Shah et al. within the broader context of the pain sciences will be illustrated in the following sections.

pH AND MUSCLE PAIN

A previous study demonstrated a positive correlation between pain and local acidity.[162] Sluka et al.[99] demonstrated that an acidic milieu without muscle damage is sufficient to cause profound changes in the properties of the "pain matrix" such that alterations in pH would be sufficient to modify the threshold sensitivity of the nociceptor. An acidic pH stimulates the production of bradykinin during local ischemia and inflammation; therefore, a local acidic milieu may explain some of the pain associated with an active trigger point. Mechanical hyperalgesia is a hallmark of a trigger point. However, ongoing nociceptive activity is not necessary to cause mechanical hyperalgesia. In a rat model, repeated injections of acidic saline boluses into one gastrocnemius muscle produced bilateral, long-lasting mechanical hyperalgesia of the paws.[99] Furthermore, the study showed that the persistent hyperalgesia was not caused by muscle tissue damage and was not maintained by continued nociceptive input from the site of muscle injury, demonstrating that secondary mechanical hyperalgesia may be maintained by neuroplastic changes in the central nervous system, such as spinal dorsal neurons and thalamic neurons.[99]

Investigators have identified specific acid sensing ion channels (ASICs) on muscle nociceptors that can be sensitized and activated by acidic pH. For example, ASIC3 knockout mice do not develop hyperalgesia following repeated bolus injections of acidic saline.[100] Hong et al.[157,163] suggest that an integrative mechanism at the spinal cord level in response to sensitized nociceptors plays a role in development of active trigger points, and should be considered in any pathogenetic hypothesis. In an expansion of Simons' integrated hypothesis, Gerwin et al.[42] propose that the acidic pH may also modulate the motor endplate by inhibiting AChE. This would result in increased concentration of ACh at the synaptic cleft, promoting sarcomere contraction and formation of the taut band characteristic of trigger points.[42]

NEUROPEPTIDES, INFLAMMATORY MEDIATORS, AND TISSUE INJURY AND PAIN

Significantly elevated levels of SP and CGRP were found in the vicinity of active trigger points. The orthodromic and antidromic release of these substances is greatly increased in response to nociceptor activation, for example by protons and BK binding to their matched receptors.[164] This dynamic phenomenon may lead to neuroplastic changes in the dorsal horn and profound changes in neuronal activity and the perception of pain. In the studies by Shah et al.,[141,142] SP and CGRP were the only two analytes in the *Active* group which had concentrations significantly below their original baselines in the recovery period following a local twitch response. These biochemical changes correspond with the commonly observed decrease in pain and local tenderness after the inactivation of a trigger point by dry needling.[159]

SP causes mast cell degranulation with the subsequent release of histamine, serotonin, and upregulation of both proinflammatory cytokines, including TNF-α and IL-6, and anti-inflammatory cytokines, including IL-4 and IL-10. TNF-α is the only cytokine prestored in the mast cell and is released immediately following mast cell degranulation. TNF-α may stimulate norepinephrine production. The finding of elevated levels of serotonin, BK, norepinephrine, and proinflammatory cytokines in active trigger points is consistent with biochemical pathways involved in tissue injury and inflammation.[141,142]

CATECHOLAMINES AND THE AUTONOMIC NERVOUS SYSTEM

Significantly elevated levels of 5-HT and norepinephrine were found in the vicinity of active trigger points, supporting the effect of the elevated TNF-α. The increased levels of norepinephrine may be associated with increased sympathetic activity in the motor endplate region of trigger points. In one study, sympathetic activity was recorded from rabbit myofascial trigger spots, which is a model of the human trigger point.[87] Intra-arterial injection of phentolamine, an α–adrenergic antagonist, decreased the spontaneous electrical activity from a locus of a myofascial trigger spot in rabbit skeletal muscle.[87] Conversely, the nicotinic ACh receptor antagonist curare had no effect on the spontaneous electrical activity. Elevated levels of norepinephrine in the local milieu of active trigger points suggest that the autonomic nervous system is involved in the pathogenesis of spontaneously painful trigger points. A study by Ge et al.[65] provided evidence of sympathetic facilitation of mechanical sensitization of trigger points. Gerwin et al.[42,92] have suggested that the presence of alpha and beta adrenergic receptors at the endplate provides a possible mechanism for autonomic interaction. Stimulation of the alpha and beta adrenergic receptors stimulated the release of ACh in the phrenic nerve of rodents.[165]

CYTOKINES AND PAIN

A unique cascade of cytokines is released following tissue injury and inflammation. For example, bradykinin stimulates the release of TNF-α which leads to the release of IL-1β and IL-6. These two cytokines stimulate the cyclooxygenase (COX) nociceptive pathway, which leads to the production of prostaglandins.[166] TNF-α also stimulates a separate nociceptive pathway via the release of IL-8, which mediates sympathetic pain by stimulating the liberation of sympathetic amines.[167]

As noted, Shah et al.[141,142] found elevated levels of TNF-α, IL-1β, IL-6, and IL-8 in the trapezius of subjects with active trigger points. A study by Schafers et al.[168] also documented the importance of cytokines in muscle pain. It was demonstrated that TNF-α produces a time- and dose-dependent muscle hyperalgesia within several hours after injection into the gastrocnemius or biceps brachii of a rat. The hyperalgesia was completely reversed by systemic treatment with the nonopioid analgesic metamizol.[168] Furthermore, TNF-α did not cause histopathological tissue damage or motor dysfunction. One day after injection of TNF-α, elevated levels of CGRP, nerve growth factor and prostaglandin E2 were found in the muscle. According to Schafers et al.,[168] TNF-α and other proinflammatory cytokines such as IL-1β may play a role in the development of muscle hyperalgesia, and the targeting of proinflammatory cytokines might be beneficial for the treatment of muscle pain syndromes.

In rat model studies, Loram et al. measured the tissue and plasma levels of cytokines following injection of carrageenan into the hind paw compared with intramuscular injection into the gastrocnemius muscle. They demonstrated, for the first time, that the initiation of primary muscle hyperalgesia is not associated with elevated levels in local muscle of TNF-α, IL-1β, or IL-6.[169] Loram et al.[169–171] also showed that IL-1β and IL-6 are elevated at a time interval when there is no hyperalgesia. One possible explanation, they suggest, is that elevated intramuscular levels of IL-1β and IL-6 induce central sensitization, but do not contribute to the initiation of hyperalgesia.[169]

Cytokines that lead to PG release via the COX pathway have been targeted for pharmacologic intervention because of their roles in the inflammatory response.[167] IL-1β is the major cytokine stimulus for central COX-2 expression during inflammation.

Loram et al. found that IL-1β was the only cytokine that reached a higher concentration in muscle than hind paw after carrageenan injection in the rat. Furthermore, IL-1β was significantly elevated 24 hours after inducing muscle inflammation at a time when secondary hyperalgesia was induced.[169] IL-1β also stimulates IL-6 production during muscle injury. Together, both cytokines are necessary for repair and regeneration of muscle.[172–174] In light of these cytokines' importance to muscle regeneration, Loram et al. suggest that pharmacologic interventions preferentially target action of IL-1β and not IL-6 in order to reduce secondary muscle hyperalgesia and still conserve the cytokines' regenerative qualities.[169]

Moreover, which cytokines and when to target them may depend on the time course of the muscle injury and inflammatory response. As mentioned, Schafers et al.[168] found that TNF-α produces a time- and dose-dependent muscle hyperalgesia within several hours after injection into rat muscle. On the other hand, Hoheisel et al.[175] found that injection of TNF-α into a rat's gastrocnemius muscle did not excite, but rather had a short desensitizing action on group IV muscle afferents. According to Hoheisel et al.,[176] the data suggest that TNF-α has a dual action when released intramuscularly. Specifically, "it suppresses neuronal excitability after release but contributes to neuronal hyperexcitability in a later phase."[176] Therefore, the elevated levels of TNF-α, IL-1β, and IL-6 found in active trigger points may mediate secondary hyperalgesia and central sensitization via the COX pathway.

A second distinct nociceptive pathway moderates the inflammatory hypernociception following tissue injury. Rat CINC-1 and its homolog in humans, IL-8, coordinate the sympathetic components of hypernociception. Loram et al.[169] demonstrated that of the four cytokines—TNF-α, IL-1β, IL-6, and CINC-1—measured in muscle after carrageenan injection, only levels of CINC-1 were elevated at the time of primary hyperalgesia. Moreover, CINC-1 and IL-8 induce a dose- and time-dependent mechanical hypernociception. Therefore, the elevated levels of IL-8 found in active myofascial trigger points may mediate inflammatory hypernociception, muscle tenderness, and pain via this pathway. Furthermore, this pathway is inhibited by β-adrenergic receptor antagonists, though not COX antagonists.[167]

CLINICAL MANAGAMENT

Trigger Point Diagnosis

As there is no medical specialty that has adopted muscle as its distinctive organ, the literature on the clinical management of patients with myofascial pain is scattered over multiple specialties and disciplines, including algology, physiatry, dentistry, otolaryngology, urology, neurology, osteopathy, orthopedics, gynecology, physical therapy, chiropractic, acupuncture, and massage therapy, among others. Because disciplines tend to have their own jargon, the term "myofascial pain" may have different meanings among different disciplines, which could potentially challenge understanding across disciplines. In dentistry, for example, the term "myofascial pain dysfunction syndrome" is commonly used for nonspecific muscle pain with or without limited mouth opening.[176] Each discipline will have to explore general and discipline-specific differential diagnoses, especially when trigger points may not be the primary dysfunction. General aspects of the differential diagnostic process may include a neurologic examination, a biomechanical assessment of posture and movement patterns, and an assessment of other possible contributing factors. Some trigger point-referred patterns are very similar to radicular pain patterns. Referred pain patterns of trigger points in the teres minor muscle or gluteus minimus muscle resemble a C8 or L5 radiculopathy, respectively.[177,178] The presence of myofascial trigger points does not rule out a radiculopathy and vice versa. Trigger points may be associated with lumbar disc lesions or contribute to symptoms of thoracic outlet syndrome.[178,180] Although much of the fibromyalgia literature suggests that myofascial pain is a regional issue, widespread pain may still be due to myofascial trigger points.[181] As part of the diagnostic process, clinicians should consider other diagnoses as well which may feature widespread pain, including but not limited to hypothyroidism, systemic lupus erythematosus, Lyme disease, babesiosis, ehrlichiosis, candida albicans infections, myoadenylate deaminase deficiency, herpes zoster, complex regional pain syndrome, hypoglycemia, parasitic diseases such as fascioliasis, amoebiasis, and *Giardia*, systemic side effects of medications, including any of the statin drugs or even glucosamine sulfate, and metabolic or nutritional deficiencies or insufficiencies of vitamin B12, vitamin D, and ferritin.[181] Having patients complete standardized pain questionnaires at the time of the initial examination allows for objective outcome measurements. Discipline-specific differential diagnoses support the notion of having a multidisciplinary approach as individual clinicians may not be familiar with diagnoses or patterns of dysfunction outside their own area or specialty.[182] Yet, the underlying mechanisms and principles of muscle dysfunction, described earlier in this chapter, apply to all disciplines.

Palpation is the criterion standard for identifying myofascial trigger points. However, there still are no research-validated criteria. Simons, Travell, and Simons[39,183–192] defined empirically-derived criteria, which have been applied to a number of interrater and intrarater reliability studies. The presence of a taut band and spot tenderness has been shown to be a reliable indicator of myofascial trigger points in one comprehensive study, while in a more recent study referred pain and a jump sign were the most reliable indicators.[183,185] The local twitch response is more difficult to elicit and has not been shown to be a reliable feature of trigger points. Occasionally, the concept of myofascial pain is challenged, because excellent interrater reliability was only achieved with experienced and well-trained clinicians. However, the fact that trigger point palpation has to be learned is no different than most other clinical skills and procedures. Palpation and, more specifically, trigger point palpation is not taught in the vast majority of medical, physical therapy, and chiropractic schools, and it should come as no surprise that clinicians do not necessarily master trigger point palpation without specific training.

Familiarity with referred pain patterns of trigger points is essential, as it will guide clinicians to clinically relevant muscles and trigger points. Recent studies have confirmed previously suggested referred pain patterns, especially in the head and neck region.[150,193–195] Other studies and case reports have described new patterns either directly from trigger points or from muscles in general.[196–198] Acupuncturists may recognize correspondences between trigger point-referred pain patterns and acupuncture meridian pathways.[199]

The physical examination for myofascial trigger points should be a standard component of the diagnostic process and does not exclude any other part of the standard examination process. In addition to trigger points, there are many other possible sources of pain. A detailed history is critical. There are several predisposing or perpetuating factors that need to be assessed in addition to possible medical diagnoses.

Mechanical perpetuating factors are relatively easy to identify by clinicians across disciplines and include forward head posture, which frequently contributes to migraines or tension-type headaches, neck pain, and upper thoracic pain,[200,201] decreased spinal mobility, structural misalignments, such as leg length discrepancies or pelvic torsions, or systemic or local hypermobility.[139,182,202–204] The combination of static and awkward postures, excessive force, and repetitive tasks predisposes a patient to the development of trigger points. Awkward postures may include prolonged wrist flexion and extension, ulnar and radial abduction, forearm supination and pronation, extended reaches beyond the shoulder-reach envelope, pinch grips that are either too wide or too narrow, habitual postures during computer tasks, among others.[112,205] Ergonomic measures often play a vital role in correction and prevention of myofascial pain problems.[205]

Psychological arousal has a direct impact on the electrical activity of myofascial trigger points, while autogenic relaxation reduces the electrical activity.[206–208] Whether specific regions of the brain, such as the anterior cingulate gyrus, which has been linked to nociceptive input from muscles, and to depression, anxiety, and anger can explain at least part of the association of psychological factors and trigger points remains to be seen.[9–11,209,210] Depression, anxiety, anger, feelings of hopelessness and helplessness, and fear avoidance are common with many chronic pain syndromes and are not specific for myofascial pain.[211,212]

Any nutritional or metabolic condition that interferes with the energy supply of muscle tissue can contribute to the development of myofascial trigger points.[181] Laboratory levels can be within the "normal" range, yet be insufficient for a given individual, which makes it more difficult to diagnose, but no less important. Common nutritional and metabolic deficiencies or insufficiencies include vitamins B1, B6, B12, and D insufficiency states, iron, magnesium, and zinc insufficiency states, and thyroid deficiency states, among others.[181] The importance of metabolic and nutritional perpetuating factors is illustrated for vitamin D.

Vitamin D deficiency is commonly observed with chronic, nonspecific musculoskeletal pain.[213] Nearly 90% of 150 subjects with musculoskeletal pain had vitamin D levels less than 20 ng/mL and 28% had less than 8 ng/mL, where levels above 30 ng/mL are considered optimal.[213] Vitamin D deficiency in adults is defined as serum 25(OH)D levels below 20 ng/mL and vitamin D insufficiency as 25(OH)D below 30 ng/mL.[214–216] Vitamin D deficiencies are endemic in northern Europe and America[215, 217,218] and are associated with muscle weakness, myofibrillar protein degradation, reduced muscle mass, osteoporosis, and decreased functional ability.[219,220] Although there are no randomized controlled studies examining the correlation between vitamin D deficiencies or insufficiencies and myofascial pain, empirical observations in a community pain management center suggest that vitamin D insufficiencies are very common among individuals with myofascial pain.[181] In the hierarchy of evidence-based medicine, clinical evidence is a valid parameter and should be included in the review of evidence.[221–223]

Physical Examination Technique

The physical examination of myofascial trigger points is performed with either a flat or pincer palpation technique. With the flat palpation technique, the taut band and trigger point are compressed in between a finger or thumb against the underlying tissue or bone (Fig. 35.8). With the pincer palpation technique, the taut band and trigger point are held in between the clinician's fingers and thumb (Fig. 35.9). The initial palpation focuses on the presence of taut bands as, by definition, trigger points are always located within a band of contractured muscle fibers. Palpation for trigger points is performed perpendicular to the fiber direction, which requires good anatomical knowledge of muscles and their fiber directions. Whether a muscle should be shortened, lengthened, or kept in a resting position depends entirely on the individual muscle, the tension in connective tissues and fascia, and available range of motion. The muscle needs to be placed in a position where the taut band can optimally be palpated. For patients with very tight and restricted muscles, the muscle may need to be placed in a relaxed position, while in hypermobile patients the muscle may need to be prestretched to be able to identify taut bands.[41] Prolonged pressure on trigger points for as long as 10–15 seconds may elicit referred pain patterns and the patient's familiar pain complaint. Local twitch responses may be

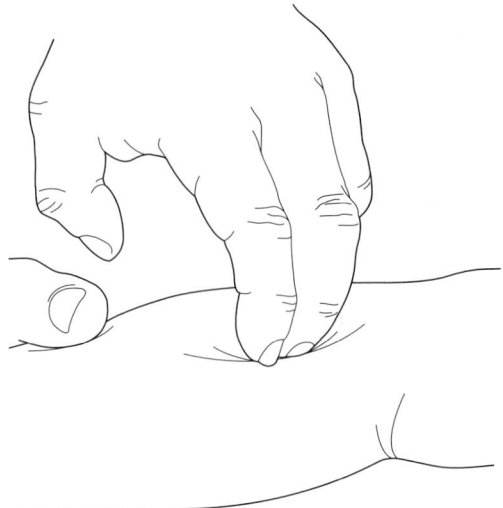

FIGURE 35.8 Flat palpation technique.

elicited by strumming the taut band, but this has little utility as part of the diagnostic process. The minimum criteria for identification of an active trigger point are the presence of a taut band with exquisite spot tenderness and patient-recognized pain.

Magnetic resonance and ultrasound elastography may become useful technologies in the future, but have not yet been utilized in clinical practice.[57,58,61] Piezoelectric and electro-hydraulic shockwave emitters are being used especially in Germany for the identification and treatment of trigger points and their specific referred pain patterns.[224,225] Both types of shockwave emitters were able to reproduce patients' familiar referred pain patterns. As endplate noise was found to be characteristic of trigger points, electromyography has been used in research studies to confirm the presence of trigger points, but in clinical practice there is no advantage to using electromyography. The limited resolution of diagnostic ultrasound has restricted its use to visualizing local twitch responses with needle penetration, but improved technology may enable clinicians and researchers to identify trigger points.[61,155,226] At this point in time, palpation remains the primary tool for the identification of trigger points.

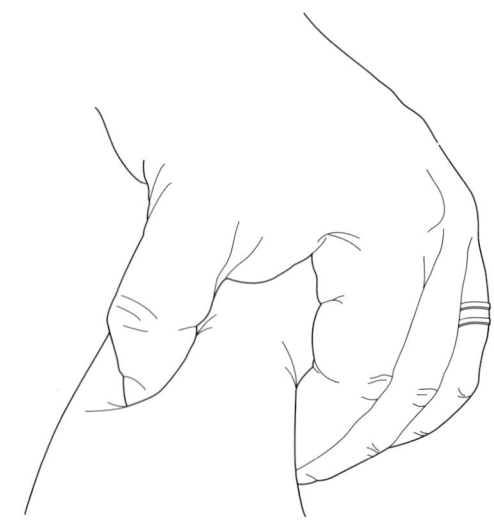

FIGURE 35.9 Pincer palpation technique.

Treatment Options

One of the first decisions to make after the initial examination is whether the patient's pain complaints have a significant myofascial component. A recent paper defined clinical prediction rules to assist in identifying patients with chronic tension-type headaches who are likely to benefit from trigger point therapy.[227] Patients with chronic tension-type headaches were examined and potential predictor variables were entered into a stepwise logistic regression model to determine the most accurate combination of variables to predict treatment success. Headache duration, headache frequency, bodily pain, and vitality were found to be predictive variables. As expected, patients with shorter and fewer headaches and those with less bodily pain were more likely to have successful outcomes. Interestingly, patients with lower vitality were found to be more responsive to intervention, which the authors could not explain based on the data or other theoretical models. If all four variables were present, the probability of success was 84%. Another interesting finding of this preliminary study was that the number of active trigger points and tenderness were not predictive of outcome.[227]

Patients with chronic pain problems may present with a combination of possible contributing factors. If metabolic or nutritional insufficiencies are suspected, additional testing may be required. It is unlikely that therapy will be successful unless such insufficiencies have been addressed adequately. The choice of treatment modalities is partially based on a clinician's bias, preferences, experience, and skills. A dentist treating a patient with facial pain and trigger points in the masseter muscle may decide to improve the patient's occlusion assuming that the muscle pain is secondary to the malocclusion. An orthopedic surgeon may manage a patient's complaint of radiating pain down the leg with epidural injections to reduce radicular pain, while a physician familiar with referred pain patterns of myofascial trigger points may decide to treat trigger points in the gluteus medius muscle with trigger point injections or myofascial release techniques. Many patients with chronic myofascial pain may benefit from a comprehensive pharmacologic management strategy, which may include nonsteroidal anti-inflammatories, opiates, antidepressants, and anticonvulsants, although these are not specific for myofascial pain.[228,229]

Patient Education

Following the initial examination, patients need to be educated about the nature and complexity of their pain. Studies have shown that patients with chronic pain gain much understanding and insight when the clinician explains the principles of peripheral and central sensitization rather than focuses on anatomical concepts such as spinal mechanics.[166,230] Excellent patient education can reduce disability and assist patients in making appropriate choices, overcoming counterproductive beliefs, and modifying dysfunctional behaviors by increasing physical activity and self-efficacy.[231,232] If the patient's pain complaint could easily be provoked by pressure on certain trigger points, it is likely that trigger point therapy will make significant improvements. However, clinicians should be cautious in promising total relief, especially for chronic pain conditions with multiple interacting aspects.

Physical Therapy

The role of physical therapy in pain management centers is often limited to instructing patients in proper stretching and strengthening exercises, stabilization programs, posture corrections, and maybe limited manual therapy interventions.[232] Relatively few physical therapists have received adequate training in pain management, and physical therapists are poorly represented in professional pain management associations.[233] It appears that few physical therapy schools have adopted a specific pain science curriculum.[234] As many as 96% of orthopedic physical therapists preferred to work with patients without chronic pain.[235] Physical therapists experienced in working with persons with chronic pain, including myofascial pain, work closely with physicians and other members of the interdisciplinary team. A comprehensive team approach may distinguish two distinct but overlapping phases. During the first phase, the emphasis is on reducing the nociceptive component of the pain problem with manual trigger point therapy, trigger point dry needling or trigger point injections, other manual therapy interventions, breathing exercises, relaxation therapy, electrotherapeutic modalities, early posture training, and physical conditioning.[206,234,236] According to Moseley, "any strategy that has an inhibitory effect on nociceptive input is probably appropriate in the short-term unless it simultaneously activates non-nociceptive threatening input."[237] During the second phase, the emphasis shifts to further improving physical functioning, cardiovascular endurance, and aerobic conditioning.

Patients need to learn self-pacing and setting appropriate and achievable goals, including physical goals, psychological goals, functional goals, and social goals.[238] An important variable is the degree of a patient's belief in their self-efficacy, which is defined as "the belief in one's capabilities to organize and execute the sources of action required to manage prospective situations."[231,239,240] Patients with a weak belief in their self-efficacy tend to avoid difficult tasks, have low aspirations, maintain a self-diagnostic focus, and emphasize personal deficiencies and adverse outcomes. They are more prone to depression and stress and give up quickly. Patients with a strong belief in their self-efficacy are more likely to set challenging goals, consider difficult tasks as challenges rather than as threats, and maintain a task-diagnostic focus. They usually are not depressed and increase their effort when faced with difficulties.

Needling Therapies

Invasive trigger point therapy can be divided into trigger point injections and trigger point dry needling. Trigger point injections are usually restricted to medical doctors and their professional support staff. The state of Maryland is the only jurisdiction in the United States where physical therapists are legally allowed to perform trigger point injections.[159] Physical therapists and physicians around the world utilize trigger point dry needling.[159] As Steinbrocker already suggested in 1944, the mechanical stimulation of trigger points is an important mechanism to explain the effects of needling therapies.[241]

Trigger point dry needling consists of superficial and deep dry needling based on the depth of needling.[159] The first comprehensive paper about deep dry needling was published in 1979 and reported that dry needling of trigger points caused immediate analgesia in almost 87% of the needle sites, which was referred to as "the needle effect."[242] In 1980, a prospective deep dry needling study of injured workers with low back pain showed that dry needling was an effective treatment for low back pain.[243] A recent Cochrane review supported the use of dry needling as an adjunct for the treatment of patients with chronic low back pain.[244] The technique used with deep dry needling is similar to the technique of trigger point injections and aims to elicit local twitch responses (Fig. 35.10).

The mechanisms and effectiveness of deep dry needling are comparable to trigger point injections.[158-160,244-249] Earlier studies suggested that dry needling would cause more postneedling soreness, but when injections are compared to dry needling using solid filament needles, there are no differences between the two methods.[224,246,249,250] Postneedling soreness occurs in most patients and can vary in duration from just a few minutes to as much as 2 days. Vasovagal reactions can occur with any needling procedure, but they are relatively rare. To avoid unnecessary

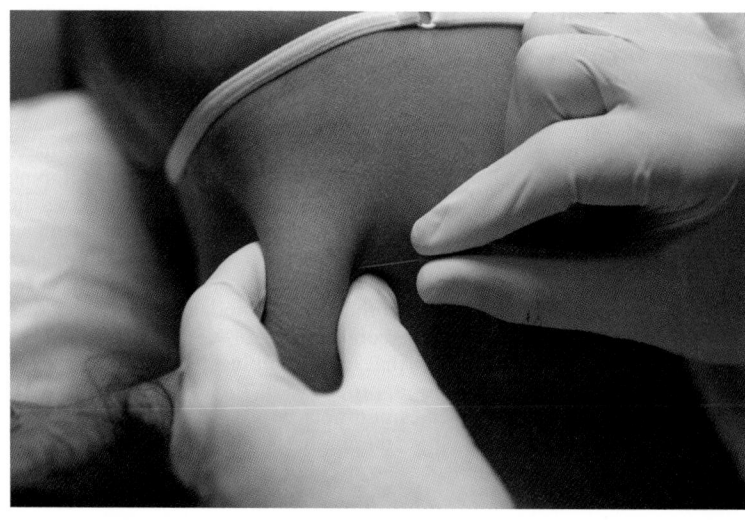

FIGURE 35.10 Trigger point dry needling of the trapezius muscle.

complications from possible vasovagal reactions, patients are needled only while lying down on the treatment table.

With the superficial dry needling technique, a solid filament needle is placed into the tissues overlying active trigger points at a depth of approximately 5–10 mm for 30 seconds. In case of any residual pain, the needle is inserted for another 2 or 3 minutes.[24,251] Local twitch responses are usually absent with superficial dry needling. The degree of available endogenous opioid peptide antagonists may determine how intensely a patient responds to the therapy. So-called weak responders may have excessive amounts of endogenous opioid peptide antagonists. A rodent model has shown that mice with deficient opioid peptide receptors did not respond well to needle-evoked nerve stimulation.[252]

Trigger point injections are administered with a variety of injectables (Fig. 35.11). Travell preferred procaine hydrochloride, which is no longer available everywhere.[30,253] The current recommendation is to use 0.25% lidocaine, which was found to be more effective than stronger concentrations.[254,255] Other anesthetics used with trigger point injections include ropivacaine, levobupivacaine, and mepivacaine, among others.[256,257] There is no scientific evidence that injections with steroids, vitamin B12, nonsteroidal anti-inflammatories, or bee venom would be beneficial, although these have been reported. Bee venom has some potential based on its antinociceptive and anti-inflammatory ef-

fects through activation of brainstem catecholaminergic neurons and activation of the alpha-2 adrenergic and serotonergic pathways of the descending inhibitory system.[258–260] Melitin, an active ingredient of bee venom, can suppress lipopolysaccharide-induced nitric oxide and the transcription of cyclooxygenase-2 (COX-2) genes and proinflammatory cytokines, including TNF-α and IL-1β in microglia.[261,262] Injections of bee venom into specific acupuncture points in several animal and human studies of knee arthritis were beneficial and reduced pain levels significantly, but there are no studies that demonstrate the effectiveness of trigger point injections with bee venom.[259,263,264] Trigger point injections with the serotonin antagonist tropisetron were found to be more effective than injections with lidocaine solution, but injectable serotonin antagonists are not available in all countries.[265,266]

There is a growing body of literature supporting the use of botulinum toxin in the treatment of myofascial trigger points, although this remains a controversial issue. Many botulinum toxin studies fail to demonstrate superiority of botulinum toxin over placebo.[267] Yet, clinicians familiar with myofascial trigger points support its use, based on the demonstrated mechanisms of botulinum toxin and empirical evidence.[268,269] Indeed, several studies have shown significant benefit of botulinum toxin injec-

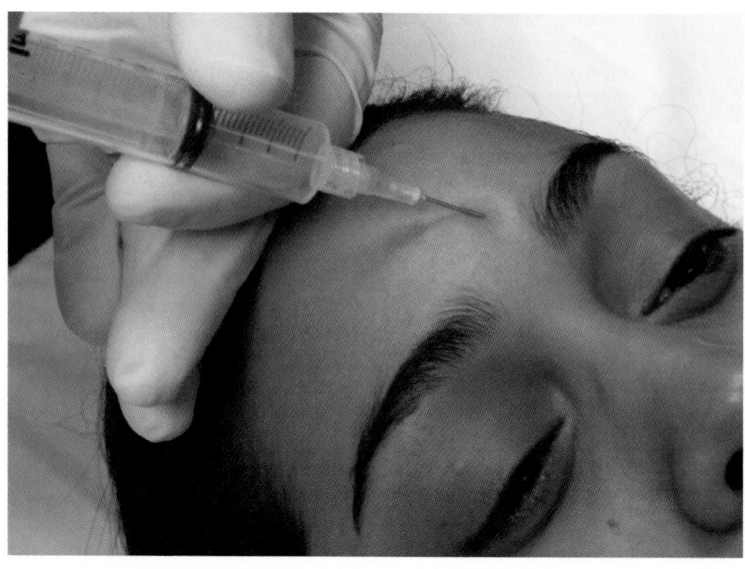

FIGURE 35.11 Trigger point injection to the frontalis muscle.

tions in the treatment of myofascial trigger points and various pain states, including migraine, tension-type headache, low back pain, and phantom pain.[270–272] Potential problems with these studies relate to the use of different dosages, varying injection sites, and the degree of familiarity with myofascial trigger points. Botulinum toxin prevents the release of ACh from the presynpatic nerve terminal.[268,273,274] ACh is released in response to evoked stimulation of the nerve or spontaneously without axonal nerve activation.[95,275,276] Botulinum toxin also has an antinociceptive effect, which in part may be due to its ability to also block the release of CGRP from the nerve terminal.[273,277–279]

Trigger point needling therapies are always part of a much broader treatment approach and should not be offered as a stand-alone intervention. Extensive training is required to gain the necessary palpation skills and kinesthetic awareness, without which trigger point needling would become a random process. Anatomical knowledge is required prior to developing the sensory-motor skills needed to visualize the tip of the needle and the pathway the needle follows inside patients' bodies.[159] Clinicians should be able to visualize a three-dimensional image of the exact location and depth of the trigger point and accurately elicit local twitch responses. The needle should not be used as a search tool except in muscles that cannot be palpated directly, such as the subscapularis or lateral pterygoid muscles. Trained clinicians can almost always identify clinically relevant trigger points, except in obese patients where certain muscles may not be accessible to palpation.[159] Eliciting local twitch responses is thought to be essential with trigger point needling to reach optimal treatment results.[160] As noted, research by Shah et al.[141,142] demonstrated that eliciting a local twitch response facilitated a normalization of the neuropeptides SP and CGRP in the local biochemical milieu of active trigger points. Myofascial trigger point injections were the second most common procedure after epidural injections in a study of Canadian pain anesthesiologists, although the art of trigger point injections and trigger point palpation are not usually covered in medical schools, and there are no formal postgraduate training programs in Canada.[280] In clinical practice, patients commonly report never having experienced local twitch responses when they were treated with trigger point injections previously.

Robinson and Arendt-Nielsen[37] suggested limiting the number of injections to no more than six during an initial treatment program with additional injections offered only as maintenance therapy. However, based on published studies, case studies, and empirical evidence, there are multiple benefits to reducing pain levels significantly before starting rigorous exercise programs.[159] Dry needling and injections can eliminate or reduce trigger point pain often in just a few sessions with a skilled clinician allowing the patient to be more successful in the conditioning phase of the rehabilitation program.[64,131,242,281–283] Patients enrolled in a stroke rehabilitation program performed significantly better in multiple variables after trigger points in their painful shoulder were treated with dry needling, compared to patients who did not get the needling therapy.[283] There are many other clinical outcome studies confirming that needling therapies are effective in inactivating trigger points and in reducing pain levels.[243,284–286]

In spite of a rapidly increasing number of clinical outcome studies, the exact mechanisms of trigger point injections and dry needling are not known.[159] Deep dry needling and trigger point injections may destroy motor endplates and cause distal axon denervations, which may trigger changes in the endplate cholinesterase and ACh receptors as part of the normal muscle regeneration process.[287,288] It is likely that trigger point needling involves central pain mechanisms, including the limbic system, the subcortical gray structures, and the descending inhibitory system. Most needling procedures are painful, possibly stretch fibroblasts in connective tissues, and activate the enkephalinergic, serotonergic, and noradrenergic inhibitory systems associated with A-δ fibers

through segmental inhibition.[289–291] Superficial dry needling is often explained in a similar fashion; however, superficial dry needling is a painless procedure, which would not activate A-δ fibers, unless the needling is combined with rotating the needle after it has been inserted.[24,159] A-δ nerve fibers are only activated by nociceptive mechanical stimulation for type I high-threshold A-δ fibers or by cold stimuli for type II A-δ fibers.[292] It is conceivable that the light stimulus of superficial dry needling activates mechanoreceptors coupled to slow conducting unmyelinated C fiber afferents and stimulates the anterior cingulate cortex with emotional and hormonal reactions representing a sense of progress, reduction of pain, and well-being.[293–295] There is also evidence that superficial dry needling may stimulate a central release of oxytocin.[295,297]

Noninvasive Treatment Options

Rickards and Fernández-de-las-Peñas et al.[298,299] published comprehensive systematic reviews of noninvasive treatment options for myofascial pain. It is beyond the scope of this chapter to describe all approaches and the reader is referred to these reviews and to a descriptive review by Dommerholt et al.[41] A wide variety of manual therapies are being used in the treatment of myofascial trigger points, such as spray and stretch, trigger point compression, muscle energy techniques, massage, etc. There is some evidence of the short-term effectiveness of manual therapies, but no conclusions can be made in relation to the medium- and long-term effectiveness.[298] Fernández-de-las-Peñas et al.[300] demonstrated that trigger point compression and transverse friction massage were equally effective in treating trigger points with a significant reduction in visual analogue scores and significant increase in the pressure pain threshold. Hou et al.[301] showed that trigger point compression reduced pain levels within minutes.

The spray and stretch technique became nearly synonymous with Travell and consists of a vapocoolant such as ethylchloride or fluoromethane sprayed over the skin overlying the muscle into the referral zone of the trigger point, followed by stretching of the muscle.[34,39,253] Because of its detrimental effect on the ozone layer, fluoromethane was recently replaced by a new "spray and stretch" product. The new product contains hydrofluorocarbons and is classified as a "volatile organic compound" and is a powerful greenhouse gas.[302] The new product's carbon dioxide equivalent or global warming potential is 1300, which means that the product has a 1300 times greater greenhouse effect than carbon dioxide.[303] Manual therapies are environmentally safe and have been shown to be more effective.[304]

Several modalities have been applied to trigger points, such as laser, ultrasound, and electrotherapy.[298,299] Laser proved to be an effective modality in most trials.[305–311] Ultrasound has mixed reviews. A recent study demonstrated a short-term decrease of the sensitivity of trigger points following ultrasound.[312] Another study of high-power static ultrasound was more beneficial than more traditionally applied ultrasound, while two other papers did not show any benefit of ultrasound.[313–315] Transcutaneous electrical stimulation is the most studied electrotherapy modality, but it remains difficult to draw any conclusions beyond short-term effects.[304,314,316–319] A prospective, randomized study of extracorporeal shockwave therapy in the treatment of athletes with acute or chronic shoulder pain, showed significantly improved isokinetic force production, a reduction in pain, and overall performance.[320]

SUMMARY

Myofascial trigger points are a very common cause of clinically observed local muscle pain, tenderness, and referred pain in patients with acute and chronic pain. However, they are also a common physical finding in asymptomatic individuals. This dichotomy challenges and behooves pain management practitioners to learn how to palpate the soft tissue and distinguish active from latent myofascial trigger points. Making this distinction is critical in order to adequately identify and treat a myofascial component of pain. Several independent and emerging lines of scientific inquiry, including histological, neurophysiological, biochemical, and somatosensory research into the nature of myofascial trigger points have revealed objective abnormalities. These findings suggest that myofascial pain consists of both motor and sensory abnormalities involving the peripheral and central nervous systems. Accordingly, active myofascial trigger points may be viewed as part of a complex series of changes in the peripheral tissue and central nervous system that occur with central sensitization, characteristic of a form of neuromuscular dysfunction. From this perspective, future clinical research studies should focus on identifying the mechanisms responsible for the pathogenesis, amplification, and perpetuation of myofascial pain syndrome. Successful treatment depends upon identifying and targeting these mechanisms and addressing the perpetuating factors that sustain this common pain syndrome.

References

1. Chaiamnuay P, Darmawan J, Muirden KD, et al. Epidemiology of rheumatic disease in rural Thailand: a WHO-ILAR COPCORD study. Community Oriented Programme for the Control of Rheumatic Disease. J Rheumatol 1998; 25(7):1382–1387.
2. Lindell L, Bergman S, Petersson IF, et al. Prevalence of fibromyalgia and chronic widespread pain. Scand J Prim Health Care 2000;18(3):149–153.
3. Vecchiet L. Muscle pain and aging. J Musculoskel Pain 2002;10:5–22.
4. McBeth J, Jones K. Epidemiology of chronic musculoskeletal pain. Best Pract Res Clin Rheumatol 2007;21(3):403–425.
5. Kellgren JH. Observations on referred pain arising from muscle. Clin Sci 1938; 3:175–190.
6. Arendt-Nielsen L, Graven-Nielsen T. Deep tissue hyperalgesia. J Musculoskeletal Pain 2002;10:97–119.
7. Sessle BJ. Acute and chronic craniofacial pain: brainstem mechanisms of nociceptive transmission and neuroplasticity, and their clinical correlates. Crit Rev Oral Biol Med 2000;11(1):57–91.
8. Wall PD, Woolf CJ. Muscle but not cutaneous C-afferent input produces prolonged increases in the excitability of the flexion reflex in the rat. J Physiol 1984;356:443–458.
9. Niddam DM, Chan RC, Lee SH, et al. Central modulation of pain evoked from myofascial trigger point. Clin J Pain 2007;23(5):440–448.
10. Niddam DM, Chan RC, Lee SH, et al. Central representation of hyperalgesia from myofascial trigger point. Neuroimage 2008;39(3):1299–1306.
11. Svensson P, Minoshima S, Beydoun A, et al. Cerebral processing of acute skin and muscle pain in humans. J Neurophysiol 1997;78(1):450–460.
12. Fields HL, Basbaum AI. Central nervous system mechanisms of pain modulation. In: Melzack R, Wall PD, eds. Textbook of Pain. 4th ed. Edinburgh: Churchill Livingstone; 1999:309–329.
13. Mense S. Nociception from skeletal muscle in relation to clinical muscle pain. Pain 1993;54(3):241–289.
14. Cooper G, Bailey B, Bogduk N. Cervical zygapophysial joint pain maps. Pain Med 2007;8(4):344–353.
15. Gunn CC. Radiculopathic pain: diagnosis and treatment of segmental irritation or sensitization. J Musculoskeletal Pain 1997;5(4):119–134.
16. Cannon WB, Rosenblueth A. The Supersensitivity of Denervated Structures: A Law of Denervation. New York: Macmillan; 1949.
17. Gunn CC. Reply to Chang-Zern Hong. J Musculoskeletal Pain 2000;8(3):137–142.
18. Byrne C, Twist C, Eston R. Neuromuscular function after exercise-induced muscle damage: theoretical and applied implications. Sports Med 2004;34(1):49–69.
19. Kirmayer LJ, Looper KJ. Abnormal illness behaviour: physiological, psychological, and social dimensions of coping with distress. Curr Opin Psychiatry 2006;19(1):54–60.
20. Barclay J. In Good Hands: The History of the Chartered Society of Physiotherapy 1894–1994. Oxford: Butterworth Heinemann; 1994.
21. Mennell J. Spray-stretch for the relief of pain from muscle spasm and myofascial trigger points. J Am Podiatry Assoc 1976;66(11):873–876.
22. Mennell J. Myofascial trigger points as a cause of headaches. J Manipulative Physiol Ther 1989;12(4):308–313.
23. Simons DG. Orphan organ. J Musculoskeletal Pain 2007;15(2):7–9.
24. Baldry PE. Acupuncture, Trigger Points, and Musculoskeletal Pain. Edinburgh: Churchill Livingstone; 2005.
25. Simons DG. Muscle pain syndromes—part I. Am J Phys Med 1975;54(6):289–311.
26. Stockman R. The causes, pathology, and treatment of chronic rheumatism. Edinburgh Med J 1904;15:107–116.
27. Cyriax J. Massage, Manipulation, and Local Anaesthesia. London: Hamish Hamilton; 1941.
28. Paris SV. A history of manipulative therapy through the ages and up to the current controversy in the United States. J Man Manip Ther 2000;8(2):66–77.
29. Wilson VP. Janet G. Travell, MD; a daughter's recollection. Tex Heart Inst J 2003;30(1):8–12.
30. Travell JG, Rinzler S, Herman M. Pain and disability of the shoulder and arm: treatment by intramuscular infiltration with procaine hydrochloride. JAMA 1942;120:417–422.
31. Travell JG, Rinzler SH. The myofascial genesis of pain. Postgrad Med 1952; 11(5):425–434.
32. Schleip R, Klingler W, Lehmann-Horn F. Active fascial contractility: fascia may be able to contract in a smooth muscle-like manner and thereby influence musculoskeletal dynamics. Med Hypotheses 2005;65(2):273–277.
33. Travell JG, Simons DG. Myofascial Pain and Dysfunction: The Trigger Point Manual. Baltimore: Williams & Wilkins; 1983.
34. Travell JG, Simons DG. Myofascial Pain and Dysfunction: The Trigger Point Manual. Baltimore: Williams & Wilkins; 1992.
35. Steindler A. The interpretation of sciatic radiation and the syndrome of low-back pain. J Bone Joint Surg Am 1940;22:28–34.
36. Simons DG. Review of enigmatic MTrPs as a common cause of enigmatic musculoskeletal pain and dysfunction. J Electromyogr Kinesiol 2004;14(1):95–107.
37. Robinson JP, Arendt-Nielsen L. Muscle pain syndromes. In: Braddom RL, ed. Physical Medicine and Rehabilitation. Philadelphia: Elsevier; 2007.
38. Harden RN, Bruehl SP, Gass S, et al. Signs and symptoms of the myofascial pain syndrome: a national survey of pain management providers. Clin J Pain 2000;16(1):64–72.
39. Simons DG, Travell JG, Simons LS. Myofascial Pain and Dysfunction: The Trigger Point Manual. 2nd ed. Baltimore: Lippincott Williams & Wilkins; 1999.
40. Simons DG, Travell JG. Myofascial trigger points, a possible explanation. Pain 1981;10(1):106–109.
41. Dommerholt J, Bron C, Franssen JLM. Myofascial trigger points: an evidence-informed review. J Man Manip Ther 2006;14(4):203–221.
42. Gerwin RD, Dommerholt J, Shah JP. An expansion of Simons' integrated hypothesis of trigger point formation. Curr Pain Headache Rep 2004;8(6):468–475.
43. McPartland JM. Travell trigger points—molecular and osteopathic perspectives. J Am Osteopath Assoc 2004;104(6):244–249.
44. McPartland JM, Simons DG. Myofascial trigger points: translating molecular theory into manual therapy. J Man Manip Ther 2006;14(4):232–239.
45. Gerwin RD. Myofascial and visceral pain syndromes: visceral–somatic pain representations. In: Bennett RM, ed. The Clinical Neurobiology of Fibromyalgia and Myofascial Pain. Binghamptom: Haworth Press; 2002;65–75.
46. Weiss JM. Pelvic floor myofascial trigger points: manual therapy for interstitial cystitis and the urgency–frequency syndrome. J Urol 2001;166(6):2226–2231.
47. Zermann DH, Ishigooka M, Doggweiler R, et al. Chronic prostatitis: a myofascial pain syndrome? Infect Urol 1999;12(3):84–92.
48. Anderson RU. Management of chronic prostatitis–chronic pelvic pain syndrome. Urol Clin North Am 2002 Feb;29(1):235–239.
49. Anderson RU, Wise D, Sawyer T, et al. Integration of myofascial trigger point release and paradoxical relaxation training treatment of chronic pelvic pain in men. J Urol 2005;174(1):155–160.
50. Doggweiler-Wiygul R. Urologic myofascial pain syndromes. Curr Pain Headache Rep 2004;8(6):445–451.
51. Jarrell J. Myofascial dysfunction in the pelvis. Curr Pain Headache Rep 2004; 8(6):452–456.
52. Hendler NH, Kozikowski JG. Overlooked physical diagnoses in chronic pain patients involved in litigation. Psychosomatics 1993;34(6):494–501.
53. Alfven G. The pressure pain threshold (PPT) of certain muscles in children suffering from recurrent abdominal pain of non-organic origin. An algometric study. Acta Paediatr 1993;82(5):481–483.
54. Zapata AL, Moraes AJ, Leone C, et al. Pain and musculoskeletal pain syndromes in adolescents. J Adolesc Health 2006;38(6):769–771.
55. Kao MJ, Han TI, Kuan TS, et al. Myofascial trigger points in early life. Arch Phys Med Rehabil 2007;88(2):251–254.
56. Cimbiz A, Beydemir F, Manisaligil U. Evaluation of trigger points in young subjects. J Musculoskeletal Pain 2006;14(4):27–35.
57. Chen Q, Basford J, An KN. Ability of magnetic resonance elastography to assess taut bands. Clin Biomech (Bristol, Avon) 2008;23:623–629.
58. Chen Q, Bensamoun S, Basford JR, et al. Identification and quantification of myofascial taut bands with magnetic resonance elastography. Arch Phys Med Rehabil 2007;88(12):1658–1661.
59. Bensamoun SF, Ringleb SI, Littrell L, et al. Determination of thigh muscle stiffness using magnetic resonance elastography. J Magn Reson Imaging 2006; 23(2):242–247.
60. Ringleb SI, Bensamoun SF, Chen Q, et al. Applications of magnetic resonance elastography to healthy and pathologic skeletal muscle. J Magn Reson Imaging 2007;25(2):301–309.
61. Sikdar S, Shah JP. Gilliams E, et al. Assessment of myofascial trigger points (MTrPs): a new application of ultrasound imaging and vibration sonoelastography. Conf Proc IEEE Eng Med Biol Soc 2008;2008:5585–5588.

62. Falla D, Farina D. Neuromuscular adaptation in experimental and clinical neck pain. *J Electromyogr Kinesiol* 2008;18(2):255–261.

63. Falla D, Farina D. Neural and muscular factors associated with motor impairment in neck pain. *Curr Rheumatol Rep* 2007;9(6):497–502.

64. Lucas KR, Polus BI, Rich PS. Latent myofascial trigger points: their effect on muscle activation and movement efficiency. *J Bodywork Movement Ther* 2004;8:160–166.

65. Ge HY, Fernández-de-las-Peñas C, Arendt–Nielsen L. Sympathetic facilitation of hyperalgesia evoked from myofascial tender and trigger points in patients with unilateral shoulder pain. *Clin Neurophysiol* 2006;117(7):1545–1550.

66. Clark KA, McElhinny AS, Beckerle MC, et al. Striated muscle cytoarchitecture: an intricate web of form and function. *Annu Rev Cell Dev Biol* 2002;18:637–706.

67. Wang K. Cytoskeletal matrix in striated muscle: the role of titin, nebulin, and intermediate filaments. *Adv Exp Med Biol* 1984;170:285–305.

68. Wang K. Titin/connectin and nebulin: giant protein rulers of muscle structure and function. *Adv Biophys* 1996;33:123–134.

69. Wang K, McClure J, Tu A. Titin: major myofibrillar components of striated muscle. *Proc Natl Acad Sci USA* 1979;76(8):3698–3702.

70. Lindstedt SL, Reich TE, Keim P, et al. Do muscles function as adaptable locomotor springs? *J Exp Biol* 2002;205(Pt 15):2211–2216.

71. Wang K, McCarter R, Wright J, et al. Viscoelasticity of the sarcomere matrix in skeletal muscles. The titin–myosin composite filament is a dual-stage molecular spring. *Biophys J* 1993;64(4):1161–1177.

72. Nagy A, Cacciafesta P, Grama L, et al. Differential actin binding along the PEVK domain of skeletal muscle titin. *J Cell Sci* 2004;117(Pt 24):5781–5789.

73. Niederlander N, Raynaud F, Astier C, et al. Regulation of the actin–myosin interaction by titin. *Eur J Biochem* 2004;271(22):4572–4781.

74. Gregorio CC, Granzier H, Sorimachi H, et al. Muscle assembly: a titanic achievement? *Curr Opin Cell Biol* 1999;11(1):18–25.

75. Wang K, Yu L. Emerging concepts of muscle contraction and clinical implications for myofascial pain syndrome [abstract]. Focus on Pain, 2000; Mesa AZ. Janet G. Travell, MD, Seminar Series.

76. Ma K, Wang K. Interaction of nebulin SH3 domain with titin PEVK and myopalladin: implications for the signaling and assembly role of titin and nebulin. *FEBS Lett* 2002;532(3):273–278.

77. McElhinny AS, Kazmierski ST, Labeit S, et al. Nebulin: the nebulous, multifunctional giant of striated muscle. *Trends Cardiovasc Med* 2003;13(5):195–201.

78. Bang ML, Mudry RE, McElhinny AS, et al. Myopalladin, a novel 145-kilodalton sarcomeric protein with multiple roles in Z-disc and I-band protein assemblies. *J Cell Biol* 2001;153(2):413–427.

79. Bang ML, Gregorio C, Labeit S. Molecular dissection of the interaction of desmin with the C-terminal region of nebulin. *J Structl Biol* 2002;137(1–2):119–127.

80. Jin JP, Wang K. Nebulin as a giant actin-binding template protein in skeletal muscle sarcomere. Interaction of actin and cloned human nebulin fragments. *FEBS Lett* 1991;281(1–2):93–96.

81. McElhinny AS, Kolmerer B, Fowler VM, et al. The N-terminal end of nebulin interacts with tropomodulin at the pointed ends of the thin filaments. *J Biol Chem* 2001;276(1):583–592.

82. Arrowsmith JE. The neuromuscular junction. *Surgery (Oxford)* 2007;25(3):105–111.

83. Hubbard DR, Berkoff GM. Myofascial trigger points show spontaneous needle EMG activity. *Spine* 1993;18(13):1803–1807.

84. Hong CZ, Yu J. Spontaneous electrical activity of rabbit trigger spot after transection of spinal cord and peripheral nerve. *J Musculoskeletal Pain* 1998;6(4):45–58.

85. Simons DG. Do endplate noise and spikes arise from normal motor endplates? *Am J Phys Med Rehabil* 2001;80(2):134–140.

86. Simons DG, Hong CZ, Simons LS. Endplate potentials are common to mid-fiber myofascial trigger points. *Am J Phys Med Rehabil* 2002;81(3):212–222.

87. Chen JT, Chen SM, Kuan TS, et al. Phentolamine effect on the spontaneous electrical activity of active loci in a myofascial trigger spot of rabbit skeletal muscle. *Arch Phys Med Rehabil* 1998;79(7):790–794.

88. Kuan TS, Chen JT, Chen SM, et al. Effect of botulinum toxin on endplate noise in myofascial trigger spots of rabbit skeletal muscle. *Am J Phys Med Rehabil* 2002;81(7):512–520.

89. Mense S, Simons DG, Hoheisel U, et al. Lesions of rat skeletal muscle after local block of acetylcholinesterase and neuromuscular stimulation. *J Appl Physiol* 2003;94(6):2494–2501.

90. Couppé C, Midttun A, Hilden J, et al. Spontaneous needle electromyographic activity in myofascial trigger points in the infraspinatus muscle: a blinded assessment. *J Musculoskeletal Pain* 2001;9(3):7–17.

91. Macgregor J, Graf von Schweinitz D. Needle electromyographic activity of myofascial trigger points and control sites in equine cleidobrachialis muscle—an observational study. *Acupunct Med* 2006;24(2):61–70.

92. Maekawa K, Clark GT, Kuboki T. Intramuscular hypoperfusion, adrenergic receptors, and chronic muscle pain. *J Pain* 2002;3(4):251–260.

93. Brückle W, Sückfull M, Fleckenstein W, et al. Gewebe-pO2-Messung in der verspannten Rückenmuskulatur (m. erector spinae). *J Rheumatol* 1990;49:208–216.

94. Henriksson KG, Bengtsson A, Lindman R, et al. Morphological changes in muscle in fibromyalgia and chronic shoulder myalgia. In: Værøy H, Merskey H, eds. *Progress in Fibromyalgia and Myofascial Pain.* Amsterdam: Elsevier; 1993:61–73.

95. Bukharaeva EA, Salakhutdinov RI, Vyskocil F, et al. Spontaneous quantal and non-quantal release of acetylcholine at mouse endplate during onset of hypoxia. *Physiol Res* 2005;54(2):251–255.

96. Chen BM, Grinnell AD. Kinetics, Ca2 + dependence, and biophysical properties of integrin-mediated mechanical modulation of transmitter release from frog motor nerve terminals. *J Neurosci* 1997;17(3):904–916.

97. Grinnell AD, Chen BM, Kashani A, et al. The role of integrins in the modulation of neurotransmitter release from motor nerve terminals by stretch and hypertonicity. *J Neurocytol* 2003;32(5–8):489–503.

98. Graven-Nielsen T, Arendt-Nielsen L. Induction and assessment of muscle pain, referred pain, and muscular hyperalgesia. *Curr Pain Headache Rep* 2003;7(6):443–451.

99. Sluka KA, Kalra A, Moore SA. Unilateral intramuscular injections of acidic saline produce a bilateral, long-lasting hyperalgesia. *Muscle Nerve* 2001;24(1):37–46.

100. Sluka KA, Price MP, Breese NM, et al. Chronic hyperalgesia induced by repeated acid injections in muscle is abolished by the loss of ASIC3, but not ASIC1. *Pain* 2003;106(3):229–239.

101. Barash IA, Peters D, Fridén J, et al. Desmin cytoskeletal modifications after a bout of eccentric exercise in the rat. *Am J Physiol Regul Integr Comp Physiol* 2002;283(4):R958–R963.

102. Fridén J, Lieber RL. Segmental muscle fiber lesions after repetitive eccentric contractions. *Cell Tissue Res* 1998;293(1):165–171.

103. Lieber RL, Shah S, Fridén J. Cytoskeletal disruption after eccentric contraction-induced muscle injury. *Clin Orthop Relat Res* 2002;(403 Suppl):S90–S99.

104. Peters D, Barash IA, Burdi M, et al. Asynchronous functional, cellular, and transcriptional changes after a bout of eccentric exercise in the rat. *J Physiol* 2003;553(Pt 3):947–957.

105. Stauber WT, Clarkson PM, Fritz VK, et al. Extracellular matrix disruption and pain after eccentric muscle action. *J Appl Physiol* 1990;69(3):868–874.

106. Thompson JL, Balog EM, Fitts RH, et al. Five myofibrillar lesion types in eccentrically challenged, unloaded rat adductor longus muscle—a test model. *Anat Rec* 1999;254(1):39–52.

107. Reitinger A, Radner H, Tilscher H, et al. Morphologische untersuchung an triggerpunkten. *Manuelle Medizin* 1996;34:256–262.

108. Windisch A, Reitinger A, Traxler H, et al. Morphology and histochemistry of myogelosis. *Clin Anat* 1999;12(4):266–271.

109. Simons DG, Stolov WC. Microscopic features and transient contraction of palpable bands in canine muscle. *Am J Phys Med* 1976;55(2):65–88.

110. Itoh K, Okada K, Kawakita K. A proposed experimental model of myofascial trigger points in human muscle after slow eccentric exercise. *Acupunct Med* 2004;22(1):2–12.

111. Chen SM, Chen JT, Kuan TS, et al. Decrease in pressure pain thresholds of latent myofascial trigger points in the middle finger extensors immediately after continuous piano practice. *J Musculoskeletal Pain* 2000;8(3):83–92.

112. Treaster D, Marras WS, Burr D, et al. Myofascial trigger point development from visual and postural stressors during computer work. *J Electromyogr Kinesiol* 2006;16(2):115–124.

113. Hägg GM. The Cinderella hypothesis. In: Johansson H, Windhorst U, Djupsjöbacka M, et al, eds. *Chronic Work-Related Myalgia.* Gävle: Gävle University Press; 2003:127–132.

114. Forsman M, Taoda K, Thorn S, et al. Motor-unit recruitment during long-term isometric and wrist motion contractions: a study concerning muscular pain development in computer operators. *Int J Ind Ergon* 2002;30(4–5):237–250.

115. Zennaro D, Laubli T, Krebs D, et al. Trapezius muscle motor unit activity in symptomatic participants during finger tapping using properly and improperly adjusted desks. *Hum Factors* 2004;46(2):252–266.

116. Febbraio MA, Pedersen BK. Contraction-induced myokine production and release: is skeletal muscle an endocrine organ? *Exerc Sport Sci Rev* 2005;33(3):114–119.

117. Gissel H. Ca2 + accumulation and cell damage in skeletal muscle during low frequency stimulation. *Eur J Appl Physiol* 2000;83(2–3):175–180.

118. Lexell J, Jarvis J, Downham D, et al. Stimulation-induced damage in rabbit fast-twitch skeletal muscles: a quantitative morphological study of the influence of pattern and frequency. *Cell Tissue Res* 1993;273(2):357–362.

119. Pedersen BK, Febbraio M. Muscle-derived interleukin-6—a possible link between skeletal muscle, adipose tissue, liver, and brain. *Brain Behav Immun* 2005;19(5):371–376.

120. Otten E. Concepts and models of functional architecture in skeletal muscle. *Exerc Sport Sci Rev* 1988;16:89–137.

121. Mense S. The pathogenesis of muscle pain. *Curr Pain Headache Rep* 2003;7(6):419–425.

122. Vyklicky L, Knotkova-Urbancova H, Vitaskova Z, et al. Inflammatory mediators at acid pH activate capsaicin receptors in cultured sensory neurons from newborn rats. *J Neurophysiol* 1998;79:670–676.

123. Jensen K, Tuxen C, Pedersen-Bjergaard U, et al. Pain and tenderness in human temporal muscle induced by bradykinin and 5-hydroxytryptamine. *Peptides* 1990;11(6):1127–1132.

124. Mense S, Simons DG. *Muscle Pain: Understanding Its Nature, Diagnosis, and Treatment.* Philadephia: Lippincott Williams & Wilkins; 2001.

125. Ambalavanar R, Dessem D, Moutanni A, et al. Muscle inflammation induces a rapid increase in calcitonin gene-related peptide (CGRP) mRNA that temporally relates to CGRP immunoreactivity and nociceptive behavior. *Neuroscience* 2006;143(3):875–884.

126. Snijdelaar DG, Dirksen R, Slappendel R, et al. Substance P. *Eur J Pain* 2000; 4(2):121–135.

127. Massaad CA, Safieh-Garabedian B, Poole S, et al. Involvement of substance P, CGRP, and histamine in the hyperalgesia and cytokine upregulation induced by intraplantar injection of capsaicin in rats. *J Neuroimmunol* 2004; 153(1–2):171–182.

128. Mense S. Pathophysiologic basis of muscle pain syndromes. In: Fischer AA, ed. *Myofascial Pain: Update in Diagnosis and Treatment*. Philadelphia: W.B. Saunders Company; 1997:23–53.

129. Marceau F, Sabourin T, Houle S, et al. Kinin receptors: functional aspects. *Int Immunopharmacol* 2002;2(13–14):1729–1739.

130. Calixto JB, Cabrini DA, Ferreira J, et al. Kinins in pain and inflammation. *Pain* 2000;87(1):1–5.

131. Giamberardino MA, Tafuri E, Savini A, et al. Contribution of myofascial trigger points to migraine symptoms. *J Pain* 2007;8(11):869–878.

132. Fernández-de-las-Peñas C, Cuadrado M, Arendt-Nielsen L, et al. Myofascial trigger points and sensitization: an updated pain model for tension-type headache. *Cephalalgia* 2007;27(5):383–393.

133. Giamberardino MA, Affaitati G, Iezzi S, et al. Referred muscle pain and hyperalgesia from viscera. *J Musculoskeletal Pain* 1999;7:61–69.

134. Vecchiet L, Giamberardino MA, Dragani L. Latent myofascial trigger points: changes in muscular and subcutaneous pain thresholds at trigger point and target level. *J Manual Medicine* 1990;5:151–154.

135. Vecchiet L, Pizzigallo E, Iezzi S, et al. Differentiation of sensitivity in different tissues and its clinical significance. *J Musculoskeletal Pain* 1998;6(1):33–45.

136. Jarrell J, Robert M. Myofascial dysfunction and pelvic pain. *Can J CME* 2003:107–116.

137. Shoskes DA, Berger R, Elmi A, et al. Muscle tenderness in men with chronic prostatitis/chronic pelvic pain syndrome: the chronic prostatitis cohort study. *J Urol* 2008;179(2):556–560.

138. Fernández-de-las-Peñas C, Fernández-Carnero J, Miangolarra-Page JC. Musculoskeletal disorders in mechanical neck pain: myofascial trigger points versus cervical joint dysfunction. *J Musculoskeletal Pain* 2005;13(1):27–35.

139. Ruiz–Saez M, Fernandez-de-las-Penas C, Blanco CR, et al. Changes in pressure pain sensitivity in latent myofascial trigger points in the upper trapezius muscle after a cervical spine manipulation in pain-free subjects. *J Manipulative Physiol Ther* 2007;30(8):578–583.

140. Hoheisel U, Mense S, Simons D, et al. Appearance of new receptive fields in rat dorsal horn neurons following noxious stimulation of skeletal muscle: a model for referral of muscle pain? *Neurosci Lett* 1993;153:9–12.

141. Shah JP, Danoff JV, Desai MJ, et al. Biochemicals associated with pain and inflammation are elevated in sites near to and remote from active myofascial trigger points. *Arch Phys Med Rehabil* 2008;89(1):16–23.

142. Shah JP, Phillips TM, Danoff JV, et al. An in vivo microanalytical technique for measuring the local biochemical milieu of human skeletal muscle. *J Appl Physiol* 2005;99:1977–1984.

143. Hoheisel U, Koch K, Mense S. Functional reorganization in the rat dorsal horn during an experimental myositis. *Pain* 1994;59(1):111–118.

144. Mense S. Referral of muscle pain: new aspects. *Amer Pain Soc J* 1994;3(1): 1–9.

145. Fukui S, Ohseto K, Shiotani M, et al. Referred pain distribution of the cervical zygapophyseal joints and cervical dorsal rami. *Pain* 1996;68:79–83.

146. O'Neill CW, Kurgansky ME, Derby R, et al. Disc stimulation and patterns of referred pain. *Spine* 2002;27(24):2776–2781.

147. Petros P, Bornstein J. Re: vulvar vestibulitis may be a referred pain arising from laxity in the uterosacral ligaments: a hypothesis based on three prospective case reports. *Aust N Z J Obstet Gynaecol* 2004;44(5):484–485.

148. Hackett GS. Referred pain from low back ligament disability. *AMA Arch Surg* 1956;73(5):878–883.

149. Bogduk N, Simons DG. Neck pain: joint pain or trigger points. In: Værøy H, Merskey H, eds. *Progress in Fibromyalgia and Myofascial Pain*. Amsterdam: Elsevier; 1993:267–273.

150. Fernandez-Carnero J, Fernández-de-las-Peñas CF, de la Llave-Rincon AI, et al. Prevalence of and referred pain from myofascial trigger points in the forearm muscles in patients with lateral epicondylalgia. *Clin J Pain* 2007;23(4): 353–360.

151. Hsieh YL, Kao MJ, Kuan TS, et al. Dry needling to a key myofascial trigger point may reduce the irritability of satellite MTrPs. *Am J Phys Med Rehabil* 2007;86(5):397–403.

152. Carlson CR, Okeson JP, Falace DA, et al. Reduction of pain and EMG activity in the masseter region by trapezius trigger point injection. *Pain* 1993;55(3): 397–400.

153. Headley BJ. Evaluation and treatment of myofascial pain syndrome utilizing biofeedback. In: Cram JR, ed. *Clinical Electromyography for Surface Recordings*. Nevada City: Clinical Resources; 1990:235–254.

154. Bajaj P, Bajaj P, Graven-Nielsen T, et al. Trigger points in patients with lower limb osteoarthritis. *J Musculoskeletal Pain* 2001;9(3):17–33.

155. Gerwin RD, Duranleau D. Ultrasound identification of the myofascial trigger point. *Muscle Nerve* 1997;20(6):767–768.

156. Hong CZ, Torigoe Y. Electrophysiological characteristics of localized twitch responses in responsive taut bands of rabbit skeletal muscle. *J Musculoskeletal Pain* 1994;2:17–43.

157. Hong CZ. Persistence of local twitch response with loss of conduction to and from the spinal cord. *Arch Phys Med Rehabil* 1994;75(1):12–16.

158. Mayoral del Moral O. Fisioterapia invasiva del síndrome de dolor miofascial. *Fisioterapia* 2005;27(2):69–75.

159. Dommerholt J, Mayoral O, Gröbli C. Trigger point dry needling. *J Man Manip Ther* 2006;14(4):E70–E87.

160. Hong CZ. Lidocaine injection versus dry needling to myofascial trigger point. The importance of the local twitch response. *Am J Phys Med Rehabil* 1994; 73(4):256–263.

161. Audette JF, Wang F, Smith H. Bilateral activation of motor unit potentials with unilateral needle stimulation of active myofascial trigger points. *Am J Phys Med Rehabil* 2004;83(5):368–374.

162. Issberner U, Reeh PW, Steen KH. Pain due to tissue acidosis: a mechanism for inflammatory and ischemic myalgia? *Neurosci Lett* 1996;208(3):191–194.

163. Hong CZ, Torigoe Y, Yu J. The localized twitch responses in responsive bands of rabbit skeletal muscle are related to the reflexes at spinal cord level. *J Musculoskeletal Pain* 1995;3:15–33.

164. Willis WD. Retrograde signaling in the nervous system: dorsal root reflexes. In: Bradshaw RA, Dennis EA, eds. *Handbook of Cell Signaling*. San Diego: Academic/Elsevier Press; 2004.

165. Bowman WC, Marshall IG, Gibb AJ, et al. Feedback control of transmitter release at the neuromuscular junction. *Trends Pharmacol Sci* 1988;9(1): 16–20.

166. Burton AK, Waddell G, Tillotson KM, et al. Information and advice to patients with back pain can have a positive effect. A randomized controlled trial of a novel educational booklet in primary care. *Spine* 1999;24(23): 2484–2491.

167. Verri WA Jr, Cunha TM, Parada CA, et al. Hypernociceptive role of cytokines and chemokines: targets for analgesic drug development? *Pharmacol Ther* 2006;112(1):116–138.

168. Schafers M, Sorkin LS, Sommer C. Intramuscular injection of tumor necrosis factor-alpha induces muscle hyperalgesia in rats. *Pain* 2003;104(3):579–588.

169. Loram LC, Fuller A, Fick LG, et al. Cytokine profiles during carrageenan-induced inflammatory hyperalgesia in rat muscle and hind paw. *J Pain* 2007 Feb;8(2):127–136.

170. Loram LC, Fuller A, Cartmell T, et al. Behavioural, histological, and cytokine responses during hyperalgesia induced by carrageenan injection in the rat tail. *Physiol Behav* 2007;92(5):873–880.

171. Loram LC, Themistocleous AC, Fick LG, et al. The time course of inflammatory cytokine secretion in a rat model of postoperative pain does not coincide with the onset of mechanical hyperalgesia. *Can J Physiol Pharmacol* 2007; 85(6):613–620.

172. Luo G, Hershko DD, Robb BW, et al. IL-1beta stimulates IL-6 production in cultured skeletal muscle cells through activation of MAP kinase signaling pathway and NF-kappa B. *Am J Physiol Regul Integr Comp Physiol* 2003; 284(5):R1249–R1254.

173. Samad TA, Moore KA, Sapirstein A, et al. Interleukin-1beta-mediated induction of Cox-2 in the CNS contributes to inflammatory pain hypersensitivity. *Nature* 2001;410(6827):471–475.

174. Tidball JG. Inflammatory processes in muscle injury and repair. *Am J Physiol Regul Integr Comp Physiol* 2005;288(2):R345–R353.

175. Hoheisel U, Unger T, Mense S. Excitatory and modulatory effects of inflammatory cytokines and neurotrophins on mechanosensitive group IV muscle afferents in the rat. *Pain* 2005;114(1–2):168–176.

176. Dworkin SF, LeResche L. Research diagnostic criteria for temporomandibular disorders: review, criteria, examinations and specifications, critique. *J Craniomandib Disord Facial Oral Pain* 1992;6:301–355.

177. Escobar PL, Ballesteros J. Teres minor. Source of symptoms resembling ulnar neuropathy or C8 radiculopathy. *Am J Phys Med Rehabil* 1988;67(3): 120–122.

178. Facco E, Ceccherelli F. Myofascial pain mimicking radicular syndromes. *Acta Neurochir Suppl* 2005;92:147–150.

179. Crotti FM, Carai A, Carai M, et al. Post-traumatic thoracic outlet syndrome (TOS). *Acta Neurochir Suppl* 2005;92:13–15.

180. Samuel AS, Peter AA, Ramanathan K. The association of active trigger points with lumbar disc lesions. *J Musculoskeletal Pain* 2007;15(2):11–18.

181. Gerwin RD. A review of myofascial pain and fibromyalgia—factors that promote their persistence. *Acupunct Med* 2005;23(3):121–134.

182. Gerwin RD, Dommerholt J. Treatment of myofascial pain syndromes. In: Boswell MV, Cole BE, eds. *Weiner's Pain Management: A Practical Guide for Clinicians*. Boca Raton: CRC Press; 2006:477–492.

183. Gerwin RD, Shannon S, Hong CZ, et al. Interrater reliability in myofascial trigger point examination. *Pain* 1997;69(1–2):65–73.

184. Donnelly JM, Palubinskas L. Prevalence and inter-rater reliability of trigger points. *J Musculoskeletal Pain* 2007;15(Suppl 13):16.

185. Bron C, Franssen J, Wensing M, et al. Interrater reliability of palpation of myofascial trigger points in three shoulder muscles. *J Man Manip Ther* 2007; 15(4):203–215.

186. Hsieh CY, Hong CZ, Adams AH, et al. Interexaminer reliability of the palpation of trigger points in the trunk and lower limb muscles. *Arch Phys Med Rehabil* 2000;81(3):258–264.

187. Lew PC, Lewis J, Story I. Inter-therapist reliability in locating latent myofascial trigger points using palpation. *Manual Ther* 1997;2(2):87–90.

188. Nice DA, Riddle DL, Lamb RL, et al. Intertester reliability of judgments of the presence of trigger points in patients with low back pain. *Arch Phys Med Rehabil* 1992;73(10):893–898.

189. Njoo KH, Van der Does E. The occurrence and inter-rater reliability of myofascial trigger points in the quadratus lumborum and gluteus medius: a prospective study in non-specific low back pain patients and controls in general practice. *Pain* 1994;58(3):317–323.

190. Sciotti VM, Mittak VL, DiMarco L, et al. Clinical precision of myofascial trigger point location in the trapezius muscle. *Pain* 2001;93(3):259–266.

191. Wolfe F, Simons DG, Fricton J, et al. The fibromyalgia and myofascial pain syndromes: a preliminary study of tender points and trigger points in persons with fibromyalgia, myofascial pain syndrome, and no disease. *J Rheumatol* 1992;19(6):944–951.

192. Al-Shenqiti AM, Oldham JA. Test–retest reliability of myofascial trigger point detection in patients with rotator cuff tendonitis. *Clin Rehabil* 2005;19(5):482–487.

193. Fernández-de-las-Peñas C, Alonso-Blanco C, Cuadrado ML, et al. Myofascial trigger points in the suboccipital muscles in episodic tension-type headache. *Man Ther* 2006;11:225–230.

194. Fernández-de-las-Peñas C, Alonso-Blanco C, Cuadrado ML, et al. Myofascial trigger points and their relationship to headache clinical parameters in chronic tension-type headache. *Headache* 2006;46(8):1264–1272.

195. Fernández-de-las-Peñas C, Ge HY, Arendt-Nielsen L, et al. Referred pain from trapezius muscle trigger points shares similar characteristics with chronic tension type headache. *Eur J Pain* 2007;11(4):475–482.

196. Cummings M. Referred knee pain treated with electroacupuncture to iliopsoas. *Acupunct Med* 2003;21(1–2):32–35.

197. Hwang M, Kang YK, Kim DH. Referred pain pattern of the pronator quadratus muscle. *Pain* 2005;116(3):238–242.

198. Hwang M, Kang YK, Shin JY, et al. Referred pain pattern of the abductor pollicis longus muscle. *Am J Phys Med Rehabil* 2005;84(8):593–597.

199. Dorsher P. Trigger points and acupuncture points: anatomic and clinical correlations. *Med Acupunct* 2006;17(3):21–25.

200. Fernández-de-las-Peñas C, Cuadrado ML, Pareja JA. Myofascial trigger points, neck mobility, and forward head posture in episodic tension-type headache. *Headache* 2007;47(5):662–672.

201. Fricton JR, Kroening R, Haley D, et al. Myofascial pain syndrome of the head and neck: a review of clinical characteristics of 164 patients. *Oral Surg Oral Med Oral Pathol* 1985;60(6):615–623.

202. Russek LN. Hypermobility syndrome. *Phys Ther* 1999;79(6):591–599.

203. Fruth SJ. Differential diagnosis and treatment in a patient with posterior upper thoracic pain. *Phys Ther* 2006;86(2):254–268.

204. Hamada H, Moriwaki K, Shiroyama K, et al. Myofascial pain in patients with postthoracotomy pain syndrome. *Reg Anesth Pain Med* 2000;25(3):302–305.

205. Khalil TM, Abdel-Moty E, Steele-Rosomoff R, et al. The role of ergonomics in the prevention and treatment of myofascial pain. In: Rachlin ES, ed. *Myofascial Pain and Fibromyalgia: Trigger Point Management.* St. Louis: Mosby-Year Book; 1994:487–523.

206. Banks SL, Jacobs DW, Gevirtz R, et al. Effects of autogenic relaxation training on electromyographic activity in active myofascial trigger points. *J Musculoskeletal Pain* 1998;6(4):23–32.

207. Lewis C, Gevirtz R, Hubbard D, et al. Needle trigger point and surface frontal EMG measurements of psychophysiological responses in tension-type headache patients. *Biofeedback Self Regul* 1994;3:274–275.

208. McNulty WH, Gevirtz RN, Hubbard DR, et al. Needle electromyographic evaluation of trigger point response to a psychological stressor. *Psychophysiology* 1994;31(3):313–316.

209. Frewen PA, Dozois DJ, Lanius RA. Neuroimaging studies of psychological interventions for mood and anxiety disorders: empirical and methodological review. *Clin Psychol Rev* 2008;28(2):229–247.

210. Graff-Guerrero A, Pellicer F, Mendoza-Espinosa Y, et al. Cerebral blood flow changes associated with experimental muscle pain stimulation in patients with major depression. *J Affect Disord* 2008;107(1–3):161–168.

211. Lidbeck J. Central hyperexcitability in chronic musculoskeletal pain: a conceptual breakthrough with multiple clinical implications. *Pain Res Manag* 2002;7(2):81–92.

212. Vlaeyen JW, Linton SJ. Fear-avoidance and its consequences in chronic musculoskeletal pain: a state of the art. *Pain* 2000;85(3):317–332.

213. Plotnikoff GA, Quigley JM. Prevalence of severe hypovitaminosis D in patients with persistent, nonspecific musculoskeletal pain. *Mayo Clin Proc* 2003;78(12):1463–1470.

214. Dawson-Hughes B, Heaney RP, Holick MF, et al. Estimates of optimal vitamin D status. *Osteoporos Int* 2005;16(7):713–716.

215. Gordon CM, DePeter KC, Feldman HA, et al. Prevalence of vitamin D deficiency among healthy adolescents. *Arch Pediatr Adolesc Med* 2004;158(6):531–537.

216. Vieth R, Bischoff-Ferrari H, Boucher BJ, et al. The urgent need to recommend an intake of vitamin D that is effective. *Am J Clin Nutr* 2007;85(3):649–650.

217. Huh SY, Gordon CM. Vitamin D deficiency in children and adolescents: epidemiology, impact, and treatment. *Rev Endocr Metab Disord* 2008;9(2):161–170.

218. MacFarlane GD, Sackrison JL Jr, Body JJ, et al. Hypovitaminosis D in a normal, apparently healthy urban European population. *J Steroid Biochem Mol Biol* 2004;89–90(1–5):621–622.

219. Holick MF. High prevalence of vitamin D inadequacy and implications for health. *Mayo Clin Proc* 2006;81(3):353–373.

220. Bischoff HA, Stahelin HB, Tyndall A, et al. Relationship between muscle strength and vitamin D metabolites: are there therapeutic possibilities in the elderly? *J Rheumatol* 2000;59(Suppl 1):39–41.

221. Moore A, McQuay H, Gray JAM. Evidence-based everything. *Bandolier* 1995;1(12):1.

222. Pencheon D. What's next for evidence-based medicine? *Evidenced-Based Healthcare Public Health* 2005;9:319–321.

223. Sackett DL, Rosenberg WM, Gray JA, et al. Evidence based medicine: what it is and what it isn't. *BMJ* 1996;312(7023):71–72.

224. Bauermeister W. Diagnose und therapie des myofaszialen triggerpunkt syndroms durch lokalisierung und stimulation sensibilisierter nozizeptoren mit fokussierten elektrohydraulische stosswellen. *Medizinisch-Orthopädische Technik* 2005;5:65–74.

225. Müller-Ehrenberg H, Licht G. Diagnosis and therapy of myofascial pain syndrome with focused shock waves (ESWT). *Medizinisch-Orthopädische Technik* 2005;5:1–6.

226. Lewis J, Tehan P. A blinded pilot study investigating the use of diagnostic ultrasound for detecting active myofascial trigger points. *Pain* 1999;79(1):39–44.

227. Fernández-de-las-Peñas C, Cleland JA, Cuadrado ML, et al. Predictor variables for identifying patients with chronic tension-type headache who are likely to achieve short-term success with muscle trigger point therapy. *Cephalalgia* 2008;28:264–275.

228. Cohen SP, Mullings R, Abdi S. The pharmacologic treatment of muscle pain. *Anesthesiology* 2004;101(2):495–526.

229. Wheeler AH. Myofascial pain disorders: theory to therapy. *Drugs* 2004;64(1):45–62.

230. Moseley L. Unraveling the barriers to reconceptualization of the problem in chronic pain: the actual and perceived ability of patients and health professionals to understand the neurophysiology. *J Pain* 2003;4(4):184–189.

231. Bandura A. Self-efficacy mechanism in physiological activation and health-promoting behavior. In: Madden JI, Matthysse S, Barchas S, eds. *Adaptation, Learning, and Affect.* New York: Raven Press; 1986.

232. Wittink H, Hoskins Michel T. *Chronic Pain Management for Physical Therapists.* Boston: Butterworth Heinemann; 2002.

233. Dommerholt J. Physical therapy in an interdisciplinary pain management center. *Pain Practitioner* 2005;14(3):32–36.

234. Scudds R, Solomon P. Pain and its management: a new pain curriculum for occupational therapists and physical therapists. *Physiother Can* 1995;47:77–78.

235. Wolff MS, Michel TH, Krebs DE, et al. Chronic pain—assessment of orthopedic physical therapists' knowledge and attitudes. *Phys Ther* 1991;71(3):207–214.

236. Chaitow L. Breathing pattern disorders, motor control, and low back pain. *J Osteop Med* 2004;7(1):33–40.

237. Moseley GL. A pain neuromatrix approach to patients with chronic pain. *Man Ther* 2003;8(3):130–140.

238. Harding VR, Simmonds MJ, Watson PJ. Physical therapy for chronic pain. *Pain Clin Updates* 1998;6(3):1–7.

239. Bandura A, Cioffi D, Taylor CB, et al. Perceived self-efficacy in coping with cognitive stressors and opioid activation. *J Pers Soc Psychol* 1988;55(3):479–488.

240. Bandura A, O'Leary A, Taylor CB, et al. Perceived self-efficacy and pain control: opioid and nonopioid mechanisms. *J Pers Soc Psychol* 1987;53(3):563–571.

241. Steinbrocker O. Therapeutic injections in painful musculoskeletal disorders. *JAMA* 1944;125:397–401.

242. Lewit K. The needle effect in the relief of myofascial pain. *Pain* 1979;6(1):83–90.

243. Gunn CC, Milbrandt WE, Little AS, et al. Dry needling of muscle motor points for chronic low-back pain: a randomized clinical trial with long-term follow-up. *Spine* 1980;5(3):279–291.

244. Furlan A, Tulder M, Cherkin D, et al. Acupuncture and dry-needling for low back pain: an updated systematic review within the framework of the cochrane collaboration. *Spine* 2005;30(8):944–963.

245. Cummings TM, White AR. Needling therapies in the management of myofascial trigger point pain: a systematic review. *Arch Phys Med Rehabil* 2001;82(7):986–992.

246. Ga H, Choi JH, Park CH, et al. Acupuncture needling versus lidocaine injection of trigger points in myofascial pain syndrome in elderly patients—a randomised trial. *Acupunct Med* 2007;25(4):130–136.

247. Garvey TA, Marks MR, Wiesel SW. A prospective, randomized, double-blind evaluation of trigger-point injection therapy for low-back pain. *Spine* 1989;14(9):962–964.

248. Jaeger B, Skootsky SA. Double blind, controlled study of different myofascial trigger point injection techniques. *Pain* 1987;4(Suppl):S292.

249. Kamanli A, Kaya A, Ardicoglu O, et al. Comparison of lidocaine injection, botulinum toxin injection, and dry needling to trigger points in myofascial pain syndrome. *Rheumatol Int* 2005;25(8):604–611.

250. Ga H, Koh HJ, Choi JH, et al. Intramuscular and nerve root stimulation vs lidocaine injection to trigger points in myofascial pain syndrome. *J Rehabil Med* 2007;39(5):374–378.

251. Baldry P. Superficial versus deep dry needling. *Acupunct Med* 2002;20(2–3):78–81.

252. Peets JM, Pomeranz B. CXBK mice deficient in opiate receptors show poor electroacupuncture analgesia. *Nature* 1978;273(5664):675–676.

253. Travell J. Basis for the multiple uses of local block of somatic trigger areas (procaine infiltration and ethyl chloride spray). *Miss Valley Med* 1949;71:13–22.

254. Iwama H, Akama Y. The superiority of water-diluted 0.25% to near 1% lidocaine for trigger-point injections in myofascial pain syndrome: a prospective, randomized, double-blinded trial. *Anesth Analg* 2000;91(2):408–409.

255. Iwama H, Ohmori S, Kaneko T, et al. Water-diluted local anesthetic for trig-

ger-point injection in chronic myofascial pain syndrome: evaluation of types of local anesthetic and concentrations in water. *Reg Anesth Pain Med* 2001; 26(4):333–336.

256. Garcia-Leiva JM, Hidalgo J, Rico-Villademoros F, et al. Effectiveness of ropivacaine trigger points inactivation in the prophylactic management of patients with severe migraine. *Pain Med* 2007;8(1):65–70.

257. Zaralidou AT, Amaniti EN, Maidatsi PG, et al. Comparison between newer local anesthetics for myofascial pain syndrome management. *Methods Find Exp Clin Pharmacol* 2007;29(5):353–357.

258. Kim HW, Kwon YB, Han HJ, et al. Antinociceptive mechanisms associated with diluted bee venom acupuncture (apipuncture) in the rat formalin test: involvement of descending adrenergic and serotonergic pathways. *Pharmacol Res* 2005;51(2):183–188.

259. Kwon YB, Kim JH, Yoon JH, et al. The analgesic efficacy of bee venom acupuncture for knee osteoarthritis: a comparative study with needle acupuncture. *Am J Chin Med* 2001;29(2):187–199.

260. Kwon YB, Lee JD, Lee HJ, et al. Bee venom injection into an acupuncture point reduces arthritis associated edema and nociceptive responses. *Pain* 2001; 90(3):271–280.

261. Son DJ, Kang J, Kim TJ, et al. Melittin, a major bioactive component of bee venom toxin, inhibits PDGF receptor beta-tyrosine phosphorylation and downstream intracellular signal transduction in rat aortic vascular smooth muscle cells. *J Toxicol Environ Health A* 2007;70(15–16):1350–1355.

262. Han S, Lee K, Yeo J, et al. Effect of honey bee venom on microglial cells nitric oxide and tumor necrosis factor-alpha production stimulated by LPS. *J Ethnopharmacol* 2007;111(1):176–181.

263. Lee JD, Park HJ, Chae Y, et al. An overview of bee venom acupuncture in the treatment of arthritis. *Evid Based Complement Alternat Med* 2005;2(1): 79–84.

264. Son DJ, Lee JW, Lee YH, et al. Therapeutic application of anti-arthritis, pain-releasing, and anti-cancer effects of bee venom and its constituent compounds. *Pharmacol Ther* 2007;115(2):246–270.

265. Ettlin T. Trigger point injection treatment with the 5-HT3 receptor antagonist tropisetron in patients with late whiplash-associated disorder. First results of a multiple case study. *Scand J Rheumatol Suppl* 2004;(119):49–50.

266. Müller W, Stratz T. Local treatment of tendinopathies and myofascial pain syndromes with the 5-HT3 receptor antagonist tropisetron. *Scand J Rheumatol Suppl* 2004;(119):44–48.

267. Ho KY, Tan KH. Botulinum toxin A for myofascial trigger point injection: a qualitative systematic review. *Eur J Pain* 2007;11(5):519–527.

268. Silberstein S. Botulinum neurotoxins: origins and basic mechanisms of action. *Pain Pract* 2004;4(Suppl 1):S19–S26.

269. Silberstein N. More than a cosmetic fix. Combined with physical therapy, botulinum toxin type A can help provide relief for chronic muscle pain. *Rehab Manag* 2007;20(1):44, 46.

270. Dodick DW, Mauskop A, Elkind AH, et al. Botulinum toxin type A for the prophylaxis of chronic daily headache: subgroup analysis of patients not receiving other prophylactic medications: a randomized double-blind, placebo-controlled study. *Headache* 2005;45(4):315–324.

271. Göbel H, Heinze A, Reichel G, et al. Efficacy and safety of a single botulinum type A toxin complex treatment (Dysport) for the relief of upper back myofascial pain syndrome: results from a randomized double-blind placebo-controlled multicentre study. *Pain* 2006;125(1–2):82–88.

272. Kern KU, Martin C, Scheicher S, et al. Auslosung von Phantomschmerzen und -sensationen durch muskulare Stumpftriggerpunkte nach Beinamputationen. *Schmerz* 2006;20(4):300–306.

273. Aoki KR. Review of a proposed mechanism for the antinociceptive action of botulinum toxin type A. *Neurotoxicology* 2005;26(5):785–793.

274. Hackett R, Kam PC. Botulinum toxin: pharmacology and clinical developments: a literature review. *Med Chem* 2007;3(4):333–345.

275. Samigullin D, Bukharaeva EA, Vyskocil F, et al. Calcium dependence of uniquantal release latencies and quantal content at mouse neuromuscular junction. *Physiol Res* 2005;54(1):129–132.

276. Wessler I. Acetylcholine release at motor endplates and autonomic neuroeffector junctions: a comparison. *Pharmacol Res* 1996;33(2):81–94.

277. Bach–Rojecky L, Lackovic Z. Antinociceptive effect of botulinum toxin type a in rat model of carrageenan and capsaicin induced pain. *Croat Med J* 2005; 46(2):201–208.

278. Mense S. Neurobiological basis for the use of botulinum toxin in pain therapy. *J Neurol* 2004;251(Suppl 1):I1–I7.

279. Luvisetto S, Marinelli S, Cobianchi S, et al. Anti-allodynic efficacy of botulinum neurotoxin A in a model of neuropathic pain. *Neuroscience* 2007;145(1):1–4.

280. Peng PW, Castano ED. Survey of chronic pain practice by anesthesiologists in Canada. *Can J Anaesth* 2005;52(4):383–389.

281. Cummings M. Myofascial pain from pectoralis major following trans-axillary surgery. *Acupunct Med* 2003;21(3):105–107.

282. Ceccherelli F, Rigoni MT, Gagliardi G, et al. Comparison between superficial and deep acupuncture in the treatment of lumbar myofascial pain: a double-blind randomized controlled study. *Clin J Pain* 2002;18:149–153.

283. Dilorenzo L, Traballesi M, Morelli D, et al. Hemiparetic shoulder pain syndrome treated with deep dry needling during early rehabilitation: a prospective, open-label, randomized investigation. *J Musculoskeletal Pain* 2004; 12(2):25–34.

284. Ga H, Choi JH, Park CH, et al. Dry needling of trigger points with and without paraspinal needling in myofascial pain syndromes in elderly patients. *J Altern Complement Med* 2007;13(6):617–624.

285. McMillan AS, Nolan A, Kelly PJ. The efficacy of dry needling and procaine in the treatment of myofascial pain in the jaw muscles. *J Orofac Pain* 1997; 11(4):307–314.

286. Tschopp KP, Gysin C. Local injection therapy in 107 patients with myofascial pain syndrome of the head and neck. *ORL J Otorhinolaryngol Relat Spec* 1996;58:306–310.

287. Gaspersic R, Koritnik B, Erzen I, et al. Muscle activity-resistant acetylcholine receptor accumulation is induced in places of former motor endplates in ectopically innervated regenerating rat muscles. *Int J Dev Neurosci* 2001;19(3): 339–346.

288. Sadeh M, Stern LZ, Czyzewski K. Changes in end-plate cholinesterase and axons during muscle degeneration and regeneration. *J Anat* 1985;140(Pt 1): 165–76.

289. Langevin HM, Bouffard NA, Badger GJ, et al. Subcutaneous tissue fibroblast cytoskeletal remodeling induced by acupuncture: evidence for a mechanotransduction-based mechanism. *J Cell Physiol* 2006;207(3):767–774.

290. Langevin HM, Bouffard NA, Badger GJ, et al. Dynamic fibroblast cytoskeletal response to subcutaneous tissue stretch ex vivo and in vivo. *Am J Physiol Cell Physiol* 2005;288(3):C747–C756.

291. Sandkühler J. The organization and function of endogenous antinociceptive systems. *Prog Neurobiol* 1996;50(1):49–81.

292. Millan MJ. The induction of pain: an integrative review. *Prog Neurobiol* 1999;57(1):1–164.

293. Lund I, Lundeberg T. Are minimal, superficial, or sham acupuncture procedures acceptable as inert placebo controls? *Acupunct Med* 2006;24(1):13–15.

294. Mohr C, Binkofski F, Erdmann C, et al. The anterior cingulate cortex contains distinct areas dissociating external from self-administered painful stimulation: a parametric fMRI study. *Pain* 2005;114(3):347–357.

295. Olausson H, Lamarre Y, Backlund H, et al. Unmyelinated tactile afferents signal touch and project to insular cortex. *Nat Neurosci* 2002;5(9):900–904.

296. Lundeberg T, Uvnas–Moberg K, Agren G, et al. Anti-nociceptive effects of oxytocin in rats and mice. *Neurosci Lett* 1994;170(1):153–157.

297. Uvnas-Moberg K, Bruzelius G, Alster P, et al. The antinociceptive effect of non-noxious sensory stimulation is mediated partly through oxytocinergic mechanisms. *Acta Physiol Scand* 1993;149(2):199–204.

298. Rickards LD. The effectiveness of non-invasive treatments for active myofascial trigger point pain: a systematic review of the literature. *Int J Osteopathic Med* 2006;9(4):120–136.

299. Fernández-de-las-Peñas C, Campo MS, Fernández-Carnero J. Manual therapies in myofascial trigger point treatment: a systematic review. *J Bodywork Movement Ther* 2005;9:27–34.

300. Fernández-de-las-Peñas C, Alonso-Blanco C, Fernández-Carnero J, et al. The immediate effect of ischemic compression technique and transverse friction massage on tenderness of active and latent myofascial trigger points: a pilot study. *J Bodywork Movement Ther* 2006;10(1):3–9.

301. Hou CR, Tsai LC, Cheng KF, et al. Immediate effects of various physical therapeutic modalities on cervical myofascial pain and trigger-point sensitivity. *Arch Phys Med Rehabil* 2002;83(10):1406–1414.

302. Energy Information Administration, Office of Integrated Analysis and Forecasting, U.S. Department of Energy. *Emissions of Greenhouse Gases in the United States 2005*. Washington, DC: U.S. Department of Energy; 2006.

303. European Environment Agency. EEA Signals 2004: a European Environment Agency update on selected issues. Copenhagen: EEA; 2004.

304. Hong CZ, Chen YC, Pon CH, et al. Immediate effects of various physical medicine modalities on pain threshold of the active myofascial trigger points. *J Musculoskeletal Pain* 1993;1(2):37–53.

305. Altan L, Bingol U, Aykac M, et al. Investigation of the effect of GaAs laser therapy on cervical myofascial pain syndrome. *Rheumatol Int* 2005;25(1): 23–27.

306. Ceccherelli F, Altafini L, Lo Castro G, et al. Diode laser in cervical myofascial pain: a double-blind study versus placebo. *Clin J Pain* 1989;5(4):301–304.

307. Gur A, Sarac AJ, Cevik R, et al. Efficacy of 904 nm gallium arsenide low level laser therapy in the management of chronic myofascial pain in the neck: a double-blind and randomized-controlled trial. *Lasers Surg Med* 2004;35(3): 229–235.

308. Hakguder A, Birtane M, Gurcan S, et al. Efficacy of low level laser therapy in myofascial pain syndrome: an algometric and thermographic evaluation. *Lasers Surg Med* 2003;33(5):339–343.

309. Ilbuldu E, Cakmak A, Disci R, et al. Comparison of laser, dry needling, and placebo laser treatments in myofascial pain syndrome. *Photomed Laser Surg* 2004;22(4):306–311.

310. Snyder-Mackler L, Barry AJ, Perkins AI, et al. Effects of helium–neon laser irradiation on skin resistance and pain in patients with trigger points in the neck or back. *Phys Ther* 1989;69(5):336–341.

311. Dundar U, Evcik D, Samli F, et al. The effect of gallium arseside aluminum laser therapy in the management of cervical myofascial pain syndrome: a double blind, placebo-controlled study. *Clin Rheumatol* 2007;26(6):930–934.

312. Srbely JZ, Dickey JP. Randomized controlled study of the antinociceptive effect of ultrasound on trigger point sensitivity: novel applications in myofascial therapy? *Clin Rehabil* 2007;21(5):411–417.

313. Gam AN, Warming S, Larsen LH, et al. Treatment of myofascial trigger-points with ultrasound combined with massage and exercise—a randomised controlled trial. *Pain* 1998;77(1):73–79.

314. Lee JC, Lin DT, Hong CZ. The effectiveness of simultaneous thermotherapy with ultrasound and electrotherapy with combined AC and DC current on

the immediate pain relief of myofascial trigger points. *J Musculoskeletal Pain* 1997;5(1):81–90.

315. Majlesi J, Unalan H. High-power pain threshold ultrasound technique in the treatment of active myofascial trigger points: a randomized, double-blind, case-control study. *Arch Phys Med Rehabil* 2004;85(5):833–836.

316. Farina S, Casarotto M, Benelle M, et al. A randomized controlled study on the effect of two different treatments (FREMS AND TENS) in myofascial pain syndrome. *Eura Medicophys* 2004;40(4):293–301.

317. Ardiç F, Sarhus M, Topuz O. Comparison of two different techniques of electrotherapy on myofascial pain. *J Back Musculoskeletal Rehabil* 2002;16: 11–16.

318. Graff-Radford SB, Reeves JL, Baker RL, et al. Effects of transcutaneous electrical nerve stimulation on myofascial pain and trigger point sensitivity. *Pain* 1989;37(1):1–5.

319. Hsueh TC, Cheng PT, Kuan TS, et al. The immediate effectiveness of electrical nerve stimulation and electrical muscle stimulation on myofascial trigger points. *Am J Phys Med Rehabil* 1997;76(6):471–476.

320. Müller-Ehrenberg H, Thorwesten L. Improvement of sports-related shoulder pain after treatment of trigger points using focused extracorporeal shock wave therapy regarding static and dynamic force development, pain relief, and sensomotoric performance. *J Musculoskeletal Pain* 2007;15(Suppl 13):33.

CHAPTER 36 ■ FIBROMYALGIA

DANIEL J. CLAUW

INTRODUCTION

Clinical practitioners commonly see patients with pain and other somatic symptoms that they cannot adequately explain based on the degree of damage or inflammation noted in peripheral tissues. In fact, this may be among the most common predicaments for which individuals seek medical attention.[1] Typically, an evaluation is performed looking for a "cause" for the pain. If none is found, these individuals are often given a diagnostic label that merely connotes that the patient has chronic pain in a region of the body, without an underlying mechanistic cause (e.g., chronic low back pain, headache, temporomandibular disorder [TMD], etc.). In other cases, the label given alludes to an underlying mechanism that may or may not be responsible for the individual's pain (e.g., "facet syndrome").

Fibromyalgia (FM) is merely the current term for individuals with chronic widespread musculoskeletal pain, for which no alternative cause can be identified. Gastroenterologists often see the exact same patients and focus on their gastroenterological complaints, and often use the terms functional GI disorder, irritable bowel syndrome (IBS), nonulcer dyspepsia, or esophageal dysmotility to explain the patient's symptoms.[2] Neurologists see these patients for their headaches and/or unexplained facial pain, urologists for pelvic pain and urinary symptoms (and use labels such as interstitial cystitis, chronic prostatitis, vulvodynia, and vulvar vestibulitis), dentists for TMD, and so on.

Until recently, these unexplained pain syndromes perplexed researchers, clinicians, and patients. However, it is now clear that:

■ Individuals will sometimes only have one of these "idiopathic" pain syndromes over the course of their lifetime. But more often, individuals with one of these entities, and their family members, are likely to have several of these conditions.[3,4] Many terms have been used to describe these coaggregating syndromes and symptoms, including functional somatic syndromes, somatization disorders, allied spectrum conditions, chronic multisymptom illnesses, medically unexplained symptoms, etc.[3,5–7]

■ Women are more likely to have these disorders than men, but the sex difference is much more apparent in clinical samples (especially tertiary care) than in population-based samples.[8,9]

■ Groups of individuals with these conditions (e.g., FM, IBS, headache, TMD, etc.) display diffuse hyperalgesia (increased pain to normally painful stimuli) and/or allodynia (pain to normally nonpainful stimuli).[10–14] This suggests that these individuals have a fundamental problem with pain or sensory processing rather than an abnormality confined to the region of the body where the person is currently experiencing pain.

■ Similar types of therapies are efficacious for all of these conditions, including both pharmacological (e.g., tricyclic compounds such as amitriptyline) and nonpharmacological treatments (e.g., exercise, cognitive behavioral therapy). Conversely, individuals with these conditions typically do not respond to therapies that are effective when pain is due to damage or inflammation of tissues (e.g., NSAIDs, opioids, injections, surgical procedures).

Until perhaps a decade or ago, these conditions were all on somewhat equal (and tenuous) scientific ground. But, within a relatively short period of time, research methods such as experimental pain testing, functional imaging, and genetics have led to tremendous advances in the understanding of several of these conditions, most notably FM, IBS, and TMD. Many in the pain field now feel that chronic pain itself is a "disease," and that many of the underlying mechanisms operative in these heretofore-considered "idiopathic" or "functional" pain syndromes may be similar whether the pain is present throughout the body (e.g., in FM) or localized to the low back, the bowel, or the bladder. Because of this, the more contemporary terms used to describe conditions such as FM, IBS, TMD, vulvodynia, and many other entities include "central pain," "neuropathic pain" (when this term is used in this setting, it is meant to imply that the pain is coming from the nervous system rather than the periphery, rather than connoting that the pain is due to nerve damage), or "nonnociceptive pain."[15,16]

The review regarding fibromyalgia below focuses on our current understanding of this disorder as one of the prototypical "central pain syndromes."

HISTORICAL PERSPECTIVE

Although the term fibromyalgia is relatively new, this condition has been described in the medical literature for centuries. Sir William Gowers coined the term *fibrositis* in 1904. During the next half century, fibrositis (as it was then called) was considered by some to be a common cause of muscular pain, by others to be a manifestation of tension or psychogenic rheumatism, and by the rheumatology community in general to be a nonentity. The current concept of fibromyalgia was established by

Smythe and Moldofsky in the mid-1970s.[17] The name change reflected the fact that there was increasing evidence that there was no *–itis* (inflammation) in the connective tissues of individuals with this condition, but instead *–algia* (pain). These authors characterized the most common tender points (regions of extreme tenderness in these individuals), and reported that patients with fibromyalgia had disturbances in deep and restorative sleep, and that selective stage 4 interruptions induced the symptoms of fibromyalgia.[18] Yunus and others then reported on the major clinical manifestations of patients with fibromyalgia seen in rheumatology clinics.[19]

The next advance in fibromyalgia was the development of the American College of Rheumatology (ACR) criteria for fibromyalgia, which were published in 1990.[20] These classification criteria require that an individual have both a history of chronic widespread pain (CWP) and 11 or more of a possible 18 tender points on examination. These ACR classification criteria were intended for research use, to standardize definitions of fibromyalgia. In this regard, the criteria have been extremely valuable. Unfortunately, many practitioners use these criteria in routine clinical practice to diagnose individual patients, and this unintended use has led to many of the current misconceptions regarding fibromyalgia, that are discussed later.

The finding of diffusely increased tenderness, as well as a lack of finding "–itis" in the muscles or other tissues of FM patients, caused the name of this entity to be changed from fibrositis to fibromyalgia. The diffuse nature of the pain and tenderness also led many groups of investigators that began to explore neural mechanisms to explain the underlying pathogenesis of these disorders.[21,22] In fact, major advances have only occurred in understanding individual syndromes within this spectrum once investigators concluded that this was not a condition caused by peripheral damage or inflammation and began to explore central, neural mechanisms of these diseases. Thus, the conditions we now understand best within this spectrum include FM, IBS (previously termed "spastic colitis" until the recognition that there was little –itis and that motility changes were not the major pathological feature), and TMD (previously termed temporomandibular joint disorder until it was recognized the problem was not largely within the joint).

EPIDEMIOLOGY

Chronic Widespread Pain

Epidemiological studies of the historical component of the ACR criteria for fibromyalgia, CWP, have been extremely instructive. CWP is typically operationalized as pain above and below the waist, involving the left and right sides of the body, and also involving the axial skeleton. Population-based studies of CWP suggest that 5% to 15% of the population has this symptom at any given point in time.[23–25] Chronic regional pain is found in 20% to 25% of the population. Both CWP and regional pain occur about 1.5 times as commonly in women than men.

Fibromyalgia

The ACR criteria for FM require that an individual has both a history of CWP, and the finding of 11 or more of 18 possible tender points on examination. Tender points represent nine paired predefined regions of the body, often over musculotendinous insertions.[20] If an individual reports pain when a region is palpated with 4 kg of pressure, this is considered a positive tender point. Between 25% and 50% of individuals who have CWP will also have 11 or more tender points, and thus meet criteria for fibromyalgia.[25,26] The prevalence of fibromyalgia is just as high

in rural or nonindustrialized societies as it is in countries such as the U.S.[27–29]

Significance of Tender Points

At the time the ACR criteria were published it was thought that there may be some unique significance to the locations of tender points. In fact, a term *control points* was coined to describe areas of the body that should not be tender in fibromyalgia, and individuals were assumed to have a psychological cause for their pain if they were tender in these regions. Since then, we have learned that the tenderness in fibromyalgia extends throughout the entire body. Thus relative to the pain threshold that a normal nonfibromyalgia patient would experience at the same points, "control" regions of the body such as the thumbnail and forehead are just as tender as in fibromyalgia tender points.[30–32] Thus, to assess tenderness in clinical practice, the practitioner can apply pressure wherever he/she wishes, and as long as they perform this exam with the same pressure in a series of patients, they can get a good sense of the overall pain threshold of any individual patient.

The tender point requirement in the ACR criteria not only misrepresents the nature of the tenderness in this condition (i.e., local rather than widespread), but also strongly influences the demographic and psychological characteristics of FM. Women are only 1.5 times more likely than men to experience CWP, but are 10 times more likely than men to have 11 or more tender points.[23] Because of this, women are approximately 10 times as likely to meet ACR criteria for fibromyalgia as men. Yet, most of the men in the population that have CWP but are not tender enough to meet criteria for FM likely have the same underlying problem as the women who meet the ACR criteria for FM.

Another unintended consequence of requiring both CWP and at least 11 tender points to be diagnosed with FM is that many individuals with fibromyalgia will have high levels of distress. Wolfe has described tender points as a "sedimentation rate for distress" because of population-based studies showing that tender points are more common in distressed individuals.[33] Distress is usually considered as a combination of somatic symptoms and symptoms of anxiety and/or depression.[33] Until recently, many assumed that because *tender points* were associated with distress, that *tenderness* (an individual's sensitivity to mechanical pressure) was associated with distress. However, recent evidence suggests that this latter association is probably due to the standard tender point technique, which consists of applying steadily increasing pressure until reaching 4 kg. In this situation, individuals who are anxious or "expectant" have a tendency to "bail out" and report tenderness. Recently, more sophisticated measures of tenderness have been developed which give stimuli in a random, unpredictable fashion, and the results of these tests are independent of psychological status.[34,35] Since tender points are associated with high levels of distress, requiring 11 or more tender points in order to diagnose someone with CWP with fibromyalgia dramatically increases the likelihood that these individuals will be female and/or and distressed, compared to individuals with CWP and <11 tender points.[25]

In fact, population-based studies suggest that the primary symptom of fibromyalgia, CWP, is only modestly associated with distress, and distress is only weakly associated with the subsequent development of CWP.[36,37] There are far more psychologically "normal" individuals who develop CWP than distressed or depressed people that do, and most individuals with CWP do not have or subsequently develop distress or depression.

In summary, although many clinicians uniquely associate fibromyalgia with women who display high levels of distress, much of this is an artifact of: (1) the ACR criteria that require 11 tender points, and (2) the fact that most studies of FM have originated from clinical samples from tertiary care centers, where healthcare seeking behaviors lead to the fact that psychological and psychiat-

TABLE 36.1

"STRESSORS" CAPABLE OF TRIGGERING FIBROMYALGIA AND RELATED CONDITIONS

- Peripheral pain syndromes
- Infections (e.g., parvovirus, EBV, Lyme disease, Q fever; not common upper respiratory infections)
- Physical trauma (automobile accidents)
- Psychological stress/distress
- Hormonal alterations (e.g., hypothyroidism)
- Drugs
- Vaccines
- Certain catastrophic events (war, but not natural disasters)

ric comorbidities are much higher.[9] When all these biases are eliminated by examining CWP in population-based studies, a clearer picture of fibromyalgia can be gleaned, and CWP becomes much like chronic musculoskeletal pain in any other region of the body.

ETIOLOGY

Genetic Factors

Research has indicated a strong familial component to the development of fibromyalgia. First degree relatives of individuals with fibromyalgia display an eightfold greater risk of developing fibromyalgia than those in the general population.[4] Family members of individuals with fibromyalgia are much more tender than the family members of controls, regardless of whether they have pain or not. Family members of fibromyalgia patients are also much more likely to have IBS, TMD, headaches, and other regional pain syndromes.[3,38,39] This familial and personal coaggregation of conditions which includes fibromyalgia was originally collectively termed *affective spectrum disorder*,[40] and more recently *central sensitivity syndromes* and chronic multisymptom illnesses.[7,41] In population-based studies, the key symptoms that often coaggregate besides pain are fatigue, memory difficulties, and mood disturbances.[7,42] Twin studies suggest that approximately half of the risk of developing CWP is due to genetic factors, and half environmental.[43]

Recent studies have begun to identify specific genetic polymorphisms that are associated with a higher risk of developing fibromyalgia. To date, the serotonin 5-HT2A receptor polymorphism T/T phenotype, serotonin transporter, dopamine 4 receptor, and COMT (catecholamine *o*-methyl transferase) polymorphisms have all been noted to be seen in higher frequency in fibromyalgia.[44–47] All of the polymorphisms identified to date involve the metabolism or transport of monoamines, compounds that play a critical role in activity of the human stress response. It is likely that there are scores of genetic polymorphisms, involving other neuromodulators as well as monoamines, which in part determine an individuals' "set point" for pain and sensory processing.

Environmental Factors

As with most illnesses that may have a genetic underpinning, environmental factors may play a prominent role in triggering the development of fibromyalgia and related conditions. Environmental "stressors" temporally associated with the development of either fibromyalgia or chronic fatigue syndrome include physical trauma (especially involving the trunk), certain infections such as Hepatitis C, Epstein Barr virus, parvovirus, Lyme disease, and emotional stress (Table 36.1). The disorder is also associated with other regional pain conditions or autoimmune disorders[22,48,49] (Figs. 36.1 and 36.2). Each of these stressors only leads to CWP or fibromyalgia in about 5% to 10% of individuals who are exposed; most individuals who experience these same infections or other stressful events regain their baseline state of health.

An example of how illnesses such as FM might be triggered occurred in the setting of the deployment of troops to liberate Kuwait during the Gulf War in 1990 and 1991. The term "Gulf War illnesses" is now commonly used to refer to a constellation of symptoms developed by some 10% to 15% of the 700,000 U.S. troops deployed to the Persian Gulf in the early 1990s. The symptoms, which include headaches, muscle and joint pain, fatigue, memory disorders, and gastrointestinal distress,[7] were seen in troops deployed from the United Kingdom (UK) and other countries as well.[50] The panels of experts who examined potential causes for these symptoms and syndromes found that the sickness could not be traced to any single environmental trigger, and noted the similarities between these individuals, and those diagnosed with fibromyalgia and chronic fatigue. Furthermore, similar syndromes involving multiple somatic symptoms have been noted in veterans of every war the U.S. or UK has been involved in during the past century.[51] This suggests that war may be an environment where individuals are simultaneously exposed to a multitude of "stressors," triggering the development of this type of illness in susceptible individuals.[52]

The previously noted relationship between individuals with other chronic rheumatic or autoimmune disorders deserves special attention, because of the relevance to practicing clinicians. As many as 25% of patients correctly diagnosed with generalized inflammatory disorders such as systemic lupus erythematosus

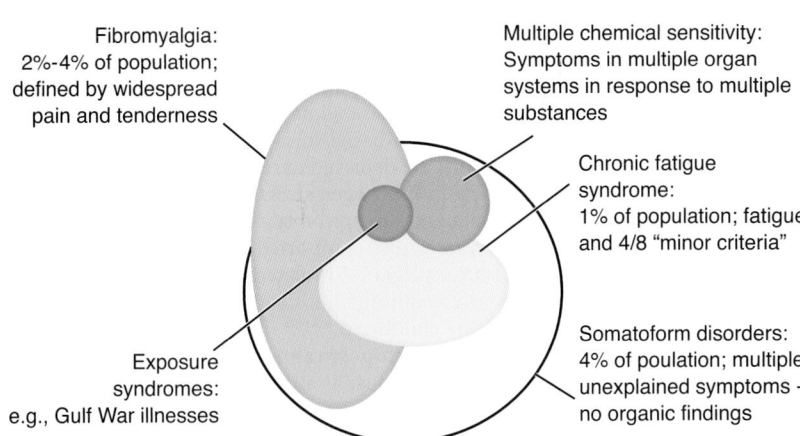

Fibromyalgia: 2%-4% of population; defined by widespread pain and tenderness

Multiple chemical sensitivity: Symptoms in multiple organ systems in response to multiple substances

Chronic fatigue syndrome: 1% of population; fatigue and 4/8 "minor criteria"

Exposure syndromes: e.g., Gulf War illnesses

Somatoform disorders: 4% of poulation; multiple unexplained symptoms - no organic findings

FIGURE 36.1 Regional or localized syndromes that overlap with fibromyalgia in prevalence, mechanisms, and treatment.

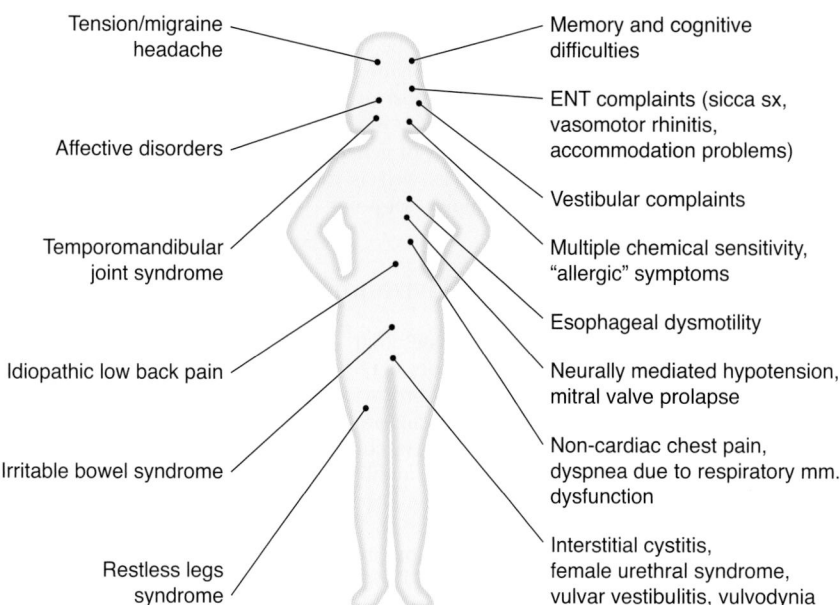

Tension/migraine headache

Affective disorders

Temporomandibular joint syndrome

Idiopathic low back pain

Irritable bowel syndrome

Restless legs syndrome

Memory and cognitive difficulties

ENT complaints (sicca sx, vasomotor rhinitis, accommodation problems)

Vestibular complaints

Multiple chemical sensitivity, "allergic" symptoms

Esophageal dysmotility

Neurally mediated hypotension, mitral valve prolapse

Non-cardiac chest pain, dyspnea due to respiratory mm. dysfunction

Interstitial cystitis, female urethral syndrome, vulvar vestibulitis, vulvodynia

FIGURE 36.2 The "systemic" conditions that overlap with fibromyalgia.

(SLE), rheumatoid arthritis (RA), and ankylosing spondylitis will also fulfill ACR criteria for FM.[53] However, in clinical practice this coexpression may go unrecognized, especially when the FM develops after the autoimmune disorder or regional pain syndrome. In this setting, when comorbid fibromyalgia goes unrecognized, patients are often unnecessarily treated more aggressively with toxic immunosuppressive drugs.

PATHOGENESIS

Role of Stressors

Once FM develops, the mechanisms responsible for ongoing symptom expression are likely complex and multifactorial. Because of the fact that disparate "stressors" can trigger the development of these conditions, the human stress response has been closely examined for a causative role. These systems are mediated primarily by the activity of the corticotropin-releasing hormone (CRH) nervous system located in the hypothalamus and locus-ceruleus-norepinephrine/autonomic (sympathetic/LC-NE) nervous system in the brainstem. Recent research suggests that although this system in humans has been highly adaptive throughout history, the stress response may be inappropriately triggered by a wide assortment of everyday occurrences that do not pose a real threat to survival, thus initiating the cascade of physiological responses more frequently than can be tolerated.[54]

The type of stress and the environment in which it occurs also have an impact on how the stress response is expressed. Victims of accidents experience a higher frequency of fibromyalgia and myofascial pain than those who cause them, which is congruent with animal studies showing that that the strongest physiological responses are triggered by events that are accompanied by a lack of control or support, and thus viewed as perceived as inescapable or unavoidable.[55] In humans, daily "hassles" and personally relevant stressors seem to be more capable of causing symptoms than major catastrophic events that do not personally impact on the individual.[56]

Two studies performed in the U.S. just before and after the terrorist attacks of September 11th point out that not all psychological stress is capable of triggering or exacerbating fibromyalgia or somatic symptoms. In one study performed by Raphael and colleagues, no difference in pain complaints or other somatic symptoms was seen in residents of New York and New Jersey who had been surveyed prior to September 11th, and then just following the terrorist attacks on the World Trade Center.[57] In another study performed in the Washington, DC, region (near the Pentagon—the other site of attack) during the same time period, patients with fibromyalgia had no worsening of pain or other somatic symptoms following the attacks, compared to just before the attack.[58]

Recent reviews regarding the role that "stressors" (e.g., infections, physical trauma, and emotional stress) or catastrophic events may have in triggering the development of fibromyalgia or related conditions have identified a number of factors that may be much more important than the intensity of the "stressor" in predicting adverse health outcomes. Female gender, worry or expectation of chronicity, and inactivity or time off work following the stressor make it more likely to trigger the development of pain or other somatic symptoms.[49] Naturally occurring catastrophic events such as earthquakes, floods, or fires are much less likely to lead to chronic somatic symptoms than similarly stressful events that are "man-made" such as chemical spills or war.[59] Being exposed to a multitude of stressors simultaneously, or over a period of time, may also be a significant risk for later somatic symptoms and or psychological sequelae. Intensely stressful events can lead to permanent changes in the activity of both mouse and human stress response systems.[54,60]

To complete this vicious circle, these changes in baseline function of the stress response (i.e., of the autonomic and neuroendocrine systems—see later) that may occur following a stressor earlier in life have been shown to predict which symptom-free individuals without chronic pain or other somatic symptoms are more likely to develop these somatic symptoms. This has been noted both in population-based studies and in experiments where healthy young adults are deprived of regular sleep or exercise.[61,62]

This theoretical link between stress, changes in stress axis activity, and subsequent susceptibility to develop somatic symptoms or syndromes is also supported by studies showing that patients with fibromyalgia and related conditions may be more likely than nonaffected individuals to have experienced physical or sexual abuse in childhood.[63–66] Twin studies have recently supported a link between posttraumatic stress disorder (PTSD) and trauma, and CWP.[67] Just as a lack of or cessation of exercise following trauma seems to be associated with a higher likelihood of developing pain or other somatic symptoms, a recent study of

Israeli war veterans with PTSD showed that those who exercised regularly were much less likely to develop CWP or fibromyalgia.[68]

Role of Neuroendocrine Abnormalities

Because of this link between exposure to "stressors" and the subsequent development of fibromyalgia, the human stress systems have been extensively studied in this condition. These studies have generally shown alterations of the hypothalamic-pituitary-adrenal (HPA) axis and the sympathetic nervous system in fibromyalgia and related conditions.[69–74] Although these studies often note either hypo- or hyperactivity of both the HPAl axis and sympathetic nervous system in individuals with fibromyalgia and related conditions, the precise abnormality varies from study to study. Moreover, these studies only find "abnormal" HPA or autonomic function in a very small percentage of patients, and there is tremendous overlap between patients and controls in many of these studies.

The inconsistency of these findings should not be surprising, since nearly all of these studies were cross-sectional studies that assumed that if HPA and/or autonomic dysfunction was found in fibromyalgia, it must have *caused* the pain and other symptoms. Data now suggest the opposite. As noted previously, there are better data suggesting that (especially HPA abnormalities) might represent a diathesis or be *due to* the pain or early life stress, rather than causing it. In fact in two recent studies examining HPA function in fibromyalgia, McLean showed that salivary cortisol levels covaried with pain levels, and that CSF levels of CRH were more closely related to an individual's pain level or a history of early life trauma than whether they were a fibromyalgia patient or control.[75,76] Since most previous studies of HPA and autonomic function in fibromyalgia failed to control for pain levels, a previous history of trauma, and PTSD or other comorbid disorders that could affect HPA or autonomic dysfunction, it is not surprising for these inconsistencies to exist.

Heart rate variability at baseline and in response to tilt table testing has been evaluated in patients with fibromyalgia as a surrogate measure of autonomic function. The consistent and reproducible finding of lower baseline heart rate variability in FM compared to controls makes it a more useful measure than tilt table testing.[73,74,77] An abnormal drop in blood pressure or excessive rate of syncope during tilt table testing has also been noted in most studies.[78–80] Moreover, recent findings also suggest that aberrations in heart rate variability may predispose to fibromyalgia symptoms,[61,62,81] possibly identifying patients at risk. Also, a recent study showed that heart rate variability was normalized following exercise therapy, suggesting that this finding might also be an epiphenomenon due in part to deconditioning.[82]

It is likely that these neurobiological alterations are shared with other syndromes that are known to be associated with HPA and/or autonomic function such as depression or PTSD. A model of susceptibility and development of these disorders, that takes into account both genetics and personality as risk factors, is illustrated in Figure 36.3. This recognizes the critical importance of stressors in "resetting stress response systems," as well as other factors including (1) the role of behavioral adaptations to these stressors such as cessation of routine exercise and (2) whether an individual is in an environment characterized by control or support.

Augmented Pain and Sensory Processing as a Hallmark of Fibromyalgia and Related Syndromes

Once fibromyalgia is established, by far the most consistently detected objective abnormalities involve pain and sensory

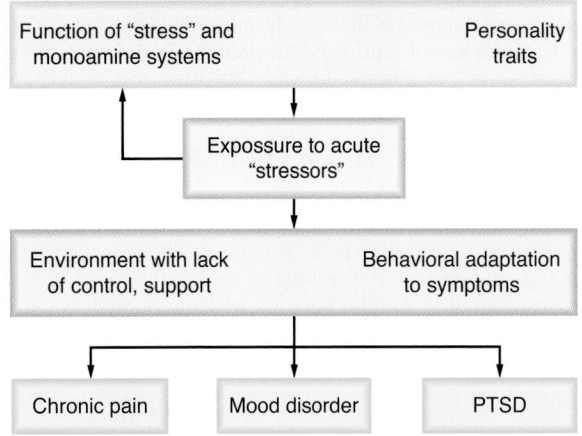

FIGURE 36.3 The hypothesized relationship between "stressors" and the development of syndromes such as fibromyalgia, PTSD, and depression.

processing systems. Since FM is defined in part by tenderness, considerable work has been performed exploring the potential reason for this phenomenon. The results of two decades of psychophysical pressure pain testing in fibromyalgia have been very instructive.

One of the earliest findings in this regard was that the tenderness in fibromyalgia is not confined to tender points, but instead extends throughout the entire body.[23,31] Theoretically, such diffuse tenderness could be either primarily due to psychological (e.g., hypervigilance, where individuals are too attentive to their surroundings), or neurobiological (e.g., the plethora of factors that can lead to temporary or permanent amplification of sensory input) factors.

Early studies typically used dolorimetry to assess pressure pain threshold, and concluded that tenderness was in large part related to psychological factors, because these measures of pain threshold were correlated with levels of distress.[23,33,83] Also, nuances such as the rate of increase of stimulus pressure, control by the operator versus by the patient, and patient distress have been shown to influence pain threshold when it is measured in this manner.[84,85]

To minimize the biases associated with "ascending" (i.e., the individual knows that the pressure will be predictably increased) measures of pressure pain threshold, Petzke and colleagues performed a series of studies using more sophisticated paradigms using random delivery of pressures.[30,35,86,87] These studies showed that: (1) the random measures of pressure pain threshold were not influenced by levels of distress of the individual, whereas tender point count and dolorimetry exams were; (2) fibromyalgia patients were much more sensitive to pressure even when these more sophisticated paradigms were used; (3) fibromyalgia patients were not any more "expectant" or "hypervigilant" than controls; and (4) pressure pain thresholds at any 4 points in the body are highly correlated with the average tenderness at all 18 tender points and 4 "control points" (the thumbnail and forehead).

Because of this close link between tenderness and fibromyalgia, this phenomenon has also been well studied as a potential relevant outcome in clinical trials of new fibromyalgia therapies. In a number of longitudinal randomized placebo-controlled trials of fibromyalgia, improvements in clinical pain have corresponded with a significant change in tender point counts or tender point index.[88] In contrast, other studies did not show a correspondence between improvements in clinical pain and tender point counts.[89–94] These discrepancies between previous studies could either be because these therapies did not improve tenderness, or because tender points are not a good measure of tenderness. Two recent studies suggest the latter because, when individuals with fibromyalgia were simultaneously assessed using tender point counts, dolorimetry, and random pressure paradigms, the random pressure paradigms showed the most responsiveness to change.[95,96]

Heat, Cold, and Electrical Stimuli

In addition to the heightened sensitivity to pressure noted in fibromyalgia, other types of stimuli applied to the skin are also judged as more painful or noxious by these patients. Fibromyalgia patients also display a decreased threshold to heat,[86,97–99] cold,[98,100] and electrical stimuli.[101] Similar but somewhat attenuated decreases in pain threshold have also been noted in individuals with CWP without 11 or more tender points.[102]

Responses to Other Sensory Stimuli

Gerster and colleagues were the first to demonstrate that fibromyalgia patients also display a low noxious threshold to auditory tones, and this finding was subsequently replicated.[103,104] However, both of these studies used ascending measures of auditory threshold, so these findings could theoretically be due to expectancy or hypervigilance. A recent study by Geisser and colleagues used an identical random staircase paradigm to test fibromyalgia patients' threshold to the loudness of auditory tones and to pressure.[96] This study found that fibromyalgia patients displayed low thresholds to both types of stimuli and the correlation between the results of auditory and pressure pain threshold testing suggested that some of this was due to shared variance, and some were unique to one stimulus or the other. The notion that fibromyalgia and related syndromes might represent biological amplification of all sensory stimuli has significant support from functional imaging studies that suggest that the insula is the most consistently hyperactive region (see later text). This region has been noted to play a critical role in sensory integration, with the posterior insula serving a purer sensory role, and the anterior insula being associated with the emotional processing of sensations.[105–107]

Specific Mechanisms That May Lead to a Low Pain Threshold in Fibromyalgia

There are two different specific pathogenic mechanisms in fibromyalgia that have been identified using experimental pain testing: (1) an absence of descending analgesic activity, and (2) increased wind-up or temporal summation.

Attenuated Diffuse Noxious Inhibitory Controls in Fibromyalgia. In healthy humans and laboratory animals, application of an intense painful stimulus for 2 to 5 minutes produces generalized whole-body analgesia. This analgesic effect, termed diffuse noxious inhibitory controls (DNIC), has been consistently observed to be attenuated or absent in groups of FM patients, compared to healthy controls.[98,108–110] Wilder-Smith and colleagues have performed studies suggesting that in IBS there is a similar decrease in descending analgesic activity.[111] A point of emphasis is that this finding of attenuated DNIC is not found in all fibromyalgia or IBS patients, but is considerably more common in patients than controls.

The DNIC response in humans is believed to be partly mediated by descending opioidergic pathways and in part by descending serotonergic-noradrenergic pathways. In fibromyalgia, the accumulating data suggests that opioidergic activity is normal or even increased, in that levels of cerebrospinal fluid (CSF) enkephalins are roughly twice as high in FM and idiopathic low back pain patients as in healthy controls.[112] Moreover, positron emission tomography (PET) data show that baseline mu-opioid receptor binding is decreased in multiple pain processing regions in

the brains of FM patients, consistent (but not pathognomonic) with the hypothesis that there is increased release of endogenous mu-opioid ligands in FM leading to high baseline occupancy of the receptors.[113]

The biochemical and imaging findings suggesting increased activity of endogenous opioidergic systems in FM are consistent with the anecdotal experience that opioids are generally ineffective analgesics in patients with FM and related conditions. In contrast, studies have shown the opposite for serotonergic and noradrenergic activity in FM. Studies have shown that the principal metabolite of norepinephrine, 3-methoxy-4-hydroxyphenethylene (MPHG), is lower in the CSF of FM patients.[114] Similarly, there are data suggesting low serotonin in this syndrome. Patients with FM were shown to have reduced serum levels of serotonin and its precursor, L-tryptophan, as well as reduced levels of the principal serotonin metabolite, 5-HIAA, in their CSF.[114,115] Further evidence for this mechanism comes from treatment studies, where nearly any type of compound that simultaneously raises both serotonin and norepinephrine (tricyclics, duloxetine, milnacipran, tramadol) has been shown to be efficacious in treating FM and related conditions.[94,116–118]

Increased Wind-up in Fibromyalgia. Experimental pain testing studies have also suggested that some individuals with fibromyalgia may have evidence of wind-up, indicative of evidence of central sensitization.[119,120] In animal models, this finding is associated with excitatory amino acid and substance P hyperactivity.[121–123] Just as with the findings regarding DNIC, these results of psychophysical pain testing are congruent with both levels of neurotransmitters in the CSF, as well as clinical trials of drugs. Four independent studies have shown that patients with FM have approximately threefold higher concentrations of substance P in CSF, when compared with normal controls[124–127] (Fig. 36.4). Other chronic pain syndromes, such as osteoarthritis of the hip and chronic low back pain, are also associated with elevated substance P levels, although chronic fatigue syndrome (which is not defined on the basis of pain) is not. Interestingly, once elevated, substance P levels do not appear to change dramatically, and do not rise in response to acute painful stimuli. Thus, high substance P appears to be a biological marker for the presence of chronic pain.

Another important neurotransmitter in pain processing, and one that likely is playing some role in FM, is glutamate. Glutamate (Glu) is a major excitatory neurotransmitter within the central nervous system, and CSF levels of glutamate are twice as high in FM patients than controls.[128] Not only are these levels elevated, but a recent study using proton spectroscopy demonstrated that the glutamate levels in the insula in fibromyalgia change in response to changes in both clinical and experimental pain when patients are treated with acupuncture.[129]

Nerve growth factor (NGF) and calcitonin gene-related peptide are additional neuropeptides that have been evaluated in FM. NGF was shown in one study to have increased levels in FM and not in FM/RA and therefore with inconclusive results.[130] CSF and serum CGRP have been studied and not found to be different in fibromyalgia patients and controls.[131,132]

Thus, a number of lines of evidence point to the fact that fibromyalgia is a state of heightened pain or sensory processing, and that this might occur because of high levels of neurotransmitters that increase pain transmission, and/or low levels of neurotransmitters that decrease pain transmission (Fig. 36.5).

Abnormalities on Functional Neuroimaging

Functional neural imaging enables investigators to visualize how the brain processes the sensory experience of pain. The primary modes of functional imaging that have been used in FM include functional magnetic resonance imaging (fMRI), single photon

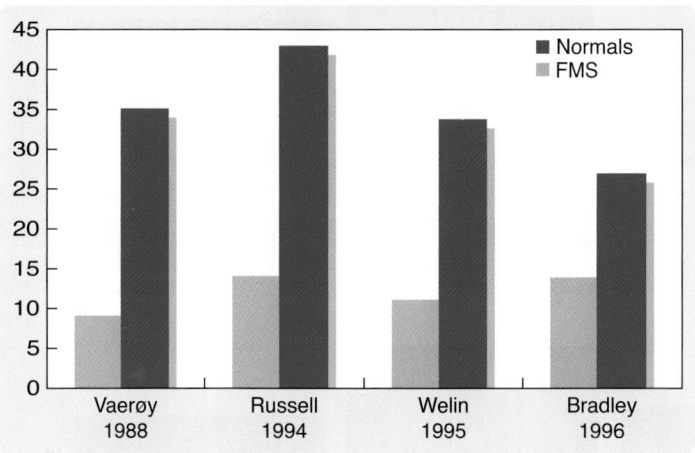

Fibromyalgia CSF Substance P

FIGURE 36.4 Levels of cerebrospinal fluid of substance P in four different studies of FM

emission computed tomography (SPECT), PET, and proton spectroscopy (H-MRS).

SPECT was the first functional neuroimaging technique to be used in fibromyalgia. SPECT imaging involves the introduction of radioactive compounds into the participant's bloodstream, which then decay over time giving a window for neural activity assessment. The first trial using SPECT imaging in FM patients was conducted by Mountz et al.[133] Their data from 10 FM patients and 7 age- and education-matched healthy controls indicated that both the caudate and the thalamus of FM patients had decreased blood flow. The findings by Mountz et al. were largely replicated in a second SPECT study by Kwiatek et al.[134] In a third SPECT trial, Guedj et al. reported a study using a more sensitive radioligand (99mTc-ECD) in FM patients and pain free controls.[135,136] Guedj et al. found hyperperfusion in FM patients within the somatosensory cortex and hypoperfusion in the anterior and posterior cingulate, the amygdala, medial frontal and parahippocampal gyrus, and the cerebellum. Finally, if these regional cerebral blood flow (rCBF) differences are relevant for fibromyalgia pathology, one could hypothesize that changes in rCBF should track with changes in pain symptoms over time. One longitudinal treatment trial used SPECT imaging to assess changes in rCBF following administration of amitriptyline within 14 FM patients.[137] After 3 months of treatment with amitriptyline, increases in rCBF in the bilateral thalamus and the basal ganglia were observed.

Since the same two regions had been implicated previously, these data suggest that amitriptyline may normalize the altered blood flow thereby reducing pain symptoms.

fMRI is a noninvasive brain imaging technique that relies on changes in the relative concentration of oxygenated to deoxygenated hemoglobin within the brain. In response to neural activity, oxygenated blood flow is increased within the local brain area. This causes a decrease in the concentration of deoxygenated hemoglobin. Since deoxygenated hemoglobin is paramagnetic, this in turn causes a change in the magnetic property of the tissue. Unlike SPECT and PET which can measure baseline levels of blood flow, the fMRI BOLD signal originates from a difference between experimental conditions and does not assess baseline blood flow. Typically in fibromyalgia trials involving fMRI, evoked pain sensations are compared to "off" conditions that have either no pain or involve an innocuous sensation.

The first study to use fMRI in fibromyalgia patients was performed by Gracely et al. In this study 16 fibromyalgia patients and 16 matched controls were exposed to painful pressures during the fMRI experiment.[138] The authors found increased neural activations (i.e., increases in the BOLD signal) in patients compared to pain free controls, when stimuli of equal pressure magnitude were administered. Regions of increased activity included the primary and secondary somatosensory cortex, the insula, and the anterior cingulate—all regions commonly observed in fMRI

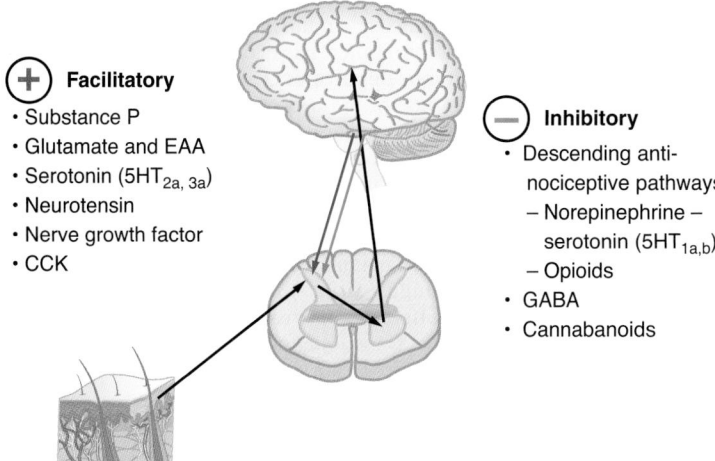

Descending Influences on Nociceptive Processing

⊕ **Facilitatory**
· Substance P
· Glutamate and EAA
· Serotonin ($5HT_{2a, 3a}$)
· Neurotensin
· Nerve growth factor
· CCK

⊖ **Inhibitory**
· Descending anti-
  nociceptive pathways
  – Norepinephrine –
    serotonin ($5HT_{1a,b}$)
  – Opioids
· GABA
· Cannabanoids

FIGURE 36.5 Neurotransmitters that are known to play either facilitatory (increase pain transmission) or inhibitory (decrease pain transmission) roles in the central nervous system.

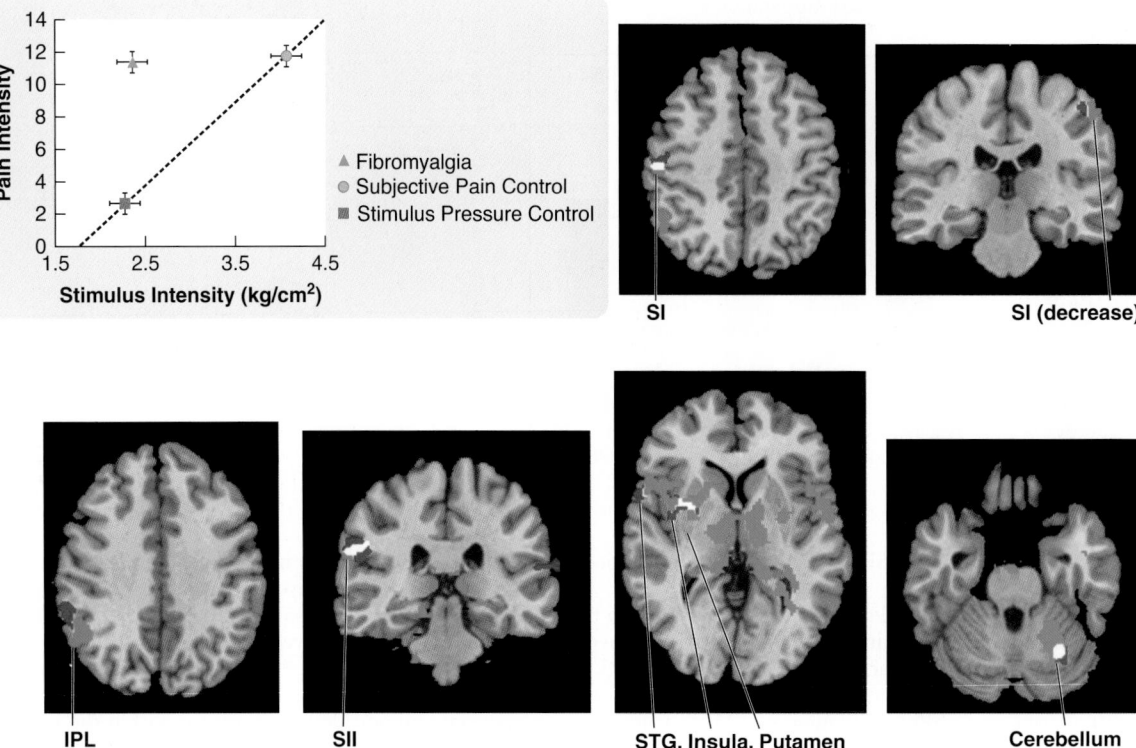

FIGURE 36.6 In *top left* panel, individuals with fibromyalgia (*red*) given a low pressure stimulus have similar levels of pain, and of neuronal activation in areas of the brain known to be involved in pain processing (*ends of arrows*) as controls given nearly twice as much pressure. Controls given the same low pressure that causes pain in fibromyalgia rate their pain as 2/20 instead of 12/20, and have no neuronal activation with this amount of pressure.

studies of healthy normal subjects during painful stimuli. Interestingly, when the pain free controls were subjected to pressures that evoked equivalent pain ratings in the FM patients, similar activation patterns were observed. These findings were entirely consistent with the "left-shift" in stimulus-response function noted with experimental pain testing, and suggest that fibromyalgia patients experience an increased gain or "volume setting" in brain sensory processing systems (Fig. 36.6). In a similar experiment, Cook et al. used painful heat stimuli during fMRI.[139] Similar to the Gracely et al. findings, the authors observed significant increases in the pain ratings of patients and augmented pain processing within the contralateral insula. fMRI has also proved useful in determining how comorbid psychological factors influence pain processing in fibromyalgia. For example, a recent study by Giesecke et al. explored the relationship between depression and enhanced evoked pain sensations in 30 patients with fibromyalgia.[140] The authors found that the anterior insula and amygdala activations were correlated with depressive symptoms, consistent with these regions being involved with affective or motivational aspects of pain processing. However, the degree of neuronal activation in areas of the brain thought to be associated with the "sensory" processing of pain (i.e., where the pain is localized and how intense it is) were not associated with levels of depressive symptoms, or the presence or absence of major depression. These data are consistent with a plethora of evidence in the pain field that there are different regions of the brain responsible for pain processing devoted to sensory intensity versus affective aspects of pain sensation, and suggest that the former and latter are largely independent of each other. In contrast, this same group showed that the presence of catastrophizing, a patient's negative or pessimistic appraisal of their pain, influences both the sensory and affective dimensions of pain on fMRI in fibromyalgia.[141]

PET has been used in several studies in fibromyalgia. In the first such study, Yunus and colleagues did not identify any differences in regional cerebral blood flow between fibromyalgia patients and controls.[142] However, Wood and colleagues used PET to show that attenuated dopaminergic activity may be playing a role in pain transmission in fibromyalgia, and Harris and colleagues showed evidence of decreased mu-opioid receptor availability (possibly due to increased release of endogenous mu-opioids) in fibromyalgia.

Event Related Potentials

Another technique that has been used to demonstrate abnormal neural responses to sensory stimuli in fibromyalgia is event related potentials. Cerebral potentials evoked by noninvasive stimulation provide a unique opportunity to investigate the functional integrity and magnitude of brain processing pathways. Expressing the ability of the human brain to discriminate, classify, and memorize the significance of exogenous stimuli, event related potentials (ERPs) have been used as a marker of cognitive function in patients with psychiatric and neurological disorders. The electrical waveforms generated can be divided into late and early components and are designated by their polarity and latency (timing of peak) after stimulus onset. Additionally, the amplitude, or the size of voltage difference between the component peak and a prestimulus baseline, is also quantified. In patients with fibromyalgia, auditory, somatosensory, and visual evoked potentials have been evaluated in a handful of studies.

Among the ERPs evaluated to date, the P300 potential (most commonly generated by an auditory consciously attended stimuli) appears to be the most promising to differentiate FM patients from controls. The P300 wave is a late cortical neuropsychological event, the latency of which reflects information processing speed while its amplitude expresses memory functions. A reduced P300 amplitude during auditory discriminated task paradigm has been significantly noted in FM patients as compared to controls in three cross-sectional studies by two different groups.[143–145] All three studies also evaluated the P300 latency, but only the largest by Alanoglu et al. noted an increase in P300 latency, a finding that may have not been found in the prior studies due to lack of power. In one study by Ozgocmen et al., ERP was performed before after-treatment, and 8 weeks of sertraline treatment led to an increase in P300 magnitude. These studies generally failed to show an association between the ERP findings and symptom severity, although there was an association noted with the total myalgic score. Although the change in the P300 potential after sertraline treatment was attractive, the authors agreed that given the corresponding significant clinical improvement in pain, fatigue, or depression, the mechanism for the change remained unclear and acknowledged it may represent regression to the mean. Larger studies by different groups with an attention to standardizing methods are essential prior to mainstream use of this marker.

Other Serological and Biochemical Abnormalities

The search for representative autoantibodies is a predictable step for a disease like fibromyalgia, often evaluated by rheumatologists and coexisting with autoimmune diseases. Antiserotonin antibody, antiganglioside antibody, and antiphospholipid antibody have been shown to be different in patients and controls, but the applicability of these findings is not yet clear.[146] Antiserotonin antibody has been shown to be increased in FM in three cross-sectional studies by two different groups. Antiganglioside antibody and antiphospholipid antibody have each been shown to be increased in FM in two cross-sectional studies by the same group. A different group evaluating antiganglioside antibody in a third cross-sectional study was unable to reproduce the results. Antithromboplastin antibody, antipolymer antibody, anti-68/84, and anti-45kDa have each been evaluated in one cross-sectional study and have shown increased levels in FM. Review of the literature suggests that ANA, antithyroid antibodies, antisilicone antibodies, and antiglutamic acid decarboxylase are not informative in FM.

This inconsistent increase in antibodies to a number of antigens may be a nonspecific finding that arises from a subtle shift in immune function in this spectrum of illness. In the closely related chronic fatigue syndrome and Gulf War illnesses, investigators have noted a shift from a TH1 to TH2 immune response, which would be expected to lead to increased production of nonspecific antibodies. Thus, any antibody or autoantibody proposed as either a diagnostic test or biomarker of FM must be carefully tested using stringent controls to ensure its authenticity.

The amino acid tryptophan and the cytokine IL-8 have both been shown to be different in patients compared to controls in a couple of studies, but none have been evaluated in longitudinal studies.[147–150] Low tryptophan, a precursor for serotonin, has been found in two of three studies by three different groups.[115,147,151] IL-8 has been consistently demonstrated in three studies by two different groups.[148–150] Moreover, IL-8 has been shown to correlate with symptoms and not to be associated with depressed FM. IL-8 levels are closely tied to autonomic function and the findings of these increased levels could be due to the dysautonomia seen in fibromyalgia and related conditions.[152] Serum IL-6 was evaluated and found to be normal in FM.[150,153]

Structural Abnormalities in Fibromyalgia

Although a few studies have found mild abnormalities in the *skeletal muscles* of fibromyalgia patients (these findings have been inconsistent and may be due to de-conditioning rather than the illness itself[154–156]), there are a few studies that suggest there may be subsets of FM patients with damage to *neural* structures. P31-spectroscopy has been used to examine muscle metabolism in FM and the results are conflicting, with one study comparing sedentary controls to FM finding no differences, and the other finding lower ATP levels among FM patients.[157,158] Studies suggest that the tenderness in fibromyalgia is not at all confined to just the muscle, so in aggregate most investigators have concluded that primary muscle disease is not a likely cause of the pain associated with fibromyalgia.

There are recent data, however, suggesting that a subset of fibromyalgia patients may have abnormalities involving small sensory nerves in the skin, indicative of a small fiber neuropathy.[159,160] There are also emerging data suggesting that there may be subtle abnormalities in brain structure seen in fibromyalgia.[161,162] Thus, if there are structural abnormalities or damage to tissues in fibromyalgia the most evidence for this is involving neural tissues.

Sleep and Activity in Fibromyalgia

In addition to pain, other symptoms very commonly seen in fibromyalgia include disturbed sleep and poor physical function. One of the first biological findings in fibromyalgia was that selective sleep deprivation led to symptoms of fibromyalgia in healthy individuals, and these findings have subsequently been replicated by several groups.[18,163] However, the electroencephalography (EEG) abnormalities that were noted in this first study and initially thought to be a marker for fibromyalgia, so-called alpha intrusions, have subsequently been found to be present in normals and in individuals with other conditions.[164,165] More recent findings on polysomnography that occur more commonly in fibromyalgia include demonstration of fewer sleep spindles, an increase in cyclic alternating pattern rate, upper airway resistance syndrome, and/or poor sleep efficiency.[166–169] However, sleep abnormalities rarely are shown to correlate with symptoms in FM, and many investigators anecdotally feel as though even identifying and treating specific sleep disorders often seen in FM patients (e.g., obstructive sleep apnea, upper airway resistance, restless leg or periodic limb movement syndromes) does not necessarily lead to improvements in the core symptoms of FM.

Actigraphy

Actigraphy, a method of motion assessment that infers sleep and wakefulness from presence of limb movements, is increasingly being used as a surrogate marker for both sleep and activity. The actigraph typically combines a movement detector and memory storage on a watch-like device. The device can be worn on wrist or ankle continuously for long periods of time. Sleep-pattern measures available via actigraphy analyses include sleep latency, wake time after sleep onset, and total sleep time; sleep architecture cannot be measured as with polysomnography. However, compared to the polysomnography, actigraphy is less expensive, invasive, and more conducive to repeated measures, resulting in extensive use in intervention studies.[170]

Actigraphy is being increasingly used in FM and is increasing and appears promising, but has not yet proven to be adequately sensitive to stand alone in clinical evaluation or treatment trials.[171–173] As a measure of sleep quality, there have been inconsistent results, with one group noting increased levels of activity at night in FM (also noted in patients with major depression) and another noting no difference. Edinger et al. used actigraphy as an outcome measure in an intervention trial comparing cognitive

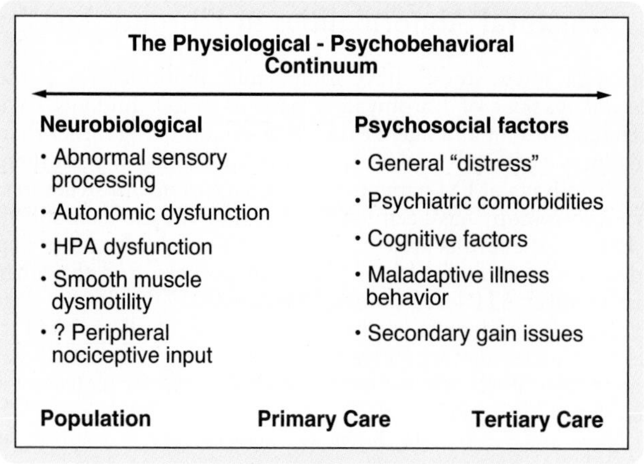

The Physiological - Psychobehavioral Continuum

Neurobiological	Psychosocial factors
• Abnormal sensory processing	• General "distress"
• Autonomic dysfunction	• Psychiatric comorbidities
• HPA dysfunction	• Cognitive factors
• Smooth muscle dysmotility	• Maladaptive illness behavior
• ? Peripheral nociceptive input	• Secondary gain issues

Population	Primary Care	Tertiary Care

FIGURE 36.7 The relationship between neurobiological factors that initiate pain and other symptoms, and psychological and behavioral factors that either preexist or develop as a result of pain, and can perpetuate or worsen symptoms. These latter factors increase in frequency as one moves from examining pain patients in the population to those seen in tertiary care centers.

behavior therapy (CBT) intervention to sleep hygiene and usual care in the treatment of insomnia.[174] Deriving an actigraphic improvement criterion, the investigators showed a greater number of patients receiving CBT had clinically significant improvement in total wake time compared to sleep hygiene therapy. No statistical difference between CBT and usual care was able to be demonstrated, even though a statistical difference between the groups was shown using sleep log data in the same study.

As an objective measure of functional status, actigraphy might hold more promise as a surrogate outcome measure, because it allows the direct recording of activity levels, rather than counting on patient self-report.[175] Kop and colleagues demonstrated that although patients with FM have SF-36 score nearly two standard deviations below the population average, they have the same average activity level as a group of sedentary controls. However, the fibromyalgia patients had much lower peak activity levels, suggesting that the problems in function that fibromyalgia report might be more due to an inability to rise to the intermittent demands of day-to-day life than overall reduced function.

Behavioral and Psychological Factors

In addition to neurobiological mechanisms, behavioral and psychological factors also play a role in symptom expression in many FM patients. The rate of current psychiatric comorbidity in patients with FM may be as high as 30% to 60% in tertiary care settings, and the rate of lifetime psychiatric disorders even higher.[3,176,177] Depression and anxiety disorders are the most commonly seen. However, these rates may be artifactually elevated by virtue of the fact that most of these studies have been performed in tertiary care centers. Individuals who meet ACR criteria for FM who are identified in the general population do not have nearly this high a rate of identifiable psychiatric conditions[9,178] (Fig. 36.7).

As already noted, population-based studies have demonstrated that the relationship between pain and distress is complex and that distress is both a cause and consequence of pain. In this latter instance, a typical pattern is that as a result of pain and other symptoms of FM, individuals begin to function less well in their various roles. They may have difficulties with spouses, children, and work inside or outside the home, which exacerbate symptoms and lead to maladaptive illness behaviors. These include isolation, cessation of pleasurable activities, reductions in activity and exercise, etc. In the worst cases, patients become involved with disability and compensation systems that almost ensure that they will not improve.[179]

The complex interaction of biological, behavioral, and psychological mechanisms is not, however, unique to FM. Nonbiological factors play a prominent role in symptom expression in all rheumatic diseases. In fact, in conditions such as RA and OA, nonbiological factors such as level of formal education, coping strategies, and socioeconomic variables account for more of the variance in pain report and disability than biological factors, such as the joint space width or sedimentation rate.[180,181]

Because of the biopsychosocial nature of fibromyalgia, several groups have attempted to identify subgroups of individuals with this condition that may present differently or respond differentially to treatment.[182,183] One of these studies examined how differential degrees of depression, maladaptive cognitions, and hyperalgesia might interact to lead to different subgroups of patients. Three identified subgroups can be usefully identified (Fig. 36.8). The first comprises approximately half of the patients who have low levels of depression and anxiety, normal cognition re-

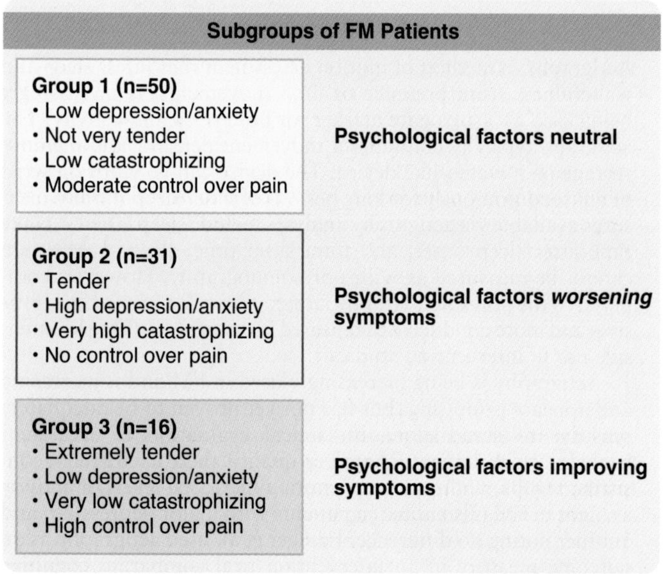

Subgroups of FM Patients

Group 1 (n=50)
• Low depression/anxiety
• Not very tender
• Low catastrophizing
• Moderate control over pain

Psychological factors neutral

Group 2 (n=31)
• Tender
• High depression/anxiety
• Very high catastrophizing
• No control over pain

Psychological factors *worsening* symptoms

Group 3 (n=16)
• Extremely tender
• Low depression/anxiety
• Very low catastrophizing
• High control over pain

Psychological factors *improving* symptoms

FIGURE 36.8 Subgroups of fibromyalgia patients based on grouping by psychological, cognitive, and neurobiological (degree of hyperalgesia) factors.

garding pain, and are mildly tender (although tender enough to meet the ACR criteria). The second subgroup, representative of a "tertiary care" fibromyalgia patient, is slightly more tender and also displayed high levels of depression. These patients also have cognitions associated with a poor prognosis in many pain conditions. These include an external locus of pain control, defined as feeling that they can do nothing about their pain, and catastrophizing, defined as having a very negative and pessimistic view of their pain. The third subgroup are the most tender, but with no negative psychological or cognitive factors. This suggests that in some "resilient" individuals, positive psychological and cognitive factor issues may actually "buffer" neurobiological factors leading to pain and other symptoms in FM.

Functional imaging studies have been instructive with regard to how these comorbid mood disorders or cognitions may be influencing pain processing in FM. Functional MRI undertaken on 30 fibromyalgia patients with variable levels of depression, with additional experimental pain testing, investigated how the presence or absence of depression influenced pain report.[140] This study found that the level of depressive symptomatology did not influence the degree of neuronal activation in brain regions responsible for coding for the sensory intensity of pain, the primary and secondary somatosensory cortices. As expected, the depressed individuals did display greater activations in brain regions known to be responsible for the affective or cognitive processing of pain, such as the amygdala and insula. Another study with similar methodology examined how the presence or absence of catastrophizing might influence pain report in FM.[141] In contrast to the results noted previously, the presence of catastrophizing was associated with increased neuronal activations in the sensory coding regions. These studies thus provide empirical evidence for the value of treatments such as cognitive behavioral therapy. This is especially the case if individuals exhibit cognitions such as catastrophizing which, independent of other factors, may be capable of increasing pain intensity.

THE EVALUATION OF INDIVIDUALS WITH CHRONIC WIDESPREAD PAIN

The evaluation of an individual with chronic pain is a complex process. In contrast to most other medical problems, simply arriving at a "diagnosis" is typically insufficient to guide treatment. This is because within any given pain diagnosis, there is tremendous heterogeneity with respect to the underlying causes and contributors to symptoms, and the most effective treatments. In particular, individuals with chronic pain can have greater or lesser peripheral nociceptive (i.e., tissue damage, inflammation) and central nonnociceptive (i.e., pain amplification, psychological factors) contributions to their pain. Therefore, the differential diagnosis of chronic pain involves identifying which of these factors are present in which individuals, so that the appropriate pharmacologic, procedural, and psychological therapies can be administered.

A careful musculoskeletal history and examination remains the most important diagnostic test for musculoskeletal pain. In other fields of medicine, advances in diagnostic testing have largely rendered a physical examination obsolete. However, in musculoskeletal medicine, technology confuses as much as it helps. For example, a high proportion of the healthy, asymptomatic population has a positive antinuclear antibody, positive rheumatoid factor, or abnormal results of imaging studies.[184–186] Worse yet, these diagnostic tests rarely tell us how "severe" the pain is, because there is typically a significant discordance between the results of laboratory or imaging studies, and the severity of pain and other symptoms that the individual is experiencing. Therefore, the musculoskeletal history and examination must

allow the clinician to arrive at the diagnosis (or at worst a very narrow differential diagnosis) and then, if necessary, further diagnostic testing should be used to confirm these findings.

DIAGNOSIS

The diagnosis of FM is illustrated in Figure 36.9. The American College of Rheumatology criteria for fibromyalgia were never intended to be used as strict diagnostic criteria for use in clinical practice. Many individuals who clearly have fibromyalgia will not have pain throughout their entire body, or will not have 11 tender points. Moreover, pain and tenderness occur across a continuum in the population, and it is impossible to know where to "draw the line" between an individual with symptoms, and someone with an "illness."[187]

History

Pain

In clinical practice, one should suspect fibromyalgia in individuals with multifocal pain that cannot be explained on the basis of damage or inflammation in those regions of the body. In most cases, musculoskeletal pain is the most prominent feature, but because pain pathways throughout the body are amplified, pain can be perceived more generally. Thus chronic headaches, sore throats, chest pain, abdominal pain, and pelvic pain are very common in individuals with fibromyalgia, and patients with chronic regional pain in any of these locations are more likely to have fibromyalgia.

Because pain is a defining feature of fibromyalgia, it is helpful to focus on the features of the pain that can help distinguish it from other disorders. The pain of fibromyalgia is typically diffuse or multifocal, often waxes and wanes, and is frequently migratory in nature. These characteristics of "central pain" are quite different from "peripheral" pain, where both the location and severity of pain are typically more constant. Patients may complain of discomfort when they are touched or when wearing tight clothing, and may experience dysesthesias or paresthesias that accompany the pain.

Nonpain Symptoms

Aside from the pain, a number of seemingly nonrelated symptoms may develop and persist. These include fatigue, sleep difficulties, weakness, problems with attention or memory, unexplainable weight fluctuations, and heat and cold intolerance. "Allergies" are reported much more commonly in fibromyalgia patients, although these excess symptoms are better considered hypersensitivities rather than true IgE-mediated immunological reactions. These patients are also more prone to nonallergic rhinitis, sinus, and nasal congestion, and lower respiratory symptoms, all of which again may be primarily attributable to neural mechanisms. Distortions in hearing, vision, and vestibular symptoms are often reported, as are sicca symptoms (sometimes so prominent that these individuals will overlap with those with Sjögren syndrome).

"Functional disorders" involving visceral organs have long been noted to be more common in fibromyalgia. These include noncardiac chest pain, heartburn and palpitations, and the frequent comorbidity of IBS. Thus, there are reports of increased echocardiographic evidence of mitral valve prolapse and esophageal dysmotility, and reduced static inspiratory and expiratory pressure on pulmonary function tests. The latter might be explained by pain in respiratory muscles. Syncope and hypotension are symptoms that may occur in FM, and in some cases will be accompanied by neurally mediated hypotension or postural orthostatic tachycardia. Pelvic complaints are common, including

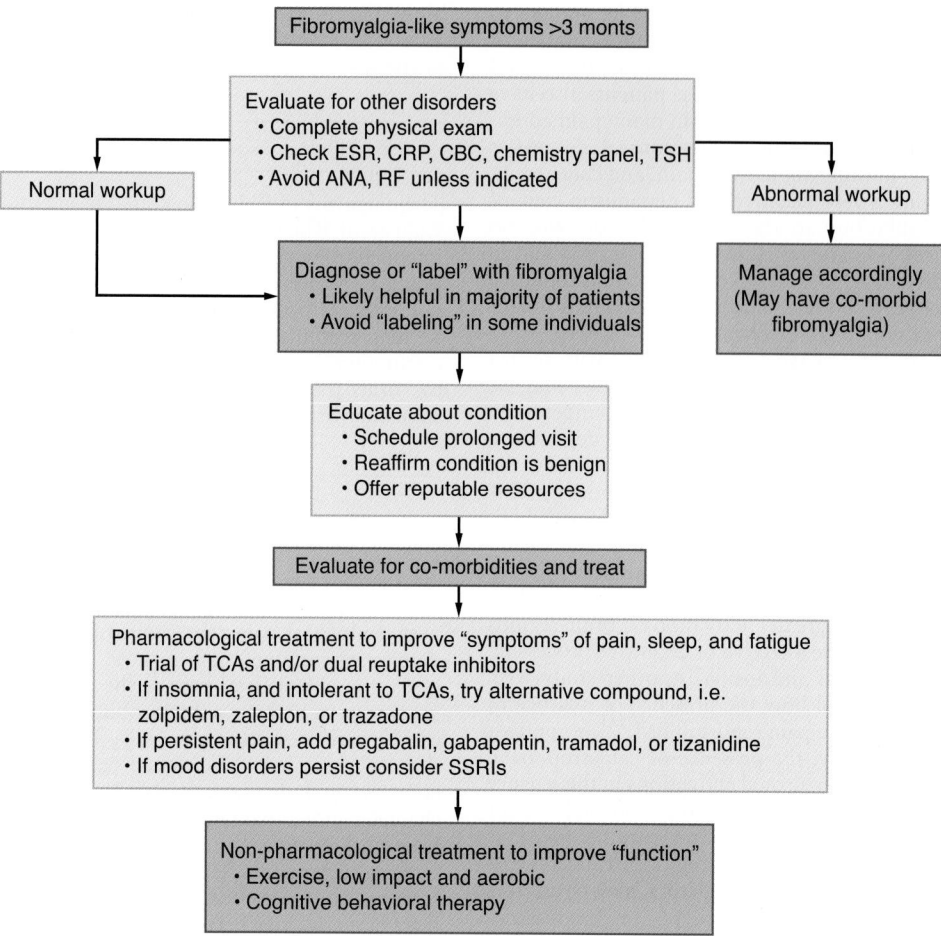

FIGURE 36.9 Algorithm for the diagnosis and treatment of fibromyalgia.

not only pain but also urinary frequency and urgency. In females the frequent comorbid diagnoses are dysmenorrhea, interstitial cystitis, endometriosis, and sensitivity disorders like vulvar vestibulitis and vulvodynia, whereas in males these same symptoms are sometimes diagnosed as chronic or non-bacterial prostatitis.

Physical Examination and Laboratory Investigations

Physical examination is often unremarkable, except for the presence of tenderness. As previously discussed, tenderness may be generalized and thus present anywhere in the body. Laboratory testing is generally not useful, except for the purpose of differential diagnosis. One factor that can help guide the intensity of the diagnostic workup is the length of time the patient has had symptoms. If the patient's symptoms have persisted for several years, minimal testing is required, whereas a more aggressive strategy should be employed for acute or subacute onset of symptoms. Simple testing should be limited to complete blood count and routine serum chemistries, along with thyroid-stimulating hormone (TSH) and ESR and/or CRP.

Serologic studies such as ANA and rheumatoid factor assays should generally be avoided unless there are historical features not seen in fibromyalgia, or abnormalities on physical examination. This represents a problem in clinical practice, because several autoimmune disorders share overlapping symptomatology with fibromyalgia. These include not only fatigue, arthralgias, and myalgias, but also such symptoms as morning stiffness and

subjective swelling of the hands and feet. Certain dermatologic features commonly seen in fibromyalgia, including malar flushing, livedo reticularis, and Raynaud-like reddening of the hands, also mimic symptoms of autoimmune disorders. This sometimes results in patients with fibromyalgia being misdiagnosed as having an autoimmune disorder such as systemic lupus erythematosus.

Aside from the many comorbid conditions already discussed, fibromyalgia may present similarly to a number of disorders or concurrently with other disorders that may confuse the diagnosis. Table 36.2 shows conditions that often mimic or present concur-

TABLE 36.2

CONDITIONS THAT SIMULATE FIBROMYALGIA

Common
Hypothyroidism
Polymyalgia rheumatica
Early in course of autoimmune disorders, e.g., rheumatoid arthritis or SLE
Sjogren's syndrome

Less common
Hepatitis C
Sleep apnea
Chiari malformation
Celiac sprue

rently with fibromyalgia. Hypothyroidism and polymyalgia rheumatica can be differentiated from fibromyalgia by results of TSH and ESR. Sleep apnea and hepatitis C also simulate fibromyalgia, and tend to present more often in men than women.

TREATMENT

Progress in the understanding of fibromyalgia has led to more therapeutic options for patients with this condition. Investigators are examining the utility of newer medications as well as nonpharmacological interventions in controlled trials (Fig. 36.10). Clinical based evidence advocates a multi-faceted program emphasizing education, certain medications, exercise, and cognitive therapy.[188]

Diagnostic Labeling

Once a physician rules out other potential disorders, an important and, at times controversial, step in the management of fibromyalgia is asserting the diagnosis. Despite some assumptions that being "labeled" with fibromyalgia may adversely affect patients, a study by White et al. indicated that patients had significant improvement in health satisfaction and symptoms after being "labeled."[178] Nonetheless, in certain select individuals (i.e., adolescents or young adults, or overtly anxious persons) the preferred route may still be not to label. Regardless, diagnosis confirmation should be ideally coupled to patient education, an intervention shown to be effective in randomized controlled trials.[188]

Pharmacological Therapy

The majority of fibromyalgia clinical trials have involved antidepressants of one class or another (Table 36.3). Trials studying the oldest class of agents, tricyclic antidepressants (TCAs), are most abundant, though several recent studies have focused on selective serotonin reuptake inhibitors and "atypical antidepressants"—a class that includes dual reuptake inhibitors and monoamine oxidase inhibitors (MAOIs).

Tricyclic Antidepressants

The most frequently studied pharmacological therapy for fibromyalgia is low doses of tricyclic compounds. Most TCAs increase

---

TABLE 36.3

PHARMACOLOGICAL THERAPIES

- **Strong evidence:** tricyclics (amitriptyline, cyclobenzaprine); dual-reuptake inhibitors (SNRI/NSRI—venlafaxine, duloxetine, milnacipran); alpha-2-delta ligands (pregabalin, gabapentin)
- **Modest evidence:** tramadol; selective serotonin reuptake inhibitors (SSRIs); dopamine agonists; gamma hydroxybutyrate (GHB)
- **Weak evidence:** growth hormone, 5-hydroxytryptamine, tropisetron, S-adenosyl-L-methionine (SAMe)
- **Not shown to be effective:** opioids, NSAIDs, corticosteroids, benzodiazepine and nonbenzodiazepine hypnotics, melatonin, guanifenesin, dehydroepiandrosterone

---

the concentrations of serotonin and/or norepinephrine (noradrenaline) by directly blocking their respective reuptake (Fig. 36.11). The effectiveness of TCAs, particularly amitriptyline and cyclobenzaprine, in treating the symptoms of pain, poor sleep, and fatigue associated with fibromyalgia is supported by several randomized, controlled trials.[94] Tolerability is a problem but can be improved by beginning at very low doses (e.g., 10 mg of amitriptyline or 5 mg of cyclobenzaprine), giving the dose a few hours before bedtime, and very slowly escalating the dose.

Selective Serotonin Reuptake Inhibitors

Because of a better side effect profile selective serotonin reuptake inhibitors (SSRIs) are frequently used in fibromyalgia. The SSRIs fluoxetine, citalopram, and paroxetine have each been evaluated in randomized, placebo-controlled trials.[188–191] In general, the results of studies of SSRIs in fibromyalgia have paralleled the experience in other pain conditions. The newer "highly selective" serotonin reuptake inhibitors (e.g., citalopram) seem to be less efficacious than the older SSRIs, which have some noradrenergic activity at higher doses.[192]

Since TCAs and high doses of certain SSRIs such as fluoxetine and sertraline that have the most balanced reuptake inhibition are the most effective analgesics, many have concluded that dual receptor inhibitors such as serotonin-NE and NE-serotonin reuptake inhibitors (SNRIs and NSRIs) may be of more benefit than pure serotonergic drugs.[192] These drugs are pharmacologically

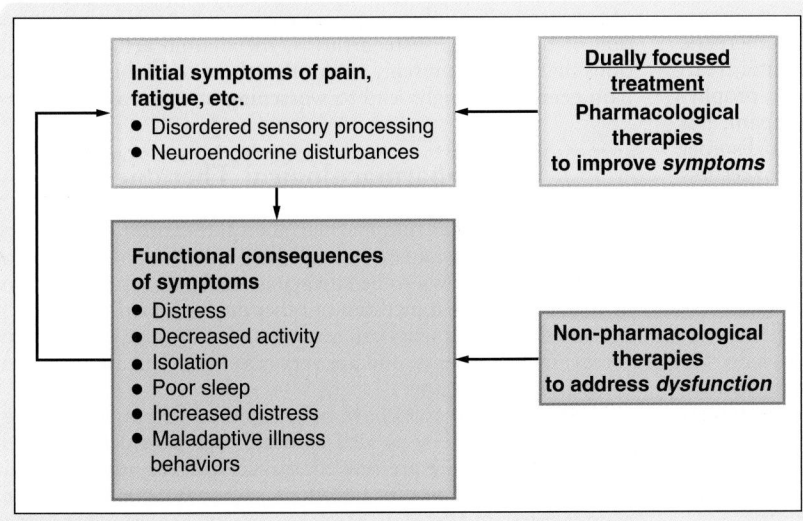

FIGURE 36.10 An example of dually focused treatment.

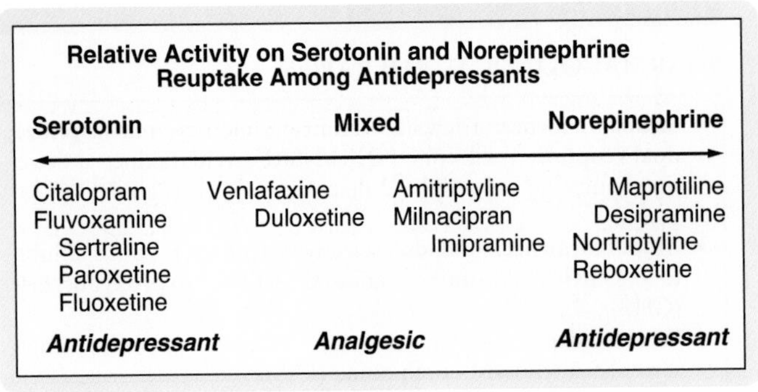

Relative Activity on Serotonin and Norepinephrine Reuptake Among Antidepressants

Serotonin	Mixed		Norepinephrine
Citalopram	Venlafaxine	Amitriptyline	Maprotiline
Fluvoxamine	Duloxetine	Milnacipran	Desipramine
Sertraline		Imipramine	Nortriptyline
Paroxetine			Reboxetine
Fluoxetine			
Antidepressant	*Analgesic*		*Antidepressant*

FIGURE 36.11 Relative activity on serotonin and norepinephrine reuptake among antidepressants.

similar to some TCAs in their ability to inhibit the reuptake of both serotonin and NE, but differ from TCAs in being generally devoid of significant activity at other receptor systems. This selectivity results in diminished side effects and enhanced tolerability. The first available SNRI, venlafaxine, has data to support its use in the management of neuropathic pain, and retrospective trial data demonstrate that this compound is also effective in the prophylaxis of migraine and tension headaches.[193] Two studies in fibromyalgia have had conflicting results, with the one using a higher dose showing efficacy.[188]

Two new SNRIs, milnacipran and duloxetine, have undergone recent multicenter trials and were shown to be effective in a number of outcome variables.[116,194] In the study evaluating milnacipran, statistically significant differences were noted in overall improvement, physical functioning, level of fatigue, and degree of reported physical impairment. In the trial of duloxetine compared to placebo, participants treated with duloxetine had decreased self-reported pain and stiffness and a reduced number of tender points. In both studies, benefits were shown to be independent of the drug effect on mood, thus suggesting that the analgesic and other positive effects of this class of drugs in fibromyalgia is not simply due to their antidepressant effects.

Other Central Nervous System Acting Drugs

Antiepileptic drugs are widely used in the treatment of various chronic pain conditions, including postherpetic neuralgia and painful diabetic neuropathy.[195] Pregabalin is a gamma-aminobutyric acid (GABA) analog and approved for the treatment of neuropathic pain. A recent randomized, double-blinded, placebo-controlled trial demonstrated efficacy of pregabalin against pain, sleep disturbances, and fatigue as compared to placebo.[196] Pregabalin is currently the only pharmacological agent approved by the Food and Drug Administration in the treatment of fibromyalgia. Gabapentin, a compound with similar pharmacology to pregabalin, is specifically indicated for the treatment of postherpetic neuralgia and studies support its use in the symptomatic treatment of a variety of pain states as well as headache prophylaxis.[195,197] Another antiepileptic compound, clonazepam, has demonstrated efficacy in treating temporal mandibular disorder and associated jaw pain and is useful in the treatment of restless leg syndrome[195] and may be of value in FM.

Sedative-hypnotic compounds are widely used by fibromyalgia patients. A handful of studies have been published on the use of certain nonbenzodiazepine hypnotics in fibromyalgia, such as zopiclone and zolpidem. These reports have suggested that these agents can improve the sleep and, perhaps, fatigue of fibromyalgia patients, though they had no significant effects on pain. On the other hand, gamma-hydroxybutyrate (also known as sodium oxybate), a precursor of GABA with powerful sedative properties, was recently shown to be useful in improving fatigue, pain, and sleep architecture in patients with fibromyalgia.[198] Note, however, that this agent is a scheduled substance due to its abuse potential.

Pramipexole is a dopamine agonist indicated for Parkinson disease that has shown utility in the treatment of periodic leg movement disorder.[199] Recent studies suggest that this compound may improve both pain and sleep in fibromyalgia patients.[200]

Tizanidine is a centrally acting alpha-2 adrenergic agonist approved by the Food and Drug Administration for the treatment of muscle spasticity associated with multiple sclerosis and stroke. Literature suggests that this agent is a useful adjunct in treating several chronic pain conditions, including chronic daily headaches and low back pain. A recent trial reported significant improvements in several parameters in fibromyalgia, including sleep, pain, and measures of quality of life.[201] Of particular interest was the demonstration that treatment with tizanidine resulted in a reduction in substance P levels within the CSF of patients with fibromyalgia.

Analgesics

There have been no adequate randomized controlled clinical trials of opiates in fibromyalgia, and many in the field (including the authors) have not found this class of compounds to be effective in anecdotal experience. Tramadol is a compound that has some opioid activity (weak mu-agonist activity) combined with serotonin/NE reuptake inhibition. This compound does appear to be somewhat efficacious in the management of fibromyalgia, as both an isolated compound and as fixed-dose combination with acetaminophen.[199].

A large number of fibromyalgia patients use nonsteroidal anti-inflammatory drugs (NSAIDs) and acetaminophen. Although numerous studies have failed to confirm their effectiveness as analgesics in fibromyalgia, there is limited evidence that patients may experience enhanced analgesia when treated with combinations of NSAIDs and other agents. This phenomenon may be a result of concurrent "peripheral" pain (i.e., due to damage or inflammation of tissues; e.g., osteoarthritis, rheumatoid arthritis) conditions that may be present, and/or that these comorbid peripheral pain generators might lead to worsening of "central" pain.

Nonpharmacological Therapies

The two best-studied nonpharmacological therapies are cognitive behavioral therapy and exercise (Table 36.4). Both of these therapies have been shown to be efficacious in the treatment of fibromyalgia, as well as a plethora of other medical conditions.[188,202] Both of these treatments can lead to sustained (e.g., greater than 1 year) improvements, and are very effective when an individual complies with therapy.

Alternative therapies have been explored by patients managing their own illness, as well as healthcare providers. As with other diseases, there are few controlled trials to advocate their general use. Trigger-point injections, chiropractic manipulation, acupuncture, and myofascial release therapy are among the more

TABLE 36.4

NONPHARMACOLOGICAL THERAPIES

- **Strong evidence:** cardiovascular exercise, cognitive behavior therapy, patient education, multidisciplinary therapy
- **Modest evidence:** strength training, acupuncture, hypnotherapy, biofeedback, balneotherapy
- **Weak evidence:** acupuncture, chiropractic, manual and massage therapy, electrotherapy, ultrasound
- **No evidence:** tender (trigger) point injections, flexibility exercise

commonly used modalities, which achieve varying levels of success. Two randomized, sham-controlled trial of acupuncture showed no difference between the two groups.[95,204] A usual-care comparison group was not studied. There is some evidence that the use of alternative therapies gives patients a greater sense of control over their illness. In instances where this sense of control is accompanied by an improved clinical state, the decision to use these therapies is between physicians and patients themselves.

PROGNOSIS

The prognosis of FM depends largely on where the individual falls on a continuum. One end of the continuum are individuals in the population with CWP, or individuals with FM that are seen in primary care, with the prognosis in these individuals being quite good.[205,206] On the other hand, individuals with FM seen in tertiary care settings do quite poorly.[207] In this latter study, there was little change in symptoms over time, and no significant change in health satisfaction, symptoms or functional disability.

With regard to function in FM, studies have reported varying disability rates from 9% to 44%.[206,208,209] Disability has been most strongly associated with functional and work status, pain, mood disturbances, coping ability, depression, pending litigation, and educational background.

General Considerations

Management strategies are similar to other chronic illnesses, where empathetic healthcare providers should develop a partnership with their patients. At one end of the continuum, there are some individuals with FM that respond to a single medication, or a graded, low-impact exercise program. At the other end of the continuum is the tertiary care patient with high levels of distress, who has no sense of control of their illness, little social support, and has looked toward disability and compensation systems to try to solve their problem. For this individual, and many in between, multimodal programs that integrate nonpharmacological (especially exercise, CBT) and pharmacological therapies are required.

References

1. Khan AA, Khan A, Harezlak J, et al. Somatic symptoms in primary care: etiology and outcome. *Psychosomatics* 2003;44(6):471–478.
2. Mayer EA, Raybould HE. Role of visceral afferent mechanisms in functional bowel disorders. *Gastroenterology* 1990;99(6):1688–1704.
3. Hudson JI, Hudson MS, Pliner LF, et al. Fibromyalgia and major affective disorder: a controlled phenomenology and family history study. *Am J Psychiatry* 1985;142(4):441–446.
4. Arnold LM, Hudson JI, Hess EV, et al. Family study of fibromyalgia. *Arthritis Rheum* 2004;50(3):944–952.
5. Wessely S, Nimnuan C, Sharpe M. Functional somatic syndromes: One or many? *Lancet* 1999;354(9182):936–939.
6. Barsky AJ, Borus JF. Functional somatic syndromes. *Ann Intern Med* 1999;130(11):910–921.
7. Fukuda K, Nisenbaum R, Stewart G, et al. Chronic multisymptom illness affecting Air Force veterans of the Gulf War. *JAMA* 1998; 280(11):981–988.
8. Drossman DA, Li ZM, Andruzzi E, et al. U.S. householder survey of functional gastrointestinal disorders. Prevalence, sociodemography, and health impact. *Dig Dis Sci* 1993;38(9):1569–1580.
9. Aaron LA, Bradley LA, Alarcon GS, et al. Psychiatric diagnoses in patients with fibromyalgia are related to health care-seeking behavior rather than to illness [see comments in *Arthritis Rheum* 1996;39(12):2086–2087]. *Arthritis Rheum* 1996;39(3):436–445.
10. Maixner W, Fillingim R, Booker D, et al. Sensitivity of patients with painful temporomandibular disorders to experimentally evoked pain. *Pain* 1995; 63(3):341–351.
11. Naliboff BD, Derbyshire SW, Munakata J, et al. Cerebral activation in patients with irritable bowel syndrome and control subjects during rectosigmoid stimulation. *Psychosom Med* 2001;63(3):365–375.
12. Giesecke T, Gracely RH, Grant MA, et al. Evidence of augmented central pain processing in idiopathic chronic low back pain. *Arthritis Rheum* 2004; 50(2):613–623.
13. Giesecke J, Reed BD, Haefner HK, et al. Quantitative sensory testing in vulvodynia patients and increased peripheral pressure pain sensitivity. *Obstet Gynecol* 2004;104(1):126–133.
14. Moshiree B, Price DD, Robinson ME, et al. Thermal and visceral hypersensitivity in irritable bowel syndrome patients with and without fibromyalgia. *Clin J Pain* 2007;23(4):323–330.
15. Clauw DJ. Fibromyalgia: update on mechanisms and management. *J Clin Rheumatol* 2007;13(2):102–109.
16. Woolf CJ. Pain: moving from symptom control toward mechanism-specific pharmacologic management. *Ann Intern Med* 2004;140(6):441–451.
17. Smythe HA, Moldofsky H. Two contributions to understanding of the "fibrositis" syndrome. *Bull Rheum Dis* 1977;28(1):928–931.
18. Moldofsky H, Scarisbrick P, England R, et al. Musculoskeletal symptoms and non-REM sleep disturbance in patients with "fibrositis syndrome" and healthy subjects. *Psychosom Med* 1975;37(4):341–351.
19. Yunus M, Masi AT, Calabro JJ, et al. Primary fibromyalgia (fibrositis): clinical study of 50 patients with matched normal controls. *Semin Arthritis Rheum* 1981;11(1):151–171.
20. Wolfe F, Smythe HA, Yunus MB, et al. The American College of Rheumatology 1990 Criteria for the Classification of Fibromyalgia. Report of the Multicenter Criteria Committee. *Arthritis Rheum* 1990;33(2):160–172.
21. Yunus MB. Towards a model of pathophysiology of fibromyalgia: aberrant central pain mechanisms with peripheral modulation. *J Rheumatol* 1992; 19(6):846–850.
22. Clauw DJ, Chrousos GP. Chronic pain and fatigue syndromes: overlapping clinical and neuroendocrine features and potential pathogenic mechanisms. *Neuroimmunomodulation* 1997;4(3):134–153.
23. Wolfe F, Ross K, Anderson J, et al. Aspects of fibromyalgia in the general population: sex, pain threshold, and fibromyalgia symptoms. *J Rheumatol* 1995;22(1):151–156.
24. Croft P, Rigby AS, Boswell R, et al. The prevalence of chronic widespread pain in the general population. *J Rheumatol* 1993;20(4):710–713.
25. Cöster L, Kendall S, Gerdle B, et al. Chronic widespread musculoskeletal pain - A comparison of those who meet criteria for fibromyalgia and those who do not. *Eur J Pain* 2008;12(5):600–610.
26. Jacobsen S, Bredkjaer SR. The prevalence of fibromyalgia and widespread chronic musculoskeletal pain in the general population. *Scand J Rheumatol* 1992;21(5):261–263.
27. Raspe H. Rheumatism epidemiology in Europe [in German]. *Soz Praventivmed* 1992;37(4):168–178.
28. Peleg R, Ablin JN, Peleg A, et al. Characteristics of fibromyalgia in Muslim Bedouin women in a primary care clinic. *Semin Arthritis Rheum* 2008;37(6): 398–402.
29. White KP, Thompson J. Fibromyalgia syndrome in an Amish community: a controlled study to determine disease and symptom prevalence. *J Rheumatol* 2003;30(8):1835–1840.
30. Petzke F, Khine A, Williams D, et al. Dolorimetry performed at 3 paired tender points highly predicts overall tenderness. *J Rheumatol* 2001;28(11): 2568–2569.
31. Granges G, Littlejohn G. Pressure pain threshold in pain-free subjects, in patients with chronic regional pain syndromes, and in patients with fibromyalgia syndrome. *Arthritis Rheum* 1993;36(5):642–646.
32. Cohen ML, Quintner J. Fibromyalgia syndrome, a problem of tautology. *Lancet* 1993;342(8876):906–909.
33. Wolfe F. The relation between tender points and fibromyalgia symptom variables: evidence that fibromyalgia is not a discrete disorder in the clinic. *Ann Rheum Dis* 1997;56(4):268–271.
34. Petzke F, Ambrose K, Gracely RH, et al. What do tender points measure? *Arthritis Rheum* 1999;42(suppl 9):S342.
35. Petzke F, Gracely RH, Khine A, et al. Pain sensitivity in patients with fibromyalgia (FM): expectancy effects on pain measurements. *Arthritis Rheum* 1999; 42(suppl 9):S342.
36. Croft P, Burt J, Schollum J, et al. More pain, more tender points: is fibromyalgia just one end of a continuous spectrum? *Ann Rheum Dis* 1996;55(7): 482–485.
37. Papageorgiou AC, Silman AJ, Macfarlane GJ. Chronic widespread pain in

the population: a seven year follow up study. *Ann Rheum Dis* 2002;61(12): 1071–1074.

38. Buskila D, Neumann L, Hazanov I, et al. Familial aggregation in the fibromyalgia syndrome. *Semin Arthritis Rheumatism* 1996;26(3):605–611.

39. Kato K, Sullivan PF, Evengard B, et al. Chronic widespread pain and its comorbidities: a population-based study. *Arch Intern Med* 2006;166(15): 1649–1654.

40. Hudson JI, Goldenberg DL, Pope HGJ, et al. Comorbidity of fibromyalgia with medical and psychiatric disorders. *Am J Med* 1993;92(4):363–367.

41. Yunus MB. Central sensitivity syndromes: a new paradigm and group nosology for fibromyalgia and overlapping conditions, and the related issue of disease versus illness. *Semin Arthritis Rheum* 2008;37(6):339–352.

42. Fukuda K, Dobbins JG, Wilson LJ, et al. An epidemiologic study of fatigue with relevance for the chronic fatigue syndrome. *J Psychiatr Res* 1997;31(1): 19–29.

43. Kato K, Sullivan PF, Evengard B, et al. Importance of genetic influences on chronic widespread pain. *Arthritis Rheum* 2006;54(5):1682–1686.

44. Bondy B, Spaeth M, Offenbaecher M, et al. The T102C polymorphism of the 5-HT2A-receptor gene in fibromyalgia. *Neurobiol Dis* 1999;6(5):433–439.

45. Offenbaecher M, Bondy B, de Jonge S, et al. Possible association of fibromyalgia with a polymorphism in the serotonin transporter gene regulatory region. *Arthritis Rheum* 1999;42(11):2482–2488.

46. Buskila D, Cohen H, Neumann L, et al. An association between fibromyalgia and the dopamine D4 receptor exon III repeat polymorphism and relationship to novelty seeking personality traits. *Mol Psychiatry* 2004;9(8):730–731.

47. Buskila D. Genetics of chronic pain states. *Best Pract Res Clin Rheumatol* 2007;21(3):535–547.

48. Buskila D, Neumann L, Vaisberg G, et al. Increased rates of fibromyalgia following cervical spine injury. A controlled study of 161 cases of traumatic injury [see comments in *Arthritis Rheum* 1997;40(11):2097; *Arthritis Rheum* 1998;41(4):758–759; *Arthritis Rheum* 1998;41(2):378–379; *Arthritis Rheum* 1998;41(1):183–184]. *Arthritis Rheum* 1997;40(3):446–452.

49. McLean SA, Clauw DJ. Predicting chronic symptoms after an acute "stressor"—lessons learned from 3 medical conditions. *Med Hypotheses* 2004; 63(4):653–658.

50. Unwin C, Blatchley N, Coker W, et al. Health of UK servicemen who served in Persian Gulf War. *Lancet* 1999;353(9148):169–178.

51. Hyams KC, Wignall FS, Roswell R. War syndromes and their evaluation: from the U.S. Civil War to the Persian Gulf War. *Ann Intern Med* 1996; 125(5):398–405.

52. Clauw DJ. The health consequences of the first Gulf War. *BMJ* 2003;327: 1357–1358.

53. Clauw DJ, Katz P. The overlap between fibromyalgia and inflammatory rheumatic diseases: when and why does it occur? *J Clin Rheumatol* 1995;1: 335–341.

54. Sapolsky RM. Why stress is bad for your brain. *Science* 1996;273(5276): 749–750.

55. Chrousos GP, Gold PW. The concepts of stress and stress system disorders. Overview of physical and behavioral homeostasis. *JAMA* 1992;267(9): 1244–1252.

56. Pillow DR, Zautra AJ, Sandler I. Major life events and minor stressors: identifying mediational links in the stress process. *J Pers Soc Psychol* 1996;70(2): 381–394.

57. Raphael KG, Natelson BH, Janal MN, et al. A community-based survey of fibromyalgia-like pain complaints following the World Trade Center terrorist attacks. *Pain* 2002;100(1–2):131–139.

58. Williams DA, Brown SC, Clauw DJ, et al. Self-reported symptoms before and after September 11 in patients with fibromyalgia. *JAMA* 2003;289(13): 1637–1638.

59. Clauw DJ, Engel CC Jr, Aronowitz R, et al. Unexplained symptoms after terrorism and war: an expert consensus statement. *J Occup Environ Med* 2003;45(10):1040–1048.

60. Heim C, Newport DJ, Bonsall R, et al. Altered pituitary-adrenal axis responses to provocative challenge tests in adult survivors of childhood abuse. *Am J Psychiatry* 2001;158(4):575–581.

61. Glass JM, Lyden A, Petzke F, et al. The effect of brief exercise cessation on pain, fatigue, and mood symptom development in healthy, fit individuals. *J Psychosom Res* 2004;57(4):391–398.

62. McBeth J, Silman AJ, Gupta A, et al. Moderation of psychosocial risk factors through dysfunction of the hypothalamic-pituitary-adrenal stress axis in the onset of chronic widespread musculoskeletal pain: findings of a population-based prospective cohort study. *Arthritis Rheum* 2007;56(1):360–371.

63. Aaron LA, Bradley LA, Alarcon GS, et al. Perceived physical and emotional trauma as precipitating events in fibromyalgia. Associations with health care seeking and disability status but not pain severity [see comments in *Arthritis Rheum* 1998 Feb;41(2):378–379; *Arthritis Rheum* 1999 Apr;42(4):828–830]. *Arthritis Rheum* 1997;40(3):453–460.

64. Alexander RW, Bradley LA, Alarcon GS, et al. Sexual and physical abuse in women with fibromyalgia: association with outpatient health care utilization and pain medication usage. *Arthritis Care Res* 1998;11(2):102–115.

65. Boisset-Pioro MH, Esdaile JM, Fitzcharles MA. Sexual and physical abuse in women with fibromyalgia syndrome. *Arthritis Rheum* 1995;38(2):235–241.

66. Drossman DA. Sexual and physical abuse and gastrointestinal illness. *Scand J Gastroenterol Suppl* 1995;208:90–96.

67. Arguelles LM, Afari N, Buchwald DS, et al. A twin study of posttraumatic stress disorder symptoms and chronic widespread pain. *Pain* 2006;124(1–2): 150–157.

68. Arnson Y, Amital D, Fostick L, et al. Physical activity protects male patients with post-traumatic stress disorder from developing severe fibromyalgia. *Clin Exp Rheumatol* 2007;25(4):529–533.

69. Crofford LJ, Pillemer SR, Kalogeras KT, et al. Hypothalamic-pituitary-adrenal axis perturbations in patients with fibromyalgia. *Arthritis Rheum* 1994;37(11):1583–1592.

70. Demitrack MA, Crofford LJ. Evidence for and pathophysiologic implications of hypothalamic-pituitary-adrenal axis dysregulation in fibromyalgia and chronic fatigue syndrome. *Ann N Y Acad Sci* 1998;840:684–697.

71. Qiao ZG, Vaeroy H, Morkrid L. Electrodermal and microcirculatory activity in patients with fibromyalgia during baseline, acoustic stimulation and cold pressor tests. *J Rheumatol* 1991;18(9):1383–1389.

72. Adler GK, Kinsley BT, Hurwitz S, et al. Reduced hypothalamic-pituitary and sympathoadrenal responses to hypoglycemia in women with fibromyalgia syndrome. *Am J Med* 1999;106(5):534–543.

73. Martinez-Lavin M, Hermosillo AG, Rosas M, et al. Circadian studies of autonomic nervous balance in patients with fibromyalgia: a heart rate variability analysis. *Arthritis Rheum* 1998;41(11):1966–1971.

74. Cohen H, Neumann L, Shore M, et al. Autonomic dysfunction in patients with fibromyalgia: application of power spectral analysis of heart rate variability [see comments in *Semin Arthritis Rheum* 2000;29(4):197–199]. *Semin Arthritis Rheum* 2000;29(4):217–227.

75. McLean SA, Williams DA, Groner KH, et al. Naturalistic evaluation of cortisol secretion and symptoms in fibromyalgia and healthy controls. *Arthritis Rheum* 2005.

76. McLean SA, Williams DA, Harris RE, et al. Momentary relationship between cortisol secretion and symptoms in patients with fibromyalgia. *Arthritis Rheum* 2005;52:3660–3669.

77. Cohen H, Buskila D, Neumann L, et al. Confirmation of an association between fibromyalgia and serotonin transporter promoter region (5- HTTLPR) polymorphism, and relationship to anxiety-related personality traits. *Arthritis Rheum* 2002;46(3):845–847.

78. Bou-Holaigah I, Calkins H, Flynn JA, et al. Provocation of hypotension and pain during upright tilt table testing in adults with fibromyalgia. *Clin Exp Rheumatol* 1997;15(3):239–246.

79. Naschitz JE, Rosner I, Rozenbaum M, et al. The capnography head-up tilt test for evaluation of chronic fatigue syndrome. *Semin Arthritis Rheum* 2000; 30(2):79–86.

80. Rosner I, Rozenbaum M, Naschitz JE, et al. Cardiovascular response to upright tilt differs in fibrolmyalgia from chronic fatigue syndrome [abstract]. *American College of Rheumatology* [Poster Session C Fibromyalgia and Soft Tissue Rheumatism I], S209. 2000.

81. McBeth J, Jones K. Epidemiology of chronic musculoskeletal pain. *Best Pract Res Clin Rheumatol* 2007;21(3):403–425.

82. Figueroa A, Kingsley JD, McMillan V, et al. Resistance exercise training improves heart rate variability in women with fibromyalgia. *Clin Physiol Funct Imaging* 2008;28(1):49–54.

83. Gracely RH, Grant MA, Giesecke T. Evoked pain measures in fibromyalgia. *Best Pract Res Clin Rheumatol* 2003;17(4):593–609.

84. Jensen K, Andersen HO, Olesen J, et al. Pressure-pain threshold in human temporal region. Evaluation of a new pressure algometer. *Pain* 1986;25(3): 313–323.

85. Petzke F, Gracely RH, Park KM, et al. What do tender points measure? Influence of distress on 4 measures of tenderness. *J Rheumatol* 2003;30(3): 567–574.

86. Petzke F, Clauw DJ, Ambrose K, et al. Increased pain sensitivity in fibromyalgia: effects of stimulus type and mode of presentation. *Pain* 2003;105(3): 403–413.

87. Petzke F, Khine A, Williams D, et al. Dolorimetry performed at 3 paired tender points highly predicts overall tenderness. *J Rheumatol* 2001;28(11): 2568–2569.

88. Färber L, Stratz T, Brückle W, et al. Efficacy and tolerability of tropisetron in primary fibromyalgia—A highly selective and competitive 5-HT3 receptor antagonist. German Fibromyalgia Study Group. *Scand J Rheumatol Suppl* 2000;113:49–54.

89. Arnold LM, Hess EV, Hudson JI, et al. A randomized, placebo-controlled, double-blind, flexible-dose study of fluoxetine in the treatment of women with fibromyalgia. *Am J Med* 2002;112(3):191–197.

90. Goldenberg D, Mayskiy M, Mossey C, et al. A randomized, double-blind crossover trial of fluoxetine and amitriptyline in the treatment of fibromyalgia. *Arthritis Rheum* 1996;39(11):1852–1859.

91. Gowans SE, de Hueck A, Voss S, et al. Effect of a randomized, controlled trial of exercise on mood and physical function in individuals with fibromyalgia. *Arthritis Rheum* 2001;45(6):519–529.

92. Jacobsen S, Danneskiold-Samsoe B, Andersen RB. Oral S-adenosylmethionine in primary fibromyalgia. Double-blind clinical evaluation. *Scand J Rheumatol* 1991;20(4):294–302.

93. Scudds RA, McCain GA, Rollman GB, et al. Improvements in pain responsiveness in patients with fibrositis after successful treatment with amitriptyline. *J Rheumatol Suppl* 1989;19:98–103.

94. Arnold LM, Keck PEJ, Welge JA. Antidepressant treatment of fibromyalgia. A meta-analysis and review. *Psychosomatics* 2000;41(2):104–113.

95. Harris RE, Gracely RH, McLean SA, et al. Comparison of clinical and evoked pain measures in fibromyalgia. *J Pain* 2006;7(7):521–527.

96. Geisser ME, Gracely RH, Giesecke T, et al. The association between experimental and clinical pain measures among persons with fibromyalgia and chronic fatigue syndrome. *Eur J Pain* 2007;11(2):202–207.

97. Gibson SJ, Littlejohn GO, Gorman MM, et al. Altered heat pain thresholds and cerebral event-related potentials following painful CO2 laser stimulation in subjects with fibromyalgia syndrome. *Pain* 1994;58(2):185–193.

98. Kosek E, Hansson P. Modulatory influence on somatosensory perception from vibration and heterotopic noxious conditioning stimulation (HNCS) in fibromyalgia patients and healthy subjects. *Pain* 1997;70(1):41–51.

99. Geisser ME, Casey KL, Brucksch CB, et al. Perception of noxious and innocuous heat stimulation among healthy women and women with fibromyalgia: association with mood, somatic focus, and catastrophizing. *Pain* 2003;102(3):243–250.

100. Kosek E, Ekholm J, Hansson P. Sensory dysfunction in fibromyalgia patients with implications for pathogenic mechanisms. *Pain* 1996;68(2–3):375–383.

101. Arroyo JF, Cohen ML. Abnormal responses to electrocutaneous stimulation in fibromyalgia. *J Rheumatol* 1993;20(11):1925–1931.

102. Carli G, Suman AL, Biasi G, et al. Reactivity to superficial and deep stimuli in patients with chronic musculoskeletal pain. *Pain* 2002;100(3):259–269.

103. Gerster JC, Hadj–Djilani A. Hearing and vestibular abnormalities in primary fibrositis syndrome. *J Rheumatol* 1984;11(5):678–680.

104. McDermid AJ, Rollman GB, McCain GA. Generalized hypervigilance in fibromyalgia: evidence of perceptual amplification. *Pain* 1996;66(2–3):133–144.

105. Tracey I, Mantyh PW. The cerebral signature for pain perception and its modulation. *Neuron* 2007;55(3):377–391.

106. Craig AD. Human feelings: why are some more aware than others? *Trends Cogn Sci* 2004;8(6):239–241.

107. Craig AD. Interoception: the sense of the physiological condition of the body. *Curr Opin Neurobiol* 2003;13(4):500–505.

108. Lautenbacher S, Rollman GB. Possible deficiencies of pain modulation in fibromyalgia. *Clin J Pain* 1997;13(3):189–196.

109. Leffler AS, Hansson P, Kosek E. Somatosensory perception in a remote pain-free area and function of diffuse noxious inhibitory controls (DNIC) in patients suffering from long-term trapezius myalgia. *Eur J Pain* 2002;6(2):149–159.

110. Julien N, Goffaux P, Arsenault P, et al. Widespread pain in fibromyalgia is related to a deficit of endogenous pain inhibition. *Pain* 2005;114(1–2):295–302.

111. Wilder–Smith CH, Robert–Yap J. Abnormal endogenous pain modulation and somatic and visceral hypersensitivity in female patients with irritable bowel syndrome. *World J Gastroenterol* 2007;13(27):3699–3704.

112. Baraniuk JN, Whalen G, Cunningham J, et al. Cerebrospinal fluid levels of opioid peptides in fibromyalgia and chronic low back pain. *BMC Musculoskeletal Disord* 2004;5(1):48.

113. Harris RE, Clauw DJ, Scott DJ, et al. Decreased central mu-opioid receptor availability in fibromyalgia. *J Neurosci* 2007;27(37):10000–10006.

114. Russell IJ, Vaeroy H, Javors M, et al. Cerebrospinal fluid biogenic amine metabolites in fibromyalgia/fibrositis syndrome and rheumatoid arthritis. *Arthritis Rheum* 1992;35(5):550–556.

115. Yunus MB, Dailey JW, Aldag JC, et al. Plasma tryptophan and other amino acids in primary fibromyalgia: a controlled study. *J Rheumatol* 1992;19(1):90–94.

116. Arnold LM, Lu Y, Crofford LJ, et al. A double-blind, multicenter trial comparing duloxetine with placebo in the treatment of fibromyalgia patients with or without major depressive disorder. *Arthritis Rheum* 2004;50(9):2974–2984.

117. Bennett RM, Kamin M, Karim R, et al. Tramadol and acetaminophen combination tablets in the treatment of fibromyalgia pain: a double-blind, randomized, placebo-controlled study. *Am J Med* 2003;114(5):537–545.

118. Gendreau RM, Thorn MD, Gendreau JF, et al. The efficacy of milnacipran in fibromyalgia. *J Rheumatol* 2005;32(10):1975–1985.

119. Staud R, Vierck CJ, Cannon RL, et al. Abnormal sensitization and temporal summation of second pain (wind-up) in patients with fibromyalgia syndrome. *Pain* 2001;91(1–2):165–175.

120. Price DD, Staud R, Robinson ME, et al. Enhanced temporal summation of second pain and its central modulation in fibromyalgia patients. *Pain* 2002;99(1–2):49–59.

121. Woolf CJ, Thompson SW. The induction and maintenance of central sensitization is dependent on N-methyl-D-aspartic acid receptor activation; implications for the treatment of post-injury pain hypersensitivity states. *Pain* 1991;44(3):293–299.

122. Woolf CJ. Windup and central sensitization are not equivalent. *Pain* 1996;66(2–3):105–108.

123. Xu XJ, Dalsgaard CJ, Wiesenfeld–Hallin Z. Spinal substance P and N-methyl-D-aspartate receptors are coactivated in the induction of central sensitization of the nociceptive flexor reflex. *Neuroscience* 1992;51(3):641–648.

124. Welin M, Bragee B, Nyberg F, et al. Elevated substance P levels are contrasted by a decrease in met-enkephalin-arg-phe levels in CSF from fibromyalgia patients. *J Musculoskeletal Pain* 1995;3(1):4.

125. Vaerøy H, Helle R, Førre O, et al. Elevated CSF levels of substance P and high incidence of Raynaud phenomenon in patients with fibromyalgia: new features for diagnosis. *Pain* 1988;32(1):21–26.

126. Russell IJ, Orr MD, Littman B, et al. Elevated cerebrospinal fluid levels of substance P in patients with the fibromyalgia syndrome. *Arthritis Rheum* 1994;37(11):1593–1601.

127. Bradley LA, Alberts KR, Alarcon GS, et al. Abnormal brain regional cerebral blood flow and cerebrospinal fluid levels of Substance P in patients and non-patients with fibromyalgia [abstract]. *Arthritis Rheum* 1996;39[9S]:1109.

128. Sarchielli P, Di Filippo M, Nardi K, et al. Sensitization, glutamate, and the link between migraine and fibromyalgia. *Curr Pain Headache Rep* 2007;11(5):343–351.

129. Harris RE, Clauw DJ. How do we know that the pain in fibromyalgia is "real"? *Curr Pain Headache Rep* 2006;10(6):403–407.

130. Giovengo SL, Russell IJ, Larson AA. Increased concentrations of nerve growth factor in cerebrospinal fluid of patients with fibromyalgia. *J Rheumatol* 1999;26(7):1564–1569.

131. Vaerøy H, Sakurada T, Førre O, et al. Modulation of pain in fibromyalgia (fibrositis syndrome): cerebrospinal fluid (CSF) investigation of pain related neuropeptides with special reference to calcitonin gene related peptide (CGRP). *J Rheumatol Suppl* 1989;19:94–97.

132. Höcherl K, Färber L, Ladenburger S, et al. Effect of tropisetron on circulating catecholamines and other putative biochemical markers in serum of patients with fibromyalgia. *Scand J Rheumatol Suppl* 2000;113:46–48.

133. Mountz JM, Bradley LA, Modell JG, et al. Fibromyalgia in women. Abnormalities of regional cerebral blood flow in the thalamus and the caudate nucleus are associated with low pain threshold levels. *Arthritis Rheum* 1995;38(7):926–938.

134. Kwiatek R, Barnden L, Tedman R, et al. Regional cerebral blood flow in fibromyalgia: single-photon-emission computed tomography evidence of reduction in the pontine tegmentum and thalami. *Arthritis Rheum* 2000;43(12):2823–2833.

135. Guedj E, Taieb D, Cammilleri S, et al. 99mTc-ECD brain perfusion SPECT in hyperalgesic fibromyalgia. *Eur J Nucl Med Mol Imaging* 2007;34(1):130–134.

136. Guedj E, Cammilleri S, Colavolpe C, et al. Predictive value of brain perfusion SPECT for ketamine response in hyperalgesic fibromyalgia. *Eur J Nucl Med Mol Imaging* 2007;34(8):1274–1279.

137. Adigüzel O, Kaptanoglu E, Turgut B, et al. The possible effect of clinical recovery on regional cerebral blood flow deficits in fibromyalgia: a prospective study with semiquantitative SPECT. *South Med J* 2004;97(7):651–655.

138. Gracely RH, Petzke F, Wolf JM, et al. Functional magnetic resonance imaging evidence of augmented pain processing in fibromyalgia. *Arthritis Rheum* 2002;46(5):1333–1343.

139. Cook DB, Lange G, Ciccone DS, et al. Functional imaging of pain in patients with primary fibromyalgia. *J Rheumatol* 2004;31(2):364–378.

140. Giesecke T, Gracely RH, Williams DA, et al. The relationship between depression, clinical pain, and experimental pain in a chronic pain cohort. *Arthritis Rheum* 2005;52:1577–1584.

141. Gracely RH, Geisser ME, Giesecke T, et al. Pain catastrophizing and neural responses to pain among persons with fibromyalgia. *Brain* 2004;127(Pt 4):835–843.

142. Yunus MB, Young CS, Saeed AS, et al. Positron emission tomography (PET) imaging of the brain in fibromyalgia syndrome (FM) [abstract]. *Arthritis Rheum* 1997;40(95):S188.

143. Alanoglu E, Ulas UH, Ozdag F, et al. Auditory event-related brain potentials in fibromyalgia syndrome. *Rheumatol Int* 2005;25(5):345–349.

144. Ozgocmen S, Yoldas T, Kamanli A, et al. Auditory P300 event related potentials and serotonin reuptake inhibitor treatment in patients with fibromyalgia. *Ann Rheum Dis* 2003;62(6):551–555.

145. Yoldas T, Ozgocmen S, Yildizhan H, et al. Auditory p300 event-related potentials in fibromyalgia patients. *Yonsei Med J* 2003;44(1):89–93.

146. Klein R, Berg PA. High incidence of antibodies to 5-hydroxytryptamine, gangliosides and phospholipids in patients with chronic fatigue and fibromyalgia syndrome and their relatives: evidence for a clinical entity of both disorders. *Eur J Med Res* 1995;1(1):21–26.

147. Russell IJ, Michalek JE, Vipraio GA, et al. Serum amino acids in fibrositis/fibromyalgia syndrome. *J Rheum* 1989;19:158–163.

148. Wallace D, Bowman RL, Wormsley SB, et al. Cytokines and immune regulation in patients with fibrositis [letter] [published erratum appears in *Arthritis Rheum* 1989 Dec;32(12):1607]. *Arthritis Rheum* 1989;32(10):1334–1335.

149. Gur A, Karakoc M, Erdogan S, et al. Regional cerebral blood flow and cytokines in young females with fibromyalgia. *Clin Exp Rheumatol* 2002;20(6):753–760.

150. Gur A, Karakoc M, Nas K, et al. Cytokines and depression in cases with fibromyalgia. *J Rheumatol* 2002;29(2):358–361.

151. Larson AA, Giovengo SL, Russell IJ, et al. Changes in the concentrations of amino acids in the cerebrospinal fluid that correlate with pain in patients with fibromyalgia: implications for nitric oxide pathways. *Pain* 2000;87(2):201–211.

152. Elenkov IJ, Wilder RL, Chrousos GP, et al. The sympathetic nerve—an integrative interface between two supersystems: the brain and the immune system. *Pharmacol Rev* 2000;52(4):595–638.

153. Wallace DJ, Linker–Israeli M, Hallegua D, et al. Cytokines play an aetiopathogenetic role in fibromyalgia: a hypothesis and pilot study. *Rheumatology (Oxford)* 2001;40(7):743–749.

154. Drewes AM, Andreasen A, Schroder HD, et al. Pathology of skeletal muscle in fibromyalgia: a histo-immuno-chemical and ultrastructural study. *Br J Rheumatol* 1993;32(6):479–483.

155. Bennett RM, Jacobsen S. Muscle function and origin of pain in fibromyalgia. *Baillieres Clin Rheumatol* 1994;8(4):721–746.

156. Geel SE. The fibromyalgia syndrome: musculoskeletal pathophysiology. *Semin Arthritis Rheum* 1994;23(5):347–353.

157. Simms RW, Roy SH, Hrovat M, et al. Lack of association between fibromyalgia syndrome and abnormalities in muscle energy metabolism. *Arthritis Rheum* 1994;37(6):794–800.

158. Park JH, Phothimat P, Oates CT, et al. Use of P-31 magnetic resonance spectroscopy to detect metabolic abnormalities in muscles of patients with fibromyalgia. *Arthritis Rheum* 1998;41(3):406–413.

159. Caro XJ, Winter EF, Dumas AJ. A subset of fibromyalgia patients have findings suggestive of chronic inflammatory demyelinating polyneuropathy and appear to respond to IVIg. *Rheumatology (Oxford)* 2008;47(2):208–211.

160. Kim SH, Kim DH, Oh DH, et al. Characteristic electron microscopic findings in the skin of patients with fibromyalgia: preliminary study. *Clin Rheumatol* 2008;27(2):219–213.

161. Sundgren PC, Petrou M, Harris RE, et al. Diffusion-weighted and diffusion tensor imaging in fibromyalgia patients: a prospective study of whole brain diffusivity, apparent diffusion coefficient, and fraction anisotropy in different regions of the brain and correlation with symptom severity. *Acad Radiol* 2007;14(7):839–846.

162. Kuchinad A, Schweinhardt P, Seminowicz DA, et al. Accelerated brain gray matter loss in fibromyalgia patients: premature aging of the brain? *J Neurosci* 2007;27(15):4004–4007.

163. Older SA, Battafarano DF, Danning CL, et al. The effects of delta wave sleep interruption on pain thresholds and fibromyalgia-like symptoms in healthy subjects; correlations with insulin-like growth factor I. *J Rheumatol* 1998;25(6):1180–1186.

164. Branco J, Atalaia A, Paiva T. Sleep cycles and alpha-delta sleep in fibromyalgia syndrome. *J Rheumatol* 1994;21(6):1113–1117.

165. Drewes AM, Svendsen L. Quantification of alpha-EEG activity during sleep in fibromyalgia: a study based on ambulatory sleep monitoring. *J Musculoskelet Pain* 1994;2(4):33–53.

166. Landis CA, Lentz MJ, Rothermel J, et al. Decreased sleep spindles and spindle activity in midlife women with fibromyalgia and pain. *Sleep* 2004;27(4):741–750.

167. Rizzi M, Sarzi–Puttini P, Atzeni F, et al. Cyclic alternating pattern: a new marker of sleep alteration in patients with fibromyalgia? *J Rheumatol* 2004;31(6):1193–1199.

168. Sarzi–Puttini P, Rizzi M, Andreoli A, et al. Hypersomnolence in fibromyalgia syndrome. *Clin Exp Rheumatol* 2002;20(1):69–72.

169. Sergi M, Rizzi M, Braghiroli A, et al. Periodic breathing during sleep in patients affected by fibromyalgia syndrome. *Eur Respir J* 1999;14(1):203–208.

170. Sadeh A, Carskadon MA, Acebo C, et al. Chronic fatigue immune dysfunction syndrome: an epidemic? [comments in *Pediatrics* 1991;88(2):195–202]. *Pediatrics* 1992;89(4 Pt 2):803–804.

171. Korszun A, Young EA, Engleberg NC, et al. Use of actigraphy for monitoring sleep and activity levels in patients with fibromyalgia and depression. *J Psychosom Res* 2002;52(6):439–443.

172. Landis CA, Frey CA, Lentz MJ, et al. Self-reported sleep quality and fatigue correlates with actigraphy in midlife women with fibromyalgia. *Nurs Res* 2003;52(3):140–147.

173. Edinger JD, Wohlgemuth WK, Krystal AD, et al. Behavioral insomnia therapy for fibromyalgia patients: a randomized clinical trial. *Arch Intern Med* 2005;165(21):2527–2535.

174. Edinger JD, Wohlgemuth WK, Krystal AD, et al. Behavioral insomnia therapy for fibromyalgia patients: a randomized clinical trial. *Arch Intern Med* 2005;165(21):2527–2535.

175. Kop WJ, Lyden A, Berlin AA, et al. Ambulatory monitoring of physical activity and symptoms in fibromyalgia and chronic fatigue syndrome. *Arthritis Rheum* 2005;52(1):296–303.

176. Boissevain MD, McCain GA. Toward an integrated understanding of fibromyalgia syndrome. I. Medical and pathophysiological aspects. *Pain* 1991;45(3):227–238.

177. Epstein SA, Kay GG, Clauw DJ, et al. Psychiatric disorders in patients with fibromyalgia. A multicenter investigation. *Psychosomatics* 1999;40(1):57–63.

178. White KP, Nielson WR, Harth M, et al. Does the label "fibromyalgia" alter health status, function, and health service utilization? A prospective, within-group comparison in a community cohort of adults with chronic widespread pain. *Arthritis Rheum* 2002;47(3):260–265.

179. Hadler NM. If you have to prove you are ill, you can't get well. The object lesson of fibromyalgia. *Spine* 1996;21(20):2397–2400.

180. Hawley DJ, Wolfe F. Pain, disability, and pain/disability relationships in seven rheumatic disorders: a study of 1,522 patients. *J Rheumatol* 1991;18(10):1552–1557.

181. Callahan LF, Smith WJ, Pincus T. Self-report questionnaires in five rheumatic diseases: comparisons of health status constructs and associations with formal education level. *Arthritis Care Res* 1989;2(4):122–131.

182. Turk DC, Okifuji A, Sinclair JD, et al. Pain, disability, and physical function-ing in subgroups of patients with fibromyalgia. *J Rheumatol* 1996;23(7):1255–1262.

183. Giesecke T, Williams DA, Harris RE, et al. Subgrouping of fibromyalgia patients on the basis of pressure-pain thresholds and psychological factors. *Arthritis Rheum* 2003;48(10):2916–2922.

184. Tan EM, Feltkamp TE, Smolen JS, et al. Range of antinuclear antibodies in "healthy" individuals. *Arthritis Rheum* 1997;40(9):1601–1611.

185. Pincus T. A pragmatic approach to cost-effective use of laboratory tests and imaging procedures in patients with musculoskeletal symptoms. *Primary Care* 1993;20(4):795–814.

186. Jensen MC, Brant–Zawadzki MN, Obuchowski N, et al. Magnetic resonance imaging of the lumbar spine in people without back pain. *N Engl J Med* 1994;331(2):69–73.

187. Wolfe F. The relation between tender points and fibromyalgia symptom variables: evidence that fibromyalgia is not a discrete disorder in the clinic. *Ann Rheum Dis* 1997;56(4):268–271.

188. Goldenberg DL, Burckhardt C, Crofford L. Management of fibromyalgia syndrome. *JAMA* 2004;292(19):2388–2395.

189. Capaci K, Hepguler S. Comparison of the effects of amitriptyline and paroxetine in the treatment of fibromyalgia syndrome. *The Pain Clinic* 2002;14(3):223–228.

190. Anderberg UM, Marteinsdottir I, Von Knorring L. Citalopram in patients with fibromyalgia—a randomized, double-blind, placebo-controlled study. *Eur J Pain* 2000;4(1):27–35.

191. Norregaard J, Volkmann H, Danneskiold–Samsoe B. A randomized controlled trial of citalopram in the treatment of fibromyalgia. *Pain* 1995;61(3):445–449.

192. Fishbain D. Evidence-based data on pain relief with antidepressants. *Ann Med* 2000;32(5):305–316.

193. Adelman LC, Adelman JU, Von Seggern R, et al. Venlafaxine extended release (XR) for the prophylaxis of migraine and tension-type headache: a retrospective study in a clinical setting. *Headache* 2000;40(7):572–580.

194. Vitton O, Gendreau M, Gendreau J, et al. A double-blind placebo-controlled trial of milnacipran in the treatment of fibromyalgia. *Hum Psychopharmacol* 2004;19(Suppl 1):S27–S35.

195. Wiffen P, Collins S, McQuay H, et al. Anticonvulsant drugs for acute and chronic pain. *Cochrane Database Syst Rev* 2000;(3):CD001133.

196. Crofford LJ, Rowbotham MC, Mease PJ, et al. Pregabalin for the treatment of fibromyalgia syndrome: results of a randomized, double-blind, placebo-controlled trial. *Arthritis Rheum* 2005;52(4):1264–1273.

197. Redillas C, Solomon S. Prophylactic pharmacological treatment of chronic daily headache. *Headache* 2000;40(2):83–102.

198. Scharf MB, Baumann M, Berkowitz DV. The effects of sodium oxybate on clinical symptoms and sleep patterns in patients with fibromyalgia. *J Rheumatol* 2003;30(5):1070–1074.

199. Bennett RM. Pharmacological treatment of fibromyalgia. *J Funct Syndr* 2001;1(1):79–92.

200. Holman AJ, Myers RR. A randomized, double-blind, placebo-controlled trial of pramipexole, a dopamine agonist, in patients with fibromyalgia receiving concomitant medications. *Arthritis Rheum* 2005; 52(8):2495–2505.

201. Russell IJ, et al. Therapy with a central alpha 2-adrenergic agonist (tizanidine) decreases cerebrospinal fluid substance P, and may reduce serum hyaluronic acid as it improves the clinical symptoms of the fibromyalgia syndrome. *Arthritis Rheum* 2002;46(9):S614.

202. Williams DA, Cary MA, Glazer LJ, et al. Randomized controlled trial of CBT to improve functional status in fibromyalgia. *Am Col Rheum* 2000;43(9):S210.

203. Levine PH, Krueger GR, Straus SE. A postviral chronic fatigue syndrome: a round table. *J Infect Dis* 1989;160(4):722–724.

204. Assefi NP, Sherman KJ, Jacobsen C, et al. A randomized clinical trial of acupuncture compared with sham acupuncture in fibromyalgia. *Ann Intern Med* 2005;143(1):10–19.

205. Littlejohn G. The fibromyalgia syndrome. Outcome is good with minimal intervention [letter]. *BMJ* 1995;310(6991):1406.

206. Macfarlane GJ, Thomas E, Papageorgiou AC, et al. The natural history of chronic pain in the community: a better prognosis than in the clinic? *J Rheum* 1996;23(9):1617–1620.

207. Wolfe F, Anderson J, Harkness D, et al. Work and disability status of persons with fibromyalgia. *J Rheumatol* 1997;24(6):1171–1178.

208. Dinerman H, Goldenberg DL, Felson DT. A prospective evaluation of 118 patients with the fibromyalgia syndrome: prevalence of Raynaud's phenomenon, sicca symptoms, ANA, low complement, and Ig deposition at the dermal-epidermal junction. *J Rheumatol* 1986;13(2):368–373.

209. Wolfe F, Anderson J, Harkness D, et al. Health status and disease severity in fibromyalgia: results of a six–center longitudinal study [see comments in *Arthritis Rheum* 1997;40(9):1553–1555]. *Arthritis Rheum* 1997;40(9):1571–1579.

CHAPTER 37 ■ PAIN OF DERMATOLOGIC DISORDERS

JOSEPH C. LANGLOIS AND JOHN E. OLERUD

INTRODUCTION

Pain is not as distinctive a feature of dermatologic disorders as is the related disorder of pruritus, which is beyond the scope of this discussion. It is well known that pruritus appears to be so intolerable that the act of scratching inflicts a transient pain with attendant structural damage to the skin. It is generally considered that the induced pain is subjectively more tolerable than the itching. Nonetheless, pain is a distinctive feature of certain dermatologic disorders and merits attention simply because of the great prevalence of skin disorders. Dermatologic disease of sufficient significance that it should be seen by a physician is present in 30% of the population in the United States. Half of all problems related to skin present to primary care physicians other than dermatologists. Of the 12 most common disorders of skin disease, only herpes simplex is attended by pain symptoms. Herpes simplex has a seroprevalence rate of 57% in a random sample of nonhospitalized U.S. civilians as reported in the NHANES data base for 1999–2004.[1] The effects of pain on the patient are best demonstrated by the impact of the persisting pain that sometimes follows herpes zoster, postherpetic neuralgia, which occasionally leads to suicide. This disease is discussed in Chapter 27, but this chapter focuses attention not only on the impact of pain but also on the need for appropriate recognition of the antecedent viral disease and on the value of immediate and appropriate treatment.

The diseases discussed in this chapter can be grouped into the categories of vasculitis, infections of viral and bacterial origin, inflammatory diseases of the subcutaneous space, and neoplasms. Some neoplasms, although benign, are specifically painful based on their neurovascular components. We discuss the causes and pathogenesis of the selected pain-related skin diseases, paying attention to symptoms and signs, methods of diagnosis, and preferred methods of treatment. For more comprehensive discussions of the individual diseases, refer to selected general textbooks of skin disease.[2–5] Because of space limitations, vasculitides and tumors are described in Table 37.1.

BASIC CONSIDERATIONS: ANATOMY AND PHYSIOLOGY OF THE SKIN

Human skin is a vast, sheet-like interface for the organism with its environment. It is adapted to the dryness of the atmosphere, resisting mechanical shearing and puncturing forces as well as the invasion of chemical and infective agents. This organ, which in aggregate covers an area of more than 2 m^2, has a mass greater than that of any other organ. It contains an extensive vascular and sweat gland system, essential for thermal regulation, and an even more extensive and finely attuned neuroreceptor network, including the varied transducers of pain and other sensations (Fig. 37.1).

The skin is covered by a thin, stratified epithelium, the epidermis, which is only 75 to 100 micrometers thick except on the palms and soles, where it is four to five times thicker. The bulk of the skin is fibroelastic dense connective tissue known as the *dermis*, which supports the extensive network of vessels and nerves as well as the specialized glandular structure of the sweat apparatus and keratinizing appendages, such as hair and nail. The subcutaneous space is a variably fatty connective tissue perforated by collagenous septa, continuous on the outermost aspects with the fibers of the dermis and continuous beneath the skin with fascial or periosteal attachments to the skeleton.

It is generally believed that the peripheral pain receptors are the finely arborized (penicillate) free nerve endings that ramify in the superficial aspects of the dermis. This network of fine C fibers has been shown to innervate the epidermis as well (see Fig. 37.1)[6–8] and has been referred to as the *cutaneous sensory nervous system*.[9] These fibers convey information from the skin to the central nervous system and thus have a sensory role. They also have an effector function in the skin, mediated by locally releasing neuropeptides. Sensory neurons express at least 17 different neuropeptides, including substance P and calcitonin gene–related peptide.[10] The cutaneous sensory nervous system appears to play an important role in the "communication" between the nervous system and the immune system, the vascular system, and the cells of the epidermis. Neuropeptides appear to participate in vital functions such as neuroinflammation and tissue repair.[6,11] They have important biological effects on a variety of cells in the skin, including keratinocytes, endothelial cells, fibroblasts, Langerhans cells, mast cells, macrophages, and smooth muscle cells.[9] It is easy to imagine how these effector functions may participate in the perpetuation of chronic skin conditions characterized by pain or itch.

The diagnosis of skin disease depends less on deductive logic than on direct observation. One should distinguish localized nodules resulting from small tumors of the skin from the large plaquelike swellings associated with acute edema and redness that mark inflammatory processes, and umbilicated small vesicles occurring in clusters on inflammatory bases that are characteristic of the herpetic viral infections. Subtle or marked defects in the integrity of the protective epidermal sheet should be noted, as manifested by denuded sites of bullae (erosions). Also to be noted are deeper defects in the integrity of the protective barrier that involve loss of the epidermis as well as of some dermis, leading to ulcer formation. Such lesions are inevitably attended by pain, unless associated with a neuropathy, which can best be explained by exposure of free nerve endings.

CLINICAL DISORDERS

Leukocytoclastic Vasculitis

Characteristic features of vasculitis are compared in Table 37.1.

Leukocytoclastic vasculitis (LV) is a common form of vasculitis that may be confined to the skin[21] or related to systemic vascu-

TABLE 37.1

CHARACTERISTICS OF CUTANEOUS VASCULITIDES

Type	Clinical signs	Pathologic features	Immuno-fluorescence findings	Granulo-matous changes	ANCA[a] cANCA	pANCA	Allergic rhinitis, asthma, eosinophilia	Pain	Comment	Treatment
Leukocy-toclastic vasculitis	Palpable purpura on lower extremities	Infiltration and destruction of postcapillary venules by polymorpho-nuclear leukocytes with leukocy-toclasis	Immunoglobu-lins and complement (C3) in small capillaries of the upper dermis (lesions <24 hr old)	−	−	−		Small lesions are usually asymptom-atic; larger papules, nodules, and ulcers are often painful	Causative factors include infections, drugs, chemicals, serum, connective tissue diseases, and malignancy	No therapy for mild cases; antihistamines, NSAIDs, dapsone, colchicine, prednisone 7- to 10-day course starting with 60 mg/day
Polyarteritis nodosa	Tender nodules, livedo reticularis, ulcers, nodules along an artery	Leukocytoclastic vasculitis of small- and medium-sized arteries	Immunoglobulins and complement in vessel walls	−	−	−	Eosinophilia sometimes	Aching pain is characteristic of the cutaneous form, aggravated by physical activity or edema	Limited cutaneous form of polyarteritis nodosa rarely progresses to systemic polyarteritis nodosa	Prednisone 1 mg/kg/day Cyclophosphamide 2 mg/kg/day[12] For hepatitis B–related polyarteritis nodosa: corticosteroids plus plasma exchange plus interferon-α[12] or lamivudine[13]
Wegener's granuloma-tosis	Papules, papulone-crotic lesions, nodules with ulceration, subcutaneous nodules, ulcers, petechiae, ecchymotic lesions, vesicles, pustules	Necrotizing vasculitis of small arteries and veins; necrotizing granulomas	Usually negative	+	44%–90%	12%–20%	Eosinophilia sometimes	Lesions can be tender	Limited form does not have renal involvement	Prednisone 1 mg/kg/day plus oral cyclophosphamide 2 mg/kg/day[12] (higher initial intravenous doses in patients with aggressive disease)[14,15]

Disease	Cutaneous lesions	Histopathology	Immunofluorescence	ANCA	ANCA titer	Laboratory	Pain/other	Systemic involvement	Treatment
Allergic granulomatosis of Churg-Strauss	Cutaneous nodules usually on scalp and extremities; Palpable purpura	Extravascular granulomas; necrotizing vasculitis of small- or medium-sized arteries and veins	Usually negative	+	As high as 70%–78% mostly pANCA	Allergic rhinitis, asthma, eosinophilia (virtually all)	Cutaneous nodules are usually tender	Serious renal involvement is infrequent; coronary arteritis and myocarditis are principal causes of death	Prednisone 1 mg/kg/day Cytotoxic drug added if needed[12]
Microscopic polyangiitis	Palpable purpura, ulcers	Necrotizing vasculitis of small vessels; sometimes small- and medium-sized arteries	Immune deposits absent (pauci-immune)	−	38%–57% (>80% overall)	Eosinophilia sometimes	Similar to leukocytoclastic vasculitis	Renal involvement frequent; pulmonary involvement common	For patients with major organ damage, prednisone 1 mg/kg/day plus oral cyclophosphamide 2 mg/kg/day[12] (higher initial intravenous doses in patients with aggressive disease)[14]
Rheumatoid vasculitis	Petechiae, palpable purpura, leg ulcerations, nail fold, and digital infarcts, gangrene	Vasculitis of small arteries, arterioles, capillaries, or venules	Immunoglobulins and complement in vessels reported in normal skin as well as in lesional skin in rheumatoid vasculitis	−	20% (rheumatoid arthritis) pANCA		Lesions are sometimes painful	Associated with relatively severe rheumatoid arthritis	For patients with severe disease: Prednisone 0.5–1 mg/kg/d combined with other agents.[16] Pulse IV cyclophosphamide and methylprednisolone[17]
Livedoid vasculitis	Livedo reticularis, purpuric macules, papules, ulcers, stellate scarring	Hyalinizing segmental vasculitis in middle and lower dermis	Immunoglobulins, complement, and fibrin in vessel walls	−			Pain may be severe		Treat coagulation defects. Aspirin 325 mg/day plus dipyridamole 50 mg tid.[18] Pentoxifylline 400 mg tid.[19] Danazol 50–100 mg bid. Therapeutic ladder as proposed by Callen[20]

[a]ANCA, antineutrophilic cytoplasmic antibodies; cANCA, ANCA of the cytoplasmic type; pANCA, ANCA of the perinuclear type; +, present; −, absent. Modified from Braverman IM. The angiitides. In: Braverman IM, ed. Skin Signs of Systemic Disease. 3rd ed. Philadelphia: WB Saunders; 1998:311.

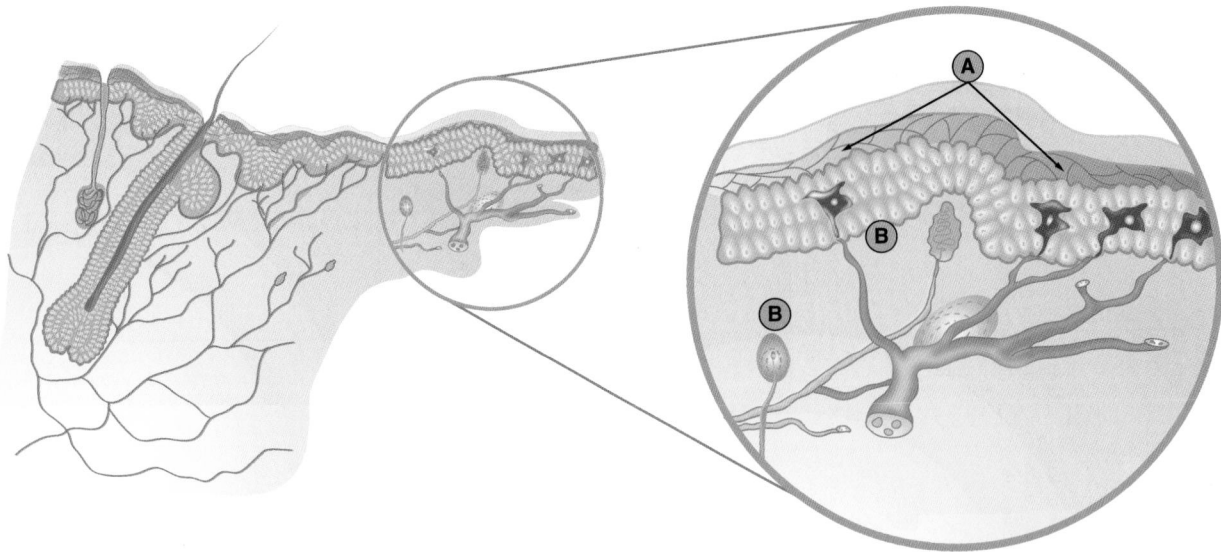

FIGURE 37.1 Schematic representations of sensory nerve formations (SNFs) for the cutaneous sensory nervous system. The SNFs depicted are the free nerve endings in the epidermis (**A**) and mechanosensors (**B**) in the dermis. Although nociception in the skin is mainly a function of free nerve endings composed of unmyelinated C fibers, more specialized SNFs for mechano- (baro-, preso-, osmo-) sensors, thermosensors, electrosensors, chemosensors, and nociosensors are also present. (Modified from Malinovsky L. Sensory nerve formations in the skin and their classification. *Microsc Res Tech* 1996;34:283–301.)

litis, connective tissue diseases, or malignancy.[22,23] LV typically affects postcapillary venules producing palpable purpura which are the clinical hallmark of the disease.[21] Although palpable purpura occurring in dependent areas (e.g., the legs and ankles in ambulatory patients and the back and sacral area in bedridden patients) is typical, a spectrum of other cutaneous lesions may occur such as papules, nodules, vesicles, bullae, pustules, ulcers, urticarial lesions, and livedo reticularis.[24,25] Purpuric lesions may often be associated with tenderness, burning, stinging, or pruritus.[21] The presence of painful skin lesions has been reported to be associated with a lower risk of systemic involvement.[26]

Histologic changes seen with LV consist primarily of infiltration of polymorphonuclear leukocytes within and/or around blood vessels and destruction of the vessel wall with fibrinoid necrosis whereas hemorrhage, nuclear dust (leukocytoclasis), endothelial changes, ulceration, necrosis, and eccrine gland necrosis are considered secondary changes.[27] The differential diagnosis of LV includes septic vasculitis and other causes of pseudovasculitis such as bacterial endocarditis, atrial myxoma with emboli, cholesterol emboli, antiphospholipid syndrome, warfarin-induced skin necrosis, calciphylaxis, and others.[28]

Etiology

Among the many reported etiologic factors associated with LV are infectious agents (e.g., streptococcus; hepatitis A, B, and C; and influenza), medications (e.g., penicillin, sulfonamides, beta-lactam antibiotics, phenothiazines, nonsteroidal anti-inflammatory drugs [NSAIDs], and streptomycin), serum sickness, anti-influenza vaccines, foodstuff allergens, chemicals (e.g., insecticides and petroleum products), connective tissue and inflammatory diseases (e.g., systemic lupus erythematosus [SLE], Sjögren's syndrome, rheumatoid arthritis, ulcerative colitis, and Behçet's disease), and malignancy (both lymphoproliferative and solid tumors).[21,24]

Pathogenesis

LV is felt to be principally caused by deposition of circulating immune complexes within the vessel walls of postcapillary venules,

activation of complement, infiltration by neutrophils, and release of lysosomal enzymes.[24] Other factors involved in the pathogenesis include histamine release, inflammatory cytokines, adhesion molecules, thrombosis of vessels, fibrinolysis, and cell-mediated immune response (late stages).[24] Endothelial cell activation and expression of E-selectin may play a role in recruiting polymorphonuclear leukocytes to the site.[29] Immunoglobulins and complement can be detected in vessel walls by direct immunofluorescence in early lesions that are less than 24 hours old (preferably less than 4 hours).[25] Patients who develop leg ulcers from LV have been reported to have an increased incidence of hypercoagulability related to factor V Leiden and lupus anticoagulant.[30]

Patients who present with LV need to be evaluated for systemic involvement particularly for involvement of kidneys, joints, gastrointestinal tract, and pulmonary and nervous systems. They may need to be reclassified depending on the type of systemic involvement according to the Chapel Hill Consensus Conference nomenclature.[31] If no systemic involvement is found, patients need to be followed over time because some patients develop systemic involvement later.

Subsets or variants of LV include urticarial vasculitis, Henoch-Schönlein purpura, and cryoglobulinemic vasculitis. Hepatitis C is an important cause of mixed cryoglobulinemic vasculitis and is responsible for the majority of cases that have an infectious etiology.[32,33]

Treatment

Any underlying infections such as group A streptococcal infections should be treated, suspect medications stopped, and other potential etiologic agents avoided. Any associated connective tissue diseases should be treated and the patient evaluated for underlying malignancy if another etiology is not found.

Specific treatment for the vasculitis should be tailored to the severity of the disease. For patients who are asymptomatic or have mild disease, options include no treatment, antihistamines, and NSAID drugs. Dapsone and colchicine may be beneficial. A prospective randomized controlled trial of colchicine showed no overall significant benefit but a few individual patients may have benefited.[34] A short course of systemic corticosteroids may be useful for an acute exacerbation of the disease. For patients with more severe and recalcitrant disease azathioprine, cyclosporine, IVIG, and plasmapheresis are considerations.[21] Tumor necrosis factor (TNF) inhibitors have been reported to both cause and treat vasculitis.[35] Rituximab has been reported to be effective in some cases but further studies are needed to determine its long term safety and effectiveness.[36]

Polyarteritis Nodosa

Polyarteritis nodosa is an uncommon form of vasculitis affecting small- and medium-sized arteries. Two forms of cutaneous involvement can occur: benign cutaneous and systemic.

Symptoms and Signs

Cutaneous polyarteritis nodosa characteristically is manifested by tender nodules, livedo reticularis, and ulcers. It may also be associated with myalgias, arthralgias, neuropathy, and fever.[37,38] Patients may have periodic flareups or exacerbations of their disease, but the long-term course of their disease is generally benign. Progression to systemic polyarteritis nodosa is rare, but has been reported. Patients need long-term follow-up to monitor for this possibility.[39]

Systemic polyarteritis nodosa may have cutaneous involvement in up to 60% patients manifested most commonly as palpable purpura, bullae, and ulcerations and less commonly as nodules, livedo reticularis, and gangrene.[37,40,41] Nodules can sometimes be palpable along the course of an artery.[42]

In both forms of polyarteritis nodosa, leukocytoclastic vasculitis affects small- and medium-sized arteries of the skin[37,38] with IgM, fibrin, or C3 demonstrable on direct immunofluorescence.[37] Angiogenic cytokines have been reported to be elevated in serum and tissue in some patients with systemic and cutaneous polyarteritis nodosa reflecting vascular injury and repair.[43]

Hepatitis B, hepatitis C, streptococcal infection, Crohn's disease, Takayatsu arteritis, tuberculosis, and relapsing polychondritis are reported associations with both cutaneous and systemic polyarteritis nodosa.[39,44,45] In addition, cutaneous polyarteritis nodosa has been reported in association with ulcerative colitis[46] as a reaction to minocycline[47] and in a single report as a reaction to conjugated estrogen.[48]

Treatment

The benign cutaneous form of polyarteritis nodosa usually responds to systemic corticosteroids alone. Response to other treatments is less predictable. Other treatments that have been used include NSAIDs, sulfapyridine, dapsone, azathioprine, colchicine, pentoxifylline, and hydroxylchloroquine.[37,38] Low dose methotrexate, cyclophosphamide, and intravenous immune globulin have also been used with variable response.[49] Patients with streptococcal induced cutaneous polyarteritis nodosa should be treated with penicillin and may need long-term prophylaxis, especially in children where streptococcal induced disease appears to be more common.[37,38,49,50] General supportive measures include rest, medications for pain, local wound care for ulcerated lesions, and antibiotics for secondary infection.

Severe systemic polyarteritis nodosa is treated with prednisone 1 mg/kg/day plus cyclophosphamide 2 mg/kg/day similar to the treatment for Wegener's granulomatosis while milder cases have been treated with prednisone alone.[12] Patients on cyclophosphamide and prednisone need to be closely monitored to keep the leukocyte count above 3000/μL and the absolute neutrophil count around 1500/μL. The prednisone is converted to an alternate day regimen after 1 month and then tapered over about 6 months. The patient is slowly tapered off the cyclophosphamide after being in remission for 1 year.[12] Close monitoring for side effects of treatment is essential. Potential side effects of cyclophos-

phamide include neutropenia, sepsis, hemorrhagic cystitis, hair loss, gonadal dysfunction, and neoplasia. Measures to prevent osteoporosis are also indicated. Pulse cyclophosphamide plus corticosteroids have been advocated to reduce the total dose and toxicity from cyclophosphamide.[51,52] Because of higher relapse rates in Wegener's granulomatosis with the same regimen, Sneller et al. strongly recommend oral daily cyclophosphamide rather than pulse therapy.[12]

Systemic polyarteritis nodosa related to hepatitis B is best treated with systemic corticosteroids in combination with plasma exchange to clear immune complexes and either interferon-α[12] or lamivudine.[13]

Wegener's Granulomatosis

Wegener's granulomatosis is an uncommon disease of unknown cause characterized by necrotizing vasculitis and granulomatous inflammation involving the upper and lower respiratory tracts, together with glomerulonephritis, although more limited forms of the disease without renal involvement may occur.[14,15] Approximately 90% of patients, when in the active stage of their disease, have antineutrophilic cytoplasmic antibodies (ANCA) of the cytoplasmic type (cANCA) directed at proteinase 3.[15] The pathogenesis of Wegener's granulomatosis is poorly understood. There is limited evidence that ANCA antibodies of the cANCA type are involved in the pathogenesis of Wegener's granulomatosis. Bacterial peptides from *Staphylococcus aureus* and other bacteria share homology with peptides of complementary proteinase 3 suggesting infection may initiate an autoimmune response.[53]

Symptoms and Signs

Cutaneous lesions occur in approximately 45% of patients and include palpable purpura, ulcers, vesicles, papules, nodules, necrotic papules, and pustules.[15,54] Pyoderma gangrenosum-like ulcerations may occur.[55] Papules, nodules, and ulcerative lesions may be tender or painful.[54,56,57] The upper airway is frequently affected and manifestations include oral ulcerations and gingival hyperplasia with petechiae.[54] Friable gingival hyperplasia with petechiae is said to be pathognomonic of Wegener's granulomatosis.[57–59] Saddle nose deformity occurs in some patients, but is a rare manifestation.[55] On biopsy of cutaneous lesions one may see small vessel vasculitis, granulomatous dermatitis, and, least commonly, granulomatous vasculitis. Not all changes may be seen in the same specimen.[60]

Treatment

The treatment of choice for Wegener's granulomatosis is daily oral cyclophosphamide, 2 mg/kg daily plus prednisone 1 mg/kg daily.[12,14,15] Some patients with aggressive disease have been given higher initial IV doses.[14,15] Daily prednisone is continued on a daily dosage for 2 to 4 weeks, then converted to an alternate-day regimen over several months and finally tapered off. Patients are kept on cyclophosphamide for 1 year after achieving remission and then tapered off in 25-mg decrements every 2 to 3 months.[15] Methotrexate and azathioprine are potential substitutes for cyclophosphamide when patients are in remission to diminish long-term toxicity from cyclophosphamide.[12] Patients on cyclophosphamide need careful monitoring to keep the leukocyte count above 3000 per μL and the absolute neutrophil count around 1500 per μL. Patients also need close monitoring for other potential side effects of cyclophosphamide including sepsis, hemorrhagic cystitis, hair loss, gonadal dysfunction, and neoplasia. The complications of prolonged corticosteroid use can also occur and measures should be implemented to prevent osteoporosis. Prophylaxis for pneumocystic pneumonia with trimethoprim-sulfamethoxazole is also recommended unless the patient is allergic to the medication.[12]

Pulsed IV cyclophosphamide has been used instead of daily oral cyclophosphamide to lower the total dose and toxicity of cyclophosphamide but there is a higher frequency of relapses[61,62] leading Sneller et al.[12] to strongly recommend daily oral cyclophosphamide over pulse therapy. For patients with milder disease on initial presentation, treatment with methotrexate and glucocorticoids may be considered.[63,12] Trimethoprim-sulfamethoxazole has been advocated by some for prevention of relapse,[64] but only felt to prevent upper airway relapse and not serious internal organ relapse by others.[12] Etanercept was found to be ineffective in maintaining remissions and was associated with increased risk of neoplasia.[65] Rituximab has shown promise in a prospective open label pilot study in inducing and maintaining remissions.[66]

Microscopic Polyangiitis

Microscopic polyangiitis is a systemic small vessel vasculitis commonly affecting the kidneys, lungs, and skin. The vasculitis affects arterioles, capillaries, venules, and sometimes small- and medium-sized arteries with few or no immune deposits evident on direct immunofluorescence (pauci-immune).[31] Positive ANCA, usually of the perinuclear type (pANCA), also referred to as myeloperoxidase-ANCA, has been reported in >80% patients.[14] There is experimental evidence to suggest that myeloperoxidase-ANCA may be involved in the pathogenesis of vasculitis.[53]

Microscopic polyangiitis as defined by the Chapel Hill Consensus Conference is distinguished from cutaneous leukocytoclastic vasculitis by the presence of systemic involvement and the absence of immune deposits on direct immunofluorescence.[31] Both of these distinguishing features are time dependent. Patients initially presenting with cutaneous leukocytoclastic vasculitis need to be followed over time to determine whether systemic involvement will occur and immune deposits in vessel walls of the skin in leukocytoclastic vasculitis typically disappear in lesions more than 24 hours old.[67]

Cutaneous involvement has been reported in 44% to 62% patients with microscopic polyangiitis.[40] Purpura is commonly reported but a variety of other cutaneous manifestations have been reported including purpuric macules and papules, vesicles, bullae, splinter hemorrhages, nodules, cutaneous necrosis, digital infarction, gangrene, pyoderma gangrenosum-like ulcerations, livedo reticularis, facial edema, urticaria, orogenital ulceration, and erythema elevatum diutinum.[40,68–73] Although not focused on specifically in reports, ischemic pain would be expected as in other forms of vasculitis, particularly with ulcers, infarction, and gangrene.

Treatment

Serious major organ involvement, such as pulmonary or renal disease, is treated with a combination of corticosteroids and cyclophosphamide similar to Wegener's granulomatosis.[12,14] Higher IV doses initially have been recommended for patients with aggressive disease.[14]

Allergic Granulomatosis of Churg-Strauss

Churg-Strauss syndrome is a rare syndrome characterized by allergic rhinitis, asthma, eosinophilia, granulomatous inflammation, and systemic vasculitis affecting small- to medium-sized arteries.[14,31] Pulmonary involvement and cardiac involvement are common with coronary arteritis and myocarditis being the principal cause of death whereas renal involvement is relatively less common and tends to be mild.[14,40] Histologically, one sees a vasculitis affecting small vessels, extravascular granulomas, tissue infiltration with eosinophils, and an absence of vascular immune deposits on direct immunofluorescence.[60] As high as 70% to 78%

of patients have positive ANCA, usually of the perinuclear type (pANCA), directed at myeloperoxidase.[14,74] Two recent reports indicated a positive ANCA in about 40% cases.[75,76] There is some evidence that ANCA antibodies of the myeloperoxidase-ANCA (pANCA) type and less convincing evidence that antibodies of the cANCA type are involved in the pathogenesis of vasculitis.[53]

Symptoms and Signs

Cutaneous lesions occur in up to 75% of patients.[77] The most common cutaneous findings are palpable purpura on the lower extremities and skin nodules.[78] Among the many other reported cutaneous manifestations are papules, plaques, petechiae, ulcers, infarcts, bullae, wheals, and livedo reticularis.[79] More recently described variations include severe digital gangrene associated with antiphospholipid antibodies[80] and purpura fulminans.[81] Pain or tenderness is characteristic of the skin nodules[82] and also likely occurs on an ischemic basis in some vasculitic lesions as well.

Treatment

The treatment of choice for Churg-Strauss syndrome is corticosteroids which usually controls the disease. For patients who do not respond or present initially with fulminant disease the addition of daily cyclophosphamide is recommended based on its success in treating other serious vasculitic disorders.[83] Pulsed IV cyclophosphamide plus corticosteroids have been recommended by some to lower the total dose and toxicity of cyclophosphamide compared to daily oral cyclophosphamide.[51,74] Careful monitoring of patients for side effects and complications of corticosteroids and cyclophosphamide is essential. Pulsed IV cyclophosphamide plus corticosteroids has also been advocated as first line therapy in patients with one or more poor prognostic factors (proteinuria >1 gm/day, creatinine >1.58 mg/dL [>140 μmol/L], cardiomyopathy, gastrointestinal involvement, and central nervous system involvement) and as second line therapy in patients who relapse on corticosteroids.[77] Patients may be switched from cyclophosphamide to a less toxic steroid sparing agent (e.g., azathioprine, when in remission).[77] There is limited information on some other reported therapies such as IVIG, plasma exchanges, rituximab, interferon alpha, and mycophenylate mofetil.[16,84,85]

Rheumatoid Vasculitis

Rheumatoid vasculitis is a systemic vasculitis that may affect vessels of different sizes including capillaries and small- and medium-sized arteries. It tends to occur in patients with more severe rheumatoid arthritis of long standing duration and high titer rheumatoid factor.[16,85,86] The diagnostic criteria as originally proposed by Scott and Bacon[17] included rheumatoid arthritis (meeting ARA criteria) plus one or more of the following: (1) mononeuritis multiplex, (2) peripheral gangrene, (3) biopsy evidence of acute necrotizing arteritis plus systemic illness such as fever or weight loss, and (4) deep cutaneous ulcers or active extra-articular disease (e.g., pleurisy, pericarditis, scleritis) if associated with typical digital infarcts or biopsy evidence of vasculitis.[17]

Histologically, one finds a vasculitis that may be leukocytoclastic, granulomatous, or lymphocytic.[84,87] IgM and/or complement was found on direct immunofluorescence in vessel walls in 6 of 7 patients by Chen et al. consistent with immune complex mediated vasculitis.[84] Immunoglobulins and complement are also commonly found in the normal skin of patients with rheumatoid arthritis and have been found to correlate with more severe extra-articular disease, vasculitis, and circulating immune complexes.[88]

Cutaneous manifestations are one of the most common features of the disease (up to 90% patients) and include petechiae, palpable purpura, hemorrhagic blisters, ulcerations, nailfold and digital infarcts, subcutaneous nodules, livedo reticularis, atrophie blanche, gangrene, maculopapular erythematous rashes, and, rarely, erythema elevatum diutinum and pyoderma gangrenosum.[16,84,85] Ulcerations and gangrene may by painful on an ischemic basis.

Treatment

Patients with isolated nailfold infarcts (Bywaters lesions) require no treatment. Patients with more severe disease are treated with systemic agents. The only placebo-controlled study to date conducted with azathioprine demonstrated no clinical benefit.[89] Prednisone 0.5 to1 mg/kg/day in combination with other agents is often used in patients with more severe disease.[16] IV pulse cyclophosphamide plus methylprednisolone was found to be more effective than other treatments in one study.[17] Patients need to be monitored closely for complications of treatment particularly neutropenia, sepsis, or both. TNF alpha inhibitors, as reviewed by Genta et al., have been reported to be effective in treating rheumatoid vasculitis but also may cause vasculitis.[16]

Livedoid Vasculitis (Livedoid Vasculopathy)

Livedoid vasculopathy is an uncommon disease characterized by livedo reticularis and purpuric papules and exquisitely painful ulcerations on the lower extremities that heal with white atrophic scars, telangiectasias, and surrounding hyperpigmentation.[25,90] Some patients have associated medical conditions. Among the most common in a recent series of patients were venous insufficiency, deep venous thrombosis, and connective tissue diseases.[90] A lengthy list of coagulation disorders have also been reported in some patients with livedoid vasculopathy and reviewed by Calamia et al.[91]

The histologic changes seen on biopsy of livedoid vasculopathy include intimal proliferation, hyalinization of the intima, fibrinoid material in the vessel wall or lumen, and varying levels of inflammation but no leukocytoclasis.[92] The histologic changes have been referred to as segmental hyalinizing vasculitis in the past.[93] Direct immunofluorescence usually demonstrates fibrin, C3, and IgM in vessel walls.[94]

A question arises as to how extensively to evaluate patients for underlying coagulation disorders. Hairston et al. recommend the following studies: complete blood cell (CBC) count, cryoglobulins, cryofibrinogens, homocyteine, ANA, anticardiolipin antibody, lupus anticoagulant, protein C and S levels, factor V Leiden gene mutation, prothrombin gene mutation (G20210A), and beta 2 glycoprotein 1 antibody.[90]

Treatment

General supportive measures for livedoid vasculopathy include avoidance of smoking, rest, antibiotics for secondary infection, local wound care for ulcerations, and pain control.

Any underlying coagulation disorders should be treated. In the absence of any specific defects a reasonable initial approach to therapy would be aspirin 325 mg/day plus dipyridamole 50 mg three times daily[18] and/or pentoxifylline 400 mg three times daily.[19] One of the authors has obtained good results with danazol 50 to 100 mg twice daily. Low-dose danazol was reported to be effective in two patients by Hsiao et al.[95] The literature on treatment of livedoid vasculopathy consists of case reports or small series with no controlled studies. Other treatments reported to be effective include low or minidose heparin,[96,97] low molecular weight heparin,[98] warfarin,[99] phenformin and ethylestranol,[100] tissue plasminogen activator,[101,102] nicotinic acid,[93] nicotinamide,[93] nifedipine,[103] PUVA therapy,[104] hyperbaric oxygen,[105] and intravenous immunoglobulin.[106] Treatment should

be individualized. The concept of a therapeutic ladder as proposed by Callen with treatments with more potentially serious side effects higher on the ladder is a sound one.[20]

OTHER VASCULAR DISORDERS

Antiphospholipid Syndrome

The antiphospholipid syndrome (APS) is an uncommon syndrome characterized by thrombotic occlusion of arteries and/or veins, complications of pregnancy (miscarriage, spontaneous abortions, and prematurity), thrombocytopenia, and positive anticardiolipin and/or lupus anticoagulant antibodies.[107–109] The anticardiolipin and/or lupus anticoagulant tests should be positive on at least two occasions at least 6 weeks apart to exclude transiently positive tests. APS may occur as a primary disorder, as a secondary disorder in patients with lupus erythematosus, and also may occur in a subset of patients with Sneddon's syndrome (livedo reticularis and multiple cerebrovascular events). Antiphospholipid antibodies in themselves are not diagnostic of antiphospholipid syndrome because they occur normally in small percentage of the normal population and have been associated with multiple other conditions.[107,110] Histologically, skin biopsies demonstrate noninflammatory thrombosis of arteries and/or veins.

Symptoms and Signs

Cutaneous manifestations of APS are common. In a recent series of 200 cases they occurred in 49% of patients with livedo reticularis, digital necrosis, subungual splinter hemorrhages, and superficial venous thrombosis being the most common.[108] Multiple other cutaneous manifestations have been reported with APS including cutaneous necrosis and gangrene, cutaneous ulcers, painful skin nodules, lesions resembling vasculitis, necrotizing vasculitis, livedoid vasculitis, anetoderma, discoid lupus erythematosus, Degos-like lesions (malignant atrophic papulosis), progressive systemic sclerosis, cutaneous T cell lymphoma, erythematous macules, petechiae, purpura, and ecchymoses.[108,110,111] Livedo reticularis is the most common skin manifestation and reported to have irregular broken circles (livedo racemosa) as opposed to the unbroken circles of physiologic cutis marmorata.[108] The cutaneous lesions of APS may be painful on an ischemic basis, particularly areas of necrosis, ulcers, and gangrene.

Diagnosis is based on the presence of either a thrombotic vascular occlusive event or a qualifying complication of pregnancy (≥1 unexplained deaths of morphologically normal fetus ≥10 weeks' gestation, ≥3 consecutive spontaneous abortions <10 weeks' gestation, or ≥1 premature birth of a morphologically normal fetus ≤34 weeks' gestation) plus the presence of either anticardiolipin or lupus anticoagulant antibodies.[107] These criteria were based on the preliminary criteria for the classification of APS published in an international consensus statement in 1999 referred to as the Sapporo criteria for the city in Japan where the conference was held.[112] These criteria were designed primarily for research purposes. Proposed revisions of the criteria were published in another international consensus statement in 2006.[113] These consensus statements provide greater detail regarding the qualifying pregnancy morbidity criteria and laboratory methods needed to confirm the diagnosis of lupus anticoagulant antibodies. The latest international consensus statement published in 2006 is remarkable for the following proposed revisions: (1) increasing the interval between repeat antiphospholipid tests from 6 weeks to 12 weeks to exclude transiently positive tests, (2) the addition of anti-beta2-glycoprotein I antibody as a qualifying antibody test, (3) more quantification of qualifying medium or high positive anticardiolipin titers (i.e., >40 GPL [IgG phospholipid units] or MPL [IgM phospholipid units] or

>99th percentile of controls), and (4) exclusion of patients if less than 12 weeks or more than 5 years separate the positive antiphospholipid antibody test and the clinical event.[113] These changes are discussed in greater detail by Kriseman et al.[109] who favor the Sapporo criteria over the more recently proposed revisions.

Treatment

The patient should be treated for any risk factors for cardiovascular events including hypertension and hyperlipidemia and advised to avoid smoking and oral contraceptives.

APS patients with a history of prior thrombosis or initially presenting with thrombosis should be treated differently depending on whether the thrombosis is venous or arterial. There is agreement that patients with venous thrombosis should be treated with warfarin with a target INR 2.0–3.0.[114,115] Arterial thrombosis may be categorized as cerebral or noncerebral. Lim et al.[114] recommend warfarin (INR 1.4–2.8) or aspirin 325 mg/day for cerebral arterial thrombosis with APS and warfarin (INR 2.0–3.0) for noncerebral arterial thrombosis. Using a different approach with analysis of more inclusive data (cohort studies, subgroup analysis, and randomized control studies) Ruiz-Irastorza et al.[115] recommend that patients with arterial thrombosis (mainly cerebral) and patients with recurrent venous thrombosis (despite adequate warfarin therapy) be treated with warfarin with a target INR 3.0–4.0. Treatment should be for life or at least long-term.[107] Asymptomatic patients incidently found to have antiphospholipid antibodies with no history of thrombosis or pregnancy complications may be offered no treatment or low-dose aspirin.[114]

For catastrophic APS (an acute severe variant with widespread microvascular occlusive events), an algorithmic approach was developed in an international consensus statement where patients presenting with non–life-threatening disease are treated with IV heparin and high-dose steroids whereas patients presenting with life-threatening disease are treated with IV heparin, high-dose steroids, and IVIG and/or plasma exchange.[116] Other therapies are then added as needed such as cyclophosphamide (for SLE flare), prostacyclin, fibrinolytics, or defibrotide.[116] Careful monitoring to detect, treat, or prevent precipitating factors is also recommended including infections, surgery, trauma, invasive procedures, underlying malignancy, SLE flares, and obstetric complications.[116,117]

Treatment and prevention of APS in pregnancy is complicated by the fact that warfarin is teratogenic. Women with APS on warfarin with a prior history of thrombosis should be switched to unfractionated heparin (UH) or low molecular weight heparin (LMWH) at full therapeutic doses.[118] They should be switched back to warfarin after the pregnancy. Women with APS based on pregnancy complications such as ≥2–3 first trimester losses, ≥1 fetal deaths, or ≥1 premature births due to placental insufficiency should be treated with low-dose aspirin and prophylactic doses of UH or LMWH.[118] The UH or LMWH is continued for 6 weeks after delivery and low-dose aspirin is continued lifelong. Pregnant women who have been incidentally found to have antiphospholipid antibodies with no prior history of thrombosis or qualifying pregnancy complications for APS are treated with low-dose aspirin during pregnancy which is continued after delivery.[118]

Multiple clinical studies have shown antimalarials to have an antithrombotic effect in patients with SLE.[115] In a recent observational prospective cohort study of 232 patients with SLE, antimalarials were protective against thrombosis and increased patient survival.[119] The role of antimalarials in treatment of APS has yet to be elucidated especially outside the setting of SLE. Other therapies that may eventually prove useful include statins and agents to inactivate complement.[115] There have been case reports of APS responding to rituximab with improvement or complete disappearance of autoimmune hemolytic anemia, thrombocytopenia, antiphospholipid antibody titers, and thrombotic episodes.[120]

Some Clinical Considerations Related to Corticosteroids and Immunosuppressive Agents

Systemic corticosteroids, corticosteroids combined with cytotoxic agents and noncorticosteroid immunosuppressive agents alone, are sometimes prescribed for serious skin disorders such as vasculitis, immunobullous disorders, connective tissue diseases, and other skin disorders. Standard measures should be taken to prevent complications—measures to prevent osteoporosis with chronic corticosteroids and measures to prevent bladder toxicity from cyclophosphamide. Chronic corticosteroids and other immunosuppressive agents have been associated with pneumocystis pneumonia (PCP) in non-HIV patients, but clear preventive guidelines have not yet been established in some of the lower risk groups for this complication. For patients with serious vasculitis some authorities recommend prophylaxis with trimethoprim-sulfamethoxazole (TMS) for all patients on chronic therapy with a combination of corticosteroids and a cytotoxic agent.[12] A recent review and meta-analysis concluded that the benefits of TMS prophylaxis outweighed the risks of serious adverse reactions requiring discontinuation of the drug when the risk of PCP was >3.5%, as for example in Wegener's granulomatosis, allogeneic bone marrow and solid organ transplants, and certain malignancies.[121] Children have a lower risk of adverse reactions to TMS so prophylaxis can be considered at lower incidence levels of PCP.[121] Other authorities monitor for depressed CD4 levels on chronic immunosuppression in non-HIV patients and institute prophylaxis for a CD4 count <300/µL.[74,122] Until more information is available, a reasonable approach would be to use TMS prophylaxis for all patients in the higher risk categories with >3.5% incidence of PCP, as in Wegener's granulomatosis, and follow CD4 counts in the lower risk categories instituting TMS prophylaxis for a CD4 count <300/µL. Patients with connective tissue diseases, polyarteritis nodosa, pemphigus, pemphigoid, and other long-term corticosteroid treatment are considered to have a <3.5% incidence of PCP.[121] It should be kept in mind, however, that PCP has been reported in patients with a CD4 counts >300/µL, so the previously noted recommendations should not prevent starting prophylaxis in other patients on a case by case basis, particularly if lymphopenic.[123,124]

Coumarin Necrosis

Coumarin necrosis is a rare reaction to warfarin and other coumarin anticoagulant derivatives that causes painful skin necrosis typically on the breasts, abdomen, buttocks, and thighs of middle-aged, obese women.[125–127]

Pathophysiology

Warfarin induced skin necrosis is believed to be caused by a temporary hypercoagulable state that occurs on initiation of warfarin treatment.[126] Protein C is a vitamin K dependent natural anticoagulant whereas factors II, VII, IX, and X are vitamin K dependent clotting (procoagulant) factors. Because of shorter half lives of protein C and factor VII, there is a relatively rapid fall in protein C and factor VII when warfarin is begun, compared to factors II, IX, and X, leading to a transient hypercoagulable state.[128] Patients who have hereditary or acquired protein C deficiency, protein S deficiency, or antithrombin III deficiency are at greater risk.[126,129] Histologically, thrombi in capillaries and venules is considered to be the primary process, but other changes related to necrosis and hemorrhage can be seen.[126,130]

Symptoms and Signs

Symptoms usually begin within the first 3 to 6 days of starting warfarin but delayed onset of warfarin induced skin necrosis has been reported.[131] One or more erythematous edematous plaques appear that develop petechiae on their surface followed by blue-black discoloration, hemorrhage, bullous formation, gangrene or necrosis, and, finally, eschar formation.[132] The lesions are very painful.

Treatment

Warfarin therapy should be discontinued and heparin substituted for warfarin. Protein C concentrate has been reported to be effective as adjunctive therapy in treating one patient with phenprocoumon (coumarin derivative) induced necrosis and, as a preventive measure, in allowing the patient to be restarted on the oral anticoagulant.[133] Avoidance of warfarin and other coumarin derivatives in the future is the most prudent approach. Restarting warfarin at low dosage under coverage of intravenous heparin has been done successfully. However, three of seven patients reported by Jillella et al.[129] experienced recurrences of their skin necrosis, so great care and caution are needed. LMWH has been recommended over chronic unfractionated heparin use if warfarin cannot be restarted because of less risk of osteoporosis, lower risk of thrombocytopenia, and there is no need to monitor partial thromboplastin time (PTT).[131]

Meticulous wound care and pain management is necessary. More than 50% of patients require surgical intervention in the form of debridement, grafting, and amputation.[130]

Calciphylaxis

Calciphylaxis is a potentially life threatening cause of painful ulcerations of the skin that occurs most commonly in patients with chronic end-stage renal disease but also rarely occurs in patients without renal failure.[134–136] It has a reported prevalence rate of 4.1% in patients undergoing hemodialysis.[137] Many but not all patients have secondary hyperparathyroidism with elevated parathyroid hormone, increased alkaline phosphatase, increased calcium, phosphorous, or calcium x phosphate ion product.[137,138] Other potential risk factors include protein C deficiency, protein S deficiency, and warfarin therapy.[139]

Histologically, there is calcification of small arteries, intimal hyperplasia, and noninflammatory thrombosis of vessels.[140] Calcification of arteries may be seen on x-rays, but is nonspecific.

Cutaneous manifestations may begin as a painful violaceous discoloration similar to livedo reticularis that evolves to indurated plaques, ulcerations, and eschar formation. Patients are at high risk for secondary infection and sepsis which is the principal cause of death. Gangrene requiring amputation may also occur.[141] Diagnosis requires clinicopathologic correlation. Preservation of pulses, proximal location of ulcers on extremities, and absence of neuropathy favors calciphylaxis over arteriosclerotic ulcers and diabetic ulcers although patients may have concomitant disease and calciphylaxis ulcers may occur on acral locations.[137]

Treatment

Measures should be taken to lower the serum calcium, serum phosphate, and calcium x phosphate product when elevated. These measures may include low calcium dialysate, noncalcium phosphate binders, and low phosphate diet.[136,142]

A number of treatments have been reported to be effective in case reports or small series. One of these is cinacalcet (Sensipar) which is a calcimimetic agent that acts by increasing the sensitivity of the calcium receptor to calcium and, thus, lowering parathyroid hormone levels.[143–145] Another agent is sodium thiosulfate—a salt that increases the solubility of calcium in the form of calcium thiosulfate.[146–148] Pamidronate, a bisphosphonate, was reported to be effective in one patient. It was tried because of experimental studies in animals where it prevented calciphylaxis and because of its anti-inflammatory properties.[149] Another bisphosphonate, etidronate, has also been reported to be effective in treating calciphylaxis.[150] Low-dose tissue plasminogen activator has been reported to be effective by relieving thrombotic occlusion of vessels.[151] Hyperbaric oxygen has also been reported to be effective by increasing the partial pressure of oxygen in ischemic tissues.[152]

Parathyroidectomy has been effective in some but not all patients. It is more likely to be beneficial in patients with marked hyperparathyroidism.[136,142]

Local wound care, pain management, and antibiotics for secondary infection are also essential. Amputation may be needed in some patients.

ULCERS

Ischemic Ulcers

Ischemic (arterial) ulcers are a cause of painful ulcerations on the lower extremities most often seen in patients with arteriosclerotic peripheral vascular disease. The ulcers typically have a dry punched out appearance and are located on the distal lower extremities at sites of trauma or pressure including the toes, feet, lateral malleoli, and pretibial areas.[153–155] There may be associated atrophic skin, loss of hair, delayed capillary filling pressure, and rubor with dependency (reactive hyperemia). The ulcer pain is worse at night and relieved by dependency. Patients also may have a history of intermittent claudication and rest pain if the obstruction is severe enough.

Histologically, arteriosclerosis affects medium and large arteries where one finds plaques with varying degrees of infiltrations with foam cells, smooth muscle cells, inflammatory cells, hemorrhage, platelets, thrombus formation, collagen deposition, and ulceration.[156] Patients may have ulcers with a mixture of venous and arterial disease. Diabetics may also have small vessel disease complicated by peripheral neuropathy leading to further trauma and injury at the site. Neuritis on an ischemic basis may also occur.

The patient should be examined for absent or diminished pulses and bruits over proximal arteries. The patient should be further evaluated with measurements to determine the ankle brachial index which consists of the ratio of the systolic blood pressure in the ankle to the systolic blood pressure in the arm as detected by hand held Doppler device. A normal ankle brachial index (ABI) is ≥ 1, <1 is abnormal, and ≤ 0.5 is severe disease.[157] Patients with calcification of arteries have a falsely elevated ABI because of noncompressibility of vessels. Other noninvasive forms of evaluation include digital pulse volume recordings, Doppler flow volume wave form analysis, duplex ultrasound, transcutaneous oximetry, stress testing, computerized tomographic angiography, magnetic resonance angiography, and toe-brachial index (to evaluate noncompressible vessels).[157,158] Digital subtraction angiography is considered the gold standard.[158]

Treatment

Measures should be taken to treat underlying causes of arteriosclerosis including cessation of smoking, control of blood pressure, hyperlipidemia, and control of diabetes.[155] Elevation of the extremity, compression and debridement of ulcers are to be avoided. Protection of the extremities from trauma with sheep-skin and foot cradling devices is helpful. Patients with claudication may benefit from an exercise program when the ulcer has healed. Adequate pain relief, local wound care, and treating any secondary infection are important. When conservative measures fail, there are a variety of nonoperative and operative revascularization procedures that may be used, including percutaneous transluminal angioplasty, stent placement, atherectomy, and bypass procedures, depending on the individual patient.[157]

Stasis Ulcers

Stasis ulcers (venous ulcers) are a common cause of painful ulcerations on the ankles typically over the medial malleoli in patients with chronic venous insufficiency.[155,159,160] Associated skin findings may include hyperpigmentation from hemosiderin deposition, varicosities, pitting edema, scars from prior ulcerations, and fibrosis and induration of tissues (lipodermatosclerosis). There may also be associated stasis dermatitis, contact dermatitis from topical medications, and secondary infection. The ulcer itself is typically shallow with irregular borders and sloping edge.[155,160]

Venous ulcers occur in the setting of chronic venous hypertension due to incompetent venous semi-lunar valves in superficial veins, communicating veins, or deep venous system or with disease of the calf muscles which act as a pump to empty the deep venous system.[153,160] The valves may be damaged by prior episodes of thrombophlebitis or be congenitally absent.[160] Obesity and peripheral edema from other causes such as pulmonary, cardiac, hepatic, or renal disease may be contributory or exacerbating factors. Pain in the ulcers is presumably on an ischemic basis.

Treatment

Elevation of the legs and support stockings will help control peripheral edema. Unna boots and other compressive wraps speed wound healing. Compression should be avoided, however, in patients with concomitant arterial disease. Local wound care may include gauzes, films, hydrogels, hydrocolloid dressings, foams, alginates and hydrofibers, or antimicrobial dressings.[161] Occlusive dressings on the wound may also relieve pain. Surgical debridement may sometimes be needed. Cultures should be taken if secondary infection is present and the patient treated with antibiotics effective for *Staphylococcus aureus* and *Streptococcus pyogenes*. Dermatitis from stasis dermatitis or contact dermatitis is treated with topical steroids and avoidance of responsible contactants. Surgical management with grafting may be necessary in refractory cases. Weight reduction and diuretics may be helpful in some obese patients. Optimization of therapy for any associated systemic conditions causing peripheral edema such as congestive heart failure or pulmonary insufficiency may also be helpful.

PAINFUL INFECTIONS

Many infections of the skin are painful. Common or selected skin infections are discussed here. For more comprehensive coverage of the topic the reader is referred to a general textbook of dermatology such as Fitzpatrick's *Dermatology in General Medicine.*

Herpes Zoster

Herpes zoster is a painful eruption caused by reactivation of the varicella virus in a dermatomal distribution.[162,163] The topic is presented and discussed in detail in Chapter 27.

Signs and Symptoms

Herpes zoster (HZ) is a painful vesicular cutaneous eruption in a dermatomal distribution that is often preceded by a 2 to 3 day prodrome of pain, paresthesias, or burning sensation in the involved dermatome. The eruption begins as erythematous macules, papules, and plaques, often grouped within a dermatome, that rapidly develop clear vesicular lesions on the surface. Lesions may become hemorrhagic or necrotic. Rarely, patients may have pain without skin lesions (zoster sine herpete). The clear vesicular blister fluid becomes cloudy which is followed by crusting and healing. In uncomplicated HZ the disease runs its course over 2 to 4 weeks with healing of lesions and subsidence of pain. Immunosuppressed patients may have delayed healing and an atypical appearance to the rash with persistent ulcerative or verrucous lesions as well as possible acyclovir resistance.[163]

Diagnosis

In the prodromal phase the disease may mimic a variety of acute medical conditions, but once the eruption appears the diagnosis becomes more straightforward. The diagnosis is confirmed by direct fluorescent antibody testing of scrapings from early vesicular lesions. Cultures can be done, but they take 2 weeks and may be negative. Postherpetic neuralgia is a serious complication of the disease that increases with age and is discussed in Chapter 27.

Treatment

Supportive care includes Burow's compresses, analgesics, and antibiotics for secondary infection when present. Antiviral therapy is indicated for all immunocompetent patients greater than 50 years old, all immunocompromised patients, and patients less than 50 years of age who have moderate to severe HZ (pain or rash), nontruncal involvement, ophthalmic zoster, Ramsay Hunt syndrome, motor nerve involvement, other neurologic involvement, or disseminated HZ. Antiviral therapy should preferably be started within the first 72 hours. Valacyclovir 1000 mg three times per day for 7 days and famciclovir 500 mg three times per day for 7 days are felt to be more effective than acyclovir 800 mg five times per day for 7–10 days because of higher blood levels and better compliance with dosing, but any of the three regimens may be used. Dosages of the medications need to be adjusted for renal insufficiency if present. For immunosuppressed patients, IV acyclovir 10 mg/kg three times per day may be needed. Valacyclovir in high dosages in immunosuppressed patients has been associated with thrombotic thrombocytopenic purpura and is best avoided under those circumstances. A 3-week course of systemic corticosteroids may provide some symptomatic relief in severe HZ if no contraindications and the patient is also receiving an antiviral agent. On May 25, 2006, the Food and Drug Administration (FDA) approved a live attenuated virus vaccine (Zostavax, Merck) for prevention of HZ in persons 60 years of age or older.[164] The vaccine was demonstrated to reduce the incidence of HZ and postherpetic neuralgia. Treatment of postherpetic neuralgia is dealt with in Chapter 27.

Herpes Simplex

Herpes simplex virus (HSV) infection is a common often painful DNA viral infection presenting as grouped vesicular lesions on an erythematous base that may be preceded by a 1 to 2 day prodrome of burning, tingling or itching.[165–168] The early clear vesicular lesions progress through stages of clouding, crusting, and then healing.

Symptoms and Signs

Primary HSV infection (no antibodies to HSV in acute phase serum) may potentially be the most severe, painful, and protracted and is often accompanied by fever, malaise, tender regional adenopathy, and a higher rate of complications.[165] "First episode" HSV may be primary infection or may be recurrent HSV where the primary infection was asymptomatic.[166] Between episodes the virus remains latent in sensory nerve ganglia and may periodically reactivate. Recurrent episodes are generally milder than the original episode and tend to become less frequent with time. Fever, stress, ultraviolet light, and certain surgical procedures may trigger reactivation of the virus (e.g., dermabrasion or laser resurfacing).

HSV infection may present in multiple clinical forms with orolabial (herpes labialis) and genital HSV being the most common. Keratoconjunctivitis, herpetic sycosis (beard area), herpetic whitlow, herpes gladiatorum, eczema herpeticum, recurrent lumbosacral HSV, and neonatal HSV are other clinical forms of the disease. HSV may also trigger recurrent episodes of erythema multiforme where HSV virus DNA can be detected in the lesions of erythema multiforme by polymerase chain reaction (PCR).[169] Immunosuppressed patients tend to have more severe and slower healing HSV infections with atypical clinical appearance such as persistent crusts, erosions, ulcerative, or vegetative lesions. Less commonly, visceral infection may occur affecting the esophagus, lungs, liver, and other organs.[165] Neonatal HSV may occur in utero, at the time of the delivery, or in the immediate few weeks after delivery. Patients may have involvement of the skin, eyes, and mouth (SEM), central nervous system (CNS), or disseminated disease. Most patients with neonatal HSV (68%) have vesicular skin lesions but a significant percentage of patients especially with CNS or disseminated disease have no skin lesions.[166]

Diagnosis

The diagnosis is most readily established by direct fluorescent antibody testing of scrapings from early vesicular lesions. Cultures should also be taken when possible from early vesicular lesions and will usually grow out within 48 to 72 hours. PCR for HSV DNA may be more sensitive than culture especially for demonstrating HSV in CNS.[165] Tzanck preparation has the advantage of obtaining immediate results but is more dependent on the experience and skill of the interpreter. It will not distinguish between HSV and herpes zoster virus. Skin biopsy will show ballooning degeneration of keratinocytes and multinucleate giant cells in the epidermis.

Treatment

Treatment with analgesics for pain, wet compresses with Burow's solution, and antibiotics for secondary infection are helpful supportive measures.

The principal antiviral medications for treatment of HSV are acyclovir, valacyclovir, and famciclovir. Valacyclovir and famciclovir have an advantage of less frequent dosing and greater bioavailability, but they are more expensive than acyclovir. Severe episodes of HSV are treated with IV acyclovir. The dosages of the medications need to be adjusted in patients with renal failure. Valacyclovir has been associated with thrombotic thrombocytopenic purpura at high dosages in immunocompromised patients and is best avoided under those circumstances. Representative treatment schedules are presented below for HSV.[165–168] A wider range of acceptable schedules and dosing is available.

First episodes of either orolabial or genital HSV infection may be treated with acyclovir 200 mg five times per day, valacyclovir 1 gm twice per day, or famciclovir 250 mg twice per day, all for 7 to 14 days.[165,166] Recurrent genital HSV may be treated with acyclovir 200 mg five times per day for 5 days, valacyclovir 500 mg twice per day for 3 to 5 days, or famciclovir 125 mg twice per day for 5 days. There is limited clinical benefit from treating recurrent orolabial HSV with intermittent topical antiviral therapy or intermittent oral antiviral drugs, although sun protective measures may be helpful on a preventative basis. If antiviral agents are used they should be initiated during the prodrome if possible.

For chronic suppression of recurrent genital HSV acyclovir 400 mg twice daily, valacyclovir 500 mg daily, valacyclovir 1 gm daily (for >9–10 recurrences per year), or famciclovir 250 mg twice daily may be used.[165,166] For chronic suppression of orolabial HSV infection, acyclovir 400 mg twice daily is usually recommended.[166] Prevention of reactivation of orolabial HSV infections with surgical procedures may be accomplished by giving valacyclovir 500 mg twice daily or famciclovir 250 mg twice daily 24 to 48 hours prior to the surgical procedure and continuing for 10 to 14 days.[165,166]

IV acyclovir 5 mg/kg every 8 hours is used for patients with severe disease in either immunocompetent patients or immunosuppressed patients. If oral antiviral agents are used in immunosuppressed patients, higher than usual doses and/or longer duration of treatment are usually recommended for initial episodes, recurrent disease, as well as for chronic suppression.[165,168] Acyclovir resistance is more likely to be encountered in immunosuppressed patients and treatment with intravenous foscarnet 40 mg/kg every 8 hours is an alternative agent that may be useful.[165]

Neonatal HSV infection is treated with IV acyclovir 60 mg/kg/day for 14 days for skin, eyes, and mouth involvement and 21 days for CNS involvement or disseminated disease.[166] Some authorities recommend oral acyclovir for 3 to 4 months following IV therapy.[165]

Erysipelas and Cellulitis

Both erysipelas and cellulitis are soft tissue infections that cause erythema, edema, warmth, and pain often on the lower extremities but other areas as well. Erysipelas is distinguished from cellulitis in being more superficial in the dermis and sharply demarcated from the surrounding normal skin, whereas cellulitis typically affects deeper tissues and is more indurated and poorly circumscribed.[170–173] Both may be associated with fever, chills, lymphangitis, and localized lymphadenopathy. Bullous formation may occur with erysipelas and rarely with cellulitis (e.g., vibrio vulnificus).[171,173] Group A streptococcus (streptococcus pyogenes) is the principal cause of erysipelas but may also cause cellulitis. Cellulitis may be caused by many other organisms as well. A break in the skin or portal of entry may sometimes be found (e.g., trauma or fissuring between the toes from tinea pedis).

The diagnosis is often made clinically before lab tests are available. Distinguishing erysipelas from cellulitis may be difficult at times. Culturing any breaks in the skin or ulcers may be helpful in recovering the organism. Culturing aspirates from the rash or skin biopsies are typically low yield procedures. Blood cultures, when positive, provide a definitive diagnosis.

Treatment

Erysipelas responds to treatment with intramuscular (IM) benzathine penicillin G or oral penicillin VK. Because *Staphylococcus aureus* may be difficult to exclude clinically, treatment with cephalexin or dicloxacillin pending culture results is prudent.

Cellulitis of the skin is often caused by *Staphylococcus aureus* and *Streptococcus pyogenes* and coverage with oral cephalexin or dicloxacillin for milder cases of infection is usually sufficient. Initial therapy is highly dependent on the history of exposure to any unusual organisms, underlying illnesses of the patient, toxicity of the patient, clinical setting (e.g., diabetic foot ulcer), and likelihood of methicillin-resistant *Staphylococcus aureus* (MRSA) which would dictate other antibiotic coverage. Seriously ill patients may need hospitalization, IV antibiotics, and infectious disease consult.

Elevation of the extremity if no arterial insufficiency is present, moist compresses (e.g., sterile saline or Burow's compresses) for any ulcers, and antifungal cream for tinea pedis are important adjunctive measures.

Furunculosis and Carbuncle

Furuncles and carbuncles are painful staphylococcal infections in hair-bearing areas that begin as a folliculitis. A furuncle occurs when infection extends down the hair follicle to the subcutaneous tissue with abscess formation producing an erythematous, painful nodule with a superimposed follicular centered pustule. A carbuncle occurs when infection spreads to multiple adjacent contiguous follicles by subcutaneous extension resulting in a larger, erythematous, painful mass with superimposed follicular pustules. Culture and sensitivity taken from the pustules should guide antibiotic therapy.[174]

Treatment

Fluctuant abscesses should be incised, drained, and cultured. Milder cases may respond to incision and drainage and moist heat alone,[175] but careful follow-up is necessary if oral antibiotics are not given. If antibiotics are needed dicloxacillin or cephalexin 250 to 500 mg four times per day for 7 to 10 days should be used to treat methicillin-sensitive *Staphylococcus aureus* (MSSA). If MRSA is suspected treat with trimethoprim-sulfamethoxazole (TMP-SMX) one double strength tablet twice daily or doxycycline 100 mg twice daily for 7 to 10 days or minocycline 100 mg twice daily for 7 to 10 days, but it should be kept in mind that these agents will not treat Group A streptococcus infection.[176] If the MRSA is resistant to erythromycin and sensitive to clindamycin, a "D test" must be done to exclude inducible clindamycin resistance before clindamycin may be used. More seriously ill patients may need hospitalization and treatment with IV antibiotics.

In patients with recurrent furunculosis, elimination of nasal staphylococcal carriage and skin colonization may be helpful although the information on efficacy is limited. Regimens include intranasal mupirocin ointment twice daily for 5 days per month, rifampin 600 mg per day for 10 days plus dicloxacillin 250 to 500 mg four times per day for 10 days for MSSA; and rifampin 600 mg per day plus either TMP-SMX one double strength tablet twice daily for 10 days or doxycycline 100 mg twice daily for 10 days or minocycline 100 mg twice daily for 10 days for MRSA.[174–176] Rifampin should never be used alone because of rapid development of resistance. Chlorhexidine may be used to cleanse the skin. Some authorities recommend an infectious disease consult before eradication of the carrier state is attempted[176] and limiting systemic antimicrobials in this situation to patients with active infection.[177]

Good hygienic measures may be helpful for patients in preventing recurrences and spread of infection to others such as frequent handwashing, keeping wounds cleanly bandaged, regular laundering of clothing in contact with the wound, regular bathing with soap, avoiding shared towels and other shared items, and cleansing of equipment and surfaces in contact with wound drainage.[177,178]

Erysipeloid

Erysipeloid is an acute painful infection of the skin caused by *Erysipelothrix rhusiopathiae*, a gram-positive rod. It is an occupational hazard of fishermen and butchers and occurs domestically in those who handle raw fish, poultry, and meat products.[179,180]

The organism gains entrance through a break in the skin to cause what has been referred to as an erysipeloid rash. A painful violaceous red, warm, raised, lesion develops usually on the hand or finger, spreads peripherally, and clears centrally. There is no ulceration or scaling. Usually the infection remains localized, but systemic infection may occur.

The treatment of choice is penicillin 2 to 3 million units daily, orally or IM for 7 to 10 days. Higher doses are needed if systemic infection occurs.[179,180]

INFLAMMATIONS

Panniculitis

Erythema Nodosum

Erythema nodosum is a common cause of septal panniculitis that typically affects young adults between 20 and 30 years of age, with M:F ratio of 1:6, although any age may be affected.[181,182] Erythema nodosum usually presents as bilateral tender, poorly circumscribed erythematous nodules, 1 to 10 cm in diameter, on the anterior tibial areas but more widespread involvement may occur.[182] The lesions typically heal over a few weeks without scarring although new lesions may continue to appear. Some patients have constitutional symptoms such as fever, malaise, arthralgias, headache, cough, abdominal pain, vomiting, or diarrhea.[181] Associated lab abnormalities may include leukocytosis and elevated erythrocyte sedimentation rate.[182]

There have been many reported causes of erythema nodosum including infections (bacterial, viral, fungal, and protozoan), medications (e.g., penicillin, sulfonamides, oral contraceptives, iodides, and salicylates), malignancy, sarcoidosis, inflammatory bowel disease, and pregnancy.[181–184] Sarcoidosis and streptococcal infections are among the most frequent causes. They were reported in 11% to 28% and 6% to 28% of cases, respectively, in two recent series.[183,184] Streptococcus infection is an important cause of erythema nodosum in children—reported in 49% cases in one series.[185] In 35% to 55% cases no etiology may be found.[183,184] Uncommon, but important, causes to exclude are mycobacterium tuberculosis, deep fungal infections (histoplasmosis, coccidioidomycosis, and blastomycosis), and malignancy (lymphoma, leukemia, and solid tumors).[181]

The pathogenesis of erythema nodosum is poorly understood and felt to be a hypersensitivity reaction to etiologic agents. Histologically, one finds inflammation of the septae between fat lobules that evolves from acute inflammation to granulomatous change followed by fibrosis. The presence of Miescher's radial granulomas with aggregates of histiocytes and neutrophils around central clefts is a characteristic feature.[186]

Treatment

Any underlying diseases or infections should be treated. Medications that are a potential cause should be discontinued. Bed rest and NSAIDs may be sufficient. In patients with more persistent or recalcitrant disease, potassium iodide 400 to 900 mg daily may be helpful. Potassium iodide is contraindicated in pregnant women, should be avoided in renal insufficiency (risk of hyperkalemia), and used cautiously, if at all, in patients with thyroid disease (risk of hyper- or hypothyroidism).[187] It should be kept in mind that both aspirin and iodides have been reported as both causing and treating erythema nodosum. A short course of systemic corticosteroids may be helpful if any underlying infectious diseases have been excluded.

Weber-Christian Disease

Weber-Christian disease, also referred to as relapsing febrile nonsuppurative nodular panniculitis, is a disease characterized by recurrent episodes of fever and crops of painful subcutaneous nodules that may be erythematous and rarely discharge oily material.[188–192] The nodules may occur on the face, trunk, and extremities but are most common on the extremities, particularly the thighs. The nodules may eventually heal with atrophy. Patients may have associated arthritis, arthralgias, myalgias, abdominal pain, and hepatosplenomegaly. Lab abnormalities described include elevated sedimentation rate, anemia, leukopenia, leukocytosis, thrombocytopenia, and circulating immune complexes. Visceral fat involvement may occur affecting the omentum, mesentery, and mediastinum, and perivisceral or intravisceral fat of the heart, kidneys, adrenals, pancreas, bone marrow, and joints. The disease may be fatal.

Histologically, one finds a lobular panniculitis with initial degeneration of fat cells and acute inflammation followed by infiltration with macrophages, foam cells, and extracellular lipid and, eventually, fibroblasts and chronic inflammatory cells corresponding to the stage of atrophy.[186]

Some of the cases of Weber-Christian disease reported in the past would be classified under different diagnostic categories today, such as cytophagic histiocytic panniculitis or alpha$_1$-antitrypsin deficiency and, possibly, lupus profundus or pancreatic panniculitis. Whether there remains a residual subset of patients with Weber-Christian disease is controversial. Some consider the Weber-Christian disease a nonspecific reaction pattern or another term for idiopathic and advise that the term be abandoned for more specific diagnoses.[193]

Treatments reported in the past to be effective include tetracycline, sulfapyridine, corticosteroids, thalidomide, antimalarials, NSAIDs, and immunosuppressive agents. Antimalarials and corticosteroids were the most effective in one series.[189]

Dercum's Disease

Dercum's disease is a rare condition of painful lipomas of the skin on the trunk and extremities in obese postmenopausal women as originally described by Dercum in 1892 who proposed the term adiposis dolorosa.[194] The condition has less frequently been reported in men. Subsequent reports also describe associated weakness, fatigue, and emotional and psychological disturbances.[195,196] Most cases are sporadic, but familial cases with autosomal dominant inheritance pattern have also been reported.[197] Histologically, one typically finds a lipoma with no distinguishing features from an ordinary lipoma.

Treatment

Weight reduction and analgesics may be helpful. Excision of individual painful tumors may also be helpful but new painful tumors may continue to appear.[198] Liposuction has also been reported to be of benefit.[199,200] Intravenous lidocaine may provide pain relief lasting from hours to months.[195,201,202]

Oral mexiletine, an oral derivative of lidocaine and antiarrythmic agent, has also been reported to be partially or completely effective.[202,203] Interferon alfa-2b was reported to provide pain relief in two patients with Dercum's disease who were being treated for hepatitis C.[204] Corticosteroids have been reported to both cause[205] and treat[206] Dercum's disease.

The pain in Dercum's disease has been characterized as both nociceptive (localized pain in lipomas aggravated by palpation) and neuropathic with allodynia (light touch perceived as painful), so approaches to management similar to other chronic pain syndromes may be beneficial.[207] With that in mind, the patient in the report was successfully treated with amitriptyline, a voltage-gated sodium channel blocker.[207]

Hidradenitis Suppurativa

Hidradenitis suppurativa is a chronic disease where recurrent painful nodules and abscesses occur in apocrine gland areas, typically the axillae, inguinal areas, and perineum, but the inframammary areas and buttocks may also be involved.[208,209]

Etiology

The etiology of hidradenitis suppurativa is felt to be follicular hyperkeratosis and occlusion, leading to acute suppurative inflammation and granulomatous changes that secondarily engulfs and destroys apocrine glands and other appendages.[210] The disease usually first appears at puberty, suggesting hormonal factors, and may occur as a part of a follicular occlusion triad of hidradenitis suppurativa, acne conglobata, and perifolliculitis capitis abscedens et suffodiens.

Symptoms and Signs

Early on, patients experience recurrent painful erythematous nodules that suppurate and eventually break down to form sinus tracts and scarring. The sinus tracts may form an extensive interconnecting network in the subcutaneous tissue with multiple openings. The disease process may be circumscribed or more diffuse. Secondary bacterial infection may occur. In addition to being physically painful, the disease may be psychologically debilitating, especially in patients with long standing disease.[211] Squamous cell cancer and amyloidosis are rare complications in patients with chronic hidradenitis suppurativa.[209]

Diagnosis

Initially, the disease appears similar to furuncles or an inflamed epidermal cyst. However, when the erythematous nodules are recurrent and lead to sinus tracts and retracted scars, the diagnosis becomes clear.

Treatment

Systemic antibiotics are often used as initial treatment such as tetracycline 250 to 500 mg four times per day or minocycline. Topical clindamycin may also be helpful. Culture and sensitivity may detect secondary bacterial infection that needs other antibiotic therapy.

When disease is limited to one or a few acutely painful erythematous nodules, intralesional triamcinolone acetonide 2.5 to 5.0 mg/mL will often relieve the pain and inflammation within a few days. If lesions are widespread or numerous, a short course of prednisone 40 to 60 mg/day tapered over 1 to 2 weeks will often cause the lesions to subside at least temporarily.

Weight reduction in obese individuals and cleansing the affected areas with antibacterial soaps such as chlorhexidine may be useful. Limited benefit has been reported with oral isotretinoin. TNF inhibitors have been reported to be beneficial in some patients. Infliximab has been reported to be effective, but some patients do not respond or response is transient and it is not without risk of significant potential side effects.[212–214] Experience with adalimumab for treating hidradenitis suppurativa is more limited. There have been two reports of patients responding to adalimumab.[215,216]

Surgical excision, with repair by flaps or grafts as needed, remains the most definitive therapy available. Not all patients are candidates for surgery. Surgical excision works best if the disease is consistently confined over time to a localized area. Liposuction has been suggested for early disease to remove apocrine glands on a preventative basis before scarring occurs.[208]

Inflamed Epidermal Cyst

Epidermal cysts are very common and typically present after puberty as whitish, sometimes pigmented, well-defined, partially compressible, subcutaneous nodules with a semi-solid feel and often with a pore opening to the surface.[217,218] They may extrude a thick whitish material with a foul odor through the pore. Most are asymptomatic, but when they are traumatized and rupture into the surrounding tissue, they incite an acute inflammatory reaction that mimics infection with pain, erythema, edema, warmth, and purulence. Initial management consists of hot compresses and incision and drainage. If secondary infection is suspected, culture and sensitivity should be done and the patient treated with an antibiotic effective for *Staphylococcus aureus* and *Streptococcus pyogenes* such as cephalexin or dicloxacillin pending culture results. Once inflammation subsides the residual cyst is excised. Some cysts are destroyed by the inflammation if severe enough.

Great care should be taken in excising previously inflamed cysts in certain locations because scar tissue may have entrapped important nerves or other structures—for example, the temporal branch of the facial nerve in the temple areas, the spinal accessory nerve in the posterior cervical triangle of the neck, or the parotid duct overlying the masseter muscle on the cheek. In these locations it may be more prudent to open the cyst, evacuate the contents, and scrape the wall of the cyst with a curette if treatment is felt to be necessary.

Although epidermal cysts typically develop after puberty, an accurate history regarding a particular cyst may not always be available. Cysts that could possibly have been present since birth should be a cause of greater concern, especially in certain locations such as the midline of the face, the midline of the scalp, or the midline of the back, since they may communicate with the central nervous system. Should one of these cysts become inflamed or infected, surgery should not be attempted without prior imaging studies such as computed tomography (CT) and magnetic resonance imaging (MRI). If a communication is found with the central nervous system, the surgery needs to be done by a neurosurgeon. Similarly, cysts present at birth on the lateral neck may be branchial cleft cysts that communicate with the pharynx. They may become infected in adult life simulating an inflamed epidermal cyst. Referral to an otolaryngologist is indicated for definitive treatment. Cysts presenting in childhood may be a sign of Gardner's syndrome, an autosomal dominant condition, associated with multiple benign tumors of the skin, osteomas, intestinal polyposis, and a high risk of colon cancer.[219] Ordinary epidermal cysts have a lining similar to normal epidermis with a granular layer, but cysts with Gardner's syndrome often have focal areas of pilomatrical differentiation.[219]

Bullous Dermatoses with Erosions

Pemphigus Vulgaris

Pemphigus vulgaris is a rare disorder and the most frequent member of a group of disorders referred to as pemphigus. Other members of the group include pemphigus foliaceous, pemphigus vegetans, pemphigus erythematosus, and paraneoplastic pemphigus. Paraneoplastic pemphigus will be discussed in the next section.

Pemphigus vulgaris is an autoimmune disorder that usually presents with painful blisters and nonhealing erosions in the mouth that eventually spread to the skin, producing flaccid blisters and bullae followed by oozing, crusted, painful erosions.[220,221] Lateral pressure on the skin adjacent to a bullous lesion causes the epidermis to shear and detach (Nikolsky sign). Uncommonly, patients may have an associated thymoma or myasthenia gravis. Drug-induced pemphigus has been reported with a variety of medications including penicillamine, rifampicin, captopril, enalapril, penicillin, and other drugs.[220,222] The bullae and blisters are caused by autoantibodies to desmosomal cadherin adhesion molecules, either desmoglein 3 with isolated mucosal pemphigus vulgaris or desmoglein 3 plus desmoglein 1 with mucocutaneous pemphigus vulgaris, whereas patients with pemphigus foliaceous have antibodies to desmoglein 1 only.[221] This leads to detachment of cells from one another (acantholysis) that is seen histologically as a suprabasilar split in the epidermis (su-

prabasilar acantholysis) in pemphigus vulgaris and subcorneal acantholysis in pemphigus foliaceous. The autoantibodies can be detected by direct immunofluorescence of perilesional skin, producing a netlike pattern on the surface of keratinocytes. Circulating autoantibodies are commonly present and detected by indirect immunofluorescence or enzyme-linked immunosorbant assay (ELISA) for antibodies to desmoglein 3 and desmoglein 1. Titers of circulating autoantibodies may correlate with disease activity but not always.

Treatment

The mainstay of treatment of pemphigus vulgaris are systemic corticosteroids often with initial starting doses of prednisone 1 mg/kg/day and increasing to 2 mg/kg/day (in divided doses), depending on response to treatment.[220] A steroid sparing agent is then added if needed, usually azathioprine or mycophenylate mofetil and, less commonly, cyclophosphamide and other agents. Pulse steroids and plasmapheresis with and without cyclophosphamide are other treatments that have been used. More recently intravenous immunoglobulin,[223,224] intravenous immunoglobulin combined with rituximab,[225] and rituximab without intravenous immunoglobulin[226–228] have shown promising results in the more treatment resistant cases. Patients need close monitoring for complications of therapy and preventive measures when possible (e.g., measures to prevent osteoporosis related to chronic corticosteroid use). Topical therapy and supportive measures for mucous membrane and cutaneous involvement are also needed.

Paraneoplastic Pemphigus

Paraneoplastic pemphigus is a rare autoimmune disorder associated with benign and malignant neoplasms. It causes a painful stomatitis similar to pemphigus vulgaris but a more polymorphic eruption on the skin.[229] The skin eruption may have features resembling pemphigus vulgaris, bullous pemphigoid, erythema multiforme, or a lichen planus-like (lichenoid) appearance. The polymorphic clinical pattern is reflected in the histology where one sees suprabasilar acantholysis, keratinocytes cell necrosis, and interface dermatitis. Direct immunofluorescence demonstrates IgG and C3 in a netlike pattern on keratinocytes similar to pemphigus vulgaris and, less frequently, a linear pattern along the epidermal basement membrane. Circulating antoantibodies detected by immunoprecipitation recognize a complex of proteins including desmoplakin I (250-kD), bullous pemphigoid antigen 1 (230-kD), envoplakin (210-kD), periplakin (190-kD), and a not further characterized 170-kD antigen.[230] Autoantibodies of paraneoplastic pemphigus can be distinguished from pemphigus vulgaris autoantibodies by their ability to react with transitional epithelium of rodent bladder, but the test is not as accurate as immunoprecipitation.[229] Paraneoplastic pemphigus associated tumors include non-Hodgkin lymphoma, chronic lymphocytic leukemia, Castleman's tumor, thymoma, spindle cell neoplasms, Waldenström's macroglobulinemia,[229] and, rarely, solid tumors including uterine carcinoma,[231] hepatocellular carcinoma,[232] bronchogenic squamous cell carcinoma,[233] and pancreatic carcinoma.[234] Mortality may be 90% or higher with some patients dying from respiratory involvement manifested as bronchiolitis obliterans.[235]

Treatment. Treatment of paraneoplastic pemphigus involves treating the underlying tumor which, in some cases, may clear the eruption but is less likely to if the tumor is malignant.[229] Variable response has been reported with prednisone alone or combined with other immunosuppressive agents. There are reports of patients responding to rituximab,[236] mycophenylate mofetil,[237] and tacrolimus topically for the stomatitis.[238]

Bullous Pemphigoid

Bullous pemphigoid is the most common of the autoimmune bullous diseases that typically affects elderly patients.[239–241] Tense bullae develop on normal or erythematous skin commonly distributed on the lower abdomen, axillae, groin, and flexor extremities. Transient oral lesions may also appear. Pruritus occurs in some patients and temporarily painful erosions after rupture of blisters and bullae. Peripheral blood eosinophilia is often an associated finding. Most cases of bullous pemphigoid are idiopathic but bullous pemphigoid-like drug eruptions have been reported with furosemide, penicillamine, nalidixic acid, sulfasalazine, captopril, penicillins, and other agents.[241]

Histologically, one finds a subepidermal bullous lesion with varying degrees of cellular infiltrate, often with eosinophils. Direct immunofluorescence demonstrates IgG and C3 in a smooth linear pattern at the epidermal basement membrane. Circulating antibodies to the epidermal basement membrane occur in approximately two thirds of patients that bind to the epidermal side of salt split skin. Two bullous pemphigoid antigens have been identified associated with the hemidesmosomal plaques at the dermal-epidermal junction. Bullous pemphigoid antigen 1 (230-kD) is an intracellular antigen and bullous pemphigoid antigen 2 (180-kD) is a transmembrane protein.[242]

Treatment. Milder cases of bullous pemphigoid or localized bullous disease may respond to high potency topical steroids alone (e.g., clobetasol 0.05% cream twice daily). Tetracycline or erythromycin 500 mg four times per day plus niacinamide 500 mg three times per day or tetracycline alone may be effective.[243,244] These treatments may also be considered in patients with more severe disease who are not good candidates for treatment with systemic corticosteroids or as adjunctive treatment with systemic steroids. Dapsone may also be effective in a subset of patients with an intense neutrophilic infiltrates on their biopsies.

Most patients with moderate to severe, generalized bullous pemphigoid are treated with prednisone 0.5 to 0.75 mg/kg/day and a steroid sparing agent is added if needed.[245] Azathioprine or mycophenylate mofetil are used most commonly. Azathioprine dosing is aided by checking thiopurine methyltransferase (TPMT) levels. Less commonly used agents are methotrexate and cyclophosphamide. For patients with severe or extensive disease, total body applications of clobetasol 0.05% cream twice daily has been shown to be superior to prednisone 1 mg/kg/day in terms of effectiveness and survival.[246] However, compliance with this regimen may be difficult in the frail elderly without assistance from family members or nursing services.[242] Topical therapy should seriously be considered in patients with extensive disease if feasible under their individual circumstances. Uncommonly used treatments for refractory disease include intravenous immune globulin, pulse steroids, and plasmapheresis.[241]

Epidermolysis Bullosa

Epidermolysis bullosa refers to a group of rare disorders that may be inherited or acquired. They all exhibit abnormal skin and sometimes mucous membrane fragility with minor trauma leading to blister formation, painful erosions, and, in some cases, scarring.[247–251] Scarring may manifest as milia or dystrophic nails or in more severe cases as pseudosyndactyly, esophageal strictures, and conjunctival scarring.

The different types of epidermolysis bullosa are differentiated from one another on the basis of whether inherited or acquired, inheritance pattern, level of split within, below or at the junction of the epidermis and dermis, distribution and severity of skin and mucous membrane involvement, scarring or nonscarring, and the affected protein and mutated gene. The inherited forms of epidermolysis bullosa demonstrate little if any inflammation on biopsy, whereas the acquired form, epidermolysis bullosa acquisita (EBA), may have an intense inflammatory infiltrate. Determining the level of the split within, below, or at the junction of the epidermis and dermis is an important part of the initial evaluation of the patient. This may be done with electron microscopy or immunofluorescent mapping with antibodies such as those to Type VII collagen, laminin, or bullous pemphigoid antigen.[252] In EBA, autoantibodies are bound in the basement membrane zone that are localized to the floor of the blister when detected by immunofluorescence on 1 molar sodium chloride (1M NaCl) split skin. EBA is often associated with other diseases such as malignancies, amyloidosis, diabetes, inflammatory bowel disease, SLE, and other autoimmune disorders, so workup of the patient for an underlying disease is indicated.[248,250]

Pathogenesis. Ultrastructural, immunohistochemical, and molecular biologic techniques have enabled the identification of affected proteins, point mutations, and corresponding ultrastructural findings in the inherited forms of epidermolysis bullosa.[252] For example, mutations in the keratins 5 and 14 are responsible for epidermolysis bullosa simplex, mutations in laminin 5 (genes LAMA3, LAMB3, and LAMC2) occur in junctional epidermolysis bullosa, and mutations in Type VII collagen (COL7A1 gene) occur in dystrophic epidermolysis bullosa.[251] EBA is an autoimmune disease with autoantibodies against type VII collagen leading to loss of or diminution of anchoring fibrils in the papillary dermis similar to the dystrophic epidermolysis bullosa phenotype.[249] Adults with EBA typically form autoantibodies to epitopes within the noncollagenous amino-terminus domain NC-1 of type VII collagen, whereas children with EBA form autoantibodies to epitopes on the NC2 or triple helical domains or both.[253]

Treatment. Avoidance of friction, pressure, trauma, and heat to skin and mucous membranes are important in the management of epidermolysis bullosa. Emollients, nutritional support, drainage of larger bullae, topical antibiotics, and nonadherent skin dressings are also important.[254] Some patients with the most severe forms of the disease may need surgical correction of pseudosyndactyly, esophageal dilation for stricture, ophthalmologic care for scarring, dental care, and monitoring for renal complications and complicating squamous cell cancer of the skin.[254] Genetic counseling is also needed with the inherited forms of the disease.

EBA is difficult to treat with no controlled studies and poor or variable response to a variety of agents. Mutasim[245] proposed an algorithm where milder cases are treated with dapsone initially followed by colchicine, then glucocorticoids, and finally cyclosporine if needed, whereas moderate to severe disease is treated initially with a combination of dapsone plus prednisone followed by cyclosporine if needed. Other treatments that have been used include other steroid sparing agents (azathioprine and mycophenylate mofetil), intravenous immune globulin, plasmapheresis, and extracorporal photochemotherapy.[245,250] Most recently, rituximab has been reported to be effective for EBA.[255,256] Childhood EBA is more responsive to treatment than in adults and will often respond to dapsone and low-dose prednisolone.[253]

Cutaneous Endometriosis

Cutaneous endometriosis is a rare condition that may cause tender nodules in the skin.[257,258] They may occur within surgical scars (e.g., cesarean section, episiotomy scars, or appendectomy scars), but also may occur as primary cutaneous endometriosis in which case they usually affect the umbilical area. Tenderness and bleeding may occur at times of menstruation. The histological appearance may correspond to different stages in the menstrual cycle but, in general, there is a poor correlation between histological appearance and the menstrual stage.[259] The range of histological findings in cutaneous endometriosis has recently been reviewed.[260] Simple surgical excision usually suffices for treatment and referral for gynecologic evaluation is also appropriate.[258]

DISORDERS OF CONNECTIVE TISSUE STRUCTURE (CARTILAGE DISORDERS)

Relapsing Polychondritis

Relapsing polychondritis (RP) is a rare, potentially life-threatening, episodic, sometimes febrile, systemic inflammatory disease affecting cartilage containing structures (e.g., ears, nose, joints, and respiratory tract) and proteoglycan rich tissues (e.g., eyes, inner ear, cardiovascular system, and kidneys).[261–264] Recurrent episodes of pain, erythema, and swelling of the ears is the most common feature of the disease occurring in up to 100% patients.[263] The earlobe is spared and eventually the ears may become "floppy" or have a "cauliflower-like" appearance as the cartilage is destroyed. Nasal chondritis may lead to a saddle nose deformity over time, sometimes without clinically apparent inflammation. Ocular involvement is common including scleritis, episcleritis, uveitis, and conjunctivitis. Proptosis, periorbital lid edema, and chemosis may simulate cellulites.[264] Other features of the disease include nonerosive polyarthritis, laryngotracheal and bronchial chondritis, cardiovascular disease (e.g., aneurysm formation, valvular heart disease, conduction abnormalities, and large vessel vasculitis), and renal disease. Pulmonary infections, systemic vasculitis, airway obstruction, and renal disease are the principal causes of death.[262] Associated diseases are not uncommon in RP including systemic vasculitis, hematologic disorders (e.g., myelodysplastic disorders, myeloma, lymphoma, and leukemia), connective tissue diseases, and other autoimmune disorders.[262] Autoantibodies to type II collagen and circulating immune complexes have been found in RP, suggesting an autoimmune pathogenesis.[265]

Cutaneous manifestations have been reported in from 17% to 50% patients.[261,266–268] In a recent series of 200 patients, 50% of patients overall were reported to have cutaneous findings.[268] When one excluded those patients with associated disease that would explain the cutaneous manifestations (e.g., psoriasis, SLE, or dermatomyositis), 35.4% of the remaining patients had cutaneous findings. Aphthosis (oral, genital, or both) was the most common manifestation. Nodules on the limbs were next in frequency that showed a septal panniculitis on biopsy in some cases and neutrophilic infiltrates suggestive of Sweet's syndrome in others. Purpura related to vasculitis, papules, pustules, superficial phlebitis, livedo reticularis, ulcerations on the limbs, and distal necrosis, in decreasing order of frequency, were also observed. Cutaneous manifestations were noted in 91% of patients with associated myelodysplasia.[268] Other reported cutaneous features of RP include urticaria, angioedema, erythema multiforme, and granulomas.[261,267]

Different sets of diagnostic criteria have been used in the published series on RP. The diagnostic criteria of McAdam et al.[266] are based on six clinical features: (1) bilateral auricular chondritis, (2) seronegative inflammatory polyarthritis, (3) nasal chondritis, (4) ocular inflammation, (5) respiratory tract chondritis, and (6) audiovestibular damage. When three or more of these criteria are present, plus histologic confirmation, the diagnosis is certain.[266] Modifications of the McAdam criteria were proposed by Damiani and Levine.[269] Under the modified criteria the diagnosis could be established with any one of the following three criteria: (1) at least three of the six clinical features of the McAdam criteria without histologic confirmation, (2) one or more of the McAdam clinical features plus histologic confirmation, or (3) chondritis in two or more separate sites with response to corticosteroids or dapsone. A third set of diagnostic criteria was used by Michet et al.[267] that included either (1) proven inflammation in the cartilaginous structures of the ear, nose, or laryngotrachea (at least two of the three sites); or (2) proven inflammation in the cartilaginous structures of the ear, nose, or laryngotrachea (just one of the three sites) plus two other manifestations (ocular involvement, seronegative arthritis, hearing loss, or vestibular involvement).

Treatment

Milder cases of RP may respond to dapsone, colchicines, and NSAIDs.[261,262,270] Acute flares and more serious involvement of vital structures are usually treated with systemic corticosteroids. Adjunctive steroid sparing agents are added if needed including azathioprine, methotrexate, or cyclophosphamide. Methotrexate was found to be the most effective in the series reported by Trentham et al.[261] Other agents that have been used include cyclosporine, penicillamine, plasma exchange, pulse steroids, anti-CD4 monoclonal antibody, and minocycline.[261,262]

Surgery and other intervention may be needed for complications of the disease including tracheostomy, cardiac valve replacement, aortic aneurysm repair, and placement of a cardiac pacemaker for conduction disturbances.[262,264] Survival has improved over time, with 94% survival in patients who have had their disease on average 8 years.[261]

Chondrodermatitis Nodularis Chronica Helicis

Chondrodermatitis nodularis chronica helicis is a common painful disorder where tender papules occur on the rim of the helix or the antihelix of the external ear.[271–273] The papules may have scaling, crusting, or ulceration suggesting the diagnosis of squamous cell cancer or basal cell cancer. Biopsy should be performed if the diagnosis is in doubt. Histopathological features may include ulceration with exudates, epidermal hyperplasia, fibrinoid dermal necrosis, mixed inflammatory cell infiltrate, thickening of the perichondrium, and degeneration of cartilage.[274] Neural hyperplasia has also been observed, on occasion, which has been suggested might explain the induction of pain by light pressure.[273]

Various treatments have been employed with different degrees of success for chondrodermatitis nodularis chronicus helicis. Injections of intralesional triamcinolone 2.5 to 5 mg/mL and surgical excision are among the most effective. If the patient sleeps habitually on one side, a pillow with a hole in it may be helpful in relieving symptoms. In one study, the results from a conservative approach by using a sponge or foam padding with a hole in it, held in place with a headband, compared favorably with surgical excision, leading the investigators to recommend this as the initial approach.[275]

NEUROVASCULAR CUTANEOUS DISEASE

Sensory Mononeuropathies

Sensory mononeuropathies are not uncommon and may affect the head, trunk, and extremities. They may manifest themselves as numbness, burning, itching, hyperesthesias, and, frequently, pain.[276] Among the more common are cheiralgia paresthetica (superficial branch of the radial nerve), meralgia paresthetica (lateral femoral cutaneous nerve), notalgia paresthetica (dorsal rami of T2-T6), and gonyalgia paresthetica (infrapateller branch of the saphenous nerve). A less common but important neuropathy to be aware of is mental nerve neuropathy which presents as unilateral numbness of the chin and lower lip (numb chin syndrome).[276–278] It is usually associated with malignancy, most commonly breast cancer or lymphoma, so thorough evaluation is needed.[277]

Notalgia paresthetica is a sensory neuropathy affecting the posterior rami of T2-T6. Patients usually complain of pruritus and less commonly pain (30%), paresthesias (28%), and hyperesthesia (12%) in a unilateral localized area on the upper back medial to the scapula.[279] Findings on examination may include hyperpigmentation and hypoesthesia.[276,280] Electromyographic evaluation may show evidence of paraspinal denervation in some cases.[281] In a study of 43 patients, 60.7% were found to have radiographic abnormalities of the spine corresponding to the nerves involved, suggesting impingement of spinal nerves.[279] Massey postulated the posterior rami of T2-T6 are subject to trauma because they traverse the multifidus spinal muscle at a right angle course.[276] A hereditary variant of notalgia paresthetica has been described and it has also been reported in MEN2A.[280] Histologically, one may find postinflammatory hyperpigmentation, lichenification, and, in some cases, macular amyloidosis possibly related to excoriation.[282]

Treatment

Treatment of notalgia paresthetica has met with variable success with such agents as topical anesthetics, capsaicin, and topical corticosteroids.[283] Oxcarbazepine (a derivative of the anticonvulsant carbamazepine with a better side effect profile) was reported to be partially effective in three of five patients treated with the medication.[284] A paravertebral block using a combination of bupivacaine and methylprednisolone led to complete resolution of symptoms for at least 1 year in one patient.[280] Recently, intralesional botulinum toxin A was reported to produce complete resolution of pruritus in two patients.[283] Gabapentin in a dose of 600 mg/day provided complete relief of symptoms in one patient with notalgia paresthetica.[285]

Fabry's Disease

Fabry's disease (FD) is a rare, X-linked recessive, lysosomal storage disease caused by deficiency of the enzyme alpha-galactosidase A, leading to accumulation of neutral glycosphingolipids, primarily globotriaosylceramide and digalactosylceramide, in endothelial cells and other cell types.[286–290] The deposits in the endothelial cells cause swelling and narrowing of the lumen that can eventually lead to ischemia, infarction, and pain.

Symptoms and Signs

Angiokeratomas are the characteristic skin lesion of FD that occur in a pattern referred to as angiokeratoma corporis diffusum (ACD) to distinguish them from other variants of angiokeratomas not associated with FD, such as isolated angiokeratomas, angiokeratomas of Mibelli on the dorsum of the fingers and toes, and angiokeratomas of the scrotum (Fordyce) that occur typically in elderly males. Individual angiokeratomas are reddish-blue to black 3 to 4 mm diameter papules that may be scaly, hyperkeratotic, or verrucous. In ACD, they are usually distributed between the umbilicus and the knees but may be widespread and affect mucous membranes as well. Angiokeratomas usually first appear in adolescence and increase in number with time.

Hypohidrosis with heat intolerance, peripheral edema, and asymptomatic eye findings are other features of the disease. The potential eye findings include tortuous retinal and conjunctival vessels, a characteristic whorled corneal opacity, and a posterior capsular cataract (Fabry cataract). The corneal opacities may be found in approximately 70% of female carriers as well and, less often, female carriers may have angiokeratomas.[291] Female carriers in general may be asymptomatic, have mild disease, or rarely severe disease manifestations.[291]

Episodic painful acroparesthesias of the hands and feet lasting from minutes to hours may be the first manifestation of the disease developing in childhood. They may be brought on by heat, cold, fatigue, exertion, or fever. Patients may be left with residual tingling or pain between attacks. Acute attacks of abdominal pain may occur simulating an acute abdomen but abdominal pain may also be chronic.[286,287]

The most serious complications of the disease relate to involvement of the kidneys, heart, and central nervous system. Untreated patients typically develop end-stage renal disease by the fifth decade. Patients may develop cardiac arrhythmias, conduction defects, left ventricular hypertrophy, transient ischemic attacks, and strokes.[286] Variants of FD have been reported that involve principally the heart or the kidneys.[286]

Histologically, ACD demonstrates dilated vessels in the papillary dermis with epidermal hyperplasia or acanthosis.[291] The abnormal lipid in the endothelial cells may be detected with a lipid stain or periodic acid-Schiff stain. Electron microscopy demonstrates membrane-bound, lamellar, or myelin-like inclusions. Examination of the urine with polarized light may show birefringent glycosphingolipids in cells with a Maltese cross appearance. The diagnosis is confirmed by finding diminished alpha-galactosidase A activity in plasma or peripheral blood leukocytes. Female carriers may have normal alpha-galactosidase A levels and, in the absence of any clinical manifestations, identification of the specific gene mutation is needed for confirmation of the diagnosis.[286]

The angiokeratomas found in FD are not unique to FD. Other storage diseases have been reported to have angiokeratomas. These include fucosidosis, mannosidosis, GM-1 gangliosidosis, aspartylglycosaminuria, sialidosis, galactosialidosis, and alpha-N-acetylgalactosaminidase deficiency.[292] Rarely, there have been reports of angiokeratoma corporis diffusum in patients without alpha-galactosidase A deficiency or other enzyme deficiencies.[293]

Treatment

Enzyme replacement therapy (ERT) with recombinant alpha-galactosidase A (agalsidase beta, Fabrazyme, Genzyme Corp.) was approved for treatment in the U.S. by the FDA in 2003.[294] ERT has been associated with improvement of neuropathic pain, relief of gastrointestinal symptoms, and stabilization of renal function and cardiomyopathy.[286] In patients with advanced disease, ERT slowed progression of renal, cardiac, and cerebrovascular disease, suggesting intervention should be early before irreversible damage occurs.[294]

Supportive therapy for cardiac, renal, neurologic and gastrointestinal symptoms is important, along with monitoring for complications in both affected males and female carriers. Genetic counseling is also important. There is no need to treat the angiokeratomas unless they are symptomatic which can be done with a variety of local destructive methods such as laser or liquid nitrogen. The angiokeratomas have not been found to be a useful surrogate marker to follow disease activity with ERT.[295]

NEOPLASMS

Both benign and malignant neoplasms may sometimes be painful because of ulceration, location on the body where they are repeatedly traumatized, or on pressure bearing surfaces such as the soles of the feet. Certain benign neoplasms are characteristically painful and bring to mind a differential diagnosis that has been reported under the acronym LEND AN EGG which includes leiomyoma, eccrine spiradenoma, neuroma, dermatofibroma, angiolipoma, neurilemmoma, endometrioma, glomus tumor, and granular cell tumor.[296] We advocate the use of the acronym ANGEL for the reasons summarized in the following text. Painful neuromas include traumatic neuromas and Morton's neuroma of the forefoot. A traumatic neuroma is a proliferative and hyperplastic reactive change to injury rather than a true neoplasm.[297] Morton's neuroma is a degenerative change in neural tissue related to chronic injury and not a true neoplasm.[298] Dermatofibromas

TABLE 37.2

CHARACTERISTIC FEATURES OF BENIGN PAINFUL CUTANEOUS NEOPLASMS

Tumor	Appearance	Usual location	Pathologic features	Comment
Glomus tumor[304,305]	Reddish-blue papule or nodule usually <1 cm in diameter	Hands and fingers especially subungually	Glomus cells with eosinophilic cytoplasm and round nuclei, blood vessels and nerve fibers	Paroxysms of pain on exposure to cold or pressure. Multiple glomus tumors (familial glomangiomas) are usually asymptomatic.
Leiomyoma[306,307]	Firm erythematous to brown intradermal papules and nodules.	Trunk and extremities.	Interlacing bundles of smooth muscle cells with cigar-shaped nuclei.	Pain on exposure to cold, pressure, trauma, emotion or may occur spontaneously. May be associated with a hereditary syndrome with renal cell cancer.
Angioleiomyoma[307,308]	Subcutaneous or deep dermal nodule or mass up to 4 cm in diameter.	Lower extremities.	Encapsulated tumor with interlacing bundles of smooth muscle cells and many small blood vessels.	Pain or tenderness with pressure. Some leiomyomas are associated with a hereditary syndrome with renal cancer.
Angiolipoma[309,310]	Subcutaneous 0.5 to 4.0 cm nodule with normal, bluish or reddish overlying skin.	Typically located on the forearm.	Encapsulated tumor with mature adipocytes, many small-caliber blood vessels, and microthrombi.	Frequently painful with pressure or when moved.
Neurilemmoma (schwannoma)[311]	2–4 cm diameter flesh-colored tumor.	Head and extremities (especially flexor) attached to a cranial or peripheral nerve.	Intraneural proliferation of schwann cells with Antoni type A or Antoni type B pattern.	Pain may be localized or radiate along the course of the nerve.
Eccrine spiradenoma[312,313]	0.3–5.0 cm firm intradermal nodule often with bluish overlying skin.	Most often on ventral surface of the skin.	Two populations of epithelial cells with eccrine differentiation. Fibrous capsule and ductal differentiation often present.	Usually tender or painful.

are common benign neoplasms that typically are not painful but pain may occur on occasion. They often exhibit the dimple sign that is elicited by exerting pressure from the sides. Cutaneous endometriosis was discussed earlier in this chapter. Endometriosis is an ectopic localization of endometrial glands that may occur by fallopian tube regurgitation, angiolymphatic invasion, transportation during surgery, or a result of local imitative metaplasia rather than a true neoplasm.[299,300] Granular cell tumors are only occasionally painful.[301] The remaining benign painful neoplasms may be remembered under the acronym ANGEL: angiolipoma, neurilemmoma, glomus tumor, eccrine spiradenoma, and leiomyoma. These tumors are all true neoplasms where pain is a characteristic feature. They are listed in Table 37.2 with their comparative features. Treatment when needed consists of complete excision which is usually curative.

Leiomyomas are deserving of further discussion because of their association with hereditary leiomyomatosis and renal cell cancer.[302,303] This is an autosomal dominant condition due to mutations in the enzyme fumarate hydratase that is associated with cutaneous leiomyomas, leiomyosarcoma (rarely), uterine fibroids (leiomyomas), and renal cell cancer. Most patients have multiple cutaneous leiomyomas but even a single leiomyoma may be a marker for the syndrome. When a patient with a cutaneous leiomyoma is encountered, a history should be taken for any personal or family history of cutaneous leiomyomas, uterine fibroids, early hysterectomy, and renal cell cancer.[303] If the history is suggestive, imaging studies of the kidneys and testing for fumarate hydratase mutations is indicated along with lifetime surveillance and examination of relatives if studies confirm the diagnosis.

Acknowledgments

The authors wish to acknowledge the contributions of Dr. George F. Odland to this chapter. He was the original primary author, and many of his touches and words remain part of the fabric of the chapter.

References

1. Xu F, Sternberg MR, Kottiri BJ, et al. Trends in herpes simplex virus type 1 and type 2 seroprevalence in the United States. *JAMA* 2006;296(8):964–973.
2. Wolff K, Goldsmith LA, Katz SI, et al. *Fitzpatrick's Dermatology in General Medicine*. 7th ed. New York: McGraw-Hill; 2008.

3. Kasper DL, Braunwald E, Faucxi AS, eds. *Harrison's Principles of Internal Medicine*. 17th ed. New York: McGraw-Hill; 2008.
4. Braverman IM, ed. *Skin Signs of Systemic Disease*. 3rd ed. Philadelphia: WB Saunders; 1998.
5. Burns T, Breathnach S, Cox N, eds. *Rook's Textbook of Dermatology*, Vol. 4. 7th ed. London: Blackwell Science Ltd; 2004.
6. Steinhoff M, Luger TA. Neurobiology of the skin. In: Wolff K, Goldsmith LA, Katz SI, eds. *Fitzpatrick's Dermatology in General Medicine*. 7th ed. New York: McGraw-Hill; 2008:895–901.
7. Hilliges M, Wang L, Johansson O. Ultrastructural evidence for nerve fibers within all vital layers of the human epidermis. *J Invest Dermatol* 1995;104(1): 134–137.
8. Reilly DM, Ferdinando D, Johnston C, et al. The epidermal nerve fibre network: characterization of nerve fibres in human skin by confocal microscopy and assessment of racial variations. *Br J Dermatol* 1997;137(2):163–170.
9. Ansel JC, Kaynard AH, Armstrong CA, et al. Skin-nervous system interactions. *J Invest Dermatol* 1996;106(1):198–204.
10. Holzer P. Local effector functions of capsaicin-sensitive sensory nerve endings: involvement of tachykinins, calcitonin gene-related peptide and other neuropeptides. *Neuroscience* 1988;24(3):739–768.
11. Otsuka M, Yoshioka K. Neurotransmitter functions of mammalian tachykinins. *Physiol Rev* 1993;73(2):229–308.
12. Sneller MC, Langford CA, Fauci AS. The vasculitis syndromes. In: Kasper DL, Braunwald E, Fauci AS, et al., eds. *Harrison's Principles of Internal Medicine*. 16th ed. New York: McGraw-Hill; 2005:2002–2014.
13. Guillevin L, Mahr A, Cohen P, et al. Short-term corticosteroids then lamivudine and plasma exchanges to treat hepatitis B virus-related polyarteritis nodosa. *Arthritis Rheum* 2004;51(3):482–487.
14. Jennette JC, Falk RJ. Small-vessel vasculitis. *N Engl J Med* 1997;337(21): 1512–1523.
15. Hoffman GS, Kerr GS, Leavitt RY, et al. Wegener granulomatosis: an analysis of 158 patients. *Ann Intern Med* 1992;116:488–498.
16. Genta MS, Genta RM, Gabay C. Systemic rheumatoid vasculitis: a review. *Semin Arthritis Rheum* 2006;36(2):88–98.
17. Scott DG, Bacon PA. Intravenous cyclophosphamide plus methylprednisolone in treatment of systemic rheumatoid vasculitis. *Am J Med* 1984;76(3): 377–384.
18. Kern AB. Atrophie blanche. Report of two patients treated with aspirin and dipyridamole. *J Am Acad Dermatol* 1982;6:1048–1053.
19. Sams WM Jr. Livedo vasculitis. Therapy with pentoxifylline. *Arch Dermatol* 1988;124:684–687.
20. Callen JP. Livedoid vasculopathy: what it is and how the patient should be evaluated and treated. *Arch Dermatol* 2006;142:1481–1482.
21. Russell JP, Gibson LE. Primary cutaneous small vessel vasculitis: approach to diagnosis and treatment. *Int J Dermatol* 2006;45(1):3–13.
22. Langford CA. 15. Vasculitis. *J Allergy Clin Immunol* 2003;111:S602–S612.
23. Gibson LE. Cutaneous vasculitis update. *Dermatol Clin* 2001;19:603–615, vii.
24. Lotti T, Ghersetich I, Comacchi C, et al. Cutaneous small-vessel vasculitis. *J Am Acad Dermatol* 1998;39:667–687.
25. Braverman IM. The angiitides. In: Braverman IM, ed. *Skin Signs of Systemic Disease*. 3rd ed. Philadelphia: WB Saunders; 1998:278–334.
26. Sais G, Vidaller A, Jugclá A, et al. Prognostic factors in leukocytoclastic vasculitis: a clinicopathologic study of 160 patients. *Arch Dermatol* 1998;134: 309–315.
27. Carlson JA, Ng BT, Chen KR. Cutaneous vasculitis update: diagnostic criteria, classification, epidemiology, etiology, pathogenesis, evaluation and prognosis. *Am J Dermatopathol* 2005;27(6):504–528.
28. Carlson JA, Chen KR. Cutaneous pseudovasculitis. *Am J Dermatopathol* 2007;29(1):44–55.
29. Sais G, Vidaller A, Jugclá A, et al. Adhesion molecule expression and endothelial cell activation in cutaneous leukocytoclastic vasculitis. An immunohistologic and clinical study in 42 patients. *Arch Dermatol* 1997;133(4):443–450.
30. Mekkes JR, Loots MA, van der Wal AC, et al. Increased incidence of hypercoagulability in patients with leg ulcers caused by leukocytoclastic vasculitis. *J Am Acad Dermatol* 2004;50(1):104–107.
31. Jennette JC, Falk RJ, Andrassy K, et al. Nomenclature of systemic vasculitides. Proposal of an international consensus conference. *Arthritis Rheum* 1994; 37(2):187–192.
32. Ferri C, La Civita L, Longombardo G, et al. Mixed cryoglobulinaemia: a cross-road between autoimmune and lymphoproliferative disorders. *Lupus* 1998;7:275–279.
33. Fiorentino DF. Cutaneous vasculitis. *J Am Acad Dermatol* 2003;48:311–340.
34. Sais G, Vidaller A, Jugclà A, et al. Colchicine in the treatment of cutaneous leukocytoclastic vasculitis. Results of a prospective, randomized controlled trial. *Arch Dermatol* 1995;131:1399–1402.
35. Guillevin L, Mouthon L. Tumor necrosis factor-alpha blockade and the risk of vasculitis. *J Rheumatol* 2004;31(10):1885–1887.
36. Chung L, Funke AA, Chakravarty EF, et al. Successful use of rituximab for cutaneous vasculitis. *Arch Dermatol* 2006;142(11):1407–1410.
37. Diaz-Perez JL, Winkelmann RK. Cutaneous periarteritis nodosa. *Arch Dermatol* 1974;110(3):407–414.
38. Daoud MS, Hutton KP, Gibson LE. Cutaneous periarteritis nodosa: a clinicopathological study of 79 cases. *Br J Dermatol* 1997;136:706–713.
39. Pak H, Montemarano AD, Berger T. Purpuric nodules and macules on the

extremities of a young woman. Cutaneous polyarteritis nodosa. *Arch Dermatol* 1998;134(2):231–232, 234–235.
40. Lhote F, Cohen P, Guillevin L. Polyarteritis nodosa, microscopic polyangiitis and Churg-Strauss syndrome. *Lupus* 1998;7(4):238–258.
41. Cohen RD, Conn DL, Ilstrup DM. Clinical features, prognosis, and response to treatment in polyarteritis. *Mayo Clin Proc* 1980;55:146–155.
42. Braverman IM. The angiitides. In: Braverman IM, ed. *Skin Signs of Systemic Disease*. 3rd ed. Philadelphia: WB Saunders, 1998:279–283.
43. Kikuchi K, Hoashi T, Kanazawa S, et al. Angiogenic cytokines in serum and cutaneous lesions of patients with polyarteritis nodosa. *J Am Acad Dermatol* 2005;53(1):57–61.
44. Coblyn JS, McCluskey RT. Case records of the Massachusetts General Hospital. Weekly clinicopathological exercises. Case 3-2003. A 36-year-old man with renal failure, hypertension, and neurologic abnormalities. *N Engl J Med* 2003:333–342.
45. Soufir N, Descamps V, Crickx B, et al. Hepatitis C virus infection in cutaneous polyarteritis nodosa: a retrospective study of 16 cases. *Arch Dermatol* 1999; 135:1001–1002.
46. Matsumara Y, Mizuno K, Okamoto H, Imamura S. A case of cutaneous polyarteritis nodosa associated with ulcerative colitis. *Br J Dermatol* 2000; 142(3):561–562.
47. Schaffer JV, Davidson DM, McNiff JM, et al. Perinuclear antineutrophilic cytoplasmic antibody-positive cutaneous polyarteritis nodosa associated with minocycline therapy for acne vulgaris. *J Am Acad Dermatol* 2001;44: 198–206.
48. Cvancara JL, Meffert JJ, Elston DM. Estrogen-sensitive cutaneous polyarteritis nodosa: response to tamoxifen. *J Am Acad Dermatol* 1998;39(4 Pt 1): 643–646.
49. Fathalla BM, Miller L, Brady S, et al. Cutaneous polyarteritis nodosa in children. *J Am Acad Dermatol* 2005;53(4):724–728.
50. Sheth AP, Olson JC, Esterly NB. Cutaneous polyarteritis nodosa of childhood. *J Am Acad Dermatol* 1994;31:561–566.
51. Gayraud M, Guillevin L, Cohen P, et al. Treatment of good-prognosis polyarteritis nodosa and Churg-Strauss syndrome: comparison of steroids and oral or pulse cyclophosphamide in 25 patients. French Cooperative Study Group for Vasculitides. *Br J Rheumatol* 1997;36:1290–1297.
52. Guillevin L, Cohen P, Mahr A, et al. Treatment of polyarteritis nodosa and microscopic polyangiitis with poor prognosis factors: a prospective trial comparing glucocorticoids and six or twelve cyclophosphamide pulses in sixty-five patients. *Arthritis Rheum* 2003;49:93–100.
53. Kallenberg CG. Antineutrophil cytoplasmic autoantibody-associated small-vessel vasculitis. *Curr Opin Rheumatol* 2007;19(1):17–24.
54. Francès C, Du LT, Piette JC, et al. Wegener's granulomatosis. Dermatological manifestations in 75 cases with clinicopathologic correlation. *Arch Dermatol* 1994;130(7):861–867.
55. Piette WW. Primary systemic vasculitis. In: Sontheimer RD, Provost TT, eds. *Cutaneous Manifestations of Rheumatic Diseases*. 2nd ed. Philadelphia: Lippincott Williams and Wilkins; 2004:184–187.
56. Hu CH, O'Loughlin S, Winkelmann RK. Cutaneous manifestations of Wegener granulomatosis. *Arch Dermatol* 1977;113:175–182.
57. Patten SF, Tomecki KJ. Wegener's granulomatosis: cutaneous and oral mucosal disease. *J Am Acad Dermatol* 1993;28:710–718.
58. Manchanda Y, Tejasvi T, Handa R, et al. Strawberry gingiva: a distinctive sign in Wegener's granulomatosis. *J Am Acad Dermatol* 2003;49:335–337.
59. Knight JM, Hayduk MJ, Summerlin DJ, et al. "Strawberry" gingival hyperplasia: a pathognomonic mucocutaneous finding in Wegener granulomatosis. *Arch Dermatol* 2000;136:171–173.
60. Carlson JA, Chen KR. Cutaneous vasculitis update: small vessel neutrophilic vasculitis syndromes. *Am J Dermatopathol* 2006;28:486–506.
61. Koldingsnes W, Gran JT, Omdal R, et al. Wegener's granulomatosis: long-term follow-up of patients treated with pulse cyclophosphamide. *Br J Rheumatol* 1998;37:659–664.
62. Guillevin L, Cordier JF, Lhote F, et al. A prospective, multicenter, randomized trial comparing steroids and pulse cyclophosphamide versus steroids and oral cyclophosphamide in the treatment of generalized Wegener's granulomatosis. *Arthritis Rheum* 1997;40:2187–2198.
63. Hoffman GS. Treatment of Wegener's granulomatosis: time to change the standard of care? *Arthritis Rheum* 1997;40(12):2099–2104.
64. Stegeman CA, Tervaert JW, de Jong PE, et al. Trimethoprim-sulfamethoxazole (co-trimoxazole) for the prevention of relapses of Wegener's granulomatosis. Dutch Co-Trimoxazole Wegener Study Group. *N Engl J Med* 1996; 335:16–20.
65. Wegener's Granulomatosis Etanercept Trial (WGET) Research Group. Etanercept plus standard therapy for Wegener's granulomatosis. *N Engl J Med* 2005;352:351–361.
66. Keogh KA, Ytterberg SR, Fervenza FC, et al. Rituximab for refractory Wegener's granulomatosis: report of a prospective, open-label pilot trial. *Am J Respir Crit Care Med* 2006;173:180–187.
67. Braverman IM. The angiitides. In: Braverman IM, ed. *Skin Signs of Systemic Disease*. 3rd ed. Philadelphia: WB Saunders; 1998:309–312.
68. Peñas PF, Porras JI, Fraga J, et al. Microscopic polyangiitis. A systemic vasculitis with a positive P-ANCA. *Br J Dermatol* 1996;134:542–547.
69. Irvine AD, Bruce IN, Walsh M, et al. Dermatological presentation of disease associated with antineutrophil cytoplasmic antibodies: a report of two contrasting cases and a review of the literature. *Br J Dermatol* 1996;134: 924–928.

70. Irvine AD, Bruce IN, Walsh MY, et al. Microscopic polyangiitis. Delineation of a cutaneous-limited variant associated with antimyeloperoxidase autoantibody. *Arch Dermatol* 1997;133:474–477.

71. Guillevin L, Durand-Gasselin B, Cevallos R, et al. Microscopic polyangiitis: clinical and laboratory findings in eighty-five patients. *Arthritis Rheum* 1999; 42:421–430.

72. Lauque D, Cadranel J, Lazor R, et al. Microscopic polyangiitis with alveolar hemorrhage. A study of 29 cases and review of the literature. *Medicine (Baltimore)* 2000;79:222–233.

73. Peco-Antic A, Bonaci-Nikolic B, Basta-Jovanovic G, et al. Childhood microscopic polyangiitis associated with MPO-ANCA. *Pediatr Nephrol* 2006;21: 46–53.

74. Cohen P, Pagnoux C, Mahr A, et al. Churg-Strauss syndrome with poor-prognosis factors: a prospective multicenter trial comparing glucocorticoids and six or twelve cyclophosphamide pulses in forty-eight patients. *Arthritis Rheum* 2007;57:686–693.

75. Sinico RA, Di Toma L, Maggiore U, et al. Prevalence and clinical significance of antineutrophil cytoplasmic antibodies in Churg-Strauss syndrome. *Arthritis Rheum* 2005;52:2926–2935.

76. Sablé-Fourtassou R, Cohen P, Mahr A, et al. Antineutrophil cytoplasmic antibodies and the Churg-Strauss syndrome. *Ann Intern Med* 2005;143:632–638.

77. Pagnoux C, Guilpain P, Guillevin L. Churg-Strauss syndrome. *Curr Opin Rheumatol* 2007;19(1):25–32.

78. Guillevin L, Cohen P, Gayraud M, et al. Churg-Strauss syndrome. Clinical study and long-term follow-up of 96 patients. *Medicine (Baltimore)* 1999;78: 26–37.

79. Davis MD, Daoud MS, McEvoy MT, et al. Cutaneous manifestations of Churg-Strauss syndrome: a clinicopathologic correlation. *J Am Acad Dermatol* 1997;37(2 Pt 1):199–203.

80. Ferenczi K, Chang T, Camouse M, et al. A case of Churg-Strauss syndrome associated with antiphospholipid antibodies. *J Am Acad Dermatol* 2007;56: 701–704.

81. Watson KM, Salisbury JR, Creamer D. Purpura fulminans — a novel presentation of Churg Strauss syndrome. *Clin Exp Dermatol* 2004;29(4):390–392.

82. Crotty CP, DeRemee RA, Winkelmann RK. Cutaneous clinicopathologic correlation of allergic granulomatosis. *J Am Acad Dermatol* 1981;5(5):571–581.

83. Langford CA, Fauci AS. The vasculitis syndromes. In: Fauci AS, Kasper DL, Longo DL, et al., eds. *Harrison's Principles of Internal Medicine.* 17th ed. New York: McGraw-Hill; 2008:2119–2131.

84. Chen KR, Toyohara A, Suzuki A, et al. Clinical and histopathological spectrum of cutaneous vasculitis in rheumatoid arthritis. *Br J Dermatol* 2002; 147(5):905–913.

85. Scott DG, Bacon PA, Tribe CR. Systemic rheumatoid vasculitis: a clinical and laboratory study of 50 cases. *Medicine (Baltimore)* 1981;60(4):288–297.

86. Lipsky PE. Rheumatoid arthritis. In: Fauci AS, Kasper DL, Longo DL, et al., eds. *Harrison's Principles of Internal Medicine.* New York: McGraw-Hill; 2005:1968–1977.

87. Magro CM, Crowson AN. The spectrum of cutaneous lesions in rheumatoid arthritis: a clinical and pathological study of 43 patients. *J Cutan Pathol* 2003; 30:1–10.

88. Rapoport RJ, Kozin F, Mackel SE, et al. Cutaneous vascular immunofluorescence in rheumatoid arthritis. Correlation with circulating immune complexes and vasculitis. *Am J Med* 1980;68(3):325–331.

89. Nicholls A, Snaith ML, Maini RN, et al. Proceedings: Controlled trial of azathioprine in rheumatoid vasculitis. *Ann Rheum Dis* 1973;32(6):589–591.

90. Hairston BR, Davis MD, Pittelkow MR, et al. Livedoid vasculopathy: further evidence for procoagulant pathogenesis. *Arch Dermatol* 2006;142: 1413–1418.

91. Calamia KT, Balabanova M, Perniciaro C, et al. Livedo (livedoid) vasculitis and the factor V Leiden mutation: additional evidence for abnormal coagulation. *J Am Acad Dermatol* 2002;46(1):133–137.

92. Barnhill RL, Busam KJ, Nousari CH, et al. Vascular diseases. In: Elder DE, Elenitsas R, Johnson BL Jr, et al., eds. *Lever's Histopathology of the Skin.* 9th ed. Philadelphia: Lippincott Williams & Wilkins; 2005:215–242.

93. Winkelmann RK, Schroeter AL, Kierland RR, et al. Clinical studies of livedoid vasculitis: (segmental hyalinizing vasculitis). *Mayo Clin Proc* 1974;49: 746–750.

94. Schroeter AL, Diaz-Perez JL, Winkelmann RK, et al. Livedo vasculitis (the vasculitis of atrophie blanche). Immunohistopathologic study. *Arch Dermatol* 1975;111(2):188–193.

95. Hsiao GH, Chiu HC. Livedoid vasculitis. Response to low-dose danazol. *Arch Dermatol* 1996;132:749–751.

96. Jetton RL, Lazarus GS. Minidose heparin therapy for vasculitis of atrophie blanche. *J Am Acad Dermatol* 1983;8:23–26.

97. Heine KG, Davis GW. Idiopathic atrophie blanche: treatment with low-dose heparin. *Arch Dermatol* 1986;122:855–856.

98. Hairston BR, Davis MD, Gibson LE, Drage LA. Treatment of livedoid vasculopathy with low-molecular-weight heparin: report of 2 cases. *Arch Dermatol* 2003;139(8):987–990.

99. Browning CE, Callen JP. Warfarin therapy for livedoid vasculopathy associated with cryofibrinogenemia and hyperhomocysteinemia. *Arch Dermatol* 2006;142:75–78.

100. Gilliam JN, Herndon JH, Prystowsky SD. Fibrinolytic therapy for vasculitis of atrophie blanche. *Arch Dermatol* 1974;109(5):664–667.

101. Klein KL, Pittelkow MR. Tissue plasminogen activator for treatment of livedoid vasculitis. *Mayo Clin Proc* 1992;67:923–933.

102. Deng A, Gocke CD, Hess J, et al. Livedoid vasculopathy associated with plasminogen activator inhibitor-1 promoter homozygosity (4G/4G) treated successfully with tissue plasminogen activator. *Arch Dermatol* 2006;142: 1466–1469.

103. Purcell SM, Hayes TJ. Nifedipine treatment of idiopathic atrophie blanche. *J Am Acad Dermatol* 1986;14(5 Pt 1):851–854.

104. Choi HJ, Hann SK. Livedo reticularis and livedoid vasculitis responding to PUVA therapy. *J Am Acad Dermatol* 1999;40(2 Pt 1):204–207.

105. Yang CH, Ho HC, Chan YS, et al. Intractable livedoid vasculopathy successfully treated with hyperbaric oxygen. *Br J Dermatol* 2003;149(3):647–652.

106. Kreuter A, Gambichler T, Breuckmann F, et al. Pulsed intravenous immunoglobulin therapy in livedoid vasculitis: an open trial evaluating 9 consecutive patients. *J Am Acad Dermatol* 2004;51(4):574–579.

107. Levine JS, Branch DW, Rauch J. The antiphospholipid syndrome. *N Engl J Med* 2002;346(10):752–763.

108. Francès C, Niang S, Laffitte E, et al. Dermatologic manifestations of the antiphospholipid syndrome: two hundred consecutive cases. *Arthritis Rheum* 2005;52(6):1785–1793.

109. Kriseman YL, Nash JW, Hsu S. Criteria for the diagnosis of antiphospholipid syndrome in patients presenting with dermatologic symptoms. *J Am Acad Dermatol* 2007;57(1):112–115.

110. Asherson RA, Cervera R. Antiphospholipid syndrome. *J Invest Dermatol* 1993;100:S21–S27.

111. Gibson GE, Su WP, Pittelkow MR. Antiphospholipid syndrome and the skin. *J Am Acad Dermatol* 1997;36:970–982.

112. Wilson WA, Gharavi AE, Koike T, et al. International consensus statement on preliminary classification criteria for definite antiphospholipid syndrome: report of an international workshop. *Arthritis Rheum* 1999;42:1309–1311.

113. Miyakis S, Lockshin MD, Atsumi T, et al. International consensus statement on an update of the classification criteria for definite antiphospholipid syndrome (APS). *J Thromb Haemost* 2006;4:295–306.

114. Lim W, Crowther MA, Eikelboom JW. Management of antiphospholipid antibody syndrome: a systematic review. *JAMA* 2006;295(9):1050–1057.

115. Ruiz-Irastorza G, Khamashta MA. The treatment of antiphospholipid syndrome: a harmonic contrast. *Best Pract Res Clin Rheumatol* 2007;21(6): 1079–1092.

116. Asherson RA, Cervera R, de Groot PG, et al. Catastrophic antiphospholipid syndrome: international consensus statement on classification criteria and treatment guidelines. *Lupus* 2003;12:530–534.

117. Asherson RA, Cervera R, Piette JC, et al. Catastrophic antiphospholipid syndrome: clues to the pathogenesis from a series of 80 patients. *Medicine (Baltimore)* 2001;80:355–377.

118. Petri M, Qazi U. Management of antiphospholipid syndrome in pregnancy. *Rheum Dis Clin North Am* 2006;32(3):591–607.

119. Ruiz-Irastorza G, Egurbide MV, Pijoan JI, et al. Effect of antimalarials on thrombosis and survival in patients with systemic lupus erythematosus. *Lupus* 2006;15:577–583.

120. Erre GL, Pardini S, Faedda R, et al. Effect of rituximab on clinical and laboratory features of antiphospholipid syndrome: a case report and a review of literature. *Lupus* 2008;17(1):50–55.

121. Green H, Paul M, Vidal L, et al. Prophylaxis of Pneumocystis pneumonia in immunocompromised non-HIV-infected patients: systematic review and meta-analysis of randomized controlled trials. *Mayo Clin Proc* 2007;82(9): 1052–1059.

122. Mansharamani NG, Balachandran D, Vernovsky I, et al. Peripheral blood CD4 + T-lymphocyte counts during Pneumocystis carinii pneumonia in immunocompromised patients without HIV infection. *Chest* 2000;118:712–720.

123. Godeau B, Coutant-Perronne V, Le Thi Huong D, et al. Pneumocystis carinii pneumonia in the course of connective tissue disease: report of 34 cases. *J Rheumatol* 1994;21:246–251.

124. Overgaard UM, Helweg-Larsen J. Pneumocystis jiroveci pneumonia (PCP) in HIV-1-negative patients: a retrospective study 2002–2004. *Scand J Infect Dis* 2007;39:589–595.

125. Koch-Weser J. Coumarin necrosis. *Ann Intern Med* 1968;68:1365–1367.

126. Bauer KA. Coumarin-induced skin necrosis. *Arch Dermatol* 1993;129(6): 766–768.

127. Chan YC, Valenti D, Mansfield AO, et al. Warfarin induced skin necrosis. *Br J Surg* 2000;87:266–272.

128. Weiss P, Soff GA, Halkin H, et al. Decline of proteins C and S and factors II, VII, IX and X during the initiation of warfarin therapy. *Thromb Res* 1987; 45(6):783–790.

129. Jillella AP, Lutcher CL. Reinstituting warfarin in patients who develop warfarin skin necrosis. *Am J Hematol* 1996;52:117–119.

130. Cole MS, Minifee PK, Wolma FJ. Coumarin necrosis—a review of the literature. *Surgery* 1988;103(3):271–277.

131. Essex DW, Wynn SS, Jin DK. Late-onset warfarin-induced skin necrosis: case report and review of the literature. *Am J Hematol* 1998;57(3):233–237.

132. DeFranzo AJ, Marasco P, Argenta LC. Warfarin-induced necrosis of the skin. *Ann Plast Surg* 1995;34(2):203–208.

133. Schramm W, Spannagl M, Bauer KA, et al. Treatment of coumarin-induced skin necrosis with a monoclonal antibody purified protein C concentrate. *Arch Dermatol* 1993;129(6):753–756.

134. Khafif RA, DeLima C, Silverberg A, et al. Calciphylaxis and systemic calcinosis. Collective review. *Arch Intern Med* 1990;150:956–959.

135. Oh DH, Eulau D, Tokugawa DA, et al. Five cases of calciphylaxis and a review of the literature. *J Am Acad Dermatol* 1999;40:979–987.
136. Guldbakke KK, Khachemoune A. Calciphylaxis. *Int J Dermatol* 2007;46(3): 231–238.
137. Angelis M, Wong LL, Myers SA, et al. Calciphylaxis in patients on hemodialysis: a prevalence study. *Surgery* 1997;122:1083–1089; discussion 1089–1090.
138. Budisavljevic MN, Cheek D, Ploth DW. Calciphylaxis in chronic renal failure. *J Am Soc Nephrol* 1996;7:978–982.
139. Wilmer WA, Magro CM. Calciphylaxis: emerging concepts in prevention, diagnosis, and treatment. *Semin Dial* 2002;15:172–186.
140. Hafner J, Keusch G, Wahl C, et al. Uremic small-artery disease with medial calcification and intimal hyperplasia (so-called calciphylaxis): a complication of chronic renal failure and benefit from parathyroidectomy. *J Am Acad Dermatol* 1995;33:954–962.
141. Ivker RA, Woosley J, Briggaman RA. Calciphylaxis in three patients with end-stage renal disease. *Arch Dermatol* 1995;131:63–68.
142. Bazari H, Jaff MR, Mannstadt M, et al. Case records of the Massachusetts General Hospital. Case7-2007: a 59-year-old woman with diabetic renal disease and nonhealing skin ulcers. *N Engl J Med* 2007;356:1049–1057.
143. Robinson MR, Augustine JJ, Korman NJ. Cinacalcet for the treatment of calciphylaxis. *Arch Dermatol* 2007;143:152–154.
144. Velasco N, MacGregor MS, Innes A, et al. Successful treatment of calciphylaxis with cinacalcet—an alternative to parathyroidectomy? *Nephrol Dial Transplant* 2006;21:1999–2004.
145. Sharma A, Burkitt-Wright E, Rustom R. Cinacalcet as an adjunct in the successful treatment of calciphylaxis. *Br J Dermatol* 2006;155:1295–1297.
146. Baker BL, Fitzgibbons CA, Buescher LS. Calciphylaxis responding to sodium thiosulfate therapy. *Arch Dermatol* 2007;143:269–270.
147. Guerra G, Shah RC, Ross EA. Rapid resolution of calciphylaxis with intravenous sodium thiosulfate and continuous venovenous haemofiltration using low calcium replacement fluid: case report. *Nephrol Dial Transplant* 2005; 20:1260–1262.
148. Ackermann F, Levy A, Daugas E, et al. Sodium thiosulfate as first-line treatment for calciphylaxis. *Arch Dermatol* 2007;143:1336–1337; author reply 1338.
149. Monney P, Nguyen QV, Perroud H, et al. Rapid improvement of calciphylaxis after intravenous pamidronate therapy in a patient with chronic renal failure. *Nephrol Dial Transplant* 2004;19:2130–2132.
150. Hanafusa T, Yamaguchi Y, Tani M, et al. Intractable wounds caused by calcific uremic arteriolopathy treated with bisphosphonates. *J Am Acad Dermatol* 2007;57(6):1021–1025.
151. Sewell LD, Weenig RH, Davis MD, et al. Low-dose tissue plasminogen activator for calciphylaxis. *Arch Dermatol* 2004;140:1045–1048.
152. Podymow T, Wherrett C, Burns KD. Hyperbaric oxygen in the treatment of calciphylaxis: a case series. *Nephrol Dial Transplant* 2001;16(11): 2176–2180.
153. Ongenae KC, Phillips TJ. Leg ulcers and wound healing. In: Arndt KA, Leboit PA, Robinson JK, et al., eds. *Cutaneous Medicine and Surgery: An integrated program in dermatology.* Philadelphia: WB Saunders; 1996:558–573.
154. Miller OF 3rd, Phillips TJ. Leg ulcers [bibliography]. *J Am Acad Dermatol* 2000;43:91–95.
155. Grey JE, Harding KG, Enoch S. Venous and arterial leg ulcers. *BMJ* 2006; 332:347–350.
156. Ross R. Atherosclerosis—an inflammatory disease. *N Engl J Med* 1999; 340(2):115–126.
157. Creager MA, Dzau VJ. Vascular diseases of the extremities. In: Fauci AS, Kasper DL, Longo DL, et al., eds. *Harrison's Principles of Internal Medicine.* 16th ed. New York: McGraw-Hill; 2005:1486–1494.
158. White C. Clinical practice. Intermittent claudication. *N Engl J Med* 2007; 356(12):1241–1250.
159. Phillips TJ, Dover JS. Leg ulcers. *J Am Acad Dermatol* 1991;25:965–987.
160. Valencia IC, Falabella A, Kirsner RS. Chronic venous insufficiency and venous leg ulceration. *J Am Acad Dermatol* 2001;44(3):401–421; quiz 422–424.
161. Fonder MA, Lazarus GS, Cowan DA, et al. Treating the chronic wound: a practical approach to the care of nonhealing wounds and wound care dressings. *J Am Acad Dermatol* 2008;58:185–206.
162. Dworkin RH, Johnson RW, Breuer J, et al. Recommendations for the management of herpes zoster. *Clin Infect Dis* 2007;44 Suppl 1:S1–S26.
163. James WD, Berger TG, Elston DM. Zoster (shingles, herpes zoster). In: James WD, Berger TG, Elston DM, eds. *Andrew's Diseases of the Skin: Clinical Dermatology.* 10th ed. Saunders Elsevier; 2006:379–384.
164. Kimberlin DW, Whitley RJ. Varicella-zoster vaccine for the prevention of herpes zoster. *N Engl J Med* 2007;356:1338–1343.
165. Corey L. Herpes simplex viruses. In: Fauci AS, Kasper DL, Longo DL, et al., eds. *Harrison's Principles of Internal Medicine.* 16th ed. New York: McGraw-Hill; 2005:1035–1042.
166. James WD, Berger TG, Elston DM. Herpes simplex. In: James WD, Berger TG, Elston DM, eds. *Andrew's Diseases of the Skin Clinical Dermatology.* 10th ed. Saunders Elsevier,; 2006:367–376.
167. Paller AS, Mancini AJ. Herpes simplex viral infection. In: Paller AS, Mancini AJ, eds. *Hurwitz Clinical Pediatric Dermatology.* 3rd ed. Elsevier Saunders; 2006:397–402.
168. Centers for Disease Control and Prevention, Workowski KA, Berman SM. Sexually transmitted diseases treatment guidelines, 2006. *MMWR Recomm Rep* 2006;55:1–94.
169. Weston WL, Brice SL. Atypical forms of herpes simplex-associated erythema multiforme. *J Am Acad Dermatol* 1998;39:124–126.
170. Bisno AL, Stevens DL. Streptococcal infections of skin and soft tissues. *N Engl J Med* 1996;334:240–245.
171. Guberman D, Gilead LT, Zlotogorski A, et al. Bullous erysipelas: a retrospective study of 26 patients. *J Am Acad Dermatol* 1999;41:733–737.
172. Weinberg AN, Swartz MN, Tsao H. Soft tissue infections: erysipelas, cellulitis, gangrenous cellulitis, and myonecrosis. In: Freedberg IM, Eisen AZ, Wolff K, et al., eds. *Fitzpatrick's Dermatology in General Medicine.* 6th ed. New York: McGraw-Hill; 2003:1883–1895.
173. Swartz MN. Clinical practice. Cellulitis. *N Engl J Med* 2004;350:904–912.
174. Lee PK, Zipoli MT, Weinberg AN, et al. Pyodermas: staphylococcus aureus, streptococcus and other gram positive bacteria. In: Freedberg IM, Eisen AZ, Wolff K, et al., eds. *Fitzpatrick's Dermatology in General Medicine.* 6th ed. New York: McGraw-Hill; 2003:1856–1878.
175. Stevens DL, Bisno AL, Chambers HF, et al. Practice guidelines for the diagnosis and management of skin and soft-tissue infections. *Clin Infect Dis* 2005; 41:1373–1406.
176. Delitt TH, Duchin J, Hofmann J. Guidelines for evaluation & management of community-associated methicillin-resistant staphylococcus aureus skin and soft tissue infections in outpatient settings. Available at: http://www.metrokc.gov/health/providers/epidemiology/MRSA-guidelines.pdf. Accessed December 2007.
177. Gorwitz RJ, Jernigan DB, Powers JH. Strategies for clinical management of MRSA in the community: summary of an experts' meeting convened by the Centers for Disease Control and Prevention. Available at: http://www.cdc.gov/ncidod/dhqp/pdf/ar/CAMRSA_ExpMtgStrategies.pdf.
178. Daum RS. Clinical practice. Skin and soft-tissue infections caused by methicillin-resistant Staphylococcus aureus. *N Engl J Med* 2007;357:380–390.
179. Swartz MN, Weinberg AN. Miscellaneous bacterial infections with cutaneous manifestations. In: Freedberg IM, Eisen AZ, Wolff K, et al., eds. *Fitzpatrick's Dermatology in General Medicine.* 6th ed. New York: McGraw-Hill; 2003: 1918–1932.
180. Varella TC, Nico MM. Erysipeloid. *Int J Dermatol* 2005;44:497–498.
181. Requena L, Yus ES. Panniculitis. Part I. Mostly septal panniculitis. *J Am Acad Dermatol* 2001;45:163–183; quiz 184–186.
182. Schwartz RA, Nervi SJ. Erythema nodosum: a sign of systemic disease. *Am Fam Physician* 2007;75(5):695–700.
183. Cribier B, Caille A, Heid E, et al. Erythema nodosum and associated diseases. A study of 129 cases. *Int J Dermatol* 1998;37:667–672.
184. Psychos DN, Voulgari PV, Skopouli FN, et al. Erythema nodosum: the underlying conditions. *Clin Rheumatol* 2000;19:212–216.
185. Kakourou T, Drosatou P, Psychou F, et al. Erythema nodosum in children: a prospective study. *J Am Acad Dermatol* 2001;44:17–21.
186. McNutt NS, Moreno A, Contreras F. Inflammatory diseases of the subcutaneous fat. In: Elder DE, Elenitsas R, Johnson BL, et al., eds. *Lever's Histopathology of the Skin.* 9th ed. Philadelphia: Lippincott Williams & Wilkins; 2005: 533–534.
187. Sterling JB, Heymann WR. Potassium iodide in dermatology: a 19th century drug for the 21st century-uses, pharmacology, adverse effects, and contraindications. *J Am Acad Dermatol* 2000;43:691–697.
188. Case records of the Massachusetts General Hospital. Weekly clinicopathological exercises. Case 17-1982. Fever and subcutaneous masses in an elderly man. *N Engl J Med* 1982;306(17):1035–1043.
189. Panush RS, Yonker RA, Dlesk A, et al. Weber-Christian disease. Analysis of 15 cases and review of the literature. *Medicine (Baltimore)* 1985;64:181–191.
190. Arnold HL, Odom RB, James WD. Weber-Christian panniculitis. In: Arnold HL, Odom RB, James WD, eds. *Andrew's Diseases of the Skin.* 8th ed. Philadelphia: WB Saunders; 1990:570–571.
191. Braverman IM. Disorders of the subcutaneous fat. In: Braverman IM, ed. *Skin Signs of Systemic Disease.* 3rd ed. Philadelphia: WB Saunders; 1998:503–506.
192. Callen JP. Miscellaneous disorders that commonly affect both skin and joints. In: Sontheimer RD, Provost TT, eds. *Cutaneous Manifestations of Rheumatic Diseases.* 2nd ed. Philadelphia: Lippincott Williams & Wilkins; 2004:229.
193. White JW Jr, Winkelmann RK. Weber-Christian panniculitis: a review of 30 cases with this diagnosis. *J Am Acad Dermatol* 1998;39:56–62.
194. Dercum FX. Three cases of a hitherto unclassified affection resembling in its grosser aspects obesity but associated with special nervous symptoms—adiposis dolorosa. *Am J Med Sci* 1892:104:521–535.
195. Iwane T, Maruyama M, Matsuki M, et al. Management of intractable pain in adiposis dolorosa with intravenous administration of lidocaine. *Anesth Analg* 1976;55:257–259.
196. Brodovsky S, Westreich M, Leibowitz A, et al. Adiposis dolorosa (Dercum's disease): 10-year follow-up. *Ann Plast Surg* 1994;33:664–668.
197. Campen R, Mankin H, Louis DN. Familial occurrence of adiposis dolorosa. *J Am Acad Dermatol* 2001:132–136.
198. Held JL, Andrew JA, Kohn SR. Surgical amelioration of Dercum's disease: a report and review. *J Dermatol Surg Oncol* 1989;15:1294–1296.
199. DeFranzo AJ, Hall JH Jr, Herring SM. Adiposis dolorosa (Dercum's disease): liposuction as an effective form of treatment. *Plast Reconstr Surg* 1990;85: 289–292.
200. De Silva M, Earley MJ. Liposuction in the treatment of juxta-articular adiposis dolorosa. *Ann Rheum Dis* 1990;49:403–404.
201. Bonatus TJ, Alexander AH. Dercum's disease (adiposis dolorosa). A case report and review of the literature. *Clin Orthop Relat Res* 1986:251–253.
202. Devillers AC, Oranje AP. Treatment of pain in adiposis dolorosa (Dercum's

disease) with intravenous lidocaine: a case report with a 10-year follow-up. *Clin Exp Dermatol* 1999;24:240–241.

203. Petersen P, Kastrup J. Dercum's disease (adiposis dolorosa). Treatment of the severe pain with intravenous lidocaine. *Pain* 1987;28:77–80.

204. Gonciarz Z, Mazur W, Hartleb J, et al. Interferon alfa-2b induced long-term relief of pain in two patients with adiposis dolorosa and chronic hepatitis C. *J Hepatol* 1997;27:1141.

205. Greenbaum SS, Varga J. Corticosteroid-induced juxta-articular adiposis dolorosa. *Arch Dermatol* 1991;127:231–233.

206. Palmer ED. Dercum's disease: adiposis dolorosa. *Am Fam Physician* 1981; 24:155–157.

207. Campen RB, Sang CN, Duncan LM. Case Records of the Massachusetts General Hospital. Case 25-2006. A 41-year old woman with painful subcutaneous nodules. *N Engl J Med* 2006:714–722.

208. Coleman WP. Hidradenitis suppurativa. In: Arndt KA, LeBoit PE, Robinson JK, et al., eds. *Cutaneous Medicine and Surgery: An Integrated Program in Dermatology*. Philadelphia: WB Saunders; 1996:481–484.

209. James WD, Berger TG, Elston DM. Hidradenitis suppurativa (acne inverse). In: James WD, Berger TG, Elston DM, eds. *Andrew's Diseases of the Skin Clinical Dermatology*. 10th ed. Saunders Elsevier; 2006:243–244.

210. Lucas S. Follicular occlusion triad (hidradenitis suppurativa, acne conglobata, and perifolliculitis capitis abscedens et suffodiens). In: Elder DE, Elenitsas R, Johnson BL, et al., eds. *Lever's Histopathology of the Skin*. 9th ed. Philadelphia: Lippincott Williams & Wilkins; 2005:555–556.

211. Wolkenstein P, Loundou A, Barrau K, et al. Quality of life impairment in hidradenitis suppurativa: a study of 61 cases. *J Am Acad Dermatol* 2007;56: 621–623.

212. Adams DR, Gordon KB, Devenyi AG, et al. Severe hidradenitis suppurativa treated with infliximab infusion. *Arch Dermatol* 2003;139:1540–1542.

213. Lebwohl B, Sapadin AN. Infliximab for the treatment of hidradenitis suppurativa. *J Am Acad Dermatol* 2003;49:S275–S276.

214. Fardet L, Dupuy A, Kerob D, et al. Infliximab for severe hidradenitis suppurativa: transient clinical efficacy in 7 consecutive patients. *J Am Acad Dermatol* 2007;56:624–628.

215. Scheinfeld N. Treatment of coincident seronegative arthritis and hidradentis suppurativa with adalimumab. *J Am Acad Dermatol* 2006;55:163–164.

216. Moul DK, Korman NJ. The cutting edge. Severe hidradenitis suppurativa treated with adalimumab. *Arch Dermatol* 2006;142:1110–1112.

217. Paller AS, Mancini AJ. Epidermal cyst. In: Paller AS, Mancini AJ, eds. *Hurwitz Clinical Pediatric Dermatology: A Textbook of Skin Disorders of Childhood and Adolescence*. 3rd ed Elsevier Saunders; 2006:236.

218. James WD, Berger TG, Elston DM. Epidermal cyst (epidermal inclusion cyst, infundibular cyst). In: James WD, Berger TG, Elston DM, eds. *Andrew's Diseases of the Skin Clinical Dermatology*. 10th ed. Saunders Elsevier; 2006: 676–677.

219. James WD, Berger TG, Elston DM. Lipomas. In: James WD, Berger TG, Elston DM, eds. *Andrew's Diseases of the Skin Clinical Dermatology*. 10th ed. Saunders Elsevier; 2006:624.

220. James WD, Berger TG, Elston DM. Pemphigus vulgaris. In: James WD, Berger TG, Elston DM, eds. *Andrew's Diseases of the Skin Clinical Dermatology*. 10th ed. Saunders Elsevier; 2006:459–463.

221. Stanley JR, Amagai M. Pemphigus, bullous impetigo, and the staphylococcal scalded-skin syndrome. *N Engl J Med* 2006;355:1800–1810.

222. Mutasim DF, Pelc NJ, Anhalt GJ. Drug-induced pemphigus. *Dermatol Clin* 1993;11:463–471.

223. Ahmed AR. Intravenous immunoglobulin therapy in the treatment of patients with pemphigus vulgaris unresponsive to conventional immunosuppressive treatment. *J Am Acad Dermatol* 2001;45:679–690.

224. Segura S, Iranzo P, Martínez-de Pablo I, et al. High-dose intravenous immunoglobulins for the treatment of autoimmune mucocutaneous blistering diseases: evaluation of its use in 19 cases. *J Am Acad Dermatol* 2007;56:960–967.

225. Ahmed AR, Spigelman Z, Cavacini LA, et al. Treatment of pemphigus vulgaris with rituximab and intravenous immune globulin. *N Engl J Med* 2006;355: 1772–1779.

226. Joly P, Mouquet H, Roujeau JC, et al. A single cycle of rituximab for the treatment of severe pemphigus. *N Engl J Med* 2007;357:545–552.

227. Cianchini G, Corona R, Frezzolini A, et al. Treatment of severe pemphigus with rituximab: report of 12 cases and a review of the literature. *Arch Dermatol* 2007;143:1033–1038.

228. Diaz LA. Rituximab and pemphigus—a therapeutic advance (editorial). *N Engl J Med* 2007;357:605–607.

229. Anhalt GJ. Paraneoplastic pemphigus. In: James WD, Cockerell CJ, Dzubow LM, eds. *Advances in Dermatology*. St Louis: Mosby; 1997:77–96.

230. James WD, Berger TG, Elston DM. Paraneoplastic pemphigus. In: James WD, Berger TG, Elston DM, eds. *Andrew's Diseases of the Skin Clinical Dermatology*. 10th ed. Saunders Elsevier; 2006:465.

231. Niimi Y, Kawana S, Hashimoto T, et al. Paraneoplastic pemphigus associated with uterine carcinoma. *J Am Acad Dermatol* 2003;48:(5 Suppl)S69–S72.

232. Hinterhuber G, Drach J, Riedl E, et al. Paraneoplastic pemphigus in association with hepatocellular carcinoma. *J Am Acad Dermatol* 2003;49:538–540.

233. Lam S, Stone MS, Goeken JA, et al. Paraneoplastic pemphigus, cicatricial conjunctivitis, and acanthosis nigricans with pachydermatoglyphy in a patient with bronchogenic squamous cell carcinoma. *Ophthalmology* 1992;99: 108–113.

234. Matz H, Milner Y, Frusic-Zlotkin M, et al. Paraneoplastic pemphigus associated with pancreatic carcinoma. *Acta Derm Venereol* 1997;77:289–291.

235. Nousari HC, Deterding R, Wojtczack H, et al. The mechanism of respiratory failure in paraneoplastic pemphigus. *N Engl J Med* 1999;340:1406–1410.

236. Borradori L, Lombardi T, Samson J, et al. Anti-CD20 monoclonal antibody (rituximab) for refractory erosive stomatitis secondary to CD20(+) follicular lymphoma-associated paraneoplastic pemphigus. *Arch Dermatol* 2001;137: 269–272.

237. Williams JV, Marks JG Jr, Billingsley EM. Use of mycophenolate mofetil in the treatment of paraneoplastic pemphigus. *Br J Dermatol* 2000;142:506–508.

238. Vecchietti G, Kerl K, Hügli A, et al. Topical tacrolimus (FK506) for relapsing erosive stomatitis in paraneoplastic pemphigus. *Br J Dermatol* 2003;148: 833–834.

239. Korman NJ. Bullous pemphigoid. In: Arndt KA, LeBoit PE, Robinson JK, et al., eds. *Cutaneous medicine and surgery An integrated program in dermatology*. Philadelphia: WB Saunders; 1996:664–673.

240. Korman NJ. Bullous pemphigoid. The latest in diagnosis, prognosis, and therapy. *Arch Dermatol* 1998;134:1137–1141.

241. James WD, Berger TG, Elston DM. Bullous pemphigoid. In: James WD, Berger TG, Elston DM, eds. *Andrew's Diseases of the Skin Clinical Dermatology*. 10th ed. Saunders Elsevier; 2006:466–469.

242. Stern RS. Bullous pemphigoid therapy—think globally, act locally. *N Engl J Med* 2002;346:364–367.

243. Berk MA, Lorincz AL. The treatment of bullous pemphigoid with tetracycline and niacinamide. A preliminary report. *Arch Dermatol* 1986;122:670–674.

244. Thomas I, Khorenian S, Arbesfeld DM. Treatment of generalized bullous pemphigoid with oral tetracycline. *J Am Acad Dermatol* 1993;28:74–77.

245. Mutasim DF. Management of autoimmune bullous diseases: pharmacology and therapeutics. *J Am Acad Dermatol* 2004;51:859–877; quiz 878–880.

246. Joly P, Roujeau JC, Benichou J, et al. A comparison of oral and topical corticosteroids in patients with bullous pemphigoid. *N Engl J Med* 2002;346: 321–327.

247. Fine JD. Epidermolysis bullosa. In: Arndt KA, LeBoit PE, Robinson JK, et al., eds. *Cutaneous medicine and surgery An integrated program in dermatology*. Philadelphia: WB Saunders; 1996:635–650.

248. Lapiere JC, Chan LS, Woodley DT. Epidermolysis bullosa acquisita. In: Arndt KA, LeBoit PE, Robinson JK, et al., eds. *Cutaneous Medicine and Surgery An integrated program in dermatology*. Philadelphia: WB Saunders; 1996: 685–690.

249. Woodley DT, Chen M. Epidermolysis bullosa: then and now. *J Am Acad Dermatol* 2004;51:S55–S57.

250. James WD, Berger TG, Elston DM. Epidermolysis bullosa acquisita. In: James WD, Berger TG, Elston DM, eds. *Andrew's Diseases of the Skin Clinical Dermatology*. 10th ed. Saunders Elsevier; 2006:473–474.

251. James WD, Berger TG, Elston DM. Epidermolysis bullosa. In: James WD, Berger TG, Elston DM, eds. *Andrew's Diseases of the Skin Clinical Dermatology*. 10th ed. Saunders Elsevier; 2006:555–559.

252. Fine JD, Eady RA, Bauer EA, et al. Revised classification system for inherited epidermolysis bullosa: Report of the Second International Consensus Meeting on diagnosis and classification of epidermolysis bullosa. *J Am Acad Dermatol* 2000;42:1051–1066.

253. Mayuzumi M, Akiyama M, Nishie W, et al. Childhood epidermolysis bullosa acquisita with autoantibodies against the noncollagenous 1 and 2 domains of type VII collagen: case report and review of the literature. *Br J Dermatol* 2006;155:1048–1052.

254. McAllister JC, Marinkovich M. Advances in inherited epidermolysis bullosa. *Adv Dermatol* 2005;21:303–334.

255. Schmidt E, Benoit S, Bröcker EB, et al. Successful adjuvant treatment of recalcitrant epidermolysis bullosa acquisita with anti-CD20 antibody rituximab. *Arch Dermatol* 2006;142:147–150.

256. Crichlow SM, Mortimer NJ, Harman KE. A successful therapeutic trial of rituximab in the treatment of a patient with recalcitrant, high-title epidermolysis bullosa acquisita (correspondence). *Br J Dermatol* 2007;156:194–196.

257. James WD, Berger TG, Elston DM. Cutaneous endometriosis. In: James WD, Berger TG, Elston DM, eds. *Andrew's Diseases of the Skin Clinical Dermatology*. 10th ed. Saunders Elsevier; 2006:628.

258. Muñoz H, Waxtein L, Vega ME, et al. An ulcerated umbilical nodule. *Arch Dermatol* 1999;135:1114–1115, 1117–1118.

259. Tidman MJ, MacDonald DM. Cutaneous endometriosis: a histopathologic study. *J Am Acad Dermatol* 1988;18:373–377.

260. Kazakov DV, Ondic O, Zamecnik M, et al. Morphological variations of scar-related and spontaneous endometriosis of the skin and superficial soft tissue: a study of 71 cases with emphasis on atypical features and types of mullerian differentiations. *J Am Acad Dermatol* 2007;57:134–146.

261. Trentham DE, Le CH. Relapsing polychondritis. *Ann Intern Med* 1998;129: 114–122.

262. Letko E, Zafirakis P, Baltatzis S, et al. Relapsing polychondritis: a clinical review. *Semin Arthritis Rheum* 2002;31:384–395.

263. Moschella SL. Miscellaneous rheumatic diseases that may involve the skin. In: Sontheimer RD, Provost TT, eds. *Cutaneous Manifestations of Rheumatic Diseases*. 2nd ed. Philadelphia: Lippincott Williams & Wilkins; 2004: 212–213.

264. Butterton JR, Collier DS, Romero JM, et al. Case records of the Massachusetts General Hospital. Case 14-2007. A 59-year-old man with fever and pain and swelling of both eyes and the right ear. *N Engl J Med* 2007:1980–1988.

265. Foidart JM, Abe S, Martin GR, et al. Antibodies to type II collagen in relapsing polychondritis. *N Engl J Med* 1978;299:1203–1207.

266. McAdam LP, O'Hanlan MA, Bluestone R, et al. Relapsing polychondritis:

prospective study of 23 patients and a review of the literature. *Medicine (Baltimore)* 1976;55:193–215.

267. Michet CJ Jr, McKenna CH, Luthra HS, et al. Relapsing polychondritis. Survival and predictive role of early disease manifestations. *Ann Intern Med* 1986;104:74–78.

268. Francès C, el Rassi R, Laporte JL, et al. Dermatologic manifestations of relapsing polychondritis. A study of 200 cases at a single center. *Medicine (Baltimore)* 2001;80:173–179.

269. Damiani JM, Levine HL. Relapsing polychondritis—report of ten cases. *Laryngoscope* 1979;89:929–946.

270. Mark KA, Franks AG Jr. Colchicine and indomethacin for the treatment of relapsing polychondritis. *J Am Acad Dermatol* 2002;46:S22–S24.

271. Long D, Maloney ME. Surgical pearl: surgical planing in the treatment of chondrodermatitis nodularis chronica helicis of the antihelix. *J Am Acad Dermatol* 1996;35:761–762.

272. Oelzner S, Elsner P. Bilateral chondrodermatitis nodularis chronica helicis on the free border of the helix in a woman. *J Am Acad Dermatol* 2003;49:720–722.

273. Cribier B, Scrivener Y, Peltre B. Neural hyperplasia in chondrodermatitis nodularis chronica helicis. *J Am Acad Dermatol* 2006;55:844–848.

274. Ioffreda MD. Inflammatory diseases of hair follicles, sweat glands and cartilage. In: Elder DE, Elenitsas R, Johnson BL, et al., eds. *Lever's Histopathology of the Skin*. 9th ed. Philadelphia: Lippincott Williams & Wilkins; 2005:500–501.

275. Moncrieff M, Sassoon EM. Effective treatment of chondrodermatitis nodularis helicis using a conservative approach. *Br J Dermatol* 2004;150:892–894.

276. Massey EW. Sensory mononeuropathies. *Semin Neurol* 1998;18:177–183.

277. Laurencet FM, Anchisi S, Tullen E, et al. Mental neuropathy: report of five cases and review of the literature. *Crit Rev Oncol Hematol* 2000;34:71–79.

278. Turner-Iannacci A, Mozaffari F, Stooler ET. Mental nerve neuropathy: case report and review. *CJEM* 2003;5:259–262.

279. Savk O, Savk E. Investigation of spinal pathology in notalgia paresthetica. *J Am Acad Dermatol* 2005;52:1085–1087.

280. Goulden V, Toomey PJ, Highet AS. Successful treatment of notalgia paresthetica with a paravertebral local anesthetic block. *J Am Acad Dermatol* 1998;38:114–116.

281. Massey EW, Pleet AB. Electromyographic evaluation of notalgia paresthetica. *Neurology* 1981;31:642.

282. Bernhard JD. Lichen simplex chronicus, prurigo nodularis, and notalgia paresthetica. In: Arndt KA, LeBoit PE, Robinson JK, et al., eds. *Cutaneous Medicine and Surgery: An Integrated Program in Dermatology*. Philadelphia: WB Saunders; 1996:208–210.

283. Weinfeld PK. Successful treatment of notalgia paresthetica with botulinum toxin type A. *Arch Dermatol* 2007;143:980–982.

284. Savk E, Bolukbasi O, Akyol A, et al. Open pilot study on oxcarbazepine for the treatment of notalgia paresthetica. *J Am Acad Dermatol* 2001;45:630–632.

285. Loosemore MP, Bordeaux JS, Bernhard JD. Gabapentin treatment for notalgia paresthetica, a common isolated peripheral sensory neuropathy. *J Eur Acad Dermatol Venereol* 2007;21:1440–1441.

286. Clarke JT. Narrative review: Fabry disease. *Ann Intern Med* 2007;146:425–433.

287. Braverman IM. Blood vessels. In: Braverman IM, ed. *Skin Signs of Systemic Disease*. 3rd ed. Philadelphia: WB Saunders; 1998:392–396.

288. Desnick RJ, Brady R, Barranger J, et al. Fabry disease, an under-recognized multisystemic disorder: expert recommendations for diagnosis, management, and enzyme replacement therapy. *Ann Intern Med* 2003;138:338–346.

289. Hopkin RJ, Grabowski GA. Lysosomal storage diseases. In: Fauci AS, Kasper DL, Longo DL, et al., eds. *Harrison's Principles of Internal Medicine*. 16th ed. New York: McGraw-Hill; 2005:2315–2319.

290. James WD, Berger TG, Elston DM. Angiokeratoma corporis diffusum (Fabry disease). In: James WD, Berger TG, Elston DM, eds. *Andrew's Diseases of the Skin Clinical Dermatology*. 10th ed. Saunders Elsevier,; 2006:538–539.

291. Larralde M, Boggio P, Amartino H, et al. Fabry disease: a study of 6 hemizygous men and 5 heterozygous women with emphasis on dermatologic manifestations. *Arch Dermatol* 2004;140:1440–1446.

292. Paller AS, Mancini AJ. Other storage disorders. In: Paller AS, Mancini AJ, eds. *Hurwitz Clinical Pediatric Dermatology A textbook of skin disorders of childhood and adolescence*. 3rd ed: Elsevier Saunders; 2006:646–647.

293. Kelly B, Kelly E. Angiokeratoma corporis diffusum in a patient with no recognizable enzyme abnormalities. *Arch Dermatol* 2006;142:615–618.

294. Banikazemi M, Bultas J, Waldek S, et al. Agalsidase-beta therapy for advanced Fabry disease: a randomized trial. *Ann Intern Med* 2007;146:77–86.

295. Ries M, Schiffmann R. Fabry disease: angiokeratoma, biomarker, and the effect of enzyme replacement therapy on kidney function. *Arch Dermatol* 2005;141:904–905; author reply 905–906.

296. Naversen DN, Trask DM, Watson FH, et al. Painful tumors of the skin: "LEND AN EGG". *J Am Acad Dermatol* 1993;28:298–300.

297. McKee PH, Calonje E, Granter SR. *Traumatic Neuroma*. In: McKee PH, Calonje E, Granter SR, eds. *Pathology of the Skin with Clinical Correlations*. 3rd ed. Philadelphia: Elsevier Mosby; 2005:1763–1764.

298. McKee PH, Calonje E, Granter SR. Morton's neuroma. In: McKee PH, Calonje E, Granter SR, eds. *Pathology of the Skin with Clinical Correlations*. 3rd ed. Elsevier Mosby; 2005:1764.

299. Choi SW, Lee HN, Kang SJ, et al. A case of cutaneous endometriosis developed in postmenopausal woman receiving hormonal replacement. *J Am Acad Dermatol* 1999;41(2 Pt 2):327–329.

300. Fair KP, Patterson JW, Murphy RJ, et al. Cutaneous deciduosis. *J Am Acad Dermatol* 2000;43:102–107.

301. Reed RJ, Argenyi Z. Granular cell tumors. In: Elder DE, Elenitsas R, Johnson BL, et al., eds. *Lever's Histopathology of the Skin*. 9th ed. Philadelphia: Lippincott Williams & Wilkins; 2005:1129–1130.

302. Launonen V, Vierimaa O, Kiuru M, et al. Inherited susceptibility to uterine leiomyomas and renal cell cancer. *Proc Natl Acad Sci U S A* 2001;98:3387–3392.

303. Rothman A, Glenn G, Choyke L, et al. Multiple painful cutaneous nodules and renal mass. *J Am Acad Dermatol* 2006;55:683–686.

304. Calonje E, Wilson-Jones, E. Glomus tumor. In: Elder DE, Elenitsas R, Johnson BL, et al., eds. *Lever's Histopathology of the Skin*. 9th ed. Philadelphia: Lippincott Williams & Wilkins; 2005:1049–1051.

305. McKee PH, Calonje E, Granter SR. Glomus tumor. In: McKee PH, Calonje E, Granter SR, eds. *Pathology of the Skin with Clinical Correlations*. 3rd ed. Elsevier Mosby; 2005:1848–1851.

306. McKee PH, Calonje E, Granter SR. Pilar leiomyoma. In: McKee PH, Calonje E, Granter SR, eds. *Pathology of the Skin with Clinical Correlations*. 3rd ed. Elsevier Mosby; 2005:1797–1799.

307. Ragsdale BD. Leiomyoma. In: Elder DE, Elenitsas R, Johnson BL, et al., eds. *Lever's Histopathology of the Skin*. 9th ed. Philadelphia: Lippincott Williams & Wilkins; 2005:1078–1081.

308. McKee PH, Calonje E, Granter SR. Angioleiomyoma. In: McKee PH, Calonje E, Granter SR, eds. *Pathology of the Skin with Clinical Correlations*. 3rd ed. Elsevier Mosby; 2005:1799–1800.

309. McKee PH, Calonje E, Granter SR. Angiolipoma. In: McKee PH, Calonje E, Granter SR, eds. *Pathology of the Skin with Clinical Correlations*. 3rd ed. Elsevier Mosby; 2005:1687–1688.

310. Ragsdale BD. Angiolipoma. In: Elder DE, Elenitsas R, Johnson BL, et al., eds. *Lever's Histopathology of the Skin*. 9th ed. Philadelphia: Lippincott Williams & Wilkins; 2005:1066–1069.

311. Reed RJ, Argenyi Z. True neoplasms of schwann cells. In: Elder DE, Elenitsas R, Johnson BL, et al., eds. *Lever's Histopathology of the Skin*. 9th ed. Philadelphia: Lippincott Williams & Wilkins; 2005:1116–1119.

312. McKee PH, Calonje E, Granter SR. Eccrine spiradenoma. In: McKee PH, Calonje E, Granter SR, eds. *Pathology of the Skin with Clinical Correlations*. 3rd ed. Elsevier Mosby; 2005:1642–1644.

313. Klein W, Chan E, Seykora JT. Eccrine spiradenoma. In: Elder DE, Elenitsas R, Johnson BL Jr, et al., eds. *Lever's Histopathology of the Skin*. 9th ed. Philadelphia: Lippincott Williams & Wilkins; 2005:903–904.

CHAPTER 38 ■ PAIN DUE TO VASCULAR CAUSES

KAJ H. JOHANSEN

INTRODUCTION

Pain in one form or another is a frequent manifestation of arterial, venous, or lymphatic problems. The nature and location of pain complaints may be virtually diagnostic of the underlying vascular condition. On the other hand, pain arising from nonvascular conditions may mimic that associated with various vascular conditions, thereby delaying or complicating diagnosis and therapy. This chapter explores the mechanisms and pathophysiology of vascular pain and its relief; it emphasizes basic neuroanatomy and neurophysiology relevant to vascular pain and includes a compilation of different vascular pain syndromes.

Because pain is a frequent presenting feature of vascular disease and its therapy, topics covered herein necessarily share an interface with numerous other chapters in this text. Information provided in this chapter is, however, intended to be supplementary or expansive upon material elsewhere rather than duplicative. For more detailed discussions of vascular pain the reader is referred to comprehensive sources on this subject.[1–4]

BASIC NEUROANATOMIC AND NEUROPHYSIOLOGIC CONSIDERATIONS

A review of the neuroanatomy and neurophysiology of vascular structures and the organs and parts they serve helps inform an understanding of the way vascular disease results in pain. This is further clarified by an understanding of how pain is stimulated peripherally and transmitted and experienced centrally.

The International Association for the Study of Pain defines pain as "an unpleasant sensory and emotional experience associated with actual or potential tissue damage, or described in terms of such damage."[5] The perception of pain is a consequence of many variables including past and current pain experiences, level of consciousness, and the patient's emotional state.

Nociceptive pain is an uncomfortable sensation associated with injurious stimulation, while *neuropathic* pain arises in the absence of such injury. From a teleologic perspective, pain's "purpose" is to signal the presence of (and presumably prevent) tissue damage and, thus, exists as one aspect of homeostasis. Only when it becomes chronic, or is a manifestation of the postoperative state, is pain unhelpful.

Pain can be characterized by its location, duration, quality, and severity or intensity. Qualities of pain include the descriptive terms "aching," "burning," "spasmodic," "radiating," "lancinating," "sharp," or "dull." Focal pain is noted at the site of injury, while diffuse pain is more characteristic of deep structures.

Radicular pain radiates along peripheral nerve pathways, not uncommonly in concert with motor or sensory neurologic deficits. Referred pain is perceived at a site remote from where the noxious stimulation is actually occurring and results from a misplaced cortical appreciation of pain. Referred pain generally follows spinal segmental innervation and must be differentiated from radicular pain, which generally follows specific dermatomal distributions. Visceral pain is dull, aching, and has an agonizing, "sickening" component.

Pain can result from numerous physical stimuli including pressure, puncture, squeeze, tension, and extreme heat or cold. Pain can also result from chemical effects such as those resulting from a marked change in pH or the presence of various mediators—histamine-like materials, serotonin, bradykinin, and other similar polypeptides. Endogenous prostanoids can lower the pain threshold as a consequence of certain stimuli; local acidosis can enhance perception of pain. Local mediators such as substance P are released at sites of injury and the neural stimulation which results can be interpreted as pain.

Nociceptive receptors are usually free nerve endings and pain is transmitted from them in the small unmyelinated A-delta and C nerve fibers. These afferent nerves' cell bodies are located in the dorsal root ganglia and their axons enter the spinal cord through the dorsal roots. These axons synapse in the dorsal grey of the cord with second-order neurons. Most pain is transmitted centrally via the crossed lateral spinothalamic tract up the cord to third-order neurons in the thalamus. The spinothalamic tract, including the periaqueductal grey region of the brainstem, is relevant to more diffuse, longer-lasting pain and, probably, neuropathic pain. Interestingly, the precise central nervous system (CNS) location for pain perception remains obscure.

Large- and medium-sized *arteries* have two types of innervation: afferent (sensory) nerves and autonomic (sympathetic) nerves. Pain is the primary sensation transmitted via nociceptive afferents in arteries and veins; position, temperature, and other such sensations do not appear to be transmitted via the innervation of blood vessels. In large- and medium-sized arteries these receptors appear to be stimulated by direct trauma (e.g., an arteriography needle), stretch (as noted with balloon dilatation or stent placement), or shear (as in arterial dissection).

Nociception in large- and medium-sized *veins* is due to pain receptors in the venous adventitia which appear to respond primarily to stretch (as in venous distention or engorgement, perhaps the consequence of downstream thrombosis or other obstruction).

Classic neuroanatomic research by Pick[6] demonstrated that sympathetic and sensory fibers enter the arterial (and venous) adventitia to form an intrinsic neural network ("adventitial plexus"), mostly composed of sensory afferents. From this plexus bundles of nonmyelinated fibers (mostly sympathetic) approach the media ("border plexus"), and extensions of this network ramify within the media ("muscular plexus").

The basis for neuropathic pain, and how it is sustained, remain obscure. Neuropathic pain also appears to be transmitted by sensory afferents but, unlike nociceptive pain, it has autonomic (sympathetic nerve) components as well. This results in the well-established (although poorly understood) role of sympathetic modulation for neuropathic pain by pharmacologic or anesthetic blockade or by sympathectomy. Recognition, diagnosis, and management of various forms of sympathetically mediated or sympathetically sustained pain (formerly termed causalgia or reflex sympathetic dystrophy [RSD] but now subsumed, by fiat of expert panels,[7] under the umbrella term *complex regional pain syndrome* [CRPS]) is discussed in detail in Chapter 25.

Most nociceptive pain is relieved when the underlying noxious stimulus is resolved. On occasion the presence or severity of nociceptive pain warrants consideration of more invasive procedures to effect pain relief. Analysis of these procedures' results, both in the near-term and chronically, has provided substantial insight into the way peripheral pain is transmitted and appreciated.

VASCULAR PAIN SYNDROMES

Pain in one form or another is a common manifestation of various vascular disorders and the location, quality, and natural history of such pain may be crucial to the diagnosis or treatment of the condition. For example, sudden tearing interscapular pain is virtually diagnostic of an acute type B thoracic aortic dissection; mitigation of this pain is a hallmark of satisfactory "medical" management of this condition by means of antihypertensive therapy with beta blockers. A compendium of the types of pain associated with various arterial, venous, and lymphatic conditions follows.

Intermittent Claudication

Claudication is one of the most common pain complaints seen by vascular specialists. The pathophysiology of arterial claudication is based on a reduction of arterial perfusion to a degree that is inadequate to meet the needs of working muscles. The most common cause is arterial occlusive disease due to generalized atherosclerosis, and the most common sites are shown in Figure 38.1. The clinical phenomenon is seen most commonly in the gastrocnemius/soleus muscle group distal to atherosclerotic occlusion of the superficial femoral artery, but can also be seen in more proximal thigh muscle groups with aortoiliac occlusive disease or in the upper extremities with chronic brachiocephalic arterial stenoses or occlusion (Fig. 38.2). Rarely, patients may note claudication of the gluteal or lumbar paraspinal muscles in association with pelvic arterial insufficiency. Claudication of the muscles of mastication is almost diagnostic of involvement of the external carotid artery by giant cell arteritis.[8]

The quality and pattern of the pain associated with intermittent claudication is stereotypical. It is absent at rest but appears following muscle exertion of a specific amount, disappearing quickly following cessation of exercise. That the phenomenon is a consequence of inadequate perfusion to working muscles is demonstrated by the parallel course of the development of symptoms and the decline in skeletal muscle perfusion as measured by Doppler arterial pressure ankle/arm indices (AAIs) during treadmill walking and by symmetrical improvement in symptoms and AAI when treadmill walking is halted (Fig. 38.3).

The pain associated with the claudication of arterial insufficiency is localized to the working muscles and is characterized as "burning," "cramping," or "aching." The muscles are not particularly tender and, because basal blood supply is adequate, no distal trophic lesions occur. At the cellular level, claudication pain likely results from a combination of ischemic neuropathy (particularly of small unmyelinated A-delta and C sensory fibers) and a localized lactic acidosis resulting from the anaerobic metabolism of ischemia, perhaps heightened by elaboration of substance P.

Several types of intermittent *pseudo*claudication exist and contribute to an important differential diagnosis among patients presenting with walking-related extremity pain. The most important and commonly seen of these alternative diagnoses is that of *neurogenic claudication*, resulting from one form or another of lumbosacral neurospinal compression syndrome—spinal stenosis, herniated disc, arachnoiditis, spondylolisthesis, and the like. Initially such patients' complaints may appear to be very similar to those of subjects with arterial insufficiency, to the extent that

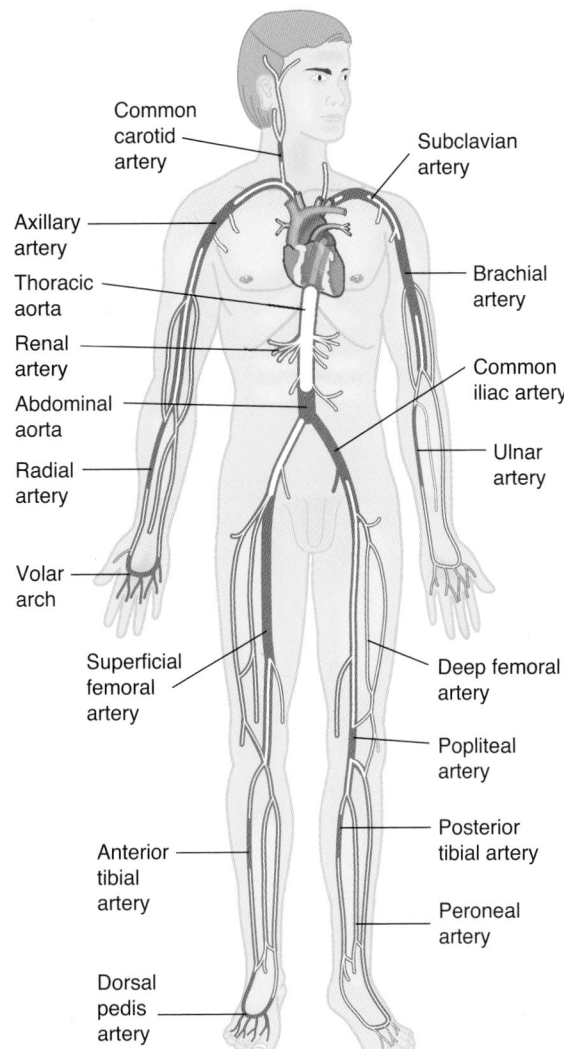

FIGURE 38.1 The most common sites for atherosclerotic occlusive arterial disease in peripheral arteries. The extent, degree, and pattern of the obstructive lesion vary considerably at each site.

they are occasionally subjected to surgical revascularization when they actually need a laminectomy (or vice versa!).

Fortunately, a careful history will frequently solve this diagnostic conundrum. Because the basis for neurogenic claudication involves compression of nerve roots by a diffuse fibrotic or inflammatory process in the region of the lower spinal cord or the cauda equina, neurogenic claudication is more commonly bilateral than that associated with arterial insufficiency. Further, the pain of neurogenic claudication is more diffuse, frequently extending from buttocks to feet, and often has a deeper, more aching or burning quality, not infrequently associated with distal paresthesias or numbness.

The subject with neurogenic claudication frequently finds relief from his/her steadily worsening symptoms by bending over while walking; when hip and leg pain forces the subject to halt, symptom relief commonly results only with sitting. Unlike the individual with arterial claudication who can walk the same distance on the level or on the treadmill over and over again with equal interspersed rest periods, the individual with neurogenic claudication who attempts to walk very far achieves shorter and shorter walking distances at the expense of longer and longer periods of sitting. Neurospinal compression may result in pain or numbness just with standing, once again and relieved by sitting.

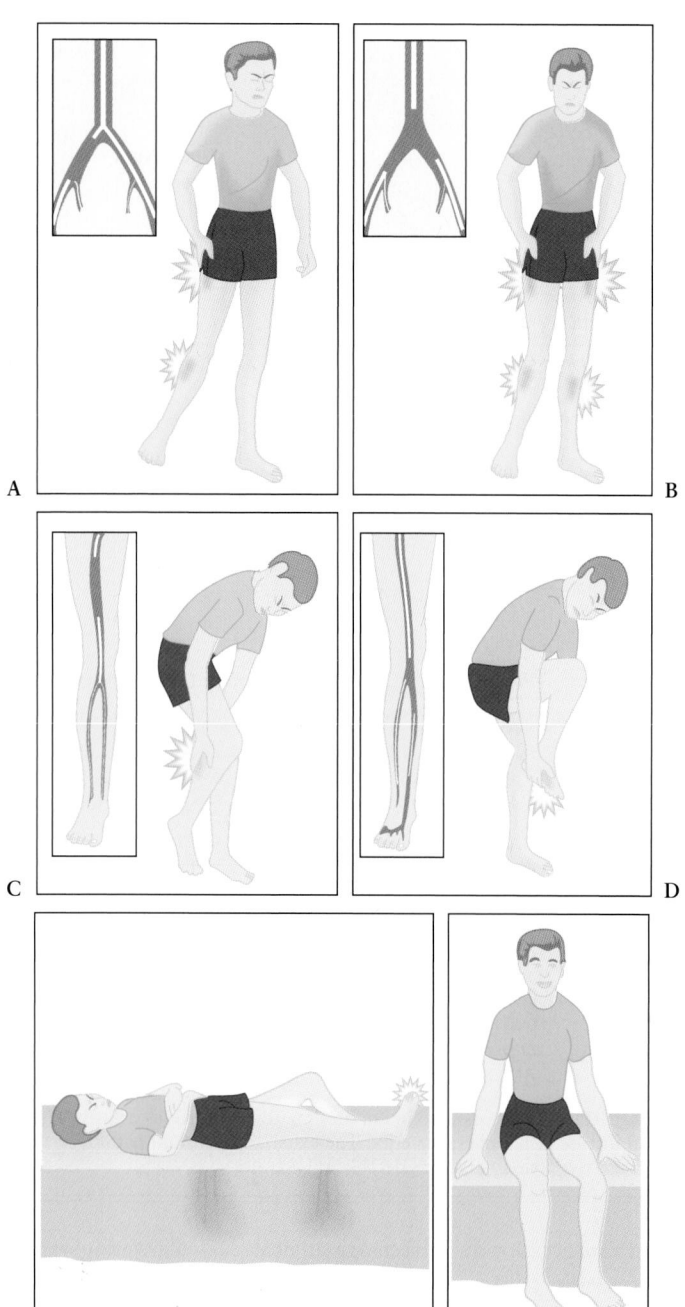

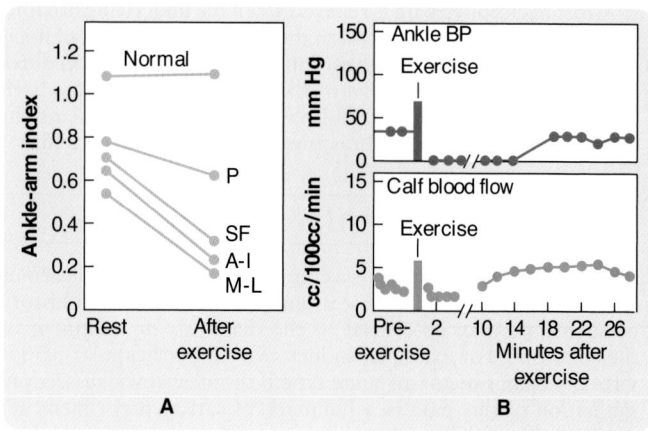

FIGURE 38.3 (**A**) Mean ankle–arm indices (ankle systolic blood pressure divided by arm [brachial] systolic blood pressure) at rest and after exercise in normal subjects and subjects with atherosclerotic occlusive disease. The location of the occlusion is indicated by the letters: *P*, popliteal artery below the knee; *SF*, superficial femoral artery; *AI*, aorta and iliac arteries; *ML*, multilevel. (**B**) Ankle pressure and calf blood flow before and after exercise in a patient with occlusion of the iliac, common femoral, and superficial femoral arteries. This patient had severe claudication and moderate rest pain. (BP, blood pressure). (Modified from Sumner DS. Practical approach to vascular laboratory testing in occlusive arterial disease. In: Rutherford RB, ed. *Vascular Surgery*, 2nd ed. Philadelphia: WB Saunders, 1984:45–56.)

FIGURE 38.2 Sites of pain (radiating lines) caused by atherosclerotic occlusive arterial disease in different parts of the arteries of the lower limbs. (**A**) Obstruction in the right common iliac artery, which produces pain in the right hip, buttock, thigh, and calf. (**B**) Obstruction in both common iliac arteries and the lower aorta, which produces pain in both hips, buttocks, thighs, and calves—the so called "Leriche syndrome." (**C**) Obstruction of the superficial femoral artery, which produces severe and incapacitating intermittent pain in the calf. (**D**) Obstruction of the popliteal and tibial arteries (and dorsal pedal arterial arch), produces pain in the foot. This foot pain can occur at rest in the distal part of the foot (**E**) when the patient lies in bed and (**F**) the rest pain is often relieved when the limb is dependent.

The pain of neurogenic claudication is felt to result from both ischemia and reactive swelling of nerve roots at their site of compression, an impression confirmed by studies utilizing intrathecal fibroscopy during treadmill walking in patients with neurogenic claudication.[9] Temporary relief of the pain of neuro-

genic claudication by various postural changes such as sitting appears to result from the fact that flexion of the hip and back relieves lumbosacral nerve root "stretch" and allows decongestion of the epidural veins in the region.[9]

Substantial diagnostic confusion can result from the fact that older patients with lower extremity claudication may have *both* atherosclerotic arterial occlusive disease *and* degenerative lumbosacral spine disease. Minimal or no change in Doppler AAI in the presence of development of lower extremity symptoms during treadmill exercise excludes arterial occlusive disease as a cause of the patient's lower extremity symptoms.

Other much less common causes of intermittent claudication include the following: proximal venous occlusive disease of the lower extremities, resulting in a characteristic sense of "bursting" discomfort and engorgement of the exercising extremity ("venous claudication")[10] as well as various forms of myositis, the most common of which is an iatrogenic muscle inflammation and necrosis which results from the administration of various statin medications to treat hyperlipidemia.[11]

Lower extremity claudication in younger individuals should bring to mind two diagnoses—*popliteal entrapment syndrome* and (when exercise-induced pain is localized to the anterolateral aspect of the leg) *chronic compartment syndrome*. The intermittent claudication seen in young people (often athletes or military recruits) associated with popliteal artery entrapment syndrome (Fig. 38.4) has the same pathophysiologic mechanism as that associated with atherosclerotic lower extremity arterial occlusive disease.[12] The cellular basis for the anterior muscle compartment pain associated with chronic compartment syndrome is ischemia resulting from diminution of the intramuscular arteriovenous pressure differential due to venous congestion and compartment tissue hypertension.[13]

Aortic and Other Large Artery Pain

A substantial number of pain receptors populate the media of large- and medium-sized arteries. As noted previously, these re-

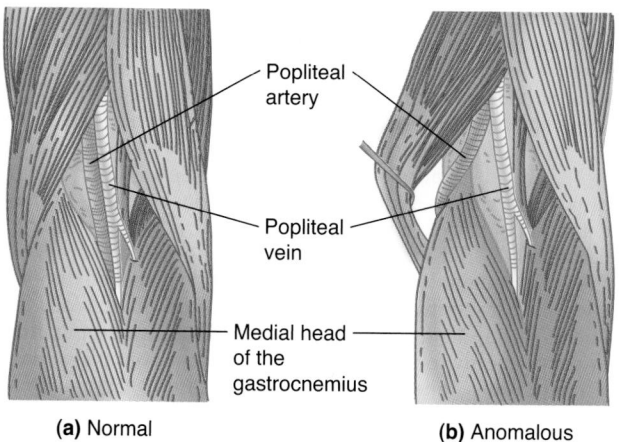

Popliteal
artery

Popliteal
vein

Medial head
of the
gastrocnemius

(a) Normal   **(b) Anomalous**

FIGURE 38.4 **(A)** The normal relationship of the popliteal artery and the two heads of the gastrocnemius muscle. **(B)** The most common anomaly, which causes popliteal artery entrapment syndrome. The popliteal artery is looped medially around and then under the medial head of the gastrocnemius. The medial hamstring muscles have been retracted for clarity. During strenuous exercise of the leg, the muscle compresses the artery, with consequent ischemia and intermittent claudication.

ceptors can respond to direct stimulation, for example by a needle or other penetrating instrument; they also may respond to stretch or shear. Sensory nerve fibers do not appear in or near the arterial intima, perhaps explaining why atherosclerosis, even when it is "inflammatory,"[14] is not painful. Chronic slow dilatation of arteries, such as occurs with abdominal aortic aneurysm (AAA), does not appear to stimulate intra-arterial pain fibers; while palpation of an AAA occasionally results in a diffuse deep sickening ache, in the author's experience this occurs with equivalent frequency following deep palpation of normal nonaneurysmal aortas. Stimulation of periaortic autonomic fibers by such palpation may contribute to this characteristic sensation.

The pain associated with aortic aneurysmal rupture, usually into the peritoneal cavity, the retroperitoneum or (rarely) the pleural space, is generally described as sudden, steady, burning, and penetrating in nature. Such pain likely arises as a consequence of nociception at several levels, including stimulation of pain fibers in the torn aorta, in the stretched or torn peritoneum or pleura and as a consequence of extravasation and hematoma expansion in an enclosed pleura or retroperitoneum (tellingly, free rupture of an AAA into the abdominal cavity is commonly characterized only by transient pain followed by rapid loss of consciousness as the patient expires from hypovolemic shock).

Pain—characteristically "tearing," "ripping," or "boring" and located in a substernal or interscapular location—is a hallmark of aortic dissection. Similar burning pain in the lateral neck characterizes extracranial carotid arterial dissection. Shearing of nociceptive receptors in the aortic or carotid media by progression of the pulsatile hematoma within the media is the likely explanation for this pain. Except for patients with Marfan or Ehlers-Danlos syndromes, whose aortic or arterial dissections may occur asymptomatically, pain is a constant consequence of arterial dissection. As previously intimated, relief of such pain with hypotensive therapy is felt to indicate satisfactory control of an aortic dissection, while persistent pain suggests that such therapy is inadequate, obligating either that such therapy be augmented or be replaced by a more invasive intervention (operation or endovascular repair).

Vasculitic inflammatory involvement of large- and medium-sized arteries is uncommon but not rare. The most common such involvement of the aorta is the development of an inflammatory aneurysm, usually of the abdominal aorta. While the pathophysiology of this process remains obscure, its presentation is stereo-

typically as a thickened "rind" of chronically inflamed fibrofatty perianeurysmal tissues, frequently with an adhesive involvement of the ureters or the duodenum which can significantly complicate open aneurysmal repair. Patients with inflammatory AAAs commonly complain of diffuse aching mid-back discomfort and their aneurysms are dully tender to palpation.

Besides the jaw claudication often associated with giant cell arteritis,[8] such patients' inflammatory vasculitis can be associated with diffuse pain and tenderness over the affected arteries—especially the superficial temporal artery; biopsy (or duplex scanning)[15] of which may be diagnostic of the underlying condition. As for inflammatory AAA and other large- and medium-sized vessel arteritis, the diffuse and poorly localized pain seen in this condition is likely due to inflammatory involvement of nociceptors found both in the arterial media and adventitia as well as in periarterial connective tissue. That the pain associated with this condition is inflammatory is borne out by its resolution following administration of anti-inflammatory agents (particularly corticosteroids).

Rest Pain, Ulcers, and Gangrene

Advanced or critical arterial insufficiency—usually in the lower extremities—displays characteristic symptoms and signs which signal impending limb loss. Indeed, all patients with rest pain, ischemic ulcers, or gangrene will require an operative intervention—either an amputation or a procedure to reestablish vascular supply to the affected area. Such patients' arterial occlusive disease is severe and multilevel ("tandem") and their mortality rate exceeds 50% over the next 5 years as a consequence of premature, aggressive coronary artery disease.

Rest pain is characterized by a diffuse, ill-localized aching or burning pain in the distal foot (occasionally the heel). It is generally initially present at night when the patient is recumbent or the leg and foot are elevated. Symptoms dissipate if the leg is hung over the edge of the bed or the subject rises and walks around. The pathophysiology of rest pain is likely that of an ischemic neuropathy, with positional malperfusion of small sensory nerves in the distal foot. The symptoms of rest pain (or other advanced arterial insufficiency) necessarily develop in the most distal small arteries, those farthest away from the heart. Thus, pain at rest does not occur proximal to the foot (with one cardinal exception: rest pain may develop with severe ischemia in the stump of a patient with a below- or above-knee amputation).

Arterial ulceration in the nondiabetic is characterized by a shallow, pallid, nonhealing erosion of the skin in the distal foot, in a similar location as that for rest pain. The pain of such ulcerations is unremitting and severe, occasionally refractory even to high-dose oral narcotic analgesic agents, and is treated only by urgent revascularization or by amputation. The pain of such ulcerations is described as aching or burning, and arises not only from the same severe ischemic neuropathy which gives rise to ischemic rest pain but also from actual necrosis of sensory nerves in the skin at the site of the arterial ulcer.

Gangrenous changes of the toes or heel are indications that tissue death has occurred. Associated pain complaints are thus a summation not only of ischemic neuropathy but of actual necrosis of sensory nerve as well as the consequences of skin and subcutaneous tissue infarction, osteomyelitis, and ascending infection. As for patients with arterial ulceration, such patients' pain may be severe and unremitting; on the other hand, in certain such patients, necrosis of sensory nerves may actually make such gangrenous distal feet insensate and anesthetic, paradoxically resulting in less pain than would be anticipated from the degree of tissue destruction present.

Atheroembolism, usually to the toes or distal foot ("blue toe syndrome"[16]) occurs because of digital or distal branch artery occlusion from debris (clot, atheroma) which has embolized into the distal circulation from a proximal source (e.g., an aortoiliac or popliteal aneurysm or an ulcerated atherosclerotic plaque). The syndrome occurs only with patent proximal arteries, and the distal limb is usually not ischemic. Pain is therefore uncommon until digital ischemia is severe enough to result in sensory nerve damage.

The diabetic foot is a special circumstance in which chronic nonhealing lower extremity and foot ulceration and toe gangrene may occur, yet the underlying pathogenesis revolves not around ischemia but rather diabetic neuropathy, foot structural changes, and diabetics' inability to combat bacterial infection. Indeed, most diabetic foot lesions are *not* ischemic[17] and revascularization is uncommonly required as part of their management. Widespread loss of distal foot and even lower leg sensation in diabetics consequent to diabetic neuropathy makes pain due to ulceration, gangrene, or infection relatively uncommon among diabetics. On the other hand, neuropathic pain is frequent (see later text).

Pain Syndromes Following Stroke

Pain is uncommon in association with cerebrovascular accident (CVA), except for patients whose cerebrovascular ischemia results from intracranial hemorrhage or tumor. Stroke survivors sometimes experience what appears to be a centrally mediated pain ipsilateral to the neurologic deficit.[18] Dejerine and Roussy first described excruciating pain involving the contralateral half of the body in a patient who had suffered a thalamic stroke and termed the condition "thalamic syndrome."[19] Similar symptoms can arise following injury anywhere along the course of the spinothalamic tracts, and this syndrome has been termed central poststroke pain (CPSP).[20]

CPSP occurs after ischemic or hemorrhagic stroke. Patients report burning or lancinating pain associated with sensory abnormalities in the painful region. Sensory abnormalities include decreased perception of sharpness and temperature, often accompanied by allodynia and hyperalgesia.[21] The pain is often constant, but may occur in paroxysms and it is usually limited to an area that is smaller than the area affected by sensory deficits. The pain is often worsened by stress and relieved by relaxation, and the pain can present an enormous burden to the patient, causing severe depression.[22]

Following thalamic stroke, CPSP is not uncommon. In a series of 100 patients with thalamic hemorrhage, 9% developed CPSP.[23] In a prospective study of 267 consecutively admitted stroke patients, CPSP occurred in 8% of the patients during the first year, with more than half of those with pain reporting moderate to severe pain.[24] In 63% of the patients, pain onset was within 1 month after stroke.

CPSP is a difficult condition to treat, and pain reduction rather than pain relief has to be the goal of the treatment. Conventional analgesics and opioids have been noted to be ineffective.[25] Numerous other types of drugs have been tried in the treatment of CPSP, but large controlled trials are lacking, and the treatment is far from being standardized. Treatment of CPSP has been reviewed in detail elsewhere.[26]

Pain Associated With Diseases Involving Small Arteries

Numerous regional or systemic disorders include involvement of small arteries. In the extremities, such conditions commonly manifest coolness, pallor, numbness, cyanosis, and pain—manifestations of Raynaud's syndrome.[27] Often such symptoms and signs result simply from abnormal arterial reactivity, such as occurs in its benign form, termed Raynaud's *disease* (seen primarily in young and middle-aged women, or as a consequence of chronic vibratory tool use, primarily in young male laborers).

Dull aching digit pain is noted by such patients during periods of extreme vasoconstriction; with the hyperemia of digital reperfusion, when vasoconstriction is replaced by vasodilatation, this dull aching pain is commonly replaced by a burning "fiery" pain as the digits are suffused via vasodilated digital arteries.

A more ominous form of small-artery involvement associated with Raynaud's syndrome (termed Raynaud *phenomenon* in this setting) results from digital arterial occlusions resulting from one or another form of various rheumatoid conditions—especially scleroderma.[28] To these individuals' diffuse pain syndrome, resulting from digital vasoconstriction and then vasodilatation, is added intractably painful fingertip ulceration or necrosis. Such patients' distal digital pain is frequently severe and unremitting, not uncommonly refractory even to large doses of opiate analgesic medications, and may require amputation for pain relief. Pathophysiologically these lesions are similar to those of advanced chronic lower extremity arterial insufficiency.

A rare form of small-artery involvement resulting in severe pain is that associated with Buerger's disease (thromboangiitis obliterans [TAO]), a condition most commonly seen in young male tobacco addicts. TAO is a nonatherosclerotic necrotizing condition of arteries, veins, and nerves themselves primarily in the extremities.[29] Because only the tibial arteries in the lower extremity, or the distal radial and ulnar arteries of the upper extremity, are commonly involved in Buerger's disease these patients have excellent arterial inflow but inadequate collateralization (Fig. 38.5), and their ability to heal refractory ulcerations or areas of gangrene is poor. These patients' foot or hand pain is described as severe, unremitting, aching, burning, and agonizing; amputation is commonly the best management.

Pain Associated With Venous Disorders

Venous disease is common and is frequently undiagnosed. This occurs in part because one major component of venous disease—deep venous thrombosis (DVT)—commonly occurs in a relatively vegetative, bland fashion associated with only minimal inflammation. Such patients' first symptom may be painless lower extremity edema or, on occasion, chest pain and cardiorespiratory collapse associated with pulmonary embolus. Pain is only inconsistently associated with superficial venous disease. Patients with primary or secondary venous varicosities may note diffuse aching or burning pain associated with their venous varicosities, a discomfort likely secondary to stretch stimulation of nociceptors in and around the venous adventitia and media or in the surrounding soft tissue.

Patients who have suffered a prior lower extremity DVT often display symptoms and signs of the postphlebitic (postthrombotic) syndrome. This condition is characterized by chronic lower extremity edema, secondary venous varicosities, and characteristic skin changes including stasis pigmentation and eczema, subcutaneous atrophy, and, in advanced stages, skin breakdown and chronic nonhealing ulcerations around the medial and lateral malleoli. These stasis ulcerations, usually relatively small and shallow but occasionally circumferential and extending from ankle to mid-leg, are, in the author's experience, notably *nonpainful*, often manifesting only mild itching or burning. When significant pain occurs in a stasis ulcer, a secondary diagnosis should be entertained—invasive infection (usually streptococcal) or (rarely) malignant transformation, ischemia, or osteomyelitis.

Superficial phlebitis generally results from chemical irritation of the intima of peripheral veins as a consequence of intravenous infusions of various agents, sterile inflammation secondary to indwelling catheters or other foreign bodies, or bacterial infection. Such phlebitis is characterized by marked localized tenderness with overlying cellulitis, a palpable "cord" along the course of the vein and, rarely, systemic toxicity. Pain is characteristically well-localized along the vein and is burning in nature, resulting

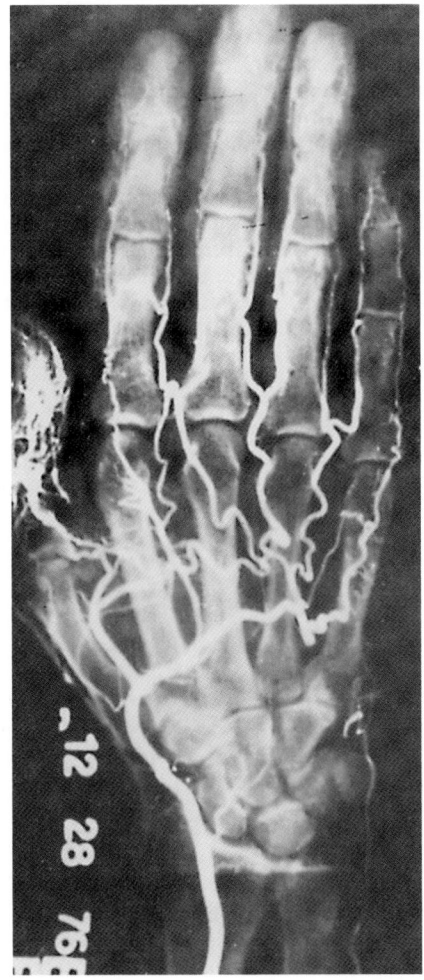

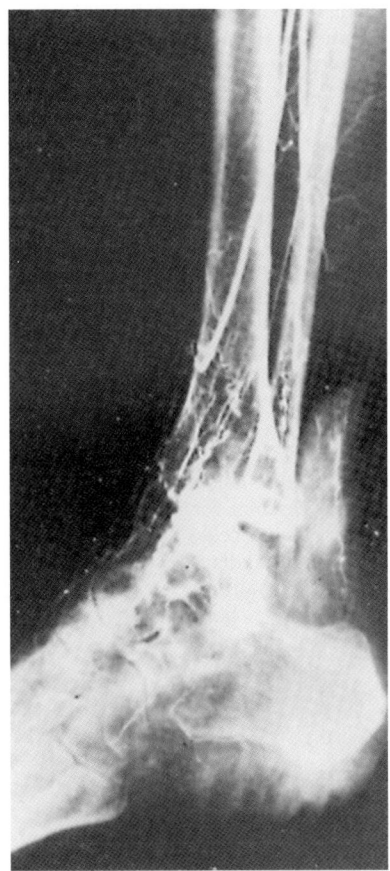

FIGURE 38.5 Angiograms of patients with thromboangiitis obliterans (Buerger's disease). (**A**) Angiogram of the hand of a patient showing lack of filling of the ulnar artery, characteristic tortuous, corkscrew-like arteries in the hand, and "skipped" areas where no contrast enters the digital arteries. (**B**) Angiogram of the distal part of the leg of a patient with thromboangiitis obliterans. The anterior and posterior tibial arteries appear normal until their abrupt occlusion at the ankle. (From deWolfe VG. Chronic occlusive arterial disease of the lower extremities. In: Spittell JA Jr, ed. *Clinical Vascular Disease*. Philadelphia: FA Davis, 1983:15–135, with permission.)

from stimulation of vein–wall nociceptive receptors. In addition, perivenous inflammation results in elaboration of acidic inflammatory or infectious mediators which stimulates perivenous nociceptors.

Pain Associated With Lymphatic Diseases

The most common lymphatic disorder is *lymphedema praecox*—idiopathic, bland nonvenous swelling, usually of a lower extremity. Other forms of lymphedema are either iatrogenic (consequent to lymphadenectomy or irradiation) or result from infections of various sorts. The lymphatics are not innervated so most forms of lymphedema are painful only when cellulitis or lymphangitis—an unfortunately common complication of lymphedema—supervenes.

Pain Associated With Amputation

Commonly performed because of intractable pain in a nonsalvageable limb, amputation itself often results in pain of various types. These can be classified as being either acute—at the time of the amputation—or chronic—occurring weeks, months, or even (upon occasion) years following the initial procedure.

Acute postamputation pain may be related to the surgical procedure itself or to incompletely understood central or neuraxial phenomena arising from the patient's preoperative pain status. Acute postamputation pain may result from the obligatory sec-

tion of major nerves during limb amputation. The incisional and wound pain that results from transtibial or transfemoral amputation commonly resolves within a week or so following amputation—sooner in many surgeons' experience if a rigid dressing is applied to the residual limb.[30]

Other relatively straightforward amputation pain issues occurring early in the postoperative period include those related to stump hematoma or ischemia or actual muscle necrosis because the amputation was performed too far distally, resulting in thrombosis of the stump's residual arterial blood supply. The latter complication generally requires re-amputation at a higher level.

Early postamputation pain problems unrelated to the wound itself include the development of diverse neuropathic phenomena, including phantom limb *sensation* or *pain*. Virtually all amputees experience the sense that the amputated limb is still present, for example, that it itches and needs to be scratched. Phantom limb *sensation* is generally considered to be benign and self-limited. Phantom limb *pain*, on the other hand, can frequently be severe and, on occasion, even incapacitating, although patients can be reassured that the phenomenon generally diminishes or disappears within months to a year following amputation. Treatment with antiseizure medications, tricyclic antidepressants, regional sympathetic blockade with long-acting local anesthetic agents, cutaneous electrical stimulation units, sympathectomy, spinal cord stimulation,[31] or even rhizotomy or distal reentry zone sectioning[32] may be of use for persistent or severe phantom limb pain.

Late postamputation pain most commonly results from a

poorly fitted limb prosthesis, and an experienced prosthetist's opinion is invaluable in this setting. Other less common but important causes of late postamputation stump pain can include progressive stump ischemia, DVT, progressive autonomic dysfunction (e.g., CRPS), or neuroma formation—the last problem best prevented by assuring that large nerves sectioned at the time of the original amputation are buried in muscle, well away from cut bone ends and the skin flap.

DIFFERENTIATING VASCULAR FROM NONVASCULAR PAIN

It is clinically self-evident that a large overlap occurs between the pain syndromes arising from vascular and nonvascular diseases. The not infrequent misdiagnosis of a ruptured AAA as ureteral or biliary colic, of an aortic dissection as a myocardial infarction or gastroesophageal reflux, or of lower extremity ischemic pain as lumbar spinal stenosis, all point to the importance of considering the entire constellation of diagnostic possibilities present in patients presenting with various forms of pain.

The scope of this chapter precludes an exhaustive discussion of those disease states in which the misdiagnosis of vascular for nonvascular disease (or, as important, the converse) can occur; the reader is referred to seminal general surgical differential diagnostic texts for further details.[33–35] Those intent on formalizing the divergence of vascular surgery from general surgery,[36,37] both in the context of resident training and as a separate specialty, must make every effort to ensure that future vascular surgeons and their general surgery colleagues experience a shared body of clinical knowledge and judgment in this context.

THE RELIEF OF VASCULAR PAIN

The relief (or at least the mitigation) of pain is the *sine qua non* of the rationale for many vascular interventions, to the extent that an ability to achieve pain relief may be tantamount to failure—either of the original diagnosis or of the intervention itself. The patient who continues to experience calf claudication after a technically successful femoral–popliteal bypass may well have needed more preoperative attention paid to the status of his lumbosacral nerve roots. The return of claudication after a period of pain-free walking suggests the progressive deterioration of the original revascularization.

Relief of several types of aortic pain can take both "medical" and surgical forms. As previously intimated, the presence of tearing central truncal pain is a hallmark of aortic dissection. All type A aortic dissections require immediate referral to a cardiothoracic surgeon for urgent intervention. However, Type B aortic dissections' natural history, as well as their indications for operative or endovascular intervention, are heavily dependent on the relief of this lesion's characteristic pain by pharmacologic therapy—specifically, the administration of beta-blocker agents, whose effect is to halt the medial hematoma's dissection by lowering systolic and mean blood pressure as well as left ventricular dV/dt.[38]

The pain associated with an expanding, leaking, or ruptured abdominal or thoracic aortic or iliac aneurysm is relieved by successful graft interposition, either by open or stent-graft means. Graft repair of aneurysms eroding into the spine commonly relieves the pain from such bony erosion. Similarly, and for obscure reasons, graft repair of inflammatory AAAs tends to resolve the characteristic inflammatory "rind" around the aorta and, with it, the diffuse, poorly localized, boring mid-abdominal-to-midback ache these patients commonly note. Interestingly, the use of corticosteroids, administered systemically or by injection, can also diminish the pain associated with an inflammatory aneu-

rysm,[39] although such therapy theoretically increases the risk of aneurysm expansion and rupture.[40]

A preponderance of pain resulting from vascular disease arises from inadequate tissue oxygenation, most commonly with exertion or other increased nutritive blood flow demands but also in basal blood flow states in which tissue viability itself is threatened. Many vascular interventions focus on restoring tissue perfusion to (or toward) normal—not only various revascularization procedures, either by open or endovascular means (Fig. 38.6), but also pharmacologic or hygienic measures as simple as the encouragement of smoking cessation or aerobic exercise or the administration of hemorheologic medications. While such inter-

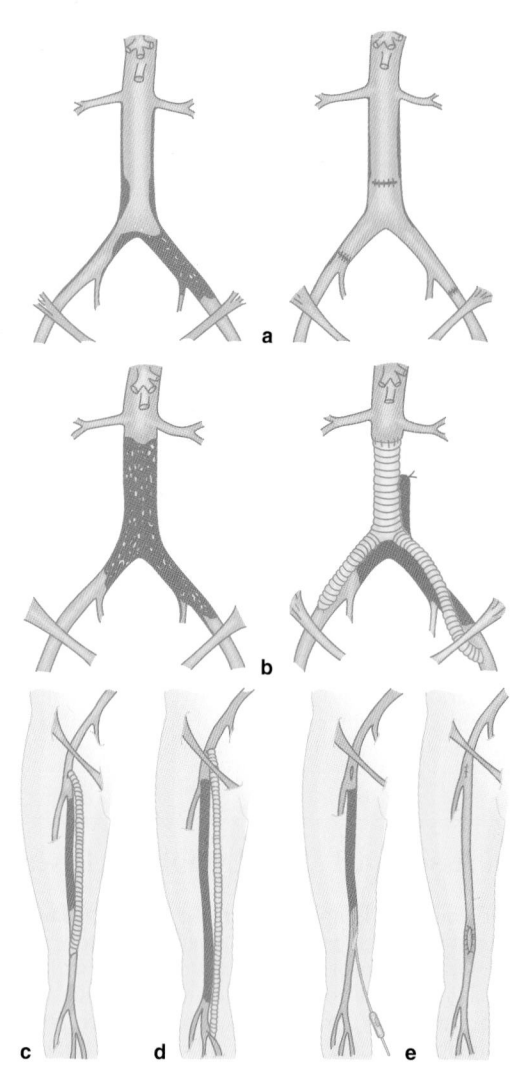

FIGURE 38.6 Various types of surgical procedures to achieve arterial revascularization. (**A**) Aortoiliac endarterectomy, which is especially useful in younger individuals with minimal deterioration of the arterial wall. This is accomplished through a transverse incision in the aortic and iliac arteries, removing the atheromatous and thrombotic cast, with subsequent reanastomosis of the iliac arteries and closure of the transverse incision in the aorta. (**B**) Endarterectomy of the proximal aorta, end-to-end aorta-graft anastomosis with oversewing of the distal aorta, and bypass graft to right external iliac artery and to the left common femoral artery. (**C**) A prosthetic bypass connecting the external iliac with the lower portion of the femoral artery. (**D**) The lower end of the prosthesis in C is grafted to the posterior tibial artery. (**E**) Endoluminal endarterectomy with vein patch arterioplasty. (Modified from Hollier LH. Principles and techniques of surgical treatment of occlusive arterial disease of the lower extremities. In: Spittell JA Jr, ed. *Clinical Vascular Disease*. Philadelphia: FA Davis, 1983:37–48.)

ventions are most commonly carried out for the symptomatic consequences of lower extremity atherosclerotic occlusive disease, the principle of relieving vascular pain by improving tissue nutrition can be relevant for nonatherosclerotic diseases of the upper extremities as well—for example, the salubrious effects seen with the administration of cilostazol in patients with various small-artery occlusive phenomena of the digits[41] or the relief of dialysis access-associated rest pain of the hand by the performance of distal revascularization/interval ligation.[42]

In unusual circumstances revascularization by conventional operative or pharmacologic means may not be feasible or may not provide tissue reperfusion adequate to relieve pain or other ischemic manifestations. In certain limited circumstances the observation, initially popularized by Leriche,[43] that sympathectomy can increase skin perfusion may offer a therapeutic alternative. Ipsilateral lumbar sympathectomy (most effectively by operative excision, although a therapeutic effect can result from phenol or absolute alcohol ablation) can heal shallow ischemic skin lesions and relieve associated ischemic rest pain, probably by the combined effects of increased skin blood flow and interruption of afferent pain fibers traveling within the lumbar sympathetic chain.[44,45] Patients subjected to such therapy have a 10% risk of developing a sometimes debilitating although transient burning pain termed postsympathectomy neuralgia.[46]

Revascularization to treat severe ischemia may not be possible, or, even if technically feasible, may not be successful in relieving pain. When tissue loss—advanced ischemic ulceration or gangrene—supervenes, amputation is indicated. However, in that subset of patients with far-advanced, refractory ischemia in which significant tissue loss has not yet developed but in which pain is severe and unremitting, Jacobs and colleagues have extensively investigated the possibility that spinal cord stimulation (SCS) might relieve pain and forestall the need for amputation as a pain-relief measure. Initial enthusiasm for this approach, based on nonrandomized studies demonstrating improved microcirculatory blood flow in subjects with advanced nonreconstructible lower extremity arterial disease,[47] has waned with publication of less favorable results of more recent prospective trials of SCS.[48] At the current time, the role of SCS in the management of subjects with advanced chronic limb ischemia appears to be restricted to those with relatively preserved microcirculatory skin perfusion.[48]

Pain associated with venous disease of various sorts is ubiquitous although rarely severe or incapacitating. The central role of vein wall distention as the proximate cause of lower extremity venous symptoms associated with saphenous or deep venous insufficiency is perhaps best demonstrated by the almost universal symptomatic improvement associated with such "low-tech" maneuvers as limb elevation or the donning of elastic support stockings. The "swollen" or "bursting" sensations associated with significant large-vessel lower extremity venous obstruction ("venous claudication") may only be effectively treated by venous bypass or by endovascular relief of proximal venous occlusions.[49] The pain associated with acute venous thrombosis, either deep or superficial, is both congestive and inflammatory and is optimally treated with limb elevation and/or compression plus anti-inflammatory medications.

The management of acute pain is central to the cultural identity of most medical specialties. Unfortunately, published research has repeatedly documented that most medical professionals have inadequate training, experience, or understanding of the proper management of acute or chronic pain. Ballantyne and Mao have recently discussed this problem as well as recent research findings which could inform a more appropriate approach to the medical management of pain.[50] Pharmacologic (or other) management of chronic or severe pain of any origin is increasingly the domain of pain specialists, frequently with an anesthesiology background, in a multidisciplinary pain clinic setting.

CONCLUSION

How best to manage the manifold types of vascular pain is a vast and incompletely illuminated topic. Vascular pain's multifactorial nature confounds simple or stereotypical prescriptions for its relief. In a large majority of cases restoration to (or toward) normalcy of the underlying arterial or venous condition will resolve or improve associated vascular pain. Chronic vascular pain is closely allied with neuritic or neuropathic abnormalities, the management of which warrants involvement of specialist consultants in chronic pain.

References

1. Loeser JD, ed. *Bonica's Management of Pain.* 3rd ed. Philadelphia: Lippincott Williams & Wilkins, 1998.
2. Wall PD, Melzack R, eds. *Textbook of Pain.* 4th ed. Edinburgh: Churchill Livingstone, 1999.
3. Raj PP, ed. *Practical Management of Pain.* 3rd ed. St. Louis: Mosby, 2000.
4. Aronoff GM, ed. *Evaluation and Treatment of Chronic Pain.* 3rd ed. Baltimore: Williams & Williams, 1998.
5. Mersky H. Classification of chronic pain: description of chronic pain syndromes and definition of pain terms. *Pain* 1986:(suppl 3):S1.
6. Pick J. *The Autonomic Nervous System: Morphological, Comparative, Clinical and Surgical Aspects.* Philadelphia: Lippincott, 1970.
7. Harden RN, Bruehl S, Galer BS, et al. Complex regional pain syndrome: are the IASP diagnostic criteria valid and sufficiently comprehensive? *Pain* 1999; 83:211–219.
8. Smetana GW, Shmerling RH. Does this patient have temporal arteritis? *JAMA* 2002; 287:92–101.
9. Binder DK, Schmidt MH, Weinstein PR. Lumbar spinal stenosis. *Semin Neurol* 2002;22:157–166.
10. Delis KT, Bountouroglou D, Mansfield AO. Venous claudication in iliofemoral thrombosis: long-term effects on venous hemodynamics, clinical status, and quality of life. *Ann Surg* 2004;239:118–126.
11. Rosenson RS. Current overview of statin-induced myopathy. *Am J Med* 2004; 116:408–416.
12. Levien LJ. Popliteal artery entrapment syndrome. *Semin Vasc Surg* 2003;16:223–231.
13. Turnipseed WD. Diagnosis and management of chronic compartment syndrome. *Surgery* 2002;132:613–617; discussion 617–619.
14. Danesh J, Whincup P, Walker M, et al. Low-grade inflammation and coronary heart disease: prospective study and updated meta-analyses. *Brit Med J* 2000: 321:199–204.
15. LeSar CJ, Meier GH, DeMasi RJ, et al. The utility of color duplex ultrasonography in the diagnosis of temporal arteritis. *J Vasc Surg* 2002;36:1154–1160.
16. Renshaw A, McCowen T, Waltke EA, et al. Angioplasty with stenting is effective in treating blue toe syndrome. *Vasc Endovascular Surg* 2002;36:155–159.
17. Reiber GE, Vileikyte L, Boyko EJ, et al. Causal pathways for incident lower-extremity ulcers in patients with diabetes from two settings. *Diabetes Care* 1999;22:157–162.
18. Widar M, Ek AC, Ahlstrom G. Coping with long-term pain after a stroke. *J Pain Symptom Manage* 2004;27:215–225.
19. Bowsher D, Leijon G, Thuomas KA. Central poststroke pain: correlation of MRI with clinical pain characteristics and sensory abnormalities. *Neurology* 1998;51:1352–1358.
20. Boivie J, Leijon G, Johansson I. Central post-stroke pain: a study of the mechanisms through analysis of the sensory abnormalities. *Pain* 1989;36:173–185.
21. Vestergaard K, Nielsen J, Andersen G, et al. Sensory abnormalities in consecutive, unselected patients with central post-stroke pain. *Pain* 1995;61:177–186.
22. Leijon G, Boivie J, Johansson I. Central post-stroke pain: neurological symptoms and pain characteristics. *Pain* 1989;36:13–25.
23. Kumral E, Kocaer T, Ertübey N, et al. Thalamic hemorrhage: a prospective study of 100 patients. *Stroke* 1995;26:964–970.
24. Andersen G, Vestergaard K, Ingeman-Nielsen M, et al. Incidence of central post-stroke pain. *Pain* 1995;61:187–193.
25. Arnér S, Meyerson BA. Lack of analgesic effect of opioids on neuropathic and idiopathic forms of pain. *Pain* 1988;33:11–23.
26. Frese A, Husstedt IW, Ringelstein EB, et al. Pharmacologic treatment of central post-stroke pain. *Clin J Pain* 2006;22:252–260.
27. Wigley FM, Raynaud's phenomenon. *N Engl J Med* 2002;347:1001–1008.
28. Pope J, Fenlon D, Thompson A, et al. Iloprost and cisaprost for Raynaud's phenomenon in progressive systemic sclerosis. *Cochrane Database Syst Rev* 2000;CD000953.
29. Ohta T, Ishioashi H, Hosaka M, et al. Clinical and social consequences of Buerger disease. *J Vasc Surg* 2004;29:176–180.
30. Smith DG, McFarland LV, Sangeorzan BJ, et al. Postoperative dressing and management strategies for transtibial amputation: critical review. *J Rehabil Res Dev* 2003;40:213–224.
31. Katayama Y, Yamamoto T, Kobayashi K, et al. Motor cortex stimulation for

phantom limb pain: comprehensive therapy with spinal cord and thalamic stimulation. *Stereotact Funct Neurosurg* 2001;77:159–162.

32. Microsurgical junctional DREZ coagulation for treatment of deafferentation syndromes. *Surg Neurol* 2001;56:259–265.
33. Greenfield LJ, ed. *Surgery: Scientific Principles and Practice.* 3rd ed. Philadelphia: Lippincott Williams & Wilkins, 2001.
34. Schwartz SL, ed. *Principles of Surgery.* 7th ed. New York: McGraw-Hill; 1999.
35. Corson JD, Williamson RCN, eds. *Surgery.* London: Mosby, 2001.
36. Veith FJ. The case for an independent American Board of Vascular Surgery. *J Vasc Surg* 2000;32:619–621.
37. Stanley JC. The discipline of vascular surgery at the close of the millennium, the American Board of Surgery Sub-Board for Vascular Surgery, and the wisdom of evolving a conjoint board of vascular surgery: one surgeon's perspective. *J Vasc Surg* 2000;31:831–835.
38. Westaby S. Management of aortic dissection. *Curr Opin Cardiol* 1995;10:505–510.
39. Stotter AT, Grigg MJ, Mansfield AO. The response of peri-aneurysmal fibrosis—the "inflammatory" aneurysm—to surgery and steroid therapy. *Eur J Vasc Surg* 1990;4;201–205.
40. Reilly JM, Savage EB, Brophy CM, et al. Hydrocortisone rapidly induces aortic rupture in a genetically susceptible mouse. *Arch Surg* 1990;125:707–709.

41. Rajagopalan S. Pfenninger D, Somers E, et al. Effects of cilostazol in patients with Raynaud's syndrome. *Am J Cardiol* 2003;92:1310–1315.
42. Diehl L, Johansen K, Watson J. Operative management of distal ischemia complicating upper extremity dialysis access. *Am J Surg* 2003;186:17–19.
43. Ewing M. The history of lumbar sympathectomy. *Surgery* 1971;70:791–796.
44. Mailis A, Furlan A. Sympathectomy for neuropathic pain. *Cochrane Database Syst Rev* 2003;CD002918.
45. AbuRahma AF, Robinson PA, Powell M, et al. Sympathectomy for reflex sympathetic dystrophy: factors affecting outcome. *Ann Vasc Surg* 1994;8:372–379.
46. Kramis RC, Roberts WJ, Gillette RG. Post-sympathectomy neuralgia: hypotheses on peripheral and central neuron mechanisms. *Pain* 1996;65:1–9.
47. Jacobs MJ, Jorning PJ, Beckers RC, et al. Post salvage and improvement of microvascular flow as a result of epidural spinal cord electrical stimulation. *J Vasc Surg* 1990:12:354–360.
48. Ubbink DT, Spincemaille GH, Prins MH, et al. Microcirculatory investigations to determine the effect of spinal cord stimulation for critical leg ischemia: the Dutch Multicenter randomized controlled trial. *J Vasc Surg* 1999;30:236–244.
49. Raju S, Owen S Jr, Neglen P. The clinical impact of iliac venous stents in the management of chronic venous insufficiency. *J Vasc Surg* 2002;35:8–15.
50. Ballantyne JC, Mao J. Opioid therapy for chronic pain. *N Engl J Med* 2003;349:1943–1953.

CHAPTER 39 ■ PAIN DUE TO THORACIC OUTLET SYNDROME

KAJ H. JOHANSEN, CYNTHIA CAMPBELL, AND GEORGE I. THOMAS

INTRODUCTION

An important and incompletely understood cause of upper extremity pain is subsumed under the rubric of "thoracic outlet syndrome" (TOS). This condition arises from compression of neurovascular structures as they enter/exit the neuraxis and the mediastinum at the base of the neck. Particularly in cases involving chronic compression of the brachial plexus, TOS can be a complicated and frustrating condition to manage, due to ongoing controversy about the underlying pathophysiology, how the diagnosis is best made, and disputes about proper and effective treatment. Many of the problems regarding TOS revolve around the uncertain natural history of the condition with and without intervention. In this chapter we discuss the various types of TOS with a particular emphasis on the neurogenic type—by far the most common, the most disputed, and also the most likely to result in pain.

ANATOMY AND PATHOPHYSIOLOGY

The thoracic outlet is the aperture through which the subclavian artery and trunks of the brachial plexus pass as they exit the neuraxis and the upper mediastinum at the base of the neck. In normal anatomic circumstances the thoracic outlet is bound by several musculotendinous and bony structures including the anterior and middle scalene muscles and, inferiorly, the first rib (Fig. 39.1). In pathologic circumstances, compression of the neurovascular bundle at the thoracic outlet is most commonly the consequence of abnormalities of the scalene muscles and/or the first rib. However, neurovascular compression can also result from the presence of a cervical rib, abnormal fibrous bands, callus

from a clavicular fracture, scarring from prior trauma or radiation therapy, or (rarely) a superior sulcus (Pancoast) tumor of the lung.

Because the subclavian vein lies anterior to the anterior scalene muscle it does not actually pass through the thoracic outlet. It is, however, located beneath (and can be compressed by) the subclavius muscle and between the clavicle and the first rib in its course toward the mediastinum.

In normal circumstances arm elevation or abduction results in a functional reduction in the caliber of the thoracic outlet aperture because of posterior rotation of the clavicle and contracture of the scalene muscles. The space between the clavicle and the first rib narrows, and below the shoulder the pectoralis minor muscle contracts.

Trauma, particularly cervical hyperextension ("whiplash") or chronic repetitive use of the upper extremities (particularly in an out-front or overhead position) may, over time, result in chronic spasm and contracture of the scalene muscles, producing both thickening of the anterior and middle scalene muscles as well as microstructural changes in muscle fiber type.[1,2]

Provocative maneuvers of the arm may result in compression of the subclavian artery and vein in up to 30% of normal individuals.[3] Reduction in the caliber of the thoracic outlet by pathophysiologic circumstances can result in extrinsic compression of the subclavian artery or vein in more than 90% of patients with TOS.

A cervical rib, abnormal bands, or residua from a clavicular fracture can result in subclavian *arterial* stricture. This may result in development of a poststenotic subclavian artery dilatation or even a subclavian artery aneurysm, mural thrombus from which may embolize into the arterial circulation of the wrist or hand.

Extrinsic compression of the subclavian vein in the costoclavicular space, perhaps involving the tendon of the subclavius muscle, can in concert with repetitive use of the upper extremity result

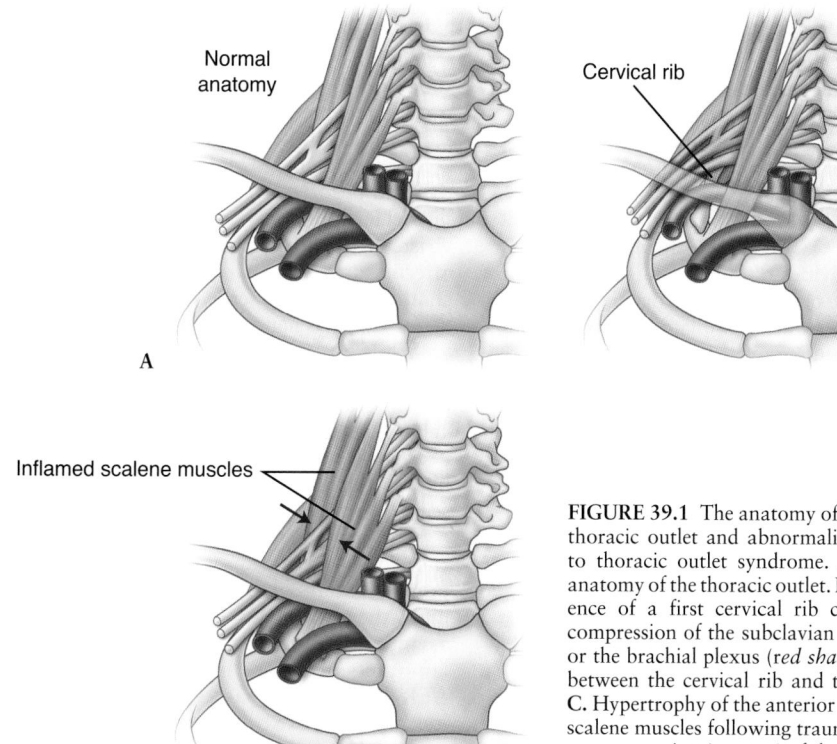

Normal anatomy

Cervical rib

A

B

Inflamed scalene muscles

C

FIGURE 39.1 The anatomy of the normal thoracic outlet and abnormalities leading to thoracic outlet syndrome. **A.** Normal anatomy of the thoracic outlet. **B.** The presence of a first cervical rib can lead to compression of the subclavian artery and/or the brachial plexus (*red shaded region*) between the cervical rib and the clavicle. **C.** Hypertrophy of the anterior and middle scalene muscles following trauma can lead to compression (*arrows*) of the subclavian artery and/or the brachial plexus.

in axillosubclavian *venous* thrombosis likely due to intimal damage and venous stasis.

CLINICAL PRESENTATION

Arterial TOS is extremely uncommon, comprising less than 1% of the totality of any TOS practice, and almost always presents as forearm or hand claudication (or other upper extremity ischemic symptoms) or evidence for distal upper extremity embolization. Physical examination demonstrates diminished or absent wrist pulses; vascular laboratory examination may show occlusion of the radial and/or ulnar arteries or their palmar or digital branches. On occasion patients may present with rest pain or gangrene of the fingers due to far-advanced ischemia from repetitive distal arterial embolic occlusion.

Physical findings in patients with *arterial* TOS are primarily those of absent or diminished pulses and/or the manifestations of distal upper extremity ischemia.

Involvement of the upper extremity venous circulation by compression of the subclavian vein at the thoracic outlet comprises approximately 5% of a TOS practice. Patients with such *venous* TOS (also termed Paget-Schroetter syndrome or "effort" thrombosis of the axillosubclavian vein) may present with aching pain distributed diffusely throughout a swollen, ruborous upper extremity. In more chronic circumstances pain and swelling may be less prominent.

Patients with *venous* TOS manifest arm swelling and discoloration; in later stages, prominent veins can be seen over the upper arm and around the shoulder.

By far the most common presentation–the overwhelming majority of the patients seen in a TOS practice–results from compression of elements of the brachial plexus, that is, *neurogenic* TOS. Patients with neurogenic TOS almost always have a prior traumatic event—a cervical hyperextension ("whiplash") injury, a fall on an outstretched arm, an object falling on the

head or the shoulder—or alternatively have a history for a repetitive stress injury, usually due to exigencies of employment. Occupational risk factors for neurogenic TOS include sustained effort with the upper extremity(s) out-front or overhead and may be seen in drywall hangers, dental hygienists, beauticians or hairdressers, grocery checkers, shelf-stockers, or clerical workers engaged in prolonged keyboarding.

Such injury- or workplace-related postures and stresses have been demonstrated to result in chronic contracture and spasm of the suspensory muscles in and around the shoulder girdle—among them the anterior and middle scalene muscles. Obesity, sedentary lifestyles and maladaptive postures—in neurogenic TOS, characterized by the head flexed on the neck and the shoulders down and forward—exacerbate chronic scalene muscle spasm.

Patients with neurogenic TOS may have few or no symptoms with the arms in a neutral position. However, they will quickly note the onset of pain and paresthesiae with the arms placed in an out-front, overhead, or abducted posture. Indeed, this presentation is so stereotypic that we do not seriously entertain the diagnosis of neurogenic TOS in the absence of a subject's indication of worsened symptoms with the arms in such provocative postures.

Symptoms characteristically evoked in neurogenic TOS patients include elevational arm aching, particularly proximally around the shoulder, the axilla and the upper arm, associated variably with numbness and tingling out the arm, distal weakness, and a limitation in range of motion of the affected upper extremity. Paresthesiae are found predominantly in a C8-T1 distribution, appropriate to impingement on the lower aspects of the brachial plexus. Indeed, 80% of patients with neurogenic TOS demonstrate pain and paresthesias radiating along an ulnar nerve distribution often into the small and ring finger as a consequence. This presumably results from upward traction on the first rib by the scalene muscles, thus selectively impacting the inferior aspects of the brachial plexus.

A significant proportion of patients with neurogenic TOS have significant headaches, primarily occipital.[4] They also may note symptoms of facial or jaw pain or pain around the ear.

Muscle pain is commonplace in neurogenic TOS, particularly around the neck and the shoulder, the scapula, and the upper arm. It is frequently difficult to discern whether such symptoms arise from neurogenic TOS itself or from concurrent soft-tissue injuries (e.g., the paraspinous or periscapular muscles: the rotator cuff in the shoulder) suffered at the same time as the injury causing the neurogenic TOS.

Patients with neurogenic TOS frequently display a series of symptoms associated with activities of daily living which, in the aggregate, strongly indicate the presence of neurogenic TOS. The presence of a strongly positive clinical template has been in our experience as predictive of the diagnosis of neurogenic TOS as the use of various provocative tests (e.g., Adson, Roos, Wright). during physical examination. Elements of our clinical template are shown in Table 39.1.

In *neurogenic* TOS objective physical findings are sparse. Such individuals have limited range of motion of the affected upper extremity and manifest diminished spontaneous (adventitial) movements of the extremity as well as an unwillingness to place (or maintain) the affected limb in various provocative postures. Muscle tenderness over the anterior and lateral neck is commonplace, as is neck muscle tightness or contracture. In the supraclavicular fossa tenderness can be elicited with palpation over the brachial plexus, often resulting in radiation of neuritic sensations into the axilla or out the arm. Occasionally a cervical rib can be palpated. Tenderness over the pectoralis minor tendon attachment at the coracoid process below the shoulder is commonplace.

More peripherally in the upper extremity, tenderness may be elicited with palpation deep in the axilla. Tenderness of the arm or forearm muscles or tendons, or evidence for peripheral nerve compression at the carpal or cubital tunnels, may be present; this is not, however, a primary manifestation of neurogenic TOS but, rather, of the concurrent upper extremity injury that may accompany neurogenic TOS ("double crush" syndrome).[5] Rarely, intrinsic hand muscle atrophy may be observed, a so-called Gilliatt hand.[6]

A series of provocative tests are commonly performed which, individually or in the aggregate, are thought by many to demonstrate the presence of neurogenic TOS. The *Adson test* is carried out with the affected arm held downward and backward: the ipsilateral wrist pulse is palpated as the head is turned toward this arm while the subject undertakes a sustained inspiration. A positive test, suggesting the presence of neurogenic TOS, results when the wrist pulse is obliterated.

The *military* or *shoulder brace position* involves retraction of the shoulders backward and downward, resulting in pulse obliteration at the wrist.

The Roos or *abduction/external rotation (AER)* ("*hands-up*") *test* involves, as described, the arms held at 90 degrees at the shoulders, the elbows flexed 90 degrees, and the hands then contracted repeatedly. A positive test involves rapid fatiguing and pain in the affected upper extremity.

Recently Sanders and colleagues have reported the high positive and negative predictive value of the *brachial plexus tension test*.[7] Here the arms are held horizontally with the elbows and wrists straight and the neck is laterally flexed *away* from the affected arm: both wrists are then extended. A positive test is characterized by a sense of tightness and pain in the ipsilateral neck as well as neuritic symptoms radiating out the affected arm.

While not a provocative test for neurogenic TOS, the *Spurling* test is important in evaluation of this condition. Because an important alternative diagnosis may be cervical radiculopathy, development of characteristic symptoms with lateral flexion of the neck *toward* the affected extremity makes neurogenic TOS less likely and neuroforaminal compression due to herniated disc, scar, or arthritis more probable.

The aforementioned provocative tests are commonly performed as part of an evaluation for neurogenic TOS. Skeptics point out that, while the sensitivity of each of these tests may be high, their specificity is very low (e.g., more than 30% of the asymptomatic population may have a positive Adson test[3]). Similar results hold for the military (shoulder brace) position. The AER ("hands-up") has a high sensitivity and much better specificity for NTOS. Experienced clinicians' view is that patients ultimately demonstrated to have neurogenic TOS will be strongly positive for many or most of these tests, individually or in the aggregate.

DIAGNOSTIC TESTS

In patients with *arterial* TOS, chest roentgenography will frequently confirm the presence of a cervical rib or callus from a clavicular fracture. A noninvasive upper extremity vascular laboratory examination will confirm the absence of (or reduction in) arterial flow at the hand and wrist level, not uncommonly in a pattern consistent with thromboembolic occlusion. Duplex scanning of the subclavian artery may demonstrate aneurysm formation with mural thrombus within. Computed tomography (CT) scan or catheter-directed arteriography may demonstrate sharp angulation of the subclavian artery over a cervical rib or around a clavicular fracture callus (Fig. 39.2); such imaging studies may also document the specific distribution of distal forearm arterial or palmar arch occlusions.

In *venous* TOS, noninvasive vascular laboratory examination will demonstrate partial or complete axillosubclavian venous thrombosis.[8] Enlarged venous collaterals around the shoulder may be displayed. Not uncommonly, upstream (arm) venous tributaries such as the basilic vein may demonstrate partial or complete thrombosis as well.

In *neurogenic* TOS chest roentgenography may demonstrate a cervical rib. We commonly perform an apical lordotic view because, with a standard chest roentgenogram, on occasion a cervical rib may be hidden as it overlies the first rib (Fig. 39.3). A chest roentgenogram may also, as for arterial TOS, demonstrate a clavicular fracture; it may also document the presence of a superior sulcus tumor causing the patient's symptoms.

Arteriography may demonstrate extrinsic narrowing or occlusion of the subclavian artery by the aforementioned anatomic stricture, particularly when the affected arm is maintained in an abducted/externally rotated posture. Imaging studies such as magnetic resonance imaging (MRI) or CT may demonstrate hypertrophied or inflamed scalene muscles, or edema or inflammation of the brachial plexus.[9,10]

TABLE 39.1

CLINICAL ELEMENTS THAT SUGGEST NEUROGENIC THORACIC OUTLET SYNDROME

Inability to drive with the hands elevated in the normal 10 o'clock/ 2 o'clock position on the steering wheel

Problems with grooming (shampooing the hair or use of a hairdryer)

Awakening at night with pain or numbness in the affected arm(s)

"Drop attacks": the tendency to drop things, often without recognizing that grip strength has diminished

Inability to carry out sustained overhead activities, for example, changing multiple light bulbs in the ceiling

Loss of handwriting legibility (with involvement of the dominant upper extremity)

Inability to remove a tight jar lid

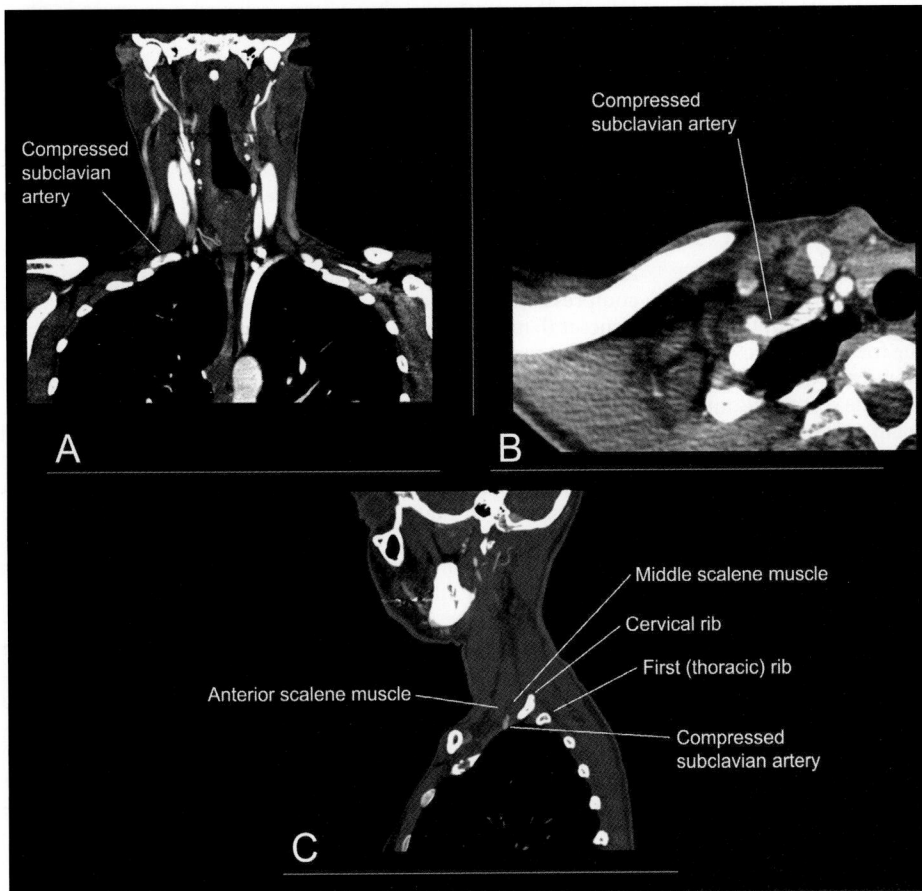

FIGURE 39.2 Computed tomography angiography with multi-planar reformatted images demonstrating compression of the subclavian artery between the insertions of the anterior and middle scalene muscles in a patient with a cervical rib. **A.** Coronal image demonstrating external compression of the subclavian artery as it passes cephalad to the cervical rib. **B.** Axial image demonstrating narrowing of the subclavian artery due to compression on the artery by the anterior scalene muscle. **C.** Sagittal, right paramedian image demonstrating compression of the subclavian artery as it passes between the insertion of the anterior and middle scalene muscles on the cervical rib. (Images courtesy of Dean Donahue, MD, Division of Thoracic Surgery, Massachusetts General Hospital, Boston, MA.)

Electrodiagnostic testing is commonly performed in patients thought to have neurogenic TOS. For patient with "true" neurogenic TOS (a rarely seen condition which results from direct brachial plexus trauma, for example, a stab or gunshot wound), specific electrodiagnostic criteria have been established—primarily, reduction in median motor and ulnar sensory nerve amplitude. In patients with the much more common "nonspecific" or "disputed"[11] neurogenic TOS, standard electromyography (EMG) or nerve conduction velocity testing is almost always normal.[12] This is not because nerve compression is not present but, rather, as demonstrated by Tender et al.,[13] because such compression occurs much more centrally, at the level of the nerve roots and proximal brachial plexus trunks—an area that is difficult to assess via nerve conduction testing.

Recently Sanders has indicated the possibility that electrodiagnostic evaluation of the median antebrachial nerve may provide useful diagnostic information in neurogenic TOS.[14]

Most significant in the diagnostic evaluation of neurogenic TOS in our practice has been the use of temporary scalene muscle inactivation, carried out by EMG-guided intrascalene injection of either bupivacaine[15] or botulinum toxin A (Botox).[16] Scalene muscle block has been demonstrated to have a sensitivity *and* specificity >90% for the presence of neurogenic TOS.[15] After installation of one of these agents into the scalene muscle, the patient with neurogenic TOS commonly notes a reduction in pain and paresthesias as well as an improvement in flexibility and range of motion in the affected arm. Headache is frequently relieved and the dysautonomic symptoms (blueish discoloration, constant aching pain, moist skin) that accompany neurogenic TOS in up to 10% of patients are relieved.

Not infrequently, after a positive block, patients become emotional and burst into tears with such novel and unanticipated relief of their symptoms (sometimes having been told by prior

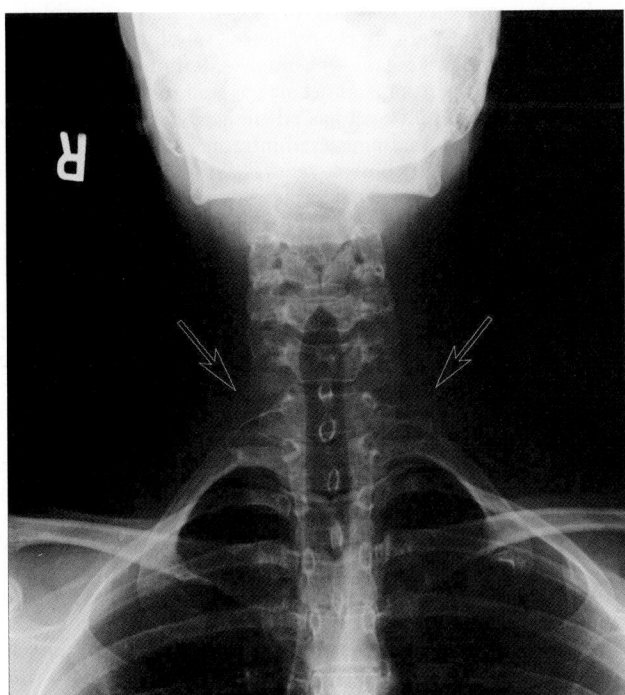

FIGURE 39.3 Chest x-ray demonstrating presence of cervical rib (*arrows*) in a patient with symptoms of thoracic outlet syndrome. (Image courtesy of Dean Donahue, MD, Division of Thoracic Surgery, Massachusetts General Hospital, Boston, MA.)

examiners that they are delusional or are malingerers). The effects start within a few minutes with bupivacaine injection and last from 15 minutes to several hours; with Botox administration (which we utilize both diagnostically and as a treatment maneuver) the onset of relief of symptoms (which occurs in more than 95% of patients who have had a positive bupivacaine block) occurs within 48 to 72 hours and lasts for 1 to 4 months.[16,17]

DIFFERENTIAL DIAGNOSIS

A number of alternative conditions present with symptoms and signs similar to those of various forms of TOS, thus complicating the diagnosis. This is most particularly true for neurogenic TOS, although on occasion arterial TOS may be written off for a time as Raynaud syndrome (or phenomenon) or some sort of dysautonomic disorder such as complex regional pain syndrome (CRPS). Venous TOS may be misdiagnosed as lymphedema or, again, some variety of sympathetic dystrophy.

In neurogenic TOS a wide range of conditions in the central nervous system or the neuraxis, most particularly multiple sclerosis but also such exotic disorders as syringomyelia, have masqueraded for a time as neurogenic TOS. Impingement on the cervical spinal cord or its nerve roots by herniated disc, arthritis, or cervical spinal stenosis can commonly present with neck, supraclavicular, shoulder, axillary, or upper extremity symptoms. Involvement of the shoulder or the scapula is a common concomitant of the injury which may initially have led to the neurogenic TOS itself. Cubital tunnel compression of the ulnar nerve in the elbow, or even carpal tunnel compression of the median nerve at the wrist, may manifest upper extremity symptoms which, on occasion, may be difficult to distinguish from those of neurogenic TOS.

Migraineurs may sometimes experience facial, jaw, or neck pain. Generalized shoulder girdle pain is a commonplace manifestation of fibromyalgia. Polymyositis, temporal (cranial) arteritis and polymyalgia rheumatica are connective tissue disorders which variably present with pain and tenderness of the muscles of the head, neck, and shoulder girdle.

The initial trauma (e.g., the "whiplash" injury suffered in a motor vehicle crash) commonly results in aches and pains and tenderness in the neck and out one or both upper extremities; it may even result in radicular symptoms which worsen with provocative postures of the arm. Such symptoms are not, however, those of neurogenic TOS, which we consider to be the consequence of *chronic* contracture of the scalene muscles. Indeed, we assert that the diagnosis of neurogenic TOS should not be invoked until at least 3 to 6 months after the initial traumatic event.

MANAGEMENT

In patients with *arterial* TOS two separate treatment goals must be met: relief of distal limb ischemia and eradication of the more proximal embolic source that resulted in the distal extremity ischemia. While repair of the proximal subclavian arterial lesion is relatively straightforward (usually aneurysmorrhaphy with a short segment of prosthetic graft material or of reversed saphenous vein), restoration of distal arterial flow is often difficult because the embolization that has occurred is chronic. The fact that the occlusion is longstanding often stymies efforts at catheter-directed thrombolysis or open arterial thrombectomy. Fortunately, if pulsatile flow can be restored to the level of the palmar arch then more distal digital tissue loss is generally avoided.

Conventional management of *venous* TOS should include systemic anticoagulation (this is, after all, a form of deep venous thrombosis and pulmonary emboli have certainly occurred as a consequence[18]) and, particularly if the onset of symptoms is recent, an attempt at catheter-directed axillosubclavian vein thrombolysis. If venous thrombus is thus relieved a stricture is often identified within the subclavian vein at the costoclavicular junction. Balloon angioplasty may frequently be carried out[19]; however, it is generally agreed that venous stenting should not be performed at this site because of the high likelihood of stent fracture between the "hammer" and "anvil" formed by the clavicle and first rib.[20]

Because of concerns about recurrent axillosubclavian venous thrombosis and chronic postthrombotic symptoms, conventional management has also commonly included not only thrombolysis and anticoagulation but staged operative thoracic outlet decompression.[21,22] Such an approach is designed to resolve the structural mechanism which led to the initial venous damage (also, by removing the costoclavicular "anvil," later stenting of the stenotic subclavian vein can be carried out if this is deemed necessary).

However, several recent natural history studies have suggested that recurrent axillosubclavian venous thrombosis is in fact quite uncommon and that the natural history of this condition is benign—enough so that thoracic outlet decompression may only rarely be warranted.[23,24] These authors argue that, far from preventing further complications, the magnitude of the dissection required for first rib resection is such that collateral vein disruption around the damaged axillosubclavian vein might paradoxically lead to worsening of the patient's venous congestive symptoms.

Early and mild-to-moderate *neurogenic* TOS should be treated by aggressive physiotherapy emphasizing postural training, abdominal breathing, and emphasis on stretching and relaxing the scalene muscles. Unfortunately, physiotherapy attempted in the early stages of neurogenic TOS is frequently misdirected, emphasizing resistance exercises; these, of course, tend only to exacerbate further scalene muscle contracture. Soon the scalene muscles are thickened and scarred, such that it is difficult to imagine much benefit from physiotherapy. Histologic studies of scalene muscle removed at this stage further support this conclusion: the muscle fibers are found to have changed from type II to type I and are interwoven with abundant fibroblasts.[1,2]

For these and other reasons, we believe that, once established, neurogenic TOS is effectively managed only by thoracic outlet decompression. Two means—chemodenervation with botulinum toxin A[16,17] or open surgical decompression of the thoracic outlet—are practiced and each has advantages and disadvantages.

Botulinum toxin, administered intramuscularly under EMG- or ultrasound-guided control, relieves symptoms of neurogenic TOS in the vast majority of subjects who have previously responded positively to a diagnostic scalene muscle block with local anesthetic. Such patients' symptoms are relieved for 1 to 4 months (mean 3 months).[17] A substantial proportion of such individuals can undergo repeat intrascalene botulinum toxin administration with attainment of another equivalent period of symptom relief.

However, scalene muscle chemodenervation, while temporarily affective at relieving symptoms of neurogenic TOS, does not appear to alter the underlying natural history of neurogenic TOS. Even when vigorous physiotherapy has been pursued during the period of time of scalene muscle denervation, durable improvement in the underlying condition is rarely detected. Tachyphylaxis to botulinum toxin is demonstrable in a substantial number of patients. The use of botulinum toxin for the treatment of thoracic outlet syndrome is not approved by the U.S. Food and Drug Administration, thus there is limited availability of this treatment. While a few of our surgery-averse patients have continued to undertake repeat botulinum toxin chemodenervation, a majority have ultimately opted for operation.

Surgical decompression of the thoracic outlet has historically been based on partial or complete excision of the first rib. The operative rationale is transparent—because the first rib is located at the bottom of the anatomic "triangle" forming the thoracic outlet and serves as the site of insertion of the anterior and middle scalene muscles which comprise the remaining two sides of the "triangle," first rib removal should effectively open this orifice. Because the short, wide first rib plays no significant role in chest wall dynamics and the scalene muscles (developmentally archaic accessory muscles of respiration) serve no significant functional role, dismantling of the musculoskeletal bounds of the thoracic outlet should have minimal impact. Large series of patients undergoing first rib resection by transaxillary,[25,26] supraclavicular,[27] or posterior[28] approaches have demonstrated significant improvements in their prior neurocompressive symptoms 75% to 90% of the time.

Patients with symptoms of neurogenic TOS who have cervical ribs have generally done well simply with resection of the cervical rib as well as the tight adhesions ("bands of Roos"[29]) commonly associated with these extrathoracic ribs.

However, based on neurogenic TOS patients' stereotypic response to bupivacaine or botulinum-mediated chemodenervation, we have rethought our operative strategy for neurogenic TOS. Because a positive response to scalene muscle block is an obligatory part of our indications for operative intervention for neurogenic TOS (a positive block has a >90% positive predictive value for a favorable outcome of operative intervention[15]), we have concluded that the pathophysiology of this condition resides in the scalene muscles and not the first rib. We now consider the rib a *victim* of the condition rather than its *cause*. Others[30,31] have reasoned similarly.

We have thus ceased performing resection of the first rib and now focus our operative efforts on radical excision of the anterior and middle scalene muscles. We have carried out more than 200 consecutive thoracic outlet decompression procedures without excising the first rib: our results (90% "excellent" or "good" results) are equivalent to those we recorded with rib excision plus total scalenectomy, but patients in whom rib salvage has occurred appear to rehabilitate substantially more rapidly than those in whom subtotal first rib resection had taken place.

We have come to believe that a separate site of brachial plexus compression, in addition to the well-accepted interscalene and costoclavicular locations, occurs beneath the pectoralis minor tendon attachment to the coracoid process, a site where tendinous impingement on the upper aspect of the axillary nerve can occur. It has long been our practice to decompress this area by dividing the pectoralis minor tendon via a small vertical infraclavicular incision separate from the supraclavicular approach through which we decompress the brachial plexus. Sanders has likewise recently adopted this approach.[32]

OUTCOMES

Patients with *arterial* TOS are generally diagnosed and managed in timely fashion due to the sensitivity of finger, hand, and upper extremity neurovascular function. Even when chronic thrombotic occlusion of distal vessels is present, upper extremity arterial collateralization is generally robust enough to maintain distal hand and finger tissue viability and function.

For *venous* TOS, the long-term outcome following first rib resection appears to be good.[21,22] However, the natural history of this condition *without* first rib resection also appears to be excellent,[23,24] leading to recent skepticism regarding whether excision of the first rib in such patients really is in fact an obligatory part of management of this condition.[33]

Published data suggest that, while thoracic outlet decompression rarely completely resolves symptoms of *neurogenic* TOS, the vast majority of patients undergoing surgical thoracic outlet decompression appear to improve and to do well. Even among a high-risk group of workmen's compensation patients undergoing surgery for neurogenic TOS following prolonged administrative delays, the vast majority felt themselves to be improved and indicated they would undergo operation again if confronted by the problem.[34]

Approximately 5% to 10% of patients who have initially undergone decompressive surgery for neurogenic TOS will display persistent or recurrent neurogenic TOS symptoms. Such individuals may be found to have a missed cervical rib, a residual stub of first rib impinging on the brachial plexus or, most frequently in our experience, adherence of scar and unresected scalene muscle to the brachial plexus.[35] In such circumstances reoperative surgery, while associated with increased risk of peripheral nerve or brachial plexus damage, may be helpful in relieving symptoms. EMG-guided scalene muscle block may be highly useful in demonstrating the presence of adherent residual scalene muscle as the inciting problem in such patients.[35]

References

1. Machleder HI, Moll F, Verity MA. The anterior scalene muscle in thoracic outlet compression syndrome: histochemical and morphometric studies. *Arch Surg* 1986;121:1141–1144.
2. Sanders RJ, Jackson CG, Banchero N, et al. Scalene muscle abnormalities in traumatic thoracic outlet syndrome. *Am J Surg* 1990;159:231–236.
3. Juvonen T, Satta J, Laitala P, et al. Anomalies at the thoracic outlet are frequent in the general population. *Am J Surg* 1995;170:33–37.
4. Raskin NH, Howard MW, Ehrenfeld WK. Headache as the leading symptom of the thoracic outlet syndrome. *Headache* 1985;25;208–210.
5. Wood VE, Biondi J. Double-crush nerve compression in thoracic-outlet syndrome. *J Bone Joint Surg Am* 1990;72:85–87.
6. Wulff CH, Gilliatt RW. F waves in patients with hand wasting caused by a single rib and band. *Muscle Nerve* 1979;2:452–457.
7. Sanders RJ, Hammond SL, Rao NM. Diagnosis of thoracic outlet syndrome. *J Vasc Surg* 2007;46:601–604.
8. Mustafa BO, Rathbun SW, Whitsett TL. Sensitivity and specificity of ultrasonography in the diagnosis of upper extremity deep vein thrombosis: a systemic review. *Arch Intern Med* 2002;162:401–404.
9. Demondion X, Boutry N, Drizenko A, et al. Thoracic outlet: anatomic correlation with MR imaging. *AJR Am J Roentgenol* 2000;175:417–422.
10. Hagspiel KD, Spinosa DJ, Angle JF, et al. Diagnosis of vascular compression at the thoracic outlet using gadolinium-enhanced high-resolution ultrafast MR angiography in abduction and adduction. *Cardiovasc Intervent Radiol* 2000;23:152–154.
11. Wilbourn AJ. The thoracic outlet syndrome is overdiagnosed. *Arch Neurol* 1990;47:328–330.
12. Komanetsky RM, Novak CB, Mackinnon SE, et al. Somatosensory evoked potentials fail to diagnose thoracic outlet syndrome. *J Hand Surg (AM)* 1996;21:662–666.
13. Tender GC, Thomas J, Thomas N, et al. Gilliatt–Sumner hand revisited: a 25-year experience. *Neurosurgery* 2004;55:883–890.
14. Machanic DI, Sanders RJ. Medial antebrachial cutaneous nerve measurements to diagnose neurogenic thoracic outlet syndrome. *Ann Vasc Surg* 2008;22:248–254.
15. Jordan SE, Machleder HI. Diagnosis of thoracic outlet syndrome using electrophysiologically guided anterior scalene blocks. *Ann Vasc Surg* 1998;12:260–264.
16. Jordan SE, Ahn SS, Freischlag JA, et al. Selective botulinum chemodenervation of the scalene muscles for treatment of neurogenic thoracic outlet syndrome. *Ann Vasc Surg* 2000;14:365–369.
17. Jordan SE, Ahn SS, Gelabart H. Combining ultrasonography and electromyography for botulinum denervation treatment of thoracic outlet syndrome: comparison with fluoroscopy and electromyography guidance. *Pain Physician* 2007;10:541–546.
18. Hingorani A, Ascher E, Lorenson E, et al. Upper extremity deep venous thrombosis and its impact on morbidity and mortality rates in a hospital-based population. *J Vasc Surg* 1997;26:853–860.
19. Sharafuddin MJ, Sun S, Hoballah JJ. Endovascular management of venous thrombotic diseases of the upper torso and extremities. *J Vasc Interv Radiol* 2002;13:975–990.
20. Bjarnason H, Hunter DW, Crain MR, et al. Collapse of a Palmaz stent in the subclavian vein. *AJR Am J Roentgenol* 1993;160:1123–1124.
21. Lee MC, Grassi CJ, Belkin M, et al. Early operative intervention after thrombolytic therapy for primary subclavian vein thrombosis: an effective treatment approach. *J Vasc Surg* 1998;27:1101–1108.
22. Sanders RJ, Cooper MA. Surgical management of subclavian vein obstruction, including six cases of subclavian vein bypass. *Surgery* 1995;118:856–863.
23. Lee WA, Hill BB, Harris JJ, et al. Surgical intervention is not required for all patients with subclavian vein thrombosis. *J Vasc Surg* 2000;32:57–67.

24. Lokanathan R, Salvian AJ, Chen JC, et al. Outcome after thrombolysis and selective thoracic outlet decompression as primary axillary vein thrombosis. *J Vasc Surg* 2001;33:783–788.
25. Sanders RJ, Monsour JU, Baer SB. Transaxillary first rib resection for the thoracic outlet syndrome. *Arch Surg* 1968;97:1014–1023.
26. Roos DB. Transaxillary approach for first rib resection to relieve thoracic outlet syndrome. *Ann Surg* 1996;163:354–358.
27. Sanders RJ, Raymer S. The supraclavicular approach to scalenectomy and first rib resection: Description of technique. *J Vasc Surg* 1985;2:751–756.
28. Tender GC, Kline DE: Posterior subscapular approach to the brachial plexus. *Neurosurgery* 2005;57(4 suppl):377–381.
29. Roos DB. Congenital anomalies associated with thoracic outlet syndrome. *Am J Surg* 1976;132:777–778.
30. Sanders RJ, Pearce WH. The treatment of thoracic outlet syndrome: a comparison of different operations. *J Vasc Surg* 1989;10:626–634.
31. Cheng SW, Reilly LM, Nelken NA, et al. Neurogenic thoracic outlet decompression: rationale for sparing the first rib. *Cardiovasc Surg* 1995;3:617–623.
32. Sanders RJ, Rao NM. Pectoralis minor obstruction of the axillary veins: report of six patients. *J Vasc Surg* 2007;45:1206–1211.
33. Johansen KH. Does spontaneous axillosubclavian vein ("effort") thrombosis oblige first rib resection? *Arch Surg* 2009. In press.
34. Franklin GM, Fulton-Kehoe D, Bradley C, et al. Outcome of surgery for thoracic outlet syndrome in Washington state workers' compensation. *Neurology* 2000;54:1252–1257.
35. Ambrad-Chelala E, Thomas GI, Johansen KH. Recurrent neurogenic thoracic outlet syndrome. *Am J Surg* 2004;187:505–510.

CHAPTER 40 ■ PAIN FOLLOWING SPINAL CORD INJURY

PHILIP J. SIDDALL AND PAUL J. WRIGLEY

INTRODUCTION

Pain presents a major challenge to those with spinal cord injury (SCI) and to those involved in their healthcare. Pain following SCI arises from a complex array of mechanisms. In addition, pain has a broad impact on physical, emotional, cognitive, and social functioning that needs to be evaluated and addressed in any management plan. Long-term sequelae involving other nonspinal musculoskeletal and visceral structures often coexist.

This chapter will provide an overview of the different types of pain presenting in people with SCI. It will examine the extent of SCI-associated pain in the community and the potential impact on the individual. The mechanisms underlying specific pains, assessment, and current treatment will also be explored.

EXTENT OF THE PROBLEM

Figures for the prevalence of pain in people with spinal cord injury vary depending on the method of survey and the way that pain is evaluated. Postal and community surveys have generally reported a prevalence of around 75% to 85%.[1-3] The figure for prospective, longitudinal studies is slightly lower. However, even these studies consistently demonstrate that around 65% of people with SCI pain have ongoing pain.[4,5] Furthermore, approximately one third of these people with pain report that the intensity of pain is severe or excruciating, indicating the importance of pain in these individuals.

The above studies address the general prevalence of pain following SCI. A few have investigated the prevalence of specific types of pain. There are several types of pain that can occur following SCI including musculoskeletal pain, visceral pain, and two distinct types of neuropathic pain that occur at and below the level of SCI. When these specific types of pain are identified, the most commonly occurring is musculoskeletal pain (58% of people at 5 years following injury) then at-level neuropathic pain (42%) and below-level neuropathic pain (34%).[5]

IMPACT OF PAIN

Loss of mobility is often considered the most serious consequence of SCI. It is interesting to note, however, that people with SCI consistently rate pain as one of the most difficult problems to manage, despite the presence of other problems that interfere with daily life.[1] Although it is sometimes difficult to attribute causality, there are a number of studies that clearly demonstrate the strong relationship between pain and poorer physical, psychological, and social functioning.[3,4,6,7] Pain may directly affect sleep and participation in activities of daily living, as well as contributing to functional disability beyond that attributable to the loss of mobility.[8-10] Pain also directly contributes to disability by limiting participation in rehabilitation and return to work.[2,10-12] Not surprisingly, these effects on functioning flow through to more global indicators of health such as reduced quality of life[13-15] and life satisfaction.[16]

The long-term prognosis for pain resolution following SCI is often poor. Many people with SCI report that despite trying a wide range of strategies, including different types of pain medications, complementary therapies, and physical therapy, their pain persists.[17] Pain may continue or worsen following injury.[3] It has also been observed that those reporting neuropathic pain 3–6 months following injury are likely to continue experiencing pain at 3–5 years.[5]

PREDISPOSING FACTORS FOR PAIN

Biological Factors

As described above, pain is a relatively common problem for people following SCI. Despite this, a clear understanding of the predisposing biological factors likely to result in pain has not been achieved. Contradictory evidence exists regarding the relationship between pain and the severity of injury (including completeness), the level of the injury, and the specific spinal cord tracts injured.[2,6,7,18-20]

Whether a complete or an incomplete injury occurs, the bulk

of clinical evidence strongly suggests that damage to the spinothalamic tracts is an important ingredient in the development of neuropathic pain following SCI. Several studies suggest that damage to spinothalamic tracts is a necessary, although not sufficient, condition for the development of neuropathic SCI pain.[21–23]

Psychological Factors

Studies have also investigated the relationship between pain and psychological factors. Indeed, some have suggested that psychosocial rather than biological factors are more closely associated with the presence and severity of pain.[4,6] These psychosocial factors include changes in mood and cognitions and social or environmental factors. Mood dysfunction is often correlated with the presence of SCI pain. Although it is often difficult to attribute causality in cross sectional studies, the presence of chronic SCI pain is consistently associated with significantly higher levels of perceived stress and depressive symptoms.[1,15,24,25]

Cognitive factors, such as catastrophic thinking about pain, self-efficacy beliefs, and acceptance, have also been demonstrated to influence pain and disability. Catastrophizing has consistently been found to be predictive of pain intensity and disability among people with SCI-related chronic pain.[25–27] Self-efficacy has also been demonstrated to be a powerful predictor of ability to perform physical tasks in people with SCI and pain.[28] One conceptualization of acceptance, re-evaluation of life values following injury, has been examined in a number of studies in SCI.[29,30] When specifically applied to those with chronic SCI-related pain, significantly lower levels of acceptance of injury as well as higher levels of helplessness were reported.[25]

Social and Environmental Factors

Comparatively little research has been done examining the contribution of social and environmental factors to the experience of pain following SCI. It has been demonstrated that social support has a positive effect on people after SCI.[27,31] However, perceived negative responses from friends, carers, and relatives may have a negative effect. Studies examining the influence of perceived responses to pain of significant others suggests that the perception of punishing responses was particularly important in the report of pain severity,[7,32] whereas negative or distracting responses were associated with increased pain-related disability.[33]

CLASSIFICATION OF PAIN FOLLOWING SPINAL CORD INJURY

Before moving on to assessment and treatment, it is important to consider the classification of SCI pain. A large number of SCI pain classification systems can be found in the SCI literature[34–37] causing confusion among researchers and clinicians. International pain and SCI associations are currently working to achieve consensus in this area. Some years ago, the Spinal Cord Injury Pain Task Force of the International Association of the Study of Pain (IASP) proposed a taxonomy of pain that attempts to provide a structure for systematically identifying the different types of SCI pain (Table 40.1).[38] This taxonomy is widely used and will therefore be employed in this chapter.

The IASP taxonomy proposes a tiered system in which pain types are firstly classified as nociceptive (musculoskeletal or visceral) or neuropathic (above-level, at-level, or below-level). The second tier classification (musculoskeletal, visceral, above-level neuropathic, at-level neuropathic, and below-level neuropathic) outlines the common types of pain encountered following SCI and is the most relevant for clinical purposes. The third tier attempts to identify the underlying pathology. Where the term "neurological level of injury" is used, this refers to the most caudal segment of the spinal cord with normal sensory and motor function bilaterally.[39]

Musculoskeletal Pain

In the acute setting following injury, nociceptive pain arises from damage to musculoskeletal structures including bones, ligaments, muscles, intervertebral discs, and facet joints. The pain is generally located in the region of preserved sensation close to the site of spinal injury although it may radiate in a somatic referred pattern. People with incomplete injuries also experience musculoskeletal pain below the neurological level. Chronic musculoskeletal pain may occur with overuse or abnormal use of structures, such as the arm and shoulder.[40,41] For mobility reasons, this type of nociceptive pain is very common in people with paraplegia and much less common in tetraplegia.[42] Pain associated with muscle spasm is another type of musculoskeletal pain commonly reported by people with incomplete injuries.

TABLE 40.1

PROPOSED CLASSIFICATION OF PAIN RELATED TO SPINAL CORD INJURY[38]

Broad type (Tier 1)	Broad system (Tier 2)	Specific structures/pathology (Tier 3)
Nociceptive	Musculoskeletal	Bone, joint, muscle trauma or inflammation Mechanical instability Muscle spasm Secondary overuse syndromes
	Visceral	Renal calculus, bowel, sphincter dysfunction, etc. Dysreflexic headache
Neuropathic	Above level	Compressive mononeuropathies Complex regional pain syndromes
	At level	Nerve root compression (including cauda equina) Syringomyelia Spinal cord trauma/ischemia Dual level cord and root trauma
	Below level	Spinal cord trauma/ischemia

Visceral Pain

Pathological processes occurring in visceral structures, such as urinary tract infection, bowel impaction, and renal calculi, also cause nociceptive pain. The level of SCI will influence the likelihood of developing these problems and the characteristics and presentation of the pain. People with thoracic injuries may experience visceral pain that is identical to those who have no spinal cord damage. However, people with cervical injuries may experience less well defined, generalized unpleasant symptoms that are difficult to localize and interpret. Despite this, pain may provide a warning for impending medical conditions, and responses to the pain by healthcare personnel can help avoid severe complications such as autonomic dysreflexia.

Above-level Neuropathic Pain

Neuropathic pain can occur above the neurological level of injury and includes pains that are not specific to SCI such as complex regional pain syndrome (previously referred to as reflex sympathetic dystrophy, causalgia, or shoulder-hand syndrome) and pain due to peripheral nerve injury (Fig. 40.1A). Although these types of pain are present in the general population, people with SCI may be more susceptible because of activities associated with wheelchair use and transfers.

At-level Neuropathic Pain

At-level neuropathic pain is defined as pain with typical neuropathic features (burning, aching, stabbing, or electric shocks) in a band within 3 dermatomes below the neurological level of injury (Fig. 40.1B). This type of pain has also been referred to as segmental, transitional zone, border zone, end zone, and girdle zone. At-level neuropathic pain is often associated with allodynia (pain from a normally non-painful stimulus) or hyperalgesia (an exaggerated pain response) in the affected dermatomes.

At-level neuropathic pain may arise from damage to spinal nerve roots (including the cauda equina) or the spinal cord itself. At times, the character of the pain may help in identifying the underlying cause. For example, unilateral pain exacerbated by spinal movement is more typical of nerve root damage than direct spinal

cord injury. The origin of the pain may be difficult to distinguish on the basis of descriptors alone. However, when possible, this allows a more specific treatment pathway to be pursued.

Direct damage to the nerve roots may occur during the initial injury or at a later date secondary to spinal column instability, degeneration or disease (e.g., facet or disc impingement). Syringomyelia (cyst formation within the spinal cord) must always be considered in the person who has delayed onset of at-level neuropathic pain especially where there is a rising level of sensory loss. Loss of pain and temperature sensation is typical, but all sensory and motor functions can be affected during syrinx formation. People typically describe a constant, burning pain that may be associated with hypersensitivity (allodynia or hyperalgesia).

Below-level Neuropathic Pain

Below-level neuropathic pain is defined as pain with typical neurological features distributed diffusely below the neurological level of SCI (Fig. 40.1C). In contrast to at-level pain, below-level pain typically begins at least 4 dermatomes levels below (caudal to) the neurological level of injury; however, the region immediately below the neurological level of injury may also be involved. This type of pain may develop many months and even years following injury, and is the most likely type of SCI pain to be described as severe or excruciating.[5] It is also referred to as central dysesthesia syndrome, central pain, SCI phantom pain, or deafferentation pain. At-level and below-level neuropathic pain may both be present and at times are difficult to separate.

Below-level neuropathic SCI pain is typically constant, varying with mood or attention and is usually unrelated to position or movement. Pain may be triggered by sudden noises or physical jarring and exacerbated by other pathology such as urinary tract infections or disturbance of bowel function. Differences in the nature of below-level neuropathic pain may be apparent between those with complete and incomplete spinal cord lesions. Incomplete injuries are more likely to have an allodynic component due to sparing of tracts conveying touch sensations.

Psychological Aspects of Pain

Some classification systems have included psychological or psychogenic as types of pain that occur following SCI. However,

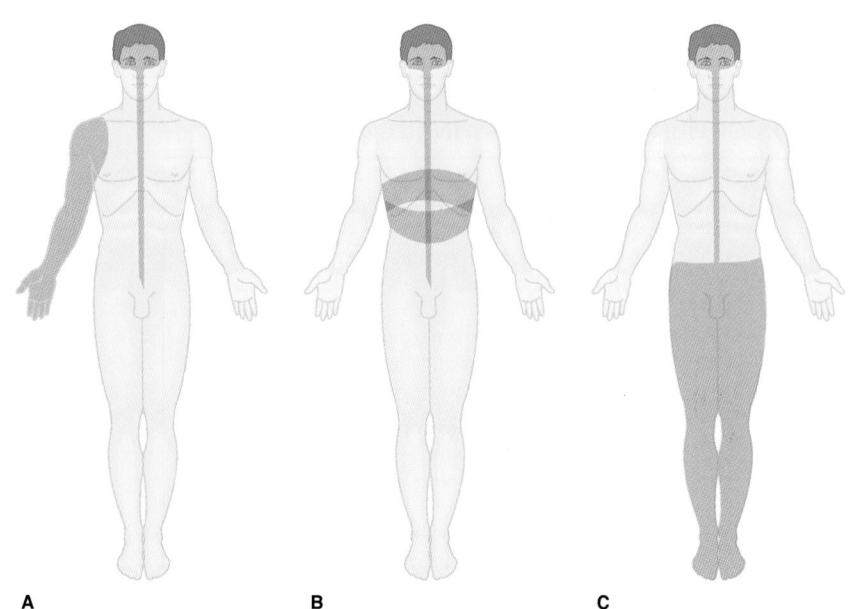

FIGURE 40.1 Typical patterns of (**A**) above-level and (**B**) at-level and (**C**) below-level neuropathic pain following a mid thoracic spinal cord injury.

A   B   C

applying a psychological label to the pain may be unhelpful. Pure psychogenic pain is extremely rare. On the other hand, it is well known that psychological factors such as mood and cognitions have a major influence on the pain experience.[6,43,44] Determining the contribution of psychological factors is an important aspect of management and will be discussed in more detail in the section on assessment.

MECHANISMS UNDERLYING PAIN IN PEOPLE WITH SPINAL CORD INJURY

Musculoskeletal Pain

Acute nociceptive pain arises from damage to structures such as bones, ligaments, muscles, intervertebral discs, and facet joints. Peripheral nociceptive mechanisms are responsible for the pain due to inflammatory mediator release, with both peripheral and central sensitization. Chronic musculoskeletal pain may occur with overuse or "abnormal" use of structures, such as the arm and shoulder and muscle spasm arising from a heightened reflex arc below the level of injury.

Visceral Pain

Pathological processes occurring in visceral structures, such as infection, impaction, and calculi formation, will generally give rise to nociceptive pain, though the quality of pain will be affected by the level of injury. As with musculoskeletal pain, visceral pain arises from afferent nociceptor activation and generally involves inflammatory processes.

Neuropathic Pain

Neuropathic pain following SCI has several clinical presentations that may reflect different underlying mechanisms. The specific mechanisms underlying at-level and below-level neuropathic pain remain unclear and therefore will be grouped together. Neuropathic pain may be due to changes occurring in the periphery, spinal cord, and brain.

Periphery

The degree to which peripheral changes influence neuropathic SCI pain remains uncertain, particularly in those with clinically complete injuries. Impingement of nerve roots may result in primary afferent functional and structural changes in a similar manner to peripheral nerve injury. People with clinically complete injuries may have residual sensory transmission through the cord that is not detectable using standard physical examination techniques (a "sensory discomplete" lesion). In this subgroup of clinically complete lesions, pain may be influenced by transmission of nociceptive impulses arising in the periphery via these residual pathways. This certainly seems to be the case in people with clinically complete injuries who report pain in the region of absent sensation that is strongly related to joint position or other nociceptive generators.

Spinal Cord

Some of the earliest investigations into SCI pain noted that blockade of the spinal cord using spinal administration of a local anesthetic immediately above the level of injury resulted in relief of pain in some people.[45] From these observations, it was proposed that neuropathic SCI pain may be due to the presence of an "irritated focus" or "neural pain generator" which was close to the rostral end of the SCI. This was supported by the finding that dorsal horn neurons immediately above the level of SCI demonstrated abnormal spontaneous neuronal activity.[46]

More recently, animal and human studies have confirmed that there are changes in the properties of nerve cells close to the site of SCI.[47] These changes include increased responsiveness to peripheral stimulation, an increase in the level of background activity and prolonged firing following a stimulus.[48–50] Further studies have demonstrated a number of changes in neurotransmitters and receptors which may lead to an increase in excitation or a reduction in inhibition and may result in the change in firing properties of these spinal neurons. These include changes in N-methyl-D-aspartate (NMDA), non-NMDA, and metabotropic glutamate receptors, sodium channels, and GABAergic, opioid, serotonergic, and noradrenergic function. In addition, SCI results in glial activation and increased cytokine and prostaglandin release as well as structural reorganization of inputs in the dorsal horn of the spinal cord.[23,51,52]

Brain

Despite the evidence supporting the concept of an "irritated focus" in the spinal cord close to the site of damage, neuropathic pain may continue despite removal of a section of the spinal cord above the level of injury.[53] This raises the question as to whether changes in the brain may also contribute to the development of pain. A number of studies in animals and humans have demonstrated brain changes associated with the presence of neuropathic pain. The precise link between these changes and the development of pain remains a matter of debate.[54] The brain changes described include alterations in thalamic neuronal firing,[55–58] expression of sodium channels,[59] biochemical changes,[60] and changes in thalamic perfusion or activity.[61,62]

Multilevel Effect

Before concluding this section on mechanisms, it is important to note that neuropathic SCI pain may be due to a combination of changes at a number of nervous system levels. For example, it has been observed that a higher proportion of patients with below-level neuropathic SCI pain have at-level sensory hypersensitivity than pain-free SCI patients.[63] When this specific group of patients were examined using magnetic resonance imaging (MRI), larger grey matter lesions were noted at the rostral end of the lesion compared to pain-free SCI patients.[64] In these patients, below-level neuropathic pain may be due to a combination of supraspinal neuroplastic changes in response to a spinothalamic lesion together with neuronal hyperexcitability at the rostral end of the injury.[23]

PATIENT ASSESSMENT

The perception and expression of pain is influenced by many factors including past experience, culture, environmental influences, and genetic makeup.[65,66] A thorough pain assessment therefore involves consideration of contributing biological, psychological, and environmental factors. An understanding of the patient's biopsychosocial system allows the clinician to develop a rational assessment of the causal links involved in the pain problem. This facilitates the development of a prioritized problem list and goal-oriented management plan. Such an approach leads to better long-term outcomes compared to unimodal treatment approaches.[67]

As is common to most clinical practice, a pain assessment first involves a careful history, followed by a focused physical examination and appropriate investigations or diagnostic procedures. The categories biological (nociceptive and neuropathic), psychological, and social can be used to summarize findings in a diagnostic framework and management template.[67]

Biological Contributors

Nociceptive. Musculoskeletal pain is suggested by descriptors such as dull and aching pain that is made worse by activity or position. If musculoskeletal pain is present, physical examination (e.g., site of tenderness, limitation of movement, muscle tone) will help to determine the structures that may be affected and the presence of inflammation or muscle spasm. In the acute phase, if skeletal damage is suspected, investigations such as radiographs, computerized tomography (CT) scan, and MRI may help to identify pathology such as a fracture, dislocation, spinal misalignment, or instability. In the chronic phase, pain and restriction in range of movement of the upper limb may suggest an overuse syndrome. The pain is described as aching and is worse with use of involved joints or pressure on the part.

Visceral pain may arise from structures in the thorax, abdomen, and pelvis. It is generally poorly localized and often described as dull, aching, and cramping. The presence of visceral pain requires a standard diagnostic approach similar to that used in the person without SCI. However, in the person with SCI, particular attention should be paid to common conditions such as urinary tract infection, obstruction from ureteric calculi, and bowel impaction. Other relatively common conditions include cholelithiasis and esophagitis.

Physical examination and appropriate investigations will help to identify the pathology that may be giving rise to the pain. However, diagnosis is often difficult when sensory inputs from visceral structures are disturbed. If investigations fail to find evidence of visceral pathology, and treatments directed at visceral pathology do not relieve the pain, consideration must be given to classifying the pain as neuropathic rather than visceral. The onset of headache and raised blood pressure in a person with an upper thoracic or cervical SCI should alert the clinician to the possibility of a visceral disturbance such as bladder distension or bowel impaction producing autonomic dysreflexia.

Neuropathic. Above-level neuropathic pain is located in the region above the neurological level of injury. Assessment depends on the description of the pain, the use of physical examination to detect the nature of any sensory disturbance, the presence of other features such as autonomic dysfunction, and the use of diagnostic techniques such as nerve conduction studies, CT scan, and MRI.

At- and below-level neuropathic pains are differentiated by their location in relation to the level of neurological injury. The value of differentiating these two types of pain lies in highlighting potentially different underlying mechanisms and, therefore, treatment approaches. As previously mentioned, at-level neuropathic pain is located adjacent to the neurological level of injury and below-level neuropathic pain is located diffusely below the neurological level of injury (see Fig. 40.1). Both types of pain are usually reported using typical neuropathic pain descriptors such as shooting, electric, and burning with tingling and allodynia. Although not definitive, nerve root pain may be suggested by a unilateral distribution.

Diagnosis is assisted by radiographic, CT, or MRI evidence of nerve root compression in the foramen by bone or disc that correlates with the location of the pain. If investigations fail to find evidence of a peripheral nerve lesion, the pain is most likely due to central changes. If there has been a recent change in the location or characteristics of the pain, MRI may be useful to determine the formation or progression of a syrinx.

Psychological and Environmental Contributors

Psychological contributors may include mood dysfunction such as depression and anxiety and maladaptive coping strategies such as fear avoidance and catastrophizing. Environmental contributors may be social or physical. Social reinforcers may arise in relationships with family, friends, or at work. Compensation issues, either financial or social (e.g., receiving an apology), may also influence pain and recovery. Physical contributors such as

wheelchair use, seating, and workplace ergonomics are also important to consider.

Obtaining a psychosocial history entails careful observation and listening, obtaining input from family, friends, and other team members. It may also require assistance from other professionals with formal training in psychological or psychiatric medicine. Psychological questionnaires may also be used to obtain baseline measures and monitor progress.

MANAGEMENT OF PAIN IN PEOPLE WITH SCI

Musculoskeletal Pain

Trauma to musculoskeletal structures may result in both pain and instability. Stabilization is the most effective treatment for pain arising from spinal instability. In this situation, pain usually resolves as healing occurs but symptomatic relief of pain may be required during the tissue healing phase.

Chronic inflammatory musculoskeletal pain may result from abnormal posture, abnormal gait, and overuse related to transfers and wheelchair use. These factors may be addressed via education, retraining, and environmental modifications, such as adaptive equipment and modification of seating. These approaches may be sufficient to eliminate the problem. In the short term, or if it is not possible to completely address the causative factors, symptomatic treatment may also be required.

In addition to correcting abnormal mechanical stresses, managing active disease processes, and modifying unhelpful psychosocial contributing factors, symptomatic pharmacological treatment of inflammatory musculoskeletal pain may be indicated. Similar principles can be used as those employed in the treatment of other degenerative and inflammatory joint conditions. Pharmacological management includes the use of simple analgesics, non-steroidal anti-inflammatory drugs (NSAIDs), local corticosteroid injections, and occasionally opioids.

Several considerations regarding the use of analgesics and NSAIDs apply in the person with SCI. NSAIDs may cause gastric erosion which is more prevalent and harder to detect in those with high spinal cord lesions. Therefore, acetaminophen is the safest first step in the treatment of musculoskeletal pain associated with SCI. If there is no response to acetaminophen, the use of "weak" opioids, such as tramadol, may be considered. While the use of "strong" opioids for acute inflammatory pain is reasonable, continued use in persistent pain remains controversial.[68] Case-by-case consideration for long term opioid therapy is reasonable, along the lines of published guidelines.[69] Opioid analgesics are known to exacerbate bowel dysfunction, and long-term use can be complicated by tolerance and dependence (both physical and psychological).

Spasticity is a common problem following SCI and has different features from muscle spasms that may occur in people who are neurologically intact. SCI results in major disruption to descending inhibitory controls with a resultant hyperreflexia and spasticity affecting muscle groups below the neurological level of injury. In addition to impairing motor function, spasticity associated with SCI may also cause pain. Spasm may be due to underlying pathology maintaining a heightened reflex arc. If so, this needs to be treated appropriately. More commonly in people with SCI, there is no underlying pathology that can be addressed and treatment once again focuses on symptomatic relief. At present, there is insufficient evidence to guide clinicians in a rational approach to the treatment of spasticity following SCI.[70] A number of approaches are traditionally used. Oral baclofen may be sufficient to control the symptoms and is the first line approach. Diazepam is an alternative approach although consideration must be given to the side effects associated with benzodiazepine use. Injection of botulinum toxin has also been suggested as an effective treatment for localized spasticity.[71] If oral agents fail to provide sufficient relief, evidence supports consideration of intrathecal baclofen administration via an infusion device.[72,73]

Visceral Pain

Identification of symptomatic urinary tract infection requires treatment with antibiotics. Obstruction from ureteric calculi may require surgical removal or lithotripsy. Bowel impaction may require disimpaction in the short term and adjustment of bowel routine in the long term. The presence of autonomic dysreflexia may constitute a medical emergency and requires immediate blood pressure reduction and treatment of the underlying trigger.

Above-level Neuropathic Pain

If there is evidence of nerve root or peripheral nerve compression, surgical decompression may be indicated. Syringomyelia may require drainage and shunting or a detethering procedure. Complex regional pain syndromes can present a difficult management problem and a more comprehensive overview of treatment is described elsewhere in this volume. Sympathetic blockade may provide complete relief of pain in some individuals but effectiveness is unpredictable.[74] Physical rehabilitation may also be helpful in some people.

At-level and Below-level Neuropathic Pain

Management of a syrinx and surgical decompression of a compromised nerve root are the two available treatments aimed at the cause of at- and below-level neuropathic pain. Most available treatments, therefore, are symptomatic in nature and aim to reduce the impact of ongoing pain. Unfortunately, there are few controlled trials examining the efficacy of treatments for at-level and below-level neuropathic pain. Available studies often have small numbers and therefore conclusions may not be reliable. Treatment is often based on findings derived from other neuropathic pain conditions. A summary of the current treatments for at- and below-level neuropathic pain is listed below according to treatment category.

Pharmacological Options

A wide range of treatment options, including anticonvulsants, tricyclic antidepressants, opioid medications and more invasive procedures, such as intrathecal drug administration, are used for the treatment of neuropathic pain following SCI.[75,76] Adequate pain control is often difficult to achieve with available treatments only providing around one third of people with a 50% reduction in their pain.[76]

Opioids. During inpatient assessment of a person with SCI, parenteral drugs may be useful in the management of pain while investigations and longer term treatments are explored. Two randomized controlled trials involving intravenous morphine[77] and alfentanil[78] have been conducted. These studies demonstrated a short-term reduction in neuropathic pain following SCI. Intravenous morphine failed to relieve spontaneous pain but reduced brush-evoked allodynia.[77] Although effective in the short term, parenteral opioid treatment is not suitable for the long term management of neuropathic SCI pain. If used, slow release opioids are preferred. Evidence for the short-term (less than 2 months) efficacy of a number of opioids has been demonstrated in other neuropathic pain states.[79] However, the evidence for use of specific oral opioids in the treatment of neuropathic SCI pain is very limited. Tolerance, dependence, and side effects such as constipation also need to be considered.

Anticonvulsant Drugs. Anticonvulsant drugs are widely used in the treatment of neuropathic pain conditions and have a broad range of actions including sodium channel blockade, enhancement of GABAergic inhibition, reduction of glutamate release, and an action on the $\alpha_2\delta$ subunit of dorsal horn voltage-gated calcium channels. This broad mix of effects may explain the different responses obtained by using members of this group. Gabapentin is widely used in the treatment of neuropathic SCI pain and anecdotally there is good support for its effectiveness in some patients. There are, however, only two small short-term controlled studies that confirm this.[80,81] In a subgroup of patients, the effectiveness of gabapentin does appear to be sustained in the longer term.[82]

Pregabalin is a newer anticonvulsant that, like gabapentin, acts via the $\alpha_2\delta$ subunit of dorsal horn voltage-gated calcium channels. A recent multicenter study of 137 people with complete and incomplete injuries examined the efficacy of pregabalin in the treatment of neuropathic pain following SCI.[83] This study demonstrated a significant positive treatment effect when compared to placebo with a mean dose after stabilization of 460 mg/day and a number needed to treat for 50% relief of 7.1. A smaller study of 33 subjects also including people with neuropathic central poststroke pain found a significant positive analgesic response to pregabalin with a lower number needed to treat of 4.0. There was no difference in relief between the brain and spinal cord injuries groups.[84]

Lamotrigine has been used and trialed for the treatment of neuropathic SCI pain as well as other neuropathic pain conditions. It has a membrane stabilizing action via inhibition of voltage-dependent sodium channels in addition to inhibiting glutamate release. In a group of subjects with neuropathic SCI pain, lamotrigine 200–400 mg daily had no statistically significant pain relieving effect. However, a subgroup of patients with incomplete injury and evoked pain demonstrated relief of spontaneous pain.[85]

Topiramate is another anticonvulsant that acts on sodium and calcium channels, potentiates GABAergic inhibition, and inhibits glutamate receptors. One randomized controlled trial has been performed in people with neuropathic SCI pain but numbers were small.[86] The efficacy of topiramate 800 mg daily in four different neuropathic pain diagnoses was examined with 9 patients receiving topiramate and 4 receiving placebo. Topiramate was significantly better than placebo in the final 2 weeks of treatment, but only on one of the two primary outcome measures (present pain index) and not on the other primary outcome measure (pain visual analog scale).

Valproate has been used for some time in the treatment of neuropathic SCI pain. However, the only published controlled trial using this drug at doses of 600–2400 mg/day failed to demonstrate any significant difference from placebo.[87] Once again, the numbers in the study were relatively small raising the possibility of a false negative result.

Carbamazepine has also been used for many years for the treatment of neuropathic SCI pain but evidence to support its use is very limited.[88] More recently, oxcarbazepine has become available and may present another alternative. However, neither of these drugs have been the subject of controlled trials for neuropathic SCI pain.

Antidepressants. Like anticonvulsants, antidepressants are widely used in the management of neuropathic pain conditions. Traditionally, the analgesic mechanism of action for tricyclic antidepressants has been thought to be due to norepinephrine and serotonin reuptake inhibition. It may be possible, however, that other actions including NMDA-receptor antagonism and sodium channel blockade also contribute.

Despite their widespread use, there is little direct evidence for the effectiveness of tricyclic antidepressants in the treatment of neuropathic SCI pain. At present, only one well designed study has been performed. This study examined a group of people with combined musculoskeletal and neuropathic SCI pain.[89] Amitriptyline at a dose of 10–125 mg/day was found to be no better than placebo. Further studies examining neuropathic SCI pain are needed to allow definitive conclusions to be made. Despite the lack of positive evidence, a trial of tricyclic antidepressants appears to be reasonable in clinical practice given supportive evidence from other neuropathic pain conditions. Tricyclic antidepressants may have a number of side effects including sedation, constipation, dry mouth, increased spasticity, and disturbance of bladder function.[89]

Selective serotonin reuptake inhibitors have now been available for some time. Although they are effective antidepressants and have a more favorable side effect profile, there remains little evidence to demonstrate superiority over tricyclic antidepressants for the treatment of neuropathic pain. The serotonin reuptake inhibitor and 5HT receptor antagonist, trazodone, has been shown in one randomized controlled trial to be no better than placebo.[90] There is increasing evidence to support the use of mixed serotonin and noradrenaline reuptake inhibitors, such as venlafaxine and duloxetine, in other neuropathic pain states. However, as yet, there is no evidence to support these agents specifically in the treatment of neuropathic SCI pain.

Drug Combinations. There are reports that combinations of anticonvulsants and tricyclic antidepressants are more effective than either administered alone.[88,91] Therefore, if a single agent is ineffective, a combination of an anticonvulsant with either a tricyclic antidepressant or an opioid may produce additional relief. However, some combinations, such as the use of tramadol and a tricyclic antidepressant, may present problems because of their combined effect on serotonin. In practice, many patients will require judicious use of a combination of agents to obtain optimum relief of pain.

Local Anesthetics. Parenteral administration of the sodium channel blocker lidocaine has been shown to reduce neuropathic SCI pain in higher doses (5 mg/kg).[92–95] Reductions in spontaneous ongoing pain, brush-evoked allodynia, and static mechanical hyperalgesia have been described. Although there is one report of long-term effectiveness with the use of lidocaine,[96] parenteral administration is generally not practical as an ongoing treatment. This interferes with its translation to long-term treatment. Mexiletine, an oral congener of lidocaine with a similar action, was not shown to be effective at a dose of 450 mg/day although, once again, the number of subjects was small (n = 11).[97]

NMDA Antagonists. Parenteral administration of the NMDA-receptor antagonist ketamine was demonstrated to be more effective than placebo and similar to fentanyl in reducing below-level neuropathic SCI pain.[78] As with lidocaine, long-term administration remains problematic and there are no effective oral alternatives available.

Propofol. The anesthetic agent and GABA_A-receptor agonist propofol is another parenteral agent that has been used for the treatment of neuropathic SCI pain. A subhypnotic dose of propofol, injected as a single intravenous bolus (0.2 mg/kg) provided less than one hour relief of spontaneous pain and allodynia in approximately half of 44 patients with SCI and poststroke pain.[98] Whether this effect would be sustained in an ongoing infusion is yet to be determined. The use of propofol would require special monitoring and a higher level of care.

Spinal Drug Administration. If oral administration fails to provide adequate analgesia, spinal administration may be considered. Evidence of efficacy is confined to case series and limited controlled trials. The approach is inherently invasive and should not be considered until more conservative measures have been thoroughly trialed. In a case series, spinal administration of morphine and clonidine[99] was found to be effective in some individuals. Combinations of morphine or clonidine with baclofen in those with spasm may provide additional benefit.[100]

In a controlled study, combined intrathecal administration of morphine and clonidine was found to be effective in a group of people with chronic at-level and below-level neuropathic SCI pain.[101] A positive response was associated with adequate drug availability above the level of SCI. People with significant scarring around the cord and cerebrospinal fluid block at the site of injury responded poorly to agents administered below the level of SCI. This study revealed a short-term reduction in pain and the long-term effectiveness of this treatment strategy remains to be established.

As mentioned previously, intrathecal baclofen is effective in managing spasticity and spasm-related pain secondary to SCI. However, the effect of baclofen on neuropathic SCI pain is less clear. Conflicting results have so far been obtained in controlled trials.[73,102]

Spinal anesthesia with subarachnoid lidocaine may also provide analgesia in SCI neuropathic pain.[103] The effect of spinal anesthesia is of course only temporary, limiting its clinical usefulness. Response to regional blockade suggests pain "generators" lie within the spinal cord or peripheral nervous system. Regional blockade has been suggested as part of the workup for techniques such as spinal cord stimulation which are more effective in peripheral neuropathic pain.[103]

Neurostimulation

Stimulation techniques, such as transcutaneous electrical nerve stimulation (TENS) and acupuncture, may be effective for some people with neuropathic pain.[17] However, positive evidence of efficacy is limited, particularly with below-level neuropathic pain.[104,105] Most studies also report a decline in efficacy over time.[76]

Other stimulation techniques are very invasive with limited evidence of efficacy. Spinal cord stimulation may provide relief although a greater effect is obtained in those with at-level neuropathic pain and incomplete lesions.[106] Deep brain stimulation seems not seem to provide long term pain relief in SCI pain.[76] Transcranial and epidural motor cortex stimulation have been tested in a few SCI pain patients with varying results.[107] A recent study using transcranial direct current stimulation (tDCS) demonstrated short-term reduction in pain following a 5 day treatment trial.[108]

Physical Approaches

Physical approaches may help to improve chronic musculoskeletal pain and may indirectly influence neuropathic SCI pain. Abnormal posture, gait, and overuse may all contribute to pain and may be addressed by physiotherapy, exercise,[109] retraining, and environmental modifications, such as the use of specialised adaptive equipment, wheelchair adjustment, and positioning. Regular exercise in people with SCI has also been demonstrated to result in improvements in both pain and mood.[110]

Surgical Approaches

Surgical approaches usually relieve pain by reversing structural problems. For example, surgery may be used to address nerve root or peripheral nerve compression, tethering of nerve roots, and syrinx formation. However, repair of a neurological lesion may not result in pain relief and may at times increase pain.

If it is not possible to address a structural problem, surgical approaches attempt to deal with the pain by destroying or disconnecting the site of abnormal neuronal activity. Several uncontrolled studies have been performed to examine efficacy of surgical approaches but have resulted in variable results. Cordotomy or cordomyelotomy have been used to a limited extent and some reports suggest effectiveness in a subgroup of patients.[111,112] Dorsal root entry zone (DREZ) lesioning, a procedure that aims to destroy hyperactive nerve cells in the dorsal horn close to the level of injury, may provide relief of neuropathic pain, although best results are obtained in those with at-level neuropathic pain.[113] DREZ lesioning guided by intramedullary recordings of spontaneous and C-fiber evoked electrical hyperactivity is suggested to be effective in relieving both at- and below-level neuropathic pain.[114,115]

Psychological and Environmental Management

Coming to terms with a spinal injury requires a huge adjustment in relationships, lifestyle, vocation, and self-image. All of these issues need to be addressed and, not surprisingly, people with a severe SCI often have significant psychological distress particularly in the acute post injury period.[7] The presence of chronic pain may be an additional factor that prevents expected rehabilitation and return to employment and function in domestic life.[10,13,15,116] Anxiety and depression are both normal responses to injury and often improve with time and the implementation of the person's inherent coping skills. In these people, formal intervention may not be required. However, for the minority who experience severe or chronic mood dysfunction impacting on their ability to function, more formal intervention should be offered.

A variety of approaches are available for managing psychological and environmental contributors to pain and distress. Pharmacological strategies such as anxiolytic and antidepressant therapy and nonpharmacological strategies such as cognitive-behavioral therapy may be used.[117,118] The effectiveness of a cognitive-behavioral approach in the management of neuropathic SCI pain has been examined with significant improvements in mood, though not pain.[118]

Relaxation and desensitization techniques are suggested to be of benefit in SCI pain and may alter the patient's attitude toward pain. More recently, the effect of movement imagery as a component of a management program for SCI neuropathic pain has been examined. In one study (using a visual illusion of walking), a reduction in neuropathic pain was noted in people following cauda equina injury.[119] In contrast, a study using imagined lower limb movements following complete SCI found an increase in pain and unpleasant phantom sensations.[120] The difference in findings appears to be related to the level and completeness of injury, with the positive responders having incomplete cauda equina injuries. The use of cognitive strategies such as movement imagery, however, may be helpful in a certain subgroup of patients and provides an interesting noninvasive alternate strategy.

Treatment Summary

Treatment guidelines need to take into consideration a broad range of issues including pain type, other medical and psychological issues, personal preference, side effects, treatment availability, and cost. As mentioned, the evidence to support many interventions in the management of SCI pain is limited, making definitive recommendations difficult to formulate. It would not be wise to provide a prescriptive approach to the management of SCI pain. However, guidelines are available that provide a general approach that may be tailored to the individual (Figs. 40.2 and 40.3).[75]

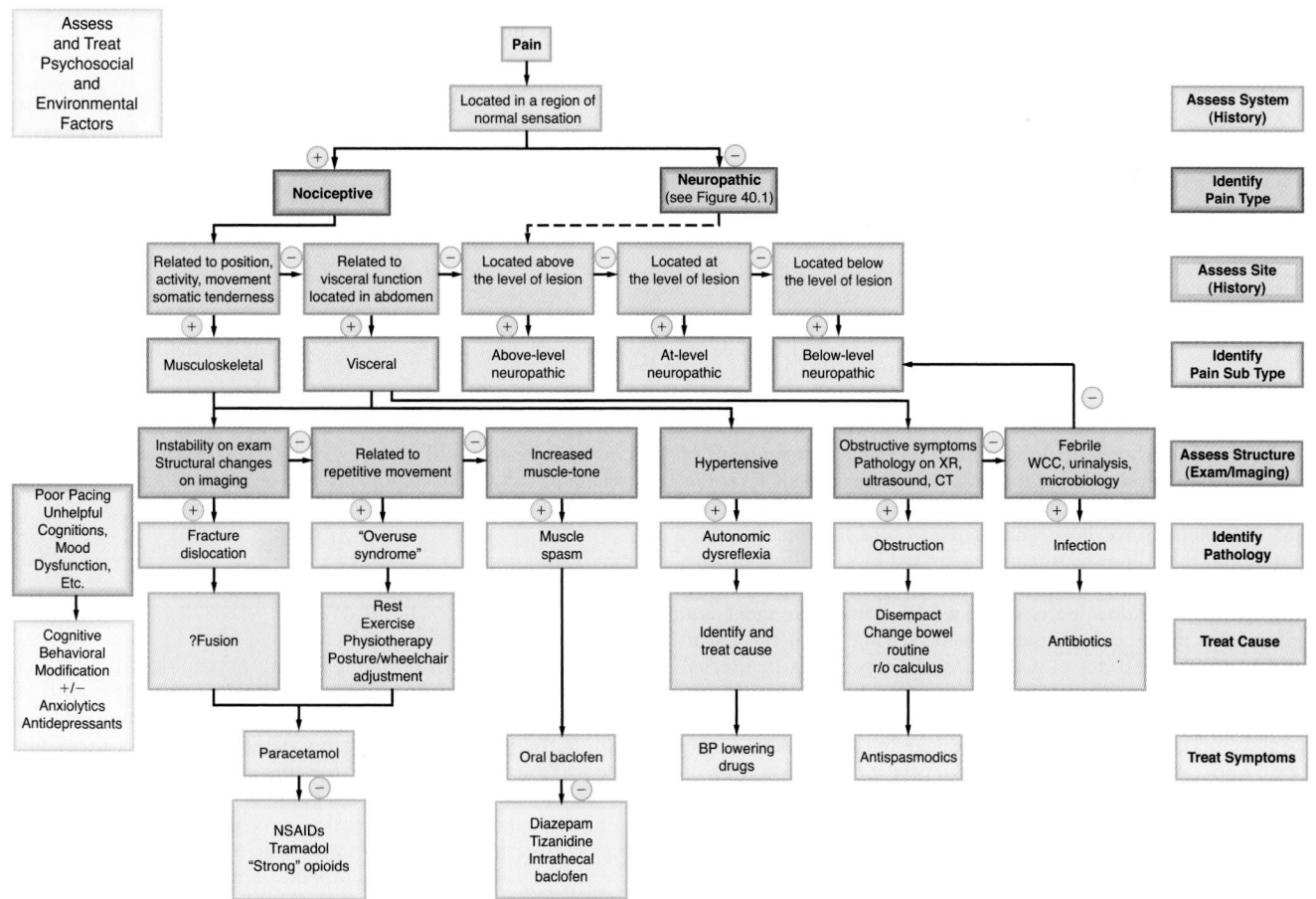

FIGURE 40.2 Assessment and treatment algorithm for the management of nociceptive pain following spinal cord injury. (Modified from Siddall PJ, Middleton JW. A proposed algorithm for the management of pain following spinal cord injury. *Spinal Cord* 2006;44:67–77.)

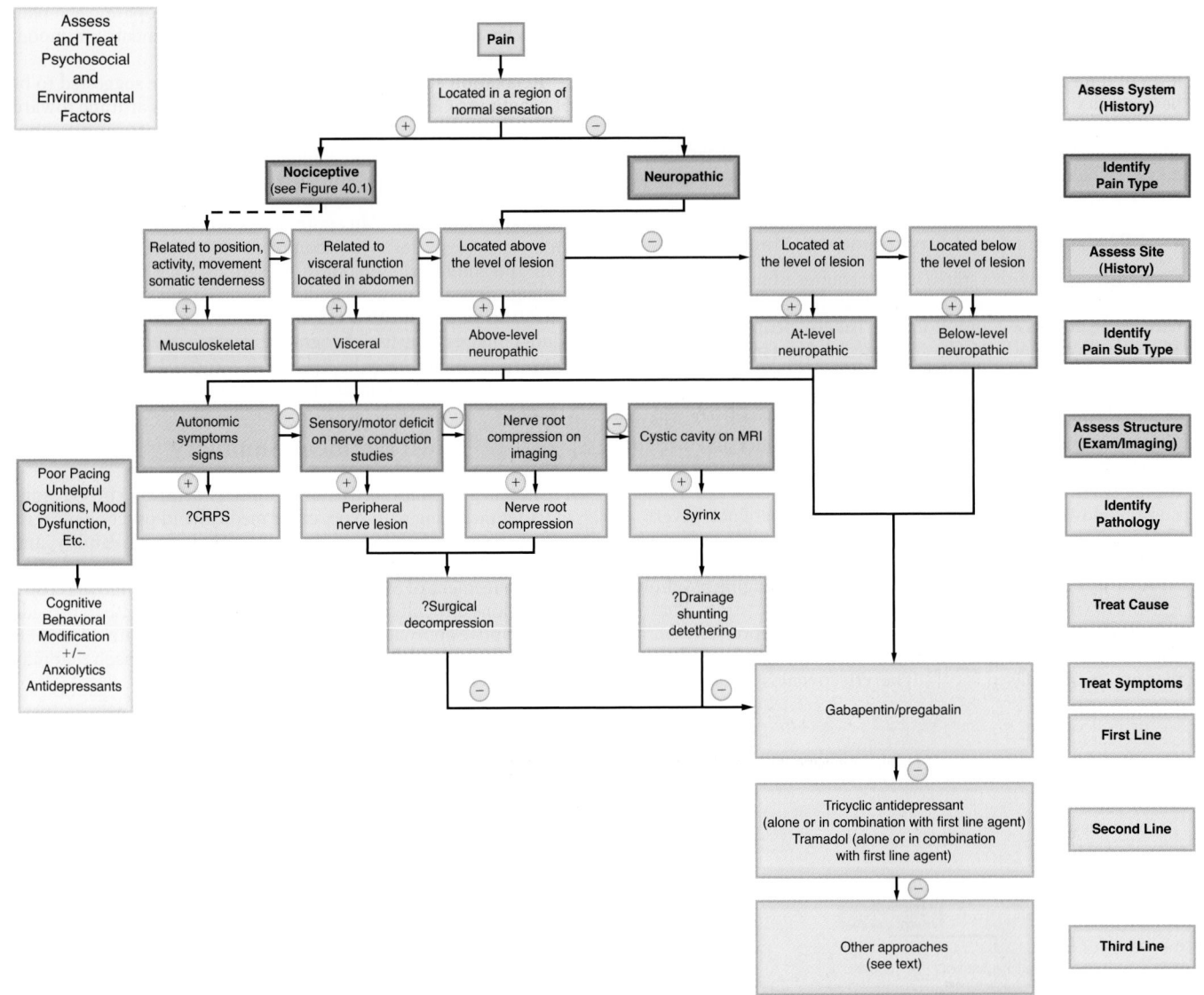

FIGURE 40.3 Assessment and treatment algorithm for the management of neuropathic pain following spinal cord injury. (Modified from Siddall PJ, Middleton JW. A proposed algorithm for the management of pain following spinal cord injury. *Spinal Cord* 2006;44:67–77.)

In this algorithm, a tri-level approach to the management of at- and below-level neuropathic SCI pain is suggested. First line treatments are those that have been validated in SCI pain; second line treatments have been validated in other neuropathic pain states; and third line treatments are limited by side effect profile, invasiveness, or lack of efficacy data. In the acute, inpatient setting, parenteral lidocaine is suggested as a first line agent and gabapentin in the subacute or chronic setting. With the recent evidence for the efficacy of pregabalin,[83] this provides an alternative to gabapentin. As a second line treatment, the use of a tricyclic antidepressant, such as amitriptyline or nortriptyline, or a weak opioid, such as tramadol, is suggested. The combination of an anticonvulsant with either a tricyclic antidepressant or an opioid may produce additional relief. However, the use of combination polypharmacy does expose the patient to greater risk. Third line treatments include many of the other treatments described above. If there is inadequate response to first and second line treatments, third line treatments may be considered. However, the likelihood of benefit must be weighed against possible adverse side effects of the treatment. In parallel with these treatments which largely focus on the biological aspects of the pain,

consideration should also be given to treatment of psychosocial issues such as mood, cognitions, and environmental factors which may be contributing to both pain and disability.

CONCLUSION

Pain provides an additional challenge to the person with SCI. It is associated with poorer physical, psychological, and social functioning. Clinicians involved in the care of people with SCI pain also face the challenge of a limited therapeutic armamentarium, particularly for neuropathic pain. Despite this, many positive treatments are available for this group. Treatments should target causative factors where possible, which may be possible in musculoskeletal and visceral pain. The majority of treatments for neuropathic pain are symptomatic in nature.

Although the current therapeutic armamentarium is limited, increasing research efforts are underway to identify better treatments, particularly for neuropathic SCI pain. Optimal management depends on systematic assessment, identification of the specific type of pain, and utilization of validated treatment options.

A carefully devised biopsychosocial assessment and treatment plan can also assist a person with SCI pain to reduce the way persistent pain interferes with their quality of life and function.

References

1. Widerström-Noga EG, Felipe-Cuervo E, Broton JG, et al. Perceived difficulty in dealing with consequences of spinal cord injury. *Arch Phys Med Rehabil* 1999;80:580–586.
2. Ravenscroft A, Ahmed YS, Burnside IG. Chronic pain after SCI. A patient survey. *Spinal Cord* 2000;38:611–614.
3. Jensen MP, Kuehn CM, Amtmann D, et al. Symptom burden in persons with spinal cord injury. *Arch Phys Med Rehabil* 2007;88:638–645.
4. Störmer S, Gerner HJ, Grüninger W, et al. Chronic pain/dysaesthesiae in spinal cord injury patients: results of a multicentre study. *Spinal Cord* 1997;35:446–455.
5. Siddall PJ, McClelland JM, Rutkowski SB, et al. A longitudinal study of the prevalence and characteristics of pain in the first 5 years following spinal cord injury. *Pain* 2003;103:249–257.
6. Richards JS, Meredith RL, Nepomuceno C, et al. Psycho-social aspects of chronic pain in spinal cord injury. *Pain* 1980;8:355–366.
7. Summers JD, Rapoff MA, Varghese G, et al. Psychosocial factors in chronic spinal cord injury pain. *Pain* 1991;47:183–189.
8. Norrbrink Budh C, Hultling C, Lundeberg T. Quality of sleep in individuals with spinal cord injury: a comparison between patients with and without pain. *Spinal Cord* 2005;43:85–95.
9. Rose M, Robinson JE, Ells P, et al. Pain following spinal cord injury: results from a postal survey. *Pain* 1988;34:101–102.
10. Widerström-Noga EG, Duncan R, Felipe-Cuervo E, et al. Assessment of the impact of pain and impairments associated with spinal cord injuries. *Arch Phys Med Rehabil* 2002;83:395–404.
11. Widerström-Noga EG, Felipe-Cuervo E, Yezierski RP. Chronic pain after spinal injury: interference with sleep and daily activities. *Arch Phys Med Rehabil* 2001;82:1571–1577.
12. Putzke JD, Richards JS, Hicken BL, et al. Interference due to pain following spinal cord injury: important predictors and impact on quality of life. *Pain* 2002;100:231–242.
13. Westgren N, Levi R. Quality of life and traumatic spinal cord injury. *Arch Phys Med Rehabil* 1998;79:1433–1439.
14. Anke AG, Stenehjem AE, Stanghelle JK. Pain and life quality within 2 years of spinal cord injury. *Paraplegia* 1995;33:555–559.
15. Rintala DH, Loubser PG, Castro J, et al. Chronic pain in a community-based sample of men with spinal cord injury: prevalence, severity, and relationship with impairment, disability, handicap, and subjective well-being. *Arch Phys Med Rehabil* 1998;79:604–614.
16. Budh CN, Osteřker AL. Life satisfaction in individuals with a spinal cord injury and pain. *Clin Rehabil* 2007;21:89–96.
17. Norrbrink Budh C, Lundeberg T. Non-pharmacological pain-relieving therapies in individuals with spinal cord injury: a patient perspective. *Complement Ther Med* 2004;12:189–197.
18. Nashold BS. Paraplegia and pain. In: Nashold BS, Ovelmen-Levitt J, eds. *Deafferentation Pain Syndromes: Pathophysiology and Treatment*. New York: Raven Press; 1991:301–319.
19. Davidoff G, Roth E, Guarracini M, et al. Function-limiting dysesthetic pain syndrome among traumatic spinal cord injury patients: a cross-sectional study. *Pain* 1987;29:39–48.
20. Berić A, Dimitrijević MR, Lindblom U. Central dysesthesia syndrome in spinal cord injury patients. *Pain* 1988;34:109–116.
21. Bowsher D. Central pain of spinal origin. *Spinal Cord* 1996;34:707–710.
22. Defrin R, Ovry A, Blumen N, et al. Characterization of chronic pain and somatosensory function in spinal cord injury subjects. *Pain* 2001;89:253–263.
23. Finnerup NB, Jensen TS. Spinal cord injury pain—mechanisms and treatment. *Eur J Neurol* 2004;11:73–82.
24. Cairns DM, Adkins RH, Scott MD. Pain and depression in acute traumatic spinal cord injury: origins of chronic problematic pain? *Arch Phys Med Rehabil* 1996;77:329–335.
25. Wollaars MM, Post MW, van Asbeck FW, et al. Spinal cord injury pain: the influence of psychologic factors and impact on quality of life. *Clin J Pain* 2007;23:383–391.
26. Turner JA, Jensen MP, Warms CA, et al. Catastrophizing is associated with pain intensity, psychological distress, and pain-related disability among individuals with chronic pain after spinal cord injury. *Pain* 2002;98:127–134.
27. Raichle KA, Hanley M, Jensen MP, et al.. Cognitions, coping, and social environment predict adjustment to pain in spinal cord injury. *J Pain* 2007;8:718–729.
28. Rudy TE, Lieber SJ, Boston JR, et al. Psychosocial predictors of physical performance in disabled individuals with chronic pain. *Clin J Pain* 2003;19:18–30.
29. Elfström M, Rydén A, Kreuter M, et al. Relations between coping strategies and health-related quality of life in patients with spinal cord lesion. *J Rehabil Med* 2005;37:9–16.
30. Elfström ML, Kreuter M, Rydén A, et al. Effects of coping on psychological outcome when controlling for background variables: a study of traumatically spinal cord lesioned persons. *Spinal Cord* 2002;40:408–415.
31. Beedie A, Kennedy P. Quality of social support predicts hopelessness and depression post spinal cord injury. *J Clin Psychol Med Settings* 2002;9:227–234.
32. Conant LL. Psychological variables associated with pain perceptions among individuals with chronic spinal cord injury pain. *J Clin Psychol Med Settings* 1998;5:71–90.
33. Stroud MW, Turner JA, Jensen MP, et al. Partner responses to pain behaviors are associated with depression and activity interference among persons with chronic pain and spinal cord injury. *J Pain* 2006;7:91–99.
34. Bryce TN, Ragnarsson KT. Epidemiology and classification of pain after spinal cord injury. *Top Spinal Cord Inj Rehabil* 2001;7:1–17.
35. Cardenas DD, Turner JA, Warms CA, et al. Classification of chronic pain associated with spinal cord injuries. *Arch Phys Med Rehabil* 2002;83:1708–1714.
36. Donovan WH, Dimitrijevic MR, Dahm L, et al. Neurophysiological approaches to chronic pain following spinal cord injury. *Paraplegia* 1982;20:135–146.
37. Siddall PJ, Taylor DA, Cousins MJ. Classification of pain following spinal cord injury. *Spinal Cord* 1997;35:69–75.
38. Siddall PJ, Yezierski RP, Loeser JD. Taxonomy and epidemiology of spinal cord injury pain. In: Yezierski RP, Burchiel KJ, eds. *Spinal Cord Injury Pain: Assessment, Mechanisms, Management Progress in Pain Research and Management*. Vol 23. Seattle: IASP Press; 2002:9–24.
39. Marino RJ, Barros T, Biering-Sorensen F, et al. International standards for neurological classification of spinal cord injury. *J Spinal Cord Med* 2003;26:S50–S56.
40. Dalyan M, Cardenas DD, Gerard B. Upper extremity pain after spinal cord injury. *Spinal Cord* 1999;37:191–195.
41. van Drongelen S, de Groot S, Veeger HE, et al. Upper extremity musculoskeletal pain during and after rehabilitation in wheelchair-using persons with a spinal cord injury. *Spinal Cord* 2006;44:152–159.
42. Curtis KA, Drysdale GA, Lanza RD, et al. Shoulder pain in wheelchair users with tetraplegia and paraplegia. *Arch Phys Med Rehabil* 1999;80:453–457.
43. Haythornthwaite JA, Benrud-Larson LM. Psychological aspects of neuropathic pain. *Clin J Pain* 2000;16(suppl 16):S101–S105.
44. Kennedy P, Frankel H, Gardner B, et al. Factors associated with acute and chronic pain following traumatic spinal cord injuries. *Spinal Cord* 1997;35:814–817.
45. Loubser PG, Clearman RR. Evaluation of central spinal cord injury pain with diagnostic spinal anesthesia. *Anesthesiology* 1993;79:376–378.
46. Loeser JD, Ward AA Jr, White LE Jr. Chronic deafferentation of human spinal cord neurons. *J Neurosurg* 1968;29:48–50.
47. Vierck CJ Jr, Siddall P, Yezierski RP. Pain following spinal cord injury: animal models and mechanistic studies. *Pain* 2000;89:1–5.
48. Hao JX, Xu XJ, Yu YX, et al. Transient spinal cord ischemia induces temporary hypersensitivity of dorsal horn wide dynamic range neurons to myelinated, but not unmyelinated, fiber input. *J Neurophysiol* 1992;68:384–391.
49. Yezierski RP, Park SH. The mechanosensitivity of spinal sensory neurons following intraspinal injections of quisqualic acid in the rat. *Neurosci Lett* 1993;157:115–119.
50. Christensen MD, Everhart AW, Pickelman JT, et al. Mechanical and thermal allodynia in chronic central pain following spinal cord injury. *Pain* 1996;68:97–107.
51. Hains BC, Waxman SG. Sodium channel expression and the molecular pathophysiology of pain after SCI. *Prog Brain Res* 2007;161:195–203.
52. Yezierski RP. Pathophysiology and animal models of spinal cord injury pain. In: Burchiel KJ, Yezierski RP, eds. *Spinal Cord Injury Pain: Assessment, Mechanisms, Management Progress in Pain Research and Management*. Vol 23. Seattle: IASP Press; 2002:117–136.
53. Melzack R, Loeser JD. Phantom body pain in paraplegics: evidence for a central "pattern generating mechanism" for pain. *Pain* 1978;4:195–210.
54. Radhakrishnan V, Tsoukatos J, Davis KD, et al. A comparison of the burst activity of lateral thalamic neurons in chronic pain and non-pain patients. *Pain* 1999;80:567–575.
55. Jeanmonod D, Magnin M, Morel A. Thalamus and neurogenic pain: physiological, anatomical, and clinical data. *Neuroreport* 1993;4:475–478.
56. Lenz FA, Kwan HC, Dostrovsky JO, et al. Characteristics of the bursting pattern of action potentials that occurs in the thalamus of patients with central pain. *Brain Res* 1989;496:357–360.
57. Gerke MB, Duggan AW, Xu L, et al. Thalamic neuronal activity in rats with mechanical allodynia following contusive spinal cord injury. *Neuroscience* 2003;117:715–722.
58. Koyama S, Katayama Y, Maejima S, et al. Thalamic neuronal hyperactivity following transection of the spinothalamic tract in the cat: involvement of N-methyl-D-aspartate receptor. *Brain Res* 1993;612:345–350.
59. Hains BC, Saab CY, Waxman SG. Changes in electrophysiological properties and sodium channel Nav1.3 expression in thalamic neurons after spinal cord injury. *Brain* 2005;128:2359–2371.
60. Pattany PM, Yezierski RP, Widerström-Noga EG, et al. Proton magnetic resonance spectroscopy of the thalamus in patients with chronic neuropathic pain after spinal cord injury. *AJNR Am J Neuroradiol* 2002;23:901–905.
61. Pagni CA, Canavero S. Functional thalamic depression in a case of reversible central pain due to a spinal intramedullary cyst. Case report. *J Neurosurg* 1995;83:163–165.

62. Ness TJ, San Pedro EC, Richards JS, et al. A case of spinal cord injury-related pain with baseline rCBF brain SPECT imaging and beneficial response to gabapentin. *Pain* 1998;78:139–143.
63. Finnerup NB, Johannesen IL, Fuglsang-Frederiksen A, et al. Sensory function in spinal cord injury patients with and without central pain. *Brain* 2003;126:57–70.
64. Finnerup NB, Gyldensted C, Nielsen E, et al. MRI in chronic spinal cord injury patients with and without central pain. *Neurology* 2003;61:1569–1575.
65. Cleeland CS. Measurement of pain by subjective report. In: Chapman CR, Loeser JD, eds. *Issues in Pain Measurement*. New York: Raven Press; 1989:391–403.
66. Mogil JS, ed. *The Genetics of Pain*. Seattle: IASP Press; 2004.
67. Gallagher RM. Rational integration of pharmacologic, behavioral, and rehabilitation strategies in the treatment of chronic pain. *Am J Phys Med Rehabil* 2005;84(suppl 3):S64–S76.
68. Large RG, Schug SA. Opioids for chronic pain of non-malignant origin—caring or crippling. *Health Care Anal* 1995;3:5–11.
69. Nicholas MK, Molloy AR, Brooker C. Using opioids with persisting noncancer pain: a biopsychosocial perspective. *Clin J Pain* 2006;22:137–146.
70. Taricco M, Pagliacci MC, Telaro E, et al. Pharmacological interventions for spasticity following spinal cord injury: results of a Cochrane systematic review. *Eura Medicophys* 2006;42:5–15.
71. O'Brien CF. Treatment of spasticity with botulinum toxin. *Clin J Pain* 2002;18:S182–S190.
72. Lewis KS, Mueller WM. Intrathecal baclofen for severe spasticity secondary to spinal cord injury. *Ann Pharmacother* 1993;27:767–774.
73. Herman RM, D'Luzansky SC, Ippolito R. Intrathecal baclofen suppresses central pain in patients with spinal lesions: a pilot study. *Clin J Pain* 1992;8:338–345.
74. Kingery WS. A critical review of controlled clinical trials for peripheral neuropathic pain and complex regional pain syndromes. *Pain* 1997;73:123–139.
75. Siddall PJ, Middleton JW. A proposed algorithm for the management of pain following spinal cord injury. *Spinal Cord* 2006;44:67–77.
76. Finnerup NB, Yezierski RP, Sang CN, et al. Treatment of spinal cord injury pain. *Pain: Clin Updates* 2001;9:1–6.
77. Attal N, Guirimand F, Brasseur L, et al. Effects of IV morphine in central pain: a randomized placebo-controlled study. *Neurology* 2002;58:554–563.
78. Eide PK, Stubhaug A, Stenehjem AE. Central dysesthesia pain after traumatic spinal cord injury is dependent on N-methyl-D-aspartate receptor activation. *Neurosurgery* 1995;37:1080–1087.
79. Attal N, Cruccu G, Haanpää M, et al. EFNS guidelines on pharmacological treatment of neuropathic pain. *Eur J Neurol* 2006;13:1153–1169.
80. Levendoglu F, Ogün CO, Ozerbil O, et al. Gabapentin is a first line drug for the treatment of neuropathic pain in spinal cord injury. *Spine* 2004;29:743–751.
81. Tai Q, Kirshblum S, Chen B, et al. Gabapentin in the treatment of neuropathic pain after spinal cord injury: a prospective, randomized, double-blind, cross-over trial. *J Spinal Cord Med* 2002;25:100–105.
82. Putzke JD, Richards JS, Kezar L, et al. Long-term use of gabapentin for treatment of pain after traumatic spinal cord injury. *Clin J Pain* 2002;18:116–121.
83. Siddall PJ, Cousins MJ, Otte A, et al. Pregabalin in central neuropathic pain associated with spinal cord injury: a placebo-controlled trial. *Neurology* 2006;67:1792–1800.
84. Vranken JH, Dijkgraaf MGW, Kruis MR, et al. Pregabalin in patients with central neuropathic pain: a randomized, double-blind, placebo-controlled trial of a flexible-dose regimen. *Pain* [advance online publication]. August 17, 2007 (DOI:10.1016/j.pain.2007.06.033).
85. Finnerup NB, Sindrup SH, Flemming WB, et al. Lamotrigine in spinal cord injury pain: a randomized controlled trial. *Pain* 2002;96:375–383.
86. Harden RN, Brenman E, Saltz S, et al. Topiramate in the management of spinal cord injury pain: a double-blind, randomized, placebo-controlled pilot study. In: Yezierski RP, Burchiel KJ, eds. *Spinal Cord Injury Pain: Assessment, Mechanisms, Management Progress in Pain Research and Management*. Vol 23. Seattle: IASP Press; 2002:393–407.
87. Drewes AM, Andreasen A, Poulsen LH. Valproate for treatment of chronic central pain after spinal cord injury. A double-blind cross-over study. *Paraplegia* 1994;32:565–569.
88. Erzurumlu A, Dursun H, Gunduz S. The management of chronic pain in spinal cord injured patients. The comparison of effectiveness of amitriptyline and carbamazepine combination and electroacupuncture application. *J Rheumatol Med Rehabil* 1996;7:176–180.
89. Cardenas DD, Warms CA, Turner JA, et al. Efficacy of amitriptyline for relief of pain in spinal cord injury: results of a randomized controlled trial. *Pain* 2002;96:365–373.
90. Davidoff G, Guarracini M, Roth E, et al. Trazodone hydrochloride in the treatment of dysesthetic pain in traumatic myelopathy: a randomized, double-blind, placebo-controlled study. *Pain* 1987;29:151–161.
91. Sandford PR, Lindblom LB, Haddox JD. Amitriptyline and carbamazepine in the treatment of dysesthetic pain in spinal cord injury. *Arch Phys Med Rehabil* 1992;73:300–301.
92. Backonja M, Gombar KA. Response of central pain syndromes to intravenous lidocaine. *J Pain Symptom Manage* 1992;7:172–178.
93. Attal N, Gaudé, V, Brasseur L, et al. Intravenous lidocaine in central pain: a double-blind, placebo-controlled, psychophysical study. *Neurology* 2000;54:564–574.
94. Finnerup NB, Biering-Sørensen F, Johannesen IL, et al. Intravenous lidocaine relieves spinal cord injury pain: a randomized controlled trial. *Anesthesiology* 2005;102:1023–1030.
95. Kvarnström A, Karlsten R, Quiding H, et al. The analgesic effect of intravenous ketamine and lidocaine on pain after spinal cord injury. *Acta Anaesthesiol Scand* 2004;48:498–506.
96. Cahana A, Carota A, Montadon ML, et al. The long-term effect of repeated intravenous lidocaine on central pain and possible correlation in positron emission tomography measurements. *Anesth Analg* 2004;98:1581–1584.
97. Chiou-Tan FY, Tuel SM, Johnson JC, et al. Effect of mexiletine on spinal cord injury dysesthetic pain. *Am J Phys Med Rehabil* 1996;75:84–87.
98. Canavero S, Bonicalzi V. Intravenous subhypnotic propofol in central pain: a double-blind, placebo-controlled, crossover study. *Clin Neuropharmacol* 2004;27:182–186.
99. Glynn CJ, Jamous MA, Teddy PJ, et al. Role of spinal noradrenergic system in transmission of pain in patients with spinal cord injury. *Lancet* 1986;2:1249–1250.
100. Middleton JW, Siddall PJ, Walker S, et al. Intrathecal clonidine and baclofen in the management of spasticity and neuropathic pain following spinal cord injury: a case study. *Arch Phys Med Rehabil* 1996;77:824–826.
101. Siddall PJ, Molloy AR, Walker S, et al. The efficacy of intrathecal morphine and clonidine in the treatment of pain after spinal cord injury. *Anesth Analg* 2000;91:1493–1498.
102. Loubser PG, Akman NM. Effects of intrathecal baclofen on chronic spinal cord injury pain. *J Pain Symptom Manage* 1996;12:241–247.
103. Loubser PG, Donovan WH. Diagnostic spinal anaesthesia in chronic spinal cord injury pain. *Paraplegia* 1991;29:25–36.
104. Nayak S, Shiflett SC, Schoenberger NE, et al. Is acupuncture effective in treating chronic pain after spinal cord injury? *Arch Phys Med Rehabil* 2001;82:1578–1586.
105. Rapson LM, Wells N, Pepper J, et al. Acupuncture as a promising treatment for below-level central neuropathic pain: a retrospective study. *J Spinal Cord Med* 2003;26:21–26.
106. Cioni B, Meglio M, Pentimalli L, et al. Spinal cord stimulation in the treatment of paraplegic pain. *J Neurosurg* 1995;82:35–39.
107. Nguyen JP, Lefaucheur JP, Decq P, et al. Chronic motor cortex stimulation in the treatment of central and neuropathic pain. Correlations between clinical, electrophysiological, and anatomical data. *Pain* 1999;82:245–251.
108. Fregni F, Boggio PS, Lima MC, et al. A sham-controlled, phase II trial of transcranial direct current stimulation for the treatment of central pain in traumatic spinal cord injury. *Pain* 2006;122:197–209.
109. Hicks AL, Martin KA, Ditor DS, et al. Long-term exercise training in persons with spinal cord injury: effects on strength, arm ergometry performance and psychological well-being. *Spinal Cord* 2003;41:34–43.
110. Latimer AE, Ginis KA, Hicks AL, et al. An examination of the mechanisms of exercise-induced change in psychological well-being among people with spinal cord injury. *J Rehabil Res Dev* 2004;41:643–652.
111. Tasker RR, DeCarvalho GT, Dolan EJ. Intractable pain of spinal cord origin: clinical features and implications for surgery. *J Neurosurg* 1992;77:373–378.
112. Pagni CA, Canavero S. Cordomyelotomy in the treatment of paraplegia pain. Experience in two cases with long-term results. *Acta Neurol Belg* 1995;95:33–36.
113. Sindou M, Mertens P, Wael M. Microsurgical DREZotomy for pain due to spinal cord and/or cauda equina injuries: long-term results in a series of 44 patients. *Pain* 2001;92:159–171.
114. Edgar RE, Best LG, Quail PA, et al. Computer-assisted DREZ microcoagulation: posttraumatic spinal deafferentation pain. *J Spinal Disord* 1993;6:48–56.
115. Falci S, Best L, Bayles R, et al. Dorsal root entry zone microcoagulation for spinal cord injury-related central pain: operative intramedullary electrophysiological guidance and clinical outcome. *J Neurosurg* 2002;97:193–200.
116. Lundqvist C, Siösteen A, Blomstrand C, et al. Spinal cord injuries: clinical, functional, and emotional status. *Spine* 1991;16:78–83.
117. Craig AR, Hancock K, Dickson H, et al. Long-term psychological outcomes in spinal cord injured persons: results of a controlled trial using cognitive behavior therapy. *Arch Phys Med Rehabil* 1997;78:33–38.
118. Budh CN, Kowalski J, Lundeberg T. A comprehensive pain management programme comprising educational, cognitive and behavioural interventions for neuropathic pain following spinal cord injury. *J Rehabil Med* 2006;38:172–180.
119. Moseley GL. Using visual illusion to reduce at-level neuropathic pain in paraplegia. *Pain* 2007;130:294–298.
120. Gustin SM, Wrigley PJ, Gandevia SC, et al. Movement imagery increases pain in people with neuropathic pain following complete thoracic spinal cord injury. *Pain* 2008;137:237–244.

CHAPTER 41 ■ EPIDEMIOLOGY, PREVALENCE, AND CANCER PAIN SYNDROMES

NEIL A. HAGEN

INTRODUCTION

Cancer is a highly prevalent and serious public health issue. It most commonly affects the elderly—the average cancer patient is aged 65 at first diagnosis—and cancer is more likely to occur in particular clinical settings, such as a life-long smokers, in obesity, and with certain environmental and heritable risks. However, there is no one who is immune from the disease, regardless of age. In North America, about 1 in 3 adults will develop cancer in their lifetime, with about a 50% fatality rate. Cancer is sufficiently prevalent that some individuals will develop more than one type of malignancy, either sequentially or concurrently. Cancer is often painful, with pain presenting as a common heralding manifestation of the disease. For example, about two thirds of women have pain at the onset or recurrence of ovarian cancer.[1] As cancer progresses, it is more likely to be associated with pain, and the pain is more likely to be severe. A range of epidemiological studies in several countries and practice settings suggests that pain from a wide variety of cancers is present in about one third of patients receiving cancer treatment and in 60% to 90% with advanced illness.[2]

Cancer treatment can also cause pain, and cancer pain is commonly classified as being either due to the underlying disease or due to its treatment. In pediatric malignancies, pain due to treatment is more common than pain from the underlying disease.[3] Cancer patients can also have pain from non–cancer-related conditions, and the causes and prevalence are similar to pain in patients without a cancer diagnosis.

There is an array of factors that contributes to the likelihood of pain being present, its severity, and the best approach to its management. Thus, in order to understand the wisest approach to the cancer patient who presents with cancer pain, the situation is best appreciated within the perspective of where the patient is in the disease trajectory and what other clinical factors are likely to be at play.

The intention of this introductory chapter is to provide a clinical context of the individual patient and to bring into focus the extensive information that follows in subsequent chapters where more detailed approaches to assessment and management will be elaborated. This chapter is divided into six sections:

■ Summary of the epidemiology of cancer pain
■ How to perform a cancer pain history
■ How to perform a physical examination of a cancer pain patient, including bedside provocative maneuvers to help identify potential underlying pain-sensitive structures
■ Problem formulation
■ Constructing an analgesic strategy
■ Managing pain in specific clinical situations

EPIDEMIOLOGY OF CANCER PAIN

Epidemiology is "the study of the relationship of the various factors determining the frequency and distribution of diseases in a human community."[4] The epidemiology of cancer pain refers to cancer pain within the population, and its delineation provides insight into the likeliest factors at play within an individual patient.

Pain Related to Extent of Disease: The Cancer Disease Trajectory

Commonly, patients with solid tumor malignancies present with an asymptomatic mass; less than 15% of patients with nonmetastatic disease describe pain from their cancer.[2] Cancer can present clinically in a wide variety of ways, including dyspnea, nausea, urinary symptoms, weakness, numbness, weight loss, and other signs and symptoms. When pain is the first symptom of cancer, there is a tendency for the cancer to be more advanced and perhaps for this reason, pain can be an independent predictor for poorer survival.

The clinician can use this information to suspect the underlying cause of pain. For example, imagine a patient with a diagnosis of melanoma who presents with a 3 day history of new onset of headache. It could be due to a benign cause (e.g., migraine) or due to malignancy (e.g., brain metastasis). Stage of cancer predicts the risk of brain metastases. In this example, the likelihood of central nervous system metastasis is much lower in the patient who has recently undergone resection of a primary melanoma in the leg, with regional lymph nodes negative, compared to the patient who has known liver and lung metastases from melanoma. About 90% of patients with melanoma have central nervous system metastases at the time of autopsy, and the report of any headache in a patient with known metastatic melanoma is ominous. If imaging studies of the brain are negative in a patient with metastatic melanoma and a new headache, the possibility of meningeal disease should be considered, along with a diagnostic dural puncture for cerebrospinal fluid analysis.

Special Needs of Particular Age Groups: Pediatric, Young Adult, Adult, Geriatric

Pain is a subjective experience, and the pain of cancer can be foreign and puzzling for the patient. Pediatric patients can lack the language and the sophistication of adults in communicating their inner world. While cancer can result in an overwhelming sense of threat at any age, the pediatric age group requires special skills and support. For instance, pediatric patients and their families become the "unit of care," far more so than with adult oncology, and specialized assessment tools must be used for this population (see Chapter 49).

Cancer pain is prevalent at all ages. However, there are several remarkable features of cancer pain within the pediatric population. First, pain from cancer treatment is highly prevalent, in part related to the high prevalence of procedures to manage hematological malignancies and other malignancies typical of this age group. Particular attention needs to be taken to diminish the fear of pain from procedures and treatment. Painful procedures include placement of intravenous catheters, repeated spinal taps, bone marrow biopsies, extensive cancer surgery, and others. Second, young patients are often proficient at managing their pain once taught an appropriate technique. Patients as young as 5 years can safely and effectively use a patient controlled analgesia device, with the overall outcome of good pain control and potentially less risk of nausea or respiratory depression compared to continuous opioid infusions.[5]

Sarcoma and hematological malignancies are common in the 16–21 age group. Rarely, young adults can present with what looks clinically to be depression, but in fact the patient has uncontrolled pain. Particular attention needs to be placed on supporting the patient to be as active and have as normal a life as possible despite the potentially disfiguring effects of cancer treatment, difficulty with cancer pain, and the many challenges of cancer treatment.

Working-aged adults with cancer pain face their own unique complexities. A need to generate income or fulfill parenting roles despite illness, financial obligations, fear of addiction, and the challenges of managing emotional distress, are all issues that need to be consciously addressed in order to provide comprehensive symptom control. Young adults often choose or have indications for more aggressive or prolonged cancer treatments. For example, aromatase inhibitors are commonly used in the adjuvant treatment of breast cancer over the course of several years; almost half of these patients describe joint pain or stiffness. Usually symptoms are mild or moderate, but nearly one quarter of patients rate their symptoms as severe.[6]

The geriatric population often has medical comorbidity, such as underlying heart, lung, renal, or cognitive impairment, and may be on a variety of medications that interact with analgesic medications. Dosages of medications such as opioids may need to be lowered because the metabolism of medication can be much slower with advanced age or underlying organ impairment. An important, emerging concept within the geriatric population is that of frailty. Factors that promote return to health or maintenance of good health—resilience—are powerful in the pediatric and young adult population; with advancing years, the ability to maintain homeostasis becomes less. Frailty is a term that describes what has become an area of intense research in the geriatric community and is a key factor in analgesic care in the older cancer population.[7] Changes in medications should generally be made more slowly and with smaller dosing increments. Attention needs to be paid to drug–drug interactions, and the clinician should be vigilant for the appearance of early signs of cognitive impairment. Because of the high prevalence of delirium in the medically ill geriatric oncology population and the difficulty in making an early diagnosis, some clinicians have advocated for the routine use of delirium screening tools.[8]

Special Needs of Particular Ethnic Groups: Communication Styles, Common Preferences, and Managing Taboos

Some ethnic groups are particularly vulnerable to specific health issues. About 90% of cancer patients in the Middle East present with advanced, incurable illness. The commonest malignancy in women in the Middle East is gynecological cancer, although cancers associated with tobacco use are increasing rapidly. Hepatoma and nasopharyngeal cancer are highly prevalent in patients who originate from Pacific Rim countries, and the higher risk persists for decades after moving to a Western country. There are some First Nations communities in North America where diabetes mellitus has reached epidemic proportions, with more than half of all adults being afflicted; cancer care can be greatly complicated by underlying diabetes. Every culture and ethnic group has a unique set of medical issues that are of particular concern.

Some countries, or parts of countries, have a lengthy history of violence and social upheaval in association with the licit or illicit drug trade, and the medical use of opioids is greatly frowned upon. Some religious cultures are believed to hold the experience of suffering to be of spiritual value. Others are commonly believed

to place a taboo on disclosure of a cancer diagnosis to the patient, relegating the burden of that knowledge and the decision making on cancer care to the eldest son.

There are approximately 6900 discrete languages spoken in the world[9] and uncountable distinct ethnic, religious, and other cultures. How is the clinician to be alert to all possible areas where culture can have a major influence on patient preferences and on patient assessment?

Basic knowledge of common beliefs within certain cultures is inarguably important, such as the prevalence of modesty as a dominant value in the Muslim faith community. Beliefs common to many cultures are complicated by the tendency in Western society for a shift in immigrant families, with increasing orientation toward secular values from one generation to the next. So when the patient who is thought to belong to a particular culture is in the physician's office along with their spouse and their adult children, which is likely to be the dominant culture? The clinician is wise to not make assumptions about what are the beliefs, values, and preferences of the patient or their family. Instead, it is far better to ask, since these issues will all have an impact on the patient's pain experience and treatment. There are many variations of beliefs within broad cultural groups, and it has been recommended in the clinical realm to instead focus on the patient and the family unit as having their own culture. It is the task of the clinician to understand and respect that culture.

If there is a taboo against disclosing a life-threatening diagnosis to the patient, the family will almost invariably make this wish abundantly clear to the clinician at an early stage. There is an emerging ethical construct that supports the clinician to respect such a request, if it is the explicit wish of the patient. If the patient indicates that another family member is to be the receiver of medical information and is to make all treatment and other decisions on the care of the patient, the patient has duly exercised their autonomy. The family, or a specific individual within the family, becomes the unit to which the authority of informed consent is conferred.[10] It is legitimate for the clinician to periodically confirm what is the preferred communication style and to whom the patient has conferred decision-making authority. Fortunately, taboos in disclosure of diagnostic information rarely interfere with obtaining information directly from the patient regarding their experience of pain and the effect of analgesic interventions.

Comorbidities Associated With Specific Cancers: Lung Disease, Liver Disease, Renal Disease, and Neurological Disease

Lung cancer is about 30 times as prevalent in life-long smokers as life-long nonsmokers. Patients with lung cancer commonly have clinically significant chronic obstructive lung disease, ischemic heart disease, or symptomatic peripheral vascular disease. If patients have pre-existing carbon dioxide retention, there is a risk the carbon dioxide retention will worsen with the use of opioids, especially with concurrent benzodiazepine use when anxiolysis is needed. Other than in the situation of life-threatening carbon dioxide retention, where very careful titration under monitored conditions may be indicated, opioids are generally not contraindicated by the presence of lung disease, and should be titrated to effect with monitoring for toxicity, similar to patients without known lung disease.

Premorbid liver disease is also prevalent in patients with specific cancer types, such as hepatoma and esophageal cancer. The major clinical features of liver disease relate to portal hypertension, with an elevated risk of episodes of gastrointestinal (GI) bleeding, ascites, and malnutrition. The capacity of the liver to metabolize medications is often less affected than other aspects of liver function, and the dose of medications commonly used in cancer pain such as opioids should not routinely be reduced.

Instead, medications should be titrated to effect. Acetaminophen should be used with caution, however, particularly in the setting of cirrhosis. The clinical presentation of liver metastases is often pain and jaundice; it is rare to encounter metabolic liver failure until almost all of the liver is replaced by cancer.

Renal disease is becoming much more prevalent in Western society, and many cancer treatments, such as platinum-based chemotherapy, are nephrotoxic. Cancer patients are at risk to accumulate medications or their active metabolites in the presence of even mild underlying renal impairment.[11] Doses of some medications used for neuropathic pain, such as gabapentin, are routinely reduced in the setting of renal impairment, but opioids are not. Instead, opioids should be titrated to effect, recognizing that a reduction in dose or increase in dosing interval may be required. In the face of end-stage disease with near-complete or total kidney failure, renally-cleared opioids (or those with active metabolites such as morphine) should be administered on an as-needed basis rather than around-the-clock.

About half of cancer patients are aged 65 years and older, an age group that has a particularly high prevalence of comorbid neurologic illness. Also, cancer and its treatments are associated with neurologic illness, such as stroke, meningitis, and other conditions. Concurrent cancer and neurologic disease affects pain management in several ways, but two deserve particular mention. First, pain assessment largely depends on an intact cognition. The widespread use of pain assessment tools such as the numeric rating scale has helped to bring some quantification to what is otherwise a subjective and often silent experience. But what if the patient is confused, and provides the wrong numbers? There is then a risk of overmedication or undermedication. The Brief Pain Inventory documents several discrete domains of the pain experience: average pain in the past 24 hours, worst pain in the past 24 hours, least pain in the past 24 hours, and so on. Study of the psychometrics of pain tools have revealed that the present pain intensity is the most reliable domain in the setting of cognitive impairment, and is the measure that should be used if there is any question of cognitive impairment. Also the information should be confirmed by other direct questions by the clinician, such as "is the pain bad, or not bad right now?" Further, cognitive impairment in cancer patients generally arises because of many contributing factors. Families are often quick to blame the pain medications. Only uncommonly are analgesics the sole or the major cause. However, in the absence of other obvious causes for delirium, rotating to a different pain medication, along with hydration and other general supportive measures, can reverse an episode of delirium even when other contributing factors are not correctable.

Cancer Pain and Substance Abuse

"Abuse" is a somewhat pejorative word, but its use has been widely accepted. Abuse has been defined in a variety of ways, but is generally taken to mean use of a recreational drug despite harm to self or others. "Addiction" is taken to be a far extreme in the spectrum of abuse, where there is an overwhelming focus on obtaining a supply, craving, and social disintegration.[12] About 15% of adult men in Western societies abuse alcohol, and only about half that proportion of adult women. A smaller proportion of the population abuses other substances, such as cocaine, methamphetamine, or cannabinoids. Some cancer patients are actively abusing psychoactive substances, and others have a past but not current history of abuse. Some active abusers are open about their lifestyle choices, and others keep it a secret.

Pain management is challenging in patients who have a prior history of substance abuse; they have more symptoms, more interference from pain, have more distress, and have more problematic drug-related behaviors than cancer pain patients who do not have a history of substance abuse.[13] Pain is common in the street-connected opioid abusing population, with about a third of patients in methadone maintenance programs describing moderate to severe chronic noncancer pain.[14] Pain can be difficult to reliably assess in cancer patients who have pre-existing chronic pain, a history of abuse of pain medications or other psychoactive compounds, and a coping strategy that has included the use of chemicals ostensibly to help them cope. There is a clash of cultures when the clinician, who believes that the pain is what the patient describes it to be, becomes aware that there may be reasons to not fully trust the patient's description. The clinician should carefully document the patient's description of her/his pain experience and obtain collateral information whenever possible. There is a role for greater reliance on diagnostic imaging to confirm clinical assessment. All patients deserve adequate pain control and to be treated with respect. However, the situation of a cancer patient with active substance abuse requires an approach that will protect the patient and their environment from things that can get in the way of successful pain management. An overall strategy for managing cancer pain in the addict is described at the end of this chapter.

Cancer Pain in Inmates

The incarcerated population has unique cancer risks, in part related to demographics.[15] Most inmates are men, are from ethnic minorities, and are less likely to be in the geriatric age group compared to the general population. Cancer risk factors are known to be highly prevalent in inmates, including smoking, drug and alcohol use, and AIDS-related illnesses. About 30% to 40% of U.S. inmates are infected with hepatitis C, and HIV infection rates are much higher than the national average.[16,17] High rates of human papillomavirus infection have been found in women inmates. A large study on the epidemiology of cancer in the incarcerated population found that the incidence of lung cancer, non-Hodgkin's lymphoma, head and neck cancers, and cervical cancer were two to three times more frequent than expected compared to age-matched controls, and death from hepatoma was more than three times the rate of controls. Survival was significantly poorer in incarcerated cancer patients compared to controls, with median survival of 21 months versus 55 months, and 5-year survival of 37% vs. about 48%.[15] In summary, compared to the general population, inmates are more likely to be affected by cancer, more likely to have cancers that are characterized by difficult to manage symptoms, and are more likely to have a past history of substance abuse or viral infection.

Inmates with cancer have been found to have a high prevalence of pain and to be undermedicated for cancer pain.[18] Drug misuse, actual drug diversion, fears held by prescribers of potential drug diversion, and lack of patient credibility have been identified as barriers to cancer pain management.

COMPONENTS OF THE COMPREHENSIVE MEDICAL EVALUATION OF A PATIENT WITH CHRONIC CANCER PAIN

An enormous amount of information is available to guide the clinician in assessing a patient with chronic cancer pain. Pain assessment tools have been extensively validated in a range of clinical settings, languages, and in different ages and disease states (see Chapter 20).

However, cancer patients are often systemically ill, and in addition to pain usually have low energy and may have a range of other symptoms. Clinicians need to find a balance between the wish to complete a comprehensive assessment and yet respect the constraints of patients' abilities to tolerate such a comprehensive evaluation. Cancer patients and their families are not always able to endure lengthy clinic visits with use of extensive bedside assessment tools, detailed psychosocial evaluations, and evaluation of other important domains.

Cancer patients and their families have many needs that compete for their time and attention. In addition to symptom control, they also are keen to learn about cancer treatment options, meet the needs of their family members such as children, and fulfill other social obligations related to their employment, completing required insurance forms, and competing financial imperatives, such as purchasing food and prescriptions. Likewise, clinicians need to attend to their many professional roles despite the constraints of competing demands for their time: they must not only assess patients but also discuss treatment options and facilitate decision-making, coordinate care, provide treatment, communicate with other team members, and attend to many other patients and other professional responsibilities. Difficulty managing the complexities of time management can not only lead to patient-related problems, such as pushing palliative and supportive care issues into the background, but also result in professional stress and burnout.

How does a clinician decide on the level of assessment of the cancer pain patient? Pragmatically, it is wisest to comprehensibly evaluate a patient at the first encounter, to the extent he/she is able to tolerate it. If necessary, the evaluation can be completed with more than one encounter. After that point, it should only be necessary to comprehensively re-evaluate if there is a major change in the clinical presentation.

The complete bedside evaluation of the patient with cancer pain includes five major components: history, physical examination, bedside provocative maneuvers, diagnosis formulation, and construction of an overall analgesic strategy.

PAIN HISTORY

Definition of Pain

Pain is defined as "an unpleasant sensory and emotional experience associated with actual or potential tissue damage, or described in terms of such damage."[19] Pain is always a subjective experience. Most nociception is mediated by nociceptors that are pain receptors found within visceral and somatic tissues. Nociceptors are present in most tissues in the body. There are some striking exceptions including most parts of the parenchyma of the central nervous system. Also, certain modalities of nociception cannot be sensed in certain parts of the body; for example, the stomach can sense stretch as an unpleasant sensation whereas when cauterized there is no pain sensation that results.

Presumably, all receptors within certain body parts will have been activated many times during a person's lifetime, such as nociceptors found in the nondominant thumb: pretty much everyone has hit their thumb with a hammer or some other blunt object, many times. Oddly, the majority of nociceptors throughout the body will never actually be activated during the entire lifetime of the individual. It should come as no surprise that patients describe their pain experience in a way that reflects their own uniqueness as a person and often, their unfamiliarity with the new pain experience.

Imagine the situation of a patient who has metastasis at the left C3 facet. Most people will never experience left C3 facet pain. The experience of nociceptors being discharged for the first time in a person's life can be puzzling, unpleasant, and difficult to describe. When experiencing a new, unfamiliar pain, patients may want to not use the word "pain" but instead use alternative descriptive words such as "discomfort," "unpleasant,","hurt," and others. The clinician should recognize that any unpleasant sensation may in fact be pain and should at all times support and legitimize the patient's experience.

Further, the pattern of pain referral may have gone unnoticed by the patient, particularly if the referred pain is less severe than the primary site of pain. If recognized, patterns of referral can greatly assist the identification of the underlying pain sensitive structure. Studies have evaluated the referral pattern in a range of tissues in many parts of the body, particularly nerves, connective tissues and ligaments, and muscles; mapping out the distribution of the resultant pain has resulted in construction of somatotopic maps. Clinicians are generally most familiar with the distribution of referred neuropathic pain along the corresponding dermatomes. *Sclerotomal pain* refers to the pattern of referred pain when the pain sensitive structure arises in connective tissues and ligaments. Stimulation of various muscles has resulted in similar although distinct patterns of referred pain, known as *myotomal pain*. Going back to the previous example of left C3 facet pain, this is a kind of sclerotomal pain and has a characteristic pattern of referral, felt draped laterally across the ipsilateral neck and projected rostrally toward the occipitonuchal junction.

Definition of Suffering

Suffering, as a human experience, needs to be distinguished from pain, per se, although the two are often interdependent: suffering is commonly present with pain and often increases as pain increases. There have been many insightful approaches to understanding suffering within the medical domain. One of the most widely accepted approaches describes suffering as a perceived threat to an individual's sense of intactness as a complete person.[20] If suffering is in part caused by pain, this definition speaks to the meaning that the person attributes to their pain. For example, at childbirth, intensity of labor pains commonly reaches 8 out of 10 or greater, and is often described as "horrible" on the McGill Categorical Scale. The sense of threat to a person's intactness as a human being during labor is generally believed to be less than the situation of pain of a similarly severe intensity caused by a life-threatening illness such as advanced cancer.

In Western countries, patients often conceptually link "pain and suffering" and may use the words interchangeably. In a comprehensive assessment of a patient with cancer pain, it is incumbent on the clinician to have an approach that is respectful of the patient's current circumstance. The clinician should not make assumptions about how much of the patient's distress is due to pain and how much is due to suffering. Remaining curious and empathic, the clinician works within the limitations of the comprehensive assessment in order to discover along with the patient as to how much of each is present, and how they might be related. There may be early clues about exigent pain as a major component of suffering: pain descriptors with a high affective component, such as "suffocating pain," have been found to predict the presence of suffering.[21]

Validated Assessment Tools

Many clinicians routinely use validated tools to support assessment of cancer patients, particularly to distinguish pain and suffering. There are several outstanding and widely used tools available. Some selected examples of the most largely used are as follows:

The Edmonton Symptom Assessment Scale, commonly referred to as the ESAS, includes 10 items: pain, tiredness, nausea, depression, anxiety, drowsiness, appetite, well-being, shortness of breath, and "other problem" (Fig. 41.1). Like many successfully applied clinical tools, it is short and has been extensively validated in a variety of countries and practice settings.

Edmonton Symptom Assessment System Graph
(ESAS)

Date																																			

Pain (10–0)

Tiredness (10–0)

Nausea (10–0)

Depression (10–0)

Anxiety (10–0)

Drowsiness (10–0)

Appetite (10–0)

Wellbeing (10–0)

Shortness of breath (10–0)

Other (10–0)

Mini-Mental (Normal _____)																																			
PPS																																			
Completed by																																			

P = patient
C = caregiver
A = caregiver-assisted

Level of Education _____

Cage Score _____

CH-0208 May 2001

FIGURE 41.1 Edmonton Symptom Assessment Scale. The full Edmonton Symptom Assessment Scale along with guidelines for its use are available at www.palliative.org. Follow the links to http://www.palliative.org/PC/ClinicalInfo/AssessmentTools/esas.pdf. The ESAS is also available in over two dozen other languages at http://www.cancercare.on.ca/index_2415.htm.   (*continues*)

Edmonton Symptom Assessment System:
Numerical Scale
Regional Palliative Care Program

Please circle the number that best describes:

No pain	0	1	2	3	4	5	6	7	8	9	10	Worst possible pain
Not tired	0	1	2	3	4	5	6	7	8	9	10	Worst possible tiredness
Not nauseated	0	1	2	3	4	5	6	7	8	9	10	Worst possible nausea
Not depressed	0	1	2	3	4	5	6	7	8	9	10	Worst possible depression
Not anxious	0	1	2	3	4	5	6	7	8	9	10	Worst possible anxiety
Not drowsy	0	1	2	3	4	5	6	7	8	9	10	Worst possible drowsiness
Best appetite	0	1	2	3	4	5	6	7	8	9	10	Worst possible appetite
Best feeling of wellbeing	0	1	2	3	4	5	6	7	8	9	10	Worst possible feeling of wellbeing
No shortness of breath	0	1	2	3	4	5	6	7	8	9	10	Worst possible shortness of breath
Other problem	0	1	2	3	4	5	6	7	8	9	10	

Patient's Name _____

Date _____ Time _____

Complete by (check one)
☐ Patient
☐ Caregiver
☐ Caregiver assisted

BODY DIAGRAM ON REVERSE SIDE

CH-0202 May 2001

FIGURE 41.1 (*continued*).

The ESAS has several strengths: it is not overly burdensome to fill out, it is an effective screening tool to identify distress due to symptoms, and it identifies symptom clusters (see below) which, if present, can make pain more difficult to manage.

The Edmonton Classification System is a tool that helps characterize pain prognosis (Fig. 41.2).

The Brief Pain Inventory, widely referred to as the BPI, deline-ates several aspects of the pain experience, including: worst pain in the past 24 hours, average pain in the past 24 hours, least pain in the past 24 hours, physical functioning, and emotional functioning. The BPI holds several advantages: it has been extensively validated, it assesses several specific dimensions of the pain experience, and it has been used for both research outcomes and for clinical care (Fig. 41.3).

Edmonton Classification System for Cancer Pain

Patient Name: _____

Patient ID No: _____

For each of the following features, circle the response that is most appropriate, based on your clinical assessment of the patient.

1.   Mechanism of Pain

No   **No** pain syndrome
Nc   Any **no**ciceptive combination of visceral and/or bone or soft tissue pain
Ne   **Ne**uropathic pain syndrome with or without any combination of nociceptive pain
Nx   Insufficient information to classify

2.   Incident Pain

Io   No incident pain
Ii   Incident pain present
Ix   Insufficient information to classify

3.   Psychological Distress

Po   No psychological distress
Pp   Psychological distress present
Px   Insufficient information to classify

4.   Addictive Behavior

Ao   No addictive behavior
Aa   Addictive behavior present
Ax   Insufficient information to classify

5.   Cognitive Function

Co   No impairment. Patient able to provide accurate present and past pain history unimpaired
Ci   Partial impairment. Sufficient impairment to affect patient's ability to provide accurate present and/or past pain history
Cu   Total impairment. Patient unresponsive, delirious or demented to the stage of being unable to provide any present and past pain history
Cx   Insufficient information to classify.

ECS-CP profile: N__ I__ P__ A__ C__   (combination of the five responses, one for each category)

Assessed by: _____   **Date:** _____

FIGURE 41.2 Edmonton Classification System. The Edmonton Classification System along with an Administration Manual are found at www.palliative.org. Follow the links to http://www.palliative.org/PC/ClinicalInfo/AssessmentTools/Edmonton%20Classification%20System%20for%20Cancer%20Pain%20(ECS-CP)%20Manual%2016%20Nov%2007%20doc.pdf.

STUDY ID #:__________ DO NOT WRITE ABOVE THIS LINE HOSPITAL #: __________

Brief Pain Inventory (Short Form)

Date: ____/____/____ Time: _______

Name: __________________ __________________ ______________

Last First Middle Initial

1. Throughout our lives, most of us have had pain from time to time (such as minor headaches, sprains, and toothaches). Have you had pain other than these every-day kinds of pain today?

   1. Yes 2. No

2. On the diagram, shade in the areas where you feel pain. Put an X on the area that hurts the most.

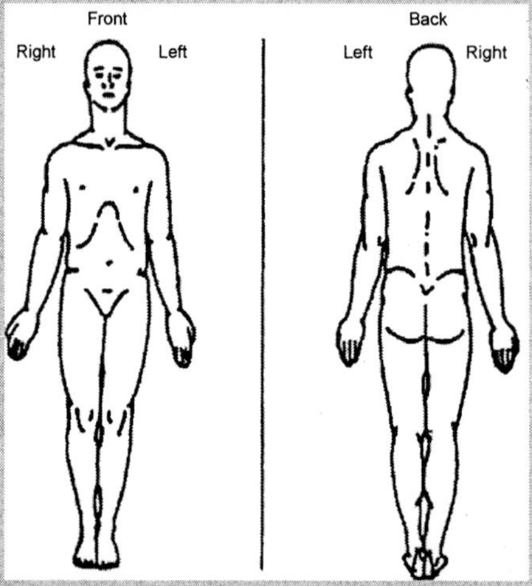

3. Please rate your pain by circling the one number that best describes your pain at its worst in the last 24 hours.

0	1	2	3	4	5	6	7	8	9	10
No Pain										Pain as bad as you can imagine

4. Please rate your pain by circling the one number that best describes your pain at its least in the last 24 hours.

0	1	2	3	4	5	6	7	8	9	10
No Pain										Pain as bad as you can imagine

5. Please rate your pain by circling the one number that best describes your pain on the average.

0	1	2	3	4	5	6	7	8	9	10
No Pain										Pain as bad as you can imagine

6. Please rate your pain by circling the one number that tells how much pain you have right now.

0	1	2	3	4	5	6	7	8	9	10
No Pain										Pain as bad as you can imagine

Page 1 of 2

FIGURE 41.3 Brief Pain Inventory. The Brief Pain Inventory is copyrighted. Permission to reproduce can be obtained from mdanderson.org/departments/prg/. The tool is available in over two dozen major languages.

(continues)

STUDY ID #:_____   DO NOT WRITE ABOVE THIS LINE   HOSPITAL #: _____

Date:____/____/____   Time:_____

Name:_____   _____   _____

　　　　　　Last　　　　　　　　　　First　　　　　　　Middle Initial

7.　What treatments or medications are you receiving for your pain?

8.　In the last 24 hours, how much relief have pain treatments or medications provided? Please circle the one percentage that most shows how much relief you have received.

0%	10%	20%	30%	40%	50%	60%	70%	80%	90%	100%
No Relief										Complete Relief

9.　Circle the one number that describes how, during the past 24 hours, pain has interfered with your:

A.　General Activity

0	1	2	3	4	5	6	7	8	9	10
Does not Interfere										Completely Interferes

B.　Mood

0	1	2	3	4	5	6	7	8	9	10
Does not Interfere										Completely Interferes

C.　Walking Ability

0	1	2	3	4	5	6	7	8	9	10
Does not Interfere										Completely Interferes

D.　Normal Work (includes both work outside the home and housework)

0	1	2	3	4	5	6	7	8	9	10
Does not Interfere										Completely Interferes

E.　Relations with other people

0	1	2	3	4	5	6	7	8	9	10
Does not Interfere										Completely Interferes

F.　Sleep

0	1	2	3	4	5	6	7	8	9	10
Does not Interfere										Completely Interferes

G.　Enjoyment of life

0	1	2	3	4	5	6	7	8	9	10
Does not Interfere										Completely Interferes

Page 2 of 2

FIGURE 41.3 *(continued)*

There are several other widely used screening tools to support assessment of cancer pain patients (see Chapter 20).

Types of Pain

Throughout the pain history, the clinician is looking for clues as to the underlying mechanism of pain. Because pain can be a foreign experience, it can be difficult to characterize in words. Patients sometimes appreciate being offered choices of words that might help describe their pain, such as burning, achy, dull, sharp, deep, and so on. Broadly, pain can be thought of as somatic, visceral, or neuropathic. The words the patient uses to describe their pain experience can guide the clinician to make inferences regarding the underlying mechanism.

Somatic pain arises from bone, muscle, ligament, subcutaneous tissue, or skin. It is often experienced as sharp or dull and is typically well localized by the patient. Less commonly, it can be referred to cutaneous sites characteristic of the tissue of origin, such as sclerotomal (connective tissue in origin) or myotomal (muscle) referred pain, as described above.

Visceral pain arises from organs such as lung, liver, or bowel and is broadly understood to arise from tissue that is embryologically mesodermal in origin. It is characteristically described as dull and achy and is usually poorly localized; typically the patient will use their entire hand to describe the location of the pain. Visceral pain is often also referred to distant sites, such as liver pain being experienced in the ipsilateral shoulder. Examination of the shoulder does not reproduce this pain.

Neuropathic pain is generally described as dull, achy, itchy, or burning. The skin can be sensitive to light touch ("allodynia")[19] and there may be brief stabbing episodes of neuralgic pain. The burning may be superficial as in the experience of scalded skin or can be deep, as if there is a feeling of having been burned deep inside. The spontaneous use of the word "burning" by the patient predicts the presence of neuropathic pain. However, the clinician should be cautious: several other pains can also be experienced as an unpleasant, burning sensation, such as muscle spasm pain—a kind of somatic pain.[22] Combinations of words, such as "burning numbness," and clinical findings such as hypesthesia, anesthesia, hyperalgesia, or allodynia in a segmental pattern within an area of pain, are of greater value in making the clinical diagnosis of neuropathic pain. For example, neuropathic pain should be diagnosed if there is significant clinical evidence such as a description of burning numbness along with tingling experienced in a distribution consistent with damage to a particular part of the nervous system; there may also be signs of motor dysfunction such as the loss of deep tendon reflexes (e.g., ankle or knee jerks) or muscle weakness; there may be bedside provocative maneuvers that reproduce the pain, such as the presence of a Tinel's sign or a positive straight leg raise maneuver. The clinician should be wary of making a diagnosis of neuropathic pain based solely on the patient's description of "burning pain," although this is an important clue to initiate further investigations.

Mixed pain is the clinical situation where there is both nociceptive (i.e., somatic and/or visceral) and neuropathic pain. A common example is chest wall pain from lung cancer; there may be poorly localized deep ache consistent with visceral (pleural) pain, sharp and well-localized somatic pain from contiguous rib invasion, and burning numbness of the overlying skin due to invasion of intercostal nerves. The term *mixed pain* has less commonly been applied to the situation of multiple mechanisms of somatic pain in the same patient—for example, painful metastasis to the humerus with contiguous muscle spasm and shoulder joint articular changes because of immobility of the painful limb. Mixed pain may benefit greatly from multiple modalities of analgesic intervention, such as simple analgesics (acetaminophen or anti-inflammatories), opioids, adjuvant analgesics in specific pain syndromes, and nondrug interventions such as heat, cold, stretch, massage, or orthotic interventions such as a joint-immobilizing splint.

Teasing out the many components of pain in the region of the body where the patient is experiencing pain will help the clinician to develop a more comprehensive approach to managing the pain and is therefore an essential part of the comprehensive pain assessment.

Presenting Complaint

The presenting complaint of the pain should contain four elements: onset, progression, focality, and accompaniments. Once the patient assessment has been completed, these four elements can be summarized in a single sentence and often represent a thumbprint of the underlying mechanism of pain.

Pain Onset

Patients are understandably often keen to tell you how long the pain has been severe. In order to characterize the nature of the underlying process, however, it is critical to also delineate the onset of pain: the time from when the pain first ever began until it became as bad as it was going to get (Table 41.1). Broadly, cancer pain unfolds in three different ways: it may have an onset of less than a day, days to weeks, or months in duration. Be wary of the tendency of pain to fluctuate, with good days and bad days, or good weeks or bad weeks; behind this background noise is the true onset of how the pain developed over time. As a guideline, pain that takes less than one day to become as bad as it is going to get is often vascular in origin. An example of this is an acute thigh hematoma from trauma to the leg or pain from hemorrhage into a site of metastasis. Pain that takes between a day and a month to reach its peak often has an inflammatory mechanism, such as a subcutaneous abscess, with each day being worse than the previous. Pain that is worse month after month, pain that is chronic, progressive, and focal, is most consistent with a diagnosis of cancer. These are only general guidelines, and there are many exceptions. However, delineating the onset of the pain, the time from when it began until it reaches its peak, can be an important clue regarding the nature of the underlying diagnosis.

Pain Progression

There are only a few common patterns of how cancer pain progresses over time. Once it has commenced, cancer pain is typically progressive and usually this progression occurs over months. A second pattern of pain is fluctuating, such as pain that is worse with standing because of metastasis to weight-bearing bone, pain worse with bladder emptying due to cancer invading the detrusor muscle, and pain that is worse at night and relieved by pacing, a classical description of pain experienced with epidural spinal cord compression. Back pain that gets worse with lying down is especially cause for concern about neuraxial tumor involvement. A third pattern of pain progression is pain that is improving: it began, peaked, and is now getting better or has resolved. This temporal profile is consistent with an underlying mechanism of pain that has been effectively treated, such as successful radiation treatment of an area of metastasis. A fourth temporal profile is intermittent episodes of pain. This temporal profile of pain can be incapacitating and can often be effectively managed with specific interventions. One example is a patient with neuropathic pain who has constant, deep, achy pain in the affected dermatome and also has superimposed spells of brief stabbing episodes of neuralgic pain. This pain is characteristically electrical in character, peaks instantly, and lasts seconds. Neuralgic pain commonly improves dramatically with anticonvulsant agents such as gabapentin, pregabalin, or carbamazepine. Another example of intermittent episodes of pain is the patient with baseline achy neuro-

TABLE 41.1

FORMULATING A PAIN PRESENTING COMPLAINT

Domain	Onset of symptoms	Progression	Focality	Accompaniments
Description	Time until peak of symptoms	Pattern of unfolding over time	Right or left; what region of the body	Symptoms that suggest what system is involved
Categories and examples	Less than a day —typically a vascular process —bleeding into a tumor —arterial embolus Between 1 day and 1 month —typically an inflammatory process —infected cancer wound —shingles pain More than 1 month —chronic, progressive and focal: likely cancer. Example: progressive neck pain due to bone metastasis —chronic, progressive and diffuse: likely toxic or degenerative. Example: peripheral neuropathy pain	Sudden and unchanging —typical of trauma Began, peaked, and now improving or resolved: —a typical monophasic course of a painful area successfully treated, such as following radiation therapy Relapsing and remitting: —a relapsing and remitting condition such as multiple sclerosis or change in lymphoma pain with steroids; Spells: —neuralgic pains are brief, electrical stabs of pain lasting seconds —seizures	Head and neck Chest Shoulder and arm Abdomen Pelvis Back Buttock and leg	Cardiac (palpitations); Pulmonary (shortness of breath, cough); Upper GI (nausea or pain on eating); Urinary (cardiac or pulmonary); Small or large bowel diarrhea or constipation Urinary (hematuria) Neurologic (confusion) Endocrine (hypoglycemia)

pathic pain with superimposed brief episodes of burning pain in the skin precipitated by light touch: allodynia.[19] Allodynia is a strong predictor of the presence of underlying neuropathic pain, and once the diagnosis is made, there are several analgesic interventions that can be effective.

Focality

In what region of the body is the pain being experienced? The medical approach to the cancer patient involves a systems approach, such as the respiratory system, the cardiac system, and so on, but it is also important to assess where pain is experienced because of referral sites away from the organ involved or due to the presence of painful distant metastases. There are several ways to classify regional pains. A simple approach is to describe seven regions of the body: head and neck, chest, shoulder and arm, abdomen, pelvis, back, and the buttock and leg region. There is commonly overlap, such as the patient who has back pain, buttock pain, and leg pain. In considering the patient who has pain in a certain region of the body, it encourages the clinician to be mindful of all potentially pain sensitive structures that could result in the experience of pain in that part of the body. The following pain history exemplifies this phenomenon.

A 47-year-old premenopausal woman presented to her oncologist with a 3 month history of progressive back pain. Two months ago, the pain progressed down the right leg into the foot, in association with tingling and loss of sensation in a distribution similar to the pain. She had a prior history of breast cancer with 3 of 12 nodes positive, treated with surgery followed by radiation therapy, chemotherapy, and was currently on aromatase inhibitors.
The regional pain exam revealed marked local spine tenderness including paraspinal muscle spasm that reproduced her back pain. Also, there were signs of active right L5 radiculopathy, including an unequivocally positive ipsilateral straight-leg raise maneuver (neuropathic pain in the right leg below the knee). An MRI of the spine revealed evidence of a large right lateral herniated L4–L5 disc and no evidence of cancer.

The presenting complaint of this cancer patient helped focus the rest of the history and the regional pain examination toward diagnoses—cancer and noncancer—that can cause chronic, progressive back pain and unilateral neurologic trouble in a leg.

Symptoms That Accompany Pain

Are there other symptoms that accompany the pain? They can be a strong indicator of the underlying disease process. Typical examples could be chest pain with breathlessness and cough, episodes of chest pain associated with palpitations, or deep achy chest pain associated with nausea after eating, a 30 pound weight loss, and dysphagia over 3 months (see Table 41.1). The symptoms that accompany the pain are a clue as to the underlying system that is involved in the disease process. Often, these other symptoms will unfold in a similar temporal profile of the underlying pain.

Formulating the Presenting Complaint

Integrating these four elements of the pain presenting complaint together within a single sentence—pain onset, progression, focality, and accompaniments—can bring clarity to an otherwise complex clinical presentation, even if the clinician has never encountered the situation previously.

A 68-year-old man presented with a 1-year history (onset) of progressive (progression) left lateral abdominal wall and flank (focality) deep ache, burning numbness of overlying skin, and a 30 pound weight loss (accompaniments).

This pain syndrome is neuropathic and potentially also visceral. This perplexing presenting complaint suggests cancer of the left flank area, as the pain is chronic, progressive, and focal. The differential diagnosis includes diabetic abdominal wall neuropathy, a rare diabetic neuropathy typically encountered in adults with early onset, mild diabetes. There are other possible causes of this presenting complaint, but postherpetic neuralgia is not likely if the presenting complaint is accurate: being inflammatory, shingles pain typically has a subacute onset, becoming maximal within days of its first appearance. This particular patient was not known to have cancer, and all investigations at the time of presentation were negative. Pain was controlled with opioids and adjuvant analgesics, and he was given appointments for follow-up computed tomography (CT) scans of the abdomen every 3 months for a year. At 9 months, he developed CT findings consistent with a left adrenal metastasis and retroperitoneal lymphadenopathy, and after biopsy demonstrating metastatic adenocarcinoma, palliative radiation therapy was effective to relieve pain. This is an example of a presenting complaint that was strongly suggestive of the underlying mechanism of pain.

Details of the Pain History

Since pain is a subjective experience, it is essential to obtain from the patient a description of the experience of pain, including the amount of pain. There is strong evidence that estimates of a patient's pain are often inaccurate; health care providers tend to underestimate pain,[23] and family caregivers often overestimate pain.[24] The input of surrogates should take second place to direct input of the patient's own experience. Estimating how much pain a patient is in, based on their facial expression or other indicators, should be approached with great caution, although behavioral cues may be the only way to assess pain in a non–self-reporting patient.

Further, extensive research evidence has indicated that there are ways to inquire of a patient that are more likely than others to get a response from the patient that is valid, reliable, and reproducible. A widely used approach is to ask the patient how much pain they are experiencing on a scale of 0 to 10, if 0 is "no pain" and 10 is the "worst pain possible." This approach has been broadly adopted within health care institutions. The clinician needs to be wary of the uncommon circumstance where the numeric rating scale turns out to be less reliable. One is delirium, a syndrome of fluctuating encephalopathy commonly encountered in cancer patients before death or in association with concurrent acute illness. When delirium is known to be present, it is appropriate to ask the patient how much pain they are experiencing using the 10 point numeric scale and record their answer, but also one should record that they have delirium. In this setting and any other settings where there is any doubt of the reliability of the patient's description, an additional method to quantify pain intensity should be used to confirm their description. A highly reliable, valid, and reproducible scale is the McGill categorical scale.[21] One asks the patient if they would describe their pain as none, mild, discomforting, distressing, horrible, or excruciating. If there is any question to the reliability of the patient's description, it is best to keep the questions simple and dichotomous, for example, "Is your pain bad, or not bad?" The more ways one poses the question, the more confident the clinician can be about the interpretation of the patient's response.

A detailed description of the many facets of the pain experience is described in detail in Chapter 20. In cancer pain, clinicians often ask the patient about their present pain intensity (on a scale of 0–10), the worst pain experienced in the past 24 hours, the least pain experienced in the past 24 hours, and the average pain.

If the patient is struggling to find words to describe their pain, the clinician should be supportive and encouraging, offering words to the patient such as burning, sharp, or crushing. If the patient spontaneously offers a word with a strong affective component, such as "suffocating" pain, the clinician should inquire about comorbidities such as concurrent dyspnea, but also recognize the possibility that such affectively loaded words may signal a more global sense of suffering. This requires further inquiry and evaluation.[21]

After delineating the intensity of the pain and the description of the pain, the clinician should find out, in detail, what part(s) of the body are affected and what the characteristics of the pain are throughout these locations. A differential description of discrete pains within the same region of the body can give a clue to as to the underlying mechanism. For example, patients with malignant brachial plexopathy often describe several different pains. There is often a deep achy, poorly localized discomfort draped over the ipsilateral shoulder, with burning pain and tingling in the ipsilateral lateral hand. There can also be pain with light touching of the area of numbness in the affected arm (allodynia), and superimposed spontaneous episodes of brief stabbing electrical pain in the arm, experienced as single jabs or brief trains (volleys) of pain. If present for several months, patients can develop pain from frozen shoulder or other articular or myofascial complications of immobility of the affected shoulder girdle region. All of these discrete pains can be elicited and described by the patient during the pain history.

The clinician then focuses on the experience of pain over time: what makes it better and what makes it worse. In particular, one seeks a description of the change of pain over time with medication (i.e., pharmacodynamics). Typically, one would expect there would be relief of pain beginning about one half hour after swallowing a short-acting opioid, peaking at approximately 60–90 minutes, and then it would wear out sometime thereafter. If the duration of analgesia is too brief (in this case less than 4 hours after taking a short acting opioid), the patient probably has end of dose failure. Identifying this phenomenon can guide the clinician to estimate the extent to which the patient is undermedicated.

Next, construct a detailed list of all prescription and nonprescription medications the patient has taken; the patient or family should be encouraged to look through the medication cabinet for all pills. The list should include the names of medications, the maximum dose that was taken, the duration that the maximum dose was taken, with what effect and what toxicity (Table 41.2). The goal is to be as confident as possible that the patient has completed an adequate trial of each of these medications and if they did not have an adequate trial, one then can consider re-embarking on a trial of that medication in a more thorough manner. By the end of this description, the clinician should have a clear understanding what sequential trials of analgesics and combination of analgesics the patient has had over time.

Depending upon the patient's past history and current social circumstances, it may be appropriate to apply certain chemical misuse/abuse/dependency risk tools, such as the CAGE (Table 41.3)or the Opioid Risk Tool (ORT). Stratifying risk allows for a structured approach to pharmacotherapy that is tailored to each patient's particular circumstances.

The clinician should also seek information about other risk factors for poor pain prognosis. This includes any history of psychiatric disorder, the presence of breakthrough pain, neuropathic pain, other psychosocial stressors, use of high dose opioids without satisfactory pain control or excessive adverse effects, and the presence of significant interference of function by pain. Interference of function refers to pain interfering with physical functions such as sleep, activities of daily living, work and social functioning, such as a parenting role, sexual relations, and emotional functioning, such as ability to engage meaningfully with those around them and ability to cope.

The clinician then embarks on a detailed medical and psychosocial history. The medical history involves a review of systems such as respiratory, cardiovascular, GI, genitourinary, musculoskeletal, dermatological, neurological, and endocrine. There is a high risk of comorbidity with particular patterns of systems dysfunction in specific cancers. An example is the high prevalence of underlying respiratory disease in a patient who has a tobacco-related malignancy or a lengthy history of tobacco use.

The elements of a psychosocial history have been described elsewhere in this book (Chapter 21).

TABLE 41.2

LIST OF MEDICATIONS TAKEN FOR PAIN

Patient name _____

Today's date _____

Name of Medication	Start Date	End Date	Maximum Daily Dose (in milligrams)	What Benefit	Side Effects	Comments

PHYSICAL EXAMINATION

The pain physical exam includes a general physical exam, a regional pain exam, more specific neurological examination guided by history, and bedside provocative maneuvers.

General Physical Examination

The general examination of the cancer patient includes a brief screening physical exam including vital signs, head and neck, respiratory system, cardiovascular system, the abdominal exam, genitourinary exam including rectal exam (as appropriate to the clinical circumstance), musculoskeletal exam, peripheral vascular exam, neurologic exam, and dermatologic exam. Particular attention is paid to document the extent of underlying malignancy; patients presenting with cancer pain may have a greater extent of disease than was previously suspected, so the clinician needs to examine the patient with a view toward stigmata of underlying organ disease.

The Regional Pain Physical Examination

The clinician approaches the regional pain examination as guided by the pain history. This approach complements but does not replace the more traditional systems approach to the physical examination described above. Seven regions of the body are: head and neck, chest, shoulder girdle and arm, abdomen, back, pelvis, and buttock and leg (Table 41.4). For example, if the patient describes pain in the head and neck, a regional pain exam is done of that part of the body. The clinician pays particular attention to look for evidence of underlying disease in that region, which may be vascular, infectious, or neoplastic in origin. The clinician looks for evidence of degenerative neck disease, with reduced range of motion of the neck, neurologic disease with ptosis suggesting ipsilateral cancer in the low cervical spine, vascular disease such as carotid artery or vertebral artery bruit, palpable muscle spasm, and other signs of an underlying pathological process.

Bedside Provocative Maneuvers

The bedside provocative maneuvers are an important part of the pain physical exam. The goal is to gently reproduce the patient's pain complaint(s). If the clinician successfully reproduces the pain, the patient may be relieved, having their subjective complaints validated. As described above, since pain is a subjective experience, often patients have the sense that others do not appreciate how serious their pain is. If the clinician is able to reproduce the pain, the patient may believe that the clinician has confirmed that it exists. Further, if the clinician is able to localize, or "touch" the pain, the patient may have greater confidence the pain can be relieved. For the clinician, being able to reproduce the pain provides insight into the underlying mechanisms or pain-sensitive structures.

For each of the seven regions of the body, there is a list of regional bedside provocative maneuvers (Table 41.5). For example, in the situation of a patient who presents with head and neck pain, the clinician would first do a general physical exam and then a regional pain exam in order to look for underlying disease processes. After this time, the clinician would systematically embark on bedside provocative maneuvers. This would include neck range of motion in six directions, including an evaluation for meningismus, palpation of the skin, assessing for allodynia, and deep palpation of underlying tissues. One continues to palpate more deeply trying to identify areas of myofascial pain or muscle spasm. One looks at typical tender points[25] and also areas that commonly develop muscle spasm in response to disease, such as the paraspinal muscles. Muscle tenderness can be sought throughout the neck, the face, the jaw, and other areas. The clinician

TABLE 41.3

CAGE TEST TO SCREEN FOR ALCOHOLISM

> **Please check the one response to each item that best describes how you have felt and behaved over your whole life.**
>
> 1. Have you ever felt you should *cut* down on your drinking?
> 2. Have people *annoyed* you by criticizing your drinking?
> 3. Have you ever felt bad or *guilty* about your drinking?
> 4. Have you ever had a drink first thing in the morning to steady your nerves or get rid of a hangover (*eye-opener*)?

TABLE 41.4

A REGIONAL APPROACH TO THE PAIN PHYSICAL EXAMINATION

Region	Syndrome	Examples of pain sensitive structures
Head and neck	somatic visceral neuropathic	paraspinal muscles focal neck myofascial pain occipitonuchal junction dentition sinuses periorbital area bone: base of skull, facial carotids orbits cervical radiculopathy
Shoulder and Arm	somatic visceral neuropathic	shoulder joint ligamentous muscle axilla apex of lung radicular pain referred from neck brachial plexus
Chest	somatic visceral neuropathic mixed pain	parietal pleura vertebral body visceral pleura thoracic nerve root chest wall: rib, muscle, nerve intradural lesion
Abdomen and Flank	somatic visceral neuropathic	flank muscle rib referred from vertebral body intra-abdominal: liver, hollow viscus, peritoneum kidney, adrenals retroperitoneal structure: pancreas intercostals nerve or intradural lesion
Back and Buttocks	somatic visceral neuropathic	bone: vertebral body, sacrum, bony pelvis paraspinal muscle cauda equina; nerve root; plexus presacral region, peritoneum cauda equina, nerve root, plexus, intercostals nerve
Pelvis	somatic visceral neuropathic	bony pelvis introitus ovaries, uterus plexus, pudendal nerve
Leg and Foot	somatic visceral neuropathic	bone: pelvis, femur, tibia muscle: gluteus, obturator ligament: insertion of biceps joint: hip, sacroiliac presacral area cauda equina, nerve root, plexus, nerve

should put on a glove and palpate the masseter musculature as well as posterior pharyngeal examination of the pterygoid muscles. Following this, bone structures should be systematically examined by palpation and percussion, including the orbit, the skull, the occipital condyle, and then down the cervical spine. Next palpate the carotid arteries (gently), the orbits, and the sinuses. Other bedside provocative maneuvers can be performed based on the clinical situation. The clinician should approach bedside provocative maneuvers as a sleuth, looking for evidence that will rule in or rule out various pain sensitive structures as being the source of the pain. Further detail on pain caused by cancer of the head and neck and oral mucositis is covered in Chapter 45.

Specific Bedside Provocative Maneuvers and Their Role in Pain Diagnosis

Spurling's Test

Spurling's test of the cervical spine is performed if there is concern the patient might have active cervical nerve root compression. It

TABLE 41.5

EXAMPLES OF BEDSIDE PROVOCATIVE MANEUVERS

Region	Structure	Provocative maneuver	Finding

Head and Neck	skin
	paraspinal muscle
	bone
	occipitonuchal
	  junction
	neck range of motion
	Spurling's maneuver
		wave hand over skin
		pinprick
		cold temperature
		gentle palpation
		gentle palpation of spinous
		  processes; deeper palpation over
		  vertebral bodies
		gentle palpation
		patient moves neck in six
		  directions
		patient laterally flexes or laterally
		  flexes and laterally rotates neck
		  (see Fig. 41.4)
			allodynia
			hyperpathia
			cold allodynia
			palpable paraspinal spasm
			tenderness
			tenderness
			pain; limited range of motion
			neuropathic pain or other
			  neuropathic symptoms or signs

Shoulder and Arm	shoulder girdle
	brachial plexus
	axilla
		active range of motion of shoulder
		passive range of motion of
		  shoulder
		examination for tender areas
		gentle percussion over Erb's point
		  in the supraclavicular fossa
		palpation
			pain
			tenderness; reduced range of
			  motion (e.g., frozen shoulder)
			bicipital tendonitis
			Tinel's sign positive tenderness

Chest	subcutaneous tissue spine	gently pinch skin palpation; percussion	unilateral lymphedema tenderness

Abdomen and Flank	organs
	abdominal wall
	retroperitoneal
	  structures (e.g.,
	  pancreas)
		gentle then deep palpation, at rest
		  then with inspiration
		Carnett's Maneuver
		Retroperitoneal stretch maneuver
		  (Fig. 41.5)
			tenderness
			worse with tension of abdominal
			  muscles (see Fig. 41.6)
			thoracic spine is not tender but
			  back pain arises with
			  retroperitoneal stretch

Back	vertebral body
	sacroiliac joint
	hips
		spine palpation and percussion
		gently press thumb into sacroiliac
		  joint
		flexion, abduction, internal then
		  external rotation; palpate hip
		  joint; palpate trochanteric bursae
			tenderness
			tenderness
			tenderness; limited range of
			  motion

Pelvis	pelvic organs rectum	internal examination rectal examination	tenderness tenderness

Buttock and Leg	low lumbar and sacral
	  nerve roots
	upper and mid lumbar
	  nerve roots
		straight leg raise maneuver
		crossed straight leg maneuver
		reverse straight leg raise maneuver
			ipsilateral neuropathic pain
			  below the knee with other
			  neurologic symptoms
			ipsilateral neuropathic pain
			  below the knee with other
			  neurologic symptoms
			ipsilateral neuropathic pain in the
			  anterior thigh with other
			  neurologic symptoms

is analogous to the straight leg raise maneuver that detects active lumbosacral radiculopathy (see below). Spurling's test consists of gentle lateral flexion of the neck for about 1 minute toward the side of the pain, followed by lateral flexion of the neck for about 1 minute away from the side of the pain. A variation is lateral flexion plus lateral rotation of the neck ("throw your ear over your shoulder"), for 1 minute to one side and then to the other. The test is positive if it results in neuropathic pain, tingling, or numbness below the elbow or loss of a previously present arm reflex such as a triceps reflex. The side and nerve root distribution of the arm pain or other neurologic impairment localizes the site of the mass that is pushing on the thecal space. Some reports have recommended axial loading be undertaken at the same time

as lateral flexion and rotation (the examiner pushes down on the top of the head).[26] We do not recommend that approach for cancer patients as there may be bone destruction and the test could be dangerous. Spurling's test can be particularly helpful to distinguish malignant brachial plexopathy (in which case the maneuver is almost invariably negative) from spinal cord compression in the cervical spine (in which case the maneuver is often positive) (Fig. 41.4). The procedure should not be undertaken if baseline pain is severe until radiographs or other imaging studies confirm that the neck is mechanically stable. Positive and negative predictive values for the test have been described for active cervical radiculopathy from benign disease but not for cancer.[26]

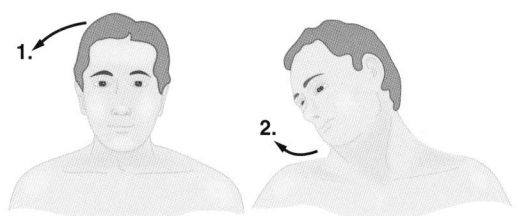

FIGURE 41.4 Spurling's test.

Dermatomal Pain

At some point, the clinician is likely to encounter an area of tenderness with pain referred to a distant site. Clinicians are familiar with dermatomal pain or radicular pain, such as L5 nerve root pain cause by a herniation of the L5–S1 disc. This pain can be provoked by a straight leg raise maneuver. The straight leg raise maneuver is a validated bedside provocative maneuver that has been carefully tested in a range of clinical situations, disease types and ages, and with a range of specific techniques to perform the test.[27] L5 radicular pain is felt down the ipsilateral buttock into the posterior part of the thigh and down the posterolateral leg into the dorsal or dorsolateral foot.

Sclerotomal Pain

There are other mechanisms for pain that may appear strikingly similar to dermatomal pain, including sclerotomal pain. A common example of sclerotomal referred pain is pain referred from the sacroiliac joint. The bedside provocative maneuver is to gently place the thumb in the sacroiliac joint and press with a few kilograms of pressure. The positive maneuver reproduces the ipsilateral paraspinal and low back pain the patient has been having. Referred sclerotomal pain goes down the ipsilateral posterior buttock and lateral leg into the ipsilateral ankle. L5 radicular pain and ipsilateral sacroiliac pain can occur in the same patient. This confusing clinical scenario may arise in a patient with active lumbosacral radiculopathy due to disc protrusion. Presumably the sacroiliac pain is a consequence of biomechanical changes that occur in a patient who is limping because of pain from the active radiculopathy. Eventually, the stress on the ipsilateral sacroiliac joint is such that it too starts to hurt. The patient may ultimately have a surgical procedure to remove herniated disc material. However, the sacroiliac pain can persist, leaving the patient with a wrong impression that the surgery was a failure. This clinical situation raises the complexity of regional pain, whereby there can be several interdependent mechanisms of pain in the same region of the body. Teasing out the various components of that regional pain will allow the clinician to direct therapeutic interventions at each.

Myotomal Pain

A third kind of referred pain is myotomal pain: pain that arises from muscles. Referred myotomal pain is generally not a great distance from the irritated muscle. One example of myotomal pain that is diagnosed based on a bedside provocative maneuver is pyriformus syndrome. In cancer patients, myotomal pain is generally not a major direct cause of referred pain, but it can occur in a similar manner as sclerotomal pain resulting from secondary mechanical dysfunction.

Myofascial Pain: How Hard Should You Press?

Myofascial pain is a term that can be used to describe specific myofascial tender point sites[25] or can be used as a more generic term for regional pain of muscular origin that is not due to primary pathology in the muscle. Myofascial pain is common in

cancer pain patients, and it can mimic other types of pathology. Identifying its presence can lead to specific therapeutic interventions, such as heat, stretch, cold and massage, trigger point injections, or regional blockade, and it is therefore important to make the diagnosis when possible. Separate from regional myofascial pain, rheumatologists have defined the systemic condition fibromyalgia in part by a series of bedside provocative maneuvers palpating for tenderness in specific areas, applying an amount of pressure that would not normally be uncomfortable. All patients experience muscle tenderness if the examiner presses hard enough. Research in muscle tenderness has identified that most commonly muscles do not hurt when the examiner presses with up to 4 kilograms of pressure using the thumb. The clinician can use a baby weigh scale to become familiar with what represents 4 kilograms or can use a bedside dolorimeter, which is a bedside tool meant to gauge how hard one is pressing. Fibromyalgia is defined through the patient's history and testing for myofascial tenderness using a standardized methodology, with the finding of at least 11 of 18 typical tender point sites. The bedside diagnosis is accurate, with a sensitivity of 88.4% and a specificity of 81.1%.[25] The bedside exam of the cancer patient, looking for regional myofascial pain unrelated to fibromyalgia, is best undertaken with a similar technique.

Back Pain

In approaching the bedside examination of the patient with back pain, the clinician needs to pay particular attention to be gentle. In examining the spine, one would first palpate in the area where the patient describes the worst pain. Push very gently, with less than a kilogram of pressure on the palpating finger on the area of the worst pain and the broad area around it, looking for paraspinal muscle spasm. If negative, one can palpate with more pressure. There are some situations where a patient appears to have severe back pain and yet the regional pain exam demonstrates that the spine is completely aligned and there is neither spinal tenderness nor palpable paraspinal muscle spasm. How can there be severe back pain but not back tenderness? Retroperitoneal tumor can cause lumbar or thoracic regional pain where there is no tenderness with even deep percussion. There may be a suggestion that the patient has a retroperitoneal cause of back pain based on the patient's posture as you enter the examination room: the patient may have adopted a so-called pain-relieving posture, such as sitting on the bed with the knees folded up into the chest. This posture results in lumbar kyphosis and subsequent relief of pain from a retroperitoneal pain-sensitive structure.

Retroperitoneal Pain Stretch Maneuver

In order to diagnose a retroperitoneal source of back pain, have the patient sit upright in the bed with the legs stretched out. This is best done in a bed in which the back of the bed can be elevated. Place a pillow into the small of the back so there is moderate thoracolumbar lordosis, and have the patient lay back down in the bed. Gently lower the back of the bed so the patient goes toward a supine direction (Fig. 41.5). Retroperitoneal tumor can cause severe back pain and is reproduced with this maneuver. Oddly, it can take a few minutes for the pain to become fully apparent as the bed is lowered and the spine is extended. The history will commonly give a suggestion that this sign may be present because the patient may describe back pain upon laying flat, with the patient having thereafter sought sleep in a recliner.

Abdominal Wall Pain

The abdominal wall is frequently a source of pain and how to examine it has been less clearly defined than examination of underlying abdominal structures. Abdominal wall pain is a common mechanism of severe idiopathic abdominal pain.[28,29] It also can be a long term sequela of abdominal surgery such as hernia repair,

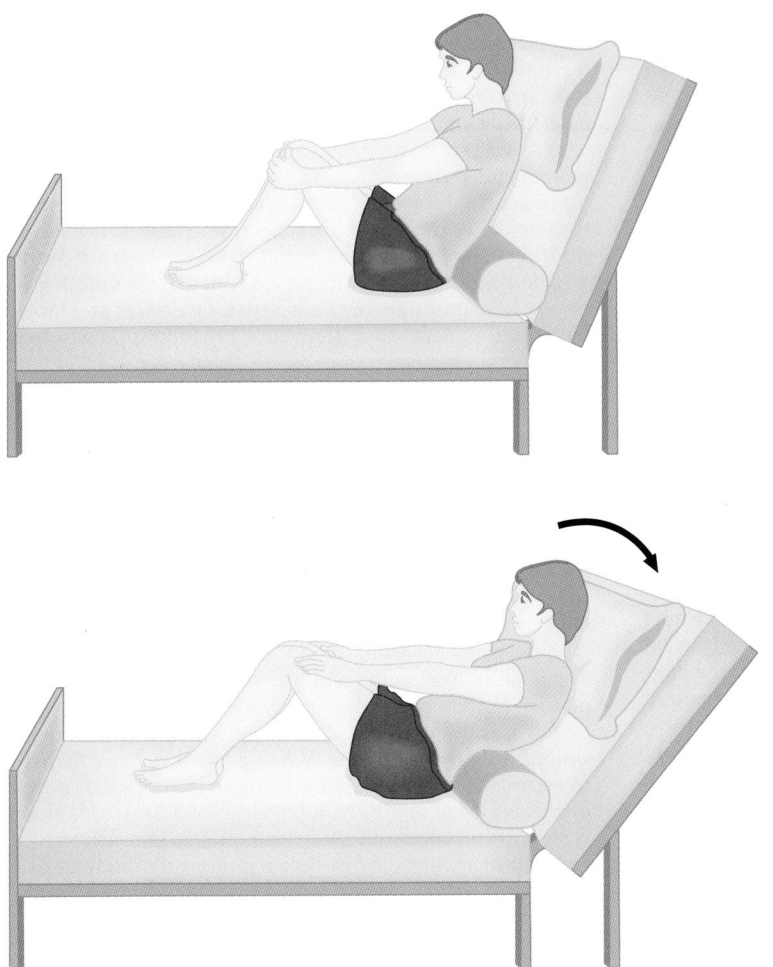

FIGURE 41.5 Retroperitoneal stretch maneuver.

open cholecystectomy, etc.[30] The distinction between an underlying and medically serious intra-abdominal source of pain from a benign abdominal wall source of pain is made through a bedside provocative test, Carnett's maneuver.

Carnett's maneuver: The patient is found to be tender upon gentle palpation, typically in the left or right lower quadrant (Fig. 41.6). If the patient tenses the abdominal wall, such as by lifting both legs a few centimeters in the air or lifting the shoulders off the bed, an inflamed visceral organ is protected from the palpating hand. Alternatively, if the pain-sensitive structure is within the abdominal wall, such as caused by a myofascial trigger point, a neuroma, a hematoma, or some other cause, pain becomes markedly worse with tensing of the abdominal wall during palpation.

Another cryptic cause of abdominal wall pain can be neuropathic pain. This can be caused by cancer invading intercostal muscles, from retroperitoneal tumor, from diabetic abdominal wall neuropathy, shingles, and other mechanisms. There are several bedside provocative maneuvers that can diagnose abdominal wall neuropathic pain. First, gently touch the normal side and then the abnormal side with a cold object, then a piece of cotton, then a pin (see Table 41.5). If any of these normally non-noxious stimuli results in pain, the patient likely has abdominal neuropathic wall pain. Sensitivity to temperature, touch, or pinprick can be one of the most dramatic bedside signs in the pain physical examination and is strong evidence of the presence of underlying neuropathic pain. The abnormal sensation can linger for up to a minute or longer, so called "after sensation." Abdominal wall neuropathic pain can be accompanied by numbness or loss of abdominal wall muscle tone.[31]

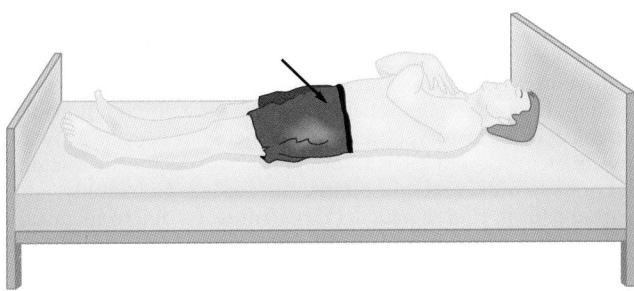

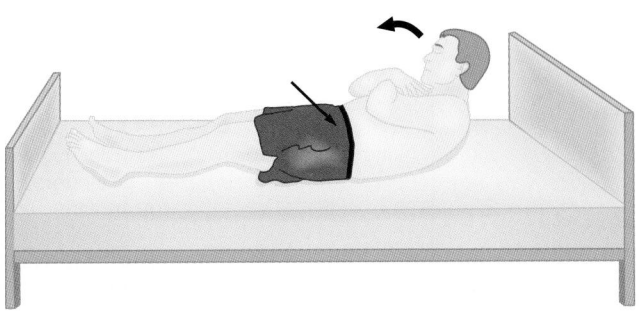

FIGURE 41.6 Carnett's maneuver.

FORMULATING A CANCER PAIN DIAGNOSIS

Syndrome Diagnosis

While it can be tempting for the clinician to make a specific diagnosis as to the underlying cause of the pain, it may be wiser to begin with a more general syndrome diagnosis. Broadly, pain can be classified into somatic, visceral, neuropathic, or mixed syndromes. Diagnosing the pain syndrome based on the characteristics, the pattern of referral, the accompaniment, and the provocative maneuvers can make it more likely that the clinician will consider a broad differential diagnosis.

The use of the taxonomy of somatic, visceral, and neuropathic pain syndromes can be challenged by closer scrutiny of their pathophysiologic basis. For example, some peripheral nerves are themselves pain sensitive structures, being innervated by nociceptors. In addition, other aspects of neuropathic pain can be nonnociceptive, that is, pain generated by a damaged nervous system. Thus, when the peripheral nervous system is invaded by cancer, there can be both nociceptive and non-nociceptive pain. A common clinical scenario is malignant brachial plexopathy. The nociceptive component generated by nociceptors within the brachial plexus is pain draped over the ipsilateral shoulder; the nonnociceptive component of the pain is commonly burning pain in the ipsilateral, numb hand. An example of a central generator of neuropathic pain is poststroke thalamic pain. Central pain caused by brain metastases is extraordinarily uncommon and may relate to the long period of time it takes for central pain to develop. However, the taxonomy remains of clinical value, and a more complex version is described in Table 41.6.

There are other causes of pain which appear nociceptive in characteristic but have a non-nociceptive mechanism. Pain purely or mostly of psychologic origin (often inappropriately termed psychogenic pain) is extraordinarily rare in the cancer population and must be used cautiously as it can either take the focus away from other equally or more important causes of pain or might stigmatize the patient as being less than genuine, truthful, or trustworthy. For this reason, the term psychogenic pain is usually avoided. An example of pain of psychologic origin would be a patient who feels pain as part of a psychotic sensory hallucination. Likewise, factitious pain is uncommon and is due to a compulsive need for unwarranted health care (different than malingering). Idiopathic pain is pain for which the cause is not evident after a detailed history, physical exam including bedside provocative maneuvers, and referral for appropriate diagnostic imaging, laboratory tests, and consultation as needed. Commonly, idiopathic pain in cancer patients turns out to be due to metastatic disease that was not evident despite extensive investigations. A

wise approach to the cancer patient with idiopathic pain is to complete investigations and then see the patient in follow-up on a regularly scheduled basis such as every 3 months. Diagnostic imaging can be repeated at that time along with a repeat clinical assessment.

The role of bedside provocative maneuvers in formulating a pain diagnosis has been described.[32] In one prospective study of 50 patients, all or much of the pain that brought the patient to the clinical venue was reproduced by a positive maneuver in 47 of 50 patients. Most commonly, pain was somatic but it could also be visceral, neuropathic, and about half the time it was mixed pain. Myopathic pain or muscle spasm pain was present in about half of all patients and allowed a broader approach to overall pain control strategies.

Pathophysiologic Diagnosis

The temporal profile of how the pain progressed over time will commonly reveal the underlying mechanism of pain (see Table 41.1). Vascular events are usually as bad as they are going to get within less than a day. An example of a vascular event is a spontaneous bleed within a tumor bed, exemplified by a patient with a vascular neoplasm, such as choriocarcinoma or melanoma, who develops a headache and accompanying neurologic symptoms that become fully established in less than a day. An inflammatory process typically takes between 1 and 30 days to be as bad as it is going to get. An example would be a tumor-related skin or deep tissue abscess. When pain takes more than a month to become as severe as it is going to get, is focal and is progressive, it is usually due to a growing mass. Needless to say, in a patient with known cancer, severe pain should be considered to be progression of malignancy in that region of the body until proven otherwise.

COMPLEMENTARY CLINICAL PERSPECTIVES IN THE CARE OF CANCER PATIENTS

Acute pain is a symptom and not a diagnosis. Chronic pain can be a symptom of ongoing tissue injury or a disease process in and of itself as previously discussed. The overall approach to a pain management strategy, therefore, is greatly shaped by the underlying pain mechanisms involved and the overall goals of care. The medical approach focuses on disease diagnosis and disease cure, the palliative approach aims to relieve, suppress, or mask pain to the greatest extent possible, the rehabilitative approach (an approach widely employed by chronic noncancer pain clinics) focuses on improved function and adaptive coping, and

---

TABLE 41.6

PAIN MECHANISMS

Nociceptive pain	Somatic	bone metastasis
	Visceral	liver pain
	Neuropathic	brachial plexopathy
	Mixed	Pancoast tumor
Non-nociceptive pain	neuropathic with peripheral generator	neuroma
	neuropathic with central generator	thalamic pain
	pain of psychological origin	psychosis presenting as pain
	factitious	compulsive need for health care
	idiopathic	advanced but cryptic cancer

the anesthetic approach has the objective to diagnose and block, such as a combination of "medical" and "palliative" approaches. With each of these perspectives, however, the goal is to relieve pain as quickly as possible, with the least toxicity possible. These various, but not mutually exclusive, approaches can be exemplified in a clinical case.

A 53-year-old man, who was previously healthy, developed a gradual onset of epigastric pain. He began to develop nausea and heartburn; symptoms worsened after eating. He developed weight loss. He seeks care from his physician 4 months after the onset of these symptoms.

The Medical Model: Pain is a Manifestation of Disease

In the medical model, pain is seen as a manifestation of an underlying illness. The general orientation is that of a systems approach, whereby the clinician focuses on the affected system. Using a rule in/rule out method, the clinician considers GI disease such as erosive esophagitis, gastritis, duodenal ulcer, and upper GI malignancy, cardiovascular disease such as a descending aortic aneurysm, and ischemic heart disease, and other neoplastic disease such as an intrathoracic malignancy with referred pain. Diagnostic tests are ordered to rule in or rule out each of these conditions. In this situation, pain is helpful in that it alerts the patient that something is wrong and needs to be investigated.

Palliative Model: Pain is Both Useless and Harmful

In this model, the underlying mechanism for pain is almost always known. The extent of underlying disease is also known and pain is both physiologically useless and potentially harmful to homeostasis. While controversial, there is some evidence that better control of cancer pain results in prolonged survival.[33,34] "Palliative" is an invented word based on the Latin for mask or cloak. The approach of the palliative model is to comprehensibly assess the whole patient, including their underlying disease, their social situation, their emotional state, and their spirituality, and then to mask or suppress the pain as much as possible. Other symptoms, such as anorexia, low energy, or nausea, should also be assessed and suppressed with medications or other approaches. Another closely related term commonly used to describe a whole-person approach to care of the cancer patient is "supportive care." An example of a palliative approach to cancer treatment is palliative chemotherapy or radiation therapy, and is discussed more fully in Chapter 48.

Rehabilitative ("Chronic Nonmalignant Pain") Model: Focus on Dysfunctional Pain Behavior and Pain-Related Deconditioning

A third model for pain diagnosis and treatment is the rehabilitation model for the management of the chronic pain syndrome and is applied in the setting of dysfunctional pain behaviors. In this scenario, pain has been investigated with findings of no underlying somatic, visceral, or neuropathic process to account for the pain or the underlying disease (e.g., arthritis) cannot be eradicated, so pain must be minimized in order to optimize quality of life. Either way, therapy is directed at reversing any chronic dysfunctional pain behaviors, and the client undergoes some form of behavior modification and functional restoration therapy.

Anesthetic Model: Diagnostic and Therapeutic Blocks

A fourth approach is the anesthetic model. In this approach, the patient undergoes a diagnostic procedure whereby local anesthetic is injected into or around suspected pain generator sites or regional blockade of sensory or autonomic nerves is performed. If the pain goes away, the patient may also undergo a series of such interventions, or in selected cases, a more definitive therapeutic block with a neurolytic agent such as phenol or alcohol. Interventional pain therapies are discussed in detail in Chapter 44.

All of the above are perspectives, and none should be adopted as the sole correct approach, but applied and integrated, depending upon clinical context. In the case history above of the patient with epigastric pain, the patient may present to his physician for assessment, and through the medical model, will have several conditions ruled out until a definitive diagnosis, such as pancreatic cancer, is made, during which time analgesics should be used to treat pain. He may undergo cancer treatment, but at the same time he may be started on long-acting opioids, with the plan of masking or suppressing the pain, or he may be referred for celiac plexus block. If this patient is having difficulty coping, or if he develops dysfunctional pain behaviors or aberrant medication use, a rehabilitative approach that focuses on behavior modification should be employed. Thus, the sage clinician can fluently move between different models of pain treatment and care depending on the clinical context and may in fact consider more than one model at the same time (Fig. 41.7).

MANAGEMENT OF PAIN IN SPECIFIC CLINICAL PRESENTATIONS

Bone Pain

Cancer-related bone pain is common. About 80% of patients who die from breast cancer will have bone metastases at the time of autopsy, and a similar prevalence has been observed in other kinds of cancer. Bone scintigraphy studies have revealed the surprising findings that bone metastases are far more numerous in any given patient than what would be expected by the pain history; about two thirds of bone metastases are painless. While the risk of pain correlates to an extent with the degree of bone destruction and whether or not the metastasis is in a weight-bearing bone, it can be difficult to predict based on imaging studies as to whether a metastatic lesion is painful or not. Oddly, bone pain can be transient and migratory; that is, very painful for several days and then appears to not be painful but other bone metastases become painful.

Typically, pain from bone metastases become worse over the course of months. However, at a point in time the pain may start to increase more quickly in a crescendo pattern, becoming worse each day. There is often severe muscle spasm in the contiguous muscles. This pattern of crescendo pain in bone metastasis predicts fracture. Crescendo back pain predicts collapse of a vertebral body; one should urgently investigate such patients for exigent or impending epidural cord compression to offer definitive treatment prior to developing their neurologic symptoms. Bone pain is described in more detail in Chapters 46 and 47.

Pain and Delirium

Delirium is a transient and potentially reversible disorder of cognition and attention.[35] Tools have been developed to assist the

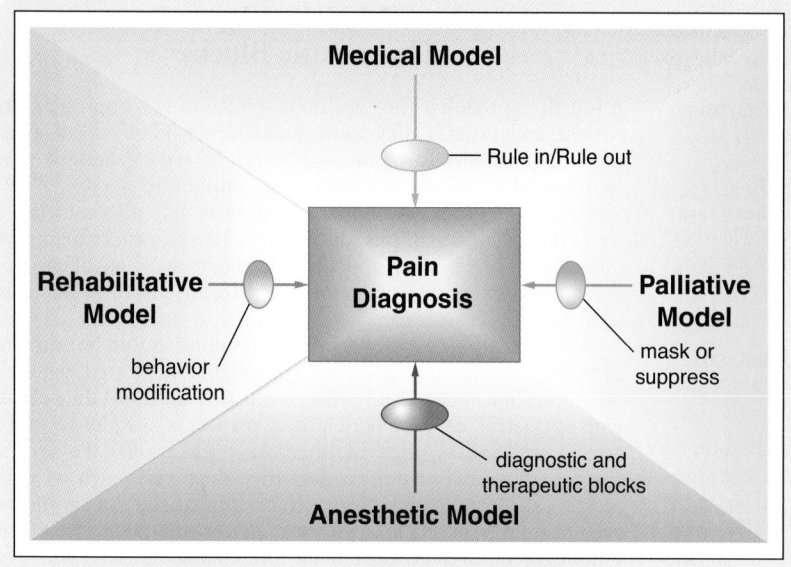

FIGURE 41.7 Complementary clinical perspectives in the care of cancer patients.

clinician to make the diagnosis as it has been found that delirium is common but the diagnosis is often delayed or missed. Since pain is a subjective symptom, there is a risk that the presence or severity of pain will be misunderstood if the diagnosis of delirium is not made.

Delirium can be caused by severe pain, pain medications, or can occur in a patient with advanced illness and organ failure who also happens to have pain. It can be challenging to distinguish between these different clinical scenarios. Almost invariably, delirium in the palliative setting is multifactorial in origin. In order to quantitate the pain, the patient's numeric rating of the pain should be dutifully recorded if possible, using tools that are intended for cognitively impaired individuals. Behaviors suggestive of pain should be sought, such as the patient grabbing the painful part of the body, the patient using other words to describe the pain, or the presence of a known destructive process in that region of the body.

Pain patients who develop delirium commonly describe a worsening of their pain, but the pain is often generalized to the whole body. In this situation, if all other potential causes of delirium have been ruled out or treated and opioids are being used, a trial of opioid dose reduction or rotation to a different opioid may be employed. Potentially reversible causes of delirium should be identified and treated, including a very wide array of possibilities such as hypercalcemia, along with hydration and other supportive measures to manage the delirium.[36] If there is clinical suspicion that the delirium may be caused by uncontrolled pain, a short-acting opioid should be considered as a test dose.

Pain and Nausea

Chronic nausea is a prevalent symptom in cancer patients, and opioids themselves can be emetogenic. Complicating this situation is the experience of patients who have both pain and nausea and are unable to take oral medications.

A wise approach to the presence of both pain and nausea is to assess each of them individually and treat any underlying cause. If there is any possibility that the opioid is causing or contributing to the nausea, this symptom should be treated aggressively and/or the patient should be rotated to a different opioid or to a nonopioid pain treatment strategy. As common as opioid-related nausea is, it is fortunate that this symptom is usually self-limiting, rarely necessitating discontinuation from opioid therapy. Alter-

native routes of administration, such as transdermal or injectable opioids, may need to be considered if the opioids are effective for pain but the patient cannot manage to take them by the oral route until habituation to this symptom occurs.

Pain and Anorexia/Cachexia/Asthenia

Anorexia/cachexia/asthenia is a common triad that accompanies many types of cancer, and when pain is also present, symptoms can be particularly difficult to manage. While fatigue is the most common symptom in cancer patients, affecting about 70% of patients, a large minority fulfill diagnostic criteria of anorexia with cachexia. Such patients may have difficulty tolerating opioids, may have concurrent nausea, or may not be able to tolerate oral opioids because of upper GI malignancy. Such patients require alternative routes of drug administration or other pain treatment strategies. Further, many interventions are available to support comprehensive assessment and management of anorexia, cachexia, and asthenia.

Pain and Bowel Disease

Slow-release opioids are about 50% absorbed in the large colon. Patients who have had a partial or complete colectomy may malabsorb slow-release opioids, as a function of the more rapid transit time. The clinician may be suspicious of this by the presence of end of dose failure of the opioid, occurring several hours before the medication would be expected to wear off. Patients may report seeing the "ghost" of slow-release tablets in their stool. Most patients who have a low colostomy (in the left lower quadrant on abdominal exam) only uncommonly malabsorb slow-release opioids, whereas patients with a right sided colostomy or ileostomy are at much higher risk. These patients should be considered for transdermal opioids or some other route of opioid administration.

Similarly, patients who have upper GI malignancy and pain can be anticipated to have nausea, obstruction, or other GI symptoms. At an early stage in their disease, they should be considered for another route of administration of analgesic medication.

Cancer Pain in the Addict

The overall strategy for pain management in the patient who carries an addiction diagnosis should be tempered according to whether the history is that of remote addiction, recent addiction, or active addiction. It must be stated that use of controlled substances for any legitimate medical purpose requires vigilance and a risk management approach that considers diversion and abuse, irrespective of the patient's diagnosis or history. However, medical judgment must be used to determine the extent of such programs relative to the patient's individual circumstances. In all situations, the clinician will want to understand if the patient is in active recovery and/or maintenance therapy, communicate with the patient's addiction counselor/therapist, and look carefully for evidence of aberrant or problematic drug-taking behavior. The patient with a remote history of substance abuse and who currently has a stable social situation and a spouse or other close family member should be managed as any other cancer pain patient. However, these patients and their family members are oftentimes very concerned about rekindling addiction and may be highly opioid phobic. Long acting oral or transdermal opioids are the preference and the dose should be titrated upward to effect, with a structured management program (e.g., frequent follow-up visits, small supplies of medicine prescribed at any given time, urine drug screens) to provide sufficient support for the patient and family. A goal should be only one prescribing physician and, once stable analgesia is achieved, there should be sufficient confidence and evidence of compliance and increasingly longer periods of time between prescribing visits. To the patient who is a recent user and in recovery, the discussion needs to be more frank and the plan of care more structured. The clinician should outline the goals of care (improved comfort and improved function), but also inquire of the patient about their level of concern regarding opioids. The physician should warn the patient to not take the opioids for any reason other than relief of pain. Together, they should agree as to how often the medication prescriptions should be refilled and by whom. Comanagement with an addiction specialist is advised if the prescribing clinician is not strongly versed in addiction medicine. Unsanctioned dose escalation is not allowed, and if necessary, the medications may need to be controlled by the spouse or other family member.

Cancer patients who are actively abusing pose particular challenges. The patient and the clinician hope that the patient can achieve relief of pain but the prescribing physician will be particularly wary of causing harm. Harm includes the risk of drug diversion or overdosing because the patient is accustomed to a less potent source of drug. Also, there is the risk that the pain medication may be stolen by those around them because of the social circumstances that often accompany addiction. There needs to be a firm, concrete framework to support clinical care. In these situations, daily dispensing of pain medication is often required, along with observed ingestion. If transdermal fentanyl patches are prescribed, which may be useful in these circumstances, the patch should be replaced under observation and then either disposed of properly or the used patch may be brought to the next prescribing visit and disposed under observation of clinicians. Liquid methadone may also be preferable over other analgesics or formulations in this circumstance.

A written agreement delineates expected behavior and the consequences of nonadherence. The agreement (sometimes referred to as an "opioid contract") should include periodic unscheduled drug screening if the patient has committed to not use other drugs. In certain jurisdictions, the prescribing physician can benefit from a state computerized prescription network whereby it can be determined if the patient is obtaining prescription medications from another legitimate source. One should avoid high doses of opioids and should also consider nonpharmacologic interventions at an earlier stage (such as palliative radiotherapy or neural blockage).

Symptom Clusters

Cancer patients commonly have more than one symptom. A large survey of medical oncology inpatients and outpatients from a U.S. Veterans Affairs medical center revealed that most had several symptoms, including low energy (62%), pain (59%), dry mouth (54%), shortness of breath (50%), and sleeping difficulty (45%).[37] Patients with "moderate" intensity pain had a median number of 11 symptoms, and as the performance status fell, the number of intense symptoms increased.[37] Other studies have confirmed that cancer patients commonly have many distressing symptoms, and as the severity of disease increases so does the number and severity of symptoms.[38]

More recently, the concept of symptom clusters has emerged as an area of intense research. Symptom clusters have been defined as three or more concurrent symptoms that are related to each other but do not necessarily share the same etiology.[39] There is evidence that the coexistence of several symptoms in the same patient is associated with worse quality of life and potentially will benefit from specific, targeted therapeutic approaches. For example, it has been suggested that release of cytokines may result in a range of symptoms related to cancer and its treatment.[40] A wide array of specific clusters has been reported. Examples posited to date include fatigue-anorexia-cachexia cluster (easy fatigue, weakness, anorexia, lack of energy, dry mouth, early satiety, weight loss, and taste changes), upper GI cluster (dizzy spells, dyspepsia, belching, bloating), neuropsychologic cluster (sleep problems, depression, and anxiety), and others.[41] Further research is needed to confirm their existence as discrete nosological entities, to delineate their underlying pathogenesis and connectedness, and to explore mechanism-based approaches to their management.[3,42,43]

Pain at the End of Life

In the final hours of life, it may not be appropriate or there may not be sufficient time to obtain a detailed history, physical examination, and diagnostic studies in order to quickly obtain relief of distressing symptoms. The actual mechanism of pain becomes increasingly less relevant as death approaches. In the instance of severe pain, one would consider subcutaneous or intravenous opioids with rapid titration to effect. Severe regional pain such as abdominal, pelvic, or lower extremity pain can be managed with neuraxial (epidural, intrathecal) local anesthetics or opioids. In a pain crisis at the end of life, the patient may be a candidate for palliative sedation.[44] Palliative sedation is appropriate when the patient is aware that they are at the end of life, other interventions are not expected to relieve pain quickly enough, and the patient or family has given their informed consent. Assessment tools that have been developed to guide the depth of sedation, such as the Ricker scale, can be used.[45] These issues are discussed further in Chapter 108.

Cancer Pain Emergencies

Occasionally, patients will present to their physician with persistent, horrible cancer pain. A cancer pain emergency has been defined as pain that is severe or excruciating (8 out of 10 on a 0 to 10 scale), for more than 6 hours.[46] Such patients typically come to an emergency room in great distress. The patient may already be on large doses of opioids, and may be dehydrated due to limited oral intake during the previous days. Often the patient will not have slept at all during that time. In such cases, the patient assessment is greatly truncated. The physician examines the patient quickly to determine whether there is evidence of a ruptured viscous, subarachnoid hemorrhage, ischemic crisis, or other catastrophe. Vital signs and cognitive status are monitored, and an intravenous access is secured. Opioid is administered with rapid upward titration using a mini bolus technique until there is relief of pain. Intravenous protocols for cancer pain emergencies have been described for morphine[46] and fentanyl,[47] and transdermal and other routes of administration of opioids have also been described.[48] Unlike conscious sedation, rapid upward titration of opioid in the setting of unrelieved cancer pain almost never results in serious toxicity. Patients appear to be able to leave the emergency room an hour or few hours after obtaining relief of pain. Only uncommonly will the cause of the cancer pain emergency be apparent. Typically the flare of pain arises in a place of known metastatic disease and the pain goes away as mysteriously as it came.

CONCLUSION

Cancer pain is common and, when present, is often severe. Fortunately, a great deal is known about its epidemiology, assessment, and management. An individualized approach to each patient offers the best opportunity to provide relief of pain and improve the quality of life at all stages of oncologic disease.

References

1. Portenoy RK, Kornblith AB, Wong G, et al. Pain in ovarian cancer patients. Prevalence, characteristics, and associated symptoms. *Cancer* 1994;74: 907–915.
2. Foley KM. Management of cancer pain. In: Devita VT, Hellman S, Rosenberg SA, eds. *Cancer: Principles and Practice of Oncology.* 7th ed. New York: Lippincott Williams and Wilkins; 2005:2615–2649.
3. Hockenberry M, Hooke MC. Symptom clusters in children with cancer. *Semin Oncol Nurs* 2007;23:152–157.
4. Friel JP, ed. *Dorland's Medical Dictionary.* 26th ed. Philadelphia: WB Saunders; 1981:451.
5. McDonald AJ, Cooper MG. Patient-controlled analgesia: an appropriate method of pain control in children. *Paediatr Drugs* 2001;3:273–284.
6. Burstein HJ, Winer EP. Aromatase inhibitors and arthralgias: a new frontier in symptom management for breast cancer survivors. *J Clin Oncol* 2007;25: 3797–3799.
7. Ahmed N, Mandel R, Fain MJ. Frailty: an emerging geriatric syndrome. *Am J Med* 2007;120:748–753.
8. Milisen K, Steeman E, Foreman MD. Early detection and prevention of delirium in older patients with cancer. *Eur J Cancer Care (Engl)* 2004;13:494–500.
9. Gordon RG Jr, ed. *Ethnologue: Languages of the World.* 15th ed. Dallas: SIL International; 2005.
10. Tse CY, Chong A, Fok SY. Breaking bad news: a Chinese perspective. *Palliat Med* 2003;17:339–343.
11. Davies G, Kingswood C, Street M. Pharmacokinetics of opioids in renal dysfunction. *Clin Pharmacokinet* 1996;31:410–422.
12. Graham AW, Schultz TK, Wilford BB, eds. *Principles of Addiction Medicine,* 2nd ed. Chevy Chase: American Society of Addiction Medicine; 1998.
13. Passik SD, Kirsh KL, Donaghy KB, et al. Pain and aberrant drug-related behaviors in medically ill patients with and without histories of substance abuse. *Clin J Pain* 2006;22:173–181.
14. Rosenblum A, Joseph H, Fong C, et al. Prevalence and characteristics of chronic pain among chemically dependent patients in methadone maintenance and residential treatment facilities. *JAMA* 2003;289:2370–2378.
15. Mathew P, Elting L, Cooksley C, et al. Cancer in an incarcerated population. *Cancer* 2005;104:2197–2204.
16. Reindollar RW. Hepatitis C and the correctional population. *Am J Med* 1999; 107(6B):100S–103S.
17. Dean-Gaitor HD, Fleming PL. Epidemiology of AIDS in incarcerated persons in the United States, 1994–1996. *AIDS* 1999;13:2429–2435.
18. Lin JT, Mathew P. Cancer pain management in prisons: a survey of primary care practitioners and inmates. *J Pain Symptom Manage* 2005;29:466–473.
19. International Association for the Study of Pain. IASP Pain Terminology Available at: http://www.iasp-pain.org/AM/Template.cfm?Section=Home&

20. template=/CM/HTMLDisplay.cfm&ContentID=4697#Pain. Accessed November 28, 2007.
20. Cassel EJ. The nature of suffering and the goals of medicine. *N Engl J Med* 1982;306:639–645.
21. Melzak R. The McGill Pain Questionnaire: major properties and scoring methods. *Pain* 1975;1:277–299.
22. Marchettini P. The burning case of neuropathic pain wording. *Pain* 2005;114: 313–314.
23. Prkachin KM, Solomon PE, Ross J. Underestimation of pain by health-care providers: towards a model of the process of inferring pain in others. *Can J Nurs Res* 2007;39:88–106.
24. Ferrell BR, Rhiner M, Cohen MZ, et al. Pain as a metaphor for illness, Part I: Impact of cancer pain on family caregivers. *Oncol Nurs Forum* 1991;18: 1303–1309.
25. Wolfe F, Smythe HA, Yunus MB, et al. The American College of Rheumatology 1990 Criteria for the Classification of Fibromyalgia. Report of the Multicenter Criteria Committee. *Arthritis Rheum* 1990;33:160–172.
26. Tong HC, Haig AJ, Yamakawa K. The Spurling test and cervical radiculopathy. *Spine* 2002;27:156–159.
27. Wisneski RJ, Garfin SR, Rothman RH. Lumbar disc disease. In: Rothman RH, Simeone FA, eds. *The Spine.* 3rd ed. Philadelphia: WB Saunders;1992: 689–699.
28. Abdominal wall tenderness test: could Carnett cut costs? *Lancet* 1991;337: 1134.
29. Hershfield NB. The abdominal wall. A frequently overlooked source of abdominal pain. *J Clin Gastroenterol* 1992;14:199–202.
30. Cunningham J, Temple WJ, Mitchell P, et al. Cooperative hernia study: pain in the postrepair patient. *Ann Surg* 1996;224:598–602.
31. Parry GJ, Floberg J. Diabetic truncal neuropathy presenting as abdominal hernia. *Neurology* 1989;39(11):1488–1490.
32. Hagen NA. Reproducing a cancer patient's pain on physical examination: bedside provocative maneuvers. *J Pain Symptom Manage* 1999;18:406–411.
33. Lillemoe KD, Cameron JL, Kaufman HS, et al. Chemical splanchnicectomy in patients with unresectable pancreatic cancer. A prospective randomized trial. *Ann Surg* 1993;217:447–455.
34. Yan BM, Myers RP. Neurolytic celiac plexus block for pain control in unresectable pancreatic cancer. *Am J Gastroenterol* 2007;102(2):430–438.
35. Lipowski ZJ. Delirium (acute confusional states). *JAMA* 1987;258: 1789–1792.
36. Lawlor PG, Fainsinger RL, Bruera ED. Delirium at the end of life: critical issues in clinical practice and research. *JAMA* 2000;284:2427–2429.
37. Chang VT, Hwang SS, Feuerman M, et al. Symptom and quality of life survey of medical oncology patients at a veterans affairs medical center: a role for symptom assessment. *Cancer* 2000;88:1175–1183.
38. Portenoy RK, Thaler HT, Kornblith AB, et al. Symptom prevalence, characteristics and distress in a cancer population. *Qual Life Res* 1994;3:183–189.
39. Dodd MJ, Miaskowski C, Paul SM. Symptom clusters and their effect on the functional status of patients with cancer. *Oncol Nurs Forum* 2001;28: 465–470.
40. Cleeland CS, Bennett GJ, Dantzer R, et al. Are the symptoms of cancer and cancer treatment due to a shared biologic mechanism? A cytokine-immunologic model of cancer symptoms. *Cancer* 2003;97:2919–2925.
41. Miaskowski C, Aouizerat BE, Dodd M, et al. Conceptual issues in symptom clusters research and their implications for quality-of-life assessment in patients with cancer. *J Natl Cancer Inst Monogr* 2007;37:39–46.
42. Fan G, Filipczak L, Chow E. Symptom clusters in cancer patients: a review of the literature. *Curr Oncol* 2007;14:173–179.
43. Chow E, Fan G, Hadi S, et al. Symptom clusters in cancer patients with brain metastases. *Clin Oncol (R Coll Radiol)* 2008;20:76–82.
44. Cherny NI. Sedation for the care of patients with advanced cancer. *Nat Clin Pract Oncol* 2006;3:492–500.
45. Riker RR, Picard JT, Fraser GL. Prospective evaluation of the Sedation-Agitation Scale for adult critically ill patients. *Crit Care Med* 1999;27: 1325–1329.
46. Hagen NA, Elwood T, Ernst S. Cancer pain emergencies: a protocol for management. *J Pain Symptom Manage* 1997;14:45–50.
47. Soares LG, Martins M, Uchoa R. Intravenous fentanyl for cancer pain: a "fast titration" protocol for the emergency room. *J Pain Symptom Manage* 2003; 26:876–881.
48. Burton AW, Driver LC, Mendoza TR, et al. Oral transmucosal fentanyl citrate in the outpatient management of severe cancer pain crises: a retrospective case series. *Clin J Pain* 2004;20:195–197.

CHAPTER 42 ■ MECHANISMS, ASSESSMENT, AND DIAGNOSIS OF PAIN DUE TO CANCER

DERMOT R. FITZGIBBON

INTRODUCTION

Cancer is a major public health problem in the United Sates and other developed countries, and pain is a very common problem associated with cancer. This chapter will review the incidence, prevalence, etiologies, and assessment strategies in cancer-related pain syndromes.

One in four deaths in the United States is due to cancer. The lifetime probability of developing cancer is higher for men (45%) than for women (38%), but women have a higher probability of developing cancer before age 60 because of the relatively early age of breast cancer onset. Recent notable trends in cancer incidence and mortality rates include stabilization of the age-standardized, delay-adjusted incidence rates for all cancers combined in men from 1995 through 2003, a continuing increase in the incidence rate by 0.3% per year in women, and a 13.6% total decrease in age-standardized cancer death rates among men and women combined between 1991 and 2004.[1]

Among men, cancers of the prostate, lung and bronchus, and colon and rectum account for about 54% of all newly diagnosed cancers. Prostate cancer alone accounts for about 29% of incident cases in men. Based on cases diagnosed between 1996 and 2002, an estimated 91% of these new cases of prostate cancer are expected to be diagnosed at local or regional stages, for which 5-year relative survival approaches 100%. The three most commonly diagnosed types of cancer among women in 2007 were cancers of the breast, lung and bronchus, and colon and rectum, accounting for about 52% of estimated cancer cases in women. Breast cancer alone accounts for 26% (178/480) of all new cancer cases among women. Approximately 559,650 Americans die from cancer, corresponding to over 1,500 deaths per day. Cancers of the lung and bronchus, prostate, and colon and rectum in men, and cancers of the lung and bronchus, breast, and colon and rectum in women continue to be the most common fatal cancers. These four cancers account for half of the total cancer deaths among men and women. Lung cancer surpassed breast cancer as the leading cause of cancer death in women in 1987. Lung cancer accounts for 26% of all female cancer deaths in 2007. Lung cancer incidence rates are declining in men and appear to be reaching a plateau in women after increasing for many decades. Colorectal cancer incidence rates decreased from 1998 through 2003 in both males and females. Female breast cancer incidence rates leveled off from 2001 to 2003 after increasing since 1980, which may reflect the saturation of mammography utilization and reduction in the use of hormone replacement therapy. Death rates for all cancer sites combined decreased by 1.6% per year from 1993 to 2003 in males and by 0.8% per year in females from 1992 to 2003. Mortality rates have continued to decrease across all four major cancer sites in men and in women, except for female lung cancer in which rates continued to increase by 0.3% per year from 1995 to 2003.[1]

There have been notable improvements over time in relative 5-year survival rates for many cancer sites and for all cancers combined. This is true for both Caucasians and African Americans. Cancers for which survival has not improved substantially over the past 25 years include uterine corpus, cervix, larynx, lung, and pancreas. For all sites of cancer (excluding basal and squamous cell skin cancers and in situ carcinomas except urinary bladder) between 1996 and 2002, the relative survival rate was 66%.[1] A National Institutes of Health (NIH) Consensus Conference on symptom management in cancer estimated that approximately 60% of patients will survive at least 5 years after diagnosis.[2] As the number of cancer survivors continues to grow, the need to address persisting symptoms and impairments due to cancer and related treatments on individuals' lives becomes increasingly important.

Prevalence data of pain in patients with cancer range from 24% to 60% in patients on active anticancer treatment[3,4] and 62% to 86% in patients with advanced cancer.[5–7] Van den Beuken-van Everdingen et al.[8] reported pain prevalence in patients with cancer according to disease stage, treatment, and survival: 64% (confidence interval [CI] 58% to 69%) in patients with metastatic, advanced, or terminal disease, 59% (CI 44% to 73%) in patients on anticancer treatment, and 33% (CI 21% to 46%) in patients who had been cured of cancer.

Some important differences exist between cancer pain patients and those that experience acute pain and/or chronic noncancer pain. Although all types of persistent pain elevate psychological distress,[9–11] alter social life,[12] disturb sleep,[13] and compromise enjoyment of life,[14] end-of-life considerations and palliative care are rarely major issues for acute and chronic noncancer pain conditions. These concerns become extremely important for the cancer pain patient with advanced disease (see Chapter 108). The complexities that emerge from the medical and psychosocial aspects of the situation necessitate a multi- and/or interdisciplinary approach to care that requires skill and sensitivity to these issues. The oftentimes rapidly changing nature of cancer pain, either in response to treatments directed at the tumor and/or progression of the tumor, mandates vigilance and potential frequent alteration of treatment strategies for pain. In addition, cancer survivors face ongoing surveillance for the possibility of disease recurrence and therefore new or changing pain complaints in these patients require careful reassessment.

As cancer treatments continue to improve survival, many oncology patients face long-term pain management issues from aggressive treatment of their disease. Different treatment strategies need to be considered when life expectancy may be decades, rather than months or years. Comprehensive cancer care requires that many health care professionals become involved with the cancer pain patient at any specific time. Similarly, successful pain management requires that those involved in cancer care support an interdisciplinary approach.

There exist several medical, psychologic, social, and cultural issues that complicate cancer pain and its management. The interaction of pain and its treatment with other common cancer symptoms such as fatigue, weakness, dyspnea, nausea, constipation, and impaired cognition magnifies the negative impact of cancer pain.[15,16] Cancer patients treated on an outpatient basis frequently have pain that is inadequately controlled, with 67% of outpatients (871 of 1308 patients) indicating that they had pain or had taken analgesic drugs daily during the preceding week, while 36% had pain severe enough to impair their ability to function.[17] Patients seen at centers that treated predominantly minorities were three times more likely than those treated elsewhere to have inadequate pain management[18] due to inadequate pain assessment, patient reluctance to report pain, and lack of staff time for pain management.[19]

ISSUES IN ASSESSMENT AND DIAGNOSIS OF CANCER PAIN

Studies from the 1990s documented inadequate treatment of pain in patients with cancer.[17,18,20,21] Despite the subsequent availability of effective pain treatments and various pain management guidelines, these deficiencies continue both in the United States and in other countries.[22–26] The most frequently identified barriers to effective management are physician underestimation of the patient's pain, inadequate pain assessment, and patient reluctance to report pain. Experienced physicians and professional organizations recognize a need for significant improvement in cancer pain assessment and treatment.[27,28] Lack of expertise by clinicians in assessing and managing cancer pain has been cited as an important cause of poor pain control.[29] Interviews of practicing physicians demonstrate knowledge deficits in the basic principles of cancer pain management.[30] Similar findings are demonstrated in nurses and nursing students.[20,31,32] Educational interventions can successfully improve cancer pain knowledge and attitudes of health care professionals.[33] However, medical education does not adequately prepare students and residents to provide adequate care for the cancer pain patient.[34,35]

In general, pain management requires a variety of assessment skills and the integration of knowledge about biobehavioral contributions to experience of pain, pharmacologic, and nonpharmacologic approaches to pain control. More specifically, safe and effective pharmacotherapy requires detailed knowledge of analgesic pharmacokinetics and pharmacodynamics, patient characteristics like individual variability and compliance with medications, side effects, and quality of life determinants. Cancer pain assessment also requires additional disease-specific knowledge of toxicities and likely outcomes of treatments. These skills must contribute to clinical judgment and decision-making, often requiring substantial individual experience.

Most studies concerning pain education of undergraduate medical students focus on knowledge, but little is known about their interviewing and pain evaluation skills. Leila et al.[36] suggested that formative assessment of both knowledge and communication skills is essential for the development of an effective pain curriculum for training medical students in pain management of chronic pain patients. Lasch et al.[37] demonstrated that for postgraduate nurses, day-long cancer pain education workshops were as effective as hands-on experience in improving cancer pain knowledge and changing attitudes. Computer simulation software may create a tool that can teach the principles and applied practice of cancer pain assessment and management, no less provide the ability to efficiently assist in the identification of specific errors in knowledge, judgment, and practice patterns of the individual.[38] Regardless of means, it can be concluded that significant improvements in pain assessment and management education are needed at all training levels and for those engaged in oncology practice in order to advance the field and assure quality care of cancer patients at all stages of disease.

PAIN AND THE CANCER PATIENT

Because pain is an unpleasant sensory and emotional experience associated with actual or potential tissue damage,[39] the sensory features and subjective qualities of pain vary, depending on its origin. Its emotional features depend in part upon the social and physical context in which pain occurs, associated cognition, and the meaning of tissue trauma for the individual, but they are almost always negative.

Sensory Component of Cancer Pain

From a sensory perspective, tumor-associated pain may be classified as nociceptive, neuropathic, or mixed. Pain is labeled nociceptive if the sustaining mechanism is believed to be related to ongoing tissue injury and is subdivided into somatic and visceral types. Pain is neuropathic if there is evidence that the pain is associated with injury to neural tissues and is sustained by aberrant somatosensory processing in the periphery or in the central nervous system. Caraceni and Portenoy[40] reported in an international survey of cancer pain characteristics and syndromes that pain inferred by the treating clinician to be nociceptive and due to somatic injury occurred in 71.6% of patients, nociceptive visceral in 34.7%, and neuropathic mechanisms occurred in 39.7%. Somatic nociceptive pain may be grouped into superficial (cutaneous) and deep. Most cutaneous pain is well-localized, sharp, pricking, or burning. Deep tissue pain usually seems diffuse and dull or aching in quality. Visceral pain is very diffuse, often referred to the body surface, perseverating, and frequently associated with a queasy quality that patients describe as "sickening."

The mechanisms of tumor involvement of the peripheral nervous system are heterogeneous and include local invasion, compression, direct infiltration, perineurial spread and rarely intraneural metastasis.[41] Compression and invasion of nerves by tumor results in the destruction of myelinated and unmyelinated fibers and of supporting tissue. Since peripheral nerves can usually evade pressure from a tumor on one side, infiltration by tumor tissue is the quintessential tissue trauma stimulus. In addition, indirect damage of unknown pathogenesis might also occur to peripheral nerves in the context of certain malignant conditions (e.g., paraneoplastic syndromes). Infiltration of tumor tissue into the perineural cleft is seen relatively often. However, this does not regularly lead to pain.[42] A massive and then painful entrapment of the nerve plexus or individual nerves occurs, especially in extensive breast carcinomas and their recurrences or in chest wall metastases of lung tumors. The perineural cleft widens tumor infiltration, and infiltration of the tumor into the nerve itself is common. Degenerative changes of the axis cylinders are sometimes visible with conventional histopathology screening methods. Primary tumors of the peripheral nerves themselves lead to painful destruction.

Compression regularly elicits pain when the affected nerve cannot give way, for example, a spinal nerve root. The process of tumor compression and invasion of nerves entails several degenerative, regenerative, and other pathophysiologic processes.[43] The whole afferent neuron is affected and goes through reactive, presumably reparative, biochemical changes. The neuron loses its neuropeptides,[44] atrophies, and may finally degenerate. This applies particularly to unmyelinated afferent neurons. The conditions in a nerve, when invaded or compressed by cancerous tissue, are probably similar to those after lesions of nerves induced by mechanical or other events. The process induces changes in the discharge properties of neurons (resting activity, response to mechanical and chemical stimulation).

Molecular Mechanism of Tumor Pain

In addition to cancer cells, tumors consist of different cell types including inflammatory cells and blood vessels that are often adjacent to primary afferent nociceptors. These cells include immune system cells such as macrophages, neutrophils, and T cells. These secrete various factors that sensitize or directly excite primary afferent neurons and include prostaglandins, tumor necrosis factor, endothelins, interleukin-1 and -6, epidermal growth factor, transforming growth factor, and platelet-derived growth factor. Receptors for many of these factors are expressed by primary afferent neurons. Endothelins (endothelin-1, -2, and -3) are a family of vasoactive peptides that are expressed at high levels by several types of tumor, including prostate cancer. Endothelins could contribute to cancer pain by directly sensitizing or exciting nociceptors as a subset of small, unmyelinated primary afferent neurons that express endothelin-A receptors.[45] Like prostaglandins, endothelins that are produced by cancer cells are also thought to be involved in regulating angiogenesis and tumor growth.[46] Consequently these factors and others from cancer and inflammatory cells, such as adenosine triphosphate, bradykinin, H^+, nerve growth factor (NGF), prostaglandins, and vascular endothelial growth factor excite or sensitize adjacent nociceptors.[47] Adjacent nociceptors such as vanilloid receptor-1 (VR1) detect extracellular H^+ and endothelin-A receptors detect endothelins released by cancer cells. NGF released by macrophages binds to the tyrosine kinase receptor TrkA.[48] Nociceptor activation results in the release of neurotransmitters, such as calcitonin gene-related peptide (CGRP), endothelin, histamine, glutamate, and substance P. Nociceptor activation also causes the release of prostaglandins from the peripheral terminals of sensory fibers, which can induce plasma extravasation, recruitment and activation of immune cells, and vasodilatation.

Other mechanisms, particularly tissue acidosis, may be involved in tumor-related pain. There are several mechanisms by which tumors could cause a decrease in pH. As inflammatory cells invade the neoplastic tissue, they release protons that generate local acidosis. The large amount of apoptosis* that occurs in the tumor environment also contributes to acidosis, as apoptotic cells release intracellular ions to create an acidic environment. This drop in pH can activate signaling by acid-sensing channels (including VR1) that are expressed by nociceptors. Tumor-induced release of protons and acidosis might be particularly important in the generation of bone cancer pain.[49] Finally, tumor-induced distention of sensory fibers may also be involved in tumor-associated nociceptive processes. Tumors are not highly innervated by sensory neurons.[50] Rapid tumor growth frequently entraps and injures nerves causing mechanical injury, compression, ischemia, or direct proteolysis. Proteolytic enzymes that are produced by the tumor cells can also cause injury to sensory and sympathetic fibers, causing neuropathic pain.

Muscle-Related Pain

Muscle-related pain may occur in a variety of settings and frequently occurs in oncology patients.[51] Because inactivity and deconditioning predisposes to muscle pain, the debilitated cancer patient may experience muscle pain. Myofascial pain syndrome (MPS) may occur independently of malignancy, or it may develop as a result of tumor-related tissue changes or treatment-related influences on soft tissues, for example, surgery and radiation therapy. The key is to identify and treat active trigger points and distinguish MPS from other pain mechanisms in the active and posttreatment cancer patient (see Chapter 35).

Muscle pain is generally described as aching and cramp-like. It can be difficult to localize and may be referred to other deep somatic structures. Muscle nociceptors are activated by tissue-threatening stimuli (pressure, ischemia), which can result in the release of local algesic substances such as bradykinin (BK), serotonin (5HT), and potassium (K^+). Kallidin found in plasma protein splits to form BK under pathological environmental changes such

as ischemia, lowered pH, and blood clotting. Following vascular damage, 5HT is released and muscle damage releases K^+. C-nociceptors, when stimulated, release somatostatin, CGRP, and substance P in the dorsal horn resulting in substance P-mediated histamine release from mast cells, causing vasodilation and increased vessel permeability releasing more BK, 5HT, and prostaglandin E2. CGRP may inhibit degradation of substance P in muscle nociceptors.

Affective Processing and Suffering

Suffering, beyond—but amplified by—the sensory dimensions of the pain experience, is not unique to cancer patients (see Chapters 7, 29, 31, 81, and 83). Suffering related to cancer is inherently emotional, unpleasant, complex, and enduring. In some patients, it often has the additional existential (or spiritual) dimension of dealing with imminent mortality.

Treating clinicians must recognize that, although suffering may be a consequence of pain, it is separate from pain and not a synonym for it. It differs from pain in that it entails additional cognitive affective states. For example, perceived helplessness (inability to cope, bankruptcy of physical, psychological, or social resources) is a key element in the suffering of most patients with incurable disease. Similarly, grief can ensue when a cancer patient perceives the loss of a psychological or social resource, a body part or desired personal appearance, a prized employment status, or a physical capability for a treasured activity. Loss often equates with perceived threat to self. In addition, suffering in the cancer patient sometimes involves a sense of separation from social support or alienation. These factors, combined with the emotional distress, fatigue, and stress associated with prolonged pain and the rigors of oncologic treatment produce a complex state that differs from manifestations of chronic pain in other patient populations. For example, Wilson et al.,[52] in a study of 381 patients with advanced cancer, found that 25% of patients were suffering at a moderate to extreme level and concluded that suffering is a multidimensional experience related most strongly to physical symptoms, but with contributions from psychological distress, existential concerns, and social–relational worries.

Psychological Factors, Depression, and Fatigue

Somatization refers to patients who transform distress and global suffering into pain and symptom expression, and health care providers frequently view pain reported by cancer patients as primarily somatogenic, whereas chronic noncancer pain in patients who lack adequate objective physical pathology is viewed as psychogenic.[53] Consequently, providers tend to treat cancer pain with pharmacologic, medical, or surgical modalities. Psychological factors are considered to be of secondary importance.[54]

As stated above, regardless of cause, but especially when unremitting, pain is a complex experience entailing physiological, sensory, affective, cognitive, and behavioral components. The final individual perception of pain is dependent on nociceptive input and psychological modifiers such as fear, anxiety, anger, and depression (Fig. 42.1).

Turk et al.[53] classified the multidimensional nature of cancer pain. They compared the adaptation of cancer patients and chronic noncancer patients to persisting pain. The majority of the cancer patients, both with (81%) and without (84%) metastatic disease, as well as the noncancer chronic pain patients (85%), fit one of three psychosocial subgroups: dysfunctional (high levels of pain, perceived interference, affective distress, and low levels of perceived control and activity), interpersonally distressed (high levels of affective distress, negative responses from significant others, and low levels of perceived support), and adaptive copers (low levels of interference and affective distress, high levels of perceived control and activity).

---

*Apoptosis is a form of cell death necessary to make way for new cells and to remove cells whose DNA has been damaged to the point at which cancerous change is liable to occur.

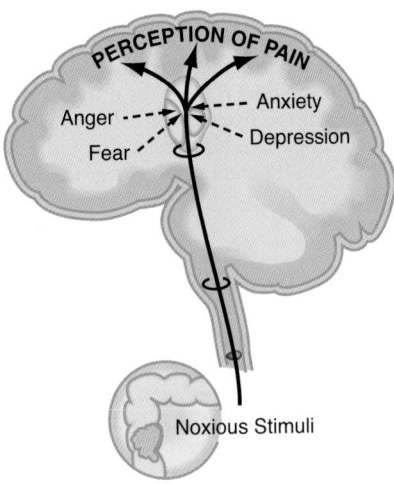

FIGURE 42.1 Individual perception of pain. Noxious stimuli are modified at supraspinal level by emotions such as anxiety, fear, and anger.

Substantial evidence suggests that psychological factors play an important role in exacerbating pain with clear origins of disease (see Chapters 29–33). For example, the belief that pain signifies disease, a commonly held belief among cancer patients,[55] is associated with elevated pain intensity.[14,56] Speigel and Bloom[56] also reported that the affective states of cancer patients, the belief that pain is an indicator for disease progression, and medication use all predict pain severity. Patients who attribute their pain to a warning of underlying disease report greater pain than patients with more nontumor-associated interpretations, despite comparable levels of disease progression.

Because of psychological factors, the relationship between pain severity and the extent of disease is rarely as linear as one might assume.[57] Research investigating the relationships between physical pathology and pain in cancer has shown inconsistent results. In one evaluative study, Twycross and Fairfield[58] reported that only 41 of 100 terminal-stage cancer patients reported pain due to disease, whereas Cleeland et al.[59] reported that the majority of patients with end-stage disease have pain of a severity that interferes with several aspects of the patient's quality of life. Front et al.[60] demonstrated that for many cancer patients, pain reports did not correspond to the presence or location of bone metastases. Turk et al.[53] found that patients with cancer-related pain reported a significantly higher level of perceived disability and inactivity due to pain than did those with pain of noncancer origin. Since the level of pain severity was comparable for the two patient groups, elevated disability may have been a consequence of the meanings patients attributed to their pain. The progression of malignant disease means further deterioration of health and impending death. Indeed, the patients with cancer-related pain appeared to be more fearful of pain and reported significantly higher levels of cognitive and behavioral fear-responses than did the patients with chronic pain not associated with cancer. These patients appeared to think and worry more about pain, avoid activities in order to prevent initiation of pain, and they generally felt more hopeless than the patients with non-cancer-related pain.

The severity of depression is correlated with pain, anxiety, disease type, and other health-related quality of life issues.[61] The interactions between cancer pain, insomnia, fatigue, and depression/anxiety are complex, warranting treatment plans that focus not only on the relief of specific symptoms to improve quality of life but also on the impact of treatment on other related symptoms. Certain cancer types are highly associated with depression and include oropharyngeal (22%–57%),[62] pancreatic (33%–50%),[63] breast (1.5%–46%),[64] and lung (11%–44%).[65,66] A less high

prevalence of depression is reported in patients with other cancers, such as colon (13%–25%),[67] gynecological (12%–23%),[68,69] and lymphoma (8%–19%).[70,71]

It is important for the physician treating cancer pain to recognize and address depression (Table 42.1). Screening for depression should focus primarily on the cognitive/affective features of depression because these are not confounded with treatment-associated toxicities. In palliative care patients, several studies have found that the single question "Are you depressed?" was the screening tool with the highest sensitivity and specificity and positive predictive value.[72,73] Untreated, depression has a significant impact on patient quality of life, health care utilization, and even disease outcome.

SOURCES OF PAIN IN THE CANCER PATIENT

Most cancer pain results from one or more of three fundamental causes (Table 42.2):

TABLE 42.1

CONSEQUENCES OF PAIN AND DEPRESSION IN CANCER PATIENTS

Impact	Comment
Suffering	Significant contribution particularly when major organic disease is present
Medical evaluation and decision-making	Depressive symptoms can complicate
Outcome and survival	Depressive disorders can adversely affect
Recovery and compliance	Depressed medically-ill patients tend to have slower recovery and poorer compliance
Suicide	Undetected and untreated depression can lead to suicide
Pain	Poorly managed pain is a common cause of reactive depression in patients with severe, life-threatening disease

TABLE 42.2

CAUSES OF PAIN IN PATIENTS WITH CANCER

Cause	Example
As a direct consequence of tumor	Involvement of bones Obstruction of hollow organs Compression of nerves
As an indirect consequence of tumors	By infections By metabolic imbalances By venous/lymphatic occlusion
As a consequence of tumor therapy	Following surgical intervention Following chemotherapy Following radiation therapy
Without relation to cancer	Migraine Diabetic neuropathy Myofascial pain problems

- direct tumor involvement
- cancer-directed therapy
- mechanisms unrelated to cancer or its treatment

Patients may present with complex patterns of pain that result from combinations of these categories, thus complicating the diagnosis. Factors influencing the pain complaint include the primary tumor type, stage of disease, tumor site, and mood factors (anxiety and depression).[11,74,75]

Many patients with advanced disease frequently have multiple pain complaints at different sites and were more common in patients with breast, lung, and prostate cancer compared with gastrointestinal cancers.[74] In a prospective study of 2266 cancer patients, Grond et al.[76] assessed localization, etiology, and pathophysiologic mechanisms of pain syndromes associated with cancer. Thirty percent of the patients presented with one, 39% with two, and 31% with three or more distinct pain syndromes. The majority of patients had pain caused by cancer (85%) or antineoplastic treatment (17%); 9% had pain related to cancer disease and 9% due to etiologies unrelated to cancer. These investigations classified pain as originating from nociceptors in bone (35%), soft tissue (45%) or visceral structures (33%), or of neuropathic origin (34%). Patients localized pain in the lower back (36%), abdominal region (27%), thoracic region (23%), lower limbs (21%), head (17%), and pelvic region (15%). Regions and systems affected by the main pain syndrome varied widely depending on the site of cancer origin, whereas the cancer site did not markedly influence the pain's temporal characteristics, intensity, or etiology.

Although a significant association exists between most cancer pain and the presence of metastases, certain tumor types are exceptions, notably breast and prostate cancers. Neither the prevalence nor the severity of pain among breast cancer patients varies directly as a function of metastatic sites of disease.[56,59] Palmer et al.[77] evaluated the sensitivity of pain as an indicator of bone metastases in patients with breast or prostate cancer. Pain was a common finding, whether or not metastatic disease was present, and it occurred in over half of the patients. Although most patients with bone metastases reported bone pain, 21% of breast and 22% of prostate patients were asymptomatic.

Cancer-directed therapy pain syndromes may result from chemotherapy and radiation therapy (see Chapter 48) or surgery. Steroid use is common in cancer care, and pain due to osteonecrosis is a well-described complication of steroid use. Morbidity is related to progressive joint damage, often leading to decreased range of motion, pain with movement, and arthritis. Weight-bearing joints are most commonly involved and the disease often requires joint replacement to restore function and relieve pain. The shoulder, elbow, wrist, hand, and vertebral bodies can also be involved. Osteonecrosis typically develops within 3 years of steroid treatment. Osteonecrosis or avascular necrosis may occur as a complication of either intermittent or continuous steroid treatment. It most commonly involves the femoral head and presents with pain in the hip, thigh, or knee that is worse with movement, with or without localized tenderness. Humeral head disease presents similarly with pain in the shoulder, upper arm, or elbow. It may occur in any bone in the body. Focal osteonecrosis may mimic bone tumor and may result from steroid therapy as well as radiation and chemotherapy. There is little correlation between the degree of bone involvement and the intensity of associated pain.

Cancer patients and, in particular, cancer survivors may experience chronic nontumor-related pain. The challenge for the treating clinician is to distinguish between tumor-associated and nontumor-associated pain. Many of the same interdisciplinary treatment paradigms apply to cancer survivors as apply to all chronic pain patients. These findings indicate that pain associated with cancer and its treatment poses a substantial management challenge for the physician. Pain can change over time, involve

multiple sites, stem from several origins, involve several causes simultaneously, and may correspond loosely or not at all to the tumor.

Several schemata exist for classifying and evaluating pain in the cancer patient and are potentially useful for diagnosis and management; refer to Chapter 41 for additional perspectives.

Influence of Tumor Type

Factors influencing the pain complaint include the primary tumor type, stage of disease, tumor site, and mood factors such as anxiety and depression.[11,74,75] When metastatic disease appears, approximately 1 in 3 patients report significant pain. As discussed above, although pain tends to reflect the presence of metastases, this may not always be the case for certain tumor types, particularly for patients with breast or prostate cancers. The prevalence and severity of pain among breast cancer patients does not appear to vary directly as a function of metastatic sites of disease.[56,57]

Pain caused by tumor may occur at the onset of disease or at an advanced stage. Although pain can be one of the early indicators of the onset of disease, pain is not a significant problem for the majority of patients in the early stages of disease, with 5% to 10% of patients with solid tumors reporting pain at a level that interferes with mood and activity. However, when it does occur, pain is often the chief concern that prompts the patient to seek medical consultation. Vuorinen et al.[78] found that 28% of newly diagnosed cancer patients reported pain. Daut and Cleeland[14] found that pain was an early symptom of cancer in 40% to 50% of patients with cancer of the breast, ovary, prostate, colon, and rectum, and in about 20% of patients with cancer of the uterus and cervix.

Knowing the natural history of the disease facilitates an understanding of the pain process and is important in determining the nature and timing of treatment. Following are descriptions of the more common pain-producing malignant diseases.

Pancreatic Cancer. Over the past 20 years, the incidence of pancreatic carcinoma in Europe and North America has remained unchanged, with an estimated 9–10 cases per 100,000 and slightly increased male:female and black:white ratios. Pancreatic cancer currently ranks as the fifth most common cause of cancer-related deaths in western countries.[79] About 90% of pancreatic tumors are adenocarcinomas with a ductal phenotype. Neuroendocrine tumors and acinar cell carcinomas represent about 2% to 5% of all pancreatic tumors. Local tumor extension almost invariably involves the peripancreatic fat tissue through direct invasion of lymphatic channels and perineural spaces. Duodenum, stomach, gallbladder, and peritoneum are infiltrated by tumors located in the pancreatic head; body and tail tumors can invade liver, spleen, and left adrenal gland. Lymphatic spread to adjacent and distant lymph nodes seems to precede hematogenous spread, which affects, in descending order, liver, peritoneum, lungs, adrenals, kidneys, bones, and brain. Thirty to 60% of patients experience pain with early, relatively limited disease and over 80% of those with advanced disease have pain.[80,81]

A number of factors contribute to the generation and maintenance of pancreatic cancer pain. Pancreatic cancer is associated with extensive macrophage infiltration.[82] Macrophage infiltration is associated with upregulation of NGF which is associated with both the extent of perineural invasion of the tumor and pain intensity.[83] Given the massive increase in inflammatory and immune cells that are known to occur as pancreatic cancer progresses and that these cells contribute to a variety of pain states, it is likely that macrophages and other inflammatory or immune cells play a role in the initiation and maintenance of pancreatic cancer pain. A second group of mechanisms that may be involved in pancreatic cancer pain is the apparent sprouting (in precancerous and early stage pancreatic cancer) and then destruction (in late stage disease) of sensory and sympathetic fibers that innervate the pancreas. With disease progression, there is a clear increase in the density of CGRP sensory fibers.[84] This increase in density of CGRP expressing fibers may represent NGF-induced sprouting, with the origin of NGF being the macrophages. With disease progression, the central area of head, body, and tail of the pancreas, where significant sprouting of CGRP fibers had previously richly innervated, gradually becomes necrotic, resulting in destruction of the distal ends of the sensory and sympathetic fibers that had innervated these regions of the pancreas.[84] As damage to even the distal ends of peripheral nerves can generate a significant neuropathic pain state, these processes of extensive sprouting and destruction of sensory and sympathetic fibers may contribute to the sensitization and activation of nerve fibers innervating the pancreas.

Pain due to pancreatic cancer is usually abdominal, typically referred to the epigastric region or the upper abdominal quadrants, but it can also involve the lower quadrants or be diffuse.[85] Back pain is associated with abdominal pain in 50% to 65% of cases, but only 5% to 10% of patients report it as their only complaint.[86] In one series, 67% of patients could not describe their pain location better than as over their "diffuse abdomen."[86] Direct infiltration of pancreatic afferent nerves, pancreatic duct obstruction with retention pancreatitis, biliary obstruction, or duodenal infiltration resulting in bowel obstruction can generate pain. Eating often aggravates the pain. Tumors of the head of the pancreas may cause epigastric pain with right flank radiation more often, whereas pain from tumors in the tail has left-sided radiation.[87] Back pain in the region of T10–L2 is very common and is the first symptom in 10% to 30% of cases. Lying flat typically exacerbates it and sitting relieves it. This pain probably comes from retroperitoneal tumor involvement, and it may not respond to celiac plexus block (see Chapter 44). It often merges with similar syndromes caused by nodal or other soft-tissue tumor involvement in the retroperitoneal region (Table 42.3).

The impact of pancreatic pain can be profound. It is commonly associated with depressed mood and contributes to the rapid decline in function that characterizes this disease.[86,88]

Complete surgical resection is the only potentially curative treatment available. However, 5-year survival is only 10% to 20%. To be resectable, tumors must show no evidence of extrapancreatic disease or direct tumor extension to the celiac axis and superior mesenteric artery, but evidence of nonobstructive superior mesenteric-protal vein confluence does not always preclude tumor resection. Optimal symptomatic treatment has a prime role in the management of metastatic disease. This may require stenting or bypass surgery for obstructive jaundice or gastric outlet/duodenal obstruction.

Ovarian Cancer. The three categories of ovarian cancer are named for their cell of origin. Ninety percent of ovarian cancers arise from cells that make up the epithelial layer that covers the surface of the ovaries. The other 2 types are germ cell tumors and stromal tumors. Stromal tumors arise in the hormonally active elements within the connective tissue stroma of the ovary. Germ cell tumors and stromal tumors each account for approximately 5% of ovarian cancers. Epithelial cancer of the ovary is the most lethal gynecologic malignancy in the United States, with approximately 22,000 new cases and 16,000 deaths occurring annually. The lifetime risk of ovarian cancer in women with a germline mutation in the gene *BRCA1* approaches 40%, whereas in women with germline mutations in *BRCA2*, the lifetime risk ranges from 10% to 20%. The symptoms of ovarian cancer are fairly nonspecific and often occur when the disease is already spread throughout the abdominal cavity. Abdominal discomfort or vague pain, abdominal fullness, bowel habit changes, early satiety, dyspepsia, and bloating are frequent presenting symptoms. Occasionally, patients may present with bowel obstruction due to intra-abdominal masses or shortness of breath due to pleural effusion. Early-stage disease is usually asymptomatic, and

---

TABLE 42.3

PANCREATIC CANCER PAIN SYNDROMES

Pain due to tumor involvement	Pain due to cancer therapies
Visceral pain: Pancreatic gland infiltration Gastric infiltration Duodenal infiltration Liver metastases: capsule distention, diaphragmatic irritation Biliary tree distention Bowel obstruction (duodenal, peritoneal carcinomatosis) Ischemic abdominal pain due to mesenteric vessel involvement	Postoperative pain syndromes: Delayed gastric emptying Wound dehiscence or nonhealing
Somatic pain: Retroperitoneal involvement (direct, nodal) Parietal peritoneum and abdominal wall involvement Abdominal distention due to ascites Bone metastases	Biliary prosthesis complications
Neuropathic pain: Radiculopathy from retroperitoneal spread or bone metastatic involvement Lumbosacral plexopathy Epidural spinal cord compression	Postchemotherapy pain syndromes: Liver chemoembolization Mucositis Postradiation pain syndromes: Radiation enteritis

From Caraceni A, Portenoy RK. Pain management in patients with pancreatic carcinoma. *Cancer* 1996;78 (3 suppl):639–653. Copyright 1996 American Cancer Society. Reprinted by permission of Wiley-Liss, Inc., a subsidiary of John Wiley & Sons, Inc.

the diagnosis is often incidental, although such patients may occasionally present with dyspareunia or pelvic pain due to ovarian torsion. Serum CA-125 level has been widely used as a marker for a possible epithelial ovarian cancer in the primary assessment of a pelvic mass. In this setting, false-positive results may derive from several conditions, especially those associated with peritoneal inflammation, such as endometriosis, adenomyosis, pelvic inflammatory disease, menstruation, uterine fibroids, or benign cysts. Malignancies other than ovarian cancer can also increase CA-125 levels, but the most marked elevations (>1500 U/mL) are generally seen with ovarian cancer. Cytoreductive surgery is the cornerstone of the initial treatment of patients with advanced ovarian cancer. Although the majority of patients with ovarian cancer achieve a clinical complete remission with first-line chemotherapy, disease will recur in most. Overall, the 5-year survival rate for patients with advanced ovarian cancer is approximately 30%. Platinum-taxane combination chemotherapy yields responses in most patients with ovarian cancer. The issue of how many treatment regimens to use in patients with advanced ovarian cancer is an area of controversy. With low response rates with subsequent chemotherapies, patients need to decide whether to continue chemotherapy or receive supportive care only.

The prevalence of pain associated with ovarian cancer resembles the prevalence rates in populations with other solid tumors.[89] Ovarian cancer spreads by intraperitoneal, lymphatic, and locally invasive pathways. Lymphatic pathways may extend from the abdominal retroperitoneum to the groin via the inguinal/femoral canals or across the diaphragm to the pleural space. Intraperitoneal spread of tumor begins with extension of tumor through the ovarian capsule, allowing implantation of tumor throughout the abdomen. Intraperitoneal metastases show a predilection for the omentum and diaphragm, but no organ is spared, and concomitant ascites is frequent. Portenoy et al.[89] noted that pain, fatigue, and psychological distress were the most prevalent symptoms in patients with advanced (stage III or IV) ovarian cancer. Patients generally describe pain as occurring in the abdomino-pelvic or lower back region, as being frequent or almost constant, and moderate to severe in intensity. Patients with advanced disease may experience pain in the lower extremities either from invasion of the lumbosacral plexus by tumor or by lymphedema secondary to iliac vessel occlusion.

Cervical Cancer. Cancer of the cervix is a frequent cancer in women worldwide. There are several histologic subtypes of cervical carcinoma. Approximately 80% of cervical cancers are squamous cell, and 15% are adenocarcinomas. The cervix drains by preureteral, postureteral, and uterosacral routes into the following regional lymph nodes: parametrial, paracervical, hypogastric (obturator), common iliac, external iliac, internal iliac, sacral, and presacral. The common sites of distant spread include the aortic (para-aortic, periaortic), lateral aortic and mediastinal nodes, lungs, and skeleton. In patients with locally advanced disease (stages IIB to IVA), 24% have para-aortic disease.[90] Identification of para-aortic nodal status allows modification of therapy (usually extended-field radiation therapy) with improved survival.[91,92] Detection of para-aortic lymph node metastases may be difficult using standard imaging techniques such as abdomino-pelvic computed tomography (CT) scanning. The sensitivity of CT scanning for identifying para-aortic nodal metastasis may be only 34%.[90] Rose et al.[93] demonstrated that positron emission tomography (PET) scanning accurately predicts both the presence and absence of pelvic and para-aortic nodal metastatic disease. Magnetic resonance imaging (MRI) has been increasingly used to evaluate tumor volume and it is superior to CT in defining the extent of disease in the cervix and parametria, making it particularly useful in planning radiation treatment fields.[94] However, MRI is relatively inaccurate in assessing lymph nodes for the presence of metastasis. Recurrent cervical cancer is almost always incurable.

Prostate Cancer. Almost all prostate cancers (95%) are adenocarcinomas. The remaining 5% of cases consist of squamous cell carcinoma, signet-ring carcinoma, transitional carcinoma, neuroendocrine carcinoma, or sarcoma. Prostate adenocarcinoma may spread locally, by direct invasion of seminal vesicles, urinary bladder, or surrounding tissues, or distantly. Distant metastases can derive from an initial lymphatic spread or from hematogenous dissemination, mainly to the bones. The Gleason system is the most widely used grading system for prostate cancer (adenocarcinoma only). Prostate cancers are stratified into five grades (1–5) on the basis of the glandular pattern and degree of differentiation. The Gleason score is derived from the sum of the most represented grade (primary grade) with the second most represented grade (secondary grade) (e.g., $3 + 4 = 7$); this correlates better with prognosis than the single Gleason grade. The Gleason system can be applied to biopsy and surgical specimens, but not to fine needle biopsy, which lack architectural data. Serum prostate-specific antigen (PSA), digital rectal examination, and transrectal ultrasonography constitute the three major diagnostic means for the detection of cancer. PSA is an organ-specific glycoprotein which originates in the cytoplasm of ductal cells of the prostate. It is responsible for liquefaction of seminal fluid. The greatest limitation of PSA is that it is tissue, and not tumor specific in the prostate. Elevated PSA levels may also be the sign of benign disorders such as benign prostatic hyperplasia or prostatitis because of the organ and not cancer specificity of this protein. Five-year relative survival varies with stage at diagnosis from 80% or more when malignancy is confined to the prostate to about 25% where bone metastases are present. The treatment of choice for advanced prostate cancer is androgen ablation, achieved via surgical (bilateral orchiectomy) or medical (LH–RH analogues) castration, which is effective, but not curative in 80% to 85% of cases. Patients progressing after hormone therapy can be treated successfully with second-line hormone therapy. Chemotherapy has a well-recognized role in the management of hormone-refractory prostate cancer. Chemotherapy combinations of taxanes plus estramustine have been tested with clinical results in the range of 33% to 46% (mean 43%) for paclitaxel and 17% to 50% (mean 32%) for docetaxel.[95] The relative role of radiotherapy in metastatic disease is to deal with isolated symptoms, which may persist despite systemic treatment.

Because of the predilection of prostate cancer to spread to bony sites, a significant proportion of patients with metastatic disease will have bone pain. Prostate cancer rarely spreads to vital organs and the disease tends to progress slowly. The only exceptions are spinal cord compression or ureteral obstruction secondary to retroperitoneal lymph node metastases.

Tumors of the prostate gland may produce local rectal, urethral, suprapubic, and penile pain as a result of expansion and inflammation of the prostate, pain referred to the back, lower extremities, and abdominal area resulting from tumor growth within the pelvis, and distant bone pain with associated neurologic dysfunction associated with long bone, vertebral, and skull metastases (Table 42.4). The regional lymph nodes of the prostate are the nodes of the true pelvis, which are the pelvic nodes below the bifurcation of the common iliac arteries. Distant lymph nodes are outside the confines of the true pelvis. They are the aortic (para-aortic, periaortic, lumbar), common iliac, inguinal, superficial inguinal (femoral), supraclavicular, cervical, scalene, and retroperitoneal nodes.

Clinical syndromes can be differentiated by the site of bony involvement, the coexistence of mechanical instability secondary to fractures, and the neurologic dysfunction caused by tumor infiltration of contiguous neurologic structures. Bone metastases to the hip and pelvis often produce local pain that is exacerbated by movement, especially during weight bearing. Local invasion of tumor from the pelvis into the sacrum may produce the syndrome of perineal pain. Patients with this syndrome complain of local and perirectal pain that is accentuated by pressure on the

TABLE 42.4

CAUSES OF PAIN IN PROSTATE CANCER

Causes of pain	Examples/clinical syndromes
Bone metastasis	Single metastasis of pelvis or long bone
	Vertebral body metastasis, spinal cord compression
	Base-of-skull metastasis, cranial nerve palsies
	Perineal pain syndromes
Soft tissue metastasis	Lumbosacral plexopathy
	Pelvic tension "myalgia"
Pelvic visceral pain	"Prostatitis" pain

From Payne R. Pain management in the patient with prostate cancer. *Cancer* 1993;71(3 suppl):1131–1137. Copyright 1996 American Cancer Society. Reprinted by permission of Wiley-Liss, Inc., a subsidiary of John Wiley & Sons, Inc.

perineal region, such as that caused by sitting or lying prone. In its most extreme form, the patient cannot sit or lie flat. Dysfunction of the parasympathetic sacral innervation to bladder and bowel impairs continence early in the course of this syndrome. Local spread of tumor from the prostate into other pelvic and abdominal structures often produces visceral and neuropathic pain. Tumor invasion of the lumbosacral plexus may occur.

Breast Cancer. Breast cancer is the most commonly diagnosed cancer and the second leading cause of cancer-related mortality among North American women. After primary treatment with breast-conserving surgery and radiation, 10% to 20% of patients will have local recurrence in the breast within 1 to 9 years. Between 10% to 25% of these will have locally extensive or metastatic disease. After radical surgery and postoperative radiation, loco-regional recurrences occur in <10%.[96] Breast cancer is a heterogeneous disease. Breast cancers are derived from the epithelial cells that line the terminal duct lobular unit. Cancer cells that remain within the basement membrane of the elements of the terminal duct lobular unit and the draining duct are classified as in situ or noninvasive. An invasive breast cancer is one in which there is dissemination of cancer cells outside the basement membrane of the ducts and lobules into the surrounding adjacent normal tissue. Breast cancer consists of the following histologic types: carcinoma, ductal, lobular, nipple, and other (undifferentiated). Increasing tumor size and nodal involvement are well-established adverse prognostic factors for patients who have early-stage breast cancer. Therapeutic strategies for individual patients with breast cancer frequently depend upon the following prognostic variables: size of the primary neoplasm, the presence and extent of axillary lymph node metastases, pathological stage of disease after primary therapy, and the presence or absence of receptor (estrogen, progesterone) activity. The breast lymphatics drain via three major routes: axillary, transpectoral, and internal mammary. Intramammary lymph nodes are considered with, and coded as, axillary lymph nodes for staging purposes. Metastases to any other lymph node are distant. Hormone receptor status is a well-established prognostic and predictive factor. The role of estrogen receptor (ER) status as a prognostic factor was confirmed in a meta-analysis of seven cooperative group adjuvant therapy trials.[97] For women who had ER-negative tumors, there was a peak annual hazard of recurrence of 18.5% at approximately 1 to 2 years after surgery that declined rapidly thereafter to a rate of 1.4% in years 8 through 12. Most breast cancers, however, are ER-positive. The human epidermal growth factor

receptor 2 (HER2) receptor is a member of the epidermal growth factor receptor family and is overexpressed in approximately 20% to 25% of human breast cancers. HER2 overexpression has historically conferred a worse prognosis compared with nonoverexpressing cohorts. HER2 status is also an important predictor of response to hormone therapy. For example, HER2-positive breast cancers are relatively resistant to tamoxifen therapy, presumably as a result of cross-talk between intracellular signaling pathways.[98] Hormone therapy with aromatase inhibitors, however, which have a unique mechanism of action compared with tamoxifen, has not demonstrated similar resistance patterns.[99]

PET scanning can be used to evaluate primary lesions, regionally metastatic, and systemic metastases of breast cancer. Combined fluorodeoxyglucose-PET (FDG-PET) and MRI provide useful treatment-planning data for patients clinically suspected of having recurrent axillary or supraclavicular breast cancer. FDG-PET helped confirm metastases in patients with indeterminate MRI findings and depicted unsuspected metastases outside the axilla.[100] FDG-PET is also superior to bone scintigraphy in the detection of osteolytic breast cancer metastases.[101]

Breast cancer can metastasize to any organ in the body: bone, lung, liver, and brain are frequent sites. Metastases usually appear within a few years but recurrence may occur, particularly in bone, many years later. Although metastatic disease may be asymptomatic, the most common site of metastases, bone, typically hurts. Between 40% and 60% of patients with metastatic breast cancer will have bony disease, and in many of these patients, the involved bones (vertebrae, femoral and humoral shafts, and the acetabular area) are those that are involved with motion. Moreover, patients with metastatic breast cancer and bone involvement as their only site of metastatic disease may have median survival expectations of 27 to 29 months, during which time pain may be the chief manifestation of disease. Even patients with pulmonary metastases have median survivals of the order of 18 to 23 months,[102] and patients with only unilateral pleural involvement on the order of 44 months.[103] Metastatic breast cancer is currently an incurable yet treatable disease. While median survival is of the order of 18 to 24 months, survival ranges from a few weeks to several years. This biological variability means that for many women, metastatic breast cancer can be viewed as a chronic relapsing and remitting disease that may respond for a time to an array of cytotoxic and endocrine therapies. However, there is no consensus on the effects of these treatments on overall survival and quality of life, on the relative efficacies of chemotherapy and endocrine therapy, on the most appropriate duration and dosages of treatment, and on the merits of combined modality treatment.

The clinician will most likely have a long relationship with the patient with metastatic breast cancer and will have the opportunity to follow the course and progression of disease. The course of disease in patients with metastatic breast cancer fits one of two patterns: an indolent course that is not immediately life-threatening or one that is rapidly progressing or with extensive vital organ disease. Knowledge of the natural history of the disease is important in determining the nature and timing of treatment.

Table 42.5 lists some of the common causes of pain in patients with breast cancer.

Lung Cancer. Lung cancer is the most common cancer in the world and the leading cause of cancer-related deaths in Western countries. Non–small-cell lung cancer (NSCLC) constitutes between 80% and 85% of all lung cancers; small-cell lung cancer (SCLC) makes up the remaining 15% to 20%. Unfortunately, at the time of diagnosis, the majority of patients already have metastatic disease, and a systemic, palliative treatment is the primary therapeutic option. Each of the two major types of lung cancer further divides into subtypes, but these categories often blend into each other or coexist. SCLCs are relatively sensitive to cytotoxic chemotherapy and radiation therapy. They are usually

TABLE 42.5

CAUSES OF PAIN IN PATIENTS WITH BREAST CANCER

Etiology	Example	Example
Tumor-related	Bone metastases	
	Neural metastases	Brachial plexopathy
		Spinal cord compression
		Meningeal carcinomatosis
		Peripheral neuropathy secondary to tumor infiltration
	Visceral metastases	Pleural
		Liver
		Bowel
		Peritoneum
Anticancer therapy	Procedure-related pain in breast	
	Postmastectomy syndrome	
	Lymphedema-related	
	Postradiation treatment	
	Peripheral neuropathy	
	Phlebitis	
	Mucositis	
	Chemical cystitis (e.g., secondary to cyclophosphamide)	
	Osteoporosis or avascular necrosis	
Pre-existing conditions	Chronic nonmalignant pain	

centrally located, but can arise peripherally. Clinically, these tumors demonstrate a rapid growth rate and early metastatic dissemination.

Before the advent of systemic therapy, local surgical or radiation therapy alone produced poor median survivals, ranging from 8 to 17 weeks and 5-year survivals of less than 1%.[104] Effective chemotherapy has allowed the control of disseminated disease and improved the median survival of patients to 1 year or more, increasing the number of long-term disease-free survivors to between 5 and 10%.[105]

SCLC tumors express many neuroendocrine markers. Individual tumors may secrete up to 10 discrete hormones.[106] Histologically, SCLCs include small-cell anaplastic carcinoma, which includes the oat cell type. Small-cell anaplastic carcinoma is an aggressive and rapidly growing neoplasm and is limited to the thorax at the time of diagnosis in only 25% of patients. Metastases occur in regional lymph nodes, lung, abdominal lymph nodes, liver, adrenal gland, bone, central nervous system (CNS), and bone marrow.

NSCLSs are a morphologically diverse group that includes squamous cell carcinoma, adenocarcinoma, and large-cell anaplastic carcinoma. Squamous cell carcinoma is less likely to metastasize early. Adenocarcinomas have become the most frequent form of lung cancer in the United States.[107] Adenocarcinoma metastasizes widely and frequently to the other lung, liver, bone, kidney, and the CNS. Large-cell anaplastic carcinoma metastasizes in a pattern quite similar to adenocarcinoma with a predilection for mediastinal lymph nodes, pleura, adrenals, CNS, and bone.

For the purposes of prognosis and for analyzing data from clinical studies, SCLC is divided into limited and extensive disease categories. Limited disease is characterized by tumor that is clinically confined to the chest, mediastinum, and ipsilateral supraclavicular lymph nodes. Ipsilateral pleural effusion represents limited disease. All other sites of metastases are defined as extensive disease.[108] The median survival for patients with limited disease is approximately 12 to 18 months; for extensive disease, it ap-

proximates 9 months.[109] During the last 10 years, several new cytotoxic agents have become available; these include taxanes (paclitaxel and docetaxel), vinorelbine, gemcitabine, and topoisomerase 1 inhibitor irinotecan. Advances in lung cancer therapy have led to modest improvements in survival of patients with early or advanced disease.[110]

Lung cancers, particularly SCLC, often entail clinical paraneoplastic syndromes. Malignancy-associated hyponatremia is commonly associated with excessive production of arginine vasopressin by tumor cells and a large fraction of new cases of syndrome of inappropriate antidiuretic hormone secretion in elderly smokers are due to SCLC. About 10% of all lung cancer patients have hypercalcemia, and of these patients 10% to 15% do not have evident bone metastases. Humoral hypercalcemia of malignancy is more common in NSCLC, and especially squamous cell carcinoma. The neurologic syndromes associated with lung cancer are rare disorders and include subacute cerebellar degeneration, optic neuritis and retinopathy, subacute necrotizing myelopathy, and peripheral neuropathy.

Pain is a common and severe symptom in patients with all types of advanced lung cancer.[111,112] Chest pain is the most common site of pain in patients with small-cell cancer. The pain complaint is often poorly localized, dull in character, may radiate to the neck or back, and exacerbates with coughing. Mercadante et al.[111] reported that patients with advanced lung cancer commonly reported chest wall (including ribs and shoulder blade) pain, followed by lower extremities and lumbar regions, then abdomen and upper extremities, and the head area. Apical lung tumors (so-called Pancoast tumors) are notorious for causing brachial plexopathy with associated neuropathic pain.[39]

Renal Cell Cancers. Renal cell carcinoma (RCC) comprises a histologically diverse group of solid tumors, together making up only about 3% of all adult neoplasms,[113] but mortality from RCC may be increasing.[114] Clear-cell and papillary RCC are the most common histologic subtypes. More than half of RCCs now present as incidental radiographic findings discovered during workup of unrelated conditions.[115] Currently, no effective serum tumor markers for diagnosis of RCC exist. Twenty-five to 30% of patients have overt metastases at the time of diagnosis. Frequent sites include the lung (50% to 60% of patients with metastases), bone (30%–40%), liver (30%–40%), and brain (5%). Unusual sites of metastases characterize renal cancer, however, and may involve virtually any organ site, including the thyroid, pancreas, skeletal muscle, and skin or underlying soft tissue. Common metastatic sites include bone, liver, lung, brain, and distant lymph nodes. The regional lymph nodes of the kidney are renal hilar, paracaval, aortic (para-aortic, periaortic, lateral aortic), and retroperitoneal. Papillary RCC are less likely to metastasize than clear cell RCC, but metastatic lesions may have a worse prognosis than clear cell metastases.

Surgical resection remains the cornerstone of treatment for RCCs. Radical nephrectomy involves resection of kidney, perirenal fat, and ipsilateral adrenal gland. The extent and benefit of lymphadenectomy is controversial. In 10% to 20% of patients, nodal involvement is found at surgery without clinically evident distant metastases.[116,117] Virtually all such patients later relapse with distant metastases despite lymphadenectomy.[117] The benefit of lymphadenectomy is limited to the prognostic information it provides, rarely providing a cure. Though RCC is extremely radioresistant, palliative radiation therapy is appropriate for brain and bone metastases. Compared to other cancers, chemotherapy is rather ineffective for RCC. Many agents have been tested with most showing response rates of less than 10%. High dose cytokine therapy with interlueukin-2 is used for advanced cases of RCC but is associated with significant toxicity. Pegylated interferon is also used for advanced cases. The most important determinant of survival is the anatomical extent of the tumor (i.e., the pathologic stage). Patients with organ-confined disease that is resected completely generally have better outcomes than those with nodal involvement or distant metastases. Twenty to 30% of patients with localized tumors relapse after radical nephrectomy. Less than 5% have local recurrences, whereas lung metastases are the most common sites of distant relapse, occurring in 50% to 60% of patients.[118,119] The median time before a relapse after nephrectomy is 15 to 18 months, and 85% of relapses occur within 3 years.[118,119] Pain is common due to bone and other metastatic spread and the poor prognosis with this disease points toward the importance of palliative care planning early on.

Colorectal Cancer. Colorectal cancer is one of the most common malignancies in the Western world and accounts for about 10% of all cancer deaths in both Europe and the United States.[113] The vast majority of these tumors are adenocarcinoma (>90%) and, to a lesser degree, carcinoid tumors, leiomyosarcomas, and lymphoma. Spread to regional lymph nodes generally correlates to depth of invasion by the primary tumor and the grade of differentiation. Nodal spread occurs in 10% to 20% of tumors confined to the bowel wall. Hematogenous spread is usually to the liver via portal venous transmission.

The liver is the prime organ for metastatic spread (65%); extra-abdominal metastases in lung (25%) and brain and bone (10%) are much less common. Most recurrences appear within 2 years (about 70%) and almost all (90%) within 5 years. Surgery is the primary modality of treatment. There is no well-defined role for radiation treatment in colon cancer. The response rates to chemotherapy (usually 5-FU) in recurrent and metastatic cancer remain poor and of limited duration. In addition to staging systems, independent prognostic factors include histologic type, histologic grade, serum carcinoembryonic antigen (CEA) level, and extramural venous invasion. Elevated CEA levels are found in a variety of cancers other than colonic, such as breast, lung, pancreas, stomach, and ovary. Ten years ago, the treatment of metastatic colorectal cancer was based on one drug only, 5-FU. With the development of drug combinations, the response rate and median overall survival have doubled, approaching 50% and

TABLE 42.6

PROGNOSTIC TUMOR MARKERS IN MALIGNANCY

Cancer	Prognostic marker
Breast	ER, HER2/neu
Prostate	PSA
Colorectal	CEA
Ovarian	CA 125
Nonseminomatous germ cell	AFP, HCG
Trophoblastic disease	HCG

AFP, alpha-fetoprotein; CA 125, cancer antigen 125; HCG, human chorionic gonadotropin

20 months, respectively.[120] Patients with nonresectable, potentially curable disease may benefit from neoadjuvant chemotherapy with the aim of inducing tumor shrinkage to the point that the disease becomes resectable. Combining CT with biologic agents might additionally improve survival in this setting. Pain is commonly caused both by local effects (e.g., obstruction) and metastatic disease (e.g., to liver).

Tumor Markers. Genomics, proteomics, and metabolomics are being used to develop molecular signatures for disease diagnosis, prognosis, and therapeutic efficacy. Tumor-associated antigens discovered by these methods are used to develop passive (humoral) as well as active immunotherapy strategies to stimulate the immune system. Development and validation of biomarkers in parallel with therapeutics can speed development times by accurate screening of patient populations and substituting surrogate markers that correlate well with clinical outcomes. A tumor marker can be defined as a molecule that indicates the likely presence of cancer or that provides information about the likely future behavior of a cancer. Markers are potentially useful in screening for early malignancy, acting as a diagnostic or prognostic aid, predicting therapeutic efficacy, maintaining surveillance following surgical removal of the primary tumor, and monitoring therapy in advanced malignancy. Examples of prognostic tumor markers in malignancy are shown in Table 42.6.

One of the main uses of tumor markers is in the postoperative follow-up of patients diagnosed with malignancy. Examples of markers used for surveillance in this fashion are listed in Table 42.7.

Markers may be used to guide treatment decisions. For example, molecular biomarkers in breast cancer may dictate therapy. Patients who are ER-positive may receive hormonal therapy in the form of tamoxifen or anastrozole, HER2 positive patients may receive immunotherapy as trastuzumab, and BRCA1 pa-

TABLE 42.7

TUMOR MARKERS USED FOR POSTOPERATIVE AND THERAPY SURVEILLANCE

Cancer	Marker
Colorectal	CEA
Breast	CA 15-3, BR 27.29, CEA
Ovarian	CA 125
Trophoblastic	HCG
Prostate	PSA
Thyroid (differentiated)	Thyroglobulin

CA 15-3, cancer antigen 15-3; BR 27.29, glycoprotein 27.29

tients chemotherapy as anthracyclines or taxanes.[121] Markers are also frequently used to monitor treatment in patients with advanced disease. Consistently increasing levels may suggest treatment failure and the need to switch to alternative treatments.

Cancer Pain Syndromes

This section is intended to complement material presented in Chapters 41, 45, and 46.

NEUROPATHIC CANCER PAIN

Neuropathic pain is a common cause of severe and difficult to control pain syndromes in patients with cancer. The most common etiologies and syndromes are discussed.

Neuropathic Pain Secondary to Cancer-Related Pathology in Cranial Nerves

Painful cranial neuralgias may occur secondary to base of skull metastases, leptomeningeal metastases, or head and neck cancers.[122] Base of skull metastases produce several well-described pain syndromes[123] and are often associated with primary tumors of the breast, lung, and prostate. Constant localized aching pain from bone destruction and neurologic deficits from progressive cranial nerve palsies are cardinal manifestations.

The middle cranial fossa syndrome presents with facial numbness, paresthesias, or dysesthetic neuropathic pain in the distribution of the second or third divisions of the trigeminal nerve. Associated motor deficits include weakness in the masseter or temporalis muscles or abducens palsy.

The jugular foramen syndrome may present as glossopharyngeal neuralgia.[123] This pain is distributed over the ear or mastoid region and may radiate to the neck or shoulder. Associated deficits include a Horner's syndrome and paresis of the palate, vocal cords, sternocleidomastoid muscle, or trapezius muscle. Some attribute this syndrome to leptomeningeal metastases[124] and local extension of head and neck malignancies.[125] It is sometimes associated with syncope.[126]

A syndrome which clinically mimics classical trigeminal neuralgia can occur secondary to tumors in the middle or posterior fossa[127–130] or from leptomeningeal metastases.[131] This association between trigeminal neuralgia and tumor is uncommon, and cancer patients with a new onset of trigeminal neuralgia should have careful imaging of the base of skull.[128] Trigeminal neuralgia secondary to tumor usually presents as a constant, dull, well-localized pain related to the underlying pathology involving bone and other somatic structures associated with paroxysmal episodes of lancinating or throbbing pain.

Squamous cell carcinomas of the face, which commonly extend by perineural spread, are an important cause of complex trigeminal syndromes.[132] Perineural spread, when present, typically involves cranial nerves V and VII because of their extensive subcutaneous distributions.[133] Glossopharyngeal neuralgia commonly results from local nerve infiltration in the neck or base of skull. It typically produces throat and neck pain, radiating to the ear and mastoid, and is aggravated by swallowing. Occasionally, syncope accompanies severe pain.[134,135]

Cervical Plexopathy

Tumor infiltration of the cervical plexus can produce several pain syndromes, depending on the pattern of nerve involvement.[136] The upper four cervical ventral rami join to form the cervical plexus. The plexus lies close to C1–C4 vertebrae. The four cutaneous branches emerge from the posterior border of the sternocleidomastoid muscle into the posterior triangle of the neck. Because sensory afferents from the cervical plexus enter the spinal tract of the trigeminal along with the sensory afferents from cranial nerves V, VII, IX, and X, nociceptive referral patterns from the face and neck overlap. Symptoms usually include local pain with lancinating or dysesthetic components referred to the retroauricular and nuchal areas (lesser and greater auricular nerves), preauricular area (greater auricular nerve), anterior neck and shoulder (transverse cutaneous and supraclavicular nerves), and the jaw.[122] Associated findings include ipsilateral Horner's syndrome or hemidiaphragmatic paralysis. CT or MRI evaluation may be necessary to rule out associated epidural cord compression. Common clinical settings include local extension of a head and neck tumor or cervical lymph node metastases. In patients with head and neck tumors who have undergone radical neck dissection followed by radiation treatment, new onset or worsening pain includes a differential diagnosis of postradical neck dissection syndrome or tumor recurrence. Infections often complicate and exacerbate pain.

Tumor-Related Mononeuropathy

The most commonly described tumor-related painful mononeuropathy is intercostal nerve injury secondary to rib metastases with local extension. Patients with tumor invasion of the sciatic notch may present with symptoms resembling sciatica.

Radicular Pain/Radiculopathy

Radiculopathy is a pattern of pain corresponding to the dermatomal territory innervated by the dorsal spinal roots. Patients with cancer-related radiculopathy may present with pain on either or both sides of the midline. The pain tends to be unilateral in the cervical and lumbosacral regions and bilateral in the thorax. In cancer patients, radiculopathy typically results from epidural tumor mass or leptomeningeal metastases. Coughing, sneezing, recumbency, and strain exacerbate the pain, which often has dysesthetic qualities. Radiculopathy may also develop secondary to leptomeningeal metastases. Clinically, leptomeningeal metastases may produce multifocal neurologic signs and symptoms at a variety of levels, including cranial neuralgias. Most commonly, they produce a generalized headache with radicular pain in the low back and buttocks.[137]

Leptomeningeal Metastases

Leptomeningeal metastasis is defined as the appearance of tumor cells in the leptomeninges or cerebrospinal fluid (CSF) distant from the site of a primary tumor. It is also known as carcinomatous meningitis, neoplastic meningitis, neoplastic meningosis, leukemic meningitis (for leukemia), lymphomatous meningitis (for lymphoma), and meningeal carcinomatosis (for carcinoma). Oncologists and neurologists have increasingly reported diffuse leptomeningeal metastases of extracranial malignant tumors.[137–139] This complication occurs most commonly with adenocarcinoma of the lung and breast, lymphomas, and melanomas.

Leptomeningeal involvement occurs in 5% to 8% of solid tumors, 5% to 29% of non-Hodgkin's lymphomas, and 11% to 70% of leukemias.[140] Meningeal involvement was once a common complication of acute lymphoblastic leukemia, prior to the advent of CNS prophylaxis. Now this problem occurs in fewer than 5% of patients. Leptomeningeal metastases develop in 1% to 8% of patients with systemic cancer,[141] and has a poor prognosis with a median survival of 3 to 6 months.[142] Untreated, the prognosis is dismal with an average survival of 6 weeks.[143]

Tumor cells may reach the leptomeninges by several mechanisms including hematogenous spread, direct extension, transport through the valveless venous plexus, extension along nerves, perineural/perivascular lymphatics, escape from choroid plexus or subependymal metastases, and iatrogenic causes. Leptomeningeal tumors can encase the spinal and cranial nerves or may directly invade them and produce demyelination and axon destruction. The major mechanism of dissemination once tumor cells reach the leptomeninges is via exfoliation into the CSF space. Leptomeningeal metastases can cause symptoms by direct compression of brain structures (by meningeal nodules causing focal symptoms), irritation of adjacent brain (seizures), blocking of CSF pathways (leading to hydrocephalus and raised intracranial pressure), ischemia, or stroke (by constriction of pial arteries), cranial and peripheral nerve palsies (by direct nerve involvement), metabolic derangements (by decreasing available glucose for brain by rapidly growing tumor cells), and by causing meningeal fibrosis.

The hallmark of the clinical presentation of leptomeningeal metastases is the simultaneous occurrence of symptoms and signs at more than one area of the neuraxis. The clinical presentation of leptomeningeal metastasis is pleomorphic and commonly affects the cerebral hemispheres, cranial nerves, or spinal cord and its roots. It is best to describe the symptoms by their location along the neuraxis. Symptoms are usually multifocal and more diffuse than one discrete lesion allows. Symptoms include headache, back and radicular pain, multiple cranial and spinal nerve involvement, and change in mental status. Pain may occur in 30% to 76% of cases.[137,144] Table 42.8 lists the frequency of spinal cord symptoms and signs in patients with leptomeningeal metastases. The most common symptom is pain (80%) and patients may report a diffuse headache (25%) or pain in a spinal, radicular, or meningeal pattern (>50%). Localizing symptoms include cranial neuropathies, mononeuritis, radiculopathy, urinary incontinence, and visual disturbance.

The diagnosis rests on finding malignant cells on CSF examination or on characteristic gadolinium-enhanced MRI findings in the appropriate clinical context. The diagnosis should ideally be based on a combination of CSF studies and neuroimaging. Careful neurologic examination is required to demonstrate multifocal involvement of the CNS, cranial nerves, and spinal roots, which constitute the clinical hallmark of the disease. CSF analysis

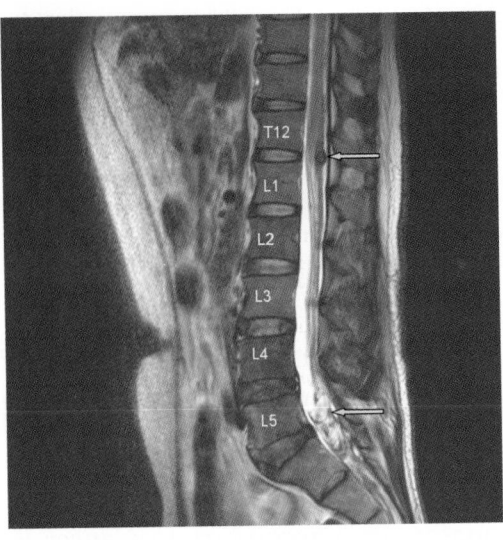

FIGURE 42.2 MRI of 50-year-old man with metastatic renal cell carcinoma. Patient presented with urinary retention and symptoms suggestive of cauda equinae syndrome. Lumbar spine (sagittal view) demonstrated diffuse leptomingeal carcinomatosis. Nodular contrast is noted particularly in the cauda equinae nerve roots (*yellow arrows*). There is also evidence of diffuse metastatic disease throughout the lumbar spine.

is almost always abnormal but only a positive cytology or demonstration of intrathecal synthesis of tumor markers is diagnostic. T1-weighted gadolinium-enhanced sequence of the entire neuraxis (brain and spine) plays an important role in supporting the diagnosis, demonstrating the involved sites and guiding treatment (Fig. 42.2). MRI images typically show enhancing nodular lesions.

Brachial Plexopathy

Most tumors involving the brachial plexus originate from the lung or breast and, as a result, invade the lower plexus. This syndrome can present from either compression or tumor infiltration of the brachial plexus from contiguous structures, such as axillary or supraclavicular nodes, or by tumors in the apex of the lung. Neuropathic pain due to tumor infiltration of the brachial plexus usually stems from lymph node metastases from breast carcinoma or lymphoma, or direct extension from lung carcinoma (i.e., Pancoast tumor). The designation of "Pancoast" tumors relates to the symptom complex or syndrome caused by a tumor arising in the superior sulcus of the lung that involves the sympathetic nerve trunks, including the stellate ganglion. Superior pulmonary sulcus syndrome associated with a Pancoast tumor is defined as progressively intense pain in the shoulder and ulnar side of the arm, associated with sensory and motor deficits and Horner's syndrome due to tumor.[39]

In brachial plexopathy, pain is usually the first symptom in 85% of patients and often precedes neurologic deficits.[145,146] The key features of malignant plexopathy are the neuropathic nature of the pain, with numbness, paresthesias, allodynia, and hyperesthesias. Typically, the pain begins in the shoulder girdle where it is often described as pressure-like or aching and may radiate to the elbow, medial forearm, and fourth and fifth fingers. It may also appear to localize at the posterior arm or elbow. The patient may report a burning quality to the pain, with hyperesthesia along the ulnar aspect of the forearm.

Involvement of the lower plexus (C7, C8, and T1) occurs when tumor arises from the lung apex; associated pain and dysesthesias involve the elbow, medial forearm, and fourth and fifth fingers. Upper plexus involvement (C5, C6), if it occurs alone, will usually

TABLE 42.8

FREQUENCY OF SPINAL CORD SYMPTOMS AND SIGNS IN PATIENTS WITH CARCINOMATOUS MENINGITIS

Symptoms or Signs	Percentage
Weakness	33
Paresthesia	31
Back pain	25
Radicular pain	19
Bowel/bladder dysfunction	13
Reflex asymmetry	67
Weakness	4
Cauda equina syndrome	33
Sensory loss	31
Positive straight leg raise	13
Decreased tone of anal sphincter	12
Nuchal rigidity	11

With permission from Zachariah B, Zachariah SB, Varghese R, Balducci L. Carcinomatous meningitis: clinical manifestations and management. *Int J Clin Pharmacol Ther* 1995;33(1):7–12.

TABLE 42.9

DIFFERENTIATING FEATURES OF BRACHIAL PLEXOPATHY INDUCED BY TUMOR INFILTRATION, RADIATION FIBROSIS, AND REVERSIBLE RADIATION INJURY

	Tumor infiltration	Radiation fibrosis	Reversible radiation injury
Incidence of pain	89%	18%	40%
Typical location of pain	Shoulder, upper arm, elbow, radiating to fourth and fifth fingers	Shoulder, wrist, hand	Hand, forearm
Nature of pain	Dull aching in shoulder; Lancinating pain in elbow and ulnar aspect of hand; Occasional dysesthesias, burning, or freezing sensations	Aching shoulder pain; Paresthesias in C5, C6 distribution in hand	Aching shoulder pain; Paresthesias in hand and forearm
Severity of pain	Moderate to severe (severe in 98% of patients)	Mild to moderate (severe in 35% of patients)	Mild
Course	Progressive neurologic dysfunction; atrophy and weakness with C7–T1 distribution; persistent pain; Homer's syndrome	Progressive weakness with C5, C6 distribution; stabilizing pain with appearance of weakness	Transient weakness and atrophy affecting C6–C7, T1; complete resolution of motor findings
CT scan findings	Circumscribed mass with diffuse infiltration of tissue planes	Diffuse infiltration of tissue planes	Normal
EMG findings	Segmental slowing; no myokymia	Myokymia	Segmental slowing; no myokymia

Modified from Foley KM. Brachial plexopathy in patients with breast cancer. In: Harris JR, Hellman S, Henderson IC, Kinne DW, eds. *Breast diseases.* Philadelphia: JB Lippincott Co, 1987.

develop into a panplexopathy. Upper plexus pain typically involves the shoulder girdle, with burning pain in the tips of both the index finger and thumb. Lung tumors can also present with pain involving the axilla and upper chest wall in the distribution of the intercostobrachial nerve.[147]

In more than 75% of patients, neurologic signs follow the appearance of dysesthesias. These signs include focal weakness, atrophy, and sensory changes in the distribution of C7, C8, and T1 roots.[146] There is usually early loss of the triceps reflex. Associated findings can include Horner's syndrome and adjacent vertebral disease. Such patients are at high risk for concurrent epidural extension.[144,148] For patients with brachial plexopathy secondary to tumor, imaging the contiguous epidural space prior to radiation treatment so that the radiation oncologist can include this area in the treatment field is recommended. A Spurling's maneuver (see Figure 41.4) can help to identify the spinal canal as the site of pathology.[149] Paraspinal involvement may help to predict epidural extension of tumor.

Neuroradiologic evaluations of choice for brachial plexopathy are CT and MRI. However, Ahmad et al.[150] demonstrated that FDG-PET scanning is a useful tool in evaluation of patients with suspected metastatic plexopathy, particularly if other imaging studies are normal. It may also be useful in distinguishing between radiation-induced and metastatic plexopathy. Electromyography (EMG) can also help distinguish malignant brachial plexopathy from radiation-induced brachial plexopathy or cervical radiculopathy (Table 42.9). In patients with brachial plexopathy, EMG usually shows fibrillation potentials and positive waves (evidence of denervation) in affected muscles. Radiation-induced brachial plexopathy is discussed below.

Lumbosacral Plexopathy

Direct tumor infiltration from adjacent soft tissues or lymph nodes or by compression from metastases in the adjacent bony

pelvis can damage the lumbosacral plexus. Most lumbosacral plexopathy reflects local extension or nodal metastases from colorectal and other pelvic tumors (cervix, uterus, bladder, prostate), sarcomas, and lymphomas, but it may also occur with metastases from breast or lung cancer or melanoma (Table 42.10).[136] Saphner et al.[151] found lumbosacral plexopathy caused by retroperitoneal lymph node metastases the most common neurologic complication in patients with advanced cervical cancer.

The cardinal clinical feature of carcinomatous plexopathy is severe, unrelenting pain.[152] The distribution of pain varies and may localize in the pelvis, low back or hip, or refer in a radicular or nonradicular pattern into the leg. The local pain is pressure-like or aching in quality. The referred pain varies with the site of plexus involvement and can be burning, crampy, or lancinating. Weeks to months after pain begins, sensory symptoms of numbness and paresthesias, as well as weakness and leg edema usually develop. A "hot and dry foot" syndrome may result from lumbo-

TABLE 42.10

COMMON NEOPLASMS BY LOCATION OF PLEXOPATHY

Tumor	Percentage
Colorectal	20
Sarcoma	16
Breast	11
Lymphoma	9
Cervix	7
All Others	37

From: Jaeckle KA. Neurological manifestations of neoplastic and radiation-induced plexopathies. *Semin Neurol* 2004;24(4):385–393.

sacral plexopathy and may reflect sympathetic fiber dysfunction.[153] The most common clinical findings on examination include leg weakness (86%), sensory loss (73%), reflex loss (64%), and leg edema (47%). Positive straight leg raising tests and sciatic notch tenderness are often present.[154]

Lumbosacral plexopathy may cause different clinical syndromes depending on the level of nerve involvement. Infiltration of the upper plexus occurs in approximately one third of patients who present with pain in the back, lower abdomen, flank, iliac crest, or anterolateral thigh. This syndrome has associated L1–L4 distribution neurologic deficits. Involvement of the lower plexus occurs in approximately one-half of patients, and presents with pain in the buttocks and perineum, with referral to the posterolateral leg and thigh. Examination may reveal associated L4–S1 neurologic deficits, leg edema, and bowel or bladder dysfunction. Sacral plexopathy can signal direct bony extension of a bony sacral lesion or a presacral mass. Numbness of the dorsal medial foot and sole with associated weakness of knee flexion, ankle dorsiflexion, and inversion is typical of lumbosacral trunk extension. Involvement of the coccygeal plexus results in sphincter dysfunction and perineal sensory loss. Panplexopathy occurs in one fifth of patients, and pain may refer anywhere in the territory of the plexus. Associated leg edema is relatively common.[153]

Jaeckle et al.[152] studied 85 cancer patients with lumbosacral plexopathy and documented pelvic tumor by CT or biopsy. They discerned three clinical syndromes: lower (L4–S1), 51%; upper (L1–L4), 31%; and panplexopathy (L1–S3), 18%. Seventy percent of patients had the insidious onset of pelvic or radicular leg pain, followed weeks to months later by sensory symptoms and weakness. The quintet of leg pain, weakness, edema, rectal mass, and hydronephrosis suggests plexopathy due to cancer. CT showed pelvic tumor in 96%. On myelography, epidural extension, usually below the conus medullaris, occurs in 45%. With treatment, only 28% of patients had objective responses on CT and 17% on examination.

In previously treated patients, the main differential diagnostic consideration is radiation-induced plexopathy (see below). Taylor et al.[155] found that MRI was more sensitive than CT for diagnosing cancer-induced lumbosacral plexopathy. Thus, MRI is the choice for the diagnostic work-up of patients with clinical and electrophysiologic evidence of plexopathy and suspected systemic cancer. Studies should include the L1 vertebral body through to the true pelvis. Neurologic findings include leg weakness, sensory loss, reflex asymmetry, focal tenderness (in the lumbar region in an upper plexopathy, sciatic notch and sacrum in a lower plexopathy, and lumbosacral region in pan-plexopathy), rectal mass, decreased sphincter tone, and positive direct and reverse straight leg raising signs.

Tumor Infiltration of the Sacrum and Sacral Nerves

Pain in a sacral distribution occurs usually as a result of the spread of bladder, gynecologic, or colonic cancer. There is dull aching midline pain and usually burning or throbbing pain in the soft tissues of the rectal or perineal region. Sitting or lying usually exacerbates the pain. With bilateral involvement, sphincter incontinence and impotence are common. There may be tenderness over the sacrum and in the regions of the sciatic notches. Sometimes there is limitation of both direct and reverse straight leg raising. Involvement of S1 and S2 roots will produce weakness of ankle plantar flexion, and the ankle jerks may be absent. There is usually sensory loss in the perianal region and in the genitalia, and this may be accompanied by hyperpathia.

Spinal and Radicular Pain

Patients perceive radicular pain as arising in a limb or thoraco-abdominal wall. The cause is ectopic activation of nociceptive afferent fibers in a spinal nerve or its roots or other neuropathic mechanisms. The pain is lancinating in quality and travels along a narrow band. It may be episodic, recurrent, or paroxysmal according to the causative lesion or any superimposed aggravating factors. While patients may experience radicular pain as a deep tissue pain, it also has a cutaneous quality in proportion to the number of cutaneous afferent fibers ectopically activated. Radicular pain differs from nociception in the axons stimulated along their course; their peripheral terminals are not the site of stimulation. Ectopic activation may occur as a result of mechanical deformation of a dorsal root ganglion, mechanical stimulation of previously damaged nerve roots, inflammation of a dorsal root ganglion, and possibly by ischemic damage to the dorsal root ganglia. Acute spine pain may be described as cramping or knife-like, but may also be merely dull or aching. It is worse with movement. Chronic spine pain without a radicular component is generally aching, dull, or burning, or any combination of these three features. It also tends to be made worse with movement.

Central Pain Syndromes Caused by Cancer

Central pain syndromes are relatively infrequent in the cancer population. While epidural spinal cord compression is almost always painful, central pain is not the predominant symptom; nociceptive input from progressive bony destruction by metastases is the usual cause of pain, with or without concurrent radicular pain from nerve root compression. Radiation myelopathy is also a possible cause of central pain syndrome.

Paraneoplastic Peripheral Neuropathy

Clinically significant peripheral neuropathy in cancer patients is common but only a small minority is paraneoplastic in origin (Table 42.11). Paraneoplastic syndrome refers to a group of disorders (caused by, or associated with, cancers) that are neither direct effects of the primary tumor mass or metastatic to the involved organs. These disorders can affect virtually any portion

TABLE 42.11

PERIPHERAL NEUROPATHY IN CANCER PATIENTS

Causes	Examples
Metastatic	Spinal cord compression Leptomeningeal metastases Metastases to peripheral nerves
Nonmetastatic	Metabolic nutritional Therapy side effects
Paraneoplastic	Subacute or chronic sensorimotor peripheral neuropathy Acute polyradiculopathy (Guillain-Barré syndrome) Mononeuritis multiplex and microvasculitis of peripheral nerve Acute brachial neuritis Autonomic neuropathy Peripheral neuropathy associated with paraproteinemia
Unrelated to cancer	Diabetes mellitus Vitamin B12 deficiency

From: Darnell RB, Posner JB. Paraneoplastic syndromes affecting the nervous system. *Semin Oncol* 2006;33(3):270–298.

of the nervous system. Most paraneoplastic syndromes stem from an autoimmune reaction to an "onconeural" antigen shared by the cancer and the nervous system.[156] The immune reaction may slow growth of the cancer, but it also damages the nervous system. Autoantibodies found in individual patients with paraneoplastic syndromes are usually associated with specific tumors. Neurologic disorders, clinically and pathologically identical to paraneoplastic syndromes, may occur in some patients without cancer, but these patients do not have paraneoplastic antibodies. Diagnosis of a paraneoplastic syndrome depends on its increased incidence in patients with cancer, the occasional response of the neurologic syndrome to treatment of the underlying cancer, or the presence of specific autoantibodies.

Antibodies as clinical markers for a paraneoplastic etiology have been available for just over 15 years, starting with the description of anti-Hu in 1985.[157] Four series totaling about 500 patients have been reported.[158–161] The most common symptoms were sensory neuronopathy, paraneoplastic limbic encephalitis, and paraneoplastic cerebellar degeneration. Cancers were diagnosed in 80% to 90% of patients and were preceded by the neurologic symptoms in 70% to 100%. The associated cancers tend to be limited and show no metastases (other than to mediastinal lymph nodes). Anti-Hu (at low titer) is also present in about 16% of patients with SCLC without neurologic symptoms.[162]

Four types of polyneuropathy constitute most of the cases of paraneoplastic peripheral neuropathy: motor, sensory, sensorimotor, and autonomic. Most paraneoplastic peripheral neuropathies are sensorimotor and axonal. A pure sensory neuronopathy, such as pathology in the dorsal root ganglion, strongly suggests a paraneoplastic syndrome associated with the anti-Hu antibody. A pure motor neuropathy subacutely developing could be the Guillain-Barré syndrome associated with Hodgkin's disease or a multifocal motor neuropathy with conduction block associated with plasma cell dyscrasias. An autonomic neuropathy is sometimes associated with the anti-Hu syndrome. Paraneoplastic disorders of the autonomic nervous system usually arise in the setting of encephalomyelitis. However, autonomic symptoms may predominate or rarely be the only symptoms or signs of a paraneoplastic neuropathy. The most common symptom is pseudo-obstruction of the bowel but anhidrosis, orthostatic hypotension, hypoventilation, sleep apnea, and cardiac arrhythmias can also present either alone or, more commonly, as part of a more widespread autonomic neuropathy. Most autonomic neuropathies are associated with SCLC and the anti-Hu syndrome. Mononeuritis multiplex suggests a vasculitis, possibly paraneoplastic in origin.

The classic paraneoplastic polyneuropathy is sensory neuropathy. Typically, patients with this disorder initially have an asymmetrical and painful sensory neuropathy, which evolves into complete loss of proprioception. The pseudoathetotic movement of the hands and severe sensory ataxia is very severe in most cases. Motor neuropathies may be acute or chronic, progressive or remitting, demyelinating, axonal or neuronal. Clinically, they are indistinguishable from the more common nonparaneoplastic motor neuropathies, unless they resolve after treatment of the cancer or are associated with a paraneoplastic antibody. These disorders include the Guillain-Barré syndrome, which occurs more frequently in patients with Hodgkin's disease than in the general population, a remitting and relapsing polyneuropathy resembling relapsing chronic inflammatory demyelinating polyneuropathy, and a subacute motor neuronopathy affecting patients with Hodgkin's disease or other lymphomas. The sensory neuropathies include a subacute pansensory neuropathy and a predominantly distal sensory neuropathy.

Paraneoplastic peripheral neuropathies are important because they may be the first sign of an otherwise occult cancer and/or because they may substantially disable the patient even when the cancer itself is asymptomatic. In about two thirds of cases, patients with paraneoplastic neurologic disorders present to the neurologist without a known tumor.

Neuropathic Pain Secondary to Therapeutic Interventions

Many pain syndromes occur in the course of or subsequent to treatment of cancer with surgery, chemotherapy, or radiation therapy. In most cases, there is injury to the peripheral nervous system or spinal cord, with pain as a major and often presenting complaint. In some cases, these syndromes occur long after the therapy is implemented, resulting in a difficult differential diagnosis between recurrent disease and a complication of therapy. Post radiation and chemotherapy pain mechanisms and syndromes are discussed in Chapter 48.

Postsurgical Neuropathic Pain

1. *Postmastectomy*: Pain can be a prominent postsurgical finding in breast cancer patients. It tends to appear in the postmastectomy period, a consequence of the disruption of normal neural pathways, or it may follow the development of lymphedema or the presence of metastases. In most situations, however, pain occurs primarily as a result of persistent restrictions in range of motion of the shoulder girdle in the region of surgery with findings of tender or trigger points in the associated muscle groups. Chronic neuropathic pain after mastectomy occurs primarily in patients whose surgery included axillary dissection,[163] although the problem can occur in women who undergo any surgical procedure on the breast from lumpectomy to radical mastectomy.[164] Postaxillary dissection pain is probably a more appropriate name than the usual postmastectomy pain for this syndrome.[165] The pain pattern typically involves paroxysms of lancinating pain against a background of burning, aching, tight constriction in the axilla, medial upper arm, and/or chest. Hyperesthesia, dysesthesia, hyperalgesia, allodynia, or hypoesthesia in the intercostobrachial nerve distribution may occur. The exact cause is unclear but various theories include dissection of the intercostobrachial nerve, intraoperative damage to axillary nerve pathways, and pain caused by neuroma formation. The intercostobrachial nerve is a cutaneous sensory branch of T1 and T2. The nerve is highly variable in size and distribution, making it difficult to avoid in these surgical procedures. Usually the pain develops shortly after surgery, but it can emerge months after surgery. Late-onset should prompt a search for other causes such as recurrent chest wall disease or bone metastases. The postmastectomy pain syndrome differs from metastatic or radiation-induced brachial plexopathy in which there is a different pattern of sensory loss, lymphedema, and usually more severe pain.

2. *Neck dissection* (also see Chapter 45): A large spectrum of surgical procedures is available for treatment of cervical lymph nodes.[166] These may be classified as radical neck dissection (RND), extended RND, modified RND, and selective neck dissection. RND for head and neck cancers can result in an iatrogenic syndrome characterized by ipsilateral face and neck pain with associated paresthesiae. Pain usually emerges weeks to months after surgery, consequent to injury to the cervical plexus or cervical nerves.[122] The most relevant functional sequel from RND is impairment of shoulder function due to sectioning the spinal accessory nerve and to the ensuing denervation of the upper trapezius muscle. Nahum et al.[167] coined the term "shoulder syndrome" to describe a clinical picture consisting of pain and limited abduction of the shoulder, full passive range of motion, and anatomic deformities such as scapular flaring, droop, and protraction. Pain is attributed to strain placed on other supporting muscles, such as the rhomboids and levator scapulae, as a consequence of shoulder drooping. A frequent ancillary sign of shoulder syndrome is sternoclavicular joint hypertrophy because of the abnormal

torque-like forces applied to the medial head of the clavicle, potentially complicated by stress fracture of the middle third of the clavicle. Recurrent tumor can also be a cause of pain that occurs or escalates after neck dissection.

3. *Thoracotomy*: Shortly following thoracotomy, a neuropathic pain can develop in the distribution of one or several intercostal nerves near the thoracotomy scar. The pain may remain stable after onset and gradually decrease over a period of months or years. Dajczman et al.[168] evaluated the prevalence and functional significance of long-term postthoracotomy pain in 56 patients who were at least 2 months postsurgery. Thirty patients (54%) with a median follow-up of 19.5 months had persistent pain; 26 others were pain-free at a median of 30.5 months postthoracotomy. Twenty-four of 44 patients (55%) who were more than 1 year after surgery, 13 of 29 patients (45%) more than 2 years, 6 of 16 (38%) more than 3 years, and 3 of 10 patients (30%) greater than 4 years postthoracotomy reported pain. Pain intensity was low, but 13 patients stated that pain "slightly" or "moderately" interfered with their lives. Five of 56 patients had sufficiently severe chronic pain to require daily analgesic use, nerve blocks, relaxation therapy, acupuncture, or referral to a pain clinic. Pain that increases with time or which first appears more than 3 months after surgery may signal recurrent tumor and should prompt further investigation. Maguire et al.[169] found two distinct patterns of nerve injury after thoracotomy and also demonstrated differences between surgical techniques. Thoracotomy with rib resection resulted in more detectable nerve damage than cautery along the top of the rib and pericostal closure. However, intercostal nerve damage at the time of operation was not associated with chronic pain or altered cutaneous sensation at 3 months postoperatively, suggesting that either the amount of intraoperative nerve damage is not indicative of long-term nerve damage or that there is a more significant cause for chronic pain other than intercostal nerve injury. In my experience, many patients experience chronic pain in the shoulder girdle region following thoracic surgical procedures not primarily from intercostal nerve damage but from a persistent inability to normally range the shoulder girdle region. In effect, these patients demonstrate persistent myofascial tenderness in the muscles of the shoulder girdle region (pectorals, trapezius, rhomboids, and deltoid).

4. *Phantom Pains*: Phantom pain disables a significant number of patients undergoing amputation of different body parts for malignancy.[170] It can have continuous or paroxysmal qualities, a burning or shooting character, and frequently invokes dysesthesias. The incidence of phantom limb pain is greater in cases where pain was present in the body part prior to amputation.[171] Phantom breast pain occurs in 13% of patients up to 1 year following mastectomy.[172] Phantom rectal pain occurs in up to 18% of patients after surgery for rectal carcinoma.[173] The reappearance or worsening of pain a long while after amputation can indicate tumor recurrence. The clinician must carefully distinguish among phantom pain, nonpainful phantom sensations, neuropathic stump pain, and nonneuropathic stump pain (see Chapter 26).

STEPWISE APPROACH TO PAIN ASSESSMENT

Assessing cancer pain is more than quantifying pain with a tool and recording it. A stepwise approach to cancer pain assessment begins with data collection and ends with a clinically relevant diagnosis which will require a thorough understanding of the various components contributing to the pain complaint. At a minimum, this involves determining the etiology of the pain and forecasting its future trajectory. It also involves determining the

TABLE 42.12

GOALS OF THE PAIN-RELATED HISTORY

Define the features of the pain
Outline the anatomical extent of the disease
Determine responses to previous disease-modifying and analgesic therapies
Clarify the impact of the pain on activity of daily living, psychological state, and familial and professional function
Determine the presence of associated symptoms that may modify the perception of pain

number of sites from which pain originates and the probable mechanisms involved. Assessment must include evaluation of the impact of pain on sleep, functional capability, activity level, and psychological well-being. In addition, the clinician must determine the nature, course, and impact of the cancer on the patient. A thorough evaluation will allow the clinician to obtain a basis for evaluating therapeutic intervention and determining the long-term goals of the patient and/or the patient's family.

The goals of the pain-related history are listed in Table 42.12. Optimal assessment includes a detailed description of these goals and classification by both pain syndrome and likely underlying mechanisms (see below).

Features of Pain History (also see Chapter 41)

Table 42.13 lists the key components to assessing the characteristics of the pain complaint.

Location

Many patients with advanced disease have multiple pains at different sites. Multiple pain complaints are more common in patients with breast, lung, and prostate cancer compared with gastrointestinal cancers.[74] Pain of tumor origin may be characterized by its location. For example, somatic pain resulting from bone metastases tends to be well-localized, while visceral pain tends to be diffuse and is often referred. Neuropathic pain may be radicular in location.

Intensity

Guidelines from the Agency for Health Care Policy and Research,[174] the American Pain Society,[175] and the American Society of Anesthesiologists[176] recommend the regular use of pain rating scales to assess pain severity and relief in all patients who commence or change treatments. These recommendations urge

TABLE 42.13

KEY COMPONENTS OF PAIN CHARACTERISTICS

Location
Intensity
Quality
Timing
Exacerbating/relieving factors
Response to previous analgesic and disease-modifying therapies
Impact of pain
Effect of pain on activities of daily living
Psychological state
Familial and professional function

clinicians to teach patients and families to use assessment tools in the home to promote continuity of pain management in all settings. Assessment tools for determining the intensity of pain are discussed above.

Quality

Tumor-associated pain can be nociceptive (somatic or visceral structures) or neuropathic in origin. Each source of pain has distinguishing qualities. For example, patients tend to describe pain that is neuropathic in origin as burning, shock-like, or shooting in quality, while they often describe pain originating from somatic structures as aching, nagging, throbbing, or sharp.

Timing

Cancer patients may have constant or intermittent pain. Constant pain is present continuously and usually fluctuates in intensity. Intermittent pain implies that pain is present for definite periods of time and that the patient is relatively pain-free between episodes of pain. Patients and their caregivers need to understand the concept of "breakthrough pain," as should health care providers. Breakthrough pain is discussed earlier in this chapter.

Exacerbating/Relieving Factors

Cancer patients with pain may experience a worsening of their pain over a wide range of activities. Commonly, patients with metastatic disease to weight-bearing bones experience an increase of their pain upon standing or sitting. Patients with breast cancer metastatic to the axillary nodes may have severe pain upon abduction of their upper extremity on positioning for external beam radiation therapy. Knowledge of these factors helps clinicians to design an appropriate pain treatment plan.

Responses to Previous Analgesic and Disease-Modifying Therapies

It is important to determine previous opioid use and benefits or side effects encountered during use. Previous unacceptable side effects to a particular opioid may limit successful future titration with the same opioid. Successful tumor shrinkage to chemotherapy or radiation therapy may indicate the need for further evaluation on tumor recurrence.

Impact of Pain

The initial pain assessment should elicit information about changes in activities of daily living, such as work and recreational activities, sleep patterns, mobility, appetite, sexual functioning, and mood. Numerous instruments, including symptom checklists and quality of life measures, may prove useful in this evaluation and are detailed in Chapter 22.

The **Memorial Pain Assessment Card** is a brief, validated measure that uses visual analog scale scores to characterize pain intensity, pain relief, and mood, and an 8-point verbal rating scale to further characterize pain intensity. The mood scale, which is correlated with measures of global psychologic distress, depression, and anxiety, is considered to be a brief measure of global symptom distress. Although this instrument does not provide detailed descriptors of pain, its brevity and simplicity may facilitate the collection of useful information while minimizing patient burden and encouraging compliance.

The **Brief Pain Inventory** measures both the intensity of pain (sensory dimension) and interference of pain in the patient's life (reactive dimension). It also queries the patient about pain relief, pain quality, and patient perception of the cause of pain. Numeric scales indicate the intensity of pain in general, at its worst, at its least, and right now. An average scale quantifies relief from current therapies. The patient marks a figure representing the body by shading the area corresponding to his or her pain. Seven items determine the degree to which pain interferes with function, mood, and enjoyment of life. Advantages of this questionnaire include that it is self-administered, easy to understand, and available in many languages.

Effects of the Pain on Activities of Daily Living

Many patients function quite effectively with a background level of mild pain that does not seriously impair or distract them.[57] As pain severity increases, the pain passes a threshold beyond which it is hard to ignore. At this point, it becomes disruptive to many aspects of the patient's life. Constant daily pain can significantly impact on a patient's daily activities. Williamson and Schulz[177] showed that as pain increased over time, restriction in activity occurred, which in turn predicted increases in depressed affect. General measures of functioning should include indicators of physical, psychological, and social functional status. Some impact factors may include interference on general activity, mood, walking, ability to work, relations with others, and sleep. The Pain Disability Index was developed as a self-report measure of general and domain-specific, pain-related disability and is considered to be reliable and valid as a brief measure of pain-related disability (Table 42.14).[178]

Maltoni et al.[179] confirmed the importance of certain clinical parameters as prognostic indicators for patients with terminal cancer (clinical experience, physical activity level, clinical symptoms relating to and unrelated to nutritional state). Performance Status Tables can help the physician assess physical activity levels (Tables 42.15 and 42.16). However, the palliative treatment of advanced cancer and the terminally ill requires a broad concept of well-being that goes beyond one based only on physical functioning.[180]

Psychological State

Psychological assessment of the cancer patient with pain is imperative and should reflect an understanding of the many factors that modulate distress, such as personality, coping, and both past and present psychiatric disorders. Knowing that the patient has received outpatient or inpatient psychiatric care helps to clarify the psychological risk. Information on how the patient handled previous painful events may provide insight into whether the patient has demonstrated chronic illness behavior.

Familial and Professional Function

The clinician must learn about the patient's familial and social resources, financial situation, and the physical environment in which he or she lives. Knowledge of the patient's and family's previous experience with cancer or other progressive medical disease may provide useful insights into the response to physical illness or the genesis of psychological symptoms. Although the influence of social factors on treatment preferences and desire for aggressive cancer therapy is still poorly defined, Yellen and Cella[181] demonstrated that positive social well-being, as well as having children living at home, predicted patient willingness to accept aggressive treatment.

Quality of Life Assessment

Prolongation of survival and maintenance or improvement of health-related quality of life (QOL) are the two important goals within the treatment of individual patients. Due to the severity of symptoms and the toxicity of treatment, QOL is a major area of concern when treating cancer patients in general and elderly patients in particular. QOL is defined as the person's evaluation of his or her well-being and functioning in different life domains.

TABLE 42.14

PAIN DISABILITY INDEX

The rating scales below are to measure the degree to which several aspects of your life are presently disrupted due to chronic pain. In other words, we would like to know how much your pain is preventing you from doing what you would normally do, or from doing it as well as you normally would. Respond to each category by indicating the **overall** impact of pain in your life, not just when the pain is at its worst. For each of the 7 categories of life activity listed, please circle the number on the scale which describes the level of disability you typically experience. A score of 0 means no disability at all, and a score of 10 signifies that all of the activities in which you would normally be involved have been totally disrupted or prevented by your pain.

(1) *Family/Home Responsibilities*

This category refers to activities related to the home or family. It includes chores or duties performed around the house (e.g., yard work) and errands or favors for other family members (e.g., driving the children to school).

0 1 2 3 4 5 6 7 8 9 10

no disability   total disability

(2) *Recreation*

This category includes hobbies, sports, and other similar leisure time activities.

0 1 2 3 4 5 6 7 8 9 10

no disability   total disability

(3) *Social Activity*

This category refers to activities which involve participation with friends and acquaintances other than family members. It includes parties, theater, concerts, dining out, and other social functions.

0 1 2 3 4 5 6 7 8 9 10

no disability   total disability

(4) Occupation

This category refers to activities that are a part of or directly related to one's job. This includes nonpaying jobs as well, such as that of a housewife or volunteer worker.

0 1 2 3 4 5 6 7 8 9 10

no disability   total disability

(5) *Sexual Behavior*

This category refers to the frequency and quality of one's sex life.

0 1 2 3 4 5 6 7 8 9 10

no disability   total disability

(6) *Self-care*

This category includes activities which involve personal maintenance and independent daily living (e.g., taking a shower, driving, getting dressed, etc.).

0 1 2 3 4 5 6 7 8 9 10

no disability   total disability

(7) *Life-support Activity*

This category refers to basic life-supporting behaviors such as eating, sleeping, and breathing.

0 1 2 3 4 5 6 7 8 9 10

no disability   total disability

TABLE 42.15

KARNOFSKY PERFORMANCE STATUS

Grade	Performance level
100	Normal, no complaints, no evidence of disease
90	Able to carry on normal activity; minor signs or symptoms of disease
80	Normal activity with effort; some signs or symptoms of disease
70	Cares for self; unable to carry on normal activity or to do active work
60	Requires occasional assistance, but is able to care for most of his or her needs
50	Requires considerable assistance and frequent medical care
40	Disabled, requires special care and assistance
30	Severely disabled, hospitalization indicated; death not imminent
20	Very sick, hospitalization necessary, active supportive treatment necessary
10	Moribund, fatal processes, progressing rapidly
0	Dead

TABLE 42.16

ECOG PERFORMANCE STATUS

Grade	Performance level
0	Fully active, able to carry on all predisease performance without restriction
1	Restricted in physically strenuous activity but ambulatory and able to carry out work of a light or sedentary nature (e.g., light housework, office work)
2	Ambulatory and capable of all self-care but unable to carry out any work activities. Up and about more than 50% of waking hours
3	Capable of only limited self-care, confined to bed or chair more than 50% of waking hours
4	Completely disabled. Cannot carry on any self-care. Totally confined to bed or chair
5	Dead

It is a subjective, phenomenological, multidimensional, dynamic, evaluative, and yet quantifiable, construct. The routine assessment of QOL may have clinical uses at the individual patient level. These uses include fostering patient-provider communication, identifying frequently overlooked problems, prioritizing problems, and evaluating the impact of palliative and rehabilitative efforts. QOL is sensitive to the treatment of pain and treatment modalities, although pain is not synonymous with poor QOL and constitutes only one important factor determining QOL. In addition, pain reduction is not always attended by the expected improvement in QOL. Two of the most widely used assessment tools in oncology are the European Organization for Research and Treatment of Cancer, Quality of Life Questionnaire Core 30 Items scale, and the Functional Assessment of Cancer Therapy—General (FACT-G).[182] FACT-G is self-reported and consists of questions on physical, functional, emotional, and social/family well-being. Patient responses are recorded on a five-point Likert-type scale (Table 42.17).

TABLE 42.17

FUNCTIONAL ASSESSMENT CANCER THERAPY—GENERAL (FACT-G)

Below is a list of statements that other people with your illness have said are important. By circling one (1) number per line, please indicate how true each statement has been for you during the past 7 days.

	Not at all	A little bit	Somewhat	Quite a bit	Very Much
PHYSICAL WELL-BEING _____					
I have a lack of energy	0	1	2	3	4
I have nausea	0	1	2	3	4
Because of my physical condition, I have trouble meeting the needs of my family	0	1	2	3	4
I have pain	0	1	2	3	4
I am bothered by side effects of treatment	0	1	2	3	4
I feel ill	0	1	2	3	4
I am forced to spend time in bed	0	1	2	3	4
				SCORE =	(MAX = 28)
SOCIAL/FAMILY WELL-BEING _____	Not at all	A little bit	Somewhat	Quite a bit	Very Much
I feel close to my friends	0	1	2	3	4
I get emotional support from my family	0	1	2	3	4
I get emotional support from my friends	0	1	2	3	4
My family has accepted my illness	0	1	2	3	4
I am satisfied with family communication about my illness	0	1	2	3	4
I feel close to my partner (or the person who is my main support)	0	1	2	3	4
Regardless of your current level of sexual activity, please answer the following question. If you prefer not to, please check this box ☐ and go to the next section.					
I am satisfied with my sex life	0	1	2	3	4
				SCORE =	(MAX = 28)
EMOTIONAL WELL-BEING _____	Not at all	A little bit	Somewhat	Quite a bit	Very Much
I feel sad	0	1	2	3	4
I am satisfied with how I am coping with my illness	0	1	2	3	4
I am losing hope in the fight against my illness	0	1	2	3	4
I feel nervous	0	1	2	3	4
I worry about dying	0	1	2	3	4
I worry that my condition will get worse	0	1	2	3	4
				SCORE =	(MAX = 24)
FUNCTIONAL WELL-BEING _____	Not at all	A little bit	Somewhat	Quite a bit	Very Much
I am able to work (include work at home)	0	1	2	3	4
My work (include work at home) is fulfilling	0	1	2	3	4
I am able to enjoy life	0	1	2	3	4
I have accepted my illness	0	1	2	3	4
I am sleeping well	0	1	2	3	4
I am enjoying the things I usually do for fun	0	1	2	3	4
I am content with the quality of my life right now	0	1	2	3	4
				SCORE =	(MAX = 28)
RELATIONSHIP WITH DOCTOR _____	Not at all	A little bit	Somewhat	Quite a bit	Very Much
I have confidence in my doctor(s)	0	1	2	3	4
My doctor is available to answer my questions	0	1	2	3	4
How much does your relationship with your doctor affect the quality of your life?	0	1	2	3	4
				SCORE =	(MAX = 12)

TABLE 42.18

COMPONENTS OF MEDICAL HISTORY: CANCER HISTORY, MEDICATIONS, PAST MEDICAL HISTORY, AND PSYCHOSOCIAL FACTORS

Cancer history	Current medications and past medical history	Psychosocial issues
Diagnosis	Previous medical and surgical illness	Family history
Chronology	Concurrent medical conditions	Social resources
Therapeutic interventions including operations and treatments	Drug reactions	Impact of disease and symptoms on patient and family
Patient's knowledge of extent of disease		Patient's and family's goals of care
Current clinical status		

General Assessment

The initial step in the general assessment of the symptomatic cancer patient is a complete medical history that reviews the cancer diagnosis, the chronology of significant cancer-related events, previous therapies, and all relevant medical, surgical, and psychiatric problems (Table 42.18). A detailed history of drug therapy should include current and prior use of prescription and nonprescription drugs, drug allergies, and previous adverse drug reactions including side effects. The patient should provide information about prior treatment modalities for each symptom. In the course of this assessment, the interviewer should document the patient's understanding of his or her current disease status. Discussion with other providers involved with the patient's care will also help determine disease status. Table 42.19 lists the different possible categories for a patient's clinical status.

A physical examination, including a neurologic evaluation, is a necessary part of the initial pain assessment (see below). A careful review of previous laboratory and imaging studies can provide information about the cause of pain and the extent of the underlying disease (see below). Evaluation of concurrent concerns includes other symptoms and related psychosocial problems. Additional investigations are often needed to clarify uncertainties in the provisional assessment. The extent of these investigations must be appropriate to the patient's general status and the overall goals of care (Table 42.20).

Associated Symptoms

Symptoms interact and therefore it is important to clarify the degree to which each symptom induces or exacerbates other physical or psychological symptoms. The evaluation should determine whether symptoms are concurrent but unrelated in etiology, concurrent and related to the same pathologic process, concurrent with the one symptom directly or indirectly a consequence of a pathologic process initiated by another symptom, or concurrent with one symptom a consequence or side effect of therapy directed against the other. Fatigue may be the most prevalent symptom reported by cancer patients.[183] Disease progression increases the number of factors diminishing QOL, as well as the prevalence and severity of physical and psychological symptoms. In addition to pain, patients with advanced cancer have fatigue, generalized weakness, dyspnea, delirium, nausea, and vomiting. These symptoms may have a major impact on both pain reporting and quality of life.

The **Memorial Symptom Assessment Scale** (MSAS) is a patient-rated instrument that was developed to provide multidimensional information about a diverse group of common symptoms. The MSAS is a reliable and valid instrument for the assessment of symptom prevalence, characteristics, and distress. This approach to comprehensive symptom assessment is helpful for clinical trials that incorporate QOL measures or studies of symptom epidemiology.[184] Portenoy et al.[185] evaluated patients with prostate, colon, breast, or ovarian cancer using the MSAS and other measures of psychological condition, performance status, symptom distress, and overall QOL. The Karnofsky Performance

TABLE 42.19

CLINICAL STATUS OF PATIENTS DEFINED BY DISEASE STATE AND TREATMENT STRATEGY

Category	Status
I	Active disease; care—palliative and supportive only
II	Active disease; treatment (e.g., chemotherapy, radiation therapy) in progress
III	Active disease, no current treatment, surveillance of tumor status
IV	No active disease; treatment of tumor in progress
V	No active disease; no current treatment, surveillance of tumor status
VI	No active disease; no current treatment, specialized care (e.g., medical oncology) not required

TABLE 42.20

COMPONENTS OF MEDICAL HISTORY: PHYSICAL EXAMINATION, INVESTIGATIONS, AND FURTHER EVALUATION

Physical examination		
Review of available laboratory and imaging data		
Further diagnostic investigations and specific assessments	Diagnostic Investigations Symptom-specific Extent of disease	Other Assessments Psychosocial Functional

Status score was less than or equal to 80 in 49.8%. Across tumor types, 40% to 80% experienced lack of energy, pain, feeling drowsy, dry mouth, insomnia, or symptoms indicative of psychologic distress. Although symptom characteristics were variable, the proportion of patients who described a symptom as relatively intense or frequent always exceeded the proportion who reported it as highly distressing. The mean ($+/-$ SD range) number of symptoms per patient was 11.5 $+/-$ 6.0 (0–25).

Laboratory and Imaging Data

Careful review of previous laboratory and imaging studies can provide important additional information. Specific radiologic or laboratory tests may help the clinician understand the pathophysiology of symptoms and their relationships to the disease. This information provides the basis for a provisional pain diagnosis that clarifies both the status of the disease and the nature of other concurrent concerns that may require therapeutic focus.

Some patients require multiple studies to evaluate the pain problem, clarify extent of disease, or to assess other symptoms. Assistance from physicians in other disciplines, nurses, social workers, psychologists, or others may prove necessary to evaluate related physical or psychosocial problems identified during the initial assessment. It is appropriate and useful to review the findings of this evaluation with the patient, family, and other appropriate persons, so that they can prioritize problems according to their importance for the patient. It is also useful to identify potential outcomes that would benefit from contingency planning, including the need for advanced medical directives, the evaluation of home care resources, and prebereavement interventions with the family.

Physical Examination

A physical examination, including a neurologic and musculoskeletal examination, is a necessary part of the initial pain assessment. The need for a thorough neurologic assessment is justified by the high prevalence of painful neurologic conditions in the cancer population.[186] The physical examination should clarify the underlying causes of the pain problem, detail the extent of the underlying disease, and discern the relation of the pain complaint to the disease.

Diagnosis

The provisional pain diagnosis includes inferences about the pathophysiology of the pain and an assessment of the pain syndrome. Evaluation of concurrent concerns includes other symptoms and related psychosocial problems. Additional investigations can often clarify uncertainties in the provisional assessment.

SUMMARY

Cancer is one of the medical conditions patients fear most. In addition to anxiety about cancer as a potentially lethal disease, patient and family expectancies that pain is an inevitable and untreatable consequence are major sources of distress. Controlling pain associated with cancer is a major health care problem. Lack of expertise by clinicians in assessing pain is an important cause of poor pain control. A stepwise approach to cancer pain assessment begins with a systemic clinical interview and ends with a clinically relevant diagnosis that outlines the mechanisms and contributing factors to the pain complaint. It involves determining the etiology of the pain and forecasting its future trajectory. It also involves determining the number of sites from which pain

originates and the probable mechanisms involved. Assessment must include evaluation of the impact of pain on sleep, functional capability, activity level, and psychological well-being. In addition, the clinician must determine the nature, course, and impact of the cancer on the patient. A thorough evaluation will allow the clinician to obtain a basis for evaluating therapeutic intervention and determining the long-term goals of the patient and/or the patient's family.

Many health care professionals may become involved with the cancer pain patient at any one time. Successful pain management requires that the person or persons responsible for pain management adopt, or at least become familiar with, an interdisciplinary approach to care.

References

1. Jemal A, Siegel R, Ward E, et al. Cancer statistics, 2007. *CA Cancer J Clin* 2007;57(1):43–66.
2. National Institutes of Health State-of-the-Science Conference Statement. Symptom Management in Cancer: Pain, Depression, and Fatigue. Bethesda, Maryland, 2002.
3. Pignon T, Fernandez L, Ayasso S, et al. Impact of radiation oncology practice on pain: a cross-sectional survey. *Int J Radiat Oncol Biol Phys* 2004;60(4):1204–1210.
4. Rietman JS, Dijkstra PU, Debreczeni R, et al. Impairments, disabilities and health related quality of life after treatment for breast cancer: a follow-up study 2.7 years after surgery. *Disabil Rehabil* 2004;26(2):78–84.
5. Bradley N, Davis L, Chow E. Symptom distress in patients attending an outpatient palliative radiotherapy clinic. *J Pain Symptom Manage* 2005;30(2):123–131.
6. Hwang SS, Chang VT, Cogswell J, et al. Study of unmet needs in symptomatic veterans with advanced cancer: incidence, independent predictors and unmet needs outcome model. *J Pain Symptom Manage* 2004;28(5):421–432.
7. Wilson KG, Graham ID, Viola RA, et al. Structured interview assessment of symptoms and concerns in palliative care. *Can J Psychiatry* 2004;49(6):350–358.
8. van den Beuken-van Everdingen MH, de Rijke JM, Kessels AG, et al. Prevalence of pain in patients with cancer: a systematic review of the past 40 years. *Ann Oncol* 2007;18(9):1437–1449.
9. Ahles TA, Blanchard EB, Ruckdeschel JC. The multidimensional nature of cancer-related pain. *Pain* 1983;17(3):277–288.
10. Carroll BT, Kathol RG, Noyes R Jr, et al. Screening for depression and anxiety in cancer patients using the Hospital Anxiety and Depression Scale. *Gen Hosp Psychiatry* 1993;15(2):69–74.
11. Glover J, Dibble SL, Dodd MJ, et al. Mood states of oncology outpatients: does pain make a difference? *J Pain Symptom Manage* 1995;10(2):120–128.
12. Strang P. Emotional and social aspects of cancer pain. *Acta Oncol* 1992;31(3):323–326.
13. Hu DS, Silberfarb PM. Management of sleep problems in cancer patients. *Oncology (Williston Park)* 1991;5(9):23–27.
14. Daut RL, Cleeland CS. The prevalence and severity of pain in cancer. *Cancer* 1982;50(9):1913–1918.
15. Coyle N, Adelhardt J, Foley KM, et al. Character of terminal illness in the advanced cancer patient: pain and other symptoms during the last four weeks of life. *J Pain Symptom Manage* 1990;5(2):83–93.
16. Grond S, Zech D, Diefenbach C, et al. Prevalence and pattern of symptoms in patients with cancer pain: a prospective evaluation of 1635 cancer patients referred to a pain clinic. *J Pain Symptom Manage* 1994;9(6):372–382.
17. Cleeland CS, Gonin R, Hatfield AK, et al. Pain and its treatment in outpatients with metastatic cancer. *N Engl J Med* 1994;330(9):592–596.
18. Cleeland CS, Gonin R, Baez L, et al. Pain and treatment of pain in minority patients with cancer. The Eastern Cooperative Oncology Group Minority Outpatient Pain study. *Ann Intern Med* 1997;127(9):813–816.
19. Anderson KO, Mendoza TR, Valero V, et al. Minority cancer patients and their providers: pain management attitudes and practice. *Cancer* 2000;88(8):1929–1938.
20. Clarke EB, French B, Bilodeau ML, et al. Pain management knowledge, attitudes and clinical practice: the impact of nurses' characteristics and education. *J Pain Symptom Manage* 1996;11(1):18–31.
21. Larue F, Colleau SM, Brasseur L, et al. Multicentre study of cancer pain and its treatment in France. *Br Med J* 1995;310(6986):1034–1037.
22. Dahl JL. Pain: impediments and suggestions for solutions. *J Natl Cancer Inst Monogr* 2004;32:124–126.
23. Cascinu S, Giordani P, Agostinelli R, et al. Pain and its treatment in hospitalized patients with metastatic cancer. *Support Care Cancer* 2003;11(9):587–592.
24. Gallagher R, Hawley P, Yeomans W. A survey of cancer pain management knowledge and attitudes of British Columbian physicians. *Pain Res Manag* 2004;9(4):188–194.
25. Jeon YS, Kim HK, Cleeland CS, et al. Clinicians' practice and attitudes toward

cancer pain management in Korea. *Support Care Cancer* 2007;15(5):463–469.

26. Enting RH, Oldenmenger WH, Van Gool AR, et al. The effects of analgesic prescription and patient adherence on pain in a Dutch outpatient cancer population. *J Pain Symptom Manage* 2007;34(5):523–531.

27. Payne R. Chronic pain: challenges in the assessment and management of cancer pain. *J Pain Symptom Manag* 2000;19(1 suppl):S12–S15.

28. Von Roenn JH, Cleeland CS, Gonin R, et al. Physician attitudes and practice in cancer pain management. A survey from the Eastern Cooperative Oncology Group. *Ann Intern Med* 1993;119(2):121–126.

29. Cleeland C. Research in cancer pain. What we know and what we need to know. *Cancer* 1991;67(3 suppl):823–827.

30. Elliott TE, Murray DM, Elliott BA, et al. Physician knowledge and attitudes about cancer pain management: a survey from the Minnesota cancer pain project. *J Pain Symptom Manage* 1995;10(7):494–504.

31. McCaffery M, Ferrell BR. Nurses' knowledge about cancer pain: a survey of five countries. *J Pain Symptom Manage* 1995;10(5):356–369.

32. Sheehan DK, Webb A, Bower D, et al. Level of cancer pain knowledge among baccalaureate student nurses. *J Pain Symptom Manage* 1992;7(8):478–484.

33. Ferrell BR, Winn R. Medical and nursing education and training opportunities to improve survivorship care. *J Clin Oncol* 2006;24(32):5142–5148.

34. Sloan PA, Donnelly MB, Schwartz RW, et al. Cancer pain assessment and management by housestaff. *Pain* 1996;67(2–3):475–481.

35. Sloan PA, Montgomery C, Musick D. Medical student knowledge of morphine for the management of cancer pain. *J Pain Symptom Manage* 1998;15(6):359–364.

36. Leila NM, Pirkko H, Eeva P, et al. Training medical students to manage a chronic pain patient: both knowledge and communication skills are needed. *Eur J Pain* 2006;10(2):167–170.

37. Lasch KE, Wilkes G, Lee J, et al. Is hands-on experience more effective than didactic workshops in postgraduate cancer pain education? *J Cancer Educ* 2000;15(4):218–222.

38. Sloan PA, LaFountain P, Plymale M, et al. Cancer pain education for medical students: the development of a short course on CD-ROM. *Pain Med* 2002;3(1):66–72.

39. Merskey H, Bogduk N. *Classification of Chronic Pain. Descriptions of Chronic Pain Syndromes and Definitions of Pain Terms.* Seattle: IASP Press, 1994.

40. Caraceni A, Portenoy RK. An international survey of cancer pain characteristics and syndromes. IASP Task Force on Cancer Pain. International Association for the Study of Pain. *Pain* 1999;82(3):263–274.

41. Grisold W, Piza-Katzer H, Jahn R, et al. Intraneural nerve metastasis with multiple mononeuropathies. *J Peripher Nerv Syst* 2000;5(3):163–167.

42. Gandhi D, Gujar S, Mukherji SK. Magnetic resonance imaging of perineural spread of head and neck malignancies. *Top Magn Reson Imaging* 2004;15(2):79–85.

43. Vega F, Davila L, Delattre JY, et al. Experimental carcinomatous plexopathy. *J Neurol* 1993;240(1):54–58.

44. Jessell T, Tsunoo A, Kanazawa I, et al. Substance P: depletion in the dorsal horn of rat spinal cord after section of the peripheral processes of primary sensory neurons. *Brain Res* 1979;168(2):247–259.

45. Pomonis JD, Rogers SD, Peters CM, et al. Expression and localization of endothelin receptors: implications for the involvement of peripheral glia in nociception. *J Neurosci* 2001;21(3):999–1006.

46. Asham EH, Loizidou M, Taylor I. Endothelin-1 and tumour development. *Eur J Surg Oncol* 1998;24(1):57–60.

47. Mantyh PW, Clohisy DR, Koltzenburg M, et al. Molecular mechanisms of cancer pain. *Nat Rev Cancer* 2002;2(3):201–209.

48. Julius D, Basbaum AI. Molecular mechanisms of nociception. *Nature* 2001;413(6852):203–210.

49. Clohisy DR, Mantyh PW. Bone cancer pain. *Cancer* 2003;97(3 suppl):866–873.

50. Mitchell BS, Schumacher U, Kaiserling E. Are tumours innervated? Immunohistological investigations using antibodies against the neuronal marker protein gene product 9.5 (PGP 9.5) in benign, malignant and experimental tumours. *Tumour Biol* 1994;15(5):269–274.

51. Twycross R. Cancer pain classification. *Acta Anaesthesiol Scand* 1997;41(1 Pt 2):141–145.

52. Wilson KG, Chochinov HM, McPherson CJ, et al. Suffering with advanced cancer. *J Clin Oncol* 2007;25(13):1691–1697.

53. Turk DC, Sist TC, Okifuji A, et al. Adaptation to metastatic cancer pain, regional/local cancer pain and non-cancer pain: role of psychological and behavioral factors. *Pain* 1998;74(2–3):247–256.

54. Turk DC, Fernandez E. On the putative uniqueness of cancer pain: do psychological principles apply? *Behav Res Ther* 1990;28(1):1–13.

55. Potter VT, Wiseman CE, Dunn SM, et al. Patient barriers to optimal cancer pain control. *Psychooncology* 2003;12(2):153–160.

56. Spiegel D, Bloom JR. Pain in metastatic breast cancer. *Cancer* 1983;52(2):341–345.

57. Serlin RC, Mendoza TR, Nakamura Y, et al. When is cancer pain mild, moderate or severe? Grading pain severity by its interference with function. *Pain* 1995;61(2):277–284.

58. Twycross RG, Fairfield S. Pain in far-advanced cancer. *Pain* 1982;14(3):303–310.

59. Cleeland CS. The impact of pain on the patient with cancer. *Cancer* 1984;54(11 suppl):2635–2641.

60. Front D, Schneck SO, Frankel A, et al. Bone metastases and bone pain in breast cancer. Are they closely associated? *JAMA* 1979;242(16):1747–1748.

61. Ell K, Sanchez K, Vourlekis B, et al. Depression, correlates of depression, and receipt of depression care among low-income women with breast or gynecologic cancer. *J Clin Oncol* 2005;23(13):3052–3060.

62. Davies AD, Davies C, Delpo MC. Depression and anxiety in patients undergoing diagnostic investigations for head and neck cancers. *Br J Psychiatry* 1986;149:491–493.

63. Joffe RT, Rubinow DR, Denicoff KD, et al. Depression and carcinoma of the pancreas. *Gen Hosp Psychiatry* 1986;8(4):241–245.

64. Sachs G, Rasoul-Rockenschaub S, Aschauer H, et al. Lytic effector cell activity and major depressive disorder in patients with breast cancer: a prospective study. *J Neuroimmunol* 1995;59(1–2):83–89.

65. Buccheri G. Depressive reactions to lung cancer are common and often followed by a poor outcome. *Eur Respir J* 1998;11(1):173–178.

66. Montazeri A, Milroy R, Hole D, et al. Anxiety and depression in patients with lung cancer before and after diagnosis: findings from a population in Glasgow, Scotland. *J Epidemiol Community Health* 1998;52(3):203–204.

67. Fras I, Litin EM, Pearson JS. Comparison of psychiatric symptoms in carcinoma of the pancreas with those in some other intra-abdominal neoplasms. *Am J Psychiatry* 1967;123(12):1553–1562.

68. Evans DL, McCartney CF, Nemeroff CB, et al. Depression in women treated for gynecological cancer: clinical and neuroendocrine assessment. *Am J Psychiatry* 1986;143(4):447–452.

69. Golden RN, McCartney CF, Haggerty JJ Jr, et al. The detection of depression by patient self-report in women with gynecologic cancer. *Int J Psychiatry Med* 1991;21(1):17–27.

70. Devlen J, Maguire P, Phillips P, et al. Psychological problems associated with diagnosis and treatment of lymphomas. II: Prospective study. *Br Med J (Clin Res Ed)* 1987;295(6604):955–957.

71. Devlen J, Maguire P, Phillips P, et al. Psychological problems associated with diagnosis and treatment of lymphomas. I: Retrospective study. *Br Med J (Clin Res Ed)* 1987;295(6604):953–954.

72. Chochinov HM, Wilson KG, Enns M, et al. "Are you depressed?" Screening for depression in the terminally ill. *Am J Psychiatry* 1997;154(5):674–676.

73. Lloyd-Williams M, Spiller J, Ward J. Which depression screening tools should be used in palliative care? *Palliat Med* 2003;17(1):40–43.

74. Twycross R, Harcourt J, Bergl S. A survey of pain in patients with advanced cancer. *J Pain Symptom Manage* 1996;12(5):273–282.

75. Vainio A, Auvinen A. Prevalence of symptoms among patients with advanced cancer: an international collaborative study. Symptom Prevalence Group. *J Pain Symptom Manage* 1996;12(1):3–10.

76. Grond S, Zech D, Diefenbach C, et al. Assessment of cancer pain: a prospective evaluation in 2266 cancer patients referred to a pain service. *Pain* 1996;64(1):107–114.

77. Palmer E, Henrikson B, McKusick K, et al. Pain as an indicator of bone metastasis. *Acta Radiol* 1988;29(4):445–449.

78. Vuorinen E. Pain as an early symptom in cancer. *Clin J Pain* 1993;9(4):272–278.

79. Rosewicz S, Wiedenmann B. Pancreatic carcinoma. *Lancet* 1997;349(9050):485–489.

80. Greenwald HP, Bonica JJ, Bergner M. The prevalence of pain in four cancers. *Cancer* 1987;60(10):2563–2569.

81. Krech RL, Walsh D. Symptoms of pancreatic cancer. *J Pain Symptom Manage* 1991;6(6):360–367.

82. Emmrich J, Weber I, Nausch M, et al. Immunohistochemical characterization of the pancreatic cellular infiltrate in normal pancreas, chronic pancreatitis and pancreatic carcinoma. *Digestion* 1998;59(3):192–198.

83. Schneider MB, Standop J, Ulrich A, et al. Expression of nerve growth factors in pancreatic neural tissue and pancreatic cancer. *J Histochem Cytochem* 2001;49(10):1205–1210.

84. Lindsay TH, Jonas BM, Sevcik MA, et al. Pancreatic cancer pain and its correlation with changes in tumor vasculature, macrophage infiltration, neuronal innervation, body weight and disease progression. *Pain* 2005;119(1–3):233–246.

85. Singh SM, Longmire WP Jr, Reber HA. Surgical palliation for pancreatic cancer. The UCLA experience. *Ann Surg* 1990;212(2):132–139.

86. Kelsen DP, Portenoy RK, Thaler HT, et al. Pain and depression in patients with newly diagnosed pancreas cancer. *J Clin Oncol* 1995;13(3):748–755.

87. Saltzburg D, Foley KM. Management of pain in pancreatic cancer. *Surg Clin North Am* 1989;69(3):629–649.

88. Passik SD, Breitbart WS. Depression in patients with pancreatic carcinoma. Diagnostic and treatment issues. *Cancer* 1996;78(3 suppl):615–626.

89. Portenoy RK, Kornblith AB, Wong G, et al. Pain in ovarian cancer patients. Prevalence, characteristics, and associated symptoms. *Cancer* 1994;74(3):907–915.

90. Heller PB, Maletano JH, Bundy BN, et al. Clinical-pathologic study of stage IIB, III, and IVA carcinoma of the cervix: extended diagnostic evaluation for paraaortic node metastasis—a Gynecologic Oncology Group study. *Gynecol Oncol* 1990;38(3):425–430.

91. Rubin SC, Brookland R, Mikuta JJ, et al. Para-aortic nodal metastases in early cervical carcinoma: long-term survival following extended-field radiotherapy. *Gynecol Oncol* 1984;18(2):213–217.

92. Vigliotti AP, Wen BC, Hussey DH, et al. Extended field irradiation for carcinoma of the uterine cervix with positive periaortic nodes. *Int J Radiat Oncol Biol Phys* 1992;23(3):501–509.

93. Rose PG, Adler LP, Rodriguez M, et al. Positron emission tomography for evaluating para-aortic nodal metastasis in locally advanced cervical cancer before surgical staging: A surgicopathologic study. *J Clin Oncol* 1999;17(1): 41–45.

94. Subak LL, Hricak H, Powell CB, et al. Cervical carcinoma: computed tomography and magnetic resonance imaging for preoperative staging. *Obstet Gynecol* 1995;86(1):43–50.

95. Kreis W, Budman D. Daily oral estramustine and intermittent intravenous docetaxel (Taxotere) as chemotherapeutic treatment for metastatic, hormone-refractory prostate cancer. *Semin Oncol* 1999;26(5 suppl 17):34–38.

96. ESMO. Recurrent or metastatic breast cancer: ESMO Clinical Recommendations for diagnosis, treatment and follow-up. *Ann Oncol* 2007;18(suppl 2): ii9–ii11.

97. Saphner T, Tormey DC, Gray R. Annual hazard rates of recurrence for breast cancer after primary therapy. *J Clin Oncol* 1996;14(10):2738–2746.

98. Schiff R, Massarweh S, Shou J, et al. Breast cancer endocrine resistance: how growth factor signaling and ER coregulators modulate response. *Clin Cancer Res* 2003;9(1 Pt 2):447S–454S.

99. Ellis MJ, Coop A, Singh B, et al. Letrozole is more effective neoadjuvant endocrine therapy than tamoxifen for ErbB-1- and/or ErbB-2-positive, ER-positive primary breast cancer: evidence from a phase III randomized trial. *J Clin Oncol* 2001;19(18):3808–3816.

100. Hathaway PB, Mankoff DA, Maravilla KR, et al. Value of combined FDG PET and MR imaging in the evaluation of suspected recurrent local-regional breast cancer: preliminary experience. *Radiology* 1999;210(3):807–814.

101. Cook GJ, Houston S, Rubens R, et al. Detection of bone metastases in breast cancer by 18FDG PET: differing metabolic activity in osteoblastic and osteolytic lesions. *J Clin Oncol* 1998;16(10):3375–3379.

102. Swenerton KD, Legha SS, Smith T, et al. Prognostic factors in metastatic breast cancer treated with combination chemotherapy. *Cancer Res* 1979; 39(5):1552–1562.

103. Smalley RV, Lefante J, Bartolucci A, et al. A comparison of cyclophosphamide, adriamycin, and 5-fluorouracil (CAF) and cyclophosphamide, methotrexate, 5-fluorouracil, vincristine, and prednisone (CMFVP) in patients with advanced breast cancer. *Breast Cancer Res Treat* 1983;3(2):209–220.

104. Cohen MH, Matthews MJ. Small cell bronchogenic carcinoma: a distinct clinicopathologic entity. *Semin Oncol* 1978;5(3):234–243.

105. Lassen U, Osterlind K, Hansen M, et al. Long-term survival in small-cell lung cancer: posttreatment characteristics in patients surviving 5 to 18+ years—an analysis of 1,714 consecutive patients. *J Clin Oncol* 1995;13(5):1215–1220.

106. Sorenson GD, Pettengill OS, Brinck-Johnsen T, et al. Hormone production by cultures of small-cell carcinoma of the lung. *Cancer* 1981;47(6):1289–1296.

107. Gazdar AF, Linnoila RI. The pathology of lung cancer—changing concepts and newer diagnostic techniques. *Semin Oncol* 1988;15(3):215–225.

108. Osterlind K, Ihde DC, Ettinger DS, et al. Staging and prognostic factors in small cell carcinoma of the lung. *Cancer Treat Rep* 1983;67(1):3–9.

109. Seifter EJ, Ihde DC. Therapy of small cell lung cancer: a perspective on two decades of clinical research. *Semin Oncol* 1988;15(3):278–299.

110. Dubey S, Powell CA. Update in lung cancer 2006. *Am J Respir Crit Care Med* 2007;175(9):868–874.

111. Mercadante S, Armata M, Salvaggio L. Pain characteristics of advanced lung cancer patients referred to a palliative care service. *Pain* 1994;59(1):141–145.

112. Sebastian P, Varghese C, Sankaranarayanan R, et al. Evaluation of symptomatology in planning palliative care. *Palliat Med* 1993;7(1):27–34.

113. Jemal A, Siegel R, Ward E, et al. Cancer statistics, 2006. *CA Cancer J Clin* 2006;56(2):106–130.

114. Murai M, Oya M. Renal cell carcinoma: etiology, incidence and epidemiology. *Curr Opin Urol* 2004;14(4):229–233.

115. Cohen HT, McGovern FJ. Renal-cell carcinoma. *N Engl J Med* 2005;353(23): 2477–2490.

116. Herrlinger A, Schrott KM, Schott G, et al. What are the benefits of extended dissection of the regional renal lymph nodes in the therapy of renal cell carcinoma. *J Urol* 1991;146(5):1224–1227.

117. Phillips E, Messing EM. Role of lymphadenectomy in the treatment of renal cell carcinoma. *Urology* 1993;41(1):9–15.

118. Rabinovitch RA, Zelefsky MJ, Gaynor JJ, et al. Patterns of failure following surgical resection of renal cell carcinoma: implications for adjuvant local and systemic therapy. *J Clin Oncol* 1994;12(1):206–212.

119. Sandock DS, Seftel AD, Resnick MI. A new protocol for the followup of renal cell carcinoma based on pathological stage. *J Urol* 1995;154(1):28–31.

120. Saletti P, Cavalli F. Metastatic colorectal cancer. *Cancer Treat Rev* 2006; 32(7):557–571.

121. James CR, Quinn JE, Mullan PB, et al. BRCA1, a potential predictive biomarker in the treatment of breast cancer. *Oncologist* 2007;12(2):142–150.

122. Vecht CJ, Hoff AM, Kansen PJ, et al. Types and causes of pain in cancer of the head and neck. *Cancer* 1992;70(1):178–184.

123. Greenberg HS, Deck MD, Vikram B, et al. Metastasis to the base of the skull: clinical findings in 43 patients. *Neurology* 1981;31(5):530–537.

124. Sozzi G, Marotta P, Piatti L. Vagoglossopharyngeal neuralgia with syncope in the course of carcinomatous meningitis. *Ital J Neurol Sci* 1987;8(3):271–275.

125. Macdonald DR, Strong E, Nielsen S, et al. Syncope from head and neck cancer. *J Neurooncol* 1983;1(3):257–267.

126. Metheetrairut C, Brown DH. Glossopharyngeal neuralgia and syncope secondary to neck malignancy. *J Otolaryngol* 1993;22(1):18–20.

127. Bullitt E, Tew JM, Boyd J. Intracranial tumors in patients with facial pain. *J Neurosurg* 1986;64(6):865–871.

128. Cheng TM, Cascino TL, Onofrio BM. Comprehensive study of diagnosis and treatment of trigeminal neuralgia secondary to tumors. *Neurology* 1993; 43(11):2298–2302.

129. Nomura T, Ikezaki K, Matsushima T, et al. Trigeminal neuralgia: differentiation between intracranial mass lesions and ordinary vascular compression as causative lesions. *Neurosurg Rev* 1994;17(1):51–57.

130. Puca A, Meglio M, Vari R, et al. Evaluation of fifth nerve dysfunction in 136 patients with middle and posterior cranial fossae tumors. *Eur Neurol* 1995; 35(1):33–37.

131. DeAngelis LM, Payne R. Lymphomatous meningitis presenting as atypical cluster headache. *Pain* 1987;30(2):211–216.

132. Clouston PD, Sharpe DM, Corbett AJ, et al. Perineural spread of cutaneous head and neck cancer. Its orbital and central neurologic complications. *Arch Neurol* 1990;47(1):73–77.

133. Catalano PJ, Sen C, Biller HF. Cranial neuropathy secondary to perineural spread of cutaneous malignancies. *Am J Otol* 1995;16(6):772–777.

134. Ferrante L, Artico M, Nardacci B, et al. Glossopharyngeal neuralgia with cardiac syncope. *Neurosurgery* 1995;36(1):58–63.

135. Weinstein RE, Herec D, Friedman JH. Hypotension due to glossopharyngeal neuralgia. *Arch Neurol* 1986;43(1):90–92.

136. Jaeckle KA. Nerve plexus metastases. *Neurol Clin* 1991;9(4):857–866.

137. Wasserstrom WR, Glass JP, Posner JB. Diagnosis and treatment of leptomeningeal metastases from solid tumors: experience with 90 patients. *Cancer* 1982;49(4):759–772.

138. Sorensen SC, Eagan RT, Scott M. Meningeal carcinomatosis in patients with primary breast or lung cancer. *Mayo Clin Proc* 1984;59(2):91–94.

139. Theodore WH, Gendelman S. Meningeal carcinomatosis. *Arch Neurol* 1981; 38(11):696–699.

140. Kesari S, Batchelor TT. Leptomeningeal metastases. *Neurol Clin* 2003;21(1): 25–66.

141. Posner JB, Chernik NL. Intracranial metastases from systemic cancer. *Adv Neurol* 1978;19:579–592.

142. Siegal T, Lossos A, Pfeffer MR. Leptomeningeal metastases: analysis of 31 patients with sustained off-therapy response following combined-modality therapy. *Neurology* 1994;44(8):1463–1469.

143. Little JR, Dale AJ, Okazaki H. Meningeal carcinomatosis. Clinical manifestations. *Arch Neurol* 1974;30(1):138–143.

144. Kaplan JG, DeSouza TG, Farkash A, et al. Leptomeningeal metastases: comparison of clinical features and laboratory data of solid tumors, lymphomas and leukemias. *J Neurooncol* 1990;9(3):225–229.

145. de Verdier HJ, Colletti PM, Terk MR. MRI of the brachial plexus: a review of 51 cases. *Comput Med Imaging Graph* 1993;17(1):45–50.

146. Kori SH, Foley KM, Posner JB. Brachial plexus lesions in patients with cancer: 100 cases. *Neurology* 1981;31(1):45–50.

147. Marangoni C, Lacerenza M, Formaglio F, et al. Sensory disorder of the chest as presenting symptom of lung cancer. *J Neurol Neurosurg Psychiatry* 1993; 56(9):1033–1034.

148. Rodichok LD, Harper GR, Ruckdeschel JC, et al. Early diagnosis of spinal epidural metastases. *Am J Med* 1981;70(6):1181–1188.

149. Yeung MC, Hagen NA. Cervical disc herniation presenting with chest wall pain. *Can J Neurol Sci* 1993;20(1):59–61.

150. Ahmad A, Barrington S, Maisey M, et al. Use of positron emission tomography in evaluation of brachial plexopathy in breast cancer patients. *Br J Cancer* 1999;79(3–4):478–482.

151. Saphner T, Gallion HH, Van Nagell JR, et al. Neurologic complications of cervical cancer. A review of 2261 cases. *Cancer* 1989;64(5):1147–1151.

152. Jaeckle KA, Young DF, Foley KM. The natural history of lumbosacral plexopathy in cancer. *Neurology* 1985;35(1):8–15.

153. Dalmau J, Graus F, Marco M. 'Hot and dry foot' as initial manifestation of neoplastic lumbosacral plexopathy. *Neurology* 1989;39(6):871–872.

154. Jaeckle KA. Neurological manifestations of neoplastic and radiation-induced plexopathies. *Semin Neurol* 2004;24(4):385–393.

155. Taylor BV, Kimmel DW, Krecke KN, et al. Magnetic resonance imaging in cancer-related lumbosacral plexopathy. *Mayo Clin Proc* 1997;72(9): 823–829.

156. Dalmau JO, Posner JB. Paraneoplastic syndromes affecting the nervous system. *Semin Oncol* 1997;24(3):318–328.

157. Graus F, Cordon-Cardo C, Posner JB. Neuronal antinuclear antibody in sensory neuronopathy from lung cancer. *Neurology* 1985;35(4):538–543.

158. Dalmau J, Graus F, Rosenblum MK, et al. Anti-Hu–associated paraneoplastic encephalomyelitis/sensory neuronopathy. A clinical study of 71 patients. *Medicine (Baltimore)* 1992;71(2):59–72.

159. Graus F, Keime-Guibert F, Reñe R, et al. Anti-Hu–associated paraneoplastic encephalomyelitis: analysis of 200 patients. *Brain* 2001;124(Pt 6): 1138–1148.

160. Lucchinetti CF, Kimmel DW, Lennon VA. Paraneoplastic and oncologic profiles of patients seropositive for type 1 antineuronal nuclear autoantibodies. *Neurology* 1998;50(3):652–657.

161. Sillevis Smitt P, Grefkens J, de Leeuw B, et al. Survival and outcome in 73 anti-Hu positive patients with paraneoplastic encephalomyelitis/sensory neuronopathy. *J Neurol* 2002;249(6):745–753.

162. Dalmau J, Furneaux HM, Gralla RJ, et al. Detection of the anti-Hu antibody in the serum of patients with small cell lung cancer—a quantitative western blot analysis. *Ann Neurol* 1990;27(5):544–552.

163. Vecht CJ. Arm pain in the patient with breast cancer. *J Pain Symptom Manage* 1990;5(2):109–117.

164. Stevens PE, Dibble SL, Miaskowski C. Prevalence, characteristics, and impact of postmastectomy pain syndrome: an investigation of women's experiences. *Pain* 1995;61(1):61–68.

165. Vecht CJ, Van de Brand HJ, Wajer OJ. Post-axillary dissection pain in breast cancer due to a lesion of the intercostobrachial nerve. *Pain* 1989;38(2): 171–176.

166. Cappiello J, Piazza C, Nicolai P. The spinal accessory nerve in head and neck surgery. *Curr Opin Otolaryngol Head Neck Surg* 2007;15(2):107–111.

167. Nahum AM, Mullally W, Marmor L. A syndrome resulting from radical neck dissection. *Arch Otolaryngol* 1961;74:424–428.

168. Dajczman E, Gordon A, Kreisman H, et al. Long-term postthoracotomy pain. *Chest* 1991;99(2):270–274.

169. Maguire MF, Latter JA, Mahajan R, et al. A study exploring the role of intercostal nerve damage in chronic pain after thoracic surgery. *Eur J Cardiothorac Surg* 2006;29(6):873–879.

170. Weinstein SM. Phantom pain. *Oncology (Huntingt)* 1994;8(3):65–70.

171. Nikolajsen L, Ilkjaer S, Kroner K, et al. The influence of preamputation pain on postamputation stump and phantom pain. *Pain* 1997;72(3):393–405.

172. Krøner K, Krebs B, Skov J, et al. Immediate and long-term phantom breast syndrome after mastectomy: incidence, clinical characteristics and relationship to pre-mastectomy breast pain. *Pain* 1989;36(3):327–334.

173. Ovesen P, Kroner K, Ornsholt J, et al. Phantom-related phenomena after rectal amputation: prevalence and clinical characteristics. *Pain* 1991;44(3): 289–291.

174. Management of cancer pain guideline overview. Agency for Health Care Policy and Research, Rockville, Maryland. *J Natl Med Assoc* 1994;86(8): 571–573, 634.

175. Quality improvement guidelines for the treatment of acute pain and cancer pain. American Pain Society Quality of Care Committee. *JAMA* 1995; 274(23):1874–1880.

176. Practice guidelines for cancer pain management. A report by the American Society of Anesthesiologists Task Force on Pain Management, Cancer Pain Section. *Anesthesiology* 1996;84(5):1243–1257.

177. Williamson GM, Schulz R. Activity restriction mediates the association between pain and depressed affect: a study of younger and older adult cancer patients. *Psychol Aging* 1995;10(3):369–378.

178. Tait RC, Chibnall JT, Krause S. The Pain Disability Index: psychometric properties. *Pain* 1990;40(2):171–182.

179. Maltoni M, Pirovano M, Scarpi E, et al. Prediction of survival of patients terminally ill with cancer. Results of an Italian prospective multicentric study. *Cancer* 1995;75(10):2613–2622.

180. Schaafsma J, Osoba D. The Karnofsky Performance Status Scale re-examined: a cross-validation with the EORTC-C30. *Qual Life Res* 1994;3(6):413–424.

181. Yellen SB, Cella DF. Someone to live for: social well-being, parenthood status, and decision-making in oncology. *J Clin Oncol* 1995;13(5):1255–1264.

182. Cella D, Chang CH, Lai JS, et al. Advances in quality of life measurements in oncology patients. *Semin Oncol* 2002;29(3 suppl 8):60–68.

183. Smets EM, Garssen B, Schuster-Uitterhoeve AL, et al. Fatigue in cancer patients. *Br J Cancer* 1993;68(2):220–224.

184. Portenoy RK, Thaler HT, Kornblith AB, et al. The Memorial Symptom Assessment Scale: an instrument for the evaluation of symptom prevalence, characteristics and distress. *Eur J Cancer* 1994;30A(9):1326–1336.

185. Portenoy RK, Thaler HT, Kornblith AB, et al. Symptom prevalence, characteristics and distress in a cancer population. *Qual Life Res* 1994;3(3):183–189.

186. Clouston PD, DeAngelis LM, Posner JB. The spectrum of neurological disease in patients with systemic cancer. *Ann Neurol* 1992;31(3):268–273.

CHAPTER 43 ■ CANCER PAIN: PRINCIPLES OF MANAGEMENT AND PHARMACOTHERAPY

DERMOT R. FITZGIBBON

INTRODUCTION

Inadequate treatment of chronic cancer pain persists despite decades of efforts to provide clinicians with information about analgesics and pain-relieving techniques. The problems associated with undertreatment of cancer pain are outlined in Table 43.1. While the reasons for inadequate treatment of cancer pain are complex, certain barriers to adequate pain relief can be identified. These barriers may be summarized as related to health care professionals; patients, families, and the public; health care implementation and reimbursement; and drug regulatory systems.

In the United States and other western nations, physicians' concerns about regulatory scrutiny and the possibility of unwarranted investigation by regulatory agencies negatively affect their prescribing of opioid analgesics to treat pain.[1] Although most U.S. state medical boards have adopted regulations, guidelines, or policy statements relating to controlled substances and pain management, some state medical boards have rejected prescribing practices that are considered acceptable by today's standards.[1]

Internationally, there are many reasons why patients receive inadequate cancer pain control.[2] Table 43.2 lists some of these reasons. To respond to these issues, the World Health Organization (WHO) advocates a strategy which includes the development of national or state policies that support cancer pain relief through government endorsement of education and drug availability; educational programs for the public, health care personnel, and regulators; and modification of laws and regulations to improve the availability of pain relieving drugs, especially opioid analgesics.

Potential solutions for inadequate control of cancer pain include the following:

1. **Education of patient and health care providers:** Many cancer patients worry that their pain will not be controlled during the course of their disease. Moreover, they report fears of drug addiction, side effects, and tolerance. Educating patients about common barriers to cancer pain treatment can be an effective pain management strategy.[3] In addition, each patient should receive a "bill of rights" indicating that the provider is committed to achieving optimal pain control. Health care providers should learn pain assessment techniques and routinely question all patients with cancer for pain prevalence and severity.

2. **Establishment of Pain Management Practice Plan:** Several guidelines address cancer pain management, including those proffered by the WHO,[4] the American Pain Society (APS),[5] the Agency for Health Care Policy and Research,[6] and the American Society of Anesthesiologists.[7] In addition, every cancer care setting should establish and follow a pain management practice plan in order to anticipate and deal with pain in the cancer patient. Physicians caring for cancer patients should maintain a list of advanced pain management referral sources and protocols and seek expert consultation when routine management strategies fail.

3. **State Cancer Pain Initiatives:** These initiatives are grass roots, multidisciplinary organizations in the United States committed to making optimal cancer pain control a reality. The first initiative began in Wisconsin,[8] and they now exist in all states

TABLE 43.1

FACTORS CONTRIBUTING TO UNDERTREATMENT OF CANCER PAIN IN UNITED STATES

Factor	Reason
Patient-related	• Pain under-reporting: —fear of disease progression —perceived lack of time or inadequate amount of time spent in physician's office discussing pain problems Poor compliance with prescribed medications
Physician-related	• Legal issues regarding overprescription or perceived overprescription of opioids. Physician reluctance to prescribe opioid analgesics has multiple causes.[49] • Difficulty assessing pain complaints • Lack of information or lack of expertise on contemporary strategies for cancer pain management • Desire to provide the patient with the latest and greatest pain management strategies may pose difficulties with untried or unproven techniques or methods.

in the United States. A Role Model Education Program has evolved from the Wisconsin Cancer Pain Initiative.[9] The key concept in the initiative movement is the provider triad: physician, nurse, and pharmacist. In most states, this program involves attendance of the triad at a day-long course covering all aspects of cancer pain management.

A clinician may achieve pain relief in the cancer patient by several means (Table 43.3). Success requires tailoring treatment to the individual patient: matching drug treatment, anesthetic, neurosurgical, psychological, and behavioral approaches to the patient's needs. Successful management requires that the person or persons responsible for pain management be familiar with all these aspects of care.

Pain Management Improvement Strategies

Many pain clinician–educators now believe that traditional medical educational approaches require complementary interventions

TABLE 43.2

INTERNATIONAL REASONS FOR INADEQUATE CANCER PAIN CONTROL

Absence of national policies on cancer pain relief and palliative care

Lack of awareness on the part of health care workers, policy makers, administrators, and the public that most cancer pain can be relieved

Shortage of financial resources and limitations of health care delivery systems and personnel

Concern that medical use of opioids will produce psychological dependence and drug abuse

Legal restrictions on the use and availability of opioid analgesics

(From World Health Organization. Cancer Pain Relief and Palliative Care. Technical Report Series 804. Geneva, Switzerland: World Health Organization; 1990.)

TABLE 43.3

APPROACHES TO PAIN MANAGEMENT IN CANCER PATIENTS

Psychological approaches (Chapters 7, 21, 29, 81–87)	Understanding Companionship Cognitive behavioral therapies
Modification of pathological process (Chapters 48, 104)	Radiation therapy Hormone therapy Chemotherapy Surgery
Drugs (Chapters 76–80)	Analgesics Antidepressants Anxiolytics Neuroleptics
Interruption of pain pathways (Chapters 97–104)	Local anesthetics Neurolytics Neurosurgery
Modification of daily activities	
Immobilization	Rest Cervical collar or corset Plastic splints or slings Orthopedic surgery

(Modified from World Health Organization. Cancer Pain Relief With a Guide to Opioid Availability. Geneva, Switzerland: World Health Organization; 1996.)

in health care systems that directly influence the routine behaviors of clinicians and patients.[9–14] This perspective echoes that advocated by the quality improvement (QI) movement.[15,16] The QI approach to pain treatment is based on the assumption that, although clinicians are concerned with patient comfort, their habits and procedures of practice do not support the achievement of effective pain relief. Although pain has received the most study, some experts believe that many symptoms of medical illness are neglected because patterns of medical practice and accountability have evolved with focus on structural disease rather than on burdens of illness, functional impairments, quality of life measures, and symptom-related distress.[17,18] QI programs designed to enhance treatment of cancer pain should include the following key elements[5]:

1. Routine assessment of pain using patient-appropriate validated tools.
2. Assure that a report of unrelieved pain raises a "red flag" that attracts clinicians' attention.
3. Make information about analgesics available in settings where physicians write orders.
4. Promise patients responsive analgesic care and urge them to communicate their pain.
5. Implement policies and safeguards for the use of modern analgesic technologies.
6. Coordinate and assess implementation of these measures.

The APS Quality of Care Committee issued guidelines for the treatment of acute and cancer pain.[5] These guidelines attempted to embody key elements for favorably influencing behaviors of both patients and clinicians. The guidelines addressed settings that used conventional pain relief methods (e.g., intermittent parenteral or oral analgesics) exclusively and those using current technology for pain management. While the guidelines focused on the assessment of pain and its treatment with analgesic drugs, they also identified that nonpharmacologic measures were an effective therapy.

Bookbinder et al.[14] studied the impact of implementing APS guidelines in a focused program at an academic cancer hospital. The program included routine monitoring of pain, staff education, and focus groups to identify organizational obstacles to effective pain management. During the first year of the program, patient satisfaction increased significantly but the "worst pain levels over the past 24 hours" remained unchanged. Results from the second and third years suggested further reduction of pain intensity on targeted hospital units. Major change did not occur until pain assessment became routine and the resulting data had convinced physicians to participate in the programs.

Pain education programs at a community level have shown mixed results. Elliott et al.[19] failed to show a significant reduction in pain prevalence, pain management index, pain intensity scores, patient and family attitude scores, and physicians' and nurses' knowledge and attitude scores. In contrast, de Wit et al.[20] reported that patients significantly increased their knowledge of pain and its mechanisms, with a decrease in pain intensity of approximately 20% to 30%.

CANCER PAIN MANAGEMENT OVERVIEW

Successful management of the cancer patient with pain ultimately depends on the ability of the clinician to accurately assess problems, identify and evaluate the components that contribute to the pain complaint, and formulate a plan for continuing care that is responsible for the evolving goals and needs of the patient and the patient's family (see Chapter 42). The formulation of an effective therapeutic strategy for the management of cancer pain requires a comprehensive assessment of the patient and the pain complaint. In general, the goals of patient care in oncology are often complex, but they broadly comprise prolonged survival and optimizing comfort and function. Adoption of these goals logically leads to a multimodality treatment approach targeted to specific problems (Fig. 43.1).

Comprehensive cancer care encompasses a continuum that progresses from disease-oriented, curative, life-prolonging treatment through symptom-oriented, supportive, and palliative care extending to terminal-phase hospice care. Pain management is, and should be, an integral component of comprehensive cancer care.[21] Designing an effective pain control strategy for the individual patient requires knowledge of the ways in which a patient's cancer, cancer therapy, and pain therapy can interact. Collaboration with different health care providers (such as medical oncologists and radiation oncologists) is essential to successful pain management.

Two important aspects of cancer affect management and include the oncologist's ability to treat the cancer and the ability to assess the components of the tumor pathophysiology that of themselves do not cause pain (the cancer's "nonpain" pathophysiology).[22] The ability to treat cancer modifies the need for pain management (successful treatment reduces the likelihood of pain)

and the appropriateness of invasive pain procedures. Cancer nonpain pathophysiology can interfere with the oral administration of medications, narrow the patient's therapeutic window for analgesic drugs, limit the effectiveness of psychological pain therapies, and complicate or preclude invasive pain-reducing procedures. In addition, cancer therapy can interfere with, or enhance, pain therapy and vice versa. Antineoplastic treatment can interfere with pain therapy by causing additional pain or by producing other adverse effects such as fatigue and gastrointestinal (GI) disturbances. Cancer treatment can enhance pain therapy by reducing the extent of cancer, by acting as an adjuvant analgesic, and, oftentimes, providing intravenous access for parenteral drug administration to patients who require it. Pain therapy can sometimes interfere with cancer therapy by increasing or complicating the adverse effects of cancer therapy (e.g., opioid-related bowel dysfunction). It can enhance cancer therapy by improving patient function or sense of well-being, and certain palliative surgical procedures may have the ancillary effect of improving organ function.

The basic principles of tumor-directed pain control include:

1. Modifying the source of pain by treating the cancer and the inflammatory effects of cancer.
2. Altering the central perception of pain, for example, by the use of analgesics, antidepressants, anxiolytics, and psychotherapy.
3. Interfering with nociceptive transmission outside of and within the central nervous system, for example, with anesthetic techniques (e.g., neurolytic celiac plexus block, neuraxial analgesia, and spinal neurolysis), or neurosurgical procedures (e.g., cordotomy and myelotomy).

The pain experienced by most cancer patients responds to direct and indirect modification of the source of the pain combined with pharmacologic and nonpharmacologic alteration of the central perception of pain.[23–25]

The guiding principle in developing pain management goals is to individualize the approach to the patient's needs. Part of the process of developing treatment goals is to take into consideration the burdens (adverse effects; opportunity costs) and benefits of different treatment options. Clinicians may find that patient treatment goals differ from their own, either because patients feel that pain is inevitable, or because patients expect pain to be relieved with minimal effort on their part. Issues that physicians should discuss with patients include expected lifestyle, cost and reimbursement issues, and concerns about opioid tolerance, addiction, and side effects. Discussing these issues in advance may uncover and address potential barriers to treatment. Moreover, treatment goals may change during the course of the patient's illness, and all health care providers interacting with the patient during the course of the illness need to keep abreast of such changes.

Patient life expectancy should influence treatment decisions. For example, if life expectancy exceeds several weeks to months, then treatment may focus on how to enable the patient to function

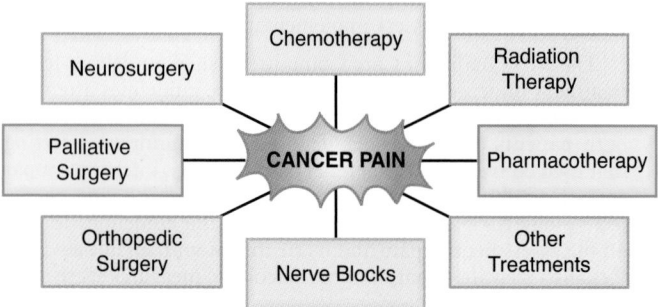

FIGURE 43.1 Multimodality therapeutic management of cancer pain. Others include psychosocial interventions, nursing care, alternative pain management strategies, and end-of-life issues.

at the highest possible level. One goal should be to relieve pain and prevent therapy from interfering with normal activities. On the other hand, those likely to die within a few days or weeks require less emphasis on maintaining an active lifestyle and more on comfort and tolerance of the side effects associated with pain therapies, allowing due attention to life closure issues. The emphasis for these patients should be on treatments that provide immediate relief, rather than those that require a long period of time to become effective. Because maintenance of mental clarity and alertness is valued by most patients, even in the last days or hours of life, patients may be willing to undergo more interventional methods of pain management to achieve better pain control.

Primary Anticancer Treatment

Pain produced by tumor infiltration may respond to antineoplastic treatment with radiation treatment and chemotherapy. These approaches to pain control are elaborated in Chapter 48.

Surgery

The surgeon treating a patient with newly diagnosed cancer must meet several responsibilities: biopsy for tissue diagnosis, adequate staging, consultation with medical and radiation oncologists for adjuvant therapy, and surgical resection. Surgery may also play a role in the relief of symptoms caused by specific problems, such as obstruction of a hollow viscus, unstable bone structures, and compression of neural tissues. A variety of surgical disciplines (e.g., general surgery, orthopedic, neurosurgical, plastic, and reconstructive) may participate in the care of the cancer patient. Beginning in the 1960s and 1970s, surgery for certain tumors such as breast, colon, and lung cancer became more conservative.

Although the development of metastatic cancer usually indicates incurable disease, curative surgical resection is possible in rare instances. These instances must meet several criteria before the surgeon can operate: the primary lesion must be controlled; there must be the potential for complete resection of the metastases; there must be no other equally effective or better antitumor therapy available; metastases should involve only one organ; one should anticipate reasonable postoperative function; expected survival should be better than if left untreated; and the patient must be able to tolerate the surgical procedure. Sometimes, excision of the primary tumor is indicated in the presence of unresectable metastatic disease. Locally advanced tumor can be very painful and unsightly, can interfere with vital functions such as breathing and swallowing, and can produce complications such as bleeding and local infection.

Stenting, Drainage Procedures, and Antibiotics

Common complications of advanced cancer include GI, hepatobiliary, and ureteric obstructions. Stents and laser treatment have a place in both upper GI and rectal obstruction due to advanced malignancy.[26–28] Endoscopic retrograde placement of ureteric stents under cystoscopic control is the most common urologic approach for the management of malignant ureteric obstruction. Difficult clinical situations may require alternative procedures such as palliative cutaneous ureterostomy, percutaneous anterograde ureteric stent placement, and a combined anterograde and retrograde technique. The insertion of internal biliary stents by endoscopic or percutaneous methods is common practice for the palliative management of obstructive jaundice caused by malignancy and most surgeons prefer this to the use of external biliary drains.[29]

The goals of antibiotic use in terminally ill patients are sometimes to prolong life and always to relieve symptoms. Treatment for cystitis, for instance, does not usually prolong life, but may relieve the patient from painful dysuria and troublesome polyuria. Antibiotics may also have pain-relieving effects when the source of pain involves infection, as illustrated by the treatment of pyonephrosis and osteitis pubis.

SYMPTOMATIC CANCER PAIN MANAGEMENT

Successful management strategies usually require a team approach focusing not only on the nociceptive processes but also on other factors that influence the final perception of pain. Figure 43.2 outlines an approach to cancer-related nociceptive and neuropathic pain.

Increasing severe pain and/or increasing and intractable side effects determine the appropriate treatment strategy. Most patients will respond satisfactorily to relatively simple oral pharmacotherapeutic strategies. When the patient requires drug treatment, therapy should comply with two basic principles: use oral analgesics and other noninvasive routes of administrations (e.g., transdermal and transmucosal) whenever possible and administer them in accordance with the principles in the WHO analgesic ladder (see below). Titrate opioid and adjuvant analgesics to maximally effective doses or to the appearance of dose-limiting side effects before considering alternative medications (e.g., opioid rotation) or more specialized (and usually) invasive approaches. As an adjunct—and occasionally as an alternative—to medication management, patients with certain pain syndromes will benefit from relatively simple anesthetic blocks, such as celiac and superior hypogastric plexus blocks, neurolytic subarachnoid and

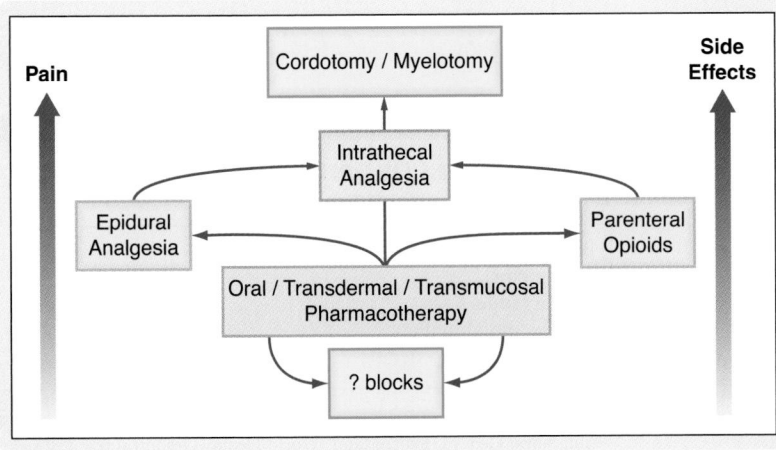

FIGURE 43.2 Tumor pain management algorithm.

intercostal blocks, and selected peripheral nerve blocks (see Chapter 44).

Severe, uncontrolled pain and/or intractable side effects require interventional pain management to achieve rapid pain control. Such interventions may include epidural analgesia and/or parenteral opioid therapy (usually intravenous or subcutaneous administration). As many of these patients have large systemic opioid requirements, it is not unusual to combine epidural and parenteral therapies. A small percentage of patients may fail these therapies and should then be treated with intrathecal drugs and/or cordotomy or myelotomy (see Chapter 44).

Occasionally, patients will have pain refractory to all interventional measures outlined. For these patients, adequate relief may only be achieved through the use of techniques such as intravenous lidocaine infusion or subanesthetic doses of ketamine. Failing these approaches, palliative sedation is an option.

World Health Organization Analgesic Ladder

In 1986, WHO proposed a method for relief of cancer pain based on a small number of relatively inexpensive drugs, including morphine.[30] This guideline has been translated into 22 languages and a total of over half a million copies have been distributed. A second edition[4] takes into account many of the advances in understanding and practice that have occurred since the mid-1980s. The groundwork for this revision was started in 1989, in the context of the meeting of a WHO Expert Committee on Cancer Pain Relief and Active Supportive Care.[2]

The WHO "analgesic ladder" is a simple and effective method for controlling cancer pain, and the proportion of cancer patients who report effective pain relief varies from 75% to 90%.[6,25,31–33] Some authors have expressed concern about the effectiveness of the WHO analgesic ladder approach and the validity of published data. Jadad et al.[34] conducted a systematic review of studies (MEDLINE from 1982 to 1995, a hand search of textbooks and meeting proceedings, reference lists, and direct contact with authors) evaluating the effectiveness of the WHO ladder as an intervention for cancer pain management. While the studies available provide useful insights into cancer pain and its treatment, they fail to predict the effectiveness of the WHO analgesic ladder in any given patient, underscoring the importance of individualized assessment and treatment plans, including mechanism-based approaches to therapy. Treatment for cancer pain should begin with a straightforward explanation to the patient of the causes of the pain or pains. Many pains respond best to a combination of drug and nondrug measures. Nevertheless, opioids, nonopioid analgesics, and adjuvant agents, alone or in combination, are the mainstay of cancer pain management (see Table 43.4).

Pharmacologic strategies for the control of tumor pain appear in Table 43.5. Table 43.6 lists the principles of pharmacotherapy endorsed by WHO.

These principles are as follows:

By Mouth

When possible, patients should take analgesic medications by mouth. However, alternative routes such as rectal, transdermal, sublingual, and parenteral (subcutaneous and intravenous) administration may better serve patients with dysphagia, uncontrolled vomiting, or GI obstruction.

By the Clock

After titration to optimal effect, patients with continuous pain should take analgesic medications on an around-the-clock (ATC) schedule. Once baseline pain is controlled, many patients will require breakthrough pain (BTP) therapy with immediate or rapid-onset opioids, since BTP is a common occurrence in cancer patients.

TABLE 43.4

A BASIC DRUG LIST FOR CANCER PAIN RELIEF

Category	Basic drugs	Alternatives
Nonopioids	acetylsalicylic acid (ASA) acetaminophen ibuprofen indomethacin	choline magnesium trisalicylate diflunisal naproxen diclofenac
Opioids for mild to moderate pain	codeine	dihydrocodeine dextropropoxyphene standardized opium tramadol
Opioids for moderate to severe pain	morphine	methadone hydromorphone oxycodone levorphanol meperidine buprenorphine
Opioid antagonist	naloxone	
Antidepressants	amitriptyline	imipramine
Anticonvulsants	carbamazepine	valproic acid
Corticosteroids	prednisolone dexamethasone	prednisone betamethasone

(From World Health Organization. Cancer Pain Relief With a Guide to Opioid Availability. Geneva, Switzerland: World Health Organization; 1996.)

TABLE 43.5

PHARMACOLOGIC STRATEGIES FOR THE CONTROL OF TUMOR PAIN

Select the appropriate analgesic drug
Prescribe the appropriate dose of that drug
Administer the drug by the appropriate route
Schedule the appropriate dosing interval
Prevent persistent pain and treat breakthrough pain
Titrate the dose of drug aggressively
Prevent, anticipate, and manage drug side effects

TABLE 43.6

THE PRINCIPLES OF DRUG THERAPY FOR CANCER PAIN

By the mouth
By the clock
By the ladder
For the individual
With attention to detail

(From World Health Organization. Cancer Pain Relief With a Guide to Opioid Availability. Geneva, Switzerland: World Health Organization; 1996.)

By the Ladder

The WHO analgesic ladder is based on the premise that most patients throughout the world will gain adequate pain relief if health care professionals learn how to use a few effective and relatively inexpensive drugs well (Fig. 43.3). Step 1 of the ladder involves the use of nonopioids. If this step does not relieve pain, add an opioid for mild to moderate pain (Step 2). When the opioid for mild to moderate pain in combination with a nonopioid fails to relieve the pain, substitute an opioid for moderate to severe pain (Step 3). Use only one drug from each of the groups at the same time. Give adjuvant drugs for specific indications (see below).

For the Individual

There are no standard doses for opioids. *The "right" dose is the dose that relieves the patient's pain with the minimum of side effects.* Combination opioid formulations (i.e., those with the nonopioid analgesic acetaminophen or a nonsteroidal anti-inflammatory drug [NSAID]) are commonly used for mild-to-moderate pain. These have a dose limit due to toxic effects of the coanalgesic.

With Attention to Detail

Carefully determine and monitor the patient's analgesic regimen. Follow-up regularly with the patient by monitoring adherence, drug efficacy, functional outcomes (activity, sleep, mood, appetite), side effects, and aberrant drug-related behaviors. Anticipate adverse effects, such as opioid-induced bowel dysfunction, and treat them prophylactically or as soon as they become problematic.

The WHO ladder advocates the use of three classes of analgesics—nonopioid, adjuvant, and opioid. Each of these classes will be considered separately.

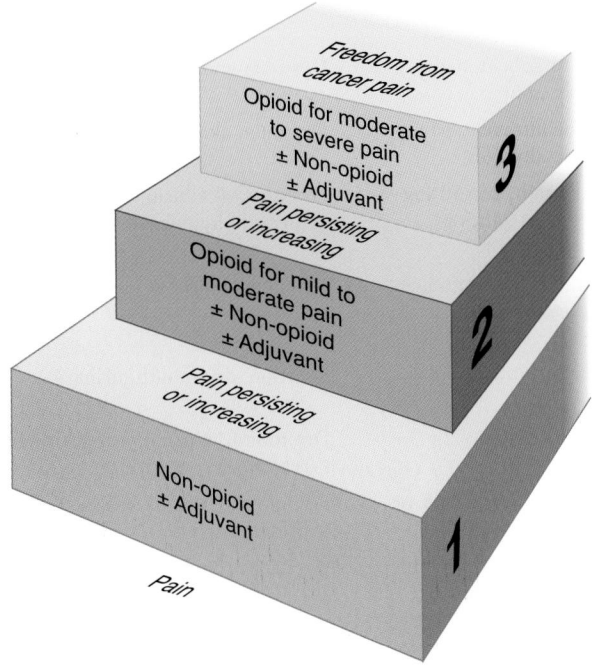

FIGURE 43.3 WHO analgesic ladder. (From World Health Organization. *Cancer pain relief with a guide to opioid availability.* Geneva, Switzerland: World Health Organization; 1996.)

NONOPIOID ANALGESICS

Nonopioid analgesic agents (also called coanalgesics) and antipyretics are essential drugs for the management of a wide variety of acute and chronic pain conditions. Clinicians should be familiar with the use, efficacy, and adverse effects of these agents. Nonopioid analgesics are important to the successful use of oral pharmacotherapy in the cancer patient with pain. These drugs may function to control pain independently (e.g., in the management of bone pain) or may help reduce the dose of opioid required for pain control (opioid-sparing effect). A wide range of drugs with varying effects and side effects are available. These medications are discussed extensively in other chapters.

Cyclooxygenase-2 (COX-2) is highly expressed during tumorigenesis and actively contributes to tumor progression,[35] and this effect involves, at least in part, induction of tumor angiogenesis.[36] Several cytokines such as reactive oxygen species and mediators of inflammatory pathway such as activation of nuclear factor-kappaB and COX-2 leads to an increase in cell proliferation, survival, and inhibition of proapoptotic pathway, ultimately resulting in tumor angiogenesis, invasion, and metastasis.[37] Increased COX-2 activity and synthesis of prostaglandins stimulates proliferation, angiogenesis, and invasiveness and inhibits apoptosis.[38] In preclinical models, selective COX-2 inhibitors possess therapeutic efficacy against established tumors, raising the possibility that COX-2 inhibitors may be used in human cancer treatment.[39] Preliminary human data suggests a potential chemoprevention role in certain cancers (breast, prostate, colon, and lung).[40] Clinical studies are currently underway to determine the benefit of this drug class taken as a sole agent or in combination with various chemotherapeutic regimens in reducing cancer risk.

Efficacy in Cancer Pain

NSAIDs are accepted as an important tool in treating cancer pain and may be combined with opioids for this purpose.[34] Although many NSAIDs are available to treat various painful conditions, it is unclear which agent is most clinically efficacious for relieving cancer-related pain and if there are clinical differences between these agents that justify their cost differences.

Eisenberg et al.[41] examined the scientific evidence on efficacy and safety of NSAIDs in the treatment of cancer-related pain. They conducted a meta-analysis of data from 25 randomized controlled trials. The studies provided data on 1545 cancer patients. Although all 25 trials reported analgesic efficacy, only the single-dose studies were comparable for analgesic efficacy analysis. Single doses of placebo produced a 15% to 36% rate of analgesia, whereas the use of NSAIDs resulted in roughly twice as much pain relief (31% versus 60%). These results support the WHO position that NSAIDs provide analgesic efficacy in patients with cancer pain.[4] The authors concluded that the meta-analysis precluded testing the hypothesis that NSAIDs are particularly effective for malignant bone pain because of a lack of comparable studies. Well-designed analgesic trials in which bone pain or pain due to other specific cancer-related syndromes assessed separately from nonbone pain are required.

Additionally, it is uncertain which opioid and NSAID combinations are the most efficacious for cancer pain or even what may be the additional benefit of combining an NSAID with an opioid in this setting. McNicol et al.[42] assessed and compared the efficacy of various NSAID and NSAID plus opioid combinations in the treatment of cancer pain. They concluded that most studies were of insufficient duration to demonstrate that the long-term use of NSAIDs is safe and effective in patients with cancer. They advised that clinicians should be as cautious in using NSAIDs in this population as they would any other population, especially given additional bleeding risks in cancer patients and the probability that a patient with cancer may be on a broad regimen of medications, some of which may increase NSAID-related toxicity.

ADJUVANT DRUGS

Adjuvant drugs may become necessary in the care of the cancer patient for one of three reasons:

- To treat the adverse effects of analgesic medications (e.g., antiemetics and laxatives)
- To enhance pain relief
- To treat concomitant psychological disturbances such as insomnia, anxiety, depression, and psychosis

Antiemetics

Much of our experience in managing opioid associated nausea and vomiting comes from the postoperative nausea and vomiting (PONV) literature. The knowledge base of PONV physiology has significantly expanded over the past decade. The mechanisms of action of pharmacologic agents (including antagonists of 5-HT3, dopaminergic, histamine H1, muscarinic cholinergic, and opioid and NK-1 receptors) for the prevention and treatment of PONV as well as chemotherapy-induced nausea and vomiting have been elucidated. Various antiemetic agents are listed in Table 43.7.

Laxatives and Opioid-Induced Bowel Dysfunction

Opioid-induced bowel dysfunction (OBD) is a distressing condition that may persist indefinitely in the clinical setting. Hard dry stool, gas distention, incomplete evacuation, and straining are common sequelae. In cancer patients, up to 90% of patients on chronic opioid therapy develop OBD.[43] Human studies have revealed that mu receptors were more consistently distributed between the myenteric and submucosal plexuses, and between the small and large intestines.[44] Exogenous mu agonists affect the GI tract in several ways. These effects appear to be central, peripheral, and local. In response to exogenous opioids, decreased motility occurs at multiple levels in the GI tract including the stomach, small intestine, and large intestine.[45] The predominant opioid effect appears to be at the local GI level. This effect appears to occur as a result of inhibition of secretions and peristalsis.[46] The goals of therapy typically are three-fold: keep stool volume maximized to trigger enterochromaffin cell serotonin release via mucosal stretch, keep stool softer and mechanically make it easier to move, and enhance peristalsis.

Fiber bulking agents are organic polymers that retain water in stool. It is important that adequate water be taken concomitantly with fiber. Without sufficient water, fiber may worsen constipation. Many practitioners recommend a combination of a stool softener with a stimulant laxative for patients on chronic opioid therapy. Stool softeners, such as docusate sodium, are detergents that allow better water penetration into stool, making

TABLE 43.7

ANTIEMETICS

Agent	Presumed primary receptor site of action	Dosage/route	Major adverse effects
Metoclopramide	D2 (primarily in GI tract) or 5HT3 (only at high doses)	5–20 mg orally or subcutaneously or iv	Dystonia, akathisia, esophageal spasm, and colic (in GI obstruction)
Haloperidol	D2 (primarily in CTZ)	0.5–4 mg orally or subcutaneously or intravenously q6hr	Dystonia and akathisia
Prochlorperazine	D2 (primarily in CTZ)	5–10 mg orally or intravenously q 6h or 25 mg rectally q6h	Dystonia, akathisia, and sedation
Chlorpromazine	D2 (primarily in CTZ)	10–250 mg orally q4h, 25–50 mg intravenously or im q4h, or 50–100 mg rectally q6h	Dystonia, akathisia, sedation, postural hypotension
Promethazine	H1, muscarinic acetylcholine receptor or D2 (primarily in CTZ)	12.5–25 mg orally or intravenously q6h or 25 mg rectally q6h	Dystonia, akathisia, and sedation
Diphenhydramine	H1	25–50 mg orally or intravenously or SQ q6h	Sedation, dry mouth, urinary retention
Scopolamine	Muscarinic acetylcholine receptor	1.5 mg transdermal patch q72h	Dry mouth, blurred vision, urinary retention, confusion
Hyoscyamine	Muscarinic acetylcholine receptor	0.125–0.25 mg SL or orally q4h or 0.25–0.5 mg SQ or iv q4h	Dry mouth, blurred vision, ileus, urinary retention, confusion
Ondansetron	5HT3	4–8 mg orally by pill or dissolvable tablet (ODT) or intravenously q4–8h	Headache, fatigue, constipation
Aprepitant	NK1	40 mg orally qd	

(Modified from Wood GJ, Shega JW, Lynch B, et al. Management of intractable nausea and vomiting in patients at the end of life: "I was feeling nauseous all of the time . . . nothing was working." *JAMA* 2007;298(10):1196–1207.)

it softer and more voluminous. Stimulant laxatives, such as senna and bisacodyl, induce peristalsis via mechanisms that are not well understood. In vitro, applying senna to intestinal mucosa leads to immediate contraction. After optimal titration of these agents, oral osmotics are commonly added to enhance laxation by pulling along water due to osmotic forces. Osmotics include sugars, such as lactulose or sorbitol, magnesium salts, such as magnesium citrate, or inert substances, such as polyethylene glycol. When unsuccessful, rescue oral and rectal interventions are also often needed. Rectal interventions include such agents as bisacodyl suppositories and phosphosoda enemas to soften, lubricate, and mobilize hard, dry, distal stool. Often synergism of multiple categories of agents is required for successful laxation.

Opioid antagonists have also been studied in the treatment of OBD. Oral naloxone given in doses between 2 mg to 4 mg three times per day was effective in improving bowel movement frequency but some patients also experienced reversal of pain relief and this reversal occurred in spite of using very low doses of naloxone relative to the total dose of opioid taken.[47] The authors suggested that patients using higher doses of opioids appear to be the most vulnerable to the analgesic effect of oral naloxone. Two peripheral opioid antagonists (alvimopan, methylnaltrexone) have been studied for opioid-induced constipation in palliative patients with advanced illnesses with insufficient response to laxative therapy (methylnaltrexone) and postoperative ileus (alvimopan) and approved for these indications by the U.S. Food and Drug Administration (FDA). Alvimopan is only approved for short-term use in hospitalized patients.

Adjuvant Analgesics

An adjuvant analgesic is a medication with primary indication other than pain relief, but it may provide or enhance analgesia in certain circumstances. In the area of cancer pain, the common adjunctive analgesics are corticosteroids, anticonvulsants, and antidepressants. These drugs play an important role for some patients who cannot otherwise attain an acceptable balance between relief and opioid side effects. Adjuvant analgesics divide broadly into general-purpose analgesics, adjuvants used for musculoskeletal pain, and those with specific use for neuropathic, bone, or visceral pain.

General Purpose Adjuvants

Corticosteroids are the most widely used general-purpose adjuvant analgesics and are available in a wide variety of formulations.[48] The painful conditions that commonly respond to steroids include increased intracranial pressure, acute spinal cord compression, superior vena cava syndrome, metastatic bone pain, neuropathic pain due to infiltration or compression, symptomatic lymphedema, and hepatic capsular distension. Patients with advanced cancer who experience pain and other symptoms that may respond to steroids usually receive relatively small doses (e.g., dexamethasone 1–2 mg bid). Using a very short course of relatively high doses (e.g., dexamethasone 100 mg intravenously followed initially by 96 mg per day in divided doses) can help manage an acute episode of very severe pain related to a neuropathic lesion (e.g., plexopathy or epidural spinal cord compression) or bony metastasis that does not respond to opioids.[49] In all cases, gradually lower the dose following pain reduction to the minimum needed to sustain relief. Topical agents (see Chapter 79) may also be useful as an adjunctive form of pharmacotherapy without increasing systemic toxicity.

Musculoskeletal Pain Adjuvants

Pain that originates from injury to muscle or connective tissue is not unusual in patients with cancer. Pharmacological and nonpharmacological approaches do not differ significantly from patients with musculoskeletal pain who do not have cancer (see Chapter 34), other than disease- or treatment-specific issues relevant to the cancer patient. Drug–drug and drug–disease interactions must always be considered and be an ongoing component of reassessment.

Neuropathic Pain Adjuvants

Neuropathic pain is a common and oftentimes very debilitating source of distress in patients with cancer because of disease and treatment (see Chapters 24–28 and 42). Most treatment strategies for cancer-related neuropathic pain are extrapolated from noncancer-related neuropathic pain (see Chapter 80). Table 43.8 summarizes those agents that are commonly used to treat neuropathic pain in cancer patients, alone or in combination with opioids. There is a wide spectrum of drug–drug and drug–disease interactions with the various adjuvant analgesics, so appropriate patient counseling and ongoing reassessment are important to optimize therapeutic outcomes and minimize adverse effects.

Xiao et al.[50] tested gabapentin as a potential analgesic for paclitaxel- and vincristine-evoked pain in an animal model. Paclitaxel- and vincristine-evoked mechano-allodynia and mechano-hyperalgesia were significantly reduced by gabapentin, but only with repeated dosing. Paclitaxel-evoked painful peripheral neuropathy was associated with an increased expression of the alpha(2)delta-1 subunit in the spinal dorsal horn, but not in the dorsal root ganglia suggesting that gabapentin's mechanisms of action for this type of neuropathy may include normalization of the nerve injury-evoked increase in calcium channel alpha(2) delta-1 subunit expression. Dunteman[51] reported on the use of oral levetiracetam titrated over days to 2 weeks in 7 patients with neoplasms involving neural structures (four invading the brachial plexus and three the lumbosacral plexus). The maximum levetiracetam dose ranged from 500 to 1500 mg bid. All patients experienced pain control improvement after the addition of levetiracetam and opioid use decreased by at least an estimated 70%, without drug-related adverse events. Like gabapentin and pregabalin, levetiracetam lacks any significant drug–drug interactions. Table 43.9 lists antiepileptic drugs currently used for neuropathic pain.

Bone Pain Adjuvants

NSAIDs, corticosteroids, calcitonin, radiopharmaceuticals, and bisphosphonates all have a potential place in the treatment of cancer-related bone pain. Chapters 46 and 48 discuss the causes and treatment of bony disease.

Visceral Pain Adjuvants

The literature offers little support for the potential efficacy of adjuvant agents for the management of bladder spasm, tenesmic pain, and colicky intestinal pain. A trial of NSAIDs may help patients with painful bladder spasms.[52] Although there is no well-established pharmacotherapy for painful rectal spasms, diltiazem can help in the management of proctalgia fugax.[53] The treatment of pain due to inoperable bowel obstruction has been described above.

Psychotropic Drugs

Many cancer patients will require a psychotropic drug. Some need it for pain relief (e.g., tricyclic antidepressants for nerve injury pain), while others need an antiemetic (e.g., haloperidol for opioid-induced nausea). Still others require an anxiolytic, such as clonazepam or alprazolam. Some require a night sedative and others an antidepressant for identifiable depression. The concurrent use of two centrally acting drugs (e.g., opioid with psychotropic drug or two psychotropic drugs together) is more likely

TABLE 43.8

NUMBERS NEEDED TO TREAT WITH VARIOUS ANALGESICS FOR DIFFERENT NEUROPATHIC PAIN STATES

Drug	Number of trials	Central pain	Peripheral pain	Painful polyneuro-pathy	Postherpetic neuralgia	Peripheral nerve injury	Trigeminal neuralgia	HIV neuro-pathy	Mixed neuro-pathic pain
TCA	16	4.0 (2.6–8.5)	2.3 (2.1–2.7)	2.1 (1.9–2.6)	2.8 (2.2–3.8)	2.5 (1.4–11)	ND		NA
SNRI	2	ND	5.1 (3.9–7.4)	5.1 (3.9–7.4)	ND	NA	ND	ND	ND
Gabapentin/ pregabalin	4	MA	4.0 (3.6–5.4)	3.9 (3–4.7)	4.6 (4.3–5.4)	NA	ND	ND	8.0 (5.9–32)
Opioids	6	ND	2.7 (2.1–3.6)	2.6 (1.7–6.0)	2.6 (2.0–3.8)	3.0 (1.5–7.4)	ND	ND	2.1 (1.5–3.3)
Tramadol	1	ND	3.9 (2.7–6.7)	3.5 (2.4–6.4)	4.8 (2.6–27)	ND	ND	NS	ND
NMDA antagonists	5	ND	5.5 (3.4–14)	2.9 (1.8–6.6)	NS	NS	ND	ND	NS
Topical lidocaine	4	ND	4.4 (2.5–17)	ND	NA	ND	ND	NA	4.4 (2.5–17)
Cannabinoids	2	6.0 (3.0–718)	ND	ND	ND	ND	ND	ND	NS
Capsaicin	11	ND	6.7 (4.6–12)	11 (5.5–317)	3.2 (2.2–5.9)	6.5 (3.4–69)	ND	NA	NA

ND, no studies done; NA, dichotomized data not available; NS, relative risk not significant.
(Modified from Finnerup NB, Otto M, Jensen TS, et al. An evidence-based algorithm for the treatment of neuropathic pain. *MedGenMed* 2007;9(2):36. Permission Pending.)

TABLE 43.9

ANTIEPILEPTIC DRUGS

Drug	Brand	Mechanism of action	Dose titration and range	Remarks
Gabapentin	Neurontin	Ca^{++} channel	100–4800 mg/d	May stop suddenly; sedation, nausea, ataxia (mostly transient by 2–4 weeks)
Pregabalin	Lyrica	Ca^{++} channel	50 mg tid; ↑ × 7 days to 100 mg tid. Max dose = 600 mg/day.	Sedation, ataxia, edema. Cognitive dysfunction.
Carbamazepine	Tegretol	Na^+ channel	400–1800 mg/d. Start low (100 mg bid).	Taper off. Check platelet count. Nausea common. Sedation, ataxia.
Oxcarbazepine	Trileptal	Na^+ channel	600–2400 mg/d. Start low (150 mg bid)	Taper off. Sedation, ataxia, nausea. Hyponatremia.
Lamotrigine	Lamictal	Na^+ channel, ↓ glutamate release	25–600 mg/d. Start low 25 mg/d. Follow package insert titration.	Taper off. Skin rash (rarely Stevens-Johnson–dose dependent); sedation, ataxia
Topiramate	Topamax	Mixed Na^+ and Ca^{++}	15–800 mg/d. Start low (15 mg bid), titrate slowly (weekly)	Taper off. Cognitive dysfunction, weight loss, fatigue.
Levetiracetam	Keppra	?	1000–4000 mg/d. Start low (250 mg bid), titrate slowly (weekly)	Somnolence, cognitive dysfunction, mood changes.

to produce sedation in ill and malnourished cancer patients than in others.

Cannabinoids

Cannabinoids, the active components of Cannabis sativa L., act in the body by mimicking endogenous substances (endocannabinoids) that activate specific cell surface receptors. The isolation of its main constituent, Delta9-tetrahydrocannabinol, and the discovery of the endocannabinoid system (cannabinoid receptors CB1 and CB2 and their endogenous ligands) resulted in studies concerning the pharmacologic activity of cannabinoids. Cannabinoids exert various palliative effects in cancer patients. In addition, cannabinoids inhibit the growth of different types of tumor cells, including glioma cells[54] and pancreatic ductal adenocarcinoma.[55] Two oral formulations of cannabinoids, dronabinol (Marinol) and nabilone (Cesamet) are approved by the FDA for use in chemotherapy-induced nausea and vomiting refractory to conventional antiemetic therapy. Cannabinoids also stimulate appetite and food intake and may have a role in the management of cancer-induced cachexia.[56] Studies of the endogenous cannabinoids (endocannabinoids) have demonstrated that they are present in most tissues and that in some pain states, such as neuropathic pain, levels of endocannabinoids are elevated at key sites involved in pain processing.[57] Abrams et al.[58] demonstrated that smoked cannabis was well tolerated and effectively relieved chronic neuropathic pain from human immunodeficiency virus (HIV)-associated sensory neuropathy. In some states, medical use of marijuana is allowed for certain conditions including HIV, cancer, multiple sclerosis, and epilepsy.

OPIOID ANALGESICS

Opioids are the mainstay of pharmacotherapy for patients with moderate or more intense pain resulting from virtually any cancer-related etiology. A detailed discussion of opioid pharmacology and principles of prescribing is found in Chapter 78.

Selection of Opioid Therapy in Cancer Pain Management

As in all patients who may have pain-related indications for opioid therapy, the effective clinical use of opioid drugs requires familiarity with drug selection, routes of administration, dosage guidelines, and potential adverse effects. Several factors must be considered if opioids are to be used effectively. These include:

- Previous opioid exposure and preference
- Severity and nature of disease
- Age of patient
- Extent of cancer, particularly hepatic and renal involvement altering normal opioid pharmacokinetics. See Table 43.10.

TABLE 43.10

EFFECTS OF RENAL FAILURE ON OPIOID PHARMACOKINETICS

Opioid	Effect
Dihydrocodeine	Decreased clearance
Dextropropoxyphene	Increased norpropoxyphene (toxic metabolite)
Morphine	Increased morphine-6-glucuronide (active metabolite)
Meperidine	Increased normeperidine (toxic metabolite)

- Concurrent disease
- Available formulations

The specific pathogenic mechanism that underlies a patient's cancer pain should not be a factor in deciding which opioid to use because the mechanism of pain does not reliably predict the response to opioid therapy.[59] This particularly applies to situations in which neuropathic mechanisms dominate the pain complaint. Opioids should be used as first-line therapy in such situations, particularly if the pain is considered moderate to severe in intensity.

Short-acting agents (e.g., morphine immediate-release [IR], hydrocodone IR, hydromorphone IR, oxycodone IR, oxymorphone IR, transmucosal fentanyl) may be favored initially because they are easier to titrate than long-acting agents (e.g., morphine controlled release [CR], oxycodone CR, oxymorphone extended release [ER], and transdermal fentanyl). Short-acting opioids are characterized by a rapid rise and fall in serum opioid levels, whereas serum levels of long-acting opioids increase slowly to therapeutic levels, remain there for an extended period, and then slowly decline.[60] In general, the clinical circumstance dictates the choice of a short- or long-acting opioid. For example, the treatment of acute or postoperative pain usually requires frequent titration, and short-acting opioids, with duration of action of 2 to 4 hours, are preferred. Conversely, the treatment of cancer pain or chronic, moderate to severe nonmalignant pain usually can be treated with a long-acting oral agent, with a duration of action of 12 to 24 hours, with less need for titration. In patients being treated with long-acting agents, short-acting opioids are usually provided as rescue medication for BTP, which is very common in patients with cancer pain. An ongoing opioid regimen should include provisions for rescue doses for the treatment of BTP. The rationale for providing rescue medication instead of increasing the dose of the ATC opioid is to prevent overmedication and associated adverse events. Often, there is a narrow therapeutic window between an opioid dosage sufficient to achieve pain relief and one that is associated with unacceptable adverse events.[61] For patients treated with a long-acting opioid, an IR or short-acting opioid formulation (often the same drug) may be used as the rescue medication. In general, the rescue drug should be started at a dose equivalent to approximately 10% of the 24-hour baseline dose and titrated upward to achieve adequate pain relief.[62] The dosing frequency of the rescue drug depends on the time to peak effect and the route of administration; in general, oral rescue doses can be administered as frequently as every 2 hours if needed, but typically tend to be given every 3 to 4 hours as needed.[63] Generally, three types of BTP should be considered—spontaneous, incident, or end-of-dose failure.[64] A key principle in treating BTP is to optimize the background pain control by appropriately adjusting the ATC opioid regimen. With end-of-dose failure, the clinician can increase the dose or shorten the dosing interval of ATC opioid or increase the dose of the rescue opioid. Similar strategies may be employed for spontaneous pain but successful management of spontaneous or incident pain may require the use of short-acting, rapid onset opioids (see oral transmucosal fentanyl).

Because of the substantial interpatient variability in opioid responsiveness, clinicians who prescribe opioids for the treatment of cancer pain should be familiar with at least three different agents appropriate for the management of moderate to severe pain.[65] The opioids used most commonly in the treatment of cancer pain are listed in Table 43.11. The pharmacology of these agents can be reviewed in Chapter 78.

The regimen for opioid medications should generally provide ATC analgesia with provision for rescue doses for the management of exacerbations of the pain not covered by the regular dosage. At all times, causes of new or uncontrolled pain should be determined and addressed by disease-modifying treatments and a gradual increase in the opioid dose until either pain control

TABLE 43.11

LONG-ACTING ORAL AND TRANSDERMAL OPIOIDS USED IN THE TREATMENT OF CANCER PAIN

Opioid	Dosing and administration	Pharmacokinetics	Most common adverse events	Comments
Hydrocodone IR	5–10 mg q4–6h	$T_{max} = 1.3$ h; $t_{1/2} = 3.8$ h	Light-headedness, dizziness, sedation, nausea	When combined with aspirin or acetaminophen, impose a dosage ceiling
Meperidine IR	50–150 mg q3–4h	Duration of action shorter than morphine	Light-headedness, dizziness, sedation, nausea	Infrequently prescribed for long-term use
Morphine IR	5–30 mg q4h	$T_{max} = 1.3$ h	Constipation, light-headedness, dizziness	Useful for initial dose titration and for BTP
Morphine ER	Based on dose of morphine IR; administered q12h	$t_{1/2} = 2$–4 h	Constipation, light-headedness, dizziness	Available in different preparations (Ms Contin, Oramorph, Kadian, Avinza)
Oxycodone IR	5–10 mg q6h	$T_{max} = 1.6$ h; $t_{1/2} = 3.5$ h	Drowsiness, light-headedness, nausea	Useful for initial dose titration and for BTP; if compounded with aspirin or acetaminophen, may impose a dosage ceiling
Oxycodone CR	Based on dose of oxycodone IR or previous opioid; administered q12h	$t_{1/2} = 4.5$ h	Constipation, nausea, somnolence	Immediate release component (approx. 30% of total dose); equianalgesic dose ratio to oxymorphone ER is 2:1
Oxymorphone IR	5–10 mg q4–6h	$T_{max} = 0.5$ h	Nausea, dizziness	Useful for initial dose titration and for BTP
Oxymorphone ER	Based on dose of oxymorphone IR or previous opioid; administered q12h	$T_{max} = 5$ h; $t_{1/2} = 9$–10 h	Nausea, dizziness	Dose and dose interval should be adjusted according to patient needs; little need for rescue medication in clinical trials
Transdermal fentanyl	One patch applied to skin q72h	$T_{max} = 34$–38 h	Nausea, vomiting	Useful for patients with GI dysfunction; poor adhesion to skin may limit use in some patients

is achieved or intolerable and unmanageable adverse effects supervene. The management of pain with opioid analgesics demands frequent patient assessment and a readiness to re-evaluate the therapeutic plan in the setting of either inadequate relief or adverse effects.

There is no single optimal or maximal dose of an opioid analgesic drug. In general, for progressive, tumor-related pain, the appropriate dose of an opioid is one that relieves a patient's pain throughout the dosing interval without causing unmanageable or intolerable adverse events.[66] The initial dose may be based on the severity of pain and known response to prior analgesic therapy, if any.[67] Aggressive upward titration to a stable dose (i.e., one that provides adequate pain relief throughout the dosing interval) is predicated on continuing assessment of the effectiveness of therapy. Patients rarely benefit from combinations of opioids given in suboptimal doses; ideally, clinicians should prescribe a single opioid analgesic and titrate to a stable dose.[67] However, it is important to recognize that there is significant interpatient variability with regard to responsiveness to different opioid drugs, and patients who respond poorly to one opioid may respond favorably to another.[68] In situations in which pain is not related to the tumor or its treatment, a dose limit should be considered.[69]

Hanks et al.[67] reported on the recommendations of the European Association for Palliative Care (EAPC) on the use of morphine and alternative opioids in cancer pain. These recommendations provide practical strategies for dealing with difficult situations (Table 43.12).

Tolerance and Hyperalgesia

Opioid tolerance is a phenomenon in which repeated exposure to an opioid results in decreased therapeutic effect of the drug or need for a higher dose to maintain the same effect. Prolonged use of opioids is known to result in antinociceptive tolerance, in which higher doses of the opioid are required to elicit the same amount of pain relief or antinociception.[70,71] In practice, physical dependence and tolerance do not prevent the effective use of these drugs in patients with cancer pain. The evidence for the development of tolerance to the analgesic effects of opioids with chronic administration has been mixed. Many of the studies were in cancer patients with severe pain and showed that they maintained a stable opioid dose (for weeks to years) even with different routes of administration.[72,73] Patients with stable disease often remain on a stable dose for weeks or months.[74] Collin et al.[75] demonstrated a relationship between tumor progression and escalation of opioid doses over time such that the development of opioid tolerance as a result of chronic opioid use was unlikely in cancer patients with pain. Although it is generally agreed that tolerance to the analgesic properties of opioids occurs in patients with malignant pain, dose escalation is thought to be mostly a result of disease progression rather than the development of pharmacodynamic tolerance.

Animal studies and anecdotal reports in humans suggest that high-dose opioid exposure can paradoxically induce hyperalgesic

TABLE 43.12

MORPHINE AND ALTERNATIVE OPIOIDS IN CANCER PAIN

1. The opioid of first choice for moderate to severe cancer pain is morphine. **C**
2. The optimal route of administration of morphine is by mouth. Ideally, two types of formulation are required: normal release (for dose titration) and modified release (for maintenance treatment). **C**
3. The simplest method of dose titration is with a dose of normal-release morphine given every 4 hours and the same dose for BTP. This "rescue" dose may be given as often as required (up to hourly) and the total daily dose of morphine should be reviewed daily. The regular dose can then be adjusted to take into account the total amount of rescue morphine. **C**
4. If pain returns consistently before the next regular dose is due the regular dose should be increased. In general, normal release morphine does not need to be given more often than every 4 hours and modified release morphine more often than 12 or 24 hours (according to the intended duration of the formulation). Patients stabilized on regular oral morphine require continued access to a rescue dose to treat BTP. **A**
5. Several countries do not have a normal release formulation of morphine, though such a formulation is necessary for optimal pain management. A different strategy is needed if treatment is started with modified release morphine. Changes to the regular dose should not be made more frequently than every 48 hours, which means that the dose titration phase will be prolonged. **C**
6. For patients receiving normal release morphine every 4 hours, a double dose at bedtime is a simple and effective way of avoiding being woken by pain. **C**
7. Several modified-release formulations are available. There is no evidence that the 12-hourly formulations (tablets, capsules, or liquids) are substantially different in their duration of effect and relative analgesic potency. The same is true for the 24-hour formulations though there is less evidence to draw on. **A**
8. If patients are unable to take morphine orally, the preferred alternative route is subcutaneous. There is generally no indication for giving morphine intramuscularly for chronic cancer pain because subcutaneous administration is simpler and less painful. **C**
9. The average relative potency ratio of oral morphine to subcutaneous morphine is between 1:2 and 1:3 (i.e., 20–30 mg of morphine by mouth is equianalgesic to 10 mg by subcutaneous injection). **C**
10. In patients requiring continuous parenteral morphine, the preferred method of administration is by subcutaneous infusion. **C**
11. Intravenous infusion of morphine may be preferred in patients:
    1. who already have an in dwelling intravenous line;
    2. with generalized edema;
    3. who develop erythema, soreness, or sterile abscesses with subcutaneous administration;
    4. with coagulation disorders;
    5. with poor peripheral circulation. **C**
12. The average relative potency ratio of oral to intravenous morphine is between 1:2 and 1:3. **A**
13. The buccal, sublingual, and nebulized routes of administration of morphine are not recommended because at the present time there is no evidence of clinical advantage over the conventional routes. **B**
14. OTFC is an effective treatment for BTP in patients stabilized on regular oral morphine or an alternative step 3 opioid. **A**
15. Successful pain management with opioids requires that adequate analgesia be achieved without excessive adverse effects. By these criteria, the application of the WHO and the EAPC guidelines (using morphine as the preferred step 3 opioid) permit effective control of chronic cancer pain in the majority of patients. In a small minority of patients, adequate relief without excessive adverse effects may depend on the use of alternative opioids, spinal administration of analgesics, or nondrug methods of pain control. **B**
16. A small proportion of patients develop intolerable adverse effects with oral morphine (in conjunction with a nonopioid and adjuvant analgesic as appropriate) before achieving adequate pain relief. In such patients, a change to an alternative opioid or a change in the route of administration should be considered. **B**
17. Hydromorphone or oxycodone, if available in both normal-release and modified-release formulations for oral administration, are effective alternatives to oral morphine. **A**
18. Methadone is an effective alternative but may be more complicated to use compared with other opioids because of pronounced interindividual differences in its plasma half-life, relative analgesic potency, and duration of action. Its use by nonspecialist practitioners is not recommended. **C**
19. Transdermal fentanyl is an effective alternative to oral morphine but is best reserved for patients whose opioid requirements are stable. It may have particular advantages for such patients if they are unable to take oral morphine, as an alternative to subcutaneous infusion. **B**
20. Spinal (epidural or intrathecal) administration of opioid analgesics in combination with local anesthetics or clonidine should be considered in patients who derive inadequate analgesia or suffer intolerable adverse effects despite the optimal use of systemic opioids and nonopioids. **B**

Level **A** evidence requires at least one randomized controlled trial as part of a body of literature of overall good quality and consistency addressing the specific recommendation (evidence levels Ia and Ib). Level **B** requires the availability of well-conducted clinical studies but no randomized clinical trials on the topic of recommendation (evidence levels IIa, IIb and III). Level **C** requires evidence obtained from expert committee reports or opinions and/or clinical experiences of respected authorities. Indicates an absence of directly applicable clinical studies of good quality (evidence level IV). Categories Ia evidence from meta-analysis of randomized controlled trials; Ib evidence from at least one randomized controlled trial; IIa evidence from at least one controlled study without randomization; IIb evidence from at least one other type of quasi-experimental study; III evidence from nonexperimental descriptive studies, such as comparative studies, correlation studies, and case-control studies; IV evidence from expert committee reports or opinions or clinical experience of respected authorities, or both. (From Hanks GW, Conno F, Cherny N et al. Morphine and alternative opioids in cancer pain: the EAPC recommendations. *Br J Cancer* 2001;84(5):587–593.)

states. Opioids such as morphine have been reported to induce hyperalgesia in humans and animals.[70] In preclinical studies, sustained opiate exposure across multiple days has been shown to reduce sensory thresholds, resulting in hypersensitivity to tactile stimulation (i.e., allodynia) and to noxious thermal stimulation (i.e., hyperalgesia).[76] Opioid-induced hyperalgesia has mostly been observed in cancer patients who receive very high and escalating opioid doses.[77] Morphine has been implicated in virtually all reported cases. Recognition of this phenomenon can be difficult in a clinical setting of cancer pain where multiple factors can confound the picture. Opioid-induced hyperalgesia should be recognized as a syndrome of neuroexcitatory effects, which includes hyperalgesia, allodynia, myoclonus, and seizures, in a setting where patients are administered large doses of systemic morphine or its structural analogues. The predominant symptom of opioid-induced hyperalgesia is severe allodynia (touch-evoked pain) and is often accompanied by myoclonus. Putting a blanket on or gently turning a bedridden patient can evoke excruciating pain. Further dose escalation will exacerbate pain complaints or symptoms. Management strategies for hyperalgesia usually require a reduction in opioid dosage and switching to a different agent, especially one that does not have known toxic metabolites.

Morphine

In a Cochrane review, Wiffen and McQuay[78] reported that oral morphine is an effective analgesic in patients who suffer pain associated with cancer and remains the criterion standard for moderate to severe pain. Oral morphine was shown to be effective over a wide dose range. In this review, it was not possible to demonstrate the superiority of one modified release product over another, either by brand or by length of time release. Some preparations have the practical advantage of a formulation as micro capsules for those who cannot readily swallow tablets. The main disadvantage of morphine in cancer patients who require high opioid doses or who have reduced renal clearance is the accumulation of active (morphine-6-glucuronide) and toxic (morphine-3-glucuronide), which may complicate the clinical picture with excessive sedation or neurotoxic adverse effects. Early signs of these effects should trigger consideration for switching to a different opioid (i.e., opioid rotation).

Oxycodone

Kalso and Vainio[79] administered morphine and oxycodone hydrochloride in a double-blind crossover study to 20 patients who were experiencing severe cancer pain. Morphine caused more nausea than oxycodone and hallucinations occurred only during morphine treatment. Otherwise, no major differences in the side effects between the two opioids were observed. Maddocks et al.[80] reported an attenuation of morphine-induced delirium in cancer patients when changed to oxycodone.

Heiskanen and Kalso[81] compared the steady-state pharmacodynamic profiles of oxycodone and morphine sulfate controlled-release in 27 patients with chronic cancer pain in a double blind, randomized, crossover design. The total opioid consumption ratio of oxycodone to morphine was 2:3 when oxycodone was administered first and 3:4 when oxycodone was administered after morphine. The total incidence of adverse experiences reported by patients was similar, but significantly more vomiting occurred with morphine, whereas constipation was more common with oxycodone. The mean daily dose of oxycodone at the end of titration was 123 mg and that of morphine 180 mg. In this study, the two opioids provided comparable pain relief. Reid et al.[82] evaluated the efficacy and tolerability of oxycodone in cancer-related pain in a systematic review of randomized controlled trials. The authors found no clinically important differences between the analgesic efficacy and the adverse effect profile of oxycodone compared with morphine. In essence, the efficacy and tolerability of oxycodone was similar to morphine, supporting its use as an opioid for cancer-related pain.

Oxymorphone

Sloan et al.[83] compared oxymorphone ER and oxycodone CR in patients ($n = 86$) with moderate to severe cancer pain. Patients were first stabilized for 3 days or longer on morphine CR or oxycodone CR. Those who attained stable pain relief for at least 3 days (three or fewer rescue doses of opioid per day) entered the first 7-day treatment period (period 1) at the stabilized dose of the titrated medication with no dosage adjustments. All patients who were treated for 7 days at their stabilized dose of either morphine CR or oxycodone CR were then crossed over to oxymorphone ER at an estimated equianalgesic dosage and treated for an additional 7 days (period 2). During periods 1 and 2, the oral IR formulation of the study medication was available as rescue medication. Each dose of rescue medication was approximately 10% of the total daily dose of scheduled medication. Similar daily pain intensity scores during the last 2 days of the initial treatment phase (morphine CR or oxycodone CR) compared with those during the last 2 days of the oxymorphone ER treatment phase indicate that equivalent analgesia was achieved after patients had been rotated to oxymorphone ER. This also suggests that the long-acting formulation can maintain drug levels in a stable fashion. Patients taking oxymorphone ER needed less breakthrough medication than patients taking morphine CR. The tolerability/safety profiles (e.g., nausea, drowsiness, and somnolence) were similar between the two drugs. There were no significant differences in daily pain intensity scores between oxymorphone ER and either morphine or oxycodone.

Hydromorphone

Hydromorphone is only available in an unmodified (i.e., IR) form. The short elimination half-life of hydromorphone necessitates at least 4-hourly administration of the drug to maintain adequate plasma levels for patients with chronic cancer pain. Therefore, its utility in cancer patients with continuous (baseline) pain is mostly in the treatment of BTP.

Methadone

Methadone is well absorbed by all routes, making it a versatile agent for cancer pain control. It has no known active metabolites and it is relatively inexpensive compared with other modified release opioid formulations. Other advantages include possibly enhanced pain relief from incomplete cross-tolerance with the potential to control pain no longer responsive to other mu-opioid receptor agonist drugs.[84–87] However, this property, along with its highly variable elimination half-life, make it a more complicated drug to use, with great potential for accidental overdose if not titrated appropriately. Prescribers must know the pharmacology of methadone very well, and patients need to be carefully counseled and cautioned to use methadone only as directed in order to prevent unintended dose accumulation.

Concomitant administration of CYP3A4 inducers will increase methadone metabolism, potentially causing a reduction in methadone plasma concentrations. This may result in the need for larger doses of methadone during the period of interaction. In addition, doses of methadone may need to be reduced when a CYP3A4 inducer is discontinued. Known inducers of CYP3A4 include rifampin, rifabutin, carbamazepine, phenytoin, phenobarbital, and abacavir. The commonly used dietary supplement for depression, St. John's Wort, has also been shown to lower the plasma concentrations of methadone.[88] Many methadone-related deaths may be due to drug interactions rather than administration of methadone alone.[89] Drugs that potentially interact with methadone include inhibitors of CYP3A4 and CYP2D6. Drugs that inhibit CYP3A4 include fluconazole, fluvoxamine, fluoxetine, paroxetine, HIV-1 protease inhibitors, and likely erythromycin and ketoconazole. In addition to CYP3A4 inhibitors affecting methadone's clearance, methadone itself acts as a CYP3A4 inhibitor and therefore has the potential to interact with other CYP3A4 substrates.[90]

Bruera et al.[91] compared the effectiveness and side effects of methadone and morphine as first-line treatment with opioids for cancer pain. Over a 4-week period, patients were randomly assigned to receive methadone (7.5 mg orally every 12 hours and 5 mg every 4 hours as needed) or morphine (15 mg sustained release every 12 hours and 5 mg every 4 hours as needed). A total of 103 patients were randomly assigned to treatment (49 in the methadone group and 54 in the morphine group). The groups had similar baseline scores for pain, sedation, nausea, confusion, and constipation. Patients receiving methadone had more opioid-related dropouts (11 of 49; 22%) than those receiving morphine (3 of 54; 6%; $p = 0.019$). The opioid escalation index at days 14 and 28 was similar between the two groups. More than three fourths of patients in each group reported a 20% or more reduction in pain intensity by day 8. The proportion of patients with a 20% or more improvement in pain at 4 weeks in the methadone group was 0.49 (95% CI, 0.34 to 0.64) and was similar in the morphine group (0.56; 95% CI, 0.41 to 0.70). The rates of patient-reported global benefit were nearly identical to the pain response rates and did not differ between the treatment groups. The authors concluded that methadone did not produce superior analgesic efficiency or overall tolerability at 4 weeks compared with morphine as a first-line strong opioid for the treatment of cancer pain.

In a Cochrane review, Nicholson[92] concluded that methadone was no more effective than morphine for cancer-related neuropathic pain and that methadone had a similar side effect profile, but these side effects may be more apparent with repeated dosing. For all these reasons, methadone is not recommended as a first-line opioid for cancer pain treatment.

Levorphanol

Like methadone, drug accumulation may follow initiation of therapy or dose escalation. Guidelines similar to those suggested for methadone may prove helpful for managing the patient requiring high doses of levorphanol.

Fentanyl

Transdermal Fentanyl

Transdermal therapeutic system fentanyl (TTS-fentanyl) patches are rectangular transparent units each comprising a protective liner and four functional layers. These layers consist of a backing layer of polyester film, a drug reservoir of fentanyl and alcohol USP gelled with hydroxyethyl cellulose, an ethylene-vinyl acetate copolymer membrane that controls the rate of fentanyl delivery to the skin surface, and a fentanyl containing silicone adhesive. The amount of fentanyl released from each system per hour is proportional to the surface area (25 mcg/hour per 10 cm^2).

The transdermal system releases fentanyl from the reservoir at a nearly constant amount per unit time. The concentration gradient existing between the saturated solution of drug in the reservoir and the lower concentration in the skin drives drug release. Fentanyl moves in the direction of the lower concentra-tion at a rate determined by the copolymer release membrane and the diffusion of fentanyl through the skin layers. While the actual rate of fentanyl delivery to the skin varies over the application period, each system is labeled with a nominal flux, which represents the average amount of drug delivered to the systemic circulation per hour across average skin. While there is variation in dose delivered among patients, the nominal flux of the systems is sufficiently accurate to allow individual titration of dosage for a given patient.

Following patch application, the skin under the system absorbs fentanyl, and a depot of fentanyl concentrates in the upper skin layers. Fentanyl then becomes available to the systemic circulation. There is a lag time of approximately 2 hours before clinically useful systemic levels of drug are achieved after applying the patch.[93] Serum fentanyl concentrations increase gradually following application, generally leveling off between 12 and 24 hours. The system delivers fentanyl continuously for up to 72 hours. After sequential 48- or 72-hour applications, patients reach and maintain steady state serum concentrations that are determined by individual variation in skin permeability and body clearance of fentanyl. A number of studies demonstrate that constant serum levels are maintained with the second transdermal system and that fluctuations of serum levels are small after the first 72 hours.[94,95]

After system removal, serum fentanyl concentrations decline gradually, falling about 50% in approximately 17 hours (range 13–22). Because of the possibility of temperature-dependent increases in fentanyl release from the system, it is important to advise patients to avoid exposing the application site to direct external heat sources, such as heating pads, heat lamps, and heated waterbeds. Prolonged exposure to heat or use in patients who are febrile can cause a toxic overdose.[96] Inter- and intraindividual variability in TTS-fentanyl absorption was reported in cancer pain patients over a 6-month period.[97] The intraindividual variability ranged from 2.8% to 75.1%. The bioavailability of fentanyl was statistically different according to patient age with patients >75 years of age absorbing 50% of the fentanyl during the selected 72-hour period and patients <65 years absorbing 66%. In spite of this variability, pain relief was reported as good to excellent in the majority of patients.

TTS-fentanyl offers the advantage of providing continuous administration of a potent opioid in the absence of needles and expensive drug-infusion pumps for the treatment of cancer pain. Several studies have investigated the management of cancer pain with TTS-fentanyl.[98–106] Pharmacokinetic studies indicate a relative steady state ("pseudo steady state") 15 hours[107] and 16–20 hours after application of the patch,[108] suggesting the possibility of early titration with TTS-fentanyl at 24-hour intervals. The long-term efficacy of TTS-fentanyl was evaluated in 51 cancer patients by Donner et al.[99] Seventy-five percent of patients had metastases. Patients used TTS-fentanyl for an average of 158 days (range, 15–855 days). Seventy-three percent of patients received treatment for a period of 3 to 12 months. The investigators discontinued TTS-fentanyl in 16% of patients because of insufficient pain relief. In these patients, the last TTS-fentanyl dosage was a mean of 233.3 mcg/hour (range, 25–700 mcg/hour). In addition, 4 patients returned to oral morphine therapy. At the start of therapy, patients needed 69.5 mcg/hour TTS-fentanyl (25–250 mcg/hour). At the end of therapy, the dosage was 167.7 mcg/hour (25–1000 mcg/hour). Most patients changed patches every 3 days, but 24% of patients required more frequent changing (varying from 48–60 hours). Pain relief was good throughout the study. Only 15% of patients did not require additional oral opioid (liquid morphine). Constipation decreased during the transdermal therapy. At the end of the study, 70% of therapy days were free of constipation. In addition, the need for laxatives decreased during therapy.

Payne et al.[104] compared pain-related treatment satisfaction, patient-perceived side effects, functioning, and well-being in 504 patients with advanced cancer who received either TTS-fentanyl or sustained-release oral forms of morphine. The mean dose of fentanyl was 84.4 mcg/hour (range, 25–400 mcg/hour). For those who received morphine, the mean 24-hour dose was 195 mg (range, 15–3000 mg). There were no significant differences between measures of pain intensity and sleep adequacy. However, patients who received TTS-fentanyl were more satisfied with their pain medication than those who received oral morphine. Patients receiving fentanyl also experienced a significantly lower frequency and impact of pain medication side effects. However, because assessment of side effects was global in nature, the investigators could not distinguish between the frequency and/or impact of individual, particular side effects. Gourlay[109] reported that open comparative studies against sustained-release formulations of morphine (morphine sulfate controlled-release, morphine sustained-release) suggest essentially equivalent effects for analgesia, measures of QOL, physical functioning, and adverse effects, except for a lower frequency of constipation and/or use of laxatives with transdermal fentanyl.

The most common formulation-unique side effects are as a consequence of the adhesive used to attach the systems to the skin and include erythema, itching, and occasional pustule formation (>1%) with an overall frequency of cutaneous side effects of approximately 10%.[109] The TTS-fentanyl system may be considered a first-line treatment modality for moderate to severe cancer pain. Appropriately used and titrated, pain control appears satisfactory with apparent high levels of patient satisfaction. In situations where compliance may be a problem, the system may have particular advantages. In addition, the system may be considered for patients who are unable to take medications by mouth.

Oral Transmucosal Fentanyl

The FDA has approved the use of transmucosal fentanyl for the management of procedure-associated pain and for the management of BTP in cancer patients. The main clinical application for this preparation is for breakthrough and incident pain in the cancer patient.[110]

Oral transmucosal fentanyl citrate (OTFC) units consist of a lozenge with a handle and are of uniform size and shape. Product manufacture involves dissolving fentanyl in a sucrose solution, pouring it into a mold, and allowing it to harden on a handle. Fentanyl is compounded in a hardened matrix form on a stick. The lozenge is available in a variety of strengths including 200, 400, 800, 1200, and 1600 mcg. In the mouth, the unit dissolves in saliva: a portion of the fentanyl diffuses across the oral mucosa, and the patient swallows the rest, which is partially absorbed in the stomach and intestine. Patients must smear the lozenge on either the buccal mucosa or under the tongue and not swallow. Smearing avoids first-pass metabolism in the liver while swallowing does not. Ideally, the lozenge should be consumed within a 15-minute period. Onset of action is very rapid (5–15 minutes). Peak analgesic effect is 20–30 minutes and duration is approximately 2 hours. Of the total available dose, 25% is absorbed transmucosally over a 15-minute period, and an additional 25% is absorbed through the gastric mucosa during the next 90 minutes.[111] Potential advantages of this drug delivery system include rapid onset analgesia, transmucosal absorption (i.e., no need to swallow), easily titrated, and ease of use. Of note, the dose of OTFC required to control BTP is not predicted by the ATC opioid dose.[112] Consequently, each patient should be titrated to a dose that is effective for control of BTP.

Farrar et al.[113] evaluated the effect of OTFC for BTP in a double-blind, randomized trial of 130 patients. All subjects started on the lowest dose of OTFC (200 mcg) and then titrated to an effective dose for BTP up to the maximum available dose (1600 mcg) over a 2-week period. All subjects who were able to achieve adequate relief with OTFC advanced to the double-blind phase, which was designed as a 10-period crossover. In this phase,

each subject received a box of 10 sequentially numbered units. Of the 10 units, seven contained fentanyl at the same dose found effective for that patient during the titration phase and three were placebo units. Instructions told patients to consume the total dose in 15 minutes and to take rescue medication after 30 minutes for inadequate pain relief. The pain types treated in the study included somatic (53%), visceral (31%), neuropathic (15%), and unknown (1%). Of the original 130 patients, 93 completed the open-label titration phase and 37 did not. Twenty patients did not complete the full 10 doses of the double-blinded phase. Eighty-six patients were included for efficacy comparisons; 6 were not because of protocol violations. In these patients, patients receiving placebo required significantly more additional rescue medication than those treated with active drug (34% vs. 15%). OTFC produced significantly larger changes in pain intensity and better pain relief than placebo at all time points (two sided $p < 0.0001$). The most frequent opioid-related adverse events reported as possibly related to OTFC were dizziness (17%), nausea (14%), somnolence (8%), constipation (5%), asthenia (5%), confusion (4%), vomiting (3%), and pruritus (3%).

OTFC was compared with morphine sulphate instant release (MSIR) for management of BTP in 134 cancer patients receiving a fixed scheduled opioid regimen in a double-blind, double-dummy, randomized, multiple crossover study.[114] OTFC was more effective than MSIR in treating BTP in terms of pain intensity, pain relief, and global performance of medication scores. In a Cochrane review, Zeppetella[115] concluded that OTFC was an effective treatment in the management of BTP.

Buccal Fentanyl

The fentanyl buccal tablet (FBT) incorporates a novel drug delivery platform, OraVescent technology (Cephalon Inc., Fraser, PA), which employs an effervescence-type reaction to enhance fentanyl absorption through the buccal mucosa and facilitate rapid systemic exposure to the analgesic. Transient pH changes accompany the effervescence reaction and increase both the rate of tablet dissolution (at a lower pH) and membrane permeation (at a higher pH) of fentanyl.[116] In a previous study of the bioavailability and pharmacokinetics of FBT compared with OTFC, a larger proportion of FBT was absorbed transmucosally (48%) compared with OTFC (22%) and T_{max} was earlier after administration of FBT (47 minutes) than OTFC (91 minutes).[117] Portenoy et al.,[118] in a randomized placebo-controlled study of FBT in patients with cancer pain, found that mean measures of the analgesic effect of buccal fentanyl separated from placebo as early as 15 minutes after administration and the extent of separation increased up to and including the 60-minute time point. A clinically significant reduction in pain intensity occurred by 15 minutes in 13% of episodes treated with fentanyl; by 30 minutes, this level of response was observed in 48% of episodes. Pain intensity decreased from a mean of 6.9 at baseline to 4.6 at 30 minutes. More recently, Slatkin et al.[119] found that most patients with cancer-related BTP experienced meaningful pain relief 10 minutes after applying FBT.

Currently, only FBT and OTFC are approved by the FDA for the management of BTP in opioid-tolerant cancer patients.

Buprenorphine

A multicenter, open-labeled, uncontrolled, prospective, observational clinical practice study involving 1223 patients with moderate to severe chronic pain demonstrated that transdermal buprenorphine was effective in alleviating cancer and noncancer pain and was overall well tolerated.[120] These patients also experienced significant improvement ($p < 0.001$) in QOL scores and reported very good to good pain relief ($p < 0.001$). The transdermal formulation of buprenorphine is not yet available in the United States.

Hydrocodone

Pure hydrocodone tablets or capsules are not available in the United States, nor is a modified release (long-acting) formulation, as of yet. It is important not to exceed toxic doses of acetaminophen or NSAID when prescribing the combination hydrocodone medications for intermittent or BTP, particularly when the patient is using other acetaminophen or NSAIDs containing drugs.

Codeine/Dihydrocodeine

The value of codeine is limited in cancer pain management by the increasing incidence of side effects at doses above 1.5 mg per kilogram of body weight.[23,121] Codeine is metabolized by CYP2D6 to morphine.[122] Patients with a deficiency of CYP2D6 enzymes or those taking inhibitors of CYP2D6, such as quinidine, cimetidine, or fluoxetine, may not be able to convert codeine into morphine and therefore may get little or no analgesic effect from codeine.[123–125]

Dihydrocodeine is an equianalgesic codeine analogue. Dihydrocodeine has active metabolites (dihydromorphine and dihydromorphine-6-glucuronide).[126] In the United States, it is available only in combination with acetaminophen or aspirin. Brands available include DHC Plus (16 and 32 mg), Panlor SS (32 mg), ZerLor (32 mg), Panlor DC (16 mg), and Synalgos DC (16 mg). Duration of effect is approximately 6 hours. When taken in higher than normal initial therapeutic doses, dihydrocodeine tends to produce euphoria.

Tramadol

Wilder-Smith et al.[127] compared the analgesic efficacy of tramadol (a dual mechanism drug with weak opioid agonist and monoamine reuptake inhibition activity) and morphine in 20 cancer patients. After 4 days, the mean daily doses were 101 +/− 58 mg of morphine and 375 +/− 135 mg of tramadol, indicating a relative potency of 4:1 with oral dosing. Side effects such as nausea and constipation were less with tramadol, but pain control was less satisfactory. Leppert and Luczak[128] reviewed the role of tramadol in cancer pain management. Overall, patients with cancer who are most likely to benefit from tramadol appear to be those with mild-to-moderate pain not relieved by acetaminophen who cannot tolerate NSAIDs and wish to avoid taking more potent opioids. In addition, tramadol also appears to have a role in reducing opioid requirements when combined with other opioids.[129]

Opioids Not Recommended for Routine Use in Cancer Pain Control

There are several opioids that should be avoided in cancer pain management, including meperidine, pentazocine, butorphanol, dezocine, and nalbuphine. Meperidine has a short half-life and its metabolite, normeperidine, is toxic.[130] Mixed agonist-antagonists such as pentazocine, butorphanol, dezocine, and nalbuphine present other problems. Although these agonist-antagonists are often classified as a kappa receptor agonist and a mu receptor antagonist, they are more accurately described as a partial agonist at both kappa and mu receptors. These agents have a low maximal efficacy and have the potential to reverse mu-receptor analgesia, and even precipitate a physical-withdrawal syndrome when taken by patients already receiving full agonists such as morphine.[131] In addition, agonist-antagonist opioids have a ceiling effect.[131,132] Propoxyphene is a poor choice for routine use because of its long half-life and the risk of accumulation of norpropoxyphene, a toxic metabolite.[133]

Long-Term Use of Opioids

Most patients with cancer are living well past 5 years after diagnosis, and many are returning to the workforce after treatment.[134] As patients live longer with cancer, concern is growing about both the health-related QOL of those diagnosed with cancer and the quality of care they receive. Cancer care progresses through stages including diagnosis, treatment, survivorship, and sometimes end-of-life care. Among the most common symptoms of cancer and treatments for cancer are pain, depression, and fatigue.[135] These symptoms may persist or appear after treatment ends.

The optimal use of opioids for long-term use in patients without active cancer should follow standard guidelines for chronic pain.[1] Posttreatment pain syndromes may evolve differently than other noncancer chronic pain syndromes, and new pain problems carry the emotional weight of possible recurrent disease. Therefore, patients in remission or putative cure who have chronic pain conditions need to be followed up with regular visits, immediate evaluation of new pain or progressive complaints, and a differential diagnosis of dose escalation that includes recurrent disease.

Opioid-Related Side Effects

Prevention or Minimizing Opioid-Related Side Effects

Appropriate dosing of opioids requires minimizing or preventing opioid-related side effects. For patients with constant pain, the early use of a long-acting opioid in preference to short-acting opioids as soon as dose titration permits may help attenuate side effects. If side effects are significant, the clinician should allow time for tolerance to develop. This may require a period of 3 to 7 days. Protecting the patient from severe side effects during this period is appropriate and will not prevent tolerance development. For example, a patient with nausea could benefit from a 1-week course of antiemetic medication at the outset of opioid therapy.

If side effects do not diminish satisfactorily over time, there are two alternatives: changing drugs and introducing supplementary medications that control the side effects. Changing from one opioid to another may enhance pain relief and reduce opioid-related side effects, particularly if incomplete cross tolerance to opioid effect is experienced.[136–140] In some cases, changing the route of administration for a particular drug, such as morphine, may eliminate certain difficult side effects.[141] It is possible to alleviate many of the most difficult side effects pharmacologically when necessary. For example, administering methylphenidate can help protect the cognitive functioning of patients using high doses of opioids.[142,143] Table 43.13 lists side effects and their treatments.

In cancer patients, certain pathophysiologic conditions commonly contribute to side effect problems or masquerade as side effect problems. For example, renal insufficiency in patients using morphine can lead to accumulation of M6G, which in turn can exacerbate side effects. Nausea is a frequent opioid toxicity, but it has other potential causes: gastric irritation, constipation or other changes in gut motility, chemotherapy, or hypercalcemia induced by bone metastases. Similarly, sedation and confusion may accompany opioid use, but other potential causes in the cancer patient, such as raised intracranial pressure, metabolic disturbances (e.g., hypercalcemia), sepsis, or concomitant drug use, merit consideration. Opioid-induced changes in mental status become less probable when the patient has been on a stable dose without recent significant dose escalation.

Opioid-induced bowel dysfunction is addressed above.

TABLE 43.13

PHARMACOLOGICAL TREATMENTS FOR OPIOID-RELATED SIDE EFFECTS

Side effect	Treatment
Constipation	Stool softener, laxative, ? opioid rotation
Sedation	Methylphenidate, modafinil
Pruritus	Diphenhydramine, hydroxyzine
Nausea	Prochlorperazine, haloperidol, metoclopramide, ondansetron, antihistamine
Dysphoria	Haloperidol, opioid rotation
Hypnagogic imagery	Haloperidol
Cognitive impairment	Methylphenidate, modafinil, opioid rotation
Respiratory depression	Naloxone
Myoclonus	Clonazepam, dose reduction, opioid rotation

Opioid Effects on Cognition, Motor Skills, and Driving Ability

A major concern that has arisen as long-term opioid therapy becomes accepted for some patients with chronic, moderate to severe pain is the effect of long-term opioid use on cognition and motor skills[144] such as driving.[145] Results have been inconsistent regarding decrements in cognitive performance. Patients with chronic pain who have been using opioids for more than 3 days exhibit relatively few differences when cognitive performance is compared with performance before taking opioids or with that of a comparable patient population not taking opioids.[146] The majority of research has revealed that the greatest potential impairment in cognitive function from opioids occurs during the first several days of use. During longer periods, impairment has been demonstrated primarily in studies that have compared patients with significant pain with healthy volunteers. The negative effects of opioids on cognition may be balanced by enhanced cognitive function with the relief of pain.[146] Questions still remain concerning the mechanisms responsible for opioid-induced cognitive impairment, interpatient variability with regard to opioid-related cognitive impairment, and the identification of predictors for cognitive impairment in patients receiving long-term opioid therapy.

The effects of opioid use specifically on driving ability has become a contentious issue, predictably because a growing number of patients are taking opioids and driving, and also because insurers may seek to assign liability in cases of motor vehicle accidents involving drivers who use opioids. Vainio et al.[147] examined the effects of continuous morphine medication on the driving ability of cancer patients. They conducted psychologic and neurologic tests, originally designed for professional motor vehicle drivers, in two groups of cancer patients who were similar apart from their experience of pain. Twenty-four patients received continuous morphine (mean 209-mg oral morphine daily) for cancer pain, and 25 were pain-free without regular analgesics. Though the results were a little worse in the patients taking morphine, there were no significant differences between the groups in intelligence, vigilance, concentration, fluency of motor reactions, or division of attention. Of the neural function tests, reaction times (auditory, visual, associative), thermal discrimination,

and body sway with eyes open were similar in the two groups; only balancing ability with closed eyes was worse in the morphine group. These results indicate that, in cancer patients receiving long-term morphine treatment with stable doses, morphine has only a slight and selective effect on functions related to driving.

Galski et al.[148] published a structured, evidence-based review on the issue of opioids and driving. Overall, the majority of studies in the evidence-based review appeared to indicate that patients who use opioids are not impaired by the opioids with regard to driving ability. Byas-Smith et al.[149] reported that many patients with chronic pain, even if treated with potent analgesics such as morphine and hydromorphone at equivalent average daily morphine doses of 118 mg, showed comparable driving ability to normal subjects.

Clearly, opioids may affect cognitive function and impair driving ability in patients who are opioid-naive or in patients who are not on stable opioid regimens. Whether some degree of cognitive tolerance develops with chronic opioid use is unknown. Other unresolved questions include the effects of different types of opioids, dose effects, and interactions with other medications on driving ability. Each of these areas deserves further study, and clinicians need to counsel patients about potentially dangerous activities on a case-by-case basis.

Some helpful guidelines are provided regarding opioid medications and driving (Table 43.14).

Opioids can cause or exacerbate confusion and these effects may range from mild impairment in concentration to frank delirium with disorientation, disorganized thinking, perceptual distortions, and hallucinations. Opioid-induced hallucinations are thought to be caused by sigma receptor activation, and they can occur in the context of intact cognitive function.[150] When this problem occurs, it is important to consider other causes of altered mental status in cancer patients (e.g., other treatments, metabolic alterations, infection, and brain metastasis). When a confusional state is due to opioids, it generally follows a recent increase in dose and will usually resolve with tolerance or as the dose is reduced. Rapid discontinuation of the opioid will result in severe pain, withdrawal symptoms, and possible exacerbation of confusion; it should be avoided. Dysphoria is probably more common than euphoria following opioid administration in patients with cancer.

Use of psychostimulants (e.g., methylphenidate, modafinil) has been reported to be helpful in overcoming daytime drowsiness and mental clouding, but their use must be monitored carefully, both for adverse effects and overuse.[151]

Opioid Rotation in Cancer Pain

Opioid rotation refers to the practice of converting from one opioid to a second when the opioid analgesic response is inadequate and/or if opioid-related adverse events are intolerable or unmanageable.[152,153] Reasons for initiating opioid rotation are listed in Table 43.15. In cancer patients, the most common reasons for opioid rotation are intolerable side effects such as cognitive failure, hallucinations, myoclonus, nausea, and uncontrollable pain.[137,154]

In all cases of opioid rotation, patients must be followed up closely to assess the adequacy of pain relief and the effect on opioid-related adverse events. As with any opioid regimen, subsequent dose adjustments will probably be necessary. Use of opioid rotation requires familiarity with a range of opioids and with the use of equianalgesic dose tables (see Chapter 78). However, it is also important to consider that the evidence to support dose ratios in standard equianalgesic tables refers largely to the context of single-dose administration; they do not necessarily reflect the clinical realities of chronic opioid administration in the treatment of cancer pain with repeated dosing of opioids. Thus, the doses shown in most standard equianalgesic dose tables may not be

TABLE 43.14

DRIVING INSTRUCTIONS FOR PATIENTS TAKING OPIOIDS

Opioid medications can cause side effects that impair your ability to drive. The final decision on whether you should drive while using opioid medications is a legal issue and should be addressed with your automobile insurance carrier. Out of concern for your safety and the safety of others, please observe the following guidelines:

- Do not drive for 4–5 days after beginning opioid treatment or after a change in opioid treatment such as a dose increase.
- Do not drive if you ever feel sedated or cognitively impaired.
- Report sedation/unsteadiness/cognitive decline to our office as soon as possible.
- Under no circumstances should you use alcohol or illicit drugs such as cannabis (marijuana) and drive.
- Avoid taking over-the-counter antihistamines, as contained in numerous cold and allergy medications.
- Do not make any changes in your medication regimen without consulting our office.

Patient Signature: _____   Date: _____

Practitioner Signature: _____   Date: _____

accurate in patients who have developed tolerance or have been taking opioids for long periods of time. In addition, the phenomenon of incomplete cross-tolerance can lead to unexpected potency in the newly introduced agent.[68]

Special care is required with methadone rotations. The process of switching from a high-dose opioid agonist to methadone is complex and should only be attempted by experienced physicians.[155] Even among experienced physicians, occasional serious toxicity can occur during the administration of methadone.[156]

TABLE 43.15

REASONS FOR UNDERTAKING OPIOID ROTATIONS

1. Reduced ability to control pain due to:
   a. Worsening of existing pain or underlying disease process
   b. Pharmacodynamic factors
   Development of opioid analgesic tolerance
   c. Pharmacokinetic factors
   Drug absorption (inability to swallow oral medications / poor vascular status or edema limiting transdermal delivery)
   Interaction with other drugs
   Changes in protein binding
   Biotransformation and metabolism (accumulation of metabolites)
   Reduced clearance—renal failure

2. Development of intolerable side effects /opioid toxicity
   a. GI (i.e., constipation, nausea, vomiting)
   b. Central nervous system (i.e., sedation, somnolence, dysphoria, hallucinations, myoclonus)
   c. Cardivascular (i.e., orthostatic hypotension due to histamine release)

3. Practical concerns
   a. Dose required to produce analgesia exceeds maximum daily dose (patients taking combination products, e.g., acetaminophen)
   b. Cost of drugs
   c. Drug availability
   d. Need for large volumes of drug to be delivered
   e. Changes in route of administration

Contrary to expectations, toxicity occurs more frequently in patients previously exposed to high doses of opioids than in patients receiving low doses. Bruera et al.[136] provide some guidelines for the conversion of patients from high-dose oral opioids to oral methadone. They recommend decreasing the previous opioid dose by one third over the first 24 hours and replacing it with methadone using an equianalgesic dose ratio. One mg of oral methadone is equal to 10 mg of oral morphine (i.e., a patient receiving 1000 mg of oral morphine per day will switch to 660 mg of oral morphine per day plus 33 mg of oral methadone during the first day). Administer methadone every 8 hours by the oral route. During the second day, if pain control is adequate, the patient requires a further one third decrease in the dose of the previous opioid. The dose of the methadone should only increase if the patient experiences moderate to severe pain. Manage transient episodes of pain with intermittent rescue doses of short-acting opioids. During day 3, discontinue the final one third of the previous opioid and maintain the patient on regular methadone every 8 hours, plus approximately 10% of the daily methadone dose as an extra dose orally for BTP. Assess pain and methadone requirements frequently until a stable methadone dose is reached. Until the equianalgesic dose ratio of parenteral and oral opioids to methadone is clearly established, patients receiving high doses of oral/parenteral opioids who require conversion to methadone should undergo this conversion only under close supervision and preferably in an inpatient environment. In general, the safe use of methadone to control cancer pain requires meticulous follow-up care and anticipatory downward dose titration.

Intravenous Opioid Therapy

Parenteral routes should be considered for patients who require rapid onset of analgesia, and for highly tolerant patients who require doses that cannot otherwise be conveniently administered.[157] Intravenous opioids allow for rapid control of pain. Ideally, patients with severe, uncontrolled pain who require intravenous therapy should start treatment in a monitored inpatient setting. High doses of intravenous opioids via patient-controlled analgesia (PCA) and/or by continuous infusion offers a means of rapidly controlling increasing severe pain. Intravenous therapy can employ any of several opioids: morphine, hydromorphone, fentanyl, sufentanil, and methadone.

Coda et al.[158] found differences in efficacy and side effects for morphine, hydromorphone, and sufentanil in bone marrow transplantation patients with severe oral mucositis pain. The pain relief achieved in all three opioid groups was nearly equivalent, while measures of side effects, especially for the combination of sedation, sleep, and mood disturbances, were statistically lower in the morphine group than in hydromorphone or sufentanil groups.

Subcutaneous Opioid Therapy

Continuous subcutaneous infusion of opioids is both an efficacious and safe method to control the chronic pain of the homebound and hospitalized patient.[159–162] Hypothetically, absorption of opioid from the subcutaneous compartment into the systemic circulation should be slow, but it is not, even for morphine.[163] Moulin et al.[164] reported equianalgesic responses in a comparison of intravenous versus subcutaneous infusions of hydromorphone. BTP control was equal in both groups and only occasionally did patients experience undue dermal irritation or recurrent infection. A wide variety of opioids are suitable for subcutaneous infusion: morphine, hydromorphone, methadone, fentanyl, and sufentanil.

Hydromorphone's solubility, its high bioavailability by continuous subcutaneous infusion (78%),[164] and the availability of a high-concentration preparation (10 mg/mL), make it a good choice for subcutaneous infusion. Parenteral hydromorphone is six times as soluble in aqueous solutions as morphine and five times as potent, allowing for smaller injection or infusion volumes in patients who require parenteral opioids.[165]

Continuous subcutaneous infusions offer a safe, simple, effective alternative to intravenous infusion when patients cannot take medications orally. Moulin et al.[164] compared the safety and efficacy of subcutaneous versus intravenous infusion of hydromorphone in cancer patients. Pain intensity, pain relief, mood, and sedation did not differ between the two techniques. The mean bioavailability of hydromorphone from subcutaneous infusion was 78% of that with intravenous infusion. Simplicity, technical advantages, and cost-effectiveness are clear advantages of continuous subcutaneous opioid infusion into the chest wall or trunk. Paix et al.[166] described the successful substitution of subcutaneous fentanyl and sufentanil for morphine, noting the benefits of sufentanil when the patient needs a very high dose of opioid that can be infused in a relatively small volume. Nelson et al.[167] compared continuous intravenous and subcutaneous morphine for chronic cancer pain and concluded that both routes were equianalgesic for most patients when administered as a continuous infusion.

Most patients will require a weekly change of the site of subcutaneous infusion.[161] The usual initial concentrations of morphine and hydromorphone are 5 mg/mL and 1 mg/mL respectively, calculated according to the hourly infusion rate. Ideally, the subcutaneous rate should not exceed 2 mL/hour although some have established considerably higher rates (rates of 20 to 80 mL/hour by adding hyaluronidase to the infusion to promote hypodermoclysis).[168] Due to a longer time to peak plasma levels after bolus injection with subcutaneous use than with intravenous use, the subcutaneous route requires a longer lockout interval (10–15 minute compared to 6–8 minute for the intravenous). PCA doses may equal 25% to 50% of the hourly infusion rate every 10 to 15 minutes as needed. Subcutaneous administration of opioids may prove impractical in patients with generalized edema, who develop erythema, soreness, or sterile abscesses with subcutaneous administration, in patients with coagulation disorders, and in patients with very poor peripheral circulation.

Intracerebroventricular Opioids

Intracerebroventricular (ICV) opioid delivery may be beneficial for highly selected cancer patients who are not obtaining adequate relief or experiencing intolerable side effects via other routes. With neurosurgical consultation, it is possible to deliver opioids directly into cerebral ventricles through ICV catheters from subcutaneous reservoirs. Morphine sulfate, the usual drug, gains a marked increase in potency when delivered ICV as compared to intrathecal or epidural infusion routes, and the ICV route appears to affect supraspinal pathways for analgesia.[169] Daily morphine doses for ICV delivery range from 50–700 mcg/day.[170,171] Generally, an implanted infusion pump, placed subcutaneously in the anterior abdominal wall and connected by subcutaneous tubing to an implanted ventricular catheter, delivers the drug. The duration of pain relief after ICV injections appears to be significantly longer than with intraspinal delivery, and some patients gain adequate relief via an implanted ventricular catheter connected to a subcutaneous Ommaya reservoir-type device with 1 to 2 injections per day.[172] This form of drug delivery is indicated for head and neck cancer pain, or, rarely, for patients with a good initial response to intraspinal infusions of opioids and subsequent development of apparent tolerance, but with limited (1–3 months) remaining survival time. The safety and side effects of ICV injections or infusions resemble those for intraspinal infusions, except that an increased risk of respiratory depression exists the first 3 days of therapy.[172]

Some refractory head and neck pain responds only to ICV opioids, but pain below the waist may be most amenable to spinal treatment. In a meta-analysis of 1587 cancer patients, Ballantyne et al.[173] compared ICV with the more common epidural and intrathecal opioid treatments in an attempt to establish the utility and safety of ICV therapy. All patients considered had intractable cancer pain that proved resistant to systemic treatment. Sedation and confusion occurred in 4% to 5% of patients receiving ICV therapy. Persistent nausea, urinary retention, and pruritus occurred more frequently with the two spinal treatments than with ICV therapy. Initial doses for ICV trial patients were in the range of 0.25 to 2.0 mg. Onset of effect was 2 to 30 minutes, and average duration of pain relief after a single dose was 12 to 48 hours. Tolerance proved less of a problem than with epidural or intrathecal therapy since the dose escalation was very gradual (the average increase in daily dosage was 0.375 mg/month). In a follow-up study, Ballantyne et al.[174] reported on 72 uncontrolled trials assessing ICV (13 trials, 337 patients), epidural catheters (31 trials, 1343 patients), and subarachnoid catheters (28 trials, 722 patients) in cancer patients. Data from these uncontrolled studies reported excellent pain relief among 73% of ICV patients compared with 72% epidural and 62% subarachnoid catheters. Unsatisfactory pain relief was low in all treatment groups. Persistent nausea, persistent and transient urinary retention, transient pruritus, and constipation occurred more frequently with epidural and subarachnoid catheters. Respiratory depression, sedation, and confusion were most common with ICV. The incidence of major infection when pumps were used with epidural and subarachnoid catheters was zero. There was a lower incidence of other complications with ICV therapy than with epidural or subarachnoid catheters.

HOME INFUSION THERAPY

Advances in pain management technology, such as ambulatory PCAs and the use of silicone subcutaneously tunneled neuraxial catheters, have expanded the scope and success of interventional pain management beyond the hospital to the home. Potential benefits of home infusion therapy include decreased health care costs, patient/caregiver convenience, and less time spent in hospital with the ability to extend interventional pain management strategies into the patient's home. A possible disadvantage to home infusion therapy may include the additional burden placed on the patient/caregiver in terms of role responsibilities and schedules. Home care agencies must have explicitly defined policies and procedures consistent with regulatory bodies and national and regional standards of practice.

A provider of infusion therapy must be a licensed pharmacy or work in conjunction with a licensed pharmacy. Skilled and qualified home nursing services are an essential component of home-based care; they are responsible for educating patients and their caregivers regarding administering the drug therapy, complying with the prescribed dosing schedule, understanding the drug delivery device being used (an infusion pump or other device), and other important information regarding the treatment regimen. Additional roles include monitoring for adverse effects, infection, displacement of catheters, and equipment malfunction.

Drug therapies commonly administered via infusion at home include antibiotics, chemotherapy, analgesics, parenteral nutrition, and immune globulin. Diagnoses commonly requiring infusion therapy include infections that are unresponsive to oral antibiotics, cancer and cancer-related pain, GI diseases or disorders which prevent normal functioning of the GI system, congestive heart failure, immune disorders, growth hormone deficiencies, and more.

Ambulatory infusion pumps are either designed to be therapy-specific, or are multi-purpose, enabling treatments such as chemotherapy, systemic antibiotics, total parenteral nutrition, hydration therapy, and opioid pain control. Recent developments in pump design include remote access capability by modem with the ability to change pump settings and download data.

Home-based PCA therapy provides select patients with the ability to deliver analgesia based on their own perception of need. PCA therapy may be superior to oral analgesia, especially in the treatment of severe oscillating pain. Patient selection criteria include intact cognition and proper supervision from a family member or health professional. A collaborative interdisciplinary approach is necessary for effective pain control for the cancer patient receiving interventional pain management at home. Collaboration between the patient, the patient's family, the home care nurse and home care agency, and the patient's physician is necessary. The physician remains responsible for determining the appropriate drug, bolus dose, background infusion rate, and lockout interval.

PCA is more commonly used in the home setting as an effective option in pain management. As discussed above, the subcutaneous and intravenous routes are the primary methods of administration. The availability of a central vascular access device such as a tunneled or peripherally inserted central catheter offers advantages over peripheral access to ensure safe and consistent administration of intravenous analgesia.

The safety and efficacy of home-based PCA opioid therapy has not been extensively reported as in-hospital use. One study,[175] however, reported on the use of morphine PCA in the home environment of 143 preterminally and terminally ill tumor patients suffering either from excruciating chronic pain or severe chronic/acute complex pain that could not be relieved adequately by oral analgesia. After initial dose adjustment, which lasted 2 to 3 days, the median morphine dose was 93 mg/day (range 12–464 mg/day). This median was 28% lower than the median dose administered orally prior to PCA therapy. During the course of treatment, morphine requirements increased by a median of 2.3 mg/day (range -29 + 52 mg/day). Most patients were treated continuously in the home care setting until death; the median duration of treatment was 27 days (range 1–437 days). Terminal morphine demands reached a median of 188 mg/day (range 15–1008 mg/day). The authors concluded that PCA was both safe and effective in the home environment, attaining excellent results in 95 (66%) patients and satisfactory pain relief in 43 (30%). PCA was considered insufficient in five (4%) cases. Side effects, in general, were considered mild: the most common being constipation, fatigue, and nausea.

Although further study is warranted, safe provision of domiciliary interventional pain management requires selection of patients who are able to manage themselves or who have responsible caregivers, effective patient and caregiver education, well-defined policies, and use of experienced and knowledgeable home care agencies and pharmacies.

COMPLEMENTARY AND ALTERNATIVE MEDICINE

Complementary and alternative medicine (CAM) therapies are used widely among cancer patients.[176] These therapies have been used as an alternative to conventional medicine (alternative medicine) and complementary to conventional medicine (complementary medicine). Most cancer patients use CAM with the hope of boosting the immune system, relieving pain, and controlling side effects related to disease or treatment. Only a minority of patients include CAM in the treatment plan with curative intent. Frequently, patients do not discuss CAM therapies with physicians.[177] Mansky and Wallerstedt[178] reported that the CAM domains of mind–body medicine, CAM botanicals, manipulative practices, and energy medicine were widely used as complementary approaches to palliative cancer care and cancer symptom management. In the area of cancer symptom management, auricular acupuncture, therapeutic touch, and hypnosis may help to manage cancer pain. Music therapy, massage, and hypnosis may have an effect on anxiety, and both acupuncture and massage may have a therapeutic role in cancer fatigue. Acupuncture and selected botanicals may reduce chemotherapy-induced nausea and emesis, and hypnosis and guided imagery may be beneficial in anticipatory nausea and vomiting. Transcendental meditation and mindfulness-based stress reduction can play a role in the management of depressed mood and anxiety. Black cohosh and phytoestrogen-rich foods may reduce vasomotor symptoms in postmenopausal women. Although there have been many trials of CAM therapies for cancer pain and a few expert reviews, there is a lack of rigorous systematic review.[179] Furthermore, studies have found that there is considerable variation in the search for CAM studies, making systematic reviews prone to bias.[180] Bardia et al.,[179] in a systematic review of CAM therapies for cancer-related pain, demonstrated a paucity of well-designed, multi-institutional trials. Most trials were of short duration, had small numbers without sample size justification, and did not report the adverse effects of CAM intervention. However, some data existed suggesting that mind–body medicine (hypnosis, imagery, and relaxation) may have some efficacy in decreasing cancer pain. Pan et al.[181] had similar conclusions regarding the role of CAM therapies in the management of pain, dyspnea, and nausea and vomiting in patients near the end of life. The heterogeneity of pain syndromes has made broad sweeping conclusions about the efficacy of acupuncture difficult. A National Institutes of Health consensus conference[182] on the use of acupuncture for pain concluded that while there have been many studies of its potential usefulness, many of these studies provide equivocal results because of design, sample size, and other factors. However, promising results have emerged, for example, showing efficacy of acupuncture in adult postoperative and chemotherapy nausea and vomiting and in postoperative dental pain. There are other situations such as addiction, stroke rehabilitation, headache, menstrual cramps, tennis elbow, fibromyalgia, myofascial pain, osteoarthritis, low back pain, carpal tunnel syndrome, and asthma, in which acupuncture may be useful as an adjunct treatment or an acceptable alternative or be included in a comprehensive management program.

CONCLUSION

Pain control is a high-priority goal of cancer care. As a very common and debilitating component of disease, aggressive treatment of pain to maximize both quality and quantity of the patient's life is an imperative.

Detailed assessment of pain and other QOL concerns is the foundation for successful pain management in the cancer patient. Typically, the pain experience is multidimensional and treatment must address physical, psychological, social, and existential components. Failure to sufficiently understand the etiology of the pain complaint will invariably result in poor pain management. Interdisciplinary collaboration is essential for comprehensive care of the cancer patient. Disciplines and specialties involved in care commonly include pain management specialists, oncologists, surgeons, psychiatrists, psychologists, physical therapists, pharmacists, nurses, and social workers. Aggressive therapy of both cancer and pain are mutually beneficial and are best done by skilled, interdisciplinary teams.

Most patients can attain adequate symptomatic relief of cancer pain using appropriate oral pharmacotherapy. The concurrent use of adjunctive or specialized therapies is sometimes necessary, however, and referral for specialized surgical, anesthetic, or psychologic intervention benefits a significant number of patients. In addition, the growth of the home care industry and hospice has broadened the possibilities of extending basic and sophisticated pain management strategies into the home.

As more patients are cured or go into long-term remission, appropriate provisions for ongoing assessment and management of chronic pain are essential.

References

1. Joranson DE, Gilson AM, Dahl JL, et al. Pain management, controlled substances, and state medical board policy: a decade of change. *J Pain Symptom Manage* 2002;23(2):138–147.
2. World Health Organization. *Cancer Pain Relief and Palliative Care*. Geneva, Switzerland: World Health Organization; 1990.
3. Devine EC, Westlake SK. The effects of psychoeducational care provided to adults with cancer: meta-analysis of 116 studies. *Oncol Nurs Forum* 1995; 22(9):1369–1381.
4. World Health Organization. *Cancer Pain Relief With a Guide to Opioid Availability*. 2nd ed. Geneva, Switzerland: World Health Organization; 1996.
5. Quality improvement guidelines for the treatment of acute pain and cancer pain. American Pain Society Quality of Care Committee. *JAMA* 1995; 274(23):1874–1880.
6. Jacox A, Carr DB, Payne R, et al. *Management of cancer pain. Clinical practice guideline No. 9*. Rockville, MD: Agency for Health Care Policy and Research, U.S. Department of Health and Human Services, Public Health Service; March 1994. AHCPR Publication No. 94-0592.
7. Practice guidelines for cancer pain management. A report by the American Society of Anesthesiologists Task Force on Pain Management, Cancer Pain Section. *Anesthesiology* 1996;84(5):1243–1257.
8. Weissman DE, Griffie J. The Palliative Care Consultation Service of the Medical College of Wisconsin. *J Pain Symptom Manage* 1994;9(7):474–479.
9. Weissman DE, Dahl JL. Update on the cancer pain role model education program. *J Pain Symptom Manage* 1995;10(4):292–297.
10. Weissman DE, Griffie J, Gordon DB, et al. A role model program to promote institutional changes for management of acute and cancer pain. *J Pain Symptom Manage* 1997;14(5):274–279.
11. Moote CA. Postoperative pain management—back to basics [in English, in French]. *Can J Anaesth* 1995;42(6):453–457.
12. Janjan NA, Martin CG, Payne R, et al. Teaching cancer pain management: durability of educational effects of a role model program. *Cancer* 1996;77(5): 996–1001.
13. Dahl JL. State cancer pain initiatives. *J Pain Symptom Manage* 1993;8(6): 372–375.
14. Bookbinder M, Coyle N, Kiss M, et al. Implementing national standards for cancer pain management: program model and evaluation. *J Pain Symptom Manage* 1996;12(6):334–347, discussion 331–333.
15. Donabedian A. Quality and cost: choices and responsibilities. *J Occup Med* 1990;32(12):1167–1172.
16. Kritchevsky SB, Simmons BP. Continuous quality improvement. Concepts and applications for physician care. *JAMA* 1991;266(13):1817–1823.
17. Max MB. Improving outcomes of analgesic treatment: is education enough? *Ann Intern Med* 1990;113(11):885–889.
18. Portenoy RK, Thaler HT, Kornblith AB, et al. Symptom prevalence, characteristics and distress in a cancer population. *Qual Life Res* 1994;3(3):183–189.
19. Elliott TE, Murray DM, Oken MM, et al. Improving cancer pain management in communities: main results from a randomized controlled trial. *J Pain Symptom Manage* 1997;13(4):191–203.
20. de Wit R, van Dam F, Zandbelt L, et al. A pain education program for chronic cancer pain patients: follow-up results from a randomized controlled trial. *Pain* 1997;73(1):55–69.
21. Levy MH. Supportive oncology: forward. *Semin Oncol* 1994;21(6):699–700.
22. Levy MH. Integration of pain management into comprehensive cancer care. *Cancer* 1989;63(11 suppl):2328–2335.
23. Jacox A, Carr DB, Payne R. New clinical-practice guidelines for the management of pain in patients with cancer. *N Engl J Med* 1994;330(9):651–655.
24. Ventafridda V, De Conno F, Panerai AE, et al. Non-steroidal anti-inflammatory drugs as the first step in cancer pain therapy: double-blind, within-patient study comparing nine drugs. *J Intern Med Res* 1990;18(1):21–29.
25. Zech DF, Grond S, Lynch J, et al. Validation of World Health Organization Guidelines for cancer pain relief: a 10-year prospective study. *Pain* 1995; 63(1):65–76.
26. Spinelli P, Dal Fante M, Mancini A. Self-expanding mesh stent for endoscopic palliation of rectal obstructing tumors: a preliminary report. *Surg Endosc* 1992;6(2):72–74.
27. Lightdale CJ. Self-expanding metal stents for esophageal and gastric cancer: a new opening. *Gastrointest Endosc* 1992;38(1):86–88.
28. Garcia C, Collins T, Ide S, et al. Nd:YAG laser as a therapeutic option in the management of gastrointestinal cancer. *Del Med J* 1993;65(6):369–373.
29. Anderson ID, Manson JM, Martin DF, et al. Relief of metastatic biliary obstruction by stent placement: is it worthwhile? *Surg Oncol* 1993;2(2): 113–117.
30. World Health Organization. *Cancer Pain Relief*. Geneva, Switzerland: World Health Organization; 1986.
31. Hanks GW, Justins DM. Cancer pain: management. *Lancet* 1992;339(8800): 1031–1036.
32. Schug SA, Zech D, Dörr U. Cancer pain management according to WHO analgesic guidelines. *J Pain Symptom Manage* 1990;5(1):27–32.
33. Grond S, Zech D, Schug SA, et al. Validation of World Health Organization guidelines for cancer pain relief during the last days and hours of life. *J Pain Symptom Manage* 1991;6(7):411–422.
34. Jadad AR, Browman GP. The WHO analgesic ladder for cancer pain management. Stepping up the quality of its evaluation. *JAMA* 1995;274(23): 1870–1873.
35. Dubois RN, Abramson SB, Crofford L, et al. Cyclooxygenase in biology and disease. *FASEB J* 1998;12(12):1063–1073.
36. Rüegg C, Dormond O. Suppression of tumor angiogenesis by nonsteroidal anti-inflammatory drugs: a new function for old drugs. *ScientificWorldJournal* 2001;1:808–811.
37. Sarkar FH, Adsule S, Li Y, et al. Back to the future: COX-2 inhibitors for chemoprevention and cancer therapy. *Mini Rev Med Chem* 2007;7(6): 599–608.
38. de Moraes E, Dar NA, de Moura Gallo CV, et al. Cross-talks between cyclooxygenase-2 and tumor suppressor protein p53: balancing life and death during inflammatory stress and carcinogenesis. *Int J Cancer* 2007;121(5): 929–937.
39. Rüegg C, Zaric J, Stupp R. Non steroidal anti-inflammatory drugs and COX-2 inhibitors as anti-cancer therapeutics: hypes, hopes and reality. *Ann Med* 2003;35(7):476–487.
40. Harris RE, Beebe-Donk J, Alshafie GA. Cancer chemoprevention by cyclooxygenase 2 (COX-2) blockade: results of case control studies. *Subcell Biochem* 2007;42:193–212.
41. Eisenberg E, Berkey CS, Carr DB, et al. Efficacy and safety of nonsteroidal antiinflammatory drugs for cancer pain: a meta-analysis. *J Clin Oncol* 1994; 12(12):2756–2765.
42. McNicol E, Strassels SA, Goudas L et al. NSAIDs or paracetamol, alone or combined with opioids, for cancer pain. *Cochrane Database Syst Rev* 2005; 1:CD005180.
43. Sykes NP. The relationship between opioid use and laxative use in terminally ill cancer patients. *Palliat Med* 1998;12(5):375–382.
44. Sternini C, Patierno S, Selmer IS, et al. The opioid system in the gastrointestinal tract. *Neurogastroenterol Motil* 2004;16(suppl 2):3–16.
45. Wood JD, Galligan JJ. Function of opioids in the enteric nervous system. *Neurogastroenterol Motil* 2004;16(suppl 2):17–28.
46. De Luca A, Coupar IM. Insights into opioid action in the intestinal tract. *Pharmacol Ther* 1996;69(2):103–115.
47. Liu M, Wittbrodt E. Low-dose oral naloxone reverses opioid-induced constipation and analgesia. *J Pain Symptom Manage* 2002;23(1):48–53.
48. Watanabe S, Bruera E. Corticosteroids as adjuvant analgesics. *J Pain Symptom Manage* 1994;9(7):442–445.
49. Loblaw DA, Laperriere NJ. Emergency treatment of malignant extradural spinal cord compression: an evidence-based guideline. *J Clin Oncol* 1998; 16(4):1613–1624.
50. Xiao W, Boroujerdi A, Bennett GJ, et al. Chemotherapy-evoked painful peripheral neuropathy: analgesic effects of gabapentin and effects on expression of the alpha-2-delta type-1 calcium channel subunit. *Neuroscience* 2007; 144(2):714–720.
51. Dunteman ED. Levetiracetam as an adjunctive analgesic in neoplastic plexopathies: case series and commentary. *J Pain Palliat Care Pharmacother* 2005; 19(1):35–43.
52. Cardozo LD, Stanton SL. A comparison between bromocriptine and indomethacin in the treatment of detrusor instability. *J Urol* 1980;123(3): 399–401.

53. Castell DO. Calcium-channel blocking agents for gastrointestinal disorders. *Am J Cardiol* 1985;55(3):210B–213B.

54. Aguado T, Carracedo A, Julien B, et al. Cannabinoids induce glioma stem-like cell differentiation and inhibit gliomagenesis. *J Biol Chem* 2007;282(9): 6854–6862.

55. Michalski CW, Oti FE, Erkan M, et al. Cannabinoids in pancreatic cancer: Correlation with survival and pain. *Int J Cancer* 2008;122(4):742–750.

56. Osei-Hyiaman D. Endocannabinoid system in cancer cachexia. *Curr Opin Clin Nutr Metab Care* 2007;10(4):443–448.

57. Jhaveri MD, Richardson D, Chapman V. Endocannabinoid metabolism and uptake: novel targets for neuropathic and inflammatory pain. *Br J Pharmacol* 2007;152(5):624–632.

58. Abrams DI, Jay CA, Shade SB et al. Cannabis in painful HIV-associated sensory neuropathy: a randomized placebo-controlled trial. *Neurology* 2007; 68(7):515–521.

59. Cherny NI. Opioid analgesics: comparative features and prescribing guidelines. *Drugs* 1996;51(5):713–737.

60. McCarberg BH, Barkin RL. Long-acting opioids for chronic pain: pharmacotherapeutic opportunities to enhance compliance, quality of life, and analgesia. *Am J Ther* 2001;8(3):181–186.

61. Coluzzi PH. Oral patient-controlled analgesia. *Semin Oncol* 1997;24(5 suppl 16):S16–S35–S42.

62. Pappagallo M, Dickerson ED, Hulka S. Palliative care and hospice opioid dosing guidelines with breakthrough pain (BP) doses. *Am J Hosp Palliat Care* 2000;17(6):407–413.

63. Cherny N, Ripamonti C, Pereira J, et al. Strategies to manage the adverse effects of oral morphine: an evidence-based report. *J Clin Oncol* 2001;19(9): 2542–2554.

64. Portenoy RK, Payne D, Jacobsen P. Breakthrough pain: characteristics and impact in patients with cancer pain. *Pain* 1999;81(1–2):129–134.

65. Cherny NJ, Chang V, Frager G, et al. Opioid pharmacotherapy in the management of cancer pain: a survey of strategies used by pain physicians for the selection of analgesic drugs and routes of administration. *Cancer* 1995;76(7): 1283–1293.

66. Levy MH. Pharmacologic treatment of cancer pain. *N Engl J Med* 1996; 335(10):1124–1132.

67. Hanks GW, Conno F, Cherny N, et al. Morphine and alternative opioids in cancer pain: the EAPC recommendations. *Br J Cancer* 2001;84(5):587–593.

68. Galer BS, Coyle N, Pasternak GW. Individual variability in the response to different opioids: report of five cases. *Pain* 1992;49(1):87–91.

69. Fitzgibbon DR, Galer BS. The efficacy of opioids in cancer pain syndromes. *Pain* 1994;58(3):429–431.

70. Ossipov MH, Lai J, King T, et al. Antinociceptive and nociceptive actions of opioids. *J Neurobiol* 2004;61(1):126–148.

71. Ossipov MH, Lai J, Vanderah TW, et al. Induction of pain facilitation by sustained opioid exposure: relationship to opioid antinociceptive tolerance. *Life Sci* 2003;73(6):783–800.

72. Arnér S, Rawal N, Gustafsson LL. Clinical experience of long-term treatment with epidural and intrathecal opioids—a nationwide survey. *Acta Anaesthesiol Scand* 1988;32(3):253–259.

73. Collett BJ. Opioid tolerance: the clinical perspective. *Br J Anaesth* 1998;81(1): 58–68.

74. Foley KM. Controversies in cancer pain. Medical perspectives. *Cancer* 1989; 63(11 suppl):2257–2265.

75. Collin E, Poulain P, Gauvain-Piquard A, et al. Is disease progression the major factor in morphine 'tolerance' in cancer pain treatment? *Pain* 1993;55(3): 319–326.

76. Gardell LR, King T, Ossipov MH, et al. Opioid receptor-mediated hyperalgesia and antinociceptive tolerance induced by sustained opiate delivery. *Neurosci Lett* 2006;396(1):44–49.

77. Angst MS, Clark JD. Opioid-induced hyperalgesia: a qualitative systematic review. *Anesthesiology* 2006;104(3):570–587.

78. Wiffen P, McQuay H. Oral morphine for cancer pain. *Cochrane Database Syst Rev* 2007;4:CD003868.

79. Kalso E, Vainio A. Morphine and oxycodone hydrochloride in the management of cancer pain. *Clin Pharmacol Ther* 1990;47(5):639–646.

80. Maddocks I, Somogyi A, Abbott F, et al. Attenuation of morphine-induced delirium in palliative care by substitution with infusion of oxycodone. *J Pain Symptom Manage* 1996;12(3):182–189.

81. Heiskanen T, Kalso E. Controlled-release oxycodone and morphine in cancer related pain. *Pain* 1997;73(1):37–45.

82. Reid CM, Martin RM, Sterne JA, et al. Oxycodone for cancer-related pain: meta-analysis of randomized controlled trials. *Arch Intern Med* 2006;166(8): 837–843.

83. Sloan P, Slatkin N, Ahdieh H. Effectiveness and safety of oral extended-release oxymorphone for the treatment of cancer pain: a pilot study. *Support Care Cancer* 2005;13(1):57–65.

84. Leng G, Finnegan MJ. Successful use of methadone in nociceptive cancer pain unresponsive to morphine. *Palliat Med* 1994;8(2):153–155.

85. Crews JC, Sweeney NJ, Denson DD. Clinical efficacy of methadone in patients refractory to other mu-opioid receptor agonist analgesics for management of terminal cancer pain. Case presentations and discussion of incomplete cross-tolerance among opioid agonist analgesics. *Cancer* 1993;72(7):2266–2272.

86. Manfredi PL, Borsook D, Chandler SW, et al. Intravenous methadone for cancer pain unrelieved by morphine and hydromorphone: clinical observations. *Pain* 1997;70(1):99–101.

87. Fitzgibbon DR, Ready LB. Intravenous high-dose methadone administered by patient controlled analgesia and continuous infusion for the treatment of cancer pain refractory to high-dose morphine. *Pain* 1997;73(2):259–261.

88. Izzo AA. Drug interactions with St. John's Wort (Hypericum perforatum): a review of the clinical evidence. *Int J Clin Pharmacol Ther* 2004;42(3): 139–148.

89. Corkery JM, Schifano F, Ghodse AH, et al. The effects of methadone and its role in fatalities. *Hum Psychopharmacol* 2004;19(8):565–576.

90. Boulton DW, Arnaud P, DeVane CL. A single dose of methadone inhibits cytochrome P-4503A activity in healthy volunteers as assessed by the urinary cortisol ratio. *Br J Clin Pharmacol* 2001;51(4):350–354.

91. Bruera E, Palmer JL, Bosnjak S, et al. Methadone versus morphine as a first-line strong opioid for cancer pain: a randomized, double-blind study. *J Clin Oncol* 2004;22(1):185–192.

92. Nicholson AB. Methadone for cancer pain. *Cochrane Database Syst Rev* 2007;4:CD003971.

93. Plezia PM, Kramer TH, Linford J, et al. Transdermal fentanyl: pharmacokinetics and preliminary clinical evaluation. *Pharmacotherapy* 1989;9(1):2–9.

94. Portenoy RK, Southam MA, Gupta SK, et al. Transdermal fentanyl for cancer pain. Repeated dose pharmacokinetics. *Anesthesiology* 1993;78(1):36–43.

95. Varvel JR, Shafer SL, Hwang SS, et al. Absorption characteristics of transdermally administered fentanyl. *Anesthesiology* 1989;70(6):928–934.

96. Frölich MA, Giannotti A, Modell JH. Opioid overdose in a patient using a fentanyl patch during treatment with a warming blanket. *Anesth Analg* 2001; 93(3):647–648.

97. Solassol I, Caumette L, Bressolle F, et al. Inter- and intra-individual variability in transdermal fentanyl absorption in cancer pain patients. *Oncol Rep* 2005; 14(4):1029–1036.

98. Donner B, Zenz M, Tryba M, et al. Direct conversion from oral morphine to transdermal fentanyl: a multicenter study in patients with cancer pain. *Pain* 1996;64(3):527–534.

99. Donner B, Zenz M, Strumpf M, et al. Long-term treatment of cancer pain with transdermal fentanyl. *J Pain Symptom Manage* 1998;15(3):168–175.

100. Grond S, Zech D, Lehmann KA, et al. Transdermal fentanyl in the long-term treatment of cancer pain: a prospective study of 50 patients with advanced cancer of the gastrointestinal tract or the head and neck region. *Pain* 1997; 69(1–2):191–198.

101. Korte W, de Stoutz N, Morant R. Day-to-day titration to initiate transdermal fentanyl in patients with cancer pain: short- and long-term experiences in a prospective study of 39 patients. *J Pain Symptom Manage* 1996;11(3): 139–146.

102. Payne R. Transdermal fentanyl: suggested recommendations for clinical use. *J Pain Symptom Manage* 1992;7(3 suppl):S40–S44.

103. Payne R, Chandler S, Einhaus M. Guidelines for the clinical use of transdermal fentanyl. *Anticancer Drugs* 1995;(6 suppl 3):50–53.

104. Payne R, Mathias SD, Pasta DJ, et al. Quality of life and cancer pain: satisfaction and side effects with transdermal fentanyl versus oral morphine. *J Clin Oncol* 1998;16(4):1588–1593.

105. Zech DF, Grond SU, Lynch J, et al. Transdermal fentanyl and initial dose-finding with patient-controlled analgesia in cancer pain. A pilot study with 20 terminally ill cancer patients. *Pain* 1992;50(3):293–301.

106. Zech DF, Lehmann KA. Transdermal fentanyl in combination with initial intravenous dose titration by patient-controlled analgesia. *Anticancer Drugs* 1995;(6 suppl 3):44–49.

107. Gourlay GK, Mather LE. Pharmacokinetics and pharmacodynamics. In: Lehmann KA, Zech D, eds. *Transdermal Fentanyl*. Berlin: Springer-Verlag; 1991: 119–140.

108. Sandler AN, Baxter AD, Katz J, et al. A double-blind, placebo-controlled trial of transdermal fentanyl after abdominal hysterectomy. Analgesic, respiratory, and pharmacokinetic effects. *Anesthesiology* 1994;81(5):1169–1180.

109. Gourlay GK. Treatment of cancer pain with transdermal fentanyl. *Lancet Oncol* 2001;2(3):165–172.

110. Fine PG, Marcus M, De Boer AJ, et al. An open label study of oral transmucosal fentanyl citrate (OTFC) for the treatment of breakthrough cancer pain. *Pain* 1991;45(2):149–153.

111. Streisand JB, Varvel JR, Stanski DR, et al. Absorption and bioavailability of oral transmucosal fentanyl citrate. *Anesthesiology* 1991;75(2):223–229.

112. Christie JM, Simmonds M, Patt R, et al. Dose-titration, multicenter study of oral transmucosal fentanyl citrate for the treatment of breakthrough pain in cancer patients using transdermal fentanyl for persistent pain. *J Clin Oncol* 1998;16(10):3238–3245.

113. Farrar JT, Cleary J, Rauck R, et al. Oral transmucosal fentanyl citrate: randomized, double-blinded, placebo-controlled trial for treatment of breakthrough pain in cancer patients. *J Natl Cancer Inst* 1998;90(8):611–616.

114. Coluzzi PH, Schwartzberg L, Conroy JD, et al. Breakthrough cancer pain: a randomized trial comparing oral transmucosal fentanyl citrate (OTFC) and morphine sulfate immediate release (MSIR). *Pain* 2001;91(1–2):123–130.

115. Zeppetella G, Ribeiro MD. Opioids for the management of breakthrough (episodic) pain in cancer patients. *Cochrane Database Syst Rev* 2006;1: CD004311.

116. Eichman JD, Robinson JR. Mechanistic studies on effervescent-induced permeability enhancement. *Pharm Res* 1998;15(6):925–930.

117. (Darvish M J Pain 2006 (suppl).

118. Portenoy RK, Taylor D, Messina J, et al. A randomized, placebo-controlled study of fentanyl buccal tablet for breakthrough pain in opioid-treated patients with cancer. *Clin J Pain* 2006;22(9):805–811.

119. Slatkin NE, Xie F, Messina J, et al. Fentanyl buccal tablet for relief of break-through pain in opioid-tolerant patients with cancer-related chronic pain. *Supportive Oncology* 2007; 5(7):327–334.

120. Muriel C, Failde I, Micó JA, et al. Effectiveness and tolerability of the bupren-orphine transdermal system in patients with moderate to severe chronic pain: a multicenter, open-label, uncontrolled, prospective, observational clinical study. *Clin Ther* 2005;27(4):451–462.

121. Levy MH. Pharmacologic management of cancer pain. *Semin Oncol* 1994; 21(6):718–739.

122. Susce MT, Murray-Carmichael E, de Leon J. Response to hydrocodone, co-deine and oxycodone in a CYP2D6 poor metabolizer. *Prog Neuropsychophar-macol Biol Psychiatry* 2006;30(7):1356–1358.

123. Ereshefsky L, Riesenman C, Lam YW. Antidepressant drug interactions and the cytochrome P450 system. The role of cytochrome P450 2D6. *Clin Pharma-cokinet* 1995;(29 suppl 1):10–18.

124. Sindrup SH, Arendt-Nielsen L, Brøsen K, et al. The effect of quinidine on the analgesic effect of codeine. *Eur J Clin Pharmacol* 1992;42(6):587–591.

125. Sindrup SH, Brøsen K. The pharmacogenetics of codeine hypoalgesia. *Phar-macogenetics* 1995;5(6):335–346.

126. Schmidt H, Vormfelde SV, Walchner-Bonjean M, et al. The role of active metabolites in dihydrocodeine effects. *Int J Clin Pharmacol Ther* 2003;41(3): 95–106.

127. Wilder-Smith CH, Schimke J, Osterwalder B, et al. Oral tramadol, a mu-opioid agonist and monoamine reuptake-blocker, and morphine for strong cancer-related pain. *Ann Oncol* 1994;5(2):141–146.

128. Leppert W, Luczak J. The role of tramadol in cancer pain treatment—a re-view. *Support Care Cancer* 2005;13(1):5–17.

129. Marinangeli F, Ciccozzi A, Aloisio L, et al. Improved cancer pain treatment using combined fentanyl-TTS and tramadol. *Pain Pract* 2007;7(4):307–312.

130. Kaiko RF, Foley KM, Grabinski PY, et al. Central nervous system excitatory effects of meperidine in cancer patients. *Ann Neurol* 1983;13(2):180–185.

131. Hoskin PJ, Hanks GW. Opioid agonist-antagonist drugs in acute and chronic pain states. *Drugs* 1991;41(3):326–344.

132. Goldstein DJ, Meador-Woodruff JH. Opiate receptors: opioid agonist-antag-onist effects. *Pharmacotherapy* 1991;11(2):164–167.

133. Davies G, Kingswood C, Street M. Pharmacokinetics of opioids in renal dys-function. *Clin Pharmacokinet* 1996;31(6):410–422.

134. Jemal A, Siegel R, Ward E, et al. Cancer statistics, 2007. *CA Cancer J Clin* 2007;57(1):43–66.

135. Statement symptom management in cancer: pain, depression, and fatigue. Paper presented at: National Institutes of Health State-of-the-Science Confer-ence; July 2002; Bethesda, Maryland.

136. Bruera E, Pereira J, Watanabe S, et al. Opioid rotation in patients with cancer pain. A retrospective comparison of dose ratios between methadone, hydro-morphone, and morphine. *Cancer* 1996;78(4):852–857.

137. de Stoutz ND, Bruera E, Suarez-Almazor M. Opioid rotation for toxicity reduction in terminal cancer patients. *J Pain Symptom Manage* 1995;10(5): 378–384.

138. Ripamonti C, Zecca E, Bruera E. An update on the clinical use of methadone for cancer pain. *Pain* 1997;70(2–3):109–115.

139. Sjøgren P, Jensen NH, Jensen TS. Disappearance of morphine-induced hyper-algesia after discontinuing or substituting morphine with other opioid ago-nists. *Pain* 1994;59(2):313–316.

140. Thomas Z, Bruera E. Use of methadone in a highly tolerant patient receiving parenteral hydromorphone. *J Pain Symptom Manage* 1995;10(4):315–317.

141. Walsh TD. Prevention of opioid side effects. *J Pain Symptom Manage* 1990; 5(6):362–367.

142. Bruera E, Miller MJ, Macmillan K, et al. Neuropsychological effects of meth-ylphenidate in patients receiving a continuous infusion of narcotics for cancer pain. *Pain* 1992;48(2):163–166.

143. Bruera E, Brenneis C, Paterson AH, et al. Use of methylphenidate as an adju-vant to narcotic analgesics in patients with advanced cancer. *J Pain Symptom Manage* 1989;4(1):3–6.

144. Jamison RN, Schein JR, Vallow S, et al. Neuropsychological effects of long-term opioid use in chronic pain patients. *J Pain Symptom Manage* 2003;26(4): 913–921.

145. Fishbain DA, Cutler RB, Rosomoff HL, et al. Can patients taking opioids drive safely? A structured evidence-based review. *J Pain Palliat Care Pharma-cother* 2002;16(1):9–28.

146. Chapman SL, Byas-Smith MG, Reed BA. Effects of intermediate- and long-term use of opioids on cognition in patients with chronic pain. *Clin J Pain* 2002;18(4 suppl):S83–S90.

147. Vainio A, Ollila J, Matikainen E, et al. Driving ability in cancer patients receiving long-term morphine analgesia. *Lancet* 1995;346(8976):667–670.

148. Galski T, Williams JB, Ehle HT. Effects of opioids on driving ability. *J Pain Symptom Manage* 2000;19(3):200–208.

149. Byas-Smith MG, Chapman SL, Reed B, et al. The effect of opioids on driving and psychomotor performance in patients with chronic pain. *Clin J Pain* 2005; 21(4):345–352.

150. Bruera E, Schoeller T, Montejo G. Organic hallucinosis in patients receiving high doses of opiates for cancer pain. *Pain* 1992;48(3):397–399.

151. Fine PG, Portenoy RK. Management of adverse effects. In: Fine PG, Portenoy RK, eds. *Clinical Guide to Opioid Analgesia*. New York: Vendome Press; 2007.

152. Mercadante S, Casuccio A, Fulfaro F, et al. Switching from morphine to methadone to improve analgesia and tolerability in cancer patients: a prospec-tive study. *J Clin Oncol* 2001;19(11):2898–2904.

153. Indelicato RA, Portenoy RK. Opioid rotation in the management of refractory cancer pain. *J Clin Oncol* 2002;20(1):348–352.

154. Ashby MA, Martin P, Jackson KA. Opioid substitution to reduce adverse effects in cancer pain management. *Med J Aust* 1999;170(2):68–71.

155. Moryl N, Santiago-Palma J, Kornick C, et al. Pitfalls of opioid rotation: substi-tuting another opioid for methadone in patients with cancer pain. *Pain* 2002; 96(3):325–328.

156. Hunt G, Bruera E. Respiratory depression in a patient receiving oral metha-done for cancer pain. *J Pain Symptom Manage* 1995;10(5):401–404.

157. Cherny NI, Portenoy RK. Cancer pain management. Current strategy. *Cancer* 1993;72(11 suppl):3393–3415.

158. Coda BA, O'Sullivan B, Donaldson G, et al. Comparative efficacy of patient-controlled administration of morphine, hydromorphone, or sufentanil for the treatment of oral mucositis pain following bone marrow transplantation. *Pain* 1997;72(3):333–346.

159. Swanson G, Smith J, Bulich R, et al. Patient-controlled analgesia for chronic cancer pain in the ambulatory setting: a report of 117 patients. *J Clin Oncol* 1989;7(12):1903–1908.

160. Drexel H, Dzien A, Spiegel RW, et al. Treatment of severe cancer pain by low-dose continuous subcutaneous morphine. *Pain* 1989;36(2):169–176.

161. Bruera E, Brenneis C, Michaud M, et al. Use of the subcutaneous route for the administration of narcotics in patients with cancer pain. *Cancer* 1988; 62(2):407–411.

162. Kerr IG, Sone M, Deangelis C et al. Continuous narcotic infusion with patient-controlled analgesia for chronic cancer pain in outpatients. *Ann Intern Med* 1988;108(4):554–557.

163. Waldmann CS, Eason JR, Rambohul E, et al. Serum morphine levels. A com-parison between continuous subcutaneous infusion and continuous intrave-nous infusion in postoperative patients. *Anaesthesia* 1984;39(8):768–771.

164. Moulin DE, Kreeft JH, Murray-Parsons N, et al. Comparison of continuous subcutaneous and intravenous hydromorphone infusions for management of cancer pain. *Lancet* 1991;337(8739):465–468.

165. Roy SD, Flynn GL. Solubility and related physicochemical properties of nar-cotic analgesics. *Pharm Res* 1988;5(9):580–586.

166. Paix A, Coleman A, Lees J, et al. Subcutaneous fentanyl and sufentanil infu-sion substitution for morphine intolerance in cancer pain management. *Pain* 1995;63(2):263–269.

167. Nelson KA, Glare PA, Walsh D, et al. A prospective, within-patient, crossover study of continuous intravenous and subcutaneous morphine for chronic can-cer pain. *J Pain Symptom Manage* 1997;13(5):262–267.

168. Hays H. Hypodermoclysis for symptom control in terminal care. *Can Fam Physician* 1985;31:1253–1256.

169. Tseng LF, Fujimoto JM. Differential actions of intrathecal naloxone on block-ing the tail-flick inhibition induced by intraventricular beta-endorphin and morphine in rats. *J Pharmacol Exp Ther* 1985;232(1):74–79.

170. Lazorthes Y. Intracerebroventricular administration of morphine for control of irreducible cancer pain. *Ann N Y Acad Sci* 1988;531:123–132.

171. Dennis GC, DeWitty RL. Long-term intraventricular infusion of morphine for intractable pain in cancer of the head and neck. *Neurosurgery* 1990;26(3): 404–407, discussion 407–408.

172. Brazenor GA. Long term intrathecal administration of morphine: a compari-son of bolus injection via reservoir with continuous infusion by implanted pump. *Neurosurgery* 1987;21(4):484–491.

173. Ballantyne JC, Carr DB, Berkey CS, et al. Comparative efficacy of epidural, subarachnoid, and intracerebroventricular opioids in patients with pain due to cancer. *Reg Anesth* 1996;21(6):542–556.

174. Ballantyne JC, Carwood CM. Comparative efficacy of epidural, subarach-noid, and intracerebroventricular opioids in patients with pain due to cancer. *Cochrane Database Syst Rev* 2005;1:CD005178.

175. Meuret G, Jocham H. Patient-controlled analgesia (PCA) in the domiciliary care of tumour patients. *Cancer Treat Rev* 1996;22(suppl A):137–140.

176. Cassileth B, Trevisan C, Gubili J. Complementary therapies for cancer pain. *Curr Pain Headache Rep* 2007;11(4):265–269.

177. Adler SR, Fosket JR. Disclosing complementary and alternative medicine use in the medical encounter: a qualitative study in women with breast cancer. *J Fam Pract* 1999;48(6):453–458.

178. Mansky PJ, Wallerstedt DB. Complementary medicine in palliative care and cancer symptom management. *Cancer J* 2006;12(5):425–431.

179. Bardia A, Barton DL, Prokop LJ, et al. Efficacy of complementary and alterna-tive medicine therapies in relieving cancer pain: a systematic review. *J Clin Oncol* 2006;24(34):5457–5464.

180. Sood A, Sood R, Bauer BA, et al. Cochrane systematic reviews in acupuncture: methodological diversity in database searching. *J Altern Complement Med* 2005;11(4):719–722.

181. Pan CX, Morrison RS, Ness J, et al. Complementary and alternative medicine in the management of pain, dyspnea, and nausea and vomiting near the end of life. A systematic review. *J Pain Symptom Manage* 2000;20(5):374–387.

182. NIH Consensus Conference. Acupuncture. *JAMA* 1998;280(17):1518–1524.

CHAPTER 44 ■ INTERVENTIONAL PAIN THERAPIES

SHANE E. BROGAN

INTRODUCTION

The World Health Organization (WHO) analgesic ladder, as described in the previous chapters on cancer pain management, is practical, easy to implement, and has been taught extensively to health professionals. However, even when the WHO approach is implemented appropriately and aggressively, 10% to 20% of patients do not attain acceptable pain control.[1–3] Traditionally, it has been this refractory group of patients that has been considered for interventional pain management, but the approach of reserving interventional management as a last resort has been called into question. This is particularly true in relation to intrathecal (IT) therapy, where a recent multicenter study suggests that early implementation of treatment leads to improved outcomes.[4] Another type of interventional therapy, namely neurolytic celiac plexus block, may be useful as an early intervention in controlling pancreatic cancer pain and other gastrointestinal system pain-producing malignancies.[5] Impediments to the appropriate use of interventional techniques include inaccessibility to experienced interventionalists and absence of up-to-date knowledge among cancer care providers of the various techniques available, including indications and timing, benefits, risks, and costs (Table 44.1).

The primary purpose of this chapter is to target this latter group of individuals. It is anticipated that a general understanding of interventional approaches to cancer pain control will lead to more appropriate and timely consideration of all potential therapeutic options.

INTRATHECAL DRUG THERAPY

IT drug delivery involves drug administration into the cerebrospinal fluid (CSF) through a small catheter. This route allows the medication to circulate in the CSF and adsorb directly onto central nervous system effector sites. This direct delivery to the central nervous system reduces the systemic toxicity of medication administered via enteral, parenteral, or transdermal routes. Opioids, among other pain modulating agents, have been successfully infused intrathecally in the treatment of cancer pain. Effective analgesia using IT opioids is typically obtained using a small fraction (i.e., 1/100th) of the systemic dose. The addition of adjunctive IT agents that have specific activity within the neuraxis, such as local anesthetics and alpha-2 agonists, may be used to improve overall effectiveness of IT opioid therapy in refractory cases.

Indications

IT therapy is usually indicated in the small proportion of cancer patients for whom comprehensive medical management has produced suboptimal pain control or unacceptable, dose-limiting, analgesic-related toxicity. Other factors may make IT therapy an attractive option, including inability to adhere to a more conventional analgesic regimen. Furthermore, cancer pain with a strong neuropathic component (e.g., plexopathy, complex regional pain syndrome) may respond better to IT therapy, particularly when adjunctive agents such as local anesthetics and clonidine are used.[6] In the setting of severe pain and the prospect of a very aggressive chemotherapy regimen, when the oral route will likely be an unreliable means of administering analgesics, strong consideration should be given to adopting an IT approach to pain management.

Some centers adopt an aggressive and early approach to the institution of IT therapy and have demonstrated more favorable outcomes compared to medical management alone. One study used a visual analog scale (VAS, on a 0–10 scale) pain intensity rating of ≥5 despite 200 mg/day or more of oral morphine or its equivalent per day, as their indication to proceed to IT therapy.[4] Patients on lower doses of opioids with moderate to severe pain were also permitted entry if opioid side effects refractory to conservative management prohibited further escalation of total opioid dose. Although the validity of the conclusions of this study has been questioned, the findings open the door to challenge precepts about this form of therapy as a last resort; certain patients may benefit from avoidance of long-term, and especially high-dose, systemic opioid therapy.

Intrathecal Drug Delivery Systems

Simple Percutaneous Intrathecal Catheter

This is a minimally invasive technique that can be done at the bedside for short-term use. It may be implemented as a trial method (i.e., to assess efficacy of IT opioids, with the intent of placing an implantable system if the trial is deemed a success), or it can be used as a definitive method of delivering IT drug when life expectancy is extremely short (i.e., days rather than weeks to months). In the setting of a patient with severe pain and only several days of expected life, this method will allow for rapid control of pain. Because the catheter is not tunneled, infection risk and mechanical failure is higher, markedly reducing successful longer term use.

Tunneled Intrathecal Catheter

Tunneled IT catheters are typically placed in the operating room under sterile conditions. A dorsally-placed catheter is tunneled subcutaneously for a variable distance and usually exits from the lateral abdominal wall. The most common system in use is the silastic DuPen Catheter (Bard Access Systems, Salt Lake City, UT).[7] With appropriate infection control measures, including the use of antimicrobial filters and meticulous exit site care, tunneled IT or epidural catheters can be used for months to years.[8,9] The catheter is usually not sutured internally, so it can be readily removed in the office if necessary. An advantage of the exteriorized system is that non-pain specialist palliative care clinicians, including those in home hospice settings, may become proficient

TABLE 44.1

OVERVIEW OF THE MORE COMMONLY PERFORMED INTERVENTIONAL CANCER PAIN THERAPIES

Intervention	Indications	Major adverse effects and risks	Comments
IT therapy (lumbar region catheter placement; see Chapter 41 for a discussion of intracerebroventricular therapy)	1) Nonhead and neck cancer pain refractory to usual pharmacotherapeutic approaches. 2) The presence of unacceptable medication side effects.	Infection, postdural puncture headache, and spinal cord injury are rare complications. Long-term use of IT opioids may be associated with suppression of the pituitary-gonadal axis.	Various delivery methods available depending on the prognosis. Cost of implanted programmable delivery system may be comparable to conventional medical therapy after several months of ongoing treatment, barring surgical complications.
Neurolytic celiac plexus block	Visceral abdominal (epigastric and referred) pain, originating from disease involving the distal stomach through the transverse colon; pancreatic cancer pain is the most typical indication.	Transient hypotension, diarrhea; very rarely, spinal cord injury.	Efficacy of up to 90% and good safety profile.
Neurolytic superior hypogastric plexus block	Visceral pain originating from the pelvic organs.	Serious adverse effects are rare.	
Spinal neurolysis	Pain refractory to other forms of therapy, particularly when IT therapy is contraindicated or inefficacious.	Dependent on level blocked. Cervical or lumbar neurolysis carries the risk of extremity motor weakness. Lumbosacral neurolysis risks bowel and bladder dysfunction, which is usually transient. Deafferentation pain at any level.	Alcohol or phenol are the typical agents used.
Vertebroplasty and kyphoplasty	Painful compression fracture of the vertebral body without involvement of the spinal canal.	Cement spread to the spinal canal causing neurologic injury; allergy to cement; pulmonary embolus.	Better outcomes are noted with fractures <6 months of age.
Image-guided tumor ablation	Painful bony metastases.	Bone instability and fracture.	Still not in widespread use, but preliminary studies are promising.

in its management with minimal training. Toward the end of life, when analgesic requirements may be rapidly escalating, hospice registered nurses can easily give IT boluses or increase the infusion rate as indicated and alter the drug(s) used with relative ease. With an implanted system (see below), drug changes are more complex than intravenous or oral dosing, and rapid dose titration is not as easily accomplished because of the need for pump reprogramming by trained specialists. Disadvantages of a tunneled system versus a self-contained implanted device are the need for an externalized pump apparatus, increased risk of infection, and the possibility of inadvertent catheter dislodgement or removal.

Implantable Drug Delivery Systems

The implanted drug delivery system (IDDS) uses a small, programmable, computerized electronic pump to deliver drug to the IT space through a catheter (Figs. 44.1 and 44.2). The pump is placed subcutaneously in the anterior abdominal wall and has a reservoir that can be refilled via a port accessed by a specialized needle through the skin. The pump is programmed by an external

hand-held device that can alter the rate of infusion and deliver boluses and also allows for a patient-controlled analgesia function. The battery life is typically 5–7 years, so it is unlikely that a replacement would be necessary during the average lifetime of the cancer patient with advanced disease. Drug refills are office-based and minimally uncomfortable. Refills are needed every 1 to 6 months depending on the drug concentration and infusion rate.

Contraindications to an IDDS are generally related to difficulties forming a suitable subcutaneous pocket for the pump, as would be the case in severe ascites, emaciation, skin infection, or other abdominal wall pathology. Patients with systemic infection, concurrent bleeding diathesis, or clotting abnormalities are poor candidates until these abnormalities are corrected or stabilized. Advantages of this system, compared to an exteriorized system, include increased patient freedom of mobility, low maintenance, and low infection risk. Disadvantages are the need for an initially more invasive surgery, high up-front costs, and the logistical problems concerning pump refills and programming. See Table

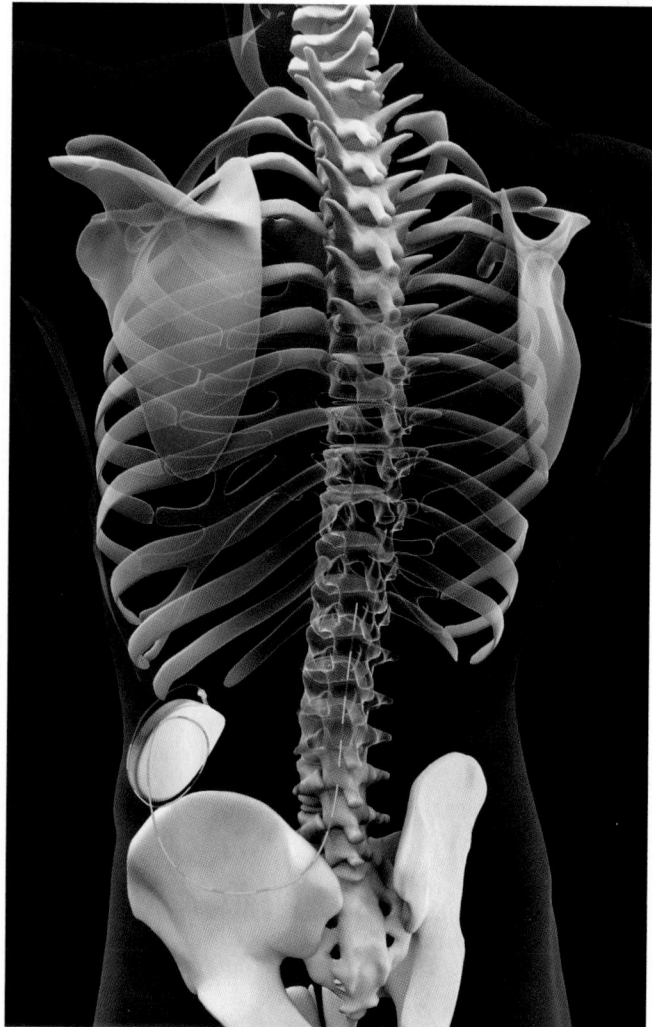

FIGURE 44.1 Schematic of an IT drug delivery system showing the pump in the anterior abdominal wall, and the catheter tunneled to the dorsal spine and into the IT space (Courtesy of Medtronic, Inc.).

44.2 for a comparison of exteriorized versus implanted pump delivery systems.

Intrathecal versus Epidural Drug Delivery

IT drug delivery has largely replaced the epidural route as the preferred neuraxial route of administration for various reasons. With all neuraxial administration of opioids, the target sites are opioid receptors of the dorsal horn of the spinal cord, which requires either direct CSF delivery or absorption of drug from the epidural space. Compared to IT delivery, epidural infusions require a ten-fold greater volume and dose of opioid in order to diffuse passively across the dura and enter the subarachnoid (IT) space. This large difference in infusion volumes and doses has a major impact both on cost and the frequency of drug reservoir changes, which necessitates breaking the system's sterility more frequently and likely results in a higher infection rate. Furthermore, treatment failure is more frequent with the epidural route, due to inadvertent catheter dislodgement and the development of epidural fibrosis which impedes diffusion of drug to the subarachnoid space.[10] Technical complication rates have been shown to be higher with long-term epidural (55%) compared to IT (5%) infusions.[11]

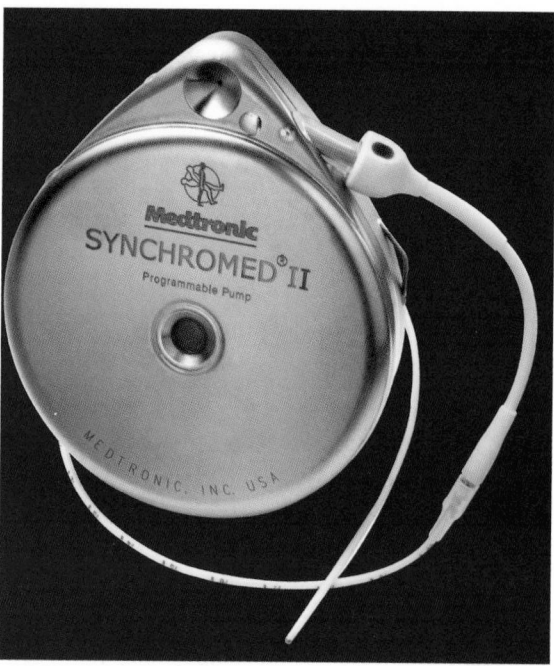

FIGURE 44.2 IT pump and catheter system. The pump is refilled percutaneously with a needle through the orifice in the center of the device (Courtesy of Medtronic, Inc.).

Notwithstanding these considerations, there remain some specific indications for epidural analgesia. Pain in a pattern involving specific, consecutive dermatomes may be blocked with local anesthetics with an appropriately positioned epidural catheter. An example of this would be a thoracic epidural catheter for isolated thoracic pain caused by rib metastases, in the setting of a short life expectancy. This technique may allow for complete analgesia using local anesthetics alone without the use of epidural opioids.

Implantable or Exteriorized Intrathecal Drug Delivery: Cost Analysis

With an IDDS, the initial costs are relatively high ($15,000–$20,000 USD). Over time, the accruing and total care costs may be less in patients with an IDDS compared to those with an exteriorized system due to greater labor-related costs (including managing mechanical failures) with externalized systems. An older study suggested that, compared to an externalized system, an IDDS will be more cost effective after approximately 3 months of therapy.[12] There are no recent cost comparisons available.

Outcome Studies

A 2002 study by Smith et al.[4] randomized 202 patients with advanced cancer to comprehensive medical management (CMM) or an IDDS plus CMM. Patients were eligible if they had a visual analog scale pain intensity rating of ≥5 at two measurements within a week of randomization, despite 200 mg/day or more of oral morphine or its equivalent. Patients on lower doses of opioids were also permitted entry if opioid side effects refractory to conservative management prohibited further escalation of total opioid dose. All patients were ≥18 years of age, had life expectancy ≥3 months, and were suitable for IDDS (no active infection, obstruction of CSF flow, or mechanical barriers). The primary outcome measure was pain control (VAS improvement ≥20%)

TABLE 44.2

COMPARISON OF INTRATHECAL DRUG DELIVERY SYSTEMS

	IDDS	Exteriorized IT delivery system
Cost	High initial cost but more cost effective after 3 months.	Lower cost for short-term use.
Indications	Refractory cancer pain and prognosis >3 months.	Refractory cancer pain with prognosis <3 months. Pain crisis requiring rapid control.
Infection risk	Early infection risk; low risk longer term.	Higher
Advantages	Patient freedom. Low maintenance.	Easier to change infusate. Easier to give boluses for aggressive symptom control. Can be removed in the office.
Disadvantages	More invasive. Requires more operator expertise in tertiary care setting.	Risk of dislodgement and failure.

combined with an improved toxicity profile, as measured by the National Cancer Institute Common Toxicity Criteria, 4 weeks after randomization. Clinical success was defined as a ≥20% reduction in VAS scores, or equal scores with a ≥20% reduction in toxicity.

At 4 weeks, both groups had an improvement in pain scores and toxicity. Sixty of 71 IDDS patients (84.5%) achieved clinical success compared with 51 of 72 CMM patients (70.8%, $p = 0.05$). IDDS patients more often achieved ≥20% reduction in both pain VAS and toxicity (57.7% [41 of 71] vs. 37.5% [27 of 72], $p = 0.02$). The mean CMM VAS score fell from 7.81 to 4.76 (39% reduction); for the IDDS group, the scores fell from 7.57 to 3.67 (52% reduction, $p = 0.055$). The mean CMM toxicity scores fell from 6.36 to 5.27 (17% reduction); for the IDDS group, the toxicity scores fell from 7.22 to 3.59 (50% reduction, $p = 0.004$). The IDDS group had significant reductions in fatigue and depressed level of consciousness ($p < 0.05$). IDDS patients also had improved survival, with 53.9% alive at 6 months compared with 37.2% of the CMM group ($p = 0.06$). The authors concluded that IT therapy, compared to CMM alone, improved clinical success by reducing drug toxicity, trended toward improving pain reduction, and possibly improved survival. It should be noted that the data were analyzed on an intent-to-treat basis, but that some crossover (5 patients) from CMM to the IDDS group did occur. When the data is interpreted on the basis of the actual treatment received, there was a significant difference between the VAS scores between groups, in favor of IT therapy.

In 2005, the same group of authors published a second paper examining the 6 month follow-up of the patients in the above mentioned trial.[13] The approach in this paper was to compare outcomes in terms of the actual treatment received (i.e., an IDDS versus CMM alone), rather than the intent-to-treat at randomization approach used in the 2002 study. Outcome measures were the same as in the initial study, but were also assessed in patients alive at 12 weeks after the initial randomization. At 4 weeks, 88.5% of IDDS patients achieved clinical success compared with 71.4% ($p = 0.02$) of non-IDDS patients, and more often achieved a ≥20% reduction in both pain VAS and toxicity (67.3% versus 36.3%; $p = 0.0003$). At 12 weeks, of the 56 patients remaining in the CMM group, 19 had received an IDDS. By 12 weeks, 82.5% of IDDS patients had clinical success compared with 77.8% ($p = 0.55$) of non-IDDS patients, and more often had a ≥20% reduction in both pain VAS and toxicity (57.9 versus 33.3%; $p = 0.01$). At 12 weeks, the IDDS VAS pain scores

decreased from 7.81 to 3.89 (47% reduction) compared with 7.21 to 4.53 for non-IDDS patients (42% reduction; $p = 0.23$). The 12-week drug toxicity scores for IDDS patients decreased from 6.68 to 2.30 (66% reduction), and for non-IDDS patients from 6.73 to 4.13 (37% reduction; $p = 0.01$). All individual drug toxicities improved with IDDS at both 4 and 12 weeks. At 6 months, only 32% of the group randomized to CMM and who did not cross over to IDDS were alive, compared with 52% to 59% for patients in those groups who received IDDS. This study concluded that an IDDS improved clinical success, reduced pain scores, relieved most toxicity of pain control drugs, and was associated with increased survival for the duration of the 6 month trial.

Pharmacology

Over a dozen different agents have been reported to be used intrathecally in the management of cancer pain, and most of these have never been approved by the U.S. Food and Drug Administration (FDA) for IT use (Table 44.3). Morphine sulphate, one of the few agents the FDA approved for IT use, is the standard first-line drug used in IT pain therapy. Additional agents are usually then added in a stepwise fashion depending on the response to morphine alone; it is not uncommon that 1–3 adjunctive agents are added to the infused solution. A recent consensus document by Stearns et al.[14] is an attempt to standardize the therapeutic approach to IT drug selection and dosing in the cancer patient (see Table 44.3).

Opioids

IT mu opioid agonists directly activate dorsal horn and brainstem opioid receptors. Morphine sulphate is FDA-approved for IT use, and it remains the first-line agent for IT analgesia. Numerous other IT opioids have been used successfully including hydromorphone, fentanyl, sufentanil, meperidine, and methadone. The choice of agent is largely idiosyncratic. Many practitioners purport that hydromorphone causes less nausea than morphine, although there are no comparative trial data to support this view. The comparatively greater lipophilicity of fentanyl and sufentanil leads to relatively rapid absorption into proximate neural structures with less CSF recirculation and migration to the brainstem. This has some theoretical advantages when a more regional anal-

TABLE 44.3

INTRATHECAL DRUGS USED IN CANCER PAIN MANAGEMENT*

Drug	Receptor	Indication	Adverse effects	Notes
Opioids Morphine Sulphate Hydromorphone Fentanyl Sufentanil	Mu opioid receptors	Nociceptive and mixed pain, first-line therapy. Neuropathic pain second-line therapy.	Sedation, respiratory depression, urinary retention, nausea, pruritus, cognitive impairment.	The lipophilic opioids like fentanyl and sufentanil are generally added when first-line treatments have failed.
Local anesthetics Bupivacaine	Neural sodium channels	Neuropathic and mixed pain, first-line therapy; nociceptive pain, second-line.	Motor weakness, hypotension, urinary retention	The chemical sympathectomy caused by IT bupivacaine may promote gastrointestinal motility.
Clonidine	Alpha-2 adrenoreceptors	Neuropathic Pain first- or second-line therapy Nociceptive pain second-line therapy.	Orthostatic hypotension, sedation, edema.	
Baclofen	Gamma-aminobutyric acid (GABA)	Coexisting spasticity; third-line for neuropathic pain.	Ataxia, sedation, auditory disturbance.	Abrupt discontinuation may cause a serious withdrawal syndrome.
Ketamine	N-methyl-D-aspartate (NMDA)	Fourth-line therapy for neuropathic pain.	Anxiety, agitation, facial flushing, delusions.	Ketamine, given intravenously at subanesthetic doses, has also been used effectively for refractory pain syndromes, especially in terminal care.[61]
Droperidol	Dopaminergic	Refractory nausea; fourth-line therapy for pain.	Extrapyramidal symptoms	
Midazolam	GABA	Neuropathic pain, fourth-line therapy.	Sedation	
Ziconotide	N-type voltage-sensitive calcium channels	Fourth-line therapy.	Cognitive, psychiatric, ataxia, nausea, elevated creatine kinase, hypotension.	Still not widely accepted as a useful intrathecal agent.

*Based on the practice guidelines published by Stearns et al.[14]

gesic effect is desired, with less risk of opioid activity (respiratory depression) at the brainstem level.

Local Anesthetics

Local anesthetics, such as bupivacaine and lidocaine, are sodium channel blockers which interrupt neural action potentials along sensory and motor nerves. When given intrathecally, local anesthetics can block incoming sensory nerves and produce complete analgesia. However, this comes at the price of motor blockade resulting in weakness, and sympathetic nervous system blockade which may result in hypotension. High doses of local anesthetics may also result in neuro- or cardiotoxicity (seizure or arrhythmia). Bupivacaine, given in doses less than 30–60 mg/day, is an excellent adjunct to IT opioids and generally causes minimal motor block. In the terminally ill patient who is bed-bound and does not object to lower extremity weakness, higher doses of local anesthetics may be used to provide profound analgesia with no cognitive side effects. Supportive means to evacuate the bowels and void urine must be anticipated.

Clonidine

Clonidine is an alpha-2 adrenergic agonist which acts at the dorsal horn by modulating the transmission of noxious sensory sig-

nals. This modulation is accomplished by mimicking the activation of descending noradrenergic pathways and inhibiting neurotransmitter release.[15] Epidural and IT clonidine has been studied extensively in postoperative pain settings and in obstetric care for labor analgesia, but little data exists from cancer pain treatment studies. It is generally considered a very useful adjunct to opioids and local anesthetics when there is a predominant neuropathic pain component.[6] Dosing is limited by side effects including sedation and hypotension. The consensus guideline by Stearns et al.[14] recommends using clonidine as a third-line agent when treating refractory cancer pain, but suggests it should be used as a second-line agent when there is a neuropathic pain component.

Other Drugs

A diverse group of drugs have been reported to be useful IT adjuncts, including baclofen, ketamine, neostigmine, midazolam, ketorolac, droperidol, and ziconotide. Droperidol is indicated for refractory nausea and vomiting. Ziconotide (formally SNX-111) is a novel snail peptide that is an N-type voltage-sensitive calcium channel blocker. Ziconotide can only be given intrathecally and appears to act at the dorsal horn to decrease afferent sensory input by mechanisms different from those of other IT drugs. Despite its FDA approval for IT use in refractory pain, ziconotide has not gained popularity due to adverse effects including cognitive impairment and psychiatric disturbance. Clinical experience has shown that most of these adverse effects are dose related and can be avoided by slow and careful titration.[16]

Contraindications and Risk Management

Absolute contraindications to IT analgesia are rare. Skin infection over the intended catheter site, bacteremia/sepsis, and uncorrectable coagulopathy represent absolute contraindications to IT catheter placement, given the respective risks of CNS infection and spinal hematoma. Oral anticoagulants need to be held until the international normalized ratio is 1.5 or less. If indicated, a low molecular weight heparin (LMWH) may be used, provided it is held for 24 hours before the catheter placement. Oral anticoagulants may be resumed shortly after postprocedure hemostasis has been established, and LMWH dosing can resume 12 hours after the procedure.[17] Hematologic relative contraindications include a lowered white cell count $\leq 2 \times 10^9$/L, an absolute neutrophil count $\leq 1000/\mu$L, or a platelet count $\leq 20 \times 10^3/\mu$L.[14] Depending on the patient circumstances, thrombocytopenia may be treated with a platelet transfusion prior to implantation. Special consideration must be given to the feasibility of implanting available pump devices in the anterior abdominal wall, particularly in emaciated patients or children. A smaller 20 milliliter capacity pump is available and may be more practical in these instances.

Complications and Side Effects

In general, most of the commonly reported drug-related adverse effects are well tolerated or readily managed with palliative or supportive interventions. The usual IT opioid side effects are similar to those experienced with the oral or transdermal route, but usually much less pronounced and include sedation, nausea, pruritus, and urinary retention. The serious complication of respiratory depression is rare, especially in opioid-tolerant patients. Local anesthetics may cause lower extremity weakness, hypotension, and bowel or bladder dysfunction. Clonidine may cause hypotension and sedation.

Meningitis is the most feared complication of IT drug delivery but it occurs infrequently when standard infection control measures are followed. Localized skin infection is more common and can usually be managed by oral antibiotics and close observation. Occasionally, catheter or pump explantation will be necessary. Guidelines about the prevention and treatment of IT drug delivery system infection have been published.[18] Typical surgical complications may develop, including seroma formation and pump pocket hematoma. These are usually self-limiting, but ongoing assessment for infection is required, and they may add to postimplant discomfort. The best prophylaxis is an appropriately sized surgical pocket with fastidious hemostasis, and this is achieved through experience.

Catheter tip inflammatory masses (granuloma) are now a well-recognized complication of IT drug delivery. These granulomatous masses can present with new onset lower extremity neurologic symptoms and are associated with high doses and high concentrations of opioid infusate. Clinicians must have a high index of suspicion for this complication; to ignore it may result in permanent neurologic damage, whereas with early recognition and minimally invasive treatment there are seldom any long-term sequelae.[19,20]

Postdural puncture headache can result from persistent cerebrospinal fluid leak around the catheter. This uncomfortable and often distressing experience is usually self-limiting, resolving spontaneously over days to weeks. Conservative management includes rest, fluids, additional analgesia, and caffeine. A headache

that persists may be treated with a fluoroscopically guided epidural blood patch, provided that there are no contraindications related to bleeding risk or leucopenia.[14]

Intrathecal Therapy and Ongoing Oncologic Care

The initiation or continuation of IT therapy need not interfere with chemotherapy or radiotherapy regimens. The superior symptom control offered by IT therapy may in fact allow patients to tolerate aggressive treatment more comfortably and increase the efficiency of the oncology suite by decreasing the amount of time spent managing complicated cancer-related symptoms. Particularly aggressive chemotherapy protocols may require that the implantation of an IT drug delivery system be strategically timed to avoid a white cell count or platelet count nadir.

Radiation therapy does affect the battery life of IDDS and may result in electrical failure. The pump may be protected by lead shielding and, if possible, radiation field avoidance. If radiation is being performed for pain control, a temporary catheter may be utilized until this therapy becomes effective, which may take up to 2 weeks (see Chapter 48).

SPINAL CHEMONEUROLYSIS

Spinal chemoneurolysis involves the destruction of nerve root axons or other spinal cord elements by chemical means, using alcohol or phenol. The destruction of selected nerve roots interrupts nociceptive pathways and can potentially create excellent analgesia in a relatively selective body area. Alcohol or phenol ablation of central neural structures has largely fallen out of favor in recent decades, mostly because of advances in the pharmacologic treatment of pain, including via the IT route as previously described. Nevertheless, it remains a useful and effective technique in developing countries with limited opioid access, and where a rapidly effective therapy, requiring little or no follow-up, is required. Like other interventional pain management techniques, intraspinal neurolysis does offer the advantage of localized pain control while minimizing the burden of systemic side effects. However, the potential adverse effects of the procedure are significant, including motor nerve root dysfunction, bowel or bladder dysfunction, and dysesthesias in the denervated dermatomes.[21] In experienced hands, these adverse effects may be minimized, but the potentially high morbidity of these problems has generally placed intraspinal neurolysis toward the end of the treatment spectrum in modern day practice.[21–25]

Spinal Chemoneurolysis Technique

Spinal chemoneurolysis, or simply neurolysis, notwithstanding its value in appropriately selected patients, is rapidly becoming a forgotten technique, and therefore physicians with experience with this treatment modality, and the ability to teach it to trainees, are becoming relatively scarce. Neurolysis is targeted at the sensory nerve root and dorsal root ganglion within the subarachnoid space while attempting to spare the more anteriorly located motor nerve roots. Neurolysis may be performed at the cervical, thoracic, or lumbo-sacral levels, with the last being the most common site of intervention. Neurolysis in the epidural space has also been described, but is less favored because of pain on injection and disappointing outcomes.[26] Knowledge of the chemical properties of alcohol and phenol is essential to the safe and effective use of each agent. The disposition of alcohol and phenol are distinctly different when deposited in the IT space (Figs. 44.3 and

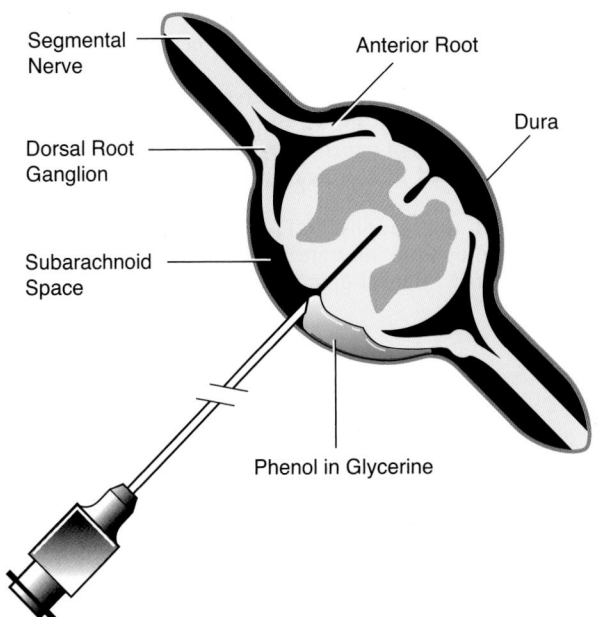

FIGURE 44.3 Lateral supine position used for injection of IT phenol, with the hyperbaric solution falling toward the sensory dorsal roots.

44.4). Alcohol is hypobaric relative to CSF, and therefore will "float" upward, whereas phenol is hyperbaric and will "sink" within the subarachnoid space relative to the position of the needle tip. These properties allow for reasonably selective targeting of nerve roots using careful patient positioning and needle placement. The patient is placed in the lateral decubitus position, with the painful side uppermost for alcohol neurolysis, and dependent for phenol neurolysis. Since it is most common for patients to be intolerant of having the painful side down (dependent), alcohol ablation is the preferred technique. For alcohol neurolysis, the patient is rolled 45 degrees away from the operator who is on the dorsal side of the patient, so that the hypobaric

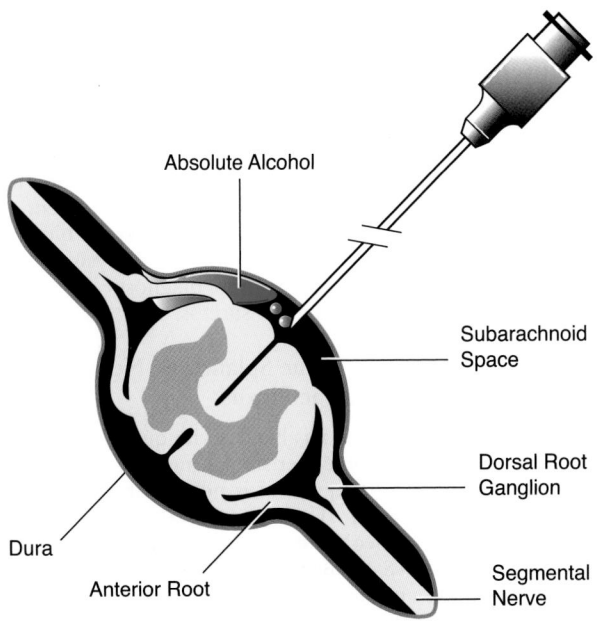

FIGURE 44.4 Lateral prone position used for injection of IT alcohol, with the hypobaric solution rising toward the sensory dorsal roots.

alcohol preferentially floats to the dorso-lateral subarachnoid space where the sensory dorsal roots reside. To treat this same anatomic location with phenol, the patient needs to be rolled toward the operator. A small bore spinal needle is advanced into the IT space at the appropriate nerve root level for the affected pain site to be treated. Recall that nerve roots and their respective dermatomal, myotomal, and sclerotomal levels do not necessarily line up anatomically. Tiny aliquots (0.1–0.2 mL) of the neurolytic agent are then injected incrementally with careful monitoring of sensory changes and dermatomal spread until the desired region is blocked. A detailed description of spinal neurolysis technique is contained within the text, *Neural Blockade*.[21]

Lumbosacral Neurolysis

Lumbosacral spinal neurolysis can provide excellent pain relief of the pelvis, perineum, rectum, and genital area in patients who have been refractory or intolerant of aggressive conventional management. Patients, who are confined to bed due to their symptom burden, or who have already had urinary and bowel diversion procedures, can expect good pain relief with an acceptable risk of complication. Prior to proceeding with lumbosacral subarachnoid neurolysis, consideration should be given instead to performing a superior hypogastric plexus block as this procedure may be equally effective yet considerably safer.

Cervical and Thoracic Neurolysis

Cervical neurolysis is seldom performed due to the technical difficulty of subarachnoid access at this level, the compactness of anatomy in this region making selective neurolysis more difficult, as well as the inherent risk of causing injury to the cervical spinal cord with consequent neurologic deficits and adverse symptoms (including pain). Thoracic neurolysis for thoracic wall pain is also technically difficult, but the consequences of motor root dysfunction are less pronounced, in that the loss of several levels of intercostal muscle function is usually well tolerated. Thoracic neurolysis does have the advantage of not placing the innervation of the bowel, bladder, and lower extremities at risk, and consequently has less risk of significant morbidity.

Adverse Effects

Studies reporting on bladder and bowel dysfunction after lumbosacral neurolysis report that about one quarter of patients develop urinary incontinence, with most resolving within 10 days.[27–29] Bowel dysfunction and lower extremity weakness was relatively less frequent. Yet, it should be noted that some of these patients may already have had urinary and bowel diversion for surgical reasons, making the decision to proceed with neurolysis somewhat easier. Other adverse effects of IT neurolysis include deafferentation pain and headache. Rare complications include infection, spinal cord damage, and posterior spinal artery thrombosis causing paraplegia.

Contraindications

IT neurolysis is contraindicated when: (1) the patient has spinal cord tumor or tumor obliteration of the subarachnoid space at the selected level; (2) skin infection is present at the needle puncture site; (3) the patient is unable to tolerate appropriate positioning; and (4) there is a primary pain source, such as a bone metastasis or fracture, that is amenable to more definitive procedural treatment.

CELIAC PLEXUS BLOCK

Chemical neurolysis of the components of the celiac plexus can be a highly effective treatment of visceral pain of the upper abdomen, and is the most commonly performed interventional cancer pain technique.

Indications

Neurolytic celiac plexus blockade (NCPB) is typically performed for cancer related *visceral* pain originating in the upper abdomen. Pain originating from the somatic nerve fibers emanating from the upper abdominal wall will not be blocked by NCPB, and therefore it is very important to distinguish between visceral versus somatic pain before contemplating this procedure. The celiac plexus carries afferent fibers from the upper abdominal organs from the stomach to the mid transverse colon, including pancreas and gallbladder. Deep visceral pain related to pancreatic adenocarcinoma and cholangiocarcinoma are typical indications for NCPB. As will be discussed later, this is a highly efficacious and safe procedure, so it should be considered early in the treatment of upper abdominal cancer pain.[30]

Anatomy of the Celiac Plexus

Understanding the path of the needle and the position of its tip in relation to the local anatomy is crucial to the safe and effective performance of any interventional procedure. The celiac plexus is a complex grouping of 1–5 ganglia of various sizes interconnected by a dense network of neural fibers. The plexus is located in the upper abdomen typically anterolateral to the aorta at the L1 vertebral level, just caudal to the take-off of the celiac artery; however, some variability has been noted, and the plexus can be found anywhere from the level of T12–L1 disc space to the level of the L2 vertebral body.[31] Just lateral to the celiac plexus are the adrenal glands, and inferiorly are the renal arteries. The celiac plexus is formed by the convergence of sympathetic preganglionic and afferent fibers from the greater (originating from the T5–T10 spinal level), lesser (T10–T11), and least (T12) splanchnic nerves. The splanchnic nerves are composed of preganglionic autonomic efferent fibers to the upper abdominal viscera that synapse in the celiac ganglia, and ascending afferent fibers capable of carrying nociceptive signals from abdominal viscera including the distal portion of the stomach, pancreas, gallbladder, and other hepatobiliary structures, the duodenum, and small intestine, and the large intestine, as far distal as the transverse colon. The splanchnic nerves travel from the spine in the posterior mediastinum, anterolateral to the thoracic vertebral bodies, and pierce the diaphragmatic crus to enter the retroperitoneal abdominal cavity. Parasympathetic preganglionic and afferent fibers originating from the vagus nerves also contribute to the celiac plexus.

General Considerations

Preparation of patients should include counseling regarding the potential adverse effects and complications of the procedure. Anticoagulants should be discontinued long enough to allow normalization of coagulation profiles. Intravenous access is mandatory so that sedation may be administered, adverse effects can be treated, and prehydration can be accomplished. The latter point is important, as celiac plexus blockade will cause splanchnic vasodilatation potentially leading to systemic hypotension, particularly in the cancer patient who may already be dehydrated and hypovolemic. An important factor to consider is whether the patient will be able to tolerate lying in the prone position; a patient

with gross ascites, even with sedation, will be unable to assume the appropriate position, and may be a better candidate for an anterior or endoscopic approach.

Tumor location within the pancreas and the degree of local tumor burden has been shown to impact NCPB outcome, with pain related to head of pancreas lesions having a more favorable outcome compared to lesions of the body and tail of the pancreas.[32]

Computed tomography (CT)-guided celiac plexus studies using a radio-opaque injectate have shown that outcome may also be affected by local anatomic distortion caused by tumor infiltration.[33,34]

Adverse Effects

NCPB is a relatively safe and well-tolerated procedure. Serious complications include transient or permanent spinal cord damage and paraplegia due to spread of the lytic injectate to the nerve roots, epidural, or IT space. Neurologic damage may also ensue after damage to an anterior spinal artery, such as the artery of Adamkiewicz, disrupting the vulnerable arterial supply of the spinal cord.[35,36] Fortunately, serious neurologic complications are very rare, with an incidence of less than 0.2% in one series of 2730 NCPBs.[37] Side effects are common and generally mild and well tolerated. NCPB will predictably cause a disruption of the sympathetic nervous supply to the proximal bowel resulting in unopposed parasympathetic (vagal) tone. This excessive parasympathetic tone will typically result in transient gastrointestinal hypermotility and diarrhea in approximately 44% of patients, a side effect that is seldom considered a problem by the patient who has been constipated due to opioid consumption and debilitation. The loss of sympathetic tone also results in splanchnic vasodilation, intravascular fluid shift to the bowel, and hypotension in approximately 38% of patients.[5] This should be anticipated and prevented with preprocedural volume enhancement and sufficient means to monitor and treat falling blood pressure (e.g., ephedrine).

Celiac Plexus Block Techniques

Numerous approaches to the celiac plexus have been described, ranging from traditional blind landmark techniques to sophisticated CT-guided methods. A 1992 study by Ischia et al.[38] compared the outcomes of the retrocrural technique, a transaortic approach, and neurolysis of the splanchnic nerves at the T12 level. No statistically significant differences ($p > 0.05$) were found among the three techniques in terms of either immediate or up-to-death results. Procedure mortality was zero with the three techniques and morbidity negligible. NCPB provided excellent pain relief in 70% to 80% of patients immediately after the block and in 60% to 75% until death.[38] Celiac plexus neurolysis may also be achieved intraoperatively at the time of diagnostic or therapeutic laparotomy, with reported good success.[39]

Posterior Approach to the Splanchnic Nerves and Celiac Plexus

The most common celiac plexus block technique is the posterior approach using a needle on either side of midline. This was first described as a blind technique, but is now performed with the help of fluoroscopy or CT. The L1 vertebral body is identified with fluoroscopy and then the c-arm is rotated obliquely so that a skin puncture site 6–8 cm (6 cm for smaller, cachectic, individuals; more toward 8 cm for obese patients) lateral to the midline will allow for coaxial needle advancement to the anterolateral aspect of the upper half of L1 vertebral body. A 15 cm or longer 20-gauge needle is then advanced toward the anterolateral shadow of the L1 vertebral body. The intention is to just miss contact with the vertebral body, as this can be quite uncomfortable for the patient. Care should be taken not to touch the L1 transverse process, as this can be mistaken for the vertebral body, giving an incorrect, and potentially dangerous, estimate of depth. This author typically performs the left side first, so if an inadvertent aortic puncture is obtained, a transaortic approach can be completed, assuring good placement anterior to the aorta and avoiding the need for a second needle placement (the transaortic approach has been advocated by some practitioners[40] as a safe, alternative technique, and involves intentionally piercing the aorta in order to provide direct chemoneurolysis to the celiac ganglia anterior to the aorta). The second needle is placed in identical manner from the right side, aiming for the space antero-lateral to the right side of the L1 vertebral body. Final needle advancements should be done under lateral fluoroscopic guidance: The left needle tip should be advanced 0.5 cm ventral to the anterior edge of the L1 vertebral body (further advancement may result in aortic puncture); the right needle tip is advanced 1 cm beyond the anterior edge of the vertebral body (Fig. 44.5). As the aorta is approached, transmitted arterial pulsations may be appreciable at the needle hub, but this is unreliable. The anatomic location of these needle tips is likely to be retrocrural, and in good position to block the splanchnic nerves as they pierce the diaphragm. Note that the celiac plexus itself is not the primary target when using the retrocrural technique, but this appears to be of little clinical significance.[38]

If an anterocrural needle position is desired, with direct lysis of the celiac plexus itself, the needles need to be further advanced through the crus of the diaphragm. The final anatomic position of the needle can only be determined by injecting several milliliters of a radio-opaque contrast agent through each needle in an antero-posterior and lateral projection. Retrocrural contrast will spread cephalad along the anterolateral aspect of the T12 and L1 vertebral bodies, while anterocrural spread will be noted in a more anterior and caudal plane. In either case, spread toward the mid-line should be present. While injecting the radio-opaque contrast, meticulous attention should also be given to avoiding: (1) vascular uptake which might result in neurolytic being delivered to the spinal cord or other organs; (2) posterior spread toward the neuroforamina, the nerve roots, and the epidural space; and (3) contrast uptake into the intima of the aorta (this is seen, under real-time fluoroscopy, as a pulsating "streaking" outlining the assumed position of the aorta). Once the needles are in a radio-graphically satisfactory position, 5–10 mL of lidocaine 2% is injected through each needle after attempting aspiration of blood, CSF, or urine and confirming proper needle placement. After several minutes, the patient is questioned about the presence of any unwanted lower extremity weakness or other neurologic

symptoms. A reduction in abdominal pain should also be noted, though this may be unreliable if the patient has received intravenous analgesics or sedatives. Finally, neurolysis is achieved by injecting 10–12 mL of ethyl alcohol (60% or higher, concentration) or phenol (6% or higher concentration) through each needle.

Anterior Approaches

Numerous anterior approaches to the celiac plexus have been described with efficacy and safety profiles comparable to those of the posterior approaches. A single needle may be placed through the anterior abdominal wall under CT guidance, potentially traversing the bowel, stomach, and pancreas, to the preaortic region where the celiac plexus elements reside.[33,41] An increasingly popular approach to the celiac plexus is via transgastric endoscopy. A needle is advanced through the endoscope under ultrasound guidance through the posterior wall of the stomach into the preaortic area in the vicinity of the celiac plexus.[42–44] This technique requires that the patient can tolerate esophago-gastroscopy.

Outcome Studies

Numerous case reports, uncontrolled case series, and several randomized controlled trials[38,39,45–47] report a preponderance of favorable outcomes with NCPB. A 1995 meta-analysis by Eisenberg et al.[5] revealed 24 papers (with 1145 patients) suitable for inclusion. Included were two randomized controlled trials, one prospective case series, and 21 uncontrolled retrospective case series. When analyzed, good to excellent pain relief was reported in 89% during the first 2 weeks after NCPB. This effect persisted after 2 weeks, with partial or complete pain relief reported in 90% of living patients at 3 months, and in 70% to 80% until death. The most frequent indication was unresectable pancreatic cancer (63%), with the balance being a variety of nonpancreatic pain sites including the stomach and esophagus. The pancreatic and nonpancreatic cases did not appear to have a significantly different outcome. The bilateral posterior approach with 15–50 mL of 50% to 100% ethyl alcohol was the most common technique used. No procedure-related mortality was reported, and adverse effects were minimal. The most common adverse effects reported were transient hypotension, diarrhea, and transient pain at the site of injection.

A recent controlled trial by Wong et al.[46] randomized 100 patients with unresectable pancreatic adenocarcinoma to either NCPB or systemic analgesia therapy (SAT) and a sham injection. A blinded observer recorded patient pain intensity, quality of

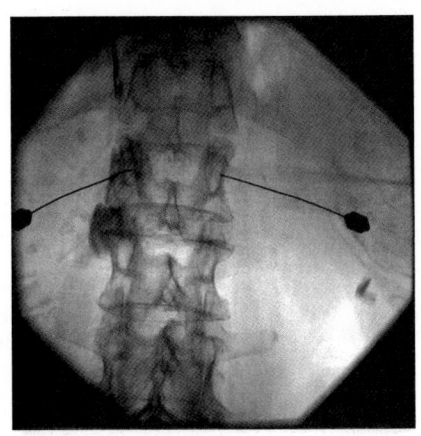

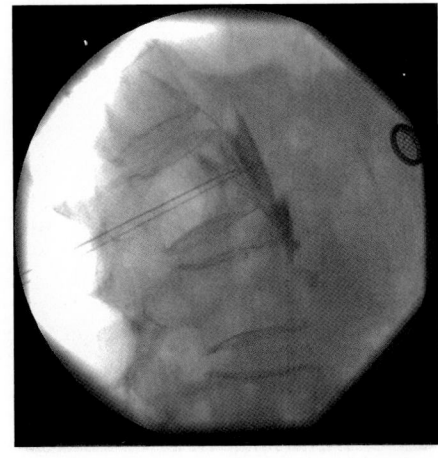

A   B

FIGURE 44.5 Fluoroscopic images of a retrocrural celiac plexus block. **A.** Antero-posterior view with the needle tips antero-lateral to the L1 vertebral body. Contrast has been injected through the left needle with spread cephalad along the course of the splanchnic nerves. **B.** Lateral fluoro-scopic view showing the needle tips advanced anterior to the anterior shadow of the L1 vertebral body and contrast spreading in the retrocrural fascial plane.

life measures, opioid consumption and related side effects, and survival time for 1 year. Baseline pain scores were relatively low, but comparable, in both groups (VAS 4.4 +/−1.7 vs. 4.1 +/−1.8, respectively). The first week after randomization, pain intensity and QOL scores were improved (pain intensity, $p <$ or $= 0.01$ for both groups; QOL, $p <0.001$ for both groups), with a more significant decrease in pain for the NCPB group ($p = 0.005$). Using repeated measures analysis, pain was found to be lower for NCPB over time ($p = 0.01$). However, opioid consumption ($p = 0.93$), frequency of opioid adverse effects (all $p>0.10$), and QOL ($p = 0.46$) were not significantly different between groups. In the first 6 weeks, fewer NCPB patients reported moderate or severe pain (pain intensity rating of$>$ or $= 5/10$) compared to opioid-only patients (14% vs. 40%, $p = 0.005$). At 1 year, 16% of NCPB patients and 6% of opioid-only patients were alive, but this was not a statistically significant difference.

While the previous study did not show a difference in life expectancy, a randomized, placebo-controlled study by Lillemoe[39] in patients with abdominal pain and unresectable pancreatic cancer demonstrated longer survival when an intraoperative chemical splanchnicectomy was performed, compared to patients who received saline. A subsequent study by Staats[47] involved additional follow-up and analysis of this same group of patients. Data on visual analog pain scores, mood, and interference with activity were collected preoperatively and every 2 months postoperatively until death. Univariate and multivariate analyses of variance showed that neurolysis, compared to the medical management, had a significant positive effect on mood scores, pain interference with activity, and had an associated increase in life expectancy (9.15+/−9.04 vs. 6.75+/−4.65 months, $p<0.05$).

SUPERIOR HYPOGASTRIC PLEXUS BLOCK

Visceral pain is common in advanced cervical, bladder, rectal, and prostate cancers. The superior hypogastric plexus is located anterior to the lower part of the L5 vertebral body and upper portion of the S1 vertebral body, posterior to the psoas fascia and peritoneum, and bounded laterally by the iliac vessels. This plexus innervates the pelvic viscera through the hypogastric nerves and inferior hypogastric plexus, and percutaneous blockade of this system (Fig. 44.6) can result in analgesia for cancer-related pelvic visceral pain. The plexus continues caudally to form the ganglion impar (this can be independently blocked to treat perineal pain) just anterior to the sacrococcygeal membrane.

The primary indication for superior hypogastric block is visceral pelvic pain that has been refractory to medical management. A local anesthetic block is typically performed first, and if good pain relief is obtained, a neurolytic block is then performed. The block is commonly performed using fluoroscopy and a bilateral posterior approach, and appropriate needle placement is confirmed with radiographic contrast. A single needle technique, traversing the L5–S1 intervertebral disc, has also been described in patients with difficult anatomy compromising the bilateral approach, with reportedly good outcomes and a favorable safety profile in a case series of eight patients.[48] No randomized studies have been published, but several prospective case series have consistently demonstrated good to excellent pain relief in over 70% of patients, reduced opioid consumption, and no significant adverse effects or complications.[49–52]

A study by Plancarte and colleagues[49] studied 227 pelvic cancer pain patients with gynecological, colorectal, or genitourinary cancer who experienced poor pain control despite the use of opioids. A bilateral percutaneous neurolytic superior hypogastric plexus block with 10% phenol was performed 1 day after a successful diagnostic block with 0.25% bupivacaine. All patients reported a VAS pain score of 7–10/10 before the diagnostic block. A positive response to a diagnostic block was obtained in 159 patients (79%). These patients then had a neurolytic block with a 72% (115/159 patients, 95% confidence interval of 65% to 79%) success rate, defined as a VAS<4/10. Sixteen (10%) of these 159 patients did require a second block if the first was suboptimal. The remaining 44 patients (28%) had moderate pain control (VAS 4–7/10) after two blocks and received supplemen-

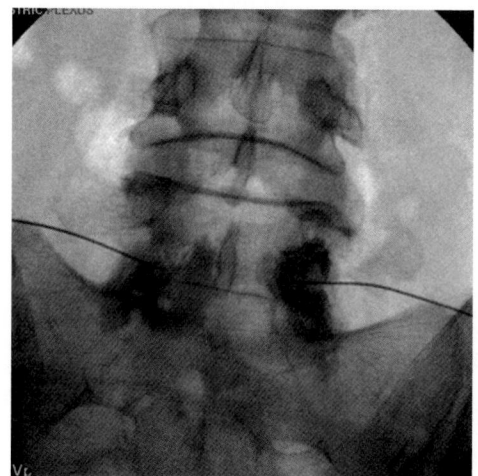
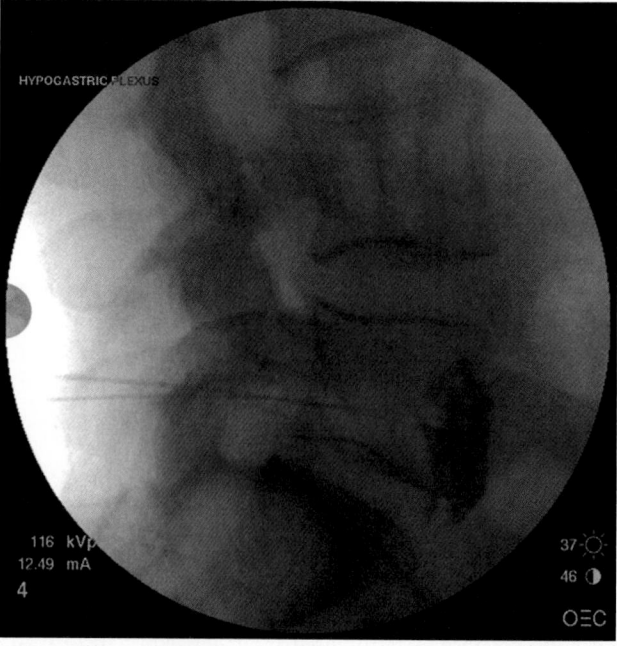

FIGURE 44.6 Anteroposterior (**A**) and lateral (**B**) fluoroscopic images of an appropriate needle position for a superior hypogastric plexus block for visceral pelvic pain. The needle tips are anterior to the anterolateral surface L5 with contrast spread in an appropriate plane to block the fibers of the plexus.

tary oral pharmacologic therapy and epidural analgesic therapy with good results. All patients experienced significant reductions in oral opioid therapy after the neurolytic blocks. No additional blocks were required by patients who had a positive response during the 3-month follow-up period. No complications related to the block were reported. This study concluded that neurolytic superior hypogastric plexus block provided both effective pain relief and a significant reduction in opioid usage (43% decrease) in 72% of the patients treated with neurolysis.

VERTEBROPLASTY AND KYPHOPLASTY

The percutaneous treatment of painful vertebral collapse secondary to metastatic tumor has emerged as a very promising therapy over the last decade. Metastatic spread to the skeleton is common, and 30% to 80% of bony metastases involve the vertebrae (see Chapter 46).[53] Vertebroplasty is a minimally invasive outpatient procedure whereby painful vertebral compression fractures are stabilized by the injection of the bone cement polymethyl methacrylate (PMMA). Access to the vertebral body is typically achieved by passing a specialized needle under fluoroscopic guidance through the pedicles bilaterally, as illustrated in Figure 44.7. Kyphoplasty differs in that the injection of cement is preceded by the attempted restoration of vertebral height by the inflation of a percutaneously placed intravertebral balloon. Kyphoplasty, compared to vertebroplasty, is technically more difficult, more uncomfortable for the patient, and considerably more expensive. However, kyphoplasty does attempt to reduce the vertebral collapse, and some authorities believe this is a worthwhile goal. A meta-analysis comparing vertebroplasty and kyphoplasty studies showed that vertebroplasty produced more significant pain relief, but had a higher risk of cement extravasation into the spinal canal.[54]

Indications

Vertebroplasty or kyphoplasty are indicated in an acute or subacute (<6 months) painful vertebral body pathologic (secondary to osteoporosis or tumor) fracture without the involvement of the spinal canal and its elements.[54,55] Careful clinical correlation between the pain symptoms and the radiographic findings should be established, as not all radiographically evident fractures are symptomatic. If there is doubt about the significance of a fracture, or in the presence of fractures at multiple levels, clinical correlation is often best achieved by examining the spine with the aid of fluoroscopy, while palpating or percussing the spinous process of the vertebrae in question to see if concordant pain can be elicited. In the case of a fracture involving the spinal canal, actual or impending neurologic deficits are best treated by a surgical approach with decompression and probable spinal fusion.

Contraindications

Absolute contraindications to vertebroplasty and kyphoplasty include asymptomatic stable fractures, clinically effective medical therapy, osteomyelitis of target vertebra, uncorrected coagulation disorders, allergy to any required component, and local or systemic infection. Relative contraindications include radicular pain or radiculopathy caused by a compressive syndrome unrelated to vertebral body collapse, a retropulsed fragment with >20% spinal canal compromise, tumor extension into epidural space, and severe vertebral body collapse (vertebra plana). The need for subsequent radiation to the area is not a contraindication, as

PMMA has been shown to be resilient to radiation at therapeutic doses.

Outcomes

Both vertebroplasty and kyphoplasty have consistently shown a significant improvement in postprocedure pain scores. In a meta-analysis by Eck et al.,[54] 168 eligible studies on vertebroplasty and kyphoplasty were assessed for their comparative analgesic efficacy and rates of complication. The mean pre- and postoperative VAS scores for vertebroplasty were 8.36 and 2.68, respectively, with a mean change of 5.68 ($p<0.001$). The mean pre- and postoperative VAS scores for kyphoplasty were 8.06 and 3.46, respectively, with a mean change of 4.60 ($p<0.001$). The pain reduction for vertebroplasty was noted to be statistically greater ($p<0.001$) compared with kyphoplasty. However, the risk of new vertebral fracture was 17.9% with vertebroplasty versus 14.1% with kyphoplasty ($p<0.01$), and the risk of cement leak was 19.7% with vertebroplasty versus 7.0% with kyphoplasty ($p<0.001$).

IMAGE-GUIDED ABLATION OF PAINFUL BONE METASTASES

Isolated bone pain secondary to metastatic tumor activity is typically treated with external beam radiation, analgesics (opioids and nonsteroidal anti-inflammatory agents), and systemic therapies including bisphosphonates, radiopharmaceuticals, corticosteroids, and chemotherapy (see Chapters 43, 46, and 48). A recent advance has been the use of radiologically-guided needle placement into selected painful metastases to provide thermal destruction using radiofrequency energy,[56] laser, and cryoablative[57,58] techniques. Another technique is percutaneous alcohol injection using selective arterial embolization[59] or direct tumor infiltration.[60]

A multicenter study by Goetz et al.[56] treated 43 patients who had failed standard therapy for painful osteolytic metastases with image-guided radiofrequency ablation. Ninety-five percent of patients had a clinically significant reduction in pain (visual analog scale decrease of ≥2, on a 10 point scale). Before treatment, the mean worst pain score was 7.9; after treatment, the average worst pain score was 4.5 ($p<0.0001$) at four weeks, 3.0 ($p<0.0001$) at 12 weeks, and 1.2 ($p<0.0005$) at 24 weeks. Pain interference scores and opioid consumption also improved during the 24 weeks of reported follow-up. Complications were seen in three patients; two were not serious, while one involved an acetabular fracture following radiofrequency ablation to this area.

OTHER TECHNIQUES

Numerous other innovative techniques have been described to control refractory cancer pain by interventional means. Neurosurgical pain control techniques are beyond the scope of this chapter, and are discussed elsewhere in this text (see Chapters 102–104). Spinal cord stimulation may be very useful in the treatment of neuropathic pain as seen in brachial plexus lesions or chemotherapy related peripheral neuropathy (see Chapters 94–96). Peripheral nerve chemical or radiofrequency neurolysis may have a role in cancer-related facial pain, extremity pain, and pain of selected dermatomes in the trunk (see Chapter 101). It is also worth mentioning that many cancer pain patients have a secondary component of myofascial pain that may be amenable

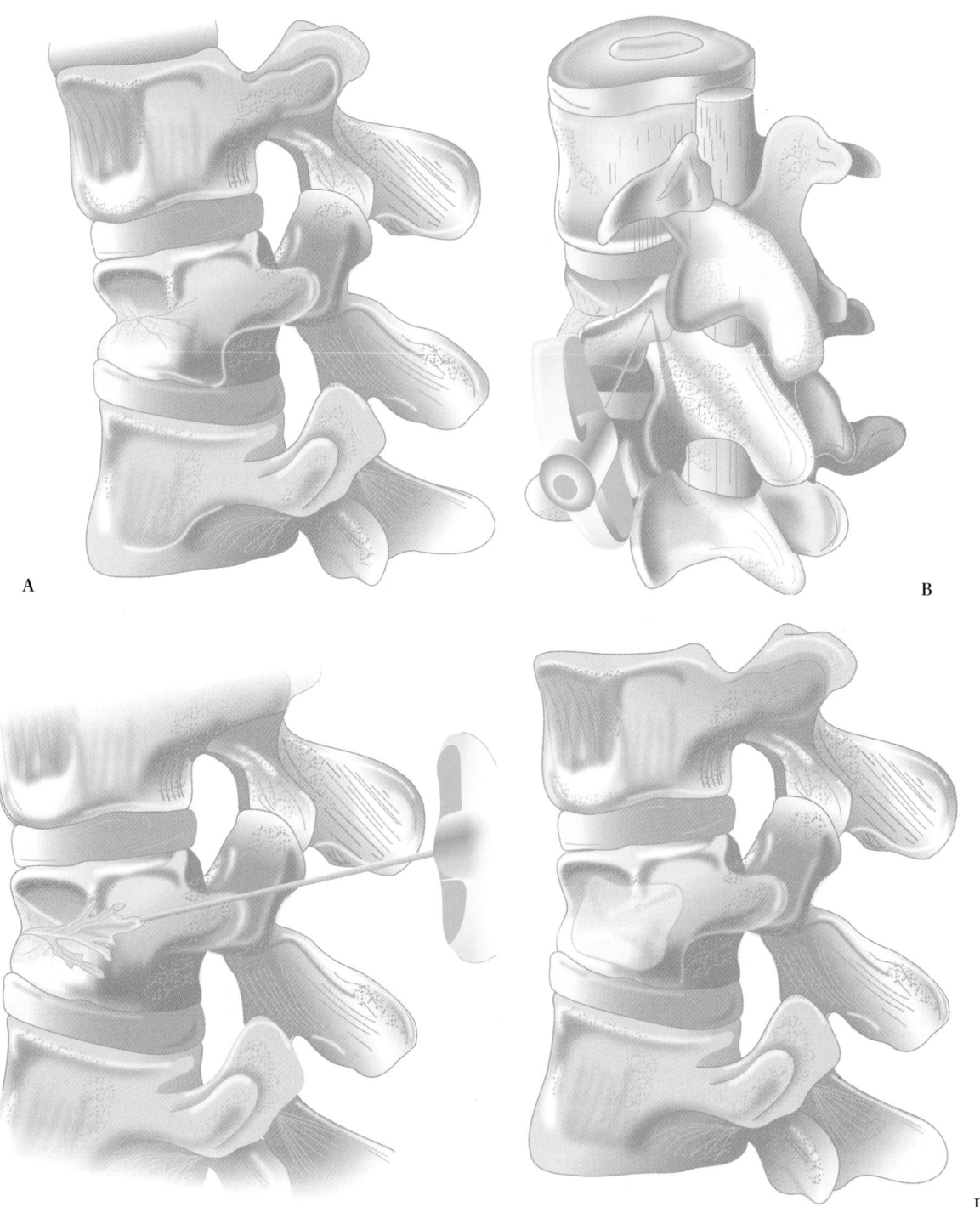

A

B

C

D

FIGURE 44.7 Vertebroplasty. **A.** Lateral projection of a lumbar vertebra with an anterior vertebral compression fracture. **B.** Oblique view illustrating a vertebroplasty canula in an appropriate position to traverse the pedicle and enter the vertebral body. **C.** Lateral projection demonstrating the canula tip appropriately placed in the vertebral body, and the injection of some cement. **D.** The completed vertebroplasty with the deposition of cement into the fracture site (redrawn courtesy of Stryker).

to trigger point injection and/or physical therapy before proceeding with more invasive techniques (see Chapter 35).

SUMMARY

Interventional therapies have a well-defined and beneficial role in the treatment of appropriately selected patients with various cancer pain syndromes. Optimizing outcomes depends upon timely referral with adequate assessment and patient selection; managing expectations of referring physicians, patients, and family members; assuring adequacy of postinterventional care; and an experienced, skilled interventionalist who will assume full responsibility for pre- and postintervention evaluation and follow-up care as indicated by the dictates of each patient's circumstances.

References

1. Cleeland CS, Gonin R, Hatfield AK, et al. Pain and its treatment in outpatients with metastatic cancer. *N Engl J Med* 1994;330(9):592–596.

2. Vainio A, Auvinen A. Prevalence of symptoms among patients with advanced cancer: an international collaborative study. Symptom Prevalence Group. *J Pain Symptom Manage* 1996;12(1):3–10.

3. Meuser T, Pietruck C, Radbruch L, et al. Symptoms during cancer pain treatment following WHO-guidelines: a longitudinal follow-up study of symptom prevalence, severity and etiology. *Pain* 2001;93(3):247–257.

4. Smith TJ, Staats PS, Deer T, et al. Randomized clinical trial of an implantable drug delivery system compared with comprehensive medical management for refractory cancer pain: impact on pain, drug-related toxicity, and survival. *J Clin Oncol* 2002;20(19):4040–4049.

5. Eisenberg E, Carr DB, Chalmers TC. Neurolytic celiac plexus block for treatment of cancer pain: a meta-analysis. *Anesth Analg* 1995;80(2):290–295.

6. Ackerman LL, Follett KA, Rosenquist RW. Long-term outcomes during treatment of chronic pain with intrathecal clonidine or clonidine/opioid combinations. *J Pain Symptom Manage* 2003;26(1):668–677.

7. Bard Access Systems. DuPen long-term epidural catheter. Available at: http://www.bardaccess.com/pdfs/ifus/ifu-dupen.pdf. Accessed .

8. Baker L, Lee M, Regnard C, et al. Evolving spinal analgesia practice in palliative care. *Palliat Med* 2004;18(6):507–515.

9. Nitescu P, Hultman E, Appelgren L, et al. Bacteriology, drug stability and exchange of percutaneous delivery systems and antibacterial filters in long-term intrathecal infusion of opioid drugs and bupivacaine in "refractory" pain. *Clin J Pain* 1992;8(4):324–337.

10. Bahar M, Rosen M, Vickers MD. Chronic cannulation of the intradural or extradural space in the rat. *Br J Anaesth* 1984;56(4):405–410.

11. Crul BJ, Delhaas EM. Technical complications during long-term subarachnoid or epidural administration of morphine in terminally ill cancer patients: a review of 140 cases. *Reg Anesth* 1991;16(4):209–213.

12. Bedder MD, Burchiel K, Larson A. Cost analysis of two implantable narcotic delivery systems. *J Pain Symptom Manage* 1991;6(6):368–373.

13. Smith TJ, Coyne PJ, Staats PS, et al. An implantable drug delivery system (IDDS) for refractory cancer pain provides sustained pain control, less drug-related toxicity, and possibly better survival compared with comprehensive medical management (CMM). *Ann Oncol* 2005;16(5):825–833.

14. Stearns L, Boortz-Marx R, Du Pen S, et al. Intrathecal drug delivery for the management of cancer pain: a multidisciplinary consensus of best clinical practices. *J Support Oncol* 2005;3(6):399–408.

15. Eisenach J, Detweiler D, Hood D. Hemodynamic and analgesic actions of epidurally administered clonidine. *Anesthesiology* 1993;78(2):277–287.

16. Rauck RL, Wallace MS, Leong MS, et al. A randomized, double-blind, placebo-controlled study of intrathecal ziconotide in adults with severe chronic pain. *J Pain Symptom Manage* 2006;31(5):393–406.

17. Horlocker TT, Wedel DJ, Benzon H, et al. Regional anesthesia in the anticoagulated patient: defining the risks (the second ASRA Consensus Conference on Neuraxial Anesthesia and Anticoagulation). *Reg Anesth Pain Med* 2003;28(3):172–197.

18. Follett KA, Boortz-Marx RL, Drake JM, et al. Prevention and management of intrathecal drug delivery and spinal cord stimulation system infections. *Anesthesiology* 2004;100(6):1582–1594.

19. Coffey RJ, Burchiel K. Inflammatory mass lesions associated with intrathecal drug infusion catheters: report and observations on 41 patients. *Neurosurgery* 2002;50(1):78–86; discussion 86–87.

20. Hassenbusch S, Burchiel K, Coffey RJ, et al. Management of intrathecal catheter-tip inflammatory masses: a consensus statement. *Pain Med* 2002;3(4):313–323.

21. Cousins M. In: Cousins MJ, Bridenbaugh PO, eds. *Neural Blockade in Clinical Anesthesia and Management of Pain.* 3rd ed. Philadelphia: Lippincott Williams & Wilkins, 1998:1022–1033.

22. Ferrer-Brechner T. Epidural and intrathecal phenol neurolysis for cancer pain. *Anesthesiol Rev* 1981;8:14–32.

23. Ferrer-Brechner T. Anesthetic techniques for the management of cancer pain. *Cancer* 1989;63(11 suppl):2343–2347.

24. Swerdlow M. Intrathecal neurolysis. *Anaesthesia* 1978;33(8):733–740.

25. Candido K, Stevens RA. Intrathecal neurolytic blocks for the relief of cancer pain. *Best Pract Res Clin Anaesthesiol* 2003;17(3):407–428.

26. Swerdlow M. Subarachnoid and extradural blocks. *Adv Pain Res Ther* 1979;2:325.

27. Ischia S, Luzzani A, Ischia A, et al. Subarachnoid neurolytic block (L5-S1) and unilateral percutaneous cervical cordotomy in the treatment of pain secondary to pelvic malignant disease. *Pain* 1984;20(2):139–149.

28. Ischia S, Luzzani A, Pacini L, et al. Lyric saddle block: clinical comparison of the results, using phenol at 5, 10, and 15 percent. *Adv Pain Res Ther* 1984;7:339.

29. Lifshitz S, Debacker LJ, Buchsbaum HJ. Subarachnoid phenol block for pain relief in gynecologic malignancy. *Obstet Gynecol* 1976;48(3):316–320.

30. de Oliveira R, dos Reis MP, Prado WA. The effects of early or late neurolytic sympathetic plexus block on the management of abdominal or pelvic cancer pain. *Pain* 2004;110:400–408.

31. Ward EM, Rorie DK, Nauss LA, et al. The celiac ganglia in man: normal anatomic variations. *Anesth Analg* 1979;58(6):461–465.

32. Rykowski JJ, Hilgier M. Efficacy of neurolytic celiac plexus block in varying locations of pancreatic cancer: influence on pain relief. *Anesthesiology* 2000;92(2):347–354.

33. De Cicco M, Matovic M, Balestreri L, et al. Single-needle celiac plexus block: is needle tip position critical in patients with no regional anatomic distortions? *Anesthesiology* 1997;87(6):1301–1308.

34. De Cicco M, Matovic M, Bortolussi R, et al. Celiac plexus block: injectate spread and pain relief in patients with regional anatomic distortions. *Anesthesiology* 2001;94(4):561–565.

35. De Conno F, Caraceni A, Aldrighetti L, et al. Paraplegia following coeliac plexus block. *Pain* 1993;55(3):383–385.

36. Woodham MJ, Hanna MH. Paraplegia after coeliac plexus block. *Anaesthesia* 1989;44(6):487–489.

37. Davies DD. Incidence of major complications of neurolytic coeliac plexus block. *J R Soc Med* 1993;86(5):264–266.

38. Ischia S, Ischia A, Polati E, et al. Three posterior percutaneous celiac plexus block techniques. A prospective, randomized study in 61 patients with pancreatic cancer pain. *Anesthesiology* 1992;76(4):534–540.

39. Lillemoe KD, Cameron JL, Kaufman HS, et al. Chemical splanchnicectomy in patients with unresectable pancreatic cancer. A prospective randomized trial. *Ann Surg* 1993;217(5):447–455, discussion 456–457.

40. Ischia S, Luzzani A, Ischia A, et al. A new approach to the neurolytic block of the coeliac plexus: the transaortic technique. *Pain* 1983;16(4):333–341.

41. Montero Matamala A, Vidal Lopez F, Inaraja Martinez L. The percutaneous anterior approach to the celiac plexus using CT guidance. *Pain* 1988;34(3):285–288.

42. Wiersema MJ, Wiersema LM. Endosonography-guided celiac plexus neurolysis. *Gastrointest Endosc* 1996;44(6):656–662.

43. Abedi M, Zfass AM. Endoscopic ultrasound-guided (neurolytic) celiac plexus block. *J Clin Gastroenterol* 2001;32(5):390–393.

44. Levy MJ, Topazian MD, Wiersema MJ, et al. Initial evaluation of the efficacy and safety of endoscopic ultrasound-guided direct ganglia neurolysis and block. *Am J Gastroenterol* 2008;103(1):98–103.

45. Mercadante S. Celiac plexus block versus analgesics in pancreatic cancer pain. *Pain* 1993;52(2):187–192.

46. Wong GY, Schroeder DR, Carns PE, et al. Effect of neurolytic celiac plexus block on pain relief, quality of life, and survival in patients with unresectable pancreatic cancer: a randomized controlled trial. *JAMA* 2004;291(9):1092–1099.

47. Staats PS, Hekmat H, Sauter P, et al. The effects of alcohol celiac plexus block, pain, and mood on longevity in patients with unresectable pancreatic cancer: a double-blind, randomized, placebo-controlled study. *Pain Med* 2001;2(1):28–34.

48. Ina H, Kobayashi MD, Imai S, et al. A new approach to the superior hypogastric plexus block: transvertebral disc (L5-S1) technique. *Reg Anesth* 1992;17(suppl 3):123.

49. Plancarte R, de Leon-Casasola OA, El-Helaly M, et al. Neurolytic superior hypogastric plexus block for chronic pelvic pain associated with cancer. *Reg Anesth* 1997;22(6):562–568.

50. Plancarte R, Amescua C, Patt RB, et al. Superior hypogastric plexus block for pelvic cancer pain. *Anesthesiology* 1990;73(2):236–239.

51. de Leon-Casasola OA, Kent E, Lema MJ. Neurolytic superior hypogastric plexus block for chronic pelvic pain associated with cancer. *Pain* 1993;54(2):145–151.

52. de Leon-Casasola OA, Plancarte-Sanchez R, Patt RB, et al. Superior hypogastric plexus block using a single needle and computed tomography guidance. *Reg Anesth* 1993;18(1):63.

53. Mercadante S. Malignant bone pain: pathophysiology and treatment. *Pain* 1997;69(1–2):1–18.

54. Eck JC, Nachtigall D, Humphreys SC, et al. Comparison of vertebroplasty and balloon kyphoplasty for treatment of vertebral compression fractures: a meta-analysis of the literature. *Spine J* 2008;8(3):488–497.

55. Heary RF, Bono CM. Metastatic spinal tumors. *Neurosurg Focus* 2001;11(6):e1.

56. Goetz MP, Callstrom MR, Charboneau JW, et al. Percutaneous image-guided radiofrequency ablation of painful metastases involving bone: a multicenter study. *J Clin Oncol* 2004;22(2):300–306.

57. Callstrom MR, Atwell TD, Charboneau JW, et al. Painful metastases involving bone: percutaneous image-guided cryoablation—prospective trial interim analysis. *Radiology* 2006;241(2):572–580.

58. Tuncali K, Morrison PR, Winalski CS, et al. MRI-guided percutaneous cryotherapy for soft-tissue and bone metastases: initial experience. *AJR Am J Roentgenol* 2007;189(1):232–239.

59. Chiras J, Adem C, Vallée JN, et al. Selective intra-arterial chemoembolization of pelvic and spine bone metastases. *Eur Radiol* 2004;14(10):1774–1780.

60. Gangi A, Kastler B, Klinkert A, et al. Injection of alcohol into bone metastases under CT guidance. *J Comput Assist Tomogr* 1994;18(6):932–935.

61. Lossignol DA, Obiols-Portis M, Body JJ. Successful use of ketamine for intractable cancer pain. *Support Care Cancer* 2005;13(3):188–193.

CHAPTER 45 ■ PAIN CAUSED BY CANCER OF THE HEAD AND NECK AND ORAL MUCOSITIS

JOEL B. EPSTEIN, MARK M. SCHUBERT, PRABHAT K. BHAMA, AND ERNEST A. WEYMULLER, JR.

INTRODUCTION

Head and neck pain in cancer patients may arise from a number of sources, including the cancer, therapy of the malignant disease, or it may be unrelated to the cancer or the cancer therapy (Table 45.1). One of the most common cancer-related, pain-producing conditions affecting the head and neck region is ulcerative oral mucositis that, when severe, can be a dose- and rate-limiting toxicity of cancer chemotherapy and radiotherapy and is the most debilitating patient-reported complication of many intensive cancer treatments. This chapter reviews the pathogenesis of mucositis mechanisms of pain in head and neck cancer, and current strategies for preventing and managing these painful conditions. Pain due to head and neck cancer and mucositis include multiple pathophysiological mechansims involved in other oncologic conditions that affect soft tissues, vascular, bone, and nervous system structures, including molecular mechanisms associated with reactive oxygen species, inflammatory mediators, neuropeptide release, and stimulation of receptors.[1-3] Phenotypic changes may occur, involving all levels of the sensory and autonomic nervous system, and are impacted by individual variables including genetic and psychosocial features. Understanding these mechanisms may lead to additional approaches to prevention and management.

TABLE 45.1

OROFACIAL PAIN IN CANCER PATIENTS

I. **Acute**
   1. Caused by disease: invasion of bone, nerve, muscle, mucosal damage; tumor pressure
   2. Caused by cancer therapy: surgery, radiation therapy, and chemotherapy
      a. Oral/dental pain: mucositis, infection (e.g., *Candida*, dental, HSV), neuropathy
   3. Unrelated conditions causing pain (e.g., myofascial pain, trauma)

II. **Chronic**
   1. Caused by persisting/progressive disease
   2. Caused by cancer therapy: surgery, radiation therapy, and chemotherapy
      a. Mucosal atrophy/xerostomia
      b. Mucosal infection
      c. Neuropathy
      d. Temporomandibular (myofascial) disorders
      e. Dental caries
      f. Osteonecrosis/mucosal necrosis
      g. Postherpetic neuralgia
   3. Unrelated conditions causing pain

HSV, herpes simplex virus.

PAIN MECHANISMS DUE TO LOCAL AND REGIONAL CANCER OF THE HEAD AND NECK

Tumor may compress and invade pain-sensitive structures and induce inflammation. Potential mechanisms of bone pain due to malignancy include periosteal pressure and stretching, compression and invasion of nerves, vascular damage, microfractures, and muscle spasm. Inflammatory mechanisms can be activated by both cancer and cancer treatments and include release of cytokines and other algogenic molecules that cause pain in the tumor environment of hypoxia and low pH. Tumors produce growth factors and cytokines that activate inflammation and nociceptive pathways. In head and neck cancer (HNC), inflammation is a major cause of pain,[2,3] initiated by reactive oxygen species (ROS), and release of mediators from tumor cells, circulating leukocytes, platelets, endothelial cells, and immune cells resident in the affected tissue and nerve fibers (sensory and sympathetic). ROS cause endothelial cell damage and increase vascular permeability, and nitric oxide (NO) induces second messenger mechanisms within neurons that may cause neuropathic pain. Further, oxidative stress activates transcription factors that cause upregulation of proinflammatory cytokines and may trigger apoptosis.

Tissue inflammation increases circulating kallikreins leading to production of bradykinin (BK) that produces pain and amplifies pain induced by serotonin (5HT). Glutamate is upregulated at sites of inflammation and affects amino-3-hydroxy-5-methyl-4-isoazolepropionic acid (AMPA), N-methyl-D-aspartate (NMDA), kainite, and metabotropic receptors. Furthermore, inflammation increases the expression and sensitivity of ion channels, such as sodium channels on nociceptors.

The low pH associated with solid tumors appears to be due to inflammation, tumor cell metabolism, and apoptosis or necrosis with release of cellular contents that may cause pain due to activation of sensory neurons through acid-sensing ion channels (ASICs). In addition, cancer-induced activation of osteoclasts results in lower pH for dissolution of bone mineral.

Tumor necrosis factor (TNF) is central in the activation of cytokines and growth factors and plays a role in inflammation, neuropathic pain, and is a key mediator in mucositis. Nerve growth factor (NGF) production is mediated by interleukin (IL)-1β and is upregulated by TNF-α. NGF activates cutaneous mast cells, leading to release of inflammatory mediators that induce pain and may also activate the sympathetic nervous system. Norepinephrine (NE) causes hyperalgesia at sites of tissue injury.

Prostaglandins (PG) synthesized by cyclo-oxygenase pathways (COX-1 and COX-2) are induced in peripheral tissues by inflammatory cytokines and growth factors. Increased levels of PGs are seen in loco-regional tumors and in metastases. PGs cause sensitization of afferents including C-polymodal nociceptors and A-δ high-threshold mechano-nociceptors and mediate hyperalgesia induced by BK and NE. COX-2 is upregulated in head and neck cancers and in mucositis.[4]

Modulation of nerve input and transmission involves presynaptic modulation of the primary signal by excitatory and inhibitory input from adjacent neurons and from descending pathways. Second order neurons and central pathways are also subject to modulation from higher centers. Modulation is mediated by interaction with receptors including AMPA, NMDA, and by neurotransmitters including substance P (SP), serotonin (5-HT), NE-A, opioid, cholecystokinin (CCK), and gamma-aminobutyric acid (GABA). Modulation is impacted by stress, learned behavior, and acute pain. Perception of pain is impacted by attention, expectation, anxiety, and depression. Mucosal changes, hyposalivation, tissue fibrosis, neurovascular changes, and recurrent cancer and secondary complications of cancer or therapy may result in chronic pain.

Neuropathic pain may result from insult to the peripheral nervous system (PNS) and/or the central nervous system (CNS), including alteration in sensory and sympathetic fibers, and may result in peripheral sensitization and central sensitization. Surgery or cytotoxic agents may lead to neuropathy due to nerve damage via crush, pressure, cut, or inflammation, resulting in ectopic firing and changes in receptive field that lead to nerve excitability and spontaneous activity (wind-up). Persistent input may also result in increased receptive fields in second order neurons and centrally. Neuronal hyperexcitability may be due to overexpression of sodium channels and activation of the NMDA receptor, which develops at voltage gated sodium channels (VGSCs).

Interactions between the sympathetic nervous system and nociceptors are thought to be associated with some of the findings in neuropathic pain. Injured C-fiber terminals may atrophy and be replaced by A-β fibers that sprout into the superficial layers of the dorsal horn and may contribute to sensory abnormalities following peripheral nerve injuries. SP in A-β fibers may be increased and lead to pain.

In addition to neuronal sensitization, TNF-α, IL-6, and IL-11 promote osteoclast formation and likely play a role in malignant bone pain. The effects of IL-1 are probably mediated by induction of NO, BK,[156] and PGs. Endothelin-1 (ET-1) may be a cause of pain in cancer involving bone. Prevention and treatment of pain based on increased understanding of pathogenesis may lead to novel approaches and improved patient outcomes.

PAIN MECHANISMS DUE TO CHEMOTHERAPY AND/OR RADIOTHERAPY

Peripheral neurotoxicity is common with a number of chemotherapeutic agents, including vinca alkaloids (vincristine, vindesine, and vinblastine). Platinum agents, including cisplatin, induce neuronal apoptosis and may lead to damage or loss of large myelinated sensory fibers; in addition, NGF and induction of lysosomal storage defects have been shown in the dorsal root ganglion (DRG). The taxanes (paclitaxel, docetaxel) cause microtubular aggregation and may increase the risk of neurotoxicity when combined with platinum agents. Other agents including noncytostatic drugs used in cancer treatment (e.g., interferon, thalidomide) or in supportive care (e.g., amphotericin-B) may also induce sensory neuropathies. Additive effects may occur from combinations of drugs.

Treatment of neuropathy generally focuses on use of centrally acting medications.[5,6] Unfortunately, strategies for prevention of neuropathy have not been documented. Amifostine and lipoic acid have been assessed in the prevention of neurotoxicity caused by platinum agents.[7,8] Melatonin was shown in one clinical trial to reduce chemotherapy induced neurotoxicity[9] and the potential role of glutamine has been examined.[10,11] Continuing study of approaches to prevent and manage neurotoxicity are needed.

Bisphosphonates are key pharmaceuticals for the treatment of malignant disease involving bone and are commonly employed for patients with multiple myeloma and metastatic breast, prostate, lung, and colon cancers. Benefits of bisphosphonate therapy include prevention of skeletally related events, hypercalcemia of cancer, and reducing bone pain associated with malignancy. Bisphosphonates inhibit osteoclast activity and thus reduce resorption of bone associated with both normal remodeling and malignancy-related bone resorption. One of the acute side effects associated with bisphosphonate administration can be bone pain, including mandible pain that may be somewhat vague, but can occasionally mimic dental pain. Since late 2002, bisphosphonates have become recognized as being associated with nonhealing bony lesions involving dentoalveolar bone. In cancer patients on bisphosphonates, the most frequent risk factor for bisphosphonate-associated osteonecrosis (BON) is dental surgery (e.g., extractions, periodontal surgery).[12–17] Pain associated with BON, when present, is usually associated with secondary infection of the soft tissues surrounding the areas of exposed bone.[154,155] Chronic BON can spread to involve nerve bundles (e.g., the inferior alveolar nerve) and produce nerve pain and numbness.

PAIN DUE TO SURGERY

Pain is a common complaint at the time of diagnosis in patients with head and neck cancer,[18] although of mild severity (visual analogue scale [VAS] ~3/10).[19] Surgical extirpation may alleviate pain, but more often, following treatment for head and neck cancer, pain increases and generally improves subsequently.[20] Furthermore, surgery on the neck is associated with shoulder and arm pain.[18]

Wittekindt et al. demonstrated that subcutaneous botulinum toxin A injections may reduce chronic neuropathic pain following neck dissection.[21] It has been theorized that the etiology of myofascial trigger points is excessive release of acetylcholine at motor end plates.[22] Botulinum toxin A achieves pain relief by preventing acetylcholine release at the neuromuscular junction. Although effective in neck dissection patients, it is unclear if this strategy has any benefit for patients who have not undergone neck dissection.

Spread of disease to regional lymph nodes is a crucial prognostic factor in head and neck cancer.[23] Treatment for cervical metastasis traditionally included radical resection of all lymph-bearing tissues in the neck, including removal of lymph nodes from levels I to V, the sternocleidomastoid (SCM) muscle, internal jugular vein (IJV), and spinal accessory nerve (SAN). This operation is known as the *radical neck dissection*, and was originally described by Crile in 1906.[24]

Based on recent studies, neck dissection has been found to have a negative impact on quality of life (QOL) and health status.[25–29] Moreover, it has been demonstrated that more extensive neck dissections are associated with higher shoulder-related disability.[27,28,30,31] Fortunately, over the latter half of the 20th century, neck dissection has evolved from solely radical neck dissection to include more conservative approaches. This has positively influenced the QOL in patients who have neoplastic disease requiring neck dissection.

The presence of shoulder and neck pain after neck dissection has been shown to be a common cause of postoperative morbidity in patients with head and neck cancer.[32] It has been postulated that mechanical overload of the shoulder secondary to change in scapular position and lack of stabilization after trapezius denervation leads to shoulder pain.[33] However, it has been demonstrated that even with preservation of the SAN, patients can have shoulder pain.[34] Moreover, pain following surgery may often be caused by tissue injury sustained during the procedure.[35]

Recently, attention has been given to the preservation of cervical sensory nerves and the effect this has on QOL. Roh and colleagues conducted a retrospective cohort study of 53 patients who underwent selective or modified radical neck dissection. The results of the study suggest that cervical sensory root branch preservation during neck dissection reduces postoperative pain and permanent sensory deficits. Additionally, the study found that dissection of level V nodal tissue (the posterior triangle of the neck) is associated with neck pain and shoulder pain.[36]

PAIN DUE TO MUCOSITIS

Oral mucositis is a frequent complication of cancer chemotherapy and radiotherapy. A five-stage model for oral mucositis has been proposed where ROS are generated during the initial phase[37–40] that results in cell damage and triggers secondary mediators, including nuclear factor-κB (NFkB) in the epithelium and connective tissue. Following upregulation of NFkB, pro-inflammatory cytokines such as TNFα, IL-1β, and IL-6 are generated, which can induce hyperalgesia. NO may also be a key factor producing pain. The ceramide pathway has been implicated in the amplification of oral mucositis and may modulate pain. Mucositis ulcerations can become secondarily colonized/infected by oral flora and further increase cytokine release and, thus, increase mucosal pain.

In addition to mucosal damage, radiation therapy damages bone by killing osteocytes, osteoclasts, and osteoblasts, and irreversibly damages endothelial cells in the vasculature throughout the radiated volume. This results in chronic hypocellular, hypovascular, and hypoxic oral soft tissue, leading to risk of soft tissue necrosis and osteonecrosis. Pain from radiation necrosis involves inflammatory and neuropathic mechanisms (see previous text) and is increased in the presence of secondary infection.

Epidemiology

Mucositis is the most common cause of oral pain during intensive treatment of cancer involving chemotherapy, radiation, or chemoradiotherapy[41–69] (Table 45.2). Oral mucositis is a common complication of myeloablative conditioning regimens used in hematopoietic cell transplant (HCT) and is virtually universal in patients treated with tumoricidal radiation therapy that includes the oropharynx. The increasing use of combined chemotherapy and radiation treatment modalities and more aggressive therapy protocols to improve cancer cure rates has increased the frequency and severity of oral complications. Changes in management include increased use of combined radiation and chemotherapy, and hyperfractionation of radiation therapy, which may result in increased toxicity.[41,43,44,46,49,52,54,57,62,69] The potential impact of targeted monoclonal antibodies and other tumor-specific targeting molecules upon mucositis is not documented, and it is not known if usage in combination with other chemotherapy may increase mucosal damage. Studies that assess mucositis as a primary or secondary outcome with targeted agents have not been conducted,[70,71] although the pattern of oral mucosal involvement and dermatologic involvement appears different than seen in traditional chemotherapy, suggesting that different mechanisms may be involved.

Advances in medical management of patients receiving intensive cancer therapies, including use of antimicrobial prophylaxis and therapy and the use of growth factors to speed hematopoietic recovery, has sharpened the focus on oral mucositis as a significant and treatment-limiting complication in cancer therapy.[72–74] Oral mucositis is also often coincident with therapy-related toxicity at other sites, including veno-occlusive disease in HCT[69] and gastrointestinal toxicity.[75] The potential for systemic infection caused by oral opportunistic and acquired flora associated with oral mucositis has been documented in several studies of leukemia and HCT patients.[76–80]

Pathogenesis

Intensive cytotoxic chemotherapy and radiation therapy directly affect the proliferation of epithelial cells and connective tissue elements leading to damage to the epithelium and submucosal tissues and potentially to loss of the mucosal barrier (Fig. 45.1 and Table 45.3). Epidermal growth factor (EGF) secretion may increase the risk of mucositis[81] and, conversely, cytokines that reduce epithelial cell proliferation have the potential to decrease the severity of tissue damage. Interaction with cytokines produced in the connective tissue such as granulocyte-macrophage colony stimulating factor (GM-CSF), TNF, IL-6 and IL-11, and others may affect tissue damage.[72–75,82,83] The oral microflora may play a role in progression of mucosal damage, as suggested in studies of gram-negative bacterial flora in radiation-induced

TABLE 45.2

FREQUENCIES OF ORAL PAIN ASSOCIATED WITH CANCER THERAPY

Acute pain during treatment	
Oropharyngeal mucositis	
Chemotherapy	15% to 70%
Bone marrow transplant	50% to 85%
Radiation therapy	Up to 100%
Postsurgical therapy	Up to 100%
Chronic pain following cancer therapy	
Mucosal pain	Up to 33%
Pain associated with mucosal infection	
Candidiasis	
After stem cell transplant	Up to 50%
After radiation therapy	20% to 33%
Herpes simplex in seropositive stem cell transplant patients	Up to 90%
Neuropathy	16%
TMD/myofascial (patients with head and neck squamous cell carcinoma)	25% to 30%

TMD, temporomandibular disorder.

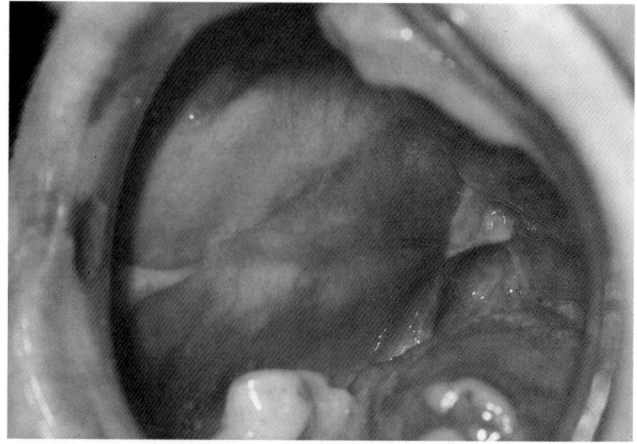

FIGURE 45.1 Mild mucositis with erythema and minor erosion of the cheek mucosa in a patient following autologous bone marrow transplant (at day +14). Mild mouth discomfort was reported.

TABLE 45.3

FACTORS CONTRIBUTING TO OROPHARYNGEAL MUCOSITIS

Direct factors	Indirect factors
Radiation therapy	Myelosuppression
Dose/fraction	Immunosuppression
Total dose/days	T-cell loss/dysfunction
Chemotherapy	B-cell loss/dysfunction
Drug/dose/schedule	Reduced secretory
Bone marrow transplant	immunoglobulin A
Chemotherapy	Infections
Irradiation	Bacterial
Salivary gland dysfunction	Plaque control
Mucosal trauma	Viral
Physical	Herpes simplex
Chemical	Varicella zoster
Thermal	Cytomegalovirus
Microbial flora	Other
Graft-versus-host disease	Fungal
Manifestations	
Prophylaxis	
Therapy	
Patient susceptibility	

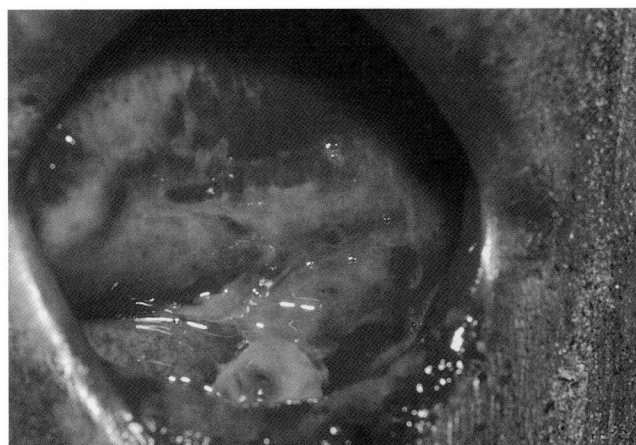

FIGURE 45.2 Severe ulcerated mucositis in a patient receiving an unrelated donor bone marrow transplant (day + 14) requiring systemic opioid analgesic.

mucositis. The outcomes of microflora-induced mucosal damage are influenced by the potential effect of cancer therapies on the hematopoietic system and, ultimately, damage to local and systemic immune function. Resolution of mucositis may be dependent on production of pluripotential growth factors affecting epithelial and connective tissues.[52,72–75] During resolution, cytokines inducing epithelial cell proliferation and migration and angiogenesis play a role.[52,84–90] Pain associated with mucositis is dependent on the degree of tissue damage, sensitization of nociceptors, and elaboration of inflammatory and pain mediators.

In head and neck cancer treated with radiation, pain intensity and pain interference scores directly correspond to mucositis and increase at week 3, often peak at week 5, and persist for weeks following the end of treatment. Concurrent chemoradiotherapy and intensified radiation protocols increase the severity and duration of oral mucositis.[91–93] However, marked improvement may be seen through 12 months posttreatment, with general functional and physical appearance measures returning toward baseline level. Follow-up of oropharyngeal cancer patients (up to 1 year) treated with radiation showed that pain is common (58.4%) and interfered with daily activities in approximately one-third of subjects.[94]

Hematopoietic Cell Transplant

Ulcerative mucositis is the most debilitating patient-reported toxicity of HCT and treatment for hematologic cancer.[54,55,60,62] Mucositis is compounded in patients with herpes simplex virus (HSV) reactivation and in those with poor oral hygiene.[53,60,65,66,95] HSV prophylaxis has altered the frequency and severity of mucosal ulceration due to HSV in HCT patients; however, even in patients given acyclovir prophylaxis, oral ulcerative mucositis occurs in up to 75% of patients.[55]

Mucositis symptoms can be increased in HCT patients with xerostomia[63] and the related oral microflora and dental plaque changes may influence the severity of mucositis.[95–101] Intensive oral hygiene has been documented to reduce the severity and duration of oral mucositis.[95] Studies have demonstrated that approximately 48% of bacteremia in the early period post-HCT

are associated with oral bacteria. Some providers are concerned about the risk of bacteremia and gingival bleeding due to brushing and flossing during the first 3 weeks post-HCT; however, septicemia is not increased in patients who continued intensive oral care.[95] Immunoglobulins and other antimicrobial proteins in the saliva are decreased after HCT conditioning, which may be an additional factor in the increased risk of mucosal infection.[75]

Clinically, oral mucositis for autologous HCT patients becomes evident approximately 2 to 5 days after marrow infusion (day + 2 to 5) with resolution in more than 90% of patients by day + 15.[55] Allogeneic HCT patients will generally show a slightly slower onset and slower resolution of mucositis. Damage to the mucosa most often presents in a bilateral pattern, primarily involving the nonkeratinized mucosa of the cheeks, lateral and ventral surfaces of the tongue, floor of the mouth, soft palate, and labial mucosa. The mucosal reaction may begin shortly after exposure to the conditioning regimen and progress to erythema and ulceration (Fig. 45.2; also see Fig. 45.1). Increased mucosal toxicity is usually seen in patients additionally conditioned for HCT with total body irradiation.[62,64,72]

Head and Neck Radiation Therapy

Tumor-related pain is commonly present at the time of diagnosis of head and neck and oral cancer (85%), although the intensity is usually not severe.[58,102] The presence and severity of pain are related to tumor stage and with bone involvement.[58] Pain occurs with treatment in all patients treated for oropharyngeal cancer and increases in severity throughout the course of radiation and persists after treatment.[41,58,67,68] Radiotherapy-related mucositis is the most frequent complication in patients during irradiation for head and neck cancers (see Table 45.1). Mucositis affects the oral tissues included in the fields of irradiation (Figs. 45.3 and 45.4). Mucositis-related pain increases during radiation treatment, and typically resolves within 1 to 2 months, or longer with combined radiation and chemotherapy. However, mucosal discomfort often continues for 6 to 12 months or longer, although the severity of pain decreases over time after treatment.[58] Chronic complaints include mucosal sensitivity attributed to mucosal atrophy (33%), musculoskeletal syndromes (temporomandibular disorder) (25%), and neurologic syndromes attributed to deafferentation (16%).[58] In another study, the most common persisting complaints after radiation treatment included xerostomia (57%), jaw pain involving the muscles of the jaw or joint pain (27%), and a 10% increased rate of dental caries.[103] Chronic complica-

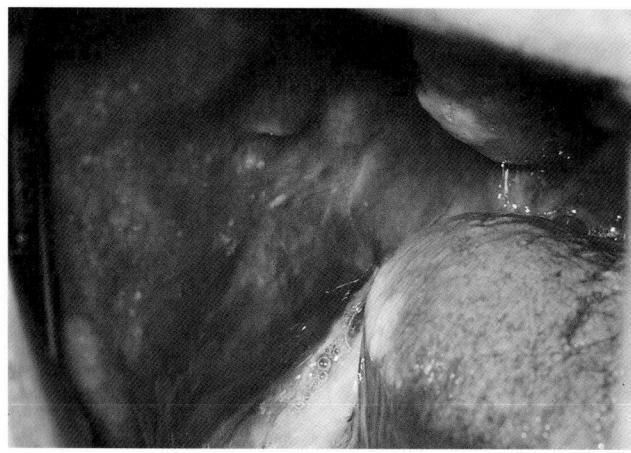 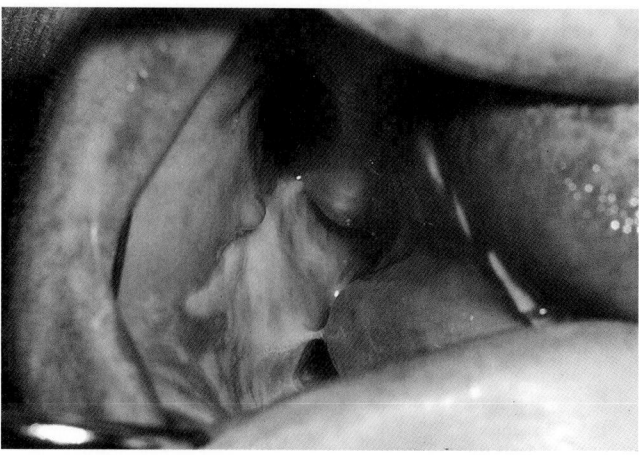

A   B

FIGURE 45.3 (A) Initial tissue reaction in a patient receiving radiation therapy (dose received 1400 cGy of planned 6000 cGy) resulting in erythema and sensitivity of the right buccal mucosa. (B) Late tissue reaction in the same patient receiving radiation therapy (total dose received 6000 cGy) resulting in oral pain and mucosal ulceration within the radiation field.

tions of radiation therapy were assessed in 676 head and neck cancer patients treated in a multicenter study and 11% had severe complications (grade 3 or 4) involving the oral mucosa, bone, or muscle.[104] These late complications were related to total radiation dose, complications in bone were more common with large radiation fields, and complications in bone and muscle were related to radiation fraction size. The severity of chronic mucosal damage may relate to severity of acute mucosal reaction.

Combined Radiation Therapy, Surgery, and/or Chemotherapy

Treatment of locally advanced head and neck carcinoma is associated with significant treatment complications affecting oral function. Hyperfractionated radiotherapy and chemotherapy improve survival, but treatment is frequently limited by the severity of oral toxicity.[41,44,46,57,105,106] Severe oral mucositis occurs in essentially all patients treated with accelerated fractionated irradiation for supraglottic cancer[1] and in those treated with combined chemotherapy and radiation therapy.[105,106] Severe mucositis may

cause considerable pain, limit or prevent oral intake, and may lead to suspension of cancer therapy.[41,106] Changes in the delivery of radiotherapy, including increasing total dose, hyperfractionation, accelerated therapy, and the combination of radiation therapy and chemotherapy, have increased the severity and duration of mucositis. Intensity modulated radiation therapy (IMRT) may not decrease ulcerated mucositis and symptoms, even though the volume of severe reaction may be reduced.[93] Mucosal reactions in patients receiving radiation treatment for head and neck cancer are currently regarded as unavoidable side effects but advances in knowledge of pathogenesis and new therapy is expected to change this view, with prophylaxis, intervention, and improved symptom management.

The importance of fungal colonization and infection in radiation mucositis is not clearly defined.[107–109] One study showed fewer cases of candidiasis in patients on fluconazole and half the number of breaks in radiation therapy than those not provided prophylaxis with fluconazole.[107] However, others have not found an association between candidiasis or oral colonization and mucositis during cancer therapy.[107,109]

Targeted chemotherapy with monoclonal antibodies and small molecules are becoming part of therapy. The impact on mucositis is not well defined, as mucositis has only been recorded with multiple toxicities and no studies have assessed mucositis using a validated scale as a primary or secondary endpoint. However, the available data suggest that oral mucositis is not more common than that seen with standard therapy and, in fact, it may occur less frequently and be less severe.[70,71,110–116] Approximately 90% of patients develop oral pain during HCT.[56]

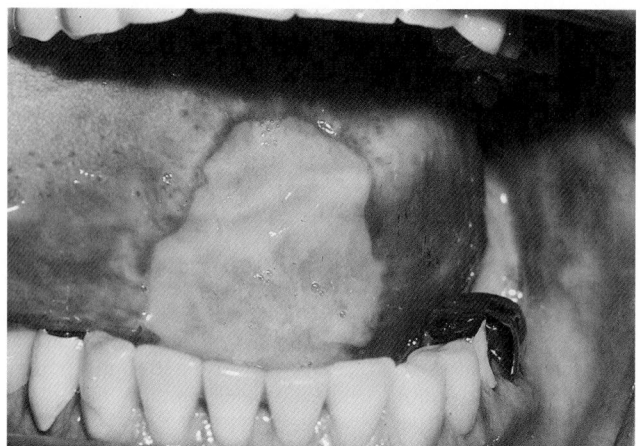

FIGURE 45.4 Localized ulcerative mucositis following brachytherapy for a squamous cell carcinoma of the middle portion of the lateral border of the tongue.

PAIN ASSESSMENT

Most studies use a VAS or 5- or 10-point scales to assess oral pain or the McGill Pain Questionnaire.[56,117] The McGill Pain Questionnaire was compared with two different factor models in patients with oral mucositis pain after HCT, and it was recommended that a single pain rating may provide a better practical measurement.[117] Many patients may be unable or unwilling to complete lengthy questionnaires, particularly when their overall condition including pain is at its worst. Notwithstanding analgesic use, most of the variance in pain report is explained by the severity of the mucositis rather than psychosocial variables.[51]

MANAGEMENT OF ORAL MUCOSITIS

Wide variation exists in quality of mucositis prevention and management studies. Many enroll a small number of patients, using outcome measures that are not validated, and may lack sensitivity. This makes assessment of outcomes difficult, mandating careful review of the methods employed in every study before generalizable conclusions can be drawn. Guidelines for the use of outcome measures and more refined study design and protocols in the management of mucositis are improving the value of more recent studies. Evidence-based guidelines[118–120] have been developed to provide guidance and will continue to evolve as new approaches to prevention and management are studied.

Development of strategies for the prevention and management of oral mucositis has been enhanced by an improved understanding of the multifactorial nature of the condition (Table 45.4). Radiation shields are recommended during standard radiation therapy. The use of midline mucosa-sparing blocks for protection of the mucosa during radiation therapy, thereby reducing mucositis, resulted in less weight loss, fewer hospitalizations for nutritional support, and a trend toward fewer treatment interruptions ($p = 0.07$) than in control patients.[48] The impact of IMRT on oral mucositis pain is not well understood, with reduced area of

TABLE 45.4

PREVENTION AND MANAGEMENT OF ORAL MUCOSITIS

Pretreatment oral/dental stabilization
Eliminate sites of infection, trauma
Dental cleaning
Good oral hygiene
Saline mouth rinses

Antimicrobial approaches
Systemic antimicrobials
Antibiotics
Antivirals acyclovir, valacyclovir, ganciclovir
Antifungal fluconazole
Topical antimicrobials
Chlorhexidine
Antimicrobial lozenges (polymyxin, tobramycin, amphotericin)

Anti-inflammatory approaches
Topical agents
Prostaglandins
Benzydamine
Corticosteroids

Biologic response modifiers
Granulocyte-macrophage colony stimulating factor
Granulocyte-colony stimulating factor
Epidermal growth factor
Transforming growth factor, interleukin-11

Miscellaneous approaches
Good oral hygiene
Saline/bicarbonate mouth rinses
Low-energy lasers
Mucosal coating agents
Vitamin supplements
Anticholinergic agents (xerogenergic agents)
Modification in cancer treatment protocols

severe tissue damage, but broader areas of low dose radiation exposure.[93]

Kepivance (palifermin; Biovitrum, Inc., Stockholm, Sweden) is the only approved agent for prevention of oral mucositis in HCT.[14,121] Further study of patients with metastatic colon cancer treated with fluorouracil-based chemotherapy showed benefit of Kepivance reducing mucositis,[122] suggesting broader potential application than currently indicated. Clinical trials to determine the prevention of mucositis in patients receiving head and neck radiation are currently under way. Benzydamine (not available in the U.S.) is recommended for use in patients receiving radiotherapy (>220 cGY/day). Oral cryotherapy is recommended for prevention of mucositis in those receiving bolus 5-FU or edatrexate treatments, or high-dose melphalan conditioning regimens for HCT. Low-energy lasers have been studied in the prevention and management of mucositis associated with HCT and head and neck radiation with consistent findings across studies.[123–125] The mechanism of action may be due to effects of cytokine release following laser exposure and enhanced epithelial cell growth, but further study is needed. Low-energy laser for prevention of mucositis has shown consistent results and further study is needed to determine the optimal delivery for clinical use.

PAIN MANAGEMENT

With only a small number of approaches documented to prevent the incidence or shorten the duration of oral mucositis, management of oral mucositis depends on palliative approaches. The use of a *stepped protocol* for pain management is currently the most appropriate approach. The elements of this protocol include the progressive utilization of: (1) basic oral care, (2) bland rinses, (3) topical anesthetic and mucosal coating agents, and (4) systemic analgesics.

Basic Oral Care

A growing body of evidence is being accrued that supports the importance of maintaining oral care protocols to remove bacterial dental plaque from teeth and periodontal tissues during intensive cancer therapies.[118,119] Patients should maintain good oral hygiene by brushing, flossing, and possibly using antimicrobial products.

Bland Oral Rinses

Although there are no studies demonstrating the effectiveness of normal saline or bicarbonate rinses in decreasing mucositis, they have been shown to reduce mucosal pain.[126,127] Frequent use of bland rinses can provide relief for mild mucositis, help remove debris, and moisturize mucosal surfaces. In a study of 40 patients undergoing radiotherapy to more than 50% of the oral cavity, half were randomized to an oral care protocol using either saline or hydrogen peroxide rinses, and the latter was associated with increased mucosal sensitivity.[128]

Topical Anesthetics and Analgesics

Topical anesthetics represent the next step up in the strategy to manage mucositis pain. While there are no studies specifically examining efficacy of various topical anesthetic agents, any agent that can be safely applied to oral mucosa to induce topical numbness that is tolerated by the patient can be used.[61] Lidocaine viscous solution is frequently recommended, but other agents that can be used include benzocaine, dyclonine, and diphenhydramine. Topical anesthetics can cause mild initial irritation, obtund taste, and diminish the gag reflex if gargled or swallowed. Swallowing of these agents to control pharyngeal pain is not generally recommended due to possible systemic side effects and toxicities if swallowed in large doses. Benzydamine has been shown to reduce mucositis and associated oral pain in radiation-induced mucositis by initially producing an anesthetic effect, but with an extended analgesic effect.[61,68] Local applications of topical anesthetic creams or gels may be especially useful for local painful mucosal ulcerations.

Topical analgesics have shown effect in mucositis pain. Initial studies of topical morphine show pain reduction in oral mucositis,[129] and doxepin in single and multidose studies has shown extended duration pain relief without burning sensation when applied to ulcerated tissue.[130]

Coating agents used as oral rinses in patients with mucositis, such as milk of magnesia and loperamide have been recommended frequently, but have not been subjected to controlled studies.[61,118] Sucralfate suspension has been studied in mucositis,[131–134] but results have been inconsistent and its use for radiation or chemotherapy mucositis are not supported.

A number of mucosal coating agents or rinses have been licensed by the FDA for the management of oral mucositis, including Gelclair (EKR Therapeutics, Bedminster, NJ), MuGard (Access Pharmaceuticals, Inc., Dallas, TX), and Caphosol (EUSA Pharma, Inc., Langhorne, PA). However, there is no or insufficient evidence to recommend their use for prevention of mucositis.[135,136]

Topical Antimicrobials

Early studies suggested that topical antimicrobials may have utility in preventing oral mucositis, but follow-up research has failed to provide evidence to support their use for prevention of mucositis.[118] Chlorhexidine has been assessed in HCT patients in a number of studies but conflicting results with its use in mucositis have been seen. The majority of follow-up studies do not demonstrate a prophylactic effect on mucositis.[137] It is important to note that the effectiveness of chlorhexidine rinsing on plaque levels, gingival inflammation, and caries risk have not been endpoints in these studies, and the use of chlorhexidine for bacterial plaque control during cancer therapy may still be useful.

Studies of antimicrobial lozenges combining agents such as polymyxin, tobramycin, and amphotericin B in head and neck radiation therapy was shown in a single center trial to be effective.[138] However, follow-up studies to duplicate the benefit of using either topical antimicrobials or b-defensin, while showing effectiveness in reducing oral microbial colonization, did not significantly impact on mucositis.[139–142]

Analgesics

Symptom management for oral mucositis often requires the use of systemic analgesics. Mucositis is the most common condition requiring the use of systemic opioid analgesics during cancer therapy.[45] A wide range of agents can be used including acetaminophen, nonsteroidal anti-inflammatory agents (NSAIDs), and opioids.

Systemic analgesics should be prescribed following the World Health Organization (WHO) analgesic ladder.[61] These recommendations include the use of nonopioid analgesics alone, or in combination with opioids and adjunctive medications, based on pain severity and effectiveness of therapy (see Chapter 39). In patients with oral mucositis pain, topical approaches should be used initially and should continue to be used in combination with systemic analgesics in order that the best pain management can be achieved with the least potent and lowest doses of systemic pain medications. Studies have shown that optimum pain control may be achieved by moving directly from WHO ladder level I analgesics to titrated doses of WHO ladder level III analgesics. Improvement in pain control is achieved by combining level III analgesics with adjuvants at lower total doses of analgesics, and therefore modification of the analgesic ladder has been discussed.[143]

A number of different delivery methods can be used for mucositis pain control. Oral, transmucosal, transdermal (patches), intravenous, and suppository routes can be used. Patient-controlled analgesia (PCA) is recommended in pain management for hospitalized cancer patients with severe mucositis.[144] A study of preteen children receiving HCT assessed morphine or hydromorphone PCA for mucositis or other painful conditions found that children successfully mastered PCA to control pain associated with HCT.[45] No instance of drug overdose or difficulty stopping the opioid was noted.[45] As has been previously voiced, addiction is not nearly so much a risk in these patients with severe and debilitating pain as is underuse and underdosing of analgesics.[61]

Anti-infective Approaches

Infection may result in direct mucosal damage, initiating or complicating mucosal pain. Acyclovir prophylaxis in HSV-seropositive HCT patients is strongly supported in the literature. Antiviral therapy prevents both HSV reactivation in HSV-seropositive HCT patients and viral shedding (seen in 2.9% of patients), in most cases.[145] Oral ulcerations may be caused by cytomegalovirus (CMV) in HCT[146] and shedding of CMV was detected in 13.3% of CMV-seropositive patients. No correlation between severity of mucositis and serologic status of HSV or CMV was seen in patients provided acyclovir prophylaxis.[145] Ganciclovir after stem cell transplant in HCT has been shown effective in suppressing CMV infection[147] and acyclovir prophylaxis has also been shown to prevent shedding of CMV by approximately half in HCT patients.[148]

Consecutive HCT patients at risk of streptococcal bacteremia were treated for 5 days with clindamycin and ceftazidime for the initial management of fever associated with severe oral mucositis.[79] Bacteremia caused by viridans streptococci occurred in 70% of patients with severe mucositis and culture results were positive a day prior to fever in approximately one-third of cases, showing that mucosal ulceration predisposes to systemic infection by oral flora. Approaches to reduce mucosal damage will reduce pain and infection risk and have been suggested as a better means of reducing systemic infection rather than via antimicrobial approaches.[79]

In a series of patients with leukemia receiving HCT, fluconazole prophylaxis was compared with no prophylaxis[109] and a trend toward reduction in oropharyngeal colonization by *Candida albicans* was seen ($p = 0.07$). However, the clinical implications are unclear since no relationship was seen between *Candida* species, antifungal prophylaxis, and mucositis, indicating that *Candida* was not involved in the etiology of mucosal damage in these patients.[108] In a randomized controlled trial, fluconazole prevented systemic fungal infections (7% of fluconazole versus 18% of placebo patients)[149] and the incidence of mucosal infection and oropharyngeal colonization by *C. albicans* was reduced.[150,151] Therefore, while *Candida* may complicate oral mucositis and cause mucosal sensitivity and systemic infection, it does not appear to be a cause of mucositis.[152]

XEROSTOMIA

Preventing mucosal toxicity will reduce the pain of oral mucositis. Mucosal toxicity is dose limiting for patients on etoposide and may be related to direct effects of myoablative doses of etoposide that are secreted in saliva.[59] Twelve patients received propantheline, an anticholinergic xerostomia-inducing agent, or placebo, and mucositis was less frequent and less severe ($p = 0.05$) in the propantheline arm. Another study investigated the effect of drug-induced xerostomia on mucositis during HCT by comparing patients with historic controls.[153] Propantheline was found to significantly reduce oral mucositis due to high-dose etoposide, although no effect was seen on esophagitis and enteritis. These findings suggest that for chemotherapeutics that are secreted in saliva, pharmacologically induced hyposalivation may decrease the exposure of the chemotherapeutic to the mucosa and thereby reduce local tissue damage.

TOPICAL APPROACHES FOR MANAGEMENT OF ORAL MUCOSITIS

Biological Response Modifiers and Cytokines

EGF in saliva was assessed in patients receiving head and neck radiation therapy.[157] The quantity of EGF in the oral environment decreased because of decreased volume of saliva and decreased in concentration per milliliter of saliva as mucositis increased throughout the course of radiation therapy.[157] These findings suggested that EGF may represent a marker of mucosal damage and has the potential to promote resolution of radiation-induced mucositis.

Mixed results have been seen with GM-CSF in several human trials.[72–75,83,84] Studies assessing granulocyte colony stimulating factor (G-CSF) have also presented mixed outcomes. These results may be due to mucositis as a secondary endpoint or toxicity report only in these studies.[52,84,85] Overall, the available and conflicting results do not provide sufficient information to recommend use of white cell growth factors for the treatment of mucositis.

Cognitive and Behavioral Interventions

Relaxation, imagery, biofeedback, hypnosis, and transcutaneous electrical nerve stimulation have been employed in the management of cancer pain with varying patient acceptance and efficacy.[61,158,159] Cognitive behavioral interventions in pediatric oncology and HCT included providing information before procedures and positive reinforcement after procedures and, less commonly, behavioral interventions such as rhythmic breathing, distraction, and imagery.[160] Psychological services were primarily available on an as-needed basis and support groups were not generally offered. Increasing emphasis on psychological support and techniques for pain management may be useful for patients during HCT.

A controlled clinical trial of psychological interventions in cancer-related pain was conducted in 94 HCT patients with oral mucositis in four groups, and relaxation and imagery training was shown to reduce pain associated with oral mucositis. However, adding cognitive-behavioral skills to relaxation and imagery did not improve pain relief.[161] The reader is referred to other chapters in this section for more detail with regard to psychological approaches to pain and an in-depth review of treatment of bone pain, use of nonopioid and opioid pharmacotherapy for cancer pain, radiopharmaceuticals, and interventional approaches to pain control in cancer.

CONCLUSION

Pain in the head and neck and oropharynx of cancer patients has a significant impact upon QOL and needs to be treated aggressively to prevent comorbidities. Cancer and cancer therapy results in release of reactive oxygen species, growth factors, cytokines, and enzymes that may cause nerve irritation or damage that may result in acute and chronic pain. Anxiety and depression compound the pain experience. Mucosal damage, particularly in the presence of immunosuppression and neutropenia, may result in risk of systemic infection (Fig. 45.5). Oropharyngeal pain in cancer patients frequently requires systemic analgesics, adjunctive medications, physical therapy, and psychological therapy, in addition to oral care and topical treatments (see Table 45.4). Good

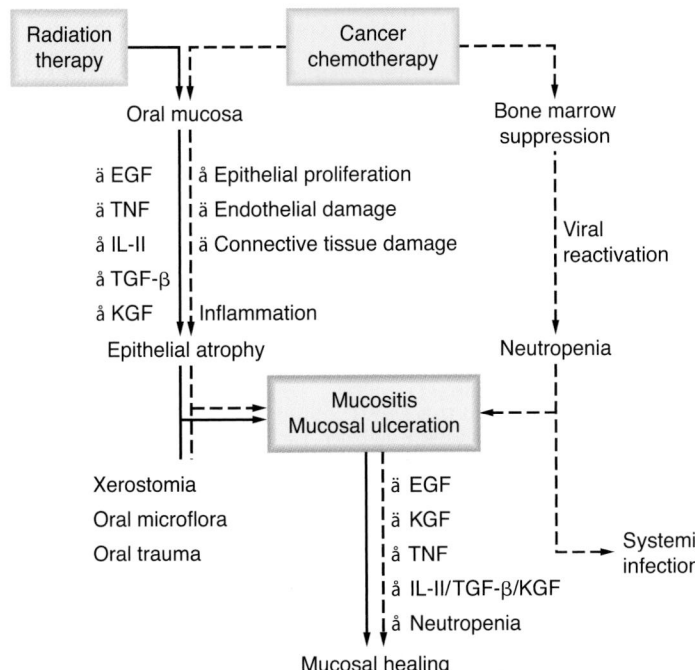

EGF - Epidermal growth factor   TGF-β - Transforming growth factor-beta
TNF - Tumor necrosis factor   KGF - Keratinocyte growth factor
IL-II - Interleukin II   AGF - Angiogenic growth factor

FIGURE 45.5 A model of the pathogenesis of oral mucositis.

TABLE 45.5

SYMPTOMATIC MANAGEMENT OF PAIN OF ORAL MUCOSITIS

Maintain good oral hygiene
Prevent mucosal damage (see Table 45.2)
Coating agents (e.g., milk of magnesia, aluminum hydroxide gel [Amphojel], sucralfate, loperamide [Kaopectate], Gelclair, Caphosol)
Topical analgesic/anti-inflammatory (benzydamine)
Topical anesthetics/analgesics
Systemic analgesics
Adjuvant systemic medications
Adjuvant cognitive/psychological support
Physical therapy (rinsing, ice chips)
Miscellaneous agents

oral hygiene including tooth brushing and dental flossing reduces the severity of oral mucositis and does not increase the risk of bacteremia.

Clinically apparent mucositis is the result of drug toxicities, tissue damage, and inflammation. The primary event is cell damage from chemotherapy, radiotherapy, or both. Secondary influences include indirect toxicities resulting in immunosuppression, neutropenia, reactivation of latent virus (herpes viruses), and opportunistic microbial (bacterial and fungal) infections. Salivary gland dysfunction caused by dehydration and direct effects of the cancer therapy on gland function may alter the local mucosal defenses. Because the etiology is multifactorial (see Table 45.3), approaches to prevention and treatment also have been multifactorial (see Table 45.4). Effective prevention and management of mucositis affect the pain experienced during cancer treatment and, when mucositis is present, symptomatic management is needed (Table 45.5).

Systemic analgesics remain an important mainstay in pain treatment along with topical analgesics and anesthetics. Pain management including adjunctive pain medications are often underutilized in head and neck cancer-related pain syndromes. Novel approaches of potential interest are agents that affect neurotransmitters of pain such as substance P and potentially reactive oxygen species, cytokine production, prostaglandins, and other neurotransmitters.

Biological response modifiers offer the potential for prevention and to speed healing. Oral care and continuing good oral hygiene is recommended prior to and during cancer therapy. Keratinocyte growth factor (Kepivance) is the only approved and recommended medication for prophylaxis of mucositis in HCT. Benzydamine is recommended in head and neck radiation therapy but it is not available in the United States. Oral cooling (cryotherapy) with ice chips is recommended for patients receiving short half-life systemic chemotherapy. Available local agents of questionable value include a coating agent (Gelclair) and a mineralizing oral solution (Caphosol). Meanwhile, a number of agents with different mechanisms of action are undergoing investigation. Of potential value is the use of xerostomic-inducing medications to reduce exposure of the oral mucosa to chemotherapeutic drugs that are secreted in saliva.

Whereas antimicrobial approaches have been shown to not prevent mucositis, there may be a positive effect on dental and gingival health and on candidiasis. Other approaches that require further study include low-energy lasers and anti-inflammatory medications.

References

1. Benoleil R, Epstein J, Eliav E, et al. Orofacial pain in cancer: part I—mechanisms. *J Dent Res* 2007;86(6):491–505.

2. Eliav E, Teich S, Benoliel R, et al. Large myelinated nerve fiber hypersensitivity in oral malignancy. *Oral Surg Oral Med Oral Pathol Oral Radiol Endod* 2002;94(1):45–50.
3. Eliav E, Tal M, Benoliel R. Experimental malignancy in the rat induces early hypersensitivity indicative of neuritis. *Pain* 2004;110(3):727–737.
4. Sonis ST, O'Donnell KE, Popat R, et al. The relationship between mucosal cyclooxygenase-2 (COX-2) expression and experimental radiation-induced mucositis. *Oral Oncol* 2004;40:170–176.
5. van Deventer H, Bernard S. Use of gabapentin to treat taxane-induced myalgias. *J Clin Oncol* 1999;17(1):434–435.
6. Wilson RH, Lehky T, Thomas RR, et al. Acute oxaliplatin-induced peripheral nerve hyperexcitability. *J Clin Oncol* 2002;20(7):1767–1774.
7. Bergstrom P, Johnsson A, Bergenheim T, et al. Effects of amifostine on cisplatin induced DNA adduct formation and toxicity in malignant glioma and normal tissues in rat. *J Neurooncol* 1999;42(1):13–21.
8. Rybak LP, Husain K, Whitworth C, et al. Dose dependent protection by lipoic acid against cisplatin-induced ototoxicity in rats: antioxidant defense system. *Toxicol Sci* 1999;47(2):195–202.
9. Lissoni P, Tancini G, Barni S, et al. Treatment of cancer chemotherapy-induced toxicity with the pineal hormone melatonin. *Support Care Cancer* 1997;5(2):126–129.
10. Jackson DV, Wells HB, Atkins JN, et al. Amelioration of vincristine neurotoxicity by glutamic acid. *Am J Med* 1988;84(6):1016–1022.
11. Jacobson SD, Loprinzi CL, Sloan JA, et al. Glutamine does not prevent paclitaxel-associated myalgias and arthralgias. *J Support Oncol* 2003;1(4):274–278.
12. Ott SM. Long-term safety of bisphosphonates. *J Clin Endocrinol Metab* 2005;90(3):1897–1899.
13. Xing L, Boyce BF. Regulation of apoptosis in osteoclasts and osteoblastic cells. *Biochem Biophys Res Commun* 2005;328(3):709–720.
14. Nasilowska-Adamska B, Rzepecki P, Manko J, et al. The influence of palifermin (Kepivance) on oral mucositis and acute graft versus host disease in patients with hematological diseases undergoing hematopoietic stem cell transplant. *Bone Marrow Transplant* 2007;40(10):983–988.
15. Ensrud KE, Barrett-Connor EL, Schwartz A, et al. Randomized trial of effect of alendronate continuation versus discontinuation in women with low BMD: results from the Fracture Intervention Trial long-term extension. *J Bone Miner Res* 2004;19(8):1259–1269.
16. Ensrud KE, Fullman RL, Barrett-Connor E, et al. Voluntary weight reduction in older men increases hip bone loss: the osteoporotic fractures in men study. *J Clin Endocrinal Metab* 2005;90(4):1998–2004.
17. Mehrotra B, Ruggiero S. Bisphosphonate complications including osteonecrosis of the jaw. *Hematology Am Soc Hematol Educ Program* 2006;356–360.
18. Chaplin J, Morton R. A prospective, longitudinal study of pain in head and neck cancer patients. *Head Neck* 1999;21(6):531–537.
19. Epstein J, Stewart K. Radiation therapy and pain in patients with head and neck cancer. *Eur J Cancer B Oral Oncol* 1993;29B(3):191–199.
20. Goodwin WJ. Salvage surgery for patients with recurrent squamous cell carcinoma of the upper aerodigestive tract: when do the ends justify the means? *Laryngoscope* 2000;110(3 Pt 2 Suppl 93):1–18.
21. Wittekindt C, Liu W, Preuss S, et al. Botulinum toxin A for neuropathic pain after neck dissection: a dose-finding study. *Laryngoscope* 2006;116(7):1168–1171.
22. Simons D, Hong C, Simons L. Endplate potentials are common to midfiber myofacial trigger points. *Am J Phys Med Rehabil* 2002;81(3):212–222.
23. Schuller D, McGuirt W, McCabe B, et al. The prognostic significance of metastatic cervical lymph nodes. *Laryngoscope* 1980;90(4):557–570.
24. Crile G, III. On the technique of operations upon the head and neck. *Ann Surg* 1906;44(6):842–850.
25. Terrell J, Ronis D, Fowler K, et al. Clinical predictors of quality of life in patients with head and neck cancer. *Arch Otolaryngol Head Neck Surg* 2004;130(4):401–408.
26. Chandu A, Sun K, DeSilva R, et al. The assessment of quality of life in patients who have undergone surgery for oral cancer: a preliminary report. *J Oral Maxillofac Surg* 2005;63(11):1606–1612.
27. Kuntz A, Weymuller EJ. Impact of neck dissection on quality of life. *Laryngoscope* 1999;109(8):1334–1338.
28. Terrell J, Welsh D, Bradford C, et al. Pain, quality of life, and spinal accessory nerve status after neck dissection. *Laryngoscope* 2000;110(4):620–626.
29. Chepeha D, Taylor R, Chepeha J, et al. Functional assessment using Constant's Shoulder Scale after modified radical and selective neck dissection. *Head Neck* 2002;24(5):432–643.
30. Rogers S, Ferlito A, Pellitteri P, et al. Quality of life following neck dissections. *Acta Otolaryngol* 2004;124(3):231–236.
31. Taylor R, Chepeha J, Teknos T, et al. Development and validation of the neck dissection impairment index: a quality of life measure. *Arch Otolaryngol Head Neck Surg* 2002;128(1):44–49.
32. van Wilgen C, Dijkstra P, van der Laan B, et al. Morbidity of the neck after head and neck cancer therapy. *Head Neck* 2004;26(9):785–791.
33. Krause H. Shoulder-arm-syndrome after radical neck dissection: its relation with the innervation of the trapezius muscle. *Int J Oral Maxillofac Surg* 1992;21(5):276–279.
34. Cheng P, Hao S, Lin Y, et al. Objective comparison of shoulder dysfunction after three neck dissection techniques. *Ann Otol Rhinol Laryngol* 2000;109(8 Pt 1):761–766.

35. Townsend CM, Sabiston DC, MD Consult LLC. *Sabiston Textbook of Surgery: The Biological Basis of Modern Surgical Practice*, 17th ed. Philadelphia: Saunders; 2004:xxv, 2388.

36. Roh J, Yoon Y, Kim S, et al. Cervical sensory preservation during neck dissection. *Oral Oncol* 2007;43(5):491–498.

37. Sonis ST. The pathobiology of mucositis. *Nat Rev Cancer* 2004;4(4): 277–284.

38. Sonis ST, Elting LS, Keefe D, et al. Perspectives on cancer therapy-induced mucosal injury: pathogenesis, measurement, epidemiology, and consequences for patients. *Cancer* 2004;100(9 Suppl):1995–2025.

39. Sonis ST, Scherer J, Phelan S, et al. The gene expression sequence of radiated mucosa in an animal mucositis model. *Cell Prolif* 2002;35(Suppl 1):93–102.

40. Sonis ST, O'Donnell KE, Popat R, et al. The relationship between mucosal cyclooxygenase-2 (COX-2) expression and experimental radiation-induced mucositis. *Oral Oncol* 2004;40(2):1706.

41. Wang CC, Nakfoor BM, Spiro IJ, et al. Role of accelerated fractionated irradiation for supraglottic carcinoma: assessment of results. *Cancer J Sci Am* 1997;3:88–91.

42. DeCosse JJ, Cennerazzo WJ. Quality-of-life management of patients with colorectal cancer. *CA Cancer J Clin* 1997;47:198–206.

43. McIlroy P. Radiation mucositis: a new approach to prevention and treatment. *Eur J Cancer Care (Engl)* 1996;5:153–158.

44. Anonymous. Preliminary results of a randomized trial comparing neoadjuvant chemotherapy (cisplatin, epirubicin, bleomycin) plus radiotherapy vs. radiotherapy alone in stage IV (> or = N2, M0) undifferentiated nasopharyngeal carcinoma: a positive effect on progression-free survival. International Nasopharynx Cancer Study Group. VUMCA I trial. *Int J Radiat Oncol Biol Phys* 1996;35:463–469.

45. Dunbar PJ, Buckley P, Gavrin JR, et al. Use of patient-controlled analgesia for pain control for children receiving bone marrow transplant. *J Pain Symptom Manage* 1995;10:604–611.

46. Ausili-Cefaro G, Marmiroli L, Nardone L, et al. Prolonged continuous infusion of carboplatin and concomitant radiotherapy in advanced head and neck cancer. A phase I study. *Am J Clin Oncol* 1995;18:273–276.

47. Pascual MJ, Maldonado J. Extramedullary toxicity in bone marrow transplantation using busulfan and cyclophosphamide conditioning. *Sangre (Barc)* 1995;40:191–197.

48. Perch SJ, Machtay M, Markiewicz DA, et al. Decreased acute toxicity by using midline mucosa-sparing blocks during radiation therapy for carcinoma of the oral cavity, oropharynx, and nasopharynx. *Radiology* 1995;197: 863–866.

49. Broun ER, Sridhara R, Sledge GW, et al. Tandem autotransplantation for the treatment of metastatic breast cancer. *J Clin Oncol* 1995;13:2050–2055.

50. Berger A, Henderson M, Nadoolman W, et al. Oral capsaicin provides temporary relief for oral mucositis pain secondary to chemotherapy/radiation therapy. *J Pain Symptom Manage* 1995;10:243–248.

51. Syrjala KL, Chapko ME. Evidence for a biopsychosocial model of cancer treatment-related pain. *Pain* 1995;61:69–79.

52. Rosenthal MA, Grigg AP, Sheridan WP. High dose busulphan/cyclophosphamide for autologous bone marrow transplantation is associated with minimal non-hemopoietic toxicity. *Leuk Lymphoma* 1994;14:279–283.

53. Carrega G, Castagnola E, Canessa A, et al. Herpes simplex virus and oral mucositis in children with cancer. *Support Care Cancer* 1994;2:266–269.

54. Cole CH, Pritchard S, Rogers PC, et al. Intensive conditioning regimen for bone marrow transplantation in children with high-risk haematological malignancies. *Med Pediatr Oncol* 1994;23:464–469.

55. Woo SB, Sonis ST, Monopoli MM, et al. A longitudinal study of oral ulcerative mucositis in bone marrow transplant recipients. *Cancer* 1993;72: 1612–1617.

56. McGuire DB, Altomonte V, Peterson DE, et al. Patterns of mucositis and pain in patients receiving preparative chemotherapy and bone marrow transplantation. *Oncol Nurs Forum* 1993;20:1493–1502.

57. Tomio L, Zorat PL, Paccagnella A, et al. A pilot study of concomitant radiation and chemotherapy integrated with locally advanced head and neck cancer. *Am J Clin Oncol* 1993;16:264–267.

58. Epstein JB, Stewart KH. Radiation therapy and pain in patients with head and neck cancer. *Eur J Cancer B Oral Oncol* 1993;29B:191–199.

59. Ahmed T, Engelking C, Szaluga J, et al. Propantheline prevention of mucositis from etoposide. *Bone Marrow Transplant* 1993;12:131–132.

60. Seto BG, Kim M, Wolinsky L, et al. Oral mucositis in patients undergoing bone marrow transplantation. *Oral Surg Oral Med Oral Pathol* 1985;60: 493–497.

61. Epstein JB, Schubert MM. Management of orofacial pain in cancer patients. *Oral Oncol Eur J Cancer* 1993;29B:243–250.

62. Chapko MK, Syrjala KL, Schilter L, et al. Chemoradiotherapy toxicity during bone marrow transplantation: time course and variation in pain and nausea. *Bone Marrow Transplant* 1989;4:181–186.

63. Schubert MM, Izutsu KT. Iatrogenic salivary gland dysfunction. *J Dent Res* 1987;66:680–688.

64. Bearman SI, Appelbaum FR, Buckner CD, et al. Regimen-related toxicity in patients undergoing bone marrow transplantation. *J Clin Oncol* 1988;6: 1562–1568.

65. Schubert MM, Peterson DE, Flournoy N, et al. Oral and pharyngeal herpes simplex virus infection after allogeneic bone marrow transplantation: analysis of factors associated with infection. *Oral Surg Oral Med Oral Pathol* 1990; 70:286–293.

66. Epstein JB, Sherlock C, Page JL, et al. Clinical study of herpes simplex virus infection in leukemia. *Oral Surg Oral Med Oral Pathol* 1990;70:38–43.

67. Epstein JB, Wong FLW. The efficacy of sucralfate suspension in the prevention of oral mucositis due to radiation therapy. *Int J Radiat Oncol Biol Phys* 1994; 28:693–698.

68. Epstein JB, Steveson-Moore P, Jackson S, et al. Prevention of oral mucositis in radiation therapy: a controlled study with benzydamine hydrochloride rinse. *Int J Radiat Oncol Biol Phys* 1989;16:1571–1575.

69. Wingard JR, Niehaus CS, Peterson DE, et al. Oral mucositis after bone marrow transplantation: a marker of treatment toxicity and predictor of hepatic veno-occlusive disease. *Oral Surg Oral Med Oral Pathol* 1991;72:419–424.

70. Bonner JA, Harari PM, Giralt J, et al. Radiotherapy plus cetuximab for squamous-cell carcinoma of the head and neck. *N Engl J Med* 2006;354(6): 567–578.

71. Bonner JA, Keene KS. Is cetuximab active in patients with cisplatin-refractory squamous cell carcinoma of the head and neck? *Nat Clin Pract Oncol* 2007; 4(12):690–691.

72. Gordon B, Spadinger A, Hodges E, et al. Effect of granulocyte-macrophage colony stimulating factor on oral mucositis after hematopoietic stem-cell transplantation. *J Clin Oncol* 1994;12:1917–1922.

73. Linch DC, Scarffe H, Proctor S, et al. Randomised vehicle-controlled dose-finding study of glycosylated recombinant human granulocyte colony-stimulating factor after bone marrow transplantation. *Bone Marrow Transplant* 1993;11:307–311.

74. Reynoso EE, Calderon E, Miranda E. GM-CSF mouthwashes to attenuate severe mucositis after high dose chemotherapy and allogeneic bone marrow transplantation (BMT) or autologous peripheral blood stem cell transplantation (APBSCT). *Ann Oncol* 1994;5(Suppl 8):1062.

75. Garfunkel AA, Tager N, Chausu S, et al. Oral complications in bone marrow transplantation patients: recent advances. *Isr J Med Sci* 1994;30:120–124.

76. Epstein JB, Gangbar SJ. Oral mucosal lesions in patients undergoing treatment for leukemia. *J Oral Med* 1987;3:205–209.

77. Schubert MM, Peterson DE, Hamilton D, et al. Changes I oral microflora following marrow transplantation. *J Dent Res* 1988;67:249.

78. Valteau D, Hartmann O, Brugieres L, et al. Streptococcal septicemia following autologous bone marrow transplantation in children treated with high-dose chemotherapy. *Bone Marrow Transplant* 1991;7:415–419.

79. Donnelly JP, Muus P, Horrevorts AM, et al. Failure of clindamycin to influence the course of severe oromucositis associated with streptococcal bacteraemia in allogeneic bone marrow transplant recipients. *Scand J Infect Dis* 1993; 25:43–50.

80. Donnelly JP, Muus P, Horrevorts AM, et al. Failure of clindamycin to influence the course of severe oromucositis associated with streptoccal bacteraemia in allogeneic bone marrow transplant recipients. *Scand J Infect Dis* 1993;25: 43–50.

81. Epstein JB, Emerton S, Guglietta A, et al. Assessment of epidermal growth factor in oral secretions of patients receiving radiation therapy for cancer. *Oral Oncol* 1997;33:359–363.

82. Chi KH, Chen CH, Chan WK, et al. Effect of granulocyte-macrophage colony-stimulating factor on oral mucositis in head and neck cancer patients after cisplatin, fluorouracil and leucovorin chemotherpy. *J Clin Oncol* 1995;13: 2620–2628.

83. Masucci G. New clinical applications of granulocyte-macrophage colony-stimulating factor. *Med Oncol* 1996;13:149–154.

84. Bültzingslöwen IV, Brennan MT, Spijkervet FK, et al. Growth factors and cytokines in the prevention and treatment of oral and gastrointestinal mucositis. *Support Care Cancer* 2006;14(6):519–527.

85. Cho SA, Park JH, Seok SH, et al. Effect of granulocyte macrophage-colony stimulating factor (GM-CSF) on FU-induced ulcerative mucositis in hamster buccal pouches. *Exp Toxicol Pathol* 2006;57(4):321–328.

86. Sonis S, Muska A, O'Brien J, et al. Alteration in the frequency, severity and duration of chemotherapy-induced mucositis in hamsters by interleukin-11. *Eur J Cancer Oral Oncol* 1995;31B: 261–266.

87. Sonis ST, Van Vugt AG, McDonald J, et al. Mitigating effects of interleukin-11 on consecutive courses of 5-fluorouracil-induced ulcerative mucositis in hamsters. *Cytokine* 1997;9:605–612.

88. Sonis ST, Van Vugt AG, Brien JP, et al. Transforming growth factor-beta 3 mediated modulation of cell cycling and attenuation of 5-fluorouracil induced oral mucositis. *Oral Oncol* 1997;33:47–54.

89. Sonis ST, Lindquist L, Van Vugt A, et al. Prevention of chemotherapy-induced ulcerative mucositis by transforming growth factor beta 3. *Cancer Res* 1994; 54:1135–1138.

90. Keith JC Jr, Albert L, Sonis ST, et al. IL-11, a pleiotropic cytokine: exciting new effects of IL-11 on gastrointestinal mucosal biology. *Stem Cells* 1994; 12(Suppl 1):89–90.

91. Bernier J, Domenge C, Ozsahin M, et al. Postoperative irradiation with or without concomitant chemotherapy for locally advanced head and neck cancer. *N Engl J Med* 2004;350(19):1945–1952.

92. List MA, Siston A, Haraf D, et al. Quality of life and performance in advanced head and neck cancer patients on concomitant chemoradiotherapy: a prospective examination. *J Clin Oncol* 1999;17(3):1020–1028.

93. Epstein JB, Beaumont JL, Gwede CK, et al. Longitudinal evaluation of the oral mucositis weekly questionnaire-head and neck cancer, a patient-reported outcomes questionnaire. *Cancer* 2007;109(9):1914–1922.

94. Epstein JB, Emerton S, Kolbinson DA, et al. Quality of life and oral function

following radiotherapy for head and neck cancer. *Head Neck* 1999;21(1): 1–11.

95. Borowski B, Benhamou E, Pico JL, et al. Prevention of oral mucositis in patients treated with high-dose chemotherapy and bone marrow transplantation: a randomised controlled trial comparing two protocols of dental care. *Eur J Cancer B Oral Oncol* 1994;30B:93–97.

96. Ferretti GA, Ash RC, Brown AT, et al. Chlorhexidine for prophylaxis against oral infections and associated complications in bone marrow transplant patients. *J Am Dent Assoc* 1987;114:461–467.

97. Spijkervet FKL, van Saene HK, van Saene JJ, et al. Effect of selective elimination of oral flora in irradiated head and neck cancer patients. *J Surg Oncol* 1991;46:167–173.

98. Samaranayake LP, Robertson AG, MacFarlane TW, et al. The effect of chlorhexidine and benzydamine mouthwashes on mucositis induced by therapeutic irradiation. *Clin Radiol* 1998;39:291–294.

99. Raether D, Walker PO, Bostrum B, et al. Effectiveness of oral chlorhexidine for reducing stomatitis. *Pediadtr Dent* 1989;11:37–42.

100. Wahlin YB, Granstrom S, Persson S, et al. Multivariate study of enterobacteria and *Pseudomonas* in saliva of patients with acute leukemia. *Oral Surg Oral Med Oral Pathol* 1991;72:300–308.

101. Dodd MJ, Larson PJ, Dibble SL, et al. Randomized clinical trial of chlorhexidine versus placebo for prevention of oral mucositis in patients receiving chemotherapy. *Oncol Nurs Forum* 1996;23:921–927.

102. Epstein JB, Jones CK. Presenting signs and symptoms of nasopharyngeal carcinoma. *Oral Surg Oral Med Oral Pathol* 1993;75:32–36.

103. Cacchillo D, Barker GJ, Barker BF. Late effects of head and neck radiation therapy and patient/dentist compliance with recommended dental care. *Spec Care Dent* 1993;13:159–162.

104. Withers HR, Peters LJ, Taylor JMG, et al. Late normal tissue sequelae from radiation therapy for carcinoma of the tonsil: patterns of fractionation study of radiobiology. *Int J Radiat Oncol Biol Phys* 1995;33:563–568.

105. Hinohira Y, Yumoto E, Takahashi H, et al. Radiotherapy combined with daily administration of low dose cisplatin for head and neck cancer. *Gan To Kagaku Ryoho* 1996;23:561–565.

106. Leyvraz S, Pasche P, Bauer J, et al. Rapidly alternating chemotherapy and hyperfractionated radiotherapy in the management of locally advanced head and neck carcinoma: four-year results of a phase I/II study. *J Clin Oncol* 1994; 12:1876–1885.

107. Gava A, Ferrarese F, Tonetto V, et al. Can the prophylactic treatment of mycotic mucositis improve the time of performing radiotherapy in head and neck tumors? *Radiol Med (Torino)* 1996;91:452–455.

108. Epstein JB, Ransier A, Lunn R, et al. Prophylaxis of candidiasis in patients with leukemia and bone marrow transplants. *Oral Surg Oral Med Oral Pathol Oral Radiol Endodosc* 1996;81:291–296.

109. Epstein JB, Frelich MM, Le ND. Risk factors for oropharyngeal candidiasis in patients who receive radiation therapy for malignant conditions of the head and neck. *Oral Surg Oral Med Oral Pathol* 1993;76:169–174.

110. Robert F, Ezekiel MP, Spencer SA, et al. Phase I study of anti-epidermal growth factor receptor antibody cetuximab in combination with radiation therapy in patients with advanced head and neck cancer. *J Clin Oncol* 2001; 19(13):3234–3243.

111. Manegold C, Gatzemeier U, Buchholz E, et al. A pilot trial of gefitinib in combination with docetaxel in patients with locally advanced or metastatic non–small-cell lung cancer. *Clin Lung Cancer* 2005;6(6):343–349.

112. Wyatt AJ, Leonard GD, Sachs DL. Cutaneous reactions to chemotherapy and their management. *Am J Clin Dermatol* 2006;7(1):46–63.

113. Koyama N, Jinn Y, Takabe K, et al. The characterization of gefitinib sensitivity and adverse events in patients with non–small-cell lung cancer. *Anticancer Res* 2006;26:4519–4526.

114. Agero LA, Dusza ST, Benvenuto-Andrade C, et al. Dermatologic side effects associated with epidermal growth factor receptor inhibitors. *J Am Acad Dermatol* 2006;55:657–670.

115. Robert F, Blumenschein G, Herbst RX, et al. PhaseI/IIa study of cetuximab with gemcitabine plus carboplatin in patients with chemotherapy-naïve advanced non–small-cell lung cancer. *J Clin Oncol* 2005;23(36):9089–9096.

116. Pinto C, Di Fabio F, Siena S, et al. Phase II study of cetuximab in combination with FOLFIRI in patients with untreated advanced gastric or gastroesophageal junction adenocarcinoma (FOLCETUX study). *Ann Oncol* 2007;18: 510–517.

117. Donaldson GW. The factorial structure and stability of the McGill Pain Questionnaire in patients experiencing oral mucositis following bone marrow transplantation. *Pain* 1995;62:101–109.

118. Keefe DM, Schubert MM, Elting LS, et al. Updated clinical practice guidelines for the prevention and treatment of mucositis. *Cancer* 2007;109(5):820–831.

119. Worthington H, Clarkson J, Eden O. Interventions for preventing oral mucositis for patients with cancer receiving treatment. *Cochrane Database Syst Rev* 2007;(4):CD000978.

120. Clarkson JE, Worthington HV, Eden OB. Interventions for treating oral mucositis for patients with cancer receiving treatment. *Cochrane Database Syst Rev* 2007;(2):CD001973.

121. Stiff PJ, Emmanouilides C, Bensinger WL, et al. Palifermin reduces patient-reported mouth and throat soreness and improves patient functioning in the hematopoietic stem-cell transplantation setting. *J Clin Oncol* 2006;24(33): 5186–5193.

122. Rosen LS, Abdi E, Daivs ID, et al. Palifermin reduces the incidence of oral

mucositis in patients with metastatic colorectal cancer treated with fluorouracil-based chemotherapy. *J Clin Oncol* 2006;24(33):5194–5200.

123. Schubert MM, Eduardo FP, Guthrie KA, et al. A phase III randomized double-blind placebo-controlled clinical trial to determine the efficacy of low level laser therapy for the prevention of oral mucositis in patients undergoing hematopoietic cell transplantation. *Support Care Cancer* 2007;15(10):1145–1154.

124. Eduardo FP, Mahnert DU, Monezi TA, et al. Cultured epithelial cells response to phototherapy with low intensity laser. *Lasers Surg Med* 2007;39(4): 365–372.

125. Corti L, Chiarion-Sileni V, Aversa S, et al. Treatment of chemotherapy-induced oral mucositis with light-emitting diode. *Photomed Laser Surg* 2006; 24(2):207–213.

126. Dodd MJ, Dibble SL, Miaskowski C, et al. Randomized clinical trial of the effectiveness of 34 commonly used mouthwashes to treat chemotherapy-induced mucositis. *Oral Surg Oral Med Oral Pathol Oral Radiol Endod* 2000; 90:39–47.

127. Dodd MJ, Miaskowski C, Greenspan D, et al. Radiation-induced mucositis: a randomized clinical trial of micronized sucralfate versus salt and soda mouthwashes. *Cancer Invest* 2003;21:21–33.

128. Feber T. Management of mucositis in oral irradiation. *Clin Oncol (R Coll Radiol)* 1996;8:106–111.

129. Cerchietti LC, Navigante AH, Korte MW, et al. Potential utility of the peripheral analgesic properties of morphine in stomatitis-related pain: a pilot study. *Pain* 2003;105(1–2):265–273.

130. Epstein JB, Epstein JD, Epstein MS, et al. Management of pain in cancer patients with oral mucositis: follow-up of multiple doses of doxepin oral rinse. *J Pain Symptom Manage* 2007;33(2):111–114.

131. Adams S, Toth B, Dudley BS. Evaluation of sucralfate as a compounded oral suspension for the treatment of stomatitis. *Clin Pharmacol Ther* 1985;2:178.

132. Pfeiffer P, Madsen EL, Hansen OM, et al. Effect of prophylactic sucralfate suspension on stomatitis induced by cancer chemotherapy. *Acta Oncol* 1990; 29:171–173.

133. Shenep JL, Kalwinsky DK, Hutson DK, et al. Efficacy of oral sucralfate suspension in prevention and treatment of chemotherapy-induced mucositis. *J Pediatr* 1988;113:758–763.

134. Epstein JB, Wong FL. The efficacy of sucralfate suspension in the prevention of oral mucositis due to radiation therapy. *Int J Radiat Oncol Biol Phys* 1994; 28:693–698.

135. Innocenti M, Moscatelli G, Lopez S. Efficacy of gelclair in reducing pain in palliative care patients with oral lesions: preliminary findings from an open pilot study. *J Pain Symptom Manage* 2002;24(5):456–457.

136. Papas AS, Clark RE, Martuscelli G, et al. A prospective, randomized trial for the prevention of mucositis in patients undergoing hematopoietic stem cell transplantation. *Bone Marrow Transplant* 2003;31(8):705–712.

137. Epstein JB, Vickers L, Spinelli J, et al. Efficacy of chlorhexidine and nystatin rinses in prevention of oral complications in leukemia and bone marrow transplantation. *Oral Surg Oral Med Oral Pathol* 1992;73:692–699.

138. Spijkervet FKL, van Saene HKF, van Saene JJ, et al. Effect of selective elimination of the oral flora on mucositis in irradiated head and neck cancer patients. *J Surg Oncol* 1991;46:161–173.

139. Stockman MA, Spijkervet FK, Burlage FR, et al. Oral mucositis and selective elimination of oral flora in head and neck cancer patients receiving radiotherapy: a double-blind randomised clinical trial. *Br J Cancer* 2003;88(7): 1012–1016.

140. El-Sayed S, Babid A, Shelley W, et al. Prophylaxis of radiation-associated mucositis in conventionally treated patients with head and neck cancer: a double-blind, phase III, randomized, controlled trial evaluating the clinical efficacy of an antimicrobial lozenge using a validated mucositis scoring system. *J Clin Oncol* 2002;20:3956–3963.

141. Trotti A, Garden A, Warde P, et al. A multinational, randomized phase III trial of iseganan HCl oral solution for reducing the severity of oral mucositis in patients receiving radiotherapy for head-and-neck malignancy. *Int J Radiat Oncol Biol Phys* 2004;58(3):674–681.

142. Giles FJ, Rodriguez R, Weisdorf D, et al. A phase III, randomized, double-blind, placebo-controlled, study of iseganan for the reduction of stomatitis in patients receiving stomatotoxic chemotherapy. *Leuk Res* 2004;28(6): 559–565.

143. Epstein JB, Elad S, Eliav E, et al. Orofacial pain in cancer: part II—Clinical perspectives and management. *J Dent Res* 2007;86(6):506–518.

144. Dunbar PJ, Chapman CR, Buckley FP, et al. Clinical analgesic equivalence for morphine and hydromorphone with prolonged PCA. *Pain* 1996;68:265–270.

145. Epstein JB, Ransier A, Sherlock CH, et al. Acyclovir prophylaxis of oral herpes virus during bone marrow transplantation. *Oral Oncol Eur J Cancer* 1996; 32(B):158–162.

146. Lloid ME, Schubert MM, Myerson D, et al. Cytomegalovirus infection of the tongue following marrow transplantation. *Bone Marrow Transplant* 1994; 14:99–104.

147. Goodrich JM, Bowden RA, Fisher L, et al. Ganciclovir prophylaxis to prevent cytomegalovirus disease after allogeneic marrow transplant. *Ann Intern Med* 1993;118:173–178.

148. Meyers JD. Prevention of cytomegalovirus infection after marrow transplantation. *Rev Infect Dis* 1989;11(Suppl 7):S1691–1705.

149. Slavin MA, Osborne B, Adams R, et al. Efficacy and safety of fluconazole prophylaxis for fungal infections after marrow transplantation—a prospective, randomized, double-blind study. *J Infect Dis* 1995;171:1545–1552.

150. Epstein JB, Truelove EL, Hanson-Huggins K, et al. Topical polyene antifun-

gals in hematopoietic cell transplant patients: tolerability and efficacy. *Support Care Cancer* 2004;12(7):517–525.

151. Worthington HV, Eden OB, Clarkson JE. Interventions for preventing oral candidiasis for patients with cancer receiving treatment. *Cochrane Library* 2005;2:1–68.

152. Belazi M, Velegraki A, Koussidou-Eremondi T, et al. Oral candida isolates in patients undergoing radiotherapy for head and neck cancer: prevalence, azole susceptibility profiles and response to antifungal treatment. *Oral Microbiol Immnol* 2004;18(6):347–351.

153. Oblon DJ, Paul SR, Oblon MB, et al. Propantheline protects the oral mucosa after high-dose ifosfamide, carboplatin, etoposide and autologous stem cell transplantation. *Bone Marrow Transplant* 1997;20:961–963.

154. Fulfaro F, Casuccio A, Ticozzi C, et al. The role of bisphosphonates in the treatment of painful metastatic bone disease: a review of phase III trials. *Pain* 1998;78(3):157–169.

155. Mannix K, Ahmedzai SH, Anderson H, et al. Using bisphosphonates to con-

trol the pain of bone metastases: evidence-based guidelines for palliative care. *Palliat Med* 2000;14(6):455–461.

156. Moller T. Skeletal metastases. *Acta Oncol* 1996;35(Suppl 7):125–136.

157. Epstein JB, Emerton S, Guglietta A, et al. Assessment of epidermal growth factor in oral secretions of patients receiving radiation therapy for cancer. *Oral Oncol* 1997;33:359–363.

158. Koerner ME. Using hypnosis to relieve pain of terminal cancer. *Hypnosis* 1977;20:39–46.

159. Barber J, Gritelson J. Cancer pain: psychological management using hypnosis. *Cancer* 1980;30:130–135.

160. McCarthy AM, Cool VA, Petersen M, et al. Cognitive behavioral pain and anxiety interventions in pediatric oncology centers and bone marrow transplant units. *J Pediatr Oncol Nurs* 1996;13:3–12.

161. Syrjala KL, Donaldson GW, Davis MW, et al. Relaxation and imagery and cognitive-behavioral training reduce pain during cancer treatment: a controlled clinical trial. *Pain* 1995;63:189–198.

CHAPTER 46 ■ CANCER-RELATED BONE PAIN

JANET ABRAHM, EDGAR ROSS, AND ROBERT J. KLICKOVICH

EPIDEMIOLOGY REVIEW

Bone pain due to cancer is caused by primary bone tumors and those malignant diseases that commonly metastasize to the bones. Metastatic bone pain most commonly results from cancers of the breast, prostate, and lung. Other malignancies involving bone are renal cell carcinoma, thyroid cancer, lymphoma, and multiple myeloma.[1] The longer these malignancies persist, the higher the probability of bone metastasis. Because current therapies are increasing survival time with most of these malignancies, there is an increasing prevalence of metastatic bone disease. Specifically, since prostate cancer is most likely to metastasize to bone rather than other organs, and patients with prostate cancer are also likely live longer than patients with other metastatic diseases, they are more likely to have more prolonged periods of pain secondary to bony invasion.[2]

Of all bony metastases, vertebral involvement is the most common. The incidence ranges from 30% to 70%.[3] Most patients with metastatic disease of the vertebrae experience back pain. Bony metastases compromise both the bone's integrity and strength. In the vertebrae, this leads to the risk of a pathologic fracture, most commonly in the elderly. Compression fractures affect between 8% and 30% of cancer patients with vertebral body involvement.[4,5] In many cases the fracture occurs without an initial traumatic event suggesting that load is an independent factor in the etiology of a pathologic fracture.[6] Other factors that can lead to pathological fractures include iatrogenic causes such as steroids, malnutrition-induced osteoporosis, bone mineral loss as a result of inactivity, and destruction of bone secondary to radiation therapy.[7]

Complications from vertebral fracture include a redistribution of load across affected vertebral bodies creating fractures at adjacent levels, an increased risk of embolic phenomena as a result of inactivity and pain, kyphosis-induced restriction in vital capacity,[8] predisposition to atelectasis, and early satiety-induced anorexia.[9] Because of this, bony metastases can contribute significantly to decreased lifespan in the patient with one or more tumor-related compression fractures.[6,10]

Pathophysiology

Over the past 10 years, animal models for bone tumor growth, bone remodeling, and bone pain have demonstrated a correlation with many features found in human bony metastatic pain. Mouse studies using murine sarcoma cells injected into the intramedullary space of the femur demonstrate mechanical as well as movement-related pain behaviors. These behaviors[11] increase with time and with tumor-induced bone destruction offering a model that appears to replicate the human experience of how metastatic bone cancer contributes to bone pain. In normal mice, a nonnoxious stimulus to the femur does not elicit the synthesis of any tissue factors, while in mice with bone cancer, a nonnoxious stimulus elicits the synthesis of substance P which binds to the neurokinin-1 receptor expressed in the spinal cord. Likewise, c-fos is not expressed at the level of the spinal cord in normal mice, but this protein is found in a population of mice with bony tumors.[12]

Both osteolytic and osteoblastic changes in bone occur in some tumor types such as lung, breast, and renal tumors. A predominance of osteolysis is found in multiple myeloma and sarcomas, leading to extreme destruction of bone. Osteoblastic lesions commonly result from metastatic prostate cancer.[13] In the prostate model, colonies of malignant prostate tissue exist along the length of the intramedullary canal divided by newly formed bone. In the sarcoma model, there is no new bone formation, only destruction, which is greatest at the proximal and distal head with little to no destruction at the mid-shaft of the bone. The prostate model also demonstrates the formation of new bone along the length of the long bone involving diaphysis, proximal, and distal end points with an increase of osteoclasts throughout the length of the intramedullary canal. These cells stimulate osteolytic remodeling inducing an inflammatory reaction mediated by macrophages. It is suspected that this macrophage induced inflammatory activity may be the basis for neuropathic type of pain found in malignancies of the bone.[12]

In those mice injected with a purely osteolytic line of cells, a greater proportion of the mouse's time was spent guarding or flinching to innocuous palpation of the mice. Human perception of allodynia or hyperpathia from lytic lesions is thought to be analogous to the mouse findings. The osteolytic model also demonstrates demineralization and destruction throughout the length of the bone involved which leads to the potential of increased pain from the loss of structural integrity.[14] In contrast, the prostate model, which includes both areas of infiltration and destruction, may result in increased stability of the bone, such that sensory receptors in the periosteum sense less distortion from palpation.[14]

Multiple studies have demonstrated that the periosteum is richly innervated by both sympathetic and sensory nerve fibers.[15,16] The periosteum receives the greatest amount of afferent sensory fibers per unit area in bone. In addition the periosteum, bone marrow and mineralized bone are innervated by both sensory and sympathetic fibers coursing with blood vessels.[17]

Osteolytic animal models demonstrate microscopic fragmentation and disruption of the bony matrix secondary to tumor growth. In the osteoblastic model, there is evidence of destructive injury as well as an increase in the density of sensory fibers compared to normal bone. An increase in specific transcription factors has also been demonstrated, including activating transcription factor-3 (ATF-3). Expression of ATF-3 is usually detectable in peripheral nerve injury models. It is also expressed in the nucleus of sensory neurons damaged by osteolytic tumor cells. However, this transcription factor is not detectable in normal sensory neuron nuclei or in sensory neurons affected by peripheral inflammation. Animal subjects with increased ATF-3 demonstrate an increase in movement-related pain behavior. Using this model gabapentin improved pain related behavior,[18] but it did not affect tumor growth, bone destruction, or changes in peripheral sensory fibers that were impacted by tumor infiltration. These changes suggest that pain experienced secondary to tumor infiltration may be caused by the destruction of normal afferent sensory fibers.[19]

Osteoclastic induced changes in pH play a role in bone pain as well. When tumor cell growth exceeds vascular supply, tumor cell death leads to a decrease in tissue pH. Additionally as tumors grow, associated inflammatory cells which may comprise as much of 80% of the tumor mass reduce local pH. This decrease of pH in the bony matrix leads to an increased absorption of bone, manifest by osteoclastic activity.[20] Excitation of sensory neurons by decreased pH in osteoclast models leads to an increased expression of pH sensing ion channels. The two major classes of these ion channels are the transient receptor potential 1 (TRPV1) and the acid-sensing ion channel-3 (ASIC-3). Administration of a TRPV antagonist within the mouse model correlates with a decrease in pain behaviors in all stages of tumor growth, suggesting a new potential therapeutic direction to reduce cancer-related bone pain.[20]

Osteoprotegerin (OPG) is a secreted soluble receptor which is one type of the tumor necrosis factor receptor (TNFR). This receptor prevents the activation of osteoclasts via a binding–sequestering of the OPG ligand. It has been demonstrated to decrease the amount of pain-related behavior in the mouse sarcoma model. The monoclonal antibody (AMG-162) can inhibit bone destruction by reducing osteoclast function. This leads to a decrease in the inflammatory mediated changes at the level of the dorsal root ganglion or higher centers which are correlated with the onset of pain from bony metastasis.[21]

Inflammatory cells associated with tumor stroma secrete a variety of compounds which may sensitize or excite afferent neurons. Compounds include prostaglandins, tumor necrosis factor-alpha, endothelins, interleukin-1 and interleukin-6, epidermal growth factor, transforming growth factor-beta, and platelet derived growth factor. Receptors for these factors are directly expressed by afferent neurons. All may play a role in bone pain, but thus far only prostaglandin- and endothelin-targeting agents have been used in the control of pain in bone cancer. Prostaglandins have a role in both sensitization and excitation of nociceptors via direct binding to the prostanoid receptor.[21]

Nerve growth factor (NGF) is a neurotrophic factor expressed in tissue following nerve injury by both the nerves injured as well as surrounding tissues. Upregulation of NGF is thought to be a component in the hyperalgesia following nerve injury. Because of this, anti-NGF antibody therapy could be effective in the control of pain related to bone cancer as it is involved in the environment of the peripheral nerves to bone and the dorsal root ganglion (DRG).[22] In the osteolytic sarcoma mouse model, anti-NGF antibody demonstrated effectiveness in attenuation of pain behaviors, and was found to be more effective than acute administration of 10 and 30 mg/kg doses of morphine sulfate.[23]

Evaluation of the Patient with Bone Cancer

The two most important imaging modalities in the evaluation of malignancy of the bone are plain radiography and nuclear bone scan.

Radiography

Radiographic studies should be ordered first in the evaluation of patients with complaints of bone pain in the context of malignancy. Radiographic patterns fall into osteolytic, osteoblastic, or mixed presentation. Osteoblastic lesions appear opaque and sclerotic. Osteolytic lesions appear more radiolucent compared to surrounding bone. Risk of fracture is greatest if more than 50% of long bone is involved.[24,25]

Bone Scan

Nuclear bone scans are most beneficial for identification of multifocal lesions.[26] Radioisotope accumulates in areas of new bone growth and is diminished in areas of metastasis secondary to decreased blood flow to the area. Cancers such as melanoma and multiple myeloma may have false negatives when reviewed on bone scan secondary to their lack of reactive bone activity.

Computed Tomography

Computed tomography (CT) offers improved spatial resolution in the evaluation of cortical bone destruction.[27] CT is most beneficial in evaluation of the three dimensional characteristics of diseased bone identified by plain radiographs and isotope scans. It is most useful in evaluation of the pelvic and shoulder girdles as well as lesions involving the spine. Additionally, CT-guided needle biopsies may provide information as to the nature of malignancy in bone.

Magnetic Resonance Imaging

Magnetic resonance imaging (MRI) provides better contrast resolution and it has advantages in defining soft tissue and marrow involvement. Also, it can define vascular relationships without contrast enhancement.[27] MRI is most beneficial in the evaluation of tumor infiltration of muscle and bone marrow, in the evaluation of spinal cord compression, and in lesions which are otherwise insufficiently imaged by the previously listed three techniques.

Treatment

The site and distribution of bone metastases and the skeletal sequelae, such as pathologic fracture and spinal cord compression, impact the patient's prognosis.[28] The focus of treatment should be directed at tumor regression, relief of cancer-related symptoms, and preservation of functional capacity. In some cases metastatic disease is so advanced as to be resistant to chemotherapy or radiotherapy. When metastatic involvement cannot be eliminated, a treatment approach that focuses on symptom management is indicated. Impaired neurologic function, pathologic fractures, and debilitating pain are the most important indications for aggressive treatment. Palliation may employ radiotherapy, radiopharmaceuticals, chemotherapy, hormone therapy, bisphosphonates, calcitonin, analgesics (opioids and antiinflammatory drugs), adjuvant analgesics (e.g., corticosteroids), and surgical treatment. Details of some of these interventions can be found in Chapters 43, 44, and 48.

Analgesic medications provide pain relief during therapy with more definitive modalities (e.g., surgical fixation, radiation therapy) as well as when malignant bone pain is resistant to other modalities of treatment. Conventional opioids or nonsteroidal anti-inflammatory drugs (NSAIDs) may not produce adequate analgesia because of incidental and intermittent nature of pain and dose-limiting side effects. NSAID use is often limited by risks of gastrointestinal (GI) bleeding and inhibition of platelet function, especially in patients with low platelet counts. In these latter patients, a cyclooxygenase-2 inhibitor (COX-2) may be preferred (see later). Renal as well as cardiovascular complications result both from selective (COX-2) and nonselective NSAIDs; these comorbidities may be exacerbated in patients undergoing cancer chemotherapy and those with advanced disease. Therefore, other more targeted pharmacotherapeutic and interventional approaches are often used, alone or in combination with traditional analgesics. The remainder of this chapter will focus on those therapies that have been studied specifically for the treatment of cancer-related bone pain to supplement material presented elsewhere in this text.

Cyclooxygenase(Cox)-2-specific Inhibitors

Cyclooxygenase-2-specific inhibitors (coxibs) have demonstrated efficacy in the treatment of chronic and acute pain when comparable to traditional (nonselective) NSAIDs without the severity of GI complication during short-term use or platelet inhibition effects.[29] The superior safety profile of coxibs in conjunction with equal efficacy of conventional NSAIDs supports their use in analgesic regimens for bone cancer. Many tumors express the COX-2 isoenzyme, which is involved in the synthesis of prostaglandins.[30] In the murine sarcoma model, acute administration of a selective COX-2 inhibitor attenuated both ongoing and movement-evoked bone cancer pain, whereas chronic inhibition of COX-2 significantly reduced ongoing and movement-evoked pain behaviors and reduced tumor burden, osteoclastogenesis, and bone destruction by >50%. COX-2 is expressed in 40% of human invasive breast cancers and bone is the primary site of metastasis in cases of breast cancer.[31,32] The role of COX-2 in murine models of breast cancer metastasis to bone demonstrated COX-2 transfection enhanced the bone metastasis, and breast cancer cells isolated and cultured from the bone metastases produced significantly more prostaglandin. Additionally, COX-2 inhibition inhibited bone metastasis in both a prevention regimen and treatment regimen suggesting COX-2 produced in breast cancer cells are significant in the progression of osteolytic bone metastases in patients with breast cancer, and that COX-2 inhibition may halt this process. Furthermore, COX-2 inhibition may benefit iatrogenically caused tumor progression.[33]

Morphine has been demonstrated to stimulate angiogenesis and tumor growth in mice. COX-2 inhibition can prevent associated tumor growth without compromise of opioid-dependent analgesia in a murine breast cancer model. Chronic morphine treatment stimulated angiogenesis in breast tumors with corresponding increased metastasis and reduced survival. Administration of a coxib prevented morphine-induced effects. Additionally, coadministration of morphine and celecoxib offered improved analgesia over either agent independently.[34]

Corticosteroids

Corticosteroids are established as analgesics in the treatment of pain secondary to metastatic bone pain. This analgesia is thought to occur through the blockade of cytokine synthesis which contributes to both inflammation and nociception.[35,36] The analgesic benefits of corticosteroids are dose-dependent and limited in their duration of activity. In a small uncontrolled study, approximately 40% of patients with metastatic prostate cancer were found to have analgesic benefit with the administration of oral corticosteroids. This was speculated to be secondary to suppression of hormone-sensitive disease that was stimulated by weak androgens of adrenal origin by negative feedback on secretion of adrenocorticotropic hormone.[37] Dexamethasone is the most commonly used agent and has the least mineralocorticoid activity. The standard dose is 12 to 24 mg per day and can be administered once daily due to the long half-life of the agent.

Bisphosphonates

Bisphosphonates are pyrophosphate analogues which bind to hydroxyapatite bone mineral surfaces acting to inhibit osteoclasts and thus bone resorption.[38] The optimal dose of the several available drugs from this pharmacological class remains to be defined since dose response appears to be a function of the disease stage.[39]

Oral clodronate given to patients with breast cancer metastatic to bone reduced the frequency of skeletal events by more than one-fourth.[40] In two randomized placebo-controlled trials comparing monthly pamidronate infusions to placebo infusions for over a 1 to 2 year period as a supplement to hormone and chemotherapy, skeletal morbidity rate could be reduced by 30% to 40%.

A recent large, randomized, multicenter trial using intravenous zoledronic acid demonstrated a reduction of 20% in the risk of developing skeletal-related events compared with pamidronate for patients with breast cancer.[41] Moreover, these trials demonstrated for the first time that a bisphosphonate significantly reduces the occurrence of skeletal events in hormone-refractory prostate cancer and in non-small cell lung cancer as well as in a range of solid tumors. Evidence is accumulating from in vitro studies that bisphosphonates are able to directly affect tumor cell growth, in addition to their effects on osteoclasts.[40]

Of the available bisphosphonates, intravenous zoledronic acid has demonstrated the broadest clinical activity and is approved in many countries for the treatment of bone metastases from all solid tumors.[42,43] The indications for bisphosphonate therapy in breast cancer patients include correction of hypercalcemia and the prevention of cancer treatment-induced bone loss.[44]

In summary, bisphosphonates are now part of usual therapeutic regimens against metastatic bone pain, and at least 50% of patients have a clinically relevant analgesic effect. Placebo-controlled trials with oral or intravenous (IV) bisphosphonates have shown that prolonged administration can reduce the frequency of skeletal-related events by 30% to 40%. The superiority of zoledronic acid compared with pamidronate has been shown by a multiple-event analysis in a large randomized trial. The short infusion time of zoledronic acid also constitutes a convenient therapy. Flu-like symptoms which are manageable with standard treatment can occur. Renal monitoring is recommended, with dose reductions for patients with renal dysfunction. Osteonecrosis of the mandible has been reported in patients receiving bisphosphonates and might be avoidable with appropriate dental care.[45]

Calcitonin

The hormone calcitonin has the potential to relieve pain and also retain bone density, thus reducing the risk of fractures. Early data suggested that calcitonin might offer added adjuvant analgesia in the treatment of bone pain related to metastatic disease.[46,47] An animal study of eel calcitonin suggests a role for it both in analgesia as well as osteoclastic activity.[48] Animals were randomly assigned to receive subcutaneously administered doses of placebo (saline), or 20 or 100 U/kg/day 7 and 14 days after having their femurs implanted with osteolytic sarcoma cells. Behavioral and pain related behaviors were assessed and radiological evaluation was followed on days 7, 14, and 21 to determine the extent of loss of bone density. Eel calcitonin dose-dependently inhibited the development of pain-related behaviors and bone destruction. This study suggested that eel calcitonin had a potential to reduce pain and advanced bone destruction in patients with bone cancer.[48]

A human clinical trial prospectively entered 22 patients to evaluate the efficacy of salmon calcitonin in controlling pain related to bone metastasis. Baseline pain control was first established via continuous subcutaneous (SC) morphine administration. In the active treatment group, increases in pain were managed with continuous subcutaneous administration of salmon calcitonin 400 IU/day. Beta-endorphin blood levels were measured prior to and after commencement of calcitonin administration at 12, 24, and 48 hours and 7 days. Pain scores, monitored by visual analogue scale, revealed significantly reduced mean pain scores in the active treatment which were also associated with an increase in beta-endorphin blood levels.[49]

Other controlled clinical trials of salmon calcitonin in the treatment of cancer-related bone pain have shown equivocal analgesic results without evidence of reducing complications due to bone metastasis or improving quality of life or survival.[50,51] Like many pain-relieving strategies, there is considerable inter-patient variability in responses. In those patients who are not responding well to other first line approaches, a trial of calcitonin may be reasonable, but close follow-up should ensure that benefits clearly outweigh harms and costs.

Opioids/Opiate Antagonists

While opioids continue to be the primary mode of controlling metastatic bone pain, new research offers a challenge as to which opioid (if any) may be most appropriate. In a murine sarcoma model of bone cancer pain, in which the progression of cancer pain and bone destruction are tightly controlled, the effects of sustained morphine treatment were evaluated. It was found that morphine enhanced, rather than diminished, spontaneous and evoked pain and that the effects were dose-dependent and naloxone-sensitive.[52] Morphine increased ATF-3 expression only in DRG cells of sarcoma mice. Morphine did not alter tumor growth in vitro or tumor burden in vivo but accelerated sarcoma-induced bone destruction and doubled the incidence of spontaneous fracture in a dose- and naloxone-sensitive manner. Furthermore, morphine increased osteoclast activity and upregulated interleukin-1 beta within the femurs of sarcoma-treated mice suggesting enhancement of sarcoma-induced osteolysis.

The results suggest that morphine may increase pain, osteolysis, bone loss, and spontaneous fracture, as well as markers of neuronal damage and expression of proinflammatory cytokines. Morphine treatment may result in "add-on" mechanisms of pain beyond those engaged by sarcoma alone. The data from this study suggests a need for increased understanding of the sequelae from prolonged morphine exposure.

Adjuvant Analgesics

The pain of bone cancer is often refractory to treatment with opioids and NSAIDs. This may be the result of neuropathic changes in involved bone tissues. In the murine model of bone cancer, tumor cells destroyed peripheral nerve fibers when invading bone marrow and mineralized bone.[53] Sensory fibers were found at and within the leading edge of the tumor, but within the deep stromal portion of the tumor, fibers displayed a discontinuous and fragmented appearance, ultimately undetectable by microscopy. In these same animals, there was expression of ATF-3. This factor is a member of the ATF/cyclic adenosine monophosphate response element binding protein family of transcription factors which are not expressed in normally functioning sensory afferent fibers, but expressed in sensory fibers of animal models following nerve injury. The expression suggests that bone-invading malignancies are concomitantly responsible for peripheral nerve injury and that there may be a pathophysiologic rationale for the use of agents typically used to control neuropathic pain in the control of bone cancer pain.[54]

NMDA Antagonism and Alpha-2 Agonists

Administration of alpha-2 agonists (dexmedetomidine and clonidine), N-methyl-D-aspartate (NMDA) antagonists (MK-801 and ketamine), and morphine were examined in a mouse sarcoma bone cancer pain model.[55] Pain-related behaviors were recorded following administration of stimulus to the site of tumor cells implantation. The respective drugs were administered 2 weeks after the implantation. As expected morphine produced a significant analgesic effect and the alpha-2 agonists produced analgesic effects with an efficacy similar to that of morphine, but only at doses that produced severe sedation. MK-801 demonstrated little analgesic effects, whereas ketamine yielded an analgesic effect with the same efficacy as morphine. The authors concluded that alpha-2 agonists produce an analgesic effect only at a sedative dose. Ketamine, but not MK-801, is associated with an analgesic response without overt side effects, suggesting that non-NMDA effects may be responsible for ketamine's analgesic efficacy in this model. Applicability of these findings to humans remains untested.

Hormonal Therapy

Progression of metastasis from breast, prostate, and uterine malignancies is dependent on hormonal stimulation for survival and growth.[56,57] Antitumor hormonal treatment deprives hormone-dependent tumor cells of an important stimulus for growth and so is a common form of adjunctive therapy in breast, prostate, and endometrial cancers.[58]

Estrogen and estrogen analogue therapy in patients with breast cancer controls symptoms in 25% to 50% of patients temporarily.[59] Hormonal manipulations improve pain in 70% of patients with widespread bone metastases from prostate cancer.[60] Therapy with estrogens is efficacious but it may take 30 to 60 days before complete palliation, and serious adverse effects may exceed overall benefits. Although hormone therapy with androgen receptor antagonists (e.g., flutamide) or antigrowth factor agents (e.g., luteinizing hormone-releasing hormone analogs of somatostatin and 5-reductase inhibitor) can be used to induce tumor regression, the palliative effect may not offer long-term benefit as hormone-refractory elements continue to proliferate and metastasize to bone.[61]

Radionucleotides

Analgesic effects from radionucleotides are not dependent on tumor destruction, per se, but are thought to result from inhibition of pain mediators from normal bone cells. Therapeutic responsiveness is greatest in osteoblastic lesions. Multiple agents have been used for palliative treatment of cancer-related bone pain, including phosphorus-32, strontium-89, yttrium-90, samarium-153, and rhenium-186.

Phosphorus-32 has been used for more than 30 years and relieves the pain from osteoblastic metastases in approximately

80% of patients treated.[62] However, myelosuppression caused by this agent has encouraged development of newer agents. Strontium-89 is a bone-seeking radionuclide, whereas samarium-153 is a bone-seeking tetraphosphonate. Both agents have been shown to have efficacy in the treatment of painful osseous metastases from prostate cancer; they have also been demonstrated to offer analgesia in breast cancer and perhaps from non-small cell lung cancer. As many as 80% of selected patients[63] with painful osteoblastic bony metastases from prostate or breast cancer may experience some pain relief following strontium-89 administration.[64] Additionally, 10% or more may become pain free and the average duration of clinical response typically ranges from 3 to 6 months with minimal myelosuppression compared to phosphorus 32.[65]

Procedural Interventions

In addition to pharmacotherapy, interventional therapies to relieve the pain associated with bone cancer can be beneficial. Procedures include intralesional injections, nerve blocks, intra-articular injections, radiofrequency rhizotomy, and vertebroplasty.

Intralesional Injection

In a study of patients with rib metastases or involvement of the ribs by multiple myeloma, infiltration of tender areas with methylprednisolone under intercostal block provided significant reduction in pain-related symptoms in over half the cases.[66] Of 20 assessable patients, 11 became pain free within 10 days with recurrence of pain in only one of these patients; in three others the pain was considerably improved. The procedure was well tolerated and there were no complications.[66] This technique has also been applied to mandibular lesions in which surgical excision of tumor runs the risk of destabilizing the affected bone.[67] This technique may be applicable to other areas of metastasis.[68] Additionally, localized injection of corticosteroid, local anesthetic and even baclofen, have been reported to offer clinically meaningful relief in areas of secondary muscular spasm.[69]

Percutaneous Vertebroplasty/Kyphoplasty

Bony metastasis to the vertebrae involve 30% to 70% of all bony lesions and compromise the strength of involved bone which can induce pathologic vertebral fractures in the absence of trauma. Additional causes include osteoporosis, malnutrition, radiation, and steroid administration. In cases of fracture secondary to pathologic bone, vertebroplasty may offer pain relief. In comparison to patients who have a nonmalignant basis for pathology of the bone such as osteoporosis, reports of analgesic benefit are not as high, but are significant with ranges reported between 50% and 80%.[70] This may be explained by the widespread nature of metastatic disease and the multifactorial nature of pain in malignant disease. The mechanism by which vertebroplasty is thought to offer pain relief are speculated to be fixation of chronically mobile bone fragments as well as thermal neurolysis secondary to the exothermic reaction of methylmethacrylate cement yielding temperatures in excess of 70° C.[71]

Rhizotomy

Minimally invasive neurodestructive techniques have been demonstrated to be effective in a number of malignancies, specifically of visceral and neuropathic nature. Techniques involve radiofrequency lesioning, cryotherapy, and chemical neurolysis using such agents as phenol, alcohol, and hypertonic saline. As we are coming to an understanding that there may be a neuropathic component to bony lesions in metastatic cancer, these techniques may offer a valuable option in the control of cancer-related bone pain. The same principles may be applied to chordoma, osteoid osteoma, or osseous metastasis. Studies of radiofrequency le-

sioning of bony and soft tissue malignancy have reported significant palliation of pain.[72–75]

Associated Processes

Avascular Necrosis

Avascular necrosis is found in survivors of cancer who have been exposed to corticosteroid therapy. Pain is usually the result of weight-bearing. In an MRI study of patients having survived childhood cancer, 67% of patients demonstrated osteonecrosis at the ankle.[76]

Postoperative Frozen Shoulder. In postthoracotomy or postmastectomy patients, there is a risk for the development of frozen shoulder. The site may become an independent locus of pain and can be complicated by complex regional pain syndrome. Adequate mobilization of the joint with sufficient analgesia should be implemented soon following surgery to prevent this chronic, painful, and debilitating complication.[77]

Granulocyte Colony-Stimulating Factor Related Pain

Granulocyte colony-stimulating factor (G-CSF) is used to stimulate the production of granulocytes in immunocompromised patients following chemotherapy and radiation. Bone pain and generalized muscle pain are a major secondary effect, lasting for 10 or more days.[78] Effective analgesia may require opioids.[79] G-CSF may induce an inflammatory reaction through undescribed distinct cellular signaling and by triggering histamine release.[80] Increased histamine levels can cause nociceptive c-fiber-mediated pain and can increase edema formation within bone leading to pain.[81] Antihistamines such as terfenadine and astemizole have anti-inflammatory properties in addition to their potency as histamine-1 antagonist and may benefit bone pain caused by G-CSF therapy.

CONCLUSION

The skeleton is the most common organ to be affected by metastatic cancer and the site of disease that produces a very high prevalence of morbidity. Skeletal morbidities include severe pain (spontaneous and incident-related), hypercalcemia, pathologic fracture, and spinal cord or nerve root compression. Currently bone pain is inadequately treated. Approximately 80% of patients experienced pain in the period before palliative therapy. Until there are breakthroughs in prevention and treatment of cancer-related bone pain, clinicians must continue to rely on conventional and modern assessment techniques, an understanding of the many causes of cancer-related pain, and the host of available therapies to optimally treat pain caused by bone metastasis.[82]

From randomized trials in advanced cancer, major skeletal related events occur on average every 3 to 6 months. The prognosis of metastatic bone disease is dependent on the primary site. In breast and prostate cancer, survival is measured in years; in lung cancer, survival may be measured in months. Severity and duration of tumor involvement in bone cancer are predictors of outcome. Duration of involvement is best estimated by measurement of bone-specific markers. Studies demonstrate a powerful correlation between the rate of bone resorption and clinical outcome, related both to skeletal morbidity and overall life expectancy. By understanding prognostic and predictive factors in individual cases, delivery of a tailored treatment according to the circumstances attending each patient leads to improved palliative and cost-effective outcomes.[83]

References

1. Buijs J T, van der Pluijm G. Osteotropic cancers: from primary tumor to bone. *Cancer Lett* 2009;273:177–193.
2. Halvorsan K, et al. In: Fisch M, Burton A, eds. *Cancer Pain Management.* New York: McGraw-Hill, 2007.
3. Jajan N, et al. Palliative radiation therapy techniques. In: Fisch M, Burton A, eds. *Cancer Pain Management.* New York: McGraw-Hill, 2007.
4. Patel B, DeGroot H. Evaluation of the risk of pathological fractures secondary to metastatic bone disease. *Orthopedics* 2001;24:612–617.
5. Bunting R, Lamont-Havers W, Schweon D, et al. Pathological fracture risk in rehabilitation of patients with bony metastases. *Clin Orthop Relat Res* 1985; 192:222–227.
6. Alberico R, et al. Neuroradiologic evaluation of the patient with cancer pain. In: de Leon Casseola O, ed. *Cancer Pain Management: Pharmacologic, Interventional, and Palliative Approaches.* Philadelphia: Elsevier, 2006.
7. Mont'Alverne F, Vallee JN, Cormier E, et al. Percutaneous vertebroplasty for metastatic involvement of the axis. *Am J Neuroradiol* 2005;26:1641–1645.
8. Sclaich C, Minne HW, Brucker T, et al. Reduced pulmonary function in patients with spinal osteoporotic fractures. *Osteoporo Int* 1998;8(3):261–267.
9. Mazanec D, Podichetty VK, Mompoint A, et al. Vertebral compression fractures: manage aggressively to prevent sequelae. *Cleve Clin J Med* 2003;70(2): 147–156.
10. Kado D, Browner WS, Palermo L, et al. Vertebral fractures and mortality in older women: a prospective study. Study of Osteoporotic Fractures Research Group. *Arch Intern Med* 1999;159(11):1215–1220.
11. Yoneda T, Hiraga T. Crosstalk between cancer cells and bone microenvironment in bone metastasis. *Biochem Biophys Res Commun* 2005;328(3): 679–687.
12. Sohara Y, Shimada H, DeClerck YA. Mechanisms of bone invasion and metastasis in human neuroblastoma. *Cancer Lett* 2005;228(1–2):203–209.
13. Clines GA, Guise TA. Mechanisms and treatment for bone metastases. *Clin Adv Hematol Oncol* 2004;2(5):295–302.
14. Chung LW, Baseman A, Assikis V, et al. Molecular insights into prostate cancer progression: the missing link of tumor microenvironment. *J Urol* 2005;173(1): 10–20.
15. Asmus SE, Parsons S, Landis SC. Developmental changes in the transmitter properties of sympathetic neurons that innervate the periosteum. *J Neurosci* 2000;20:1495–1504.
16. Bjurholm A. Neuroendocrine peptides in bone. *Int Orthop* 1991;15:325–329.
17. McMahon S, et al. Inflammatory mediators and modulators of pain. In: McMahon S, Koltzenburg M, eds. *Wall and Melzack's Textbook of Pain.* 5th ed. London: Elsevier, 2006.
18. Lipton A. Management of bone metastases in breast cancer. *Curr Treat Options Oncol* 2005;6(2):161–171.
19. Sarantopoulos C. Advances in the therapy of cancer pain: from novel experimental models to evidence-based treatments. *SIGNA VITAE* 2007;2(suppl 1): S23–S41.
20. Yin JJ, Pollock CB, Kelly K. Mechanisms of cancer metastasis to the bone. *Cell Res* 2005;15(1):57–62.
21. Lipton A. Pathophysiology of bone metastases: how this knowledge may lead to therapeutic intervention. *J Support Oncol* 2004;2(3):205–220.
22. Eaton CL, Coleman RE. Pathophysiology of bone metastases from prostate cancer and the role of bisphosphonates in treatment. *Cancer Treat Rev* 2003; 29(3):189–198.
23. Mantyh P. Pain due to bone metastases: new research issues and their clinical implications. In: de Leon Casseola O, ed. *Cancer Pain Management: Pharmacologic, Interventional, and Palliative Approaches.* Philadelphia: Elsevier, 2006.
24. Riccio AI, Wodajo FM, Malawer M. Metastatic carcinoma of the long bones. *Am Fam Physician* 2007;76(10):1489–1494.
25. Coleman RE. Clinical features of metastatic bone disease and risk of skeletal morbidity. *Clin Cancer Res* 2006;12(20 Pt 2):6243s–6249s.
26. Mentzel H, Kentouche K, Sauner D, et al. Comparison of whole-body STIR-MRI and 99mTc-methylene-diphosphonate scintigraphy in children with suspected multifocal bone lesions. *Eur Radiol* 2004;14(12):2297–2302.
27. Edeiken J, Karasick D. Imaging in bone cancer. *CA Cancer J Clin* 1987;37: 239–245.
28. James SL, Davies AM. Post-operative imaging of soft tissue sarcomas. *Cancer Imaging* 2008;8:8–18.
29. Jayr C. Analgesic effects of cyclooxygenase 2 inhibitors. *Bull Cancer* 2004; 91(suppl 2):S125–131.
30. Sabino MA, Ghilardi JR, Jongen JL, et al. Simultaneous reduction in cancer pain, bone destruction, and tumor growth by selective inhibition of cyclooxygenase-2. *Cancer Res* 2002;62(24):7343–7349.
31. Singh B, Berry JA, Shoher A, et al. COX-2 involvement in breast cancer metastasis to bone. *Oncogene* 2007;31;26(26):3789–3796.
32. Singh B, Berry JA, Shoher A, et al. COX-2 induces IL-11 production in human breast cancer cells. *J Surg Res* 200;131(2):267–275.
33. Farooqui M, Li Y, Rogers T, et al. COX-2 inhibitor celecoxib prevents chronic morphine-induced promotion of angiogenesis, tumour growth, metastasis and mortality, without compromising analgesia. *Br J Cancer* 2007;97(11): 1523–1531.
34. Clezardin P, Teti A. Bone metastasis: pathogenesis and therapeutic implications. *Clin Exp Metastasis* 2007;24(8):599–608.
35. Mercadante S. Malignant bone pain: pathophysiology and treatment. *Pain* 1997;69:1–18.
36. MacDonald N. Principles governing the use of cancer chemotherapy in palliative medicine. In: Doyle D, Hanks GW, MacDonald N, eds. *Oxford Textbook of Palliative Medicine.* Oxford: Oxford Medical Publications, 1993;105–111.
37. Tannock I, Gospodarowicz M, Meakin W, et al. Treatment of metastatic prostatic cancer with low dose prednisone: evaluation of pain and quality of life as pragmatic indices of response. *J Clin Oncol* 1989;7;590–597.
38. Vitte C, Fleisch H, Guenther HL. Bisphosphonates induce osteoblasts to secrete an inhibitor of osteoclast-mediated resorption. *Endocrinology* 1996;137: 2324–2333.
39. Body JJ, Mancini I. Bisphosphonates for cancer patients: why, how, and when? *Support Care Cancer* 2002;10(5):399–407.
40. Costa L. Biphosphonates: reducing the risk of skeletal complications from bone metastasis. *Breast* 2007;16 (suppl 3):S16–S20.
41. Coleman RE. Optimising treatment of bone metastases by Aredia(TM) and Zometa(TM). *Breast Cancer* 2000;7(4):361–369.
42. Santini D, Fratto ME, Vincenzi B, et al. Zoledronic acid in the management of metastatic bone disease. *Expert Opin Biol Ther* 2006;6(12):1333–1348.
43. Rosen L. Zoledronic acid versus pamidronate in the treatment of skeletal metastases in patients with breast cancer orosteolytic lesions of multiple myeloma: a phase III, double-blind, comparative trial. *Cancer J* 2001;7(5):377–387.
44. Pavlakis N, Schmidt RL, Stockler M. Bisphosphonates for breast cancer. *Cochrane Database Syst Rev* 2002;(1):CD003474.
45. Lipton A. *Clin Breast Cancer* 2007;1(suppl 7):S14–S20.
46. Gennari C. Analgesic effect of calcitonin in osteoporosis. *Bone.*2002;30(suppl 5):67S–70S.
47. Visser E. A review of calcitonin and its use in the treatment of acute pain. *Acute Pain* 2005;7(4):185–189.
48. Keiichi O. Calcitonin inhibits pain and bone destruction in a model of bone cancer pain. *Anesthesiology* 2004;101:A1037.
49. Mystakidou K, Befon S, Hondros K, et al. Continuous subcutaneous administration of high-dose salmon calcitonin in bone metastasis: pain control and beta-endorphin plasma levels. *J Pain Symptom Manage* 1999;18(5):323–330.
50. Tsavaris N, Kopterides P, Kosmas C, et al. Analgesic activity of high-dose intravenous calcitonin in cancer patients with bone metastases. *Oncol Rep* 2006;16(4):871–875.
51. Martinez-Zapata MJ, Roque M, Alonso-Coello P, et al. Calcitonin for metastatic bone pain. *Cochrane Database Syst Rev* 2006;3:CD003223.
52. King T, Vardanyan A, Majuta L, et al. Morphine treatment accelerates sarcoma-induced bone pain, bone loss, and spontaneous fracture in a murine model of bone cancer. *Pain* 2007;132(1–2):154–168.
53. Hortobagyi GN. Moving into the future: treatment of bone metastases and beyond. *Cancer Treat Rev* 2005;31(suppl 3):9–18.
54. Donovan-Rodriguez T, Dickenson AH, Urch CE. Gabapentin normalizes spinal neuronal responses that correlate with behavior in a rat model of cancer-induced bone pain. *Anesthesiology* 2005;102(1):132–140.
55. Saito O, Aoe T, Kozikowski A, et al. Ketamine and N-acetylaspartylglutamate peptidase inhibitor exert analgesia in bone cancer pain. *Can J Anaesth* 2006; 53(9):891–898.
56. Sant'Agnese PA. The prostatic endocrine-paracrine regulation system and neuroendocrine differentiation in prostatic carcinoma: a review and future direction in basic reseaerch. *J Urol* 1992;152:2.
57. Wood BC. Hormone treatments in the common hormone-dependent carcinomas. *Palliat Med* 1993;7:257–272.
58. Mike S, Harrison C, Coles B, et al. Chemotherapy for hormone-refractory prostate cancer. *Cochrane Database Syst Rev* 2006;(4):CD00524.
59. Reale C, Turkiewicz AM, Reale CA. Antalgic treatment of pain associated with bone metastases. *Crit Rev Oncol Hematol* 2001;37:1–11.
60. Lattouf JB, Saad F. Preservation of bone health in prostate cancer. *Curr Opin Support Palliat Care* 2007;1(3):192–197.
61. Pelger RC, Soerdjbalie-Maikoe V, Hamdy NA. Strategies for management of prostate cancer-related bone pain. *Drugs Aging* 2001;18(12):899–911.
62. Silberstein EB. The treatment of painful osseous metastases with phosphorus-32-labeled phosphates. *Semin Oncol* 1993;20(3 Suppl 2):10–21.
63. Oosterhof GO, Roberts JT, de Reijke SA, et al. Strontium(89) chloride versus palliative local field radiotherapy in patients with hormonal escaped prostate cancer: a phase III study of the European Organisation for Research and Treatment of Cancer, Genitourinary Group. *Eur Urol* 2003;44(5):519–526.
64. Robinson K. Strontium 89 therapy for the palliation of pain due to osseous metastases. *JAMA* 1995;2;274(5):420–424.
65. Kraeber-Bodéré F. Treatment of bone metastases of prostate cancer with strontium-89 chloride: efficacy in relation to the degree of bone involvement. *Eur J Nucl Med* 2000;10:1487–1493.
66. Rowell NP. Intralesional methylprednisolone for rib metastases: an alternative to radiotherapy? *Palliat Med* 1988;2(2):153–155.
67. Adornato M, Paticoff KA. Intralesional corticosteroid injection for treatment of central giant-cell granuloma. *J Am Dent Assoc* 2001;132(2):186–190.
68. Lin P, Frink SJ. Intralesional treatment of bone tumors. *Operative Techniques in Orthopaedics* 2004;14(4):251–258.
69. Sis T, Wong C. Difficult problems and their solutions in patients with cancer pain of the head and neck areas. *Curr Rev Pain* 2000;4(3):206–214.

70. Alberico R, et al. Vertebroplasty and kyphoplasty. In: de Leon Casseola O, ed. *Cancer Pain Management: Pharmacologic, Interventional, and Palliative Approaches.* Philadelphia: Elsevier, 2006.

71. Fourney D, Schomer DF, Nader R, et al. Percutaneous vertebroplasty and kyphoplasty for painful vertebral body fractures in cancer patients. *J Neurosurg Spine* 2003 Jan;98(suppl 1):21–30.

72. Dupuy D, Ahmed M, Rodrigues B, et al. Percutaneous radiofrequency ablation of painful osseous metastases: a phase II trial. *Proc Am Soc Clin Oncol* 2001; 20:385a.

73. Locklin MA, Berger A, et al. Palliation of soft tissue cancer pain with radiofrequency ablation. *J Natl Cancer Inst* 2001;93:648–649.

74. Wood B, Fojo A, Levy EB, et al. Radiofrequency ablation of painful neoplasms as a palliative therapy: early experience. *J Vasc Interv Radiol* 2000;11S:207.

75. Goetz M, Callstrom MR, Charboneau JW, et al. Percutaneous image-guided radiofrequency ablation of painful metastases involving bone: a multicenter study. *J Clin Oncol* 2004;22(2):300–306.

76. Larkin K. Practical aspects of cancer pain and symptom management and pediatric palliative care. In: Fisch M, Burton A, eds. *Cancer Pain Management.* New York: McGraw-Hill, 2007.

77. Cherny N. The assessment of cancer pain. In: McMahon S, Koltzenburg M, eds. *Wall and Melzack's Textbook of Pain.* 5th ed. London: Elsevier, 2006.

78. Kubista E, Glaspy J, Holmes FA, et al. Bone pain associated with once-per-cycle pegfilgrastim is similar to daily filgrastim in patients with breast cancer. *Clin Breast Cancer* 2003;6:391–398.

79. Gudi R, Krishnamurthy M, Patcher BR. Astemizole in the treatment of granulo-cyte colony-stimulating factor-induced bone pain. *Ann Intern Med* 1995; 123(3):236–237.

80. Konig B, Konig W. Effect of growth factors on Escherichia coli-hemolysin-induced mediator release from human inflammatory cells. Involvement of the signal transduction pathway. *Infect Immun* 1994;62:2085–2093.

81. Bennett A. The role of biochemical mediators in peripheral nociception and bone pain. *Cancer Surv* 1988;7:55–67.

82. Slatkin N. Cancer-related pain and its pharmacologic management in the patient with bone metastasis. *J Support Oncol* 2006;4(2 Suppl 1):15–21.

83. Coleman RE. Clinical features of metastatic bone disease and risk of skeletal morbidity. *Clinical Cancer Research* 2006;12(20 Pt 2):6243s–6249s.

CHAPTER 47 ■ CANCER-RELATED VISCERAL PAIN

JANET ABRAHM, EDGAR ROSS, AND ROBERT J. KLICKOVICH

EPIDEMIOLOGY REVIEW

In 2004, 1.4 million Americans were diagnosed with cancer. This number equals approximately 4000 new diagnoses per day. In the same year, over 500,000 American deaths were attributed to cancer, accounting for 22% overall mortality.[1] Currently, more than 10 million individuals in the United States carry the burden of a cancer diagnosis, which is 3% of the population.[2] Approximately 50% of patients who carry a diagnosis of cancer report pain as a symptom of the disease process. This percentage increases to 75% of patients reporting pain in the advanced stages of disease.[3,4]

After patients come to terms with the diagnosis of cancer and the implications of their disease, most patients and their families will express concern about the pain and suffering they will experience as their disease progresses. Commonly asked questions include: how much pain will there be and can it be controlled?[4] Unfortunately, despite evidence that cancer pain can be controlled, it is managed poorly in many cases. Multiple factors limit adequate treatment of cancer pain, including misperceptions of disease processes, misconceptions regarding pain medications and procedures, professionals inadequately trained in pain management, failure to consult specialists trained in contemporary pain management methods, and social stigma around opioid use, including fears of addiction by patients, family members, and professional health care providers.[5] Also, many common cancers in the advanced stages of disease, when pain is highly prevalent, are incurable and survival may be measured in months, not years. While health care professionals may only measure survival duration as a meaningful treatment outcome, patients and families may measure outcomes in terms of improvement in quality of life, alleviation of pain, and relief of other associated symptoms related to cancer and treatment.[6]

Since pain syndromes arise from cancer therapies (including chemotherapy, radiation therapy, or surgery), patients who survive their primary malignancy may be left with pain secondary to an iatrogenic process. Chemotherapy may induce a painful peripheral neuropathy. Neuropathy is well described with vin-cristine, platinum, taxanes, thalidomide, bortezomib, and other agents. Pain secondary to radiation may appear years to decades after completion of radiotherapy. Pain syndromes following surgery may present after mastectomy, amputation, thoracotomy, or other surgical approaches to malignancies (see Chapters 41, 42, 45, and 48).[7]

CHARACTERISTICS OF VISCERAL PAIN

Anatomy and Physiology

Visceral pain is caused by disorders of internal organs such as the stomach, kidney, gallbladder, urinary bladder, and intestines as well as changes in the central nervous system. Pain can result from distension, impaction, ischemia, inflammation, or traction on the mesentery, and can be associated with symptoms such as nausea, fever, malaise, and pain.[8] Growth of visceral tumors disrupts normal physiological processes secondary to compression and invasion of adjacent structures. Progression of disease may be asymptomatic until a critical event manifests (e.g., obstruction of a hollow viscus). Under these conditions, the first symptom a patient may experience is pain.[9–11]

Visceral pain is unique in quality of presentation when compared to pain that arises from musculoskeletal structures of the body. Visceral pain is usually vague in its presentation and may be confused by referral to a variety of somatic locations. Symptoms may seem out of proportion to physical examination and imaging.[12] Additionally, visceral pain may be attributable both to the malignancy itself and to chemotherapeutic and radiation therapies. Increased pain following symptomatic relief may suggest the local recurrence of disease or a new locus of disease requiring repeat evaluation of the patient.[13]

Some features of visceral nociception may offer a better understanding of the experience of patients with visceral pain. Visceral pain is more frequently accompanied by an autonomic response than is somatic pain or pain from skin injury. There is a poor correlation between the extent of visceral tissue damage and the severity of pain experienced. The diffuse nature of visceral pain and its referral to superficial structures is due to the convergence of visceral and somatic afferents on the same dorsal horn neurons. Visceral pain is poorly localized because of poor representation within the primary somatosensory cortex. The majority of visceral afferents are specific to motor or reflex responses with few neural afferents that are specialized for pain transmission. Those afferents that are specialized for pain are sparsely distributed throughout the viscera; both high-threshold nociceptors and "silent" nociceptors are invoked in the pain experience.[11]

Studies have demonstrated multiple visceral pain mechanisms as well as the mechanisms by which one class of visceral pain may relate to other sources of malignant pain. There are four primary classes of visceral pain:

1. Mechanical: caused by stretch of visceral structures (bowel lumen or hepatic capsule)
2. Ischemic: caused by tumor invasion or compression of visceral blood supply
3. Inflammatory: humoral mediators of inflammation released secondary to tumor infiltration of visceral structures
4. Neuropathic: compression or invasion of neural structures supplying the viscera.[13]

Surgery, chemotherapy, or radiation therapy of cancer can also be responsible for iatrogenic damage of the viscera, associated visceral structures, or nerves. Applying a stimulus that causes tissue damage (e.g., cutting, burning, or pinching) to skin or muscle reliably produces the perception of pain but these stimuli do not reliably evoke reports of pain when applied to visceral structures. Pain secondary to distension of a hollow viscous, such as in the case of bowel obstruction, does not necessarily produce a similar perception when applied to surface structures. In controlled studies, visceral pain can be consistently demonstrated by mechanical distension of hollow organs using distending fluids or balloon devices.[14] These modalities of inducing pain most closely reproduce the natural or pathophysiological processes causing pain. Mechanical distension can be specifically applied to a given organ structure in isolation of other structures, mimicking processes involving the gastrointestinal, biliary, and urinary tracts which may occur from tumor obstruction (or adhesions) in these sites. Distension of organ capsules, such as the splenic, renal, or hepatic capsule, has also been demonstrated to produce profound pain. On the other hand, gentle or slow but progressive distension or obstruction may not produce pain until a critical point in which ischemia or rupture result. Torsion or stretch on mesenteric structures or omentum may produce states of ischemia, infarct, and inflammatory response producing reports of severe pain.[15]

Inflammatory processes in visceral structures may produce pain as a result of ischemic response, but some tumors may produce inflammatory mediators with no inciting ischemic event. Both prostaglandin E2 and serotonin have been demonstrated as independent chemical stimuli in the production of pain as malignancy invades adjacent structures.[16–18] Experimental studies have demonstrated that the application of inflammatory chemical stimuli can evoke pain behaviors, yet specific mechanical means of eliciting pain have been limited in their translation to studies of other visceral structures.[19]

Ischemic pain has also been described as occurring secondary to occlusion of visceral vasculature or by compression of visceral structures by tumor growth. When tumor growth exceeds vascular supply, necrosis may result, inducing a variety of inflammatory processes.[18] Inflammatory mediators, such as hydrogen ions, kinins, prostanoids, leukotrienes, or other cytokines, are initiators of visceral pain. These chemical agents also sensitize neurologic afferents of organ structures amplifying nociception associated with mechanical stimuli. In general, healthy viscera are typically insensate to pain while superficial structures are continually sensate.[19] When diseased, however, visceral organs produce pain severe enough to be incapacitating to other physical activity. Superficial pain may provoke physical activity. Pain from surface structures of the body evokes reflexive motion in the classic "fight or flight" response, whereas the sensation of visceral pain discourages motion or physical activity. Anecdotal evidence supports an association between pain of visceral origin and emotional response and is commonly held to be more anxiety provoking than pain from somatic structures. Some argue that this anxiety comes from a patient's inability to visualize the cause of the pain.[20] Anxiety scales are reported higher in patients with visceral pain ratings of 2 on a scale of 10 when compared to a higher-rated pain experience with visible cause on a superficial structure.[21] Furthermore, some symptomatology is more common in patients with visceral pain. Perception of both nausea and dyspnea are more commonly associated with pain of a visceral organ. An autonomic response to visceral pain is far more common than to pain of superficial structures.[22,23]

Psychological processing of visceral pain is distinct from that related to somatic pain. There are a low number of visceral nociceptors compared with somatic nociceptors. There is a lack of specialization of visceral afferents. Many visceral afferents are polymodal nociceptors. Viscera have convergence with somatic afferents on dorsal horn lamina resulting in referred pain. Viscera have unique ascending tracts through the dorsal column.[24] Viscera have poor representation within the primary somatosensory cortex. Viscera have significant input through the medial thalamus to the limbic cortex, amygdala, anterior cingulate, and insular cortex.[25] Viscera also have a close association with autonomic nerves. The perception of visceral pain may be disproportionate to pathology exhibited by physical examination or imaging. As an example, a small nephrolith may offer some of the most severe pain states whereas extensive cancer metastasis may evoke little or no discomfort. Disorders such as chronic pancreatitis demonstrate very little correlation between laboratory studies and flares in pain perception. Disorders such as irritable bowel syndrome and noncardiac chest pain syndrome appear to lack a definitive histopathologic basis for the discomfort and pain.[26,27]

Many models exist for visceral pain including intraperitoneal injection of a chemical, distension of hollow organs (cecum, colon, rectum), distension of the gallbladder and associated biliary system, distention or chemical stimulation of the bladder and other urinary tract structures, as well as distension, compression, or traction on reproductive organs. However, lesions studied in one organ are limited in that they are specific to a given stimulus and do not necessarily translate to application in other visceral structures.[28]

Sensitization

Sensitization occurring secondary to the repeated presentation of visceral stimuli has been noted in human psychophysical studies as well as animal studies. Repeated presentation of the same visceral stimuli produces increasing strength of response in neuronal, cardiovascular, and visceromotor reflex responses. Inflammation of visceral structures increases the magnitude of response to a given mechanical stimulus and decreases the stimulation thresholds for the evocation of nociceptive responses. Inflammation of visceral structures significantly modifies behavioral, neuronal, autonomic, and motor responses to visceral stimulation in experimental models. This model mirrors clinical circumstances, since inflammation in visceral structures frequently leads to reports of pain.[29]

Painful conditions such as mucositis, esophagitis, gastritis, pancreatitis, and colitis all exhibit mucosal inflammatory changes. The inflammatory sensitization may take place at primary afferents. These afferents are normally nonreactive to most stimuli and have been described as "silent" in non-pathological states. However, in the context of an inflammatory tissue response, they become spontaneously active and highly reactive to mechanical stimuli. Silent afferents may comprise 50% of the neuronal sample in a visceral organ, but are infrequently noted in superficial or cutaneous structures. Lack of baseline sensitivity in normal viscera may be secondary to sparsity of visceral afferentation. There are fewer afferents per unit area than similar measures of cutaneous afferents. Because of this sparse innervation, increased activity may be necessary to cross a threshold for perception. Spinal neurons responsive to visceral stimuli also change their responsiveness to visceral stimuli in the presence of inflammation. The cause of this behavior is unknown. Increased afferent activity, altered intrinsic properties of dorsal horn neurons, and altered modulatory influences or some combination may all serve a role in the process. Dorsal column pathways have been demonstrated to play a role in visceral nociception, but not in cutaneous nociception. The results of multiple studies suggest that visceral pain requires a sensitization process both in the periphery and the spinal cord. However, somatic central sensitization characterized by "wind up" of interneurons within the dorsal horn does not occur with visceral pain.[30]

Localization

Visceral pain is classically thought of as deep and diffuse in presentation. Localization of the pain generator can be difficult to identify by physical examination. Superficial pain, in contrast, can be elicited by examination with precise localization and with consideration to the site of the body examined; pain locus can be identified within millimeters. Moreover, surface pain loci reliably localize to the same site, never migrating to other body areas, in the absence of neural injury.

Visceral pain is characterized as migratory in its presentation, often perceived in several loci simultaneously or migrating regionally in spite of localization of pathology. This is evident in the presentation of appendicitis. Furthermore, the perception of pain associated with visceral pathology is not normally localized to the organ itself but to somatic structures that receive afferent inputs at the same spinal segments as the visceral afferent entry. For this reason, visceral pain is classically described as either unlocalized pain or as referred pain that may have two separate features. Sensation of the diseased viscera is transferred to a surface site (e.g., an ischemic myocardium can be felt in neck and arms) or additional sites may become hypersensitive to inputs applied directly to those other sites (e.g., flank muscle becomes sensitive to palpation with urolithiasis). This latter phenomenon is referred to as secondary somatic hyperalgesia.

Psychophysical studies of internal organ sensation have been very focused on a given organ using simple stimuli correlating the given stimuli to a given organ with perception at the respective site of stimulus. Other psychophysical studies using visceral stimuli have examined the referred sensations described by subjects. These studies have often failed to contrast referred pain to a body surface with cutaneous sensations at the same surface. Patient illustrations of referred sensations tend to extend over large surface areas, whereas studies using cutaneous stimuli generate pinpoint localization to highly precise sites.

The phenomenon of secondary somatic hyperalgesia produced by visceral pathology has been compared to sites of sensitivity with lesions produced by herpes zoster. These initial studies were fundamental to the development of dermatomal mapping. In visceral disease processes, multiple dermatomes have been identified suggesting that secondary somatic hyperalgesia is widely distributed (i.e., poorly localized).

Recent psychophysical studies have attempted to compare visceral with nonvisceral pain. In one study, the sensation produced with balloon distension of the esophagus was compared to thermal stimulation of the mid-chest skin. Subjects perceived larger areas of sensation for esophageal distension than for intensity-matched heat-evoked sensation on body maps. Temporally, there was also a difference. A rapid response was noted with heat stimulus whereas there was poor correlation with the esophageal stimulus and the perception of the sensation. Intense visceral discomfort remained after discontinuation of the distending apparatus but not after discontinuation of the cutaneous stimulation. Visceral sensation was concluded to be diffuse both spatially and temporally. Corollary observation of cerebral blood flow identified that similar cerebral areas were activated by both stimuli.

When evaluating the patient in visceral pain with malignancy, the early presentation may be misleading with vague midline discomfort. It may be poorly localized and accompanied by both an emotional response and autonomic event. Later in the evolution of disease process, patients may complain of somatic or referred pain hypersensitivity at the spinal level of the visceral nociceptor terminus. Referred pain is sharp and localized. It is often associated with allodynia and muscle spasm. Furthermore, visceral hypersensitivity may induce the perception of pain in another organ receiving innervation from the same spinal segment.

Visceral Afferentation

Visceral primary afferents differ significantly from cutaneous primary afferents in both number and pattern of distribution. Visceral sensory pathways are organized into nerve fascicles and cell body groupings extending from prevertebral regions to contact viscera predominately via perivascular pathways. Cell bodies of visceral primary afferent nerve fibers are located in the visceral dorsal root ganglia of the thoracic and upper lumbar spine, but the peripheral axons of these neurons follow a circuitous path to visceral organs passing via the paravertebral sympathetic chain and ganglia as well as nerve fascicles that are termed the cardiac and splanchnic nerves. The splanchnic nerves are divided into the greater, lesser, least, thoracic, and lumbar divisions. The pelvic nerves arise from dorsal root ganglia at sacral levels, accepting sympathetic chain input before innervating urogenital structures.

Visceral sensory processing also differs from cutaneous sensory processing because visceral neuronal synapses exist at cell bodies of prevertebral ganglia such as the celiac ganglion, superior mesenteric ganglion, and pelvic ganglion, producing changes in local visceral function outside central control. The gastrointestinal tract is also supplied by an independent enteric nervous system relating to functions of digestion and absorption. In the pelvis, structures receive dual innervation with afferents from lower thoracic-upper lumbar segments and from sacral segments. Testicle and ovary embryologically originate in the superior aspect of the abdomen and, therefore, receive thoracic innervation. The urinary bladder has a similar thoracolumbar innervation with sensory inputs extending up to the T10 level, but also receives sacral inputs (the pelvic nerve) with other tissues originating from sacral dermatomes (rectum, genital structures).

Pelvic organs also receive efferent and afferent connections from the vagus nerve and local ganglionic circuitry, resulting in a complex and diffuse neuroanatomy. Afferents with endings in a focal visceral site may have cell bodies in the dorsal root ganglia of 10 or more spinal levels in a bilaterally distributed fashion. In contrast, cutaneous afferents from a particular body surface arise from only 3 to 5 unilaterally located dorsal root ganglia.

Visceral receptors are located in mucosa, serosa, and muscle of hollow organs as well as visceral mesentery. They are not reported in parenchyma of solid organs. The specialized receptors that discriminate a variety of stimuli in somatic structures are absent in viscera. The mesentery, however, does contain Pacinian corpuscles. Hollow organs contain specialized low-threshold and high-threshold mechanoreceptors. Low-threshold receptors serve a basic regulatory function whereas high-threshold receptors are activated only with noxious mechanical stimuli. Visceral nociception results from summation of nociceptive input to regulatory low-threshold receptors and noxious high-threshold and silent nociceptors rather than activation of stimulus-specific nociceptors.[31]

Ascending Pathways

Visceral afferent fiber activation causes an increase in nitric oxide synthase in the dorsal horn of the spinal cord, causing expression of the oncogene C-fos in laminae I, V, VII, X of the dorsal horn within the thoracolumbar spine. Similar upregulation is seen in the amygdala and paraventricular hypothalamic nuclei, and consequent elevation in norepinephrine production within the locus ceruleus.

Features of visceral pain processing differing from somatic processing include dorsal column ascending secondary sensory afferents, the spinal trigeminal to parabrachioamygdaloid tract, and the spinohypothalamic pathway. In the visceral system, both ventrolateral and dorsal column postsynaptic neurons have a role in nociception. Ascending tracts synapse at the lateral thalamus first, then limbic centers, then somatosensory cortex. While somatic nociception is represented somatotopically within the primary somatosensory cortex, visceral pain is represented in the secondary somatosensory cortex and poorly represented within the primary somatosensory cortex. Visceral pain is well represented in the limbic system, including anterior cingulate gyrus, insular cortex, and amygdala, suggesting a basis for the strong emotional component of visceral pain. While visceral pain elicits decreased patient activity, nausea, and hypotension, somatic pain elicits agitation, reactive activity, and hypertension. Nociceptive activity within the gastrointestinal tract induces inhibition of dorsal motor neurons of the vagus within the medulla leading to gastroparesis and nausea.

VISCERAL PAIN SYNDROMES

Although most pain associated with malignancy is diffuse and chronic, most acute pain syndromes in cancer are secondary to diagnostic or therapeutic interventions. Some tumors generate an acute onset of pain, which may be the result of a perforation of a hollow viscus or rupture of a visceral capsule. Any sudden onset of pain warrants a comprehensive pain assessment. Below is a list of possible pain syndromes that may be encountered by the health care provider.

Oral Mucosa

Paraneoplastic Pemphigus

Paraneoplastic pemphigus is a mucocutaneous disorder accompanying non-Hodgkin's lymphoma and chronic lymphocytic leukemia. It is characterized by widespread shallow ulcers, hemorrhagic crusting of the lips, conjunctival bullae, and may be accompanied by pulmonary lesions, occurring secondary to autoantibodies directed against desmoplakins and desmogleins.[32]

Oropharyngeal Mucositis and Stomatitis

Mucositis and stomatitis should be distinguished as two separate processes (also see Chapter 45). Oral mucositis is an inflammation of oral mucosa resulting from chemotherapeutic agents or ionizing radiation, manifesting as erythema or ulcerations. Stomatitis is any inflammatory condition of oral tissue, including mucosa, dentition, periapices and periodontium, including inflammation secondary to infection of oral tissues. Mucositis appears 7 to 10 days after initiation of high-dose cancer therapy and is generally self-limited when uncomplicated by infection,

resolving 2 to 4 weeks after completion of chemotherapy. In order to standardize assessment, a variety of scales have been created to grade the level of stomatitis by characterizing alterations in lips, tongue, mucous membranes, gingiva, teeth, pharynx, quality of saliva, and voice. The clinical syndrome usually involves the oropharynx but may involve other gastrointestinal mucosal surfaces such as the esophagus, stomach, or intestine, producing such symptoms as odynophagia, dyspepsia, or diarrhea. Any mucosal damage may become superinfected with microorganisms, most commonly Candida albicans and herpes simplex.[33]

Radiotherapy may also induce mucositis. Doses of radiation in excess of 4000 cGy frequently cause ulceration with pain lasting several weeks following treatment.[34] Acute pain associated with radiotherapy can be caused by acute radiation toxicity causing inflammation and ulceration of skin or mucous membranes. The syndrome produced is dependent upon the exposed field.[35,36]

Mediastinum

5-Fluorouracil-induced Anginal Chest Pain

In patients receiving 5-fluorouracil (5-FU) infusions, ischemic chest pain may develop. Painful events are more common in patients with a history of coronary artery disease and are likely secondary to coronary vasospasm.

Pleura

Lung tumors, with or without chest wall involvement, may produce visceral pain. In a large case series of patients with lung malignancies, pain was found to be unilateral in 80% of patients and bilateral in 20% of patients. Patients with hilar tumors reported sternal or scapular pain. Patients with tumors involving the upper and lower lobe experienced referral of pain into the shoulder and lower chest, respectively.[37,38] Additionally, some lung malignancies generate ipsilateral facial pain, thought to be secondary to noxious stimulation of vagal afferent neurons.[39-42]

Pancoast Syndrome

Pancoast syndrome is caused by malignant neoplasms of the superior sulcus of the lung with destructive lesions of the thoracic inlet and involvement of the brachial plexus and cervical sympathetic nerves (stellate ganglion).[43] Patients report severe pain in the shoulder region radiating toward the axilla and scapula along the ulnar aspect of the muscles of the hand, and patients may also develop atrophy of hand and arm muscles, Horner syndrome (ptosis, miosis, hemianhidrosis, enophthalmos), and compression of the blood vessels with edema.[44] Ninety-five percent of patients have either squamous cell or adenocarcinomas. Small cell carcinoma is found in fewer than 5% percent of cases in most series. Along with these symptoms and signs, additional predictors of poor prognosis are weight loss, supraclavicular fossa or vertebral body involvement, disease stage, and surgical treatment.[45,46]

These bronchopulmonary tumors may invade the bony structures of the chest. The first or second thoracic vertebra or the first, second, or third ribs may be invaded. One review has described rib erosion in 50% of patients. The tumor may invade the first or second thoracic vertebral bodies or intervertebral foramina, extending to the spinal cord and resulting in cord compression. The subclavian vein or artery may also be invaded. Advanced tumors may involve the recurrent laryngeal nerve, phrenic nerve, or superior vena cava.

Pancreas

Midline Retroperitoneal Syndrome

The most common cancer-related causes of upper abdominal retroperitoneal pain are pancreatic cancer and retroperitoneal lymphadenopathy, particularly celiac lymphadenopathy. These disease processes elicit afferent activity via injury to deep somatic structures of the posterior abdominal wall, distortion of pain-sensitive connective tissue, vascular and ductal structures, as well as local inflammation and direct infiltration of the celiac plexus. Patients report pain in the epigastrium, in the low thoracic region of the back, or both. Pain is described as diffuse, dull and boring, exacerbated with recumbency, and improved by sitting forward. Computed tomography (CT), magnetic resonance imaging, or ultrasound scanning of the abdomen may reveal the disease process.

Pancreatic Cancer

Patients with pain secondary to unresectable pancreatic cancer report severe abdominal pain radiating into the back. This pain is often refractory to analgesics, even strong opioids. Pain may be accompanied by obstructive jaundice (yellowing of the skin and eyes, itching, dark urine, clay-colored stool) and occurs more frequently when the cancer is located at the head of the pancreas. Other associated symptoms may include weight loss, anorexia, fatigue, and a change in bowel habits (constipation or diarrhea). Controlled trials support the use of neurolytic celiac plexus block with superior results in terms of pain relief over analgesics alone (see Chapter 44 and discussion of celiac plexus block below).[48]

Liver Pain

Hepatic Distension Syndrome

The liver has many nociceptive structures including the liver capsule, blood vessels, and biliary tract. Afferents from these structures travel via the celiac plexus, the phrenic nerve, and the lower right intercostal nerves. Hepatic metastasis typically causes pain when the tumor stretches the capsule. Patients with intrahepatic metastases or hepatomegaly secondary to cholestasis may report discomfort in the right subcostal region or right mid-back or flank.[49] Patients may experience referred pain to the right neck, shoulder, or scapula.[50] Patients describe the pain as a dull ache exacerbated by movement, pressure in the abdomen, and deep inspiration. Associated symptoms include anorexia and nausea.

Physical examination reveals a hard, irregular subcostal mass, which is dull to percussion, and descends with inspiration. Diagnostic ultrasound or CT may reveal a space-occupying lesion.

Analgesics are the first line of therapy for pain control with drug selection and titration a function of the extent of hepatic compromise. Corticosteroids reduce hepatic edema and liver pain. If a tumor is chemosensitive, chemotherapy may be the treatment of choice. Hormone therapy may decrease hepatomegaly from liver metastasis but may take several months to accomplish a goal of pain relief. As with pancreatic cancer, celiac plexus block may provide definitive relief. Two randomized controlled trials have demonstrated hepatic irradiation to be effective in palliation of hepatic pain in 80% of patients with a reduction of systemic symptoms in half as many patients.[51]

Intestinal Pain

Chronic Intestinal Obstruction

In patients with abdominal or pelvic cancers, intestinal obstruction causes diffuse abdominal pain. Pain may be secondary to smooth muscle contraction, mesenteric tension, and ischemia of the bowel wall. Obstruction may be due to tumor, autonomic neuropathy, ileus, metabolic abnormality, or medication. Pain may be continuous or intermittent (colicky) and may be associated with vomiting, anorexia, and constipation.

Peritoneal Carcinomatosis

The peritoneal cavity, enclosed by visceral and parietal peritoneum, is the largest potential space in the body. Any pathologic process involving the peritoneal cavity can easily disseminate throughout this space by means of unrestricted movement of fluid and cells. Primary malignant diseases arising from the peritoneal cavity include malignant mesothelioma, cystic mesothelioma, and primary peritoneal carcinoma. Carcinomatosis can cause peritoneal inflammation, mesenteric tethering, and malignant adhesions and ascites, all of which can trigger nociceptive activity. Patients most commonly report abdominal pain and distension. Mesenteric tethering and tension appear to cause a diffuse abdominal or low-back pain. Tense malignant ascites can produce diffuse abdominal discomfort and a distinct stretching pain in the anterior abdominal wall. Adhesions can also cause obstruction of a hollow viscus, with intermittent colicky pain.[52] CT scanning may demonstrate evidence of ascites, omental infiltration, and peritoneal nodules.

Radiation Enteritis

Acute radiation enteritis may develop in as many as 50% of patients receiving pelvic or abdominal radiotherapy. Patients with small intestinal involvement complain of cramping abdominal pain and have associated nausea and diarrhea. Patients receiving pelvic radiotherapy may develop proctocolitis, associated with pain, tenesmus, diarrhea, mucous discharge, and bleeding. These symptoms may resolve shortly after completion of therapy or may last as long as 6 months.

Intraperitoneal Chemotherapy Pain

Approximately 25% of patients receiving intraperitoneal chemotherapy may develop transient mild to moderate abdominal pain and complain of fullness or bloating.[53] A second group of patients (approximately 25%) may experience pain severe enough to require opioid analgesia or discontinuation of therapy. Pain is secondary to chemical serositis or infection. Infectious peritonitis is accompanied by fever and leukocytosis in blood and peritoneal fluid.

Pelvic Pain

Malignancy-related pelvic pain not due to bone metastases is most often secondary to presacral recurrence of rectal carcinoma or secondary to pelvic recurrence of cervical cancer. Lumbosacral plexus infiltration is common, resulting in severe pain with a significant neuropathic contribution. Analgesics or interventional therapies should be implemented according to protocols and guidelines (see Chapter 43).

Malignant Perineal Pain

Perineal pain may be secondary to tumors of the colon or rectum, female reproductive tract, and distal genitourinary system. A report of perineal pain following therapeutic resolution of malignancy may be a precursor of recurrence and should prompt complete evaluation.[54] Pain preceding evidence of disease may be secondary to microscopic perineural invasion of an insidious malignant process. Patients report pain to be constant and aching, exacerbated with sitting or standing. Associated symptoms may include tenesmus or bladder spasm.[55] If tumor invades musculature of the pelvis, patients may complain of a constant aching in the pelvis, which is exacerbated with standing. Examination of the pelvic floor may demonstrate tumor.

Ureteral Obstruction

Patients with tumor involving the pelvis may have pain due to tumor compression or infiltration of the distal ureter.[6] Obstruction of the proximal ureter is less common and is associated with retroperitoneal lymphadenopathy, an isolated retroperitoneal metastasis, mural metastases or intraluminal metastases. Cancers of the cervix, ovary, prostate, and rectum are most commonly associated with this complication. Other rare causes of ureteral obstruction include retroperitoneal fibrosis resulting from radiotherapy or graft versus host disease. Pain is described as dull chronic discomfort in the flank often with associated radiation into the inguinal region or genitalia.[6] However, patients may have obstruction without evidence of pain.

Ovarian Cancer Pain

Patients experiencing severe chronic abdominal or pelvic pain may be experiencing the harbinger of ovarian cancer. It is the most common presenting symptom and most common symptom of recurrence.[6] Two-thirds of patients experience pain in the 2 weeks prior to the onset or recurrence of the disease. In patients who have been previously treated, it is an important symptom of potential recurrence.[6]

Tumor-related Gynecomastia

In patients complaining of breast pain or tenderness, there is a risk of occult tumor of the testes or lung. Human chorionic gonadotrophin (HCG) secreting tumors of testis, including malignant and benign types as well as other HCG secreting tumors, may produce breast tenderness or gynecomastia.[56] Approximately 10% of patients diagnosed with testicular cancer complain of gynecomastia or breast tenderness.[57]

Intravesical Chemotherapy or Immunotherapy

Patients receiving intravesical Bacillus Calmette-Guérin (BCG) therapy for urinary bladder transitional cell carcinoma experience a syndrome of bladder irritability. Patients report urinary frequency and painful micturition. In rare cases, patients receiving BCG therapy may develop a painful polyarthritis.[58] Other intravesical chemotherapies, such as doxorubicin, may also cause a painful chemical cystitis.[59]

Corticosteroid-induced Perineal Discomfort

In patients receiving high-dose corticosteroid therapy, some may report an uncomfortable sensation of burning perineal pain.[60]

Adrenal

Adrenal Pain Syndrome

Patients with adrenal metastases of considerable size, common in lung cancer, may develop unilateral flank pain or abdominal pain. Patients report pain from this condition as highly variable, describing it as dull and aching to severe in presentation.[61]

Vascular Obstruction

Hypercoagulability with thrombosis is the most frequent complication associated with malignancy and the second most frequent cause of mortality in malignant disease. A thrombotic event may occur in advance of the diagnosis of cancer by months or years; therefore, thrombosis should be considered as a marker for occult malignancy. Chemotherapy and hormone therapy are associated with an increased thrombotic risk. Additionally, deep vein thrombosis (DVT) is a more common postoperative complication in patients with malignancies than in other postoperative populations.

Hypercoagulability in malignancy is secondary to tumor cell expression of tissue factor and cancer procoagulant. Apoptosis of malignant cells or penumbra of nonmalignant cells affected by invading malignant tissue activates normally dormant tissue factor, initiating a coagulation cascade and formation of thrombus. Tumor proliferation, chemotherapy, hormonal therapy, radiation therapy, and hematopoietic growth factors all increase apoptotic activity and increase the risk of thrombus. Factors contributing to the formation of thrombus include cytokine release, acute phase reaction, and neovascularization. Tumors associated with higher risk of hypercoagulability include tumors of the pelvis, pancreas, stomach, breast, and brain.

Venous Thrombosis

Patients with DVT most often present with pain and swelling of the lower extremity. Patients often report that pain is mild, dull and crampy, or a diffuse perception of pressure or heaviness. The calf is most often involved, but the sole of the foot, heel, thigh, groin, or pelvis may be the site of thrombus and pain. Exacerbating factors include standing or walking. Physical examination may reveal signs of DVT, including swelling, warmth, dilation of superficial veins, tenderness along venous tracts, and pain with stretching of the affected limb. Rarely, a patient may present with ischemia of the lower extremity or in worse cases, a gangrenous limb. This presentation may occur in the absence of arterial or capillary occlusion (phlegmasia cerulea dolens). Signs include severe pain, extensive edema, and cyanosis of the affected leg. Mortality varies, but may be as high as 40% secondary to ischemia of the affected extremity or progression of thrombus to cause pulmonary emboli.

Only 2% of DVT cases involve the upper extremity with a low rate of associated pulmonary embolism. On physical examination, upper extremity DVT most often presents with edema, dilated collateral circulation, and pain.[62] In patients with malignancy, central venous catheterization is the most frequent cause[63] along with extrinsic compression by tumor.[64]

Superior Vena Cava Obstruction

For patients with lung cancer and lymphoma, superior vena cava (SVC) obstruction develops with extrinsic compression of the SVC by tumor expansion or by enlarged mediastinal lymph nodes.[63] Intravascular catheters are an iatrogenic cause,[65] especially with left-sided ports where the catheter tip rests in the upper portion of the vessel. Physical examination reveals facial swelling, dilated neck veins, and dilated chest wall veins. Less common patient reports of symptoms associated with SVC obstruction include chest pain, headache, and mastalgia.[66]

Acute Mesenteric Vein Thrombosis

Acute thrombosis of the mesenteric veins is most commonly associated with hypercoagulability secondary to malignancy and more rarely secondary to venous compression by lymphadenopathy, extension of venous thrombosis, or iatrogenic hypercoagulable states.

Pain Syndromes Related to Intravenous Chemotherapeutic Agents

Chemotherapeutic agents may cause vascular pain secondary to venous spasm, chemical phlebitis, vesicant extravasation, and anthracycline-associated flare. Venospasm pain is not secondary to inflammation or phlebitis. Attenuation of symptoms may come from application of a warm compress or reduction of chemotherapeutic infusion rate.

Agents causing chemical phlebitis include amsacrine, dacarbazine, carmustine and vinorelbine, potassium chloride, and hyperosmolar solutions. The pain and erythema associated with chemical phlebitis should be monitored closely as it shares many of the early features of vesicant cytotoxic extravasation that in later stages presents as desquamation and ulceration of cutaneous structures.

Venous flare reaction is often associated with the use of anthracycline or doxorubicin and presents with local urticaria, pain, or stinging.

Hepatic Artery Infusion Pain

Patients receiving cytotoxic infusions directly into the hepatic artery often report diffuse abdominal pain.[65] Pain is attributed to gastric ulceration, gastric erosion, or cholangitis. With no persistence of complications, resolution of pain occurs with completion of therapy.

Complex Visceral Pain Syndromes

Nontraumatic rupture of a visceral tumor may cause sudden, severe abdominal or pelvic pain and is most commonly associated with hepatocellular carcinoma.[67] Metastases from other tumors also cause visceral ruptures (e.g., kidney rupture from a metastasis from adenocarcinoma of the colon[68] or metastasis-induced perforated appendicitis.[69] Torsion of pedunculated visceral tumors may cause cramping abdominal pain.[70]

Postradiation Visceral Pain

Postradiation therapy pain syndromes often involve both somatic and visceral structures, regardless of the target organ. Late effects, including connective tissue fibrosis, neural damage, and secondary malignancies, can occur long after completion of radiotherapy. A recent large retrospective cohort study revealed an association between previous pelvic radiation and hip fractures, with an increase in lifetime fracture rate from 17% (control) to 27% (radiation group). Pelvic pain after radiotherapy may be due to pelvic insufficiency fracture, enteritis, visceral dysfunction, or neural damage. Chronic pelvic pain has been reported as a consequence of prostate brachytherapy. Twenty percent of patients receiving brachytherapy have been reported to complain of dysuria 1 year after treatment.

Radiation Enteritis and Proctitis

In 2% to 10% of patients receiving pelvic or abdominal radiation therapy, chronic enteritis and proctocolitis may occur.[71] The rectum and distal colon are more frequently sites of involvement. Onset may be as early as 3 months or as late as 30 years.[72] Presentations may include proctitis (bloody diarrhea, tenesmus, and cramping pain), obstruction due to stricture formation, or fistulae to the bladder or vagina.[6] Small bowel radiation damage typically causes colicky abdominal pain, which can be associated with chronic nausea or malabsorption. Barium studies may demonstrate a narrow tubular bowel segment resembling Crohn's disease or ischemic colitis. Endoscopy and biopsy may be needed to identify recurrent cancer.

Burning Perineum Syndrome

Perineal discomfort may develop 6–18 months following pelvic radiotherapy. Patients complain of burning pain in the perianal region and may involve the vagina or scrotum. For those patients with postabdominoperineal resection, phantom anus pain and recurrent tumor should be considered.

Radiation Cystitis

Radiation therapy used in the treatment of tumors of the pelvic organs (prostate, bladder, colon/rectum, uterus, ovary, and vagina/vulva) may produce chronic radiation cystitis.[6] Symptoms of radiation injury to the bladder may be as minor as temporary irritation with voiding or asymptomatic hematuria, or as severe as gross hematuria, a contracted nonfunctional bladder, persistent incontinence, and fistula formation. Other signs and symptoms may include frequency, urgency, dysuria, hematuria, incontinence, hydronephrosis, pneumaturia, and fecaluria.[6]

Postchemotherapy Visceral Pain

Painful peripheral neuropathy is frequently a dose-limiting side effect of some chemotherapeutic regimens. Once the therapy is stopped, the neuropathic pain will resolve with or without symptomatic treatment. However, in a small number of patients, the neuropathy does not resolve and may continue to be intensely painful. Prevalence during treatment varies from agent to agent, with the intensity of treatment (dose intensity and cumulative dose), with other concurrent therapies such as surgery and radiotherapy, and with the use of combination chemotherapy. Estimates of prevalence range from 4% to 76% during chemotherapy treatment.

TREATMENT

In general, treatment for cancer-related visceral pain syndromes should adhere to standard cancer pain treatment guidelines (e.g., WHO Analgesic Ladder; American Pain Society Guidelines). The reader is referred to Chapters 43, 44, and 48 for details of various pharmacotherapeutic, radiotherapeutic, and interventional treatment modalities. Therapies that target visceral pain mechanisms with some specificity that are not covered in detail in other chapters are elaborated below.

N-Methyl-D-Aspartate Receptor Antagonists

Ketamine, which blocks N-Methyl-D-Aspartate (NMDA) receptors, can influence visceral hypersensitivity. Primary visceral hypersensitivity is attributed to a reduction in peripheral nociceptive thresholds. Two central processes mediate secondary visceral hypersensitivity: (a) plasticity of activated C-fibers; and (b) convergence of afferents at multiple levels and maintained by glutamate release that binds to NMDA receptors. NMDA receptor activation results in nitric oxide synthase expression, nitric oxide production, and prostaglandin production.

Through these mechanisms (and perhaps others) ketamine has been found to be useful in the management of pain states that are either poorly responsive to opioids and other analgesics, or when there are dose-limiting adverse effects to other pain treatments. Ketamine use has been described, with variable success, in adults, pediatric patients, via intrathecal, parenteral, and oral routes, and in inpatient as well as outpatient settings.[73–82]

Corticosteroids

Dexamethasone inhibits neuronal nitric oxide synthase gene expression. It has been effective in treating visceral pain and bowel obstruction.[83]

Gabapentin

Gabapentin has been demonstrated to reduce glutamate levels and reduces hypersensitivity associated with celiac pain.[84]

Procedural Intervention

Ganglion Impar Block

The ganglion impar is a solitary retroperitoneal structure located at the level of the sacrococcygeal junction. This unpaired ganglion marks the end of two sympathetic chains. The ganglion receives sympathetic and parasympathetic fibers at the lumbar and sacral levels, providing sympathetic innervation to portions of the pelvic viscera and genitalia.[85] Visceral pain in the perineal area associated with malignancies may be effectively treated with neurolysis of the ganglion impar (also know as Walther's ganglion).[86] Patients who will benefit from this block frequently present with a vague, poorly localized pain that is frequently accompanied by sensations of burning and urgency. The ganglion impar block is useful to the management of sympathetically mediated pain in the perineum, rectum, and genitalia. It has been primarily used for malignancy; however, it has been used for treatment of associated syndromes such as radiation enteritis, proctalgia fugax, and reflex sympathetic dystrophy.

The ganglion impar is close in proximity to the rectum. There is increased risk of contamination through the needle track as the needle is removed. Infection and fistula are possible complications in patients who are already immunocompromised or have received radiation to the perineum.

Thoracic Sympathetic Ganglion Block

Preganglionic fibers of the thoracic sympathetics exit with respective thoracic paravertebral nerves from the intervertebral foramen. After exiting the intervertebral foramen, thoracic paravertebral nerves branch looping dorsal through the same foramen to provide innervation to the spinal ligaments, meninges, and respective vertebra. The paravertebral nerve at this level also affects the thoracic sympathetic chain through myelinated preganglionic fibers of the white rami communicantes. Preganglionic and postganglionic fibers synapse at the level of thoracic sympathetic ganglia. Postganglionic fibers provide sympathetic innervation to the vasculature, sweat glands, and pilomotor muscles of the skin as well as the cardiac plexus and terminate in distal ganglia as they course up and down the thoracic sympathetic trunk.[87]

Block of the thoracic sympathetic ganglion is useful for evaluation of sympathetically mediated pain to the thoracic and upper abdominal viscera, the thorax, and the chest wall. Differential blockade may serve as a prognostic indicator of the benefit to be expected from lesioning of the thoracic sympathetic ganglion. The block has been used in the past to treat intractable abdominal pain as well as intractable cardiac pain. It has also been demonstrated to be effective in the treatment of acute herpes zoster, postherpetic neuralgia, and phantom breast pain following mastectomy. Thoracic sympathetic chain destruction may be used to relieve pain in pain syndromes that have been improved by local anesthetic block.[88]

Because of the close proximity to the pleural space of the exiting nerve roots at the thoracic level from sympathetic ganglion, pneumothorax is a possible complication. The pleural space lies lateral and anterior to the thoracic sympathetic chain. The lower cervical ganglion fuses with the first thoracic ganglion to make the stellate ganglion. Caudad in the thoracic chain, thoracic ganglia move further anterior resting along the posterolateral surface of the vertebral body. Other possible complications include accidental injection of the epidural, subdural, and subarachnoid space. Infection is of greater concern in patients with malignancy because of their immunocompromised state.

Interpleural Catheters

The role of interpleural analgesia (IPA) in both acute and chronic pain management is still undergoing clinical scrutiny. Original work with this technique showed that IPA could provide analgesia in patients with subcostal incisions and fractured ribs.

The technique for insertion of an interpleural catheter is relatively easy, and an epidural tray can be utilized. Local anesthetics (0.5% bupivacaine or 2% lidocaine) have been traditionally utilized via intermittent bolus or a continuous infusion. Interpleural phenol has been described as an alternative for the treatment of visceral pain associated with esophageal cancer. This may be an effective technique to treat visceral pain associated with cancer of the esophagus, liver, biliary tree, stomach, and pancreas.

For analgesia associated with cancer, continuous infusions of bupivacaine or intermittent bolus doses of bupivacaine may also provide adequate analgesia. Higher concentrations of bupivacaine increase the risk of toxicity.

Complications are secondary to needle or catheter injury or are secondary to the neurolytic agent injected in the interpleural space. Pneumothorax may occur in 2% of patients, and lung injury has been reported when a rigid catheter is used. Phrenic nerve palsy may occur following this block resulting in respiratory failure. Thus, bilateral blocks should be avoided. Doses of phenol should be limited; systemic effects from drug absorption may occur since the pleural membranes are highly vascularized.

Surgery

Referral for surgical options should be pursued with diagnosis and treatment of pain in malignancy at any time during the course of care. Surgical objectives in the palliation of cancer include staging of disease, control of disease, control of pain and associated symptoms, reconstruction, and rehabilitation.[89] Patients interested in and capable of tolerating surgical options should be referred to a surgeon for consideration of options, even if there are nonsurgical options available. If no intervention is recommended, the patient will have an understanding for the surgical referral and have a sense of closure with regard to the variety of options available for palliation. Surgical consult is particularly valuable in the areas of wound management, complicated issues with regard to nutrition, and discussion of progression of disease.[88]

There is no standard set of procedures for the palliation of malignant visceral pain. The operations available are a reflection of the subjective pain experience of the patient, the specific stage of the disease, and the anatomic effects of the disease. Often, other distressing symptoms may be the reason for surgical management as well as the complaints of pain. The given surgical option should palliate as many symptoms as possible without altering benefit/risk ratios.[88] The most important preoperative measure involves reassurance to the patient that preparation is complete and that postoperative analgesia has been considered. This is best achieved with close coordination with the partnering anesthesia team and preoperative consultation regarding analgesic options. Furthermore, the operative encounter may be the foundation for continued postoperative pain management options.

Malignancy presenting with pain is likely to be advanced in nature. Resection of an organ or portion of an organ for management of pain is reasonable even in the case of uncontrollable disease, especially if the disease is resectable or partially resectable. There is little data, however, comparing the efficacy of resection with nonoperative approaches.

In visceral disease, surgical resection has proven effective for the relief of dysphagia, odynophagia, and chest pain in patients with esophageal carcinoma; the relief of painful ulceration in those with gastric carcinoma; and the preemptive control of jaundice, pain, and duodenal obstruction in those with pancreatic carcinoma.[88]

Surgery can promote comfort as well as eliminate pain. Mechanical bowel obstruction may be expected in as many as 15% of cancer patients. Pain is a reflection of the severity of the distension, the nature of the primary neoplasm, and the level of obstruction. Resection has also been offered on occasion for relief of pain associated with carcinoma of the kidney. In some situations, nephrectomy may be considered to prevent pain, hematuria, and constitutional effects of the disease. In patients with large bladder masses, total or partial organ resection may be a consideration in cases where more conservative options have been considered. Stent placement may relieve severe pain secondary to malignant ureteral obstruction by tumors of the prostate, cervix, bladder, and colon. If stent placement is not an option, percutaneous nephrostomy may be effective.[88]

Debulking of functional tumors of the liver may be beneficial in patients with carcinoid to decrease such symptoms as flushing and diarrhea. Debulking has also been used in patients with metastatic gastrinoma, ovarian cancer, and large and small bowel malignancies.

Finally, drainage of ascites which may develop in as many as half of cancer patients may relieve associated symptoms such as bloating, diffuse abdominal pain, dyspnea, nausea, early satiety, and gastric reflux.

CONCLUSION

Failure to assess and treat cancer pain, whether of somatic, visceral, neuropathic, or mixed types is still a common problem among patients in all stages of malignant disease. Barriers to adequate care have been discussed in previous chapters. Notwithstanding needed improvements in clinician education, access to pain and supportive care specialists, among other needed systems improvements, and similar to other causes of cancer pain, relief of pain in patients with visceral malignancies or treatment-related visceral pain syndromes should be organized as part of a comprehensive interdisciplinary approach to care. Visceral pain cannot be exclusively managed with pharmacotherapy, and the resources of several medical and supportive care disciplines should be considered with each patient so that pain management can be tailored to the individual requirements of each patient according to his or her unique constellation of clinical and social circumstances.

References

1. Goudas LC, Bloch R, Gialeli-Goudas M, et al. The epidemiology of cancer pain. *Cancer Invest* 2005;23(2):182–190.
2. Burton AW, Cleeland CS. Cancer pain: progress since the WHO guidelines. *Pain Pract* 2001;1(3):236–242.
3. Nicholas D, et al. Cultural and family issues. In: De Leon Casseola O, ed. *Cancer Pain Management: Pharmacologic, Interventional, and Palliative Approaches.* Philadelphia: Elsevier; 2006.
4. Mantyh P. Cancer pain: causes, consequences and therapeutic opportunities. In: McMahon S, Koltzenburg M, eds. *Wall and Melzack's Textbook of Pain.* 5th ed. London: Elsevier; 2006.
5. Passik S. Psychiatric issues in cancer pain management. In: Fisch M, Burton A, eds. *Cancer Pain Management.* New York: McGraw-Hill; 2007.
6. Paice J. Cancer pain. In: Von Roenn J, ed. *Current Diagnosis and Treatment Pain.* New York: Lange Medical Books; 2006.
7. Cherny N. The assessment of cancer pain. In: McMahon S, Koltzenburg M, eds. *Wall and Melzack's Textbook of Pain.* 5th ed. London: Elsevier; 2006.
8. Al-Chaer ER, Traub RJ. Biological basis of visceral pain: recent developments. *Pain* 2002;96(3):221–225.
9. Bielefeldt K. Visceral pain: basic mechanisms. In: McMahon S, Koltzenburg M, eds. *Wall and Melzack's Textbook of Pain.* 5th ed. London: Elsevier; 2006.
10. Ness T. Visceral pain. In: De Leon Casseola O, ed. *Cancer Pain Management: Pharmacologic, Interventional, and Palliative Approaches.* Philadelphia: Elsevier; 2006.
11. Gebhart G. Visceral pain mechanisms. In: Chapman CR, Foley K, eds. *Current and Emerging Issues in Cancer Pain: Research and Practice.* Lippincott–Raven; 1993. Also available at http://www.painresearch.utah.edu/cancerpain/ch07.html.
12. Chang V. Assessment of pain and other symptoms. In: de Leon Casseola O, ed. *Cancer Pain Management: Pharmacologic, Interventional, and Palliative Approaches.* Philadelphia: Elsevier; 2006.
13. Reddy S. Pain following mastectomy, thoracotomy, and radical neck dissection.

14. Ness T. Visceral pain. In: Von Roenn J, ed. *Current Diagnosis and Treatment Pain.* New York: Lange Medical Books; 2006.
15. Davis M, et al. Management of visceral pain due to cancer related intestinal obstruction. In: In: de Leon Casseola O, ed. *Cancer Pain Management: Pharmacologic, Interventional, and Palliative Approaches.* Philadelphia: Elsevier; 2006.
16. Cervero F. Visceral hyperalgesia revisited. *Lancet* 2000;356(9236):1127–1128.
17. Sarkar S, Hobson AR, Hughes A, et al. The prostaglandin E2 receptor-1 (EP-1) mediates acid-induced visceral pain hypersensitivity in humans. *Gastroenterology* 2003;124(1):18–25.
18. Gebhart GF. Pathobiology of visceral pain: molecular mechanisms and therapeutic implications. IV. Visceral afferent contributions to the pathobiology of visceral pain. *Am J Physiol Gastrointest Liver Physiol* 2000;278(6): G834–G838.
19. Helmlinger G, Sckell A, Dellian M, et al. Acid production in glycolysis-impaired tumors provides new insights into tumor metabolism. *Clin Cancer Res* 2000; 8(4):1284–1291.
20. Bueno L, Fioramonti J. Visceral perception: inflammatory and non-inflammatory mediators. *Gut* 2002;51:i19–i23.
21. Houghton LA, Calvert EL, Jackson NA, et al. Visceral sensation and emotion: a study using hypnosis. *Gut* 2002;51(5):701–704.
22. Strigo IA, Bushnell MC, Boivin M, et al. Psychophysical analysis of visceral and cutaneous pain in human subjects. *Pain* 2002;97(3):235–246.
23. Nishino T, Shimoyama N, Ide T, et al. Experimental pain augments experimental dyspnea, but not vice versa in human volunteers. *Anesthesiology* 1999; 91(6):1633.
24. Lémann M, Dederding JP, Flourié B, et al. Abnormal perception of visceral pain in response to gastric distension in chronic idiopathic dyspepsia. *Dig Dis Sci* 19991;36(1):1249–1254.
25. Yamada T, Alpers DH, Laine L, et al, eds. *Textbook of Gastroenterology.* 3rd ed. Philadelphia: Lippincott Williams & Wilkins; 1999.
26. Honoré P, Kamp EH, Rogers SD, et al. Activation of lamina I spinal cord neurons that express the substance P receptor in visceral nociception and hyperalgesia. *J Pain* 2002;3(1):3–11.
27. Chadwick VS, Chen W, Shu D, et al. Activation of the mucosal immune system in irritable bowel syndrome. *Gastroenterology* 2002;122(7):1778–1783.
28. Ouatu-Lascar R, Fitzgerald RC, Triadafilopoulos G. Differentiation and proliferation in Barrett's esophagus and the effects of acid suppression. *Gastroenterology* 1999;117(2):327–335.
29. McMahon S, Dmitrieva N, Koltzenburg M. Visceral pain. *Br J Anaesth* 1995; 75(2):132–144.
30. Anand P, Aziz Q, Willert R, et al. Peripheral and central mechanisms of visceral sensitization in man. *Neurogastroenterol Motil* 2007;19(s1):29–46.
31. Eide PK. Wind-up and the NMDA receptor complex from a clinical perspective. *Eur J Pain* 2000;4(1):5–15.
32. Menétrey D, de Pommer J. Origins of spinal ascending pathways that reach central areas involved in visceroception and visceronociception in the rat. *Eur J Neurosci* 1991;3(3),249–255.
33. Burrton A. Chronic pain in the cured cancer patient. In: Fisch M, Burton A, eds. *Cancer Pain Management.* New York: McGraw-Hill; 2007.
34. Worthington H, Clarkson JE, Eden OB. Interventions for preventing oral mucositis for patients with cancer receiving treatment. *Cochrane Database Syst Rev* 2007;(4):CD000978.
35. Epstein J, Stewart K. Radiation therapy and pain in patients with head and neck cancer. *Eur J Cancer B Oral Oncol* 1993;29B(3):191–199.
36. Rider CA. Oral mucositis: a complication of radiotherapy. *J Colo Dent Assoc* 1991;69(3):23–25.
37. Worthington HV, Clarkson JE, Eden OB, et al. Interventions for treating oral mucositis for patients with cancer receiving treatment. *Cochrane Database Syst Rev* 2001;(1):CD001973.
38. Marangoni C, Lacerenza M, Formaglio F, et al. Sensory disorder of the chest as presenting symptom of lung cancer. *J Neurol Neurosurg Psychiatry* 1993; 56(9):1033–1034.
39. Marino C, Zoppi M, Morelli F, et al. Pain in early cancer of the lungs. *Pain* 1986;27(1):57–62.
40. Capobianco DJ. Facial pain as a symptom of nonmetastatic lung cancer. *Headache* 1995;35(10):581–585.
41. Des Prez RD, Freemon FR. Facial pain associated with lung cancer: a case report. *Headache* 1983;23(1):43–44.
42. Schoenen J, Broux R, Moonen G. Unilateral facial pain as the first symptom of lung cancer: are there diagnostic clues? *Cephalalgia* 1992;12(3):178–179.
43. Shakespeare TP, Stevens M. Unilateral facial pain and lung cancer. *Australas Radiol* 1996;40(1):45–46.
44. D'Silva K. Pancoast syndrome. Available at http://www.emedicine.com/med/topic3418.htm. Accessed January 26, 2007.
45. Kori SH, Foley KM, Posner JB. Brachial plexus lesions in patients with cancer: 100 cases. *Neurology* 1981;31(1):45–50.
46. Kori SH. Diagnosis and management of brachial plexus lesions in cancer patients. *Oncology* 1995;9(8):756–760, discussion 765.
47. Komaki R, Putnam JB Jr, Walsh G, et al. The management of superior sulcus tumors. *Semin Surg Oncol* 2000;18(2):152–164.
48. Wong G, et al. Palliation of pain in adenocarcinoma of the pancreas. In: Cam-

eron J, ed. *American Cancer Society Atlas of Clinical Oncology: Pancreatic Cancer*. Hamilton, Ontario: BC Decker, Inc.; 2001.

49. Warshaw A, Fernández-del Castillo C. Pancreatic carcinoma. *N Engl J Med* 1992;326(7):455–465.

50. Borgelt B, Gelber R, Brady LW, et al. The palliation of hepatic metastases: results of the Radiation Therapy Oncology Group pilot study. *Int J Radiat Oncol Biol Phys* 1981;7:587–591.

51. Mulholland MW, Debas H, Bonica JJ. Diseases of the liver, biliary system and pancreas. In: Bonica JJ, ed. *The Management of Pain*. 2nd ed. Lea and Febiger; 1990:1214–1223.

52. Dawson LA. Radiation therapy for liver metastases. *ASCO Educational Book* 2008;1:161–164.

53. Averbach AM, Sugarbaker PH. Recurrent intra-abdominal cancer with intestinal obstruction. *Int Surg* 1995;80(2):141–146.

54. Almadrones L, Yerys C. Problems associated with the administration of intraperitoneal therapy using the Port-A-Cath system. *Oncol Nurs Forum* 1990; 17(1):75–76.

55. Boas RA, Schug SA, Acland RH. Perineal pain after rectal amputation: a 5-year follow-up. *Pain* 1993;52(1):67–70.

56. Rigor BM Sr. Pelvic cancer pain. *J Surg Oncol* 2000;75(4):280–300.

57. Cantwell BM, Richardson PG, Campbell SJ. Gynaecomastia and extragonadal symptoms leading to diagnosis delay of germ cell tumours in young men. *Postgrad Med J* 1991;67(789):675–677 (see comments in *Postgrad Med J* 1991; 67[794]:1082).

58. Tseng A Jr, Horning SJ, Freiha FS, et al. Gynecomastia in testicular cancer patients. Prognostic and therapeutic implications. *Cancer* 1985;56(10): 2534–2538.

59. Kudo S, Tsushima N, Sawada Y, et al. Serious complications of intravesical bacillus Calmette–Guerin therapy in patients with bladder cancer (in Japanese). *Nippon Hinyokika Gakkai Zasshi* 1991;82(10):1594–1602.

60. Berger MS, Cooley ME, Abrahm JL. A pain syndrome associated with large adrenal metastases in patients with lung cancer. *J Pain Symptom Manage* 1995; 10(2):161–166.

61. Perron G, Dolbec P, Germain J, et al. Perineal pruritus after i.v. dexamethasone administration. *Can J Anesth* 2003;50(7):749–750.

62. Berger MS, Cooley ME, Abrahm J. A pain syndrome associated with large adrenal metastases in patients with lung cancer. *J Pain Symptom Manage* 1995; 10(2):161–166.

63. Burihan E, de Figueiredo LF, Francisco Júnior J, et al. Upper-extremity deep venous thrombosis: analysis of 52 cases. *Cardiovasc Surg* 1993;1(1):19–22.

64. Bona RD. Central line thrombosis in patients with cancer. *Curr Opin Pulm Med* 2003;9(5):362–366.

65. Wudel LJ Jr, Nesbitt JC. Superior vena cava syndrome. *Curr Treat Options Oncol* 2001;2(1):77–91.

66. Morales M, Llanos M, Dorta J. Superior vena cava thrombosis secondary to Hickman catheter and complete resolution after fibrinolytic therapy. *Support Care Cancer* 1997;5(1):67–69.

67. Kemeny MM. Continuous hepatic artery infusion (CHAI) as treatment of liver metastases. Are the complications worth it? *Drug Saf* 1991;6(3):159–165.

68. Miyamoto M, Sudo T, Kuyama T. Spontaneous rupture of hepatocellular carcinoma: a review of 172 Japanese cases. *Am J Gastroenterol* 1991;86(1):67–71.

69. Wolff JM, Boeckmann W, Jakse G. Spontaneous kidney rupture due to a metastatic renal tumour. Case report. *Scand J Urol Nephrol* 1994;28(4):415–417.

70. Ende DA, Robinson G, Moulton J. Metastasis-induced perforated appendicitis: an acute abdomen of rare aetiology. *Aust N Z J Surg* 1995;65(1):62–63.

71. Andreasen DA, Poulsen J. Intra-abdominal torsion of the testis with seminoma (in Danish). *Ugeskrift Laeger* 1997;159(14):2103–2104 (see comments in *Ugeskr Laeger* 1997;30;159[27]:4281–4282).

72. Saltz L. *Colorectal Cancer: Multimodality Management*. Humana Press; 2002:655.

73. Nussbaum ML, Campana TJ, Weese JL. Radiation-induced intestinal injury. *Clin Plast Surg* 1993;20(3):573–580.

74. Finkel JC, Pestieau SR, Quezado ZM. Ketamine as an adjuvant for treatment of cancer pain in children and adolescents. *J Pain* 2007;8(6):515–521.

75. Bell RF, Eccleston C, Kalso E. Ketamine as adjuvant to opioids for cancer pain. A qualitative systematic review. *J Pain Symptom Manage* 2003;26(3):867–875.

76. Chung WJ, Pharo GH. Successful use of ketamine infusion in the treatment of intractable cancer pain in an outpatient. *J Pain Symptom Manage* 2007;33 (1):2–5.

77. Fitzgibbon EJ, Viola R. Parenteral ketamine as an analgesic adjuvant for severe pain: development and retrospective audit of a protocol for a palliative care unit. *J Palliat Med* 2005;8(1):49–57.

78. Fitzgibbon EJ, Hall P, Schroder C, et al. Low dose ketamine as an analgesic adjuvant in difficult pain syndromes: a strategy for conversion from parenteral to oral ketamine. *J Pain Symptom Manage* 2002;23(2):165–170.

79. Mannion S, O'Brien T. Ketamine in the management of chronic pancreatic pain. *J Pain Symptom Manage* 2003;26(6):1071–1072.

80. Prommer E. Ketamine to control pain. *J Palliat Med* 2003;6(3):443–446.

81. Mercadante S, Arcuri E, Tirelli W, et al. Analgesic effect of intravenous ketamine in cancer patients on morphine therapy: a randomized, controlled, double-blind, crossover, double-dose study. *J Pain Symptom Manage* 2000;20(4): 246–252.

82. Gordon DB, Sehgal N, Schroeder ME, et al. Treatment of pain crisis at end of life from severe lower extremity venous outflow obstruction with hyperalgesia and allodynia. *J Pain* 2002;3(3):244–248.

83. Kotlinska–Lemieszek A, Luczak J. Subanesthetic ketamine: an essential adjuvant for intractable cancer pain. *J Pain Symptom Manage* 2004;28(2):100–102.

84. Warr DG. Chemotherapy- and cancer-related nausea and vomiting. *Curr Oncol* 2008;15(suppl 1):S4–S9.

85. Pelham A, Lee MA, Regnard CB. Gabapentin for coeliac plexus pain. *Palliat Med* 2002;16(4):355–356.

86. Waldman S. *Ganglion of Walther (Impar) Block*. Atlas of Interventional Pain Management. Philadelphia: Saunders; 2003.

87. Plancarte R, de Leon Casasola OA, El-Helaly M, et al. Presacral blockade of the ganglion of Walther. *Anesthesiology* 1990;73:A751.

88. Dunn, G. Selected surgical approaches. In: Simpson K, Budd K, eds. *Cancer Pain Management: A Comprehensive Approach*. Oxford: Oxford University Press; 2000.

89. Thoracic sympathetic ganglion block. In: Waldman S, ed. *Atlas of Interventional Pain Management*. Philadelphia: Saunders; 2003.

90. Dunn GP. Surgical palliative care: an enduring framework for surgical care. *Surg Clin North Am* 2005;85(2):169–190.

CHAPTER 48 ■ RADIOTHERAPY AND CHEMOTHERAPY IN CANCER PAIN MANAGEMENT

AJIT S. AHLUWALIA, NORA A. JANJAN, AND CAMERON MUIR

INTRODUCTION

"Cancer pain is best controlled by removing the cancer or causing it to regress."[1] These words of the renowned oncologist and palliative medicine specialist Dr. Neil MacDonald are a useful framework from which to consider the role of palliative chemotherapy and radiotherapy in the management of symptomatic disease. About 50% of cancers are still cured by surgery and only 10% by other modalities. In the year 2007, 1,444,920 new cancer cases were diagnosed and about 559,650 cancer-related deaths occurred. The trends in cancer incidence and mortality shows a 13.6% decrease in the cancer death rate between the years 1991 and 2004.[2] This trend can be attributed to the persistent efforts in research and encouraging advances in the field of oncology. On the heels of this trend is the significant burden of symptoms like pain related to oncologic disease and its treatments.

Cancer has a negative impact on almost all cancer patients' activities of daily living. Quality of life measurements have been shown to predict survival and add to the prognostic information derived from the Karnofsky Performance Status (KPS) and extent of disease. Physical symptoms including pain, dry mouth, constipation, change in taste, lack of appetite and energy, feeling bloated, nausea, vomiting, weight loss, and feeling drowsy or dizzy often portend a poorer prognosis.[3] Palliative care is an integral component of cancer treatment with a goal to effectively and efficiently relieve symptoms and maintain the maximum functional and emotional well-being for the duration of the patient's life.[4–10]

Palliative chemotherapy has been an ambiguous term, mostly used to refer to chemotherapy given to patients in whom the likelihood of cure was minimal. In the true sense, palliative chemotherapy would mean chemotherapy delivered with an aim to relieve symptoms, improve quality of life, or both, regardless of stage of disease or likelihood of remission or cure. The primary outcomes of most studies involving disease-modifying chemotherapeutic agents, however, do not have symptom relief as an end point and only recently are the end points related to quality of life becoming part of these studies. Reduction in the size of tumor, which is the intended goal of chemotherapy, should intuitively decrease cancer pain. However, since therapeutic benefits of chemotherapy are limited by their own toxicities, their risks versus benefits need to be weighed as part of treatment planning and decision-making on a case-by-case basis.

Palliative radiation is instrumental in the management of bone pain related to bone metastasis. Seventy percent of metastatic bone lesions are painful and debilitating. The goal of treatment is to relieve pain, restore functional ability, and prevent pathological fractures.[11,12] The location of the metastasis can be a limitation in the effectiveness of a palliative intervention. Metastatic involvement of weight-bearing bones and those used in functional activities are often less likely to respond completely to palliative interventions due to applied mechanical forces put upon them. Pain relief is achieved in 73% of spine metastases, 88% of limb lesions, 67% of pelvic metastases, and 75% of metastases to other parts of the skeleton.[13]

Poorer health is a more frequent finding in lung, breast, prostate, and colon cancer patients as these primary tumor types tend to metastasize to the bones and viscera more aggressively.[14–16] After bone metastases are diagnosed, the median survivals are 12 months for breast cancer, 6 months for prostate cancer, and 3 months for lung cancer. In breast cancer, the survival decreases to only 9 months if visceral metastases are also present.[15,16] In prostate cancer, the distribution of bone metastases on scintigraphy also has prognostic significance. The rate of survival is significantly longer when the metastases are restricted to the pelvis and lumbar spine, as well as among patients who respond to salvage hormone therapy,[17–19] but lower if metastatic involvement is outside the pelvis and lumbar spine irrespective of response to salvage hormone therapy. The median length of survival is critical to evaluating response to and determining the appropriate recommendations for palliative therapy.

Economically, bone pain related to cancer results in increased utilization of health care resources and cost.[20,21] The economic implications provide a strong impetus to develop novel palliative approaches. Palliative medicine approaches are also providing patients with a positive treatment option both to augment conventional treatments or as the primary modality when disease modifying therapy for cancers fail to produce effect.[22]

RADIOTHERAPY

Role of Radiotherapy

Despite the establishment of multiple palliative medicine programs in the country and the proven efficacy of palliative radio-therapy for symptoms, radiotherapy is underutilized.[12] Even with relatively short life expectancy (weeks to months), palliative radiotherapy may be helpful, but in a survey completed in 2002, less than 3% of the patients in hospice care received radiation with a palliative intent.[23] The most common barriers to radiotherapy include radiotherapy expense, transportation difficulties, short life expectancy, and educational deficiencies among the specialties caring for patients with oncologic disease. Although the focus of this chapter is on pain management, this section will review the many indications for palliative radiotherapy, since symptoms—including pain—rarely occur alone, but rather in tandem.

Bone Disease

In the years 2000–2004, the annual prevalence of bone metastasis was estimated to be 256,137, and the rates were highest in multiple myeloma and lung cancer. The direct cost for patients with bone metastasis was $75,329 and the incremental cost was $44,442 compared to patients with cancer without bone metastasis. The national cost burden for patients with skeletal metastasis was estimated at $12.6 billion which is 17% of the $74 billion total direct medical cost estimated by NIH.[24] Although more abbreviated radiation courses may result in cost savings, the response to therapy must be critically analyzed to ensure that treatment efficacy is not compromised. Ineffective therapy may prove more costly than a more prolonged and effective radiation schedule because of the continued need for analgesics and the functional limitations caused by unrelieved pain and disability.[25,26]

Multidisciplinary evaluation of patients with metastatic disease to the bone allows comprehensive management of the associated symptoms, determines the risk for pathologic fracture, and helps coordinate administration of a wide range of available antineoplastic therapies (also see Chapter 46).[10] Bone metastases can be treated with localized, systemic, or both kinds of therapies.[11,24–38] Because radiation provides treatment only to a localized symptomatic site of disease, it is frequently used in coordination with systemic therapies such as chemotherapy, hormonal therapy, and bisphosphonates. Radiopharmaceuticals provide another systemic option that treats diffuse symptomatic bone metastases. Because the radiation is deposited directly at the involved area in the bone, radiopharmaceuticals, such as strontium 89, can also be used to treat bone metastases when symptoms recur in a previously irradiated site.[39–54] Radiopharmaceuticals can also act as an adjuvant to localized external beam irradiation and reduce the development of other symptomatic sites of disease.

Control of cancer-related pain with the use of analgesics is imperative to allow comfort during and while awaiting response to therapeutic interventions. Pain represents a sensitive measure of disease activity. Close follow-up should be performed to ensure control of cancer and treatment-related pain, and to initiate diagnostic studies to identify progressive or recurrent disease. Pain, risk for pathologic fracture, and spinal cord compression are the most common indications to treat bone metastases with localized therapy including radiation and surgery.

Clinical Applications

Radiotherapy can be delivered with curative or palliative intent. Curative treatment attempts to render the patient disease free of either primary or metastatic disease. Treatment with palliative intent is intended to control the symptoms of disease when the disease cannot be eradicated. A number of clinical, prognostic, and therapeutic factors must be considered to determine the most optimal treatment regimen for a course of palliative radiotherapy. Although any site of disease can be effectively palliated, treatment of bone metastases is one of the most common indications for palliative irradiation with external beam therapy.[11,26,29]

The limited radiation tolerance of the normal tissues, such as the spinal cord, that are adjacent to a bone metastasis make it impossible to administer a large enough dose of radiation to completely eradicate most tumors. Palliative radiation should result in sufficient tumor regression to relieve symptoms for the duration of the patient's life. Palliative radiotherapy is often combined with chemotherapy and/or surgery to optimize therapeutic outcomes from tumor-related pain, bleeding, visceral obstruction, or lymphatic and vascular obstruction. Common sites include respiratory system structures, pelvis, skin and subcutaneous tissues, brain, and all bony structures. Potential relief of symptoms is a more important determinant for palliative radiation than whether lesions result from locally advanced or metastatic disease. Symptoms that recur after palliative radiation most commonly result from localized regrowth of tumor in the radiation field.

The palliative interventions recommended depend on the patient's clinical status, burden of disease, and location of the symptomatic site. For either locally advanced or metastatic disease, these factors are indexed to the relative effectiveness, durability, and morbidity of each palliative intervention. Each patient's prognosis represents the single most important factor in deciding the approach to palliative therapy.

Because patients with metastatic disease have a limited life expectancy, the number of radiation fractions prescribed for treatment with palliative intent depends on prognosis and not primary histology, so a lower total dose is given with palliative radiation over 1 to 2 weeks (hypofractionated radiation schedule). Based on the radiation tolerance of normal tissues, a low daily radiation dose (1.8 to 2.0 Gy) is given with conventional radiation; in contrast, large daily radiation fractions are given with hypofractionated radiation schedules. Hypofractionated radiation schedules for palliative therapy can range from 2.5 Gy per fraction administered over 3 weeks for a total dose of 35 Gy to a single 8-Gy dose of radiation. Most frequently, 30 Gy is administered in 10 fractions over 2 weeks.[10,11,28–32,55–60] Especially among patients with short life expectancies, many centers administer 20 Gy in 1 week because the rates of pain relief, mobility, and frequency of pathologic fractures are similar to more protracted radiation schedules.

RESPONSE OF TUMORS TO RADIOTHERAPY

Trachea, Bronchi, and Lungs

Locally advanced primary or metastatic involvement of the lung often requires palliative intervention because cure is possible in only a few of these cases. A variety of symptoms, some of them emergent, can manifest because of tumor involvement of the lung.[61] Pain can result from tumor invasion of the ribs and nerve roots of the chest wall. Vertebral involvement can be associated with spinal cord compression. Lower respiratory tract obstruction, bleeding, and pneumonitis can result from tracheobronchial tumor growth. Mediastinal infiltration can cause superior vena cava syndrome. All of these clinical presentations can be palliated with external beam radiation that encompasses the disease that is evident on diagnostic images and that treats pain referred along involved nerve roots. Radiation schedules that administer 30 Gy in 10 fractions over 2 weeks, two fractions of 8.5 Gy 1 week apart, or one fraction of 10 Gy (depending upon the patient's life expectancy and ability to tolerate multifraction therapy) are typically prescribed to previously unirradiated sites. Hemoptysis and chest pain can be effectively palliated; dyspnea and dysphagia are not as effectively relieved. If the area has been previously irradiated, techniques that exclude critical anatomic structures, such as the spinal cord, are applied. Other approaches can be used when the symptomatic site is well localized and accessible. Brachytherapy, which applies radioactive sources next to tumors, can be used to treat bronchial obstruction and bleeding by placing a radioactive source directly against the tumor under bronchoscopic guidance. In these cases, large doses of radiation can be delivered over a few minutes by a high-dose rate brachytherapy unit.

Pelvis

Hemorrhage with or without obstruction or compression of viscera, lymphatics, vascular structures, and nerves commonly occurs with locally advanced or metastatic disease in the pelvis. Treatment may require emergent radiotherapeutic, surgical interventions, or both. Hemorrhage is commonly associated with tumors involving the rectum and genitourinary tracts. As with tumors in the lung, radiation is an effective means of stopping active bleeding. Colorectal cancers are often diagnosed among patients with unexplained bleeding. In patients that have locally advanced tumors with months to years of life expectancy, 40 Gy in 2.5 Gy fractions to 50 Gy in 2 Gy fractions have been used with the intent to stop bleeding, render the patient operable, and provide a chance for cure. With extensive metastatic disease, 30 Gy in 10 fractions or 20 Gy in 5 fractions is used to palliate symptoms of bleeding and obstruction. Colorectal tumor involvement may also result in obstruction requiring stent placement to maintain the integrity of the visceral lumen while administering radiation. Diverting colostomy is occasionally required but is reported to have been avoided after chemohypofractionated irradiation.[61]

Tumors involving the cervix can hemorrhage and require emergent radiotherapeutic intervention. Superficial radiographs are applied directly to the bleeding cervix through a cone to treat the bleeding site and do not compromise later radiation of other pelvic structures. Usually, radiation doses between 5 and 10 Gy are administered in 1 to 3 applications of cone therapy. Brachytherapy also can be used to treat gynecologic tumors, especially in the vagina, cervix, and endometrium.

Bladder cancers or tumors that secondarily invade the bladder can also result in significant bleeding that can be palliated by external beam radiation. Urinary obstruction commonly occurs with locally advanced pelvic cancers, especially with bladder, rectum, prostate, and cervical cancers. Occasionally, placement of a urinary stent, urostomy, or nephrostomy is required until sufficient tumor regression can be accomplished by radiation to reestablish integrity of the urinary tract.[61] As with the bowel and gynecologic tracts, a bladder fistula, resulting from either the tumor itself or from tumor regression, is a concern.

The pelvic lymph nodes and major blood vessels may become obstructed by tumor. This most frequently is seen when tumors arise in pelvic structures, but can also occur with pelvic metastases from breast and other cancers. Lymph-vascular obstruction results in painful edema that is refractory to diuretic and other therapies. Other than pain and functional interference, when severe, fluid and electrolyte imbalances can occur. Pelvic radiation can relieve lymph-vascular obstruction through tumor regression.

Pelvic tumors can also invade the sacral plexus and result in intractable pain. Tumor can track along nerve roots and can be associated with bony invasion of the sacrum. Pain caused by visceral, lymph-vascular, or both kinds of obstructions often respond more rapidly to palliative radiation than the more refractory neuropathic pain seen with sacral plexus involvement. Other radiotherapeutic approaches, such as brachytherapy, are extremely limited when the cancer persists or recurs after external beam radiation. Interventional pain management techniques are frequently required to control pain associated with sacral plexus involvement (see Chapter 44).

Skin and Subcutaneous Tissues

Tumors can cause ulceration of the skin and subcutaneous tissues that are often painful and distressing because of constant drainage. Representing a source for the development of sepsis in immunocompromised patients, localized radiation can be applied to destroy tumor and allow re-epithelialization of the skin. Radiation that treats only the skin and subcutaneous tissues (electron beam therapy) is generally used to avoid radiation side effects to underlying uninvolved normal structures. Although usually 10 radiation treatments are given, the course of radiation can be abbreviated further, ranging from 1 to 5 days. Occasionally, these lesions are treated with brachytherapy. The radioactive sources can be placed in a mold that sits on top of the tumor and delivers treatment over a few minutes (high-dose rate) or a few days (low-dose rate).

Brain Metastases

Radiation is used to relieve the symptoms of headache, seizure, nausea and vomiting, and neurologic dysfunction associated with brain metastases. In patients with good performance status, surgery or radiosurgery followed by postoperative whole brain radiation is the preferred approach. Radiation is generally with a total of 30 Gy in 10 fractions or 20 Gy in 5 fractions.[62]

BONE METASTASES

There are two major sets of experience with palliative radiation for bone metastases. The Radiation Therapy Oncology Group (RTOG) conducted a prospective trial that included a variety of treatment schedules. To account for prognosis, patients were stratified on the basis of whether they had a solitary or multiple sites of bony metastases. The initial analysis of the study concluded that low-dose, short-course treatment schedules were as effective as high-dose protracted treatment programs.[63] For solitary bone metastases, no difference existed in the relief of pain when 20 Gy using 4-Gy fractions was compared with 40.5 Gy delivered as 2.7 Gy-fractions. Relapse of pain occurred in 57% of patients at a median of 15 weeks after completion of therapy for each dose level. In patients with multiple bone metastases, the following dose schedules were compared: 30 Gy at 3 Gy per fraction, 15 Gy given as 3 Gy per fraction, 20 Gy using 4 Gy per fraction, and 25 Gy using 5 Gy per fraction. No difference was identified in the rates of pain relief among these treatment schedules. Partial relief of pain was achieved in 83% and complete relief occurred in 53% of the patients studied. More than 50% of these patients developed recurrent pain, the fracture rate equaled 8%, and the median duration of pain control was 12 weeks for all the radiation schedules used for multiple bony metastases. Prognostic factors for response included the initial pain score and site of the primary cancer.

In a reanalysis of the data, a different definition for complete pain relief was used and excluded the continued administration of analgesics. Using this definition, the relief of pain was significantly related to the number of fractions and the total dose of radiation that was administered.[64] Complete relief of pain was achieved in 55% of patients with solitary bone metastases who received 40.5 Gy at 2.7 Gy per fraction as compared with 37% of patients who received a total dose of 20 Gy given as 4 Gy per fraction. A similar relationship was observed in the reanalysis of patients who had multiple bone metastases. Complete relief of pain was achieved in 46% of patients who received 30 Gy at 3 Gy per fraction versus 28% of patients treated to 25 Gy using 5-Gy fractions. In most cases, the interval to response was 4 weeks for both complete and minimal relief of symptoms.

Three important issues are identified from the RTOG experience. First, the results of the reanalysis demonstrate the importance of defining what represents a response to therapy. Second, this revised definition of response showed that the total radiation dose did influence the degree that pain was relieved.[63,64] The response rates and the radiobiologically equivalent doses are listed from the reanalysis in (Table 48.1) for each of the treatment schedules used. Patients treated with total doses of 40 Gy or more had a 75% rate of complete pain relief versus a 62% rate of complete pain relief for patients treated with total doses of less than 40 Gy.[13,65] Third, the RTOG experience identified the amount of time that was needed to experience relief of pain after

---

TABLE 48.1

DOSE RESPONSE EVALUATION FROM THE REANALYSIS OF THE RADIATION THERAPY ONCOLOGY GROUP BONE METASTASES PROTOCOL

	Dose per fraction (Gy)	Total dose (Gy)	Tumor dose at 2 Gy per fraction†	Complete response rate (%)‡	p Value
Solitary bone metastases					p < 0.0003
	2.7	40.5	42.9	55	
	4.0	20.0	23.3	37	
Multiple bone metastases					p < 0.0003
	3.0	30.0	32.5	46	
	3.0	15.0	16.2	36	
	4.0	20.0	23.3	40	
	5.0	25.0	31.25	28	

†The radiobiological equivalent dose if administered at 2 Gy per fraction.
‡The complete response rate using the definition that excludes the use of analgesics and that accounts for retreatment.

TABLE 48.2

PERCENTAGE OF PATIENTS WHO RESPONDED TO RADIATION RELATIVE TO TIME, DESIGNATED IN WEEKS AFTER COMPLETION OF RADIATION THERAPY†

Total dose (Gy)	Dose per fraction (Gy)	Tumor dose at 2 Gy per fraction	Weeks after radiation			
			<2 (%)	2–4 (%)	4–12 (%)	12–20 (%)
Solitary metastases						
40.5	2.7	42.9	7	29	53	77
20	4	23.3	16	50	66	82
Multiple metastases						
30	3	32.5	19	48	73	84
15	3	16.2	34	70	84	93
20	4	23.3	28	53	75	88
25	5	31.25	22	41	72	80

†This prospective trial, conducted by the Radiation Therapy Oncology Group, randomized radiation dose and number of fractions and stratified the randomization on the basis of solitary or multiple bone metastases.[63,64] Also listed is the radiobiological equivalent dose if administered at 2 Gy per fraction.

radiation for bone metastases (Table 48.2). It is important to note that only one-half of the patients who were going to respond had relief of symptoms at 2 to 4 weeks after radiation.[63,64] This underscores the need for continued analgesic support after completing radiation. Consistently, it took 12 to 20 weeks after radiation to accomplish the maximal level of relief. That period of time may reflect the time needed for reossification. Radiographic evidence of recalcification is observed in approximately one-fourth of cases, and in 70% of cases, recalcification is seen within 6 months of completing radiation treatments.[28,30,31,66] Recalcification is the basis of stabilization and prevention of fractures in the future. For pain relief, a short course of radiation is adequate; however, a longer schedule is recommended for adequate recalcification.[67,68] Again, clinical context, with a focus on life expectancy, is a key determinant of radiation type, dose, and fractionation schedule.

SINGLE FRACTION RADIATION

A single large radiation fraction is reportedly as effective in relieving pain as other radiation schedules that have more treatments. Radiobiologically, a single 8-Gy fraction would give the same side effects to late reacting tissues (i.e., tissues such as the spinal cord that do not regenerate) as if 18 Gy were given over nine treatments at 2 Gy per fraction.[69] Because tumors and acute reacting tissues, such as the esophagus and other mucosal structures, respond differently than the late reacting tissues, the radiobiologically equivalent dose to the tumor for a single 8-Gy fraction would be 12 Gy if 2 Gy fractions were used. The most common dose fractionation schedule used for palliative radiation in the United States is 30 Gy over 10 fractions. Radiobiologically, this is equivalent to 36 Gy at 2 Gy per fraction for late reacting tissues and 32.5 Gy to the tumor. When a single dose of radiation was compared with a radiation schedule with multiple radiation fractions, no difference was reported in either how quickly symptoms resolved or the duration of pain relief.[10,24,32,55,58,60,65,70–78] Pain relief was achieved in 80% after treatment and 50% of patients at 6 months irrespective of the number of fractions.[65,70–78,80,81] Complete response rates after a single 8-Gy fraction total 15% at 2 weeks, 23% at 4 weeks, 28% at 8 weeks, and 9% at 12 weeks postradiation.

Despite the radiobiological differences in the dose administered, the similarities in response may be caused by tumor regression and reossification that occurs at 3 months. The RTOG experience showed that the maximum response to therapy was seen consistently at 3 months and was independent of dose administered.[63,64] The disparity in the relationship between radiation dose and clinical response may also be attributed to limited follow-up in the single fraction study because a significant proportion of patients in the study were lost to follow-up after 3 months.[70–73] With longer follow-up, the response to a single radiation fraction may not prove to be as durable as multiple fractions that give high total radiation doses.[80–82] These data demonstrate that prognosis needs to be linked to variables such as site irradiated, total radiation dose, and reirradiation.[83]

A shorter radiation schedule, such as a single fraction, is advantageous for patients with poor prognostic factors. First, it is easier for patients with a poor KPS to complete therapy. Second, response rates are equal to single and multifraction therapy at 3 months because median survival is less than 6 months among patients with poor prognostic factors.[10,32,55,57,65,70–78] The option of retreatment after a single fraction of radiation may also provide an advantage among patients with good prognostic factors as a means to periodically reduce tumor burden and control symptoms in noncritical anatomic sites. Higher radiation doses that provide more durable pain relief are considered warranted for patients with good prognostic factors who require treatment over the spine and other critical sites.[10,11,13,29,32,55,56,60,80–82,84–90]

The projected length of survival is the critical issue to determine the optimal radiation dose and schedule for palliative radiation. In one study, only 12 of 243 patients were alive at the time of analysis, with approximately 50% alive at 6 months, 25% at 1 year, 8% at 2 years, and 3% at 3 years after palliative radiation. For breast cancer patients, the survival rates at these time points after palliative radiation were 60%, 44%, 20%, and 7%, respectively. For prostate cancer, the survival rates were 60% at 6 months, 24% at 1 year, and there were no patients who survived 2 years.[59] This survival difference may be an important observation because unrelieved pain and the resultant sequelae of immobility may contribute to mortality as well as morbidity.[3,17,18,20,91–93]

Reirradiation for persistent or recurrent pain is often precluded when higher radiation doses are administered. Because the radiobiological dose is relatively low when a single fraction of radiation is administered, reirradiation is generally possible.[69–73,80–83] Reirradiation was necessary in 25% of patients who received a single 8-Gy radiation fraction, but all of these patients were reported to respond to the second dose of radiation.[65,70–78] Pain relief in patients with reirradiation was better in patients with longer duration of pain-free interval after the initial radiation (≥4 months), had better performance status (KPS 1 or 2) and had a single bone metastasis.[94]

Acute radiation toxicities are a function of the dose per fraction, total dose, and the area and volume of tissue irradiated. If mucosal surfaces, such as the upper respiratory and digestive tract, bowel, and bladder, can be excluded from the radiation portals, acute radiation side effects can be significantly reduced. The radiation schedule used for palliative radiation is therefore influenced by the radiation tolerance of adjacent normal tissues as well as prognosis.

PATHOLOGIC FRACTURE

The most significant morbidities of bone metastases relate to pathologic fracture and spinal cord compression. Pain that persists or that recurs after palliative radiation should be evaluated to exclude progression of disease, possible extension of disease outside the radiation portal that results in referred pain, and bone fracture. It is unclear whether osteolytic metastases are more likely to fracture than osteoblastic lesions, because osteoblastic lesions, by definition, have an osteolytic component so that new bone can be formed.[95] Reduced cortical strength can result in compression, stress, or microfractures associated with reduced cortical strength. Serial radiography is useful in following posttreatment disease progression and fractures.[30,95] Pathologic fractures occur in 8% to 30% of patients with bone metastases.[95–101] Proximal long bones are more commonly involved than distal bones. Consequently, pathologic fractures occur 50% of the time in the femur and 15% in the humerus (Fig. 48.1). The femoral neck and head are the most frequent locations for pathologic fracture because of the propensity for metastases to involve proximal bones and the stress of weight placed on this part of the femur. More than 80% of pathologic fractures occur in breast (50%), kidney, lung, and thyroid cancers.

Approximately 10% to 30% of metastatic lesions in long bones develop a pathologic fracture that requires surgical intervention. Patients with pathologic fracture caused by bone metastases have clinical outcomes after surgical repair that are comparable with patients sustaining a traumatic fracture.[97–99,102] Poor prognosis is associated with hypercalcemia and ongoing severe pain from other metastatic bone lesions. Therefore, in those cases, the decision for surgical intervention should be even more carefully weighed, based upon a relative benefit to burden analysis.[97]

Treatment of pathologic fracture or impending fracture depends on the bone involved and the clinical status of the patient. Indications for surgical intervention of pathologic fracture or impending fracture include these factors: (a) an expected survival of more than 6 weeks; (b) an ability to accomplish internal stability of the fracture site; (c) no coexistent medical conditions that preclude early mobilization; (d) metastases involving weight-bearing bones; and (e) lytic lesions more than 2 to 3 cm in size or metastases that destroy more than 50% of the cortex.[97–101] Intramedullary stabilization without resection of metastases using locking nails meets the requirements of palliative therapy. This procedure is less invasive and allows early weight bearing.[102] Postoperative radiation is often given after surgical fixation of a pathologic fracture to reduce risk of progressive disease in the bone that could result in instability of the internal fixation.[98]

SPINAL CORD COMPRESSION

Metastatic spinal cord compression (MSCC) is the most dreaded complication of cancer. Pain is the initial symptom in approximately 90% of patients with spinal cord compression.[103] Paraparesis or paraplegia occurs in more than 60%, sensory loss is noted in 70% to 80%, and 14% to 77% have bladder, bowel, or both kinds of disturbances.[56,84,85,104] Six predictive risk factors are associated with MSCC: the inability to walk, increased deep tendon reflexes, compression fractures on radiographs of spine, bone metastases present, bone metastases diagnosed more than 1 year earlier, and age less than 60 years. Patients with no risk factors had a 4% chance of developing cord compressions and a patient with all six risk factors present had an 87% chance of developing cord compression.[105,106] Breast, lung, and prostate cancer comprised 21%–24% risk of developing cord compression.[105,106,107]

The clinical course of spinal cord compression resulting from malignant melanoma is similar to that resulting from breast or prostate cancer. The time from the original diagnosis of melanoma to the development of metastatic spinal disease averages 32 months, and the average time is reported to be 27 months from diagnosis of skeletal metastases to spinal cord compression. The extent of the epidural mass influences prognosis because a complete spinal block results in greater residual neurologic impairment than a partial block. Median survival among patients with spinal cord compression is 7 months, with a 36% probability for a 1-year survival. For specific types of cancers, the mean survival time is 14 months for breast cancer, 12 months in prostate cancer, 6 months in malignant melanoma, and 3 months in lung cancer once epidural spinal cord compression is diagnosed.[14,84,96] After the diagnosis of epidural spinal cord compression, the overall survival time averages 12 months, with a median survival time of 5 months. The vertebral column is involved by metastatic tumor in 40% of patients who die of cancer. Approximately 70% of vertebral metastases involve the thoracic spine, 20% the lumbosacral region, and 10% the cervical spine.

Weakness can signal the rapid progression of symptoms, and 30% of patients with weakness become paraplegic within 1 week. Rapid development of weakness, defined as occurring in less than 2 months, most commonly occurs in lung cancer, whereas breast and prostate cancers can progress more slowly. Neurologic deficits can develop within a few hours in up to 20% of patients with spinal cord compression.[84–90,108,109] The severity of weakness at presentation is the most significant factor for recovery of function. The slower the rate of development of motor deficits, the better the functional outcome.[104,110] If no neurologic deficits are present in a magnetic resonance imaging (MRI) scan proven spinal carcinoma, then radiation can preserve function. Patients with neurologic symptoms should be treated within 24 hours.[111,112] Ninety percent of patients who are ambulatory at presentation are ambulatory after treatment. Only 13% of paraplegic patients regain function, particularly if paraplegia is present for more than 24 hours before the initiation of therapy. Notwithstanding the high mortality associated with MSCC, more than 30% of patients who develop spinal cord compression are alive 1 year later, and 50% of these patients remain ambulatory if the syndrome is recognized and treated appropriately.

Pain can be present for months to just days prior to the onset of other neurologic dysfunction. Unlike degenerative joint disease, which primarily occurs in the low cervical and low lumbar regions, pain caused by epidural spinal cord compression can occur anywhere in the spinal axis and is aggravated by recumbency. Any cancer patient with back pain, especially with known metastatic involvement of the vertebral bodies, should be assessed for spinal cord compression. The risk of spinal cord compression exceeds 60% among patients with back pain and plain film evidence of vertebral collapse caused by metastatic cancer.[56,84–90,113–117]

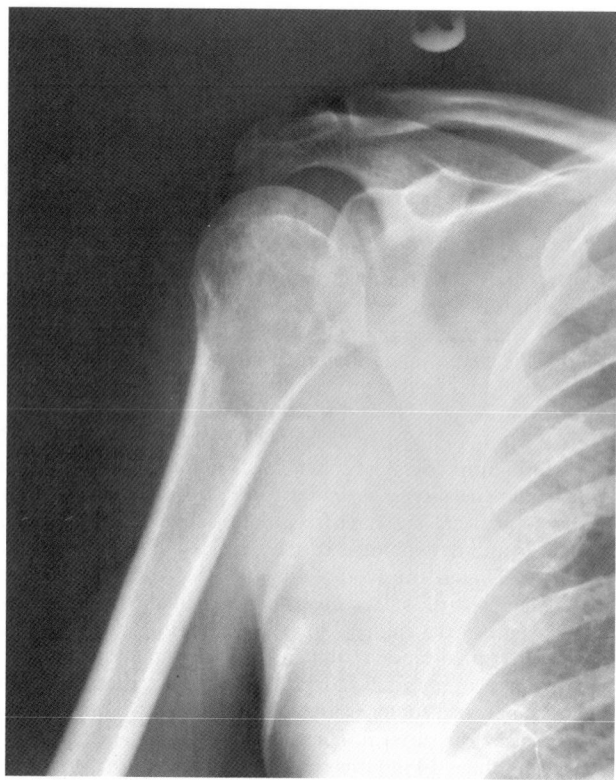

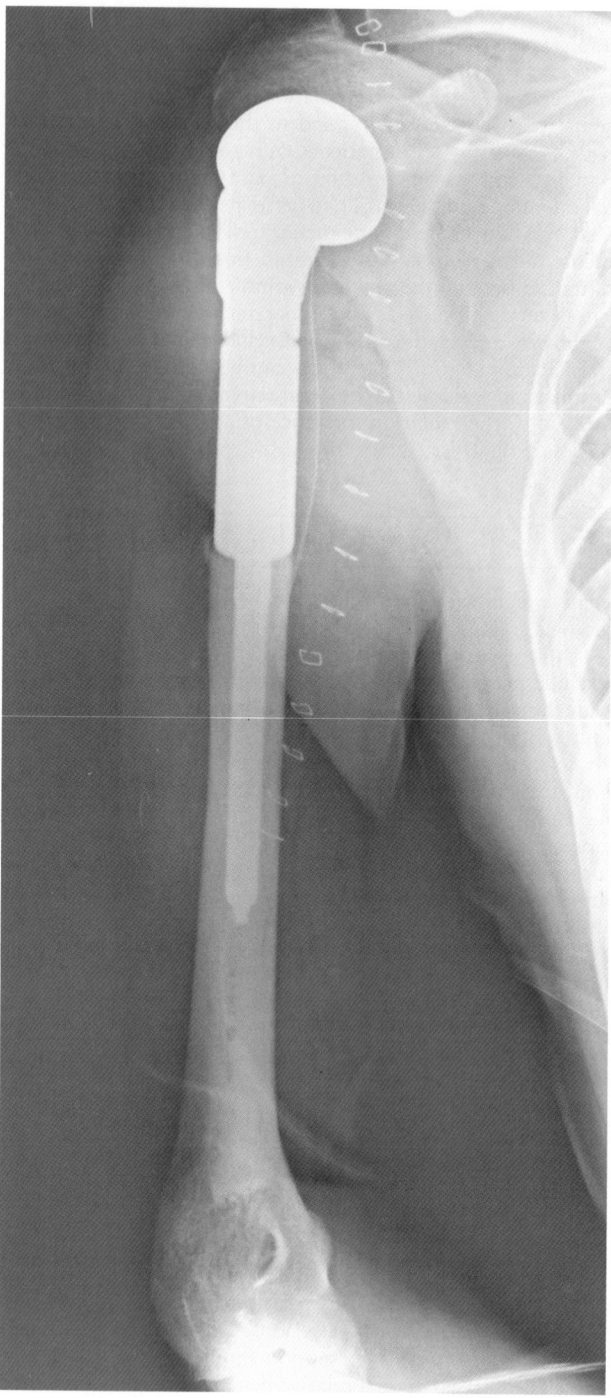

FIGURE 48.1 (**A**) An extensive lytic lesion in the proximal humerus. (**B**) Prophylactic internal fixation performed to prevent pathologic fracture. This patient, who complained primarily of pain in the hip, would have been placed on crutches to reduce stress on the involved femur. A bone scan and radiography, obtained to exclude other sites of metastatic involvement, identified this lesion in the humerus. The humerus would have certainly fractured if all the patient's weight had been displaced to the upper extremities with crutches.

Radiographic determination of the involved spinal levels is critical to radiation treatment planning. Plain film radiography shows involvement of more than one spinal level in approximately one-third of patients. If the results of MRI, tomographic studies, and surgical findings are included, more than 85% of patients have multiple sites of vertebral involvement.[84–90,108,113,116] For patients with known malignancy, a whole spine MRI is recommended as the preferred diagnostic modality.[104,118,119] With plain radiography, the destruction of the pedicles is the most common finding that identifies spine metastases. In contrast, computed tomography (CT) shows that the initial anatomic location of metastases is in the posterior portion of the vertebral body and that destruction of the pedicles occurs only in combination with involvement of the vertebral body

(Fig. 48.2).[116] Symptomatic patients with a normal vertebral contour and osteoblastic changes on plain film and bone scan should also be evaluated for spinal cord compression (Fig. 48.3). Osteoblastic bony expansion, commonly seen in both prostate and breast cancers, can result in spinal cord compromise as well as osteolytic vertebral compression fractures.[115]

Emergency treatment of spinal cord compression includes corticosteroids, radiotherapy, neurosurgical intervention, or combinations of these three therapies. Radiotherapy is the treatment of choice for most cases of spinal cord compression and is a radiotherapeutic emergency (Fig. 48.4). Spinal cord compression resulting from metastatic tumor can be prevented or effectively treated when diagnosed early.[84–90,108,111,113] Radiotherapy with shorter courses (e.g., 1 fraction with 8 Gy or 5 fractions with 4

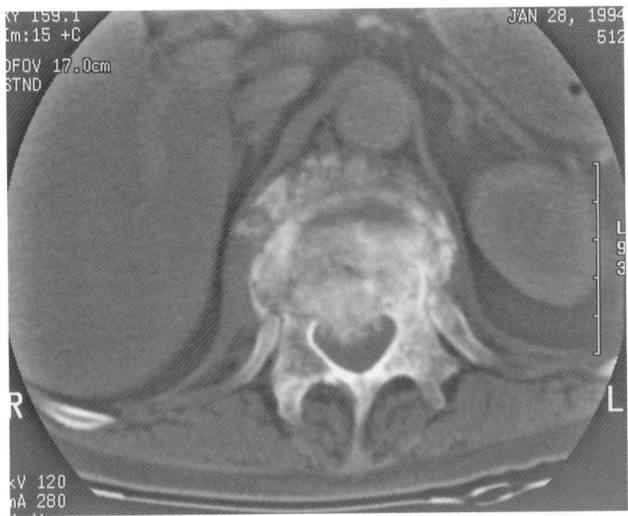

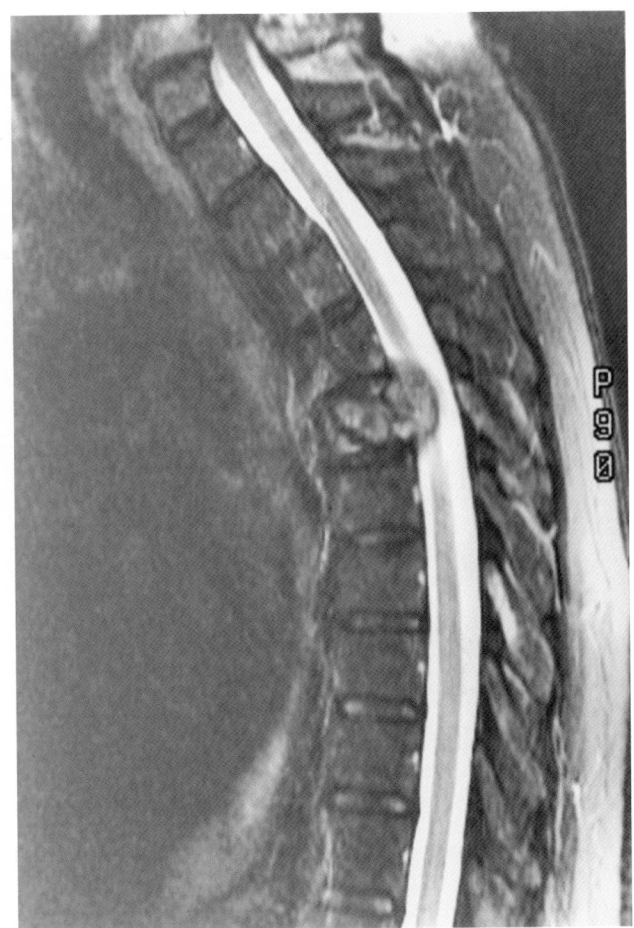

FIGURE 48.2 (A) CT scan showing involvement of the posterior aspect of the vertebral body resulting in partial spinal cord compression. (B) MRI showing involvement of the posterior aspect of the vertebral body resulting in partial spinal cord compression.

Gy) is as effective as a longer course (e.g., 30 Gy in 10 fractions) but the longer courses have lower recurrence rates. A scoring system for survival based on prognostic factors can guide the type of radiation course.[120] Patients with longer estimated survival time may benefit from the longer course of radiation.

Neurosurgical intervention for MSCC involves spinal cord decompression accomplished by a laminectomy and is indicated in a variety of clinical presentations.[84–86,88–90,117,120–123] These situations include: rapid neurologic deterioration in the setting of tumor progression in a previously irradiated area in order to provide stabilization of the spine, tumor-induced paraplegia in patients with otherwise limited disease and good probability of survival, and to establish a diagnosis. Adjuvant radiotherapy is often given to treat microscopic residual disease after neurosurgical intervention.[84,85,88,108] A statistically significant improvement in functional outcome has been reported with laminectomy and radiotherapy in treatment of epidural spinal cord compression over either modality alone.[104,121–123] In paraparetic patients who undergo laminectomy and radiation, 82% regain the ability to walk, 68% have improved sphincter function, and 88% have relief of pain. With radiation alone, 65% regained ambulation, 26% had improved sphincter function, and 70% had improvement of pain.[87,89,90,108,113,122] Laminectomy, however, carries risks associated with surgery and anesthesia. Pain may worsen after laminectomy if operative procedures fail to stabilize the spine. Vertebral collapse may occur because of cancer or vertebral instability after cancer therapy (Fig. 48.5).

Paravertebral masses are most commonly associated with lung cancer and are rare in prostate cancer. Overall, approximately 20% of patients with epidural cord compression have an associated paravertebral mass. Surgical resection combined with radia-

tion therapy has been suggested to improve functional outcome when a paravertebral mass is associated with spinal cord compression.[96,124,125] The overall survival is worse with lung cancer and sarcoma than with breast and renal cancer.[123]

Radiation Tolerance of the Spinal Cord

Radiation tolerance is based on the dose per fraction, total dose, and the volume of tissue treated. The dose per fraction is the most important factor in the tolerance of tissues to radiation. Clinical and experimental experience has failed to demonstrate any difference in radiosensitivity in different segments of the spinal cord.[126] The risk of radiation myelitis in the cervicothoracic spine is less than 5% when 6000 cGy is administered at 172 cGy per fraction or 5000 cGy is given with daily fractions of 200 cGy per fraction. Especially among patients who have received chemotherapy, the total dose to the spinal cord is generally limited to 4000 cGy administered at 200 cGy per fraction to minimize any risk of irreversible radiation injury to the spinal cord. The total dose is also an extremely important factor defining the radiation tolerance of the spinal cord. A steep curve based on total radiation dose predicts the risk of developing radiation myelopathy; a small increase in total radiation dose can result in a large increased risk for radiation myelopathy.[126,127,128] Retreatment of a previously irradiated segment of spinal cord results in high risk for radiation-induced myelopathy because other neurologic pathways cannot compensate for an injury to a specific level of the spinal cord.

The radiation tolerance of the spinal cord can be compromised

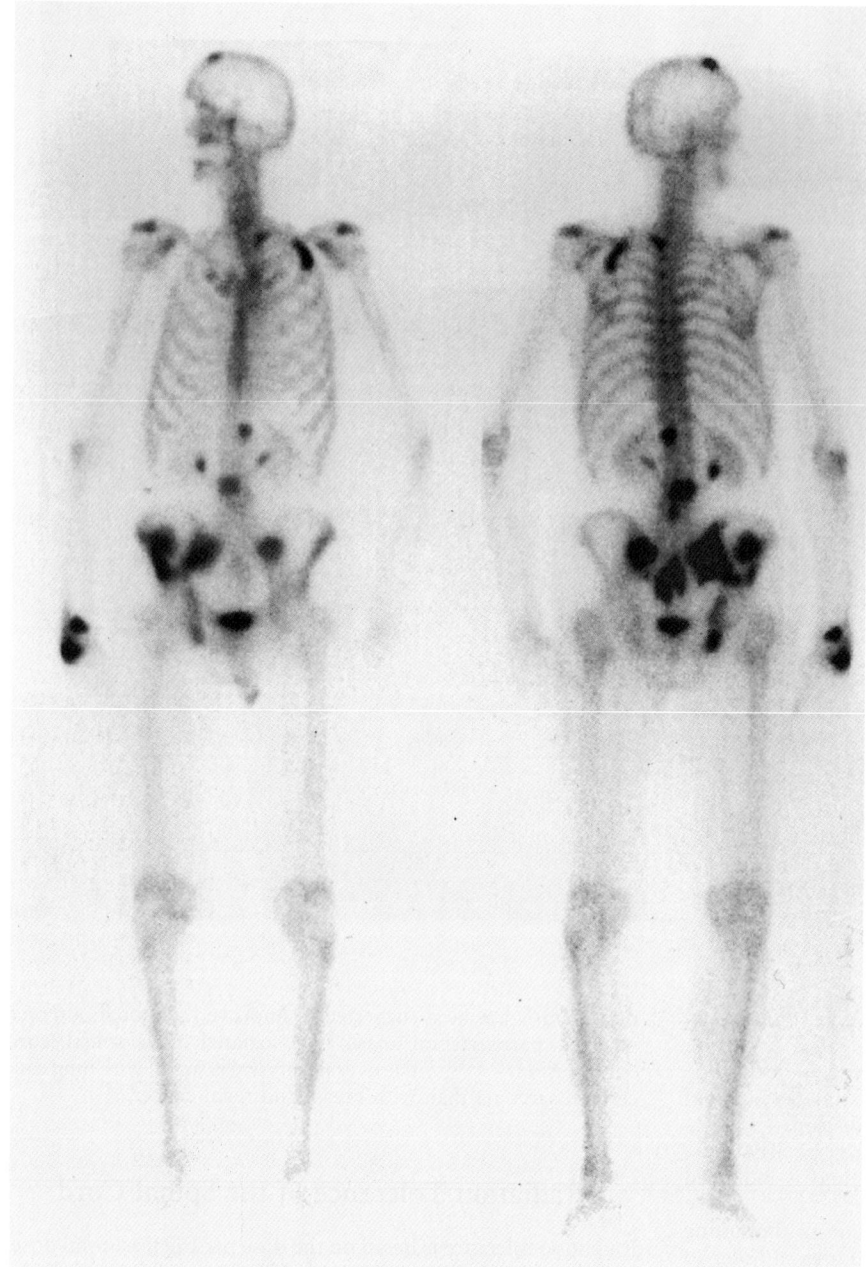

FIGURE 48.3 Bone scan that demonstrates multifocal disease involvement. Metastatic involvement in weight-bearing areas such as the pelvis and lower lumbar area significantly affects mobility.

by prior injury. Difficulty arises in differentiating pathologic and radiotherapeutic injury when there has been spinal cord compression. Vasogenic edema of the spinal cord and nerve roots can be caused by compression injury. Metastatic epidural compression results in vasogenic spinal cord edema, venous hemorrhage, loss of myelin, and ischemia. Vasogenic edema results in an increased synthesis of prostaglandin E, which can be myelotoxic. Inhibition of this inflammatory pathway is one of the putative benefits of corticosteroids or nonsteroidal antiinflammatory therapy. Other consequences of pathologic compression include hemorrhage, loss of myelin, and ischemia.[126–129]

Two separate mechanisms of radiation injury result from white matter damage and vasculopathies. White matter damage is associated with diffuse demyelination and swollen axons that can be focally necrotic and have associated glial reaction. Vascular damage has been shown experimentally to be age dependent and can result in hemorrhage, telangiectasia, and vascular necro-

sis.[126–129] Six major types of injuries have been shown experimentally to result from radiation to the spinal column. Five of these occur in the spinal cord and one in the dorsal root ganglia. The most severe spinal lesions, all of which are caused by vascular damage and result in neurologic dysfunction, include white matter necrosis, hemorrhage, and segmental parenchymal atrophy. The two less severe spinal lesions included focal fiber loss and scattered white matter vacuolation caused by damage to glial cells, axons, the vasculature, or all three; these less severe sequelae are seen with lower total doses of radiation and are less likely to result in neurologic dysfunction. In dorsal root ganglia, radiation damage included intracytoplasmic vacuoles and loss of neurons and satellite cells that could affect sensory function. These findings are distinct from the demyelination of the posterior columns associated with the self-limiting Lhermitte's syndrome.[129] Meningeal thickening and fibrosis can also be observed after radiation, but the clinical significance of this is unknown. Ependymal and nerve root damage from radiation is rare.

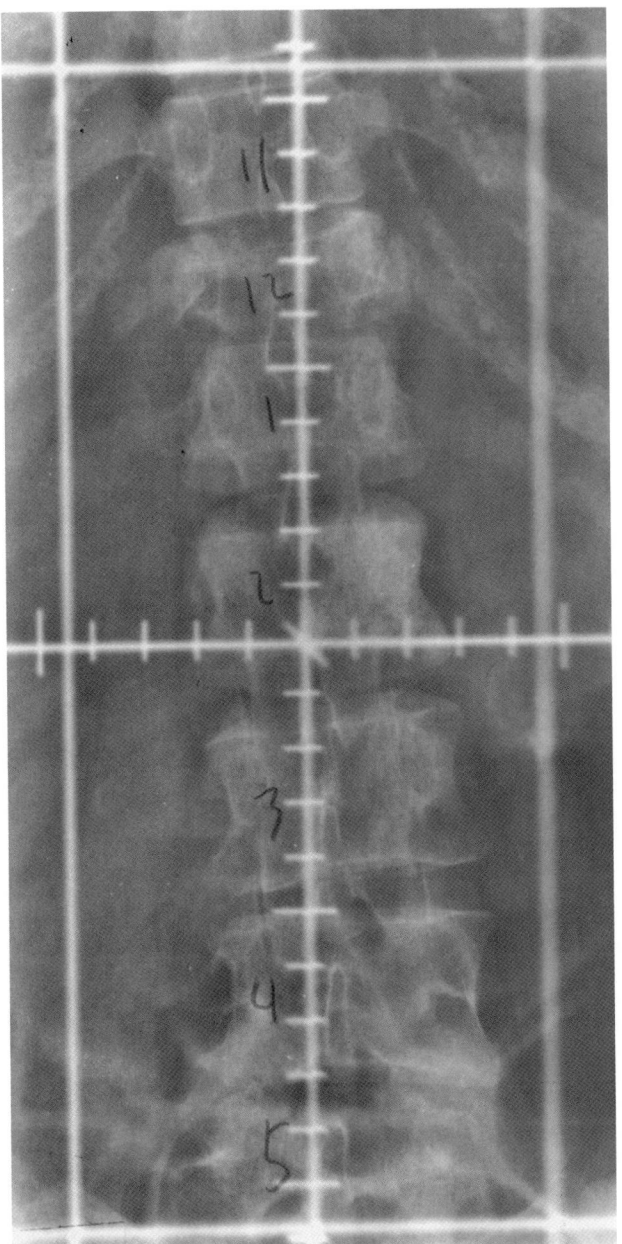

FIGURE 48.4 Typical radiation portal to treat multifocal areas of disease involvement in the vertebral bodies and epidural region.

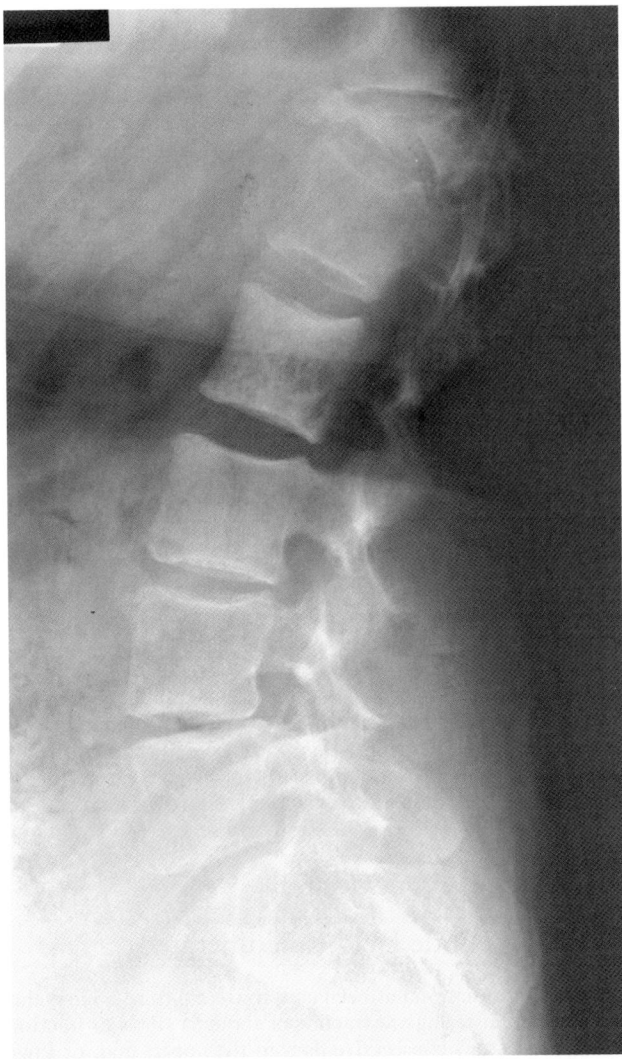

FIGURE 48.5 Compression fracture of the twelfth thoracic vertebral body following an initial pain-free interval after palliative radiation. Vertebral weakness with rapid tumor regression resulted in a compression fracture that caused recurrent back pain because of spinal instability.

Clinical Management

Persistent pain after radiotherapy for vertebral metastases should be investigated to exclude the possibility of progressive disease inside or outside the radiation portal or mechanical spinal instability because of a vertebral compression fracture. Changes seen in the bone marrow on MRI after palliative radiotherapy initially include decreased cellularity, edema, and hemorrhage, followed by fatty replacement and fibrosis. These well-defined changes on MRI after radiotherapy can be distinguished from those seen with progressive malignant disease.[116,130–134]

Prior radiation portals may affect the ability to radiate spine metastases, especially in breast and lung cancer patients. Standard radiation portals currently used for breast cancer therapy infrequently treat the spinal axis. The upper thoracic and lower cervical region, however, may be irradiated in a field encompassing the supraclavicular nodes and axillary apex if significant axillary node involvement is documented. With techniques used in the past for breast cancer, the thoracic spine would receive a significant dose of radiation from a field that treated the internal mammary lymph nodes.[113] Treatment of the mediastinum in lung cancer generally includes the majority of the thoracic spine treated to the maximum dose tolerated by the spinal cord.[125] Unfortunately, previous radiation of the spine as part of definitive therapy does not reduce the risk for subsequent spinal cord compression as a consequence of persistent or recurrent disease.

Surgical decompression is often the only available option for therapy because previously administered radiation may preclude further radiotherapy in the region of the malignant spinal cord compression. This is often the case in lung cancer because metastases are located in the thoracic spine in over 70% of cases, and many of these patients have received mediastinal irradiation.[125] Early involvement by the radiotherapist in the management of patients with suspected spinal cord involvement is important to allow time to obtain prior radiotherapy records, determine if further radiation is possible, and expedite the safest, most efficacious clinical decision-making process.

Based on clinical and radiographic grounds, leptomeningeal carcinomatosis must also be considered in the diagnostic evaluation. Leptomeningeal carcinomatosis occurs more commonly than clinically diagnosed. For example, only one-half of breast cancer patients with leptomeningeal carcinomatosis are diagnosed before death.[84,90,113,135,136] Performing a lumbar puncture is a relative barrier to the diagnosis; at least three cerebrospinal fluid samples are necessary to cytologically exclude the diagnosis of leptomeningeal disease because in 10% to 40% of patients the initial cerebrospinal fluid sample fails to document tumor cells.[135] MRI can identify leptomeningeal disease among patients with normal cerebrospinal fluid cytology and is sensitive and specific in locating regions of nodular leptomeningeal involvement. Except in the case of nodular leptomeningeal involvement, in which localized radiotherapy may be of benefit as an adjuvant, intrathecal chemotherapy is generally the treatment of choice.[136]

TREATMENT OF DIFFUSE BONE METASTASES

Wide field radiotherapy, systemic radionuclides, and bisphosphonates have been used to treat patients with disseminated bone metastases. These approaches are useful in augmenting the therapeutic effect of localized radiation and in preventing asymptomatic bony lesions from progressing. Although usually not a significant consideration in localized irradiation, adequate bone marrow reserve is required for wide field radiotherapy and systemic radionuclides. Bone marrow scans can be performed to determine the volume of functioning marrow and assess the feasibility of delivering wide field radiotherapy or radionuclides.[10,27,43,44,47,130]

Wide Field Radiotherapy

Hemibody irradiation has been used to treat diffuse bone metastases by administering one fraction of about 6–10 Gy or fractions of 3 Gy for 2 to 5 consecutive days to the upper, mid, or lower body. Delivering 3 Gy on 2 consecutive days is equianalgesic to doses of 3 Gy on 5 days for all primary cancers except prostate cancer. Fractioning reduces the need for premedication with prednisone, hydrocortisone, normal saline, or dextrose in half normal saline with potassium chloride and antinausea medication like ondansetron, prochlorperazine, and metoclopromide[34,35] and allows for higher total doses to be delivered, but the effect on pain is equivalent to single dose radiation.[137–139] Response rates are consistently reported to be greater than 70%, and more than 20% of patients have complete relief of pain. In prostate and breast cancer patients, the overall response rate is 80%, and complete relief of pain is 30%, respectively.[140–142] Approximately one-half of patients experience relief of pain within 48 hours of treatment, and the overall response rates equal 80% for all types of primary tumors. About 70% of the patients treated did not require further palliative irradiation for recurrent bone pain over the duration of their lives.[138]

An RTOG study demonstrated that hemibody radiation reduced the time to disease progression and decreased the need for subsequent palliative radiation of bone metastases at 1 year of follow-up when compared with local field irradiation alone. These results from the RTOG study are consistent with other reported experience using hemibody irradiation.[140–142] Median survival after hemibody irradiation is significantly better among patients who present with a good performance status. Approximately 90% of patients with a complete response and 70% of patients with a partial response had a good to excellent performance status before radiotherapy. Prior systemic therapy does not influence response to wide field radiotherapy. Symptomatic

bone metastases that are refractory to chemotherapy or hormonal therapy are reported to have complete response of 70% and partial response rates of 24% with hemibody radiation. Symptoms are palliated in 88% of cases when a previously treated area is reirradiated. Premedication prevents nausea, and partial shielding minimizes lung dose and the risk for radiation pneumonitis. Hematologic depression is limited. Toxicity is observed in less than 10% of patients, whereas 50% experience stabilization of disease at 1 year.

Hemibody radiation may be an important palliative option among patients with diffuse lytic bone metastases that are refractory to other therapies. However, it is not routinely used for the treatment of focal metastases on account of the potential toxicity to the visceral structures and the difficulties in treatment setup. Concerns regarding the permanent effects on bone marrow reserve also exist relative to the subsequent need for chemotherapy.

Radiopharmaceuticals

An alternative to hemibody irradiation for the treatment of widely disseminated bone metastases is the use of systemic radioisotopes. The most commonly used radiopharmaceutical in the treatment of bone metastases is strontium 89. Strontium 89 combines with the calcium component of hydroxyapatite in osteoblastic lesions. Many studies report effective palliation of pain lasting more than 6 months in 60% to 80% of patients with breast and prostate cancers.[39–44,46,48,49,53] Improvements in functional status and quality of life have been observed, and approximately 20% of patients have complete resolution of pain. Pain control has been reported to be superior among patients with disseminated prostate cancer treated both with strontium 89 and local radiotherapy as compared with localized irradiation alone.[42] Myelotoxicity resulting in 25% reduction of platelet and white blood cell counts represents the only significant toxicity associated with strontium 89, which is usually transient and reversible within 12 weeks.[40,44,47,143,144] Hematotoxicity is more pronounced in patients with pretreatment platelet counts of less than or equal to 60×10^3, white blood cell counts of less than or equal to 2.5×10^3, or greater than or equal to 30% involvement of the red marrow–bearing bone. The radiation dose absorbed by the bone marrow is 2 to 50 times less than the dose administered by strontium 89 to the osteoblastic lesion. Radiation doses to metastatic bony lesions with strontium 89 can range from 3 to more than 300 Gy.

Clinical response to strontium 89 is comparable with wide field radiotherapy. Response to strontium 89 therapy has been documented both subjectively and objectively. Subjective response, manifested as symptomatic improvement, was reported by more than 80% of prostate cancer patients using a validated self-reporting tool. Objective evidence of response was documented by reductions in alkaline and acid phosphatase levels that corresponded with a decrease in evidence of active metastatic disease on sequential bone scans.[40–43,46,49,145] Prior therapies for prostate cancer, including local radiation therapy and systemic chemotherapy or hormone therapy, do not influence toxicity or affect clinical response to strontium 89. Administered as an adjuvant to localized external beam radiotherapy in metastatic prostate cancer, strontium 89 has been shown to improve pain relief, reduce analgesic requirements, and delay progression of disease in prospective randomized clinical trials. Quality-of-life assessments demonstrated increased physical activity along with improved pain relief after strontium 89 was administered in conjunction with localized external beam radiation therapy.[146,147] Cost-benefit analysis has also suggested an advantage to the administration of strontium 89 with reductions in costs of hospitalization for tertiary care.[42,43,53]

Several other radiopharmaceuticals are available for clinical application including samarium 153, gallium nitrate, phosphorus

TABLE 48.3

PHYSICAL CHARACTERISTICS AND CLINICAL DATA FOR RADIONUCLIDES

Radionuclide	Half-life (days)	Beta energy (MeV)	Gamma energy (keV)	Response rate (%)	Duration of response (mo)	Toxicity
^{32}P	14.26	1.7	0	77	5.1	Moderate
^{89}Sr	50.53	1.5	0	80	3–6	Low
^{117m}Sn	13.61	0.16 1.1	159	NR	NR 1.3	NR
^{186}Re	3.78	0.9 0.8	137	77	—	Low
^{153}Sm	1.95	0.7 0.6	103	65	4	Low

^{32}P, Phosphorus 32,; ^{83}Sr, Strontium-89-Chloride,; ^{117m}Sn, ^{117m}Sn(4+)diethylenetriaminepentaacetic acid; ^{186}Re, Rhenium-186; ^{153}Sm, Samarium-153; NR, No Response
Modified from Lam MG, de Klerk JM, van Rijk PP, et al. Bone seeking radiopharmaceuticals for palliation of pain in cancer patients with osseous metastases. *Anticancer Agents Med Chem* 2007;7(4):381–397; Liepe K, Kotzerke J. A comparative study of 188Re-HEDP, 186Re-HEDP, 153Sm-EDTMP and 89Sr in the treatment of painful skeletal metastases. *Nucl Med Commun* 2007 Aug;28(8):623–630; and Bouchet LG, Bolch WE, Goddu SM, et al. Considerations in the selection of radiopharmaceuticals for palliation of bone pain from metastatic osseous lesions. *J Nucl Med* 2000 Apr;41(4):682–687.

32, and rhenium 186.[39,44,45,47,51,52,54,149] The therapeutic mechanism of action relates to the physical and biological half-life in the bony lesion, the mean energy, and the delivered dose of the radiopharmaceutical. Table 48.3 summarizes some of the physical characteristics and clinical data for various radionuclides. Phosphorus 32 and strontium 89 emit pure beta rays (little penetration in tissue), whereas rhenium 186 and samarium 153 emit both beta rays and relatively high-energy gamma-ray photons that penetrate tissue for some distance (103 to 159 keV).

Because samarium 153 has a gamma-ray component, it is possible to directly image the distribution of the radiation dose. The scans after injection of samarium 153 are comparable to diagnostic scans obtained with technetium 99m. The mean skeletal uptake is over 50% of the dose.[52] Nonskeletal sites receive negligible radiation doses, and complete clearance of radionuclide other than that absorbed by bone occurs within 6 to 8 hours of administration.[51] In a double-blind placebo-controlled clinical trial, samarium 153 has been shown to be an effective agent in palliating painful bone metastases in breast cancer patients. Pain relief occurred within 1 week and lasted at least 16 weeks after administration.[46,149,150] Approximately 65% of patients responded within the first 4 weeks, and 43%–72% had relief of pain of at least 16 weeks' duration. No significant bone marrow toxicities have been observed. Recommended doses range between 1.0 and 1.5 mCi per kg. In more than one-third of patients, multiple administrations are possible.[54,151] These observations suggest potential suitability of this form of palliative therapy for patients with both intermediate and limited life expectancies who are not tolerating or responding favorably to other pain-relieving treatments.

Selectively concentrating in bone, the mechanism of action of rhenium 186 is similar to that of technetium diphosphonate 99m, which is used in diagnostic bone scans. This characteristic allows direct imaging of the deposition of rhenium 186 in bony metastases. The metastatic lesion receives a highly concentrated dose of radiation after the administration of rhenium 186, whereas the radiation dose to the marrow is limited to 0.75 Gy.[39,48] Thrombocytopenia appears to be the dose-limiting toxicity but is mild, allowing therapy to be repeated.[143,152]

Phosphorus 32 has 77% of patients experiencing significant relief of pain.[39,148] The response rates and duration of response with phosphorus 32 are similar to wide field radiation and strontium 89. However, the main disadvantage of phosphorus 32 is severe hematologic toxicity.

Clinical trials are ongoing to compare the conventional radiopharmaceuticals with newer radiopharmaceuticals and their effect in combination with bisphosphonates and chemotherapy.[49] There is prolonged survival benefit in patients with hormone refractory prostate cancer if radiopharmaceuticals and chemotherapy are used in combination.[153] Although bone marrow toxicity is relatively limited in the doses of radiopharmaceuticals currently administered either alone or in combination with other agents, future dose intensity studies may require hematologic support with colony-stimulating factors.

Sequential radiography and bone scans after hormonal and radiopharmaceutical therapy for breast and prostate cancers demonstrate an osteoblastic response that reflects remodeling of the bone in osteolytic osseous metastases.[30,31] Approximately one-third of patients have evidence of increased tracer uptake on bone scans (flare) obtained 8 to 16 weeks after treatment. Of these patients with a flare response on bone scan, 72% experience a response to the treatment. By comparison, only 36% have a response to treatment when a limited response or no flare response is observed.

Relapse of disease has been associated with an increase in the osteolytic component. Osteoclast resorption in bone metastases is associated with the release of acid and acid-dependent proteases that dissolve the organic matrix of the bone. Gallium nitrate has been shown to inhibit accelerated bone turnover among patients with widespread bone metastases and has been clinically applied in the treatment of hypercalcemia. Preferentially accumulating in the cortical surface, which is the most metabolically active region of the bone, gallium nitrate acts to inhibit osteoclast resorption. Additionally, gallium nitrate increases the absorption of calcium and phosphorus and the incorporation of collagen into the bone.

CHEMOTHERAPY

Role of Chemotherapy

Chemotherapy can be used as an adjuvant to radiotherapy and/ or surgery or as part of a combined antineoplastic regimen for primary treatment. In patients with cancers like lymphomas, Wilms' tumor, rhabdomyosarcoma, and small cell lung cancer, chemotherapy is used alone as the primary therapy.[154] Systemic chemotherapy has the advantage of ubiquitous distribution throughout the body, wherever the bloodstream might take a cancer cell. Thus, adjuvant chemotherapy is used in patients who appear cured after surgery but are suspected of having residual disease or micrometastasis. Adjuvant chemotherapy has proven effective in node-positive breast cancer, Duke's B2 and C colorectal carcinoma, stage III ovarian carcinoma, testicular carcinoma, non-small cell lung cancer, Wilms' tumor, osteogenic sarcoma, and anaplastic astrocytomae.[154]

Neoadjunct chemotherapy is used as initial chemotherapy in cancers that would be only partially curable by surgery or radiation. It is often administered with anal cancer, bladder cancer, esophageal cancer, laryngeal cancer, locally advanced non-small cell lung cancer, and osteogenic sarcoma. The goals of this therapy are to: (a) decrease the size of the tumor to be removed or radiated; (b) increase the likelihood that the tumor will be surgically extirpable; and (c) decrease the likelihood of micrometastatic spread/seeding at the time of surgery.[154] Systemic chemotherapy is the primary treatment for disseminated/metastatic malignant disease.

Based on the mechanisms mentioned above, the goal of systemic chemotherapy is to interrupt the division of rapidly dividing cancer cells. It is usually administered in multiple (usually 4 to 6) cycles every 3 to 4 weeks. The timing and dosing of chemotherapy are established to maximize malignant cell kill, while at the same time not exceeding the body's ability to regenerate the normally rapidly dividing cells that are "innocent bystanders" of the cytotoxic effects of chemotherapy, namely the bone marrow progenitors, gastrointestinal epithelial cells, and hair follicles. The predominant effect of chemotherapy on the intestinal tract occurs in the first few days to a week after administration, whereas the peak effect on the blood progenitor cells occurs 10 to 14 days post-therapy. Thus, patients only require prophylactic antiemetics for the days around therapy, but they "nadir" their blood counts, with variable risks of infection and bleeding, approximately 2 weeks after receiving treatment.

Regardless of the setting of administration (primary, adjuvant, neoadjuvant, or combined modality), substantial evidence suggests that combination chemotherapy with agents that have different mechanisms of action as well as different (noncumulative) toxicities yields significantly higher efficacy than single-agent chemotherapy. On the basis of an extensive review of in vivo and in vitro laboratory research and clinical experiences acquired during the 1950s and 1960s, DeVita and Schein[155] developed a set of basic principles of combination chemotherapy for cancer patients, and these are still the guiding principles today. Among the most important of these principles are the following: (a) all of the component drugs in a combination must have activity against the neoplasm being treated; (b) drugs must be administered at dosages close to the minimum effective dosage for each drug as a single agent, or beyond if possible; (c) drugs that interrupt the synthesis of cellular macromolecules at several sites can be combined for additive or synergistic effects on the various synthetic pathways; (d) drugs in combination should have as little cross-toxicity as possible; and (e) mechanisms of tumor cell resistance to two agents in combination must not be similar.[155]

Clinical Applications

Conventionally, efficacy of chemotherapy is defined by an objective decrease in the radiographic size of the tumor (usually by CT). A complete response (CR) represents total disappearance of all observable disease for a minimum of 1 to 3 months, depending on the criteria used,[156,157] whereas a partial response (PR) represents a decrease in measurable tumor size by at least 50%. Overall response rate (RR) for a given regimen is the combination of CR + PR, and a significant RR translates into an improved survival of responders compared with nonresponders. It also translates into relief of pain related to the tumor mass—although pain relief from chemotherapy has rarely been the end point of clinical trials (Table 48.4). Currently, there are some forms of cancers, such as pediatric tumors, lymphomas, testicular cancer, and ovarian cancer, where complete remission and cure have been realized.[158]

Despite progress, there remain many patients whose malignancies are resistant to chemotherapy. They have progressive disease either shortly after the completion of therapy or, in some cases, during the time of active therapy. The category that falls between an objective response and progressive disease, in which the tumor neither shrinks nor grows in the face of active anticancer therapy, is referred to as *stable disease*. Whether or not there is any pain-relieving benefit to the administration of chemotherapy in the setting of stable disease is undetermined. Although there is speculation about the role of chemotherapy in altering peripheral sensory nerve function, thereby producing analgesia,[159] as well as relieving pain by altering the "tumor-host milieu,"[159] these hypotheses have been tested in limited trials, wherein assessment of the analgesic or symptom outcomes is a primary end point of therapy.[160–167] One of the significant barriers to these types of studies is the lack of a universally adopted system for evaluating pain along with other variables of disease progression or remission. Although some systems have been developed, they remain underused and underappreciated.[168–171] In the absence of empirically proven outcomes, clinical observations suggest that "systemically administered cytotoxic drugs do not relieve cancer pain in the absence of tumor regression."[159] Tumor regression is a function of responsiveness to a given chemotherapeutic regimen. Tumor variables that determine the course of chemotherapy and prognosis for response rate include histologic type (squamous cell carcinoma, adenocarcinoma, germ cell, lymphoma, etc.), grade (high, intermediate, low), and the degree of differentiation (well differentiated, poorly differentiated). Careful assessment of the overall performance status of patients will help to determine their ability to tolerate systemic chemotherapy and endure the likely associated toxicities.

In general, the more rapidly growing the tumor, the more frequent its cellular division; therefore, the cells are more *potentially* responsive to cytotoxic therapy: In these cases, intervention can lead to increased pain control, long-term survival, and, potentially, cure. Those rapidly growing tumors that are chemotherapy-resistant tend to be imminently fatal. Table 48.5 summarizes the most common malignancies and their likelihood of response to chemotherapy. Of the most common solid tumors (lung, colorectal, prostate, and breast), all except breast carcinoma are minimally responsive to current chemotherapeutic regimens. This and other evidence provides a basis for reviewing the palliative benefits of chemotherapy.

RESPONSE OF TUMORS TO CHEMOTHERAPY

Curable by Chemotherapy

Compared with other solid tumor types, Hodgkin's and non-Hodgkin's lymphomas (NHL) tend to respond better than most to combination chemotherapy. For Hodgkin's lymphoma, there are several active regimens, but the preferred treatment regimen of doxorubicin, bleomycin, vinblastine, and dacarbazine is highly active and produces a complete remission rate that varies from 98% for early-stage disease (overall survival of more than 93% at 6 years) to 82% for advanced stage disease (overall survival of

TABLE 48.4

EFFICACY OF CHEMOTHERAPY IN RELIEVING PAIN

Primary cancer	Source or site of pain	Degree of pain relief
Breast	Tumor ulceration	+ + +
	Chest wall infiltration	+ + +
	Bone metastasis	+ +
	Lymphedema of arm	+
Prostate	Bone metastases	+ + + +
Lymphomas	Para-aortic adenopathy→back pain	+ + +
	Superior vena cava obstruction	+ + +
	Spinal cord compression	+ + +
Leukemia	Periosteal irritation/invasion	+ + +
Myeloma	Medullary pressure	+ + +
Testicle	Para-aortic adenopathy→back pain	+ +
Oral/pharyngeal	Tumor ulceration	+ +
	Invasion of nerves	+ +
Lung	Pancoast syndrome	+
Colorectal	Low abdominal	
Cervical	Perineal pain	+
Bladder	Low back	
Intracranial tumors	Increased cerebrospinal fluid pressure→severe headache	
	(a) with corticosteroids	+ + +
	(b) without corticosteroids	+

+ + + +, complete relief; + + +, very good, but incomplete relief; + +, moderate relief; +, little or no relief.
Modified from Bonadonna G, Molinari R. Role and limits of anticancer drugs in the treatment of advanced cancer pain. In: Bonica JJ, Ventafridda V, eds. *Advances in Pain Research and Therapy*. Vol 2. New York: Raven Press; 1979,131–144.

73% at 6 years).[172–174] The therapeutic effect of this combination regimen is rapid, even in advanced cases, providing prompt pain relief in those patients who have pain (although this has never been a primary end point of clinical trials), with observed resolution of other symptoms and signs as well. In NHLs, there is a larger variability based on histology, with high-grade NHL being significantly more responsive to therapy than low-grade types. For high-grade NHL, treatment with a variety of combination chemotherapy regimens (e.g., bleomycin, doxorubicin, cyclophosphamide, vincristine, and prednisone; cyclophosphamide, doxorubicin, vincristine, and prednisone; or others with antibody therapies with rituximab) produces a 79% event-free survival.[175–177] Again, no studies of NHL have examined pain as a primary end point, although pain remits in concert with active disease. Similar results are also obtained in carcinoma of the testicle with platinum, etoposide, and bleomycin, in Wilms' tumor, and in the leukemias (especially the lymphoblastic types).[178]

Chemotherapy Has Significant Activity

Breast Cancer

In moderately chemosensitive tumors, the results obtained with the various chemotherapeutic combinations are less favorable (30% to 60% response rates), and in general, the therapeutic effect is slower in onset. Small cell lung cancer, for example, tends to be quite aggressive, and combination chemotherapy regimens with cisplatin and etoposide or cyclophosphamide, doxorubicin, and vincristine can induce an objective response in approximately 60% of cases, with CR occurring in approximately 10%. Again, this and other studies have not attempted to quantify relief from pain or dyspnea in small cell lung cancer.

The course of recurrent or metastatic breast cancer follows two dominant pathways. The hormone receptor–positive tumors tend to occur in older (postmenopausal) women and follow a more indolent course when treated with hormone therapy, with bone as the most common metastatic site. The hormone receptor–negative tumors tend to occur in younger (premenopausal) women and follow a more aggressive course, with visceral and soft tissue involvement that is usually responsive to chemotherapy.[179] Conventional chemotherapy includes cyclophosphamide, methotrexate, and prednisone and has been shown to improve quality of life. Anthracycline-containing regimens have been shown to be superior to cyclophosphamide, methotrexate, and prednisone. Single agents that contain taxanes (docetaxel, paclitaxel, and protein-bound paclitaxel), capecitabine, gemcitabine, or vinorelbine have been shown to be as effective in improving survival and quality of life as combination chemotherapy in metastatic breast cancer.[180–182] Trastuzumab, alone or in combination in Her-2/neu positive patients, has been shown to increase survival. Yet again, it is noteworthy that given the prevalence of recurrent breast cancer, few studies have specifically addressed quality of life issues,[179] and that even fewer address symptomatic benefits of therapy.

A British study evaluating patients with advanced breast cancer who received first-line palliative chemotherapy (a variety of regimens) did have primary palliative (subjective patient-centered) outcomes that were assessed by using the Rotterdam Symptom Checklist. In this study, one-fourth of the patients

TABLE 48.5

RESPONSIVENESS OF CANCER TO CHEMOTHERAPY

Cure of advanced cancer
Choriocarcinoma
Acute lymphoblastic leukemia
Malignant lymphoma (Hodgkin's disease, diffuse high grade or
    intermediate grade non-Hodgkin's lymphoma)
Hairy cell leukemia
Testicular cancer
Childhood solid tumors (embryonal rhabdomyosarcoma, Ewing's
    sarcoma, Wilms' tumor)
Acute myelocytic leukemia
Acute lymphocytic leukemia
Acute promyelocytic leukemia

Significant palliative, some cure of advanced disease
Ovarian cancer
Bladder cancer
Small cell lung cancer
Gastric cancer

Palliation, probably increased survival
Breast cancer
Multiple myeloma
Head and neck cancer
Non-small cell lung cancer

Adjunct treatment with increased cure
Breast cancer
Colon cancer
Osteogenic sarcoma
Early stage large cell lymphoma

Adapted from Joseph R. Bertino, William Hait. Principles of cancer
therapy. In: Goldman L, Ausiello D. *Cecil Textbook of Medicine*. 22nd ed.
Philadelphia: WB Saunders; 2004:1137–1150.

(26%) felt better after having received chemotherapy, with statistically significant decreases in psychological distress, pain, and improvement in lack of energy and sense of tiredness. As might be expected, feeling better correlated with disease response ($p = 0.03$).[183]

Head and Neck Cancer

Head and neck cancer is one of the most challenging disease sites to treat. Cisplatin and fluorouracil make the tumor more responsive to radiotherapy, and this is the standard accepted multimodal regimen that has been shown to increase survival. In fact, studies have shown that combination chemotherapy with cisplatin and fluorouracil, hydroxyurea and fluorouracil, and taxanes like pacletaxel and cisplatin followed by radiation have all increased survival by 50% to 60%.[184] Chemotherapy with a single agent like cisplatin or carboplatin followed by radiation is also being investigated.[185] These aggressive regimens have potential toxicities and twice-a-day radiotherapy with concomitant chemotherapy have shown improved locoregional control, survival, and improved quality of life.[186]

Ovarian Cancer

Finally, ovarian cancer is one of the more sensitive malignancies to cytotoxic chemotherapy.[187,188] Combination regimens in which a platinum-based agent (cisplatin or carboplatin) is used achieve overall response rates of 60% to 80%. Newer agents,

most notably the taxanes, also have significant activity in ovarian cancer, with overall response rates of 20% to 40%. The combination of carboplatin and paclitaxel has demonstrated superior response rates and has become the standard of care for ovarian cancer amenable to chemotherapy.[187,188] Doyle et al.[189] showed that although objective responses are low with palliative chemotherapy, active palliation with chemotherapy is associated with substantive improvement in patients' emotional function and global quality of life.

Chemotherapy has Minor Activity

Many of the adenocarcinomas (lung, colorectal, esophageal, pancreatic, and prostate), malignant melanoma, malignant brain tumors, and sarcoma of bone and soft tissue are poorly responsive to chemotherapy, so long-term alteration of the course of disease is rarely obtained with chemotherapeutic drugs. In this group of tumors, anticancer modalities are rarely effective in reducing the size of the tumor (achieving neither PR nor CR), and as a result, the associated pain and other symptoms are unlikely to be affected significantly by chemotherapy. There are many factors responsible for the limited efficacy of chemotherapy in these tumors. First, the cellular biology of these solid tumors that often produce pain is such that they have limited response to current drug regimens. Second, the size of the tumor is inversely related to the incidence of satisfactory drug penetration into the mass. Thus, the larger the mass, the poorer the cytotoxic response. Furthermore, given that these tumors generally do not exhibit long-term responses to first-line therapy, additional therapy with second- or third-line drug treatments often yields a minimal (usually less than primary therapy) response rate. Finally, in certain target sites (e.g., head and neck, pelvis) prior radical surgery and/or prior radiation therapy impair the vascular supply to the tumor bed, thus interfering with delivery of an effective drug concentration to the target site.

Since this group represents the most challenging to demonstrate objective response rates to chemotherapy, it is the ideal patient population in which to demonstrate a purely palliative benefit of chemotherapy, represented by decreases in pain, dyspnea, and fatigue and increases in performance status, appetite, and weight gain. A few investigators have pursued these outcome measures with meaningful results. The initial Food and Drug Administration approval of gemcitabine was granted not by data showing its benefits on overall survival or objective response rate, but by improvements in pain control, weight gain, and performance status in patients with pancreatic cancer.[190]

Non-small cell lung cancer is the most prevalent cancer type, and combinations of chemotherapeutic drugs like vinorelbine, gemcitabine, docetaxel, and paclitaxel provide modest survival and probable quality-of-life benefit in a significant number of patients when contrasted with best supportive care.[191–193] These agents show response rates in the 11% to 25% range when combined with platinum-based therapy. No study has examined the effects of therapy on pain or dyspnea, although a few have evaluated improvements in performance status and weight gain.[194] However, oral topotecan has been shown to improve pain, dyspnea, sleep, and fatigue, as well as increased survival, in patients with recurrent small cell lung cancer compared with best supportive care.[38]

In the realm of gastrointestinal malignancies, the role of chemotherapy is limited.[195] The fluoropyrimidines (5-FU and its derivatives) are the conventional agents with demonstrated efficacy in gastrointestinal malignancies. 5-FU has resulted in disappointingly low response rates of approximately 20%. In a large study of more than 400 patients conducted by the North Central Cancer Treatment Group,[196] 70% of patients who received 5-FU/low-dose leucovorin had improvements in performance status and weight gain; there was no assessment of pain as a primary end point. The combination of 5-FU and leucovorin with newer agents like oxaliplatin (FLOFIRI) and irinotecan (FOLFOX) have shown improvement in quality of life.[36,197,198]

In pancreatic cancer, the approval of gemcitabine for pancreatic cancer was based on the palliative end point of "clinical benefit" over the conventional 5-FU therapy. In this study, clinical benefit was defined by a composite of pain, performance status, and weight gain.[190] This was one of the first studies to directly assess the primary end point of pain via patient report of pain intensity together with analgesic consumption. Several recent systematic reviews have shown that gemcitabine-based combinations have shown improved survival as well as quality of life.[199,200]

Prostate cancer is yet another prevalent disease that is poorly responsive to conventional chemotherapy. There is more palliative end-point evidence supporting the use of chemotherapy in prostate cancer than any other disease, in part because it is a slow-growing tumor that tends to cause significant pain and disability for a prolonged period of time. The most widely discussed study is Tannock's Canadian study[201] which used mitoxantrone and prednisone for hormone-refractory metastatic prostate cancer where the primary end point was pain relief. In this study, pain relief was again defined differently from previous studies as a "2-point decrease in pain as assessed by a six-point pain scale. . .without an increase in analgesic medication and maintained for two consecutive evaluations at least 3 weeks apart."[201] They found that this chemotherapy combination produced a positive effect above the benefit of prednisone alone in 29% of patients, with a 50% decrease in analgesic requirements. Other studies suggest the positive impact of docetaxel-based chemotherapy in providing relief of pain in hormone-refractory metastatic prostate cancer.[202,203]

Finally, soft tissue sarcomas demonstrate a response rate of approximately 35% to combination chemotherapy with doxorubicin and ifosfamide, with no studies assessing quality of life or symptomatic benefit from chemotherapy in this disease.[37]

DECISION MAKING ABOUT CHEMOTHERAPY

The diagnosis of cancer is often quite traumatic for both the patient and the family. On the one hand, the administration of chemotherapy is, by definition, cytotoxic—to malignant cells as well as normal host cells. On the other hand, the risks of not treating the disease are also quite significant. Given the fact that pain is a prevalent feature of both early- and advanced-stage cancer—present in nearly 50% of patients with early-stage disease and in 70% to 90% of cases of advanced cancer—the challenge is to strike a balance between therapeutic and toxic (including fatal) effects of chemotherapy. Thus, it is imperative that an interdisciplinary team of clinicians with expertise in oncologic surgery, radiation therapy and medical oncology, nursing, palliative medicine, and pharmacology evaluate patients to determine the treatment plan that is likely to provide the greatest cumulative benefit for the patient. If, as ought to be the ideal, the patient is always to be kept at the center of the decision-making process, then studies that assess patient-centered outcomes (pain, dyspnea, fatigue, appetite, weight loss, performance status, anxiety, well-being, and other quality of life measures) for chemotherapy merit a higher priority. Newer targeted therapies need to be evaluated for benefits related to reduction of symptom burden from neoplastic disease. Although it is generally accepted that patients with a poor performance status do not usually benefit from systemic chemotherapy, it is not known whether patients with, for example, lung cancer have improvements in dyspnea as a result of chemotherapy.

An additional challenge for the medical oncologist is decision making if first-line chemotherapy fails to control the tumor. For some disease types, there is clear objective benefit from second-line therapy. For many, however, second-line therapy is more likely to lead to enhanced cumulative toxicities rather than objective tumor response. A sensitive and thoughtful discussion with the patient and the family regarding the goals and priorities of care is needed. Emphasis must be placed on the ability to successfully manage the symptoms of progressive advanced disease with nonchemotherapeutic modalities when burdens are likely to outweigh benefits.

SIDE EFFECTS AND COMPLICATIONS

Toxicities and the predictable side effects of each of the chemotherapeutic agents are listed in Table 48.6. Perhaps the most common painful sequela of chemotherapy administration is a toxic peripheral neuropathy manifested as painful paresthesias, hyporeflexia, and, less frequently, sensory or motor loss or autonomic dysfunction.[157] The drugs most commonly associated with this complication are the plant alkaloids, especially vincristine; antimetabolites; the taxanes, especially paclitaxel; platinum-based compounds like cisplatin; vinorelbine, procarbazine, and interferon.[204–208] In some cases, the painful peripheral neuropathy not only limits the dosing of anticancer therapy, but also significantly affects quality of life and can be more difficult to treat than the more common nociceptive pain syndromes associated with the disease.

Dermatologic complications can occur from extravasation of chemotherapeutic agents into the subcutaneous tissues. This is especially problematic with drugs like vinca alkaloids, anthracyclines, and taxanes that cause severe local pain and ulceration with progressive tissue destruction.[207]

Another painful complication of cancer and its therapy is acute herpes zoster and postherpetic neuralgia, which occur with increased frequency in patients with cancer—especially in those receiving chemotherapy or immunosuppressive drugs. Lastly, although the palliative benefits of glucocorticoids on mood, pain (as an antiinflammatory coanalgesic), and appetite are well known, chronic steroid therapy can cause myopathy, as well as necrosis of the femoral and humeral heads.[209] Furthermore, one should be aware of the fact that withdrawal of glucocorticoids can cause a sense of decreased well-being, with increased pain, decreased energy, and apathy called *pseudorheumatism*.[210]

ENDOCRINE THERAPY

In the 1890s, Beatson[211] was the first to demonstrate hormonal control of breast cancer when he induced regression of metastatic tumor by ovariectomy. In 1941, Huggins and Hodges[212] reported the successful use of exogenous estrogen administration for prostatic carcinoma. Since then, several other tumors have been shown to respond to hormonal manipulation, which is achieved either by ablating endocrine glands or by administration of an exogenous hormone or hormone antagonist.

Mechanism of Action

The mechanism of action of these agents has been clarified by the demonstration that receptors that bind with estrogen exist in the cytosol of normal and malignant cells.[213] Hormones bind to receptors in the cytoplasm and sterically alter the shape of the receptive protein itself, which, after transport to the cell nucleus, interacts with DNA, and results in altered messenger RNA production and protein synthesis.[213] After this interaction, cytoplasmic receptor concentration is restored and the cycle can be repeated. Estrogen receptors can be quantitated as 8S and 4S proteins.[213] Primary tumors in humans have estrogen receptor

TABLE 48.6

COMMONLY USED CYTOTOXIC ANTICANCER AGENTS

Class (Drug)*	Bone marrow	Nausea, vomiting suppr.	Other toxicity	Indications
A. ALKYLATING AGENTS				
Mechlorethamine (Mustargen)	4+	3+	Vesicant to skin, phlebitis	Hodgkin's disease, non-Hodgkin's lymphoma, lung cancer, mycosis fungoides
Cyclophosphamide (Cytoxan)	3+	2+	Alopecia and cystitis, SIADH	Lymphomas; breast, lung, and ovarian cancer; myeloma; leukemias; head and neck cancer
Ifosfamide (Ifex)	3+	2+	Cystitis, nephrotoxicity, CNS toxicity	Germ cell tumors, sarcoma, non-Hodgkin's lymphoma, cervical and lung cancer
Melphalan (Alkeran)	3+	1+	Persistent thrombocytopenia on long use, pulmonary toxicity	Breast and ovarian cancer, myeloma
Busulfan (Myeleran)	3+	1+	Pigmentation, pulmonary fibrosis, hepatotoxicity	Pre–bone-marrow transplantation, chronic myelogenous leukemia
Chlorambucil (Leukeran)	3+	0	Pancytopenia with long-term use hepatotoxicity	Chronic lymphocytic leukemia, nodular lymphomas
CCNU (Lomustine)	4+	2+	Cumulative marrow suppression, chronic renal failure, pulmonary toxicity	Brain tumors, lung and colon cancer, lymphomas
BCNU (Carmustine)	4+	4+	Chronic renal failure, pulmonary fibrosis, tanning of skin, nephrotoxicity	Hodgkin's disease, non-Hodgkin's lymphoma, myeloma, brain tumors
MeCCNU (Semustine)	4+	2+	Pronounced thrombocytopenia, chronic renal failure	Colon and gastric cancer, brain tumors, lymphomas
Streptozocin (Streptozotocin, Zanosar)	0	2+	Hepatotoxicity, renal tubular acidosis, renal failure	Islet cell tumors of pancreas, Hodgkin's disease, carcinoid tumors
Cisplatin (cis-platinum, Platinol)	1+	3+	Nephrotoxicity, ototoxicity, peripheral neuropathy	Testicular tumors, ovarian and lung cancer, lymphomas
Temozolomide (Temodar)			Photosensitivity	Melanoma, brain tumors
B. ANTIMETABOLITES				
Methotrexate: high dose with rescue	1+	2+ ⎤	Fatigue, buccal ulcerations, hepatotoxicity, lung disease	Breast, lung, cervical, and head and neck cancers, sarcomas, acute lymphocytic leukemia, meningeal leukemia, carcinomatosis
Methotrexate: no rescue	4+	1+ ⎬		
	1+	0 ⎦		
5-Fluorouracil (5-FU)	3+	2+	Mucositis, diarrhea, photophobia, alopecia, cerebellar ataxia, myocardial ischemia	Colon, breast, ovarian, gastric, pancreatic, head and neck cancer
6-Mercaptopurine (Purinethol)	2+	1+	Hepatotoxicity, skin rashes	For maintenance phase of acute lymphocytic leukemia
6-Thioguanine	2+	1+	Cholestasis, hepatotoxicity	Acute myelogenous leukemia and ALL

(continues)

TABLE 48.6

CONTINUED

Class (Drug)*	Toxicities‡			Indications
	Bone marrow	Nausea, vomiting suppr.	Other toxicity	
Cytarabine (cytosine arabinoside, Cytosar-U)	4+	2+	Mucositis, alopecia, hepatotoxicity, pancreatitis, cerebral dysfunction, corneal damage, pulmonary edema, "Ara-C syn"	Acute myelogenous leukemia, non-Hodgkin's lymphoma, meningeal leukemia, carcinomatosis
Hydroxyurea	3+	1+	Megaloblastosis	Alternate to busulfan for chronic myelogenous leukemia, rapid reduction of high WBC in acute or chronic myelogenous leukemia, cervical, head, and neck cancers
Fludarabine (Fludara)	3+	1+	Neurologic and pulmonary toxicity	CLL
C. PLANT ALKALOIDS AND INHIBITORS OF CHROMATIN FUNCTION				
Vinblastine (Velban)	3+	1+	Mild peripheral neuropathy	Hodgkin's disease, head and neck tumors, testicular tumors, breast, bladder, and renal cancer
Vincristine (Oncovin)	1+	1+	Local necrosis, peripheral neuropathy (paresthesias, etc.), alopecia, ileus, motor weakness, SIADH	Lymphomas, acute lymphocytic leukemia, childhood sarcomas, breast cancer
Etoposide (VP-16)	1–2+	1+	Mucositis, bronchospasm, hypotension with rapid IV infusion, CNS toxicity.	Small cell lung cancer, breast cancer, lymphomas (relapsed), testicular cancer, choriocarcinoma
Docetaxel (Taxotere)	3+	1+	Hypersensitivity reaction, fluid retention, neuropathy, arthralgias	Breast, prostate, lung ovarian, esophageal, gastric, bladder cancer
Paclitaxel (Taxol)	3+	1+	Hypersensitivity reaction, neuropathy, arthralgias, cardiotoxicity	Metastatic breast cancer, lung, ovarian, esophageal, gastric cancer
Irinotecan (Camptosar)	2+	2+	Diarrhea	Colorectal cancer
Vinorelbine (Navelbine)	2+	2+	Hyperbilirubinemia, asthenia, neuropathy	Lung cancer
D. ANTIBIOTICS AND NONCOVALENT DNA BINDING DRUGS				
Doxorubicin (Adriamycin)	4+	2+	Mucositis, alopecia, myocardiopathy, red urine	Breast, lung, ovarian, pancreatic, gastric, and thyroid cancer, leukemia and lymphomas, sarcomas
Bleomycin (Blenoxane)	1+	1+	Pneumonitis, mucositis, pulmonary fibrosis, alopecia, skin changes, hypersensitivity reaction	Head and neck tumors, cervical carcinoma, lymphoma
Dactinomycin (Cosmegen)	3+	2+	Mucositis, phlebitis, diarrhea, alopecia, skin changes	Wilms' tumor, gestational, trophoblastic neoplasia, soft tissue sarcoma, childhood solid tumors

(continues)

TABLE 48.6

CONTINUED

Class (Drug)*	Toxicities‡			Indications
	Bone marrow	Nausea, vomiting suppr.	Other toxicity	
Daunorubicin (Cerubidine)	4+	2+	Mucositis, hepatotoxicity, myocardiopathy	Acute nonlymphatic and lymphatic leukemias, childhood solid tumors
Mithramycin (Mithracin)	3+	3+	Hemorrhage, skin flushing, thrombocytopenia, hypocalcemia	Malignant hypercalcemia, testicular tumor (salvage therapy)
Mitomycin C (Mutamycin)	3+	2+	Mucositis, pneumonitis, renal failure	Breast, lung, colon, gastric, pancreatic, and bladder carcinoma
E. MISCELLANEOUS				
Gemcitabine (Gemzar)	2+	2+	Pain, fever, rash	Pancreatic cancer
Procarbazine (Matulane)	3+	2+	Side effects of monoamine oxidase inhibitors, skin rash	Lung and testicular cancer, brain tumors, lymphoma
L-Asparaginase (Elspar)	0	2+	Pancreatitis, CNS toxicity, hypofibrinogenemia	Acute myelogenous leukemia, T-cell lymphoma
Hexamethylmelamine	1+	3+	Anorexia, central and peripheral neuropathy	Ovarian and small cell lung carcinoma
F. TARGETED THERAPIES				
Imatinib (Gleevec)	2+		Fluid retention, hypophosphatemia	CLL, gastrointestinal stromal tumors
Bortezomib (Avastin)	2+		neuropathy, asthenia, hypotension	Relapsed multiple myeloma
Erlotinib (Tarceva)	1+		Rash, diarrhea, interstitial lung disease	2nd and 3rd line non-small cell lung cancer
Lenalidomide (Revimid)	2+		Diarrhea, pruritus, rash fatigue, leg cramps	Myelodysplasia, myelomas
Nexavar (Sorafenib)	1+		Rash, hand and foot fatigue, diarrhea, hair loss	Renal cell carcinoma
Rituximab (Rituxan)	1+		Hypersensitivity reaction, Lymphopenia	Relapsed low grade non-Hodgkin's lymphoma
Thalidomide (Thalomid)	1+		Teratogenicity, sedation, constipation, neuropathy, rash	Myeloma
Trastuzumab (Herceptin)	0		Hypersensitivity reaction	Metastatic or adjunct Her-2/neu-positive breast cancer

ALL, acute lymphoblastic leukemia; CLL, chronic lymphocytic leukemia; WBC, white blood cells
*The names of drugs in parentheses represent proprietary names and in some instances other generic names.
‡Degree of toxicity: 4 + marked, 3 + severe, 2 + moderate, 1 + minimal or mild, 0 none.
Modified from Perry MC. Principles of cancer therapy. In: Goldman L, Ausiello D, eds. *Cecil Textbook of Medicine*. 23rd ed. Philadelphia: WB Saunders; 2008:1370–1387.

values that range from zero to almost 1000 fmol per mg cytosol protein. Receptors also exist for progesterones and androgens, and receptors for corticosteroids have been identified in the cytosol of leukemic cells.[213]

Hormonal ablation can be achieved by surgical means, as occurs with oophorectomy, adrenalectomy, and hypophysectomy; by irradiation of the ovaries or ablating the pituitary gland with the various radioactive compounds; by injecting alcohol; or by surgical extirpation. Medical adrenalectomy can be achieved by administering aminoglutethimide, a potent inhibitor of the conversion of cholesterol to pregnenolone in the adrenal gland.[213] Hormone additive therapy is achieved by the administration of estrogens, progestins, androgens, antiestrogens, corticosteroids, and thyroid hormones. Table 48.7 lists the hormonal agents used

TABLE 48.7

HORMONALLY ACTIVE AGENTS IN CANCER TREATMENT

Agents	Toxicity	Indications
Estrogen		
Diethylstilbestrol	Feminization of men, fluid retention, thromboembolic phenomenon, induction of endometrial cancer	Breast and prostate cancer
Estradiol	Feminization of men, fluid retention, thromboembolic phenomenon, induction of endometrial cancer	Breast and prostate cancer
Antiestrogens		
Tamoxifen (Nolvadex)	Hot flashes, nausea, vomiting, vaginal bleeding or discharge, hypercalcemia, visual disturbances, thrombocytopenias, endometrial cancer, rare liver dysfunction	Adjunct and metastatic cancer
Progestins		
Medroxyprogesterone (Provera, Depo-provera)	Weight gain, thromboembolic phenomena, fetal hazard	Breast and endometrial cancer
Megestrol acetate (Megace)	Weight gain, thromboembolic phenomena, fetal hazard	Breast and endometrial cancer
Aromatase Inhibitors		
Aminoglutethimide	Dizziness and rash	Breast and prostate cancer
Letrozole (Femara)	Hot flashes, arthralgias	Adjunct and metastatic breast cancer in postmenopausal women
Anastrazole (Arimidex)	Hot flashes, arthralgias	Adjunct and metastatic breast cancer in postmenopausal women
Exemestane (Aromasin)	Hot flashes, arthralgias	Metastatic breast cancer in postmenopausal women
Gonadotropin Releasing Hormone Analogues		
Leuprolide (Lupron, Lupron Depot)	Increased bone pain, hot flashes, thromboembolic phenomena	Prostate and breast cancer
Goserelin (Zoladex)	Worsening bone pain, hot flashes	Breast and prostate cancer
Antiandrogens		
Flutamide (Eulexin)	Worsening bone pain, hot flashes, gynecomastia	Prostate cancer (usually in conjunction with LHRH antagonist)
Bicalutamide (Casodex)	Worsening bone pain, hot flashes, gynecomastia	Prostate cancer (usually in conjunction with LHRH antagonist)
Nilutamide (Nilandron)	Worsening bone pain, hot flashes, gynecomastia, visual disturbances, interstitial pneumonitis	Prostate cancer (usually in conjunction with LHRH antagonist)
Androgens		
Fluoxymesterone (Halotestin)	Masculinization in women, hepatotoxicity	Breast cancer
Glucocorticoids		
Dexamethasone (Decadron)	Cushingoid appearance, hyperglycemia, fluid retention, osteoporosis, muscular weakness, peptic ulcer disease, cataracts, psychosis, aseptic necrosis	ALL, lymphomas, myeloma, CLL
Prednisone (Deltasone)	Cushingoid appearance, hyperglycemia, fluid retention, osteoporosis, muscular weakness, peptic ulcer disease, cataracts, psychosis, aseptic necrosis	ALL, lymphomas, myeloma, CLL

ALL, acute lymphoblastic leukemia; CLL, chronic lymphocytic leukemia
Adapted from Perry MC. Principles of cancer therapy. In: Goldman L, Ausiello D, eds. *Cecil Textbook of Medicine.* 23rd ed. Philadelphia: WB Saunders; 2008:1370–1387 and Goetz MP, Erlichman C, Loprinzi CL. Pharmacology of endocrine manipulation. In: DeVita VT, Rosenberg SA, eds. *Cancer: Principles and Practices of Oncology.* 7th ed. Philadelphia: Lippincott Williams & Wilkins; 2006:457–469.

in the treatment of various cancers and side effects. Such hormone changes can cause complex endocrine effects, such as pituitary inhibition of luteinizing hormone, follicle-stimulating hormone, and prolactin, as well as changes in endogenous steroid hormone production.[213]

Endocrine Therapy for Relief of Cancer Pain

At the First International Symposium on Cancer Pain[214] and at another symposium held subsequently,[215] Pannuti and colleagues presented a comprehensive summary of the results reported by a number of oncologists. Table 48.8 contains mean data presented by Pannuti et al.[214,215] that provide an overview of the response to hormonal therapy of patients with four types of cancers. These reports were some of the first in which the efficacy of hormonal therapy on pain relief was correlated with the efficacy of these agents on tumor remission. Unfortunately, a significant number of reports on advanced cancer had no discrete data on pain relief but only measurements of volume reduction of tumor size. Pannuti and colleagues[214] further pointed out that there was no uni-

versally accepted rating system or qualification of pain relief on the part of oncologists, and this obviously led to heterogeneous results that could not be compared.

As can be noted in Table 48.8, Pannuti et al.[214] gave progestin therapy in the form of high doses of injectable medroxyprogesterone acetate (MAP-HD) and noted pain relief in 83% of breast cancer patients with predominantly bone metastasis, although only 45% had objective evidence of tumor remission. Patients with estrogen receptor (ER) and progesterone receptor (PR) positive tumors have greater pain relief.[216] In view of the corticosteroid-like side effects from these large doses of MAP-HD, it is possible that much of the subjective response was due to nonspecific steroid action. Hypophysectomy has been proven to provide a high degree of pain relief.[217,218] With regard to advanced cancer of the prostate, MAP-HD and hypophysectomy produced the highest degree of pain relief. For hypophysectomy, pain relief was significant, even in the absence of tumor remission. With regard to renal carcinoma, androgens and progestins (particularly in the form of MAP-HD) provided pain relief and tumor remission in approximately 40% of the patients.

Although ovarian carcinoma contains steroid receptors, very

TABLE 48.8

RESULTS WITH HORMONAL THERAPY IN ADVANCED CANCER

Agent or technique, by type of tumor	Number of reports	Tumor remission (% of tumors)		Pain relief (% of patients)
		Objective	Subjective	
Breast				
Androgens	7	14	37	44
Antiestrogens	2	24	43	33
Progestins (other than MAP)	3	32	50	44
MAP-LD	4	28	51	21
MAP-HD	4	45	ND	83
Corticosteroids	2	4	16	12
L-DOPA	1	33	33	33
Hypophysectomy Surgical	4	30	42	82
Chemical (alcohol injection)	2	30	ND	90
Adrenalectomy	2	36	41	44
Prostate				
Estrogens (DES-P)	3	42	76	81
Cyproterone acetate (CP)	2	80	ND	80
MAP-LD	1	ND	ND	75
MAP-HD	2	ND	100	100
Surgical hypophysectomy	3	ND	35	71
Adrenalectomy	3	20	ND	71
Orchidectomy	1	ND	71	ND
Clear Cell Renal Cancer				
Progestins (other than MAP)	2	8	53	ND
Androgens	1	ND	100	ND
MAP-LD	2	8	53	75
MAP-HD	2	ND	100	86
Corticosteroids	1	ND	100	ND
Endometrial				
MAP-LD	2	35	75	ND
17-Hydroxyprogesterone	2	33	70	ND

DES-P, diethylstilbestrol diphosphate; HD, high dose (1000–1500 mg/day); LD, low dose (<500 mg/day); MAP, medroxyprogesterone acetate; ND, no data available.
Modified from Pannuti F, Martoni A, Rossi AP, et al. The role of endocrine therapy for relief of pain due to advanced cancer. In: Bonica JJ, Ventafridda V, eds. *Advances in Pain Research and Therapy.* Vol 2. New York: Raven Press; 1979:145–166 and Pannuti F. Hormonal treatment. In: Twycross RF, Ventafridda V, eds. *The Continuing Care of Terminal Cancer Patients.* New York: Pergamon Press; 1980:79–89.

little objective response to hormone therapy has been demonstrated.[214] Subjective response to the tumor occurred in some patients with progestin therapy, but no information is available concerning pain relief. Well-differentiated papillary thyroid carcinoma, found particularly in women younger than the age of 40, is likely to be dependent on thyroid-stimulating hormone, and pituitary thyroid-stimulating hormone secretion can be suppressed by thyroxine administration, but no data are available concerning pain relief.

Side Effects

Endocrine therapy is generally much better tolerated than chemotherapy. None of these agents produces bone marrow suppression. Corticosteroids and high doses of medroxyprogesterone acetate (MPA), given for long periods of time, are associated with classic Cushingoid side effects, and parenteral MPA can cause administration site abscess.[214] Sex hormones, particularly estrogens, can cause intermittent uterine bleeding, which can be upsetting, especially for postmenopausal women. Androgens cause virilization and increased libido in some women. Estrogen given to men causes alopecia, testicular atrophy, gynecomastia, loss of libido, and impotence. Long-term administration of estrogen is also associated with a decrease in mortality from cardiac and cerebrovascular disease—presumably on the basis of favorable effects on lipoproteins—whereas androgens are thought to increase the risk of cardiovascular disease. Adrenalectomy causes side effects similar to those of estrogens, with the exception of the excess cardiovascular complications. Surgical adrenalectomy and hypophysectomy are both major operative procedures and carry a small but significant mortality risk (see Table 48.7).

References

1. MacDonald N. The role of medical and surgical oncology in the management of cancer pain. In: Foley KM, Bonica JJ, Ventafridda V, eds. *Advances in Pain Research and Therapy.* Vol 16. New York: Raven Press; 1990:27–39.
2. Jemal A, Siegel R, Ward E, et al. Cancer statistics, 2007. *CA Cancer J Clin* 2007;57(1):43–66.
3. Chang VT, Thaler HT, Polyak TA, et al. Quality of life and survival—the role of multidimensional symptom assessment. *Cancer* 1998;83(1):173–179.
4. Jacox A, Carr DB, Payne R. New clinical practice guidelines for the management of pain in patients with cancer. *N Engl J Med* 1994;330(9):651–655.
5. Brescia FJ, Portenoy RK, Ryan M, et al. Pain, opioid use, and survival in hospitalized patients with advanced cancer. *J Clin Oncol* 1992;10(1):149–155.
6. Porzsolt F. Goals of palliative cancer therapy: scope of the problem. *Cancer Treat Rev* 1993;19(suppl A):3–14.
7. Rubens RD. Approaches to palliation and its evaluation. *Cancer Treat Rev* 1993;19(suppl A):67–71.
8. Porzsolt F, Tannock I. Goals of palliative cancer therapy. *J Clin Oncol* 1993;11(2):378–381.
9. Cella DF, Tulsky DS. Quality of life in cancer: definition, purpose, and method of measurement. *Cancer Invest* 1993;11(3):327–336.
10. Janjan NA. Radiation for bone metastases—conventional techniques and the role of systemic radiopharmaceuticals. *Cancer* 1997;80(suppl 8):1628–1645.
11. Powers WE, Ratanatharathorn V. Palliation of bone metastases. In: Perez CA, Brady LW, eds. *Principles and Practice of Radiation Oncology.* 3rd ed. Philadelphia: Lippincott–Raven; 1998:2199–2219.
12. McCloskey SA, Tao ML, Rose CM, et al. National survey of perspectives of palliative radiation therapy: role, barriers, and needs. *Cancer J* 2007;13(2):130–137.
13. Arcangeli G, Micheli A, Arcangeli F, et al. The responsiveness of bone metastases to radiotherapy: the effect of site, histology, and radiation dose on pain relief. *Radiother Oncol* 1989;14(2):95–101.
14. Greenwald HP, Bonica JJ, Bergner M. The prevalence of pain in four cancers. *Cancer* 1987;60(10):2563–2569.
15. Sherry MM, Greco FA, Johnson DH, et al. Breast cancer with skeletal metastases at initial diagnosis—distinctive clinical characteristics and favorable prognosis. *Cancer* 1986;58(1):178–182.
16. Sherry MM, Greco FA, Johnson DH, et al. Metastatic breast cancer confined to the skeletal system. An indolent disease. *Am J Med* 1986;81(3):381–386.
17. Lai PP, Perez CA, Lockett MA. Prognostic significance of pelvic recurrence and distant metastasis in prostate carcinoma following definitive radiotherapy. *Int J Radiat Oncol Biol Phys* 1992;24(3):423–430.
18. Yamashita K, Denno K, Ueda T, et al. Prognostic significance of bone metastases in patients with metastatic prostate cancer. *Cancer* 1993;71(4):1297–1302.
19. Knudson G, Grinis G, Lopez-Majano V, et al. Bone scan as a stratification variable in advanced prostate cancer. *Cancer* 1991;68(2):316–320.
20. Cohen HJ. Cancer and the functional status of the elderly. *Cancer* 1997;80(10):1883–1886.
21. Delea T, Langer C, McKiernan J, et al. The cost of treatment of skeletal-related events in patients with bone metastases from lung cancer. *Oncology* 2004;67(5–6):390–396.
22. Grootjans-Geerts I. Palliative care is more than palliative antitumour treatment and symptom management. *Ned Tijdschr Geneeskd* 2007;151(12):679–680.
23. Lutz S, Spence C, Chow E, et al. Survey on use of palliative radiotherapy in hospice care. *J Clin Oncol* 2004;22(17):3581–3586.
24. Schulman KL, Kohles J. Economic burden of metastatic bone disease in the U.S. *Cancer* 2007;109(11):2334–2342.
25. Dale RG, Jones B. Radiobiologically based assessments of the net costs of fractionated radiotherapy. *Int J Radiat Oncol Biol Phys* 1996;36(3):739–746.
26. Janjan NA. Radiotherapeutic approaches to cancer pain management. *Highlights Oncol Pract* 1997;14(4 suppl 11):103–113.
27. Nielsen OS, Munro AJ, Tannock IF. Bone metastases: pathophysiology and management policy. *J Clin Oncol* 1991;9(3):509–524.
28. Mercadante S. Malignant bone pain: pathophysiology and treatment. *Pain* 1997;69(1–2):1–18.
29. Awan AM, Weichselbaum RR. Palliative radiotherapy. *Hematol Oncol Clin North Am* 1990;4(6):1169–1181.
30. Hortobagyi GN, Libshitz HI, Seabold JE. Osseous metastases of breast cancer—clinical, biochemical, radiographic, and scintigraphic evaluation of response to therapy. *Cancer* 1984;53(3):577–582.
31. Vogel CL, Schoenfelder J, Shemano I, et al. Worsening bone scan in the evaluation of antitumor response during hormonal therapy of breast cancer. *J Clin Oncol* 1995;13(5):1123–1128.
32. Rose CM, Kagan AR. The final report of the expert panel for the radiation oncology bone metastasis work group of the American College of Radiology. *Int J Radiat Oncol Biol Phys* 1998;40(5):1117–1124.
33. Hanks GE. The crisis in health care costs in the United States: some implications for radiation oncology. *Int J Radiat Oncol Biol Phys* 1992;23(1):203–206.
34. Rubin P, Salazar O, Zagars G, et al. Systemic hemibody irradiation for overt and occult metastases. *Cancer* 1985;55(suppl 9):2210–2221.
35. Rostom AY, El-Hussainy G, Kandil A, et al. Tumor lysis syndrome following hemi-body irradiation for metastatic breast cancer. *Ann Oncol* 2000;11(10):1349–1351.
36. Lièvre A, Mitry E. Chemotherapy for colorectal cancers. *J Chir* (Paris) 2003;140(1):52–55.
37. Budd GT. Palliative chemotherapy of adult soft-tissue sarcomas. *Semin Oncol* 1995;22(Suppl 3):30–34.
38. O'Brien ME, Ciuleanu TE, Tsekov H, et al. Phase III trial comparing supportive care alone with supportive care with oral topotecan in patients with relapsed small-cell lung cancer. *J Clin Oncol* 2006;24(34):5441–5447.
39. Holmes RA. Radiopharmaceuticals in clinical trials. *Semin Oncol* 1993;20(3 suppl 2):22–26.
40. Manoso MW, Healey JH. Metastatic cancer to the bone. In: DeVita VT, Hellman S, Rosenberg SA, eds. *Cancer: Principles and Practice of Oncology.* Philadelphia: Lippincott Williams & Wilkins; 2005:2373–2374.
41. Porter AT, McEwan AJB, Powe JE, et al. Results of a randomized phase III trial to evaluate the efficacy of strontium 89 adjuvant to local field external beam irradiation in the management of endocrine resistant metastatic prostate cancer. *Int J Radiat Oncol Biol Phys* 1993;25(5):805–813.
42. Porter AT, McEwan AJB. Strontium 89 as an adjuvant to external beam radiation improves pain relief and delays in disease progression in advanced prostate cancer: results of a randomized controlled trial. *Semin Oncol* 1993;20(3 suppl 2):38–43.
43. Robinson RG, Preston DF, Baxter KG, et al. Clinical experience with strontium 89 in prostatic and breast cancer patients. *Semin Oncol* 1993;20(3 suppl 2):44–48.
44. Robinson RG, Preston DF, Schiefelbein M, et al. Strontium 89 therapy for the palliation of pain due to osseous metastases. *JAMA* 1995;274(5):420–424.
45. Krishnamurthy GT, Swailem FM, Srivastava SC, et al. Tin-117m(4+)DTPA: pharmacokinetics and imaging characteristics in patients with metastatic bone pain. *J Nucl Med* 1997;38(2):230–237.
46. Serafini AN, Houston SJ, Resche I, et al. Palliation of pain associated with metastatic bone cancer using samarium-153 lexidronam: a double-blind placebo-controlled clinical trial. *J Clin Oncol* 1998;16(4):1574–1581.
47. Rogers CL, Speiser BL, Ram PC, et al. Efficacy and toxicity of intravenous strontium-89 for symptomatic osseous metastases. *Brachyther Int* 1998;14:133–142.
48. de Klerk JMH, Zonnenberg BA, van het Schip AD, et al. Dose escalation study of rhenium-186 hydroxyethylidene bisphosphonate in patients with metastatic prostate cancer. *Eur J Nucl Med* 1994;21(10):1114–1120.
49. Sciuto R, Maini CL, Tofani A, et al. Radiosensitization with low-dose carboplatin enhances pain palliation in radioisotope therapy with strontium-89. *Nucl Med Commun* 1996;17(9):799–804.
50. Bolger JJ, Dearnaley DP, Kirk D, et al. Strontium-89 (metastron) versus external beam radiotherapy in patient with painful bone metastases secondary to

prostatic cancer: preliminary report of a multicenter trial. *Semin Oncol* 1993; 20(suppl 2):32–33.

51. Eary JF, Collins C, Stabin M, et al. Samarium 153-EDTMP biodistribution and dosimetry estimation. *J Nucl Med* 1993;34(7):1031–1036.

52. Bayouth JE, Macey DJ, Kasi LP, et al. Dosimetry and toxicity of samarium-153-EDTMP administered for bone pain due to skeletal metastases. *J Nucl Med* 1994;35(1):63–69.

53. McEwan AJB, Amyotte GA, McGowan DG, et al. A retrospective analysis of the cost-effectiveness of treatment with metastron in patients with prostate cancer metastatic to bone. *Eur Urol* 1994;26(suppl 1):26–31.

54. Alberts AS, Smit BJ, Louw WKA, et al. Dose response relationship and multiple dose efficacy and toxicity of samarium-153-EDTMP in metastatic cancer to bone. *Radiother Oncol* 1997;43(2):175–179.

55. Bates T, Yarnold JR, Blitzer P, et al. Bone metastasis consensus statement. *Int J Radiat Oncol Biol Phys* 1992;23(1):215–216.

56. Bates T. A review of local radiotherapy in the treatment of bone metastases and cord compression. *Int J Radiat Oncol Biol Phys* 1992;23(1):217–221.

57. Madsen EL. Painful bone metastases: efficacy of radiotherapy assessed by the patients: a randomized trial comparing 4 Gy × 6 versus 10 Gy × 2. *Int J Radiat Oncol Biol Phys* 1983;9(12):1775–1779.

58. Niewald M, Tkocz HJ, Abel U, et al. Rapid course radiation therapy vs. more standard treatment: a randomized trial for bone metastases. *Int J Radiat Oncol Biol Phys* 1996;36(5):1085–1089.

59. Gaze MN, Kelly CG, Kerr GR, et al. Pain relief and quality of life following radiotherapy for bone metastases: a randomised trial of two fractionation schedules. *Radiother Oncol* 1997;45(2):109–116.

60. Ben-Josef E, Shamsa F, Williams AO, et al. Radiotherapeutic management of osseous metastases: a survey of current patterns of care. *Int J Radiat Oncol Biol Phys* 1998;40(4):915–921.

61. Kagan AR. Palliation of visceral recurrences and metastases. In: Perez CA, Brady LW, eds. *Principles and Practice of Radiation Oncology*. 3rd ed. Philadelphia: Lippincott–Raven; 2004:2405–2411.

62. Kagan AR. Palliation of brain and spinal cord metastases. In: Perez CA, Brady LW, eds. *Principles and Practice of Radiation Oncology*. 4th ed. Philadelphia: Lippincott–Raven; 2004,2373–2384.

63. Tong D, Gillick L, Hendrickson FR. The palliation of symptomatic osseous metastases: final results of the study by the Radiation Therapy Oncology Group. *Cancer* 1982;50(5):893–899.

64. Blitzer PH. Reanalysis of the RTOG study of the palliation of symptomatic osseous metastasis. *Cancer* 1985;55(7):1468–1472.

65. Arcangeli G, Giovinazzo G, Saracino B, et al. Radiation therapy in the management of symptomatic bone metastases: the effect of total dose and histology on pain relief and response duration. *Int J Radiat Oncol Biol Phys* 1998; 42(5):1119–1126.

66. Ford HT, Yarnold JR. Radiation therapy: pain relief and recalcification. In: Stoll BA, Parbhoo S, eds. *Bone Metastases: Monitoring and Treatment*. New York: Raven; 1983:343–354.

67. Koswig S, Budach V. Remineralization and pain relief in bone metastases after different radiotherapy fractions (10 times 3 Gy vs. 1 time 8 Gy): a prospective study. *Strahlenther Onkol* 1999;175(10):500–508.

68. Koswig S, Buchali A, Böhmer D, et al. Palliative radiotherapy of bone metastases: a retrospective analysis of 176 patients. *Strahlenther Onkol* 1999; 175(10):509–514.

69. Barton M. Tables of equivalent dose in 2 Gy fractions: a simple application of the linear quadratic formula. *Int J Radiat Oncol Biol Phys* 1995;31(2): 371–378.

70. Barak F, Werner A, Walach N, et al. The palliative efficacy of a single high dose of radiation in treatment of symptomatic osseous metastases. *Int J Radiat Oncol Biol Phys* 1987;13(8):1233–1235.

71. Cole DJ. A randomized trial of a single treatment versus conventional fractionation in the palliative radiotherapy of painful bone metastases. *Clin Oncol* 1989;1(2):59–62.

72. Hoskin PJ, Price P, Easton D, et al. A prospective randomised trial of 4 Gy or 8 Gy single doses in the treatment of metastatic bone pain. *Radiother Oncol* 1992;23(2):74–78.

73. Price P, Hoskin PJ, Easton D, et al. Prospective randomised trial of single and multifraction radiotherapy schedules in the treatment of painful bone metastases. *Radiother Oncol* 1986;6(4):247–255.

74. Amichetti M, Orru P, Madeddu A, et al. Comparative evaluation of two hypofractionated radiotherapy regimens for painful bone metastases. *Tumori* 2004;90(1):91–95.

75. Wu JS, Wong R, Johnston M, et al. Cancer Care Ontario Practice Guidelines Initiative Supportive Care Group: meta-analysis of dose-fractionation radiotherapy trials for the palliation of painful bone metastases. *Int J Radiat Oncol Biol Phys* 2003;55(3):594–605.

76. Steenland E, Leer JW, van Houwelingen H, et al. The effect of a single fraction compared to multiple fractions on painful bone metastases: a global analysis of the Dutch Bone Metastasis Study. *Radiother Oncol* 1999;52(2):101–109.

77. Nielsen OS, Bentzen SM, Sandberg E, et al. Randomized trial of single dose versus fractionated palliative radiotherapy of bone metastases. *Radiother Oncol* 1998;47(3):233–240.

78. Hartsell WF, Scott CB, Bruner DW, et al. Randomized trial of short- versus long-course radiotherapy for palliation of painful bone metastases. *J Natl Cancer Inst* 2005;97(11):798–804.

79. Falkmer U, Jarhult J, Wersall P, et al. A systematic overview of radiation therapy effects in skeletal metastases. *Acta Oncol* 2003;42(5–6):620–633.

80. Chow E, Harris K, Fan G. Palliative radiotherapy trials for bone metastases: a systematic review. *J Clin Oncol* 2007;25(11):1423–1436.

81. Sze WM, Shelley M, Held I, et al. Palliation of metastatic bone pain: single fraction versus multifraction radiotherapy—a systematic review of the randomised trials. *Cochrane Database Syst Rev* 2004;(2):CD004721.

82. Sze WM, Shelley MD, Held I, et al. Palliation of metastatic bone pain: single fraction versus multifraction radiotherapy—a systematic review of randomised trials. *Clin Oncol (R Coll Radiol)* 2003;15(6):345–352.

83. Mithal NP, Needham PR, Hoskin PJ. Retreatment with radiotherapy for painful bone metastases. *Int J Radiat Oncol Biol Phys* 1994;29(5):1011–1014.

84. Boogerd W, van der Sande JJ. Diagnosis and treatment of spinal cord compression in malignant disease. *Cancer Treat Rev* 1993;19(2):129–150.

85. Byrne TN. Spinal cord compression from epidural metastases. *N Engl J Med* 1992;327(9):614–619.

86. Grant R, Papadopoulos SM, Greenberg HS. Metastatic epidural spinal cord compression. *Neurol Clin* 1991;9(4):825–841.

87. Maranzano E, Latini P, Checcaglini F, et al. Radiation therapy in metastatic spinal cord compression. A prospective analysis of 105 consecutive patients. *Cancer* 1991;67(5):1311–1317.

88. Janjan NA. Radiotherapeutic management of spinal metastases. *J Pain Symptom Manage* 1996;11(1):47–56.

89. Loblaw DA, Laperriere NJ. Emergency treatment of malignant extradural spinal cord compression: an evidence-based guideline. *J Clin Oncol* 1998; 16(4):1613–1624.

90. Boogerd W. Central nervous system metastasis in breast cancer. *Radiother Oncol* 1996;40(1):5–22.

91. Stafford RS, Cyr PL. The impact of cancer on the physical function of the elderly and their utilization of health care. *Cancer* 1997;80(10):1973–1980.

92. Reuben DB, Mor V, Hiris J. Clinical symptoms and length of survival in patients with terminal cancer. *Arch Intern Med* 1988;148(7):1586–1591.

93. Rutten EH, Crul BJ, van der Toorn PP, et al. Pain characteristics help to predict the analgesic efficacy of radiotherapy for the treatment of cancer pain. *Pain* 1997;69(1–2):131–135.

94. Hayashi S, Hoshi H, Iida T. Reirradiation with local-field radiotherapy for painful bone metastases. *Radiat Med* 2002;20(5):231–236.

95. Huber S, Ulsperger E, Gomar C, et al. Osseous metastases in breast cancer: radiographic monitoring of therapeutic response. *Anticancer Res* 2002; 22(2B):1279–1288.

96. Paterson AHG. Bone metastasis in breast cancer, prostate cancer, and myeloma. *Bone* 1987;8(suppl 1):17–22.

97. Bunting RW, Boublik M, Blevins FT, et al. Functional outcome of pathologic fracture secondary to malignant disease in a rehabilitation hospital. *Cancer* 1992;69(1):98–102.

98. Townsend PW, Smalley SR, Cozad SC, et al. Role of postoperative radiation therapy after stabilization of fractures caused by metastatic disease. *Int J Radiat Oncol Biol Phys* 1995;31(1):43–49.

99. Heisterberg L, Johansen TS. Treatment of pathologic fractures. *Acta Orthop Scand* 1979;50(6 Pt 2):787–790.

100. Fidler M. Incidence of fracture through metastases in long bones. *Acta Orthop Scand* 1981;52(6):623–627.

101. Oda MAS, Schurman DJ. Monitoring of pathological fracture. In: Stoll BA, Parbhoo S, eds. *Bone Metastases: Monitoring and Treatment*. New York: Raven; 1983:271–288.

102. Piatek S, Westphal T, Bischoff J, et al. Intramedullary stabilisation of metastatic fractures of long bones. *Zentralbl Chir* 2003;128(2):131–138.

103. Helweg-Larsen S, Sorensen PS. Symptoms and signs in metastatic spinal cord compression: a study of progression from first symptom until diagnosis in 153 patients. *Eur J Cancer* 1994;30A(3):396–398.

104. Loblaw DA, Perry J, Chambers A, et al. Systematic review of the diagnosis and management of malignant extradural spinal cord compression: the Cancer Care Ontario Practice Guidelines Initiative's Neuro-Oncology Disease Site Group. *J Clin Oncol* 2005;23(9):2028–2037.

105. Talcott JA, Stomper PC, Drislane FW, et al. Assessing suspected spinal cord compression: a multidisciplinary outcomes analysis of 342 episodes. *Support Care Cancer* 1999;7(1):31–38.

106. Loblaw DA, Smith K, Lockwood G, et al. The Princess Margaret Hospital experience of malignant spinal cord compression. *Proc Am Soc Clin Oncol* 2003;22:119.

107. Loblaw DA, Laperriere NJ, Mackillop WJ. A population-based study of malignant spinal cord compression in Ontario cancer patients. *Clin Oncol (R Coll Radiol)* 2003;15(4):211–217.

108. Boogerd W, van der Sande JJ, Kröger R. Early diagnosis and treatment of spinal metastases in breast cancer: a prospective study. *J Neurol Neurosurg Psychiatry* 1992;55(12):1188–1193.

109. Rades D, Stalpers LJ, Veninga T, et al. Evaluation of functional outcome and local control after radiotherapy for metastatic spinal cord compression in patients with prostate cancer. *J Urol* 2006;175(2):552–556.

110. Rades D, Heidenreich F, Karstens JH. Final results of a prospective study of the prognostic value of the time to develop motor deficits before irradiation in metastatic spinal cord compression. *Int J Radiat Oncol Biol Phys* 2002; 53(4):975–979.

111. Lövey G, Koch K, Gademann G. Metastatic epidural spinal compression: prognostic factors and results of radiotherapy. *Strahlenther Onkol* 2001; 177(12):676–679.

112. Nagata M, Ueda T, Komiya A, et al. Treatment and prognosis of patients

with paraplegia or quadriplegia because of metastatic spinal cord compression in prostate cancer. *Prostate Cancer Prostatic Dis* 2003;6(2):169–173.

113. Turner S, Marosszeky B, Timms I, et al. Malignant spinal cord compression: a prospective evaluation. *Int J Radiat Oncol Biol Phys* 1993;26(1):141–146.

114. Peteet J, Tay V, Cohen G, et al. Pain characteristics and treatment in an outpatient cancer population. *Cancer* 1985;57(6):1259–1265.

115. Wada E, Yamamoto T, Furuno M, et al. Spinal cord compression secondary to osteoblastic metastasis. *Spine* 1993;18(10):1380–1381.

116. Algra PR, Heimans JJ, Valk J, et al. Do metastases in vertebrae begin in the body or the pedicles? Imaging study in 45 patients. *AJR Am J Roentgenol* 1992;158(6):1275–1279.

117. Landmann C, Hünig R, Gratzi O. The role of laminectomy in the combined treatment of metastatic spinal cord compression. *Int J Radiat Oncol Biol Phys* 1992;24(4):627–631.

118. Husband DJ, Grant KA, Romaniuk CS. MRI in the diagnosis and treatment of suspected malignant spinal cord compression. *Br J Radiol* 2001;74(877):15–23.

119. Loughrey GJ, Collins CD, Todd SM, et al. Magnetic resonance imaging in the management of suspected spinal canal disease in patients with known malignancy. *Clin Radiol* 2000;55(11):849–855.

120. Rades D, Dunst J, Schild SE. The first score predicting overall survival in patients with metastatic spinal cord compression. *Cancer* 2008;112(1):157–161.

121. Patchell R, Tibbs PA, Regine F, et al. A randomized trial of direct decompressive surgical resection in the treatment of spinal cord compression caused by metastasis. *Proc Am Soc Clin Oncol* 2003;21(23 suppl):237s.

122. Patchell RA, Tibbs PA, Regine WF, et al. Direct decompressive surgical resection in the treatment of spinal cord compression caused by metastatic cancer: a randomised trial. *Lancet* 2005;366(9486):643–648.

123. Klimo P Jr, Thompson CJ, Kestle JR, et al. A meta-analysis of surgery versus conventional radiotherapy for the treatment of metastatic spinal epidural disease. *Neuro Oncol* 2005;7(1):64–76.

124. Kim RY, Smith JW, Spencer SA, et al. Malignant epidural spinal cord compression associated with a paravertebral mass: its radiotherapeutic outcome on radiosensitivity. *Int J Radiat Oncol Biol Phys* 1993;27(5):1079–1083.

125. Bach F, Agerlin N, Sorensen JB, et al. Metastatic spinal cord compression secondary to lung cancer. *J Clin Oncol* 1992;10(11):1781–1787.

126. Jeremic B, Djuric L, Mijatovic L. Incidence of radiation myelitis of the cervical spinal cord at doses of 5500 cGy or greater. *Cancer* 1991;68(10):2138–2141.

127. Powers BE, Thames HD, Gillette SM, et al. Volume effects in the irradiated canine spinal cord: do they exist when the probability of injury is low? *Radiother Oncol* 1998;46(3):297–306.

128. Tong XQ, Sugimura H, Kisanuki A, et al. Multiple fractionated and single-dose irradiation of bone marrow: evaluation by MR and correlation with histopathological findings. *Acta Radiol* 1998;39(6):620–624.

129. Wen PY, Blanchard KL, Block CC, et al. Development of Lhermitte's sign after bone marrow transplantation. *Cancer* 1992;69(9):2262–2266.

130. Steiner RM, Mitchell DG, Rao VM, et al. Magnetic resonance imaging of diffuse bone marrow disease. *Radiol Clin North Am* 1993;31(2):383–409.

131. Algra PR, Bloem JL, Tissing H, et al. Detection of vertebral metastases: comparison between MR imaging and bone scintigraphy. *Radiographics* 1991;11(2):219–232.

132. Le Bihan DJ. Differentiation of benign versus pathologic compression fractures with diffusion-weighted MR imaging: a closer step toward the "holy grail" of tissue characterization? *Radiology* 1998;207(2):305–307.

133. Sugimura H, Kisanuki A, Tamura S, et al. Magnetic resonance imaging of bone marrow changes after irradiation. *Invest Radiol* 1994;29(1):35–41.

134. Yankelevitz DF, Henschke C, Knapp PH, et al. Effect of radiation therapy on thoracic and lumbar bone marrow: evaluation with MR imaging. *AJR Am J Roentgenol* 1991;157(1):87–92.

135. Bach F, Bjerregaard B, Soletormos G, et al. Diagnostic value of cerebrospinal fluid cytology in comparison with tumor marker activity in central nervous system metastases secondary to breast cancer. *Cancer* 1993;72(8):2376–2382.

136. Russi EG, Pergolizzi S, Gaeta M, et al. Palliative radiotherapy in lumbosacral carcinomatous neuropathy. *Radiother Oncol* 1993;26(2):172–173.

137. Salazar OM, DaMotta NW, Bridgman SM, et al. Fractionated half-body irradiation for pain palliation in widely metastatic cancers: comparison with single dose. *Int J Radiat Oncol Biol Phys* 1996;36(1):49–60.

138. Salazar OM, Sandhu T, da Motta NW, et al. Fractionated half-body irradiation (HBI) for the rapid palliation of widespread, symptomatic, metastatic bone disease: a randomized phase III trial of the International Atomic Energy Agency (IAEA). *Int J Radiat Oncol Biol Phys* 2001;50(3):765–775.

139. Scarantino CW, Caplan R, Rotman M, et al. A phase I/II study to evaluate the effect of fractionated hemibody irradiation in the treatment of osseous metastases—RTOG 88-22. *Int J Radiat Oncol Biol Phys* 1996;36(1):37–48.

140. Salazar OM, Rubin P, Hendrickson FR, et al. Single dose half-body irradiation for palliation of multiple bone metastases from solid tumors. Final Radiation Therapy Oncology Group Report. *Cancer* 1986;58(1):29–36.

141. Poulter CA, Cosmatos D, Rubin P, et al. A report of RTOG 8206: a phase III study of whether the addition of single dose hemibody irradiation to standard fractionated local field irradiation is more effective than local field irradiation alone in the treatment of symptomatic osseous metastases. *Int J Radiat Oncol Biol Phys* 1992;23(1):207–214.

142. Skolyszewski J, Sas-Korczynska B, Korzeniowski S, et al. The efficiency and

143. Liepe K, Runge R, Kotzerke J. Systemic radionuclide therapy in pain palliation. *Am J Hosp Palliat Care* 2005;22(6):457–464.

144. Liepe K, Kotzerke J. A comparative study of 188Re-HEDP, 186Re-HEDP, 153Sm-EDTMP, and 89Sr in the treatment of painful skeletal metastases. *Nucl Med Commun* 2007;28(8):623–630.

145. Bauman G, Charette M, Reid R, et al. Radiopharmaceuticals for the palliation of painful bone metastasis: a systemic review. *Radiother Oncol* 2005;75(3):258–270.

146. Baczyk M, Milecki P, Baczyk E, et al. The effectiveness of strontium 89 in palliative therapy of painful prostate cancer bone metastases. *Ortop Traumatol Rehabil* 2003;5(3):364–368.

147. Lam MG, de Klerk JM, van Rijk PP, et al. Bone seeking radiopharmaceuticals for palliation of pain in cancer patients with osseous metastases. *Anticancer Agents Med Chem* 2007;7(4):381–397.

148. Bauman G, Charette M, Reid R, et al. Radiopharmaceuticals for the palliation of painful bone metastasis—a systemic review. *Radiother Oncol* 2005;75(3):258–270.

149. Sartor O, Reid RH, Hoskin PJ, et al. Samarium-153-Lexidronam complex for treatment of painful bone metastases in hormone-refractory prostate cancer. *Urology* 2004;63(5):940–945.

150. Dolezal J, Vizda J, Odrazka K. Prospective evaluation of samarium-153-EDTMP radionuclide treatment for bone metastases in patients with hormone-refractory prostate cancer. *Urol Int* 2007;78(1):50–57.

151. Sartor O, Reid RH, Bushnell DL, et al. Safety and efficacy of repeat administration of samarium Sm-153 lexidronam to patients with metastatic bone pain. *Cancer* 2007;109(3):637–643.

152. Lam MG, de Klerk JM, van Rijk PP, et al. Bone seeking radiopharmaceuticals for palliation of pain in cancer patients with osseous metastases. *Anticancer Agents Med Chem* 2007;7(4):381–397.

153. Ricci S, Boni G, Pastina I, et al. Clinical benefit of bone-targeted radiometabolic therapy with 153Sm-EDTMP combined with chemotherapy in patients with metastatic hormone-refractory prostate cancer. *Eur J Nucl Med Mol Imaging* 2007;34(7):1023–1030.

154. Edward Chu, DeVita VT. Principles of medical oncology. In: DeVita VT, Rosenberg SA, eds. *Cancer: Principles and Practice of Oncology.* 7th ed. Philedelphia: Lippincott; 2006:296–306.

155. DeVita VT, Schein PS. The use of drugs in combination for the treatment of cancer: rationale and results. *N Engl J Med* 1973;288(19):998–1006.

156. Papageorgio C, McLeod H. Chemotherapy: principles and pharmacology. In: Govindan R. *Washington Manual of Oncology.* Philadelphia: Lippincott Williams & Wilkins; 2002,11–47.

157. Perry MC. Chemotherapy, toxicity, and the clinician. *Semin Oncol* 1982;9(1):1–4.

158. Bonadonna G, Molinari R. Role and limits of anticancer drugs in the treatment of advanced cancer pain. In: Bonica JJ, Ventafridda V, eds. *Advances in Pain Research and Therapy.* Vol 2. New York: Raven Press; 1979:131–138.

159. MacDonald N. The role of medical and surgical oncology in the management of cancer pain. In: Foley KM, Bonica JJ, Ventafridda V, eds. *Advances in Pain Research and Therapy.* Vol 16. New York: Raven Press; 1990:27–39.

160. Ellis PA, Smith IE, Hardy JR, et al. Symptom relief with MVP (mitomycin C, vinblastine, and cisplatin) chemotherapy in advanced non-small-cell lung cancer. *Br J Cancer* 1995;71(2):366–370.

161. Hardy JR, Noble T, Smith IE. Symptom relief with moderate dose chemotherapy (mitomycin-C, vinblastine, and cisplatin) in advanced non-small cell lung cancer. *Br J Cancer* 1989;60(5):764–766.

162. Tummarello D, Graziano F, Isidori P, et al. Symptomatic, stage IV, non-small-cell lung cancer (NSCLC): response, toxicity, performance status change, and symptom relief in patients treated with cisplatin, vinblastine, and mitomycin-C. *Cancer Chemother Pharmacol* 1995;35(3):249–253.

163. Middleton GW, Smith IE, O'Brien ME, et al. Good symptom relief with palliative MVP (mitomycin-C, vinblastine, and cisplatin) chemotherapy in malignant mesothelioma. *Ann Oncol* 1998;9(3):269–273.

164. Andreopoulou E, Ross PJ, O'Brien ME, et al. The palliative benefits of MVP (mitomycin C, vinblastine, and cisplatin) chemotherapy in patients with malignant mesothelioma. *Ann Oncol* 2004;15(9):1406–1412.

165. Socinski MA, Morris DE, Masters GA, et al. Chemotherapeutic management of stage IV non-small cell lung cancer. *Chest* 2003;123(suppl 1):226S–243S.

166. Saxena AK, Kumar S. Management strategies for pain in breast carcinoma patients: current opinions and future perspectives. *Pain Pract* 2007;7(2):163–177.

167. von Plessen C, Bergman B, Andresen O, et al. Palliative chemotherapy beyond three courses conveys no survival or consistent quality-of-life benefits in advanced non-small-cell lung cancer. *Br J Cancer* 2006;95(8):966–973.

168. Bruera E, MacMillan K, Hanson J, et al. The Edmonton staging system for cancer pain. *Pain* 1989;37(2):203–209.

169. Anderson KO. Assessment tools for the evaluation of pain in the oncology patient. *Curr Pain Headache Rep* 2007;11(4):259–264.

170. Caraceni A. Evaluation and assessment of cancer pain and cancer pain treatment. *Acta Anaesthesiol Scand* 2001;45(9):1067–1075.

171. Cleeland CS, Ryan KM. Pain assessment: global use of the Brief Pain Inventory. *Ann Acad Med Singapore* 1994;23(2):129–138.

172. Canellos GP, Anderson JR, Propert KJ, et al. Chemotherapy of advanced Hodgkin's disease with MOPP, ABVD, or MOPP alternating with ABVD. *N Engl J Med* 1992;327(21):1478–1484.

173. DeVita VT Jr, Hubbard SM. Hodgkin's disease. *N Engl J Med* 1993;328(8): 560–565.
174. Hoppe RT, Advani RH, Bierman PJ, et al. Hodgkin disease/lymphoma: clinical practice guidelines in oncology. *J Natl Compr Canc Netw* 2006;4(3): 210–230.
175. Hennessy BT, Hanrahan EO, Daly PA. Non-Hodgkin lymphoma: an update. *Lancet Oncol* 2004;5(6):341–353.
176. Maloney DG. Immunotherapy for non-Hodgkin's lymphoma: monoclonal antibodies and vaccines. *J Clin Oncol* 2005;23(26):6421–6428.
177. Weingart O, Rehan FA, Schulz H, et al. Sixth biannual report of the Cochrane Haematological Malignancies Group—focus on non-Hodgkin lymphoma. *J Natl Cancer Inst* 2007;99(17):E1.
178. Djulbegovic B, Sullivan DM. *Decision Making in Oncology: Evidence-Based Management.* New York: Churchill Livingstone; 1997,21–72, 343–350.
179. Overmoyer BA. Chemotherapeutic palliative approaches in the treatment of breast cancer. *Semin Oncol* 1995;22(suppl 3):2–9.
180. Tannock IF, Boyd NF, DeBoer G, et al. A randomized trial of two-dose levels of cyclophosphamide, methotrexate, and fluorouracil chemotherapy for patients with metastatic breast cancer. *J Clin Oncol* 1988;6(9):1377–1387.
181. Muss HB. Breast cancer and differential diagnosis of benign lesions. In: Golgman L, Ausiello D, eds. *Cecil Textbook of Medicine.* 23rd ed. Philadelphia: WB Saunders; 2008,1501–1510.
182. Guarneri V, Conte PF. The curability of breast cancer and the treatment of advanced disease. *Eur J Nucl Med Mol Imaging* 2004;31(suppl 1):S149–S161.
183. Ramirez AJ, Towlson KE, Leaning MS, et al. Do patients with advanced breast cancer benefit from chemotherapy? *Br J Cancer* 1998;78(11):1488–1494.
184. Garden AS, Harris J, Vokes EE, et al. Preliminary results of Radiation Therapy Oncology Group 97-03: a randomized phase ii trial of concurrent radiation and chemotherapy for advanced squamous cell carcinomas of the head and neck. *J Clin Oncol* 2004;22(14):2856–2864.
185. Robbins KT, Kumar P, Harris J, et al. Supradose intra-arterial cisplatin and concurrent radiation therapy for the treatment of stage IV head and neck squamous cell carcinoma is feasible and efficacious in a multi-institutional setting: results of Radiation Therapy Oncology Group Trial 9615. *J Clin Oncol* 2005;23(7):1447–1454.
186. Magné N, Marcy PY, Chamorey E, et al. Concomitant twice-a-day radiotherapy and chemotherapy in unresectable head and neck cancer patients: a long-term quality of life analysis. *Head Neck* 2001;23(8):678–682.
187. Markman M. The use of chemotherapy as palliative treatment for patients with advanced ovarian cancer. *Semin Oncol* 1995;22(suppl 3):25–29.
188. Fung-Kee-Fung M, Oliver T, Elit L, et al. Optimal chemotherapy treatment for women with recurrent ovarian cancer. *Curr Oncol* 2007;14(5):195–208.
189. Doyle C, Crump M, Pintilie M, et al. Does palliative chemotherapy palliate? Evaluation of expectations, outcomes, and costs in women receiving chemotherapy for advanced ovarian cancer. *J Clin Oncol* 2001;19(5):1266–1274.
190. Burris HA, Moore MJ, Andersen J, et al. Improvements in survival and clinical benefit with gemcitabine as first-line therapy for patients with advanced pancreatic cancer: a randomized trial. *J Clin Oncol* 1997;15:2403–2413.
191. Bunn PA, Kelly K. New chemotherapeutic agents prolong survival and improve quality of life in non-small cell lung cancer: a review of the literature and future directions. *Clin Cancer Res* 1998;5:1087–1100.
192. Clegg A, Scott DA, Sidhu M, et al. A rapid and systematic review of the clinical effectiveness and cost-effectiveness of paclitaxel, docetaxel, gemcitabine, and vinorelbine in non-small-cell lung cancer. *Health Technol Assess* 2001;5(32): 1–195.
193. Khuri FR. Docetaxel for locally advanced or metastatic non-small-cell lung cancer: current data and future directions as front-line therapy. *Oncology (Williston Park)* 2002;16(suppl 6):53–62.
194. Adelstein DJ. Palliative chemotherapy for non-small cell lung cancer. *Semin Oncol* 1995;22(suppl 3):35–39.
195. Pelley RJ. Role of chemotherapy in the palliation of gastrointestinal malignancies. *Semin Oncol* 1995;22(suppl 3):45–52.
196. Poon MA, O'Connell MJ, Moertel CG, et al. Biochemical modulation of fluorouracil: evidence of significant improvement of survival and quality of life in patients with advanced colorectal carcinoma. *J Clin Oncol* 1989;7(10): 1407–1417.
197. Ajani JA, Moiseyenko VM, Tjulandin S, et al. Quality of life with docetaxel plus cisplatin and fluorouracil compared with cisplatin and fluorouracil from a phase III trial for advanced gastric or gastroesophageal adenocarcinoma: the V-325 Study Group. *J Clin Oncol* 2007;25(22):3210–3216.
198. Michael M, Hedley D, Oza A, et al. The palliative benefit of irinotecan in 5-fluorouracil-refractory colorectal cancer: its prospective evaluation by a Multicenter Canadian Trial. *Clin Colorectal Cancer* 2002;2(2):93–101.
199. Yip D, Karapetis C, Strickland A, et al. Chemotherapy and radiotherapy for inoperable advanced pancreatic cancer. *Cochrane Database Syst Rev* 2006; (3):CD002093.
200. Sultana A, Smith CT, Cunningham D, et al. Meta-analyses of chemotherapy for locally advanced and metastatic pancreatic cancer. *J Clin Oncol* 2007; 25(18):2607–2615.
201. Tannock IF, Osoba D, Stockler MR, et al. Chemotherapy with mitoxantrone plus prednisone or prednisone alone for symptomatic hormone-resistant prostate cancer: a Canadian randomized trial with palliative endpoints. *J Clin Oncol* 1996;14(6):1756–1764.
202. Tannock IF, de Wit R, Berry WR, et al. Docetaxel plus prednisone or mitoxantrone plus prednisone for advanced prostate cancer. *N Engl J Med* 2004; 351(15):1502–1512.
203. Mike S, Harrison C, Coles B, et al. Chemotherapy for hormone-refractory prostate cancer. *Cochrane Database Syst Rev* 2006;(4):CD005247.
204. Overmoyer BA. Chemotherapeutic palliative approaches in the treatment of breast cancer. *Semin Oncol* 1995;22(suppl 3):2–9.
205. Young DF, Posner JD. Nervous system toxicity of chemotherapeutic agents. In: Vinken TJ, Bruyn GW, eds. *Handbook of Clinical Neurology.* Amsterdam: North Holland; 1980:91–129.
206. Verstappen CC, Heimans JJ, Hoekman K, et al. Neurotoxic complications of chemotherapy in patients with cancer: clinical signs and optimal management. *Drugs* 2003;63(15):1549–1563.
207. Nakane M. Neurotoxicity and dermatologic toxicity of cancer chemotherapy. *Gan To Kagaku Ryoho* 2006;33(1):29–33.
208. Visovsky C. Chemotherapy-induced peripheral neuropathy. *Cancer Invest* 2003;21(3):439–451.
209. Solomon L. Drug-induced arthropathy and necrosis of the femoral head. *J Bone Joint Surg Br* 1973;55(2):246–261.
210. Rotstein J, Good RA. Steroid pseudorheumatism. *Arch Intern Med* 1957; 99(4):545–555.
211. Beatson GT. On the treatment of inoperable cases of carcinoma of the mammae: suggestions for a new method of treatment with illustrative cases. *Lancet* 1896;2:104–107.
212. Huggins C, Hodges VC. Studies on prostatic cancer. *Cancer Res* 1941;1: 293–297.
213. Goetz MP, Erlichman C, Loprinzi CL. Pharmacology of endocrine manipulation. In: DeVita VT, Rosenberg SA, eds. *Cancer: Principles and Practice of Oncology.* 7th ed. Philadelphia: Lippincott Williams & Wilkins; 2006, 457–466.
214. Pannuti F, Martoni A, Rossi AP, et al. The role of endocrine therapy for relief of pain due to advanced cancer. In: Bonica JJ, Ventafridda V, eds. *Advances in Pain Research and Therapy.* Vol 2. New York: Raven Press; 1979,145–166.
215. Pannuti F. Hormonal treatment. In: Twycross RF, Ventafridda V, eds. *The Continuing Care of Terminal Cancer Patients.* New York: Pergamon Press; 1980,79–89.
216. Sonoo H, Shimozuma K, Kurebayashi J, et al. Systemic therapy, pain relief, and quality of life of breast cancer patients with bone metastasis. *Gan To Kagaku Ryoho* 1995;22(suppl 1):10–15.
217. Romanelli P, Esposito V, Adler J. Ablative procedures for chronic pain. *Neurosurg Clin N Am* 2004;15(3):335–342.
218. Liscák R, Vladyka V. Radiosurgical hypophysectomy in painful bone metastases of breast carcinoma [Article in Czech]. *Casopis Lekaru Ceskych* 1998; 137(5):154–157.

CHAPTER 49 ■ CANCER PAIN IN CHILDREN

JACQUELINE CASILLAS AND LONNIE K. ZELTZER

OVERVIEW OF CHILDHOOD CANCER

Epidemiology

There are approximately 12,400 children diagnosed with cancer each year in the United States.[1] As recently as the 1970s, a diagnosis of cancer during childhood was considered a uniformly fatal disease. However, through enrollment in clinical trials available through the cooperative pediatric oncology group(s), there is now an overall 80% survival rate across the major 12 diagnostic categories of childhood cancer. *The International Classification of Childhood Cancers*, Third Edition (ICCC-3) include: (1) leukemias, myeloproliferative and myelodysplastic diseases, (2) lymphomas, (3) central nervous system neoplasms, (4) neuroblastoma and other peripheral nervous cell tumors, (5) retinoblastoma, (6) renal tumors, (7) hepatic tumors, (8) malignant bone tumors, (9) soft tissue and other extraosseous sarcomas (e.g., rhabdomyosarcoma), (10) germ cell tumors, (11) other malignant epithelial neoplasms and malignant melanomas (e.g., thyroid and nasopharyngeal carcinomas), and (12) other, unspecified malignant neoplasms.[2] Certain types of cancer are more common in specific age groups of children. For example, acute leukemias, neuroblastoma, and renal tumors are more common in the younger age groups (ages 2–6 years), whereas the malignant bone tumors and lymphomas are more common during the adolescent years.

Treatment

Despite the low incidence rates of pediatric malignancies, there is a rapidly growing population of childhood cancer survivors reaching public health epidemic rates. This is due to better supportive care and use of aggressive, multimodal treatment strategies of chemotherapy, radiation, and surgery. Because the majority of pediatric cancer patients are enrolled in cooperative group clinical trials, there is a very uniform approach to treatment through the use of nationally available standardized treatment protocols.[3] There are "roadmaps" that are followed by the treating pediatric oncologists and communicated to the family and patient so that they know when to expect the next cycle of chemotherapy, including when the next invasive procedure can be anticipated to occur. As a result, there may be certain periods of higher anxiety, resulting in greater pain for pediatric cancer patients during the cancer treatment continuum as they anticipate the upcoming procedures. However, with careful planning, an effective pain management regimen can be developed and implemented.

Survivorship

The end result of the aggressive treatment regimens for pediatric cancer patients is a success story for the 21st century. The current estimated survival rate for a pediatric cancer patient is 80%. However, despite these advances for 5-year survival rates, there continues to be a high risk for the development of chronic health conditions (late effects) years after the cancer treatment is completed. Complications of treatment include risk for second malignant neoplasms, cardiac and/or pulmonary dysfunction, skeletal problems, and neurocognitive deficits.[4] There is nearly a 75% risk of childhood cancer patients having a chronic health problem by 30 years postdiagnosis.[5] Another important childhood cancer statistic that impacts the field of pain management is the current estimated prevalence rate of childhood cancer survivors; this number of survivors within the United States is over 300,000.[1] Thus, given this rapidly growing population of childhood cancer survivors, it is important to be familiar with the unique challenges faced both during and after completion of treatment for cancer during childhood because the population of survivors continues to increase in numbers and has unique pain management issues, as this chapter will further elucidate.

PAIN IN CHILDREN: HOW DOES THIS DIFFER FROM THAT IN ADULTS?

The model of pain for the adult population is a comprehensive one consisting not only of a physical domain but also psychological and social domains—the biopsychosocial model. In children, the biopsychosocial model of pain is more complex because the developmental level of the child needs to be considered in this model. Childhood is a period in which there are complex and rapid neurodevelopmental changes occurring from birth to young adulthood. Children grow and develop through five stages of development: (1) infancy, (2) toddlerhood, (3) preschool period, (4) school age period, and (5) adolescence. These levels of development are important because they directly impact the assessment and management of pain in children. For example, it was previously believed that newborns and infants could not experience pain because of immature neurological systems and only as the child developed could pain be experienced. However, ongoing basic research has dispelled this myth and newborns and infants can experience pain and mount a stress response to noxious stimuli. Furthermore, a noxious stimulus transmitted through neural afferent systems to a newborn brain may even be experienced as more painful than for an adult because the pain inhibitory system is not fully developed at birth.

Infants–Preschool

From birth through early childhood, a normal developmental assessment evaluates five main areas: gross motor skills, fine motor skills, language skills, personal/social skills, and cognitive skills. Changes occurring in these areas impact the pain assessment and emotional response of the child to the painful stimuli. For example, the language skills of a 2-year-old include a 50-word vocabulary and two-word sentences. During this period, if the child is not able to effectively communicate the pain sensation and inadequate pain treatment occurs, then there can be more fear and anxiety with each subsequent painful procedure. One year later, at 3 years of age, there is an expected 250-word vocabulary, three-word sentences, and speech is intelligible to strangers 75% of the time. This child may be able to more effectively communicate with their parents and doctors and have a treatment for the pain initiated more promptly, a factor related to these enhanced communication skills that can serve to decrease anxiety for future procedures.

School Age–Adolescence

A school-age child will have a progressive ability to effectively communicate with the health care team. In turn, the providers must clearly communicate with the child about their treatment plan in order to minimize the anxiety children can experience from medical interventions. During adolescence, normal development of increasing desire for autonomy necessitates direct communication by the health care team, not only with parents, but also directly with the adolescent based on the adolescent's desire for independent decision-making (when possible). However, in all levels of normal development, the impact of illness can cause a pediatric patient to regress and become more dependent on their parents to support their physical and emotional needs, with parents often providing the primary input to the health care team about children's pain and effectiveness of pain management. When possible, it is always helpful for the health care team to also attempt to get the child and adolescent's self-report of pain.

PEDIATRIC CANCER PAIN

The vast majority of pediatric cancer patients do not have a chronic medical condition at the time of diagnosis and therefore have not experienced chronic or recurrent episodic pain. Instead, they have mainly interfaced with the health care system for well child checks with the associated immunization schedules and for acute, intermittent self-limiting infections or minor injuries. Thus, it is not surprising that the diagnosis and rapid initiation of treatment of the cancer can overwhelm a child with fear and anxiety because of the number of invasive, painful medical procedures that are required, but for which the child is not psychologically prepared. In addition, acute pain associated with the first medical procedure at the time of diagnosis can set the expectations of pain to be experienced by the child for all future procedures. Studies have demonstrated that even posttraumatic stress symptoms can be experienced by childhood cancer survivors due to memory recall of invasive procedures during treatment, and these painful memories continue beyond the treatment into the survivorship period.[6]

Pain Evaluation and Treatment Plans for Children with Cancer

The importance of eliciting and listening to all details of the pain narrative of the pediatric cancer patient is critical. Again, what is asked of the child and expected of the child is dependent on the developmental level of the child. For the school-aged child or adolescent, the pain assessment should occur early on, where there is the support of family, and in a nonthreatening environment. In tertiary care centers that care for large numbers of pediatric cancer patients, there are child life services available that serve as another resource to help elucidate a clear description of the pain narrative. For the infant or toddler, the health care provider is dependent upon the parents' narratives of the painful experience because they are the source of safety and communica-

tion for the young child. Across the entire developmental continuum of pediatrics, the physical examination is critical to provide additional information about physical factors that contribute to the experience of pain. During the physical examination, it is also critical for the health care provider to recognize and identify psychosocial factors, such as parental fear or anxiety, that can also increase the suffering associated with pain for the pediatric cancer patient. After a careful history and physical examination, a targeted treatment plan can then be developed. Further details of treatment plans for the various etiologies of pain in the pediatric cancer population will be discussed in the sections below.

ETIOLOGIES FOR PAIN IN PEDIATRIC CANCER PATIENTS

There are seven main categories of reasons for pain in children with cancer that include: (1) pain associated with medical procedures used for cancer diagnosis and treatment, (2) pain associated with bone marrow infiltration by malignant disease, (3) neuropathic pain and pain due to central nervous system tumors, (4) bone pain and amputation, (5) visceral pain, (6) pain associated with bone marrow transplantation, and (7) stress and other symptoms.

Pain Related to Medical Procedures

Invasive, painful procedures for the childhood cancer patient include diagnostic tests such as bone marrow biopsies, lumbar punctures (LPs), surgery for tissue biopsy, venipunctures for diagnosis and/or treatment administration, and access to a subcutaneous central venous port-a-catheter. Not only does the pediatric cancer patient face many painful stimuli repeatedly, but these pain-evoking procedures can occur in a relatively short period of time (within a few days, weeks, or months). In addition to the physical pain that invasive procedures cause related to tissue damage by insertion of a needle or device through the skin and/or bone, the procedures themselves produce a great deal of psychological distress, including fear and anxiety.[7] This anxiety can result in a quick recall of the procedure that will impact future pain management for all future painful procedures. Children with acute lymphoblastic leukemia (ALL) on current treatment protocols, for example, receive lumbar punctures on a regular basis ranging from once weekly to once every 3 months (which is considered a less intensive period of treatment). The initial LPs that are done at time of diagnosis and for the initial induction treatment therefore set the stage for the pain anticipated and experienced for children during their 2 to 3 years of ongoing chemotherapy. Studies in ALL cancer patients have clearly demonstrated that children do have accurate memories of their painful procedures. The more negative a memory a child had about a previous LP, the higher the likelihood of increasing distress related to future LPs.[8]

There may also be specific groups of pediatric cancer patients that are at higher risk for distress due to painful, invasive procedures. Early studies have suggested that differences in reactions to painful stimuli can be attributed, at least in part, to a child's temperament, including the dimensions of distractibility and persistence.[9–12] Chen has shown that having a higher level of pain sensitivity (i.e., *pain perception*) is associated with greater anxiety and pain both prior to and during an LP procedure.[13] In addition, the psychological stress and corresponding coping experienced by the parent can affect the child's coping responses to the painful stressor. It has been shown that mothers of childhood cancer survivors do experience posttraumatic stress symptoms well into the survivorship period years after their child was treated for cancer.[14] Thus, given that a child is dependent on their parents for both physical and emotional support throughout the cancer care continuum, a child can be at increased risk for distress due to pain if their caretaker is not able to soothe or provide a safe, consistent environment because of their own maladaptive coping.

Treatment Plans for Painful Invasive Procedures

Pain Assessment

Various methods of identifying and quantifying pain in children have been employed by both researchers and health care providers and fall into three categories: physiologic, behavioral or observation, and self-report. For example, for infants and young children who are not able to verbally express their feelings, pain is often assessed by physiologic parameters that include elevations in heart rate and blood pressure. Similarly, health care providers often use behavioral cues such as facial expressions and/or stiffening of the body to indicate that an infant or preverbal child is experiencing pain. Even with physiologic parameters and behavioral cues to assist a health care provider with identifying pain in a child, it has been found that health care providers may underestimate a child's pain experience. Thus, it has been suggested that screening tools, such as visual analog scale pain scores (when developmentally possible, likely by age 4 because of the sufficient personal and social skills to interact with a health care provider), should be employed to identify at-risk children.[15,16]

Various other pain assessment tools have been evaluated regarding their effectiveness to identify pain and distress in children. One such example is the use of dolls with different facial expressions to identify pain in a culturally diverse group of children with cancer undergoing the invasive medical procedure of subcutaneously accessing a port-a-cath.[17] This tool may be helpful for a young child because a doll is nonthreatening and is a familiar object that can cognitively engage a young child. von Baeyer and Spagrud have completed a systematic review of observational measures of pain used for children between 3 and 18 years and have included the level of scientific evidence to support their use.[18] In this review they have identified two scales for use in assessing pain intensity associated with medical procedures: Face, Legs, Arms, Cry, Consolability (FLACC) and the Children's Hospital of Eastern Ontario Pain Scale (CHEOPS).[19,20] In addition, for the older child, visual analog scales are used most commonly in the clinical setting when the self-report of pain can be provided. Thus, when the child experiences pain from a procedure, the first step is to complete a comprehensive pain assessment that includes the child's and parent's pain narrative, pain measurement scales where developmentally appropriate, and all in combination with the physical changes that can help accurately quantitate the pain experience.

Pharmacologic Treatments

Up-front treatment plans for first-time invasive procedures for a pediatric cancer patient include the use of pharmacologic treatment of the pain. A child's first LP, for example, should include the integration of pediatric pain service and/or pediatric anesthesia team so that effective systemic anesthesia (in addition to local) can be administered; appropriate physiologic monitoring can also be done to minimize risk from the pharmacologic intervention. Propofol can be considered if a patient has a central line because induction occurs rapidly with this anesthetic and can be easily titrated to produce a deep sedation to eliminate painful stimulation the child experiences during the procedure.[9] Local anesthetic, such as lidocaine, should be administered even when the patient is receiving conscious sedation so that the total dose of propofol to be administered can be minimized and pain control can be maximized. When deciding upon the use of bolus versus a continuous infusion of propofol, there is data to suggest that bolus dosing can result in a more rapid recovery after completion of the invasive procedure because it results in a cumulative lower dose of the anesthetic.[21]

Nonpharmacologic Treatments

Importantly, there are also several cognitive–behavioral interventions that can be employed to minimize the anxiety associated with painful procedures. These can include an emphasis on the family-centered care model, which includes the parent being present with the patient while undergoing induction anesthesia and at the time the pediatric cancer patient regains consciousness. Child life services can assist with preparing the patient to understand the various mechanical procedures that will occur, betadine/alcohol prepping, palpation of landmarks, application of the local anesthetic agent, etc. Relaxation therapies that can be used for painful procedures include focused attention, such as mindfulness meditation, and hypnosis/guided imagery.[22,23] For example, guided imagery has been shown to lower postoperative pain ratings, decrease hospitalization stays, and decrease anxiety in pediatric patient populations. [24]

Distraction methods are also another category of cognitive-behavioral therapies employed to decrease the pain experience during invasive medical therapies. They include use of bubbles, music therapy, mutual storytelling, pop-up books, videos, and simple conversation so that the attention is taken away from the procedure and focused onto another target. For example, by offering music therapy to the adolescent who may feel a lack of control due to the required invasive procedure, the opportunity to exert some autonomy over the painful experience (such as through singing) can occur through the freedom of expression of his/her feelings about the procedure as well as the change in focus of attention.[25,26]

Pain Due to Bone Marrow Infiltration

The acute leukemias, ALL and acute myelogenous leukemia (AML), are the most common diagnostic category of pediatric cancer.[28] The rapid growth of the leukemic blasts within the bone marrow commonly results in the experience of diffuse bone pain. The clinical presentation of the bone pain, however, is variable depending on the age of the patient. Very young children, such as toddlers who are most commonly affected by ALL, may present with a limp or inability to walk. A school-age child who is able to provide a pain narrative may report diffuse, not well localized, total body pain. An adolescent patient may have back pain that he or she associates with a sports injury and may localize the pain to a specific area in a long bone. There are also solid tumors, such as neuroblastoma, which most commonly presents during the toddler years, that can metastasize to both the bone marrow and bone and can also present as a limp or, alternatively, as localized pain to a specific bony area.

Treatment Plans for Pain Due to Bone Marrow Infiltration or Bony Metastases

Pain Assessment

Given the importance of pain narrative from a patient, the assessment of bone marrow infiltration pain in an infant or toddler becomes even more complex because the clinician is required to move beyond the traditional communication dyad of the doctor–patient relationship to one that is a triad doctor–child–parent relationship. For example, a toddler with bone pain due to leukemic infiltration who cannot clearly verbalize his or her painful experience often requires the parent to report the painful experience on behalf of the child. Thus, the pain is often described as total body pain because the toddler no longer has the strength to walk. The physical examination is critical to supplement the parent's narrative because there may be additional physical factors contributing to the leukemic bone pain. For example, there may be point tenderness on examination that is due to an occult bone fracture from cortical thinning related to the acute leukemia that would require more than chemotherapy to treat the bone pain. However, whenever possible, it is critical to ask the child himself or herself about the pain.

Pharmacologic Treatments: Chemotherapy and Radiation Therapy

The most effective method of eradication of pain due to bone marrow infiltration begins with treatment of the primary disease. For ALL, induction chemotherapy regimens generally place children into remission within a 1-month treatment course.[28] For most standard risk ALL patients, by day 7 of treatment, there is a significant reduction in the leukemic burden to less than 25% of the bone marrow being affected. This decrease in leukemic burden results in marked improvement in the bone pain. Adolescents with acute leukemias, however, often have more resistant disease and may have longer periods of acute pain due to the persistence of blasts within the bone marrow and may require analgesics throughout the induction chemotherapy regimen.[29] For patients with bony metastases from solid tumors, such as neuroblastoma, effective treatment may also include local radiation therapy to the affected site.

Pharmacologic Treatment: Analgesic Therapy

Pharmacologic regimens for the treatment of pain from bone marrow infiltration for both children and adolescents includes the use of opioids, such as morphine or hydromorphone. These opioid analgesics may be administered through bolus dosing regimens if the pain is not constant. However, for those patients experiencing constant pain, the delivery of the opioid should include the use of patient-controlled analgesia (PCAs). PCAs are extremely effective at reducing pain because there is no lag time in the delivery of the analgesic, there can be both continuous and demand delivery, and there are lock-out mechanisms for total doses given, thereby increasing the safety profile. Hospitals have different protocols in place for the use of PCAs where some do not allow for their use in very young children because it requires a parent or nurse to administer the boluses and is no longer "patient-controlled." Alternatively, other hospitals, such as those with well-integrated pain management services within their pediatric oncology division, do allow for the use of parent-controlled or nurse-controlled PCAs for the younger or cognitively impaired child.[9] Often, health care providers will use adjuvant pain medications, such as acetaminophen or nonsteroidal anti-inflammatory agents (NSAIDs), together with opioid analgesics to optimize pain control and minimize the side effects of opioids, such as respiratory depression at high doses.[30] However, in the patient with bone marrow infiltration there is also bone marrow suppression and resultant thrombocytopenia. As a result, the use of NSAIDs is not recommended for these patients because of the NSAIDs' antiplatelet effects that may place the pediatric cancer patient at increased risk for hemorrhage secondary to both the quantitative and qualitative platelet defects.

Neuropathic Pain

Pediatric cancer patients can experience neuropathic pain for a variety of reasons, including nerve invasion, inflammation of a nerve root due to the malignancy or infectious process, and/or from cancer treatment side effects. These etiologies include: (1) chemotherapy-related peripheral neuropathies, such as with vin-

cristine neurotoxicity; (2) neural compression or invasion by tumors, such as pelvic Ewing's sarcomas; and (3) infectious related, such as herpes zoster reactivation due to immune suppression. Vincristine is a vinca-alkaloid chemotherapeutic agent used as an effective cytotoxic agent for many types of pediatric malignancies including leukemias, lymphomas, and various solid tumors. Vincristine binds to tubulin and inhibits microtubule formation and disrupts the formation of the mitotic spindle, which is thought to be one of the mechanisms by which it causes peripheral neuropathies, including jaw pain, leg pain, and abdominal pain.[31] In addition, direct injury of the nerve can occur with soft tissue sarcomas arising in the pelvis, such as Ewing's sarcoma or rhabdomyosarcoma, and the child may present with complaints of abdominal pain, lower extremity weakness, and/or bladder and bowel dysfunction.

Treatment Plans for Neuropathic Pain

Pharmacologic Treatments

The medications that can be used for neuropathic pain include the use of tricyclic antidepressants (TCAs), such as amitriptyline, anticonvulsant medications, such as gabapentin, and local anesthetics, including the topical application of the 5% lidocaine patch.[32,33] Although there has been clinical observation and scientific evidence that TCAs are effective at treating neuropathic pain, not all types of antidepressants have been shown to be effective. A Cochrane review of the adult pain literature, for example, has recommended that future research on the treatment of neuropathic pain should include the assessment of effectiveness for other "naturally occurring" antidepressants such as St. Johns Wort and L-tryptophan because there is currently insufficient data to support their use or disuse.[34] Opioids, including methadone, can also be used for severe neuropathic pain that has not been effectively treated with TCAs or anticonvulsant medications.[35] However, methadone is also associated with a heightened risk profile that has not been studied widely in children. In general, opioid-based regimens are often less effective in treating neuropathic pain. Thus, when considering the use of opioids for neuropathic pain, one should first try to maximize the total recommended daily dose of the TCAs and antineuroleptic agents, such as gabapentin, given their relatively low toxicity profile before initiating a long-term opioid regimen.

Nonpharmacologic Treatments

Mechanical approaches are also important to consider in the treatment regimen for neuropathic pain. These include the use of physical therapy and acupuncture. Physical therapy can be considered for those patients who have neuropathic pain, particularly due to vincristine because this agent can also cause motor weakness. Although physical therapy can be an effective therapeutic modality, there are several barriers to its utilization in cancer patients,[36] such as financial and/or insurance barriers. A pediatric cancer patient may be fatigued and not want to engage in exercises. With persistence and coupling of the child to a therapist who can gently but firmly encourage the patient to participate regularly in the recommended exercise regimen, physical therapy can be an effective, nonpharmacologic modality to supplement pharmacologic regimens that are insufficient at relieving the neuropathic pain.

Pain Associated With Central Nervous System Tumors

Central nervous system (CNS) tumors are the most common form of solid tumors diagnosed during childhood. Because of the mass effect of the brain tumor, the child often presents with symptoms of headaches due to increased intracranial pressure. To decrease the intracranial pressure and thereby treat the pain/headache for the child, different therapeutic approaches can be used. For some brain tumors that are locally invasive without metastatic potential, such as low grade gliomas (astrocytomas), complete surgical removal is the treatment of choice. Often, the child will be placed on a corticosteroid pulse postoperatively to decrease associated cerebral edema. If the child continues to have headaches postoperatively, nonsteroidal anti-inflammatory drugs (NSAIDs), such as ibuprofen, can be considered if there is no plan for chemotherapy and/or radiation therapy. If an NSAID is used in the pain treatment regimen, a histamine H_2-receptor antagonist to inhibit stomach acid production is also required.

For malignant brain tumors with metastatic potential, such as medulloblastomas, chemotherapy and radiation therapy are included in addition to the surgical treatment regimen. Not all primary resections of malignant brain tumors result in complete surgical removal of the tumor, so pain may persist due to residual disease. Opioids, such as morphine sulfate (MS), administered intravenously are the preferred pharmacologic medication of choice. When using high dose or prolonged courses of opioids for the treatment of central nervous system pain from brain tumors the treatment plan must also include a bowel regimen to reduce the likelihood of constipation. Constipation may already be a significant problem for the child prior to the use of opioids because certain types of chemotherapeutic agents used to treat CNS tumors, such as vincristine, can cause severe impaired gut peristalsis. There are several different classes of medications that can be used to treat or prevent constipation including polyethylene glycol (often preferable because it is a tasteless and odorless powder that can be mixed with any liquid), senakot (a stimulant laxative), docusate (a lubricating laxative), milk of magnesia (which contains magnesium hydroxide, an osmotic laxative) and/ or mineral oil (a lubricant).

Benzodiazepines, such as midazolam, can also be used indirectly for the treatment of pain due to CNS tumors even though this class of medications does not have direct analgesic effect. Their mechanism of action for the treatment of pain in children includes decrease in anxiety, decrease in muscle spasm that may occur postoperatively, and facilitation of night sleep.[37] Postoperatively after the resection of the CNS tumor, the child may remain within the intensive care unit (ICU) because of the need for monitoring intracranial pressure. In this setting, benzodiazepines may be used as a continuous infusion or with frequent bolus dosing so that agitation is minimized.[38] Benzodiazepines are often used concomitantly with opioid analgesics in the ICU setting when significant postoperative pain is reported, observed, or expected.

Pain Associated With Primary Malignant Bone Tumors

Primary malignant bone tumors, such as osteosarcoma or Ewing's sarcoma, can result in significant pain for the childhood cancer patient. Bone pain from osteosarcoma, for example, is due to both destruction of normal trabecular bone pattern from direct tumor invasion in combination with intense soft tissue inflammation from the periosteal new bone formation. Thus, the pain can often be very severe and often requires the use of opioid analgesic medications. NSAIDs could also be considered but should be used with caution given that there is a higher risk for bleeding in the patient receiving chemotherapy because of the bone marrow suppression and resultant thrombocytopenia. Cognitive development is also a consideration in developing the pain management regimen for pediatric cancer patients with bone tumors. Given that the most common primary malignant bone tumors, osteosarcoma and Ewing's sarcoma, often occur during adolescence, patient-controlled analgesia (PCA) can be considered when frequent bolus dosing is required for treatment of acute pain. For continued longer-term pain associated with bone tumors for home pain management, oral methadone is a good opioid of choice because of its long half-life and its effects on both opioid and NMDA receptors.

Phantom Limb Pain

Amputation and limb-salvage procedures may be used as surgical approaches to achieve local control of a bone tumor and each can result in a chronic pain syndrome coined *phantom limb pain*. Phantom limb pain is experienced when the pediatric patient continues to have pain appearing to come from where the affected amputated limb used to be. There are multiple possible etiologies for the occurrence of phantom limb pain that include possible damage to the nerve endings in the surgical stump with abnormal regrowth postoperatively leading to abnormal painful discharges to spinal cord and brain. There may also be abnormalities in the central nervous system response to the loss of limb in which there may be loss of inhibitory sensory input from the amputated limb. Phantom limb pain is often a severe pain and very challenging to treat. Systematic analyses of studies to effectively treat chronic postoperative phantom limb pain have not clearly demonstrated an effective treatment option in randomized control trials.[39,40] Central strategies, such as hypnotherapy, aimed at altering metabolic activity in pain perception areas of the brain, such as the anterior cingulate cortical area, may be more effective than peripheral strategies or opioids (see Chapters 26 and 54).

Pharmacologic Treatments

The first important principal in treatment of phantom limb pain is to effectively treat the bone pain preoperatively before the amputation. This can include the use of anesthetic techniques, such as epidurals, with the use of opioids or local anesthetic to prevent dorsal horn sensitization.[41] Following the surgical amputation, treatment of the acute postoperative pain must be initiated promptly in attempt to minimize the development of a chronic pain syndrome. Strategies for the acute postoperative pain for amputees include focal or epidural blocks given that by blocking the specific group of nerves (i.e., a plexus or ganglion) one can block the sensation of pain to the affected area. Given that long-term opioid use is not usually effective for phantom limb pain syndrome, gabapentin has been tried given its low toxicity profile. It should be noted, however, that randomized control trials have not demonstrated its effectiveness when compared to placebo control.[42] Similarly, amitriptyline has been used to pharmacologically treat chronic pain syndromes but has not been proven effective when compared to placebo in an amputee population.[43]

Nonpharmacologic Treatment

Complementary and alternative medicine (CAM) options for the treatment of chronic pain due to phantom limb pain include the use of hypnotherapy, massage, and acupuncture.[44–46] Hypnotherapy, for example, focuses on calming of the nervous system. Through the use of guided imagery techniques during hypnosis, there is a modification of the sensation and perception of the painful stimuli. Neuroimaging research has demonstrated that specific areas of the brain have decreased arousal. Thus, it is thought that there is a reinterpretation of the chronic pain experience.[47]

Visceral Pain

The four major etiologies of visceral pain include: (1) organ invasion with capsular wall stretching, (2) organ compression, (3) hollow organ obstruction (e.g., ureter or bowel), and (4) tumor regrowth within the organ or peritoneal cavity bleeding.

Treatment Plans for Visceral Pain Due to Organ Invasion

For visceral pain due to organ invasion with capsular wall stretching or tumor regrowth the primary treatment to decrease the pain is to decrease the tumor size. For solid organ abdominal malignancies, such as Wilms' tumor (a primary renal tumor), treatment employs a multimodal approach including surgery, chemotherapy, and/or radiation therapy. Surgical resection of the abdominal tumor can result in significant postoperative pain, so where technically possible, laparoscopic surgery consisting of small incisions into the abdominal wall musculature should be considered. Removal of the diseased organ is often not possible through laparoscopic surgery and so it is critical to promptly initiate the treatment of the pain due to a large abdominal wall incision with opioid analgesics to expedite postoperative recovery. Clinicians can be hesitant to use opioid analgesic medications postoperatively because of the concern that their use may have a further impact on slowed bowel function that occurs because of bowel surgery. If postoperative abdominal pain is not treated effectively, however, several additional postoperative complications can occur. These include longer and more intense pain, which, in turn, inhibits mobility and places the patient at risk for pulmonary atelectasis and/or infection.

Regional pain blocks are also a consideration for the treatment of visceral pain due to tumor invasion of a solid organ or nerve plexus. They can be used in the pediatric population with knowledgeable pediatric anesthesia consultation. Regional anesthetic blocks include epidurals or fluoroscopically guided celiac plexus blocks and can be very effective for pain control for unresponsive abdominopelvic tumors, such as bladder rhabdomyosarcoma or neuroblastoma. These types of anesthetic approaches allow targeted pain control within a specific neural plexus while minimizing the sedating effects that a high dose, systemic opioid infusion may cause. There have been recent reports of newer radiographic techniques to facilitate the correct placement of celiac plexus blocks in children, including three-dimensional rotational angiography.[48]

Treatment Plans for Pain Due to Intestinal Obstruction

Visceral abdominal pain can also be due to intestinal obstruction from the tumor mass. The sporadic form of Burkitt's lymphoma, for example, commonly involves the ileocecal region and can result in intestinal obstruction because of the extremely rapid growth of these cancer cells. Because Burkitt's is a type of non-Hodgkin lymphoma, surgery is not an effective treatment and emergency treatment of the abdominal obstruction consists of chemotherapy and/or radiation therapy. Chemotherapy can work quickly and effectively at reducing or eliminating the abdominal obstruction. Thus, bolus doses of opioid analgesics may only be required briefly while awaiting the tumor kill by the cytoreductive chemotherapeutics. Induction chemotherapy for rapidly growing tumors, particularly Burkitt's lymphoma, can result in tumor lysis syndrome and thus careful management of fluids and electrolytes is critical and must be considered in the treatment plan.

For all etiologies of visceral abdominal pain, it is important to initiate treatment of the pain early in an attempt to prevent visceral hyperalgesia and subsequent central pain. Visceral hyperalgesia results from an insult, such as tumor invasion or surgical manipulation, to the celiac plexus consisting of the hepatic plexus, splenic plexus, gastric plexuses, pancreatic plexus, supra/renal plexuses, testicular plexus, superior mesenteric plexus, and the inferior mesenteric plexus. If the treatment of the visceral pain is not initiated promptly or is ineffective, then the ongoing nociception ultimately results in central pain that can be very difficult to treat. Given that the visceral pain sensation consists of a feedback system from the abdominal neural plexus to the central nervous system, cognitive–behavioral therapies (CBT),

including those that promote coping and reduction of anxiety, also reduce pain perception and must be included. There are questionnaires available that can be used to systematically assess children's pain coping strategies, and this information can then be factored into the treatment plan.[49] CBT includes the use of distraction, relaxation strategies, and also specific comfort measures for young infants such as use of a pacifier, oral sucrose, and swaddling.

Pain Associated With Bone Marrow Transplantation

Pediatric cancer patients requiring bone marrow transplantation (BMT) as part of their treatment regimen are considered a high-risk group of patients for the development of acute and chronic pain given the intensity of this treatment regimen. Cancer diagnoses that may require BMT, either allogeneic or autologous, for curative therapy include ALL, AML, myelodysplastic syndrome, and neuroblastoma. Pediatric cancer patients who have received a BMT have unique risk factors for the development of acute pain, including mucositis, graft-versus-host disease (GVHD), and tissue erosive infectious complications. Thus, pain management is critical in the care of the BMT patient and, if not treated adequately, can result in decreased quality of life.

Mucositis

Although mucositis occurs when chemotherapy alone is given, mucositis is often more prolonged and severe for the BMT patient.[50] There is often a longer period for stem cell recovery extending beyond the 7 to 10 day nadir occurring postexposure to chemotherapy. The grading scale for describing the severity of oral mucositis established by the World Health Organization (WHO) begins with mild, grade I mucositis, in which the oral mucosa is red and tender, to severe, grade IV mucositis in which the pediatric cancer patient is unable to eat and maintain his or her own nutrition.[51] The severity of the mucositis often corresponds to the description of the severity of the pain by the patient. Grade I mucositis may only require bolus dosing of an opioid analgesic. In the BMT setting, however, mucositis pain often requires use of an opioid PCA given the chronicity of the pain (over a several week period) and the extensive tissue injury involving the entire gastrointestinal tract. An effective approach to PCA delivery of the opioid analgesic is to have a low basal rate that is augmented with the demand dosing for breakthrough pain.[52] If the demand dosing is frequent, resulting in a lock out of demand dose administration, then an increase in the basal rate is warranted. The pediatric BMT patient may require several weeks use of an opioid PCA because the pain from mucositis can be severe and occur over a prolonged time period of several weeks while awaiting engraftment. However, when engraftment occurs and counts recover, the PCA can often be weaned off quickly. The caveat to this is that there may be withdrawal symptoms, including agitation and/or diarrhea, and a methadone taper should be considered.

Additional Treatments for Pain Due to Mucositis

Topical agents, such as lidocaine, which can be "swished and spit" can also help decrease the chronic pain from mucositis. Mucositis can be complicated by a secondary candidal infection presenting as white plaques overlaying the erythematous oral mucosa tissue. Treatment of the thrush with topical antifungal agents such as nystatin is also an important adjuvant therapy for treatment of mucositis pain (see Chapter 45).

Graft-Versus-Host Disease (GVHD)

GVHD is a unique complication of childhood cancer patients who undergo BMT. GVHD occurs due to the host (recipient) cells appearing foreign to the engrafted hematopoietic stem cells.

There are two forms of GVHD, consisting of acute and chronic GVHD. Acute GVHD occurs within the first 100 days of the BMT, causing dermatitis, enteritis, and/or hepatitis. Acute GVHD can be clinically manifested by skin rash, right upper quadrant pain, and/or diarrhea and abdominal pain. The skin rash can range from mild erythema of the palms and soles of the feet to bullous desquamation in the severe form. Chronic GVHD occurs 100 days beyond the hematopoietic stem cell infusion and is thought to be an autoimmune process. Chronic GVHD primarily has skin manifestations that include scleroderma-type changes often accompanied by joint stiffness and immobility.

Treatment Plans for GVHD

Treatment of pain due to acute gut GVHD, often presenting as crampy abdominal pain due to the diffuse enteritis, requires the use of an opioid analgesic in the form of a PCA. If the BMT patient has been on a PCA due to mucositis pain, the basal dose can be titrated up to meet the demand from the additional painful stimuli from the GVHD. Conversely, chronic GVHD is often an outpatient disease and requires a chronic pain management plan because the autoimmune process can cause muscle and organ invasion, resulting in chronic neuropathic pain. In the setting of chronic pain, oral opioid use may be required until the neuropathic pain is adequately treated with alternative agents, including anticonvulsants such as gabapentin or tricyclic antidepressants. Nonpharmacologic therapies, including the use of acupuncture, massage therapy, and other relaxation strategies, should also be considered.

Other Factors Important to Pain Assessment and Development of the Treatment Plan for the BMT Pediatric Patient

There can be significant anxiety experienced by the pediatric patient due to prolonged hospitalization, up to and even beyond 3 months in duration for successful outcomes post-BMT. Thus, both pharmacologic and psychological services to decrease anxiety for the child are critical. Facilitation of night sleep is also important and may require the use of amitriptyline, diphenhydramine, or trazodone. Other symptoms that can decrease a child's pain tolerance include nausea, vomiting, diarrhea, and pruritis, and these symptoms should be treated or prevented as well. Lastly, if there are surgical interventions or other painful procedures required as part of the supportive care of the BMT patient, such as chest tube placement, careful attention to and pharmacologic treatment of associated pain must occur. Distraction methods can also be considered adjunctively because they have been reported as effective methods for the pediatric cancer patient and include the use of bubbles and hand-held video games.[53]

OVERVIEW OF OPIOID ANALGESIA IN CHILDREN

Opioid and non–opioid analgesia in children include the use of typical mu opioid agonists (e.g., morphine sulfate [MS] and methadone) NSAIDs, atypical opioid analgesics (e.g., tramadol), and ketamine. Opioid rotation is commonly used as a means of optimizing analgesia while minimizing opioid-related adverse effects. It has been shown that in the pediatric cancer population opioid monotherapy is the *most* effective method for treating moderate to severe pain.[54] It is not effective, however, for *all* pediatric cancer patients due to various etiologies including opioid-induced tolerance and opioid-induced hyperalgesia.[55] The analgesic response to any given opioid dose depends on the tolerance of the patient. An opioid tolerant patient will require a higher dose for the same analgesic response when compared to the opioid naïve patient. Adverse effects of opioid analgesics, for both the opioid

naïve as well as the opioid tolerant patient, include somnolence, constipation, pruritis, nausea, vomiting, urinary retention, and sweating.

Dependence and Addiction

There can also be barriers to the use of high dose or long-term use of opioid analgesia in children due to parents' and health care providers' concerns regarding the risk of dependence or addiction.[56] Some of the more common symptoms of withdrawal in a child with physiologic opioid dependence include severe dysphoria, diarrhea, anxiety, restlessness, and chills and usually occur when the opioid analgesic is stopped abruptly. The symptoms observed in pediatric patients can vary from those observed in adults. For example, an infant can have a high pitched cry and inability to be soothed with a pacifier, bottle, or swaddling. A toddler's signs of withdrawal may include only diarrhea and temperature instability. Conversely, addiction is a complex behavior characterized by the compulsive use of a drug and psychological craving. Addiction is not commonly seen in the pediatric population but may be observed in the older adolescent who has complex psychosocial issues resulting in maladaptive coping to pain.

Tolerance to Opioids

Given that tolerance to opioid analgesics can limit their clinical effectiveness, various approaches can be used to prevent or reverse tolerance in children who require prolonged exposure to high-dose opioids. One proposed approach to prevent tolerance includes the use of N-methyl-D-aspartate (NMDA) antagonists concomitantly with the opioid. Ketamine has been studied and shown to have a role in mitigating opioid-induced tolerance in children and adolescents who experience cancer pain. Finkel et al. have used ketamine at lower doses than used for anesthetic purposes. Specifically, they used ketamine from 0.1 to 1.0 mg/kg/hour in patients who had signs of opioid tolerance or had severe side effects such as profound sedation.[57] With this regimen, they found that adjuvant ketamine infusions used in combination with opioid analgesics (including morphine, methadone, and hydromorphone) resulted in improved pain control. Tramadol hydrochloride is an atypical opioid that has a weak affinity for the μ-opioid receptor, as well as being a weak inhibitor of serotonin and noradrenaline reuptake. The advantage of tramadol is that it has negligible respiratory depression.[58] It is hepatically metabolized and renally excreted, factors that must be taken into consideration when using this medication in the pediatric cancer patient because chemotherapy can result in hepatotoxicity. The active metabolite is O-demethyltramadol (M1) and recent pharmacokinetic studies in children have demonstrated that it is possible to produce enough of the active metabolite to achieve adequate pain relief.[59] Safe dosing regimens for children ≥12 months of age include 1–2 mg/kg per oral route of administration every 4 to 6 hours with a maximum dose of 8 mg/kg/day.[60]

There are several new unique delivery systems of opioid analgesics and ketamine being tested that might prove useful in the pediatric cancer population to avoid the fear and pain associated with injections. Currently, oral transmucosal delivery of fentanyl citrate (including the trade names of Actiq [a lozenge on a handle] and Fentora [an effervescent tablet]) are the only two formulations that are commercially available with indications for the treatment of breakthrough pain in opioid tolerant adult patients.[61]

Another noninvasive method of opioid drug delivery includes the use of fentanyl transdermal therapeutic (TTS) systems. One practical advantage is that when the oral route of tablet, capsule, or liquid administration is contraindicated or not well-tolerated by a child, the transdermal drug delivery method allows for an alternative route. There are emerging numbers of pharmacokinetic studies on the use of TTS in children compared to adult dosing regimens as discussed in a recent review by Zernikow et el.[69] In this critical review, they discuss the approximate conversion factor of 45 mg per day of MS to fentanyl TTS 12.5ug/hour for initial therapy for children and adolescents requiring long-term morphine therapy. The data supporting the transdermal route over traditional MS is minimal but there are studies emerging that demonstrate child and parent satisfaction with the TTS delivery system of fentanyl in both pain relief and quality of life in the pediatric palliative care setting.[62]

PALLIATIVE CARE FOR CHILDREN WITH CANCER

A chapter on pain management for children with cancer is not complete without highlighting the important topic of palliative care given that overall 20% of children will not be cured of their disease. The WHO's definition of palliative care is "the active total care of patients whose disease is not responsive to curative treatment. Control of pain, other symptoms, and psychological, social, and spiritual problems is paramount. The goal of palliative care is achievement of the best possible quality of life for patients and their families."[63] The "other symptoms" in addition to pain that can be experienced by the child without the option of curative therapy include fatigue, dyspnea, poor appetite, nausea, vomiting, constipation, and/or diarrhea.[64] Thus, symptom control for children facing end of life is imperative. Studies have demonstrated that when the multidisciplinary approach of palliative care is employed, families and patients report improved satisfaction with their care, improved informed decision making, and a decrease in the number of emergency room visits and inpatient admissions.[65]

The American Academy of Pediatrics (AAP) has put forth a policy statement promoting the use of palliative care at the end of life for children with life-limiting disease. Their statement highlights that palliative care can improve the quality of life for terminal patients and their families through the treatment of symptoms and by addressing the psychological, social, or spiritual aspects of facing a noncurable disease.[66] Despite this policy statement on the importance of the provision of palliative care services for children with life-threatening disease, there are barriers that currently exist and thereby impede its implementation across the U.S. health care system. First, there can be differences in parents' understanding of prognosis of their child's illness when compared to their health care providers' knowledge, a discrepancy that in turn can impact a parental informed decision for end-of-life care, including pain management.[67] Secondly, for parents whose children have an incurable cancer diagnosis, they rate doctor–patient communication as the principal determinant of high-quality physician care. Conversely, physicians' care ratings depend on biomedical rather than doctor–patient relationship aspects of care.[68] It is, therefore, critical for physicians caring for the dying child to listen to the concerns of the patient and the parent particularly for those related to descriptions of pain. By listening to a patient's description of pain and thereby classifying the etiology of the pain one can determine the best therapeutic approach (as discussed above). By being aggressive with symptom management, the pain and suffering at the end-of-life for a terminal pediatric cancer can be minimized.[69]

Pediatric palliative care requires evaluation and re-evaluation of symptoms. In addition to the assessment of pain, the provider needs to assess for symptoms of fatigue, dyspnea, anxiety, nausea, and sleep patterns. There should also be the assessment of caretaker function and support because fatigue or anxiety in the primary caretaker can in turn affect the symptoms associated with pain manifested by the child. Treatment of other end-of-life symp-

toms, such as dyspnea, can require the use of MS to decrease the sensation of air hunger. If the child is heavily sedated and the family or caretaker has minimal awake time with the child, psychostimulants (e.g., methylphenidate, modafinil) can be used in the morning to override some of the sedative side effects of high-dose opioids needed for pain. In addition, nondrug therapies, such as music therapy or hypnotherapy, can be used concurrently with pain medications. The pediatric palliative care model as described above can be delivered both in the inpatient setting as well as in the home if pediatric hospice services are available. In either setting, the goal of maximizing quality of life for the quantity of time that remains for a child without curative therapy should be emphasized. It should be noted that many clinicians now consider palliative care to begin with a serious diagnosis, such as cancer, even if the likelihood for cure is high, because some children even with low-risk cancers, like ALL in the young child, will die. Thus, a focus on maximizing quality of life and reducing distressing symptoms should be as important a focus in the child with cancer as is the aim for cure.

COMPLEMENTARY AND ALTERNATIVE MEDICINE (CAM) IN THE PEDIATRIC CANCER PATIENT

There are multiple nonpharmacologic therapies that can be employed for pain management in the pediatric cancer patient (Table 49.1). These include massage therapy, yoga, hypnotherapy, meditation, biofeedback, relaxation, spirituality, acupuncture, botanicals, physical therapy, and energy therapies including the use of magnets. The definition of complementary and alternative medicine (CAM) is those interventions that are not generally provided by U.S. hospital clinics, nor widely taught in medical school.[70] Thus, although these CAM techniques may not be familiar territory for physicians trained within the United States, there is an emerging body of literature discussing the state-of-the-science of CAM use in both adult and pediatric populations.[71] In addition, the latest literature in medical education has documented a clear trend of higher usage rates of CAM by anesthesia training programs across the United States.[72] Thus, CAM interventions should be considered as adjuvant therapy for the treatment of pediatric cancer pain.

Acupuncture

Acupuncture consists of inserting fine needles into the skin's surface, or using heat, pressure, or other stimulation in areas that correspond to specific points along "meridians" (i.e., energy channels within the body). These meridians in which the body's life forces (spiritual, emotional, mental, and physical) flow can be out of balance and cause the physical sensations of pain, imbal-

TABLE 49.1

COMPLEMENTARY AND ALTERNATIVE MEDICINE THERAPIES TO BE CONSIDERED IN THE TREATMENT OF PEDIATRIC CANCER PAIN

- Acupuncture
- Hypnotherapy
- Massage
- Biofeedback
- Botanicals
- Magnets
- Spirituality/religiosity
- Therapeutic yoga

ance, and sickness. Insertion of the needles into specific points along meridians through the practice of acupuncture helps to restore the balance of forces within the body and thereby eliminate the pain by achieving a flow of energy or Qi (pronounced chi). Although the practice of acupuncture is more widely accepted within Eastern societies, the use of acupuncture for treatment of pain has been increasing across the United States.[73,74] Approximately half of the states within the United States require licensure for the practice of acupuncture. For those states that do not regulate the practice, the health care provider should ask for certification by the National Commission for the Certification of Acupuncturists (see Chapter 93).

There is a growing body of literature evaluating its effectiveness for alleviating pain.[75,76] The available literature on the use and effectiveness of acupuncture in the treatment of pain in the pediatric population suggests it being an acceptable treatment modality for adolescents with chronic pain, as well as being an effective modality for other common symptoms experienced by the childhood cancer patient, including headache, nausea, and vomiting.[77–79] Nonetheless, acupuncture has not been widely disseminated into pain treatment regimens for the pediatric population. One reason is the preexisting beliefs by health care practitioners in the United States that children are afraid of needles and thus they do not make referrals for acupuncture.[80,81] On the contrary, it has been shown that for those children who have been referred to acupuncture for various chronic pain syndromes, over two-thirds report that it was a positive experience and an effective modality for treatment of their pain.[82] Acupuncture, therefore, can be considered as a possible adjuvant treatment modality for neuropathic pain in the pediatric cancer patient.

Hypnotherapy

Hypnosis is a cognitive strategy that helps the child achieve a narrowed focus of attention, relax, and learn how to dissociate from the current sensory environment. Liossi and others in randomized controlled studies of children with cancer undergoing medical procedures have shown hypnotherapy to be effective in reducing procedure-related pain and anxiety.[83–85] In addition, a recent review article by Wood and Bioy provides a succinct review on the effectiveness of this technique, an understanding of the physiologic effect of hypnosis, and the practical application of its use to treat pain in children.[86] For example, Rainville and colleagues have demonstrated, through the use of positive emission tomography (PET) changes, in regional cerebral blood flow, when hypnosis is used.[87] In hypnotic states, there is increased blood flow to the occipital cortical areas. This increase in blood flow to the occipital region is thought to result in a reduction of inhibitory processes that occur normally during high levels of attention.[88] Thus, hypnosis results in an acceptance of specific, altered sensations, thereby mediating changes in perception of the painful experience.

Several studies on the effect of hypnosis for symptom management in children, including the effect on pain perception, anxiety, and nausea/vomiting have been completed. Early studies have demonstrated the feasibility of being able to hypnotize children.[89] Subsequent studies by Zeltzer et al. have demonstrated the effectiveness of hypnosis in decreasing other symptoms experienced by pediatric cancer patients, including nausea.[90] More recent studies have demonstrated the effectiveness of hypnosis in decreasing pain and anxiety in children undergoing the invasive painful procedures of lumbar punctures and bone marrow biopsies.[91] Thus, there continues to be increasing evidence of both the feasibility of administration and the effectiveness of hypnosis in the pediatric population, and it should be considered when a pediatric cancer patient is undergoing invasive, painful procedures. As the review paper by Wood and Bioy discusses, practical considerations of using hypnosis include the child's age (as younger children are more responsive to the hypnosis when compared to adolescents), cognitive development, and therapeutic relationship with his or her provider.[92]

Massage

Massage is the practice of light body stroking or deep tissue stroking that is thought to work by increasing serotonin and reducing cortisol. The basic principle of massage is that when muscles are overworked, there is a release of waste products that accumulate in the area that can be relieved using the hands of the therapist to manipulate muscles and surrounding tissues. Massage therapy has been used as an adjuvant therapy in pain management with a number of studies demonstrating its effectiveness. For example, it has been shown that when massage therapy was used in addition to a standard pharmacologic regimen for postoperative pain management, the experimental group demonstrated decreased pain intensity, pain unpleasantness, and anxiety when compared to the control group.[92] Massage therapy is also a CAM modality that can be easily instituted at the bedside for the cancer patient.[93] There are few studies to date completed in the pediatric population on the use and effectiveness of massage therapy. Nonetheless, the studies that have been completed do demonstrate decreased pain in the group receiving a standardized massage protocol.[94] In a study of children with ALL, a daily massage over a 1-month period was found to have an impact on the immune system as demonstrated by an increased white blood cell count, as well as an improvement in children's negative affect.[95] Studies have also demonstrated the positive effect in decreasing anxiety in an ethnically diverse sample (Latino) of children with pain due to arthralgias.[96] Given the promising application of massage therapy to decrease pain in children, future research is warranted to evaluate the effectiveness of the healing powers of touch (i.e., massage) in a randomized controlled trial for pediatric cancer patients.

Biofeedback

Biofeedback involves measuring physiologic parameters, including blood pressure, heart rate, skin temperature, sweating, and muscle tension, and conveying the changes that occur while the child is learning breathing and imagery strategies to alter these bodily processes. This bodily feedback information can be provided through the use of computer-generated, audio-generated, or other forms of visual-generated systems with skin temperature or muscle contraction being the most commonly measured parameter. The basic concept of biofeedback is that by providing physiologic information to a patient who is usually unaware of these bodily processes, while also teaching the child cognitive and breathing strategies that alter these processes, the child can learn to reduce muscle tension and autonomic arousal, thereby reducing pain. For children, it provides proof that the mind can affect the body by being able to gain physiologic control of the part of the nervous system that is activated by pain or stress.

Studies on the use of biofeedback have primarily been focused on adult patients, particularly those with headaches. Meta-analysis of this mind–body approach for the treatment of headache pain indicates that it is effective when used alone or in combination with other CAM modalities.[97] Studies completed in pediatric patients again are limited in number, but those that have been completed also have focused on the treatment of pediatric migraine headache. Similar to the adult literature, meta-analysis on the use of biofeedback, as well as other behavioral methodologies to treat headache in children, demonstrate that it can be considered as an important adjunct to the pain treatment regimen.[98] Given that there are minimal side effects and there is data suggesting its effectiveness, biofeedback can also be considered as another adjunctive therapy to pain management in the pediatric cancer patient. There is no license to practice biofeedback although the majority of practitioners have other medical licensures, such as registered nursing (RN), physical therapy (PT) or marriage and family therapy (MFT). Hospitals and clinics with pediatric pain programs can often provide referral lists of biofeedback therapists.

Botanicals

The use of herbal or alternative medicines requires at least brief mention in the treatment of cancer pain given the increasing frequency of use within the U.S. population with or without data suggesting its effectiveness.[99] The studies that have evaluated the use of herbal medicine in pediatric patients have been for the treatment of otalgia and have been completed outside the United States.[100] One such study evaluating the use of the naturopathic ear drop, Otikon, concluded that it was as effective as anesthetic ear drops for acute otitis media associated with ear pain.[101] Thus, given the paucity of studies documenting effectiveness of botanicals, this CAM option cannot be recommended in the treatment of pediatric cancer pain. The lesson that must be taken away, however, is that it is important for practitioners to ask if botanicals (including megavitamins and herbs) are being used by the parent to help treat their child's pain because there may be drug interactions that may interfere with the cancer treatment regimen.

Magnets

The use of magnets to treat chronic pain is another CAM modality that has been under investigation in adult populations. Interestingly, despite the lack of clear data documenting the effectiveness, one study documented that magnet use was the second most common CAM modality used by adult patients with arthritis, second only to the use of a chiropractor.[101] The basic mechanism of magnet use is that they produce a type of energy, a magnetic field, that can affect the pain sensation, although the exact mechanism by which pain reduction occurs has not been identified. There are various magnet products for use in health care including shoe insoles, shoe inserts, mattress pads, bandages, belts, pillows, bracelets, and headwear.[102] Despite all of these various health care products, there are limited data documenting the effectiveness of this CAM modality. A recent systematic review and meta-analysis of randomized trials demonstrated no significant difference in pain reduction.[103] There may be a placebo effect for the patient who places a magnet on the body in the form of a bracelet or bandage.[104] The only reports in the literature of magnets in pediatric populations refer to the dangers of magnet ingestions resulting in gastrointestinal injuries.[105] Thus, the use of magnets to treat young pediatric cancer patients is another CAM modality that cannot be recommended at this point in time and may be associated with risk of ingestion by a young child.

Spirituality/Religiosity

Spirituality (i.e., religiosity) is an important domain that must be considered when conceptualizing the model of palliative care for children with pain.[106] Spirituality must be discussed as another CAM modality because it is commonly used by cancer patients to cope with their diagnosis, aggressive treatment plans, and the associated painful experiences. Spirituality has been shown to be an important coping mechanism for adult cancer patients. For example, it has been shown that breast cancer patients who rate their spirituality as high have lower rates of depression although no effect on pain ratings.[107] Similarly, when mothers of childhood cancer patients were asked to rate their religiosity concomitantly with the measurement of depression using the Beck Depression Inventory-II, it was shown that those mothers who reported lower levels of religious beliefs and behaviors had higher rates of depressive symptoms.[108] It has therefore been recommended that health care providers consider—when they have patients practicing prayer or prayer-like behaviors—to include a discussion on the benefit of this behavior at improving health through the mind–body connection.[109] In addition, given that most major medical centers caring for children with cancer have access to a chaplain or spiritual support, consulting this service should be considered (where appropriate) when developing a pain management plan for the pediatric cancer patient.

Therapeutic Yoga

Therapeutic yoga, including Iyengar yoga, has been used in children to reduce pain, anxiety, and correct health problems. Iyengar yoga, for example, uses poses (asanas) and breathing to correct body structure, enhance internal organ function, facilitate mindful awareness, and achieve a sense of mind–body–spiritual wellbeing. Studies conducted in adolescents have demonstrated the practice of yoga results in improvement of mood, a decrease in the stress hormones, and decreased pain and disability.[110] In the practice of Iyengar yoga, a teacher who has studied for a minimum of 5 years teaches various poses to a child that can be beneficial in decreasing pain. For the pediatric cancer patient with unique needs, including an impaired immune system, private yoga lessons are preferred over group lessons, with therapeutic Iyengar yoga our preferred method of yoga because of extensive teacher training, the use of supportive props, and selection of specific poses based on the needs of the child.

SUMMARY

Although pediatric cancer statistics are currently at an all time high with an overall survival rate of 80%, cancer-related morbidity, including the risk for the development of significant acute and chronic pain, persists. Thus, a comprehensive approach to pain management in the pediatric cancer patient, especially through empowerment of the child through a mind–body therapeutic approach to their pain management, is critical. There are several pharmacologic treatments that can be used to treat the various types of pediatric cancer pain including opioid analgesia, NMDA antagonist agents, NSAIDs, atypical opioid medications, tricyclic antidepressants, and anticonvulsants. Integration of CAM modalities as an adjuvant or alternative to pharmacologic interventions is also important because there can be limitations in the traditional pharmacologic approach to pain, particularly for chronic pain syndromes. Although not all CAM therapies have a long track record in the scientific literature regarding their effectiveness, it does not mean these options should be excluded from pain management consideration, but rather a discussion with families of the strengths and limitations of such approaches is warranted.

In summary, the foundation to the pain evaluation and treatment plans for children with cancer is a focus on the whole child. The importance of eliciting and listening to all details of the pain narrative of the pediatric cancer patient is critical. Child self-report will be dependent on the developmental level of the child and child pain evaluation encompasses the parental role in the pain experience, a proxy reporter of the pain narrative. For both the child and the parents, the pain assessment should occur early on, in a nonthreatening environment, where the strong triad relationship between the pediatric cancer patient, the parent and the health care provider can be an effective one. In this family-centered care approach, the common goal of alleviating the child's pain can be achieved through education, empowerment, and the provision of mind–body therapeutics.

References

1. (http://seer.cancer.gov – sect_29_table.012pgs.pdf)
2. Steliarova-Foucher E, Stiller C, Lacour B, et al. International Classification of Childhood Cancer, Third Edition. *Cancer* 2005;103:1457–1467.
3. Cure Search Children's Oncology Group Webpage. [Internet]. http://www.childrensoncologygroup.org/. Accessed 2009.
4. Hudson MM, Mertens AC, Yasui Y, et al. Health status of adult long-term survivors of childhood cancer: a report from the Childhood Cancer Survivor Study. *JAMA* 2003;290:1583–1592.
5. Oeffinger KC, Mertens AC, Sklar CA, et al. Chronic health conditions in adult survivors of childhood cancer. *N Engl J Med* 2006;355:1572–1582.
6. Stuber Ml, Kazak AE, Meeske, K, et al. Predictors of posttraumatic stress symptoms in childhood cancer survivors. *Pediatrics* 1997;100;958–964.

7. Jay SM, Elliot CH, Ozolins M, et al. Behavioral management of children's distress during painful medical procedures. *Behav Res Ther* 1985;23:513–520.

8. Chen E, Zeltzer LK, Craske MG, et al. Children's memories for painful cancer treatment procedures: implications for distress. *Child Dev* 2000;71:933–947.

9. Schechter NL, Bernstein BA, Beck A, et al. Individual differences in children's response to pain: role of temperament and parental characteristics. *Pediatrics* 1991;87:171–177.

10. Goldsmith HH, Buss AH, Plomin R, et al. Roundtable: what is temperament? Four approaches. *Child Dev* 1987;58:505–529.

11. Broom ME, Rehwaldt M, Fogg L. Relationships between cognitive behavioral techniques, temperament, observed distress, and pain reports in children and adolescents during lumbar puncture. *J Pediatr Nurs* 1998;13:48–54.

12. Helgadóttir HL, Wilson ME. Temperament and pain in 3 to 7-year-old children undergoing tonsillectomy. *J Pediatr Nurs* 2004;19:204–213.

13. Chen E, Craske MG, et al. Pain-sensitive temperament: does it predict procedural distress and response to psychological treatment among children with cancer? *J Pediatr Psychol* 2000;25:269–278.

14. Stuber ML, Kazak AE, Meeske K, et al. Is posttraumatic stress a viable model for understanding responses to childhood cancer? *Child Adolesc Psychiatr Clin N Am* 1998;7:169–182.

15. Van Hulle Vincent C. Nurses' knowledge, attitudes, and practices: regarding children's pain. *MCN Am J Matern Child Nurs* 2005;30:177–183.

16. Vetter TR, Heiner EJ. Disconcordance between patient self-reported visual analog scale pain scores and observed pain-related behavior in older children after surgery. *J Clin Anesth* 1996;8:371–375.

17. Badr Zahr LK, Puzantian H, Abboud M, et al. Assessing procedural pain in children with cancer in Beirut, Lebanon. *J Pediatr Oncol Nurs* 2006;23:311–320.

18. von Baeyer CL, Spagrud LJ. Systematic review of observational (behavioral) measures of pain for children and adolescents aged 3 to 18 years. *Pain* 2007;127:140–150.

19. McGrath PJ, Hohnson G, Goodman JT, et al. CHEOPS: A behavioral scale for rating postoperative pain in children. In: Fields HL, Dubner R, Cervero F, eds. *Advances in Pain Research and Therapy.* Vol. 9. New York: Raven Press; 1985:395–402.

20. Merkel SI, Voepel-Lewis T, Shayevitz JR, et al. The FLACC: a behavioral scale for scoring postoperative pain in young children. *Pediatr Nurs* 1997;23:293–297.

21. Klein SM, Hauser GJ, Anderson BD, et al. Comparison of intermittent versus continuous infusion of propofol for elective procedures in children. *Pediatr Crit Care Med* 2003;4:78–82.

22. Ott MJ. Mindfulness meditation in pediatric clinical practice. *Pediatr Nurs* 2002;28:487–490.

23. Yuan-Chi L, Lee ACC, Kemper KJ, et al. Use of complementary and alternative medicine in pediatric pain management service: a survey. *Pain Medicine* 2005;6:452–458.

24. Lambert SA. The effects of hypnosis/guided imagery on the postoperative course of children. *J Dev Behav Pediatr* 1996;17:307–310.

25. Chetta HD. The effect of music and desensitization on preoperative anxiety in children. *J Music Ther* 1981;18:74–87.

26. Avers L, Mathur A, Kamat D. Music therapy in pediatrics. *Clin Pediatr* 2007;46:575–579.

27. Jemal A, Thomas A, Murray T, et al. Cancer statistics, 2002. *CA Cancer J Clin* 2002;52:23–47.

28. Reaman GH. Pediatric cancer research from past successes through collaboration to future transdisciplinary research. *J Pediatr Oncol Nurs* 2004;21:123–127.

29. Albritton K, Bleyer WA. The management of cancer in the older adolescent. *Eur J Cancer* 2003;39:2584–2599.

30. Guindon J, Walczak JS, Beaulieu P. Recent advances in the pharmacological management of pain. *Drugs* 2007;67:2121–2133.

31. Ozyurek H, Turker H, Akbalik M, et al. Pyridoxine and pyridostigmine treatment in vincristine-induced neuropathy. *Pediatr Hematol Oncol* 2007;24:447–452.

32. Finnerup NB, Otto M, Jensen TS, et al. An evidence-based algorithm for the treatment of neuropathic pain. *Med Gen Med* 2007;15;9:36. Review.

33. Collins JJ, Kerner J, Sentivany S, et al. Intravenous amitriptyline in pediatrics. *J Pain Symptom Manage* 1995;10:471–475.

34. Saarto T, Wiffen PJ. Antidepressants for neuropathic pain. *Cochrane Database Syst Rev* 2007 Oct 17;(4):CD005454.

35. Altier N, Dion D, Boulanger A, et al. Management of chronic neuropathic pain with methadone: a review of 13 cases. *Clin J Pain* 2005;21:364–369.

36. Silver J, Mayer RS. Barriers to pain management in the rehabilitation of the surgical oncology patient. *J Surg Oncol* 2007;95:427–435.

37. Richtsmeier AJ, Barkin RL, Alexander M. Benzodiazepines for acute pain in children. *J Pain Symptom Manage* 1992;7:492–495.

38. Tobias JD, Rasmussen GE. Pain management and sedation in the pediatric intensive care unit. *Pediatr Clin North Am* 1994;41:1269–1292.

39. Halbert J, Crotty M, Cameron ID. Evidence for the optimal management of acute and chronic phantom pain: a systematic review. *Clin J Pain* 2002;18:84–92.

40. Mishra S, Bhatnagar S, Singhal AK. High-dose morphine for intractable phantom limb pain. *Clin J Pain* 2007;23:99–101.

41. Baron R, Maier C. Phantom limb pain: are cutaneous nociceptors and spinothalamic neurons involved in the signaling and maintenance of spontaneous and touch-evoked pain? A case report. *Pain* 1995;60:223–228.

42. Nikolajsen L, Finnerup NB, Kramp S, et al. A randomized study of the effects of gabapentin on postamputation pain. *Anesthesiology* 2006;105:1008–1015.

43. Robinson LR, Czerniecki JM, Ehde DM, et al. Trial of amitriptyline for relief of pain in amputees: results of a randomized controlled study. *Arch Phys Med Rehabil* 2004;85:1–6.

44. Douglas DB. Hypnosis: useful, neglected, available. *Am J Hosp Palliat Care* 1999;16:665–670.

45. Leskowitz ED. Phantom limb pain treated with therapeutic touch: a case report. *Arch Phys Med Rehabil* 2000;81:522–524.

46. Bradbrook D. Acupuncture treatment of phantom limb pain and phantom limb sensation in amputees. *Acupunct Med* 2004;22:93–97.

47. Rainville P, Hofbauer RK, Bushnell MC, et al. Hypnosis modulates activity in brain structures involved in the regulation of consciousness. *J Cogn Neurosci* 2002;14(6):887–901.

48. Goldschneider KR, Racadio JM, Weidner NJ. Celiac plexus blockade in children using a three-dimensional fluoroscopic reconstruction technique: case reports. *Reg Anesth Pain Med* 2007;32:510–515.

49. Varni JW, Waldron SA, Gragg RA, et al. Development of the Waldron/Varni pediatric pain coping inventory. *Pain* 1996;67:141–150.

50. Silverman S Jr. Diagnosis and management of oral mucositis. *J Support Oncol* 2007;5(suppl 1):13–21.

51. Stiff PJ. Coding for mucositis. [Internet]. 2005; http://www.cdc.gov/nchs/ppt/icd9/att_mucositis_sep05.ppt/. Accessed 2009.

52. Friedrichsdorf SJ, Finney D, Bergin M, et al. Breakthrough pain in children with cancer. *J Pain Symptom Manage* 2007;34:209–216.

53. Windich-Biermeier A, Sjoberg I, Dale JC, et al. Effects of distraction on pain, fear, and distress during venous port access and venipuncture in children and adolescents with cancer. *J Pediatr Oncology Nurs* 2007;24:8–19.

54. Zernikow B, Smale H, Michel E, et al. Paediatric cancer pain management using the WHO analgesic ladder—results of a prospective analysis from 2265 treatment days during a quality improvement study. *Eur J Pain* 2006;10:587–595.

55. Angst MS, Clark JD. Opioid-induced hyperalgesia: a qualitative systematic review. *Anesthesiology* 2006;104:570–587.

56. Von Roenn JH, Cleeland CS, Gonin R, et al. Physician attitudes and practice in cancer pain management. A survey from the Eastern Cooperative Oncology Group. *Ann Intern Med* 1993;119:121–126.

57. Finkel JC, Pestieau SR, Quezado ZM. Ketamine as an adjuvant for treatment of cancer pain in children and adolescents. *J Pain* 2007;8:515–521.

58. Payne KA, Roelofse JA. Tramadol drops in children: analgesic efficacy, lack of respiratory effects, and normal recovery times. *Anesth Prog* 1999;46:91–96.

59. Garrido MJ, Habre W, Rombout F, et al. Population pharmacokinetic/pharmacodynamic modelling of the analgesic effects of tramadol in pediatrics. *Pharm Res* 2006;23:2014–2023. Epub 2006 Aug 9.

60. Payne KA, Roelofse JA, Shipton EA. Pharmacokinetics of oral tramadol drops for postoperative pain relief in children aged 4 to 7 years—a pilot study. *Anesth Prog* 2002;49:109–112.

61. Mystakidou K, Tsilika E, Tsiatas M, et al. Oral transmucosal fentanyl citrate in cancer pain management: a practical application of nanotechnology. *Int J Nanomedicine* 2007;2:49–54.

62. Noyes M, Irving H. The use of transdermal fentanyl in pediatric oncology palliative care. *Am J Hosp Palliat Care* 2001;18:411–416.

63. http://www.who.int/cancer/palliative/definition/en/. Accessed 2009.

64. Wolfe J, Grier HE, Klar N, et al. Symptoms and suffering at the end of life in children with cancer. *N Engl J Med* 2000;342:326–333.

65. Jennings PD. Providing pediatric palliative care through a pediatric supportive care team. *Pediatr Nurs* 2005;31:195–200.

66. Bioethics CO, Committee on Hospital Care. Palliative Care for Children. *Pediatrics* 2000;106(2):351–357.

67. Wolfe J, Klar N, Grier HE, et al. Understanding of prognosis among parents of children who died of cancer: impact on treatment goals and integration of palliative care. *JAMA* 2000;284:2469–2475.

68. Mack JW, Hilden JM, Watterson J, et al. Parent and physician perspectives on quality of care at the end of life in children with cancer. *J Clin Oncol* 2005;23:9155–9161. Epub 2005 Sep 19.

69. Calabrese CL. ACT—for pediatric palliative care. *Pediatr Nurs* 2007;33:532–534.

70. Eisenberg DM, Kessler RC, Foster C, et al. Unconventional medicine in the United States: prevalence, costs, and patterns of use. *N Engl J Med* 1993;328:246–252.

71. Tsao JC, Zeltzer LK. Complementary and alternative medicine approaches for pediatric pain: a review of the state-of-the-science. *Evid Based Complement Alternat Med* 2005;2:149–159.

72. Lin YC, Lee AC, Kemper KJ, et al. Use of complementary and alternative medicine in pediatric pain management service: a survey. *Pain Med* 2005;6:452–458.

73. Itoh K, Kitakoji H. Acupuncture for chronic pain in Japan: a review. *Evid Based Complement Alternat Med* 2007;4:431–438.

74. Kundu A, Berman B. Acupuncture for pediatric pain and symptom management. *Pediatr Clin North Am* 2007;54:885–889.

75. Tulder MW VA, Cherkin DC, Berman B, et al. Acupuncture for low back pain. *Cochrane Database Syst Rev* 2000;(2):CD001351.

76. Wang SM, Kain ZN, White PF. Acupuncture analgesia: II. Clinical considerations. *Anesth Analg* 2008;106:611–621.

77. Tsao JC, Meldrum M, Kim SC, et al. Treatment preferences for CAM in children with chronic pain. *Evid Based Complement Alternat Med* 2007;4:367–374.

78. Gottschling S, Meyer S, Gribova I, et al. Laser acupuncture in children with headache: a double-blind, randomized, bicenter, placebo-controlled trial. *Pain* 2008;137:405–412.

79. Reindl TK, Geilen W, Hartmann R, et al. Acupuncture against chemotherapy-induced nausea and vomiting in pediatric oncology. Interim results of a multi-center crossover study. *Support Care Cancer* 2006;14(2):172–176. Epub 2005 Jul 14.

80. Kemper KJ, Sarah R, Silver-Highfield E, et al. On pins and needles? Pediatric pain patients' experience with acupuncture. *Pediatrics* 2000;105:941–947.

81. Liossi C, Hatira P. Clinical hypnosis versus cognitive behavioral training for pain management with pediatric cancer patients undergoing bone marrow aspirations. *Int J Clin Exp Hypn* 1999;47:104–116.

82. Liossi C, Hatira P. Clinical hypnosis in the alleviation of procedure-related pain in pediatric oncology patients. *Int J Clin Exp Hypn* 2003;51:4–28.

83. Liossi C, White P, Hatira P. Randomized clinical trial of local anesthetic versus a combination of local anesthetic with self-hypnosis in the management of pediatric procedure-related pain. *Health Psychol* 2006;25:307–315.

84. Wood C, Bioy A. Hypnosis and pain in children. *J Pain Symptom Manage* 2008;35(4):437–446. Epub 2008 Feb 4.

85. Rainville P, Hofbauer RK, Paus T, et al. Cerebral mechanisms of hypnotic induction and suggestion. *J Cogn Neurosci* 1999;11:110–125.

86. Rainville P, Hofbauer RK, Bushnell MC, et al. Hypnosis modulates activity in brain structures involved in the regulation of consciousness. *J Cogn Neurosci* 2002;14:887–901.

87. LeBaron S, Zeltzer LK, Fanurik D. Imaginative involvement and hypnotizability in childhood. *Int J Clin Exp Hypn* 1988;36:284–295.

88. Zeltzer LK, Dolgin MJ, LeBaron S,et al. A randomized, controlled study of behavioral intervention for chemotherapy distress in children with cancer. *Pediatrics* 1991;88:34–42.

89. Butler LD, Symons BK, Henderson SL, et al. Hypnosis reduces distress and duration of an invasive medical procedure for children. *Pediatrics* 2005;115:e77–e85.

90. Mitchinson AR, Kim HM, Rosenberg JM, et al. Acute postoperative pain management using massage as an adjuvant therapy: a randomized trial. *Arch Surg.* 2007;142:1158–1167; discussion 1167.

91. Gatlin CG, Schulmeister L. When medication is not enough: nonpharmacologic management of pain. *Clin J Oncol Nurs* 2007;11:699–704.

92. Field T, Hernandez-Reif M, Seligman S, et al. Juvenile rheumatoid arthritis: benefits from massage therapy. *J Pediatr Psychol* 1997;22:607–617.

93. Field T, Cullen C, Diego M, et al. Leukemia immune changes following massage therapy. *J Bodyw Mov Ther* 2001;5:271–274.

94. Zebracki K, Holzman K, Bitter KJ, et al. Brief report: use of complementary and alternative medicine and psychological functioning in Latino children with juvenile idiopathic arthritis or arthralgia. *J Pediatr Psychol* 2007;32:1006–1010. Epub 2007 Jul 11.

95. Sierpina V, Astin J, Giordano J. Mind-body therapies for headache. *Am Fam Physician* 2007;76:1518–1522.

96. Andrasik F. Behavioral treatment of migraine: current status and future directions. *Expert Rev Neurother* 2004;4:403–413.

97. Eisenberg DM, Davis RB, Ettner SL, et al. Trends in alternative medicine use in the United States, 1990–1997: results of a follow-up national survey. *JAMA* 1998;280:1569–1575.

98. Sarrell EM, Cohen HA, Kahan E. Naturopathic treatment for ear pain in children. *Pediatrics* 2003;111:e574–e579.

99. Sarrell EM, Mandelberg A, Cohen HA. Efficacy of naturopathic extracts in the management of ear pain associated with acute otitis media. *Arch Pediatr Adolesc Med* 2001;155:796–799.

100. Rao JK, Mihaliak K, Kroenke K, et al. Use of complementary therapies for arthritis among patients of rheumatologists. *Ann Intern Med* 1999;131:409–416.

101. Pittler MH, Brown EM, Ernst E. Static magnets for reducing pain: systematic review and meta-analysis of randomized trials. *CMAJ* 2007 Sep 25;177:736–742.

102. Carter R, Aspy CB, Mold J. The effectiveness of magnet therapy for treatment of wrist pain attributed to carpal tunnel syndrome. *J Fam Pract* 2002;51:38–40.

103. Centers for Disease Control and Prevention (CDC). Gastrointestinal injuries from magnet ingestion in children—United States, 2003–2006. *MMWR Morb Mortal Wkly Rep* 2006 Dec 8;55:1296–1300.

104. Donnelly JP, Huff SM, Lindsey ML, et al. The needs of children with life-limiting conditions: a health care-provider-based model. *Am J Hosp Palliat Care* 2005;22:259–267.

105. Aukst-Margetić B, Jakovljević M, Margetić B, et al. Religiosity, depression, and pain in patients with breast cancer. *Gen Hosp Psychiatry* 2005;27:250–255.

106. Elkin TD, Jensen SA, McNeil L, et al. Religiosity and coping in mothers of children diagnosed with cancer: an exploratory analysis. *J Pediatr Oncol Nurs* 2007;24:274–278.

107. Krebs K. The spiritual aspect of caring—an integral part of health and healing. *Nurs Adm Q* 2001;25:55–60.

108. Woolery A, Myers H, Sternlieb B, et al. A yoga intervention for young adults with elevated symptoms of depression. *Altern Ther Health Med* 2004;10:60–63.

109. Kuttner L, Chambers CT, Hardial J, et al. A randomized trial of yoga for adolescents with irritable bowel syndrome. *Pain Res Manag* 2006;11:217–223.

110. Centers for Disease Control and Prevention (CDC). Trends in childhood cancer mortality—United States, 1990–2004. *MMWR Morb Mortal Wkly Rep* 2007;56:1257–1261.

CHAPTER 50 ■ ACUTE PAIN MANAGEMENT IN CHILDREN

CHRISTINE GRECO AND CHARLES B. BERDE

INTRODUCTION

Nociception alerts the organism to potential or actual sources of harm. Nociceptive functions are active at birth even in preterm neonates, and the experience of pain or pleasure has a powerful impact on learning and neurologic development.[1] Fitzgerald and coworkers,[1] using neurobiological studies in infant rats and psychophysical studies in infant humans, showed that the infant nervous system is in many respects hyperresponsive to noxious stimuli compared to the mature nervous system. Infant rats and humans withdraw their limbs from milder mechanical or thermal stimuli compared to older rats or humans. Infant rats and humans develop hyperalgesia following tissue injury, with evidence for spinal sensitization even in preterm neonates.

While in the 1980s there was a growing acceptance that peripheral and spinal mechanisms of nociceptive are active in preterm and term neonates, controversy persisted regarding maturation of supraspinal mechanisms and regarding how to view pain as conscious experience or suffering in neonates. Recent studies have examined correlates of brain activation using near-infrared spectroscopy, which is sensitive to regional changes in blood flow. A noxious stimulus to the heel (performed for clinically-indicated blood sampling) evoked increased signal overlying the contralateral, but not ipsilateral, cerebral cortex, which has been interpreted as a specific pattern of activation not solely dependent on global changes in autonomic arousal and blood pressure. These and other lines of evidence suggests that painful stimulation reaches the brain in neonates, though they do not per se establish the nature of pain viewed as conscious experience or suffering in neonates. Additional discussion follows later in the chapter regarding potential consequences of either untreated pain or pain treatment in critically ill neonates.[1]

Care of infants and children with acute pain has changed considerably over the past 25 years, and available evidence suggests that undertreatment of acute pain has become less prevalent in economically developed countries over this time period. Changes in practice appear to be the combined result of a series of developments in basic research, in clinical trials, and in advocacy by parents as well as by clinicians, as listed in Table 50.1.

TABLE 50.1

SOME PROMINENT FACTORS POSSIBLY CONTRIBUTING TO INCREASED AWARENESS OF AND TREATMENT OF PAIN IN INFANTS AND CHILDREN OVER THE PAST 25 YEARS

1. Studies demonstrating maturation of nociceptive pathways in infant animals and in infant humans
2. Clinical trials demonstrating improved outcomes of neonates undergoing surgery under adequate anesthesia
3. Pharmacologic studies examining pharmacokinetic, pharmacodynamic, and clinical outcomes of analgesics in infants and children
4. Development of acute pain services in pediatric tertiary centers
5. Advocacy by parents

PAIN ASSESSMENT IN INFANTS AND CHILDREN

Assessing pain in infants and children is a fundamental but challenging aspect of pediatric care. Uniform assessment of pain should be part of the standard of care for hospitals caring for children. Typical adult pain measures are not applicable to preverbal children and young children. Infants and very young children are dependent on adult caregivers to adequately interpret their behavior and other signs in determining whether they have pain. Methods of measuring pain in preverbal patients and in toddlers (ages 2 and 3) generally involve combinations of behavioral observation (including facial expression, crying, limb postures, and consolability) and physiologic parameters (including oxygen saturation and heart rate and a variety of other indices of autonomic arousal). Preschool and early school-aged children (i.e., ages 3 or 4–8) are generally able to give some degree of self-report, and pain scales in this age group add self-report measures to other parameters. Fear and anxiety in children may complicate pain assessment and, in some cases, either overrate or underrate pain. For this reason, many behavioral scales are taken to be measures of "distress," which combines pain, fear, and anxiety. For example, a 2-year-old child fearful of having a relatively painless ear examination may appear to have extreme pain based on behavioral measures. A 7-year-old child may deny pain because of the fear of having to receive a "shot" if he admits to having pain. Valid and reliable pain measures have been developed for children based on developmental levels reflecting a child's ability to communicate and understand concepts of pain. In general, behavioral measures tend to underrate persistent pain relative to self-report.

Pain assessment in infants, neonates, and premature infants is especially challenging. Previously, infants were not thought to be fully capable of experiencing pain which led in part to inadequate efforts of treating pain in infants. Numerous studies have examined the response of neonates and preterm infants to pain and have shown various response patterns including changes in stress hormones levels, observed behavioral responses, and alterations in heart rate, heart rate variability, oxygen saturation, and other physiologic responses.[2-5] Studies have shown that neonates who are subjected to heel lancing for blood sampling consistently swipe the foot being lanced with the unaffected foot, indicating that neonates have the ability to localize to the site of pain.[6,7] Other data have shown that hospitalized infants display graded responses of heart rate, oxygen saturation, mean arterial pressure, and behavioral state with varying degrees of pain intensity, indicating that infants have the ability to distinguish severity of pain.[8] Pain assessment scales for infants are typically composite pain scores consisting of behavioral parameters such as facial grimacing, posture, and crying combined with more objective data such as heart rate, blood pressure, and oxygen saturation. Pain ratings may be erroneous in critically ill infants, since sepsis, hypotension, respiratory failure, and other conditions will change many of the physiologic and behavioral parameters in composite pain scales. The Crying Requires Oxygen Increased Vital Signs Expres-

DATE/TIME						
Crying – Characteristic cry of pain is high pitched. 0 – No cry or cry that is not high pitched 1 – Cry is high pitched but baby is easily consolable 2 – Cry is high pitched but baby is inconsolable						
Requires O2 for SaO2 < 95% - Babies experiencing pain manifest decreased oxygenation. Consider other causes of hypoxemia, e.g., oversedation, atelectasis, pneumothorax. 0 – No oxygen required 1 - < 30% oxygen required 2 - > 30% oxygen required						
Increased vital signs (BP and HR) – Take BP last as this may awaken child making other assessments difficult. 0 – Both HR and BP unchanged or less than baseline 1 – HR or BP increased but increase in < 20% of baseline 2 – HR or BP is increased > 20% over baseline						
Expression – The facial expression most often associated with pain is a grimace. A grimace may be characterized by brow lowering, eyes squeezed shut, deepening nasolabial furrow, or open lips and mouth. 0 – No grimace present 1 – Grimace alone is present 2 – Grimace and non-cry vocalization grunt is present						
Sleepless – Scored based upon the infant's state. 0 – Child has been continuously asleep 1 – Child has awakened at frequent intervals 2 – Child has been awake constantly						
TOTAL SCORE						

FIGURE 50.1 Crying Requires oxygen Increased vital signs Expression Scale (CRIES).

sion Scale (CRIES) scale and the Premature Infant Pain Profile have been validated for infants and premature infants (Figs. 50.1 and 50.2).[9,10]

Concrete thinking and stages of cognitive and language development of preschool-age children can present difficulties in pain assessment. Many toddlers, when ill, hospitalized, or confronted with strangers, refuse to cooperate with self-report or formal testing of pain. Involving parents or other familiar caregivers in the assessment of pain for toddlers can provide useful information. Studies comparing parents' to clinicians' ratings have sometimes shown good agreement, sometimes shown disparities.[11]

The Children's Hospital of Eastern Ontario Pain Scale (CHEOPS) and the Behavioral Observational Pain Scale (BOPS) have been validated for assessing postoperative pain in toddlers and young children.[12,13] The Face Legs Activity Cry Consolability (FLACC) scale is a very widely used scale involving the five items in the title, each scored from 0–2 to give a composite score ranging from 0–10 (Fig. 50.3).[14] The FLACC scale has become widely used because it is quick, versatile, and its components appears reasonable for a wide range of patient groups, including infants and older patients with developmental disabilities.[14,15]

Several validated self-report pain scores have been developed for children 4 years and older, including photos or drawings of faces where numerical anchors signify gradations of pain and a slide rule device where increasing color intensity indicates increasing pain intensity (Figs. 50.4 and 50.5).[16] Young children are able to differentiate pain intensity when presented with facial expressions, although more than five choices of facial expressions interfere with the child's ability to reliably indicate pain. Most older school-age children and adolescents have the cognitive and emotional maturity to use adult numerical visual analogue scales, nevertheless, pain, illness, hospitalization, and separation from

Indicator	Finding	Points
Gestational age	≥ 36 weeks	0
	32 weeks to 35 weeks 6 days	1
	28 weeks to 31 weeks 6 days	2
	< 28 weeks	3
Behavioral state	Active/awake, eyes open, facial movements	0
	Quiet/awake, eyes open, no facial movements	1
	Active/sleep, eyes closed, no facial movements	2
	Quiet/sleep, eyes closed, no facial movements	3
Hear rate maximum	0–4 beats per minute increase	0
	5–14 beats per minute increase	1
	15–24 beats per minute increase	2
	≥ 25 beats per minute increase	3
Oxygen saturation	0 to 2.4% decrease	0
	2.5 to 4.9% decrease	1
	5.0 to 7.4% decrease	2
	7.5 decrease or more	3
Brow bulge	None (≤ 9% of time)	0
	Minimum (10–39% of time)	1
	Moderate (40–69% of time)	2
	Maximum (≥ 70% of time)	3
Eye squeeze	None (≤ 9% of time)	0
	Minimum (10–39% of time)	1
	Moderate (40–69% of time)	2
	Maximum (≥ 70% of time)	3
Nasolabial furrow	None (≤ 9% of time)	0
	Minimum (10–39% of time)	1
	Moderate (40–69% of time)	2
	Maximum (≥ 70% of time)	3

FIGURE 50.2 Premature Infant Pain Scale.

parents cause some older children and teenagers to regress emotionally, making scales used for younger children, such as faces scale, more applicable. There has been considerable dispute regarding relative merits of different presentations of face-type scales.[14,17–21]

ANALGESIC PHARMACOLOGY IN INFANTS AND CHILDREN

Age-related differences in analgesic pharmacology involve a combination of pharmacokinetic and pharmacodynamic factors. Neonates and young children have delayed maturation of hepatic enzymes involved in the metabolism of analgesics such as opioids and amide local anesthetics, increasing the risk of drug accumulation and toxicity. Most neonates and young infants will have considerable maturation of hepatic enzyme systems involved in biotransformation and conjugation by the age of 6 months, although enzyme maturation rates can vary considerably; examples will be cited below. Neonates and young infants have decreased plasma concentrations of albumin and α-1 acid glycoprotein which leads to decreased protein binding and greater concentra-

tions of unbound, pharmacologically active drug. Neonates also have reduced glomerular filtration rates in the first few weeks of life resulting in slower elimination of many renally excreted drugs and many active metabolites of drugs that have undergone hepatic metabolism. A number of specific age-related differences in pharmacokinetics and in drug actions and risks will be detailed with each drug class below.[22,23]

NONOPIOID ANALGESICS

Nonopioid analgesics refer to aspirin, acetaminophen, nonsteroidal anti-inflammatory drugs (NSAIDs), and selective cyclooxygenase (COX-2) inhibitors. Many of these analgesics were thought of as primarily peripherally active; however, analgesia does occur from a combination of peripheral as well as central actions involving inflammatory processes in the spinal cord and brain, especially involving activation of microglia. Nonopioid analgesics are often first-line drugs used for mild–moderate pain in infants and children since they do not produce respiratory effects and are generally nonsedating.

DATE/TIME						
Face						
0 – No particular expression or smile						
1 – Occasional grimace or frown, withdrawn, disinterested						
2 – Frequent to constant quivering chin, clenched jaw						
Legs						
0 – Normal position or relaxed						
1 – Uneasy, restless, tense						
2 – Kicking or legs drawn up						
Activity						
0 – Lying quietly, normal position, moves easily						
1 – Squirming, shifting back and forth, tense						
2 – Arched, rigid or jerking						
Cry						
0 – No cry (awake or asleep)						
1 – Moans or whimpers, occasional complaint						
2 – Crying steadily, screams or sobs, frequent complaints						
Consolability						
0 – Content, relaxed						
1 – Reassured by occasional touching, hugging or being talked to, distractable						
2 – Difficult to console or comfort						
TOTAL SCORE						

FIGURE 50.3 Face Legs Activity Cry Consolability Scale (FLACC).

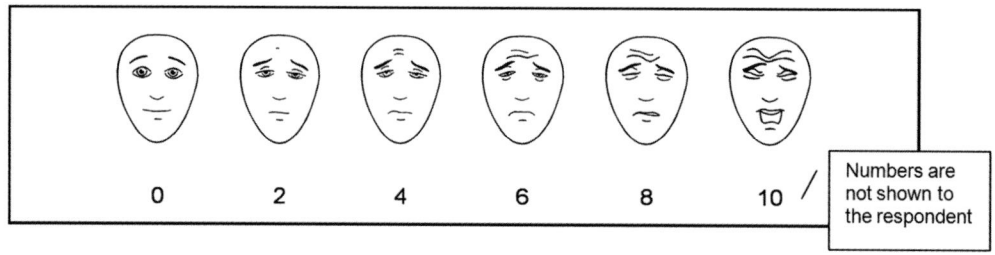

FIGURE 50.4 Faces pain scale. (From Hicks CL, von Baeyer CL, Spafford PA, et al. The Faces Pain Scale-Revised: toward a common metric in pediatric pain measurement. *Pain* 2001;93(2):173–183. Used with permission from IASP®.)

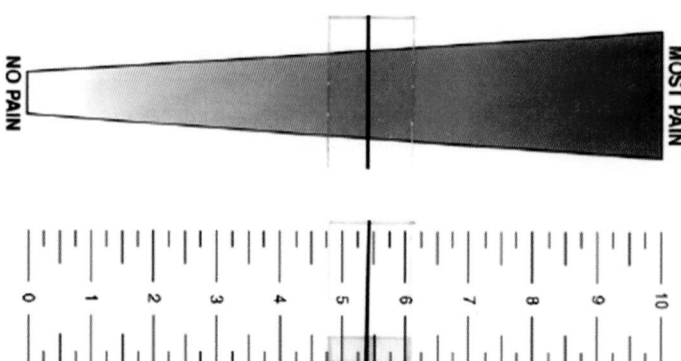

FIGURE 50.5 Color Analogue Scale.

Ontogeny of Prostanoid Biosynthesis and Cyclo-oxygenases

A variety of prostanoids are produced during fetal life, and COX inhibition can alter essential functions, including patency of the ductus arteriosus. Recent studies by Ririe and coworkers[24] in infant rats suggest that COX-mediated processes in spinal microglia are quite immature at birth. These studies raise the question of whether commonly used analgesics acting on COX isoforms might be ineffective in infants due to this delayed maturation of a prominent site of action.

Aspirin and Other Salicylates

The use of aspirin in children has diminished significantly, in part because of its association with Reye Syndrome. The elimination of aspirin is reduced in infants. In our practice, aspirin is almost never prescribed as an analgesic; its use is confined to situations in which antiplatelet actions are required. Nonacetylating salicylates such as choline magnesium salicylate have been used in children with arthritis and other forms of pain. Adult studies indicate that the nonacetylating salicylates are associated with relatively reduced risks of gastropathy and bleeding compared to traditional NSAIDs.[25] Elixir formulations are available.

Acetaminophen

Acetaminophen is the most commonly used analgesic and has been safely used in children of all ages. It is typically used for mild to moderate pain and is commonly combined with opioids to provide additional analgesic effect. The mechanisms underlying acetaminophen's analgesic and antipyretic actions remain controversial. Multiple central targets of acetaminophen's actions have been described, including COX-2 isoenzyme (type 3 as well as type 2) inhibition, on endogenous cannabinoid receptors, and on TRPV1 receptors. Clinically, acetaminophen by itself appears to produce minimal gastropathy, minimal effect on platelet function, and much milder anti-inflammatory actions compared to NSAIDs. Acetaminophen combined with NSAIDs can produce additional analgesic benefits, with synergism in some models, and with potential for exacerbation of some toxicities. For example, in adults chronically receiving NSAIDs, daily administration of higher dose, but not lower dose, acetaminophen increased the relative risk of gastropathy. The elimination of acetaminophen is primarily through glucuronidation and sulfation and elimination rates are similar among infants, children, and adults.[26] Various formulations are available with different concentrations. Inadvertent dosing errors have led to reports of fulminant hepatic failure among infants and children.[27] Typical oral dosing is 10–15 mg/kg/dose. The maximum daily dosing is 40 mg/kg/day for premature infants, 75 mg/kg/day for term infants, and 100mg/kg/day for children. Rectal dosing can be used for children who are unable to tolerate oral dosing, although absorption of rectal dosing can be variable.[28,29] Maximal concentration after rectal dosing occurs at approximately 2–3 hours. Typical rectal dosing is 30–45 mg/kg initially followed by 20 mg/kg every 6 hours.[28,29]

Nonsteroidal Anti-inflammatory Drugs (NSAIDs)

NSAIDs are commonly used for mild–moderate pain and for fever control in children. They are often combined with opioids to augment analgesic efficacy and to potentially reduce opioid use and opioid side effects. The use of several NSAIDs in postsurgical patients has been shown to reduce opioid use by approximately 30% to 40%. NSAIDs produce their anti-inflammatory effect by reversibly inhibiting COX-1 and COX-2 isoforms and inhibiting the conversion of arachidonic acid to prostanoids.[30] The clearance of ibuprofen, ketorolac, and several other NSAIDs is more rapid in toddlers and preschool children compared to adults.[31]

Based on epidemiologic studies and pooled data from clinical trials, NSAIDs have a generally good safety margin in children and in infants from roughly age 6 months onward, particularly with short-term use. The incidence of side effects is quite low in children receiving NSAIDs for postoperative pain relief. A large scale study in children administered short-term use of ibuprofen showed a very low overall risk of severe side effects.[32] The risks of renal and hepatic toxicities are increased in states of decreased renal and hepatic blood flow such as with significant surgical blood loss. There are limited safety data on the use of NSAIDs among neonates and young infants. Indomethacin has been used for closure of patent ductus arteriosis in neonates. Elimination of indomethacin is slower in neonates and has the associated risk of hyponatremia and renal toxicity in this age group.[33] Much of the safety data for long-term use of NSAIDs in children is based on experience in treating juvenile rheumatoid arthritis (JRA.) Long-term use is associated with a higher incidence of mild gastrointestinal distress but significant gastropathy and gastrointestinal bleeding in children is less common when compared to adults.

Although NSAIDs inhibit platelet aggregation and can prolong bleeding time, clinically significant bleeding is uncommon in healthy children. The use of NSAIDS after tonsillectomy procedures remains somewhat controversial. Children requiring tonsillectomy often have obstructive sleep apnea and are at increased risk of hypoventilation and apnea with opioids, making nonopioid analgesics an attractive alternative. Nausea and vomiting are also common after tonsillectomy, and opioids exacerbate these problems. Life-threatening bleeding can occur after tonsillectomy in the immediate postoperative period and for approximately 7–10 days after the patient has been discharged from the hospital. Most individual clinical trials are not sufficiently large to achieve sufficient statistical power to address this risk.[34]

Two meta-analyses came to different conclusions. One found no significant increase in bleeding, while the other reported a three-fold increase in bleeding episodes of sufficient severity to require reoperation.[35,36] While NSAIDs are widely used following tonsillectomy in many centers worldwide, the prevailing practice at this institution is to avoid them before and after this operation.

An additional concern with NSAID use is impaired bone healing after orthopaedic surgeries that involve osteoclast activation and new bone formation. In vitro studies, animal models, and some case-control studies in adults suggest a higher incidence of impaired bone healing and nonunion with NSAID use.

However, compared to adults, children are less likely to have impairment of bone formation with similar orthopaedic procedures. For surgeries requiring a high degree of active bone formation, our view is that it is generally reasonable to avoid NSAIDs. For surgeries with lower risk of nonunion, or for selected patients with greater than average risks or side effects from opioids, judicious use of NSAIDs for brief time periods may be considered.

Selective COX-2 inhibitors were developed with the advantage of a lower incidence of gastrointestinal symptoms and slightly decreased effect on platelet function in randomized control trials in adult patients compared to traditional NSAIDs. The risk of nephropathy with selective COX-2 inhibitors is similar to that of traditional NSAIDs.[37] Anti-inflammatory and analgesic effects of COX-2 inhibitors are also similar to those of traditional NSAIDs. COX-2 inhibitors have been associated with cardiovascular complications in adults with both short-term and long-term use. Rofecoxib and valdecoxib have been withdrawn from the market in response to these reports of cardiovascular complica-

TABLE 50.2

DOSING GUIDELINES FOR NONOPIOID ANALGESICS

	Dose <60 kg	Dose >60 kg
Acetaminophen	10–15 mg/kg q 4 h PO	650–1000 mg q 4 h PO
Naproxen	5 mg/kg q 12 h PO	250–500 mg q 12 h PO
Ibuprofen	6–10 mg/kg q 6–8 h PO	400–600 q 6 h PO
Celecoxib	2–4 mg/kg q 12 h PO	100–200 mg q 12hrs PO
Ketorolac	0.5 mg/kg q6–8 h intravenously, not for >5 d	30 mg q 6–8 h intravenously, not for >5 d

PO, orally; q, every.
Dosing guidelines listed herein refer to children >1 year of age.
Further modifications in dosing are required for use of these agents in term and preterm neonates and in infants. Modifications are detailed in the text.

tions in adults. The cardiovascular risk of COX-2 inhibitors in infants and children remains unclear. The use of COX-2 inhibitors may be considered in children with JRA who experience good analgesia with traditional NSAIDs, but who have significant gastrointestinal symptoms, or in children with bleeding disorders, such as hemophilia, to achieve analgesia with less risk of bleeding than with traditional NSAIDs. Surprisingly, two trials of COX-2 inhibitors for analgesia after tonsillectomy were disappointing. One study found better analgesia with ibuprofen compared to placebo.[38] Some studies suggest that COX-2 inhibitors might be less likely to interfere with active bone formation. Please see Table 50.2 for dosing guidelines of common nonopioid analgesics.

OPIOIDS

Opioids are among the most widely used of analgesics for treating moderate to severe pain in infants and children. As with adults, they are extremely useful, but require careful patient selection, titrated dosing, and active treatment of side effects.

Ontogeny of Opioid Actions

The ontogeny of opioid actions has been studied in human clinical trials, in case series, and in a number of infant animal models. Infant animal models have provided useful information, though there are marked differences among species in opioid actions. Age-related differences in analgesia and side effects involve pharmacokinetics as well as pharmacodynamics. As previously discussed, opioids (except for remifentanil) have prolonged actions in neonates and infants due to immature hepatic enzyme systems and immature renal excretion of active metabolites. Effects of hepatic and renal dysfunction on opioid clearance are discussed in a separate section below. Additional factors that influence opioid pharmacokinetics include developmental changes in expression of P-glycoproteins both in the gastrointestinal tract and in the blood–brain barrier and changes in protein binding.

Pharmacodynamic studies of opioids in neonates and younger infants have examined analgesia and side effects, with a major emphasis on measures of respiratory depression. These studies are made difficult by a number of factors, including the imprecision inherent in observational pain measures in neonates, on the state-dependence of behavioral responses, on the confounding effects of critical illness on measures, and on the variability of painful stimuli. Major sites of opioid actions, including the periaqueductal grey matter and descending pathways, containing the dorsilateral funiculus, appear immature in infant rats. Conversely, opioids administered systemically or via the epidural route show strong analgesic responses in infant rats at developmental stages

corresponding to preterm neonates. In human studies, opioids have given mixed results in studies of procedural pain in neonates, and studies randomly assigning ventilated neonates to receive morphine infusions versus placebo infusions (with both groups receiving morphine for painful procedures) have not shown clear advantages in the morphine infusion groups.[39,40]

Children who are at particular risk for respiratory depressant effects of opioids include those with tonsillar hypertrophy associated with obstructive sleep apnea, children with certain neurologic conditions, and children with craniofacial abnormalities as well as neonates and young infants. Neonates and infants, particularly premature infants, have an increased risk of apnea and hypoventilation in response to opioids on a pharmacodynamic as well as pharmacokinetic basis. Careful dosing, cardiorespiratory monitoring, and close nursing observation are warranted for neonates and younger infants receiving opioids.

Codeine

Codeine is an opioid typically used orally to treat mild–moderate pain; it is available as an elixir and in pill form. For reasons to be detailed below, our opinion is that codeine is in general a suboptimal choice as an analgesic in children in most settings.[41] Codeine is essentially a prodrug: it is extensively metabolized in the liver and a portion of it is demethylated to morphine, which accounts for the analgesic effect.[42] A study of children undergoing surgery receiving a fairly large dose of codeine found that roughly one third of the subjects generated undetectable blood concentrations of morphine, which would result in no discernible analgesic effect. Conversely, there are genotypes associated with ultrarapid metabolism of codeine to morphine; in these subjects, standard recommended codeine doses can produce apnea. Standard dosing is 0.5–1 mg/kg every 4 hours. Dose escalation beyond this range appears to generate a higher incidence of side effects, particularly nausea and vomiting. In standard doses, codeine is a very weak analgesic. Studies in adult patients comparing efficacy of codeine to ibuprofen have shown that 30–45 mg codeine has less analgesic effect than 600 mg of ibuprofen. Because of the relatively high incidence of the impaired inability to demethylate codeine and the higher incidence of side effects, other oral opioids such as oxycodone, morphine, hydromorphone, and hydrocodone are preferred to codeine, especially in patients with moderate–severe pain. Intramuscular codeine has the double disadvantage of being a weak and inconsistent analgesic delivered by a noxious route.

Codeine is often dispensed in combination with acetaminophen to increase efficacy. When prescribing codeine combined with acetaminophen, care is required to avoid inadvertent administration of toxic doses of acetaminophen, particularly when increased dosages are prescribed for pain or when patients are taking other over-the-counter preparations containing acetaminophen. Codeine is also used commonly prescribed as an antitussive.

Oxycodone

Oxycodone can be used for moderate pain in doses of 0.05–0.1 mg/kg every 4 hours and for moderate to severe pain in starting doses of 0.1–0.2 mg/kg every 4 hours. Although historically prescribed in smaller doses, oxycodone dosing can be escalated as needed much like any of the so-called "strong opioids." Oxycodone is generally well-tolerated by children either alone or in combination with acetaminophen. Our impression is that it is associated with fewer side effects than codeine when used to treat moderate–severe pain. Oxycodone is metabolized in the liver to oxymorphone, which is metabolically active.[43] Since oxymorphone is renally eliminated, it can accumulate in patients with renal failure. Oxycodone is commonly used in children postoperatively when transitioning from parenteral opioids to oral opioids in preparation for discharge.

A sustained-release preparation of oxycodone is available for use in the treatment of chronic pain. It has a bioavailability of approximately 60% and reaches peak analgesic effect after 60–90 minutes. Sustained-release oxycodone was originally marketed as a long-acting opioid that would avoid the stigma and addiction potential of other long-duration opioids, such as sustained-release morphine or methadone. Oxycodone is no longer devoid of such stigma, and diversion for abuse has been a major public health issue in the United States.[44]

Morphine

Morphine is often the first-line opioid chosen for parenteral use in children. It has a long track record in pediatrics, has received extensive pharmacologic study at all age groups, is inexpensive, and can be administered via oral, sublingual, intravenous, subcutaneous, rectal, and neuraxial routes.

The duration of morphine's clinical effects are related in a complex manner to distribution into and out of the central nervous system, hepatic metabolism, and excretion of active metabolites, including morphine-6-glucuronide. Morphine primarily undergoes glucuronidation in the liver to morphine-3-glucuronide, which has predominantly excitatory actions, and morphine-6-glucuronide, which has analgesic, sedative, and respiratory depressant actions similar to that of morphine. Since morphine-6-glucuronide is renally eliminated, it can accumulate in patients with renal failure, producing delayed sedation and hypoventilation. In addition, accumulation of morphine-3-glucuronide can contribute to delirium, agitation, and seizures. Other opioids such as fentanyl and methadone should be considered for patients with severely reduced glomerular filtration rate or renal failure. The elimination half-life of morphine in older children and adults is approximately 3–4 hours. The elimination half-life is approximately 7 hours in full-term newborns and even longer in premature infants. Long-acting preparations of morphine are typically used for children with sickle cell pain, cancer pain, and other types of chronic pain.

Dosing of morphine in children, as with all opioids, should be titrated to effect and individualized based on severity of pain, underlying medical conditions, age, side effects, and weight. See Table 50.3 for dosing guidelines for oral and parenteral morphine.

Hydromorphone

Hydromorphone is a commonly used opioid for acute pain management in children for both parenteral and oral use. Like morphine, it is used in children for patient-controlled analgesia (PCA), continuous infusions, oral dosing, intermittent intravenous boluses, and epidural analgesia. Hydromorphone can provide effective analgesia in children with cancer pain and mucositis. In steady-state dosing, hydromorphone is 5–6 times more potent than morphine when given intravenously in children.[45]

While hydromorphone is commonly prescribed to patients with renal insufficiency, this practice is not evidence-based. Hydromorphone is metabolized to glucuronides that can also accumulate in patients with renal insufficiency. Information on metabolism of hydromorphone in neonates and young infants is very sparse.

Methadone

Methadone is a long-acting opioid with a slow elimination and prolonged duration of analgesia.[46,47] The elimination half-life is highly variable, ranging from 6–30 hours. Methadone has a high oral bioavailability of 70% to 100%. Due to these unique properties, methadone is convenient to use as a prolonged duration opioid. Intermittent intravenous dosing at prolonged intervals (e.g., every 4, 6, or 8 hours) can provide a basal level of analgesia similar to that achieved by continuous infusions or frequent intravenous boluses of other opioids.[48]

Methadone is available as an elixir and is often used in place of sustained-release opioid preparations to treat chronic pain in young children or in children unable to swallow pills. Conversely, methadone requires careful titration and vigilance to avoid overdosage, both because of extreme pharmacokinetic variability and for pharmacodynamic reasons detailed below.

Methadone is prepared as a racemic mixture of l- and d-isomers. The l-isomer acts as a μ-receptor agonist; the d-isomer acts as an antagonist at the N-methyl-D-aspartate (NMDA) receptors in the brain and spinal cord. Antagonism at the NMDA receptors results in analgesia and reduced hyperalgesia, as well as partially reversing tolerance to opioids.[49]

The NMDA antagonism of methadone is also a rationale for its use in the treatment of neuropathic pain. The combined μ-agonist and NMDA antagonist actions of methadone result in incomplete cross tolerance. Thus, the dose conversion ratios between methadone and morphine and other mu opioids are different for opioid-naïve versus opioid-tolerant patients. For opioid-naïve patients, the average daily intravenous methadone requirement is roughly one third of the corresponding intravenous morphine requirement; however, average daily methadone requirements for opioid-tolerant patients may be as little as 10% to 15% of the total daily morphine dosing.[50] This is particularly relevant when converting morphine to methadone for children with advanced cancer and when weaning nonventilated infants and children following prolonged opioid therapy, especially following intensive care. Careful titration and frequent patient assessment for respiratory depression is warranted in dosing methadone. For patients showing signs of oversedation or respiratory depression, it is often necessary to hold multiple doses of methadone because of its prolonged duration of action. For opioid-naïve patients, methadone has been used in our practice for acute, postoperative pain management as an every 4 hour "sliding scale" where, following initial loading doses, dosing for little/no pain is 0.025 mg/kg, dosing for moderate pain is 0.05 mg/kg, and dosing for severe pain is 0.075 mg/kg. After the first 24 hours of "sliding scale" dosing, patients can be typically transitioned to a more regular dosing schedule. For adults, there is a very convenient website that rapidly permits equipotent conversions among opioids via multiple routes of administration, with allowances for degrees of opioid tolerance.[51] It remains to be studied whether these conversion ratios are reasonable guides for dosing conversion in children.[52]

TABLE 50.3

INITIAL DOSING GUIDELINES FOR OPIOIDS

Drug	Equianalgesic Doses and Intervals		Parenteral Dosing — Usual Starting Intravenous or Subcutaneous Doses			Oral Dosing — Usual Starting Oral Doses and Intervals	
	Parenteral	Oral	Child <50 kg	Child >50kg	Ratio	Child <50kg	Child >50kg
Codeine	120 mg	200 mg	NR	NR	1:2	0.5–1.0 mg/kg every 3–4 h	30–60 mg every 3–4 h
Morphine	10 mg	30 mg (long-term) 60 mg (single dose)	Bolus: 0.1 mg/kg every 2–4 h; Infusion: 0.03 mg/kg/h	Bolus: 5–8 mg every 2–4 h; Infusion: 1.5 mg/hr	1:3 (long-term) 1:6 (single dose)	Immediate release: 0.3 mg/kg every 3–4 h; Sustained release: 20–35 kg, 10–15 mg every 8–12h; 35–50 kg, 15–30 mg every 8–12 h	Immediate release: 15–20 mg every 3–4 h; Sustained release: 30–45 mg every 8–12 h
Oxycodone	NA	15–20 mg	NA	NA	NA	0.1–0.2 mg/kg every 3–4 h	5–10 mg every 3–4 h
Methadone*	10 mg	10–20 mg	0.1 mg/kg every 4–8 h	5–8 mg every 4–8 h	1:2	0.1–0.2 mg/kg every 4–8 h	5–10 mg every 4–8 h
Fentanyl	100 mg (0.1 mg)	NA	Bolus: 0.5–1.0 mg/kg every 1–2 h; Infusion: 0.5–2.0 mg/kg/h	Bolus: 25–50 mg every 1–2 h; Infusion: 25–100 mg/h	NA	NA	NA
Hydromorphone	1.5–2 mg	6–8 mg	Bolus: 0.02 mg every 2–4 h; Infusion: 0.006 mg/kg/h	Bolus: 1 mg every 2–4 h; Infusion: 0.3 mg/h	1:4	0.04–0.08 mg/kg every 3–4 h	2–4 mg every 3–4 h
Meperidine†	75–100 mg	300 mg	Bolus 0.5–1.0 mg/kg every 2–3 h	Bolus: 50–75 mg every 2–3 h	1:4	2–3 mg/kg every 3–4 h	100–150 mg every 3–4 h

NA, not applicable; NR, not recommended.

Doses are for patients over 6 months of age. In infants under 6 months, initial per kilogram doses should begin at roughly 25% of the per kilogram doses recommended here. Higher doses are often required for patients receiving mechanical ventilation. All doses are approximate and should be adjusted according to clinical circumstances. Recommendations are adapted from previous summary tables, including those of a consensus statement from the World Health Organization and the International Association for the Study of Pain.

*Methadone requires additional vigilance because it can accumulate and produce delayed sedation. If sedation occurs, doses should be withheld until sedation resolves. Thereafter, doses should be substantially reduced, the interval between doses should be extended to 3 to 12 hours, or both.

†The use of meperidine should generally be avoided if other opioids are available, especially with long-term use, because its metabolite can cause seizures.

Adapted from Berder CB, Sethna NF. Analgesics for the treatment of pain in children. *N Engl J Med* 2002;347(14):1094–1103.

Fentanyl

Fentanyl has a rapid onset and brief duration of action after single-dose administration, and it is often used for brief painful procedures in children such as lumbar punctures, bone marrow aspirations, fracture reductions, and dressing changes. Fentanyl is also used for PCA in children with acute and chronic pain and in highly selected situations as a transdermal patch for children with chronic pain.

Fentanyl primarily undergoes glucuronidation in the liver to inactive metabolites, making it a preferred opioid for patients with renal or liver failure. Fentanyl is 50–100 times more potent than morphine with single-dose administration and roughly 30–50 times more potent with continuous infusions. The action of fentanyl after single-dose administration is terminated by rapid redistribution; however, after prolonged infusion or repeated boluses, the termination of fentanyl effect is determined more by elimination than redistribution and results in a prolonged duration of action. Continuous infusions or repeated boluses in neonates can cause a particularly prolonged effect. Rapid administration is associated with glottic and chest wall rigidity, which can be especially pronounced in neonates and young infants. Neuromuscular blockade and assisted ventilation are usually necessary for treatment, particularly in neonates and young infants. Naloxone may sometimes be effective in reversing fentanyl-induced rigidity, but this action is not reliable.

For brief painful procedures, incremental doses of fentanyl at 0.5–1 mcg/kg every 1–3 minutes usually provide effective analgesia. Cardiorespiratory monitoring and immediate availability of airway equipment and personnel skilled in airway management are necessary. Oral transmucosal fentanyl has also been used for brief painful procedures in children and for breakthrough cancer pain. The oral transmucosal dose is partially absorbed across the buccal mucosa and partially swallowed; overall, the bioavailability is approximately 50%. It is generally well-tolerated by children although almost 90% of children experience facial pruritus. Additionally, the peak analgesic effect after a standard 15–20 mcg/kg dose is 30–45 minutes, which may be limiting for some procedures. Transdermal fentanyl is used in children with cancer pain and other forms of chronic pain requiring regular opioid dosing. It is indicated in a small subgroup of children who are unable to swallow pills, who have limited intravenous access, or for children who have experienced side effects with a number of other opioids. Approximately 12–24 hours are necessary to achieve steady state plasma levels after applying the transdermal fentanyl patch, and it is therefore not indicated for acute fluctuations in pain intensity. Additional short-acting opioids are necessary to treat breakthrough pain. Transdermal fentanyl is indicated for opioid-tolerant patients who have relatively constant pain. Adverse events have been reported among opioid-naïve patients who were treated with transdermal fentanyl for acute post-surgical pain. There has been a series of manufacturing problems that have led to inconsistent delivery for some batches of transdermal fentanyl. We emphasize here that transdermal fentanyl is not recommended for opioid-naïve patients.[53]

Meperidine

Meperidine is a synthetic opioid roughly one tenth the potency of morphine when administered intravenously. It has some anticholinergic actions as well. It is metabolized to normeperidine which can cause seizures, hallucinations, and agitation, particularly with repeated dosing. Metabolism in infants is quite variable.[54] Life-threatening reactions can occur with the use of meperidine in patients taking monoamineoxidase inhibitors, leading to hyper-reflexia, seizures, hemodynamic instability, and death.

Meperidine does have the unique property in subanalgesic doses of treating rigors associated with blood product transfusions or shivering following general anesthesia. Because of the serious adverse effects of meperidine and because it offers no particular advantage for pain control, its use should generally be limited to the treatment of rigors or shivering.

OPIOID ADMINISTRATION IN INFANTS AND CHILDREN

As in adult patients, there are several means for systemic opioid delivery in pediatric patients. The choice of which method depends to a certain extent on available resources, coexisting medical conditions, types of pain, patients' mobility, and other factors.

Regardless of method of opioid delivery, protocols for safe opioid administration should be in place to detect excess sedation, signs of respiratory depression, and impending respiratory failure. Protocols should include regular nursing assessments, documentation of vital signs and levels sedation, and, where appropriate, use of electronic cardiorespiratory monitoring. Patients who should be considered for cardiorespiratory monitoring include infants who are younger than 6 months, infants who have a history of apnea and bradycardia or prematurity, and opioid-naïve children who require a continuous opioid infusion. Children at increased risk for airway obstruction while receiving opioids such as those with tonsillar hypertrophy and obstructive sleep apnea or children with craniofacial abnormalities should also be considered for cardiorespiratory monitoring. There is considerable variation in practices regarding methods to detect and prevent opioid-induced respiratory depression. Many recommendations are based on reasonable extrapolation from physiologic considerations. Nevertheless, evidence to quantify the risk reduction from specific forms of monitoring is quite sparse.

Intermittent Intravenous Bolus Dosing

In clinical care areas other than the intensive care units or the postanesthesia care units, in our institution, most intermittent bolus dosing of opioids are administered as an infusion over 20 minutes rather than "intravenous push." Although a slow administration is thought of as a somewhat safer method of intermittent dosing, careful monitoring and repeated patient assessments remain important during and after the opioid infusion. Intermittent systemic boluses cause wide fluctuations in plasma opioids concentrations. Patients therefore experience probably few side effects but increased pain just prior to their next bolus opioid dose. After the dose is administered, patients experience pain relief often with excessive side effects as the plasma–opioid concentration reaches supratherapeutic levels. To avoid wide variations in plasma concentrations with resultant fluctuations in analgesia and side effects, continuous infusions and PCA are commonly used.

Continuous Opioid Infusions

Continuous opioid infusions offer the advantage of providing steady state plasma levels and results in good analgesia in infants and children who experience relatively constant levels of pain intensity. Additional intermittent boluses are necessary for periods of increased pain, such as endotracheal tube suctioning or chest physiotherapy. Recommended starting infusion rates have been adjusted for age, based on both pharmacokinetic considerations, on studies of respiratory responses, and on clinical outcome studies. Starting infusion rates for morphine have been recommended as around 0.025 mg/kg/hour for children and infants >6 months of age, with reductions to 0.015 mg/kg/hour from 1–6 months, ranging down to 0.005 mg/kg/hour for preterm neonates at 32 weeks postconception. These recommendations should be taken as population averages; individual rates should be adjusted according to clinical conditions, expected intensity of painful stimuli, and behavioral and physiologic signs.

Patient, Nurse, and Parent-Controlled Analgesia

PCA is widely used among pediatric centers for variety of acute painful conditions such as cancer pain, sickle cell pain from vaso-occlusive crises, and acute postoperative pain. Most children 6 years of age and older have the cognitive ability to understand cause and effect relationships of pushing the PCA button and obtaining pain relief. In rare cases, experienced children younger than 6 who have had long-standing pain are able to use PCA. For most children younger than 6 years, PCA has a higher failure rate, in part because of a lack of development of understanding of a causal connection between button-pressing and delivery of medication to provide pain relief. However, nurse-controlled analgesia (NCA) has been shown to provide effective analgesia with good patient, parent, and caregiver satisfaction in younger children. NCA is also used for children with cognitive and physical limitations who are unable to use the PCA.[55–57] In our hospital, NCA is the most common method of systemic opioid administration following major surgery in infants and in children with cognitive or physical limitations to self-administration.

Commonly used opioids for PCA/NCA are morphine, hydromorphone, and fentanyl. Use of a basal infusion along with PCA boluses has been a subject of controversy and some controlled studies in adults and children. In some studies, a basal infusion improves pain scores, patient satisfaction, and the quality of nighttime sleep. In other studies, a basal infusion increased surrogate measures of hypoventilation, including brief respiratory pauses. Our view is that the recommendations regarding addition of a basal infusion depend on patient medical conditions and risk factors, on psychologic factors, on expected intensity of painful stimuli, and on history of previous opioid use. For example, we commonly omit a basal infusion for children who have received a regional block intraoperatively, for children with increased respiratory risks, or for those undergoing surgical procedures expected to be only moderately, but not severely, painful. Conversely, we generally include a basal infusion for patients who are opioid tolerant or those with pain due to cancer or sickle cell disease, and in these subjects we generally aim to adjust the basal infusion to provide at least 50% of daily opioid requirements. For those undergoing very painful operations, such as scoliosis surgery, open lateral thoracotomy, or major hip surgery, we generally maintain a basal infusion at least through the first postoperative night.

Parent-controlled analgesia is widely accepted for use among children with advanced cancer or children in palliative care. However, use in the setting of acute postoperative pain or opioid-naïve children is controversial. There have been several serious adverse events reported, including apnea and death with the use of parent-controlled analgesia in children with risk factors and with insufficient protocols for patient observation. Our view is that parent-controlled analgesia for opioid-naïve children should be restricted to institutions which have formal programs for parent education, protocols for frequent assessments by nurses, and protocols for cardio-respiratory monitoring. Please see Table 50.4 for PCA dosing.

TABLE 50.4

TYPICAL STARTING DOSES FOR PATIENT-CONTROLLED ANALGESIA

Drug	Bolus dose (μg/kg)	Continuous rate (μg/kg/h)	4-hour limit (μg/kg)
Morphine	20	4–15	300
Hydromorphone	5	1–3	60
Fentanyl	0.25	0.15	4

The usual lockout interval is 7 minutes.

Treatment of Opioid Side Effects

Opioids are alike in that all produce side effects including nausea, vomiting, constipation, pruritus, urinary retention, respiratory depression, and sedation. In some cases, severe side effects are as distressing to children as pain. Although children may have particular side effects with individual opioids, there are few data to suggest that side effects differ greatly among the more commonly used opioids.

Kehlet[58] and others have argued for multimodal approaches to postoperative analgesia that emphasize opioid-sparing, in part because of the detrimental impact of opioid side effects on the course of postoperative recovery.

There is an important role for standardized protocols for treatment of opioid side effects and for rapid institution of therapy for many patients. Nevertheless, along with prompt intervention, there is a role for clinical assessment and for consideration of a differential diagnosis. Two examples: (1) a patient may be itching due to opioids, but could also have itching as part of an allergic response to a variety of other medications or physiologic processes, and (2) a patient with advanced cancer, worsening back pain, and increasing opioid dosing may have urinary retention due to the opioid, but urinary retention could also be a harbinger of impending compression of the spinal cord or caudal equina. Clinicians need to balance prompt intervention with consideration of alternative diagnoses underlying these symptoms.

Opioid side effects occur by actions at both peripheral and central sites. For example, opioid-induced nausea and vomiting involves activation of receptors in the brainstem, as well as in the gastrointestinal tract.[59] Similarly, some opioids may produce itching by peripheral histamine release, but the observation of profound itching with very small doses of intrathecal morphine supports the view that a predominant mechanism of opioid-induced itching is neurogenic and central, involving an imbalance of afferent signaling and neurotransmission in the spinal dorsal horn and nucleus caudalis.

Traditionally, treatment of opioid side effects has emphasized antagonists at nonopioid-receptors such as the use of antagonists of dopamine or serotonin receptors for treatment of nausea and vomiting or use of antihistamines for treatment of itching. These drugs may generate their own side effects, including extra pyramidal reactions from dopamine antagonists (phenothiazines, butyrophenones, metoclopramide), headache from serotonin antagonists (ondansetron, granisetron), and sedation, constipation, and urinary retention from antihistamines (diphenhydramine, hydroxyzine). Extra pyramidal reactions from dopamine antagonists may be prophylaxed or treated with antihistamines or central muscarinic anticholinergics, though prophylactic coadministration of antihistamines further complicates management In our experience, extrapyramidal reactions may be misdiagnosed by some clinicians as seizures. Even among patients who do not have overt extrapyramidal signs, occasional patients report extreme dysphoria following administration of these agents. Dopamine antagonists and serotonin antagonists are partially effective in treatment of opioid-induced nausea and vomiting, but the numbers-needed-to-treat are higher than commonly believed by clinicians. The evidence for effectiveness of antihistamines in the treatment of opioid-induced itching is quite weak.[60] Local hives or itching at a site of opioid injection does not imply an allergic response.

There is a growing body of evidence supporting treating opioid side-effects, especially nausea, vomiting, and itching, at least in inpatients postoperatively, by ultra-low dose infusions of opioid antagonists such as naloxone.[61] Low dose naloxone infusions are not simply reversing opioid actions altogether, rather they are exploiting a differential dose response for reversing side effects versus reversing analgesia, in part due to differential binding to opioid receptors coupled to G-stimulatory versus G-inhibitory proteins. We could not identify studies that would guide low dose naloxone infusions for side effect treatment in highly opioid-tolerant patients, though a preliminary report in patients with sickle cell disease suggested that a slightly higher naloxone infusion rate of 1 mcg/kg/hour might be recommended.[62] Nalbuphine is widely used for treatment of opioid-induced itching and nausea, though one pediatric study showed no benefit compared to placebo.[63]

A related approach is to design opioid antagonists that are constrained to different body compartments. Methylnaltrexone is a quaternized opioid antagonist that has access to the area postrema (which lacks a blood brain barrier), but which is excluded from prominent sites of central analgesic action, such as the periaqueductal grey matter. Alvimopan is an enterally constrained opioid antagonist that blocks opioid actions in the gastrointestinal tract, with minimal uptake in the portal vein and efficient first-pass hepatic clearance of the small quantities that do reach the liver. Available evidence suggests that these two approaches hold promise for more effective treatment of opioid side effects, including nausea, vomiting, constipation, and other forms of postoperative gastrointestinal dysfunction. Pediatric studies are unavailable.

Constipation is commonly seen in patients requiring opioids even for short-term use. It is such a prevalent side effect of opioids that one should consider a proactive approach of prescribing laxatives for patients expected to require more than just few doses of opioids. Please see Table 50.5 for management of common opioid side effects in children.

Local Anesthetics and Regional Anesthesia in Infants and Children

Local anesthetics are widely used for a range of indications in infants and children, including topical analgesia for needle procedures, cutaneous infiltration for minor procedures, wound infiltration for surgery, peripheral and plexus blocks, and epidural and spinal anesthesia and analgesia. Work over the past 30 years has examined pharmacokinetics, safety, and clinical outcomes of local anesthesia in infants and children.

Pharmacokinetic information is available for many of the commonly used local anesthetics. Amino amides, including lidocaine, bupivacaine, and ropivacaine, have reduced clearance in neonates and younger infants due to immaturity of hepatic metabolism. In the case of lidocaine, the predominant hepatic metabolite, MEGX, can accumulate in neonates, with a resultant risk of seizures. The amino ester chloroprocaine is rapidly metabo-

TABLE 50.5

MANAGEMENT OF COMMON OPIOID SIDE EFFECTS

Side effect	Comments	Drug dosage
Nausea	Consider switching to different opioid Use antimetics Exclude other processes (e.g., bowel obstruction)	Ondansetron 10–30 kg: 1–2 mg intravenously q 8 h >30 kg: 2–4 mg intravenously q 8 h Naloxone infusion 0.25–1 mcg/kg/h Metoclopramide 0.1–0.2 mg/kg PO/intravenously q 6 h
Pruritus	Exclude other causes (e.g., drug allergy) Consider switching to different opioid Use antipruritics	Nalbuphine 10–20 mg/kg/dose intravenously q 6 h Naloxone infusion 0.25–1 mcg/kg/h Diphenhydramine 0.25–0.5 mg/kg PO/intravenously q 6h
Sedation	Add nonsedating analgesic (e.g., ketorolac) and reduce opioid dose Consider switching to different opioid	Methylphenidate 0.05–0.2 mg/kg PO bid (morning and midday dosing) Dextroamphetamine 5–10 mg every day
Constipation	Regular use of stimulant and stool softener laxatives	Naloxone infusion 0.25–1 mcg/kg/h Ducosate Child: 10–40 mg PO daily Adults: 50–200 mg PO daily Dulcolax Child: 5 mg PO/PR daily Adult: 10 mg PO/PR daily Methylnaltrexone, alvimopam dosing is extrapolated from adults

bid, twice a day; PO, orally; PR, rectally; q, every

lized by plasma esterases even in neonates and may be useful if prolonged infusions are required in neonates.[64]

Cutaneous Analgesia

Needle procedures are a prominent source of distress for infants and children. A number of local anesthetic formulations can produce good analgesia for superficial needle procedures. Several approaches can accelerate transfer across the skin, including eutectic mixtures, heating elements, iontophoresis, and jet injection. Selection among approaches may depend in part on local availability, cost, desired onset time, and impact of vasodilatation or vasoconstriction on the planned procedures.[65,66]

Wound Infiltration

Infiltration of the layers of surgical wounds is a simple approach to providing postoperative analgesia. This may be accomplished by one-time infiltration before wound closure or by placement of wound catheters for prolonged infusions of local anesthetics. With single injection of currently available local anesthetics, duration of analgesia is rarely longer than 4–6 hours. (Disclaimer: one of the authors [CBB] conducts research on the development of prolonged-duration local anesthetics.)

EPIDURAL ANALGESIA IN INFANTS AND CHILDREN

Epidural analgesia has widespread use in infants and children for postoperative pain management, and can be considered in selected cases for children with cancer pain, and for certain chronic pain conditions such as complex regional pain syndrome. While epidural infusions can provide outstanding analgesia for children, they require specific expertise both in the techniques of placement and in management, and in our view they should not be undertaken without a system of pediatric-specific management protocols.

A unique difference between adults and children concerns the fact that most pediatric regional anesthesia, including epidural analgesia, is performed after induction of general anesthesia or sedation, since many children will not tolerate having some needle procedures while awake. While the safety track record of placement of epidural needles and catheters has been good in several published pediatric case series, there remains some controversy regarding the risk-benefit ratio.[67–69]

Placing a lumbar epidural catheter in an anesthetized child is generally considered to be safe among experienced pediatric anesthesia providers. There is more controversy over direct needle placement of thoracic epidurals in anesthetized children, particularly in infants. As an alternative to direct thoracic needle placement in infants, a common technique is to advance an epidural catheter from the caudal space to the desired surgical dermatome. Several studies have shown success in placing thoracic epidural catheters in infants using this technique.[70] Since neonates and infants have an increased risk of amide local anesthetic toxicity, proper placement of the epidural catheter tip is crucial in order to provide optimal analgesia while using safe local anesthetic infusion rates.

For anesthetized patients who are receiving direct thoracic placement or for cephalad advancement of catheters to thoracic levels from the caudal route, our own strong personal preference is to encourage some method of objective confirmation of positioning whenever possible. Three methods can be used in different situations: (1) electrical nerve stimulation using Tsui's technique,[71](2) radiographic confirmation, especially using fluoros-

copy, and (3) ultrasound. Confirming the location of intended caudal-to-thoracic epidural catheter tip placement is strongly recommended since failure rates as high as 30% have been reported using a "blind" technique. As described by Tsui,[71] electrical stimulation employs a saline-filled, wire-wrapped catheter, with twitches seen at the myotomal level of the catheter tip in a current range generally between 2 and 15 mA. This technique also confirms that a catheter is not subarachnoid (in which case, bilateral twitches in a broad distribution are seen at a current <0.5–1 mA) and not threaded out from a nerve root foramen (in which case unilateral twitches in a narrow distribution may be seen at a current <1.5 mA). In brief, as catheters are advanced cephalad, one sees the following progression of twitches: ankle dorsi- or plantar-flexion (lumbosacral junction), knee extension (mid-lumbar), hip flexion (upper lumbar), abdominal or flank muscle contractions without hip flexion (thoracic above T12), intercostal muscle contractions (midthoracic), and hand twitches (around C8–T1).

Our experience with combined use of nerve stimulation and fluoroscopy also suggests that Tsui's[71] method gives a reasonable prediction of sidedness. If we are placing an epidural for one-sided surgery (e.g., hip osteotomy or lateral thoracotomy), we are comfortable with bilateral twitches, or preferentially ipsilateral twitches, but our practice is to reposition the catheter if the twitches are predominantly wrong-sided. Studies in adults and our own experience suggest that sidedness matters to clinical effectiveness.[72]

Confirming location of the epidural catheter tip in infants can be accomplished by obtaining a chest radiograph after injecting a small volume of radiocontrast dye or through the use of a radio-opaque epidural catheter which can easily be seen on plain chest radiograph or fluoroscopy. An additional method of confirming epidural catheter tip location is to advance the catheter from the caudal space under direct visualization using fluoroscopy.

Ultrasound guidance can be used in guiding and confirming placement of epidural catheters in neonates and younger infants, though this technique requires two operators and significant experience in ultrasound techniques. Neuraxial structures, such as ligamentum flavum, dura, and epidural space, as well as depth from skin to epidural space, can be clearly visualized using ultrasound, in part because of incomplete ossification of the vertebrae in neonates and younger infants.[73]

In clinical areas outside of the operating room, it is sometimes necessary to check position of an epidural catheter when patients appear to be uncomfortable despite generally adequate rates of continuous epidural infusions. This can be particularly challenging in infants and preverbal patients. One method is to inject a small volume of approximately 0.5 mL of radiocontrast dye into the epidural catheter which then can be detected on plain radiograph. Another method that we use frequently in our institution is a "chloroprocaine test" as detailed below.

Drugs and Drug Dosing Used for Epidural Analgesia

Continuous epidural analgesia in infants and children generally consists of dilute solutions of local anesthetics combined with fentanyl, hydromorphone, or α2 agonists such as clonidine.

Bupivacaine is the most commonly used amide local anesthetic for epidural analgesia because it has long duration of action with slightly greater selectivity of sensory block compared to motor block. Pharmacokinetic studies of bupivacaine in children over the age of 6 months have reported good safety for infusion rates of bupivacaine of below 0.4 mg/kg/hour with plasma bupivacaine levels in a safe range of <2–3 μg/mL.[74] Neonates have reduced clearance of bupivacaine; pharmacokinetic studies in neonates receiving continuous bupivacaine infusions have shown a continuous rise in plasma bupivacaine levels after the first 48 hours.

As a result of various pharmacokinetic studies, we use a maximum dose of 0.4 mg/kg/hour of bupivacaine for continuous epidural infusions in children over the age of 6 months. For children less than 4–6 months of age, we restrict the dose of bupivacaine to 0.2 mg/kg/hour. Because of the limitations in dosing of bupivacaine in young infants, it is reasonable to use adjuvants to epidural infusions which will have a synergistic effect with bupivacaine such as opioids and clonidine in order to maximize analgesia.

Ropivacaine is a long-acting amide local anesthetic shown in adults to have less central nervous system and cardiac toxicity and slightly more sensory selectivity when compared to bupivacaine. Pharmacokinetic studies in infants and children receiving single boluses of epidural ropivacaine show that as with bupivacaine, clearances for ropivacaine are reduced in infants. In different studies, clearances for ropivacaine have ranged from around 4–8.5 mL • min-1 • kg-1 with generally lower values in younger infants. Data to support a less extensive motor block for ropivacaine have been mixed. Overall, infusion rates of 0.4 mg/kg/hour in older infants and children and 0.2–0.3 mg/kg/hour in neonates and younger infants appear quite safe. It is plausible that slightly higher rates than these will be shown to be safe as well.[75–77]

Chloroprocaine is used as an alternative to amide local anesthetics for continuous epidural infusions in neonates and very young infants to avoid the limitations of reduced clearance of amide local anesthetics and to safely permit sufficient epidural infusion rates for optimal analgesia. Even in neonates, chloroprocaine is rapidly metabolized with an elimination half-life of less than 6 minutes, making it an attractive choice for continuous epidural infusions in neonates. Studies of continuous epidural chloroprocaine infusions in term and preterm infants have shown good sensory blockade with no signs of neurotoxicity.[64]

Compared to infusions of ropivacaine or bupivacaine, higher weight-scaled infusion rates of chloroprocaine are required to achieve similar degrees of blockade. For preterm and term infants, we use 1.5% chloroprocaine infused at around 0.5 mL/kg/hour for midthoracic epidural catheters and 0.6–0.7 mL/kg/hour for lumbar and lower thoracic catheters. Even for neonates, our preference is to include additives in most of these infusions, but at roughly a ten-fold lower concentration compared to those recommended above for infusions used for older children with bupivacaine or ropivacaine. For example, fentanyl is often included at a concentration of 0.2 mcg/mL and clonidine is often included at a concentration of 0.04 mcg/mL.

We also use chloroprocaine to test previously placed epidural catheters as a second loading dose. The rationale for using chloroprocaine rather than lidocaine or other amide local anesthetics for a second loading dose is based on the concern that since most patients will have had intraoperative infusions of amide local anesthetics, additional amide local anesthetics as a bolus test dose may cause serum amide local anesthetic levels to reach toxic levels. Injecting approximately 0.5 mL/kg of 3% chloroprocaine (up to a maximum total dose of around 18 mLs for patients >50 kg) incrementally into the epidural catheter should result in some evidence of sensory and motor block, thereby confirming position of the catheter in the epidural space. If the patient is tachycardic or hypertensive due to pain, then these parameters generally trend more toward normal values within 5–10 minutes if the catheter is in an epidural location, and the patient shows behavioral signs of improved analgesia. Once proper position of the epidural catheter has been confirmed, then good analgesia should be able to be obtained through the use of appropriate epidural solutions and infusion rates. In many cases, if the chloroprocaine test shows epidural positioning, a next step would be to give a small loading dose of epidural hydromorphone (e.g., about 5 mcg/kg), followed by addition of hydromorphone to the subsequent epidural infusion. Because of its hydrophilicity and cephalad spread, hydro-

morphone can help rescue a situation in which the catheter tip is at a level below the dermatomal level of the surgery.

Neuraxially-administered opioids have a synergistic analgesic effect when combined with local anesthetics. Due to the hydrophilic property of hydromorphone, there is a slight preference to using hydromorphone for postoperative analgesia for more extensive surgical procedures involving several dermatomes. However, due to more rostral spread of hydromorphone, the risk of respiratory depression is greater, and generally we restrict the use of epidural hydromorphone to infants over the age of 4 months, or to younger infants with considerable degrees of opioid tolerance. Fentanyl and hydromorphone are most commonly used for epidural analgesia since epidural morphine offers no particular advantage but may be associated with higher incidence of side effects. All neuraxially-administered opioids can cause side effects including nausea, vomiting, urinary retention, pruritus, sedation, respiratory depression, and constipation. The incidence of vomiting in patients receiving epidural fentanyl has been reported to be between 28% and 52% depending on the population studied and concentration of epidural fentanyl. Nausea, vomiting, and other side effects from epidural opioids are treated much in the same way that side effects from parenteral opioids are treated. Low-dose naloxone infusions significantly reduce opioid side effects without reversing opioid-induced analgesia; the recommended starting dose for naloxone in treating opioids-induced nausea or pruritus is 0.25 μg/kg/hour, though higher naloxone infusion rates are currently under study.

Clonidine is often added to epidural local anesthetic infusions to enhance analgesia without increasing nausea, vomiting, pruritus, or respiratory depression. Studies of combinations of epidural clonidine with local anesthetics in children have shown a low side effect profile.[78]

Controlled trials of single doses of clonidine administered caudally with bupivacaine have showed variable prolongation of analgesia by approximately 50% to 75% than epidural bupivacaine alone. Pharmacokinetic studies of single-dose epidural clonidine in children show wide variation in plasma concentration as well as wide variation in the time for clonidine absorption from the epidural space. Increasing a single dose of epidural clonidine from 1–5 μg/kg with local anesthetics to local anesthetics alone in children 1 year of age and older showed variable prolongation of analgesia, greater sedation without respiratory depression, and reductions in heart rate and blood pressure which were not clinically significant. Other studies have not shown significant prolongation of single-shot caudal analgesia with clonidine doses as high as 2 mcg/kg.[79]

While some clinicians perform single-shot caudal blocks routinely with clonidine doses in the range of 2 mcg/kg, our view is that this dose frequently results in prolonged sedation, especially if other sedatives or systemic opioids are administered as well. Our practice for children 1 year of age and older is to use 0.5–1 μg/kg, to a maximum of 15 μg as a single-bolus for caudal blocks and roughly 0.12–0.16 μg/kg/hour (0.3–0.4 mL/kg/hour of a solution containing 0.4 mcg/mL) added to continuous epidural local anesthetic infusions (except for neonates, where lower doses and concentrations are used, as noted above). Please see Table 50.6 for recommended doses for epidural infusions.

PERIPHERAL NERVE BLOCKS IN CHILDREN

Peripheral nerve blocks (PNB) provide reliable and safe postoperative pain management. A report by the French Language Society of Pediatric Anesthesiologists showed that among 24,000 regional blocks in children, the complication rate for PNB was 0 in 1000.[68]

In a retrospective review of 339 continuous PNBs in children

TABLE 50.6

RECOMMENDED EPIDURAL INFUSION RATES

Solution	(mL/kg/hr)*		
	<1 month	1–4 months	>4 months †
Bupivacaine 0.1% +/− Fentanyl 2 mCg/mL +/− Clonidine 0.4 mCg/mL	rarely used	0.2	0.4
Ropivacaine 0.1% +/− Fentanyl 2 mCg/mL +/− Clonidine 0.4 mCg/mL	rarely used	0.3	0.4–0.5
Bupivacaine 0.1% + hydromorphone 10 mCg/mL	rarely used	rarely used	0.3–0.4
Ropivacaine 0.1% + hydromorphone 10 mCg/mL	rarely used	rarely used	0.3–0.4
Chloroprocaine 1.5% + Fentanyl 0.2 mCg/mL +/− Clonidine 0.04 mCg/mL	0.5 (mid thoracic) 0.6–0.7 (lumbar and low thoracic)	0.5 (mid thoracic) 0.6–0.7 (lumbar and low thoracic)	rarely used rarely used

*Infusion rates and solutions should be modified according to clinical circumstances. Little information is available on how best to adjust these rates based on degrees of prematurity.
Rates shown reflect upper end of usual infusion rates, based largely on both systemic accumulation of local anesthetics and on expected extent of sensory and/or motor blockade. Solutions containing hydrophilic opioids such as hydromorphone may pose a higher risk for delayed respiratory depression, so appropriate frequency of observation and continuous electronic monitoring is recommended. Higher concentrations of opioids may be considered for selected patients who are opioid tolerant.
†Weight scaled infusion rates should plateau at values recommended for patients weighing around 45 kg, such as maximum infusion rates for larger patients should rarely exceed 15 mL/hr.

over a 4 year period, no major adverse events were noted. Forty-five percent had minor adverse events; most commonly catheter leakage or dislodgement and nausea and vomiting. Two patients were noted to have fever and local inflammatory signs, however culture of the catheter was negative for both patients. Only 1.6% reported failure of pain relief. A general trend in clinical trials of PNB is the observation of very good analgesia with a very low side effect profile that compares favorably to either systemic opioids or epidural infusions. In a randomized trial comparing popliteal block versus epidural analgesia for foot and ankle surgery, popliteal block resulted in superior analgesia with reduced incidences of nausea, vomiting, and urinary retention.[80]

The use of ultrasound has been shown in some studies to increase the duration of analgesia with reduced volumes of local anesthetic solutions.[81] Advantages of ultrasound guidance include direct visualization of nerves and other structures such as arteries which may reduce the likelihood of intraneural or intravascular injection and direct visualization of local anesthetic spread. Combining the use of ultrasound with peripheral nerve stimulation is sometimes used when advancing catheters for continuous use to further confirm catheter placement. The addition of clonidine to PNBs in children has been shown to significantly increase duration of sensory blockade by approximately 4 hours; however, the incidence of motor blockade was also significantly increased.[82]

Like epidural anesthesia, the placement of PNB may require general anesthesia or deep sedation for most younger children. Motivated older children and adolescents will often require only minimal sedation; it is often helpful to apply a topical anesthetic to the anticipated needle insertion site to minimize pain from needle insertion. Indications for using peripheral nerve blocks as the sole anesthetic technique include risk of malignant hyperthermia, risk of postoperative apnea, and patient preference.

Recommendations regarding dosing of local anesthetics for PNB in children vary among authors. Where immediate onset is required, one group has recommended 0.5 cc/kg of a mixture of 1% lidocaine with 1:200,000 epinephrine and 0.5% ropivacaine. Several groups employ continuous perineural infusions with 0.1–0.15 mL/kg/hour of ropivacaine in a concentration range between 0.1% to 0.2%.

Supraclavicular

A supraclavicular block is applicable to all surgeries of the upper extremity excluding shoulder surgery. A continuous catheter technique is often used in the treatment of complex regional pain syndrome in children. Supraclavicular block has been successfully used as the sole anesthetic for children younger than 12 years of age undergoing closed reduction of arm fractures.[83] (Using 1.5% lidocaine with epinephrine, the mean time to sensory blockade was 2.3 minutes with duration of block 3.5 hours).

The trunks of the brachial plexus are located between the anterior and medial scalene muscles in the interscalene groove. Using ultrasound guidance, the first rib and subclavian artery should be located, with the pleura located just beneath the first rib. The anterior and middle scalene muscles are then located as they insert onto the first rib cephalad to the subclavian artery. The brachial plexus is located between the anterior and middle scalene muscles and superficial and lateral to the subclavian artery. Under direct ultrasound visualization, the needle is inserted from a lateral to medial direction toward the plexus, with particular attention to avoiding directing the needle medial to the anterior scalene muscles or caudally beneath the first rib to prevent pneumothorax. Only a single injection is required due to the close proximity of the trunks of the plexus in this region. If using a continuous catheter technique, we typically recommend tunnelling supraclavicular catheters, particularly for patients requiring aggressive postoperative physical therapy and for catheters of longer duration such as in the treatment of complex regional pain syndrome.

Infraclavicular

Infraclavicular block is indicated for all distal upper extremity surgeries such as syndactyly repair and repairs of open forearm fractures. In the infraclavicular region, the plexus is located posterior to the pectoralis major and minor. The cords of the brachial plexus are located medial, lateral, and posterior to the axillary artery. Under direct ultrasound visualization with the ultrasound probe medial and caudal to the coracoid process, the pectoralis muscles and the axillary artery and vein should be identified. The axillary vein is located caudal to the axillary artery. The needle is inserted under direct ultrasound visualization and advanced laterally; once the sheath surrounding the plexus is reached, spread of local anesthetic should be visualized spreading to the cords of the plexus.

Sciatic Nerve Block

The sciatic nerve block is useful in providing analgesia for a variety of surgical procedures of the of lower leg or foot, for painful physical therapy following surgery, and for treatment of complex regional pain syndrome affecting the lower leg or foot. One study showed excellent pain relief and excellent rehabilitation with no adverse events using a continuous infusion of 0.2% ropivacaine at 0.1 mL/kg/hour for 96 hours.[84]

In the study of foot and ankle surgery by Dadure et al.,[84] the children with continuous popliteal nerve blocks received a continuous infusion of 0.2% ropivacaine at 0.1 cc/kg/hour and a 100% satisfaction rate was reported.

Studies in adult patients comparing continuous sciatic nerve block with PCA have shown superior analgesia, reduced morphine use, and reduced frequency of nausea, vomiting, and sedation for adult patients with continuous popliteal sciatic catheters. Two commonly used approaches for sciatic nerve block in children are the subgluteal approach and the popliteal approach. A single-injection technique is indicated after relatively minor surgery when postoperative pain is expected to be mild and of short duration. A continuous catheter technique will provide prolonged analgesia after more extensive surgical procedures.

Sciatic-Subgluteal Approach

Since patients will need to be positioned in the prone position for a subgluteal approach to a sciatic nerve block, younger children will require general anesthesia for placement. Cooperative older children and adolescents can often tolerate the procedure in a prone procedure with sedation. The technique described below uses ultrasound guidance with peripheral nerve stimulation for further confirmation. With the patient in a prone position, ultrasound is used to locate the sciatic nerve; a line marking the midpoint between the ischial tuberosity and the greater trochanter can be useful in estimating position of the sciatic nerve. Under visualization, an insulated 17-gauge stimulating needle is advanced approximately 1–2 cm below the midpoint mark and is directed medially and superiorly. Initially, twitching of the gluteal muscles can be observed but will disappear as the needle advances further. Dorsi- and plantar-flexion of the foot is observed with stimulation of the sciatic nerve. A 20-gauge stimulating catheter is advanced approximately 3 cm beyond the tip of the needle; angling the needle slightly caudally may facilitate advancing the catheter. Further nerve stimulation of the catheter confirms proper catheter placement.[85]

Popliteal Approach

Block of the sciatic nerve can also be achieved at the level of the popliteal fossa. The sciatic nerve divides into the tibial and common peroneal nerves in the popliteal fossa, proximal to the popliteal fossa crease. For this block, patients can be positioned either prone or supine with the hip and knee flexed. Our general preference is to use the prone approach when catheter placement is being considered, since it makes it easier to maintain sterility and to perform tunneling of the catheter. Ultrasound is used to locate the structures in the popliteal fossa; the popliteal artery and vein are located deep and proximal to the sciatic nerve. The course of the sciatic nerve should be seen and the point at which the sciatic nerve bifurcates should be located. The tendon of the biceps femoris is located laterally and the tendons of the semimembranosus and semitendinosus muscles are located medially. Ultrasound viewing and needle advancement can be performed using several approaches, including an in-plane approach, with the needle advancing in a lateral-to-medial direction, or an out of plane approach, with the needle advancing in a sagittal direction. Injection of local anesthetic should show local anesthetic spread around the tibial and common peroneal nerves.[81]

A multiple regression model estimated that the depth of needle insertion (mm) to reach the sciatic nerve in the popliteal fossa in children was -0.86 height (cm) $+ 1.60$ weight (kg) $+26$ with a minimal distance of 13 mm.[86] For catheter placement, ultrasound can be used alone or in combination with stimulating needles and catheters. An 18-gauge insulated stimulating needle can be advanced under ultrasound to the sciatic nerve. Muscle twitching of the toes or foot movement confirms proper needle placement. A 20-gauge stimulating catheter is then advanced approximately 3–5 cm beyond the needle. Stimulation of the catheter should reconfirm proper placement.

Femoral Block

A femoral nerve block provides effective analgesia for knee surgery, for surgery on the anterior thigh such as a muscle biopsy, and for femur surgery or fractures. It will also provide analgesia to the medial lower extremity below the knee by blocking the saphenous nerve. Compared to PCA morphine and epidural analgesia, continuous femoral nerve block provides more effective analgesia with fewer side effects. Results indicate that using ultrasound guidance produced prolonged duration of sensory blockade with less volume of local anesthetic compared to using nerve stimulation. The typical landmarks for a femoral nerve block are the inguinal crease and the femoral arterial pulse. The femoral nerve is located lateral and deep to the femoral artery as it courses below the inguinal ligament. With the patient positioned in a supine position, ultrasound is used to locate the position of the femoral vein, artery, and nerve in the inguinal crease. Under ultrasound visualization, an insulated block needle is inserted just lateral to the arterial pulse and directed slightly cephalad. Proper placement of the needle should be seen on ultrasound, positioned *alongside* the femoral nerve. Nerve stimulation is an alternative method to confirm proper placement of the needle. With proper needle placement, twitching of the quadriceps and patella should be seen. Quadriceps movement alone without signs of patellar movement is due to stimulation of the sartorius muscle and does not confirm proper needle placement. If the femoral nerve is not readily located, it will be necessary to redirect the needle slightly laterally. When placing a catheter for continuous femoral block, the needle is angled slightly more cephalad and the catheter is advanced. If using nerve stimulation, twitching of the quadriceps and patella will indicate correct catheter placement. Infection rates for continuous femoral catheters appear to be low when used for short-term use. In a study examining bacterial colonization and infection rates in continuous femoral catheters, 57% of catheters had positive bacterial colonization with staphylococcus epidermis as the most common organism. However, there were no septic complications or serious infections for catheters in place for 48 hours.[87]

PAINFUL CONDITIONS IN PEDIATRIC HOSPITAL CARE

Cancer Pain

Infants and children with cancer experience pain from cancer treatment such as painful mucositis, postamputation pain, and peripheral neuropathies as well as from tumor spread causing bone pain, neuropathic pain, or headaches from raised intracranial pressure. Repeated painful needles procedures such as bone marrow biopsies and lumbar punctures are a great source of pain and distress. Several surveys have shown that as successful chemotherapeutic protocols, radiation therapy, and surgical techniques have advanced, cancer treatment and painful procedures account for greater sources of cancer pain in infants and children.

Frequent diagnostic and painful procedures are common for infants and children with cancer. For minor needle procedures, such as intravenous line insertions and assessing implanted vascular access ports, topical analgesia should be routinely used. A number of approaches to cutaneous analgesia have been used, including local anesthetic creams or patches, with or without physical methods to accelerate transit of drug across the stratum corneum. Cognitive–behavioral interventions such as hypnosis and other relaxation techniques have also been shown to be effective for procedural pain. Children can also apply these techniques to nausea, headaches, and other symptoms. Conscious sedation or general anesthesia is typically used for more invasive needle procedures such as bone marrow biopsies and lumbar punctures. Safe sedation protocols have been developed by the American Academy of Pediatrics and are widely used by pediatric oncologists and other pediatric subspecialists for procedural sedation. Pediatric anesthesiologists are consulted for patients with risk factors that place them at increased risk for conscious sedation, for patients who fail conscious sedation, or for more invasive procedures such as central line insertions. Brief general anesthesia is typically used for children who require daily radiation therapy. There is ongoing controversy regarding choice of drugs and safety practices for sedation by nonanesthesiologists.

Mucositis is a common side effect in children receiving chemotherapy or radiation; it is especially severe and prolonged with bone marrow transplantation. Initially, pain from mucositis is often treated with topical agents although evidence for efficacy in the prevention and treatment of mucositis has been mixed. Opioids are used for pain that persists despite topical agents. Data supports the safety and efficacy of opioid infusions and PCA for the treatment of mucositis.[55,88] Since many children with mucositis will require opioids for weeks, our practice is to eventually administer approximately 60% of the total daily opioid dose as a basal rate in order to provide sustained analgesia. NCA is used for young children.

Although a majority of children have resolution of the cancer pain after initial chemotherapy induction protocols, some children will continue to experience visceral, somatic, and neuropathic pain due to tumor invasion of solid organs, bone, nerves, and plexuses. Opioids are provided by the oral route whenever feasible. It is common practice to use a long-acting opioid, either methadone elixir or tablets or capsules of a sustained-release preparation of morphine, hydromorphone, or oxycodone, along with short-acting opioids for rescue or breakthrough pain. Currently, methadone is the most widely available long-acting opioid available as an elixir formulation. Several sustained-release

opioids are available as capsules containing microbeads. Although they are recommended for use in adults sprinkled specifically on apple sauce immediately prior to use, the package inserts recommend against this use in children. If the microbeads are chewed, crushed, or left in contact with liquids for extended periods of time, they release their contents, negating the sustained-release feature and giving the potential for overdosage. Some patients with rapidly escalating pain or patients unable to tolerate oral opioids may require opioids via parenteral routes, including intravenous and subcutaneous routes. Continuous infusions and PCA or NCA allow rapid titration for escalating pain. In the setting of neuropathic cancer pain, we frequently prescribe anticonvulsants and antidepressants, largely by extrapolation from adult practice. Fatigue, somnolence, sleep disturbance, and depressed mood are a commonly overlapping group of symptoms in children with advanced cancer. Opioids and other sedating medications may contribute to these symptoms, but they may exist even in children not receiving opioids or sedatives. Along with treating specific or remediable causes of these symptoms, our common practice, again extrapolated from adult clinical trials, is to consider a trial of a stimulant such as methylphenidate.

A subgroup of children with cancer pain will have persistent pain despite massive dose escalation. Many of these children will have unremitting neuropathic pain associated with tumor extension to the epidural space, onto a plexus, or along the course of major nerves. One approach to persistent pain in this setting is to add a low-dose ketamine infusion. At rates below 0.2 mg/kg/ hour, dysphoria and dissociation are relatively uncommon.[89]

Oral ketamine has been used as well, with a provisional dose ratio of about 3:1 compared to intravenous dosing in steady state. In selected cases of refractory pain, our practice is to use regional anesthetic techniques, and we most commonly in this setting favor implanted intrathecal ports with the catheter generally advanced to the dorsal horn level appropriate to the patient's location of greatest pain.[90] Note that for tumors predominantly in the pelvis, lumbar spine, or lower extremities, this implies having the catheter tip advanced up to around T11. The choice of drugs for these infusions must be individualized, based on the nature of the patient's pain, and quality of life issues, including considerations of weakness, bowel and bladder dysfunction, sedation, etc. In the majority of cases, we have found it necessary to include small doses of local anesthetics along with opioids, and in some cases we have included other additives such as clonidine or ketamine. There is a small subgroup of children for whom it appears that the most feasible option for achieving relief of pain, distress, or terminal dyspnea is to provide sedation using a range of agents, including benzodiazepines, barbiturates, or other drugs.[91]

The principle of double-effect is widely cited in discussions of opioid administration in palliative care. As noted by Quill, Dresser, and Brock,[92] there are some conceptual and practical difficulties in the application of this principle for opioid titration in palliative care; these difficulties become even greater in the use of sedatives in end-of-life care. An alternative view, favored by these authors, concerns an emphasis on patient autonomy and choice in decision-making.[92]

Central principles in treating cancer pain in children includes basing decision-making on consideration of patients' and their families' goals and hopes, collaborative care, emphasis on frequent pain assessments, individualized drug dosing, and proactive treatment of opioid side effects.

Children with Developmental Disabilities

Children with cognitive and developmental disabilities such as cerebral palsy and neurodegenerative disorders present unique challenges in assessing and managing pain. Many children with disabilities experience daily pain associated with muscle spasms, hip dislocation, and other musculoskeletal pains and undergo frequent painful invasive procedures such as scoliosis repair, tendon releases, and surgical treatment of gastroesophageal reflux. Children may have little or no cognitive deficits but significant motor and communication impairments, making pain assessment especially difficult. Often, parents and caretakers are able to distinguish subtle behavioral signs indicating pain. A number of pain assessment tools such as FLACC tool, and the Noncommunicating Children's Pain Checklist have been used for children with cognitive and developmental disabilities. In comparing several pain assessment tools for children with cognitive limitations, physicians and nurses rated the FLACC as having higher clinical utility.[17,93]

Other children with severe cognitive impairment will have persistent agitation and screaming without a clear etiology and are admitted to the hospital for diagnostic evaluation and therapeutic trials. Patients should be evaluated for treatable causes of pain such as fractures, hip dislocations, esophagitis, and constipation. In some cases where no underlying cause can be eventually identified, therapeutic trials of anticonvulsants and antispasmodics may provide relief.[94]

Pain Associated with Sickle Cell Vaso-Occlusive Episodes

Pain is a common consequence of sickle cell disease due to acute vaso-occlusive episodes as well as pain from compression fractures, avascular necrosis, acute cholecystitis, splenic sequestration, and stroke. Painful vaso-occlusive episodes are the most common cause of pain in children with sickle cell disease and can occur in children as young as 6 months of age as fetal hemoglobin and its protection against vaso-occlusive crises decreases. Children can demonstrate a range of severity and frequency of vaso-occlusive episodes, from occasional episodes managed at home with oral analgesics to baseline daily pain with frequent exacerbations requiring numerous hospitalizations and systemic opioids administration. PCA is commonly used for severe pain in hospitalized patients, along with NSAIDs. Larger opioid boluses may be necessary than are typically used for postoperative pain management for patients with extreme pain or for patients who are opioid tolerant. Often, basal infusions are necessary, particularly at night to permit periods of uninterrupted sleep. Published case series indicate that even with generous PCA parameters, pain scores remain high for a high percentage of patients.[95]

CONCLUSION

Evidence is available to support safe and effective treatment of acute pain in infants, children, and adolescents in a majority of circumstances. Analgesic pharmacology has received extensive study in pediatrics over the past 25 years. Individual analgesics often provide incomplete relief in standard doses, and there is a rationale for analgesic combinations and multimodal analgesia in many situations. Opioids can provide good analgesia at all ages, but with a spectrum of side effects that require active treatment and with specific requirements for observation and monitoring according to age and patient condition-related risk factors. Techniques have been developed for neuraxial and peripheral regional anesthesia at all ages. There is a growing emphasis on ultrasound, nerve stimulation, selective use of fluoroscopy, and other approaches to provide objective confirmation of needle and/or catheter positioning. Pediatric acute pain management, whether by an acute pain service or by other delivery models, can be improved by system-wide approaches that emphasize systematic assessment of pain and other symptoms, communication, clinician education, clarification of responsibilities, and protocols for analgesic administration, side effect management, and monitoring.

References

1. Fitzgerald M, Walker SM. Infant pain management: a developmental neurobiological approach. *Nat Clin Pract Neurol* 2009;5(1):35–50.
2. Anand KJ, Hickey PR. Pain and its effects in the human neonate and fetus. *N Engl J Med* 1987;317(21):1321–1329.
3. Anand KJ, Hickey PR. Halothane-morphine compared with high-dose sufentanil for anesthesia and postoperative analgesia in neonatal cardiac surgery. *N Engl J Med* 1992;326(1):1–9.
4. Stevens BJ, Johnston CC. Physiological responses of premature infants to a painful stimulus. *Nurs Res* 1994;43(4):226–231.
5. Anand KJ. Neonatal stress responses to anesthesia and surgery. *Clin Perinatol* 1990;17(1):207–214.
6. Andrews K, Fitzgerald M. Cutaneous flexion reflex in human neonates: a quantitative study of threshold and stimulus-response characteristics after single and repeated stimuli. *Dev Med Child Neurol* 1999;41(10):696–703.
7. Franck LS. A new method to quantitatively describe pain behavior in infants. *Nurs Res* 1986;35(1):28–31.
8. Porter FL, Wolf CM, Miller JP. Procedural pain in newborn infants: the influence of intensity and development. *Pediatrics* 1999;104(1):e13.
9. Krechel S, Bildner J. CRIES: a new neonatal postoperative pain measurement score. Initial testing of validity and reliability. *Paediatr Anaesth* 1995;5(1): 53–61.
10. Stevens B, Johnston C, Petryshen P, et al. Premature Infant Pain Profile: development and initial validation. *Clin J Pain* 1996;12(1):13–22.
11. Zhou H, Roberts P, Horgan L. Association between self-report pain ratings of child and parent, child and nurse and parent and nurse dyads: meta-analysis. *J Adv Nurs* 2008;63(4):334–342.
12. Hesselgard K, Larsson S, Romner B, et al. Validity and reliability of the Behavioural Observational Pain Scale for postoperative pain measurement in children 1–7 years of age. *Pediatr Crit Care Med* 2007;8(2):102–108.
13. McGrath PJ, Johnson G, Goodman JT. CHEOPS: a behavioral scale for rating postoperative pain in children. *Adv Pain Res Ther* 1985;9:395–402.
14. Merkel SI, Voepel-Lewis T, Shayevitz JR, et al. The FLACC: a behavioral scale for scoring postoperative pain in young children. *Pediatr Nurs* 1997;23(3): 293–297.
15. Malviya S, Voepel-Lewis T, Burke C, et al. The revised FLACC observational pain tool: improved reliability and validity for pain assessment in children with cognitive impairment. *Paediatr Anaesth* 2006;16(3):258–265.
16. Hicks CL, von Baeyer CL, Spafford PA, et al. The Faces Pain Scale-Revised: toward a common metric in pediatric pain measurement. *Pain* 2001;93(2): 173–183.
17. Voepel-Lewis T, Malviya S, Tait AR. Validity of parent ratings as proxy measures of pain in children with cognitive impairment. *Pain Manag Nurs* 2005; 6(4):168–174.
18. Voepel-Lewis T, Malviya S, Tait AR, et al. A comparison of the clinical utility of pain assessment tools for children with cognitive impairment. *Anesth Analg* 2008;106(1):72–78, table of contents.
19. Voepel-Lewis T, Merkel S, Tait AR, et al. The reliability and validity of the Face, Legs, Activity, Cry, Consolability observational tool as a measure of pain in children with cognitive impairment. *Anesth Analg* 2002;95(5):1224–1229, table of contents.
20. Grossi E, Borghi C, Cerchiari EL, et al. Analogue chromatic continuous scale (ACCS): a new method for pain assessment. *Clin Exp Rheumatol* 1983;1(4): 337–340.
21. Stinson JN, Kavanagh T, Yamada J, et al. Systematic review of the psychometric properties, interpretability and feasibility of self-report pain intensity measures for use in clinical trials in children and adolescents. *Pain* 2006;125(1–2): 143–157.
22. Alcorn J, McNamara PJ. Ontogeny of hepatic and renal systemic clearance pathways in infants: part I. *Clin Pharmacokinet* 2002;41(12):959–998.
23. Anderson BJ, Holford NH. Mechanism-based concepts of size and maturity in pharmacokinetics. *Annu Rev Pharmacol Toxicol* 2008;48:303–332.
24. Ririe DG, Eisenach JC. Effect of cyclooxygenase-1 inhibition in postoperative pain is developmentally regulated. *Anesthesiology* 2004;101(4):1031–1035.
25. Furst DE. Are there differences among nonsteroidal antiinflammatory drugs? Comparing acetylated salicylates, nonacetylated salicylates, and nonacetylated nonsteroidal antiinflammatory drugs. *Arthritis Rheum* 1994;37(1):1–9.
26. Strassburg CP, Strassburg A, Kneip S, et al. Developmental aspects of human hepatic drug glucuronidation in young children and adults. *Gut* 2002;50(2): 259–265.
27. Heubi JE, Barbacci MB, Zimmerman HJ. Therapeutic misadventures with acetaminophen: hepatoxicity after multiple doses in children. *J Pediatr* 1998; 132(1):22–27.
28. Birmingham PK, Tobin MJ, Henthorn TK, et al. Twenty-four–hour pharmacokinetics of rectal acetaminophen in children: an old drug with new recommendations. *Anesthesiology* 1997;87(2):244–252.
29. Montgomery CJ, McCormack JP, Reichert CC, et al. Plasma concentrations after high-dose (45 mg.kg-1) rectal acetaminophen in children. *Can J Anaesth* 1995;42(11):982–986.
30. Boynton CS, Dick CF, Mayor GH. NSAIDs: an overview. *J Clin Pharmacol* 1988;28(6):512–517.
31. Kauffman RE, Lieh-Lai MW, Uy HG, et al. Enantiomer-selective pharmacokinetics and metabolism of ketorolac in children. *Clin Pharmacol Ther* 1999; 65(4):382–388.

32. Kokki H, Hendolin H, Maunuksela EL, et al. Ibuprofen in the treatment of postoperative pain in small children. A randomized double-blind-placebo controlled parallel group study. *Acta Anaesthesiol Scand* 1994;38(5):467–472.

33. Van Overmeire B, Smets K, Lecoutere D, et al. A comparison of ibuprofen and indomethacin for closure of patent ductus arteriosus. *N Engl J Med* 2000; 343(10):674–681.

34. Rusy LM, Houck CS, Sullivan LJ, et al. A double-blind evaluation of ketorolac tromethamine versus acetaminophen in pediatric tonsillectomy: analgesia and bleeding. *Anesth Analg* 1995;80(2):226–229.

35. Krishna S, Hughes LF, Lin SY. Postoperative hemorrhage with nonsteroidal anti-inflammatory drug use after tonsillectomy: a meta-analysis. *Arch Otolaryngol Head Neck Surg* 2003;129(10):1086–1089.

36. Marret E, Flahault A, Samama CM, et al. Effects of postoperative, nonsteroidal, antiinflammatory drugs on bleeding risk after tonsillectomy: meta-analysis of randomized, controlled trials. *Anesthesiology* 2003;98(6):1497–1502.

37. Krämer BK. Cyclo-oxygenase-2 and renal function. *Nephrol Dial Transplant* 2001;16(1):180–183.

38. Pickering AE, Bridge HS, Nolan J, et al. Double-blind, placebo-controlled analgesic study of ibuprofen or rofecoxib in combination with paracetamol for tonsillectomy in children. *Br J Anaesth* 2002;88(1):72–77.

39. Lynn AM, Nespeca MK, Bratton SL, et al. Intravenous morphine in postoperative infants: intermittent bolus dosing versus targeted continuous infusions. *Pain* 2000;88(1):89–95.

40. Lynn AM, Nespeca MK, Opheim KE, et al. Respiratory effects of intravenous morphine infusions in neonates, infants, and children after cardiac surgery. *Anesth Analg* 1993;77(4):695–701.

41. Williams DG, Hatch DJ, Howard RF. Codeine phosphate in paediatric medicine. *Br J Anaesth* 2001;86(3):413–421.

42. Sindrup SH, Brosen K. The pharmacogenetics of codeine hypoalgesia. *Pharmacogenetics* 1995;5(6):335–346.

43. Kokki H, Rasanen I, Reinikainen M, et al. Pharmacokinetics of oxycodone after intravenous, buccal, intramuscular and gastric administration in children. *Clin Pharmacokinet* 2004;43(9):613–622.

44. Friedman RA. The changing face of teenage drug abuse—the trend toward prescription drugs. *N Engl J Med* 2006;354(14):1448–1450.

45. Collins JJ, Geake J, Grier HE, et al. Patient-controlled analgesia for mucositis pain in children: a three-period crossover study comparing morphine and hydromorphone. *J Pediatr* 1996;129(5):722–728.

46. Berde CB, Beyer JE, Bournaki MC, et al. Comparison of morphine and methadone for prevention of postoperative pain in 3- to 7-year-old children. *J Pediatr* 1991;119(1 Pt 1):136–141.

47. Fredheim OM, Moksnes K, Borchgrevink PC, et al. Clinical pharmacology of methadone for pain. *Acta Anaesthesiol Scand* 2008;52(7):879–889.

48. Shaiova L, Berger A, Blinderman CD, et al. Consensus guideline on parenteral methadone use in pain and palliative care. *Palliat Support Care* 2008;6(2): 165–176.

49. Chang G, Chen L, Mao J. Opioid tolerance and hyperalgesia. *Med Clin North Am* 2007;91(2):199–211.

50. Benitez-Rosario MA, Salinas-Martin A, Aguirre-Jaime A, et al. Morphine-methadone opioid rotation in cancer patients: analysis of dose ratio-predicting factors. *J Pain Symptom Manage* 2009;37(6):1061–1068.

51. The Clinician's Ultimate Reference. Narcotic analgesic converter. Available at: http://www.globalrph.com/narcoticonv.htm. Accessed June 12, 2009.

52. Pereira J, Lawlor P, Vigano A, et al Equianalgesic dose ratios for opioids. A critical review and proposals for long-term dosing. *J Pain Symptom Manage* 2001;22(2):672–687.

53. Zernikow B, Michel E, Anderson B. Transdermal fentanyl in childhood and adolescence: a comprehensive literature review. *J Pain* 2007;8(3):187–207.

54. Pokela ML, Olkkola KT, Koivisto M, et al. Pharmacokinetics and pharmacodynamics of intravenous meperidine in neonates and infants. *Clin Pharmacol Ther* 1992;52(4):342–349.

55. Anghelescu DL, Burgoyne LL, Oakes LL, et al. The safety of patient-controlled analgesia by proxy in pediatric oncology patients. *Anesth Analg* 2005;101(6): 1623–1627.

56. Monitto CL, Greenberg RS, Kost-Byerly S, et al. The safety and efficacy of parent-/nurse-controlled analgesia in patients less than six years of age. *Anesth Analg* 2000;91(3):573–579.

57. Voepel-Lewis T, Marinkovic A, Kostrzewa A, et al. The prevalence of and risk factors for adverse events in children receiving patient-controlled analgesia by proxy or patient-controlled analgesia after surgery. *Anesth Analg* 2008;107(1): 70–75.

58. Kehlet H. Postoperative opioid sparing to hasten recovery: what are the issues? *Anesthesiology* 2005;102(6):1083–1085.

59. Berde C, Nurko S. Opioid side effects—mechanism-based therapy. *N Engl J Med* 2008;358(22):2400–2402.

60. Kjellberg F, Tramer MR. Pharmacological control of opioid-induced pruritus: a quantitative systematic review of randomized trials. *Eur J Anaesthesiol* 2001; 18(6):346–357.

61. Maxwell LG, Kaufmann SC, Bitzer S, et al. The effects of a small-dose naloxone infusion on opioid-induced side effects and analgesia in children and adolescents treated with intravenous patient-controlled analgesia: a double-blind, prospective, randomized, controlled study. *Anesth Analg* 2005;100(4):953–958.

62. Koch J, Manworren R, Clark L, et al. Pilot study of continuous co-infusion of morphine and naloxone in children with sickle cell pain crisis. *Am J Hematol* 2008;83(9):728–731.

63. Nakatsuka N, Minogue SC, Lim J, et al. Intravenous nalbuphine 50 microg × kg(-1) is ineffective for opioid-induced pruritus in pediatrics. *Can J Anaesth* 2006;53(11):1103–1110.

64. Henderson K, Sethna NF, Berde CB. Continuous caudal anesthesia for inguinal hernia repair in former preterm infants. *J Clin Anesth* 1993;5(2):129–133.

65. Schechter NL, Zempsky WT, Cohen LL, et al. Pain reduction during pediatric immunizations: evidence-based review and recommendations. *Pediatrics* 2007; 119(5):e1184–e1198.

66. Zempsky WT. Pharmacologic approaches for reducing venous access pain in children. *Pediatrics* 2008;122(suppl 3):S140–S153.

67. Drasner K. Thoracic epidural anesthesia: asleep at the wheal? *Anesth Analg* 2004;99(2):578–579.

68. Giaufre E, Dalens B, Gombert A. Epidemiology and morbidity of regional anesthesia in children: a one-year prospective survey of the French-Language Society of Pediatric Anesthesiologists. *Anesth Analg* 1996;83(5):904–912.

69. Llewellyn N, Moriarty A. The national pediatric epidural audit. *Paediatr Anaesth* 2007;17(6):520–533.

70. Bösenberg AT, Bland BA, Schulte-Steinberg O, et al. Thoracic epidural anesthesia via caudal route in infants. *Anesthesiology* 1988;69(2):265–269.

71. Goobie SM, Montgomery CJ, Basu R, et al. Confirmation of direct epidural catheter placement using nerve stimulation in pediatric anesthesia. *Anesth Analg* 2003;97(4):984–988, table of contents.

72. Borghi B, Agnoletti V, Ricci A, et al. A prospective, randomized evaluation of the effects of epidural needle rotation on the distribution of epidural block. *Anesth Analg* 2004;98(5):1473–1478, table of contents.

73. Rapp HJ, Folger A, Grau T. Ultrasound-guided epidural catheter insertion in children. *Anesth Analg* 2005;101(2):333–339, table of contents.

74. Luz G, Wieser C, Innerhofer P, et al. Free and total bupivacaine plasma concentrations after continuous epidural anaesthesia in infants and children. *Paediatr Anaesth* 1998;8(6):473–478.

75. Bosenberg AT, Thomas J, Cronje L,et al. Pharmacokinetics and efficacy of ropivacaine for continuous epidural infusion in neonates and infants. *Paediatr Anaesth* 2005;15(9):739–749.

76. Hansen TG, Ilett KF, Lim SI, et al. Pharmacokinetics and clinical efficacy of long-term epidural ropivacaine infusion in children. *Br J Anaesth* 2000;85(3): 347–353.

77. McCann ME, Sethna NF, Mazoit JX, et al. The pharmacokinetics of epidural ropivacaine in infants and young children. *Anesth Analg* 2001;93(4):893–897.

78. De Negri P, Ivani G, Visconti C, et al. The dose-response relationship for clonidine added to a postoperative continuous epidural infusion of ropivacaine in children. *Anesth Analg* 2001;93(1):71–76.

79. Wheeler M, Patel A, Suresh S, et al. The addition of clonidine 2 microg.kg-1 does not enhance the postoperative analgesia of a caudal block using 0.125% bupivacaine and epinephrine 1:200,000 in children: a prospective, double-blind, randomized study. *Paediatr Anaesth* 2005;15(6):476–483.

80. Dadure C, Bringuier S, Nicolas F, et al. Continuous epidural block versus continuous popliteal nerve block for postoperative pain relief after major podiatric surgery in children: a prospective, comparative randomized study. *Anesth Analg* 2006;102(3):744–749.

81. Oberndorfer U, Marhofer P, Bosenberg A, et al. Ultrasonographic guidance for sciatic and femoral nerve blocks in children. *Br J Anaesth* 2007;98(6): 797–801.

82. Cucchiaro G, Ganesh A. The effects of clonidine on postoperative analgesia after peripheral nerve blockade in children. *Anesth Analg* 2007;104(3): 532–537.

83. Pande R, Pande M, Bhadani U, et al. Supraclavicular brachial plexus block as a sole anaesthetic technique in children: an analysis of 200 cases. *Anaesthesia* 2000;55(8):798–802.

84. Dadure C, Motais F, Ricard C, et al. Continuous peripheral nerve blocks at home for treatment of recurrent complex regional pain syndrome I in children. *Anesthesiology* 2005;102(2):387–391.

85. van Geffen GJ, Gielen M. Ultrasound-guided subgluteal sciatic nerve blocks with stimulating catheters in children: a descriptive study. *Anesth Analg* 2006; 103(2):328–333, table of contents.

86. Konrad C, Johr M. Blockade of the sciatic nerve in the popliteal fossa: a system for standardization in children. *Anesthesia & Analgesia* 1998;87:1256–1258.

87. Cuvillon P, Ripart J, Lalourcey L, et al. The continuous femoral nerve block catheter for postoperative analgesia: bacterial colonization, infectious rate and adverse effects. *Anesth Analg* 2001;93:1045–1049.

88. Ruggiero A, Barone G, Liotti L, et al. Safety and efficacy of fentanyl administered by patient controlled analgesia in children with cancer pain. *Support Care Cancer* 2007;15(5):569–573.

89. Finkel JC, Pestieau SR, Quezado ZM. Ketamine as an adjuvant for treatment of cancer pain in children and adolescents. *J Pain* 2007;8(6):515–521.

90. Clemente CD. *Anatomy: A Regional Atlas of the Human Body*. 3rd ed. Baltimore-Munich: Urban & Schwarzenberg; 1987.

91. Berde C, Wolfe J. Pain, anxiety, distress, and suffering: interrelated, but not interchangeable. *J Pediatr* 2003;142(4):361–363.

92. Quill TE, Dresser R, Brock DW. The rule of double effect—a critique of its role in end-of-life decision making. *N Engl J Med* 1997;337(24):1768–1771.

93. von Baeyer CL, Spagrud LJ. Systematic review of observational (behavioral) measures of pain for children and adolescents aged 3 to 18 years. *Pain* 2007; 127(1–2):140–150.

94. Hauer JM, Wical BS, Charnas L. Gabapentin successfully manages chronic unexplained irritability in children with severe neurologic impairment. *Pediatrics* 2007;119(2):e519–e522.

95. Jacob E, Miaskowski C, Savedra M, et al. Quantification of analgesic use in children with sickle cell disease. *Clin J Pain* 2007;23(1):8–14.

CHAPTER 51 ■ ACUTE PAIN IN ADULTS

ROBERT W. HURLEY, STEVEN P. COHEN, AND CHRISTOPHER L. WU

INTRODUCTION

Acute pain is the normal and predicable neurophysiologic response to noxious mechanical, thermal, or chemical stimuli; is generally time-limited; and resolves with the cessation of the noxious stimuli. The etiology, more often than not, is known or understood. It is typically associated with invasive procedures, trauma, or medical diseases. The pain sensation is usually limited to the area of trauma or damage or the area that immediately surrounds it. Perhaps most importantly, the painful sensations associated with such an injury are expected to resolve over time when adequate wound healing has occurred. In contrast, chronic pain persists beyond either the course of an acute injury or illness or its expected time for healing and repair. Acute pain states can then be further divided by duration, etiology, mechanism, intensity, and/or symptoms. In this chapter, acute pain will be discussed using postsurgical or postprocedural and posttraumatic pain as models.

A revolution in the management of acute pain has occurred over the past few decades. Widespread recognition of the undertreatment of acute pain by clinicians, economists, and health policy experts has led to the development of a national clinical practice guideline for acute pain management by the Agency for Healthcare Quality and Research (formerly the Agency for Health Care Policy and Research) of the U. S. Department of Health and Human Services. This landmark document includes acknowledgment of the historic inadequacies in perioperative pain management, importance of good pain control, need for accountability for adequate provision of perioperative analgesia by health care institutions, and a statement on the need for involvement of specialists in appropriate cases. In addition, several professional societies, including the American Society of Anesthesiologists,[1,2] and the Joint Commission on Accreditation of Healthcare Organizations (JCAHO), have developed clinical practice guidelines for acute pain management or provided new pain management standards.

With their knowledge of and familiarity with pharmacology, various regional techniques, and the neurobiology of nociception, perioperative physicians such as anesthesiologists are continually on the forefront of clinical and research advances in acute pain, especially acute postoperative pain management. Anesthesiologists have traditionally been leaders in the development of acute postoperative pain services, application of evidence-based practice to acute postoperative pain, and creation of innovative approaches to acute pain management. However, the treatment of acute pain (including postprocedural pain) needs to involve a multidisciplinary approach similar to that which has evolved in the treatment of chronic pain. The physical and psychosocial effects of acute pain, though time-limited by definition, remain a significant morbidity that can affect patients' quality of recovery.

ACUTE AND CHRONIC EFFECTS OF ACUTE PAIN

Uncontrolled acute pain may produce a range of detrimental acute and chronic effects. Attenuation of periprocedural patho-physiology that occurs during a procedure or surgery through reduction of nociceptive input into the central nervous system (CNS) and optimization of periprocedural analgesia may decrease complications and facilitate the patient's recovery during the immediate postprocedural period[3] and after discharge from the hospital.

The perioperative period is associated with a variety of pathophysiological responses that may be initiated or maintained by peripheral nociceptive input. Although these responses may have had a beneficial purpose in nature, the same response to the modern day surgery may actually be harmful. Uncontrolled perioperative pain may therefore be considered a major morbidity for the patient. Furthermore, attenuation of postprocedural or acute medical pain may decrease perioperative morbidity and mortality.[4]

The transmission of pain stimuli from the periphery to the spinal cord and supraspinally results in the neuroendocrine stress response. The dominant neuroendocrine response to pain involves hypothalamic–pituitary–adrenocortical and sympatho-adrenal interaction, resulting in increased sympathetic tone, increased catecholamine and catabolic hormone secretion including cortisol, adrenocorticotropic hormone, antidiuretic hormone, glucagon, aldosterone, renin, angiotensin II; and decreased secretion of anabolic hormones. The outcome of these changes includes sodium and water retention and increased levels of blood glucose, free fatty acids, ketone bodies, and lactate. A hypermetabolic, catabolic state results as metabolism and oxygen consumption are increased, and metabolic substrates are mobilized from storage depots. The negative nitrogen balance and protein catabolism may impede the patient's recovery and contribute to morbidity or mortality. Sympathetic activation may increase myocardial oxygen consumption and decrease myocardial oxygen supply, which may be important in the development of myocardial ischemia and infarction.[4,5] Sympathetic activation may also delay return of postprocedural gastrointestinal motility that may develop into an ileus.

Postprocedural acute pain may initiate several detrimental spinal reflex pathways. Respiratory function can be markedly diminished, especially with acute pain involving the upper abdomen, flank, and/or thorax. Reflex inhibition of phrenic nerve activity is an important component of this decreased pulmonary function.[4,5] However, control of acute pain is also important, because patients with poor pain control may have poor inspiratory effort, have an inadequate cough, and be more likely to develop pulmonary complications.[4]

NEUROBIOLOGY OF ACUTE PAIN

The neurobiology of pain is extremely complex, with redundancy and plasticity such that there is no "final common pathway" for the process of nociception. However, understanding the neurobiology of pain is crucial when contemplating which nociceptive processes to target in the treatment of acute pain. Identification of new molecular and cellular processes involved in the process of nociception has increased the number of potential targets for analgesic therapies.

Primary Afferents and Peripheral Nerve Neurotransmitters

A variety of mechanical, thermal, or chemical stimuli can result in the sensation of pain. Information about these painful or noxious stimuli is carried to higher brain centers by receptors and neurons that are distinct from those that carry innocuous somatic sensory information. This topic will be covered at length in Chapters 3 and 4. In brief, small diameter Aδ and C fibers primarily transmit nociceptive information, but subsets of Aδ and C fibers are thermo receptors that transmit nonpainful cold and warm information, respectively.[6] Neurotransmission by the Aδ and C fibers is performed by numerous peptides and amino acids. Substance P (SP) was the first peptide to be defined as specific to the small diameter primary afferents and is released by noxious thermal, mechanical, and chemical stimulation of the periphery.[7–9] Exogenous application of SP into the spinal cord of rats results in dorsal horn neuronal activation[10] and behavioral responses consistent with pain.[11] Neurokinin-1 (NK-1), the receptor for SP, is found on superficial and deep neurons in the dorsal horn of the spinal cord consistent with their role in pain transmission.[12] Other peptides present in the small diameter afferents include calcitonin growth-related protein (CGRP), galanin, vasoactive intestinal polypeptide (VIP) and somatostatin (SST); however, their role in the modulation of nociceptive transmission is less well understood. In addition to these peptides, the excitatory amino acid glutamate is also present within small diameter primary afferents, released by noxious stimulation[13] and activates the second order dorsal horn neurons.[14] The effects of glutamate are predominantly mediated by three receptor classes: alpha-amino-3-hydroxy-5-methyl-4-isoxazolepropionic acid (AMPA)/Kainate, N-methyl-D-aspartate (NMDA), and metabotropic glutamate receptors (mGluR). AMPA receptors are found on postsynaptic neurons predominantly within the superficial dorsal horn.[15] NMDA receptors are found both pre- and postsynaptically (i.e., on nociceptive primary afferents and apposing second order neurons within the superficial and deep dorsal horn).[16] Metabotropic GluR receptors are predominantly found postsynaptically on the cell body and dendrites of dorsal horns neurons.

The primary afferent's presynaptic nerve terminal in the dorsal horn of the spinal cord represents a site for a therapeutic intervention. Primary afferent fibers transmit the pain signal to the spinal cord and possess numerous receptor systems that can reduce this transmission by reducing transmitter release such as the alpha$_2$-adrenergic, glycinergic, serotoninergic, opioidergic, and GABAergic receptors[17–19] as well as ion channels sensitive to local anesthetics and anticonvulsants including voltage gated calcium, sodium, and potassium channels.

Spinal Cord and Supraspinal Structures

Aδ and C fiber neurons synapse primarily within Lamina I, II, and V of the dorsal horn of the spinal cord. These primary afferents release neurotransmitters and neuropeptides that activate the second order projection neurons of the spinal cord. Pain transmission through the spinal cord may be modulated by an endogenous descending pain inhibitory system and may be influenced by exogenously administered medications. The primary components of this descending pain inhibition system is the "triad" of the periaqueductal gray (PAG), the rostral ventromedial medulla (RVM), and the dorsal lateral pontine tegmentum (DLPT), which includes the locus coeruleus (LC) and the A7 nuclei. The PAG is an important site for the production of analgesia following systemic administration of opioids. The endogenous opioid [Met^5]-enkephalin is present within this nucleus[20] and opioid receptors of each subtype are present in this region.[21] The PAG provides dense projections to the RVM[22] and brainstem noradrenergic nuclei LC and A7.[23] Although each of these regions has direct projections to the spinal cord, it has been proposed that their projections to the RVM are important components in the modulation of pain by these regions.[24] The RVM can function as a relay nucleus in the production of antinociception by more rostral midbrain structures (PAG), but it also has a primary role in the suppression of nociceptive transmission at the level of the spinal cord. The suppression of nociceptive reflex behavior is thought to be mediated by the axons of RVM neurons that descend within the dorsolateral funiculus and terminate bilaterally in laminae I, II, V, VI, and VII of the spinal cord. Anatomical studies have shown these axons terminate coincident with spinothalamic tract cells and interneurons of the dorsal horn that are related to pain transmission.[25,26] Consistent with the anatomical terminations of the RVM axons, physiological studies have shown that stimulation of the RVM results in the inhibition of a population of pain-specific neurons within the dorsal horn.[27,28] Spinally projecting neurons of the RVM possess numerous neurotransmitters including serotonin, enkephalin, GABA, glutamate, and substance P.[29–31] The DLPT contains all of the noradrenergic neurons that project to the RVM and the spinal cord.[32,33] In animal models, electrical stimulation of the DLPT sites produces analgesia[34,35] and the analgesia produced by the activation of these nuclei is mediated by the alpha$_2$ adrenergic receptor.[35,36] The pain physician can pharmacologically manipulate each of these neurotransmitter systems to modulate pain transmission throughout the central nervous system.

PREVENTION

Preemptive Analgesia

The development of central and/or peripheral sensitization after traumatic injury or surgical incision can result in the amplification of acute pain. Preventing the establishment of altered central processing by analgesic treatment may, in the short term, result in the reduction of postprocedural or traumatic pain and accelerated recovery. In the long term, the benefits may include a reduction in the development of chronic pain and an improvement in the patient's quality of recovery and satisfaction. Although experimental animal studies convincingly confirm the ability of preemptive and preventative analgesia to decrease postinjury pain, the results of clinical trials are mixed.[37–39]

The precise definition of preemptive versus preventative analgesia is one of the major controversies in this area of medicine and contributes to the question of whether preemptive analgesia is clinically relevant. Definitions of "preemptive analgesia" include 1) any attempt to give medications prior to surgical incision, 2) administration of medications during the intraoperative or intraprocedural period, or 3) administration of medications during the intraoperative and postoperative period.[40] The first two definitions are relatively narrow and may contribute to the lack of a detectable effect of preemptive analgesia in clinical trials. For the purpose of this text, preemptive analgesia is defined as an analgesic intervention started before the noxious stimulus arises in order to block peripheral and central pain transmission. "Preventative analgesia" most closely resembles the third definition and encompasses an attempt to block pain transmission prior to the injury (incision), during the noxious insult (surgery itself) and following the injury and throughout the recovery period. Unfortunately, few trials have examined the concept of preventative analgesia in a rigorous fashion. Preemptive analgesia abiding by the first one of the above three definitions have been loosely examined. Although some argue that the timing of the intervention[37–39] may not be as clinically important as other aspects of preemptive analgesia including intensity and duration of the intervention, this notion may be based on semantic confusion or poor study design. For example, an intervention administered before surgical incision is not necessarily preemptive if it is incomplete or insufficient such that the development of peripheral or central sensitization would not be prevented. Incisional and inflammatory injuries are important in initiating and maintaining both peripheral and central sensitization. Confining the definition of preemptive analgesia to only the immediately preoperative or intraoperative (incisional) period may not be clinically relevant or appropriate because the inflammatory response may last well into the postoperative period and continue to maintain this sensitization. Other methodological and study design issues also may complicate the question of whether preemptive analgesia is clinically relevant. A variety of agents and techniques[37–39] have been used to study preemptive analgesia. Using the broader definition of preemptive analgesia termed preventative analgesia that covers the preoperative, the intraoperative and postoperative periods, the combination of experimental data and positive clinical trials strongly suggests that preventative analgesia is a clinically relevant phenomenon. Furthermore, it has been suggested that simple preoperative therapy such as the inclusion of a single dose of the anticonvulsant, gabapentin, can reduce postoperative pain and opioid use with minimal side effects in a number of different surgeries.[41] Maximal clinical benefit is observed when there is complete blockade of noxious stimuli with extension of this blockade into the postoperative period. Recent preclinical and clinical studies provide substantial evidence that central sensitization and persistent pain after surgical incision is predominantly maintained by the incoming barrage of sensitized peripheral pain fibers throughout the perioperative period.[42] By preventing central sensitization and the peripheral input maintaining it, preventative analgesia along with intensive multimodal analgesic interventions could theoretically reduce acute postprocedure pain/hyperalgesia and chronic pain after surgery or trauma.[43] In a systematic review of clinical trials examining preemptive or preventative analgesic approaches, Katz[44] reported an analgesic benefit of preventative analgesia but no such benefit with the preemptive strategy.

Multimodal Approach to Perioperative Recovery

A multimodal approach to analgesia is broad definition which may include a combination of interventional analgesic techniques (epidural catheter or peripheral nerve catheter analgesia) and systemic pharmacologic therapies (nonsteroidal anti-inflammatory agents [NSAID] or opioid administration), multiple systemic pharmacologic therapies (the combination of NSAIDs, opioids, and anticonvulsants) and/or the multiple pharmacologic therapies delivered through the interventional catheter (local anesthetics plus opioids or other adjuvants). Postprocedural or posttraumatic pain is best managed through a multimodal approach.[45] Regardless of the manner technique employed; the principles of a multimodal strategy include sufficient diminution of the patient's pain to instill a sense of control over their pain, enable early mobilization, allow early enteral nutrition, and attenuate the perioperative stress response. A secondary goal of this approach is to maximize the benefit (analgesia) while minimizing the risk (side effects of the medication being used). These goals are often achieved through the use of regional anesthetic techniques and a combination of analgesic agents. The use of epidural anesthesia and analgesia is an integral part of the multimodal strategy because of the superior analgesia and physiologic benefits conferred by epidural analgesia.[3,46]

A multimodal approach to the management of acute pain to control postinjury pathophysiology and facilitate rehabilitation may result in accelerated recovery and decreased length of hospitalization.[47] A multimodal approach involving a combination of neuraxial analgesia and systemic analgesics during the recovery from radical prostatectomy resulted in reduced use of opioids; reduce pain scores and a decreased length of stay.[48] A recent meta-analysis examining the use of epidural analgesia following colorectal surgery found superior pain relief, faster return of bowel function and higher initial costs but lower total costs in those who received epidural analgesia as a sole regimen.[49] Although this study was supportive of the use of epidural analgesia as a sole regimen, it did not show decreased length of stay for patients in the epidural group. Multimodal analgesia in the form of systemic administration of multiple analgesics from different classes has also been found to provide adequate analgesia with low side effects as compared to epidural analgesia alone.[50] Patients undergoing major abdominal or thoracic procedures and who participate in a multimodal strategy have a reduction in hormonal and metabolic stress, preservation of total-body protein, shorter times to tracheal extubation, lower pain scores, earlier return of bowel function, and earlier fulfillment of intensive care unit discharge criteria.[47,51] By integrating the most recent data and techniques from surgery, anesthesiology and pain treatment, the multimodal approach may be seen as an extension of "clinical pathways" or "fast track protocols" by revising traditional care programs into effective postoperative rehabilitation pathways.[47] This approach may potentially decrease perioperative morbidity, decrease the length of hospital stay, and improve patient satisfaction without compromising safety. However, the widespread implementation of these programs requires multidisciplinary collaboration, change in the traditional principles of postoperative care, additional resources, and expansion of the traditional acute pain service, which may be difficult in the current economic climate.

TREATMENT METHODS

Many options are available for the treatment of acute pain, including systemic (i.e., opioid and nonopioid adjuvant) analgesics and regional (i.e., neuraxial and peripheral) analgesic techniques. By considering patients' preferences and an individualized assessment of the risks and benefits of each treatment modality, the clinician can optimize the analgesic regimen for each patient. Essential aspects for postoperative monitoring for patients receiving various postoperative analgesic treatment methods are listed in Table 51.1.

Systemic Analgesic Techniques

Opioids

Opioid analgesics are the gold standard treatments for postprocedural, traumatic and acute medical pain. These agents generally exert their analgesic effects through *mu* opioid receptors in the CNS and the periphery following an inflammatory injury, including surgical incision.[52] A theoretical advantage of opioid analgesics is that there is no analgesic ceiling. Another advantage is that opioids may be administered multiple routes including subcutaneous, transcutaneous, transmucosal, and intramuscular routes. Opioids also may be administered at specific anatomic sites such as the intrathecal (subarachnoid) or epidural space (see "Single-Dose Neuraxial Opioids" and "Continuous Epidural Analgesia" sections below). Unfortunately, the effectiveness of opioids is limited by side effects including nausea, vomiting, sedation, or the most concerning, respiratory depression. The repetitive use of opioids may induce the development of tolerance.

The most common routes of systemic opioid analgesic administration in the acute pain setting are oral (PO), intravenous (IV), and intramuscular (IM). Commonly, parenteral administration of medications is necessary in the acute pain setting because the patient is unable to tolerate oral intake. Possible parenteral routes of administration include IV, IM, transdermal (TD), and iontophoretic/transdermal (ITD). The treatment of moderate to severe acute pain often requires rapid and reliable onset of analgesia. To achieve this, the preferred medication route has tradition-

TABLE 51.1

MONITORING AND DOCUMENTATION OF POSTOPERATIVE ANALGESIA

Analgesic Medication*
Name, concentration, and dose of drug
Settings of PCA device: demand dose, lockout interval, continuous infusion
Limits set (e.g., 1-hour limits on dose administered)
Supplemental or breakthrough analgesics

Routine Monitoring
Amount of drug administered including number of unsuccessful and successful doses
Vital signs: temperature, heart rate, blood pressure, respiratory rate, 0–10 pain score
Analgesia
Pain at rest and with activity, percent pain relief
Use of breakthrough medication

Common Side Effects
Cardiovascular: hypotension, bradycardia, or tachycardia
Pulmonary: respiratory rate
Gastrointestinal: Nausea and vomiting, pruritis, urinary retention
Neurological: motor and sensory function, level of sedation

Instructions Provided
Treatment of side effects
Parameters for triggering notification of covering physician
Contact information should be provided (24 hours/7 days per week) if problems occur
Emergency analgesic treatment if PCA device fails

*Postoperative analgesia includes systemic opioids and regional analgesic techniques. This list incorporates some of the important elements of preprinted orders, documentation, and intravenous PCA and epidural analgesia daily care described in the ASA Practice Guidelines for Acute Pain Management.
CNS, central nervous system; PCA, patient-controlled analgesia.

ally been IV or IM. The development of ITD fentanyl and the validation of its efficacy in postoperative patients may expand the parenteral administration possibilities.[53] Traditional transdermal fentanyl is not ideal for the use in the acute pain setting because of its slow onset of analgesia. The full analgesic benefit of this medication can be up to 24–36 hours after application to the skin. The other important criterion for acute pain management includes reliable and predictable analgesia. Unfortunately, there is wide intersubject and intrasubject variability in serum concentration and analgesic response after systemically administered opioids in the treatment of postoperative pain.[54] The IM route of administration may result in a wider variability than the IV or ITD routes and therefore may be a less ideal alternative. However, because it possesses a rapid onset time, it may be the best alternative to those who do not have the option of ITD or do not have immediate IV access.

The transition from parenteral to oral administration of opioids usually occurs after the patient is able to tolerate oral intake and his/her pain has been stabilized with parenteral opioids. The conversion from IV or IM medications can be performed by converting the parenteral opioid into the 24-hour "parenteral morphine equivalents (PME)" and converting this into the oral equivalent of the short- and long-acting opioid of choice. The division of long-acting versus short-acting medica-

TABLE 51.2

GUIDELINES FOR EQUIANALGESIC DOSING OF OPIOID AGONISTS IN MILLIGRAMS[#]

Medication	Parenteral (IV, SC, IM)	Oral	Transdermal
Codeine	120	200	n/a
Fentanyl	0.1	n/a	5.5 mcg/hr
Hydrocodone	n/a	20	n/a
Hydromorphone	1.5	7.5	n/a
Levorphanol	2	4	n/a
Meperidine	75	300	n/a
Methadone (opioid naïve)	5	10	n/a
Morphine	10	30	n/a
Oxycodone	n/a	20	n/a
Oxymorphone	1	10	n/a
Tramadol	n/a	100	n/a

*Methadone conversion is dependent on starting dose of morphine equivalent secondary to atypical pharmacokinetics and dynamics (see Table 51-7)
#Equianalgesic doses are approximate and are intended to serve only as an estimate of opioid requirements. Actual doses may vary, in part because of wide interpatient variability in response to opioids. Doses should be individualized and gradually titrated to effect. IV, intravenous; IM, intramuscular; SC, subcutaneous, n/a, not applicable.

tions is highly dependent on the patient, the nature of their pain, the diurnal variation of their pain, but a general rule is 50% of the daily requirement can be provided as a sustained preparation and 50% as a immediate release breakthrough preparation. Numerous "standard" tables exist for these conversions that are based on pharmacokinetic data and physician experience. Other sources of conversion tables or calculators are available commercially and for educational use on the Internet including Epocrates and the Hopkins Opioid Program (www.hopweb.org), respectively (Table 51.2 and 51.3).

Tramadol. Tramadol is a synthetic opioid that exhibits weak μ-agonist activity and inhibits reuptake of norepinephrine and serotonin. Although tramadol exerts its analgesic effects primarily through central mechanisms, it may exhibit peripheral local anesthetic properties.[55] Tramadol is effective for treating moderate postoperative pain and comparable in analgesic efficacy to aspirin (650 mg) and acetaminophen (1000mg) (see Table 51.4). The advantages of tramadol for mild to moderate acute pain treatment include the relative lack of respiratory depression,

TABLE 51.3

METHADONE CONVERSION BASED ON PATIENT HISTORY OF OPIOID CONSUMPTION

Current Oral Morphine Equivalent (OME) (mg)	Methadone Equianalgesic Conversion (mg)
<100	OME / 4
101–300	OME / 8
301–600	OME / 10
601–800	OME / 12
801–1000	OME / 15
>1000	OME / 20

major organ toxicity, or depression of gastrointestinal motility; and it has a low potential for abuse.[56] Common side effects with an overall incidence ranging from 1.6% to 6.1% include dizziness, drowsiness, sweating, nausea, vomiting, dry mouth, and headache.[57] Tramadol should be used with caution in patients with seizures or increased intracranial pressure and in those taking monoamine oxidase inhibitors or serotonin reuptake inhibitors, including most antidepressants.[58]

Nonsteroidal Anti-Inflammatory Agents

NSAIDs such as aspirin, ibuprofen, and naproxen exert their analgesic effect through the inhibition of the cyclooxygenase (COX) and synthesis of prostaglandins (PG). COX enzymes and PGs are important inflammatory mediators and may play an important role in the generation and maintenance of peripheral and central sensitization. Nonselective nonsteroidal anti-inflammatory drugs (NSAIDs) inhibit both cyclooxygenase (COX) I and II enzymes and thereby decrease the production of prostaglandin E_2 (PGE_2) and other prostaglandins derived from arachidonic acid. Prostaglandins act at peripheral, as well as central sites to alter nociceptive thresholds.[58] For example, administration of PGE_2 directly into the hindpaw[59] or onto the spinal cord[60] of animals produces peripheral edema and hyperalgesia. Several studies have highlighted the importance of a peripheral site of action for NSAIDs. Administration in the periphery of monoclonal antibodies to PGE_2 is associated with a decrease in paw edema and hyperalgesia.[61] More recently, studies have highlighted a central component for NSAID action. In the spinal cord, PGE_2 can act presynaptically to increase the release of glutamate from primary afferent C-fibers[60,62] and postsynaptically to directly excite dorsal horn neurons by activation of nonselective cation currents.[63] Both effects promote the development and maintenance of central sensitization and enhanced pain states. The systemic administration of NSAIDs reduces inflammation and the behavioral correlate of central/peripheral sensitization—hyperalgesia.[64]

NSAIDs provide effective analgesia for mild to moderate acute pain and are a useful supplement to opioids for treatment of moderate to severe pain. The NSAID may provide some opioid-sparing properties through an additive or synergistic analgesic effect. NSAIDs such as ketorolac, which can be administered either orally or parenterally, are considered an integral part of a multimodal analgesic regimen by producing analgesia through different mechanisms than opioids or local anesthetics. As with opioids, NSAIDs by themselves do not appear to have a significant impact on mortality or major morbidity when compared to other analgesic agents. However, NSAIDs may improve analgesia and patient-oriented outcomes (e.g., satisfaction and quality of life) in part by reducing opioid analgesic requirements, decreasing opioid-related side effects, and facilitating patient recovery.[65,66] When given in addition to systemic opioids, NSAIDs will improve postoperative analgesia and reduce opioid requirements by up to 50%, which may reduce opioid-related side effects and facilitate return of gastrointestinal function, reduce nausea, decrease respiratory depression and improve patient satisfaction. However, not all studies note a decrease in opioid-related side effects with concurrent NSAID use.[67]

An analgesic benefit of aspirin over placebo has been shown for the 650 mg and 1000 mg doses (Table 51.4). The number of patients needed to treat for at least a 50% reduction in pain (NNT) was 4.4(4.0–4.9) and 4.0 (3.2–5.4), respectively. Single-dose aspirin (650 mg) produced significantly more drowsiness and gastric irritation than placebo, with a number-needed-to-harm (NNH) of 28 (19–51) and 38 (22–174) respectively. The authors also found that the type of pain model, pain measurement, sample size, quality of study design, and study duration had no significant impact on the results.[68] Similar NNT were obtained for naproxen 400–500 mg in postoperative pa-

TABLE 51.4

RELATIVE EFFICACY OF SINGLE DOSE ORAL ANALGESICS

Medication	NNT*	95% CI
Aspirin (650 mg)	4.4	4.0–4.9
Aspirin (1000 mg)	4.0	3.2–5.4
Ibuprofen (400 mg)	2.7	2.5–3.0
Ibuprofen (600 mg)	2.4	1.9–3.3
Diclofenac (50 mg)	2.3	2.0–2.7
Ketorolac (10 mg)	2.6	2.3–3.1
Celecoxib (200 mg)	3.5	2.9–4.4
Celecoxib (400 mg)	2.1	1.8–2.5
Acetaminophen (650 mg)	5.3	4.1–7.2
Acetaminophen (1000 mg)	3.8	3.4–4.4
Tramadol (50 mg)	7.1	4.6–18.0
Tramadol (100 mg)	4.8	3.4–8.2
Codeine (60 mg)	9.1	6.0–23.4
Oxycodone (15 mg)	2.4	1.5–4.9
Codeine (60 mg) + Acetaminophen (650 mg)	3.6	2.9–4.5
Codeine (60 mg) + Acetaminophen (1000 mg)	2.2	1.7–2.9
Oxycodone (5 mg) + Acetaminophen (325 mg)	2.5	2.0–3.2

*NNT in this case refers to the number of patients who must be treated to obtain more than 50% pain relief for moderate-to-severe postoperative pain. NNT conveys statistical and clinical significance, is useful to compare treatment efficacy for different interventions, and summarizes treatment effects in a clinically relevant way. A lower mean NNT number implies greater analgesic efficacy in this example.
CI, confidence interval; NNT, number needed to treat

tients.[69,70] The COX-II selective inhibitor, celecoxib, when given at 200mg has a NNT of 4.5 when compared to placebo in postoperative patients.[71] Neither naproxen nor celecoxib were associated with an increase in adverse events.

Acetaminophen is commonly used for acute pain management as an alternative to NSAIDs, but its site of action at the molecular level is still controversial and not well defined. There are, however, some lines of evidence supporting its role in the inhibition of cyclooxygenase. Acetaminophen has been demonstrated to inhibit a variant of COX-II enzymes in vivo[72] and be similar to the COX-II selective inhibitors: it inhibits prostaglandin synthesis in intact cells at low concentrations of added arachidonic acid further suggesting that it may inhibit COX-II function.[73] It has also been suggested that the molecular target of acetaminophen is a splice variant of COX-I, named as COX-III,[74] but its low expression level and activity suggests that this selective interaction is unlikely to be clinically relevant.[75] This suggests that acetaminophen inhibits COX-II activity in vivo and that its analgesic effect may be a function of decreased peripheral PGE_2 synthesis in addition to centrally mediated analgesic effects of acetaminophen on descending serotoninergic pathways.[76]

Acetaminophen is very effective in the treatment of acute pain, especially that of postprocedural pain. The number of patients needed to treat for at least a 50% reduction in pain over 4–6 hours (NNT) for 1000 mg of acetaminophen is 4.4, which is similar to that of 650 mg of aspirin or 100 mg of ibuprofen.[77] However, it was less effective than higher dose ibuprofen (400 mg) or diclofenac (50 mg) with NNTs of 2.3 and 2.4, respectively. Fortunately, acetaminophen is rarely associated with adverse effects in the short term, however is associated with hepatotoxicity after chronic use or overdose. In countries outside of the United States, intravenous propacetamol, the prodrug of acetaminophen or acetaminophen itself is administered to postoperative patients who are not able to tolerate oral analgesics. In clinical trials conducted in patients with moderate to severe pain after orthopedic and gynecologic surgery, the analgesic efficacy of propacetamol was similar to that of NSAIDs[78,79] While providing fast and significant pain relief as well as a significant opioid-sparing effect,[78,80] it is not associated with the increased incidence of nausea, vomiting, and respiratory depression observed with opioids or the deleterious gastrointestinal, hematological, cardiovascular, and renal effects associated with NSAIDs and selective COX-II inhibitors. Lack of inhibition of COX-I peripherally by acetaminophen may explain its favorable safety effect.[81] These results have been replicated with intravenous acetaminophen in patients recovering from major orthopedic surgery.[82]

Excitatory Amino Acids

The excitatory amino acid neurotransmitter, glutamate, has a central role in the transmission of nociceptive signals from the periphery to the supraspinal structures and in the modulation of those signals in brainstem and spinal cord through descending bulbospinal tracts. The NMDA receptor, in particular, has been shown to have a crucial role in the development of persistent pain states including neuropathic pain.[83] Although this receptor represents an obvious target for the production of analgesia, pharmacologic antagonism has met with little clinical success. Intravenous administration of the NMDA antagonist ketamine produced a reduction in neuropathic pain; however this came at the cost of high incidence of side effects.[84] Ketamine has had better results in the treatment of cancer pain as both a direct analgesic, and by improving opioid-based analgesia.[85,86] Clinical trials of dextromethorphan and memantine have failed to show any beneficial effect when compared to placebo.[87,88] The role of NMDA antagonists in acute postprocedural or posttraumatic pain has met with less disappointing but somewhat mixed results. In one study, the addition of low-dose ketamine (0.25mg/kg) to postoperative pain management with morphine was not found to be beneficial.[89] The addition of ketamine did not reduce the patient's pain scores, opioid consumption, need for rescue analgesia or increase in the quality of recovery. However, the use of low-dose (subanesthetic doses) of ketamine has been successfully used to reduce morphine requirements, need for rescue analgesia and pain scores in patients recovering from abdominal surgery, orthopedic surgery, and trauma.[90–93]

Anticonvulsants

Anticonvulsants, including gabapentin, carbamazepine, lamotrigine, and pregabalin, have traditionally used for the treatment of chronic neuropathic conditions. Gabapentin is an anticonvulsant that was developed as a spasmolytic and adjunct for the treatment of generalized or partial epileptic seizures resistant to conventional therapies. Although it was originally designed as a structural analog of the inhibitory neurotransmitter gamma-aminobutyric acid (GABA), it does not bind to GABA receptors and the mechanism of action of this class of drugs is not fully understood.[94] It is likely that its analgesic effects result from an action at the $alpha_2delta_1$ accessory unit of voltage-dependent Ca_2 channels for which it has substantial affinity[95] and which are upregulated in the dorsal root ganglia and spinal cord after peripheral nerve injury[96] as can be produced by surgical incision.[97,98] Gabapentin may produce analgesia by binding to and inhibiting presynaptic voltage-dependent Ca_2 channels, decreasing calcium influx and thereby inhibiting the release of neurotransmitters including glutamate from the primary afferent nerve fibers that synapse on and activate pain responsive neurons in the spinal cord.[99]

In clinical studies, several open-label single center and multicenter, double-blind trials established that gabapentin was also effective for the treatment of chronic pain conditions, including postherpetic neuralgia, diabetic neuropathy, central pain, phantom pain, malignant pain, trigeminal neuralgia, and human immunodeficiency virus–related neuropathy, which may be difficult to treat with more conventional therapies.[100–105] The role of gabapentin in the treatment of acute pain is more controversial. Although in animal and human models of acute pain the administration of gabapentin produces no analgesia, when it is administered prior to a variety of surgical procedures, patients report decreased pain and decreased opioid use postoperatively.[41] A recent study by Gilron et al. [106] also showed synergism between gabapentin and morphine in patients suffering from neuropathic pain. This synergistic effect may have played a role in the decreased pain scores of those receiving gabapentin because concomitant opioids were routinely administered in the postoperative period. Unfortunately, there is little evidence in the literature regarding the use of the anticonvulsant medications for the management of acute pain. In one trial, postoperative administration of gabapentin was found to have no benefit for patient's status post total abdominal hysterectomy in the acute postoperative period but was beneficial in the reduction of chronic pain associated with the surgery in the same patients.[107] Therefore, with the exception of the well-documented effectiveness of carbamazepine in the treatment of the acute exacerbation of trigeminal neuralgia, there is no evidence for the effectiveness of anticonvulsants in the treatment of acute pain not related to an operation or trauma.

Alpha-Adrenergic Medications

Alpha-adrenergic receptors are widely distributed throughout the CNS and peripheral nervous system (PNS). Alpha$_1$ receptors play an essential role in the regulation of vascular tone, but no significant role in nociception. Activation of alpha$_2$ receptors produces analgesia. They are linked to an inhibitory G-protein on the presynaptic terminus of Aδ and C fibers and are activated by descending noradrenergic tracts from the brainstem locus coeruleus (LC) and A7, which hyperpolarizes the primary afferent and reduces afferent transmitter release and pain transmission. However, depending on the particular alpha$_2$ receptor subtype 2a, 2b, or 2c, different physiologic consequences may occur. The alpha$_{2b}$ subtype produces hemodynamic responses (hypotension), while the alpha$_{2a}$ receptor is responsible analgesia.[108,109] Clonidine is the prototypic alpha$_2$ agonist used for analgesia, although it has substantial hemodynamic side effects because of its lack of absolute alpha subtype selectivity. A newer agent, dexmedetomidine (DEX), is a more selective alpha$_2$ receptor agonist that is analgesic and sedating with fewer cardiovascular effects.[110,111]

In experimental models of acute transient pain, systemically administered clonidine had no analgesic benefit.[112] In studies of postoperative patients, intravenous clonidine has been found to augment the local anesthetic block of the psoas compartment for hip surgery.[113] However, the benefit was short lived and provided approximately 7 hours of additional analgesia. Preoperative and perioperative administration of systemic clonidine has been found to have a very modest analgesic (and anxiolytic) effect following abdominal hysterectomy.[114,115] Perioperative use of systemic clonidine has been found to reduce overall opioid requirements following spinal surgery when given as a bolus of 3 mcg/kg and followed by an infusion of 0.3 mcg/kg/hour; however, modest changes in blood pressure and heart were also noted.[116]

Dexmedetomidine, though more selective for alpha$_2$ receptors and more subtype selective (alpha$_{2a}$), does not produce significant analgesia in human experimental models of acute heat or electrical pain at doses that produce modest to severe sedation.[117] In one study, dexmedetomidine infusion reduced healthy volunteer's cold pressor–induced pain by 30% at doses that produced sedation and memory loss but did not produce hemodynamic perturbations.[110] Preoperative administration of dexmedetomidine reduced postoperative opioid consumption but had no effect on postprocedure pain scores or recovery time.[118] Perioperative administration reduces opioid requirements after thoracotomy[119] and tubal ligation[120] but resulted in significant sedation and heart rate instability in some patients.

Serotoninergic Medications

Serotoninergic receptors found in the spinal dorsal horn have a complex relationship to the modulation of nociceptive transmission. Three of the subtypes of serotoninergic receptors play a role in nociceptive transmission, $5HT_1$ and $5HT_2$ hyperpolarize neurons within the dorsal horn and inhibit pain transmission, whereas $5HT_4$ receptors depolarize dorsal horn neurons and augment the transmission of nociceptive information.[121] Presynaptic terminals of descending neurons from the RVM appear to appose $5HT_1$ and $5HT_2$ receptors of primary afferents and interneurons in the spinal cord producing a reduction in pain like behavior in animals following activation of the RVM. Unfortunately, no subtype specific serotoninergic agonists are available for human use for analgesia. Interestingly, a recent study found that activation of the $5HT_4$ receptor in the brainstem eliminates the respiratory depression associated with administration the opioid fentanyl,[122] thus having an indirect but very beneficial effect on the treatment of pain.

The only clinically available serotonergic agonists or indirect serotoninergic agonists consist of the selective serotonin reuptake inhibitors (SSRIs) that are primarily used for the treatment of depression and anxiety disorders. Unfortunately, the data regarding the use of SSRIs in acute pain are lacking or negative. The lack of clinical studies assessing the analgesic value of this class is likely due to the lack of analgesic benefit of this class of drugs in the treatment of chronic pain.[123]

Nonselective Noradrenergic and Serotoninergic Medications

Although the group of nonselective noradrenergic and serotoninergic reuptake inhibitor medications, the tricyclic antidepressants (TCA) does not carry a FDA indication for pain, they are a mainstay of treatment of a variety of neuropathic and nonneuropathic chronic pain states. TCAs suppress nociceptive transmission independent of their effects upon depressed affect in the psychological domain. The exact mechanism of analgesic action remains unclear. As a class of agents, TCAs act to inhibit the reuptake and destruction or storage of biogenic amines including norepinephrine and serotonin. One possible mechanism is the accentuation of the descending serotoninergic and noradrenergic bulbospinal pathways on the spinal cord dorsal horn, by acting locally on $5HT_1$, $5HT_2$ and a$alpha_2$ receptors. Interestingly, selective serotonin reuptake inhibitors have little if any analgesic potential,[124] yet the TCAs with the greatest analgesic efficacy as those that have their greatest effect upon serotonin reuptake.[125] Alternate mechanisms including histamine receptor blockade,[126] calcium channel blockade,[127] antagonism of the NMDA receptor,[128] anti-inflammatory effects,[129] and blockade of sodium channels[130] have been suggested.

The results for TCAs in experimental models of acute pain are somewhat mixed. The secondary amine, desipramine, which has the greatest norepinephrine reuptake inhibitor selectivity, has no effect on pain scores in a capsaicin-induced mechanical allodynia model.[131] In contrast, imipramine the tertiary amine precursor to desipramine produced a reduction in pain resulting from noxious stimulation of the nasal mucosa.[132] A single study found that the administration of the tertiary tricyclic amine, amitriptyline, during the acute stage of herpes zoster decreased the prevalence of postherpetic neuralgia.[133] TCAs have not been found to be effective in the treatment of postoperative pain.[134,135]

The role of the selective serotonin and norepinephrine reuptake inhibitors, duloxetine and venlafaxine, has not been fully elucidated. Like the TCAs, these drugs have been used successfully to treat chronic pain conditions. However, there is no evidence for the effect or lack of effect on acute pain relief from duloxetine and the one study examining the use of venlafaxine for postoperative pain was negative.[136] The atypical antidepressant bupropion has not been investigated in trials of acute pain; however, it is not effective in the treatment of nonneuropathic chronic back pain.[137]

Intravenous Patient-Controlled Analgesia

Various factors, including the interpatient and intrapatient variability in analgesic needs, variability in serum drug levels (especially with intramuscular injections), and administrative delays, may contribute to inadequate postoperative analgesia. There may be difficulty in compensating for these factors with the use of a traditional PRN analgesic regimen. By circumventing some of these issues, intravenous patient-controlled analgesia (IVPCA) optimizes delivery of analgesic opioids and minimizes the effects of pharmacokinetic variability among individual patients. IV PCA is based on the premise that a negative-feedback loop exists, when pain is experienced, analgesic medication is self-administered, and when pain is reduced, there are no further demands. When the negative-feedback loop is violated, excessive sedation or respiratory depression may occur.[138] Although some equipment-related malfunctions have been reported, the PCA device itself is relatively free of problems, and most problems related to PCA use result from user or operator errors.[138]

A PCA device can be programmed for several variables, including the demand (bolus) dose, lockout interval, and background infusion (Table 51.5). The optimal demand or bolus dose is integral to intravenous PCA analgesic efficacy because an insufficient demand dose may result in inadequate analgesia, whereas an excessive demand dose may result in a higher incidence of undesirable side effects such as respiratory depression.[139] Although the optimal demand dose is uncertain, available data suggest that the optimal demand dose for morphine is 1 mg and that for fentanyl is 40 µg for opioid-naïve patients; however, the actual dose for fentanyl is often less in clinical practice.[138,139] The lockout interval may also affect the analgesic efficacy of intravenous PCA and is a safety feature of intravenous PCA. Although the optimal lockout interval is unknown, most intervals range from 5 to 10 minutes, and varying the interval within this range appears to have no effect on analgesia or side effects.[138] Most PCA devices allow the addition of a continuous or background infusion in addition to the demand dose. Initially, routine use of a background infusion was thought to confer certain advantages, including improved analgesia especially during sleep; however, subsequent trials failed to demonstrate any analgesic benefits of a background infusion in opioid-naïve patients.[140] Although the routine use of continuous or background infusions in intravenous PCA in adult opioid-naïve patients is not recommended, there may be a role for use of a background infusion for opioid-tolerant or pediatric patients. A Cochrane database meta-analysis revealed that IV PCA (compared to PRN opioids) provided significantly greater analgesia and patient satisfaction; however, patients who had IV PCA used more opioids with a higher incidence of pruritus but no difference in the incidence of other adverse events compared to PRN opioids.[141]

The incidence of opioid-related adverse events from intravenous PCA does not appear to differ significantly from that administered intravenously, intramuscularly, or subcutaneously. The rate of respiratory depression associated with intravenous PCA is low (<0.5%) and does not appear to be higher than that with systemic or neuraxial opioids.[142,143] Factors that may be associ-

TABLE 51.5

INTRAVENOUS PATIENT-CONTROLLED ANALGESIA REGIMENS FOR ACUTE PAIN

Medication	Pharmacodynamics	Bolus *	Lockout interval (min)
Morphine	*Mu* opioid receptor agonist	0.5–2.5 mg	5–10
Fentanyl	*Mu* opioid receptor agonist	10–20 mcg	5–10
Hydropmorphone	*Mu* opioid receptor agonist	0.5–0.25 mg	5–10
Alfentanil	*Mu* opioid receptor agonist	0.1–0.2 mg	5–8
Sufentanil	*Mu* opioid receptor agonist	2–5 mcg	4–10
Methadone	*Mu* opioid receptor agonist NMDA receptor antagonist	0.5–2.5 mg	8–20
Meperidine	*Mu* opioid receptor agonist	5–25 mg	5–10
Oxymorphone	*Mu* opioid receptor agonist	0.2–0.4 mg	8–10
Buprenorphine	*Mu* opioid receptor partial agonist *Kappa* opioid receptor antagonist	0.03–0.1 mg	8–20
Nalbuphine	*Mu* opioid receptor antagonist *Kappa* opioid receptor agonist	1–5 mg	5–15
Pentazocine	*Mu* opioid receptor antagonist *Kappa* opioid receptor agonist	5–15 mg	5–15

*All doses are for adult patients. The anesthesiologist should proceed with titrated intravenous loading doses if necessary to establish initial analgesia. Individual patient's requirements vary widely, with smaller doses typically given for elderly or compromised patients. Continuous infusions are not initially recommended for opioid-naïve adult patients.

ated with occurrence of respiratory depression with intravenous PCA include use of a background infusion, advanced age, concomitant administration of sedative or hypnotic agents, and co-existing pulmonary disease such as sleep apnea.[142,143]

Regional Analgesic Techniques

A variety of neuraxial and peripheral regional analgesic techniques may be employed for the effective treatment of acute pain. The majority of these techniques were initially developed for the management of acute postoperative pain; however, their application is appropriate for the treatment of any severe acute pain. In general, epidural and peripheral techniques when local anesthetics are used can provide superior analgesia compared with systemic opioids,[144] and use of these techniques may even reduce morbidity and mortality in the postoperative population.[4,5] However, there are risks associated with the use of these techniques, and a risk versus benefit analysis of these techniques should be performed on an individual basis in to determine the appropriateness of neuraxial or peripheral regional techniques for each patient, especially in light of some of the controversies about the use of these techniques in the presence of anticoagulation.

Single-Dose Neuraxial Opioids

A single dose of opioid may provide significant analgesia when administered as a sole or adjuvant analgesic agent when administered intrathecally or epidurally. One of the most important factors in determining the clinical pharmacology for a particular opioid is its degree of lipid solubility. Once inside the cerebrospinal fluid (CSF) through direct intrathecal injection or gradual migration from the epidural space, hydrophilic opioids (i.e., morphine and hydromorphone) tend to remain within the CSF and produce a delayed but longer duration of analgesia along with a generally higher incidence of side effects due to its cephalad spread. Neuraxial administration of lipophilic opioids, such as fentanyl and sufentanil, tends to provide rapid onset of analgesia, and the rapid clearance from the CSF may limit cephalad spread and development of certain side effects such as delayed respiratory depression but not pruritis.[145] The site of analgesic action for hydrophilic opioids is overwhelmingly spinal, but the primary site of action (spinal versus systemic) for single-dose neuraxial lipophilic opioids is not as certain.[146]

The differences in pharmacokinetics between lipophilic and hydrophilic opioids may influence the choice of opioid in an attempt to optimize analgesia and minimize side effects for a particular clinical situation. Single-dose intrathecal administration of a lipophilic opioid may be useful in situations (e.g., ambulatory surgical patients) in which rapid analgesic onset (minutes) combined with a moderate duration of action (<4 hours) and minimal risk of respiratory depression is needed.[147] Single-dose hydrophilic opioid administration provides effective postoperative analgesia and may be useful in patients monitored on an inpatient basis for which a longer duration of analgesia would be beneficial.

Single-dose epidural administration of lipophilic and hydrophilic opioids is used to provide analgesia, with considerations generally similar to those discussed with single-dose intrathecal administration of opioids. A single bolus of epidural fentanyl may be administered to provide rapid postoperative analgesia; however, diluting the epidural dose of fentanyl (typically 50 to 100 μg) in at least 10 mL of preservative-free normal saline is suggested to decrease the onset and prolong the duration of analgesia, possibly as a result of an increase in the initial spread and diffusion of the lipophilic opioid.[148] Single-dose epidural morphine is effective for postoperative analgesia and may decrease postoperative patient morbidity in selected patients.[149,150] Use of a single-dose hydrophilic opioid may be especially helpful in

TABLE 51.6

RECOMMENDED DOSAGE FOR NEURAXIAL ADMINISTRATION OF OPIOIDS

Medication	Intrathecal Single Dose	Epidural Single Dose	Epidural Continuous Infusion
Fentanyl	5–25 mcg	50–100 mcg	25–100 mcg/hr
Morphine	0.1–0.3 mg	1–5 mg	0.1–1 mg/hr
Morphine-extended release	Not recommended	5–15 mg	Not recommended
Hydromorphone	0.005–0.1 mg	0.5–1 mg	0.1–0.2 mg/hr
Sufentanil	2–10 mcg	1–50 mcg	10–20 mcg/hr
Alfentanil	Not recommended	0.5–1 mg	0.2 mg/hr
Methadone	Not recommended	4–8 mg	0.3–0.5 mg/hr

Doses are based on the use of the neuraxial opioid alone. No continuous intrathecal infusions are provided. Lower doses may be effective when administered to elderly patients. Units vary across medications for single dose (mcg versus mg) and continuous infusions (mcg/hr versus mg/hr).

providing postoperative epidural analgesia when the epidural catheter's location is not congruent with the surgical incision (e.g., lumbar epidural catheter for thoracic surgery). Lower doses of epidural morphine may be required for elderly patients and thoracic catheter sites. Commonly used dosages for intrathecal and epidural administration of neuraxial opioids are provided in Table 51.6.

An extended-release formulation of (single-dose) epidural morphine (Depo-Dur™) encapsulated within liposomes resulting in up to 48 hours of analgesia has been introduced.[151] The greatest benefit of liposomal morphine is its extended release formulation and the prolonged duration of effect which may be important with the increasing use of long acting low molecular weight heparin medications for postoperative patients for thrombosis prophylaxis. Liposomal morphine exhibits a dose dependent increase in analgesia, but unfortunately also a dose-dependent increase in adverse events including respiratory depression. This formulation is relatively new and therefore no long term data have been developed looking at patient outcomes including overall adverse event rates or any reduction in thrombosis rates as compared to traditional epidural catheter based long term management. As with traditional single-dose neuraxial opioids, clinicians should provide a lower dose of liposomal extended-release morphine in the elderly or those with decreased physiologic reserve or coexisting diseases, and liposomal extended-release morphine has not been approved for use in pediatric patients.

Continuous Epidural Analgesia

Analgesia delivered through an indwelling epidural catheter is a generally safe and effective method for management of acute pain.[152] Postoperative epidural analgesia can provide superior analgesia compared with systemic opioids.[46]

Epidural Medications. Epidural infusions of local anesthetic alone may be used for postoperative analgesia, but in general, they are not as effective in controlling pain as local anesthetic–opioid epidural analgesic combinations.[46] The rationale for using local anesthetic only epidural infusions has been to avoid the side effects of epidural opioids. Unfortunately, this practice results in a significant failure rate of the technique including regression of sensory block providing inadequate analgesia and relatively high incidence of motor block and hypotension. These outcomes can lead to decreased patient and provider satisfaction in the technique.

Opioids may be used alone for postoperative epidural infusions in order to avoid the motor block or hypotension from

local anesthetic induced sympathetic blockade.[152] This advantage might be desirable in patients following abdominal aortic aneurysm operations as well as surgery with large fluid shifts in patients with significant cardiac or cerebrovascular disease. There are differences between continuous epidural infusions of lipophilic (e.g., fentanyl, sufentanil) and hydrophilic (e.g., morphine, hydromorphone) opioids. The analgesic site of action (spinal versus systemic) for continuous epidural infusions of lipophilic opioids is not clear, although several randomized clinical trials suggest that it is systemic[155] because there were no differences in plasma concentrations, side effects, or pain scores between those who received intravenous or epidural infusions of fentanyl. Although some data suggest a benefit from epidural of lipophilic opioids when compared to IV administration,[154] the overall advantage of administering continuous epidural infusions of lipophilic opioids alone is marginal at best. Hydrophilic opioids are quite different because of their relative lack of diffusion into the systemic circulation; the primary site of their analgesic action is spinal.[155] Hydrophilic opioids can distribute throughout the cerebrospinal fluid therefore the continuous infusion of these opioids may be especially useful for providing postoperative analgesia when the site of catheter insertion is not congruent with the site of surgery. Continuous epidural infusions of hydrophilic opioids provide superior analgesia compared with traditional PRN administration of systemic opioids.[156]

The combination of local anesthetics and opioids in a continuous epidural infusion may have advantages over infusions using a local anesthetic or opioid alone. Compared with a local anesthetic or opioid alone, a local anesthetic–opioid combination provides superior postoperative analgesia including improved dynamic pain relief, limits regression of sensory block, and possibly decreases the dose of local anesthetic administered,[157] although the incidence of side effects may or may not be diminished.[152] Continuous epidural infusion of a local anesthetic–opioid combination also provides superior analgesia compared with intravenous PCA with opioids.[46] It is unclear whether the analgesic effect of the local anesthetic and opioid in the epidural analgesia is additive or synergistic. Experimental studies demonstrate a synergistic effect between local anesthetics and opioids[158]; however, clinical trials suggest an additive effect[159] and the lack of improvement in side effects when used in combination supports the clinical experimental data.

The choice of local anesthetic for continuous epidural infusions varies. In general, bupivacaine or ropivacaine over lidocaine is chosen because of the differential and preferential clinical sensory blockade with minimal impairment of motor function.[160]

The concentrations used for postoperative epidural analgesia (≤0.125% bupivacaine or ≤0.2% ropivacaine) are lower than those used for intraoperative anesthesia. The choice of opioid also varies, although many clinicians choose to use a lipophilic opioid (fentanyl, 2 to 5 μg/mL, or sufentanil, 0.5 to 1 μg/mL) to allow for rapid titration of analgesia.[152,155] However, the use of the lipophilic opioid may just provide greater analgesia than local anesthetics alone; it is not clear whether use of these highly permeable medications does not simply provide a stable systemic concentration of opioid. The use of a hydrophilic opioid (morphine, 0.05 to 0.1 mg/mL, or hydromorphone, 0.01 to 0.05 mg/mL) as part of a local anesthetic–opioid epidural analgesic regimen may is more consistent with the goal of spinal delivery of opioid and also provides effective postoperative analgesia.[155]

A variety of adjuvant medications may be added to epidural infusions to enhance analgesia while minimizing side effects, but none has gained widespread acceptance. Two of the more studied adjuvants are clonidine and epinephrine. Clonidine mediates its analgesic effects primarily through its action at alpha$_2$ receptors in the spinal cord, and the epidural dose typically used ranges from 5 to 20 μg/hour.[161,162] The clinical application of clonidine is limited by its side effects: hypotension, bradycardia, and sedation.[161,162] Hypotension and bradycardia are both dose dependent. Epinephrine may improve epidural analgesia, can increase sensory block, and is generally administered at a concentration of 2 to 5 μg/mL[163] but it is also associated with a worsened motor block.[164] Epidural epinephrine added to local anesthetics is also associated with longer stage two labor and decrease APGAR scores in parturient.[164] Epidural administration of NMDA antagonists, such as ketamine, has been performed on a limited basis. Lauretti et al[165] found no analgesic benefit when ketamine was added to the clonidine epidural infusion following orthopedic surgery. This contrasts with another trial showing a pre-emptive analgesic benefit of epidural ketamine prior to a thoracotomy incision.[166] The theoretical explanation for the latter result is that ketamine attenuates the development of central sensitization and might potentiate the analgesic effect of epidural opioids. The caveat to this is that the safety of neuraxial ketamine infusions is controversial and may result in neuronal apoptosis.[167] Further safety and analgesic data are needed to justify its use.

Side Effects of Neuraxial Analgesic Drugs. Many medication-related (opioid and local anesthetic) side effects can occur with use of postoperative epidural analgesia. However, before automatically ascribing the cause to the epidural analgesic regimen, it is important to first consider other causes of the most common adverse effects of epidural analgesia namely hypotension, respiratory insufficiency/depression. These can include low intravascular volume, bleeding, and low cardiac output for hypotension and cerebrovascular accident, pulmonary edema, and evolving sepsis. Standing orders and nursing protocols for analgesic regimens, neurological, hemodynamic and respiratory monitoring; treatment of side effects; and physician notification about critical parameters should be standard for all patients receiving neuraxial and other types of postoperative analgesia.

Local anesthetics used in an epidural analgesic regimen may block sympathetic fibers and contribute to postoperative hypotension. Although the incidence of postoperative hypotension with postoperative epidural analgesia may be as high as approximately 7%, the average is closer to 0.7% to 3%.[168] Strategies to treat noncritical hypotension due to epidural analgesia include decreasing the overall dose of local anesthetic administered, or use of opioid-alone epidural since it is unlikely that neuraxial opioid alone would contribute to postoperative hypotension.[152]

Use of local anesthetics for postoperative epidural analgesia may also contribute to lower extremity motor block in approximately 2% to 3% of patients[168] and this may contribute to development of pressure sores in the heels.[169] A lower concentration of local anesthetics and catheter-incision congruent placement of epidural catheters for abdominal or thoracic procedures may decrease the incidence of motor block.[170] Although motor block resolves in most cases after stopping the epidural infusion for approximately 2 hours, persistent or increasing motor block needs to be promptly evaluated, and spinal hematoma, spinal abscess, and intrathecal catheter migration should be considered as part of the differential diagnosis.

Nausea and vomiting associated with neuraxial administration of a single dose opioid occurs in approximately 20% to 50% of patients,[171] and the cumulative incidence among those receiving continuous infusions of opioids may be as high as 45% to 80%.[172] Clinical and experimental data suggest that the incidence of neuraxial opioid–related nausea and vomiting is dose dependent.[173] Nausea and vomiting from neuraxial opioids may be related to the cephalad migration of opioid within the CSF to the area postrema in the medulla.[171] Use of fentanyl alone or in combination with a local anesthetic in an epidural infusion is associated with a lower incidence of nausea and vomiting compared with infusions using morphine.[172,174] A variety of agents have been successfully used to treat neuraxial opioid–induced nausea and vomiting, including naloxone, droperidol, metoclopramide, dexamethasone, and transdermal scopolamine.[175,176]

Pruritus is one of the most common side effects of epidural or intrathecal administration of opioids, with an incidence of approximately 60% compared with about 15% to 18% for epidural local anesthetic administration or systemic opioids.[177] Although the cause of neuraxial opioid–induced pruritus is uncertain, it does not appear to be associated with peripheral histamine release but may be related to central activation of an "itch center" in the medulla or opioid receptors in the trigeminal nucleus or nerve roots with cephalad migration of the opioid[171] or through the activation of a separate population of primary afferents that mediate nonhistamine itch.[178] It is unclear whether the incidence of neuraxial opioid–related pruritus is dose dependent because a quantitative systematic review[177] suggests no evidence of a relationship, whereas other clinical and experimental studies indicate a significant correlation.[179] Use of an epidural infusion of fentanyl alone or as part of a local anesthetic–opioid combination appears to be generally associated with a lower incidence of pruritus compared with morphine.[174] A variety of agents have been evaluated for the prevention and treatment of opioid-induced pruritus. Intravenous naloxone, naltrexone, nalbuphine, and droperidol appear to be efficacious for the pharmacologic control of opioid-induced pruritus.[177] Although pruritus is a common side effect, it often mild, it is relatively easy to treat.[180]

Neuraxial opioids used in appropriate doses are not associated with a higher incidence of respiratory depression than that seen with systemic administration of opioids. The incidence of respiratory depression associated with neuraxial administration of opioids is dose dependent and typically ranges from 0.1% to 0.9%.[181] The incidence of respiratory depression with continuous infusions of epidural opioids appears to be no greater than that seen after systemic opioid administration.[181] Although some institutions require patients with continuous epidural infusions of hydrophilic opioids to receive monitoring in an intensive care unit setting, many large-scale trials have demonstrated the relative safety (incidence of respiratory depression <0.9%) of this technique on regular hospital wards.[182] Neuraxial lipophilic opioids are thought to cause less <u>delayed</u> respiratory depression than hydrophilic opioids, although administration of lipophilic opioids may be associated with significant, <u>early</u> respiratory depression.[183] Delayed respiratory depression is primarily associated with the cephalad spread of the hydrophilic opioids, which typically occurs within 12 hours after injection.[184] Risks factors for respiratory depression with neuraxial opioids include increasing dose, increasing age, concomitant use of systemic opioids or sedatives, and possibly prolonged or extensive surgery, presence of comorbidities, and thoracic surgery.[184] Treatment with naloxone and airway management, if necessary, is effective in 0.1–to 0.4-mg increments; however, the clinical duration of action is relatively short compared with the respiratory-depressant effect of neuraxial opioids, and a continuous infusion of naloxone (0.5 to 5 µg/kg/hour) may be needed.[185]

Urinary retention associated with neuraxial administration of opioids is the result of an interaction with the opioid receptors in the spinal cord that decreases the detrusor muscle's strength of contraction.[171] The incidence of urinary retention seems to be higher with neuraxially administered opioids than that given systemically. Urinary retention does not appear to depend on opioid dose and may be treated with the use of low-dose naloxone, although at the risk of reversing the analgesic effects.[185] Epidural administration of local anesthetics is also associated with urinary retention, with a reported rate of approximately 10% to 30%.[186] Higher epidural infusion rates of local anesthetics (with a greater extent of sensory block and higher incidence of motor block) may be associated with a higher incidence of urinary retention.[187]

Patient-Controlled Epidural Analgesia. Epidural analgesia has been traditionally delivered as a fixed rate or continuous infusion (CEI); however, the administration of epidural analgesia through a patient-controlled device (PCEA) has become more common. Like intravenous PCA, PCEA allows for individualization of postoperative analgesic requirements and may have several advantages over CEI, including lower drug use and greater patient satisfaction.[188] PCEA also provides superior analgesia compared with intravenous PCA. PCEA is a safe and effective technique for acute analgesia in hospitalized. Observational data from two series of more than 1000 patients each reveal that more than 90% of patients with PCEA receive adequate analgesia, with a median pain score of 1 (of a possible 10) at rest and 4 with activity.[168,189] Incidences of side effects are 1.8% to 16.7% for pruritus, 3.8% to 14.8% for nausea, 13.2% for sedation, 4.3% to 6.8% for hypotension, 0.1% to 2% for motor block, and 0.2% to 0.3% for respiratory depression.[168, 189] These rates are comparable to those reported with CEI, with an incidence of 10.2% to 22% for pruritus, 3.1% to 22% for nausea, 7.4% for sedation, 0.7% to 6.6% for hypotension, 3% for motor block, and 0.1% to 1.6% for respiratory depression.[182,190] The optimal PCEA analgesic solution and delivery parameters are unclear. Use of a continuous or background infusion in addition to the demand dose is more common with PCEA than with intravenous PCA and may provide analgesia superior to the use of a demand dose alone.[191] In general, most acute pain specialists are gravitating toward a variety of low-concentration local anesthetic–opioid combinations (Table 51.7) in an attempt to improve analgesia while minimizing side effects.

Outcome Studies of Epidural Analgesia. Use of perioperative epidural anesthesia and analgesia, especially with a local anesthetic–based analgesic solution, can attenuate the pathophysiological response to surgery and may be associated with a reduction in mortality and morbidity compared with analgesia with systemic (opioid) agents.[4,5] A meta-analysis of randomized data (141 trials enrolling 9559 subjects) demonstrated that perioperative use of neuraxial anesthesia and analgesia versus general anesthesia and systemic opioids reduced overall mortality (primarily in orthopedic patients) by approximately 30%.[192] In a Medicare database analysis of 68,000 surgical patients, postoperative epidural-based analgesia was associated with a decrease in overall mortality.[193] Furthermore, use of epidural analgesia can decrease the incidence of postoperative gastrointestinal, pulmo-

TABLE 51.7

NEURAXIAL PATIENT-CONTROLLED ANALGESIA REGIMENS FOR ACUTE PAIN

Location of Incision	Analgesic Solution	Continuous Rate (ml/hr)	Demand Dose (ml)	Lockout interval (min)
General regimen	0.05% Bupivacaine + 4 mcg/ml fentanyl	4–10	2–6	10
	0.0625% Bupivacaine + 5 mcg/ml fentanyl	4–6	3–4	10–15
	0.1% Bupivacaine + 5 mcg/ml fentanyl	6	2	10–15
	0.2% Ropivacaine + 5 mcg/ml fentanyl	5	2	20
Thoracic	0.0625% to 0.125% Bupivacaine + 5 mcg/ml fentanyl	3–4	2–3	10–15
Abdominal	0.0625% Bupivacaine + 5 mcg/ml fentanyl	4–6	3–4	10–15
	0.125% Bupivacaine + 0.5 mcg/ml sufentanil	3–5	2–3	12
	0.1% to 0.2% Ropivacaine + 2 mcg/ml fentanyl	3–5	2–5	10–15
Lower extremity	0.0625% to 0.125% Bupivacaine + 5 mcg/ml fentanyl	4	2	10

Patient-controlled epidural analgesic regimens commonly used at the Johns Hopkins Hospital

nary, and possibly cardiac complications.[4,5] By inhibiting sympathetic outflow, decreasing the total opioid dose, and attenuating a spinal reflex inhibition of the gastrointestinal tract,[4] postoperative thoracic epidural analgesia can facilitate return of gastrointestinal motility without contributing to bowel dehiscence.[194] Randomized clinical trials demonstrate that use of postoperative thoracic epidural analgesia with a local anesthetic–based analgesic solution allows earlier return of gastrointestinal function and fulfillment of discharge criteria.

Perioperative use of epidural analgesia with a local anesthetic–based regimen in patients undergoing abdominal and thoracic surgery decreases postoperative pulmonary complications by preserving postoperative pulmonary function by providing superior analgesia and attenuating a spinal reflex inhibition of diaphragmatic function.[4] A meta-analysis of 48 randomized clinical trials and another large, randomized clinical trial demonstrated that use of thoracic epidural analgesia with a local anesthetic–based regimen decreased the incidence of pulmonary infections and complications.[195,196] However, patients who receive postoperative epidural opioids, intercostal blocks, wound infiltration, or intrapleural analgesia do not have a significant decrease in the incidence of pulmonary complications.

Use of postoperative thoracic, but not lumbar, epidural analgesia may decrease the incidence of postoperative myocardial infarction,[192] possibly by attenuating the stress response by improving postoperative analgesia, and providing a favorable redistribution of coronary blood flow.[198] The finding that only thoracic epidural analgesia decreases the incidence of postoperative myocardial infarction corroborates experimental data on the physiologic benefits of thoracic epidural analgesia, such as a reduction in the severity of myocardial ischemia or size of infarction, attenuation of sympathetically mediated coronary vasoconstriction, and improvement of coronary flow to areas at risk for ischemia.[198]

Although postoperative epidural analgesia appears to decrease postoperative gastrointestinal, pulmonary, and possibly cardiac morbidity, the benefits of postoperative epidural analgesia are not as clear for other areas such as postoperative coagulation, cognitive dysfunction and immune function. Despite the fact that many randomized clinical trials and meta-analyses show that use of *intra*-operative regional anesthesia decreases the incidence of hypercoagulable-related events such as deep venous thrombosis, pulmonary embolism, or vascular graft failure[192,199] evidence of a beneficial effect of *post*operative epidural analgesia in decreasing the incidence of hypercoagulable-related events is not compelling.

The ability of postoperative epidural analgesia to attenuate postoperative pathophysiology and improve outcomes also depends on the type of drugs used (opioids versus local anesthetics). Maximal attenuation of perioperative pathophysiology occurs with use of a local anesthetic-based epidural analgesic solution. The use of a local anesthetic–based or local anesthetic/opioid combination versus opioid-alone analgesic solution is associated with an earlier recovery of gastrointestinal motility after abdominal surgery and less frequent occurrence of pulmonary complications. Epidural analgesia is not a generic entity because different catheter locations and analgesic regimens may differentially affect perioperative morbidity.

Use of postoperative epidural analgesia may be associated with an improvement in postoperative analgesia and patient-reported outcomes such as patient satisfaction and health-related quality of life (HRQL).[200] Compared with systemic opioids, epidural local anesthetics consistently provide superior analgesia.[46] The data on the analgesic superiority of postoperative epidural analgesia reflect those seen with epidural analgesia during labor.[201] Although the concept of satisfaction is complex and difficult to measure accurately, the analgesic benefits of postoperative epidural analgesia may contribute to greater patient satisfaction and improve HRQL.[200]

Risks of Epidural Analgesia. The benefits of perioperative epidural anesthesia-analgesia must be weighed against the risks of this technique. Risks and benefits should be evaluated for each patient. There are complications associated with placement of an epidural catheter, with several risks associated with indwelling epidural catheters including epidural hematoma and abscess should be discussed in the context of postprocedure and/or acute pain management with epidural analgesia. The concurrent use of anticoagulants and of neuraxial anesthesia and analgesia has always been a relatively controversial issue but has been highlighted over the past decade with the increased incidence of spinal hematomas after the introduction of low-molecular-weight heparin in North America in 1993. Traditionally, the incidence of spinal hematoma is estimated at approximately 1 in 150,000 for epidural block, with a lower incidence of 1 in 220,000 for spinal blocks. Before its introduction in North America, low-molecular-weight heparin was used in Europe without significant problems; however, the incidence of spinal hematoma rose to as high as 1 in 40,800 for spinal anesthetics and 1 in 6600 for epidural anesthetics (1 in 3100 for postoperative epidural analgesia) in the United States between 1993 and 1998.[202] The estimate of the higher incidence of spinal hematomas after epidural catheter removal is based in part on the Food and Drug Administration's MedWatch data, which suggest that epidural catheter removal may be a traumatic event, although this is still a relatively controversial issue.[203] Different types and classes of anticoagulants have different pharmacokinetic properties that affect the timing of neuraxial catheter or needle insertion and catheter removal. Despite a number of observational and retrospective studies investigating the incidence of spinal hematoma in the setting of various anticoagulants and neuraxial techniques, there is no definitive conclusion regarding the absolute safety of neuraxial anesthesia and anticoagulation. The American Society of Regional Anesthesia and Pain Medicine (ASRA) lists a series of consensus statements based on the available literature for administration (insertion and removal) of neuraxial techniques in the presence of various anticoagulants, including oral anticoagulants (warfarin), anti-platelet agents, fibrinolytics-thrombolytics, standard unfractionated heparin, and low-molecular-weight heparin.[204,205] These guidelines will be updated shortly to include the newer long-acting anticoagulants that have been approved since the consensus guidelines were composed. Two of the newer agents, Fondaparinux and Dabigatran etexilate have half-lives of 17 and 14–17 hours respectively. It has been recommended to delay insertion of an epidural catheter until two half-lives have past to de crease the risk of epidural hematoma.[206] The ASRA consensus statements include the concepts that the timing of neuraxial needle or catheter insertion or removal should reflect the pharmacokinetic properties of the specific anticoagulant, that frequent neurological monitoring is essential, that concurrent use of multiple anticoagulants may increase the risk of bleeding, and that the analgesic regimen should be tailored to facilitate neurological monitoring, which may be continued in some cases for 24 hours after epidural catheter removal. An updated version of the ASRA consensus statements on neuraxial anesthesia and anticoagulation can be found on their web site (www.asra.com), and some of these statements address the newer anticoagulants.

Infection associated with postoperative epidural analgesia may result from exogenous or endogenous sources.[152] Serious infections such as epidural abscess and meningitis associated with epidural analgesic are rare (<1 in 1,000, <1:50,000, respectively).[207] Epidural infections are associated with many sources of the bacteria including needle contamination, catheter contamination, epidural medication contamination, lack of the use of in-line bacterial filters, duration of catheter implantation and patient predisposing factors for infection.[208] The use of epidural analgesia in the general surgical population with a typical duration of postoperative catheterization (approximately 2–4 days) is generally not associated with epidural abscess formation.[168] A trial of postoperative epidural analgesia (mean catheterization of 6.3 days) in more than 4000 surgical cancer patients did not reveal any abscesses. Even though serious infectious complications appear to be rare after short-term (<4 days) epidural infusions, there may be a relatively higher incidence of superficial inflammation or cellulitis (4% to 14%) and even higher rate of catheter colonization (20% to 35%), with the proportion of positive cultures increasing with the duration of catheterization; however, catheter colonization rate may not be a good predictor of epidural space infection.[209]

Peripheral Regional Analgesia

The use of peripheral regional analgesic techniques as a single injection or continuous infusion can provide superior analgesia for acute pain when compared with systemic opioids and may even result in improvement in various outcomes.[210] A variety of wound infiltration and peripheral regional techniques (e.g., brachial plexus, lumbar plexus, femoral, sciatic-popliteal, and scalp nerve blocks) can be used to provide postprocedural and acute analgesia. Peripheral nerve regional analgesic techniques may have several advantages over systemic opioids including superior analgesia and decrease in opioid-related side effects and over neuraxial techniques including decreased risk of epidural hematoma formation.[211] A one-time injection of local anesthetic for peripheral regional techniques may be used primarily for intraoperative anesthesia or as an adjunct for postprocedure analgesia but can be used for acute traumatic pain management such as long bone fractures or rib fractures. Compared with placebo, peripheral nerve blocks with local anesthetics provide superior analgesia and are associated with decreased opioid use, decreased opioid-related side effects, and improvement in patient satisfaction.[210] The duration of postoperative analgesia resulting from the local anesthetic in the peripheral nerve block varies but may last up to 24 hours after injection. Continuous infusions of local anesthetics can be administered through peripheral nerve catheters. The use of continuous infusions or patient-controlled peripheral analgesia results in superior analgesia decreased opioid-related side effects, and greater patient satisfaction in comparison with systemic opioids.[211] Unfortunately, the optimal parameters including the local anesthetic, the medication concentration, the inclusion of opioid or other adjuvant medications, or continuous versus PCA versus intermittent boluses for peripheral analgesia have not been determined.

Several nonepidural regional analgesic techniques can be used for management of postoperative thoracic pain, including paravertebral and intercostal blocks, interpleural (intrapleural) analgesia, and cryoanalgesia. The most promising technique appears to be the thoracic paravertebral block, which has been used for thoracic, breast, and upper abdominal surgery and for treatment of rib fracture pain.[212] The possible sites of analgesia for the thoracic paravertebral block include direct somatic nerve, sympathetic nerve, and epidural blockade. The thoracic paravertebral block can be administered as a single injection or continuous infusion through a catheter may provide equal or superior analgesia compared with thoracic epidural analgesia, and is a valuable alternative to thoracic epidural analgesia.[213] The analgesic efficacy of interpleural analgesia is controversial.[214] In a meta-analysis of randomized-controlled trials examining interpleural analgesia, no difference was observed between interpleural analgesia and placebo injections. Interpleural analgesia appears to be inferior to epidural and paravertebral analgesia for postoperative

pain control, preservation of lung function after thoracotomy, and reduction of postoperative pulmonary complications.[214] Intercostal blocks may provide short-term postoperative analgesia and may be repeated postoperatively; however, the incidence of pneumothorax increases with each intercostal nerve blocked (1.4% per nerve, with an overall incidence of 8.7% per patient).[215] Like interpleural analgesia, intercostal blocks do not reduce the incidence of pulmonary complications postoperatively compared to epidural analgesia. Cryoanalgesia can be used for postoperative analgesia after thoracotomy but, like interpleural analgesia and intercostal blocks, does not appear to provide any analgesic advantage over epidural analgesia and is not effective for other types of postoperative pain.[216]

Intra-articular Analgesia

Local peripheral administration of opioids including intra-articular injections after knee procedures may provide analgesia for up to 24 hours after surgery.[217] Peripheral opioid receptors are found on the peripheral terminals of primary afferent nerves and are upregulated during inflammation of peripheral tissues.[52] The results of the several randomized clinical trials investigating this topic are summarized.[217] Use of a higher dose of intra-articular morphine (5 mg versus 1 mg) results in superior analgesia; however, there may be no advantage in the degree of analgesia provided between intra-articular and systemic opioids. The systemic absorption and action of intra-articular morphine injection have not yet been excluded. Intra-articular injection of local anesthetics may provide a limited duration of postoperative analgesia, but the clinical benefit from intra-articular local anesthetics injections is unclear.[218]

ANALGESIA IN SPECIAL POPULATIONS

This chapter has provided a general approach to the principles and practice of acute pain management, but this approach may not be applicable to certain populations that may have unique anatomic, physiologic, pharmacologic, affective, and cognitive issues. The management of acute pain should be tailored to the specific needs of a particular population. Although each topic by itself could merit a separate chapter in some textbooks, the general principles and essence of the issues associated with each population are outlined, and references are made to other more extensive sources.

War Trauma

The treatment of traumatic battlefield pain is largely a function of the type and acuity of injury, stability of the patient, level of treatment (Table 51.8), availability of resources, and patient diagnosis. The chain of casualty evacuation is built up levels or echelons of care, which were developed in WWII to facilitate the rapid evacuation of wounded soldiers based on their medical condition and needs. In order to maximize efficiency and ensure the continued availability of resources, healthcare providers at each level provide no more care than that which is necessary to either return the soldier to duty or safely evacuate the casualty to the next highest level. For first level treatment, pain management consists of parenteral morphine or NSAIDs or acetaminophen, which some units dispense to individual soldiers as part of "wound packs."[219] COX-2 inhibitors possess the advantage of having minimal inhibitory effects on platelet function, which can prolong bleeding. One concern about NSAIDs is the possible increased incidence of renal failure in dehydrated and hypovolemic soldiers,[220] but this risk is mitigated by the young age, and lack of concomitant medical problems and medication usage in most

TABLE 51.8

LEVELS OF CARE IN A WAR ZONE

Level (Echelon)	Location	Type of medical unit	Primary functions/ personnel
First	Combat Zone	Battalion Aid Station	Pain relief, stabilization and preparation for medical evacuation. Self care/ Corpsmen care/ Buddy care
Second	Combat Zone	Mobile Field Surgical Teams or Forward Surgical Teams	Resuscitation and surgical stabilization by surgeons, anesthetists, and nurses.
Third	Controlled Area of Combat Zone	Combat Support Hospital or Mobile Army Surgical Hospital	Medical and surgical care. Broad array of physicians and nurses.
Fourth	Communication Zone	Military Medical Centers in United States or overseas.	Medical and surgical care. May provide definitive treatment (in United States) or rehabilitation services in retained active duty personnel.
Fifth	United States	VA Hospitals	Definitive long-term treatment and rehabilitation in wounded or medically boarded soldiers.

deployed soldiers. Acetaminophen may be marginally safer than NSAIDs, but is generally less effective as an analgesic.[221]

Morphine is the standard opioid analgesic used for battlefield pain control, having been first administered orally in the War of 1812 and parenterally in the U. S. Civil War. Intramuscular morphine can be given on the battlefield or battalion aid station (BAS), ideally by a medical corpsman, or alternatively by a colleague or the soldier himself. Although IM administration generally provides rapid and reliable analgesia, the liabilities of this delivery mode include variable absorption during shock and with certain wounds, and the risk of infection. Intravenous administration is more reliable than IM use, but is often impractical and requires specialized equipment and trained personnel.[222] The U. S. military is currently investigating the feasibility of providing oral transmucosal fentanyl citrate (OTFC) in "wound packs" to small, highly disciplined units that tend to operate independently without the benefit of an organized, medical support system (e.g. Special Forces). The pharmacokinetics of transmucosal delivery are comparable to that of IM administration, with therapeutic blood levels being reached within 10–15 minutes, and peak plasma concentration occurring about 20 minutes after administration.[223] Approximately 25% of OTFC is absorbed via the oral mucosa, with another 25% being slowly absorbed through the gastrointestinal tract.[223] The pharmacokinetics of OTFC appears to be independent of age, unaffected by multiple dose regimens, and less prone to hemodynamic variations,[224,225] which may make it an ideal drug for battlefield analgesia. Kotwal et al.[226] recently reported using high dose (1600 mcg) OTFC to treat 22 soldiers with acute orthopedic injuries in an out-of-hospital setting in Operation Iraqi Freedom (OIF). Excellent pain relief without the need for additional analgesia was reported in 19 patients, with minor, self-limiting side effects occurring in 8 soldiers. One patient, who received a repeat dose of fentanyl followed by subsequent intravenous opioids, experienced respiratory depression re-

quiring reversal with naloxone 4 hours following administration. Other rapidly acting analgesics that may someday be used in lieu of parenteral opioids include intranasal butorphanol, intranasal ketamine and fentanyl buccal tablets.

Second level medical treatment facilities include mobile field surgical teams and forward surgical teams (FST), whose providers include surgeons, anesthetists and nurses. The primary functions of FSTs are resuscitation and stabilization, with the typical duration of stay being measured in hours. Pain control at this echelon of care generally involves oral opioid and nonopioid analgesics, and intravenous opioids, which can be safely monitored by nurses and other personnel trained in postanesthesia recovery. Patient-controlled analgesia may be used at these facilities as resources dictate, but is often unavailable.

Care at third level military treatment facilities includes intensive care units and medical wards, which may administer continuous infusions of opioid and nonopioid (e.g. Ketamine and epidural infusions of local anesthetics) analgesics for acute and subacute injuries. When pain management–trained anesthesiologists have been deployed to CSH, more advanced interventions such as sympathetic and paravertebral blocks have been performed. Recently, anesthesiologists have begun to employ peripheral nerve catheters for intermediate-term pain control (Table 51.9).[227,228] In addition to providing safe and titratable pain relief, peripheral nerve catheters can be used for anesthesia in patients requiring repeat surgery or wound debridement. With proper maintenance and monitoring, tunneled peripheral nerve catheters can be reliably used for up to 3 weeks after placement. The limitations of peripheral nerve catheters at CSH include shortage of personnel, speed of exodus, infection risk, and concerns about compartment syndrome.

To a lesser degree, care at this level also focuses on reducing the long-term sequelae of acute injuries. The U. S. military has attempted to reduce the incidence of chronic pain following

TABLE 51.9

ADVANTAGES OF PERIPHERAL NERVE CATHETERS FOR WAR INJURIES

Can provide anesthesia for repeat surgery or wound debridement
Can provide excellent, limb-specific analgesia
Stable hemodynamics
Minimal side effects
Reduced need for opioid and other analgesics
Improved alertness
Requires only simple, easily transportable equipment

trauma or surgery by the preventive use of neuropathic pain medications such as gabapentin. When used preemptively before surgical procedures associated with a high incidence of severe acute and chronic pain, gabapentin and other drugs used to treat neuropathic pain have been shown to reduce both perioperative pain scores and opioid requirements.[41] At fourth and fifth echelon treatment centers, acute and chronic pain management is similar to that delivered in civilian trauma centers and pain management clinics, as outlined in this and other chapters.

In summary, pain management in the operational setting is fraught with a unique set of challenges almost unimaginable in civilian pain treatment facilities. Because of wide variations in medical resources and personnel, there is no "optimal" pain treatment for war injuries. Instead, treatment should be individually tailored based on a patient's injury, hemodynamic condition, available resources, and the ability to monitor treatment response. In modern warfare, the most common cause of soldier attrition is not battle-related injury, but rather acute and recurrent non–battle-related injuries, similar to those encountered in civilian pain treatment facilities and primary care offices. Recent evidence suggests that high return-to-unit rates can be obtained by the deployment of aggressive pain management capabilities in mature theaters of operation.

Ambulatory Surgical Patients

The percentage of surgical procedures being performed on an outpatient basis continues to increase. There is an increase in the number of outpatient surgical procedures and in the complexity of operations being performed and comorbidities of the surgical outpatients. Optimizing treatment of postoperative and postdischarge pain is especially important in patients undergoing outpatient surgery because inadequate control of postoperative pain is one of the leading causes of prolonged stays or readmission after outpatient surgery.[229] Although there has been much effort to minimize symptoms such as pain and nausea in the postanesthesia care unit and subsequent (phase II) recovery area to facilitate discharge after outpatient surgery, increasing data suggest that postdischarge pain is common and may interfere with patients' recovery and the overall health-related costs of outpatient surgery.[230,231] Despite the advances in surgical techniques that minimize surgical trauma and postoperative pain, the incidence of moderate to severe postdischarge pain is still approximately 25% to 35%[232] and can be especially troublesome for certain patients, such as those undergoing tubal ligation and orthopedic procedures.[233] After discharge, poorly controlled nausea and vomiting may interfere with the intake of oral analgesics. In light of these considerations, the traditional reliance on opioid analgesia may not be appropriate for patients undergoing ambulatory surgery because of the opioid-related side effects that may delay hospital discharge and postdischarge recovery after outpatient surgery. A multimodal or "balanced" analgesic approach using a combination of opioid and nonopioid analgesic adjuvant medications including NSAIDs or acetaminophen; and local anesthetics wound

infiltration or regional anesthetic techniques may be more appropriate in this surgical population. The use of local anesthetics has decreased postoperative pain, and the drugs can be administered as peripheral nerve blocks, tissue infiltration, wound instillation, or topical analgesics. Similar results have been achieved using systemic NSAIDs and acetaminophen.

Although multimodal analgesia may be especially effective in the immediate postoperative period, not all of the options may be routinely available after the patient is discharged to home. For example, use of local anesthetics in peripheral nerve blocks, tissue infiltration, or wound instillation may be effective in the immediate postoperative period; however, a single dose of local anesthetic rarely provides more than 24 hours of analgesia. Realistically, most outpatients rely on a combination of short-acting analgesics including an opioid and acetaminophen or NSAID for postoperative pain control after hospital discharge.[55] Routine use of acetaminophen, especially when an NSAID is added to the regimen, is recommended to maximize postoperative analgesia,[234] although it is important to remember that when acetaminophen is used as a co-analgesic agent in combination products this limits the number of combination analgesic tablets that the patient may consume because of liver toxicity. The future of postoperative pain control in ambulatory surgical patients may include postdischarge (home) use of continuous infusion of local anesthetic solutions or even use of long acting, "sustained-release" local anesthetics or opioids.

Elderly Patients

The elderly population, which is expected to increase by 33% over the next 2 decades, accounts for approximately 12.5% of the total U. S. population and 38% of all health care spending (approximately 5% of the U. S. gross domestic product). There are changes in the physiology, pharmacodynamics, pharmacokinetics, and processing of nociceptive information that may influence the effectiveness of postoperative pain control in the elderly. There may be communication, affective, cognitive, social, and ideological barriers to effective postoperative pain control in this group. The elderly generally have decreased physiologic reserves and increased co-morbidities compared with younger counterparts, which may result in a higher incidence of postoperative complications such as postoperative delirium, especially in the presence of severe or uncontrolled postoperative pain.

There is a clinically significant reduction in the intensity of pain perception or symptoms with increasing age.[235,236] For instance, silent myocardial ischemia is more common in the elderly, who may instead present with other angina equivalents. Experimental studies demonstrate a decrease in Aδ and C-fiber nociceptive function, delay in central sensitization, increase in pain thresholds, and decrease in sensitivity to low-intensity noxious stimuli.[237,238] However, elderly patients may have an increased response to higher-intensity noxious stimuli, decreased pain tolerance, and decreased descending modulation (i.e., serotonin and noradrenergic), which may contribute to the relatively high incidence of chronic pain in elderly patients.[237,239] Despite the methodological issues in available studies evaluating age-related differences in the perception of pain, there appears to be a clinically relevant decrease in pain perception with increasing age. However, this should not be interpreted that elderly patients experience less pain than younger patients when they do report the presence of pain.

The physiologic and pharmacokinetic effects of aging on acute pain management are complex, and the clinical implications include the slow titration of opioids that produces longer circulation times, smaller total doses because of increased sensitivity, and expectation of a longer duration of action due to reduced clearance. In general, analgesic requirements decrease with increasing age. Age has been shown to be the best predictor for postoperative requirements of intravenously and neuraxially administered morphine.[240] Similar to that seen in younger patients, there is large inter-patient variability in postoperative analgesic requirements. Use of intravenous PCA in the elderly is appropriate to compensate for the wide interpatient variability, although postoperative titration of intravenous morphine can also allow successful and safe administration to elderly patients. Age per se is not an impediment to effective postprocedure or acute pain use of intravenous PCA or PCEA.[241] Use of postoperative epidural analgesia for elderly patients, especially in those with decreased physiologic reserves, may attenuate perioperative pathophysiology and is reported to improve postoperative outcomes such as facilitating return of gastrointestinal function after abdominal surgery, decreasing the incidence of myocardial ischemia, lowering pain scores, and decreasing pulmonary complications.

Postoperative pain management in the elderly may be especially challenging because of some of the affective, cognitive, social, and ideological barriers. Health care providers treating geriatric patients tend to have an unfounded level of fear of complications associated with treating perioperative pain as reflected by the inadequate treatment of pain in elderly patients, even relative to younger patients.[239] Elderly patients may also contribute to inadequate pain control by their own reluctance to report pain or take opioid medications. Elderly patients have a higher incidence of affective or cognitive impairments such as depression or dementia that may interfere with effective pain management.[239] One of the most devastating complications in the elderly surgical patient is postoperative delirium, which is associated with increased mortality rates and longer hospital stays.[242] The cause of postoperative delirium is unknown, although it is believed to result from an imbalance of neurotransmitters, particularly acetylcholine and serotonin, in the presence of decreased neurophysiologic reserve and inflammatory mediators.[243,244] Although the cause of postoperative delirium is multifactorial, uncontrolled postoperative pain may be an important contributor to its development.[245] Higher pain scores predict a decline in mental status and an increased risk of delirium.[246] A multimodal analgesic approach may be useful in elderly patients but must be used with caution because adverse drug reactions in the elderly increase as the number of medications administered increases. Although the benefits of intra-operative regional anesthetic techniques on postoperative cognitive function are unclear, the postoperative or acute pain use of epidural analgesia may diminish postoperative or pain-related delirium in part through superior analgesia and a decrease in pulmonary complications.

Opioid-Tolerant Patients

Postprocedural or acute pain may be difficult to manage in the opioid-tolerant patient because the standard approaches used for assessment and therapy in opioid-naïve patients is inadequate for opioid-tolerant patients. Although opioid-tolerant patients typically require higher doses of analgesic medications in the immediate postprocedure period, many health care providers still do not provide adequate postprocedural pain relief, in part because of the fear of addiction or medication-related side effects. In dealing with patients with chronic opioid use, health care providers often mistakenly interchange several pharmacologic terms (i.e., tolerance, physical dependence, and addiction), a practice that may contribute to misunderstanding and inappropriate treatment decisions.

Tolerance refers to the pharmacologic property of an opioid in which an increasing amount is needed to maintain a given level of analgesia. Physical dependence is another pharmacologic property of opioids characterized by the occurrence of a withdrawal syndrome on abrupt discontinuation of the opioid or administration of an antagonist. Tolerance and physical dependence are pharmacologic properties of opioids and not synonymous with the aberrant psychological state or behaviors associated with addiction, a chronic disorder characterized by the compulsive use

of a substance resulting in physical, psychological, or social harm to the user and continued use despite that harm. The exaggerated fear of addiction contributes to the under-treatment of postprocedural and acute pain by health care providers; however, the data suggest that there is minimal risk of iatrogenic addiction with use of opioids for pain control in patients who do not have a prior history of addiction.[247,248] Several principles for pain assessment and treatment can be applied in the postprocedural or acute pain opioid-tolerant patient. The physician should expect high self-reported pain scores[249]; base treatment decisions on objective pain assessment (e.g., ability to deep breathe, cough, ambulate) in conjunction with patients' self-reported pain scores; recognize the need to identify and treat two major problems, maintenance of a basal opioid requirement and control of incisional/procedural/acute pain; and recognize that detoxification is usually not an appropriate goal in this period. Likewise, several general strategies can be employed for the treatment of postprocedural or acute pain in the opioid-tolerant patient. The physician can create a treatment plan early and discuss it with the patient, procedural team, and nursing staff; replace the patient's baseline or basal opioid requirements; anticipate an increase in postprocedural analgesic requirements; maximize the use of adjuvant drugs; consider use of regional analgesic techniques; and plan for the transition to an oral regimen.[249] Although chronic pain patients are not synonymous with opioid-tolerant patients, many of these patients are opioid-tolerant, and the same general principles and strategies may be applied to chronic pain patients who are opioid-tolerant. Recognizing and treating nonnociceptive sources of distress may be especially important for chronic pain patients. Although there is no specific threshold or timeframe for when a patient becomes opioid tolerant, after an opioid-tolerant patient is identified, a strategy for acute pain control should be created and discussed with the patient. This may include anticipation or arrangement for a longer than normal length of hospital stay, consultation with the anesthesiology or pain service, and confirmation of the patient's daily opioid intake to facilitate calculation of the patient's basal or maintenance opioid requirement in the hospitalized period. Administration of a PRN analgesic regimen alone for opioid-tolerant patients is highly discouraged because replacing the basal opioid requirement in the acute period can optimize pain relief and possibly prevent opioid withdrawal. Basal opioid requirements can be administered systemically (typically intravenously or transdermally) until the patient can tolerate an oral analgesic regimen.[138] For example, 50% to 100% of the patient's baseline opioid requirement can be administered as a continuous infusion as part of an intravenous PCA regimen, with a demand dose to cover the additional incisional pain. Conversion tables (Table 51.2 and 51.3) may facilitate equi-analgesic conversion of opioids; however, these tables provide only estimations to assist health care providers in initiating opioid titration.[250] Opioid-tolerant patients generally require increased postoperative analgesic levels, including a larger demand dose.[249] Patients may require frequent adjustment (e.g., two to three times each day) of the intravenous PCA demand dose or continuous infusion, depending on the analgesic requirements. There is individual variability in response to different opioids, and if a decision is made to switch opioids, the choice of opioid may not as important as using an equi-analgesic dose. Patients may experience different side effects with different opioids, and rotating to another opioid may be reasonable if the patient is not tolerating the first opioid.[251] Adjuvant agents such as NSAIDs should be administered on a regularly scheduled basis to optimize analgesic efficacy and possibly provide an opioid-sparing effect. Use of regional analgesic techniques with neuraxial opioids may provide excellent analgesia in opioid-tolerant patients while preventing withdrawal symptoms.[252] After the patient is tolerating oral intake, the conversion from intravenous opioids to a form of oral or transdermal administration that would be more suitable for discharge to home may be initiated.

Opioid-tolerant patients typically can be converted to a combination of a regularly administered, controlled-release formulation of opioid such as sustained-release morphine or transdermal fentanyl and a short-acting, immediate-release opioid on a PRN basis. Although the conversion of intravenous opioid to an oral or transdermal form can be accomplished over a period of 1–2 days in opioid-tolerant patients, this process may take several days in extremely difficult cases. Converting from an intravenous to oral or transdermal form of opioid is not an exact science, and available conversion tables can serve only as a rough guide because of significant inter-patient and intra-patient variability in the sensitivity to opioids, lack of complete cross-tolerance between opioids which may lead to greater than anticipated potency of a new opioid, and changes in the levels of pain, which may rapidly decrease in the immediate postoperative period.[250]

Obesity, Obstructive Sleep Apnea, and Sleep

Patients with obesity and obstructive sleep apnea (OSA) may be at higher risk for postoperative complications. Obesity and OSA are separate disease states, but there is some association between the two, because OSA occurs in a relatively higher percentage of obese than non-obese patients.[253] Although some data suggest that epidural analgesia may decrease postoperative complications in the obese patient,[254] the optimal postoperative analgesic and monitoring regimen for patients with OSA is not clear. Data suggest that sleep is disrupted in the immediate postoperative period and may influence postoperative morbidity and patient-oriented outcomes.

Obesity is defined as a body mass index (BMI) of more than 30 kg/m^2, with morbid and super-morbid obesity defined as a BMI of more than 35 kg/m^2 and 55 kg/m^2, respectively. The prevalence of obesity has increased to include approximately 22.5% of the U. S. population.[255] Although obese patients do not necessarily have OSA, obesity is the most important physical characteristic associated with OSA. Approximately 60% to 90% of OSA patients are obese, and at least 5% of morbidly obese patients have OSA, which is defined as more than five episodes per hour of cessation of airflow for more than 10 seconds despite continued ventilatory effort.[253] It is estimated that approximately 4% of men and 2% of women (18 million Americans overall) have OSA and that up to 95% of persons with OSA are underdiagnosed.[253] Patients with OSA are generally at higher risk for chronic cognitive impairment, pulmonary hypertension, cardiomyopathy, systemic hypertension, and possibly for myocardial infarction.[256,257] The pathophysiology of airflow obstruction is related primarily to upper airway pharyngeal collapse, including the retro-palatal, retro-glossal, and retro-epiglottic pharynx, during sleep, especially during rapid eye movement (REM) sleep.[253] During these obstructive episodes, OSA patients may exhibit hypoxia, bradyarrhythmias or tachyarrhythmias; myocardial ischemia, abrupt decreases in left ventricular stroke volume and cardiac output, or increases in pulmonary and systemic blood pressure.[257] Based on our understanding of the pathophysiology of OSA, it is easy to see how acute pain management can be difficult in this population. Patients with OSA are at higher risk for respiratory arrest.[258] Use of sedative doses of benzodiazepines and opioids may result in frequent hypoxemia and apnea, which may be especially dangerous in the OSA patient.[258] Avoiding respiratory depressants by optimizing use of NSAIDs and epidural analgesia with a local anesthetic–based regimen may attenuate the risk for respiratory depression and arrest because the use of epidural and systemic opioids is associated with sudden postoperative respiratory arrest.[259]

The American Society of Anesthesiologists Task Force on Perioperative Management of Patients with Obstructive Sleep Apnea created guidelines that include acute pain management in patients with OSA.[260] Although the consultants acknowledged that the conclusions regarding postoperative analgesic options were based on insufficient literature evaluating the effects of various analgesic techniques, the presence of equivocal literature regarding the use of epidural opioids compared with intramuscular or intravenous opioids in reducing respiratory depression, and insufficient literature regarding the addition of a basal infusion to systemic patient-controlled opioids, the consultants nevertheless recommended that regional techniques rather than systemic opioids should be used in an attempt to reduce the likelihood of adverse outcomes in patients at increased peri-operative risk from OSA.[260] In addition, the consultants recommended the exclusion of opioids from neuraxial postoperative analgesia to reduce peri-operative risk, and the use of NSAIDs to reduce adverse outcomes through their opioid-sparing effect. The consultants were equivocal regarding whether avoiding a basal infusion of opioids in patients with OSA reduces the likelihood of adverse outcomes.[260] Unfortunately, there is a paucity of randomized clinical trial data to provide definitive high-quality evidence-based recommendations in the provision of postoperative analgesia for OSA patients.

GENDER OR SEX DIFFERENCES IN ANALGESIA

A large body of data has been collected in the past 20 years concerning differences between the sexes in response to pain, including pain thresholds, and in the tolerance and response to acute pain treatment. However, the exact differences as well as their relevance are far from clear. According to the International Association for the Study of Pain (IASP), "pain is an unpleasant sensory and emotional experience arising from actual or potential tissue damage or described in terms of such damage." This definition does not differentiate between "pain" as a woman experiences it from "pain" as a man experiences it and thus fundamental questions still remain.

Females report more severe pain, more frequent bouts of pain, more anatomically diffuse and longer-lasting pain than males with similar disease processes, even when male and female specific disorders including male urologic and female gynecologic pain are excluded from the analysis. Females have a higher prevalence of pain related to musculoskeletal or to visceral origin, as well as pain related to autoimmune disease (Table 51.10).[262] Substantial amounts of the accumulated data rely heavily on the subjective signs of the pain experience. These are highly influenced by sociocultural variables that have little to do with a biological difference of pain threshold or perception between women and men. An inherent reporting bias exists in the epidemiological research related to the incidence of pain in the sexes. Females are more likely to visit a physician and are more likely to report pain as a symptom than males[263,264] reviewed in[265] which can therefore lead to an overestimation of the differences between the sexes.

In a meta-analysis of studies examining sex differences in pain response in healthy subjects less than 60 years old, the authors found women report higher pain severity at lower thresholds and have less tolerance to noxious stimulation than males.[266] In a large multicenter trial, Rolke and colleagues[236] used quantitative sensory testing (QST) to determine sensory detection thresholds and pain thresholds for thermal and mechanical noxious stimuli. Females had lower pain thresholds, with the greatest disparities for sex differences found for heat pain threshold, followed by cold pain and pain to blunt pressure.

Many other physiological, socio-cultural, and psychological variables have been identified as contributing to the differences between the two sexes with regard to pain. One factor includes the end point being examined, such as pain threshold vs. pain tolerance.[266–268] Pool and colleagues[269] showed that pain tolerance is highly malleable and strongly influenced by the subject's "gender" norms. Males who are highly identified with the "male" role tolerate higher levels of noxious stimuli, but those males who do not have this belief tolerate noxious stimuli at the same level

TABLE 51.10

SEX PREVALENCE OF CLINICAL PAIN SYNDROMES OR DISEASES

Bodily area		Prevalence	
		Female > Male	Female < Male
Head	*Headache*	Chronic tension	Cluster
		Migraine with aura	Migraine without aura
		Postdural puncture	Posttraumatic
		Cervicogenic	War injury
		Temporal arteritis	
		Occipital neuralgia	
	Oral	Odontalgia	Para-trigeminal syndrome
		Burning mouth	Trigeminal postherpetic
		Temporomandibular disorder	neuralgia
		Trigeminal neuralgia	
Extremities	*Arms*	Carpal tunnel syndrome	Brachial plexus neuropathy
		Raynaud's disease	War Injuries
		CRPS Type I	CRPS Type II
		Scleroderma	
	Legs	Chronic venous insufficiency	Meralgia paraesthetica
		Peroneal muscular atrophy	Gout
		Piriformis syndrome	Intermittent claudication
		Raynaud's disease	CRPS Type II
		CRPS type I	
Viscera	*Bowel*	Chronic constipation	Duodenal ulcer
		Irritable bowel syndrome	
		Proctalgia fugax	
	Esophagus	Esophagitis	
	Pancreas		Pancreatic disease
	Gall Bladder	Postcholecystectomy pain	
Autoimmune		Lupus erythematosus	Reiter's syndrome
		Multiple sclerosis	
		Rheumatoid arthritis	

as females. The age of the subject also modifies the pain threshold. Advancing age is positively associated with pain threshold.[235,236] Pickering and colleagues[268] found that the difference in score between males and females decreased with advancing age. The significant sex difference seen in thermal and mechanical threshold and in tolerance in younger volunteers became non-significant in volunteers greater than 40 years old.

As discussed above, the sex difference in humans is neither a universal nor a large effect. Furthermore, no difference between sexes is found in at least one-third of the published studies, and effect sizes are often in the small to moderate range.[266] Other investigators have sought objective measures of pain as a result of the numerous factors that have been shown to influence and in some cases abolish the pain threshold and tolerance differences between the sexes. Paulson and colleagues[267] used positron emission tomography (PET) to investigate regional brain activation after a painful somatic thermal stimulus in healthy normal volunteer male and female subjects. They reported that females had significantly greater activation of the contralateral prefrontal cortex, the contralateral insula and the thalamus compared to males suggesting sexual dimorphism in response to pain. Unfortunately, this study reflected a difference in brain activation that was more likely the result of different pain intensities rather than a true sex difference. In a later study also using PET technology, the pain intensity was matched between the sexes and the results were the opposite of the earlier study — males had greater activation than females.[270] Finally, a study using matched pain intensity and

functional magnetic resonance imaging (fMRI) showed no sex-based difference in brain activation.[271] Other PET studies have described sex differences in responses to visceral pain from rectal balloon distension, although principally with chronic visceral pain patients.[272,273] However, the differences reported were predominantly in the direction of greater activation in men. These studies were replicated using fMRI with similar results of a male predominance of neuronal activation in pain-related areas of the brain.[272]

Pain thresholds in humans vary by internal factors such as sex, gender, female menstrual phase and psychological variables including catastrophizing, anxiety, and depression. External factors also affect the outcome including testing environment, sex, and gender of the examiner, and the modality of the noxious stimuli. In the largest study assessing the role of sex on pain thresholds using multiple modalities, it was found that females had lower pain thresholds in thermal and mechanical pain testing.[236] Unfortunately, this subjective difference has not been consistently supported by other confirmatory techniques including PET or fMRI brain imaging. Awareness of the possible differences between males and females in response to pain is the only clinical application of the present data with no guidance for particular situations.

Unlike the abundance of literature addressing the question of drug-induced sex differences in experimental pain in rodents, the human literature is not as voluminous. The majority of the literature addresses the response to *mu* opioid receptor agonists and the remainder addresses *kappa* opioid receptor agonists. There has not been testing of other clinically available medications on humans in models of experimental pain. In multiple studies, either no difference[274-276] was noted between sexes or females had a significantly greater response to the medication.[277-279] Although initial studies attributed the difference to pharmacokinetic differences,[280] the metabolism of morphine to morphine-6-glucuronide (M6G), more recent work by Romberg and colleagues[275] demonstrate that no sex differences exist in M6G concentrations. In order to further exclude pharmacokinetic explanations for the sex differences, the same investigative group, subsequently published findings using the potent synthetic *mu* opioid receptor agonist alfentanil. The subject's response to alfentanil did not differ based on their sex.[281]

The human response to *kappa* opioid receptor agonists is somewhat variable. In a postsurgical model of pain, females had a greater analgesic response to kappa agonist-antagonist medications including pentazocine, nalbuphine, and butorphanol.[282-284] However, in experimental models of pain either no difference between males and females was noted[285] or males had an increased sensitivity to the medications.[286] Mogil and colleagues[286] suggest that the increased responsiveness to *kappa* opioid receptors agonists may be related to the absence of the MC1r gene. In an elegant study, this group studied women with fair skin and red hair who often have a functional reduction in MC1r. The women with a genetically proven loss of function polymorphisms experienced an accentuated analgesic response to pentazocine. Their analgesic response was indistinguishable from the male subjects in the study.[286] This finding has led to the proposal that the MC1r gene product acts as an anti-opioid and therefore when removed unmasks the true *kappa* opioid effect. This enhanced effect would be inconsistent with the finding that females have an increased response to *kappa* opioid receptor agonists in clinical models of pain (e.g. postoperative) because fair-skinned redheaded females represent only a minority of women in general. Unfortunately, it does not explain the lack of difference or the greater analgesic response of females to *mu* opioids in clinical and experimental models or *kappa* opioids in experimental models of pain.

Unfortunately, the data with regard to opioid analgesics garnered from human trials is not sufficient to guide clinical practice. The studies, so far, do not justify the conclusion that males or females have a greater responsiveness to *mu* or *kappa* opioid receptor agonists and therefore they should continue to receive similar acute pain management until more definitive studies are conducted.

ACUTE PAIN SERVICES

Although dedicated individuals can improve postoperative pain control for a few patients, more comprehensive perioperative pain management programs (i.e., acute pain services) developed specifically to treat this problem can address the needs for all patients within an institution. The organizational aspects of such comprehensive services are considerable, necessary for effective and safe care, and may include issues such as education; administration, nursing, and documentation (Table 51.11). With skills in regional anesthetic techniques and knowledge of the neurobiology of nociception and the pharmacology of analgesics and local anesthetics, anesthesiologists have been leaders in postoperative pain relief and development of acute pain services. Provision of perioperative analgesia, along with other services such as critical care medicine and preoperative evaluation, is highly compatible with the emerging identity of anesthesiologists as perioperative physicians and enhances the role of anesthesiologists as valued consultants outside the operating room.

TABLE 51.11

ORGANIZATIONAL ASPECTS OF AN ACUTE PAIN SERVICE

Educational Activity
Health care providers: Anesthesiologists, Surgeons, Nurses, Pharmacists
Hospital administrators
Patients and families
Research
Residency-fellowship teaching

Administrative Activity
Economic issues
Evaluation of equipment
Human resources: pain service personnel, administrative-secretarial support
Institutional administrative activity
Quality improvement and assurance

Nursing
Continuing education and training
Defining of roles in patient care
Nursing policies and procedures
Pain service nursing

Documentation
Educational packages
Policies and procedures
Preprinted forms
Bedside pain management assessment flow sheet
Daily consultation notes

Although there are several models for the development of acute pain services[287,288] the key organizational aspects are similar. Development and maintenance of acute pain services require a commitment and financial support at the national and local level. In the United States, there appears to be a dichotomy at the national and third-party payer level between the call for improved postoperative pain control with the introduction of practice guidelines or expanded roles for acute pain services and decreased reimbursement for the provision of such services. Because there are financial burdens associated with the establishment of an acute pain service, high-volume or larger hospitals are more likely have acute pain services and have access to more high-tech analgesic techniques such as epidural analgesia.[289,290] Whether acute pain services actually improve outcomes is unclear. Two systematic reviews have examined the impact of acute pain services on patients outcomes[291] and while systematic reviews suggest that the introduction of acute pain services is associated with a decrease in pain scores, the effect of acute pain services on the incidence of analgesic-related side effects such as nausea and vomiting, satisfaction, and overall costs or cost reductions are uncertain.[291] Despite the direct costs (e.g., personnel, equipment, medication) associated with managing an acute pain service, there is no available properly conducted pharmaco-economic study to examine the cost-effectiveness of an acute pain service. Use of postoperative epidural analgesia in the context of acute pain services may decrease the cost of patient care through shorter intensive care unit stays and a decreased rate of complications.[5] Despite the costs associated with implementation of an acute pain service and acute pain management practice guidelines, acute pain services provide a valuable service at the individual, institutional, and societal levels.

LONG-TERM IMPACT OF ACUTE PAIN

Chronic postsurgical pain [CPSP] is a largely unrecognized problem which may occur in 10% to 50% of postoperative patients (depending on type of surgery) with 2% to 10% of these patients experiencing severe CPSP.[292] Poorly controlled acute postoperative pain or acute pain in general may be an important predictive factor in the development of chronic pain.[43,293] Increasing experimental and clinical evidence suggests that the transition from acute to chronic pain occurs very quickly and that long-term behavioral and neurobiological changes occur much earlier than previously anticipated.[294] CPSP is relatively common after procedures such as limb amputation (30% to 83%), thoracotomy (22% to 67%), sternotomy (27%), breast surgery (11% to 57%), and gallbladder surgery (up to 56%).[43] Although studies suggest that the severity of acute postoperative pain may be an important predictor in the development of CPSP, a causal relationship between severity of acute postoperative pain and subsequent CPSP has not been definitively established and other factors may be more important in predicting the development of CPSP.

Control of acute pain may improve long-term recovery or patient-oriented outcomes including quality of life or return of function. Patients whose pain is controlled in the early postoperative period (especially with use of continuous epidural or peripheral catheter techniques) may be able to actively participate in postoperative rehabilitation, which may improve short- and long-term recovery after surgery.[295] In a recent study, a multimodal approach to acute analgesia using either epidural or spinal analgesia reduced the patient's area of hyperalgesia and allodynia in the acute phase and diminished their long-term pain as well.[296] Another study examined the showed that acute postoperative pain was an important risk factor for the development of chronic pain.[297] Optimizing treatment of acute postoperative pain can improve health-related quality of life (HRQL) [200]. Postsurgical chronic pain that develops as a result of poor acute pain control can interfere with patients' activities of daily living and reduce a person to a less functional status.

References

1. American Society of Anesthesiologists Task Force on Acute Pain Management. Practice guidelines for acute pain management in the perioperative setting. A report by the American Society of Anesthesiologists Task Force on Pain Management, Acute Pain Section. *Anesthesiology* 1995;82:1071–1081.
2. American Society of Anesthesiologists Task Force on Acute Pain Management. Practice guidelines for acute pain management in the perioperative setting: an updated report by the American Society of Anesthesiologists Task Force on Acute Pain Management. *Anesthesiology* 2004;100:1573–1581.
3. Kehlet H, Holte K. Effect of postoperative analgesia on surgical outcome. *Br J Anaesth* 2001;87:62–72.
4. Liu S, Carpenter RL, Mulroy MF, et al. Intravenous versus epidural administration of hydromorphone. Effects on analgesia and recovery after radical retropubic prostatectomy. Anesthesiology 1995;82:682–688.
5. Wu CL, Fleisher LA. Outcomes research in regional anesthesia and analgesia. *Anesth Analg* 2000;91:1232–1242.
6. Darian-Smith I. Thermal sensibility. In: Darian-Smith I, ed. *Handbook of Physiology*. Bethesda: Am Physiol Soc 1984:879–914.
7. Oh SB, Tran PB, Gillard SE, et al. Chemokines and glycoprotein120 produce pain hypersensitivity by directly exciting primary nociceptive neurons. *J Neurosci* 2001;21:5027–5035.
8. Oku R, Satoh M, Takagi H. Release of substance P from the spinal dorsal horn is enhanced in polyarthritic rats. *Neurosci Lett* 1987;74:315–319.
9. Tiseo PJ, Adler MW, Liu-Chen LY. Differential release of substance P and somatostatin in the rat spinal cord in response to noxious cold and heat; effect of dynorphin A(1-17). *J Pharmacol Exp Ther* 1990;252:539–545.
10. Salter MW, Henry JL. Responses of functionally identified neurones in the dorsal horn of the cat spinal cord to substance P, neurokinin A, and physalaemin. *Neuroscience* 1991;43:601–610.
11. Malmberg AB, Yaksh TL. Hyperalgesia mediated by spinal glutamate or substance P receptor blocked by spinal cyclooxygenase inhibition. *Science* 1992;257:1276–1279.
12. Stucky CL, Galeazza MT, Seybold VS. Time-dependent changes in Bolton-Hunter-labeled 125I-substance P binding in rat spinal cord following unilateral adjuvant-induced peripheral inflammation. *Neuroscience* 1993;57:397–409.
13. Jeftinija S, Jeftinija K, Liu F, et al. Excitatory amino acids are released from rat primary afferent neurons in vitro. *Neurosci Lett* 1991;125:191–194.
14. Aanonsen LM, Lei S, Wilcox GL. Excitatory amino acid receptors and nociceptive neurotransmission in rat spinal cord. *Pain* 1990;41:309–321.
15. Dougherty PM, Palecek J, Paleckova V, et al. The role of NMDA and non-NMDA excitatory amino acid receptors in the excitation of primate spinothalamic tract neurons by mechanical, chemical, thermal, and electrical stimuli. *J Neurosci* 1992;12:3025–3041.
16. Liu H, Wang H, Sheng M, et al. Evidence for presynaptic N-methyl-D-aspartate autoreceptors in the spinal cord dorsal horn. *Proc Natl Acad Sci U S A* 1994;91:8383–8387.
17. Glaum SR, Miller RJ, Hammond DL. Inhibitory actions of *mu*- and *delta*-opioid receptor agonists on excitatory transmission in lamina II neurons of adult rat spinal cord. *J Neurosci* 1994;14:4965–4971.
18. Hammond DL, Ruda MA. Developmental alterations in nociceptive threshold, immunoreactive calcitonin gene-related peptide and substance P, and fluoride-resistant acid phosphatase in neonatally capsaicin-treated rats. *J Comp Neurol* 1991;312:436–450.
19. Stone LS, Broberger C, Vulchanova L, et al. Differential distribution of alpha2A and alpha2C adrenergic receptor immunoreactivity in the rat spinal cord. *J Neurosci* 1998;18:5928–5937.
20. Beitz AJ. The organization of afferent projections to the midbrain periaqueductal gray of the rat. *Neuroscience* 1982;7:133–159.
21. Mansour A, Fox CA, Akil H, et al. Opioid-receptor mRNA expression in the rat CNS: anatomical and functional implications. *Trends Neurosci* 1995;18:22–29.
22. Beitz AJ, Mullett MA, Weiner LL. The periaqueductal gray projections to the rat spinal trigeminal, raphe magnus, gigantocellular pars alpha and paragigantocellular nuclei arise from separate neurons. *Brain Res* 1983;288:307–314.
23. Bajic D, Proudfit HK. Projections of neurons in the periaqueductal gray to pontine and medullary catecholamine cell groups involved in the modulation of nociception. *J Comp Neurol* 1999;405:359–379.
24. Gebhart GF. Recent developments in the neurochemical bases of pain and analgesia. *NIDA Res Monogr* 1983;45:19–35.
25. Basbaum AI, Clanton CH, Fields HL. Three bulbospinal pathways from the rostral medulla of the cat: an autoradiographic study of pain modulating systems. *J Comp Neurol* 1978;178:209–224.
26. Skagerberg G, Björklund A. Topographic principles in the spinal projections of serotonergic and non-serotonergic brainstem neurons in the rat. *Neuroscience* 1985;15:445–480.
27. Duggan AW, Griersmith BT. Inhibition of the spinal transmission of nociceptive information by supraspinal stimulation in the cat. *Pain* 1979;6:149–161.
28. Light AR, Casale EJ, Menetrey DM. The effects of focal stimulation in nucleus raphe magnus and periaqueductal gray on intracellularly recorded neurons in spinal laminae I and II. J. *Neurophysiol* 1986;56:555–571.
29. Antal M, Petko M, Polgar E, et al. Direct evidence of an extensive GABAergic innervation of the spinal dorsal horn by fibres descending from the rostral ventromedial medulla. *Neuroscience* 1996;73:509–518.
30. Bowker RM, Abbott LC, Dilts RP. Peptidergic neurons in the nucleus raphe magnus and the nucleus gigantocellularis: their distributions, interrelationships, and projections to the spinal cord. *Prog Brain Res* 1988;77:95–127.
31. Menetrey D, Basbaum AI. The distribution of substance P-, enkephalin- and dynorphin- immunoreactive neurons in the medulla of the rat and their contribution to bulbospinal pathways. *Neuroscience* 1987;23:173–187.
32. Clark FM, Proudfit HK. The projection of noradrenergic neurons in the A7 catecholamine cell group to the spinal cord in the rat demonstrated by anterograde tracing combined with immunocytochemistry. *Brain Res* 1991;547:279–288.
33. Kwiat GC, Basbaum AI. The origin of brainstem noradrenergic and serotonergic projections to the spinal cord dorsal horn in the rat. *Somatosens Mot Res* 1992;9:157–173.
34. Proudfit HK. In: Fields HL, Besson JM, eds. Progress in brain research. New York: Elseiver; 1988;77:357–370.
35. Yeomans DC, Proudfit HK. Antinociception induced by microinjection of substance P into the A7 catecholamine cell group in the rat. *Neuroscience* 1992;49:681–691.
36. Yeomans DC, Clark FM, Paice JA, et al. Antinociception induced by electrical stimulation of spinally projecting noradrenergic neurons in the A7 catecholamine cell group of the rat. *Pain* 1992;48:449–461.
37. Moiniche S, Kehlet H, Dahl JB. A qualitative and quantitative systematic review of preemptive analgesia for postoperative pain relief: the role of timing of analgesia. *Anesthesiology* 2002;96:725–741.
38. Dahl JB, Moiniche S. Pre-emptive analgesia. *Br Med Bull* 2004;71:13–27.
39. Ong CK, Lirk P, Seymour RA, et al. The efficacy of preemptive analgesia for acute postoperative pain management: a meta-analysis. *Anesth Analg* 2005;100:757–773, table of contents.
40. Kissin I. Preemptive analgesia. *Anesthesiology* 2000;93:1138–1143.
41. Hurley RW, Cohen SP, Williams KA, et al. The analgesic effects of perioperative gabapentin on postoperative pain: a meta-analysis. *Reg Anesth Pain Med* 2006;31:237–247.

42. Pogatzki-Zahn EM, Zahn PK. From preemptive to preventive analgesia. *Curr Opin Anaesthesiol* 2006;19:551–555.
43. Perkins FM, Kehlet H. Chronic pain as an outcome of surgery. A review of predictive factors. *Anesthesiology* 2000;93:1123–1133.
44. Katz J, McCartney CJ. Current status of preemptive analgesia. *Curr Opin Anaesthesiol* 2002;15:435–441.
45. Kehlet H. Multimodal approach to control postoperative pathophysiology and rehabilitation. *Br J Anaesth* 1997;78:606–617.
46. Block BM, Liu SS, Rowlingson AJ, et al. Efficacy of postoperative epidural analgesia: a meta-analysis. *JAMA* 2003;290:2455–2463.
47. Kehlet H, Wilmore DW. Multimodal strategies to improve surgical outcome. *Am J Surg* 2002;183:630–641.
48. Ben-David B, Swanson J, Nelson JB, et al. Multimodal analgesia for radical prostatectomy provides better analgesia and shortens hospital stay. *J Clin Anesth* 2007;19:264–268.
49. Gendall KA, Kennedy RR, Watson AJ, et al. The effect of epidural analgesia on postoperative outcome after colorectal surgery. *Colorectal Dis* 2007;9:584–598; discussion 598–600.
50. Chilvers CR, Nguyen MH, Robertson IK. Changing from epidural to multimodal analgesia for colorectal laparotomy: an audit. *Anaesth Intensive Care* 2007;35:230–238.
51. Taqi A, Hong X, Mistraletti G, et al. Thoracic epidural analgesia facilitates the restoration of bowel function and dietary intake in patients undergoing laparoscopic colon resection using a traditional, nonaccelerated, perioperative care program. *Surg Endosc* 2007;21:247–252.
52. Stein C. The control of pain in peripheral tissue by opioids. *New Engl J Med* 1995;332:1685–1690.
53. Viscusi ER, Reynolds L, Tait S, et al. An iontophoretic fentanyl patient-activated analgesic delivery system for postoperative pain: a double-blind, placebo-controlled trial. *Anesth Analg* 2006;102:188–194.
54. Gourlay GK. Sustained relief of chronic pain. Pharmacokinetics of sustained release morphine. *Clin Pharmacokinet* 1998;35:173–190.
55. Pang WW, Huang PY, Chang DP, et al. The peripheral analgesic effect of tramadol in reducing propofol injection pain: a comparison with lidocaine. *Reg Anesth Pain Med* 1999;24:246–249.
56. Budd K, Langford R. Tramadol revisited. *Br J Anaesth* 1999;82:493–495.
57. Edwards JE, McQuay HJ, Moore RA. Combination analgesic efficacy: individual patient data meta-analysis of single-dose oral tramadol plus acetaminophen in acute postoperative pain. *J Pain Symptom Manage* 2002;23:121–130.
58. Svensson CI, Yaksh TL. The spinal phospholipase-cyclooxygenase-prostanoid cascade in nociceptive processing. *Annu Rev Pharmacol Toxicol* 2002;42:553–583.
59. Moncada S, Ferreira SH, Vane JR. Prostaglandins, aspirin-like drugs, and the oedema of inflammation. *Nature* 1973;246:217–219.
60. Ferreira SH, Lorenzetti BB. Intrathecal administration of prostaglandin E2 causes sensitization of the primary afferent neuron via the spinal release of glutamate. *Inflamm Res* 1996;45:499–502.
61. Portanova JP, Zhang Y, Anderson GD, et al. Selective neutralization of prostaglandin E2 blocks inflammation, hyperalgesia, and interleukin 6 production in vivo. *J Exp Med* 1996;184:883–891.
62. Malmberg AB, Yaksh TL. Cyclooxygenase inhibition and the spinal release of prostaglandin E2 and amino acids evoked by paw formalin injection: a microdialysis study in unanesthetized rats. *J Neurosci* 1995;15:2768–2776.
63. Baba H, Kohno T, Moore KA, et al. Direct activation of rat spinal dorsal horn neurons by prostaglandin E2. *J Neurosci* 2001;21:1750–1756.
64. Buritova J, Besson JM. Peripheral and/or central effects of racemic-, S(+)-, and R(-)-flurbiprofen on inflammatory nociceptive processes: a c-Fos protein study in the rat spinal cord. *Br J Pharmacol* 1998;125:87–101.
65. Crews JC. Multimodal pain management strategies for office-based and ambulatory procedures. *JAMA* 2002;288:629–632.
66. Jin F, Chung F. Multimodal analgesia for postoperative pain control. *J Clin Anesth* 2001;13:524–539.
67. Grass JA, Sakima NT, Valley M, et al. Assessment of ketorolac as an adjuvant to fentanyl patient-controlled epidural analgesia after radical retropubic prostatectomy. *Anesthesiology* 1993;78:642–648; discussion 621A.
68. Edwards JE, Oldman AD, Smith LA, et al. Oral aspirin in postoperative pain: a quantitative systematic review. *Pain* 1999;81:289–297.
69. Mason L, Edwards J, Moore RA, et al. Single dose oral indometacin for the treatment of acute postoperative pain. *Cochrane Database Syst Rev* 2004:CD004308.
70. Mason L, Edwards JE, Moore RA, et al. Single dose oral naproxen and naproxen sodium for acute postoperative pain. *Cochrane Database Syst Rev* 2004:CD004234.
71. Barden J, Edwards JE, McQuay HJ, et al. Single dose oral celecoxib for postoperative pain. *Cochrane Database Syst Rev* 2003:CD004233.
72. Simmons DL, Botting RM, Robertson PM, et al. Induction of an acetaminophen-sensitive cyclooxygenase with reduced sensitivity to nonsteroid anti-inflammatory drugs. *Proc Natl Acad Sci U S A* 1999;96:3275–3280.
73. Graham GG, Scott KF. Mechanisms of action of paracetamol and related analgesics. *Inflammopharmacology* 2003;11:401–413.
74. Chandrasekharan NV, Dai H, Roos KL, et al. COX-3, a cyclooxygenase-1 variant inhibited by acetaminophen and other analgesic/antipyretic drugs: cloning, structure, and expression. *Proc Natl Acad Sci U S A* 2002;99:13926–13931.
75. Graham GG, Scott KF. Mechanism of action of paracetamol. *Am J Ther* 2005;12:46–55.
76. Pelissier T, Alloui A, Caussade F, et al. Paracetamol exerts a spinal antinociceptive effect involving an indirect interaction with 5-hydroxytryptamine3 receptors: in vivo and in vitro evidence. *J Pharmacol Exp Ther* 1996;278:8–14.
77. Moore A, Ed. Oxford league table of analgesics in acute pain. London: Bandolier, 2003.
78. Varrassi G, Marinangeli F, Agro F, et al. A double-blinded evaluation of propacetamol versus ketorolac in combination with patient-controlled analgesia morphine: analgesic efficacy and tolerability after gynecologic surgery. *Anesth Analg* 1999;88:611–616.
79. Zhou TJ, Tang J, White PF. Propacetamol versus ketorolac for treatment of acute postoperative pain after total hip or knee replacement. *Anesth Analg* 2001;92:1569–1575.
80. Hernandez-Palazon J, Tortosa JA, Martinez-Lage JF, et al. Intravenous administration of propacetamol reduces morphine consumption after spinal fusion surgery. *Anesth Analg* 2001;92:1473–1476.
81. Bonnefont J, Alloui A, Chapuy E, et al. Orally administered paracetamol does not act locally in the rat formalin test: evidence for a supraspinal, serotonin-dependent antinociceptive mechanism. *Anesthesiology* 2003;99:976–981.
82. Sinatra RS, Jahr JS, Reynolds LW, et al. Efficacy and safety of single and repeated administration of 1 gram intravenous acetaminophen injection (paracetamol) for pain management after major orthopedic surgery. *Anesthesiology* 2005;102:822–831.
83. Woolf CJ, Salter MW. Neuronal plasticity: increasing the gain in pain. *Science* 2000;288:1765–1769.
84. Eide, PK, Jorum E, Stubhaug A, et al. Relief of post-herpetic neuralgia with the N-methyl-D-aspartic acid receptor antagonist ketamine: a double-blind, cross-over comparison with morphine and placebo. *Pain* 1994;58:347–354.
85. Block BM, Hurley RW, Raja SN. Mechanism-based therapies for pain. *Drug News Perspect* 2004;17:172–186.
86. Cherry DA, Plummer JL, Gourlay GK, et al. Ketamine as an adjunct to morphine in the treatment of pain. *Pain* 1995;62:119–121.
87. Gilron I, Booher SL, Rowan MS, et al. A randomized, controlled trial of high-dose dextromethorphan in facial neuralgias. *Neurology* 2000;55:964–971.
88. Nikolajsen L, Gottrup H, Kristensen AG, et al. Memantine (a N-methyl-D-aspartate receptor antagonist) in the treatment of neuropathic pain after amputation or surgery: a randomized, double-blinded, cross-over study. *Anesth Analg* 2000;91:960–966.
89. Gillies A, Lindholm D, Angliss M, et al. The use of ketamine as rescue analgesia in the recovery room following morphine administration—a double-blind randomised controlled trial in postoperative patients. *Anaesth Intensive Care* 2007;35:199–203.
90. Adam F, Chauvin M, Du Manoir B, et al. Small-dose ketamine infusion improves postoperative analgesia and rehabilitation after total knee arthroplasty. *Anesth Analg* 2005;100:475–480.
91. Galinski M, Dolveck F, Combes X, et al. Management of severe acute pain in emergency settings: ketamine reduces morphine consumption. *Am J Emerg Med* 2007;25:385–390.
92. Heidari SM, Saghaei M, Hashemi SJ, et al. Effect of oral ketamine on the postoperative pain and analgesic requirement following orthopedic surgery. *Acta Anaesthesiol Taiwan* 2006;44:211–215.
93. Webb AR, Skinner BS, Leong S, et al. The addition of a small-dose ketamine infusion to tramadol for postoperative analgesia: a double-blinded, placebo-controlled, randomized trial after abdominal surgery. *Anesth Analg* 2007;104:912–917.
94. Suman-Chauhan N, Webdale L, Hill DR, et al. Characterisation of [3H]gabapentin binding to a novel site in rat brain: homogenate binding studies. *Eur J Pharmacol* 1993;244:293–301.
95. Gee NS, Brown JP, Dissanayake VU, et al. The novel anticonvulsant drug, gabapentin (Neurontin), binds to the alpha2delta subunit of a calcium channel. *J Biol Chem* 1996;271:5768–5776.
96. Newton RA, Bingham S, Case PC, et al. Dorsal root ganglion neurons show increased expression of the calcium channel alpha2delta-1 subunit following partial sciatic nerve injury. *Brain Res Mol Brain Res* 2001;95:1–8.
97. Zahn PK, Brennan TJ. Incision-induced changes in receptive field properties of rat dorsal horn neurons. *Anesthesiology* 1999;91:772–785.
98. Zahn PK, Brennan TJ. Primary and secondary hyperalgesia in a rat model for human postoperative pain. *Anesthesiology* 1999;90:863–872.
99. Shimoyama M, Shimoyama N, Hori Y. Gabapentin affects glutamatergic excitatory neurotransmission in the rat dorsal horn. *Pain* 2000;85:405–414.
100. Backonja M, Beydoun A, Edwards KR, et al. Gabapentin for the symptomatic treatment of painful neuropathy in patients with diabetes mellitus: a randomized controlled trial. *JAMA* 1998;280:1831–1836.
101. Hahn K, Arendt G, Braun JS, et al. A placebo-controlled trial of gabapentin for painful HIV-associated sensory neuropathies. *J Neurol* 2004;251:1260–1266.
102. Mellick, LB and Mellick, GA. Successful treatment of reflex sympathetic dystrophy with gabapentin. *Am J Emerg Med* 1995;13:96.
103. Rosenberg JM, Harrell C, Ristic H, et al. The effect of gabapentin on neuropathic pain. *Clin J Pain* 1997;13:251–255.
104. Rowbotham M, Harden N, Stacey B, et al. Gabapentin for the treatment of postherpetic neuralgia: a randomized controlled trial. *JAMA* 1998;280:1837–1842.

105. Werner MU, Perkins FM, Holte K, et al. Effects of gabapentin in acute inflammatory pain in humans. *Reg Anesth Pain Med* 2001;26:322–328.
106. Gilron I, Bailey JM, Tu D, et al. Morphine, gabapentin, or their combination for neuropathic pain. *N Engl J Med* 2005;352:1324–1334.
107. Fassoulaki A, Stamatakis E, Petropoulos G, et al. Gabapentin attenuates late but not acute pain after abdominal hysterectomy. *Eur J Anaesthesiol* 2006;23:136–141.
108. Kamibayashi T, Maze M. Clinical uses of alpha2 -adrenergic agonists. *Anesthesiology* 2000;93:1345–1349.
109. Stone LS, MacMillan LB, Kitto KF, et al. The α_{2a} adrenergic receptor subtype mediates spinal analgesia evoked by α_2 agonists and is necessary for spinal adrenergic-opioid synergy. *J Neurosci* 1997;17:7157–7165.
110. Hall JE, Uhrich TD, Barney JA, et al. Sedative, amnestic, and analgesic properties of small-dose dexmedetomidine infusions. *Anesth. Analg* 2000;90:699–705.
111. Pandharipande PP, Pun BT, Herr DL, et al. Effect of sedation with dexmedetomidine vs lorazepam on acute brain dysfunction in mechanically ventilated patients: the MENDS randomized controlled trial. *JAMA* 2007;298:2644–2653.
112. Eisenach JC, Hood DD, Curry R. Intrathecal, but not intravenous, clonidine reduces experimental thermal or capsaicin-induced pain and hyperalgesia in normal volunteers. *Anesth Analg* 1998;87:591–596.
113. Mannion S, Hayes I, Loughnane F, et al. Intravenous but not perineural clonidine prolongs postoperative analgesia after psoas compartment block with 0.5% levobupivacaine for hip fracture surgery. *Anesth Analg* 2005;100:873–878, table of contents.
114. Dimou P, Paraskeva A, Papilas K, et al. Transdermal clonidine: does it affect pain after abdominal hysterectomy? *Acta Anaesthesiol Belg* 2003;54:227–232.
115. Hidalgo MP, Auzani JA, Rumpel LC, et al. The clinical effect of small oral clonidine doses on perioperative outcomes in patients undergoing abdominal hysterectomy. *Anesth Analg* 2005;100:795–802, table of contents.
116. Marinangeli F, Ciccozzi A, Donatelli F, et al. Clonidine for treatment of postoperative pain: a dose-finding study. *Eur J Pain* 2002;6:35–42.
117. Angst MS, Ramaswamy B, Davies MF, et al. Comparative analgesic and mental effects of increasing plasma concentrations of dexmedetomidine and alfentanil in humans. *Anesthesiology* 2004;101:744–752.
118. Unlugenc H, Gunduz M, Guler T, et al. The effect of pre-anaesthetic administration of intravenous dexmedetomidine on postoperative pain in patients receiving patient-controlled morphine. *Eur J Anaesthesiol* 2005;22:386–391.
119. Wahlander S, Frumento RJ, Wagener G, et al. A prospective, double-blind, randomized, placebo-controlled study of dexmedetomidine as an adjunct to epidural analgesia after thoracic surgery. *J Cardiothorac Vasc Anesth* 2005;19:630–635.
120. Aho MS, Erkola OA, Scheinin H, et al. Effect of intravenously administered dexmedetomidine on pain after laparoscopic tubal ligation. *Anesth Analg* 1991;73:112–118.
121. Cardenas CG, Del Mar LP, Cooper BY, et al. 5HT4 receptors couple positively to tetrodotoxin-insensitive sodium channels in a subpopulation of capsaicin-sensitive rat sensory neurons. *J Neurosci* 1997;17:7181–7189.
122. Manzke T, Guenther U, Ponimaskin EG, et al. 5-HT4(a) receptors avert opioid-induced breathing depression without loss of analgesia. *Science* 2003;301:226–229.
123. Max MB, Lynch SA, Muir J, et al. Effects of desipramine, amitriptyline, and fluoxetine on pain in diabetic neuropathy. *N Engl J Med* 1992;326:1250–1256.
124. Kishore-Kumar R, Schafer SC, Lawlor BA, et al. Single doses of the serotonin agonists buspirone and m-chlorophenylpiperazine do not relieve neuropathic pain. *Pain* 1989;37:223–227.
125. McQuay HJ, Tramer M, Nye BA, et al. A systematic review of antidepressants in neuropathic pain. *Pain* 1996;68:217–227.
126. Rumore MM, Schlichting DA. Clinical efficacy of antihistaminics as analgesics. *Pain* 1986;25:7–22.
127. Dickenson AH, Matthews EA, Suzuki, R. Neurobiology of neuropathic pain: mode of action of anticonvulsants. *Eur J Pain* 2002;6(Suppl A):51–60.
128. Eisenach JC, Gebhart GF. Intrathecal amitriptyline acts as an N-methyl-D-aspartate receptor antagonist in the presence of inflammatory hyperalgesia in rats. *Anesthesiology* 1995;83:1046–1054.
129. Seltzer Z, Tal M, Sharav Y. Autotomy behavior in rats following peripheral deafferentation is suppressed by daily injections of amitriptyline, diazepam, and saline. *Pain* 1989;37:245–250.
130. Brau ME, Dreimann M, Olschewski A, et al. Effect of drugs used for neuropathic pain management on tetrodotoxin-resistant Na(+) currents in rat sensory neurons. *Anesthesiology* 2001;94:137–144.
131. Wallace MS, Barger D, Schulteis G. The effect of chronic oral desipramine on capsaicin-induced allodynia and hyperalgesia: a double-blinded, placebo-controlled, crossover study. *Anesth Analg* 2002;95:973–978, table of contents.
132. Hummel T, Hummel C, Friedel I, et al. A comparison of the antinociceptive effects of imipramine, tramadol and anpirtoline. *Br J Clin Pharmacol* 1994;37:325–333.
133. Bowsher D. The effects of pre-emptive treatment of postherpetic neuralgia with amitriptyline: a randomized, double-blind, placebo-controlled trial. *J Pain Symptom Manage* 1997;13:327–331.
134. Levine JD, Gordon NC, Smith R, et al. Desipramine enhances opiate postoperative analgesia. *Pain* 1986;27:45–49.
135. Max MB, Zeigler D, Shoaf SE, et al. Effects of a single oral dose of desipramine on postoperative morphine analgesia. *J Pain Symptom Manage* 1992;7:454–462.
136. Reuben SS, Makari-Judson G, Lurie SD. Evaluation of efficacy of the perioperative administration of venlafaxine XR in the prevention of postmastectomy pain syndrome. *J Pain Symptom Manage* 2004;27:133–139.
137. Semenchuk MR, Sherman S, Davis B. Double-blind, randomized trial of bupropion SR for the treatment of neuropathic pain. *Neurology* 2001;57:1583–1588.
138. Macintyre PE. Safety and efficacy of patient-controlled analgesia. *Br J Anaesth* 2001;87:36–46.
139. Camu F, Van Aken H, Bovill JG. Postoperative analgesic effects of three demand-dose sizes of fentanyl administered by patient-controlled analgesia. *Anesth Analg* 1998;87:890–895.
140. Dawson PJ, Libreri FC, Jones DJ, et al. The efficacy of adding a continuous intravenous morphine infusion to patient-controlled analgesia (PCA) in abdominal surgery. *Anaesth Intensive Care* 1995;23:453–458.
141. Hudcova J, McNicol E, Quah C, et al. Patient-controlled opioid analgesia versus conventional opioid analgesia for postoperative pain. *Cochrane Database Syst Rev* 2006:CD003348.
142. Etches RC. Respiratory depression associated with patient-controlled analgesia: a review of eight cases. *Can J Anaesth* 1994;41:125–132.
143. Looi-Lyons LC, Chung FF, Chan VW, et al. Respiratory depression: an adverse outcome during patient-controlled analgesia therapy. *J Clin Anesth* 1996;8:151–156.
144. Dolin SJ, Cashman JN, Bland JM. Effectiveness of acute postoperative pain management: I. Evidence from published data. *Br J Anaesth* 2002;89:409–423.
145. Hamber EA, Viscomi CM. Intrathecal lipophilic opioids as adjuncts to surgical spinal anesthesia. *Reg Anesth Pain Med* 1999;24:255–263.
146. Liu SS, Bernards CM. Exploring the epidural trail. *Reg Anesth Pain Med* 2002;27:122–124.
147. Liu SS, McDonald SB. Current issues in spinal anesthesia. *Anesthesiology* 2001;94:888–906.
148. Birnbach, DJ, Johnson, MD, Arcario, T, et al. Effect of diluent volume on analgesia produced by epidural fentanyl. *Anesth Analg* 1989;68:808–810.
149. Beattie WS, Buckley DN, Forrest JB. Epidural morphine reduces the risk of postoperative myocardial ischaemia in patients with cardiac risk factors. *Can J Anaesth* 1993;40:532–541.
150. Tsui SL, Law S, Fok M, et al. Postoperative analgesia reduces mortality and morbidity after esophagectomy. *Am J Surg* 1997;173:472–478.
151. Gambling D, Hughes T, Martin G, et al. A comparison of Depodur, a novel, single-dose extended-release epidural morphine, with standard epidural morphine for pain relief after lower abdominal surgery. *Anesth Analg* 2005;100:1065–1074.
152. Wheatley RG, Schug SA, Watson D. Safety and efficacy of postoperative epidural analgesia. *Br J Anaesth* 2001;87:47–61.
153. Loper KA, Ready LB, Downey M, et al. Epidural and intravenous fentanyl infusions are clinically equivalent after knee surgery. *Anesth Analg* 1990;70:72–75.
154. Salomaki TE, Laitinen JO, Nuutinen LS. A randomized double-blind comparison of epidural versus intravenous fentanyl infusion for analgesia after thoracotomy. *Anesthesiology* 1991;75:790–795.
155. de Leon-Casasola OA, Lema MJ. Postoperative epidural opioid analgesia: what are the choices? *Anesth Analg* 1996;83:867–875.
156. Malviya S, Pandit UA, Merkel S, et al. A comparison of continuous epidural infusion and intermittent intravenous bolus doses of morphine in children undergoing selective dorsal rhizotomy. *Reg Anesth Pain Med* 1999;24:438–443.
157. Sitsen E, van Poorten F, van Alphen W, et al. Postoperative epidural analgesia after total knee arthroplasty with sufentanil 1 mug/mL combined with ropivacaine 0.2%, ropivacaine 0.125%, or levobupivacaine 0.125%: a randomized, double-blind comparison. *Reg Anesth Pain Med* 2007;32:475–480.
158. Vercauteren M, Meert TF. Isobolographic analysis of the interaction between epidural sufentanil and bupivacaine in rats. *Pharmacol Biochem Behav* 1997;58:237–242.
159. Camann W, Abouleish A, Eisenach J, et al. Intrathecal sufentanil and epidural bupivacaine for labor analgesia: dose-response of individual agents and in combination. *Reg Anesth Pain Med* 1998;23:457–462.
160. Zaric D, Nydahl PA, Philipson L, et al. The effect of continuous lumbar epidural infusion of ropivacaine (0.1%, 0.2%, and 0.3%) and 0.25% bupivacaine on sensory and motor block in volunteers: a double-blind study. *Reg Anesth* 1996;21:14–25.
161. Curatolo M, Schnider TW, Petersen-Felix S, et al. A direct search procedure to optimize combinations of epidural bupivacaine, fentanyl, and clonidine for postoperative analgesia. *Anesthesiology* 2000;92:325–337.
162. Paech MJ, Pavy TJ, Orlikowski CE, et al. Postoperative epidural infusion: a randomized, double-blind, dose-finding trial of clonidine in combination with bupivacaine and fentanyl. *Anesth Analg* 1997;84:1323–1328.
163. Niemi G, Breivik H. Adrenaline markedly improves thoracic epidural analgesia produced by a low-dose infusion of bupivacaine, fentanyl, and adrenaline after major surgery: a randomised, double-blind, cross-over study with and without adrenaline. *Acta Anaesthesiol Scand* 1998;42:897–909.
164. Soetens FM, Soetens MA, Vercauteren MP. Levobupivacaine-sufentanil with

or without epinephrine during epidural labor analgesia. *Anesth Analg* 2006;
103:182–186, table of contents.

165. Lauretti GR, Rodrigues AM, Paccola CA, et al. The combination of epidural
clonidine and S(+)-ketamine did not enhance analgesic efficacy beyond that
for each individual drug in adult orthopedic surgery. *J Clin Anesth* 2005;17:
79–84.

166. Ozyalcin NS, Yucel A, Camlica H, et al. Effect of pre-emptive ketamine on
sensory changes and postoperative pain after thoracotomy: comparison of
epidural and intramuscular routes. *Br J Anaesth* 2004;93:356–361.

167. Vranken JH, Troost D, de Haan P, et al. Severe toxic damage to the rabbit
spinal cord after intrathecal administration of preservative-free S(+)-keta-
mine. *Anesthesiology* 2006;105:813–818.

168. Liu SS, Allen HW, Olsson GL. Patient-controlled epidural analgesia with
bupivacaine and fentanyl on hospital wards: prospective experience with
1,030 surgical patients. *Anesthesiology* 1998;88:688–695.

169. Smet IG, Vercauteren MP, De Jongh RF, et al. Pressure sores as a complication
of patient-controlled epidural analgesia after cesarean delivery. Case report.
Reg Anesth 1996;21:338–341.

170. Liu SS, Moore JM, Luo AM, et al. Comparison of three solutions of
ropivacaine/fentanyl for postoperative patient-controlled epidural analgesia.
Anesthesiology 1999;90:727–733.

171. Chaney MA. Side effects of intrathecal and epidural opioids. *Can J Anaesth*
1995;42:891–903.

172. White MJ, Berghausen EJ, Dumont SW, et al. Side effects during continuous
epidural infusion of morphine and fentanyl. *Can J Anaesth* 1992;39:576–582.

173. Kelly MC, Carabine UA, Mirakhur RK. Intrathecal diamorphine for analgesia
after caesarean section. A dose finding study and assessment of side-effects.
Anaesthesia 1998;53:231–237.

174. Ozalp G, Guner F, Kuru N, et al. Postoperative patient-controlled epidural
analgesia with opioid bupivacaine mixtures. *Can J Anaesth* 1998;45:938–
942.

175. Choi JH, Lee J, Choi JH, et al. Epidural naloxone reduces pruritus and nausea
without affecting analgesia by epidural morphine in bupivacaine. *Can J Anaesth* 2000;47:33–37.

176. Moscovici R, Prego G, Schwartz M, et al. Epidural scopolamine administration in preventing nausea after epidural morphine. *J Clin Anesth* 1995;7:
474–476.

177. Kjellberg F, Tramer MR. Pharmacological control of opioid-induced pruritus:
a quantitative systematic review of randomized trials. *Eur J Anaesthesiol*
2001;18:346–357.

178. Johanek LM, Meyer RA, Hartke T, et al. Psychophysical and physiological
evidence for parallel afferent pathways mediating the sensation of itch. *J Neurosci* 2007;27:7490–7497.

179. Ko MC, Naughton NN. An experimental itch model in monkeys: characterization of intrathecal morphine-induced scratching and antinociception. *Anesthesiology* 2000;92:795–805.

180. Macario A, Scibetta WC, Navarro J, et al. Analgesia for labor pain: a cost
model. *Anesthesiology* 2000;92:841–850.

181. de Leon-Casasola OA, Parker BM, Lema MJ, et al. Epidural analgesia versus
intravenous patient-controlled analgesia. Differences in the postoperative
course of cancer patients. *Reg Anesth* 1994;19:307–315.

182. Rygnestad T, Borchgrevink PC, Eide E. Postoperative epidural infusion of
morphine and bupivacaine is safe on surgical wards. Organisation of the
treatment, effects and side-effects in 2000 consecutive patients. *Acta Anaesthesiol Scand* 1997;41:868–876.

183. Katsiris S, Williams S, Leighton BL, et al. Respiratory arrest following intrathecal injection of sufentanil and bupivacaine in a parturient. *Can J Anaesth*
1998;45:880–883.

184. Mulroy MF. Monitoring opioids. *Reg Anesth* 1996;21:89–93.

185. Wang JJ, Ho ST, Tzeng JI. Comparison of intravenous nalbuphine infusion
versus naloxone in the prevention of epidural morphine-related side effects.
Reg Anesth Pain Med 1998;23:479–484.

186. Curatolo M, Petersen-Felix S, Scaramozzino P, et al. Epidural fentanyl, adrenaline and clonidine as adjuvants to local anaesthetics for surgical analgesia:
meta-analyses of analgesia and side-effects. *Acta Anaesthesiol Scand* 1998;
42:910–920.

187. Turner G, Blake D, Buckland M, et al. Continuous extradural infusion of
ropivacaine for prevention of postoperative pain after major orthopaedic surgery. *Br J Anaesth* 1996;76:606–610.

188. Sia AT, Chong JL. Epidural 0.2% ropivacaine for labour analgesia: parturi-
ent-controlled or continuous infusion? *Anaesth Intensive Care* 1999;27:
154–158.

189. Wigfull J, Welchew E. Survey of 1057 patients receiving postoperative patient-
controlled epidural analgesia. *Anaesthesia* 2001;56:70–75.

190. Burstal R, Wegener F, Hayes C, et al. Epidural analgesia: prospective audit
of 1062 patients. *Anaesth Intensive Care* 1998;26:165–172.

191. Komatsu H, Matsumoto S, Mitsuhata H. Comparison of patient-controlled
epidural analgesia with and without night-time infusion following gastrec-
tomy. *Br J Anaesth* 2001;87:633–635.

192. Rodgers A, Walker N, Schug S, et al. Reduction of postoperative mortality
and morbidity with epidural or spinal anaesthesia: results from overview of
randomised trials. *BMJ* 2000;321:1493.

193. Wu CL, Hurley RW, Anderson GF, et al. Effect of postoperative epidural
analgesia on morbidity and mortality following surgery in medicare patients.
Reg Anesth Pain Med 2004;29:525–533; discussion 515–529.

194. Holte K, Kehlet H. Epidural analgesia and risk of anastomotic leakage. *Reg
Anesth Pain Med* 2001;26:111–117.

195. Ballantyne JC, Carr DB, deFerranti S, et al. The comparative effects of postoperative analgesic therapies on pulmonary outcome: cumulative meta-analyses
of randomized, controlled trials. *Anesth Analg* 1998;86:598–612.

196. Rigg JR, Jamrozik K, Myles PS, et al. Epidural anaesthesia and analgesia and
outcome of major surgery: a randomised trial. *Lancet* 2002;359:1276–1282.

197. Norris EJ, Beattie C, Perler BA, et al. Double-masked randomized trial comparing alternate combinations of intraoperative anesthesia and postoperative
analgesia in abdominal aortic surgery. *Anesthesiology* 2001;95:1054–1067.

198. Liu S, Carpenter RL, Neal JM. Epidural anesthesia and analgesia. Their role
in postoperative outcome. *Anesthesiology* 1995;82:1474–1506.

199. Christopherson R, Beattie C, Frank SM, et al. Perioperative morbidity in
patients randomized to epidural or general anesthesia for lower extremity
vascular surgery. Perioperative Ischemia Randomized Anesthesia Trial Study
Group. *Anesthesiology* 1993;79:422–434.

200. Carli F, Mayo N, Klubien K, et al. Epidural analgesia enhances functional
exercise capacity and health-related quality of life after colonic surgery: results
of a randomized trial. *Anesthesiology* 2002;97:540–549.

201. Halpern SH, Leighton BL, Ohlsson A, et al. Effect of epidural vs parenteral
opioid analgesia on the progress of labor: a meta-analysis. *JAMA* 1998;280:
2105–2110.

202. Schroeder DR. Statistics: detecting a rare adverse drug reaction using spontaneous reports. *Reg Anesth Pain Med* 1998;23:183–189.

203. Vandermeulen EP, Van Aken H, Vermylen J. Anticoagulants and spinal-
epidural anesthesia. *Anesth Analg* 1994;79:1165–1177.

204. Horlocker TT, Wedel DJ. Neurologic complications of spinal and epidural
anesthesia. *Reg Anesth Pain Med* 2000;25:83–98.

205. Horlocker TT, Wedel DJ, Benzon H, et al. Regional anesthesia in the anticoagulated patient: defining the risks (the second ASRA Consensus Conference
on Neuraxial Anesthesia and Anticoagulation). *Reg Anesth Pain Med* 2003;
28:172–197.

206. Rosencher N, Bonnet MP, Sessler DI. Selected new antithrombotic agents and
neuraxial anaesthesia for major orthopaedic surgery: management strategies.
Anaesthesia 2007;62:1154–1160.

207. Moen V, Dahlgren N, Irestedt L. Severe neurological complications after central neuraxial blockades in Sweden 1990–1999. *Anesthesiology* 2004;101:
950–959.

208. Christie IW, McCabe S. Major complications of epidural analgesia after surgery: results of a six-year survey. *Anaesthesia* 2007;62:335–341.

209. Simpson RS, Macintyre PE, Shaw D, et al. Epidural catheter tip cultures:
results of a 4-year audit and implications for clinical practice. *Reg Anesth
Pain Med* 2000;25:360–367.

210. Wang H, Boctor B, Verner J. The effect of single-injection femoral nerve block
on rehabilitation and length of hospital stay after total knee replacement. *Reg
Anesth Pain Med* 2002;27:139–144.

211. Liu SS, Salinas FV. Continuous plexus and peripheral nerve blocks for postoperative analgesia. *Anesth Analg* 2003;96:263–272.

212. Karmakar MK. Thoracic paravertebral block. *Anesthesiology* 2001;95:
771–780.

213. Kaiser AM, Zollinger A, De Lorenzi D, et al. Prospective, randomized comparison of extrapleural versus epidural analgesia for postthoracotomy pain. *Ann
Thorac Surg* 1998;66:367–372.

214. Pettersson N, Perbeck L, Brismar B, et al. Sensory and sympathetic block
during interpleural analgesia. *Reg Anesth* 1997;22:313–317.

215. Shanti CM, Carlin AM, Tyburski JG. Incidence of pneumothorax from intercostal nerve block for analgesia in rib fractures. *J Trauma* 2001;51:536–539.

216. Miguel R, Hubbell D. Pain management and spirometry following thoracotomy: a prospective, randomized study of four techniques. *J Cardiothorac Vasc
Anesth* 1993;7:529–534.

217. Kalso E, Smith L, McQuay HJ, et al. No pain, no gain: clinical excellence and
scientific rigour—lessons learned from IA morphine. *Pain* 2002;98:269–275.

218. Moiniche S, Mikkelsen S, Wetterslev J, et al. A systematic review of intra-
articular local anesthesia for postoperative pain relief after arthroscopic knee
surgery. *Reg Anesth Pain Med* 1999;24:430–437.

219. Wedmore IS, Johnson T, Czarnik J, et al. Pain management in the wilderness
and operational setting. *Emerg Med Clin North Am* 2005;23:585–601,
xi–xii.

220. Nakahura T, Griswold W, Lemire J, et al. Nonsteroidal anti-inflammatory
drug use in adolescence. *J Adolesc Health* 1998;23:307–310.

221. Towheed TE, Judd MJ, Hochberg MC, et al. Acetaminophen for osteoarthritis. *Cochrane Database Syst Rev* 2003:CD004257.

222. Jowitt MD, Knight RJ. Anaesthesia during the Falklands campaign. The land
battles. *Anaesthesia* 1983;38:776–783.

223. Streisand JB, Varvel JR, Stanski DR, et al. Absorption and bioavailability of
oral transmucosal fentanyl citrate. *Anesthesiology* 1991;75:223–229.

224. Egan TD, Sharma A, Ashburn MA, et al. Multiple dose pharmacokinetics of
oral transmucosal fentanyl citrate in healthy volunteers. *Anesthesiology* 2000;
92:665–673.

225. Kharasch ED, Hoffer C, Whittington D. Influence of age on the pharmacokinetics and pharmacodynamics of oral transmucosal fentanyl citrate. *Anesthesiology* 2004;101:738–743.

226. Kotwal RS, O'Connor KC, Johnson TR, et al. A novel pain management strategy for combat casualty care. *Ann Emerg Med* 2004;44:121–127.

227. Buckenmaier CC 3rd, Auton AA, Flournoy WS. Continuous peripheral nerve block catheter tip adhesion in a rat model. *Acta Anaesthesiol Scand* 2006;50:694–698.

228. Buckenmaier CC 3rd, Shields CH, Auton AA, et al. Continuous peripheral nerve block in combat casualties receiving low-molecular weight heparin. *Br J Anaesth* 2006;97:874–877.

229. Twersky R, Fishman D, Homel P. What happens after discharge? return hospital visits after ambulatory surgery. *Anesth Analg* 1997;84:319–324.

230. Wu CL, Berenholtz SM, Pronovost PJ, et al. Systematic review and analysis of postdischarge symptoms after outpatient surgery. *Anesthesiology* 2002;96:994–1003.

231. Wu CL, Raja SN. Optimizing postoperative analgesia: the use of global outcome measures. *Anesthesiology* 2002;97:533–534.

232. Hendolin HI, Paakonen ME, Alhava EM, et al. Laparoscopic or open cholecystectomy: a prospective randomised trial to compare postoperative pain, pulmonary function, and stress response. *Eur J Surg* 2000;166:394–399.

233. Chung F, Mezei G, Tong D. Adverse events in ambulatory surgery. A comparison between elderly and younger patients. *Can J Anaesth* 1999;46:309–321.

234. Romsing J, Moiniche S, Dahl JB. Rectal and parenteral paracetamol, and paracetamol in combination with NSAIDs, for postoperative analgesia. *Br J Anaesth* 2002;88:215–226.

235. Lariviere M, Goffaux P, Marchand S, et al. Changes in pain perception and descending inhibitory controls start at middle age in healthy adults. *Clin J Pain* 2007;23:506–510.

236. Rolke R, Baron R, Maier C, et al. Quantitative sensory testing in the German Research Network on Neuropathic Pain (DFNS): standardized protocol and reference values. *Pain* 2006;123:231–243.

237. Gibson SJ, Helme RD. Age-related differences in pain perception and report. *Clin Geriatr Med* 2001;17:433–456, v–vi.

238. Gregoratos G. Clinical manifestations of acute myocardial infarction in older patients. *Am J Geriatr Cardiol* 2001;10:345–347.

239. Gloth FM 3rd. Geriatric pain. Factors that limit pain relief and increase complications. *Geriatrics* 2000;55:46–48, 51–54.

240. Macintyre PE, Jarvis DA. Age is the best predictor of postoperative morphine requirements. *Pain* 1996;64:357–364.

241. Gagliese L, Jackson M, Ritvo P, et al. Age is not an impediment to effective use of patient-controlled analgesia by surgical patients. *Anesthesiology* 2000;93:601–610.

242. Marcantonio ER, Flacker JM, Michaels M, et al. Delirium is independently associated with poor functional recovery after hip fracture. *J Am Geriatr Soc* 2000;48:618–624.

243. Flacker JM, Lipsitz LA. Neural mechanisms of delirium: current hypotheses and evolving concepts. *J Gerontol A Biol Sci Med Sci* 1999;54:B239–246.

244. Flacker JM, Lipsitz LA. Serum anticholinergic activity changes with acute illness in elderly medical patients. *J Gerontol A Biol Sci Med Sci* 1999;54:M12–16.

245. Schor JD, Levkoff SE, Lipsitz LA, et al. Risk factors for delirium in hospitalized elderly. *JAMA* 1992;267:827–831.

246. Lynch EP, Lazor MA, Gellis JE, et al. The impact of postoperative pain on the development of postoperative delirium. *Anesth Analg* 1998;86:781–785.

247. Aronoff GM. Medical treatment of opiate addiction. *JAMA* 2000;283:2931–2932.

248. Savage SR. Long-term opioid therapy: assessment of consequences and risks. *J Pain Symptom Manage* 1996;11:274–286.

249. Rapp SE, Ready LB, Nessly ML. Acute pain management in patients with prior opioid consumption: a case-controlled retrospective review. *Pain* 1995;61:195–201.

250. Anderson R, Saiers JH, Abram S, et al. Accuracy in equianalgesic dosing: conversion dilemmas. *J Pain Symptom Manage* 2001;21:397–406.

251. Woodhouse A, Ward ME, Mather LE. Intra-subject variability in post-operative patient-controlled analgesia (PCA): is the patient equally satisfied with morphine, pethidine and fentanyl? *Pain* 1999;80:545–553.

252. de Leon-Casasola OA, Myers DP, Donaparthi S, et al. A comparison of postoperative epidural analgesia between patients with chronic cancer taking high doses of oral opioids versus opioid-naive patients. *Anesth Analg* 1993;76:302–307.

253. Benumof JL. Obstructive sleep apnea in the adult obese patient: implications for airway management. *J Clin Anesth* 2001;13:144–156.

254. Rawal N, Sjostrand U, Christoffersson E, et al. Comparison of intramuscular and epidural morphine for postoperative analgesia in the grossly obese: influence on postoperative ambulation and pulmonary function. *Anesth Analg* 1984;63:583–592.

255. Flegal KM, Carroll MD, Kuczmarski RJ, et al. Overweight and obesity in the United States: prevalence and trends, 1960–1994. *Int J Obes Relat Metab Disord* 1998;22:39–47.

256. Findley LJ, Barth JT, Powers DC, et al. Cognitive impairment in patients with obstructive sleep apnea and associated hypoxemia. *Chest* 1986;90:686–690.

257. Roux F, D'Ambrosio C, Mohsenin V. Sleep-related breathing disorders and cardiovascular disease. *Am J Med* 2000;108:396–402.

258. Cullen DJ. Obstructive sleep apnea and postoperative analgesia—a potentially dangerous combination. *J Clin Anesth* 2001;13:83–85.

259. Garpestad E, Katayama H, Parker JA, et al. Stroke volume and cardiac output decrease at termination of obstructive apneas. *J Appl Physiol* 1992;73:1743–1748.

260. Gross JB, Bachenberg KL, Benumof JL, et al. Practice guidelines for the perioperative management of patients with obstructive sleep apnea: a report by the American Society of Anesthesiologists Task Force on Perioperative Management of patients with obstructive sleep apnea. *Anesthesiology* 2006;104:1081–1093; quiz 1117–1088.

261. Wizeman TM, Pardue ML. *Exploring the Biological Contributions to Human Health: Does Sex Matter?* Washington, DC: National Academy Press; 2001.

262. Holdcroft A, Berkley KJ. Sex and gender difference in pain and its relief. In: Wall P, Melzack R, eds. *Textbook of Pain.* 5th ed. Philadelphia: Elsevier; 2005.

263. Bingefors K, Isacson D. Epidemiology, co-morbidity, and impact on health-related quality of life of self-reported headache and musculoskeletal pain—a gender perspective. *Eur J Pain* 2004;8:435–450.

264. Isacson D, Bingefors K. Epidemiology of analgesic use: a gender perspective. *Eur J Anaesthesiol* 2002;26(Suppl):5–15.

265. Myers CD, Riley JL 3rd, Robinson ME. Psychosocial contributions to sex-correlated differences in pain. *Clin J Pain* 2003;19:225–232.

266. Riley JL 3rd, Robinson ME, Wise EA, et al. Sex differences in the perception of noxious experimental stimuli: a meta-analysis. *Pain* 1998;74:181–187.

267. Paulson PE, Minoshima S, Morrow TJ, et al. Gender differences in pain perception and patterns of cerebral activation during noxious heat stimulation in humans. *Pain* 1998;76:223–229.

268. Pickering G, Jourdan D, Eschalier A, et al. Impact of age, gender, and cognitive functioning on pain perception. *Gerontology* 2002;48:112–118.

269. Pool GJ, Schwegler AF, Theodore BR, et al. Role of gender norms and group identification on hypothetical and experimental pain tolerance. *Pain* 2007;129:122–129.

270. Derbyshire SW, Nichols TE, Firestone L, et al. Gender differences in patterns of cerebral activation during equal experience of painful laser stimulation. *J Pain* 2002;3:401–411.

271. Moulton EA, Keaser ML, Gullapalli RP, et al. Sex differences in the cerebral BOLD signal response to painful heat stimuli. *Am J Physiol Regul Integr Comp Physiol* 2006;291:R257–267.

272. Berman SM, Naliboff BD, Suyenobu B, et al. Sex differences in regional brain response to aversive pelvic visceral stimuli. *Am J Physiol Regul Integr Comp Physiol* 2006;291:R268–276.

273. Naliboff BD, Berman S, Chang L, et al. Sex-related differences in IBS patients: central processing of visceral stimuli. *Gastroenterology* 2003;124:1738–1747.

274. Fillingim RB, Ness TJ, Glover TL, et al. Morphine responses and experimental pain: sex differences in side effects and cardiovascular responses but not analgesia. *J Pain* 2005;6:116–124.

275. Romberg R, Olofsen E, Sarton E, et al. Pharmacokinetic-pharmacodynamic modeling of morphine-6-glucuronide-induced analgesia in healthy volunteers: absence of sex differences. *Anesthesiology* 2004;100:120–133.

276. Wasan AD, Davar G, Jamison R. The association between negative affect and opioid analgesia in patients with discogenic low back pain. *Pain* 2005;117:450–461.

277. Pud D, Yarnitsky D, Sprecher E, et al. Can personality traits and gender predict the response to morphine? An experimental cold pain study. *Eur J Pain* 2006;10:103–112.

278. Sarton E, Olofsen E, Romberg R, et al. Sex differences in morphine analgesia: an experimental study in healthy volunteers. *Anesthesiology* 2000;93:1245–1254.

279. Zacny JP. Characterizing the subjective, psychomotor, and physiological effects of a hydrocodone combination product (Hycodan) in non-drug-abusing volunteers. *Psychopharmacology (Berl)* 2003;165:146–156.

280. Murthy BR, Pollack GM, Brouwer KL. Contribution of morphine-6-glucuronide to antinociception following intravenous administration of morphine to healthy volunteers. *J Clin Pharmacol* 2002;42:569–576.

281. Olofsen E, Romberg R, Bijl H, et al. Alfentanil and placebo analgesia: no sex differences detected in models of experimental pain. *Anesthesiology* 2005;103:130–139.

282. Gear RW, Gordon NC, Heller PH, et al. Gender difference in analgesic response to the kappa-opioid pentazocine. *Neurosci Lett* 1996;205:207–209.

283. Gear RW, Miaskowski C, Gordon NC, et al. Kappa-opioids produce significantly greater analgesia in women than in men. *Nat Med* 1996;2:1248–1250.

284. Gordon NC, Gear RW, Heller PH, et al. Enhancement of morphine analgesia by the GABAB agonist baclofen. *Neuroscience* 1995;69:345–349.

285. Fillingim RB, Gear RW. Sex differences in opioid analgesia: clinical and experimental findings. *Eur J Pain* 2004;8:413–425.

286. Mogil JS, Wilson SG, Chesler EJ, et al. The melanocortin-1 receptor gene mediates female-specific mechanisms of analgesia in mice and humans. *Proc Natl Acad Sci U S A* 2003;100:4867–4872.

287. Rawal N. 10 years of acute pain services—achievements and challenges. *Reg Anesth Pain Med* 1999;24:68–73.

288. Bardiau FM, Braeckman MM, Seidel L, et al. Effectiveness of an acute pain service inception in a general hospital. *J Clin Anesth* 1999;11:583–589.

289. Merry A, Judge MA, Ready B. Acute pain services in New Zealand hospitals; a survey. *N Z Med J* 1997;110:233–235.

290. Carr DB, Miaskowski C, Dedrick SC, et al. Management of perioperative pain in hospitalized patients: a national survey. *J Clin Anesth* 1998;10:77–85.

291. Lee A, Chan S, Chen PP, et al. Economic evaluations of acute pain service programs: a systematic review. *Clin J Pain* 2007;23:726–733.
292. Kehlet H, Jensen TS, Woolf CJ. Persistent postsurgical pain: risk factors and prevention. *Lancet* 2006;367:1618–1625.
293. Macrae WA. Chronic pain after surgery. *Br J Anaesth* 2001;87:88–98.
294. Carr DB, Goudas LC. Acute pain. *Lancet* 1999;353:2051–2058.
295. Capdevila X, Barthelet Y, Biboulet P, et al. Effects of perioperative analgesic technique on the surgical outcome and duration of rehabilitation after major knee surgery. *Anesthesiology* 1999;91:8–15.
296. Lavand'homme P, De Kock M. The use of intraoperative epidural or spinal analgesia modulates postoperative hyperalgesia and reduces residual pain after major abdominal surgery. *Acta Anaesthesiol Belg* 2006;57:373–379.
297. Poleshuck EL, Katz J, Andrus CH, et al. Risk factors for chronic pain following breast cancer surgery: a prospective study. *J Pain* 2006;7:626–634.

CHAPTER 52 ■ REGIONAL ANESTHESIA TECHNIQUES FOR ACUTE PAIN MANAGEMENT

STEVE MELTON AND SPENCER S. LIU

INTRODUCTION

This chapter focuses on regional anesthesia techniques for acute postoperative pain management. Central neuraxial, paravertebral, and peripheral nerve blocks including single-shot injections, continuous perineural catheters, and ultrasound-guided techniques are discussed. Included in this discussion are the indications, mechanisms of action, side effects and complications of regional anesthetic techniques, and the associated outcomes and evidence in the application of these techniques for acute postoperative pain management.

BLOCK PREPARATION

Whether performing regional anesthetic techniques in the operating room or a separate block-area, all patients should have an intravenous (IV) infusion line, standard monitors (continous pulse oximetry, electrocardiogram, intermittent noninvasive blood pressure), supplemental oxygen, and appropriate sedation for the procedure. Airway management and medications for emergency cardiopulmonary resuscitation, including intralipid infusion, should be immediately available. All regional anesthetic techniques are performed using strict aseptic technique.

CENTRAL NEURAXIAL

Subarachnoid and epidural analgesia are commonly practiced regional anesthesia techniques for acute postoperative pain management. As a means of postoperative pain control, single-shot techniques with perispinal additives and/or continuous or patient-controlled catheter techniques with local anesthetics and/or perispinal additives may be used. The practice of neuraxial anesthesia requires an appreciation of both surface and underlying spinal anatomy, including the relationship between the cutaneous dermatomes, spinal nerves, and vertebrae.[1]

Subarachnoid Analgesia

Indications

Spinal analgesia may be used for postoperative analgesia following obstetric, gynecologic, hernia repair, genitourinary, and or-thopedic surgeries of the lower extremity. Additionally, spinal analgesia offers postoperative pain control for cardiac, abdominal, vascular, spine, and thoracic surgery. Obstetric analgesia will not be included in our discussion. Intrathecal (IT) additives including fentanyl, sufentanil, morphine, hydromorphone, and clonidine are discussed below.

Technique

Subarachnoid block may be performed with the patient in the sitting, lateral (Fig. 52.1), or prone position through a midline or paramedian approach (Fig. 52.2). After patient positioning, the appropriate interspace is identified, prepped, and draped in sterile fashion. Local anesthetic is infiltrated at the needle insertion site. The introducer needle is placed midline and advanced in the midline plane with slight cephalad angulation through the supraspinous ligament and into the interspinous ligament. The depth to the subarachnoid space must be anticipated to avoid inadvertent dural puncture with the introducer needle in thin patients. The spinal needle is then advanced through the introducer, stabilizing the introducer with the nondominant hand. As the needle passes through the ligamentum flavum, an increase in resistance is appreciated, followed by a loss of resistance, with a characteristic "pop" indicating penetration of the dura and entry into the subarachnoid space. The spinal needle stylet is removed, and free cerebrospinal fluid (CSF) flow is confirmed through the needle. If free CSF flow is not visualized, the hub of the needle may be rotated 90 degrees, followed by slight advancement of the needle if necessary. If CSF free flow is unable to be confirmed, the needle is slowly withdrawn in slight increments, with 90 degree rotation at each increment to allow for free CSF flow. Upon obtaining free flow of CSF, the dorsal aspect of the nondominant hand is firmly placed against the patient's back with the index finger and thumb stabilizing the spinal needle hub for injection. In the dominant hand, the syringe with local anesthetic and additive is attached to the spinal needle hub and injected. If redirection of the spinal needle is necessary secondary to bone contact, paresthesia, or failure to obtain CSF, the anatomy should be re-evaluated and the introducer repositioned as necessary at the same or a new level. If a paresthesia is encountered at any time, needle advancement or injection should be stopped, and resolution of paresthesia confirmed before and during subsequent advancement and or injection.

The paramedian-lateral and paramedian-lateral oblique approaches offer alternatives to the midline approach in patients

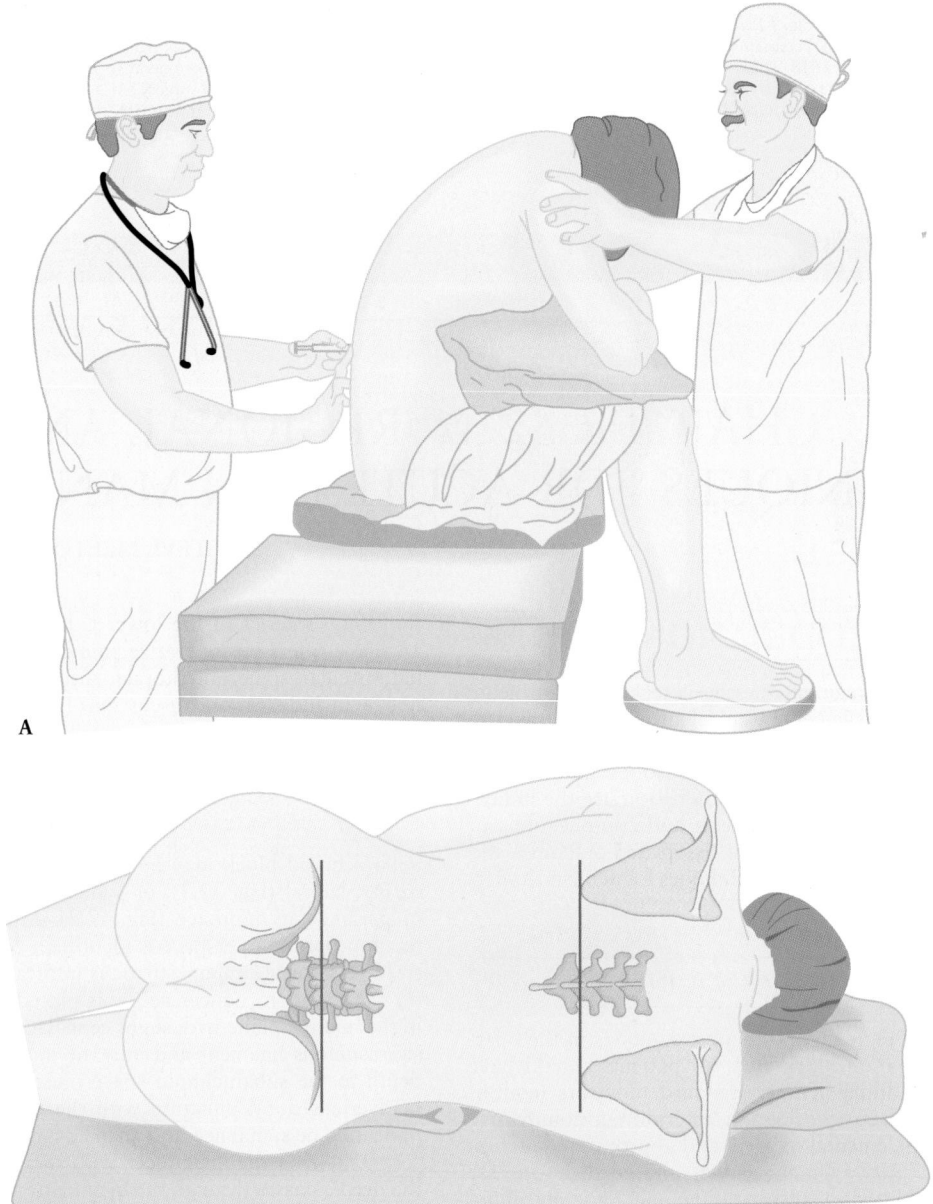

FIGURE 52.1 Sitting (**A**) and lateral (**B**) position position for neuraxial block. A line drawn between the superior aspects of the iliac crests will cross the L4 spinous process or L4-L5 interspace. A line drawn between the inferior angles of the scapulae will cross the T7 spinous process.

with narrow interspinous spaces for both subarachnoid and epidural blocks.

For the paramedian-lateral approach, the spinal introducer insertion site is approximately one fingerbreadth lateral to the insertion site of the midline approach. The introducer is oriented with slight medial and cephalad direction to allow the spinal needle to bypass the supraspinous and interspinous ligaments, pass through the triangular-shaped ligamentum flavum, and enter the subarachnoid space at the midline (see Fig. 52.2).

Using the paramedian-lateral oblique approach, the caudad spinous process of the desired interspace is identified. The needle is inserted approximately one fingerbreadth lateral to this point and directed with cephalomedial orientation to bypass the supraspinous and interspinous ligaments, pass through the triangular-shaped ligamentum flavum, and enter the subarachnoid space at the midline. Alternatively, the needle is initially oriented perpendicular to the skin in all planes and advanced with the intent to

contact lamina. Upon contact with lamina, the needle is walked off the superior edge of the lamina and advanced through the ligamentum flavum to enter the subarachnoid space (see Fig. 52.2).

Intrathecal Opioids

The advantages of IT opioids lay in the absence of sympathetic blockade and postural hypotension, potentially easier ambulation of patients, and avoidance of cardiovascular collapse or convulsions—the major complications of local anesthetic blockade.

Mechanism of Action

IT opioids selectively decrease nociceptive afferent input from A-delta and C-fibers without affecting dorsal root axons or so-

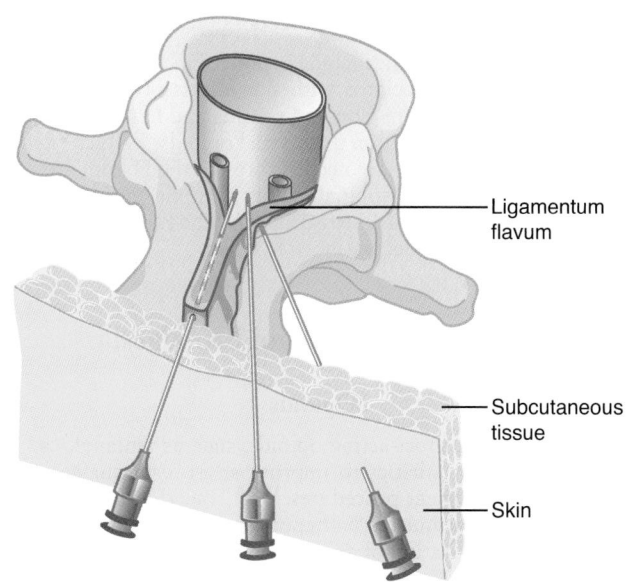

FIGURE 52.2 Midline, paramedian-lateral, and paramedian-lateral oblique approaches to the subarachnoid and epidural space.

matosensory evoked potentials.[2] Opioid receptors in the ventral medial medullary reticular formation may be involved in activation of bulbospinal noradrenergic pathways. Additionally, a descending inhibitory pathway projecting through the dorsolateral funiculus may reinforce other analgesic mechanisms.[3,4]

A single-dose injection of neuraxial opioids can provide effective postoperative analgesia as a sole analgesic agent or in combination with other agents such as local anesthetics or alpha-2 agonists. The analgesic profile of neuraxially administered opioids is primarily dependent on the degree of lipophilicity versus hydrophilicity of the agent. Hydrophilic opioids, such as morphine and hydromorphone, produce a longer duration of analgesia as compared to lipophilic opioids such as fentanyl or sufentanil. The pharmacokinetic differences in analgesia between hydrophilic and lipophilic opioids should be tailored to the surgical procedure and venue (inpatient versus outpatient) to optimize analgesia and minimize side effects. A single IT injection of a hydrophilic opioid such as morphine, which provides 12 to 18 hours of postoperative analgesia, is appropriate for surgical inpatients with appropriate monitoring of side effects. For outpatient postoperative analgesia, however, utilizing a lipophilic opioid such as fentanyl, with a rapid analgesic onset and short duration of action, is more appropriate, minimizing the risk of delayed respiratory depression.[5]

Morphine/Hydromorphone. Hydrophilic opioids such as morphine and hydromorphone provide excellent selective spinal analgesia because of a small volume of distribution and slow clearance from the spinal cord.[6] However, slow spinal cord penetration and prolonged duration in the CSF caused by hydrophilicity also results in slow onset (>30 minutes), prolonged duration of action (6 or more hours), and risk of delayed respiratory depression from rostral spread in CSF.

Sufentanil. Sufentanil is a lipophilic opioid. Lipophilic opioids have a more favorable clinical profile of fast onset (minutes), modest duration (1–4 hours), and little risk of delayed respiratory depression. Clinical studies suggest that IT administration of sufentanil may produce selective spinal analgesia; however, laboratory studies suggest that systemic uptake followed by supraspinal analgesia may be the dominant mechanism of action. Because of the extreme lipid solubility of sufentanil, it has a very large volume of distribution in the spinal cord with rapid clearance into

the spinal cord vasculature and epidural space in pig models.[6] This laboratory finding implies that very little spinal sufentanil is available for interaction with spinal cord opioid receptors because of sequestration in lipid soluble white matter and systemic redistribution. Thus, there is little support for the spinal administration of sufentanil in order to achieve selective spinal analgesia.

Fentanyl. Fentanyl is a lipophilic opioid, and thus, has a more favorable clinical profile of fast onset (minutes), modest duration (1–4 hours), and little risk of delayed respiratory depression.[2] Fentanyl, however, is less lipid soluble than sufentanil and will maintain modest spinal selectivity when injected intrathecally.[6,7] Dose-response data indicate that spinal fentanyl alone provides dose-dependent analgesia with a minimally effective dose of approximately 10 mcg.[8] Risk of early respiratory depression is also dose dependent, with significant risk occurring with doses greater than 25 mcg.[9] Thus, the best risk-benefit dose range would be limited to easily treated pruritus (~60%) [10,11] while minimizing the risk of early respiratory depression and urinary retention.[9,10,12]

Side Effects

Side effects of neuraxial opioids are caused by the presence of drug in either the CSF or systemic circulation. More common side effects include depression of ventilation, pruritis, nausea, vomiting, urinary retention, and sedation.[13]

Depression of Ventilation. The most feared side effect is respiratory depression and arrest. It has been demonstrated that the risk of respiratory depression is dose related,[14] with few instances of clinically significant depression reported at doses less than 0.4 mg of IT morphine.[15] Respiratory depression, however, has been noted at even smaller doses on rare occasions.[16] The incidence of respiratory depression is less than 1% for opioids regardless of route of administration.[17] Respiratory depression typically occurs within minutes to hours for lipophilic opioids (fentanyl, sufentanil) with early respiratory depression (minutes) not being reported with a hydrophilic opioid such as morphine. For morphine, delayed respiratory depression characteristically occurs 6 to 12 hours after administration but has been reported up to 19 hours after IT injection.[18] Clinically significant respiratory depression has never been reported beyond 19 hours after IT morphine administration. The following factors may contribute to the development of respiratory depression after IT opioid administration: opioid-naïve state, concurrent use of systemic opioids or sedatives, increasing age, and sleep or obstructive sleep apnea. Frequent monitoring of patients who have received IT opioid is recommended; however, the need for an intensive care-like unit setting for postoperative monitoring of these patients is controversial.[19]

Pruritis. The most common side effect after IT opioids is pruritis. Although IT opioid-induced pruritis is likely due to cephalad migration of the drug and interaction with opioid receptors in the trigeminal nucleus located superficially in the medulla,[18] the exact etiology is unclear. Itching is not histamine-related nor is it related to systemic absorption of the drug. The incidence has been reported anywhere from 20% to 100% in various studies and may be dose-dependent.[18,20–22] It appears that patients who receive morphine have a higher incidence of pruritis than those who receive fentanyl.[18,23]

Nausea and Vomiting. Nausea and vomiting are also common and troubling side effects after IT opioid injection. Although the incidence is lower than that seen with pruritis, patients may require treatment more frequently. Nausea occurs in approximately 20% to 40% of patients receiving IT opioids. Nausea usually occurs within 4 hours of injection and may be more likely when

IT morphine is utilized.[18] The mechanism is likely due to the cephalad migration of drug and subsequent interaction with opioid receptors in the area postrema.[18,24] Although the mechanism is not related to systemic absorption, the incidence is comparable to IV and epidural administration.

Urinary Retention. Urinary retention following IT opioids is much more common than after equivalent doses given intravenously. Urinary retention induced by IT opioids is not dose-related, may be more frequent when IT morphine is administered, and is likely related to opioid receptor-induced inhibition of sacral parasympathetic nervous system outflow, resulting in detrusor relaxation and an increase bladder capacity.[18]

Sedation. Sedation is a dose-dependent side effect of IT opioids that occurs with all opioids.[25] The difference in levels of sedation from IT, IV, and epidural routes is not well documented, but appears to be common regardless of route of delivery. The incidence may be higher with sufentanil than other opioids.[18,26,27]

Intrathecal Clonidine

Research has demonstrated the antinociceptive properties and the mechanisms involved in the production of spinal analgesia after administration of alpha-2 adrenergic drugs. Clonidine is the best characterized alpha-2 adrenergic agonist and provides dose-dependent analgesia.[28]

Mechanism of Action

Clonidine's analgesic activity is mediated through pre- and post-synaptic alpha-2 receptors localized in the superficial layers of the spinal dorsal horn. Clonidine attenuates nociceptive input from A-delta and C-fibers and acts synergistically with spinal local anesthetics.[29] Additionally, neuraxial placement of clonidine inhibits spinal substance P release and nociceptive neuron firing produced by noxious stimulation.[13]

Side Effects

Side effects of IT clonidine include hypotension, bradycardia, and sedation. It is not associated with side effects of spinal opioids such as respiratory depression and pruritus and has less potential for causing urinary retention than spinal opioids.[30] Much smaller bolus doses of clonidine are needed through the IT route to produce potent and long-lasting analgesia than via the epidural or systemic routes. Doses of 15 to 30 mcg may be equally efficacious as larger doses while decreasing side effects.

Clinical Subarachnoid Analgesia

Opioids

Highly lipophilic, short-acting opioids, such as fentanyl, can be added to local anesthetics to improve short-term analgesia for inpatient or outpatient procedures.[31–33] The addition of 10 mcg fentanyl to bupivacaine 0.5% (hyperbaric) significantly improves the quality and duration of analgesia, with no further advantage occurring if the dose is increased up to 40 mcg.[34] Hydrophilic opioids, however, provide extended postoperative analgesia in the inpatient setting. Dose response trials demonstrate that low doses of hydrophilic opioids maximize postoperative analgesia with a lower incidence of side effects (Table 52.1) For example, Cole et al.[35] demonstrated that 0.3 mg of IT morphine significantly reduces pain and patient-controlled analgesia (PCA) requirements compared to placebo following knee arthroplasty with no significance difference in hypoxemia and apnea between groups. For opioid-tolerant patients, higher doses are probably acceptable, while doses of less than 0.3 mg may be ideal for opioid-naïve individuals.[36] IT opioids have been used for cardiac surgery with improved analgesia; however, concerns with bleeding complications in patients who are receiving heparin and studies demonstrating prolonged extubation times may have limited its use.[19] Alhashemi et al.[37] demonstrated that 250 mcg is the optimal dose of IT morphine to provide significant postoperative analgesia without delaying tracheal extubation after coronary

---

TABLE 52.1

DOSE RESPONSE STUDIES OF INTRATHECAL MORPHINE

Author	Surgery	Study Design	Dose Range	Optimal Dose
Jacobson 98	Ortho	RCT	0, 0.3, 2.5	0.3–1
Boezaart 99	Ortho	RCT	0.2, 0.3, 0.4	0.3
Kirson 89	GU	RCT	0, 0.1, 0.2	0.1
Sarma 93	GYN	RCT	0, 0.1, 0.3, 0.5	0.3
Yamaguchi 90	GI	RCT	0, 0.04, 0.06, 0.08, 0.1, 0.12, 0.15, 0.20	0.06–0.12
Jiang 91	OB	RCT	0, 0.025, 0.05, 0.075, 0.1, 0.125	0.075–0.125
Milner 96	OB	RCT	0.1, 0.2	0.1
Kelly 98	OB	RCT	0, 0.125, 0.25, 0.375	—
Palmer 99	OB	RCT	0, 0.025, 0.05, 0.075, 0.1, 0.2, 0.3, 0.4, 0.5	0.1
Sarvela 02	OB	RCT	0.1, 0.2	0.1

Table adapted from Richman, Wu. Intrathecal opioid injections for postoperative pain. In: Fishman SM, Benzon H, Raja SN, et al., eds. *Benzon Essentials of Pain Medicine and Regional Anesthesia.* New York: Churchill Livingstone; 2005.

artery bypass graft surgery. IT opioid combinations provide superior analgesia versus systemic opioids in patients undergoing vascular and thoracic procedures. Compared to those who received IV PCA morphine, patients who received a mixture of either 20 mcg of sufentanil with 0.2 mg of morphine or 50 mcg of sufentanil with 0.5 mg of morphine have improved pain control with minimal side effects other than an increased frequency of urinary retention.[5,38] Although epidural analgesia with local anesthetics and opioids is likely superior to IT opioids in decreasing pulmonary complications after thoracotomy,[39] IT opioids may be a good alternative to epidural analgesia in situations where an epidural catheter cannot be maintained.[19]

Clonidine

Studies demonstrate that intrathecal clonidine at doses from 15 to 150 mcg improve postoperative analgesia while minimizing side effects. Coadministration of 25 to 75 mcg of clonidine with morphine 250 mcg to a bupivacaine spinal anesthetic demonstrated decreased 24h IV morphine consumption and improved 24h visual analog scale (VAS) scores as compared to 250 mcg intrathecal morphine added to bupivacaine spinal anesthetic alone.[40–42]

Epidural Analgesia

Indications. Epidural analgesia provides segmental analgesia. Continuous catheters allow flexibility in the depth and duration of analgesia. Epidural analgesia is effective for thoracic, abdominal, gynecologic, urologic, and orthopaedic surgery of the lower extremity. Obstetric analgesia will not be included in our discussion.

Block Technique.
Epidural. Epidural blockade may be performed with the patient in the sitting or lateral (see Fig. 52.1) position through a midline or paramedian approach. After patient positioning, the appropriate interspace is identified, prepped, and draped in sterile fashion. Local anesthetic is infiltrated at the needle insertion site. Using the midline approach, the epidural needle is oriented in the same plane as the spinous processes with slight cephalad angulation toward the interlaminar space. The epidural needle is directed through the skin wheal and slowly advanced through the supraspinous and interspinous ligaments to enter the ligamentum flavum. Upon entering the ligamentum flavum, a subtle change of resistance is appreciated. The ligamentum flavum is usually reached at a depth of 3.5 to 5 cm from the skin in the normal adult. When the resistance of the ligamentum flavum is appreciated, the stylet is removed from the epidural needle and a loss-of-resistance syringe containing either air and/or 3 cc of saline with a small air bubble is attached to the hub. Constant pressure is applied to the plunger of the syringe as the needle is slowly advanced. Alternatively, intermittent pressure is applied to the plunger between small, gentle advances of the epidural needle. Upon entering the epidural space, there is a sudden, significant loss of resistance to plunger displacement. The dorsal aspect of the nondominant hand is firmly placed against the patient's back with the index finger and thumb stabilizing the hub for injection. A test dose of 3 cc of a local anesthetic with 1:200,000 epinephrine is injected, and the patient is observed for signs and symptoms of IT or intravascular injection. The local anesthetic should be administered in 5 mL increments until the appropriate total dose is given. A 20-gauge radio-opaque catheter with 1 cm graduations is passed through the epidural needle. The catheter is advanced 4–5 cm beyond the needle tip into the epidural space. The needle is then withdrawn over the catheter and the catheter secured to the patient's back.

Alternatively, a paramedian-lateral or paramedian-lateral oblique approach to the epidural space may be used. For this approach, the epidural needle insertion site is approximately one fingerbreadth lateral to the insertion site of the midline approach.

The epidural needle is directed with slight cephalomedial orientation to allow the needle to bypass the supraspinous and interspinous ligaments as the needle is advanced to enter the triangular-shaped ligamentum flavum. Upon entering the ligamentum flavum, the loss-of-resistance technique is used to enter the epidural space at the midline (see Fig. 52.2).

Using the paramedian-lateral oblique approach, the caudad spinous process of the desired interspace is identified. The epidural needle is inserted approximately one fingerbreadth lateral to this point and directed with cephalomedial orientation to bypass the supraspinous and interspinous ligaments as the needle is advanced to enter the ligamentum flavum. Upon entering the ligamentum flavum, the loss-of-resistance technique is used to enter the epidural space at the midline. Alternatively, the needle is initially oriented perpendicular to the skin in all planes and advanced with the intent to contact lamina. Upon contact with lamina, the needle is walked off the superior edge of the lamina and advanced through the ligamentum flavum using the loss-of-resistance technique to enter the epidural space at the midline (see Fig. 52.2).

While the paramedian approach may be used for both lumbar and thoracic epidurals, it is extremely advantageous in the mid-thoracic vertebrae (T4–T10) where the steep angle of the spinous processes limits midlines access to the interlaminar foramen (Fig. 52.3).

Combined spinal epidural technique. The benefits of both spinal and epidural anesthesia/analgesia may be obtained using the combined spinal epidural (CSE) technique. Using the epidural technique as described above, the epidural needle is advanced into the epidural space. After loss of resistance to plunger displacement indicating entrance into the epidural space, the plunger is carefully removed and a spinal needle is passed through the epidural needle until the characteristic "pop" is felt, indicating penetration of the dura and entry into the subarachnoid space (Fig. 52.4). After free CSF flow is confirmed, the dorsal aspect of the nondominant hand is firmly placed against the patient's back with the index finger and thumb stabilizing the hub for injection. Local anesthetic with additive is injected and the spinal needle is withdrawn. A 20-gauge radio-opaque catheter with 1 cm graduations is passed through the epidural needle. The catheter is advanced 4–5 cm beyond the needle tip into the epidural space. The needle is then withdrawn over the catheter, and the catheter secured to the patient's back. Prior to dosing the catheter a test dose should be administered through the catheter.

Epidural Opioids

Epidural opioids as a single injection or continuous infusion are an important postoperative analgesic option.

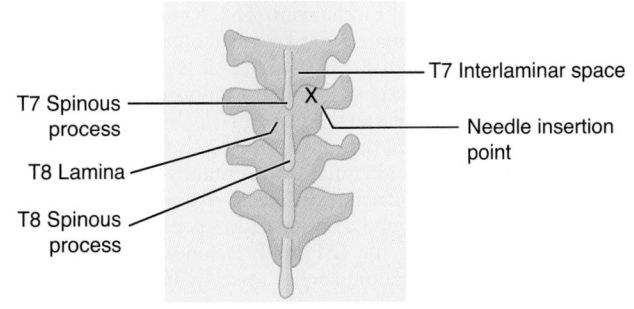

FIGURE 52.3 Surface and underlying anatomy for thoracic epidural block.

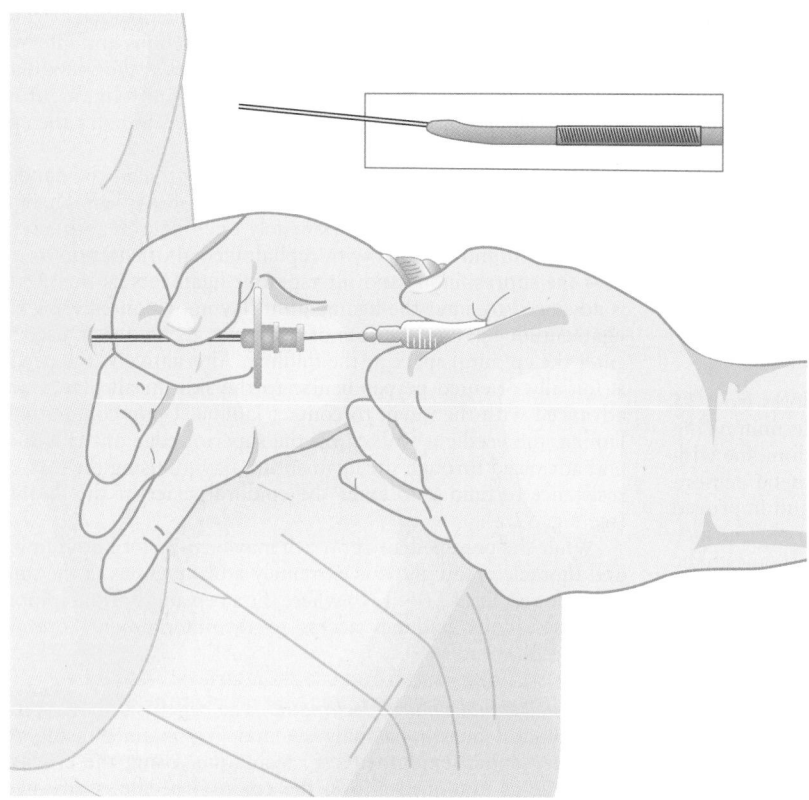

FIGURE 52.4 Combined spinal epidural technique.

Mechanism of Action

There are two mechanisms by which epidurally administered opioids can act to produce analgesia: spinal and supraspinal/systemic analgesia. Supraspinal analgesia is mediated by the systemic uptake of epidurally administered opioids and their subsequent redistribution to the brainstem. Spinal analgesia produced from epidurally administered opioids is achieved via diffusion through the spinal meninges into the CSF. Once inside the CSF, epidurally administered opioids interact with spinal opioid receptors located in lamina II of the spinal cord dorsal horn and achieve antinociception via presynaptic reduction of afferent neurotransmitter release and postsynaptic hyperpolarization of dorsal horn neurons.[42] A key pharmacologic property of an epidurally administered opioid that determines its analgesic and side effect profile is the extent of its lipophilicity. After single-dose epidural administration, lipophilic opioids, such as fentanyl and sufentanil, have a faster onset but shorter duration of action when compared to that of more hydrophilic opioids, such as morphine and hydromorphone. Furthermore, the extent of lipophilicity affects the side effect profile. Lipophilic opioids with relatively rapid clearance from the CSF limit the development of delayed respiratory depression.[2] Epidural opioids do not predominately produce analgesia through a spinal mechanism. The degree to which lipophilic opioids produce analgesia via a spinal or supraspinal mechanism is still somewhat controversial.[42,43] It is generally thought that lipophilic opioids (especially when administered in a continuous infusion) will produce analgesia primarily by systemic uptake and redistribution of the lipophilic opioid to brainstem opioid receptors.[42] On the other hand, it is clear that hydrophilic opioids primary site of analgesic action is selectively spinal.[44,45] Epidurally administered hydrophilic opioids, after penetrating the dural membrane and entering the CSF, will remain within the CSF to produce spinal analgesia and spread rostrally in the CSF (due in part to its low lipid solubility) to act at the brainstem.[45] An opioid administered in the epidural space will also diffuse into the surrounding tissues including epidural fat and veins. Opioids that diffuse into fat are no longer available to bind to opioids receptors and thus unavailable for analgesic affect.

Morphine. A single epidural dose of a hydrophilic opioid such as morphine is especially efficacious for prolonged postoperative analgesia. Epidural morphine, when administered as a single bolus, has been shown to provide effective postoperative analgesia for major abdominal and vascular surgery.[46] The dose of epidural morphine may need to be reduced for elderly patients and thoracic epidural catheter sites.[47]

Extended-Release Epidural Morphine. Extended-release epidural morphine (EREM) consists of a lipid-based delivery system designed to provide 48 hours of pain relief without the need for an indwelling epidural catheter.

The absence of an indwelling catheter offers potential advantages over continuous epidural infusions, particularly in patients being treated with anticoagulation therapy. EREM is approved by the U.S. Food and Drug Administration at dose levels of 10–20 mg, noting that older patients may require less medication than younger patients. EREM is not recommended in patients over 65 years of age in doses exceeding 15mg. The side effect profile of EREM is consistent with that of other epidurally administered opioids analgesics. Close monitoring of respiratory function is indicated in all patients having received EREM.[48–50]

Fentanyl. A single epidural bolus of a lipophilic opioid like fentanyl may be administered to provide a rapid (onset within 5 to 10 minutes) but relatively transient (up to 4 hours) postoperative analgesia. Diluting the epidural dose of fentanyl (typically 50 to 100 mcg) in at least 10 mL of preservative-free normal saline may hasten onset and prolong the duration of analgesia possibly as a result of an increase in the initial spread and diffusion of fentanyl.[51] Combining a hydrophilic opioid such as morphine and a lipophilic opioid such as fentanyl in a single epidural injection combines the short onset time produced by the lipophilic opioid and the long duration of analgesia produced by the hydrophilic opioid.[52]

Hydromorphone. Lumbar epidural morphine and hydromorphone afford comparable analgesia, but the occurrence of moderate to severe pruritus on the first postoperative day is reduced by the use of hydromorphone.[53]

Side Effects

Respiratory Depression. Respiratory depression associated with epidural administration of opioids is dose-dependent and the incidence is typically reported from 0.1% to 0.9%.[17,25,54–57] The incidence of respiratory depression with epidural opioids (when used in appropriate doses), whether single injection or continuous infusion, is not higher than that seen with systemic administration of opioids.[17,54] Factors that may increase the risk of developing respiratory depression in patients who have received epidural opioid include thoracic surgery, presence of comorbidities, increasing age, an opioid-naïve state, and concomitant use of systemic opioids and sedatives.[54]

Nausea and Vomiting. Nausea and vomiting occurs in 20% to 50% of patients after a single dose of epidural opioids,[58–60] and the overall incidence in those receiving continuous infusion of epidural opioids is reported at 45% to 80%.[61–63] The development of opioid-induced nausea and vomiting after the administration of epidural opioids appears to be dose-dependent.[21,64,65] Nausea and vomiting from epidural opioids is the result of interaction with opioid receptors in the area postrema and chemotactic trigger zone of the medulla.

Pruritis. The etiology of epidural opioid-induced pruritus is unclear and may be related to activation of an "itch-center" in the medulla and interaction with opioid receptors in the trigeminal and upper cervical spinal cord with cephalad migration of the opioid; however, opioid-induced pruritus does not appear to be associated with peripheral histamine release.[18] Pruritus from epidural opioid administration may occur in as many as 60% of patients as compared to a 15% to 18% incidence with systemic opioid use.[66,67] It is not clear whether pruritus from epidural opioid administration is a dose-dependent relationship.[68]

Urinary Retention. Administration of epidural opioids may result in urinary retention, which is related to a decrease in detrusor muscle strength contraction secondary to spinal opioid receptor activation.[18] The 70% to 80% incidence of urinary retention from epidurally administered opioids appears to be much higher than the 18% incidence of urinary retention associated with systemically administered opioids.[18,66] The development of urinary retention does not appear to be dose dependent.[69]

Epidural Clonidine

Mechanism of Action

Clonidine induces dose-dependent spinal cord antinociception, primarily through stimulation of alpha-2 adrenoceptors in the dorsal horn, mimicking the activation of descending inhibitory pathways.

Side Effects

Side effects associated with commonly used doses of epidural clonidine include hypotension, bradycardia, and sedation.[70] It is not associated with side effects of spinal opioids such as respiratory depression and pruritus.

Clinical Effects

In healthy volunteers, the reduction in pain intensity after epidural clonidine correlates with its concentrations in the CSF, but not in the serum.[28] In a review of clonidine in combination with epidural opioids as compared to clonidine or epidural opioids alone, the trials[71–73] provided weak and scattered evidence that administering clonidine with an opioid spinally is more effective than either clonidine or the opioid used alone for acute pain management.[74] Walker et al [74] attributed these results to the marginal doses of epidural clonidine used in these trials (range: 70 to 300 mcg) and to the small number of patients enrolled per study group.

Epidural Infusions

Continuous infusions of epidural local anesthetic and/or opioids will provide superior postoperative analgesia when compared to parenteral opioids for a variety of surgical procedures (Table 52.2).

Epidural Combined Local Anesthetic and Opioid Infusion

Although continuous infusions of epidural opioids may be used alone and are effective in controlling postoperative pain, continuous infusions of epidural opioids are more commonly administered in conjunction with a local anesthetic. This combination may confer analgesic advantages over infusions using either a local anesthetic alone or opioid alone, although the incidence of side effects may or may not be diminished.[18,75,76] The choice of opioid varies among clinicians: many will choose to use a lipophilic opioid (fentanyl, 2 to 5 mcg/mL, or sufentanil, 0.5 to 1 mcg/mL) as part of a patient-controlled epidural analgesia (PCEA) regimen to allow for rapid titration of analgesia[55,60]; however, use of a hydrophilic opioid (morphine, 0.05 to 0.1 mg/mL, or hydromorphone, 0.01 to 0.05 mg/mL) as part of a local anesthetic-opioid epidural analgesic regimen may also provide effective postoperative analgesia.[55]

While these studies support improved analgesic efficacy with the combination of a local anesthetic and an opioid compared with either drug alone, another study found no difference in analgesic efficacy between the combination versus either single drug.[77] Most studies indicate that combination therapy reduces dose requirements for either local anesthetic or the opioid as compared to when they are administered as single drugs alone. This dose reduction is associated with reduced local anesthetic-related side effects including hypotension and motor block and reduced opioids-related side effects including sedation, vomiting, and pruritus (Table 52.3).

Complications of Neuraxial Techniques. Despite the analgesic benefits conferred by neuraxial techniques, there are many risks associated with these techniques. Postoperative backache occurs in approximately 11% and 30% of patients undergoing spinal and epidural anesthesia, respectively.[78] While there are many factors that influence the incidence of postdural puncture headache, the overall incidence has been reported to be 6.7% for males and 8.6% for nonpregnant females.[79,80] Serious events related to neuraxial blocks include cardiac arrest, respiratory failure, seizures, infection, bleeding, and neurologic complications (Tables 52.4 and 52.5). The rate of neurologic complications after central nerve blockade is 0.4%, including radiculopathy/neuropathy, cauda equine syndrome, paraplegia, and intracranial events.[81] Prospective data collected over a 16-year period at a large tertiary teaching institution with a nonobstetric general surgical population identified 8210 epidural catheters inserted for postoperative analgesia. Epidural abscess was rare (<0.1%), and spinal hema-

TABLE 52.2

ANALGESIA BY SURGICAL SITE, EPIDURAL SITE, AND EPIDURAL INFUSION

*Epidural analgesia is superior to parenteral opioids for rest and incident pain.

Surgery	Epidural Site	Epidural Infusion		Epidural Mean VAS (mm)	Parenteral Mean VAS (mm)	P Value
Thoracic	Thoracic	Local anesthetic +/− opioid	Rest	21.9	11.3	S
			Incident	36.2	24.7	S
		Opioid only	Rest	12.1	11.5	NS
			Incident	41.3	35.5	S
	Lumbar	Opioid only	Rest	19.4	13.7	S
			Incident	1 study		
Abdominal	Thoracic	Local anesthetic +/− opioid	Rest	18.9	9.0	S
			Incident	39.6	27.4	S
		Opioid only	Rest	26.5	20.0	S
			Incident	50.0	43.1	S
	Lumbar	Local anesthetic +/− opioid	Rest	23.1	6.9	S
			Incident	46.7	26.9	S
		Opioid only	Rest	23.2	15.5	S
			Incident	51.8	41.9	S
Pelvic and Cesarean Delivery	Thoracic	Local anesthetic +/− opioid	Rest	1 study		S
			Incident	52.4	37.3	S
	Lumbar	Local anesthetic +/− opioid	Rest	21.3	12.4	S
			Incident	38.3	32.0	S
		Opioid only	Rest	21.8	16.0	S
			Incident	49.1	31.5	S
Lower Extremity	Lumbar	Local anesthetic +/− opioid	Rest	31.3	26.5	S
			Incident	60.2	25.6	S
		Opioid only	Rest	25.4	16.0	S

NS, nonsignificant; S, significant; VAS, visual analog scale.
*Mean VAS include both rest and incident pain. Weighted mean difference between epidural analgesia and parenteral opioids (positive numbers favor epidural analgesia) were rounded.
Table modified from Block BM, Liu SS, Rowlingson AJ, et al. Efficacy of postoperative epidural analgesia. *JAMA* 2003;290:2455–2463.

TABLE 52.3

SIDE EFFECT RATES ASSOCIATED WITH EPIDURAL INFUSIONS COMPARED TO PARANTERAL OPIOIDS

Side Effect	Epidural Site	Epidural Infusion	Patients at Risk	Incidence Rates		P Value
				Epidural	Parenteral	
Nausea or Vomiting	Thoracic	Local anesthetic +/− opioid	717	26	25	NS
		Opioid only	191	5	9	S
	Lumbar	Local anesthetic +/− opioid	321	42	72	S
		Opioid only	704	60	38	S
Pruritis	Thoracic	Local anesthetic +/− opioid	717	2	0	S
		Opioid only	191	7	0	S
	Lumbar	Local anesthetic +/− opioid	321	2	0	S
		Opioid only	704	38	6	S
Motor Block or Numbness	Thoracic	Local anesthetic +/− opioid	717	2	1	NS
		Opioid only	191	0	0	NS
	Lumbar	Local anesthetic +/− opioid	321	1	0	S
		Opioid only	704	7	0	S
Hypotension	Thoracic	Local anesthetic +/− opioid	702	14	2	S
		Opioid only	190	0	0	NS
	Lumbar	Local anesthetic +/− opioid	350	8	14	S
		Opioid only	698	1	3	S

NS, nonsignificant; S, significant.
Table modified from Block BM, Liu SS, Rowlingson AJ, et al. Efficacy of postoperative epidural analgesia. *JAMA* 2003;290:2455–2463.

TABLE 52.4

NUMBER AND INCIDENCE OF SERIOUS EVENTS RELATED TO NEURAXIAL BLOCKS (EXCLUDING OBSTETRIC CASES)

	Spinal (35,439 performed)	Epidural (5561 performed)
Cardiac Arrest	9 (2.5) (0.0–5.1)	0 (0.0–0.5)
Respiratory Failure	2 (0.6) (0.0–2.0)	0 (0.0–0.5)
Seizures	1 (0.3) (0.0–1.4)	1 (1.8) (0.0–9.0)
Peripheral Neuropathy	9 (2.5) (0.0–5.1)	0 (0.0–0.5)
Cauda Equina Syndrome	3 (0.8) (0.0–2.3)	0 (0.0–0.5)
Central Neurologic Event	0 (0.0–0.8)	0 (0.0–0.5)
Meningitis	1 (0.3) (0.0–1.4)	1 (1.8) (0.0–9.0)
Death	3 (0.8) (0.0–2.3)	0 (0.0–0.5)

Values are expressed as n (n/10,000) (95% CI) when applicable.
Table modified from Auroy Y, Benhamou D, Barques L, et al. Major complications of regional anesthesia in France. The SOS regional anesthesia hotline service. *Anesthesiology* 2002;97(5):1274–1280.

toma was very rare (<0.05%).[82] The American Society of Regional Anesthesia and Pain Medicine (ASRA) consensus statement concludes that patients taking antiplatelet drugs or receiving subcutaneous unfractionated heparin for deep vein thrombosis prophylaxis are not viewed as being at increase risk of spinal hematoma; however, when taken in combination, these patients may be at increased risk. Patients receiving fractionated low-molecular-weight heparin, thrombolytic, fibrinolytic, or "fully anticoagulated" patients (elevated protime or prothrombin time) are considered to be at increased risk of neuraxial bleeding, and the ASRA consensus statement recommendations should be followed.[83]

PERIPHERAL NERVE BLOCKS

Introduction

Single injection and continuous peripheral nerve blocks (CPNBs) for postoperative pain management to be discussed in this chapter include interscalene, supraclavicular, infraclavicular, axillary, lumbar plexus, femoral, sciatic, popliteal, ankle, and paravertebral blocks. Common ultrasound-guided techniques are included. Indications, outcomes, side effects, and complications are reviewed.

Single injection peripheral nerve blocks provide superior pain control with decreased side effects as compared to opioids. Single injection block techniques, despite their efficacy, provide only a finite length of postoperative analgesia.[84] Efforts to prolong the analgesia of peripheral nerve block local anesthetic solutions with the addition of adjuncts, including but not limited to morphine,[85–87] fentanyl,[88–90] sufentanil,[91,92] buprenorphine,[86,93,94] tramadol,[95,96] ketamine,[97] and clonidine[98–104] have been investigated. Crucial to all investigations of perineural analgesia adjuncts is the inclusion of systemic control groups, providing evidence for or against a peripheral perineural site of action as opposed to a systemic effect of an adjunct administered peripherally. We will review those studies when available for applicable blocks.

Continuous perineural infusion of local anesthetic with or without adjuvants provides the ability to extend the duration and benefits of single injection techniques. CPNBs may be used to extended postoperative analgesia for more painful surgeries and to facilitate early, intense postoperative rehabilitation. Although PCEA and IV PCA provide adequate pain management for inpatients with postoperative pain, these techniques are unsuitable for postoperative pain management after outpatient surgical procedures. The use of CPNBs as a means of postoperative pain management may provide faster inpatient discharge,[105–108] and allow procedures otherwise requiring inpatient hospitalization for pain management to be performed in the outpatient setting.[84,106–111] There is strong evidence that home CPNBs improve postoperative analgesia and patient satisfaction, while decreasing supplemental opioid requirements and opioid-related side effects.[110] Data suggests the risk of injury in patients discharged with an insensate extremity is relatively small,[112] and that doses of local anesthetic associated with home infusion regimens are very unlikely to be associated with systemic local anesthetic toxicity.[113] Appropriate patient selection, education, and follow-up are crucial when sending these patients home and prescribing outpatient infusions in an unmonitored environment.[111] Perhaps the greatest testament to the viability, efficiency, safety, and effectiveness of ambulatory CPNBs are reports of their successful use as a viable and important long-term analgesic technique in the military, from evacuation to rehabilitation, providing patients with anesthesia and analgesia for multiple, sequential operations over an extended period of time.[114,115]

A meta-analysis of randomized controlled trials (RCTs) to determine the analgesic efficacy of postoperative perineural catheter analgesia compared with opioids found a statistically and clinically significant improvement in postoperative pain control with peripheral nerve catheters compared to opioids and a decrease in opioid related side effects. These improvements were noted through postoperative day 3. When analyzed according to catheter location (i.e., interscalene, femoral, etc.) and type of pain assessment (resting versus maximal), CPNB provided superior postoperative analgesia compared with opioids, with fewer side effects, improved patient satisfaction, better sleep patterns, improved rehabilitation, and shorter hospital stays. CPNB did not generally obviate the needs for opioids entirely.[116]

Ultrasound guidance for regional anesthetic techniques may offer benefits for the practicioner skilled in its application. A safe and successful ultrasound-guided nerve block requires (1) appropriate imaging and detection of target nerve and adjacent anatomic structures, (2) proficiency in tracking needle advancement in real time, and (3) assessment of local anesthetic spread around the target nerve.[117] Future, large, multicentered trials are necessary to evaluate the impact of ultrasound guidance on regional anesthetic techniques for acute pain management.

Upper Extremity Nerve Blocks

Peripheral nerve blockade following upper extremity surgery avoids the limitations associated with the use of IV PCA. Ambula-

TABLE 52.5

AGGREGATE ESTIMATED RATE OF OCCURRENCE OF NEUROLOGIC COMPLICATIONS AFTER NEURAXIAL BLOCKADE

	Estimated rate of occurrence	Lower CI (n = 10,000)	Upper CI (n = 10,000)	Q value	P Value
Spinal anesthesia					
Radiculopathy/ Neuropathy (6 studies)	3.78	1.06	13.50	168.70	S
Cauda Equina Syndrome (4 studies)	0.11	0.03	0.37	20.59	S
Intracranial Event (2 studies)	0.03	0.00	0.20	1.66	NS
Paraplegia (4 studies)	0.06	0.02	0.20	5.38	NS
Epidural Anesthesia					
Radiculopathy/ Neuropathy (9 studies)	2.19	0.88	5.44	142.30	S
Cauda Equina Syndrome (4 studies)	0.23	0.14	0.39	2.30	NS
Intracranial Event (2 studies)	0.07	0.03	0.21	0.24	NS
Paraplegia (4 studies)	0.09	0.04	0.22	2.23	NS

CI, 95% confidence interval; NS, nonsignificant (nonsignificance indicates absence of heterogenicity between studies); S, significant;.
Estimated rate of occurrence was calculated using a random effects general linear model.
Table modified from Brull R, McCartney CJ, Chan VW, et al. Neurological complications after regional anesthesia: contemporary estimates of risk. *Anesth Analg* 2007;104:965–974.

tory perineural catheters allow for early inpatient discharge or surgery in the outpatient setting. Additionally, peripheral nerve block analgesic techniques may improve early rehabilitation (Table 52.6).

Interscalene Block

Indications. The interscalene block (ISB) is performed at the level of the roots and trunks. It provides both brachial (C5–C7) and cervical plexus (C3-C4) blockade; however, incomplete anesthesia of the inferior trunk (C8,T1) is not uncommon. As a result of phrenic nerve (C3–C5) blockade, there is a 100% incidence of ipsilateral hemidiaphragmatic paresis with the interscalene approach.[118] Thus, this approach should be avoided in patients with pre-existing pulmonary disease who are unable to tolerate a potential 25% reduction in pulmonary function.[119] Side effects after interscalene block may include a transient Horner's syn-

TABLE 52.6

UPPER EXTREMITY PERIPHERAL NERVE BLOCK DOSING

Local Anesthetic (20–40 mL)	Anesthesia (hrs)	Analgesia (hrs)
3% 2-Chloroprocaine (+HCO3 + epinephrine)	1.5	2.0
1.5% Mepivacaine (+HCO3)	2–3	2–4
1.5% Mepivacaine (+HCO3 + epinephrine)	2.5–4	3–6
2% Lidocaine (+ HCO3 + epinephrine)	3–6	5–8
0.5% Ropivacaine (+epi)	6–8	8–12
0.75% Ropivacaine (+epi)	8–10	12–18
0.5% Bupivacaine (+ epi)	8–10	16–18

Continuous infusion ropivacaine 0.2% or dilute concentration of bupivacaine or levobupivacaine; 6–8 mL/hour with a 2–4 mL hourly bolus.
Table modified from Hadzic A, Vloka JD. *Peripheral Nerve Blocks, Principles and Practice.* Columbus, OH: McGraw-Hill; 2004.

drome and recurrent laryngeal nerve block resulting in hoarseness. The transient and benign nature of these side effects should be discussed with the patient prior to block placement. The ISB performed as a single-shot injection or continuous catheter technique provides postoperative analgesia for operations on the shoulder, clavicle, or upper arm.

Landmarks. The patient is positioned supine or with the head of the bed slightly elevated. The head is gently turned toward the nonoperative side. The clavicular head of the sternocleidomastoid muscle is identified. Having the patient briefly lift their head will accentuate this landmark. At the C6 level, the anterior scalene muscle is palpated along the posterior border of the sternocleidomastoid clavicular head. The fingers are rolled laterally over the anterior scalene muscle into the groove between the anterior and middle scalene muscles. The "interscalene groove" at the C6 level is the initial needle insertion site. The external jugular vein which often overlies the sternocleidomastoid muscle at this point must be avoided (Fig. 52.5).

Needles. Insulated needles used: 24-gauge, 2.5 cm or 22-gauge, 5 cm. Insulated Tuohy needles for catheter placement: 18-gauge, 3.8 cm or 5 cm. Catheters are inserted 5 cm beyond the needle tip.

Technique.
Nerve stimulation. The nerve stimulator is initially set at 1.0 mA. After cleaning the area with antiseptic solution, using sterile technique, the needle is introduced slowly in a caudad, posterior, and medial direction (Fig. 52.6). The brachial plexus is rarely deeper than 2 cm from the skin. An evoked motor response in the deltoid, biceps, triceps, forearm, or hand at 0.5 mA or less indicates acceptable needle tip position for local anesthetic injection. An evoked motor response of the trapezius muscle indicates posterior needle tip position and a response of the diaphragm indicates anterior needle tip position.

Ultrasound. Ultrasound visualization of the brachial plexus at the interscalene groove may be approached by imaging in the axial oblique plane with a linear, high-frequency ultrasound probe, identifying sonoanatomic landmarks from a medial to lateral direction at the C6 level. The roots/trunks of the brachial plexus are seen in cross section between the anterior and middle scalene muscles as round hypoechoic structures. Alternatively, placing the probe in the supraclavicular fossa in the coronal oblique plane obtains the perivascular position of the brachial plexus around the hypoechoic subclavian artery in cross section

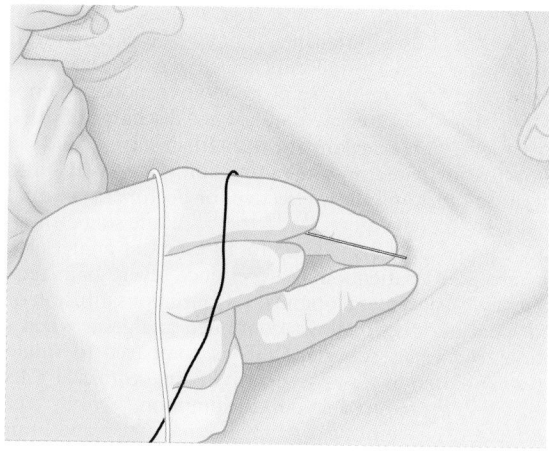

FIGURE 52.6 Needle orientation for interscalene block of the brachial plexus.

just above the hyperechoic first rib. At this level, the trunks/proximal divisions appear lateral and superior to the subclavian artery. Upon scanning the cephalad, the brachial plexus can be followed to its position between the anterior and middle scalene muscles at the C6 level (Fig. 52.7). Introducing the block needle from the lateral end of the ultrasound probe in-plane with the beam allows direct visualization of needle tip advancement and local anesthetic spread. Alternatively, the needle may be introduced in the middle of the ultrasound probe, out-of-plane with the beam, providing a cross-sectional image of the needle tip when it is beneath the ultrasound beam. While the in-plane technique is generally preferred for single-shot injections and provides tunneling for continuous catheter placement, the out-of-plane technique may provide more optimal needle orientation for continuous catheter advancement.

Clinical Effects. ISB for postoperative analgesia as compared to opioids, suprascapular nerve block, subacromial bursa block, or intra-articular administration of local anesthetics for shoulder surgery demonstrated reduction in pain visual analog scores

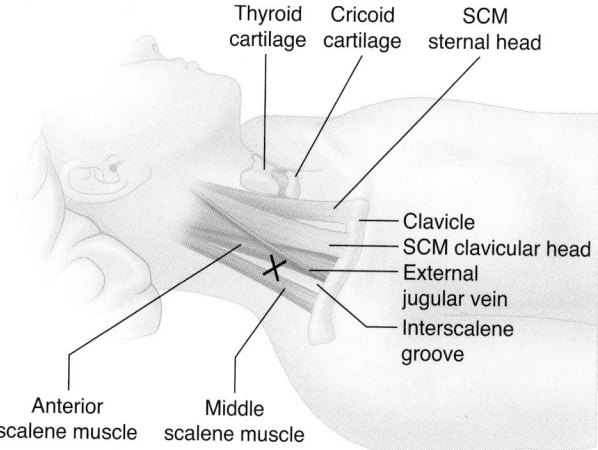

FIGURE 52.5 Landmarks for the interscalene approach to the brachial plexus. X, needle insertion site.

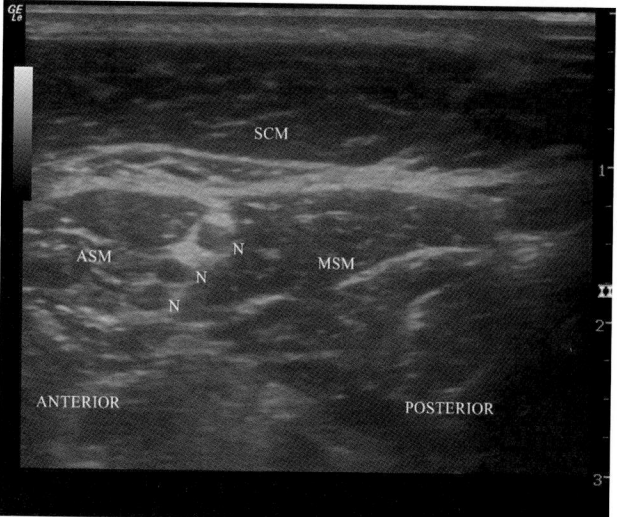

FIGURE 52.7 Sonographic landmarks for ultrasound-guided interscalene nerve block. ASM, anterior scalene muscle; MSM, middle scalene muscle; N, nerve trunk SCM, sternocleidomastoid muscle.

(VAS),[120–123] delayed time until first analgesic use [120] and reduced total opioid requirements.[120,121,124] Furthermore, the use of ISB demonstrated a reduced incidence of postoperative nausea and vomiting,[120,121] improved postoperative mood,[122] improved sleep the night after surgery,[125] quickened discharge of the ambulatory patient,[120] reduced inpatient length of stay,[125] and lowered rates of unanticipated hospital admission.[121,126,127] Continuous interscalene block (CISB) is effective for postoperative analgesia for major shoulder surgery.[105,108,128–130] While single-shot injection techniques may provide up to 18 hours of analgesia, upon block resolution patients may experience severe pain requiring treatment with parenteral opioids. + Continuous infusion of perineural local anesthetic allows continued analgesia when single injection techniques subside. CISB as compared to single-shot injection and opioids for postoperative pain, decreased VAS pain scores,[105,131–136] reduced opioid consumption,[105,132,133] reduced side effects,[131,135] improved rehabilitation,[105,108] and improved patient satisfaction.[105,131,132,135] Likewise, CISB for outpatient infusions[105,108,133,137–142] provided reliable postoperative analgesia enabling prompt hospital discharge,[105] decreasing average and maximum VAS pain scores,[133,137,138] reducing opioid consumption,[105,138] decreasing side effects,[138] improving sleep,[110] and diminishing breakthrough pain upon single-shot block resolution.[143] Ilfeld et al.[108] reported in a subset of patients without major comorbidities that it may be feasible to convert total shoulder arthroplasty into an ambulatory procedure discharging patients with a continuous interscalene infusion as part of a multimodal analgesic regimen provided at home.

Supraclavicular Block

Indications. The supraclavicular block of the brachial plexus is performed at the level of the trunks and divisions. Due to the compact arrangement of the brachial plexus at the supraclavicular level, this block provides a complete block of the brachial plexus. A supraclavicular brachial plexus block performed as a single injection or continuous catheter technique provides postoperative analgesia for operations on the humerus, elbow, forearm, wrist, or hand.

Landmarks. The patient is positioned supine or, if using the ultrasound technique, the head of the bed may be elevated. The head is gently turned toward the nonoperative side. The clavicular head of the sternocleidomastoid muscle is identified. Having the patient briefly lift their head will accentuate this landmark. At the C6 level, the anterior scalene muscle is palpated along the posterior border of the sternocleidomastoid clavicular head. The fingers are rolled laterally over the anterior scalene muscle into the groove between the anterior and middle scalene muscles. The fingers are then moved inferiorly down the interscalene groove until they are approximately 1 cm from the clavicle (Fig. 52.8).

This is the initial needle insertion site. The subclavian artery can often be palpated just caudad to this point and must be avoided.

Needles. Insulated needle used: 22-gauge, 5 cm. Insulated Tuohy needle for catheter placement:18-gauge, 5 cm. Catheters are inserted 5 cm beyond the needle tip.

Technique.

Nerve stimulation. The nerve stimulator is initially set at 1.0 mA. After cleaning the area with antiseptic solution, using sterile technique, the needle is directed slightly lateral to the parasagital plane and parallel to the plane of the bed (Fig. 52.9). The needle should never be directed medial to the parasagital plane in order to avoid the dome of the pleura. The brachial plexus at the supraclavicular level is usually reached at a depth of 4–5 cm from the skin. Flexion of the fingers or thumb at 0.5 mA or less indicates acceptable needle tip position for local anesthetic injection. Biceps contraction or forearm pronation indicates lateral needle tip position. Pectoralis muscle contraction indicates anterior needle tip position. Latissimus dorsi contraction indicates posterior needle tip position. Bright-red blood with aspiration indicates anterior needle-tip position with entrance of the needle into the subclavian artery.

Ultrasound. Ultrasound visualization of the brachial plexus at the supraclavicular level is achieved with placement of a linear, high-frequency ultrasound probe in the supraclavicular fossa in the coronal oblique plane. This image obtains the perivascular position of the brachial plexus around the hypoechoic subclavian artery in cross section just above the hyperechoic first rib (Fig. 52.10). At this level, the trunks/divisions appear lateral and superior to the subclavian artery. Introducing the block needle from the lateral end of the ultrasound probe and advancing in line with the plane of the beam allows direct visualization of needle tip advancement and local anesthetic spread.

Clinical Effects. Few studies have investigated the postoperative analgesic efficacy of single injection or continuous supraclavicular block with placebo or IV PCA with opioids. Up to 17 hours of analgesia has been reported following single-shot injection of bupivacaine or ropivacaine for upper limb surgery.[144,145] Supraclavicular catheters for patients undergoing surgery or physiotherapy of the upper limb for treatment of reflex sympathetic dystrophy associated with painful shoulder provided effective postoperative analgesia for 24 to 48 hours.[146]

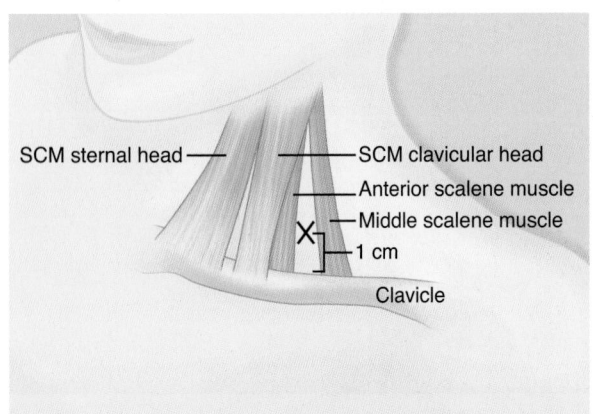

FIGURE 52.8 Landmarks for the supraclavicular approach to the brachial plexus. X, needle insertion site.

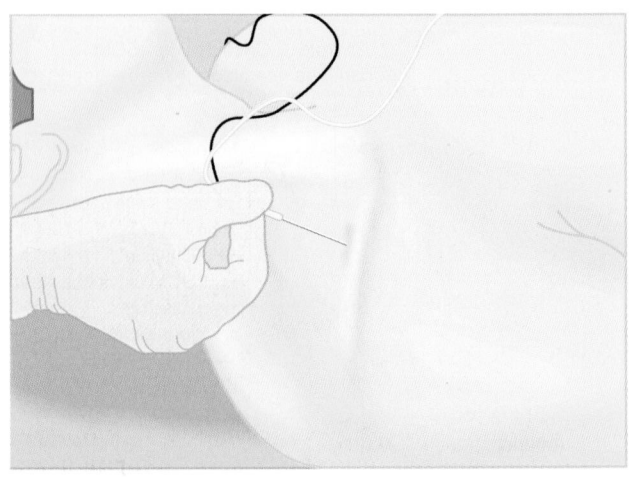

FIGURE 52.9 Needle orientation for supraclavicular block of the brachial plexus.

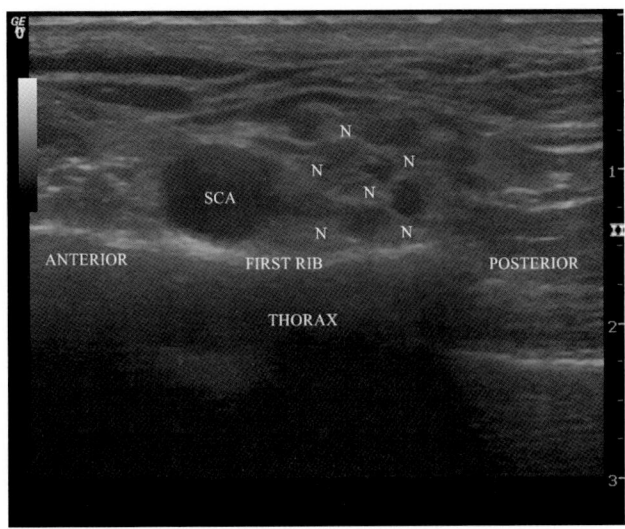

FIGURE 52.10 Sonographic landmarks for ultrasound-guided supraclavicular nerve block. N, divisions of the brachial plexus; SCA, subclavian artery.

Infraclavicular Block

Indications. The infraclavicular block targets the brachial plexus at the level of the cords. The lateral, posterior, and medial cords are named for their position around the axillary artery. The infraclavicular approach to the brachial plexus can be performed as a single-shot or continuous catheter technique to provide postoperative analgesia for operations on the elbow, forearm, wrist, or hand. Perineural catheters at this level are very stable due to limited movement at the catheter insertion site below the clavicle.

Landmarks. With the operative arm at the patient's side or abducted and externally rotated, the coracoid process is palpated. The needle insertion site is 2 cm medial and 2 cm caudad from the coracoid process (Fig. 52.11).

Needles. Insulated needle used: 21-gauge, 10 cm. Insulated Tuohy needle for catheter placement:18-gauge, 10 cm. Catheters are inserted 5 cm beyond the needle tip.

Technique.
Nerve stimulation. The nerve stimulator is initially set at 1.0 mA. After cleaning the area with antiseptic solution, using sterile technique, the needle is oriented perpendicular to all planes and directed posteriorly. Initial advancement of the needle will elicit pectoralis muscle contraction contraction from direct muscle stimulation. Finger and/or thumb flexion at 0.5 mA or less indicates acceptable needle tip position for local anesthetic injection. Biceps contraction or forearm pronation indicates lateral needle tip position. If initial needle advancement fails to elicit the appropriate motor-evoked response, the needle should be redirected slightly caudad within the parasagittal plane.

Ultrasound. A linear or curvilinear, low-frequency ultrasound probe is placed in the parasagittal plane at the deltopectoral groove. At this level, the hyperechoic cords of the brachial plexus, the hypoechoic pulsatile axillary artery, and the hypoechoic compressible axillary vein can be identified in cross section, deep to the pectoralis major and minor muscles (Fig. 52.12). Introducing the block needle from the superior end of the ultrasound probe and advancing in line with the plane of the beam allows direct visualization of needle tip advancement and local anesthetic spread. While the cords of the brachial plexus can be difficult to visualize, needle tip placement posterior to the artery with local anesthetic spread circumferentially around the artery indicates a high likelihood of success. Subsequent medial and/or lateral redirection of the needle may be necessary to achieve circumferential local anesthetic spread.

Clinical Effects. Hadzic et al.,[147] comparing single-shot infraclavicular block to general anesthesia, demonstrated superior immediate postoperative analgesia, but the use of short-acting local anesthetic resulted in similar VAS pain scores and opioid consumption at 24 and 48 hours. Continuous infraclavicular blocks for postoperative pain management demonstrated decreased opi-

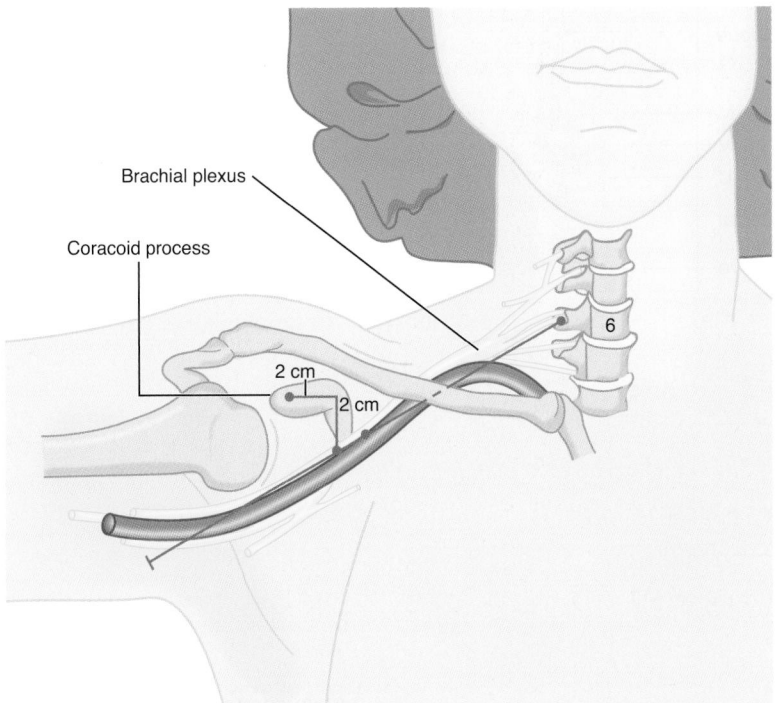

Brachial plexus

Coracoid process

2 cm

2 cm

6

FIGURE 52.11 Landmarks for the infraclavicular approach to the brachial plexus.

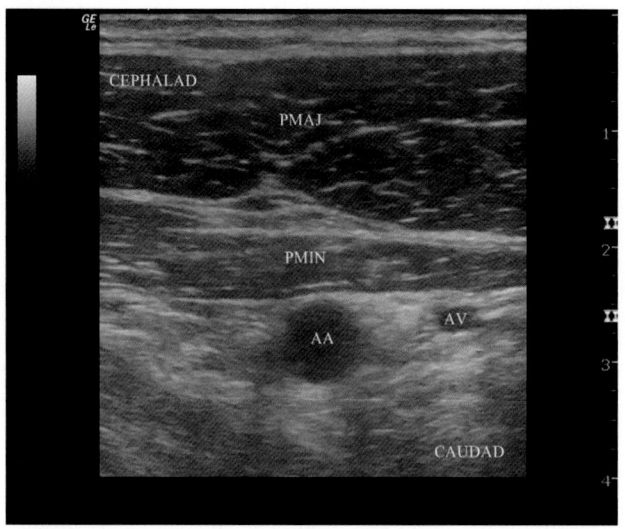

FIGURE 52.12 Sonographic landmarks for ultrasound-guided infraclavicular nerve block. AA, axillary artery; AV, axillary vein; PMAJ, pectoralis major muscle; PMIN, pectoralis minor muscle.

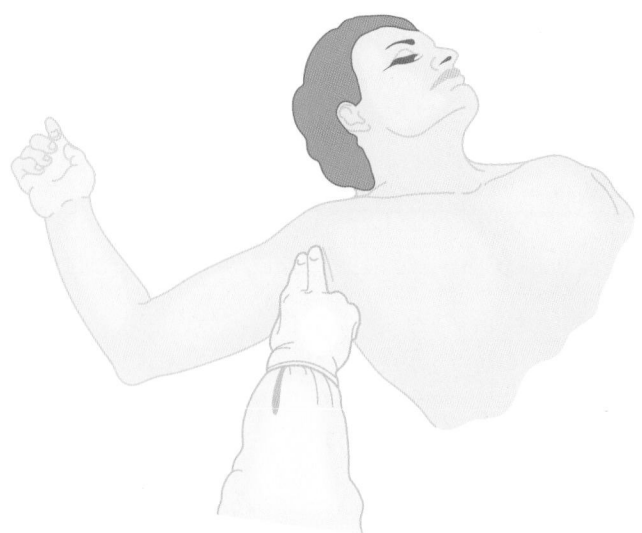

FIGURE 52.14 Position and axillary artery palpation for axillary nerve block.

oid consumption, decreased average and maximum VAS pain scores, decreased side effects, and improved patient satisfaction as compared to opioids.[148–150] In a subset of patients without major comorbidities, it is feasible to convert total elbow arthroplasty into an ambulatory procedure using a continuous infraclavicular block as part of a multimodal analgesic regimen provided at home.[109]

Axillary Nerve Block

Indications. The axillary nerve block targets the terminal branches of the brachial plexus. It is performed as a single injection or continuous catheter technique to provide anesthesia and postoperative analgesia for operations on the hand, wrist, and forearm. At the level of the axilla, the musculocutaneous nerve is often located within the belly of the coracobrachialis, separated from the median, ulnar, and radial nerves (Fig. 52.13). Thus, an additional musculocutaneous nerve block is recommended to provide analgesia of the entire forearm.

Landmarks. The patient is positioned supine with the operative arm abducted 90 degrees and externally rotated. The axillary artery is palpated at its most proximal point in the axilla (Fig. 52.14). The coracobrachialis muscle is palpated medial to the biceps muscle.

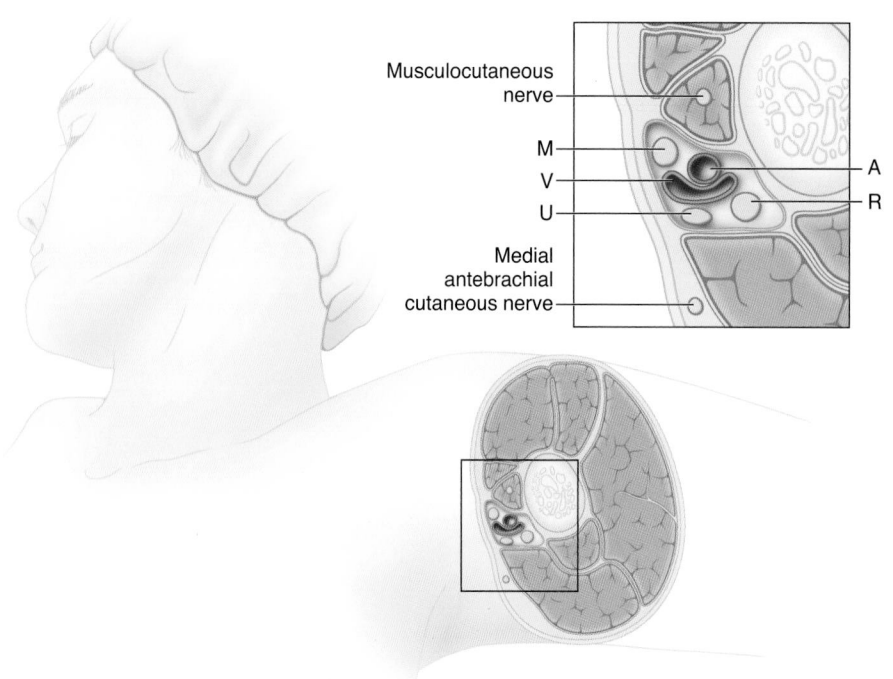

FIGURE 52.13 Axilllary cross section.

Needles. Insulated needle used: 22-gauge, 5 cm. Insulated Tuohy needle for catheter placement: 18-gauge, 5 cm. Catheters are introduced 5 cm beyond the needle tip.

Technique.
Nerve stimulation and transarterial.

MEDIAN, ULNAR, AND RADIAL NERVES. The nerve stimulator is initially set at 1.0 mA. After cleaning the area with antiseptic solution, using sterile technique, the needle is inserted superior to the point of maximal axillary artery palpation, entering at a 30 to 45 degree angle to the skin. Finger flexion and/or thumb opposition at 0.5 mA or less indicates appropriate needle tip position for local anesthetic injection. An evoked motor response of the musculocutaneous nerve cannot be accepted. Again, at the level of the axilla, the musculocutaneous nerve is often found traveling independently within the belly of the coracobrachialis, separated from the median, ulnar, and radial nerves (see Fig. 52.14). Aspiration of bright-red blood indicates the needle has entered the axillary artery. At this point, the transarterial technique should be used and nerve stimulation abandoned. Using the transarterial technique, the needle should be advanced slowly with continuous aspiration until blood can no longer be aspirated. Incremental local anesthetic injection after negative aspiration at this location will provide blockade of the plexus. Intermittent purposeful re-entry of the block needle into the vessel after stopping local anesthetic injection can confirm needle tip location just beyond the artery. After needle re-entry into the vessel indicated by positive aspiration of blood, the needle is again slowly advanced beyond the vessel with continuous aspiration until blood can no longer be aspirated. At this point, local anesthetic injection is resumed.

MUSCULOCUTANEOUS NERVE. The nerve stimulator is set at 2.0 mA. After cleaning the area with antiseptic solution, using sterile technique, the needle is inserted into the coracobrachialis muscle at the midhumeral level to block the musculocutaneous nerve (Fig. 52.15). The needle is fanned through the coracobrachialis muscle until vigorous biceps contraction from musculocutaneous nerve stimulation is elicited, as opposed to unintentional direct stimulation of the biceps muscle itself. It is not necessary to dial down the current. Ten mL of local anesthetic is injected.

Ultrasound. Using a linear, high-frequency ultrasound probe at the axillary fold in an abducted and externally rotated arm, terminal branches of the brachial plexus can be identified in cross section. They appear as round to oval hypo- or hyperechoic structures approximately 1 cm from the skin surface in close proximity to the hypoechoic axillary artery (Fig. 52.16). The terminal branches are variable in their position around the artery; however, the radial nerve is most commonly identified in a posterior position, the median nerve in an anterior position, and the ulnar nerve in a medial position. The musculocutaneous nerve is identified within the coracobrachialis muscle (Fig. 52.17). Introducing the block needle from the lateral end of the ultrasound probe and advancing in line with the plane of the beam allows direct visualization of needle tip advancement and local anesthetic spread.

Clinical Effects. Postoperative analgesic advantages of single injection axillary nerve block include extended time to first requested analgesic,[151] decreased opioid use,[151,152] and decreased VAS pain scores.[151] There was no difference in pain, opioid consumption, adverse effects, or patient satisfaction identified at 24

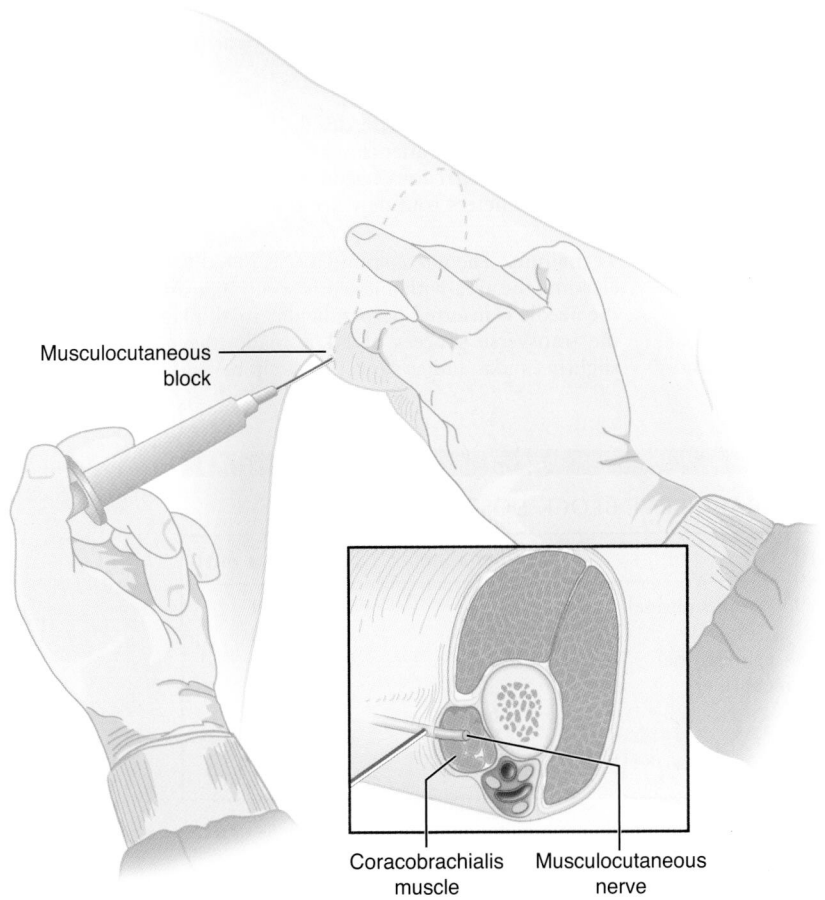

Musculocutaneous block

Coracobrachialis muscle   Musculocutaneous nerve

FIGURE 52.15 Musculocutaneous nerve block.

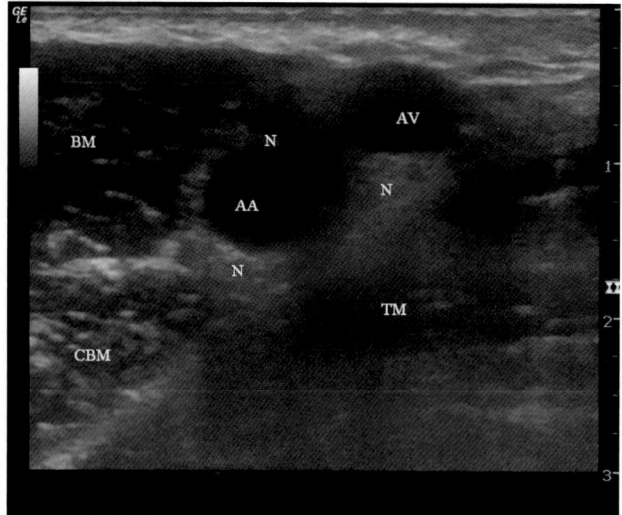

FIGURE 52.16 Sonographic landmarks for ultrasound-guided axillary nerve block. AA, axillary artery; AV, axillary vein; BM, biceps muscle; CBM, corachobrachialis muscle; N, terminal branch of brachial plexus; TM, triceps muscle.

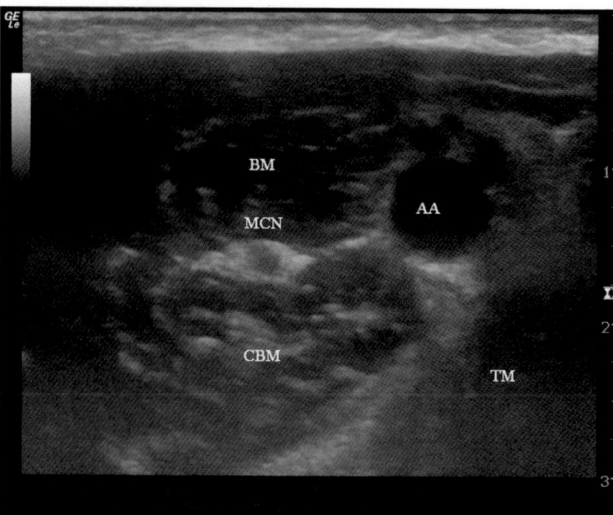

FIGURE 52.17 Sonographic landmarks for ultrasound-guided musculocutaneous nerve block. AA, axillary artery; BM, biceps muscle; CBM, corachobrachialis muscle; MCN, musculocutaneous nerve; TM, triceps muscle.

hours in these studies,[151,152] likely due to the short-acting local anesthetic used. Continuous axillary nerve blocks have demonstrated successful postoperative analgesia with home catheters after hand surgery.[141,153]

Lower Extremity Peripheral Nerve Blocks

Peripheral nerve blockade following lower extremity surgery avoids the limitations associated with the use of IV PCA and PCEA. Peripheral nerve blocks of the lower extremity allow reduced side effects, regional analgesia techniques in the setting of anticoagulation, and ambulatory catheters for early patient discharge or surgery in the outpatient setting. Additionally, peripheral nerve block analgesic techniques may improve early rehabilitation (Table 52.7).

Posterior Lumbar Plexus Block

Indications. The lumbar plexus is formed within the psoas major muscle by the ventral rami of L1–L4 with a variable contribution from T12. At the L4-L5 level, the terminal nerves of the lumbar plexus are formed including the lateral femoral cutaneous, femo-

ral, and obturator nerves. Posterior lumbar plexus block (LPB) as a single injection or continuous catheter technique is effective for postoperative pain management following procedures of the hip, knee, and femur.

Landmarks. The patient is placed in the Sims' position. The intersection of the intercristal line with a line drawn from the posterior superior iliac spine (PSIS) parallel to the vertebral spinous processes determines the initial needle insertion point. In most patients, this corresponds to 5 cm lateral from the midline (Fig. 52.18).

Needles. Insulated needle used: 21-gauge, 10 cm. Consider a 15-cm needle in patients with an increased body mass index (BMI). Insulated Tuohy needle for catheter placement: 18-gauge, 10 cm. Catheters routinely are inserted 5–10 cm.

Technique. The nerve stimulator is initially set at 1.5 mA. After cleaning the area with antiseptic solution, using sterile technique, the needle is inserted perpendicular to all planes. If contact with the transverse process of L4 is made, the needle is redirected slightly caudal and advanced 1–2 cm beyond the transverse pro-

TABLE 52.7

LOWER EXTREMITY PERIPHERAL NERVE BLOCK DOSING

Local Anesthetic (20–40 mL)	Anesthesia (hrs)	Analgesia (hrs)
3% 2-Chloroprocaine (+HCO3 + epinephrine)	1.5	2.0
1.5% Mepivacaine (+HCO3)	2–3	2–4
1.5% Mepivacaine (+HCO3 + epinephrine)	2.5–4	3–6
2% Lidocaine (+ HCO3 + epinephrine)	3–6	5–8
0.5% Ropivacaine (+ epi)	6–8	8–12
0.75% Ropivacaine (+ epi)	8–10	12–18
0.5% Bupivacaine (+ epi)	8–10	16–18

Continuous infusion ropivacaine 0.2% or dilute concentration of bupivacaine or levobupivacaine; 8–10 mL/hour or 5 mL/hour with 5 mL hourly bolus or 8 mL/hour with 4 mL Q30min bolus.
Table modified from Hadzic A, Vloka JD. *Peripheral Nerve Blocks, Principles and Practice.* Columbus, OH: McGraw-Hill: 2004.

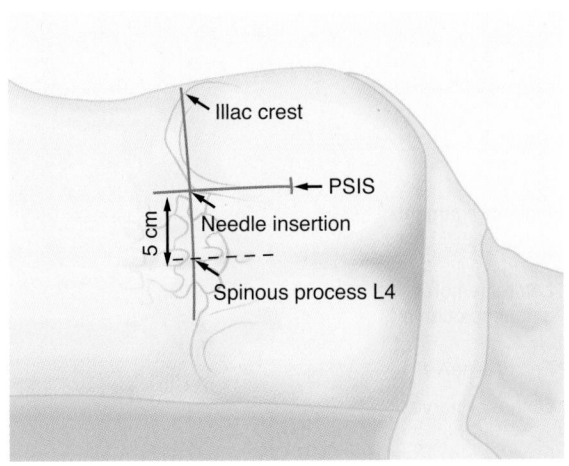

FIGURE 52.18 Landmarks for posterior LPB.

cess. The lumbar plexus is usually encountered at a depth of 6–10 cm. An evoked motor response of the quadriceps muscle at 0.5 mA indicates acceptable needle tip position for local anesthetic injection. An evoked motor response of the adductor muscles indicates medial needle tip position. Elicitation of hamstring contraction, foot dorsiflexion, or plantarflexion indicates stimulation of the lumbosacral trunk and caudomedial needle tip position in relation to the lumbar plexus. If initial passes fail to elicit an evoked motor response providing feedback for needle position, the needle should be withdrawn to the skin level and redirected in 5 to 10 degress increments cephalad, and then caudad. Susequent to these maneuvers, the needle is withdrawn to skin and cautiously redirected medial in 5 to 10 degree increments. The operator must remember that slight variations in the needle angle at the skin translate to larger variations at the needle tip as the needle depth increases. Medial placement of the needle tip may increase the potential risk of unitential central neuraxial anesthesia.

Clinical Effects. A single injection posterior lumbar plexus block provides 6 to 12 hours of postoperative analgesia. Continuous lumbar plexus block (CLPB) improves analgesia and patient satisfaction as compared to parenteral opioids and side effects as compared to epidural analgesia. Continuous catheters are beneficial for anterior cruciate ligament repair (ACLR), total hip arthroplasty (THA), and total knee arthroplasty (TKA). For TKA, the addition of a single injection sciatic nerve block improves analgesia. CLPBs and continous femoral nerve blocks (CFNBs) demonstrate similar analgesic efficacy for TKA. Given the potential risks associated with LPB, CFNB might be the continuous technique of choice for TKA. The results of a prospective study suggest that for a subset of patients without major comorbidities, it might be feasible to convert THA into an overnight-stay procedure using an ambulatory continuous psoas compartment nerve block as part of a multimodal analgesic regimen provided at home.[106]

Femoral Nerve Block

Indications. A femoral nerve block (FNB) will reliably block the femoral and lateral femoral cutaneous nerves, but inconsistently block the obturator nerve. Single-shot or continuous FNBs provide postoperative analgesia for operations on the knee and femur.

Landmarks. With the patient supine, the femoral artery pulse is palpated at the level of the femoral crease. The initial needle

insertion site is approximately one fingerbreadth lateral to the femoral artery pulse (Fig. 52.19).

Needles. Insulated needle used: 22-gauge, 5 cm. Insulated Tuohy needle for catheter placement: 18-gauge, 10 cm. The catheter is inserted 5 cm beyond the needle tip.

Technique.
Nerve stimulation. The nerve stimulator is initially set at 1.0 mA. Initial needle insertion is approximately one fingerbreadth lateral to the femoral artery pulse. After cleaning the area with antiseptic solution, using sterile technique, the needle is directed perpendicular to the skin or slightly cephalad. An evoked motor response of the quadriceps with a current of 0.5 mA or less indicates acceptable needle tip position for local anesthetic injection. The femoral nerve is superficial, rarely beyond 3 cm from the skin. An evoked motor response of the sartorius muscle indicates stimulation of the anterior division of the femoral nerve, necessitating deeper needle advancement to obtain the appropriate motor response.

Ultrasound. Using a linear, high-frequency ultrasound probe at the infrainguinal location, the femoral nerve will appear in cross section as a hyperechoic triangular structure just lateral to the femoral artery, medial to the iliacus muscle, inferior to the fascia iliaca, and superior to the psoas muscle (Fig. 52.20). Introducing the block needle from the lateral end of the ultrasound probe and advancing in line with the plane of the beam allows direct visualization of needle tip advancement and local anesthetic spread. The femoral nerve lies deep to the fascia iliaca and outside of the femoral sheath which contains the femoral artery, vein, and lymphatics (Fig. 52.21). This is an important consideration when evaluating needle tip position and local anesthetic spread. Local anesthetic will be visualized spreading beneath the fascia iliaca, circumferentially around the femoral nerve. While the in-plane technique is generally preferred for single-shot injections and provides tunneling for continuous catheter placement, the out-of-plane technique may provide more optimal needle orientation for continuous catheter advancement.

Clinical Effects. FNB improves analgesia after ACLR.[154,155] Further improvement has been demonstrated with the addition of a sciatic nerve block.[156] CFNB extends the duration of analgesia for ACLR.[156] FNB provides improved analgesia for TKA, and one study demonstrated improvement with rehabilitation.[157] Studies did not all agree that sciatic nerve block in addition to FNBs further improve postoperative analgesia for TKA.[158–162] Some studies question whether CFNB offers additional benefit after TKA.[163,164] A majority of studies suggest that extended pain relief is achieved with CFNB. Additionally, CFNB has demonstrated improved rehabilitation after TKA.[165,166] Given the potential risks associated with LPBs, CFNB might be the continuous technique of choice for TKA. The addition of a single injection sciatic nerve block to CFNBs further improves postoperative analgesia after TKA and additional improvement is seen with combined continuous femoral and sciatic nerve blocks[160,161]; however, concerns with compartment syndrome or perioperative nerve injury may necessitate postoperative examination by the surgical team.[160] In these circumstances, it is possible to dose a catheter previously placed, when the surgery team has completed their exams or the observation period has ended. CFNB provided equivalent analgesia and rehabilitation performance as epidural with fewer side effects.[166]

Sciatic Nerve Block: Classic Labat Approach

Indications. The sciatic nerve, the largest nerve in the body, is formed from the convergence of the L4–S3 ventral rami at the

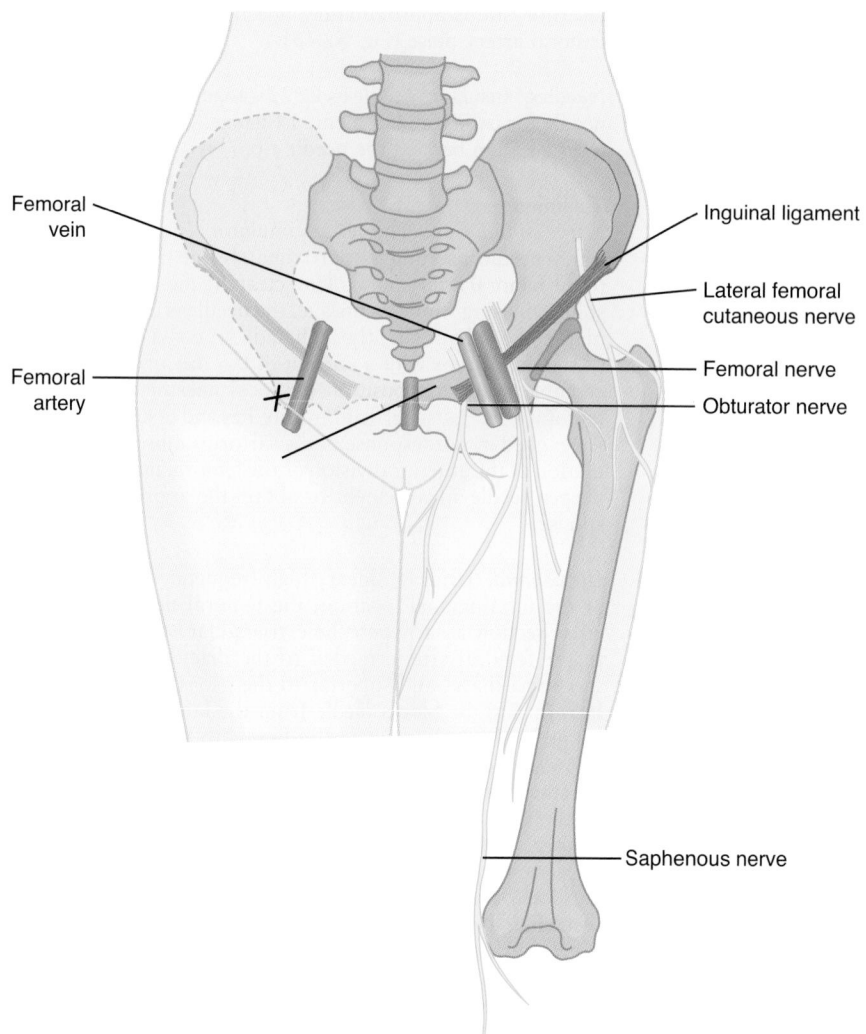

FIGURE 52.19 Landmarks for femoral nerve block. X, needle insertion site.

inferior border of the piriformis muscle. The sciatic nerve consists of two nerves, the tibial and common peroneal nerves, bound together by epineurium. Usually, these nerves separate distal to the midthigh level; however, separation may occur prior to entering the gluteal region with the peroneal division passing through or superior to the piriformis muscle. A sciatic nerve block as a single injection or continuous catheter technique provides analgesia for operations on the foot and ankle, excluding the saphenous nerve sensory distribution. Additionally, a sciatic nerve block as a single injection or continuous catheter technique can be an important addition to a femoral or lumbar plexus block in providing analgesia for knee surgery.

Landmarks. The patient is placed in the Sims' position. A line is drawn from the greater trochanter to the PSIS. A second line is drawn from the greater trochanter to the patient's sacral hiatus. A third line is drawn perpendicular from the midpoint of the first line to its intersection with the second line. This point of intersection is the initial needle insertion site. Alternatively, a single line is drawn from the greater trochanter to the PSIS, and a second line is drawn perpendicular from the midpoint of this line to a point 5 cm medial. This point represents the initial needle insertion site (Fig. 52.22).

Needles. Insulated needle used for the majority of patients: 21-gauge, 10 cm. Consider 15-cm needle in patients with in-

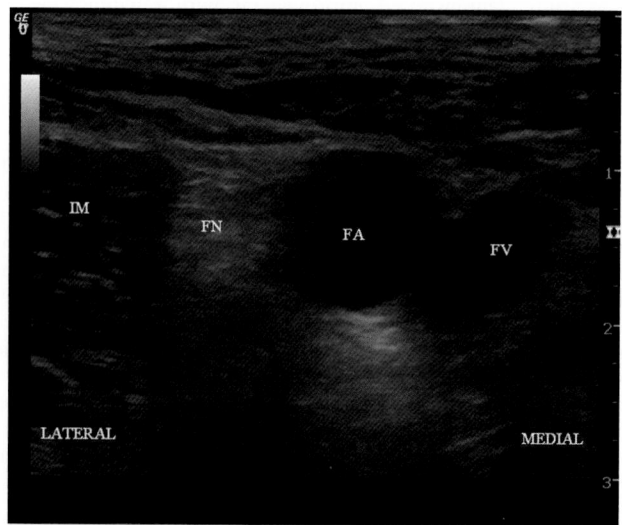

FIGURE 52.20 Sonographic landmarks for ultrasound-guided femoral nerve block. FA, femoral artery; FI, fascia iliaca; FN: femoral nerve; FV: femoral vein; IM, iliacus muscle; PM: psoas muscle.

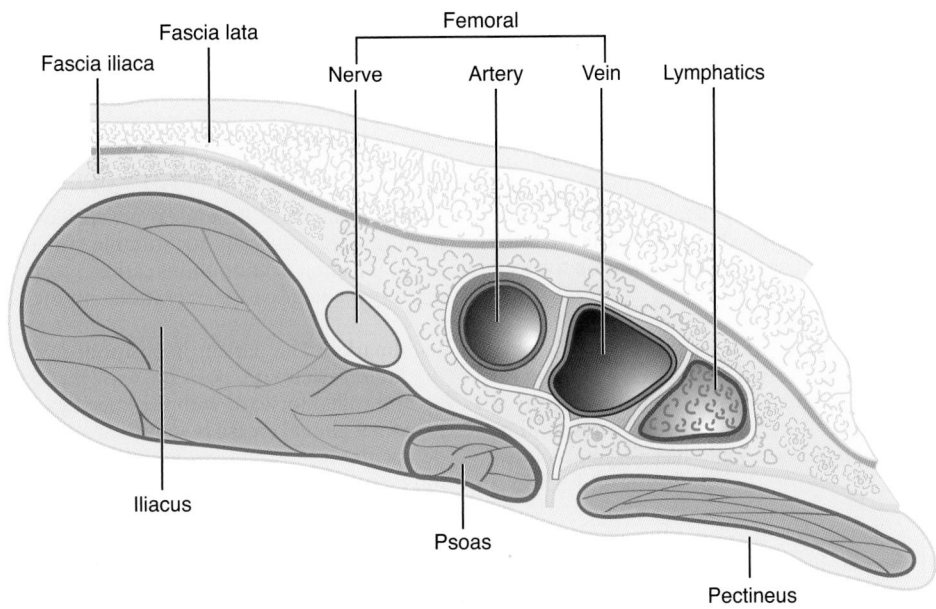

FIGURE 52.21 Transverse section of superior thigh. The femoral sheath containing the femoral artery, vein, and lymphatics lies deep to the fascia lata. The femoral nerve lies outside of the femoral sheath and deep to the fascia iliaca.

creased BMI. Insulated Tuohy needle for catheter placement: 18-gauge, 10 cm. Catheters are inserted 5 cm beyond the needle tip.

Technique. The nerve stimulator is initially set at 1.0 to 1.5 mA. The foot on the side to be blocked should be free, allowing unobstructed movement with nerve stimulation and direct visualiza-

tion of response. After cleaning the area with antiseptic solution, using sterile technique, the needle is inserted perpendicular to all planes. Initial needle advancement will often elicit direct gluteus maximus and/or piriformis muscle contraction. With further needle advancement, plantarflexion/inversion or dorsiflexion/eversion of the foot at 0.5 mA of current or less indicates accept-

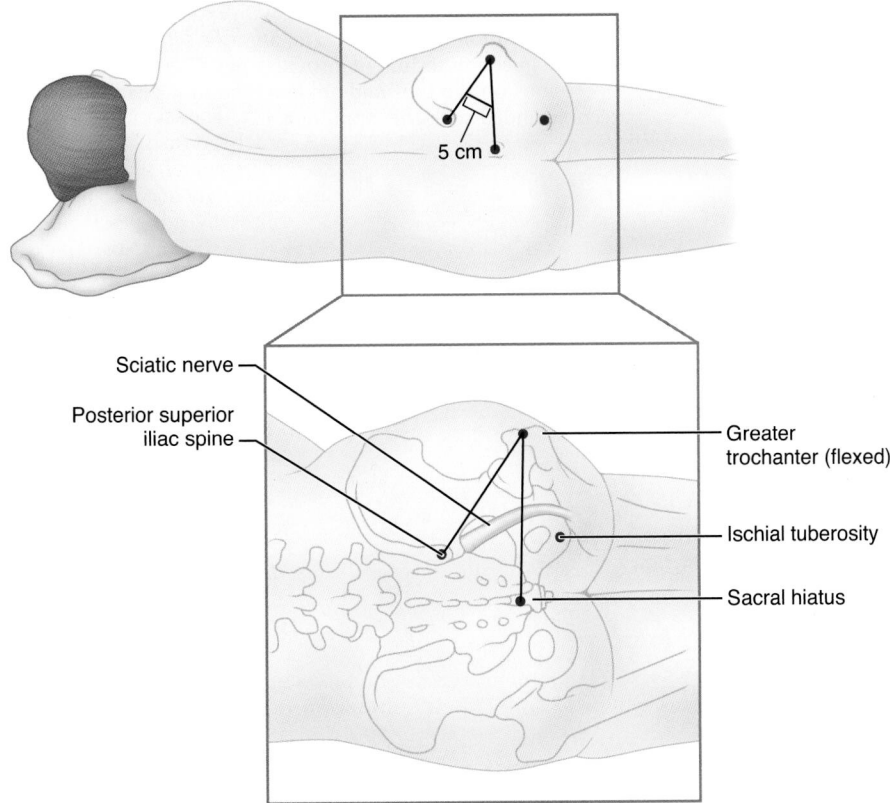

FIGURE 52.22 Landmarks for classic Labat's sciatic nerve block.

able needle tip position for local anesthetic injection. Hamstring muscle contraction indicates medial needle tip position.

Sciatic Nerve Block: Raj Approach

Indications. The Raj approach targets the sciatic nerve at a shallow location in an easily palpable groove between the semitendinosus and biceps femoris muscles. Patient positioning and monitoring of stimulation response, however, require assistance. The Raj approach as a single injection or continuous catheter technique provides postoperative analgesia for operations on the foot and ankle.

Landmarks. The patient is positioned supine and with the help of an assistant the operative leg is raised 90 degrees. Midpoint on a line connecting the greater trochanter to the ischial tuberosity is the initial needle insertion site. This point should correspond to the groove between the semitendinosus and biceps femoris muscles (Fig. 52.23).

Needles. Insulated needle used: 21-gauge, 10 cm. Insulated Tuohy needle for catheter placement: 18-gauge, 10 cm. Catheters are inserted 5 cm beyond needle tip.

Technique. The nerve stimulator is initially set at 1.0 to 1.5 mA. After cleaning the area with antiseptic solution, using sterile technique, the needle is directed perpendicular to all planes. Plantarflexion/inversion of the foot at 0.5 mA or less indicates acceptable needle tip position for local anesthetic injection.

Dorsiflexion/eversion of the foot indicates lateral needle tip position, and direct adductor muscle contraction indicates medial needle tip position.

Sciatic Nerve Block: Infragluteal-Parabiceps Approach

Indications. The infragluteal-parabiceps sciatic nerve block is performed using easily identifiable soft tissue landmarks. As a single injection or continuous catheter technique, it provides postoperative analgesia for operations on the foot and ankle.

Landmarks. The patient is positioned prone or alternatively in the lateral decubitus position with the extremity to be blocked up and rolled forward with the knee flexed 90 degrees. The most proximal gluteal crease is identified and marked. The lateral border of the biceps femoris muscle is identified and marked at it intersects the gluteal crease. The initial needle insertion site is 1 cm distal to the gluteal crease at the lateral border of the biceps femoris muscle (Fig. 52.24).

Needles. Insulated needles used: 22-gauge 5 cm or 21-gauge 10 cm. Insulated Tuohy needle for catheter placement: 18-guage, 5 or 10 cm. Catheters are inserted 5 cm beyond the needle tip.

Technique. The nerve stimulator is initially set at 1.0 to 1.5 mA. After cleaning the area with antiseptic solution, using sterile technique, the needle is inserted with slight cephalad and anterior orientation within the parasagital plane. Plantarflexion/inversion of the foot at 0.5 mA or less indicates acceptable needle tip position for local anesthetic injection. Dorsiflexion/eversion of the foot indicates the lateral needle tip position.

Sciatic Nerve Block: Anterior Approach

Indications. The anterior approach to the sciatic nerve, requiring minimal positioning of the surgical extremity for block placement, is advantageous for patients experiencing pain with movement of the extremity and/or those with external fixators in place, making positioning difficult. The anterior sciatic nerve block as a single injection technique provides postoperative analgesia for operations on the foot and ankle. Continuous catheters are not recommended with this approach.

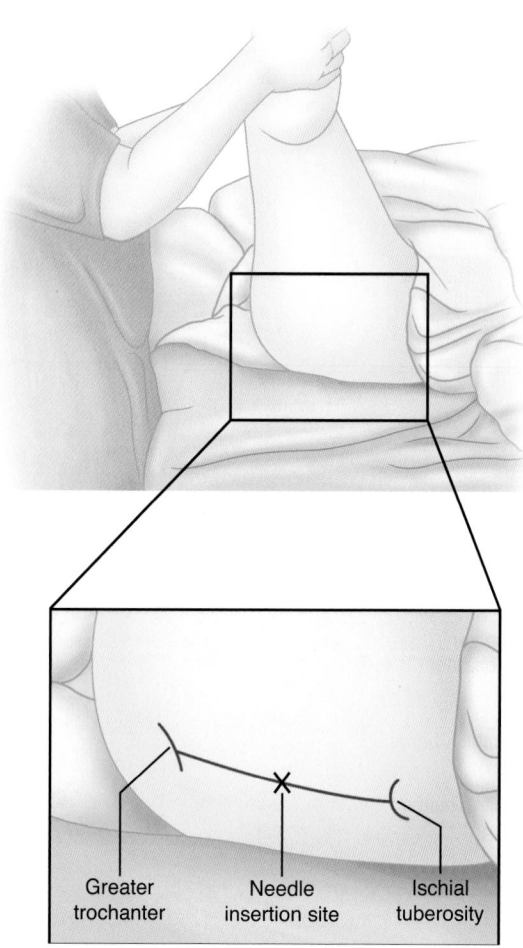

FIGURE 52.23 Patient position and landmarks for sciatic nerve block using Raj approach.

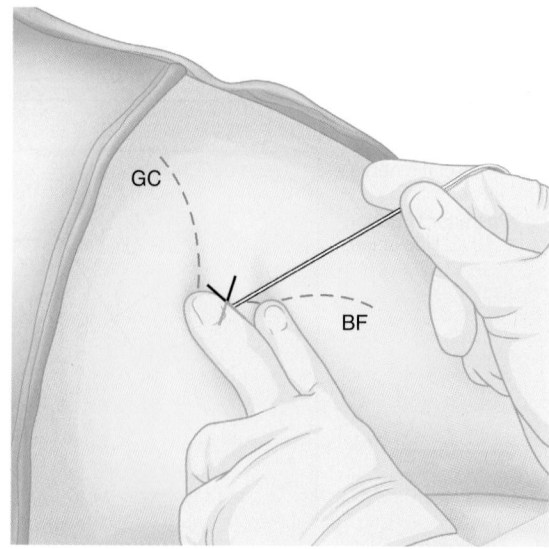

FIGURE 52.24 Landmarks and needle orientation for infragluteal-parabiceps sciatic nerve block.

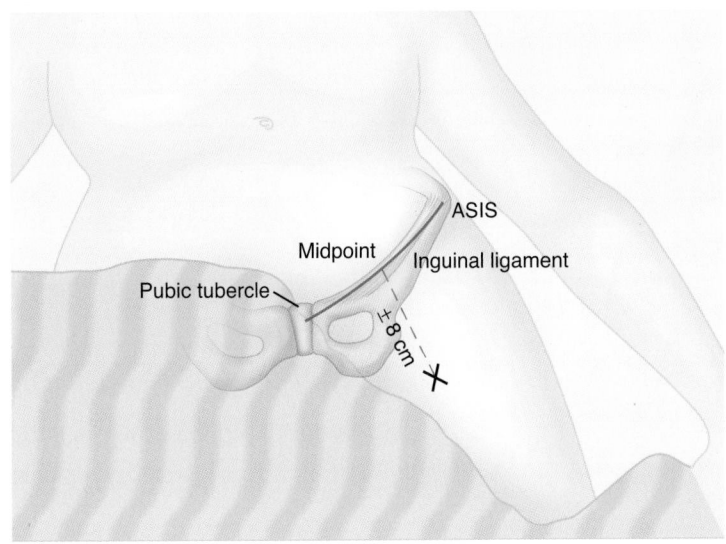

FIGURE 52.25 Landmarks for anterior approach to sciatic nerve block. X, needle insertion site.

Landmarks. The patient is positioned supine. A line is drawn from the anterior superior iliac spine to the pubic tubercle and marked at its midline. A second line is drawn perpendicular to first line from its midpoint to a point 8 cm caudally which represents the initial needle insertion site (Fig. 52.25). Alternatively, the femoral artery pulse is identified along the femoral crease. A line is drawn perpendicular to the femoral crease to a point 4 to 5 cm distal from the femoral artery pulse. This point 4 to 5 cm distal from the femoral artery pulse, along the line drawn perpendicular to the femoral crease, is the initial needle insertion site.

Needles. Insulated needle used: 21-gauge, 15 cm.

Technique.
Nerve stimulation. The nerve stimulator is initially set at 1.5 mA. After cleaning the area with antiseptic solution, using sterile technique, the needle is inserted perpendicular to all planes and advanced until the femur is contacted. The needle tip is then redirected slightly medial until plantarflexion/inversion of the foot is elicited at a current of 0.5 mA or less, indicating acceptable needle tip position for local anesthetic injection. If subsequent medial passes continue to contact bone, internal rotation of the leg will displace the lesser trochanter, optimizing the anterior approach to the sciatic nerve. Dorsiflexion/eversion of the foot indicates lateral needle tip position.

Ultrasound. Using a curvilinear, high-frequency ultrasound probe placed in the transverse plane at the medial aspect of the upper midthigh, the sciatic nerve will appear in cross section as a hyperechoic circle or triangular structure medial to the femur and deep to the adductor magnus muscle (Fig. 52.26). Introducing the block needle from the lateral end of the ultrasound probe and advancing in line with the plane of the beam allows direct visualization of needle tip advancement and local anesthetic spread.

Sciatic Nerve Block: Popliteal Approach

Indications. The popliteal nerve block as a distal block of the sciatic nerve preserves hamstring function and facilitates ambulation. It can be performed from a posterior or lateral approach. A disadvantage of either approach is that the tibial and common peroneal components of the sciatic nerve may separate prior to reaching the popliteal fossa, potentially resulting in an incomplete block if local anesthetic does not spread to each division. Popliteal nerve block using a single injection or continuous catheter tech-

nique provides postoperative analgesia for operations on the foot and ankle.

Landmarks: Posterior Popliteal Approach. The patient is positioned prone with the operative foot slightly elevated and free so that the motor evoked response is unobstructed. The popliteal crease is identified and marked. The tendons of the biceps femoris and semitendinosus muscles are identified and accentuated by having the patient bend the knee against resistance. The needle insertion site is marked approximately 7 cm proximal to the popliteal crease, midpoint between the biceps femoris and semitendinosus tendons (Fig. 52.27).

Needles. Insulated needles used: 22-gauge, 5 cm or 21-gauge 10 cm. Insulated Tuohy needle for catheter placementL 18-gauge, 5 cm. Catheters are inserted 5 cm beyond the needle tip.

Technique.
Nerve stimulation. The nerve stimulator is initially set at 1.0 to 1.5 mA. After cleaning the area with antiseptic solution, using sterile technique, the needle is inserted slightly cephalad in the parasagittal plane. Plantarflexion/inversion of the foot at 0.5 mA or less indicates acceptable needle tip position for local anesthetic

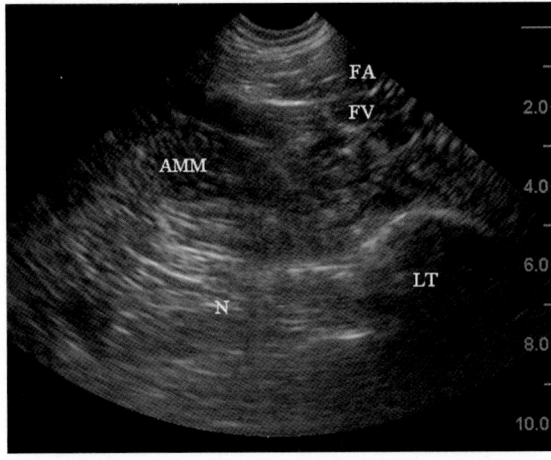

FIGURE 52.26 Sonographic landmarks for ultrasound-guided anterior sciatic nerve block. AMM, adductor magnus muscle; FA: femoral artery; FV: femoral vein; LT: lesser trochanter; N: sciatic nerve.

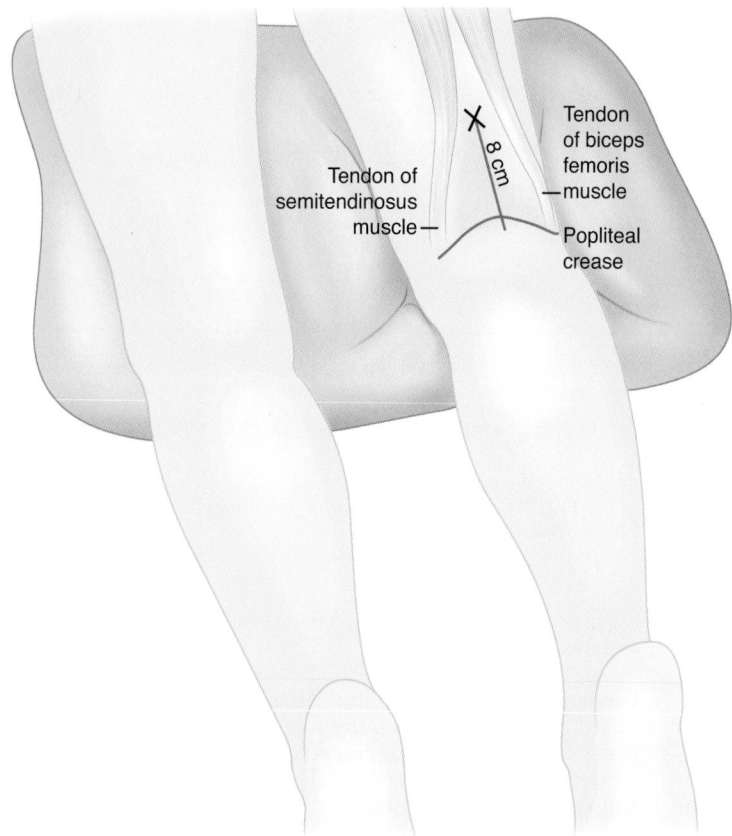

FIGURE 52.27 Landmarks for posterior popliteal nerve block. X, needle insertion site.

injection. Dorsiflexion/eversion of the foot indicates lateral needle tip position. Motor response of the semitendinosus mucle indicates medial needle tip insertion, and the needle should be redirected laterally. Motor response of the biceps femoris muscle indicates lateral needle tip insertion, and the needle should be redirected medially. Aspiration of blood indicates medial needle tip position.

Ultrasound. Using a linear,-low frequency ultrasound probe placed in a transverse plane in the popliteal fossa at the level of the popliteal crease, the popliteal artery can be imaged in cross section. The tibial nerve can be found posterior and medial to the popliteal artery and the common peroneal lateral to the artery Fig. 52.28). Both components of the sciatic nerve appear as round to oval hyperechoic structures. Slowly moving the ultrasound probe proximally will demonstrate the common peroneal nerve moving medial to join the tibial nerve (Fig. 52.29). At the level these nerves join, introducing the block needle from the lateral end of the ultrasound probe and advancing in line with the plane of the beam allows direct visualization of needle tip advancement and local anesthetic spread.

Landmarks: Lateral Popliteal Approach. The patient is placed in the supine position with the legs placed in the neutral position. The foot of the operative leg is slightly elevated so that it remains free and the motor evoked response unobstructed. The popliteal crease is noted and marked at its lateral extension. The groove between the vastus lateralis and biceps femoris is palpated and accentuated by having the patient lift his or her foot off the table. The needle insertion site is 8 to 10 cm cephalad to the popliteal crease within the groove (Fig. 52.30).

Needles. Insulated needle used: 21-gauge, 10 cm. Insulated Tuohy needle for catheter placement: 18-gauge, 10 cm. Catheters are inserted 5 cm beyond the needle tip.

Technique.
Nerve stimulation. The nerve stimulator is initially set at 1.0 to 1.5 mA. After cleaning the area with antiseptic solution, using sterile technique, the needle is advanced parallel to the bed to contact the femur. The needle is then withdrawn to the skin and redirected 30 degrees posterior (Fig. 52.31). If initial passes fail, subsequent attempts are made more anteriorly or posteriorly. Plantarflexion/inversion of the foot at 0.5 mA or less indicates acceptable needle tip position for local anesthetic injection. Dorsiflexion/eversion of the foot indicates lateral needle tip posi-

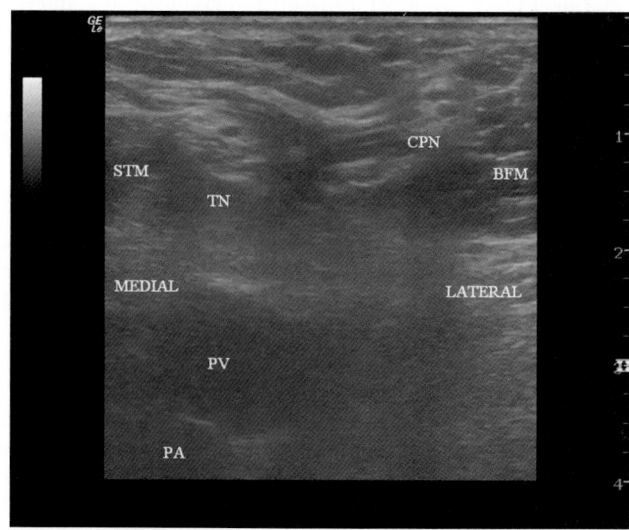

FIGURE 52.28 Ultrasound image just cephalad to popliteal crease. BFM, biceps femoris muscle; CPN: common peroneal nerve; PA, popliteal artery; PV: popliteal vein; STM, semitendinosus muscle; TN, tibial nerve.

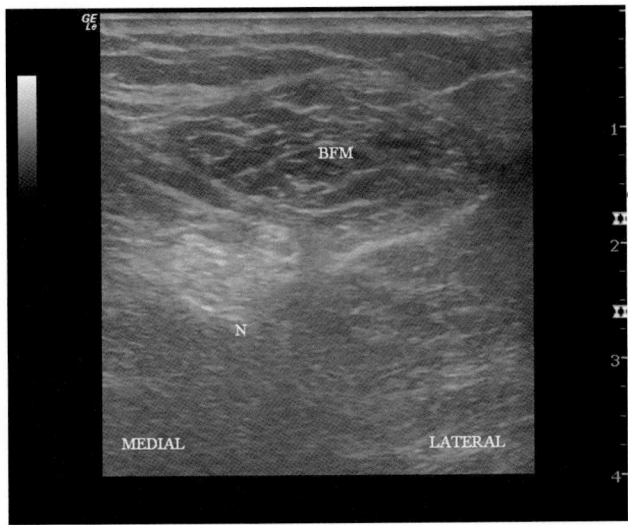

FIGURE 52.29 Sonographic landmarks for popliteal nerve block. BFM, biceps femoris muscle; N, junction of common peroneal and tibial components of sciatic nerve.

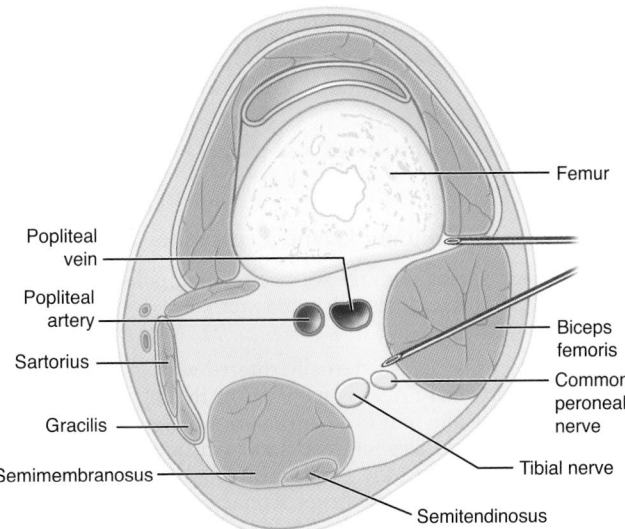

FIGURE 52.31 Anatomy of lateral politeal approach.

tion. Motor response of the hamstring suggests medial needle tip placement. Aspiration of blood indicates anterior and medial needle tip position.

Ultrasound. The patient is placed in the lateral position or alternatively in the supine position with the leg elevated to allow placement of a linear, low-frequency ultrasound probe in the transverse plane in the popliteal fossa at the level of the popliteal crease. At this point, the popliteal artery can be imaged in cross section. The hyperechoic tibial nerve can be seen in cross section posterior and medial to the popliteal artery, and the hyperechoic common peroneal nerve can be seen in cross section lateral to the artery (see Fig. 52.28). Slowly moving the ultrasound probe proximally will image the common peroneal nerve moving medial to join the tibial nerve (see Fig. 52.29). At this level, introducing the block needle from the lateral end of the ultrasound probe or from a more traditional lateral approach allows the needle tip to be advanced toward the sciatic nerve in line with the plane of the beam. This allows direct visualization of needle tip advancement and local anesthetic spread.

Clinical Effects. For outcomes associated with the addition of single injection or continuous sciatic nerve blocks to femoral or posterior lumbar plexus blocks, please refer to those sections. Sciatic nerve blockade by means of the classic posterior approach,

the modified subgluteal posterior approach, or the lateral popliteal approach with 30 mL of 0.75% ropivacaine provides postoperative analgesia for up to 16 hours with similar time to resolution of motor block and patient satisfaction.[167]

Popliteal nerve block can provide analgesia for up to 20 hours after foot and ankle procedures[168] with a high level of patient satisfaction.[169] In patients undergoing foot and ankle procedures, polpiteal nerve block provided a significant increase in analgesic duration as compared to ankle block and subcutaneous local anesthetic infiltration.[170] Postoperative analgesia with popliteal nerve block provided 18 hours of analgesia as compared to 11.5 hours with the ankle block and 6.3 hours with local infiltration.

Continuous popliteal nerve blocks for postoperative analgesia reduce supplemental opioid requirements and opioid related side effects.[171,172] Additional benefits include improved sleep,[173] reduced hospital length of stay,[171] reduced outpatient admissions,[171] reduced perioperative costs,[171] and high patient satisfaction.[171,173] One small study examined the ability of continuous sciatic analgesia to allow conversion of inpatient foot surgery to outpatient surgery,[171] and although more patients in the perineural analgesia group were able to be discharged home, the difference was not statistically significant.

Ankle Block

Indications. The ankle is innervated by four branches of the sciatic nerve (posterior tibial, deep peroneal, common peroneal,

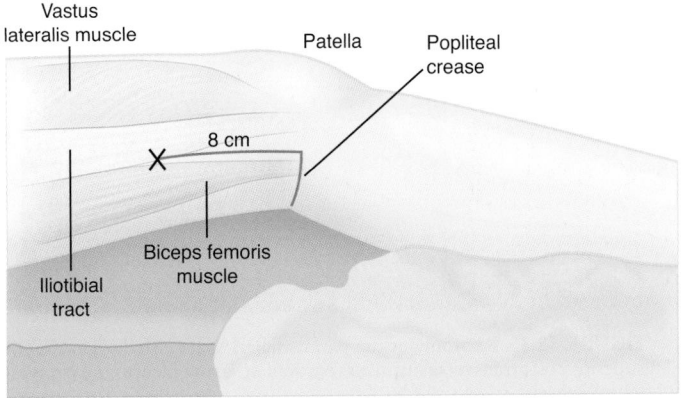

FIGURE 52.30 Landmarks for lateral politeal nerve block. X, needle insertion site.

sural) and one branch of the femoral nerve (saphenous). The ankle block provides analgesia for operations on the forefoot and facilitates early ambulation.

Needles. Needle used: 22–25-gauge, 3.7 cm, 1.5 inch. If using nerve stimulate for tibial nerve, a 22-gauge, 5 cm insulated needle is used.

Landmarks and Technique

Place patient supine with the leg resting on a pillow so that the foot is free to rotate internally and externally.

Tibial nerve. The leg is externally rotated with the knee flexed. The posterior tibial artery is palpated at the inferior border of the medial malleolus and 1 to 2 cm anterior to the Achilles tendon (Fig. 52.32). After cleaning the area with antiseptic solution, using sterile technique, the needle is directed posterior to the artery and advanced until the flexor retinaculum is pierced or bone contact with the tibia is made. If bone is contacted, the needle is withdrawn slightly prior to injection. Ten mL of local anesthetic without epinephrine is injected after negative aspiration. If a nerve stimulation technique is used, the nerve stimulator is initially set at 2 mA. Flexion of the great toe indicates acceptable needle tip position for local anesthetic injection. It is not necessary to dial down the current.

Deep peroneal nerve. Block of the deep peroneal nerve is accomplished by asking the patient to extend the foot and first toe against resistance. This allows palpation of the extensor digitorum and extensor hallucis longus tendons above the ankle joint at the level of the malleoli. After cleaning the area with antiseptic solution, using sterile technique, the needle is directed perpendicular to the skin, medial to the anterior tibial artery and between the tendons until the extensor retinaculum is penetrated or bone contact with the tibia is made (see Fig. 52.32). If bone is contacted, the needle is withdrawn slightly prior to injection. After a negative aspiration, 2 to 4 mL of local anesthetic without epinephrine is injected deep to the fascia.

Superficial peroneal, saphenous, and sural nerves. After cleaning the area with antiseptic solution, using sterile technique, the saphenous, sural, and superficial peroneal nerves are blocked with a subcutaneous ring of local anesthetic just proximal to the malleoli extending across the anterior portion of the ankle from the lateral aspect of the Achilles tendon to the medial malleolus (see Fig. 52.32).

Clinical Effects. In patients undergoing foot and ankle procedures, polpiteal nerve block provided a significant increase in analgesic duration as compared to ankle block and subcutaneous local anesthetic infiltration.[170] Postoperative analgesia with popliteal nerve block provided 18 hours of analgesia as compared to 11.5 hours with the ankle block and 6.3 hours with local infiltration.

Paravertebral Blocks

The paravertebral space is an anatomically triangular area whose borders are defined by the parietal pleura or iliopsoas muscle anterolaterally; the superior costotransverse ligament (thoracic levels) posteriorly; the vertebra, vertebral disk, and intervertebral foramina medially; and the heads of the ribs superiorly and inferiorly (Fig. 52.33). Within this space, the spinal root emerges from the intervertebral foramina and divides into dorsal and ventral rami. Paravertebral blocks provide segmental anesthesia and analgesia (Table 52.8).

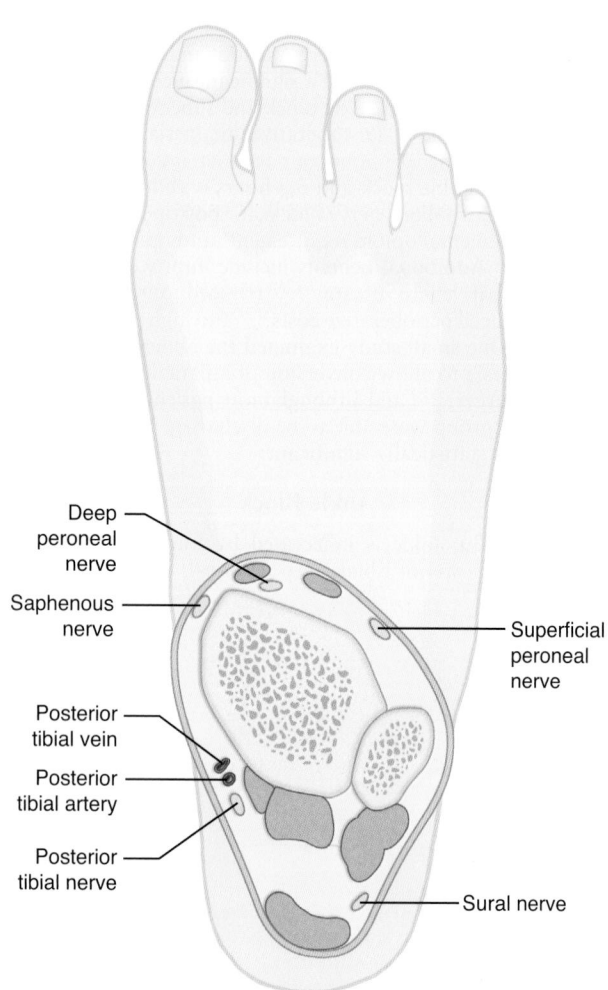

FIGURE 52.32 Landmarks for ankle block.

Deep peroneal nerve
Saphenous nerve
Superficial peroneal nerve
Posterior tibial vein
Posterior tibial artery
Posterior tibial nerve
Sural nerve

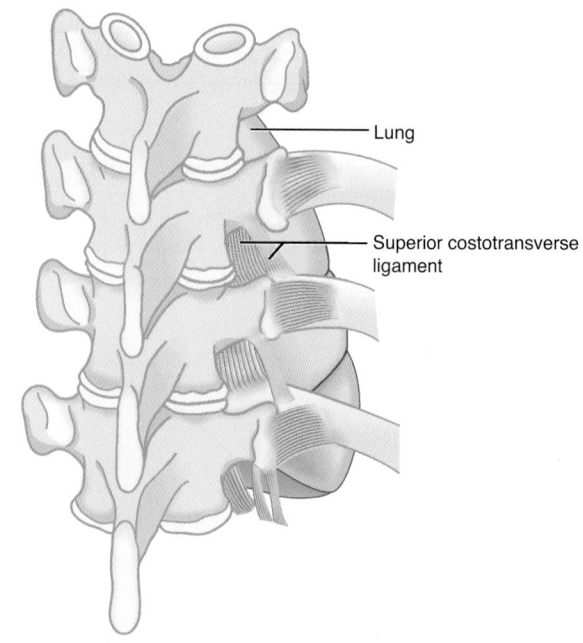

Lung
Superior costotransverse ligament

FIGURE 52.33 Anatomy of the paravertebral space. Medial portion of superior costotransverse ligament removed at arrow identifying paravertebral space.

TABLE 52.8

LOWER THORACIC/LUMBAR PARAVERTEBRAL BLOCK DOSING

Local Anesthetic (3–5 mL at each space for multiple-injection technique or 15–20 mL for single-injection technique)	Anesthesia (hrs)	Analgesia (hrs)
1.5% Mepivacaine (plus HCO3; plus epinephrine)	2–3	3–4
2% Lidocaine (plus HCO3 + epinephrine)	2–3	3–4
0.5% Ropivacaine	3–5	8–12
0.75% Ropivacaine	4–6	12–18
0.5% Bupivacaine (plus epinephrine)	4–6	12–18
0.5% L-Bupivacaine (plus epinephrine)	4–6	12–18

Continuous infusion ropivacaine 0.2% or dilute concentration of bupivacaine or levobupivacaine; 10 mL/hour or 5–6 mL/hour with 4–5 Q30 min boluses.
Table modified from Hadzic A, Vloka JD. *Peripheral Nerve Blocks, Principles and Practice.* Columbus, OH: McGraw-Hill; 2004.

Indications

Paravertebral nerve blocks (PVBs) using single injection or a continuous catheter techniques provide anesthesia and analgesia to the chest and abdomen. PVBs are highly versatile, serving as the primary anesthetic for breast surgery, herniorrhaphy, soft tissue mass excisions, and harvesting of iliac crest bone grafts. PVBs are also an effective analgesic adjunct in laproscopic surgery, cholecystectomy, nephrectomy, appendectomy, thoracotomy, thoracoscopy, obstretric analgesia, minimally invasive cardiac surgery, and hip surgery.

Landmarks

The patient is placed in the sitting position with the neck and back flexed and the shoulders forward. The spinous processes correlating to the levels to be blocked are identified and marked. Additional marks are then made 2.5 cm laterally on the side to be blocked from the midpoint of the superior aspect of each spinous process (Fig. 52.34). In the thoracic area, due to the steep angulation of the spinous processes, the transverse process is located lateral to the spinous process of the vertebral body above it. Thus, the spinous process of the vertebra above the level to be blocked is identified. In the lumbar area, the transverse process is located lateral to the spinous process of the same vertebral body. Thus, the spinous process of the level to be blocked is identified.

Needles

A 22-gauge Tuohy needle with extention tubing is used. An 18-gauge insulated Tuohy needle with hemostasis valve/sideport as-

sembly and 50 mm tubing is used. Catheters are placed 2–2.5 cm beyond the needle tip into paravertebral space.

Technique

After cleaning the area with antiseptic solution, skin wheals of local anesthetic are raised at each needle insertion site. The needle is inserted perpendicular to the back in all planes, parallel to the neuroaxis, and advanced until it contacts the transverse process, paying careful attention to limit the initial attempt to a predetermined appropriate depth. The transverse process is usually contacted at a depth of 2–5 cm from the skin. If the transverse process is not contacted at an appropriate depth, the needle tip is assumed to lie between adjacent transverse processes, requiring redirection of the needle cephalad and then caudad, parallel to the neuroaxis. Upon successful contact with the transverse process, the depth is noted. The needle is then withdrawn to the subcutaneous tissue and redirected caudad to "walk off" the inferior border of the transverse process, passing the needle 1 cm beyond the depth at which the transverse process was contacted at the thoracic level or 0.5 cm beyond the depth at which the transverse process was contacted at the lumbar level due to the thin lumbar transverse processes. Caudad redirection of the needle is important to minimize the possibility of a pneumothorax by preventing initial inadvertent contact with the rib from being interpreted as the transverse process. If initial inadvertent contact with the rib is mistaken for the transverse process, caudad redirection will correctly identify the transverse process with subsequent contact of periosteum at a more superficial level; however, cephalad redirection at this point will lead to penetration of the pleura. At the thoracic levels, it is common to appreciate a subtle loss of resistance as the needle passes through the superior costotransverse ligament into the paravertebral space. In the lumbar region, there is no superior costotransverse ligament. If a distinct loss of resistance is sensed here, the needle has likely pierced the psoas fascia and the needle should be withdrawn to a more shallow depth.

Clinical Effects

Single-shot injection PVBs are effective regional analgesic techniques for minor and major breast cancer procedures as well as cosmetic and reconstructive breast augmentation[174–179] providing up to 23 hours of analgesia,[174] with reduction in pain VAS scores,[177,180] opioid consumption,[176,177,180] pain with movement,[177] postoperative nausea and vomiting (PONV),[176,177,180] and hospital length of stay.[176,181] In doing so, PVBs have improved postoperative pain management and side effects facilitat-

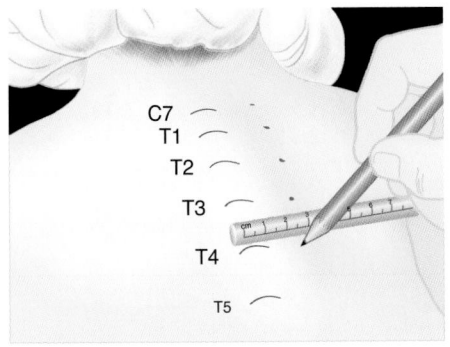

FIGURE 52.34 Identifying landmarks for paravertebral blocks.

TABLE 52.9

NUMBER AND INCIDENCE OF SERIOUS EVENTS RELATED TO UPPER EXTREMITY PERIPHERAL NERVE BLOCKS (EXCLUDING OBSTETRIC CASES)

	Peripheral Neuropathy	Respiratory Failure	Seizures	Cardiac Arrest	Death
Interscalene Block (3459 performed)	1 (2.9) (0.0–14.5)	0 (0.0–8.7)	0 (0.0–8.7)	0 (0.0–8.7)	0 (0.0–8.7)
Supraclavicular Block (1899 performed)	0 (0.0–15.9)	0 (0.0–15.9)	1 (5.3) (0.0–26.3)	0 (0.0–15.9)	0 (0.0–15.9)
Axillary Block (11,024 performed)	2 (1.8) (0.0–6.3)	0 (0.0–2.7)	1 (0.9) (0.0–4.5)	0 (0.0–2.7)	0 (0.0–2.7)

Values are expressed as n (n/10,000) (95% CI).
Table modified from Auroy Y, Benhamou D, Barques L, et al. Major complications of regional anesthesia in France. The SOS regional anesthesia hotline service. *Anesthesiology* 2002;97(5):1274–1280.

TABLE 52.10

NUMBER AND INCIDENCE OF SERIOUS EVENTS RELATED TO LOWER EXTREMITY PERIPHERAL NERVE BLOCKS (EXCLUDING OBSTETRIC CASES)

	Cardiac Arrest	Respiratory Failure	Seizures	Peripheral Neuropathy	Death
Posterior LPB (394 performed)	1 (25.4) (0.0–126.9)	2 (50.8) (0.0–177.7)	1 (25.4) (0.0–126.9)	0 (0.0–76.1)	1 (25.4) (0.0–126.9)
Femoral Block (10,309 performed)	0 (0.0–2.9)	0 (0.0–2.9)	0 (0.0–2.9)	3 (2.9) (0.0–7.8)	0 (0.0–2.9)
Sciatic Nerve Block (8507 performed)	0 (0.0–3.5)	0 (0.0–3.5)	2 (2.4) (0.0–8.2)	2 (2.4) (0.0–8.2)	0 (0.0–3.5)
Popliteal Sciatic Nerve Block (952 performed)	0 (0.0–31.5)	0 (0.0–31.5)	0 (0.0–31.5)	3 (31.5) (0.0–84.0)	0 (0.0–31.5)

Values are expressed as n (n/10,000) (95% CI).
Table modified from Auroy Y, Benhamou D, Barques L, et al. Major complications of regional anesthesia in France. The SOS regional anesthesia hotline service. *Anesthesiology* 2002;97(5):1274–1280.

TABLE 52.11

AGGREGATE ESTIMATED RATE OF OCCURRENCE OF NEUROPATHY AFTER PERIPHERAL NERVE BLOCKADE

	Estimated rate of occurrence (n = 100)	Lower CI (n = 100)	Upper CI (n = 100)	Q value	P value
Brachial Plexus Blockade					
Interscalene Block (7 studies)	2.84	1.33	5.98	90.71	S
Supraclavicular Block (1 study)	0.03	0.00	0.42	NA	NA
Axillary Block (10 studies)	1.48	0.52	4.11	315.57	S
Midhumeral Block (2 studies)	0.02	0.00	0.09	0.28	NS
Lumbar Plexus Blockade					
Postlumbar Plexus Block (3 studies)	0.19	0.02	1.93	6.18	S
Femoral Nerve Block (4 studies)	0.34	0.04	2.81	57.51	S
Sacral Plexus Blockade					
Sciatic Nerve Block (3 studies)	0.41	0.02	9.96	38.71	S
Popliteal Nerve Block (4 studies)	0.24	0.10	0.61	0.96	NS

CI, confidence interval; NA, not analyzed; NS, no significant difference; S, significant difference.
Tile estimated rate of occurrence was calculated using a random effects general linear model (see text).
Table modified from Brull R, McCartney CJ, Chan VW, et al. Neurological complications after regional anesthesia: contemporary estimates of risk. *Anesth Analg* 2007;104:965–974.

ing these surgeries in the outpatient surgical setting[174,176] with tremendous potential for cost savings.[174] A recent retrospective analysis suggests that paravertebral anesthesia and analgesia for breast cancer surgery may reduce the risk of recurrence or metastasis during the initial years of follow-up. Additionally, single-shot injection PVBs provide effective postoperative analgesia for inguinal hernia repair,[180,182,183] providing up to 14 hours of postoperative analgesia with delayed time to the first dose of opioid up to 22–24 hours[180,182] with one study reporting a zero incidence of PONV.[180]

Continuous PVB for analgesia after breast cancer surgery has been reported.[184] Continuous PVB for postthoracotomy analgesia provides analgesia of similar or better quality than epidural analgesia,[185–188] with a lower incidence of side effects, including urinary retention,[185] hypotension,[188] and PONV.[187] Additional reports exist on the safe and effective use of single injection and continuous catheter techniques for cardiac[189–191] and vascular surgery.[192]

Complications of Peripheral Nerve Blocks

While complications after regional anesthesia are uncommon, the exceedingly large number of patients needed to investigate a true incidence of these complications limits such a study.[81] Potential risks of peripheral nerve blocks are block specific and include, but are not limited to, local pain, discomfort, bruising, bleeding, infection, transient neuropathy, permanent neuropathy, paralysis, seizures, pneumothorax, respiratory failure, cardiac arrest, and death (Tables 52.9 and 52.10).[81] The incidence of neurologic deficit after surgery associated with peripheral nerve block is unclear. Determining the incidence of block-related nerve injury is limited by a variety of factors. Among such factors are inconsistent follow-up, the use of self-reporting and survey analysis of complications, the lack of standardized documentation of preoperative and postoperative neurologic function, the absence of routine postoperative neurodiagnostic testing, and the limited ability of these tests to

determine the precise etiology of nerve injury, including surgical factors such as tourniquet duration, tourniquet inflation pressure, retractor injuries, and stretch injuries producing neurologic deficits.[193] Horlocker et al.[194] reported that 89% of neurologic deficits after 1614 axillary nerve blocks were related to the surgical procedure itself.[194] Four percent of patients undergoing shoulder arthroplasty sustain brachial plexus injuries in the absence of PNB.[195] Prospective analyses of more than 70,000 patients using carefully conducted survey studies suggest incidence rates of 0.02%.[194,196] Other studies report nerve injury rates from 0% to 10% after single-shot upper extremity blocks and rates less than 0.5% for lower extremity blocks. Reports with CPNB techniques report a similar incidence. Capdevilla et al.[197] demonstrated a 0.21% incidence of nerve injuries after 1416 upper and lower extremity CPNBs, as did Swenson et al.[129] in a similar analysis of 620 CPNBs. A report on neurologic outcomes occurring after 1065 consecutive peripheral nerve blocks over a 1-year period from a single institution followed for up to 12 months reported the incidence of block-related neuropathy was 0.22% (Tables 52.11 and 52.12).[198]

The reported incidence of clinical pneumothorax in a prospective study of over 500 interscalene blocks was 0.2%.[199] In data gathered prospectively from 1001 subclavian perivascular brachial plexus blocks with a nerve stimulator, no clinical pneumothorax was reported.[200] Greengrass et al.[201] reported a 0.035%–0.5% incidence of pneumothorax with paravertebral blocks.

The associated risk of bleeding following peripheral regional anesthetic techniques in the setting of prophylactic or therapeutic anticoagulation remains undefined. In the context of LPBs, this issue is especially important as all of the cases involving PNBs and bleeding in association with anticoagulation in the 2003 ASRA consensus statement were associated with LPBs.[83,202,203] Case reports of retroperitoneal hematoma have been in the setting of low-molecular-weight heparin use. For this reason, LPBs have

TABLE 52.12

CHARACTERISTICS OF PERIOPERATIVE NERVE INJURY AFTER PERIPHERAL NERVE BLOCK

Author Date	Number of Patients	Study Design	SS vs. CC	Block Type UE	Block Type LE	Incidenc (F/U time)	Recovery (@m)	Deficit
Auroy 2002	50,223	P (Survey)	SS	All	All	0.02% (NST)	42 (6m)	Neuropathy
Auroy 1997	21,278	P (Survey)	SS	All	All	0.02% (48 hours)	100%	Neuropathy
Fanelli 1999	3996	P (Survey)	SS	ISB, AX	FB, SB	1.7% (1 month)	99% (3m)	Neuropathy
Klein 2002	2382	P	SS	All	FB, SB	0.25% (7 days)	100% (3m)	Paresthesia, Numbness
Stan 1995	1995	P	SS	AX		0.2% (NST)	100% (2m)	Sensory, Paresthesia
Horlocker 1999	1614	R	SS	AX		8.4% (2 weeks)	100% (5m)	Pain, Numbness
Candido 2005	693	P	SS	ISB		8.5% (2 days–1 month)	97% (4m)	Pain, Paresthesia, Hypesthesia, IS pain
Bishop 2005	568	R	SS	ISB		23% (2 weeks)	91% (6m)	Sensory, Neuropathy
Davis 1991	543	R	SS	BP		0% (NST)		NST
Borgeat 2001	520	P	B	ISB		14% (10 days)	99% (6m)	Paresthesia, Dysesthesia
Capdevila 2005	1416	P	CC	All	All	0.2% (24 hours)	100% (3m)	Femoral Nerve Lesions (n = 3)
Singelyn 1999	1142	P	CC		FNC	0.1% (1 week)	64% (NST)	Dysesthesia, Motor Weakness
Borgeat 2003	700	P	CC	ISC		8% (10 days)	100% (7m)	Paresthesia, Pain, Dysesthesia
Swenson 2006	620	P	CC	ISC	FNC,SC, PC	0.3% (1week)	100% (2m)	Weakness, Sensory loss
Bergman 2003	405	P	CC	AXC		1% (postop)	100% (NST)	Pain, Numbness

AX, axillary; B, both single-shot and continuous catheter; BP, brachial plexus block; CC, continuous catheter; FB, femoral block; FC, femoral nerve catheter; F/U, follow-up; ISB, interscalene block; ISC, interscalene catheter; m, months; NST, not stated; P, prospective; PC, popliteal catheter; R, retrospective; SB, sciatic block; SC, sciatic catheter; SS, single-shot.
Table includes largest studies with neurologic outcome data to assess; some incidence values reflect all neurologic deficits, regardless of surgical or block-related etiology, while others reflect only block-related deficits
Table modified from O'Connor CJ. Nerve injury after peripheral nerve blockade. *ASRA News* 2007:3–5.

TABLE 52.13

ENOXAPARIN ANTICOAGULATION GUIDELINES FOR SINGLE INJECTION PERIPHERAL NERVE BLOCK AND CONTINUOUS PERIPHERAL NERVE BLOCK AT WALTER REED ARMY MEDICAL CENTER

Definitions
- Prophylactic enoxaparin: 30 mg twice daily or 40 mg once daily.
- Therapeutic enoxaparin: 1 mg/kg twice daily or 1.5 mg/kg once daily.
- CPNB: continuous PNB (catheter).
- Single injection PNB (no catheter).

Prophylactic Enoxapatin
- Wait 10–12 hours to place/pull catheter or administer single injection block.

Therapeutic Enoxaparin
- Do not place CPNB catheters until 24 hours after last enoxaparin dose. Do not place lumbar plexus catheters if therapeutic enoxaparin will continue.
- Single injection PNBs are administered at the discretion of the staff anesthesiologist 12–24 hours after the last enoxaparin dose.

CPNB catheter is in place and enoxaparin increased from prophylactic to therapeutic dose
- Lumbar plexus catheter: recommend removal of the catheter 24 hours after last enoxaparin dose.
- Other catheters including thoracic paravertebral CPNB (the thoracic paravertebral spaces are relatively avascular): recommend continuation of CPNB therapy.
- Consider adding neurologic checks (motor function) to daily anesthesia note for patients with catheter(s) on therapeutic enoxaparin.

Catheter Removal Guidelines
- Prophylactic enoxaparin: remove the catheter 10–12 hours after the last enoxaparin dose.
- Therapeutic enoxaparin: remove the catheter ~24 hours after the last enoxaparin dose.
- Hold the next enoxapmin dose until ~2 hours after pulling a CPNB catheter.

Table modified from Buckenmaier CC, Shields CH, Auton AA, et al. Continuous peripheral nerve block in combat casulties receiving low-molecular weight heparin. *Br J Anaesth* 2006;97:874–877.

reportedly been managed more conservatively in the setting of low-molecular-weight heparin use as compared to other PNB techniques.[203,204] In a report collectively involving 305 CPNB catheters placed in 187 patients in the setting of enoxaparin use, amounting to 3082 catheter days, there were no catheter-related bleeding complications (see Tables 52.10 and 52.13).[204] Additional data is necessary to make definitive recommendations regarding nonneuraxial regional techniques in the anticoagulated

patient. Conservatively, the ASRA Consensus Statements on Neuraxial Anesthesia and Anticoagulation may be applied to plexus and peripheral techniques. However, this may be more restrictive than necessary.[83]

Major infectious adverse events are rare. Among 969 catheters (68%) submitted for culture in a multicenter study by Capdevila,[197] 278 had positive bacterial colonization (28.7%) with a single organism in 242 cases. Three percent of patients had

TABLE 52.14

RANDOMIZED CONTROLLED TRIALS USING ANALGESIC ADJUNCTS TO PERIPHERAL NERVE BLOCKS

Author	Technique	Adjunct	Local Anesthetic	Result	Systemic Control	Adverse Effects	Overall
Bourke (1993)	Axillary	Morphine 100 μg/kg	Lidocaine 1.5% with epi 5 mcg/mL	Morphine group consumed less analgesics	Yes	NA	Positive
Racz (1991)	Axillary	Morphine 5 mg	Lidocaine 1% + Bupivacaine 0.5% 40 mL (1:1)	No difference	Yes	No	Negative
Kardash (1995)	Supraclavicular	Fentanyl 75 mg	Mepivacaine 1.5% 30 mL + Epi 5 mcg/mL	No difference	Yes	NA	Negative
Singelyn (1992)	Axillary	Clonidine 150 mg	Mepivacaine 1% 40 mL + Epi 5 mcg/mL	Prolonged analgesia with clonidine	Yes	No	Positive
Kapral (1999)	Axillary	Tramadol 100 mg	Mepivacaine 1% 40 mL	Prolonged sensory/motor block	Yes	No	Positive
Candido (2001)	Axillary	Buprenorphine 0.3 mg	1% Mepivacaine, Tetracaine 0.2% 40 mL (1:1) + Epi 5 mcg/ml	Prolonged postoperative analgesia 2X control	Yes		Positive
Culebras (2001)	Interscalene	Clonidine 150mcg	Bupivacaine 0.5% 40 mL	No difference in postoperative analgesia	Yes	↓BP ↓ HR	Negative
Lee (2002)	Interscalene	Ketamine 30 mg	Ropivacaine 0.5% 30 ml	No difference in postoperative analgesia	Yes	Yes	Negative
Mannion (2005)	Posterior Lumbar Plexus	Tramadol 1.5 mg/kg	Levobupivacaine 0.5% 0.4 mL/kg	No difference	Yes	No	Negative
Couture (2004)	Femoral	Clonidine 1 mcg/kg	Bupivacaine 0.5% 30 mL	No difference	Yes	No	Negative

BP, blood pressure; HR, heartrate; NA, not applicable.
Table modified from Murphy DB, McCartney CJ, Chan VW. Novel analgesic adjuncts for brachial plexus block: a systematic review. *Anesth Analg* 2000;90: 1122–1128.

local inflammatory signs. The bacterial species most frequently found were coagulase-negative staphylococcus (61%) and gram-negative bacillus (21.6%). A *Staphylococcus aureus* psoas abscess (0.07%) was reported in one diabetic woman who had a femoral catheter after a total knee replacement. No bacteremia was found. Risk factors for local inflammation/infection were postoperative monitoring in intensive care, catheter duration greater than 48 hours, male sex, and absence of antibiotic prophylaxis.[197]

Analgesic Adjuncts for Peripheral Nerve Blocks

Efforts to prolong analgesia of PNB local anesthetic solutions with the addition of adjuncts, including but not limited to morphine,[89–91] fentanyl,[92–94] sufentanil,[95,96] buprenorphine,[90,97,98] tramadol,[99,100] ketamine,[101] and clonidine[107,108] have been investigated. A recent systematic qualitative review of double-blind RCTs on the benefit of clonidine as an adjunct to PNBs demonstrated that clonidine improved duration of analgesia when used as an adjunct to intermediate-acting local anesthetics for axillary nerve blocks. Studies to date do not allow for definitive conclusions regarding clonidine as an adjunct for other upper and lower extremity single injection and continuous nerve blocks.[205] Crucial to all investigations of perineural analgesia adjuncts is the inclusion of systemic control groups, providing evidence for or against a peripheral perineural site of action as opposed to a systemic effect of an adjunct administered peripherally (Table 52.14).

References

1. Barash PG, Cullen BF, Stoelting RK. *Clinical Anesthesia.* 4th ed. Philadelphia: Lippincott Williams & Wilkins; 2001: xvi,1576.
2. Hamber EA, Viscomi CM. Intrathecal lipophilic opioids as adjuncts to surgical spinal anesthesia. *Reg Anesth Pain Med* 1999;24(3):255–263.
3. Kovelowski CJ, Ossipov MH, Hruby VJ, et al. Lesions of the dorsolateral funiculus block supraspinal opioid delta receptor mediated antinociception in the rat. *Pain* 1999;83(2):115–122.
4. Grabow TS, Hurley RW, Banfor PN, et al. Supraspinal and spinal delta(2) opioid receptor-mediated antinociceptive synergy is mediated by spinal alpha(2) adrenoceptors. *Pain* 1999;83(1):47–55.
5. Liu N, Kuhlman G, Dalibon N, et al. A randomized, double-blinded comparison of intrathecal morphine, sufentanil and their combination versus IV morphine patient-controlled analgesia for postthoracotomy pain. *Anesth Analg* 2001;92(1):31–36.
6. Ummenhofer WC, Arends RH, Shen DD, et al. Comparative spinal distribution and clearance kinetics of intrathecally administered morphine, fentanyl, alfentanil, and sufentanil. *Anesthesiology* 2000;92(3):739–753.
7. Bernards CM, Hill HF. Physical and chemical properties of drug molecules governing their diffusion through the spinal meninges. *Anesthesiology* 1992;77(4):750–756.
8. Reuben SS, Dunn SM, Duprat KM, et al. An intrathecal fentanyl dose-response study in lower extremity revascularization procedures. *Anesthesiology* 1994;81(6):1371–1375.
9. Varrassi G, Celleno D, Capogna G, et al. Ventilatory effects of subarachnoid fentanyl in the elderly. *Anaesthesia* 1992;47(7):558–562.
10. Liu S, Chiu AA, Carpenter RL, et al. Fentanyl prolongs lidocaine spinal anesthesia without prolonging recovery. *Anesth Analg* 1995;80(4):730–734.
11. Vaghadia H, McLeod DH, Mitchell GW, et al. Small-dose hypobaric lidocaine-fentanyl spinal anesthesia for short duration outpatient laparoscopy. I. A randomized comparison with conventional dose hyperbaric lidocaine. *Anesth Analg* 1997;84(1):59–64.
12. Cornish PB. Respiratory arrest after spinal anesthesia with lidocaine and fentanyl. *Anesth Analg* 1997;84(6):1387–1388.
13. Stoelting RK. *Pharmacology and Physiology in Anesthetic Practice.* 3rd ed. Philadelphia: Lippincot Williams & Wilkins; 1999.
14. Clergue F, Montembault C, Despierres O, et al. Respiratory effects of intrathecal morphine after upper abdominal surgery. *Anesthesiology* 1984;61(6):677–685.
15. Boezaart AP, Eksteen JA, Spuy GV, et al. Intrathecal morphine. Double-blind evaluation of optimal dosage for analgesia after major lumbar spinal surgery. *Spine* 1999;24(11):1131–1137.
16. Krenn H, Jellinek H, Haumer H, et al. Naloxone-resistant respiratory depression and neurological eye symptoms after intrathecal morphine. *Anesth Analg* 2000;91(2):432–433.
17. Etches RC. Respiratory depression associated with patient-controlled analgesia: a review of eight cases. *Can J Anaesth* 1994;41(2):125–132.
18. Chaney MA. Side effects of intrathecal and epidural opioids. *Can J Anaesth* 1995;42(10):891–903.

19. Fishman SM, Benzon HT, Raja SN, et al. *Essentials of Pain Medicine and Regional Anesthesia.* 2nd ed. Philadelphia: Elsevier Churchill Livingstone; 2005.
20. Sarvela J, Halonen P, Soikkeli A, et al. A double-blinded, randomized comparison of intrathecal and epidural morphine for elective cesarean delivery. *Anesth Analg* 2002;95(2):436–440, table of contents.
21. Kelly MC, Carabine UA, Mirakhur RK. Intrathecal diamorphine for analgesia after caesarean section. A dose finding study and assessment of side-effects. *Anaesthesia* 1998;53(3):231–237.
22. Slappendel R, Weber EW, Benraad B, et al. Itching after intrathecal morphine. Incidence and treatment. *Eur J Anaesthesiol* 2000;17(10):616–621.
23. Ozalp G, Güner F, Kuru N, et al. Postoperative patient-controlled epidural analgesia with opioid bupivacaine mixtures. *Can J Anaesth* 1998;45(10):938–942.
24. Cousins MJ, Mather LE. Intrathecal and epidural administration of opioids. *Anesthesiology* 1984;61(3):276–310.
25. Bailey PL, Rhondeau S, Schafer PG, et al. Dose-response pharmacology of intrathecal morphine in human volunteers. *Anesthesiology* 1993;79(1):49–59; discussion 25A.
26. Nelson KE, Rauch T, Terebuh V, et al. A comparison of intrathecal fentanyl and sufentanil for labor analgesia. *Anesthesiology* 2002;96(5):1070–1073.
27. Gautier PE, De Kock M, Fanard L, et al. Intrathecal clonidine combined with sufentanil for labor analgesia. *Anesthesiology* 1998;88(3):651–656.
28. Eisenach JC, De Kock M, Klimscha W. Alpha(2)-adrenergic agonists for regional anesthesia. A clinical review of clonidine (1984-1995). *Anesthesiology* 1996;85(3):655–674.
29. Chiari A, Eisenach JC. Spinal anesthesia: mechanisms, agents, methods, and safety. *Reg Anesth Pain Med* 1998;23(4):357–362; discussion 384–387.
30. Gentili M, Bonnet F. Spinal clonidine produces less urinary retention than spinal morphine. *Br J Anaesth* 1996;76(6):872–873.
31. Ben-David B, Soloman E, Levin H, et al. Intrathecal fentanyl with small-dose dilute bupivacaine: better anesthesia without prolonging recovery. *Anesth Analg* 1997;85(3):560–565.
32. Roussel JR, Heindel L. Effects of intrathecal fentanyl on duration of bupivacaine spinal blockade for outpatient knee arthroscopy. *AANA J* 1999;67(4):337–343.
33. Kuusniemi KS, Pihlajamäki KK, Pitkänen MT, et al. The use of bupivacaine and fentanyl for spinal anesthesia for urologic surgery. *Anesth Analg* 2000;91(6):1452–1456.
34. Seewal R, Shende D, Kashyap L, et al. Effect of addition of various doses of fentanyl intrathecally to 0.5% hyperbaric bupivacaine on perioperative analgesia and subarachnoid-block characteristics in lower abdominal surgery: a dose-response study. *Reg Anesth Pain Med* 2007;32(1):20–26.
35. Cole PJ, Craske DA, Wheatley RG. Efficacy and respiratory effects of low-dose spinal morphine for postoperative analgesia following knee arthroplasty. *Br J Anaesth* 2000;85(2):233–237.
36. Urban MK, Jules-Elysee K, Urquhart B, et al. Reduction in postoperative pain after spinal fusion with instrumentation using intrathecal morphine. *Spine* 2002;27(5):535–537.
37. Alhashemi JA, Sharpe MD, Harris CL, et al. Effect of subarachnoid morphine administration on extubation time after coronary artery bypass graft surgery. *J Cardiothorac Vasc Anesth* 2000;14(6):639–644.
38. Mason N, Gondret R, Junca A, et al. Intrathecal sufentanil and morphine for post-thoracotomy pain relief. *Br J Anaesth* 2001;86(2):236–240.
39. Ballantyne JC, Carr DB, deFerranti S, et al. The comparative effects of postoperative analgesic therapies on pulmonary outcome: cumulative meta-analyses of randomized, controlled trials. *Anesth Analg* 1998;86(3):598–612.
40. Strebel S, Gurzeler JA, Schneider MC, et al. Small-dose intrathecal clonidine and isobaric bupivacaine for orthopedic surgery: a dose-response study. *Anesth Analg* 2004;99(4):1231–1238, table of contents.
41. Sites BD, Beach M, Biggs R, et al. Intrathecal clonidine added to a bupivacaine-morphine spinal anesthetic improves postoperative analgesia for total knee arthroplasty. *Anesth Analg* 2003;96(4):1083–1088, table of contents.
42. Bernards CM. Understanding the physiology and pharmacology of epidural and intrathecal opioids. *Best Pract Res Clin Anaesthesiol* 2002;16(4):489–505.
43. Cooper DW. Can epidural fentanyl induce selective spinal hyperalgesia? *Anesthesiology* 2000;93(4):1153–1154.
44. Bernards CM. Rostral spread of epidural morphine: the expected and the unexpected. *Anesthesiology* 2000;92(2):299–301.
45. Angst MS, Ramaswamy B, Riley ET, et al. Lumbar epidural morphine in humans and supraspinal analgesia to experimental heat pain. *Anesthesiology* 2000;92(2):312–324.
46. Connelly NR, DuBose R, Brull SJ. Use of single-dose epidural morphine in a patient undergoing an abdominal aortic aneurysm resection. *J Clin Anesth* 1990;2(4):272–275.
47. Ready LB, Chadwick HS, Ross B. Age predicts effective epidural morphine dose after abdominal hysterectomy. *Anesth Analg* 1987;66(12):1215–1218.
48. Hartrick CT, Martin G, Kantor G, et al. Evaluation of a single-dose, extended-release epidural morphine formulation for pain after knee arthroplasty. *J Bone Joint Surg Am* 2006;88(2):273–281.
49. Viscusi ER, Martin G, Hartrick CT, et al. Forty-eight hours of postoperative pain relief after total hip arthroplasty with a novel, extended-release epidural morphine formulation. *Anesthesiology* 2005;102(5):1014–1022.
50. Gambling D, Hughes T, Martin G, et al. A comparison of Depodur, a novel, single-dose extended-release epidural morphine, with standard epidural mor-

phine for pain relief after lower abdominal surgery. *Anesth Analg* 2005; 100(4):1065–1074.

51. Birnbach DJ, Johnson MD, Arcario T, et al. Effect of diluent volume on analgesia produced by epidural fentanyl. *Anesth Analg* 1989;68(6):808–810.

52. Dottrens M, Rifat K, Morel DR. Comparison of extradural administration of sufentanil, morphine and sufentanil-morphine combination after caesarean section. *Br J Anaesth* 1992;69(1):9–12.

53. Chaplan SR, Duncan SR, Brodsky JB, et al. Morphine and hydromorphone epidural analgesia. A prospective, randomized comparison. *Anesthesiology* 1992;77(6):1090–1094.

54. Mulroy MF. Monitoring Opioids. *Reg Anesth* 1996;21(6 Suppl):89–93.

55. de Leon-Casasola OA, Parker B, Lema MJ, et al. Postoperative epidural bupivacaine-morphine therapy. Experience with 4,227 surgical cancer patients. *Anesthesiology* 1994;81(2):368–375.

56. de Leon-Casasola OA, Parker BM, Lema MJ, et al. Epidural analgesia versus intravenous patient-controlled analgesia. Differences in the postoperative course of cancer patients. *Anesthesiology* 1994;19(5):307–315.

57. Ready LB, Loper KA, Nessly M, et al. Postoperative epidural morphine is safe on surgical wards. *Anesthesiology* 1991;75(3):452–456.

58. Tzeng JI, Hsing CH, Chu CC, et al. Low-dose dexamethasone reduces nausea and vomiting after epidural morphine: a comparison of metoclopramide with saline. *J Clin Anesth* 2002;14(1):19–23.

59. Wang JJ, Tzeng JI, Ho ST, et al. The prophylactic effect of tropisetron on epidural morphine-related nausea and vomiting: a comparison of dexamethasone with saline. *Anesth Analg* 2002;94(3):749–753; table of contents.

60. Wheatley RG, Schug SA, Watson D. Safety and efficacy of postoperative epidural analgesia. *Br J Anaesth* 2001;87(1):47–61.

61. Gedney JA, Liu EH. Side-effects of epidural infusions of opioid bupivacaine mixtures. *Anaesthesia* 1998;53(12):1148–1155.

62. Nakata K, Mammoto T, Kita T, et al. Continuous epidural, not intravenous, droperidol inhibits pruritus, nausea, and vomiting during epidural morphine analgesia. *J Clin Anesth* 2002;14(2):121–125.

63. Biasi D, Caramaschi P, Carletto A, et al. Symmetric multiple lipomatosis with Charcot's joint and neuropathic ulcer. Description of a clinical case. *Minerva Med* 1993;84(3):135–139.

64. Milner AR, Bogod DG, Harwood RJ. Intrathecal administration of morphine for elective Caesarean section. A comparison between 0.1 mg and 0.2 mg. *Anaesthesia* 1996;51(9):871–873.

65. Kirson LE, Goldman JM, Slover RB. Low-dose intrathecal morphine for postoperative pain control in patients undergoing transurethral resection of the prostate. *Anesthesiology* 1989;71(2):192–195.

66. Walder B, Schafer M, Henzi I, et al. Efficacy and safety of patient-controlled opioid analgesia for acute postoperative pain. A quantitative systematic review. *Acta Anaesthesiol Scand* 2001;45(7):795–804.

67. Kjellberg F, Tramèr MR. Pharmacological control of opioid-induced pruritus: A quantitative systematic review of randomized trials. *Eur J Anaesthesiol* 2001;18(6):346–357.

68. Ko MC, Naughton NN. An experimental itch model in monkeys: characterization of intrathecal morphine-induced scratching and antinociception. *Anesthesiology* 2000;92(3):795–805.

69. O'Riordan JA, Hopkins PM, Ravenscroft A, et al. Patient-controlled analgesia and urinary retention following lower limb joint replacement: prospective audit and logistic regression analysis. *Eur J Anaesthesiol* 2000;17(7):431–435.

70. Armand S, Langlade A, Boutros A, et al. Meta-analysis of the efficacy of extradural clonidine to relieve postoperative pain: an impossible task. *Br J Anaesth* 1998;81(2):126–134.

71. van Essen EJ, Bovill JG, Ploeger EJ. Extradural clonidine does not potentiate analgesia produced by extradural morphine after meniscectomy. *Br J Anaesth* 1991;66(2):237–241.

72. Rockemann MG, Seeling W, Brinkmann A, et al. Analgesic and hemodynamic effects of epidural clonidine, clonidine/morphine, and morphine after pancreatic surgery—a double-blind study. *Anesth Analg* 1995;80(5):869–874.

73. Carabine UA, Milligan KR, Mulholland D, et al. Extradural clonidine infusions for analgesia after total hip replacement. *Br J Anaesth* 1992;68(4):338–343.

74. Walker SM, Goudas LC, Cousins MJ, et al. Combination spinal analgesic chemotherapy: a systematic review. *Anesth Analg* 2002;95(3):674–715.

75. Hjortsø NC, Lund C, Mogensen T, et al. Epidural morphine improves pain relief and maintains sensory analgesia during continuous epidural bupivacaine after abdominal surgery. *Anesth Analg* 1986;65(10):1033–1036.

76. Vercauteren M, Meert TF. Isobolographic analysis of the interaction between epidural sufentanil and bupivacaine in rats. *Pharmacol Biochem Behav* 1997; 58(1):237–242.

77. Torda TA, Hann P, Mills G, et al. Comparison of extradural fentanyl, bupivacaine and two fentanyl-bupivacaine mixtures of pain relief after abdominal surgery. *Br J Anaesth* 1995;74(1):35–40.

78. Seeberger MD, Lang ML, Drewe J, et al. Comparison of spinal and epidural anesthesia for patients younger than 50 years of age. *Anesth Analg* 1994; 78(4):667–673.

79. Wu CL, Rowlingson AJ, Cohen SR, et al. Gender and post-dural puncture headache. *Anesthesiology* 2006;105(3):613–618.

80. Vandam LD, Dripps RD. Long-term follow-up of patients who received 10,098 spinal anesthetics; syndrome of decreased intracranial pressure (headache and ocular and auditory difficulties). *J Am Med Assoc* 1956;161(7):586–591.

81. Brull R, McCartney CJ, Chan VW, et al. Neurological complications after regional anesthesia: contemporary estimates of risk. *Anesth Analg* 2007;104(4):965–974.

82. Cameron CM, et al. A review of neuraxial epidural morbidity: experience of more than 8,000 cases at a single teaching hospital. *Anesthesiology* 2007;106(5):997–1002.

83. Horlocker TT, Wedel DJ, Benzon H, et al. Regional anesthesia in the anticoagulated patient: defining the risks (the second ASRA Consensus Conference on Neuraxial Anesthesia and Anticoagulation). *Reg Anesth Pain Med* 2003;28(3):172–197.

84. Grant SA, Nielsen KC, Greengrass RA, et al. Continuous peripheral nerve block for ambulatory surgery. *Reg Anesth Pain Med* 2001;26(3):209–214.

85. Racz H, Gunning K, Della Santa D, et al. Evaluation of the effect of perineuronal morphine on the quality of postoperative analgesia after axillary plexus block: a randomized double-blind study. *Anesth Analg* 1991;72(6):769–772.

86. Viel EJ, Eledjam JJ, De La Coussaye JE, et al. Brachial plexus block with opioids for postoperative pain relief: comparison between buprenorphine and morphine. *Reg Anesth* 1989;14(6):274–278.

87. Flory N, Van-Gessel E, Donald F, et al. Does the addition of morphine to brachial plexus block improve analgesia after shoulder surgery? *Br J Anaesth* 1995;75(1):23–26.

88. Kardash K, Schools A, Concepcion M. Effects of brachial plexus fentanyl on supraclavicular block. A randomized, double-blind study. *Reg Anesth* 1995; 20(4):311–315.

89. Karakaya D, Büyükgöz F, Bariş S, et al. Addition of fentanyl to bupivacaine prolongs anesthesia and analgesia in axillary brachial plexus block. *Reg Anesth Pain Med* 2001;26(5):434–438.

90. Nishikawa K, Kanaya N, Nakayama M, et al. Fentanyl improves analgesia but prolongs the onset of axillary brachial plexus block by peripheral mechanism. *Anesth Analg* 2000;91(2):384–387.

91. Bazin JE, Massoni C, Groslier D, et al. Brachial plexus block: effect of the addition of sufentanil to local anesthetic mixture on postoperative analgesia duration [Article in French]. *Ann Fr Anesth Reanim* 1997;16(1):9–13.

92. Bouaziz H, Kinirons BP, Macalou D, et al. Sufentanil does not prolong the duration of analgesia in a mepivacaine brachial plexus block: a dose response study. *Anesth Analg* 2000;90(2):383–387.

93. Candido KD, Franco CD, Khan MA, et al. Buprenorphine added to the local anesthetic for brachial plexus block to provide postoperative analgesia in outpatients. *Reg Anesth Pain Med* 2001;26(4):352–356.

94. Candido KD, Winnie AP, Ghaleb AH, et al. Buprenorphine added to the local anesthetic for axillary brachial plexus block prolongs postoperative analgesia. *Reg Anesth Pain Med* 2002;27(2):162–167.

95. Kapral S, Gollmann G, Waltl B, et al. Tramadol added to mepivacaine prolongs the duration of an axillary brachial plexus blockade. *Anesth Analg* 1999;88(4):853–856.

96. Mannion S, O'Callaghan S, Murphy DB, et al. Tramadol as adjunct to psoas compartment block with levobupivacaine 0.5%: a randomized double-blinded study. *Br J Anaesth* 2005;94(3):352–356.

97. Lee IO, Kim WK, Kong MH, et al. No enhancement of sensory and motor blockade by ketamine added to ropivacaine interscalene brachial plexus blockade. *Acta Anaesthesiol Scand* 2002;46(7):821–826.

98. Casati A, Magistris L, Fanelli G, et al. Small-dose clonidine prolongs postoperative analgesia after sciatic-femoral nerve block with 0.75% ropivacaine for foot surgery. *Anesth Analg* 2000;91(2):388–392.

99. Couture DJ, Cuniff HM, Maye JP, et al. The addition of clonidine to bupivacaine in combined femoral-sciatic nerve block for anterior cruciate ligament reconstruction. *AANA J* 2004;72(4):273–278.

100. Mannion S, Hayes I, Loughnane F, et al. Intravenous but not perineural clonidine prolongs postoperative analgesia after psoas compartment block with 0.5% levobupivacaine for hip fracture surgery. *Anesth Analg* 2005;100(3):873–878, table of contents.

101. Singelyn FJ, Gouverneur JM, Robert A. A minimum dose of clonidine added to mepivacaine prolongs the duration of anesthesia and analgesia after axillary brachial plexus block. *Anesth Analg* 1996;83(5):1046–1050.

102. Singelyn FJ, Dangoisse M, Bartholomée S, et al. Adding clonidine to mepivacaine prolongs the duration of anesthesia and analgesia after axillary brachial plexus block. *Reg Anesth* 1992;17(3):148–150.

103. Eledjam JJ, Deschodt J, Viel EJ, et al. Brachial plexus block with bupivacaine: effects of added alpha-adrenergic agonists: comparison between clonidine and epinephrine. *Can J Anaesth* 1991;38(7):870–875.

104. Iskandar H, Benard A, Ruel-Raymond J, et al. The analgesic effect of interscalene block using clonidine as an analgesic for shoulder arthroscopy. *Anesth Analg* 2003;96(1):260–262, table of contents.

105. Ilfeld BM, Vandenborne K, Duncan PW, et al. Ambulatory continuous interscalene nerve blocks decrease the time to discharge readiness after total shoulder arthroplasty: a randomized, triple-masked, placebo-controlled study. *Anesthesiology* 2006;105(5):999–1007.

106. Ilfeld BM, Gearan PF, Enneking FK, et al. Total hip arthroplasty as an overnight-stay procedure using an ambulatory continuous psoas compartment nerve block: a prospective feasibility study. *Reg Anesth Pain Med* 2006;31(2):113–118.

107. Ilfeld BM, Gearan PF, Enneking FK, et al. Total knee arthroplasty as an overnight-stay procedure using continuous femoral nerve blocks at home: a prospective feasibility study. *Anesth Analg* 2006;102(1):87–90.

108. Ilfeld BM, Wright TW, Enneking FK, et al. Total shoulder arthroplasty as an

outpatient procedure using ambulatory perineural local anesthetic infusion: a pilot feasibility study. *Anesth Analg* 2005;101(5):1319–1322.

109. Ilfeld BM, Wright TW, Enneking FK, et al. Total elbow arthroplasty as an outpatient procedure using a continuous infraclavicular nerve block at home: a prospective case report. *Reg Anesth Pain Med* 2006;31(2):172–176.

110. Ilfeld BM, Enneking FK. Continuous peripheral nerve blocks at home: a review. *Anesth Analg* 2005;100(6):1822–1833.

111. Klein SM, Evans H, Nielsen KC, et al. Peripheral nerve block techniques for ambulatory surgery. *Anesth Analg* 2005;101(6):1663–1676.

112. Klein SM, Nielsen KC, Greengrass RA, et al. Ambulatory discharge after long-acting peripheral nerve blockade: 2382 blocks with ropivacaine. *Anesth Analg* 2002;94(1):65–70, table of contents.

113. Knudsen K, Beckman Suurküla M, Blomberg S, et al. Central nervous and cardiovascular effects of i.v. infusions of ropivacaine, bupivacaine and placebo in volunteers. *Br J Anaesth* 1997;78(5):507–514.

114. Stojadinovic A, Auton A, Peoples GE, et al. Responding to challenges in modern combat casualty care: innovative use of advanced regional anesthesia. *Pain Med* 2006;7(4):330–338.

115. Buckenmaier CC, McKnight GM, Winkley JV, et al. Continuous peripheral nerve block for battlefield anesthesia and evacuation. *Reg Anesth Pain Med* 2005;30(2):202–205.

116. Richman JM, Liu SS, Courpas G, et al. Does continuous peripheral nerve block provide superior pain control to opioids? A meta-analysis. *Anesth Analg* 2006;102(1):248–257.

117. Marhofer P, Chan W. Ultrasound-guided regional anesthesia: current concepts and future trends. *Anesth Analg* 2007;104(5):1265–9, tables of contents.

118. Urmey WF, Talts KH, Sharrock NE. One hundred percent incidence of hemidiaphragmatic paresis associated with interscalene brachial plexus anesthesia as diagnosed by ultrasonography. *Anesth Analg* 1991;72(4):498–503.

119. Urmey WF, McDonald M. Hemidiaphragmatic paresis during interscalene brachial plexus block: effects on pulmonary function and chest wall mechanics. *Anesth Analg* 1992;74(3):352–357.

120. Al-Kaisy A, McGuire G, Chan VW, et al. Analgesic effect of interscalene block using low-dose bupivacaine for outpatient arthroscopic shoulder surgery. *Reg Anesth Pain Med* 1998;23(5):469–473.

121. Brown AR, Weiss R, Greenberg C, et al. Interscalene block for shoulder arthroscopy: comparison with general anesthesia. *Arthroscopy* 1993;9(3):295–300.

122. Kinnard P, Truchon R, St-Pierre A, et al. Interscalene block for pain relief after shoulder surgery. A prospective randomized study. *Clin Orthop Relat Res* 1994;304:22–24.

123. Singelyn FJ, Lhotel L, Fabre B. Pain relief after arthroscopic shoulder surgery: a comparison of intraarticular analgesia, suprascapular nerve block, and interscalene brachial plexus block. *Anesth Analg* 2004;99(2):589–592, table of contents.

124. Laurila PA, Löppönen A, Kanga-Saarela T, et al. Interscalene brachial plexus block is superior to subacromial bursa block after arthroscopic shoulder surgery. *Acta Anaesthesiol Scand* 2002;46(8):1031–1036.

125. Arciero RA, Taylor DC, Harrison SA, et al. Interscalene anesthesia for shoulder arthroscopy in a community-sized military hospital. *Arthroscopy* 1996;12(6):715–719.

126. D'Alessio JG, Rosenblum M, Shea KP, et al. A retrospective comparison of interscalene block and general anesthesia for ambulatory surgery shoulder arthroscopy. *Reg Anesth* 1995;20(1):62–68.

127. Chelly JE, Greger J, Al Samsam T, et al. Reduction of operating and recovery room times and overnight hospital stays with interscalene blocks as sole anesthetic technique for rotator cuff surgery. *Minerva Anestesiol* 2001;67(9):613–619.

128. Tuominen M, Haasio J, Hekali R, et al. Continuous interscalene brachial plexus block: clinical efficacy, technical problems and bupivacaine plasma concentrations. *Acta Anaesthesiol Scand* 1989;33(1):84–88.

129. Swenson JD, Bay N, Loose E, et al. Outpatient management of continuous peripheral nerve catheters placed using ultrasound guidance: an experience in 620 patients. *Anesth Analg* 2006;103(6):1436–1443.

130. Boezaart AP, de Beer JF, du Toit C, et al. A new technique of continuous interscalene nerve block. *Can J Anaesth* 1999;46(3):275–281.

131. Borgeat A, Tewes E, Biasca N, et al. *Patient-controlled interscalene analgesia with ropivacaine after major shoulder surgery: PCIA vs PCA. Br J Anaesth* 1998;81(4):603–605.

132. Kean J, Wigderowitz CA, Coventry DM. Continuous interscalene infusion and single injection using levobupivacaine for analgesia after surgery of the shoulder. A double-blind, randomised controlled trial. *J Bone Joint Surg Br* 2006;88(9):1173–1177.

133. Klein SM, Grant SA, Greengrass RA, et al. Interscalene brachial plexus block with a continuous catheter insertion system and a disposable infusion pump. *Anesth Analg* 2000;91(6):1473–1478.

134. Borgeat A, Schäppi B, Biasca N, et al. Patient-controlled analgesia after major shoulder surgery: patient-controlled interscalene analgesia versus patient-controlled analgesia. *Anesthesiology* 1997;87(6):1343–1347.

135. Borgeat A, Kalberer F, Jacob H, et al. Patient-controlled interscalene analgesia with ropivacaine 0.2% versus bupivacaine 0.15% after major open shoulder surgery: the effects on hand motor function. *Anesth Analg* 2001;92(1):218–223.

136. Lehtipalo S, Koskinen LO, Johansson G, et al. Continuous interscalene brachial plexus block for postoperative analgesia following shoulder surgery. *Acta Anaesthesiol Scand* 1999;43(3):258–264.

137. Ilfeld BM, Enneking FK. A portable mechanical pump providing over four days of patient-controlled analgesia by perineural infusion at home. *Reg Anesth Pain Med* 2002;27(1):100–104.

138. Ilfeld BM, Morey TE, Wright TW, et al. Continuous interscalene brachial plexus block for postoperative pain control at home: a randomized, double-blinded, placebo-controlled study. *Anesth Analg* 2003;96(4):1089–1095, table of contents.

139. Nielsen KC, Greengrass RA, Pietrobon R, et al. Continuous interscalene brachial plexus blockade provides good analgesia at home after major shoulder surgery-report of four cases. *Can J Anaesth* 2003;50(1):57–61.

140. Capdevila X, Macaire P, Aknin P, et al. Patient-controlled perineural analgesia after ambulatory orthopedic surgery: a comparison of electronic versus elastomeric pumps. *Anesth Analg* 2003;96(2):414–417, table of contents.

141. Rawal N, Allvin R, Axelsson K, et al. Patient-controlled regional analgesia (PCRA) at home: controlled comparison between bupivacaine and ropivacaine brachial plexus analgesia. *Anesthesiology* 2002;96(6):1290–1296.

142. Russon K, Sardesi AM, Ridgway S, et al. Postoperative shoulder surgery initiative (POSSI): an interim report of major shoulder surgery as a day case procedure. *Br J Anaesth* 2006;97(6):869–873.

143. Wilson AT, Nicholson E, Burton L, et al. Analgesia for day-case shoulder surgery. *Br J Anaesth* 2004;92(3):414–415.

144. Vaghadia H, Chan V, Ganapathy S, et al. A multicentre trial of ropivacaine 7.5 mg × ml(−1) vs bupivacaine 5 mg × ml(−1) for supra clavicular brachial plexus anesthesia. *Can J Anaesth* 1999;46(10):946–951.

145. Cox CR, Checketts MR, Mackenzie N, et al. Comparison of S(-)-bupivacaine with racemic (RS)-bupivacaine in supraclavicular brachial plexus block. *Br J Anaesth* 1998;80(5):594–598.

146. Pham-Dang C, Gunst JP, Gouin F, et al. A novel supraclavicular approach to brachial plexus block. *Anesth Analg* 1997;85(1):111–116.

147. Hadzic A.Arliss J, Kerimoglu B, et al. A comparison of infraclavicular nerve block versus general anesthesia for hand and wrist day-case surgeries. *Anesthesiology* 2004;101(1):127–132.

148. Ilfeld BM, Morey TE, Enneking FK. Infraclavicular perineural local anesthetic infusion: a comparison of three dosing regimens for postoperative analgesia. *Anesthesiology* 2004;100(2):395–402.

149. Ilfeld BM, Morey TE, Enneking FK. Continuous infraclavicular perineural infusion with clonidine and ropivacaine compared with ropivacaine alone: a randomized, double-blinded, controlled study. *Anesth Analg* 2003;97(3):706–712.

150. Ilfeld BM, Morey TE, Enneking FK. Continuous infraclavicular brachial plexus block for postoperative pain control at home: a randomized, double-blinded, placebo-controlled study. *Anesthesiology* 2002;96(6):1297–1304.

151. McCartney CJ, Burll R, Chan VW, et al. Early but no long-term benefit of regional compared with general anesthesia for ambulatory hand surgery. *Anesthesiology* 2004;101(2):461–467.

152. Chan VW, Peng PW, Kaszas Z, et al. A comparative study of general anesthesia, intravenous regional anesthesia, and axillary block for outpatient hand surgery: clinical outcome and cost analysis. *Anesth Analg* 2001;93(5):1181–1184.

153. Mezzatesta JP, Scott DA, Schweitzer SA, et al. Continuous axillary brachial plexus block for postoperative pain relief. Intermittent bolus versus continuous infusion. *Reg Anesth* 1997;22(4):357–362.

154. Mulroy MF, Larkin KL, Batra MS, et al. Femoral nerve block with 0.25% or 0.5% bupivacaine improves postoperative analgesia following outpatient arthroscopic anterior cruciate ligament repair. *Reg Anesth Pain Med* 2001;26(1):24–29.

155. Edkin BS, Spindler KP, Flanagan JF. Femoral nerve block as an alternative to parenteral narcotics for pain control after anterior cruciate ligament reconstruction. *Arthroscopy* 1995;11(4):404–409.

156. Williams BA, Kentor ML, Vogt MT, et al. Femoral-sciatic nerve blocks for complex outpatient knee surgery are associated with less postoperative pain before same-day discharge: a review of 1,200 consecutive cases from the period 1996-1999. *Anesthesiology* 2003;98(5):1206–1213.

157. Wang H, Boctor B, Verner J. The effect of single-injection femoral nerve block on rehabilitation and length of hospital stay after total knee replacement. *Reg Anesth Pain Med* 2002;27(2):139–144.

158. Cook P, Stevens J, Gaudron C. Comparing the effects of femoral nerve block versus femoral and sciatic nerve block on pain and opiate consumption after total knee arthroplasty. *J Arthroplasty* 2003;18(5):583–586.

159. Davies AF, Segar EP, Murdoch J, et al. Epidural infusion or combined femoral and sciatic nerve blocks as perioperative analgesia for knee arthroplasty. *Br J Anaesth* 2004;93(3):368–374.

160. Ben-David B, Schmalenberger K, Chelly JE. Analgesia after total knee arthroplasty: is continuous sciatic blockade needed in addition to continuous femoral blockade? *Anesth Analg* 2004;98(3):747–749, table of contents.

161. Pham Dang C, Gautheron E, Guilley J, et al. The value of adding sciatic block to continuous femoral block for analgesia after total knee replacement. *Reg Anesth Pain Med* 2005;30(2):128–133.

162. Allen HW, Liu SS, Ware PD, et al. Peripheral nerve blocks improve analgesia after total knee replacement surgery. *Anesth Analg* 1998;87(1):93–97.

163. Hirst GC, Lang SA, Dust WN, et al. Femoral nerve block. Single injection versus continuous infusion for total knee arthroplasty. *Reg Anesth* 1996;21(4):292–297.

164. Salinas FV, Liu SS, Mulroy MF. The effect of single-injection femoral nerve

block versus continuous femoral nerve block after total knee arthroplasty on hospital length of stay and long-term functional recovery within an established clinical pathway. *Anesth Analg* 2006;102(4):1234–1239.

165. Singelyn FJ, Deyaert M, Joris D, et al. Effects of intravenous patient-controlled analgesia with morphine, continuous epidural analgesia, and continuous three-in-one block on postoperative pain and knee rehabilitation after unilateral total knee arthroplasty. *Anesth Analg* 1998;87(1):88–92.

166. Capdevila X, Barthelet Y, Biboulet P, et al. Effects of perioperative analgesic technique on the surgical outcome and duration of rehabilitation after major knee surgery. *Anesthesiology* 1999;91(1):8–15.

167. Taboada M, Alvarez J, Cortés J, et al. The effects of three different approaches on the onset time of sciatic nerve blocks with 0.75% ropivacaine. *Anesth Analg* 2004;98(1):242–247, table of contents.

168. Rongstad K, Mann R, Prieskorn D, et al. Popliteal sciatic nerve block for postoperative analgesia. *Foot Ankle Int* 1996;17(7):378–382.

169. Singelyn FJ, Gouverneur JM, Gribomont BF. Popliteal sciatic nerve block aided by a nerve stimulator: a reliable technique for foot and ankle surgery. *Reg Anesth* 1991;16(5):278–281.

170. McLeod DH, Wong DH, Vaghadia H, et al. Lateral popliteal sciatic nerve block compared with ankle block for analgesia following foot surgery. *Can J Anaesth* 1995;42(9):765–769.

171. White PF, Issioui T, Skrivanek GD, et al. The use of a continuous popliteal sciatic nerve block after surgery involving the foot and ankle: does it improve the quality of recovery? *Anesth Analg* 2003;97(5):1303–1309.

172. Singelyn FJ, Aye F, Gouverneur JM. Continuous popliteal sciatic nerve block: an original technique to provide postoperative analgesia after foot surgery. *Anesth Analg* 1997;84(2):383–386.

173. Ilfeld BM, Morety TE, Wang RD, et al. Continuous popliteal sciatic nerve block for postoperative pain control at home: a randomized, double-blinded, placebo-controlled study. *Anesthesiology* 2002;97(4):959–965.

174. Weltz CR, Greengrass RA, Lyerly HK. Ambulatory surgical management of breast carcinoma using paravertebral block. *Ann Surg* 1995;222(1):19–26.

175. Greengrass R, O'Brien F, Lyerly K, et al. Paravertebral block for breast cancer surgery. *Can J Anaesth* 1996;43(8):858–861.

176. Coveney E, Weltz CR, Greengrass R, et al. Use of paravertebral block anesthesia in the surgical management of breast cancer: experience in 156 cases. *Ann Surg* 1998;227(4):496–501.

177. Pusch F, Freitag H, Weinstabl C, et al. Single-injection paravertebral block compared to general anaesthesia in breast surgery. *Acta Anaesthesiol Scand* 1999;43(7):770–774.

178. Klein SM, Bergh A, Steele SM, et al. Thoracic paravertebral block for breast surgery. *Anesth Analg* 2000;90(6):1402–1405.

179. Terheggen MA, Wille F, Borel Rinkes IH, et al. Paravertebral blockade for minor breast surgery. *Anesth Analg* 2002;94(2):355–359, table of contents.

180. Naja MZ, el Hassan MJ, Oweidat M, et al. Paravertebral blockade vs general anesthesia or spinal anesthesia for inguinal hernia repair. *Middle East J Anesthesiol* 2001;16(2):201–210.

181. Naja MZ, Ziade MF, Lonnqvist PA. Nerve-stimulator guided paravertebral blockade vs. general anaesthesia for breast surgery: a prospective randomized trial. *Eur J Anaesthesiol* 2003;20(11):897–903.

182. Klein SM, Greengrass RA, Weltz C, et al. Paravertebral somatic nerve block for outpatient inguinal herniorrhaphy: an expanded case report of 22 patients. *Reg Anesth Pain Med* 1998;23(3):306–310.

183. Weltz CR, Klein SM, Arbo JE, et al. Paravertebral block anesthesia for inguinal hernia repair. *World J Surg* 2003;27(4):425–429.

184. Buckenmaier CC 3rd, Klein SM, Nielsen KC, et al. Continuous paravertebral catheter and outpatient infusion for breast surgery. *Anesth Analg* 2003;97(3):715–717.

185. Matthews PJ, Govenden V. Comparison of continuous paravertebral and ex-

tradural infusions of bupivacaine for pain relief after thoracotomy. *Br J Anaesth* 1989;62(2):204–205.

186. Perttunen K, Nilsson E, Heinonen J, et al. Extradural, paravertebral and intercostal nerve blocks for post-thoracotomy pain. *Br J Anaesth* 1995;75(5):541–547.

187. Richardson J, Sabanathan S, Jones J, et al. A prospective, randomized comparison of preoperative and continuous balanced epidural or paravertebral bupivacaine on post-thoracotomy pain, pulmonary function and stress responses. *Br J Anaesth* 1999;83(3):387–392.

188. Casati A, Alessandrini P, Nuzzi M, et al. A prospective, randomized, blinded comparison between continuous thoracic paravertebral and epidural infusion of 0.2% ropivacaine after lung resection surgery. *Eur J Anaesthesiol* 2006;23(12):999–1004.

189. Cantó M, Sánchez MJ, Casas MA, et al. Bilateral paravertebral blockade for conventional cardiac surgery. *Anaesthesia* 2003;58(4):365–370.

190. Ganapathy S, Murkin JM, Boyd DW, et al. Continuous percutaneous paravertebral block for minimally invasive cardiac surgery. *J Cardiothorac Vasc Anesth* 1999;13(5):594–596.

191. Dhole S, Mehta Y, Saxena H, et al. Comparison of continuous thoracic epidural and paravertebral blocks for postoperative analgesia after minimally invasive direct coronary artery bypass surgery. *J Cardiothorac Vasc Anesth* 2001;15(3):288–292.

192. Richardson J, Vowden P, Sabanathan S. Bilateral paravertebral analgesia for major abdominal vascular surgery: a preliminary report. *Anaesthesia* 1995;50(11):995–998.

193. O'Connor C. Nerve injury after peripheral nerve blockade. *ASRA News* 2007:3–5.

194. Horlocker TT, Kufner RP, Bishop AT, et al. The risk of persistent paresthesia is not increased with repeated axillary block. *Anesth Analg* 1999;88(2):382–387.

195. Lynch NM, Cofield RH, Silbert PL, et al. Neurologic complications after total shoulder arthroplasty. *J Shoulder Elbow Surg* 1996;5(1):53–61.

196. Fanelli G, Casati A, Garancini P, et al. Nerve stimulator and multiple injection technique for upper and lower limb blockade: failure rate, patient acceptance, and neurologic complications. Study Group on Regional Anesthesia. *Anesth Analg* 1999;88(4):847–852.

197. Capdevila X, Pirat P, Bringuier S, et al. Continuous peripheral nerve blocks in hospital wards after orthopedic surgery: a multicenter prospective analysis of the quality of postoperative analgesia and complications in 1,416 patients. *Anesthesiology* 2005;103(5):1035–1045.

198. Watts SA, Sharma DJ. Long-term neurological complications associated with surgery and peripheral nerve blockade: outcomes after 1065 consecutive blocks. *Anaesth Intensive Care* 2007;35(1):24–31.

199. Borgeat A, Ekatodramis G, Kalberer F, et al. Acute and nonacute complications associated with interscalene block and shoulder surgery: a prospective study. *Anesthesiology* 2001;95(4):875–880.

200. Franco CD, Vieira CE. 1,001 subclavian perivascular brachial plexus blocks: success with a nerve stimulator. *Reg Anesth Pain Med* 2000;25(1):41–46.

201. Greengrass R, Buckenmaier CC 3rd. Paravertebral anaesthesia/analgesia for ambulatory surgery. *Best Pract Res Clin Anaesthesiol* 2002;16(2):271–283.

202. Klein SM, D'Ercole F, Greengrass RA, et al. Enoxaparin associated with psoas hematoma and lumbar plexopathy after lumbar plexus block. *Anesthesiology* 1997;87(6):1576–1579.

203. Weller RS, Gerancher JC, Crew JC, et al. Extensive retroperitoneal hematoma without neurologic deficit in two patients who underwent lumbar plexus block and were later anticoagulated. *Anesthesiology* 2003;98(2):581–585.

204. Buckenmaier CC 3rd, Shields CH, Auton AA, et al. Continuous peripheral nerve block in combat casualties receiving low-molecular weight heparin. *Br J Anaesth* 2006;97(6):874–877.

205. McCartney CJ, Duggan E, Apatu E. Should we add clonidine to local anesthetic for peripheral nerve blockade? A qualitative systematic review of the literature. *Reg Anesth Pain Med* 2007;32(4):330–338.

CHAPTER 53 ■ BURN PAIN

SAM R. SHARAR AND DAVID R. PATTERSON

INTRODUCTION

If burn injuries in themselves are not the most painful type of trauma a person can sustain, then they likely reach this status once the nature of their treatment is considered. Contemporary treatment of burn injuries involves a multitude of invasive and rehabilitative procedures that continue—often on a daily basis—for days, weeks, or months. Each intervention is critical to achieving optimal wound healing and long-term physical/occupational function, yet has the potential for inflicting more pain, on a repeated basis, than that of the initial trauma. Burn injuries are

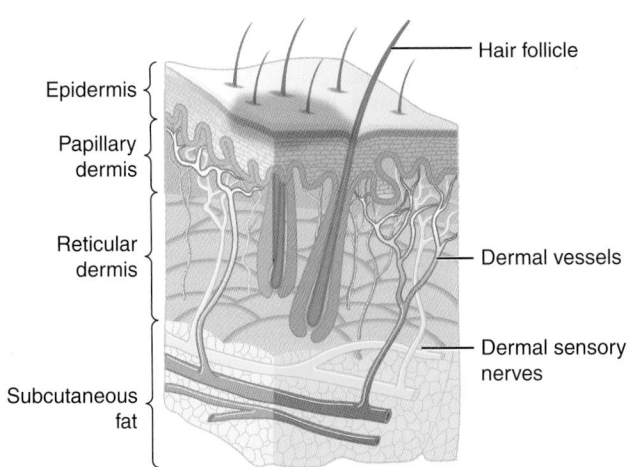

FIGURE 53.1 Anatomic layers of skin. Graphic representation of skin layers including the outer epidermis, the thin papillary dermis, the collagen-dense reticular dermis, and the deep subcutaneous fat. The dermal sensory neurons of mechanoheat receptors and dermal capillaries are shown, relative to a first-degree burn injury (confined to the outer epidermal skin layer). (Reproduced with permission from Sharar SR, Patterson DR, Wiechman-Askay S. Burn pain. In: Waldman SD ed. *Pain Management*. Philadelphia: Saunders-Elsevier, 2007:240–256.)

rehabilitation challenges with issues such as scarring, contractures, amputations, psychological adjustment, and pain. Despite this increased challenge to provide effective pain relief, there has long been substantial evidence that pain from burn injuries is undertreated, particularly in children.[3,4] Further, the magnitude of pain reported after burn injury and during burn care correlates strongly with long-term adverse psychological outcome in this patient population.[5,6] Thus, there are humane, medical, and economic reasons to better control burn pain in a practical and cost-effective fashion. Associated with this emphasis, a recent review of research presented at the American Burn Association annual meeting reported that the research category of "pain/anxiety/patient comfort" was the third most popular of 10 burn-related clinical and laboratory research areas.[7]

THE NATURE OF BURN PAIN

Treating the human suffering from burn pain is challenging, from the perspectives of both the patient and clinician. It is well known that a burn injury results in one of the most intense types of sensory nociception imaginable, attributable to the unique tissue injury that results from a thermal insult to the dermal sensory organs and a resulting acute inflammatory response that, at least in the early postburn period, is related to the depth of tissue injury (Figs. 53.1 and 53.2). First-degree burns (e.g., sunburn) are characterized by tissue injury that is limited to the epidermal skin layer and an inflammatory response in the superficial dermal layers and results in hyperemia (manifest as erythema), an intact epidermis (no skin blistering), and sensitization of dermal sensory organelles producing hyperalgesia and mild to moderate pain. Second-degree or *partial thickness* burns involve tissue injury that extends to variable depths into the dermis; *superficial second degree* burns involve only the upper, papillary dermis and are more likely to heal spontaneously, while *deep second degree* burns involve the deeper, collagen-dense reticular dermis and are

pervasive in both industrial nations and developing countries around the world, and affect individuals across a wide demographic span. In the United States, it is estimated that 1.25 million people annually sustain burn injuries, resulting in 51,000 acute hospitalizations and 5,500 deaths.[1] As death rates for burn injuries have recently declined (33% between 1985 and 1995[2]), due primarily to improved surgical care, more patients with large burns are surviving and pose unique physical and psychological

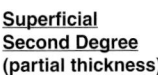
First Degree

Example: sunburn
Physical exam: erythema, painful, + capillary refill
Injury: damaged epidermis, inflamed papillary dermis
Treatment: spontaneous healing in 3–4 days

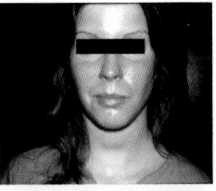
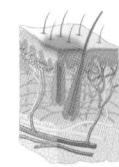

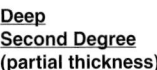
Superficial Second Degree (partial thickness)

Example: scald burn
Physical exam: pink, painful, + capillary refill, blisters, moist
Injury: damaged epidermis and papillary dermis
Treatment: spontaneous healing in 7–10 days

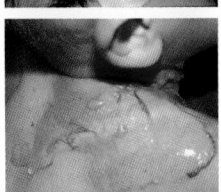
Hyperemia
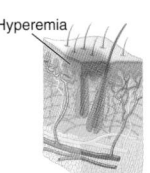

Deep Second Degree (partial thickness)

Example: scald, grease burn
Physical exam: mottled red/white, ± painful, − capillary refill
Injury: damaged epidermis and papillary/reticular dermis
Treatment: spontaneous healing or excision/grafting

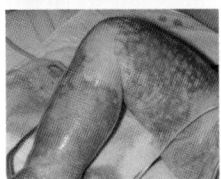
Hyperemia Stasis
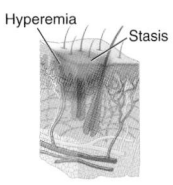

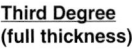
Third Degree (full thickness)

Example: flame, contact burn
Physical exam: white/black, painless, dry, charred, leathery, − capillary refill
Injury: damaged epidermis, dermis, ± subcutaneous fat
Treatment: excision/grafting

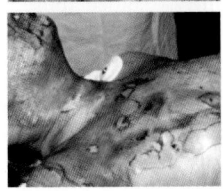
Coagulation
Hyperemia Stasis
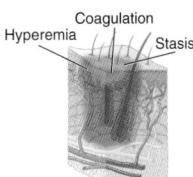

FIGURE 53.2 Definitions and examples of partial- and full-thickness burn injuries. Superficial and deep skin burns are defined, including clinical characteristics (etiology, physical exam findings, tissue injury, and usual treatment), photographic examples, and graphic representations of tissue injury (including zones of hyperemia, stasis, and coagulation). (Reproduced with permission from Sharar SR, Patterson DR, Wiechman-Askay S. Burn pain. In: Waldman SD ed. *Pain Management*. Philadelphia: Saunders-Elsevier, 2007:240–256.)

more likely to require surgical treatment. Because second-degree burns consistently injure and/or inflame sensory receptors in the dermis, these burns are associated with marked hyperalgesia and produce moderate to severe pain. Third-degree burns are characterized by complete destruction of the dermis, including its sensory and vascular structures, such that, although pain may still be a presenting symptom, hypalgesia to cutaneous stimulation, a leathery skin texture, and lack of capillary refill are common. Complaints of acute pain with third-degree burns are typically minimal but can be variable and are universally present with respect to the transition zone between burned and unburned skin. All burn injuries involving the dermis (i.e., second- and third-degree) result in sensitized and reorganized states of both peripheral mechanoheat receptors and dorsal horn neurons. Models of these cellular alterations provide a conceptual framework for understanding how such peripheral neuronal injuries that are present after a burn can cause acute and subacute pain, hyperalgesia and chronic pain, and are described in detail elsewhere.[8,9]

As noted previously, in addition to the significant pain caused by the burn injury itself, the major clinical analgesic challenge results from procedural and postoperative pain associated with contemporary burn care, involving a series of aggressive procedures that stimulate nociceptive peripheral afferent fibers on a daily basis for days, weeks, or months after the initial injury. In the typical treatment paradigm, a burn injury will first be assessed as to its depth and then treated accordingly. Shallow burns will be left to heal on their own, and full thickness thermal injuries will typically be excised and covered with a skin graft. Burns of indeterminate depth in many burn centers will undergo a series of wound débridements and dressing changes, typically on a daily basis, until burn depth can be more accurately determined. Burn care-related pain can be anticipated and treated, to a large degree, based on the clinical setting in which the pain occurs. Wound débridement, limb/joint mobility exercises, therapeutic skin stretching, and other medical procedures result in *procedural pain*, which is of high intensity but limited duration. Patients who are between procedures and have minimal physical activity, continue to experience *resting pain* that is relatively less intense, but almost constant in duration. When pain control interventions fail to control resting pain, patients will experience *breakthrough pain*. Finally, because surgical interventions are a frequent treatment for severe burn injuries, *postoperative pain* is an additional type of pain to be considered. Each of these four types of burn pain has specific treatment strategies, as described later in this chapter.

In addition to the four clinical settings described, burn pain varies somewhat temporally with the phase of treatment, most often divided into the resuscitative, healing, and remodeling phases.[9] In the *resuscitative phase* immediately after the injury, the patient is stabilized hemodynamically and initial wound treatments are performed. This phase is usually of short duration (e.g., hours), but depending on the size of injury can last up to 72 hours, as in the case of large surface area burns. Initial wound care in this phase is often intensely painful and, in the rush of treating life-threatening events, analgesia may be unintentionally de-emphasized. Pain in the *healing phase* is characterized by repeated episodes of burn wound care and dressing changes, wound examinations, needle sticks for intravenous access or blood sampling, and surgical procedures including débridement and grafting. The healing phase can last from days to several weeks depending on the severity of the burn and progress of the systemic response to the injury. It has been reported that hyperalgesia is more severe during this phase, independent of the size and degree of the burn. In the *remodeling phase* the systemic and local inflammatory responses decrease, wound healing is nearing completion, and rehabilitative activities gain emphasis. Depending on the characteristics of the wound scar, this phase is characterized by reductions in resting pain, but ongoing episodic procedural pain associated with physical and occupational therapy sessions. It is important to note that the duration and sequence of these phases can vary depending on the clinical progress of wound treatment. For example, a patient who has progressed to the re-

modeling phase can return to the healing phase after a surgical procedure recreates an open wound (e.g., burn site or skin graft donor site).

Although the clinical and temporal settings of burn care can provide some prediction as to the pain a patient might experience, the magnitude and quality of a given individual's pain experience have proven extremely difficult to anticipate. The sensory and affective qualities of burn pain have received scant attention in the literature, and few studies have addressed pain patterns over the course of hospitalization. For example, Choiniere and colleagues observed the evolution of burn pain experienced over the course of hospitalization and found that it varied substantially both within and across patients over time.[10] They also reported that burn pain was not accurately predicted by social–demographic factors or burn size (the latter finding is contrary to the inaccurate assumptions of many clinicians inexperienced in treating burns). Similarly, patient pain reports do not correlate with the quantity of opioid analgesics received, a finding first published in 1981[11] and still reported over two decades later.[4] This unpredictable and often opioid-resistant nature of burn pain has been hypothetically linked to underlying sensory nerve damage,[12,13] and contributes to the difficulty of effectively treating burn pain.

Although capturing the pain experience of an individual patient will likely continue to prove elusive for the reasons listed, it remains important to continue to treat burn pain aggressively. Not only can burn recovery (like that from any trauma) be hindered by the presence of acute pain,[14–16] burn pain has been reported to influence posthospitalization emotional recovery more than the size of the burn, the duration of hospitalization, or even the patient's preinjury mental health. Ptacek and Patterson[5] reported that inpatient pain scores in adults correlated more strongly with distress and quality of life scores at 1 month after discharge than did any other independent variable studied, a finding that persisted at 1-year and 2-year follow-up periods.[6] Similarly, Saxe et al. reported that the amount of morphine received by burn-injured children may impact their subsequent development of posttraumatic stress disorder.[17] Future studies will likely further substantiate the practical utility of adequately treating burn pain.

PSYCHOLOGICAL FACTORS

It is well known that pain processing is largely subjective and that the degree to which pain is interpreted as a threat will influence how much patients will suffer. A burn injury is a form of trauma that has dire emotional consequences for many survivors, and the threat value of the injury will likely have an impact on the amount of pain they perceive. Moreover, the nature of a patient's preinjury psychological makeup also has a great deal to do with how much pain they will perceive. In considering psychological factors, it is then important to consider the preinjury status of patients, as well as their emotional adjustment during and after hospitalization.

Burn injuries often occur when people are at risk because of low social resources or because of personality and/or psychiatric factors. The estimates of preinjury psychological problems in some studies of burn patients are so high that injuries of this type should be considered to be, in part, a symptom of social ills.[18] Estimated rates of psychiatric diagnoses in patients admitted for burn care have ranged from 25% to 75%, with the most prevalent diagnoses including depression, character disorder, and substance abuse.[18] In addition, the nature in which the burn injury occurred is often cause for concern: suicide attempts, child and elder abuse (or neglect), adult battering, and juvenile fire-setting are all, unfortunately, common sources of the injury. Psychological disturbances that predate the burn injury have the potential to increase complications, lengthen hospital stays, and lead to more serious long-term adjustment problems.[19–21] A number of these preinjury complications have direct relevance to pain control. Patients with drug and alcohol histories may show lower pain tolerance, higher drug seeking behaviors, and greater tolerance to opioid analgesics. DSM-IV Axis II character disorders can present a particular challenge to clinicians. Patients with such personality predispositions may not only show drug-seeking but also dramatic acting out behaviors, manipulation, staff-splitting, and low frustration tolerance. Patients with borderline personality disorders, in particular, engage in parasuicide behavior and self-mutilation. All of these factors might complicate pain control, in addition to making the patient's overall management a challenge.

Both the burn care environment and psychological reactions to burn injuries contribute to pain and complications in its management. Patients with large unhealed burn areas or other significant medical complications are usually placed in intensive care units. In the critical care setting, delirium and other psychotic reactions are common[21,22] with infections, alcohol withdrawal, and metabolic complications being the most frequent etiologies.[23] Poor communication from altered mental status or endotracheal intubation may further impede pain assessment. Anxiety is commonly reported by burn-injured patients, both at greater levels than reported to be tolerable and for prolonged periods throughout hospitalization.[24] As a result, anxiety assessment tools specific for burn-injured patients have been reported and validated and may predict burn pain and postdischarge functional capacity better than other anxiety assessment tools.[25] As hospitalization persists and patients show greater mental capacity, depression becomes increasingly common and is well known to interact with pain.[26] Depressive symptoms have a prevalence as high as 54% during postburn hospitalization[27] and are a significant predictor of physical health at 2 months postdischarge.[28] Posttraumatic stress disorder is another complication that can negatively impact pain control. One potential symptom of acute and posttraumatic stress disorder is withdrawal, and this reaction can lead to staff underestimating patients' pain (through a lack of observed emotion or verbosity).[29]

The manner in which the burn environment and patients' personality factors can amplify pain is particularly notable in children, for whom the burn unit environment can be extremely strange and frightening. There is little opportunity for the burn staff to prepare children psychologically for the repeated medical procedures they must endure, and conditioned anxiety to the stimuli associated with burn care can be expected. Children will also often demonstrate regression and behavioral acting out in response to hospitalization, making pain control during procedures a particular challenge. It should be noted that although many burn centers have pediatric-specific pain protocols, their emphasis is appropriately on safety; hence, they are often not aggressive enough to adequately address pain or prevent procedural anxiety in every child. As previously mentioned, aggressive treatment of pain may serve to reduce the subsequent development of posttraumatic stress disorder in children.[17] A comprehensive review of issues specific to pediatric burn pain can be found elsewhere.[30]

There is growing evidence that although pain was once thought to be a problem only during the early phases (e.g., resuscitative and healing phases) of burn care, a significant number of patients experience ongoing pain long after hospital discharge. For example, a long-term, neuropathic pain syndrome has been recently described in burned patients, presenting approximately 4 months after the initial injury[31] and persisting for an average of 13 months. Similarly, in a survey of 358 respondents of a burn survivor support group,[32] 52% reported ongoing pain, 66% said that it interfered with their rehabilitation, and 55% said the pain interfered with their daily lives. Respondents in this study also reported that thoughts of the accident and depression made their pain worse. The pathophysiology and ideal treatment for such chronic, postburn pain is currently unknown and an area of current study. Furthermore, patients may show persistent depression, anxiety, or posttraumatic stress disorder that can interfere with pain control, with both depression and anxiety predicting worse outcomes in pain, fatigue, and physical functioning assessments up to 2 years postdischarge.[33] Sleep problems are prevalent, yet frequently overlooked in postdischarge phase, and may reflect inadequate pain treatment.[34] When psychological or pain problems persist long after hospital discharge the possibility of social or financial disincentives should be entertained. Although some patients will certainly have internally generated psychological problems, for others, the issues will persist because of such factors as litigation or the desire to avoid returning to an undesirable job.

GENERALIZED TREATMENT PARADIGM FOR BURN PAIN

Because burn pain is highly variable and cannot be reliably predicted by either clinical assessment of the patient or their burn wound, we recommend a structured approach to burn analgesia that incorporates both pharmacologic and nonpharmacologic therapies, targets specific pain issues unique to the burn patient, and can be tailored to anticipated variations in patient need and institutional capability. One clear goal of such a paradigm is to avoid the undertreatment of burn pain, an unfortunate reality in the settings of adult[35] and pediatric[3,36] burn care, and more historically described for other acute pain settings.[37] Perry and colleagues[38] noted that burn staff members failed to medicate patients adequately with opioids, despite education regarding the low risks for addictive and other side effects. These investigators offered a psychodynamic conceptualization of this issue, proposing that staff members who were required to perform repeated and painful procedures on these patients had a need for patients to demonstrate pain as a means to create a psychological distance between themselves and the realities of burn care. Alternatively, the fear of creating psychological dependence on opioids may explain the reluctance of some burn care staff to aggressively treat burn pain. However, there is currently no evidence that opioid addiction occurs more commonly in burn patients than in other populations requiring opioids for acute pain (~1/3000).[39]

In the generalized burn pain management paradigm, selection of an analgesic regimen is individualized and based on two broad categories: (1) the clinical need for analgesia (i.e., treatment of background vs. procedural vs. postoperative pain), and (2) limitations imposed by the patient (e.g., presence of intravenous [IV] access, endotracheal tube, or opioid tolerance) or by clinical facilities (available monitoring capabilities and personnel). The presence or absence of IV access directly influences analgesic drug choice, particularly in children in whom IV access may be problematic. Patients who are endotracheally intubated and ventilated are "protected" from the risk of opioid-induced respiratory depression; thus, opioids may be more generously administered in these individuals, as is often indicated for complex burn debridement procedures in patients with more extensive or severe burn injuries. Individual differences in opioid efficacy should be considered in all patients, including opioid tolerance in patients requiring prolonged opioid analgesic therapy or in those with preexisting substance abuse histories. Due to the development of drug tolerance with prolonged medical use or recreational abuse of opioids (both commonly seen in burn patients), opioid analgesic doses needed for burn analgesia may significantly exceed those recommended in standard dosing guidelines. One clinically relevant consequence of drug tolerance is the potential for opioid withdrawal to occur during inpatient burn treatment. Thus, the period of inpatient burn care is not an appropriate time to institute deliberate opioid withdrawal or detoxification measures in the substance-abusing patient, because such treatment ignores the very real analgesic needs of these patients. Similarly, when reductions in analgesic therapy are considered as burn wounds heal, reductions should occur by careful taper, in order to prevent acute opioid withdrawal syndrome.

Institutional capability to provide adequate monitoring (pulse oximetry, independent patient observer, etc.) as required for "moderate sedation" (as defined by the American Society of Anesthesiologists, Table 53.1)[40] may also dictate which agents

TABLE 53.1

AMERICAN SOCIETY OF ANESTHESIOLOGISTS CONTINUUM OF DEPTH OF SEDATION

	Minimal sedation (anxiolysis)	Moderate sedation/ analgesia (conscious sedation)	Deep sedation/analgesia	General anesthesia
Responsiveness	Normal response to verbal stimulation	Purposeful* response to verbal or tactile stimulation	Purposeful* response following repeated or painful stimulation	Unrousable even with painful stimulus
Airway	Unaffected	No intervention required	Intervention may be required	Intervention often required
Spontaneous ventilation	Unaffected	Adequate	May be inadequate	Frequently inadequate
Cardiovascular function	Unaffected	Usually maintained	Usually maintained	May be impaired

* Reflex painful withdrawal from a painful stimulus is NOT considered a purposeful response.
Approved by the American Society of Anesthesiologists House of Delegates on October 13, 1999, and amended on October 27, 2004.
(Reproduced with permission from American Society of Anesthesiologists Task Force on Sedation and Analgesia by Non-anesthesiologists. Practice guidelines for sedation and analgesia by non-anesthesiologists. *Anesthesiology* 2002;96:1004–1017.)

are used for procedural analgesia, as some of the more potent opioids (e.g., fentanyl) and anesthetic agents (e.g., ketamine, propofol) may unpredictably result in potentially dangerous levels of sedation ("deep sedation" or "general anesthesia"). The use of potent opioids and anxiolytics should only occur in settings with adequate monitoring, personnel, and resuscitation equipment appropriate for the degree of sedation anticipated. For many burn wound débridement procedures and most rehabilitative therapy sessions in the hospital ward or outpatient clinic setting, opioid analgesia with "minimal sedation" is sufficient and no special monitoring is required. Larger or more potent doses of opioids, or the concurrent use of anxiolytic sedatives (e.g., benzodiazepines) may produce more pronounced sedation ("moderate sedation"), but could also progress to "deep sedation" where patient–staff communication and/or patient consciousness are lost. Current guidelines of the Joint Commission on Accreditation of Healthcare Organizations (JCAHO),[41] as well as adult[40] and pediatric[42] physician specialty professional organizations, dictate both general and specific levels of monitoring (e.g., continuous pulse oximetry, presence of an independent observer specifically responsible for monitoring ventilation and vital signs) for patients requiring each of these levels of procedural analgesia and sedation.

Because nociception at the burn site is the predominant mechanism of pain and suffering in these patients during the resuscitative and healing phases, pharmacologic treatment with potent opioids, anxiolytics, and other agents (e.g., ketamine) is the first line of therapy. However, nonpharmacologic methods of treating burn pain are also extremely useful. Some nonpharmacologic pain control techniques should be second nature to the staff and integrated into standard care (e.g., minimizing the number and intrusiveness of dressing changes, limb elevation, brief educational approaches). Other, more novel nonpharmacologic analgesic techniques are more practically implemented after a stable pharmacologic regimen is established or may require special expertise (e.g., hypnosis). To reinforce a consistent approach to analgesic management, particularly in centers where house staff physicians or nursing staff may rotate or change frequently, the establishment of succinct yet detailed institutional guidelines may help physicians and nurses with choosing and administering analgesics that target specific analgesic needs,[43,44] as shown in Table 53.2. To maximize simplicity and utility, it is recommended that such guidelines be safe and effective over a broad range of ages, be explicit in their dosing recommendations, have a limited formulary to maximize staff familiarity, and allow the bedside nurse to continuously evaluate efficacy and safety.[44] In addition, the regular use of a weight-based pediatric medication worksheet (placed at the bedside and in the patient record), containing all

analgesic and resuscitation drugs likely to be administered, provides a supplemental safeguard against accidental overdose, particularly in the young pediatric age group.[45]

In recent years, a number of comprehensive reviews of burn pain management that emphasize such a systematic and multidisciplinary approach to burn pain management have been published,[9,30,46,47] including practice guidelines from the American Burn Association.[48] The reader is referred to these sources for additional perspective and detail.

PHARMACOLOGIC APPROACHES

In describing pharmacologic approaches for burn analgesia, three consistent observations can be made. First, for patients with injuries extensive enough to require hospitalization, pain from the burn itself is severe. Thus, potent opioids form the cornerstones of pharmacologic pain control in these patients, leaving few indications for the mild to moderate analgesia provided by nonsteroidal antiinflammatory drugs (NSAIDs) or acetaminophen, with notable exceptions of the rehabilitative phase of care and outpatient treatment. Second, because burn pain has well-defined components described previously—background, procedural, and postoperative pain—pharmacologic choices for analgesia should target each pain pattern individually. Finally, because burn pain will vary somewhat unpredictably throughout hospitalization due to surgical intervention, activity levels, etc., analgesic regimens should be continuously evaluated and reassessed to avoid problems of under- or over-medication.[6] Pain assessment is facilitated by the regular use of standardized, self-report scales for adults and older children, and observational scoring systems for the very young, as described in Chapter 20. A reliance on nurse assessment of patients' burn pain can be problematic, however, as it is well documented that nurses' and patients' assessment of burn pain and analgesia are not always comparable,[35,49,50] with nursing staff typically underestimating the need for analgesic therapy.

Opioids

Opioid agonists are the most commonly used analgesics in the treatment of burn pain, in part because (1) they are effective, (2) the benefits and risks of their use are familiar to the majority of care providers, and (3) they provide some dose-dependent degree of sedation that can be advantageous to both burn patients and staff, particularly during burn wound care procedures. The wide

TABLE 53.2

HARBORVIEW MEDICAL CENTER/UNIVERSITY OF WASHINGTON BURN CENTER BURN ANALGESIA AND SEDATION GUIDELINES FOR ADULTS

	ICU No PO intake	ICU taking PO	Ward large open areas	Ward small open areas/predischarge
Background pain	continuous morphine sulfate (IV) drip	scheduled methadone or MS Contin	scheduled methadone or MS Contin	scheduled NSAIDs/acetaminophen or scheduled oxycodone or none
Procedural pain	morphine sulfate (IV) or fentanyl (IV)	oxycodone, fentanyl IV, or fentanyl Actiq	oxycodone, fentanyl IV, Nitrox (IH) or fentanyl Actiq	oxycodone
Breakthrough pain (PRN dosing)	morphine sulfate (IV) or fentanyl (IV)	oxycodone	oxycodone	NSAIDs/acetaminophen or oxycodone
Background anxiolysis	scheduled lorazepam (IV) or continuous lorazepam (IV)	scheduled lorazepam	none or scheduled lorazepam	none
Procedural anxiolysis	lorazepam or midazolam	lorazepam	none or lorazepam	none
Discharge or transfer pain medications	N/A	For transfer to ward: wean drips, establish PO pain meds early, anticipate dose tapering as needs decrease	oxycodone for procedural pain; methadone taper or MS Contin taper if applicable	oxycodone or NSAIDs for procedural pain

Medications are to be given orally unless otherwise specified. Exception: fentanyl Actiq is given transmucosal.
Analgesic and anxiolytic choices are simplified to a minimum number of agents to encourage staff familiarity, and are targeted to specific pain and anxiety needs. Therapy can be individualized to include agents not in this guideline when clinically indicated. This chart is laminated and prominently displayed in all patient care areas. IH, inhalation; IV, intravenous; NSAIDs, nonsteroidal antiinflammatories; Nitrox, 50% nitrous oxide/ 50% oxygen inhaled.

spectrum of opioids available for clinical use (see Chapter 78) provides dosing flexibility (i.e., variable routes of administration, variable duration of action) that is ideal for the targeted treatment of burn pain. The pharmacokinetics of opioids in burn patients are not consistently different from nonburn patients,[51,52] although decreased volume of distribution and clearance, and increased elimination half-life have been reported for morphine.[53] Similarly, pharmacodynamic potency of opioids has inconsistently been reported as increased[54] and decreased[53] in burn patients.

The route of opioid administration is an important consideration in burn patients, with the principal choice between IV, oral, or transmucosal administration dictated by the severity of burn (critically ill patients require IV access and may have abnormal gut function) and high risk of burn patients for developing IV catheter-related sepsis (hence, physician reluctance to maintain long-term IV access).[55] Intramuscular opioid administration is avoided because of the need for repeated, painful injections and because of variable vascular absorption due to unpredictable compartmental fluid shifts and muscle perfusion in burn patients, particularly in the resuscitative phase. Patient-controlled analgesia (PCA) with IV opioids offers the burn patient a safe and efficient method of achieving more flexible analgesia for both background and procedural analgesia. PCA also offers the patient some degree of control over his/her medical care, this being a major issue for burn patients whose waking hours are often completely scheduled with care activities ranging from wound care to physical and rehabilitation therapy. Some studies comparing PCA opioid use to other routes of administration in the burn population have shown potential benefits of PCA.[56,57] The PCA administration of potent, short-acting opioids (e.g., fentanyl,[58] alfentanil,[59] remifentanil) for procedural analgesia may also have

a useful role in burn analgesic management, but this has not been extensively investigated.

Because IV access is infrequently present in hospitalized burn patients outside of the critical care setting (for reasons noted previously), oral and transmucosal opioid delivery are frequently employed. For background pain, long-acting oral opioids (e.g., methadone) or sustained release opioids are often utilized. However, the latter agents are not available in appropriate dose ranges for pediatric patients, so a reliance on shorter acting oral opioids is often necessary. For background pain control in this population, the use of regularly scheduled oral opioids is recommended over pro re nata (PRN) dosing, so that more stable plasma opioid concentrations and analgesic effects may be obtained.[60] Similarly, the use of short-acting oral opioids is common for anticipated procedural pain, emphasizing early administration of the drug so that adequate plasma levels and associated analgesia are present prior to beginning the procedure. Alternatively, oral transmucosal administration of opioids is reported in burn patients to be particularly advantageous in those patients without IV access and in children, in both the inpatient[61] and outpatient clinic[62] settings.

Nonopioids

The list of nonopioid analgesics in widespread use for the treatment of burn pain is relatively extensive, although clinical evidence to support such use is variably found in the published literature. Oral NSAIDs and acetaminophen, as outlined previously, are only mild analgesics and exhibit a ceiling effect in their dose-response relationship, rendering them unsuitable for the treatment of typical, severe burn pain. However, they are of benefit in treating minor burns, particularly in the outpatient setting. Topical application of NSAIDs on burn wounds can theoretically inhibit nociception at the injury site with minimal systemic uptake,[63] yet does not result in significant analgesia.[64] The opioid agonist-antagonist drugs (e.g., nalbuphine, butorphanol) produce "mixed" actions at the opiate receptor level, theoretically providing analgesia (agonist property) with lesser side effects (antagonist properties), but also exhibit ceiling effects. Although studies have shown this class of drugs to be effective in treating burn pain,[65] experience with them is both limited and suggestive of efficacy in patients with only relatively mild burn pain.

Antidepressants, anticonvulsants, antipsychotics, and alpha-2-agonists have been proposed as potential analgesic agents for burn pain[66] based on their known mechanisms of action in other pain states, yet have not been studied extensively in the setting of burns. As neuropathic pain can occur in patients with healed burns,[13,31,32] these agents may have specific application in this setting, as suggested by a preliminary reports with a variety of nonopioid agents including gabapentin,[67,68] dexmedetomidine,[69] clonidine,[70] and haloperidol.[71]

Anxiolytics

Current, aggressive therapies for cutaneous burn wounds, together with the persistent and repetitive qualities of background and procedural pain, make burn care an experience that is likely to engender anxiety in both adult and pediatric patients. It is also recognized that anxiety can exacerbate acute pain.[14] This has led to the common practice of using anxiolytic drugs in combination with opioid analgesics, a practice has persisted since the 1980s.[72] A recent survey of North American burn centers reported that up to 39% of hospitalized pediatric burn victims regularly receive anxiolytics as part of their pain and sedation management regimen.[73] Intuitively, this practice is particularly useful in premedicating patients for daily wound care procedures, due to the anticipatory anxiety experienced by these patients prior to and during debridement. Although previously shown that benzodiazepine therapy improves postoperative pain scores in nonburn settings,[74] it is also reported that low-dose benzodiazepine administration significantly reduces burn wound care pain reports.[75] It appears that the patients most likely to benefit from this therapy are not those with high trait (premorbid) anxiety, but rather those with high state (at the time of the procedure) anxiety or those with high baseline pain scores.

Anesthetics

Inhaled nitrous oxide is an analgesic agent safe for administration by nonanesthesia personnel to achieve moderate sedation. It provides safe and effective analgesia without loss of consciousness for moderately painful procedures in other healthcare settings (e.g., dentistry), and is also a commonly used, although less well-studied agent for the treatment of burn pain.[76,77] It is typically used as a 50% mixture in 50% oxygen, and is self-administered by an awake, cooperative, spontaneously breathing patient via a mouthpiece or mask. A secondary benefit of nitrous oxide use, like that of PCA opioid administration, is the element of control given to the patient for his/her care. Nitrous oxide is less useful with critically ill or uncooperative patients. It has also been implicated in a very small, but measurable incidence of toxicity issues (e.g., spontaneous abortion, bone marrow suppression) to patients or staff exposed for prolonged periods,[78,79] although not in the setting of burn pain treatment.

Although it is obvious that general anesthesia is required for the surgical excision and grafting of deep burn wounds, it is not uncommon to encounter specific wound care procedures that are on a scale below that of surgical burn care, yet are nevertheless difficult to perform on a conscious patient, particularly a child. These procedures are ideally suited for deep sedation or general anesthesia and include (1) the removal of hundreds of skin staples from recently grafted wounds, (2) meticulous wound care of recently grafted, and often tenuous skin on the face or neck, and

(3) wound care procedures in variably cooperative children. Historically, IV, intramuscular, or oral ketamine have been used for these procedures,[80–82] and there is limited evidence that ketamine administration acutely after experimental skin burns may prevent hyperalgesia and "wind-up."[8] More recently, some high-volume burn centers have developed specific training and skill retention programs in ketamine administration by nonanesthesiologists, and report that satisfactory sedation for bedside procedures can be achieved in children with a low incidence of side effects.[84] However, ketamine is a dose-dependent anesthetic that can produce deep sedation and general anesthesia in an unpredictable manner; thus, appropriate patient monitoring is requisite, and nonanesthesiologists administering the drug must have specialized training and airway management skills, as well as anesthesiologist back-up. In addition, its use is limited by the potential risk of associated emergence delirium reactions (5% to 30% incidence), particularly in the elderly.

The extension of full anesthetic care capabilities with anesthesiology staffing outside of the operating room and into the burn unit has been successfully implemented in some specialized burn centers.[85,86] This has been facilitated by the recent introduction into clinical anesthetic practice of a variety of drugs with a rapid onset and short duration of action, a more rapid awakening/recovery, and fewer associated side effects—ideal qualities for agents to be used for procedural burn wound care. These agents include IV propofol and remifentanil, and inhaled sevoflurane and desflurane. Propofol is particularly advantageous, and can be titrated to effect both in terms of level of consciousness and duration of action using continuous IV infusion techniques.[87] The provision of brief, dense analgesia/anesthesia in a comprehensively monitored setting by individuals specifically trained to provide the service appears safe and efficient, both in terms of allowing wound care to proceed rapidly under ideal conditions for patient and nursing staff, and in terms of cost-effective use of the operating room only for true surgical burn care procedures.

Local anesthetics are of obvious use in regional blockade for wound care procedures, but have also been used for burn pain analgesia as a topical gel or IV infusion. Topical local anesthetic use on the burn wound is controversial. Prilocaine-lidocaine cream (EMLA) has no effect on burn pain in volunteers,[88] however, topical 5% lidocaine applied at 1 mg/cm[2] offers analgesic benefit without associated side effects.[89] Topical lidocaine use is significantly tempered by reports of local anesthetic-induced seizures due to enhanced systemic absorption at the open wound site.[90] The analgesic benefit of an IV lidocaine bolus (1 mg/kg) and 3-day continuous infusion (40 mg/kg/min) has also been reported acute burn injuries,[91] although whether its mechanism is due to antiinflammatory or analgesic actions is unclear. Neuraxial administration of local anesthetics (and/or opioids) via epidural catheter would seem to be of benefit in patients with lower extremity burns, resulting in both analgesia (particularly during procedural burn care) and sympathectomy (of theoretical benefit to wound healing). However, such use has only been reported anecdotally.[92] A major drawback of this technique is the use of an indwelling catheter in patients densely colonized with infectious organisms at the wound site, thus increasing the risk for epidural abscess formation.[93] Nonneuraxial regional blocks have recently been reported to be of benefit for the pain associated with surgical skin donor site preparation on the anterolateral thigh, both a single injections[94] and as continuous infusions.[95]

Pharmacologic Options for Background Pain Management

Because background pain is relatively constant, it is best treated with mild-to-moderately potent analgesics administered so that plasma drug concentrations remain relatively constant throughout the day. Examples include the continuous IV infusion of fentanyl or morphine (± PCA), the oral administration of long-acting opioids with prolonged elimination (methadone) or prolonged enteral absorption (sustained-release morphine, sustained release oxycodone), or oral administration on a regular schedule of short-acting oral analgesics (oxycodone, hydromorphone, codeine, acetaminophen). Background pain generally decreases with time as the burn wounds (and associated donor sites) heal, so that analgesics can be slowly tapered (in the absence of significant analgesic tolerance).

Pharmacologic Options for Procedural Pain Management

In contrast to background pain, procedural pain is significantly more intense, but shorter in duration; therefore, analgesic regimens for procedural pain are best comprised of moderately-to-highly potent opioids that have a short duration of action, with a sedation target level of moderate sedation. IV access is helpful in this setting, with ketamine and short-acting opioids (fentanyl, alfentanil) offering a potential advantage over more longer-acting agents (morphine, hydromorphone). In the absence of IV access, orally administered opioids (morphine, hydromorphone, oxycodone, codeine) are commonly used, although their relatively long durations of action (2–6 hours) may potentially limit postprocedure recovery for other rehabilitative or nutritional activities. Oral ketamine, oral transmucosal fentanyl, and nitrous oxide are agents of particular use when IV access is not present, due to their rapid onsets and short durations of action. Finally, when a particularly painful dressing change or one that requires extreme cooperation in a noncompliant patient (e.g., face débridement in a young child) is anticipated, the provision of brief deep sedation or general anesthesia with appropriate patient monitoring, administered by anesthesiologists or appropriately trained nonanesthesiologists may be helpful.

Pharmacologic Options for Postoperative Pain Management

Postoperative pain deserves special mention because of the increased analgesic needs that should be anticipated following burn excision and grafting. This is particularly true when donor sites have been harvested, as these are often the principal source of increased postoperative pain complaints, rather than the grafted burn. Typically, this increased analgesic need is limited to 1–4 days following surgery before returning to preoperative levels.

NONPHARMACOLOGIC APPROACHES

Cognitive Interventions and Coping Styles

In terms of pain control, cognitions can be thought of as behaviors that can be modified and that may influence the amount of pain that patients experience. Although such approaches are common in chronic pain control, there are few studies of cognitive–behavioral interventions in patients with burn injuries.[96,97] In understanding such interventions, it is important to emphasize that burn injuries are unexpected and have far-reaching consequences for patients. Further, as noted previously, the aggressive procedural medical care typically associated with burn injuries adds further stress and uncertainty through the daily demands of surgery, rehabilitation, dependency on caregivers, and pain. Such uncertainty often leads to feelings of helplessness in both adult and pediatric burn patients. It is almost impossible to predict the style with which an individual patient reacts and responds to such stress; however, if one is able to determine some characteristics of the patient's cognitive style, this insight can be useful in choosing the most appropriate psychologically based interventions.

Burn patients bring different cognitive styles in the manner in which they respond to stressful medical procedures. One critical distinction lies in how much information patients desire regarding their injury and care. Whereas some patients will seek out as much information as possible, others would just as soon leave their care to healthcare professionals.[98,99] In applying cognitive interventions to burn patients, it will behoove the clinician to be aware of how they cope with stressful medical procedures. Paramount to such thinking is whether the patient will approach procedures with a tendency toward cognitive avoidance, in which case they will distract or dissociate themselves from painful stimuli. This is in contrast to patients who tend to respond to acute pain by focusing on the procedures. Such patients may take a hypervigilant stance toward pain and may find distractions difficult. Patients often fall into position along a continuum of coping styles, from an approach coping style to an avoidance coping style. If one can determine where they fall along this continuum, it is easier to determine what type of psychological intervention will be most useful[47] (Fig. 53.3).

If patients fall on the avoidance end of the continuum, too much information and focus on the details of care procedures will likely make them more anxious. In contrast, distraction will likely be useful for patients who possess this coping style. In the burn unit, simple distraction is more likely to be of benefit with brief procedures such as blood draws or line placements, and studies have reported that music can be effective for such simple distraction with burn pain.[100] Children at certain development levels may benefit from not seeing their wounds or by being more engaged by the clinicians. Such distraction will be less effective with older children or adults during the more extensive wound care procedures. In such instances, engaging patients in deep relaxation with distracting imagery will likely be more useful, although imagery often requires substantially more training time for both patients and staff. A particularly elaborate form of distraction involves the use of computer-generated immersive virtual reality (see later).

In contrast, when patients cope with painful procedures by

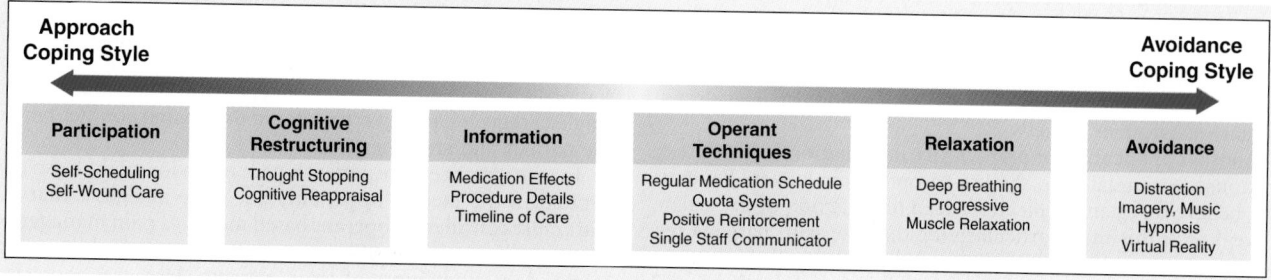

FIGURE 53.3 Control coping continuum and associated nonpharmacological techniques. The spectrum of coping styles from approach to avoidance is depicted, including specific clinical interventions for patients whose coping styles fall on different positions along the continuum (see text for details).

carefully focusing on them and even participating in their own care (i.e., approach coping style), they are usually less viable candidates for distraction techniques. Such patients may benefit by reappraisal techniques. Rather than focusing away from pain, reappraisal techniques might encourage patients to attend to their nociception. They can then be encouraged to differentiate sensory from affective components of pain, as well as evaluate the meaning of the sensation. As is the case with chronic pain, patients may benefit from being taught to differentiate "hurt from harm" with respect to their pain sensations.[101] It is also useful to teach such patients that increased pain sensation is usually a positive sign with respect to burn wound healing. Specifically, full thickness burns often destroy nerve endings and the capacity for nociception, but as these burn wounds heal, skin buds emerge which are highly enervated and sensitive to pain and temperature. Teaching patients the latter two principles will likely be useful to them independent of their cognitive styles in response to acute pain. Further, with enough focus on pain sensations, some patients are able to gain the sense that they are able to modify them, and thus be in more control of their perceptions.

PREPARATORY INFORMATION

Providing patients with information about impending procedures can provide a powerful means of mitigating pain and anxiety. Such interventions have been found to enhance pain control with acute pain from a variety of different procedures.[102] Patients may be provided with preparatory information (what steps will be taken during a procedure) or sensory information (what they will likely feel). The use of preparatory information has not been studied with burn patients, but there is evidence that it can be useful with a variety of medical procedures such as cardiac catheterization, endoscopies, cast removal, and surgery.[103–105] Unfortunately, burn injuries often do not easily lend themselves to such interventions. Certainly, it is not possible to anticipate that a burn injury will occur and medical procedures are often performed quickly, and in an invasive matter. There is little time to prepare patients, and this can be particularly difficult for children. In addition, with some medical procedures in nonburn settings, understanding what will occur may reduce anxiety and pain associated with those procedures. Unfortunately, the frequent challenge with burn care is that the procedures are very painful, invasive, and truly threatening, unlike many other types of medical procedures that simply have the appearance of being threatening.

Preparation is particularly relevant to two phenomena associated with burn care. First of all, nociceptive input may often increase as a burn wound heals. As mentioned earlier, full thickness burn injuries may not be that painful, while healing injuries with new skin buds may be particularly sensitive. Care providers should take care to communicate to such patients that increased pain is actually a sign that the wound is healing, information that may help allay patient anxiety. The second beneficial instance of preparatory information involves informing patients' family members of important medical issues. For example, burn patients often show periods of delirium when in the intensive care unit, a clinical phenomenon that can be frightening to both patients and their family members. Letting them know in advance that such confusion is a common and usually benign occurrence can mitigate subsequent anxiety.

Another application of preparatory information is to address irrational fears related to the use of opioid analgesics. Patients may believe that pain medications lead to addiction or are a sign of weakness; this may particularly be the case with patients recovering from an alcohol or chemical dependency. Information about the negligible rates of opioid addiction among burn patients can be useful in this regard. Also, it is useful to let patients know that adequate analgesia likely promotes recovery. Certainly, our own research indicates that high levels of pain are one of the most significant predictors of posthospital adjustment.[5,6] It can also be explained that poor pain control may actually lead to more potential substance abuse, as opposed to protocols that manage pain aggressively on an a priori basis.

BEHAVIORAL INTERVENTIONS

Behavioral interventions might seem more applicable to chronic pain conditions, yet have surprising relevance to burn pain treatment. The application of such principles to burn can be divided into classical (stimulus) and operant (respondent) strategies. Stimulus conditioning applications have to do with the patient's state prior to wound care. Certainly, decreasing the patient's level of arousal through relaxation training, or any other means available, can minimize the ensuing cycle between anxiety and nociception. With children, the stimulus context of painful procedures can be particularly relevant. Children (and many adults) will often show heightened anxiety and fear just by being exposed to the stimuli associated with painful procedures (e.g., nursing scrubs, procedures rooms). If the threatening nature of the wound care environment can be reduced, pain control can be enhanced by virtue of stimulus–response principles. As a nonburn example, some children's hospitals have instituted the creative approach of having a magnetic resonance imaging (MRI) scan tunnel appear as a cave in a jungle environment (rather than the morgue-like drawer such equipment more typically seems to resemble). What follows from this logic is that the burn-injured child's room should be considered a safe environment in which painful procedures do not occur.

Operant (reinforcement) principles are also highly applicable to burn pain management. One application has to do with medication scheduling. The tendency in many acute care settings is to simply medicate patients on an "as-needed" or PRN schedule, an approach that is nonsensical for several reasons in burn care. Certainly, the notion of waiting until the patient hurts does not make sense from a pharmacologic perspective.[3,60,106] However, operant principles would also suggest that PRN medication schedules reinforce patients' pain complaints, both in terms of the euphoria-producing properties of opioid analgesics and the attention received from caregivers. Providing opioid analgesics on a regular schedule that reflects their pharmacokinetic properties will minimize the potential for operant factors to exacerbate the pain problem. For emotionally dependent or anxious patients, as-needed pain scheduling can actually create a paradigm for creating more pain behaviors and pain perception.[101]

A regular analgesic drug administration schedule is particularly important with patients who have substance abuse histories. Such patients may demonstrate frequent pain complaints and/or drug seeking behaviors on the burn unit. The tendency of such patients to approach multiple caregivers for analgesics has the potential to create "staff splitting" and resentment (i.e., countertransference) toward the patients. Accordingly, the burn unit staff may hold punitive attitudes about the patient's substance abuse history and/or the excessive nature of his or her pain complaints. Regularly scheduled medications will often minimize such conflict, as well as provide more transparent management of the patient's pain. In addition, channeling communications and negotiations about changing doses or types of medication through a single caregiver can be very useful in decreasing conflict between the patient and staff members.

In rare instances, the patient's pain behavior might be so exaggerated in the face of apparently adequate analgesia that burn staff must consider an operant based model of pain management. Effective burn team members are trained to be highly attentive to the pain complaints of their patients. However, occasional patients may show excessive complaints based on such factors as strong dependency needs or somatic tendencies. As in any case, it is important that such patients receive adequate doses of analgesics. However, operant approaches, in which discussions of pain are minimized and patients are distracted from their complaints,[101] may become the prominent intervention. In other words, there would be discussions with the patient that medications changes will be limited to circumscribed periods and, in between such times, the patient will be encouraged to focus away from the issue of pain.

Burn rehabilitation involves continuously increasing activity levels, and patients may become simply overwhelmed with the pain associated with such movements. The quota system[107] represents a useful application of operant principles to burn care in such instances. The repeated, invasive nature of burn care has the potential to create a state of learned helplessness in patients.[108] The quota system uses rest as a reinforcement for activity, and keeps activity levels well within the patient's level of physical endurance. Ehde and colleagues have reported that with overwhelmed, seemingly unmotivated patients, it is useful to encourage the burn team to reduce their overall demands, take baseline behaviors, and gradually increase demands on what the patient's baseline behavior suggests is within their range of tolerance.[107] Such interventions can create steady increases in activity in patients who have been overwhelmed by care, and also a sense of mastery, as they are able to see steady improvement in their activities.

Avoiding the rewarding of escape behavior during procedures is a final application of operant principles. With children, it is particularly essential to do all the interventions possible to enhance pain control during procedures such as adequate analgesics and anxiolytics, sufficient emotional preparation, optimizing the wound care environment, and including parents when appropriate. Children also do better if allowed to have control of their wound care procedures, perhaps by doing their own dressing removal.[108] However, there are times when it is important to set firm limits during wound care by following through with procedures; otherwise, pain behaviors can exacerbate. Establishing this balance can certainly be a challenge for caregivers since it is not appropriate to force treatment when children are inadequately medicated. The point here is that once all that can be done that is possible in terms of analgesia, the timing of when a child can refuse or rest during wound care becomes an important issue in operant management.

HYPNOSIS

In terms of randomized controlled studies, hypnosis is one of the areas where the most evidence exists for psychologically based interventions in burn care. In 1987 there were at least 14 papers published on this subject,[109] and such investigations continue.[110] A recent review by Patterson and Jensen[111] indicates that burn pain constitutes some of the best evidence in the literature that hypnosis can be effective. Further, a number of additional reports have focused on the use of hypnosis to treat complications from burns other than pain, although with few exceptions, these reports have been anecdotal.[109,112]

There are a number of reasons why burn patients appear to be such good candidates for hypnotic based pain control interventions[113] First, because burn patients are in high levels of pain, they are motivated to engage in hypnosis, a technique that they might ordinarily resist. In support of this, patients with high levels of initial pain seem to show a better analgesic response to hypnosis.[114,115] Second, patients with unanticipated traumatic injuries, such as burns, may be more cooperative because of the dependency that might often be a normal reaction to trauma care (i.e., a willingness to allow others to take care of one). Third, the dissociation that may accompany a burn injury may also be a factor that moderates hypnotizability. Certainly, dissociative tendencies have been related to hypnosis,[116] as well as the acute stress disorder is a typical early reaction to burn injuries. Finally,

and on a more simplistic level, hypnosis is most effective when it can be applied to a predictable, discreet event—a description that characterizes most burn wound care procedures, as painful as they are.

Ewin[117,118] has published anecdotal data to suggest that hypnosis used early in burn care can not only enhance pain control, but might even facilitate wound healing. This work has received a great deal of attention, but also criticism given the lack of controlled studies to support the underlying premise.[119] The question of whether hypnosis can have such powerful effects when used early in burn care will hopefully be the subject of future controlled studies. However, it would be of great utility to determine what effects aggressive pain interventions of any modality have when used very early in the patient's care.

There have been two recent publications describing the delivery of hypnosis through immersive virtual reality technology (see later) in order to treat burn pain.[120,121] The advantage of this approach is that the clinician can rely on technology to achieve hypnotic induction and suggestion; thus, extensive training for hypnosis is not required. Although these reports are anecdotal, their preliminary results with this technology demonstrate analgesic effects that are equivalent to those obtained when a "live" clinician is used.

VIRTUAL REALITY

Immersive virtual reality is a particularly attention-grabbing distraction technique, and is designed to give users the illusion of going inside a computer-generated virtual environment (Fig. 53.4). Virtual reality appears to provide significant cognitive distraction to users because it is interactive and places significant cognitive demand on patients through the provision of multisensory input (visual, aural, and sometimes tactile). In addition, it utilizes a head-mounted display that blocks visual and aural input to the user from the immediate and often frightening, real world burn care environment. Thus, virtual reality may exert its analgesic effect by diverting conscious attention away from concurrent nociceptive stimulation, resulting in an attenuated subjective pain experience. Functional brain imaging studies have shown the virtual reality results in pain reduction that is similar to that of systemic opioid administration, both in terms of magnitude of

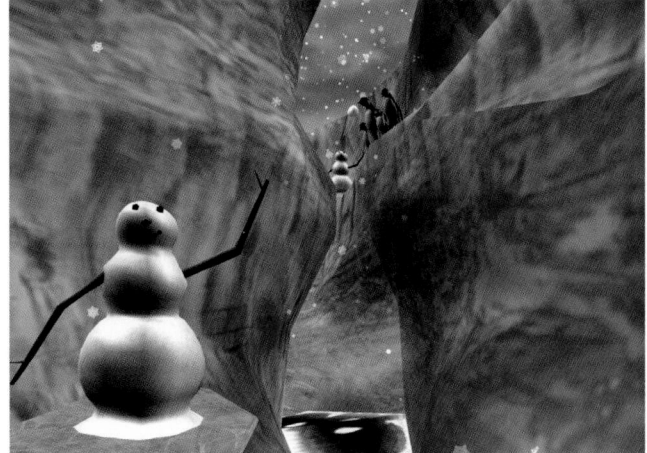

FIGURE 53.4 Virtual reality environment "SnowWorld." as seen by the patient/user. Snow/ice motif and blue/white/lavender colors suggest a cool temperature setting in direct contrast to the hot setting in which most burn injuries occur. Virtual igloos, penguins, and snowmen on canyon walls facilitate user interaction with the virtual world through user-targeted shooting of virtual snowballs at these virtual objects.

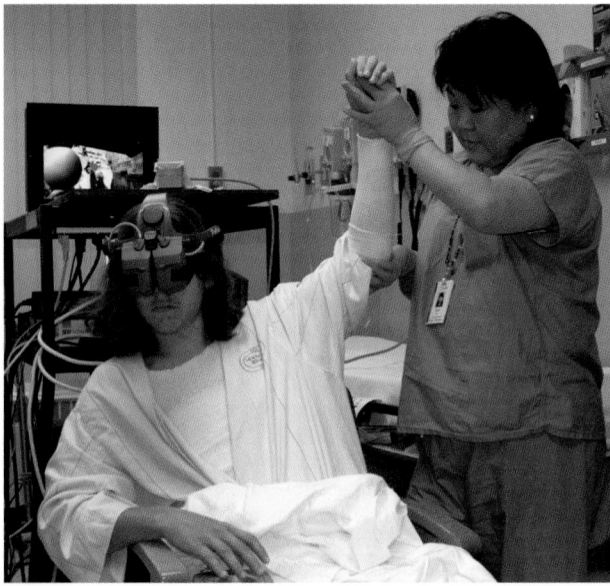

FIGURE 53.5 Clinical use of virtual reality distraction during burn wound care. A burn patient undergoes postburn skin stretching and passive joint range-of-motion while experiencing immersive virtual reality analgesia. Both auditory and visual stimulation are provided through a lightweight head-mounted display that can track the users position in the virtual environment by assessment of head position, and user interaction with objects in the virtual environment is controlled by manual trackball.

analgesia and brain activity changes, and is also additive to opioid analgesia when administered concurrently.[122] The use of adjunctive, immersive virtual reality was first reported to provide clinically meaningful pain relief in the setting of burn wound débridement,[123] with findings subsequently replicated in larger populations of burn patients.[124,125] Virtual reality analgesia is also advantageous for the less severe pain associated with certain types of postburn rehabilitation activities[126] (Fig. 53.5), and has been combined with hypnotic suggestion (as noted previously) to provide nonpharmacologic analgesia for burn wound care.[120,121]

CONCLUSION

Effective treatment of burn injuries requires an appreciation of the unique patterns of nociception caused by this trauma and their interaction with psychological factors. Aggressive use of opioid analgesics tailored to the nature of the pain (e.g., procedural, background, postoperative) serves as the cornerstone of a multifaceted approach to burn pain. Procedural pain often involves consideration of a variety of supplemental pharmacologic approaches, ranging from mild sedation to general anesthesia. Nonpharmacologic approaches should be woven into the structure of burn care as adjuncts to pharmacologic analgesia (i.e., multimodal analgesia). The under-treatment of burn pain remains an unfortunate reality, particularly since adequate analgesia may facilitate recovery and posthospital adjustment, as well as represent a more humane course of treatment.

Acknowledgment

The authors' work was supported in part by funding from the National Institutes of Health (AR054115, GM042725).

References

1. Brigham PA, McLoughin E. Burn incidence and medical care use in the United States: estimates, trends, and data sources. *J Burn Care Rehabil* 1996;17: 95–107.
2. Esselman PC, Thombs BD, Magyar-Russell G, et al. Burn rehabilitation: state of the science. *Am J Phys Med Rehabil* 2006;85:383–413.
3. Melzack R. The tragedy of needless pain. *Sci Am* 1990;262:27–33.
4. Carrougher GJ, Ptacek JT, Sharar SR, et al. Comparison of patient satisfaction and self-reports of pain in adult burn-injured patients. *J Burn Care Rehabil* 2003;24:1–8.
5. Ptacek JT, Patterson DR, Montgomery BK, et al. Pain, coping, and adjustment in patients with severe burns: preliminary findings from a prospective study. *J Pain Symptom Manage* 1995; 10:446–455.
6. Patterson DR, Tininenko J, Ptacek JT. Pain during burn hospitalization predicts long-term outcome. *J Burn Care Res* 2006;27:719–726.
7. Loor MM, Vern TZ, Latenser BA, et al. Trends in burn research as reflected in American Burn Association presentations, 1998 to 2003. *J Burn Care Rehabil* 2005;26:397–404.
8. Silbert BS, Osgood PF, Carr DB. Burn pain. In Yaksh TL, et al., (eds). *Anesthesia: Biologic Foundations*. Philadelphia: Lippincott-Raven; 1997:759–773.
9. Summer GJ, Puntillo KA, Miaskowski C, et al. Burn injury pain: the continuing challenge. *J Pain* 2007;8:533–548.
10. Choinière M, Melzack R, Rondeau J, et al. The pain of burns: characteristics and correlates. *J Trauma* 1989;29:1531–1539.
11. Perry S, Heidrich G, Ramos E. Assessment of pain by burn victim patients. J Clin Beh Res 1981;2:322–326.
12. Atchison NE, Osgood PF, Carr DB, et al. Pain during burn dressing change in children: relationship to burn area, depth, and analgesic regimens. *Pain* 1991;47:41–45.
13. Choiniere M, Melzack R, Papillon J. Pain and paresthesia in patients with healed burns: an exploratory study. *J Pain Symptom Manage* 1991;6: 437–444.
14. Chapman CR. Psychological factors in postoperative pain and their treatment. In: Smith G, Covino BG, eds. *Acute Pain*. London: Butterworths; 1985:22–41.
15. Chien S. Role of the sympathetic nervous system in hemorrhage. *Physiol Rev* 1967; 47:214–288.
16. Mackersie RC, Karagianes TG. Pain management following trauma and burns. *Crit Care Clin* 1990; 7:433–449.
17. Saxe G, Stoddard F, Courtney D, et al. Relationship between acute morphine and the course of PTSD in children with burns. *J Am Acad Child Adolesc Psychiatry* 2001;40:915–921.
18. Patterson DR, Everett JJ, Bombardier CH, et al. Psychological effects of severe burn injuries. *Psychol Bull* 1993;113:362–378.
19. Berry CC, Wachtel TL, Frank HA. An analysis of factors which predict mortality in hospitalized burn patients. *Burns Incl Therm Inj* 1982;9:38–45.
20. Brezel BS, Kassenbrock JM, Stein JM. Burns in substance abusers and in neurologically and mentally impaired patients. *J Burn Care Rehabil* 1988;9: 169–171.
21. Steiner H, Clark WR Jr. Psychiatric complications of burned adults: a classification. *J Trauma* 1977;17:134–143.
22. Andreasen NJ, Norris AS, Hartford CE. Incidence of long-term psychiatric complications in severely burned adults. *Ann Surg* 1971;174:785–793.
23. Blank K, Perry S. Relationship of psychological processes during delirium to outcome. *Am J Psychiatry* 1984;141:843–847.
24. Carrougher GJ, Ptacek JT, Honari S, et al. Self-reports of anxiety in burn-injured hospitalized adults during routine wound care. *J Burn Care Rehabil* 2006;27:676–681.
25. Aaron LA, Patterson DR, Finch CP, et al. The utility of a burn-specific measure of pain anxiety to prospectively predict pain and function: a comparative analysis. Burns 2001; 27:329–334.
26. Romano JM, Turner JA. Chronic pain and depression: does the evidence support a relationship? *Psychol Bull* 1985;97:18–34.
27. Thombs BD, Bresnick MG, Magyar-Russell G. Depression in survivors of burn injury: a systematic review. *Gen Hosp Psychiatry* 2006;28:494–502.
28. Thombs BD, Bresnick MG, Magyar-Russell G, et al. Symptoms of depression predict change in physical health after burn injury. *Burns* 2007;33:292–298.
29. Perry SW. Undermedication for pain on a burn unit. *Gen Hosp Psych* 1984; 6:308–316.
30. Stoddard FJ, Sheridan RL, Saxe GN, et al. Treatment of pain in acutely burned children. *J Burn Care Rehabil* 2002;23:135–156.
31. Schneider JC, Harris NL, El Shami A, et al. A descriptive review of neuropathic-like pain after burn injury. *J Burn Care Res* 2006;27:524–528.
32. Dauber A, Osgood PF, Breslau AJ, et al. Chronic persistent pain after severe burns: a survey of 358 burn survivors. *Pain Med* 2002;3:6–17.
33. Edwards RR, Smith MT, Klick B, et al. Symptoms of depression and anxiety as unique predictors of pain-related outcomes following burn injury. *Ann Behav Med* 2007;34:313–322.
34. Jaffe SE, Patterson DR. Treating sleep problems in patients with burn injuries: practical considerations. *J Burn Care Rehabil* 2004;25:294–305.
35. Choinière M, Melzack R, Girard N, et al. Comparisons between patients' and nurses' assessment of pain and medication efficacy in sever burn injuries. *Pain* 1990;40:143–152.
36. Schechter NL, Allen DA, Hanson K. Status of pediatric pain control: a com-

parison of hospital analgesic usage in children and adults. *Pediatrics* 1986; 77:11–15.

37. Angell M. The quality of mercy. *N Engl J Med* 1982;306:98–99.

38. Perry S, Heidrich G, Ramos E. Assessment of pain in burn patients. *J Burn Care Rehabil* 1981;2:322–326.

39. Porter J, Jick H. Addiction rare in patients treated with narcotics. *N Engl J Med* 1980;302:123.

40. American Society of Anesthesiologists Task Force on Sedation and Analgesia by Non-Anesthesiologists. Practice guidelines for sedation and analgesia by non-anesthesiologists. *Anesthesiology* 2002;96:1004–1017.

41. Joint Commission on the Accreditation of Healthcare Organizations (JCAHO). *Pain Management Across the Continuum of Care: The Patient's Experience*. Oakbrook Terrace, IL: Joint Commission Resources; 2000.

42. American Academy of Pediatrics, American Academy of Pediatric Dentistry, Coté CJ, Wilson S, Work Group on Sedation. Guidelines for monitoring and management of pediatric patients during and after sedation for diagnostic and therapeutic procedures: an update. *Pediatrics* 2006;118:2587–2602.

43. Cortiella J, Marvin JA. Management of the pediatric burn patient. *Nurs Clin North Am* 1997;32:311–329.

44. Sheridan RL, Hinson M, Nackel A, et al. Development of a pediatric burn pain and anxiety management program. *J Burn Care Rehabil* 1997;18:455–459.

45. Gibbons J, Honari SR, Sharar SR, et al. Opiate-induced respiratory depression in young pediatric burn patients. *J Burn Care Rehabil* 1998;19:225–229.

46. Patterson DR, Hoffman HG, Weichman SA, et al. Optimizing control of pain from severe burns: a literature review. *Am J Clin Hypn* 2004;47:43–54.

47. Sharar SR, Patterson DR, Wiechman-Askay S. Burn pain. In: Waldman SD, ed. *Pain Management*. Philadelphia, PA: Saunders-Elsevier; 2007:240–256.

48. Faucher L, Furukawa K. Practice guidelines for the management of pain. *J Burn Care Res* 2006;27:659–668.

49. Iafrati NS. Pain on burn unit: patient vs. nurse perceptions. *J Burn Care Rehabil* 1986; 7:413–416.

50. Marvin JA. Pain assesment versus measurement. *J Burn Care Rehabil* 1995; 16:348–357.

51. Perry S, Inturrisi C. Analgesia and morphine disposition in burn patients. *J Burn Care Rehabil* 1983;4:276–279.

52. Herman RA, Veng-Pedersen P, Miotto J, et al. Pharmocokinetics of morphine sulfate in patients with burns. *J Burn Care Rehabil* 1994;15:95–103.

53. Furman WR, Munster AM, Cone EJ. Morphine pharmacokinetics during anesthesia and surgery in patients with burns. *J Burn Care Rehabil* 1990;11: 391–394.

54. Silbert BS, Lipkowski AW, Cepeda MS, et al. Enhanced potency of receptor-selective opioids after acute burn injury. *Anesth Analg* 1991;73:427–433.

55. Franceschi D, Gerding RL, Phillips G, et al. Risk factors associated with intravascular catheter infections in burn patients: a prospective, randomized study. *J Trauma* 1989;29:811–816.

56. Choiniere M, Grenier R, Paquette C. Patient-controlled analgesia: a double-blind study in burn patients. *Anaesthesia* 1992;47:467–472.

57. Rovers J, Knighton J, Neligan P, et al. Patient-controlled analgesia in burn patients: a critical review of the literature and case report. *Hosp Pharm* 1994; 29:108–111.

58. Prakash S, Fatima T, Pawar M. Patient-controlled analgesia with fentanyl for burn dressing changes. *Anesth Analg* 2004;99:552–555.

59. Sim KM, Hwang NC, Chan YW, et al. Use of patient-controlled analgesia with alfentanil for burn dressing changes: a preliminary report of five patients. *Burns* 1996;22:238–241.

60. Patterson DR, Ptacek JT, Carrougher G, et al. The 2002 Lindberg Award. PRN vs. regularly scheduled opioid analgesics in pediatric burn patients. *J Burn Care Rehabil* 2002; 23:424–430.

61. Sharar SR, Bratton SL, Carrougher GJ, et al. A comparison of oral transmucosal fentanyl citrate and oral hydromorphone for inpatient pediatric burn wound care. *J Burn Care Rehabil* 1998;19:516–521.

62. Sharar SR, Carrougher GJ, Selzer K, et al. A comparison of oral transmucosal fentanyl citrate and oral oxycodone for pediatric outpatient wound care. *J Burn Care Rehabil* 2002;23:27–31.

63. Alvi R, Jones S, Burrows D, et al. The safety of topical anaesthetic and analgesic agents in a gel when used to provide pain relief at split skin donor sites. *Burns* 1998;24:54–57.

64. Møiniche S, Pedersen JL, Kehlet H. Topical ketorolac has no antinociceptive or anti-inflammatory effect in thermal injury. *Burns* 1994;20:483–496.

65. Lee JJ, Marvin JA, Heimbach DM. Effectiveness of nalbuphine for relief of burn debridement pain. *J Burn Care Rehabil* 1989;10:241–246.

66. Pal SK, Cortiella J, Herndon J. Adjunctive methods of pain control in burns. *Burns* 1997;23:404–412.

67. Cuignet O, Pirson J, Soudon O, et al. Effects of gabapentin on morphine consumption and pain in severely burned patients. *Burns* 2007;33:81–86.

68. Gray P, Williams B, Cramond T. Successful use of gabapentin in acute pain management following burn injury: a case series. *Pain Med* 2008;9:371–376.

69. Walker J, Maccallum M, Fischer C, et al. Sedation using dexmedetomidine in pediatric burn patients. *J Burn Care Res* 2006;27:206–210.

70. Kariya N, Shindoh M, Nishi S, et al. Oral clonidine for sedation and analgesia in a burn patient. *J Clin Anesth* 1998;10:514–517.

71. Ratcliff SL, Meyer WJ III, Cuervo LJ, et al. The use of haloperidol and associated complications in the agitated, acutely ill pediatric burn patient. *J Burn Care Rehabil* 2004;25:472–478.

72. Perry S, Heidrich G. Management of pain during debridement: a survey of U.S. burn units. *Pain* 1982;13:267–280.

73. Martin-Herz SP, Patterson DR, Honari S, et al. Pediatric pain control practices of North American Burn Centers. *J Burn Care Rehabil* 2003;24:26–36.

74. Egan KJ, Ready LB, Nessly M, et al. Self-administration of midazolam for postoperative anxiety: a double blinded study. *Pain* 1992;49:3–8.

75. Patterson DR, Ptacek JT, Carrougher GJ, et al. Lorazepam as an adjunct to opioid analgesics in the treatment of burn pain. *Pain* 1997;72:367–374.

76. Baskett PJF, Hyland J, Deane M, et al. Analgesia for burns dressing in children. *Br J Anaesth* 1969;41:684–688.

77. Filkins SA, Cosgrav P, Marvin JA. Self-administered anesthesia: a method of pain control. *J Burn Care Rehabil* 1981;2:33–34.

78. American Society of Anesthesiologists. Report of an ad hoc committee on the effect of trace anesthetics on the health of operating room personnel. Occupational disease among operating room personnel: a national study. *Anesthesiology* 1974;41:321–340.

79. Nunn JF, Chanarin I, Tanner AG, et al. Megaloblastic bone marrow changes after repeated nitrous oxide anaesthesia. *Br J Anaesth* 1986;58:1469–1470.

80. Demling RH, Ellerbe S, Jarrett F. Ketamine anesthesia for tangenital excision of burn eschar: a burn unit procedure. *J Trauma* 1978;18:269–270.

81. Ward CM, Diamond AW. An appraisal of ketamine in the dressing of burns. *Postgrad Med J* 1976;5:222–223.

82. Humphries Y, Melson M, Gore D. Superiority of oral ketamine as an analgesic and sedative for wound care procedures in the pediatric patient with burns. *J Burn Care Rehabil* 1997;18:34–36.

83. Warncke T, Stubhaug A, Jørum E. Ketamine, an NMDA receptor antagonist, suppresses spatial and temporal properties of burn-induced secondard hyperalgesia in man: a double-blind crossover comparison with morphine and placebo. *Pain* 1997;72:99–106.

84. Owens VF, Palmieri TL, Comroe CM, et al. Ketamine: a safe and effective agent for painful procedures in the pediatric burn patient. *J Burn Care Res* 2006;27:211–216.

85. Dimick P, Helvig E, Heimbach D, et al. Anesthesia-assisted procedures in a burn intensive care unit procedure room: benefits and complications. *J Burn Care Rehabil* 1993;14:446–449.

86. Powers PS, Cruse CW, Daniels S, et al. Safety and efficacy of debridement under anesthesia in patients with burns. *J Burn Care Rehabil* 1993;14: 176–180.

87. Tosun Z, Esmaoglu A, Coruh A. Propofol-ketamine vs propofol-fentanyl combinations for deep sedation and analgesia in pediatric patients undergoing burn dressing changes. *Paediatr Anaesth* 2008;18:43–47.

88. Pedersen JL, Callesen T, Møiniche S, et al. Analgesic and anti-inflammatory effects of lignocaine-prilocaine (EMLA) cream in human burn injury. *Br J Anaesth* 1996;76:806–810.

89. Brofeldt BT, Cornwell P, Doherty D, et al. Topical lidocaine in the treatment of partial-thickness burns. *J Burn Care Rehabil* 1989;10:63–68.

90. Wehner D, Hamilton GC. Seizures following topical application of local anesthetics to burn patients. *Ann Emerg Med* 1984;13:456–458.

91. Jönsson A, Cassuto J, Hanson B. Inhibition of burn pain by intravenous lignocaine infusion. *Lancet* 1991;338:151–152.

92. Punja K, Graham M, Cartotto R. Continuous infusion of epidural morphine in frostbite. *J Burn Care Rehabil* 1998;19:142–145.

93. Still JM, Abramson R, Law EJ. Development of an epidural abscess following staphylococcal septicemia in an acutely burned patient 1995;38:958–959.

94. Cuignet O, Mbuyamba J, Pirson J. The long-term analgesic efficacy of a single-shot fascia iliaca compartment block in burn patients undergoing skin grafting procedures. *J Burn Care Rehabil* 2005;26:409–415.

95. Cuignet O, Pirson J, Boughrouph J, et al. The efficacy of continuous fascia iliaca compartment block for pain management in burn patients undergoing skin grafting procedures. *Anesth Analg* 2004;98:1077–1081.

96. Everett JJ, Patterson DR, Chen ACN. Cognitive and behavioral treatments for burn pain. *Pain Clinic* 1990;3:133–145.

97. Fauerbach JA, Lawrence JW, Haythornthwaite JA, et al. Coping with the stress of a painful medical procedure. *Behav Res Ther* 2002;40:1003–1015.

98. Thompson SC. Will it hurt less if I can control it? a complex answer to a simple question. *Psychol Bull* 1981;90:89–101.

99. Strickland BR. Internal-external expectancies and health-related behaviors. *J Consult Clin Psychol* 1978;46:1192–1211.

100. Prensner JD, Yowler CJ, Smith LF, et al. Music therapy for assistance with pain and anxiety management in burn treatment. *J Burn Care Rehabil* 2001; 22:83–88.

101. Fordyce WE. *Behavioral Methods for Chronic Pain and Illness*. St. Louis: Mosby Year Book, Inc.; 1976.

102. Tan S. Cognitive and cognitive-behavioural methods for pain control: a selective review. *Pain* 1982;12:201–228.

103. Kendall PC, Williams I, Pechacek TF, Graham LF, Shisslak C, Herzoll N. Cognitive-behavioural and patient education interventions in cardiac catheterization procedures: the Palo Alto medical psychology project. *J Consulting Clin Psychol* 1979;47:49–58.

104. Johnson JE, Morrisey JF, Leventhal H. Psychological preparation for an endoscopic examination. *Gastrointest Endosc* 1973;19:180–182.

105. Johnson JE, Kirchhoff KT, Endress MP. Altering children's distress behaviour during orthopedic cast removal. *Nurs Res* 1975;24:404–410.

106. Paice JA, Noskin GA, Vanagunas A, et al. Efficacy and safety of scheduled dosing of opioid analgesics: a quality improvement study. *J Pain* 2005;6: 639–643.

107. Ehde DM, Patterson DR, Fordyce WE. The quota system in burn rehabilitation. *J Burn Care Rehabil* 1998;19:436–439.

108. Kavanagh CK, Lasoff E, Eide Y, et al. Learned helplessness and the pediatric burn patient: dressing change behavior and serum cortisol and beta-endorphin. *Adv Pediatr* 1991;38:335–363.

109. Patterson DR, Questad KA, Boltwood MD. Hypnotherapy as a treatment for pain in patients with burns: research and clinical considerations. *J Burn Care Rehabil* 1987;8:263–268.

110. Frenay MC, Faymonville ME, Devlieger S, et al. Psychological approaches during dressing changes of burned patients: a prospective randomised study comparing hypnosis against stress reducing strategy. *Burns* 2001;27:793–799.

111. Patterson DR, Jensen MP. Hypnosis and clinical pain. *Psychol Bull* 2003;129:495–521.

112. Wakeman JR, Kaplan JZ. An experimental study of hypnosis in painful burns. *Am J Clin Hypn* 1978;21:3–12.

113. Patterson DR, Adcock RJ, Bombardier CH. Factors predicting hypnotic analgesia in clinical burn pain. *Int J Clin Exp Hypn* 1997;45:377–395.

114. Patterson DR, Everett JJ, Burns GL, et al. Hypnosis for the treatment of burn pain. *J Consult Clin Psychol* 1992;60:713–717.

115. Patterson DR, Ptacek JT. Baseline pain as a moderator of hypnotic analgesia for burn injury treatment. *J Consult Clin Psychol* 1997;65:60–67.

116. Spiegel H, Spiegel D. *Trance and Treatment*. Washington, DC: American Psychiatric Press; 1978.

117. Ewin D. Hypnosis in burn therapy. In: Burrows GD, Dennerstein L, eds. *Hypnosis*. Amsterdam: Elsevier; 1979.

118. Ewin DM. Emergency room hypnosis for the burned patient. *Am J Clin Hypn* 1986;29:7–12.

119. Van der Does AJ, Van Dyck R. Does hypnosis contribute to the care of burn patients? *Gen Hosp Psychiatry* 1989;11:119–124.

120. Patterson DR, Tininenko JR, Schmidt AE, et al. Virtual reality hypnosis: a case report. *Int J Clin Exp Hypn* 2004;52:27–38.

121. Patterson DR, Wiechman SA, Jensen M, Sharar SR. Hypnosis delivered through immersive virtual reality for burn pain: a clinical case series. *Int J Clin Exp Hypn* 2006;54:130–142.

122. Hoffman HG, Richards TL, Van Oostrom T, et al. The analgesic effects of opioids and immersive virtual reality distraction: evidence from subjective and functional brain imaging assessments. *Anesth Analg* 2007;105:1776–1783.

123. Hoffman HG, Doctor JN, Patterson DR, et al. Use of virtual reality for adjunctive treatment of adolescent burn pain during wound care: a case report. *Pain* 2000;85:305–309.

124. Das DA, Grimmer KA, Sparnon AL, et al. The efficacy of playing a virtual reality game in modulating pain for children with acute burn injuries: a randomized controlled trial. *BMC Pediatr* 2005;5:1.

125. van Twillert B, Bremer M, Faber AW. Computer-generated virtual reality to control pain and anxiety in pediatric and adult burn patients during wound dressing changes. *J Burn Care Res* 2007;28:694–702.

126. Sharar SR, Carrougher GJ, Nakamura D, et al. Factors influencing the efficacy of virtual reality distraction analgesia during postburn physical therapy: preliminary results from 3 ongoing studies. *Arch Physical Med Rehabil* 2007;88:S43–S49.

CHAPTER 54 ■ PERSISTENT PAIN IN CHILDREN

NEIL L. SCHECHTER, TONYA M. PALERMO, GARY A. WALCO, AND CHARLES B. BERDE

Persistent pain problems in children, as in adults, may stem from a wide variety of causes. They may be associated with ongoing illnesses such as cancer or sickle cell disease (SCD), may be the residua of pathologic processes that have resolved but have sensitized the peripheral or central nervous system such as postinfectious myalgias, or may represent a nonprogressive disorder whose main manifestation is pain such as headaches, widespread musculoskeletal pain, or functional abdominal pain. Regardless of the etiology of the pain, its assessment, its impact, and often the modalities used to treat are remarkably similar and often distinct from approaches used to address acute pain. For example, while the broader context of pain, including an array of genetic, developmental, environmental, and individual factors, is rarely a major focus of assessment in acute pain, these factors are essential to consider when pain is recurrent or persistent. Likewise, treatment goals may shift from pain eradication in acute pain to pain reduction, rehabilitation, and improved coping in chronic pain.

In this chapter, we will describe the epidemiology of chronic pain, define its impact on children and families, and offer general approaches to its evaluation and treatment. Discussion of cancer pain is contained elsewhere in this volume as are more detailed descriptions of specific pain problems.

EPIDEMIOLOGY OF CHRONIC PAIN IN CHILDREN

The epidemiology of the various chronic pain problems in children is often hard to ascertain primarily due to variability in the methodologies in the available research. While this fact is an issue for adults as well, the limitations of the pediatric literature in the area of chronic pain, the often more complex diagnostic criteria which must factor in developmental change, child variants of adult disorders, and the limitations in the child's ability to report symptoms give us pause as we sift through data on the prevalence of persistent pain syndromes in children. A sample of the epidemiology of selected persistent pain problems in children follows.

Musculoskeletal Pain

One of the most common sites for pain in children and adolescents is the musculoskeletal system, including joint pain, bone pain, and muscle pain. Discomfort may arise from disease processes (e.g., inflammation associated with arthritis), it may be related to central pain processing difficulties (e.g., juvenile fibromyalgia syndrome or Pain Associated Disability Syndrome), or may be related to trauma or injury, typically focusing on a specific area of the body (e.g., back pain or neck pain).

Arthritis

Estimates of the prevalence of juvenile arthritis have shifted a good deal over the years due to a number of factors, including diagnostic difficulties, changes in the classification schemas used, differences in research methodology, cohort effects, and factors occurring with the passage of time. Estimates of prevalence range from 10–220 cases per 100,000. Recent estimates suggest that 294,000 children between 0 and 17 years of age are being affected by "arthritis or other rheumatic conditions".[1]

Regarding pain in this population, Schanberg et al.[2] found that children with polyarticular juvenile arthritis had pain an average of 73% of the days. Although for most children this pain was in the mild to moderate range, 31% reported pain in the severe range.

Nonrheumatologic Musculoskeletal Pain

A number of studies have tried to identify the prevalence of musculoskeletal pain in children and adolescents not associated with arthritis or other rheumatologic conditions. De Inocencio[3] reported on a review of 6500 office visits of children 3 to 14 years of age and found that 6.1% were for musculoskeletal complaints, the majority of which were for arthralgias and soft tissue pain. Common etiologies included trauma as well as mechanical or overuse pathology.

More generally, many children and adolescents report significant episodes of chronic nonspecific pain at least once in their lifetime, including limb pain (4.2% to 33.6%), knee pain (up to 18.5%) and back pain (7.6% to 34%).[4] Mikkelsson et al.[5] followed third and fifth graders over 1 year and found that pain occurring at least once per week persisted in 52.4%, with neck pain having the highest persistence. Thus, although the range of prevalence rates is very broad, it is clear that specific and pervasive musculoskeletal pain is quite common in children and adolescents. It also appears that overall the prevalence and cumulative incidence of these symptoms increase with age, and are more common and appear slightly earlier in females compared to males.

Complex Regional Pain Syndrome (CRPS). There are few studies reporting on the prevalence of CRPS in children and adolescents. Available data indicates a very high female to male ratio (about 6:1) and more common occurrences in the lower extremity than upper.[6] In a more recent study of children presenting to a pediatric pain program in Australia, Low et al.[7] reported that patients were 90% girls, with lower limbs affected in 85% of cases, and most typically (80% of the time) precipitated by minor trauma.

Fibromyalgia Syndrome. The prevalence of fibromyalgia syndrome in children and adolescents is difficult to determine. Mikkelsson et al.[8] used a structured pain questionnaire in a large sample of Finnish third and fifth grade children and found that 22 of them (1.25% overall) met criteria for fibromyalgia syndrome. In a retrospective review of patients referred to a pediatric rheumatology clinic between 1989 and 1995, 7% were diagnosed with fibromyalgia syndrome.[9] Female gender predominance is also a well-replicated finding.[10] Although various studies have shown correlates to the presence of the syndrome, such as joint hypermobility,[11] temperament,[12] familial aggregation,[13] and psychiatric symptoms,[8] causal relationships have not been shown.

Temporomandibular Disorders (TMD). TMD pain is often underrecognized in children and adolescents. In a prospective study of 11-year-olds, 7% were assigned a diagnosis of TMD.[14] It appears that precursors to these difficulties may be found in children as young as 7 years and progress throughout childhood. Significant correlates include bruxism and tooth-grinding, as well as bite and tooth positioning.[15]

Headache

Another area of inquiry that has received a good deal of attention is headache in childhood, particularly in adolescence. In a recent review by Hershey et al.,[16] it was concluded that up to 75% of children have had significant headaches by the age of 15 years, with up to 28% of adolescents describing symptoms consistent with migraine headaches. In general, meta-analytic reviews suggest a gradual increase in headache incidence over childhood with 37% to 51% of children reporting a significant headache by 7 years and up to 82% by 15 years.[17]

The distinction between migraine and tension type headache is often complex, particularly in pediatric headache. For example, when applying International Classification of Headache Disorders-II criteria to a large sample of German children age 7–14, Kröner-Herwig and colleagues[18] found that 7.5% of the headaches could be classified as migraine, 18.5% as tension-type, and the majority were unclassifiable. Virtanen et al.[19] found that among children who were classified as having migraines at age 6 years, half were unchanged at age 13, while for 32%, there was a shift toward tension-type headaches. Other authors found a similar lack of stability in headache type over time with headache types shifting or disappearing entirely. Therefore, the precise relationship between various types of headaches in children remains unclear.

In addition, various authors report close relationships between headache pain and other difficulties, including neck pain,[20] back pain,[21] abdominal pain,[22] sleep disturbances,[23] fatigue,[24] epilepsy,[25,26] epistaxis,[27] psychiatric difficulties, and risk of suicide.[28–30]

In summary, headaches in children appear to be quite common. Precisely what differentiates migraine headache from tension-type headaches is difficult to discern at times, although recent shifts in diagnostic criteria and increased awareness of the syndromes should be helpful. Headaches increase in frequency and severity with age with a clear shift around the time of puberty, are more common and problematic in females, and health-related quality of life (HRQOL) may be significantly impacted.[31]

Chronic Abdominal Pain

Chronic abdominal pain accounts for 2% to 4% of pediatric visits. Hyams et al.[32] found that 75% of middle school and high school students reported abdominal pain, while 21% reported it was severe enough to affect activities and 8% visited a physician for it. Like other pain problems, various definitions and correlates of persistent abdominal pain (recurrent abdominal pain, chronic abdominal pain, functional abdominal pain (FAP), nonorganic abdominal pain, and psychogenic abdominal pain) have led to varying perspectives in its prevalence. The Rome II criteria for abdominal pain not due to gastrointestinal pathology have become the commonly accepted nosology. The categories are now functional dyspepsia, irritable bowel syndrome, FAP syndrome, and abdominal migraine.[33] A revision of these criteria, Rome III, was published in 2006, which further differentiates FAP from FAP syndrome.[34]

It appears that the roots of nonspecific abdominal pain may be identified quite early in development based on chart reviews of a cohort of children followed from birth to 5 years. Chitkara et al.[35] found an incidence of abdominal pain of unknown origin of 4.5/1000 person years leading to repeated visits to the pediatrician. Finally, as was the case with prior pain problems, there is growing evidence the difficulties with chronic abdominal pain early in life are associated with the risk of future abdominal pain, other pain problems (e.g., headache), and broader somatic concerns later in childhood and beyond.[36,37]

Disease- or Treatment-Related Pain

Sickle Cell Disease

For many years, the focus of pain management in children and adolescents with SCD were episodes of vaso-occlusion. Dampier and colleagues[38] gathered pain diary data in children and adolescents with SCD. They found that vaso-occlusive pain is experienced on 2% of days in preschool-age children and on 5% to 10% of days in school-age children and young adolescents. School-age children tended to have less intense pain than adolescents, and girls tended to report a higher number of painful sites than boys. Subsequent data[39] showed that 40% to 50% of school-age children experience one pain episode a month, while about 10% experience more than two episodes a month. While the majority of these episodes lasted one day or less, about 5% of episodes in older children last longer than 2 weeks.

More recently, however, it is clear that children with SCD are affected by a number of recurrent chronic pain concerns beyond those related to vaso-occlusion. Although Niebanck et al.[40] found that overall the prevalence of tension type and migraine headaches in children with SCD approximates that of healthy peers, they found that headache was more common in younger children with SCD and that there were relationships noted between frequency of headache and frequency of vaso-occlusion. This suggests that factors related to SCD may increase the risk of headache pain. In addition, sequelae of splenic sequestration may lead to ongoing visceral pain in the left upper quadrant and irreversible joint damage, such as related to aseptic necrosis, may cause ongoing discomfort.

Cystic Fibrosis

Koh et al.[41] evaluated 46 children with cystic fibrosis (CF) and found that nearly half of the sample described pain occurring at least weekly with primary locations of the abdominal and pelvic region, chest, head, and neck. Although most children reported mild pain intensity and relatively short duration, a small subgroup reported moderately intense pain in the chest that was of longer duration. Pain in this group was thought to be musculoskeletal in nature, related to pulled or torn intercostal muscles, costochondritis, pleuritis, pneumothorax, or rib fracture. A web-based study of adolescents and young adults with CF found that about half experienced moderate daily pain of 2 hours duration or less, with disability highest in areas of recreation, occupation, and social activities.[42]

Phantom Limb

Phantom pain occurs when a limb has been amputated and the individual continues to feel pain in a part of the body that is no longer there. In an early attempt to ascertain the prevalence of such conditions in children, Krane and Heller[43] conducted a retrospective survey of 5- to 19-year-olds who had undergone limb amputation in the preceding 10 years. Amputations were secondary to congenital deformity, trauma/infection, or cancer. Phantom sensations were experienced in all patients, and the overwhelming majority stated they experienced phantom pain as well. Melzack et al.[44] reported that phantom limbs are experienced by 20% of those with congenital limb deficiencies and 50% of those who underwent amputation before age 6 years. Phantom pain was reported in 20% and 42% of these groups, respectively. Using diary data, Wilkins et al.[45] found recurrent episodes of phantom pain due to congenital limb deficiencies, surgery, and trauma, with an average intensity of 6.43 out of 10.

Additional Considerations

The above review should make it clear that there is an array of chronic and recurrent pain problems that affect children and adolescents. It is unwise, therefore, to focus on "chronic" or "recurrent" pain as a unified entity, but rather as diverse syndromes, perhaps with certain common factors. As will be discussed below, a broad biopsychosocial perspective is deemed optimal, which embraces genetic, developmental, and environmental influences.

In the remainder of this chapter, we will discuss the impact of persistent pain on children and offer a general approach to evaluating and managing it. A more detailed review on a number of more common entities will be offered as well. Additional information on many of these problems is available in other sections of this volume, such as Chapters 25, 49, 57, and 61.

IMPACT OF PERSISTENT PAIN ON CHILDREN AND FAMILIES

Recurrent and chronic pain can have a major impact on the daily lives of children, adolescents, and their families. While some children experiencing pain symptoms have minimal day to day impairment, other children exhibit psychologic problems and have significant activity limitations due to pain. The children who seek treatment for their chronic pain symptoms likely represent the group which is experiencing the most impairment.[46] For many children, chronic pain has been associated with poorer HRQOL, psychosocial difficulties, academic problems, and disruptions in peer and family relationships.[47,48]

Disability or activity limitation that results from chronic pain is a separate concept from pain itself, and it is equally important to consider in assessment and management of pediatric pain patients.[49] Disability refers to those areas in an individual's life that are limited due to pain.[50] The domains of functioning that seem to be particularly impacted by chronic pediatric pain are participation in physical and social activities, school and academics, sleep, and family functioning. Specifically, chronic pain has been associated with more frequent school absences and academic difficulties.[51,52] Missed schooling can have direct effects on academic performance and school success as well as important effects on socialization and maintenance of peer relationships. Difficulties with peer relationships have been found in children with chronic pain, with one study of children with juvenile fibromyalgia reporting that children were more isolated, less well-liked, and less socially accepted than their healthy peers.[53]

Pain can also interfere with the quality and quantity of children's sleep, with over half of children and adolescents with chronic pain reporting sleep difficulties.[48] These problems typically include difficulty initiating sleep, maintaining sleep, and early morning awakening. Sleep problems have been shown to correlate with depressive symptoms.[54] Sleep deprivation can also reduce children's abilities to cope with pain and enhance pain sensitivity.[55] For example, in children with SCD, high daily pain was associated with poor sleep quality that night, which in turn predicted high pain levels the following day.[56]

Activities limited due to pain vary depending on the level of pain children experience. Higher levels of pain intensity and longer pain duration have been associated with greater activity limitations and impairment.[57–59] Specific domains of activity restriction have also been associated with pain level. In one study of children with SCD, while children decreased participation in all activities (school, play, sports, social) when pain was high, they were able to maintain school attendance and social activities when pain levels were low.[58] Future research is needed to better understand the relationship between pain and activity restriction among different populations.

Persistent pain also has a substantial impact on the emotional status of children and adolescents. In general, children with recurrent pain experience more stress and feel less cheerful and more depressed compared to children without pain.[60] Chronic pain is associated with psychiatric comorbidity, particularly anxiety and mood disorders, at least in some selected populations. For example, in a sample of children seen in primary care for recurrent abdominal pain, 79% of children met criteria for an anxiety disorder and 43% for a depressive disorder.[61] Children and adolescents with chronic pain have also demonstrated lower levels of self-esteem, more internalizing (e.g., somatization) and externalizing behaviors,[62,63] and higher levels of neuroticism and fear of failure compared to healthy children.[64] Moreover, children's coping style (particularly maladaptive coping) and catastrophizing behaviors are associated with increased psychologic problems and physical limitations.[65] In one study of children with mixed chronic pain conditions, maladaptive coping was correlated with depression and disability, with children with musculoskeletal pain having the most difficulty coping and greatest physical impairment.[47]

HRQOL refers to an individual's perception of the impact a disease or condition has on his or her physical health status, psychologic functioning, and emotional well-being. Youth with chronic pain and their parents report lower HRQOL than healthy children. For example, in one study of adolescents with recurrent headache, participants with head pain reported lower HRQOL in physical, social, and psychologic functioning domains compared to headache-free adolescents.[66] Similarly, in another study examining HRQOL in children with FAP, both children and their parents reported significantly lower HRQOL compared to healthy participants, with parents of children with FAP reporting the lowest quality of life ratings overall.[67]

Chronic pain also has a negative impact on family life. Parents often experience significant financial burden due to the evaluation and management of their child's recurrent and chronic pain, including direct costs of pain treatment such as hospitalization, doctor's visits, and costs of medications. Indirect costs include parental time off work, transportation costs, childcare, and incidental costs totaling over $15,000 per child per year.[68] The stress of chronic pain on families is also associated with increased levels of family conflict and poorer family functioning. Previous studies have shown more family problems in children with chronic headaches compared to healthy children[69] and that poorer family environments are associated with increased headache-related disability.[70,71] Moreover, frequent quarreling within families significantly increased the occurrence of weekly and monthly head pain in children and adolescents.[18]

Parenting children with chronic pain is also related to problems with emotional functioning, particularly elevated levels of parental depression, anxiety, and parenting stress.[72] One study of mothers of adolescents with chronic pain found that mothers reported feelings of guilt, inadequacy, and uncertainty in parenting competence due to their child's pain.[73] Chronic pain in children has also been associated with increased restrictions on parental socialization and high levels of parental strain, anger, and hostility.[74]

ASSESSMENT

Accurate pain assessment is critical for individualizing pain treatment strategies and to assess treatment progress in achieving important goals of pain reduction and increased function. Measurement of aspects of recurrent and chronic pain require tools that measure the frequency, intensity, duration, time course, and activity interference due to pain. Validated measures have been developed to capture most of these domains.[75,76] Diaries are often used in the clinical management of children with recurrent and chronic pain to provide information for evaluation purposes and to document treatment progress. Pain diaries may be useful for obtaining estimates of intensity, frequency, and duration of pain as well as possible patterns (e.g., differences between school days and nonschool days) and triggers (e.g., exams, performance stress, etc.). If a diary is used, it should be for a short time only to understand more about the pain. Prolonged use of a diary may unduly focus attention to the pain and subsequently increase pain complaints.

A critical area to assess is function. Measures such as the Functional Disability Inventory,[50] the Pediatric Quality of Life Inventory,[77] the Child Activity Limitations Interview,[78] and the Bath Adolescent Pain Questionnaire[79] all provide information about child functioning in normal daily activities. These measures are all brief and can be administered easily to document children's functional disability at baseline and treatment progress.

Psychosocial assessment is an important component in the assessment of a child with chronic pain in order to evaluate psychologic, social, and family functioning which may contribute to pain or pain-related disability. Psychosocial assessment may consist of clinical interviews, administration of standardized psychologic measures, and observation of child and family members. A detailed clinical interview should cover developmental, behavioral, and psychiatric concerns in the patient's and family's history. Potential stressors and areas of maladaptive coping should be inquired about as well as a comprehensive school history, and history of peer and social relationships. Ideally, a separate psychosocial assessment is conducted with child and parent alone in order to obtain their individual perspectives. Many outpatient pediatric pain clinics use intake questionnaire packets that cover demographics, developmental history, and other aspects of psychologic functioning in order to consistently obtain this information in the evaluation of new patients. Review of intake packets may then provide details that serve as a springboard for more focused clinical interviews or additional psychologic assessments during the intake visit.

Depending upon the particular presenting concerns, standardized psychologic measures may be administered to screen for mental health diagnoses, in particular, anxiety and depressive symptoms, to assess coping behaviors, and family functioning. A variety of standardized instruments can be used in the clinical setting with the advantage of obtaining a quick assessment of children's psychologic functioning given the limited time available for in-depth psychologic evaluation in the medical setting. For example, screening for anxiety and depression can be accomplished using scales such as the Children's Depression Inventory,[80] the Revised Manifest Children's Anxiety Scale,[81] or the Revised Child Anxiety and Depression Scale.[82] When psychologic measures are used to screen for psychologic distress, it is important to consider the limitations of self-report and in particular that children may want to present themselves in a favorable light (social desirability response bias), which has been described in children and adolescents with chronic pain.[83]

Parental and family functioning has also been a major area of focus in pediatric chronic pain assessment.[84] Parental response to pain behaviors can be assessed using the Adult Response to Child pain behaviors,[85] and family functioning can be evaluated using a variety of measures such as the Family Assessment Device.[86] For a comprehensive review of measures available to assess parental impact of chronic pain, see Eccleston et al.[75]

There are also measures of child coping that have been validated on pediatric chronic pain samples including the Pain Response Inventory[87] and the Pain Coping Questionnaire.[88] Measures of specific areas of coping, including catastrophizing, are available such as the Pain Catastrophizing Scale, child version PCS-C.[89]

CLINICAL EVALUATION OF THE CHILD WITH CHRONIC PAIN

Background

The evaluation of a child with chronic pain is often complex and time-consuming, yet it often falls unfortunately on the already

overburdened shoulders of the office-based primary care practitioner. The typical child with chronic pain has been evaluated by many practitioners from multiple disciplines. If the source of the pain is obvious such as previously or newly identified organic disease (e.g., ulcerative colitis, SCD, cancer), the focus is on addressing the underlying illness while simultaneously treating the associated pain. In other situations, the source of the pain may be known but not amenable to direct treatment and therefore the focus must be solely on the pain itself (e.g., persistent postoperative, posttraumatic, or postviral pain). For both of these groups of children, there is no need for an extensive search for an explanation for their pain, and the clinician can focus on its treatment.

The more challenging situation and the emphasis of the majority of this chapter occurs when no obvious pathophysiologic source of the pain has yet been identified. The child is suffering, the parents are frustrated, and no treatable disease process has emerged to explain the pain. In these situations, the clinician must attempt to identify those children who may have an as yet undiagnosed underlying progressive disease process and separate them from those who have chronic pain syndromes, which although uncomfortable, do not represent life-threatening illness. This is not an easy task, given the inherent vagueness of the symptoms, the inadequacies of children as historians, and the vast differential diagnosis.

It is critical, however, in the attempt to rule out potentially serious or life-threatening causes of pain, that physicians avoid an endless search for the underlying etiology of the discomfort. Continued laboratory investigation often convinces the child and family that there must be a biological explanation for the problem and suggests to them that the "answer" may be found in the next laboratory test. Clinicians often report that they are ordering additional tests "for the sake of completeness" and both clinicians and families often find it difficult to draw a diagnostic line in the sand where all are content with extent of the investigation. Konijnenberg and colleagues[90] highlighted this problem in a series of papers in which 17 different pediatricians reviewed the medical records of 134 children with unexplained chronic pain. There was disagreement on diagnostic approach in over a third of the patients and on the primary cause of the pain in over one half.[90] Unfortunately, this diagnostic uncertainty leads to further excessive and expensive laboratory and imaging studies. It is particularly unfortunate if, after completing an extensive battery of tests, which are negative, the doctor implies that the problem must be psychologic and refers the child to a mental health professional.

Therefore, one of the most critical aspects of the evaluation of the child with unexplained chronic pain is the acceptance by child, family, and provider that medical investigation has been sufficient to allow the primary focus of the encounter to be on the management of the pain, regardless of its etiology.

History

General

The traditional elements of the pain history for adults are applicable to chronic pain in children. Although younger children are developmentally less capable of presenting a coherent narrative, they certainly are capable of reporting on specific aspects of their pain. These include pain intensity (with the aid of developmentally appropriate tools), radiation, exacerbating and relieving factors, and quality of the pain. For chronic pain, which tends to occur in older children and adolescents, as mentioned earlier, a strong focus of the interview should involve the impact of the pain on the child's functioning—school attendance and work quality, social relationships, and mood. Roth-Isigkeit and colleagues[48] studied 750 German schoolchildren and found that 30% to 40% reported restrictions in daily living secondary to pain. Chalikidis'[91] study of chronic pain in Australian youth revealed that 71% of children had difficulty sleeping and over 90% were unable to be involved in sports. Improvement in function may occur well before decreased pain intensity and is therefore an important marker of response to treatment.

It is important to be aware of the child's medical history. Emerging data from multiple streams suggest that early exposure to painful stimuli (e.g., multiple surgeries, stormy neonatal course, multiple painful procedures) potentially predisposes the infant to changes in nociception. An extensive body of work by Fitzgerald and colleagues[92–95] in rat pups has demonstrated long lasting hypersensitivity to pain from early tissue injury. Grunau and coworkers,[96–99] in a series of papers, compared toddlers who were born prematurely to babies of normal gestation and birth weight and found differences in pain sensitivity and somatization. Far less pronounced but measurable differences between the groups were found even when the children had reached 8–10 years. Anand[100] has even suggested that there are increased rates of ADHD, substance abuse, and anxiety in children who have been exposed to repeated neonatal pain and stress.

Another essential element to query is the history of pain problems in the family. Although some authors, such as Borge,[101] question whether chronic pain symptoms run in families, on the whole, the majority of studies have suggested that parent and family history of pain are predictors of child pain. This pattern has been identified in children with rheumatologic disease,[102] recurrent abdominal pain, migraine, and fibromyalgia. The mediators of this phenomenon are unclear. They may be physiologic (such as altered pain thresholds) or psychologic (e.g., social modeling of catastrophizing behavior) or most likely a combination of both. Eccleston and colleagues[65] report that parents who have chronically ill children are often anxious and depressed (60% and 40%) and these symptoms may be a response to parenting a sick child or may predate the child's illness. They have identified factors that are associated with a higher level of emotional distress in parents of children with chronic pain. These include depression in the child, long duration of pain, and young age of the child. Regardless of the mediators for this phenomenon, it is essential that family history of pain be examined, as data are fairly conclusive that children of parents with chronic pain are at risk for somatic and emotional issues. The child's pain cannot be adequately addressed if the parent's pain is not recognized.

Psychologic and social factors should be explored in every child with chronic pain, regardless of its suspected etiology. Such an exploration does not imply causation, but there is a transactional relationship between chronic pain and anxiety and depression. Many families may become angry when psychologic issues are raised and assume that the physician is ignoring the very genuine pain the child may be experiencing. The family should understand that all pain, particularly chronic pain, has physiologic and psychologic components and any comprehensive treatment program addresses all domains. Questions regarding anxiety, depression, and excessive irritability should be posed to both the child and his or her family. The use of existing standardized questionnaires has been described earlier in this chapter.

The child's school experience should also be explored.[103] As stated earlier, increased school absenteeism is commonly reported in most chronic pain syndromes,[104] widespread musculoskeletal pain,[5] and abdominal pain.[105] Certainly, learning disabilities and attentional problems may be a source of stress which may increase the child's awareness of discomfort and cause it to be intolerable. Likewise, social difficulties and bullying may similarly increase stress and concomitant pain. Frequent absences themselves may be a source of distress for the child. School with its academic and social demands is stressful for many children. Reintegrating after frequent or prolonged absences, however, when the child still may feel vulnerable and have to deal with accumulated work, loss of contact with peers, and complex social encounters ("Where have you been?" "What is wrong with you?" "You don't look like you have a disease.") let alone the school environment, can be so overwhelmingly stressful as to preclude the child from returning. These factors, however, should not be construed as the "cause" of the pain per se but may have a role in amplifying the child's interpretation of the pain signal. Therefore, frank discussion about the child's grades and competencies, social skills, friendships, and existing school accommodations should be part of the history gathering. A detailed discussion regarding school and chronic pain is contained in the treatment section of this chapter.

Specific

The previously described information is important when gathering the history of any chronic pain problem. There are specific questions, however, associated with each chronic pain condition that may help us determine if the pain fits the traditional syndrome or may represent a problem which requires additional investigation. The red flags in history and physical examination which suggest ongoing progressive disease for three common chronic pains (headache, widespread musculoskeletal pain, and functional gastrointestinal pain) are discussed in specific sections on these entities at the end of this chapter.

Physical Evaluation

Information gathered from the physical examination in conjunction with the history can help differentiate a chronic pain syndrome from pain secondary to an underlying disease. The child's general appearance (sickly or well appearing) may be helpful, although individuals who are in pain for a prolonged period of time may look pale and wan. It is essential to monitor growth parameters as chronic illness may well impede growth. There is an association between chronic pain and postural orthostatic tachycardia syndrome and therefore heart rate should be obtained both supine and standing.

The child should be asked to localize his or her pain. The differential diagnosis and intervention strategies are very different for generalized discomfort versus highly localized pain. Specific discussion of the examination of the back, abdomen, and joints are beyond the scope of this review but regardless of the origin of the pain, the clinician should obtain general impressions of the child's mood, cooperativeness, irritability, and eye contact. The child's gait and posture should be noted.

Emerging literature supports the association of chronic musculoskeletal pain with hypermobility. This may be secondary to central sensitization which may be induced by constant subluxation and slippage or may have other etiologies. Regardless of the origin, a Beighton score should be calculated on all children with chronic musculoskeletal pain.[106] Preliminary research suggests an association with cervical hypermobility and headache as well.[107]

Clinical Formulation

The task for the clinician is to examine the data that emerged from the history and physical and determine whether or not there are sufficient red flags to warrant further investigation for progressive disease. If there are, the child and family should be informed that the investigation is ongoing. If there are not, the clinician should report to the child and family that the child most likely has a chronic pain syndrome. In either situation, the pain should be treated appropriately although the approach, both philosophically and practically, will vary between the two. If the pain is thought to be a manifestation of a time-limited disease process, although the approach will be multifactorial, there will often be an emphasis on more aggressive pharmacologic intervention while the disease process runs its course. If the pain is associated with a chronic condition or represents a chronic pain syndrome, the emphasis is more typically on coping and function with supplemental analgesia.

Feedback With Family

The initial feedback session with the child and family after the evaluation has been completed sets the tone for the subsequent relationship. If the child has ongoing disease, the pain care physician should be part of a coordinated effort to address the child's problems. If it is decided that additional interventions to address an underlying disease process are not necessary, care coordination remains critical and one health care provider should assume that responsibility. Chronic pain patients often see multiple traditional as well as alternative health care providers and may acquire extensive medical records. Case management is a critical role.

Regardless of the etiology of the pain, it is imperative that the clinician informs the family that he or she is familiar with the symptom complex, even if the exact problem is not clearly defined. Chronic pain treatment has key dimensions that should be addressed such as sleep, school, and physical and social activities regardless of the etiology of the pain. It is also essential for chronic pain that the family be aware that pain persistence does not have the warning protective function that it does in acute pain. The notion that the pain "hurts" but is not causing "harm" is essential to convey to alleviate familial anxiety.

The current conceptualization of chronic pain in children is that it results from the interplay between biologic vulnerabilities and psychologic and environmental variables. Biologic vulnerability may result from abnormalities of sensory processing which may stem from peripheral tissue damage or inflammation. This burst of nociceptor activity increases the strength of the connection between the nociceptor and the spinal cord neurons. This may yield enhanced responsiveness and excitability in the central nervous system known as "central sensitization." Such hyperresponsiveness is associated with decreased pain thresholds and hyperalgesia and has been linked to functional gastrointestinal disorders as well as fibromyalgia in adults. It may well be that many chronic pain conditions are associated with central sensitization or autonomic dysregulation.[108–110]

As mentioned, however, there are psychologic and environmental variables that amplify or dampen that vulnerability. Multiple studies, as previously mentioned, support the relationship of abdominal and musculoskeletal pain as well as headache with internalizing symptoms such as anxiety and depression. The massive stress of school, the loss of normal opportunities to socialize with friends, and the impact of the immobilization and sleep deprivation often accompanying chronic pain further contribute to that relationship.

All of this must be conveyed to the family in a supportive, nonjudgmental manner. Their acceptance of a multidisciplinary approach is fundamental to its success.

Treatment

General Principles of Treatment

A number of general principles have evolved to define the treatment of chronic pain in children. If there is a specific identified etiology, direct measures to address it should be undertaken. For children with an identified etiology as well as those without, a multimodal approach focusing on function is key. Initially, the family should be informed that the child will be carefully monitored through frequent scheduled appointments. A symptom diary may provide interim data between appointments. This monitoring reassures anxious parents that someone will be watching their child if new symptoms emerge which suggest a previously unrecognized disease process. This approach has been labeled "watchful waiting." If the pain problem does not evolve significantly over time, it mitigates against an ongoing progressive disease. Any monitoring should focus not only on pain intensity but also on function (sleep, mood, school attendance, etc.).

Interventions typically employed to address chronic pain must allow the child to return to a "normal" life. As a result, drugs which significantly alter the child's sensorium are inadvisable as are prolonged hospital or home stays. Drugs which reduce central sensitization such as amitriptyline and gabapentin are often the mainstay of pharmacologic treatment regardless of the etiology of the chronic persistent pain. Other antidepressants and anticonvulsants are frequently used, but few are approved for use in children. Analgesics may be helpful but the risk of rebound headache or abdominal pain secondary to excessive nonsteroidal usage is genuine. Opioids are occasionally necessary. Long-acting opioids should always be prescribed with a short-acting breakthrough opioid.

Physical therapy is of particular value in musculoskeletal pain syndromes such as fibromyalgia but is valuable in any pain syndrome in which the child's activity level has been diminished and he or she has become deconditioned. A graded exercise program increases the child's feelings of well-being and provides reassurance and confidence as the child regains lost abilities. Other physical and occupational therapy modalities such as desensitization, transcutaneous electrical nerve stimulation, and stretching or strengthening particular muscle groups are also helpful. Biofeedback, a technique to gain conscious control of physiologic functions which are typically beyond voluntary control through the use of a computer, has demonstrated efficacy in headache reduction but may be helpful for other chronic pain conditions.

There is a strong body of evidence that suggests that psychologic interventions are effective for chronic pain treatment in children. Multiple reviews and meta-analyses attest to the strength of the impact of these approaches which include cognitive-behavioral as well as psychotherapeutic strategies.[111,112] Although many of the cognitive-behavioral strategies were developed to help coping with procedures, many such as meditation, hypnosis, reframing, and help with coping and avoiding catastrophization all have efficacy in chronic pain as well. A psychotherapist can function as a life coach, helping the child with strategies that might soften the impact of school re-entry, decrease anxiety, and provide advice to parents who are overwhelmed.

School is the work of childhood and chronic pain is often associated with frequent school absence. Parents often need help ushering the crying, complaining children off to school when the path of least resistance is to allow them to remain in bed. Specific criteria for school attendance should be developed. In general, school attendance should be mandatory except for those times when the child has a fever. This eliminates parental vacillation and second thoughts and allows them to be consistent and to shift the blame to the health care provider. Modification can be made for work load, length of day, extended time, physical education attendance, etc., but the child should develop the rhythm of daily school attendance. More detailed information on the importance of school and school reintegration is offered later in this chapter.

There are certainly situations where the parent's response is detrimental to the child's coping. Occasionally, parents may be so insistent on identifying an etiology that the child is dragged to a continuous parade of specialists, subjected to unnecessary procedures, and school absence is promoted. There is emerging literature which suggests that children whose parents are overly apologetic or overly solicitous report more pain than children whose parents are matter of fact.

In summary, the treatment of chronic pain in children needs to address the pain itself as well as the life context in which that pain is occurring. As a result, analgesia often needs to be coupled with antidepressants and/or anticonvulsants. Sleep, school, coping, activity level, and family functioning all are important dimensions of the treatment of chronic pain.

SPECIFIC INTERVENTIONS FOR CHRONIC/PERSISTENT PAIN

Children who receive care in a multidisciplinary pediatric pain clinic are typically offered a multicomponent treatment plan which often involves psychologic therapy, physical therapy, and medication management. Philosophically, most programs incorporate a rehabilitation approach in which pain is accepted as a symptom that will be diminished but might not be entirely eradicated. Therefore, the focus is typically on improving function and quality of life. The specific structure of each program differs depending on local factors with some providing inpatient rehabilitation while others are solely outpatient. Many new programs are developing in the United States and abroad. Zeltzer and Schlank[113] list many pediatric pain programs in the United States, Canada, and internationally.

Pharmacologic Interventions

Pediatric analgesic pharmacology is summarized in greater detail elsewhere in this volume (see Chapter 50). The current discussion emphasizes specific uses of analgesics in the setting of chronic persistent pain, as opposed to acute pain. Pharmacotherapy of chronic pain in children and adolescents requires patience and balance of risks, benefits, and side effects. For most patients coming to a chronic pain clinic, pharmacotherapy should not be used in isolation, but only as a component of a multimodal treatment program. In considering a medication trial, clinicians' discussions with patients and parents strike a difficult balance. The aims of drug therapy and expected benefits should be outlined. Side effects and risks should be discussed in a manner that is honest, but tailored to the style of the individual patient and family. There is a growing literature on how patients hear risk discussions.[114]

Discussions of side effects do have the potential to generate nocebo (negative placebo) effects.

For some conditions, treatments can be specific and mechanism-driven. For example, for children with rheumatoid arthritis, pharmacotherapy is largely directed at underlying inflammatory processes, and for most patients, treatment of inflammation serves to treat the pain. Similarly, pharmacotherapy for migraine and for specific subtypes of chronic abdominal pain may be directed at underlying mechanisms in some cases.

Acetaminophen and nonsteroidal anti-inflammatory drugs (NSAIDs) are widely used for pediatric acute pain management, and NSAIDs are an integral component of management of chronic inflammatory disorders. Daily use of either of these classes of medications can produce rebound headaches. There is comparatively little studied on chronic daily administration of acetaminophen in children. Chronic administration of NSAIDs in children with rheumatoid arthritis has been associated with gastropathy and nephropathy, but overall with a lower risk than has been reported in adults.

A majority of trials of cyclooxygenase (COX)-2 inhibitors in children have involved short term use. A recent 3-month trial comparing celecoxib to naproxen showed equal efficacy and no statistically significant difference in adverse events.[115]

Opioids have been extensively studied for pediatric acute pain management and for pain in children with cancer. As with adults, there is little consensus regarding which children with chronic noncancer pain have a favorable risk-benefit ratio for long-term opioid analgesia. Overall, prospective studies on adults in pain clinic populations with nonlife-shortening conditions have not shown good effect of long-term use of opioids on either pain

scores or measures of quality of life or functioning. Those who defend chronic opioid therapy in adults may argue that these studies did not address ideal patient subgroups. With children and adolescents, there are additional concerns. First, opioid tolerance and opioid-induced hyperalgesia are likely to proceed more rapidly for children compared to adults.[116,117] Secondly, long-term opioid administration may have detrimental effects on endocrine function. Thirdly, with many chronic medical conditions in childhood, longevity is difficult to predict, and advances in treatment have changed prognosis for many chronic illnesses of childhood and young adult life. For these reasons, we do use opioids on a long-term basis for a small subset of children with chronic pain not due to life-limiting illnesses, but we do so with some caution and with consideration of alternatives. There is a theoretical argument in favor of selection of either methadone or buprenorphine for long-term opioid therapy in younger patients, based on a hypothesis that relates the development of tolerance and hyperalgesia to differential activation of receptor-mediated activation of second messenger systems versus receptor-mediated endocytosis.

For adults with many forms of chronic pain, especially neuropathic pain disorders, there is evidence for efficacy of several anticonvulsant and antidepressant medications. We will cite some limited pediatric information below, but at present most information regarding efficacy must be extrapolated from clinical trials in adults. In adults, these medications are side effect prone, inconsistently effective; they generally produce partial, rather than complete, pain relief. In adults, there are very few randomized controlled trials (RCTs) that compare one antidepressant to another,[118] or that compare an antidepressant to an anticonvulsant. There is remarkably sparse evidence for selecting one medication over another in general for adults with chronic pain, except for specific conditions that are uncommon in pediatrics, such as trigeminal neuralgia.

One publication is cited here mainly to recommend caution in its interpretation. The authors use an "indirect meta-analysis" to compare duloxetine to the anticonvulsants gabapentin and pregabalin for treatment of neuropathic pain in adults. What is actually done is to use outcomes from active treatment groups in studies comparing duloxetine to placebo to the active treatment groups in studies comparing gabapentin or pregabalin to placebo.[119]

For antidepressants in trials for neuropathic pain in adults, numbers needed to treat (NNTs) range from 2–4 for trials involving tricyclics (mostly with "global improvement" as an endpoint) to as high as 5 for trials involving duloxetine with 50% pain relief as a primary endpoint. Overall, tricyclics appear to be more effective than selective serotonin reuptake inhibitors (SSRIs) for neuropathic pain in adults.

For children and adolescents, we commonly choose nortriptyline as a first line tricyclic. We encourage starting at a very low dose (e.g., 10 mg every night for adolescents and older children and 5 mg every night for younger children). The rate of dose escalation is determined by clinical circumstances and side effects. For an outpatient who experiences no adverse symptoms, dosing might be increased every 3 days until there is good analgesia or he or she reaches a dose around 40 or 50 mg daily. Dosing is occasionally even more rapid for inpatients with severe neuropathic cancer pain. Conversely, if the child does experience side effects, dose escalation proceeds more slowly. If there is no indication of analgesia or side effects by the time dosing is escalated to 50 mg/daily (and if we are convinced that the child is taking the medication), we will often obtain a blood level prior to further dose escalation. Clearance of tricyclics in children is enormously variable. An electrocardiogram is widely recommended either prior to initiating treatment or after dose escalation. We adhere to this recommendation while recognizing that there is little evidence that electrocardiography can identify patients at risk for sudden cardiac events.

There are a number of clinical trials and case series on antidepressants for migraine prophylaxis in pediatrics, including amitriptyline, nortriptyline, and trazodone, though many have involved open label designs or crossover comparisons to other drugs.[120,121]

There is a widely quoted case series on the SSRI citalopram for treatment of recurrent abdominal pain in children. While there is apparent improvement in a large percentage of patients, this should be interpreted with great caution because of the open-label and uncontrolled design of the study.[122]

There has been extensive controversy regarding potential risks of antidepressants in triggering suicidal ideation and completed suicide among adolescents. What is clear to us is that these medications require close monitoring for changes in a child's mood and behavior. Prescribing should begin in low doses, doses should be escalated in a gradual and stepwise manner, and there should be a system for frequent reassessments, ideally including regular phone calls in between clinic visits. For guidance of families, there is a well-written statement on the National Institutes of Mental Health website.[123]

Anticonvulsants are also widely used for treatment of neuropathic pain in adults. As with antidepressants, side effects are common, treatment responses tend to be partial rather than full, and NNTs generally range from as low as 3 to over 5.

Gabapentin emerged as a widely prescribed medication for neuropathic pain in the 1990s, in part because of the widespread belief that it was safer or easier to prescribe compared to other anticonvulsants. There is a remarkable dearth of trials comparing anticonvulsants to each other for neuropathic pain in adults.

As with tricyclics, our recommendation for gabapentin dosing is to start with small doses and escalate slowly, particularly in ambulatory patients. Different clinicians begin adolescents in a dose range from 100 mg daily to 300 mg daily. Our preference is to start for a few days with night-time-only dosing, to begin morning and then afternoon dosing after about 3 days, and to escalate every few days as tolerated until there is pain relief, significant side effects, or dosing reaches a range around 1800 mg daily over a period of about 3 weeks. Again, some patients tolerate escalation with no side effects, and others may tolerate daily doses as low as 300 mg. We commonly recommend giving half the daily dose at night, with one quarter in the morning and one quarter in the afternoon. As with tricyclics, dose escalation of gabapentin may be considerably more rapid for children with advanced cancer and refractory neuropathic pain.[124]

In our view, if trials of gabapentin or pregabalin produce minimal benefit or problematic side effects, there is reason to consider trials of anticonvulsants with different mechanisms. In particular, for peripheral neuropathic pain, we often try anticonvulsants with actions on sodium channels, such as oxcarbazepine.[125,126]

In our practice, topiramate is used primarily for migraine prophylaxis. Among the anticonvulsants, topiramate has a relatively high risk for neurocognitive side effects, especially effects on memory, word-finding, and mental clarity.[127]

Some of our colleagues have tended to select anticonvulsants rather than antidepressants as first-line agents because of the aforementioned controversy regarding suicidal ideation and suicide attempts with antidepressants in pediatrics. Unfortunately, anticonvulsants may increase these risks as well. An analysis of placebo-controlled trials of anticonvulsants for a range of indications found increased frequencies of suicidal ideation and attempts in the active drug groups compared to control groups, and this increased risk was apparently not limited to a particular drug class or a particular patient group.[128]

Psychological Interventions

Although there is a well-established evidence base for the effectiveness of psychologic treatments for chronic pain in adults,[129] there is a more limited evidence base in children and adolescents. The first systematic review of published RCTs of psychologic therapy for children and adolescents with chronic pain (with a subset meta-analysis of pain relief) was published several years ago.[111] These authors concluded that although there were few published RCTs, strong evidence emerged that psychologic therapies, principally relaxation and cognitive-behavioral therapy (CBT), are effective in reducing the severity and frequency of chronic pain in children and adolescents.

The CBT interventions included in these studies primarily involved brief, standardized treatments where children were taught specific coping skills (e.g., positive self-statements, relaxation) in the outpatient setting. A number of limitations, however, were noted in the pediatric chronic pain trials included in this review, particularly the relatively small numbers of trials (especially for nonheadache chronic pain), small sample sizes, and lack of non-pain outcomes such as function, mood, and disability.

Teaching parents appropriate strategies for managing their child's pain-related behaviors (e.g., reinforcing adaptive coping, discouraging maladaptive pain behaviors) is beneficial in treatment, and these strategies are increasingly being incorporated into psychologic therapies. For example, in a recent study, a cognitive-behavioral family intervention was compared to standard pediatric care for recurrent abdominal pain.[130] Children in the cognitive-behavioral family intervention group received five 40-minute sessions and were trained in relaxation skills and positive self-talk, and parents were taught to limit secondary gains from children's sick behaviors. The standard medical care group received customary medical treatment consisting of follow-up office visits, education, support, and medications as deemed appropriate by the treating physician. Children who received the cognitive-behavioral intervention reported significantly less pain after treatment, and at 1-year follow-up compared to children receiving standard care, providing support for the use of cognitive-behavioral family interventions in children with abdominal pain.[130]

Research has also shown that including parental behavior management strategies in conjunction with children's CBT can lead to improvements in parents' psychologic functioning. In one study using an interdisciplinary cognitive-behavioral program to treat adolescents with chronic pain, both youth and their parents obtained significant reductions in levels of anxiety, depression, and stress immediately following treatment and at a 3-month follow-up.[72]

Studies utilizing minimal therapist contact and self-administered treatments for chronic pain are the largest treatment advance to make CBT more accessible to children and families. These self-administered treatments focus on relaxation, and CBT for children with headaches have produced equal or better results as equivalent therapist-led treatments.[131–133] Importantly, self-administered treatments are more than three times more cost-effective compared to in-office treatments,[134] making such CBT interventions ideal for pediatric pain patients to be implemented on a large scale.[135]

More recently, two small pilot studies have been published using innovative technologies to deliver minimal therapist contact psychologic treatments for children with chronic or recurrent pain. Hicks and colleagues[136] evaluated the efficacy of distance CBT delivered via the internet and telephone for children ages 9 to 16 years with recurrent pain. They found significant reduction in pain levels for children receiving the distance treatment versus a standard medical care control group. In another recent study of a minimal therapist-contact treatment for recurrent pain, Connelly and colleagues[137] evaluated a CD-ROM pain management program (focused on relaxation training) in children ages 7–12 years with recurrent headache. They also found significant improvements in headache activity (less intense and frequent pain) in children who received the 4-week CD-ROM intervention versus children receiving standard care. These studies are important for demonstrating feasibility in the delivery of CBT to children with recurrent pain using computer technologies and hold promise for future treatment developments in this area.

Pilot studies are emerging in the application of acceptance and commitment therapy (ACT) to children with chronic pain.[138] ACT is an increasingly popular form of CBT that emphasizes the importance of accepting pain symptoms and working toward valued goals, using interventions such as exposure, cognitive defusion, and mindfulness. Parents are also integrated into treatment using similar interventions emphasizing exposure to previously avoided private experiences, acceptance, and defusion exercises. In a pilot study of adolescents with idiopathic chronic pain, Wicksell and colleagues[138] reported that after 7–10 treatment sessions, patients showed a 63% reduction in functional disability, a 68% drop in school absences, 27% reduction in internalizing/catastrophizing symptoms, and a 46% decrease in pain intensity. Reductions were sustained at 3- and 6-month follow-ups. ACT appears promising, and it is anticipated that larger scale studies will be forthcoming using this approach to treat children and adolescents with chronic pain.

Complementary and alternative medicine (CAM) interventions are becoming increasingly popular in the treatment of chronic pain and have been successful in helping children and adults manage pain symptoms.[139] CAM refers to therapies (e.g., hypnosis, acupuncture, yoga, and biofeedback) commonly used in conjunction with conventional medical treatment. Biofeedback is one type of CAM therapy effective in the treatment of persistent pediatric pain. Biofeedback involves connecting a patient to a machine that monitors physiologic responses (e.g., muscle tension, heart rate). One form of feedback, thermal biofeedback, involves using electronic instruments (e.g., a temperature probe on the finger) to measure temperature, and a computer monitor to display reinforcing information back to the patient. Using relaxation approaches, patients can use the objective biofeedback information to learn to increase peripheral temperature.

Biofeedback, especially thermal biofeedback, has undergone empirical evaluation in children with migraine and tension headache, and there is evidence to recommend biofeedback and/or relaxation to any child who suffers from headaches.[140] Recently, biofeedback has been evaluated in children with chronic abdominal pain.[141,142] While results from these studies suggest that biofeedback is effective in reducing pain, RCTs using larger sample sizes are needed. Like CBT, research shows that incorporating parenting strategies into biofeedback treatment may increase the effectiveness of treatment. Children whose parents received behavior management strategies in combination with the child's standard biofeedback treatment demonstrated more clinically significant improvement in headache pain and showed greater reductions in headache frequency than those who received biofeedback alone.[143,144]

School and Social Reintegration

School and social functioning are impaired in many children with chronic pain. In industrialized societies, school is the work of children. Numerous studies have documented that children with chronic pain have difficulties with consistent school attendance and making progress with academic work, although there may also be specific impairments in peer and social relationships that are amplified in the school setting. On average, children with chronic pain miss more school days than do children with other chronic health conditions, and they often identify school as the most problematic stressor.[49] For example, Stang and Osterhaus[104] estimated that several hundred thousand school days are missed each month as a result of pediatric headache alone. In a sample of children with SCD-related pain, Shapiro and colleagues[145] reported that on average, children missed 21% of school days, which is the equivalent of 6–8 weeks of the school year.

There is also evidence that children with chronic pain may experience problems with social competence and peer relationships in the school setting. In one study, adolescents with juvenile fibromyalgia syndrome were perceived as being less popular, more isolated, and withdrawn compared to matched classroom comparison peers.[47] Moreover, these adolescents were less well liked, were selected less often as a best friend, and had fewer reciprocated friendships. Negative peer interactions were explored in one study,[146] finding that children with chronic abdominal pain had higher levels of relational victimization in comparison to pain-free peers.

The school setting may also be perceived as stressful due to problematic interactions with teachers and perceptions that adults are not supportive of children with chronic pain. In a study using vignettes, teachers' attributions about the causes of chronic pain revealed a lack of knowledge of the biopsychosocial framework and a primary perception that pain was either physical or psychologic.[147] Teachers responded more positively to students when medical evidence supporting the pain problem was available, and responses were associated with parental attitudes toward the school. Teachers were more likely to report children who were entitled to accommodations if parents approached the school in a collaborative manner rather than using a confrontational approach.[148]

There is variability in how children and families respond to impairments that may arise in the school setting. Some children and adolescents have worked out accommodations that allow them to have reduced class time, in-home tutoring, or online courses. Several mechanisms in public education laws can be used in this regard including individualized education plans and section 504 plans for other health impairments. Some families opt to remove their child from the school setting and engage in home schooling.

Regardless of the exact setting where school is to occur, addressing the impairments in school and social functioning is a primary focus of treatment for the child with persistent pain. Some children and adolescents have spent extensive time outside of their usual school and social settings and therefore graded plans for reintegration into these settings are needed. In the context of CBT, parent management guidelines have been implemented in clinical settings and in treatment studies focused on operant techniques. In general, parents are encouraged to establish a reduction of attention paid to pain symptoms in favor of increased attention paid to functional improvement. Such guidelines often include recommendations to reduce status checks; that is, allowing the child to communicate directly about pain symptoms, rather than having the parent repeatedly check in with the child about his or her pain level. Most parents experience tremendous relief in being released from the role of documenting the child's pain level. Often the focus on pain intensity and a specific numerical value (e.g., 8 out of 10) provides little in the way of adaptive coping behaviors and may lead to difficulties making decisions to reintegrate in school and social settings because of lack of change in pain levels.

Formal operant systems can be devised with families where children earn points or rewards for school attendance and participation in other social activities. The goal is to shift the pattern of contingencies so that the child experiences reinforcement for their efforts in school or social activities. An example of a point system would include specifying a target activity such as attendance at school for 4 hours each day, and then developing rewards for reaching the goal (such as full computer and television privileges) and consequences for failure to achieve the goal (such as removal of access to computer and television). Psychologists and other members of the pain team can work in treatment with children and parents to develop clear, graded plans for increasing activity. Typically, an explanation to children and parents is provided that functional improvement often precedes rather than follows pain relief. It is important to start at the same place as the child in terms of their perceived ability to sit in a chair and focus on school work for an operant system to be successful. Sometimes, very short time periods of school attendance (e.g., 1 hour) will need to be built upon gradually, and the child will need to have some control over his or her schedule. For example, it can be helpful to have the child choose what time of the day (and what classes) he or she would like to begin with upon the reintegration to school.

Carrying out a graded plan for increasing school and social functioning requires considerable effort from the parents who must arrange transportation and other logistics with getting the child to the school setting at specific times. Clinicians need to communicate sensitively to parents about their role and make clear the logical sequence of the plan to ensure its success. Additional interventions may be needed to assist children with problems related to peer relationships, interactions with teachers, or specific problems related to the school setting. There are not yet any published treatment studies evaluating school-related interventions for children with chronic pain.

Sleep

Sleep difficulties are commonly reported by children and adolescents with chronic pain. For example, in a large epidemiological study of children with chronic pain in the community,[48] over half reported some sleep problems. Self-reported sleep problems have also been documented in clinical samples of children and adolescents with juvenile rheumatoid arthritis (JRA),[149] headache,[23] SCD,[56,150] and CRPS.[151] Most commonly, children and adolescents with chronic pain describe difficulties falling asleep, frequent night and early morning awakening, and excessive daytime sleepiness.[152]

Important consequences of sleep problems have also been identified, including decrements in children's HRQOL, mood, and physical functioning.[54,153] Day-to-day variability in pain, mood, and sleep have been examined in children with SCD[150] finding that negative mood partially explained the relationship between more intense pain and poor quality sleep on the same and subsequent days. Other studies have demonstrated that depression is a strong predictor of poor sleep quality and insomnia symptoms in adolescents with chronic pain.[154]

Despite the known prevalence and significant impact of sleep problems on youth with chronic pain, there has been very limited attention to either the assessment or management of sleep problems. This is in contrast to the adult pain population where insomnia related to chronic pain has long been recognized among the most costly forms of illness in terms of prescription medications and lost work productivity.[155,156]

In clinical practice, it can be very informative to assess sleep problems in all pediatric patients with chronic pain and to offer specific sleep interventions to those patients with significant sleep disturbances. In particular, a detailed history of sleep patterns should be obtained to identify problems related to insufficient sleep duration, poor sleep habits, phase delays, or difficulties falling asleep or staying asleep. Insufficient sleep duration is common during adolescence with reported sleep in healthy samples of about 7 hours per night,[157] although optimal developmental sleep requirements for adolescents have been estimated at 9 hours per night.[158] In chronic pain samples, similar restricted sleep of about 7 hours per night has been reported.[154,159] Poor sleep habits including use of caffeine in the evening, lack of consistent bedtime routines, and the presence of electronics in the bedroom can also be clear barriers to children receiving adequate sleep duration. Children with chronic pain may also develop a high level of vigilance and arousal at bedtime and a high focus on pain when the distractions of the day are not present. These children may de-

scribe negative thoughts, worries, and somatic tension that interfere with falling asleep.

Interventions may be needed to help children increase their duration of sleep, to modify problematic sleep habits, and to teach behavioral strategies to reduce insomnia symptoms. Although interventions are being evaluated for adults with chronic pain and secondary sleep problems,[160] only one published study has separately evaluated a sleep intervention in a pediatric pain population. In this study by Bruni and colleagues,[161] the benefits of sleep hygiene education (e.g., education about age appropriate sleep duration, keeping consistent weekday and weekend sleep schedules) were assessed in a group of children and adolescents with migraine headaches and sleep problems. These investigators found that children who received sleep hygiene education obtained an improvement in migraine attacks (lower frequency and shorter duration) compared to children in a control group who did not receive sleep hygiene education. The development and evaluation of treatments for comorbid sleep disturbances in youth with chronic pain is an important clinical need.

SPECIFIC ENTITIES

Functional Gastrointestinal Pain

The conceptual framework through which we view chronic abdominal pain has evolved over the years, as has the definition. At this point, chronic abdominal pain is defined as long-lasting intermittent or constant abdominal pain that is either functional or organic (disease-based). Red flags for organic disease include pain that awakens the child from sleep, nocturnal diarrhea, persistent vomiting, weight loss, persistent right upper or lower quadrant pain, or dysphagia. If the history and concomitant physical examination do not suggest underlying pathology then, more than likely, the patient has one of the FAP syndromes. FAP is defined by a lack of demonstrable evidence of a pathologic condition and typically has a minimum of 3 months duration which, according to the Rome II criteria, need not be consecutive.[162,163] FAP is further subcategorized as functional dyspepsia (pain in the upper abdomen), irritable bowel syndrome (pain associated with alteration in bowel movements), abdominal migraine (intense pain with features of migraine such as anorexia, nausea, vomiting, and occurring paroxysmally), and FAP syndrome in which the symptoms do not fit any of the other functional syndromes and in which the pain is nearly continuous and has no relation to physiologic events such as eating, menses, or defecation.

In addition to the general strategies for addressing chronic pain, there are unique approaches to addressing the various categories of functional gastrointestinal pain in children. An evidence-based review of the literature completed prior to the development of the Rome III criteria identified only 10 randomized controlled intervention studies to address recurrent abdominal pain. It found that there was evidence to support the efficacy of famotidine, pizotifen, CBT, biofeedback, and peppermint oil enteric coated capsules. Dietary interventions such as increasing fiber had mixed results.[142]

The Rome III committee endorsed specific treatments for each of the subtypes of functional gastrointestinal pain recognizing the limitations of the literature. For functional dyspepsia, they suggested treatment with antisecretory agents such as H2 blockers or proton pump inhibitors are appropriate for pain predominant symptoms while prokinetics seem appropriate for symptoms dominated by discomfort such as bloating. For irritable bowel syndrome, they suggested peppermint oil. Antidepressants and serotonergic agents had limited support in pediatrics despite their efficacy in adults. For abdominal migraine, avoidance of potential triggers such as caffeine was advised. Treatment with the preventative agents used for migraine (cyproheptadine, sumatriptan) seems appropriate when paroxysms are frequent. Pizotifen has been studied in children and found to be effective. Finally, for functional gastrointestinal pain syndrome, reduction of psychosocial stressors, behavioral treatment, and antidepressants such as citalopram appear most effective.[34,162,163]

Headache

A critical goal of the evaluation of pediatric headache is to determine whether the headache is primary or secondary headache.[163] Primary headaches include migraine, tension type headache, and cluster headaches. They are classified by their features as compared to secondary headaches which are classified by the underlying disorder responsible for them. Secondary headaches are those attributed to head and neck trauma, intracranial vascular and nonvascular disorders, substance administration or withdrawal, infection, or pain associated with disorders of the eyes, cranium, ears, sinuses, or teeth. Red flags in the history which suggest secondary headache are sudden onset of a severe headache, headache associated with systemic illness, new headache type in a patient with cancer or human immunodeficiency virus, sudden onset of the "worst headache in your life," a pattern of gradually increasing headache pain and frequency, or headache in a child under 3. Positive answers to these questions clearly demand additional investigation as well as imaging studies.[164]

The distinctions between different types of primary headache[165,166] are often blurred in children, and headache type may change with age. Zebenholzer and colleagues[167] found that in a 1.5-year period, 30% of children were headache free, 20% had swapped headache type, and 50% continued having the same type of headache. Such fluidity makes diagnosis complex and treatment is often empiric. Criteria for the diagnosis of migraine in children require 5 or more headaches that last between 1 and 48 hours (shorter duration than in adults), are bilateral or unilateral, have a pulsating quality, and are aggravated by physical activities. They are typically accompanied by nausea and vomiting and photophobia and phonophobia which tend not to occur simultaneously in adults.[168] Tension headaches are typically categorized by their frequency: infrequent (less than once monthly), frequent (greater than once per month but less than 15 days per month), and chronic daily headache (basically every day). These headaches are typically bilateral, are not pulsating, and not aggravated by physical activity, without nausea and vomiting or photophobia or phonophobia.

The general approach to headache treatment is similar to that of other chronic pains. Reassurance is critical. Maintaining regular school attendance is a cornerstone. For headache, it appears that maintenance of regular routines (arise and bedtimes, mealtimes, etc.) is helpful, as is regular exercise.[169] There is limited evidence to generally support a specific diet or dietary exclusion, although there may well be individuals for whom food is an important trigger.[166]

There are strong data that behavioral interventions are effective at reducing headache burden regardless of the headache type. These include biofeedback, progressive muscle relaxation, distraction, and hypnosis. In a systematic review of the RCTs of psychologic interventions for chronic pain (12 headache and one recurrent abdominal pain trial), Eccleston and colleagues[111] reported the odds ratio for a 50% reduction in pain was 9.62, indicating the success of psychologic interventions. Hermann,[170] in another review, found in particular that thermal biofeedback was more effective in the treatment of migraine headaches than other psychologic modalities and the more commonly used prophylactic drug regimens. A more recent review of the literature concurred and suggested that psychologic treatments were effective in children under 12. In particular, biofeedback and relaxation training either alone or in combination produced significant

reductions in headache pain. The findings, although still positive, were less dramatic for tension or mixed headache diagnoses.[171]

The literature on pharmacologic treatment of pediatric headache, in particular, migraine, is less persuasive. Subcommittees of the American Academy of Neurology and the Child Neurology Society reviewed the evidence for acute and preventative treatment. They found that ibuprofen was effective in the acute treatment of migraine and acetaminophen was probably effective. They endorsed the use of sumatriptan nasal spray but did not find convincing evidence to support the use of any other oral or subcutaneous triptan.

Regarding preventive therapy, they felt that the lack of sufficient or contradictory evidence prevented them from endorsing the use of cyproheptadine, amitriptyline, divalproex sodium, topiramate, levetiracetam, propranolol, or trazodone. They were not discounting the possibility that these medications might be beneficial but merely stating that there was inadequate information available to judge their efficacy at the present time.[172] Clinicians may well have had positive experiences with these medications for specific patients.

There is emerging literature on the use of specific vitamins and minerals for headache prevention. High dose riboflavin (400 mg per day) has been found to reduce migraine frequency and appears safe. There have been no trials in children or adolescents.[173] Similarly, high dose magnesium has been shown to reduce headache frequency.[174]

In summary, there is convincing evidence that cognitive-behavioral approaches are beneficial in primary pediatric headaches, regardless of etiology. Lifestyle changes which reduce stress are noninvasive and make empiric sense although they have been infrequently studied. The evidence on analgesic and preventative medications is not as plentiful or as methodologically sound but a number of analgesics, 5-HT receptor agonists, anticonvulsants, antidepressants, beta blockers, and calcium channel blockers have been shown to be efficacious in adults and have been used with success in children.

Widespread Musculoskeletal Pain

The differential diagnosis of musculoskeletal pain is vast. Two questions can help sort out the chronic pain syndromes (such as fibromyalgia) from progressive disease. The first concerns the diffuseness of the symptom. Is the pain localized or widespread? The second concerns the child's general well-being. Does the child appear well or unwell? If the pain is localized and the child is well, the differential diagnosis includes "growing pains," CRPS, mechanical pain, pauciarticular juvenile rheumatoid arthritis, and spondyloarthropathy. If the child is unwell, the infectious arthritides should be considered. If the pain is diffuse and the child is unwell, malignancies or autoimmune diseases top the list. If the child is well, hypermobility and fibromyalgia should be considered. Red flags in the history that help us include pain in the morning, swelling, nocturnal pain not relieved by analgesics, poor growth, or bony tenderness.[175]

The distinction between fibromyalgia and other widespread musculoskeletal problems is somewhat arbitrary, particularly in children. Intriguingly, a number of studies have identified an increased association between fibromyalgia and hypermobility. Therefore, there may be more linkages between these groups than is presently assumed.[176,177] It is also important to address syndromes that are associated with hypermobility such as Ehlers-Danlos or Marfan syndromes which may have other problems associated with them.

Treatment for widespread musculoskeletal pain, whether based on fibromyalgia, hypermobility, or Ehlers-Danlos syndrome, usually has physical therapy at its cornerstone.[178] There is the attempt to restore the normal range of movement, even if the joint is hypermobile, strengthen the surrounding musculature to add to joint stability, and improve the general level of fitness in the individual. Premedicating with an analgesic prior to therapy may be warranted as pain may promote noncompliance with the prescribed regimen. Improving the child's level of fitness may help with sleep promotion and improve his or her general sense of well-being. Bulbena and others have reported an association between hypermobility and anxiety disorder in adults and believe that the tissue disorder is a predisposing factor for trait anxiety.[179–181] Even in children without hypermobility who have chronic musculoskeletal pain, cognitive-behavioral and, if necessary, pharmacologic interventions which reduce catastrophizing and panic and promote coping are often appropriate. Finally, it is possible that the repeated microtrauma that hypermobility causes in joints and ligamentous structures and associated pain leads to disordered sensory processing. Disordered sensory processing has been identified in many individuals with widespread musculoskeletal pain. Regardless of its origin, anticonvulsants and/or antidepressants may have a role in dampening central sensitization and therefore in the management of chronic musculoskeletal pain. Eccleston and colleagues[72] report on their multidisciplinary program which emphasizes family oriented CBT, physical activity, goal setting, pacing, relaxation, and communication. It appears that models which address the disordered sensory processing and its manifestations holistically are most likely to be successful.

Complex Regional Pain Syndromes (CRPS)

CRPS1, also known as reflex sympathetic dystrophy (RSD) involves limb pain with neuropathic descriptors (allodynia, paresthesias, dysesthesias) and variable combinations of neurovascular disturbances (coldness, mottling, nonarticular swelling, cyanosis or rubor, delayed capillary refill), sudomotor disturbances, motor abnormalities (spasms, dystonia, "jumping movements"), and trophic changes, including atrophy, abnormal hair growth, or joint contractures. Where these findings occur with clinical signs of injury to a nameable nerve trunk, the terms CRPS2 or causalgia are used. For purposes of current discussion, we will use the term RSD/CRPS to refer to these disorders inclusively.

CRPS in children and adolescents has distinct epidemiological features. It is much more common in girls than boys, it is uncommon before age 6, the apparent onset is most common from around ages 10–12, and the lower extremities are affected much more commonly than the upper extremities.[182]

For a majority of children with CRPS, an effective treatment program emphasizes patient and parent education about the nonprotective character of the pain, intensive rehabilitation that involves active exercise, resumption of weight-bearing, desensitization, and psychologic interventions based primarily on individual and family-based CBT. For some children, this can be accomplished on an outpatient basis.[183] For others who fail to improve with outpatient treatment, a next step is to do this type of multidisciplinary rehabilitation program in an inpatient or intensive day-hospital program.[184]

In adult pain medicine practice, at least in the United States, there is a considerable emphasis on early use of nerve blocks and other invasive approaches, especially sympathetic nerve blocks, spinal cord stimulation, operative, chemical, or radiofrequency sympathectomies, and more recently intravenous ketamine infusions in the treatment of RSD/CRPS. In our view, these approaches are not evidence-based in adults, and they are even less supported by evidence for children and adolescents. In a previous case series, even though some of the patients did receive regional anesthetic interventions and even though some reported benefit, there was no clear association between the duration of symptoms prior to blockade and the eventual benefit.[185]

Some pediatric case series report marked improvement in function and pain scores with no use of nerve blocks.[184] Overall, most case series suggest a good long-term prognosis for the majority of children and adolescents with CRPS. Hence, in our view, the initial therapeutic approach should be to emphasize intensive rehabilitation whenever possible.

We do make selective use of regional anesthetic approaches for patients who fail to progress despite a very good rehabilitation program and for selected patients with very severe limb swelling, dystonia, or very limited limb movement. In general, our preference is to use combined somatic-sympathetic blockade using continuous catheter approaches rather than selective sympathetic blockade or other repeated single-shot blocks. For lower extremity CRPS confined to a stocking distribution in the lower leg, our practice is to place continuous popliteal fossa sciatic perineural catheters under combined ultrasound-nerve-stimulation guidance.[186]

For lower extremity involvement in a wider distribution, we place an epidural catheter using fluoroscopy and/or nerve stimulation guidance to ensure proper dermatomal level and sidedness. For upper extremity CRPS, brachial plexus catheters are placed in either supraclavicular or infraclavicular sites using combined ultrasound and nerve stimulation guidance. For all forms of continuous regional anesthesia, catheters are placed with meticulous attention to sterile technique in the operating room, and they are tunneled to facilitate skin care and to reduce the chances for dislodgment. Prophylactic antibiotics are used. Patients are typically admitted to the hospital for infusions and intensive rehabilitation for periods of 5–8 days. While outpatient rehabilitation assisted by peripheral blockade has been described, in our view there is merit to inpatient admission to optimize intensive rehabilitation during the course of the infusions. In addition, our preference is to run higher infusion rates at nighttime and lower rates during the day to facilitate "cycle-breaking" at night and active mobilization during the day.

Evidence is lacking for efficacy of many types of analgesic medications commonly prescribed for adults with CRPS. Pediatric data are limited to case reports and uncontrolled case series. We do try tricyclic antidepressants and anticonvulsants for many of these patients. Responses are inconsistent.

Back Pain

Back pain is very common in adults, and a major contributor to absence from the workplace. Persistent back pain is relatively common in adolescents but uncommon in younger children, and in younger children, its occurrence mandates earlier consideration of a range of diagnostic possibilities, including infections (osteomyelitis, pyelonephritis, intervertebral discitis), tumors, and congenital anomalies of the spine and central nervous system (tethered spinal cord, diastematomyelia).[187,188]

In specialist referral practice, back pain in adolescents is commonly seen in athletes, dancers, gymnasts, and cheerleaders, and in children who are significantly overweight. For many patients with features suggestive of muscular pain and a normal neurologic exam, initial treatment should emphasize resumption of daily activities, a moderate exercise program including core stabilization and postural exercises, and avoidance of high impact, high velocity, or repetitive stresses on the spine. For patients with significant obesity, dietary counseling may be appropriate. Axial low back pain that worsens with back extension is commonly seen with spondylolysis and spondylolisthesis.[189,190] There is some support for bracing in the treatment of these conditions.[191]

Symptomatic lumbar disc disease is uncommon in children and relatively less common in adolescents. In our referral practice, lumbar disc disease is most commonly seen in adolescent athletes. There is an extensive literature on the advantages and disadvantages of operative treatment for lumbar radiculopathy in adults; pediatric literature is mostly limited to relatively small case series, and, with few exceptions, to relatively short-term follow-up. We recently reviewed experience with fluoroscopically-guided epidural steroid injections for lumbar radiculopathy in children and adolescents. A majority of patients reported reductions in pain and improvements in straight-leg raising, and the safety profile was excellent. In 2–5 year follow-up, less than 40% of patients in this case series came to discectomy.[192]

BARRIERS TO CARE

Most health care systems are stymied by the complicated care necessary to address the issues raised by children with chronic pain. The family's search for a satisfying answer may cause them to solicit multiple opinions for the pain problem. Additionally, children with chronic pain often report pain in more than one site and, as a result, multiple specialists are often involved in their care, each one focusing on one particular pain complaint. For example, headache and abdominal pain are frequent fellow travelers. The family may seek the opinion of a neurologist for the headache and a gastroenterologist for the abdominal pain. They may seek out alternative providers such as chiropractors, acupuncturists, or naturopaths as well. Laboratory and imaging studies are frequently performed in multiple settings. The primary care provider who typically provides care coordination must collate the records, reconcile often disparate opinions, be alert to the possibility of interactions among the drugs prescribed by the myriad of involved physicians, and be on the front line to address each new symptom and concern without overmedicalizing it. Care coordination is, therefore, a critical time consuming and often unreimbursed aspect of the care for children with chronic pain and its absence is a barrier to adequate treatment.

Another problem is the lack of facilities and practitioners capable of addressing both the biologic and psychologic dimensions of chronic pain. In the outpatient arena, few individuals are comfortable addressing both realms, and multidisciplinary teams, an alternative, are often not viable economically. Inpatient facilities are rarely geared to individuals who may have both psychologic and physical problems. A busy inpatient unit with desperately ill children is not the appropriate setting for a child with chronic pain, as it tends to overmedicalize the problem. Likewise, the typical psychiatric ward is often unprepared to deal with the patient who is moaning in pain and may have an as yet undiagnosed medical illness.

Finally, the inherent vagueness and poignancy of the symptom of persistent pain often leads families to seek out additional opinions and to feel that their search is never quite completed. This can create uneasiness between provider and patient which may interfere with the therapeutic alliance.

CONCLUSION

Persistent pain is a relatively common experience for children and may stem from a variety of causes: ongoing organic disease, persistence of pain which resulted from organic disease, as well as disorders whose primary manifestation is pain. Regardless of its origin, however, it has significant impact on the child and his or her family. In general, the goal of the clinician is to identify red flags for organic disease and if not present, focus on symptom reduction and increasing function. Specific attention should be given to sleep, mood, school, activity, and family functioning. Typical interventions include analgesia, physical therapy, cognitive-behavioral strategies, and other medications targeted to

specific symptoms. Success in the management of chronic pain should be monitored by improvement in function and not specifically through immediate reduction in pain intensity.

References

1. Helmick CG, Felson DT, Lawrence RC, et al. Estimates of the prevalence of arthritis and other rheumatic conditions in the United States. Part I. *Arthritis Rheum* 2008;58:15–25.
2. Schanberg LE, Anthony KK, Gil KM, et al. Daily pain and symptoms in children with polyarticular arthritis. *Arthritis Rheum* 2003;48:1390–1397.
3. De Inocencio J. Epidemiology of musculoskeletal pain in primary care. *Arch Dis Child* 2004;89:431–434.
4. McGrath PA. Chronic pain in children. In: Crombie IK, Croft PR, Linton SJ, et al, eds. *Epidemiology of Pain*. Seattle: IASP Press; 1999:81–101.
5. Mikkelsson M, Salminen JJ, Kautiainen H. Non-specific musculoskeletal pain in preadolescents. Prevalence and 1-year persistence. *Pain* 1997;73:29–35.
6. Wilder RT, Berde CB, Wolohan M, et al. Reflex sympathetic dystrophy in children. Clinical characteristics and follow-up of seventy patients. *J Bone Joint Surg* 1992;74:910–919.
7. Low AK, Ward K, Wines AP. Pediatric complex regional pain syndrome. *J Pediatr Orthop* 2007;27:567–572.
8. Mikkelsson M, Sourander A, Piha J, et al. Psychiatric symptoms in preadolescents with musculoskeletal pain and fibromyalgia. *Pediatrics* 1997;100:220–227.
9. Siegel DM, Janeway D, Baum J. Fibromyalgia syndrome in children and adolescents: clinical features at presentation and status at follow-up. *Pediatrics* 1998;101:377–382.
10. Eraso RM, Bradford NJ, Fontenot CN, et al. Fibromyalgia syndrome in young children: onset at age 10 years and younger. *Clin Exp Rheumatol* 2007;25:639–644.
11. Gedalia A, Press J, Klein M, et al. Joint hypermobility and fibromyalgia in schoolchildren. *Ann Rheum Dis* 1993;52:494–496.
12. Conte PM, Walco GA, Kimura Y. Temperament and stress response in children with juvenile primary fibromyalgia syndrome. *Arthritis Rheum* 2003;48:2923–2930.
13. Buskila D, Neumann L, Hazanov I, et al. Familial aggregation in the fibromyalgia syndrome. *Semin Arthritis Rheum* 1996;26:605–611.
14. LeResche L, Mancl LA, Drangsholt MT, et al. Predictors of onset of facial pain and temporomandibular disorders in early adolescence. *Pain* 2007;129:269–278.
15. Magnusson T, Egermarki I, Carlsson GE. A prospective investigation over two decades on signs and symptoms of temporomandibular disorders and associated variables. A final summary. *Acta Odontol Scand* 2005;63:99–109.
16. Hershey AD, Winner P, Kabbouche MA, et al. Headaches. *Curr Opin Pediatr* 2007;19:663–669.
17. Lewis DW, Ashwal S, Dahl G, et al. Practice parameter: evaluation of children and adolescents with recurrent headaches: report of the Quality Standards Subcommittee of the American Academy of Neurology and the Practice Committee of the Child Neurology Society. *Neurology* 2002;59:490–498.
18. Kröner-Herwig B, Heinrich M, Morris L. Headache in German children and adolescents: a population-based epidemiological study. *Cephalalgia* 2007;27:519–527.
19. Virtanen R, Aromaa M, Rautava P, et al. Changing headache from preschool age to puberty. A controlled study. *Cephalalgia* 2007;27:294–303.
20. Laimi K, Salminen JJ, Metsähonkala L, et al. Characteristics of neck pain associated with adolescent headache. *Cephalalgia* 2007;27:1244–1254.
21. Grimmer K, Nyland L, Milanese S. Repeated measures of recent headache, neck and upper back pain in Australian adolescents. *Cephalalgia* 2006;26:843–851.
22. Galli F, D'Antuono G, Tarantino S, et al. Headache and recurrent abdominal pain: a controlled study by means of the Child Behaviour Checklist (CBCL). *Cephalalgia* 2007;27:211–219.
23. Gilman DK, Palermo TM, Kabbouche MA, et al. Primary headache and sleep disturbances in adolescents. *Headache* 2007;47:1189–1194.
24. Ghandour RM, Overpeck MD, Huang ZJ, et al. Headache, stomachache, backache, and morning fatigue among adolescent girls in the United States: associations with behavioral, sociodemographic, and environmental factors. *Arch Pediatr Adolesc Med* 2004;158:797–803.
25. Stevenson SB. Epilepsy and migraine headache: is there a connection? *J Pediatr Health Care* 2006;20:167–171.
26. Wirrell EC, Hamiwka LD. Do children with benign rolandic epilepsy have a higher prevalence of migraine than those with partial epilepsies or nonepilepsy controls? *Epilepsia* 2006;47:1674–1681.
27. Jarjour IT, Jarjour LK. Migraine and recurrent epistaxis in children. *Pediatr Neurol* 2005;33:94–97.
28. Egger HL, Angold A, Costello EJ. Headaches and psychopathology in children and adolescents. *J Am Acad Child Adolesc Psychiatry* 1998;37:951–958.
29. Pakalnis A, Gibson J, Colvin A. Comorbidity of psychiatric and behavioral disorders in pediatric migraine. *Headache* 2005;45:590–596.
30. Wang SJ, Juang KD, Fuh JL, et al. Psychiatric comorbidity and suicide risk in adolescents with chronic daily headache. *Neurology* 2007;68:1468–1473.

31. Brna P, Gordon K, Dooley J. Canadian adolescents with migraine: impaired health-related quality of life. *J Child Neurol* 2008;23:39–43.

32. Hyams JS, Burke G, Davis PM, et al. Abdominal pain and irritable bowel syndrome in adolescents: a community-based sample. *J Pediatr* 1996;129: 220–226.

33. Rasquin-Weber A, Hyman PE, Cucchiara S, et al. Childhood functional gastrointestinal disorders. *Gut* 1999;45(suppl2):II60–II68.

34. Rasquin A, Di Lorenzo C, Forbes D, et al. Childhood functional gastrointestinal disorders: child/adolescent. *Gastroenterology* 2006;130(5):1527–1537.

35. Chitkara DK, Talley NJ, Weaver AL, et al. Incidence and presentation of common functional gastrointestinal disorders in children from birth to 5 years: a cohort study. *Clin Gastroenterol Hepatol* 2007;5:186–191.

36. Ramchandani PG, Hotopf M, Sandhu B, et al. The epidemiology of recurrent abdominal pain from 2 to 6 years of age: results of a large, population-based study. *Pediatrics* 2005;116:46–50.

37. Størdal K, Nygaard EA, Bentsen BS. Recurrent abdominal pain: a five-year follow-up study. *Acta Paediatr* 2005;94:234–236.

38. Dampier C, Ely E, Brodecki D, et al. Characteristics of pain managed at home in children and adolescents with sickle cell disease by using diary self-reports. *J Pain* 2002;3:461–470.

39. Dampier C, Setty BNY, Eggleston B, et al. Vaso-occlusion in children with sickle cell disease: clinical characteristics and biologic correlates. *J Pediatr Hematol Oncol* 2004;26:785–790.

40. Niebanck AE, Pollock AN, Smith-Whitley K, et al. Headache in children with sickle cell disease: prevalence and associated factors. *J Pediatr* 2007;151: 67–72.

41. Koh JL, Harrison D, Palermo TM, et al. Assessment of acute and chronic pain symptoms in children with cystic fibrosis. *Pediatr Pulmonol* 2005;40: 330–335.

42. Hubbard PA, Broome ME, Antia LA. Pain, coping, and disability in adolescents and young adults with cystic fibrosis: a Web-based study. *Pediatr Nurs* 2005;31:82–86.

43. Krane EJ, Heller LB. The prevalence of phantom sensation and pain in pediatric amputees. *J Pain Symptom Manage* 1995;10:21–29.

44. Melzack R, Israel R, Lacroix R, et al. Phantom limbs in people with congenital limb deficiency or amputation in early childhood. *Brain* 1997;120: 1603–1620.

45. Wilkins KL, McGrath PJ, Finely GA, et al. Prospective diary study of nonpainful and painful phantom sensations in a preselected sample of child and adolescent amputees reporting phantom limbs. *Clin J Pain* 2004;20:293–301.

46. Hunfeld JA, Perquin CW, Duivenvoorden HJ, et al. Chronic pain and its impact on quality of life in adolescents and their families. *J Pediatr Psychol* 2001;26:145–153.

47. Kashikar-Zuck S, Goldschneider KR, Powers SW, et al. Depression and functional disability in chronic pediatric pain. *Clin J Pain* 2001;17:341–349.

48. Roth-Isigkeit A, Thyen U, Stoven H, et al. Pain among children and adolescents: restrictions in daily living and triggering factors [electronic version]. *Pediatrics* 2005;115:e152–e162.

49. Palermo TM. Impact of recurrent and chronic pain on child and family daily functioning: a critical review of the literature. *J Dev Behav Pediatr* 2000;21: 58–69.

50. Walker LS, Greene JW. The functional disability inventory: measuring a neglected dimension of child health status. *J Pediatr Psychol* 1991;16:39–58.

51. Breuner CC, Smith MS, Womack WM. Factors related to school absenteeism in adolescents with recurrent headache. *Headache* 2004;44:217–222.

52. Lynch AM, Kashikar-Zuck S, Goldschneider KR, et al. Psychosocial risks for disability in children with chronic back pain. *J Pain* 2006;7:244–251.

53. Kashikar-Zuck S, Lynch AM, Graham TB, et al. Social functioning and peer relationships of adolescents with juvenile fibromyalgia syndrome. *Arthritis Rheum* 2007;57:474–480.

54. Palermo TM, Kiska R. Subjective sleep disturbances in adolescents with chronic pain: Relationship to daily functioning and quality of life. *J Pain* 2005;6:201–207.

55. Lewin DS, Dahl RE. Importance of sleep in the management of pediatric pain. *J Dev Behav Pediatr* 1999;20:244–252.

56. Valrie CR, Gil KM, Redding-Lallinger R. Brief report: sleep in children with sickle cell disease: an analysis of daily diaries utilizing multilevel models. *J Pediatr Psychol* 2007;32:857–861.

57. Langeveld JH, Koot HM, Passchier J. Headache intensity and quality of life in adolescents. How are changes in headache intensity in adolescents related to changes in experienced quality of life? *Headache* 1997;3:37–42.

58. Maikler VE, Broome ME, Bailey P, et al. Children's and adolescents' use of pain diaries for sickle cell pain. *J Soc Pediatr Nurs* 2001;6:161–169.

59. Tkachuk GA, Cottrell CK, Gibson JS, et al. Factors associated with migraine-related quality of life and disability in adolescents: a preliminary investigation. *Headache* 2003;43:950–955.

60. Langeveld JH, Koot HM, Loonen MC, et al. A quality of life instrument for adolescents with chronic headache. *Cephalalgia* 1996;16:183–196; discussion 137.

61. Campo JV, Perel J, Lucas A, et al. Citalopram treatment of pediatric recurrent abdominal pain and comorbid internalizing disorders: an exploratory study. *J Am Acad Child Adolesc Psychiatry* 2004;43:1234–1242.

62. Vaalamo I, Pulkkinen L, Kinnunen T, et al. Interactive effects of internalizing and externalizing problem behaviors on recurrent pain in children. *J Pediatr Psychol* 2002;27:245–257.

63. Varni JW, Rapoff MA, Waldron SA, et al. Chronic pain and emotional distress in children and adolescents. *J Dev Behav Pediatr* 1996:17:154–161.

64. Merlijn VP, Hunfeld JA, van der Wouden JC, et al. Psychosocial factors associated with chronic pain in adolescents. *Pain* 2003;101:33–43.

65. Eccleston C, Crombez G, Scotford A, et al. Adolescent chronic pain: patterns and predictors of emotional distress in adolescents with chronic pain and their parents. *Pain* 2004;108:221–229.

66. Nodari E, Battistella PA, Naccarella C, et al. Quality of life in young Italian patients with primary headache. *Headache* 2002;42:268–274.

67. Youssef NN, Murphy TG, Langseder AL, et al. Quality of life for children with functional abdominal pain: a comparison study of patients' and parents' perceptions. *Pediatrics* 2006;117:54–59.

68. Sleed M, Eccleston C, Beecham J, et al. The economic impact of chronic pain in adolescence: methodological considerations and a preliminary costs-of-illness study. *Pain* 2005;119:183–190.

69. Anttila P, Sourander A, Metsähonkala L, et al. Psychiatric symptoms in children with primary headache. *J Am Acad Child Adolesc Psychiatry* 2004;43: 412–419.

70. Larsson B, Sund AM. Emotional/behavioural, social correlates and one-year predictors of frequent pains among early adolescents: influences of pain characteristics. *Eur J Pain* 2007;11:57–65.

71. Logan DE, Scharff L. Relationships between family and parent characteristics and functional abilities in children with recurrent pain syndromes: an investigation of moderating effects on the pathway from pain to disability. *J Pediatr Psychol* 2005;30:698–707.

72. Eccleston C, Malleson PN, Clinch J, et al. Chronic pain in adolescents: evaluation of a programme of interdisciplinary cognitive behaviour therapy. *Arch Dis Child* 2003;88:881–885.

73. Smart S, Cottrell D. Going to the doctors: the views of mothers of children with recurrent abdominal pain. *Child Care Health Dev* 2005;31:265–273.

74. Liakopoulou-Kairis M, Alifieraki T, Protagora D, et al. Recurrent abdominal pain and headache—psychopathology, life events and family functioning. *Eur Child Adolesc Psychiatry* 2002;11:115–122.

75. Eccleston C, Jordan AL, Crombez G. The impact of chronic pain on adolescents: a review of previously used measures. *J Pediatr Psychol* 2006;31: 684–697.

76. Stinson JN, Kavanagh T, Yamada J, et al. Systematic review of the psychometric properties, interpretability and feasibility of self-report pain intensity measures for use in clinical trials in children and adolescents. *Pain* 2006;125: 143–157.

77. Varni JW, Seid M, Rode CA. The PedsQL: measurement model for the pediatric quality of life inventory. *Medical Care* 1999;37:126–139.

78. Palermo TM, Witherspoon D, Valenzuela D, et al. Development and validation of the Child Activity Limitations Interview: a measure of pain-related functional impairment in school-age children and adolescents. *Pain* 2004;109: 461–470.

79. Eccleston C, Jordan A, McCracken LM, et al. The Bath Adolescent Pain Questionnaire (BAPQ): development and preliminary psychometric evaluation of an instrument to assess the impact of chronic pain on adolescents. *Pain* 2005;118:263–270.

80. Kovacs M. The Children's Depression Inventory (CDI). *Psychopharmacol Bull* 1985:21:995–998.

81. Reynolds CR, Richmond BO. What I think and feel: a revised measure of children's manifest anxiety. *J Abnorm Child Psychol* 1978;6:271–280.

82. Chorpita BF, Moffitt CE, Gray, J. Psychometric properties of the revised child anxiety and depression scale in a clinical sample. *Behav Res Ther* 2005;43: 309–322.

83. Logan DE, Claar RL, Scharff L. Social desirability response bias and self-report of psychological distress in pediatric chronic pain patients. *Pain* 2008; 136:366–372.

84. Palermo TM, Chambers CT. Parent and family factors in pediatric chronic pain and disability: an integrative approach. *Pain* 2005;119:1–4.

85. Walker LS, Levy RL, Whitehead WE. Validation of a measure of protective parent responses to children's pain. *Clin J Pain* 2006;22:712–716.

86. Miller IW, Epstein NB, Bishop DS, et al. The Mcmaster family assessment device: Reliability and validity. *J Marital Fam Ther* 1985;11:345–356.

87. Van Slyke DA, Smith CA, Walker LS, et al. Development and validation of the children's pain beliefs questionnaire. Paper presented at the 6th Florida Conference on Child Health Psychology, 1997.

88. Reid G., Gilbert CA, McGrath PJ. The Pain Coping Questionnaire: preliminary validation. *Pain* 1998;76:83–96.

89. Crombez G, Bijttebier P, Eccleston C, et al. The child version of the pain catastrophizing scale (PCS-C): a preliminary validation. *Pain* 2003;104: 639–646.

90. Konijnenberg AY, DeGraeff-Meeder ER, Kimpen JL, et al. Children with unexplained chronic pain: do pediatricians agree regarding the diagnostic approach and presumed primary cause? *Pediatrics* 2004:114:1220–1226.

91. Chalkiadis GA. Management of chronic pain in children. *Med J Aust* 2001; 175:476–479.

92. Torsney C, Fitzgerald M. Age-dependent effects of peripheral inflammation upon the electrophysiological properties of neonatal rat dorsal horn neurons: development of hyperalgesia and allodynia. *J Neurophysiol* 2002;87:1311–1317.

93. Fitzgerald M, Howard R. The neurobiological basis of pediatric pain. In: Schechter N, Berde C, Yaster M, eds. *Pain in Children and Adolescents*. 2nd ed. Philadelphia: Lippincott Williams & Wilkins, 2003:19–42.

94. Fitzgerald M, Millard C, McIntosh N. Cutaneous hypersensitivity following peripheral tissue damage in newborn infants and its reversal with topical analgesia. *Pain* 1989;39:31–36.

95. Pattinson D, Fitzgerald M. The neurobiology of infant pain: development of excitatory and inhibitory neurotransmission in the spinal dorsal horn. *Reg Anesth Pain Med* 2004;29:36–44.

96. Grunau RV, Whitfield MF, Petrie JH. Pain sensitivity and temperament in extremely low-birth-weight premature toddlers and preterm and full-term controls. *Pain* 1994;58:341–346.

97. Grunau RE, Whitfield MF, Petrie JH, et al. Early pain experience, child and family factors, as precursors of somatization: A prospective study of extremely premature and fullterm children. *Pain* 1994;56:353–359.

98. Grunau RE. Early pain in preterm infants. A model of long-term effects. *Clin Perinatol* 2002;29:373–394.

99. Grunau RE, Whitfield MF, Petrie J. Children's judgements about pain at age 8–10 years: do extremely low birthweight (< or = 1000 g) children differ from full birthweight peers? *J Child Psychol Psychiatry* 1998;39:587–594.

100. Anand KJ, Scalzo FM. Can adverse neonatal experiences alter brain development and subsequent behavior? *Biol Neonate* 2000;77:69–82.

101. Borge AI, Nordhagen R Recurrent pain symptoms in children and parents. *Acta Paediatr* 2000;89:1479–1483.

102. Schanberg LE, Anthony KK, Gil KM. Family pain history predicts child health status in children with chronic rheumatic disease. *Pediatrics* 2001;108:E47.

103. Chan ECC, Piira T, Betts G. The school functioning of children with chronic and recurrent pain. *Pediatr Pain Lett* 2005;7:11–16.

104. Stang PE, Osterhaus JT. Impact of migraine in the United States: data from the National Health Interview survey. *Headache* 1993;33:29–35.

105. Walker LS, Guite JW, Duke M, et al. Recurrent abdominal pain: a potential precursor or irritable bowel syndrome in adolescents and young adults. *J Pediatr* 1998;132:1010–1015.

106. Grahame R. The revised (Brighton 1998) criteria for the diagnosis of benign joint hypermobility syndrome (BJHS). *J Rheumatol* 2000;27:1777–1779.

107. Rozen TD, Roth JM, Denenberg N. Cervical spine joint hypermobility: a possible predisposing factor for new daily persistent headache. *Cephalalgia* 2006;26:1182–1185.

108. Moshiree B, Zhou Q, Price DD, et al. Central sensitization in visceral pain disorders. *Gut* 2006;55:905–908.

109. Verne GN, Price DD. Irritable bowel syndrome as a common precipitant of central sensitization. *Curr Rheumatol Rep* 2002;4:322–328.

110. Ji RR, Kohno T, Moore KA, et al. Central sensitization and LTP: do pain and memory share similar mechanisms? *Trends Neurosci* 2003;26:696–705.

111. Eccleston C, Morley S, Williams A, et al. Systematic review of randomized controlled trials of psychological therapy for chronic pain in children and adolescents with a subset meta-analysis of pain relief. *Pain* 2002;22:157–165.

112. Walco GA, Sterling CM, Conte PM, et al. Empirically supported treatments in pediatric psychology: disease related pain. *J Pediatr Psychol* 1999;24:155–167.

113. Zeltzer L, Schlank C. *Conquering Your Child's Chronic Pain*. New York: HarperCollins; 2005.

114. Moore RA, Derry S, McQuay HJ, et al. What do we know about communicating risk? A brief review and suggestion for contextualising serious, but rare, risk, and the example of cox-2 selective and non-selective NSAIDs. *Arthritis Res Ther* 2008;10(1):R20.

115. Foeldvari I, Szer IS, Zemel LS, et al. A prospective study comparing celecoxib with naproxen in children with juvenile rheumatoid arthritis. *J Rheumatol* 2009;36(1):174–182.

116. Buntin-Mushock C, Phillip L, Moriyama K, et al. Age-dependent opioid escalation in chronic pain patients. *Anesth Analg* 2005;100:1740–1745.

117. Wang Y, Mitchell J, Moriyama K, et al. Age-dependent morphine tolerance development in the rat. *Anesth Analg* 2005;100:1733–1739.

118. Sindrup SH, Bach FW, Madsen C, et al. Venlafaxine versus imipramine in painful polyneuropathy: a randomized, controlled trial. *Neurology* 2003;60:1284–1289.

119. Quilici S, Chancellor J, Löthgren M, et al. Meta-analysis of duloxetine vs. pregabalin and gabapentin in the treatment of diabetic peripheral neuropathic pain. *BMC Neurol* 2009;9:6.

120. Levinstein B. A comparative study of cyproheptadine, amitriptyline, and propranolol in the treatment of adolescent migraine. *Cephalalgia* 1991;11:122–123.

121. Hershey AD, Powers SW, Bentti A-L, et al. Effectiveness of amitriptyline in the prophylactic management of childhood headaches. *Headache* 2000;40:539–549.

122. Campo JV, Perel J, Lucas A, et al. Citalopram treatment of pediatric recurrent abdominal pain and comorbid internalizing disorders: an exploratory study. *J Am Acad Child Adolesc Psychiatry* 2004;43(10):1234–1242.

123. National Institute of Mental Health. Antidepressant Medications for Children and Adolescents: Information for Parents and Caregivers. Available at: http://www.nimh.nih.gov/health/topics/child-and-adolescent-mental-health/antidepressant-medications-for-children-and-adolescents-information-for-parents-and-caregivers.shtml. Accessed March 15, 2009.

124. Straube S, Derry S, McQuay HJ, et al. Enriched enrollment: definition and effects of enrichment and dose in trials of pregabalin and gabapentin in neuropathic pain. A systematic review. *Br J Clin Pharmacol* 2008;66(2):266–275.

125. Lalwani K, Shoham A, Koh JL, et al. Use of oxcarbazepine to treat a pediatric patient with resistant complex regional pain syndrome. *J Pain* 2005;6(10):704–706.

126. Sindrup SH, Jensen TS. Pharmacologic treatment of pain in polyneuropathy. *Neurology* 2000;55(7):915–920.

127. Shapiro RE. Topiramate for migraine prevention: a randomized controlled trial. *J Pediatr* 2004;145(3):419–420.

128. U.S. Food and Drug Administration. Information for Healthcare Professionals Suicidal Behavior and Ideation and Antiepileptic Drugs. Available at: http://www.fda.gov/Drugs/DrugSafety/PostmarketDrugSafetyInformationforPatientsandProviders/ucm100192.htm. Accessed

129. Morley S, Eccleston C, Williams A. Systematic review and meta-analysis of randomized controlled trials of cognitive behaviour therapy and behaviour therapy for chronic pain in adults, excluding headache. *Pain* 1999;80:1–13.

130. Robins PM, Smith SM, Glutting JJ. A randomized controlled trial of a cognitive-behavioral family intervention for pediatric recurrent abdominal pain. *J Pediatr Psychol* 2005;30:397–408.

131. Burke EJ, Andrasik F. Home- vs. clinic-based biofeedback treatment for pediatric migraine: results of treatment through one-year follow-up. *Headache* 1989;29:434–440.

132. Kroener-Herwig B, Denecke H. Cognitive-behavioral therapy of pediatric headache: are there differences in efficacy between a therapist-administered group training and a self-help format? *J Psychosom Res* 2002;53:1107–1114.

133. McGrath PJ, Humphreys P, Keene D, et al. The efficacy and efficiency of a self-administered treatment for adolescent migraine. *Pain* 1992;49:321–324.

134. Larsson B, Daleflod B., Hkansson L et al. Therapist-assisted versus self-help relaxation treatment of chronic headaches in adolescents: a school-based intervention. *J Child Psychol Psychiatry* 1987;28:127–136.

135. Larsson B. Behavioural treatment of somatic disorders in children and adolescents. *Eur Child Adolesc Psychiatry* 1992;1:68–81.

136. Hicks CL, von Baeyer CL, McGrath PJ. Online psychological treatment for pediatric recurrent pain: a randomized evaluation. *J Pediatr Psychol* 2006;31:724–736.

137. Connelly M, Rapoff MA, Thompson N, et al. Headstrong: a pilot study of a CD-ROM intervention for recurrent pediatric headache. *J Pediatr Psychol* 2006;31:737–747.

138. Wicksell RK, Melin L, Olsson GL. Exposure and acceptance in the rehabilitation of adolescents with idiopathic chronic pain—a pilot study. *Eur J Pain* 2007;11:267–264.

139. Davis MP, Darden PM. Use of complementary and alternative medicine by children in the United States. *Arch Pediatr Adolesc Med* 2003;157:393–396.

140. Tsao JC, Zeltzer LK. Complementary and alternative medicine approaches for pediatric pain: a review of the state-of-the-science. *Evid Based Complement Alternat Med* 2005;2:149–159.

141. Humphreys PA, Gevirtz RN. Treatment of recurrent abdominal pain: components analysis of four treatment protocols. *J Pediatr Gastroenterol Nutr* 2000;31:47–51.

142. Weydert JA, Ball TM, Davis MF. Systematic review of treatments for recurrent abdominal pain. *Pediatrics* 2003;111:e1–e11.

143. Allen KD, Shriver MD. Role of parent-mediated pain behavior management strategies in biofeedback treatment of childhood migraines. *Behav Ther* 1998;29:477–490.

144. Kröner-Herwig B, Mohn U, Pothmann R. Comparison of biofeedback and relaxation in the treatment of pediatric headache and the influence of parent involvement on outcome. *Appl Psychophysiol Biofeedback* 1998:23:143–157.

145. Shapiro BS, Dinges DF, Orne EC, et al. Home management of sickle cell-related pain in children and adolescents: natural history and impact on school attendance. *Pain* 1995;61:139–144.

146. Greco LA, Freeman KE, Dufton L. Overt and relational victimization among children with frequent abdominal pain: links to social skills, academic functioning, and health service use. *J Pediatr Psychol* 2007;32:319–329.

147. Logan DE, Catanese SP, Coakley RM, et al. Chronic pain in the classroom: teachers' attributions about the causes of chronic pain. *J Sch Health* 2007;77:248–256.

148. Logan DE, Coakley RM, Scharff L. Teachers' perceptions of and responses to adolescents with chronic pain syndromes. *J Pediatr Psychol* 2007;32:139–149.

149. Bloom BJ, Owens JA, McGuinn M, et al. Sleep and its relationship to pain, dysfunction, and disease activity in juvenile rheumatoid arthritis. *J Rheumatol* 2002;29:169–173.

150. Valrie CR, Gil KM, Redding-Lallinger R, et al. Daily mood as a mediator or moderator of the pain-sleep relationship in children with sickle cell disease. *J Pediatr Psychol* 2008;33:317–322.

151. Meltzer LJ, Logan DE, Mindell JA. Sleep patterns in female adolescents with chronic musculoskeletal pain. *Behav Sleep Med* 2005;3:193–208.

152. Palermo TM, Fonareva I. Commentary: Sleep in children and adolescents with chronic pain. *Pediatr Pain Lett* 2006;8:11–15.

153. Long AC, Krishnamurthy V, Palermo TM. Sleep disturbances in school-age children with chronic pain. *J Pediatr Psychol* 2008;33:258–268.

154. Palermo TM, Putnam J, Armstrong G, et al. Adolescent autonomy and family functioning are associated with headache-related disability. *Clin J Pain* 2007;23:458–465.

155. Smith MD, McGhan WF. Insomnia: costs to lose sleep over. *Bus Health* 1997;15:57–58, 60.

156. Stoller MK. Economic effects of insomnia. *Clin Ther* 2004;16:873–897; discussion 854.

157. Wolfson AR, Carskadon MA. Sleep schedules and daytime functioning in adolescents. *Child Dev* 1998;69:875–887.

158. Carskadon MA, Wolfson AR, Acebo C, et al. Adolescent sleep patterns, circadian timing, and sleepiness at a transition to early school days. *Sleep* 1998; 21:871–881.

159. Tsai SY, Labyak SE, Richardson LP, et al. Actigraphic sleep and daytime naps in adolescent girls with chronic musculoskeletal pain. *J Pediatr Psychol* 2008; 33:307–311.

160. Morin CM, Gibson D, Wade J. Self-reported sleep and mood disturbance in chronic pain patients. *Clin J Pain* 1998;14:311–314.

161. Bruni O, Galli, F, Guidetti V. Sleep hygiene and migraine in children and adolescents. *Cephalalgia* 1999;25:57–59.

162. Di Lorenzo C, Colletti RB, Lehmann HP, et al, and the AAP Subcommittee on Chronic Abdominal Pain and NASPGHAN Committee on Abdominal Pain. Chronic abdominal pain in children: a technical report of the American Academy of Pediatrics and the North American Society for Pediatric Gastroenterology, Hepatology and Nutrition. *J Pediatr Gastroenterol Nutr* 2005; 40:245–261.

163. Headache Classification Subcommittee of the International Headache Society. The International Classification of Headache Disorders: 2nd ed. *Cephalalgia* 2004;24(Suppl 1):9–160.

164. Lipton RB, Bigal ME, Steiner TJ, et al. Classification of primary headaches. *Neurology* 2004;63:428–435.

165. Guidetti V, Galli V. Recent development in paediatric headache. *Curr Opinion Neurol* 2001;14:335–340.

166. Lewis DW. Headaches in children and adolescents. *Am Fam Physician* 2002; 65:625–632.

167. Zebenholzer K, Wöber C, Kienbacher C, et al. Migrainous disorder and headache of the tension type not fulfilling the criteria: a follow-up study in children and adolescents. *Cephalalgia* 2000;20:611–616.

168. Winner P, Wasiewski W, Gladstein J, et al. Multicenter prosective evaluation of proposed pediatric migraine revision to the HIS criteria. Pediatric Headache Committee of the American Association for the Study of Headache. *Headache* 1998;37:545–548.

169. Marcus DA. Reducing headache disability in children and adolescents. *Am Fam Physician* 2002;554, 557.

170. Hermann C, Kim M, Blanchard EB. Behavioral and prophylactic pharmacological intervention studies of pediatric migraine: ans exploratory meta-analysis. *Pain* 1995;60:239–256.

171. Cvengros JA, Harper D, Shevell M. Pediatric headache: an examination of process variables in treatment. *J Child Neurol* 2007;22:1172–1181.

172. Lewis D, Ashwal S, Hershey A, et al, and the American Academy of Neurology Quality Standards Subcommittee and the Practice Committee of the Child Neurology Society. Practice parameter: pharmacological treatment of migraine headache in children and adolescents: report of the American Academy of Neurology Quality Standards Subcommittee and the Practice Committee of the Child Neurology Society. *Neurology* 2004;63:2215–2224.

173. Schoenen J, Jacquy J, Lenaerts M. Effectiveness of high dose riboflavin n migraine prophylaxis. A randomized controlled trial. *Neurology* 1998;50: 466–470.

174. Peikert A, Wilimzig C, Köhne-Volland R. Prophyllaxis of migraine with oral magnesium: results of prospective, multi-center, placebo-controlled and double-blind randomized study. *Cephalalgia* 1996;16:257–263.

175. Malleson PN, Beauchamp RD. Rheumatology: 16. Diagnosing musculoskeletal pain in children. *CMAJ* 2001;165:183–188.

176. Karaaslan Y, Haznedaroglu S, Oztürk M. Joint hypermobility and primary fibromyalgia: a clinical enigma. *J Rheumatol* 2000;27:1774–1776.

177. Fitzcharles MA. Is hypermobility a factor in fibromyalgia. *J Rheumatol* 2000; 27:1587–1589.

178. Keer R, Grahame R. *Hypermobility Syndrome: Recognition and Management for Physiotherapists.* Edinburgh: Butterworth Heineman; 2003.

179. Bulbena A, Duro JC, Porta M, et al. Anxiety disorders in the joint hypermobility syndrome. *Psychiatry Res* 1993;46:59–68.

180. Bulbena A, Agulló A, Pailhez G, et al. Is joint hypermobility related to anxiety in a nonclinical population also? *Psychosomatics* 2004;45:432–437.

181. Martín-Santos R, Bulbena A, Porta M, et al. Association between joint hypermobility syndrome and panic disorder. *Am J Psychiatry* 1998;155: 1578–1583.

182. Wilder RT. Management of pediatric patients with complex regional pain syndrome. *Clin J Pain* 2006;22:443–448.

183. Lee BH, Scharff L, Sethna NF, et al. Physical therapy and cognitive-behavioral treatment for complex regional pain syndromes. *J Pediatr* 2002;141:135–140.

184. Sherry DD, Wallace CA, Kelley C, et al. Short- and long-term outcomes of children with complex regional pain syndrome type I treated with exercise therapy. *Clin J Pain* 1999;15:218–223.

185. Wilder RT, Berde CB, Wolohan M, et al. Reflex sympathetic dystrophy in children. Clinical characteristics and follow-up of seventy patients. *J Bone Joint Surg Am* 1992;74:910–919.

186. Dadure C, Motais F, Ricard C, et al. Continuous peripheral nerve blocks at home in the treatment of recurrent complex regional pain syndrome I in children. *Anesthesiology* 2005;102:387–391.

187. Jones GT, Watson KD, Silman AJ, et al. Predictors of low back pain in British schoolchildren: a population-based prospective cohort study. *Pediatrics* 2003; 111(4 Pt 1):822–828.

188. Pellisé F, Balagué F, Rajmil L, et al. Prevalence of low back pain and its effect on health-related quality of life in adolescents. *Arch Pediatr Adolesc Med* 2009;163(1):65–71.

189. Micheli LJ, Wood R. Back pain in young athletes. Significant differences from adults in causes and patterns. *Arch Pediatr Adolesc Med* 1995;149(1):15–18.

190. Purcell L, Micheli L. Low back pain in young athletes. *Sports Health: A Multidisciplinary Approach* 2009:1(3);212–222.

191. Kurd MF, Patel D, Norton R, et al. Nonoperative treatment of symptomatic spondylolysis. *J Spinal Disord Tech* 2007;20(8):560–564.

192. Berde CB, Stein JM, Moody PA, et al. Epidural steroid injections for radiculopathy +/− back pain in children and adolescents. Society for Pediatric Anesthesia Annual Meeting Abstracts; March 2007, p. 94.

CHAPTER 55 ■ PAIN IN THE OLDER PERSON

PAUL ARNSTEIN AND KEELA HERR

OVERVIEW

Medical science continues to expand its capacity to forestall death. As a result, people are living longer but increasingly spend their final years with daily, unrelenting pain.[1–3] Pain is emerging as a more formidable foe than death, whose conquest will demand stretching the limits of our technology and ability to provide compassionate care. The number of pain-producing surgical interventions and outpatient procedures is increasing, as is the prevalence of chronic diseases like arthritis, diabetes, and cancer.[4] Because of its increasing incidence, high economic costs, and negative impact on quality of life of patients and their families,[5] uncontrolled pain has become a public health priority.

Those over age 65 make up the fastest growing segment of our population, as the number of older adults in the United States doubled to 35 million between 1960 and 2000. Estimates have that number doubling again in less than 30 years as the "baby boomers" permeate this age group. The number of centurions are growing at an even faster pace, as their numbers have doubled between 1990 and 2006.[6] Longevity is being enjoyed around the world, but "it is very hard to be reflective, perceptive, and wise when. . .everything hurts." [7] Although not all older adults have severe or ongoing pain, a majority do when they seek health care services.[8–12]

The Prevalence of Pain in Older Adults

Delineating the prevalence of pain with advancing age is a challenge because epidemiologic studies differ in the age cut-points, methods of data collection, and the types of pain studied. A national telephone-based survey in the United States asked people of all ages about current, recent, and persistent discomforts. Older adults reported similar prevalence rates of current pain as their younger counterparts. Among respondents over age 65 who had current pain, almost 60% indicated that it lasted for at least a year. This was significantly more than their younger and middle-aged counterparts (37% and 44%, respectively).[3] Despite evidence that the incidence of persistent* pain peaks in the middle years,[13] other studies support that over age 60 people are twice as likely as younger counterparts[14]; and by 80, adults are three times more likely to have persistent pain than those under 18 years of age.[15]

PAIN IN THE OLDER PERSON

Impact of Pain on Functioning and Quality of Life

Overall, 25% to 50% of community-dwelling seniors are estimated to have pain that interferes with normal function.[16] Residents of long-term care facilities have even higher rates of impaired functioning from unresolved pain with estimates as high as 80%.[17] Unrelieved pain interferes with nutrition and sleep, which may contribute to the overall decline in health and function observed in people with pain. Combined with impaired physical health, the decline in social and recreational activities produces emotional distress, contributing to depression[18] which is capable of worsening both pain and disability.

Physiologically, aging alters functions, including a degeneration of peripheral neuronal structure[19] that slows transduction and transmission involved in signaling pain.[13] Once pain is established, the lower density of descending inhibitory circuits[20] and an impaired ability to recover from hyperalgesic or allodynic states[21] is attributed to aging. The decline in function of the endogenous antinociceptive mechanisms as well as the capacity to reverse spinal and supraspinal sensitization[22] places older patients at greater risk for developing persistent pain following an illness, surgery, or trauma.[23]

Physiologic changes in the cardiovascular system increase myocardial demand, producing tachycardia, hypertension, and a risk of hypercoagulation in response to pain. Combined, these increase the risk of cardiac damage during a heart attack.[24] Hormonal, metabolic,[25,26] and immunologic suppression resulting from pain can worsen the primary disorder[27] and/or increase the risk of infections, poor healing,[28] atelectasis, or pneumonia.[29]

Severe acute postoperative pain also appears to put the older adult at risk for the development of persistent pain.[30,31] Prospective studies of older adults after hip surgery demonstrated the link between more postoperative pain and prolonged length of stays with more complications, poorer participation in rehabilitation therapies, and poorer functional outcomes at 6 months.[10] Avoiding opioids or using subtherapeutic doses actually increases the risk of delirium. Cognitively intact patients with undertreated pain are nine times more likely to develop delirium than patients whose pain is adequately treated.[32]

Psychologically, similar patterns of beliefs about pain and coping strategies are seen across adulthood.[13] Affective distress, like anxiety and depression, is linked to higher pain intensity levels regardless of age as pain and decreased physical/mental functioning occur when pain is severe or persistent. Although a decline

in functional abilities, strength, and balance can occur with aging, the rate and extent of deterioration is more pronounced in those with pain.[33–35]

Undertreatment of Pain in Older Persons

Given these potentially serious pain-related consequences, evidence that pain is commonly undertreated or untreated in older adults is disturbing. Among those with pain, a significant portion of those over age 65 do not receive analgesics, including over a quarter of older adults with cancer pain,[36] almost 30% of institutionalized elders,[12,37] 40% of elders with hip fracture in the Emergency Department,[8] and 40% to 80% of elders living with pain in the community.[38–40]

The diagnosis and treatment of pain in older persons is more difficult in those who present with multiple medical problems and a history that reveals many potential sources of pain. Although there is an undeniable need to prevent harm from pain-relieving treatments, this focus must be balanced with a concerted effort to avoid pain-induced harm. Guidelines for the assessment, treatment, and monitoring of older patients with pain have been widely distributed advocating for individualized approaches to pain and balancing concerns for the safety and efficacy of treatments.[40–42]

It is time to replace unrealistic fears and mistaken beliefs with guidelines that delineate prudent, safe, effective use of available treatments. Perhaps the greatest opportunity for improvement is halting the practices of using placebos as a proxy for mind/body therapy[43] or recommending treatments such as acetaminophen alone for severe pain knowing that would be ineffective for the types of discomfort experienced.[44]

Change in Pain Threshold and Tolerance

Over a dozen studies have investigated the effect of aging on pain threshold with some inconsistency in findings.[13] Although inconclusive due to methodological heterogeneity, evidence supports an age-related increase in thresholds to thermal, pressure, and electrical stimulation.[22,45] Although it is possible that ischemic pain thresholds are lower,[13] other research concludes that pain thresholds consistently differ in the direction of elevated thresholds with age whether or not levels of statistical significance are achieved.[22]

Age differences in the perception of painful stimuli have been assessed using direct, indirect, and multimethod forms of testing. Despite a contrary finding,[46] older persons rate mild suprathreshold thermal stimuli as less intense and unpleasant than do younger subjects.[47,48] At higher intensities, however, older adults rate the stimulus as more intense and unpleasant than do younger subjects.[49] This pattern supports the notion that with advancing age, pain threshold increases while tolerance of pain decreases.

Several other investigators have also found a lower tolerance for experimentally-induced pain in older adults. Conflicting research exists here as well, with some investigators failing to find a difference in pain tolerance attributable to age.[50,51] It is likely that in addition to age, interacting attributes such as gender, genetics, affect, motivation, social, and cultural factors play a role in determining the amount of pain any individual would tolerate in the context of a research study. In clinical settings, comorbid conditions, numerous psychosocial factors, and medications are likely to further influence pain threshold/tolerance levels.

Clinical Presentation of Acute Pain

Although common characteristics of acute pain (e.g., pattern, onset, duration) are relevant, an important distinction in older

---

*The terms chronic pain and persistent pain are often used interchangeably to denote pain that lasts for more than 3 months. Persistent pain is used in this text to avoid negative connotation often associated with the label "chronic pain," as is recommended by the American Geriatrics Society.

adults is that pain may be absent or atypical in acute infectious, metabolic, or traumatic disorders. Acute myocardial infarction (MI) almost always presents with severe chest pain in younger adults. In older adults, however, it may be asymptomatic, referred in an atypical pattern, or present with vague signs like confusion, restlessness, aggression, anorexia, and fatigue.[52] Up to 30% of older adults with MI report an absence of acute symptoms, while another 30% (especially women) have an atypical presentation.[53] Similar age patterns have been documented in the presentation of different gastrointestinal disorders.[54,55]

Persistent Pain

Older adults may be more vulnerable to the development of persistent pain after an acute illness or injury. A clear example is the risk of developing postherpetic neuralgia. Increasing age is the greatest predictor of postherpetic neuralgia, with one study calculating that adults over age 50 were 15 times more likely to have pain 1 month after the initial shingles reactivation than younger counterparts.[56] Among patients over age 70, half have pain for at least 1 year, compared to 3% of those under 60 years old.[57]

The risk of developing persistent pain after a low back strain, surgery, or trauma is not clearly linked to age[58]; however, persistent musculoskeletal pain clearly increases with advancing age. Osteoarthritis of the knee, hip, foot, back, neck, and shoulder account for a majority of cases.[59] Conditions with widespread persistent pain, like fibromyalgia, peak in prevalence in the seventh decade, then decline.[60-62] This decline in pain with advanced age may be related to the tendency of people living with regional or widespread pain to die at a younger age than their pain-free counterparts.[63]

Cancer Pain

Older adults make up the largest proportion of cancer patients, with many reporting moderate to severe pain.[64] Among institutionalized older adults with cancer, risk factors for higher levels of pain include being widowed, deemed terminal, and having impaired physical or mental functioning.[36] It could be argued that some of the impaired functioning was actually a consequence of intense pain, known to have a detrimental effect on physical, psychologic, social, and spiritual functioning.[65]

Older adults are at risk for inadequate pain control because of either their own reluctance to take analgesics or that of professionals who prescribe and administer these medically necessary drugs.[36,66] It is unconscionable that 26% of older adults with daily cancer pain do not receive any analgesics.[36] The greatest risk of cancer pain is during active treatment of the disease and at the end of life, which can be prevented or effectively relieved in a majority of cases.[67] Even metastatic bone pain, the most common cause of persistent cancer pain,[68] has analgesic and adjuvant options that are underutilized.

ASSESSMENT OF PAIN IN THE OLDER PERSON

Clinical Evaluation of Pain

Without self-report, pain often goes undetected and subsequently untreated. Thus, methods of assessment must be used to identify pain in all patients. Like patients in other age groups, self-report of pain is the criterion standard for assessment. The numeric rating scale, verbal descriptor scale, and faces pain scale are the most established tools for the alert, cognitively intact older adults.

The Iowa Pain Thermometer demonstrated comparable results to these scales and was most preferred by a sample of older adults.[69]

There is some evidence, however, that these one-dimensional scales are ineffective screening tools for a substantial segment of the population, including older persons. Krebs and colleagues[70] found in a primary care setting that about 40% of patient visits were for pain and over a third of patients were seeking care because of disabling pain. Routine use of the numeric rating scale revealed a "no pain" score for 28% of those presenting for pain and 21% of patients with pain-related disability.[70] Examining the Minimum Data Set that is required for all U.S. nursing home residents, 94% scored "0" on the pain scale, despite research that consistently estimates between 45% to 80% of residents have pain.[71]

These scales can be used more effectively in older persons by addressing sensory deficits (uses eyeglasses, hearing aids, large font/bold print written tools, etc.) and determining understanding of the scale before using it.[72] Responder burden can be reduced by using simply worded tools with few items (e.g., numeric rating scale or verbal descriptor scale when possible). Showing the older adult a printed version while explaining the assessment tool is recommended.[72] The revised Faces Pain Scale is preferred by some older adults[73] and validated versions are available in 31 languages.[74] The Brief Pain Inventory (BPI) is useful in many settings as it records dimensions of pain in addition to intensity (e.g., interference with functionality). A short version of BPI was recently validated to facilitate assessing older adults in long-term care settings.[75]

It is useful to adopt a few validated tools for use in clinical settings to accommodate needs of different patients. When a patient has difficulty understanding the first-line scale, back-up methods are available. It is critical to allow sufficient time for older patients to process questions and formulate responses before accepting or rejecting one tool as the best. Once the best pain assessment tool for a particular patient is found, all team members (including caregivers) need to use it consistently for all pain assessments. Follow-up assessments after interventions intended to relieve pain should be conducted at intervals aligned with anticipated peak of desired or adverse effects, as "current pain" measures are more accurate than pain recall. In addition to evaluating analgesic effects, assessing adverse effects evaluate the safety of the treatment.

Evaluation of Pain in Research

The verbal descriptor scale, numeric pain rating scale, revised faces pain scale, and Iowa Pain Thermometer have high completion rates, good validity, and acceptable reliability for use in researching older adults with pain. The visual analog scale, however, is more difficult for older adults to complete[76] and has more measurement error,[77] with as many as 30% of cognitively intact elders unable to use this scale.[78] To get a more comprehensive measure of the effect of treatments, the Initiative on Methods, Measurement, and Pain Assessment in Clinical Trials (IMMPACT) group recommends measuring pain intensity, physical, and emotional functioning, as well as the participant's perception of overall improvement.[79] Visit the group's website at www.IMMPACT.org for useful tools and recommendations.

The McGill Pain Questionnaire (MPQ) measures the sensory, affective, evaluative, and miscellaneous components of pain.[80] Although older adults consistently rate sensory and affective components of their pain lower than younger counterparts, the validity, reliability, and subscale distinctions of the MPQ are similar in young and older persistent pain populations.[13] The short form of the MPQ (SF-MPQ)[81] is similarly appropriate, with no apparent age-related measurement errors.[78] An expanded and revised version of this short form (SF-MPQ-2) has been validated and is in the process of being published. The revised faces pain scale is the tool for measuring intensity preferred by many older adults, including those who are from ethnic minorities or those with mild–moderate cognitive impairment.[73,82]

Nonverbal, Cognitively Impaired Older Adults

When the patient is unable to reliably self-report the presence or nature of pain due to severe cognitive impairment or critical illness, clinicians rely on a combination of assessment strategies to fill this void. Measures of pain behaviors are often combined with surrogate reports from those who know the patient best and the patient's response to analgesics. Even if the patient is unconscious, intubated, or chemically paralyzed, the clinician's understanding of the pain typically associated with the medical conditions/procedures allows them to make assumptions, termed "Assume Pain is Present" to guide pain prevention and treatment interventions regardless of cognitive/verbal abilities.[83,84] A good history and physical examination provides information on pain-related diagnoses and conditions that support a judgment of pain present.

A large number of behavioral pain assessment tools have been developed for use in this population in the last decade; however, there is a lack of consensus about recommending one tool for use with all patients. The characteristics of the specific patient sample and the setting are important in selecting an appropriate behavioral measure. Readers are referred to the following website for information and critiques of existing English behavioral tools: http://prc.coh.org/elderly.asp. For example, The Pain Assessment in Advanced Dementia tool rates pain (0–10 scale) based on breathing, vocalizations, facial expressions, body movements, and consolability and may be useful for repeated observations of patients that present with common pain-related behaviors.[83] However, this instrument will miss or underestimate pain in patients whose presentation of pain is manifested as a change in daily activities, interpersonal interactions, or mental changes and use of a tool that incorporates these factors, such as the Pain Assessment Checklist for Seniors with Limited Ability to Communicate, may be more appropriate when monitoring for more subtle changes in behavior suggestive of pain.[85] Adding surrogate reporting of pain by people who know the patient best or observing the response to empirical treatment with analgesics has merit in this population.[84]

Behavioral Indicators of Pain

Among the behaviors displayed by people unable to communicate their pain, facial expression is often the first or most common indication of pain,[86] and it may be the only one. Common facial expressions suggestive of pain include grimacing, clenched teeth, and tightly shut eyes. Other common behavioral indicators of pain are:

- Vocalizations, such as moaning, groaning, crying or screaming
- Immobilization, guarding, holding, or rubbing the hurt body part
- Stiff or awkward movements (e.g., limping)
- Mental status changes including depressed mood, irritability, or confusion
- Changes in interpersonal interactions, ranging from withdrawn to aggressive
- Changes in activity patterns or routines

Purposeless body movements, such as tossing and turning in bed or flailing extremities, can also indicate pain. The patients should be observed for evidence of pain-related behaviors unique to that individual during activities known to be painful (e.g., injections, dressing changes, repositioning).

PHARMACOLOGIC TREATMENT OF PAIN IN OLDER PERSONS

Pharmacokinetics and Pharmacodynamics Associated With Aging

With the exception of the rectal route, the rate of medication absorption is typically not affected by aging. The pattern of drug distribution does change because of less total body water, and more body fat is seen in older adults. This favors the distribution and accumulation of lipophilic (fentanyl) agents, while decreasing that of hydrophilic (morphine) drugs. The decline in serum protein concentrations with age can increase the bioavailability of drugs, like nonsteroidal anti-inflammatory drugs (NSAIDs), that are highly protein-bound.[11,13] This effect is magnified when patients take multiple medications that displace NSAIDs from protein binding sites, further increasing free serum concentration of the active analgesic.

This protein binding can also slow the metabolism and excretion of NSAIDs that is already compromised due to the smaller size, lower blood flow, and reduced function of the liver with age. These hepatic changes, combined with fewer drug-metabolizing enzymes, increase drug elimination time and slow the metabolism required to produce active metabolites. Reductions in renal size, glomerular filtration rate, and renal blood flow raise the risk of side effects and toxicity to drugs that accumulate due to slowed elimination of the unchanged drug as well as active and toxic metabolites.[11] NSAIDs can further contribute to this slowed clearance by lowering renal blood flow and glomerular filtration rate through its antiprostaglandin effect.

Pharmacodynamic changes have also been noted with aging. The density and sensitivity of mu receptors change and often increase sensitivity to both the desired and undesired effects of opioids.[11,13] Combined with other age-related changes in the neurologic and pulmonary systems, there is a greater risk of sedation and respiratory depression with the initial administration of opioid analgesics. These collective pharmacokinetic and pharmacodynamic changes warrant using lower doses and longer dosing intervals with advanced age, especially with known hepatic or renal impairment.

Safe, Effective Use of Nonsteroidal Anti-Inflammatory Drugs in the Older Person

Acetaminophen is considered the safest nonopioid analgesic and is the first-line analgesic of choice for older patients[16] when pain is mild or moderate. Compared to other nonopioids, it has similar or lower analgesic potency without gastroduodenopathy or an effect on platelet function. When combined with warfarin, over-anticoagulation can result.[87] Persistent excessive use of acetaminophen may impair renal function and cause hepatotoxicity, especially in patients with chronic alcoholism and liver disease or in patients who drink three or more alcoholic beverages per day. Dosage limits of 2–3 g per day will minimize the risk of renal or hepatic toxicity. However, because acetaminophen is included in many drug compounds, care must be taken to avoid inadvertent exposure.

Concerned that medication-related problems are a leading cause of hospitalization and death among older adults, Dr. Mark Beers and a team of leading gerontologists developed a list of 48 medications and drug classes that should be avoided in older adults, regardless of frailty. As a class, all NSAIDs (both nonselective and COX-2 selective) made the list with a "high severity" designation, as did the individual agents indomethacin and ketorolac.[88] An estimated 10% to 20% of older adults are prescribed NSAIDs, which account for 3300 deaths and 41,000 hospitalizations in the United States annually,[89] mostly from gastrointestinal (GI) bleeding. Within the class, ibuprofen appears to have the best efficacy and GI safety among widely available oral NSAIDs. Diclofenac sodium and naproxen have intermediate (doubled) risks, while piroxicam and ketorolac have the greatest (four-fold) risk of GI ulcerations or bleeds.[90,91]

NSAIDs will also worsen established hypertension, congestive heart failure, and renal impairment. Renal dysfunction, a history of aspirin hypersensitivity, serious skin disorders (e.g., Stevens-Johnson syndrome), anticoagulant therapy, a history of organ transplantation, blood disorders (e.g., coagulopathy, neutropenia), hypertension, or congestive heart failure often disqualifies patients as candidates for NSAID therapy. The risk of taking NSAIDs when patients are on warfarin, digoxin, anticonvulsants, or oral antidiabetic agents needs to be carefully considered and avoided when possible.

The COX-2 selective NSAIDs appear to have less risk of GI ulcerations and bleeding in the elderly than do nonselective NSAIDs.[91] However, the GI safety advantages of COX-2 selective NSAIDs are significantly reduced when used in combination with low-dose aspirin in high doses, with multiple NSAIDs, or after a year of continuous therapy. The COX-2 inhibitors have no advantages in regard to renal function compared to nonselective agents.

The occurrence of rare but serious cardiovascular events and skin problems prompted a withdrawal of rofecoxib from the worldwide market in September of 2004. Valdecoxib was later voluntarily withdrawn from the market amid evidence of similar problems. In a retrospective analysis of a large cancer prevention study, rofecoxib has been found to double the risk of endpoints that include fatal and nonfatal heart attacks, strokes, and deaths from unknown causes. These events declined slowly, remaining significantly elevated for at least a year after rofecoxib was discontinued.[92] Celecoxib remains on the U.S. market, with other COX-2 agents available elsewhere, awaiting the definitive research delineating whether these risks are drug-specific or a drug-class effect.

Safe Nonsteroidal Anti-Inflammatory Drug Product Selection and Monitoring Use

The decision to use a NSAID in the management of persistent pain in older adults requires individualization considering comorbidities, concomitant medications, and associated risk factors with benefits outweighing the risks. If short-term NSAID therapy is considered and GI risk is considered low, it may be reasonable to select ibuprofen or naproxen.

Prolonged NSAID therapy should be used with extreme caution, and baseline and periodic monitoring for these potential problems and occult GI bleeding is recommended. Given an analgesic ceiling, patients are started at a low dose and asked to record the analgesic effect for 1–2 weeks before increasing the dose. If, after titrating to a higher dose, there is no analgesic advantage, return to the lower dose.

To lessen the risk of GI and renal toxicity, urge the patient to drink a full glass of water with the NSAID and maintain adequate hydration throughout therapy. If therapy extends over a few weeks or longer, a gastroprotective drug, such as a proton pump inhibitor (PPI) or misoprostol, is advised.[93] For patients at highest GI risk (history of ulcers), the use of a COX-2 inhibitor with a PPI is considered.[93] Patients who are taking aspirin for cardioprotective purposes need special consideration since some NSAIDs (e.g., ibuprofen) inhibit its cardioprotective actions and increase GI risk. In general, NSAIDs with the highest safety margin should be used in the lowest effective dose for the shortest duration after acetaminophen is deemed inadequate or contraindicated.[94]

Other options for high-risk patients include nonacetylated salicylates or topical NSAIDs and may have better safety margins than more traditional options.[95,96] Choline magnesium trisalicy-late has advantages of minimal GI toxicity, no effects on platelets, a twice daily dosing regimen and is available in pill or liquid form.[96] Topical agents are particularly beneficial when pain is localized as it places a higher concentration at the target tissue, has fewer systemic side effects, and enjoys a high degree of acceptance by many older persons. Topical options include an expanding variety of NSAIDs, opioids (e.g., morphine gel), adjuvant, and experimental options.[97]

Safe, Effective Use of Opioids in the Older Person

Potential Risks of Opioid Analgesics

Opioid therapy is the cornerstone of treatment for moderate and severe levels of pain. Opioids must be used cautiously in older adults who have increased sensitivity to their effects,[98] especially in the presence of renal or hepatic dysfunction.[99] The most serious risk is respiratory depression, which occurs infrequently when opioids are dosed and titrated cautiously.[16] Respiratory depression is more common with acute or intermittent therapy rather than long-term opioid therapy. The greatest risk is during the first day of opioid therapy and during periods of dose escalation. At greatest risk are patients with pre-existing respiratory dysfunction, including chronic obstructive pulmonary disease, emphysema, kyphoscoliosis, severe obesity, or cor pulmonale. Especially concerning is the tendency of older adults to experience oxygen desaturations at night due to sleep apnea.[99] As many as 30% of older adults with sleep apnea who take opioids are at risk for these respiratory effects.[100] Methadone in particular is associated with a higher risk for sleep-related problems.[101]

Opioids can also cause peripheral vasodilatation which may produce orthostatic hypotension and a corresponding risk of falling. Endocrine and immune system suppression occurs with opioids, the significance and reversibility of which in the older adults is currently being investigated.[102,103]

Still, long-term use of opioids poses a lower risk of life-threatening events than sustained NSAID therapy.[16] The most common side effects, with the exception of constipation, diminish over the first couple of weeks of therapy. Several days at a steady dose without visual or cognitive impairment should be evident before advising patients to resume driving or other potentially dangerous activities. Reluctance to prescribe opioid drugs has probably been overinfluenced by political and social pressures to control illicit drug use.[16] Although substance abuse, diversion, and addiction disorders do occur in older adults,[104] many are deprived prescriptions or refuse them because of overstated risks.

One active area of research is that of opioid-induced hyperalgesia, a phenomenon linked to high-dose, long-term opioid therapy. Over the course of treatment, patients become more sensitive to pain or develop new areas of pain in addition to a loss of the drug's original potency.[105] Awareness of this phenomenon has stimulated much debate and research into the best ways to treat patients on long-term opioids. One strategy is to limit the dose and duration of opioid therapy; another is to switch patients to a different opioid. The incidence, effects, and prevention strategies pertaining to opioid-induced hyperalgesia in the older adult remain to be elucidated.

Opioids to Avoid in Older Adults

The revised Beers Criteria do not identify the class of opioids as high risk, but do list propoxyphene, meperidine, and pentazocine as drugs to avoid in older adults.[88] Pentazocine often leads to central nervous system excitement, confusion, and agitation, and its use should be avoided in frail older patients. Propoxyphene is no more effective than acetaminophen, yet has been associated with the same adverse effects as other opioid drugs. A year-long prospective study of over 350,000 older adults found a two-fold increased risk of hip fractures among older adults taking propoxyphene compared to nonusers, with a dose-response relationship.[106] Propoxyphene typically is combined with high-dose acetaminophen, adding liver toxicity to its list of potential problems.

Although the duration of meperidine analgesia is 4 hours or less, its toxic metabolite normeperidine has approximately a 30 hour half-life, which is even longer with impaired renal function. At doses of 600 mg per day or when used for more than 48 hours, the risk of neurotoxicity-induced seizure is high. Normeperidine can also cause tremulousness, dysphoria, myoclonus, and a potentially fatal interaction with monoamine oxidase inhibitors.[107] Methadone did not make the most recent Beers Criteria list of medications to avoid in older adults, but due to its complex pharmacokinetics, its link to hypertension and sleep apnea, caution is advised in older adults.[101,108] It should be used only by clinicians with considerable clinical experience with this drug.[16,109] Despite these disadvantages, methadone is a valuable tool that helps carefully selected and monitored patients with refractory pain at a relatively low cost.

Safe Product Selection and Use of Opioids

Oxycodone and morphine are probably the best first-line opioid agents for an opioid naïve patient with acute pain. The adage, start low–go slow, would have the prudent clinician starting as low as 2.5 mg oxycodone, 5 mg oral morphine, or 1–2 mg parenteral morphine, and then basing adjustments on the individual response. Morphine can be titrated more quickly than other agents, but generally the short-acting opioids are titrated on a daily basis and long-acting formulations can be safely titrated once or twice a week.[109] Hydrocodone is another reasonable first-line option; however, it is available only in fixed-dose combinations with acetaminophen and has less than ideal pharmacokinetic properties for older adults. Tramadol is commonly chosen, but it has low potency and an association with seizures that requires cautious patient selection and attention to potential drug-drug interactions.[109]

In Europe, buprenorphine is emerging as a potential first-line opioid with desirable pharmacokinetic and pharmacodynamic properties in older adults. Labeling and prescribing restrictions in the United States preclude it from being used widely; however, it merits consideration for expanded use in the future. Buprenorphine is a potent opioid with partial mu-agonist and kappa-antagonist activity.[110] The absorption, distribution, metabolism, and excretion of buprenorphine, as well as the ceiling to its respiratory depressant effects, make it a good choice for older adults. The transdermal buprenorphine patch is ideally suited for older adults, although it is not yet commercially available in the United States.[111]

Safe, Effective Use of Adjuvants in the Older Person

Adjuvant analgesics include a variety of agents with analgesic activity whose primary use and indication is other than for pain. Many of these adjuvants are used "off-label" and have been found clinically useful for specific pain conditions.[112] These drugs may be used alone or in combination with analgesics to treat persistent pain conditions, particularly neuropathic pain. Amitriptyline is the best studied adjuvant for pain, but it should be avoided in the elderly due to its cardiac, anticholinergic, and sedative effects.[88] Nortriptyline or desipramine are better choices with a 75% lower incidence of side effects at comparable doses.[112] Duloxetine, a selective serotonin and norepinephrine reuptake inhibitor, has approved labeling for certain pains and appears to be a better tolerated antidepressant for older adults.

Antiepileptic drugs are first-line agents to treat neuropathic pain in older persons.[113,114] Gabapentin and pregabalin have labeled indications for specific neuropathic pain disorders. Lower toxicity and fewer drug-drug interactions increase these drugs' usefulness in the older population. Due to a risk of somnolence, mental clouding, and dizziness, dosing should be initiated as low as 100 mg at bedtime and cautiously titrated upward. Carbamazepine also has U.S. Food and Drug Administration-approved labeling for trigeminal neuralgia, but like many older antiepileptic agents, drug-drug interaction, liver, and hematologic toxicity make them less than ideal in older adults.

Many other adjuvant drugs can be used in the older adult for their coanalgesic effect or to offset side effects of pain relievers. They may be selected for their general ability to reduce pain, such as a local anesthetic, or based on targeted (e.g., alpha-2-adrenergic, GABA-B) receptors where they work.[113] Targets vary considerably based on the underlying pathology; however, for each agent selected, they must start at a low dose, with careful titration, and have frequent monitoring to establish their safety and efficacy before adding, subtracting, or adjusting other medications.

ADDITIONAL TREATMENTS FOR PAIN OF OLDER PERSONS

Pharmacologic management is the foundation of pain treatment in most settings; however, alone, medication(s) often fall short of providing optimal pain reduction and functional improvement. In addition to medical management, there are many other approaches to pain relief that add benefit to the treatment plan. In conventional medicine, there are physical or psychosocial (cognitive/behavioral) modalities often provided by a physical therapist, physiatrist, or psychologist. Additional complementary and alternative medicine (CAM) approaches are also utilized for the prevention and control of pain. Integrated, multidisciplinary pain treatment programs are likely the most beneficial in optimizing the outcomes when pain is complex and refractory to initial treatment attempts.

Physical Modalities

Physical approaches to pain control range from highly technical interventional approaches to simple applications of heat/cold, orthotics, electrical stimulation, or therapeutic exercise. Among modalities offered by physical therapists, active techniques, like therapeutic exercise and aquatic therapy, work better for older adults than passive approaches like superficial heat, transcutaneous electrical nerve stimulation, and acupuncture.[115] The dry and fragile skin of some older adults may contribute to discomfort, irritation, or even tearing of skin when removing pads. Therefore, good hydration, extra gel, or cream at the electrode site and caution when removing the pads from the skin may improve tolerance of that modality. Caution to protect the skin of older adults also comes into play with the topical application of heat and cold or during massage techniques.[116]

Interventional approaches can provide significant benefit to older adults whose severe, disabling pain is not responsive to less invasive measures. Proper selection and precise performance of the specific procedure is needed, as is vigilant monitoring of patient response. For many nerve blocks, the major life-threatening complication is intravascular injection, thus many providers will use fluoroscopic verification of needle placement before injections.[117] Older adults are more likely to have contraindications to certain injections, such as anticoagulation, uncontrolled diabetes, and progressive neurologic disorders. New innovations like the X-Stop (Medtronic Spine, LLC, Memphis, TN), kyphoplasty, and vertebroplasty interventions are providing less invasive options for vertebral disorders (e.g., spinal stenosis, vertebral compression fractures) that are more common in older adults.[118]

Psychosocial Approaches to Pain Control

Psychosocial (cognitive/behavioral) modalities may focus on altering the patient's thoughts, feelings, or behaviors in a way that reduce pain, stress, and emotional distress. Specific techniques include education and counseling, distraction, coping skills training, and facilitating emotional disclosure. There are a variety of techniques such as relaxation, imagery, and hypnotherapy that help people. Although older adults are less likely to be referred for these forms of therapy, they benefit from cognitive-behavioral therapy,[119] relaxation, and biofeedback training.[120] Despite limited research, it appears that older patients with persistent pain benefit substantially from coping skills training.[121–123]

Older adults do better when interventions are tailored to meet their specific needs (multimodal presentation, addressing needs of visual or auditory impairment, involving spouses/caregivers, etc.).[119] Although these and other psychosocial modalities help many older persons, there are some who may be physically or mentally inappropriate candidates for specific techniques.[116]

Complementary and Alternative Medicine Approaches to Pain Control

A variety of CAM approaches are used by older adults to relieve pain. Patients may use the terms holistic, natural, home remedy, or "Eastern Medicine" to refer to these techniques. Given that more than 60% of persons over age 50 use CAM approaches, professionals need to ask patients about their use of these methods in a nonjudgmental manner that encourages honest, full disclosure. The National Center for Complementary and Alternative Medicine[124] recognizes five categories of approaches: Alternative Medical Systems, Mind-body Medicine, Biologically-based Therapy, Manipulative and Body-based Practices, and Energy-based Medicine. Back pain is the most common condition for which CAM approaches are used, with pain accounting for 6 out of the top 10 reasons people use these approaches.[125]

Perhaps some people turn to CAM to give them a greater sense of control or to feel less dependent on a doctor, a pill, or a procedure. Close to 40% of patients however, seek CAM therapies because of a failure to benefit from conventional medicine or a lack of access to medicine due to costs.[125] Many older persons have embraced the use of biological therapies such as glucosamine/chondroitin, S-adenosyl-L-methionine, and Devil's claw, which have potency comparable to NSAIDs with less toxicity. However, some herbal remedies have been tainted with drugs or heavy metals.[126,127] More commonly, interactions between medications and herbal remedies occur.[128]

Multidisciplinary Pain Treatments

Multidisciplinary pain treatment programs are underutilized for older adults with pain[129]; although studies have not found age-related differences in treatment expectations, acceptance, compliance, or drop-out rates.[130] Subtle, and likely unintentional, age biases prevent many qualifying older adults from being admitted to these programs.[130] Multidisciplinary pain clinics have better outcomes in terms of pain reduction, functional improvement, and lower health care utilization than those who receive only single-modality interventions.[131] Although the cost-benefit ratio has not clearly been delineated for older adults, there is no compelling evidence to suggest that they should be denied such treatment. In fact, the potential adverse effects of untreated pain and/or polypharmacy suggest that multidisciplinary treatment should be considered for all geriatric patients with significant pain complaints.

CONCLUSION

Certainly, there are risks when treating older adults with severe or persistent pain. In fact, the undertreatment of pain is an important risk that can contribute to physical harm, mental despair, and social isolation during what has been dubbed "the golden years." Although much remains to be learned, we currently have sufficient knowledge to improve the way pain is assessed and treated, while refining methods to further improve the safety and efficacy of pain relief efforts.

Clear consistent assessment methods are needed by choosing and using tools validated for older adults. The patient's understanding of the tool should be validated so that meaningful information is gathered and recorded. When planning interventions, a shared decision-making approach is appropriate, where patients and their loved ones are informed of the risks, benefits, and variable responses typical for particular treatment options. This shared decision-making engages the patient as an active participant in the treatment process and educates them about desired and undesired effects that may be encountered and need to be recorded.

Cautious drug and dose selection is needed for the older adult. Lower starting doses and longer dosing intervals are justified until the patient's response to analgesics is known. Monitoring the patient's response early in therapy for side effects, drug (or herbal) interactions, and toxicity is important, especially for those with comorbid conditions that add risks. Continued monitoring for older adults on sustained treatment is important as several late-onset toxicities (e.g., GI bleed, hypertension, liver/renal impairment, opioid-induced hyperalgesia) may not emerge until months or years of therapy have passed.

The prudent use of nonoperative interventions (e.g., nerve blocks) and nondrug or CAM therapies should be considered for older adults with persistent pain. Given the breadth of options available to treat pain, allowing it to go untreated in older adults is erroneous. Whereas not all treatments are good options for older adults, failing to treat pain is unacceptable, especially for those who are so vulnerable to the harmful effects of unrelieved pain.

References

1. Desbiens NA, Mueller–Rizner N, Connors AF Jr, et al. Pain in the oldest-old during hospitalization and up to one year later. *J Am Geriatr Soc* 1997;45(10):1167–1172.
2. Looi Y, Audisio R. A review of the literature on post-operative pain in older cancer patients. *Eur J Cancer* 2007;43(15):2222–2230.
3. Center for Disease Control (CDC). Health, United States, 2006 with Chartbook on pain in Americans. Hyattsville, MD; 2006. Library of Congress Catalog No.76-641496. Available at http://www.cdc.gov/nchs/data/hus/hus06.pdf. Accessed September 21, 2007.
4. Center for Disease Control (CDC). Health, United States, 2007 with Chartbook on trends in the health of Americans. Hyattsville, MD; 2006. Library of Congress Catalog No.76-641496. Available at http://www.cdc.gov/nchs/data/hus/hus07.pdf. Accessed September 21, 2007.
5. Gerstle DS, All AC, Wallace DC. Quality of life and chronic nonmalignant pain. *Pain Manag Nurs* 2001;2(3):98–109.
6. United States Department of Health and Human Services (USDHHS). A profile of older Americans, 2007. Available at http://www.agingcarefl.org/aging/AOA-2007profile.pdf. Accessed November 11, 2008.
7. Medling PS. Foreword. In: Gibson SJ, Weiner DK, eds. *Pain in Older Persons.* Seattle, IASP Press; 2005:xi–xiv.
8. Herr K, Titler M. Acute pain assessment and pharmacological management practices for the older adult with a hip fracture: review of emergency department trends. *J Emerg Nurs* 2009;35(4):312–320.
9. D'Avolio DA, Feldman J, Mitchell P, et al. Access to care and health-related quality of life among older adults with nonurgent emergency department visits. *Geriatr Nurs* 2008;29(4):240–246.

10. Morrison RS, Magaziner J, McLaughlin MA, et al. The impact of post-operative pain on outcomes following hip fracture. *Pain* 2003;103(3):303–311.

11. Strassels SA, McNicol E, Suleman R. Pharmacotherapy of pain in older adults. *Clin Geriatr Med* 2008;24(2):275–298, vi–vii.

12. Won AB, Lapane KL, Vallow S, et al. Persistent nonmalignant pain and analgesic prescribing patterns in elderly nursing home residents. *J Am Geriatr Soc* 2004;52(6):867–874.

13. Gagliese L, Melzack R. Pain in the Elderly. In: McMahon SB, Koltzenburg M, eds. *Wall and Melzack's Textbook of Pain.* 5th ed. London, Elsevier Churchill Livingstone; 2006:1169–1179.

14. Herr K. Chronic pain: challenges and assessment strategies. *J Gerontol Nurs* 2002;28(1):20–27; quiz 54–55.

15. Weiner D, Peterson B, Keefe F. Chronic pain-associated behaviors in the nursing home: resident versus caregiver perceptions. *Pain* 1999;80(3):577–588.

16. American Geriatrics Society. AGS panel on persistent pain in older persons. Clinical practice guidelines: the management of persistent pain in older persons. *J Am Geriatr Soc* 2002;50(6 suppl):S205–224.

17. Ferrell BA, Ferrell BR, Osterweil D. Pain in the nursing home. *J Am Geriatr Soc* 1990;38:409–414.

18. Williamson GM, Schulz R. Activity restriction mediates the association between pain and depressed affect: a study of younger and older adult cancer patients. *Psychol Aging* 1995;10(3):369–378.

19. Verdu E, Ceballos D, Vilches JJ, et al. Influence of aging on peripheral nerve function and regeneration. *J Peripher Nerv Syst* 2000;5(4):191–208.

20. Iwata K, Tsuboi Y, Shima A, et al. Central neuronal changes after nerve injury: neuroplastic influences of injury and aging. *J Orofac Pain* 2004;18(4):293–298.

21. Crisp T, Giles JR, Cruce WL, et al. The effects of aging on thermal hyperalgesia and tactile-evoked allodynia using two models of peripheral mononeuropathy in the rat. *Neurosci Lett* 2003;339(2):103–106.

22. Edwards RR. Age-associated differences in pain perception and pain processing. In: Gibson SJ, Weiner DK, eds. *Pain in Older Persons.* Seattle, IASP Press; 2005:45–65.

23. Gagliese L, Ferrell M. The neurobiology of aging, nociception and pain: an integration of animal and human experimental evidence. In: Gibson SJ, Weiner DK, eds. *Pain in Older Persons.* Seattle, IASP Press; 2005:25–44.

24. Pavlin DJ, Cen C, Penaloza DA, et al. Pain as a factor complicating recovery and discharge alter ambulatory surgery. *Anesth Analg* 2002;95(3):627–634.

25. Greisen J, Juhl CB, Grofte T, et al. Acute pain induces insulin resistance in humans. *Anesthesiology* 2001;95(3):578–584.

26. Lvungqvist O, Nygren J, Soop M, et al. Metabolic postoperative management: novel concepts. *Curr Opin Crit Care* 2005;11(4):295–299.

27. Page GG, Ben–Eliyahu S, Yirmiya R, et al. Morphine attenuates surgery-induced enhancement of metastatic colonization in rats. *Pain* 1993;54(1):21–28.

28. Rittner HL, Brack A, Stein C. Pain and the immune system. *Br J Anaesth* 2008;101(1):40–44.

29. Desai PM. Pain management and pulmonary dysfunction. *Crit Care Clin* 1999;15(1):151–166.

30. Macrae WA. Chronic post-surgical pain: 10 years on. *Br J Anaesth* 2008;101(1):77–86.

31. Grass JA. The role of epidural anesthesia and analgesia in postoperative outcome. *Anesthesiol Clin North America* 2000;18(2):407–428, viii.

32. Morrison RS, Magaziner J, Gilbert M, et al. Relationship between pain and opioid analgesics on the development of delirium following hip fracture. *J Gerontol A Biol Sci Med Sci* 2003;58(1):76–81.

33. Messier SP, Glasser JL, Ettinger WH, et al. Declines in strength and balance in older adults with chronic knee pain: a 30-month longitudinal, observational study. *Arthritis Rheum* 2002;47(2):141–148.

34. Rejeski WJ, Miller ME, Foy C, et al. Self-efficacy and the progression of functional limitations and self-reported disability in older adults with knee pain. *J Gerontol B Psychol Sci Soc Sci* 2001;56(5):S261–265.

35. Scudds RJ, Robertson JM. Pain factors associated with physical disability in a sample of community-dwelling senior citizens. *J Gerontol A Biol Sci Med Sci* 2000;55(7):M393–399.

36. Bernabei R, Gambassi G, Lapane K, et al. Management of pain in elderly patients with cancer. SAGE (Systematic Assessment of Geriatric Drug Use via Epidemiology) Study Group. *JAMA* 1998;279(23):1877–1882.

37. Lichtenberg PA, McGrogan AJ. Chronic pain in elderly psychiatric inpatients. *Clin Biofeedback Health Int* 1987;10:3–7.

38. Pahor M, Guralnik JM, Wan JY, et al. Lower body osteoarticular pain and dose of analgesic medications in older disabled women: the Women's Health and Aging Study. *Am J Public Health* 1999;89(6):930–934.

39. Woo J, Ho S C, Lau J, et al. Musculoskeletal complaints and associated consequences in elderly Chinese aged 70 and over. *J Rheumatol* 1994;21(10):1927–1931.

40. AGS Panel on Chronic Pain in Older Persons. The management of chronic pain in older persons. *J Am Geriatr Soc* 1998;46:635–651.

41. Jacox A, Carr DB, Payne R, et al. *Management of Cancer Pain. Clinical Practice Guideline No. 9.* Rockville, MD: Agency for Healthcare Research and Quality; 1994. AHCPR 94–0592.

42. Lawhorne L, Passerini J, Cranmer K, et al. *Chronic Pain Management in the Long-Term Care Setting.* Columbia, MD: American Medical Directors Association; 1999.

43. Sherman R, Hickner J. Academic physicians use placebos in clinical practice and believe in the mind-body connection. *J Gen Intern Med* 2008;23(1):7–10.

44. Tilburt JC, Emanuel EJ, Kaptchuk TJ, et al. Prescribing "placebo treatments": results of national survey of US internists and rheumatologists. *BMJ* 2008;337:a1938.

45. Gibson SJ, Farrell M. A review of age differences in the neurophysiology of nociception and the perceptual experience of pain. *Clin J Pain* 2004;20(4):227–239.

46. Heft MW, Cooper BY, O'Brien KK, et al. Aging effects on the perception of noxious and non-noxious thermal stimuli applied to the face. *Aging (Milano)* 1996;8(1):35–41.

47. Chakour MC, Gibson SJ, Bradbeer M, et al. The effect of age on A delta- and C-fiber thermal pain perception. *Pain* 1996;64(1):143–152.

48. Gibson SJ, Gorman MM, Helme RD. Assessment of pain in the elderly using event-related cerebral potentials. In: Bond MR, Charlton JE, Woolf CJ, eds. *Proceedings of the Sixth World Congress on Pain.* New York: Elsevier; 1991:527–533.

49. Harkins SW, Price DD, Martelli M. Effects of age on pain perception: thermonociception. *J Gerontol* 1986;41(1):58–63.

50. Edwards RR, Fillingim RB. Age-associated differences in responses to noxious stimuli. *J Gerontol A Biol Sci Med Sci* 2001;56(3):M180–185.

51. Neri M, Agazzani E. Aging and right–left asymmetry in experimental pain measurement. *Pain* 1984;19(1):43–48.

52. Tresch DD. Management of the older patient with acute myocardial infarction: difference in clinical presentations between older and younger patients. *J Am Geriatr Soc* 1998;46(9):1157–1162.

53. Mehta RH, Rathore SS, Radford MJ, et al. Acute myocardial infarction in the elderly: differences by age. *J Am Coll Cardiol* 2001;38(3):736–741.

54. Cooper GS, Shlaes DM, Salata RA. Intraabdominal infection: differences in presentation and outcome between younger patients and the elderly. *Clin Infect Dis* 1994;19(1):146–148.

55. Hilton D, Iman N, Burke GJ, et al. Absence of abdominal pain in older persons with endoscopic ulcers: a prospective study. *Am J Gastroenterol* 2001;96(2):380–384.

56. Choo PW, Galil K, Donahue JG, et al. Risk factors for postherpetic neuralgia. *Arch Intern Med* 1997;157(11):1217–1224.

57. Jung BF, Johnson RW, Griffin DR, et al. Risk factors for postherpetic neuralgia in patients with herpes zoster. *Neurology* 2004;62(9):1545–1551.

58. Turk DC. The role of demographic and psychosocial factors in transition from acute to chronic pain. In: Jensen TS, Turner JA, Wiesenfeld–Hallin Z, eds. *Proceedings of the 8th World Congress on Pain.* Seattle: IASP Press; 1997:185–214.

59. Pickering G. Age differences in clinical pain states. In: Gibson SJ, Weiner DK, eds. *Pain in Older Persons.* Seattle: IASP Press; 2005:67–85.

60. Bergman S, Herrström P, Högström K, et al. Chronic musculoskeletal pain, prevalence rates and sociodemographic associations in a Swedish population study. *J Rheumatol* 2001;28(6):1369–1377.

61. Thomas E, Peat G, Harris L, et al. The prevalence of pain and pain interference in a general population of older adults: cross sectional findings from the North Staffordshire Osteoarthritis Project (NorStOP). *Pain* 2004;110(1–2):361–368.

62. Wolfe F, Ross K, Anderson J, et al. The prevalence and characteristics of fibromyalgia in the general population. *Arthritis Rheum* 1995;38(1):19–28.

63. Macfarlane GJ, McBeth J, Silman AJ. Widespread body pain and mortality: prospective population study. *BMJ* 2001;323(7314):662–665.

64. Stein WM, Miech RP. Cancer pain in the elderly hospice patient. *J Pain Symptom Manage* 1993;8(7):474–482.

65. Ferrell BR, Ferrell BA, Ahn C, et al. Pain management for elderly patients with cancer at home. *Cancer* 1994;74(suppl 7):2139–2146.

66. Cleeland CS, Gonin R, Hatfield AK, et al. Pain and its treatment in outpatients with metastatic cancer. *N Engl J Med* 1994;330(9):592–596.

67. Miaskowski C, Cleary J, Burney R, et al. *Guideline for the Management of Cancer Pain in Adults and Children, APS Clinical Practice Guideline Series.* No.3. Glenview, IL: American Pain Society; 2005.

68. Mercadante S. Malignant bone pain: pathophysiology and treatment. *Pain* 1997;69(1–2):1–18.

69. Ware LJ, Epps C, Herr K, et al. Evaluation of the revised faces pain scale, verbal descriptor scale, numeric rating scale, and Iowa pain thermometer in older minority adults. *Pain Manag Nurs* 2006;7(3):117–125.

70. Krebs EE, Carey TS, Weinberger M. Accuracy of the pain numeric rating scale as a screening test in primary care. *J Gen Intern Med* 2007;22(10):1453–1458.

71. Rahman A. Debate looms on CMS use of pain measure in nursing homes. *Aging Today* 26;2005:3,12.

72. Hadjistavropoulos T, Herr K, Turk DC, et al. An interdisciplinary expert consensus statement on assessment of pain in older persons. *Clin J Pain* 2007;23(suppl 1):S1–43.

73. Li L, Liu, X, Herr K. Postoperative pain intensity assessment: a comparison of four scales in Chinese adults. *Pain Med* 2007;8(3):223–234.

74. von Baeyer CL, Piira T. The Faces Pain Scale—Revised (FPS-R) around the world: translation and adaptation for use in many cultures. *Pain Res Manag* 2003;8(suppl B):57B.

75. Auret JA, Toye C, Goucke R, et al. Development and testing of a modified version of the pain inventory for use in residential aged care facilities. *J Am Geriatr Soc* 2008;56:301–306.

76. Herr K, Mobily P. Comparison of selected pain assessment tools for use with the elderly. *Appl Nurs Res* 1993;6(1):39–46.

77. Chibnall JT, Tait RC. Pain assessment in cognitively impaired and unimpaired older adults: a comparison of four scales. *Pain* 2001;92(1–2):173–186.

78. Gagliese L, Melzack R. Age differences in the quality of chronic pain: a preliminary study. *Pain Res Manag* 1997;2:157–162.

79. Dworkin RH, Turk DC, Wyrwich KW, et al. Interpreting the clinical importance of treatment outcomes in chronic pain clinical trials: IMMPACT recommendations. *J Pain* 2008;9(2):105–121.

80. Melzack R. The McGill Pain Questionnaire: major properties and scoring methods. *Pain* 1975;1(3):277–299.

81. Melzack R. The short-form McGill Pain Questionnaire. *Pain* 1987;30(2):191–197.

82. Herr K, Bjoro K, Decker S. Tools for assessment of pain in non-verbal older adults with dementia: a state-of-the-science review. *J Pain Symptom Manage* 2006;31(2):170–192.

83. Warden V, Hurley AC, Volicer L. Development and psychometric evaluation of the Pain Assessment in Advanced Dementia (PAINAD) scale. *J Am Med Dir Assoc* 2003;4(1):9–15.

84. Herr K, Coyne PJ, Key T, et al. Pain assessment in the nonverbal patient: position statement with clinical practice recommendations. *Pain Manag Nurs* 2006;7(2):44–52.

85. Fuchs–Lacelle S, Hadjistavropoulos T. Development and preliminary validation of the Pain Assessment Checklist for Seniors with Limited Ability to Communicate (PACSLAC). *Pain Manag Nurs* 2004;5(1):37–49.

86. Kunz M, Mylius V, Schepelmann K, et al. Impact of age on the facial expression of pain. *J Psychosom Res* 2008;64(3):311–318.

87. Hylek EM, Heiman H, Skates SJ, et al. Acetaminophen and other risk factors for excessive warfarin anticoagulation. *JAMA* 1998;279:657–662.

88. Fick DM, Cooper JW, Wade WE, et al. Updating the Beers criteria for potentially inappropriate medication use in older adults. *Arch Intern Med* 2003;163(22):2716–2724.

89. Griffin MR. Epidemiology of nonsteroidal anti-inflammatory drug-associated gastrointestinal injury. *Am J Med* 1998;104(3A):S23–S29, discussion S41–S42.

90. Ong CKS, Lirk P, Tan CH, et al. An evidence-based update on nonsteroidal anti-inflammatory drugs. *Clin Med Res* 2007;5(1):19–34.

91. Silverstein FE, Faich G, Goldstein JL, et al. Gastrointestinal toxicity with celecoxib vs nonsteroidal anti-inflammatory drugs for osteoarthritis and rheumatoid arthritis: the CLASS study: a randomized controlled trial. Celecoxib Long-term Arthritis Safety Study. *JAMA* 2000;284(10):1247–1255.

92. Baron JA, Sandler RS, Bresalier RS, et al. Cardiovascular events associated with rofecoxib: final analysis of the APPROVe trial. *Lancet* 2008;372(9651):1756–1764.

93. Graham DY, Agrawal NM, Campbell DR, et al. NSAID-Associated Gastric Ulcer Prevention Study Group. Ulcer prevention in long-term users of nonsteroidal anti-inflammatory drugs: results of a double-blind, randomized, multicenter, active- and placebo-controlled study of misoprostol vs lansoprazole. *Arch Intern Med* 2002;162(2):169–175.

94. Simon LS, Lipman AG, Jacox A, et al. *Guideline for the Management of Pain in Osteoarthritis, Rheumatoid Arthritis, and Juvenile Chronic Arthritis*. 2nd ed. Glenview, IL: American Pain Society; 2002.

95. Amar PJ, Schiff ER. Acetaminophen safety and hepatotoxicity—where do we go from here? *Expert Opin Drug Saf* 2007;6(4):341–355.

96. Coyle N. Pharmacologic management of adult cancer pain. *Oncology (Williston Park)* 2007;21(suppl 2 Nurse Ed):10–22; discussion 26.

97. McCleane G. Topical analgesic agents. *Clin Geriatr Med* 2008;24(2):299–312.

98. Fine PG, Portenoy RK. *A Clinical Guide to Opioid Analgesia*. New York, Vendome Healthcare; 2007.

99. Johnson SJ. Opioid Safety in patients with renal or hepatic dysfunction. *Pain Treatment Topics, 2007*. Available at http://pain-topics.org/pdf/Opioids-Renal-Hepatic-Dysfunction.pdf. Accessed November 10, 2008.

100. Hutchison R, Rodriguez L. Capnography and respiratory depression. *Am J Nurs* 2008;108(2):35–39.

101. Webster LR, Choi Y, Desai H, et al. Sleep-disordered breathing and chronic opioid therapy. *Pain Med* 2008;9(4):425–432.

102. Govitrapong P, Suttitum T, Kotchabhakdi N, et al. Alterations of immune functions in heroin addicts and heroin withdrawal subjects. *J Pharmacol Exp Ther* 1998;286(2):883–889.

103. Ogrin C, Schussler GC. Suppression of thyrotropin by morphine in a severely stressed patient. *Endocr J* 2005;52(2):265–269.

104. Boddiger D. Drug abuse in older US adults worries experts. *Lancet* 2008;372(9650):1622.

105. DuPen A, Shen D, Ersek M. Mechanisms of opioid-induced tolerance and hyperalgesia. *Pain Manag Nurs* 2007;8(3):113–121.

106. Kamal–Bahl SJ, Stuart BC, Beers MH. Propoxyphene use and risk for hip fractures in older adults. *Am J Geriatr Pharmacother* 2006;4(3):219–226.

107. Forman WB. Opioid analgesic drugs in the elderly. *Clin Geriatr Med* 1996;12(3):489–500.

108. Forman JP, Rimm EB, Curhanet GC. Frequency of analgesic use and risk of hypertension among men. *Arch Intern Med* 2007;167(4):394–399.

109. American Medical Association (AMA). Assessing and treating pain in older adults [serial online]. Pain Management Module 5. 2007. Available at http://www.ama-cmeonline.com/pain_mgmt/module05/index.htm. Accessed November 17, 2008.

110. Pergolizzi J, Böger RH, Budd K, et al. Opioids and the management of chronic severe pain in the elderly: consensus statement of an International Expert Panel with focus on the six clinically most often used World Health Organization Step III opioids (buprenorphine, fentanyl, hydromorphone, methadone, morphine, oxycodone). *Pain Pract* 2008;8(4):287–313.

111. Likar R, Vadlau EM, Breschan C, et al. Comparable analgesic efficacy of transdermal buprenorphine in patients over and under 65 years of age. *Clin J Pain* 2008;24(6):536–543.

112. Lussier D, Portenoy RK. Adjuvant analgesics. In: Doyle D, Hanks G, Cherny NI, et al., eds. *Oxford Textbook of Palliative Medicine*. 3rd ed. Oxford: Oxford University Press; 2004:349–377.

113. Lynch ME, Watson CPN. The pharmacotherapy of chronic pain: a review. *Pain Res Manag* 2006;11(1):11–38.

114. McClain BC, Green CR. Pediatric and geriatric medication considerations. In: Tollison CD, Satterwaite JR, Tollison JW, eds. *Practical Pain Management*. Philadelphia: Lippincott Williams & Wilkins; 2001:288–313.

115. Scudds RJ, Scudds, RA. Physical therapy approaches to the management of pain in older adults. In: Gibson SJ, Weiner DK, eds. *Pain in Older Persons*. Seattle: IASP Press; 2005:223–237.

116. Rakel B, Herr K. Assessment and treatment of postoperative pain in older adults. *J Perianesth Nurs* 2004;19(3):194–208.

117. Bernstein C, Lateef B, Fine P. Interventional pain management procedures in older patients. In: SJ Gibson, DK Weiner, eds. *Pain in Older Persons*. Seattle: IASP Press; 2005:263–281.

118. Lavelle W, Lavelle ED, Smith HS. Interventional techniques for back pain. *Clin Geriatr Med* 2008;24(2):345–368.

119. Waters S, Woodward JT, Keefe F. Cognitive-behavioral therapy for pain in older adults. In: Gibson SJ, Weiner DK, eds. *Pain in Older Persons*. Seattle: IASP Press; 2005:239–261.

120. Puder RS. Age analysis of cognitive-behavioral group therapy for chronic pain outpatients. *Psychol Aging* 1988;3(2):204–207.

121. Nicholson NL, Blanchard EB. A controlled evaluation of behavioral treatment of chronic headache in the elderly. *Behav Ther* 1993;24:395–408.

122. Keefe FJ, Caldwell DS, Williams DA, et al. Pain coping skills training in the management of osteoarthritis knee pain I: a comparative study. *Behav Ther* 1990;21:49–62.

123. Keefe FJ, Caldwell DS, Williams DA, et al. Pain coping skills training in the management of osteoarthritis knee pain II: follow up results. *Behav Ther* 1990;21:435–447.

124. Panel on Definition and Description. CAM Research Methodology Conference. Defining and describing complementary and alternative medicine. *J Altern Ther Health Med* 1997;3(2):49–57.

125. National Center for Complementary and Alternative Medicine. Use of CAM in the United States 2007. Available at http://nccam.nih.gov/news/camuse.pdf. Accessed October 13, 2008.

126. Saper RB, Phillips RS, Sehgal A, et al. Lead, mercury, and arsenic in US- and Indian-manufactured Ayurvedic medicines sold via the Internet. *JAMA* 2008;300(8):915–923.

127. Koh HL, Woo SO. Chinese proprietary medicine in Singapore: regulatory control of toxic heavy metals and undeclared drugs. *Drug Saf* 2000;23(5):351–362.

128. Prestwood K. Complementary and alternative medicine for the treatment of pain in older adults. In: Gibson SJ, Weiner DK, eds. *Pain in Older Persons*. Seattle: IASP Press; 2005:285–307.

129. Katz B, Scherer S, Gibson SJ. Multidisciplinary pain management clinics for older adults. In: Gibson SJ, Weiner DK, eds. *Pain in Older Persons*. Seattle: IASP Press; 2005:309–326.

130. Kee WG, Middaugh SJ, Redpath S, et al. Age as a factor in admission to chronic pain rehabilitation. *Clin J Pain* 1998;14(2):121–128.

131. Sorkin BA, Rudy TE, Hanlon RB, et al. Chronic pain in old and young patients: differences appear less important than similarities. *J Gerontol* 1990;45(2):P64–68.

CHAPTER 56 ■ OBSTETRIC PAIN

CYNTHIA A. WONG

HISTORICAL NOTES

Childbirth pain is arguably the most severe pain most women will endure in their lifetimes. The modern era of childbirth analgesia began in 1847 when Dr. James Young Simpson administered ether to a woman in childbirth and later, in the same year, chloroform. The use of analgesia for childbirth aroused violent opposition from some physicians, the public, and the clergy.[1] Simpson was labeled a heretic, blasphemer, and an agent of the devil. The furor died down somewhat in 1853, when John Snow successfully administered chloroform to Queen Victoria for the birth of her eighth child.

In the ensuing years, public opinion regarding obstetric analgesia began to change, thus forcing the medical community to offer analgesia. Women enthusiastically embraced labor analgesia. Fanny Longfellow, the wife of poet Henry Wadsworth Longfellow and the first woman in the United States to receive labor analgesia in the modern era, wrote that "This is certainly the greatest blessing of this age."[2] Pain began to lose its theological connections.[3] It was no longer considered punishment for sin or divine retribution. Instead, disease and pain were considered biologic processes that could be studied and treated.

Following this auspicious beginning in the 19th century, however, childbirth analgesia was largely neglected by the medical community. The next major step occurred in the early 20th century when *Dämmerschlaf*, or "twilight sleep," was introduced in Europe.[4] The combination of scopolamine and morphine was enthusiastically accepted by women, but not by the medical profession. Medical professionals expressed concern about the effect of childbirth analgesia on the progress of labor. In addition, with the advent of twilight sleep, physicians began to appreciate that anesthetics cross the placenta and had potentially adverse effects on the newborn. This was the stimulus for Virginia Apgar, an anesthesiologist, to develop an evaluation tool to assess neonatal well-being in 1953.[5] A salutary effect of the Apgar score was that scientific studies comparing the effects of different anesthetic techniques on neonatal outcome were now possible.

Regional anesthesia was first introduced in 1884, when Carl Koller described the use of cocaine to anesthetize the eye.[6] Descriptions of regional anesthesia, including spinal, lumbar epidural, caudal, paravertebral, and pudendal nerve blocks, were published in the obstetric literature between 1900 and 1930.[3] In the 1930s and 1940s, John G. P. Cleland contributed to our understanding of the innervation of the uterus and applied this knowledge to regional anesthesia in the care of the obstetric patient.[7] Continuous neuraxial analgesia, as it is practiced today, had its birth in 1943, when Robert A. Hingson and Waldo B. Edwards published the first report of continuous caudal analgesia for childbirth.[8] Flexible, disposable catheters replaced the original malleable needles, and refinements were made, and continue to be made, in technique, drugs, doses, and delivery techniques.

Although other regional nerve block and systemic analgesic techniques are often used for analgesia, women continue to request neuraxial labor analgesia for childbirth at ever increasing rates. In the most recent survey performed in 2001, over 60% of women in large maternity hospitals in the United States received neuraxial analgesia during labor.[9] Similarly, spinal or epidural anesthesia accounts for over 95% of the anesthetics for elective cesarean deliveries. Multimodal analgesic therapy, which often includes a regional technique component, is the norm for postcesarean analgesia. This chapter will summarize the physiology of childbirth pain, physiologic changes of pregnancy that influence the provision of analgesic and anesthetic care, specific labor analgesic techniques, the effects of analgesia on the mother and infant, and the treatment of nonobstetric pain during pregnancy and lactation.

PAIN OF CHILDBIRTH

Although it is a common observation that parturients vary in the amount of pain and suffering associated with labor and vaginal delivery, few well-designed studies on the prevalence, intensity, and quality of labor pain have been performed. Melzack et al.[10] used the McGill Pain Questionnaire to assess childbirth pain. The mean total pain rating index (PRI) was 34 for nulliparous and 30 for parous women. Significant differences were also found between nulliparas and parous women in the sensory qualities of pain. Labor pain scores were 8 to 10 points higher than those associated with cancer pain, phantom limb pain, and postherpetic neuralgia (Fig. 56.1A), although there was a wide range of scores ranging from mild to excruciating (Fig. 56.1B).

Childbirth Pain Mechanisms and Pathways

Most data support the concept that the pain of the first stage of labor originates predominantly in the cervix and the lower uterine segment, rather than the body of the uterus. Dilation of the cervix and lower uterine segment results in distension, stretching, and tearing of tissues. During the late first stage and second stage of labor, the descent of the fetus and intense stretching and tearing of the tissues of the vagina and perineum become additional sources of pain.

Based on animal and human studies, Cleland concluded that the sensory afferents from the uterus and cervix that transmit pain during the first stage of labor enter the spinal cord at T11 and T12 (Fig. 56.2).[7] He demonstrated that these visceral sensory afferents are intermingled with sympathetic efferents by demonstrating that bilateral paravertebral lumbar sympathetic blockade abolished the pain of the first stage of labor. Second stage pain from descent of the fetus in the birth canal is primarily somatic in nature and is transmitted through sacral nerves to the S2 through S4 segments of the spinal cord.

Bonica[11] used a series of discrete nerve blocks of various nociceptive pathways, including paracervical, segmental epidural, caudal, and transsacral blocks, to further refine our knowledge of the nerve pathways that transmit labor pain to the central nervous system. He demonstrated that the upper part of the cervix and lower uterine segment are supplied by afferents that accompany the sympathetic nerves through the uterine and cervical plexus, the inferior, middle, and superior hypogastric plexuses, and the aortic plexuses. The nociceptive afferents then pass to

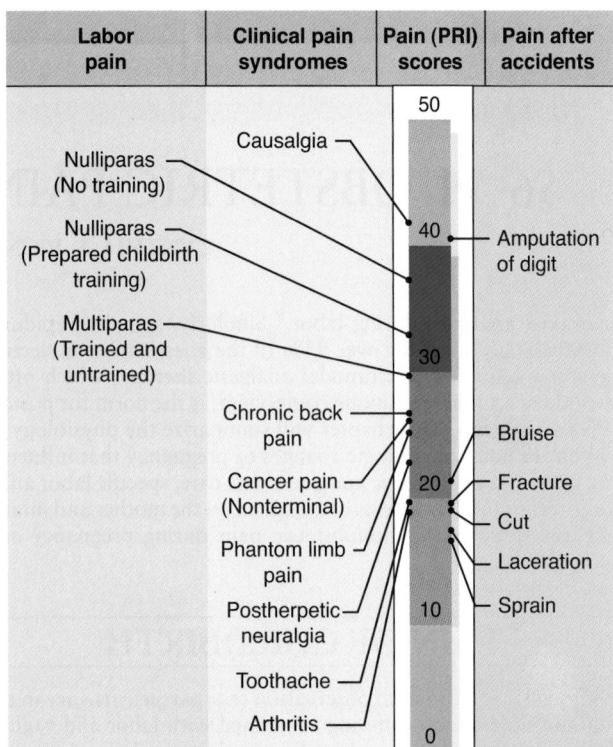

A

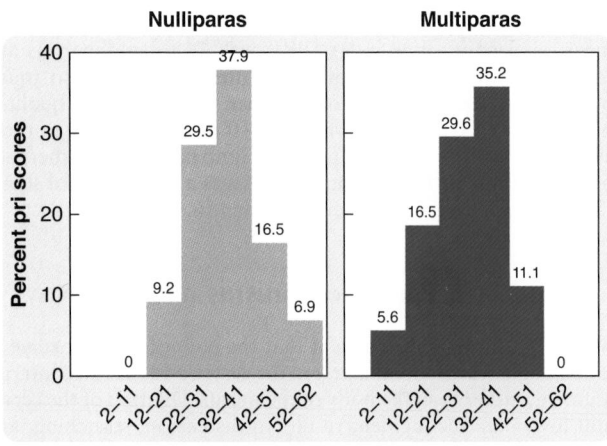

Intervals within the PRI range

B

FIGURE 56.1 **A.** Comparison of pain scores using the McGill Pain Questionnaire obtained from women during labor and from patients in general hospital clinics and an emergency department. The PRI represents the sum of the rank values for all words chosen from 20 sets of pain descriptions. **B.** Distribution of PRI scores from nulliparous and parous women in six intervals of the total PRI range. (Redrawn after Melzack R. The myth of painless childbirth (the John J. Bonica lecture). *Pain* 1984;19(4): 321–337, with permission.)

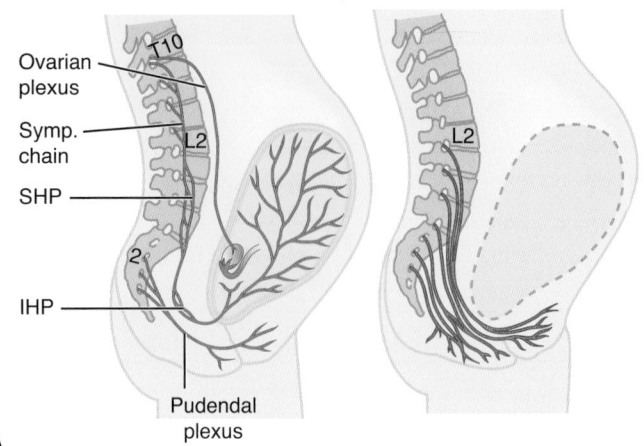

A   B

FIGURE 56.2 Schematic depiction of the peripheral nociceptive pathways involved in the pain of childbirth. **A.** The uterus, including the lower uterine segment and cervix, is supplied by afferents that pass from the uterus to the spinal cord by accompanying sympathetic nerves through the cervical plexus, the superior and inferior hypogastric plexuses (SHP, IHP), the lumbar and lower thoracic sympathetic chain, and to the T11, T12, and L1 nerve roots. The vagina and perineum are supplied by afferents that travel to the spinal cord via the pudendal nerve to the S2 through S4 nerve roots. **B.** The nerves involved in the transmission of nociceptive impulses are provoked by noxious stimulation of pelvic structures.

roots of the lumbosacral plexus. The pain may be severe if the fetus is in an abnormal position.

Visceral C-fibers transmitting pain during the first stage of labor terminate in the spinal cord in a loose network of synapses in the ipsilateral, superficial, and deep dorsal horn and the ventral horn, as well as crossing the midline to the contralateral dorsal horn with extensive rostrocaudal extension.[12] In contrast, somatic afferent fibers tend to terminate in the ipsilateral superficial laminae of the dorsal horn with minimal rostrocaudal fiber extension. This explains the diffuse localization of visceral first stage labor pain compared to somatic second stage labor pain. It may also explain why the neuraxial administration of lipid soluble opioids in early labor provides complete analgesia, as these drugs penetrate deeply into the spinal cord.

Understanding the anatomic basis of the transmission of labor pain underlies the current treatment of labor pain using regional anesthesia techniques. The visceral pain of the first stage of labor can be blocked with bilateral cervical plexus, lumbar sympathetic blocks, or central neuraxial blockade. The somatic pain caused by descent of the fetus in the birth canal can be blocked with bilateral pudendal nerve blocks or neuraxial blockade.

Our current understanding of the neurophysiologic basis of labor pain is superficial at best. Better understanding of the pain pathways, neurotransmitters, and receptors involved in labor pain will open up new avenues for the treatment of labor pain in the future.

Factors That Affect the Pain of Childbirth

In addition to physiologic factors such as intensity, duration, pattern of contractions, and descent of the fetus, the amount or degree of pain and suffering associated with childbirth is influenced by physical, psychologic, emotional, and motivational factors.

Physical factors that are associated with the severity and duration of childbirth pain include age, parity,[13] history of previous pain or dysmenorrhea, fatigue, the condition of the cervix at the onset of labor, and the relationship between the size and position of the fetus to the size of the birth canal. Generally, an older nullipara experiences longer and more painful labor than a

the lumbar sympathetic chain and course cephalad through the lower thoracic sympathetic chain via the rami communicantes of the T10, T11, T12, and L1 spinal segments. Finally, they pass through the dorsal roots of these nerves to make synaptic contact with the interneurons of the dorsal horn.

Typical of pain arising from viscera, the pain of the first stage of labor is often referred to the T10 through L1 dermatomes. Additionally, during the late first stage and second stage of labor, some parturients experience referred pain to the lower lumbar and sacral dermatomes as a result of stimulation of pain-sensitive structures within the pelvic cavity and pressure on one or more

younger nullipara.[10] The cervix of parous women begins to soften even before the onset of labor and is less sensitive than that of the nullipara. The intensity of uterine contractions in early labor tends to be higher in nulliparous compared to parous women, whereas the reverse is true as labor advances. Pain is greater in the presence of dystocia caused by a contracted pelvis, a large baby, or abnormal presentation or position. Women who go on to require cesarean delivery following a period of labor have more breakthrough pain[14] and require more epidural[14] and systemic[15] analgesia during labor than women who deliver vaginally.

Psychologic factors, such as fear, apprehension, and anxiety, also influence the degree of pain and suffering during childbirth.[16] The presence of family members[17] or birthing companions[18] during labor and delivery may decrease anxiety and positively affect the progress of labor. Education, intense motivation, and cultural influences can influence the affective and behavioral dimensions of pain, although they probably minimally affect actual pain sensation. Bonica[19] observed women who had had predelivery training in psychoprophylaxis manifested little or no pain behavior during childbirth, although when questioned the next day, most of them indicated the process had been quite painful. Jewish health providers rated the labor pain of Jewish women higher than that of Bedouin women who were delivering in the same institution,[20] whereas the level of pain assessed by the women themselves was not different.

Effects of Pain on the Mother and Fetus

Labor and vaginal delivery produce tissue damage and, similar to tissue injury from other causes, result in pain and local segmental, suprasegmental, and cortical responses. These responses include marked stimulation of the respiration and circulation, as well as the hypothalamic, autonomic centers of neuroendocrine function, limbic structures, and psychodynamic mechanisms of anxiety and apprehension. These may have a deleterious impact on the mother, fetus, and newborn. Many of these responses are mitigated by effective pain relief.

The pain of childbirth is a powerful respiratory stimulus, resulting in a marked increase in minute ventilation and oxygen consumption during contractions.[21] Compensatory periods of hypoventilation between contractions cause transient maternal hypoxemia and, potentially, fetal hypoxemia (Fig. 56.3). Maternal hyperventilation causes severe respiratory alkalosis and a left shift of the maternal oxyhemoglobin dissociation curve, thus diminishing oxygen transfer to the fetus. The pain and stress of labor activates the sympathetic nervous system, resulting in an increase in plasma catecholamine concentrations, cardiac output and blood pressure (Fig. 56.4). Epinephrine and norepinephrine levels increase by 200% to 600% during unmedicated labor,[22] and this increase is associated with a decrease in uterine blood flow. Pain and anxiety and the accompanying increased catecholamine levels may contribute to prolonged or dysfunctional labor.[23] Epinephrine is a tocolytic, and physicians have long observed that an apparent dysfunctional labor pattern can be corrected with effective analgesia.[24] Finally, unrelieved severe pain can produce serious mental health disturbances that may interfere with maternal–fetal bonding, future sexual relationships, and contribute to postpartum depression,[10] and, rarely, posttraumatic stress disorder.

The healthy parturient easily tolerates the large increase in cardiac work, but parturients with heart disease, severe preeclampsia, or pulmonary hypertension may not tolerate these changes without adverse outcome. Similarly, the healthy fetus tolerates the changes in uterine blood flow; however, these changes may be deleterious in the setting of uteroplacental insufficiency (e.g., preeclampsia, intrauterine growth retardation).

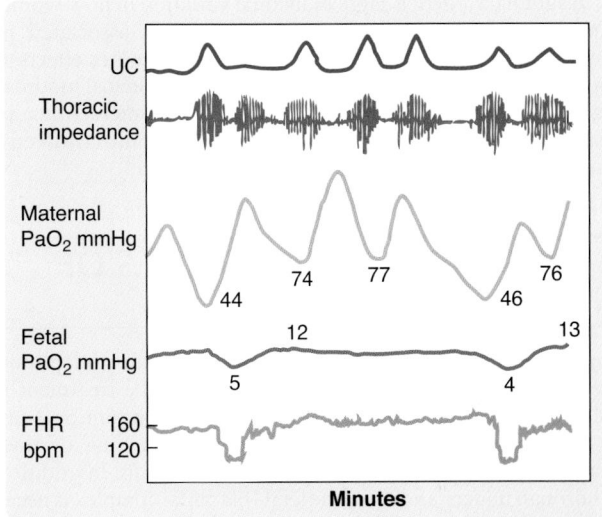

FIGURE 56.3 Continuous recording of uterine contractions (UC), maternal thoracic impedance, maternal transcutaneous oxygen tension (PaO_2), fetal oxygen tension, and fetal heart rate (FHR) in a nullipara breathing room air 120 minutes before spontaneous delivery. Marked hyperventilations during uterine contractions were followed by hypoventilation or apnea between contractions. After the first and fourth contractions, the maternal PaO_2 fell to 44 and 46 mm Hg, with a consequent decrease in fetal PaO_2, and variable decelerations, which reflect fetal hypoxemia. (Redrawn after Huch A, Huch R, Schneider H, et al. Continuous transcutaneous monitoring of fetal oxygen tension during labour. *Br J Obstet Gynaecol* 1977;84[Suppl 1]:1–39.)

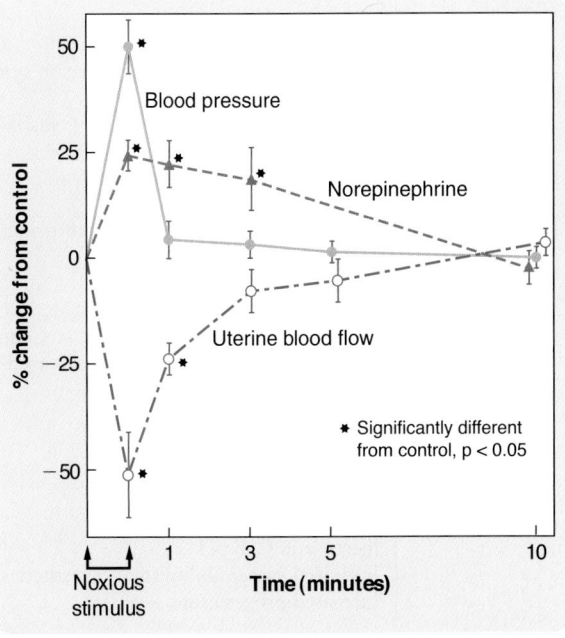

FIGURE 56.4 Effect of noxious stimulus (application of an electric current to the skin) on maternal arterial blood pressure, norepinephrine blood level, and uterine blood flow in a pregnant ewe. The increase in arterial pressure is transient and the decay in norepinephrine level is more protracted and is reflected by a mirror image decrease in uterine blood flow. (Redrawn after Shnider SM, Wright RG, Levinson G, et al. Uterine blood flow and plasma norepinephrine changes during maternal stress in the pregnant ewe. *Anesthesiology* 1979;50(6):524–527, with permission.)

In summary, there is large individual variation in how women experience childbirth pain and suffering. Pain associated responses to noxious stimuli during childbirth are net effects of highly complex interactions of various neural systems, modulating influences, and psychologic factors. These interactions are responsible for the complex physiologic, behavioral, and affective responses that characterize the pain of childbirth.

PHYSIOLOGIC CHANGES OF PREGNANCY

Pregnancy is associated with significant anatomic and physiologic changes. Many of these changes impact the treatment of pain during pregnancy, parturition, and the puerperium. Safe care of these women requires a thorough understanding of these changes and their impact on the treatment of pain. In addition, a thorough understanding of the fetal–placental complex is necessary for the safe care of the fetus and neonate. These changes and their anesthetic implications are summarized in Table 56.1 and discussed below.

Respiratory Changes

Pregnancy is associated with anatomic and physiologic changes involving the airway, lung volumes, ventilation, and the dynamics of breathing. Capillary engorgement, an increase in upper airway soft tissue mass, and enlargement of the breasts contribute to making endotracheal intubation more difficult in pregnant compared to nonpregnant women.[25] Failed intubation and pulmonary aspiration (often associated with difficult airway management) are the most common causes of anesthesia-related maternal mortality.[26] Therefore, in addition to the ability to provide complete analgesia, continuous neuraxial labor analgesia has the added benefit of avoiding the need for general anesthesia and endotracheal intubation should emergency cesarean delivery be required.

Oxygen consumption, carbon dioxide production, and minute ventilation increase during pregnancy.[27] Functional residual capacity (FRC) decreases[28] and closing capacity may exceed FRC in supine pregnant women at term. Obesity, recumbency, and anesthesia (neuraxial or general) further decrease FRC.

During parturition, minute ventilation and oxygen consumption increase markedly, and hyperventilation results in P_aCO_2

TABLE 56.1

PHYSIOLOGIC CHANGES OF PREGNANCY AND ANESTHETIC IMPLICATIONS

Physiologic change	Anesthetic implication
Respiratory	
Increase in O_2 requirement and CO_2 production	Greater risk of desaturation after induction of general anesthesia
Decrease in FRC	Greater risk of desaturation after induction of general anesthesia
Cardiovascular	
Hyperdynamic: increased reliance on sympathetic nervous system	Increase in incidence and severity of hypotension after neuraxial analgesia/anesthesia
Decreased responsiveness to vasoactive agents	Require higher doses of vasopressors to correct hypotension
Aortocaval compression	More profound hypotension with parturient in the supine position
Aortocaval compression and engorgement of azygous veins	Less epidural space and decreased egress of drugs from the epidural space result in lower requirement for epidural drugs
Central nervous system	
Increased lumbar lordosis and decreased thoracic kyphosis	Decreased size of lumbar interspinous space and altered movement of anesthetic agents within CSF
Rotation of pelvis	Tuffier's line more cephalad
Widening of the pelvis	Spine more "head-down" in lateral position
Decrease in CSF volume	Decrease in local anesthetic dose requirements
Decrease in CSF specific gravity	Altered baricity of spinal anesthetic solutions
Increase in CSF pH	Change in proportion of un-ionized drug
Increased susceptibility to all anesthetics	Decrease in anesthetic dose requirements
Increased progesterone levels	Increased pain threshold
Pharmacokinetics	
Altered volume of distribution	Change in drug pharmacokinetics
Altered protein binding of drugs	Change in drug pharmacokinetics
Increased renal blood flow	Change in drug elimination
Altered hepatic microsomal enzyme activity	Change in drug metabolism

values as low as 10 to 15 mm Hg.[29] Maternal aerobic oxygen requirements exceed oxygen consumption resulting in a progressive maternal lactic acidemia.[30]

Cardiovascular Changes

The cardiovascular system is hyperdynamic during pregnancy. Total blood volume increases by approximately 50% during pregnancy,[31] as does cardiac output (Fig. 56.5).[27] Plasma volume increases more than red cell mass, resulting in the physiologic anemia of pregnancy.[31] Organ perfusion is markedly increased, particularly perfusion of the uterus. Systolic blood pressure falls minimally, whereas diastolic pressure decreases by approximately 20%.[27] Both return to prepregnant levels at term. Hemodynamic stability is more highly dependent on sympathetic nervous system activity[32] and arterial responsiveness to vasopressors is reduced.[33]

Aortocaval Compression

At term, compression of the aorta and vena cava by the gravid uterus in the supine position results in decreased right ventricular preload and a 10% to 20% decrease in cardiac output compared to the standing position.[34] Vena cava compression begins as early as 13 to 16 weeks' gestation and is nearly complete at term (Fig. 56.6).[35] Partial aortic compression in the supine position results in decreased blood flow to the pelvis and lower extremities. Aortic compression is completely relieved by the lateral position,[36] whereas partial caval decompression is still present.[35] However, in the lateral position, collateral circulation through the azygous system maintains venous return and cardiac output.[37] The left lateral position is superior to the right lateral position for maintenance of venous return.[38]

During labor, cardiac output increases due to increased central blood volume secondary to autotransfusion during uterine systole and because of increased sympathetic nervous system activity. Due to the adverse effects of aortocaval compression, parameters of fetal well-being deteriorate when parturients labor in the supine compared to lateral position.[39] Adverse effects may be more profound in the parturient with neuraxial blockade induced sympathetic blockade.

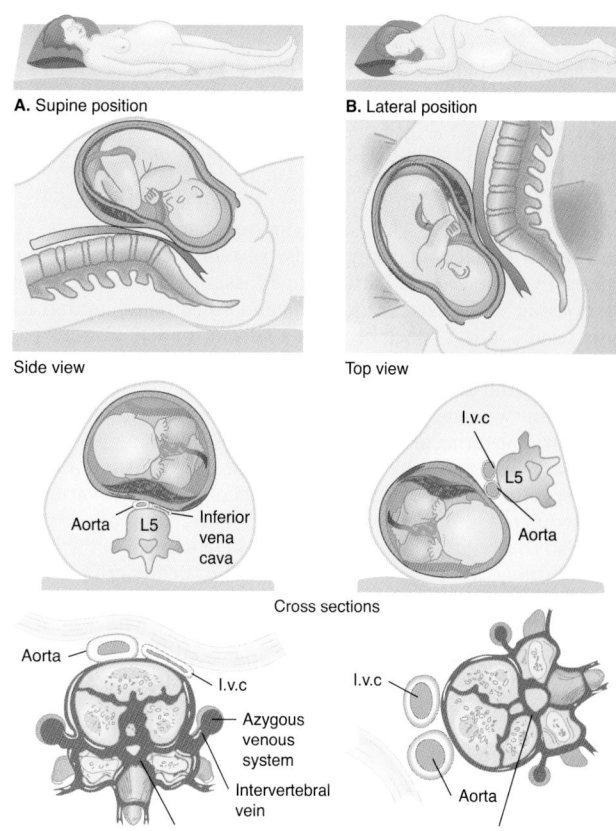

FIGURE 56.6 Effect of the pregnant uterus on the inferior vena case (I.r.c.) and the aorta in the supine position (*left*) and the lateral position (*right*). The marked aortocaval compression in the supine position causes venous blood to be diverted to and through the vertebral venous plexus, which becomes engorged and reduces the size of the epidural and subarachnoid spaces. (Redrawn after Bonica JJ. Obstetric analgesia and anesthesia, 2nd ed. Seattle: University of Washington Press; 1980:8, with permission.)

Implications for Labor Analgesia

Shunting of lower extremity blood through the azygous system results in venous engorgement in the epidural space. This functionally reduces the size of the epidural and subarachnoid spaces, thus reducing the amount of anesthetic necessary to produce neuroblockade. Sympathetic blockade in the term parturient (e.g., as a consequence of neuraxial analgesia/anesthesia) results in a marked decrease in blood pressure compared to nonpregnant control subjects.[40] Pregnant women may require higher doses of vasopressors compared to nonpregnant individuals to treat hypotension.[33]

Central Nervous System Changes

Anatomy of the Spinal Column and Analgesic Implications

Anatomic and physiologic changes in the nervous system alter responses to pain and susceptibility to both general and regional anesthesia. Specifically, anatomic changes in the spinal canal may affect neuraxial anesthesia techniques. The epidural and vertebral foraminal veins are enlarged, resulting in an increased risk of intravascular injection. Additionally, there is decreased nonvascular space in the spinal canal and decreased egress of epidural anesthetic agents from the epidural space. Engorged epidural veins[41] and increases in abdominal pressure[42] are associated with

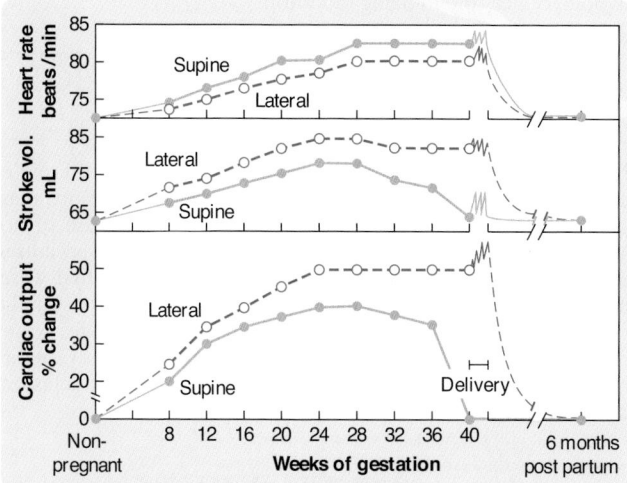

FIGURE 56.5 Changes in heart rate, stroke volume, and cardiac output during pregnancy and in the puerperium. (Redrawn after Bonica JJ. Obstetric analgesia and anesthesia, 2nd ed. Seattle: University of Washington Press; 1980:5, with permission.)

a decrease cerebral lumbosacral cerebral spinal fluid (CSF) volume.

Anatomic changes also occur to the ligamentous and bony structures of the vertebral column. The hormonal changes of pregnancy may cause the ligamentum flavum to feel less dense and "softer" in pregnant women compared to nonpregnant patients; thus, it may be more difficult to feel the passage of the epidural needle through the ligamentum flavum. Progressive accentuation of lumbar lordosis during pregnancy alters the relationship of surface anatomy to the vertebral column. The line joining the iliac crests (Tuffier's line) assumes a more cephalad relationship to the vertebral column and accentuated lumbar lordosis results in less space between adjacent lumbar spinous processes. The apex of the lumbar lordosis is shifted caudad during pregnancy, and the typical thoracic kyphosis in women is reduced in pregnant women.[43] This may influence the spread of hypo- or hyperbaric intrathecal anesthetic solutions in supine patients.

Subarachnoid dose requirements may also be affected by the lower specific gravity of CSF in pregnant compared with nonpregnant women[44] and the higher CSF pH.[45] Widening of the pelvis may lead to a relative head-down position in women in the lateral position; thus, affecting movement of hypo- or hyperbaric anesthetic solutions in the CSF. Because of the gravid uterus, it may be more difficult for a pregnant woman to achieve flexion of the lumbar spine. Finally, labor pain may make it difficult for women to assume and maintain an ideal position while the anesthesiologist initiates neuraxial anesthesia.

Neurohormonal Changes and Analgesic Implications

Pregnancy-induced neurohumoral changes may alter responses to pain. Lower plasma substance P concentrations[46] and higher CSF progesterone levels[47] are found in pregnancy. In a rat model, the pregnancy-associated increased concentration of plasma β-endorphin was associated with an increased tolerance to visceral stimulation and this effect was reversed by naloxone.[48] Pain thresholds are increased during pregnancy[49] and labor.[50] Both peripheral and central nervous tissue from pregnant animals (including human) appears to be more susceptible to many different analgesic and anesthetic agents, including local anesthetics, volatile anesthetic agents, and thiopental. Possible mechanisms of enhanced neural blockade during pregnancy include potentiation of the analgesic effect of endogenous analgesic systems, hormone-related changes in the actions of spinal cord neurotransmitters, increased permeability of the neural sheath, or other pharmacodynamic or pharmacokinetic differences between pregnant and nonpregnant women.[51]

Together, these anatomic and physiologic changes result in a 25% reduction in the segmental dose requirement for spinal anesthesia,[47] and a similar segmental dose reduction for epidural anesthesia.[52]

Pharmacokinetic Changes

Pregnancy alters disposition of drugs by several mechanisms. Volume of distribution may be altered. For example, the elimination half-life of thiopental is markedly prolonged secondary to a large increase in the volume of distribution.[53] Plasma protein concentration decreases, leading to altered drug binding.[54] For example, lidocaine is less protein bound during pregnancy, resulting in a higher free fraction in the blood.[55] Increased renal blood flow and glomerular filtration and altered hepatic microsomal activity change renal and hepatic drug clearance.

Uteroplacental Unit

Blood flow to the uterus increases markedly during pregnancy, from 50 to 100 mL/minute before pregnancy, to 700 to 900 mL/

minute at term. Uterine blood flow (UBF) is directly related to uterine perfusion pressure and indirectly related to uterine vascular resistance.

$$UBF = \frac{uterine\ arterial\ -\ uterine\ venous\ pressure}{uterine\ vascular\ resistance}$$

UBF is not autoregulated; therefore, decreases in uterine arterial pressure (systemic hypotension), increases in venous pressure (caval compression, uterine contraction or increase in uterine tone, Valsalva maneuver), or increases in uterine vascular resistance (increase in uterine vasoconstriction relative to systemic vasoconstriction) result in decreased UBF.

The net effect on UBF of any therapeutic intervention depends on relative changes in systemic and uterine vessels and effect on uterine tone. Labor analgesia may directly and indirectly affect UBF, both positively and negatively. For example, neuraxial analgesia may increase UBF as a result of decreased sympathetic outflow (secondary to both pain relief and direct sympathetic blockade), and decreased maternal hyperventilation. Conversely, neuraxial analgesia-induced maternal hypotension may decrease UBF. Additionally, neuraxial analgesia may be associated with transient uterine hypertonus secondary to an acute decrease in circulating epinephrine levels[56] and loss of its tocolytic effects.[57] Uterine hypertonus may also result from high concentrations of local anesthetic in uterine tissue, for example, after a paracervical block.[58]

Transfer of Drugs Across the Placenta

Most drugs administered to the mother cross the placenta to the fetus to some degree. Placental transfer depends on a number of factors, including plasma drug concentration and electrochemical gradients across the placenta, molecular weight, lipid solubility, degree of ionization, membrane surface area and thickness (changes during pregnancy), maternal and fetal blood flow, placental binding and metabolism, and degree of maternal and fetal protein binding. Direct drug teratogenicity may manifest as death, structural abnormalities, growth restriction, and functional deficiencies. Teratogenic potential is influenced by the timing of exposure, drug dose, duration of exposure, and genetic predisposition.[59] The risk of structural teratogenicity is greatest during the period of organogenesis (day 31 to 71 after the first day of the last menstrual period). Functional or behavioral teratogenicity may result from drug exposure during pregnancy, and even after birth, as the central nervous system continues to develop during this period. Nondrug teratogens include hypoxia, hypercarbia, hyperthermia, hypoglycemia, and ionizing radiation.

NONPHARMACOLOGIC METHODS OF LABOR ANALGESIA

Nonpharmacologic methods to relieve the pain and suffering of childbirth include childbirth education, emotional support, massage, aromatherapy, audiotherapy, and therapeutic use of hot and cold. More specialized techniques that require specialized training or equipment include hydrotherapy, intradermal water injections, biofeedback, transcutaneous electrical nerve stimulation (TENS), acupuncture or acupressure, and hypnosis. Many of these techniques are inadequately studied in that study quality is poor and sample size is small,[60,61] and therefore, conclusions about efficacy are not possible.

Antenatal Childbirth Education

Childbirth education is widely practiced. Unfortunately, studies of childbirth education lack scientific rigor. Study results are inconsistent as to whether participation in childbirth education classes influences outcomes, such as use of analgesia, duration of labor, mode of delivery, and incidence of nonreassuring fetal status.

Labor Support

Emotional support is commonly provided by the parturient's husband or a friend. "Continuous labor support" refers to the nonmedical support of the parturient by a trained person.[61] Prospective, controlled trials and several systematic analyses have concluded that women who receive continuous labor support have shorter labors, fewer operative deliveries, fewer analgesic interventions, and greater satisfaction.[62]

Hydrotherapy

Hydrotherapy is the immersion of the parturient in warm water (deep enough to cover the abdomen) during labor (not birth). Systematic reviews of randomized controlled trials have concluded that women experience less pain and use less analgesia without change in the duration of labor, rate of operative delivery, or neonatal outcome.[63]

Intradermal Water Injections

Intradermal water injection consists of the injection of 0.05 to 0.1 mL of sterile water, using an insulin or tuberculin syringe, at 4 sites on the lower back: over each posterior superior iliac crest, and 1 cm medial/3 cm caudad to these injections (Fig. 56.7). The technique is used to treat back pain during labor. The injections themselves are acutely painful for about 20 to 30 seconds, but as the injection pain fades, so does lower back pain.[61] Randomized controlled trials have found that the technique is effective in reducing severe back pain during labor without any known side effects to the mother and fetus, although the rate of use of other analgesic modalities does not appear different from control groups.[61]

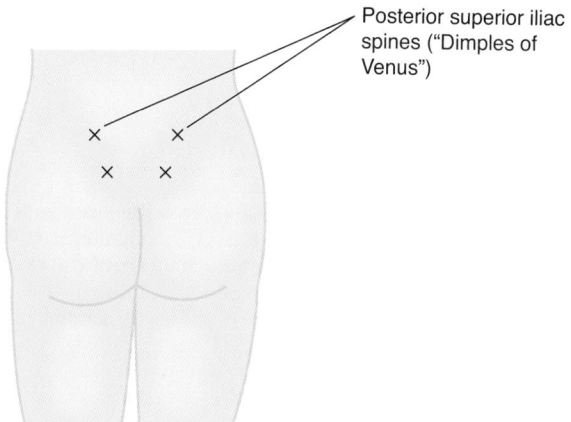

Posterior superior iliac spines ("Dimples of Venus")

FIGURE 56.7 Placement of intradermal water blocks: four intradermal injections of 0.05 to 0.1 mL of sterile water to form four small blebs over each posterior superior iliac spine and 3 cm below and 1 cm medial to each spine. The exact locations of the injections do not appear to be critical to the block success. (Redrawn after Simkin P, Bolding A. Update on nonpharmacologic approaches to relieve labor pain and prevent suffering. *J Midwifery Womens Health* 2004;49(6):489–504, with permission.)

Hypnosis

Self-hypnosis for treatment of childbirth pain has been practiced for several centuries. Hypnosis requires prenatal training of the mother, and sometimes her partner, by a trained hypnotherapist. A meta-analysis of five randomized controlled trials that included 749 women found the use of pharmacologic analgesia methods was decreased in the hypnosis compared to control groups.[64] Data were inconclusive or limited regarding progress of labor and neonatal outcomes.

Transcutaneous Electrical Stimulation

TENS involves the application of low-intensity, high-frequency electrical impulses to the skin of the lower back. The buzzing, electrical current sensation caused by the TENS unit may reduce the mother's awareness of contraction pain. Studies of TENS are inconsistent, but in general, labor pain does not appear to be lessened, nor is the use of other analgesic modalities.[61]

Acupuncture and Acupressure

Acupuncture is a component of traditional Chinese medicine that has gained popularity in Western cultures in recent years. In three randomized controlled trials conducted in Scandinavian countries, women randomized to acupuncture versus control (no or "false" acupuncture) reported modestly lower pain scores and lower use of epidural and systemic opioid analgesia.[65,66] Whether these results can be replicated in other Western societies requires further study.

SYSTEMIC ANALGESIA

Inhalational Analgesia

Inhalation analgesia for labor and vaginal delivery is unusual in the United States, but is more common in other countries. The only inhaled anesthetic agent currently in common use is nitrous oxide. It is available in the United Kingdom as Entonox (The Linde Group, Munich, Germany), a mixture of 50% nitrous oxide and 50% oxygen. Special equipment is required to ensure the safe administration of the drug without contamination of the labor room. The mother must be taught to breathe the mixture correctly, so that peak brain nitrous oxide concentrations coincide with peak contraction pain. Studies are conflicting as to whether nitrous oxide provides benefit to the parturient.[67] The intermittent use of nitrous oxide, however, appears safe for the fetus and neonate, as there is negligible fetal accumulation and neonatal respiration or neurobehavioral scores are not depressed.[68] Concomitant use of nitrous oxide and systemic opioids, however, may increase the risk of maternal hypoxemia.

Volatile halogenated anesthetic agents have been used in the past for labor analgesia. Analgesia, however, is incomplete, as doses that provide significant analgesia are also associated with significant maternal sedation. Theoretically, the newer volatile agents, desflurane and sevoflurane, have an advantage compared to the older agents (e.g., methoxyflurane, halothane), because their lower blood–gas solubility coefficient results in more rapid onset and offset. In a small study, pain relief scores were significantly higher in women who received sevoflurane compared to nitrous oxide, and women preferred sevoflurane.[69] Sedation scores, however, were also higher with sevoflurane, and whether or not volatile agents interfere with the progress of labor (they inhibit uterine contractility) remains to be determined.

Parenteral Opioid Analgesia

Systemic opioid analgesia, administered by the subcutaneous, intramuscular, or intravenous route, is widely used around the world either as the sole analgesic modality or prior to the administration of regional labor analgesia. The use of systemic opioids for labor analgesia lacks rigorous scientific study. There is a high incidence of side effects (e.g., sedation, nausea, and vomiting), and analgesia is incomplete, at best, during active labor. In fact, existing data suggest that opioids provide little significant analgesia.[70,71] Meperidine is the most commonly used systemic opioid; however, there are few studies comparing opioids and little scientific evidence that any one opioid is better than another. All have similar, dose-related, maternal and fetal side effects. Maternal side effects include nausea, vomiting, delayed gastric emptying, dysphoria, and respiratory depression. All opioids cross the placenta. In utero, opioids may result in a slower fetal heart rate and decreased beat-to-beat variability.[72] The likelihood of neonatal respiratory depression depends on the dose and timing of administration.

Patient-Controlled Intravenous Analgesia

Patient-controlled intravenous analgesia (PCIA) has theoretical advantages to nurse-administered opioid analgesia, including superior analgesia with smaller drug doses, resulting in a lower incidence of side effects. PCIA studies have been reported using meperidine, nalbuphine, fentanyl, and more recently, remifentanil with and without a background infusion. Remifentanil has the theoretical advantage of rapid onset and offset compared to the other opioids. Bolus doses have ranged from 0.2 to 1 µg/kg with lock-out intervals from 1 to 5 minutes,[73–76] and infusion rates from 0.025 to 0.1 µg/kg/minute.[75] However, as with other systemic opioid techniques, it is unclear whether remifentanil PCIA can provide satisfactory analgesia without an unacceptably high incidence of side effects.[73,76]

NEURAXIAL ANALGESIA

Neuraxial labor analgesia is the most effective method of pain relief during childbirth and the only method that provides complete analgesia without maternal or fetal sedation. The use of neuraxial analgesia for childbirth has increased dramatically in the United States over the past 40 years.[9] The most common techniques are continuous lumbar epidural analgesia and combined spinal-epidural analgesia. Single-shot spinal, continuous spinal, and caudal analgesia are occasionally used.

Contraindications to neuraxial analgesia and anesthesia include patient refusal, infection at the puncture site, pre-existing coagulopathy, and lack of experienced anesthesia providers. Relative contraindications include hemorrhage or other causes of hypovolemia, untreated systemic infection, preload-dependent disease states, and lumbar spine pathology. The anesthesiologist should weigh the risk and benefits of a neuraxial procedure for each patient independently and the specific neuraxial analgesic technique should be tailored to individual patient needs. The risks and benefits of the procedure should be discussed with each parturient, preferably early in labor. The advantages and disadvantages of specific neuraxial techniques are listed in Table 56.2.

TABLE 56.2

ADVANTAGES AND DISADVANTAGES OF SPECIFIC NEURAXIAL TECHNIQUES FOR LABOR ANALGESIA

	Analgesia technique				
	Continuous epidural	Combined spinal-epidural	Single-shot spinal	Continuous spinal	Caudal
Advantages	• Continuous technique • No dural puncture • Ability to convert to epidural anesthesia	• Rapid onset • Early sacral block • Low dose of anesthetic • Complete early labor analgesia with opioid only†	• Rapid onset • Technically easier • Early sacral block	• Rapid onset • Early sacral block • Low dose of anesthetic • Continuous technique • Ability to convert to spinal anesthesia	• Ability to access epidural space in patient with lumbar epidural pathology
Disadvantages	• Slow onset • Requires greater mass of anesthetic* • Delayed sacral blockade/sacral sparing	• Requires dural puncture • Delayed diagnosis of malfunctioning epidural catheter	• Requires dural puncture • Limited duration of analgesia	• Requires dural puncture with large gauge needle‡ • Potential for accidental intrathecal injection of epidural dose of anesthetic agents	• Requires large volume/mass of anesthetic to block T10 dermatome†‡‡

*Greater vascular absorption of anesthetic agents and greater likelihood for accidental intravascular injection of a toxic amount of local anesthetic.
†Large doses of epidural opioid may provide near complete analgesia for early labor, but at the expense of significant systemic absorption and with accompanying side effects.
‡Increased risk of PDPH.
‡‡May not be able to achieve T4 sensory blockade necessary for cesarean delivery.

Epidural Analgesia

Lumbar epidural analgesia has been the mainstay of regional labor analgesia. Placement of an epidural catheter allows analgesia to be maintained until after delivery. Additionally, it allows conversion to epidural anesthesia should cesarean delivery be necessary. No dural puncture is required. Randomized studies consistently demonstrate that pain scores are lower and patients are more satisfied with epidural analgesia compared to nonneuraxial analgesia.[77,78] Injection of anesthetics in the lumbar epidural space allows spread of the anesthetic solution both cephalad and caudad. Neural blockade to the T10 dermatome is necessary to relieve uterine and cervical pain, whereas blockade of the sacral dermatomes is necessary to block the pain of vaginal and perineal distention.

Compared to spinal analgesic techniques, the onset of epidural analgesia is significantly slower (15–20 minutes compared to 2–5 minutes), particularly the onset of sacral analgesia. It may take several hours of lumbar epidural infusion, or several bolus injections of local anesthetic into the lumbar epidural space, to achieve sacral analgesia. This is particularly disadvantageous in a rapidly laboring parturient who requires rapid onset of sacral analgesia for the late first and second stages of labor. In addition, epidural compared to spinal analgesia requires significantly more drug(s) to attain comparable analgesia, thus increasing the risk of systemic toxicity. Finally, there is significantly more systemic absorption of anesthetic agents, and therefore, maternal and fetal plasma drug concentrations are higher with epidural compared to spinal analgesia.

Lumbar epidural analgesia is initiated in either the sitting or lateral position. The epidural space is identified with a 17- or 18-gauge epidural needle, usually using a loss-of-resistance to air or saline technique. A flexible catheter is passed through the needle approximately 4 to 5 cm into the epidural space, the epidural needle is removed, and the catheter is secured. A test dose is frequently administered to rule out intrathecal or intravascular catheter placement. The most common test dose is lidocaine 15 mg/mL with epinephrine 5 μg/mL, 3 mL. No matter whether a test dose is injected, drugs should be injected incrementally into the epidural space, as no test is 100% sensitive and catheters may migrate during use. Pregnant women are very difficult to resuscitate from local anesthetic cardiac toxicity.

Analgesia is initiated by bolus injection of anesthetic(s) through the epidural needle, catheter, or both. Analgesia is maintained with intermittent bolus injections or a continuous infusion. The catheter is removed after delivery when there is no further need for analgesia/anesthesia.

Drugs for Initiation of Epidural Analgesia

Drugs commonly used for epidural labor analgesia are listed in Table 56.3. Local anesthetics, primarily bupivacaine, have been the mainstay of epidural analgesia for many years. The amount of epidural local anesthetic required for satisfactory analgesia increases as labor progresses.[79] Low bupivacaine concentrations (≤1.25 mg/mL) provide excellent analgesia with minimal motor block. The ED$_{50}$ of bupivacaine 1.25 mg/mL was lower than the ED$_{50}$ of bupivacaine 2.5 mg/mL, suggesting that the use of low concentrations is associated with less overall drug requirement.[80] Bupivacaine is highly protein bound with minimal placental transfer,[81] and duration of analgesia is approximately 2 hours. Onset to peak effect is approximately 20 minutes. Lidocaine and 2-chloroprocaine have shorter latency, but their duration of analgesia is shorter, limiting their usefulness for routine labor analgesia. In addition, lidocaine is less protein bound than bupivacaine and therefore has a higher umbilical vein/maternal vein ratio.[82] Controlled studies, however, have found no difference in neonatal neurobehavioral scores between epidural lidocaine, bupiva-

TABLE 56.3

TYPICAL DRUGS FOR INITIATION OF EPIDURAL LABOR ANALGESIA*

Drug	Concentration	
Local anesthetics†		Dose (Volume)
Bupivacaine	1.00–1.25 mg/mL	10–15 mL
Ropivacaine	1.0–2.0 mg/mL	10–15 mL
Opioids†		Dose (Mass)
Fentanyl	—	50–100 μg
Sufentanil	—	5–10 μg
Adjuvants		
Epinephrine	1.25–5.00 μg/mL	—
Clonidine‡	—	60–75 μg‡‡

*The actual drug dose will depend on the stage of labor (women in advanced labor require higher doses), the progress of labor (women with rapid progress of labor will require higher doses), and whether or not an anesthetic containing test dose has been administered.
†Local anesthetics and opioids are commonly administered together, in which case a lower dose of each is required.
‡Clonidine is not approved for use in obstetric patients in the United States.
‡‡This dose should be combined with local anesthetics, as higher doses used alone cause sedation and hypotension.

caine, and 2-chloroprocaine.[83,84] 2-Chloroprocaine is most useful for rapidly converting epidural *analgesia* to epidural *anesthesia* for urgent operative delivery.

Ropivacaine is a homologue of bupivacaine, formulated as a single levorotatory enantiomer. Its onset and duration of action are similar to bupivacaine,[85] but it has less potential for cardiac toxicity. Although potency studies suggest that ropivacaine is approximately 40% less potent than bupivacaine,[86] clinical studies comparing low concentrations of ropivacaine and bupivacaine for labor analgesia suggest that they are equipotent in terms of sensory blockade for labor analgesia.[87,88] However, ropivacaine may be associated with less motor blockade than equipotent doses of bupivacaine.[89] Levobupivacaine, the S-enantiomer of bupivacaine, is not available in the United States. Similar to ropivacaine and bupivacaine in its onset and duration of action, it is less cardiotoxic than bupivacaine and is associated with less motor blockade compared to bupivacaine.[87,89]

Opioids, particularly the lipid-soluble opioids, fentanyl and sufentanil, are commonly added to local anesthetics for epidural analgesia. Epidural opioids and local anesthetics interact synergistically to provide analgesia.[90,91] The addition of opioids shortens latency, allows for decreased concentration of local anesthetic, thus decreasing motor block, and prolongs analgesia. While epidural opioids alone can provide moderate analgesia for early labor, analgesia is incomplete, and the necessary dose is accompanied by bothersome side effects (e.g., pruritus, nausea, vomiting, maternal sedation, neonatal respiratory depression). Combining local anesthetics with opioids allows for effective analgesia while minimizing the side effects of both drugs.

Fentanyl and sufentanil are ideal for labor analgesia because of their rapid onset (5 to 10 minutes). Their short duration of action (60 to 90 minutes) is overcome by maintaining analgesia with a continuous epidural infusion. Doses commonly used for epidural analgesia initiation and maintenance have been shown to be safe for both the mother and neonate.[92,93] Morphine has a much slower onset (30 to 60 minutes) and longer duration of action (12 to 24 hours) than fentanyl or sufentanil. The long duration of action is not beneficial, as the bothersome side effects of morphine (pruritus, nausea, and vomiting) continue to be present after delivery.

Adjuvants for epidural labor analgesia include epinephrine and clonidine. Epidural epinephrine may contribute to analgesia by decreasing the uptake of local anesthetics and opioids from the epidural space secondary to vasoconstriction,[94] and by binding to spinal cord α_2-adrenergic receptors.[95] Clonidine also binds to α_2-adrenergic receptors and has been shown to supplement epidural labor analgesia. It is not approved for use in obstetric patients in the United States, however, because of the risks of sedation and hypotension.

Combined Spinal-Epidural Analgesia

Combined spinal-epidural (CSE) analgesia has become increasingly popular in the past decade. There are advantages and disadvantages to CSE compared to traditional epidural analgesia (see Table 56.2). Onset of analgesia is significantly faster compared to epidural analgesia.[96] Complete analgesia for early labor can be accomplished with the intrathecal injection of lipid soluble opioids without the addition of local anesthetics, thus avoiding motor blockade and decreasing the risk of hypotension. This is ideal for patients who wish to ambulate, or for those with preload dependent conditions such as stenotic heart lesions. The effective opioid dose is significantly less than for systemic or epidural administration. Therefore, systemic drug absorption is minimal, as are direct fetal effects. The addition of local anesthetic to a lipid soluble opioid results in sacral analgesia within several minutes. This is a decided advantage compared to lumbar epidural analgesia, as sacral analgesia is difficult to accomplish after a single lumbar epidural dose of local anesthetic. Therefore, CSE analgesia provides more complete analgesia for women in advanced stages of labor or women whose labor is progressing rapidly. Finally, use of the CSE technique may decrease the incidence of failed epidural analgesia (e.g., a nonfunctioning epidural catheter).[97,98]

There are several undesirable side effects of CSE analgesia. The incidence of pruritus is higher with intrathecal versus epidural opioids.[99] Dural puncture is required to initiate CSE analgesia. The risk of postdural puncture headache (PDPH) may be minimally higher with the CSE compared to pure epidural technique (estimated excess rate of 3 in 1000).[100] However, a more serious concern is that dural puncture in the obstetric patient may be a risk factor for postpartum neuraxial infection, a rare but potentially life-threatening complication.[101]

Another potential drawback of CSE analgesia is that it will be unclear for 1 to 2 hours after initiation of analgesia as to whether the epidural catheter is properly sited in the epidural space. Therefore, if a functioning epidural catheter is critical to the safe care of the patient (e.g., in the presence of a nonreassuring fetal heart rate pattern or an anticipated difficult airway), then CSE analgesia may not be the technique of choice.

Several techniques for CSE analgesia/anesthesia have been described, including using two skin punctures in two interspaces, two punctures in one interspace, and the needle-through-needle technique.[100] The most common CSE technique for labor analgesia is the needle-through-needle technique in a midlumbar interspinous space. The epidural space is identified with an epidural needle in the standard fashion. The epidural needle then functions as an introducer needle as a long spinal needle is passed through it until the dura is punctured. The intrathecal drug(s) is injected through the spinal needle, the spinal needle is withdrawn, and an epidural catheter is threaded through the epidural needle. Analgesia is maintained via the epidural catheter, as with traditional epidural analgesia.

Drugs for Initiation of Combined Spinal-Epidural Analgesia

CSE labor analgesia is usually initiated with a lipid soluble opioid (fentanyl or sufentanil) or a combination of opioid and local anesthetic (Table 56.4). Morphine is not commonly used because of its long latency and long duration of action (a disadvantage, as women usually deliver before regression of side effects). However, morphine has been successfully combined with intrathecal bupivacaine and fentanyl in order to shorten latency and increase duration of analgesia.[102] This combination of drugs may be particularly useful in settings where continuous epidural infusion techniques are impractical.[102] Meperidine is unique among the opioids in that it has weak local anesthetic properties. However, meperidine was associated with a significantly higher incidence of nausea and vomiting compared to combined fentanyl-bupivacaine.[103]

Intrathecal opioids can provide complete analgesia early in labor when the pain stimuli are primarily visceral. Onset of analgesia occurs within 5 minutes[96] and lasts 70 to 100 minutes.[104] The reported ED_{95} of intrathecal fentanyl varies from 14[105] to 23 μg.[106] The relative potency ratio of intrathecal sufentanil to fentanyl for labor analgesia is 4.4:1.[104] When administered at twice the ED_{50}, the duration of sufentanil analgesia was 25 minutes longer than fentanyl, although the incidence of side effects was not different.[104] The duration of action of intrathecal opioids is dose-related, although fentanyl doses greater than 25 μg do not increase duration of analgesia and are associated with a higher incidence of side effects.[105]

In the late first stage and second stage of labor, local anesthetic must be added to the opioid in order to block somatic stimuli from the vagina and perineum. The local anesthetic works synergistically with the opioid; thus, lower doses of both drugs can be used.[107,108] Bupivacaine is most commonly combined with fentanyl or sufentanil. The ED_{95} of bupivacaine combined with sufentanil 1.5 μg was 3.3 mg,[109] and was 1.66 mg when combined with fentanyl 15 μg.[110] Bupivacaine doses between 1.25 to 2.5 mg are commonly used. Levobupivacaine and ropivacaine are not approved for intrathecal use in the United States. They are less potent than bupivacaine for intrathecal labor analgesia.[109]

Bupivacaine without opioid is not commonly used for labor analgesia. Doses high enough to provide analgesia are associated

---

TABLE 56.4

DRUGS FOR THE INITIATION OF INTRATHECAL LABOR ANALGESIA

Drug(s)*	Opioid dose (μg)	Bupivacaine dose (mg)
Fentanyl	15–25	—
Sufentanil	5–7.5	—
Bupivacaine-fentanyl	10–15	1.25–2.5
Bupivacaine-sufentanil	1–2.5	1.25–2.5
Bupivacaine-fentanyl-morphine†	Fentanyl 12.5–25	2.0–2.5
	Morphine 200–250	

*Opioids alone provide complete analgesia for early labor, but the addition of local anesthetics is required for late first stage and second stage analgesia.
†The combination of bupivacaine-fentanyl-morphine may be advantageous in the settings where continuous epidural infusions for maintenance of analgesia are impractical and single-shot techniques are an alternative.

with significant motor blockade and lower doses either do not provide satisfactory analgesia or are associated with an unacceptably short duration of action.[108]

Maintenance of Epidural Analgesia

Epidural analgesia may be maintained with intermittent bolus injection, continuous epidural infusion, or patient controlled epidural analgesia (PCEA), with or without a background infusion. Continuous epidural infusions result in less need for bolus injections[111,112] and increased patient satisfaction,[113] but higher total drug dose[111,113] compared to intermittent injections. However, the infusion of lower concentration-bupivacaine at a higher rate may result in similar analgesia with less motor block and no increase in total dose.[113,114] Common infusion solutions and protocols are listed in Table 56.5.

PCEA allows for both a continuous epidural infusion and patient-titrated bolus injections. PCEA resulted in greater patient satisfaction[115,116] and a lower average hourly dose of bupivacaine (and therefore less motor block),[116,117] and less need for physician intervention.[117] The protocols for PCEA vary widely, and it is unclear whether this affects analgesia and outcome. At one extreme, most of the hourly dose is administered via a background infusion which the parturient may supplement with self-administered boluses. At the other extreme, there is no background infusion and the entire dose is self-administered via intermittent boluses. Bupivacaine consumption is higher with background infusions compared to a pure PCEA technique without a background infusion.[118] Although data are conflicting as to whether a background infusion improves analgesia, it may be helpful in selected parturients (e.g., nulliparas with long labors).[119] Solutions for PCEA generally mimic those used for continuous infusions (see Table 56.5). The parturient administered bolus dose is 5 to 10 mL, the lock-out interval is 10 to 20 minutes, and the background infusion varies from 0 to 15 mL. Commonly, 30% to 50% of the hourly dose is administered as a background infusion.

The bolus administration of epidural anesthetic solution appears to result in improved analgesia with a lower total drug dose. Investigators have recently demonstrated that timed (automated) intermittent boluses (5 to 10 mL every 30 to 60 minutes) administered via a programmable pump result in improved parturient satisfaction, less drug use, longer duration of analgesia, and less breakthrough pain compared to a continuous infusion of the same mass of drug per unit time.[120–122] There may be better distribution of anesthetic solution within the epidural space when large volumes are injected as a bolus compared to a slow infusion.

TABLE 56.5

DRUG SOLUTIONS FOR MAINTENANCE OF EPIDURAL LABOR ANALGESIA*

Drug solution	Local anesthetic concentration (mg/mL)	Opioid concentration (μg/mL)
Bupivacaine-fentanyl	0.625–1.25	2–4
Bupivacaine-sufentanil	0.625–1.25	0.20–0.33
Ropivacaine-fentanyl	0.8–1.5	2–4
Ropivacaine	2.0	—

*Continuous infusions rate: 10–15 mL/hour. PCEA parameters: PCEA bolus 5–10 mL, lockout interval 10–20 min, background infusion 0–15 mL/hour (commonly 30%–50% of hourly dose requirement).

Other Central Neuraxial Techniques

Single-Shot and Continuous Spinal Analgesia

In general, single-shot spinal analgesia is not useful for most laboring patients because of its limited duration of action. It may be indicated in parturients who require analgesia/analgesia shortly before anticipated delivery or in settings where continuous epidural analgesia is not possible. Drugs for single-shot spinal analgesia mimic those used for the initiation of CSE analgesia (see Table 56.4).

Continuous spinal analgesia is currently not practical for most parturients. The available catheters (essentially epidural catheters) require a large gauge introducer needle and are therefore associated with an unacceptably high incidence of PDPH. However, the placement of a continuous spinal catheter is a management option in patients with inadvertent dural puncture with an epidural needle or when rapid analgesia is necessary in an obese patient. Continuous spinal labor analgesia is commonly maintained with the same solution used for epidural analgesia, but at a rate of 1 to 2 mL/hour.

Caudal Analgesia

Continuous caudal epidural analgesia is used infrequently in the practice of modern obstetric anesthesia. Large volumes of local anesthetic are required for first stage analgesia and result in higher maternal plasma concentrations of drug. There is a risk of needle/catheter misplacement and direct injection into the fetus. However, this technique is an option in patients in whom access to the lumbar spinal canal is not possible (e.g., fused lumbar spine).

Side Effects of Neuraxial Analgesia

Common side effects of neuraxial labor analgesia include hypotension and pruritus. Other side effects include urinary retention, delayed gastric emptying (after opioid techniques, but not pure local anesthetic techniques), oral herpes simplex virus recrudescence, shivering, maternal hyperthermia, and fetal bradycardia.

Hypotension

Blockade of the sympathetic nervous system by local anesthetics causes vasodilation, increased venous capacitance, decreased preload, and decreased cardiac output. Hypotension may result in decreased uteroplacental perfusion and fetal heart rate decelerations or bradycardia. Therefore, maternal blood pressure and fetal heart rate should be monitored for 15 to 30 minutes after the induction of neuroblockade. Although intravenous volume expansion prior to initiating neuraxial analgesia has traditionally been used to reduce the incidence and degree of hypotension, it is not clear that this has any real benefit with modern low-dose neuraxial labor analgesia techniques.[123] The mother should be positioned in the full lateral position after initiation of neuraxial blockade and hypotension should be treated with small bolus doses of intravenous vasopressor.

Pruritus

Pruritus is common side effect of neuraxial opioid administration. It is more common after intrathecal (as high as 100%) compared to epidural administration, and the incidence and severity are dose related.[106,108] The cause is unknown, but it is not thought to be histamine-related. Pruritus may be generalized or localized to the nose, face, or chest and is typically self-limited. Concomitant local anesthetic administration decreased the incidence and severity of pruritus compared to fentanyl alone,[124] whereas the addition of epinephrine worsened the pruritus.[125] The one-time administration of naloxone (40 to 80 µg) or nalbuphine (2.5 to 5 mg) is usually effective for the treatment of pruritus induced by fentanyl or sufentanil. A naloxone infusion may be required for the treatment of morphine-induced pruritus.

Fetal Bradycardia

Fetal bradycardia, not associated with maternal hypotension, occurs after initiation of both epidural and CSE analgesia. Clark and colleagues[57] hypothesized that this may be due to the acute decrease in plasma epinephrine levels following the initiation of neuraxial analgesia.[56] Epinephrine is a tocolytic, and the acute decrease in maternal plasma concentration may result in temporary imbalance of uterine tocolytic/tocodynamic forces, resulting in uterine hypertonus, decreased uterine perfusion, and ultimately, fetal bradycardia. Nitroglycerin has been used successfully to treat uterine hypertonus associated with the initiation of neuraxial analgesia.[126]

Maternal Hyperthermia

Epidural labor analgesia greater than 6 hours is associated with maternal fever.[127,128] The mechanism is unclear, but may be a result of increased heat production (e.g., shivering), decreased heat loss (inhibition of sweating in area of neuroblockade or less heat loss via respiratory tract because of lack of hyperventilation), or alterations in temperature regulation induced by epidural analgesia.

Complications of Neuraxial Analgesia

Complications of neuraxial labor analgesia include inadequate or failed analgesia, inadvertent dural puncture, subdural injection, respiratory depression, high- or total-spinal anesthesia, systemic local anesthetic toxicity, needle or catheter trauma to central nervous system tissue (spinal cord and nerve roots), direct tissue local anesthetic toxicity (cauda equina syndrome, arachnoiditis), pneumocephalus, spinal or epidural hematoma, spinal or epidural abscess, and meningitis.

Inadvertent Dural Puncture

Inadvertent dural puncture with an epidural needle occurs in 1.5% of obstetric patients receiving epidural analgesia or anesthesia, and 52% will develop a PDPH.[129] This is a particularly troublesome complication of epidural analgesia because women are usually quickly mobile after childbirth with the need to care for their newborn infants. A therapeutic epidural blood patch with autologous blood remains the gold standard treatment. Between 34% to 68% of women get complete relief,[130–132] whereas 7% to 16% of women get no relief. The volume of autologous blood that provides the best outcome with fewest side effects is not well studied, but anesthesiologists generally inject between 15 and 20 mL of autologous blood.

Other treatment modalities for the prevention and treatment of PDPH have not proven effective (e.g., epidural saline infusion, caffeine, prophylactic blood patch) or are inadequately studied (placement of an intrathecal catheter).

Respiratory Depression

Severe respiratory depression or arrest has been reported after the intrathecal injection of sufentanil in laboring women.[133] The risk appears to be increased when intrathecal opioids are administered before or after systemic opioids. Respiratory depression is opioid dose-dependent.[106] It generally occurs within 2 hours after the intrathecal administration of fentanyl and sufentanil. In contrast, respiratory depression after epidural and intrathecal morphine usually presents 6 to 12 hours after administration of drug.

OTHER REGIONAL ANALGESIC TECHNIQUES

Neuraxial analgesia is the most effective and flexible analgesic technique for labor and delivery. However, some parturients may not be candidates for neuraxial analgesia or may not want it. Other nerve blocks may provide acceptable, albeit less flexible, analgesia.

Paracervical Block

A paracervical block blocks transmission of visceral afferent nerve impulses from the uterus and cervix through the paracervical (Frankenhäuser's) ganglion. Advantages include excellent analgesia for the first stage of labor, before fetal descent, without somatic sensory or motor block. However, the block is not continuous, and it does not relieve somatic pain caused by distension of the pelvic floor, vagina, or perineum.

Serious maternal complications are unusual; however, serious fetal complications are not uncommon. Inadvertent direct fetal scalp injection can result in fetal systemic local anesthetic toxicity and may be more likely to occur with advanced cervical dilation (>8 cm). Fetal bradycardia is the most common fetal complication. The etiology is unclear. Recommendations to reduce complications include (1) perform the block only in parturients with no evidence of uteroplacental insufficiency, (2) perform the block when the cervix is dilated <8 cm, (3) monitor uterine activity and fetal heart rate continuously, (4) after injecting local anesthetic on one side, wait 5 to 10 minutes before injecting anesthetic on the second side, and (5) consider using 2-chloroprocaine.[134]

Lumbar Sympathetic Block

Paravertebral lumbar sympathetic blockade interferes with transmission of visceral afferent nerve impulses from the uterus and cervix at the level of the L2 to L3 sympathetic chain. Similar to a paracervical block, it provides analgesia for the first stage, but not the second stage of labor. Disadvantages include a technique that is not continuous and that is technically difficult to learn and perform and requires bilateral injections. Advantages include that it is associated with less fetal bradycardia than a paracervical block, it provides first stage analgesia without any motor block, it is useful for patients with previous back surgery,[135] and the progress of labor is accelerated compared to epidural analgesia.[136]

Pudendal Block

A pudendal nerve block interrupts pain signals from vaginal, vulvar, and perineal distension. It provides satisfactory analgesia for spontaneous vaginal and low- or outlet-forceps delivery, but not mid-forceps delivery or exploration of the upper vagina, cervix, or uterine cavities. Bilateral success rate may be as low as 50%.[137] The pudendal nerve can be blocked via the transperineal or transvaginal route. Most obstetricians in the United States employ the transvaginal route immediately before delivery. However, earlier pudendal nerve blocks (just before or after complete cervical dilation) provide better analgesia, do not increase the incidence of instrumental delivery,[138] and allow for a repeat block should the initial block fail.

Maternal and fetal complications of pudendal nerve block are rare. Fetal complications include fetal trauma and/or direct fetal injection of local anesthetic.[139]

Perineal Infiltration

Perineal infiltration is often used immediately before delivery to provide anesthesia for an episiotomy or repair. It provides no motor relaxation. Five to 10 mL of local anesthetic are injected into the posterior fourchette. Perineal infiltration may be complicated by direct injection of local anesthetic into the fetal scalp resulting in neonatal local anesthetic toxicity.[140]

EFFECTS OF ANALGESIA ON THE PROGRESS OF LABOR

There has been much controversy concerning the effect of neuraxial labor analgesia on the progress of labor and mode of delivery. Early investigators noted that regional analgesia appeared to be an effective treatment for dysfunctional labor.[24,141] Observational studies, however, have uniformly found an association between neuraxial analgesia, prolonged labor, and operative delivery. A number of randomized controlled trials have compared neuraxial labor analgesia to systemic opioid analgesia and most found no difference in the rate of cesarean delivery between groups.[142,143] The probable explanation for observed association between epidural analgesia and cesarean delivery is that women who have more pain during labor (and thus more likely to request analgesia) have a higher risk of cesarean delivery.[14,15] Fetal macrosomia, malposition, and dysfunctional labor are associated with more painful labor and a higher rate of cesarean delivery.

Another concern is whether neuraxial analgesia adversely affects the first stage of labor, particularly when administered in the latent phase. Again, observational studies suggest that early labor initiation of neuraxial analgesia is associated with an increased rate of cesarean delivery. Randomized controlled trials, however, uniformly demonstrated that early labor initiation of neuraxial compared to systemic opioid analgesia does not adversely affect the outcome of labor,[77,144,145] and in fact, may result in faster labor.[144,145]

Randomized controlled trials comparing neuraxial to systemic opioid analgesia have assessed the risk of instrumental vaginal delivery and duration of labor as secondary outcomes. Systematic review of these trials have found that the duration of the first stage of labor may be prolonged by approximately 30 minutes, the duration of the second stage of labor may be prolonged by approximately 15 minutes, and the rate of instrumental forceps delivery may be increased.[142,143] Several groups of investigators have demonstrated that neuraxial analgesia with bupivacaine 2.5 mg/mL results in a higher instrumental vaginal delivery rate compared to low dose bupivacaine-opioid techniques.[99,146] Thus, it is the responsibility of the anesthesiologist to use a regional technique that minimizes motor block in order to decrease the risk of instrumental vaginal delivery.

NONOBSTETRIC DRUG THERAPY DURING PREGNANCY AND LACTATION

The management of pain during pregnancy is complicated by the need to limit the transfer of drugs across the placenta, particularly during the first trimester, as well as the necessity of limiting radiation exposure. Key management concepts (Table 56.6) include assessment of risk versus benefit. For example, withholding seizure medications at the risk of recurrent seizures is not sensible. In general, using older drugs with a longer history is advisable, as well as using the minimum effective dose. Drugs with an active metabolite should be avoided if possible, and nerve blocks are preferable to systemic analgesia.

TABLE 56.6

PRINCIPLES OF DRUG ADMINISTRATION DURING PREGNANCY AND LACTATION

Pregnancy
- Assess risk versus benefit
- Consider gestational age of fetus
- Use older drugs
- Use the minimum effective dose
- Avoid drugs with active metabolites
- Consider nerve blocks
- Consider nonpharmacologic therapies
- Use ultrasound and MRI for imaging

Lactation
- Assess risk versus benefit
- Choose the safest drug
- Use minimum effective dose
- Use drugs with no active metabolite
- If drug may present risk to neonate, measure neonatal drug concentration
- Give maternal dose just after feeding
- Consider age of infant (maturity of metabolic pathways)

Most drugs administered to the mother cross into breast milk, although neonatal drug exposure is much smaller than fetal exposure. Principles of drug administration during lactation are listed in Table 56.6. Drugs undergo first pass metabolism in the neonatal gut, and neonatal exposure is generally 1% to 2% of the maternal dose.[147] Determinants of drug transfer to milk and neonatal exposure include maternal plasma concentration, drug pKa (breast milk is slightly acidotic compared to plasma), volume of milk, and the maturity of neonatal drug metabolism and elimination pathways.[148] Hepatic drug-metabolizing enzymes appear to mature at different rates but are generally impaired in the neonate compared to the adult.[148] Glomerular filtration rate does not reach adult values until 2.5 to 5 months of age.

Drug Classification During Pregnancy and Lactation

The United States Food and Drug Administration introduced a 5-category pregnancy drug classification in 1979 (Categories A, B, C, D, X). This classification has some major limitations.[149] There are very few controlled studies in humans in which lack of fetal harm has been demonstrated. Animal studies do not translate well to humans, as teratogenicity is markedly species specific. Therefore, the safety status of most drugs is largely unknown. All new drugs are classified as Category C (either animal studies have revealed adverse effects but no controlled studies in women have been reported, or studies in women and animals are not available), and this does not help the practitioner or patient assess the drug's safety during pregnancy. Several Internet databases offer information on drug use during pregnancy and lactation,[149] as well as a well-known reference book.[59] Some drug companies maintain pregnancy registries for specific drugs.

The American Academy of Pediatrics has categorized drugs in terms of safety to the nursing infant.[150] Most drugs, including most analgesics, are listed as compatible with breastfeeding.

Analgesic Drugs During Pregnancy and Lactation

Acetaminophen is the first line analgesic during pregnancy for the treatment of mild pain. Low-dose aspirin is considered safe; however, higher doses should be avoided as they may be associated with an increased risk for placental abruption and other bleeding problems and fetal gastroschisis.[149] Nonsteroidal anti-inflammatory drugs (NSAIDs) may cause constriction of the ductus arteriosus and may have adverse effects on fetal renal function, leading to oligohydramnios. Therefore, indomethacin and ibuprofen are not recommended for use for more than 2 days beyond the first trimester.[149] Opioids are considered safe during pregnancy, although there is a potential for neonatal abstinence syndrome after delivery.

Acetaminophen is also considered safe for nursing infants, as are NSAIDs. However, aspirin should be used with caution during lactation because of the slow elimination of salicylates by neonates and resultant drug accumulation.[149,150] Opioids are considered safe during lactation.[150] However, meperidine should be avoided, as normeperidine has a markedly prolonged half-life in the newborn[151] and accumulation may result in neurobehavioral depression and seizures.

References

1. Cohen J. Doctor James Young Simpson, Rabbi Abraham De Sola, and Genesis Chapter 3, verse 16. *Obstet Gynecol* 1996;88(5):895–898.
2. Wagenknecht E. *Selected Letters and Journals of Fanny Appleton Longfellow (1817–1861).* New York: Longmans, Green; 1956.
3. Caton D. The history of obstetric anesthesia. In: Chestnut DH, Polly LS, Tsen LC, et al. ed. *Obstetric Anesthesia Principles and Practice.* 4th ed. Philadelphia: Elsevier Mosby; 2009:3–12.
4. von Steinbüchel R. Vorläufige Mitteilung über die Anwendung des Skopolamin-Morphium-Injektionen in der Geburtshilfe. *Zentrallblatt Gyn* 1902;30:1304–1306.
5. Apgar V. A proposal for a new method of evaluation of the newborn infant. *Curr Res Anesth Analg* 1953;32(4):260–267.
6. Koller C. On the use of cocaine for producing anaesthesia on the eye. *Lancet* 1884;2:990–992.
7. Cleland JGP. Paravertebral anesthesia in obstetrics. *Surg Gynecol Obstet* 1933;57:51–62.
8. Hingson RA, Edwards WB. Continuous caudal analgesia: An analysis of the first ten thousand confinements thus managed with the report of the authors' first thousand cases. *JAMA* 1943;123:538–546.
9. Bucklin BA, Hawkins JL, Anderson JR, et al. Obstetric anesthesia workforce survey: twenty-year update. *Anesthesiology* 2005;103(3):645–653.
10. Melzack R. The myth of painless childbirth (the John J. Bonica lecture). *Pain* 1984;19(4):321–337.
11. Bonica JJ. The nature of pain in parturition. *Clin Obstet Gynaecol* 1975;2:499–516.
12. Pan PH, Eisenach JC. The pain of childbirth and its effect on the mother and the fetus. In: Chestnut DH, Polly LS, Tsen LC, et al. ed. *Obstetric Anesthesia. Principles and Practice.* 4th ed. Philadelphia: Elsevier Mosby; 2009:387–403.
13. Sheiner E, Sheiner EK, Shoham-Vardi I. The relationship between parity and labor pain. *Int J Gynaecol Obstet* 1998;63(3):287–288.
14. Hess PE, Pratt SD, Soni AK, et al. An association between severe labor pain and cesarean delivery. *Anesth Analg* 2000;90(4):881–886.
15. Alexander JM, Sharma SK, McIntire DD, et al. Intensity of labor pain and cesarean delivery. *Anesth Analg* 2001;92(6):1524–1528.
16. Lang AJ, Sorrell JT, Rodgers CS, et al. Anxiety sensitivity as a predictor of labor pain. *Eur J Pain* 2006;10(3):263–270.
17. Henneborn WJ, Cogan R. The effect of husband participation on reported pain and probability of medication during labor and birth. *J Psychosom Res* 1975;19(3):215–222.
18. Kennell J, Klaus M, McGrath S, et al. Continuous emotional support during labor in a US hospital. A randomized controlled trial. *JAMA* 1991;265(17):2197–2201.
19. Bonica JJ. *Principles and Practice of Obstetric Analgesia and Anesthesia.* Philadelphia: FA Davis; 1969.
20. Sheiner EK, Sheiner E, Shoham-Vardi I, et al. Ethnic differences influence care giver's estimates of pain during labour. *Pain* 1999;81(3):299–305.
21. Bonica JJ. Maternal respiratory changes during pregnancy and parturition. In: Marx GF, ed. *Parturition and Perinatology.* Philadelphia: FA Davis; 1973:1–19.
22. Shnider SM, Wright RG, Levinson G, et al. Uterine blood flow and plasma norepinephrine changes during maternal stress in the pregnant ewe. *Anesthesiology* 1979;50(6):524–527.
23. Lederman RP, Lederman E, Work B Jr, et al. Anxiety and epinephrine in multiparous labor: Relationship to duration of labor and fetal heart rate pattern. *Am J Obstet Gynecol* 1985;153(8):870–877.
24. Moir DD, Willocks J. Management of incoordinate uterine action under continuous epidural analgesia. *Br Med J* 1967;3(5562):396–400.
25. Samsoon GLT, Young JR. Difficult tracheal intubation: a retrospective study. *Anaesthesia* 1987;42(5):487–490.
26. Hawkins JL, Koonin LM, Palmer SK, et al. Anesthesia-related deaths during obstetric delivery in the United States, 1979–1990. *Anesthesiology* 1997;86(2):277–284.
27. Spätling L, Fallenstein F, Huch A, et al. The variability of cardiopulmonary adaptation to pregnancy at rest and during exercise. *Br J Obstet Gynaecol* 1992;99(suppl 8):1–40.
28. Alaily AB, Carrol KB. Pulmonary ventilation in pregnancy. *Br J Obstet Gynaecol* 1978;85(7):518–524.
29. Hägerdal M, Morgan CW, Sumner AE, et al. Minute ventilation and oxygen consumption during labor with epidural analgesia. *Anesthesiology* 1983;59(5):425–427.
30. Jouppila R, Hollmén A. The effect of segmental epidural analgesia on maternal and foetal acid-base balance, lactate, serum potassium and creatine phosphokinase during labour. *Acta Anaesth Scand* 1976;20(3):259–268.
31. Lund CJ, Donovan JC. Blood volume during pregnancy. Significance of plasma and red cell volumes. *Am J Obstet Gynecol* 1967;98(3):394–403.
32. Kuo CD, Chen GY, Yang MJ, et al. Biphasic changes in autonomic nervous activity during pregnancy. *Br J Anaesth* 2000;84(3):323–329.
33. Annibale DJ, Rosenfeld CR, Kamm KE. Alterations in vascular smooth muscle contractility during ovine pregnancy. *Am J Physiol* 1989;256(5 Pt 2):H1282–H1288.
34. Clark SL, Cotton DB, Pivarnik JM, et al. Position change and central hemodynamic profile during normal third-trimester pregnancy and post partum. *Am J Obstet Gynecol* 1991;164(3):883–887.
35. Kerr MG, Scott DB, Samuel E. Studies of the inferior vena cava in late pregnancy. *Br Med J* 1964;1(5382):532–533.
36. Abitbol MM. Aortic compression by pregnant uterus. *N Y State J Med* 1976;76(9):1470–1475.
37. Clark SL, Cotton DB, Lee W, et al. Central hemodynamic assessment of normal term pregnancy. *Am J Obstet Gynecol* 1989;161(6 Pt 1):1439–1442.
38. Kuo CD, Chen GY, Yang MJ, et al. The effect of position on autonomic nervous activity in late pregnancy. *Anaesthesia* 1997;52(12):1161–1165.
39. Abitbol MM. Supine position in labor and associated fetal heart rate changes. *Obstet Gynecol* 1985;65(4):481–486.
40. Assali NS, Prystowsky H. Studies on autonomic blockade. I. Comparison between the effects of tetraethylammonium chloride (TEAC) and high selective spinal anesthesia on blood pressure of normal and toxemic pregnancy. *J Clin Invest* 1950;29(10):1354–1366.
41. Hirabayashi Y, Shimizu R, Fukada H, et al. Soft tissue anatomy within the vertebral canal in pregnant women. *Br J Anaesth* 1996;77(2):153–156.
42. Hogan QH, Prost R, Kulier A, et al. Magnetic resonance imaging of cerebrospinal fluid volume and the influence of body habitus and abdominal pressure. *Anesthesiology* 1996;84(6):1341–1349.
43. Hirabayashi Y, Shimizu R, Fukuda H, et al. Anatomical configuration of the spinal column in the supine position. II. Comparison of pregnant and non-pregnant women. *Br J Anaesth* 1995;75(1):6–8.
44. Richardson MG, Wissler RN. Density of lumbar cerebrospinal fluid in pregnant and nonpregnant humans. *Anesthesiology* 1996;85(2):326–330.
45. Hirabayashi Y, Shimizu R, Saitoh K, et al. Acid-base state of cerebrospinal fluid during pregnancy and its effect on spread of spinal anaesthesia. *Br J Anaesth* 1996;77(3):352–355.
46. Dalby PL, Ramanathan S, Rudy TE, et al. Plasma and saliva substance P levels: the effects of acute pain in pregnant and non-pregnant women. *Pain* 1997;69(3):263–267.
47. Datta S, Hurley RJ, Naulty JS, et al. Plasma and cerebrospinal fluid progesterone concentrations in pregnant and nonpregnant women. *Anesth Analg* 1986;65(9):950–954.
48. Iwasaki H, Collins JG, Saito Y, et al. Naloxone-sensitive, pregnancy-induced changes in behavioral responses to colorectal distention: pregnancy-induced analgesia to visceral stimulation. *Anesthesiology* 1991;74(5):927–933.
49. Gintzler AR, Liu NJ. The maternal spinal cord: biochemical and physiological correlates of steroid-activated antinociceptive processes. *Prog Brain Res* 2001;133:83–97.
50. Ohel I, Walfisch A, Shitenberg D, et al. A rise in pain threshold during labor: a prospective clinical trial. *Pain* 2007;132(suppl 1):S104–S108.
51. Lauretti GR. Mechanisms of labor pain. In: Norris MC, ed. *Obstetric Anesthesia.* 2nd ed. Philadelphia: Lippincott Williams & Wilkins; 1999:235–249.
52. Bromage PR. Spread of analgesic solutions in the epidural space and their site of action: a statistical study. *Br J Anaesth* 1962;34:161–178.
53. Morgan DJ, Blackman GL, Paull JD, et al. Pharmacokinetics and plasma binding of thiopental. II. Studies at cesarean section. *Anesthesiology* 1981;54(6):474–480.
54. Wood M, Wood AJJ. Changes in plasma drug binding and alpha1-acid glycoprotein in mother and newborn infant. *Clin Pharmacol Ther* 1981;29(4):522–526.
55. Fragneto RY, Bader AM, Rosinia F, et al. Measurements of protein binding of lidocaine throughout pregnancy. *Anesth Analg* 1994;79(2):295–297.
56. Shnider SM, Abboud T, Artal R, et al. Maternal catecholamines decrease during labor after lumbar epidural anesthesia. *Am J Obstet Gynecol* 1983;147(1):13–15.
57. Clark VT, Smiley RM, Finster M. Uterine hyperactivity after intrathecal injection of fentanyl for analgesia during labor: a cause of fetal bradycardia? *Anesthesiology* 1994;81(4):1083.
58. Fishburne JI, Greiss FC, Hopkinson R, et al. Responses of the gravid uterine vasculature to arterial levels of local anesthetic agents. *Am J Obstet Gynecol* 1979;133(7):753–761.

59. Briggs GG, Freeman RK, Yaffe SJ. *Drugs in Pregnancy and Lactation.* 7th ed. Philadelphia: Lippincott Williams & Wilkins; 2005.

60. Huntley AL, Coon JT, Ernst E. Complementary and alternative medicine for labor pain: a systematic review. *Am J Obstet Gynecol* 2004;191(1):36–44.

61. Simkin P, Bolding A. Update on nonpharmacologic approaches to relieve labor pain and prevent suffering. *J Midwifery Womens Health* 2004;49(6):489–504.

62. Hodnett ED, Gates S, Hofmeyr GJ, et al. Continuous support for women during childbirth. *Cochrane Database Syst Rev* 2007;3:CD003766.

63. Cluett ER, Nikodem VC, McCandlish RE, et al. Immersion in water in pregnancy, labour and birth. *Cochrane Database Syst Rev* 2004;2:CD000111.

64. Smith CA, Collins CT, Cyna AM, et al. Complementary and alternative therapies for pain management in labour. *Cochrane Database Syst Rev* 2006;4:CD003521.

65. Skilnand E, Fossen D, Heiberg E. Acupuncture in the management of pain in labor. *Acta Obstet Gynecol Scand* 2002;81(10):943–948.

66. Ramnerö A, Hanson U, Kihlgren M. Acupuncture treatment during labour–a randomised controlled trial. *BJOG* 2002;109(6):637–644.

67. Clyburn P. The use of Entonox for labour pain should be abandoned. *Int J Obstet Anesth* 2001;10(1):27–29.

68. Stefani SJ, Hughes SC, Shnider SM, et al. Neonatal neurobehavioral effects of inhalation analgesia for vaginal delivery. *Anesthesiology* 1982;56(5):351–355.

69. Yeo ST, Holdcroft A, Yentis SM, et al. Analgesia with sevoflurane during labour: ii. Sevoflurane compared with Entonox for labour analgesia. *Br J Anaesth* 2007;98(1):110–115.

70. Bricker L, Lavender T. Parenteral opioids for labor pain relief: a systematic review. *Am J Obstet Gynecol* 2002;186(5 Suppl Nature):S94–S109.

71. Nelson KE, Eisenach JC. Intravenous butorphanol, meperidine, and their combination relieve pain and distress in women in labor. *Anesthesiology* 2005;102(5):1008–1013.

72. Hill JB, Alexander JM, Sharma SK, et al. A comparison of the effects of epidural and meperidine analgesia during labor on fetal heart rate. *Obstet Gynecol* 2003;102(2):333–337.

73. Olufolabi AJ, Booth JV, Wakeling HG, et al. A preliminary investigation of remifentanil as a labor analgesic. *Anesth Analg* 2000;91(3):606–608.

74. Blair JM, Dobson GT, Hill DA, et al. Patient controlled analgesia for labour: a comparison of remifentanil with pethidine. *Anaesthesia* 2005;60(1):22–27.

75. Balki M, Kasodekar S, Dhumne S, et al. Remifentanil patient-controlled analgesia for labour: optimizing drug delivery regimens. *Can J Anaesth* 2007;54(8):626–633.

76. Volmanen P, Akural EI, Raudaskoski T, et al. Remifentanil in obstetric analgesia: a dose-finding study. *Anesth Analg* 2002;94(4):913–917.

77. Chestnut DH, Vincent RD Jr, McGrath JM, et al. Does early administration of epidural analgesia affect obstetric outcome in nulliparous women who are receiving intravenous oxytocin? *Anesthesiology* 1994;80(6):1193–1200.

78. Ramin SM, Gambling DR, Lucas MJ, et al. Randomized trial of epidural versus intravenous analgesia during labor. *Obstet Gynecol* 1995;86(5):783–789.

79. Capogna G, Celleno D, Lyons G, et al. Minimum local analgesia concentration of extradural bupivacaine increases with progression of labor. *Br J Anaesth* 1998;80(1):11–13.

80. Lyons GR, Kocarev MG, Wilson RC, et al. A comparison of minimum local anesthetic volumes and doses of epidural bupivacaine (0.125% w/v and 0.25% w/v) for analgesia in labor. *Anesth Analg* 2007;104(2):412–415.

81. Belfrage P, Berlin A, Raabe N, et al. Lumbar epidural analgesia with bupivacaine in labor. Drug concentration in maternal and neonatal blood at birth and during the first day of life. *Am J Obstet Gynecol* 1975;123(8):839–844.

82. Kennedy RL, Bell JU, Miller RP, et al. Uptake and distribution of lidocaine in fetal lambs. *Anesthesiology* 1990;72(3):483–489.

83. Kuhnert BR, Harrison MJ, Linn PL, et al. Effects of maternal epidural anesthesia on neonatal behavior. *Anesth Analg* 1984;63(3):301–308.

84. Abboud TK, Kim KC, Noueihed R, et al. Epidural bupivacaine, chloroprocaine, or lidocaine for cesarean section—maternal and neonatal effects. *Anesth Analg* 1983;62:914–919.

85. Katz JA, Bridenbaugh PO, Knarr DC, et al. Pharmacodynamics and pharmacokinetics of epidural ropivacaine in humans. *Anesth Analg* 1990;70(1):16–21.

86. Polley LS, Columb MO, Naughton NN, et al. Relative analgesic potencies of ropivacaine and bupivacaine for epidural analgesia in labor: implications for therapeutic indexes. *Anesthesiology* 1999;90(4):944–950.

87. Beilin Y, Guinn NR, Bernstein HH, et al. Local anesthetics and mode of delivery: bupivacaine versus ropivacaine versus levobupivacaine. *Anesth Analg* 2007;105(3):756–763.

88. Lee BB, Ngan Kee WD, Ng FF, et al. Epidural infusions of ropivacaine and bupivacaine for labor analgesia: a randomized, double-blind study of obstetric outcome. *Anesth Analg* 2004;98(4):1145–1152.

89. Lacassie HJ, Habib AS, Lacassie HP, et al. Motor blocking minimum local anesthetic concentrations of bupivacaine, levobupivacaine, and ropivacaine in labor. *Reg Anesth Pain Med* 2007;32(4):323–329.

90. Vercauteren M, Meert TF. Isobolographic analysis of the interaction between epidural sufentanil and bupivacaine in rats. *Pharmacol Biochem Behav* 1997;58(1):237–242.

91. Polley LS, Columb MO, Wagner DS, et al. Dose-dependent reduction of the minimum local analgesic concentration of bupivacaine by sufentanil for epidural analgesia in labor. *Anesthesiology* 1998;89(3):626–632.

92. Bader AM, Fragneto R, Terui K, et al. Maternal and neonatal fentanyl and

93. bupivacaine concentration after epidural infusion during labor. *Anesth Analg* 1995;81:829–832.

93. Porter JS, Bonello E, Reynolds F. The effect of epidural opioids on maternal oxygenation during labour and delivery. *Anaesthesia* 1996;51(10):899–903.

94. Salinas FV. Pharmacology of drugs used for spinal and epidural anesthesia and analgesia. In: Wong CA, ed. *Spinal and Epidural Anesthesia.* New York: McGraw-Hill; 2006:76–109.

95. Curatolo M, Petersen-Felix S, Arendt-Nielsen L, et al. Epidural epinephrine and clonidine: segmental analgesia and effects on different pain modalities. *Anesthesiology* 1997;87(4):785–794.

96. D'Angelo RD, Anderson MT, Phillip J, et al. Intrathecal sufentanil compared to epidural bupivacaine for labor analgesia. *Anesthesiology* 1994;80(6):1209–1215.

97. Pan PH, Bogard TD, Owen MD. Incidence and characteristics of failures in obstetric neuraxial analgesia and anesthesia: a retrospective analysis of 19,259 deliveries. *Int J Obstet Anesth* 2004;13(4):227–233.

98. Norris MC. Are combined spinal-epidural catheters reliable? *Int J Obstet Anesth* 2000;9(1):3–6.

99. Nageotte MP, Larson D, Rumney PJ, et al. Epidural analgesia compared with combined spinal-epidural analgesia during labor in nulliparous women. *N Engl J Med* 1997;337(24):1715–1719.

100. Cook TM. Combined spinal-epidural techniques. *Anaesthesia* 2000;55(1):42–64.

101. Reynolds F. Infection as a complication of neuraxial blockade. *Int J Obstet Anesth* 2005;14(3):183–188.

102. Minty RG, Kelly L, Minty A, et al. Single-dose intrathecal analgesia to control labour pain: is it a useful alternative to epidural analgesia? *Can Fam Physician* 2007;53(3):437–442.

103. Booth JV, Lindsay DR, Olufolabi AJ, et al. Subarachnoid meperidine (Pethidine) causes significant nausea and vomiting during labor. The Duke Women's Anesthesia Research Group. *Anesthesiology* 2000;93(2):418–421.

104. Nelson KE, Rauch T, Terebuh V, et al. A comparison of intrathecal fentanyl and sufentanil for labor analgesia. *Anesthesiology* 2002;96(5):1070–1073.

105. Palmer CM, Cork RC, Hays R, et al. The dose-response relation of intrathecal fentanyl for labor analgesia. *Anesthesiology* 1998;88(2):355–361.

106. Herman NL, Choi KC, Affleck PJ, et al. Analgesia, pruritus, and ventilation exhibit a dose-response relationship in parturients receiving intrathecal fentanyl during labor. *Anesth Analg* 1999;89(2):378–383.

107. Stocks GM, Hallworth SP, Fernando R, et al. Minimum local analgesic dose of intrathecal bupivacaine in labor and the effect of intrathecal fentanyl. *Anesthesiology* 2001;94(4):593–598.

108. Wong CA, Scavone BM, Loffredi M, et al. The dose-response of intrathecal sufentanil added to bupivacaine for labor analgesia. *Anesthesiology* 2000;92(6):1553–1558.

109. Van de Velde M, Dreelinck R, Dubois J, et al. Determination of the full dose-response relation of intrathecal bupivacaine, levobupivacaine, and ropivacaine, combined with sufentanil, for labor analgesia. *Anesthesiology* 2007;106(1):149–156.

110. Whitty R, Goldszmidt E, Parkes RK, et al. Determination of the ED95 for intrathecal plain bupivacaine combined with fentanyl in active labor. *Int J Obstet Anesth* 2007;16(4):341–345.

111. Bogod DG, Rosen M, Rees GA. Extradural infusion of 0.125% bupivacaine at 10 ml h-1 to women during labor. *Br J Anaesth* 1987;59(3):325–330.

112. Lamont RF, Pinney D, Rodgers P, et al. Continuous versus intermittent epidural analgesia. A randomised trial to observe obstetric outcome. *Anaesthesia* 1989;44(11):893–896.

113. Hicks JA, Jenkins JG, Newton MC, et al. Continuous epidural infusion of 0.075% bupivacaine for pain relief in labour. A comparison with intermittent top-ups of 0.5% bupivacaine. *Anaesthesia* 1988;43(4):289–292.

114. Ewen A, McLeod DD, MacLeod DM, et al. Continuous infusion epidural analgesia in obstetrics. A comparison of 0.08% and 0.25% bupivacaine. *Anaesthesia* 1986;41(2):143–147.

115. Gambling DR, McMorland GJ, Yu P, et al. Comparison of patient-controlled epidural analgesia and conventional intermittent "top-up" injections during labor. *Anesth Analg* 1990;70(3):256–261.

116. Curry PD, Pacsoo C, Heap DG. Patient-controlled epidural analgesia in obstetric anaesthetic practice. *Pain* 1994;57(1):125–128.

117. van der Vyver M, Halpern S, Joseph G. Patient-controlled epidural analgesia versus continuous infusion for labour analgesia: a meta-analysis. *Br J Anaesth* 2002;89(3):459–465.

118. Vallejo MC, Ramesh V, Phelps AL, et al. Epidural labor analgesia: continuous infusion versus patient-controlled epidural analgesia with background infusion versus without a background infusion. *J Pain* 2007;8(12):970–975.

119. Halpern S. Recent advances in patient-controlled epidural analgesia for labour. *Curr Opin Anaesthesiol* 2005;18(3):247–251.

120. Wong CA, Ratliff JT, Sullivan JT, et al. A randomized comparison of programmed intermittent epidural bolus with continuous epidural infusion for labor analgesia. *Anesth Analg* 2006;102(3):904–909.

121. Lim Y, Sia AT, Ocampo C. Automated regular boluses for epidural analgesia: a comparison with continuous infusion. *Int J Obstet Anesth* 2005;14(4):305–309.

122. Fettes PD, Moore CS, Whiteside JB, et al. Intermittent versus continuous administration of epidural ropivacaine with fentanyl for analgesia during labour. *Br J Anaesth* 2006;97(3):359–364.

123. Hofmeyr G, Cyna A, Middleton P. Prophylactic intravenous preloading for regional analgesia in labour. *Cochrane Database Syst Rev* 2004;4:CD000175.

124. Asokumar B, Newman LM, McCarthy RJ, et al. Intrathecal bupivacaine

reduces pruritus and prolongs duration of fentanyl analgesia during labor: a prospective, randomized controlled trial. *Anesth Analg* 1998;87(6): 1309–1315.

125. Douglas MJ, Kim JH, Ross PL, et al. The effect of epinephrine in local anaesthetic on epidural morphine-induced pruritus. *Can Anaesth Soc J* 1986;33(6): 737–740.

126. Mercier FJ, Dounas M, Bouaziz H, et al. Intravenous nitroglycerine to relieve intrapartum fetal distress related to uterine hyperactivity: a prospective observational study. *Anesth Analg* 1997;84(5):1117–1120.

127. Camann WR, Hortvet LA, Hughes N, et al. Maternal temperature regulation during extradural analgesia for labour. *Br J Anaesth* 1991;67(5):565–568.

128. Lieberman E, Lang JM, Frigoletto F Jr, et al. Epidural analgesia, intrapartum fever, and neonatal sepsis evaluation. *Pediatrics* 1997;99(3):415–419.

129. Choi PT, Galinski SE, Takeuchi L, et al. PDPH is a common complication of neuraxial blockade in parturients: a meta-analysis of obstetrical studies. *Can J Anaesth* 2003;50(5):460–469.

130. Stride PC, Cooper GM. Dural taps revisited. A 20-year survey from Birmingham Maternity Hospital. *Anaesthesia* 1993;48(3):247–255.

131. Williams EJ, Beaulieu P, Fawcett WJ, et al. Efficacy of epidural blood patch in the obstetric population. *Int J Obstet Anesth* 1999;8(2):105–109.

132. Banks S, Paech M, Gurrin L. An audit of epidural blood patch after accidental dural puncture with a Tuohy needle in obstetric patients. *Int J Obstet Anesth* 2001;10(3):172–176.

133. Hughes SC. Respiratory depression following intraspinal narcotics: expect it! *Int J Obstet Anesth* 1997;6(3):145–146.

134. Chestnut DH. Alternative regional anesthetic techniques: Paracervical block, lumbar sympathetic block, pudendal block, and perineal infiltration. In: Chestnut DH, Polly LS, Tsen LC, et al. ed. *Obstetric Anesthesia. Principles and Practice.* 4th ed. Philadelphia: Elsevier Mosby; 2009:493–503.

135. Suelto MD, Shaw DB. Labor analgesia with paravertebral lumbar sympathetic block. *Reg Anesth Pain Med* 1999;24(2):179–181.

136. Leighton BL, Halpern SH, Wilson DB. Lumbar sympathetic blocks speed early and second stage induced labor in nulliparous women. *Anesthesiology* 1999; 90(4):1039–1046.

137. Scudamore JH, Yates MJ. Pudendal block—a misnomer? *Lancet* 1966; 1(7427):23–24.

138. Zador G, Lindmark G, Nilsson BA. Pudendal block in normal vaginal deliveries. Clinical efficacy, lidocaine concentrations in maternal and foetal blood, foetal and maternal acid-base values and influence on uterine activity. *Acta Obstet Gynecol Scand Suppl* 1974;1974:34:51–64.

139. Chase D, Brady JP. Ventricular tachycardia in a neonate with mepivacaine toxicity. *J Pediatr* 1977;90(1):127–129.

140. De Praeter C, Vanhaesebrouch P, De Praeter N, et al. Episiotomy and neonatal lidocaine intoxication. *Eur J Pediatr* 1991;150(9):685–686.

141. Climie CR. The place of continuous lumbar epidural analgesia in the management of abnormally prolonged labour. *Med J Aust* 1964;2:447–450.

142. Leighton BL, Halpern SH. The effects of epidural analgesia on labor, maternal, and neonatal outcomes: a systematic review. *Am J Obstet Gynecol* 2002; 186(5 Suppl Nature):S69–S77.

143. Sharma SK, McIntire DD, Wiley J, et al. Labor analgesia and cesarean delivery: an individual patient meta-analysis of nulliparous women. *Anesthesiology* 2004;100(1):142–148; discussion 6A.

144. Wong CA, Scavone BM, Peaceman AM, et al. The risk of cesarean delivery with neuraxial analgesia given early versus late in labor. *N Engl J Med* 2005; 352(7):655–665.

145. Ohel G, Gonen R, Vaida S, et al. Early versus late initiation of epidural analgesia in labor: does it increase the risk of cesarean section? A randomized trial. *Am J Obstet Gynecol* 2006;194(3):600–605.

146. Comparative Obstetric Mobile Epidural Trial (COMET) Study Group UK. Effect of low-dose mobile versus traditional epidural techniques on mode of delivery: a randomised controlled trial. *Lancet* 2001;358(9275):19–23.

147. Berlin CM, Briggs GG. Drugs and chemicals in human milk. *Semin Fetal Neonatal Med* 2005;10(2):149–159.

148. Spigset O, Hägg S. Analgesics and breast-feeding: safety considerations. *Paediatr Drugs* 2000;2(3):223–238.

149. Hansen WF, Peacock AE, Yankowitz J. Safe prescribing practices in pregnancy and lactation. *J Midwifery Womens Health* 2002;47(6):409–421.

150. American Academy of Pediatrics Committee on Drugs. Transfer of drugs and other chemicals into human milk. *Pediatrics* 2001;108(3):776–789.

151. Kuhnert BR, Kuhnert PM, Philipson EH, et al. Disposition of meperidine and normeperidine following multiple doses during labor. II. Fetus and neonate. *Am J Obstet Gynecol* 1985;151(3):410–415.

CHAPTER 57 ■ PAIN AND SICKLE CELL DISEASE

SAMIR K. BALLAS

INTRODUCTION

Historical Milestones

Historically, sickle cell disease (SCD) evolved through four periods: (1) the tribal medicine period in Africa, (2) the period of clinical recognition by Western medicine, (3) the period of biochemical/cellular research, and (4) the period of molecular characterization and treatment. Thus, this evolution progressed from bedside to bench, eventually returning to the bedside.

SCD was known in Africa before the twentieth century. Inhabitants of West Africa realized that the disease was hereditary and gave it specific names such as Chwechwechwe, Ahotutuo, Nwiiwii, and Nuidudui.[1] These names are characterized by alliteration of letters that seemingly signified the recurrent clinical manifestations of the disease and the crying sounds by children in pain.

Dr. James Herrick of Chicago[2] ushered in the clinical period with a report of SCD in 1910. He described a young black student from Grenada in the West Indies who presented with cough and fever. This case report is significant because it documented "peculiar elongated and sickle-shaped red blood corpuscles in a case of severe anemia," and this left no doubt that the patient had a severe variety of sickle cell syndrome, probably sickle cell anemia (SS).[2]

Between 1910 and 1949, there was a plethora of descriptions of the various clinical features of SCD by physicians, most notably by Mason[3] who coined the term SS and by Diggs[4] who noted that the hallmark of SS is recurrent and painful vascular occlusive crisis interspersed with periods of stable state with no signs or symptoms other than those due to chronic hemolytic anemia.

The biochemical/cellular period in the history of SCD was ushered in by Pauling and his associates[5] who introduced the concept of SS as a molecular disease. They demonstrated that hemoglobin isolated from red cells of patients with SCD differed electrophoretically from the hemoglobin of normal persons and that the hemoglobin of those with sickle cell trait was a mixture of normal and sickle hemoglobin. Neel[6] showed that the inheritance of SS followed simple Mendelian genetics. Ingram[7] reported that the only difference between normal and sickle hemoglobin was the replacement of glutamic acid by valine. The work of several groups established the subunit structure and primary sequences of the subunits ($\alpha\beta,\gamma,\delta$) of human hemoglobin and localized the sickle mutation to the sixth residue of the β-globin chain

($\beta 6^{Glu \rightarrow Val}$). The interaction of the sickle mutation with other hemoglobin abnormalities clarified the spectrum of sickle cell syndromes. The advent of DNA technology in the 1970s and the 1980s paved the way for the molecular period including the molecular diagnosis of sickle cell disorders, prenatal diagnosis, and the identification of α-genotypes and β^s haplotypes and their effect on the clinical picture of SCD. By the 1980s, it had become clear that SCD is a highly heterogeneous disorder not only at the clinical level but also at the cellular and molecular levels. The recent success of the human genome project initiated studies to determine epistatic genes that may modify the phenotypic expressions of SCD.[8]

Hematologic Aspects of Sickle Cell Disease

Hemoglobinopathies are inherited disorders of the structure and/or function of the hemoglobin molecule that have no established cure in adult patients. Cure has been achieved in selected children with SS by using allogeneic bone marrow transplantation, stem cells, or cord blood transplantation.[9-14] Hemoglobinopathies are broadly divided into two major groups: structural variants and thalassemias. Structural variants are, most commonly, the result of single base mutations in the globin genes. Thalassemias are characterized by decreased synthesis of globin chains.

Nature of the Sickle Mutation

The most common structural variant of normal hemoglobin is the sickle hemoglobin (Hb S) followed by hemoglobin C (Hb C). Both of these hemoglobins are the result of single base mutation in the sixth codon of exon l of the β-globin gene responsible for the synthesis of the β-globin chain of the hemoglobin molecule. In case of Hb S, the mutation is the result of a single base change (GAG → GTG) in the sixth codon of exon 1 of the β-globin gene responsible for the synthesis of the β-globin polypeptide of the Hb molecule ($\alpha_2\beta_2$). This change, in turn, results in replacement of the normal glutamic acid with valine at position 6 of the β-globin chain and the formation of sickle Hb.[7,15] In case of Hb C, the mutation is the result of a single base change (GAG →

TABLE 57.2

MAJOR SICKLE CELL SYNDROMES ARRANGED IN ORDER OF DECREASING SEVERITY

Disease	Abbreviation
Sickle Cell Anemia	SS
Sickle-β^0-Thalassemia	S-β^0-Thal
Hb SC Disease	Hb SC
Hb SO Arab	Hb SO Arab
Sickle-β^+-Thalassemia	S-β^+-Thal

AAG) in the same codon as the Hb S; this change results in replacement of the normal glutamic acid with lysine at position 6 of the β-globin chain and the formation of Hb C. These mutations change the net charge of the variant hemoglobin thus allowing their separation by electrophoresis.

Structural variants of hemoglobin are inherited in an autosomal codominant manner according to Mendelian principles. Thus, if one parent is normal and the other has SS, then all children will have sickle cell trait.

Sickle cell syndromes, collectively referred to as SCD, comprise a group of clinically significant hemoglobinopathies in which the sickle gene is inherited from at least one parent. SS is the homozygous state where the sickle gene is inherited from both parents. Sickle cell syndromes also result from the coinheritance of the sickle gene with hemoglobin (Hb)C gene giving rise to HbSC diseases, with β-thalassemia genes (β^0 or β^+) giving rise to sickle -β^0-thalassaemia or sickle -β^+-thalassemia respectively or with other β-globin structural variants giving rise to other combinations such as HbSO Arab, HbSD disease, and so on. Tables 57.1 and 57.2 list major types of sickle cell syndromes commonly seen in the United States. Certain complications of SCD may be more common in one category than another. Thus, frequent painful crises, severe anemia that requires blood transfusion and acute chest syndrome (ACS), are more common in SS than other types of SCD. Sickle retinopathy, on the other hand, is more common in HbSC disease than in SS. It must be emphasized that the order of severity outlined in Table 57.2 is based

TABLE 57.1

MAJOR TYPES OF SICKLE CELL SYNDROME AND THEIR TYPICAL HEMATOLOGICAL PARAMETERS

Disease	Abbreviation	Genotype	Hb(g/dL)	Retic(%)	MCV(fl)	Hb A%	Hb A_2*%	Hb S%	Hb F%
Sickle Cell Anemia									
1. No α-Gene Deletion	SS	β^S/β^S; αα/αα	7.0–8.0	10–20	85–110	0	2.5–3.5	75–96	1–20
2. Deletion of 2 α-Genes	SS, α-Thal	β^S/β^S; −α/−α	9.0–10.0	6–12	70–80	0	3.0–4.4	75–94	1–20
Sickle- β^0- Thalassemia	S-β^0-Thal	β^S/β^o thal	7.0–10.0	6–15	60–70	0	4.0–6.0	70–90	1–20
Sickle-β^+- Thalassemia	S-β^+-Thal	β^S/β^+ thal	>10.0	5–10	60–70	10–20	4.0–6.0	65–85	1–15
Hb SC disease	SC	β^S/β^c	>10.0	5–10	75–85	0	45–50	50	1–6
Sickle Cell Trait	AS	β^A/β^S	12–16	1.0–2.0	>82	55–57	2.5–3.5	40	<1.0

Hb, Hemoglobin; MCV, Mean Corpuscular Volume; Retic, Reticuloyte Count.
*Hb A_2 and Hb C have the same electrophoretic mobility at alkaline pH and are not separable on routine analysis; they can be separated, however, by High Pressure Liquid Chromatography (HPLC).
(Note that all disorders may be associated with variable degrees of α-gene deletions.)

TABLE 57.3

UNIQUE FEATURES OF SICKLE-α-THALASSEMIA ($\beta^S/\beta^S - \alpha/-\alpha$) COMPARED WITH SS WITHOUT α-GENE DELETION (β^S/β^S; $\alpha\alpha/\alpha\alpha$)

Milder anemia
Increased HbA_2 level
Splenomegaly in adults
Increased prevalence of avascular necrosis
Increased prevalence of retinopathy
Decreased prevalence of cerebrovascular accidents
Decreased prevalence of leg ulcers
Less tissue damage

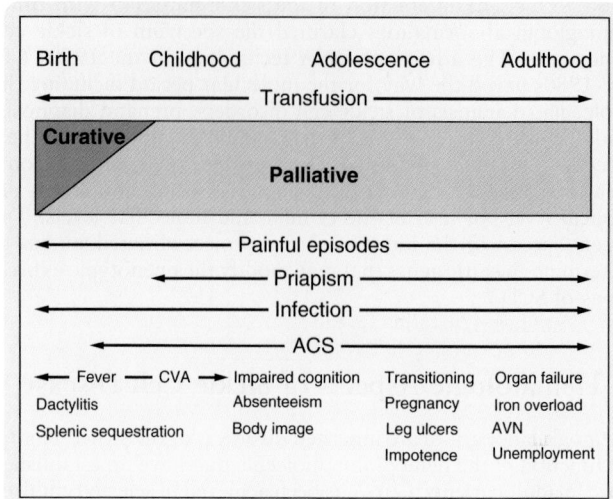

FIGURE 57.1 Sequence of complications of SS from birth through adult life. Cure is possible in selected children. The mainstay of management in most patients is palliative, with pain management being most important. ACS, acute chest syndrome; AVN, avascular necrosis; CVA, cerebrovascular accident. (Modified from Ballas SK. Sickle cell disease: current clinical management. *Semin Hematol* 2001;38:308, with permission.)

on population statistics. Thus, if one compares the overall clinical picture of 100 patients with SS, for example, with that of 100 patients with HbSC disease then the latter will be milder as far as frequency of painful episodes, morbidity, and mortality are concerned. On the individual basis, however, the scheme of Table 57.2 does not always apply. Thus, an individual patient with SS may have a mild disease whereas an occasional patient with S-β^+-thalassemia may have a severe disease.

Genotypes

Sickle cell syndromes can also be divided into subcategories depending on the α genotypes and β haplotypes.[16-18] About 65% of patients with SS have normal α genotypes ($\beta^s\beta^s$; $\alpha\alpha/\alpha\alpha$), 30% have one α gene deleted ($\beta^s\beta^s$; $-\alpha/\alpha\alpha$), and the remaining 5% have two α genes deleted ($\beta^s\beta^s$; $-\alpha/-\alpha$). The effect of α gene deletion on the clinical picture of sickle cell syndromes is controversial. Generally speaking, α gene deletion is associated with milder anemia[19] and less blood transfusion. The increased hemoglobin level associated with α gene deletion however, increases the blood viscosity, which is often accompanied by increased frequency of painful crises[20,21] and vaso-occlusive episodes such as avascular necrosis.[22,23] The effect of α gene deletion on the clinical picture is best illustrated in SS with two α gene deletions ($\beta^s\beta^s$; $-\alpha/-\alpha$). Table 57.3 lists the unique features of this type of SCD.[24,25] It is noteworthy that HbA_2 is elevated in SS with two α gene deletions, a finding that confuses this diagnosis with S-β^0-thalassemia that is, typically, also associated with elevated HbA_2 levels. The clinical picture, family history, hematologic data, and molecular diagnostics can differentiate the two diagnoses.[25]

β-Haplotypes refer to the nucleotide sequence 5' and 3' to the sickle gene. Three major types have been described in Africans and African Americans.[17] These are the Senegalese (Sen), Benin (Ben), and Central African Republic (CAR) haplotypes. The significance of these haplotypes pertains to their effect on HbF production. It has been established that the higher the HbF level, the milder is the SS.[21,26] Again, these conclusions are based on population data and may not apply to an individual patient.

Sickle cell syndromes are multisystem disorders that have protean clinical manifestations. Management of these syndromes includes the following approaches: (1) management of anemia and its sequelae; (2) management of painful episodes; (3) management of infections; (4) management of organ damage; and (5) management with experimental therapeutic modalities. This chapter will focus on the pathogenesis and management of acute and chronic sickle cell pain syndromes.

PATHOPHYSIOLOGY

SCD is a quadrumvirate of: (1) pain syndrome; (2) anemia and its sequelae; (3) organ failure including infection; and (4) comorbid

conditions. Pain, however, is the insignia of SCD and dominates its clinical picture throughout the life of the patients (Fig. 57.1). Pain also may precipitate or be itself precipitated by the other three components of the quadrumvirate. Management of sickle pain must be within the framework of the disease as a whole and not in isolation. The pain associated with SCD is often perplexing to treat. There is no doubt as to the original pathology, yet because of the complex biopsychosocial accompaniments to SCD, opioid-seeking behavior can easily be misinterpreted as inappropriate. In order not to miss catastrophic complications, a complaint of pain should always be taken seriously. There are anecdotes of patients with SCD who were dismissed from certain programs only to be found dead at home within 24 hours or less after dismissal or to be admitted to other hospitals with serious complications.[27] Sickle pain could be the prodrome of a serious and potentially fatal complication of SCD in some patients.

Vaso-occlusion

The most important pathophysiologic event in SS that explains most of its clinical manifestations is vaso-occlusion which may involve both the micro- and macrovasculature.[28-31] Factors that culminate in vaso-occlusion are listed in Table 57.4.[9,31-34] The primary process that leads to vascular occlusion is the polymerization of sickle Hb upon deoxygenation which, in turn, results in distortion of the shape of red blood cells (RBCs), cellular dehydration, and decreased deformability and stickiness of RBC that promotes their adhesion to vascular endothelium (Fig. 57.2). Progress in the pathogenesis of vascular occlusion pertains to cellular dehydration and adhesion to endothelial cells described below.

Red Blood Cell Dehydration

Cellular dehydration is secondary to loss of potassium (K^+) and water. Two major transport mechanisms seem to play a significant role in cellular dehydration. The first mechanism is the potassium chloride (KCl) cotransport pathway activated by acidifica-

TABLE 57.4

DETERMINANTS THAT CONTRIBUTE TO VASCULAR
OCCLUSION IN SICKLE CELL DISEASE

Microrheology
    RBC factors
        Polymerization of deoxy HbS
        Cellular dehydration
        Dense cells
        Fetal hemoglobin
        α-Genotype, β-haplotypes, Hb variants
        Sickling–unsickling cycles
        RBC deformability and mechanical fragility

    Factors extrinsic to RBC
        Adhesion to vascular endothelia
        Inflammatory mediators and reperfusion injury
        White blood cells
        Hemostatic factors
        Vascular factors

Macrovascular occlusion

Whole blood rheology
    Hematocrit
    Plasma components
    Vascular tone

Other factors
    Epistatic genes
    The environment

tion and cell swelling.[35–37] This pathway is most active in reticulocytes and is a feature of low-density sickle cells (reversibly sickled cells). Reticulocyte dehydration appears to contribute to the generation of dense sickle cells directly without going through repetitive cycles of oxygenation-deoxygenation.[38]

The second transport system that mediates cellular dehydration is the calcium (Ca^{2+}) activated K^{+} channel or the Gardos pathway, which seems to be activated by Ca^{2+} reflux-induced deoxygenation.[35–37,39–41] Although much of the intracellular Ca^{2+} in sickle cells is sequestered in endocytic vesicles,[42–44] transient reflux of Ca^{2+} during deoxygenation-induced sickling seems to be responsible for stimulating the Gardos pathway. Unlike the KCl cotransport, the Gardos pathway seems to be most active in the dense fraction of sickle RBCs. However, in most patients, both transport systems are operative.

It should be noted, however, that the exact mechanism by which polymerization of sickle Hb leads to cellular dehydration is not fully delineated to date. Further research in this area may refine current approaches to molecular therapy.

Adhesion to Vascular Endothelium

Adhesion of sickle RBCs to vascular endothelium appears to be a pathophysiologic contributor to vaso-occlusion. Sickle RBCs adhere to cultured endothelial cells in vitro under both static and dynamic conditions whereas normal cells do not.[45–48] These findings suggest that sickle RBCs have sticky surfaces that promote their attachment to monolayers of cultured endothelial cells. These in vitro observations have been documented to occur also in ex vivo perfusion studies in rats[49] and transgenic mice.[50] Both cellular and plasma factors have been reported to affect adhesion of sickle RBCs to vascular endothelium. Thus, young deformable sickle RBCs appear to be more adherent to vascular endothelium than are dense, rigid, irreversibly sickled cells.[48,51,52]

Adherence of sickle RBCs to vascular endothelium results in

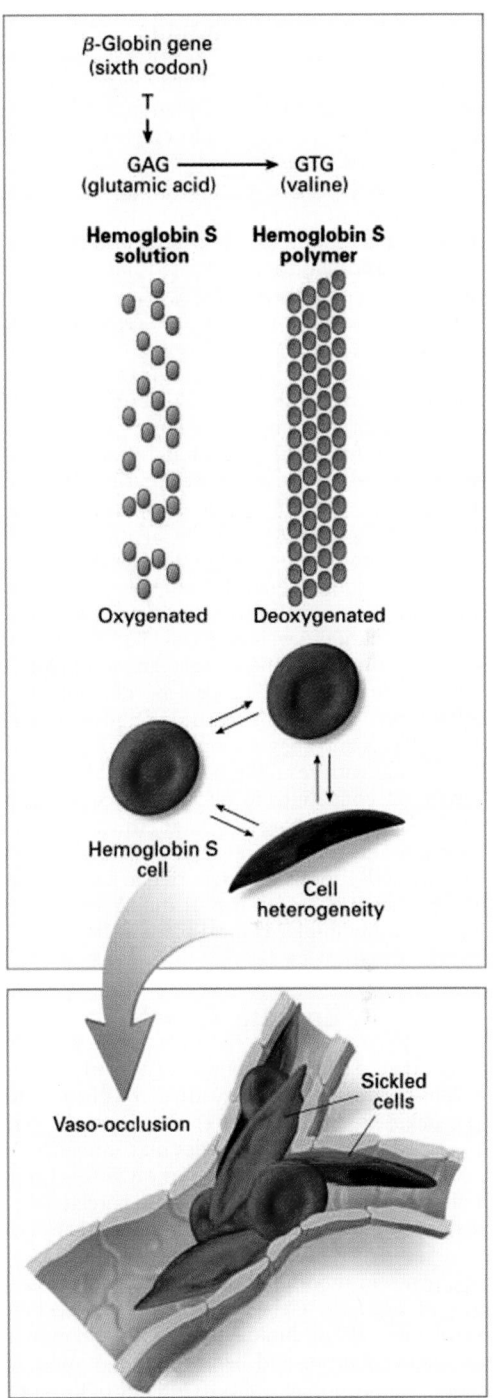

FIGURE 57.2 Pathophysiology of SCD. In hemoglobin S, a substitution of T for A in the sixth codon of the β-globin gene leads to the replacement of a glutamic acid residue by a valine residue. On deoxygenation, hemoglobin S polymers form, causing cell sickling and damage to the membrane. Some sickle cells adhere to endothelial cells, leading to vaso-occlusion. (Reproduced from Steinberg MH. Management of sickle cell disease. *New Engl J Med* 1999;340:1022, with permission.)

intimal hyperplasia in larger vessels that may lead to vascular occlusion and tissue infarction.[53,54] Hebbel et al.[45] reported strong correlation between the degree of adhesion of SS RBC to endothelial cells in vitro and the severity of the disease in patients with SS or other variants of SCD. Hypofibronectinemia seems also to be related to disease severity: the lower the level of plasma fibronectin, the more severe the disease.[55]

Tissue Damage

Recent in vivo studies in transgenic mice suggest that vaso-occlusion results in the creation of an inflammatory state.[56,57] The sequence of events seems to be as follows: (1) reticulocytes carrying the $\alpha_4\beta_1$ receptor adhere to endothelial cells; (2) this is followed by logjam where there is propagation of occlusion caused by the accumulation of rigid deoxygenated mature RBCs proximal to the site of adhesion; (3) the obstruction eventually clears leading to reperfusion and its associated injury; and (4) a new cycle of adhesion starts thus creating a vicious cycle of occlusion and reperfusion. Evidence of reperfusion injury includes: (1) inflammatory response in the vascular bed of the transgenic mouse with increased leukocyte rolling, adhesion, and emigration after 3 hours of mild hypoxia followed by reperfusion; (2) local production of free radicals; and (3) the complete inhibition of (1) and (2) after the infusion of monoclonal murine anti-P-selectin antibody, before reoxygenation.[56] Restoration of oxygen to ischemic tissue seems to result in the generation of free radicals associated with inflammatory endothelial and tissue damage.

Sickle RBCs from patients with a high level of Hb F seem to be less adherent to vascular endothelium than those from patients with low Hb F levels. Specifically, Setty et al.[58] found that pediatric SS patients with high levels of F cells had a concomitant decrease in the number of CD36+, very late antigen (VLA) 4+, and CD71+ erythrocytes, and hence, less adherent RBCs. Moreover, Hb F seems to affect the exposure of phosphatidylserine on the surface of RBCs and coagulation activation. In vivo cycles of sickling/unsickling with resulting membrane changes and microvesicle formation contribute to phosphatidylserine exposure.[59] Phosphatidylserine-exposing RBCs in the transgenic sickle mouse[60] were found to have shortened RBC survival. Children with SS and high HB F levels were reported to have less phosphatidylserine-exposing RBCs and, hence, milder hemolytic anemia suggesting a possibly milder clinical picture.[61]

Epistatic Genes

Other factors that may also affect the severity of SS include gene modifiers (epistatic genes) that may affect the phenotypic expression of the sickle mutation. Styles et al.[62] reported that specific human leucocyte antigen (HLA) alleles may influence the risk of stroke in SS. Adekile et al.[63] found that the 677 C→T mutation of the methyltetrahydrofolate reduction gene is relatively frequent among Kuwaiti patients with SS, but did not find any correlation with disease severity or prevalence of avascular necrosis. The role of epistatic genes in modifying the phenotypic expression is an active area of research. Genes that modulate the biochemical pathways of nitric oxide biology, oxidants, inflammation, cell adhesion, vasoregulation, and hemostasis may modulate SCD, and single-nucleotide polymorphisms in some of those genes have already been associated with sickle cell subphenotypes.[8] Future research may enable us to decipher the intricate pathophysiology of SS and its complications and usher in newer therapeutic venues.

In addition to the factors discussed above, there is growing evidence that psychosocial and environmental factors may precipitate vaso-occlusion and affect the frequency and severity of painful episodes. Physical stress, trauma, dehydration, and infections are known precipitating factors.

TYPES OF SICKLE PAIN

Sickle cell pain can be classified in a number of ways.[64–66] Pathophysiologically, sickle cell pain could be nociceptive or neuropathic; temporally, it could be acute or chronic; anatomically, it could be somatic, visceral, unilateral, bilateral, localized, or dif-

TABLE 57.5

ETIOLOGIC CLASSIFICATION OF SICKLE CELL PAIN

Acute pain syndromes
  Acute painful sickle cell crises
  ACS
  Acute abdominal pain syndromes
    Right upper quadrant syndrome
    Left upper quadrant syndrome
  Hand-Foot syndrome (dactylitis)
  Priapism
  AMF

Chronic pain syndrome
  With objective signs
    Avascular (aseptic) necrosis
    Arthropathies
    Vertebral body collapse
    Leg ulcers
    Chronic osteomyelitis
  Without objective signs
    Intractable chronic pain

Neuropathic pain syndromes unique/common in SCD
  Mental nerve neuropathy
  Ischemic optic neuropathy
  Spinal cord infarction
  Other neuropathies

Pain syndromes secondary to therapy
  Postoperative pain
  Loose prosthesis (shoulders/hips)

Pain syndromes due to comorbid conditions
  Trauma
  Peptic ulcer disease
  Migraine headache
  Arthritides (septic, rheumatoid, degenerative, collagen)
  Other conditions

fuse; pathologically, it could be mild, moderate, or severe; and etiologically, it could be due to the disease itself or secondary to therapy or to comorbid conditions. The etiologic classifications of sickle pain are listed in Table 57.5 and includes acute pain syndromes, chronic pain syndromes, neuropathic pain syndromes, pain secondary to therapy, and pain due to comorbid conditions.

ACUTE SICKLE CELL PAIN SYNDROMES

The Acute Painful Sickle Cell Crises

Vaso-occlusion is the de facto prerequisite for the development of the acute sickle cell painful crises. Tissue damage consequent to vaso-occlusion initiates a number of complex biochemical, neurologic, electrochemical, and inflammatory events that incite nociception and pain. The inflammatory response to vaso-occlusion may enhance sympathetic activity via neuroendocrine pathways triggering release of norepinephine, which in the setting of tissue injury causes more tissue ischemia, thus creating a vicious cycle. It is the combination of ischemic tissue damage and secondary inflammatory response that accounts for the extreme severity of the pain in SCD (Fig. 57.3). Tissue injury generates several major pain mediators[67–70] including, but not limited to, interleukin-1, bradykinin, K^+, hydrogen (H^+), histamine, substance P, and calcitonin gene-related peptide (CGRP). Inter-

Sequence of Events in The Sickle Cell Painful Crisis

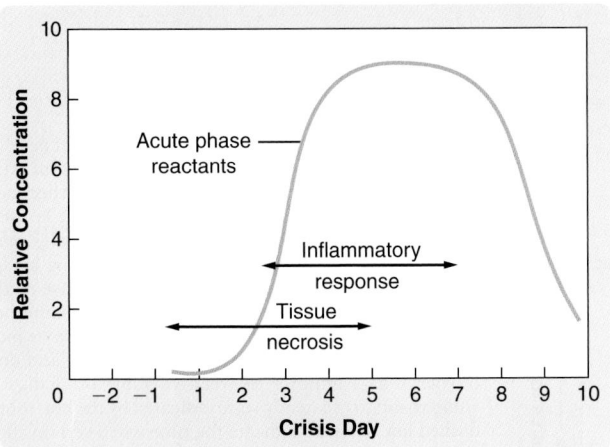

FIGURE 57.3 Sequence of events during the evolution of painful crisis. Tissue necrosis consequent to ischemia elicits an inflammatory response that is associated with an increase in the serum level of acute-phase reactants. (Modified from Ballas SK. Sickle cell disease: clinical management. *Baillieres Clinical Haematology* 1998;11:193, with permission.)

keukin-1 (IL-1) is an endogenous pyrogen and also upregulates the cyclooxygenase gene leading to synthesis of prostaglandins E_2 and I_2. Bradykinin, K^+, H^+, and histamine activate nociceptive afferent nerve fibers and evoke a pain response. Prostaglandins sensitize peripheral nerve endings and facilitate the transmission of painful stimuli along A-δ and C fibers that reach the cerebral cortex via the spinal cord and the thalamus. Moreover, activated nociceptors release stored substance P, which itself facilitates the transmission of painful stimuli. Bradykinin, substance P, and CGRP also cause vasodilatation and extravasations of fluids that can lead to local swelling and tenderness. The pathway for pain stimuli is subject not only to activators, sensitizers, and facilitators, but also to inhibitors. Serotonin, enkephalin, β-endorphin, and dynorphin are endogenous central pain inhibitors. Thus, in a given patient, the net outcome of tissue ischemia may be severe or mild pain, depending on the extent of tissue damage and the net balance of pain stimulators versus pain inhibitors. This may explain, in part, the considerable variation in the frequency and severity of painful sickle crises among patients, and longitudinally in the same patient.

Predisposing Factors

There are at least three sets of predisposing factors that predict the frequency and severity of the acute painful sickle cell crisis. These are genetic, cellular, and environmental (or epigenetic) factors. Genetic factors include Hb F level, the coexistence of α-gene deletion, β-thalassemia, β-haplotypes, and epistatic gene modifiers as was mentioned above. They also include gender, since males constitute about 60% to 66% of admissions to the hospital.[71,72] Females, however, have longer hospital stays per admission than males.[71] Cellular factors with decreased RBC deformability and increased number of dense cells in the steady state have a salutary effect, most likely because these are associated with more severe anemia and hence relatively decreased whole blood viscosity.[19,73] Patients with SS and relatively high hemoglobin level are more likely to experience more frequent crises than those patients with SS and lower Hb level. Decreased level of vitamin A (less than 30 ug/dL) and nocturnal hypoxia are environmental factors amenable to preventative therapy.[74,75]

Precipitating Factors

Like other acute episodes of illness, the acute sickle cell painful crisis has precipitating features. Major reported factors that seem

to precipitate vaso-occlusive crises include dehydration, stress of any kind (physical, traumatic, physiologic, emotional), infection, acidosis, sleep apnea, and pregnancy.[64,65] Nevertheless, most painful episodes are not preceded by an obvious precipitating factor. Gill et al.[76] reported that daily mood and stress predict painful events, utilization of health care facilities, and work activity in adults with SCD. In a retrospective study, Smith et al.[77] found a complex relationship between temperature changes, temperature extremes, and their relationship to emergency department (ED) visits and hospital admissions for sickle cell painful crises in adults. The most relevant finding of this study was an inconsistent confirmation of a relationship between daily ambient temperature and ED visits or hospital admissions for sickle cell crises. Jones et al.[78] studied retrospectively the number of admissions with acute pain and SCD to King's College Hospital, London, together with daily meteorological records collected locally. Data from 1400 days and 1047 separate admissions were analyzed. Increased admissions were significantly associated with increased wind speed and low humidity, but showed no relationship to temperature, rainfall, or barometric pressure. The strongest effect was for maximum wind speed/humidity ratio with 464 admissions on days in the lowest two quartiles of this parameter and 582 in the highest quartiles. The effect of high wind and low humidity is likely to be related to skin cooling. Anecdotally, many patients report that sudden changes in temperature seem to precipitate acute painful episodes.

Phases of the Acute Painful Crisis

The clinical picture of sickle cell pain is protean in nature. Typically, acute painful episodes affect long bones and joints with the low back being the most frequently reported site of pain.[64,79] Other regions of the body, including the scalp, face, jaw, abdomen, and pelvis, may be involved. A severe acute sickle cell painful episode has been defined as one that requires treatment in a medical facility with parenteral opioids for 4 or more hours.[80,81] The occurrence of three or more such crises indicates that the affected patient has severe SCD. Descriptors most often used to characterize sickle cell pain include throbbing, sharp, dull, stabbing, and shooting in decreasing order of frequency.

The concept that the painful crisis evolves along phases was first introduced by Ballas and Smith[82] and Akinola et al.[83] who independently and almost simultaneously described the presence of two phases of the uncomplicated painful crisis in prospective longitudinal studies of adults with SCD. Akinola et al.[83] studied 20 patients over 16 months, and Ballas and Smith[82] studied 117 painful crises affecting 36 patients with SS over 6 years. In both studies, the initial phase was associated with increasing pain, decreased RBC deformability, increase in the number of dense cells, red cell distribution width (RDW), hemoglobin distribution width (HDW), reticulocyte count, leukocytosis, and decrease in the number of platelets. The second phase was characterized by established pain of maximum severity and gradual reversal of the abnormalities of the first phase. Later, Ballas[84] revised the description of the painful crisis and refined its evolution into four phases by including observations by several other investigators (Fig. 57.4, Table 57.6). The phases were called prodromal, initial, established, and resolving phases. Beyer et al.[85] found that the painful crisis also evolves along phases in children but the phases were broken down into seven and were labeled differently. Jacob et al.[86] studied 40 crises affecting 27 children over 9 months. Their findings supported previous observations related to changes during the evolution of painful episodes that may be occurring in phases. Although the phases were given different names, the concepts were similar.

The evolution of the uncomplicated painful crises along phases allows the observer to determine the presence of objective signs of its occurrence. To that end there are two extremely important prerequisites for finding objective signs. First, the availability of

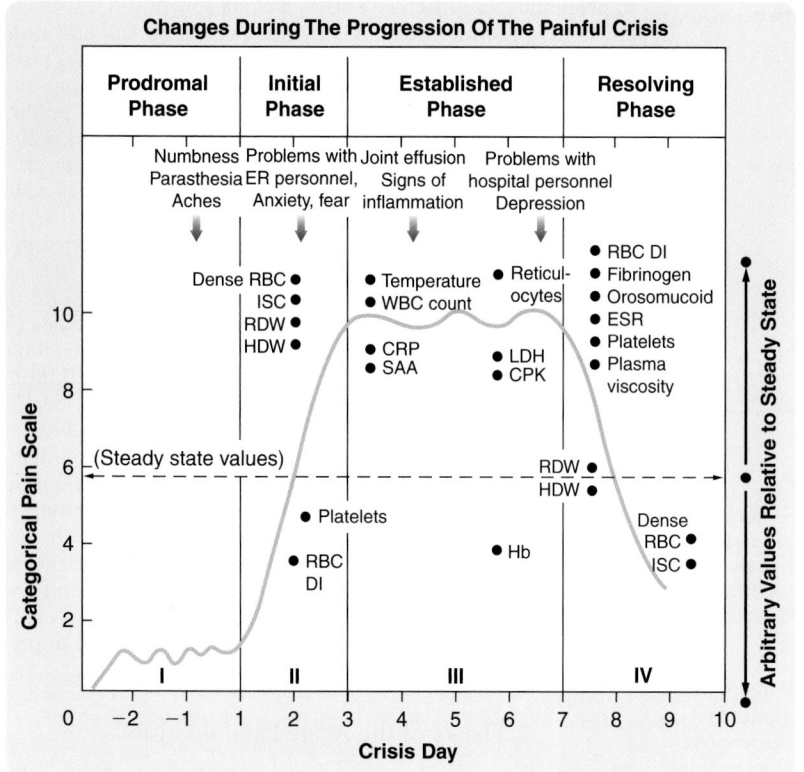

FIGURE 57.4 A typical profile of the events that develop during the evolution of a severe sickle cell painful crisis in an adult in the absence of overt infection or other complications. Such events are usually treated in the hospital with an average stay of 9–11 days. Pain becomes most severe by day 3 of the crisis and starts decreasing by day 6 or 7. The Roman numerals refer to the phase of the crisis: I, prodromal phase; II, initial phase; III, established phase; and IV, resolving phase. Dots on the X axis indicate the time when changes became apparent, and dots on the Y axis indicate the relative value of change in comparison to the steady state indicated by the horizontal dashed line. Arrows indicate the time when certain clinical signs and symptoms may become apparent. Values shown are those reported at least twice by different investigators; values that were anecdotal, unconfirmed, or that were not reported to occur on a specific day of the crisis are not shown. CPK, creatinine phosphokinase; CRP, C-reactive protein; ESR, erythrocyte sedimentation rate; Hb, hemoglobin; HDW, hemoglobin distribution width; ISC, irreversibly sickled cells; LDH, lactate dehydrogenase; RBC DI, red cell deformability index; RDW, red cell distribution width; SAA, serum amyloid A. (Modified from Ballas SK. The sickle cell painful crisis in adults: phases and objective signs. *Hemoglobin* 1995;19:327, with permission.)

steady state data. A steady state is best defined as a point in time in the history of a patient not preceded by an acute painful crisis or comorbid conditions for at least 1 month, not followed by a painful crisis within 2 days and in the absence of previous blood transfusion for at least 3 or, even better, 4 months. The second prerequisite to identify objective signs is to do serial lab determinations. Some parameters change at variable points in the progression of a painful crisis (see Fig. 57.4, Table 57.7). The presence of phases allows the provider to monitor the progress of the crisis and manage it rationally, thereby avoiding the conflicts that may arise between patients and providers about the authenticity of pain.

TABLE 57.6

PHASES OF THE ACUTE SICKLE CELL PAINFUL CRISIS

Phase	Possible synonym(s)	Duration
Prodromal	Precrisis	Up to 2 days before crisis
Initial	First Evolving Infarctive	Days 1 and 2 of the crisis
Established	Second Postinfarctive Inflammatory	Days 3–7 of crisis
Resolving	Last Healing Recovery Postcrisis	Post day 7 of crisis

From Ballas SK. Sickle cell pain. In: *Progress in Pain Research and Management.* Vol. 11. Seattle, WA: IASP Press; 1998, with permission.

Consequence of the Crisis

The decrease in Hb level with the concomitant increase in reticulocyte count seems likely to be due to the hyperhemolysis that sometimes occurs during uncomplicated painful crises. This has been confirmed[87] by the finding of decreased RBC survival during the evolution of the painful crisis in selected patients (Fig. 57.5). The increase in platelet count, fibrinogen, and blood viscosity as the crisis resolves indicates a hypercoagulable state that may cause recurrence of the crisis. This may explain, in part, why about 16% of patients are readmitted to the hospital with a painful crisis within 1 week after discharge.[71,82] Other possible causes of readmission include premature discharge or the development of an opioid withdrawal syndrome after discharge. More recently, Ballas and Lusardi[71] and Jacob et al.[88] reported a decrease in analgesic efficacy after the fourth to sixth hospital day in some patients. These patients continued to have relatively high pain scores by the time they were discharged and were most likely to be readmitted within 1 week after discharge. The reasons for loss of analgesic efficacy are not known. Possible etiologies include inadequate pain management, increase in the levels of acute phase reactants that bind to opioids and make them unavailable to induce pain relief, the development of tolerance to opioids, hyperalgesia, or adaptations at opioid receptor sites.[65,66] Patients with frequent painful crises that require hospital admission seem to have more morbidity and mortality than otherwise.

The above data suggest that special attention has to be paid at the resolving phase of the painful crises. Measures should be considered to avoid the possibility of hospital readmission soon after discharge. Providers should consider continuing aggressive pain therapy during hospitalization; if needed, rule out the possibility of tolerance and consider opioid rotation, designing discharge instructions that avoid causing withdrawal after discharge. To that end, the establishment of a postdischarge clinic to evaluate patients within a few days after discharge to ensure compliance with discharge instructions is recommended.

TABLE 57.7

MAJOR CHANGES IN OBJECTIVE SIGNS DURING THE EVOLUTION OF THE SICKLE CELL PAINFUL CRISIS

Prodromal phase	Initial phase	Established phase	Resolving phase
Decreasing RBC deformability	*Decreasing* RBC deformability Platelets	*Peak* Temperature WBC count Dense cells ISC RDW HDW Reticulocytes LDH CRP SAA	*Peak* Fibrinogen Orosomucoid ESR
Increasing Dense RBC	*Increasing* Temperature WBC count Dense cells ISC RDW HDW ESR LDH CRP Fibrinogen Orosomucoid SAA	*Nadir* RBC deformability Hb *Increasing* Fibrinogen Orosomucoid Plasma viscosity ESR	*Decreasing* Temperature WBC count Dense cells ISC RDW HDW CRP *Increasing* RBC deformability Plasma viscosity Platelets

CRP, C-reactive protein; ESR, erythrocyte sedimentation rate; Hb, hemoglobin; HDW, hemoglobin distribution width; ISC, irreversibly sickled cells; LDH, lactate dehydrogenase; RDW, red cell distribution width; SAA, serum amyloid A; WBC, white blood cells.
From Ballas SK. Sickle cell pain. In: *Progress in Pain Research and Management.* Vol. 11. Seattle, WA: IASP Press; 1998, with permission.
(Note: Parameters shown are those reported at least twice by different investigators.)

Acute Chest Syndrome

In 1979, Charache et al.[89] introduced the term ACS to define acute episodes of fever, chest pain, increased leukocytosis, and pulmonary infiltrates (Fig. 57.6) in adult patients with SS, most of whom probably had pulmonary infarction. More recently, the definition of ACS was expanded to include hypoxemia, cough, shortness of breath, wheezing, chills, and worsening anemia.[90] Moreover, the current definition of ACS stresses that the infiltrates must be "new," when compared with a previous chest ra-

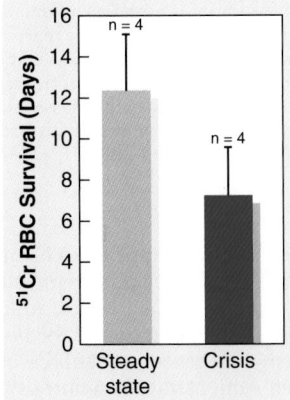

FIGURE 57.5 RBC survival decreases significantly during the evolution of the sickle cell painful crisis.

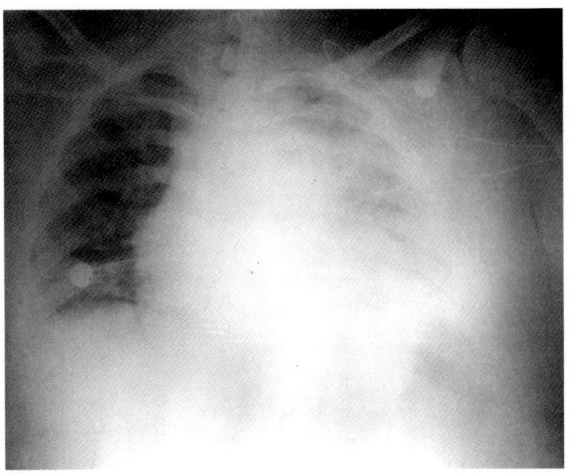

FIGURE 57.6 Chest radiograph showing diffuse pulmonary infiltrates of a patient with ACS.

diograph. If a previous radiograph is not available, the infiltrate should be considered as new and treated as such. The signs and symptoms of ACS vary from very mild to very severe and even life-threatening. Another feature of ACS that is not included in the definition is the presence of blister cells in peripheral blood.[91] ACS is second only to acute painful episodes as a cause of hospitalization of patients with SCD and also the most common complication of surgery and anesthesia.[92] ACS is the most common cause of death and is closely associated with acute painful episodes especially in adults.[93,94] Although ACS is usually self-limited and resolves with treatment, it can be associated with respiratory failure with a mortality rate of about 1.8% in children and 4.8% in adults.[95,96]

Risk factors for developing ACS are listed in Table 57.8.[97,98] The incidence of acute syndrome is highest in SS, followed by S-β^0-thalassemia, Hb SC disease and S-β^+-thalassemia in decreasing order of frequency. The single most important preventative factor is a high level of Hb F due either to endogenous genetic factors or to exogenous induction, for example with hydroxyurea.[80,97,99–101] The mean corpuscular volume (MCV) of RBCs, platelet count, and α-thalassemia bear no relation to ACS.[90,98] Known etiologies of ACS include infection, especially community-acquired pneumonia, pulmonary infarction as a result of in situ sickling, fat-bone marrow embolism, or pulmonary embolism. Infection is commonly caused by chlamydia, mycoplasma, respiratory syncytial virus, coagulase-positive *Staphylococcus aureus*, *S. pneumoniae*, *Mycoplasma hominis*, parvovirus, and rhinovirus in decreasing order of frequency.[95] Adhesion of sickled RBCs to endothelial cells of small- or medium-sized pulmonary vessels may result in occlusion of microvascular flow and consequent pulmonary infarction.[101–103] This sequence of events is supported by dynamic imaging studies but confirmatory clinical data are not available. Pulmonary thromboembolism is uncommon as a cause of ACS despite the presence of a hypercoagulable state in sickle cell disease.[104] It seems that this hypercoagulable state plays a more important role in stimulating cellular adhesion and activating the inflammatory system than in initiating the thrombotic cascade.[49,105] There is no definite evidence of the prevalence of pulmonary embolism (PE) in hospitalized patients with SCD. Stein et al.[106] determined the prevalence of deep vein thrombosis (DVT) and PE in hospitalized patients with and without SCD. They found high prevalence of PE in patients with SCD compared with non-SCD African American patients of the same age, although the prevalence of DVT was comparable in both groups. Stein et al.[106] suggested that their findings are compatible with the concept that thrombosis in situ mimics PE and might be present in many SCD patients. On the other hand, their data suggest that PE is not rare in patients with SCD, indicating that PE might be an etiologic factor in patients with SCD who develop respiratory symptoms. In such patients, imaging studies may clarify the exact diagnosis. Pulmonary fat-bone marrow embolism

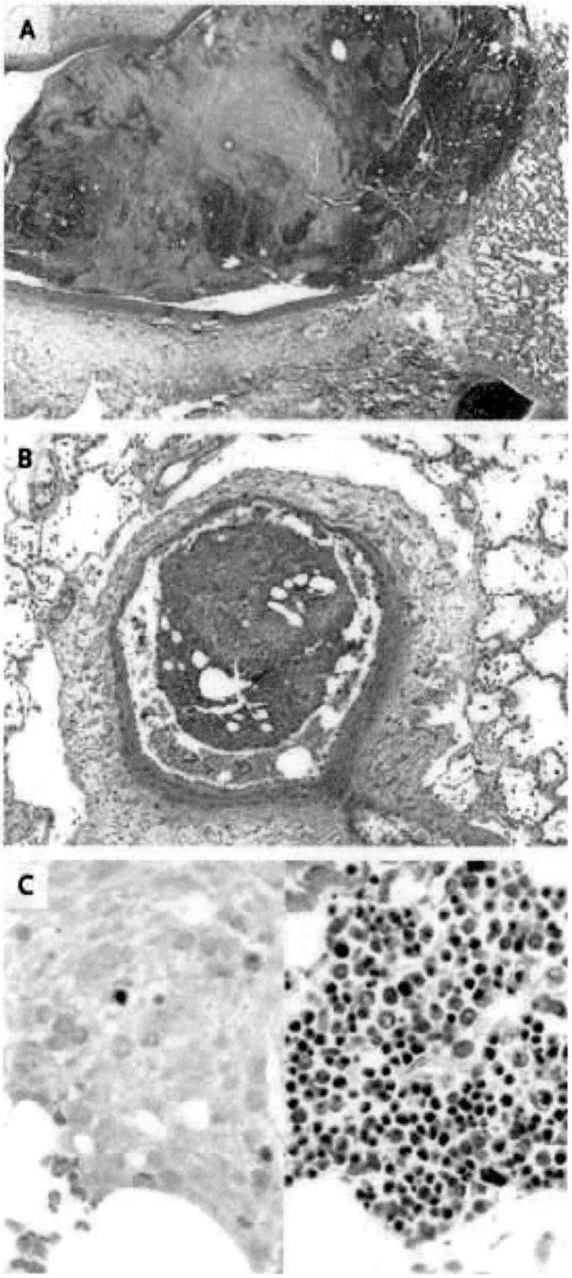

FIGURE 57.7 Photomicrographs of Lung and Bone Marrow (Hematoxylin and Eosin). Bone marrow emboli, consisting of particles of bone marrow surrounded by fibrin, are present in small pulmonary arteries (Panels A and B). In Panel C, a section of bone marrow shows the absence of cellular detail, indicating infarction (*left*), as compared with a section of normal bone marrow from the same patient (*right*). (Medoff BD, Shepard JA, Smith RN, et al. Case records of the Massachusetts General Hospital. Case 17-2005. A 22-year-old woman with back and leg pain and respiratory failure. *New Engl J Med* 2005;352:2432, with permission.)

(Fig. 57.7) in patients with SS appears to be more common than previously thought.[98,104] The characteristic clinical picture is of severe bone pain, usually in long bones, followed by dyspnea, hypoxia, and fever. Tissue infarction of the bone marrow within the long bones seems to generate a source of fat and necrotic tissue that has been demonstrated on autopsy.

The exact mechanism by which fat or bone marrow reaches the lung during painful sickle cell crises is not well known. A probable cause is "retrograde embolization."[107] According to

---

TABLE 57.8

RISK FACTORS FOR ACUTE CHEST SYNDROME

High white blood cell count	Rib infarction
High hemoglobin level	Pregnancy
High pain rate	Aseptic necrosis of the hips
SS	Analgesics
S-α-Thalassemia	Acute anemic events
Fever	Cold weather
Age	

From Ballas SK. Sickle cell anemia. *Drugs* 2002;62:1158, with permission.

this hypothesis, obstruction of vascular channels within the bone by conglomerates of sickled RBCs leads to bone marrow infarction and necrosis of the hematopoietic elements and fat. The increased intramedullary pressure disrupts the endothelium of the engorged vessels, thus allowing the retrograde movement of necrotic bone marrow and fat into adjacent intramedullary sinusoids which directly communicate with arterioles and veins, in turn spreading the necrotic material systemically. Concurrent with tissue damage, the secretary phospholipase A$_2$ (sPLA$_2$) is activated and cleaves membrane phospholipids to form several mediators of inflammation including free fatty acids.[108] The latter causes damage to pulmonary endothelium culminating in a leak syndrome which, if severe, may be similar to adult respiratory distress syndrome. Elevated levels of PLA$_2$ is both a marker and probably a predictor of ACS.[95,108]

Diagnostic work-up of ACS should include serial chest radiographs, induced deep sputum and blood cultures, monitoring arterial blood gases, monitoring hemoglobin level, ventilation, and perfusion scans, and ruling out thrombophlebitis in the pelvis or lower extremities. The diagnosis of fat embolism entails the identification of fat-laden macrophages in blood, urine, induced deep sputum, or better bronchoalveolar lavage fluid obtained by bronchoscopy.[96,104] Blister cells have been described in the peripheral blood of patients with SCD and ACS.[91]

Management of ACS includes oxygen, incentive spirometry, antibiotics, simple blood transfusion or exchange transfusion, judicious use of analgesics, careful hydration, and possibly vasodilators. Incentive spirometry prevents splinting and atelectasis, and may actually prevent ACS in patients who have rib infarction.[109] Intravenous (IV) antibiotics are indicated since it is difficult to rule out pneumonia or infected lung infarcts. A combination of a third generation cephalosporin and a macrolide or a fluoroquinolone should be used to cover typical and atypical pathogens. Simple transfusion or exchange transfusion is indicated in patients with worsening respiratory function. The beneficial effects of blood transfusion may not be due simply to decreasing the proportion of sickled RBCs and other mechanisms may be involved. These include: (1) an immunomodulatory mechanism by which inflammatory cytokines (IL-8, in particular) bind to the Duffy antigen present on transfused RBCs, but often absent on RBCs of African Americans,[110] and (2) the albumin that is present in transfused units or used in blood exchange may bind free fatty acids, thus neutralizing their damaging effect on the pulmonary endothelium.

Although IV corticosteroids in children with ACS may be beneficial,[111] their use in adults with ACS is controversial. Huang et al.[112] reported 2 adult patients with SCD whose clinical picture deteriorated and was complicated by worsening pain, fat embolism, and coma after corticosteroid therapy. Adults, unlike children, have more adipose tissue that may hypertrophy with corticosteroids, increasing the chances of fat embolization. Moreover, corticosteroids may induce or worsen avascular necrosis, which is more common in adults than in children.

Excessive use of opioid analgesics may precipitate ACS because of their depressive effects on respiration. Recent reports[95] recommend the use of nonsteroidal anti-inflammatory drugs (NSAIDs). This recommendation should be considered carefully. Opioids have a few systemic adverse effects, and careful monitoring of their use ensures their safety. They should be discontinued if the respiratory rate is less than 10 per minute, and their adverse effects can be quickly reversed with opioid antagonists. NSAIDs, on the other hand, have considerable systemic adverse effects that may not be readily obvious. NSAIDs decrease the level of prostaglandins and prostacyclin that are essential in modulating the vascular tone of smooth muscle and renal blood flow. Thus, NSAIDs may worsen the clinical picture of acute syndrome as a result of vasoconstrictive effects and bronchospasm.

Preliminary reports on the use of nitric oxide (NO), a vasodilator, in patients with SCD support a possible role of this agent in the management of ACS.[113] Another recent investigational approach to treat ACS includes the use of purified poloxamer 188, which is a nonionic surfactant. It is hypothesized that this agent reduces blood viscosity, prevents adhesion of RBCs to vascular endothelium, and improves microvascular blood flow.[114,115] Ballas et al.[116] performed a Phase I evaluation of purified poloxamer 188 in the management of ACS. Forty-three patients with SCD and ACS were treated with doses up to 2960 mg/day by continuous IV infusion. The maximum tolerated dose has not been identified. No evidence of renal toxicity or other limiting adverse events were found. One adult patient died due to sepsis and adult respiratory distress syndrome, which were unrelated to treatment. Poloxamer 188 seems to be safe in patients with ACS, and preliminary data suggest that it may shorten its duration and the length of hospitalization in a dose-related manner. Children appear to benefit more than adults. The data and safety profile justify further studies with purified poloxamer 188 in the treatment of ACS.

Because ACS is relatively frequent in hospitalized patients with SS and in view of the need to monitor arterial blood gases in its management, it is important to establish baseline blood gases and pulmonary function tests for all patients. These determinations will be of value in evaluating patients who present with acute onset of pulmonary signs and symptoms.

Acute Abdominal Pain Syndromes

The abdomen is the second most common site of pain in SCD after musculoskeletal pain (including chest wall). The cause may be intra-abdominal pathology or pain referred from the lungs with pneumonia or from the lower ribs and the femoral heads with avascular necrosis. Specific pain syndromes due to SCD are listed in Table 57.9.[64]

An acute abdominal sickle cell painful crisis is characterized by severe, usually generalized, abdominal pain and signs of peritoneal irritation. It may also be accompanied by fever, leukocytosis, and markedly elevated levels of lactate dehydrogenate (LDH). Clinically, a severe abdominal crisis may closely mimic an acute abdomen and may lead to an exploratory laparotomy in search of surgically correctable pathology. Patients with SCD who arrive at the ED with an acute abdominal crisis may be misdiagnosed with acute appendicitis or acute cholecystitis and undergo laparotomy and often "prophylactic" appendectomy and/or cholecystectomy.[64,84]

TABLE 57.9

DIFFERENTIAL DIAGNOSIS OF ABDOMINAL PAIN IN SICKLE CELL DISEASE

Left upper quadrant syndrome
   Splenic sequestration
   Acute pancreatitis

Right upper quadrant syndrome
   Calculus cholecystitis
   Acute viral hepatitis
   Hepatic sequestration
   Hepatic crisis
   Intrahepatic cholestasis

Other acute abdominal episodes
   Abdominal crisis (pseudo-acute surgical abdomen)
   Bowel infarction
   Girdle syndrome

From Ballas SK. Sickle cell pain. In: *Progress in Pain Research and Management*. Vol. 11. Seattle, WA: IASP Press; 1998, with permission.

The abdominal pain has been attributed to enlarged mesenteric and retroperitoneal lymph nodes, bone marrow hyperplasia, infarction of the vertebral bodies, hepatobiliary disease, splenic disease, or mesenteric arterial thrombosis.[117,118] The abdominal pain seen in crisis may persist for several days, although protracted episodes lasting longer than 5 days are not unusual.[119] Differentiation from other causes of acute abdominal pain may be difficult.

Pain in the trunk in association with abdominal distention has been referred to as girdle syndrome.[120,121] It is thought to result from sickling in the mesenteric blood supply. Fluid levels may be visible on radiographs of the abdomen. Mild cases are self-limiting over a 2- to 5-day period and are treated symptomatically with IV fluids since gut absorption is impaired. More severe cases have associated involvement of the liver and lungs, and in very severe cases multiorgan failure including ACS should be considered. Such patients may have markedly distended loops of bowel and require nasogastric suction and exchange transfusion. Infarction of segments of gut can occur, and surgical intervention may be required.

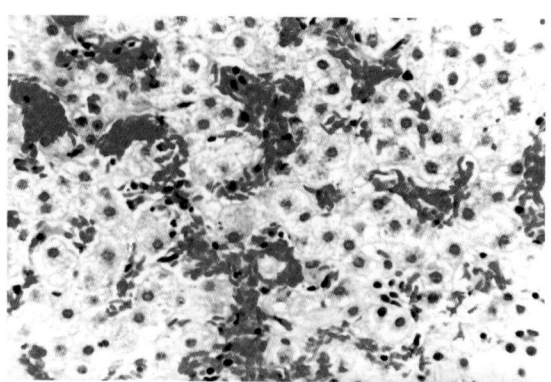

FIGURE 57.8 Liver biopsy from a patient with SS and hepatic crisis showing engorgement of hepatic sinusoids with sickled erythrocytes. (Ballas SK. Sickle cell pain. *Progress in Pain Research and Management*. Vol. 11. Seattle, WA: IASP Press; 1998, with permission.)

Right Upper Quadrant Syndrome

Chronic hyperbilirubinemia, cholelithiasis, and gallbladder disease are common in patients with SCD. At least two thirds of patients with SS have hepatomegaly and 75% have cholelithiasis. About 90% of patients with cholelithiasis undergo cholecystectomy either prophylactically or after an episode of acute calculus cholecystitis. Most cholecystectomies are currently performed by laparoscopy, a much simpler procedure than laparotomy, and are associated with less morbidity.[122,123]

A genetic basis for the hyperbilirubinemia pertains to mutations in UDP-glucuronyl transferase 1(UGT1A1), the enzyme that catalyses bilirubin glucuronidation. It seems that genetic polymorphism of the UGT 1A enzyme affects the metabolism of bilirubin. The bilirubin level as well as gallstone formation appear to be significantly higher in patients with the 7/7 genotype compared with the 6/6 genotype of the enzyme. Similar findings were reported in patients with Hb E-thalassemia.[124,125]

Vasavda et al.[126] determined the linear effects of α-thalassemia, the UGT1A1, and haem oxygenase (HMOXI) polymorphisms on bilirubin levels and cholelithiasis in 263 patients with SCD. Regression analysis showed that serum bilirubin levels and the incidence of gallstones were strongly associated with the number of UGT1A1 (TA) repeats in all subjects (p <0.0001 and p <0.01, respectively). While HMOXI genotype had no effect, coinheritance of α-thalassemia reduced serum bilirubin levels in all SCD patients independently of the number of UGT1A1 (TA) repeats. Each additional (TA) repeat was associated with an increase in mean serum bilirubin levels of 21% and cholerlithiasis risk of 87% in SCD.

Hepatic crisis (also called sickle cell intrahepatic cholestasis) is manifested by the sudden onset of right upper quadrant pain, progressive hepatomegaly, increasing bilirubin levels (mostly indirect), and prolongation of prothrombin and partial thromboplastin times.[127] The levels of liver enzymes (γ-glutamyl transpeptidase [γGT] and alanine amino transferase [ALT]) are also increased but not to those levels seen in acute viral hepatitis. Liver biopsy shows engorgement of hepatic sinusoids with sickled erythrocytes (Fig. 57.8). Hepatic crises vary in severity from minor episodes to sever life-threatening situations. Children and adults may suffer from either form; adults, however, have a higher frequency of the severe form. Total blood exchange is a recommended form of therapy. Blood exchange is indicated if the total bilirubin level increases progressively to values greater than 50 g/L. At that level, the prothrombin time values are usually prolonged. Blood exchange should be total in nature that is, remove whole blood and replace it with RBCs and fresh frozen plasma in order to correct the coagulation abnormality.[128]

Left Upper Quadrant Syndrome

Acute Splenic Sequestration Crisis. The spleen is the first organ to suffer from the destructive effects of sickle microvasculopathy that eventually lead to functional asplenia and autosplenectomy. During infancy, the spleen is enlarged in about 75% of patients with sickle anemia. Children between the ages of 5 months and 2 years are most vulnerable to splenic sequestration that varies in severity from mild to life-threatening episodes. In its full blown picture, acute splenic sequestration is characterized by a pentad of: (1) rapid fall in hemoglobin level, (2) rise in reticulocyte count, (3) fall in platelet count, (4) sudden increase in spleen size associated with acute pain and tenderness in the left upper quadrant, and (5) signs and symptoms of hypovolemia.[129,130] Minor episodes may resolve spontaneously but severe episodes can be fatal and may be mistaken for the sudden infant death syndrome. Fibrosis occurs by the age of 8 years and the risk for splenic sequestration decreases.[131,132] Nevertheless, older children and adults with persistent splenomegaly in certain sickle cell syndromes (SS with two a-gene deletions, Hb SC disease, and sickle -β-thalassemia) continue to be vulnerable for relatively milder episodes of splenic sequestration and for splenic infarction or splenic hemorrhage.[133] Severe splenic sequestration that could be life-threatening, however, has been described in adults with SS.[134–137]

The pathophysiologic mechanisms that lead to acute splenic sequestration are not well understood. One possible mechanism is acute obstruction of the venous flow from the spleen with a resultant damming effect associated with sudden enlargement of the spleen due to pooling of RBCs and platelets.[138,139] The acidotic environment of the spleen, due to its sluggish circulation, stimulates sickling, increases viscosity, and contributes to further obstruction of blood flow. Infection can cause more vascular engorgement in addition to rapid acceleration of sickling. Obstruction of venous flow may be related to abnormal rheologic properties of sickle erythrocytes.[140] Moreover, scanning electron microscopy has demonstrated trapping rigid sickle cells in the splenic cords of patients with SS.[141]

Treatment of acute splenic sequestration consists of rapid restoration of intravascular volume and oxygen-carrying capacity. This goal is achieved by the transfusion of sickle-negative RBCs at a rate of 15–20 mL/kg with careful monitoring to avoid sudden overexpansion of blood volume that may precipitate pulmonary edema. After successful treatment, the spleen usually shrinks within a few days and gradually regains its baseline size.

Acute episodes of splenic sequestration tend to recur within a few months to a year after the initial sequestration crisis. Splenectomy has been recommended for patients who survive the initial severe episode.[30] The onset of splenic sequestration correlates with the increased risk for septicemia from *Streptococcus pneumoniae* and *Haemophilus influenza* type b, and it is recommended that all patients with sickle cell syndromes receive pneumococcal and *H. influenza* vaccines. It is important to educate the family about acute splenic sequestration so they can be alert for early symptoms and seek immediate medical intervention. The spleen is the major organ that produces immunoglobulin M (IgM). Patients with autosplenectomy typically have low levels of IgM, a finding that is similar to those patients with anatomic splenectomy.[142]

Hand–Foot Syndrome (Dactylitis)

This acute pain syndrome occurs most commonly in infants and young children between the ages of 6 months and 2 years with a few case reports up to 7 years. The clinical picture is characterized by acute painful swelling of one or more extremities. It is caused by inflammation due to ischemic infarction of the bone of the affected extremity resulting in swelling, redness, and pain in affected areas. Fever and leukocytosis may be present. The episode is usually self-limiting and resolves within 1 week, but recurrent attacks are common. Treatment is symptomatic and if the attack persists, acute osteomyelitis should be ruled out.[64,65]

Priapism

Priapism occurs when sickle cells congest the copra and prevent emptying of blood from the penis. It can result from tricorporal involvement (both of the corpora cavernosa and the corpus spongiosum) or bicorporal involvement (both corpora cavernosa). The latter is more common, especially in children, and is not usually associated with impotence. There are two major clinical presentations of priapism: acute and chronic.[143] The acute presentation is characterized by a prolonged painful erection that persists beyond several hours, responds poorly to exchange transfusion, and frequently requires surgical intervention. Acute priapism may be followed by complete or partial impotence. The chronic form of priapism is characterized by repetitive, reversible, painful erections called "stuttering" priapism. It usually occurs after intercourse or it may awaken patients early in the morning. Stuttering priapism responds well to diazepam or pseudoephedrine. Patients who become impotent may benefit from psychologic counseling and the insertion of penile implants. A practical and relatively simple approach to manage outpatients with priapism has been recently reported.[105] Specifically, aspiration of the corpora cavernosa followed by irrigation with a dilute epinephrine solution was effective in producing detumescence in most patients. Patients who do not respond to this approach are potential candidates for exchange transfusion and/or surgery.[128]

An association between priapism, leg ulceration, nitric oxide resistance, pulmonary hypertension, and death was reported by Kato et al.[144] The hallmark of this association seems to be an elevated level of LDH, a marker of hyperhemolysis.

Acute Multiorgan Failure

This is a catastrophic life-threatening complication of SCD in the context of acute sickle cell painful crisis that may even occur in patients with otherwise mild SCD.[145,146] Fever, rapid decrease in hemoglobin level and platelet count, nonfocal encephalopathy, and rhabdomyolysis are associated with acute multiorgan failure (AMF). Prompt and aggressive simple blood transfusion or blood exchange transfusion could be life saving with rapid recovery of organ failure in most cases. AMF may occur in patients with a history of relatively mild disease with little or no evidence of

chronic organ damage and may be recurrent. High hemoglobin levels in the steady state may be a predisposing factor.

Differential diagnosis of AMF includes ACS and drug overdose. AMF is initially heralded by a rapid fall in hemoglobin and platelet counts from baseline. Aspartate aminotransferase (AST), ALT, total and direct bilirubin, serum creatinine, and creatine phosphokinase are elevated by the third or fourth day of an acute sickle cell painful crisis.

CHRONIC SICKLE CELL PAIN

There are two types of chronic sickle cell pain: chronic pain due to obvious pathology (leg ulcers and avascular necrosis) and intractable chronic pain with no obvious objective signs.

Avascular Necrosis

Avascular necrosis (also called ischemic necrosis or osteonecrosis) is the most commonly observed complication of SCD after the number of painful crises in adults. Although it tends to be most severe and disabling in the hip area, it is a generalized bone disorder in that the femoral and humeral heads as well as the vertebral bodies may be equally affected. Figure 57.9 shows a "fish mouth" or step-like depression seen in some patients with SCD and is probably caused by avascular necrosis or infarction of the central portion of the vertebral body and may lead to vertebral collapse.[64] The limited terminal arterial blood supply and the paucity of collateral circulation make these three areas especially vulnerable to sickling and subsequent bone damage. Patients with SS and α-gene deletion have a higher incidence of avascular necrosis because the relatively high hematocrit increases blood viscosity and thus, enhances microvasculopathy in the aforementioned an-

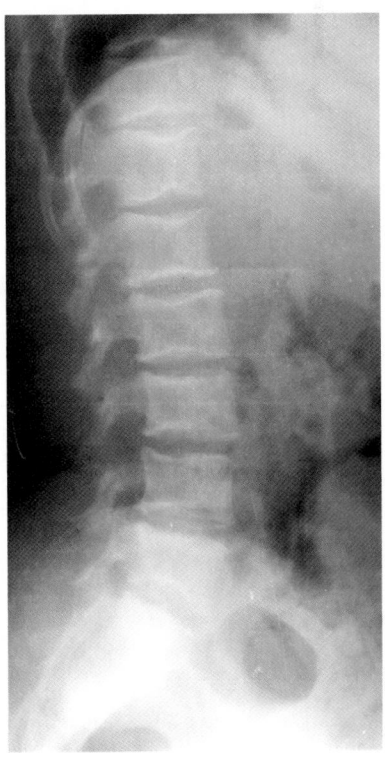

FIGURE 57.9 "Step-like" or "fish mouth" deformity of the lumbar vertebrae of a patient with SS. (Ballas SK. Sickle cell pain. *Progress in Pain Research and Management.* Vol. 11. Seattle, WA: IASP Press; 1998, with permission.)

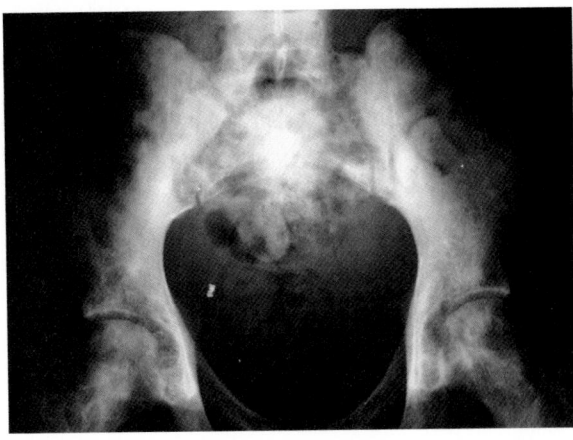

FIGURE 57.10 Avascular necrosis of the femoral head in SCD. Sickle cell pain. (Ballas SK. Sickle cell pain. *Progress in Pain Research and Management.* Vol. 11. Seattle, WA: IASP Press; 1998, with permission.)

atomic sites.[147,148] The MCV and AST levels are negatively correlated with vascular necrosis.[148]

Figure 57.10 shows an example of the radiologic picture of avascular necrosis of the hips in sickle cell disease. Ficat et al.[149] proposed a four-stage radiographic classification as summarized in Table 57.10. Knowing the stage of the disease is important in choosing the most appropriate therapeutic approach. At the time of diagnosis of avascular necrosis, 47.4% of the patients showed stage II disease, 29.6% showed stage III, and 23% showed stage IV.[148]

Medical treatment of avascular necrosis is symptomatic and includes providing nonopioid and/or opioid analgesics for pain relief as well as physical therapy. Advanced forms of the disease (stage III or IV) require total bone replacement. Core decompression in the management of avascular necrosis appears to be effective if done in the early stages of avascular necrosis.[150] This, however, was not supported by a prospective randomized multicenter study comparing physical therapy alone with core decompression and physical therapy for femoral head avascular necrosis in 46 patients with SCD.[151] Physical therapy alone appeared to be as effective as hip core decompression followed by

physical therapy in improving hip function and postponing the need for additional surgical intervention at a mean of 3 years of treatment. Results of hip arthroplasty in patients with SS are not as encouraging as results of arthroplasty performed for arthritic hip.[152] Placement of an internal prosthesis may be difficult owing to the presence of hard sclerotic bone in patients with SCD. Other problems associated with hip arthroplasty in these patients include an increased incidence of infection,[153,154] a failure rate of about 50%, and a high morbidity due to loosening of both cemented and uncemented prostheses. Recent techniques of arthroplasty may improve the life expectancy of hip prostheses.[155]

Leg Ulcers

Leg ulceration is a painful and sometimes disabling complication of SS that occurs in 5% to 10% of adult patients. The most common site for the appearance of leg ulcers is the distal third of the leg, especially on the inner area, just above the ankle and over the medial malleoli (Fig. 57.11). Ulceration involves the skin and underlying tissues of the involved areas. The deeper the ulcer, the more severe. Leg ulcers are classified into stages depending on their depth and net surface area (Table 57.11). Severe pain may necessitate the use of opioid analgesics. Leg ulcers are more common in males and older patients, and less common in patients with α-gene deletion, high total Hb level, or high levels of Hb F.[24] Leg ulcers seem to be more common in patients who are also carriers of the CAR β-gene cluster haplotype.[156] As was mentioned earlier, leg ulceration can be associated with priapism, pulmonary hypertension, and death in a subtype of SCD characterized by high levels of LDH as a marker of hyperhemolysis.

Treatment of leg ulcers includes wound care using wet to dry dressings soaked in saline or Burow's solution. With aggressive daily localized treatment, many ulcers heal within a few months. Leg ulcers that persist beyond 6 months may require blood transfusion or skin grafting, although results of the latter treatment have been disappointing. Because leg ulcers may recur after minimal trauma, protective stockings or leggings with nonelastic (special Velcro) lower-extremity orthoses with ankle straps, to be worn during working hours, appears to be an effective preventative measure.[157] Principles of management include education, protection, infection control, débridement, and compression bandages. Débridement may be achieved surgically or medically

---

TABLE 57.10

RADIOLOGICAL CLASSIFICATION OF AVASCULAR NECROSIS

Imaging findings		Clinical symptoms
Stage I	Normal plain radiograph Normal CT Abnormal MRI with marrow and bone necrosis	Usually no pain
Stage II	Sclerosis and lytic areas on radiography Necrosis on CT and MRI	Pain not always present
Stage III	Flattening of femoral head, widening of the joint space and cresent sign on radiograph. Cresent sign on MRI	Pain present especially with weight bearing, relieved with rest.
Stage IV	Collapse of the femoral head and narrowing of the joint space; osteoarthritis	Pain at rest, joint stiffness and weakness, secondary arthritis

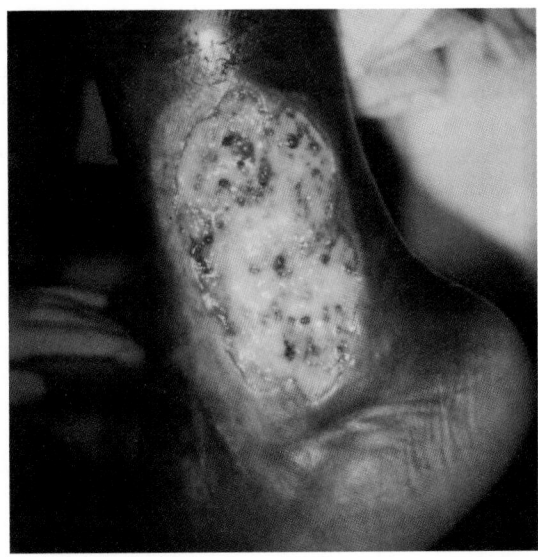
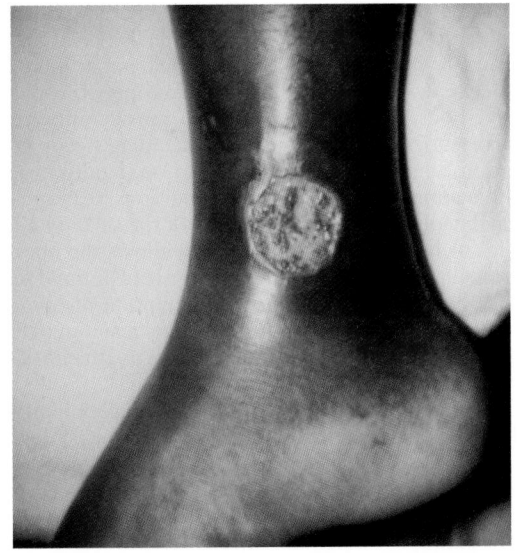

A   B

FIGURE 57.11 Leg ulcers in a patient with SS. (Ballas SK. Sickle cell pain. *Progress in Pain Research and Management*. Vol. 11. Seattle, WA: IASP Press; 1998, with permission.)

by using agents, such as a papain/urea/chlorophyllin ointment (Panafil), that facilitate débridement by enzymatic digestion of necrotic tissue. The efficacy of blood transfusion or exchange transfusion, hyperbaric oxygen, and skin grafting is anecdotal. Recent advances in management include the use of platelet-derived growth factor, prepared either autologously (Procuren), or by recombinant technology (Regranex) and the use of cultured skin grafts.

The relationship between leg ulcers in patients with SS and hydroxyurea is not clear. Early reports[158] suggested that hydroxyurea seems to have a salutary effect on leg ulcers. Recent reports[159] indicated that that hydroxyurea used in treatment of myeloproliferative disorders is associated with increased incidence of leg ulcers. To date, there is no evidence whether hydroxyurea is beneficial or harmful in the management of leg ulcers in patients with SS. Ferster and colleagues[160] recently reported their experience with a group of 93 children and young adults with SCD treated with hydroxyurea for a median follow-up of 3.5 years. Leg ulcers did not complicate the clinical picture of these patients.

TABLE 57.11

STAGES OF THE SEVERITY OF LEG ULCERATION

Stage 1: Nonblanchable erythema of intact skin; the heralding lesion of skin ulceration. In individuals with darker skin, discoloration of the skin, warmth, edema, induration, or hardness may also be indicators.

Stage 2: Partial thickness skin loss involving epidermis, dermis, or both. The ulcer is superficial and presents clinically as an abrasion, blister, or shallow crater.

Stage 3: Full thickness skin loss involving damage to or necrosis of subcutaneous tissue that may extend down to, but not through, underlying fascia. The ulcer presents clinically as a deep crater with or without undermining of adjacent tissue.

Stage 4: Full thickness skin loss with extensive destruction, tissue necrosis, or damage to muscle, bone, or supporting structures (e.g., tendon, joint capsule). Undermining and sinus tracts may also be present.

Chronic Pain Without Objective Signs

The second type of chronic pain in SCD is intractable chronic pain without obvious pathology where the only complaint is the patient's self-report of unremitting pain. Failure to treat recurrent severe acute painful crises aggressively, extensive surgery, or severe emotional stress may all contribute to the development of an intractable chronic pain syndrome. The pathophysiology of this transition is not well understood. Possibilities include recruitment and activation of dormant afferent nerve fibers that transmit stimuli and result in "central sensitization" whereby the pain threshold is lowered to a degree that ambient innocuous events cause severe pain—a condition referred to as allodynia.[64,65,70] Moreover, central sensitization changes the way the brain and nervous system respond to pain; new pathways develop that can lead to the sensation of chronic pain.[70,161] Once chronic pain sets in, it usually becomes independent of the usual inciting events. Nevertheless, chronic pain syndrome continues to be punctuated with superimposed acute painful crises due to vaso-occlusion.

Neuropathic Pain

Neuropathic pain is characterized as burning, tingling, shooting, lancinating, and numbing. These symptoms may occur in the presence or absence of obvious central or peripheral nerve injury. A number of reported neuropathic pain syndromes seem to be associated with, and due to, the disease itself. These include mental nerve neuropathy,[162,163] trigeminal neuralgia,[164] acute proximal median mononeuropathy,[165] entrapment neuropathy,[166] acute demyelinating polyneuropathy,[166] ischemic optic neuropathy,[167] orbital infarction,[168] orbital apex syndrome,[169] and spinal cord infarction.[170]

MANAGEMENT OF SICKLE CELL PAIN

Effective management of sickle cell pain is complex and entails a thorough understanding of the issues that are associated with the treatment of pain in an incurable chronic disease.[64–66,171,172] Major prerequisites for an effective and rational management of sickle cell pain pertain to the patient, the pathophysiology of the disease, the pharmacology of analgesics, and the attitude of the health care providers. A patient is a unique human entity. The more a provider knows the patient, the more effective pain management becomes. Knowledge of the patient should not be limited to age, sex, precise diagnosis, complications, and previous pain management methods. It should also take into consideration the biopsychosocial fabric of the patient's life, including his or her level of education, employment status, occupation, family structure, source of income, ethnicity, housing conditions, fears, religion, beliefs, habits, hobbies, and perception of the severity and prognosis of his or her disease. This approach allows the physician to individualize pain management and avoid unfounded generalizations about patients and their consumption of opioid analgesics. Such generalizations, for instance, may result in oversedation of a patient naïve to opioids, or in undertreatment of a patient too tolerant to them.

Sickle cell pain, like other types of pain, is a complex human experience that is strongly affected not only by pathophysiologic factors but also by psychologic, social, cultural, and spiritual ones. It is, however, consequent to tissue damage generated by the sickling process and occlusion of the microvasculature, as was described in the pathophysiology section. An important aspect of effective management of sickle cell pain is the intent of the care provider. Do the providers in question endeavor to treat patients in an empathetic manner by listening to, respecting, and believing them? Or do they stigmatize them as drug addicts demonstrating drug-seeking behavior and thereby justify the expulsion of some patients from their system?

Perhaps the difficulty of treating sickle cell pain can best be addressed with reference to a clinical anecdote. The patient is a young African American male who makes frequent visits to the ED for painful episodes and is labeled as an addict. The connection of the disease with race results in many ramifications that impact on care. Disparities in care arise because of the wide cultural gulf between health care providers who are predominantly white and the predominantly black patient group.[172–175] Communication and stereotyping complicate pain assessment and treatment. Frequent flyers in the ED often become labeled as drug seekers, regardless of their diagnosis or the chronicity of their disease. Concerns about addiction are justified in the SCD population since these patients carry many associated risks, including disease chronicity and dismal prognosis, comorbid psychiatric disease including depression and anxiety, young age, and unremitting pain. Yet the approach needs to be one not of avoiding opioids, but rather recognizing the risk while providing adequate pain management (with opioids if necessary) under controlled conditions that aim to minimize risk.

Nonpharmacologic Management of Pain

Nonpharmacologic management of pain includes cutaneous stimulation (transcutaneous electrical nerve stimulation), heat, cold, and vibration, distraction, relaxation, massage, music, guided imagery, self-hypnosis, self-motivation, acupuncture, and biofeedback. Although there are no well-controlled clinical trials of the efficacy of these methods in the management of sickle cell pain, there are many anecdotal reports of their efficacy in pain management, both by patients and providers.

Pharmacologic Management of Pain

Pharmacologic management of pain includes three major classes of compounds: nonopioids, opioids, and adjuvants.[64,65,171] Nonopioids include acetaminophen, NSAIDs, topical agents, and corticosteroids. Most clinically useful opioid analgesics are agonists at the mu-opioid receptor, although the mixed agonist/antagonist buprenorphine and the partial agonist pentazocine have achieved some popularity, especially in Europe. Adjuvants commonly used

in the management of sickle cell pain include antihistamines, benzodiazepines, antidepressants, anticonvulsants, and phenothiazines. Aspects of these pharmacologic agents that pertain to SCD will be discussed here.

Nonopioids and Sickle Cell Disease

Acetaminophen. This drug has been implicated in papillary necrosis of the kidney and in hepatoxicity with a dose that exceeds 4 g/day or with the recommended dose in patients with liver disease.[176–178] Since patients with SCD are at risk for renal and hepatic complications, the dosage given to them and their renal and hepatic functions have to be monitored carefully.

NSAIDs. These drugs are well-tolerated by most patients. Care has to be taken if the patients are sensitive to them, if the renal function is impaired, and if the patient has pulmonary complications, especially ACS. NSAIDs should not be given to patients with impaired renal function. NSAIDs occasionally cause bronchospasm and may worsen or precipitate ACS.[178]

Opioids and Sickle Cell Disease

Depending on point of view, opioids may be considered first-line treatment for severe acute sickle cell pain. There is certainly no alternative to opioids for the treatment of severe pain, although nonopioid and nonmedical treatments should be added whenever possible as opioid-sparing adjuncts. Specific considerations for choice of opioid in SCD patients are outlined here.

Meperdine. This should be avoided whenever possible. If it has to be given, the dose has to be adjusted in the presence of abnormal renal function, and the patient has to be monitored for early signs of neurotoxicity such as myoclonus, tremors, and hyper-excitability.[64,65]

Morphine. The major metabolite of morphine (6-morphine glucuronide) is excreted in the kidney. Accordingly, the dose of morphine has to be monitored in the presence of renal failure. Other recently reported side effects of morphine include increased risk of ACS in patients with SCD,[179,180] acceleration of renal injury,[181] and retinopathy[182] in transgenic sickle mice. In a retrospective study of hospitalized children with SCD, Buchanan et al.[180] reported that patients on morphine were more likely to develop ACS and had longer hospital stays than patients receiving nalbuphine hydrochloride (Nubain).

Methadone. Methadone is associated with several potential toxicities, including cardiotoxicity due to prolongation of the QTc interval with arrhythmia that could be fatal. In treating sickle cell pain with methadone, the provider should follow the adage "start low and go slow." Most reported fatalities due to methadone are due to overaggressive introduction of methadone to patients who have never before received the drug. This is a reflection of the drug's unusual and unpredictable pharmacokinetics. Another important point in using methadone is to be aware of the side effects of other drugs used in combination with methadone. Patients with SCD often receive antibiotics or antidepressants which also prolong the QTc interval. The EKG of such patients should be carefully monitored.[70,161]

Adjuvants and Sickle Cell Disease

Antidepressants that are known to cause priapism should not be used in patients with history of priapism. These include trazodone, selective serotonin reuptake inhibitors, and tricyclic antidepressants in decreasing order of risk to cause priapism.[70,161]

Pain Management of Outpatients[64,65,171]

Management of patients with SCD as outpatients in the clinic or office is extremely important and is the basis on which future treatments and interventions are based. Patients should be followed by the same providers in order to maintain continuity of care. The most important aspect of outpatient management is in the collection of baseline data that include detailed medical history, physical exam, known complications, medications, and comprehensive laboratory data. Management of exacerbations in the ED or in the hospital depends heavily on knowing the steady state parameters of the patient in question. As was mentioned earlier, a steady state is a point in time in the history of a patient that is not preceded by an acute painful episode or comorbid conditions for at least 1 month or more and that is not associated with blood transfusion within the previous 3–4 months. It is highly desirable that patients be seen and evaluated in the office or clinic by a social worker and a psychologist or psychiatrist. It is in the outpatient setup that details of care in general and in the ED, day unit, and hospital in particular are explained and discussed. The pros and cons of all medications the patient is taking will be reviewed. Prescriptions will be given as needed. Vaccines will be administered when required.

Treatment of sickle cell pain as a chronic pain condition using round the clock long-acting opioids has been advocated by some clinicians.[183,184] They claim that such regimens stabilize the disease, reduce the number and frequency of acute exacerbations and crises, reduce ED visits, and reduce length of hospital stay.

In the outpatient setting, patients should be empowered to cope with their disease and be authorities on its manifestations that apply to them individually. This includes education about SCD, its genetic basis, inheritance and family counseling; adherence to regular schedule of medical follow-up; avoidance of situations that exert an adverse effect on their disease and adoption of those activities of daily living that are beneficial to them; knowing their rights and responsibilities as patients with SCD when dealing with care providers, medical facilities, and the workplace; and participation in local support groups and communication with community leaders and advocates.

Management and follow-up of outpatients in the office and clinic should culminate in an individualized treatment plan for each patient. Such a plan should summarize pertinent aspects of the medical history, physical exam, laboratory data, complications, and treatment plans as outpatients, in the day unit, emergency room, and the hospital. In some places, the treatment plan may be transformed into an identification card to be carried by the patient and presented to case provider as needed.[185]

Pain Management in the Day Unit

The major advantage of treating sickle cell painful crisis in the day unit (or day hospital) is that the patients do not have to wait for a long time before they receive treatment.[186] In the day unit, analgesic therapy is usually initiated within 15–20 minutes after arrival to the unit. Adult patients are admitted to the day unit if they have an uncomplicated painful crisis based on inclusion and exclusion criteria protocol. After thorough assessment, treatment is initiated with IV hydration and a loading dose of opioid analgesic followed by assessment within 30 minutes. After the initial assessment, the patient may be medicated with 25% to 75% of the loading dose of opioid analgesic depending on the level of pain relief and sedation. The patient's vital signs are assessed every 30 minutes for the first 2 hours of treatment, and then hourly thereafter. If the respiratory rate falls below 10 breaths per minute, systolic blood pressure below 90 mm Hg, and/or sedation, the opioid is withheld and the patient is closely monitored. The duration of treatment usually lasts an average of 6 hours.

Pain Management in the Emergency Department[64,65,171]

Treatment of acute sickle cell painful episodes in the ED follows similar principles of thorough assessment, treatment with analgesics/adjuvants, coordination of cure, monitoring, outcome, and disposition.

The major problem in the ED is the length of waiting time to initial analgesia, which could be up to several hours. Needless to say, waiting while in pain constitutes a stressful situation that could worsen the painful crises and render it no longer amenable to resolution and discharge from the ED, but to hospital admission. Many EDs are in the process of determining and implementing strategies that could shorten the time to initial treatment.

Specific treatment in the ED should be based on the history or the computerized version of the treatment plan, if available. Usually, analgesics are given individually every 2 hours for a total of three doses. Adjuvants may also be given intravenously or orally as needed. If the pain is resolved or reduced to a level with which the patient is comfortable, the patient is discharged with instructions for follow-up by the primary care physician and/or hematologist. Otherwise, the patient will be admitted to the hospital.

Management of Sickle Cell Pain in the Hospital[64,65,171,187]

Prerequisites for rational management of the acute sickle cell painful crisis in the hospital include knowledge of the patient, knowledge of the nature of sickle cell pain, and knowledge of the pharmacology of analgesics in general and opioids in particular. To that end, it is desirable to have patients with crises admitted to the care of providers (preferably hematologists) who are familiar with these prerequisites and with the principles of pain management. Patient-controlled analgesia (PCA) is a useful method of delivering opioid analgesics in hospitalized patients.[187] Successful management of the acute painful crisis in the hospital should include the following steps:

- Multidimensional assessment to determine the location of pain, its intensity, its quality, precipitating factors, modifying factors, triggers, and to determine mood, relief, and sedation. A major component of assessment is to listen and believe the patient without a judgmental attitude.
- Choice of analgesics (opioids/nonopioids), adjuvants, and hydration, if needed; such choices are individualized based upon the past medical history and the assessment of the patient in question. If the acute painful episode is superimposed on chronic pain for which the patient is taking long-acting/controlled-release opioids with short-acting opioids for breakthrough pain, keep the long-acting/controlled-release opioids the same and discontinue the oral short-acting ones.
- Determination of the route and method of administration of short-acting analgesics. These, again, should be individualized; parenteral analgesics are usually administered either on a fixed schedule or via a PCA pump.
- Titration of the dose of analgesics to achieve relief with which the patient is comfortable.
- Maintenance of the dose that achieves adequate relief. Consider opioid rotation (i.e., change the opioid chosen) initially to an equianalgesic or lower dose of a different opioid if the first opioid does not achieve or maintain relief.
- Plan to treat breakthrough pain, neuropathic pain, and side effects of the crisis or the analgesics, if present.
- Tapering the dose of analgesics once the patient uses the PCA pump less frequently or the intensity of pain decreases by two or more points.
- Gradual switching to oral analgesics using tables of equianalgesic dose as an initial guide. One example would be to decrease the parenteral dose by 25% and replace it with an equianalgesic oral dose. The latter should be adjusted according to its effect to achieve pain relief with which the patient is comfortable.
- Prevention of withdrawal by using either clonidine patch or methadone.
- Plan for discharge and follow-up.

Details of these steps may vary among patients, providers, and institutions. It should be emphasized that desirable outcome of management of the acute painful crisis in the hospital depends on early and aggressive treatment of pain without delay, avoidance of hasty and premature discharge from the hospital, and having a plan for follow-up after discharge, preferably within a week or less.

Specific Approaches to Treatment

There are five approaches to the treatment of SCD: supportive therapy, symptomatic treatment, preventative therapy, abortive therapy, and curative therapy (Table 57.12). Most important among these that have the potential to ameliorate or cure the disease include Hb F induction, RBC rehydration, bone marrow/stem cell transplantation, and gene therapy.

It has been the hope of patients with SCD, their families, and providers that there will be therapy that will either cure or markedly alter the natural history of this disease. With better understanding of the pathology of SCD and coordination of multiple therapies that attack different pathologic mechanisms of the disease, this goal seems likely. Although the long-term safety and efficacy of these novel therapies have not been well studied, there is good potential for at least some of them to achieve the desired goal.

Induction of Hb F. High levels of Hb F have a beneficial effect in patients with SS. Platt et al.[21] has shown that there is a significant inverse correlation between the frequency of painful crises and Hb F levels greater than 4% (i.e., the higher the Hb F, the milder the disease). Hb F interferes with the polymerization of sickle Hb and the higher (and the more pancellular) it is, the lower the intracellular concentration of sickle Hb. However, there are exceptions to this rule in that there are patients with high Hb F levels and severe disease and vice versa.

Agents that have been shown to increase the level of Hb F in humans are listed in Table 57.13. Among these, hydroxyurea as monotherapy seems to be the least toxic and most effective.[80,81,188] Moreover, hydroxyurea is the only drug studied for

---

TABLE 57.13

AGENTS THAT AUGMENT FETAL HEMOGLOBIN PRODUCTION

Cell-cycle specific agents
Azacytidine
Cytosine arabinoside
Myleran
Hydroxyurea
Decitabine

Short chain fatty acids
Arginine butyrate—IV
Isobutyramide—PO
Phenylacetate—PO
    Phenylbutyrate—PO
    Valproic acid—PO

Recombinant human erythropoietin (rHuEPO) combination therapy
Hydroxyurea + rHuEPO
Other combinations

IV, intravenous; PO, oral
From Ballas SK. Sickle cell anemia. *Drugs* 2002;62:1165, with permission.

---

efficacy in a relatively large scale, placebo-controlled, randomized clinical trial. All the other agents listed in Table 57.13 have been reported anecdotally to increase Hb F levels. None of the others was used in a controlled phase III clinical trial to date.

Hydroxyurea is a cell-cycle specific cytotoxic agent that inhibits ribonucleotide reductase. The molecular mechanism(s) by which hydroxyurea increases the production of Hb F is (are) unknown. Possible mechanisms include perturbations in cellular kinetics and/or recovery from cytotoxicity, recruitment of early erythroid progenitors and recruitment of primitive erythroid progenitors (BFU-E) that lead to production of Hb F-containing reticulocytes (F-reticulocytes). Long-term hydroxyurea therapy with the maximum tolerated dose (mean dose 21.3 mg/kg) with respect to myelosuppression raises Hb F by as much as 15% to 20% (mean 14.9%, range 1.9% to 26.3%).

In the randomized, placebo-controlled, double blind multi-center study of hydroxyurea (MSH) study, among 299 adult patients with SS with three or more painful crises per year, hydroxyurea resulted in a significant ($p < 0.001$) reduction in the incidence of painful crises, ACS, and transfusion requirement.[80,81] Hydroxyurea improved the quality of life of the patients taking it.[189] There was no difference between the placebo and hydroxyurea arms in the incidence of death, stroke, or hepatic sequestration. Maximum tolerated doses of hydroxyurea were not required to reduce the incidence of painful episodes. Although an increase in Hb F seems to be the obvious and logical explanation for the salutary effects of hydroxyurea, other reasons for its beneficial effects include changes in RBC volume, cellular hydration, the cell membrane, and a direct effect on endothelial cells.

Follow-up of patients who continued to take hydroxyurea after the termination of the MSH study had less mortality than those who did not take hydroxyurea.[190] Adverse effects of hydroxyurea are listed in Table 57.14. Toxic effects are dose- and time-dependent. Careful monitoring of blood counts every 2 weeks after starting hydroxyurea can prevent these. Later, the frequency of monitoring of blood counts and blood chemistries can be decreased to once every 1 to 2 months once the patient is in a stable condition and receiving an acceptable maintenance dose. Anemia is a rare toxic effect of hydroxyurea; in fact, in the MSH study, most patients who took hydroxyurea experienced

---

TABLE 57.12

CURRENT APPROACHES TO MANAGEMENT OF SICKLE CELL DISEASE

  I. Supportive therapy
     Folic acid
     Immunization (Adults)
     Psychologic support

 II. Symptomatic treatment
     Analgesia/adjuvants for pain
     Blood transfusion
     Antibiotics
     Surgery

III. Preventative therapy
     Prophylactic antibiotics (infants and children)
     Immunizations (infants and children)
     Avoidance of known precipitating factors
     Hb F induction (Hydroxyurea)
       Purified poloxamer 188
     RBC rehydration (investigational)

IV. Abortive therapy
     ? Nitric oxide

 V. Curative therapy
     Transplantation
     Bone marrow, stem cells, cord blood
     Gene therapy (experimental, transgenic mice)

TABLE 57.14

SIDE EFFECTS OF HYDROXYUREA

Toxic side effects
Myelosuppression
Leukopenia
Thrombocytopenia
Anemia

Idiosyncratic adverse effects
Nausea
Vomiting
Pruritus
Skin rash
Hair loss
Leg ulcers

Effects reported in animals
Carcinogenesis
Teratogenesis

Long-term effects
Unknown

Adapted from Ballas SK. Sickle cell anemia. *Drugs* 2002;62:1155, with permission.

an increase in their Hb levels. It is unfortunate to note that it seems that hydroxyurea is underutilized in the treatment of patients with SS. There may be many patients who meet the criteria for treatment with hydroxyurea but are not receiving it.[191] The idiosyncratic effects of hydroxyurea occur in some patients but not others. However, the incidence of these effects was similar between the placebo and hydroxyurea in the MSH study.[80] In animal studies, hydroxyurea had carcinogenic and teratogenic effects.[192–194] To date, however, no carcinogenic effect has been reported in patients with polycythemia vera and erythrocytosis due to congenital heart disease treated with hydroxyurea.[195,196]

The following limitations should be considered when using hydroxyurea to prevent painful crises in patients with SCD. Firstly, hydroxyurea was approved in the United States by the Food and Drug Administration for the prevention of crises in patients with SS and not in other types of SCD. Secondly, the long-term effects of hydroxyurea in patients with SCD are not known and, finally, some patients do not respond to hydroxyurea. Methods to identify these nonresponders are being studied in order to improve the selection process for hydroxyurea therapy. In some patients, combining hydroxyurea with other agents that augment Hb F production may be indicated.

Purified Poloxamer 188 (Flocor)

This is a nonionic surfactant that is thought to reduce blood viscosity and to prevent adhesion of RBCs to vascular endothelium, thus improving microvascular blood flow. It appeared to be a promising agent in preventing or reducing the frequency of acute sickle painful crises. A randomized, double-blind, placebo-controlled, intention-to-treat trial using purified poloxamer 188 (Flocor) was conducted between March 1998 and October 1999 in 40 medical centers in the United States.[197] Two-hundred and fifty-five patients with SCD (ages 9–53) who had a painful episode severe enough to require hospitalization and opioid analgesics for the treatment of pain were enrolled in the study. A decrease in the duration of painful episodes and an increase in the proportion of patients who achieved resolution of the symptoms were observed when the purified poloxamer 188-treated patients were compared with the patients receiving placebo. The differ-

ence between these groups was significant but relatively small. In subgroup analysis, a more significant effect on both parameters was observed in children and patients who were receiving concomitant hydroxyurea. It is important to confirm both of these observations in further prospective trials.

Red Blood Cell Rehydration

Polymerization of deoxy Hb results in cellular dehydration which, in turn, increases the intracellular concentration of sickle Hb that leads to further polymerization, thus creating a vicious cycle. Major mechanisms by which water is lost from sickle cells include the Ca^{2+}-activated K^+ channel (Gardos channel) and the KCl cotransport channel. Activation of these channels result in K^+ and water loss from sickle erythrocytes with consequent dehydration. A decrease in the intracellular concentration of sickle Hb, even small decreases, can slow the polymerization of sickle Hb to a point where RBCs can exit from the capillaries (decreased transit time) before the sickle Hb polymerizes (increased delay time for polymerization). Hydroxyurea achieves this goal by decreasing the effective concentration of sickle Hb and diluting it with Hb F, which does not participate in polymerization. Another approach to inhibit polymerization is to rehydrate sickle RBCs and restore their normal water content.[198,199]

A selective approach to specifically rehydrate sickle RBCs by inhibiting the Gardos pathway has been tried by using oral clotrimazole.[198] In 5 patients treated with 20 mg/kg/day of clotrimazole, the RBC Gardos channel was inhibited, cell K^+ content increased, RBCs were rehydrated, and a very modest increase in hemoglobin levels was noted. The effects of clotrimazole on cellular rehydration, however, were very modest compared with those seen in hydroxyurea. A phase III randomized, double-blind, placebo-controlled trial, however, failed to show that Gardos channel inhibitors decreased the frequency of acute sickle cell painful crisis (unpublished data). Oral magnesium pidolate also reduces RBC dehydration in patients with SCD by inhibiting the KCl cotransport channel.[199] Clinical trials using myasthenia gravis are underway at the present.

Bone Marrow/Stem Cell/Cord Blood Transplantation

Although transplantation therapy was initially limited for children,[9–12] the procedure has been extended to older adolescents and young adults in recent studies. Thus, Panepinto et al.[13] in the United States reported outcomes after myeloablative hematopoietic cell transplantation (HCT) from HLA-matched sibling donors in 67 patients with SCD transplanted between 1989 and 2002. The most common indications for transplantation were stroke and recurrent vaso-occlusive crisis in 38% and 37% of patients, respectively. The median age at transplantation was 10 years (range 2–27 years). Twenty-seven percent of patients had a poor performance score at transplantation. Ninety-four percent received busulfan and cyclophosphamide-containing conditioning regimens, and bone marrow was the predominant source of donor cells. Most patients achieved hematopoietic recovery, and no deaths occurred during the early posttransplant period. Rates of acute and chronic graft-versus-host disease (GVHD) were 10% and 22%, respectively. Sixty-four of 67 patients are alive with 5-year probabilities of disease-free and overall survival of 85% and 97%, respectively. Nine patients had graft failure with recovery of sickle erythropoiesis, 8 of whom had recurrent sickle-related events.

Similarly, Bermaudin et al.[14] from France reported outcomes of related myeloablative stem cell transplantation from HLA-matched sibling donors in 87 consecutive patients (2–27 years old) with severe SCD between November 1988 and December 2004. Cerebral vasculopathy was the principal indication for transplantation in 55 patients (63%). All the patients received grafts from a sibling donor after a myeloablative conditioning regimen (CR). The only change in the CR during the study period was the introduction of antithymocyte globulin (ATG) in March 1992. The rejection rate was 22.6% before the use of ATG, but 3% thereafter. With a median follow-up of 6 years (range, 2.0 to 17.9 years), the overall and event free survival (EFS) rate were 93.1% and 86.1%, respectively. GVHD was the main cause of transplantation related mortality (TRM). Importantly, cord blood transplant recipients did not develop GVHD. No new ischemic lesions were detected after engraftment, and cerebral velocities were significantly reduced. The outcome improved significantly with time: the EFS rate among the 44 patients receiving transplants after January 2000 was 95.3%.

These studies confirm and extend earlier reports that HCT from HLA-matched related donors after myeloablative conditioning (especially with ATG) offer a very high survival rate, with few transplant-related complications and the elimination of sickle-related complications in the majority of patients who undergo this therapy.

Gene Therapy

Gene therapy, in simple terms, is the introduction of new genes into healthy or abnormal cells either in vitro or in vivo. Gene therapy in SS is limited at present to investigational laboratory procedures and the use of transgenic mouse models to determine the most effective and safest method of altering the genetic information in hematopoietic stem cells.[200] Research in this area has advanced at a faster rate than previously expected, and gene therapy may be available for trial in selected patients with sickle cell disease in the near future.

CONCLUSION

SCD is an inherited disorder of hemoglobin structure that has no established cure in adults at the present. Cure has been achieved in selected patients with bone marrow/stem cell/cord blood transplantation from HLA-matched donors in the majority of cases after myeloablative conditioning regimen.

SCD is almost synonymous with pain, and the acute sickle cell painful crisis is the insignia or hallmark and the number one cause of hospitalization. Advances in the pathophysiology of SCD focused on the sequence of events that occur between polymerization of deoxy hemoglobin S and vaso-occlusion. Adhesion of sickle RBCs to endothelial cells, cellular dehydration, inflammatory response, reperfusion injury, and tissue damage appear to be important pathophysiologic events that culminate in the perception of pain.

The acute sickle cell painful crisis evolves along four phases: prodromal, initial, established, and resolving phases. Several clinical and laboratory changes occur during the painful crisis provided the findings are compared to well-established baseline data. The resolving acute painful crisis may culminate in a hypercoagulable state that could precipitate another crisis in some patients. Hospital readmission seems to occur within 1 week in about 16% of patients after discharge from the hospital.

Serious and potentially fatal complications of SCD such as ACS and AMF occur within 3 or 4 days after the onset of an acute crisis, Other types of acute sickle pain include priapism, dactylitis, hepatic crisis, and splenic sequestration.

Chronic pain and neuropathic pain do occur in SCD, and their pathophysiologic events and management are similar in other types of chronic pain. Although management of SS continues to be primarily palliative in nature, there have been promising preventative and curative approaches to therapy. Pain management should be individualized and coupled with the proper utilization of opioid and nonopioid analgesics in order to achieve adequate pain relief. Early recognition and treatment of organ failure minimizes morbidity and improves outcome. The use of hydroxyurea decreases the morbidity and mortality of SCD. Cure

is possible in selected children and young adults with bone marrow or cord blood transplantation. Future research seems to focus on refining the molecular and cellular approaches to therapy including gene therapy and mechanisms that rehydrate sickle RBCs and/or prevent their adhesion to vascular endothelium.

References

1. Konotey–Ahulu FID. *The Sickle Cell Disease Patient*. London: Macmillan; 1991.
2. Herrick JB. Peculiar elongated and sickle-shaped red blood corpuscles in a case of severe anemia. *Arch Intern Med* 1910;6:517–521.
3. Mason VR. Sickle cell anemia. *JAMA* 1922;79:1318–1320.
4. Diggs LW. Sickle cell crisis. *Am J Clin Pathol* 1965;44:1–19.
5. Pauling L, Itano HA, Singer SJ, et al. Sickle cell anemia, a molecular disease. *Science* 1949;110:543–548.
6. Neel JV. The inheritance of the sickling phenomenon with particular reference to sickle cell disease. *Blood* 1951;6:389–412.
7. Ingram VM. A specific chemical difference between the globins of normal human and sickle-cell anemia haemoglobin. *Nature* 1956;178:792–794.
8. Steinberg MH. Predicting clinical severity in sickle cell anaemia. *Br J Haematology* 2005;129:465–481.
9. Walters MC, Patience M, Leisenring W, et al. Bone marrow transplantation for sickle cell disease. *N Engl J Med* 1996;335:369–376.
10. Gore L, Lane PA, Quinones RR, et al. Successful cord blood transplantation for sickle cell anemia from a sibling who is human leukocyte antigen-identical: implications for comprehensive care. *J Pediatr Hematol Oncol* 2000;22: 437–440.
11. Adamkiewicz TV, Mehta PS, Boyer MW, et al. Transplantation of unrelated placental blood cells in children with high-risk sickle cell disease. *Bone Marrow Transplant* 2004;34:405–411.
12. Mazur M, Kurtzberg J, Halperin E, et al. Transplantation of a child with sickle cell anemia with an unrelated cord blood unit after reduced intensity conditioning. *J Pediatr Hematol Oncol* 2006;28:840–844.
13. Panepinto JA, Walters MC, Carreras J, et al. Matched-related donor transplantation for sickle cell disease: report from the Center for International Blood and Transplant Research. *Br J Haematol* 2007;137:479–485.
14. Bernaudin F, Soccie G, Kuentz M, et al. Long-term results of related myeloablative stem-cell transplantation to cure sickle cell disease. *Blood* 2007; 110:2749.
15. Ingram VM. Gene mutations in human haemoglobin: the chemical difference between normal and sickle cell haemoglobin. *Nature* 1975;180:326–328.
16. Steinberg MH, Embury SH. Thalassemia in blacks: genetic and clinical aspects and interactions with the sickle hemoglobin gene. *Blood* 1986;68:985–990.
17. Pagnier J, Mears JG, Dunda–Belkodja O, et al. Evidence for the multicentric origin of the sickle cell hemoglobin gene in Africa. *Proc Natl Acad Sci U S A* 1984;81:1771–1773.
18. Powars DR. Sickle cell anemia βˢ-gene-cluster haplotypes as prognostic indicators of vital organ failure. *Semin Hematol* 1991;28:202–208.
19. Ballas SK, Larner J, Smith ED, et al. Rheological predictors of the severity of the painful sickle cell crisis. *Blood* 1988;72:1216–1223.
20. Baum K, Dun DT, Maude GH, et al. The painful crisis of homozygous sickle cell disease. A study of risk factors. *Arch Intern Med* 1987;147:1231–1234.
21. Platt OS, Thorington BD, Brambilla DJ, et al. Pain in sickle cell disease: rates and risk factors. *N Engl J Med* 1991;325:11–16.
22. Ballas SK, Talacki CA, Rao VM, et al. The prevalence of avascular necrosis in sickle cell anemia: correlation with alpha-thalassemia. *Hemoglobin* 1989; 13:649–655.
23. Milner PF, Kraus AP, Sebes JL, et al. Sickle cell disease as a cause of osteonecrosis of the femoral head. *N Engl J Med* 1991;325:1476–1481.
24. Koshy M, Entsuah R, Koranda A, et al. Leg ulcers in patients with sickle cell disease. *Blood* 1989;75:1403–1408.
25. Ballas SK, Gay RN, Chehab FF. Is Hb A2 elevated in adults with sickle-α-thalassemia (Bˢ/Bˢ; −α/−α)? *Hemoglobin* 1997;21:405–420.
26. Steinberg MH, Hsu H, Nagel RL, et al. Gender and haplotype effects upon hematological manifestations of adult sickle cell anemia. *Am J Hematol* 1995; 48:175–181.
27. Ballas SK, Branden Z. Misinterpretation of pain escalation in an adult patient with sickle cell anemia defers accurate diagnosis. *Pain Digest* 1997;7: 208–210.
28. Boros L, Thomas C, Weiner WJ. Large cerebral vessel disease in sickle cell anemia. *J Neurol Neurosurg Psychiatry* 1976;39:1236–1239.
29. Powars ER, Wilson B, Imbus C, et al. The natural history of stroke in sickle cell disease. *Am J Med* 1978;65:461–471.
30. Serjeant GR, Serjeant BE. *Sickle Cell Disease*. 3rd ed. New York: Oxford University Press; 2001.
31. Embury SH, Hebbel RP, Mohandas N, et al, eds. *Sickle Cell Disease: Basic Principles and Clinical Picture*. New York: Raven Press; 1994.
32. Powars DR. Sickle cell anemia and major organ failure. *Hemoglobin* 1990; 14:573–598.
33. Hebbel RP. Beyond hemoglobin polymerization: the red blood cell membrane and sickle disease pathophysiology. *Blood* 1991;77:214–237.

34. Francis RB, Johnson CS. Vascular occlusion in sickle cell disease: current concepts and unanswered questions. *Blood* 1991;77:1404–1405.

35. Brugnara C, Bunn HF, Tosteson DC. Regulation of erythrocytes cation and water content in sickle cell anemia. *Science* 1986;232:388–390.

36. Joiner CH. Cation transport and volume regulation in sickle red blood cells. *Am J Physiol* 1993;264(2 pt 1):C251–C270.

37. Mueller BU, Brugnara C. Prevention of red cell dehydration: a possible new treatment for sickle cell disease. *Pediatr Pathol Mol Med* 2001;20:15–25.

38. Lew VL, Freeman CJ, Ortiz OE, et al. A mathematical model of the volume, pH and ion content regulation in reticulocytes: application to the pathophysiology of sickle cell dehydration. *J Clin Invest* 1991;87:100–112.

39. Brugnara C, Kopin AS, Bunn HF, et al. Regulation of cation content and cell volume in hemoglobin erythrocytes from patients with homozygous hemoglobin C disease. *J Clin Invest* 1985;75:1608–1617.

40. Brugnara C. Inhibition of K transport by divalent cations in sickle erythrocytes. *Blood* 1987;70:1810–1815.

41. Brugnara C, Gee B, Armsby CC, et al. Therapy with oral clotrimazole induces inhibition of the Gardos channel and reduction of erythrocyte dehydration in patients with sickle cell disease. *J Clin Invest* 1996;97:1227–1234.

42. Lew VL, Hockaday A, Sepulveda MI, et al. Compartment of sickle cell calcium in endocytic inside-out vesicles. *Nature* 1985;315:586–588.

43. Rhoda MD, Apova M, Beuzard Y, et al. Compartmentation of Ca^{2+} in sickle cells. *Cell Calcium* 1985;6:397–411.

44. Rubin E, Schlegal RA, Williamson P. Endocytosis in sickle erythrocytes: a mechanism for elevated intracellular Ca^{2+} levels. *J Cell Physiol* 1986;126:53–59.

45. Hebbel RP, Boogaerts MAB, Eaton JW, et al. Erythrocyte adherence to endothelium in sickle cell anemia: a possible determinant of disease severity. *N Engl J Med* 1980;302:992–995.

46. Hebbel RP, Yamada O, Moldow CF, et al. Abnormal adherence of sickle cell erythrocytes to cultured vascular endothelium: possible mechanism for microvascular occlusion in sickle cell disease. *J Clin Invest* 1980;65:154–160.

47. Hoover R, Rubin R, Wise G, et al. Adhesion of normal and sickle erythrocytes to endothelial monolayer cultures. *Blood* 1979;54:872–876.

48. Barbarino GA, McIntire LV, Eskin SG, et al. Rheological studies of erythrocyte-endothelial cell interactions in sickle cell disease. *Prog Clin Biol Res* 1987;240:113–127.

49. Fabry ME, Kaul DK. Sickle cell vaso-occlusion. *Hematol Oncol Clin North Am* 1991;5:375–398.

50. Kaul DK, Fabry ME, Costantini F, et al. In vivo demonstration of red cell-endothelial interaction, sickling and altered microvascular response to oxygen in the sickle transgenic mouse. *J Clin Invest* 1995;96:2845–2853.

51. Kaul DK, Fabry ME, Nagel RL. Microvascular sites and characteristics of sickle cell adhesion to vascular endothelium in shear flow conditions: pathophysiological implications. *Proc Natl Acad Sci U S A* 1989;86:3356–3360.

52. Mohandas N, Evans E. Adherence of sickle erythrocytes to vascular endothelial cells: requirement for both cell membrane changes and plasma factors. *Blood* 1984;64:282–287.

53. Stockman JA, Nigro MA, Mishkin MM, et al. Occlusion of large cerebral vessels in sickle cell anemia. *N Engl J Med* 1972;287:846–850.

54. Rothman SM, Fulling KH, Nelson JS. Sickle cell anemia and central nervous system infarction: a neuropathological study. *Ann Neurol* 1986;20:684–690.

55. Emeribe AO, Udoh AE, Etukudoh MH, et al. Hypofibronectinaemia and severity of sickle cell anemia. *Br J Haematol* 2000;111:1194–1197.

56. Kaul DK, Hebel RP. Hypoxia/reoxygenation causes inflammatory response in transgenic sickle mice but not in normal mice. *J Clin Invest* 2000;106:411–420.

57. Platt OS. Sickle cell anemia as an inflammatory disease. *J Clin Invest* 2000;106:337–338.

58. Setty BN, Kulkarni S, Dampier CD, et al. Fetal hemoglobin in sickle cell anemia: relationship to erythrocyte adhesion markers and adhesion. *Blood* 2001;97:2568–2573.

59. Zwaal RFA, Schroit AJ. Pathophysiologic implications of membrane phospholipid asymmetry in blood cells: a review. *Blood* 1997;89:1121–1132.

60. de Jong K, Emerson RK, Butler J, et al. Short survival of phosphatidylserine exposing red blood cells in murine sickle cell anemia. *Blood* 2001;98:1577–1584.

61. Setty BN, Kulkarni S, Rao AK, et al. Fetal hemoglobin in sickle cell disease: relationship to erythrocyte phosphatidylserine exposure and coagulation activation. *Blood* 2000;96:1119–1124.

62. Styles LA, Hoppe C, Klitz W, et al. Evidence for HLA-related susceptibility for stroke in children with sickle cell disease. *Blood* 2000;95:3562–3567.

63. Adekile AD, Kutlar F, Haider MZ, et al. Frequency of the 677 C→T mutation of the methylenetetrahydrofolate reduction gene among Kuwati sickle cell patients. *Am J Hematol* 2001;66:263–266.

64. Ballas SK. *Sickle Cell Pain. Progress in Pain Research and Management.* Vol. 11. Seattle, WA: IASP Press; 1998.

65. Benjamin LJ. Nature and treatment of the acute painful episode in sickle cell disease. In: Steinberg MH, et al., eds. *Disorders of Hemoglobin: Genetics, Pathophysiology, and Clinical Management.* Cambridge: Cambridge University Press; 2001:671–710.

66. Benjamin LJ, Payne R. Pain in sickle cell disease: a multidimensional construct. In: Pace B, ed. *Renaissance of Sickle Cell Disease Research in the Genomic Era.* London: Imperial College Press; 2007:99–118.

67. Fields HL. *Pain.* New York: McGraw-Hill; 1987.

68. Cousins MJ. Acute post operative pain. In: Wall PD, Melzack R, eds. *Textbook of Pain.* 3rd ed. New York: Churchill Livingstone; 1994:357–385.

69. Katz N, Ferrante FM. Nociception. In: Ferrante FM, VadeBoncoeur TR, eds. *Post Operative Pain Management.* New York: Churchill Livingstone; 1993:17–67.

70. McMahon SB, Koltzeninburg M, eds. *Wall and Melzack's Textbook of Pain.* 5th ed. Philadelphia: Elsevier, Churchill Livingstone; 2006.

71. Ballas SK, Lusardi M. Hospital readmission for adult acute sickle cell painful episodes: frequency, etiology, and prognostic significance. *Am J Hematol* 2005;79:17–25.

72. Udezue E, Girshab AM. Differences between males and females in adult sickle cell pain crisis in eastern Saudi Arabia. *Ann Saudi Med* 2004;24:179–182.

73. Lande WM, Andrews DL, Clark MR, et al. The incidence of painful crisis in homozygous sickle cell disease: correlation with red cell deformability. *Blood* 1988;72:2056–2059.

74. Schall JI, Zemel BS, Kawchak DA, et al. Vitamin A status, hospitalizations, and other outcomes in young children with sickle cell disease. *J Pediatr* 2004;145:99–106.

75. Hargrave DR, Wade A, Evans JP, et al. Nocturnal oxygen saturation and painful sickle cell crises in children. *Blood* 2003;101:846–848.

76. Gil KM, Carson JW, Porter LS, et al. Daily mood and stress predict pain, health care use, and work activity in African American adults with sickle-cell disease. *Health Psychol* 2004;23:267–274.

77. Smith WR, Coyne P, Smith VS, et al. Temperature changes, temperature extremes, and their relationship to emergency department visits and hospitalizations for sickle cell crisis. *Pain Managt Nurs* 2003;4:106–111.

78. Jones S, Duncan S, Thomas N, et al. Windy weather and low humidity are associated with an increased number of hospital admissions for acute pain and sickle cell disease in an urban environment with a maritime temperate climate. *Br J Haematol* 2005;131:530–533.

79. Ballas SK, Delengowski A. Pain measurement in hospitalized adults with sickle cell painful episodes. *Annals Clin Lab Sci* 1993;23:358–361.

80. Charache S, Terrin ML, Moore RD, et al. Effect of hydroxyurea on the frequency of painful crises in sickle cell anemia. *N Engl J Med* 1995;332:1317–1322.

81. Charache S, Barton FB, Moore RD, et al. Hydroxyurea and sickle cell anemia: clinical utility of a myelosuppressive "switching" agent: the Multi-center Study of Hydroxyurea in Sickle Cell Anemia. *Medicine (Baltimore)* 1996;75:300–326.

82. Ballas SK, Smith ED. Red blood cell changes during the evolution of the sickle cell painful crisis. *Blood* 1992;79:2154–2163.

83. Akinola NO, Stevens SME, Franklin IM, et al. Rheological changes in the prodromal and established phases of sickle cell vaso-occlusive crisis. *Br J Haematol* 1992;81:598–602.

84. Ballas SK. The sickle cell crises in adults: phases and objective signs. *Hemoglobin* 1995;19:323–333.

85. Beyer J, Simmons L, Woods GM, et al. A chronology of pain/comfort in children with sickle cell disease. *Arch Pediatr Adolesc Med* 1999;153:913–920.

86. Jacob E, Beyer JE, Miaskowski C, et al. Are there phases to the vaso-occlusive painful episode in sickle cell disease? *J Pain Symptom Manage* 2005;29:392–400.

87. Ballas SK, Marcolina MJ. Hyperhemolysis during the evolution of uncomplicated acute painful episodes in patients with sickle cell anemia. *Transfusion* 2006;46:105–110.

88. Jacob E, Miaskowski C, Savedra M, et al. Changes in intensity, location, and quality of vaso-occlusive pain in children with sickle cell disease. *Pain* 2003;102:187–193.

89. Charache S, Scott JC, Charache P. Acute chest syndrome in adults with sickle cell anemia. *Arch Intern Med* 1979;139:67–69.

90. Vichinsky EP, Styles LA, Colangelo LH, et al. Acute chest syndrome in sickle cell disease: clinical presentation and course. Cooperative study of sickle cell disease. *Blood* 1997;89:1787–1792.

91. Karayalcin G, Imran M, Rosner F. "Blister cells." Association with pregnancy, sickle cell disease and pulmonary infarction. *JAMA* 1972;219:1727–1729.

92. Vichinsky EP, Haberkern CM, Neumayr L, et al. A comparison of conservative and aggressive transfusion regimens in the perioperative management of sickle cell disease. *N Engl J Med* 1995;333:206–213.

93. Thomas AN, Pattison C, Serjeant GR. Causes of death in sickle cell disease in Jamaica. *Br Med J Res Educ* 1982;285:633–635.

94. Vichinsky E. Comprehensive care in sickle cell disease: its impact on morbidity and mortality. *Semin Hematol* 1991;28:220–226.

95. Claster S, Vichinsky E. Acute chest syndrome in sickle cell disease: pathophysiology and management. *J Intensive Care Med* 2000;15:59–166.

96. Vichinsky EP, Neumayr LD, Earles AN, et al. Causes and outcomes of the acute chest syndrome in sickle cell disease. *N Engl J Med* 2000;342:1855–1865.

97. Ballas SK. Acute chest syndrome in sickle cell anemia [editorial]. *J Intensive Care Med* 2000;15:123–125.

98. Castro O, Brambilla DJ, Thorington BD, et al. The acute chest syndrome in sickle cell disease: incidence and risk factors. The Cooperative Study of Sickle Cell Disease. *Blood* 1994;84:643–649.

99. Platt OS, Brambilla DJ, Rosse WF, et al. Mortality in sickle cell disease. Life expectancy and risk factors for early death. *N Engl J Med* 1994;330:1639–1644.

100. Stuart MJ, Setty BN. Acute chest syndrome of sickle cell disease: a new light on an old problem. *Curr Opin Hematol* 2001;8:111–122.

101. Stuart MJ, Setty BN. Sickle cell acute chest syndrome: pathogenesis and rationale for treatment. *Blood* 1999;94:1555–1560.

102. Sugihara K, Sugihara T, Mohandas N, et al. Thrombospondin mediates adherence of CD36+ sickle reticulocytes to endothelial cells. *Blood* 1992;80:2634–2642.

103. Haynes J, Taylor AE, Dixon D, et al. Microvascular hemodynamics in the sickle red blood cell perfused isolated rat lung. *Am J Physiol* 1993;264(2 Pt 2):H484–489.

104. Vichinsky E, Williams R, Das M, et al. Pulmonary fat embolism: a distant cause of severe acute chest syndrome in sickle cell anemia. *Blood* 1994;83:3107–3112.

105. Marthedakis E, Ewatt DH, Cavander JD, et al. Outpatient penile aspiration and epinephrine irrigation for young patients with sickle cell anemia. *Blood* 2000;95:78–82.

106. Stein PD, Beemath A, Meyers FA, et al. Deep venous thrombosis and pulmonary embolism in hospitalized patients with sickle cell disease. *Am J Med* 2006;119(10):897, e7–11.

107. Simkin PA, Downey DJ. Hypothesis: retrograde embolization of marrow fat may cause osteonecrosis. *J Rheumatol* 1987;14:870–872.

108. Styles LA, Schalkwijk CG, et al. Phospholipase A2 levels in acute chest syndrome of sickle cell disease. *Blood* 1996;87:2573–2578.

109. Rucknagel DL, Kalinyak KA, Gelfand MJ. Rib infarcts and acute chest syndrome. *Lancet* 1991;337:831–833.

110. Abboud MR, Taylor EC, Habib D, et al. Elevated serum and bronchoalveolar lavage fluid levels of IL-8 and G-CSF associated with the acute chest syndrome in patients with sickle cell disease. *Br J Haematol* 2000;111:482–490.

111. Bernini JC, Rogers ZR, Sandler ES, et al. Beneficial effect of intravenous dexamethasone in children with mild to moderately severe acute chest syndrome complicating sickle cell disease. *Blood* 1998;92:3082–3089.

112. Huang JC, Gay RN, Khella SL. Sickling crisis, fat embolism, and coma after steroids. *Lancet* 1994;344:951–952.

113. Atz AM, Wessel DL. Inhaled nitric oxide in sickle cell disease with acute chest syndrome. *Anesthesiology* 1997;87:988–990.

114. Adams-Graves P, Kedar A, Koshy M, et al. RheothRx (Poloxamer 188) injection for the acute painful episode of sickle cell disease. *Blood* 1997;90:2041–2046.

115. Hunter RL, Papadea C, Gallagher CJ, et al. Increased whole blood viscosity during coronary artery bypass surgery. Studies to evaluate the effects of soluble fibrin and poloxamer 188. *Thromb Haemost* 1990;63:6–12.

116. Ballas SK, Files B, Luchtman-Jones L, et al. Secretory phospholipase A$_2$ levels in patients with sickle cell disease and acute chest syndrome. *Hemoglobin* 2006;30:165–170.

117. Leivy FE, Schnabel TG. Abdominal crisis in sickle anemia. *Am J Med Sci* 1932;183:381–391.

118. Gage TP, Gagner JM. Ischemic colitis complicating sickle cell crisis. *Gastroenterology* 1983;84:171–174.

119. Lukens JN. Sickle cell disease. *Dis Mon* 1981;27:1–56.

120. Brozovic M, Davies SC, Brownell AI. Acute admissions of patients with sickle cell disease who live in Britain. *Br Med J (Clin Res Ed)* 1987;294:1206–1208.

121. Davies SC, Brozovic M. The presentation, management and prophylaxis of sickle cell disease. *Blood Rev* 1989;3:29–44.

122. Haberkern CM, Neumayr LD, Orringer EP, et al. Cholecystectomy in sickle cell anemia patients: perioperative outcome of 364 cases from the National Preoperative Transfusion Study. *Blood* 1997;89:1533–1542.

123. Vecchio R, Cacciola E, Murabito P, et al. Laparoscopic cholecystectomy in adult patients with sickle cell disease. *G Chir* 2001;22:45–48.

124. Passon RG, Howard TA, Zimmerman SA, et al. Influence of bilirubin uridine diphosphate-glucuronosyltransferase 1A promotor polymorphisms on serum bilirubin levels and cholelithiasis in children with sickle cell anemia. *J Pediatr Hematol Oncol* 2001;23:448–451.

125. Premawardhena A, Fisher CA, Fathlu F, et al. Genetic determinants of jaundice and gallstones in haemoglobin E β-thalassemia. *Lancet* 2001;357:1945–1946.

126. Vasavda N. Menzel S, Kondaveeti S, et al. The linear effects of alpha-thalassemia, the UGT141 and HMOX1 polymorphisms on cholelithiasis in sickle cell disease. *Br J Haematol* 2007;138(2):263–270.

127. Sheehy TW, Law DE, Wade BH. Exchange transfusion in sickle cell intrahepatic cholestasis. *Arch Intern Med* 1980;140:1364–1366.

128. Talacki CA, Ballas SK. Modified method of exchange transfusion in sickle cell disease. *J Clin Apher* 1990;5:183–187.

129. Edmond AM, Collis R, Darvill D, et al. Acute splenic sequestration in homozygous sickle cell disease: natural history and management. *J Pediatr* 1985;107:201–206.

130. Solanki DL, Kletter GG, Castro O. Acute splenic sequestration in adults with sickle cell disease. *Am J Med* 1986;80:985–990.

131. Powars DR. Natural history of sickle cell disease—the first ten years. *Semin Hematol* 1975;12:267–285.

132. Topley JM, Rogers DW, Steven MCG, et al. Acute splenic sequestration and hypersplenism in the first five years in homozygous sickle cell disease. *Arch Dis Child* 1981;56:765–769.

133. Moll S, Orringer EP. Case report: splenomegaly and splenic sequestration in an adult with sickle cell anemia. *Am J Med Sci* 1996;312:299–302.

134. De Ceulaer K, Serjeant GR. Acute splenic sequestration in Jamaican adults with homozygous sickle cell disease: a role of alpha thalassaemia. *Br J Haematol* 1991;77:563–564.

135. Bowcock SJ, Nwabueze ED, Cook AE, et al. Fatal splenic sequestration in adult sickle cell disease. *Clin Lab Haematol* 1988;10:95–99.

136. Sarma PSA. Acute splenic sequestration crisis in a young woman with homozygous sickle cell anemia. *Postgrad Med J* 1989;65:105–107.

137. Koduri PR. Acute splenic sequestration crisis in adults with sickle cell anemia. *Am J Hematol* 2007;82:174–175.

138. Altman KL, Watman RN, Solomon K. Surgically induced splenogenic anemia in the rabbit. *Nature* 1951;168:827.

139. Itzchak Y, Glickman MG, Gottschalk A, et al. Hemodynamic and morphologic evaluation of the spleen after splenic vein ligation in the dog. *Invest Radiol* 1978;13:155–160.

140. Jensen WW, Lessin LS. Membrane alterations associated with hemoglobinopathies. *Semin Hematol* 1970;4:409–426.

141. Barnhart MI, Henry RL, Lushner JM. *Sickle Cell*. 2nd ed. Kalamazoo, MI: The Upjohn Company; 1976:15–35.

142. Ballas SK, Burka ER, Lewis CN, et al. Serum immunoglobulin levels in patients with sickle cell syndromes. *Am J Clin Pathol* 1980;73:394–396.

143. Powars DR, Johnson CS. Priapism. *Hematol Oncol Clin North Am* 1996;10:1363–1372.

144. Kato GJ, McGowan V, Machado RF, et al. Lactate dehydrogenase as a biomarker of hemolysis-associated nitric oxide resistance, priapism, leg ulceration, pulmonary hypertension, and death in patients with sickle cell disease. *Blood* 2006;107:2279–2285.

145. Hassell KL, Eckman JR, Lane PA. Acute multiorgan failure syndrome: a potentially catastrophic complication of severe sickle cell pain episodes. *Am J Med* 1994;96:155–162.

146. Athanasou NA, et al. Vascular occlusion and infarction in sickle crisis and the sickle chest syndrome. *J Clin Pathol* 1985;38:659–664.

147. Ballas SK, Talacki CA, Rao VM, et al. The prevalence of avascular necrosis in sickle cell anemia: correlation with a-thalassemia. *Hemoglobin* 1989;13:649–655.

148. Milner PF, Kraus AP, Sebes JL, et al. Sickle cell disease as a cause of osteonecrosis of the femoral head. *N Engl J Med* 1991;325:1476–1481.

149. Ficat RP. Idiopathic bone necrosis of the femoral head. *J Bone Joint Surg Br* 1985;67-B:3–9.

150. Styles K, Vichinsky E. Core decompression in avascular necrosis of the hip in sickle cell disease. *Am J Hematol* 1996;52:103–107.

151. Neumayr LD, Aguilar C, Earles AN, et al. Physical therapy alone compared with core decompression and physical therapy for femoral head osteonecrosis in sickle cell disease. Results of a multicenter study at a mean of three years after treatment. *J Bone Joint Surg Am* 2006;88:2573–2582.

152. Saito S, Saito M, Nishina T, et al. Long term total hip arthroplasty for osteonecrosis of the femoral head: a comparison with osteoarthritis. *Clin Orthop* 1989;244:198–207.

153. Hanker GJ, Amstutz HC. Osteonecrosis of the hip in sickle cell diseases. *J Bone Joint Surg* 1988;70:499–506.

154. Clarke JH, Jinnah RH, Brooker AF, et al. Total replacement of the hip for avascular necrosis in sickle cell disease. *J Bone Joint Surg Br* 1989;71:465–470.

155. Learmonth ID, Young C, Rorabeck C. The operation of the century: total hip replacement. *Lancet* 2007;370:1508–1519.

156. Powars DR, Chan LS, Schroeder WA. The variable expression of sickle cell disease is genetically determined. *Semin Hematol* 1990;27:360–376.

157. Ballas SK, Park CH, Jacobs SR. The spectrum of painful episodes in adult sickle cell disease. *Pain Digest* 1995;5:73–89.

158. Orringer EP, Fowler VG, Teague MT, et al. *A Possible Role for Hydroxyurea Therapy. Book of Abstracts of the 17th Annual Sickle Cell Disease Conference*. Nashville, TN: Mehary Medical College; 1992:81.

159. Weinlich G, Fritsch P. Leg ulcers in patients tested with hydroxyurea for myeloproliferative disorders: what is the trigger? *Br J Haematol* 1999;141:171–172.

160. Ferster A, Tahrir P, Vermylen C, et al. Five years of experience with hydroxyurea in children and young adults with sickle cell disease. *Blood* 2001;97:3628–3632.

161. Loeser JD, Butler SH, Chapman CR, et al. *Bonica's Management of Pain*. 3rd ed. Philadelphia: Lippincott Williams & Wilkins; 2001.

162. Konotey-Ahulu FID. Mental nerve neuropathy: a complication of sickle cell crisis. *Lancet* 1972;2:388.

163. Kirson LE, Tomaro AJ. Mental nerve paresthesia secondary to sickle cell crisis. *Oral Surg Oral Med Oral Pathol* 1979;48:509–512.

164. Asher SW. Multiple cranial neuropathies, trigeminal neuralgia, and vascular headaches in sickle cell disease: a possible common mechanism. *Neurology* 1980;30:210–211.

165. Shields RW Jr, Harris JW, Clark M. Mononeuropathy I sickle cell anemia: anatomical and pathophysiological basis for its rarity. *Muscle Nerve* 1991;14:370–374.

166. Ballas SK, Reyes PE. Peripheral neuropathy in adults with sickle cell disease. *Am J Pain Med* 1997;71:53–58.

167. Salvin ML, Barondes MJ. Ischemic optic neuropathy in sickle cell disease. *Am J Ophthalmol* 1988;105:212–213.

168. Blank JP, Gill FM. Orbital infarction in sickle cell disease. *Pediatrics* 1981;67:879–881.

169. Al-Rashid RA. Orbital apex syndrome secondary to sickle cell anemia. *J Pediatr* 1979;95:426–427.

170. Rothman SM, Nelson JS. Spinal cord infarction in a patient with sickle cell anemia. *Neurology* 1980;30:1072–1076.

171. Benjamin LJ, Dampier CD, Jacox A, et al. *Guideline for the Management of Acute and Chronic Pain in Sickle Cell Disease. APS Clinical Practice Guidelines Series No. 1.* Glenview, IL: American Pain Society; 1999.

172. Dunlop RJ, Bennett KC. Pain management for sickle cell disease. *Cochrane Database Syst Rev* 2006;19(2): CD003350.

173. Todd KH, Green C, Bonham VL Jr, et al. Sickle cell disease related pain: crisis and conflict. *J Pain* 2006;7:453–458.

174. Green CR, Anderson KO, Baker TA, et al. The unequal burden of pain: confronting racial and ethnic disparities in pain. *Pain Med* 2003;4:277–294.

175. Labbe E, Herbert D, Haynes J. Physicians' attitude and practices in sickle cell disease pain management. *J Palliat Care* 2005;21:246–251.

176. Lipton RB, Stewart WF, Ryan RE, et al. Efficacy and safety of acetaminophen, aspirin and caffeine in alleviating migraine headache pain. *Arch Neurol* 1998; 55:210–217.

177. Sunshine A, Olson NZ. Non-narcotic analgesics. In: *Textbook of Pain.* 2nd ed. New York: Churchill Livingstone; 1989:670–685.

178. Ferrante MF. Non-steroidal anti-inflammatory drugs. In: *Postoperative Pain Management.* New York: Churchill Livingstone; 1993:133–143.

179. Kopecky EA, Jacobson S, Joshi P, et al. Systemic exposure to morphine and the risk of acute chest syndrome in sickle cell disease. *Clin Pharmacol Ther* 2004;75:140–146.

180. Buchanan ID, Woodward M, Reed GW. Opioid selection during sickle cell pain crisis and its impact on the development of acute chest syndrome. *Pediatr Blood Cancer* 2005;45:716–724.

181. Weber ML, Hebbel RP, Gupta K. Morphine induces kidney injury in transgenic sickle cell mice [abstract]. *Blood* 2005;106(suppl 1):884a–885a.

182. Gupta K, Chen C, Lutty GA, et al. Morphine exaggerates retinopathy in transgenic sickle mice [abstract no. 209]. *Blood* 2005;106(suppl 1):64a–65a.

183. Shaiova L, Wallenstein D. Outpatient management for sickle cell pain with chronic opioid pharmacotherapy. *J Natl Med Assoc* 2004;96:984–986.

184. Brookoff D, Polomano R. Treating sickle cell pain like cancer pain. *Ann Intern Med* 1992;116:364–368.

185. Ballas SK. The treatment of pain in adults with sickle cell disease. *Am J Hematol* 1990;34:49–54.

186. Benjamin LJ, Swinson GI, Nagel RL. Sickle cell anemia day hospital: an approach for the management of uncomplicated painful crises. *Blood* 2000;95: 1130–1137.

187. van Beers EJ, van Tuijn CF, Nieuwerk PT, et al. Patient-controlled analgesia versus continuous infusion of morphine during vaso-occlusive crisis in sickle cell disease, a randomized controlled trial. *Am J Hematol* 2007;82:955–960.

188. Charache S, Dover GJ, Moore RD, et al. Hydroxyurea: effects on hemoglobin F production in patients with sickle cell anemia. *Blood* 1992;79:2555–2565.

189. Ballas SK, Barton FB, Waclawiw MA, et al, and the Investigators of the Multicenter Study of Hydroxyurea in Sickle Cell Anemia. Hydroxyurea and sickle cell anemia: effect on quality of life. *Health Qual Life Outcomes* 2006;4:59.

190. Steinberg MH, Barton F, Castro O, et al. Effect of hydroxyurea on mortality and morbidity in adult sickle cell anemia: risks and benefits up to 9 years of treatment. *JAMA* 2003;289:1645–1651.

191. Lanzkron S, Haywood C Jr, Segal JB, et al. Hospitalization rates and costs of care of patients with sickle-cell anemia in the state of Maryland in the era of hydroxyurea. *Am J Hematol* 2006;81(12):927–932.

192. Evenson DR, Jost LK. Hydroxyurea exposure alters mouse testicular kinetics and sperm chromatin structure. *Cell Prolif* 1993;26:147–159.

193. DePass LR, Weaver EV. Comparison of tertogenic effects of aspirin and hydroxyurea in the Fischer 344 and Wistar strains. *J Toxicol Environ Health* 1982;10:297–305.

194. Ferm VH. Severe developmental malformations: malformations induced by urethane and hydroxyurea in the hamster. *Arch Pathol* 1966;81:174–177.

195. Fruchtman SM, Kaplan ME, Peterson P, et al. Acute leukemia (AL), hydroxyurea (HO) and polycythemia vera (PV): an analysis of risk and the Polycythemia Vera Study Group [abstract]. *Blood* 1994;84(suppl 1):518a.

196. Triadou P, Maier–Redelsperger M, Krishnamoorty R, et al. Fetal hemoglobin variations following hydroxyurea treatment in patients with cyanotic congenital heart disease. *Nouv Rev Fr Hematol* 1994;36:367–372.

197. Orringer EP, Casella JF, Ataga KI, et al. Purified poloxamer 188 for treatment of acute vaso-occlusive crisis in sickle cell disease: a randomized controlled trial. *JAMA* 2001;286:2099–2106.

198. Brugnara C, de Franceschi L, Alper SL. Inhibition of Ca(2 +)-dependent K+ transport and cell dehydration in sickle erythrocytes by clotrimazole and other imidazole derivatives. *J Clin Invest* 1993;92:520–526.

199. DeFranceschi L, Bachir D, Galacteros F, et al. Oral magnesium supplements reduce erythrocyte dehydration in patients with sickle cell disease. *J Clin Invest* 1997;100:1847–1852.

200. Pawliuk R, Westerman KA, Fabry ME, et al. Correction of sickle cell disease in transgenic mouse models by gene therapy. *Science* 2001;294(5550): 2368–2371.

CHAPTER 58 ■ PAIN IN HUMAN IMMUNODEFICIENCY VIRUS DISEASE

WILLIAM BREITBART AND ALBERTO CORTES-LADINO

INTRODUCTION

With the introduction of highly active antiretroviral therapies (i.e., combination therapies including protease inhibitors) the face of the acquired immunodeficiency syndrome (AIDS) epidemic, particularly for those who can avail themselves of and/or tolerate these new therapies, is indeed changing. Death rates from AIDS in the United States have dropped dramatically in the last several years, and rates of serious opportunistic infections and cancers are declining. Despite these hopeful developments, the future is still unclear, and millions of patients with human immunodeficiency virus (HIV) disease worldwide will continue to die of AIDS and suffer from the enormous burden of physical and psychologic symptoms. Even with advances in AIDS therapies, pain continues to be an important palliative care issue for patients with HIV disease. As the epidemiology of the AIDS epidemic changes in the United States, the challenge of managing pain in AIDS patients

with a history of substance abuse is becoming an ever growing challenge. Studies conducted between 1990 and 1995 have documented that pain in individuals with HIV infection or AIDS is highly prevalent, diverse, and varied in syndromal presentation, associated with significant psychologic and functional morbidity, and alarmingly undertreated.[1-11] Pain management needs to be more integrated into the total care of patients with HIV disease. Responses from a self-referred sample of AIDS outpatients indicate that AIDS patients experience many distressing physical and psychologic symptoms along with a high level of distress.[12] This chapter describes the prevalence and types of pain syndromes encountered in patients with HIV disease and reviews the psychologic and functional impact of pain as well as the barriers to adequate pain treatment in this population. Finally, principles of pain management, with particular emphasis on the management of pain in HIV-infected patients with a history of substance abuse, are outlined.

PREVALENCE OF PAIN IN ACQUIRED IMMUNODEFICIENCY SYNDROME

Estimates of the prevalence of pain in HIV-infected individuals have been reported to range from 30% to over 90%, with the prevalence of pain increasing as disease progresses,[1,2,4,5,9,13–15] particularly in the latest stages of illness.

Studies suggest that approximately 30% of ambulatory HIV-infected patients in early stages of HIV disease (pre-AIDS; Category A or B disease) experience clinically significant pain, and as many as 56% have had episodic painful symptoms of less clear clinical significance.[1,4,7,9,16] In a prospective cross-sectional survey of 438 ambulatory AIDS patients in New York City, 63% reported frequent or persistent pain of at least 2 weeks duration at the time of assessment.[1] The prevalence of pain in this large sample increased significantly as HIV disease progressed, with 45% of AIDS patients with Category A3 disease, 55% of those with Category B3, and 67% of those with Category C1, 2, or 3 disease reporting pain. Patients in this sample of ambulatory AIDS patients also were more likely to report pain if they had other concurrent HIV-related symptoms (e.g., fatigue, wasting), had received treatment for an AIDS-related opportunistic infection, or if they had not been receiving antiretroviral medications (e.g., AZT, ddI, ddC, d4t).

In a study of pain in hospitalized patients with AIDS in a public hospital in New York City, over 50% of patients required treatment for pain, with pain being the presenting complaint in 30% and the second most common presenting problem after fever.[5] In a French multicenter study, 62% of hospitalized patients with HIV disease had clinically significant pain.[4] Schofferman and Brody[17] reported that 53% of patients with far-advanced AIDS cared for in a hospice setting had pain, while Kimball and McCormack[14] reported that up to 93% of AIDS patients in their hospice experienced at least one 48-hour period of pain during the last 2 weeks of life.

Larue and colleagues[18] demonstrated that patients with AIDS being cared for by hospice at home had prevalence rates and intensity ratings for pain that were comparable to, and even exceeded, those of cancer patients. Breitbart and colleagues[2] reported that ambulatory AIDS patients in their New York City sample reported a mean pain intensity on average of 5.4 (on the 0–10 numerical rating scale of the Brief pain Inventory) and a mean pain at its worst of 7.4. In addition, as with pain prevalence, the intensity of pain experienced by patients with HIV disease increases significantly as disease progresses. AIDS patients with pain, like their counterparts with cancer pain, typically describe an average of 2.5 to 3 concurrent pains at a time.[2,3]

Frich and Borgbjerg[19] concluded that the incidence of disturbing pain in AIDS is high, specifically in the extremities, gastrointestinal (GI) tract, and head. In a study of 95 AIDS patients, the overall incidence of pain was 88%, and 69% of the patients suffered from pain which interfered with daily activity to a degree described as moderate to severe. In AIDS patients approaching end of life, 93% of patients reported experiencing pain and discomfort at some time during the last 2 weeks of life. This percentage may be even higher if some pain and discomfort went unrecognized. Most patients experienced at least one 48-hour period of pain and discomfort during the last 2 weeks of life; furthermore, 88% received some sort of opioid analgesia with the majority experiencing some relief.[14]

IMPACT OF HIGHLY ACTIVE ANTIRETROVIRAL THERAPY ON MEDICAL CARE, PALLIATIVE CARE, AND QUALITY OF LIFE

Brechtl and colleagues[20] assessed the impact of highly active antiretroviral therapy (HAART) on a wide range of clinical outcomes and psychologic variables in patients with advanced HIV/AIDS. Data on 70 patients with CD4 + cell counts below 300 cc and a projected survival greater that 1 month was collected at baseline and after 1 and 3 months. In addition to standard clinical and laboratory markers, a series of observer-rated and self-report instruments were used to measure pain and symptom distress, psychologic well-being, depression, and physical functioning abilities. The only psychosocial measure that improved significantly with treatment was depression. Ratings of pain intensity, physical and psychologic symptom distress, and overall quality of life did not change. These results suggest that despite the improvements in CD4 + cell count and HIV viral load, body weight, albumin, and ferritin, the benefits of HAART treatment on pain and symptom distress and psychosocial well-being are less clear.[20]

PAIN SYNDROMES IN HUMAN IMMUNODEFICIENCY VIRUS/ ACQUIRED IMMUNODEFICIENCY SYNDROME—OVERVIEW

Pain syndromes encountered in AIDS are diverse in nature and etiology. The most common pain syndromes reported in studies to date include painful sensory peripheral neuropathy, pain due to extensive Kaposi's sarcoma (KS), headache, oral and pharyngeal pain, abdominal pain, chest pain, arthralgias and myalgias, as well as painful dermatologic conditions.[1,3,5,7,9,13,17,18,21,22] In a sample of 151 ambulatory AIDS patients who underwent a research assessment which included a clinical interview, neurologic examination, and review of medical records,[3] the most common pain diagnoses included headaches (46% of patients, 17% of all pains), joint pains (arthritis, arthralgias, etc., 31% of patients, 12% of all pains), painful polyneuropathy (distal symmetrical polyneuropathy, 28% of patients, 10% of all pains), and muscle pains (myalgia, myositis, 27% of patients, 12% of all pains). Other common pain diagnoses included skin pain (KS, infections, 25% of patients; 30% of homosexual males in the sample had pain from extensive KS lesions), bone pain (20% of patients), abdominal pain (17% of patients), chest pain (13%), and painful radiculopathy (12%). Patients in this sample had a total of 405 pains (averaging three concurrent pains), with 46% of patients diagnosed with neuropathic type pain, 71% with somatic pain, 29% with visceral pain, and 46% with headache (classified separately because of controversy as to pathophysiology). When pain type was classified by pains (as opposed to patients), 25% were neuropathic pains, 44% were nociceptive-somatic, 14% were nociceptive-visceral, and 17% were idiopathic type pains. Patients in this study with lower CD4 + cell counts were significantly more likely to be diagnosed with polyneuropathy and headache. Hewitt and colleagues[3] demonstrated that while pains of a neuropathic nature (e.g., polyneuropathies, radiculopathies) certainly comprise a large proportion of pain syndromes encountered in AIDS patients, pains of a somatic and/or visceral nature are also extremely common clinical problems. A review performed by O'Neill and Sherrard[7] showed that HIV therapies including didanosine, stavudine, and zalcitabine have become a major cause of neuropathic pain, which influences the high prevalence of pain among HIV patients.

Pain syndromes seen in HIV disease can be categorized into three types (Table 58.1): (1) those directly related to HIV infection or consequences of immunosuppression; (2) those due to AIDS therapies; and (3) those unrelated to AIDS or AIDS therapies.[3,11] In studies to date, approximately 45% of pain syndromes encountered are directly related to HIV infection or consequences of immunosuppression; 15% to 30% are due to therapies for HIV- or AIDS-related conditions, as well as diagnostic procedures; and the remaining 25% to 40% are unrelated to HIV or its therapies.[3]

TABLE 58.1

PAIN SYNDROMES IN AIDS PATIENTS

I PAIN RELATED TO HIV/AIDS
  HIV Neuropathy
  HIV Myelopathy
  Kaposi's Sarcoma
  Secondary Infections (intestines, skin)
  Organomegaly
  Arthritis/Vasculitis
  Myopathy/Myositis

II PAIN RELATED TO HIV/AIDS THERAPY
  Antiretrovirals, Antivirals
  Antimycobacterials, PCP Prophylaxis
  Chemotherapy (Vincristine)
  Radiation
  Surgery
  Procedures (bronchoscopy, biopsies)

III PAIN UNRELATED TO AIDS
  Disc Disease
  Diabetic Neuropathy

In three reviews of the literature, Breitbart,[23] Douaihy et al.,[24] and Markus and Fincham[25] discussed the assessment and management of HIV-/AIDS-related pain and its impact on quality of life and presented a multidisciplinary approach with specific recommendations to treat psychosocial issues associated with HIV and the pain syndromes related.

PAIN IN WOMEN WITH HUMAN IMMUNODEFICIENCY VIRUS/ ACQUIRED IMMUNODEFICIENCY SYNDROME

The Memorial Sloan Kettering group has reported on the experience of pain in women with AIDS.[3,26] While preliminary in nature, these studies suggest that women with HIV disease experience pain more frequently than men with HIV disease and report somewhat higher levels of pain intensity. This may in part be a reflection of the fact that women with AIDS-related pain are twice as likely to be undertreated for their pain compared to men.[2] Women with HIV disease have unique pain syndromes of a gynecologic nature specifically related to opportunistic infectious processes and cancers of the pelvis and genitourinary tract.[27] Women with AIDS were significantly more likely to be diagnosed with radiculopathy and headache in one survey.[3] In a pilot survey of aberrant drug-taking attitudes and behaviors of a mixed group of 52 cancer patients and a group of 111 women with HIV/AIDS, Passik et al.[28] reported that patients would consider engaging in aberrant behaviors, or would possibly excuse them in others, if pain or symptom management were inadequate.

PAIN IN CHILDREN WITH HUMAN IMMUNODEFICIENCY VIRUS/ ACQUIRED IMMUNODEFICIENCY SYNDROME

Children with HIV infection also experience pain.[29] HIV-related conditions in children that are observed to cause pain include meningitis and sinusitis (headaches), otitis media, shingles, cellulitis and abscesses, severe candida dermatitis, dental caries, intestinal infections, such as *Mycobacterium avium intracellulare* (MAI) and cryptosporidium, hepatosplenomegaly, oral and esophageal candidiasis, and spasticity associated with encephalopathy that causes painful muscle spasms. Oleske and colleagues[30] have reported that pain in HIV-infected children carries an increased mortality.

SPECIFIC PAIN SYNDROMES ENCOUNTERED IN PATIENTS WITH HUMAN IMMUNODEFICIENCY VIRUS DISEASE

The following section reviews, in detail, the various painful manifestations of HIV disease. The authors acknowledge the important review by O'Neill and Sherrard[7] that formed the basis of this section on specific pain syndromes in HIV disease.

Gastrointestinal Pain Syndromes

Many of the opportunistic infections and HIV-associated neoplasms may present as pain referable to the GI tract. Generally, the pain will be alleviated by specific treatment of the causative diseases. Adequate analgesia should be provided during diagnostic assessment.[7]

Oropharyngeal Pain

Oral cavity and throat pain is very common, accounting for approximately 20% of the pain syndromes encountered in one study.[5] The sources of oral cavity pain have been well described.[7,31,32] Oropharyngeal candidiasis occurs in up to 75% of HIV-positive individuals and, although frequently asymptomatic, it is the most common cause of oral cavity pain. Bacterial infections are mainly seen as necrotizing gingivitis and can arise in HIV-positive patients in spite of maintaining a good standard of oral hygiene.[7] Dental abscesses occur more commonly in HIV-infected individuals than in the general population. Oral ulcerations are extremely common and can be the result of herpes simplex virus (HSV), cytomegalovirus (CMV), Epstein-Barr virus (EBV), atypical and typical mycobacterial infection (MAI), cryptococcal infection, or histoplasmosis. Frequently, no infectious agent can be identified, and these painful aphthous ulcers are a clinically challenging problem.[7] Up to 75% of patients with cutaneous KS also have intraoral lesions, most commonly on the palate, although these seldom cause pain.[7]

Esophageal Pain

About one third of patients with HIV disease experience esophageal symptoms such as dysphagia or pain upon swallowing (odynophagia) often due to esophageal candidiasis. Esophageal candidiasis occurs in between 25% and 75% of patients with HIV disease[33–35] and may present as dysphagia or odynophagia. Ulcerative esophagitis, which can be quite painful, is usually a result of CMV infection but can be idiopathic. Infectious causes of esophagitis include HSV, EBV, Mycobacteria, Cryptosporidium, and *Pneumocystis carinii*.[33,34,36–39] KS and lymphoma both have been reported to invade the esophagus resulting in dysphagia, pain, and ulceration.[7] Zidovudine has also been reported to be a cause of esophageal ulceration.[40]

Abdominal Pain

Abdominal pain is the primary site of pain in 12%–25% of patients with HIV disease.[3,5,41] Infectious causes of abdominal pain predominate and include cryptosporidiosis, shigella, salmonella and Campylobacter enteritis, CMV, ileitis, and MAI. Perforation of the small and large intestine secondary to CMV infection has been described.[41] Repeated intussusception of the small intestine has been seen in association with Campylobacter infection.[42] Lymphoma in the GI tract can present with abdominal pain and intestinal obstruction.[43] KS spreads to the GI tract of 40% to 50% of AIDS patients with cutaneous lesions.[44] Rarely, intestinal KS may cause obstruction, bleeding, perforation, and diarrhea.[45] Other causes of abdominal pain in HIV positive patients[7] include ileus, organomegaly, spontaneous aseptic peritonitis, toxic shock, herpes zoster, and Fitzhugh-Curtis syndrome (perihepatitis in association with tubal gonococcal or chlamydia infection).

Biliary Tract and Pancreatic Pain

Cholecystitis may occur in HIV-infected patients as a result of opportunistic infection; CMV and cryptosporidiosis are the most common infectious agents. Extrahepatic biliary tract obstruction secondary to KS or MAI infection has been reported.[7] Sclerosing cholangitis (CMV, cryptosporidiosis), also known as AIDS cholangiopathy, is another cause of right upper quadrant or epigastric pain.[46] Opportunistic liver infections (CMV, MAI, fungal infections) as well as drug-induced hepatic toxicities (ddI, pentamidine) are sources of hepatitis and abdominal or right upper quadrant pain.[47]

Pancreatitis is often related to adverse effects of HIV-related therapies, in particular the antiretroviral agents didanosine (ddI) and dideoxycytidine (ddC). Between 7% to 10% of patients on ddI develop pancreatitis, and lower rates are reported with other antiretrovirals. Intravenous pentamidine is also associated with pancreatitis. Infectious causes of pancreatitis include CMV, MAI, and cryptococcal infection.[48] Rarely, lymphoma or KS may involve the pancreas resulting in pancreatitis.

Anorectal Pain

Painful anorectal diseases are common, occurring in about one third of homosexual men with HIV disease.[49] Infectious causes of anorectal pain include perirectal abscesses, CMV proctitis, fissure-in-ano, and HSV infection. A small increase has been noted in anal/anorectal carcinoma in HIV-positive homosexual men.[50]

Chest Pain Syndromes

Chest pain is a common complaint in patients with HIV disease, comprising approximately 13% of the pain syndromes encountered in a sample of ambulatory AIDS patients.[3] Sources of chest pain in patients with HIV disease are similar to those encountered in the general population (i.e., cardiac, esophageal, lung and pleura, and chest wall); the etiologies may be somewhat unique (i.e., opportunistic infections) cancers. In immunosuppressed patients, infectious causes of chest pain should be considered, particularly in the presence of fever and some localizing sign such as dysphagia, dyspnea, or cough. Infectious causes of chest pain include Pneumocystis pneumonia (with or without a pneumothorax), esophagitis (CMV, candidiasis, HSV), pleuritis/pericarditis (viral, bacterial, tuberculous), and postherpetic neuralgia. Opportunistic cancers (KS, lymphoma) invading the esophagus, pericardium, chest wall, lung, and pleura may be sources of chest pain.

Rarely, pulmonary embolus or bacterial endocarditis may be the cause of chest pain.

NEUROLOGIC PAIN SYNDROMES IN ACQUIRED IMMUNODEFICIENCY SYNDROME

Pain syndromes originating in the nervous system include headache, painful peripheral neuropathies, radiculopathies, and myelopathies. The HIV virus is highly neurotropic, invading central nervous system (CNS) and peripheral nervous system structures early in the course of HIV disease. As many as 40% to 75% of patients with late-stage AIDS have a neurologic complication[51–54] either directly due to HIV itself (e.g., AIDS dementia, HIV peripheral neuropathy, HIV myelopathy), or secondary to opportunistic infection (e.g., CNS toxoplasmosis, CMV neuropathy), cancer (e.g., CNS lymphoma), or medication side effects (toxic neuropathies due to ddI, ddC [zalcitabine], D$_4$T [stavudine], or AZT [zidovudine]-induced headache). Headache is a frequent symptom in HIV-infected patients and may be an important indication of disease of the CNS including opportunistic infections and cancers. Rarely, cerebrovascular events (e.g., thalamic stroke) occurring in hypercoagulable states can result in central pain syndromes.

Headache

Headache is extremely common, reported by approximately 40% to 50% of patients with HIV disease, particularly in later stages of illness.[3,55] Headache poses a diagnostic dilemma for physicians in that the underlying cause may range from benign stress and tension to life threatening CNS infection.[7] The differential diagnosis of headache in patients with HIV disease includes HIV encephalitis and atypical aseptic meningitis, opportunistic infections of the nervous system, AIDS-related CNS neoplasms, sinusitis, tension, migraine, and AZT-induced headache.[56] Toxoplasmosis and cryptococcal meningitis are the two most commonly encountered opportunistic infections of the CNS in patients with HIV disease.[53] Cerebral toxoplasmosis usually presents with persistent headache, sometimes associated with focal signs, change in mental status, or seizures. Diagnosis is based on radiologic imaging (magnetic resonance imaging is more sensitive than computed tomography) with a characteristic appearance of multiple deep ring-enhancing lesions and a clinical response to a trial of empiric treatment for toxoplasmosis. A brain biopsy is sometimes necessary to establish a definitive diagnosis and to differentiate cerebral toxoplasmosis from cerebral lymphoma. Cryptococcal meningitis usually presents with symptoms of headache, neck stiffness, and recurring fever, although focal neurologic signs may occur. Other opportunistic infections of the CNS that can present as headache in the AIDS patient include CMV, HSV and herpes zoster, progressive multifocal leukoencephalopathy (papovavirus), Candida albicans, mycobacterium tuberculosis, Mycobacterium avium intracellulare, and neurosyphilis. Headache related to sinus infection is common in immunocompetent patients with HIV disease who present with headache but have no focal neurologic signs. Opportunistic cancers of the CNS include CNS lymphoma, metastatic systemic lymphoma, and metastatic intracranial KS. These can present, particularly in the immunocompromised patient with HIV disease, with signs of increased intracranial pressure with or without focal neurologic signs, as well as fever and meningismus. More benign causes of headache in the patient with HIV disease include AZT-induced headache, occurring in 15% to 30% of patients, tension headache, migraine with or without aura, and unclassifiable or idiopathic headache.[57] Evers and colleagues[58] concluded that the progressing immunologic deficiency of HIV-infected patients seems to influence the pain processing of headache in different ways. During that natural course of infection, the migraine frequency significantly decreased, while the frequency of tension type headaches increased.[58]

NEUROPATHIES ENCOUNTERED IN HUMAN IMMUNODEFICIENCY VIRUS-INFECTED PATIENTS

Pain syndromes of a neuropathic nature occur in approximately 40% of AIDS patients with pain.[3] While several types of peripheral neuropathy have been described in patients with HIV/AIDS (Table 58.2), the most common painful neuropathy encountered is the predominantly sensory neuropathy of AIDS, affecting up to 30% of people with HIV infection.[51,54,59,60] Other potentially painful neuropathies encountered in HIV/AIDS patients, however, can be caused by viral and nonviral infectious processes (mononeuritis multiplex, including polyneuritis cranialis, polyradiculopathy of the lower limbs-cauda equina syndrome, and plexopathies caused by CMV, HZV, and MAI), immune mediated inflammatory demyelination (acute and chronic Guillain-Barré syndrome), a variety of medical conditions (diabetic neuropathy, postherpetic neuralgia, entrapment neuropathies), nutritional deficiencies (B6, B12), toxins (alcohol), and HIV-related therapies (e.g., ddl, ddC). Several antiretroviral drugs, such as ddI, ddC, and D4T, and chemotherapy agents used to treat KS (vincristine), as well as a number of medications used in the treatment of *Pneumocystis carinii* pneumonia (PCP), mycobacterial infection, and other HIV-associated infections can cause painful toxic neuropathy.[7,61,62]

TABLE 58.2

NEUROPATHIES ENCOUNTERED IN HIV/AIDS INFECTED PATIENTS

I PREDOMINANTLY SENSORY NEUROPATHY OF AIDS

II IMMUNE-MEDIATED
    Inflammatory demyelinating polyneuropathies (IDPs)
        Acute (Guillain-Barré syndrome)
        Chronic (CIDP)

III INFECTIOUS
    Cytomegalovirus polyradiculopathy
    Cytomegalovirus multiple mononeuropathy
    Herpes Zoster
    MAI

IV TOXIC/NUTRITIONAL
    Alcohol, Vitamin deficiencies (B6, B12)
    Antiretrovirals:
        ddI (didanosine), ddC (zalcitabine), D4T (stavudine)
    Antivirals:
        Foscarnet
    PCP prophylaxis:
        Dapsone
    Antibacterial:
        Metronidazole
    Antimycobacterials:
        INH (isoniazid), rifampin, ethionamide
    Antineoplastics:
        Vincristine, vinblastine

V OTHER MEDICAL CONDITIONS:
    Diabetic neuropathy
    Postherpetic neuralgia

Predominantly Sensory Neuropathy of Acquired Immunodeficiency Syndrome

The most frequently encountered neuropathy is a symmetrical predominantly sensory painful peripheral neuropathy. This is a late manifestation, occurring most often in patients with an AIDS-defining illness but has been reported earlier in the course of the disease.[51] Prevalence in hospice populations ranges from 19% to 26%.[17,63,64] It is the only peripheral sensory neuropathy which has been postulated to be a direct result of HIV infection of the peripheral nervous system.[51] It has been reported by Zhou and colleagues[65] that in subjects with advanced HIV-1 infection, epidermal nerve fiber density assessment correlates with the clinical and electrophysiologic severity of distal sensory polyneuropathy. The predominant symptom in about 60% of patients is pain in the soles of the feet. Paraesthesia is frequent and usually involves the dorsum of the feet in addition to the soles. Most patients have signs of peripheral neuropathy (most commonly, absent or reduced ankle jerks and elevated thresholds to pain and vibration sense), and while the signs progress, the symptoms often remain confined to the feet.[51,66,67] Although the patient's complaints are predominantly sensory, electrophysiologic studies demonstrate both sensory and motor involvement.

A qualitative study of 19 patients using a grounded-theory approach was designed to assess the impact distal symmetrical peripheral neuropathy has on persons with AIDS. Themes in the debilitation continuum included isolating the symptom cluster, inventing and testing interventions, and assimilating the annoyance. Their results suggested that only individualized interventions presented favorable results.[68]

Immune-Mediated Neuropathies

Acute Guillain-Barré syndrome has been described in association with seroconversion (group-I infection) but may occur at any time. Both acute and chronic inflammatory demyelinating polyneuropathies are predominantly motor, and sensory abnormalities are rare.[60] Mononeuritis multiplex presents with sensory or motor deficits in the distribution of multiple spinal, cranial, or peripheral nerves[52] and may progress into a chronic inflammatory demyelinating polyneuropathy.[60]

Infectious Neuropathies

Polyradiculopathies (associated with CMV infection) often present with radicular pain and follow a distinct course.[69] The onset is usually subacute and the deficit initially confined to sacral and lumbar nerve roots. Both sensory and motor functions are involved, and there is usually early involvement of sphincters. Progression is relentless.[60] An analysis by Harrison and colleagues[70] of pain related to herpes zoster identified three variables related to pain: extent of lesion healing, extension of lesion crusting, and the number of new vesicles. Harrison et al.,[70] showed that the significance of baseline pain due to herpes zoster was a predictor of return to daily life functioning. Furthermore, the significance of pain at presentation and at 1 month were significant predictors of chronic pain.[70]

Toxic/Nutritional Neuropathies

Toxic and nutritional neuropathies in patients with HIV disease have been reported with the following: alcohol, vitamin deficiencies (B6, B12), antiretroviral drugs such as ddI, ddC, and D4T, antivirals such as foscarnet, PCP prophylaxis such as dapsone, antibacterial drugs such as metronidazole, antimycobacterial drugs such as isoniazid, rifampin, and ethionamide, and antineo-plastics such as vincristine and vinblastine.[61,67]

Painful Neuropathies According to Stage of Human Immunodeficiency Virus Infection

The type of neuropathy varies with the stage of infection. The acute or seroconversion phase of HIV disease is associated with mononeuritides, brachial plexopathy, and acute demyelinating polyneuropathy. The latent or asymptomatic phase (CD4+ T lymphocytes >500/mm^3) is characterized by acute and chronic demyelinating polyneuropathies. The transition phase (200–500 CD4+ cells) is characterized by herpes zoster (shingles) and mononeuritis multiplex. The late phase of HIV disease (<200 CD4+ cells) is characterized by HIV predominantly sensory polyneuropathy, CMV polyneuropathy, mononeuritis multiplex, autonomic neuropathy, mononeuropathies secondary to meningeal disease, and antiretroviral induced toxic neuropathies.[61]

RHEUMATOLOGIC PAIN SYNDROMES

In studies conducted by the Memorial Sloan-Kettering group,[3] over 50% of pain syndromes were classified as rheumatologic in nature including various forms of arthritis, arthropathy, arthralgia, myopathy, myositis, and myalgias. In another study, 72% of patients with different stages of HIV infection had painful symptoms involving the musculoskeletal system.[71]

Arthritis and Arthropathies

HIV disease has been associated with several types of painful arthritis and arthropathies including nonspecific arthralgias, reactive arthritis, psoriatic arthritis, HIV-associated arthritis, and, rarely, aseptic arthritis.[72,73] The most frequently reported arthritis is a reactive arthritis or Reiter's syndrome.[72–74] Acute HIV infection may present with a polyarthralgia in association with a mononucleosis-like illness. There is also a syndrome of acute severe and intermittent articular pain, often referred to as HIV-associated painful articular syndrome, which commonly affects the large joints of the lower limbs and shoulders. Psoriasis and psoriatic arthritis have been reported in patients with HIV infection.[75,76] The arthritis is typically seen in conjunction with the skin changes of psoriasis, and authors suggest it may follow a disease course that proves refractory to conventional therapy.[7] An HIV-associated arthritis has also been described,[77] which typically presents as an oligoarthritis affecting the joints of the lower limbs. Synovial fluid is noninflammatory, and biopsy shows a mild chronic synovitis. There is no associated infection to suggest a reactive arthritis, and the patients reported have been HLA-B27 negative. It appears that this arthritis is caused by the HIV virus itself.[72] Septic arthritis has been reported in patients with HIV disease, including arthritis due to bacterial infections and infections with *Cryptococcus neoformans* and *Sporothrix schenckii*.[72,73]

Myopathy and Myositis

Muscle pain is very common in patients with HIV disease. Several types of myopathy and myositis have been described in HIV-infected patients including HIV-associated myopathy or polymyositis, necrotizing noninflammatory myopathy in association with zidovudine and without zidovudine, pyomyositis, and microsporidiosis myositis.[78–84] Polymyositis may occur at any stage of HIV infection, is thought to be the result of direct viral infec-

tion of muscle cells,[73] and may present with a subacute onset of proximal muscle weakness and myalgia.[78] Electromyographic evidence of myopathy, a raised serum creatinine kinase, and biopsy evidence of polymyositis are common in symptomatic patients. Drugs used in the treatment of HIV disease may also be associated with the development of myalgia[56] and myositis.[79,85] Zidovudine has been particularly implicated. In these patients, symptoms frequently improve following discontinuation of zidovudine therapy.[7]

THE IMPACT OF PAIN ON QUALITY OF LIFE

Pain, in patients with HIV disease, has a profound negative impact on physical and psychologic functioning, as well as overall quality of life.[4,8] In a study of the impact of pain on psychologic functioning and quality of life in ambulatory AIDS patients,[4,8] depression was significantly correlated with the presence of pain. In addition to being significantly more distressed, depressed, and hopeless, those with pain were twice as likely to have suicidal ideation (40%) as those without pain (20%). HIV-infected patients with pain were more functionally impaired.[8] Such functional interference was highly correlated to levels of pain intensity and depression. Patients with pain were more likely to be unemployed or disabled and reported less social support. Larue and colleagues[4] reported that HIV-infected patients with pain intensities greater than 5 (on a 0–10 NRS) reported significantly poorer quality of life during the week preceding their survey than patients without pain. Pain intensity had an independent negative impact on HIV patients' quality of life, even after adjustment for treatment setting, stage of disease, fatigue, sadness, and depression. Singer and colleagues[9] also reported an association between the frequency of multiple pains, increased disability, and higher levels of depression. Psychologic variables, such as the amount of control people believe they have over pain, emotional associations, and memories of pain, fears of death, depression, anxiety, and hopelessness, contribute to the experience of pain in people with AIDS and can increase suffering.[8,86] The Memorial group also reported that negative thoughts related to pain were associated with greater pain intensity, psychologic distress, and disability in ambulatory patients with AIDS.[87] Those AIDS patients who felt that pain represented a progression of their HIV disease reported more intense pain than those who did not see pain as a threat. Vogel and colleagues[88] assessed 504 ambulatory AIDS patients in order to measure symptom distress, physical and psychosocial functioning, and demographic and disease-related factors. As opposed to those who reported sexual contact as a means of transmission, patients who reported intravenous drug use as HIV transmission indicated higher levels of distress as well as physical symptom distress.[12] Furthermore, Vogel and colleagues[88] showed that both the number of symptoms and symptom distress were highly associated with psychologic distress and poorer quality of life.

Rosenfeld, Breitbart, and colleagues assessed hastened death, its prevalence, and predictors in more than 370 patients with advanced AIDS, and measures for depression, hopelessness, spiritual well-being, social support, pain, and physical symptoms were administered. The most significant variables associated with high desire of death were hopelessness and depression.[88b]

MANAGEMENT OF PAIN IN ACQUIRED IMMUNODEFICIENCY SYNDROME

Assessment Issues

The initial step in pain management is a comprehensive assessment of pain symptoms. The health professional working in the AIDS setting must have a working knowledge of the etiology and treatment of pain in AIDS. This would include an understanding of the different types of AIDS pain syndromes discussed above, as well as a familiarity with the parameters of appropriate pharmacologic treatment. A close collaboration of the entire health care team is optimal when attempting to adequately manage pain in the AIDS patient. A careful history and physical examination may disclose an identifiable syndrome (e.g., herpes zoster, bacterial infection, or neuropathy) that can be treated in a standard fashion.[89,90] A standard pain history[91,92] may provide valuable clues to the nature of the underlying process and indeed may disclose other treatable disorders. A description of the qualitative features of the pain, its time course, and any maneuvers that increase or decrease pain intensity should be obtained. Pain intensity (current, average, at best, at worst) should be assessed to determine the need for weak versus potent analgesics and as a means to serially evaluate the effectiveness of ongoing treatment. Pain descriptors (e.g., burning, shooting, dull, or sharp) will help determine the mechanism of pain (somatic, nociceptive, visceral nociceptive, or neuropathic) and may suggest the likelihood of response to various classes of traditional and adjuvant analgesics (nonsteroidal anti-inflammatory drugs [NSAIDs], opioids, antidepressants, anticonvulsants, oral local anesthetics, corticosteroids, etc.).[93–95] Additionally, detailed medical, neurologic, and psychosocial assessments (including a history of substance use or abuse) must be conducted. Where possible, family members or partners should be interviewed and included in the pain management treatment plan. Patient and family education pamphlets on the management of HIV/AIDS pain are available. During the assessment phase, pain should be aggressively treated while pain complaints and psychosocial issues are subject to an ongoing process of re-evaluation.[92]

PAIN MEASUREMENT AND ASSESSMENT TOOLS

An important element in assessment of pain is the concept that assessment is continuous and needs to be repeated over the course of pain treatment. The use of readily available, simple, and clinically validated pain self-report measures or tools can make this process simpler and more reliable. There are essentially four aspects of pain experience in AIDS that require ongoing assessment and evaluation which can be aided by these tools: (1) pain intensity; (2) pain relief; (3) pain-related functional interference (e.g., mood state, general, and specific activities); and (4) monitoring of intervention effects.

Three commonly used self-report pain intensity assessment tools include: (1) a simple descriptive pain intensity scale; (2) a 0–10 numeric pain intensity scale; and (3) the Visual Analog Scale (VAS) for Pain Intensity. A Pain Faces scale is used in children and in non-English speaking or illiterate populations. The Memorial Pain Assessment Card (MPAC)[96] is a helpful clinical tool that allows patients to report their pain experience. The MPAC consists of visual analog scales that measure pain intensity, pain relief, and mood. The Brief Pain Inventory (BPI)[97] is another pain assessment tool that has been widely used in cancer and AIDS pain research and clinical settings. The BPI has a useful Pain Interference Subscale that assesses pain's interference in seven domains of quality of life and function. There are many other pain assessment tools available for adults and children.

Joint Commission on Accreditation of Healthcare Organization Pain Standards

Effective January 1, 2001, the Joint Commission on Accreditation of Healthcare Organizations (JCAHO) established new pain management standards for accreditation.[98] These new standards

---

TABLE 58.3

JOINT COMMISSION ON ACCREDITATION OF HEALTHCARE ORGANIZATION'S PAIN STANDARDS

- Recognize the right of patients to appropriate assessment and management of pain;
- Assess the existence and, if so, the nature and intensity of pain in all patients;
- Record the results of the assessment in a way that facilitates regular reassessment and follow-up;
- Determine and assure staff competency in pain assessment and management, and address pain assessment and management in the orientation of all new staff;
- Establish policies and procedures which support the appropriate prescription or ordering of effective pain medications;
- Educate patients and their families about effective pain management; and address patient needs for symptom management in the discharge planning process.

Source: www.jcaho.org/standard/pm_hap.html.
HRSA. Available at: www.hrsa.gov. Accessed May 5, 2001.

---

state that: (1) individuals served have the right to appropriate assessment and referral for a provision of management of pain and (2) that pain must be assessed in all individuals. The pain standards are available at www.jointcommission.org/standards/. Some key concepts of the JCAHO standards are listed in Table 58.3. The pain assessment tools and measures described above can be useful in helping organizations and practitioners comply with these standards. General principles of assessment and management described in this chapter may also be helpful. Other sources for help in meeting the pain standards include such resources as Building an Institutional Commitment to Pain Management: The Mayday Resource Manual for Improvement.[99] This resource is an excellent compilation of resource material to promote institutional support of pain management; all of the sample resource tools are available on a disc.

Multimodal Approach

Federal guidelines developed by the Agency for Health Care Policy and Research (AHCPR) for the management of cancer pain also address the issue of management of pain in AIDS and state that, "The principles of pain assessment and treatment in the patient with HIV positive/AIDS are not fundamentally different from those in the patient with cancer and should be followed for patients with HIV-positive/AIDS."[93] In contrast to pain in cancer, pain in HIV disease may more commonly have an underlying treatable cause.[7]

Optimal management of pain in AIDS is multimodal and requires pharmacologic, psychotherapeutic, cognitive-behavioral, anesthetic, neurosurgical, and rehabilitative approaches. A multidimensional model of AIDS pain, which recognizes the interaction of cognitive, emotional, socioenvironmental, and nociceptive aspects of pain suggests a model for multimodal intervention.

Pharmacotherapies for Pain in Acquired Immunodeficiency Syndrome

The World Health Organization (WHO)[95] has devised guidelines for analgesic management of cancer pain that the AHCPR has endorsed for the management of pain related to cancer or AIDS.[92] These guidelines, also known widely as the "WHO Analgesic Ladder," have been well validated.[100] This approach advocates selection of analgesics based on severity of pain, as well as the type of pain (i.e., neuropathic versus non-neuropathic pain). For mild-to-moderate severity pain, nonopioid analgesics such as NSAIDs and acetaminophen are recommended. For pain that is persistent and moderate to severe in intensity, opioid analgesics of increasing potency should be utilized. Adjuvant agents, such as laxatives and psychostimulants, are useful in preventing as well as treating opioid side effects such as constipation or sedation, respectively. Adjuvant analgesic drugs, such as the antidepressant analgesics, are suggested for considered use, along with opioids and NSAIDs, in all stages of the analgesic ladder (mild, moderate, or severe pain), but have their most important clinical application in the management of neuropathic pain.

This WHO approach, while not yet validated in AIDS, has been recommended by the AHCPR and clinical authorities in the field of pain management and AIDS.[5,7,9,17,62,93,101] Clinical reports describing the successful application of the principles of the WHO Analgesic Ladder to the management of pain in AIDS, with particular emphasis on the use of opioids, have also recently appeared in the literature.[6,14,17,102–105]

Nonopioid Analgesics

The nonopioid analgesics (Table 58.4) are prescribed principally for mild-to-moderate pain or to augment the analgesic effects of opioid analgesics in the treatment of severe pain. The use of NSAIDs in patients with AIDS must be accompanied by heightened awareness of toxicity and adverse effects. NSAIDs are highly protein-bound, and the free fraction of available drug is increased in AIDS patients who are cachectic, wasted, and hypoalbuminic, often resulting in toxicities and adverse effects. Patients with AIDS are frequently hypovolemic, on concurrent nephrotoxic drugs, and experiencing HIV nephropathy and so are at increased risk for renal toxicity related to NSAIDs. The antipyretic effects of the NSAIDs may also interfere with early detection of infection in patients with AIDS.

The major adverse effects associated with NSAIDs include gastric ulceration, renal failure, hepatic dysfunction, and bleeding. The nonacetylated salicylates, such as salsalate, sodium salicylate, and choline magnesium salicylate, theoretically have fewer GI side effects and might be considered in cases where GI distress is an issue. Prophylaxis for NSAID-associated GI symptoms include H2 antagonist drugs (cimetidine 300 mg three or four times a day or ranitidine 150 mg twice a day), misoprostol 200 mg four times a day, omeprazole 20 mg once a day, or an antacid. Patients should be informed of these symptoms, issued guaiac cards with reagent, and taught to check their stool weekly. NSAIDs effect kidney function and should be used with caution. NSAIDs can cause a decrease in glomerular filtration, acute and chronic renal failure, interstitial nephritis, papillary necrosis, and hyperkalemia.[106] In patients with renal impairment, NSAIDs should be used with caution, since many (i.e., ketoprofen, fenoprofen, naproxen, and carprofen) are highly dependent on renal function for clearance. The risk of renal dysfunction is greatest in patients with advanced age, pre-existing renal impairment, hypovolemia, concomitant therapy with nephrotoxic drugs, and heart failure. Prostaglandins modulate vascular tone, and their

TABLE 58.4

ORAL ANALGESICS FOR MILD TO MODERATE PAIN IN AIDS

Analgesic (by class)	Starting Dose (mg)	Duration (hrs)	Plasma Half-life (hrs)	Comments
NONSTEROIDAL				
Aspirin	650	4–6	4–6	The standard for comparison among nonopioid analgesics
Ibuprofen	400–600	—	—	Like aspirin, can inhibit platelet function
Choline magnesium trisalicylate	700–1500	—	—	Essentially no hematologic or GI side effects
Celecoxib	100–200	11	11	Decrease dose by 50% in moderate hepatic impairment
WEAKER OPIOIDS				
Codeine	32–65	3–4	—	Metabolized to morphine, often used to suppress cough in patients at risk of pulmonary bleed
Oxycodone	5–10	3–4	—	Available as a single agent and in combination with aspirin or acetaminophen
Proxyphene	65–13	4–6	—	Toxic metabolite norpropoxy accumulates with repeated dosing

inhibition by the NSAIDs can cause hypertension as well as inter-ference with the pharmacologic control of hypertension.[107] Caution should be used in patients receiving B-adrenergic antagonists, diuretics, or angiotensin-converting enzyme inhibitors. Several studies have suggested that there is substantial biliary excretion of several NSAIDs, including indomethacin and sulindac. In patients with hepatic dysfunction, these drugs should be used with caution. NSAIDs, with the exception of the nonacetylated salicylates (e.g., sodium salicylate, choline magnesium trisalicylate), produce inhibition of platelet aggregation (usually reversible, but irreversible with aspirin). NSAIDs should be used with extreme caution, or avoided, in patients who are thrombocytopenic or who have clotting impairment. The role of cyclooxygenases (COX)-2 antagonists, such as celecoxib, play in T-cell proliferation in HIV patients on combination antiretroviral therapy has been well described, suggesting these types of medications as potential therapeutic targets in HIV infection.[108,109] The overexpression of COX has been linked to the development and progression of several types of cancer including astrocytomas, breast, ovarian, and colorectal, and it has been reported that the inhibition of COX-2 suppresses growth and induces apoptosis in human esophageal adenocarcinoma cells.[110]

COX-2 inhibitors have an analgesic action equal to that of conventional NSAIDs, but with fewer GI complications and have been widely used for rheumatic diseases.[111] COX-2 inhibitors are associated with an increased risk of adverse cardiovascular events, including myocardial infarction, stroke, and new onset or worsening of pre-existing hypertension, GI irritation, ulceration, bleeding, and perforation, and are contraindicated for the treatment of perioperative pain in the setting of coronary artery bypass graft.[112]

OPIOID ANALGESICS

Opioid analgesics are the mainstay of pharmacotherapy of moderate to severe intensity pain in the patient with HIV disease (Table 58.5). Several reports describing the safe and effective use of opioid drugs in the management of moderate to severe pain in populations of patients with HIV disease (including patients with a history of injection drug use (IDU) as their HIV transmission factor) have begun to appear in the literature.[14,102–105,113] Kaplan and colleagues[113] conducted a multicenter study in which 44 patients with moderate to severe AIDS-related pain were treated with sustained release oral morphine in an open-label prospective study of patients treated for up to 18 days. Pain intensity decreased by 65% in the completed patients, quality of life was good in 80%, acceptability of therapy was 96% in the com-

TABLE 58.5

OPIOID ANALGESICS FOR MODERATE TO SEVERE PAIN IN AIDS

Analgesic	Equi-analgesic route	Dose (mg)	Analgesic onset (hrs)	Duration (hrs)	Plasma half-life (hrs)	Comments
Morphine	PO IM, IV, SC	30–60* 10	1–1.5 0.5–1	4–6 3–6	2–3	Standard of comparison for the narcotic analgesics. *30 mg for repeat around-the-clock dosing; 60 mg for single dose or intermittent dosing.
Morphine	PO	90–120	1–1.5	8–12	—	Now available in long acting sustained release forms.
Oxycodone	PO PO	20–30 20–40	1 1	3–6 8–12	2–3 2–3	In combination with aspirin or acetaminophen it is considered a weaker opioid, as a single agent it is comparable to the strong opioids, like morphine. Available in immediate release and sustained release preparation.
Hydromorphone	PO IM, IV	7.5 1.5	0.5–1 0.25–.05	3–4 3–4	2–3 2–3	Short half-life; ideal for elderly patients. Comes in suppository and injectable forms.
Methadone	PO IM, IV	20 10	2–1 0.5–1	4–8 —	15–30 15–30	Long half-life; tends to accumulate with initial dosing, requires careful titration. Good oral potency.
Levorphanol	PO IM	4 2	0.5–1.5 0.5–1	3–6	12–16 12–16	Long half-life; requires careful dose titration in first week. Note that analgesic duration is only 4 hours.
Meperidine	PO IM	300 75	0.5–1.5 0.5–1	3–6 3–4	3–4 3–4	Active toxic metabolite, or meperidine, tends to accumulate (plasma half-life is 12–16 hours), especially with renal impairment and in elderly patients causing delirium, myoclonus and seizures.
Fentanyl transdermal system	TD IV	0.1 0.01	12–18	48–72 —	20–22 —	Transdermal patch is convenient, bypassing GI analgesia until depot is formed. Not suitable for rapid titration

IM, intramuscular; IV, intravenous; PO, per oral; SC, subcutaneous; TD, transdermal.

pleted patients, 92% of side effects were resolved, and total morphine dose remained stable through the course of the study. In a pilot study, Lefkowitz and Newshan[103] reported similar findings on the effectiveness and safety of the transdermal fentanyl patch in a small sample of patient with AIDS-related pain. With transdermal fentanyl, pain severity scores decreased, mean pain relief scores increased, and daily functioning measures improved significantly.[103] Furthermore, Lefkowitz and Newshan[103] reported transdermal fentanyl was effective for chronic pain in chemically dependent and nonchemical dependent AIDS patients. In persons with AIDS near the end of life, the use of opioid analgesia remains common practice. The medical records of 185 adult AIDS patients receiving hospice care were reviewed by Kimball and McCormick.[14] Most patients (93%) experienced at least one 48-hour period of discomfort during the last two weeks of life; the majority (88%) received some form of opioid analgesia. Of these patients, 62% experienced some relief of pain thereafter.[14]

Principles that are useful in guiding the appropriate use of opioid analgesics for pain[94,100,114] include the following: (1) choose an appropriate drug; (2) start with lowest dose possible; (3) titrate dose; (4) use "as needed" doses selectively; (5) use an appropriate route of administration; (6) be aware of equivalent analgesic doses; (7) use a combination of opioid, nonopioid, and adjuvant drugs; (8) be aware of tolerance; and (9) understand physical and psychologic dependence. Rotate opioids to restore analgesic efficacy when necessary. In choosing the appropriate opioid analgesic for cancer pain, Portenoy[94] highlights the following important considerations: (1) opioid class; (2) "weak" versus "strong" opioids; (3) pharmacokinetic characteristics; (4) duration of analgesic effect; (5) favorable prior response; and (6) opioid side effects.

Opioid analgesics are divided into two classes, the agonists and the agonist-antagonists, based on their affinity to opioid receptors. Pentazocine, butorphanol, and nalbuphine are examples of opioid analgesics with mixed agonist-antagonist properties. These drugs can reverse opioid effects and precipitate an opioid withdrawal syndrome in patients who are opioid-tolerant or dependent. They are of limited use in the management of chronic pain in AIDS. Oxycodone (in combination with either aspirin or acetaminophen), hydrocodone, and codeine are the so-called "weaker" opioid analgesics and are indicated for use in Step 2 of the WHO ladder for mild-to-moderate intensity pain. More severe pain is best managed with morphine or another of the stronger opioid analgesics, such as hydromorphone, methadone, levorphanol, or fentanyl. Oxycodone, as a single agent without aspirin or acetaminophen, is available in immediate and sustained-release forms and is considered a "stronger" opioid in these forms.

The oral route has often been described as the preferred route of administration of opioid analgesics from the perspectives of convenience and cost. However, the transdermal route of administration has gained rapid acceptance among clinicians and patients. Patients with HIV infection are burdened with the task of taking anywhere from 20–40 tablets of medication per day and often need to follow complicated regimens where medication has to be taken on an empty stomach, etc. In a study on patient-related barriers to pain management in AIDS patients,[115] the vast majority of AIDS patients endorse a preference to utilize a pain intervention that required a minimal number of additional pills (e.g., sustained-release preparations of oral opioids) or interventions that did not require taking pills at all (i.e., transdermal opioid system). Immediate release oral morphine or hydromorphone preparations require that the drug be taken every 3 to 4 hours. Longer-acting, sustained-release oral morphine preparations and oxycodone preparations are available that provide up to 8–12 hours or more of analgesia, minimizing the number of daily doses required for the control of persistent pain. Rescue doses of immediate-release, short-acting opioid are often necessary to supplement the use of sustained-release morphine or oxy-

codone, particularly during periods of titration or pain escalation. The transdermal fentanyl patch system (Duragesic, Ortho-McNeil Inc., Raritan, NJ) also has applications in the management of severe pain in AIDS.[103,105] Each transdermal fentanyl patch contains a 48–72 hour supply of fentanyl, which is absorbed from a depot in the skin. Levels in the plasma rise slowly over 12–18 hours after patch placement, so dosage forms are available. As with sustained-release morphine preparations, all patients should be provided with oral or parenteral rapidly acting short duration opioids to manage breakthrough pain. The transdermal system is convenient and can minimize the reminders of pain associated with repeated oral dosing of analgesics. In AIDS patients, it should be noted that the absorption of transdermal fentanyl could be increased with fever, resulting in increased plasma levels and shorter duration of analgesia from the patch.

It is important to note that opioids can be administered through a variety of routes: oral, rectal, transdermal, intravenous, subcutaneous, intraspinal, and even intraventricularly.[105] There are advantages and disadvantages as well as indications for use of these various routes. Further discussion of such alternative delivery routes as the intraspinal route, etc., are beyond the scope of this chapter; however, interested readers are directed to Chapter 45 and the Agency for Health Care Policy and Research Clinical Practice Guideline: Management of Cancer Pain.[93]

Opioid Side Effects

While the opioids are extremely effective analgesics, their side effects are common and can be minimized if anticipated in advance. Sedation is a common CNS side effect, especially during the initiation of treatment. Sedation usually resolves after the patient has been maintained on a steady dosage. Persistent sedation can be alleviated with a psychostimulant, such as dextroamphetamine, pemoline, or methylphenidate. All are prescribed in divided doses in early morning and at noon. Additionally, psychostimulants can improve depressed mood and enhance analgesia.[116,117] Delirium, of an either agitated or somnolent variety, can also occur while on opioid analgesics and is usually accompanied by attentional deficits, disorientation, and perceptual disturbances (visual hallucinations and more commonly illusions). Myoclonus and asterixis are often early signs of neurotoxicity that accompany the course of opioid induced delirium. Meperidine, when administered chronically in patients with renal impairment, can lead to a delirium due to accumulation of the neuroexcitatory metabolite normeperidine.[118] Opioid-induced delirium can be alleviated through the implementation of three possible strategies: (1) lowering the dose of the opioid drug presently in use; (2) changing to a different opioid; or (3) treating the delirium with low doses of high potency neuroleptics, such as haloperidol. The third strategy is especially useful for agitation and clears the sensorium.[119] For agitated states, intravenous haloperidol in doses starting at between 1 mg and 2 mg is useful, with rapid escalation of dose if no effect is noted. GI side effects of opioid analgesics are common. The most prevalent are nausea, vomiting, and constipation.[94] Concomitant therapy with prochlorperazine for nausea is sometimes effective. Since all opioid analgesics are not tolerated in the same manner, switching to another narcotic can be helpful if an antiemetic regimen fails to control nausea. Constipation caused by narcotic effects on gut receptors is a problem frequently encountered, and it tends to be responsive to the regular use of senna derivatives. A careful review of medications is imperative, since anticholinergic drugs such as the tricyclic antidepressants can worsen opioid-induced constipation and can cause bowel obstruction. Respiratory depression is a worrisome but rare side effect of the opioid analgesics. Respiratory difficulties can almost always be avoided if two general principles are adhered to: (1) start opioid analgesics in low doses in opioid-naive patients; and (2) be cognizant of relative potencies when switching opioid analgesics, routes of administration, or both.

Opioid rotation is a useful strategy to improve pain management especially in long-term treatment. Accumulation of toxic metabolites can lead to the development of symptoms that include hallucinations, myoclonus, nausea and vomiting, and persisting pain. Several strategies of opioid rotation using equianalgesic doses have been reported to be useful in managing pain while decreasing the tolerance as well as the frequency and severity of opioid toxicity.[120-122]

Adjuvant Analgesics

Adjuvant analgesics are the third class of medications frequently prescribed for the treatment of chronic pain and have important applications in the management of pain in AIDS (Table 58.6). Adjuvant analgesic drugs are used to enhance the analgesic efficacy of opioids, treat concurrent symptoms that exacerbate pain, and provide independent analgesia. They may be used in all stages of the analgesic ladder. Commonly used adjuvant drugs include antidepressants, neuroleptics, psychostimulants, anticonvulsants, corticosteroids, and oral anesthetics.[93,120,121]

Antidepressants

The current literature supports the use of antidepressants as adjuvant analgesic agents in the management of a wide variety of chronic pain syndromes, including cancer pain, postherpetic neuralgia, diabetic neuropathy, fibromyalgia, headache, and low back pain.[122-127] The antidepressants are analgesic through a number of mechanisms that include antidepressant activity,[123] potentiation or enhancement of opioid analgesia,[128-130] and direct analgesic effects.[131] The leading hypothesis suggests that both serotonergic and noradrenergic properties of the antidepressants are probably important and that variations among individuals in pain (as to the status of their own neurotransmitter systems) is an important variable.[90] Other possible mechanisms of antidepressant analgesic activity that have been proposed include adrenergic and serotonin receptor effects,[132] adenosinergic effects,[133] antihistaminic effects,[132] and direct neuronal effects, such as inhibition of paroxysmal neuronal discharge and decreasing sensitivity of adrenergic receptors on injured nerve sprouts.[134]

There is substantial evidence that the tricyclic antidepressants in particular are analgesic and useful in the management of chronic neuropathic and non-neuropathic pain syndromes. Amitriptyline is the tricyclic antidepressant most studied and has been

TABLE 58.6

PSYCHOTROPIC ADJUVANT ANALGESIC DRUGS FOR AIDS PAIN

Generic name	Approximate daily dosage range (mg)	Route	Generic name	Approximate daily dosage range (mg)	Route
TRICYCLIC ANTIDEPRESSANTS			**PHENOTHIAZINES**		
Amitriptyline	10–150	PO,IM	Fluphenazine	1–3	PO,IM
Nortriptyline	10–150	PO	Methotrimeprazine	10–20 q6h	IM,IV
Imipramine	15.5–150	PO,IM			
Desipramine	10–150	PO	**BUTYROPHENONES**		
Clomipramine	10–150	PO	Haloperidol	1–3 PO	PO,IV
Doxepin	12–150	PO,IM	Pimozide	2–6 BID	PO
HETEROCYCLIC AND NONCYCLIC ANTIDEPRESSANTS			**ANTIHISTAMINES**		
Trazodone	125–300	PO	Hydroxyzine	50 q4h–q6h	PO
Maprotiline	50–300	PO			
			ANTICONVULSANTS		
SEROTONIN REUPTAKE INHIBITORS			Carbamazepine	200 tid–400 TID	PO
Fluoxetine	20–80	PO	Phenytoin	300–400	PO
Paroxetine	10–60	PO	Valproate	500 tid–1000 TID	PO
Sertraline	50–200	PO	Oxcarbazepine	300 bid–1800 daily‡‡	PO
Citalopram	10–60	PO	Pregabalin	50 tid–150 BID‡‡	PO
Escitalopram	10–60	PO	Gabepentin	1800–3600 daily‡‡	PO
			Felbamate	1200–3600 daily‡‡	PO
NEWER AGENTS			Lamotrigine	100–400 daily‡‡	PO
Nefazodone	300–600*	PO			
Venlafaxine	75–225†	PO	**ORAL LOCAL ANESTHETICS**		
Duloxetine	60‡	PO	Mexiletine	600–900	PO
			CORTICOSTEROIDS		
PSYCHOSTIMULANTS			Dexamethasone	4–16	PO,IV
Methylphenidate	2.5–20 BID	PO			
Dextroamphetamine	2.5–20 BID	PO	**BENZODIAZEPINES**		
Pemoline	13.75–75 BID	PO	Alprazolam	0.25–2.0 TID	PO
Modafinil	100–400	PO	Clonazepam	0.5–4 BIC	PO

BID, twice a day; IM, intramuscular; IV, intravenous; PO, per oral; q6h, every 6 hours; QID, four times a day; TID, three times a day.
*Monitor liver function; if AST, ALT increase by 3x, discontinue and do not reintroduce.
†Adjust dose for renal impairment.
‡Adjust for renal impairment. Not recommended in hepatic impairment.
‡‡Adjust dose for renal impairment.

proved effective as an analgesic in a large number of clinical trials addressing a wide variety of chronic pain syndromes, including neuropathy, cancer pain, fibromyalgia, and others.[90,123,126,135–137] Other tricyclics that have been shown to have efficacy as analgesics include imipramine,[138,139] desipramine,[89,140] nortriptyline,[141] clomipramine,[142,143] and doxepin.[144]

The heterocyclic and noncyclic antidepressant drugs, such as trazodone, mianserin, maprotiline, and the newer serotonin-specific reuptake inhibitors (SSRIs), fluoxetine and paroxetine, may also be useful as adjuvant analgesics for chronic pain syndromes.[90,116,126,131,138,140,145–150] Fluoxetine, a potent antidepressant with specific serotonin reuptake inhibition activity,[148] has been shown to have analgesic properties in experimental animal pain models[149] but failed to show analgesic effects in a clinical trial for neuropathy.[140] Several case reports suggest fluoxetine may be a useful adjuvant analgesic in the management of headache[150] and fibrositis.[151] Paroxetine, a newer SSRI, is the first antidepressant of this class shown to be a highly effective analgesic in a controlled trial for the treatment of diabetic neuropathy.[138] Newer antidepressants such as sertraline, venlafaxine, and nefazodone may also eventually prove to be clinically useful as adjuvant analgesics. Nefazodone, for instance, has been demonstrated to potentiate opioid analgesics in an animal model.[152] Based on the post hoc result of three multicenter randomized, double-blind, placebo-controlled, parallel-group studies, the serotonin-norepinephrine reuptake inhibitor duloxetine appears to be well tolerated in the treatment of diabetic peripheral neuropathic pain.[93]

Given the diversity of clinical syndromes in which the antidepressants have been demonstrated to be analgesic, trials of these drugs can be justified in the treatment of virtually every type of chronic pain.[121] The established benefit of several of the antidepressants in patients with neuropathic pains,[135,138] however, suggests these drugs may be particularly useful in populations such as cancer and AIDS patients, where an underlying neuropathic component to the pain(s) often exists.[121] While studies of the analgesic efficacy of these drugs in HIV-related painful neuropathies have not yet been conducted, they are widely applied clinically using the model of diabetic and postherpetic neuropathies.

While antidepressant drugs are analgesic in both neuropathic and non-neuropathic pain models, their clinical use is most commonly in combination with opioid drugs, particularly for moderate to severe pain. Antidepressant adjuvant analgesics have their most broad application as "coanalgesics," potentiating the analgesic effects of opioid drugs.[93] The "opioid sparing" effects of antidepressant analgesics has been demonstrated in a number of trials, especially in cancer populations with neuropathic as well as non-neuropathic pain syndromes.[126,127]

The dose and time course of onset of analgesia for antidepressants when used as analgesics appears to be similar to their use as antidepressants.

There is compelling evidence that the therapeutic analgesic effects of amitriptyline are correlated with serum levels, as are the antidepressant effects, and that analgesic treatment failure is due to low serum levels.[135] A high-dose regimen of up to 150 mg of amitriptyline or higher is suggested.[135] The proper analgesic dose for paroxetine is likely in the 40–60 mg range, with the major analgesic trial utilizing a fixed dose of 40 mg.[138] There is anecdotal evidence to suggest that the debilitated medically ill (cancer and AIDS patients) often respond (for depression or pain) to lower doses of antidepressant than are usually required in the physically healthy, probably because of impaired metabolism of these drugs.[120] As to the time-course of onset of analgesia, a biphasic process appears to occur. There are immediate or early analgesic effects that occur within hours or days, and these are probably mediated through inhibition of synaptic reuptake of catecholamines. In addition, there are later, longer analgesic effects that peak over a 2 to 4 week period that are probably due to receptor effects of the antidepressants.[135,136]

Neuroleptics and Benzodiazepines

Neuroleptic drugs, such as methotrimeprazine, fluphenazine, haloperidol, and pimozide, may play a role as adjuvant analgesics[141,153–155] in AIDS patients with pain; however, their use must be weighed against what appears to be an increased sensitivity to the extrapyramidal side effects of these drugs in AIDS patients with neurologic complications.[156] Anxiolytics, such as alprazolam and clonazepam, may also be useful as adjuvant analgesics, particularly in the management of neuropathic pains.[157–159]

Psychostimulants

Psychostimulants, such as dextroamphetamine, methylphenidate, pemoline, and modafinil, may be useful antidepressants in patients with HIV infection or AIDS who are cognitively impaired.[117,158] Psychostimulants also enhance the analgesic effects of the opioid drugs.[160] Psychostimulants are also useful in diminishing sedation secondary to narcotic analgesics, and they are potent adjuvant analgesics. Bruera et al.[117] demonstrated that a regimen of 10 mg methylphenidate with breakfast and 5 mg with lunch significantly decreased sedation and potentiated the effect of narcotics in patients with cancer pain. Methylphenidate has also been demonstrated to improve functioning on a number neuropsychologic tests, including tests of memory, speed, and concentration, in patients receiving continuous infusions of opioids for cancer pain.[117] Dextroamphetamine has also been reported to have additive analgesic effects when used with morphine in postoperative pain.[161] In relatively low doses, psychostimulants stimulate appetite, promote a sense of well-being, and improve feelings of weakness and fatigue in cancer patients.

Pemoline is a unique alternative psychostimulant that is chemically unrelated to amphetamine but may have similar usefulness as an antidepressant and adjuvant analgesic in AIDS patients.[117] Advantages of pemoline as a psychostimulant in AIDS pain patients include the lack of abuse potential, the lack of federal regulation through special triplicate prescriptions, the mild sympathomimetic effects, and the fact that it comes in a chewable tablet form that can be absorbed through the buccal mucosa and thus can be used by AIDS patients who have difficulty swallowing or who have intestinal obstruction. Clinically, pemoline is as effective as methylphenidate or dextroamphetamine in the treatment of depressive symptoms and in countering the sedating effects of opioid analgesics. There are no studies of the capacity of pemoline to potentiate the analgesic properties of opioids. Pemoline should be used with caution in patients with liver impairment, and liver function tests should be monitored periodically with longer-term treatment. The U.S. Food and Drug Administration (FDA) suggests that patients sign an informed consent document which outlines the potential liver toxicities of pemoline when pemoline is prescribed.

Modafinil, a novel psychostimulant that has shown efficacy in treating excessive daytime sleepiness associated with narcolepsy, has recently demonstrated potential for the treatment of depression and fatigue.[162] Modafinil needs further study; however, it appears to be a promising alternative to other psychostimulants in patients who cannot tolerate or have contraindications to the use of other stimulants. Modafinil has minimal cardiovascular effects, does not cause tolerance or dependence, has a low abuse potential, and does not require a special triplicate prescription.

Anticonvulsant Drugs

Selected anticonvulsant drugs appear to be analgesic for the lancinating dysesthesias that characterize diverse types of neuropathic pain.[122] Clinical experience also supports the use of these agents in patients with paroxysmal neuropathic pains that may not be lancinating, and to a far lesser extent, in those with neuropathic pains characterized solely by continuous dysesthesias. Although most practitioners prefer to begin with carbamazepine because of the extraordinarily good response rate observed in trigeminal neuralgia, this drug must be used cautiously in AIDS patients with thrombocytopenia, those at risk for marrow failure, and those whose blood counts must be monitored to determine disease status. If carbamazepine is used, a complete blood count should be obtained prior to the start of therapy, after 2 and 4 weeks, and then every 3–4 months thereafter. A leukocyte count below 4000 is usually considered to be a contraindication to treatment, and a decline to less than 3000, or an absolute neutrophil count of less than 1500 during therapy, should prompt discontinuation of the drug. Other anticonvulsant drugs may be useful for managing neuropathic pain in AIDS patients, including phenytoin, clonazepam, valproate, and gabapentin.[121] Several newer anticonvulsants have been used in the treatment of neuropathic pain. These drugs can be rapidly titrated and well tolerated and include gabapentin, pregabalin, oxcarbazepine, lamotrigine, and felbamate.

Although not fully understood, anticonvulsant medications are commonly used in the treatment of several chronic pain states. Pregabalin is FDA-approved for neuropathic pain associated with diabetic neuropathy. A randomized placebo-controlled trial reported by Dworkin et al.[163] demonstrated that pregabalin at doses of 300 mg or 600 mg daily significantly reduced pain by 30% after 8 weeks of treatment. It has also been used for pain in patients with fibromyalgia.[164] Gabapentin is also FDA-approved for the treatment of postherpetic neuralgia. In a multicenter, double-blind, randomized, placebo-controlled 7-week trial, gabapentin at doses of 1800 mg and 2400 mg daily was superior to placebo in postherpetic neuralgia patients.[165] Oxcarbazepine has shown in small clinical trials to be effective in the management of trigeminal neuralgia and diabetic neuropathy.[166,167] There is evidence that lamotrigine can be used to treat effectively HIV neuropathy, trigeminal neuralgia, spinal cord injury pain, and poststroke pain.[168–170]

Corticosteroids

Corticosteroid drugs have analgesic potential in a variety of chronic pain syndromes, including neuropathic pains and pain syndromes resulting from inflammatory processes.[92] Like other adjuvant analgesics, corticosteroids are usually added to an opioid regimen. In patients with advanced disease, these drugs may also improve appetite, nausea, malaise, and overall quality of life. Adverse effects include neuropsychiatric syndromes, GI disturbances, and immunosuppression.

Baclofen

Baclofen is a GABA-agonist that has proven efficacy in the treatment of trigeminal neuralgia.[171] On this basis, a trial of this drug is commonly employed in the management of paroxysmal neuropathic pains of any type. Dosing is generally undertaken in a manner similar to the use of the drug for its primary indication: spasticity. A starting dose of 5 mg two to three times per day is gradually escalated to 30–90 mg per day, and sometimes higher if side effects do not occur. The most common adverse effects are sedation and confusion.

Oral Local Anesthetics

Local anesthetic drugs may be useful in the management of neuropathic pains characterized by either continuous or lancinating dysesthesias. Controlled trials have demonstrated the efficacy of tocainide[172] and mexiletine,[173] and there is clinical evidence that suggests similar effects from flecainide[174] and subcutaneous lidocaine.[175] It is reasonable to undertake a trial with oral local anesthetics in patients with continuous dysesthesias who fail to respond adequately to, or who cannot tolerate, the tricyclic antidepressants and with patients with lancinating pains refractory to trials of anticonvulsant drugs and baclofen. Mexiletine is preferred in the United States.[92] Paice and colleagues[176] studied 26 subjects in order to test the efficacy of topical capsaicin in the management of HIV-associated pain. Results suggest that capsaicin is ineffective in relieving pain with HIV-associated distal symmetrical peripheral neuropathy; however, capsaicin has been shown to be effective in relieving pain associated with other neuropathic pain syndromes.[176]

DRUG INTERACTIONS: ANALGESICS AND ANTIHUMAN IMMUNODEFICIENCY VIRUS DRUG THERAPIES

Many of the available anti-HIV drugs have the potential to interact with other medications prescribed for pain, depression, anxiety, or other medical conditions. These drug interactions can be dangerous, resulting in drug toxicities due to elevated levels of medication or drug ineffectiveness because of the lowering of drug levels in the serum. Opioid analgesics can interact with certain anti-HIV drug therapies, and these interactions should be kept in mind when prescribing opioids. The protease inhibitor ritonavir can increase the levels of several opioid drugs including codeine, hydrocodone, oxycodone, methadone, and fentanyl. Patients on ritonavir should not be prescribed meperidine or propoxyphene because of increased risk of serious toxicity. Antidepressant and anticonvulsant analgesics can also interact primarily with ritonavir. Ritonavir can increase the serum levels of bupropion (bupropion, bupropion hydrochloride, fluoxetine, trazodone, and desipramine), resulting in increased drug toxicities (e.g., seizures with bupropion). Both ritonavir and saquinavir may increase levels of anticonvulsants such as phenobarbital, phenytoin, carbamazepine, and clonazepam.

NONPHARMACOLOGIC INTERVENTIONS

A variety of physical and psychologic therapies may also prove useful in the management of HIV-related pain (Table 58.7). Phys-

TABLE 58.7

NONPHARMACOLOGIC INTERVENTIONS

PHYSICAL THERAPIES
Cutaneous stimulation (superficial heat, cold, and massage)
Transcutaneous electrical nerve stimulation
Acupuncture
Bedrest

PSYCHOLOGIC THERAPIES
Relaxation, imagery, biofeedback, distraction, and reframing
Hypnosis
Patient education

NEUROSURGICAL PROCEDURES
Nerve blocks
Cordotomy

TABLE 58.8

EXERCISE 1: SLOW RHYTHMIC BREATHING FOR RELAXATION

1. Breathe in slowly and deeply.
2. As you breathe out slowly, feel yourself beginning to relax; feel the tension leaving your body.
3. Now breathe in and out slowly and regularly, at whatever rate is comfortable for you. You may wish to try abdominal breathing.
4. To help you focus on your breathing and breathe slowly and rhythmically: (1) breathe in as you say silently to yourself, "in, two, three"; (2) breathe out as you say silently to yourself, "out, two, three."
   Or
   Each time you breathe out, say silently to yourself a word such as "peace" or "relax."
5. Do steps 1 through 4 only once or repeat steps 3 and 4 for up to 20 minutes.
6. End with a slow deep breath. As you breathe out say to yourself, "I feel alert and relaxed."

Adapted from McCaffery and Beebe, 1989.[193]

ical interventions range from bedrest and simple exercise programs to the application of cold-packs or heat to affected sites. Other nonpharmacologic interventions include whirlpool baths, massage, the application of ultrasound, and transcutaneous electrical nerve stimulation. Increasing numbers of AIDS patients have resorted to acupuncture to relieve their pain, with anecdotal reports of efficacy.

Several psychologic interventions have demonstrated potential efficacy in alleviating HIV-related pain, including hypnosis, relaxation, and distraction techniques such as biofeedback and imagery and cognitive-behavioral techniques (see Tables 58.8 and 58.9 for sample relaxation and distraction exercises). Where non-

TABLE 58.9

EXERCISE 2: PEACEFUL DISTRACTION

Something may have happened to you a while ago that brought you peace and comfort. You may be able to draw on that past experience to bring you peace or comfort now. Think about these questions.

1. Can you remember any situation, even when you were a child, when you felt calm, peaceful, secure, hopeful, or comfortable?
2. Have you ever daydreamed about something peaceful? What were you thinking of?
3. Do you get a dreamy feeling when you listen to music? Do you have any favorite music?
4. Do you have any favorite poetry that you find uplifting or reassuring?
5. Have you ever been religiously active? Do you have favorite readings, hymns, or prayers? Even if you haven't heard or thought of them for many years, childhood religious experiences may still be very soothing.

Additional points: Very likely some of the things you think of in answer to these questions can be recorded for you, such as your favorite music or a prayer. Then, you can listen to the tape whenever you wish. Or, if your memory is strong, you may simply close your eyes and recall the events or words.

Adapted from McCaffery and Beebe, 1989.[193]

pharmacologic and standard pharmacologic treatments fail, anesthetic and even neurosurgical procedures (such as nerve block, cordotomy, and epidural delivery of analgesics) are additional options available to the patient who appreciates the risks and limitations of these procedures.

UNDERTREATMENT OF PAIN IN ACQUIRED IMMUNODEFICIENCY SYNDROME

Reports of dramatic undertreatment of pain in AIDS patients have appeared in the literature.[2,4–6] These studies suggest that all classes of analgesics, particularly opioid analgesics, are underutilized in the treatment of pain in AIDS. The Memorial Group[2] has reported that less than 8% of ambulatory AIDS patients reporting pain in the severe range (8–10 on a NRS of pain intensity) received a strong opioid, such as morphine, as recommended by published guidelines (i.e., the WHO Analgesic Ladder). In addition, 18% of patients with "severe" pain were prescribed no analgesics whatsoever, 40% were prescribed a nonopioid analgesic (e.g., NSAID), and only 22% were prescribed a "weak" opioid (e.g., acetaminophen in combination with oxycodone). Utilizing the Pain Management Index (PMI),[177] a measure of adequacy of analgesic therapy derived from the Brief Pain Inventory's record of pain intensity and strength of analgesia prescribed, these investigators further examined adequacy of pain treatment. Only 15% of the sample received adequate analgesic therapy based on the PMI. This degree of undermedication of pain in AIDS (85%) far exceeds published reports of undermedication of pain (using the PMI) in cancer populations of 40%.[178] Larue and colleagues[4] report that in France, 57% of patients with HIV disease reporting moderate to severe pain did not receive any analgesic treatment at all, and only 22% received a "weak" opioid.

While opioid analgesics are underutilized, it is also clear that adjuvant analgesic agents, such as the antidepressants, are also dramatically underutilized.[2,4–6] Breitbart and colleagues[2] report that less than 10% of AIDS patients reporting pain received an adjuvant analgesic drug (e.g., antidepressants, anticonvulsants) despite the fact that approximately 40% of the sample had neuropathic type pain. This class of analgesic agents is a critical component of the WHO Analgesic Ladder, particularly in managing neuropathic pain, and is vastly underutilized in the management of HIV-related pain.

BARRIERS TO PAIN MANAGEMENT IN ACQUIRED IMMUNODEFICIENCY SYNDROME

A number of different factors have been proposed as potential influences on the widespread undertreatment of pain in AIDS, including patient, clinician, and health care system related barriers.[2,115,179] Sociodemographic factors, which have been reported to be associated with undertreatment of pain in AIDS, include gender, education, and substance abuse history.[1] Women, less educated patients, and patients who reported IDU as their HIV risk transmission factor are significantly more likely to receive inadequate analgesic therapy for HIV-related pain.

Breitbart and colleagues[115] surveyed 200 ambulatory AIDS patients utilizing a modified version of the Barriers Questionnaire (BQ),[180] which assesses a variety of patient-related barriers to pain management (resulting in patient reluctance to report pain or take opioid analgesics). Results of this study demonstrated that patient-related barriers (as measured by BQ scores) were significantly correlated with undertreatment of pain (as measured by the PMI) in AIDS patients with pain. Additionally, BQ scores were significantly correlated with higher levels of psychologic distress and depression, indicating that patient-related barriers contributed to undertreatment for pain and poorer quality of life. The most frequently endorsed BQ items were those concerning the addiction potential of opioids, side effects and discomfort related to opioid administration, and misconceptions about tolerance. While there were no age, gender, or HIV risk transmission factor associations with BQ scores, nonwhite and less educated patients scored higher on the BQ. Several additional AIDS specific patient-related barriers examined[115,179] reveal that 66% of patients are trying to limit their overall intake of medications (i.e., pills) or utilize nonpharmacologic interventions for pain, 50% of patients cannot afford to fill a prescription for analgesics or have no access to pain specialists, and about 50% are reluctant to take opioids for pain out of a concern that family/friends/physicians will assume they are misusing or abusing these drugs.

In a survey of approximately 500 AIDS care providers,[181] clinicians (primarily physicians and nurses) rated the barriers to AIDS pain management they perceived to be the most important in the care of AIDS patients. The most frequently endorsed barriers were those regarding lack of knowledge about pain management or access to pain specialists and concerns regarding the use and addiction potential of opioid drugs in the AIDS population. The top five barriers endorsed by AIDS clinicians included: lack of knowledge regarding pain management (51.8%); reluctance to prescribe opioids (51.5%); lack of access to pain specialists (50.9%); concern regarding drug addiction and/or abuse (50.5%); and lack of psychologic support/drug treatment services (43%). Patient reluctance to report pain and patient reluctance to take opioids were less commonly endorsed barriers, with about 24% of respondents endorsing those barriers. In contrast, past surveys of oncologists rated patient reluctance to report pain or take opioids as two of the top four barriers. Like AIDS care providers, oncologists also endorsed highly a reluctance to prescribe opioids, even to a population of cancer patients with a significantly lower prevalence of past or present substance abuse disorders. Both oncologists and AIDS care providers report they have inadequate knowledge of pain management and pain assessment skills.

Pain Management and Substance Abuse in Acquired Immunodeficiency Syndrome

Individuals who inject drugs are among the AIDS exposure categories with the highest rate of increase over the past 5 years, especially in large urban centers. Pain management in the substance-abusing AIDS patient is perhaps the most challenging of clinical goals. Fears of addiction and concerns regarding drug abuse affect both patient compliance and physician management of pain and use of narcotic analgesics, often leading to the undermedication of HIV-infected patients with pain.

Studies of patterns of chronic narcotic analgesic use in patients with cancer, burns, and postoperative pain, however, have demonstrated that, although tolerance and physical dependence commonly occur, addiction (i.e., psychological dependence and drug abuse) is rare and almost never occurs in individuals who do not have histories of drug abuse.[182–184] More relevant to the clinical problem of pain management in AIDS patients, however, is the issue of managing pain in the growing segment of HIV-infected patients who have a history of substance abuse or who are actively abusing drugs. The use, specifically of opioids for pain control in patients with HIV infection and a history of substance abuse, raises several difficult pain treatment questions, including how to treat pain in people who have a high tolerance to narcotic analgesics, how to mitigate this population's drug-seeking and potentially manipulative behavior, how to deal with patients who may offer unreliable medical histories or who may not comply

with treatment recommendations, and how to counter the risk of patients spreading HIV while high and disinhibited.

Perhaps of greatest concern to clinicians is the possibility that they are being lied to by a substance abusing AIDS patient complaining of pain. Clinicians must rely on a patient's subjective report, which is often the best or only indication of the presence and intensity of pain, as well as the degree of pain relief achieved by an intervention. Physicians who believe they are being manipulated by drug-seeking patients often hesitate to use an appropriate opioid regimen. The fear is that the clinician is being "duped" into prescribing narcotic analgesics which will then be abused or sold. Clinicians do not want to contribute to or help sustain addiction. This leads to an immediate defensiveness on the part of the clinician and an impulse to avoid prescribing opioids and even to avoid full assessment of a pain complaint. Because concerns are often raised regarding the credibility of AIDS patients' report of pain, particularly where there is a history of IDU, Breitbart and colleagues[184b] conducted a study of 516 ambulatory AIDS patients in which they compared the report of pain experience and the adequacy of pain management among patients with and without a history of substance abuse. This study found that there were no significant differences in the report of pain experience (i.e., pain prevalence, pain intensity, and pain-related functional interference) among patients who reported IDU as their HIV transmission risk factor and those who reported other transmission factors (non-IDU). Furthermore, there were no differences in the report of pain experience among patients who acknowledged current substance abuse, those in methadone maintenance, and those who were in drug free recovery. The description of HIV-related pain was comparable among IDU and non-IDU groups. What was different was the treatment received by these two groups. Patients in the IDU group were significantly more undermedicated for pain compared to the non-IDU group. A survey of 211 HIV-infected patients was conducted in order to assess pain reporting in HIV-infected patients with and without intravenous drug use.[185] It was demonstrated by Martin and colleagues[185] that non-IDU patients showed a strong correlation between pain and disease stage, CD4+ levels, and mortality rates. Intravenous drug users, however, did not display the same correlation between pain and disease parameters. Finally, Martin et al.[185] concluded that pain was more prominent in IDU compared to non-IDU, suggesting the need to differentiate risk groups in pain-related studies. Unfortunately, the existence or severity of pain cannot be objectively proven. The clinician must accept and respect the report of pain in spite of the possibility of being duped and proceed in the evaluation, assessment, and management of pain.

Experience from the cancer pain literature suggests that it is possible to adequately manage pain in substance abusers with life-threatening illness and to do so safely and responsibly utilizing opioid analgesics and several sound principles of pain management outlined here (Table 58.10).[101,186–188] Most clinicians experienced in working with this population of patients recommend that practitioners set clear and direct limits. While this is an important aspect of the care of intravenous drug-using people with HIV disease, it is by no means the whole answer. As much as possible, clinicians should attempt to eliminate the issue of drug abuse as an obstacle to pain management by dealing directly with the problems of opiate withdrawal and drug treatment. Clinicians should err on the side of believing patients when they complain of pain and should utilize knowledge of specific HIV-related pain syndromes to corroborate the report of a patient perceived as being unreliable. Messiah and colleagues[189] sought to demonstrate whether physicians were able to accurately identify IDUs and treat them appropriately. The results suggest that identification of active IDU may be partially based on incorrect interpretations of subjective cues.[189]

The clinician must be familiar with and understand the current terminology relevant to substance abuse and addiction. It is important to distinguish between the terms *tolerance*, *physical de-*

TABLE 58.10

AN APPROACH TO PAIN MANAGEMENT IN SUBSTANCE ABUSERS WITH HIV DISEASE

1. Substance abusers with HIV disease deserve pain control; we have an obligation to treat pain and suffering in all of our patients.
2. Accept and respect the report of pain.
3. Be careful about the label *substance abuse*; distinguish between tolerance, physical dependence, and addiction (psychological dependence or drug abuse).
4. Not all *substance abusers* are the same; distinguish between active users, individuals in methadone maintenance, and those in recovery.
5. Individualize pain treatment.
6. Utilize the principles of pain management outlined for all patients with HIV disease and pain (WHO Analgesic Ladder).
7. Set clear goals and conditions for opioid therapy: set limits, recognize drug abuse behaviors, make consequences clear, use written contracts, and establish a single prescriber.
8. Use a multidimensional approach: pharmacologic and non-pharmacologic interventions, attention to psychosocial issues, team approach.

pendence, and *addiction* or *abuse* (psychologic dependence). Tolerance is a pharmacologic property of opioid drugs defined by the need for increasing doses to maintain an (analgesic) effect. Physical dependence is characterized by the onset of signs and symptoms of withdrawal if narcotic analgesics are abruptly stopped or a narcotic antagonist is administered. Tolerance usually occurs in association with physical dependence. Addiction or abuse (also often termed psychologic dependence) is a psychologic and behavioral syndrome in which there is drug craving, compulsive use (despite physical, psychologic, or social harm to user), other aberrant drug-related behaviors, and relapse after abstinence.[101] The term "pseudoaddiction" has been coined to describe the patient who exhibits behavior that clinicians associate with addiction, such as requests for higher doses of opioids, but in fact is due to uncontrolled pain and inadequate pain management.[190]

The clinician must also distinguish between the "former" addict who has been drug free for years, the addict in a methadone maintenance program, and the addict who is actively abusing illicit and/or prescription drugs. Actively using addicts and those on methadone maintenance with pain must be assumed to have some tolerance to opioids and may require higher starting and maintenance doses of opioids. Preventing withdrawal is an essential first step in managing pain in this population. In addition, "active" addicts with AIDS will understandably require more in the way of psychosocial support and services to adequately deal with the distress of their pain and illness. Former addicts may pose the challenge of refusing opioids for pain because of fears of relapse. Such patients can be assured that opioids, when prescribed and monitored responsibly, may be an essential part of pain management, and the use of the drug for pain is quite different from its use when they were abusing similar drugs. Some authorities emphasize the importance of conducting a comprehensive pain assessment in order to define the pain syndrome. Specific pain syndromes often respond best to specific interventions (i.e., neuropathic pains respond well to antidepressants or anticonvulsants). Adequate assessment of the cause of pain is essential in all AIDS patients and particularly in the substance abuser. It is critical that adequate analgesia be provided while diagnostic studies are underway. Often, treatments directed at the underlying disorder causing pain are very effective as well.

For example, headache from CNS toxoplasmosis responds well to primary treatments and steroids.

When deciding on an appropriate pharmacologic intervention in the substance abuser, it is advisable to follow the WHO Analgesic Ladder. This approach advocates selection of analgesics based on severity of pain; however, clinicians also often take into account the nature of the pain syndrome in selecting analgesics. For mild to moderate pain, NSAIDs are indicated. The NSAIDs are continued with adjuvant analgesics (antidepressants, anticonvulsants, neuroleptics, steroids) if a specific indication exists. Patients with moderate to severe pain, or those who do not achieve relief from NSAIDs, are treated with a "weak" opioid, often in combination with NSAIDs and adjuvant drugs, if indicated.

It has been pointed out that it is critical to apply appropriate pharmacologic principles for opioid use. Data by Kaplan et al.[191] suggest that AIDS patients with prior drug use history benefited from opioid analgesia but required substantially more morphine than nonusers. One should avoid using agonist-antagonist opioid drugs. The use of as needed dosing often leads to excessive drug-centered interactions with staff that are not productive. While patients should not necessarily be given the specific drug or route they want, every effort should be made to give patients more of a sense of control and a sense of collaboration with the clinician. Often, a patient's report of beneficial or adverse effects of a specific agent are useful to the clinician.

The management of pain in substance abusing AIDS patients requires a team approach. Early involvement of pain specialists, psychiatric clinicians, and substance abuse specialists is critical. Nonpharmacologic pain interventions should be appropriately applied, not as a substitute for opioids but as an important adjunct. Realistic goals for treatment must be set, and problems related to inappropriate behavior around the handling of prescriptions and interactions with staff should be anticipated.

Hospital staff must be educated and made aware that such difficult patients evoke feelings that if acted on could interfere with providing good care. Clear limit setting is helpful for both the patient and treating staff. Sometimes, written rules about what behaviors are expected and what behaviors are not tolerated and the consequence should be provided. The use of urine toxicology monitoring, restrictions of visitors, and strict limits on amount of drug per prescription can all be very useful. It is important to also remember that rehabilitation or detoxification from opioids is not appropriate during an acute medical crisis and should not be attempted at that time. Once more stable medical conditions exist, referral to a drug rehabilitation program may be very useful. Constant assessment and re-evaluation of the effects of pain interventions must also take place in order to optimize care. Special attention should be given to points in treatment where routes of administration are changed or where opioids are being tapered. It must be made clear to patients what drugs and/or regimen would be introduced to control pain when opioids are tapered or withdrawn, and what options are available if that nonopioid regimen is ineffective.[192]

Finally, it is important to recognize that substance abusers with AIDS are quite likely to have comorbid psychiatric symptoms as well as multiple other physical symptoms which can all contribute to increased pain and suffering. Adequate attention must be paid to these physical and psychologic symptoms for pain management to be optimized.

CONCLUSION

Pain in AIDS, even in this era of protease inhibitors and decreased AIDS death rates, is a clinically significant problem contributing greatly to psychologic and functional morbidity. Pain can be adequately treated and so must be a focus of palliative care in the AIDS patient.

Substance abusers and women are particularly undertreated segments of the AIDS pain population and need special attention. Managing pain in AIDS patients with a history of substance abuse is a particularly challenging problem which AIDS care providers will be facing with increasing frequency.

References

1. Breitbart W, McDonald MV, Rosenfeld B, et al. Pain in ambulatory AIDS patients. I: pain characteristics and medical correlates. *Pain* 1996;68(2–3): 315–321.
2. Breitbart W, Rosenfeld BD, Passik SD, et al. The undertreatment of pain in ambulatory AIDS patients. *Pain* 1996;65(2–3):243–249.
3. Hewitt DJ, McDonald M, Portenoy RK, et al. Pain syndromes and etiologies in ambulatory AIDS patients. *Pain* 1997;70(2–3):117–123.
4. Larue F, Fontaine A, Colleau SM. Underestimation and undertreatment of pain in HIV disease: multicentre study. *BMJ* 1997;314(7073):23–28.
5. Lebovits AH, Lefkowitz M, McCarthy D, et al. The prevalence and management of pain in patients with AIDS: a review of 134 cases. *Clin J Pain* 1989; 5(3):245–248.
6. McCormack JP, Li R, Zarowny D, et al. Inadequate treatment of pain in ambulatory HIV patients. *Clin J Pain* 1993;9(4):279–283.
7. O'Neill WM, Sherrard JS. Pain in human immunodeficiency virus disease: a review. *Pain* 1993;54(1):3–14.
8. Rosenfeld B, Breitbart W, McDonald MV, et al. Pain in ambulatory AIDS patients. II: impact of pain on psychological functioning and quality of life. *Pain* 1996;68(2–3):323–328.
9. Singer EJ, Zorilla C, Fahy-Chandon B, et al. Painful symptoms reported by ambulatory HIV-infected men in a longitudinal study. *Pain* 1993;54(1): 15–19.
10. Breitbart W. Pharmacotherapy of pain in AIDS. In: Wormser G, ed. *A Clinical Guide to AIDS and HIV.* Philadelphia: Lippincott-Raven; 1996:359–378.
11. Breitbart W, ed. Pain in AIDS. In: Jensen TS, Turner JA, Wiesenfeld-Hallin Z, eds. *Proceedings in the 8th World Congress on Pain—Progress in Pain Research and Management.* Vol 8. Seattle, WA: IASP Press; 1997:63–100.
12. Vogl D, Rosenfeld B, Breitbart W, et al. Symptom prevalence, characteristics, and distress in AIDS outpatients. *J Pain Symptom Manage* 1999;18:253–262.
13. Breitbart W, Passik S, Bronaugh T, et al., eds. Pain in the ambulatory AIDS patient: prevalence and psychosocial correlates. In: *Proceedings of the 38th Annual Meeting, Academy of Psychosomatic Medicine, Atlanta, Georgia, October 17–20, 1991.* Chicago: Academy of Psychosomatic Medicine; 1991:60.
14. Kimball LR, McCormick WC. The pharmacologic management of pain and discomfort in persons with AIDS near the end of life: use of opioid analgesia in the hospice setting. *J Pain Symptom Manage* 1996;11(2):88–94.
15. Schofferman J, Brody R. Pain in far advanced AIDS. In: Foley K, Bonica JJ, Ventrafridda V, eds. *Proceedings of the Second International Congress on Pain: Vol 16, Advances in Pain Research and Therapy.* New York: Raven Press; 1990:379–386.
16. Selwyn P. Palliative care for patient with human immunodeficiency virus/acquired immune deficiency syndrome. *J Palliat Med* 2005;8(6):1248–1268.
17. Schofferman J, Brody R. Pain in far advanced AIDS. In: Foley KM, Bonica JJ, Ventafridda V, eds. *Advances in Pain Research and Therapy.* New York: Raven Press; 1990:379–386.
18. Larue F, Brasseur L, Musseault P, et al. Pain and HIV infection: a French national survey. *J Palliat Care* 1994;10:95.
19. Frich LM, Borgbjerg FM. Pain and pain treatment in AIDS patients: a longitudinal study. *J Pain Symptom Manage* 2000;19(5):339–347.
20. Brechtl JR, Breitbart W, Galietta M, et al. The use of highly active antiretroviral therapy (HAART) in patients with advanced HIV infection: impact on medical, palliative care, and quality of life outcomes. *J Pain Symptom Manage* 2001;21(1):41–51.
21. Breitbart W Dibiase L. Current perspectives on pain in AIDS. *Oncology (Williston Park)* 2002;6:818–829, 834–835.
22. Penfold J, Clark AJ. Pain syndromes in HIV infection. *Can J Anaesth* 1992; 39(7):724–730.
23. Breitbart W. Pain. In: O'Neill JF, Selwyn P, Schietinger H, eds. *A Clinical Guide to Supportive and Palliative Care for HIV/AIDS.* Washington, DC: U.S. Department of Health Resources and Services; 2003:85–122.
24. Douaihy AB, Stowell KR, Kohnen S, et al. Psychiatric aspects of comorbid HIV/AIDS and pain, part 1. *AIDS Read* 2007;17(6):310–314.
25. Markus MB, Fincham JE. Helminths, HIV/AIDS and tuberculosis. *S Afr Med J* 2000;90(9):834, 836.
26. Breitbart W, McDonald M, Rosenfeld B, et al., eds. Pain in women with AIDS [Abstract]. Proceedings of the 14th Annual Meeting of the American Pain Society, Los Angeles, CA, 1995.
27. Marte C, Allen M. HIV-related gynecologic conditions: overlooked complications. *Focus: A Guide to AIDS Research and Counseling* 1991;7(1):1–3.
28. Passik SD, Kirsh KL, McDonald MV, et al. A pilot survey of aberrant drug-taking attitudes and behaviors in samples of cancer and AIDS patients. *J Pain Symptom Manage* 2000;19(4):274–286.
29. Strafford M, Cahill C, Schwartz T, et al. Recognition and treatment of pain in pediatric patients with AIDS. *J Pain Symptom Manage* 1991;6:146.
30. Oleske J. Pain Relief for Children with HIV/AIDS: A Global Imperative. In: WHO, ed; 2007:1–3.
31. Cook GC. The mouth in human immunodeficiency virus (HIV) infection. *Q J Med* 1990;76(279):655–657.
32. Rabeneck L, Popovic M, Gartner S, et al. Acute HIV infection presenting with painful swallowing and esophageal ulcers. *JAMA* 1990;263(17):2318–2322.
33. Bonacini M, Young T, Laine L. The causes of esophageal symptoms in human immunodeficiency virus infection. A prospective study of 110 patients. *Arch Intern Med* 1991;151(8):1567–1572.
34. Connolly GM, Hawkins D, Harcourt-Webster JN, et al. Oesophageal symptoms, their causes, treatment, and prognosis in patients with the acquired immunodeficiency syndrome. *Gut* 1989;30:1033–1039.
35. Eisner MS, Selwyn P. Etiology of odynophagia and dysphagia in patients with the acquired immunodeficiency syndrome. *Arthritis Rheum* 1990;31:A446.
36. de Silva DG. Tumour necrosis factor. *Ceylon Med J* 1990;35(4):151–153.
37. Goodman P, Pinero SS, Rance RM, et al. Mycobacterial esophagitis in AIDS. *Gastrointest Radiol* 1989;14(2):103–105.
38. Kazlow PG, Shah K, Benkov KJ, et al. Esophageal cryptosporidiosis in a child with acquired immune deficiency syndrome. *Gastroenterology* 1986;91(5): 1301–1303.
39. Kitchen VS, Helbert M, Francis ND, et al. Epstein-Barr virus associated oesophageal ulcers in AIDS. *Gut* 1990;31(11):1223–1225.
40. Edwards P, Turner J, Gold J, et al. Esophageal ulceration induced by zidovudine. *Ann Intern Med* 1990;112(1):65–66.
41. Barone JE, Gingold BS, Arvanitis ML, et al. Abdominal pain in patients with acquired immune deficiency syndrome. *Ann Surg* 1986;204(6):619–623.
42. Balthazar EJ, Reich CB, Pachter HL. The significance of small bowel intussusception in acquired immune deficiency syndrome. *Am J Gastroenterol* 1986; 81(11):1073–1075.
43. Davidson T, Allen-Mersh TG, Miles AJ, et al. Emergency laparotomy in patients with AIDS. *Br J Surg* 1991;78(8):924–926.
44. Friedman SL, Wright TL, Altman DF. Gastrointestinal Kaposi's sarcoma in patients with acquired immunodeficiency syndrome. Endoscopic and autopsy findings. *Gastroenterology* 1985;89(1):102–108.
45. Potter DA, Danforth DN Jr, Macher AM, et al. Evaluation of abdominal pain in the AIDS patient. *Ann Surg* 1984;199(3):332–339.
46. Cello JP. Acquired immunodeficiency syndrome cholangiopathy: spectrum of disease. *Am J Med* 1989;86(5):539–546.
47. Bonacini M. Hepatobiliary complications in patients with human immunodeficiency virus infection. *Am J Med* 1992;92(4):404–411.
48. Wilcox CM, Forsmark CE, Grendell JH, et al. Cytomegalovirus-associated acute pancreatic disease in patients with acquired immunodeficiency syndrome. Report of two patients. *Gastroenterology* 1990;99(1):263–267.
49. Wexner SD, Smithy WB, Milsom JW, et al. The surgical management of anorectal diseases in AIDS and pre-AIDS patients. *Dis Colon Rectum* 1986; 29(11):719–723.
50. Rabkin CS, Blattner WA. HIV infection and cancers other than non-Hodgkin lymphoma and Kaposi's sarcoma. *Cancer Surv* 1991;10:151–160.
51. Cornblath DR, McArthur JC. Predominantly sensory neuropathy in patients with AIDS and AIDS-related complex. *Neurology* 1988;38(5):794–796.
52. Dalakas MC, Pezeshkpour GH. Neuromuscular diseases associated with human immunodeficiency virus infection. *Ann Neurol* 1988;23 Suppl: S38–S48.
53. Levy RM, Bredesen DE, Rosenblum ML. Opportunistic central nervous system pathology in patients with AIDS. *Ann Neurol* 1988;23 Suppl:S7–S12.
54. Snider WD, Simpson DM, Nielsen S, et al. Neurological complications of acquired immune deficiency syndrome: analysis of 50 patients. *Ann Neurol* 1983;14(4):403–418.
55. Goldstein J. Headache and acquired immunodeficiency syndrome. *Neurol Clin* 1990;8(4):947–960.
56. Richman DD, Fischl MA, Grieco MH, et al. The toxicity of azidothymidine (AZT) in the treatment of patients with AIDS and AIDS-related complex. A double-blind, placebo-controlled trial. *N Engl J Med* 1987;317(4):192–197.
57. Lipton RB, Feraru ER, Weiss G, et al. Headache in HIV-1-related disorders. *Headache* 1991;31(8):518–522.
58. Evers S, Wibbeke B, Reichelt D, et al. The impact of HIV infection on primary headache. Unexpected findings from retrospective, cross-sectional, and prospective analyses. *Pain* 2000;85(1–2):191–200.
59. Levy RM, Bredesen DE, Rosenblum ML. Neurological manifestations of the acquired immunodeficiency syndrome (AIDS): experience at UCSF and review of the literature. *J Neurosurg* 1985;62(4):475–495.
60. Parry GJ. Peripheral neuropathies associated with human immunodeficiency virus infection. *Ann Neurol* 1988;23 Suppl:S49–S53.
61. Griffin JW, Wesselingh SL, Griffin DE, et al. Peripheral nerve disorders in HIV infection. Similarities and contrasts with CNS disorders. In: Price RW, Perry SW, eds. *HIV, AIDS and the Brain.* New York: Raven Press; 1994: 159–182.
62. Lefkowitz M, Breitbart W. Chronic pain and AIDS. In: Wiener RH, ed. *Innovations in Pain Medicine.* Orlando, FL: Paul Deutsch Press; 1992:2–3.
63. Moss V. Palliative care in advanced HIV disease: presentation, problems and palliation. *AIDS* 1990;4(Suppl 1):S235–S242.
64. Singh S, Fermie P, Peters W, eds. Symptom control for individuals with advanced HIV infection in a subacute residential unit: which symptoms need palliating? Paper presented at: International Conference on AIDS/III STD World Congress; July 19–24, 1992; Amsterdam, the Netherlands.
65. Zhou L, Kitch DW, Evans SR, et al. Correlates of epidermal nerve fiber densi-

ties in HIV-associated distal sensory polyneuropathy. *Neurology* 2007; 68(24):2113–2119.

66. Lange DJ, Britton CB, Younger DS, et al. The neuromuscular manifestations of human immunodeficiency virus infections. *Arch Neurol* 1988;45(10): 1084–1088.

67. Simpson DM, Wolfe DE. Neuromuscular complications of HIV infection and its treatment. *AIDS* 1991;5(8):917–926.

68. Ownby KK, Dune LS. The processes by which persons with HIV-related peripheral neuropathy manage their symptoms: a qualitative study. *J Pain Symptom Manage* 2007;34(1):48–59.

69. Fuller GN, Jacobs JM, Guiloff RJ. Association of painful peripheral neuropathy in AIDS with cytomegalovirus infection. *Lancet* 1989;2(8669):937–941.

70. Harrison RA, Soong S, Weiss HL, et al. A mixed model for factors predictive of pain in AIDS patients with herpes zoster. *J Pain Symptom Manage* 1999; 17(6):410–417.

71. Berman A, Espinoza LR, Diaz JD, et al. Rheumatic manifestations of human immunodeficiency virus infection. *Am J Med* 1988;85(1):59–64.

72. Espinoza LR, Aguilar JL, Berman A, et al. Rheumatic manifestations associated with human immunodeficiency virus infection. *Arthritis Rheum* 1989; 32(12):1615–1622.

73. Kaye BR. Rheumatologic manifestations of infection with human immunodeficiency virus (HIV). *Ann Intern Med* 1989;111(2):158–167.

74. Winchester R, Bernstein DH, Fischer HD, et al. The co-occurrence of Reiter's syndrome and acquired immunodeficiency. *Ann Intern Med* 1987;106(1): 19–26.

75. Espinoza LR, Berman A, Vasey FB, et al. Psoriatic arthritis and acquired immunodeficiency syndrome. *Arthritis Rheum* 1988;31(8):1034–1040.

76. Johnson TM, Duvic M, Rapini RP, et al. AIDS exacerbates psoriasis. *N Engl J Med* 1985;313(22):1415.

77. Rynes RI, Goldenberg DL, DiGiacomo R, et al. Acquired immunodeficiency syndrome-associated arthritis. *Am J Med* 1988;84(5):810–816.

78. Dalakas MC, Pezeshkpour GH, Gravell M, et al. Polymyositis associated with AIDS retrovirus. *JAMA* 1986;256(17):2381–2383.

79. Gorard DA, Henry K, Guiloff RJ. Necrotizing myopathy and zidovudine. *Lancet* 1988;331:1050–1051.

80. Ledford DK, Overman MD, Gonzalvo A, et al. Microsporidiosis myositis in a patient with the acquired immunodeficiency syndrome. *Ann Intern Med* 1985;102(5):628–630.

81. Nelson MR, Daniels D, Dean R, et al. Staphylococcus aureus psoas abscess in a patient with AIDS. *Int J STD AIDS* 1992;3(4):294.

82. Panegyres PK Ran N, Kakulas BA, et al. Necrotizing myopathy and zidovudine. *Lancet* 1988;331:1050–1051.

83. Watts RA, Hoffbrand BI, Paton DF, et al. Pyomyositis associated with human immunodeficiency virus infection. *Br Med J (Clin Res Ed)* 1987;294(6586): 1524–1525.

84. Wolf RF, Sprenger HG, Mooyaart El, et al. Nontropical pyomyositis as a cause of subacute, multifocal myalgia in the Acquired Immunodeficiency Syndrome. *Arthritis Rheum* 1990;33(11):1728–1732.

85. Bessen LJ, Greene JB, Louie E, et al. Severe polymyositis-like syndrome associated with zidovudine therapy of AIDS and ARC. *N Engl J Med* 1988;318(11): 708.

86. Breitbart W. Suicide risk and pain in cancer and AIDS patients. In: Chapman R, Foley KM, eds. *Current Emerging Issues in Cancer Pain: Research and Practice*. New York: Raven Press; 1993:49–65.

87. Payne D, Jacobsen P, Breitbart W, eds. Negative thoughts related to pain are associated with greater pain, distress and disability in AIDS pain. Paper presented at: American Pain Society, 13th Scientific Meeting; Miami, FL; 1994.

88a. Vogl D, Rosenfeld B, Breitbart W, et al. Symptom prevalence, characteristics, and distress in AIDS outpatients. *J Pain Symptom Manage*.

88b. Breitbart W, Rosenfeld B, Passik S, et al. A comparison of pain report and adequacy of analgesic therapy in ambulatory AIDS patients with and without a history of substance abuse. *Pain* 1997;1–2:235–243.

89. Kishore-Kumar R, Max MB, Schafer SC, et al. Desipramine relieves postherpetic neuralgia. *Clin Pharmacol Ther* 1990;47(3):305–312.

90. Watson CP, Chipman M, Reed K, et al. Amitriptyline versus maprotiline in postherpetic neuralgia: a randomized, double-blind, crossover trial. *Pain* 1992;48(1):29–36.

91. Foley KM. The treatment of cancer pain. *N Engl J Med* 1985;313(2):84–95.

92. Portenoy R, Foley K. Management of cancer pain. In: Holland J, Rowland J, eds. *Handbook of Psychooncology*. New York: Oxford University Press; 1989:369–382.

93. Jacox A, Carr DB, Payne R, et al. *Clinical Practice Guideline Number 9: Management of Cancer Pain*. Rockville, MD: Agency for Health Care Policy and Research, U.S. Department of Health and Human Services, Public Health Service; 1994:139–141.

94. Portenoy RK. Pharmacologic approaches to the control of cancer pain. *J Psychosocial Oncology* 1990;8:75–107.

95. WHO, ed. *Cancer Pain Relief*. Geneva, Switzerland: Author; 1986.

96. Fishman B, Pasternak S, Wallenstein SL, et al. The Memorial Pain Assessment Card. A valid instrument for the evaluation of cancer pain. *Cancer* 1987; 60(5):1151–1158.

97. Daut RL, Cleeland CS, Flanery RC. Development of the Wisconsin Brief Pain Questionnaire to assess pain in cancer and other diseases. *Pain* 1983;17(2): 197–210.

98. Acello B. Meeting JCAHO standards for pain control. *Nursing* 2000;30(3): 52–54.

99. Wisconsin Cancer Pain Initiative. Building an Institutional Commitment to Pain Management: The Mayday Resource Manual for Improvement Available at: www.aacpi.org. Accessed: May 5, 2001.

100. Ventafridda V, Caraceni A, Gamba A. Field testing of the WHO Guidelines for Cancer Pain Relief: summary report of demonstration projects. In: Foley KM, Bonica JJ, Ventafridda V, eds. *Proceedings of the Second International Congress on Pain*. New York: Raven Press; 1990:155–165.

101. American Pain Society (APS). *Principles of Analgesic Use in the Treatment of Acute Pain and Cancer Pain*. 2nd ed. Skokie, IL: American Pain Society; 1992.

102. Anand A, Carmosino L, Glatt AE. Evaluation of recalcitrant pain in HIV-infected hospitalized patients. *J Acquir Immune Defic Syndr* 1994;7(1): 52–56.

103. Lefkowitz M, Newshan G, ed. An evaluation of the use of Duragesic for chronic pain in patients with AIDS. Presented at: American Pain Society 16th Annual Meeting; October 23–26, 1997; New Orleans, LA.

104. Newshan G, Wainapel S. Pain characteristics and their management in persons with AIDS. *J Assoc Nurses AIDS Care* 1993;4(2):53–59.

105. Patt RB, Reddy SR. Pain and the opioid analgesics: alternate routes of administration. *PAACNOTES* 1993:453–458.

106. Murray MD, Brater DC. Adverse effects of nonsteroidal anti-inflammatory drugs on renal function. *Ann Intern Med* 1990;112(8):559–560.

107. Radeck K, Deck C. Do nonsteroidal anti-inflammatory drugs interfere with blood pressure? *J Gen Intern Med* 1987;2:108–112.

108. Johansson CC, Bryn T, Aandahl EM, et al. Treatment with type-2 selective and non-selective cyclooxygenase inhibitors improves T-cell proliferation in HIV-infected patients on highly active antiretroviral therapy. *AIDS* 2004; 18(6):951–952.

109. Kvale D, Ormaasen V, Kran AM, et al. Immune modulatory effects of cyclooxygenase type 2 inhibitors in HIV patients on combination antiretroviral treatment. *AIDS* 2006;20(6):813–820.

110. Aggarwal BB, Shishodia S, Sandur SK, et al. Inflammation and cancer: how hot is the link? *Biochem Pharmacol* 2006;72(11):1605–1621.

111. Bolten WW. [Symptomatic therapy of rheumatic diseases. How they reduce pain and thereby save costs] [in German]. *MMW Fortschr Med* 2002; 144(33–34):30–36.

112. Lexi-Comp, Inc. Available at: www.lexi.com. Accessed 2008.

113. Kaplan R, Conant M, Cundiff D, et al. Sustained-release morphine sulfate in the management of pain associated with acquired immune deficiency syndrome. *J Pain Symptom Manage* 1996;12(3):150–160.

114. Foley K, Inturrisi C. Analgesic drug therapy in cancer pain. In: Payne R, Foley K, eds. *Cancer Pain Medical Clinics of North America*. Philadelphia: WB Saunders; 1987:207–232.

115. Breitbart W, Passik S, McDonald MV, et al. Patient-related barriers to pain management in ambulatory AIDS patients. *Pain* 1998;76(1–2):9–16.

116. Breitbart W, Mermelstein H. Pemoline. An alternative psychostimulant for the management of depressive disorders in cancer patients. *Psychosomatics* 1992;33(3):352–356.

117. Bruera E, Chadwick S, Brenneis C, et al. Methylphenidate associated with narcotics for the treatment of cancer pain. *Cancer Treat Rep* 1987;71(1): 67–70.

118. Kaiko RF, Foley KM, Grabinski PY, et al. Central nervous system excitatory effects of meperidine in cancer patients. *Ann Neurol* 1983;13(2):180–185.

119. Breitbart W. Psychiatric management of cancer pain. *Cancer* 1989;63(11 Suppl):2336–2342.

120. Breitbart W. Psychotropic adjuvant analgesics for cancer pain. *Psycho-Oncology* 1992;7:133–145.

121. Portenoy R. Adjuvant analgesics in pain management. In: Doyle D, Hanks GWC, MacDonald N, eds. *Oxford Textbook of Palliative Medicine*. 2nd ed. New York: Oxford University Press; 1998:361–390.

122. Butler S. Present status of tricyclic antidepressants in chronic pain therapy. In: Benedetti C, Chapman CR, Moricca G, eds. *Advances in Pain Research and Therapy*. Vol 7. New York: Raven Press; 1986:173–196.

123. France RD. The future for antidepressants: treatment of pain. *Psychopathology* 1987;20(Suppl 1):99–113.

124. Getto CJ, Sorkness CA, Howell T. Issues in drug management. Part I. Antidepressants and chronic nonmalignant pain: a review. *J Pain Symptom Manage* 1987;2(1):9–18.

125. Magni G, Arsie D, De Leo D. Antidepressants in the treatment of cancer pain. A survey in Italy. *Pain* 1987;29(3):347–353.

126. Ventafridda V, Bonezzi C, Caraceni A, et al. Antidepressants for cancer pain and other painful syndromes with deafferentation component: comparison of amitriptyline and trazodone. *Ital J Neurol Sci* 1987;8(6):579–587.

127. Walsh TD. Controlled study of imipramine and morphine in chronic pain due to advanced cancer. In: Foley K, ed. *Advances in Pain Research and Therapy*. New York: Raven Press; 1986:155–165.

128. Botney M, Fields HL. Amitriptyline potentiates morphine analgesia by a direct action on the central nervous system. *Ann Neurol* 1983;13(2):160–164.

129. Malseed RT, Goldstein FJ. Enhancement of morphine analgesia by tricyclic antidepressants. *Neuropharmacology* 1979;18(10):827–829.

130. Ventafridda V, Bianchi M, Ripamonti C, et al. Studies on the effects of antidepressant drugs on the antinociceptive action of morphine and on plasma morphine in rat and man. *Pain* 1990;43(2):155–162.

131. Spiegel K, Kalb R, Pasternak GW. Analgesic activity of tricyclic antidepressants. *Ann Neurol* 1983;13(4):462–465.

132. Gram L. Receptors, pharmacokinetics and clinical effects. In: Burrows G, ed. *Antidepressants*. Amsterdam, the Netherlands: Elsevier; 1983:81–95.

133. Merskey H, Hamilton JT. An open label trial of the possible analgesic effects of dipyridamole. *J Pain Symptom Manage* 1989;4(1):34–37.

134. Devor M. Nerve pathophysiology and mechanisms of pain in causalgia. *J Auton Nerv Syst* 1983;7(3–4):371–384.

135. Max MB, Culnane M, Schafer SC, et al. Amitriptyline relieves diabetic neuropathy pain in patients with normal or depressed mood. *Neurology* 1987; 37(4):589–596.

136. Pilowsky I, Hallett EC, Bassett DL, et al. A controlled study of amitriptyline in the treatment of chronic pain. *Pain* 1982;14(2):169–179.

137. Sharav Y, Singer E, Schmidt E, et al. The analgesic effect of amitriptyline on chronic facial pain. *Pain* 1987;31(2):199–209.

138. Sindrup SH, Gram LF, Brosen K, et al. The selective serotonin reuptake inhibitor paroxetine is effective in the treatment of diabetic neuropathy symptoms. *Pain* 1990;42(2):135–144.

139. Young RJ, Clarke BF. Pain relief in diabetic neuropathy: the effectiveness of imipramine and related drugs. *Diabet Med* 1985;2(5):363–366.

140. Max MB, Lynch SA, Muir J, et al. Effects of desipramine, amitriptyline, and fluoxetine on pain in diabetic neuropathy. *N Engl J Med* 1992;326(19): 1250–1256.

141. Gomez-Perez FJ, Rull JA, Dies H, et al. Nortriptyline and fluphenazine in the symptomatic treatment of diabetic neuropathy. A double-blind cross-over study. *Pain* 1985;23(4):395–400.

142. Langohr HD, Stohr M, Petruch F. An open and double-blind cross-over study on the efficacy of clomipramine (Anafranil) in patients with painful mono- and polyneuropathies. *Eur Neurol* 1982;21(5):309–317.

143. Tiegno M, Pagnoni B, Calmi A, et al. Chlorimipramine compared to pentazocine as a unique treatment in post-operative pain. *Int J Clin Phamacol Res* 1987;7:141–143.

144. Hameroff SR, Cork RC, Scherer K, et al. Doxepin effects on chronic pain, depression and plasma opioids. *J Clin Psychiatry* 1982;43(8 Pt 2):22–27.

145. Costa D, Mogos I, Toma T. Efficacy and safety of mianserin in the treatment of depression of women with cancer. *Acta Psychiatr Scand Suppl* 1985;320: 85–92.

146. Davidoff G, Guarracini M, Roth E, et al. Trazodone hydrochloride in the treatment of dysesthetic pain in traumatic myelopathy: a randomized, double-blind, placebo-controlled study. *Pain* 1987;29(2):151–161.

147. Eberhard G, von Knorring L, Nilsson HL, et al. A double-blind randomized study of clomipramine versus maprotiline in patients with idiopathic pain syndromes. *Neuropsychobiology* 1988;19(1):25–34.

148. Feighner JP. A comparative trial of fluoxetine and amitriptyline in patients with major depressive disorder. *J Clin Psychiatry* 1985;46(9):369–372.

149. Hynes MD, Lochner MA, Bemis KG, et al. Fluoxetine, a selective inhibitor of serotonin uptake, potentiates morphine analgesia without altering its discriminative stimulus properties or affinity for opioid receptors. *Life Sci* 1985; 36(24):2317–2323.

150. Diamond S, Freitag FG. Do non-steroidal anti-inflammatory agents have a role in the treatment of migraine headaches? *Drugs* 1989;37(6):755–760.

151. Geller SA. Treatment of fibrositis with fluoxetine hydrochloride (Prozac). *Am J Med* 1989;87(5):594–595.

152. Pick CG, Paul D, Eison MS, et al. Potentiation of opioid analgesia by the antidepressant nefazodone. *Eur J Pharmacol* 1992;211(3):375–381.

153. Beaver WT, Wallenstein SL, Houde RW, et al. A comparison of the analgesic effects of methotrimeprazine and morphine in patients with cancer. *Clin Pharmacol Ther* 1966;7(4):436–446.

154. Lechin F, van der Dijs B, Lechin ME, et al. Pimozide therapy for trigeminal neuralgia. *Arch Neurol* 1989;46(9):960–963.

155. Maltbie AA, Cavenar JO Jr, Sullivan JL, et al. Analgesia and haloperidol: a hypothesis. *J Clin Psychiatry* 1979;40(7):323–326.

156. Breitbart W, Marotta RF, Call P. AIDS and neuroleptic malignant syndrome. *Lancet* 1988;2(8626–8627):1488–1489.

157. Caccia MR. Clonazepam in facial neuralgia and cluster headache. Clinical and electrophysiological study. *Eur Neurol* 1975;13(6):560–563.

158. Fernandez F, Levy JK. Psychiatric diagnosis and pharmcotherapy of patients with HIV infection. In: Tasman A, Goldfinger SM, Kaufman KR, eds. *Review of Psychiatry*. Vol. 9. Washington, DC: American Psychiatric Press; 1990: 614.

159. Swerdlow M, Cundill JG. Anticonvulsant drugs used in the treatment of lancinating pain. A comparison. *Anaesthesia* 1981;36(12):1129–1132.

160. Bruera E, Brenneis C, Paterson AH, et al. Use of methylphenidate as an adjuvant to narcotic analgesics in patients with advanced cancer. *J Pain Symptom Manage* 1989;4(1):3–6.

161. Forrest WH Jr, Brown BW Jr, Brown CR, et al. Dextroamphetamine with morphine for the treatment of postoperative pain. *N Engl J Med* 1977; 296(13):712–715.

162. Menza MA, Kaufman KR, Castellanos A. Modafinil augmentation of antidepressant treatment in depression. *J Clin Psychiatry* 2000;61(5):378–381.

163. Dworkin RH, Corbin AE, Young JP, Jr, et al. Pregabalin for the treatment of postherpetic neuralgia: a randomized, placebo-controlled trial. *Neurology* 2003;60(8):1274–1283.

164. Crofford LJ. The relationship of fibromyalgia to neuropathic pain syndromes. *J Rheumatol Suppl* 2005;75:41–45.

165. Rice AS, Maton S. Gabapentin in postherpetic neuralgia: a randomised, double blind, placebo controlled study. *Pain* 2001;94(2):215–224.

166. Zakrzewska JM, Patsalos PN. Oxcarbazepine: a new drug in the management of intractable trigeminal neuralgia. *J Neurol Neurosurg Psychiatry* 1989; 52(4):472–476.

167. Dogra S, Beydoun S, Mazzola J, et al. Oxcarbazepine in painful diabetic neuropathy: a randomized, placebo-controlled study. *Eur J Pain* 2005;9(5): 543–554.

168. Simpson DM, McArthur JC, Olney R, et al. Lamotrigine for HIV-associated painful sensory neuropathies: a placebo-controlled trial. *Neurology* 2003; 60(9):1508–1514.

169. Sindrup SH, Jensen TS. Pharmacotherapy of trigeminal neuralgia. *Clin J Pain* 2002;18(1):22–27.

170. Vestergaard K, Andersen G, Gottrup H, et al. Lamotrigine for central poststroke pain: a randomized controlled trial. *Neurology* 2001;56(2): 184–190.

171. Fromm GH. Trigeminal neuralgia and related disorders. *Neurol Clin* 1989; 7(2):305–319.

172. Lyndstrom P, Lindbloom T. The analgesic tocainide for trigeminal neuralgia. *Pain* 1987;28:45–50.

173. Chabal C, Jacobson L, Mariano A, et al. The use of oral mexiletine for the treatment of pain after peripheral nerve injury. *Anesthesiology* 1992;76(4): 513–517.

174. Dunlop R, Davies R, Hockley J, et al. Letter to the editor. *Lancet* 1989;1: 420–421.

175. Brose WG, Cousins MJ. Subcutaneous lidocaine for treatment of neuropathic cancer pain. *Pain* 1991;45(2):145–148.

176. Paice JA, Ferrans CE, Lashley FR, et al. Topical capsaicin in the management of HIV-associated peripheral neuropathy. *J Pain Symptom Manage* 2000; 19(1):45–52.

177. Zelman D, Cleeland C, Howland E. Factors in appropriate pharmacological management of cancer pain: a cross-institutional investigation. *Pain* 1987;4 Suppl:S136.

178. Cleeland CS, Gonin R, Hatfield AK, et al. Pain and its treatment in outpatients with metastatic cancer. *N Engl J Med* 1994;330(9):592–596.

179. Passik S, Breitbart W, Rosenfeld B, et al., eds. AIDS specific patient-related barriers to pain management. Presented at: 13th Annual Meeting of the American Pain Society; November 10–13, 1994; Miami, FL.

180. Ward SE, Goldberg N, Miller-McCauley V, et al. Patient-related barriers to management of cancer pain. *Pain* 1993;52(3):319–324.

181. Breitbart W, Kaim M, Rosenfeld B. Clinicians' perceptions of barriers to pain management in AIDS. *J Pain Symptom Manage* 1999;18(3):203–212.

182. Kanner RM, Foley KM. Patterns of narcotic drug use in a cancer pain clinic. *Ann N Y Acad Sci* 1981;362:161–172.

183. Perry S, Heidrich G. Management of pain during debridement: a survey of U.S. burn units. *Pain* 1982;13(3):267–280.

184a. Porter J, Jick H. Addiction rare in patients treated with narcotics. *N Engl J Med* 1980;302(2):123.

184b. Rosenfeld B, Breitbart W, Gibson C, et al. Desire for hastened death among patients with advanced AIDS. *Psychosomatics* 2006;47(6):504–512.

185. Martin C, Pehrsson P, Osterberg A, et al. Pain in ambulatory HIV-infected patients with and without intravenous drug use. *Eur J Pain* 1999;3(2): 157–164.

186. Macaluso C, Weinberg D, Foley K. Opioid abuse and misuse in a cancer pain population. *J Pain Symptom Manage* 1988;3:54.

187. McCaffery M, Vourakis C. Assessment and relief of pain in chemically dependent patients. *Orthop Nurs* 1992;11(2):13–27.

188. Portenoy R, Payne R. Acute and chronic pain. In: Lowinson J, Ruiz P, Millman R, eds. *Comprehensive Textbook of Substance Abuse*. Baltimore, MD: Williams and Wilkins; 1992:691–721.

189. Messiah A, Loundou AD, Maslin V, et al. Physician recognition of active drug use in HIV-infected patients is lower than validity of patient's self-reported drug use. *J Pain Symptom Manage* 2001;21(2):103–112.

190. Weissman DE, Haddox JD. Opioid pseudoaddiction—an iatrogenic syndrome. *Pain* 1989;36(3):363–366.

191. Kaplan R, Slywka J, Slagle S, et al. A titrated morphine analgesic regimen comparing substance users and non-users with AIDS-related pain. *J Pain Symptom Manage* 2000;19(4):265–273.

192. Swica Y, Breitbart W. Treating pain in patients with AIDS and a history of substance use. *West J Med* 2002;176(1):33–39.

193. McCaffery and Beebe, 1989.

CHAPTER 59 ■ THE TREATMENT OF CHRONIC PAIN IN PATIENTS WITH HISTORY OF SUBSTANCE ABUSE

HOWARD A. HEIT AND DOUGLAS L. GOURLAY

INTRODUCTION

Chronic pain has no positive physiologic value, while acute pain is an adaptive, beneficial response necessary for the preservation of tissue integrity.[1] Recurrent migraine headache, painful peripheral neuropathy, or metastatic bone cancer serves no useful physiologic purpose. In addition, pain is the most common complaint presenting to the primary health care professional and should be treated in all populations.[2]

The U.S. Census Bureau reported in July 2007 that the nation's population had reached 301 million. Approximately 16% to 23% (50 to 70 million) of the population suffers pain which is under-treated or not treated at all.[2] Three percent to 16% of the American population may have the disease of addiction.[3] This incidence and percentage of chronic pain and addiction is most likely representative of most developed countries. Furthermore, in certain subsets of the general population, the incidence of pain may be considerably greater as has been reported in methadone maintenance treatment programs.[4] Opioids may be indicated in a small percentage of these patients with moderate to severe pain. However, this population may be at increased risk for relapse even in the context of a comprehensive treatment plan that includes "rational pharmacotherapy." In addition, regulatory scrutiny often leaves the health care professional in a position of real or perceived vulnerability when prescribing a controlled substance (CS). This may put both health care professionals and their patients at risk of a suboptimal outcome for an often treatable medical condition.

The use of controlled substances including opioids in persons who may suffer from concurrent substance use disorders presents challenges to the health care professional. Success in the treatment of either condition requires an approach that encompasses the biopsychosocial needs of the patient. Pain management necessitates the need for appropriate boundary setting within the doctor-patient relationship. Unfortunately, it is impossible to determine beforehand, with any degree of certainty, who will become problematic users of prescription medications. By recognizing the need to carefully assess all patients, in a biopsychosocial model, stigma can be reduced, patient care improved, and overall risk contained.[5]

The goals of this chapter are to address the complex issues associated with the treatment of pain in persons with problematic behavior and to offer the health care professional an approach that may reduce risk and, hopefully, improve outcome.

PRINCIPLE OF BALANCE

Health care professionals who treat patients at the interface of pain and addiction and officials who formulate and enforce regulations must understand the central principle of "balance" as it relates to the use of any CS including opioids.

That principle provides for a system of controls to reduce the risk of diversion, abuse, or trafficking of opioids, balanced against the assurance of the availability of opioids for legitimate medical and scientific purposes and accessibility of opioids to all who need them for the relief of pain.[6] Health care professionals must embrace this principle as should our patients, dispensing pharmacists, and community.

By applying the principle of balance, it stands to reason that health care professionals should be able to treat pain in patients with the disease of addiction who are willing to simultaneously address both conditions. One can successfully treat acute pain in the face of an active addiction, but one will not achieve the stated goals in chronic pain management with an untreated substance use disorder.[7] Mutual support programs such as Alcoholics Anonymous and Narcotics Anonymous are quite clear in terms of their position on the management of any medical condition: these are side issues and should not interfere with the 12 steps and traditions of their respective programs. Inappropriate use of prescription medications, even when legitimately prescribed by a licensed professional, can interfere in the recovery process. For this reason, patients "in recovery" from drug or alcohol misuse need to ensure that their physicians are knowledgeable in the recovery process or have guidance from someone with such knowledge involved in their care.

The Importance of the Definitions

Using precise definitions at the interface of pain and addiction medicine will allow health care providers to improve their clinical practice of pain management (Table 59.1).[8–10]

Confusion between physical dependence and addiction may contribute to the under-treatment of chronic pain. Ballantyne et al. have expressed concern over the apparent separation of physical and psychological dependence in the diagnosis of addiction as if to suggest that these are entirely separable phenomena.[11] Although the following definitions share many elements in common, "continued use despite harm" remains the behavioral marker in the chronic pain patient that will define, over time, an addictive disorder, if present.[12] Physical dependence does not mean addiction,[12a] nor is it necessarily devoid of psychological components. Physical dependence and addiction can coincide, but physical dependence is neither necessary nor sufficient to make a diagnosis of addiction. Physical dependence is an expected, neuropharmacological adaptation that occurs as a result of chronic exposure to an agonist class of drug. Addiction is a much more complex biobehavioral phenomenon.[8–10]

Physical dependence is a natural, expected neuroadaptive response that can occur with opioids, alcohol, benzodiazepines, corticosteroids, antidepressants, diabetic agents, cardiac medications, and many other medications used in clinical medicine. Abrupt cessation of these medications can produce a withdrawal syndrome that can include, but is not limited to, nausea, vomiting,

TABLE 59.1

DEFINITIONS

1. Addiction is a primary, chronic, neurobiologic disease with genetic, psychosocial, and environmental factors influencing its development and manifestations. It is characterized by behaviors that include one or more of the following: impaired control over drug use, compulsive use, and continued use despite harm and craving.*
2. Physical dependence is a state of adaptation that is manifested by a drug-class-specific withdrawal syndrome that can be produced by abrupt cessation, rapid dose reduction, decreasing blood level of the drug, and/or administration of an antagonist.*
3. Tolerance is a state of adaptation in which exposure to a drug induces changes that result in a diminution of one or more of the drugs' effects over time.*
4. Pseudoaddiction is a syndrome that causes patients to seek additional medications due to inadequate pharmacotherapy being prescribed. Typically when the pain is treated appropriately, the inappropriate behavior ceases.†
5. Pseudotolerance is the need to increase medication such as opioids for pain when other factor(s) are present, such as disease progression, new disease, increased physical activity, lack of compliance, change in medication formulation, drug interaction, addiction, and/or deviant behavior.‡
6. Iatrogenic addiction occurs when a patient, with a negative personal or family history for alcohol or drug addiction or abuse, is appropriately prescribed a controlled substance and subsequently in the therapeutic course meets the diagnostic criteria for addiction to that substance.**
7. Misuse is use of a medication (for a medical purpose) other than as directed or as indicated, whether willful or unintentional, and whether harm results or not.§
8. Abuse is any use of an illicit drug with the intentional self-administration of a medication for nonmedical purpose such as altering one's state of consciousness (e.g., getting high). Note that licit substances (e.g., alcohol) can also be abused.§
9. Diversion is the intentional removal of a medication from legitimate distribution and dispensing channels.§
10. Aberrant behavior is when the patient steps outside the boundaries of the agreed upon treatment plan which is established as early as possible in the doctor-patient relationship.¶

*American Academy of Pain Medicine, American Pain Society, and American Society of Addiction Medicine. Definitions Related to the Use of Opioids for the Treatment of Pain. Glenview, IL: American Academy of Pain Medicine, 2001.
†Weissman DE, Haddox JD. Opioid pseudoaddiction—an iatrogenic syndrome. *Pain* 1989;36(3):363–366.
‡Pappagallo M. The concept of pseudotolerance to opioids. *J Pharm Care Pain Symptom Control* 1998;6:95–98.
**Authors' definition.
§Katz NP, Adams EH, Chilcoat H, et al. Challenges in the development of prescription opioid abuse-deterrent formulations. *Clin J Pain* 2007;23(8): 648–660.
¶Gourlay DL, Heit HA. Pain and Addiction: Managing risk through comprehensive care. *J Addict Dis* 2008;27(3):23–30.

diaphoresis, diarrhea, abdominal cramps, seizures, anhedonia, dysphoria, and in some cases even death.[8–10] For example, a heroin addict may be both physically dependent and addicted to the narcotic, while the pain patient taking opioids is physically dependent, but not addicted. Both will experience some degree of withdrawal if the drug is abruptly stopped. In the pain patient, physical dependence with withdrawal may also be associated with withdrawal-mediated hyperalgesia.[13]

Iatrogenic addiction is not clearly defined in the literature.[14]

The true incidence of iatrogenic addiction to opioids is not known.[14] It is therefore important to set limits and boundaries for all patients before writing the first prescription.[5]

It is only by careful evaluation and rational pharmacotherapeutic management of the pain that concurrent diagnoses such as addiction or pseudoaddiction can be confirmed. While a diagnosis of addiction is made prospectively over time, a diagnosis of pseudoaddiction is usually made retrospectively.[7] When reasonable limits and boundaries are placed on a patient and they continue to step out of bounds, addiction or pseudoaddiction should be considered.

Health care professionals with improved understanding of the definitions on the basic scientific and clinical levels will be better able to evaluate and treat chronic pain patients with or without the disease of addiction.

BASIC SCIENCE OF THE DISEASE OF ADDICTION

Drugs of misuse act at local cellular and membrane sites that are within a neurochemical system that is called the reward and withdrawal pathway (Fig. 59.1).[15] This pathway is in the mesolimbic dopamine system, and it involves, among other structures, the ventral tegmental area, nucleus accumbens, amygdala, and prefrontal cortex of the primitive brain. Addiction is a neurobiological disease that causes disruption of this pathway. This disruption is mediated via receptor sites and neurotransmitters. Central to this reward and withdrawal pathway is the neurotransmitter dopamine, which has been shown to be relevant not only to drug reward, but to food, drink, sex, and social reward.[16,17] Disruption of this neurochemical pathway by drugs of abuse may lead to addiction. Drug withdrawal can intensify with repeated drug use and can persist during prolonged periods of drug abstinence, a symptom complex known as the protracted abstinence syndrome.[18] This sensitization of a neural process related to drug cravings or to environmental stimuli such as sights, smells, and sounds associated with drugs (referred to as cues) leads to the progressive increase in drug-seeking behavior that characterizes addiction. Such sensitization appears to increase the attractiveness of the drug taking and that of the drug-associated stimuli.[19]

One of the most common reasons for relapse is stress.[15] It stands to reason that if a chronic pain patient is in recovery from drug or alcohol use and his or her pain is inadequately treated, he or she may turn to the inappropriate use of licit or illicit drugs.

The health care professional must recognize addiction as a treatable albeit irreversible brain disease[20,21]; it is a distinct medical condition that may or may not be associated with the patient's pain syndrome.

Opioids can cause physical dependence and, upon abrupt discontinuation, withdrawal as a result of up regulation of the cyclic aminophosphorase (cAMP) pathway at the locus ceruleus.[18] This is a normal physiologic response to this class of medications. It should be noted that most of the medications capable of producing physical dependence are not associated with the disease of addiction.

Tolerance is also a natural, expected physiologic response that can occur with exposure to certain classes of drugs, especially alcohol and opioids. The *key* to this definition is that all other factors remain stable so that just the physiologic response to the drug can be evaluated.[8] In fact, tolerance is neither good nor bad. It occurs at different rates, to different effects, in different patients, over time. So while there is relatively rapid tolerance to the cognitive blunting effects of the opioid class of drug, tolerance to the constipating effects of opioids rarely occurs. Unappreciated disease progress that is associated with dose escalation is termed pseudotolerance and is a term that was coined to describe the apparent loss of analgesic effect in cancer patients with unrecog-

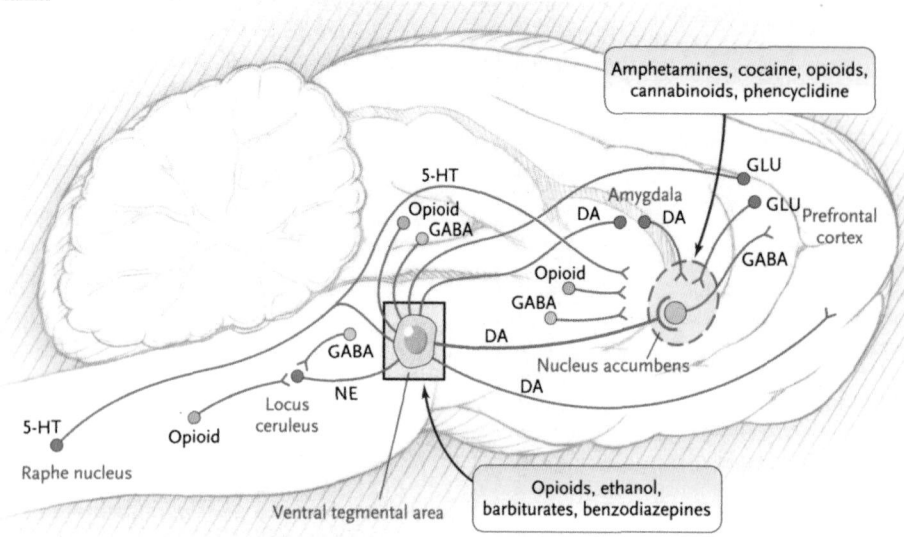

FIGURE 59.1 Common reward pathway: mesocorticolimbic dopamine (DA) system. (Reproduced from Cami J, Farre M. Drug addiction. *N Engl J Med* 2003; 349(10):975–986, with permission.)

nized increases in tumor burden.[22] Pharmacodynamic tolerance involves adaptations that occur at both the site of the drug action (e.g., receptor and ion channel), as well as in related systems more distal to it. For example, pharmacodynamic tolerance to opioids is evident at both the level of the opioid receptor in the locus ceruleus (primary) and in the dopaminergic reward pathways afferent to the site of this discrete drug action (secondary).[19] Both persons addicted to heroin and chronic pain patients taking opioids can exhibit tolerance to the drug.

Binary Concept of Pain and Addiction

In the past, the literature has suggested that pain conditions and addictive disorders might be dichotomous phenomena.[5,7,23] It has been said that in the context of a "legitimate" pain diagnosis, which usually meant a condition that made sense to the assessing health care professional, the likelihood of there being an addictive disorder was so small as to not even merit investigation. Unfortunately, if the patient had an obvious substance use disorder, very real and treatable pain conditions were often ignored. With time, this thinking was tempered somewhat to suggest that in the absence of a current or past personal or family history of a substance use disorder, the risk of addiction was very low indeed.[5] This dichotomous approach to pain and addiction has not served patients, health care professionals, or society well.

In reality, there is nothing about a genuine pain condition that is protective against having a concurrent substance use disorder; however, untreated pain, as a stressor, should be considered in the assessment of relapse risk.[15] While there are some data in the animal literature to suggest that acute pain may blunt the euphoric reward of some drugs including opioids,[24,25] the ability to generalize this phenomenon to the human population and more importantly, the sustainability of this "protection" has yet to be established. Patients with a substance use disorder are often disproportionate consumers of health care resources, especially in the context of trauma.[26,27] The presence of a preexisting substance use disorder is not mitigated by a concurrent pain problem; it is complicated by it.

While there is no evidence in the literature to suggest that those patients without past histories or increased risk of substance use disorders become addicted as a result of rational pharmacotherapy for the treatment of any medical condition, including chronic pain, there is little credible evidence to the contrary either. Perhaps more relevant questions to ask are whether rational phar-

macotherapeutic management of acute or chronic pain can reactivate a previously dormant substance use disorder or express an as yet unidentified genetic predisposition toward substance misuse or addiction. In the authors' opinion, the answer to both questions is very likely, "Yes."[7]

Risk, of course, varies with circumstance. For example, the prevalence of alcoholism in the hospitalized general medical population is estimated at 19% to 26%,[28] while in the trauma subset, the prevalence rises to 40% to 62%.[27] Regardless of what the actual risk is, it is clear that no one specific marker can reliably identify the at-risk pain patient, so careful boundary setting for all patients is strongly recommended.[5]

Not all aberrant behavior reflects drug misuse or addiction. Some individuals who do not meet the diagnostic criteria for addiction may also use medications and other drugs problematically. This group is sometimes referred to as "chemical copers."[29] These individuals lack the skills commonly acquired during childhood and adolescence and tend to turn to external sources for support in dealing with life's problems. More often than not, however, these patients suffer from complex, multidimensional problems that may only be partially responsive to even optimum pharmacotherapy in the absence of a biopsychosocial treatment plan. Unidimensional problems may respond to unidimensional pharmacologic solutions. Multidimensional problems, however, may transiently respond to pharmacologic interventions, but rarely in a sustainable fashion.[7]

It is only by aggressive investigation and rational pharmacotherapeutic management of the pain that this diagnosis can be made. The diagnosis of addiction is often made prospectively over time. When the patient's behavior remains aberrant despite the appropriate management of the underlying painful condition with reasonably set limits, substance misuse or addiction should be considered. In contrast, the diagnosis of pseudoaddiction is made retrospectively in that with appropriate management of pain, aberrant behavior is reduced or eliminated.[5,7] When reasonable limits and boundaries are placed on a patient and yet the patient continues to step out beyond these limits, addiction and pseudoaddiction should be in the differential diagnosis.

Boundary setting may include interval dispensing and contingency prescribing. Interval dispensing requires the patient to see other members of the health care team, such as a staff member of the prescriber or the pharmacist on a more frequent basis than the actual prescriber. Thus, interval dispensing can be a simple and effective means to help patients keep from "borrowing from tomorrow to pay for today," thereby reducing the risk of running out of medications early. With contingency prescribing, receiving the next prescription is contingent on something such as bringing bottles in for "pill counts" or mandatory attendance at all appointments.

Pain and Opioid Addiction—A Continuum Approach

While pain and addiction can and sometimes do exist as comorbid conditions, they may also be present as part of a dynamic continuum with pain at one end of the spectrum and addiction at the other (Fig. 59.2).[7,23] In cases where the identified substance of misuse is one in which there can be no doubt about the medical appropriateness of its use, such as with alcohol or cocaine, a comorbid pain and substance use disorder should be considered. However, when the drug in question can arguably be both the problem and the solution, depending on the health care professionals' training and perspective, a continuum model may better apply.[7,23] With chronic pain, appropriateness of ongoing opioid use should be periodically evaluated, especially when there is little or no objective evidence of improvement in pain relief or function.

In cases in which pain and addiction coexist either as a continuum or comorbid condition, it is important to identify which aspect of the illness is dominant. Failure to treat both conditions, when present, will undoubtedly lead to frustration and poor outcomes in both domains. It is equally important to realize that this continuum is dynamic, with substance use disorder symptoms becoming dominant during periods of stress even after years of stable recovery.[7,23]

Separating the "Motive" from "Behavior" when Dealing with Pain and Addiction

One of the greatest challenges facing practitioners treating complex pain patients is dealing with the patient who explains his or her aberrant behavior in terms of his or her chronic pain. Not infrequently, the health care professional will hear the patient say, "But I'm not an addict, I'm a pain patient" when challenged with explaining why he has run out of medication early, yet again. Of course, interpreting such behavior can be challenging.[30] The differential diagnosis is long and includes dependence, pseudo-addiction, true addiction, comorbid psychopathology, "chemical coping,"[29] and even criminal behavior such as diversion.[7] More often than not, the patient and/or patient's family can identify and are willing to discuss the aberrant behavior in the context of a "problem," rather than as evidence of a possible substance use disorder.

Take for example the patient who has unilaterally escalated his or her daily dose of medication, necessitating an early return for prescription renewal. While this may occur occasionally for quite legitimate reasons, repeated unilateral dose increases reflect behavior that must be carefully evaluated. In such a case, it may be more useful to focus on the problematic behavior (running out early) rather than the motive behind the behavior (i.e., addiction/abuse, chemical coping, etc.) when exploring this with the patient. Once the problematic behavior is identified and a remedial course of action selected, the ease with which the patient adheres to this "solution" will help to identify which aspect of the aberrant behavior differential is likely at work. Patients whose problematic behavior remains unchanged despite conservative efforts likely suffer from more complex problems that would best be referred to a substance-use-disorder professional or other clinician with greater experience and resources to assess and manage these more challenging cases. Non-forensic, patient-centered urine drug testing (UDT), which is discussed in Chapter 60, can be a very useful tool in these cases.[5,31,32]

In the case of criminal behavior, such as diversion of the prescribed medications, the behavior and motive behind it are clearly unacceptable. In the authors' opinion, this is cause to sever the doctor-patient relationship and dismiss the patient from the practice. Dismissing patients for such criminal behavior is unlikely to be construed as abandonment in most jurisdictions.

Opioids for Analgesia or Opioid-Stabilizing Effect?

Not all pain syndromes are equally responsive to opioids.[33] Neuropathic pain may be less opioid responsive, often requiring higher doses.[34] In cases in which a patient is physically dependent on opioids, as one would expect with prolonged use of this class of drug, it can sometimes be useful to consider the appropriateness of continuation of opioid therapy, especially when treatment goals of improved function and decreased pain remain unmet.

Most pain is, to some degree, opioid responsive. Yet, despite years of experience with opioid therapy, it remains unclear who in advance will achieve a sustained response.

When the patient and clinician define the need to remain on opioid therapy not by how well the patient is doing but rather by how poorly things go when they try to reduce or discontinue the drug, it is time to reexamine the therapeutic role of opioids. When opioid levels in a physically dependent pain patient become inadequate, early withdrawal may occur. In the context of opioid-abstinence-induced hyperalgesia, it would be expected that the pain complaint might worsen.[13] It is something of a myth that patients who no longer need opioids always come off them easily. In any trial of therapy, including opioid pharmacotherapy, there must be a clear exit strategy in addition to an entrance, stabilization, and maintenance strategy before writing the first prescription.[7,35] This is not to say that those patients who are clearly benefiting from opioid pharmacotherapy should be weaned from these medications on the assumption that they "may no longer need them," but rather that not all persons who have inadequate pain relief or function while on opioids should remain on this class of drugs. In fact, some persons with poorly controlled pain while on opioid therapy may improve with a carefully executed opioid taper. The term taper is used here rather than detoxification, which is a term more commonly associated with the disease of addiction. Pain patients are "tapered," and addiction patients are "detoxed." In some jurisdictions, this can be a critical distinction in medicolegal terminology.

Recommendations for Terminating Opioid Therapy

A trial of opioid therapy is just that: a trial. In some cases, a decision to discontinue opioids is made. While the optimum case is one in which both the clinician and the patient feel this is the appropriate course to take, not infrequently it is the clinician

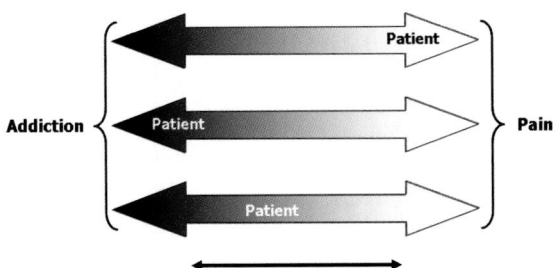

FIGURE 59.2 Pain and addiction continuum. (Adapted from Heit HA, Gourlay D. Chronic pain and addiction. In: Pasricha PJ, Willis WD, Gebhart GF, eds. *Chronic Abdominal and Visceral Pain: Theory and Practice.* New York: Taylor and Francis, 2006:231–244, with permission.)

TABLE 59.2

CAGE-AID (ALCOHOL INCLUDING DRUGS) QUESTIONNAIRE[40]

- Have you tried to <u>C</u>ut down or <u>C</u>hange your pattern of drinking or drug use?
- Have you been <u>A</u>nnoyed or <u>A</u>ngry by others' concern about your drinking or drug use?
- Have you felt <u>G</u>uilty about the consequences of your drinking or drug use?
- Have you had a drink or used a drug in the morning (<u>E</u>ye-opener) to decrease hangover or withdrawal symptoms?

alone who has made this decision. Discontinuation of the opioid class of drugs should, when possible, be done respecting that the patient may have become physically dependent. While no one taper schedule should be considered the criterion standard, it is important to bear the following in mind. The speed with which the dose can be reduced at the beginning of the taper does not necessarily predict the speed with which the patient will be able to finish. As a general rule, a taper that most patients will tolerate well is to drop the dose 10% every 1 to 2 weeks until the patient reaches the bottom third, and then reduce the dose by 5% every 2 to 4 weeks until completed. During the taper, worsening pain scores, especially in the morning, may indicate too rapid a dose reduction, frustrating the efforts at tapering the drug. It is important to remember that opioid termination should not be synonymous with termination of care, although for some patients, the net effect is that they will seek care elsewhere if opioids are not being prescribed.

The purpose of effective pain management in any patient population, including those suffering from substance use disorders, is to reduce pain while improving function. When a drug appears to do more harm than good and yet continues to be used, an active addictive disorder must be considered. While risk can never be eliminated, it can usually be managed. Failure to identify pain

and addiction, where they exist, can render even the most ardent efforts at pain management ineffective and frustrating.

ASSESSMENT TOOLS

There are multiple assessment tools that are available for health care professionals to stratify the risk of drug/alcohol abuse or addiction.[36a] These tools may be used in pain management, especially if one is considering the use of controlled substances. The following tools have been proposed to help the clinician identify the "at risk" patient for aberrant behavior, including the Alcohol Use Disorders Identification Test (AUDIT),[36] the Screener and Opioid Assessment for Patients with Pain (SOAPP),[37,38] the CAGE-AID (Alcohol Including Drugs) (Table 59.2),[39,40] and the Opioid Risk Tool (ORT).[41] The CAGE Questionnaire has a sensitivity and specificity such that if the patient answers two out of four questions positively on it there is a current diagnosis of alcohol misuse or drug dependency with a sensitivity of 77% to 94% and a specificity of 79% to 97%.[40]

ORT is a five-question clinical interview or patient questionnaire to assess patients at risk for aberrant behavior with prescription opioids prior to treatment initiation. It quantifies the level of risk for patients in an easy-to-use format. Its scoring is based on gender, family history of substance abuse, personal history of substance abuse, age, history of sexual abuse, and psychological disease (Table 59.3).[41]

An increased risk does not mean that any given patient will behave aberrantly, and for those that do, not all behavior is equally important in terms of meaning. However, for those patients at increased risk, the need for closer monitoring should be evident. It is also important to note that on initial evaluation of all patients, the health care professional should always ask respectfully and in a nonjudgmental manner about a history of drug or alcohol abuse/addiction, physical or sexual abuse, or any current or past history of mental disorders. This information allows the treating health care professional to formulate the appropriate treatment plan with boundary settings. It also offers the opportunity to bring another member(s) into the treatment team

TABLE 59.3

STRATIFYING RISK: OPIOID RISK TOOL

	Female	Male
Five-question clinical interview to assess patients		
Specifically developed to screen patients with chronic pain who will be using opioids		
Quantifies the level of risk for patient	**Family history of substance abuse**	
	Alcohol	[ ]1	[ ]3
	Illegal drugs	[ ]2	[ ]3
	Prescription drugs	[ ]4	[ ]4

	Female	Male
Three risk categories	**Personal history of substance abuse**	
• Low: 0–3 points	Alcohol	[ ]3	[ ]3
• Moderate: 4–7 points	Illegal drugs	[ ]4	[ ]4
• High: 8 points and above	Prescription drugs	[ ]5	[ ]5
	Age (if between 16–45)	[ ]1	[ ]1
	History of preadolescent sexual abuse	[ ]3	[ ]0
	Psychological disease	
	Attention deficit disorder, obsessive-compulsive disorder, bipolar, schizophrenia	[ ]2	[ ]2
	Depression	[ ]1	[ ]1
	Scoring Total: _____	

Adapted from Webster LR, Webster RM. Predicting aberrant behaviors in opioid-treated patients: preliminary validation of the Opioid Risk Tool. *Pain Med* 2005;6(6):432–442.

to begin to address the biopsychosocial issues of the patient. This increases the chances of the patient reaching his or her goals of pain management.

UNIVERSAL PRECAUTIONS IN PAIN MEDICINE

The heightened interest in pain management is making the need for appropriate boundary setting within the clinician-patient relationship even more apparent. Unfortunately, it is impossible to determine beforehand, with any degree of certainty, who will become problematic users of prescription medications. With this in mind, a parallel can be drawn between the chronic pain management paradigm and our past experience with problems identifying the "at-risk" individuals from an infectious disease model.

The term "universal precautions," as it applies to infectious disease, came out of the realization that it was impossible for a health care professional to reliably assess risk of infectivity during an initial assessment of a patient.[42] Lifestyle, history, and even aberrant behavior such as injection drug use were unreliable indicators that led to patient stigmatization and increased health care professional risk. It was only after research into the prevalence of such diseases as hepatitis B, hepatitis C, and HIV that we realized the safest and most reasonable approach to take was to apply an appropriate minimum level of precaution to *all* patients to reduce the risk of transmission of potentially life threatening infectious disease to health care professionals. Fear was replaced by knowledge and with knowledge came the practice we now know as Universal Precautions (UP) in infectious disease.

UP, in pain medicine, is a risk management term introduced in 2005 which proposes adopting a minimum level of inquiry and care applicable to *all* patients presenting with chronic pain. UP offers an assessment and ongoing management scheme for all chronic pain patients.[5] It recognizes the need to carefully assess all patients within a multidimensional biopsychosocial model, including history of and present aberrant behaviors that might be associated with drug or alcohol use. By applying careful and reasonably set limits in the clinician-patient relationship, it is possible to triage chronic pain patients into three categories according to risk as presented later in this chapter.[7]

UP were introduced as a means to open up a dialogue between the pain management and addiction communities around the assessment and management of risk. They were not proposed as complete but rather as a good starting point for those treating chronic pain. It is important to note that UP are not simply about opioid therapy, but rather stress the importance of assessing and, where necessary, managing treatable comorbid conditions including substance use disorders.[43] As with UP in infectious disease, by applying the following recommendations, patient care may be improved, stigma reduced, and overall risk contained.[5]

The Ten Principles of Universal Precautions in Pain Medicine

The ten principles of UP are listed in Table 59.4. Treatable causes for pain should be identified where they exist and therapy directed toward the pain generator. In the absence of specific objective findings, pain can and should be treated. Any comorbid conditions, including substance use disorders and other psychiatric illness, must also be identified and addressed. A complete inquiry into personal and family history of substance misuse is essential to adequately assess and treat any patient. A sensitive and respectful assessment of risk should not be seen in any way as diminishing a patient's complaint of pain. Patient-centered urine drug testing (UDT) should be discussed with all patients regardless of what medications they are currently taking. In the authors' opinion,

TABLE 59.4

THE TEN PRINCIPLES OF UNIVERSAL PRECAUTIONS

1. Diagnosis with appropriate differential
2. Psychological assessment including risk of addictive disorders
3. Informed consent (verbal or written/signed)
4. Treatment agreement (verbal or written/signed)
5. Pre/post intervention assessment of pain level and function
6. Appropriate trial of opioid therapy $+/-$ adjunctive medication
7. Reassessment of pain score and level of function
8. Regularly assess the "Four A's" of pain medicine *Analgesia, Activity, Adverse reactions, and Aberrant behavior*[47]
9. Periodically review pain and comorbidity diagnoses, including addictive disorders
10. Documentation

Adapted from Gourlay D, Heit H, Almarhezi A. Universal Precautions in Pain Medicine: A rational approach to the management of chronic pain. *Pain Med* 2005;6(2)107–112.

the prescription of controlled substances to patients who are "philosophically opposed" to UDT is relatively contraindicated.

Informed consent is part of an initial evaluation. Health care professionals must discuss with and answer any questions about the proposed treatment plan including anticipated benefits and foreseeable risks. The specific issues of addiction, physical dependence, and tolerance should be explored at a level appropriate to the patient's understanding.

Written opioid agreements facilitate the documentation of informed consent, patient education, and compliance in the management of chronic pain.[44] A well-written agreement establishes the responsibilities of clinician to patient and vice versa. It outlines the treatment plan and documents informed consent. The opioid agreement establishes boundaries and consequences for nonadherence. Noncompliance with the agreement can aid in the diagnosis of the disease of addiction or substance misuse, which would often require a change in the treatment plan.

Opioid agreements have the potential to improve the therapeutic relationship.[44–46] The agreement, whether written and signed or informal, must be part of an environment of care that emphasizes honest and open communication. A practice policy for all patients prescribed opioids to sign a medication management agreement is often a simple and effective way to approach this sometimes uncomfortable issue. In the authors' opinion, the agreement should be reasonable, readable and flexible. Sometimes such agreements are called opioid contracts. However, these rarely reach the level of legally binding contracts, and as such are better referred to as medication management agreements. Where written agreements are used, both the patient and clinicians should sign two copies. The patient should be offered a copy to share with whomever he or she thinks appropriate. Effective agreements clearly define both the clinician's and patient's responsibilities (Table 59.5).[44–46]

Pre- and post-intervention assessment of pain level and function must emphasize that any treatment plan begins with a "trial of therapy." This is particularly true when controlled substances are contemplated or used. Without a documented assessment of preintervention pain scores and level of function, it may be difficult to demonstrate success in any medication trial. The ongoing assessment and documentation of goals met will support the continuation of any mode of therapy. Failure to meet these goals should necessitate reevaluation and possible change in the treatment plan.

An appropriate trial of opioid therapy, generally with adjunctive medication, may be warranted in moderate to severe pain. Although opioids should not routinely be thought of as treatment of first choice, they must also not be considered as agents of last

TABLE 59.5

TREATMENT AGREEMENT FOR OPIOID MAINTENANCE THERAPY FOR NONCANCER/CANCER PAIN

- Goals of therapy
- Single prescriber if possible
- Informed consent on all opioid risks
- Definition of addiction, tolerance, and physical dependence
- Need for patient disclosure of substance abuse history, psychiatric history including history of sexual, physical or emotional abuse, and medications currently prescribed
- Need for complete, honest self-report of pain relief, side effects, and function at each medical visit
- Establishment of regular medical visits
- Requirement for prescription renewal only during regular office hours
- Conditions of noncompliance (for example, evidence of drug hoarding or use of any illegal drug may cause termination of the clinician-patient relationship)
- Use of the word "may" instead of "will" in the agreement, so clinical judgment can be used in each situation
- Patient consent to random urine drug tests and pill counts
- Permission for the practice to contact appropriate sources to obtain or provide information about the patient's care or actions
- Where appropriate recovery program for substance misuse or addiction (patients must agree to concurrent assessment and treatment of their substance use disorder)

Adapted from Heit H. Creating and Implementing Opioid Agreements. *Disease Management Digest* 2003;7(1):2–3.

TABLE 59.6

TRIAGE OF THE CHRONIC PAIN PATIENT

Group I—primary care patients
This group has no past or current history of substance use disorders. They have a noncontributory family history with respect to substance use disorders and lack major or untreated psychopathology. This group clearly represents the majority of patients who will present to the primary care practitioner.

Group II—primary care patients with specialist support
In this group, there may be a past history of a treated substance use disorder or a significant family history of problematic drug use. They may also have a past or concurrent psychiatric disorder. These patients, however, are not actively addicted but do represent increased risk which may be managed in consultation with appropriate specialist support. This consultation may be formal and ongoing (comanaged) or simply with the option for referral back for reassessment should the need arise.

Group III—specialty pain management
This group of patients represents the most complex cases to manage due to an active substance use disorder or major, untreated psychopathology. These patients are actively addicted and pose significant risk to both themselves and to the practitioners who often lack the resources or experience to manage them. The prescription of controlled substances should generally be left to those persons with the experience and resources to manage the active addict.

Adapted from Gourlay D, Heit H, Almarhezi A. Universal Precautions in Pain Medicine: A rational approach to the management of chronic pain. *Pain Med* 2005;6(2):107–112.

resort. Pharmacologic regimens must be individualized based on subjective as well as objective clinical findings. The appropriate combination of agents, including opioids and adjunctive medications, may be seen as "rational pharmacotherapy" and provide a stable therapeutic platform from which to base treatment changes.

Regular reassessment of the patient's pain score and level of function, combined with corroborative support from family or other knowledgeable third parties, will help document the rationale to continue or modify the current therapeutic trial. The routine assessment of the "Four A's" of pain medicine, Analgesia, Activity, Adverse effects, and Aberrant behavior, will help to direct therapy and support pharmacologic options taken.[47] It may also be useful to document a fifth A: Affect (Personal communication, E. Covington, November 23, 2005). The prescriber should periodically review pain diagnosis and comorbid conditions, including substance use disorders. Underlying illnesses evolve. Diagnostic tests change with time. In the pain and addiction continuum, it is not uncommon for a patient to move from a dominance of one disorder to the other. As a result, treatment focus may need to change over the course of time. If an addictive disorder predominates, aggressive treatment of an underlying pain problem will likely fail if not coordinated with treatment for the concurrent addictive disorder.

Careful and complete documentation of the initial evaluation and at each follow up is both medicolegally indicated and in the best interest of all parties. Thorough documentation, combined with an appropriate doctor-patient relationship, will reduce medicolegal exposure and risk of regulatory sanction. If you do not document it, it did not happen.

Patient Triage

One of the goals in the initial assessment of a pain patient is to obtain a reasonable assessment of risk of a concurrent substance use disorder or major psychopathology. In this context, patients can be stratified into three basic groups. The UP triage scheme offers a practical framework to help determine which patients they may safely manage in the primary care setting, those comanaged with specialist support, and those who should be referred on for management of their chronic pain condition in a specialist setting (Table 59.6).[5]

It is important to remember that Groups II and III can be dynamic; Group II becoming Group III with relapse to active addiction, while Group III patients can move to Group II with appropriate treatment. In some cases, as more information becomes available to the practitioner, the patient who was originally thought to be low risk (Group I) may become Group II or even Group III. It is important to continually reassess risk over time.

TREATING THE PAIN PATIENT ON OPIOID AGONIST TREATMENT

The treatment of pain in a patient on opioid agonist treatment (OAT) with methadone or sublingual (S/L) buprenorphine for the disease of opioid addiction can be particularly challenging. In some cases, the controlled substance prescribed for pain can be the solution, the problem, or both.[7]

Methadone and S/L buprenorphine (with or without naloxone) can be used for the dual purpose of treating the disease of addiction and pain, but they pose an interesting challenge for the prescriber. For appropriate prescribing of these medications, their unique pharmacokinetic and pharmacodynamic properties must be understood. This allows for proper patient selection and evaluation in order to optimize outcomes in the treatment of pain, addiction, or the comorbid conditions of pain and addiction.

In the disease of addiction, the dose of methadone or S/L buprenorphine is usually given once a day. In the clinical experience of the authors, methadone and buprenorphine are best dosed every 6–8 hours for the most effective treatment of opioid responsive pain.[48] However, it should be noted that this dosing schedule for S/L buprenorphine for analgesia is not documented in the peer review literature.[48]

Buprenorphine's high receptor affinity may interfere with effectiveness of other full mu analgesics. As with other partial mu-agonists, buprenorphine is contraindicated in opioid-dependent patients since it may precipitate severe withdrawal.[49,50]

Pain management for patients who are using S/L buprenorphine for the disease of addiction requires a specialized approach. The literature suggests that to treat pain in a patient on OAT with S/L buprenorphine, one must discontinue the S/L buprenorphine and do a reinduction of the drug after the acute pain syndrome resolves.[51] This may not be necessary in some instances. In certain circumstances, the patient may be spared the discomfort of having to go into withdrawal as the full mu-agonist is discontinued and he or she is rotated back to S/L buprenorphine. In most cases, the pain can simply be managed by titrating the S/L dose upward to effect with a 6–8 hour dosing regimen up to maximum dose of 32 mg/day.[48] If breakthrough medication is needed, consider using one with high potency such as fentanyl or hydromorphone because of their high affinity to the opioid receptor.[48] In the authors' opinion, rapid onset opioid formulations should be used with caution in this population and primarily for acute pain (with tightly set boundaries as per UP with limited "pill load"[35] prescribed between evaluations of the acute pain) (see Chapter 60). It is important to remember that it is always possible to add a full mu-agonist to a patient who is maintained on buprenorphine without fear of precipitating withdrawal. The reverse is, however, not true.

The patient who is on OAT and requires chronic pain management should agree to the principles of UP and be placed in the appropriate group for risk stratification (Group II or Group III) and monitored accordingly.

THE TREATMENT OF PAIN AND SUFFERING IN OUR SOCIETY

There is a debate over whether opioids are "good" or "bad" and whether or not they should be available. Of course, opioids are "good" when used appropriately and "bad" when they are misused. They should be made available to the patients who need them, but only with appropriate monitoring and oversight individualized to each case.[52] The chronic pain population is incredibly heterogeneous and varies tremendously in terms of vulnerability to addiction and misuse. The best way to accomplish the goal of keeping opioids available to those who need them is for all stakeholders involved in legitimate opioid therapy to openly address the complexity of the issue and to do so in a collaborative fashion.[52]

Major stakeholders in achieving an appropriate balance in the treatment of pain and the prevention of drug abuse and diversion are health care professionals, patients, third-party payers, regulatory bodies, law enforcement, pharmaceutical industry, and the media. If these groups reconcile themselves to the need for thoughtful and unemotional dialogue, opioid treatment can remain a viable option while efforts are made to stem the tide of prescription drug misuse and addiction. Everyone has a stake in this complex issue. We are all aging and many of us will have pain. Societal solutions are needed now so that we can all enjoy the comfort of knowing that safe and effective pain treatment will be there for us if we need it. It is the responsibility of all to make this a reality.[52]

One wonders if pain patients are being held to a higher standard regarding compliance with their treatment plan. For example, in the treatment of any chronic illness such as diabetes mellitus, 100% adherence to the treatment plan, while desirable, is obviously not achieved in the majority of patients. In fact, a recent review indicates that approximately 20% to 50% of patients are not adherent to recommended medical therapy.[53] The failure to comply is a complex interplay of a multitude of biopsychosocial factors including but not limited to patient motivation. To expect 100% compliance with any pharmacotherapeutic agent, including CS, is to ignore this fact.

CONCLUSION

The purpose of effective pain management in any patient population, including those suffering from substance use disorders, is to reduce pain while improving function. While achieving this goal may be more difficult in patients with substance use disorders, it is not impossible. Risk can never be eliminated, but it can usually be managed. By approaching these patients within a biopsychosocial model using the information presented in this chapter, the health care professional can give the patient the best quality of life possible given the reality of his or her clinical situation.

References

1. Oaklander A. The pathology of pain. *Neuroscientist* 1999;5(5):302–310.
2. Krames ES, Olson K. Clinical realities and economic considerations: patient selection in intrathecal therapy. *J Pain Symptom Manage* 1997;14(suppl 3):S3–S13.
3. Savage SR. Long-term opioid therapy: assessment of consequences and risks. *J Pain Symptom Manage* 1996;11(5):274–286.
4. Rosenblum A, Joseph H, Fong C, et al. Prevalence and characteristics of chronic pain among chemically dependent patients in methadone maintenance and residential treatment facilities. *JAMA* 2003;289(18):2370–2378.
5. Gourlay DL, Heit HA, Almahrezi A. Universal precautions in pain medicine: a rational approach to the management of chronic pain. *Pain Med* 2005;6(2):107–112.
6. Joranson DE, Gilson AM, Ryan KM, et al. *Achieving Balance in Federal and State Pain Policy: A Guide to Evaluation.* 2nd ed. Madison, WI: University of Wisconsin Comprehensive Cancer Center; 2003. Available at: http://www.medsch.wisc.edu/painpolicy. Accessed December 19, 2004.
7. Gourlay DL, Heit H. Pain and addiction: managing risk through comprehensive care. *J Addict Dis* 2008;27(3):23–30.
8. Heit HA. Addiction, physical dependence, and tolerance: precise definitions to help clinicians evaluate and treat chronic pain patients. *J Pain Palliat Care Pharmacother* 2003;17(1):15–29.
9. American Academy of Pain Medicine, American Pain Society, American Society of Addiction Medicine. *Definitions Related to the Use of Opioids for the Treatment of Pain.* Glenview, IL: American Academy of Pain Medicine; 2001.
10. Savage SR, Joranson DE, Covington EC, et al. Definitions related to the medical use of opioids: evolution towards universal agreement. *J Pain Symptom Manage* 2003;26(1):655–667.
11. Ballantyne JC, LaForge KS. Opioid dependence and addiction during opioid treatment of chronic pain. *Pain* 2007;129(3):235–255.
12. Inturrisi CE. Clinical pharmacology of opioids for pain. *Clin J Pain* 2002;18(suppl 4):S3–S13.
12a. Heit HA, Gourlay DL. *DSM-V and the definitions: Time to get it right. Pain Medicine* 2009;10(5):784–786.
13. Li X, Clark JD. Hyperalgesia during opioid abstinence: mediation by glutamate and substance p. *Anesth Analg* 2002;95(4):979–984.
14. Wasan AD, Correll DJ, Kissin I, et al. Iatrogenic addiction in patients treated for acute or subacute pain: a systematic review. *J Opioid Manag* 2006;2(1):16–22.
15. Koob GF, Le Moal M. Drug addiction, dysregulation of reward, and allostasis. *Neuropsychopharmacology* 2001;24(2):97–129.
16. Nestler EJ, Landsman D. Learning about addiction from the genome. *Nature* 2001;409(6822):834–835.
17. Nestler EJ. Molecular basis of long-term plasticity underlying addiction. *Nat Rev Neurosci* 2001;2(2):119–128.
18. Kasser CL, Geller A, Howell EH, et al. Principles of detoxification. In: Graham AW, Schultz TK, eds. *Principles of Addiction Medicine.* 2nd ed. Chevy Chase, MD: American Society of Addiction Medicine; 1998.
19. Nestler EJ, Hyman SE, Malenka RC. *Reinforcement and Addictive Disorders. Molecular Neuropharmacology: A Foundation for Clinical Neuroscience.* New York: McGraw-Hill; 2001.
20. Leshner AI. Addiction is a brain disease, and it matters. *Science* 1997;278(5335):45–47.
21. Wise RA. Addiction becomes a brain disease. *Neuron* 2000;26(1):27–33.
22. Pappagallo M. The concept of pseudotolerance to opioids. *J Pharm Care Pain Symptom Control* 1998;6:95–98.

23. Heit H, Gourlay D. Chronic pain and addiction. In: Pasricha P, Willis W, Gebhart G, eds. *Chronic Abdominal and Visceral Pain: Theory and Practice.* New York: Taylor and Francis; 2006:231–244.

24. Ozaki S, Narita M, Narita M, et al. Suppression of the morphine-induced rewarding effect and G-protein activation in the lower midbrain following nerve injury in the mouse: involvement of G-protein-coupled receptor kinase 2. *Neuroscience* 2003;116(1):89–97.

25. Ozaki S, Narita M, Narita M, et al. Suppression of the morphine-induced rewarding effect in the rat with neuropathic pain: implication of the reduction in mu-opioid receptor functions in the ventral tegmental area. *J Neurochem* 2002;82(5):1192–1198.

26. Graham AW. Screening for alcoholism by life-style risk assessment in a community hospital. *Arch Intern Med* 1991;151(5):958–964.

27. Reyna TM, Hollis HW Jr, Hulsebus RC. Alcohol-related trauma. The surgeon's responsibility. *Ann Surg* 1985;201(2):194–197.

28. Moore RD, Bone LR, Geller G, et al. Prevalence, detection, and treatment of alcoholism in hospitalized patients. *JAMA* 1989;261(3):403–407.

29. Bruera E, Moyano J, Seifert L, et al. The frequency of alcoholism among patients with pain due to terminal cancer. *J Pain Symptom Manage* 1995;10(8):599–603.

30. Passik SD, Kirsh KL, Whitcomb L, et al. Pain clinicians' rankings of aberrant drug-taking behaviors. *J Pain Palliat Care Pharmacother* 2002;16(4):39–49.

31. Gourlay D, Heit H, Caplan Y. *Urine Drug Testing in Primary Care: Dispelling the Myths & Designing Strategies.* 3rd ed. Available online at: http://www.familydocs.org/assets/Professional_Development/CME/UDT.pdf. Accessed March 7 2006.

32. Heit HA, Gourlay DL. Urine drug testing in pain medicine. *J Pain Symptom Manage* 2004;27(3):260–267.

33. Dellemijn P. Are opioids effective in relieving neuropathic pain? *Pain* 1999;80(3):453–462.

34. Scadding JW. Treatment of neuropathic pain: historical aspects. *Pain Med* 2004;5(suppl 1):S3–S8.

35. Gourlay DL, Heit HA. Universal Precautions Revisited: Managing the Inherited Pain Patient. *Pain Medicine* 2009;10(52):S115–S123.

36. Saunders JB, Aasland OG, Babor TF, et al. Development of the Alcohol Use Disorders Identification Test (AUDIT): WHO Collaborative Project on Early Detection of Persons with Harmful Alcohol Consumption—II. *Addiction* 1993;88(6):791–804.

36a. Passik SD, Kirsh KL, Kasper D. Addiction-related assessment tools and pain management: instruments for screening, treatment planning, and monitoring compliance. *Pain Medicine* 2008;9(S2):S145–S166.

37. Butler SF, Budman SH, Fernandez K, et al. Validation of a screener and opioid assessment measure for patients with chronic pain. *Pain* 2004;112(1–2):65–75.

38. Akbik H, Butler SF, Budman SH, et al. Validation and clinical application of the Screener and Opioid Assessment for Patients with Pain (SOAPP). *J Pain Symptom Manage* 2006;32(3):287–293.

39. Brown RL, Rounds LA. Conjoint screening questionnaires for alcohol and other drug abuse: criterion validity in a primary care practice. *Wis Med J* 1995;94(3):135–140.

40. Fiellin DA, Reid MC, O'Connor PG. Outpatient management of patients with alcohol problems. *Ann Intern Med* 2000;133(10):815–827.

41. Webster LR, Webster RM. Predicting aberrant behaviors in opioid-treated patients: preliminary validation of the Opioid Risk Tool. *Pain Med* 2005;6(6):432–442.

42. Centers for Disease Control and Prevention. Recommendations for prevention of HIV transmission in health-care settings. *MMWR* 1987;36 (suppl 2S):1–16.

43. Gourlay D, Heit H. Universal precautions: a matter of mutual trust and responsibility. *Pain Med* 2006;7(2):210–211.

44. Fishman SM, Bandman TB, Edwards A, et al. The opioid contract in the management of chronic pain. *J Pain Symptom Manage* 1999;18(1):27–37.

45. Fishman SM, Kreis PG. The opioid contract. *Clin J Pain* 2002;18(suppl 4):S70–75.

46. Heit HA. Creating and implementing opioid agreements. *Dis Manag Digest* 2003;7(1):2–3.

47. Passik SD, Weinreb HJ. Managing chronic nonmalignant pain: overcoming obstacles to the use of opioids. *Adv Ther* 2000;17(2):70–83.

48. Heit HA, Gourlay DL. Buprenorphine: new tricks with an old molecule for pain management. *Clin J Pain* 2008;24(2):93–97.

49. Clark NC, Lintzeris N, Muhleisen PJ. Severe opiate withdrawal in a heroin user precipitated by a massive buprenorphine dose. *Med J Aust* 2002;176(4):166–167.

50. Sporer KA. Buprenorphine: a primer for emergency physicians. *Ann Emerg Med* 2004;43(5):580–584.

51. Center for Substance Abuse Treatment. *Clinical Guidelines for the Use of Buprenorphine in the Treatment of Opioid Addiction.* Treatment Improvement Protocol (TIP) Series 40. DHHS Publication No. (SMA) 04-3939. Rockville, MD: Substance Abuse and Mental Health Services Administration, 2004.

52. Passik SD, Heit H, Kirsh KL. Reality and responsibility: a commentary on the treatment of pain and suffering in a drug-using society. *J Opioid Manag* 2006;2(3):123–127.

53. Kripalani S, Yao X, Haynes RB. Interventions to enhance medication adherence in chronic medical conditions: a systematic review. *Arch Intern Med* 2007;167(6):540–550.

CHAPTER 60 ■ COMPLIANCE MONITORING IN CHRONIC PAIN MANAGEMENT

DOUGLAS L. GOURLAY AND HOWARD A. HEIT

INTRODUCTION

The pain management practitioner faces several challenges in the safe and effective management of chronic pain. One of these relates to the important issue of monitoring compliance with a previously agreed upon course of therapy. Unfortunately, in today's medicolegal climate, the need for pain practitioners to take steps to reduce the risk of diversion and misuse of controlled substances (CS) has become apparent. While the debate continues as to what degree prescribers contribute to the overall source of CS that reaches the street,[1–3] there should be no debate about the prescriber's responsibility to ensure a decreased need for these drugs by addressing demand reduction strategies in all susceptible individuals. All pain patients are not potential diverters; all aberrant behavior does not represent drug addiction or misuse.[4] However, we tend to adopt a more casual attitude toward prescription drugs, including opioids, despite the fact that there is a disturbing trend toward prescription drug abuse by adolescents and others who have found their family medicine chests a ready supply of abuseable drugs.[5] Whether this is because of an implicit sense of safety associated with prescription products or due to a simple comparison with typical illicit drugs of abuse found on the street is unclear. What is clear is that once the prescription medication is no longer used for its original therapeutic indication, it may become available for the growing prescription drug abuse problem.[5] Only recently have we begun to formally examine strategies to deal with this problem.[5]

A considerable effort has been expended in teaching clinicians how to initiate pharmacotherapy ("entrance strategy") but, unfortunately, there has not been an equal effort expended in teaching the technique of terminating these medications ("exit strategy"), some of which may have considerable withdrawal syndromes associated with their rapid taper or abrupt discontinuation.

The challenge today is not identifying aberrant behavior; it is in interpreting what it means.[4] More importantly, there has been little written in the literature to guide prescribers in the appropriate steps to take once such behavior is identified. This chapter will explore some of these issues and offer suggestions as to their management.

For the purposes of this chapter, compliance monitoring may be defined as those steps taken by a prescriber to ensure that treatment plans are adhered to and prescribed medications are appropriately used. Many factors contribute to a patient's failure to adhere to an agreed upon treatment plan.[6] To expect 100% adherence, even when controlled substances are involved, is to ignore this fact.[6]

Compliance monitoring should begin with an individual assessment of risk. As outlined in Chapter 59, it is unwise to assume that you can assess risk, with any degree of certainty, at the first visit. Risk assessment and management is best performed over time. Treatment agreements, interval and contingency prescribing, pill counts, and urine drug testing can all play important parts in helping to manage risk and improve outcomes.[7–12]

Urine drug testing (UDT), which is a tool providing objective evidence of clinical stability in an otherwise largely subjective branch of medicine, should play a key role in any practitioner's patient care plan. As with the diabetic patient who self reports optimum glycemic control at a follow-up visit, the clinician still performs a HgBA$_1$C test (which is a measure of glycemic control over time) as an objective measure of treatment success. Since hyperglycemia is not illegal, there is little prejudice created in the clinician's mind when the objective test is at odds with the patient's self report. Just as with HgBA$_1$C, the clinician can use a discordant urine drug test result to motivate change on the part of the patient and to monitor healthy changes already made. This chapter will discuss the basics of clinical urine drug testing.

Compliance monitoring should be based on the initial visit then subsequent assessments of risk over time. A variety of tools have been developed to help the clinician with this important task.[13–18] Regardless of the tool used, the result is only an estimate of the risk of the patient engaging in aberrant behavior. It is not a contraindication for the prescribing of controlled substances but might cause a prudent clinician to seek formal consultation with or referral to other appropriate health care professionals who have sufficient experience and resources to manage these often challenging cases.[7]

INTERPRETING ABERRANT BEHAVIOR

Even with the most reasonable treatment plan, a patient's ability to comply is based on a multitude of potentially conflicting factors. When a patient fails to comply with recommendations in a previously agreed upon treatment plan, the treating clinician needs to have an approach that allows the patient and prescriber to adequately address these issues. Not all aberrant behavior represents abuse, addiction, or criminal intent. Similarly, what may seem like reasonable treatment goals for any given patient may be more difficult for some patients to comply with than others, even in the context of a previously signed treatment agreement. When a patient steps out of previously defined limits and boundaries, the clinician should examine this behavior in the context of a "Golden Moment" where the patient may actually begin to see things for the way they are, rather than the way he or she wished they were.[18a] In this way, both clinician and patient can improve their level of communication that is inherent in all positive therapeutic relationships. Rather than simply dismissing the patient for breaking the treatment agreement, which can perpetuate the patient's revolving-door approach to health care, both parties become better educated to move forward in a strengthened therapeutic relationship based on mutual trust and honesty. This ap-

proach best serves the mutual interests of patient, practitioner, and the community in which they live.

Some patients however are not ready to undertake this level of personal growth; they may need to seek care elsewhere. It is important to remember that it is generally better for a patient to abandon a reasonable and prudent course of therapy than it is for that patient to be dismissed from the practice. While it may be necessary and appropriate to discontinue the prescription of controlled substances such as the opioid class of medication, this should rarely be seen as equivalent to dismissal from care, although a drug-seeking patient may interpret the two as being the same.

Potential Treatment Traps in Compliance Monitoring

Borrowing from Tomorrow to Pay for Today

For most patients, problematic prescription drug use does not involve parenteral misuse or diversion. For those patients who do exhibit aberrant behavior such as running out of medications early, the most common problem relates to simply taking more than prescribed. The concept of *borrowing from tomorrow to pay for today* is something that many patients can relate to.[4] In these circumstances, prescribing smaller quantities of medications, to be dispensed by the pharmacist on an interval basis, can assist the patient with treatment adherence. Patients who need more oversight than weekly medication pickup should likely be referred on for more formal assessment of potential comorbid conditions such as substance use disorders or other significant psychopathology.

Avoiding Excessive Pill Loads

In the management of chronic pain, medications must be carefully titrated to their optimum dose. Traditional teaching for a trial of opioid therapy suggests using immediate-release medications to establish drug responsiveness followed by conversion to modified-release medication, typically in a two or three times daily dosing schedule with a suitable amount of immediate-release medication for breakthrough pain management. While the literature continues to suggest that patients do better on modified-release opioids for the baseline treatment of chronic pain, there are no long-term perspective studies in the literature to confirm this most important clinical point.[19–22] By definition, a successful trial is one in which the patient is clearly improved either in terms of pain relief, functional restoration, or ideally both. Properly chosen patients often do well with this approach. Some, however, improve initially but lack the sustainable relief seen with opioid-responsive pain. In these cases, there is often seen a gradual dose escalation with diminishing returns as the side effect profile begins to overtake the therapeutic effect. For some patients, efficacy is measured by the subtle cognitive effects transiently seen with a new drug or drug dose rather than the marked reduction in pain scores and improved function typically seen with treatment-responsive pain. Unfortunately, tolerance to these effects can develop quickly, leading to significant dose escalation. Sometimes, in an effort to reduce drug use, the prescriber provides the patient with smaller dose tablets in the hopes the patient will be able to titrate the dose down, thereby reducing the overall dose taken and the adverse effects often seen with higher medication levels.

For example, a patient who is using 80 mg of controlled-release oxycodone in an every 8-hour dosing schedule may request 20 mg tablets rather than the 80 mg tablets, indicating that they often feel they don't need to take the entire dose to keep their pain under control. In an effort to reduce the total daily dose, the 80 mg tablets are changed to 20 mg tablets. In this case now, instead of receiving 3 tablets per day, 21 tablets per week, the patient receives 12 tablets per day (to be used "as directed" in a 3 times daily divided dose). This is a total of 84 tablets per week. In a monthly prescription, this amounts to 336 tablets. While some patients may achieve the desired goal of dose reduction, others will ultimately begin to redistribute the controlled-release drug, often taking the medication more frequently during the day than the agreed upon 8-hour interval. With such large quantities of tablets available, *borrowing from tomorrow to pay for today* can become a problem.[4] In such cases when patients have asked for smaller unit doses as just described, it can be revealing to ask the patient to bring in their extra medications at the next visit. It is a minority of patients who are able to comply with this request, indicating that they use the medication up eventually! In these cases, closer inquiry may show that the duration of action for the modified-release drug is really only 3 or 4 hours, necessitating 6 or more dosing intervals per day to achieve "stability." Clearly the use of a modified-release medication in the same fashion as an immediate-release preparation is inappropriate. In a sense, the patient can be legitimately advised that the "clever delivery system" has failed them. In these cases, the answer is not to dose more frequently with the controlled-release preparation but, rather, to consider rotating to another modified-release system or to a truly long-acting medication such as methadone.

URINE DRUG TESTING IN PAIN MEDICINE

Urine drug testing (UDT) is a useful tool in pain management that provides valuable objective information to assist in diagnostic and therapeutic decision making.[11] Results of UDT provide confirmation of the agreed upon treatment plan (adherence/compliance); UDT can diagnose relapse or drug misuse as early as possible and, finally, can be used to advocate for the patient with third party interests.[12]

To assess compliance, the clinician may look for the presence of prescribed medications as evidence of their use. Not finding the prescribed drug or finding unprescribed or illicit drugs in the urine merits further discussion with the patient while recognizing that laboratory error and test insensitivity can result in misleading data. Bingeing by the patient can result in unexpected negative urine reports if the patient runs out of medication prior to sample collection. Therefore, these results by themselves cannot be relied on to prove drug diversion and may be consistent with addiction, pseudoaddiction, or the use of an opioid for nonalgesic purposes—so-called chemical coping.[23] The purpose of UDT should be explained to the patient at the initial evaluation. UDT should be used, like all other diagnostic tests, to improve patient care. UDT can also enhance the relationship between clinicians and patients by providing documentation of adherence to mutually agreed upon treatment plans.[11,12]

Reports of unprescribed or illicit substances in the urine aid in the assessment and diagnosis of drug misuse or addiction. UDT results can be used to encourage change to more functional behaviors, while supporting the positive changes previously made. Thus, the appropriate use of a UDT result requires documentation in the medical record and an understanding on the part of both the patient and the clinician of how these results are to be used.[24]

In the pain management setting, the presence of an illicit or unprescribed drug does not necessarily negate the legitimacy of the patient's pain complaints, but it may suggest a concurrent disorder such as drug abuse or addiction. While acute pain can be treated in a patient with an active addictive disorder, it is improbable that one can successfully treat chronic pain in a patient with untreated addiction. The patient must be willing to accept assessment and treatment of both disorders to receive adequate outcomes in either.[25] Thus the diagnosis of a concurrent addictive disorder, when it exists, does nothing to negate a legitimate pain disorder but rather, it complicates it. In some cases, the very nature of the patient's diagnosis may change as a result of information gained through drug testing.

Specimen Choice

Urine has been the preferred biologic specimen for determining the presence or absence of most drugs since the 1970s.[26] This is in part due to the increased window of detection of 1 to 3 days for most drugs and/or their metabolites.[27] When compared to serum samples, the relatively noninvasive nature of sample collection, ease of storage, and low cost of testing favor urine as the specimen of choice.

Whom to Test

The question of whom to test is made easier by having a uniform practice policy that helps reduce individual stigma. Beyond this, any risk of patient profiling based on racial, cultural, or other physical appearances is eliminated. Careful explanation of the purpose of testing normally allays patient concerns.[11]

Frequency of Testing

Testing frequency is a function of many factors, some of which are patient based and others are a function of the practice. For example, in a pain practice where the patient referral base is typically more complex, a policy of testing all patients on admission and thereafter to be determined by clinical assessment of risk is recommended. On the other hand, in the average primary care setting, where the prevalence of substance-use-disordered individuals should be no greater than the population as a whole, it may be sufficient to discuss urine drug testing with all patients and reserve actual testing to a behaviorally triggered paradigm. Unfortunately, this latter approach does subject the patient and practitioner to the risk of missing a potentially treatable comorbid disorder (substance misuse/addiction).[2,28,29] As time moves forward, the use of urine drug testing is fast becoming a standard of care. What is becoming clear is that the risk to the patient and practitioner alike is a function of what is done with the data thus obtained and not fundamentally in the data itself.[29]

Testing Strategies

The literature is clear that there is often a disconnect between the reason a urine drug test was ordered, the results obtained, and, most importantly, the clinical consequences to the patient as a results of these tests. The fundamental problem is a lack of testing strategy or plan for the clinician to use in response to results obtained. So, for the cocaine-misusing, chronic noncancer pain patient who refuses to give up the use of this drug, the clinical course correction necessary may, for the sake of safety, simply involve the termination of the use of controlled substances such as the opioid class of drug. On the other hand, in the palliative care case where there may be a moral imperative to the continued use of controlled substances for pain management, the decision to move this person into a more supervised setting for medication management might be made based on this new information.

The clinician must know the drugs for which to test, appropriate methods to use, and the expected use of the results obtained.[30a] If the purpose of testing is to find unprescribed or illicit drug use, Gas Chromatography/Mass Spectroscopy (GC/MS) and Liquid Chromatograph/Mass Spectroscopy (LC/MS) or similar

TABLE 60.1

RETENTION TIMES AND DETECTION WINDOWS OF COMMON ANALYTES

Drug	Approximate retention time
Amphetamines	48 hours
Barbiturates	Short acting (e.g., secobarbital) 24 hours Long acting (e.g., phenobarbital) 2–3 weeks
Benzodiazepines	3 days if therapeutic dose ingested Up to 4–6 weeks after extended dosage (i.e., one or more years)
Cocaine	
Metabolite	2–4 days
Ethanol	2–4 hours
Methadone	Approximately 3 days
Opiates	2 days
Propoxyphene	6–48 hours
Cannabinoids	Moderate smoker (4 times/week) 5 days Heavy smoker (smoking daily) 10 days Retention time for chronic smokers may be 20–28 days
Phencyclidine	Approximately 8 days Up to 30 days in chronic users (mean value = 14 days)

Interpretation of retention time must take into account variability of urine specimens, drug metabolism and half-life, patient's physical condition, fluid intake, and method and frequency of ingestion. These are general guidelines only.

technologies are the most specific for identifying individual drugs or their metabolites.[30] Caution must be exercised when interpreting UDT results in a pain practice. True negative urine results for prescribed medication may indicate a pattern of bingeing rather than drug diversion. Time of last use of the drug(s) can be helpful in the interpretation of negative UDT results. Table 60.1 lists retention times/detection windows of common analytes.

A routine UDT screening panel should test for the following drugs/drug classes:

- cocaine
- amphetamines/methamphetamine
- opioids
- methadone
- marijuana
- benzodiazepines

To reduce the risk of an undetected substituted or adulterated test sample, random urinary creatinine, pH, and temperature should be included in the test panel to assist with interpretation and to increase specimen reliability. The temperature of a urine sample within 4 minutes of voiding should be between 90°F and 100°F.[31] Urinary pH undergoes physiologic fluctuations throughout the day, but should remain within the range of 4.5 to 8.0.[31] Urinary creatinine varies with daily water intake and hydration; normal human urine has a creatinine concentration greater than 20 mg/dL. Values lower than 20 mg/dL indicate dilution and findings lower than 5 mg/dL are inconsistent with human urine.[31,32] Test results outside of these ranges should be discussed with the patient and/or the laboratory, as necessary.[11]

The detection time of most drugs or their metabolites in urine is usually 1 to 3 days, which is influenced by several factors including but not limited to dose, route of administration, me-

tabolism, urine concentration, and pH.[30,33] Chronic use of a lipid-soluble drug such as marijuana may extend the window of detection to a week or more.[31,34] Benzodiazepines and their metabolites differ widely in their elimination half-lives, which affect their clinical effect, excretion, and detection.[35] See Table 60.1.

The method chosen to detect a particular drug will depend on the reason for undertaking the test. Immunoassay drug tests are most commonly used. They are designed to classify substances as either present or absent and are generally highly sensitive. In pain management, specific drug identification using more sophisticated identification tests is often needed. Combined techniques such as GC/MS make accurate identification of a specific drug and/or its metabolites possible. When the patient is being prescribed drugs from several different classes of compounds, such as is often the case with many pain patients, specific drug identification is strongly recommended.

Immunoassay drug tests for natural opioids are very responsive to morphine and codeine, but do not distinguish between the two. UDT by immunoassay also shows a low sensitivity for semisynthetic/synthetic opioids such as oxycodone and fentanyl.[35,36] A negative result does not exclude their use. Even though an immunoassay may be negative for consumed oxycodone, it should be positive on GC/MS if the drug was used within the window of detection. The clinical importance of this fact with urine drug testing cannot be overstated, since compliant patients may have been dismissed from pain management practices secondary to false-negative immunoassay test when looking specifically for prescribed medication. More recently, drug-specific immunoassay tests have been developed for such drugs as oxycodone or methadone, which are semisynthetic and synthetic drugs, respectively. The previous detection of an analyte, especially semisynthetic drugs, does not ensure future detection, even when dose and dosing interval have not changed.[11] This is especially true when the drug concentration is "peri-threshold" as would be the case when the concentration is 302 ng/mL and the cutoff is 300 ng/mL. Small changes in the state of hydration could easily make the sample "negative" one day and positive another.

The presence of a prescribed drug in the urine sample makes monitoring of that class of drugs impossible by immunoassay technique alone. Specific drug identification by chromatographic testing (i.e., GC/MS, LC/MS) is also necessary to identify which member of the detected class is responsible for the positive screen.[11]

The clinician also must understand the basic metabolism of commonly prescribed drugs, especially opioids, so he or she will be able to appropriately interpret a urine drug test result that is positive for the prescribed medication and/or its metabolite(s). For example, codeine is a prodrug that has no intrinsic analgesic activity but is metabolized to morphine and other compounds for its analgesic properties. See Figure 60.1 for basic opioid metabolic pathways.

The amount of drug and/or metabolite(s) (i.e., ng/dL) within a urine sample should not be used to extrapolate backward and make specific determinations regarding compliance with prescribed medication. Software and laboratory products have not been scientifically validated and reported in the peer review literature to give this information at this time. Interpreting UDT beyond the current scientific knowledge may possibly put clinicians and patients at medical and/or legal risk.[36b,37,37a] In addtion, UDT can not diagnose addiction, physical dependence, or diversion and should always be verified and correlated with the clinical picture. Health care professionals should use UDT results in conjunction with other clinical information when deciding to continue with or adjust the established boundaries of the treatment plan.

Dealing with Unexpected Urine Toxicology Results

Unlike drug testing that is forensically based, such as workplace testing, drug testing in clinical practice must be used to improve

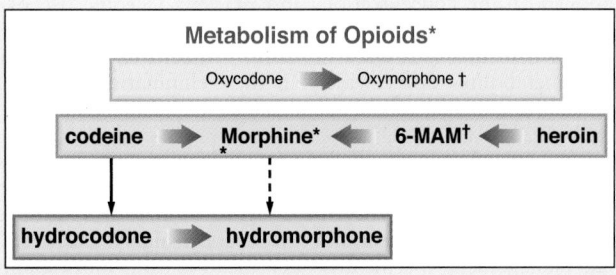

FIGURE 60.1 Basic opioid metabolic pathways. *Not comprehensive pathways, but may explain the presence of apparently unprescribed drugs; †6-MAM: 6-monoacetylmorphine; an intermediate metabolite. (From *D Gourlay, HA Heit, Y Caplan. *Urine Drug Testing in Clinical Practice: Dispelling the Myths & Designing Strategies.* 3rd ed.; †Sloan PA, Barkin RL. Oxymorphone, and oxymorphone extended release: a pharmacotherapeutic review. *J Opioid Manag* 2008;4(3):131–144; **Cone EJ, Heit HA, Caplan YH, et al. Evidence of morphine metabolism to hydromorphone in pain patients chronically treated with morphine. *J Anal Toxicol* 2006;30(1):1–5.)

patient care. Unfortunately, these test results may come back unexpectedly negative for a prescribed drug or positive for an unprescribed one. The first step in interpreting contested results is to contact the lab to ensure that no clerical errors have been made. Occasionally, a negative urine is falsely reported as positive either due to a simple clerical error (i.e., lab wrote positive when they meant negative) or the patient has taken some other product or medication that is causing an unexpected result. In some cases, more definitive testing recommended by the lab will give answers to these questions, but they should never be ignored. There must be a process to follow that ultimately includes discussing the unexpected result with the patient.[11,12]

Unfortunately, drug tests may yield results that appear to be at odds with the patient's apparent level of clinical stability. Once confirmed as accurate, it is important to speak with the patient, carefully documenting the results and ensuing discussion in the medical record. When the patient acknowledges recreational use of prohibited substances, he or she should at least be advised of the clinical consequences of continued use including referral on to a specialist in substance use disorders or, if the patient indicates an unwillingness to stop using, discontinuation of the prescription of any controlled substances. When the patient indicates that he or she will no longer use, the patient should be tested more frequently and, when possible, randomly in order to ensure that this drug use has indeed stopped.[11,12] There are far more illicit/unprescribed drug users who *think* they are recreational users than actually *are* recreational users.

Decision to Terminate Opioid Therapy

The decision to change therapeutic direction should ideally be one made through mutual consultation and agreement between the patient and the physician. Unfortunately, occasions arise when the decision to discontinue a particular therapeutic agent or class of drugs must be made unilaterally. When it is clear that mutually agreed upon therapeutic goals have not been met, the trial of therapy should be considered a failure and an exit strategy implemented. One commonly held myth is that patients who no longer need opioid therapy come off these agents easily. This is often untrue. In fact, many articles have been written about pharmacologic efforts at attenuating the withdrawal symptoms associated with opioid withdrawal.[38–41] Unfortunately, most of these articles are contained in the addiction medicine literature: The pain management literature has been surprisingly quiet on this issue. Interestingly, many medications other than the opioid class of drugs can pose significant challenges to the

prescriber and patient alike when the decision is made to discontinue a course of therapy.[42–47]

As a general rule, it is better to taper a drug than to abruptly discontinue it. Furthermore, the ease with which a patient is able to reduce a large dose to a smaller one may not predict the ease with which the patient ultimately discontinues the drug altogether. For this reason, a reasonable taper schedule for drugs with a known discontinuation syndrome is to reduce the agent by ~10% every 1 to 2 weeks until the last one-third of the dose is reached, at which point the agent should be reduced by ~5% every 2 to 4 weeks until the agent is stopped. When withdrawal symptoms present themselves, it may be helpful to temporarily suspend the taper until these symptoms resolve. In some cases, certain therapeutic agents can be used to blunt the withdrawal process, especially toward the end of the taper. In the case of opioid withdrawal, the alpha-agonist clonidine can be useful to offset the hyperadrenergic symptoms associated with opioid withdrawal.[48]

When the decision is made to discontinue a certain class of medication, it is important to remember that this should not be misinterpreted as discontinuation of treatment. Unfortunately for some patients, discontinuation of a certain drug may result in their abandoning the practitioner who has made the decision to no longer provide this medication. From a medicolegal perspective, it is easier to defend against an assertion of "patient-abandonment" by a patient who has fired a practitioner who has made a patient-centered decision to alter treatment based on sound medical judgement, than it is to formally discharge the patient from your practice.

In conclusion, it is important to remember that a patient's failure to adhere rigorously to a previously agreed upon treatment protocol should not be interpreted as definitive evidence of a substance use disorder or worse, criminal intent. Patients fail to comply for a complex variety of reasons that must be assessed on an individual basis. Remember, aberrant behavior is much easier to identify than it is to interpret. By separating the motive from the behavior in assessing and interpreting departures from the agreed upon treatment plan, a patient-centered approach to problem solving can be implemented.[4]

References

1. Joranson DE, Gilson AM. Drug crime is a source of abused pain medications in the United States. *J Pain Symptom Manage* 2005;30(4):299–301.
2. Katz NP, Adams EH, Benneyan JC, et al. Foundations of opioid risk management. *Clin J Pain* 2007;23(2):103–118.
3. Joranson DE, Gilson AM. A much-needed window on opioid diversion. *Pain Med* 2007;8(2):128–129.
4. Gourlay D, Heit H. Pain and addiction: managing risk through comprehensive care. *J Addict Dis* 2008;27(3):8.
5. *National Drug Control Strategy Annual Report.* Chapter 1: Stopping drug use before it starts. Rockville, MD: Office of National Drug Control Policy; 2008: 17–19.
6. Kripalani S, Yao X, Haynes RB. Interventions to enhance medication adherence in chronic medical conditions: a systematic review. *Arch Intern Med* 2007; 167(6):540–550.
7. Gourlay D, Heit H. Universal precautions: a matter of mutual trust and responsibility. *Pain Med* 2006;7(2):210–211; author reply 212.
8. Fishman SM, Bandman TB, Edwards A, et al. The opioid contract in the management of chronic pain. *J Pain Symptom Manage* 1999;18(1):27–37.
9. Fishman SM, Kreis PG. The opioid contract. *Clin J Pain* 2002;18(Suppl 4): S70–75.
10. Heit H. Creating and implementing opioid agreements. *Dis Manage Digest* 2003;7(1):2–3.
11. Heit HA, Gourlay DL. Urine drug testing in pain medicine. *J Pain Symptom Manage* 2004;27(3):260–267.
12. Gourlay D, Heit H, Caplan Y. Urine Drug Testing in Primary Care: dispelling the myths & designing strategies. 2006 [cited 2006 March 7]; 3rd edition: [Monograph for California Academy of Family Physicians]. Available at: http://www.familydocs.org/assets/Professional_Development/CME/UDT.pdf.
13. Saunders JB, Aasland OG, Babor TF, et al. Development of the Alcohol Use Disorders Identification Test (AUDIT): WHO Collaborative Project on Early Detection of Persons with Harmful Alcohol Consumption—II. *Addiction* 1993; 88(6):791–804.

14. Butler SF, Budman SH, Fernandez K, et al. Validation of a screener and opioid assessment measure for patients with chronic pain. *Pain* 2004;112(1–2):65–75.

15. Akbi H, Butler SF, Budman SH, et al. Validation and clinical application of the Screener and Opioid Assessment for Patients with Pain (SOAPP). *J Pain Symptom Manage* 2006;32(3):287–293.

16. Brown RL, Rounds LA. Conjoint screening questionnaires for alcohol and other drug abuse: criterion validity in a primary care practice. *Wis Med J* 1995; 94(3):135–140.

17. Fiellin DA, Reid MC, O'Connor PG, Outpatient management of patients with alcohol problems. *Ann Intern Med* 2000;133(10):815–827.

18. Webster LR, Webster RM. Predicting aberrant behaviors in opioid-treated patients: preliminary validation of the Opioid Risk Tool. *Pain Med* 2005;6(6): 432–442.

18a. Gourlay DL, Heit HA. Universal precautions revisited: managing the inherited pain patient. *Pain Med* 2009;10 Suppl 2:S115–S123.

19. Dole VP. Implications of methadone maintenance for theories of narcotic addiction. *JAMA* 1988;260(20):3025–3029.

20. Brookoff D. Abuse potential of various opioid medications. *J Gen Intern Med* 1993;8(12):688–690.

21. Zacny JP. Should people taking opioids for medical reasons be allowed to work and drive? *Addiction* 1996;91(11):1581–1584.

22. Haythornthwaite JA, Menefee LA, Quatrano–Piacentini AL, et al, Outcome of chronic opioid therapy for non-cancer pain. *J Pain Symptom Manage* 1998; 15(3):185–194.

23. Bruera E, Moyano J, Seifert L, et al. The frequency of alcoholism among patients with pain due to terminal cancer. *J Pain Symptom Manage* 1995;10(8): 599–603.

24. Passik SD, Schreiber J, Kirsh KL, et al. A chart review of the ordering and documentation of urine toxicology screens in a cancer center: do they influence patient management? *J Pain Symptom Manage* 2000;19(1):40–44.

25. Gourlay D, Heit H, Almarhezi A. Universal precautions in pain medicine: a rational approach to the management of chronic pain. *Pain Medicine* 2005; 6(2):107–112.

26. Caplan YH, Goldberger BA. Alternative specimens for workplace drug testing. *J Anal Toxicol* 2001;25(5):396–399.

27. Conigliaro C, Reyes C, Schultz J. Principles of screening and early intervention. 3rd ed. In: Graham A, et al, eds. *Principles of Addiction Medicine.* Chevy Chase, MD: American Society of Addiction Medicine; 2003:323–336.

28. Katz NP, Sherburne S, Beach M, et al. Behavioral monitoring and urine toxicology testing in patients receiving long-term opioid therapy. *Anesth Analg* 2003; 97(4):1097–1102, table of contents.

29. Katz N, Fanciullo GJ. Role of urine toxicology testing in the management of chronic opioid therapy. *Clin J Pain* 2002;18(Suppl 4):S76–S82.

30. Vandevenne M, Vandenbussche H, Verstraete A. Detection time of drugs of abuse in urine. *Acta Clin Belg* 2000;55(6):323–333.

30a. Reifield GM, Chronister CW, Goldberger BA, et al. Unexpected urine drug test results in a hospice patient on high dose morphine therapy. Clin Chem. In Press.

30b. Gourlay DL, Heit HA. Letter to the editor. *Clin Chem.* In Press.

31. Cook JD, Caplan YH, LoDico CP, et al. The characterization of human urine for specimen validity determination in workplace drug testing: a review. *J Anal Toxicol* 2000;24(7):579–588.

32. Lipman A, Jackson K. Opioids. In: Warfield C, Bajwa Z, eds. *Principles and Practice of Pain Management.* New York: McGraw Hill; 2003.

33. Casavant MJ. Urine drug screening in adolescents. *Pediatr Clin North Am* 2002;49(2):317–327.

34. Huestis MA, Mitchell JM, Cone EJ. Detection times of marijuana metabolites in urine by immunoassay and GC-MS. *J Anal Toxicol* 1995;19(6):443–449.

35. Simpson D, Braithwaite RA, Jarvie DR, et al. Screening for drugs of abuse (II): Cannabinoids, lysergic acid diethylamide, buprenorphine, methadone, barbiturates, benzodiazepines and other drugs. *Ann Clin Biochem* 1997;34(Pt 5): 460–510.

36. Shults T, St. Clair S. *The Medical Review Officer Handbook.* Triangle Park, NC: Quadrangle Research; 1999.

36b. Nafziger AN, Bertino JS. Utility and application of urine drug testing in chronic pain management with opioids. *Clin J Pain* 2009;25(1):73–79.

37. Shutlz T. *MRO Alert.* Triangle Park, NC: Quadrangle Research; 1–4.

37a. Gourlay DL, Heit HA. The art and science of urine drug testing. *Clin J Pain.* In press.

38. Stock C, Shum JH. Buprenorphine:a new pharmacotherapy for opioid addictions treatment. *J Pain Palliat Care Pharmacother* 2004;18(3):35–54.

39. Bisaga A, Comer SD, Ward AS, et al. The NMDA antagonist memantine attenuates the expression of opioid physical dependence in humans. *Psychopharmacology (Berl)* 2001;157(1):1–10.

40. Bickel WK, Stitzer ML, Liebson IA, et al. Acute physical dependence in man: effects of naloxone after brief morphine exposure. *J Pharmacol Exp Ther* 1988; 244(1):126–132.

41. Fishman SM, Wilsey B, Mahajan G, et al. Methadone reincarnated: novel clinical applications with related concerns. *Pain Med* 2002;3(4):339–348.

42. Tran KT, Hranicky D, Lark T, et al. Gabapentin withdrawal syndrome in the presence of a taper. *Bipolar Disord* 2005;7(3):302–304.

43. Hirose S. Restlessness related to SSRI withdrawal. *Psychiatry Clin Neurosci* 2001;55(1):79–80.

44. Mareth TR, Brown TM. SSRI withdrawal. *J Clin Psychiatry* 1996;57(7):310.

45. Kotzalidis G, de Pisa E, Patrizi B, et al., Similar discontinuation symptoms for withdrawal from medium-dose paroxetine and venlafaxine after nine years in the same patient. *J Psychopharmacol* 2008;22(5):581–584.

46. Campagne DM. Venlafaxine and serious withdrawal symptoms: warning to drivers. *MedGenMed* 2005;7(3):22.

47. Johnson H, Bouman WP, Lawton J. Withdrawal reaction associated with venlafaxine. *BMJ* 1998;317(7161):787.

48. Lowenson J, ed. *Substance Abuse.* 4th ed. Philadelphia: Lippincott Williams and Wilkins; 2005.

CHAPTER 61 ■ HEADACHE

PETER J. GOADSBY

INTRODUCTION

Headache is a remarkably common problem even in general medicine or neurology and, by definition, has a substantial pain component. Books are devoted to the topic and interested readers are directed to recent editions for more detail on the subjects covered here.[1-5] The headache disorders are classified by the International Classification of Headache disorders,[6] now in its second edition, as being either primary, where the headache syndrome is itself the problem, or secondary, where the headache syndrome is driven by other pathological processes. This chapter is designed to cover the primary headaches with a broad view. Facial neuralgias and facial pain syndromes are covered elsewhere in this book. Where a primary headache causes face pain, and most primary headaches can do this, it will be included here for completeness. The chapter will cover the broad principles, the generic anatomy and physiology of head pain, and then discuss in turn the currently defined primary headache syndromes. There is much opportunity in headache to make patients significantly better and much research advancement in this very exciting area of medicine.

GENERAL PRINCIPLES

A general system for headache nosology is outlined in Table 61.1. The clinical challenge remains that while life-threatening headache is relatively uncommon in Western society, it occurs and its detection requires suitable awareness by the doctors of its clinical markers (Table 61.2). Primary headache, in contrast, often confers considerable disability over time and while not life-threatening, certainly robs patients of a decent quality of life.

Primary Headache Syndromes

The primary headaches are a group of remarkable disorders in which headache and associated features are seen in the absence of any exogenous cause. First, the general anatomy and physiology will be described as it applies to most of the syndromes. Then, the primary headache syndromes will be addressed and finally the chronic daily headache (CDH) syndromes will be explicitly mentioned as they drive so much disability.

Anatomy and Physiology

The most common *disabling* primary headaches, migraine and cluster headache, have been studied extensively in recent times and they are now relatively well understood insofar as neurological disorders that involve the brain are concerned. The word disabling is emphasized as the author takes the view that there are not sufficient, clear data to imply that tension-type headache provides a substantial and disabling community problem.[7] This is largely due to the probable inclusion of patients with migraine in many cohorts that have studied tension-type headache. In experimental animals, the detailed anatomy of the connections of the pain-producing intracranial extracerebral vessels and the dura mater has built on the classical human observations of Wolff,[8] and Feindel, Penfield, and McNaughton.[9,10] It is these structures, and not the brain itself, that primarily generate, or are perceived to generate, head pain.

The key structures involved are:

■ The large intracranial vessels and dura mater
■ The peripheral terminals of the trigeminal nerve that innervate these structures
■ The central terminals and second order neurons of the caudal trigeminal nucleus and dorsal horns of C_1 and C_2 (trigemino-cervical complex)
■ Higher center processing in the thalamus, ventroposteromedial and posterior thalamus, and cortex
■ Modulatory centers in the diencephalon and brainstem, such as periaqueductal grey matter, locus coeruleus and parts of the hypothalamus

The innervation of the large intracranial vessels and dura mater by the trigeminal nerve is known as the trigeminovascular system. The cranial parasympathetic autonomic innervation provides the basis for symptoms such as lacrimation and nasal stuffiness, which are prominent in the trigeminal autonomic cephalalgias,[11,12] although they may also be seen in migraine. It is clear from human functional imaging studies that vascular changes in migraine and cluster headache are driven by these neural vasodilator systems so that these headaches should be regarded as *neurovascular*.[13] The concept of a primary *vascular* headache should be abandoned since it neither explains the pathogenesis of what are complex central nervous system disorders, nor does it necessarily predict treatment outcomes. The term *vascular headache*

COMMON CAUSES OF HEADACHE

Primary headache		Secondary headache	
Type	Prevalence (%)	Type	Prevalence (%)
Migraine	16	Systemic infection	63
Tension-type	69	Head injury	4
Cluster headache	0.1	Subarachnoid hemorrhage	<1
Idiopathic stabbing	2	Vascular disorders	1
Exertional	1	Brain tumor	0.1

Olesen J, Tfelt-Hansen P, Ramadan N, et al. *The Headaches.* Philadelphia: Lippincott Williams & Wilkins; 2005.

TABLE 61.2

WARNING SIGNS IN HEAD PAIN

- Sudden onset pain
- Fever
- Marked change in pain character or timing of attacks
- Neck stiffness
- Pain associated with higher center complaints
- Pain associated with neurological disturbance, such as clumsiness or weakness
- Pain associated with local tenderness, such as of the temporal artery

has no place in modern medical practice when referring to primary headache.

Migraine is an episodic syndrome of headache with sensory sensitivity, such as to light, sound, and head movement, probably due to dysfunction of aminergic brainstem/diencephalic sensory control systems (Fig. 61.1). The first of the migraine genes has

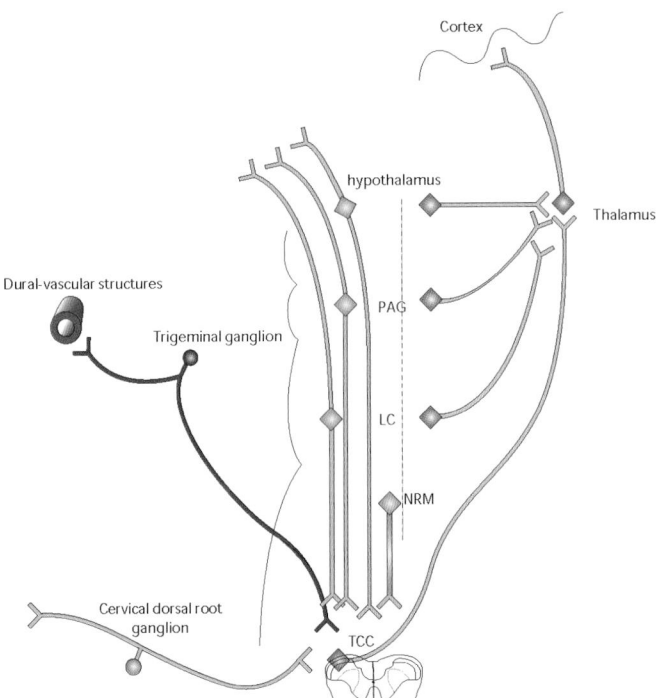

FIGURE 61.1 Pathophysiology of Migraine. Diagram of some structures involved in the transmission of trigeminovascular nociceptive input and the modulation of that input that form the basis of a model of the pathophysiology of migraine.[102] Afferents from dural-vascular structures innervated predominantly by branches of the first (ophthalmic division) of the trigeminal nerve whose cell bodies are found in the trigeminal ganglion (Vg) project to second order neurons in the trigeminocervical complex (TCC). The TCC extends from trigeminal nucleus caudalis to the caudal portion of the dorsal horn of the C_2 spinal cord. Input from cervical structures, such as joints or muscles, project through cell bodies in the upper cervical dorsal root ganglia (DRGs) to the TCC. TCC neurons project to ventrobasal thalamus (thalamus) and then to cortex. Sensory modulation can occur by descending influences onto the TCC that largely respect the midline (*dashed line*), such as those from hypothalamus, midbrain periaqueductal grey (PAG), pontine locus coeruleus (LC), and nucleus raphe magnus (RVM). These influences are cartooned as being direct but both direct and indirect projections are recognized. In addition, sensory modulation can occur from at least LC; PAG and hypothalamic projects to thalamus nuclei as ascending systems again that largely respect the midline.

been identified for familial hemiplegic migraine, and includes mutations in the *CACNA1A* gene for the $Ca_V2.1$ (α_{1A}) subunit of the neuronal P/Q voltage-gated calcium channel,[14] the Na/K ATP pump α_2 subunit gene *ATP1A2*,[15] and the voltage-gated sodium channel *SCN1A*.[16] These findings and the clinical features of migraine suggest it might be part of the spectrum of diseases known as channelopathies, or now ionopathies: disorders involving dysfunction of ion channel fluxes.[17] Functional neuroimaging has suggested that brainstem regions in migraine (Fig. 61.2), and the posterior hypothalamic region, in cluster headache (Fig. 61.3), are good candidates for specific involvement in primary headache.[13]

Secondary Headache

It is imperative to establish in the patient presenting with any form of head pain whether there is an important secondary headache. Perhaps the most crucial clinical feature to elicit is the length of the history. Patients with a short history require prompt attention and may require prompt investigation and management. Patients with a longer history generally require time and patience rather than alacrity. There are some important general features, including associated fever or sudden onset of pain (see Table 61.2). Patients with a history of recent onset headache or neurological signs need a positive diagnosis of a benign disorder or require brain imaging with computed tomography (CT) or magnetic resonance imaging (MRI). Patients with a history of recurrent headache over a period of 1 year or more, fulfilling IHS criteria for migraine (Table 61.3) and with a normal physical examination, have positive brain imaging findings in only about 1/1000 images.[18] In general, it should be noted that brain tumor is a rare cause of headache, and rarely a cause of isolated long-term histories of headache. A notable exception to the general rules about secondary headache is pituitary tumor, which can trigger underlying primary headache biologies, and should always be considered, especially in the differential diagnosis of trigeminal autonomic cephalalgias.[19]

The management of secondary headache is generally self-evident: treatment of the underlying condition, such as an infection or mass lesion. One notable exception is the condition of chronic posttraumatic headache in which pain persists for long periods after head injury. This is an interesting problem that may be seen after central nervous system infection, both blunt and surgical trauma, intracranial bleeds, and other precipitants, using the term "trauma" in its broader context to mean a biological insult. While the syndrome is generally self-limiting up to 3–5 years after the event, treatment of the headache may be required if it is disabling (see CDH discussion below).

Migraine

Clinical Features

Migraine is an episodic brain disorder that affects about 12% to 15% of the population,[20,21] and can be highly disabling.[22] It has been estimated to be the most costly neurological disorder in the European community at more than €27 billion per year,[23] and its cost to the U.S. economy is a staggering $19.6 billion per year.[24] Migraine presents with headache generally accompanied by features, such as sensitivity to light, sound, or movement, and often with nausea, or less often vomiting (see Table 61.3). None of the features is compulsory, and indeed given that the migraine aura, visual disturbances with flashing lights or zig-zag lines moving across the fields or other neurological symptoms, is reported in only about 25% of patients, a high index of suspicion is required to diagnose migraine. In a controlled study of patients presenting to primary care physicians with a main complaint of headache

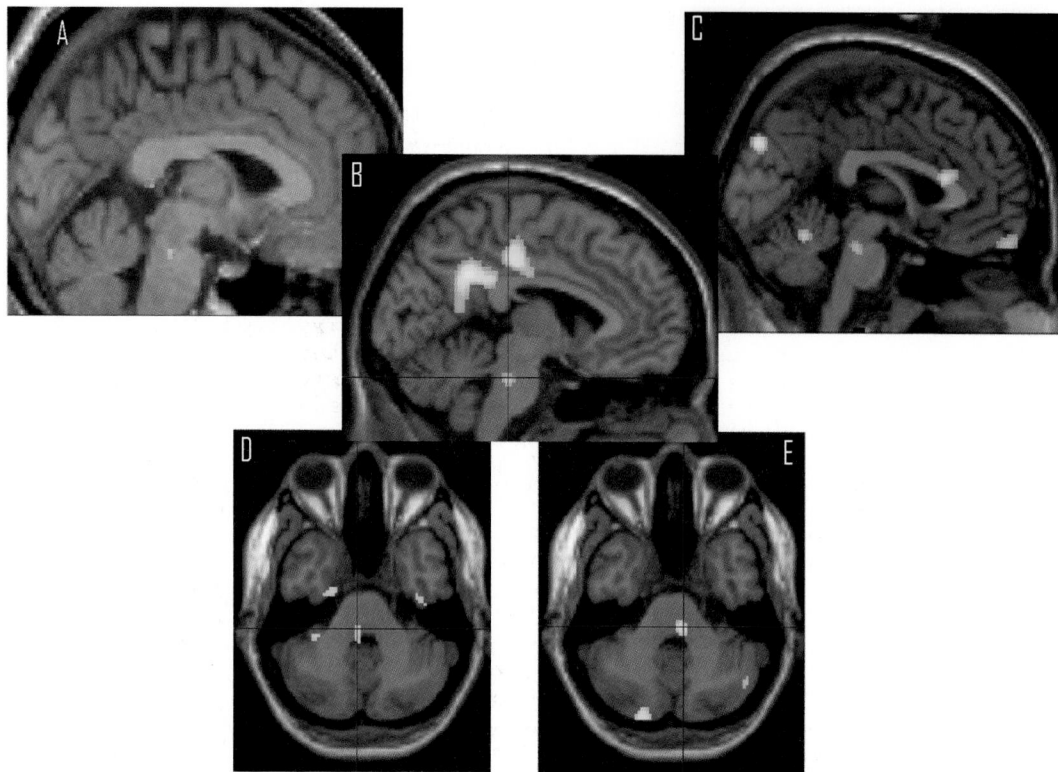

FIGURE 61.2 Activations identified on positron emission tomography in migraine. Consistently, there is dorso-lateral pons activation in episodic migraine without aura, triggered by nitroglycerin (**A**)[103] or spontaneously studied (**B**),[104] and in chronic migraine (**C**).[25] Moreover, there is lateralization to the right (**D**) and left (**E**) in this structure that parallels the unilateral presentation of the pain.[105]

over the previous 3 months, migraine was the diagnosis on more than 90% of occasions,[7] thus a high index of suspicion is well rewarded. A headache diary can often be helpful in making the diagnosis; although, in reality the diary usually helps more in assessing disability or recording how often patients use acute attack treatments. Phenotyping remains an essentially clinical art mixing experience and an understanding of the problems likely to present—*good headache histories are taken not given*. In differentiating the two main primary headache syndromes seen in clinical practice, *migraine at its most simple level is headache with associated features, and tension-type headache is headache that is featureless;* furthermore *most disabling headache presentations in primary care are probably migrainous in biology.* By features here is meant throbbing pain, sensitivity to sensory stimuli (visual, auditory, olfactory), or to head movement itself.

Frequent Migraine

If headache with associated features describes migraine attacks, then *headachy* describes the migraine sufferer over their lifetime. It is important to realize that the word migraine can both describe the attacks using standard criteria (see Table 61.3), and describe the disorder itself, which is more than just the attacks. The migraine sufferer inherits a tendency to have headache that is amplified at various times by their interaction with their environment, the much-discussed triggers. The brain of the migraineur seems more sensitive to sensory stimuli and to change, and this tendency is notably amplified in females during their menstrual cycle. Migraine sufferers may have headache when they oversleep, when tired, when they skip meals, when they overexert, when stressed, or when they relax from a stressor. They are less tolerant to change

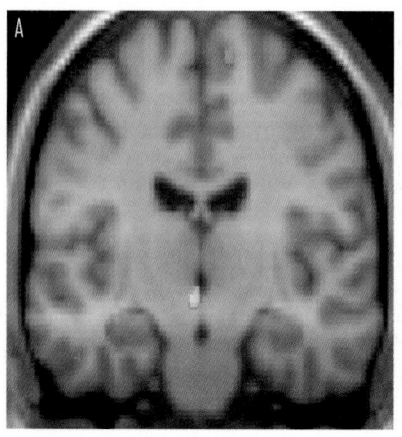

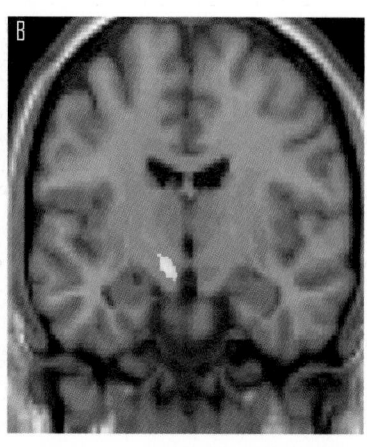

FIGURE 61.3 Activations on positron emission tomography in the posterior hypothalamic grey matter in patients with acute cluster headache (**A**). The activation demonstrated is lateralized to the side of the pain.[42] When comparing the brains of patients with cluster headache with a control population using an automatic anatomical technique known as voxel-based morphometry (VBM) that employs high-resolution T1 weighted MRI, a similar region is demonstrated (**B**) and has increased grey matter.[43]

TABLE 61.3

SIMPLIFIED DIAGNOSTIC CRITERIA FOR MIGRAINE

Repeated attacks of headache lasting 4–72 hours that have these features, normal physical examination and no other reasonable cause for the headache

At least 2 of:	At least 1 of:
• unilateral pain • throbbing pain • aggravation by movement • moderate or severe intensity	• nausea/vomiting • photophobia and phonophobia

Adapted from the IHS Classification[6]

and part of successful management is to advise them to maintain regularity in their lives in the knowledge of this fluctuating biology. It is this biology that marks migraine and in clinical practice must override the phenotype of individual headaches. It has been said that migraine can never occur daily; this is simply not correct. Chronic migraine very definitely occurs and is probably the largest part of the group of headaches known collectively as CDH that presents to doctors (see below). After making a diagnosis, the second step in the clinical process is to be sure that the disease burden has been captured: how much headache does the patient have and more important, what can the patient not do? What is their degree of disability? One can ask the patient directly to get a flavor for this, keep a diary, or get a quick but accurate estimate using the Migraine Disability Assessment Scale (MIDAS), which is well-validated and very easy to use in practice (Fig. 61.4).

Principles of Management of Migraine

After diagnosis, the management of migraine begins with an explanation of some aspects of the disorder to the patient.

- Migraine is an inherited tendency to have headache; this is caused by the patient's genes, therefore it cannot be cured *but*;
- Migraine can be modified and controlled by lifestyle adjustment and the use of medicines;
- Migraine is not life-threatening or associated with serious illness with the exception of females who smoke and use estrogenic oral contraceptives, but migraine can make life a misery;
- Migraine management takes time and cooperation when, for example, a headache diary has to be collected, or inquiry made concerning the disability.

INSTRUCTIONS: Please answer the following questions about ALL your headaches you have had over the last 3 months. Write your answer in the box next to each question. Write zero if you did not do the activity in the last 3 months (Please refer to the calendar below, if necessary)

1. On how many days in the last 3 months did you miss work or school because of your headaches? .... |__|__| days

2. How many days in the last 3 months was your productivity at work or school reduced by half or more because of your headaches (*Do not include days you counted in question 1 where you missed work or school*)? .... |__|__| days

3. On how many days in the last 3 months did you **not** do household work because of your headaches? .... |__|__| days

4. How many days in the last 3 months was your productivity in household work reduced by half or more because of your headaches (*Do not include days you counted in question 3 where you did not do household work*)? .... |__|__| days

5. On how many days in the last 3 months did you miss family, social, or leisure activities because of your headaches? .... |__|__| days

A. On how many days in the last 3 months did you have a headache? (If a headache lasted more than one day, count each day) .... |__|__| days

B. On a scale of 0 - 10, on average how painful were these headaches?

   (*where 0 = no pain at all, and 10 = pain as bad as it can be*) .... |__|__|

Version 3.0   © Innovative Medical Research 1997

FIGURE 61.4 Migraine Disability Assessment Score (MIDAS) Questionnaire.

Nonpharmacological Management of Migraine

This approach aims to help the migrainous patient identify things making the problem worse and encourage them to modify these. Patients need to know that the brain sensitivity to triggers in migraine varies. Patient associations are often very helpful in supporting migraineurs to identify triggers. The knowledge that there is variability will remove considerable frustration on the patient's part, and will ring true to most as they have had the experience. The crucial lifestyle advice is to explain to the patient that migraine is a state of brain sensitivity to change. This implies that the migraine sufferer needs to regulate their lives: healthy diet, regular exercise, regular sleep patterns, avoiding excess caffeine and alcohol and, as far as practical, modifying or minimizing changes in stress. The balanced life with less highs and lows will benefit most migraine sufferers.

Preventive Treatments of Migraine

The patient needs to understand they have an inherited, incurable, but manageable problem. To start a preventive, they need to have sufficient disability to wish to take a medicine to reduce the affects of the disease on their life. The basis of considering preventive treatment from a medical viewpoint is a combination of acute attack frequency and attack tractability that is conferring an unacceptable degree of disability. Patients with attacks unresponsive to abortive medications are easily considered for prevention, while patients with simply treated attacks may be less obvious candidates. Another important consideration is disease progress. If a patient diary shows a clear trend of an increasing frequency of attacks it is better to initiate a preventive than wait for the problem to worsen.

A simple rule for frequency might be that for 1–2 headaches a month there is usually no need to start a preventive, for 3–4 it may be needed but not necessary, and for 5 or more per month prevention should definitely be considered. Options available for treatment are covered in detail in Table 61.4 and vary somewhat by country. One problem with preventives is that they have fallen into use for migraine from other indications and often bring unwanted or intolerable side effects. It is not clear how preventives work although it seems likely that they modify the brain sensitivity that underlies migraine. Another key clinical point is that generally each drug should be started at a low dose and gradually increased to a reasonable maximum if there is going to be a clinical effect.

Little has been done in terms of systematic study of patients with more intractable forms of migraine. Neuromodulation or neurostimulation approaches are promising, including stimulation of the occipital nerve, and functional imaging studies show that central processing of pain signals in migraine in the thalamus may be modified by such therapies.[25] This is an exciting and developing area.[26]

Acute Attack Therapies of Migraine

Acute attack treatments for migraine can be usefully divided into disease nonspecific treatments, analgesics and nonsteroidal anti-inflammatory drugs (NSAIDs), and disease specific treatments, ergot-related compounds, and triptans (Table 61.5). It is important to be aware that most acute attack medications seem to have a propensity to aggravate headache frequency and can induce a state of refractory daily, near-daily, or medication-overuse headache. As evidence is gathered, this seems to occur in patients with migraine: either a previous clear history or a family or personal history of headacheyness.[27] Codeine-containing compound analgesics are particularly troublesome when available in over-the-counter (OTC) preparations. One should advise patients with migraine to avoid taking acute attack medicines on more than two days a week. A proportion of patients who stop taking regular analgesics will have substantial improvement in their headache with a reduction in frequency; however, for some it will not make any difference. It is crucial to emphasize to the patient that standard preventive medications often simply do not work in the presence of regular analgesic use.

Treatment strategies: Given the array of options to control an acute attack of migraine, how does one start? The simplest approach to treatment has been described as *Stepped Care*. In this model, all patients are treated, assuming no contraindications, with the simplest treatment, such as aspirin 900 mg or paracetamol (acetaminophen) 1000 mg with an antiemetic. Aspirin is an effective strategy, has been proven so in double-blind controlled clinical trials, and is best used in its most soluble formulations. The alternative would be a strategy known as *Stratified Care*, by which the physician determines, or stratifies, treatment at the start based on likelihood of response to levels of care. An intermediate option may be described as stratified care by attack. The latter is what many headache authorities suggest and what patients often do when they have the options.[28] Patients use simpler options for their less severe attacks relying on more potent options when their attacks or circumstances demand them.

Nonspecific Acute Migraine Attack Treatments. Simple drugs, such as aspirin and acetaminophen, are cheap and can be effective. Dosages should be adequate and the addition of domperidone (10 mg orally) or metoclopramide (10 mg orally) can be very helpful. NSAIDs can very useful when tolerated. Their success is often limited by inappropriate dosing, and adequate doses of naproxen (500–1000 mg orally or rectally, with an antiemetic), ibuprofen (400–800 mg orally[29]), or tolfenamic acid (200 mg orally[30]) can be extremely effective.

Specific Acute Migraine Attack Treatments. When simple analgesic measures fail or more aggressive treatment is required, the specific antimigraine treatments are required (Table 61.6). While ergotamine remains a useful treatment, it can no longer be considered the treatment of choice in acute migraine.[31] There are particular situations in which ergotamine is very helpful, but its use must be carefully controlled as ergotamine overuse produces dreadful headache in addition to a host of vascular problems. The triptans, serotonin 5-HT$_{1B/1D}$ receptor agonists, have revolutionized the life of many patients with migraine and are clearly the most powerful option available to stop a migraine attack. They can be rationally applied by considering their pharmacological, physicochemical, and pharmacokinetic features,[32] as well as the formulations that are available.[28] Recent data suggests that combining a triptan with an NSAID can improve efficacy and reduce headache recurrence.[33]

Tension-Type Headache

Clinical Features

As its name suggests, tension-type headache (TTH) is the headache form most seeking of understanding. TTH is diagnosed often, and while the phenotype is common, much of the disabling headache that goes under the name TTH is likely to be chronic migraine in terms of its biology. TTH has two forms: episodic TTH, where attacks occur on less than 15 days a month, and chronic TTH, where attacks, on average over time, are seen on 15 days or more a month. The International Headache Society (IHS) seeks to subdivide episodic tension-type headache into an infrequent variety, arguably of little impact on the patient's life, and a more frequent but nonchronic version. Patients with the chronic form are part of the broader clinical syndrome of CDH, but chronic tension-type headache and CDH are not equal concepts.

TTH has been defined by the IHS both for its episodic and chronic forms, although the admixture of symptoms allowed has

TABLE 61.4

PREVENTIVE TREATMENTS IN MIGRAINE*

Drug	Dose	Selected side effects
Pizotifen	0.5 mg to 2 mg daily	Weight gain Drowsiness
β-Blocker propranolol	40 mg to 120 mg b.d.	Reduced energy Tiredness Postural symptoms *Contraindicated in asthma*
Tricyclics • amitriptyline • dosulepin (dothiepin) • nortriptyline	25 mg to 75 mg nocte	Drowsiness *note*: some patients are very sensitive and may only need a total dose of 10 mg, although generally 1–1.5 mg/kg body weight is required
Anticonvulsants • Valproate • Topiramate • Gabapentin	400–600 mg twice daily 50–200 mg/day 900–3600 mg daily	Drowsiness Weight gain Tremor Hair loss Fetal abnormalities Hematological or liver abnormalities Paraesthesia Cognitive dysfunction Weight loss Care with a family history of glaucoma Nephrolithiasis Dizziness Sedation
Methysergide	1–6 mg daily	Drowsiness Leg cramps Hair loss Retroperitoneal fibrosis (1 month drug holiday is required every 6 months)
Flunarizine	5–15 mg daily	Drowsiness Weight gain Depression Parkinsonism
Single studies† • Lisinopril • Candesartan	20 mg daily 16 mg daily	Cough Dizziness
Nutraceuticals‡ • Riboflavin • Coenzyme Q10 • Butterbur • Feverfew	400 mg daily 100 mg three times daily 75 mg twice daily 6.25 mg three times daily	GI upset
No Convincing Controlled Evidence • Verapamil		
Controlled Trials to demonstrate no effect • Nimodipine • Clonidine • SSRIs: fluoxetine		

*Commonly used preventives are listed with reasonable doses and common side effects. The local national formulary should be consulted for detailed information.
†Compounds not widely considered mainstream but with a positive randomized control trial against placebo
‡Nonpharmaceuticals with at least one positive randomized controlled trial against placebo.

TABLE 61.5

ORAL ACUTE MIGRAINE TREATMENTS

Nonspecific treatments	Specific treatments
(often used with anti-emetic/ prokinetics, such as domperidone (10 mg) or metoclopramide (10 mg))	
- Aspirin (900 mg)	- *Ergot derivatives*
- Acetaminophen (Paracetamol 1000 mg)	• ergotamine (1–2 mg)
- *NSAIDs*	- *Triptans*
• naproxen (500–1000 mg)	• sumatriptan (50 or 100 mg)
• ibuprofen (400–800 mg)	• naratriptan (2.5 mg)
• tolfenamic acid (200 mg)	• rizatriptan (10 mg)
	• zolmitriptan (2.5 or 5 mg)
	• eletriptan (40 or 80 mg)
	• almotriptan (12.5 mg)
	• frovatriptan (2.5 mg)

consistency problems. A useful clinical approach is to diagnose TTH when the headache is completely featureless: no nausea, no vomiting, no photophobia, no phonophobia, no osmophobia, no throbbing, and no aggravation with movement. Such an approach neatly divides migraine, which has one or more of these features and is the main differential diagnosis, from TTH.

Pathophysiology

The pathophysiology of TTH is poorly understood. This results from the fact that the name implies to most that it is a product of *nervous tension*, for which there is no clear evidence, and the definitions employed have undoubtedly admitted patients with migraine to the studies. Moreover, the concept that TTH in some way involves muscle contraction is incorrect since the evidence is that muscle contraction is no more likely than it is in migraine.[34] It seems likely that TTH is due to a primary disorder of central nervous system pain modulation alone in contrast with migraine, which is a more generalized disturbance of sensory modulation.

Management

Adopting the clinical approach to TTH outlined above results in diagnosing a headache form that is usually less disabling, more often described by patients as irritating. Its episodic form is generally amenable to simple analgesics, paracetamol (acetaminophen), aspirin, or other NSAIDs, which can be purchased OTC. There are clear clinical studies to demonstrate that triptans in TTH alone are not helpful, although germane to the above discussion, triptans are effective in TTH where the patient also has migraine.[35] For chronic TTH, amitriptyline is the only treatment with clear evidence of efficacy[36–38]; the other tricyclics, selective serotonin reuptake inhibitors, or the benzodiazepines have not been shown in controlled trials to be effective. Similarly, there is no controlled evidence for the use of electromyograph biofeedback, relaxation therapy, or acupuncture. Botulinum toxin has been shown reasonably clearly to be ineffective.[39] Stress management has been shown to be an effective approach in a controlled trial.[38]

Trigeminal-Autonomic Cephalalgias

Cluster Headache

Cluster headache is a rare form of primary headache with a population frequency of approximately 0.1%.[40] As a clinical anchor,

TABLE 61.6

STRATIFICATION OF ACUTE SPECIFIC MIGRAINE TREATMENTS

Clinical situation	Treatment options
Failed analgesics/ NSAIDs	*First tier* Sumatriptan 50 mg or 100 mg po Almotriptan 12.5 mg po Rizatriptan 10 mg po Eletriptan 40 mg po Zolmitriptan 2.5 mg po *Slower effect/better tolerability* Naratriptan 2.5 mg po Frovatriptan 2.5 mg po *Infrequent headache* Ergotamine 1–2 mg po Dihydroergotamine nasal spray 2 mg
Early nausea or difficulties taking tablets	Zolmitriptan 5 mg nasal spray Sumatriptan 20 mg nasal spray Rizatriptan 10 mg MLT wafer Zolmitriptan 2.5 mg rapidly
Headache recurrence	Ergotamine 2 mg (most effective pr/ usually with caffeine) Naratriptan 2.5 mg po Almotriptan 12.5 mg po Eletriptan 40 mg
Tolerating acute treatments poorly	Naratriptan 2.5 mg Almotriptan 12.5 mg
Early vomiting	Zolmitriptan 5 mg nasal spray Sumatriptan 25 mg pr Sumatriptan 6 mg sc
Menstrually-related headache	*Prevention* Ergotamine po nocte Estrogen patches *Treatment* Triptans Dihydroergotamine nasal spray
Very rapidly developing symptoms	Zolmitriptan 5 mg nasal spray Sumatriptan 6 mg sc Dihydroergotamine 1 mg imi

it is about as common as multiple sclerosis in the United Kingdom,[41] and must be regarded as a disorder best managed by neurologists or headache specialists. It is perhaps the most painful condition of humans; in the cohort of more than 10 patients seen by the author, not a single one has had a more painful experience, including childbirth, multiple fractures of the limbs, or renal stones. It is one of a group of conditions known now as trigeminal-autonomic cephalalgias (TACs), and thus needs to be differentiated from other TACs[11] and the short lasting headaches without cranial autonomic symptoms, such as lacrimation or conjunctival injection (Table 61.7).

The core feature of cluster headache is periodicity, be it circadian or in terms of active and inactive bouts over weeks and months (Table 61.8). The typical cluster headache patient is male, with a 3:1 predominance, with bouts of one to two attacks of relatively short duration unilateral pain every day for eight to ten weeks a year. They are generally perfectly well between attacks. Patients with cluster headache tend to move about during attacks, pacing, rocking, or even rubbing their head for relief. The pain is usually retro-orbital boring and very severe. It is associated with ipsilateral symptoms of cranial (parasympathetic) autonomic activation: a red or watering eye, the nose running or

TABLE 61.7

CLUSTER HEADACHE, OTHER TACS, AND SHORT-LASTING HEADACHES

Trigeminal autonomic cephalalgias (TACs)*	Other short-lasting headaches
• Cluster headache • Paroxysmal hemicrania • SUNCT/SUNA† syndrome	• Primary stabbing headache • Trigeminal neuralgia • Primary cough headache • Primary exertional Headache • Primary sex headache • Hypnic headache

*Beware of pituitary tumor-related headache in the differential diagnosis of these TACs.
†Short-lasting unilateral neuralgiform headache attacks with conjunctival injection and tearing/cranial autonomic features.

blocking, or cranial sympathetic dysfunction (eyelid droop). Cluster headache is likely to be a disorder involving central pacemaker regions of the posterior hypothalamus and perhaps other neurons of this region (see Fig. 61.2).[42,43]

The TACs (cluster headache, paroxysmal hemicrania, and SUNCT syndrome) present a distinct group to be differentiated from short-lasting headaches that do not have prominent cranial autonomic syndromes, notably trigeminal neuralgia, idiopathic

TABLE 61.8

DIAGNOSTIC CRITERIA FOR CLUSTER HEADACHE

3.1 Diagnostic criteria:
  A. At least 5 attacks fulfilling B–D
  B. Severe or very severe unilateral orbital, supraorbital and/or temporal pain lasting 15 to 180 minutes if untreated
  C. Headache is accompanied by at least one of the following:
    1. Ipsilateral conjunctival injection and/or lacrimation
    2. Ipsilateral nasal congestion and/or rhinorrhea
    3. Forehead and facial sweating
    4. Ipsilateral eyelid edema
    5. Ipsilateral forehead and facial sweating
    6. Ipsilateral miosis and/or ptosis
    7. A sense of restlessness or agitation
  D. Attacks have a frequency from 1 every other day to 8 per day
  E. Not attributed to another disorder

3.1.1 *Episodic cluster headache*
  Description: Occurs in periods lasting 7 days to 1 year separated by pain-free periods lasting 1 month or more
  Diagnostic criteria:
  A. All fulfilling criteria A–E of 3.1.
  B. At least 2 cluster periods lasting from 7–365 days and separated by pain-free remissions of ≥1 month

3.1.2 *Chronic cluster headache*
  Description: Attacks occur for more than 1 year without remission or with remissions lasting less than 1 month
  Diagnostic criteria:
  A. All alphabetical headings of 3.1
  B. Attacks recur over >1 year without remission periods or with remission periods <1 month

Headache Classification Committee of The International Headache Society. The International Classification of Headache Disorders: second edition. *Cephalalgia* 2004;24(Suppl 1):1–160.

(primary) stabbing headache, and hypnic headache.[44] By determining the cycling pattern, length of attack, frequency of attack, and timing of the attacks, most patients can be usefully classified. The importance of clinical classification of this group is threefold. First, the clinical phenotype determines the likely secondary causes that must be considered and appropriate investigations ordered. Secondly, the appropriate classification gives clarity to the patient with a clear diagnosis and allows the physician to draw on available literature to comment on natural history. Thirdly, the correct diagnosis determines therapy that can be very different in these conditions, being very good if the diagnosis is correct but largely ineffective if it is not (Table 61.9).

Managing Cluster Headache

Cluster headache is managed using acute attack treatments and preventive agents. Acute attack treatments are usually required by all cluster headache patients at some time, while preventives can seem almost life-saving for the patients with chronic cluster headache and are often needed to shorten the active periods in patients with the episodic form of the disorder.

Preventive Treatments. The options for preventive treatment in cluster headache depend on the bout length (Table 61.10). Patients with short bouts require medicines that act quickly but will not necessarily be taken for long periods, whereas those with long bouts or those with chronic cluster headache require safe, effective medicines that can be taken for long periods. Verapamil is now widely considered as the first-line preventive treatment when the bout is prolonged or in chronic cluster headache. By contrast, limited courses of oral corticosteroids or methysergide can be very useful strategies when the bout is relatively short.

Verapamil has been suggested as a useful option for the last decade and compares favorably with lithium. What has clearly emerged from clinical practice is the need to use higher doses than had initially been considered and certainly higher than those used in cardiological indications. Although most patients will start on doses as low as 40–80 mg twice daily, doses up to 960 mg daily are often required. Side effects, such as gingival hyperplasia, constipation, and leg swelling, are recognized as are cardiac dysrhythmias. Verapamil can cause heart block by slowing conduction in the atrioventricular (AV) node, monitored clinically by the PR interval on the electrocardiogram (EKG). Given that the effects on the AV node take up to 10 days to manifest, 2 week intervals are recommended between dose changes on the first exposure, with EKGs prior to the next escalation, and routine 6 monthly EKGs after the dose is established.[45]

Acute Attack Treatment. Cluster headache attacks often peak rapidly and thus require a treatment with quick onset. Many patients with acute cluster headache respond very well to treatment with oxygen inhalation. This should be given as 100% oxygen at 10–12 L/minutes for 15–20 minutes.[46] It is important to have a high flow and high oxygen content. Injectable sumatriptan 6 mg is effective, rapid in onset,[47] and has no evidence of tachyphylaxis.[48] Sumatriptan 20 mg[49] and zolmitriptan 5 mg[50,51] nasal sprays are effective in acute cluster headache in controlled trials, and offer a useful option. Sumatriptan is not effective when given preemptively as 100 mg orally three times daily,[52] and there is no evidence that it is useful when used orally in the acute treatment of cluster headache; indeed, it can be associated with medication overuse headache problems.[53]

Surgical Treatment. The surgical treatment of cluster headache has been completely transformed by the introduction of neurostimulation therapies. Surgical treatment of cluster headache is reserved for the most refractory patients, typically with chronic cluster headache. Destructive procedures, such as pterygopalati-

TABLE 61.9

DIFFERENTIAL DIAGNOSIS OF SHORT-LASTING HEADACHES

Feature	Cluster headache	Paroxysmal hemicrania	SUNCT/SUNA*	Primary stabbing headache	Trigeminal neuralgia*	Hypnic headache
Gender	M>F 3:1	F = M	M>F	F>M	F>M	M = F
Pain						
-type	Boring/ throbbing	Boring/ throbbing	Stabbing/ throbbing	stabbing	stabbing	throbbing
-severity	very severe	very severe	very severe	severe	very severe	moderate
-cranial location	any	any	any	any	V2/V3>V1	generalized
Duration	15–180 min	1–45 min	15–600 s	secs-3 min	<5 s	15–30 mins
Frequency	1–8 per day	1–40 per day	1/d–30/hr	any	any	1–3/night
Autonomic	+	+	+	−	−	−
Alcohol	+	One-third	−	−	−	−
Cutaneous trigger to attacks	−	−	+	−	+	−
Indomethacin	−	+	−	+	−	−

SUNCT, short-lasting unilateral neuralgiform headache attacks with conjunctival injection and tearing; SUNA, short-lasting unilateral neuralgiform headache attacks with cranial autonomic symptoms.
*SUNCT/SUNA generally has no refractory period to trigger additional attacks, while this is a very common feature of trigeminal neuralgia.

nectomy or radiofrequency lesions of the trigeminal ganglion, have been used. The former is without clear effects and the latter is helpful but often at significant cost, including ocular complications or anesthesia dolorosa. Trigeminal rhizotomy has also been employed, with all the complications of radiofrequency lesions and the occasional death.[54] Set against this, the functional imaging work describing activations in the posterior hypothalamic region[42] directly lead to deep brain stimulation approaches in the same region that seem highly effective.[55] Occipital nerve stimulation is a further very promising and a largely noninvasive approach to the management of intractable chronic cluster headache,[56,57] which may become the surgical treatment of choice in this setting over the next 5 to 10 years.

Paroxysmal Hemicrania

Sjaastad and Dale[58] first reported eight cases of a frequent unilateral severe but short-lasting headache without remission, coining the term chronic paroxysmal hemicrania (CPH). The mean daily

TABLE 61.10

PREVENTIVE MANAGEMENT OF CLUSTER HEADACHE

Short-term prevention	Long-term prevention
Episodic cluster headache	*Episodic cluster headache and prolonged Chronic cluster headache*
• Prednisolone	• Verapamil
• Methysergide	• Lithium
• Verapamil	• Methysergide
• Greater occipital nerve injection	• Melatonin
• Daily nocturnal ergotamine	• ?Topiramate
	• ?Gabapentin

?, unproven but promising.

frequency of attacks varied from 7 to 22 with the pain persisting from 5 to 45 minutes on each occasion. The site and associated autonomic phenomena were similar to cluster headache, but the attacks of CPH were suppressed completely by indomethacin.

The essential features of paroxysmal hemicrania that we have seen from a substantial cohort of patients are[59]:

■ unilateral very severe pain;
■ short-lasting attacks typically 20 minutes in length;
■ very frequent attacks (usually more than 5 a day);
■ marked autonomic features ipsilateral to the pain;
■ robust, quick (less than 72 hours), and excellent response to indomethacin.

The pathophysiology of paroxysmal hemicrania is marked by activations on positron emission tomography (PET) in the contralateral posterior hypothalamus and contralateral ventral midbrain.[60] The posterior hypothalamic activity is shared with cluster headache, short-lasting unilateral neuralgiform headache attacks with conjunctival injection and tearing (SUNCT), and hemicrania continua, while the ventral midbrain activity is only seen in hemicrania continua, which remarkably is also an indomethacin-sensitive primary headache.[13]

The therapy of paroxysmal hemicrania (PH) may be complicated by gastrointestinal side effects seen with indomethacin, in which topiramate may be helpful.[61] Secondary PH is more likely if the patient requires high doses (>200 mg/day) of indomethacin and raised cerebrospinal fluid (CSF) pressure should be suspected in apparent bilateral PH. It is worth noting that indomethacin reduces CSF pressure by an unknown mechanism.[62] It is appropriate to image patients, with MRI if practical, when a diagnosis of PH is being considered.

Short-Lasting Unilateral Neuralgiform Headache Attacks with Conjunctival Injection and Tearing or Cranial Autonomic Activation (SUNCT/SUNA)

Sjaastad and colleagues[63] reported three male patients whose brief attacks of pain in and around one eye were associated with sudden conjunctival injection and other autonomic features of cluster headache. The attacks lasted only 15–60 seconds and recurred 5–30 times per hour, and could be precipitated by chewing or eating certain foods, such as citrus fruits. They were not abolished by indomethacin. Brain imaging has suggested that they share with cluster headache and paroxysmal hemicrania the feature on activation studies of involvement of the posterior hypothalamic region.[64] Of the patients recognized with this problem, males dominate slightly and the paroxysms of pain may last between 5 and 300 seconds, although longer duller interictal pains are recognized, as are longer attacks with a saw-tooth pattern.[65] The conjunctival injection seen with SUNCT is often the most prominent autonomic feature and tearing may be very obvious. If one of either conjunctival injection or tearing are absent, or neither are present but another cranial autonomic symptom is seen, the term SUNA is used. The two key clinical features of SUNCT/SUNA are the attacks being triggerable with no refractory period to triggering. The latter serves as a very useful distinction between SUNCT/SUNA and trigeminal neuralgia. SUNCT/SUNA can be treated very often with lamotrigine and, if that is unhelpful, topiramate or gabapentin.[66] Carbamazepine often has a useful but incomplete effect. Given what has been reported, cranial MRI with pituitary and posterior fossa views is highly recommended when SUNCT/SUNA is considered as a diagnosis.

Other Primary Headaches

Primary Stabbing Headache

Short-lived jabs of pain, defined by the Headache Classification Committee of the IHS as primary stabbing headache,[6] are well documented in association with most types of primary headache.

The essential clinical features are:

- Pain confined to the head, although rarely is it facial;
- Stabbing pain lasting from 1 to many seconds and occurring as a single stab or a series of stabs;
- Recurring at irregular intervals (hours to days).

These pains have been called ice-pick pains or jabs and jolts. They generally respond to indomethacin (25–50 mg, two to three times daily). The symptoms tend to wax and wane and, after a period of control on indomethacin, it is appropriate to withdraw treatment and observe the outcome. Most patients will not want treatment when the nature of the problem is explained and they are reassured that the attacks are not sinister in any way.

Primary Cough Headache

Sharp pain in the head on coughing, sneezing, straining, laughing, or stooping has long been regarded as a symptom of organic intracranial disease, commonly associated with obstruction of the CSF pathways. The presence of an Arnold-Chiari malformation or any lesion causing obstruction of CSF pathways or displacing cerebral structures must be excluded before cough headache is assumed to be benign. Cerebral aneurysm, carotid stenosis, and vertebrobasilar disease may also present with cough or exertional headache as the initial symptom. The term "Benign Valsalva's maneuver-related headache" covers the headaches provoked by coughing, straining, or stooping but *cough headache* is more succinct and so widely used it is unlikely to be displaced.

The essential clinical features of primary cough headache are:

- Bilateral headache of sudden onset, lasting minutes, precipitated by coughing;
- May be prevented by avoiding coughing;
- Diagnosed only after structural lesions, such as posterior fossa tumor, have been excluded by neuroimaging.

Indomethacin is the medical treatment of choice in cough headache. Raskin[67] followed up an observation of Sir Charles Symonds, reporting that some patients with cough headache are relieved by lumbar puncture.[68] This is a simple option when compared to prolonged use of indomethacin. The mechanism of this response remains unclear.

Primary Exertional Headache

The relationship of this form of headache to cough headache is unclear and certainly much is shared. Indeed the relationship to migraine also requires delineation.

The clinical features are:

- Pain specifically brought on by physical exercise;
- Bilateral and throbbing in nature at onset and may develop migrainous features in those patients susceptible to migraine;
- Lasts from 5 minutes to 24 hours;
- Prevented by avoiding excessive exertion, particularly in hot weather or at high altitude.

The acute onset of headache with straining and breath holding, as in weightlifter's headache, may be explained by acute venous distension. The development of headache after sustained exertion, particularly on a hot day, is more difficult to understand. Anginal pain may be referred to the head, probably by central connections of vagal afferents and may present as exertional headache, so-called cardiac cephalgia.[69] The link to exercise is the important clinical clue. Pheochromocytoma may occasionally be responsible for exertional headache. Intracranial lesions or stenosis of the carotid arteries may have to be excluded as discussed for benign cough headache. Headache may be precipitated by any form of exercise and often has the pulsatile quality of migraine. The most obvious form of treatment is to take exercise gradually and progressively whenever possible. Indomethacin at daily doses varying from 25 to 150 mg is generally very effective in benign exertional headache. Indomethacin 50 mg, ergotamine 1–2 mg orally, dihydroergotamine by nasal spray, or methysergide 1–2 mg orally given 30–45 minutes before exercise are useful prophylactic measures.

Primary Sex Headache

Sex headache may be precipitated by masturbation or coitus and usually starts as a dull bilateral ache while sexual excitement increases, suddenly becoming intense at orgasm. The term orgasmic cephalgia is not accurate since not all sex headaches require orgasm. Two types of primary sex headache are recognized: a dull ache in the head and neck that intensifies as sexual excitement increases, and a sudden severe ("explosive") headache occurring at orgasm. Low CSF volume headache may also be precipitated by a sexual activity and is considered as a form of new daily persistent headache (see below).

The essential clinical features of sex headache are:

- Precipitation by sexual excitement;
- Bilateral at onset;
- Prevented or eased by ceasing sexual activity before orgasm.

Headaches developing at the time of orgasm are not always benign and consideration of a diagnosis of subarachnoid headache is essential. Sex headache affects men more often than women and may occur at any time during the years of sexual activity. It may develop on several occasions in succession and then not trouble the patient again, despite any obvious change in sexual technique. In patients who stop sexual activity when headache is first noticed, it may subside within a period of five minutes to two hours, and it is recognized that more frequent orgasm can aggravate established sex headache. About one-third of the patients with sex headache have a history of exertional headaches, but there is no excess of cough headache in patients with sex headache. In about 50% of patients, sex headache will settle in 6 months. Migraine is reported in about 25% of patients with sex headache.

Primary sex headaches are usually irregular and infrequent in occurrence, so management can often be limited to reassurance and advice about ceasing sexual activity if a milder, warning headache develops. When the condition recurs regularly or frequently, it can be prevented by the administration of propranolol; the dosage required varies from 40–200 mg daily. An alternative is the calcium channel blocking agent diltiazem 60 mg three times daily, which this author finds particularly useful in such patients. Ergotamine (1–2 mg) or indomethacin (25–50 mg) taken about 30–45 minutes prior to sexual activity can also be helpful.

Hypnic Headache

This syndrome was first described by Raskin in patients aged 67 to 84 who had headache of a moderately severe nature that typically came on a few hours after going to sleep.[70] These headaches last from 15 to 30 minutes, are typically generalized, although may be unilateral, and can be throbbing. Patients may report falling back to sleep only to be awoken by a further attack a few hours later with up to three repetitions of this pattern over the night. In Dodick's series of 19 patients, 16 (84%) were female and the mean age at onset was 61, ±9 years.[71] Headaches were bilateral in two-thirds and unilateral in one-third and in 80% of cases mild or moderate. Three patients reported similar headaches when falling asleep during the day. None had photophobia or phonophobia, and nausea is unusual.

Patients with this form of headache generally respond to a bedtime dose of lithium carbonate (200–600 mg) and in those that do not tolerate this verapamil or methysergide at bedtime may be alternative strategies. Dodick and colleagues[71] reported that one to two cups of coffee or caffeine 60 mg orally at bedtime was helpful. This is a simple approach that is effective in about one-third of patients. An important secondary cause of hypnic headache is hypertension which should be carefully pursued and appropriately investigated as treatment of the blood pressure will arrest the headache problem.[72]

Primary Thunderclap Headache

Sudden onset severe headache may occur in the absence of sexual activity and the differential diagnosis includes the sentinel bleed of an intracranial aneurysm, cervicocephalic arterial dissection, and cerebral venous thrombosis. Headaches of explosive onset may also be caused by the ingestion of sympathomimetic drugs or tyramine-containing foods in a patient who is taking monoamine oxidase inhibitors, and can also be a symptom of pheochromocytoma. Whether thunderclap headache can be the presentation of an unruptured cerebral aneurysm is unclear. Day and Raskin[73] reported a woman with three episodes of sudden onset very severe headache who was found to have an unruptured aneurysm of the internal carotid artery, with adjacent areas of segmental vasospasm. In the absence of CT scan or CSF evidence of subarachnoid hemorrhage, studies indicate that such patients do very well, and there indeed seems to be a form of benign or primary thunderclap headache.

Wijdicks, Kerkhoff, and van Gijn[74] followed up 71 patients whose CT scans and CSF findings were negative for an average of 3.3 years. Twelve patients had further such headache, and 31 (44%) later had regular episodes of migraine or tension-type headache. Factors identified as precipitating the headache were sexual intercourse in 3 cases, coughing in 4, and exertion in 12, while the remainder had no obvious cause. A history of hypertension was found in 11 and of previous headache in 22. Markus[75] compared the presentation of 37 patients with subarachnoid hemorrhage and 189 with a similar thunderclap headache and normal CSF examination and could not discern any characteristic to distinguish the two conditions.

Investigation of any sudden onset severe headache, be it in the context of sexual excitement or isolated thunderclap headache, should be driven by the clinical context. The first presentation should be vigorously investigated with radiograph, CT, and CSF examination, and where possible MRI, magnetic resonance venography, or magnetic resonance angiography. Formal cerebral angiography should be reserved for when no primary diagnosis is forthcoming, and the clinical situation is particularly suggestive of intracranial aneurysm. Bearing in mind the entity of diffuse multifocal reversible cerebral vasospasm,[76] which may be seen in apparent primary thunderclap headache without there being an intracranial aneurysm, caution in interpretation of findings is crucial.

Hemicrania Continua

Two patients were initially reported with this syndrome, a woman aged 63 years and a man of 53, who developed unilateral headache without obvious cause. Both patients were relieved completely by indomethacin while other NSAIDs were of little or no benefit. Newman and colleagues[77] reviewed the 24 previously reported cases and added 10 of their own, including some with pronounced autonomic features resembling cluster headache. They divided their case histories into remitting and unremitting forms. Of the 34 patients reviewed, 22 were women and 12 men with the age of onset ranging from 11 to 58 years. The symptoms were controlled by indomethacin 75–150 mg daily. The essential features of hemicrania continua are:

■ Unilateral pain;
■ Pain is continuous but with exacerbations that may be severe;
■ Complete resolution of pain with indomethacin;
■ Exacerbations may be associated with autonomic features.

Apart from analgesic overuse as an aggravating factor, and a report in a human immunodeficiency virus-infected patient, the status of secondary hemicrania continua is unclear. Antonaci and colleagues[78] proposed the "indotest" by which the intramuscular injection of indomethacin 50 mg could be used as a diagnostic tool. In hemicrania continua, pain was relieved in 73 ±66 minutes and the pain-free period was 13 ±8 hours. A placebo-controlled modification of this test is preferred where possible to the open-label version. Using the latter method in conjunction with PET, it has been shown that there is activation of the contralateral posterior hypothalamus and ipsilateral dorsal rostral pons in association with the headache of hemicrania continua, as well as activation of the ipsilateral ventrolateral midbrain.[79] The alternative is a trial of oral indomethacin, initially 25 mg three times daily, then 50 mg three times daily, and then 75 mg three times daily. One should allow up to 2 weeks for any dose to have a useful effect. Acute treatment with sumatriptan has been employed and reported to be of no benefit. Cyclo-oxygenase II (COX-II) antagonists seem effective, although undesirable now, and topiramate is helpful in some patients, as is greater occipital nerve injection.

Chronic Daily Headache

Each of the above primary headache forms can occur very frequently. When a patient experiences headache on 15 days or more a month, one can apply the broad diagnosis of CDH. CDH is not one thing, but a collection of very different problems with different management strategies.[5] Crucially, not all daily headache is simply tension-type headache (Table 61.11). This is a very common clinical misconception in headache, confusing the clinical phenotype with the headache *biotype*. Population-based estimates of daily headache are remarkable, demonstrating that about 5% of Western populations have daily or near daily headache.[80] Daily headache may again be primary or secondary, and it seems clinically useful to consider the possibilities in this way when making management decisions (see Table 61.11). It should

TABLE 61.11

CLASSIFICATION OF CHRONIC DAILY HEADACHE

Primary		Secondary
>4 hr daily	<4 hr daily	
Chronic migraine*	Chronic cluster headache†	Posttraumatic • head injury • iatrogenic • postinfectious
CTTH*	Chronic paroxysmal hemicrania	Inflammatory, such as • Giant cell arteritis • Sarcoidosis • Behçet's syndrome
Hemicrania continua*	SUNCT	Chronic cerebrospinal fluid infection
NDPH*	Hypnic headache	Substance abuse headache

*May be complicated by analgesic overuse. In the case of substance abuse headache, the headache is completely resolved after the substance abuse is controlled.[6] Clinical experience suggests that many patients continue to have headache even after cessation of analgesic use. The residual headache probably represents the underlying headache biology.
†Chronic cluster headache patients may have more than 4 hours per day of headache. The inclusion of the syndrome here is to emphasize that, by and large, the attacks themselves are less than 4 hours in duration.

be said that population-based studies bear out clinical practice in that a large group of refractory daily headache patients overuse various OTC preparations.

Chronic Migraine

While it is widely accepted that some of the primary headaches (tension-type headache, cluster headache, and paroxysmal hemicrania) have chronic varieties, this question seems to have become unnecessarily troublesome for migraine. Few headache authorities would argue that migraine can never be chronic in terms of frequency, but the issue of whether patients with frequent headache, some of which fulfils standard criteria for migraine and some for tension-type headache, have a single migrainous biology is a very vexed one. Given that tension-type headache describes a phenomenology that is indistinct at best, it seems unlikely that all its phenotypes will have a single biological generator.

The concept behind chronic migraine is that some patients who inherit a migrainous biology end up with CDH. The typical patient will have daily headache of a dull, nonspecific type, punctuated by more severe attacks that would often, in isolation, fulfil standard criteria for migraine. In headache speciality clinics, this group is dominant, with about 90% of patients in referral headache clinics having chronic migraine usually with analgesic overuse. It could be suggested that they have a biologically more difficult problem and this is the basis for their overrepresentation in referral centers.

If one applies the concepts outlined for tension-type headache (see above) then the diagnosis of chronic tension-type headache (CTTH) is made when the patient has 15 days or more a month of entirely featureless generalized dull or pressure-like pain. When *any* of the attacks on *some* days have migrainous features: nausea, photophobia, phonophobia, throbbing, or aggravation with movement, then chronic migraine is more likely to be the diagnosis. Clearly both chronic migraine and CTTH exist. Moreover, some patients must simply have CTTH and episodic migraine coexisting; however, it is simply impossible on clinical or other grounds to determine who they are. The approach outlined over-diagnoses chronic migraine, taking that to be a biological entity, and underdiagnoses the coexistence of CTTH and episodic migraine. The converse would be true; if one diagnoses them all as CTTH and episodic migraine, then chronic migraine is missed. In clinical practice, the concept of chronic migraine is particularly helpful. Given that the lifestyle advice is identical for both CTTH and migraine, and that the range of therapeutic options for preventive treatment in migraine is so much greater, the clinician loses absolutely nothing diagnosing chronic migraine, and the patient has much to gain. For research there are other imperatives.

Management

The management of CDH can be very rewarding. Most patients overusing analgesics respond very sensibly when the problem is explained.

The keys to managing CDH are:

▪ Exclude treatable causes (see Table 61.11)
▪ Obtain a clear analgesic history
▪ Make a diagnosis of the primary headache type involved

Medication Overuse

Medication overuse is defined as consuming an acute attack therapy on 10 days or more per month. It is essential that analgesic overuse be reduced and eliminated if one is to see the underlying headache phenotype and commence to manage the problem. Patients can reduce their use either by, as an example, 10% every week or two, depending on their circumstances, or if they wish, and there is no contraindication, by immediate cessation of use. Either approach can be facilitated by first keeping a careful diary over a month or two to be sure of the size of the problem. A small dose of an NSAID, such as naproxen 500 mg twice daily if tolerated, will take the edge off the pain as the analgesic use is reduced, as does a greater occipital nerve injection. It is a useful aside that NSAID overuse does not seem to be a common issue in daily headache when they are dosed once or twice daily, whereas with more frequent dosing problems may develop. When the patient has reduced their analgesic use substantially, a preventive should be introduced. It must be emphasized that preventive therapies most often simply do not work in the presence of analgesic overuse. Thus, the patient must reduce the analgesics or the entire attempt to use the preventive is largely wasted, although this helpful rule must have some limitations that require study. The most common cause of intractability to treatment is the use of a preventive when analgesics continue to be used regularly. For some patients, this is very difficult and often one must be blunt that some degree of pain is inevitable in the first instance if the problem is to be controlled.

Some patients with medication overuse will require admission for detoxification. Broadly, this consists of two groups: those who fail outpatient withdrawal or those who have a significant complicating medical indication, such as brittle diabetes mellitus, or complicating medicines, such as opioids or barbiturates, where withdrawal may be problematic as an outpatient. When such patients are admitted, acute medications are withdrawn completely on the first day, unless there is some contraindication. Antiemetics, such as domperidone oral or suppositories, and fluids are administered as required, as well as clonidine for opioid withdrawal symptoms. For acute intolerable pain during the waking hours, aspirin (1 g intravenously) is useful and at night chlorpromazine by injection, after ensuring adequate hydration. If the patient does not settle over 3–5 days, a course of intravenous dihydroergotamine (DHE) can be employed as Raskin described.[81] As time goes by, one feels that DHE is indispensable in this setting. Often 5-HT$_3$ receptor antagonists, such as ondansetron or granisetron, will be required with DHE as it is essential to ensure that the patient does not have significant nausea.

Preventive Treatments

Tricylics, amitriptyline, doselupin (dothiepin), or nortriptyline, at doses up to 1 mg/kg, are very useful in patients with chronic migraine. Tricyclics are started in low dose (10–25 mg) daily and best given 12 hours prior to when the patient wishes to wake up to avoid excess morning sleepiness. The other very useful medications for these patients are the anticonvulsants, such as valproate, topiramate, and gabapentin. For valproate, doses up to 1500 mg daily are used, starting at 200 mg twice daily increasing to 400 mg or 600 mg twice daily as tolerated over 2 to 4 week intervals. The blood count and liver enzymes should be checked at baseline and the various side effects explained to patients, especially the fetal abnormalities to females. The efficacy of topiramate in chronic migraine is now established by placebo-controlled studies.[82,83] One can start at 25 mg nightly and increase by 25 mg every 10–14 days to aim for 50 mg twice daily. For gabapentin, the dose is 1800 to 3600 mg daily; it is very well tolerated, although probably less effective from a population viewpoint.

New Daily Persistent Headache

New daily persistent headache (NDPH) is a clinically useful concept with a range of important possible causes because some are very treatable (Table 61.12). From a nosological point of view, all that is mentioned here could be placed within various categories of the IHS classification,[6] and indeed the IHS refers to primary NDPH. However, the term as employed here serves both patients and clinicians by highlighting a group of conditions, some of which are curable, and encompasses the IHS term under the primary featureless form of NDPH.[84]

The patient with NDPH presents with a history of headache on most, if not all, days. The onset of headache is abrupt, often moment-to-moment, but at least in less than a few days where three is suggested as an upper limit. The typical history is for the patient to recall the exact day and circumstances, so from one moment to the next a headache develops that never leaves them. This presentation triggers certain key questions about the onset and behavior of the pain. The pressing issues arise from considering the secondary headache possibilities. Although subarachnoid hemorrhage is listed for some logical consistency, as the headache may certainly come on from one moment to the next, it is not likely to produce diagnostic confusion in this group of patients. Suffice it to say that subarachnoid hemorrhage is so important that it must always be considered if only to be excluded, either by history or appropriate investigation.

Primary New Daily Persistent Headache. Case series of primary NDPH showed it to occur in both males and females.[85] Migrainous features are common, with unilateral headache in about one-third and throbbing pain in about one-third. Nausea was reported

TABLE 61.12

DIFFERENTIAL DIAGNOSIS OF NEW DAILY PERSISTENT HEADACHE

Primary	Secondary
• Migrainous-type • Featureless (tension-type)	• Subarachnoid hemorrhage • Low cerebrospinal fluid volume headache • Raised cerebrospinal fluid pressure headache • Posttraumatic headache* • Chronic meningitis

*Includes postinfective forms.

in about half the patients, as was photophobia and phonophobia observed. A number of these patients have a previous history of migraine but not more than one might expect given the population prevalence of migraine.[85,86] It is remarkable that the initial report noted that 86% of patients were headache-free at 24 months. It is general experience amongst those interested in headache management that primary NDPH is perhaps the most intractable and least therapeutically rewarding form of headache. In general, one can classify the dominant phenotype, migraine, or tension-type headache, and treat with preventives according to that subclassification.

Secondary New Daily Persistent Headache. The secondary causes of the syndrome of NDPH are worthy of consideration, as they have distinctive clinical pictures that can guide investigation (see Table 61.12).

Low Cerebrospinal Fluid Volume Headache

The syndrome of persistent, low CSF volume headache is an important diagnosis not to miss. The more immediately obvious version of this problem is encountered commonly after lumbar puncture. In that situation, the headache usually settles rapidly with bedrest. In the chronic situation, the patient typically presents with a history of headache from one day to the next. The pain is generally not present on waking, worsens during the day, and is relieved by lying down. Recumbency usually improves the headache in minutes, and it takes only minutes to an hour for the pain to return when the patient is upright again. The patient may give a history of an index event: lumbar puncture, epidural injection, or a vigorous Valsalva, such as with lifting, straining, coughing, clearing the Eustachian tubes in an aeroplane, or multiple orgasms. Patients may volunteer, or a history may be obtained, that soft drinks with caffeine provide temporary respite. Spontaneous leaks are recognized, and the clinician should not be put off the diagnosis if the headache history is typical when there is no obvious index event. As time passes from the index event, the postural nature may be less obvious; certainly cases whose index event was several years prior to the eventual diagnosis are recognized. The term low volume rather than low pressure is used, since there is no clear evidence at which point the pressure can be called low. While low pressures, such as 0 to 5 cm, are often identified, a pressure of 16 cm CSF has been recorded with a documented leak. One should be aware of the possibility of the development of subdural collections in patients with low CSF volume headaches, which makes imaging before any invasive studies all the more important.

The investigation of choice is MRI with gadolinium (Fig. 61.5), which produces a striking pattern of diffuse pachymeningeal enhancement,[87] although in about 10% of cases a leak can be documented without enhancement.[88] The finding of diffuse meningeal enhancement is so typical that in clinical context, immediate treatment is appropriate. It is also common to see Chiari malformations on MRI with some degree of descent of the cerebellar tonsils. This is important since surgery in such settings simply worsens the headache problem. It seems appropriate that any patient being considered for such surgery for a headache indication should be reviewed by a neurologist first. To investigate further, CSF pressure may be determined, or preferably a leak sought with indium-labeled CSF. In CSF studies that can demonstrate the site, early emptying of tracer into the bladder or lack of progression of tracer over the cerebral convexities.

Treatment is bedrest in the first instance. False positive transient improvement in persistent low CSF volume headache with chiropractic and other similar therapies is recognized where the treatment necessitates the patient lying down for a prolonged period for the therapy. Intravenous caffeine (500 mg in 500 mL saline administered over two hours) is the standard and often very efficacious treatment. The ECG should be checked for any

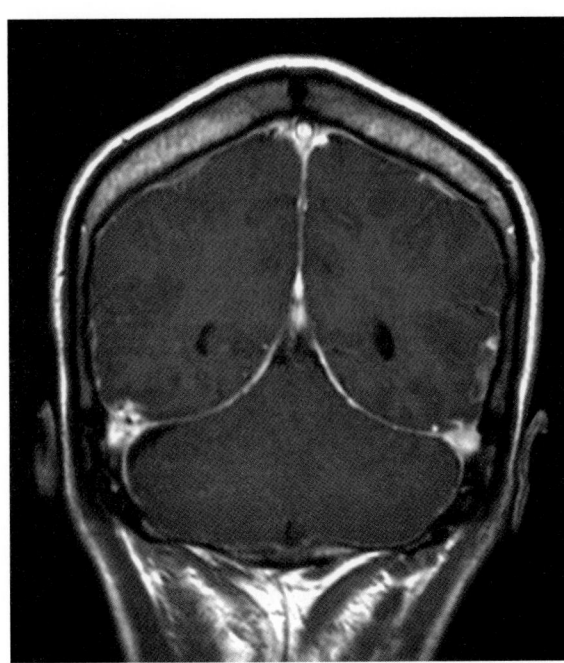

FIGURE 61.5 MRI showing diffuse meningeal enhancement after gadolinium administration in a patient with low cerebrospinal fluid volume (pressure) headache.

arrhythmia prior to administration. A reasonable practice is to carry out at least two infusions separated by 4 weeks after obtaining the suggestive clinical history and MRI with enhancement. Since intravenous caffeine is safe, and can be curative by an unknown mechanism, it spares many patients the need for further tests. If that is unsuccessful, an abdominal binder may be helpful. If a leak can be identified, either by the radioisotope study, CT myelogram, or spinal T2-weighted MRI, an autologous blood patch is usually curative. In more intractable situations, theophylline is a useful alternative that offers outpatient management, although its onset of action is rather slow. An important phenotypically identical headache can be seen in the Postural Orthostatic Tachycardia Syndrome (POTS)[89] and should be considered when investigating this group of patients.

Raised Cerebrospinal Fluid Pressure Headache

As is the case for low CSF pressure states, raised CSF pressure as a cause of headache is well recognized by neurologists. Brain imaging can often reveal the cause, such as raised pressure due to a space-occupying lesion. The particular setting in which patients enter the spectrum of NDPH are those with idiopathic intracranial hypertension who present with headache without visual problems, particularly with normal fundi. It is recognized that intractable chronic migraine can be triggered by persistently raised intracranial pressure.[90] These patients typically give a history of generalized headache that is present on waking, and gets better as the day goes on. It is generally worse with recumbency. Visual obscurations are frequently reported. Fundal changes on raised intracranial pressure would make the diagnosis relatively straightforward but it is in those without such changes that the history must drive investigation. Patients often report a curious whooshing sensation in the occipital region.

Brain imaging is mandatory if raised pressure is suspected, and it is most simple in the long run to obtain an MRI and include MRV. The CSF pressure should be measured by lumbar puncture taking care to do so when the patient is symptomatic, so that both the pressure and response to removal of CSF can be determined. A raised pressure and improvement in headache with removal of

CSF is diagnostic of the problem. The fields should be formally documented even in the absence of overt ophthalmic involvement. Initial treatment can be with acetazolamide (250 to 500 mg twice daily). The patient may respond in weeks with improvement in headache. If this is not effective, topiramate has many actions that may be useful in this setting: carbonic anhydrase inhibition, weight loss, and neuronal membrane stabilization probably through actions on phosphorylation pathways. A small number of severely disabled patients who do not respond to medical treatment will come to intracranial pressure monitoring and even shunting. This is exceptional and not undertaken without careful work-up.

Posttraumatic Headache

The issue of posttraumatic headache is vexing. The Headache Classification Committee accepts the existence of such a syndrome.[6] Much of the scientific discussion becomes marred by the often-quoted medico-legal morass concerning delayed effects of head injury. The term is used here to indicate trauma in a very broad way. NDPH may be seen after a blow to the head but more commonly after an infective episode, typically viral, or even malarial meningitis. A recent series identified one-third of all patients with NDPH reported the headache starting after a flu-like illness. The patient may note a period in which they had a significant infection: fever, neck stiffness, photophobia, and marked malaise. The headache starts during that period and never stops. Investigation reveals no current cause for the headache. It has been suggested that some patients with this syndrome have a persistent Epstein-Barr infection,[91] but this syndrome is anything but clearly delineated. A complicating factor will often be that the patient had a lumbar puncture during that illness, so a persistent low CSF volume headache needs to be considered first. Posttraumatic headache may be seen after carotid artery dissection, subarachnoid hemorrhage, and following intracranial surgery for a benign mass. The underlying theme seems to be that a traumatic event involving the dura mater can trigger a headache process that lasts for many years after that event.

The treatment of this form of NDPH is substantially empirical. Tricyclics, notably amitriptyline, and anticonvulsants, valproate, topiramate, and gabapentin, have been used with good effects. The monoamine oxidase inhibitor phenelzine may also be useful in carefully selected patients. On the positive side, the headache seems to run a limited course of 3 to 5 years in most patients, so will eventually settle.

Other Important Forms of Secondary Headache (Table 61.13)

Giant Cell Arteritis

This is an important cause of headache because delay in steroid treatment may result in blindness due to retinal artery ischemia.

TABLE 61.13

OTHER SECONDARY HEADACHES

- Giant cell arteritis
- Cervicogenic headache
- Raeder's paratrigeminal neuralgia[97]
- Tolosa-Hunt syndrome[98,99]
- Headache as a presentation of cervical dystonia[5]
- Headache in temporomandibular dysfunction
- Cardiac cephalalgia[69]
- Headache with endocrine disturbance, particularly pituitary tumor[19]
- Neck-tongue syndrome[100]
- Red-Ear syndrome[101]

It is also known as temporal arteritis or cranial arteritis. Patients are usually elderly with focal tenderness of the scalp, which may be provoked markedly by resting the head on the pillow. Jaw claudication provoked by chewing is a characteristic but relatively uncommon feature. Constitutional symptoms are common, particularly weight loss, malaise, or polymyalgia rheumatica. An elevated erythrocyte sedimentation rate is a strong pointer to the diagnosis. The temporal artery may be tenderly inflamed, swollen, or pulseless. On suspicion of this diagnosis, steroid treatment should be started pending the result of temporal artery biopsy. Treatment is very often long-term and requires careful monitoring for reactivation and the side effects of corticosteroids.

Cervicogenic Headache

It is a time-honored concept that the neck is responsible for much headache. Unfortunately, as with much of history, the good story is often ruined by the facts. While there is little doubt that there is a rich overlap between the innervation of intracranial pain-producing structures by the ophthalmic division of the trigeminal nerve and the posterior fossa and high cervical innervation by branches especially of the C_2 dorsal root,[92] causality is another issue. The Headache Classification Committee recognizes that head pain can arise from the neck and labels this cervicogenic headache.[6] The term has been used by others to define a syndrome[93] that is so poorly described as to be useless in practice.[94] Most patients with neck discomfort and headache referred to specialty practice have migraine. They will have neck stiffness or discomfort as a premonitory symptom that can clearly persist in all stages of the attack.[95] They may respond to local therapies, such as greater occipital nerve injection;[96] however, this implies no more than triggering, and is to be expected. The pursuit of neck pathology and the treatment of patients who have migraine by manipulative or physical means has no support in the controlled literature, and is rarely of long-lasting value. This not to say that the patient with clear neck pathology and pain does not exist; they do, and are very well treated by therapy aimed at the responsible neck pathology.

References

1. Lance JW, Goadsby PJ. *Mechanism and Management of Headache*. 7th ed. New York: Elsevier; 2005.
2. Silberstein SD, Lipton RB, Goadsby PJ. *Headache in Clinical Practice*. 2nd ed. London: Martin Dunitz; 2002.
3. Olesen J, Tfelt-Hansen P, Welch KM, et al. *The Headaches*. Philadelphia: Lippincott Williams & Wilkins; 2005.
4. Lipton RB, Bigal ME. *Migraine and Other Headache Disorders*. 1st ed. New York: Marcel Dekker, Taylor, and Francis Books, Inc.; 2006.
5. Goadsby PJ, Dodick D, Silberstein SD. *Chronic Daily Headache for Clinicians*. Hamilton, Canada: BC Decker Inc.; 2005.
6. Headache Classification Subcommittee of the International Headache Society. The international classification of headache disorders: 2nd edition. *Cephalalgia* 2004;24(Suppl 1):9–160.
7. Tepper SJ, Dahlof CG, Dowson A, et al. Prevalence and diagnosis of migraine in patients consulting their physician with a complaint of headache: data from the landmark study. *Headache* 2004;44(9):856–864.
8. Wolff HG. *Headache and Other Head Pain*. 1st ed. New York: Oxford University Press; 1948.
9. Feindel W, Penfield W, McNaughton F. The tentorial nerves and localization of intracranial pain in man. *Neurology* 1960;10:555–563.
10. McNaughton FL, Feindel WH. Innervation of intracranial structures: a reappraisal. In: Rose FC, ed. *Physiological Aspects of Clinical Neurology*. Oxford: Blackwell Scientific Publications; 1977:279–293.
11. Goadsby PJ, Lipton RB. A review of paroxysmal hemicranias, SUNCT syndrome, and other short-lasting headaches with autonomic features, including new cases. *Brain* 1997;120(Pt 1):193–209.
12. May A, Goadsby PJ. The trigeminovascular system in humans: pathophysiological implications for primary headache syndromes of the neural influences on the cerebral circulation. *J Cereb Blood Flow Metabol* 1999;19(2):115–127.
13. Cohen AS, Goadsby PJ. Functional neuroimaging of primary headache disorders. *Expert Rev Neurother* 2006;6(8):1159–1172.
14. Ophoff RA, Terwindt GM, Vergouwe MN, et al. Familial hemiplegic migraine and episodic ataxia type-2 are caused by mutations in the Ca^{2+} channel gene CACNL1A4. *Cell* 1996;87(3):543–552.
15. De Fusco M, Marconi R, Silvestri L, et al. Haploinsufficiency of ATP1A2 encoding the Na^+/K^+ pump alpha2 subunit associated with familial hemiplegic migraine type 2. *Nat Genet* 2003;33(2):192–196.
16. Dichgans M, Freilinger T, Eckstein G, et al. Mutation in the neuronal voltage-gated sodium channel SCN1A causes familial hemiplegic migraine. *Lancet* 2005;366(9483):371–377.
17. Goadsby PJ, Kullmann DK. Another migraine gene. *Lancet* 2005;366(9483):345–346.
18. American Academy of Neurology. Practice parameter: the utility of neuroimaging in the evaluation of headache patients with normal neurologic examinations (summary statement). Report of the Quality Standards Subcommittee of the American Academy of Neurology. *Neurology*.1994;44(7):1353–1354.
19. Levy M, Matharu MS, Meeran K, et al. The clinical characteristics of headache in patients with pituitary tumors. *Brain* 2005;128(Pt 8):1921–1930.
20. Lipton RB, Stewart WF, Diamond S, et al. Prevalence and burden of migraine in the United States: data from the American Migraine Study II. *Headache* 2001;41(7):646–657.
21. Steiner TJ, Scher AI, Stewart WF, et al. The prevalence and disability burden of adult migraine in England and their relationships to age, gender, and ethnicity. *Cephalalgia* 2003;23(7):519–527.
22. Menken M, Munsat TL, Toole JF. The global burden of disease study—implications for neurology. *Arch Neurol* 2000;57(3):418–420.
23. Andlin-Sobocki P, Jonsson B, Wittchen HU, et al. Cost of disorders of the brain in Europe. *Eur J Neurol* 2005;12(Suppl 1):1–27.
24. Stewart WF, Ricci JA, Chee E, et al. Lost productive time and cost due to common pain conditions in the US workforce. *JAMA* 2003;290(18):2443–2454.
25. Matharu MS, Bartsch T, Ward N, et al. Central neuromodulation in chronic migraine patients with suboccipital stimulators: a PET study. *Brain* 2004;127(Pt 1):220–230.
26. Goadsby PJ. Neurostimulation in primary headache syndromes. *Expert Rev Neurother* 2007;7(12):1785–1789.
27. Goadsby PJ. Is medication-overuse headache a distinct biological entity? *Nat Clin Pract Neurol* 2006;2(8):401.
28. Goadsby PJ, Lipton RB, Ferrari MD. Migraine—current understanding and treatment. *N Engl J Med* 2002;346(4):257–270.
29. Kellstein DE, Lipton RB, Geetha R, et al. Evaluation of a novel solubilized formulation of ibuprofen in the treatment of migraine headache: a randomized, double-blind, placebo-controlled, dose-ranging study. *Cephalalgia* 2000;20(4):233–243.
30. Myllylä VV, Havanka H, Herrala L, et al. Tolfenamic acid rapid release versus sumatriptan in the acute treatment of migraine: comparable effect in a double-blind, randomized, controlled, parallel-group study. *Headache* 1998;38(3):201–207.
31. Tfelt-Hansen P, Saxena PR, Dahlof C, et al. Ergotamine in the acute treatment of migraine—a review and European consensus. *Brain* 2000;123(Pt 1):9–18.
32. Goadsby PJ. The pharmacology of headache. *Prog Neurobiol* 2000;62(5):509–525.
33. Brandes JL, Kudrow D, Stark SR, et al. Sumatriptan-naproxen for acute treatment of migraine: a randomized trial. *JAMA* 2007;297(13):1443–1454.
34. Schoenen J, Wang W. Tension-type headache. In: Goadsby PJ, Silberstein SD, eds. *Headache*. 1st ed. Oxford: Butterworth-Heinemann; 1997:177–200.
35. Lipton RB, Stewart WF, Cady R, et al. 2000 Wolfe Award. Sumatriptan for the range of headaches in migraine sufferers: results of the Spectrum Study. *Headache* 2000;40(10):783–791.
36. Diamond S, Baltes BJ. Chronic tension headache—treated with amitriptyline—a double-blind study. *Headache* 1971;11(3):110–116.
37. Göbel H, Hamouz V, Hansen C, et al. Chronic tension-type headache: amitriptyline reduces clinical headache-duration and experimental pain sensitivity but does not alter pericranial muscle activity readings. *Pain* 1994;59(2):241–249.
38. Holroyd KA, O'Donnell FJ, Stensland M, et al. Management of chronic tension-type headache with tricyclic antidepressant medication, stress-management therapy, and their combination: a randomized controlled trial. *JAMA* 2000;285(17):2208–2215.
39. Silberstein SD, Göbel H, Jensen R, et al. Botulinum toxin type A in the prophylactic treatment of chronic tension-type headache: a multicentre, double-blind, randomized, placebo-controlled, parallel-group study. *Cephalalgia* 2006;26(7):790–800.
40. Sjaastad O, Bakketeig LS. Cluster headache prevalence. Vågå study of headache epidemiology. *Cephalalgia* 2003;23(7):528–533.
41. Ford HL, Gerry E, Johnson M, et al. A prospective study of the incidence, prevalence, and mortality of multiple sclerosis in Leeds. *J Neurol* 2002;249(3):260–265.
42. May A, Bahra A, Buchel C, et al. Hypothalamic activation in cluster headache attacks. *Lancet* 1998;352(9124):275–278.
43. May A, Ashburner J, Buchel C, et al. Correlation between structural and functional changes in brain in an idiopathic headache syndrome. *Nat Med* 1999;5(7):836–838.
44. Goadsby PJ. Pathophysiology of cluster headache: a trigeminal autonomic cephalgia. *Lancet Neurol* 2002;1(4):251–257.
45. Cohen AS, Matharu MS, Goadsby PJ. Electrocardiographic abnormalities in patients with cluster headache on verapamil therapy. *Neurology* 2007;69(7):668–675.
46. Cohen AS, Matharu MS, Burns B, et al. Randomized double-blind, placebo-controlled trial of high-flow inhaled oxygen in acute cluster headache. *Cephalalgia* 2007;27:1188.
47. Treatment of acute cluster headache with sumatriptan. The Sumatriptan Cluster Headache Study Group. *N Engl J Med* 1991;325(5):322–326.

48. Ekbom K, Waldenlind E, Cole JA, et al. Sumatriptan in chronic cluster headache: results of continuous treatment for eleven months. *Cephalalgia* 1992; 12(4):254–256.

49. van Vliet JA, Bahra A, Martin V, et al. Intranasal sumatriptan in cluster headache: randomized placebo-controlled double-blind study. *Neurology* 2003;60(4):630–633.

50. Cittadini E, May A, Straube A, et al. Effectiveness of intranasal zolmitriptan in acute cluster headache. A randomized, placebo-controlled, double-blind crossover study. *Arch Neurol* 2006;63(11):1537–1542.

51. Rapoport AM, Mathew NT, Silberstein SD, et al. Zolmitriptan nasal spray in the acute treatment of cluster headache: a double-blind study. *Neurology* 2007;69(9):821–826.

52. Monstad I, Krabbe A, Micieli G, et al. Preemptive oral treatment with sumatriptan during a cluster period. *Headache* 1995;35(10):607–613.

53. Paemeleire K, Bahra A, Evers S, et al. Medication-overuse headache in cluster headache patients. *Neurology* 2006;67(1):109–113.

54. Jarrar RG, Black DF, Dodick DW, et al. Outcome of trigeminal nerve section in the treatment of chronic cluster headache. *Neurology* 2003;60(8): 1360–1362.

55. Leone M, Franzini A, Broggi G, et al. Long-term follow-up of bilateral hypothalamic stimulation for intractable cluster headache. *Brain* 2004;127(Pt 10): 2259–2264.

56. Burns B, Watkins L, Goadsby PJ. Treatment of medically intractable cluster headache by occipital nerve stimulation: long-term follow-up of eight patients. *Lancet* 2007;369(9567):1099–1106.

57. Magis D, Allena M, Bolla M, et al. Occipital nerve stimulation for drug-resistant chronic cluster headache: a prospective pilot study. *Lancet Neurol* 2007;6(4):314–321.

58. Sjaastad O, Dale I. A new (?) clinical headache entity "chronic paroxysmal hemicrania" 2. *Acta Neurol Scand* 1976;54(2):140–159.

59. Cittadini E, Matharu MS, Goadsby PJ. Paroxysmal hemicrania: a prospective clinical study of thirty-one cases. *Brain* 2008:131(Pt 4):1142–1155.

60. Matharu MS, Cohen AS, Frackowiak RS, et al. Posterior hypothalamic activation in paroxysmal hemicrania. *Ann Neurol* 2006;59(3):535–545.

61. Cohen AS, Goadsby PJ. Paroxysmal hemicrania responding to topiramate. *J Neurol Neurosurg Psychiat* 2007;78(1):96–97.

62. Jensen K, Ohrström J, Cold GE, et al. The effects of indomethacin on intracranial pressure, cerebral blood flow, and cerebral metabolism in patients with severe head injury and intracranial hypertension. *Acta Neurochir (Wien)* 1991;108(3-4):116–121.

63. Sjaastad O, Saunte C, Salvesen R, et al. Shortlasting, unilateral, neuralgiform headache attacks with conjunctival injection, tearing, sweating, and rhinorrhea. *Cephalalgia* 1989;9(2):147–156.

64. May A, Bahra A, Buchel C, et al. Functional magnetic resonance imaging in spontaneous attacks of SUNCT: short-lasting neuralgiform headache with conjunctival injection and tearing. *Ann Neurol* 1999;46(5):791–794.

65. Cohen AS, Matharu MS, Goadsby PJ. Short-lasting unilateral neuralgiform headache attacks with conjunctival injection and tearing (SUNCT) or cranial autonomic features (SUNA). A prospective clinical study of SUNCT and SUNA. *Brain* 2006;129(Pt 10):2746–2760.

66. Cohen AS, Matharu MS, Goadsby PJ. Suggested guidelines for treating SUNCT and SUNA. *Cephalalgia* 2005;25:1200.

67. Raskin NH. The cough headache syndrome: treatment. *Neurology* 1995; 45(9):1784.

68. Symonds C. Cough headache. *Brain* 1956;79(4):557–568.

69. Lance JW, Lambros J. Unilateral exertional headache as a symptom of cardiac ischemia. *Headache* 1998;38(4):315–316.

70. Raskin NH. The hypnic headache syndrome. *Headache* 1988;28(8):534–536.

71. Dodick DW, Mosek AC, Campbell JK. The hypnic ("alarm clock") headache syndrome. *Cephalalgia* 1998;18(3):152–156.

72. Gil-Gouveia R, Goadsby PJ. Secondary "hypnic headache." *J Neurol* 2007; 254(5):646–654.

73. Day JW, Raskin NH. Thunderclap headache: symptom of unruptured cerebral aneurysm. *Lancet* 1986;2(8518):1247–1248.

74. Wijdicks EFM, Kerkhoff H, van Gijn J. Long-term follow up of 71 patients with thunderclap headache mimicking subarachnoid haemorrhage. *Lancet* 1988;2(8602):68–70.

75. Markus HS. A prospective follow-up of thunderclap headache mimicking subarachnoid haemorrhage. *J Neurol Neurosurg Psychiatry* 1991;54(12): 1117–1125.

76. Dodick DW, Brown RD, Britton JW, et al. Nonaneurysmal thunderclap headache with diffuse, multifocal, segmental, and reversible vasospasm. *Cephalalgia* 1999;19(2):118–123.

77. Newman LC, Gordon ML, Lipton RB, et al. Episodic paroxysmal hemicrania: two new cases and a literature review. *Neurology* 1992;42(5):964–966.

78. Antonaci F, Pareja JA, Caminero AB, et al. Chronic paroxysmal hemicrania and hemicrania continua. Parenteral indomethacin: the 'indotest.' *Headache* 1998;38(2):122–128.

79. Matharu MS, Cohen AS, McGonigle DJ, et al. Posterior hypothalamic and brainstem activation in hemicrania continua. *Headache* 2004;44(88): 747–761.

80. Scher A, Stewart WF, Liberman J, et al. Prevalence of frequent headache in a population sample. *Headache* 1998;38(7):497–506.

81. Raskin NH. Repetitive intravenous dihydroergotamine as therapy for intractable migraine. *Neurology* 1986;36(7):995–997.

82. Silberstein SD, Lipton RB, Dodick DW, et al. Efficacy and safety of topiramate for the treatment of chronic migraine: a randomized, double-blind, placebo-controlled trial. *Headache* 2007;47(2):170–180.

83. Diener HC, Bussone G, van Oene JC, et al. Topiramate reduces headache days in chronic migraine: a randomized, double-blind, placebo-controlled study. *Cephalalgia* 2007;27(7):814–823.

84. Goadsby PJ, Boes CJ. New daily persistent headache. *J Neurol Neurosurg Psychiat* 2002;72(suppl 6):ii6–ii9.

85. Vanast WJ. New daily persistent headaches: definition of a benign syndrome. *Headache* 1986;26:317.

86. Li D, Rozen TD. The clinical characteristics of new daily persistent headache. *Cephalalgia* 2002;22(1):66–69.

87. Mokri B, Piepgras DG, Miller GM. Syndrome of orthostatic headaches and diffuse pachymeningeal gadolinium enhancement. *Mayo Clin Proc* 1997; 72(5):400–413.

88. Mokri B, Atkinson JLD, Dodick DW, et al. Absent pachymeningeal gadolinium enhancement on cranial MRI despite symptomatic CSF leak. *Neurology* 1999;53(2):402–404.

89. Mokri B, Low PA. Orthostatic headaches without CSF leak in postural tachycardia syndrome. *Neurology* 2003;61(7):980–982.

90. Mathew NT, Ravishankar K, Sanin LC. Coexistence of migraine and idiopathic intracranial hypertension without papilledema. *Neurology* 1996;46(5): 1226–1230.

91. Diaz-Mitoma F, Vanast WJ, Tyrrell DLJ. Increased frequency of Epstein–Barr virus excretion in patients with new daily persistent headaches. *Lancet* 1987; 1(8530):411–415.

92. Bartsch T, Goadsby PJ. Anatomy and physiology of pain referral in primary and cervicogenic headache disorders. *Headache Curr* 2005;2:42–48.

93. Antonaci F, Fredriksen T, Sjaastad O. Cervicogenic headache: clinical presentation, diagnostic criteria, and differential diagnosis. *Curr Pain Headache Rep* 2001;5(4):387–392.

94. Goadsby PJ. A critical view of cervicogenic headache. In: Sjaastad O, Fredriksen TA, Bono G, Nappi G, eds. *Cervicogenic Headache.* London: Smith-Gordon; 2004:131–136.

95. Giffin NJ, Ruggiero L, Lipton RB, et al. Premonitory symptoms in migraine: an electronic diary study. *Neurology* 2003;60(6):935–940.

96. Afridi SK, Shields KG, Bhola R, et al. Greater occipital nerve injection in primary headache syndromes—prolonged effects from a single injection. *Pain* 2006;122(1-2):126–129.

97. Goadsby PJ. Raeder's syndrome: "paratrigeminal" paralysis of oculopupillary sympathetic. *J Neurol Neurosurg Psychiat* 2002;72(3):297–299.

98. Tolosa E. Periarteritic lesions of the carotid siphon with the clinical features of a carotid infraclinoidal aneurysm. *J Neurol Neurosurg Psychiat* 1954;17(4): 300–302.

99. Hunt WE, Meagher JN, LeFever HE, et al. Reader's syndrome: "paratrigeminal" paralysis of oculo-pupillary sympathetic. *Neurolgy (Minneap)* 1961;11: 56–62.

100. Bogduk N. An anatomical basis for the neck–tongue syndrome. *J Neurol Neurosurg Psychiat* 1981;44(3):202–208.

101. Lance JW. The red ear syndrome. *Neurology* 1996;47(3):617–620.

102. Goadsby PJ. Can we develop neurally acting drugs for the treatment of migraine? *Nat Rev Drug Disc* 2005;4(9):741–750.

103. Bahra A, Matharu MS, Buchel C, et al. Brainstem activation specific to migraine headache. *Lancet* 2001;357(9261):1016–1017.

104. Afridi S, Giffin NJ, Kaube H, et al. A positron emission tomographic study in spontaneous migraine. *Arch Neurol* 2005;62(8):1270–1275.

105. Afridi S, Matharu MS, Lee L, et al. A PET study exploring the laterality of brainstem activation in migraine using glyceryl trinitrate. *Brain* 2005;128(Pt 4):932–939.

CHAPTER 62 ■ NONCARDIAC CHEST PAIN

RONNIE FASS

INTRODUCTION

Noncardiac chest pain (NCCP) is defined as recurring angina-like retrosternal chest pain of noncardiac origin. A patient's history and characteristics do not reliably distinguish between cardiac and esophageal causes of chest pain.[1] This is compounded by the fact that patients with a history of coronary artery disease (CAD) may also experience chest pain of noncardiac origin. The heightened awareness about the potentially devastating ramifications of chest pain may drive patients to seek medical attention despite a negative cardiac workup.[2] Furthermore, almost half of NCCP patients are not convinced by their negative cardiac diagnosis, and reassurance alone has proved to be an ungratifying therapeutic strategy.[3] Compared to patients with cardiac angina, those with NCCP are usually younger, less likely to have typical symptoms, and more likely to have a normal resting electrocardiogram.[4] Additionally, levels of anxiety of NCCP patients seen in a rapid access chest pain clinic significantly exceeded those of patients with cardiac angina and remained above community norms for at least 2 months after clinic visit.[5] NCCP patients view their condition as significantly less controllable and less understandable than those whose pain is of cardiac origin.[5]

NCCP may be the manifestation of nongastrointestinal (GI) or GI-related disorders (Fig. 62.1). An important step toward understanding of the underlying mechanisms of NCCP was the recognition that gastroesophageal reflux disease (GERD) is the most common contributing factor for chest pain. While chest pain has been considered an atypical manifestation of GERD, it is an integral part of the limited repertoire of esophageal symptoms. In patients with non–GERD-related NCCP, esophageal motility disorders and functional chest pain of presumed esophageal origin are the main underlying mechanism for symptoms. The Rome III Committee uses the term "functional chest pain of presumed esophageal origin" to describe recurrent episodes of substernal chest pain of visceral quality with no apparent explanation (Table 62.1). As with all other functional esophageal disorders, GERD and esophageal dysmotility should also be ruled out before the diagnosis is established.[6]

Up to 20% of the patients with functional chest pain exhibit other functional disorders, primarily irritable bowel syndrome (27%) and abdominal bloating (22%).[7] The mechanisms responsible for functional chest pain include abnormal mechanophysical properties of the esophagus, central and peripheral hypersensitivity, and psychological comorbidity (Table 62.2). The latter may include depression, anxiety, and somatization.

EPIDEMIOLOGY

Information about the epidemiology of NCCP in the United States and around the world is relatively scarce. The mean annual

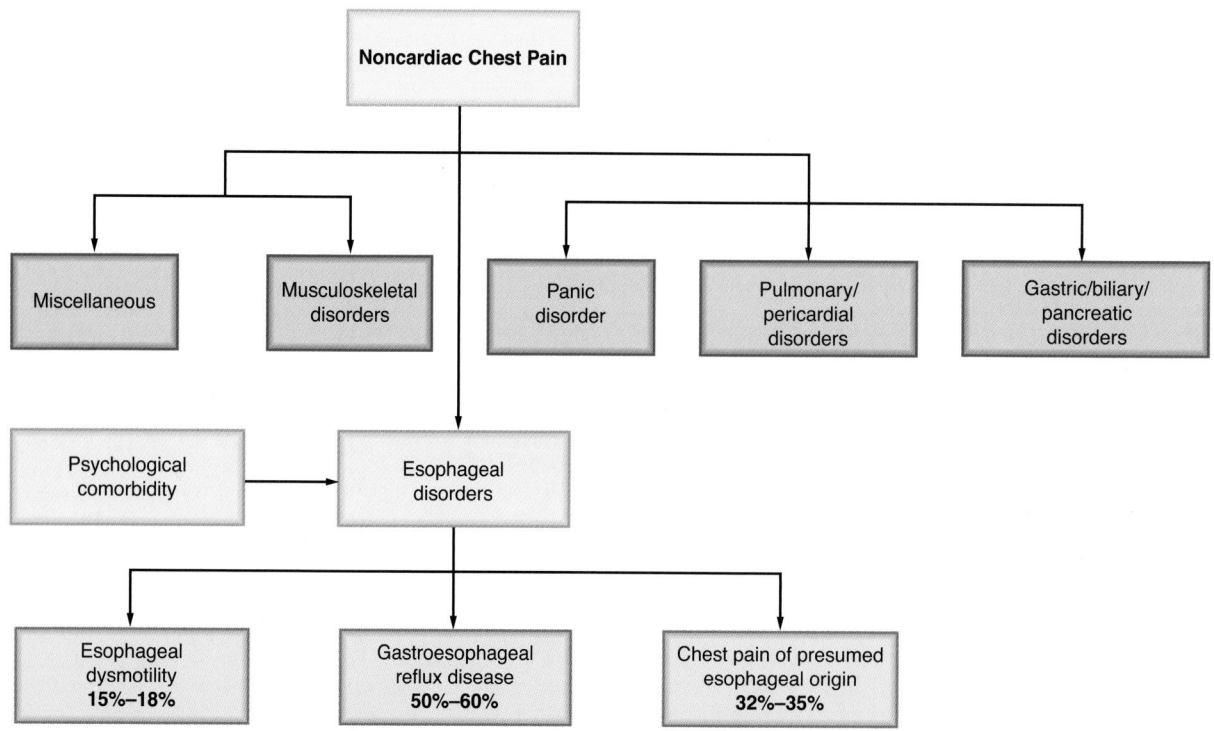

FIGURE 62.1 The different underlying mechanisms of NCCP.

TABLE 62.1

ROME III DIAGNOSTIC CRITERIA FOR FUNCTIONAL CHEST PAIN OF PRESUMED ESOPHAGEAL ORIGIN

Must include all of the following:
- Midline chest pain or discomfort that is not of burning quality
- Absence of evidence that gastroesophageal reflux is the cause of the symptom
- Absence of histopathology-based esophageal motility disorders

Criteria fulfilled for the last 3 months with symptoms onset at least 6 months prior to diagnosis.

TABLE 62.2

THE MAIN DIFFERENT PROPOSED UNDERLYING MECHANISMS OF FUNCTIONAL CHEST PAIN OF PRESUMED ESOPHAGEAL ORIGIN

- Abnormal mechanophysical properties
  - Hyperactive
  - ↓ Compliance
- Visceral hypersensitivity
  - Peripheral and central sensitization
  - Altered central processing of visceral stimuli (altered autonomic activity)
- Psychological abnormalities
  - Panic attack
  - Anxiety
  - Depression

prevalence of NCCP in the general population is approximately 25%, making NCCP the most common atypical/extraesophageal manifestation of GERD. A recent nationwide population-based study from South America[8] found that the annual prevalence of NCCP was 23.5% and that NCCP has been equally reported by both genders. In this study, frequent typical GERD symptoms (at least once a week) were significantly and independently associated with NCCP. Another recent published epidemiological study demonstrated that the annual prevalence of NCCP in a Chinese population was 19%.[9]

Whilst females with NCCP tend to consult health care providers more often than men, the disorder affects both genders equally.[10] Additionally, females are more likely to present to hospital emergency departments with NCCP than males. However, there are no gender differences regarding chest pain intensity, although women tend to use terms like "burning" and "frightening" more often than men.[11]

Epidemiological studies report a decrease in the prevalence of NCCP with increasing age. Women under 25 years of age and those between 45 and 55 years of age have the highest prevalence rates.[12] Patients with NCCP are younger, consume greater amounts of alcohol, smoke more, and are more likely to suffer from anxiety than their counterparts with ischemic heart disease. Patients with NCCP continued to seek treatment on a regular basis after the diagnosis was established for both chest pain and other unrelated symptoms, but few were in contact with hospital services.[13]

A recent U.S.-based survey revealed that cardiologists manage by themselves about half of the patients diagnosed with NCCP. Of those NCCP patients that were referred, 45.9% were sent back to the primary care physician (PCP), and only 29.3% to a gastroenterologist (Fig. 62.2).[14]

In a survey of PCPs, Wong et al.[15] demonstrated that most NCCP patients were diagnosed and treated by PCPs (79.5%), without being referred to a gastroenterologist (Fig. 62.2). The most preferred subspecialty for the initial diagnostic evaluation

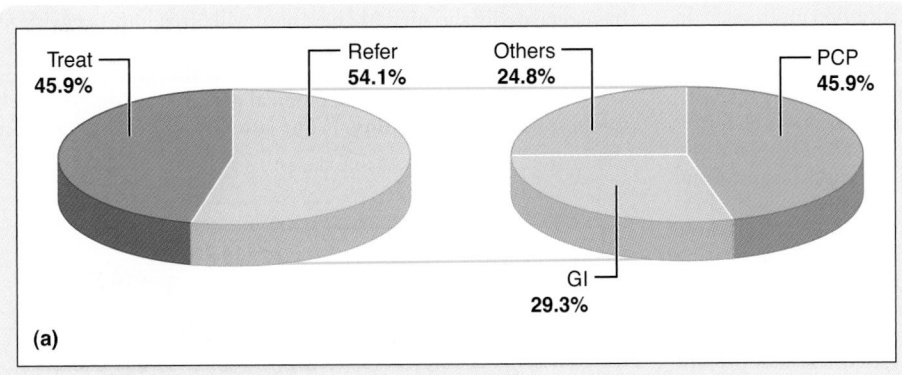

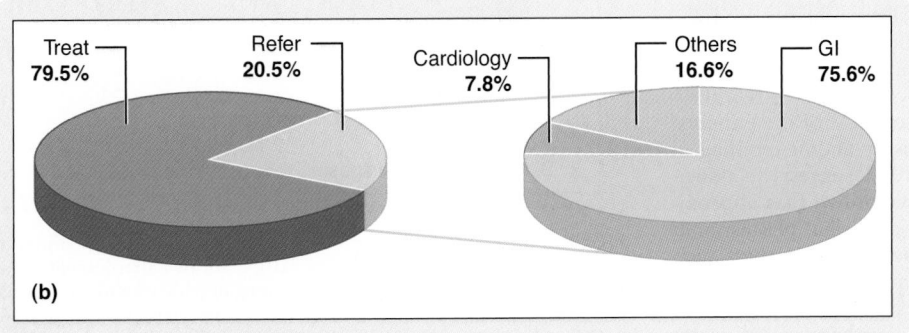

FIGURE 62.2 (A) A survey of 246 cardiologists determined that approximately half self-managed NCCP patients. (From Wong WM, Risner-Adler S, Beeler J, et al. Noncardiac chest pain: the role of the cardiologist—a national survey. *J Clin Gastroenterol* 2005;39:858–862, with permission.) **(B)** A similar survey of 205 primary care physicians demonstrated that the majority self-managed NCCP patients. (Redrawn after Wong WM, Risner-Adler S, Beeler J, et al. Noncardiac chest pain: the role of the cardiologist—a national survey. *J Clin Gastroenterol* 2005;39:858–862.)

of a patient presenting with chest pain was cardiology (62%), followed by gastroenterology (17%). However, the mean percentage of such referrals was only 22%. The most preferred subspecialty for the further management of NCCP was gastroenterology (76%), followed by cardiology (8%). However, the mean percentage of the actual referral rate was 29.8% for gastroenterologists and 14% for cardiologists.[15] Eslick and Talley[16] assessed the types of health care professionals consulted for chest pain. In their study, the main health care professionals seen were PCPs (85%), cardiologists (74%), and gastroenterologists (30%).

NATURAL HISTORY

The long-term prognosis of NCCP patients is excellent and very few eventually succumb to CAD or other cardiovascular-related disorders. In a study that followed 46 NCCP patients over a period of 11 years, only 4.3% died from a cardiovascular-related event.[17] However, most of the NCCP patients continue to report episodes of long-term chest pain. In the previous study, 75% of the surviving NCCP patients continued to report chest pain 11 years later, and 34% reported chest pain symptoms weekly.[17] Furthermore, studies have demonstrated that many NCCP patients have long-term impaired functional status and utilize health care resources because of their chest pain.[18] In one study, the rates of work absenteeism and interruption to daily activities were 29% and 63%, respectively, over a 1-year period.[16]

PATHOPHYSIOLOGY

Gastroesophageal Reflux Disease

The most common cause of NCCP is GERD. Locke and colleagues have found that NCCP is more commonly reported by patients who experience heartburn symptoms at least weekly (37%) as compared with those who have infrequent heartburn (less than once a week) (30.7%) and those without any symptoms of GERD (7.9%).[10] In this study 5% of the individuals with NCCP reported severe or very severe heartburn symptoms.[10] In another community-based study the authors demonstrated that 53% of all patients with NCCP experience heartburn and 58% acid regurgitation.[12] Beedassy et al. evaluated 104 patients with NCCP and documented that 48% had an abnormal pH test.[19] While 52 patients reported chest pain during the pH study, only in 21% of them did the chest pain coincide with an abnormal pH test. Interestingly, only 10 of the 52 NCCP patients with chest pain during the pH test had a positive symptom index.[19] Of these 10 patients, however, 80% had an abnormal pH test indicating that patients with a positive symptom index are significantly more likely to have an abnormal pH test.[19] In contrast, Dekel et al. found that a positive symptom index is a relatively uncommon phenomenon in NCCP patients regardless if GERD was present or absent.[20] The authors pointed out that the low incidence of a positive symptom index in NCCP patients is due to a very low number of reported chest pain episodes during the pH study.

By using 24-hour esophageal pH monitoring and/or endoscopy, GERD can be demonstrated in up to 60% of all patients with NCCP.[21] However, esophageal mucosal injury is relatively uncommon in NCCP, affecting only up to 25% of the patients. The presence of an abnormal acid exposure and/or esophageal mucosal inflammation in patients with NCCP suggests an association with GERD. However, studies have shown that approximately 80% of the NCCP patients with abnormal pH test and/or endoscopy report marked improvement in their chest pain when proton pump inhibitors (PPI) are administered.[21-23]

It is still unclear why GERD leads to chest pain alone in some subjects and heartburn alone in others. Furthermore, it is not uncommon that some patients may experience both chest pain and heartburn as a result of gastroesophageal reflux. As with GERD, less than 5% of all acid reflux events are perceived by NCCP patients and, thus, result in chest pain, regardless of whether mucosal injury is present. The latter observation underscores the importance of peripheral and central factors in modulating perception of intra-esophageal stimuli, through brain–gut interactions, and thus the generation of chest pain.[24] Exposure to acid has been demonstrated to sensitize esophageal sensory afferents to subsequent mechanical stimuli, such as intra-esophageal balloon distension, raising the role of visceral hypersensitivity as an important mediating physiological mechanism.

Linked Angina

It is well known that the esophagus and the heart share similar sensory innervation and several studies have demonstrated that acidification of the distal esophagus may influence the flow of the coronary circulation.[25-27] Chauhan et al. have shown a reduction in coronary artery blood flow in response to acid perfusion into the distal esophagus in patients with syndrome X. Syndrome X is defined as typical chest pain and electrocardiographic changes suggestive of myocardial ischemia on stress test, but patent coronary arteries on angiogram.[24] The reduction in coronary blood flow was also associated with typical anginal pain, suggesting the presence of an esophagocardiac inhibitory reflex.[28] These findings were later confirmed by Rosztoczy et al. who showed a decrease in coronary artery blood flow in 19 out of 42 (45%) patients undergoing acid perfusion of the esophagus.[29]

Esophageal Dysmotility

Though often entertained as an etiology of NCCP in the absence of GERD, the role of esophageal dysmotility in NCCP is likely very limited. More than 70% of the patients with non–GERD-related NCCP have normal esophageal motility (Fig. 62.3).[29,30] Esophageal dysmotility when documented by esophageal manometry is rarely associated with reports of chest pain.[31] Studies have repeatedly shown that chest pain will often improve without any normalization of the esophageal motor disorder. Unlike GERD, in which PPIs are highly effective in alleviating symptoms, we are still devoid of pharmacological agents that can effectively treat esophageal dysmotility.[30] The latter further complicates our

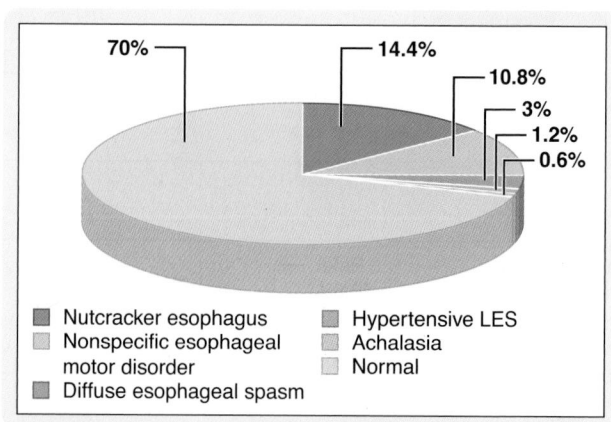

FIGURE 62.3 Distribution of esophageal motility abnormalities in NCCP patient without GERD (N = 910). (Redrawn after Katz PO, Dalton CB, Richter JE, et al. Esophageal testing of patients with noncardiac chest pain or dysphagia. Results of three years' experience with 1161 patients. *Ann Intern Med* 1987;106(4):593–597, with permission.)

ability to determine any relationship between chest pain and manometric findings. That being said, esophageal motility disorders still can be demonstrated in 30% of the patients with non–GERD-related NCCP.[30] Dekel et al. demonstrated, via the Clinical Outcomes Research Initiative Database, that hypotensive lower esophageal sphincter (LES) was the most common (61%) esophageal motor disorder found in patients with NCCP.[30] It has been suggested that this is due to an increased rate of GERD in these patients. Spastic esophageal motility disorders were shown to be the second most common cause with nutcracker esophagus affecting 10%, hypertensive LES affecting 10%, and diffuse esophageal spasm affecting 2% of the NCCP cases with esophageal dysmotility.[29] However, in another study of non–GERD-related NCCP, Katz et al. reported that nutcracker esophagus was the most common motor disorder documented during esophageal manometry followed by nonspecific esophageal motility disorders, diffuse esophageal spasm, hypertensive LES, and achalasia (Fig. 62.3).

The high prevalence of nutcracker esophagus in NCCP patients is intriguing. Nutcracker esophagus is defined manometrically as high amplitude contractions in the distal esophagus (>180 mm Hg) in the presence of a normally functioning LES. The general significance of nutcracker esophagus and specifically its role in NCCP has been an area of intense controversy.[32] Achem et al. demonstrated improvement in chest pain symptoms of patients with NCCP and nutcracker esophagus who received antireflux medical therapy.[32] In this study, esophageal manometry normalized only in a minority of the patients thus indicating that the underlying etiology of the chest pain was likely GERD rather than the nutcracker esophagus.[32] As a result of the weak correlation between documented esophageal dysmotility during manometry and chest pain, some have postulated that motility disorders serve more as a marker for a presently poorly understood esophageal abnormality which contributes to the underlying etiology of NCCP.[33] Consequently, one may argue that esophageal motor disorders, with the exception of achalasia, may have no direct etiological role in symptom generation of patients with NCCP and thus should not be pursued diagnostically or therapeutically.

Sustained Esophageal Contractions

High-frequency intraluminal ultrasonography, a technique useful for the evaluation of smooth muscle contraction, has been employed to assess the esophageal motor corollary of chest pain in NCCP patients.[34] By using high-frequency intraluminal ultrasonography, Balaban et al. have shown a close correlation between longitudinal muscle contractions and reports of chest pain.[34] When evaluating the 10 participating subjects, the authors demonstrated esophageal longitudinal muscle contractions preceding 18 of 24 spontaneous chest pain events. These muscle contractions cannot be detected by conventional esophageal pressure recordings that solely evaluate the esophageal circular muscle.[34] Balaban et al. further showed that edrophonium-induced chest pain was also preceded by sustained esophageal muscle contractions.[34] The authors also demonstrated that swallow-associated contractions of the longitudinal muscles lasted an average of 6.4 seconds whereas contractions associated with chest pain lasted a mean of 68.0 seconds.[35] Pehlivanov et al. demonstrated that the duration of the sustained esophageal muscle contractions might be correlated with the type of symptom perceived by patients. Shorter durations of these contractions were associated more with heartburn while longer durations were linked more with chest pain.[35] Furthermore, sustained esophageal muscle contractions were observed in patients who reported heartburn that was unrelated to an acid reflux event giving further credence to the hypothesis that sustained esophageal contractions are responsible for the generation of esophageal-related symptoms such as chest pain.[34] Unfortunately, high-frequency intraluminal ultraso-

nography is highly operator dependent and consequently may not always be an objective evaluative tool. None of the initial studies have been replicated by other investigators. While sustained esophageal muscle contractions appear to be predictable markers for chest pain, it is still unclear if they are the direct underlying mechanism or just an epiphenomenon.[36]

Visceral Hypersensitivity

The underlying mechanisms responsible for non–GERD-related NCCP remain to be fully elucidated. Numerous studies have consistently documented alteration in pain perception regardless of whether esophageal dysmotility was present or absent (Table 62.2).

Visceral hypersensitivity is a phenomenon in which the conscious perception of visceral stimulus is enhanced independent of the intensity of the stimulus.[37] Peripheral and central mechanisms have been proposed to be responsible for visceral hypersensitivity in patients with NCCP. It has been hypothesized that peripheral sensitization of esophageal sensory afferents leads to subsequently heightened responses to physiologic or pathologic stimuli of the esophageal mucosa.[37] Additionally, central sensitization at the brain level or the dorsal horn of the spinal cord may modulate afferent neural function and thus enhance perception of intraluminal stimuli.[21] What causes peripheral or central sensitization remains to be determined. Studies have shown that acute tissue irritation results in subsequent peripheral and central sensitization which is manifested as increased background activity of sensory neurons, the lowering of nociceptive thresholds, changes in stimulus response curves, and enlargements of receptive fields.[38] Peripheral sensitization involves the reduction of esophageal pain threshold and an increase in the transduction processes of primary afferent neurons.[39] Esophageal tissue injury, inflammation, spasm, or repetitive mechanical stimuli can all sensitize peripheral afferent nerves. The presence of esophageal hypersensitivity can be subsequently demonstrated long after the original stimulus is no longer present and the esophageal mucosa has healed. However, it is still unclear what factors are pivotal for the persistence of such esophageal hypersensitivity.

Several studies have demonstrated that patients with non–GERD-related NCCP have lower perception thresholds for pain. Richter et al. used balloon distension protocol in the distal esophagus and found that 50% of the patients with NCCP developed pain at volumes of 8 mL or less in comparison with 9 mL or more in healthy subjects who developed pain (Fig. 62.4).[40] The authors found no difference in the pressure-volume curve of the two groups as well as no difference in esophageal motility.[40] When the balloon was inflated to 10 mL, patients with a history of NCCP were more likely to experience pain (18/30) than the control subjects (6/30).[39] Barish et al. evaluated 50 patients with NCCP and 30 healthy volunteers using a graded balloon distension protocol.[39] Of the patients with NCCP, 56% (28/50) experienced their "typical" chest pain during balloon distension as compared with 20% (6/30) of the normal controls.[39] Of those with NCCP who experienced pain, 86% reported pain at volumes less than 80 mL.[41] There was no difference in esophageal tone between the two groups.

Rao et al. used impedance planimetry to evaluate 24 patients with NCCP and 12 healthy controls and demonstrated that during balloon distension those with NCCP had lower perception thresholds for first sensation, moderate discomfort, and pain in comparison to healthy controls.[41] Typical chest pain was reproduced in 83% of the NCCP patients.[41] In addition, the reactivity of the esophagus to balloon distension was increased in those with NCCP as was the pressure elastic modulus. Rao et al.[42] also performed graded balloon distensions of the esophagus using impedance planimetry in 16 consecutive patients with NCCP (normal esophageal evaluation) and 13 healthy control subjects.

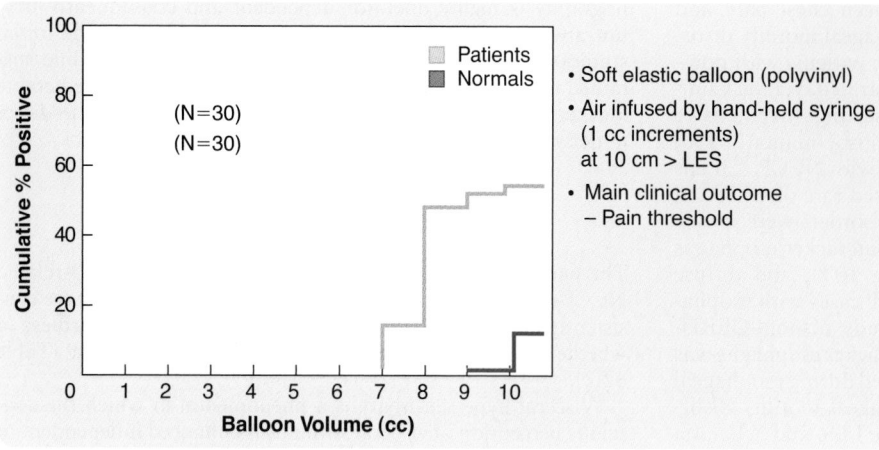

FIGURE 62.4 Pain thresholds in NCCP patients versus normal controls using a balloon distension protocol. (Redrawn after Richter JE, Barish CF, Castell DO. Abnormal sensory perception in patients with esophageal chest pain. *Gastroenterology* 1986;91(4):845–852, with permission.)

Patients who experienced chest pain during the balloon distension were subsequently restudied after receiving intravenous atropine. Balloon distensions reproduced chest pain at lower sensory thresholds than controls in most NCCP subjects. Similar findings were documented after atropine administration despite relaxed and more deformable esophageal wall. Thus, the investigators concluded that hypersensitivity, rather than motor dysfunction, is the predominant mechanism for functional chest pain (Fig. 62.5).

Sarkar et al.[43] recruited 19 healthy volunteers and 7 patients with NCCP. Hydrochloric acid was infused into the distal esophagus during a period of 30 minutes. Sensory responses to electrical stimulation were monitored within the acid-exposed distal esophagus and the nonexposed proximal esophagus both before and after infusion. In the healthy subjects, acid infusion into the distal esophagus lowered the pain threshold in the upper esophagus. Patients with NCCP already had a lower resting esophageal pain threshold than healthy subjects. After acid perfusion, their pain threshold in the proximal esophagus fell farther and for a longer duration than was the case for the healthy subjects (Fig. 62.6). Additionally, there was a decrease in the pain threshold of the anterior chest wall after acid infusion. This study demonstrated the development of secondary visceral hypersensitivity in the proximal esophagus by repeated acid exposure of the distal esophagus. The concurrent visceral and somatic pain hypersensitivity is, most likely, caused by central sensitization (increase in excitability of spinal cord and supraspinal neurons induced by activation of esophageal nociceptors in the area of the tissue injury). The patients with NCCP demonstrated both visceral hypersensitivity at the site of insult and at a distant, secondary site

in the esophagus. However, it is unclear from the study what mechanism is responsible for the exaggerated secondary hypersensitivity and what initiates central sensitization in patients with NCCP. It is interesting to note that other studies[44] in NCCP, using similar human model of acute tissue irritation by acid infusion, showed no significant effect on pain thresholds.

Borjesson et al. also demonstrated that patients with NCCP have reduced sensitivity to esophageal balloon distension during simultaneous transcutaneous electrical nerve stimulation (TENS) as compared with healthy controls.[36,44] This further supports the role of visceral hypersensitivity in NCCP and suggests that the phenomenon is probably due to central sensitization.[45]

Mehta et al. also demonstrated that acid infusion into the distal esophagus reduces esophageal pain thresholds for balloon distension in patients with NCCP not previously sensitive to balloon distension or acid infusion.[46]

In one study, subjects underwent perfusion of the distal esophagus with either normal saline or 0.1N hydrochloric acid.[46] Perceptual responses to intraluminal esophageal balloon distension using an electronic barostat were recorded. Perfusion with acid was associated with a reduced sensation threshold (innocuous perception) and tended to reduce the pain threshold (aversive sensation). The study demonstrated short-term sensitization of mechanosensitive afferent pathways by transient exposure to acid. It was suggested that in patients with NCCP, acid reflux induces sensitization of the esophagus and this may subsequently alter the way in which otherwise normal esophageal distensions are perceived.[47]

Sarkar et al. evaluated 14 patients with GERD-related NCCP and 8 healthy controls. All subjects underwent an esophageal

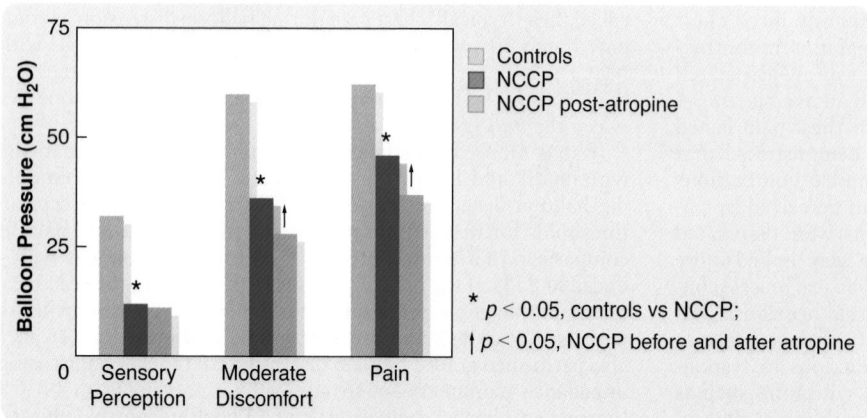

FIGURE 62.5 Mean pressure thresholds in controls and in patients with NCCP before and after atropine was given. (Redrawn after Rao S, Hayek B, Summers RW. Functional chest pain of esophageal origin: hyperalgesia or motor dysfunction. *Am J Gastroenterol* 2001; 96(9):2584–2589, with permission.)

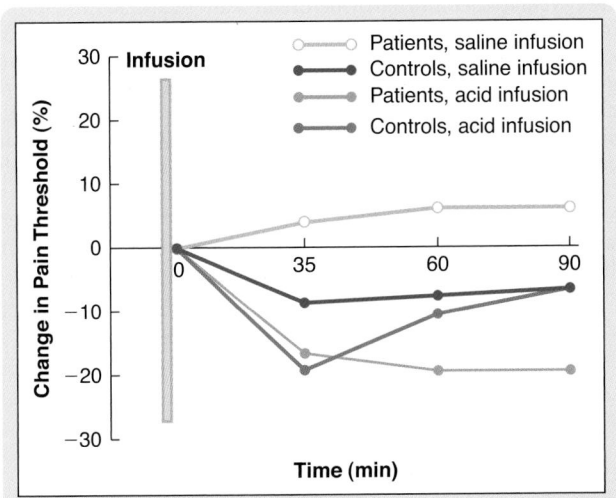

FIGURE 62.6 Mean change in pain threshold in the upper esophagus after 5 minutes infusion of acid or saline into the lower esophagus (NCCP vs. control). (Redrawn after Sarkar S, Aziz Q, Woolf CJ, et al. Contribution of central sensitization to the development of non-cardiac chest pain. *Lancet* 2000;356(9236):1154–1159, with permission.)

electrical stimulation protocol in the proximal esophagus and those with NCCP demonstrated lower perception thresholds for pain than normal controls.[47] After a 6-week course of high-dose PPI (omeprazole 20 mg twice daily), however, there was an increase in the perception thresholds for pain during electrical stimulation in the group of patients with NCCP (Fig. 62.7).[47] This study demonstrated that patients with NCCP and evidence of GERD have a component of esophageal hypersensitivity that is responsive to high-dose PPI therapy.[47]

In another small study that enrolled 22 NCCP patients with documented nutcracker esophagus, the authors demonstrated that stepwise balloon distensions reproduced pain symptoms at a lower threshold in 90% of the NCCP patients as compared

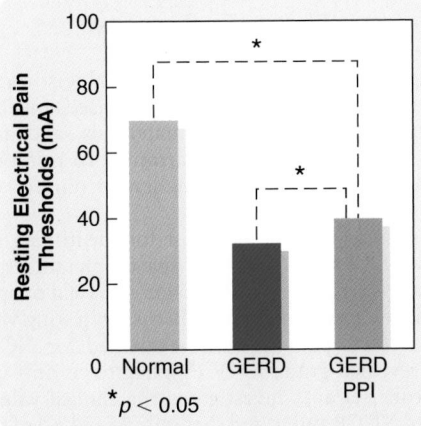

FIGURE 62.7 Patients with chest pain and occult GERD demonstrate visceral hypersensitivity that may be partially responsive to acid suppression with a PPI. (Redrawn after Sarkar S, Thompson DG, Woolf CJ, et al. Patients with chest pain and occult gastroesophageal reflux demonstrate visceral pain hypersensitivity which may be partially responsive to acid suppression. *Am J Gastroenterol* 2004;99(10):1998–2006, with permission.)

with 20% of the healthy controls.[48] It was concluded that patients with NCCP and nutcracker esophagus also exhibit visceral hypersensitivity. Additionally, the latter is the likely main underlying mechanism for patients' symptoms, rather than the presence of the high amplitude contractions (nutcracker esophagus). Unfortunately, the presence of GERD in these patients was not determined in this study.

Abnormal Cerebral Processing of Visceral Stimulation

Positron emission tomography (PET) and functional magnetic resonance imaging (fMRI) have been increasingly used to evaluate brain–gut relationship in patients with esophageal disorders, primarily GERD and NCCP.

Kern et al. demonstrated, via fMRI, that slow infusion of 0.1N hydrochloric acid evokes a cerebral cortical response primarily in the posterior cingulate, parietal, and anteromesial frontal lobes prior to inducing heartburn.[49] Aziz et al., using PET scanning and a distal esophageal balloon distension protocol, examined the human brain loci involved in the process of esophageal sensation.[50] Both nonpainful and painful esophageal balloon distensions elicited bilateral activation along the central sulcus, the insular cortex, and the frontal and parietal operculum.[50] Painful esophageal balloon distensions, however, elicited an increased activation of these brain areas in addition to activation of the right anterior insular cortex (important in affective processing) and the anterior cingulate gyrus (important in pain processing and generating an affective and cognitive response to pain).[51]

During the early 1990s, investigators suggested that NCCP patients demonstrated altered central processing of intra-esophageal stimuli.[51] Investigators have used cerebral-evoked potentials as an objective measurement to assess the subjective sensation of pain of NCCP patients.[52] In response to esophageal balloon distension, evoked potential quality scores and amplitude of the major peaks increased significantly with increased sensation, both in NCCP patients and healthy controls. However, in the patients, quality score and amplitude of all four peaks of the evoked potentials were lower and latencies of two of the four peaks were longer than in the controls. The volumes of air required to produce the various sensations were lower in the patients. The investigators concluded that the results suggest that increased perception of esophageal distension in NCCP patients is caused by altered central processing of intra-esophageal events. Kamath et al. studied the effect of esophageal electrical stimulation on cortical evoked potentials in patients with NCCP. The authors demonstrated that in patients with NCCP the evoked potentials were of greater amplitude and the peak latencies were slightly longer than in controls.[37] The authors concluded that increased perception of esophageal stimulation in NCCP reflects an altered cortical processing of visceral sensation.

Hollerbach et al. studied 20 subjects (8 with NCCP, 12 healthy) and demonstrated an abnormal cerebral processing of esophageal stimuli in patients with NCCP. Cortical-evoked responses were lower in intensity during electrical esophageal stimulation in patients with NCCP in comparison to the healthy controls. Because of the smaller cortical-evoked potentials, it was hypothesized that the increased perception of esophageal stimuli might in fact be the result of enhanced cerebral processing of visceral sensory input rather than hypersensitive responses of visceral afferent pathways.[37]

Altered Autonomic Activity

Tougas et al. have performed several studies exploring autonomic nervous system function and its role in the pathogenesis of NCCP.

In one study, the investigators assessed autonomic activity, using spectral analysis of heart rate variability, before and during distal esophageal acidification of patients with NCCP and matched healthy controls.[53] Of those with NCCP, 68% developed angina-like symptoms during the esophageal acidification. These patients had a higher baseline heart rate and a lower baseline vagal activity than patients without acid sensitivity. During acid infusion, vagal cardiac outflow increased in acid-sensitive patients as compared with patients without acid sensitivity.[53] Additionally, Tougas et al. have also documented increased vagal activity in patients with NCCP during other intra-esophageal stimuli, both mechanical and electrical. These studies indicate that autonomic dysregulation may be present in at least a subset of patients with NCCP.[54] The authors further hypothesized that increased perception of esophageal stimulation may also reflect an exaggerated brainstem response. However, Tougas has hypothesized that in most cases in which both central and autonomic factors are involved, central factors will likely lead to autonomic dysregulation.[54]

Psychological Comorbidity

Studies have demonstrated that central factors, such as stress, psychological disorders, and others play an important role in enhancing perception of intraesophageal stimuli.[55] Stress has been noted to be an important factor in the generation and exacerbation of both functional and organic gastrointestinal disorders, including NCCP.[55] Certain stressful life events have been associated with the onset or symptom exacerbation of functional bowel disorders. Daily experiences of stress appear to have an important modulating effect on perception of intraluminal events and may alter perception thresholds for pain.[56]

Between 17% and 43% of the patients with NCCP are estimated to suffer from some type of psychological abnormality.[56] Psychological comorbidity can modulate esophageal perception and cause subjects to perceive low-intensity esophageal stimuli as being painful.[13,57–60] Anxiety, depression, neuroticism, and hypochondriac behavior have all been described in NCCP patients.[61–64] The findings, however, have been inconsistent when NCCP patients were compared to subjects with CAD, with some authors reporting increased anxiety and depression in NCCP patients while others reporting no significant difference between the two disorders.[65] In a recent study of 167 patients with NCCP and 32 with chest pain and CAD, there was no significant difference in the incidence of depression, anxiety, or neuroticism between the two groups.[65] The authors stated that the discrepancy of their results with previous findings might be secondary to different inclusion criteria or an overall low prevalence of current major depression.[65] The study also did find that panic disorder was more common in NCCP patients (41%) as compared to those with CAD.[66]

Among all esophageal symptoms, chest pain was shown to closely correlate with psychometric abnormalities. In some patients, chest pain is part of a host of symptoms that characterize panic attack.[66] Panic attack is a common cause for emergency room visits due to chest pain. In a large study that encompassed 441 consecutive ambulatory patients presenting with chest pain to the emergency department of a heart center, 25% were diagnosed as suffering from a panic attack.[67] While the reason for the observed association between NCCP and panic disorder remained to be fully understood, hyperventilation was demonstrated to precipitate chest pain in 15% of the patients with NCCP.[67] Additionally, it was demonstrated that hyperventilation could provoke reversible esophageal manometric abnormalities such as esophageal spasm (4%) and a nonspecific esophageal motor disorder (22%).[68] Furthermore, studies have demonstrated that hyperventilation may precipitate a panic attack.[69]

Anxiety and depression influence reports of pain and thus contribute to the pathophysiology of NCCP. Lantinga et al.[70]

found that patients with NCCP had higher levels of neuroticism and psychiatric comorbidity before and after cardiac catheterization than did patients with CAD. This finding appears to have prognostic significance because these patients display less improvement in pain, more frequent pain episodes, greater social maladjustment, and more anxiety at 1-year follow-up than individuals with relatively low initial levels of psychosocial disturbances. In a large epidemiological study from England, a significant relationship between NCCP and psychiatric disorders was demonstrated in young adults.[71] Two independent variables were associated with chest pain: parental illness and fatigue during childhood.[14]

DIAGNOSIS OF NONCARDIAC CHEST PAIN

GERD-Related NCCP

There is no gold standard for diagnosing GERD-related NCCP. The currently available diagnostic tests to detect GERD in patients with NCCP include barium swallow, upper endoscopy, the acid perfusion test, ambulatory 24-hour esophageal pH monitoring, and the PPI test.

Barium Esophagram

Barium esophagram has very little use in the diagnosis of GERD. Barium esophagram has a low sensitivity (20%) for diagnosing GERD in general due to lack of anatomical and mucosal abnormalities in most of the GERD patients.[73] Furthermore, the significance of barium reflux during the procedure as a diagnostic for GERD is questionable. Johnston et al. found that the proportion of patients with an abnormal 24-hour esophageal pH study was similar to the proportion of patients with a normal 24-hour esophageal pH study who had spontaneous barium reflux during the test.[73] Additionally, spontaneous barium reflux has been demonstrated in up to 20% of healthy subjects.[74]

The role of barium esophagram is unclear in patients with GERD-related NCCP, primarily due to the rare presence of esophageal mucosal abnormalities. However, one may consider performing a barium esophagram as the initial diagnostic test in patients who report dysphagia in addition to chest pain.

Upper Endoscopy

Once a patient is referred to a gastroenterologist for evaluation of NCCP, if any alarm symptoms (decreased appetite, weight loss, dysphagia, odynophagia, hematemesis, and anemia) are present, an upper endoscopy is warranted to rule out mucosal abnormalities such as benign or malignant tumors, esophageal ulceration, or peptic stricture.

Upper endoscopy is the best test for identifying esophageal mucosal involvement in GERD (erosive esophagitis, stricture, ulcers, and Barrett esophagus). The diagnostic yield of upper endoscopy, esophageal manometry, and Bernstein testing was assessed in 100 consecutive patients being evaluated for NCCP. Upper endoscopy revealed grade II–IV esophagitis in only 24 patients (24%).[75] Frober et al.[76] investigated the clinical value of upper endoscopy in NCCP and found that only 15 (31%) of the patients had esophageal mucosal injury, with all but one having grade I erosive esophagitis.

Recently, Dickman et al.[77] evaluated upper GI findings in patients with noncardiac chest pain versus those with GERD using a national endoscopic database (Table 62.3). Of the NCCP group, 28.6% had hiatal hernia, 19.6% erosive esophagitis, 4.4% Barrett esophagus, and 3.6% stricture/stenosis. The prevalence of

TABLE 62.3

THE VALUE OF UPPER ENDOSCOPY IN CHEST PAIN PATIENTS AS COMPARED TO THOSE WITH REFLUX-RELATED SYMPTOMS USING A LARGE MULTICENTER CONSORTIUM

Findings	Chest pain group N = 3688 (%)	Reflux group N = 32,981 (%)	P Value
Barrett esophagus	163 (4.4%)	3,016 (9.1%)	<0.0001
Esophageal inflammation	715 (19.4%)	9,153 (27.8%)	<0.0001
Hiatal hernia	1,053 (28.6%)	14,775 (44.8%)	<0.0001
Normal	1,627 (44.1%)	12,801 (38.8%)	<0.0001
Stricture/stenosis	132 (3.6%)	1,223 (3.7%)	0.69

(From Dickman R, Mattek N, Holub J, et al. Prevalence of upper gastrointestinal tract findings in patients with noncardiac chest pain versus those with gastroesophageal reflux disease (GERD)-related symptoms: results from a national endoscopic database. *Am J Gastroenterol* 2007;102:1173–1179, with permission.)

these findings was significantly lower in the NCCP group as compared to the GERD group. The authors concluded that most of the endoscopic findings in NCCP patients were GERD related but less common as compared to GERD patients. Thus, the value of upper endoscopy in NCCP is very limited, because the findings are primarily related to GERD. Potentially, the test is indicated as a screening tool for Barrett esophagus in this specific patient population.

Ambulatory 24-hour Esophageal pH Monitoring

Ambulatory 24-hour esophageal pH monitoring with symptom correlation is still commonly used to evaluate patients with NCCP.[78] Approximately 50% to 60% of the NCCP patients have abnormal esophageal acid exposure or a positive symptom index alone. However, the presence of abnormal distal esophageal acid exposure during pH testing does not necessarily mean that the patient's chest pain is GERD related. Hewson et al.[78] examined 100 consecutive patients with NCCP and detected abnormal acid exposure in 48% of the patients. Of the 83 patients who had spontaneous chest pain during the study, 37 (46%) had abnormal reflux parameters and 50 (60%) had a normal study but a positive symptom index (calculated as the percentage of symptoms that are associated with acid reflux events). The authors concluded that 24-hour esophageal pH testing with symptom index (SI) is the single best test for evaluating patients with NCCP. In contrast, Dekel et al.[20] demonstrated that a positive SI is a relatively uncommon phenomenon in NCCP patients because most of the patients do not experience chest pain during the pH study.

The pH test is invasive, inconvenient to patients, costly, and not readily available for many physicians. Additionally, the yield of the test in NCCP has not been rigorously assessed. This is compounded by the rarity of chest pain symptoms during the test in many patients, making it difficult to determine the relationship between patients' symptoms and acid reflux events.[79]

Because of the introduction of the PPI therapeutic trial, the role of 24-hour esophageal pH testing in NCCP has markedly changed in the last decade. Presently, the test is commonly used to assess NCCP patients who failed an empirical therapy with a PPI.

The Wireless pH System

The wireless Bravo (Medtronic, Shoreview, MN) pH monitoring system is a "catheterless" pH system. It involves the attachment of a radiotelemetry pH capsule to the wall of the esophagus (peroral or transnasal). It simultaneously measures pH and transmits data to a pager-sized receiver clipped onto the patient's belt, thereby circumventing the need for a nasally placed pH catheter, which is uncomfortable for many patients.[80] Unlike the traditional pH catheter system, the wireless pH system can collect data for up to 48 hours. The system was found to be well tolerated and reliable, and it provided reproducible results.[81]

Prakash and Clouse[82] found that by extending the recording time to 48 hours, using the wireless pH system, the number of subjects recording symptoms during the test increased by 6.8% and the number of symptoms available for association with an acid reflux event was doubled. The study also demonstrated that patients with NCCP benefited the most from extending the duration of the pH test. In another study, the same authors demonstrated that the wireless pH system increased the detection of NCCP patients with abnormal pH test and/or positive reflux-symptom association probabilities.[83]

The Proton Pump Inhibitor Test

The PPI test (or short therapeutic trial) is defined as a short course of high dose PPI for diagnosing GERD. This is a simple and noninvasive diagnostic tool for GERD. It is readily available and at the disposal of every PCP. Additionally, it increases the role of PCPs in evaluating and treating patients with different manifestations of GERD. It also offers significant cost savings when compared to the other diagnostic tests for GERD.

Empirical therapy with PPIs (usually offers 2–3 months of treatment with PPI) has often been used by physicians as the initial treatment of patients with typical or atypical manifestations of GERD. However, it is both impractical and costly for patients to complete several months or longer of acid suppression therapy before determining whether the medication is of benefit or not.[21]

The doses used in the PPI test have ranged from 40 mg to 80 mg daily for omeprazole; 30 mg to 60 mg daily for lansoprazole; and 40 mg daily for rabeprazole, over duration of treatment of 1 to 28 days, in patients with symptoms suggestive of GERD or NCCP.[88–101] In patients with laryngeal manifestations of GERD, the doses ranged from 40 mg to 80 mg omeprazole daily and the duration of treatment from 1 to 4 weeks.[84–87] By far, the most commonly used PPI in most of the PPI test trials is omeprazole, which has led to the term the "omeprazole test."[88–97] However, studies using other PPIs demonstrated that they are equally efficacious as short therapeutic trials.[98–100]

An important factor in determining the sensitivity of a PPI test is the definition of a positive test. In most studies, a symptom score cutoff was used: if the symptom assessment score for heartburn, chest pain, or other symptoms improved by more than 50% to 75% (depending on the study) relative to baseline, the test was considered positive. As with any diagnostic test, the optimal cutoff is critical in defining test accuracy.[101] The symptom score cutoff values that were used among studies that evaluated PPI tests for GERD were chosen arbitrarily. Rarely, studies calculated the Receiver Operator Curve (ROC) by varying the percentage reduction in the symptom tested to ascertain the optimal value for detecting patients with GERD.[88,92,101] This cutoff point provides the greatest sensitivity, specificity, positive predictive value, and accuracy of the short therapeutic trial tested.

As with any other test, the sensitivity of a PPI test depends on the prevalence of the disease in the patient population that is evaluated. Obviously, the PPI test has minimal utility in patients with erosive esophagitis, in whom acid reflux is almost always the underlying cause. However, as the likelihood of a particular syndrome being attributable to reflux decreases, the potential value of a PPI test increases.

The diagnostic accuracy of the PPI test is limited by the lack of gold standard for the diagnosis of GERD. In the absence of gold standard, studies evaluating the PPI test have used a combination of upper endoscopy and ambulatory 24-hour esophageal pH monitoring as the closest one can get to a gold standard. Factors that may determine the sensitivity of the PPI test include type of antireflux medication used, dosage, treatment duration, definition of a positive test (symptom score cutoff, change in symptom grading, receiver operating characteristics curve analysis), and the GERD-related symptom evaluated.

Only one study attempted to compare the accuracy of the PPI test (omeprazole test) to 24-hour esophageal pH monitoring in diagnosing GERD.[102] The study used the presence of erosive esophagitis as indicative of GERD in patients who are not on aspirin or nonsteroidal anti-inflammatory drugs (NSAIDs). Thirty-five patients were included, and they underwent both pH testing and the PPI test (omeprazole 40 mg before breakfast and 20 mg before dinner). The PPI test was significantly more sensitive than total acid contact time during pH testing (83% vs. 60%, p <0.03). The sensitivity of the pH test increased to 80% only after adding patients with positive SI, and patients with abnormal acid contact time, in the supine and/or erect positions despite normal total acid contact time. The authors concluded that the PPI test was at least as sensitive as ambulatory 24-hour esophageal pH monitoring in diagnosing GERD in patients with documented erosive esophagitis.

In different studies, the sensitivity of the PPI test for GERD-related NCCP ranged from 69% to 95% and the specificity from 67% to 86%.[88,95–97,103,104] The dosages of PPIs used ranged from 60 mg to 80 mg daily for omeprazole,[88,95–97] 30 mg to 90 mg for lansoprazole,[103,105] and 40 mg for rabeprazole.[106] The trial duration ranged from 1 to 28 days.[88,95–97,103,105,106]

In a double-blind placebo-controlled trial, 37 patients with NCCP were randomized to either placebo or high-dose omeprazole (40 mg before breakfast and 20 mg before dinner) for 7 days.[88] After a washout period and repeated baseline symptom assessment, patients crossed over to the opposite arm. The PPI test was considered positive if the chest pain improved by at least 50% after treatment. The combination of upper endoscopy and 24-hour esophageal pH monitoring was used as the gold standard. Sixty-two percent (23/37) of the patients had evidence of GERD: 7 had abnormal esophageal acid exposure by pH testing only, 8 had erosive esophagitis only, and 8 had both. Of the GERD-positive group, 78.3% had a positive PPI test and 22.7% had a positive placebo response. In contrast, of the GERD-negative group, 14.2% had a positive PPI test and 7.1% had a positive placebo response. Thus, the calculated sensitivity was 78.3%, specificity 85.7%, and the positive predictive value was 90%.[88] When different reductions in chest pain were evaluated as previously mentioned, the greater accuracy of predicting

GERD-related NCCP was obtained with 65% symptom reduction, producing a sensitivity of 85.7% and specificity of 90.9%.[88] Using similar design, other investigators confirmed the usefulness of the PPI test for diagnosing GERD-related NCCP.[97,103] Furthermore, subsequent studies demonstrated that short therapeutic trials with PPIs other than omeprazole achieved similar efficacy for the diagnosis of GERD-related NCCP.[105,106] A study in the Chinese population showed that the PPI test, using lansoprazole 30 mg daily for a period of 4 weeks, was useful in diagnosing endoscopy-negative GERD-related NCCP.[103]

As with the PPI test in patients with classic GERD symptoms, the PPI test in NCCP has been recently scrutinized by two meta-analyses. In the first meta-analysis of randomized controlled trials (parallel group and crossover design), the authors evaluated the pooled risk ratio for continued chest pain after PPI therapy; overall number needed to treat; and pooled sensitivity, specificity, and diagnostic odds ratio for the PPI test versus reference standards.[107]

Eight studies were included in the PPI efficacy analysis. The pooled risk ratio for continued chest pain after PPI therapy was 0.54 (95% confidence interval [CI], 0.41–0.71). The overall number needed to treat was 3 (95% CI, 2–4). The pooled sensitivity, specificity, and diagnostic odds ratio for the PPI test versus 24-hour pH monitoring and upper endoscopy were 80%, 73%, and 13.83 (95% CI, 5.48–34.91), respectively. All studies were small, and there was evidence of publication bias or other small study effects. The authors concluded that PPI therapy reduces symptoms in NCCP and may be useful as a diagnostic test in identifying abnormal esophageal acid reflux. However, in this meta-analysis, the authors included a potpourri of diagnostic and therapeutic trials with a PPI in patients with NCCP. Many of these trials have little in common and often used different clinical endpoints. Of the eight studies that were included in the PPI efficacy analysis, two (25%) were published only in an abstract form.[95,106] Additionally, one study[108] focused on the value of the pH testing-derived parameter—the SI in patients with NCCP. The usage of an open label PPI test in this study was a secondary endpoint. Another study[103] was done exclusively in Chinese patients with nonerosive reflux disease-related NCCP. Furthermore, the latter study included a standard dose PPI given during a period of 1 month. One study[109] was an open label, empirical therapy in patients with NCCP, using omeprazole 40 mg in the evening during a period of 6 weeks. The studies differ significantly from each other in many clinical aspects, affecting the quality and reliability of the meta-analysis.

Wang et al. have also performed a meta-analysis of the PPI test in patients with NCCP.[110] Unlike the previous meta-analysis, the authors found only six studies that met inclusion criteria. The overall sensitivity and specificity of a PPI test were 80% (95% CI, 71% to 87%) and 74% (95% CI, 64% to 83%), respectively, compared with 19% (95% CI, 12% to 29%) and 77% (95% CI, 62% to 87%), respectively, in the placebo group. The PPI test showed significant higher discriminative power, with a summary diagnostic odds ratio of 19.35 (95% CI, 8.54–43.84) compared to 0.61 (95% CI, 0.20–1.86) in the placebo group. Thus, the authors concluded that the use of PPI treatment as a diagnostic test for detecting GERD in patients with NCCP has an acceptable sensitivity and specificity and could be used as an initial approach by PCPs to detect GERD in selected patients with NCCP.

There is evidence that when using the PPI test, there is a significant correlation between the extent of esophageal acid exposure in the distal esophagus as determined by ambulatory 24-hour esophageal pH monitoring and the change in symptom intensity score after treatment, suggesting that the higher the esophageal acid exposure, the greater the response to the PPI test in patients with GERD-related NCCP.[22]

Economic analysis also showed that the PPI test for GERD-related NCCP is a cost-saving approach primarily due to significant reduction in the usage of various costly, invasive diagnostic tests.[88]

In patients with NCCP, the PPI test was evaluated using a cost minimization analysis.[88] The PPI test was found to save $573 per average patient with NCCP undergoing diagnostic evaluation. The test was associated with an 81% reduction in the number of upper endoscopies and 79% reduction in the number of ambulatory 24-hour esophageal pH tests. This significant reduction is due to the high positive predictive value of the PPI test for patients with GERD-related NCCP.

When a decision-analytic model utilizing Bayesian analysis was developed to compare the costs and outcomes of alternative diagnostic strategies for NCCP, noninvasive strategies utilizing the PPI test as the initial step resulted in significant cost savings as compared to invasive strategies. These cost savings were a direct result of a significant reduction in the utilization of invasive diagnostic tests that are of unproven utility in the diagnosis and subsequent management of patients with NCCP.[111]

Multichannel Intraluminal Impedance

The combination of an impedance catheter and a pH probe provides a unique opportunity to study physiologic and pathologic events within the esophagus and their relationship to symptoms. In addition, the recording assembly can disclose the characteristics of the gastric refluxate (acidic, weakly acidic, alkaline, gas, liquid, and mixed gas and liquid). The specific value of the multichannel intraluminal impedance plus pH sensor and the documentation of weakly acidic reflux in patients with NCCP remains to be elucidated.

The combined multichannel intraluminal impedance and manometry testing has been useful in determining bolus transport patterns, bolus transit parameters, and bolus clearance in patients with esophageal motor disorders and a variety of symptoms including chest pain.[112] The true value of this technique has not been specifically evaluated in patients with NCCP.

Esophageal Dysmotility

In approximately a third of the patients with non–GERD-related NCCP, various esophageal motility abnormalities have been described.[29,30,113] Thus, in NCCP, esophageal manometry is commonly performed if GERD has been excluded as the underlying cause.[8] The role of esophageal manometry in NCCP has evolved over the last few years, primarily due to lack of effective treatment for the various esophageal motility abnormalities. This was compounded by clinical evidence that patients with non–GERD-related NCCP reported symptom improvement on pain modulators regardless if esophageal dysmotility was present or absent (except for achalasia).[114] Consequently, the role of esophageal manometry in non–GERD-related NCCP appears to be limited to identifying the small number of patients with achalasia.[31]

Esophageal Manometry

Esophageal manometry is the best tool to detect motility disorders of the esophagus. Evaluation of the amplitude of the esophageal contraction wave, its configuration, and propagation as well as the function of the upper and lower esophageal sphincters may be provided.[115]

The relationship between motility abnormalities diagnosed in NCCP patients and chest pain remains controversial. In a large retrospective study of patients with NCCP, only 28% were found to have esophageal dysmotility during esophageal manometry.[29] Nutcracker esophagus was the most common motility disorder (48%) followed by nonspecific esophageal motility disorder (36%), diffuse esophageal spasm (10%), hypertensive LES (4%), and achalasia (2%).

In NCCP patients with esophageal dysmotility, some have stipulated that esophageal spasm, for example, may be the cause of chest pain either by distending the proximal segment of the esophagus (leading to activation of mechanoreceptors) or by producing myoischemia (activation of chemoreceptors).[116] However, in patients with NCCP, documented esophageal manometry abnormalities are rarely associated with symptoms. Therefore, some have suggested that maybe these abnormalities are not the direct cause of patients' chest pain but rather a marker of an underlying motor disorder.[117] Consequently, documenting the presence of an esophageal motility disorder during esophageal manometry (except achalasia) does not conclusively prove that it is the underlying cause of patients' chest pain. This should not be surprising, as this test assesses patients in a fasting, supine state, free of exogenous influences, and with a rapid succession of wet and/or dry swallows.

The role of high-resolution esophageal manometry in evaluating NCCP patients remains unknown.

Provocative Testing

In order to enhance the value of esophageal manometry in providing a definitive diagnosis, pharmacological provocative agents have been used to elicit chest pain while monitoring changes in esophageal amplitude contractions.

Edrophonium (Tensilon) Test

The edrophonium (Tensilon) test has been used pharmacologically to induce esophageal dysmotility and chest pain in patients with NCCP. Edrophonium is an anticholinesterase that increases cholinergic activity at muscarinic receptors.[118] The pharmacologic action of this short-acting drug is manifested within 30 to 60 seconds after injection and lasts an average of 10 minutes. The aim of the edrophonium test is to induce greater esophageal body amplitude contractions in the hope of provoking the patient's typical chest pain.[119] The test is performed by injection of either 80 mg/kg or 10 mg edrophonium intravenously (IV), immediately followed by 5 to 10 swallows of 5 to 10 mL of water over a period of 5 to 10 minutes. The pain occurs during swallowing within 5 minutes after the administration of the drug and disappears as the drug is quickly metabolized.[20] Overall, the side effects are minimal, and the antidote atropine is rarely required. Side effects include increased salivation, nausea, vomiting, and abdominal cramps.

The sensitivity of the edrophonium test is relatively low. Studies have shown that the edrophonium test is positive in approximately 30% of patients with normal baseline esophageal manometry.[120,121] Consequently, the usage of the edrophonium test has declined in the last decade.

Ergonovine Stimulation Test

The ergonovine stimulation test has been demonstrated to induce augmentation of esophageal contractions and chest pain in patients with NCCP. Ergonovine is a sympathomimetic agent of the ergot alkaloid group. The drug is reportedly as effective as edrophonium in the provocation of chest pain in NCCP patients, but the side effects are more common and could potentially be fatal (coronary artery spasm). Thus, ergonovine is rarely used today in clinical practice in the evaluation of NCCP.[20]

Pentagastrin Stimulation Test

Pentagastrin directly stimulates esophageal smooth muscle, especially in patients with primary esophageal dysmotility. Its sensitivity to inducing pain in patients with NCCP is low, and presently the drug is no longer used for NCCP provocative testing.[20]

SENSORY TESTING OF THE ESOPHAGUS

The esophagus, like the rest of the viscera, receives dual sensory innervation, traditionally referred to as parasympathetic and sympathetic because the sensory nerves are anatomically associated with the autonomic nervous system, but more properly based on the actual nerves, vagal and spinal (Fig. 62.8).[122] The vagal afferent neurons compose 80% of the vagal trunk and have cell bodies in the nodose ganglia.[123] Vagal afferents whose receptive fields are located in the esophageal smooth muscle layer are sensitive to mechanical distension, whereas polymodal (responding to multiple modalities of stimuli) vagal afferents with receptive fields in the mucosa are sensitive to various chemical or mechanical intraluminal stimuli, which, under normal circumstances, are not associated with conscious perception.[124] In general, vagal afferents do not play a direct role in visceral pain transmission at the level of the gut, except for certain types of vagal afferents that appear to have a pain modulatory effect.[125] Recent reports suggest that vagal afferents may also play a role in perception of esophageal distension.[125,126] In contrast, spinal afferents, which have their cell bodies in the dorsal root ganglia, are primarily acting as nociceptors and are central to the perception of discomfort and pain.[127] Spinal afferents with receptive fields in the muscle layer and serosa are primarily mechanosensitive. The intraepithelial nerve endings of spinal afferent are likely to be involved in mediating acid-induced pain during topical exposure to intraluminal acid.[21,128] Many of the afferents contain calcitonin gene-related peptide and substance P, which are neurotransmitters that are important in mediating visceral nociception.[123]

Data regarding cortical loci involved in processing of esophageal sensation in humans are relatively scarce.[129] Nonpainful esophageal balloon distensions elicit bilateral activation along the central sulcus, the insular cortex, and the frontal and parietal operculum.[50] In contrast, painful esophageal balloon distensions result in intense activation of the same areas and additional activation of the right anterior insular cortex (important in affective processing) and anterior cingulate gyrus (important in pain processing and generating an affective and cognitive response to pain).[135–137] Nonpainful infusion of 0.1N hydrochloric acid resulted in cerebral cortical activity that was concentrated in the posterior cingulate and the parietal and anteromesial frontal lobes.[49] The superior frontal lobe regions activated corresponded to Brodmann area 32, the insula, the operculum, and the anterior cingulate.

Chest pain symptoms may represent an activation of a common pathway in response to different intraesophageal stimuli. Different intraesophageal stimuli (e.g., acid and balloon distension) may elicit similar symptoms in different patients or different symptoms in the same patient.[21,130] Thus, esophageal symptoms such as heartburn or chest pain are not stimulus specific.

A recent study demonstrated that chest pain and heartburn may be provoked in normal subjects during esophageal balloon distension either in the proximal or distal portion of the esophagus.[21] Volume thresholds for heartburn and chest pain in both esophageal locations were similar, suggesting that, for a specific volume, some patients develop chest pain and others heartburn. Furthermore, volume thresholds for both chest pain and heartburn did not differ significantly at each esophageal location and between locations. In this study, esophageal balloon distension reproduced typical heartburn symptoms in some patients with documented GERD and chest pain in others. This study clearly demonstrates that balloon distension may result in different types of esophageal symptoms.

The mechanism by which an esophageal stimulus causes heartburn in some patients and chest pain in others remains poorly understood. Balaban and colleagues[34] have demonstrated a temporal correlation between sustained contractions of the esophageal longitudinal muscle and both spontaneous and provoked esophageal chest pain. In a subsequent study that assessed the temporal relationship between sustained esophageal longitudinal muscle contractions and heartburn,[35] the investigators suggested that shorter duration of the sustained esophageal contraction was associated with heartburn and longer duration with chest pain.

Perception of intraesophageal events, either physiologic or pathologic, is a complicated process that involves central and peripheral mechanisms. Several studies have shown that most intraesophageal stimuli are not perceived by subjects.[131] For example, less than 20% of all acid reflux events result in GERD symptoms, regardless of whether mucosal injury is present.[131] It is yet to be elucidated what factors determine perception of an intraesophageal event, leading to symptom generation. In GERD, it has been demonstrated that the actual hydrogen ion concentration (H+) of the refluxate, the summation of several short reflux events, the distribution of acid along the esophagus (proximal migration), or the nadir or duration of acid reflux events.[129] Several studies have demonstrated that fat and other nutrients can modulate perception of intraluminal events that are mediated by gut neurotransmitters, hormones, or enzymes. Meyer and colleagues have shown that intraduodenal fat significantly shortened latency to onset of heartburn and intensified the perception of

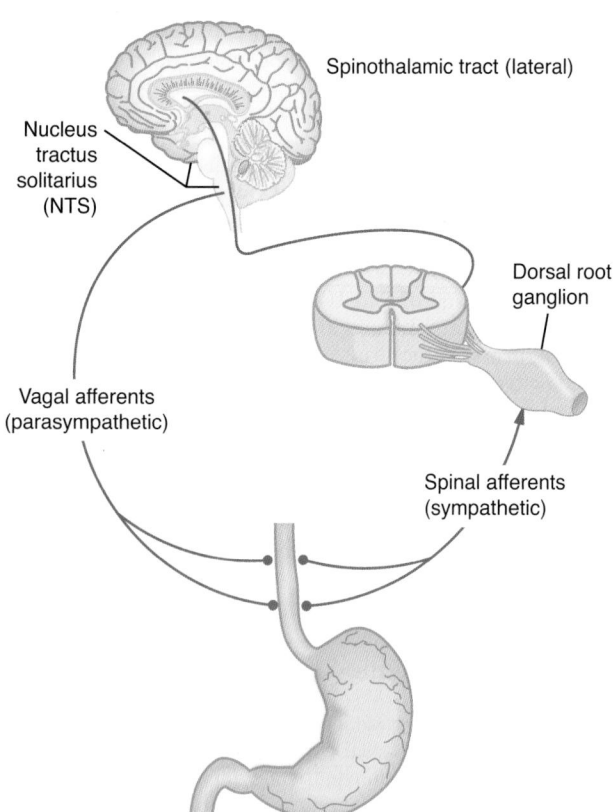

FIGURE 62.8 Esophageal sensory afferent pathways. (Redrawn after Fass R. Sensory testing of the esophagus. *J Clin Gastroenterol* 2004;38(8): 628–641, with permission.)

acid-induced heartburn in subjects with GERD who underwent intraesophageal acid perfusion.[132]

Central neural mechanisms seem to have an important role in modulating esophageal perception also.[133] Psychological comorbidity (e.g., anxiety and depression) can modulate esophageal perception and cause subjects to perceive low-intensity esophageal stimuli (pathologic or physiologic) as being painful.[134] Another important factor is stress that seems to enhance perception of intraesophageal stimuli by reducing perception thresholds for pain.[135] Stress has recently emerged as an important factor in symptom generation and exacerbation of both functional and organic GI disorders.[136] Traditionally, stress is considered a domain of psychology and, thus, commonly lumped together with the role of psychiatric comorbidity.[55] However, recent developments in the understanding of brain–gut interactions in functional bowel disorders resulted in reassessment of the role of chronic stress in the pathophysiology and management of GI disorders such as NCCP. Certain stressful life events have been associated with the onset or symptom exacerbation of functional bowel disorders. In addition, daily experiences of stress seem to have an important modulating effect on perception of intraluminal events.

Other central factors, such as sleep quality, may also alter perception of intraesophageal events.[136a] Further research is needed to better define the brain–gut (or gut–brain) relationship as it relates to symptom generation in esophageal disorders.

Acid Perfusion Test (Bernstein Test)

The acid perfusion test was introduced as an objective method to identify esophageal chemosensitivity to acid.[137] A nasogastric tube was passed through the nares of a fasting, sitting subject and into the stomach.[137,138] After the gastric content was aspirated, the tube was withdrawn until it measured 30 cm from the nares to the tip.[138] This maneuver assumed that the solution would be delivered at a level near the junction of the upper and middle thirds of the esophagus. The tube was connected to an IV bottle. A control administration of 0.9% NaCl was perfused for 10 to 15 minutes at a rate of 6 to 7.5 mL per minute. This was followed by administration of 0.1N hydrochloric acid, at a similar rate, for 30 minutes or until discomfort was induced.[138] If symptoms appeared, the test was discontinued and saline solution was given.

The acid perfusion test was originally devised to distinguish between chest pain of cardiac and esophageal origin. However, since the initial description, many modifications have been made to the original Bernstein test. Although the basic principle of the test remained similar, many investigators have tried different acid perfusion rates, concentrations, and durations in the hope of increasing the sensitivity of the test.[78,139–145] Furthermore, some have even suggested the addition of bile salts to the acid solution.[146]

Many attempts were made to change the test from a qualitative to a quantitative tool. Time to onset of symptoms during acid perfusion was used to compare the extent of chemosensitivity to acid between GERD and Barrett patients.[147] Fass and colleagues[21] placed a manometry catheter 10 cm above the upper border of the LES to ensure sufficient exposure of the esophageal mucosa to acid. Saline was infused initially for 2 minutes and then without the patient's knowledge 0.1N hydrochloric acid was infused for 10 minutes at a rate of 10 mL per minute. Patients were instructed to report whenever their typical symptoms were reproduced. Esophageal chemosensitivity was assessed by both the latency until typical symptom perception was induced (expressed in seconds) and the total sensory intensity rating reported by the subject at the end of acid perfusion by using a verbal descriptor scale. The scale consisted of a 20-cm vertical bar flanked by descriptors of increasing intensity (no sensation, faint,

very weak, weak, very mild, mild, moderate, barely strong, slightly intense, strong, intense, very intense, and extremely intense). Placement of words along the side of the scale was determined from their relative log intensity rating in a normative study.[148] The validity of these scales for assessing the perceived intensity of visceral sensations has been confirmed.[149]

An acid perfusion test intensity score (cm $\times$ seconds) was then calculated as follows: $I \times T/100$, where I is the total intensity rating at the end of acid perfusion and T is the duration of report of typical symptom perception during the test. For convenience, the score was divided by 100.

The test is highly specific but the sensitivity ranges from 6% to 60%.[150–157] A negative test has no clinical relevance and does not exclude esophageal origin.

Presently, the acid perfusion test is rarely performed in clinical practice because of its limited diagnostic value in NCCP and other esophageal disorders. Because of the low sensitivity and the emergence of noninvasive and highly sensitive modalities, such as the PPI test and empirical therapy with a PPI, many authors have considered the acid perfusion test to be obsolete.[78,158,159]

Electrical Stimulation

Electrical stimulation of the esophagus has been used by several research groups to study visceral perception and cortical responses to different intensities of intraesophageal stimuli. The technique has yet to be standardized and published protocols are difficult to compare.

Electrical stimulation of the esophageal mucosa is performed by using a 5-mm stainless steel electrode attached to a standard manometric catheter assembly.[160] The electrode is made from fine stainless steel wire wrapped around the end of the catheter and fixed with surgical silk.[161] The electrodes are connected to an electrical stimulator. The catheter assembly is then passed through the nostril and the electrode is placed in the esophagus. Electrical stimuli are applied repeatedly in a series of 24 stimuli (duration 200 μs at 0.2 Hz). A reference electrode is placed on the abdominal wall, 5 cm below the xiphoid process. Electrical stimulation of the upper and lower esophagus can be achieved by 2 pairs of silver/silver chloride bipolar ring electrodes located at 5 and 20 cm proximal to the tip of the catheter.[43]

The ascending stimulus paradigm includes stimuli that are delivered at a frequency of 0.2 Hz at intensities between 0 and 100 mA.[43] Severity and qualitative perceptual responses are usually assessed by a verbal descriptor.[162] Descriptors are used in ascending order of severity. Sensory threshold is the intensity (measured in mA) at which the participant reports faint sensation, and pain threshold is the intensity at which the participant reports an intense sensation.[43] A somewhat different stimulus paradigm is used in patients who undergo recording of cerebral evoked responses to esophageal electrical stimulation.[37]

Intraluminal Ultrasonography

High-frequency intraluminal ultrasonography has been introduced as a novel modality to study the relationship between esophageal motor events and symptoms. The technique has been a useful tool for evaluating smooth muscle contractions.[33] Esophageal ultrasonography can be performed continuously using a catheter-based probe, which allows direct visualization of changes in smooth muscle conformation.[34] The capability of intraluminal ultrasonography to evaluate changes in the thickness of the longitudinal muscle of the esophagus has been used to determine the relationship between esophageal symptoms and motor changes of the esophageal wall. Although the technique has yet to be standardized, investigators have used an esophageal catheter assembly that included a 12.5-MHz ultrasound transducer, solid-state pressure catheter, and monopolar antimony pH catheter.[34] The ultrasound transducer was placed 5 cm above the LES. The 24-hour recordings were analyzed every 2 seconds for a period of 2 minutes before and 30 seconds after the onset of the studied symptom. Rules for image analysis remain at the discretion of the investigator. Because of the limited number of centers that are proficient with this technique, image analysis is primarily operator dependent and interobserver and intraobserver agreements have yet to be determined.

Using intraluminal ultrasonography, Balaban and colleagues demonstrated that most chest pain episodes in patients with NCCP were preceded by sustained thickening of the esophageal smooth muscle wall due to longitudinal muscle contraction that was not detected by esophageal manometry catheter.[34] The same muscular changes were noted after edrophonium-induced chest pain. The authors suggested that the duration rather than the magnitude of the longitudinal muscle contraction is the determining factor for generating esophageal pain. In this study, swallow-associated longitudinal muscle contractions lasted an average of 6.4 seconds, whereas contractions associated with chest pain persisted for a mean of 68.0 seconds. Similar studies in patients with GERD revealed that the mean duration of sustained longitudinal muscle contractions during heartburn was 44.9 seconds.[35] The motor changes were also observed in patients who reported heartburn that was unrelated to acid reflux events, further supporting the investigator's hypothesis that this sustained esophageal muscle contraction is responsible for generation of esophageal symptoms, such as chest pain and heartburn.

Even though high-frequency intraluminal ultrasonography has been a valuable research tool to assess the biomechanics of the human esophagus, its exact role in evaluating esophageal-related symptoms has not been fully elucidated.[163] Initial studies provided intriguing data, but other investigators have yet to replicate these findings. Additionally, sustained contractions of the esophageal longitudinal muscle may represent an epiphenomenon that occurs with symptoms, rather than being the trigger for symptoms.

Balloon Distension

Balloon distension has been used primarily for research purposes to determine perception thresholds for pain. This modality has been used extensively in studies of various functional bowel disorders, most notably irritable bowel syndrome, functional dyspepsia, and NCCP.[40,164,165]

More than 40 years ago, intraesophageal balloon distension in humans was reported to produce pain referred to the chest.[166] Early data indicated that, in patients with documented ischemic heart disease, balloon distension of the esophagus produced pain indistinguishable from anginal pain, but without ECG changes.[167] This may be explained by convergence of sensory pathways at the level of spinal cord or in the midbrain. Despite this similarity in pain, it seems that esophageal balloon distension itself has no effect on coronary function or blood flow.[168]

Balloon distension was reintroduced during the mid-1980s in a seminal study that evaluated perception thresholds for pain in patients with NCCP.[40] The latex balloon was attached to a manometric catheter and filled with air. The balloon was positioned 10 cm above the LES and distended in a stepwise fashion using a handheld syringe.

A further development in the balloon distension technique was the introduction of a pump that was powered by compressed air.[39] The pump ensured inflations at a predetermined rate, which was difficult to achieve with a handheld syringe. However, neither system was able to provide concomitant pressure measurements that could have been helpful to determine whether the balloon remained within the esophageal lumen during each inflation. This was particularly critical in protocols that inflated bal-

loons within the distal portion of the esophagus. Fass and colleagues[21] demonstrated that balloon distension in the esophagus resulted in phasic esophageal contractions that increased with increase in balloon volume. These powerful contractions, in association with shortening of the esophagus, may propel the balloon into the stomach without being recognized by the subject or the investigator. Concomitant pressure measurements would have been helpful to detect the migration of the balloon into the gastric fundus by demonstrating a sudden decrease in intraluminal pressure despite continued increase in the balloon's volume.

The introduction of the electronic barostat, a computer-driven volume-displacement device, has helped to ensure proper location of the balloon, regardless of inflation paradigm that was used.[169] The basic principle of the barostat is to maintain a constant pressure within the balloon/bag in the lumen despite muscular contractions and relaxations.[113,169] To maintain a constant pressure, the barostat aspirates air with contractions and injects air with relaxations. Presently, many prefer the use of a polyethylene bag to that of a latex balloon. Bags are infinitely compliant and show no increase in intra-bag pressure until about 90% of the maximum bag volume has been achieved.[169,170] In contrast, latex balloons resist inflation and thus show a rapid increase in intra-balloon pressure with small volumes of distension.[21,169,171] When the pressure increases above the elastance threshold, the balloon becomes plastic and accommodates large volumes of air with very little change in pressure.[169,170] For tubular organs in the GI tract, such as the esophagus, experts recommend the use of a cylindrical bag (rather than the spherical) with a fixed length.[21,169]

Barostats have been used extensively in studies evaluating rectosigmoid and gastric perception thresholds for pain. However, this technique has been rarely used to assess esophageal mechanosensitivity in humans. Unlike the rectum and the stomach, the esophagus does not serve as a storage organ, but rather as a conduit. Consequently, intraesophageal distensions do not mimic a normal, physiologic stimulus and thus perceptual responses to such a stimulus may have no scientific merit. This factor, in addition to the patient's difficulties in tolerating balloon distension, which commonly results in poor recruitment rates as well as the potential for esophageal perforation, have made esophageal balloon distensions by a barostat a less attractive research tool.

Various distension protocols have been used in different studies. Like any other technique that assesses esophageal sensation, balloon distension has yet to be standardized. Slow ramp distension is an ascending method that involves slow (rate varies from one study to another) increase in volume or pressure of the balloon usually until the desired perceptual response has been reported by the subject.[21,46,172] In contrast, phasic distensions are rapid inflations of the balloon that can be delivered in random sequence or double random staircase.[21,46] The latter includes two series of distension stimuli (staircases), and the computer alternates between the two staircases on a random basis.[21,169,172] With the tracking method, the barostat is programmed to deliver a series of intermittent phasic stimuli separated by interpulse rest period within an interactive stimulus tracking procedure.[21,173,174] If the subject indicates a sensation below the tracked intensity then the following stimulus will increase in pressure. If the subject reports the desired sensation, then the following pressure step is randomized to stay the same or decrease. The random element is placed to mask the relationship between ratings and subsequent stimulus change, and, therefore, decrease potential scaling bias.[39]

Quantification of perceptual responses depends on the characteristics of the mechanoreceptors in a specific region of the GI tract. Volume or pressure distension can be considered the most physiologic stimuli.[165,175] The most reliable reports of esophageal sensory thresholds are obtained during volume distension. Although the overall pressure-volume curve is linear, the pressure at any given volume may vary because of the presence or absence of a superimposed esophageal phasic contractions.[21] Despite this physiologic phenomenon, other investigators rely primarily on pressure when performing balloon studies in the esophagus.

Commonly, qualitative and quantitative perceptual responses are evaluated during balloon distension studies. Qualitative perceptual responses include symptom reports in response to balloon distension, such as chest pain, heartburn, bloating, and fullness, among others.[21,176] Heartburn is a common sensation that occurs during balloon distension and may mimic the patient's typical heartburn symptom.[176] Quantitative perceptual responses are commonly obtained during slow-ramp distension and include the minimal distension volume or pressure at which the individual first reports moderate sensation (innocuous sensation), discomfort, and pain (aversive sensation).[21] Discomfort threshold is commonly defined as the first unpleasant esophageal sensation, and pain threshold is defined as the first sensation of pain.[21]

Pitfalls that may modify perceptual responses to balloon distension include the following: increased rate of balloon distension results in reported perception at lower volumes or pressures[177]; longer durations of balloon distension are more likely to elicit sensation than shorter durations[177]; elderly subjects demonstrate diminished visceral pain perception and female patients seem to have lower perception thresholds for pain compared with male patients[178–180]; and the proximal esophagus has been suggested to be more sensitive to chemical and mechanical stimuli than the distal esophagus.[21,181] Additionally, reduced sensitivity to intraluminal stimuli has been demonstrated in specific patient populations, such as those with Barrett mucosa or esophageal stricture.[147,182,183] A recent study demonstrated the development of secondary hypersensitivity in the adjacent portion of the esophagus that was not sensitized by a chemical stimulus (acid).[43]

Balloon studies are primarily designed to assess the presence of visceral hypersensitivity in various esophageal disorders. Early studies demonstrated that pain develops with balloon distension more frequently in NCCP patients than in normal control subjects and that their pain occurs at smaller volumes.[39,40,184] Short-term sensitization of mechanosensitive afferent pathways by transient exposure to irritants has been shown in both humans and animal models of visceral hypersensitivity.[45,185] Human studies that evaluated the effect of esophageal acid perfusion on perception of esophageal distension in healthy control subjects and patients with GERD had varying results.[45,73,186,187]

Mehta and colleagues[45] reported that perfusion of the esophagus with 0.1N hydrochloric acid for 30 minutes resulted in enhanced sensitivity to esophageal balloon distension. Similarly, Sarkar and colleagues[187] reported that acid perfusion into the distal esophagus was associated with the development of mechanical hypersensitivity in the proximal esophagus, which had not been exposed to acid, suggesting the development of secondary visceral hypersensitivity. Peghini and coworkers[73] found a lowering of the pain threshold to distension only in those individuals who were symptomatic during acid perfusion.[186] In contrast, De-Vault[186] reported that a 15-minute acid perfusion had no significant effect on pain perception during esophageal distension. The mechanisms underlying the sensitizing effect of acute tissue irritation on visceral afferent pathways have been well characterized in the form of peripheral and central sensitization.[127] Such sensitization manifests as increased background activity of sensory neurons, the lowering of nociceptive thresholds, changes in stimulus response curves, and enlargement of receptive fields. During a noxious event, a series of counter-regulatory mechanisms are activated that are aimed at containing the development of both the acute and any long-lasting sensitization.[127]

Studies evaluating balloon distensions in patients with chronic acid exposure or esophageal mucosal injury are scarce. Fass and colleagues demonstrated that mild to moderate chronic tissue injury in GERD differentially affects mechanosensitive and chemosensitive afferent pathways.[21] GERD patients showed enhanced perception of acid perfusion but not of esophageal distension. Chemosensitivity but not mechanosensitivity was correlated

with reflux symptoms and with the degree of endoscopically shown tissue injury at baseline. Trimble and coworkers evaluated patients with heartburn and excess reflux defined by abnormal upper endoscopy or 24-hour esophageal pH monitoring and compared them with patients with heartburn and a normal 24-hour pH test. The results demonstrated that the latter group had lower volume thresholds for perception of esophageal balloon distension and discomfort.[134] This study suggests that patients with typical heartburn who lack any evidence of excess acid are highly sensitive to mechanical stimuli.

Balloon distension has been commonly used to assess the effect of various drugs on esophageal sensory perception. Imipramine, octreotide, and nifedipine have all been shown to increase perception thresholds for pain in normal controls or patients with NCCP.[188–192]

Esophageal-Evoked Potentials

Cerebral evoked potentials reflect electrical activity of the brain in response to visual, auditory, somatosensory, and visceral stimuli. There is a clear relationship between stimulus frequency, using esophageal electrical stimulation, and amplitude of cerebral evoked potentials.[193] Studies have demonstrated that a significant and progressive decrease of evoked potential amplitudes is associated with increasing stimulus frequency. This suggests a rapid attenuation of the cerebral autonomic responses with increased frequency of electrical stimulation.[193] Furthermore, a stimulus intensity-response relationship has been shown in brain response to increasing stimulus intensity, which is probably explained by increased recruitment of afferent fibers.[193,194]

Balloon distension and electrical stimulation protocols have been used in studies assessing cerebral-evoked potentials in response to esophageal stimulation. It is unclear if one of the sensory testing methods is better than the other.

Esophageal balloon distension triggers a characteristic triphasic evoked potential.[195] Two negative peaks (N1 and N2) and 1 positive peak (P1) can be demonstrated. Latency is the time in milliseconds from the stimulus to the peak. There is a considerable intersubject variability but almost no intrasubject variability when recording cerebral-evoked potentials. Studies in normal subjects have shown significantly shorter latencies during balloon distension in the proximal esophagus as compared with the distal esophagus.[196]

Assessment of patients with NCCP, using the esophageal balloon distension paradigm, revealed that amplitude and quality of cerebral-evoked potentials increased with increasing sensation, while the latencies remained stable.[195] Additionally, the amplitude and quality of evoked potentials were lower in NCCP patients as compared with controls. Similar levels of sensation were produced by lower balloon volumes in NCCP patients.[193]

Esophageal stimulation and cerebral-evoked potentials may provide clues to the pathway and type of neurons involved in nociception.[197] Additionally, cerebral-evoked potentials were used to identify brain areas that are responsible for esophageal pain sensation.[198,199]

Brain Imaging

In addition to cortical-evoked potentials, other techniques have been increasingly used to evaluate the brain–gut relationship in patients with esophageal disorders. These techniques include PET and fMRI. The GI is intricately connected to the central nervous system by pathways that are continuously sampling and modulating gut function.[200]

PET scanning is an established method to study the functional neuroanatomy of the human brain.[201,202] Radio-labeled compounds allow the study of biochemical and physiologic processes involved in cerebral metabolism.[200] Tomographic images represent spatial distribution of radioisotopes in the brain. Regional cerebral blood flow is studied with labeled water (H215O) and glucose metabolism with 18Fl-labeled fluorodeoxyglucose. Unlike PET, fMRI does not require radioisotopes and, hence, is considered a safer imaging technique. fMRI detects increases in oxygen concentration in areas of heightened neuronal activity.[195, 201,203] This imaging technique is best suited for locating the site but not the sequence or duration of neuronal activity. Overall, fMRI provides both anatomic and functional information.

Thus far, only a few studies have attempted to assess the cortical process of esophageal sensation in humans. Aziz and colleagues examined the human brain loci involved in the process of esophageal sensation using PET and distal esophageal balloon distension in eight healthy volunteers.[50] Nonpainful stimuli elicited bilateral activation along the central sulcus, insular cortex, and the frontal and parietal operculum. Painful stimuli resulted in intense activation of the same areas and additional activation of right anterior insular cortex and anterior cingulate gyrus. The former is important in affective processing while the latter is important in pain processing and generating an affective and cognitive response to pain.[204–206] In another study, Kern and colleagues evaluated activation of cerebral cortical responses to esophageal mucosal acid exposure by using an fMRI.[49] Ten healthy subjects underwent intraesophageal perfusion of 0.1N hydrochloric acid over 10 minutes. None of the study subjects reported GERD symptoms during acid perfusion. Cerebral cortical activity was concentrated in the posterior cingulate, parietal, and anteromesial frontal lobes. The superior frontal lobe regions activated in this study corresponded to Brodmann area 32, the insula, the operculum, and the anterior cingulate.

Further studies are needed to assess cerebral activation in patients with different esophageal disorders. In addition, it would be of great interest to determine whether there are differences in central processing of an intraesophageal stimulus in patients with NCCP, nonerosive reflux disease, or functional heartburn. It is also important to begin to examine the role of psychophysiologic states such as stress, anxiety, and depression and their effects on central nuclei involved with perception of esophageal stimuli.

Sensory Testing—Pitfalls in Study Design

Surprisingly, many studies using esophageal sensory testing to evaluate sensory perception thresholds are afflicted with design flaws that make interpretation of the results very difficult. Studies using balloon distension paradigms in the distal esophagus, without simultaneously measuring intra-esophageal pressure, are inherently flawed because of the tendency of the balloon to migrate into the stomach due to esophageal contraction and shortening in response to distension of the balloon. Other common pitfalls include using different rates of balloon distension or acid perfusion, different balloon distension paradigms, or more commonly using an inappropriate control group. For example, a study that compares esophageal sensory testing of patients with Barrett esophagus versus normal controls, and uses a younger control group, is likely to bias the study results. Patients with Barrett esophagus are commonly older, and age per se (being older) increases perception thresholds for pain.[182] Thus, it will be difficult to discern if the Barrett epithelium or the difference in age is responsible for patients' alteration in pain perception.

Studies that evaluate esophageal sensory testing in irritable bowel syndrome (IBS) patients, as compared with normal controls and use a more gender diverse control group, are also hard to interpret. IBS patients are commonly women and a control group that is composed of a significant number of men may bias the results toward the IBS group unrelated to the underlying disorder (IBS). Men, as compared with women, demonstrate an increase of perception thresholds for pain in response to esophageal stimuli.

Ensuring a similar study protocol and age as well as gender matched control group will reduce the potential bias in esophageal sensory testing studies. However, because of lack of standardization in study design, comparison between studies remains a difficult task.

TREATMENT

Treatment for NCCP should be targeted toward the specific underlying mechanism responsible for the patient's symptoms. Table 62.4 provides a general treatment plan for NCCP.

GERD-Related NCCP

Lifestyle modifications include elevation of the head of the bed, weight loss, smoking cessation, and avoidance of alcohol, coffee, fresh citrus juice, and other food products as well as medications that can exacerbate reflux such as opioids, benzodiazepines, and calcium-channel blockers.[207, 208] While these lifestyle modifications are commonly advocated as first line treatment in GERD patients, there is no evidence to support their efficacy in GERD-related NCCP. Regardless, enthusiasm about lifestyle modifications is very high among physicians, and thus it is highly likely that GERD-related NCCP subjects will be instructed to follow them.

The efficacy of histamine (H$_2$) receptor antagonists in controlling symptoms in patients with GERD-related NCCP has been shown to range from 42% to 52%.[209] In one study, cimetidine (unknown dose) and antacids were shown to be effective in only 42% of the patients with GERD-related NCCP who were followed for a period of 2 to 3 years.[210] Stepping down GERD therapy from a PPI to an H$_2$ receptor antagonist has been disappointing in GERD-related NCCP patients.

Omeprazole (Prilosec) 20 mg twice daily or placebo was administered over a period of 8 weeks to GERD-related NCCP patients in the only double-blind placebo-controlled trial that

---

TABLE 62.4

TREATMENT PLAN FOR NCCP

GERD-related NCCP	PPIs, double dose for at least 2 months
Dysmotility-related NCCP	• Achalasia: Medical, endoscopic, and surgical therapy • Nutcracker esophagus: Treat for GERD first. If no response, pain modulator • Spastic motility disorder: Pain modulator
Chest pain of presumed esophageal origin	Pain modulators, low dose, and at bedtime (long term)

has been performed.[211] Patients who received omeprazole had a significant reduction in both the number of days with chest pain and in their chest pain severity scores compared to the patients who received placebo. Thus far, most of the studies assessing the efficacy of PPIs in NCCP primarily utilized omeprazole. However, it is likely that all other PPIs would demonstrate similar efficacy. In fact, a recent open-label study with esomeprazole (Nexium) administered 40 mg once daily over a period of 1 month demonstrated complete resolution of symptoms in 57.1% of subjects with either NCCP or laryngeal manifestations of GERD.[212] In another open-label study, 85% of NCCP patients reported symptom relief or improvement after receiving PPI twice daily (different brands) for a period of 3 months.[213]

A retrospective review of patients' files revealed that PPIs reduce the number of chest pain episodes, emergency department visits, and hospitalizations due to chest pain in subjects with documented CAD.[214] It is likely that GERD-related symptoms contribute to the medical-seeking behavior of this patient population.

Patients with GERD-related NCCP should be treated with at least double the standard dose of PPI until symptoms remit, followed by dose tapering to determine the lowest PPI dose that can control symptoms. As with other extraesophageal manifestations of GERD, NCCP patients may require more than 2 months of therapy for optimal symptom control. Long-term maintenance PPI treatment has been shown to be highly effective.[215] Borzecki and colleagues[216] developed a decision tree to compare empiric treatments for NCCP patients with H_2 receptor antagonists or standard-dose PPI for 8 weeks with initial investigations (upper endoscopy or upper GI series). Empiric treatment was more cost-effective in the initial investigation strategy, with a cost of $849 per patient versus $2,187 per patient.

The value of antireflux surgery in GERD-related NCCP is unclear. Several studies have demonstrated a significant improvement in symptoms following laparoscopic fundoplication in patients with GERD-related NCCP. For instance, Patti and associates reported improvement in chest pain symptoms following laparoscopic fundoplication in 85% of patients with GERD-related NCCP.[217] In addition, Farrell and coworkers reported that 90% of NCCP patients who underwent antireflux surgery experienced improvement in chest pain and 50% reported complete symptom resolution.[218] In contrast, So and colleagues reported that after laparoscopic fundoplication, relief of atypical GERD symptoms (e.g., chest pain) was less satisfactory than relief of typical GERD symptoms (e.g., heartburn).[219] In their study, the authors evaluated symptom improvement with a questionnaire given 3 months and 12 months after antireflux surgery. Overall, heartburn was relieved in 93% of patients, whereas only 48% of patients reported relief of chest pain symptoms.

Non–GERD-Related NCCP

The treatment of non–GERD-related NCCP is primarily based on esophageal pain modulation (Table 62.5). An important development in this field was the recognition that NCCP patients with spastic esophageal motor disorders (except achalasia), as docu-

TABLE 62.5

THERAPEUTIC MODALITIES OF NON-GERD-RELATED NCCP

- Muscle relaxants (nitrates, calcium channel blockers)
- Botulinum toxin injection
- Pain modulators (trazodone, TCAs, SSRIs, theophylline)
- Surgery for motility disorders
- Cognitive-behavioral therapy/hypnotherapy

mented by esophageal manometry, are more likely to respond to pain modulators than to muscle relaxants. Unfortunately, no large, well-designed studies to assess pain modulators in patients with non–GERD-related NCCP have been performed thus far.

Several recent studies have shown that most NCCP patients are managed by cardiologists and PCPs who appear to know little about the role and treatment of esophageal hypersensitivity in NCCP.[15,14,220] Even gastroenterologists appeared somewhat uninformed about the role of visceral hypersensitivity in NCCP.[221]

Nitroglycerin and long-acting nitrates cause relaxation of GI smooth muscles by stimulating cyclic guanosine monophosphate (GMP)-dependent pathways. Several open-label studies have reported that nitrates improve symptoms and esophageal motility patterns in patients with chest pain and esophageal dysmotility. Several investigators reported symptomatic improvement in patients with diffuse esophageal spasm (DES), accompanied by normalization of esophageal motility during treatment with nitrates.[222,223] In one small study, five patients with DES experienced a 4-year clinical and manometric remission.[224] However, other studies have failed to demonstrate similar efficacy.[225,226] Long-acting nitrates in doses of 10 to 20 mg two to three times daily, as well as short-acting, sublingual nitrates for acute episodes of chest pain in NCCP patients, were used in these studies.

Overall, studies that evaluated the value of nitrates in NCCP have been limited by small numbers of patients and inconsistent results in regard to drug efficacy. A placebo-controlled trial that excludes patients with GERD has yet to be performed.

Since calcium plays an important role in esophageal muscle contraction, the role of calcium channel blocking agents in patients with NCCP and esophageal spastic motility disorders has been the focus of investigation. Nifedipine (10–30 mg, by mouth, three times a day) decreases the amplitude and duration of esophageal contractions in patients with nutcracker esophagus after only 2 weeks.[121] Unfortunately, the effect of the drug disappeared after 6 weeks of treatment with the complete recurrence of symptoms. Davies and associates used a placebo-controlled trial to assess the efficacy of nifedipine in the prevention of symptomatic episodes of esophageal spasm in eight NCCP patients over a 6-week period.[227] The authors were unable to find statistically significant differences in symptom improvement between the two therapeutic arms. In contrast, symptom improvement was noted in 20 NCCP patients with various esophageal motility disorders, including hypertensive LES, nutcracker esophagus, DES, and vigorous achalasia, treated with nifedipine (10 mg, by mouth, three times a day).[228] Nifedipine was also found to significantly decrease LES resting pressure, with a direct correlation to the plasma levels of drug.[229]

Diltiazem (60–90 mg, by mouth, four times a day) for 8 weeks significantly improved mean chest pain scores and esophageal motility studies in patients with nutcracker esophagus when compared to placebo.[230, 231] However, in a study evaluating eight patients with DES, the effect of diltiazem in relieving chest pain was not different from the effect of placebo, probably due to the small number of patients who participated in the study.[232]

Other calcium channel blockers have been evaluated in patients with primary esophageal motor disorders including verapamil, fendiline, nimodipine (Nimotop; Bayer, West Haven, CT), and nisoldipine (Sular; Sciele, Alpharetta, GA), with various effects on LES resting pressure and esophageal amplitude contractions. Regardless, calcium channel blockers appear to have a transient esophageal motor effect that translates to a short-lived improvement in symptoms, compounded by a variety of side effects such as hypotension, bradycardia, and pedal edema.

Sildenafil (Viagra; Pfizer, New York, NY) is a potent selective inhibitor of cyclic GMP-specific PDE5 (phosphodiesterase 5), which inactivates nitric oxide–stimulated GMP. Intracellular accumulation of the latter induces smooth muscle relaxation. The drug has been shown to improve esophageal motility in patients with nutcracker esophagus or hypertensive LES by lowering LES resting pressure, reducing distal esophageal amplitude contractions, and prolonging the duration of LES relaxation.[233, 234] However, thus far, there have been no studies that specifically addressed NCCP patients, so the value of this compound in NCCP remains unknown. Additionally, the usage of this compound in NCCP will likely be limited by its cost and side effects.

The antispasmodic cimetropium bromide has been shown to be efficacious in eight NCCP patients with nutcracker esophagus when taken intravenously,[235] but clinical data regarding the efficacy of an oral formulation are still lacking. Hydralazine, an antihypertensive compound that directly dilates peripheral vessels, was shown to improve chest pain and dysphagia by decreasing the amplitude and duration of esophageal contractions in a small study of only five patients.[226] Overall, evidence to support the therapeutic benefit of anticholinergic agents for the treatment of NCCP remains very limited.

Pain Modulators

Visceral hypersensitivity is thought to be the primary underlying mechanism of patients with non–GERD-related NCCP, regardless of the presence or absence of esophageal motor disorder. Consequently, drugs that can alter esophageal pain perception have become the mainstay of therapy in these patients.

Several drugs have been shown to have a pain modulatory or a visceral analgesic effect, thus alleviating chest pain symptoms. These drugs include tricyclic antidepressants (TCAs), selective serotonin reuptake inhibitors (SSRIs), theophylline, and trazodone.

Several studies have demonstrated that antidepressants have a visceral analgesic effect,[236] but they also appear to inhibit calcium channels and thus may have an additional muscle relaxant-like effect.[237] TCAs have both central neuromodulatory and peripheral visceral analgesic effects. Several clinical trials have found favorable TCA-related effects on esophageal pain perception in both healthy subjects and patients with NCCP.

Imipramine, administered at a dose of 75 mg daily, significantly increases the pain threshold of healthy men during intraesophageal balloon distension as compared to baseline.[238] In another study, 60 patients with NCCP and normal coronary angiography were randomized to receive clonidine (0.2 mg daily), imipramine (50 mg nightly), or placebo for a period of 3 weeks. Patients who received imipramine had a significant (52%) reduction in the frequency of chest pain episodes, independent of cardiac, esophageal, or psychiatric test results, suggesting that imipramine has a visceral analgesic effect on chest pain.[239] In contrast, amitriptyline failed to show an effect on both perception and esophageal compliance in subjects undergoing balloon distension protocol.[240]

Because of their anticholinergic side effects, TCAs are commonly administered at nighttime. Based on our experience, it is recommended that TCA doses are slowly titrated to a maximum of 50 mg daily. The incremental increase in dosing should be based on symptom improvement and development of side effects.

Trazodone (100–150 mg, by mouth, four times a day) for 6 weeks showed a significant improvement in the symptoms of patients with NCCP and esophageal dysmotility as compared to placebo.[241] However, esophageal motility abnormalities remained unchanged. A small, open-label study reported symptom control and improved esophageal motility in patients with NCCP and DES following treatment with both trazodone and clomipramine.[242]

A randomized trial assessing the effect of sertraline in patients with NCCP demonstrated a significant reduction in pain scores, regardless of concomitant improvement in psychological scores.[243] In addition, a recent study demonstrated that citalopram, given 20 mg intravenously in a single dose, reduced chemical and mechanical esophageal hypersensitivity without altering esophageal motility.[244]

Octreotide, a synthetic analog of somatostatin, has been shown to increase rectal and sigmoid perception thresholds for pain in IBS subjects, as well as healthy subjects.[245,246] It has been postulated that the effect of octreotide is mediated by the activation of somatostatin receptors at the spinal cord and/or the supraspinal level.

Octreotide, administered 100 mg subcutaneously, was found to significantly increase perception thresholds for pain as compared to placebo in healthy subjects undergoing intraesophageal balloon distension.[247] Unfortunately, due to cost and the lack of an oral formulation, octreotide is rarely utilized for NCCP in clinical practice.

Theophylline, a xanthine derivative, has been shown to inhibit adenosine-induced angina-like chest pain and adenosine-induced pain in other regions of the body.[248] A study using an esophageal balloon distension protocol and impedance demonstrated that intravenous theophylline increased thresholds for sensation and pain in 75% of patients with functional chest pain.[249] Similar results were documented in functional chest pain patients receiving oral theophylline for a period of 3 months. In another study, the same authors showed that oral doses of theophylline 200 mg twice daily was more effective than placebo in preventing chest pain in 19 patients with functional chest pain (Fig. 62.9).[250]

Alprazolam has been shown in a study to ameliorate chest pain at a mean dose of 4.3 mg daily in patients with NCCP and panic disorder.[251] In this study, 15 out of 20 patients reported at least a 50% reduction in panic attack episodes and a corresponding decline in the frequency of chest pain episodes. Clonazepam, given 1 to 4 mg daily, was also shown to be effective in the treatment of patients with NCCP and panic disorder.[252] The treatment of a functional disorder such as NCCP with benzodiazepines has been greatly discouraged, primarily due to the likelihood of becoming addicted to this class of drugs.

Serotonin (5-HT) is a neurotransmitter present in the central nervous system, enteric neurons, and particularly in enterochromaffin cells in the GI tract. It is involved in visceral perception and motor activity processes in the gastrointestinal tract.[253] Ondansetron, a 5-HT3 receptor antagonist that is used as an antiemetic, has been shown to increase esophageal perception thresholds for pain in patients with NCCP.[253] The selective 5-HT4 receptor agonist tegaserod has been demonstrated to reduce both chemoreceptor sensitivity to acid and mechanoreceptor sensitivity to balloon distension in patients with functional heartburn.[254] Thus far, there are no studies assessing the value of tegaserod in patients with non–GERD-related NCCP.

Endoscopic Treatment and Surgery for NCCP

Botulinum toxin (BOTOX; Allergan, Irvine, CA) interacts selectively with cholinergic neurons to inhibit the release of acetylcholine at the presynaptic terminals. Botulinum toxin injection into the LES has been used in several uncontrolled trials that included patients with NCCP and documented esophageal spastic motility disorder. Injecting botulinum toxin into the LES in a small, uncontrolled study resulted in 50% reduction of chest pain episodes in 72% of the subjects for a mean duration of 7.3 months (Fig. 62.10).[255]

Laparoscopic fundoplication relieves heartburn and acid regurgitation in most patients with GERD, but its effect on chest pain is less clear. DeMeester and associates[210] identified a temporal correlation between chest pain and acid reflux events in 12 of 23 patients with NCCP. Chest pain resolved in all 12 patients treated either by surgery (8 patients) or acid-reducing agents

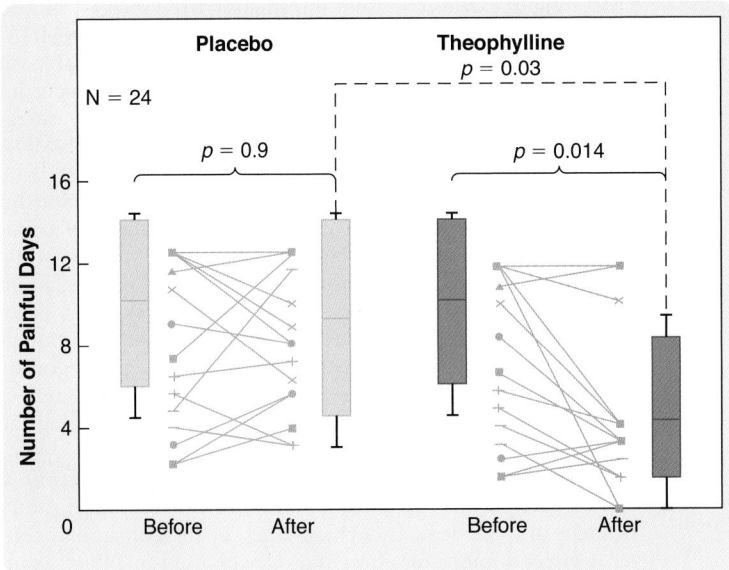

FIGURE 62.9 The effect of oral theophylline versus placebo on the number of painful days in each individual with non-GERD-related NCCP at baseline and after drug administration (200 mg twice daily for 4 weeks). (Redrawn after Rao SS, Mudipalli RS, Remes-Troche JM, et al. Theophylline improves esophageal chest pain—a randomized, placebo-controlled study. *Am J Gastroenterol* 2007;102:930–938, with permission.)

(4 patients). Patti and coworkers[217] reviewed patients who complained of chest pain in addition to heartburn and acid regurgitation. Overall, chest pain improved in 85% of these patients after undergoing laparoscopic fundoplication for GERD. Improvement in chest pain increased to 96% in patients whose chest pain correlated with GERD most of the time. Farrell and colleagues[218] evaluated the effectiveness of antireflux surgery for patients with atypical manifestations of GERD. Chest pain improved in 90% of patients after laparoscopic fundoplication, with symptom resolution in 50% of patients. Although surgical studies demonstrated a high success rate of antireflux surgery in GERD-related NCCP patients, the patients included were carefully selected.

Very few studies to date have specifically evaluated the value of endoscopic treatment for GERD in patients with GERD-related NCCP. Liu et al., who treated 18 NCCP patients with endoluminal gastroplication, demonstrated short-term symptomatic response (6 months) in 72% of them.[256] During long-term

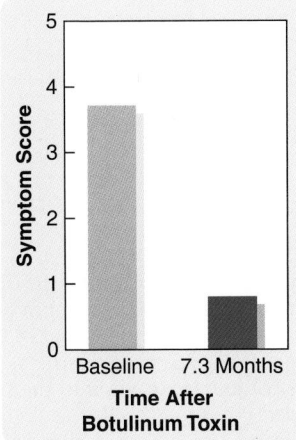

FIGURE 62.10 The effect of botulinum toxin injection in 29 non-GERD-related NCCP patients with spastic esophageal motility disorder. (Redrawn after Miller L, Pullela S, Parkman H, Smith. Treatment of chest pain in patients with noncardiac, nonreflux, nonachalasia spastic esophageal motor disorders using botulinum toxin injection into the gastroesophageal junction. *Am J Gastroenterol* 2002;97(7):1640–1646, with permission.)

follow-up (1–3 years) 75% of nonresponders became symptom free, and 40% of responders became symptomatic.

Psychological Treatment

Psychological comorbidity, mainly depression and anxiety, is common in patients with NCCP. Psychotherapy may be helpful in the treatment of patients with NCCP, particularly those who also have hypochondriasis, anxiety, or panic disorder.

Several studies have demonstrated that patients with NCCP who are treated with cognitive-behavioral therapy report significant improvement in quality of life and reduction in chest pain symptoms. Additionally, cognitive-behavioral therapy has been successfully used for the treatment of NCCP patients without an existing panic disorder.[257] A study evaluating patients who were treated with cognitive-behavioral therapy reported that 48% of these patients remained pain free at 12-month follow-up, as compared to only 13% of the patients in the nonintervention group. Other psychological interventions that have been suggested to be effective in patients with NCCP include reassurance, education, relaxation techniques, breathing training, and biofeedback. Biofeedback was assessed in a study that compared it to primary care visits only in patients with NCCP.[258] Patients in the biofeedback group demonstrated a significantly lower symptom frequency and severity. However, a large group of patients assigned to the biofeedback arm (52%) did not complete the study.

Hypnotherapy has been recently evaluated in the treatment of NCCP patients. Jones and colleagues[259] reported an 80% improvement in symptoms, with a significant reduction in pain intensity, among patients who were receiving 12 sessions of hypnotherapy, compared to only a 23% symptom improvement in the control group (Fig. 62.11). The study concluded that hypnotherapy appears to have a role in treating NCCP and that further studies are needed.

Future Therapy

Future research in NCCP will continue to focus on mechanisms for pain and will attempt to identify new therapeutic modalities aimed to reduce visceral pain. Research will likely concentrate primarily on the role of central and peripheral sensitization in enhancing perception of intra-esophageal stimuli. Furthermore,

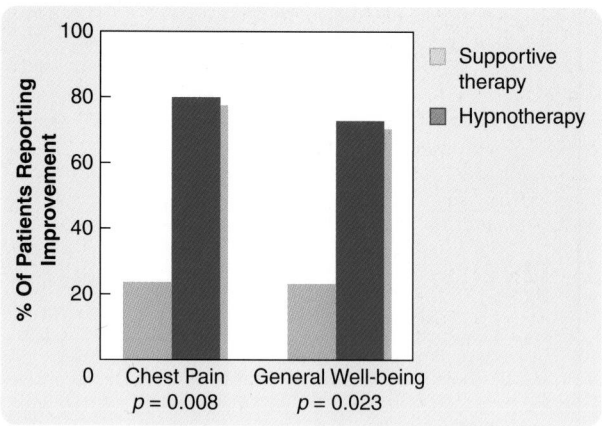

FIGURE 62.11 Percentage of patients reporting a global improvement in chest pain or general well-being with either hypnotherapy (N = 15) or supportive therapy (N = 13). (Redrawn after Jones H, Cooper P, Miller V, Smith. Treatment of non cardiac chest pain: a controlled trial of hypnotherapy. *Gut* 2006;55:1403–1408, with permission.)

currently available treatments for other functional GI disorders, such as IBS and nonulcer dyspepsia, may be tested in NCCP as well.

The serotonin-related drugs, such as 5-HT3 receptor antagonists and 5-HT4 receptor agonists, appear to have a pain-modulatory effect, probably by altering the initiation, transmission, or

processing of extrinsic sensory information from the gastrointestinal tract. Phosphorylation of N-methyl-D-aspartate (NMDA) receptors expressed by dorsal horn neurons leads to central sensitization via an increase in their excitability and subsequent increase in receptive field size.[43] Potentially, this central sensitization may be prevented or even reversed by antagonism of NMDA receptors within the spinal cord.

Potential targets that are currently under consideration include vanilloid receptor ion channels, acid-sensing ion channels, sensory neuron-specific Na + channels, P2X purinoceptors, cholecystokinin (CCK) receptors, bradykinin and prostaglandin receptors, glutamate receptors, tachykinin, and calcitonin gene-related peptide receptors as well as peripheral opioid and cannabinoid receptors.[260,261] The peripheral opioid receptor agonists are of high interest because they may offer visceral analgesic effect without crossing the blood-brain barrier and thus affecting the CNS.

Spinal afferents, which may play a role in visceral nociception, express tachykinins that include substance P, neurokinins A and B, and neuropeptide K. Tachykinin receptor antagonists may confer a visceral analgesic effect that can be used in PPI-resistant patients. Neurokinin (NK)-1, NK-2, and NK-3 receptor antagonists were only evaluated in preclinical trials. Cholecystokinin receptor antagonists may alter visceral pain perception.[262]

Another important area that is likely to attract future attention when treating patients with NCCP is complementary and alternative therapeutic modalities that can interfere with the mind and body axis. Figure 62.12 provides a proposed management algorithm for NCCP.

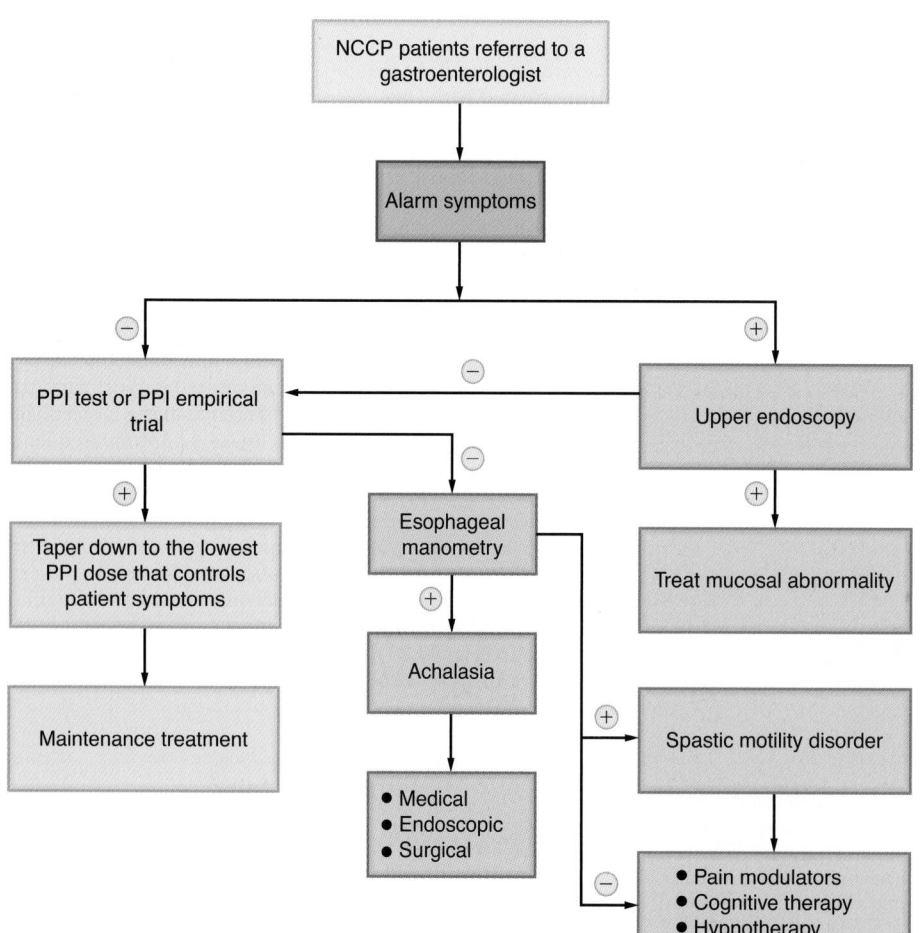

FIGURE 62.12 Proposed management algorithm for NCCP. (Redrawn after Fass R, Navarro-Rodriguez T. *J Clin Gastroenterol* 2008;42(5):636–646, with permission.)

References

1. Jerlock M, Welin C, Rosengren A, et al. Pain characteristics in patients with unexplained chest pain and patients with ischemic heart disease. *Eur J Cardiovasc Nurs* 2007;6:130–136.

2. Ockene IS, Shay MJ, Alpert JS, et al. Unexplained chest pain in patients with normal arteriograms. *N Engl J Med* 1980;303:1249–1252.

3. Dumville JC, MacPherson H, Griffith K, et al. Non-cardiac chest pain: a retrospective cohort study of patients who attended a Rapid Access Chest Pain Clinic. *Fam Pract* 2007;24:152–157.

4. Sekhri N, Feder GS, Junghans C, et al. How effective are rapid access chest pain clinics? Prognosis of incident angina and non-cardiac chest pain in 8762 consecutive patients. *Heart* 2007;93:458–463.

5. Robertson N, Javed N, Samani N, et al. Psychological morbidity and illness appraisals of patients with cardiac and non-cardiac chest pain attending a Rapid Access Chest Pain Clinic: a longitudinal cohort study. *Heart* 2008;94:e12.

6. Drossman DA, Corazziari E, Delvaux M, et al. *Rome III: The Functional Gastrointestinal Disorders.* 3rd ed. McLean, VA: Degnon Associates, Inc; 2006.

7. Mudipalli RS, Remes-Troche JM, Andersen L, et al. Functional chest pain: esophageal or overlapping functional disorder. *J Clin Gastroenterol* 2007;41:264–269.

8. Chiocca JC, Olmos JA, Salis GB, et al. Prevalence, clinical spectrum, and atypical symptoms of gastro-oesophageal reflux in Argentina: a nationwide population-based study. *Aliment Pharmacol Ther* 2005;22(4):331–342.

9. Wong WM, Lai KC, Lam KF, et al. Prevalence, clinical spectrum, and health care utilization of gastro-oesophageal reflux disease in a Chinese population: a population-based study. *Aliment Pharmacol Ther* 2003;18(6):595–604.

10. Locke GR 3rd, Talley NJ, Fett SL, et al. Prevalence and clinical spectrum of gastroesophageal reflux: a population-based study in Olmsted County, Minnesota. *Gastroenterology* 1997;112(5):1448–1456.

11. Mousavi S, Tosi J, Eskandarian R, et al. Role of clinical presentation in diagnosing reflux-related non-cardiac chest pain. *J Gastroenterol Hepatol* 2007;22:218–221.

12. Eslick GD, Jones MP, Talley NJ. Non-cardiac chest pain: prevalence, risk factors, impact, and consulting: a population-based study. *Aliment Pharmacol Ther* 2003;17:1115–1124.

13. Tew R, Guthrie E, Creed F, et al. A long-term follow-up study of patients with ischemic heart disease versus patients with nonspecific chest pain. *J Psychosom Res* 1995;39(8):977–985.

14. Wong WM, Risner-Adler S, Beeler J, et al. Noncardiac chest pain: the role of the cardiologist—a national survey. *J Clin Gastroenterol* 2005;39:858–862.

15. Wong WM, Beeler J, Risner-Adler S, et al. Attitudes and referral patterns of primary care physicians when evaluating subjects with noncardiac chest pain: a national survey. *Dig Dis Sci* 2005;50(4):656–661.

16. Eslick G, Talley N. Non-cardiac chest pain: predictors of health care seeking, the types of health care professional consulted, work absenteeism and interruption of daily activities. *Aliment Pharmacol Ther* 2004;20(8):909–915.

17. Potts S, Bass C. Psychological morbidity in patients with chest pain and normal or near-normal coronary arteries: a long-term follow-up study. *Psychol Med* 1995;254:339–347.

18. Eslick GD. Noncardiac chest pain: epidemiology, natural history, health care seeking, and quality of life. *Gastroenterol Clin North Am* 2004;33(1):1–23.

19. Beedassy A, Katz PO, Gruber A, et al. Prior sensitization of esophageal mucosa by acid reflux predisposes to a reflux-induced chest pain. *J Clin Gastroenterol* 2000;31(2):121–124.

20. Dekel R, Martinez-Hawthorne SD, Guillen RJ, et al. Evaluation of symptom index in identifying gastroesophageal reflux disease-related noncardiac chest pain. *J Clin Gastroenterol* 2004;38(1):24–29.

21. Fass R, Malagon I, Schmulson M. Chest pain of esophageal origin. *Curr Opin Gastroenterol* 2001;17:376–380.

22. Fass R, Fennerty MB, Johnson C, et al. Correlation of ambulatory 24-hour esophageal pH monitoring results with symptom improvement in patients with noncardiac chest pain due to gastroesophageal reflux disease. *J Clin Gastroenterol* 1999;28(1):36–39.

23. Barlow JD, Gregersen H, Thompson DG. Identification of the biomechanical factors associated with the perception of distension in the human esophagus. *Am J Physiol Gastrointest Liver Physiol* 2002;282(4):G683–G689.

24. Chauhan A, Petch MC, Schofield PM. Cardio-oesophageal reflex in humans as a mechanism for "linked angina." *Eur Heart J* 1996;17(3):407–413.

25. Kaski JC. Cardiac syndrome X and microvascular angina. In: Kaski JC, ed. *Chest Pain with Normal Coronary Angiograms: Pathogenesis, Diagnosis and Management.* London, UK: Kluwer Academic Publishers; 1999:1–12.

26. Kaski JC, Rosano GM, Collins P, et al. Cardiac syndrome X: clinical characteristics and left ventricular function. Long-term follow-up study. *J Am Coll Cardiol* 1995;25(4):807–814.

27. Kaski JC. Pathophysiology and management of patients with chest pain and normal coronary arteriograms (cardiac syndrome X). *Circulation* 2004;109(5):568–572.

28. Rosztoczy AI, Vass A, Wittmann T, et al. Esophageal acid stimulation combined with transesophageal echocardiography shows high clinical impact in the establishment of esophago-cardiac reflex. *Gastroenterology* 2003;124(Suppl 4):A534, #T1618

29. Katz PO, Dalton CB, Richter JE, et al. Esophageal testing of patients with noncardiac chest pain or dysphagia. Results of three years' experience with 1161 patients. *Ann Intern Med* 1987;106(4):593–597.

30. Dekel R, Pearson T, Wendel C, et al. Assessment of oesophageal motor function in patients with dysphagia or chest pain—the Clinical Outcomes Research Initiative experience. *Aliment Pharmacol Ther* 2003;18(11–12):1083–1089.

31. Fass R, Winters GF. Evaluation of the patient with noncardiac chest pain: is gastroesophageal reflux disease or an esophageal motility disorder the cause? *Medscape Gastroenterol* 2001;3(6):1–10.

32. Achem SR, Kolts BE, Wears R, et al. Chest pain associated with nutcracker esophagus: a preliminary study of the role of gastroesophageal reflux. *Am J Gastroenterol* 1993;88(2):187–192.

33. Nguyen HN, Silny J, Matern S. Multiple intraluminal electrical impedancometry for recording of upper gastrointestinal motility: current results and further implications. *Am J Gastroenterol* 1999;94(2):306–317.

34. Balaban DH, Yamamoto Y, Liu J, et al. Sustained esophageal contraction: a marker of esophageal chest pain identified by intraluminal ultrasonography. *Gastroenterology* 1999;116(1):29–37.

35. Pehlivanov N, Liu J, Mittal RK. Sustained esophageal contraction: a motor correlate of heartburn symptom. *Am J Physiol Gastrointest Liver Physiol* 2001;281(3):G743–G751.

36. Lembo AJ. Visceral hypersensitivity in noncardiac chest pain. *Gastroenterol Clin North Am* 2004;33(1):55–60.

37. Hollerbach S, Bulat R, May A, et al. Abnormal cerebral processing of oesophageal stimuli in patients with noncardiac chest pain (NCCP). *Neurogastroenterol Motil* 2000;12(6):555–565.

38. Handwerker HO, Reeh PW. Nociceptors: chemosensitivity and sensitization by chemical agents. In: Willis WD Jr, ed. *Hyperalgesia and Allodynia.* New York: Raven Press; 1992:107.

39. Barish CF, Castell DO, Richter JE. Graded esophageal balloon distention. A new provocative test for noncardiac chest pain. *Dig Dis Sci* 1986;31(12):1292–1298.

40. Richter JE, Barish CF, Castell DO. Abnormal sensory perception in patients with esophageal chest pain. *Gastroenterology* 1986;91(4):845–852.

41. Rao S, Gregersen H, Hayek B, et al. Unexplained chest pain: the hypersensitive, hyperreactive, and poorly compliant esophagus. *Ann Intern Med* 1996;124(11):950–958.

42. Rao S, Hayek B, Summers RW. Functional chest pain of esophageal origin: hyperalgesia or motor dysfunction. *Am J Gastroenterol* 2001;96(9):2584–2589.

43. Sarkar S, Aziz Q, Woolf CJ, et al. Contribution of central sensitisation to the development of non-cardiac chest pain. *Lancet* 2000;356(9236):1154–1159.

44. Börjesson M, Pilhall M, Eliasson T, et al. Esophageal visceral pain sensitivity: effects of TENS and correlation with manometric findings. *Dig Dis Sci* 1998;43(8):1621–1628.

45. Mehta AJ, De Caestecker JS, Camm AJ, et al. Sensitization to painful distension and abnormal sensory perception in the esophagus. *Gastroenterology* 1995;108(2):311–319.

46. Hu WH, Martin CJ, Talley NJ. Intraesophageal acid perfusion sensitizes the esophagus to mechanical distension: a Barostat study. *Am J Gastroenterol* 2000;95(9):2189–2194.

47. Sarkar S, Thompson DG, Woolf CJ, et al. Patients with chest pain and occult gastroesophageal reflux demonstrate visceral pain hypersensitivity which may be partially responsive to acid suppression. *Am J Gastroenterol* 2004;99(10):1998–2006.

48. Mujica VR, Mudipalli RS, Rao SS. Pathophysiology of chest pain in patients with nutcracker esophagus. *Am J Gastroenterol* 2001;96(5):1371–1377.

49. Kern MK, Birn RM, Jaradeh S, et al. Identification and characterization of cerebral cortical response to esophageal mucosal acid exposure and distention. *Gastroenterology* 1998;115(6):1353–1362.

50. Aziz Q, Andersson JL, Valind S, et al. Identification of human brain loci processing esophageal sensation using positron emission tomography. *Gastroenterology* 1997;113(1):50–59.

51. DeVault KR, Castell DO. Esophageal balloon distention and cerebral evoked potential recording in the evaluation of unexplained chest pain. *Am J Med* 1992;92(5A):20S–26S.

52. Kamath MV, May A, Hollerbach S, et al. Effects of esophageal stimulation in patients with functional disorders of the gastrointestinal tract. *Crit Rev Biomed Eng* 2000;28(1–2):87–93.

53. Tougas G, Spaziani R, Hollerbach S, et al. Cardiac autonomic function and oesophageal acid sensitivity in patients with non-cardiac chest pain. *Gut* 2001;49(5):706–712.

54. Tougas G. The autonomic nervous system in functional bowel disorders. *Gut* 2000;47(Suppl 4):iv78–iv80.

55. Mayer EA. The neurobiology of stress and gastrointestinal disease. *Gut* 2000;47(6):861–869.

56. Aziz Q. Acid sensors in the gut: the taste of things to come. *Eur J Gastroenterol Hepatol* 2001;13(8):885–888.

57. Bass C, Wade C. Chest pain with normal coronary arteries: a comparative study of psychiatric and social morbidity. *Psychol Med* 1984;14(1):51–61.

58. Channer KS, Papouchado M, James MA, et al. Anxiety and depression in patients with chest pain referred for exercise testing. *Lancet* 1985;2(8459):820–823.

59. Costa PT Jr. Influence of the normal personality dimension of neuroticism

on chest pain symptoms and coronary artery disease. *Am J Cardiol* 1987; 60(18):20J–26J.

60. McCroskery JH, Schell RE, Sprafkin RP, et al. Differentiating anginal patients with coronary artery disease from those with normal coronary arteries using psychological measures. *Am J Cardiol* 1991;67(7):645–646.

61. Flugelman MY, Weisstub E, Galun E, et al. Clinical, psychological, and thallium stress studies in patients with chest pain and normal coronary arteries. *Int J Cardiol* 1991;33(3):401–408.

62. Mayou R, Bryant B, Forfar C, et al. Non-cardiac chest pain and benign palpitations in the cardiac clinic. *Br Heart J* 1994;72(6):548–553.

63. Chignon JM, Lepine JP, Ades J. Panic disorder in cardiac outpatients. *Am J Psychiatry* 1993;150(5):780–785.

64. Tennant C, Mihailidou A, Scott A, et al. Psychological symptom profiles in patients with chest pain. *J Psychosom Res* 1994;38(4):365–371.

65. Dammen T, Ekeberg O, Arnesen H, et al. Personality profiles in patients referred for chest pain. Investigation with emphasis on panic disorder patients. *Psychosomatics* 2000;41(3):269–276.

66. Potokar JP, Nutt DJ. Chest pain: panic attack or heart attack? *Int J Clin Pract* 2000;54:110–114.

67. Fleet RP, Dupuis G, Marchand A, et al. Panic disorder in emergency department chest pain patients: prevalence, comorbidity, suicidal ideation, and physician recognition. *Am J Med* 1996;101:371–380.

68. Stollman NH, Bierman PS, Ribeiro A, et al. CO_2 provocation of panic: symptomatic and manometric evaluation in patients with noncardiac chest pain. *Am J Gastroenterol* 1997;92:839–842.

69. Cooke RA, Anggiansah A, Wang J, et al. Hyperventilation and esophageal dysmotility in patients with noncardiac chest pain. *Am J Gastroenterol* 1996; 91:480–484.

70. Lantinga LJ, Sprafkin RP, McCroskery JH, et al. One-year psychosocial follow-up of patients with chest pain and angiographically normal coronary arteries. *Am J Cardiol* 1988;62:209–213.

71. Hotopf M, Mayou R, Wadsworth M, et al. Psychosocial and developmental antecedents of chest pain in young adults. *Psychosom Med* 1999;61:861–867.

72. Orlando RC. Esophageal perception and noncardiac chest pain. *Gastroenterol Clin N Am* 2004;33:25–33.

73. Johnston BT, Troshinsky MB, Castell JA, et al. Comparison of barium radiology with esophageal pH monitoring in the diagnosis of gastroesophageal reflux disease. *Am J Gastroenterol* 1996;91:1181–1185.

74. Eslick GD, Fass R. Noncardiac chest pain: evaluation and treatment. *Gastroenterol Clin North Am* 2003;32:531–552.

75. Hsia PC, Maher KA, Lewis JH, et al. Utility of upper endoscopy in the evaluation of noncardiac chest pain. *Gastrointest Endosc* 1991;37:22–26.

76. Frobert O, Funch-Jensen P, Jacobsen NO, et al. Upper endoscopy in patients with angina and normal coronary angiograms. *Endoscopy* 1995;27:365–370.

77. Dickman R, Mattek N, Holub J, et al. Prevalence of upper gastrointestinal tract findings in patients with noncardiac chest pain versus those with gastroesophageal reflux disease (GERD)-related symptoms: results from a national endoscopic database. *Am J Gastroenterol* 2007;102:1173–1179.

78. Hewson EG, Sinclair JW, Dalton CB, et al. Twenty-four-hour esophageal pH monitoring: the most useful test for evaluation of noncardiac chest pain. *Am J Med* 1991;90:576–583.

79. Paterson WG. Canadian Association of Gastroenterology Practice Guidelines: management of noncardiac chest pain. *Can J Gastroenterol* 1998;12: 401–407.

80. Faybush EM, Fass R. Gastroesophageal reflux disease in noncardiac chest pain. *Gastroenterol Clin North Am* 2004;33:41–54.

81. Pandolfino JE, Richter JE, Ours T, et al. Ambulatory esophageal pH monitoring using a wireless system. *Am J Gastroenterol* 2003;98:740–749.

82. Prakash C, Clouse RE. Value of extended recording time with wireless pH monitoring in evaluating gastroesophageal reflux disease. *Clin Gastroenterol Hepatol* 2005;3:329–334.

83. Prakash C, Clouse RE. Wireless pH monitoring in patients with non-cardiac chest pain. *Am J Gastroenterol* 2006;101:446–452.

84. Metz D, Childs M, Ruiz C, et al. Pilot study of the oral omeprazole test of reflux laryngitis. *Otolaryngol Head Neck Surg* 1997;116:41–46.

85. Ours T, Kavuru M, Schilz R, et al. A prospective evaluation of esophageal testing and a double-blind, randomized study of omeprazole in a diagnostic and therapeutic algorithm for chronic cough. *Am J Gastroenterol* 1999;94: 3131–3138.

86. Jaspersen D, Diehl K, Geyer P, et al. Diagnostic omeprazole test in suspected reflux-associated chronic cough. *Pneumologie* 1999;53:438–441.

87. Kiljander T, Salomaa E, Heitanen E, et al. Chronic cough and gastro-oesophageal reflux: a double-blind placebo-controlled study with omeprazole. *Eur Respir J* 2000;16:633–638.

88. Fass R, Fennerty M, Ofman J, et al. The clinical and economic value of a short course of omeprazole in patients with noncardiac chest pain. *Gastroenterology* 1998;115:42–49.

89. Schenk B, Kuipers E, Klinkenberg-Knol E, et al. Omeprazole as a diagnostic tool in gastroesophageal reflux disease. *Am J Gastroenterol* 1997;92: 1997–2000.

90. Schindlbeck NE, Klauser AG, Voderholzer WA, et al. Empiric therapy for gastroesophageal reflux disease. *Arch Intern Med* 1995;155(16):1808–1812.

91. Johnsson F, Weywadt L, Solhaug J, et al. One-week omeprazole treatment in the diagnosis of gastro-oesophageal reflux disease. *Scand J Gastroenterol* 1998;33:15–20.

92. Fass R, Ofman JJ, Gralnek IM, et al. Clinical and economic assessment of the omeprazole test in patients with symptoms suggestive of gastroesophageal reflux disease. *Arch Intern Med* 1999;150:2161–2168.

93. Bate C, Riley S, Chapman R, et al. Evaluation of omeprazole as a cost-effective diagnostic test for gastro-oesophageal reflux disease. *Aliment Pharmacol Ther* 1999;13:59–66.

94. Juul-Hansen P, Rydning A, Jacobsen C, et al. High-dose proton-pump inhibitors as a diagnostic test of gastro-esophageal reflux disease in endoscopic-negative patients. *Scand J Gastroenterol* 2001;36:806–810.

95. Squillace SJ, Young MF, Sanowski RA. Single dose omeprazole as a test for noncardiac chest pain [abstract]. *Gastroenterology* 1993;107:A197.

96. Young MF, Sanowski RA, Talbert GA, et al. Omeprazole administration as a test for gastroesophageal reflux [abstract]. *Gastroenterology* 1992;102:192.

97. Pandak WM, Arezo S, Everett S, et al. Short course of omeprazole: a better first diagnostic approach to noncardiac chest pain than endoscopy, manometry, or 24-hour esophageal pH monitoring. *J Clin Gastroenterol* 2002;35(4): 307–314.

98. Xia HH, Lai KC, Lam SK. Symptomatic response to lansoprazole predicts abnormal acid reflux in endoscopy-negative patients with non-cardiac chest pain. *Aliment Pharmacol Ther* 2003;17:369–377.

99. Bautista J, Fullerton H, Briseno M, et al. The effect of an empirical trial of high-dose lansoprazole on symptom response of patients with non-cardiac chest pain—a randomized, double-blind, placebo-controlled, crossover trial. *Aliment Pharmacol Ther* 2004;19:1123–1130.

100. Dickman R, Emmons S, Cui H, et al. The effect of a therapeutic trial of high-dose rabeprazole on symptom response of patients with non-cardiac chest pain: a randomized, double-blind, placebo-controlled, crossover trial. *Aliment Pharmacol Ther* 2005;22(6):547–555.

101. Fass R. Empirical trials in treatment of gastroesophageal reflux disease. *Dig Dis* 2000;18:20–26.

102. Fass R, Ofman JJ, Sampliner RE, et al. The omeprazole test is as sensitive as 24-h oesophageal pH monitoring in diagnosing gastro-oesophageal reflux disease in symptomatic patients with erosive oesophagitis. *Aliment Pharmacol Ther* 2000;14(4):389–396.

103. Xia HH, Lai KC, Lam SK, et al. Symptomatic response to lansoprazole predicts abnormal acid reflux in endoscopy-negative patients with non-cardiac chest pain. *Aliment Pharmacol Ther* 2003;17:369–377.

104. Maev IV, Iurenev GL, Burkov SG, et al. Rabeprazole test and comparison of the effectiveness of course treatment with rabeprazole in patients with gastroesophageal reflux disease and non-coronary chest pain. *Klin Med (Mosk)* 2007;85(2):45–51.

105. Fass R, Pulliam G, Hayden CW. Patients with noncardiac chest pain (NCCP) receiving an empirical trial of high dose rabeprazole, demonstrate early symptom response—a double blind, placebo-controlled trial [abstract]. *Gastroenterology* 2001;129(A-221):1162.

106. Fass R, Fullerton H, Hayden CW, et al. Patients with noncardiac chest pain (NCCP) receiving an empirical trial of high dose rabeprazole, demonstrate early symptom response—a double blind, placebo-controlled trial [abstract]. *Gastroenterology* 2002;122:A-580-A-1, W1175.

107. Cremonini F, Wise J, Moayyedi P, et al. Meta-analysis: diagnostic and therapeutic use of proton pump inhibitors in noncardiac chest pain. *Am J Gastroenterol* 2005;100:1226–1232.

108. Dekel R, Martinez-Hawthorne S, Guillen R, et al. Evaluation of symptom index in identifying gastroesophageal reflux disease-related noncardiac chest pain. *J Clin Gastroenterol* 2004;38:24–29.

109. Chambers J, Cooke R, Anggiansah A, et al. Effect of omeprazole in patients with chest pain and normal coronary anatomy: initial experience. *Int J Cardiol* 1998;65(1):51–55.

110. Wang W, Huang J, Zheng G, et al. Is proton pump inhibitor testing an effective approach to diagnose gastroesophageal reflux disease in patients with noncardiac chest pain? *Arch Intern Med* 2005;165(11):1222–1228.

111. Ofman JJ, Gralnek IM, Udani J, et al. The cost-effectiveness of the omeprazole test in patients with noncardiac chest pain. *Am J Med* 1999;107:219–227.

112. Savarino E, Tutuian R. Combined multichannel intraluminal impedance and manometry testing. *Dig Liver Dis* 2008;40:167–173.

113. Azpiroz F, Malagelada JR. Physiological variations in canine gastric tone measured by electronic barostat. *Am J Physiol* 1985;248:G229–G237.

114. Clouse RE, Lustman PJ, Eckert TC, et al. Low-dose trazodone for symptomatic patients with esophageal contraction abnormalities. A double-blind, placebo-controlled trial. *Gastroenterology* 1987;92:1027–1036.

115. Knippig C, Fass R, Malfertheiner P. Tests for the evaluation of functional gastrointestinal disorders. *Dig Dis* 2001;19:232–239.

116. Shrestha S, Pasricha PJ. Update on noncardiac chest pain. *Dig Dis* 2000; 18(3):138–146.

117. DiMarino AJ Jr, Allen ML, Lynn RB, et al. Clinical value of esophageal motility testing. *Dig Dis* 1998;16(4):198–204.

118. London RL, Ouyang A, Snape WJ Jr, et al. Provocation of esophageal pain by ergonovine or edrophonium. *Gastroenterology* 1981;81:10–14.

119. Nostrant TT. Provocation testing in noncardiac chest pain. *Am J Med* 1992; 92:56S–64S.

120. Lee CA, Reynolds JC, Ouyang A, et al. Esophageal chest pain. Value of high-dose provocative testing with edrophonium chloride in patients with normal esophageal manometries. *Dig Dis Sci* 1987;32:682–688.

121. Richter J, Dalton C, Buice R, et al. Nifedipine: a potent inhibitor of contractions in the body of the human esophagus. Studies in healthy volunteers and

patients with the nutcracker esophagus. *Gastroenterology* 1985;89(3): 549–554.

122. Gebhart GF, Bielefeldt K. Visceral pain. In: Bushnell MC, Basbaum AI, eds. *The Senses: A Comprehensive Reference*, vol. 5, Pain. San Diego, CA: Academic Press; 2008:543–570.

123. Goyal RK, Hirano I. The enteric nervous system. *N Engl J Med* 1996;334(17): 1106–1115.

124. Grundy D, Scratcherd T. Sensory afferents from the gastroinestinal tract. In: Schultz SG, Wood JD, Rauner BB, eds. *Handbook of Physiology*. New York: Oxford University; 1989:593–620.

125. Randich A. Visceral nerve stimulation and pain modulation. In: Joshn LR, ed. *Physiology of the Gastrointestinal Tract*. 3rd ed. Amsterdam: Elsevier; 1993:126–139.

126. Tougas G, Fitzpatrick D, Upton ARM, et al. The cortical evoked responses produced by balloon distention and electrical stimulation of the esophagus involve different vagal fibers [abstract]. *Gastroenterology* 1993;104.

127. Mayer EA, Gebhart GF. Basic and clinical aspects of visceral hyperalgesia. *Gastroenterology* 1994;107(1):271–293.

128. Rodrigo J, Hernandez CJ, Vidal MA, et al. Vegetative innervation of the esophagus. III. Intraepithelial endings. *Acta Anat (Basel)* 1975;92:242–285.

129. Fass R, Tougas G. Functional heartburn—the stimulus, the pain and the brain. *Gut* 2002;51:885–892.

130. Takeda T, Liu J, Gui O, et al. Heartburn not chest pain, is the most common symptoms in response to esophageal distension in normal subjects [abstract]. *Gastroenterology* 2001;120(Suppl 5):A-222, #1167.

131. Baldi F, Ferrarini F, Longanesi A, et al. Acid gastroesophageal reflux and symptom occurrence. Analysis of some factors influencing their association. *Dig Dis Sci* 1989;34(12):1890–1893.

132. Meyer JH, Lembo AJ, Elashoff JD, et al. Duodenal fat intensifies the perception of heartburn. *Gut* 2001;49:624–628.

133. Fass R. Focused clinical review—nonerosive reflux disease. *Medscape Gastroenterol* 2001;3:1–13.

134. Trimble KC, Pryde A, Heading RC. Lowered oesophageal sensory thresholds in patients with symptomatic but not excess gastro-oesophageal reflux: evidence for a spectrum of visceral sensitivity in GORD. *Gut* 1995;37:7–12.

135. Fass R, Naliboff BD, Fass SS, et al. The effect of auditory stress on perception of intraesophageal acid in patients with GERD. *Gastroenterology* 2008;134: 696–705.

136a. Schey R, Dickman R, Parthasarathy S, et al. Sleep deprivation is hyperalgesic in patients with gastroesophageal reflux disease. *Gastroenterology* 2007; 133(6):1787–1795.

136. Fass R, Malagon I, Pulliam G, et al. Gender differences in perceptual and emotional ratings of intra-esophageal stimuli in GERD patients undergoing auditory-induced stress [abstract]. *Gastroenterology* 2002;122:A187.

137. Bernstein LM, Baker LA. A clinical test for esophagitis. *Gastroenterology* 1958;34(5):760–781.

138. Bernot R, Norton RA. The esophageal acid perfusion test. *Lahey Clin Found Bull* 1965;14:58–63.

139. Fisher RS, Cohen S. Gastroesophageal reflux. *Med Clin North Am* 1978;62: 3–20.

140. Breen KJ, Whelan G. The diagnosis of reflux oesophagitis: an evaluation of five investigative procedures. *Aust N Z J Surg* 1978;48:156–161.

141. Behar J, Biancani P, Sheahan DG. Evaluation of esophageal tests in the diagnosis of reflux esophagitis. *Gastroenterology* 1976;71:9–15.

142. Battle WS, Nyhus LM, Bombeck CT. Gastroesophageal reflux: diagnosis and treatment. *Ann Surg* 1973;177:560–565.

143. Howard PJ, Maher L, Pryde A, et al. Symptomatic gastro-oesophageal reflux, abnormal oesophageal acid exposure, and mucosal acid sensitivity are three separate, though related, aspects of gastro-oesophageal reflux disease. *Gut* 1991;32:128–132.

144. Kaul B, Petersen H, Grette K, et al. The acid perfusion test in gastroesophageal reflux disease. *Scand J Gastroenterol* 1986;21:93–96.

145. Price SF, Smithson KW, Castell DO. Food sensitivity in reflux esophagitis. *Gastroenterology* 1986;75:240–243.

146. Bachir GS, Leigh-Collis J, Wilson P, et al. Diagnosis of incipient reflux esophagitis: a new test. *South Med J* 1981;74:1072–1074.

147. Johnson DA, Winters C, Spurling TJ, et al. Esophageal acid sensitivity in Barrett's esophagus. *J Clin Gastroenterol* 1987;9:23–27.

148. Gracely RH, McGrath F, Dubner R. Ratio scales of sensory and affective verbal pain descriptors. *Pain* 1978;5:1–18.

149. Silverman DH, Munakata JA, Ennes H, et al. Regional cerebral activity in normal and pathological perception of visceral pain. *Gastroenterology* 1997; 112:64–72.

150. Vantrappen G, Janssens J, Ghillebert G. The irritable oesophagus—a frequent cause of angina-like pain. *Lancet* 1987;1(8544):1232–1234.

151. Soffer EE, Scalabrini P, Wingate DL. Spontaneous noncardiac chest pain: value of ambulatory esophageal pH and motility monitoring. *Dig Dis Sci* 1989;34(11):1651–1655.

152. Peters L, Maas L, Petty D, et al. Spontaneous noncardiac chest pain. Evaluation by 24-hour ambulatory esophageal motility and pH monitoring. *Gastroenterology* 1988;94:878–886.

153. Nevens F, Janssens J, Piessens J, et al. Prospective study on prevalence of esophageal chest pain in patients referred on an elective basis to a cardiac unit for suspected myocardial ischemia. *Dig Dis Sci* 1991;36(2):229–235.

154. Hewson EG, Dalton CB, Richter JE. Comparison of esophageal manometry, provocative testing, and ambulatory monitoring in patients with unexplained chest pain. *Dig Dis Sci* 1990;35:302–309.

155. Ghillebert G, Janssens J, Vantrappen G, et al. Ambulatory 24 hour intraesophageal pH and pressure recordings versus provocation tests in the diagnosis of chest pain of oesophageal origin. *Gut* 1990;31(7):738–744.

156. De Caestecker JS, Pryde A, Heading RC. Comparison of intravenous edrophonium and oesophageal acid perfusion during oesophageal manometry in patients with non-cardiac chest pain. *Gut* 1988;29:1029–1034.

157. Richter JE. Provocative tests in esophageal diseases. In: Scarpignato C, Galmiche JP, eds. *Functional Evaluation in Esophageal Diseases*. Basel: Karger; 1994.

158. Eslick GD, Fass R. Non-cardiac chest pain: evaluation and treatment. *Gastroenterol Clin N Am* 2003;32:531–552.

159. Hewson EG, Sinclair JW, Dalton CB, et al. Acid perfusion test: does it have a role in the assessment of non cardiac chest pain? *Gut* 1989;30:305–310.

160. Hollerbach S, Klamath MV, Fitzpatrick D, et al. The cerebral response to electrical stimuli in the oesophagus is altered by increasing stimulus frequencies. *Neurogastroenterol Motil* 1997;9:129–139.

161. Tougas G, Hudoba P, Fitzpatrick D, et al. Cerebral-invoked potential responses following direct vagal and esophageal electrical stimulation in humans. *Am J Physiol* 1993;294:G486–G491.

162. Heft MW, Parker SR. An experimental basis for revising the graphic rating scale for pain. *Pain* 1984;19:153–161.

163. Takeda T, Kssab G, Liu J, et al. A novel ultrasound technique to study the biomechanics of the human esophagus in vivo. *Am J Physiol Gastrointest Liver Physiol* 2002;282:G785–G793.

164. Ritchie J. Pain from distention of the pelvic colon by inflating a balloon in the irritable colon syndrome. *Gut* 1973;14:125–132.

165. Mertz H, Walsh JH, Sytnik B, et al. The effect of octreotide on human gastric compliance and sensory perception. *Neurogastroenterol Motil* 1995;7: 175–185.

166. Kramer P, Hollander W. Comparison of experimental esophageal pain with clinical pain of angina pectoris and esophageal disease. *Gastroenterology* 1955;29:719–743.

167. Lipkin M, Sleisenger MH. Studies of visceral pain: measurements of stimulus intensity and duration associated with the onset of pain in esophagus, ileum, and colon. *J Clin Invest* 1958;37:28–34.

168. Yakshe PN, et al. Does provocative esophageal testing influence coronary blood flow or coronary flow reserve? Preliminary results of concurrent esophageal and cardiac testing [abstract]. *Gastroenterology* 1993;104:A227.

169. Whitehead WE, Delvaux M, Team TW. Standardization of barostat procedures for testing smooth muscle tone and sensory thresholds in the gastrointestinal tract. *Dig Dis Sci* 1997;42:223–241.

170. Toma TD, Zighelboim J, Phillips SF, et al. Methods for studying intestinal sensitivity and compliance: in vitro studies of balloons and a barostat. *Neurogastroenterol Motil* 1996;8:19–28.

171. Khan MI, Feinle C, Read DW. Investigating gastric and sensory response to distention: comparative studies using flaccid bags and latex balloons. *2nd United European Gastroenterology Meeting* 1992:13:175.

172. Sun WM, Read NW, Prior A, et al. Sensory and motor responses to rectal distention vary according to rate and pattern of balloon inflation. *Gastroenterology* 1990;99:1008–1015.

173. Munakata J, Naliboff B, Harraf F, et al. Repetitive sigmoid stimulation induces rectal hyperalgesia in patients with irritable bowel syndrome. *Gastroenterology* 1997;112:55–63.

174. Whitehead WE, Crowell MD, Shone D, et al. Sensitivity to rectal distention: validation of a measurement system [abstract]. *Gastroenterology* 1993;104: A600.

175. Lembo T, Niazi M, Mayer EA. Do mucosal mechanoreceptors contribute to rectal hyperalgesia in IBS patients? [abstract]. *Gastroenterology* 1993;104: A540.

176. Pehlivanov M, Liu J, Mittal R. Sustained esophageal contraction: a motor correlate of heartburn symptom [abstract]. *Gastroenterology* 1999;116: A1062.

177. Nguyen P, Castell DO. Stimulation of esophageal mechanoreceptors is dependent on rate and duration of distention. *Am J Physiol* 1994;267:G115–G118.

178. Lasch H, Castell DO, Castell JA. Evidence of diminished visceral pain with aging: studies using graded intraesophageal balloon distention. *Am J Physiol* 1997;272:G1–G3.

179. Fass R, Pulliam G, Johnson C, et al. Symptom severity and oesophageal chemosensitivity to acid in old and young patients with gastro-oesophageal reflux. *Age Aging* 2000;29(2):125–130.

180. Nguyen P, Lee SD, Castell DO. Evidence of gender differences in esophageal pain threshold. *Am J Gastroenterol* 1995;90:901–905.

181. Niemantsverdriet EC, Timmer R, Breumelhof R, et al. Regional differences in esophageal acid sensitivity studied with pH-controlled segmental acid perfusion [abstract]. *Gastroenterology* 1997;112:A237.

182. Grade A, Pulliam G, Johnson C, et al. Reduced chemoreceptor sensitivity in patients with Barrett's esophagus may be related to age and not to the presence of Barrett's epithelium. *Am J Gastroenterol* 1997;92:2040–2043.

183. Winwood PJ, Mavrogiannis CC, Smith CL. Reduced sensitivity to intraoesophageal acid in patients with reflux-induced strictures. *Scand J Gastroenterol* 1993;28:109–112.

184. Clouse RE, McCord GS, Lustman PJ, et al. Clinical correlates of abnormal sensitivity to intraesophageal balloon distension. *Dig Dis Sci* 1991;36(8): 1040–1045.

185. Garrison DW, Chandler MJ, Foreman RD. Viscerosomatic convergence onto feline spinal neurons from esophagus, heart and somatic fields: effects of inflammation. *Pain* 1992;49:373–382.

186. DeVault KR. Acid infusion does not affect intraesophageal balloon distention-induced sensory and pain thresholds. *Am J Gastroenterol* 1997;92:947–949.

187. Sarkar S, Woolf CJ, Aziz Q, et al. Secondary hyperalgesia is induced by acid in the healthy human oesophagus [abstract]. *Gut* 1997;41:A26.

188. Cannon RO III, Quyyumi AA, Mincemoyer R, et al. Imipramine in patients with chest pain despite normal coronary angiograms. *N Engl J Med* 1994; 330:1411–1417.

189. Peghini PL, Katz PO, Castell DO. Imipramine decreases oesophageal pain perception in human male volunteers. *Gut* 1998;42:807–813.

190. Castell DO, Wood JD, Frieling T, et al. Cerebral electrical potentials evoked by balloon distension of the human esophagus. *Gastroenterology* 1990;98: 662–666.

191. DeVault KR. Nifedipine does not alter barostat determined esophageal smooth muscle tone [abstract]. *Gastroenterology* 1995;108:A591.

192. Smout AJ, DeVore MS, Dalton CB, et al. Effects of nifedipine on esophageal tone and perception of esophageal distension. *Dig Dis Sci* 1992;37:598–602.

193. DeVault KR. Provocative tests for pain of esophageal origin. In: Castell DO, Richter JE, eds. *The Esophagus*. 3rd ed. Philadelphia: Lippincott Williams & Wilkins; 1999:135–143.

194. Hollerbach S, Kamath MV, Chen Y, et al. The magnitude of the central response to esophageal electrical stimulation is intensity dependent. *Gastroenterology* 1997;112(4):1137–1146.

195. Smout AJ, DeVore MS, Castell DO. Cerebral potentials evoked by esophageal distension in human. *Am J Physiol* 1990;259:G955–G959.

196. Frieling T, Enck P, Wienbeck M. Cerebral responses evoked by electrical stimulation of rectosigmoid in normal subjects. *Dig Dis Sci* 1989;34:202–205.

197. DeVault KR, Beacham S, Castell DO, et al. Esophageal sensation in spinal cord-injured patients: balloon distension and cerebral evoked potential recording. *Am J Physiol* 1996;271:G937–G941.

198. Franssen H, Weusten BL, Wieneke GH, Smout AJ. Source modeling of esophageal evoked potentials. *Electroencephalogr Clin Neurophysiol* 1996;100: 85–95.

199. Aziz Q, Furlong PL, Barlow J, et al. Topographic mapping of cortical potentials evoked by distension of the human proximal and distal oesophagus. *Electroencephalogr Clin Neurophysiol* 1995;96:219–228.

200. Aziz Q, Thompson DG. Brain-gut axis in health and disease. *Gastroenterology* 1998;114(3):559–578.

201. Hartshorne MF. Positron emission tomography. In: Orrison WW, Lewine JD, Sanders JA, Hartshorne MR, eds. *Functional Brain Imaging*. St. Louis, MO: Mosby-Year Book; 1995:187–212.

202. Aine CJ. A conceptual overview and critique of functional neuroimaging techniques in humans: I. MRI/FMRI and PET. *Crit Rev Neurobiol* 1995;9: 229–309.

203. Sanders JA, Orrison WW. Functional magnetic resonance imaging. In: Orrison WW, Lewine JD, Sanders JA, Hartshorne MF, eds. *Functional Brain Imaging*. St. Louis, MO: Mosby-Year Book; 1995:239–326.

204. Vogt BA, Sikes RW, Vogt LJ. Anterior cingulate cortex and the medial pain system. In: Vogt BA, Gabriel M, eds. *Neurobiology of Cingulate Cortex and Limbic Thalamus*. Boston: Birkhauser; 1994:313–344.

205. Talbot JD, Marrett S, Evans AC, et al. Multiple representations of pain in human cerebral cortex. *Science* 1991;251:1355–1358.

206. Minshohima S, Maorrow TJ, Koeppe RA. Involvement of insular cortex in central autonomic regulation during painful thermal stimulation. *J Cereb Blood Flow Metab* 1995;15:1355–1358.

207. Fass R, Bautista J, Janarthanan S. Treatment of gastroesophageal reflux disease. *Clin Cornerstone* 2003;5(4):18–29.

208. Kitchin L, Castell D. Rationale and efficacy of conservative therapy for gastroesophageal reflux disease. *Arch Intern Med* 1991;151(3):448–454.

209. Fang J, Bjorkman D. A critical approach to noncardiac chest pain: pathophysiology, diagnosis, and treatment. *Am J Gastroenterol* 2001;96(4):958–968.

210. DeMeester T, O'Sullivan G, Bermudez G, et al. Esophageal function in patients with angina-type chest pain and normal coronary angiograms. *Ann Surg* 1982;196(4):488–498.

211. Achem S, Kolts B, MacMath T, et al. Effects of omeprazole versus placebo in treatment of noncardiac chest pain and gastroesophageal reflux. *Dig Dis Sci* 1997;42:2138–2145.

212. Louis E, Jorissen L, Bastens B, et al. Atypical symptoms of GORD in Belgium: epidemiological features, current management and open label treatment with 40 mg esomeprazole for one month. *Acta Gastroenterol Belg* 2006;69(2): 203–208.

213. Dore MP, Pedroni A, Pes GM, et al. Effect of antisecretory therapy on atypical symptoms in gastroesophageal reflux disease. *Dig Dis Sci* 2007;52:463–468.

214. Liuzzo JP, Ambrose JA, Diggs P. Proton-pump inhibitor use by coronary artery disease patients is associated with fewer chest pain episodes, emergency department visits, and hospitalizations. *Aliment Pharmacol Ther* 2005;22: 95–100.

215. Fass R, Malagon I, Schmulson M. Chest pain of esophageal origin. *Curr Opin Gastroenterol* 2001;17:376–380.

216. Borzecki A, Pedrosa M, Prashker M. Should noncardiac chest pain be treated empirically? A cost-effectiveness analysis. *Arch Intern Med* 2000;160: 844–852.

217. Patti M, Molena D, Fisichella P, et al. Gastroesophageal reflux disease (GERD) and chest pain. Results of laparoscopic antireflux surgery. *Surg Endosc* 2002;16(4):563–566.

218. Farrell T, Richardson W, Trus T, et al. Response of atypical symptoms of gastro-oesophageal reflux to antireflux surgery. *Br J Surg* 2001;88(12): 1649–1652.

219. So J, Zeitels S, Rattner D. Outcomes of atypical symptoms attributed to gastroesophageal reflux treated by laparoscopic fundoplication. *Surgery* 1998; 124(1):28–32.

220. Cheung TK, Lim PWY, Wong BC. Noncardiac chest pain—an Asia-Pacific survey on the views of primary care physicians. *Dig Dis Sci.* 2007;52: 3043–3048.

221. Cheung TK, Lim PWY, Wong BCY. The view of gastroenterologists on noncardiac chest pain in Asia. *Aliment Pharmacol Ther* 2007;26:597–603.

222. Orlando R, Bozymski E. Clinical and manometric effects of nitroglycerin in diffuse esophageal spasm. *N Engl J Med* 1989;289(1):23–25.

223. Millaire A, Ducloux G, Marquand A, et al. Clinical effects and effects on esophageal motility. *Arch Mal Coeur Vaiss* 1989;82(1):63–68.

224. Swamy N. Esophageal spasm: clinical and manometric response to nitroglycerine and long acting nitrites. *Gastroenterology* 1977;72(1):23–27.

225. Kikendall J, Mellow M. Effect of sublingual nitroglycerin and long-acting nitrate preparations on esophageal motility. *Gastroenterology* 1980;79(4): 703–706.

226. Mellow M. Effect of isosorbide and hydralazine in painful primary esophageal motility disorders. *Gastroenterology* 1982;83(2):364–370.

227. Davies H, Lewis M, Rhodes J, et al. Trial of nifedipine for prevention of oesophageal spasm. *Digestion* 1987;36(2):81–83.

228. Nasrallah S, Tommaso C, Singleton R, et al. Primary esophageal motor disorders: clinical response to nifedipine. *South Med J* 1985;78(3):312–315.

229. Konrad-Danlhoff I, Baunack A, Ramsch K, et al. Effect of the calcium antagonists nifedipine, nirendipine, nimodipine and nisoldipine on oesophageal motility in man. *Eur J Pharmacol* 1991;41:313–316.

230. Richter J, Spurling T, Cordova C, et al. Effects of oral calcium blocker, diltiazem, on esophageal contractions. Studies in volunteers and patients with nutcracker esophagus. *Dig Dis Sci* 1984;29(7):649–656.

231. Cattau E Jr., Castell D, Johnson D, et al. Diltiazem therapy for symptoms associated with nutcracker esophagus. *Am J Gastroenterol* 1991;86(3): 272–276.

232. Drenth J, Bos L, Engels L. Efficacy of diltiazem in the treatment of diffuse oesophageal spasm. *Aliment Pharmacol* Ther 1990;4(4):411–416.

233. Lee LI, Park H, Kim TH, et al. The effect of sildenafil on esophageal motor function in healthy subjects and patients with nutcracker esophagus. *Neurogastroenterol Motil* 2003;15:617–623.

234. Bortolotti M, Pandolfo N, Giovannini M, et al. Effect of sildenafil on hypertensive lower esophageal sphincter. *Eur J Clin Invest* 2002;32:682–685.

235. Bassoti G, Gaburri M, Imbimbo B, et al. Manometric evaluation of cimetropium bromide activity in patients with the nutcracker oesophagus. *Scand J Gastroenterol* 1988;29(9):1079–1084.

236. Egbunike I, Chaffee B. Antidepressants in the management of chronic pain syndromes. *Pharmacotherapy* 1990;10(4):262–270.

237. Becker B, Morel N, Vanbellinghen A, et al. Blockade of calcium entry in smooth muscle cells by the antidepressant imipramine. *Biochem Pharmacol* 2004;68(5):833–842.

238. Peghini P, Katz P, Castell D. Imipramine decreases oesophageal pain perception in human male volunteers. *Gut* 1998;42(6):807–813.

239. Cannon RO 3rd, Quyyumi AA, Mincemoyer R, et al. Imipramine in patients with chest pain despite normal coronary angiograms. *N Engl J Med* 1994; 330:1411–1417.

240. Gorelick A, Koshy S, Hooper F, et al. Differential effects of amitriptyline on perception of somatic and visceral stimulation in healthy humans. *Am J Physiol* 1998;275(3 Pt 1):G460–G466.

241. Clouse RE, Lustman PJ, Eckert TC, et al. Low-dose trazodone for symptomatic patients with esophageal contraction abnormalities. A double-blind, placebo-controlled trial. *Gastroenterology* 1987;92(4):1027–1036.

242. Handa M, MIne K, Yamamoto H, et al. Antidepressant treatment of patients with diffuse esophageal spasm: a psychosomatic approach. *J Clin Gastroenterol* 1999;28(3):228–232.

243. Varia I, Logue E, O'Connor C, et al. Randomized trial of sertaline in patients with unexplained chest pain of noncardiac origin. *Am Heart J* 2000;140: 367–372.

244. Broekaert D, Fischler B, Sifrim D, et al. Influence of citalopram, a selective serotonin, reuptake inhibitor, on oesophageal hypersensitivity: a double-blind, placebo-controlled study. *Aliment Pharmacol Ther* 2006;23(3):365–370.

245. Bradette M, Delvaux M, Staumont G, et al. Octreotide increases thresholds of colonic visceral perception in IBS patients without modifying muscle tone. *Dig Dis Sci* 1994;39(6):1171–1178.

246. Schwetz I, Naliboff B, Munakata J, et al. Anti-hyperalgesic effect of octreotide in patients with irritable bowel syndrome. *Aliment Pharmacol Ther* 2004; 19(10):123–131.

247. Johnston B, Shils J, Leite L, et al. Effects of octreotide on esophageal visceral perception and cerebral evoked potentials induced by balloon distension. *Am J Gastroenterol* 1994;94 (1):65–70.

248. Crea F, Pupita G, Galassi A, et al. Role of adenosine in pathogenesis of anginal pain. *Circulation* 1990;81(1):164–172.

249. Rao SS, Mudipalli RS, Mujica VR, et al. An open-label trial of theophylline for functional chest pain. *Dig Dis Sci* 2002;47:2763–2768.

250. Rao SS, Mudipalli RS, Remes-Troche JM, et al. Theophylline improves esophageal chest pain—a randomized, placebo-controlled study. *Am J Gastroenterol* 2007;102:930–938.

251. Beitman B, Basha I, Trombka L, et al. Pharmacotherapeutic treatment of panic disorder in patients presenting with chest pain. *J Fam Pract* 1989;28(2):177–180.

252. Wulsin L, Maddock R, Beitman B, et al. Clonazepam treatment of panic disorder in patients with recurrent chest pain and normal coronary arteries. *Int J Psychiatry Med* 1999;29(1):97–105.

253. Tack J, Sarnelli G. Serotonergic modulation of visceral sensation: upper gastrointestinal tract. *Gut* 2002;51(Suppl 1):i77–i80.

254. Rodriguez-Stanley S, Zubaidi S, Proskin H, et al. Effect of tegaserod on esophageal pain threshold, regurgitation, and symptom relief in patients with functional heartburn and mechanical sensitivity. *Clin Gastroenterol Hepatol* 2006;Apr;4(4):442–450.

255. Miller L, Pullela S, Parkman H, et al. Treatment of chest pain in patients with noncardiac, nonreflux, nonachalasia spastic esophageal motor disorders using botulinum toxin injection into the gastroesophageal junction. *Am J Gastroenterol* 2002;97(7):1640–1646.

256. Liu JL, Carr-Locke DL, Osterman MT, et al. Endoscopic treatment for atypical manifestations of gastroesophageal reflux disease. *Am J Gastroenterol* 2006;101:440–445.

257. van Peski-Oosterbaan A, Spinhoven P, van Rood Y, et al. Cognitive-behavioral therapy for noncardiac chest pain: a randomized trial. *Am J Med* 1999;106(4):424–429.

258. Ryan M, Gervirtz R. Biofeedback-based psychophysiological treatment in a primary care setting: an initial feasibility study. *Appl Psychophysiol Biofeedback* 2004;29(2):79–93.

259. Jones H, Cooper P, Miller V, et al. Treatment of non-cardiac chest pain: a controlled trial of hypnotherapy. *Gut* 2006;55:1403–1408.

260. Holzer P. Gastrointestinal afferents as targets of novel drugs for the treatment of functional bowel disorders and visceral pain. *Eur J Pharmacol* 2001;429(1–3):177–193 Review.

261. Zheng Y, Medda BK, Banerjee B, *et al.* Prevention of gastroesophageal reflux-induced ulceration by selective TPRV1 receptor antagonist in rats [abstract]. *Gastroenterology* 2007;132(Suppl S1):A275.

262. Scarpignato C, Pelosini I. Management of irritable bowel syndrome: novel approaches to the pharmacology of gut motility. *Can J Gastroenterol* 1999;13(Suppl A):50A–65A.

CHAPTER 63 ■ ABDOMINAL, PERITONEAL, AND RETROPERITONEAL PAIN

EMERAN MAYER AND HENG WONG

INTRODUCTION

Abdominal pain can result from multiple peripheral and central causes, including injury to or inflammation of the gut, noxious (mechanical or chemical) viscerosensory stimuli, or central pain amplification. Whereas the former causes are generally associated with acute pain, the latter mechanism plays a prominent role in many chronic abdominal pain conditions, including functional gastrointestinal (GI) disorders (FGIDs) and chronic pancreatitis.

Abdominal pain can be divided into visceral and somatic components, which can occur in isolation or in combination during an episode of pain. Somatic and visceral pain have different characteristics which are clinically significant. Somatic pain arises from stimulation of the parietal peritoneum and accurately localizes to a specific part of the abdomen, while visceral pain has a diffuse nature and is experienced over a large portion of the abdomen. The teleological reason for this dichotomy is that somatic pain allows an organism to identify, appraise, and avoid a noxious stimulus. While this does not apply specifically in the case of peritoneal irritation, the parietal peritoneum has a similar embryological origin as somatic structures and therefore receives somatic innervation. In the case of a noxious visceral stimulus, the organism is unable to avoid the stimulus, and there is no functional reason to be able to accurately localize the site of visceral irritation. The responses to a visceral insult are largely autonomic and not consciously mediated by the organism. For example, during an episode of infective gastroenteritis, the response by way of vomiting and diarrhea is an attempt to expel the pathogen or toxin. In the case of ureteric obstruction by a calculus, the peristaltic contractions occur in an attempt to clear the obstruction.

KEY FEATURES IN THE DIAGNOSIS OF ABDOMINAL PAIN

Abdominal pain is a common problem experienced by children and adults alike and, as its potential causes are protean, diagnosis can often be a challenge. However, clinicians can frequently narrow down the potential causes to a few by taking a detailed history and performing a physical examination. In this section, the key features which help the decision-making process will be discussed.

First and foremost, it is crucial to distinguish between acute and chronic abdominal pain. While chronic pain reflects a chronic underlying disease process, the same cannot be said for acute pain. For example, an episode of acute pain may represent the first presentation of a chronic disease process such as the initial symptoms of functional dyspepsia. Alternatively, acute pain may represent a recurrence of a chronic disease which occurs intermittently and is interspersed with asymptomatic periods. A classic example would be that seen in irritable bowel syndrome (IBS) when patients may have symptom-free periods that may last from months to years. Lastly, it is also important to note that patients with chronic abdominal pain can also develop an unrelated acute cause of abdominal pain. For example, in a patient with IBS, an episode of acute abdominal pain may be due to a recurrence of IBS or may occur from an unrelated cause such an episode of diverticulitis or ureteric stone.

In this chapter, acute abdominal pain will be defined as acute pain of a nonrecurrent nature, while chronic abdominal pain will refer to either constant or recurrent pain that has occurred over a 3-month period. It must be emphasized that the distinction between acute and chronic abdominal pain is not always clear

TABLE 63.1

EXTRA-ABDOMINAL CAUSES OF ABDOMINAL PAIN

Cardiopulmonary
Ischemic heart disease
Pericarditis
Pneumonia
Pneumothorax
Pulmonary empyema
Pulmonary embolism/infarction

Neurological
Radiculopathy
Herpes zoster
Tabes dorsalis

Hematological
Henoch-Schönlein purpura
Sickle cell crises

Metabolic/endocrinological
Acute intermittent porphyria
Addison's disease
Diabetic ketoacidosis
Hypercalcemia
Lead poisoning
Uremia

Miscellaneous
Familial Mediterranean fever
Narcotic withdrawal
Fractured ribs

as discussed in the preceding paragraph, and that this definition merely provides a framework for the discussion of the diagnosis of abdominal pain.

Lastly, one must bear in mind that there are a number of extra-abdominal causes presenting as abdominal pain that must be considered when evaluating both acute and chronic abdominal pain. Some of these causes are listed in Table 63.1.

Acute Abdominal Pain

Acute abdominal pain may occur as a result of life-threatening conditions, such as perforated viscera, to relatively benign diagnoses, such as acute gastroenteritis (Table 63.2). The main features relevant to the diagnosis of acute abdominal pain are discussed in this section and an example of the application of such information is illustrated in Figure 63.1.

Site of Pain

The location of pain is largely dependent on whether the pain originates from visceral or somatic structures. Pain from structures with somatic innervation, such the peritoneum, localize accurately to a specific location of the abdomen as the parietal peritoneum receives dense innervation by somatic spinal afferents. On the other hand, pain that originates from the viscera localizes poorly, is inconsistently localized in different patients, and is often experienced over a large portion of the abdomen. This is due to the relatively small number of mechanically sensitive spinal afferents innervating viscera which converge with somatic inputs onto the same spinal neurons at several spinal segments. In general, the perceived site of visceral pain corresponds to the embryological origin to the viscera: the embryological fore-

gut (stomach, duodenum, pancreas, biliary tree), midgut (jejunum and ileum, ascending colon), and hindgut (descending, sigmoid, rectum) localize to the epigastrium, periumbilical area, and suprapubic region respectively.

The localization of visceral pain is illustrated in a study by Doran,[1] in which balloon distention of the bile duct of postcholecystectomy patients leads to epigastric pain in the majority of patients (47%), consistent with the expected localization of visceral pain of foregut origin. However, pain was described in the right upper quadrant and in the back in 18% and 16% of patients, respectively. Furthermore, 19% of patients experienced no pain at all.[1] This variation is seen in clinical practice where patients with acute choledocholithiasis frequently have epigastric pain, but a significant proportion have right upper quadrant pain.

In acute abdominal pain, there can be activation of both somatic and visceral pain afferents. For example, in acute appendicitis, the initial pain is poorly localized in the central abdomen even though the appendix is physically located in the right iliac fossa. At this stage, inflammation is limited to the appendix, and pain is transmitted predominantly via visceral afferents. Subsequently, as the inflammation progresses and involves the parietal peritoneum, the pain from acute appendicitis then becomes localized accurately to the right iliac fossa.

Abdominal pain may radiate to a site distant from the abdomen. Typical examples include the pain seen in acute cholecystitis, when right upper quadrant pain may be referred to the shoulder or scapula or in acute pancreatitis when epigastric pain may be referred to the back. This occurs when there is convergence of visceral and somatic afferents onto a common dorsal horn neuron in the spinal cord. Sensitization of dorsal horn neurons distal to the site of predominant visceral afferent input can result in a situation where visceral pain may be perceived to originate from the area supplied by the corresponding somatic afferent. Activation of the visceral afferent therefore results in the perception of pain in the area supplied by the somatic afferent.

Chronology

The chronology or temporal characteristics of pain provide valuable information on the etiology of the pain. A sudden onset of severe pain which is rapidly progressive usually indicates life-threatening pathology for which urgent treatment is required. Examples include perforation of viscera or major vascular events, such as embolic mesenteric ischemia or a dissecting aortic aneurysm, which can progress over minutes. Progression of pain can also occur relatively slowly over hours or days, such as that seen in acute appendicitis.

The classification of abdominal pain into constant or colicky pain is very useful. Pain due to parietal inflammation and capsule distension is usually constant, while pain from obstruction of viscera with peristaltic activity tends to be colicky.

The frequency of the colic can also help in narrowing the possible causes of pain. Colicky pain from the small and large bowel usually occurs repeatedly over seconds or minutes, while the time course of biliary or renal colic may occur over hours to days. The chronology of the different types of abdominal pain is illustrated in Figure 63.2.

Aggravating/Relieving Factors

Factors which aggravate or alleviate the pain are also useful in the clinical evaluation of abdominal pain. Parietal pain is worsened by movement, which includes deep inspiration and coughing. However, one needs to distinguish parietal pain from muscular pain of the abdominal wall, which is also worsened by movement. In contrast, patients with intestinal obstruction or renal colic tend to writhe about in an attempt to find relief of pain without success. Posture can exacerbate or relieve certain types of abdominal pain. For example, pain from retroperitoneal

TABLE 63.2

CAUSES OF ACUTE ABDOMINAL PAIN AND ASSOCIATED FEATURES

Diagnosis	Location	Onset	Chronology	Aggravating/ relieving factors	Associated features
Parietal Inflammation					
Acute cholecystitis	• Right upper quadrant, sometimes epigastric • Localized • Radiates to shoulder/ scapula	Rapid	Constant	Aggravated by food and deep inspiration	• Fever • Leukocytosis
Acute cholangitis	• Right upper quadrant/ epigastric • Localized • Radiates to scapula/back	Rapid	Constant, pain may be colicky if no parietal involvement	Aggravated by food	• Fever; shaking chills • Jaundice • Leukocytosis • Hyperbilirubinemia • Abnormal liver function test (LFT): cholestatic or mixed pattern
Acute pancreatitis	• Epigastric/periumbilical • Localized • Radiates directly through to mid-back	Rapid	Constant	Aggravated by supine position Relieved by sitting up and adopting fetal position	• May have history of heavy alcohol intake, prior pancreatitis, hyperlipidemia, or on certain drugs • Fever • Vomiting prominent • Leukocytosis • Hyperamylasemia
Acute appendicitis	• Periumbilical initially, then right lower quadrant • Diffuse pain initially, then localized	Gradual	Usually constant, may be colicky initially	When localized to right lower quadrant, aggravated by movements, coughing	• Fever • Leukocytosis
Acute diverticulitis	• Usually left lower quadrant, may be right lower quadrant in right-sided disease • Localized	Gradual	Constant	Aggravated by movement if severe	• Bloody stools • Fever • Leukocytosis
Perforated viscus	• Generalized pain	Sudden	Constant	Aggravated by movement	• Fever • Rigid abdomen; rebound tenderness • Absent bowel sounds • Leukocytosis
Spontaneous bacterial peritonitis	• Generalized, but some patients do not have pain	Gradual	Constant	None	• Significant ascites • Stigmata of chronic liver disease • May have fever but this may be low grade or absent in patients with chronic liver disease • Leukocytosis, may be normal in advanced liver disease • Peritoneal fluid—increased cell count, low albumin

(continued)

TABLE 63.2

CONTINUED

Diagnosis	Location	Onset	Chronology	Aggravating/ relieving factors	Associated features
Visceral Inflammation Infectious enterocolitis	• Variable, usually below umbilicus • Diffuse	Rapid	Colicky	• Aggravated by food, may be partially relieved by defecation	• Diarrhea, may be bloody depending on pathogen • Tenesmus • Leukocytosis • Stool tests for bacteria parasites or *C. difficile* may be positive
Vascular Acute ischemic colitis	• Periumbilical/ lower abdomen • Diffuse	Sudden (if caused by embolus) or rapid	May be constant or colicky	Aggravated by food	• Bloody stools • Pain out of proportion to physical examination • Atrial fibrillation, left-sided cardiac murmurs • Leukocytosis
Dissecting aortic aneurysm	• Epigastric/ periumbilical • Diffuse	Sudden	Constant	None	• Described as "tearing pain" • Radiates to back • Unequal femoral pulses • Expansile abdominal mass • Bruit over abdomen • Hypotensive
Splenic infarct	• Left upper quadrant	Sudden	Constant	None	• Rub may be auscultated over spleen • Risk factors for embolic events
Visceral Obstruction Intestinal obstruction (volvulus, intussusception, adhesions, cancer, strangulated hernia)	• Central, may be generalized • Diffuse	Gradual/rapid depending on etiology	Colicky	Aggravated by food	• Vomiting is prominent • "Tinkling" bowel sounds

Condition	Location	Onset	Nature	Aggravating factors	Associated features
Choledocholithiasis	• Epigastric/right upper quadrant • Diffuse	Rapid	Colicky, episodes usually last hours	Aggravated by food	• Jaundice • Increased bilirubin • Abnormal LFT: cholestatic or mixed pattern
Ureteric stones	• Either flank • Diffuse	Rapid	Colicky	None	• Hematuria • Radiates to testes or inner thigh or groin
Acute urinary retention	• Suprapubic • Localized	Rapid	Constant	Aggravated by movements/cough	• Palpable bladder • Prostatomegaly or fecal impaction may be present
Capsule Distention Liver congestion (heart failure, Budd-Chiari, alcoholic hepatitis)	• Right upper quadrant • Localized	Gradual	Constant	None	• Heavy alcohol intake • Jaundice • Hepatomegaly • Features of heart failure • Absent hepatojugular reflux in Budd-Chiari • Abnormal LFT • May have exquisite tenderness to palpation over liver
Pyelonephritis	• Either flank • Localized	Gradual	Constant	None	• Fever • Hematuria • Increased cell count in urine
Ectopic pregnancy	• Right lower quadrant or left lower quadrant • Localized	Gradual (sudden if ruptured)	Constant	None	• Amenorrhea • Nonmenstrual vaginal bleeding • Adnexal mass • Pregnancy test positive
Tubo-ovarian abscess	• Right lower quadrant or left lower quadrant • Localized	Gradual	Constant	None	• Fever • Adnexal mass • Leukocytosis

With permission from Wong and Mayer.[147]

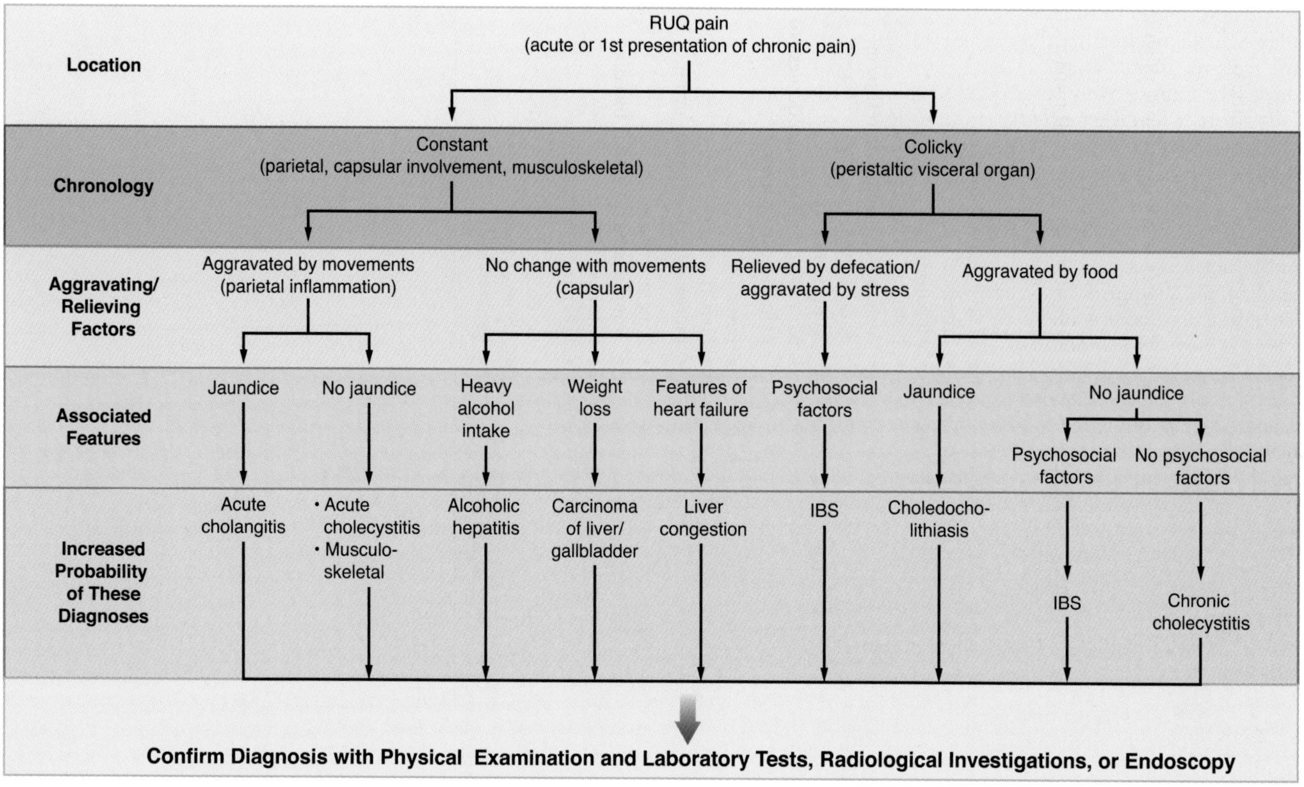

Location	RUQ pain (acute or 1st presentation of chronic pain)							
Chronology	**Constant** (parietal, capsular involvement, musculoskeletal)				**Colicky** (peristaltic visceral organ)			
Aggravating/ Relieving Factors	Aggravated by movements (parietal inflammation)		No change with movements (capsular)			Relieved by defecation/ aggravated by stress	Aggravated by food		
Associated Features	Jaundice	No jaundice	Heavy alcohol intake	Weight loss	Features of heart failure	Psychosocial factors	Jaundice	No jaundice	
								Psychosocial factors	No psychosocial factors
Increased Probability of These Diagnoses	Acute cholangitis	• Acute cholecystitis • Musculo-skeletal	Alcoholic hepatitis	Carcinoma of liver/ gallbladder	Liver congestion	IBS	Choledocho-lithiasis	IBS	Chronic cholecystitis

Confirm Diagnosis with Physical Examination and Laboratory Tests, Radiological Investigations, or Endoscopy

FIGURE 63.1 Example of diagnostic workup for acute right upper quadrant pain (with permission from Wong and Mayer[147]).

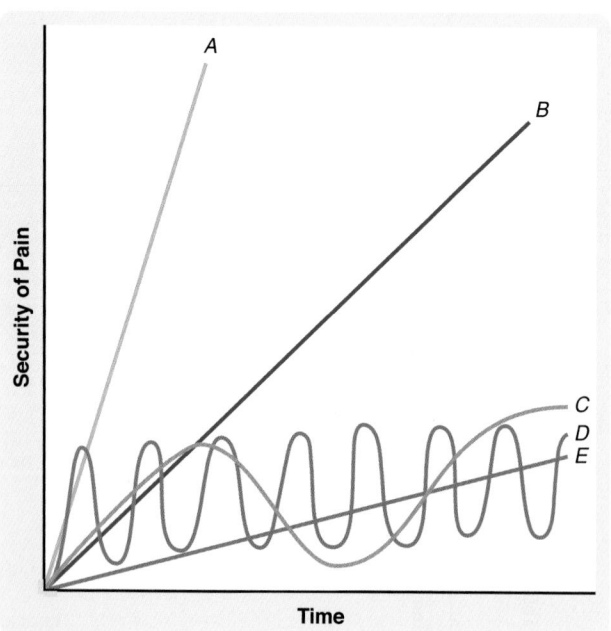

FIGURE 63.2 Typical chronologies of abdominal pain. (**A**) Pain of sudden onset that progresses very rapidly (e.g., rupture of aortic aneurysm). (**B**) Pain that occurs with rapid onset (e.g., acute pancreatitis). (**C**) Colicky pain with long time course (e.g., choledocholithiasis). (**D**) Colicky pain with short time course (e.g., small bowel obstruction). (**E**) Pain that occurs gradually (e.g., acute appendicitis). (With permission from Wong and Mayer.[147])

structures, such as the pancreas, is worsened in the supine position and relieved by leaning forward or assuming a fetal position.

Pain from the GI tract may be exacerbated by intake of food. However, it is important to distinguish between exacerbation of pain directly related to food intake, and nausea or loss of appetite. Many causes of abdominal pain may cause nausea and avoidance of food, while food intake may not necessarily worsen the pain. Examples would be abdominal pain due to liver congestion and ureteric obstruction. The temporal relationship between food intake and the exacerbation of pain should also be considered in the evaluation. For example, pain from the upper GI tract worsens within minutes after food intake, while pain from the small bowel or colon may worsen after hours of food intake. However, it is important to note that pain within minutes of food intake may also occur from colonic contractions due to the gastro-colic reflex. In this clinical scenario, the pain is frequently accompanied by the urge to defecate. On the other hand, food may relieve upper GI lesions, and this usually occurs from the buffering of acid in conditions such as gastroduodenal ulcers or gastroesophageal reflux disorder.

The relief of pain after vomiting suggests pathology in the stomach or proximal small bowel, while relief after defecation or flatulence suggests colonic disease.

Quality

The quality of pain is generally not helpful in the clinical setting as the description of pain is frequently subjective. A useful exception is the "tearing" pain of a dissecting aortic aneurysm. In patients with a previously known cause of abdominal pain, a similar quality experienced during the current episode is useful in the diagnosis. For example, in a patient with a history of acute diverticulitis, the development of a similar episode of pain would point toward another episode of diverticulitis, whereas a different type of pain would suggest an alternative diagnosis.

The description of the severity of pain is also often subjective and is of little diagnostic value. However, if the pain is associated with features of autonomic activation, such as sweatiness and nausea, the pain is likely to be severe. This is particularly useful in situations when the pain is episodic and the patient is asymptomatic at the time of giving the history of pain. Examples include the pain of renal colic and choledocholithiasis.

Associated Factors

Certain features associated with abdominal pain are particularly useful in the diagnosis of acute pain. Patients with abdominal pain and jaundice are likely to have hepatobiliary pathology, while patients with abdominal pain and hematemesis are likely to have an upper GI lesion. The presence of abdominal pain and bloody stools suggest distal colonic pathology. Frank hematuria associated with loin pain suggests ureteric obstruction from renal calculi. Fever is often associated with acute abdominal pain of organic origin, but not with chronic functional abdominal pain or with an acute exacerbation of chronic functional abdominal pain. Weight loss is not a feature of acute abdominal pain, and, if present, there is a likely chronic element to the abdominal pain. Vomiting is commonly associated with many causes of acute abdominal pain, but is rare in functional pain syndromes (despite the common presence of nausea). In obstruction of the proximal small intestine, vomiting is particularly prominent with onset immediately following food intake. In the later stages of large bowel obstruction, the vomitus may look feculent. Abdominal pain associated with heavy alcoholic intake may be related to alcoholic hepatitis or acute pancreatitis.

Past Medical History

A patient's past medical history provides valuable clues in assessing acute abdominal pain. For example, patients with hyperuricemia may be more prone to the formation of renal calculi and the development of renal colic. Patients with atherosclerosis and hypertension would have a higher risk of having an aortic aneurysm and mesenteric ischemia. In patients with poorly controlled diabetes mellitus, one needs to consider the possibility of diabetic ketoacidosis as a cause of acute abdominal pain. In patients with previous abdominal surgery, adhesion colic with intestinal obstruction may occur.

Drug History

Certain medications may be related to the development of abdominal pain. For example, patients taking nonsteroidal anti-inflammatory drugs (NSAIDs) have an increased likelihood of peptic ulcer disease, and patients taking bisphosphonates may develop gastro-esophageal reflux disease. Recent ingestion of antibiotics in patients with bloody diarrhea may point to a diagnosis of pseudomembranous colitis.

Physical Examination

By the time the physical examination is performed, the physician would have determined from the history a list of likely causes of abdominal pain. The physical examination serves to narrow down the possibilities even further.

The physical examination should always start with a general inspection of the patient as the initial appearance helps the clinician determine if the patient is gravely ill and requires immediate treatment. Drowsiness, diaphoresis, and tachypnea are features that point toward a life-threatening condition that demands attention. The vital signs must be taken to exclude hypotensive shock, which may be due to sepsis or hypovolemia. Patients who are curled tightly in the fetal position and lying still are likely to have peritoneal irritation, while patients who writhe about are more likely to have visceral pain. The presence of cachexia suggests an underlying chronic cause of the acute abdominal pain.

The presence of jaundice is an important finding, as this would indicate a hepatobiliary source of the pain. Stigmata of chronic liver disease such as palmar erythema, spider naevi, and Dupuytren's contracture should be sought as this would point toward a hepatic cause of pain and possibly a pancreatic source, since chronic liver disease and pancreatitis often coexist in patients with high alcohol intake. The abdomen may also be grossly distended with intestinal obstruction or with severe ascites. The abdomen should also be inspected carefully for scars, hernia, or bruises.

Palpation of the abdomen should begin at a site distant from that of the presenting pain as this allows the patient to get accustomed to the physical examination, and hence reduce voluntary guarding. Careful palpation will often identify organomegaly and mass lesions and can localize areas of tenderness. Involuntary guarding is due to a reflex contraction of the abdominal muscles following pressure on inflamed peritoneum. Its presence suggests peritonitis, but in practice it is difficult to distinguish peritonitis from voluntary guarding by the patient. With severe peritonitis, the abdomen will feel "board-like" from generalized abdominal wall contraction. Rebound tenderness is another feature of peritonitis and is elicited by gradually applying pressure on the abdomen and suddenly removing the examining hand. Pain on percussion also occurs in peritonitis, and the pain can be brought on by coughing or movement. Percussion is useful in a distended abdomen as it can distinguish between grossly dilated bowel and ascites. Absent bowel sounds on auscultation suggests ileus, which is often present in peritonitis, while tinkling bowel sounds are heard in intestinal obstruction. Bruits may be heard over a hepatoma or an aortic aneurysm.

Rectal examination is an integral part of the physical examination and should always be performed. The presence of bloody stools indicates lower colonic pathology while melena suggests upper GI pathology. A vaginal examination should also be performed to exclude adnexal masses and pelvic inflammatory disease. A systemic examination is also essential as causes of abdominal pain may be associated with pathology in other systems. For example, the presence of atrial fibrillation and left-sided cardiac murmurs predispose to embolic mesenteric ischemia. In addition, the systemic examination may detect extra-abdominal causes of abdominal pain, such as pneumothorax and pneumonia.

Chronic Abdominal Pain

While chronic abdominal pain is rarely life-threatening and seldom requires emergency treatment, chronic abdominal pain can be disabling and significantly affect an individual's health-related quality of life. Although functional GI disorders account for the majority of chronic abdominal pain, mortality and complications can occur as a result of organic GI disease. The challenge is therefore to distinguish functional conditions from chronic organic GI disease. Certain features pointing to organic disease include weight loss, prolonged fever, bloody or melenic stools, steatorrheic stools, jaundice, a strong family history of carcinoma, a palpable mass on physical examination, or anemia (particularly iron deficiency anemia) on laboratory investigation.

The approach to the patient with chronic abdominal pain is similar to that highlighted above for acute abdominal pain. However, certain features such as psychosocial factors, comorbid conditions, and extraintestinal manifestations may be more relevant in chronic abdominal pain. Application of the relevant features in coming to a diagnosis of chronic abdominal pain is illustrated in Figure 63.3. Some of the common causes of chronic abdominal pain are listed in Table 63.3.

Site of Pain

Chronic abdominal pain has even more inconsistent localization than acute abdominal pain, particularly in functional GI disor-

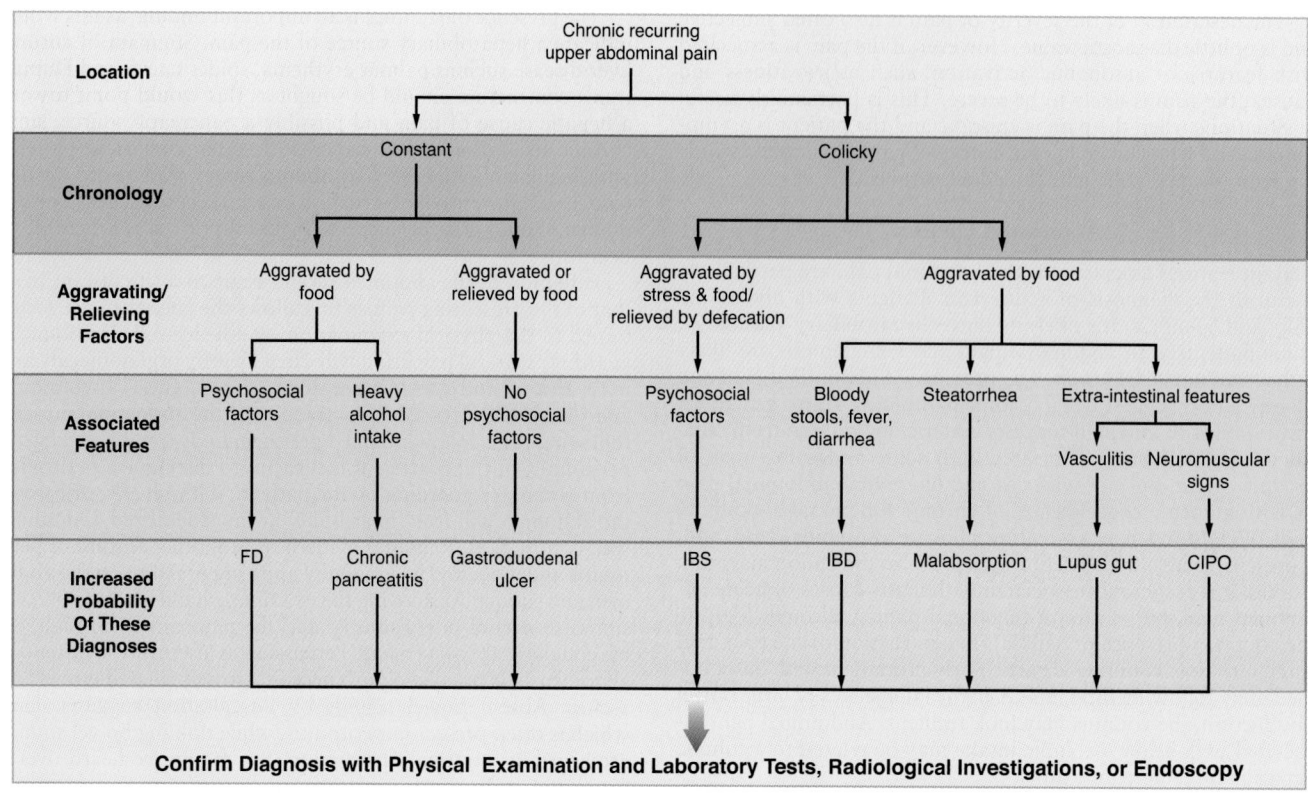

FIGURE 63.3 Example of diagnostic workup for chronic upper abdominal pain. (With permission from Wong and Mayer.)[147]

ders. The atypical pain referral areas in chronic abdominal pain occurs as a result of sensitization, both centrally and peripherally, and the recruitment of previously silent nociceptors. For example, chronic pancreatitis may present as back pain, while patients with FGID tend to report abdominal pain that is diffuse and in atypical regions of their abdomens or even in extra-abdominal sites. For example, patients may experience sigmoid pain to the left upper quadrant or right lower quadrant, and gastric pain at the right upper quadrant. In rare cases, patients report radiation of abdominal pain into the lower extremities, the back, or the entire side of their body. This alteration in viscerosomatic referral area has been reproduced experimentally. When intraluminal balloons were distended at different sites in the colon or stomach, patients with IBS or functional dyspepsia (FD) localized pain to different and larger areas in the abdomen compared to healthy controls.[2]

Pain from carcinoma tends to occur late in the disease. The pain in carcinoma of the solid abdominal organs (e.g., liver, pancreas, kidney) is due to stretching of the organ capsule from tumor growth or from tumor invasion of the capsule, and small early lesions therefore do not usually cause pain. As the pain is secondary to stimuli to the capsule, the pain is well localized. Pain from carcinoma of the GI tract occurs only when the tumor has resulted in a luminal obstruction or has invaded adjacent tissues.

Chronology

Functional GI disorders tend to undergo periods of exacerbation and remission over time, the exception being Functional Abdominal Pain Syndrome (FAPS) where the pain may be constant. In contrast, the pain from advanced carcinoma of the solid visceral organs is constant, and in the absence of intervention is invariably progressive, usually over weeks to months. It is frequently assumed that lower abdominal pain that occurs monthly in relation to menses is related to the pelvic organs. However, GI transit has been reported to be related to the phase of the menstrual cycle,

and both healthy individuals and IBS patients have reported increased GI symptoms during menses compared to other menstrual phases. In functional GI disorders, abdominal discomfort, particularly bloating, is frequently better in the morning on awakening and worse in the evening. The reason for this observation is not clear, but it may be related to the beneficial effects of sleep, as good sleep has been associated with fewer symptoms the following day.

Aggravating/Relieving Factors

Food Intake. A significant number of patients with chronic pain arising from the GI tract report that their symptoms are exacerbated by food intake. This symptom aggravation may be related to specific food items (oily foods, milk products, spicy food), to the volume of food ingestion, to food intake in general, or may even be triggered solely by the thought, smell, or sight of food prior to any food entering the GI tract. Food-induced exacerbation of symptoms is more characteristic for FD and gastroesophageal reflux disease (GERD), than for IBS. Unlike other FGIDs, pain from FAPS is characteristically not affected by food intake.

Bowel Movement. The association of chronic abdominal pain to bowel movements suggests the involvement of the lower GI tract. This point is important to elicit in the history and may help with the diagnosis, particularly if the pain is at an atypical site. This association between chronic abdominal pain and bowel movements is part of the diagnostic criteria of IBS. In patients with IBS, the abdominal pain is associated with a change in stool consistency or stool frequency, and is typically relieved with defecation.

Stress. A history of aversive early life events, such as loss of the primary caregiver, divorce of parents, or a history of physical or sexual trauma, greatly enhances an individual's vulnerability for

(*Text continues on page 913*)

TABLE 63.3

CAUSES OF CHRONIC ABDOMINAL PAIN

Diagnosis	Location	Chronology	Aggravating/relieving factors	Associated features	Psychosocial factors	Extra-abdominal/comorbid diagnosis
Inflammatory Erosive reflux esophagitis	• Epigastric/retrosternal • Diffuse	Severe: persistent Mild: remits/relapses	• Aggravated by • Supine position • Food	• Acid brash • Drug history -NSAIDs -Alendronate -Calcium channel blockers -α and β blockers -Anticholinergics -Tricyclics	None	Extraesophageal • Asthma • Laryngitis • Sore throat • Recurrent bronchitis/pneumonia • Chronic cough • Dental erosions • Sinusitis Comorbid • Scleroderma • Diabetes mellitus • Zollinger-Ellison syndrome • Obesity • Pregnancy
Gastroduodenal ulcer	• Epigastric/right upper quadrant • Localized	Persistent	• Aggravated or relieved by food	• Drug history • NSAIDs • Steroids • Anemia, often iron deficient	Smoking	Comorbid • Zollinger Ellison syndrome • Hypercalcemia
Crohn's disease	• Variable depending on site of disease • Diffuse	Remits/relapses	• Aggravated by food	• Fever • Bloody diarrhea, tenesmus, urgency (colonic disease) • Fistula • Intestinal obstruction • Anemia • Leukocytosis	Smoking	Extra-abdominal • Arthritis • Pyoderma gangrenosum • Erythema nodosum • Uveitis • Episcleritis • Thrombosis Comorbid • Ankylosing spondylitis • Primary sclerosing cholangitis
Eosinophilic gastroenteritis	• Usually central, may be generalized if eosinophilic ascites	Remits/relapses	• Aggravated by food	• Mucosal pattern: vomiting, diarrhea • Muscular pattern: vomiting, distension • Serosal pattern: ascites • Eosinophilia	None	Extra-abdominal • Pleural effusion

(continued)

TABLE 63.3

CONTINUED

Diagnosis	Location	Chronology	Aggravating/ relieving factors	Associated features	Psychosocial factors	Extra-abdominal/ comorbid diagnosis
Lupus gut	• Variable depending on site of disease • Diffuse	Remits/relapses	• Aggravated by food	• Diarrhea • Fever • Anemia • Antinuclear antigen/ double-stranded DNA positive • Decreased C3/C4	Cerebral lupus may mimic psychiatric disease	Extra-abdominal • Malar rash • Vasculitic rash • Arthritis • Digital infarcts • Cardio-pulmonary disease • Glomerulonephritis • Cerebral lupus
Celiac disease	• Central • Diffuse	Persistent	• Aggravated by fatty food (malabsorption)	• Steatorrhea • Weight loss (good appetite) • Anemia (usually iron or folate deficiency) • Antiendomysial antibody positive • Antitissue transglutaminase antibody positive	None	Extraintestinal • Osteopenia • Aphthous stomatitis • Hyposplenism • Fatty liver • Infertility • Epilepsy • Polyneuropathy Comorbid • Dermatitis herpetiformis • Type 1 diabetes mellitus • Primary biliary cirrhosis • Autoimmune hepatitis • Down's syndrome • Autoimmune thyroiditis • IgA deficiency
Malabsorption (e.g., tropical sprue, small bowel bacterial overgrowth)	• Central • Diffuse	Persistent	• Aggravated by fatty food	• Steatorrhea • Travel history (tropical sprue) • Previous GI surgery (bacterial overgrowth)	None	Comorbid (bacterial overgrowth) • Small bowel hypomotility, e.g., CIPO
Ulcerative colitis	• Lower abdomen • Diffuse	Remits/relapses	• Aggravated by food	• Pain not prominent unless severe colitis • Fever • Bloody diarrhea, tenesmus, urgency • Anemia • Leukocytosis	None	Extra-abdominal • Arthritis • Pyoderma gangrenosum • Erythema nodosum • Uveitis • Episcleritis • Thrombosis

Condition	Site / character of pain	Course	Aggravating / relieving factors	Associated features		Comorbid / Extra-abdominal
Chronic pancreatitis	• Epigastric • Localized • Radiates to back and flanks	Remits/relapses	Aggravated by • Supine position • Food Relieved by sitting forward	• Recurrent pancreatitis • Weight loss • Steatorrhea • Amylase may or may not be raised	None	Comorbid • Primary sclerosing cholangitis • Ankylosing spondylitis Extra-abdominal • Diabetes mellitus Comorbid • Hypertriglyceridemia
Chronic cholecystitis	• Epigastric/right upper quadrant • Diffuse • Radiates to scapula	Remits/relapses	Aggravated by food	None	None	None
Malignancy Advanced colorectal carcinoma	• Obstructed—central, lower abdomen, diffuse • Extraluminal invasion—variable, localized	Progressive	Aggravated by food (obstructed)	• Family history of cancer • Weight loss • Change in bowel habit • Bloody stools • Anemia, often iron deficient	None	Extra-abdominal • Metastases • Anemia (particularly iron deficiency) • Paraneoplastic phenomena
Hepatoma	• Right upper quadrant • Localized	Progressive	None	• Family history of cancer • Weight loss • History and signs of chronic liver disease • Jaundice • Abdominal mass • Anemia • Abnormal LFT • Increased alpha-fetoprotein	None	Extra-abdominal • Metastases • Anemia • Paraneoplastic phenomena
Gallbladder carcinoma	• Right upper quadrant • Localized	Progressive	None	• Weight loss • Abdominal mass • Anemia	None	Extra-abdominal • Metastases • Anemia • Paraneoplastic phenomena

(continued)

TABLE 63.3

CONTINUED

Diagnosis	Location	Chronology	Aggravating/ relieving factors	Associated features	Psychosocial factors	Extra-abdominal/ comorbid diagnosis
Pancreatic carcinoma	• Epigastric • Localized	Progressive	None	• Family history of cancer • Weight loss • Jaundice (if head of pancreas involved) • Abdominal mass • Abnormal LFT with cholestatic pattern (if head of pancreas involved)	None	Extra-abdominal • Metastases • Anemia • Paraneoplastic phenomena
Renal carcinoma	• Either loin • Localized	Progressive	None	• Family history of cancer • Weight loss • Hematuria • Abdominal mass • Anemia	None	Extra-abdominal • Metastases • Anemia • Paraneoplastic phenomena
Functional Nonerosive reflux disease	• Epigastric/ retrosternal • Diffuse	Remits/relapses	Aggravated by stress, supine position, fatty food	• Acid brash • Drug history -NSAIDs -Alendronate -Calcium channel blockers -α and β blockers -Anticholinergics • Normal hemoglobin (Hb) and white cell count (WCC)	• Smoking • Alcohol • Depression, bipolar disorder, schizophrenia, borderline personality	Extra-abdominal • Asthma • Laryngitis Comorbid • Scleroderma • Diabetes mellitus • Zollinger Ellison syndrome • Obesity • Pregnancy
Nutcracker esophagus	• Epigastric/ retrosternal • Diffuse	Remits/relapses	Aggravated by stress	• Dysphagia • Normal Hb and WCC	• Anxiety, depression, somatization	Comorbid • GERD
Diffuse esophageal spasm	• Epigastric/ retrosternal • Diffuse	Remits/relapses	Aggravated by food, hot/cold liquids	• Dysphagia • Normal Hb and WCC	None	None
FD	• Right upper quadrant/ epigastric/ left upper quadrant	Remits/relapses	Aggravated by stress, food	• Vomiting, bloating • Normal Hb and WCC	• Anxiety, depression, Early life stress	Extra-abdominal • Backache • Headache Comorbid • IBS

	Site	Course	Relation to food/stress	Clinical features	Psychological	Extra-abdominal/Comorbid

Chronic intestinal pseudo-obstruction (CIPO)	• Diffuse/localized depending on subtype
	• Central
	• Diffuse
		Mild: remits/relapses
		Severe: persistent
			Aggravated by food	• Dysphagia
				• Constipation
				• Abdominal distention
				• Bloating
				• History of malignancy (paraneoplastic phenomenon)
				• Family history of CIPO
				• Drug history
				  • Tricyclics
				  • Narcotics
				  • Anticholinergics
				  • Phenothiazines
				• Orthostatic hypotension
				• Normal Hb and WCC
					None	Extra-abdominal
						• Urinary symptoms
						• Neuromuscular symptoms/signs
						Comorbid
						• Diabetes mellitus
						• Multiple sclerosis
						• Scleroderma
						• Muscular dystrophy
						• Amyloidosis

IBS	• Variable • Diffuse	Remits/relapses	Aggravated by stress, food	• Diarrhea, constipation or alternating habit • Mucus par rectum • Bloating • Normal Hb and WCC	• Anxiety, depression, hypochondriasis, panic, phobia, neuroticism, somatization, posttraumatic stress disorder • Early life stress	Extra-abdominal • Dyspareunia • Impotence • Insomnia • Fatigue • Backache • Dysmenorrhea • Urinary frequency Comorbid • Functional dyspepsia • Fibromyalgia • Interstitial cystitis • Chronic prostatitis • Chronic pelvic pain syndrome • Migraine
FAPS	• Variable • Diffuse	Persistent	Aggravated by stress	• No change in bowel habit • Onset associated with stressful event/abuse • Normal Hb and WCC	• Anxiety, depression, somatization	None

(continued)

TABLE 63.3

CONTINUED

Diagnosis	Location	Chronology	Aggravating/ relieving factors	Associated features	Psychosocial factors	Extra-abdominal/ comorbid diagnosis
Chronic Infection						
Esophageal candidiasis	• Epigastric/ retrosternal • Diffuse	Persistent	Aggravated by swallowing	• Oral candidiasis	None	Comorbid • Immunosuppression (drug-induced, HIV)
Cytomegalovirus infection	• Variable depending on site of disease • Diffuse	Persistent	Aggravated by swallowing (esophagus)	• Bloody diarrhea (colon)	None	Comorbid • Immunosuppression (drug-induced, HIV)
Tuberculosis (TB) enterocolitis	• Variable depending on site of disease • Diffuse	Persistent	Aggravated by food	• Weight loss • Bloody stools • Change of bowel habit • Fever • Abdominal mass • Fistulae • Travel to endemic area • Exposure to patient with TB • Monocytosis	None	Extra-abdominal • Pulmonary TB • Rash (erythema nodosum) Comorbid • Immunosuppression (drugs, HIV) • Malnutrition
TB peritonitis	• Generalized	Persistent	None	• Weight loss • Ascites • Fever • Travel to endemic area • Exposure to patient with TB • Monocytosis • Peritoneal fluid—increased cell counts, stain positive for acid-fast bacilli	None	Extra-abdominal • Pulmonary TB • Rash (erythema nodosum) Comorbid • Immunosuppression (drugs, HIV) • Malnutrition
Miscellaneous						
Chronic mesenteric ischemia	• Variable • Diffuse	Remits/relapses	Aggravated by food	• Bloody stools • Anemia	None	Comorbid • Atherosclerotic disease
Adhesions	• Variable • Diffuse	Remits/relapses	Aggravated by food	• Previous abdominal/ pelvic surgery	None	None

With permission from Wong and Mayer.[147]

FGIDs later in life, a typical example being IBS. Apart from increasing susceptibility to FGIDs, stress is also associated with the initial onset or exacerbation of symptoms in FGIDs and common examples of severe stressors include bereavement, divorce proceedings, or financial distress. However, the role of stress in symptom exacerbation is not limited to functional GI pain, but has also been reported in inflammatory bowel disease (IBD) and GERD.[3] For example, a population-based study found that 64% of patients with GERD had exacerbation of symptoms with stress, and GERD patients who are chronically anxious and exposed to long periods of stress are more likely to exhibit stress-induced symptom exacerbation. Stress has also been reported to be associated with exacerbations in patients with IBD.

Psychiatric Comorbidity. Psychiatric comorbidity is strongly associated with FGIDs and should be evaluated when assessing a patient with chronic abdominal pain. It is not uncommon for patients with FGIDs to have a history of anxiety and depression. In a subset of IBS patients who develop IBS-like symptoms following an enteric infection (i.e., postinfectious IBS [PI-IBS], hypochondriasis, anxiety, neuroticism, and somatization) have been reported to be risk factors predisposing to the development of PI-IBS.[4]

Lifestyle Factors

Lifestyle may be relevant in the assessment of chronic abdominal pain. For example, a history of heavy alcohol intake may lead to chronic pancreatitis and alcoholic liver cirrhosis, which is in itself a risk factor for hepatoma. Sexual orientation or intravenous drug abuse may be related to the probability of chronic hepatitis B or C and human immunodeficiency virus (HIV), which are risk factors for hepatoma and opportunistic infections, respectively. Travel to the tropics may predispose to chronic infections such as tuberculosis of the abdomen, giardiasis, and tropical sprue.

Quality of Pain

As in the assessment of acute abdominal pain, the quality of pain is generally unhelpful in evaluating chronic abdominal pain, an exception being the "burning" sensation that is typical of GERD. Heartburn is defined as "a burning feeling rising from the stomach or lower chest up toward the neck" and when heartburn is a major or sole symptom, GERD is the cause in at least 75% of patients.[5] However, distension (and possibly contractions) of the distal esophagus can also be experienced as a burning sensation. In patients with a known history of recurrent chronic abdominal pain, the quality of pain is useful in assessing if the pain is due to another recurrence or if the pain is from an alternative cause.

Associated Factors

One of the challenges in the assessment of chronic abdominal pain is to distinguish FGIDs from organic disease. Factors that point to an organic disease and deserve detailed investigations include the presence of fever, jaundice, bloody stools, or significant weight loss. Persistent fever is not a feature of FGIDs, and when present, one needs to search for chronic infections, inflammatory disease, or malignancy. Jaundice would point toward pathology of the hepatobiliary system while the chronic passage of bloody stools mandates colonic evaluation. While weight loss can be present in severe FGIDs, one needs to exclude organic disease before making the diagnosis of FGIDs. It is commonly thought that abdominal pain that wakes a patient from sleep is of an organic origin, but it has been reported that nocturnal pain is a common symptom in patients with FGIDs.[6]

Nongastrointestinal Symptoms

Patients with FGIDs, particularly IBS, commonly have associated chronic pain conditions such as migraine, fibromyalgia, chronic fatigue, interstitial cystitis, dysmenorrhea, and dyspareunia. In some of these patients, the extra-GI symptoms may be more distressing than the GI symptoms. The identification of extra-GI symptoms is valuable in the overall management of patients with FGIDs. In IBD, extraintestinal manifestations may be present. These include erythema nodosum, pyoderma gangrenosum, sacroiliitis, and uveitis. Patients with lupus gut may have a malar rash and vasculitic skin lesions.

Drug History

In addition to the risk of acute peptic ulcers, chronic NSAID usage is associated with NSAID colitis. The frequent use of antispasmodics and antidiarrheal agents to treat colicky abdominal pain can lead to the development of chronic constipation and subsequent constipation colic. This needs to be recognized, as continued use of antispasmodic agents would only temporarily alleviate the symptoms and lead to worsening of the underlying constipation. Similarly, chronic use of opiate analgesics can lead to chronic constipation.

Family History

The family history is particularly useful in evaluating chronic abdominal pain as there is a genetic predisposition to inflammatory disorders such as IBD and celiac disease, as well as carcinoma. FGIDs are also more common in patients who have a family history, and this predisposition is thought to be due to both genetic and environmental factors.

Physical Examination

The presence of spider naevi and palmar erythema would alert the clinician to the possibility of liver pathology or alcohol-related disease. In patients with advanced malignancy, masses may be palpable in the abdomen. The presence of blood on rectal examination would indicate organic disease rather than functional disorders. In FGIDs, the physical examination does not usually add more information than that obtained from the history.

FUNCTIONAL GASTROINTESTINAL DISORDERS

General Considerations

FGIDs comprise a wide a spectrum of GI disorders in both the adult and pediatric population. Unlike organic disease, FGIDs are currently classified purely by symptoms, and the diagnosis of FGIDs requires the absence of pathology that may account for the symptoms. The use of symptom-based diagnosis has been validated in a study in which the use of the Rome criteria demonstrated a positive predictive value of 98% in IBS when alarm features such as weight loss, blood in stools, use of antibiotics, nocturnal symptoms, a family history of colon cancer, and abnormalities on physical examination were absent.[7] However, the lack of a discriminatory value between abdominal pain and discomfort in some of these symptom-based criteria puts into question their ability to identify a homogenous group of disorders. For example, chronic abdominal discomfort (in the form of urgency) relieved by bowel movement, but without associated pain, is a nonspecific symptom occurring in different types of organic colitis, such as collagenous and microscopic colitis. Unless these diagnoses are ruled out by biopsies from the colonic mucosa with specialized histological examinations, a large number of these organic conditions will be included under the Rome criteria for IBS.[8] Another problem with symptom-based criteria is the difficulty in classifying FGIDs which have similar symptoms such as those encountered in FD and GERD.

Some FGIDs are characterized by pain or discomfort (e.g., IBS, FD, and FAPS), while others are characterized by altered bodily functions such as functional diarrhea, functional constipation, and aerophagia. This section will focus on FGIDs in the adult population in which chronic abdominal pain is a prominent feature.

Despite the benign prognosis of FGIDs, the health-related quality of life in FGID patients can be affected significantly by their symptoms. For example, the reduction in health-related quality of life in IBS has been reported to be similar to that for patients with diabetes mellitus or renal failure. Similarly, the health-related quality of life in FD was poorer than that experienced by patients with chronic liver disease.[9]

Pathophysiology

Despite considerable progress in the understanding of epidemiological, clinical, and some pathophysiological aspects of FGIDs over the past decade, there is currently no general agreement on the relative contribution of central and peripheral mechanisms involved in the pathophysiology of these disorders. However, a consensus is evolving around the following general concepts: (a) FGIDs are currently defined by symptom criteria, but each diagnostic category may comprise heterogeneous group of pathophysiologies, presenting with similar symptoms. Different subsets of patients may therefore show alterations in GI motility, secretion, gut immune function, or dysregulation of the brain-gut axis, either in isolation or in combinations thereof[10]; (b) despite this heterogeneity, the FGIDs share certain features, which are characteristic for functional disorders in general. These include enhanced stress sensitivity which is associated with autonomic nervous system and hypothalamic-pituitary-adrenal axis dysfunction, comorbidity with psychiatric and chronic pain disorders, greater prevalence in women, and enhanced perception of visceral events. These features have been conceptualized in terms of alterations in the emotional motor system (EMS), a set of parallel output pathways from the brain coordinating autonomic, neuroendocrine, and pain modulatory responses associated with anxiety, anger, and other emotions.[11]

Enhanced Perception of Visceral Pain

A common feature in patients with FGIDs associated with pain or discomfort appears to be an alteration in the perception of visceral afferent stimuli ("visceral hypersensitivity") in which a normally innocuous stimulus, such as contractions or distensions of the gut, leads to the sensation of pain or discomfort. The stimuli may be spontaneous peristaltic activity or from distension by luminal contents such as gas, ingested food/liquids, or feces. Visceral hypersensitivity may be quantified as lowered discomfort thresholds, increased intensity, and affective stimulus ratings, and atypical viscerosomatic referral areas (the somatic area of the body at which a subject localizes a visceral stimulus) in which the referral area is both atypical in location and of a larger area. It has been reported that patients with IBS, FD, or noncardiac chest pain have reduced perception thresholds to balloon distension of the rectosigmoid, stomach, and esophagus, respectively.[10,12]

Fifty to 70% of IBS patients have been reported to have a lower perception threshold for pain and discomfort in response to rectal, sigmoid, and left colonic balloon inflation.[10] When other measures of visceral hypersensitivity (i.e., reported intensity of pain and altered viscerosomatic referral area) were grouped with lowered perception thresholds to rectal balloon distension, 94% of IBS patients showed evidence for altered visceral perception.[13] Visceral hypersensitivity may be relevant clinically as there is a

correlation between the experimentally observed pain thresholds and the reported severity of the symptom of pain in IBS.[10]

Similarly, increased sensitivity to gastric distension has been reported in FD and may be relevant clinically as the pain reproduced on gastric distension was associated with nausea and bloatedness, similar to that of FD which occurred after a meal.[14] The reduction in threshold to gastric distension was observed in 34% to 65% of FD subjects compared to controls.[15,16] Using combined measurements of viscerosomatic referral areas and gastric distension thresholds, 87% of FD subjects had evidence for altered perception of gastric stimuli.[15]

This perceptual abnormality appears to be unique to FGIDs, since it is not observed in patients with mild, uncomplicated chronic inflammatory disorders of the upper or lower gut. For example, abdominal pain is not a prominent feature in ulcerative colitis despite extensive chronic inflammation of the colonic mucosa. In contrast to FGIDs, patients with ulcerative colitis,[17] chronic organic dyspepsia,[15] and GERD[18] had no difference in mechanical visceral hypersensitivity compared to controls. It has been suggested that in chronic inflammatory conditions, patients are able to activate adaptive endogenous central pain modulation pathways, while patients with FGIDs have a compromised ability to activate these adaptive mechanisms.[19] It has been reported that IBS patients have a reduced ability to activate descending endogenous pain modulation mechanisms in response to rectal balloon inflation.[20]

Stress Sensitivity

Stress sensitivity is a key feature of FGIDs and may play an important role in both the etiology of and symptom exacerbation in IBS, FD, and FAPS. It is also present in affective disorders and other chronic pain disorders such as fibromyalgia and interstitial cystitis, and may be the reason for the common coexistence of these disorders with FGIDs.

Etiology

IBS patients report more lifetime stressful events including severe abuse history[10] and early childhood aversive events than controls.[21] Poor quality of life has also been reported to predispose to the onset of IBS.[22] PI-IBS is a subset of IBS in which patients with infective gastroenteritis develop persistent symptoms even after the initial infection has resolved. In these patients, the presence of sustained psychological stressors before, during, or after the period of infection increases the probability of developing PI-IBS.[4] Aversive events in childhood experiences may also predispose to other FGIDs, such as FD[23] and FAPS.[24] The onset of pain in FAPS is frequently associated with stressful events such as bereavement of a spouse or close relation or stillbirth during pregnancy.[24] It is currently assumed that early life stress may interact with genetic predisposition to determine the vulnerability of an individual to adult stressors and subsequent development of FGIDs (Fig. 63.4).

Symptom Exacerbation

Psychosocial stressors are commonly associated with exacerbation of symptoms in FGIDs. For example, stressful events are more likely to lead to abdominal pain and change in stool pattern in IBS patients compared to healthy controls, and stress has been correlated with bowel symptoms and physician visits.[25] A detailed history will identify sustained or traumatic stressful life events preceding symptom exacerbation in the majority of IBS patients even though patients may not offer this information initially. Studies in experimental animal models support the concept of acute stress-induced visceral hypersensitivity and it has been reported that auditory stress enhances perception of visceral stimuli in IBS patients.[26] Several studies reported an association be-

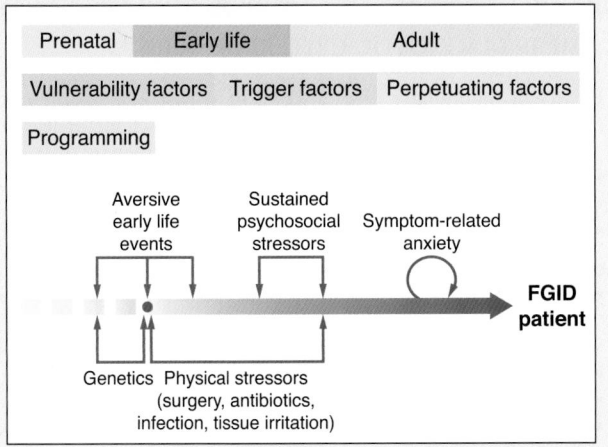

Prenatal	Early life		Adult
Vulnerability factors	Trigger factors		Perpetuating factors
Programming			

FIGURE 63.4 Putative role of stress in the pathophysiology of functional GI disorders. Upper section: (1) The top bar indicates the phases in life from prenatal to adulthood. (2) The second bar indicates the role of different factors in the etiology of FGIDs in relation to the different phases of life. Vulnerability factors are thought to mediate their effects in utero until early life. Trigger factors manifest in early life to adulthood and lead to FGIDs. Perpetuating factors (such as symptom-related fears and anxiety) play a role in the chronicity of FGIDs. (3) The third bar indicates the role of an individual's programming by prenatal environmental influences. Lower section: Various vulnerability, trigger, and perpetuating factors interact with genetic predispositions to result in the development of chronic FGIDs. (With permission from Wong and Mayer.[147])

tween stress and FD,[27,28] but this has not been demonstrated in other studies.[29]

In addition to its effects on the etiology and symptom exacerbation of IBS, a history of emotional, physical, or sexual abuse, stressful life events, chronic social stress, and maladaptive coping style have been shown to adversely affect the illness experience and treatment outcome.[10] Similarly, a history of physical or sexual abuse in FAPS is associated with poorer health status, medical refractoriness, increased health care visits, and increased diagnostic and therapeutic procedures.[30]

TREATMENT OF ABDOMINAL PAIN

General Principles in the Treatment of Acute Abdominal Pain

Acute abdominal pain generally signals visceral pathology that may require immediate surgery or medical intervention. The treatment of an organic cause of acute abdominal pain is dependent on the specific diagnosis as treatment is targeted against the underlying pathophysiology, such as surgery in perforated viscera and in acute appendicitis or acid suppression in peptic ulcer disease, and is beyond the scope of this chapter. One of the hallmarks of acute abdominal pain is that it will subside with effective treatment of the underlying pathology.

General Principles in the Treatment of Chronic Abdominal Pain

The treatment of chronic abdominal pain is targeted against the underlying pathophysiology if an organic cause of the pain can be identified. However, in the majority of cases, chronic abdomi-

nal pain occurs as a result of FGIDs for which the treatment is much less satisfactory. Treatment for functional abdominal pain disorders is tailored for symptom relief rather than specific disease processes (which are largely unknown), and treatment is often suboptimal. This section will focus on the management of FGIDs and will discuss general therapeutic principles as well as specific treatment modalities for the respective FGID.

Doctor-Patient Relationship and Patient Education

The doctor-patient relationship is of utmost importance in the treatment of FGIDs and cannot be overemphasized. The physician must listen to and determine the patient's understanding of the illness and related concerns as patients frequently seek validation from the physician that their symptoms are real. It is likely that many patients have been told previously that their symptoms are "all in their head" and their worries brushed aside. The reason for many patients with FGIDs to visit a physician is a flare of their usual symptoms, and it is important to identify such trigger factors, in particular various psychosocial stressors.

A thorough explanation of the symptoms and relationship to FGIDs should be given to the patient, including the natural history and benign prognosis of the disorder as many patients have inappropriate coping styles, incorrect beliefs about their symptoms, and a significant amount of anxiety related to their symptoms. It has been reported that patients who are not properly informed tend to have more health care visits, and that symptoms are reduced when diagnostic and prognostic information are explained to the patient. The physician must then set realistic short- and long-term goals, including methods of adapting to symptoms that are not amenable to treatment.

Lastly, the patient must be involved in the treatment; the keeping of a symptom diary is an example. Apart from providing the patient with a sense of empowerment, the symptom diary can help identify lifestyle or dietary factors that exacerbate symptoms, and modifications based on this information may provide symptomatic relief to the patient that is cost-effective and devoid of drug side effects.

Dietary Modification

Patients with FGIDs often complain that certain types of food exacerbate their symptoms. Food sensitivity of symptoms may be related to conditioned fear responses related to anticipatory anxiety, food intake in general, volume of the meal, or sensitivities to certain food items. For example, some FD patients may get a worsening of symptoms with large meals, while some IBS patients report symptom exacerbation with fatty food, gas-producing foods, alcohol, and caffeine. In the latter category, the offending agents tend to differ from person to person, and it is useful for the patient to maintain a symptom diary in order to determine their individual food sensitivities.

Pharmacological Agents

Pharmacological therapy in FGIDs can be broadly classified into peripheral and central agents. Peripherally targeted drugs are aimed at a wide range of presumed (but largely unproven) pathophysiologies including altered GI motility and secretion, visceral hypersensitivity, and altered intestinal flora. Categories of drugs include antispasmodics, prokinetics, visceral analgesics, antibiotics, and probiotics. Centrally targeted drugs are given based on the following rationales: (a) reduction of central mechanisms which modulate visceral afferent signals, pain, and emotions (the targets of these treatments are central stress and emotion-generating circuits involving various neurotransmitter systems, such as substance P/neurokinin receptors, corticotropin releasing factor [CRF]/CRF$_1$ receptors, serotonin/5-HT$_3$ receptors, and norepinephrine/alpha-2 receptors); and (b) treatment of psychiatric comorbidity, in particular anxiety disorders and depression.

Altered central processing of peripheral afferent input from the viscera appears to be a feature shared by different FGIDs and centrally acting drugs, such as low-dose tricyclic antidepressants (TCAs), selective serotonin reuptake inhibitors (SSRIs), combined serotonin and norepinephrine reuptake inhibitors (SNRI), and compounds used in the treatment of neuropathic pain, such as gabapentin, carbamazepine, and lamotrigine, may be useful in selected patients. However, evidence from high-quality randomized, controlled trials to support the use of the majority of these agents is lacking, and use is largely based on personal clinical experience. Furthermore, in the case of antidepressants, it is unclear if reported benefits are secondary to drug-induced improvement in mood and affect, or represent a direct effect on the brain-gut axis.

The observation that much lower doses of TCAs are required and a shorter lag time to onset of therapeutic effect is present in treating functional GI symptoms (as well as chronic pain in a variety of other disorders) suggests that their action may be mediated in part by their various postsynaptic effects, rather than their inhibitory effect on the reuptake of serotonin and norepinephrine. Interestingly, in addition to their presumed central mechanisms of action, TCAs have also been found to have an analgesic effect on visceral afferent neurons as well as an effect on neuropathic pain.

Patients frequently use anxiolytics and sedatives, and many of the popular IBS drugs in the past were combinations of such centrally acting drugs with "antispasmodics." There appears to be a small benefit of benzodiazepines over placebo in the treatment of IBS, but the risk of physical dependence potentially outweighs the benefits of this class of drugs for chronic therapy.

Psychological Therapy

Several trials have shown the benefit of different forms of psychological therapy for FGIDs,[10,31–35] while others did not reveal any advantage compared to standard medical treatment.[36,37] A major problem with conducting studies on the efficacy of psychological therapy is the inability to blind the therapists to the treatment arms. Similarly, blinding the subjects to treatment arms is difficult. A related problem is a lack of a credible placebo treatment arm seen in many of the studies on psychological therapies. For example, studies often employed standard medical treatment or the monitoring of symptoms while awaiting therapy as their placebo arms. However, these placebo arms are associated with a negative expectancy as the subjects were often referred to these trials when they failed standard medical treatment and were not expected to improve while waiting for therapy. Therefore, the placebo effect of psychological therapy cannot be clearly separated from its true effects. This is particularly relevant in FGIDs where the improvements to placebo occur in up to 50% of patients. Lastly, unlike pharmacological therapy, psychological therapy is dependant largely on the skills of the therapist, and results obtained in one center may not be reproducible in another center.

IRRITABLE BOWEL SYNDROME

IBS is defined as abdominal pain or discomfort that is associated with defecation or a change in bowel habits, and requires the absence of detectable organic disease that may explain the symptoms. The recently revised Rome III diagnostic criteria used in the diagnosis of IBS are listed in Table 63.4. Given the high prevalence of IBS in the general population, comorbidity of organic GI syndromes with IBS is to be expected. Such comorbidity has been reported for ulcerative, microscopic, and collagenous colitis, and celiac disease. This comorbidity has important implications for the treatment of these patients when IBS-like symptoms persist despite optimal management of the underlying organic disease.

TABLE 63.4

ROME III DIAGNOSTIC CRITERIA FOR IBS[38]

Recurrent abdominal pain or discomfort at least 3 days per month in the last 3 months (but with symptom onset for at least 6 months) associated with 2 or more of the following:
- Improvement with defecation
- Onset associated with a change in frequency of stool
- Onset associated with a change in form (appearance) of stool.

Symptoms that cumulatively support the diagnosis of IBS
- Abnormal stool frequency: ≤3 bowel movements per week or >bowel movements per week
- Abnormal stool form: lumpy/hard stool or loose/watery stool
- Defecation straining
- Urgency
- Feeling of incomplete bowel movement
- Passing mucus
- Bloating or feeling of abdominal distention

IBS is further subdivided into IBS with diarrhea (IBS-D), IBS with constipation (IBS-C), or IBS with mixed bowel habits (IBS-M), depending on the predominant bowel habit. When patients do not fulfill any of the criteria for IBS-D, IBS-C, or IBS-M, they are classified as unspecified IBS. Lastly, there is another subset termed PI-IBS which includes patients who develop persistent IBS symptoms despite the resolution of infection from a bout of bacterial gastroenteritis.

Epidemiology

IBS is a common disorder and the worldwide prevalence range is about 10% to 20%.[38,39] Like many related functional pain disorders, it is more common in women with a female:male ratio of 2–2.5:1.[40] It is generally assumed that IBS most commonly presents between the ages of 30 and 50 years; however, recent surveys indicated that IBS is also common in the pediatric population where such symptoms have traditionally been referred to as recurrent abdominal pain.

The socioeconomic burden attributed to IBS is significant, with IBS patients taking three times as many days of sick leave than individuals without IBS,[40] and 8% of IBS subjects retiring early because of their symptoms.[41] It accounts for 12% and 19% of the patient load in primary care and gastroenterology clinics, respectively. In the United States, IBS was estimated to account for $1.6 billion in direct and $19.2 billion in indirect costs.[10]

Symptoms

The location of abdominal symptoms in IBS is highly variable and is diffuse because it is related to the visceral component of abdominal pain and there is an altered central perception of pain, as discussed previously. The pain is frequently aggravated by emotion or stress, poor sleep, and after food intake, but these aggravating factors cannot be elicited in all patients. By definition, abdominal symptoms are relieved by defecation. If symptoms are unrelated to defecation or food intake, and if patients indicate that symptoms are constant and not relievable by any physiological intervention, the differential diagnosis of FAPS should be considered. It is important to note that weight loss is uncommon in IBS (in the absence of depression or eating disorders), and its presence mandates investigation of an underlying organic cause. IBS symptoms occur mainly during wakefulness, but may also awaken patients from sleep.

Symptom severity in IBS varies widely from mild to very severe. The majority of patients in population-based surveys fall into the mild symptom category, while the majority of chronic specialty clinic attendees report their symptoms as severe. Even though present in mildly symptomatic patients as well, the latter group of patients tends to have a higher prevalence of coexisting psychiatric disorders and health-seeking behavior. The presence of coexisting depression predicts a poorer response to both pharmacological and psychological treatment.[34]

IBS symptoms tend to recur frequently as it has been reported that in a 12-week period, IBS patients experience an average of 12 episodes of symptom exacerbation with intervening periods of remission. However, taken over a long time course, the natural history of IBS is that of periods of exacerbation followed by periods of remission. Two longitudinal studies done 1 year and 5 years apart have shown that about 40% of IBS subjects become asymptomatic at the end of the respective studies.[42,43] In a more recent population-based longitudinal study, 55% of subjects who initially reported symptoms of IBS did not report these symptoms at the time of the final survey.[44] Although the IBS symptoms resolved in the majority of subjects, transitions to other complexes of GI symptoms, such as functional dyspepsia, were also observed.

Psychiatric Comorbidity

Psychiatric disorders, such as anxiety disorders (e.g., generalized anxiety disorder, panic disorder, and posttraumatic stress syndrome), depression, somatization, hypochondriasis, and phobias,[45,46] commonly coexist with IBS. The prevalence of coexisting psychiatric disorders varies with the target population studied, and has been reported to range from 40% to over 90% in tertiary referral centers. The high comorbidity seen in such referral centers is likely to reflect an overestimate as patients with coexisting psychiatric disorders, in particular depression, tend to exhibit greater health care-seeking behavior. It has been suggested that individuals with IBS who do not consult physicians regarding their symptoms ("IBS nonconsulters") may be similar psychologically to the healthy controls.[10,47] However, several population-based surveys tend to contradict this conclusion, demonstrating the presence of more GI symptoms in individuals with affective disorders[45,48] and that somatization and interpersonal sensitivity were independently associated with FGIDs.[48] Regardless of psychiatric comorbidity, stress still plays an important role in IBS nonconsulters, as their symptoms show greater reactivity to stress than healthy controls[25] and total life event stress was independently associated with FGIDs.[48]

Comorbid Conditions/Extraintestinal Manifestations

IBS is associated with several chronic functional pain syndromes. Population-based studies have reported that 13% to 30% and 6% of IBS patients have fibromyalgia and migraine, respectively. In contrast, non-IBS patients had a prevalence of 4% to 5% and 2% for fibromyalgia and migraine, respectively.[49,50] Similarly, 25% of patients with chronic widespread pain had IBS, compared to 5% of controls.[51] IBS also frequently coexists with chronic fatigue syndrome and 63% of patients with chronic fatigue syndrome have IBS symptoms.[52] Interstitial cystitis, chronic prostatitis, and chronic pelvic pain are also common in IBS patients. The association between IBS and comorbid conditions, such as fibromyalgia, chronic fatigue syndrome, migraine headaches, and interstitial cystitis, occurs more commonly in females.[53] This is partially explained by the greater prevalence of such non-GI pain disorders in women. For example, the sex ratio for interstitial cystitis is 10:1.

IBS patients often complain of extraintestinal symptoms such as dyspareunia, fatigue, loss of energy, impotence, urinary frequency, backache, and dysmenorrhea.[54,55] These extraintestinal symptoms are clinically relevant and patients with FGIDs consult primary care physicians for non-GI complaints three times more than healthy subjects.[56] In addition, extraintestinal symptoms, such as loss of libido, poor sleep, and increased fatigue, rather than the GI symptoms per se, may play a prominent role in negatively influencing the patient's health-related quality of life.[57] Like comorbid conditions in IBS, extraintestinal symptoms are more common in females.[53]

Pathophysiology

Even though IBS is the most common and best studied FGID, there is no general agreement on the pathophysiology and the relative contributions of the peripheral and central components. Numerous putative pathophysiologies have been described in the literature but these abnormalities frequently involve only a proportion but not all IBS patients. This may be due to the problem of heterogeneity inherent in symptom-based diagnostic groups as discussed earlier. Moreover, some studies did not segregate IBS patients into the subsets of IBS-C, IBS-D, or IBS-M, and there is evidence that the underlying pathophysiology may differ among these patients.

Evidence for Peripheral Mechanisms

Altered Gastrointestinal Motility. There are quantitative but not qualitative differences in GI motility in IBS compared to controls. These differences appear to be present in only 25% to 75% of IBS subjects, are frequently not reproducible in different laboratories, and currently cannot be used as diagnostic markers.[10] However, differences in GI motility may play a role in determining the predominant bowel habit in IBS subgroups. For example, colonic transit is accelerated in IBS-D[58] and high amplitude propagating contractions occur more frequently in IBS-D subjects than controls. The increased frequency of high amplitude propagating contractions may be clinically relevant as they were correlated with abdominal pain[59] and may be the mechanism underlying urgency and diarrhea. Exaggerated or prolonged colonic motility responses to food intake ("gastrocolonic response") may be present in the subset of patients who report an exacerbation of abdominal pain by food intake. It is important to differentiate these patients with GERD or FD for whom the treatment is different.

Mucosal Inflammation. Evidence for mucosal inflammation in the pathophysiology of IBS was based on early studies on PI-IBS. Even after resolution of the initial infection, changes in intestinal permeability, as well as increases in intraepithelial lymphocytes and enteroendocrine cells, could be detected in PI-IBS.[4,60] However, mucosal changes alone do not fully account for the pathogenesis of PI-IBS as clinical symptoms have not been found to correlate with the observed mucosal inflammatory changes, the majority of patients with bacterial gastroenteritis do not develop IBS symptoms postinfection, and the prevalence of IBS is not greater in countries with endemic GI infections.[61] There is good evidence that concurrent central factors, such as comorbid psychiatric diagnoses and the presence of concurrent psychological stressors at the time of GI infection,[4,62] contribute to the probability of developing PI-IBS.

More recently, it has been reported that patients meeting current diagnostic criteria for IBS can have increased inflammatory cells on mucosal biopsies which were detected by immunohistochemistry but not by conventional histology. These patients had increased intraepithelial lymphocytes and increased CD3+ and CD25+ cells in the lamina propria.[8] In addition, increased mucosal mast cells in the colonic mucosa of IBS patients have also been reported.[63] In patients with severe intractable abdominal pain meeting current diagnostic criteria for IBS, surgical biopsies of the ileum revealed the presence of lymphocytic infiltrates within the myenteric plexus and longitudinal muscle hypertrophy.[64] Fecal calprotectin, a surrogate marker of inflammation, is increased in the large majority of patients with proven organic GI disease, but it has also been detected in a small subset of IBS patients.[65]

Activation of immune cells in the intestinal mucosa has been considered as a possible mechanism underlying chronic sensitization of peripheral visceral afferent pathways.[66] A small subset of patients with IBD, especially those with ulcerative colitis who are in clinical remission, exhibit IBS-like symptoms and have demonstrable changes in colonic motility. It has been suggested that the inflammatory process may induce long-term changes in the enteric nervous system and possibly extrinsic sensory afferents, resulting in IBS-like symptoms.[66] However, rectal balloon studies of ulcerative colitis patients with mild disease and without IBS-like symptoms did not reveal evidence for visceral hypersensitivity.[17] Moreover, in Crohn's disease patients with isolated small bowel disease, rectal distension thresholds were elevated, consistent with the activation of endogenous antinociceptive pathways.[67] Taken together with the clinical observation that pain is not a major feature in ulcerative colitis despite extensive mucosal inflammation, these findings may be explained by the hypothesis that the majority of IBD patients are able to activate adaptive mechanisms (descending antinociceptive pathways) which modulate afferent activity from the chronically inflamed gut, but these mechanisms may be inadequate in a minority of patients who develop IBS-like symptoms subsequently.[68]

A mast cell-nerve interaction has been implicated because more mast cells were observed to be in close proximity to nerve endings in IBS patients compared with controls. Furthermore, there was a positive correlation between the nerve-to-mast cell proximity and rate of degranulation of mast cells, suggestive of a functional purpose of the close spatial relationship of the mast cell and nerve ending. This interaction was also reported to be clinically significant, as there was a correlation between the proximity of mast cells to nerve endings and symptoms of abdominal pain and discomfort.[69] Although the observations of the mast cell-nerve interaction can be interpreted to suggest a role of mast cells in the sensitization of colonic nerve endings, it is also possible that activity of the nerve endings result in mast cell degranulation. It has been reported that stress is associated with the degranulation of mast cells in the jejunum in humans.[70]

Altered Intestinal Flora. There is some recent data suggesting that the bacterial flora may be altered in patients with IBS and that these alterations may differ between IBS groups according to predominant bowel habit.[71] It has been proposed that small bacterial overgrowth may be involved in the pathophysiology of IBS and treatment with nonabsorbable antibiotics (neomycin, rifaximin) may be associated with IBS symptom relief.[72–74] Qualitative changes in colonic flora, such as a decrease in Bifidobacterium, have been described in IBS patients. There may be a functional role of the Bifidobacterium as a recent study on the use of Bifidobacteria infantis as a probiotic reported a beneficial effect on IBS symptoms compared to placebo.[75,76]

Evidence for Central Alterations

Altered Modulation of Visceral Pain. Enhanced perception of visceral events may be a common abnormality shared by several FGIDs, in particular IBS, FD, noncardiac chest pain, and FAPS. The pathophysiologic mechanisms responsible for this visceral hypersensitivity are not known, even though various animal models exist to support a possible role for both peripheral as well as central mechanisms. As discussed previously, low-grade immune activation of the intestinal mucosa has been suggested

to play a role in maintaining a chronic state of peripheral and central sensitization, even though this has never been demonstrated in patients. On the other hand, compelling evidence from brain-imaging studies suggests a central component to visceral hypersensitivity.[77] Studies in IBS patients suggest normal activation of viscerosensory regions, such as the insular cortex, during controlled rectal distension, but altered activation of pain modulation regions, including subregions of the anterior cingulate cortex and the periaqueductal gray.[78,79] Abnormal activation of areas associated with emotional and autonomic responses to stimuli (e.g., ventromedial prefrontal cortex, infragenual cingulated cortex, and perigenual ACC) and subcortical areas (e.g., amygdala, dorsal pons, and hypothalamus) have also been reported in IBS patients.[80] These central abnormalities are clinically relevant as brain imaging studies showed an effect of alosetron, a $5HT_3$ receptor antagonist with proven efficacy in IBS-D, on areas such as the amygdala and dorsal pons that correlated with an improvement in IBS symptoms.[81] Similarly, amitriptyline is effective in the treatment of IBS and has been reported to alter activity in the anterior cingulate cortex.[82]

Altered activation of anterior cingulate subregions has also been reported in patients with fibromyalgia,[83,84] supporting the general notion that different functional pain disorders may share central abnormalities consistent with central pain amplification.

Autonomic Nervous System. Converging results from animal, experimental, and human studies suggest that stress-induced activation of central autonomic circuits play an important role in the regulation of gut motility, secretion, and immune modulation. Acute stress-induced activation of contractions and secretions of the hindgut is mediated by sacral parasympathetic pathways, and increased activation of these pathways in IBS patients has been demonstrated in response to severe laboratory stressors.[85] Evidence suggesting tonic hyperactivity of the sympathetic nervous system comes from studies in female IBS patients who have been shown to have elevated urine catecholamine levels[86] and higher plasma norepinephrine levels during sleep. Abnormalities of the autonomic activity of the heart in IBS patients have also been demonstrated.

Psychoneuroendocrine Axis. The central nervous system is able to influence inflammation in the periphery as anxiety has been reported to be associated with higher levels of TNF-alpha in monocytes from IBS patients compared to controls. This may be mediated via the hypothalamic-pituitary-adrenal axis as abnormalities of this axis have been described in IBS. During infusions of corticotropin-releasing hormone, IBS patients had an exaggerated adrenocorticotropic hormone (ACTH) and cortisol response, and the ACTH response correlated with plasma IL-6.[87] Under conditions of stress, IBS patients were reported to have higher cortisol levels compared to controls in one study[88] but this difference was not seen in another study.[89]

Treatment

Symptomatic treatment (usually aimed at normalizing bowel habits or decreasing abdominal pain) by a reassuring health care provider typically provides relief for patients with mild symptoms who are seen in primary care settings. However, the treatment of patients who have more severe symptoms remains challenging. Only a small number of pharmacologic and psychological treatments are supported by well-designed randomized, controlled trials involving patients with IBS. Treatment of IBS with currently available drugs usually is targeted to the management of individual symptoms, such as constipation, diarrhea, and abdominal pain.

Tricyclic Antidepressants

Low doses of TCAs (e.g., nortriptyline or amitriptyline 10–50 mg at bedtime) are generally used in the treatment of IBS, even though definitive evidence for their effectiveness from well controlled clinical trials is lacking. Doses should be started as low as 5 mg once daily, and gradually advanced to a maximum of 75 mg once daily. The therapeutic effect should be expected within days to 2 weeks of starting the TCA. If no beneficial effect is observed at 75 mg once daily or if significant side effects are experienced, the TCA should be discontinued. Due to the significant side effects of this class of drugs at the higher dose range, doses should not be escalated into the antidepressant dose range (e.g., 100–200 mg every night). To maximize compliance, the patient should be informed about the rationale of the treatment choice (i.e., goal is the treatment of pain and not psychiatric symptoms) and informed about the much lower risk for side effects at the low-dose range, compared to full psychiatric doses. The choice and dose of TCA should be individualized in every patient. For example, TCAs with prominent anticholinergic effects (amitriptyline) may be most useful in the patient with prominent abdominal pain and diarrhea-predominant bowel habit (utilizing their peripheral anticholinergic effect on gut motility and secretion) and in the patient with sleep problems (utilizing their sedative effect).

The efficacy of antidepressants in FGIDs was studied in a meta-analysis by Jackson et al.[90] Data were obtained from nine trials of IBS patients and three trials of FD patients. TCAs were used in all studies apart from one study in which a tetracyclic antidepressant was used. Both high and low doses of the antidepressants were used in these studies. Overall, there was a significant benefit of antidepressants on global GI symptoms and standardized pain scores with a number needed to treat (NNT) of 3.2 (i.e., 3.2 patients needed to be treated to improve symptoms in 1 patient).[90]

A large randomized, placebo-controlled trial of the TCA desipramine in IBS (median dose: 100 mg) reported that by an intention-to-treat basis, there was no significant benefit of desipramine over placebo. However, if the results were analyzed on a per protocol basis and excluded patients who withdrew from the study, there was a significant effect in IBS patients (NNT = 5.2). Moreover, this effect was greater in patients who had detectable plasma levels of desipramine in whom the NNT was 4.3. This suggests that, while desipramine is useful, the side effects are bothersome and compliance with TCAs is an issue. Since doses well beyond 75 mg were used in this study, it is unclear if the observed beneficial effects on IBS symptoms were secondary to a decrease in anxiety. However, consistent with the notion that the TCAs' effect on pain is not related to their antidepressant effects, IBS patients with depression did not show any benefit in the measured composite outcome with desipramine in this trial.[34] Subgroup analyses showed that desipramine was more effective for IBS patients with moderate symptoms, history of physical or sexual abuse, and diarrhea.

Selective Serotonin Reuptake Inhibitors

SSRIs are better tolerated than TCAs in terms of their side-effect profile, but the role of SSRIs in the treatment of IBS has never been demonstrated in large well-controlled clinical trials, even though evidence exists from several smaller trials. Creed et al.[33] reported that paroxetine 20 mg once daily for 3 months improved the physical component of the health-related quality of life at 1 year compared to routine care, and also improved abdominal pain and the mental component of the health-related quality of life at 3 months, although these effects were not sustained at 1 year. The main limitation of this trial was that no placebo drug was administered to patients in the control arm in which routine care was provided, and the efficacy of paroxetine may be contributed by a placebo effect. Other smaller trials examined the role of SSRIs compared to placebo and, while some reported beneficial effects,[91–93] others reported no significant benefit.[94] In the absence of evidence from large well-controlled trials, it would be reasonable to use SSRIs in selected patients, particularly those with psychiatric comorbidity.

Antispasmodics

Antispasmodic medications relax the smooth muscle of the intestines, thereby relieving contractility. They comprise anticholinergic agents, calcium channel blockers, and opioid receptor antagonists. Although antispasmodic medications are frequently used in the treatment of IBS, evidence from well-controlled clinical trials for this class of medication is lacking. A meta-analysis of several low quality studies reported a possible benefit of smooth muscle relaxants such as mebeverine, trimebutine, octylonium bromide, pinaverium bromide, and cimetropium bromide over placebo.[95] The problems with most of the studies were small numbers, lack of adequate blinding, and short duration.

Antispasmodic medications are frequently combined with anxiolytic or sedative agents in the treatment of IBS. However, the evidence is not strong and the data supporting the use of this combination is derived from small studies.[96]

Serotonin Receptor Targeted Drugs

Serotonin (5-HT) receptor antagonists and agonists have been developed and used in the treatment of IBS-D and IBS-C, respectively.

Alosetron is a selective 5-HT$_3$ receptor antagonist that has been demonstrated to improve symptoms in female IBS-D patients. The exact sites of action of alosetron are not known, but it probably interacts with both peripheral and central targets. It has been reported in a placebo-controlled trial using functional positron emission tomography brain imaging that alosetron reduces resting activity in limbic structures, in particular the amygdala.[81] Moreover, alosetron did not reduce activity in the insula, the viscerosomatic cortex.[97] This suggests that alosetron may not have a direct antinociceptive effect, but that it acts on limbic pain modulation circuits. Unfortunately, alosetron was associated with ischemic colitis in 0.1% to 1% of patients and was subsequently withdrawn from the market in 2000. It has recently been reintroduced for restricted use.

Tegaserod is a partial 5-HT$_4$ receptor agonist which has been extensively evaluated and demonstrated to be efficacious in the treatment of female IBS-C patients. However, it was recently reported to be associated with an increased incidence of cardiovascular events compared to placebo and has recently been withdrawn from the market.

Psychotherapy

Psychotherapy has been reported to be useful in patients with severe IBS.[31,33] Interestingly, coexistent depression appears to predict a worse outcome with psychotherapy,[33] suggesting that psychotherapy may exert a positive effect independent of coexisting psychiatric comorbidity. It was reported that subjects with a history of sexual abuse did better than those without abuse. The significance of this observation is not known, but it is notable that a history of abuse was also a predictor of better response with desipramine as discussed above.[34]

Cognitive-Behavioral Therapy

Cognitive-behavioral therapy (CBT) is the best-studied psychological treatment for IBS.[31,98] Cognitive techniques (typically administered in a group or an individual format in 4 to 15 sessions) are aimed at changing catastrophic or maladaptive thinking patterns underlying the perception of somatic symptoms. Behavioral techniques aim to modify dysfunctional behaviors through relaxation techniques, contingency management (rewarding healthy behaviors), or assertion training. Some randomized, controlled trials have also shown reductions in IBS symptoms with the use of gut-directed hypnosis, which involves relaxation, change in beliefs, and self-management.[99] Data from head-to-head comparisons of psychotherapy with pharmacotherapy for IBS or psychotherapy plus pharmacotherapy with pharmacotherapy alone are lacking. The magnitude of improvement that has been reported with psychological treatments seems to be similar to or greater than that reported with medications studied specifically for bowel symptoms in IBS, although comparisons are limited by, among other things, the lack of a true placebo control in trials of psychotherapies. In a meta-analysis of 17 randomized trials of cognitive treatments, behavioral treatments, or both for IBS (including hypnosis), as compared with control treatments, those patients who were randomly assigned to CBT were significantly more likely to have a reduction in GI symptoms of at least 50% (odds ratio, 12; 95% CI, 6 to 260), and the estimated number needed to treat with CBT or hypnotherapy for one patient to have improvement was estimated to be two.[98] In several studies, coexisting depression was a predictor of poor response to CBT.[33,34] It has been postulated that the presence of depression may reflect a more severe illness or that depressed subjects may be less willing or able to engage in psychological therapy or to be compliant to an antidepressant regimen.[33]

Hypnotherapy

Hypnotherapy may improve symptoms in patients with severe IBS in the short term,[100,101] as well as in the long term over a period of at least 5 years.[102] The beneficial effects of hypnotherapy were observed in both depressed and nondepressed subjects. However, male subjects with IBS-D and subjects over 50 years old did not respond as well as other IBS subjects.[101,103] A recent systematic review reported that hypnotherapy may be beneficial in the treatment of IBS, but the main problem with current data is that the trials comprised small number of patients.[104] The mechanism(s) underlying the beneficial effects of hypnotherapy in IBS are not known but may involve changes in brain responses to painful stimuli,[105,106] reduction of central pain amplification, and normalization of colonic motility.

FUNCTIONAL DYSPEPSIA

As with other FGIDs, the diagnosis of FD is based on the exclusion of organic diseases and the presence of a set of key symptoms. FD is defined as the presence of symptoms thought to originate from the upper GI tract for which there is no detectable organic disease that can explain the symptoms. These symptoms include epigastric pain, epigastric burning, postprandial fullness, or early satiation. Symptoms of bloating and nausea may be experienced by FD patients, but they appear to be less specific and are not considered cardinal symptoms of FD.[107] The Rome III criteria for FD are listed in Table 63.5.

TABLE 63.5

ROME III DIAGNOSTIC CRITERIA FOR FD[91]

1. One or more of:
   - Bothersome postprandial fullness
   - Early satiation
   - Epigastric pain
   - Epigastric burning

AND

2. No evidence of structural disease (including at upper endoscopy) that is likely to explain the symptoms

*The criteria must be fulfilled for the last 3 months with symptom onset at least 6 months before diagnosis.

TABLE 63.6

ROME III DIAGNOSTIC CRITERIA FOR FD SUBGROUPS[91]

Postprandial distress syndrome
One or both of the following:
1. Bothersome postprandial fullness, occurring after ordinary sized meals, at least several times per week
2. Early satiation that prevents finishing a regular meal, at least several times per week

*The criteria must be fulfilled for the last 3 months with symptom onset at least 6 months before diagnosis.

Supportive criteria:
1. Upper abdominal bloating or postprandial nausea or excessive belching can be present
2. Epigastric pain syndrome may coexist

Epigastric pain syndrome
One or both of the following:
1. Pain or burning localized to the epigastrium of at least moderate severity at least once per week
2. The pain is intermittent
3. Not generalized or localized to other abdominal or chest regions
4. Not relieved by defecation or passage of flatus
5. Not fulfilling criteria for gallbladder and sphincter of Oddi disorders

*The criteria must be fulfilled for the last 3 months with symptom onset at least 6 months before diagnosis.

Supportive criteria:
1. The pain may be of a burning quality but without a retrosternal component
2. The pain is commonly induced or relieved by ingestion of a meal but may occur while fasting
3. Postprandial distress syndrome may coexist

The symptoms of FD overlap with atypical manifestations of GERD, and previous studies on FD may have inadvertently included patients with atypical GERD symptoms, especially since 24-hour pH measurements are not frequently used to exclude GERD patients. This may be particularly relevant in the context of large community-based studies or questionnaire-based studies. It is therefore important to be mindful of this possibility when reviewing research literature on FD.

Several attempts have been made to subdivide FD into distinct subsets on the basis of predominant symptoms. In the Rome III criteria, symptoms have been divided into meal-related (Postprandial Distress Syndrome) and meal-unrelated (Epigastric Pain Syndrome). These proposed subsets of FD are defined in Table 63.6. The clinical utility of these subgroups is controversial, since there is considerable overlap between them. Moreover, the concept of distinct pathophysiologies correlating with distinct symptom patterns has not been confirmed.

Epidemiology

FD is a common disorder with an estimated prevalence of 15% to 20%.[108] Unlike IBS, there does not appear to be a sex-related difference in prevalence.[109] The socioeconomic burden of FD is significant, as FD patients take three times as much sick leave as patients with duodenal ulcers.[110] Two to 5% of primary care visits and more than 10% of primary care drug expenditure in the United Kingdom are related to FD.[111,112] Approximately 1 out of 2 individuals with FD seek health care for their symptoms at some time in their life.[113] It is therefore not surprising that in the United Kingdom, the annual indirect and direct cost of dyspepsia to society is US $1.46 billion and US $730 million, respectively.[114]

Comorbidity With Irritable Bowel Syndrome

FD and IBS frequently coexist in patients, and a third of FD patients have concurrent symptoms of IBS[115] while approximately 40% of IBS patients also report FD symptoms. Frequently, pain or discomfort in the upper abdomen is assumed to be related to the upper GI tract, but on detailed questioning, the "dyspepsia" may be related to bowel disturbances. As discussed earlier, the localization of visceral pain, especially in FGIDs, is often imprecise. In a 1-year follow-up of patients with IBS or dyspepsia, 22% of IBS patients reported a change in their symptom profile to that of FD, and 16% of FD patients reported a change to an IBS symptom profile.[116] This transition of patients between different diagnostic categories (e.g., IBS and FD), which has also been demonstrated in a recent 12-year longitudinal study,[44] puts into question the concept that these symptom-based entities are really distinct syndromes.

Psychiatric Comorbidity

Anxiety, depression, and neuroticism appear to be more common in FD clinic patients.[117] Similar to the situation in IBS, this association in clinic attenders may be biased, as anxiety has been reported to be associated with health-seeking behavior in FD. Compared to patients with nonlife-threatening organic GI disease, FD patients have higher anxiety, but not depression or neuroticism scores.[118]

Pathogenesis

The pathophysiology of FD is not fully understood, and both central and peripheral mechanisms have been proposed. While enhanced perception of gastric stimuli may be a key central mechanism, the role of gastric acid, acute and chronic gastric mucosal infections, and gastroduodenal dysmotility remains to be determined.

Visceral Hypersensitivity

As with IBS patients, visceral hypersensitivity is common in FD and a significant subset of FD patients (34%–65%) report pain and discomfort at lower volumes of gastric distension compared to healthy control subjects[15,16] or compared to patients with dyspepsia from organic causes.[15] Chemical sensitivity to capsaicin has also been reported in FD patients.[119]

Central pain amplification is likely to contribute to the observed gastric hypersensitivity. For example, the presence of lipids in the duodenum increases the sensitivity of FD patients to gastric balloon distension compared to controls.[120] This abnormal modulation of gastric perception thresholds to distension by lipid in a distant site supports the concept of a centrally mediated mechanism. Furthermore, it has been reported that in response to gastric balloon distension, about half the patients with FD experienced altered viscerosomatic referral patterns.[15]

IBS coexists with FD in a substantial proportion of patients, and studies show that sensitivity to balloon distension in the small intestine was similar in IBS and FD.[121] These findings support the concept that IBS and a subset of FD patients share similar pathophysiologic mechanisms.

Gastric Acid

Several large multicenter studies have demonstrated that only a small subset of FD patients (10%–15%) benefited from acid suppression therapy.[122,123] This suggests that such patients either represent a subgroup of patients characterized by hypersensitivity to intraduodenal or intra-antral acid[124,125] or that they suffer from atypical manifestations of GERD.[126] There is some recent evidence against the latter as it was reported that responsiveness to acid suppression therapy in FD did not correlate with abnormal 24-hour pH studies.[127]

Helicobacter Pylori

Chronic *H. pylori* infection has been postulated to be related to sensitization of visceral afferent pathways. Two large prospective studies have reported improvement of symptoms in FD following eradication of *H. pylori*.[128,129] However, three other trials failed to demonstrate a beneficial effect from *H. pylori* eradication.[130–132] Furthermore, no differences in perceptual responses to controlled gastric distension have been observed between FD patients with and without *H. pylori* infection.[133] A recent meta-analysis reported that the relative risk reduction at 12 months with *H. pylori* eradication was 9% compared with placebo, and 15 patients needed to be treated for 1 patient to benefit.[134] Chronic *H. pylori* infection may be related to dyspeptic symptoms in a small subset of FD subjects, and *H. pylori* eradication in patients with FD has been recommended by a consensus conference.[135]

Presumed Postinfectious Functional Dyspepsia

About 20% of patients with FD develop symptoms after an acute episode of presumed gastroenteritis based on symptoms such as fever, myalgia, vomiting, or diarrhea.[136] A similar observation has been reported in patients following *Giardia* infection.[137] This is analogous to the group of PI-IBS patients who develop persistent symptoms of IBS following a bout of gastroenteritis. Patients with presumed postinfectious FD were younger and had lower body mass index than those with unspecified-onset FD.[136] A greater proportion of patients with presumed postinfectious FD patients had impaired gastric accommodation but not hypersensitivity to distension when compared to patients with unspecified-onset FD.[136]

Gastroduodenal Motility

Forty percent of FD subjects have evidence of impaired gastric accommodation.[138,139] It has been suggested that impaired gastric accommodation may cause rapid transit of food from the proximal stomach, resulting in early antral distension, which in turn results in dyspeptic symptoms. There is limited data that improved gastric accommodation by sumatriptan resulted in a reduction of meal-induced symptoms.[140] In addition, postprandial antral hypomotility has been demonstrated in manometric studies in about half of FD subjects and this abnormality correlates with delayed gastric emptying, which has been demonstrated in a third of FD subjects.[141] A correlation between delayed gastric emptying and dyspeptic symptoms of postprandial fullness has been reported in FD patients.[142]

Treatment

In general, therapy of patients with FD can be directed at peripheral and central targets. The peripheral targets are based on the proposed pathophysiological abnormalities outlined above. Central nervous system-directed therapy is analogous to that used in the treatment of IBS.

Acid suppression therapy is safe and may have a beneficial

effect over placebo in approximately 10% of patients meeting current symptom criteria for FD. It is currently assumed that the subset of responsive patients comprises those with either atypical GERD or with duodenal hypersensitivity to gastric acid. The choice of acid suppressive agents is open to debate, and both histamine (H2) receptor antagonists and proton pump inhibitors have been reported to be more effective than placebo.[143] A small subset of FD patients improve with eradication of *H. pylori* and the likelihood of a positive response is comparable to that with acid suppression. This form of treatment is reasonable given that the treatment is of short duration and can also reduce the risk of subsequent peptic ulcer disease, atrophic gastritis, and gastric cancer.[135] There are no well-designed clinical trials in defined populations of FD patients supporting the use of prokinetic drugs. The use of low dose TCAs has not been as extensively evaluated in FD compared to IBS. Small studies have reported a beneficial effect of TCAs in the treatment of FD.[15,144] A recent small study looking at a combination of melitracen (TCA) and flupentixol (an antipsychotic drug) reported a significant benefit over placebo in FD patients.[145] The benefits of psychological therapy on FD are not well established, but may be a reasonable option in patients who do not respond to pharmacotherapy.

FUNCTIONAL ABDOMINAL PAIN SYNDROME

FAPS is defined as a continuous or near continuous abdominal pain that is present for at least 6 months, is poorly related to gut function, and is associated with some loss of daily activities.[146] The diagnostic criteria for FAPS are listed in Table 63.7.

The main feature that distinguishes FAPS from IBS and FD is that the abdominal pain in FAPS is present all or most of the time, while the abdominal pain in IBS and FD is generally related to physiological events such as defecation or food intake, respectively. The abdominal pain in FAPS is constant and generally referred to the entire abdomen rather than a specific location. Sometimes atypical referral patterns to extra-abdominal regions (thighs, chest, and back) and to an entire side of the body are reported.

Epidemiology

FAPS is uncommon compared to IBS with a prevalence of 0.5% to 2%. FAPS is more common in women with the highest prevalence in the fourth decade of life. Like IBS, FAPS is responsible for a disproportionately large portion of health care resources and high work absenteeism. Patients with FAPS tend to have about three times as many days of sick leave and number of physician visits as subjects without bowel symptoms.[24]

TABLE 63.7

ROME III DIAGNOSTIC CRITERIA FOR FAPS[146]

Must include all of the following:
- Continuous or nearly continuous abdominal pain
- No or only occasional relationship of pain with physiological events (e.g., eating, defecation, or menses)
- Some loss of daily functioning
- The pain is not feigned
- Insufficient symptoms to meet criteria for another functional gastrointestinal disorder that would explain the pain

*The criteria must be fulfilled for the last 3 months with symptom onset at least 6 months before diagnosis.

Psychiatric Comorbidity

The psychiatric comorbidity seen in FAPS is prominent and bears many similarities to that in IBS. The majority of FAPS patients have psychiatric diagnoses of anxiety, depression, and somatization.[146] Unresolved losses, such as demise of a spouse or parent, personally meaningful surgery (e.g., hysterectomy), or termination of pregnancy, are common in FAPS.

Pathophysiology

The pathophysiology of FAPS is poorly understood and literature in this area is scarce. As there is no definite relationship to physiological events like eating, defecation, or menses in FAPS, a neurologic etiology is likely. The abnormal viscerosomatic referral patterns could result from either sensitization of primary afferent origin or from increased resting activity of spinal, thalamic, or cingulate neurons, all of which have large receptive fields. The epidemiological and psychosocial similarities between IBS and FAPS and the frequent history of IBS in a patient with FAPS suggest shared pathophysiological mechanisms such as alteration of central pain modulation pathways.

Treatment

There are no well-controlled clinical trial results that would guide the treatment of FAPS, which is largely empirical. Treatment options include the use of TCAs, SSRIs, SNRIs, and anticonvulsants (e.g., gabapentin, carbamazepine, and lamotrigine).

References

1. Doran FSA. The sites to which pain is referred from the common bile-duct in man and its implication for the theory of referred pain. *Brit J Surg* 1967; 54(7):599–606.
2. Mayer EA, Gebhart GF. Basic and clinical aspects of visceral hyperalgesia. *Gastroenterology* 1994;107(1):271–293.
3. Mayer EA. The neurobiology of stress and gastrointestinal disease. *Gut* 2000; 47(6):861–869.
4. Gwee KA, Leong YL, Graham C, et al. The role of psychological and biological factors in postinfective gut dysfunction. *Gut* 1999;44(3):400–406.
5. Dent J, Brun J, Fendrick AM, et al. An evidence-based appraisal of reflux disease management—the Genval Workshop Report. *Gut* 1999;44(Suppl 2): S1–S16.
6. Fass R, Fullerton S, Tung S, et al. Sleep disturbances in clinic patients with functional bowel disorders. *Am J Gastroenterol* 2000;95(5):1195–2000.
7. Vanner SJ, Depew WT, Paterson WG, et al. Predictive value of the Rome Criteria for diagnosing the irritable bowel syndrome. *Am J Gastroenterol* 1999;94(10):2912–2917.
8. Chadwick VS, Chen W, Shu D, et al. Activation of the mucosal immune system in irritable bowel syndrome. *Gastroenterology* 2002;122(7):1778–1783.
9. Haag S, Senf W, Hauser W, et al. Impairment of health-related quality of life in functional dyspepsia and chronic liver disease: the influence of depression and anxiety. *Aliment Pharmacol Ther* 2008;27(7):561–571.
10. Drossman DA, Camilleri M, Mayer EA, et al. AGA technical review on irritable bowel syndrome. *Gastroenterology* 2002;123(6):2108–2131.
11. Holstege G, Bandler R, Saper CB, et al. *The Emotional Motor System*. Amsterdam: Elsevier; 1996:3–6.
12. Mayer EA, Naliboff BD, Chang L. Evolving pathophysiological model of functional gastrointestinal disorders: implications for treatment. *Eur J Surg Suppl* 2002;168(Suppl 587):3–9.
13. Mertz H, Naliboff B, Munakata J, et al. Altered rectal perception is a biological marker of patients with irritable bowel syndrome. *Gastroenterology* 1995; 109(1):40–52.
14. Schmulson M, Mayer EA. Gastrointestinal sensory abnormalities in functional dyspepsia. *Baillieres Clin Gastroenterology* 1998;12(3):545–550.
15. Mertz H, Fullerton S, Naliboff B, et al. Symptoms and visceral perception in severe functional and organic dyspepsia. *Gut* 1998;42:814–822.
16. Tack J, Caenepeel P, Fischler B, et al. Symptoms associated with hypersensitivity to gastric distension in functional dyspepsia. *Gastroenterology* 2001; 121(3):526–535.
17. Chang L, Munakata J, Mayer EA, et al. Perceptual responses in patients with inflammatory and functional bowel disease. *Gut* 2000;47(4):497–505.

18. Fass R, Naliboff B, Higa L, et al. Differential effect of long-term esophageal acid exposure on mechanosensitivity and chemosensitivity in humans. *Gastroenterology* 1998;115(6):1363–1373.

19. Bradesi S, McRoberts JA, Anton PA, et al. Inflammatory bowel disease and irritable bowel syndrome: separate or unified? *Curr Opin Gastroenterol* 2003; 19(4):336–342.

20. Wilder-Smith CH, Schindler D, Lovblad K, et al. Brain functional magnetic resonance imaging of rectal pain and activation of endogenous inhibitory mechanisms in irritable bowel syndrome patient subgroups and healthy controls. *Gut* 2004;53(11):1595–1601.

21. Lowman BC, Drossman DA, Cramer EM, et al. Recollection of childhood events in adults with irritable bowel syndrome. *J Clin Gastroenterol* 1987; 9(3):324–330.

22. Ford AC, Forman D, Bailey AG, et al. Irritable bowel syndrome: a 10-yr natural history of symptoms and factors that influence consultation behavior. *Am J Gastroenterol* 2008;103(5):1229–1239.

23. Talley NJ, Fett SL, Zinsmeister AR, et al. Gastrointestinal tract symptoms and self-reported abuse: a population-based study. *Gastroenterology* 1994; 107(4):1040–1049.

24. Drossman DA. Chronic functional abdominal pain. *Am J Gastroenterol* 1996; 91(11):2270–2281.

25. Whitehead WE, Crowell MD, Robinson JC, et al. Effects of stressful life events on bowel symptoms: subjects with irritable bowel syndrome compared with subjects without bowel dysfunction. *Gut* 1992;33(6):825–830.

26. Dickhaus B, Mayer EA, Firooz N, et al. Irritable bowel syndrome patients show enhanced modulation of visceral perception by auditory stress. *Am J Gastroenterol* 2003;98(1):135–143.

27. Bennett E, Beaurepaire J, Langeluddecke P, et al. Life stress and non-ulcer dyspepsia: a case-control study. *J Psychosom Res* 1991;35(4–5):579–590.

28. Haug TT, Wilhelmsen I, Berstad A, et al. Life events and stress in patients with functional dyspepsia compared with patients with duodenal ulcer and healthy controls. *Scand J Gastroenterol* 1995;30(6):524–530.

29. Talley NJ, Piper DW. Major life event stress and dyspepsia of unknown cause: a case control study. *Gut* 1986;27(2):127–134.

30. Drossman DA, Talley NJ, Leserman J, et al. Sexual and physical abuse and gastrointestinal illness. Review and recommendations. *Ann Intern Med* 1995; 123(10):782–794.

31. Brandt LJ, Bjorkman D, Fennerty MB, et al. Systematic review on the management of irritable bowel syndrome in North America. *Am J Gastroenterol* 2002;97(11 Suppl):S7–S26.

32. Calvert EL, Houghton LA, Cooper P, et al. Long-term improvement in functional dyspepsia using hypnotherapy. *Gastroenterology* 2002;123(6): 1778–1785.

33. Creed F, Fernandes L, Guthrie E, et al. The cost-effectiveness of psychotherapy and paroxetine for severe irritable bowel syndrome. *Gastroenterology* 2003; 124(2):303–317.

34. Drossman DA, Toner BB, Whitehead WE, et al. Cognitive-behavioral therapy versus education and desipramine versus placebo for moderate to severe functional bowel disorders. *Gastroenterology* 2003;125(1):19–31.

35. Soo S, Moayyedi P, Deeks J, et al. Psychological interventions for non-ulcer dyspepsia. *Cochrane Database Syst Rev* 2001;4:CD002301.

36. Boyce PM, Talley NJ, Balaam B, et al. A randomized controlled trial of cognitive behavior therapy, relaxation training, and routine clinical care for the irritable bowel syndrome. *Am J Gastroenterol* 2003;98(10):2209–2218.

37. Corney RH, Stanton R, Newell R, et al. Behavioural psychotherapy in the treatment of irritable bowel syndrome. *J Psychosom Res* 1991;35(4–5): 461–469.

38. Longstreth GF, Thompson WG, Chey WD, et al. Functional bowel disorders. *Gastroenterology* 2006;130(5):1480–1491.

39. Longstreth GF, Thompson WG, Chey WD, et al. Functional bowel disorders. In: Drossman DA, Corazziari E, Delvaux M, et al., eds. ROME III: *The Functional Gastrointestinal Disorders*. McLean, VA: Degnon Associates; 2006: 487–556.

40. Drossman DA, Li Z, Andruzzi E, et al. U.S. householder survey of functional gastrointestinal disorders. Prevalence, sociodemography and health impact. *Dig Dis Sci* 1993;38(9):1569–1580.

41. Rees GA, Davies GJ, Parker M, et al. Gastrointestinal symptoms and diet of members of an irritable bowel self-help group. *J R Soc Health* 1994;114(4): 182–187.

42. Kay L, Jorgensen T, Jensen KH. The epidemiology of irritable bowel syndrome in random population: prevalence, incidence, natural history and risk factors. *J Intern Med* 1994;236(1):23–30.

43. Talley NJ, Weaver AL, Zinsmeister AR, et al. Onset and disappearance of gastrointestinal symptoms and functional gastrointestinal disorders. *Am J Epidemiol* 1992;136(2):165–177.

44. Halder SL, Locke GR 3rd, Schleck CD, et al. Natural history of functional gastrointestinal disorders: a 12-year longitudinal population-based study. *Gastroenterology* 2007;133(3):799–807.

45. Mayer EA, Craske MG, Naliboff BD. Depression, anxiety and the gastrointestinal system. *J Clin Psychiatry* 2001;62(Suppl 8):28–36.

46. Walker EA, Katon WJ, Jemelka RP, et al. Comorbidity of gastrointestinal complaints, depression, and anxiety in the epidemiologic catchment area (ECA) study. *A J Med* 1992;92(Suppl 1A):26S–30S.

47. Talley NJ, Howell S, Poulton R. The irritable bowel syndrome and psychiatric disorders in the community: is there a link? *Am J Gastroenterol* 2001;96(4): 1072–1079.

48. Locke GR 3rd, Weaver AL, Melton LJ 3rd, et al. Psychosocial factors are linked to functional gastrointestinal disorders: a population based nested case-control study. *Am J Gastroenterol* 2004;99(2):350–357.

49. Cole JA, Rothman KJ, Cabral HJ, et al. Migraine, fibromyalgia, and depression among people with IBS: a prevalence study. *BMC Gastroenterol* 2006; 6:26.

50. Sperber AD, Atzmon Y, Neumann L, et al. Fibromyalgia in the irritable bowel syndrome: studies of prevalence and clinical implications. *Am J Gastroenterol* 1999;94:3541–3546.

51. Kato K, Sullivan PF, Evengard B, et al. Chronic widespread pain and its comorbidities: a population-based study. *Arch Intern Med* 2006;166(15): 1649–1654.

52. Gomborone JE, Gorard DA, Dewsnap PA, et al. Prevalence of irritable bowel syndrome in chronic fatigue. *J R Coll Physicians Lond* 1996;30(6):512–513.

53. Chang L, Heitkemper MM. Gender differences in irritable bowel syndrome. *Gastroenterology* 2002;123(5):1686–1701.

54. Chaudhary NA, Truelove SC. The irritable colon syndrome: a study of the clinical features, predisposing causes, and prognosis in 130 cases. *Q J Med* 1962;31:307–322.

55. Whorwell PJ, McCallum M, Creed FH, et al. Non-colonic features of irritable bowel syndrome. *Gut* 1986;27(1):37–40.

56. Sandler RS, Drossman DA, Nathan HP, et al. Symptom complaints and health care seeking behavior in subjects with bowel dysfunction. *Gastroenterology* 1984;87(2):314–318.

57. Spiegel BM, Gralnek IM, Bolus R, et al. Clinical determinants of health-related quality of life in patients with irritable bowel syndrome. *Arch Intern Med* 2004;164(16):1773–1780.

58. Cann PA, Read NW, Brown C, et al. Irritable bowel syndrome: relationship of disorders in the transit of a single solid meal to symptom patterns. *Gut* 1983;24(5):405–411.

59. Chey WY, Jin HO, Lee MH, et al. Colonic motility abnormality in patients with irritable bowel syndrome exhibiting abdominal pain and diarrhea. *Am J Gastroenterol* 2001;96(5):1499–1506.

60. Spiller RC, Jenkins D, Thornley JP, et al. Increased rectal mucosal enteroendocrine cells, T-lymphocytes, and increased gut permeability following acute Campylobacter enteritis and in post-dysenteric irritable bowel syndrome. *Gut* 2000;47(6):804–811.

61. Bradesi S, Schwetz I, Mayer EA, et al. Inflammation induced altered nerve function in the gut—does it play a role in GI symptom generation? In Holtmann G, Talley NJ, eds. *Gastrointestinal Inflammation and Disturbed Gut Function*. London: Kluwer Academic Publishers; 2003:109–119.

62. Neal KR, Hebden J, Spiller R. Prevalence of gastrointestinal symptoms six months after bacterial gastroenteritis and risk factors for development of the irritable bowel syndrome: postal survey of patients. *BMJ* 1997;314:779–782.

63. O'Sullivan M, Clayton N, Breslin NP, et al. Increased mast cells in the irritable bowel syndrome. *Neurogastroenterol Motil* 2000;12(5):449–457.

64. Tornblom H, Lindberg G, Nyberg B, et al. Full-thickness biopsy of the jejunum reveals inflammation and enteric neuropathy in irritable bowel syndrome. *Gastroenterology* 2002;123(6):1972–1979.

65. Tibble JA, Sigthorsson G, Foster R, et al. Use of surrogate markers of inflammation and Rome criteria to distinguish organic from nonorganic intestinal disease. *Gastroenterology* 2002;123(2):450–460.

66. Collins SM. A case for an immunological basis for irritable bowel syndrome. *Gastroenterology* 2002;122(7):2078–2080.

67. Bernstein CN, Niazi N, Robert M, et al. Rectal afferent function in patients with inflammatory and functional intestinal disorders. *Pain* 1996;66(2–3): 151–161.

68. Schwetz I, Bradesi S, Mayer EA. Current insights into the pathophysiology of irritable bowel syndrome. *Curr Gastroenterol Rep* 2003;5(4):331–336.

69. Barbara G, Stanghellini V, De Giorgio R, et al. Activated mast cells in proximity to colonic nerves correlate with abdominal pain in irritable bowel syndrome. *Gastroenterology* 2004;126(3):693–702.

70. Santos J, Saperas E, Nogueiras C, et al. Release of mast cell mediators into the jejunum by cold pain stress in humans. *Gastroenterology* 1998;114:640–648.

71. Kassinen A, Krogius-Kurikka L, Mäkivuokko H, et al. The fecal microbiota of irritable bowel syndrome patients differs significantly from that of healthy subjects. *Gastroenterology* 2007;133(1):24–33.

72. Lin HC. Small intestinal bacterial overgrowth: a framework for understanding irritable bowel syndrome. *JAMA* 2004;292(7):852–858.

73. Pimentel M, Chow EJ, Lin HC. Normalization of lactulose breath testing correlates with symptom improvement in irritable bowel syndrome. A double-blind, randomized, placebo-controlled study. *Am J Gastroenterol* 2003;98(2): 412–419.

74. Sharara AI, Aoun E, Abdul-Baki H, et al. A randomized double-blind placebo-controlled trial of rifaximin in patients with abdominal bloating and flatulence. *Am J Gastroenterol* 2006;101(2):326–333.

75. Whorwell PJ, Altringer L, Morel J, et al. Efficacy of an encapsulated probiotic Bifidobacterium infantis 35624 in women with irritable bowel syndrome. *Am J Gastroenterol* 2006;101(7):1581–1590.

76. O'Mahony L, McCarthy J, Kelly P, et al. Lactobacillus and bifidobacterium in irritable bowel syndrome: symptom responses and relationship to cytokine profiles. *Gastroenterology* 2005;128(3):541–551.

77. Mayer EA, Naliboff BD, Craig AD. Neuroimaging of the brain–gut axis: from

basic understanding to treatment of functional GI disorders. *Gastroenterology* 2006;131(6):1925–1942.

78. Berman S, Munakata J, Naliboff B, et al. Gender differences in regional brain response to visceral pressure in IBS patients. *Eur J Pain* 2000;4(2):157–172.

79. Naliboff BD, Derbyshire SWG, Munakata J, et al. Cerebral activation in irritable bowel syndrome patients and control subjects during rectosigmoid stimulation. *Psychosom Med* 2001;63(3):365–375.

80. Chang L. Brain responses to visceral and somatic stimuli in irritable bowel syndrome: a central nervous system disorder? *Gastroenterol Clin North Am* 2005;34(2):271–279.

81. Berman SM, Chang L, Suyenobu B, et al. Condition-specific deactivation of brain regions by 5-HT3 receptor antagonist alosetron. *Gastroenterology* 2002;123(4):969–977.

82. Morgan V, Pickens D, Gautam S, et al. Amitriptyline reduces rectal pain related activation of the anterior cingulate cortex in patients with irritable bowel syndrome. *Gut* 2005;54(5):601–607.

83. Chang L, Berman S, Mayer EA, et al. Brain responses to visceral and somatic stimuli in patients with irritable bowel syndrome with and without fibromyalgia. *Am J Gastroenterol* 2003;98(6):1354–1361.

84. Gracely RH, Petzke F, Wolf JM, et al. Functional magnetic resonance imaging evidence of augmented pain processing in fibromyalgia. *Arthritis Rheum* 2002;46(5):1333–1343.

85. Welgan P, Meshkinpour H, Beeler M. Effect of anger on colon motor and myoelectric activity in irritable bowel syndrome. *Gastroenterology* 1988;94(5 Pt 1):1150–1156.

86. Heitkemper M, Jarrett M, Cain K, et al. Increased urine catecholamines and cortisol in women with irritable bowel syndrome. *Am J Gastroenterol* 1996; 91(5):906–913.

87. Dinan TG, Quigley EM, Ahmed SM, et al. Hypothalmic-pituitary-gut axis dysregulation in irritable bowel syndrome: plasma cytokines as a potential marker? *Gastroenterology* 2006;130(2):304–311.

88. Walter SA, Aardal-Eriksson E, Thorell LH, et al. Pre-experimental stress in patients with irritable bowel syndrome: high cortisol values already before symptom provocation with rectal distensions. *Neurogastroenterol Motil* 2006;18(12):1069–1077.

89. Elsenbruch S, Lucas A, Holtmann G, et al. Public speaking stress-induced neuroendocrine responses and circulating immune cell redistribution in irritable bowel syndrome. *Am J Gastroenterol* 2006;101(10):2300–2307.

90. Jackson JL, O'Malley PG, Tomkins G, et al. Treatment of functional gastrointestinal disorders with antidepressant medications: a meta-analysis. *Am J Med* 2000;108(1):65–72.

91. Tack J, Broekaert D, Fischler B, et al. A controlled cross-over study of the selective serotonin reuptake inhibitor citalopram in irritable bowel syndrome. *Gut* 2006;55(8):1095–1103.

92. Vahedi H, Merat S, Rashidioon A, et al. The effects of fluoxetine in patients with pain and constipation-predominant irritable bowel syndrome: a double-blind randomized-controlled study. *Aliment Pharmacol Ther* 2005;22(5):381–385.

93. Tabas G, Beaves M, Wang J, et al. Paroxetine to treat irritable bowel syndrome not responding to high-fiber diet: a double-blind, placebo-controlled trial. *Am J Gastroenterol* 2004;99(5):914–920.

94. Talley NJ, Kellow JE, Boyce P, et al. Antidepressant therapy (imipramine and citalopram) for irritable bowel syndrome: a double-blind, randomized, placebo-controlled trial. *Dig Dis Sci* 2008;53(1):108–115.

95. Poynard T, Naveau S, Mory B, et al. Meta-analysis of smooth muscle relaxants in the treatment of irritable bowel syndrome. *Aliment Pharmacol Ther* 1994; 8(5):499–510.

96. Mertz H. Irritable bowel syndrome. *N Engl J Med* 2003;349(22):2136–2146.

97. Mayer EA, Berman S, Derbyshire SW, et al. The effect of the 5-HT3 receptor antagonist, alosetron, on brain responses to visceral stimulation in irritable bowel syndrome patients. *Aliment Pharmacol Ther* 2002;16(7):1357–1366.

98. Lackner JM, Mesmer C, Morley S, et al. Psychological treatments for irritable bowel syndrome: a systematic review and meta-analysis. *J Consult Clin Psychol* 2004;72(6):1100–1113.

99. Whorwell PJ. Review article: the history of hypnotherapy and its role in the irritable bowel syndrome. *Aliment Pharmacol Ther* 2005;22(11–12):1061–1067.

100. Whorwell PJ, Prior A, Faragher EB. Controlled trial of hypnotherapy in the treatment of severe refractory irritable-bowel syndrome. *Lancet* 1984; 2(8414):1232–1234.

101. Whorwell PJ, Prior A, Colgan SM. Hypnotherapy in severe irritable bowel syndrome: further experience. *Gut* 1987;28(4):423–425.

102. Gonsalkorale WM, Miller V, Afzal A, et al. Long-term benefits of hypnotherapy for irritable bowel syndrome. *Gut* 2003;52(11):1623–1629.

103. Gonsalkorale WM, Houghton LA, Whorwell PJ. Hypnotherapy in irritable bowel syndrome: a large-scale audit of a clinical service with examination of factors influencing responsiveness. *Am J Gastroenterol* 2002;97(4):954–961.

104. Wilson S, Maddison T, Roberts L, et al. Systematic review: the effectiveness of hypnotherapy in the management of irritable bowel syndrome. *Aliment Pharmacol Ther* 2006;24(5):769–780.

105. Faymonville ME, Roediger L, Del Fiore G, et al. Increased cerebral functional connectivity underlying the antinociceptive effects of hypnosis. *Brain Res Cogn Brain Res* 2003;17(2):255–262.

106. Schulz-Stubner S, Krings T, Meister IG, et al. Clinical hypnosis modulates functional magnetic resonance imaging signal intensities and pain perception in a thermal stimulation paradigm. *Reg Anesth Pain Med* 2004;29(6):549–556.

107. Tack J, Talley NJ, Camilleri M, et al. Functional gastroduodenal disorders. *Gastroenterology* 2006;130(5):1466–1479.

108. Locke GR 3rd. Prevalence, incidence and natural history of dyspepsia and functional dyspepsia. *Baillieres Clin Gastroenterol* 1998;12(3):435–442.

109. Chang L, Toner BB, Fukudo S, et al. Gender, age, society, culture, and the patient's perspective in the functional gastrointestinal disorders. *Gastroenterology* 2006;130(5):1435–1446.

110. Nyren O, Adami HO, Gustavson S, et al. The "epigastric distress syndrome": a possible disease entity identified by history and endoscopy in patients with nonulcer dyspepsia. *J Clin Gastroenterol* 1987;9(3):303–309.

111. Knill-Jones RP. Geographical differences in the prevalence of dyspepsia. *Scand J Gastroenterol Suppl* 1991;182:17–24.

112. Logan R, Delaney B. ABC of the upper gastrointestinal tract: implications of dyspepsia for the NHS. *BMJ* 2001;323(7314):675–677.

113. Koloski NA, Talley NJ, Boyce PM. Predictors of health care seeking for irritable bowel syndrome and nonulcer dyspepsia: a critical review of the literature on symptom and psychosocial factors. *Am J Gastroenterol* 2001;96(5):1340–1349.

114. Moayyedi P, Mason J. Clinical and economic consequences of dyspepsia in the community. *Gut* 2002;50(Suppl 4):iv10–iv2.

115. Talley NJ. Spectrum of chronic dyspepsia in the presence of the irritable bowel syndrome. *Scand J Gastroenterol Suppl* 1991;182:7–10.

116. Agréus L, Svärdsudd K, Nyrén O, et al. Irritable bowel syndrome and dyspepsia in the general population: overlap and lack of stability over time. *Gastroenterology* 1995;109(3):671–680.

117. Talley NJ, Fung LH, Gilligan IJ, et al. Association of anxiety, neuroticism, and depression with dyspepsia of unknown cause. A case-control study. *Gastroenterology* 1986;90(4):886–892.

118. Langeluddecke P, Goulston K, Tennant C. Psychological factors in dyspepsia of unknown cause: a comparison with peptic ulcer disease. *J Psychosom Res* 1990;34(2):215–222.

119. Hammer J, Fuhrer M, Pipal L, et al. Hypersensitivity for capsaicin in patients with functional dyspepsia. *Neurogastroenterol Motil* 2008;20(2):125–133.

120. Barbera R, Feinle C, Read NW. Abnormal sensitivity to duodenal lipid infusion in patients with functional dyspepsia. *Eur J Gastroenterol Hepatol* 1995; 7(11):1051–1057.

121. Holtmann G, Goebell H, Talley NJ. Functional dyspepsia and irritable bowel syndrome: is there a common pathophysiological basis? *Am J Gastroenterol* 1997;92(6):954–959.

122. Bolling-Sternevald E, Carlsson R, Aalykke C, et al. Self-administered symptom questionnaires in patients with dyspepsia and their yield in discriminating between endoscopic diagnoses. *Dig Dis* 2002;20(2):191–198.

123. Talley NJ, Meineche-Schmidt V, Pare P, et al. Efficacy of omeprazole in functional dyspepsia: double-blind, randomized, placebo-controlled trials (the Bond and Opera studies). *Aliment Pharmacol Ther* 1998;12(11):1055–1065.

124. Misra SP, Broor SL. Is gastric acid responsible for the pain in patients with essential dyspepsia? *J Clin Gastroenterol* 1990;12(6):624–627.

125. Samsom M, Verhagen MA, VanBerge-Henegouwen GP, et al. Abnormal clearance of exogenous acid and increased acid sensitivity of the proximal duodenum in dyspeptic patients. *Gastroenterology* 1999;116(3):515–520.

126. Farup PG, Hovde O, Torp R, et al. Patients with functional dyspepsia responding to omeprazole have a characteristic gastro-oesophageal reflux pattern. *Scand J Gastroenterol* 1999;34(6):575–579.

127. Bolling-Sternevald E, Lauritsen K, Aalykke C, et al. Effect of profound acid suppression in functional dyspepsia: a double-blind, randomized, placebo-controlled trial. *Scand J Gastroenterol* 2002;37(12):1395–1402.

128. McCarthy C, Patchett S, Collins RM, et al. Long-term prospective study of Helicobacter pylori in nonulcer dyspepsia. *Dig Dis Sci* 1995;40(1):114–119.

129. McColl K, Murray L, El-Omar E, et al. Symptomatic benefit from eradicating Helicobacter pylori infection in patients with nonulcer dyspepsia. *N Engl J Med* 1998;339(26):1869–1874.

130. Blum A, Talley NJ, O'Morain C, et al. Lack of effect of treating *helicobacter pylori* infection in patients with nonulcer dyspepsia. Omeprazole plus Clarithromycin and Amoxicillin Effect One Year after Treatment (OCAY) Study Group. *N Engl J Med* 1998;339(26):1875–1881.

131. Greenberg PD, Cello JP. Lack of effect of treatment for *Helicobactor pylori* on symptoms on nonulcer dyspepsia. *Arch Intern Med* 1999;159(19):2283–2288.

132. Talley NJ, Janssens J, Lauritsen K, et al. Eradication of *Helicobacter pylori* in functional dyspepsia: randomised double blind placebo controlled trial with 12 months' follow up. The Optimal Regimen Cures Helicobacter Induced Dyspepsia (ORCHID) Study Group. *BMJ* 1999;318(7187):833–837.

133. Holtmann G, Talley N, Goebell H. Association between *H. pylori*, duodenal mechanosensory thresholds, and small intestinal motility in chronic and unexplained dyspepsia. *Dig Dis Sci* 1996;41(7):1285–1291.

134. Moayyedi P, Soo S, Deeks J, et al. Systematic review and economic evaluation of *Helicobacter pylori* eradication treatment for non-ulcer dyspepsia. Dyspepsia Review Group. *BMJ* 2000;321(7262):659–664.

135. Malfertheiner P, Megraud F, O'Morain C, et al. Current concepts in the management of *Helicobacter pylori* infection—the Maastricht 2–2000 Consensus Report. *Aliment Pharmacol Ther* 2002;16(2):167–180.

136. Tack J, Demedts I, Dehondt G, et al. Clinical and pathophysiological characteristics of acute-onset functional dyspepsia. *Gastroenterology* 2002;122(7):1738–1747.

137. Dizdar V, Gilja OH, Hausken T. Increased visceral sensitivity in Giardia-induced postinfectious irritable bowel syndrome and functional dyspepsia. Effect of the 5HT3-antagonist ondansetron. *Neurogastroenterol Motil* 2007; 19(12):977–982.

138. Kim DY, Delgado–Aros S, Camilleri M, et al. Noninvasive measurement of gastric accommodation in patients with idiopathic nonulcer dyspepsia. *Am J Gastroenterol* 2001;96(11):3099–3105.

139. Tack J, Piessevaux H, Caenepeel P, et al. Role of impaired gastric accommodation to a meal in functional dyspepsia. *Gastroenterology* 1998;115(6): 1346–1352.

140. Tack J, Caenepeel P, Corsetti M, et al. Role of tension receptors in dyspeptic patients with hypersensitivity to gastric distention. *Gastroenterology* 2004; 127(4):1058–1066.

141. Stanghellini V, Tosetti C, Paternico A, et al. Risk indicators of delayed gastric emptying of solids in patients with functional dyspepsia. *Gastroenterology* 1996;110(4):1036–1042.

142. Sarnelli G, Caenepeel P, Geypens B, et al. Symptoms associated with impaired gastric emptying of solids and liquids in functional dyspepsia. *Am J Gastroenterol* 2003;98(4):783–788.

143. Talley NJ. Update on the role of drug therapy in non-ulcer dyspepsia. *Rev Gastroenterol Disord* 2003;3(1):25–30.

144. Otaka M, Jin M, Odashima M, et al. New strategy of therapy for functional dyspepsia using famotidine, mosapride and amitriptyline. *Aliment Pharmacol Ther* 2005;21(Suppl 2):42–46.

145. Hashash JG, Abdul-Baki H, Azar C, et al. Clinical trial: a randomised controlled cross-over trial of flupenthixol + melitracen in functional dyspepsia. *Aliment Pharmacol Ther* 2008;27(11):1148–1155.

146. Clouse RE, Mayer EA, Aziz Q, et al. Functional abdominal pain syndrome. In: Drossman DA, Corazziari E, Delvaux M, et al., eds. *Rome III: The Functional Gastrointestinal Disorders.* 3rd ed. McLean, Virginia: Degnon Associates, Inc.; 2006:557–594.

147. Wong HY, Mayer EA. A clinical perspective on abdominal pain. In: McMahon S, Koltzenburg M, eds. *Wall and Melzack's Textbook of Pain.* 5th ed. New York: Churchill Livingstone; 2005.

CHAPTER 64 ■ PELVIC PAIN IN FEMALES

KATY VINCENT AND JANE MOORE

INTRODUCTION

Pelvic pain is common in women, frequently leading to disability, social disruption, and loss of economic productivity. Many women do not seek help, often having lived with the pain since adolescence and accepting it as normal. In New Zealand, only 34% of a community sample of women aged between 18 and 50 years reported no pelvic pain, with 55.2% reporting dysmenorrhea, 25.4% chronic pelvic pain (CPP), and 19.7% dyspareunia.[1] In the United States, 14.7% of women of the same age range reported CPP with estimated outpatient medical costs of $881.5 million per year, 15% reporting work absenteeism, and 45% reduced productivity.[2] Similarly in the United Kingdom, 24% of 18 to 49 year olds reported CPP[3] and 37 of every 1000 women consulting their general practitioner presented with CPP[4]; this was comparable to asthma (37/1000) and back pain (41/1000) and higher than migraine (21/1000).

Pelvic pain is a frustrating symptom for both the patient and the doctor. Presentation can be variable, involving many organ systems, and severity can fluctuate over time. The frequent lack of an obvious initial diagnosis in both acute and chronic pelvic pain means that women frequently undergo large numbers of investigations and often unnecessary surgical procedures with associated morbidity and mortality. There is often a long interval between presentation and diagnosis with 25% remaining without a diagnosis after 3 to 4 years and more than 30% of women having had their pain for more than 5 years.[4]

The aim of this chapter is to provide an overview of the common causes of pelvic pain as well as to detail some of the less well known, but easily treated causes with up-to-date evidence and a clear rationale for investigation and treatment. Because of the complexity of the innervation of the pelvis and the anatomical proximity of pelvic viscera, there is frequently overlap between what has traditionally been considered the domain of gynecology, urology, or gastroenterology. Therefore, some conditions will only be briefly discussed here when they are considered in more detail in other chapters of this book.

We discuss acute and chronic pelvic pain separately as, although there are overlaps, presentation and management are often very different. The Royal College of Obstetricians and Gynecologists' (RCOG) definition of CPP will be used: "intermittent or constant pain in the lower abdomen or pelvis of at least 6 months' duration, not occurring exclusively with menstruation or intercourse and not associated with pregnancy."[5] In addition, we also consider pelvic pain in pregnancy, dysmenorrhea, and mittelschmerz, and that associated with the complications of assisted conception. Finally, we discuss dyspareunia and the vulval pain syndromes which frequently coexist with other pelvic pain and whose etiology and management may be similar.

ACUTE PELVIC PAIN

Introduction

The maxim that "acute pelvic pain in a woman of reproductive age is an ectopic pregnancy until proven otherwise" needs always to be borne in mind as ruptured ectopic pregnancies are associated with high morbidity and mortality and the consequences of a missed diagnosis are severe. However, there are many other causes of acute pain in the lower abdominal/pelvic area that also need to be considered in the differential diagnosis. Many of these are not gynecological (Table 64.1), though the symptom fre-

TABLE 64.1

NONGYNEACOLOGICAL CAUSES OF ACUTE PELVIC PAIN

Appendicitis
IBS
Constipation
Inflammatory bowel disease
Mesenteric adenitis
Diverticulitis
Strangulation of a hernia
Urinary tract infection
Renal/bladder calculi

TABLE 64.2

RISK FACTORS FOR AN ECTOPIC PREGNANCY

Past history of PID
Progesterone-only contraceptive pill
Previous ectopic pregnancy
Previous tubal surgery
IVF
Endometriosis
Uterotubal anomalies
Fetal exposure to diethylstilbestrol

TABLE 64.3

INVESTIGATION OF ACUTE PELVIC PAIN

Urinary/serum hCG
MSU
Triple swabs (high vaginal, cervical, and endocervical *Chlamydia*)
Urethral swab
FBC, G&S (Xmatch if ectopic suspected)
CRP
Pelvic US–TA or TV as appropriate
Abdominal radiograph ($+/-$ contrast)
Pelvic MRI
Diagnostic laparoscopy

CRP, C-Reactive protein; FBC, full blood count; G&S, group & save; MSU, midstream urine; TA, transabdominal; TV, transvaginal; US, ultra sound

quently presents, or is referred, to the gynecologist. Unless the patient is extremely unwell, assessment should begin as always with a detailed history followed by examination and appropriate investigations.

Overview of Assessment

Where at all possible, the history should be taken in private, allowing the woman (whatever her age) to have with her only those people she requests to be present. A detailed history of the pain should be taken and associated bowel and urinary symptoms and vaginal discharge/bleeding should be enquired about directly. It is also important to ascertain with accuracy the date of her last menstrual period (LMP) and whether this was normal, as well as a contraceptive history and any recent episodes of unprotected sexual intercourse (UPSI). In all cases, but particularly with adolescents, these areas need to be approached sensitively. The presence of any risk factors for ectopic pregnancy (Table 64.2) should be established and the woman's obstetric history ascertained. With an acute exacerbation of a chronic pain, it is important to enquire whether any precipitating factors (either physical or psychological) are present. At all times, clinicians should be alert to the possibility of assault and know where to access appropriate help locally if required.

Initial examination should ascertain that she is hemodynamically stable before examining the abdomen. The exact site of the pain should be established and evidence of an acute abdomen or abdominal/pelvic masses looked for. Pelvic pain in a sexually active woman (especially with a positive pregnancy test) should prompt a gentle digital internal examination, looking specifically for adnexal tenderness/masses and cervical excitation. Any discharge should be noted and appropriate swabs taken. If vaginal bleeding is present, a speculum examination should also be performed. Rectal examination may be indicated depending on the history. Again, privacy should be ensured, although a chaperone is recommended.[6]

All women should have a urinary pregnancy test, but otherwise investigations should be prompted by the history and examination findings rather than routinely ordered. Initially, investigations should be kept to a minimum in the case of an acute exacerbation of CPP. Investigations that might be considered are listed in Table 64.3.

Gynecological Factors

Pelvic Inflammatory Disease

Pelvic inflammatory disease (PID) is a common cause of acute pelvic pain and the incidence is increasing. It is an upper genital tract infection and can include one or more of the following: endometritis, salpingitis, tubo-ovarian abscess, and pelvic perito-

nitis. Prompt treatment and effective contact tracing are important as long-term sequelae include CPP, subfertility, and ectopic pregnancy. While infection usually ascends from the cervix, cervical swabs can be negative even when pathogenic organisms are isolated from the fallopian tubes. The pain is thought to be due to inflammation, tissue destruction, irritation of peritoneal surfaces, and distortion of anatomy. Right upper quadrant pain and perihepatic adhesions occur in the Fitz-Hugh-Curtis syndrome, which is seen in 10% to 20% of women with PID.[7,8] Clinical features of PID lack sensitivity and specificity, but include lower abdominal pain and tenderness, deep dyspareunia, abnormal vaginal/cervical discharge, cervical excitation and adnexal tenderness, and fever.[9] Evidence of acute infection will not always be seen on diagnostic laparoscopy and therefore this investigation should be reserved for cases where alternative pathology needs to be excluded or if a pelvic mass is seen on ultrasound (US).[10] Where there is a high index of suspicion, it is recommended that empirical antibiotic treatment should be commenced once swabs have been taken without waiting for culture results or performing further investigations.[10] A number of different organisms are associated with PID, including *Chlamydia trachomatis*, *Neisseria gonorrhoea*, *Mycoplasma genitalium*, and anerobes.[9] The most commonly implicated organisms vary geographically and therefore local guidelines for appropriate antibiotic treatment regimens should always be consulted. There are now high rates of quinolone-resistant gonorrhoea in the Unites States and, since April 2007, fluoroquinolone antibiotics have no longer been recommended for the treatment of PID there,[11] though this is not yet the case in the United Kingdom. Antibiotic treatment is usually continued for 14 days (with intravenous doses converted to oral once apyrexial), and therefore patient compliance can be an issue. The presence of an intrauterine contraceptive device (IUCD) only increases the risk of developing PID in the first few weeks after insertion. Leaving the device in situ while mild PID is being treated does not appear to affect the outcome. In severe cases, however, it is recommended that the IUCD be removed.[10]

When there is definite evidence of a pelvic abscess or severe disease, surgery is recommended (either laparoscopy or laparotomy), to drain the abscess and divide adhesions.[10] Depending on location, it may also be possible to drain pelvic collections under US guidance. This has been shown to be effective with fewer complications than surgery.[12]

To prevent reinfection, contact tracing and treatment of all sexual partners from 6 months prior to presentation is recommended.[10] This may be best done through a local genitourinary medicine (GUM) clinic, which will have experience of contact tracing and counselling about the long-term consequences of sexually transmitted infections. If admission is not required and appropriate facilities exist, it may be more effective to refer the woman to a GUM clinic immediately, to be seen the same day, before treatment is started. Sexual intercourse should be avoided until both the patient and her partner have completed a full course of treatment.

Adnexal Pathology

The adnexae comprise the fallopian tubes and the ovaries, the overlying peritoneum, and accompanying blood vessels. Common adnexal problems causing pain are discussed here.

Adnexal Torsion. Unlike the testes, it is rare for a normal adnexa to undergo torsion. However, the ovaries and the distal ends of the fallopian tubes hang free and, if enlarged by an ovarian cyst or hydrosalpinx for example, are able to twist and cause ischemia and thus pain, with necrosis ensuing if the torsion is not resolved. Initially, the pain may be a dull ache which comes and goes; however, once necrosis occurs, the pain becomes constant and severe and may be accompanied by pyrexia, nausea, leucocytosis, and raised inflammatory markers. Clinically, a tender pelvic mass will be found on internal examination and this can be confirmed with US. Management is surgical, ideally by urgent laparoscopy. If the adnexae appear healthy, then the torsion can be untwisted and the cyst/hydrosalpinx dealt with appropriately; however, if the tissues are gangrenous, it is recommended that the whole mass is removed intact without first attempting to resolve the torsion.

Other Ovarian Cyst Accident. As well as undergoing torsion, an ovarian cyst (either functional or pathological) can also cause pain by rupturing or by hemorrhaging into itself.

Ruptured cysts usually cause acute pain followed by a generalized dull ache; however, if enough fluid/blood is released into the pelvis to irritate the diaphragm, then shoulder pain may also be present. Diagnosis is usually clinical, although, an US may show fluid in the pelvis and the absence of a previously noted ovarian cyst. Pregnancy must always be excluded (usually with a urinary pregnancy test), but if the pain is resolving and the woman is hemodynamically stable, then management is conservative, providing symptom relief. However, if she is unstable or a significant amount of fluid is present in the pelvis, laparoscopy may be required. In this instance, it is obviously important to be sure the diagnosis is correct and that an ectopic pregnancy, for example, has not been missed.

Hemorrhage into a cyst may be self-limiting or require surgery. Again this decision should be based on the clinical picture.

In all these cases, if there is any doubt as to the nature of the cyst, then surgery should be performed so that tissue for histology can be obtained.

Hematometra/Hematocolpos

A relatively rare cause of acute, or acute-on-chronic, pelvic pain is a hematometra or hematocolpos (literally blood in the uterus or blood in the cervix). This can be primarily from a congenital anomaly or secondary to procedures such as transcervical resection of the endometrium if cervical stenosis occurs. With congenital anomalies where a bifid uterus exists with one blind ending horn, it is possible to have normal menstrual flow from one horn and a gradually increasing hematometra in the other.

Diagnosis is by US or magnetic resonance imaging (MRI) and management is surgical, which may be as simple as cervical dilatation or incising an imperforate hymen. The discovery of a congenital müllerian anomaly should prompt a thorough investigation of the renal and urogenital system as many of these anomalies coexist.[13]

Acute Exacerbation of Chronic Pelvic Pain

An emergency presentation with acute pelvic pain can be an exacerbation of a much more chronic problem. Often the patient is known to the department, but for others the sudden worsening of chronic pain can be the final straw that causes the woman to present for the first time. As well as organizing appropriate analgesia (remaining alert to the possibility of an opioid addiction) and treating any associated symptoms, a careful search for the factor(s) precipitating the exacerbation should be made. This may be disease-related, such as an ovarian cyst accident; treatment-related, such as reactivation of endometriosis by add-back hormone replacement therapy (HRT) or constipation secondary to increased analgesia use; or lifestyle-related, such as increased activity worsening musculoskeletal pain or a bereavement worsening psychological status. If such precipitating factors can be identified, they should be discussed with the patient. Coping strategies can be taught to prevent future emergency presentations, which may also be reduced by easy access to a health care professional who knows the woman well.

Complications Specific to Pregnancy

A number of complications specific to pregnancy can present with pelvic pain and need always to be borne in mind in a woman of reproductive age. It is also worth noting, however, that the physiological and anatomical adaptations of pregnancy can alter the presenting features of many nonpregnancy-related conditions such as appendicitis. When treating pain in a possibly ongoing pregnancy, nonsteroidal anti-inflammatory drugs (NSAIDs) are contraindicated because of effects on implantation, fetal renal function, and premature closure of the ductus arteriosus. Acetaminophen (paracetamol) and opioids, however, are safe. Reassurance and explanation are perhaps more important than ever in these cases to avoid anxiety about the pregnancy further clouding the clinical picture.

Ectopic Pregnancy

An ectopic pregnancy is one in which the conceptus implants outside the uterine cavity. Most commonly, this is within the fallopian tube (98.3%) but more rarely can be in the abdominal cavity, on the ovary, or on the cervix. The incidence is approximately 1 in 100 pregnancies[14]; however, this is likely to increase with the increasing incidence of pelvic infection and assisted conception. Rarely, a heterotopic pregnancy can occur, which is effectively a twin pregnancy in two different sites (e.g., one intrauterine and one ectopic pregnancy). These cases can be easily missed with false reassurance given once the intrauterine pregnancy is seen on US. With the rising prevalence of assisted conception techniques the incidence of heterotopic pregnancies is increasing.[15]

Classically, presentation is with a period of amenorrhoea followed by brown vaginal loss and then onset of pelvic pain. Realistically, however, presentation is varied, ranging from asymptomatic (an incidental finding at routine scan), through any combination of pain and/or old or fresh vaginal bleeding, to collapse secondary to hypovolemia. Initial pain is thought to be secondary to stretching of the peritoneum covering the distended fallopian tube; however, with rupture of the tube, peritonitis occurs and tracking of the blood up to the diaphragm can cause shoulder tip pain.

In the collapsed patient with a positive pregnancy test, diagnosis is assumed and resuscitation commenced with surgery performed immediately when she is stable. At the opposite extreme, in a hemodynamically stable woman with minimal symptoms, diagnosis can be difficult. In early pregnancy an intrauterine gestation may not be visible even with transvaginal US (TVUS). A combination of serial human chorionic gonadotrophin (hCG) levels and repeated US may be required to determine the location and viability of the pregnancy. If a high index of suspicion is present or the woman is isolated socially, this observation may best be done as an inpatient; however, in the majority of cases, early pregnancy clinics facilitate safe outpatient management.

Appropriate management depends on the severity of presentation. With an unstable patient, urgent laparotomy or laparoscopy should be performed depending on the skills of the available surgeon. With a stable patient, the majority of cases should be able to be managed laparoscopically, reducing postoperative pain, recovery time, and hospital stay. Some units now manage appropriate cases medically using methotrexate; however, this is not without risks and requires careful surveillance and a motivated patient.[16]

However the pregnancy is managed, the risks of an ectopic pregnancy in the future are considerably higher than in the background population, and the woman should be counselled about this prior to discharge and advised to get an early scan in her next pregnancy. It should not be forgotten that a pregnancy has been lost and many women/couples value the opportunity to talk this through either at the time or at a later date.

Miscarriage

Miscarriage is defined as pregnancy loss prior to viability (currently considered to be 24 weeks) and occurs in 10% to 20% of clinical pregnancies.[17] Because of connotations of blame, the medical term abortion should no longer be used when pregnancy loss is spontaneous. The different types of miscarriage are shown in Table 64.4. Bleeding is not always the presenting feature. Classically, bleeding precedes pain in a miscarriage as opposed to an ectopic pregnancy where the pain occurs first. As this is not reliable, all pain or bleeding in early pregnancy should be referred to an early pregnancy unit for further assessment and management. Management may be expectant, medical (using prostaglandin analogues ± antiprogesterone) or surgical (evacuation of retained products of conception [ERPC]). If the woman is hemodynamically unstable or the bleeding is very heavy, then surgery is recommended; otherwise the choice of management should be made by the woman. Nonsurgical options are associated with longer periods of bleeding, but avoid the risks of a general anesthetic and may allow the woman to feel more in control. Contrary to previous beliefs, there is no increase in infection rate with expectant management.[18] All nonimmunized, Rhesus-negative women who miscarry after 12 weeks' gestation should be given prophylaxis with anti-D immunoglobulin. Prior to 12 weeks, anti-D immunoglobulin should be given for medical or surgical evacuation or if the bleeding is very heavy and associated with pain.[17] The negative psychological impact of early pregnancy loss can be enormous, both for the woman and her family, and therefore counselling and support should be offered. Ideally, this should be at a local level, although national support groups also exist.

TABLE 64.4

TYPES OF MISCARRIAGE[125]

Threatened	May be continuing to bleed Viable pregnancy
Inevitable	Bleeding Cervical os open
Complete	Bleeding settled All products of conception passed
Incomplete	May be continuing to bleed Products still present
Delayed	No/minimal bleeding Fetal demise, all products still present
Anembryonic pregnancy	May have bleeding Gestational sac present but no fetal pole

Fibroid Degeneration

Uterine fibroids (leiomyomas) are benign tumors of the uterus which are found in approximately 20% of women of reproductive age. They are usually asymptomatic and are more common in older women and women of African origin. They possess estrogen receptors and are thus stimulated to grow during pregnancy. As their blood supply is mainly peripheral, central areas can suffer from ischemia if enlargement is rapid, causing pain. This is known as red degeneration. The pain is generally well localized with tenderness over the area of the fibroid only (as opposed to placental abruption where the whole uterus is tender and woody hard) and may be accompanied by a mild pyrexia and leukocytosis. Opioid analgesia is often required and admission may be necessary, if only for observation and fetal monitoring if there is any doubt about the diagnosis.

Ovarian Cyst Accident

As in the nonpregnant state, hemorrhage into or rupture or torsion of an ovarian cyst can occur during pregnancy. In general, presentation and management are as for the nonpregnant woman; however, symptoms can be masked and nonspecific during pregnancy. Rupture of a cyst can present with severe pain and shock, and in early pregnancy laparoscopy may be necessary to exclude ectopic pregnancy. However, if pain is resolving and no other symptoms are present, conservative management is recommended.

If surgical management is required beyond early pregnancy, laparotomy may have to be considered because of the risks and technical difficulties of a laparoscopy with an enlarged uterus.

Ligamentous Stretch

As the uterus enlarges, it moves out of the pelvis and becomes an abdominal organ. During this process, the supporting round ligaments are stretched and cause pain in the late first/early second trimester in 10% to 30% of pregnancies. Management is by simple analgesia and reassurance; however, it is important to ensure that other causes of pain are not missed, such as rupture of a heterotopic pregnancy or acute appendicitis.

Urinary Retention and Uterine Incarceration

Uterine retroversion occurs in up to 15% of pregnancies in the first trimester but by 15 weeks gestation spontaneous anteversion almost always occurs. It is reported that retroversion persists into the second trimester in 1 in 3000 pregnancies.[19] Rarely, it may not be noticed until a cesarean section is performed at term; however, it can become impacted and present with urinary frequency, urgency, abdominal pain, and urinary retention. Pelvic adhesions secondary to infection or endometriosis and posterior wall fibroids can predispose to incarceration. Diagnosis can be aided by US or MRI (Fig. 64.1); however, fetal parts may be palpable vaginally and an enlarged bladder abdominally. Gentle manual decompression is usually possible after emptying the bladder with a Foley catheter. Intermittent catheterization is occasionally necessary for a few days subsequently, but an indwelling catheter is not recommended because of the risk of infection.[20] If asymptomatic retroversion persists until term, delivery should be by cesarean section and a classical incision is often required.[19]

Complications of Assisted Conception

Ovarian Hyperstimulation Syndrome

Ovarian hyperstimulation syndrome (OHSS) is a serious and sometimes fatal complication of assisted conception techniques.

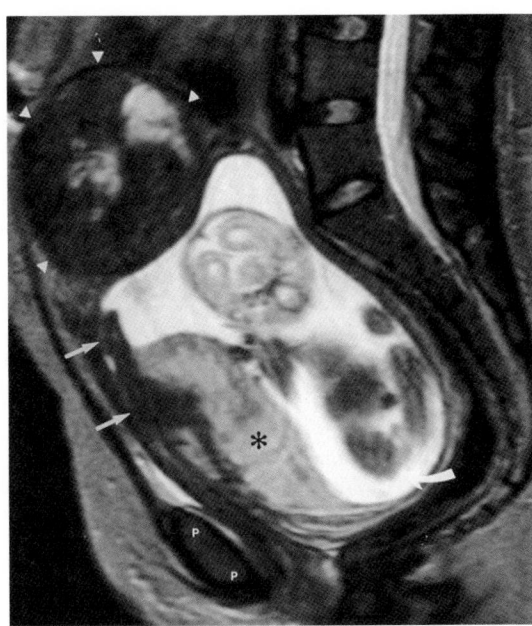

FIGURE 64.1 MRI of persistent retroversion of the uterus at 20 weeks gestation. The uterine fundus containing the breech (*curved arrow*) can be seen in the Pouch of Douglas. The placenta (*) is attached to the posterior uterine wall with a large intramural fibroid (*arrowheads*) superiorly on the lower portion of the anterior wall, and the cervix (*arrows*) just below, above the level of the symphysis pubis (*P*). (From Hamoda H, Chamberlain PF, Moore NR, et al. Conservative treatment of an incarcerated gravid uterus. *BJOG* 2002;109:1074–1075, with permission.)

It is a systemic disease secondary to the release of vasoactive products from the hyperstimulated ovaries. It can be subdivided into early, within 9 days of the ovulatory hCG dose, or late and is classified according to severity (Table 64.5). Mild disease has been reported to complicate up to 33% of in vitro fertilization (IVF) cycles, while the severe form can occur in up to 8%. OHSS is more likely in women with polycystic ovaries, young women,

and in cycles where conception occurs, especially of multiple pregnancies.[21] Presentation is variable depending on severity (see Table 64.5) but should always be borne in mind in a woman with abdominal/pelvic pain who has recently undergone assisted conception. Mild and moderate disease can be managed on an outpatient basis, but more severe forms or concerns about a worsening condition require admission. In general, management involves symptom control: analgesia with either acetaminophen (paracetamol) or codeine but avoiding NSAIDs, and antiemetics suitable for early pregnancy (e.g., prochlorperazine, metoclopramide); continuing progesterone luteal support but stopping hCG support and avoiding strenuous exercise and sexual intercourse because of the risk of ovarian torsion. In severe cases, multidisciplinary management is advised to deal with issues of fluid balance and thromboembolic risk (0.7% to 10%).[22] Paracentesis may be necessary, but should always be done under US guidance because of the risk of injury to enlarged, vascular ovaries. Importantly, women should be reassured that pregnancy may continue normally despite OHSS.[21]

Pelvic Infection

Pelvic infection can occur after investigation of tubal patency with a hysterosalpingogram (HSG) or laparoscopy and dye test, or after oocyte retrieval. Prior to such investigations being arranged, all women should have cervical swabs performed and any infection should be treated with an appropriate antibiotic regimen. Oocyte retrieval is usually performed transvaginally under US guidance. Rates of pelvic infection secondary to this procedure vary between units and published series but are generally low, between 0% to 1%.[23] Initial management is with antibiotics and US to exclude a pelvic abscess. Progressive worsening of symptoms or failure to improve should prompt a further search for a pelvic collection and consideration of the possibility of bowel damage, for which laparoscopy or laparotomy would be required.

DYSMENORRHEA

Dysmenorrhea is defined as pain with menstruation and is thus separate from CPP. It is common, with estimates of prevalence ranging from 20% to 90%. It has a major social and economic impact and is the leading cause of school and work absenteeism in young women.[24] Traditionally it has been subdivided into primary and secondary dysmenorrhea. Primary (functional) dysmenorrhea is not associated with other pathology, is thought to be because of overproduction of prostaglandins and leukotrienes in the myometrium causing strong, painful contractions of the uterus, and is common in adolescents.[25] It is frequently considered to be a "normal" part of development and assumed to improve with age or after pregnancy, though this has not been shown to be true in longitudinal studies. Secondary dysmenorrhea is associated with other pathology (Table 64.6) and therefore

---

TABLE 64.5

SYMPTOMS AND SIGNS OF OVARIAN HYPERSTIMULATION SYNDROME (ADAPTED FROM JENKINS ET AL.[21])

Mild OHSS	Abdominal bloating Mild abdominal pain Ovarian size usually <8 cm
Moderate OHSS	Moderate abdominal pain Nausea ± vomiting US evidence of ascites Ovarian size usually 8–12 cm
Severe OHSS	Clinical ascites (occasionally hydrothorax) Oliguria Hematocrit >45% Hypoproteinemia Ovarian size usually >12 cm
Critical OHSS	Tense ascites or large hydrothorax Hematocrit >55% White cell count >25000/mL Oligo/anuria Thromboembolism Acute respiratory distress syndrome

---

TABLE 64.6

CAUSES OF DYSMENORRHEA

Endometriosis
Adenomyosis
Müllerian anomalies
PID
Fibroids
Cervical stenosis
Pelvic venous congestion
Intrauterine device

often occurs with other symptoms such as dyspareunia and menorrhagia. It is traditionally considered to affect women in their thirties and over but it is worth remembering that children as young as 10 years old have been shown to have biopsy-proven endometriosis,[26] and congenital uterine anomalies probably occur in around 4% of the population, increasing to 10% in adolescents with pelvic pain.[25] Clinically, therefore, we find this distinction to be unhelpful, and will consider dysmenorrhea as a symptom which deserves to be treated and investigated as appropriate, no matter what age the patient.

Initial assessment should include a detailed history, including risk factors for pathology associated with dysmenorrhea and other symptoms. In young girls who are not sexually active and without associated symptoms, a pelvic examination is not necessary before commencing empirical treatment. If there are concerns about structural anomalies, an abdominal US can offer reassurance, but cannot diagnose or exclude endometriosis.

Nonsteroidal Anti-Inflammatory Drugs

Many women, especially teenagers, self-medicate for their dysmenorrhea and NSAIDs are often the drugs of choice. NSAIDs act by inhibiting cyclo-oxygenase and therefore reduce prostaglandin production and associated uterine contractions. Mefenamic acid has been shown to also inhibit the lipoxygenase pathway.[27] Systematic reviews have concluded that NSAIDs are an effective treatment for dysmenorrhea but that there is insufficient evidence to determine which, if any, is the most effective.[28] A greater improvement of symptoms can be obtained if treatment is started 24 hours prior to the onset of bleeding and, if a loading dose of twice the regular dose is used initially, followed by regular doses as needed.[29]

Hormonal Treatments

The combined oral contraceptive pill (COCP) has been used as a treatment for dysmenorrhea for many years. It acts to inhibit ovulation and limit endometrial growth, reducing progesterone and subsequent prostaglandin and leukotriene production.[25] A number of trials have shown a significant improvement in dysmenorrhea with COCP use, both high[30] and lower dose formulations.[31] Tricycling the COCP (i.e., taking three packets of pills back-to-back without having a withdrawal bleed in between packets) has also been shown to reduce symptoms as well as decreasing the frequency of menstruation[32] and thus may be a good alternative to other forms of longer term contraception in some women.

Depot medroxyprogesterone acetate (DMPA), a long-acting injectable contraceptive, also reliably inhibits ovulation in both its intramuscular and subcutaneous formulations[33] and amenorrhea is common. In one study, 64% of adolescents reported an improvement in dysmenorrhea symptoms with DMPA[34]; however, concerns about loss of bone mineral density (BMD) limit its prolonged use in adolescence. For women also requiring long-term contraception, a levonorgestrel releasing intrauterine system (LNG-IUS) is another alternative. The majority of women are amenorrheic with the system in place and, even for those who continue to bleed, menses tend to be lighter and less painful, though bleeding can be erratic for the first 6 months. In some instances, this may be the most appropriate option for nulliparous young adults, in which case a brief general anesthetic may be necessary for insertion. For severe symptoms, a therapeutic trial of a Gonadotrophin Releasing Hormone agonist (GnRH agonist) (see below) could also be considered.

Surgical Treatments

Surgery for dysmenorrhea should only be considered as an investigation for other pathologies if there is no response to medical treatment (e.g., diagnostic laparoscopy) or as a last resort. Systematic reviews suggest that there is insufficient evidence to support the use of surgical nerve interruption[35] (either laparoscopic uterine nerve ablation [LUNA] or presacral neurectomy [PSN]) in dysmenorrhea, and the rates of complications are high.

Nonpharmacological Interventions

A number of other interventions have been studied to improve dysmenorrhea with varying success. Both high-frequency transcutaneous electrical nerve stimulation (TENS) and acupuncture have shown benefit in some studies[36] as has topical heat therapy[37]; however, psychological interventions have not been shown to be beneficial in pure dysmenorrhea.[38] As always, the role of education and validation of symptoms cannot be emphasized strongly enough, and this is particularly true for adolescents.

MITTELSCHMERZ

Mittelschmerz (literally "middle pain" in German) is one-sided, lower abdominal pain that occurs at or around ovulation. It can last from minutes to 48 hours and requires no treatment other than simple analgesics. It is thought to occur in approximately 50% of women at some point. What causes the pain is not known exactly, but possible suggestions include tubal, uterine, or cecal spasm, increased tension in the ovary or Graafian follicle, or peritoneal irritation due to leak of blood or fluid from the follicle. However, the latter is probably unlikely as in one study, 33 out of 34 women experienced the pain prior to follicular rupture (as confirmed with US)[39] and pain is on the same side as follicular rupture in only 86% of women.[40] Mittelschmerz probably causes most concern when a woman recommences ovulation after a long period of treatment with an ovulation inhibitor. Because it is not expected, the sudden, acute pain can then lead to investigation for other conditions such as appendicitis or an ovarian cyst accident. Similar, but more severe, pain can occur with trapped ovary syndrome and endometriosis, as discussed below.

CHRONIC PELVIC PAIN

Introduction

CPP is a symptom, not a diagnosis. As will be seen, the causes are diverse, often multifactorial, and not always evident on routine examinations or even laparoscopy. As well as the economic impact already alluded to, CPP has major psychological, social, and cultural consequences not only for the woman but for her partner, family, and society as a whole. It is acknowledged that it is frequently poorly managed, yet it is as common as migraine and back pain and affects all races and social classes.

Factors Associated with Chronic Pelvic Pain

A number of factors are thought to be associated with CPP and should be explored during the consultation at an appropriate point.

Social

CPP is seen in women of all social classes with no variation in prevalence depending on marital or employment status.[41] However, social support can be an important factor in how a woman deals with her pain and social isolation can make the situation very difficult. It is easy to see how a vicious circle is set up with pain leading to the loss of the woman's social role and thus her self-esteem, causing isolation and contributing to further pain.

Abuse

Although frequently alluded to, the relationship between physical or sexual abuse and CPP is still not clear. The majority of studies are retrospective and only target women who have already developed the symptom. It appears that women in secondary care with any chronic pain condition are more likely to report a history of childhood abuse than pain-free women. When CPP is considered, sexual abuse is more commonly reported than in other pain conditions. It could be, however, that childhood sexual abuse is a predisposing factor for the development of depression, anxiety, and somatization which may then lead to the development of CPP.[5] In a rare prospective study,[42] children who had been abused were followed until their twenties and were not found to have an increase in medically unexplained symptoms when compared to a population who were not known to have been abused. However, those with unexplained symptoms were more likely to report their abuse. Thus, a revealed abuse history should not be assumed to be the cause of the pain, but failure to respond to treatments should perhaps prompt an exploration of these areas if a good therapeutic relationship already exists.

Psychological

Women with CPP display an increased incidence of "negative" psychological features, such as depression, anxiety, and catastrophisation.[43] This is common with other chronic pain conditions, such as fibromyalgia and irritable bowel syndrome (IBS). However, it is not possible to know whether these factors predispose a woman to develop CPP, contribute to a perpetuation of the pain, or are a consequence of years of living with pain and attempts to justify its severity or even existence to friends, family, and health care professionals. What is known is that psychological state can alter the experience of pain, and this is the area that should be emphasized to the woman when a referral to a psychologist is suggested. Improving sleep patterns alone can both improve mood and have a significant effect on ability to function.

Personality

Similarly, whether personality types predispose to the development of chronic pain conditions or merely alter the way in which they are dealt with is not known. Some personality traits can make recovery more difficult. "Driven types," for example, are unable to pace themselves and do too much on a "good day" so that on the following day, symptoms are worse again. On the other hand, those who take easily to the "sick role" can be hard to persuade to engage in therapeutic options and may also fail to respond. Women with diagnosed personality disorders should be managed in conjunction with a psychiatrist.

Overview of Assessment

The initial assessment of a woman with CPP is very important. Complete recovery at follow-up is associated with a favorable patient rating of the quality of the initial consultation.[44] The woman needs to be given time to tell her story, without interruptions, but with the support of whomever she would like to be present (which may be no one but the doctor). The extra time taken to listen to the history in the patient's own words may well give valuable information about the context of the pain, its effects on her life, and her beliefs about its cause and prognosis. In fact,

---

TABLE 64.7

WHAT WOMEN WOULD LIKE FROM THE CPP CONSULTATION[45]

Personal care
To be understood and taken seriously
Explanation
Reassurance

an explanation for the pain has been shown to be one of things women with CPP most want out of their consultation (Table 64.7).[45] The process of telling her story and of the examination can, in itself, be therapeutic. Once a cycle of chronic pain has been set up, it is unlikely that a single cause for the pain will be identified, and the clinician should be alert for any contributing factors that may be revealed.

History

A detailed history of the pain should be taken including when and how it began, its associations, such as bowel, bladder, and psychological symptoms, and the effects of posture and movement. The circumstances surrounding the start of the pain and whether they recently changed should be discussed, as should the reasons why she has presented now. Cyclicity of symptoms or exacerbation with intercourse need to be established as does her current and future fertility aspirations. Relevant information may well be gleaned from her obstetric history, and a contraceptive and smear history should also be taken. It should be ascertained that no "red flag" symptoms, such as rectal bleeding or weight loss, exist. While a history of past or present abuse (verbal, physical, or sexual) may also be present, it may not be appropriate to discuss this at the first consultation. If abuse is revealed, these experiences need to be accepted as stated, and it is important to know where to access specialist help locally should this be required.[5]

Examination

Examination requires more time than is routine in gynecology and, as it is the time when the patient is most vulnerable, new information is often revealed at this point.[46] The decision as to whether to have a chaperone present is a personal one that will depend upon both the doctor's and patient's wishes. However, the presence of a third person may alter the dynamic and prevent certain information being revealed. Examination should begin, as always, with observation. This includes evidence of skin alterations or damage and posture, but also of both the patient's attitude to the examination and the doctor's response to this. Evidence of altered sensation (hypersensitivity or allodynia) should be sought before abdominal palpation is performed. The effect of movement should be assessed, which might suggest musculoskeletal pain. The extent to which an internal examination is performed will depend on the history. With marked vaginismus, anything more than a gentle, one finger examination may be inappropriate. Altered sensation on the vulva and perineum should be looked for and pelvic floor muscle tone assessed if possible. Rectal examination should only be performed if there is a clear indication in the history.

Investigations

Investigations should be guided by the history, but care should be taken to avoid over-investigation initially. Many women will have already seen a number of doctors, often of many specialities, and had a variety of frequently invasive investigations. One particularly useful strategy is to ask the woman to keep a detailed pain diary over 1 to 2 months. This can reveal information about the timing of the pain and its associations to the doctor and to the patient.[5]

Therapeutic Trial

Very cyclical symptoms are usually gynecological in origin, although pain perception itself may vary with the menstrual cycle as can symptoms of both interstitial cystitis (IC) and IBS. Where symptoms are markedly cyclical, a therapeutic trial of a GnRH analogue should be considered before a laparoscopy is performed.[5] This group of drugs, given initially as monthly subcutaneous injections, cause a prolonged activation of the GnRH receptor leading to an initial worsening of symptoms (the "initial flare"). This is followed by a reduction in luteinizing hormone (LH) and follicle stimulating hormone (FSH), such that serum estradiol levels are suppressed by 21 days and remain at levels equivalent to postmenopausal women with continued dosing. Common adverse effects are shown in Table 64.8. The most common complaints of hot flushes and emotional symptoms are often well tolerated if pain is relieved. The biggest concern, however, is the loss of BMD which can be up to 6% after 6 months of treatment.[47] If the trial is successful, then treatment can continue with the addition of low-dose combined HRT, and this combination has been shown to be safe and effective for up to 2 years.[47] After this time, many women are not prepared to continue with monthly injections (though three monthly preparations exist and can be effective in some women) and seek alternative management options. However, in those that would like to continue with treatment, there is now evidence from small studies that the combination is safe for up to 10 years, with one of these women having stopped treatment to conceive and then recommenced treatment after delivery.[48]

Diagnostic Laparoscopy

If no relief is gained from a therapeutic trial of GnRH analogue or if there are other indications such as subfertility or a pelvic mass, diagnostic laparoscopy should be performed. However, laparoscopy is not without risks with large series quoting approximately 3% risk of minor complications and 0.6–1.8/1000 risk of major complications such as bowel perforation and vascular damage.[49] Furthermore, although it was initially thought that a negative laparoscopy would reassure a woman, more recent studies have shown this not to be the case[50] and it may reaffirm her beliefs that the doctors do not believe her and think the pain is of psychological origin.

Empirical Treatment

Even if no clear cause of the pain can be found on investigation, the pain should still be treated empirically. Analgesia or hormonal treatments may be appropriate, but it is often worth considering drugs such as amitriptyline, gabapentin, and pregabalin in addition. These drugs are effective in neuropathic pain and may have a role in reducing visceral hypersensitivity.[51] Topical capsaicin cream on the skin of the abdomen (not the vulva) may be useful for hyperalgesia and allodynia. Nonpharmacological treatments such as acupuncture, TENS, chiropractic, and osteopathic manipulations may be beneficial, and pain management techniques and support groups can also be of value.[52]

The Importance of Visceral Hyperalgesia in Chronic Pelvic Pain

Visceral hyperalgesia (and subsequent viscero-visceral/viscerosomatic referral) is thought to have an important role in CPP.[53] It can be the primary pain generator, perpetuating factor, or cause of secondary symptoms. Visceral hyperalgesia should therefore always be borne in mind, especially when symptoms from multiple organs are present or where there is no clear demonstrable cause. This area is covered in more detail in Chapters 3, 4, and 65. Sex steroid hormones are known to act at multiple sites throughout the peripheral and central nervous system, and it is

---

TABLE 64.8

HORMONAL TREATMENTS FOR ENDOMETRIOSIS RELATED PAIN[126]

Treatment	Main adverse effects
COCP[127] (continuous or tricycling)	Thromboembolic disorders, altered serum lipid profile, hypertension, skin reactions, migraine, intermenstrual bleeding, depression, altered libido
Danazol[128]	Deepening of voice, acne, hirsutism, clitoral hypertrophy, vaginal dryness, hematological disturbances, altered serum lipid profile, thromboembolic disorders, depression, weight gain, altered libido, muscle cramps
Gestrinone[129]	Headache, depression, weight gain, voice changes, acne, hirsutism, intermenstrual spotting, gastrointestinal disturbances, muscle cramps
Progestogens (e.g., medroxyprogesterone acetate)[129]	Depression, weight gain, altered libido, acne, vaginal bleeding, breast tenderness, thromboembolic disorders, gallbladder disease, worsening of ovarian cysts
LNG-IUS[130]	Irregular vaginal bleeding, depression, weight gain, reduced libido, breast tenderness, vaginal discharge, uterine perforation, ovarian cysts
GnRH agonists[131]	Initial flare in symptoms, bruising/pain at injection site, depression, emotional lability, reduced libido, vaginal dryness, hot flushes, headache, pituitary apoplexy
GnRH antagonists	Same as for GnRH agonists except that no initial flare occurs

thus not surprising that these symptoms often show cyclicity and can respond to hormonal manipulation.

Gynecological Factors in Chronic Pelvic Pain

Endometriosis

Endometriosis is defined as "the presence of endometrial-like tissue outside the uterus, which induces a chronic, inflammatory reaction."[53a] While it is a common cause of CPP and dysmenorrhea, it is also a common incidental finding in asymptomatic women. Therefore, it is imperative that a detailed history and examination are undertaken even in a woman who has previously been diagnosed with endometriosis, as it may not be the sole cause of, or even related to, her pain.

Endometriosis is a complex condition, with much still unknown about its etiology, natural history, and incidence. In 1927, Sampson suggested it was due to retrograde menstruation.[54] However, this process can be demonstrated in more than 90% of women, therefore a combination of retrograde menstruation and an altered immune environment,[55] allowing implantation and the development of a nerve and blood supply, is currently considered to be the most likely etiology. In order to make a definitive diagnosis of endometriosis, direct visualization of ectopic endometrial implants must occur,[56] preferably with biopsy and histological confirmation.

The prevalence of endometriosis is difficult to establish, as the vast majority of implants are in the pelvic cavity (though extrapelvic disease does occur) and not every woman will have a laparoscopy or laparotomy. Clinical presentation can be variable (Table 64.9), and to confuse matters further, the extent of disease seen at laparoscopy correlates poorly with the severity of symptoms.[57]

Although laparoscopy and lesion histology is the criterion standard diagnostic test, current guidelines recommend that if the history and clinical examination are suggestive of endometriosis, a definitive diagnosis is not required before commencing empirical treatment.[56] There are a large variety of treatment options currently available for endometriosis, and the appropriate treatment(s) should be decided in discussion with the woman depending on her specific constellation of symptoms and current and future fertility wishes. A full discussion of these options is beyond the scope of this chapter; however, an overview of the management of endometriosis-related pain (but not infertility) is given below. More detailed reviews can be found elsewhere.[58-60]

Medical Management of Endometriosis. As with dysmenorrhea, traditionally NSAIDs have been used to treat pain secondary to endometriosis. However, there is no evidence to suggest that they have any greater effect than placebo.[61] Women need to also be informed of the inhibitory effect of NSAIDs on ovulation when taken midcycle. The enzyme cyclo-oxygenase 2 (COX-2) is involved in both pain and inflammation, and specific COX-2 inhibitors have shown promising results in human studies of endometriosis-related pain.[62] However, because of concerns over the safety of this class of drugs,[63] they cannot currently be recommended.

The majority of endometriotic tissue is hormonally sensitive, and hormonal suppression has been shown to reduce endometriosis-associated pain.[56] The available hormonal treatments are shown in Table 64.8. They all appear to be equally effective at controlling endometriosis-related pain but have differing adverse effect profiles. In general, however, symptoms return over time after stopping the treatment. For example, in one study, the median time to recurrence of pain was 6.1 months after stopping danazol and 5.2 months after a GnRH analogue.[64]

Over recent years, it has become apparent that endometriotic deposits express aromatase and are thus able to synthesize estradiol,[65] possibly explaining why some women continue to have symptoms while in a hypoestrogenic state. Recent small trials of nonsteroidal aromatase inhibitors (AI) in combination with hormonal treatments have shown promising results, especially as the women concerned were refractory to other treatments.[66] AI, such as anastrazole and letrozole, are used in the treatment of postmenopausal women with estrogen-sensitive breast cancers and are known to have a mild adverse effect profile, though, as with GnRH analogues, there are concerns about loss of BMD.[67]

The recent discovery that endometriotic implants in a rat model develop a sensory and autonomic innervation[68] may explain some of the pain symptoms suffered by women with endometriosis which were previously thought to be due to scarring and inflammation. It is possible that a neuropathic component to the pain may exist, and therefore in women who only show a partial response to hormonal treatment, the addition of a drug such as amitriptyline or gabapentin may be beneficial.

Surgical Management of Endometriosis. As can be seen from the discussion of medical treatments, these options only keep the disease suppressed but do not affect a cure: once treatment is stopped, symptoms may recur. Complete surgical excision of disease can be performed and has been shown to significantly reduce pain scores, improve sexual function, and improve quality of life. In one series, for example, 67% of women reported an improvement following surgery, 8% felt their symptoms to be unchanged, 25% were worse, but only 33% required further surgery during the 5-year follow-up period.[69] However, particularly with deeply infiltrating endometriosis (DIE), there are significant risks associated with surgery (including bowel perforation, fistula formation, and ureteric damage), and this should therefore only be undertaken at specialist centers by a multidisciplinary team with the necessary expertise.[56] However, if a diagnostic laparoscopy is being undertaken and mild disease is seen, then current recommendations are that this should be excised or ablated at the time.[56] Neither pre- nor postoperative hormonal treatment have been shown to improve outcome measures including pain scores[70] and therefore cannot be recommended. However, the LNG-IUS did significantly reduce the risk of recurrence of moderate–severe dysmenorrhea at 1 year[71] and is therefore worth considering.

Adenomyosis

Adenomyosis is defined as the presence of endometrial glands and stroma within the myometrium.[72] Typically, the surrounding myometrium is hypertrophic and hyperplastic. Very little research has been undertaken on adenomyosis specifically, with much of the management being extrapolated from that of endometriosis—a condition with which it has many similarities but also a number of differences. Previously, the diagnosis was made histologically after hysterectomy, and it was a common finding in women undergoing hysterectomy for menorrhagia. It is now

TABLE 64.9

SYMPTOMS AND SIGNS OF ENDOMETRIOSIS

Symptoms	Signs
Dysmenorrhea	Fixed, retroverted uterus
Dyspareunia	Enlarged ovary
Dyschezia	Uterosacral nodules
CPP	Rectovaginal nodules
Infertility	
Hematuria	
Hematochezia	
Chronic fatigue	

possible to make the diagnosis radiologically with MRI or TVUS.[73] In experienced units, these two methods are equally accurate, but MRI is less user-dependent and usually considered to be the investigation of choice. However, a relatively high rate of false positives will be seen, with, for example, uterine contractions being falsely diagnosed as adenomyosis. Without reliable diagnostic criteria, clinical trials of treatments are difficult and a true prevalence is unknown.

There appear to be two distinct forms of the condition: diffuse, where endometrial cells are widely distributed throughout the myometrium, and focal, where a discrete collection of cells are seen, also known as an adenomyoma.[74] Surgical excision of the former is not possible, thus treatment options are limited to either medical management or hysterectomy. While some cases of focal disease may be amenable to surgical management, it is possibly not as responsive to hormonal treatment. In a similar manner to fibroids, it has been suggested that it might be possible to embolize adenomyotic tissue. So far, this has not proved to be successful, but promising preliminary results are emerging with the use of focused US to ablate the abnormal tissue.[75]

Adenomyosis is thought to cause menorrhagia, metrorrhagia, dysmenorrhea, and infertility, although some authorities dispute its effect on fertility.[76] It is thought to occur secondary to a breach in the integrity of the myometrial-endometrial junction, such as occurs in pregnancy, especially those complicated by abnormal placentation and surgery (including ERPC and cesarean section), or after blunt trauma to the abdomen. As with endometriosis, the ectopic endometrial tissue is hormone sensitive and has been shown to express aromatase.[77] GnRH agonists, Danazol, and the LNG-IUS have all been shown to be successful in the treatment of adenomyosis, though all have side effects. Perhaps the most promising of these is the LNG-IUS because of its mild adverse effect profile and apparent tolerability by patients. Unfortunately, no studies have been done on AI and adenomyosis to date.

Adhesions

Adhesions are a common finding in women with and without pelvic pain. They are formed after trauma to the visceral or parietal peritoneum and so can be secondary to surgery, infection, and endometriosis. Between 70% and 85% are thought to occur after surgery[78] and are thus iatrogenic. The relationship between adhesions and pain is still unclear. A prospective, blinded randomized controlled trial of 116 women with CPP undergoing laparoscopy and followed for 1 year showed there to be no benefit of adhesiolysis over diagnostic laparoscopy alone.[79] In another prospective, randomized trial at 9–12 months follow-up, there was no significant difference in pain between the groups who had or had not undergone adhesiolysis at laparotomy. However, in a subgroup analysis of this data, those women who had dense, vascular adhesions involving the bowel did have a significant improvement in pain after adhesiolysis.[80] Therefore, although adhesiolysis cannot be recommended in general as a treatment for CPP, in those women who have severe adhesions involving the bowel, it may be successful.

There are two other distinct cases where adhesions are known to cause pain: trapped ovary syndrome and ovarian remnant syndrome. In the former, a retained ovary becomes trapped in dense adhesions after hysterectomy, while in the latter, a small piece of ovary is unintentionally left behind at oophorectomy and again becomes trapped in adhesions. In both cases, the pain is cyclical and can be suppressed with a GnRH analogue. It may be possible to surgically remove the ovary/remnant; however, with distorted anatomy this is not without risk, and some women may prefer to remain on the combination of GnRH analogue and low-dose HRT instead.[5]

Chronic Pelvic Inflammatory Disease

Chronic inflammation with scar tissue and distortion of pelvic structures can be seen in women who have had repeated episodes of acute PID or those in whom infection has been asymptomatic initially (as is frequently the case with *Chlamydia*). US may demonstrate features of chronic salpingitis, such as dilated fallopian tubes and poor mobility,[81] and severe adhesions may be seen at laparoscopy. These can be divided surgically, especially if they are causing anatomical distortion. However, although this may improve fertility as has been discussed, it may not have any effect on the pain. Chronic inflammation can cause sensitization of peripheral nerves, and therefore a trial of amitriptyline or gabapentin/pregabalin may be indicated, especially if there are other symptoms suggesting a generalized visceral hypersensitivity syndrome. An exploration of the woman's attitudes to and beliefs about her pain may be beneficial. Guilt about earlier sexual behavior or concerns about current or future fertility may be revealed.

Pelvic Venous Congestion

Congestion of dilated pelvic veins has been suggested to be a cause of pelvic pain with menstrual exacerbation.[82] In one study of women with unexplained CPP, dilated pelvic veins were found in 30%,[83] but they are also found in at least 10% of the general population with increasing incidence in multiparous women. There is therefore some doubt as to whether the condition causes pain or is an incidental finding. One trial suggested continuous medroxyprogesterone acetate in combination with psychological support to be a successful treatment; however, no benefit was obtained after stopping treatment.[84] Embolization of ovarian veins or hysterectomy and bilateral oophorectomy have also been advocated as treatments.[85]

Gastrointestinal Factors in Chronic Pelvic Pain

As with acute pelvic pain, CPP secondary to a nongynecological cause can present to gynecologists because of the site of the pain and its presumed etiology. It is therefore important that a detailed history of bowel function and its relation to and/or effect on the pain is taken. The gastrointestinal (GI) tract can be both the initial pain generator and the cause of secondary symptoms in a visceral hypersensitivity syndrome. IBS and constipation are very common and may be provoked by other conditions or medication, and thus need to always be borne in mind. DIE frequently presents with bowel symptoms; however, it is important to remember that similar symptoms can be the presenting features of GI tract malignancies and inflammatory bowel disease and to fully investigate any "red flag" symptoms, such as rectal bleeding or unexplained weight loss.

Irritable Bowel Syndrome

IBS is a functional disorder of the GI tract and is discussed in detail in Chapter 63. We have mentioned it here, however, to draw attention to the fact that cyclical changes in the severity of symptoms are seen. Healthy, pain-free women frequently show alterations in their bowel habit around menstruation, possibly secondary to prostaglandin release, and this is often amplified in women with IBS.[86] It has been shown that rectal sensitivity to balloon distension varies with the menstrual cycle in women with IBS, but not in those without.[87] Interestingly, in women whose IBS is clearly cyclical even without evidence of other gynecological symptoms, the use of GnRH analogue treatment to suppress endogenous hormone production has been shown to be successful.[88]

Constipation

Constipation is a common cause of pelvic pain and can be easily avoided. It may be due to poor diet, lack of exercise, or reduced fluid intake; however, it is frequently iatrogenic, secondary to opioid use. It is therefore important to emphasize the need for fluid intake and dietary fiber, as well as prescribing laxatives whenever such analgesics are required.

Urological Factors in Chronic Pelvic Pain

Pain originating in the urinary tract will also often be pelvic and therefore present to gynecologists. Again, symptoms may be cyclical or associated with symptoms in other organs. This coexistence of symptoms and the common embryological origin of the structures involved have led to the suggestion of a "urogenital pain syndrome," including some or all of interstitial cystitis, vulvodynia, urethral syndrome, coccyodynia, and perineal pain.[89]

Interstitial Cystitis

Interstitial cystitis is characterized by pelvic pain and urinary urgency and frequency which may be associated with other symptoms, particularly dyspareunia sometimes relieved by voiding.[90] Frequently, women give a history of repeated urinary tract infections but with negative cultures. The etiology is unknown but is likely to be multifactorial and leads to chronic inflammation of the bladder wall. Hunner's ulcers or glomerulations may be seen at cystoscopy, but are not pathognomonic and, in 10% of patients, cystoscopic findings will be normal.[89] In these women, painful bladder syndrome may be a more appropriate diagnosis as bladder inflammation is not present. Multidisciplinary treatment regimens are likely to be most successful, including a combination of dietary modification, pharmacological agents such as pentosan polysulfate sodium, and physical therapy.

Urethral Syndrome

Urethral syndrome is also characterized by urinary urgency, frequency, dysuria, and suprapubic/lower back pain without any obvious cause. Dysfunction of the pelvic floor may be involved as success is often achieved with skeletal muscle relaxants or electrostimulation and biofeedback. Because of similarities in presentation to prostatitis in men, a chronic low-grade infection of the paraurethral glands has been suggested to be a possible cause. If tenderness can be elicited just lateral to the urethra through the anterior vaginal wall, this may be a possibility and a prolonged course of antibiotics may be justified.[91]

Musculoskeletal Factors in Chronic Pelvic Pain

Dysfunction in the musculoskeletal system can be both the primary cause of CPP or secondary to pathology elsewhere. Though it may not be the first thought in a gynecological consultation, it is surprisingly common, with one retrospective study suggesting that 75% of 132 nonconsecutive patients with CPP had musculoskeletal abnormalities.[92] It is therefore important that the musculoskeletal system is appropriately assessed and any issues dealt with in order that a good response to treatment occurs. A detailed description of appropriate assessment is not possible here, but can be found elsewhere.[93] Some of the important musculoskeletal factors to be borne in mind are discussed briefly below, and in more detail in Chapters 34 and 35.

Fibromyalgia

Two of the 18 tender points of fibromyalgia are in the gluteal muscles in the upper outer quadrants of the buttocks. Pain here can easily be confused with the lower back pain often described by women with CPP. Furthermore, fibromyalgia may have cyclical exacerbations[94] and therefore symptoms are often assigned to a gynecological cause.

Trigger Points

Trigger points are frequently found in abdominal and pelvic floor muscles causing or exacerbating both CPP and dyspareunia. These can be the primary pain generator or can be secondary, either to other musculoskeletal abnormalities such as sacroiliac joint dysfunction or to repeated episodes of visceral pain as occurs in adenomyosis. The continued presence of a trigger point can explain a partial response to treatment of the underlying pathology and is an indication for a careful reexamination of the patient at her follow-up visit.

Pelvic Floor Abnormalities

In women, pelvic floor abnormalities can be secondary to postural alterations caused by pain or other musculoskeletal conditions, viscero-muscular referral patterns, or trauma as occurs during childbirth or certain surgical procedures. Unilateral or bilateral pelvic floor abnormalities can cause CPP, dyspareunia (with secondary vaginismus), perineal pain, and dyschezia yet are frequently overlooked. In a woman with dyspareunia, demonstrating that pressure on a tender, tense pelvic floor muscle recreates her pain during intercourse can help toward relieving concerns about her reproductive organs. Good response to treatment is frequently obtained from physiotherapy and recent studies on the injection of botulinum toxin into the pelvic floor muscles have shown promising results.[95]

Hernia

Acute obstruction of a hernia will cause acute pain; however, a number of different types of hernias can also be responsible for CPP, though the exact mechanism by which they cause pain is debated. Most commonly these include inguinal, femoral, and obturator hernias. Imaging modalities such as computed tomography or MRI may be useful in making the diagnosis if a clear examination finding is not present. Surgical repair is usually the recommended treatment, and this can either be open or laparoscopic with both having their own advantages and disadvantages.[96]

Sacroiliac Joint Pain

The sacroiliac joint (SIJ) is the largest axial joint in the body. A network of muscles support the joint and deliver regional muscular forces to the pelvic bones. The associated ligaments are weaker in women to allow mobility and facilitate parturition. The innervation of the joint is still debated, but probably includes fibers from L2-S4.[97] It is widely accepted that SIJ dysfunction causes lower back pain, and pelvic pain appears to occur in a significant percent of patients. In general, the pain is unilateral (unless both joints are affected) and below the L5 spinous process, sometimes radiating down as far as the foot.[98] SIJ dysfunction and pain can occur for a number of reasons, including pregnancy, trauma, and prolonged bending and lifting. A number of possible treatments exist with varying degrees of success. Conservative options include physiotherapy and joint stabilization which have been shown to be successful in some series.[97] Intra-articular joint injections under radiological guidance have been shown to produce good to excellent pain relief in most studies. Surgical fusion of the joint may be required in some cases, though adequately powered, prospective studies are lacking.

Neurological Factors in Chronic Pelvic Pain

It has already been mentioned that in many conditions causing pelvic pain, secondary sensitization of the peripheral or central nervous system can occur, perpetuating or increasing pain and extending referral areas and involving other organ systems.[99]

There are also situations where damage to a nerve or nerve roots can be the primary cause of the pain. The specific nerve(s) involved will determine the precise distribution of pain and associated symptoms; however, a number of general features are usually associated with a neuropathy. Classically, the pain is shooting, burning, or stabbing in nature. Initially at least, the pain will be in a clearly defined area, though secondary changes may blur this. Trophic skin changes may also be present. Symptoms may be exacerbated or relieved by movements which stretch/relax the nerve or increase/decrease compression by surrounding structures. Local anesthetic blockade of the specific nerve may relieve the pain entirely; however, it is also possible that pain can be worsened by this procedure, perhaps because the injected fluid volume worsens compression. Because of the complex innervation of the pelvis, there are many different neuropathies that can occur. We will discuss in detail here only the most common, pudendal neuropathy; however, a careful consideration of innervation patterns may point to an unusual neuropathy in a woman whose symptoms cannot otherwise be explained. We also consider neuropathies secondary to a Pfannenstiel incision because of the prevalence of this procedure in obstetrics and gynecology. More information on other pelvic neuropathies can be found elsewhere.[100]

Pudendal Neuropathy

The pudendal nerve arises from the sacral plexus in the ventral rami of sacral nerves 2, 3, and 4 (S2-S4), and exits the pelvis through the greater sciatic foramen between the piriformis and coccygeus muscles. It then winds around the sacrospinous ligament and passes through Alcock's canal to enter the pelvis again through the lesser sciatic foramen before branching into the clitoral, superficial perineal, deep perineal, and posterior rectal branches (Fig. 64.2).[101] It can be seen that there are many points where nerve entrapment could occur and many situations in which this nerve could be damaged including surgery and childbirth.[102]

Pain is felt in the distribution of the nerve and is exacerbated by sitting and relieved to a variable extent by standing or lying on the unaffected side. Perineal sensation is usually preserved as is muscle tone, though pain may be recreated during rectal examination. Local anesthetic nerve blocks may be successful and can also aid with diagnosis; however, they may have to be repeated regularly. While surgical decompression may be an option, damage to the nerve may not be reversible.

Neuropathy Secondary to a Pfannenstiel Incision

A Pfannenstiel incision is a low transverse abdominal incision which was first described in 1900.[103] It is commonly used for cesarean sections and many benign gynecological procedures but more rarely in general surgery. Aesthetically, it is more pleasing to the woman, being below the "bikini" line. It also has a number of advantages over other abdominal incisions, including lower incisional hernia rates, fewer wound infections, less hematoma formation, and less direct postoperative pain.[104] However, the ilioinguinal and iliohypogastric nerves have a superficial course and are relatively easily injured by a Pfannenstiel incision. In the literature, the reported incidence of nerve damage after a Pfannenstiel incision is 3.7%[104]; however, the true incidence may well be higher as many cases are not reported or diagnosed. Typically, the pain is burning or lancinating near the incision and radiates to the area supplied by the nerve with associated sensory impairment. The nerves can be damaged in a number of ways: direct nerve trauma with neuroma formation, suture incorporation of the nerve during fascial closure, and constriction of the nerve during scar or wound healing.[105] Optimal treatment is still unclear. In many cases, the symptoms resolve over time without treatment. The nerve can be blocked with local anesthetic, which will at least confirm the diagnosis even if the pain is not entirely removed. In some cases surgery is required; even in these cases, however, long-term recovery is good.[105] Education is clearly required, about both careful surgical technique to reduce the incidence of nerve entrapment and the presentation, such that diagnosis and treatment occur more rapidly.

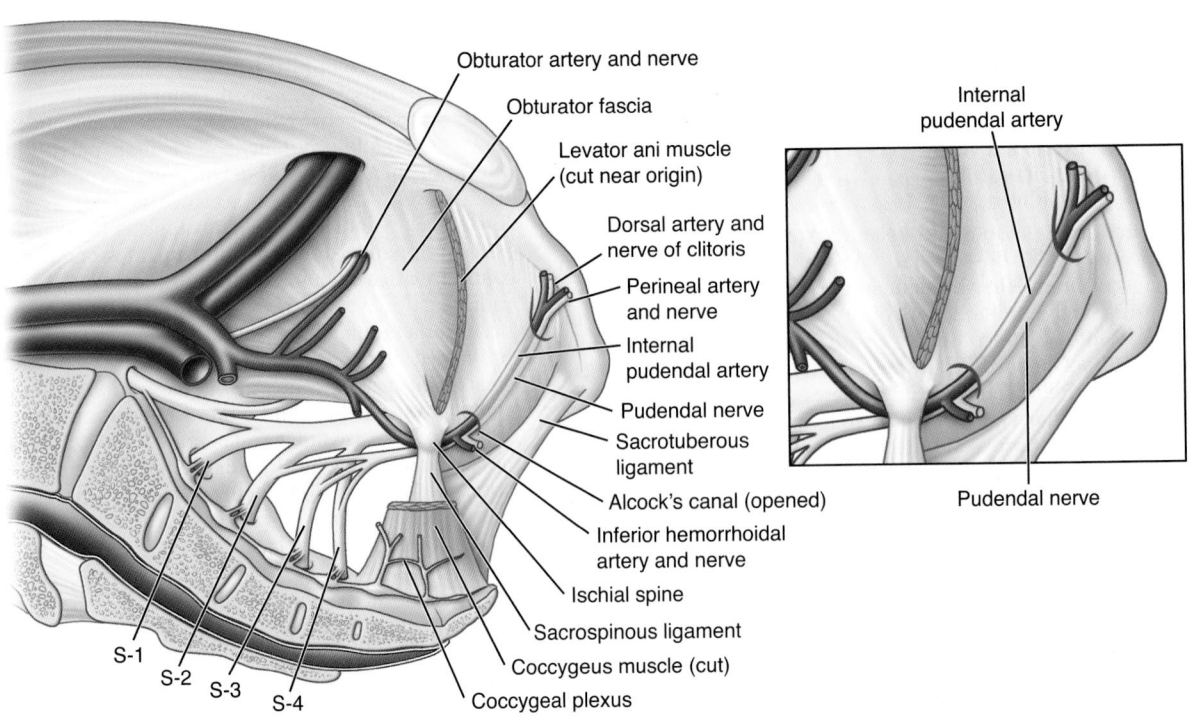

FIGURE 64.2 Course of the pudendal nerve.

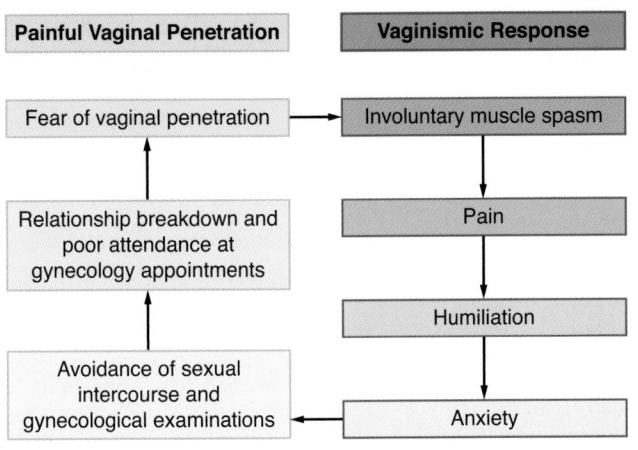

FIGURE 64.3 Cycle of vaginismus. (Adapted from Butcher J. Female sexual problems II: sexual pain and sexual fears. *BMJ* 1999;318: 110–112.)

DYSPAREUNIA

Overview

Dyspareunia is defined as genital pain just before, during, or after sexual intercourse. It can be subdivided into primary, having always occurred in association with intercourse, and secondary, having developed after a period of pain-free sexual activity. Perhaps more usefully, it can also be divided into superficial, with pain only on entry, and deep, thought to be associated with organic pathology.[106] As with so many pain conditions, these subdivisions are oversimplistic and frequently clinically unhelpful. Whatever the initial trigger for an episode of painful intercourse, fear of further pain can set up a cycle of muscular tension and vaginismus (Fig. 64.3) ensuring that future episodes will be painful, reinforcing that fear. Furthermore, the psychological consequences of an inability to have pain-free intercourse on both the woman and her partner should not be underestimated. Psychological morbidity can worsen the experience. However, dyspareunia should not be assumed to be psychological in origin just because no pathology is evident at initial examination.

Possible causes of dyspareunia are listed in Table 64.10. Superficial vulval pain is a common cause of dyspareunia and is discussed in detail in the following section. If superficial dyspareunia occurs after childbirth, time should be taken to explore the woman's fantasies and to reassure her. Occasionally, hypoestrogenism may be the cause, but it is very rare for surgery to be required in these cases. Deep dyspareunia can be secondary to many abdominopelvic pathologies, but is also often positional. If a woman complains of pain on contact with the cervix, this may be due to inadequate arousal and failure of the upper vagina to balloon and therefore move the cervix out of reach.[107] Whatever the ini-

tial cause of pain, vaginismus is a frequent sequela and is therefore discussed here in more detail.

Vaginismus

The term "vaginismus" was first used in 1862[108] and is now thought to be one of the commonest female sexual problems. The true prevalence is unknown; however, it is identified in 10% to 20% of women requesting help for sexual dysfunction.[109] Definitions vary as to whether spasm of the muscles surrounding the lower third of the vagina is included or whether it is difficulty in allowing vaginal entry, often associated with involuntary pelvic muscle contraction.[110] Though pain with intercourse is usually the presenting feature, there is often fear of any object being placed in the vagina, thus tampons are not used and gynecological examinations not well tolerated. Some women are so fearful that they avoid smear tests and other essential health checks.

Vaginismus is thought to occur as a conditioned response secondary to adverse physical or psychological stimuli. Early traumatic experiences are thought to predispose to the condition, including traumatic sexual experiences, unsympathetic gynecological examinations, and assault,[110] although a history of abuse (physical or sexual) is not usually associated with vaginismus.[111] A background of religious orthodoxy has however, been shown to be associated.[112] Psychosexual fantasies often coexist such as that the vagina is too small to accommodate a penis or that it is a delicate, fragile organ which will be damaged during intercourse.[110] These can arise secondary to comments made inadvertently, for example at the time of episiotomy repair, and clinicians should therefore think carefully about what is said at vulnerable times. Male sexual dysfunction can develop as a consequence of vaginismus,[113] although the reverse can also occur with vaginismus arising secondary to a male partner's impotence.

Treatment should be individualized to the specific woman/couple and her/their desires. For most women, successful vaginal penetrative intercourse and an improved sexual experience for both partners is the aim. However, in some instances the woman may not feel comfortable with intercourse even after the vaginismus has resolved. Current guidelines suggest that the basis of treatment should be to enable the woman to become more comfortable with her genitals, followed by graded exposure to different types of vaginal penetration in order to overcome her fear of penetration.[110] At all times during treatment, the woman should feel that she is in control and the extent to which her partner is involved should be her decision, though involvement should be encouraged. For some couples, fertility is the ultimate aim and an appropriate referral may need to be made.

A number of different approaches are described, one of which is a combination of behavioral and desensitization exercises using relaxation and graded vaginal trainers. Education is also important, and there may be a need for exploration of fantasies before they can be dispelled.[110] Hypnotherapy,[113] physiotherapy using biofeedback, amitriptyline, and local injections with botulinum toxin[114] have all been reported to have good results. If physical

TABLE 64.10

CAUSES OF DYSPAREUNIA

Vulval	Vaginal	Pelvic	Musculoskeletal	Systemic
Vulvodynia	Vaginismus	Endometriosis	Pelvic floor tension	Hypoestrogenism
Vestibulodynia	Congenital abnormality	IBS	Pelvic floor trigger point	Inadequate arousal
Herpes simplex	Inadequate lubrication	IC/urethral syndrome		Psychological
Postepisiotomy	Radiation vaginitis	Chronic PID		Abuse history
		Adnexal pathology		

causes have been excluded, treatment is usually highly successful with some authors reporting up to 100% success.[110]

Vulval Pain Syndromes

Although not truly pelvic pain, the vulval pain syndromes (vulvodynia and vestibulodynia) exhibit many features which are similar to CPP, and the two can coexist in a urogenital pain syndrome. Much of what has already been discussed in relation to the assessment and multidisciplinary management of CPP is just as relevant for vulval pain. It is therefore appropriate to include a brief overview of these conditions in a chapter devoted to pelvic pain in females.

As with CPP, there is frequently a delay between presentation and diagnosis, and many unsuccessful, often inappropriate and sometimes damaging treatments may have already been tried.[115] It is therefore not surprising that many of these women report anger and frustration and that psychological morbidity is more prevalent than in asymptomatic women.[116] There is no evidence to suggest that these psychological features are a cause rather than a consequence of the conditions. Because vulval pain syndromes are almost invariably associated with dyspareunia in sexually active women, sexual dysfunction is also common, with secondary problems such as vaginismus and anorgasmia developing. However, there is no evidence of higher rates of previous sexual or physical abuse in these women as compared to healthy controls.[117]

The vulval pain syndromes were first described in the late 1800s[118]; however, there has been confusion surrounding their nomenclature, etiology, and management ever since. Further difficulties occur as vulval pain can present to gynecologists, dermatologists, or genitourinary medicine specialists, each of whom historically had different preferred treatments. The International Society for the Study of Vulvovaginal Disease (ISSVD), a multispecialty society, is working to redress this and has recently reclassified these syndromes as either vulvodynia (which can be localized or generalized, and provoked or unprovoked) or vestibulodynia.[119] These terms replace dysesthetic vulvodynia and vestibulitis. Many women will, however, present with symptoms of both conditions.

The ISSVD defines vulvodynia as "vulvar discomfort, most often described as burning pain, occurring in the absence of relevant visible findings or a specific, clinically identifiable, neurologic disorder."[119] The term vestibulodynia has replaced vestibulitis as there is no evidence of inflammation and is defined by the ISSVD as "provoked vulval dysesthesia localized to the vestibule."[119] Pain can also occur on urination and defecation.

By definition, therefore, a thorough history and examination with appropriate investigations should be undertaken to exclude other causes of vulval pain, such as those listed in Table 64.11, before a label of a vulval pain syndrome is given. To date, the true prevalence remains unknown, with the large reported variation in numbers of women attending clinics likely due to variation in the type of clinic and known interests of the consultants. However, as more specialized vulval clinics become established, the number of referrals for vulval pain syndromes continues to increase. The etiology remains unknown, but is likely to be multifactorial.[115] Although it is unlikely that irritation from topical agents (e.g., antifungal agents, bubble bath, etc.) is the precipitating factor, their use may well exacerbate symptoms and should be discouraged. Examination will reveal either focal or generalized pain in response to light touch with a cotton-tipped swab, but is otherwise unremarkable.

A number of treatments have been shown to be successful; however, treatment needs to be carefully tailored to the individual patient and a multidisciplinary approach is usually of benefit. Basic advice on vulval care should be given, recommending careful hygiene but with avoidance of perfumed products and over-

TABLE 64.11

CAUSES OF SECONDARY VULVAL PAIN

Infection
Candida albicans
Herpes simplex

Inflammation
Lichen sclerosus
Eczema
Contact dermatitis
Psoriasis
Crohn's disease

Iatrogenic
Postepisiotomy
Postsurgical scar

Hormonal
Hypoestrogenism

Trauma

Rare
Symptomatic dermographism
Aphthous ulceration
Bullous disorders
Sacral meningeal cysts
Pudendal nerve entrapment

drying. Though topical products in general should be avoided, fragrance-free emollient creams can be soothing and local anesthetic gel such as topical lidocaine can be particularly useful prior to intercourse acting as both a pain reliever and a lubricant.[115] There is no evidence to suggest that topical corticosteroids, antifungal preparations, or testosterone are helpful and only minimal evidence to support the use of topical estrogens.[119] Recent work has suggested a central component to vulvodynia which may explain the success of drugs such as amitriptyline and gabapentin in the condition.[120] One study quotes a 47% complete response to tricyclic antidepressants in a cohort of 33 women with either generalized or localized vulvodynia.[121]

Whether tension in the pelvic floor muscles (a common finding in women with vulvodynia) is involved in perpetuating the pain remains unknown; however, physiotherapists can be very successful in treating vulval pain syndromes. In one series, 71% of women had a greater than 50% improvement in symptoms, 62% experienced improvement in sexual functioning, and 50% had an increase in quality of life.[122]

Surgery should be considered as a last resort. However, it can be successful in a subgroup of women and should not be dismissed entirely. In general, it appears to be less successful in women with coexisting vaginismus and more successful in women who had a good response to lidocaine gel preoperatively. Postoperative psychosexual counseling and the use of dilators and physical therapy have been shown to improve outcome.[119]

As with other chronic pain syndromes, the value of patient support groups, such as the Vulval Pain Society, should not be underestimated as the vulval pain syndromes are a particularly isolating group of disorders. The effect of the conditions on relationships can be devastating and, unlike conditions such as endometriosis which are coming more and more into the public's awareness, vulval pain is still seen as a taboo subject and not discussed.

CONCLUSION

Research in many fields over recent years has led to an improved understanding of both the basic science of visceral pain and of many of the conditions causing pelvic pain. However, time to listen to and explore a woman's story as well as to perform a careful examination must be invested in order to make the best use of this knowledge. Sociological research has identified the recurrent theme of the social meaninglessness of pain without a medical diagnosis[123] and encouraged us to consider chronic pain in a biopsychosociocultural context.[124] The more recent move toward multidisciplinary CPP clinics is a positive step forward in these respects and acknowledges that the secondary consequences of the pain (be they musculoskeletal, psychological, gastrointestinal, sexual, etc.) must also be managed in order to facilitate a full recovery.

References

1. Grace VM, Zondervan KT. Chronic pelvic pain in New Zealand: prevalence, pain severity, diagnoses, and use of the health services. *Aust N Z J Public Health* 2004;28(4):369–375.
2. Mathias SD, Kuppermann M, Liberman RF, et al. Chronic pelvic pain: prevalence, health-related quality of life, and economic correlates. *Obstet Gynecol* 1996;87(3):321–327.
3. Zondervan KT, Yudkin PL, Vessey MP, et al. The community prevalence of chronic pelvic pain in women and associated illness behaviour. *Br J Gen Pract* 2001;51(468):541–547.
4. Zondervan KT, Yudkin PL, Vessey MP, et al. Prevalence and incidence of chronic pelvic pain in primary care: evidence from a national general practice database. *Br J Obstet Gynaecol* 1999;106(11):1149–1155.
5. Kennedy SH, Moore J. *The Initial Management of Chronic Pelvic Pain.* London: RCOG; 2005. Guideline No. 41.
6. Crowley P, Calder A, Lamont L, et al. *Gynaecological Examinations: Guidelines for Specialist Practice.* London: RCOG; 2002.
7. Curtis AH. A cause of adhesion in the right upper quadrant. *JAMA* 1930; 94:1221–1222.
8. Fitz-Hugh T Jr. Acute gonococcic peritonitis of the right upper quadrant in women. *JAMA* 1934;102:2094–2096.
9. Bevan CD, Johal BJ, Mumtaz G, et al. Clinical, laparoscopic, and microbiological findings in acute salpingitis: report on a United Kingdom cohort. *Br J Obstet Gynaecol* 1995;102:407–414.
10. Ross J, Stewart P. *Management of Acute Pelvic Inflammatory Disease.* London: RCOG; 2003. Report No. 32.
11. Rio C, Hall G, Hook EW 3rd, et al. Update to CDC's sexually transmitted diseases treatment guidelines, 2006: fluoroquinolones no longer recommended for treatment of gonococcal infections. *MMWR Morb Mortal Wkly Rep* 2007;56(14):332–336.
12. Aboulghar MA, Mansour RT, Serour GI. Ultrasonographically guided transvaginal aspiration of tuboovarian abscesses and pyosalpinges: an optional treatment for acute pelvic inflammatory disease. *Am J Obstet Gynecol* 1995; 172:1501–1503.
13. Creighton SM. Common congenital anomalies of the female genital tract. *Rev Gynaecol Prac* 2005;5(4):221–226.
14. Bakken IJ, Skjeldestad FE. Time trends in ectopic pregnancies in a Norwegian county, 1970–2004: a population-based study. *Hum Reprod* 2006;21(12): 3132–3136.
15. Braude P, Rowell P. Assisted conception. III—problems with assisted conception. *BMJ* 2003;327(7420):920–923.
16. Kelly AJ, Sowter MC, Trinder J. *The Management of Tubal Pregnancy.* London: RCOG; 2004 Report No. 21.
17. Hinshaw K, Fayyad A, Munjuluri P. *The Management of Early Pregnancy Loss.* London: RCOG; 2006. Report No. 25.
18. Jurkovic D. Modern management of miscarriage: is there a place for nonsurgical treatment? *Ultrasound Obstet Gynecol* 1998;11:161–163.
19. Hamoda H, Chamberlain PF, Moore NR, et al. Conservative treatment of an incarcerated gravid uterus. *BJOG* 2002;109(9):1074–1075.
20. Yohannes P, Schaefer J. Urinary retention during the second trimester of pregnancy: a rare cause. *Urology* 2002;59(6):946.
21. Jenkins JM, Drakeley AJ, Mathur RS. *The Management of Ovarian Hyperstimulation Syndrome.* London: RCOG; 2006. Report No. 5.
22. Stewart JA, Hamilton PJ, Murdoch AP. Thromboembolic disease associated with ovarian stimulation and assisted conception techniques. *Hum Reprod* 1997;12:2167–2173.
23. Ludwig AK, Glawatz M, Griesinger G, et al. Perioperative and postoperative complications of transvaginal ultrasound-guided oocyte retrieval: prospective study of >1000 oocyte retrievals. *Hum Reprod* 2006;21(12):3235–3240.
24. French L. Dysmenorrhea. *Am Fam Physician* 2005;71(2):285–291.
25. Harel Z. Dysmenorrhea in adolescents and young adults: etiology and management. *J Pediatr Adolesc Gynecol* 2006;19(6):363–371.
26. Goldstein DP, deCholnoky C, Leventhal JM, et al. New insights into the old problem of chronic pelvic pain. *J Pediatr Surg* 1979;14(6):675–680.
27. Boctor AM, Eickholt M, Pugsley TA. Meclofenamate sodium is an inhibitor of both the 5-lipoxygenase and cyclooxygenase pathways of the arachidonic acid cascade in vitro. *Prostaglandins Leukot Med* 1986;23(2–3):229–238.
28. Marjoribanks J, Proctor ML, Farquhar C. Nonsteroidal anti-inflammatory drugs for primary dysmenorrhoea. *Cochrane Database Syst Rev* 2003;4: CD001751.
29. DuRant RH, Jay MS, Shofitt T. Factors influencing adolescents' responses to regimens of naproxen for dysmenorrhoea. *Am J Dis Child* 1985;139: 489–493.
30. Proctor ML, Roberts H, Farquhar CM. Combined oral contraceptive pill (OCP) as treatment for primary dysmenorrhoea. *Cochrane Database Syst Rev* 2001;2:CD002120.
31. Davis ARMD, Westhoff CMD, O'Connell KMD, et al. Oral contraceptives for dysmenorrhea in adolescent girls: a randomized trial. *Obstet Gynecol* 2005;106(1):97–104.
32. Sulak PJM, Cressman BEM, Waldrop ER, et al. Extending the duration of active oral contraceptive pills to manage hormone withdrawal symptoms. *Obstet Gynecol* 1997;89(2):179–183.
33. Jain J, Dutton C, Nicosia A, et al. Pharmacokinetics, ovulation suppression and return to ovulation following a lower dose subcutaneous formulation of Depo-Provera(R). *Contraception* 2004;70(1):11–18.
34. Harel Z, Biro FM, Kollar LM. Depo-provera in adolescents: effects of early second injection or prior oral contraception. *J Adolesc Health* 1995;16(5): 379–384.
35. Proctor M, Latthe P, Farquhar C, et al. Surgical interruption of pelvic nerve pathways for primary and secondary dysmenorrhoea. *Cochrane Database Syst Rev* 2005;4:CD001896.
36. Proctor ML, Smith CA, Farquhar CM, et al. Transcutaneous electrical nerve stimulation and acupuncture for primary dysmenorrhoea. *Cochrane Database Syst Rev* 2002;1:CD002123.
37. Akin MD, Weingand KW, Hengehold DA, et al. Continuous low-level topical heat in the treatment of dysmenorrhea. *Obstet Gynecol* 2001;97(3):343–349.
38. Proctor ML, Murphy PA, Pattison HM, et al. Behavioural interventions for primary and secondary dysmenorrhoea. *Cochrane Database Syst Rev* 2007; 3:CD002248.
39. O'Herlihy C, Robinson HP, de Crespigny LJ. Mittelschmerz is a preovulatory symptom. *Br Med J* 1980;280:986.
40. Marinho AO, Sallam HN, Goessens L, et al. Ovulation side and occurrence of mittelschmerz in spontaneous and induced ovarian cycles. *Br Med J (Clin Res Ed)* 1982;284(6316):632.
41. Zondervan K, Barlow DH. Epidemiology of chronic pelvic pain. *Bailliere's Clin Obstet Gynaecol* 2000;14(3):403–414.
42. Raphael KG, Widom CS, Lange G. Childhood victimization and pain in adulthood: a prospective investigation. *Pain* 2001;92:283–293.
43. Newton-John T. The psychology of pain. In: MacLean A, Stones RW, Thornton S, eds. *Pain in Obstetrics and Gynaecology.* London: RCOG Press; 2001; 59–69.
44. Selfe SA, Matthews Z, Stones RW. Factors influencing outcome in consultations for chronic pelvic pain. *J Womens Health* 1998;7(8):1041–1048.
45. Price J, Farmer G, Harris J, et al. Attitudes of women with chronic pelvic pain to the gynaecological consultation: a qualitative study. *BJOG* 2006; 113(4):446–452.
46. Skrine R, Mountford H, eds. *Psychosexual Medicine: An Introduction.* London: Arnold; 2001.
47. Sagsveen M, Farmer JE, Prentice A, et al. Gonadotrophin-releasing hormone analogues for endometriosis: bone mineral density. *Cochrane Database Syst Rev* 2003;4:CD001297.
48. Bedaiwy MA, Casper RF. Treatment with leuprolide acetate and hormonal add-back for up to 10 years in stage IV endometriosis patients with chronic pelvic pain. *Fertil Steril* 2006;86(1):220–222.
49. Chapron C, Querleu D, Bruhat MA, et al. Surgical complications of diagnostic and operative gynaecological laparoscopy: a series of 29,956 cases. *Hum Reprod* 1998;13(4):867–872.
50. Onwude JL, Thornton JG, Morley S, et al. A randomised trial of photographic reinforcement during postoperatve counselling after diagnostic laparoscopy for pelvic pain. *Eur J Obstet Gynecol Reprod Biol* 2004;112(1):89–94.
51. Kuiken SD, Tytgat GN, Boeckxstaens GE. Drugs interfering with visceral sensitivity for the treatment of functional gastrointestinal disorders: the clinical evidence. *Aliment Pharmacol Ther* 2005;21(6):633–651.
52. Stones RW, Mountfield J. Interventions for treating chronic pelvic pain in women. *Cochrane Database Syst Rev* 2000;4:CD000387.
53. Berkley K. Multiple mechanisms of pelvic pain: lessons from basic research. In: MacLean A, Stones RW, Thornton S, eds. *Pain in Obstetrics and Gynaecology.* London: RCOG Press; 2001;26–39.
53a. Kennedy S, Berggvist A, Chapron C, et al. ESHRE guideline for the diagnosis and treatment of endometriosis. *Hum Reprod* 2005;20(10):2698–2704.
54. Sampson JA. Peritoneal endometriosis due to the menstrual dissemination of endometrial tissue into the peritoneal cavity. *Am J Obstet Gynecol* 1927;14: 422–469.
55. Kyama C, Debrock S, Mwenda J, et al. Potential involvement of the immune system in the development of endometriosis. *Reprod Biol Endocrinol* 2003; 1(1):123.

56. Kennedy S, Moore J. *The Investigation and Management of Endometriosis.* London: RCOG; 2006.

57. Chapron C, Fauconnier A, Dubuisson JB, et al. Deep infiltrating endometriosis: relation between severity of dysmenorrhoea and extent of disease. *Hum Reprod* 2003;18(4):760–766.

58. Crosignani P, Olive DL, Bergqvist A, et al. Advances in the management of endometriosis: an update for clinicians. *Hum Reprod Update* 2006;12(2):179–189.

59. Chapron C, Vercellini P, Barakat H, et al. Management of ovarian endometriomas. *Hum Reprod Update* 2002;8(6):591–597.

60. Chapron C, Chopin N, Borghese B, et al. Surgical management of deeply infiltrating endometriosis: an update. *Ann N Y Acad Sci* 2004;1034:326–337.

61. Allen C, Hopewell S, Prentice A. Nonsteroidal anti-inflammatory drugs for pain in women with endometriosis. *Cochrane Database Syst Rev* 2005;4:CD004753.

62. Cobellis L, Razzi S, Simone SD, et al. The treatment with a COX-2 specific inhibitor is effective in the management of pain related to endometriosis. *Eur J Obstet Gynaecol Reprod Biol* 2004;116(1):100–102.

63. Juni P, Nartey L, Reichenbach S, et al. Risk of cardiovascular events and rofecoxib: cumulative meta-analysis. *Lancet* 2004;364:2021–2029.

64. Miller JD, Shaw RW, Casper RFJ, et al. Historical prospective cohort study of the recurrence of pain after discontinuation of treatment with danazol or a gonadotropin-releasing hormone agonist. *Fertil Steril* 1998;70(2):293–296.

65. Kitawaki J, Kusuki I, Koshiba H, et al. Detection of aromatase cytochrome P-450 in endometrial biopsy specimens as a diagnostic test for endometriosis. *Fertil Steril* 1999;72:1100–1106.

66. Attar E, Bulun SE. Aromatase inhibitors: the next generation of therapeutics for endometriosis? *Fertil Steril* 2006;85(5):1307–1318.

67. Howell A, Cuzick J, Baum M, et al. Results of the ATAC (Arimidex, Tamoxifen, Alone or in Combination) trial after completion of 5 years' adjuvant treatment for breast cancer. *Lancet* 2005;365(9453):60–62.

68. Berkley KJ, Dmitrieva N, Curtis KS, et al. Innervation of ectopic endometrium in a rat model of endometriosis. *Proc Natl Acad Sci USA* 2004;101(30):11094–11098.

69. Abbott JA, Hawe J, Clayton RD, et al. The effects and effectiveness of laparoscopic excision of endometriosis: a prospective study with 2–5 year follow-up. *Hum Reprod* 2003;18(9):1922–1927.

70. Yap C, Furness S, Farquhar C. Pre and post operative medical therapy for endometriosis surgery. *Cochrane Database Syst Rev* 2004;3:CD003678.

71. Vercellini P, Frontino G, De Giorgi O, et al. Comparison of a levonorgestrel-releasing intrauterine device versus expectant management after conservative surgery for symptomatic endometriosis: a pilot study. *Fertil Steril* 2003;80(2):305–309.

72. Ferenczy A. Pathophysiology of adenomyosis. *Hum Reprod Update* 1998;4:312–322.

73. Dueholm MA, Lundorf EB. Transvaginal ultrasound or MRI for diagnosis of adenomyosis. *Curr Opin Obstet Gynecol* 2007;19(6):505–512.

74. Bergeron C, Amant F, Ferenczy A. Pathology and pathophysiology of adenomyosis. *Best Prac Res Clin Obstet Gynaecol* 2006;20:511–521.

75. Rabinovici J, Stewart EA. New interventional techniques for adenomyosis. *Best Prac Res Clin Obstet Gynaecol* 2006;20(4):617–636.

76. Fedele L, Bianchi S, Frontino G. Hormonal treatments for adenomyosis. *Best Prac Res Clin Obstet Gynaecol* 2008;22(2):333–339.

77. Urabe M, Yamamoto T, Kitawaki J, et al. Estrogen biosynthesis in human uterine adenomyosis. *Acta Endocrinol (Copenh)* 1989;121(2):259–264.

78. Peters AA, Bakkum EA, Hellebrekers BW. Clinical significance of adhesions in patients with chronic pelvic pain. In: MacLean A, Stones RW, Thornton S, eds. *Pain in Obstetrics and Gynaecology.* London: RCOG Press; 2001;214–223.

79. Swank DJ, Swank-Bordewijk SC, Hop WC, et al. Laparoscopic adhesiolysis in patients with chronic abdominal pain: a blinded randomised controlled multi-centre trial. *Lancet* 2003;361:1247–1251.

80. Peters AA, Trimbos-Kemper GC, Admiraal C, et al. A randomized clinical trial on the benefit of adhesiolysis in patients with intraperitoneal adhesions and chronic pelvic pain. *BJOG* 1992;99(1):59–62.

81. Timor-Tritsch IE, Lerner JP, Monteagudo A, et al. Transvaginal sonographic markers of tubal inflammatory disease. *Ultrasound Obstet Gynecol* 1998;12(1):56–66.

82. Beard RW, Reginald PW, Wadsworth J. Clinical features of women with chronic lower abdominal pain and pelvic congestion. *Br J Obstet Gynaecol* 1988;95:153–161.

83. Gültaplý NZ, Kurt A, Ýpek A, et al. The relation between pelvic varicose veins, chronic pelvic pain and lower extremity venous insufficiency in women. *Diagn Interv Radiol* 2006;12(1):34–38.

84. Farquhar CM, Rogers V, Franks S, et al. A randomized controlled trial of medroxyprogesterone acetate and psychotherapy for the treatment of pelvic congestion. *BJOG* 1989;96(10):1153–1162.

85. Beard RW, Kennedy RG, Gangar KF, et al. Bilateral oophorectomy and hysterectomy in the treatment of intractable pelvic pain associated with pelvic congestion. *BJOG* 1991;98(10):988–992.

86. Whorwell PJ. Abdominal pain. In: MacLean A, Stones RW, Thornton S, eds. *Pain in Obstetrics and Gynaecology.* London: RCOG Press; 2001;209–213.

87. Houghton LA, Lea R, Jackson N, et al. The menstrual cycle affects rectal sensitivity in patients with irritable bowel syndrome but not healthy volunteers. *Gut* 2002;50:471–474.

88. Palomba S, Orio F, Manguso F, et al. Leuprolide acetate treatment with and without coadministration of tibolone in pre-menopausal women with menstrual cycle-related irritable bowel syndrome. *Fertil Steril* 2005;83(4):1012–1020.

89. Wesselmann U, Magora F, Ratner V. Pain of urogenital origin. *Pain Clin Updates* 2000;8(5):1–8.

90. Dell JR. Interstitial cystitis/painful bladder syndrome: appropriate diagnosis and management. *J Womens Health* 2007;16(8):1181–1187.

91. Gittes RF, Nakamura RM. Female urethral syndrome: a female prostatitis? *West J Med* 1996;164:435–438.

92. King PM, Myers CA, Ling FW, et al. Musculoskeletal factors in chronic pelvic pain. *J Psychosom Obstet Gynecol* 1991;12:87–98.

93. Prendergast SA, Weiss J. Screening for musculoskeletal causes of pelvic pain. *Clin Obstet Gynecol* 2003;46(4):773–782.

94. Macfarlane TV, Blinkhorn A, Worthington HV, et al. Sex hormonal factors and chronic widespread pain: a population study among women. *Rheumatology (Oxford)* 2002;41(4):454–457.

95. Jarvis SK, Abbott JA, Lenart MB, et al. Pilot study of botulinum toxin type A in the treatment of chronic pelvic pain associated with spasm of the levator ani muscles. *Aust N Z J Obstet Gynaecol* 2004;44:46–50.

96. Perry CP, Echeverri JDV. Hernias as a cause of chronic pelvic pain in women. *JSLS* 2006;10:212–215.

97. Cohen SP. Sacroiliac joint pain: a comprehensive review of anatomy, diagnosis, and treatment. *Anesth Analg* 2005;101(5):1440–1453.

98. Dreyfuss P, Michaelsen M, Pauza K, et al. The value of medical history and physical examination in diagnosing sacroiliac joint pain. *Spine* 1996;21(22):2594–2602.

99. Bajaj P, Bajaj P, Madsen H, et al. Endometriosis is associated with central sensitization: a psychophysical controlled study. *J Pain* 2003;4(7):372–380.

100. Perry CP. Peripheral neuropathies and pelvic pain: diagnosis and management. *Clin Obstet Gynecol* 2003;46(4):789–796.

101. Moore KL. *Clinically Oriented Anatomy.* 3rd ed. Baltimore: Williams & Wilkins; 1992.

102. Robert R, Prat-Pradal D, Labat JJ, et al. Pudendal nerve entrapment. *Surg Radiol Anat* 1998;20:93–98.

103. Pfannenstiel HJ. Über die Vortheile des suprasymphysären Fascien-querschnitts für die gynäkologischen Köliotomien, zugleig ein Beitrag zu der Indikationsstellung der Operationswege. *Gynäkologie* 1900;97:1735–1756.

104. Luijendijk RW, Jeekel J, Storm RK, et al. The low transverse Pfannenstiel incision and the prevalence of incisional hernia and nerve entrapment. *Ann Surg* 1997;225(4):365–369.

105. Whiteside JL, Barber MD, Walters MD, et al. Anatomy of ilioinguinal and iliohypogastric nerves in relation to trocar placement and low transverse incisions. *Am J Obstet Gynecol* 2003;189(6):1574–1578.

106. Butcher J. Female sexual problems II: sexual pain and sexual fears. *BMJ* 1999;318:110–112.

107. Reamy KJ. Meeting sexual dysfunction again for the first time. *J Sex Marital Ther* 2001;27:197–201.

108. Sims MJ. On vaginismus. *Trans Obstet Soc London* 1861;3:356–367.

109. Schnyder U, Schnyder-Luthi C, Balinari P, et al. Therapy for vaginismus: in vivo versus in vitro desensitization. *Can J Psychiatry* 1998;43:941–944.

110. Crowley T, Richardson D, Goldmeier D. Recommendations for the management of vaginismus: BASHH Special Interest Group for Sexual Dysfunction. *Int J STD AIDS* 2006;17:14–18.

111. Meana M, Binik YM, Khalife S, et al. Biopsychosocial profile of women with dyspareunia. *Obstet Gynecol* 1997;90:583–589.

112. Stanley E. Vaginismus. *BMJ* 1981;282:1435–1437.

113. Al-Sughayir MA. Vaginismus treatment. Hypnotherapy versus behaviour therapy. *Neurosciences* 2005;10(2):163–167.

114. Ghazizadeh S, Nikzad M. Botulinum toxin in the treatment of refractory vaginismus. *Obstet Gynecol* 2004;104:922–925.

115. Nunns D. Vulval pain syndromes. *Br J Obstet Gynaecol* 2000;107:1185–1193.

116. Nunns D, Mandal D. Psychological and psychosexual aspects of vulval vestibulitis. *Genitourin Med* 1997;73:541–544.

117. Edwards L, Mason M, Phillips M, et al. Childhood sexual and physical abuse: incidence in patients with vulvodynia. *J Reprod Med* 1997;42:135–139.

118. Skene AJC. *Treatise on the Diseases of Women.* New York: Appleton and Company; 1889.

119. Haefner HK, Collins ME, Davis GD, et al. The vulvodynia guideline. *J Low Genit Tract Dis* 2005;9(1):40–51.

120. Pukall CF, Strigo IA, Binik YM, et al. Neural correlates of painful genital touch in women with vulvar vestibulitis syndrome. *Pain* 2005;115(1–2):118–127.

121. Munday PE. Response to treatment in dysaesthetic vulvodynia. *J Obstet Gynaecol* 2001;6:610–613.

122. Hartmann EH, Nelson C. The perceived effectiveness of physical therapy treatment on women complaining of chronic vulvar pain and diagnosed with either vulvar vestibulitis syndrome or dysesthetic vulvodynia. *J Womens Health* 2001;25:513–18.

123. Grace VM. Mind/body dualism in medicine: the case of chronic pelvic pain without organic pathology: a critical review of the literature. *Int J Health Serv* 1998;28(1):127–151.

124. Grace VM. Chronic pelvic pain: sociocultural perspectives. In: MacLean A, Stones RW, Thornton S, eds. *Pain in Obstetrics and Gynaecology.* London: RCOG Press; 2001;12–25.

125. Hinshaw K, Fayyad A, Munjuluri P. *The Management of Early Pregnancy Loss.* London: RCOG; 2006.
126. *British National Formulary.* No. 57 London: BMJ Publishing; 2007.
127. Moore J, Kennedy S, Prentice A. Modern combined oral contraceptives for pain associated with endometriosis. *Cochrane Database Syst Rev* 2000;2: CD001019.
128. Selak V, Farquhar C, Prentice A, et al. Danazol for pelvic pain associated with endometriosis. *Cochrane Database Syst Rev* 2007;4:CD00068.
129. Prentice A, Deary AJ, Bland E. Progestagens and anti-progestagens for pain

associated with endometriosis. *Cochrane Database Syst Rev* 2000;2: CD002122.
130. Lockhat FB, Emembolu JO, Konje JC. The efficacy, side effects and continuation rates in women with symptomatic endometriosis undergoing treatment with an intra-uterine administered progestogen (levonorgestrel): a 3-year follow-up. *Hum Reprod* 2005;20(3):789–793.
131. Prentice A, Deary AJ, Goldbeck-Wood S, et al. Gonadotrophin-releasing hormone analogues for pain associated with endometriosis. *Cochrane Database Syst Rev* 2000;2:CD000346.

CHAPTER 65 ■ PELVIC PAIN IN MALES

ANDREW BARANOWSKI

INTRODUCTION

This chapter is about pain *perceived* to be in the male pelvis—the pelvic pain syndromes. For the purpose of this chapter, the pelvis will be considered as the anatomical bony pelvis, the structures both within and adjacent to it, including the male external genitalia, nervous system structures, and soft tissue/muscular structures; that is, the pelvis in its broadest sense. Although this chapter will focus primarily upon the male urogenital pelvic pain syndromes, the importance of other systems, particularly the musculoskeletal and nervous systems, will be emphasized when appropriate.

There are many well-recognized, well-defined pathologies that may result in pain perceived within the male urogenital system, such as infections of the organs, infiltration of somatic and nervous tissue by cancer, and referred sensations from the musculoskeletal system; however, for less-defined pathologies, the mechanisms underlying the pains have been less widely appreciated outside of pain medicine. The mechanisms for this second group, which is probably the majority of male pelvic pain patients, involve neurological mechanisms and, in particular, central sensitization that may involve the whole neuroaxis.

The latest classification approaches have taken this dichotomy of mechanisms into account. To emphasize the differences, those conditions where the main mechanisms are related to central sensitization are known as the pelvic pain syndromes and they are considered separately from those conditions with ongoing nociceptive, acute pain mechanisms, such as those due to chronic infection. The pelvic pain syndromes are defined by their symptoms and signs and often by the presence of central sensitization and the subsequent visceral hyperalgesia, viscerovisceral hyperalgesia, and viscerosomatic hyperalgesia. Often an important part of the process of diagnosing the pelvic pain syndromes is excluding other pathologies.

Classification of the pelvic pain syndromes involves terminology, phenotype, and taxonomy. The phenotype describes the condition in terms of symptoms, signs, and, where possible, mechanisms. Incorporating the phenotype into a hierarchy of phenotypes produces a taxonomy that allows comparisons between phenotypes. This approach enables appropriate prognosis and treatment. The terminology used can be very emotive and careful description of the meaning of the terms is often required. The classification of pelvic urogenital pain has been rapidly evolving over the past 10 years and is likely to continue to do

so.[1,2,3,4,5,6,7,8] This ongoing change in classification reflects our increasing knowledge, but also has caused problems for research and evidence-based treatment. The classification will be covered in depth as it is the key to understanding male pelvic pain syndromes.

The central nervous system mechanisms of central sensitization and the psychological responses that result in the chronic pain syndrome are covered in other chapters within this book; those processes that are specific to urogenital pain will be expanded upon in this chapter. There are some obvious differences between the male and female urogenital systems that will result in specific pain syndromes; however, it is important to recognize that there is much overlap as well. Those differences due to gender and sex are covered in Chapter 7.

This chapter supports that in most men with chronic pain perceived in the pelvic organs, the cause of the pain is not often due to classical pathologies of infection or infiltration, but more commonly due to chronic pain mechanisms involving a number of systems with referred pain, functional consequences (e.g., urinary and fecal incontinence, urinary hesitance, impotence), and chronic pain psychological responses.[8]

TAXONOMY AND PHENOTYING CHRONIC PELVIC PAIN

A realization has occurred that pain **perceived** within the pelvis may be associated with classical pathology of the pelvic structures OR that it may result secondary to central nervous system pain mechanisms. It is the latter conditions that this chapter will primarily concentrate on.

Classical Pathologies

Classical pathologies include infection, inflammation, degeneration, and neoplastic and autoimmune mechanisms of any of the pelvic or adjacent pelvic structures (referred pain). In the case of classical pathology, chronic persistent pain is the result of ongoing local pathology, persistent nociception activation with peripheral sensitization, and possibly a central sensitization process. Treatment will primarily be focused on managing the underlying pathology and the use of analgesics where required. Removing the peripheral cause should resolve the pain.

Pelvic Pain Syndromes and Nonpelvic Pain Syndromes

Most of the recent attempts at classification, taxonomy, and phenotyping have tried to separate out the classical pathologies from those conditions without classical pathology that have become known as the pelvic pain syndromes.[3,7,9] The pelvic pain syndromes are the conditions where there is no peripheral stimulus maintaining the pain experience. In its attempt to separate out the pelvic pain syndromes from those with a nociceptive cause, the European Association for Urology (EAU) in their 2004 classification system called those conditions associated with classical pathology as "well-defined" conditions and The European Society for the Study of Interstitial Cystitis (ESSIC) called them "confusable diseases."[3,9] Both of those terms have a disadvantage. The term well-defined suggests that the pain syndromes are poorly defined; however, as an understanding of chronic pain mechanisms (including visceral pain mechanisms) and central sensitization develops, this is clearly not the case. ESSIC used the term "confusable" to separate out the pain syndromes from those conditions that might be confused with the pain syndromes, a very difficult concept. In future classifications, one way forward is that chronic pelvic urogenital pain syndromes will become a differential diagnosis with the classical pathologies, and the taxonomy will be divided into pelvic pain syndromes and nonpelvic pain syndromes.[10] The emphasis is thus on the pelvic pain syndromes, which is probably correct as in most patients classical disease processes are not present. Table 65.1 illustrates the division of chronic pelvic pain into pain syndromes and nonpelvic pain syndromes. Table 65.2 provides the definitions for chronic pelvic pain and the pelvic pain syndromes.

Male Urogenital Pain Syndromes

Traditionally, pelvic pain conditions would be classified into those of the male, female, or both. This approach is currently being reconsidered, as the mechanisms discussed above may be common to both sexes with the only difference being the sex organ that the pain is perceived in. However, as there has been a lot of research looking at the end organ pain syndromes and their treatment, this is summarized below as relevant for the male.

Male Specific Pelvic Pain Syndromes

The unique male pelvic pain syndromes are those where the pain is **perceived** in the male sex organs. Table 65.3 summarizes these conditions. The definitions serve to emphasize that classical pathologies are absent.

Subclassification of the Pelvic Pain Syndromes by Organ

Much discussion has been had about whether it is appropriate to divide the pelvic pain syndromes by the end organ that the pain is perceived in. Many would rather maintain a more generic approach and keep to the term pelvic pain syndrome to cover all pains perceived within the pelvis and not associated with a classical pathology. The EAU approach (Table 65.1) uses a progressive step-by-step approach to classification.[3,10] That is, classification starts at the left end of the table if pain is perceived within the

pelvis or the external sex organs. Further subclassification only occurs if there are distinct localizing factors within an end organ. Such an approach to taxonomy is very similar to that used to classify life and the animal and plant kingdoms. For instance, we would progress from animal to mammal to elephant only as the evidence allowed. The primary localizing factor for pelvic pain is pain produced by local physical stimulation, such as palpation. If an end organ is clearly associated with the area of perceived pain, then the pain may be labelled with that end organ name as in Table 65.1. If more than one organ is deemed to be involved then either two names may be given to the condition, or it may be more appropriate to consider the pain in more generic terms as a pelvic pain syndrome.

The Importance of Taxonomy and Phenotyping

The above taxonomy (hierarchical classification of conditions) and phenotyping (identifying of the physical characteristics—symptoms and signs—and mechanisms of the diseases within the taxonomy) is important.

Appropriate taxonomy and phenotyping is a prerequisite for epidemiology, diagnosis, management, and prognosis. With traditional management of pelvic pain there has been a tendency to use inappropriate treatments with inappropriate expectations; the result is increased distress and a worse prognosis.[8]

Currently, it is not unusual for inappropriate treatments to be instigated due to a failure to understand the pain syndromes.[1] For example, classic mismanagement would be the recurrent use of antibiotics, or the use of surgery for the complaint of pain. Whereas surgery may have a role for functional reasons (e.g., incontinence), there is a serious debate about its use for pain management. Appropriate taxonomy and phenotyping allows appropriate expectation of both the patient and those providing medical care. Unfortunately, many patients and doctors have inappropriate expectations for treatments aimed at cure. This produces distress and the increased distress is associated with a worse prognosis.[11,12]

An appropriate taxonomy and phenotyping encourages interdisciplinary and multidisciplinary management. In the case of most pelvic pain syndromes, where there may be a reduction in symptoms with appropriate treatment, cure is often not possible. The best outcomes in terms of reduced disability and improved quality of life will come from a symptom management approach involving multiple interdisciplinary teams (e.g., urology, pain medicine, neurology) and multiple members of the team (e.g., nurses, doctors, psychologists, physiotherapists). This is a standard approach for other pain syndromes and should be the standard approach for the urogenital/pelvic pain syndromes.

EPIDEMIOLOGY

Epidemiology requires a clear understanding of the disease that is being studied. Unfortunately, as the phenotyping and taxonomy of male pelvic pain is ongoing, clear-cut epidemiological data for specific pelvic urogenital pain syndromes are not available.

Incidence/Prevalence

Prostate Pain Syndrome

Male pain perceived deep within the pelvis is usually labelled as prostatitis, despite the absence of infection and, frequently, the absence of inflammation within fluids extracted from the prostate. The NIH classification[4] of *prostatitis* includes pain perceived in the prostate without evidence of inflammation or infection and

TABLE 65.1

THE DIVISION OF CHRONIC PELVIC PAIN INTO PELVIC PAIN SYNDROMES AND NONPELVIC PAIN SYNDROMES[10]

AXIS I Region	Axis II System	Axis III End organ as pain syndrome as identified from Hx, Ex, and Ix	Axis IV referral characteristics	Axis V temporal characteristics	Axis VI character	VII Associated symptoms	VIII Psychological symptoms
Chronic Pelvic Pain	Pelvic pain syndrome	Urological	Bladder pain syndrome (See Table 65.2 on ESSIC classification)	Suprapubic	ONSET	Aching	URINARY	Cognitive
			Urethral pain syndrome	Inguinal	Acute	Burning	Frequency	Behavioral
			Prostate pain syndrome — Type A inflammatory*** — Type B noninflammatory	Urethral	Chronic	Stabbing	Nocturia	Emotional
			Scrotal pain syndrome — Testicular pain syndrome — Epididymal pain syndrome — Postvasectomy pain syndrome	Penile/clitoral	ONGOING	Electric	Hesitance	
			Penile pain syndrome	Perineal	Sporadic	Other**	Poor flow	
		Gynecological	Vaginal pain syndrome	Rectal	Cyclical		Pis en deux	
			Vulvar pain syndrome — Generalized vulvar pain syndrome — Localized vulvar pain syndrome — Vestibular pain syndrome — Clitoral pain syndrome	Back	Continuous		Urge	
			Other — Endometriosis associated pain syndrome	Buttocks	TIME		Urgency	
		Anorectal	Anorectal pain syndrome		Filling		Incontinence	
		Neurological	Pudendal pain syndrome		Emptying		Other**	
		Muscular	Pelvic floor muscle pain syndrome		Immediate post		GYNECOLOGICAL e.g., Menstrual	
	Nonpelvic pain syndromes	Neurological Urological	Pudendal neuralgia		Late post		SEXUAL e.g., Female dyspareunia	
					PROVOKED		impotence	
							Anorectal Incontinence Constipation***	
							MUSCULAR Hyperalgesia Dysfunction	
							CUTANEOUS Allodynia	

TABLE 65.2

DEFINITIONS OF PELVIC PAIN

- *Chronic pelvic pain* is nonmalignant pain perceived in structures related to the pelvis of either men or women. In the case of documented nociceptive pain that becomes chronic, the pain must have been continuous or recurrent for at least 6 months. If nonacute pain mechanisms and central sensitization mechanisms are well documented, then the pain may be regarded as chronic, irrespective of the time period. In all cases, there often are associated negative cognitive, behavioral, sexual, and emotional consequences.[3,10]

- *Pelvic pain syndrome* is the occurrence of persistent or recurrent episodic pelvic pain associated with symptoms suggestive of lower urinary tract, sexual, bowel, or gynecological dysfunction. There is no proven infection or other obvious pathology.[3,10]

has reinforced this misnomer. Therefore, most of the data relating to pain perceived within the prostate stems from the prostatitis literature. As well as pain, these patients often have urinary urge (constant need to void as a result of a sensory disturbance), frequency (secondary to the urge), hesitancy and poor flow, but they do not have urgency (need to void because of a fear of incontinence).

Several studies have looked at the demographic distribution of the disease. Prostatitis appears to be more common in men younger than 50 years of age, though there may be a second cohort aged greater than 74 years.[13,14] The Nickel et al. study[14] identified 9.7% of men as having "chronic prostatitis-like" symptoms as defined by the NIH Chronic Prostatitis Symptom Index. This index includes urinary "irritative" and "obstructive" symptoms as well as measures of quality of life, as these are frequently disrupted.[15]

Scrotal Pain Syndrome

Testicular pain in isolation and without obvious cause is well defined as an example of chronic visceral pain. It is essential to rule out pain referred to the testis, such as from an adductor enthesitis or from the spine. Thoraco pathology with or without involvement of the nerve roots may also produce pain perceived in the testis.

Despite being well defined, the testicular pain syndrome is poorly researched and information about its incidence is scanty. The majority of the information stems from postvasectomy surgery, where the incidence may be as high as 19% following this operation. Once more the problem appears to be more frequent in younger men.[16,17,18,19]

Penile Pain Syndrome

There are very few data on this condition, which also appears to be unusual in the pain clinic. The condition must not be confused with the penile pain of pudendal neuralgia or pain sensation referred from the bladder or urethra. This condition is also quite different from the psychiatric obsession associated with the sex organs that can occur in certain patients. A painful penis without obvious cause has been seen to follow circumcision and may represent a central sensitization process.

Precipitating Factors

Very little is known about the factors that predispose men to urogenital pain syndromes.[20,21] In certain, but probably only a small proportion of, cases some form of trauma or infection may be the precipitating factor. Surgical trauma in the form of vasectomy may result in testicular pain.[22] Recurrent minor injury may be a predisposing factor, as for any pain syndrome.

The role of the pudendal nerve is disputed by different experts in the field. There is no doubt that pudendal neuralgia (pain associated with pudendal nerve damage) exists.[23] The mechanism(s) presumably will be the same as for all nerves and the pain would be perceived in the appropriate dermatome. Depending on the site of damage the pain may be perceived in the anus, peri-

TABLE 65.3

PHENOTYPE CLASSIFICATION OF THE MALE PELVIC UROGENITAL PAIN SYNDROMES

- *Penile pain syndrome* is the occurrence of pain within the penis that is not primarily in the urethra, with the absence of proven infection or other obvious pathology.[3,10]

- *Prostate pain syndrome* is the occurrence of persistent or recurrent episodic prostate pain, which is associated with symptoms suggestive of urinary tract and/or sexual dysfunction. There is no proven infection or other obvious pathology.[3,10] (This definition of prostate pain syndrome was adapted from the National Institutes of Health [NIH] consensus definition and classification of prostatitis[4] and includes those conditions that they term "chronic pelvic pain syndrome." Using their classification system, prostate pain syndrome may be further subdivided into: type A, inflammatory, and type B, noninflammatory.)

- *Scrotal pain syndrome* is the occurrence of persistent or recurrent episodic scrotal pain that is associated with symptoms suggestive of urinary tract or sexual dysfunction. There is no proven epididymo-orchitis or other obvious pathology.[3,10]

- *Testicular pain syndrome* is the occurrence of persistent or recurrent episodic pain localized to the testis on examination that is associated with symptoms suggestive of urinary tract or sexual dysfunction. There is no proven epididymo-orchitis or other obvious pathology (this is a more specific definition than scrotal pain syndrome).[3,10]

- *Postvasectomy pain syndrome* is a scrotal pain syndrome that follows vasectomy.[3,10]

- *Epididymal pain syndrome* is the occurrence of persistent or recurrent episodic pain localized to the epididymis on examination that is associated with symptoms suggestive of urinary tract or sexual dysfunction. There is no proven epididymo-orchitis or other obvious pathology (more specific definition than scrotal pain syndrome).[3,10]

neum, deeper within the pelvis, the bladder base, or the penis.[24] Whether the sexual function and the central sensitization of the sexual process imparts any specific properties on the damaged pudendal nerve is not known. As may be expected, the nerve damage may be associated with a range of sensory abnormalities such as dysesthesia, allodynia, or numbness. The pudendal nerve is suggested to be at risk from recurrent injuries (such as cycling or long hours of sitting) and from acute trauma, including surgical interventions, such as for cancer or orthopedics.[25,26,27,28] Sitting while working at a computer appears to be a predisposing factor among young men (personal observation).

The role of the musculature is also highly debated.[29,30,31,32,33,34,35,36] In general, it is now well accepted that the pelvic muscles (including the core muscles of the abdomen and spine) may be involved in the pelvic pain syndromes and that these muscles are subject to the same causes as any other muscle. Trauma, as during sports injury, birth injury for women, and accidents may produce a muscle-based pain. Stress is said to be responsible for pelvic muscle tension and hence pain in certain cases, though it must be appreciated that chronic pain will also be associated with psychological responses and even psychiatric disorders.[37,38,39]

The role of negative sexual encounters (NSE) continues to be disputed.[40,41] The prevalence of childhood male sexual abuse may be as high as 16% in some countries; in the UK it has been estimated as 5%. Three percent of male adults may also have had an NSE. Victims of torture are frequently subjected to sexual abuse. What is not clear is the relationship of this abuse to male urogenital pain syndromes. In our editorial,[8] it was suggested that there is little sound evidence to support NSEs as a cause of chronic urogenital pain in patients. However, there is no doubt that in a patient who has suffered a NSE, that incident may require management in its own right.

There are now several articles that indicate that the psychological status of the patient is relevant to the pelvic pain experience. Patients exhibiting high distress associated with catastrophizing and poor coping strategies do less well.[42,43,44,45]

MECHANISMS

Differences Between Visceral and Somatic Pains

In a proportion of patients with pain perceived to be in the pelvis, ongoing classical visceral pain mechanisms may be involved. A number of these mechanisms are listed in Table 65.4 and com-

TABLE 65.4

DIFFERENCES BETWEEN VISCERAL AND SOMATIC PAINS

	Visceral pain mechanism	Somatic pain mechanisms
Effective painful stimuli	Stretching, distension, ischemia, inflammation, producing poorly localized pain	Mechanical, thermal, chemical, and electrical stimuli, producing well localized pain
Summation	Widespread stimulation produces a significantly magnified pain	Widespread stimulation produces a modest increase in pain
Autonomic involvement	Autonomic features (e.g., nausea and sweating) frequently present	Autonomic features less frequent
Referred pain	Pain perceived at a site distant to the cause of the pain is common.	Pain is well localized
Referred hyperalgesia	Referred cutaneous and muscle hyperalgesia common as is involvement of other viscera. **This is very important.**	Hyperalgesia tends to be localized
Innervation	Low density, unmyelinated C fibers and thinly myelinated Aδ	Dense innervation with a wide range of nerve fibers
Primary afferent physiology	Intensity coding. As stimulation increases afferent firing increases with an increase in sensation and ultimately pain	Two fiber coding; there are separate well defined peripheral nerves for nociceptive pain and normal sensation. For pain to be perceived, under normal circumstances without central sensitization, the smaller C and Aδ associated nociceptors have to be activated.
Silent afferents	50%–90% of visceral afferents are silent until the time they are switched on. These fibers are very important in the central sensitization process.	Little evidence for silent afferents
Central mechanisms	Play an important part in the hyperalgesias, viscerovisceral, visceromuscular and musculovisceral hyperalgesias. Sensations not normally perceived become perceived and nonnoxious sensations become painful	Responsible for the allodynia and hyperalgesia of chronic somatic pain
Abnormalities of function	Central mechanisms associated with visceral pain may be responsible for organ dysfunction	Somatic pain associated with somatic dysfunction
Central pathways and representation	As well as classical pathways, there is evidence for a separate dorsal horn pathway and central representation	Classical pain pathways

pared to somatic pain mechanisms. In certain patients with persistent pelvic pain, chronic central sensitization mechanisms are predominant.

Peripheral Mechanisms[46,47,48,49]

Sensitization of visceral afferents and activation of silent afferents by endogenous mediators, including nerve growth factor (NGF), is considered pivotal for the development of visceral pain. NGF is able to both directly activate primary afferents and indirectly activate them (such as through the regulation of the expression of bradykinin[50]). Multiple tachykinins are implicated in both the normal control of bladder contraction and in the heightened stimulation and sensitization of the afferent loop of the micturition reflex after inflammation. Similar mechanisms are known for the other organs. ATP released from hollow organs, such as when the bladder is distended, acts upon purinergic P2X3 receptors found on visceral afferents and on small diameter DRG neurons. Once more these mechanisms may be involved in normal function as well as pain. Voltage gated ion channels (tetrodotoxin resistant sodium channel, NaV1.8) are also implicated in the visceral pain states.

Central Mechanisms[51,52,53,54,55]

In visceral pain excitatory amino-acid receptors such as N-methyl-D-aspartate (NMDA) and alpha-amino-3-hydroxy-5-methyl-4-isoxazoleproprionic acid (AMPA) play a vital role in the production of viscerovisceral, musculovisceral, and visceromuscular hyperalgesia. Both clinical studies and basic science support that central mechanisms activated as a result of an insult in one organ can result in non-noxious sensations being perceived and noxious sensations becoming more painful both in the same organ and in different organs and the muscles. Such mechanisms explain why many patients have multiple end organ sensitivities. For example, patients with the bladder pain syndrome may also have muscle trigger points and anorectal sensitivity (e.g., irritable bowel syndrome). Once triggered, the changes in the central nervous system can persist for great lengths of time.

Muscles and Pelvic Pain

As with any pain syndrome, muscle tenderness and trigger points may be implicated as a source of pain in the urogenital pain syndromes. Central mechanisms are of great importance in the pathogenesis of these muscle hyperalgesias. The muscles involved may form a part of the spinal, abdominal, or pelvic complex of muscles. It is not unknown for adjacent muscles of the lower limbs and the thorax to become involved. Pain may be well localized to the trigger points but is more often associated with classical referral patterns. As well as trigger points, inflammation of the attachments to the bones (enthesitis) and of the bursa (bursitis) may be found.[56,57,58,59]

Numerous events have been suggested as causative factors. A local infection, such as a bladder infection, may produce local muscle spasm and subsequent muscle associated pain. Renal stones are clearly associated with spinal muscle hyperalgesia.[60] The onset of pain may be due to some form of minor strain or may be associated with a more obvious injury, such as those associated with sports.[61] Certain postures will affect the different muscles in different ways and, consequently, may either exacerbate the pain or reduce it. Stress has been implicated as being both an initiator of pelvic myalgia and as a maintenance factor; as a consequence, negative sexual encounters may also have a precipitating effect.[62]

Pelvic Muscle Pain Syndromes[63,64]

The following are some examples of pelvic muscle pain syndromes.

Piriformis.[65,66] This muscle originates from the anterior part of the sacrum and inserts onto the greater trochanter. The muscle produces external rotation of the leg. It starts within the pelvis, leaving it by the greater sciatic foramen. It is the relationship of the piriformis at this level to the nerves that allows the possibility of nerve irritation by the piriformis (see below). Pain associated with this muscle refers to the buttock and is worse on passive internal rotation or active external rotation against resistance. Trigger points are usually identified at the level of the greater sciatic foramen.

Obturator Internus.[67,68] This muscle arises from the inner surface of the anterolateral wall of the pelvis, where it covers the majority of the foramen ovale and is attached to the obturator membrane, the inferior rami of the pubis, and the ischium. It leaves the pelvis via the lesser sciatic notch to attach to the greater trochanter. It may develop trigger points deep in its body (detected by internal pelvic examination) or in its external part. Pain may refer anteriorly, deep within the pelvis, and to the genitalia and/or posteriorly to the rectum and buttocks. Bursitis may occur as the muscle passes out of the pelvis and around the ischium. This muscle may be associated with pudendal nerve irritation (see below).

Levator Ani.[69] The levator ani is inserted into the inner surface of the anatomical lesser pelvis and is composed of three parts—iliococcygeus, puborectalis, and pubococcygeus. The muscles form a sling with fibers uniting in the midline, and blending with the sphincters of the pelvic organs (Fig. 65.1). Trigger points produce a range of referral patterns from the anus to the penis and into the testis. It has been suggested that levator plate hyperalgesia, trigger points, and referred pain are responsible for the prostate pain syndrome.[70,71]

The relationship of these muscles to the pelvic organs results in a wide range of other symptoms, such as urinary urge with associated frequency. Pain may be exacerbated by use of the muscles, such as during intercourse, ejaculation, voiding of urine, and defecation.

Coccygeus.[71] The coccygeus originates from the spine of the ischium and inserts into the coccyx.

Psoas.[72] The psoas originates from the transverse process of the lumbar vertebrae; leaving the pelvis below the inguinal ligament, it inserts into the lesser trochanter of the femur. Pain can refer to the back, pelvis, and groin.

Spinal and Abdominal Muscle Pain Syndromes

The spinal and abdominal muscle pain syndromes often have a close relationship with the pelvic muscle pain syndromes. Muscle pains may be seen to spread from the site of the original pain (either the pelvis or the spinal/abdominal muscles) to involve adjacent muscles. Sometimes this progression may be picked up from the history; in other patients it may be impossible to separate out the history around what appears to be total body pain. Kinesophobia and subsequent immobility are predisposing factors to the spread of muscle pain.[73,74] Stress and tension are also negative prognostic factors.

The thoracolumbar junction is an important source of referred pain to the buttocks, hips, groin, and testicles.[75]

As in the pelvic muscle pain syndromes, spasm of the abdominal and spinal musculature may be associated with local nerve irritation, such as the genitofemoral nerve with psoas spasm and

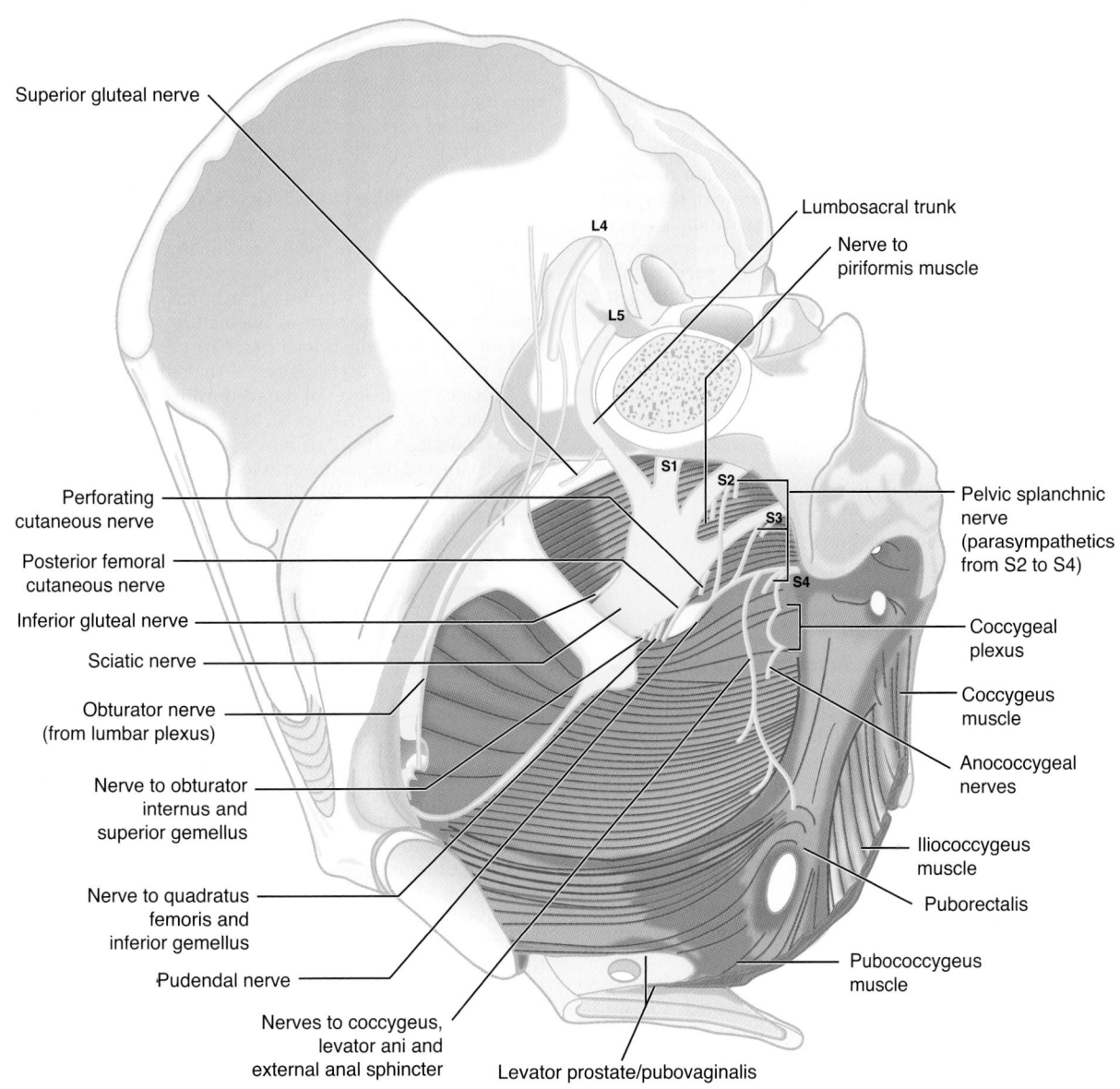

FIGURE 65.1 Male pelvic anatomy.

the anterior cutaneous branches of the intercostals nerves as they transgress the rectus abdominis. Disease at the thoracolumbar junction may result in L1 and or T12 root irritation and, consequently, pain perceived in the groin and testicles.

Pelvic Nerves and Pain

It is well established that nerve injury may be associated with a range of symptoms that include dysesthesia, allodynia, hyperalgesia, and constant or intermittent pain. The mechanisms are well established (see other chapters in this book). In some cases the onset of pain is clearly associated with the nerve damage. However, in many cases arriving at the diagnosis of peripheral nerve injury generated pain can be difficult. This is particularly so for the urogenital pains:

1. Due to the difficulty in identifying the nerves and examining their relevant dermatomes.
2. Pelvic dermatomes overlap widely and, consequently, signs of nerve injury are difficult to identify.

3. Many pelvic nerves are primarily sensory or autonomic and as a result there is little somatic motor data available to aid the diagnosis of nerve damage.
4. Even when there are motor fibers present, significant nerve damage has to be present for there to be abnormal neurophysiology and the muscles are difficult to access.
5. Referred sensations (including cutaneous dysesthesia, allodynia, and hyperalgesias) from the muscle hyperalgesias, tendonitis, and enthesitis are common and frequently confuse the picture.

Peripheral Nerve Pain Syndromes

Nerves and the Male Genitalia. The afferents from the skin of the male genitals pass via a complex of multiple sensory nerves and this makes the diagnosis of nerve injury as a cause of pain difficult. The anterolateral part of the scrotum has afferents primarily associated with the genitofemoral nerve; there is some possible involvement of the ilioinguinal and iliohypogastric nerves. The posterior scrotal branches of the pudendal nerve transmit sensation from the posterior scrotum. The penis shaft is innervated on its dorsal surface by the genitofemoral, ilioinguinal, and iliohypogastric nerves, and the ventral surface by the perineal branches of the posterior femoral cutaneous nerve and cutaneous branches of the pudendal nerve. The glans penis is associated with the dorsal nerve of the penis, the terminal branch of the pudendal nerve. All the nerves that are associated with the scrotum may also receive afferents from the testis, though classically the nerves from the testis are usually associated with the genitofemoral nerve. The superficial branches of the pudendal's superficial perineal nerve and the perineal branch of the posterior femoral cutaneous nerve receive afferents from the perineal skin. Deeper afferents from the perineum and from some of the pelvic organs pass to the pudendal nerve via its deep perineal branch.

The course of the afferents from the pelvic organ is well described in most anatomy books as are the sources of innervation. For the aims of this chapter the involvement of the pudendal nerve must be emphasized. It must also be recognized that the pelvic plexus is both associated with the parasympathetic and sympathetic nerves and that, as well as efferents associated with these pathways, afferents may travel back to both the sacral roots and the thoracolumbar roots with these autonomic nerves. Sites for injury and for possible intervention may thus include the ganglion impar, superior hypogastric plexus, inferior hypogastric plexus, and lumbar sympathetic trunk, as well as more central spinal root areas.

Pain Arising from Damage to the Anterior Groin Nerves. The iliohypogastric nerve arises from L1 and its anterior branch supplies the skin above the pubis where its lateral cutaneous branch is distributed to the anterolateral part of the buttock. Nerve damage may be associated with surgical trauma during operations on the groin or loin. More proximal lesions are rare, but should be considered as they may represent sepsis or neoplastic infiltration.

The ileo-inguinal nerve is smaller than the iliohypogastric nerve; arising from L1, it is distributed to the skin of the groin and mons pubis. Nerve damage may be associated with surgical trauma during operations on the groin or loin. More proximal lesions are rare, but should be considered as they may also represent sepsis or neoplastic infiltration.

The genitofemoral nerve arises from L1 and L2. It passes through the psoas, then down it to emerge through the deep inguinal ring. Its genital branch supplies the cremaster and a part of the antero and lateral scrotum. The femoral branch passes close to the external iliac artery, the deep circumflex iliac artery and the femoral artery to be distributed to the upper part of the femoral triangle. As the two branches of the genitofemoral nerve may separate at any level, sensory phenomena associated with nerve damage will depend upon the level of the lesion and individual variability. Genitofemoral neuralgia may suggest a vascular aneurysm, local sepsis, or be associated with loin or groin surgery.

Lateral cutaneous nerve of the thigh arises from L2 and L3 and passes to eventually leave the abdomen behind or through the inguinal ligament at a variable distance medial to the anterior superior iliac spine. In the thigh it divides into an anterior branch that supplies the anterolateral skin of the thigh, approximately 10 cm down from the inguinal ligament to the knee. The posterior branch supplies the skin more laterally from the greater trochanter, down to midthigh.

Obturator nerves L2, L3, and L4 descend through the psoas, around the pelvis closely approximated to the obturator internus muscle and obturator vessels to leave the pelvis via the obturator foramen. This nerve has significant motor innervation; its cutaneous branch is distributed primarily to the inner thigh.

Pain Arising from Damage to the Posterior Triangle Nerves. The posterior triangle area is the area defined by the upper border of the piriformis superiorly, the lower border of quadratus femoris inferiorly, the greater trochanter laterally, and the lateral border of the sacrum, lateral border of the sacrotuberal ligament, and lateral border of the ischial tuberosity medially. It is in this region that the sciatic nerve, the posterior femoral cutaneous nerve (this branches into the posterior cutaneous perineal branch as well as the cluneal nerves), the nerve to obturator internus muscle, and the pudendal nerve can be found; they pass deep to the piriformis and superficial to the superior gemellus and obturator internus muscles.

The pudendal nerve has its roots at the S2, S3, and S4 levels. It has three main branches, the inferior anal/rectal nerve, the superficial perineal nerve (which terminates as cutaneous branches in the perineum and posterior aspect of the scrotum), and the deep perineal nerve, which is distributed to the pelvic structures (possibly innervating parts of the bladder, prostate, and urethra) and terminates as the dorsal nerve of the penis, innervating the glans penis. It has been suggested that the pudendal nerve may be damaged at the level of the piriformis muscle, the sacrospinal ligament, or within Alcock's canal, medial to the obturator internus muscle. The site of injury will determine the site of perceived pain and the nature of associated symptoms (e.g., the more distal the damage, the less likely the anal region will be involved). There is also a school of thought that suggests that the fine nerve endings of the pudendal may become trapped in the muscle planes producing neuropathic pain, possibly with mechanisms similar to complex regional pain syndrome.[24,76]

FUNCTIONAL PROBLEMS AND MALE PELVIC PAIN

In addition to pain, many patients with urogenital pain syndromes suffer with abnormalities of organ function. The exact mechanisms involved may not be clear. It is well described that certain drugs (Table 65.5) and surgical interventions can produce organ dysfunction.

The mechanisms, both central and peripheral, involved in the production of the pain may also be the cause of some of the functional disorders. Certainly those functions that are reliant on voluntary control may be affected by changes in sensory perception. The sensation of urge perceived with a more or less empty bladder may be associated with urinary frequency and, similarly, the sensation of rectal fullness may be associated with frequent attempts to defecate. Because of convergence of visceral afferent input within the central nervous system abnormalities of sensation perceived primarily in one organ may result in functional abnormalities further afield[77,78,79] and widespread muscle spasm.[78,80] Abnormal visceral motor function may also occur.[81]

TABLE 65.5

DRUGS PRESCRIBED IN PAIN CLINICS AND SOME OF THEIR EFFECT ON ORGAN FUNCTION

Drugs	Effects
Opioids, including tramadol	Constipation Urinary hesitance Reduced sexual desire and erectile ability
Antidepressants	Constipation Urinary hesitance and retention Reduce orgasmic sensation Delay or inhibit ejaculation
Anticonvulsants	Carbamazepine may block testosterone production with subsequent: testicular atrophy, gynecomastia, galactorrhea May inhibit ejaculation

The role of the neuro-endocrine and neuro-immune systems is poorly understood. The effect of these conditions on fertility is also poorly understood.

PSYCHOLOGICAL CONSEQUENCES OF MALE PELVIC PAIN

The effect of gender on illness and illness behavior is clearly established; however, there is little research on the effect of illness on gender identity and sexual psychology. One may assume that disorders of the male urogenital system will be prone to produce problems within both of these areas with a risk that the male either fails to achieve meaningful relationships or that established relationships have an increased chance of breaking down. All chronic pain is associated with depression and cognitive behavioral problems. The severity of the pain appears to be the main determinant. Depression and catastrophizing are poor prognostic factors. Trip et al.'s paper and more recent work by the same group[45] are key studies. Problems with work, relationships, sex, and loss of meaning of life appeared to be as equally important as the pain itself. For the successful management of a patient with chronic pelvic pain, a multidisciplinary team approach is essential (see below).

MALE UROGENITAL PELVIC PAIN SYNDROMES-TREATMENT

Sex Differences and Therapies

There are some fundamental differences between males and females that may affect drug pharmacokinetics and pharmacodynamics. In contrast to women, men usually have greater muscle mass, lower percentage body fat, and less fluctuations in hormones. Other genetic-related factors may be at play. Men appear to require significantly more morphine than women per kg body weight[82] and women seem to achieve statistically significantly more analgesia with kappa agonists (nalbuphine, buprenorphine, and pentazocine) than do men. The effect of sex differences on other therapies is poorly researched.

Specific Pain Syndrome Treatments

A more complex review can be obtained in the current EAU guidelines for chronic pelvic pain.[10]

Prostate Pain Syndrome

Because the exact nature of this condition is poorly understood, specific drug treatment options do not exist. Most patients will receive one or more courses of antibiotics. The use of antibiotics remains controversial. However, the current EAU guidelines[10] indicate that "because some patients have been observed to improve with antimicrobial therapy[83,84,85,86] a trial treatment with antibiotics is recommended." They go on to say that "patients responding to antibiotics should be maintained on the medication for 4 to 6 weeks or even longer. If relapse occurs after discontinuation, continuous low-dose antimicrobial therapy should be reintroduced and sustained if effective. Long-term results with trimethoprim-sulphamethoxazole have remained poor."[87,88,89] Results of therapy with quinolone, including norfloxacin,[90] ciprofloxacin,[91,92] and ofloxacin,[93,94,95] appear to be more encouraging.

Symptom control is primarily aimed at reducing spasm in the bladder outflow system (smooth and/or striated muscles) or the use of simple analgesics.[96,97]

Striated muscle relaxants may help if there is pelvic floor muscle spasm or in the presence of pelvic floor muscle trigger points.[84]

There are some studies that demonstrate an improvement of symptoms in patients with NIH III a/b prostatitis when alpha adrenoceptor blockers are used. Alpha adrenoceptors are found in the bladder neck and prostate and alpha adrenoceptor blockers are conventionally used to improve flow in the presence of lower urinary tract obstructive symptoms.[98,99,100,101] Whether improvement in pain is due to improving urinary outflow is not known.

Analgesics are often considered the mainstay of symptomatic management. Simple analgesics containing paracetamol are often first line, unfortunately in many cases with little benefit. Nonsteroidal anti-inflammatory medications can be considered but should only be used long term if there is evidence of inflammation. Opioids should only be used if one or the other of the national guidelines has been followed (e.g., The British Pain Society guidelines).

Studies have looked at the role of hormone manipulation with the 5-alpha-reductase inhibitor finasteride. In a small percentage of patients finasteride has been found efficacious with an improvement in voiding and a reduction in pain.[84,102,103] The role for anticholinergics is debatable. Meares has suggested they may be beneficial in reducing urinary urgency.[104]

Prospective studies on the effects of phytotherapy and pentosanpolysulphate (PPS) need to be undertaken; there have been some positive case reports.[105]

There is little evidence for immune modulation using cytokine inhibitors.[106,107]

There are advocates for therapies, such as biofeedback, relaxation exercises, lifestyle changes (e.g., diet, discontinuing bike riding, changing a work station), acupuncture, massage therapy, chiropractic therapy, and meditation.[84,96] Pelvic floor exercises and biofeedback pelvic floor training, independent of other influences, may benefit this group of patients.[109] The debate about exercise versus trigger point therapy continues with very little research.[109] It appears that managing the associated muscle hyperalgesia is important, whether it is the primary problem or secondary. If we draw comparisons with other musculoskeletal-related pain syndromes, managing the patient as a whole appears appropriate. The physical treatment options should probably consist of exercises, postural/core work, trigger point release, and pacing. Maintaining the locus of control with the patient is important.

Heat therapy, such as transrectal hyperthermia[110,111,112] and transurethral thermotherapy,[113,114,115] has been reported to produce favorable results in some patients. Generally, the evidence is weak and the treatments rarely used.

Scrotal/Testicular/Epididymal Pain Syndromes

There is very limited research on this condition and, as a result, the evidence for efficacy is limited.[8] Some groups have advocated the use of antibiotics but, as with the prostate pain syndrome, there appears to be limited supporting evidence in the absence of an identified infection.

If urinary symptoms are present then those symptoms may be managed as in the prostate pain syndrome. Similarly, the use of NSAIDs may have a role if inflammation is present. Analgesics, including opioids and neuropathic analgesics, may be tried; the effect must be monitored and appropriate guidelines adhered to.

There is still debate as to what scrotal contents may be associated with pain. However, there is a suggestion that in the presence of a hydrocele, spermatocele, or varicocele, on average 50% of patients may see benefit from surgery.[116,117,118] In the absence of such a lesion, the role of surgery is debatable and may even be detrimental.[8]

In the scrotal pain syndrome, microsurgical testicular denervation has been advocated; however, the number of studies are limited and not double blind for technical reasons.[119,120] The results of epididymectomy and orchidectomy are considered even worse (though 20% and 60% success rates, respectively, have been suggested).[121,122] It should be of concern that these procedures are still undertaken despite the fact that pain may be increased by the procedure.

Nerve blocks (L1 dorsal root renal/sympathectomy, groin blocks, and pudendal/perineal [posterior triangle] blocks) are regularly used in the treatment of scrotal pain syndrome. As well as a possible therapeutic role (for which there are no supporting studies), they are also important for the differential diagnosis process. Although the evidence for therapeutic benefit is limited, the risks are either small or extremely rare.

Generic Treatment Approach

Urogenital pain syndromes should be managed with the same general approach that is used for any of the pain syndromes. Where possible, the consultation and therapeutic procedure environment should be purpose-built, allowing privacy and comfort (many of these patients would prefer to stand or lie for the consultation). Anatomical models and diagrams, including drawings or photographs of genitalia, that will facilitate the consultation should be available. As well as doctors, nurses skilled in the management of this group of patients should be at hand to reinforce the discussion from the consultation.

Psychology and Sexual Counselling

In view of the psychological consequences of urogenital pain, experienced pain management psychologists should be at hand. The full range of their skills utilized for chronic pain management will be required, but psychosexual counselling and relationship work is often required as well. For the sexual problems, we operate a system where the medical and nursing staff undertake the medical management of the sexual problems but also provide medical information on normality and variants to enable the patient to place their sexual problems in context. Psychological interventions are instigated early and often while physical treatments are ongoing—the aim is to support and prevent psychological and sexual problem deterioration. Under such circumstances both the patient and the psychologist have to be able to work with this model of early psychology and ongoing physical treatment.

Trigger Point Therapy

As discussed above, trigger points and hyperalgesic muscles should be managed as appropriate with treatment options that include drugs, stretching, exercise, relaxation, and injections. Injections into pelvic trigger points are no different than injections into muscles elsewhere, but require the expertise of a specialist with skills using imaging such as CT, ultrasound, or possible procedural MRI. The agent injected is not agreed upon, but usually is a local anesthetic and steroid mixture. Botulinum toxin injections into some of the deeper pelvic muscles has been advocated.[123,124]

Nerve Blocks

Nerve blocks may have a role in the management of specific nerve injuries but may also serve to relax muscles. Nerve blocks may be therapeutic or diagnostic.

Surgery

Surgery was discussed above and, in view of the risks with minimal proven benefit, should not be undertaken without a good surgical reason. If the surgery is significant, psychological evaluation and intervention should be considered first.[125,126]

Drugs

Centrally Acting Analgesics. Chong and Hester[127] summarized the current knowledge in relation to the role of targeting neuropathic pain in urogenital pain syndromes. There is a debate as to when and whether such drugs have a role in the management of the pelvic pain syndromes. Tricyclic and tetracyclic antidepressant drugs may have a role if there are neuropathic qualities to the pain. The best evidence is for amitriptyline. SSRIs and SNRIs are also considered to have a role. Venlafaxine has the strongest evidence but is troubled with cardiac side effects. Duloxetine may have an advantage where stress incontinence is a problem.

Gabapentin and pregabalin have become very popular in the management of chronic pelvic pain and several studies have suggested they may have a role (still to be published). Other antiepileptics could be considered, as for the management of any neuropathic pain.

Opioids should be considered providing appropriate precautions are undertaken and guidelines adhered to.

Neuromodulation

The evidence base for neuromodulation in chronic pelvic/urogenital pain is limited. However, some very good guidelines do exist for the use of neuromodulation in peripheral nerve injury and complex regional pain syndrome.[128] Hence, one would expect neuromodulation to help certain urogenital pain conditions. Case history reports support this. The main problem is achieving stimulation in the appropriate area, and although some specialists do claim to gain benefit by stimulating the lower thoracic region, it appears that most specialist implanters would now stimulate the sacral roots either by a lumbar retrograde or trans-sacral approach. The stimulation is thus preganglionic/ganglionic and not dorsal horn or true peripheral sensory nerve only. The trans-sacral approach is easy to trial and also has the benefit of some excellent guidelines for bowel and bladder dysfunction neuromodulation.[129,130] It is our policy to try transforaminal/trans-sacral neuromodulation first, and if that fails to reduce the pain, but the patient wishes to try other approaches, we then try lumbar retrograde or lumbar anterograde approaches.

OVERVIEW AND CONCLUSION

Male urogenital pain may arise from the specific male urogenital organs. However, there is a strong literature pointing out that in many men the pain may arise from other sources but is perceived in the male sex organs. It is now well established that when a man presents with urogenital pelvic pain, the nervous system, musculoskeletal system, and other organs should be looked at as potential sources of the pain. The role of the central nervous system in altering afferent perception and producing efferent dysfunction is now well understood. The central nervous system is also key as a cause for the widespread distribution of the pain syndrome. Often multiple organs and systems are involved. The nervous system may also be key in the association between the pelvic pain syndromes and systemic disorders such as fibromyalgia and chronic fatigue syndrome. In view of this complex of interacting mechanisms, a single therapeutic option is rarely rewarding. Antibiotics and surgery for pain are also rarely rewarding. Multimodal approaches to pain management appear to provide the best results. Management should not only be aimed at the pain, but also the other sensory symptoms and functional disorders. The more distressed the patient, the worse the prognosis; hence, early pain management and early psychological, sexual, and relationship support is crucial to a good outcome.

References

1. Abrams P, Baranowski AP, Berger RE, et al. A new classification is needed for pelvic pain syndromes—are existing terminologies of spurious diagnostic authority bad for patients? *J Urol* 2006;175(6):1989–1990.

2. Abrams P, Cardozo L, Fall M, et al. The standardisation of terminology of lower urinary tract function: report from the Standardisation Sub-committee of the International Continence Society. *Neurourol Urodyn* 2002;21(2):167–178.

3. Fall M, Baranowski AP, Fowler CJ, et al. EAU guidelines on chronic pelvic pain. *Eur Urol* 2004;46(6):681–689.

4. Gillenwater, JY, Wein AJ. Summary of the National Institute of Arthritis, Diabetes, Digestive and Kidney Diseases Workshop on Interstitial Cystitis, National Institutes of Health, Bethesda, Maryland, August 28–29, 1987. *J Urol* 1988;140(1):203–206.

5. Kreiger JN, Nyberg L, Nickel JC. NIH consensus definition and classification of prostatitis. *JAMA* 1999;82:236–237.

6. Hanno P, Baranowski AP, Rosamilia A, et al. *International Continence Society guidelines on chronic pelvic pain*. International Consultation on Incontinence (ICI) (2005).

7. van de Merwe JP, Nordling J, Bouchelouche P, et al. Diagnostic criteria, classification, and nomenclature for painful bladder syndrome/interstitial cystitis: an ESSIC proposal. *Eur Urol* 2008;53:60–67.

8. Baranowski AP, Abrams P, Berger RE, et al. Urogenital pain—time to accept a new approach to phenotyping and, as a consequence, management. *Eur Urol* 2008;53:33–36.

9. Van de Merwe JP, Nordling J. Interstitial cystitis: definitions and confusable diseases. ESSIC meeting 2005 Baden. *Eur Urol Today* 2006;March:6–7& 16–17.

10. Fall M, Baranowski AP, Elneil S, et al. Guidelines on chronic pelvic pain. In: *EAU Guidelines*. Edition presented at the 23rd EAU Annual Congress, Milan, 2008.

11. Tripp D, Nickel CJ, Wang Y, et al. Catastrophizing and pain-contingent rest predict patient adjustment in men with chronic prostatitis/chronic pelvic pain syndrome. *J Pain* 2006;7(10):697–708.

12. Rothrock NE, Lutgendorf S, Kreder KJ. Coping strategies in patients with interstitial cystitis: relationships with quality of life and depression. *J Urol* 2003;169:233–236.

13. Roberts RO, Lieber MM, Rhodes T, et al. Prevalence of a physician-assigned diagnosis of prostatitis: the Olmsted County study of urinary symptoms and health status among men. *Urology* 1998;51(4):578–584.

14. Nickel JC, Downey J, Hunter D, et al. Prevalence of prostatitis-like symptoms in a population based study using the National Institutes of Health chronic prostatitis symptom index. *J Urol* 2001;165,842–845.

15. Litwin MS, McNaughton-Collins M, Fowler FJ Jr., et al. The National Institutes of Health chronic prostatitis symptom index: development and validation of a new outcome measure. Chronic Prostatitis Collaborative Research Network. *J Urol* 1999;162(2):369–375.

16. Granitsiotis P, Kirk D. Chronic testicular pain: an overview. *Eur Urol* 2004; 45(4):430–436.

17. Ahmed I, Rasheed S, White C, et al. The incidence of post-vasectomy chronic testicular pain and the role of nerve stripping (denervation) of the spermatic cord in its management. *Br J Urol* 1997;79(2):269–270.

18. McMahon AJ, Buckley J, Taylor A, et al. Chronic testicular pain following vasectomy. *Br J Urol* 1992;69(2):188–191.

19. Ahmed I, Rasheed S, White C, et al. The incidence of post-vasectomy chronic testicular pain and the role of nerve stripping (denervation) of the spermatic cord in its management. *Br J Urol* 1997;79(2):269–270.

20. Wesselmann U, Burnett AL, Heinberg LJ. The urogenital and rectal pain syndromes. *Pain* 1997;73(3):269–294.

21. Nickel JC, Siemens DR, Nickel KR, et al. The patient with chronic epididymitis: characterization of an enigmatic syndrome. *J Urol* 2002;167(4):1701–1704.

22. Davis BE, Noble MJ, Weigel JW, et al. Analysis and management of chronic testicular pain. *J Urol* 1990;143(5):936–939.

23. Labat JJ, Robert R, Bensignor M, et al. Les névralgies du nerf pudendal (honteux interne). Considérations anatomo-cliniques et perspectives thérapeutiques. *J Urol (Paris)* 1990;96:239–244.

24. Robert R, Prat-Pradal D, Labat JJ, et al. Anatomic basis of chronic perineal pain: role of the pudendal nerve. *Surg Radiol Anat* 1998;20:93–98.

25. Kao JT, Burton D, Comstock C, et al. Pudendal nerve palsy after femoral intramedullary nailing. *J Orthop Trauma* 1993;7:58–63.

26. Lyon T, Koval KJ, Kummer F, et al. Pudendal nerve palsy induced by fracture table. *Orthop Rev* 1993;22:521–525.

27. Alevizon SJ, Finan MA. Sacrospinous colpopexy: management of postoperative pudendal nerve entrapment. *Obstet Gynecol* 1996;88:713–715.

28. Ricchiuti VS, Haas CA, Seftel AD, et al. Pudendal nerve injury associated with avid bicycling. *J Urol* 1999;162:2099–2100.

29. Glazer HI. Dysesthetic vulvodynia. Long term follow-up after treatment with surface electromyography-assisted pelvic floor muscle rehabilitation. *J Reprod Med* 2000;45:798–802.

30. Wise D. *A Headache in the Pelvis: A New Understanding and Treatment for Prostatitis and Chronic Pelvic Pain Syndromes*, 3rd ed. National Center for pelvic Pain; 2005.

31. Fon LJ, Spence RA. Sportsman's hernia. *Br J Surg* 2000;87(5):545–552.

32. Davis BE, Noble MJ, Weigel JW, et al. Analysis and management of chronic testicular pain. *J Urol* 1990;143(5):936–939.

33. Hetrick DC, Ciol MA, Rothman I, et al. Musculoskeletal dysfunction in men with chronic pelvic pain syndrome type III: a case-control study. *J Urol* 2003; 170(3):828–831.

34. Clemens JQ, Nadler RB, Schaeffer AJ, et al. Biofeedback, pelvic floor re-education, and bladder training for male chronic pelvic pain syndrome. *Urology* 2000;56(6):951–955.

35. Carter JE. Abdominal wall and pelvic myofascial trigger points. In: Howard FM, ed. *Pelvic Pain, Diagnosis and Management*. Philadelphia: Lippincott Williams & Wilkins, 2000, 314–358.

36. Slocumb JC. Neurological factors in chronic pelvic pain: trigger points and the abdominal pelvic pain syndrome. *Am J Obstet Gynecol* 1984;149:536–543.

37. Egan KJ, Krieger JN. Psychological problems in chronic prostatitis patients with pain. *Clin J Pain* 1994;10:218–226.

38. Berghuis JP, Heiman JR, Rothman I, et al. Psychological and physical factors involved in chronic idiopathic prostatitis. *J Psychosom Res* 1996;41(4):313–325.

39. Wenninger K, Heiman JR, Rothman I, et al. Sickness impact of chronic nonbacterial prostatitis and its correlates. *J Urol* 1996;155(3):965–968.

40. Royal College of Obstetricians and Gynaecologists. *The initial management of chronic pelvic pain*. Guideline No. 41. April 2005.

41. Savidge CJ, Slade P. Psychological aspects of chronic pelvic pain. *J Psychosom Res* 1997;42(5):433–444.

42. Vlaeyen JW, Linton SJ. Fear-avoidance and its consequences in chronic musculoskeletal pain: a state of the art. *Pain* 2000;85:317–332.

43. Newton-John T, Brooke S. Treating sexual dysfunction in chronic pain patients. In: Gifford, L, ed. *Topical Issues in Pain 2*. Cornwall: CNS Press Ltd., 2000.

44. Tripp DA, Nickel JC, Wang Y, et al. Catastrophizing and pain-contingent rest predict patient adjustment in men with chronic prostatitis/chronic pelvic pain syndrome. *J Pain* 2006;7(10):697–708.

45. Tripp DA, Nickel JC, Wang Y, et al. Biopsychosocial factors in quality of life in CP/CPPS. *BJU Int* 2008;101:59-64.

46. Nazif O, Teichman JM, Gebhart GF. Neural upregulation in interstitial cystitis. *Urology* 2007;69(4 suppl):24–33.

47. Pezet S, McMahon SB. Neurotrophins: mediators and modulators of pain. *Annu Rev Neurosci* 2006;29:507–538.

48. McMahon SB, Jones NG. Plasticity of pain signaling: role of neurotrophic factors exemplified by acid-induced pain. *J Neurobiol* 2004;61(1):72–87.

49. Pontari MA, Ruggieri MR. Mechanisms in prostatitis/chronic pelvic pain syndrome. *J Urology* 2004;172(3):839–845.

50. Petersen M, Segond von Banchet G, Heppelmann B, et al. Nerve growth factor regulates the expression of bradykinin binding sites on adult sensory neurons via the neurotrophin receptor p75. *Neuroscience* 1998;83(1):161–168.

51. Giamberardino MA. Visceral pain. *Pain* 2005: Clinical Updates, XIII (6):1–6.

52. Roza C, Laird JM, Cervero F. Spinal mechanisms underlying persistent pain and referred hyperalgesia in rats with an experimental ureteric stone. *J Neurophysiol* 1998;79(4):1603–1612.

53. Vecchiet L, Giamberardino MA, de Bigontina P. Referred pain from viscera: when the symptom persists despite the extinction of the visceral focus. *Adv Pain Res Ther* 1992;20:101–110.

54. Melzack R, Coderre TJ, Katz J, et al. Central neuroplasticity and pathological pain. *Ann N Y Acad Sci* 2001;933:157–174.

55. McMahon SB, Dmitrieva N, Koltzenburg M. Visceral pain. *Br J Anaesth* 1995;75(2):132–144.

56. Akermark C, Johansson C. Tenotomy of the adductor longus tendon in the treatment of chronic groin pain in athletes. *Am J Sports Med* 1992;20:640–643.

57. Taylor DC, Meyers WC, Moylan JA, et al. Abdominal musculature abnormalities as a cause of groin pain in athletes. *Am J Sports Med* 1991;3:239–242.

58. Slocumb JC. Neurological factors in chronic pelvic pain: trigger points and the abdominal pelvic pain syndrome. *Am J Obstet Gynecol* 1984;149:536–543.

59. Gajraj NM. Botulinum toxin A injection of the obturator internus muscle for chronic pelvic pain. *J Pain* 2005;6(5):333–337.

60. Giamberardino MA, de Bigontina P, Martegiani C, et al. Effects of extracorporeal shock-wave lithotripsy on referred hyperalgesia from renal/ureteral calculosis. *Pain* 1994;56:77–83.

61. Lloyd-Smith R, Bernard AM, Herry JY, et al. Survey of overuse and traumatic hip and pelvic injuries in athletes. *Phys Sports Med* 1985;10:131–141.

62. Savidge CJ, Slade P. Psychological aspects of chronic pelvic pain. *J Psychosom Res* 1997;42(5):433–444.

63. Weiss JM. Pelvic floor myofascial trigger points: manual therapy for interstitial cystitis and the urgency-frequency syndrome. *J Urol* 2001;166:2226–2231.

64. Prendergast SA, Weiss JM. Screening for musculoskeletal causes of pelvic pain. *Clin Obstet Gynecol* 2003;46:773–782.

65. Fishman LM, Schaefer MP. The piriformis syndrome is underdiagnosed. *Muscle Nerve* 2003;28:646–649.

66. McCrory P. The "piriformis syndrome"—myth or reality? *Br J Sports Med* 2001;35:209–210.

67. Cox JM, Bakkum BW. Possible generators of retrotrochanteric gluteal and thigh pain: the gemelli-obturator internus complex. *J Manipulative Physiol Ther* 2005;28(7):534–538.

68. Meknas K, Christensen A, Johansen O. The internal obturator muscle may cause sciatic pain. *Pain* 2003;104:375–380.

69. Salvati EP. The levator syndrome and its variant. *Gastroenterol Clin North Am* 1987;16:71–78.

70. Segura, JW, Opitz JL, Greene LF. Prostatosis, prostatitis or pelvic floor tension myalgia? *J Urol* 1979;122:168–169.

71. Hetrick DC, Ciol MA, Rothman I, et al. Musculoskeletal dysfunction in men with chronic pelvic pain syndrome type III: a case-control study. *J Urol* 2003; 170:828–831.

72. Ingber RS. Iliopsoas myofascial dysfunction: a treatable cause of "failed" low back syndrome. *Arch Phys Med Rehabil* 1989;70(5):382–386.

73. Nederhand MJ, Hermens HJ, Ijzerman MJ, et al. The effect of fear of movement on muscle activation in posttraumatic neck pain disability. *Clin J Pain* 2006;22(6):519–525.

74. Klaber Moffett JA, Jackson DA, Richmond S, et al. Randomised trial of a brief physiotherapy intervention compared with usual physiotherapy for neck pain patients: outcomes and patients' preference. *BMJ* 2005;330(7482):75.

75. Maigne R. Le syndrome de la jonction dorso-lombaire. Douleur lombaire basse, douleur pseudo-viscérale, pseudo douleur de hanche et pseudo douleur pubienne. *Sem Hop (Paris)* 1981;57:545–554.

76. Ramsden CE, McDaniel MC, Harmon RL, et al. Pudendal nerve entrapment as source of intractable perineal pain. *Am J Phys Med Rehabil* 2003;82: 479–484.

77. Cervero F, Laird JM. Understanding the signalling and transmission of visceral nociceptive events. *J Neurobiol* 2004;61(1):45–54.

78. Procacci P, Maresca M. Clinical approach to visceral sensation. In: Cervero F, Morrison JFB, eds. *Visceral Sensation. Progress in Brain Research.* Amsterdam: Elsevier, 1986;67:21–28.

79. Melzack R, Coderre TJ, Katz J, et al. Central neuroplasticity and pathological pain. *Ann N Y Acad Sci* 2001;933:157–174.

80. Vecchiet L, Giamberardino MA, Dragani L et al. Pain from renal/ureteral calculosis: evaluation of sensory thresholds in the lumbar area. *Pain* 1989; 36:289–295.

81. Laird JM, Roza C, Cervero F. Effects of artificial calculosis on rat ureter motiliy: peripheral contribution to the pain of ureteric colic. *Am J Physiol* 1997;272:1409–1416.

82. Chia YY, Chow LH, Hung CC, et al. Gender and pain upon movement are associated with the requirements for postoperative patient-controlled iv analgesia: a prospective survey of 2,298 Chinese patients. *Can J Anaesth* 2002; 49:249–255.

83. Brunner H, Weidner W, Schiefer HG. Studies on the role of Ureaplasma urealyticum and Mycoplasma hominis in prostatitis. *J Infect Dis* 1983;147: 807–813.

84. Olavi L, Make L, Imo M. Effects of finasteride in patients with chronic idiopathic prostatitis: A double-blind, placebo-controlled, pilot study. *Eur Urol* 1998;33:24–34.

85. de la Rosette JJ, Karthaus HF, van Kerrebroeck PE, et al. Research in 'prostatitis syndromes': the use of alfuzosin (a new alpha 1-receptor-blocking agent) in patients mainly presenting with micturition complaints of an irritative nature and confirmed urodynamic abnormalities. *Eur Urol* 1992;22:222–227.

86. de la Rosette JJ, Debruyne FM. Nonbacterial prostatitis: a comprehensive review. *Urol Int* 1991;46:121–125.

87. Drach GW. Trimethoprim sulfamethoxazole therapy of chronic bacterial prostatitis. *J Urol* 1974;111:637–639.

88. McGuire EJ, Lytton B. Bacterial prostatitis: treatment with trimethoprim-sulfamethoxazole. *Urology* 1976;7:499–500.

89. Meares EM. Long-term therapy of chronic bacterial prostatitis with trimethoprim-sulfamethoxazole. *Can Med Assoc J* 1975;112:22–25.

90. Schaeffer AJ, Darras FS. The efficacy of norfloxacin in the treatment of chronic bacterial prostatitis refractory to trimethoprim-sulfamethoxazole and/or carbenicillin. *J Urol* 1990; 144:690–693.

91. Childs SJ. Ciprofloxacin in treatment of chronic bacterial prostatitis. *Urology* 1990;35:15–18.

92. Weidner W, Schiefer HG, Brähler E. Refractory chronic bacterial prostatitis: a re-evaluation of ciprofloxacin treatment after a median followup of 30 months. *J Urol* 1991;146:350–352.

93. Cox CE. Ofloxacin in the management of complicated urinary tract infections, including prostatitis. *Am J Med* 1989;87:61S–68S.

94. Pust RA, Ackenheil-Koppe HR, Gilbert P, et al. Clinical efficacy of ofloxacin (tarivid) in patients with chronic bacterial prostatitis: preliminary results. *J Chemother* 1989;1(suppl 4):869–871.

95. Remy G, Rouger C, Chavanet P, et al. Use of ofloxacin for prostatitis. *Rev Infect Dis* 1988;10(suppl 1):173–174.

96. Nickel JC, Weidner W. Chronic prostatitis: current concepts and antimicrobial therapy. *Infect Urol* 2000;13:22.

97. Nickel JC. Prostatitis: evolving management strategies. *Urol Clin North Am* 1999;26:737–751.

98. Barbalias GA, Meares EM Jr., Sant GR. Prostatodynia: clinical and urodynamic characteristics. *J Urol* 1983;130:514–517.

99. Osborn DE, George NJ, Rao PN, et al. Prostatodynia—physiological characteristics and rational management with muscle relaxants. *Br J Urol* 1981;53: 621–623.

100. de la Rosette JJ, Karthaus HF, van Kerrebroeck PE, et al. Research in 'prostatitis syndromes': the use of alfuzosin (a new alpha 1-receptor-blocking agent) in patients mainly presenting with micturition complaints of an irritative nature and confirmed urodynamic abnormalities. *Eur Urol* 1992;22:222–227.

101. Neal DE Jr., Moon TD. Use of terazosin in prostatodynia and validation of a symptom score questionnaire. *Urology* 1994;43:460–465.

102. Golio G. The use of finasteride in the treatment to chronic nonbacterial prostatitis. Abstracts of the 49th Annual Meeting of the Northeastern Section of the American Urological Association, Phoenix, AZ: 1997;128.

103. Holm M, Meyhoff HH. Chronic prostatic pain. A new treatment option with finasteride? *Scand J Urol Nephrol* 1997;31:213–215.

104. Meares EJ. Prostatitis and related disorders. In: Walsh PC, Retik AB, Stamey TA, Vaughan EDJ, eds. *Campbell's Urology.* Philadelphia: WB Saunders, 1992:807.

105. Wedrén H. Effects of sodium pentosanpolysulphate on symptoms related to chronic non-bacterial prostatitis. A double-blind randomized study. *Scand J Urol Nephrol* 1987;21:81–88.

106. Canale D, Scaricabarozzi I, Giorgi P, et al. Use of a novel non-steroidal anti-inflammatory drug, nimesulide, in the treatment of abacterial prostatovesiculitis. *Andrologia* 1993;25:163–166.

107. Canale D, Turchi P, Giorgi PM, et al. Treatment of abacterial prostato-vesiculitis with nimesulide. *Drugs* 1993;46(suppl 1):147–150.

108. Hetrick DC, Glazer H, Liu YW, et al. Pelvic floor electromyography in men with chronic pelvic pain syndrome: a case-control study. *Neurol Urodyn* 2006;25(1):46–49.

109. Kamihira O, Sahashi M, Yamada S, et al. [Transrectal hyperthermia for chronic prostatitis.] *Nippon Hinyokika Gakkai Zasshi* 1993;84:1095–1098.

111. Kumon H, Ono N, Uno S, et al. [Transrectal hyperthermia for the treatment of chronic prostatitis.] *Nippon Hinyokika Gakkai Zasshi* 1993;84:265–271.

112. Montorsi F, Guazzoni G, Bergamaschi F, et al. Is there a role for transrectal microwave hyperthermia of the prostate in the treatment of abacterial prostatitis and prostatodynia? *Prostate* 1993;22:139–146.

113. Shaw TK, Watson GM, Barnes DG. Microwave hyperthermia in the treatment of chronic abacterial prostatitis and prostatodynia: Results of a double-blind placebo controlled trial. *J Urol* 1993;149:405A.

114. Nickel JC, Sorenson R. Transurethral microwave thermotherapy of nonbacterial prostatitis and prostatodynia: initial experience. *Urology* 1994;44: 458–460.

115. Nickel JC, Sorensen R. Transurethral microwave thermotherapy for nonbacterial prostatitis: a randomized double-blind sham controlled study using new prostatitis specific assessment questionnaires. *J Urol* 1996;155:1950–1954; discussion 1954–1955.

116. Gray CL, Powell CR, Amling CL. Outcomes for surgical management of orchalgia in patients with identifiable intrascrotal lesions. *Eur Urol* 2001;39: 455–459.

117. Yaman O, Ozdiler E, Anafarta K, et al. Effect of microsurgical subinguinal varicocele ligation to treat pain. *Urology* 2000;55:107–108.

118. Padmore DE, Norman RW, Millard OH. Analyses of indications for and outcomes of epididymectomy. *J Urol* 1996;156:95–96.

119. Heidenreich A, Olbert P, Engelmann UH. Management of chronic testalgia by microsurgical testicular denervation. *Eur Urol* 2002;41:392–397.

120. Choa RG, Swami KS. Testicular denervation. A new surgical procedure for intractable testicular pain. *Br J Urol* 1992;70:417–419.

121. Padmore DE, Norman RW, Millard OH. Analyses of indications for and outcomes of epididymectomy. *J Urol* 1996;156:95–96.

122. Sweeney P, Tan J, Butler MR, et al. Epididymectomy in the management of intrascrotal disease: a critical reappraisal. *Br J Urol* 1998;81:753–755.

123. Thomson AJ, Jarvis SK, Lenart M, et al. The use of botulinum toxin type A (BOTOX) as treatment for intractable chronic pelvic pain associated with spasm of the levator ani muscles. *BJOG* 2005;112(2):247–249.

124. Bennett JD, Miller TA, Richards RS. The use of Botox in interventional radiology. *Tech Vasc Interv Radiol* 2006;9(1):36–39.

125. Naja MZ, Al-Tannir MA, Maaliki H, et al. Nerve-stimulator-guided repeated pudendal nerve block for treatment of pudendal neuralgia. *Eur J Anaesthesiol* 2006;23(5):442–444.

126. Robert R, Labat JJ, Bensignor M et al. Decompression and transposition of the pudendal nerve in pudendal neuralgia: a randomized controlled trial and long-term evaluation. *Eur Urol* 2005;47(3):403–408.

127. Chong MS, Hester J. Pharmacotherapy for neuropathic pain with special reference to urogenital pain. In: Baranowski AP, Abrams P, Fall M, eds. *Urogenital Pain in Clinical Practice.* Marcel Dekker, Inc., 2007.

128. Spinal cord stimulation for the management of pain (2005), http://www.britishpainsociety.org/pub_professional.htm#spinalcord

129. Urge incontinence and urinary frequency http://www.nice.org.uk/guidance/index.jsp?action=download&o=30827

130. Faecal incontinence http://www.nice.org.uk/guidance/index.jsp?action=download&o=30919

CHAPTER 66 ■ CRANIAL NEURALGIAS

ANITA H. HICKEY, STEVEN SCRIVANI, AND ZAHID BAJWA

INTRODUCTION

Since the last edition of this book was written, advancements in various diagnostic capabilities have improved our understanding of the etiology and pathogenesis of the neuralgias of the face, head, and neck. Recent modifications in the nomenclature have also occurred which reflect a more accurate organization and classification of the cranial neuralgias and facial pain. Although the nomenclature of these severe and often incapacitating pain syndromes remains controversial, immense efforts have been made to scientifically categorize these syndromes based on causal factors, when known, or strict diagnostic criteria, when causal factors are not known.[1-3] Although not perfect, this classification system continues to be refined and to serve as a valuable instrument to further advance the scientific understanding and treatment of these disorders.[4] The importance of accurate diagnosis and classification of these conditions is particularly critical as it pertains to treatment of many of the neuralgias for which successful medical and surgical treatments have been developed.

Cranial neuralgias refer to paroxysmal pain in the distribution of a specific cranial nerve. Previous classifications separated facial pain into "typical," "atypical," and "secondary" neuralgias. Because a great portion of the current literature continues to utilize these terms, it is important to understand the meaning of both the previously used nomenclature and the revised nomenclature.[2] Other features ascribed to the previous classification system are described in Table 66.1.

The revised classification system utilizes the terms "classical" and "symptomatic." The term classical refers to trigeminal neuralgia (TN) of unknown etiology. Classical rather than primary has been applied to those patients with a typical history even though a vascular or other source of compression or demyelination may be discovered during its course. The term symptomatic or secondary can then be reserved for those patients in whom a neuroma, tumor, multiple sclerosis (MS), or other cause has been demonstrated.

The term persistent idiopathic facial pain has replaced atypical facial pain in the taxonomy. This change reflects a lack of known mechanisms, continued recognition of the potential contribution of multiple etiologic factors to this syndrome, and an emerging knowledge of the pathophysiology of diffuse pain syndromes previously not well understood.[5-8]

This chapter is organized around the current classification of neuralgias of the cranial nerves and associated disorders. We cover most of these but particularly emphasize TN as this single disorder is best studied amongst cranial neuralgias and offers the

TABLE 66.1

CHARACTERISTICS OF FACIAL PAIN SYNDROMES

Feature	Typical Neuralgia	Atypical Neuralgia Unilateral Facial Pain	Persistent Idiopathic Facial Pain (Formerly Atypical Facial Pain)
Frequency	Intermittent: every few moments to once a day or less	Constant, can fluctuate	Constant, not much variation
Pain-free Intervals	Always	Rarely	Never
Description	Electric shock, stabbing, shooting	Burning, aching, can have superimposed shocks	Burning, aching
Location	Unilateral; usually trigeminal, rarely nervus intermedius, glossopharyngeal, vagus, upper cervical	Trigeminal or upper cervical. Unilateral, rarely bilateral	Not restricted to specific cranial nerve distribution. Intraoral or facial. Can extend to neck. Starts unilateral. May progress to bilateral
Sensory Changes	None or mild hypesthesia	Often hypesthesia	Common hypesthesia Dysesthesia, paresthesias
Precipitating Factors	Triggered by nonnoxious stimulation, often in anterior face and remote from face	Rarely triggered; trigger usually in area of pain	Not triggered
Autonomic Changes	None	Rarely present	None
Local Tenderness	None	Rare	Rare
Causative Factors	Vascular compression of nerve in subarachnoid space; rarely MS	Tumor, infection, trauma or mechanical impingement on nerve; MS, often no cause found	None known
Common age at onset (year)	>50	30	Variable
Gender	60% female	75% female	90% female

most reports of diverse clinical experiences. Emphasis will also be made on updates in classification, diagnosis, and treatment of cranial neuralgias. A narrative bridge from past literature and understanding is included to enhance the reader's understanding of more recent research, insights, and therapeutic approaches.

CLASSICAL TRIGEMINAL NEURALGIA

History

TN was described as early as the first century AD in the writings of Aretaeus (Fig. 66.1). Treatments at that time included bloodletting and the application of bandages containing arsenic, mercury, hemlock, cobra, and bee venom as well as other poisons. Eleventh century Arab physician Jurjani advanced the vascular compression theory as the causative factor of the severe pain and spasm of this syndrome.[9] The first clinical descriptions of TN in the European literature has been ascribed to Johannes Bausch in 1672 and John Locke in 1677. French physician Nicolaus André, who in 1756 described five cases of "unbearably painful twitch," is credited with first recognizing this condition as a unique medical entity. It was André who coined the term tic douloureux ("painful spasm"). English physician John Fothergill similarly published a full account of the syndrome and presented the paper to the Medi-

cal Society of London in 1773 and thus the disorder has sometimes been referred to him.[9–11] Other historical names for TN include prosopalgia and neuralgia of the fifth.

In a treatise on neuralgia published by Massachusetts physician E.P. Hurd in 1890, the following description of the clinical presentation of TN is found: "Probably no more atrocious suffering is known. . .During the attack, the patients utter loud outcries, toss about on their beds and smite their heads. The muscles of the affected side of the face are often the seat of rapid contractions, convulsive shocks, which have given to this disease one of the names by which it is known,(tic douloureux). These contractions may be limited to single groups of muscles, as the zygomaticae, or the frontal part of the occipito-frontales. . .then the paroxysmal shocks diminish in frequency and intensity, and all becomes calm; the storm has passed, to be renewed again under the same form in a time not far distant."[12]

In the nineteenth century, susceptibility to this condition was thought to be secondary to hereditary factors (with "the ancestors of the neuralgic subject being either neuralgic or sufferers from hysteria, epilepsy, or other neurosis"), in combination with other factors such as disease, intemperance, or insufficient diet. Medical treatment was ineffective until the introduction of trichloroethylene inhalation in the 1920s. Prior to this, treatment in the late 1800s focused on advocating a nutritious diet, adequate sleep, hydrotherapy, vigorous exercise, and moderation in all things. Patients were advised to avoid strain, reading, and brain work, which were felt to be instrumental in initiating an attack, as well

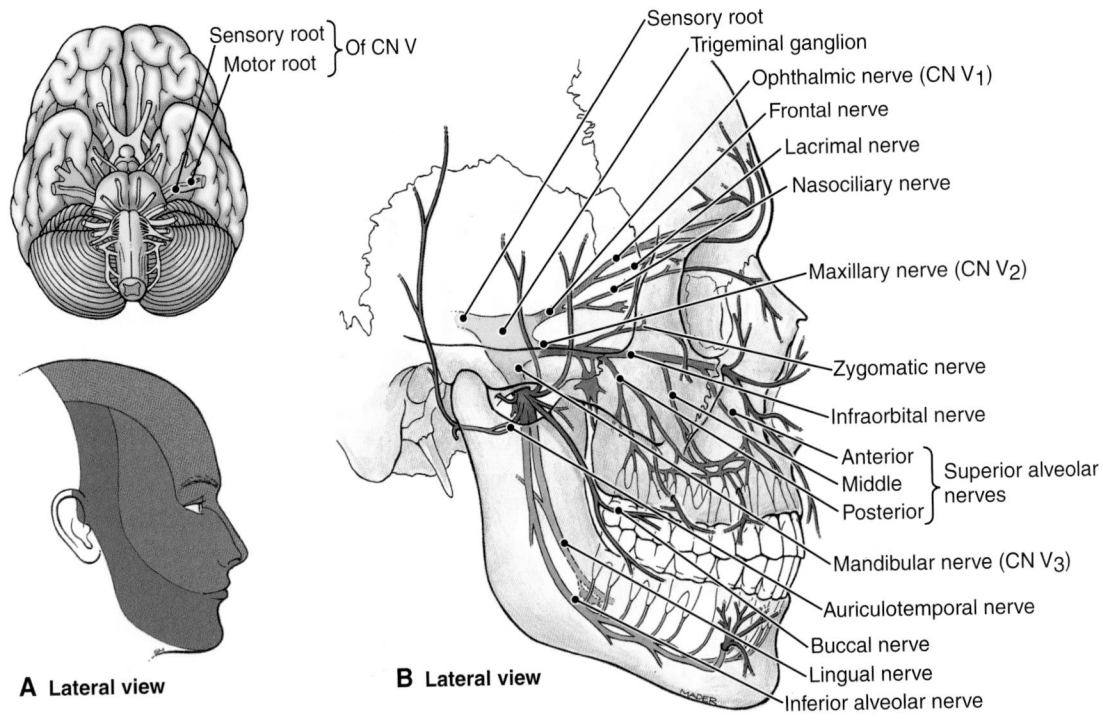

A Lateral view

B Lateral view

■ Ophthalmic nerve (CN V$_1$)
■ Maxillary nerve (CN V$_2$)
■ Mandibular nerve (CN V$_3$)

FIGURE 66.1 Distribution of the trigeminal nerve (cranial nerve V). The trigeminal nerve gives rise to three divisions: V1, the ophthalmic nerve, V2, the maxillary nerve, and V3, the mandibular nerve. Each division provides sensory innervations to the skin, subcutaneous tissue, and dura mater. The sensory fibers from each division pass through an autonomic ganglion and project the postsynaptic parasympathetic fibers from that ganglion (V1 for the ciliary ganglion, V2 for the pterygopalatine ganglion, and V3 for the submandibular and otic ganglia). V3 additionally supplies motor innervations to four pairs of muscles: temporal, masseter, lateral and medial pterygoid muscles. (From Moore KL, Dalley AF. *Clinically Oriented Anatomy*. 5th ed. Baltimore: Lippincott Williams & Wilkins; 2006.)

as alcohol, tobacco, and other stimulants. Successful nonsurgical treatment for TN was reported by such notable nineteenth century physicians as Wilhelm Erb and Duchenne de Boulogne. These included the use of electrotherapy in the form of interrupted current and galvanism.[11,12]

Although early attempts at surgical treatment of TN by Mareschal, surgeon to King Louis XIV of France, around 1750 and Veillard and Dussans in 1768 were unsuccessful, Bell and Magendie's clarification of the anatomy and function of the trigeminal and facial nerves in the early nineteenth century is thought to have contributed to subsequent effective surgical treatments for facial pain. Successful neurectomy of the inferior maxillary nerve was reported by Dr. Joseph Pancoast of Philadelphia in 1840 and in 1851. Dr. J. M. Carnochan described successful resection of the maxillary nerve and removal of Meckel's ganglion from the foramen rotundum to the infraorbital foramen. Subsequent surgical advances in technique were made by Horsley, Taylor, and Coleman in 1891 (middle fossa approach) and Hartley and Krause in 1892 (subtemporal approach). Cushing's modification to this approach, reported in 1900, involved approaching the trigeminal ganglion from below the middle meningeal artery. His contribution was credited with decreasing the mortality rate of the surgery to 5%. In 1921, Frazier suggested electrical stimulation to clearly define and spare the motor root, and in 1928, Stookey recommended differential sectioning of the sensory fibers of only the affected divisions of the trigeminal nerve. In 1925, Dandy reported a novel lateral suboccipital or cerebellar approach which preserved the motor root and was associated with little blood loss. Because of his posterior fossa approach, he was able to observe vascular loops impinging on the root entry zone (REZ) in many patients and inferred that this was the cause of trigeminal neuralgia.[11,12]

In 1967, Peter Jannetta reported use of the posterior fossa approach with the aid of an operating microscope.[13,14] He was able to confirm Dandy's observations of vascular loops compressing the REZ and subsequently performed a large series of successful surgical treatment of patients with TN using a technique that became known as microvascular decompression (MVD). MVD involves decompression of the nerve by moving the offending vascular loop(s), which are then restrained with nonabsorbent Teflon felt. Due to its low complication and high success rates, MVD has become the surgical procedure of choice for the treatment of intractable trigeminal neuralgia. The history of the medical and surgical treatments for TN has recently been thoroughly reviewed by Cole, Liu, and Apfelbaum.[1,11,12]

Epidemiology

Several epidemiological studies have collected data on the incidence of TN during the last 60 years. Although there is some variation in the reported incidence, in all cases it continues to be reported as a rare neurologic disorder. A U.K. study by Brewis et al.[15] published in 1966 reported an incidence of 2 per 100,000. This number was thought to be low due to lack of inclusion of patients seen by otolaryngologists. U.S. studies by Kurtzke[16] in 1982 and Katusic et al.[17] in 1990 reported an incidence of 4 and 4.8, respectively (age and sex adjusted per 100,000 per year). A prospective U.K. study by MacDonald et al.[18] reported an incidence of 8 per 100,000 per year. The most recently published epidemiological study was also performed in the United Kingdom and reported an incidence of 26 per 100,000 per year between January 1992 and April 2002.[19] This study reviewed patients diagnosed with TN by general practitioners rather than those referred to specialists.

The incidence of TN has consistently been found to be higher in females with a 1.74:1 female/male ratio. Onset is usually after age 40 with peak occurrence between ages 50 and 80. Occurrence

in patients younger than age 40 should raise suspicion of secondary causes such as tumor or MS. TN occurs rarely in children.[20,21]

Etiology and Pathophysiology

The various pathologic findings reported and complex theories advanced in the TN literature attempt to explain the combination of unique clinical features of TN such as:

- Stereotyped paroxysms of lancinating pain which occur in a limited part of the trigeminal territory
- Separation of the trigger area from the painful region
- Nonnoxious triggers
- Absence of sensory or motor deficit
- Characteristic response of TN to antiepileptic medications

New diagnostic techniques are now challenging theories that were previously advanced to resolve the many questions which remain regarding the etiology and pathophysiology of TN.

Observation of surgical findings led to the twentieth century vascular compression theory of TN. This theory was proposed when Dandy, Gardner, and Miklos and recognized the presence of a groove or distortion of the trigeminal nerve root by vessels, or rarely tumors. Jannetta produced convincing evidence that this was the cause of TN by his large series of effective microvascular decompression surgeries using the operating microscope. He also demonstrated the absence of trigeminal nerve compression in patients undergoing suboccipital craniotomy for other reasons and in a series of fresh cadaver studies.[11,13,14] Jannetta's[22] review of 4400 operative procedures from 1969 to 1999 revealed a rostroventral superior cerebellar artery loop compressing the trigeminal nerve either at the brainstem or distally to be the most common cause of vascular compression. Compression by the posterior inferior cerebellar, vertebral, and anterior inferior cerebellar arteries has been also been found. Other reported causes of compression of the trigeminal nerve have included meningiomas, epidermoid cysts, arachnoid cysts, and schwannomas arising from the nerve root itself.[23] Malis[24] proposed petrous ridge and fibrous dural band compression as a cause of TN and demonstrated successful alleviation of TN in a case series of 43 patients undergoing decompression of these fibrous bands.

Kerr[25] and King further argued a peripheral versus a central mechanism for TN. Kerr's[25] peripheral hypothesis, based on epidemiology, surgical resections, and cadaver and animal studies, suggested that the paroxysmal neuralgic pain of TN with associated trigger zones is consistent with minor mechanical or pulsatile compression superimposed upon predisposing axonal degenerative changes due to hypertension, atherosclerosis, or disease such as MS. He also noted that with aging, replacement of the bony roof of the carotid canal with connective tissue is known to occur. He argued that that these degenerative bony changes would permit pulsatile contact with areas of the ventral ganglion which correlate with the anatomic area in which most trigger zones are known to occur.[14,25]

King argued a central etiology for TN based on injections of alumina gel into the spinal nucleus of the fifth nerve in cats which resulted in a syndrome of dysesthesia of the face with over reaction to tactile stimulation.[21,25] Calvin et al.[26] proposed electrophysiologic mechanisms which required both peripheral and central events to produce the symptoms of TN. Fromm and colleagues[27] published studies which implicated an initial peripheral injury followed by failure of central inhibitory mechanisms as causative factors leading to the onset of TN.

The compression theory of TN, described by the findings of Dandy, Gardner, Miklos, Jannetta, and others, postulates a mechanism for production of the complex of TN symptoms that involves degenerative changes to the central peripheral myelin transitional zone of the trigeminal nerve, due to either direct or indirect effects of compression along the course of the nerve from the pons to its entry into Meckel's cave.[28] Recent ultrastructure analysis of trigeminal root biopsy specimens of patients with TN obtained during surgery for microvascular decompression support this theory. They reveal axonopathy, axonal loss, demyelination, and axon apposition without intervening glial processes consistent with the "ignition hypothesis" of TN. This model correlates the above pathophysiologic changes with the paroxysmal symptoms of TN based on similar foci of nerve root demyelination and juxtaposition of axons which have been demonstrated in patients with MS and TN together with experimental studies which indicate that this anatomic arrangement favors the ectopic generation of spontaneous nerve impulses and their ephaptic conduction to adjacent fibers. These studies also demonstrate that spontaneous nerve activity is likely to be increased by deformity of the nerve and frequently associated pulsatile vasculature.[29–32]

More conclusive evidence supporting both peripheral and central etiologies of TN can be found in recent electrophysiological studies. One such recent study has revealed evidence of peripheral damage to small A delta fibers of the trigeminal nerve near the REZ in the brainstem. Findings revealed demyelination and axonal degeneration or isolated advanced axonal damage on the symptomatic side in patients with classic TN (CTN). In patients with CTN and concomitant chronic facial pain, facilitation of central trigeminal processing at the supraspinal level was found. This is consistent with divergent results of MVD in these two groups of patients. Outcome data from MVD in patients with CTN shows excellent or good pain relief in 97% immediately postoperatively and in 80% of those with 5-year follow-up. In patients with TN and concomitant persistent facial pain, previously defined as "atypical," only 51% show good or excellent pain relief at 5 years.[33,34] Pre- and postoperative electrophysiological recording sessions revealed that relief of pain correlates with normalization of previously prolonged trigeminal reflex responses. Electrophysiological testing has also been able to differentiate CTN from symptomatic TN (STN) with a high degree of sensitivity and specificity (92% and 95%).[34,35] Although not practical for routine patient diagnostic purposes, this research is helpful in understanding the decreased response rates in these distinct groups of patients.

Symptoms and Signs

Clear and concise criteria are essential in establishing a diagnosis and conducting research for TN. This is particularly true for a condition such as TN where there is no objective laboratory test to confirm the clinical diagnosis. White and Sweet[36,37] helped to achieve these goals by publishing precise and succinct criteria which facilitated early and accurate clinical recognition of TN and facilitated subsequent research (Table 66.2). The International Headache Society recently established new clinical diagnostic criteria for TN as part of the International Classification

---

TABLE 66.2

SWEET CRITERIA

1. The pain in TN is paroxysmal.
2. The pain in TN may be provoked by light touch to the face.
3. The pain in TN is confined to the trigeminal zone.
4. The pain in TN is unilateral.
5. In a patient with TN, the clinical sensory examination is normal.

TABLE 66.3

INTERNATIONAL CLASSIFICATION OF HEADACHE DISORDERS, SECOND EDITION, DIAGNOSTIC CRITERIA FOR CLASSICAL AND SYMPTOMATIC TRIGEMINAL NEURALGIA

ICHD-II Diagnostic Criteria for Classical TN
A. Paroxysmal attacks of pain lasting from a fraction of a second to 2 minutes, affecting one or more divisions of the trigeminal nerve and fulfilling criteria B and C
B. Pain has at least one of the following characteristics:
   1. Intense, sharp, superficial, or stabbing
   2. Precipitated from trigger areas or by trigger factors
C. Attacks are stereotyped in the individual patient
D. There is no clinically evident neurologic deficit
E. Not attributed to another disorder

ICHD-II Diagnostic Criteria for Symptomatic TN
Pain indistinguishable from CTN but caused by a demonstrable structural lesion other than vascular compression.
A. Paroxysmal attacks of pain lasting from a fraction of a second to 2 minutes, with or without persistence of aching between paroxysms, affecting one or more divisions of the trigeminal nerve and fulfilling criteria B and C
B. Pain has at least one of the following characteristics:
   1. Intense, sharp, superficial, or stabbing
   2. Precipitated from trigger areas or by trigger factors
C. Attacks are stereotyped in the individual patient
D. A causative lesion, other than vascular compression, has been demonstrated by special investigations and/or posterior fossa exploration

There may be sensory impairment in the distribution of the appropriate trigeminal division. STN demonstrates no refractory period after a paroxysm unlike CTN.

---

of Headache Disorders, Second Edition (ICHD-II) (Table 66.3),[2] which have gained wide acceptance and reflect a significant advance that should further promote communication and stimulate research regarding TN.

CTN has well-described pathognomonic features which differentiate it from other types of facial pain. It is characterized by intense paroxysmal, electrical pain which may be accompanied by muscular spasms on the affected side of the face. The attacks generally last from fractions of a second to 2 minutes and are followed by a refractory period during which no pain can be triggered. Pain is abrupt in onset and termination. Between paroxysms, "the patient is in dreaded fear of the next flash of pain."[38] Occurrence of spontaneous remission of pain for weeks, months, or years is another feature of TN which may complicate accurate assessment of therapies.[39]

The pain of TN is limited to the distribution of one or more divisions of the trigeminal nerve and occurs most frequently in V2, V3, or a combination of V2 and V3. First division pain is rare in TN.[40] The pain of TN occurs on the right side of the face more often than the left with predominance ranging from 59% to 66%. Reviews have reported a 3% to 5% occurrence of bilateral pain. Pain rarely occurs on both sides simultaneously. Rather, the painful spasms occur on one side for weeks or months and then, following a period of remission, occur on the opposite side.[38,41–43] Pain occurring on both sides simultaneously or the presence of an abnormal neurologic exam should raise concerns of a secondary etiology such as tumor or MS.[44,45]

Trigger zones, or areas of the face or head that upon nonnoxious stimulation elicit a TN episode, are also a characteristic feature of TN. In two large series of patients with TN, trigger zones were reported to be present in 91%.[36,46] Trigger zones may be

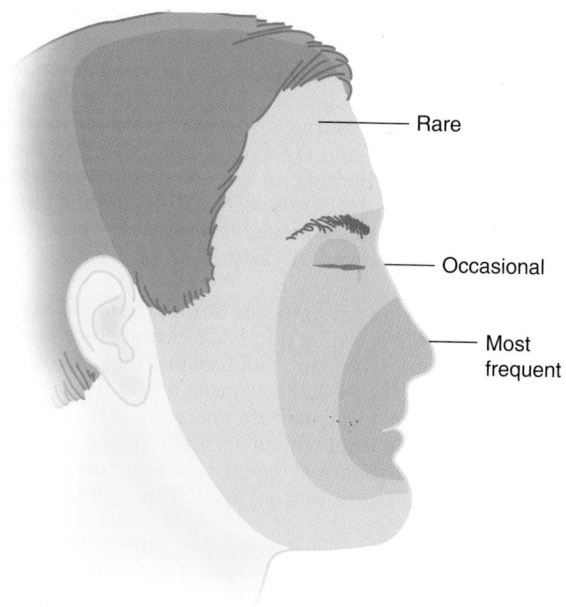

- Rare
- Occasional
- Most frequent

FIGURE 66.2 The most likely sites of triggering for tic douloureux are in the anterior face.

found in more than one division of the trigeminal nerve. The pain can also be triggered in a different zone from the trigger. The central part of the face near the nose and lips is the area in which triggers most often occur (Fig. 66.2). Touch and vibration have been found to be the most effective stimuli.[47] Attacks are reported to be set off by washing the face, shaving, talking, chewing, brushing of the hair and scalp, or a light breeze on the face of a patient. This can lead to poor hygiene, weight loss, dehydration, and social withdrawal. The ICHD-II criteria also list precipitation of pain paroxysms by "trigger areas" or "trigger factors." These triggers may include stimuli outside of the trigeminal distribution, such as a limb movement, and may include other sensory stimulation such as bright lights, loud noises, or tastes.[2]

Over time, some patients with CTN develop a persistent background pain in addition to their paroxysmal pain. This presentation is referred to as atypical TN in much of the past and current literature. Many studies report that these patients are significantly less responsive to pharmacologic and interventional therapies than those with CTN. This may be due to central facilitation of trigeminal nociceptive processing in these patients in accordance with recent electrophysiological findings.[33]

Pre-TN is an additional syndrome reported initially in 1949 by Symonds.[48] In these patients, a dull aching or burning pain involving a part of the upper or lower jaw develops for hours, days, or weeks and may be triggered by jaw movements or liquids. They may have several bouts of this pain with remissions for weeks, months, or years followed by sudden onset of the paroxysmal pain of CTN. Carbamazepine and/or baclofen have been effective in most cases. Unfortunately, some patients undergo multiple dental procedures before the syndrome is recognized as an early sign of TN.[48–50]

Differential Diagnosis

The diagnosis of TN is made essentially upon clinical information. Differentiating CTN from STN and other causes of facial pain is of great relevance in treating underlying disease or lesions and for instituting effective medical or surgical therapy. This requires a thorough history to obtain the patient's detailed description of defining characteristics, frequency and duration of pain,

exacerbating factors, presence or absence of triggers, and associated symptoms. A complete physical exam is necessary to confirm the presence or absence of neurologic deficits. Appropriate tests, including more advanced testing with computed tomography (CT) or magnetic resonance imagining/angiography (MRI/MRA) is often indicated to confirm the suspected diagnosis and exclude secondary causes.

Since TN is itself a rare disease, rare presentations of other disease processes fulfilling the diagnostic criteria of TN may require close examination. Rare cases of sinusitis presenting as CTN involving first and second division of the trigeminal nerve have been reported with one report of fatal progression in a diabetic patient.[51,52] Since involvement of the ophthalmic branch occurs in less than 5% of TN patients, a high degree of suspicion is indicated in such cases.

As the example above illustrates, it is important to differentiate CTN and STN since STN may be secondary to a progressive lesion or disease process. Expedient treatment of the underlying disease process or lesion in these cases may limit patient morbidity and mortality and improve overall patient outcome. Although most patients with malignant and benign tumors present with sensory deficit or persistent idiopathic facial pain, the literature does contain reports of patients with tumors initially presenting with TN and no neurologic deficits.[53,54].

MS is a common cause of symptomatic TN which should be considered in any person under 50 who presents with TN. Brainstem auditory evoked potential and blink reflex testing are sensitive methods for examining patients with TN. When the patient's neurologic exam is abnormal or if the patient does not respond to standard medical therapy, increasingly sensitive methods of CT or MRI/MRA result in accurate diagnosis in almost all cases.[55–59]

The cranial neuralgias covered in greater depth later in this chapter must also be differentiated from TN. Glossopharyngeal neuralgia presents with paroxysmal, electrical pain, spontaneous remissions, and triggers associated with swallowing, chewing, coughing, and talking in some patients. Pain occurs most frequently in the ear, tonsils, larynx, and tongue and may radiate to the neck, shoulder, or face. In less than 10% of cases there is an association with TN. Glossopharyngeal neuralgia is also rarely found in patients with MS.[60]

Intense and stabbing pain localized in the depth of the ear canal is also described in by patients with geniculate ganglion or nervus intermedius neuralgia, a rare disorder affecting the sensory branch of the facial nerve. Other cranial neuralgias which may be confused with TN include "tic convulsif" and hemifacial spasm.

Patients with tic convulsif present with severe otalgia combined with unilateral facial spasm. This rare neuralgic disease is thought to be due to vascular compression of the sensory and motor components of the facial nerve at their junction with the brainstem. Hemifacial spasm is a neuralgia involving the facial nerve which is characterized by intermittent, involuntary, irregular, unilateral contractions of muscles supplied by the ipsilateral facial nerve.[61–63]

Cluster headache pain is unilateral and usually occurs in the ocular, frontal, and temporal areas (though it may occur in the infraorbital and maxillary regions). It usually presents initially in men who are between 18 and 40 years old. Pain is severe, constant, stabbing, burning, and throbbing with associated ipsilateral ptosis, miosis, tearing, and rhinorrhea. Bouts often occur for several weeks to months with 1–3 attacks in a 24-hour period. Patients will not infrequently be woken from sleep with an attack. Pain-free intervals of several months may occur between bouts of attacks. These headaches tend to respond to ergot preparations, prednisone, and methysergide.[64]

Pain arising from a group of disorders known as trigeminal autonomic cephalgias may also be confused with TN. These include cluster headaches, chronic paroxysmal hemicranias, and short-lasting unilateral neuralgiform headaches with conjunctival injection and tearing (SUNCT). Knowledge of their epidemiology and a careful history will assist with accurate diagnosis.[65]

Chronic paroxysmal hemicrania usually occurs in women. It generally involves the ocular, frontal, and temporal areas. Occasionally, it may involve the occipital, infraorbital, aural, mastoid, and nuchal areas on the same side. Attacks vary in frequency in duration but may last 5–45 minutes. Pain is excruciating and is associated with ipsilateral conjunctival injection, lacrimation, nasal stuffiness, and rhinorrhea. These headaches respond well to indomethacin.[66]

SUNCT is a rare syndrome which typically affects males between age 23 and 77 years of age. It is characterized by unilateral burning, stabbing, or electric pain which is usually near the eye. Episodes generally last from 15 to 120 seconds and multiple episodes can occur daily. Patients present with cutaneously triggered attacks in up to 75% of cases. These attacks are differentiated from TN by lack of a refractory period and presence of associated conjunctival injection, tearing, rhinorrhea, and facial sweating or flushing. As in TN, primary and secondary forms occur. Secondary forms may be due to cerebellopontine angle arteriovenous malformation, infection, and pituitary tumors.[65,67,68]

Painful ophthalmoplegia such as seen in Tolosa-Hunt syndrome, ocular diabetic neuropathy, ophthalmic herpes zoster, and ophthalmoplegic migraine must also be differentiated from TN.

Tolosa-Hunt syndrome is a painful ophthalmoplegia caused by granulomatous inflammation in the cavernous sinus. It is characterized by episodic unilateral or bilateral orbital pain associated with paralysis of one or more of the third, fourth, or sixth cranial nerves. Involvement of the V2 and V3 divisions of the trigeminal nerve, the optic nerve, and the facial nerve has been reported. The pain is typically described as steady gnawing or boring. Spontaneous resolution may be followed by remissions and relapses of symptoms. Involvement of the optic, facial, acoustic, or trigeminal nerves has been reported. Treatment with corticosteroids results in resolution of pain and paresis in most cases within 72 hours. Failure of response to steroids or recurrence of symptoms should prompt further work-up.[2]

Ocular diabetic neuropathy may present as eye and forehead pain associated with ocular cranial nerve paresis (usually cranial nerve III). As in other diabetic neuropathies, pain improves with glucose control, treatment with tricyclics, and anticonvulsant medications.[2]

Herpes zoster (HZ) involving the trigeminal ganglion affects the ophthalmic division in the majority of cases. Ophthalmic herpes may be accompanied by palsies of the third, fourth, and/or sixth cranial nerves or with facial palsy. Burning pain, sometimes accompanied by neuralgic pain, is typically followed by vesicular eruption within 7 days. Pain may resolve or persist as postherpetic neuralgia.[2]

Ophthalmoplegic migraine is a rare clinical entity presenting as recurrent migraine like headaches accompanied by paresis of one or more of the ocular cranial nerves in the absence or other intracranial lesion. There may be a latent period of up to 4 days from onset of headache to onset of ocular cranial nerve paresis. Demonstration on MRI of thickening and enhancement of the cisternal part of the occulomotor nerve in these patients suggests the etiology of recurrent demyelinating neuropathy.[2]

Other common causes of facial pain include pain caused by sinusitis or other inflammatory conditions involving the eyes, tumors of the nose or sinuses, disorders of the teeth, jaws, or related structures such as temporomandibular joint (TMJ) pain and posttraumatic pain of the peripheral branches of the trigeminal nerve.

Sinusitis presents with pain involving the periocular, frontal, nasal, and maxillary areas. It is generally described as deep and constant and is associated with purulent discharge, fever, and fullness of the nose and ears. CT reveals opacification of the sinuses. In older patients or immunocompromised individuals, tumors or mycoses should be ruled out.[69]

Pain related to the teeth is often triggered by chewing or by hot, cold, sweet, and sour substances. It may have occasional sharp and shooting characteristics but usually will also have a diffuse, continuous aching, throbbing, or burning component which is difficult to localize. This type of pain is also differentiated from TN by lack of trigger zones or periods of spontaneous remissions. TMJ pain and myofascial pain related to the jaw is described as aching, burning, or cramping pain associated with use of the jaw or muscles of mastication. Clicking and other signs of joint dysfunction are associated features.[70,71] These topics are discussed in further detail in Chapter 67 on facial pain within this text.

Trauma to peripheral branches of the trigeminal nerve after surgery, blunt or penetrating trauma, or dental procedures generally presents as constant pain with burning, tingling, or stabbing components as well as a dull background pain. One study comparing patients with facial pain after nerve injury to patients with pain of spontaneous origin found decreased temperature and tactile thresholds and abnormal temporal summation of pain in patients with nerve injury but not in patients with spontaneous pain.[72]

Persistent idiopathic facial pain is typically described as a continuous, dull ache that is poorly localized. It fluctuates in intensity and is generally unresponsive to analgesics. It occurs most frequently in women with a mean age of 44.6 years and range of 17–87 years. Most of these patients have multiple diagnoses including depression, headache, neck and back pain, and irritable bowel disease. Neurologic and radiologic exams are normal by definition. These patients often have undergone multiple dental procedures.[73]

Treatment

Treatment—Medical Management

The use of the antiepileptic medications for the treatment of TN was first suggested by Bergougan in 1942.[74] His trial of phenytoin in these patients was based on Trousseau's theory that the paroxysmal pain of TN was similar to the paroxysmal brain activity occurring in patients with epilepsy.[75]

Medical therapy of TN is largely based on the efficacy of drugs that have undergone double-blind evaluation. This is particularly important in light of the need to obtain expedient relief of the excruciating pain of the paroxysms suffered by these patients with proven therapies. The occurrence of unpredictable periods of prolonged spontaneous remission in patients with TN creates a greater likelihood of attributing successful treatment of this disease to ineffective agents. Surgical consultation should be sought early for patients with structural lesions and in patients refractory to medical treatment. For patients unresponsive to medical therapy who are not surgical candidates due to coexisting medical conditions, treatment with radiation or percutaneous therapies, as described in the following paragraphs, may be effective.

Of the medications studied in the treatment of TN, carbamazepine is considered the drug of choice according to the European Federation of Neurological Societies and the Quality Standards Subcommittee of the American Academy of Neurology.[76] Current evidence suggests that oxcarbazepine should be the first line agent in patients with intolerable side effects or inadequate pain control with carbamazepine.[77] The combination of carbamazepine with baclofen or lamotrigine has been shown to be effective in cases where patients do not respond to carbamazepine alone or in whom it loses efficacy.[77]

Carbamazepine is a tricyclic antiepileptic that is metabolized at the same site targeted by the tricyclic antidepressant imipramine in the cytochrome P450 isoenzyme center. Carbamazepine slows the recovery rate of voltage-gated sodium channels, modulates activated calcium channel activity, and activates the descending inhibitory modulation system. Although it is one of the oldest antiepileptic drugs and many new drugs in this class exist with fewer side effects and fewer drug-drug interactions, four placebo-controlled studies and a systematic review have established its effectiveness in reducing the intensity and frequency of attacks and the number of triggers with a combined number needed to treat of 1.7.[78–82]

Although carbamazepine has been shown to have an initial response rate of over 70% in TN patients, one long term study which evaluated its efficacy over a 16-year period reported that by 5–16 years only 22% of participants continued to have effective relief with 44% requiring additional or alternative treatment.[83] The recommended starting dose is 100 to 200 mg twice daily with gradual increase by 200 mg until pain relief or intolerable side effects occur. The typical maintenance dose of carbamazepine is 600 to 1200 mg daily in divided doses. Side effects occur in up to 40% of patients initially but generally subside in most patients after a few weeks. The biologic half-life of carbamazepine is 30–35 hours when first administered. This decreases to 12 hours with autoinduction of liver enzymes which occurs after a few weeks. Since pain relief appears to be closely related to serum level, slow-release formulations may be effective in maintaining serum drug concentration.[84]

The efficacy of carbamazepine is limited by side effects that include drowsiness, dizziness, constipation, nausea, and ataxia. More severe adverse effects include rashes, leucopenia, abnormal liver function, and rarely, aplastic anemia and hyponatremia due to inappropriate secretion of antidiuretic hormone. Compared with placebo, it has a number needed to harm of 3 for minor side effects and 24 for major side effects. Monitoring of complete blood count, liver function, and sodium is recommended.[85–87]

Oxcarbazepine is the 10-keto analogue of carbamazepine. A large double-blind, crossover trial comparing oxcarbazepine with carbamazepine and three multicenter, double-blind randomized trials comparing oxcarbazepine to carbamazepine revealed equal efficacy with fewer adverse effects. Tolerability was reported as "good" to "excellent" by 62% of patients receiving oxcarbazepine, compared with 48% of patients receiving carbamazepine.[86,88]

Lamotrigine also decreases repetitive firing of sodium channels by slowing the recovery rate of voltage-gated channels. In a small, double-blind, crossover, randomized controlled trial evaluating patients on carbamazepine or phenytoin who were refractory to treatment with these medications, lamotrigine (400 mg) versus placebo increased the number of patients who improved after 4 weeks of treatment.[89] A case series also suggests its efficacy as monotherapy for TN. Side effects include dizziness, constipation, nausea, and drowsiness. Stevens-Johnson's syndrome has been reported to occur in 1 in 10,000 patients taking lamotrigine. Its utility as a single agent may be limited by its long titration schedule.[90,91]

Phenytoin is one of our oldest anticonvulsants with a molecular structure similar to the barbiturates. It acts by blocking sodium channels in rapidly discharging neurons and by inhibiting presynaptic glutamate release. Although it is has been used longer than any other antiepileptic drug in the treatment of TN, there are no controlled trials supporting its efficacy. Uncontrolled observations report that it is effective in relieving symptoms in 23 of 30 patients when 3–5 mg/kg was given intravenously for acute therapy.[92–94] Phenytoin interacts with many drugs including digoxin and warfarin. Severe rashes can occur in 1 of 10 to 20 patients. There is also a possibility of hyperglycemia, hepatotoxicity, gingival hyperplasia, and megaloblastic anemia. Fosphenytoin, a prodrug of phenytoin that is better tolerated intravenously, also appears to be effective in acutely ill patients.[95]

Baclofen is an analog of the neurotransmitter gamma-aminobutyric acid. Its effectiveness in the treatment of TN may be due to depression of excitatory synaptic transmission in the spinal trigeminal nucleus.[96] In three small randomized controlled trials, baclofen was shown to be effective as both monotherapy and add-on therapy to carbamazepine in the treatment of patients with TN. The starting dose is 5 to 10 mg three times a day, with gradual titration to a maintenance dose of 50 to 60 mg per day. Sedation, dizziness, and dyspepsia can occur with treatment. The dose should be adjusted in patients with decreased renal function since baclofen is excreted primarily by the kidneys. Baclofen has central nervous system and cardiovascular depressant effects and thus careful titration should occur in patients on other sedating medications and on antihypertensive agents. Antidiabetic medications may need to be adjusted secondary to increases in blood glucose. Baclofen should be discontinued slowly since seizures and hallucinations have been reported with upon withdrawal.[97–99]

Other medications that have shown efficacy in recent trials include subcutaneous sumatriptan and intranasal lidocaine. Two randomized, placebo-controlled crossover studies with a total of 38 patients show significant relief of painful paroxysms of TN after subcutaneous sumatriptan but not placebo. Continuation of oral sumatriptan, 50 mg orally twice a day, resulted in continuous analgesia following the subcutaneous injection in one of the studies.[100,101] Intranasal 8% lidocaine spray was examined in 25 patients with V2 division TN in a randomized controlled trial crossover study resulting in moderate or better pain relief in 23 of 25 subjects receiving lidocaine spray and 1 subject receiving placebo. Relief lasted from 0.5–24 hours.[102]

Uncontrolled observations and case studies have shown efficacy in the treatment of TN with valproic acid, clonazepam, and pimozide.[103–106] The efficacy of pimozide is severely limited by its significant side effects which include parkinsonism, mental retardation, and memory impairment. The newer anticonvulsant drugs gabapentin and topiramate have been shown to be effective in the treatment of neuropathic pain; however, there are no controlled studies of their effectiveness in the treatment of TN. Small case series report their effectiveness in the treatment of symptomatic TN secondary to MS.[107–109] A small prospective randomized study and a case report demonstrated relief of TN symptoms with injection of botulinum toxin (16–100 units).[110,111] A six patient retrospective analysis and an eight patient prospective trial of intravenous lidocaine, in doses ranging from 2 to 5 mg/kg/hour, resulted in partial or complete relief of TN pain paroxysms provoked by vibratory symptoms.[112,113]

In summary, the current literature supports carbamazepine as first-line therapy for TN, although data also supports use of oxcarbazepine as first-line therapy, particularly in patients refractory to carbamazepine monotherapy or who have intolerable side effects. Those patients who do not respond to monotherapy may benefit from combination therapy with gabapentin, lamotrigine, topiramate, or baclofen. The newer anticonvulsant medication, pregabalin, has been shown to be effective in treating neuropathic pain; however, its use has not been reported in patients with TN. Intravenous phenytoin, fosphenytoin, or lidocaine, subcutaneous sumatriptan, or botulinum toxin injections may be effective in refractory cases of TN or for abortive treatment of severe, frequent acute attacks which may affect the patient's ability to eat or drink. Infusions should be conducted in a carefully monitored setting with appropriate medical attention and emergency equipment available. Due to reports of spontaneous intermittent or permanent remissions of TN, periodic withdrawal of medications is warranted in patients who have prolonged pain-free periods on oral medications.

Treatment—Nerve and Neurolytic Blockade

Local anesthetic injection or infusion has been used for diagnostic purposes and for temporizing treatment in patients with unbearable pain refractory to medical therapy and/or awaiting MVD.[114] No controlled studies of nerve blockade for relief of TN have been reported and controlled studies are needed to validate this approach. Small case series include significant reduction of pain and triggers in 5 elderly patients for a median of 2 months subsequent to injection of the infraorbital nerve in patients with second division TN using a combination of 4% tetracaine dissolved in 0.5% bupivacaine. Another study looking at relief of pain following injection of the infraorbital nerve reported greater than 3 months of relief with 4% tetracaine and 0.5% bupivacaine (compared to 3 days or less with 0.5% bupivacaine or 1% mepivacaine alone).[115,116] A combination of ketamine, morphine, and bupivacaine produced similar pain relief and duration as reported following a series of injections of symptomatic peripheral trigeminal nerve branches in patients with TN.[117]

A case report of stimulator-guided mandibular and maxillary division nerve blockade using a combination of lidocaine, bupivacaine, clonidine, and fentanyl at monthly intervals for 1 year in 2 patients describes prolongation of relief after 3 months and pain-free status with no recurrence at 9 month follow-up. No sensory or motor disturbances were reported.[118] Peripheral injections are of value in elderly patients who have not responded to medical or other surgical therapies. Standard precautions to avoid intravascular injection of drugs should be taken and care should be taken when performing V2 and V3 blockade as total brainstem anesthesia with respiratory arrest following extraoral trigeminal V2–V3 blocks has been reported.[119]

Careful aspiration, fluoroscopic guidance when available, utilizing contrast (when no contraindication exists), and digital subtraction can decrease the risk of intravascular or intrathecal injection. As with intravenous infusions, injections should be performed in a monitored setting with appropriate medical attention and readily available emergency equipment.

Alcohol, phenol, or glycerol injection has long been reported in the treatment of TN. Percutaneous gangliolysis using glycerol is discussed under surgical techniques. A retrospective case audit of patients who received peripheral alcohol injections for TN from 1994–1999 found a mean duration of effect of 11 months.[120] Effectiveness of peripheral alcohol injections in TN is believed to be comparable to peripheral cryotherapy. Glycerol injections provided a mean of 7 months of pain relief.[121] A retrospective analysis of 157 cases of intractable idiopathic TN treated with peripheral glycerol injections reported an initial 98% success rate with 60 patients having recurrent pain between 25 and 36 months. The study reports complete or near complete pain relief in 154 patients at 4 years (with inclusion of patients with recurrent pain who were reinjected).[122] Postinjection facial swelling, discomfort, and numbness are reported complications of alcohol injections. More serious complications occurred in 3 of 413 injections over a 20-year period.[123] A small case series of 60 peripheral injections in 18 patients of the infraorbital, supraorbital, and mandibular nerves using 10% phenol in glycerol reported 87% initial marked or total pain relief and a median of 9 months of continued relief. Most patients with recurrent pain requested a repeated procedure rather than surgery or a ganglion nerve block. No serious complications or dysesthetic pain were reported. In patients with facial sensory loss, sensation was recovered within 6 months and was well tolerated.[124]

Treatment—Surgical

Surgical therapies are aimed at either damaging or destroying pain transmitting nerve fibers or relieving pressure on the nerve from vascular loops, fibrous bands, or mass lesions. Radiation therapy may relieve pain in patients who are not surgical candidates and who are refractory to medical management of TN.

Microvascular Decompression. MVD is performed under general anesthesia using a microscope to visualize the trigeminal nerve as it leaves the pons via a suboccipital craniectomy. Compression of the nerve by a vein or artery is relieved by repositioning the artery or coagulating the vein. Although MVD is inva-

sive, it is associated with the best long-term outcome and overall mortality and complication rates are low. A recent analysis of long-term follow-up data of 1324 patients with TN who underwent MVD between 1976 and 2000 revealed an increase in the postoperative cure rate from 92.9% to 96.7% in patients operated on after 1986. Recurrence rate decreased from 10.2% to 6.5% in the patients operated on between 1986 and 2000 compared to the patients who underwent MVD between 1976 and 1986.[125] Barker[126] recently reported results of 1185 patients who underwent MVD over a 20-year period. It was noted that the rate of complications was significantly reduced and no deaths occurred after 1980 when intraoperative monitoring of brainstem evoked response was used. Female sex, symptoms lasting more than 8 years, venous compression of the terminal REZ, and the lack of immediate postoperative cessation of pain were significant predictors of eventual recurrence.[126] In a retrospective comparative analysis of 225 patients who underwent MVD and 206 having undergone percutaneous trigeminal radiofrequency rhizotomy, 64% of patients who underwent MVD remained completely pain free 20 years postoperatively versus 50% risk of recurrence of pain 2 years after radiofrequency rhizotomy.[127] Hospital and surgeon volume was found to be a significant factor affecting morbidity in a study conducted from 1996–2000 by Kalkanis and associates.[128] The overall mortality rate was 0.3% with volume and mortality not statistically related. The rate of discharge other than to home was 3.8%, with hospitals and/or surgeons who performed the surgeries at low volumes being 5.1% as compared to 1.6% for high volume.[128] Percutaneous rhizotomy or gangliolysis is useful in treating the elderly or debilitated patient who is refractory or intolerant to medical therapy and for whom surgery is not warranted due to risk factors. Gangliolysis is performed under fluoroscopic guidance by placing a needle percutaneously through the foramen ovale and advancing it to the trigeminal cistern.

The three techniques currently used for gangliolysis include percutaneous radiofrequency ablation/thermocoagulation, trigeminal ganglion compression, and retrogasserian glycerol rhizolysis. Percutaneous radiofrequency trigeminal gangliolysis involves the use of radiofrequency to create anatomically distinct lesions in cycles of 45–90 seconds at 60° to 90° C. Percutaneous trigeminal ganglion compression is performed under general anesthesia utilizing a Fogarty catheter that is inserted via a 14-gauge catheter into the trigeminal cistern and inflated with radiocontrast to compress the gasserian ganglion. Careful observation of heart rate and blood pressure is required due to the possibility of severe bradycardia and hypotension which may require treatment with atropine and vasopressors. Percutaneous glycerol rhizolysis is performed in a sitting position. After confirmation of needle location with radiocontrast, 0.1 to 0.4 mL of anhydrous glycerol is injected into the cistern of Meckel's cave.

A recent systematic review of radiofrequency ablation/thermocoagulation techniques for the treatment of TN demonstrated complete pain relief without medication in a median of 88% in patients undergoing radiofrequency thermocoagulation at 6-month follow-up.[129] This dropped to 61% at the 3-year follow-up. Retrospective analysis of patients undergoing percutaneous glycerol rhizolysis showed complete pain relief in 84% of patients with or without medication at 6 months following treatment. This dropped to a median of 54% at 3-year follow-up. There is insufficient data to compare pain relief from percutaneous balloon compression of the gasserian ganglion with the other ablative techniques.[129]

Complications with any of the ablative techniques described above have been noted to include dysesthetic disturbances in 4% to 10% of patients treated. Up to 30% of patients treated with radiofrequency thermocoagulation experienced significant permanent sensory loss. Other complications included corneal numbness and keratitis, anesthesia dolorosa, transient masseter weakness, cranial nerve deficits, and vascular injuries. The complication rate was highest in patients undergoing radiofrequency thermocoagulation though most complications were transient.[129]

Ablative procedures are less invasive than MVD and are generally associated with a high initial response rate. Recurrence is common, however, and the incidence of facial numbness is higher than with MVD. Patients who have a recurrence of TN after an ablative procedure can successfully undergo MVD.[126]

Peripheral Neurectomy. Surgical destruction of the peripheral branches of the trigeminal nerve is indicated for patients who have failed medical therapy, who have failed gangliolysis, or who have severe cardiopulmonary disease and are unable to tolerate a suboccipital craniectomy and MVD. Duration of good to excellent relief varies from less than 1 year to a range of 2–5 years in reported series. The median pain-free period among 88 patients in one series was 41 months with a mean of 52.5 months. A more recent analysis of 40 patients reported excellent to good results in all patients for a period of time ranging from 2–5 years.[130,131] The procedure can be repeated; however, the risk of neuroma as well as diminished success is increased. Dense numbness in the distribution of the eradicated nerve results following neurectomy.

Cryoablation of the peripheral branches of the trigeminal nerve can be performed using a 1.4 to 2 mm probe which incorporates a nerve stimulator to test both sensory and motor function as well as a thermistor to identify temperature at the tip of the probe. A 3.5 to 5.5 mm ice ball is produced which results in disruption of the nerve structure with wallerian degeneration while leaving the myelin sheath and endoneurium intact (axonotmesis).[132] The use of cryotherapy to successfully treat patients with TN has been reported by several authors to provide analgesia for periods ranging from 6–13 months. There was no permanent sensory loss although, in one review, up to one third of patients developed atypical facial pain following the procedure.[133–135]

Stereotactic Radiosurgery. The first radiosurgical device was developed in the 1950s by Professor Lars Leksell at the Karolinska Institute in Stockholm. This work resulted in the development of the gamma knife which is able to precisely irradiate small intracranial targets with gamma ray photons. The patient's head is immobilized by the use of an external metal frame which is attached to the skull by four screws. A large helmet with 201 fixed ports allows radiation from radioactive cobalt-60 sources to converge on the intracranial target. The goal of radiosurgical treatment for TN is the delivery of energy to the proximal trigeminal root with minimal injury to surrounding structures.[136,137] Improved targeting with MRI has resulted in pain-free results in 21.8% to 75% of patients and pain improvement in 65% to 88%. Gamma knife surgery (GKS) produces lesions aimed at target area with the use of a stereotactic frame.[138] Data on radiosurgery for TN is predominantly observational and of generally poor quality.[139–141]

In a recent outcome study reviewing 151 patients treated with GKS, patient age, right-sided pain, and previous neurectomy correlated with pain-free outcome. One study found that treatment response did not correlate with the dose of radiation.[142] Treatment response correlated with vascular compression of the trigeminal nerve, as visualized on high resolution MRI, in some[143] but not all[142,144] reports. Pain relief with GKS occurs after a lag time of about 1 month.[145,146] A systematic review of these data found that approximately 75% of patients report complete relief within 3 months, and 50% of patients can permanently stop drug therapy after surgery. Sensory disturbances (e.g., numbness, paresthesias, and dysesthesias) are the most frequent complications.[146] Although radiosurgery is less effective than MVD, it is an effective, minimally invasive treatment option for patient's refractory to medical therapy who are not surgical candidates or who wish to forego the risks of surgery. Patients who fail to respond to radiosurgery or who have recurrence of symptoms may respond to repeat treatment.[147,148]

Linear accelerator radiosurgery is an alternative to the gamma knife developed in the mid 1980s. Unlike the radioactive cobalt-based gamma knife, linear systems use x-ray beams generated from a linear accelerator. This system also uses a metal head frame which is attached to the patient's skull. Recent developments include intensity modulated radiation therapy, which employs computer-controlled "beam-shaping" to more precisely conform the beam to the shape of the target.[149] A case series of 22 patients who had failed medical therapy and either declined or were unsuitable to undergo a surgical procedure found that radiosurgery by this technique was safe and effective.[150]

CyberKnife radiosurgery is a more recently developed system to incorporate a miniature linear accelerator mounted on a flexible, robotic arm. This system offers targeting accuracy without the need for the invasive head frame and is able to treat tumors anywhere in the body. While GKS has the advantage of over 30 years of clinical use, recent observational studies using the CyberKnife system for the treatment of CTN report a 92.7% initial success for pain relief at a median latency to pain relief of 7 days. Long-term response rate at 11 months was 78%.[151] Larger study groups and longer follow-up is needed to further evaluate long-term pain relief and complications.

SYMPTOMATIC TRIGEMINAL NEURALGIA

STN is differentiated from CTN through demonstration by special studies of a causative lesion other than vascular compression. Sensory impairment and bilaterality may be present as well as lack of a refractory period after a paroxysm.[2] MS and benign or malignant neoplasms are the most common cause of STN, although fungal infection and bacterial sinusitis with intracranial extension, scrub typhus, hardened felt from previous microvascular decompression surgery, and TN as the first manifestation of mixed connective tissue disorder have also been reported.[151–156]

Multiple Sclerosis

MS is an inflammatory autoimmune systemic disease which is characterized by demyelinating lesions and plaques within the central nervous system. Widespread neuronal loss with periods of remyelination may be associated with periods of remission.

MS affects women more than men with a cumulative ratio of females to males of 1.77 to 1.0. Median and mean age of onset of MS is 23.5 and 30 years of age, respectively.[157] TN occurs in up to 2% of patients with MS although this represents only about 0.5% of patients presenting with TN.[158,159] These patients can present with symptoms which mimic CTN but often present with bilateral symptoms and persistent background facial pain.[159]

The pathophysiology of TN in MS continues to be debated. Although demyelinating lesions affecting the trigeminal REZ have been found on autopsy and on MRI, 24 MS patients out of a series of 851 studied at one institution were found to have entry zone lesions which were clinically silent.[160,161]

Although MVD was once thought to be contraindicated in MS patients with STN, a recent report of MVD performed in 35 MS patients with severe neurovascular compression at the REZ resulted in a 39% excellent and 22% fair to good long-term pain relief. Seventy-four percent of these patients had demyelinating lesions affecting the brainstem trigeminal pathway on the painful side in addition to neurovascular compression.[162] In a series of five patients with STN and MS who were refractory to medical treatment and had undergone multiple unsuccessful percutaneous procedures, those patients undergoing MVD combined with partial sectioning of the nerve did better than those undergoing MVD alone.[163]

In general, patients with STN secondary to MS respond less favorably to medical and interventional therapies and may require significantly more treatment than their cohorts with CTN.[164]

Neoplasm

The presentation of CTN does not rule out the presence of a tumor. Some authors advocate advanced imaging of all patients presenting with CTN due to delayed neurologic symptoms in patients with space-occupying lesions.[155] Among 2972 patients diagnosed with TN at the Mayo Clinic between 1976–1990, tumors were the cause of facial pain in 296 patients. Sex and pain distributions paralleled those in CTN; however, patients presenting with tumors were younger than those with CTN. Delay in tumor diagnosis averaged 6.3 years. The development of neurologic deficits prompted further imaging and diagnosis of tumor in 47% of these patients. These patients were often successfully treated medically for many years prior to onset of neurologic symptoms.[165,166]

Meningioma and epidermoid and acoustic neuroma are the most frequent posterior fossa tumors associated with STN. In a review of 161 and 80 consecutive posterior fossa tumors from 1993–1999 and 1979–2003 at separate institutions, cranial nerve dysfunction was the most common neurologic sign on admission. Intracranial hypertension and disturbance of gait also presented in up to 44% of these patients.[167,168] Twenty cases of TN caused by contralateral tumors of the posterior fossa have been reported. Only 4 of these cases symptomatically conformed to CTN. The mechanism of contralateral tumor causing TN is thought to be distortion and displacement of the brain stem and compression of the contralateral Meckel's cave.[169,170]

Pain in all three divisions of the trigeminal nerve is the first symptom of a tumor in Meckel's cave in over 65% of cases. The most common cavernous sinus tumors are trigeminal schwannomas and meningiomas. Tumors in this location make up only 0.5% of all intracranial tumors.[171] Case reports of metastatic disease to Meckel's cave presenting as TN include colorectal cancer, esophageal cancer, breast cancer, renal cell carcinoma, and lymphoma.[171–175] Primary melanoma, adenocarcinoma, and lymphoma involving Meckel's cave and associated with TN have also been reported.[176–179] TN with subacute onset of numbness in one or more divisions of the trigeminal nerve is thought to be associated with rapidly expanding tumor in this region.[175]

Other reported causes of symptomatic TN include platybasia (a skull base deformity),[180] sarcoid granuloma of the trigeminal nerve, and infarction of the REZ of the trigeminal nerve in the pons.[181–182] TN has also been seen in adults and children as the only manifestation of Chiari type I malformations.[183–185] Patients with hydrocephalus from remote causes such as a lumbar myxopapillary ependymoma and a quadrigeminal arachnoid cyst have also presented with TN.[186,187] Shunting and relief of hydrocephalus resulted in resolution of symptoms in these cases.

Five to 10% of TN has been reported to be STN secondary to brain tumors.[188] Although persistent pain, numbness, palsies, and gait disturbances along with other neurologic signs often differentiate these patients from those with CTN, delay in the presentation of neurologic deficits is not infrequent. Expedient work-up including advanced imaging is indicated in cases of TN with new onset of neurologic signs such as numbness or palsies.

Herpes Zoster and Postherpetic Neuralgia

Etiology

Acute HZ results from the reactivation of the varicella zoster virus which is referred to as "chicken-pox" in children or "shingles" in adults. The virus remains dormant in the dorsal root ganglia of cranial or spinal nerves after resolution of the original infection. As cellular immunity wanes with disease, chemotherapy, or age, the virus is reactivated and is transported along peripheral nerves producing an acute neuritis. Viral replication results in direct nerve sheath and neuronal injury. Destruction of tissue and inflammation result in excitation of nociceptors and dorsal horn sensitization. The dorsal horns of patients who do not develop postherpetic neuralgia show less tissue damage and more rapid resolution of inflammatory changes.[189]

Epidemiology

The rate of HZ and the rate of HZ-associated complications increase with age, with 68% of cases occurring in those aged 50 years and older. Postherpetic neuralgia occurs in 18% of adult patients with HZ and in 33% of those aged 79 years and older.[190]

In HZ involving the trigeminal nerve, neuronal spread of the virus occurs along the ophthalmic (first) and less frequently the maxillary (second) division of the fifth cranial nerve. Vesicular eruptions usually occur at the terminal points of sensory innervation, causing extreme pain. HZ involving the ophthalmic ganglion of the trigeminal nerve, or zoster ophthalmicus, accounts for as many as 10% to 25% of HZ cases. Nasociliary involvement will most likely cause ocular inflammation. Inflammation of the eye can lead to impairment of vision and in some cases temporary blindness. Such cases are considered emergent and prompt treatment is required to prevent chronic inflammation or long-term vision loss.

Contiguous spread of the virus may lead to the involvement of other cranial nerves, resulting in optic neuropathy (cranial nerve II) or isolated cranial nerve palsies (cranial nerve III, IV, or VI).

Symptoms and Signs

Acute HZ typically presents with a prodrome consisting of hyperesthesia, paresthesias, burning dysesthesias, or pruritus along the affected dermatome(s). This prodrome is usually accompanied by fever and general malaise. It generally lasts 1 to 2 days but may precede the appearance of skin lesions by up to 3 weeks. Manifestation of prodromal symptoms without development of the characteristic rash may occur in some patients. This presentation is known as "zoster sine herpete," and may delay correct diagnosis and treatment.

Following the prodromal period, a vesicular skin rash appears along the affected nerve. Involvement of the trigeminal nerves characteristically respects the vertical midline. The vesicles will discharge fluid and begin to scab over after about 1 week. The pain is extreme during the inflammatory stage. Vesicles at the tip of the nose are known as Hutchinson's Sign and signal a 75% likelihood of ocular sequelae which may include follicular conjunctivitis, epithelial and/or interstitial keratitis, dendritic keratitis, uveitis, scleritis chorioretinitis, optic neuropathy, and palsies of the third, fourth, or sixth cranial nerves.

Pain that persists beyond healing of the rash but which resolves within 4 months of onset is referred to as subacute herpetic neuralgia. Postherpetic neuralgia refers to pain persisting longer than 4 months from initial onset of rash.[191] Affected patients usually report constant, severe, burning, lancinating pain in the distribution of the affected nerve(s). Patients may also complain of pain in response to nonnoxious stimuli (allodynia). Even the slightest pressure from clothing, bed sheets, or a slight breeze may elicit severe pain.

Diagnosis

The diagnosis of acute HZ is essentially clinical, based on the characteristic unilateral appearance of a vesicular rash limited to the distribution of a specific nerve or nerve root. As discussed in the section on signs and symptoms above, this is preceded most commonly by a painful prodrome characterized by burning dysesthesias or paresthesias along the affected dermatome. The criterion standard of laboratory diagnosis is polymerase chain reaction testing together with direct identification of varicella zoster virus in culture. Immunocompromised patients may benefit from IgG- and IgA-anti varicella zoster virus antibodies.[192,193]

Treatment

The goals of treatment of acute HZ include treatment of the acute viral infection, treatment of the severe acute pain associated with HZ infection, and prevention of postherpetic neuralgia.

Acute HZ infection should be treated with antiviral medication within 72 hours of vesicular eruption to reduce the duration and severity of pain associated with the infection. The use of antivirals may produce a moderate reduction in the risk of development of postherpetic neuralgia. Oral steroids may also be beneficial in reducing the severe pain of acute HZ.[194]

Acute treatment of acute HZ with neuropathic analgesics (i.e., anticonvulsants or tricyclic antidepressants) starting within 48 hours of onset of rash may also reduce acute pain and incidence of postherpetic neuralgia.[195–198] Patients with ocular involvement should have immediate evaluation and treatment of ophthalmic complications by a specialist.

The varicella zoster vaccine approved in May 2006 by the U.S. Food and Drug Administration was found to reduce the incidence of shingles by 51% in a randomized double-blind study. Pain was reduced by 61% in those who received the vaccine but still developed the infection, and postherpetic neuralgia was reduced by two thirds compared with placebo.[199]

Nutritional counseling may also be indicated in populations at risk for HZ. In a review of 243 HZ cases, it was determined that individuals, particularly those over age 60, who ate less than one serving of fruit or vegetables weekly had a three-fold greater risk of HZ compared to those who ate more than three servings daily independent of vitamin supplement intake.[200] An association between deficiency of vitamin A (a key immune modulator involved in the synthesis of lymphocytes, neutrophils, cytokines, and immunoglobulins) and increased risk of HZ has also been observed.[201]

Systematic reviews of the literature have concluded that pharmacologic therapies shown to be more effective than placebo for postherpetic neuralgia include tricyclic antidepressants, opioids, gabapentin, pregabalin, tramadol, capsaicin, and lidocaine 5% patch. Intrathecal methylprednisolone was shown to be of benefit in patients refractory to pharmacologic therapies.[202,203] Safety and tolerability should be considered when selecting pharmacologic treatments. Older patients may have more intolerable side effects at standard doses and thus may require smaller doses and more gradual titration. They may also be on multiple medications for coexisting medical conditions with potential for drug-drug reactions.

Sympathetic blockade, including stellate ganglion block, has commonly been used to provide pain relief of variable duration in both acute HZ and in postherpetic neuralgia. Although a recent review of sympathetic blocks in the treatment of acute HZ and postherpetic neuralgia found the evidence to be inconclusive due to lack of properly controlled studies, it found available data to suggest that sympathetic blocks may provide considerable pain relief during acute HZ but appear to provide only short-term relief in postherpetic neuralgia.[204]

NERVUS INTERMEDIUS NEURALGIA

Nervus intermedius neuralgia is an uncommon disorder affecting the sensory branch of the facial nerve (cranial nerve VII) (Fig.

66.3). It is located between the motor component of the facial nerve and the vestibulocochlear nerve (cranial nerve VIII). Sensory fibers contained in the nervus intermedius nerve carry afferent sensory input from the skin of the external auditory meatus, mucous membranes of the nasopharynx and nose, and taste from the anterior two-thirds of the tongue, floor of the mouth, and the palate. The geniculate ganglion contains the cell bodies of the sensory fibers of the nervus intermedius. Compression of the geniculate ganglion therefore can also result in nervus intermedius neuralgia.

The cell bodies of parasympathetic axons within the nervus intermedius are contained within the superior salivatory nucleus. These axons synapse with neurons which supply parasympathetic innervations to the lachrymal gland as well as the submandibular and sublingual glands.

Nervus intermedius neuralgia involves severe pain deep in the ear which may radiate to the outer ear, mastoid, or eye region. The syndrome was reported as "Tic Douloureux of the sensory filaments of the facial nerve" by Clark and Taylor in 1909.[205] Rare cases continue to be reported.

Etiology

Vascular compression is suggested as the cause of many cases of nervus intermedius neuralgia. Jannetta described relief of nervus intermedius and other cranial neuralgias following MVD in 1976.[206] He more recently reviewed 14 cases of nervus intermedius neuralgia, which, after failed conservative treatment, went on to MVD. Over 71% experienced an excellent outcome, over 21% experienced partial relief, and 7% had no relief following MVD. Good long-term results were seen in 90% of patients.

In a 1991 review of 18 cases of "primary otalgia" seen over a 15-year period, vascular loops, adhesions, thickened arachnoid, and benign osteoma were among abnormalities involving the nervus intermedius. The authors reported decompression of cranial nerves V, IX, X, the tympanic nerve, and the chorda tympani in addition to the nervus intermedius in many of these cases.[207,208] Nonetheless, the existence of nervus intermedius as a unique entity has been questioned due to the similarity of its presentation to that of glossopharyngeal neuralgia.

Symptoms and Signs

The pain of nervus intermedius neuralgia is sharp, lancinating, and paroxysmal. Painful attacks are unilateral and can be triggered by cold, noise, swallowing, or touch. Patients may also experience symptoms such as increased salivation, bitter taste, tinnitus, and vertigo during paroxysms. Patients with nervus intermedius neuralgia may also rarely have pain in the trigeminal distribution. This may be due to cross compression of cranial nerve V in addition to the nervus intermedius (as has been seen on surgical exploration).[209]

Diagnosis

Sensation is supplied to the area of the ear by the cranial nerves V, VII, VIII, IX, and X and the second and third cervical nerves. A thorough history should be taken to ascertain the exact distribution and character of the pain as well as any triggers or precipitating factors. A comprehensive examination should rule out other causes of otalgia before the diagnosis of geniculate ganglion neuralgia can be made. This should include examinations of the nose, paranasal sinuses, mouth, teeth, nasopharynx, pharynx, and larynx to rule out other causes of pain, audiogram, auditory evoked response potentials, and vestibular tests. MRI with gadolinium enhancement of the brain, cerebellopontine angle, and

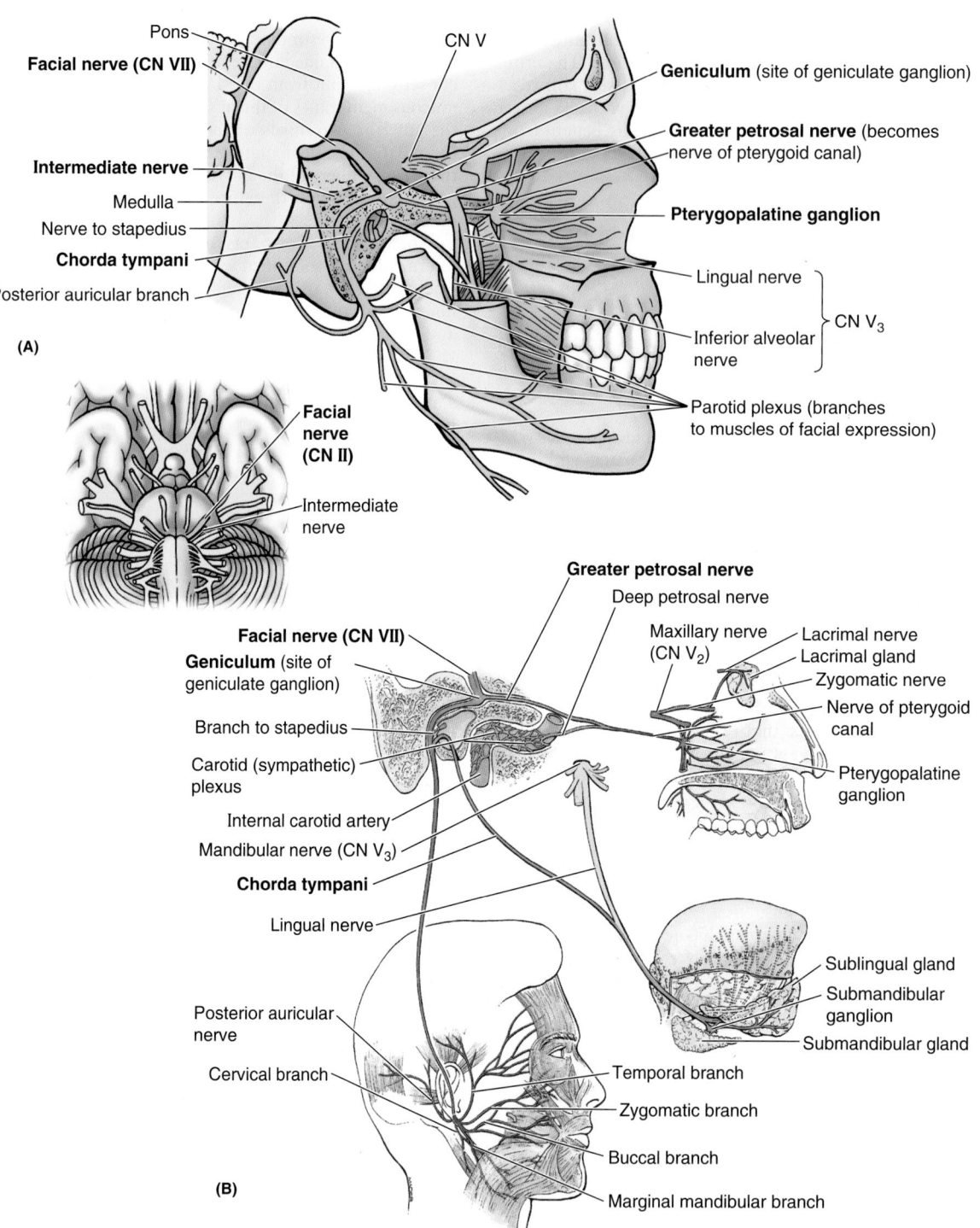

FIGURE 66.3 A, B. Distribution of the facial nerve (cranial nerve VII). The facial nerve emanates from the brainstem between the pons and the medulla. The motor part of the facial nerve arises from the facial nerve nucleus in the pons and divides into five branches after coursing through the petrous temporal bone, the internal auditory meatus, the facial canal, the stylomastoid foramen, and the parotid gland. It is responsible for muscles of facial expression and supplies preganglionic parasympathetic fibers to ganglia of the head and neck. It also supplies taste sensation to the anterior two thirds of the tongue, partial afferent innervations of the oropharynx, as well as a some cutaneous sensation around the auricle. (From Moore KL, Dalley AF. *Clinically Oriented Anatomy.* 5th ed. Baltimore: Lippincott Williams & Wilkins; 2006.)

facial nerve and MRA should be performed. As described above, vascular compression or other pathology may involve more than one of the cranial nerves in the middle fossa.

As described in the previous section, nervus intermedius neuralgia can be caused by HZ infection. The pain from acute HZ involving the geniculate ganglion is usually constant and burning as opposed to the lancinating paroxysmal pain of nervus intermedius neuralgia. Onset of the pain from acute HZ is generally followed by a vesicular eruption involving the ear drum and external auditory canal.

Treatment

Pharmacologic treatment of nervus intermedius neuralgia is similar to that of TN. When conservative management fails, a thorough work-up to exclude other causes of pain should be investigated. The nervus intermedius or geniculate ganglion cannot be injected with local anesthetic or other solution; however, blockade of other nerves supplying the area of the ear can be anesthetized to exclude them as causes of the otalgia. Surgical management consists of MVD or section of the nervus intermedius. Excision of the nervus intermedius and geniculate ganglion has also been advocated along with selective retrolabyrinthine V nerve section in extreme cases.[208]

GLOSSOPHARYNGEAL NEURALGIA

Glossopharyngeal neuralgia is a rare neuralgia with a reported relative frequency of 0.75% to 1% compared to TN.[210,211] It is defined as paroxysmal pain in the areas supplied by cranial nerves IX and X. The glossopharyngeal or ninth cranial nerve exits the upper medulla just rostral to the vagus nerve. Sensory fibers carried in the glossopharyngeal nerve supply the posterior one third of the tongue, the tonsils, pharynx, the middle ear, and the carotid body. The glossopharyngeal nerve also supplies parasympathetic fibers to the parotid gland via the otic ganglion, motor fibers to the stylopharyngeus muscle, and contributes to the pharyngeal plexus. The symptoms associated with glossopharyngeal neuralgia can be better understood upon review of its branches, which include the tympanic nerve, stylopharyngeal nerve, tonsillar nerve, nerve to the carotid sinus, branches to the posterior third of the tongue, lingual branches, and a communicating branch to the vagus nerve (Fig. 66.4).

Etiology

Classical or idiopathic and secondary or symptomatic forms of glossopharyngeal neuralgia exist similar to TN. Symptomatic causes include tumors, peritonsillar abscess, carotid aneurysm, Chiari type I malformations, and Eagle syndrome (in which cranial nerve IX is compressed against an ossified stylohyoid ligament).[212–214] Idiopathic glossopharyngeal neuralgia occurs most commonly from vascular compression of cranial nerve IX (often in association with cranial nerve X) at the nerve REZ. The vertebral artery or posterior inferior cerebellar arteries are most often implicated on surgical exploration.

Symptoms and Signs

The character of pain in the patient with glossopharyngeal neuralgia is similar to that of TN. The unbearable, electrical, lancinating pain is located unilaterally in the ear, larynx, tonsillar fossa, or base of the tongue. It is rarely bilateral. It may radiate toward the ear, the angle of the jaw, or the upper and lateral aspect of the neck. Paroxysms of pain are often triggered by swallowing, yawning, coughing, or talking.

Diagnosis

A careful history and physical exam is essential in the evaluation of a patient suspected of suffering from glossopharyngeal neuralgia. MRI/MRA should be performed to rule out a mass lesion or vascular pathology. An ossified stylohyoid ligament (consistent with Eagle syndrome) may be identified on roentgenogram. As in TN, the paroxysms of glossopharyngeal neuralgia may last from seconds to minutes. Dozens of attacks may occur daily with episodes lasting from weeks to months followed by periods of remission. The patient is generally free from pain between attacks although dull background pain may persist. Investigation should also exclude MS in younger patients with bilateral symptoms or neurologic deficits. The branch of the glossopharyngeal nerve to the carotid sinus is involved in maintenance of blood pressure and is thought to play a role in some profound cardiac arrhythmias or even asystole which occur in some patients in association with pain paroxysms. The differential diagnosis includes geniculate or nervus intermedius neuralgia. Rare glossopharyngeal zoster has been reported.[215]

Treatment

The pharmacologic treatment of glossopharyngeal neuralgia is similar to TN. When conservative therapy has failed, surgical exploration and vascular decompression has been shown to be highly effective on long-term follow-up with a low complication rate.[216,217] When a source of neurovascular compression is not found, successful relief of symptoms has been obtained with section of the glossopharyngeal nerve together with the upper fibers of the vagus nerve.[218,219]

VAGAL NEURALGIA

The two sensory branches of the vagus nerve, the auricular branch and the superior laryngeal nerve, are involved in this rare neuralgia (Fig. 66.5). The auricular branch of the vagus nerve, or Alderman's nerve, divides into two branches: the posterior auricular nerve and the nerve supplying the auricula and posterior part of the external acoustic meatus. The superior laryngeal nerve descends behind the internal carotid artery and divides into the internal and external laryngeal nerves. The internal laryngeal nerve supplies sensation to the base of the tongue, epiglottis, and the larynx to above the vocal cords. The external laryngeal nerve supplies the cricothyroid muscle, the inferior pharyngeal constrictor, and communicates with the superior cardiac nerve behind the common carotid artery.

Etiology

Idiopathic or classic vagal neuralgia is characterized by lack of a known precipitating lesion or by vascular compression of the upper fibers of the vagal nerve as they leave the brainstem. Secondary or symptomatic vagal neuralgia involving the superior laryngeal branch has been reported to be secondary to multiple causes including deviation of the hyoid bone, lateral pharyngeal diverticulum, and as a complication following carotid endarterectomy.[220–222]

Symptoms and Signs

Vagal neuralgia is characterized by severe pain paroxysms in the submandibular region, throat, and/or under the ear. Attacks are

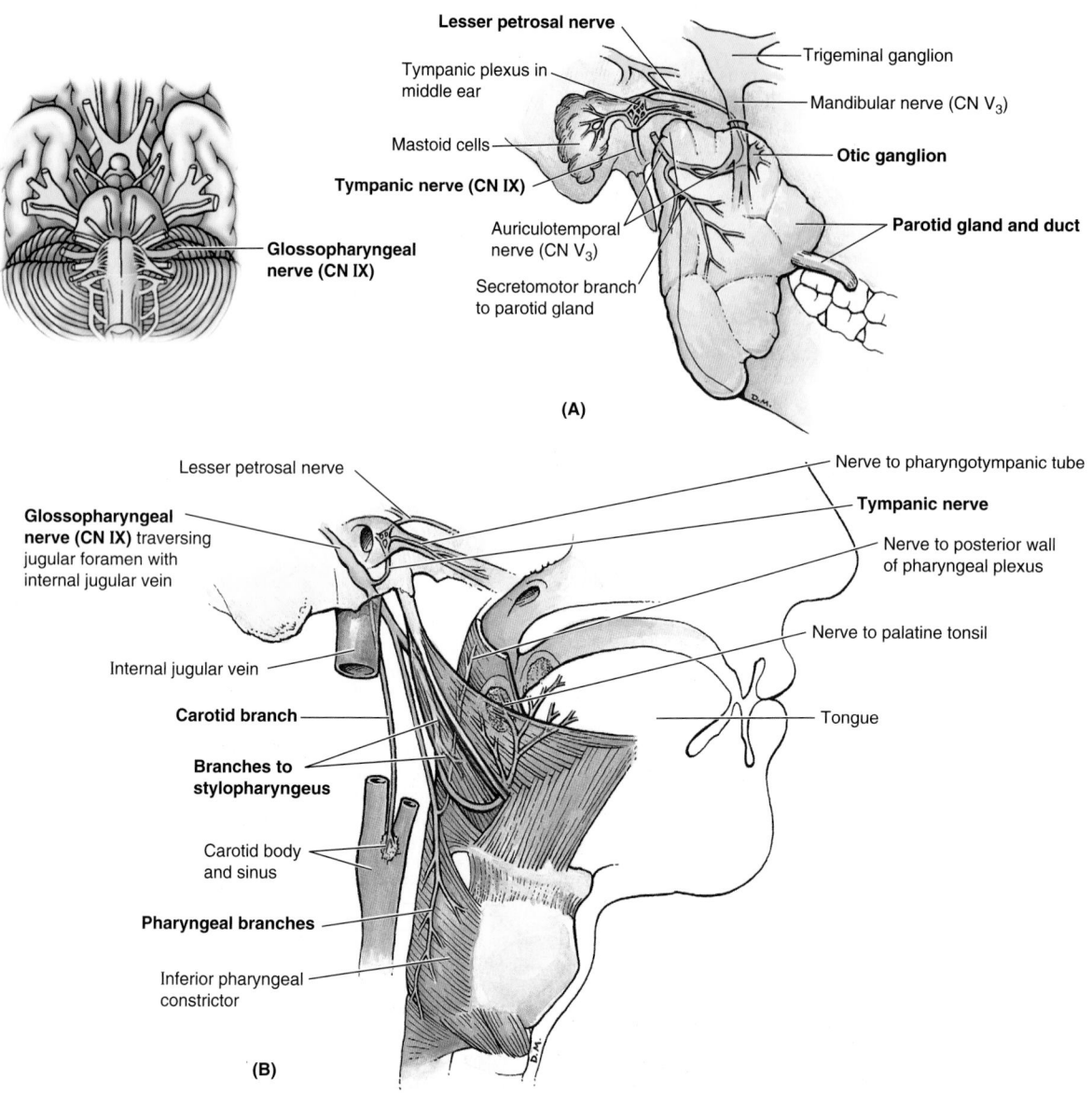

FIGURE 66.4 Distribution of the glossopharyngeal nerve. **A.** The glossopharyngeal nerve exits the skull via the jugular foramen between the internal jugular vein and internal carotid artery, lateral and ventral to the vagus and accessory nerves. It receives general sensory fibers via the tympanic nerve, the nerve to the palatine tonsils, and pharyngeal nerve branches. It receives special sensory fibers (taste) from the posterior one third of the tongue and visceral sensory fibers from the carotid bodies and carotid sinus. **B.** The parasympathetic component of the glossopharyngeal nerve supplies the postsynaptic innervations to the parotid gland via the otic ganglion. The glossopharyngeal nerve is responsible for the afferent limb of the gag reflex and thus the gag reflex is absent in patients with damage to the glossopharyngeal nerve. The efferent limb of the gag reflex is supplied by the vagus nerve. (From Moore KL, Dalley AF. *Clinically Oriented Anatomy.* 5th ed. Baltimore: Lippincott Williams & Wilkins; 2006.)

triggered by swallowing, talking, yawning, coughing, or straining and turning the head. A trigger zone is generally present in the larynx or lateral aspect of the throat overlying the hyoid bone. Compression of the vagus nerve has also reported to be associated with intractable hiccups, coughing, spontaneous gagging, and dysphagia.[223,224]

Diagnosis

The diagnosis of vagal neuralgia is based on a thorough history to define the distinct characteristics and precipitating factors of

the patient's pain. A careful exam of the head and neck should be performed to rule out other pathology. MRI/MRA should be performed to rule out compressive mass lesions or neurovascular compression. Hoarseness of speech and a trigger point superolateral to the thyroid cartilage may be noted on exam of the patient. Differential diagnosis includes glossopharyngeal neuralgia, geniculate neuralgia, and carotidynia.

Treatment

Pharmacologic therapy of vagal neuralgia is identical to that of TN. Successful treatment of superior laryngeal neuralgia with

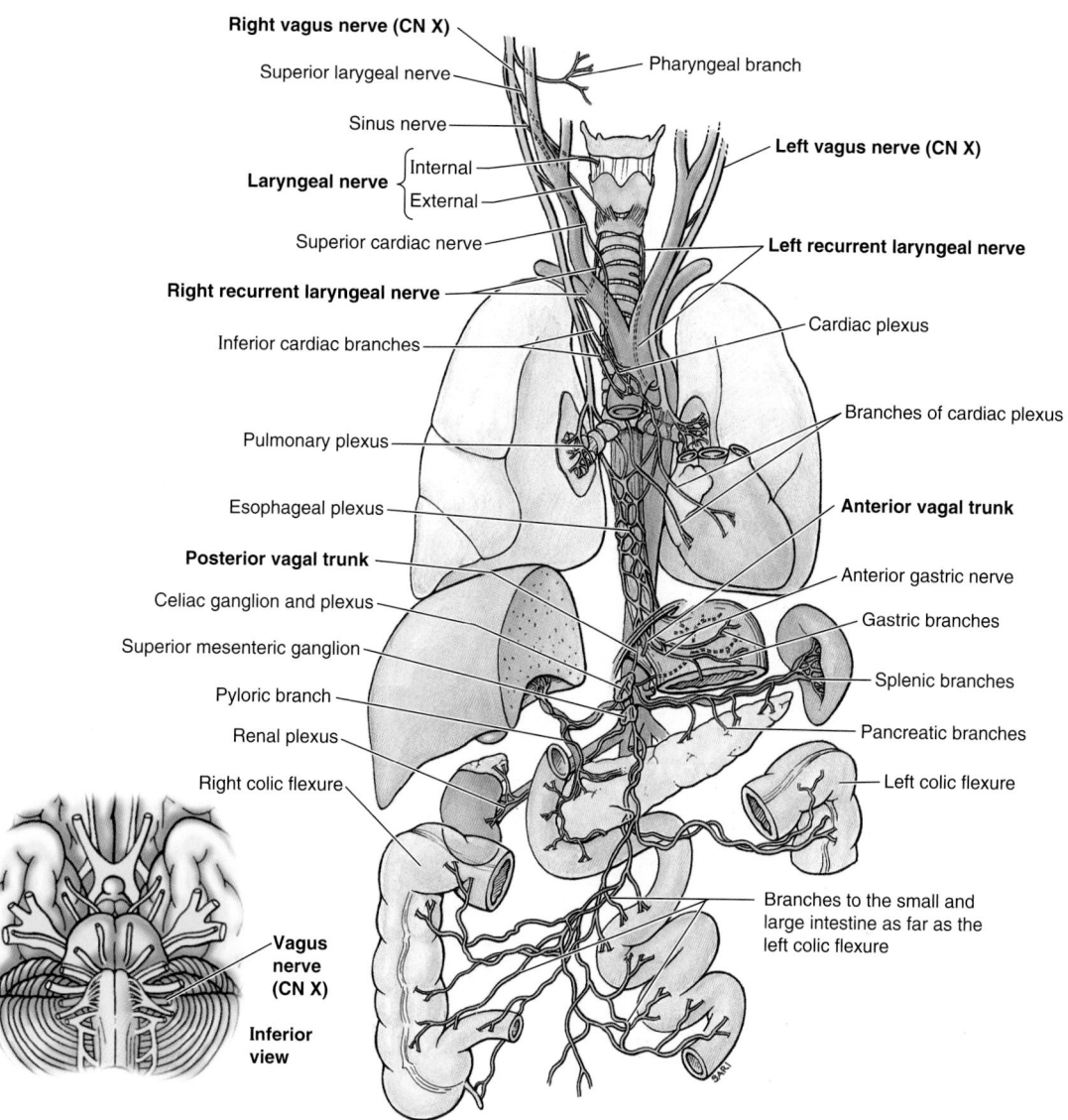

FIGURE 66.5 Distribution of the vagal nerve (cranial nerve X). The vagus nerve originates in the brainstem and courses through the jugular foramen to extend into the head, neck, thorax, and abdomen where it provides efferent motor parasympathetic innervation to viscera as well as afferent innervation that delivers information about the state of organs to the brain. (From Moore KL, Dalley AF. *Clinically Oriented Anatomy.* 5th ed. Baltimore: Lippincott Williams & Wilkins; 2006.)

high concentration lidocaine injections after carbamazepine treatment failure has been reported.[225] Surgical treatment following pharmacologic therapy failure warrants consideration. MVD has been successful when neurovascular compression of the vagus is identified. When no compressive lesion is identified, relief of pain can be obtained following section of the glossopharyngeal nerve and the upper rootlets of the vagal nerves. The medial aspect of the descending trigeminal tract has also been sectioned in refractory cases to produce loss of pain and temperature sensation in the pharynx.[226]

OTHER TERMINAL BRANCH NEURALGIAS

Rare neuralgias involving branches of the trigeminal nerve have been reported. These include supraorbital neuralgia, nasociliary neuralgia, infraorbital neuralgia, and nummular headache. Injury

or entrapment of other peripheral branches of the trigeminal nerve such as the lingual, alveolar, or mental nerves may result in pain in the area supplied by that branch.

Supraorbital neuralgia is characterized by paroxysmal or constant pain in the region of the supraorbital notch. It is unilateral and radiates to the medial aspect of the forehead in the area supplied by the supraorbital nerve. It can be caused by injury or entrapment of the supraorbital nerve at its outlet. The pain is transiently relieved by injection of a small volume of local anesthetic at the supraorbital notch. Medical treatment is often unsuccessful when entrapment of the nerve is present. Successful treatment with cryoablation and surgical release of the nerve at its outlet has been reported.[227,228]

Nasociliary neuralgia, or Charlin's neuralgia, is a rare condition characterized by stabbing pain lasting seconds to hours in one side of the nose. The pain radiates to the medial frontal region and is triggered by touching the lateral aspect of the ipsilateral nostril. Temporary relief from pain following local anesthetic blockade of the nasociliary nerve is diagnostic. Inflammatory cutaneous lesions and chronic sinusitis have been implicated as secondary causes of nasociliary neuralgia.[229,230] Relief following surgical section of the nasociliary nerve, turbinectomy, and septoplasty has been described.[231]

Infraorbital neuralgia has been reported most frequently in association with posttraumatic entrapment syndromes.[232] If pain is not successfully alleviated by reduction of zygomatic fracture and mobilization of surrounding soft tissue and bone, pharmacologic therapy with antiepileptic agents alone or combined with antidepressants such as the tricyclics or serotonin norepinephrine reuptake inhibitors may be effective.

Nummular headache is thought to be neuralgia related to a terminal cutaneous branch of the trigeminal nerve. It has been described as a primary disorder characterized by head pain felt exclusively in a small round area generally 2–6 cm in diameter. The pain is not attributed to another disorder and neurologic and neuroimaging exams are normal by definition. A constant background pain may be described as well as exacerbations which are spontaneous or triggered by combing the hair or touch in the affected area. In patients refractory to pharmacologic therapy, reduction of pain was reported for an average of 14 weeks after initial and repeat injection with botulinum toxin A.[233]

In all cases of idiopathic neuralgia of the terminal branches of the trigeminal nerve, a careful history and physical exam to rule out other causes of facial pain the is imperative. Age less than 40 and presence of neurologic deficit should prompt further diagnostic radiologic exams to rule out compressive lesions.

OTHER CRANIAL NEURALGIA-RELATED CAUSES OF PAIN: ANESTHESIA DOLOROSA

Etiology

Anesthesia dolorosa is defined as perception of pain in an area that is anesthetic. It is a dreaded complication of trigeminal nerve surgery, including partial nerve sections, MVD, percutaneous gangliolysis, neurolytic injections, and stereotactic radiosurgery. It has also been reported after penetrating cranial injury.[234] The area of persistent and painful anesthesia is in the distribution of the injured nerve.

Symptoms and Signs

The patient with anesthesia dolorosa complains of burning, pulling, or stabbing pain which can also include a sharp, stinging, shooting, or electrical component. The pain often increases with cold or with rapid temperature changes.

Diagnosis

As it pertains to the head and face, anesthesia dolorosa typically involves the territory of a specific branch or branches of the trigeminal nerve or the occipital nerve. Quantitative sensory testing may be used to confirm lack of sensation.

Treatment

There are no controlled trials evaluating pharmacologic therapy for anesthesia dolorosa. Empiric treatment of pain by clinical characteristics has led to use of anticonvulsants in patients with lancinating and electrical pain, tricyclic antidepressants and serotonin norepinephrine reuptake inhibitors in patients with burning

pain, and intravenous lidocaine and ketamine infusions in patients unresponsive to other pharmacologic therapy.[235,236] Motor cortex stimulation was the recommended surgical treatment of choice for facial anesthesia dolorosa according to authors of a recent review of the literature on central and neuropathic pain over the last 15 years. Motor cortex stimulation may act by replacing nociceptive with nonnociceptive sensory input at the cortical, thalamic, brainstem, and spinal level. It may also interfere with the emotional component of nociceptive perception.[237] In a prospective study of 10 patients undergoing trial and treatment with motor cortex stimulation, patients with facial weakness and sensory loss regained both strength and discriminative sensation during stimulation.[238] Multicenter randomized studies are now in progress to further evaluate this modality of treatment. Anesthesia dolorosa did not appear to respond to deep brain stimulation according to one 15-year series of 141 patients.[239]

CONCLUSION

Knowledge of the features of neuralgic pain, a thorough understanding of the unique characteristics and specific anatomic distribution of each cranial nerve, and a familiarity with the distinctive features of other pain syndromes involving the structures of the head and neck is essential to establishing a diagnosis of trigeminal or other cranial neuralgias. Although the cranial neuralgias are rare when compared with other neuropathic pain syndromes, the extreme suffering encountered in patients who present with these syndromes, together with the need to distinguish between classical and symptomatic presentations, mandates advanced neuroimaging in all cases to rule out progressive processes such as intracranial tumors, infection, or MS. Pharmacologic, surgical, and percutaneous therapies for the cranial neuralgias have continued to advance with development of new agents and techniques which are associated with fewer side effects and complications. Improved monitoring in the case of surgical and percutaneous therapies have also been instrumental in reducing patient morbidity and mortality.

References

1. Burchiel KJ. A new classification for facial pain. *Neurosurgery* 2003;53: 1164–1166.
2. International Headache Society. The International Classification of Headache Disorders, 2nd edition. *Cephalalgia* 2004;24(suppl 1):1–160.
3. Nurmikko TJ, Eldridge PR. Trigeminal neuralgia—pathophysiology, diagnosis and current treatment. *Br J Anaesth* 2001;87(1)117–132.
4. Zebenholzer K, Wöber C, Vigl M, et al. Facial pain and the second edition of the International Classification of Headache Disorders. *Headache* 2006; 46(2):259–263.
5. Jääskeläinen SK, Forssell H, Tenovuo O. Electrophysiological testing of the trigeminofacial system: aid in the diagnosis of atypical facial pain. *Pain* 1999; 80:191–200.
6. Nielsen LA, Henriksson KG. Mechanisms in chronic musculoskeletal pain (fibromyalgia): the role of central and peripheral sensitization and pain disinhibition. *Best Pract Res Clin Rhematol* 2007;21(3):465–480.
7. Burchiel KJ. Trigeminal neuropathic pain. *Acta Neurochir Suppl (Wien)* 1993;58:145–149.
8. Merskey H, Bogduk N. *Classification of Chronic Pain. Descriptions of Chronic Pain Syndromes and Definitions of Pain Terms.* Seattle: IASP Press: 1994:59–71.
9. Cowan JA, Brahma B, Sagher O. Surgical treatment of trigeminal neuralgia: comparison of microvascular decompression, percutaneous ablation, and stereotactic radiosurgery. Surgical management of chronic pain. *Tech Neurosurg* 2003;8(3):157–167.
10. Block A, Kremer EF, Fernandez E. *Handbook of Pain Syndromes: Biopsychosocial Perspectives.* Mahwah, NJ: Lawrence Erlbaum Associates; 1999; 435–436.
11. Cole CD, Liu JK, Apfelbaum RI. Historical perspectives on the diagnosis and treatment of trigeminal neuralgia. *Neurosurg Focus* 2005;18(5):1–10.
12. Hurd EP. *A Treatise on Neuralgia.* Detroit, MI: George S. Davis; 1890.
13. Jannetta P. Neurovascular compression in cranial nerve and systemic disease. *Ann Surg* 1980;192:518–525.
14. Jannetta PJ. Arterial compression of the trigeminal nerve at the pons in patients with trigeminal neuralgia. *J Neurosurg* 1967:17:159–180.

15. Brewis M, Poskanzer DC, Rolland C, et al. Neurological disease in an English city. *Acta Neurol Scand* 1966;42(suppl 24):1–89.
16. Kurtzke JF. The current neurologic burden of illness and injury in the United States. *Neurology* 1982;32:1207–1214.
17. Katusic S, Beard CM, Bergstralh E, et al. Incidence and clinical features of trigeminal neuralgia, Rochester, Minnesota, 1945–1984. *Ann Neurol* 1990; 27(1)89–95.
18. MacDonald BK, Cockerell OC, Sander JW, et al. The incidence and lifetime prevalence of neurological disorders in a prospective community based study in the UK. *Brain* 2000;123:664–676.
19. Hall GC, Carroll D, Parry D, et al. Epidemiology and treatment of neuropathic pain: the UK primary care perspective. *Pain* 2006;122(1–2):156–162.
20. Lopes PG, Castro ES Jr, Lopes LH. Trigeminal neuralgia in children: two case reports. *Pediatr Neurol* 2002;26(4):309–310.
21. Ramanathan M, Parameshwarman AA, Jayakumar N, et al. Reactivation of trigeminal neuralgia following distraction osteogenesis in an 8-year-old child: report of a unique case. *J Indian Soc Pedod Prev Dent* 2007;25(1):49–51.
22. Love S, Coakham HB. Trigeminal neuralgia: pathology and pathogenesis. *Brain* 2001;124(12):2347–2360.
23. McLaughln MR, Jannetta PJ, Clyde BL, et al. Microvascular decompression of cranial nerves: lessons learned after 4400 operations. *J Neurosurg* 1999; (90):1–8.
24. Malis LI. Retrous ridge compression and its surgical correction. *J Neurosurg* 2007;107:220–224.
25. Kerr FW. Evidence for a peripheral etiology of trigeminal neuralgia. *J Neurosurg* 2007;107:225–231.
26. Calvin WH, Loeser JD, Howe JF. A neurophysiological theory for the pain mechanism of tic douloureux. *Pain* 1977;3:147–154.
27. Fromm GH, Chattha AS, Terrence CF, et al. Role of inhibitory mechanisms in trigeminal neuralgia. *Neurology* 1981;31:683–687.
28. Selçuk P, Kurtkaya O, Uzün I, et al. Microanatomy of the central myelin-peripheral myelin transition zone of the trigeminal nerve. *Neurosurgery* 2006; 59:354–359.
29. Devor M, Govrin-Lippmann R, Rappaport ZH. Mechanism of trigeminal neuralgia: an ultrastructural analysis of trigeminal root specimens obtained during microvascular decompression surgery. *J Neurosurg* 2002;96(3):532–543.
30. Rappaport ZH. An electron-microscopic analysis of biopsy samples of the trigeminal root taken during microvascular decompressive surgery. *Stereotact Funct Neurosurg* 1997;68(1–4 Pt 1):182–186.
31. Love S, Gradidge T, Coakham HB. Trigeminal neuralgia due to multiple sclerosis: ultrastructural findings in trigeminal rhizotomy specimens. *Neuropathol Appl Neurobiol* 2001;27(3):238–244.
32. Obermann M, Yoon MS, Ese D, et al. Impaired trigeminal nociceptive processing in patients with trigeminal neuralgia. *Neurology* 2007;69:835–841.
33. Watson JC. From paroxysmal to chronic pain in trigeminal neuralgia implications of central sensitization. *Neurology* 2007;69:817–818.
34. Cruccu G, Biasiotta A, Galeotti F, et al. Diagnostic accuracy of trigeminal reflex testing in trigeminal neuralgia. *Neurology* 2006;66:139–141.
35. Leandri M. Early trigeminal evoked potentials in tumours at the base of the skull and trigeminal neuralgia. *Electroencephalogr Clin Neurophysiol* 1988; 71(2):114–124.
36. White JC, Sweet WH. *Pain and the Neurosurgeon.* Springfield, IL: Charles C. Thomas; 1969.
37. White JC, Sweet WH. *Pain, Its Mechanisms and Neurosurgical Control.* Springfield, IL: Charles C. Thomas; 1969.
38. Davies EW, Naffziger HC. Major trigeminal neuralgia. An analysis of two hundred and forty-five cases. *Calif Med* 1948;68:130–134.
39. Rushton JG, MacDonald HN. Trigeminal neuralgia: special considerations of nonsurgical treatment. *JAMA* 1957;165:437.
40. Wilkins R. Trigeminal neuralgia: introduction. In: Wilkins R, Rengachary S, eds. *Neurosurgery.* New York: Mc Graw-Hill; 1985:2337–2344.
41. Peet MM, Schneider RC. Trigeminal neuralgia: a review of six hundred and eighty-nine cases with a follow-up study on sixty-five per cent of the group. *J Neurosurg* 1957;9:367–377.
42. Harris W. An analysis of 1,433 cases of paroxysmal trigeminal neuralgia (trigeminal-tic) and the en-results of gasserian alcohol injection. *Brain* 1940; 63:209–224.
43. Ruge D, Brochner R, Davis L. A study of the treatment of 637 patients with trigeminal neuralgia. *J Neurosurg* 1958; 15:528–536.
44. Jackson EM, Bussard GM, Hoard MA, et al. Trigeminal neuralgia: a diagnostic challenge. *Am J Emerg Med* 1999;17:597–600.
45. Gass A, Kitchen N, MacManus DG, et al. Trigeminal neuralgia in patients with multiple sclerosis: lesion localization with magnetic resonance imaging. *Neurology* 1997;49:1142–1144.
46. Albrecht K, Krump J. Diagnosis, differential diagnosis and possibilities for treatment of trigeminal neuralgia: with special reference to the conservative treatment with hydantoin drugs and vitamin B12, [in German]. *Munch Med Wochenschr* 1954;96:985.
47. Kugelberg E, Lindblom U. The mechanism of pain in trigeminal neuralgia. *J Neurol Neurosurg Psychiat* 1959;22:36.
48. Symonds C. Facial pain. *Ann R Coll Surg Engl* 1949;4:206.
49. Mitchell RG. Pre-trigeminal neuralgia. *Br Dent J* 1980;149:167.
50. Fromm GH, Graff-Radford SB, Terrence CF, et al. Pre-trigeminal neuralgia. *Neurology* 1990;40:1493–1495.
51. Sawaya RA. Trigeminal neuralgia associated with sinusitus. *ORL J Otorhinolaryngol Relat Space* 2000;62:160–163.
52. Lin YW, Lin SK, Weng IH. Fatal paranasal sinusitis presenting as trigeminal neuralgia. *Headache* 2006;46(1):174–178.
53. Cheng TM, Cascino TL, Onofrio BM. Comprehensive study of diagnosis and treatment of trigeminal neuralgia secondary to tumors. *Neurology* 1993;43: 2298–2302.
54. Mathews ES, Scrivani SJ. Percutaneous stereotactic radiofrequency thermal rhizotomy for the treatment of trigeminal neuralgia. *Mt Sinai J Med* 2000; 67:288–299.
55. Metzer SW. Trigeminal neuralgia secondary to tumor with normal exam, responsive to carbamazepine. *Headache* 1991;31(3):164–166.
56. Cruccu G, Biasiotta A, Galeotti F, et al. Diagnostic accuracy of trigeminal reflex testing in trigeminal neuralgia. *Neurology* 2006;66(1):139–141.
57. Jamjoom AB, Jamjoom ZA, al-Fehaily M, et al. Trigeminal neuralgia related to cerebellopontine angle tumors. *Neurosurg Rev* 1996;19(4):237–241.
58. Meng L, Yuguang L, Feng L, et al. Cerebellopontine angle epidermoids presenting with trigeminal neuralgia. *J Clin Neurosci* 2005;12(7):784–786.
59. Tanaka T, Morimoto Y, Shiiba S, et al. Utility of magnetic resonance cisternography using three-dimensional fast asymmetric spin-echo sequences with multiplanar reconstruction: the evaluation of sites of neurovascular compression of the trigeminal nerve. *Oral Surg Oral Med Oral Pathol Oral Radiol Endod* 2005;100(2):215–225.
60. Laha RK, Jannetta PJ. Glossopharyngeal neuralgia. *J Neurosurg* 1977;47: 316–320.
61. Yentür EA, Yegül I. Nervus intermedius neuralgia: an uncommon pain syndrome with an uncommon etiology. *J Pain Symptom Manage* 2000;19(6): 407–408.
62. Yeh HS, Tew JM Jr. Tic convulsif, the combination of geniculate neuralgia and hemifacial spasm relieved by vascular decompression. *Neurology* 1984; 34(5):682–683.
63. Samii M, Günther T, Iaconetta G, et al. Microvascular decompression to treat hemifacial spasm: long-term results for a consecutive series of 143 patients. *Neurosurgery* 2002;50(4):712–718.
64. Goadsby PJ. Pathophysiology of cluster headache: a trigeminal autonomic cephalgia. *Lance Neurol* 2002;1(4):251–257.
65. Bussone G, Usai S. Trigeminal autonomic cephalgias: from pathophysiology to clinical aspects. *Neurol Sci* 2004;25(suppl 3):S74–S76.
66. Boes CJ, Swanson JW. Paroxysmal hemicrania, SUNCT and hemicrania continuea. *Semin Neurol* 2006;26(2):260–270.
67. Cohen AS, Matharu MS, Goadsby PJ. Short-lasting unilateral neuralgiform headache attacks with conjunctival injection and tearing (SUNCT) or cranial autonomic features(SUNA)-a prospective clinical study of SUNCT and SUNA. *Brain* 2006;129(10):2746–2760.
68. Bigal ME, Lipton RB. The differential diagnosis of chronic daily headaches: an algorithm-based approach. *J Headache Pain* 2007;8(5):263–272.
69. Rosenfeld RM. Clinical practice guideline on adult sinusitis. *Otolaryngol Head Neck Surg* 2007;137(3):365–377.
70. Zakrzewska JM. *Trigeminal Neuralgia. Major Problems in Neurology:28.* London, England: WB Saunders Company Ltd; 1995:63–72.
71. Israel HA, Scivani SJ. The interdisciplinary approach to oral, facial and head pain. *J Am Dent Assoc* 2000;131(7):919–926.
72. Eide PK, Rabben T. Trigeminal neuropathic pain: pathophysiological mechanisms examined by quantitative assessment of abnormal pain and sensory perception. *Neurosurgery* 1998;43(5)1103–1110.
73. Lang E, Kaltenhäuser M, Seidler S, et al. Persistent idiopathic facial pain exists independent from somatosensory input from the painful region: findings from quantitative sensory functions and somatotopy of the primary somatosensory cortex. *Pain* 2005;118(1–2):80–91.
74. Bergougan M. Cures hereuses de nevralgies faciales essentielles par le diphenyl-hydantoinate de soude. *Rev Laryng Otol Rhino* 1942;63:34.
75. Trousseau A. De la nevralgie epileptiforme. *Arch Gen Med* 1853;1:33.
76. Jorns TP, Zakrzewska JM. Evidence-based approach to the medical management of trigeminal neuralgia. *Br J Neurosurg* 2007;21(3):253–261.
77. Cruccu G, Groneth G, Alkne J, et al. AAN-EFNS guidelines on trigeminal neuralgia management. *Eur J Neurol* 2008;15(10):1013–1028.
78. Campbell FG, Graham JG, Zilkha KJ. Clinical trial of carbamazepine (tegretol) in trigeminal neuralgia. *J Neurol Neurosurg Psychiatry* 1966;29: 265–267.
79. Rockliff BW, Davis EH. Controlled sequential trials of carbamazepine in trigeminal neuralgia. *Arch Neurol* 1966;15:129–136.
80. Killian JM, Fromm GH. Carbamazepine in the treatment of neuralgia. *Arch Neurol* 1968;19:129–136.
81. Nichol CF. A four year double-blind study of tegretol in facial pain. *Headache* 1969;9:54–57.
82. Wiffen P, Collins S, McQuay H, et al. Anticonvulsant drugs for acute and chronic pain. *Cochrane Database Syst Rev* 2005;3:CD001133.
83. Taylor JC, Brauer S, Espir ML. Long-term treatment of trigeminal neuralgia. *Postgrad Med J* 1981;57:16–18.
84. Tomson T, Ekbom K. Trigeminalneuralgia: time course of pain in relation to carbamazepine dosing. *Cephalgia* 1981;1:91–97.
85. Hart RG, Easton DJ. Carbamazepine and hematologic monitoring. *Ann Neurol* 1982;11:309–312.
86. Liebel JT, Menger N, Langohn H. Oxcarbaepine in der Behandlung der Trigeminusneuralgie. *Nervenheilkunde* 2001;20:461–465.
87. Gronseth G, Gruccu G, Alksne J, et al. The diagnostic evaluation and treat-

ment of trigeminal neuralgia.(An evidence based review: Report of the Quality Standards Subcommittee of the American Academy of Neurology and the European Federation of Neurological Societies). *Neurology* 2008;71(15):1183–1190.

88. Beydoun A, Schmidt D, D'Souza J. Oxcarbazepine versus carbamazepine in trigeminal neuralgia: a meta-analysis of three double blind comparative trials. *Neurology* 2002;58(suppl 3):02.083.

89. Zakrezewsk JM, Chaudhry Z, Nurmikko TJ, et al. Lomotrigine (lamictal) in refractory trigeminal neuralgia: results from a double-blind placebo controlled crossover trial. *Pain* 1997;73:223–230.

90. Leandri M, Lundardi G, Inglese M, et al. Lamotrigine in trigeminal neuralgia secondary to multiple sclerosis. *J Neurol* 2000;247:556–558.

91. Canaveo S, Bonicalzi V, Ferroli P, et al. Lamotrigine control of idiopathic trigeminal neuralgia. [letter]. *J Neurol Neurosurg Psychiatry* 1995;59:646.

92. Iannone A, Baker AB, Morrell F. Dilantin in the treatment of trigeminal neuralgia. *Neurology* 1958;8:126–128.

93. Braham J, Saia A. Phenytoin in the treatment of trigeminal and other neuralgias. *Lancet* 1960;2:892–893.

94. McCleane GJ. Intravenous infusion of phenytoin relieves neuropathic pain: a randomized, double-blinded, placebo-controlled, crossover study. *Anesth Analg* 1999;89:985–988.

95. Cheshire WP. Fosphenytoin: an intravenous option for the management of acute trigeminal neuralgia crisis. *J Pain Symptom Manage* 2001;21:506–510.

96. Fromm GH. Terrence CF, Chattha AS, et al. Baclofen in trigeminal neuralgia: its effect on the spinal trigeminal nucleus: a pilot study. *Arch Neurol* 1980;37:768–771.

97. Fromm GH, Terrence CF, Chattha AS. Baclofen in the treatment of trigeminal neuralgia: double-blind study and long-term follow-up. *Ann Neurol* 1984;15:240–244.

98. Fromm GH, Terrence CF. Comparison of L-baclofen and racemic baclofen in trigeminal neuralgia. *Neurology* 1987;37:1725–1728.

99. Parekh S, Shah K, Kotdawalla H, et al. Baclofen in carbamazepine resistant trigeminal neuralgia-a double blind clinical trial. *Cephalgia* 1989;9:392–393.

100. Kanai A, Saito M, Hoka S. Subcutaneous sumatriptan for refractory trigeminal neuralgia. *Headache* 2006;46(4):577–582.

101. Kanai A, Suzuki A, Osawa S, et al. Sumatriptan alleviates pain in patients with trigeminal neuralgia. *Clin J Pain* 2006;22(8):677–680.

102. Kanai A, Suzuki A, Kobayashi M, et al. Intranasal lidocaine 8% spray for second division trigeminal neuralgia. *Br J Anaesth* 2007;98:(2):275.

103. Peiris JB, Perera GL, Devendra SV, et al. Sodium valproate in trigeminal neuralgia. *Med J Aust* 1980;2:278.

104. Karlov VA, Savitskaia ON. [Comparative effectiveness of antiepileptic preparations in the treatment of patients with trigeminal neuralgia]. *Zh Nevropatol Psikhiatr Im S S Korsakova* 1980;80:530–535.

105. Court JE, Kase CS. Treatment of tic douloureux with a new anticonvulsant (clonazepam). *J Neurol Neurosurg Pshychiatry* 1976;39:297–299.

106. Lechin F, vad der Dijs B, Lechin ME, et al. Pimozide therapy for trigeminal neuralgia. *Arch Neurol* 1989;46:960–963.

107. Wiffen PJ, McQuay HJ, Edwards JE, et al. Gabapentin for acute and chronic pain. *Cochrane Database Syst Rev* 2005;3:CD005452.

108. Gilron I, Booher SL, Rowan JS, et al. Topiramate in trigeminal neuralgia: a randomized, placebo-controlled multiple cross-over pilot study. *Clin Neuropharacol* 2001;24:109–112.

109. Zvartau-Hind M, Din MU, Gilani A, et al. Topiramate relieves refractory trigeminal neuralgia in MS patients. *Neurology* 2000;55:1587–1588.

110. Türk U, Ihan S, Alp R, et al. Botulinum toxin and intractable trigeminal neuralgia. *Clin Neuropharacol* 2005;28(4):161–162.

111. Allam N, Brasis-Neto JP, Brown G, et al. Injections of botulinum toxin type a produce pain alleviation in intractable trigeminal neuralgia. *Clin J Pain* 2005;21(2):182–184.

112. Kugelberg E, Lindblom U. The mechanism of the pain in trigeminal neuralgia. *Neurol Neurosurg Psychiatry* 1959;22:36–43.

113. Galer BS, Miller KV, Rowbotham MC. Response to intravenous lidocaine infusion differs based on clinical diagnosis and site of nervous system injury. *Neurology* 1993;43:1233–1235.

114. Umino M, Kohase H, Ideguchi S, et al. Long-term pain control in trigeminal neuralgia with local anesthetics using and indwelling catheter in the mandibular nerve. *Clin J Pain* 2002;18(3):196–199.

115. Radwan IA, Saito S, Goto F. High-concentration tetracaine for the management of trigeminal neuralgia: quantitative assessment of sensory function after peripheral nerve block. *Clin J Pain* 2001;17(4):323–326.

116. Goto F, Ishizaki K, Yoshikawa D, et al. The long lasting effects of peripheral nerve blocks for trigeminal neuralgia using high concentration of tetracaine dissolved in bupivacaine. *Pain* 1999;79(1):101–103.

117. Chang FS, Huang GS, Cherng CH, et al. Repeated peripheral nerve blocks by the co-administration of ketamine, morphine, and bupivacaine attenuate trigeminal neuralgia, [letter]. *Can J Anesh* 2003;50(2):201–202.

118. Naja MZ, Al-Tannir M, Ziade MF, et al. Repeated nerve blocks with clonidine, fentanyl and bupivacaine for trigeminal neuralgia. *Anaesthesia* 2006;61:70–71.

119. Nique TA, Bennett CR. Inadvertent brainstem anesthesia following extraoral trigeminal V2-V3 blocks. *Oral Surg Oral Med Oral Pathol* 1981;51(5):468–470.

120. McLeod NM, Patton DW. Peripheral alcohol injections in the management of trigeminal neuralgia. *Oral Surg Oral Med Oral Pathol Oral Radiol Endod* 2007;104(1):12–17.

121. Fardy MJ, Zakrzewska JM, Patton DW. Peripheral surgical techniques for the management of trigeminal neuralgia-alcohol and glycerol injections. *Acta Neurochir (Wien)* 1994;129(3–4):181–184.

122. Erdem E, Alkan A. Peripheral glycerol injections in the treatment of idiopathic trigeminal neuralgia: retrospective analysis of 157 cases. *J Oral Maxillofac Surg* 2001;59(10):1176–1180.

123. Fardy MJ, Patton DW. Complications associated with peripheral alcohol injections in the management of trigeminal neuralgia. *Br J Oral Maxillofac Surg* 1994;32(6):387–391.

124. Wilkenson HA. Trigeminal nerve peripheral branch phenol/glycerol injections for tic douloureux. *J Neurosurg* 1999;90(5):828–832.

125. Kondo A. Microvascular decompression surgery for trigeminal neuralgia. *Stereotact Funct Neurosurg* 2001;77(1–4):187–189.

126. Barker FG, Jannetta PJ, Bissonette PAC, et al. The long-term outcome of microvascular decompression for trigeminal neuralgia. *N Engl J Med* 1996;334(17):1077–1083.

127. Tronnier VM, Rasche D, Hamer J, et al. Treatment of idiopathic trigeminal neuralgia: comparison of long-term outcome after radiofrequency rhizotomy and microvascular decompression. *Neurosurgery* 2001;48(6):1261–1267.

128. Kalkanis SN, Eskandar EN, Carter BS, et al. Microvascular decompression surgery in the United States, 1996–2000: mortality rates, morbidity rates, and the effects of hospital and surgeon volumes. *Neurosurgery* 2003;52:1251–1261.

129. Lopez BC, Jamlyn PJ, Zakrzewska JM. Systematic Review of ablative neurosurgical techniques for the treatment of trigeminal neuralgia. *Neurosurgery* 2004;54:973–983.

130. Quinn JH, Weil T. Trigeminal neuralgia: treatment by repetitive neurectomy. Supplemental report. *J Oral Surg* 1975;33(8):591–595.

131. Murali R, Rovit RL. Are peripheral neurectomies of value in the treatment of trigeminal neuralgia? An analysis of new cases and cases involving previous radiofrequency gasserian thermocoagulation. *J Neurosurg* 1996;85(3):435–437.

132. Trescott AM. Cryoanalgesia in interventional pain management. *Pain Physician* 2003;6:345–360.

133. Jakrewska JM. Cryotherapy in the management of paroxysmal trigeminal neuralgia. *J Neurol Neurosurg Psychiatry* 1987;50(4):485–487.

134. Pradel W. Cryosurgical treatment of genuine trigeminal neuralgia. *Br J Oral Maxillofac Surg* 2002;40(3):244–247.

135. Zakrzewska JM, Nally FF. The role of cryotherapy (cryoanalgesia) in the management of paroxysmal neuralgia: a six year experience. *Br J Oral Maxillofac Surg* 1988;26(1):18–25.

136. Hoh DJ, Liu CY, Pagnini PG, et al. Chained lightning, part I: exploitation of energy and radiobiological principles for therapeutic purposes. *Neurosurgery* 2007;61(1):14–27.

137. Hoh DJ, Liu CY, Chen JC, et al. Chained lightning, part II: neurosurgical principles, radiosurgical technology, and the manipulation of energy beam delivery. *Neurosurgery* 2007;61(3):433–446.

138. Young RF, Vermeulen SS, Grimm P, et al. Gamma knife radiosurgery for treatment of trigeminal neuralgia: idiopathic and tumor related. *Neurology* 1997;48:608–614.

139. Pollock BE, Phong LK, Gorman DA, et al. Stereotactic radiosurgery for idiopathic trigeminal neuralgia. *J Neurosurg* 2002;97:347–353.

140. Petit JH, Herman JM, Nagda S, et al. Radiosurgical treatment of trigeminal neuralgia: evaluating quality of life and treatment outcomes. *Int J Radiat Oncol Biol Phys* 2003;56:1147–1153.

141. Lopez BC, Hamlyn PJ, Zakrzewska JM. Stereotactic radiosurgery for primary trigeminal neuralgia: state of evidence and recommendations for future reports. *J Neurol Neurosurg Psychiatry* 2004;75(7):1019–1024.

142. Cheuk AV, Chin LS, Pitit JH, et al. Gamma knife surgery for trigeminal neuralgia: outcome, imaging, and brainstem correlates. *Int J radiat Oncol Biol Phys* 2004;60:537–541.

143. Brisman R, Khandji AG, Mooij RB. Trigeminal nerve-blood vessel relationship as revealed by high-resolution magnetic resonance imaging and its effect on pain relief after gamma knife radiosurgery for trigeminal neuralgia. *Neurosurgery* 2002;50:1261–1266.

144. Shaya M, Jawahar A, Caldito G, et al. Gamma knife radiosurgery for trigeminal neuralgia: a study of predictors of success, efficacy, safety and outcome at LSUHSC. *Surg Neurol* 2004;61:529–534.

145. Nurmikko TJ, Edridge PR. Trigeminal neuralgia—pathophysiology, diagnosis and current treatment. *Br J Anaesth* 2001;87:117–132.

146. Sheehan J, Pan HC, Stroila M, et al. Gamma knife surgery for trigeminal neuralgia: outcomes and prognostic factors. *J Neurosurg* 2005;102:434–441.

147. Shetter AG, Rogers CL, Ponce R, et al. Gamma knife radiosurgery for recurrent trigeminal neuralgia. *J Neurosurg* 2002;97:536–538.

148. Pollock BE, Foote RL, Link MJ, et al. Repeat radiosurgery for idiopathic trigeminal neuralgia. *Int J Radiat Oncol Biol Phys* 2005;61:192–195.

149. Frighetto L, De Salles AA, Smith ZA, et al. Noninvasive linear accelerator radiosurgery as the primary treatment for trigeminal neuralgia. *Neurology* 2004;62:660–662.

150. Chen JC, Girvigian M, Greathouse H, et al. Treatment of trigeminal neuralgia with linear accelerator radiosurgery: initial results. *J Neurosurg* 2004;101(suppl 3):346–350.

151. Lim M, Villavicencio AT, Burneikiene S, et al. CyberKnife for idiopathic trigeminal neuralgia. *Neurosurg Focus* 2005;18(5):E9.

152. Kiya K, Sacoda K, Gen M, et al. A case of aspergillotic meningoencephalitis

associated with trigemininal neuralgia. *No Shinkei Geka* 1982;10(8): 861–866.

153. Suzuki K, Iwabucchi N, Kuramochi S, et al. Aspergillus aneurysm of the middle cerebral artery causing a fatal subarachnoid hemorrhage. *Inter Med* 1995;34(6):550–553.

154. Arai M, Nakamura A, Shichi D. [Case of tsutsugamushi disease (scub typhus) presenting with fever and pain indistinguishable from trigeminal neuralgia]. *Rinsho Shinkeigaku* 2007;47(6)362–364.

155. Vitali AM, Sayer FT, Honey CR. Recurrent trigeminal neuralgia secondary to Teflon felt. *Acta Neuochir (Wien)* 2007;149(7):719–722.

156. Hojaili B, Barland P. Trigeminal neuralgia as the first manifestation of mixed connective tissue disorder. *J Clin Rheumatol* 2006;12(3):145–147.

157. Irizarry MC. Multiple sclerosis. In: Cudkowicz ME, Irizarry MC, eds. *Neurologic Disorders in Women*. Boston: Butterworth-Heinemann; 1997:85.

158. Solaro C, Brichetto G, Amato MP, et al. The prevalence of pain in multiple sclerosis: a multicenter cross sectional study. *Neurology* 2004;16(5):919–921.

159. Rovitt RL. *Trigeminal Neuralgia*. Baltimore: Williams & Wilkins; 1990.

160. da Silva CJ, da Roch AJ, Mendes MF, et al. Trigeminal involvement in multiple sclerosis: magnetic resonance imaging findings with clinical correlation in a series of patients. *Mult Scler* 2005;11(3):282–285.

161. van der Meijs AH, Tan IL, Barkhof F. Incidence of enhancement of the trigeminal nerve on MRI in patients with multiple sclerosis. *Mult Scler* 2002;8(1): 64–67.

162. Broggi G, Ferroli P, Franzini A, et al. Operative findings and outcomes of microvascular decompression for trigeminal neuralgia in 35 patients affected by multiple sclerosis. *Neurosurgery* 2004;55(4):830–838.

163. Resnick DK, Jannetta PJ, Lunsford LD, et al. Microvascular decompression for trigeminal neuralgia in patients with multiple sclerosis. *Surg Neurol* 1996; 46(4):358–361.

164. Cheng JS, Sanchez-Mejia RO, Limbo M, et al. Management of medically refractory trigeminal neuralgia in patients with multiple sclerosis. *Neurosurg Focus* 2005;18(5):e13.

165. Puca A, Meglio M. Typical trigeminal neuralgia associated with posterior cranial fossa tumors. *Ital J Neurol Sci* 1993;14(7):549–452.

166. Cheng TM, Cascino TL, Onofrio BM. Comprehensive study of diagnosis and treatment of trigeminal neuralgia secondary to tumors. *Neurology* 1993; 43(11):2298–2302.

167. Roberti F, Sekhar LN, Kalavakonda C, et al. Posterior fossa meningiomas: surgical experience in 161 cases. *Surg Neurol* 2001;56(1):8–20.

168. Lobato RD, Gonzaáez P, Alday R, et al. Meningiomas of the basal posterior fossa. Surgical experience in 80 cases. *Neurocirugia (Astur)* 2004;15(6): 525–542.

169. Haddad FS, Taha JM. An unusual cause for trigeminal neuralgia: contralateral meningioma of the posterior fossa. *Neurosurgery* 1990;26(6):1033–1038.

170. Florensa R, Llovet J, Pou S, et al. Contralateral trigeminal neuralgia as a false localizing sign in intracranial tumors. *Neurosurgery* 1987;20(1):1–3.

171. Mewes H, Schroth I, Deinsberger W, et al. Pain of the trigeminal nerve as the first symptom of metastasis from an oesoguscarcinoma in Meckel's cave—case report [in German]. *Zentralbl Neurochir* 2001;62(2):65–68.

172. Mastronardi L, Lunardi P, Osman FJ, et al. Metastatic involvement of the Meckel's cave and trigeminal nerve. A case report. *J Neurooncol* 1997;32(1): 87–90.

173. Nakano I, Iwwsuki K, Kondo A. Solitary metastatic breast carcinoma in a trigeminal nerve mimicking a trigeminal neuroma. Case report. *J Neurosurg* 1996;85(4):677–680.

174. Hirota N, Fujimoto T, Takahashi M, et al. Isolated trigeminal nerve metastases from breast cancer: an unusual cause of trigeminal mononeuropathy. *Surg Neurol* 1998;49(5):558–561.

175. Kuntzer T, Bogousslavsky J, Rilliet B, et al. Herald facial numbness. *Eur Neurol* 1992;32(5):297–301.

176. Inatomi Y, Inoue T, Nagata S, et al. Trigeminal neuralgia caused by the metastasis of malignant lymphoma to the trigeminal nerve: a case report. *No Shinkei Geka* 1998;26(5):401–405.

177. Falavigna A, Borba LA, Ferraz FA, et al. Primary melanoma of Meckel's cave: case report. *Arq Neuropsiquiatr* 2004;62(2A):353–356.

178. Tacconi L, Arulampalam T, Johnston F, et al. Adenocarcinoma of Meckel's cave: case report. *Surg Neurol* 1995;44(6):553–555.

179. Abdel Aziz KM, van Loveren HR. Primary lymphoma of Meckel's cave mimicking trigeminal schwannoma: case report. *Neurosurgery* 1999;44(4): 859–862.

180. Kanpolat Y, Tatli M, Ugur HC, et al. Evaluation of platybasia in patients with idiopathic trigeminal neuralgia. *Surg Neurol* 2007;67(1):78–81.

181. Quinones-Hinojosa A, Chang EF, Khan SA, et al. Isolated trigeminal nerve sarcoid granuloma mimicking trigeminal schwannoma: case report. *Neurosurgery* 2003;52(3):700–705.

182. Golby AJ, Norbash A, Silverberg GD. Trigeminal neuralgeia resulting from infarction of the root entry zone of the trigeminal nerve: case report. *Neurosurgery* 1998;43(3):620–622.

183. Ivánez V, Moreno M. [Trigeminal neuralgia in children as the only manifestation of Chiari I malformation]. *Rev Neuro* 1999;28(5):485–487.

184. Rosetti P, Ben Taib NO, Brotchi J, et al. Arnold Chiari Type I malformation presenting as a trigeminal neuralgia: case report. *Neurosurgery* 1999; 44(5): 1122–1123.

185. Teo C, Nakaji P, Serisier D, et al. Resolution of trigeminal neuralgia following third ventriculostomy for hydrocephalus associated with Chiari I malformation: case report. *Minim Invasive Neurosurg* 2005;48(3):302–305.

186. Schwartz NE, Rosenberg S, So YT. Action at a distance: a lumbar spine tumor presenting as trigeminal neuralgia. *Clin Neurol Neurosurg* 2006;108(8): 806–808.

187. Ohnishi YI, Fujimoto Y, Taniguchi M, et al. Neuroendoscopically assisted cyst-cysternal shunting for a quadrigeminal arachnoid cyst causing typical trigeminal neuralgia. *Minim Invasive Neurosurg* 2007;50(2):124–127.

188. Uzumi N, Hasegawa J, Kaoru K, et al. Pain relief by stellate ganglion block in a case with trigeminal neuralgia caused by a cerebellopontine angle tumor. *Anesth Prog* 2002;49:88–91.

189. Wu CL, March A, Dworkin RH. The role of sympathetic nerve blocks in acute herpes zoster and postherpetic neuralgia. *Pain* 2007;87:121–129.

190. Wollan PC, St Sauver JL, Kurland MJ, et al. A population-based study of the incidence and complication rates of herpes zoster before zoster vaccine introduction. *Mayo Clin Proc* 2007;82(11):1341–1349.

191. Dworkin RH, Portenoy RK. Pain and its persistence in herpes zoster. *Pain* 1996;67:241.

192. Sampathkumar P, Drage LA, Martin DP. Herpes zoster(shingles) and post herpetic neuralgia. *Mayo Clin Proc* 2009;84(3):274–280.

193. Gross G, Schöfer H, Wassilew S, et al. Herpes zoster guideline of the German Dermatology Society (DDG). *J Clin Virol* 2003;26(3):277–289.

194. Schmader K. Management of herpes zoster in elderly patients. *Infect Dis Clin Pract* 1995;4:293–299.

195. Crooks RJ, Jones DA, Fiddian AP. Zoster associated chronic pain: an overview of clinical trials with acyclovir. *Scand J Infect Dis Suppl* 1991;80:62–68.

196. Whitley RJ, Weiss H, Gnann J, et al. Acyclovir with and without prednisone for treatment of herpes zoster. A randomized, placebo-controlled trial. The Institute of Allergy and Infectious Diseases Collaborative Antiviral Study Group. *Ann Intern Med* 1996;125:376–383.

197. Bowsher D. The effects of pre-emptive treatment of postherpetic neuralgia with amitriptyline: a randomized, double-blind, placebo controlled trial. *J Pain Symptom Manage* 1997;13:327–331.

198. Kuraishi Y, Takasaki I, Nojima H, et al. Effects of the suppression of acute herpetic pain by gabapentin and amitriptyline on the incidence of delayed postherpetic pain in mice. *Life Sci* 2004;74:2619–2626.

199. Oxman MN, Levin MJ, Johnson GR, et al. A vaccine to prevent herpes zoster and postherpetic neuralgia in older adults. *N Engl J Med* 2005;352(22): 2271–2284.

200. Thomas SL, Wheeler JG, Hall AJ. Micronutrient intake and the risk of herpes zoster: a case-control study. *Int J Edidemiol* 2006;35:307–314.

201. High KP, Legault C, Sinclair JA, et al. Low plasma concentrations of retinol and alpha-tocopherol in hematopoietic stem cell transplant recipients: the effect of mucositis and the risk of infection. *Am J Clin Nutr* 2002;76: 1358–1366.

202. Alper BS, Lewis PR. Treatment of postherpetic neuralgia: a systematic review of the literature. *J Fam Pract* 2002;51:121–128.

203. Hempenstal K, Nurmikko TJ, Johnson RW, et al. Analgesic therapy in postherpetic neuralgia: a quantitative systematic review. *PLoS Med* 2005;2:e164.

204. Wu CL, March A, Dworkin RH. The role of sympathetic nerve blocks in acute herpes zoster and postherpetic neuralgia. *Pain* 2007;87:121–129.

205. Clark LP, Taylor AS. True tic douloureux of the fibers of the sensory filaments of the facial nerve. *JAMA* 1909; 53:2144–2146.

206. Jannetta PJ. Microsurgical approach to the trigeminal nerve for tic douloureux. *Prog Neurosurg* 1976;7:180–200.

207. Lovely TJ, Jannetta PJ. Surgical management of geniculate neuralgia. *Am J Otol* 1997;18(4):512–517.

208. Rupa V, Sauders RR, Weider DJ. Geniculate neuralgia: the surgical management of primary otalgia. *J Neuosurg* 1991;75(4):505–511.

209. Pulek JL. Geniculate neuralgia: long-term results of surgical treatment. *Ear Nose Throat J* 2002;81(1):30–33.

210. Bohm E, Strann RR. Glossopharyngeal neuralgia. *Brain* 1962;85:371–388.

211. Chawla JC, Falconer MA. Glossopharyngeal and vagal neuralgia. *Br Med J* 1967;3:529–531.

212. Bryun GW. Glossopharyngeal neuralgia. In: Vinkin PJ, Gruyn GW, Klawans HL, eds. *Handbook of Clinical Neurology*. Amsterdam: Elsevier; 1985: 459–473.

213. Fini G, Gasparini G, Filippini F, et al. The long stylid process syndrome or Eagle's syndrome. *J Craniomaxillofac Surg* 2000;28:123–127.

214. Soh KB. The glossopharyngeal nerve, glossopharyngeal neuralgia and the Eagle's syndrome-current concepts and management. *Singapore Med J* 1999;40: 659–665.

215. Nakagawa H, Nagasao M, Kusuyama T, et al. A case of glossopharyngeal zoster diagnosed by detecting viral antigen in the pharyngeal mucous membrane. *J Laryngol Otol* 2007;121(2):163–165.

216. Sampson JH, Grossi PM, Asaoka K, et al. Microvascular decompression for glossopharyngeal neuralgia: long-term effectiveness and complication avoidance. *Neurosurgery* 2004;54(4):884–889.

217. Zhao K, Zuo H, Zhang L, et al. [Long-term follow-up results of microsurgical treatment for glossopharyngeal neuralgia]. *Zhonghua Wai Ke Za Zhi* 2000; 38(8):598–600.

218. Resnick DK, Jannetta PJ, Bissonnette D, et al. Microvascular decompression for glossopharyngeal neuralgia. *Neurosurgery* 1995;36:64–68.

219. Patel A, Kassam A, Horowitz M, et al. Microvascular decompression in the management of glossopharyngeal neuralgia: analysis of 217 cases. *Neurosurgery* 2002;50:705–710.

220. Kodama S, Oribe K, Suzuki M. Superior laryngeal neuralgia associated with deviation of the hyoid bone. *Auris Nasus Larynx* 2007;35(3):429–431.

221. Bagatzounis A, Geyer G. [Lateral pharyngeal diverticulum as a cause of superior laryngeal nerve neuralgia] *Laryngorhinootologie.* 1994;73(4):219–221.

222. O'Neill BP, Aronson AE, Pearson BW, et al. Superior laryngeal neuralgia: carotidynia or just another pain in the neck? *Headache* 1982;22(1):6–9.

223. Johnson DL. Intractable hiccups: treatment by microvascular decompression of the vagus nerve. Case Report. *J Neurosurg* 1993;78(5):813–816.

224. Resnick DK, Jannetta PJ. Hyperactive rhizopathy of the vagus nerve and microvascular decompression. Case report. *J Neurosurg* 1999;90(3):580–582.

225. Takahashi SK, Suzuki M, Izuha A, et al. Two cases of idiopathic superior laryngeal neuralgia treated by superior laryngeal nerve block with a high concentration of lidocaine. *J Clin Anesth* 2007;19(3):237–238.

226. Kunc Z. Treatment of essential neuralgia of the ninth nerve with selective tractotomy. *J Neurosurg* 1965;23:494–500.

227. Trescott AM. Headache management in an interventional pain practice. *Pain Physician* 2000;3(2):197–200.

228. Sjaastad O, Stolt-Nielsen A, Pareja JA, et al. Supraorbital neuralgia. On the clinical manifestation and a possible therapeutic approach. *Headache* 1999;39(3):204–212.

229. Lambert WC, Okorodudu AO, Schwartz RA. Cutaneous nasociliary neuralgia. *Acta Derm Venereol* 1985;65(3):257–258.

230. Spokoinaia VA. Neuralgia of the trigeminal nerve and pterygopalatine ganglion as a complication of paranasal sinusitis [in Russian]. *Vestn Otorinolaringol* 1989;4:49–53.

231. Ahao Y, Li H, Cai Q, et al. Partial middle turbinectomy and folded for nasociliary neuralgia by transnasal endoscopic surgery, [in Chinese]. *Lin Chauang Er Bi yan Hou Ke Za Zhi* 2004;18(2):91–92.

232. Rath EM. Surgical treatment of maxillary nerve injuries. The infraorbital nerve. *Atlas Oral Maxillofac Surg Clin North Am* 2001;9(2):31–41.

233. Mathew NT, Kailasam J, Meadors L. Botulinum toxin type A for the treatment of nummular headache: four case studies. *Headache* 2007;48(3):442–447.

234. Tatli M, Keklikci U, Aluclu U, et al. Anesthesia dolorosa caused by penetrating cranial injury. *Eur Neurol* 2006;56(3):162–165.

235. Stillman M. Clinical approach to patients with neuropathic pain. *Cleve Clin J Med* 2006;73(8):726–739.

236. Wallace MS. Pharmacologic treatment of neuropathic pain. *Curr Pain Headache Rep* 2001;5:138–150.

237. Lazorthes Y, Sol JC, Fowo S, et al. Motor cortex stimulation for neuropathic pain. *Acta Neurochir Suppl* 2007;97(Pt 2):37–44.

238. Brown JA, Pilitsis JG. Motor cortex stimulation for central and neuropathic facial pain: a prospective study of 10 patients and observations of enhanced sensory and motor function during stimulation. *Neurosurgery* 2005;56(2):290–297.

239. Levy RM, Lamb S, Adams JE. Treatment of chronic pain by deep brain stimulation: long term follow-up and review of the literature. *Neurosurgery* 1987;21(6):885–893.

CHAPTER 67 ■ FACIAL PAIN

STEVEN J. SCRIVANI, NOSHIR R. MEHTA, DAVID A. KEITH, M. ALAN STILES, RAYMOND J. MACIEWICZ, AND RONALD J. KULICH

INTRODUCTION

Facial pain syndromes are common in clinical practice. Many of these syndromes are also unique, given the complex anatomy and specialized sensory innervation of the head, face, and neck, and so can pose diagnostic challenges.

The common descriptive terms for facial pain complaints are frequently misleading. To avoid confusion, clinicians should be familiar with the International Headache Society's Diagnostic Classification for Head, Face, and Neck Pain Disorders (Tables 67.1 through 67.6).[1] Clinicians need to be able distinguish among painful conditions that arise from structural pathology, headache syndromes, oral and facial structures, temporomandibular joint disorders, myofascial pain disorders, and primary cranial neuralgias.

ORGANIZATION OF THE TRIGEMINAL NOCICEPTIVE SYSTEM

Although nociceptive transmission in the trigeminal and spinal systems is similar, the two systems have important differences. In the perioral region, the trigeminal divisions contain afferents that subserve the dermatomes, which include the lips, teeth, gingival, anterior two thirds of the tongue, upper pharynx, uvula, and soft palate. In addition to this cutaneous distribution, the trigeminal nerve contains afferents that provide sensory innervation to a variety of deep structures in the head, including the muscles of mastication and facial expression, the nasal and oral mucosa, the cornea, tongue, tooth pulp, temporomandibular joint, dura mater, intracranial vessels, external auditory meatus, and ear (partially, and with cranial nerves VII, IX, and X).

The trigeminal system carries somatosensory information from these cutaneous and deep afferent structures as well as from specialized organs that have principally nociceptive innervation.

TABLE 67.1

INTERNATIONAL HEADACHE SOCIETY INTERNATIONAL CLASSIFICATION OF HEADACHE DISORDERS II

14 CATEGORIES
- The Primary Headaches: 1–4
- The Secondary Headaches: 5–12
- Cranial Neuralgias, central and primary facial pain and other headache disorders: 13–14

Adapted from Headache Classification Subcommittee of the International Headache Society. The International Classification of Headache Disorders: 2nd edition. *Cephalalgia.* 2004;24(Suppl 1):9–160.

TABLE 67.2

THE PRIMARY HEADACHES (1–4)

1. Migraine
   *without aura
   *with aura
2. Tension-type headache
3. Cluster headache and other trigeminal autonomic cephalalgias
4. Other primary headaches

TABLE 67.3

THE SECONDARY HEADACHES (5–12)

5. Attributed to head and/or neck trauma
6. Attributed to cranial or cervical vascular disorder
7. Attributed to nonvascular intracranial disorder
8. Attributed to a substance or its withdrawal
9. Attributed to infection
10. Attributed to disorder of homeostasis
11. Headache or facial pain attributed to disorder of cranium, neck, eyes, ears, nose, sinuses, teeth, mouth, or other facial or cranial structures
12. Attributed to psychiatric disorder

TABLE 67.4

HEADACHE OR FACIAL PAIN ATTRIBUTED TO DISORDERS OF CRANIUM, NECK, EYES, EARS, NOSE, SINUSES, TEETH, MOUTH, OR OTHER FACIAL OR CRANIAL STRUCTURES (11.1–8)

11.1—Cranial bones
11.2—Neck
11.3—Eyes
11.4—Ears
11.5—Rhinosinusitis (Sinus disorders)
11.6—Teeth, jaws, or related structures
11.7—TMJ disorders (TMD)
11.8—Other

TABLE 67.5

CRANIAL NEURALGIAS, CENTRAL AND PRIMARY FACIAL PAIN, AND OTHER HEADACHES (13.1–19)

13.1—Trigeminal neuralgia
13.2—Glossopharyngeal neuralgia
13.8—Occipital neuralgia
13.12—Constant pain caused by compression, irritation, or distortion of cranial nerves or upper cervical roots by *structural lesions*

TABLE 67.6

CRANIAL NEURALGIAS, CENTRAL AND PRIMARY FACIAL PAIN, AND OTHER HEADACHES (13.1–19)

13.15—Head or facial pain attributed to herpes zoster
postherpetic neuralgia

13.18—Central causes of facial pain
anesthesia dolorosa
central poststroke pain
facial pain attributed to multiple sclerosis
persistent idiopathic facial pain
burning mouth syndrome

Most nociceptive afferents relay through the trigeminal brainstem complex, with oral and perioral structures represented more rostrally than peripheral sites on the face.[2] In addition, nociceptive afferents from the other cranial nerves and the upper cervical spinal segments (C2–C4) also are relayed through the trigeminal brainstem complex.

In the subnucleus caudalis, cells relaying nociceptive signals (nociceptive-specific cells and wide–dynamic-range cells) are primarily localized to analogous regions of lamina I and V in the spinal cord. Deep afferents also converge on cells that also receive cutaneous nociceptive input, providing a substrate for referred pain in the head, face, and neck through the trigeminal system. Finally, the trigeminal nociceptive relay cells are strongly modulated by central pathways (descending opioidergic, noradrenergic, and serotonergic) that may dynamically modulate nociception under a variety of environmental situations and behavioral states.[2]

Although the trigeminal dermatomes do not generally overlap those supplied by the adjacent cervical spinal nerves and other cranial nerves, they overlap extensively in the spinal afferent system. Three adjacent spinal roots must be injured to render any one region anesthetic. In the trigeminal system, under normal conditions, a section of one trigeminal division renders almost the entire dermatome anesthetic. Because the peripheral sensory nerves overlap so little with the trigeminal system, nerve lesions may result in more pronounced central somatosensory changes than those evoked by similar lesions in spinal nerves. These changes may partly underlie trigeminal neuropathic pain disorders. Additionally, the trigeminal system may be developmentally and functionally distinct as a result of three hypothetical factors: (1) it innervates highly specialized tissues that are engaged in highly specialized functions; (2) it experiences two developmentally unique events: one programmed pain event and one programmed denervation event (eruption and exfoliation of teeth); and (3) it can be affected by dental surgery procedures performed with local anesthesia, which alters the afferent input into the system. These factors may also influence the development of chronic facial pain.

DIAGNOSTIC EVALUATION

Pain in the mouth or face is one of the most common presenting symptoms in clinical practice. The majority of symptoms are related to dental disease and, in most cases, the cause can readily be established, the problem dealt with expeditiously, and the pain eliminated. However, in a few patients, pain may be persistent and defy attempts at treatment. Intractable oral and facial pains can be diagnostically challenging, given the many potential causes of pain, the anatomic complexity of the region, and the psychosocial importance of the face and mouth. A rigorous protocol for evaluating these patients includes a thorough history and an appropriate clinical examination (see Chapter 24).

A detailed history should always be obtained before examining the patient or ordering special tests or imaging studies because the history will establish a diagnosis in a majority of cases.

Chief Complaint

The patient's description of the pain may provide clues to its cause. Primary neuralgias are frequently described as sharp and lancinating, secondary neuralgias have a burning quality, vascular headaches are throbbing, and muscle pain is described as a deep and dull ache. The patient may not be able to give all these descriptions at the first interview, and corroborating information from relatives and friends may be needed to build a general picture of the pain as it affects the patient. Each pain complaint should be listed in order of severity.

History of Present Complaint

The intensity of the pain needs to be measured against the patient's own experience of pain, need for medication, and effect on lifestyle. For example, does the pain interfere with work, sleep, or social activities? How severe is it on a 10-point scale? Does it fluctuate over time? The origin of the pain should be determined by asking the patient to indicate the site of the pain or the site of its maximum intensity. Its anatomic distribution should be accurately traced in terms of local anatomy.

The patient should be encouraged to remember the events surrounding the onset of the pain, even if it was several years ago. Any other instance of similar pain should be ascertained, even though the patient may not associate these with the present problem. The time relations of the pain should be clarified in terms of duration and frequency of attacks, as well as possible remissions.

Aggravating factors should be determined. Is the pain aggravated by the ingestion of specific foods or beverages, by lying down, during times of stress, talking, brushing the teeth, shaving, applying make-up, or by other identifiable factors? In addition, relieving factors (e.g., lying down, sleeping, heat, and cold) are important clues.

The effects of previous treatments need to be clarified. Which medications have helped? Has surgery altered the nature of the pain? Has endodontic treatment or extraction affected the pain? Finally, the presence or absence of associated factors (e.g., swelling of the face, flushing, tearing, nasal congestion, or facial weakness) needs to be ascertained.

Medical History

Take a detailed history of the patient and the reported pain. Especially, note any trauma to the head, face, and mouth. Identify current and past medications, relevant family history, and the use of over-the-counter medications, supplements, and alternative or complementary therapies. Identify any jaw habits, such as clenching, grinding, posturing the jaw, or gum chewing, including occupational or vocational habits (e.g., playing a wind instrument, scuba diving, and so on). A comprehensive psychosocial history is imperative for all patients with chronic pain disorders (see Chapter 21). Establish the details of any pending or planned disability claims or litigation (see Chapter 22).

Physical Examination

The purpose of the physical examination is to discover any possible anatomic or physiologic basis for the pain; therefore, it is important to proceed systematically. Patients with facial pain should have a complete head and neck examination, not an examination directed by a presumed diagnosis.

Neurologic Function

The most important evaluations are of those of the cranial nerves (CN) V (trigeminal) and VII (facial) and the upper cervical nerves (C2–C4). The three divisions of the trigeminal nerve—supraorbital, infraorbital, and inferior alveolar nerves—supply the majority of sensation to the mouth and face. Examine the skin distribution of all three divisions, as well as the intraoral distribution of the second and third divisions. Directional sense, two-point discrimination, and sensory perception with von Frey hairs may help with the diagnosis. Heat, cold, and taste may need to be tested in certain situations. Pain to pressure over the six foramina may indicate trigeminal involvement. Corneal and gag reflexes should be assessed. The size and strength of the masticatory muscles reflect the motor division of CN V. Facial nerve function can be assessed by asking the patient to whistle, purse the lips, smile, close the eyes, and frown.

Upper cervical nerve sensation can be assessed on the scalp for C2 and at the angle of the jaw and upper neck for C3. Pressure over the midsuperior nuchal line directly affects the greater occipital nerve and may reproduce the headache in occipital neuralgia.

Because of the overlap of CNs V, VII, IX, and X and their convergence on the spinal trigeminal nucleus, a more detailed examination of these nerves may be necessary. CN IV and VI nerve palsies may indicate increased intracranial pressure.

Muscle Function

Pain in the masticatory muscles, face, posterior cervical spine, and upper back (the suprascapular and pectoral girdle) are common causes of head, face, and neck pain, so the neck, shoulder, and masticatory muscles should be thoroughly assessed. The size of the muscles can be assessed visually (e.g., temporal hollowing, masseteric hypertrophy). The muscles should be palpated, trigger points noted, and head and neck posture should be assessed. A more thorough evaluation of the masticatory muscles includes measuring the maximum interincisal opening and lateral and protrusive excursions. Tremors and fasciculation should also be noted.

Temporomandibular Joint

Palpate the lateral pole of the mandibular condyle for tenderness with the mouth open and closed. Course and fine crepitation should be noted and joint noises auscultated. Clicks and pops and the position in the opening or closing cycle should be observed. Determining whether or not these are eliminated by separating the teeth with a tongue blade or by posturing the jaw forward will help focus on the functional importance of these joint noises.

Intraoral Examination

Note how the maxillary and mandibular teeth interdigitate when the mouth is closed (dental occlusion) as well as the state of the dentition and oral hygiene. Look for evidence of wear on the teeth, excessive toothbrush abrasion, or palatal erosion from repetitive vomiting. The health of the oropharyngeal mucosa should be recorded, as well as the moistness of the mucosa and pooling of saliva. The parotid and submandibular glands can be milked to evaluate the quality and quantity of saliva expressed. The tongue and soft palate should be centered midline and freely mobile. Excessive draping of the soft palate, as seen in sleep apnea, should be noted.

Diagnostic Imaging (see Chapter 19)

Periapical dental films and panoramic maxillofacial radiographs are inexpensive, readily available, do not expose patients to excessive radiation, and offer detailed information about the teeth and jaws. Computed tomography (CT) can provide more detailed images of the bony structures of the jaws, temporomandibular joints, and base of the skull. Three-dimensional imaging can be helpful in some instances. Magnetic resonance imaging (MRI) is best for evaluating the soft tissues and can be used for assessing the deep oro- and nasopharyngeal anatomy and the internal anatomy of the temporomandibular joints. In addition, the brain can be evaluated with MRI with and without gadolinium contrast. MRI studies can help determine whether the vasculature is impinging on the trigeminal ganglion, which can cause trigeminal neuralgia.

Bone scan with technetium-99m will highlight areas of metabolic activity within the bone and can help identify areas of infection, tumor extension and continued growth, or degenerative change in the temporomandibular joint.

Laboratory Studies

Routine blood tests include complete blood count and differential to exclude anemia and blood dyscrasias. Erythrocyte sedimentation rate may be elevated in temporal arteritis. Rheumatoid factor and Lyme titer may be helpful in evaluating temporomandibular joint disease.

FACIAL PAIN DISORDERS

Pain Attributed to Disorders of the Oral Cavity

Facial Pain of Dental Origin (Odontogenic)

Tooth pulp has a specialized and possibly exclusively nociceptive innervation.[3] In contrast, periodontal tissues are innervated by a wide variety of sensory afferents. Pain of dental origin is extremely variable and can simulate nearly any pain syndrome. Dental pain may be spontaneous or induced in various ways, and it can be intermittent or continuous (Table 67.7). Because of the extreme variability of toothache, all pains about the mouth and the face should be considered to be of dental origin until proven otherwise.

Dental pain is typically provoked by thermal or mechanical stimulation of the damaged tooth, but it can also be provoked by light touch, tooth-tooth contact (in eating and talking), and pressure. Dental pain is usually described as an aching sensation and sometimes as throbbing. When mild, it may be felt only as a tenderness or soreness. When severe, it may have a burning or electric- or shock-like quality.

Patients often cannot localize pain arising solely from the dental pulp. They often cannot determine whether the offending tooth is mandibular or maxillary, much less which tooth is involved. The pain is felt diffusely in the teeth, jaws, face, and head.[4] Clinical and radiographic findings of dental decay, fractured dental restoration, tooth fracture, or abscess drainage (fistula) may confirm dental pain as the source of the complaint (Tables 67.8 and 67.9).

Reversible and Irreversible Pulpitis. Dental pain occurs most commonly secondary to dental caries, which represent a loss of integrity of tooth enamel. When enamel integrity is sufficiently breached, sensitivity to cold or sweet stimulus may result. Carious progression occurs more rapidly with dentinal involvement. At this stage, the vital dental pulp is exposed to the oral environment, and inflammatory changes in the pulpal tissue are evident histologically.

TABLE 67.7

DENTAL AND ORAL SURGICAL CONDITIONS

Dentoalveolar Pathology
  *pulpal
  *periodontal
Odontogenic and Nonodontogenic Pathology
Trigeminal Neuralgia and "Equivalents"
Headache and Neck pain
Temporomandibular Disorders
Oral Mucous Membrane Disease
Oral Manifestations of Systemic Disease
Neuropathic Pain (Persistent Idiopathic Facial Pain)
"Burning Mouth/Tongue Syndrome"

TABLE 67.8

FEATURES OF ODONTOGENIC PAIN

Presence of etiologic factors for an odontogenic origin of pain
Unilateral pain
Localized pain (diagnosis-specific)
Pain qualities (sharp, dull, aching, throbbing)
Sensitivity to temperature
Sensitivity to pressure, palpation, percussion
Pain reduction by local anesthetic injection?

The pulpal inflammatory process is initially reversible. Reversible pulpitis is characterized by inflammation of the pulp that may recover or heal when the insult is removed. Continued stimuli jeopardizes the pulp's ability to respond and repair itself. Irreversible pulpitis can be distinguished from reversible pulpitis by the duration of symptoms. Both require a stimulus to initiate the pain; however, the duration of pain is measured in seconds in reversible pulpitis but in minutes or hours in irreversible pulpitis. Spontaneous odontogenic pain most frequently marks pulpal death or necrosis. Pain elicited with heat is most commonly associated with pulpal necrosis.[5] The general clinical characteristics displayed by toothache of pulpal origin are described in Table 67.8.

Cracked Tooth. Incomplete fractures of a vital tooth may trigger intermittent pain when biting on the offending tooth. Risk factors include older age, extensive dental restoration, and parafunctional habits, such as teeth grinding. Unfortunately, the cracks are often difficult to find and do not appear on all radiographs. The pain is often confused with that of pulpitis or trigeminal neuralgia, which may result in unnecessary treatment (see Table 67.9). Careful clinical examination, including staining or meticulous bite tests on each tooth cusp, may be useful.[6,7]

Acute dental pain typically responds to local treatments (e.g., ice packs and reduced mechanical stimulation) or systemic nonsteroidal anti-inflammatory drugs (NSAIDs). Opioid analgesics (and combinations) are also indicated, depending on the extent of the pain. In many cases, treatment with antibiotics is appropriate and palliative until a definitive dental intervention is performed. Definitive dental procedures are generally curative.

Disorders of the Periodontium (Periodontal Disease)

Chronic periodontal disease is an immune-mediated inflammatory process initiated by pathogenic oral microorganisms,[8,9] destroying either focal or generalized areas of tooth-supporting structures and the surrounding bone. Chronic periodontitis is generally not a chronically painful disorder. Typically, patients notice gingival sensitivity and tenderness or gingival enlargement secondary to inflammation and bleeding with brushing or probing examination. A tooth with lost bone support may have lost the gingival attachment surrounding the necks and soft tissue of the root, which may result in tooth sensitivity, tenderness, and mobility. In acute periodontal infection, tenderness to the touch, erythema, and bleeding may be evident. An acute periodontal abscess may cause swelling and purulence (see Table 67.9). When inflammation or infection (i.e., acute pericoronitis) occurs in the soft tissue or bone around an erupting or partially erupted tooth (particularly third molars, otherwise known as wisdom teeth), similar signs and symptoms may be seen, with pain as a primary complaint.

The pain of periodontal disorders also generally responds to NSAIDs, opioid analgesics, or combination analgesics. An acute abscess may also have to be locally incised and drained. Areas of generalized periodontitis may be treated with tooth scaling and

TABLE 67.9

ODONTIC PAIN

Diagnosis	Pulpitis	Peridontal	Cracked Tooth	Dentinal
Diagnostic Features	Spontaneous and/or evoked deep/diffuse pain in compromised dental pulp. Pain may be sharp, throbbing, or dull.	Localized deep continuous pain in compromised periodontium (e.g., gingiva, periodontal ligament) exacerbated by biting or chewing.	Spontaneous or evoke brief sharp pain in a tooth with history of trauma or restorative work (e.g., crown, root canal).	Brief, sharp pain evoked by different kinds of stimulus to the dentin (e.g., hot or cold drinks).
Diagnostic Evaluation	Look for deep caries and recent or extensive dental work. Pain provoked/exacerbated by percussion, thermal, or electric stimulation of affected tooth. Dental radiographs helpful (periapical).	Tooth percussion over compromised periodontium provokes pain. Look for inflammation or abscess (e.g., periodontitis, apical dental radiographs helpful (bitewings, periapical).	Presence of tooth fracture may be detectable by radiograph. Percussion should elicit pain. Dental radiographs are helpful (periapical taken from different angles).	Exposed dentin or cementum due to recession of periodontium. Possible erosion of dentinal structure. Cold stimulation reproduces pain.
Treatment	Medication: NSAIDs, nonopiate analgesics. Dentistry: remove carious lesion, tooth restoration, endodontic treatment, or tooth extraction.	Medication: NSAIDs, nonopiate analgesics, antibiotics, mouthwashes. Dentistry: drainage and débridement of periodontal pocket, scaling and root planning, periodontal surgery, endodontic treatment, or tooth extraction.	Medication: NSAIDs, nonopiate analgesics. Dentistry: depends on level of the tooth fracture-restoration, treatment, or extraction of the tooth.	Medication: mouthwash (fluoride), desensitizing toothpaste. Dentistry: fluoride or potassium salts, tooth restoration, endodontic treatment. Patient education, diet, tooth brushing force and frequency, proper toothpaste.

curettage of the gingival pocketing and possibly local or systemic antibiotic therapy.

Acute Necrotizing Ulcerative Gingivitis

Acute necrotizing ulcerative gingivitis (ANUG) is an aggressively destructive process. The diagnostic triad includes pain, ulcerated or "punched out" interdental papillae, and gingival bleeding. Secondary signs include fetid breath, pseudomembrane formation, "wooden teeth" feeling, foul metallic taste, tooth mobility, lymphadenopathy, fever, and malaise. The cause of ANUG is poorly understood. It appears to be an opportunistic infection in a host of lowered resistance. The most important predisposing factor is human immunodeficiency virus infection and the second, a history of necrotizing gingivitis. Other contributing factors include poor oral hygiene, unusual emotional stress, poor diet, inadequate sleep, recent illness, alcohol use, tobacco use, and various infections, such as malaria, measles, and intestinal parasites. Treatment consists primarily of bacterial control. Chlorhexidine oral rinses, professional débridement and scaling, and adjunctive antibiotic therapy with a soft diet rich in protein, vitamins, and fluids are important in treating and preventing the disease.[10]

Oral Mucous Membrane Disorders

Diseases of the oral mucosa are numerous and have a variety of local and systemic causes. Typically, these diseases present with pain and oral mucosal lesions, including vesicles, bullae, erosions, erythema, or red and white patches (Table 67.10). Pain may be a symptom of the primary disease process, secondary to an associated process (i.e., infection), or related to damaged oral mucosa

(i.e., mouth movements, chewing foods, thermal, chemical) and is often treated with both systemic and local analgesic agents.

Disorders of the Maxilla and Mandible

Numerous disorders of the bony substrate of the jaws may present with pain. These disorders are generally classified as being of odontogenic or nonodontogenic origin, cystic, cystic-like, or tumor, and benign or malignant (either primary or metastatic disease). Often, additional historical or examination findings warrant further evaluation (i.e., swelling, mass, discoloration, numbness, weakness, bleeding, drainage, tooth loss, or mobility). Pain can be treated symptomatically until a definitive diagnosis is established and definitive therapy is initiated (Table 67.11).

Salivary Gland Disorders

Disorders of the three major pairs of salivary glands (parotid, submandibular, and sublingual) and many hundreds of minor salivary glands in the mouth may also produce pain as a primary or associated symptom. These disorders are often accompanied by other signs and symptoms (including swelling, drainage, cervical adenopathy, or generalized signs of systemic infection), depending on the cause of the disorder. Disorders of the parotid gland can locally extend to produce otologic symptoms or CN (V, VII, or IX) involvement. Disorders of the submandibular gland may result in symptoms of impaired swallowing or impairment of CNs V, IX, XII (Table 67.12).

Burning Mouth-Tongue Syndrome (Oral Burning)

Burning mouth-tongue syndrome (BMS) is an idiopathic pain condition of the oral mucous membranes akin to idiopathic neu-

TABLE 67.10

COMMON PAINFUL MUCOSAL CONDITIONS

Infections
Herpetic stomatitis
Varicella zoster
Candiasis
Acute necrotizing gingivostomatitis

Immune/Autoimmune
Allergic reactions (toothpaste, mouthwashes, topical medications)
Erosive lichen planus
Benign mucous membrane pemphigoid
Aphthous stomatitis and aphthous lesions
Erythema multiform
Graft versus host disease

Traumatic and Iatrogenic Injuries
Factitial, accidental (burns: chemical, solar, thermal)
Self-destructive (rituals, obsessive behaviors)
Iatrogenic (chemotherapy, radiation)

Neoplasia
Squamous cell carcinoma
Mucoepidermoid carcinoma
Adenocystic carcinoma
Brain tumors

Neurologic
Burning mouth syndrome and glossodynia
Neuralgias
Postviral neuralgias
Posttraumatic neuropathies
Dyskinesias and dystonias

Nutritional and Metabolic
Vitamin deficiencies (B_{12}, folate)
Mineral deficiencies (iron)
Diabetic neuropathy
Malabsorption syndromes

Miscellaneous
Xerostomia, secondary to intrinsic or extrinsic conditions
Referred pain from esophageal or oropharyngeal malignancy
Mucositis secondary to esophageal reflux
Angioderma

ropathic pain syndromes. It can be focal (inside of the lips and tongue) or generalized and is typically described as a constant, bilateral, burning, painful sensation. The syndrome generally affects middle-aged or older women and has been attributed to numerous oral disorders (i.e., mucous membrane disease, Sjögren

TABLE 67.11

ODONTOGENIC AND NONODONTOGENIC DISORDERS

Odontogenic Cysts and Tumors
Nonodontogenic Cysts and Tumors
Metabolic Bone Disease
Metastatic Bone Disease
Neurogenic Tumors
Vascular Lesions—Hemangiomas and Vascular malformations

TABLE 67.12

SALIVARY GLAND DISEASE

Inflammatory
Noninflammatory
Infectious
Obstructive
Immunologic (Sjogren's Syndrome)
Tumors
Others (Red herrings)

syndrome-dry mouth, fungal infections) and systemic diseases (i.e., vitamin deficiencies, diabetes mellitus, immune connective tissue disorders, vasculitides). More recent evidence suggests that BMS is more likely a neuropathic pain disorder of either peripheral or central origin. Some recent taste-testing data and functional brain imaging studies support this hypothesis (Table 67.13).[11–15] Current treatments for BMS focus on this hypothesis and use both topical (oral mucosa) and systemic antineuropathic pain medications (see neuropathic pain section below); however, there is little evidence that such treatments are effective.

Pain Attributed to Disorders of the Eye

Pain in and around the eye is a common presenting problem (Table 67.14). Most ophthalmologic conditions producing eye pain are associated with obvious ocular symptoms, signs, or histories that implicate the eye as the origin of pain. Several facial pain and headache syndromes present with "eye pain" as the chief symptom (Table 67.15). In addition, during the history and physical examination, several signs and symptoms warn of more serious eye disease and even of potential life-threatening problems (Table 67.16).

History and Ocular Examination

A complete ocular history should include any prior visual loss, ophthalmic diseases (e.g., corneal infections, uveitis, and glaucoma), use of contact lenses, recent or remote ocular surgery, and ocular trauma. In addition to noting the specific features of pain when taking the history for eye pain, such as time of onset, severity, exacerbating and palliating factors, radiation, quality, duration, and frequency, ask about the specific location of pain; for example, intraocular, retrobulbar, periocular, or frontal and associated symptoms, such as tearing, loss of vision, double vision, photophobia, and discharge.[16]

Simple instruments are required to perform the basic eye examination, in which the pain specialist can triage patients with eye pain and identify those who require formal ophthalmologic consultation. Such equipment includes a near vision card (Snellen card), a hand light, and a direct ophthalmoscope. The Snellen card is used to check the visual acuity (VA). The VA should be tested using the patient spectacle correction and each eye should be tested individually. The pupil response to light, the regularity of the pupil, and relative afferent papillary defect should be evaluated using a hand light. Also, examine extraocular motility examination and the eyelids. Use a hand light to assess the conjunctiva for chemosis, injections, and foreign bodies and the cornea for keratitis, corneal foreign bodies, and lacerations. Evaluation of the optic nerve using the direct ophthalmoscope should be sufficient to exclude gross optic atrophy, fundoscopic abnormalities, and papilledema.

Ocular and Orbital Causes of Eye Pain

Although a large percentage of patients with headache attribute their pain to their refractive errors and present with many pairs

TABLE 67.13

TRIGEMINAL NEUROPATHIC PAIN DISORDERS

Diagnosis	Trigeminal neuralgia	Deafferentation pain	Acute and postherpetic neuralgia	Burning mouth syndrome
Diagnostic features	Brief severe lancinating pain evoked by mechanical stimulation of trigger zone (pain free between attacks). Usually unilateral, affects the V2/V3 areas (rarely V1). Possible pain remission periods (for months/years).	Spontaneous or evoked pain with prolonged after-sensation after tactile stimulation. Trigger zone due to surgery (tooth extraction) or trauma. Positive and negative descriptors (e.g., burning, nagging, boring).	Pain associated with herpetic lesions, usually in the V1 dermatoma. Spontaneous pain (burning and tingling), but may present as dull and aching. Occasional lancinating evoked pain.	Constant burning pain of the mucous membranes of the tongue, mouth. Hard or soft palate or lips. Usually affects women age >50 years.
Diagnostic evaluation	MRI for evidence of tumor or vasocompression of the trigeminal tract or root (cerebropontine angle). Rule-out multiple sclerosis, especially in young adults.	Etiologic factors such as trauma or surgery in the painful area. Order MRI if the area is intact to rule-out peripheral or central lesions.	Small cutaneous vesicles or scarring, usually affecting V1. Loss of normal skin color. Corneal ulceration can occur. Sensory changes in affected area (e.g., hyperesthesia, dysesthesia).	Rule-out salivary gland dysfunction (xerostomia) or tumor, Sjögren's, candidiasis, geographic or fissured tongue, and chemical or mechanical irritations. Nutrition and menopause.
Treatment	Medication: anticonvulsants (e.g., carbamazepine, gabapentin); antidepressants (e.g., amitriptyline, nortriptyline, desipramine); nonopiate analgesics, botulinum toxin. Combination of baclofen and anticonvulsants can produce good results. Surgery: microvascular decompression of trigeminal root, ablative surgeries (e.g., rhizotomy, gamma knife).	Medication: anticonvulsants (e.g., carbamazepine, gabapentin); antidepressants; nonopiate analgesics; topical agents (e.g., lidocaine 5% patches). Surgery: ablative surgeries (e.g., rhizotomy, gamma knife).	Medication: acyclovir (acute phase) anticonvulsants, antidepressants; nonopiate analgesics; topical agents (e.g., lidocaine 5% patches). Surgery: ablative surgeries (e.g., rhizotomy, gamma knife).	Medication: anticonvulsants, benzodiazepines, antidepressants; nonopiate analgesics; topical agents (e.g., lidocaine, mouth washes). Cognitive-behavior: biofeedback, relaxation, coping skills.

of "incorrect" glasses, correcting the refractive errors helps few patients. The eye is rarely the source of headache localized to the eye and orbit without clinical signs, such as red eye, or symptoms, such as decreased vision or a history of eye trauma. If the basic eye history and examination are normal, an intraocular cause for the pain is less likely. However, in some ocular causes of eye pain, the eye is superficially normal. The pain specialist should be able to recognize the features of these uncommon causes of eye pain.

Ocular Causes for Eye Pain with a White Eye ("Quite Eye") Other causes of eye pain include acute angle-closure glaucoma, anterior or posterior uveitis, posterior scleritis, intraocular tumors, optic neuritis, and corneal disorders (Tables 67.17 and 67.18).

Glaucoma. Glaucoma may cause acute or chronic eye pain. Glaucoma is a broad term for a large array of clinical disorders that are characterized by damage to the optic nerve with visual field defects generally associated with elevated intraocular pressure. Pain in glaucoma is entirely a function of the rate of rise of intraocular pressure, so only acute forms are likely to be painful.[17] The aqueous humor is produced by the ciliary body in the posterior chamber; it flows through the pupillary aperture and exits the anterior chamber through the trabecular meshwork in the anterior chamber angle. Disorders of elevated intraocular pressure are of two types: open angle, in which the aqueous humor can flow through the trabecular meshwork, and angle-closure, in which the iris or some other structure is physically blocking access to the trabecular meshwork. These types are further subdivided into primary and secondary forms.[18]

Primary open-angle glaucoma is the most common type of glaucoma and is almost always entirely asymptomatic. Therefore, this form of glaucoma is rarely the cause of ocular pain in patients with a "quite eye."[18] Interestingly, the miotic eye drops used to treat primary open-angle glaucoma are more likely to cause eye and brow ache. In contrast, acute angle-closure glaucoma is associated with severe, acute eye pain. Fortunately, it is far less common than primary open-angle glaucoma. Even though patients with angle-closure glaucoma can have a normal appearing eye, they typically present with a red eye, edematous cornea, blurred vision, a pupil that is often partially dilated, irregularly shaped, and poorly reactive to light, and intense eye pain.[19,20] The pain may radiate widely and often is associated with nausea and vomiting. Teeth have been extracted to treat this disorder, as well as laparotomies for the accompanying gastrointestinal complaints.

TABLE 67.14

PARANASAL, PERIOCULAR, PERIAURICULAR, AND HEAD AND NECK CANCER PAIN

Diagnosis	Paranasal sinus pain	Periocular pain	Periauricular pain	Head and neck cancer
Diagnostic features	Bilateral or unilateral throbbing or pressure frontal area pain, exacerbated by leaning forward or palpitation over the sinus.	Pain or tenderness with or without eye movements, deep orbital pain, and referred pain.	Diffuse aching or sudden pain with or without aural discharge (e.g., otitis media).	Variety of symptoms. Pain may be due to tumor, nerve compression, secondary infection, secondary myofascial pain, deafferentation, radiotherapy, chemotherapy.
Diagnostic evaluation	History of chronic allergies, frequent upper respiratory infections, sinusitis, headaches of various types, sinus surgery Refer to ear, nose, and throat specialist for endoscopic and/or CT study (e.g., sinus opacification).	Examine eyelids, lacrimal function, conjunctiva, and sclera. Ophthalmoscopy and ophthalmology referral. Rule-out primary headache, temporal arteritis, orbital pseudotumor.	The area is innervated by multiple cranial and cervical nerves so complete functional and structural exam necessary (e.g., inspect tympanic membrane, TMJ, and myofascial). CT and MRI invaluable for mastoiditis and cholesteatoma.	Complete evaluation by multidisciplinary team, CT, MRI, endoscopy, biopsy and surveillance. Treatment coordination by oncologist.
Treatment	Ear, nose, and throat specialist evaluation/treatment Medication: sinusitis-topical decongestants; systemic antibiotics. Chronic sinus pain-NSAIDs; nonopiate analgesics; topical agents (lidocaine spray); anticonvulsants, antidepressants; botulinum toxin. Surgery	Proper ophthalmologic evaluation and treatment. Medication: NSAIDs; nonopiate analgesics; systemic antibiotics, topical corticosteroids, botulinum toxin across forehead and glabellar areas in selected cases. Surgery	Proper ear, nose, and throat specialist evaluation and treatment. Medication: NSAIDs; nonopiate analgesics; systemic antibiotics, topical corticosteroids, botulinum toxin in selected cases. Surgery	Oncologist evaluation and treatment. Medication: anticonvulsants, antidepressants, opiate or nonopiate analgesics, topical agents, muscles relaxants. Surgery: ablative surgeries.

TABLE 67.15

HEADACHE AND FACIAL PAIN SYNDROMES WITH EYE PAIN

Cluster headache and cluster-tic syndrome
Paroxysmal hemicrania
SUNCT syndrome
Trigeminal neuralgia
Sphenopalatine neuralgia (Sluder's neuralgia)
Ice-pick headache
Ice cream headache
Hypnic headache
Eye pain, headache and lung cancer
Nonorganic pain and headache (psychosomatic and psychiatric disorders)

TABLE 67.16

RED FLAGS FOR A PATIENT WITH EYE PAIN

New visual acuity defect, color vision defect, or visual field loss
Relative afferent pupillary defect
Extraocular muscle abnormality, ocular misalignment, or diplopia
Proptosis
Lid retraction or ptosis
Conjunctival chemosis, injection, or redness
Corneal opacity
Hyphema or hypopyon
Iris irregularity
Nonreactive pupil
Fundus abnormality
Recent ocular surgery (<3 months)
Recent ocular trauma

TABLE 67.17

PAIN IN OR AROUND THE EYE: "QUITE EYE" AND NORMAL EXAM

Cluster headache and cluster-tic syndrome
Paroxysmal hemicrania
SUNCT/SUNA syndrome
Migraine and tension-type headache
Ice-pick headache/Ice cream headache/Valsalvaa headache
Trigeminal neuralgia
Sinus disease (acute)
Teeth, jaws (TMD)
Carotid disease
Temporal arteritis
Eye pain, headache, and lung cancer

Early diagnosis of this disease is important; key features are summarized in Table 67.17.[21,22] This disease is easily diagnosed, and patients should be referred immediately to an ophthalmologist because it can usually be quickly reversed.

Corneal Disorders. Corneal abrasion is a scraping away or denuding of the corneal surface by external forces on the corneal surface. Eye pain caused by corneal disease is typically described as "scratchy" or a "foreign body sensation." Corneal epithelial defects typically occur after trauma, after ultraviolet light keratitis, in contact lens wearers, or from corneal infections. Some patients with corneal disease may present with no conjunctival signs and with an apparently normal eye; however, most patients have some visible external findings such as red eye, corneal opacity, or abrasion. A corneal abrasion can cause photophobia and excruciating eye pain that often radiates to other parts of the head and face.[17,20] Corneal abrasions are best seen by placing a drop of fluorescein in the eye and looking through a slit lamp using a cobalt blue light. If the cornea is abraded, antibiotic ointment should be applied.[16,23] However, most abrasions are self-limited and heal within 24 to 48 hours.[23]

Uveitis. The uveal tracts are the pigmented middle ocular tissue, iris, ciliary body, and choroids. Uveitis could have a pure anterior involvement iritis, which occurs in half the cases. These patients may present with eye pain, photophobia, and decreased vision with a relatively quite appearing eye. The other patients with uveitis have posterior involvement chorioretinitis with inflammation of the ciliary body, the choroids, or both. Posterior uveitis is more likely to cause visual loss than anterior uveitis.[24,25]

TABLE 67.18

PAIN IN OR AROUND THE EYE: "QUITE EYE" AND OPHTHALMOLOGIC FINDINGS

<u>Ocular processes</u>—glaucoma, corneal disease, uveitis, scleritis, intraocular tumors, ocular ischemia, hemorrhage
<u>Processes affecting the optic nerve</u>—optic neuritis, ischemic, compressive or infiltrative optic neuropathy
<u>Orbital processes</u>—tumor, infection, inflammatory, vascular, posttraumatic
<u>Cavernous sinus/retro-orbital processes</u>—aneurysm, tumor, thrombosis, infection, inflammatory, C-C fistula, posttraumatic
<u>Intracranial processes</u>—tumor, pseudotumor cerebri, infection, inflammatory, vascular, intracranial pressure changes

Scleritis. Inflammation of the deeper layers of the eye wall, known as scleritis, usually presents with severe, intense, and boring pain.[23–25] The pain is often localized to the eye but may radiate into the sinuses, jaw, or frontal region. The sclera may appear thin or have a bluish hue, and the globe is usually tender. About half the cases are idiopathic, with other causes including herpes simplex virus, herpes zoster, and collagen vascular disease.[23]

Intraocular Tumors. Primary intraocular tumors typically do not cause pain, but orbital extension of tumors may produce trigeminal involvement (neuropathic pain). Intraocular tumors may also produce pain by secondary inflammatory reaction (uveitis) or elevated intraocular pressure induced by the tumor.

Ocular Causes of Eye Pain with a Red (Inflamed) Eye.[16,23]

Conjunctivitis. Conjunctivitis, or "pink eye," is the most common cause of a red, irritated eye. Because the conjunctiva has fewer pain fibers than the cornea, conjunctivitis is generally less painful than corneal epithelial defects, and visual acuity is usually only slightly reduced. The three most common types of conjunctivitis are viral, allergic, and bacterial. The viral type is often associated with an upper respiratory tract infection, cold, or sore throat, with adenovirus infection being the most common viral cause. The condition is characterized by a watery discharge, mild foreign-body sensation, and photophobia. Bacterial infection tends to produce more mucopurulent exudates. Allergic conjunctivitis is extremely common and is often mistaken for infectious conjunctivitis. Itching, redness, and epiphora are typical. The palpebral conjunctiva may become hypertrophic with giant excrescences called cobblestone papillae. Irritation from contact lenses or any chronic foreign body can also induce formation of cobblestone papillae.

Keratoconjunctivitis Sicca. Also known as "dry eye," keratoconjunctivitis sicca produces a burning, foreign-body sensation, as well as injection and photophobia. In mild cases, the eye appears surprisingly normal, but tear production, as measured by wetting of a filter paper (a Schrimer strip), is deficient. A variety of systemic drugs, including antihistamines, anticholinergic, and psychotropic medications, cause dry eye by reducing lacrimal secretion. Disorders that involve the lacrimal gland directly, such as sarcoidosis or Sjögren syndrome, also cause dry eye. Patients may develop dry eye after radiation therapy if the treatment field includes the orbit.

Blepharitis. Blepharitis refers to inflammation of the eyelids. The most common form occurs in association with acne rosacea or seborrheic dermatitis. The eyelid margins are usually colonized heavily by staphylococci. Upon close inspection, they appear greasy, ulcerated, and crusted with scaling debris that clings to the lashes. A chalazion is a painless, granulomatous inflammation of the meibomian gland that produces a pea-like nodule within the eyelid. Basal cell, squamous cell, or meibomian gland carcinoma should be suspected for any nonhealing, ulcerative lesion of the eyelids.

Dacryocystitis. Dacryocystitis is inflammation of the lacrimal drainage system and usually occurs after obstruction of the system. It can produce epiphora and ocular injection. Gentle pressure over the lacrimal sac evokes pain and reflux of mucous or pus from the tear puncta.

Herpes Simplex Infection. Primary ocular infection is generally caused by herpes simplex type 1, rather than type 2. It manifests as a unilateral follicular blepharoconjunctivitis and is easily confused with adenovirus conjunctivitis, unless vesicles appear on the periocular skin or conjunctiva. A dendritic pattern of corneal epithelial ulceration revealed by fluorescein staining is pathognomonic for herpes infection but is seen in only a minority of primary infections. Recurrent ocular infection arises from reactivation of the latent herpes virus.

Herpes Zoster Infection. Herpes zoster recurrence from reactivation of latent varicella virus causes a dermatomal pattern of painful vesicular dermatitis, which is covered in detail elsewhere in this text.

Disorders with Eye and Periocular Pain as the Primary Presentation. Several facial pain syndromes present with prominent ophthalmologic signs and symptoms (Table 67.19). The more common ones are discussed below.

Primary Headache Disorders (see Chapter 61). Many of the primary headache disorders can present with frontotemporal area head pain or sometimes with periorbital and eye pain (migraine, tension-type headache). Some of these disorders have a primary presenting symptom of pain in and around the eye (cluster headache, paroxysmal hemicrania, conjunctival injection and tearing [SUNCT], and short-lasting unilateral neuralgiform headache attacks with autonomic symptoms [SUNA]). In addition to the pain, other signs and symptoms consistent with the diagnosis of a headache disorder are often present (i.e., aura, autonomic phenomenon, etc.).

Carotid Artery Disease. Head, face, and neck pain are frequently reported by patients with subarachnoid hemorrhage, intracranial aneurysms, arteriovenous malformations, and carotid and vertebral artery dissections. Patients describe headache, eye pain, facial pain, and neck pain. Associated symptoms may also be present, depending on the vascular source of the pain.

Subarachnoid hemorrhage can also present with meningismus, neck pain, nausea, altered consciousness, and seizure. The headache and facial pain is highly variable, ranging from mild pain to the "first and worst headache of my life."

Aneurysms can present with head and face pain with cranial nerve palsies, visual disturbances and sudden blindness, and retinal abnormalities. Imaging and lumbar puncture are often warranted for the diagnosis before definitive treatment.[26]

The primary symptom of carotid artery dissection is often headache, either alone or with other symptoms. Frequently, carotid artery dissection also presents with eye pain, facial pain, and neck pain. The headache can be focal or diffuse, whereas the facial pain is generally ipsilateral. Other findings may be pulsatile tinnitus, visual disturbance, central retinal artery occlusion, and Horner syndrome.

Orbital Inflammatory Pseudotumor. Orbital inflammatory pseudotumor is a pain syndrome thought to be caused by idiopathic orbital inflammation, which presents typically with eye pain and other orbital findings (proptosis, injection, chemosis, or ophthalmoplegia). The pain may be either unilateral or bilateral.[16,20,23] Imaging (CT or MRI) typically shows evidence of idiopathic inflammation, enlargement, and contrast enhancement of orbital structures suggesting pathologic involvement. Orbital biopsy may be required to exclude other causes.

Idiopathic Intracranial Hypertension ("Pseudotumor Cerebri"). Idiopathic intracranial hypertension ("pseudotumor cerebri") and facial pain occur primarily in young, obese women of childbearing age. The common presenting findings are daily headache, transient visual obscurations (seconds), pulsatile intracranial noises, and double vision.[16,20] Typically, visual acuity and color representation are preserved, but many patients have optic nerve-related, visual-field defects (e.g., enlarged blind spots, generalized constriction, and inferior nasal field loss). Several predisposing factors have been identified, including the use of oral contraceptives, anabolic steroids, tetracycline, and vitamin A.

Tolosa-Hunt syndrome. Tolosa-Hunt syndrome is an idiopathic inflammatory granulomatous process involving the cavernous sinus. Patients present with painful, steroid-responsive ophthalmoplegia and have episodic, unilateral orbital, or retro-orbital pain. The ophthalmoplegia (CN II, III, IV, VI) occurs simultaneously or within the first 2 weeks after the onset of pain. Facial sensation and visual acuity may be diminished.[16,27] Other pathologic conditions should be excluded by physical examination or neuroimaging. Tolosa-Hunt syndrome is thought to be caused a nonspecific, granulomatous inflammatory infiltrative process with no obvious specific pathologic trigger in the region of the posterior superior orbital fissure, orbital apex, or cavernous sinus. The syndrome typically responds quickly (within 72 hours) to treatment with steroids.

Raeder's Paratrigeminal Syndrome (Paratrigeminal Oculo-Sympathetic Syndrome). This uncommon facial pain syndrome presents with first division trigeminal neuropathic pain, sensory loss, or both, sympathetic dysfunction (miosis, ptosis, or both), but with normal forehead sweating (compared to Horner syndrome). The symptom cluster is localized to the middle cranial fossa medial to the trigeminal ganglion and lateral to the anterior clinoid process. Neuroimaging is necessary and important and, if negative, should be repeated over a period of time to avoid missing an underlying abnormality. This syndrome is not specific to any known pathologic condition.[20]

Herpes Zoster Ophthalmicus (Postherpetic Neuralgia). Herpes zoster ophthalmicus is caused by reactivation of latent herpes zoster virus in the gasserian ganglion, which typically involves the ophthalmic division of the trigeminal nerve. Ocular symptoms can occur after zoster eruption in any branch of the trigeminal nerve but are particularly common when vesicles form on the nose, reflecting nasociliary nerve involvement (Hutchinson's sign). Cranial neuropathies can also occur, usually weeks after the skin eruptions.

Temporal Arteritis. Temporal arteritis presents with periorbital or temporal headache, facial pain, and occasional neck pain. There may be "jaw claudication," scalp tenderness, and visual loss. The headache is mild to severe and of acute or gradual onset; the patient is typically without a history of headache or of changes in headache pattern. Occulomotor disturbances, dizziness, vertigo, and hearing impairment and cervical myelopathy may be present, and very frequently, the superficial temporal artery is thickened, nodular, and pulseless.

Patients with temporal arteritis are generally male, smokers, and over age 50. The disorder may be associated with polymyalgia rheumatica, especially in elderly patients. If untreated or inad-

---

TABLE 67.19

FACIAL PAIN SYNDROMES WITH PREDOMINANT OPHTHALMOLOGIC FINDINGS

Ocular motor nerve palsy
Carotid artery disease
Orbital inflammatory pseudotumor
Increased intracranial pressure and pseudotumor cerebri
Intracranial hemorrhage and stroke
Intracranial arteriovenous malformation
Trigeminal neuropathies
Tolosa-Hunt syndrome
Raeder's paratrigeminal syndrome
Gradenigo's syndrome
Postherpetic neuralgia

equately treated, it may result in unilateral or bilateral blindness, brainstem strokes, and transient ischemic attacks. A careful history and physical examination gives a high index of suspicion for this diagnosis. Additionally, blood studies (elevated Erythrocyte sedimentation rate, C-reactive protein) and temporal artery biopsy may be necessary. However, biopsies can have false negatives as a result of skipped lesions; therefore, bilateral biopsies are often recommended. Treatment consists of immediate high-dose corticosteroids.

Temporomandibular Disorders

Temporomandibular disorder (TMD) typically presents with facial pain, limited and dysfunctional mandibular movements, temporomandibular joint noises (clicking, popping, crepitus), and a change in the way the teeth meet on mouth closure. In addition, reports of eye and periorbital pain, ear pain and stuffiness, headache, neck pain, dizziness, and limitation of neck movement are often present. For a more detailed description of evaluation and treatments for TMD, see the section on TMD in this chapter.

Pain Referred to the Eye from Intracranial Disease

Pain from intracranial diseases, especially those involving the dura and cavernous sinus, may be referred to the eye and orbit. The ophthalmic division of the trigeminal nerve serves the eye and the orbit. Interestingly, a tentorial-dural branch joins the ophthalmic division in the cavernous sinus, receiving sensory innervations from much of the intracranial dura, the arteries at the skull base, and the major venous structures. Inflammation, neoplasm, or ischemia involving intracranial structures may cause pain, which is often referred to as the ipsilateral eye. Therefore, eye pain that remains unexplained after a thorough ophthalmic evaluation may require neuroimaging to rule out an intracranial disorder.[16,23,28]

Pain Attributed to Disorders of the Ear

Otalgia is defined as pain localizing to the ear. Primary otalgia is pain that originates from the ear (see Table 67.14). Referred otalgia does not have a distinct otologic cause and is also called secondary, nonotogenic otalgia. Although earache is a frequent symptom, systematic population-based studies of the epidemiology of the different forms of pain associated with diseases of the ears have not been conducted. However, 97% of cases of otitis media present with earache,[29] and otalgia was found to be referred in as many as 50% of adults in a general medicine population.[29] An analysis of the symptoms of nasopharyngeal carcinomas revealed that deafness and earache, encountered in 85% of patients, were the most common symptoms beside swelling of the throat.[30]

The cranial and cervical nerves supply sensory innervation to the ear. The auriculotemporal branch of the mandibular division of the trigeminal nerve supplies sensation to the anterior aspect of the auricle helix (including the tragus), the anterior aspect of the external auditory canal, and the anterior aspect of the lateral tympanic membrane. The great auricular nerve derived from the cervical nerve plexus (C2 and C3) innervates the remaining parts of the lateral surface of the auricle and the medial surface as well. Afferents from facial, glossopharyngeal, and vagus nerves supply the posterior aspect of the external auditory canal, the posterior aspect of the lateral tympanic membrane, the posteromedial aspect of the auricle, and a patch of skin on the mastoid process. The middle ear receives sensory afferents primarily from the glossopharyngeal nerve as part of the tympanic plexus. The sensory afferents of the tympanic plexus are largely formed by Jacobson's branch of the glossopharyngeal nerve. The vestibulocochlear nerve does not mediate pain afferents from the inner ear because it does not carry pain fibers. Therefore, marked inner ear pathology may develop without otalgia (see Table 67.14).[30,31]

In the ear's embryologic development, the otic vesicles come to rest between branchial nerves 1, 2, 3, and 4. The sensory and motor nerves of these arches are CNs V, VII, IX, and X, respectively.[32–34]

Four distinct regions of afferent innervations of the head and neck sites refer pain to the ear: (1) the inferior gingiva, floor of the mouth, inferior buccal mucosa, and the anterior two thirds of the tongue, all of which are innervated by the third branch of CN V; (2) the tonsillar fossae, lateral bases of the tongue, and some of the inferior nasopharynx innervated by branches of CN IX; (3) the posterolateral oropharynx, hypopharynx, medial base of the tongue, and occasionally a small portion of the inferior nasopharynx innervated by mixed branches of CNs IX and X; and (4) the supraglottic larynx and lingual and laryngeal surfaces of the epiglottis innervated solely by branches of CN X.[32–34]

Otalgia may have otologic (primary) or nonotologic (secondary) causes. A systemic approach to diagnosis is necessary to prevent overlooking a serious condition and to establish the diagnosis and proper therapy.

Primary Otalgia

Primary otalgia is pain with a cause in the ear. Usually, it can be diagnosed by examination of the pinna, auditory canal, and tympanic membrane.

Pinna

Primary pinna pain may be caused by injuries or trauma, such as lacerations, burns, frostbite, or infections. Persistent minor lesions should be biopsied to rule out underlying malignancy.

External Auditory Canal

Otitis externa, sometimes referred to as "swimmer's ear," is an inflammation of the external auditory meatus with resulting edema, otorrhea, pruritus, and otalgia. The otalgia of otitis externa is mediated by sensory afferents of the auriculotemporal nerve, the complex of facial glossopharyngeal and vagus nerves, and the cervical nerves. External otitis arises from acute inflammation after an ear trauma, inadequate cleansing of the external auditory canal, or lengthy contact with liquids in bacterially contaminated water, especially in lakes or swimming pools. Ear wax buildup also may be responsible for earache and pressure in the ear.

The diagnosis is based on physical examination of the external auditory canal for edema, erythema, debris (desquamated epithelium), and otorrhea. Physical findings may be minimal, with only slight edema or hyperemia. In such cases, a history of recent water exposure or preceding ear instrumentation may be useful. Management includes suctioning of any debris or fluids from the external auditory canal, treatment with antibiotic and steroid otic drops, and dry ear precautions.[29,35]

Malignancy must be considered when evaluating a patient with otalgia and an apparent refractory otitis externa. A primary neoplasm of the external auditory canal will too often be misdiagnosed as an otitis externa, potentially resulting in a costly delay in treatment. Patients with malignant otitis externa may have severe otalgia, a severe form of otitis externa that has involved the bone and marrow of the skull base. It is usually found in diabetics or otherwise immunocompromised patients, so this diagnosis must be carefully considered in these patients with otalgia. Timely diagnosis and prompt referral of a patient with malignant otitis externa is crucial because progression from bone involvement to death is rapid.[29,35]

Middle Ear

Infection of the middle ear, otitis media, is likely the most common cause of primary otalgia.[36] The pain from inflamed mucosa in these patients is mediated by way of the glossopharyngeal nerve, which supplies sensation to the middle ear and medial aspect of the tympanic membrane. An acute infection of the mucous membrane of the middle ear usually stems from an infection of the upper air passages with dysfunction of the eustachian tube. Rhinitis and adenoid inflammation may also be causes of acute otitis media. The tympanic membrane will be red and swollen. Occasionally, a purulent discharge is present.

Gradenigo syndrome, defined as the triad of otalgia, otorrhea, and abducens nerve palsy, results from bacterial infection of the petrous apex air cells. Such an infection causes dysfunction of the abducens nerve because it passes through a dural tunnel in proximity to the petrous apex. These complications must be considered in a patient with otalgia and a history of recent otitis media.

Other Primary Causes

Primary neoplasms arising from within the ear or skull base may cause primary otalgia. Such lesions may originate from the skin of the external ear or from glandular tissues of the external or middle ear. A careful otologic and CN examination will help make the diagnosis. The sternocleidomastoid muscle attaches to the mastoid process, and overuse or spasm may manifest as a dull, aching otalgia.

Secondary (Referred) Otalgia

In the absence of otologic factors, the pain is termed secondary, nonotologic, or referred otalgia. The classic definition of referred pain is pathology in one part of the body that gives rise to pain in another nonpathologic site. Referred ear pain may result from pathologic factors involving the sensory supply of the CN V, IX, and X and the spinal nerves C2 and C3. Irritation of the sensory branch of the facial nerve (CN VII) is not true reflex or referred pain. It is usually the initial symptom of Bell palsy or Ramsay Hunt syndrome, and the diagnostic finding of facial paralysis usually occurs within 24 to 48 hours after the onset of pain.[33,34]

Trigeminal Nerve Referred Pain. Pain referred to the ear from the second and third divisions of the trigeminal nerve is usually located anterior to the tragus and along the anterior wall of the external auditory canal, which is supplied by the auriculotemporal nerve. Any disease process involving the anterior two thirds of the tongue, the floor of the mouth, gingiva, mandible, anterior half of the palate, teeth, infratemporal fossa, paranasal sinuses, and the submandibular or parotid glands may result in trigeminal-nerve referred pain. The most common otalgia of fifth nerve origin are dental disorders.

Glossopharyngeal Nerve (CN IX) Referred Pain. Referred pain over the glossopharyngeal nerve may result from infections, ulcerations, and tumors of the palatine tonsil, nasopharynx, eustachian tube, posterior half of the palate, and the posterior third of the tongue. This pain is usually felt deep in the ear, in contrast to the more superficially located pain mediated by the trigeminal nerve. Such ear pain is frequently the only symptom after tonsillectomy and adenoidectomy.

Vagus Nerve (CN X) Referred Pain. Ulcerative lesions due to malignancy or chronic infections in the larynx or hypopharynx may irritate the superior laryngeal branch of the vagus nerve, causing pain referred to the ear.

Spinal Nerves C2 and C3 Referred Pain. Pain in the mastoid area and over the posterior portion of the pinna is mediated by the great auricular nerve, which is derived from the spinal nerves C2 and C3. The most common cause of cervical pain is trauma to the cervical spine. Cervical arthritis, cervical disks, cervical tumors, and muscle traction headache should be considered in the

differential diagnosis. The differential diagnosis for referred otalgia is extensive: the more common causes are described below.

Temporomandibular Disorders. In addition to otalgia, otologic manifestations of temporal mandibular joint (TMJ) disorders can include aural fullness, tinnitus, and vertigo.[4,6,37] A study of approximately 450 patients with TMJ pain found that otalgia was the presenting symptom in 48%.[34] In this study, the TMJ syndrome (and hence otalgia) was successfully managed with conservative therapies such as heat, massage, patient education, occlusal splints, and pain control.

Eagle Syndrome. Eagle syndrome is defined as otalgia, facial pain, sore throat, globus, or dysphagia secondary to elongation of the styloid process or ossification of the stylohyoid ligament. The abnormal styloid process may produce pain through different mechanisms, one of which is direct compression and irritation of the trigeminal, facial, glossopharyngeal, or vagus nerves. The styloid process is typically 20 to 30 mm long. However, 4% of the population has a styloid process longer than 30 mm and of these, only 4% are symptomatic. The degree to which an elongated styloid process causes pain is somewhat poorly defined and controversial.[6,38]

Gastroesophageal Reflux Disease. A large number of symptoms have been linked to extraesophageal reflux of gastric contents, including laryngitis, hoarseness, pharyngitis, bronchospasm, laryngospasm, and chronic cough.[39] Gastroesophageal reflux disease (GERD) can cause otalgia by irritating the upper aerodigestive tract in the sensory distribution of the glossopharyngeal and vagus nerves. Because these nerves also innervate the ear, irritation and damage from acidic gastric secretions may be perceived as originating within the ear. The reflux of gastric secretions can also potentially extend superiorly to the eustachian tubes, irritating the ear directly. The diagnosis of reflux-related otalgia should be considered in all patients with otalgia, a normal otoscopic exam, and other symptoms of GERD. Consultation with a gastroenterologist may be beneficial in managing these patients.[39,40]

Neoplastic Process (see Table 67.14). Malignancies of the upper aerodigestive tract and tumors in various sites of the head and neck can cause otalgia. Tumors on the anterior aspect of the tongue can also manifest as otalgia if they affect the chorda tympani branch of the facial nerve. Nasal and sinus malignancies may present with otalgia secondary to eustachian tube dysfunction or direct neural involvement. In the latter case, the otalgia is mediated by the afferents from the posterior lateral nasal nerves by way of the sphenopalatine ganglion, which is associated with the second division of the trigeminal nerve. Lesions arising from the infratemporal fossa can cause otalgia by involvement of Arnold's nerve (the auricular branch of vagus nerve) or Jacobson's nerve (the tympanic branch of the glossopharyngeal nerve). Many of these patients face a costly delay in diagnosis if malignancy is not considered as a cause.

Treatment of referred otalgia must be directed specifically to the relevant local causes. Such causes may include pulpitis, periapical dental abscess, glossitis, sinusitis, benign or malignant growth in the mouth or sinuses, dental malocclusion, Ramsay Hunt syndrome, tonsils, hypopharynx, or larynx inflammation, or growths in the nasopharynx or eustachian tube.

Pain Attributed to Disorders of the Nose and Paranasal Sinuses (see Table 67.14)

These disorders are grouped together because the paranasal sinuses communicate with the nasal passages through small ostia. Most important among these disorders is sinusitis as it is commonly linked to headache by physicians and the general public alike. "Sinus trouble" as a cause of headache is a source of many controversies, including how to name them: "sinus headache," "rhinosinusitis headache," and "sinogenic facial pain" are used to refer to the same disorder.

Rhinosinusitis

Rhinosinusitis is the inflammation of the nasal passages (rhinitis) and one or more of the paranasal sinuses (maxillary, ethmoid, frontal, or sphenoid). The term is more accurate than "sinusitis" because rhinitis usually precedes sinusitis, the mucosa of the nose and sinuses are contiguous, both conditions may involve nasal obstruction and discharge.[41,42]

Sinusitis is overdiagnosed as a cause of headache and facial pain because of the belief that pain over the sinuses must be related to the sinus. Many of the 60% of patients with unrecognized migraine attribute their symptoms to sinusitis.[41,43] Rhinosinusitis is an uncommon cause of facial pain: more than 80% of patients with purulent secretions visible on nasal endoscopy have no facial pain, most patients with nasal polyposis do not have pain, and facial pain persists in a large proportion of patients after endoscopic sinus surgery.[44-47] Paradoxically, sinus disease also tends to be underestimated, and a potentially dangerous condition, sphenoid sinusitis, is frequently missed.[48]

Clinical Features. Diagnostic criteria for rhinosinusitis are defined in the ear, nose, and throat literature.[49] In this diagnostic scheme, rhinosinusitis is subdivided into acute, recurrent acute, subacute, chronic, and acute exacerbations of chronic. Acute sinusitis lasts from 1 day to 4 weeks, subacute sinusitis from 4 to 12 weeks, and chronic sinusitis for more than 12 weeks. Headache is considered a minor criterion for the diagnosis of acute rhinosinusitis, and headache in the absence of other diagnostic criteria is not considered to be diagnostic of sinusitis.[41,50,51]

Key points in the history of pain secondary to rhinosinusitis are exacerbations of pain during an upper respiratory tract infection, an association with rhinological symptoms, pain that worsens when flying or skiing, and pain in response to medical treatment. Rhinosinusitis usually presents with facial tenderness and pain, nasal congestion, and purulent nasal discharge. Common signs and symptoms include anosmia or hyposmia, pain on mastication, and halitosis. Most cases of infectious rhinosinusitis that last less than 7 days are viral. Acute bacterial sinusitis in adults most often presents with 7 or more days of purulent anterior rhinorrhea, nasal congestion, postnasal drip, facial or dental pain or pressure, and cough, frequently at nighttime. Although approximately 50% of adults have fever and 60% of children have headache, headache, facial pain, and fever often are of little value in diagnosing sinusitis. Williams et al.[52] found that maxillary toothache was highly specific in making the diagnosis of rhinosinusitis: 93% of their patients with toothache had rhinosinusitis. However, only 11% of their patients had maxillary toothache.[52,53]

The headaches associated with rhinosinusitis are usually continuous. The location of the pain and the position that improves the headache varies on the sinus involved (Table 67.20).

Pain in acute maxillary sinusitis is usually in the cheek, gums, and maxillary teeth on the affected side. Acute frontal sinusitis causes frontal headache with tenderness over the sinus and on the medial side of the orbital floor, under the supraorbital ridge, where the frontal sinus is thinnest. Frontal sinusitis can result in brain abscess, meningitis, subdural or epidural abscess, osteomyelitis, orbital edema, and orbital cellulitis. Acute ethmoid sinusitis typically produces pain in between the eyes. Coughing, straining, and lying supine can worsen the pain, whereas keeping the head upright lessens it. Complications of ethmoid sinusitis include meningitis, orbital cellulites, and cavernous sinus thrombosis.[54]

TABLE 67.20

INTERNATIONAL HEADACHE SOCIETY CRITERIA FOR ACUTE SINUS HEADACHE

- Diagnostic criteria: pain in one or more regions of the head, face, ears, or teeth.
- Clinical, laboratory, or imaging evidence of acute rhinosinusitis (e.g., purulence in the nasal cavity, nasal obstruction, fever, CT, MRI, or fiberoptic nasal endoscopy findings).
- Simultaneous onset of headache and rhinosinusitis.
- Headache lasts <7 days after remission or successful treatment of acute rhinosinusitis.

It is necessary, therefore, to differentiate headaches caused by rhinosinusitis from so-called "sinus headaches," which are chronic headache attacks fulfilling the criteria for migraine without aura with prominent autonomic symptoms in the nose or migraine without aura triggered by nasal changes.

Acute sphenoid sinusitis, which accounts for only 3% of all cases of acute sinusitis, is frequently misdiagnosed.[48] Although sphenoid sinusitis rarely causes headache, it can lead to marked morbidity and mortality and so must be identified early and managed aggressively.

As mentioned above, the cavernous sinus is lateral to the sphenoid sinus. The cavernous sinus contains the internal carotid arteries and the third, fourth, fifth, and seventh CNs. The maxillary division of the CN V may indent the wall of the sphenoid sinus. The sphenoid walls can be extremely thin, and sometimes the sinus cavity is separated from the adjacent structure by just a thin mucosal barrier. Because of this proximity, infection may spread to these structures and present as a central nervous system infection or neurologic catastrophe.[48,54]

Headache is always present in acute sphenoid sinusitis and it may be frontal, occipital, or temporal and most commonly is a combination of these locations. Periorbital pain is common and vertex pain is rare. Nasal pain and discharge are present in only 30% of cases, and fever occurs in more than 50% of patients. Also, pain or paresthesias in the facial distribution of the fifth nerve and photophobia or eye tearing suggest sphenoid sinusitis.[48] The headache and associated symptoms may lead to a misdiagnosis of migraine, meningitis, trigeminal neuralgia, or brain tumor. A severe, intractable, new-onset headache that interferes with sleep and is not relieved by simple analgesics should raise the suspicion of sphenoid sinusitis. Neuroimaging is necessary for a definitive diagnose. Complications include bacterial meningitis, cavernous sinus thrombosis, subdural abscess, ophthalmoplegia, and pituitary insufficiency.[48,54]

Acute sinus headache is defined by the International Headache Society (IHS) diagnostic criteria in the setting of an infectious process requiring verification through imaging and confirmation by response to appropriate antibiotics. The IHS established the following diagnostic criteria for acute sinus headache (rhinosinusitis headache) (see Table 67.20)[1]:

A. Purulent discharge in the nasal passage, either spontaneous or by suction
B. Pathologic findings on radiographic examination, CT, or transillumination
C. Simultaneous onset of headache and sinusitis
D. Headache location (see Table 67.3 for location of pain with infection of corresponding paranasal sinus)
E. The disappearance of the headache after treatment for acute sinusitis

These criteria may not be valid for diagnosing sphenoid sinusitis because the purulent discharge is often missing and headache may precede sinus drainage. The IHS has not validated chronic sinusitis as a cause of headache or facial pain unless it relapses into an acute stage.

Obviously, the term "acute sinus headache" or what is referred to as "rhinosinusitis headache" in this chapter does not address the primary headache disorder with secondary nasal symptomatology, commonly referred to as "sinus headache."[41,55,56]

Plain sinus radiographs can diagnose acute maxillary or frontal sinusitis but are often inadequate for ethmoid or sphenoid sinusitis. CT is the optimal imaging study to assess the paranasal sinuses. The mucosa of the normal, noninfected sinus approximates the bone so closely that it cannot be visualized on CT. Therefore, any soft tissue seen within a sinus is abnormal. CT may reveal mucosal thickening, sclerosis, clouding, or air-fluid levels. Scans of the sinuses without contrast in the coronal plain are highly sensitive for detecting nasal and paranasal sinus disease, including disease in the ethmoid and sphenoid sinuses.[57] The prevalence of reversible sinus abnormalities visualized by CT in patients who have the common cold is high. This fact suggests that CT may not be specific for bacterial infections. Anterior ethmoid sinus infection is found in every patient who had frontal or maxillary sinusitis.

MRI is more sensitive than CT in detecting fungal infections. In MRI, T2-weighted images are highly sensitive for detecting retained fluid and inflamed tissue of the sinuses, a fact that may lead to exaggerating the importance of otherwise unremarkable sinus disease, such as mild inflammation, small polyps, and retention cysts. Transillumination and ultrasonography of the sinuses have low sensitivity and specificity for detecting similar findings. Diagnostic endoscopy with the flexible fiberoptic rhinoscope permits direct visualization of the nasal passages and sinus drainage areas.[58]

Differential Diagnosis. Migraine and tension-type headache are often confused with true sinus headache because of their similar locations.[43,55,56] Some patients, in addition to having all the features of migraine without aura, have head pain in the face, associated congestion of the nose, and headache triggered by weather changes. These patients do not have purulent nasal discharge or other diagnostic criteria of acute rhinosinusitis. The diagnostic criteria of rhinosinusitis and migraine are similar. Although facial pressure or pain, facial congestion, and nasal blockages are considered major criteria for rhinosinusitis, headache and fatigue are minor criteria, meaning that these symptoms have less diagnostic value but are not necessarily less frequent or less intense. In migraine, the seminal emphasis for diagnosis is the severity, quality, and location of a headache associated with gastrointestinal or sensory symptoms. Nasal symptoms, including congestion, facial pressure or pain, and rhinorrhea, are commonly reported symptoms associated with migraines but are often ignored because they are not considered essential for the diagnosis of migraine. Therefore, it is important to differentiate headaches caused by rhinosinusitis from headaches fulfilling the criteria of migraine without aura with prominent autonomic symptoms in the nose or of migraine without aura triggered by nasal changes, the so-called "sinus headaches" (Table 67.21).[43,55,56]

Management (see Table 67.21). Acute rhinosinusitis causes excruciating pain; therefore, analgesia is important. In one study, analgesia successfully treated nearly 80% of patients with maxillary sinusitis.[59]

Emergency treatment goals are to facilitate drainage of the congested nasal sinuses and to eliminate the pathogenic bacteria. Steam and saline prevent crusting of secretions in the nasal cavity and facilitate mucociliary clearance. Locally active decongestants provide symptomatic relief by shrinking inflamed and swollen nasal mucosa. Oral decongestants should be used if prolonged treatment (>3 days) is necessary. These agents are α-adrenergic agonists that reduce nasal blood flow without the risk of rebound

TABLE 67.21

AN OTOLARYNGOLOGY, NEUROLOGY, ALLERGY, AND PRIMARY CARE CONSENSUS ON DIAGNOSIS AND TREATMENT OF SINUS HEADACHE

Diagnostic Recommendations:

Stable pattern of recurrent, self-limiting headache associated with rhinogenic symptoms are most likely migraine

Prominent rhinogenic symptoms associated with fever, purulent discharge with headache as one of several complaints (pain) is likely rhinogenic in origin

MRI or CT as appropriate based on headache history, patterns, changes, and physical signs

Referral to headache specialist for new onset, frequent headache, headache associated with neurological symptoms or signs, or headache that does not respond to appropriate therapy (migraine or rhinogenic)

Therapeutic Recommendations:

Migraine with no evidence of infection should be given a trial of migraine-specific medication and scheduled for follow-up evaluation

Noninfectious rhinogenic symptoms with headache as a minor complaint should be provided with a trial of nasal steroids and/or selective antihistamines and/or oral decongestants

Adapted from Levine HL, Setzen M, Cady RK, et al. An otolaryngology, neurology, allergy, and primary care consensus on diagnosis and treatment of sinus headache. *Otolaryngol Head Neck Surg* 2006;134(3):516–523.

vasodilation. Mucoevacuant (guaifenesin) and intranasal steroids may improve the symptoms, but antihistamines are not helpful.[60]

Most patients with rhinosinusitis respond to treatment with antibiotics. Amoxicillin is the first choice, unless the patient has been treated within the previous month or lives in an area that has a high prevalence of β-lactamase–resistant H influenza. There is no clear evidence that culturing purulent secretions contribute to managing acute rhinosinusitis, but obtaining a culture and defining its antibiotic sensitivity may help, particularly if there are orbital or intracranial complications.

Acute frontal and sphenoid sinusitis require immediate referral to an otolaryngologist for treatment to avoid intracranial complications. Consultation should also be considered when the symptoms are not relieved with at least two consecutive 2-week courses of antibiotics.[59]

Sometimes rhinosinusitis does not respond to medical treatment and surgical intervention is necessary to relieve worsening and excruciating pain. The goal of surgery is to improve sinus drainage by enlarging the orifices, removing obstructive anatomic structures, or both. Endoscopic sinus surgery alleviates the facial pain in 75% to 83% of cases,[44,60] producing greater improvement in headache than in facial pain.

Isolate Rhinogenic Disorders Causing Headache

Rhinogenic headache and facial pain can be caused by septal impaction or contact, rhinitis (allergic or vasomotor) and nasal polyps, trauma, intranasal tumors, and septal hematoma. In patients without evidence of acute or chronic sinusitis, nasal polyps, or a tumor, Chow[61] found that pain was caused by a septal spur in 12 of 18 patients who had rhinologic sources for their primary symptom of facial pain or headache.

Deviated Nasal Septum. A deviated nasal septum can produce symptoms similar to those of nasal obstruction. Symptoms may be marked if the deviation is in the region of the nasal valve. However, deflection of the nasal septum is not important as a possible cause of headache.

Inflammatory Rhinitis. Inflammatory rhinitis is accompanied by rhinorrhea, fever, pain affecting the middle part of the face and the distribution of the first and second trigeminal branches, and symptoms of an infection of the upper respiratory tract. Inflammatory rhinitis differs from allergic rhinitis in having more neutrophils on a nasal swab, whereas allergic rhinitis will show an increase in eosinophilic leucocytes.

Allergic Rhinitis. As a rule, allergic rhinitis does not cause primary pain, but it may give rise to acute sinusitis in which facial pain is a secondary development.

Vasomotor Rhinitis. The symptoms of vasomotor rhinitis are similar to those of allergic rhinitis but with less sneezing, and the patient does not test positive for allergies. The pathophysiology involves an imbalance between the parasympathetic and sympathetic autonomic nerve supply of the nasal mucosa. The former predominates, the increased vascularity causing nasal obstruction.

Pain Attributed to Temporomandibular Disorders

TMD are defined as a subgroup of craniofacial pain disorders that involve the TMJ, the masticatory muscle system, and the associated head, face, and neck musculoskeletal complex (muscles, ligaments, and joints).[62] Patients with TMD most frequently present with pain, limited or asymmetric mandibular motion, and TMJ sounds. The pain or discomfort is located around the jaw, TMJ, and the muscles of mastication. Commonly associated symptoms include ear pain and stuffiness, tinnitus, dizziness, eye pain, neck pain, arm and shoulder pain, and dysfunction and headache. In some cases, the onset is acute and symptoms are mild and self-limiting. Other patients experience chronic TMD with persistent pain in association with a combination of physical, behavioral, psychologic, and psychosocial symptoms similar to those of other chronic pain syndromes.

An estimated 75% of the U.S. adult population has experienced one or more of the signs and symptoms of TMD.[63] Epidemiologic studies indicate a prevalence of 40% to 75% of adults having at least one sign of joint dysfunction and approximately 33% of persons having at least one symptom of TMD.[64,65] Some signs appear to be relatively common in the general population; TMJ sounds and deviation on opening occur in approximately 50% of healthy people.[66] Other signs are relatively rare; limited mouth opening and occlusal changes occur in fewer than 5% of the population.[67] These disorders are disorders of middle-aged adults (ages 20 to 50), with women seeking care more than men (female:male ratio ranges from 3:1 to 9:1).[68] Despite large numbers of people experiencing signs and symptoms of TMD over their lifetime, only 5% to 10% of these individuals are believed to actually need treatment.

Temporomandibular Disorders: A Triad of Dysfunctions

At least three distinct and separate dysfunctions create or affect the symptoms described by the TMD patient[69]:

I. Muscle disorders (myofascial pain dysfunction) are related to muscle dysfunction, often leading to muscle spasms, pain, and dysfunction. This type of dysfunction can occur in any skeletal muscle. The triggering area lies in the fascial coverings and attachment zones of the muscles, thus the term myofascial. This syndrome is sometimes incorrectly referred to as myofacial pain dysfunction.
II. Temporomandibular joint articular disorder (TMJD) is related to specific problems in the TMJs. These problems may

range from joint sounds to locking, pain, and degenerative changes of the joints themselves. Invariably, muscle dysfunction is a secondary effect of true TMJD.
III. Cervical spinal dysfunction is related to the spinal column, vertebrae, and the associated ligaments and muscles. The majority of symptoms not directly related to the jaw muscles are triggered or affected by this syndrome.

TMDs are classified in the eleventh major category of the IHS's *Classification and Diagnostic Criteria for Headache Disorders, Cranial Neuralgias, and Facial Pain* as headache or facial pain associated with disorders of the cranium, neck, eyes, ears, nose, sinuses, teeth, mouth, or other facial or cranial structures (see Table 67.3).[1] The American Academy of Orofacial Pain adopted a part of this classification and broadened it to include a more focused classification of TMD (Tables 67.22 and 67.23). In this classification, TMDs are broadly divided into two major groups: the masticatory muscle disorders and the articular disorders.[70] The masticatory muscle disorders include myofascial pain, myositis, myospasm, local myalgia, myofibrotic contracture, and neoplasia. The articular disorders include congenital and developmental disorders, disc derangement disorders, temporomandibular dislocation, inflammatory disorders, osteoarthritis, ankylosis, and fracture. The most common muscle disorders are localized myalgia and myofascial pain syndrome. The most common articular disorders are disc derangement disorders and osteoarthritis.

Treatment of TMD has included, among other therapies, oral orthopedic jaw appliances, occlusal adjustment, prosthetic reconstruction, orthodontic correction, biofeedback, biobehavioral stress management, psychotherapy, nutritional guidance, physical therapy, acupuncture, pharmacotherapy, and surgical management. Each of these techniques is supported by some degree of success and therefore merits notice. However, the key to successful treatment is an accurate diagnosis, which relies on knowing the symptoms and their probable causes on an interdisciplinary approach (Table 67.24).

TABLE 67.22

TEMPOROMANDIBULAR JOINT ARTICULAR DISORDERS

Congenital or developmental
  Aplasia
  Hypoplasia
  Hyperplasia
  Neoplasia

Disc derangement disorders
  Disc displacement with reduction
  Disc displacement without reduction

Temporomandibular joint dislocation

Inflammatory disorders
  Capsulitis/synovitis
  Polyarthritides

Osteoarthritis (noninflammatory)
  Primary osteoarthritis
  Secondary osteoarthritis

Ankylosis

Fracture

TABLE 67.23

MASTICATORY MUSCLE DISORDERS

11.7.2.1—Local myalgia
11.7.2.2—Myofascial pain
11.7.2.3—Centrally mediated myalgia
11.7.2.4—Myospasm
11.7.2.5—Myositis
11.7.2.6—Myofibrotic contracture
11.7.2.7—Neoplasia

Clinical Presentation

The most common symptom of TMD is muscle pain. It is usually accompanied by restricted movement. Patients often also present with reduced jaw opening, as well as impaired range of motion in the cervical vertebrae, shoulders, and arms. Other commonly associated symptoms of TMD are listed below.

Headache. Symptoms of TMD-related bilateral head and face pain involve multiple postural muscles, the muscles of mastication, or both. The pain is typically of moderate intensity, dull and aching in quality, and described as deep and constant.[71–75] Pain is often exacerbated by use of the affected muscles. Morning headaches may be related to nocturnal bruxism or sleep disorders,[76] whereas increasing pain during the day may be related to masticatory muscle use or head posture.[77]

Front of Head. Patients reporting pain in the front of the head often refer to it as "sinus headache." The pain is usually accompanied by pressure along the upper anterior teeth, bridge of the nose, and behind the eyes. Chronic front of the head pain and facial pain generally indicate a primary headache disorder, not chronic sinus disease. These symptoms can also be caused by a reduced posterior occlusal dimension, causing heavy incisal contact, resulting in pain of pressure in the anterior vortex of the face. A band-like feeling of the front of the head can also be brought about by posterior neck muscle contractions or muscle tension of the frontalis muscle.

Side of the Head. Temporal headaches are mainly related to muscle contraction and fiber spasm of the temporalis muscle. The temporalis muscle has three groups of muscle fibers: anterior, middle, and posterior. The anterior fibers bring the lower jaw up and forward, and the middle and posterior fibers swing the jaw to full closure and retract the mandible.

Clenching, grinding, or biting on objects while the jaw is displaced anteriorly (edge-to-edge) generally creates pain in the anterior temporal group (i.e., the patient has pain in the "temple" area). Individuals who work at desk jobs with their heads forward and down tend to clench and grind in this position because gravity

TABLE 67.24

TEMPOROMANDIBULAR DISORDERS

Diagnosis	TMJ Articular disorders	Muscle disorders	Myofascial disorders
Diagnostic features	Pain localized in the preauricular area during jaw function. Usually presence of painful click or crepitus during mouth opening. Limited opening (<35 mm), deviated or painful jaw movements.	Tenderness of the masticatory muscles. Dull, aching pain exacerbated by jaw function or palpation.	Diffused dull or aching pain affecting multiple groups of muscles of the head and neck region, as well as other parts of the body.
Diagnostic evaluation	Internal derangement of the TMJ with abnormal function of the disc-condyle complex, and/or degeneration of the joint surface. Palpation is painful. Possible joint swelling in acute phases. MRI, CT, etc., of the joint may rule-out tumors and advanced degenerative stages.	Tenderness during palpation of the masticatory muscles and tendons. Possible limited range of jaw movement and during passive stretching exam. Can be associated with a parafunctional habit (bruxism-early morning pain).	Presence of trigger or tender points in one or more groups of muscles. Pain can radiate to distant areas with stimulation or not of the trigger points. Rule out presence of lupus erythematosus.
Treatment	Patient education and self-care. Medication: NSAID, nonopiate analgesics. Physical Therapy: exercise program. Occlusal splints Oral maxillofacial surgery: arthrocentesis, arthroscopic surgery, open surgery	Patient education and self-care. Medication: topical and systemic NSAIDs., nonopiate analgesics, muscle-relaxants, antidepressants, (usually tricyclic antidepressants), anxiolytics, anticonvulsants, botulinum toxin, trigger point injections, and vapocoolant spray. Physical therapy: transcutaneous electrical nerve stimulation, massage, exercise program. Occlusal splints Cognitive-behavior: biofeedback, relaxation, coping skills.	Same as muscle disorders.

has a greater affect on the mandible. This condition is further aggravated by habits such as pencil or pen biting, pipe smoking, or gum chewing.

Clenching or grinding during sleep or clenching with the jaw in a posterior position tends to tire the middle and posterior group of fibers, and the pain is more posteriorly located. Generally, the temporalis is affected in any dysfunction of the lower jaw.

Back of Head. Deep, dull pain, constant and aggravating in the back of the head, is usually a result of spasms of the trapezius and sternocleidomastoid muscles. These muscles are long and strong, and under tension, they pull on their bony attachments to the skull—the occiput and mastoid areas. This pulling leads to soreness in the bone and to deep dull pain radiating up the back of the head and down the neck. The muscle tension may be independent of, or secondarily related to, displacement of the cervical and upper thoracic vertebrae.

Face Pain. Pain in the sides of the face or pain described by the patient as "sinus" pain in the zygomatic or orbital area may also have a musculoskeletal origin.[69] Clenching, acute or chronic stress, and reduction of dental height related to the loss of posterior teeth combined with daytime tooth clenching and acute or chronic stress can create muscle trigger points or muscle fatigue. Patients are often aware of this condition after meals and report "a heavy and tired feeling" in the jaw muscles. Face pain related to sinuses and other pathologies are discussed separately in this chapter.

Eye Pain. Orbital pain symptoms are often described as unilateral, constant, and "boring." Orbital pain is frequently seen in patients with TMD that includes pain involving the eye and periorbital region.[69,78–80] Patients with a history of trauma, chronic upper cervical vertebral subluxations, or nerve root impingements related to the occiput and the atlantoaxial region may present with orbital symptoms. In addition, entrapment of the greater occipital nerve at the occiput level can also produce this type of pain, which is often diagnosed as occipital neuralgia. Orbital pain often responds to physical medicine, along with changes in head posture and mandibular position through the use of dental bite appliances.

Ear Symptoms. Pain, stuffiness, and tinnitus may have a musculoskeletal cause.[81,82] Mandibular posture in relationship to the maxilla affects the masticatory elevator muscles. The medial pterygoid muscles help stabilize the left-to-right balance of the mandible on tooth closure. Innervation from the nerve to the medial pterygoid also supplies the middle ear muscles. The tensor tympani and tensor palati are actually one muscle with a raphe that wraps around the hamulus notch of the maxilla. Growth and development problems related to the proper expansion of the maxilla can affect eustachian tube function and can precipitate middle ear infections in children, as well as ear stuffiness with changes in pressure in the ear in adults. Maxillary and mandibular dysfunctions aid in the development and maintenance of such symptoms.

Tinnitus and other types of ear sounds may also have a peripheral musculoskeletal cause. Specifically, cervical and mandibular postural factors are found in patients with tinnitus. A combination of physical medicine and dental jaw appliance therapy has been effective in some cases where trauma or aberrations in childhood growth and development have affected the proper expansion of the maxilla.

Sharp, jabbing ear pain upon movement of the mandible is often seen in patients who have an internal derangement of the TMJ. Usually this derangement presents unilaterally and ipsilateral to the joint in question.

Ear pain and symptoms such as stuffiness in the absence of positive otologic findings are among the most common reasons to evaluate the patient for dental and maxillomandibular imbalance. Treatment often alleviates or reduces the impact of the symptoms on the patient.[83–88]

Temporomandibular Joint Symptoms. Pain and sounds related to the TMJs are very common.[89,90] Patients commonly report clicking or grating noises in the "jaw joints." Generally, clicking is not accompanied by pain. Grating noises are usually unilateral and accompanied by pain radiating to the ear on movement. These noises may be related to trauma or bruxism in the presence of missing posterior teeth, resulting in injury or anterior disc displacement without reduction "locking" of the temporomandibular joint.

Clicking. Much has been written about clicking of the TMJs. Clicks can be classified as immediate-opening clicking, midopening clicking, late-opening clicking, and reciprocal clicking.

The reason for the click, however, remains the same. When the mouth opens, the condyle hits the back of, and "clicks under," the articulator disc. This situation can happen at any point during movement, depending on the relative position of the condyle and disc.

Typically, the articular disc is attached to the head of the condyle on the medial and lateral poles. The superior head of the lateral pterygoid is inserted into the anterior portion of the disc and soft, elastic tissue borders the disc posteriorly.

This arrangement holds the articular disc in position with the condyle in various jaw movements. If the joint is anatomically healthy, there cannot be a click. Tearing or stretching of the articulator attachments are a prerequisite for clicking.

Clicking can be caused by acute trauma, such as an automobile accident, whiplash, or a blow to the face. It can also be caused by chronic microtrauma, such as loss of posterior vertical dimension of occlusion or loss of teeth.

Dental interventions can also create this problem by retruding the condyle posteriorly during reconstruction or orthodontic retrusion. Difficult extractions can also affect the joint-disc assembly.

Grating Sounds. Grating sounds generally occur in a later stage of TMJ articular dysfunction, along with articular cartilage degeneration. The disc is either torn and shredded or missing completely. The grating is caused by bone-to-bone friction and usually indicates osteoarthritic degenerative changes in the joint.

Locking of the Joint. The jaw lock mainly occurs after clicking has been evident for a while. The articular disc, which is biconcave under normal circumstances, loses its shape and becomes spherical or ball-like if anteriorly displaced for a period of time. In this case, the condyle cannot travel normally along the anterior wall of the glenoid fossa. The patient perceives this restriction as an inability to open the mouth fully. Sometimes the cartilage may fold on itself with the same clinical effect.

Hypermobility. Increased movement in the jaw comes when the TMJ ligaments are stretched or torn. This loss of integrity allows excessive movement, sometimes to the point of anterior open dislocation in a wide opening movement, such as yawning.

Treatment is often a combination of dental therapies, jaw appliance therapy, and physical medicine and can be supplemented with treatment for bruxism and stress management through biofeedback relaxation and sleep medicine.

Neck Pain. Neck stiffness and pain are commonly part of the TMD complex.[91–93] Trauma, poor posture, and musculoskeletal tension can have chronic effects on the cervical spine, creating pain, stiffness, and trigger point flare up in the muscles of the head and neck. The trigeminal and cervical nerves help maintain head, neck, and jaw posture.[94] Mastication and jaw function rely on all the anterior and posterior cervical muscles. In addition, mandibular and head postures interact to maintain the airway space during function and sleep.

Studies of maxillomandibular position and the cervical spine have shown that reductions of the vertical dimension of the teeth and a deep bite can adversely affect cervical muscle function, leading to chronic stiffness, pain, and reduced range of motion.[95] It is therefore important to assess the dental factors in patients with chronic neck pain.

Arm and Back Symptoms. Patients presenting with TMD may also commonly present with shoulder pain: pain radiating down the arm that may or may not be accompanied by tingling and or numbness. Physical examination often reveals thoracic outlet syndrome, costoclavicular syndrome, vertebral subluxations or nerve impingement of the brachial plexus, and even previously undiagnosed rotator cuff injuries.[96]

Temporomandibular Joint Articular Disorders
(see Tables 67.22 to 67.24)

The TMJ is a synovial diarthrodial joint that allows the temporal bone to articulate with the condylar head of the mandible. The joint allows for sliding as well as hinge movement of the mandible during functional mastication. The condyles are not perfectly round but are wider medio–laterally than anterior–posteriorly. Individual variations follow functional loads and depend on the thickness of connective tissue layers covering the articulating surfaces.[97,98]

The condyles travel within their respective mandibular fossae. Each mandibular fossa or glenoid fossa forms the temporal component of the TMJ. This component is a concave area on the inferior border of the squamous part of the temporal bone and is also referred to as the articular fossa.[99]

Between the bones that form the TMJ are interposing discs or articular cartilages.[100] Each articular disc is formed of dense fibrous connective tissue and divides the joint cavity into two separate compartments: the upper discotemporal space and the lower discomandibular space. Both compartments are lubricated by synovial fluid.[101] The inferior surface of the disc is concave to match the articular surface of the condyle, whereas the superior surface of the disc is convex to follow the concave surface of the articular fossa. The articular disc is firmly attached to the medial and lateral poles of the condyle. The lateral ligamentous attachments are relatively thin and weak compared to the medial pole attachments and tend to tear more frequently than the medial ligamentous attachments. This weakness is the reason for more anterior medial than lateral disc displacements.

Viewed sagittally, the articular disc is divided into three parts: a thicker anterior section called the anterior band, a middle thinner intermediary zone, and a broader posterior band that is the thickest of the three (Fig. 67.1). The thinner intermediary zone, along with the two broader anterior and posterior zones, gave the articular cartilage its classic bowtie appearance on MRI (Fig. 67.2).

In the adult, the central part of the articular disc is avascular and lacks innervations, which allows for changes in the central thin part of the disc to occur without pain. The articular disc has a relatively random arrangement of type I collagen fibers, elastic fibers, and glycosaminoglycans comprised of chondroitin sulfate, dermatan sulfate, and hyaluronic acid. The discs allow for rotation in the upper joint compartment and translation in the lower joint compartment.[102] Thus, rotation is approximately the first 22.5 mm of mouth opening, and translation from that point to full mouth opening ranges from 45 to 55 mm between the front teeth.[102]

In each joint, the anterior part of the articular cartilage attaches to the superior head of the lateral pterygoid muscle, and the inferior head of the lateral pterygoid muscle attaches into the fovea of the condyle. In humans, this attachment of the superior head of the lateral pterygoid is variably inserted into 40% to 60% of the articular disc.[103] The posterior part of the articular cartilage blends into loose retrodiscal tissue consisting of blood vessels, loose connective tissue, and nerves.

On mouth closure, the retrodiscal tissue is squeezed like a sponge and allows the condyle to be fully seated in its fossa. As the mouth opens and the condyles move forward in their respective fossa, the blood vessels in the retrodiscal tissues expand to fill the void left by the translating condyles and their interposing articular cartilages. This act of a sponge being squeezed and then being filled is repeated during jaw function. This region can be injured if the mouth suddenly opens and closes as a result of a blow or injury to the mandible. This injury can lead to bleeding in the joint space, followed by pain and limitation of movement.

Congenital or Developmental Disorders. Congenital or developmental disorders, such as aplasia, hypoplasia, hyperplasia, and neoplasia, can be odontogenic or nonodontogenic and primarily present as esthetic and functional problems. Neoplastic lesions, such as osteomas and osteoblastomas of the bone, produce pain in more advanced stages,[104] as do other primary tumors, such as chondroblastoma and benign giant cell tumors. The most common metastatic tumors are squamous cell carcinoma, nasopharyngeal tumors, and parotid gland tumors, such as adenoid cystic carcinomas.[105]

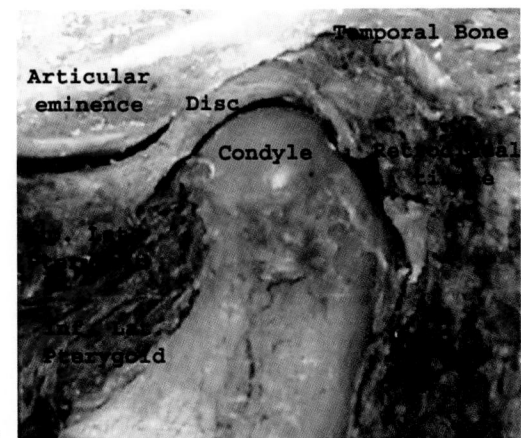
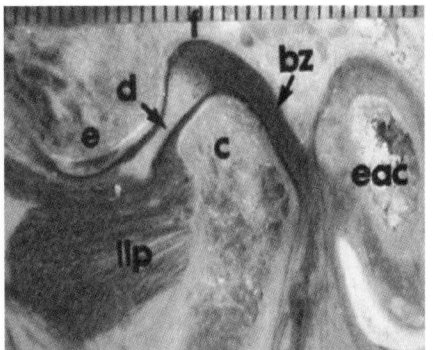

FIGURE 67.1 A,B. Gross anatomy of the TMJ as seen in sagittal sections. bz, bilaminar zone of disc; c, mandibular condyle; d, intra-articular disc; e, eminence; eac, external auditory canal; f, glenoid fossa; llp, lower head of the lateral pterygoid muscle.

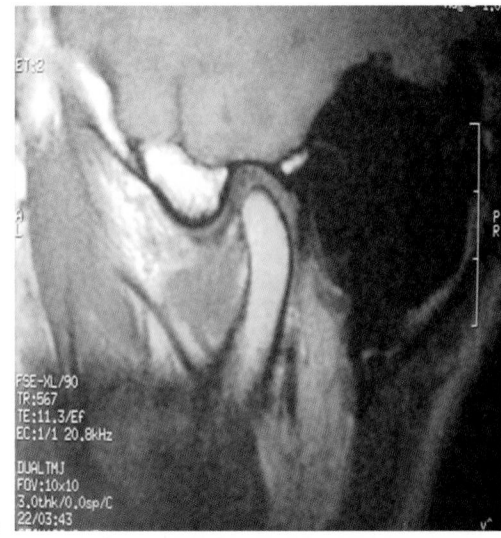 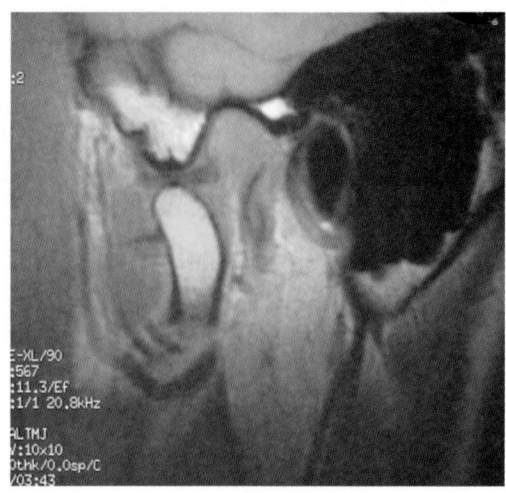

FIGURE 67.2 T1-weighted MRIs of a normal temporomandibular joint in (**A**) closed mouth position and (**B**) open mouth position.

Disc derangement disorders or articular disc displacements, by far the most common TMJ articular disorders, are characterized by an abnormal position of the articular disc relative to the head of the condyle or temporal fossa. Disc displacement is usually marked by a "clicking or popping" sound in the TMJ when the mouth is opened and closed. Pain is initially not part of the presenting symptoms, as long as there is full function. Disc displacements suggest torn or stretched collateral discal ligaments that bind the disc to the condyle.

Disc displacements are usually anterior or anteromedial, although posterior and lateral displacements have been described. Anterior or anteromedial displacement may be related in part to the fact that the thinnest discal attachments are on the lateral pole of the condyle, as well as the medial direction of pull by the lateral pterygoid and the inward condylar movement during mouth opening.[106]

Disc Displacement With Reduction. A clicking sound on mouth opening and closing is classified as disc displacement with reduction. The term reduction describes the process of the misaligned disc temporarily coming back (or slipping back) to its proper interposition between the condyle and fossa during full mouth opening (see Fig. 67.2). On closing the mouth, the disc again

displaces as the teeth come closer together. This repetitive, ongoing displacement on opening and closing produces a reciprocal noise (clicks) and is hence termed "reciprocal clicking." Given the very common nature of its occurrence, this displacement may actually represent a stage of physiologic accommodation that need not be treated. Where displacement progresses, the incidence of intermittent "locking" may increase as a result of the momentary impedance of the disc as it follows the path of the condyle. This stage generally occurs as a sequel of a chronic clicking condition in patients who tend to clench and grind their teeth at night (nocturnal parafunction) and who have missing posterior teeth with subsequent overclosure of the bite. The teeth act as the doorstop for the TMJs and support the ultimate position of the TMJ on full closure. Good dental vertical dimension without shift on closure is essential in reducing the risk factors for progression. Bite appliance therapy is effective in treating muscular as well as disc displacement problems.[107–109]

Disc Displacement Without Reduction. Progression to the next stage is sometimes referred to as a "closed lock." In this stage, the disc has been permanently displaced, and its shape has been deformed so that it prevents the condyle of the mandible from translating to a full open position (Fig. 67.3). Jaw opening is

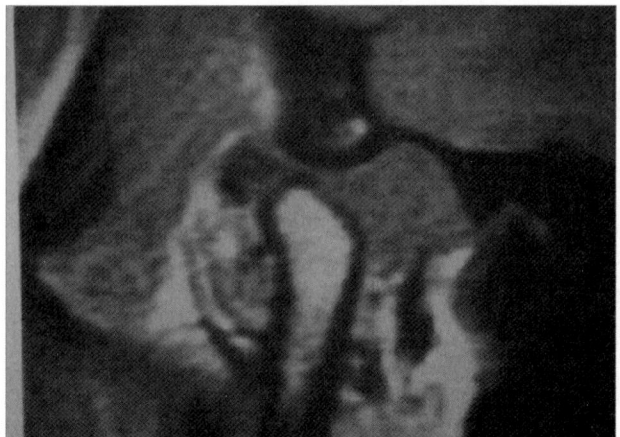 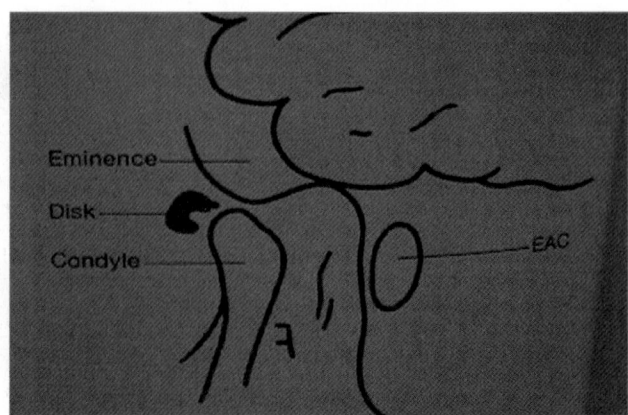

FIGURE 67.3 TMJ disk displacement without reduction.

usually limited to 22 to 25 mm, or about the length of the tips of two fingers inserted between the upper and lower incisors. Pain may reduce chewing capacity, the mandible deviates to the side of the lock, the joint becomes inflamed, and normal occlusion or "bite" may be disrupted. MRI is the standard for assessing the soft tissue of the articular cartilage and its displacement, whereas CT is generally done to assess hard tissue for chronic osteoarthritic or bony changes.[110,111]

Temporomandibular Joint Dislocation. In TMJ dislocation, or open lock or condylar subluxation, the condyle translates beyond the anterior eminence of the articular fossa and becomes trapped in this open-mouth position. Chronic hypertranslation can usually be managed by having the patient physically manipulate the jaw back into position. The patient learns to relax the jaw-closing muscles and to slip the condyle back into position. The most common subluxation occurs during yawning or opening the mouth widely when eating.

If the problem is related to trauma or a sudden acute translation, the subluxation is considered to be an acute dislocation. Acute dislocation requires medical intervention in which the muscles are relaxed by anesthesia, analgesics, or injected into the muscles and joint, followed by manipulating the joint downward and backward to let it slip past the anterior eminence of the glenoid fossa. Follow-up with anti-inflammatory medication, ice, and rest or a dental appliance may be necessary until the acute stage passes.[112]

Inflammatory Disorders. Capsulitis and synovitis are relatively common in the TMJ secondary to macro- or microtrauma, irritation, or infections. These insults are accompanied by pain on movement and inflammation with extreme tenderness of the TMJ or on distraction of the joints. MRI may show effusions in the T2-weighted signal, the teeth may not be brought together completely, and pain may occur in the ear.

Joint inflammation may also be a result of systemic polyarthritis. Symptoms are similar to those in other joints of the body and are secondary to connective tissue diseases that affect the same population of patients.

Osteoarthritis (Noninflammatory). Primary osteoarthritis is a degenerative condition of the joints characterized by hard-tissue abrasion and degradation of the articular surface of the condyle related to overload. The condition is frequently seen in patients with a long history of missing and unreplaced teeth or in patients with dentures due to remodeling effects. Remodeling is usually slow and generally painless in the early stages. Slow progression may remain relatively benign over the life span of the patient.

Primary osteoarthritis is usually identified by radiography, such as a dental panoramic image, tomography, or a dental CT scan and grating (crepitus) noises in the joint during movement (Figs. 67.4 and 67.5). Secondary osteoarthritis is usually associated with a single prior event, such as trauma or infection, or by rheumatoid arthritis. An idiopathic degenerative condition primarily affecting adolescent girls is termed condylysis. It is seen as a sudden lysis of the condyle, which can creates a shift of the jaw to the affected side and an anterior open bite. The cause of condylysis is not clear but the condition is associated with young women with rheumatoid arthritis.[113]

Ankylosis. Ankylosis is usually related to joint trauma, with subsequent bleeding and restricted mandibular movement. Ankylosis maybe fibrous or bony in nature. Fibrous ankylosis usually is seen in the upper joint compartment as a result of adhesions forming after a joint bleed and prolonged immobility. The jaw still opens slightly, usually enough to accommodate 1 or 2 fingers placed horizontally between the central incisors. Bony ankylosis has no movement associated with it. Both conditions may require surgical release and postsurgical mobilization.[114]

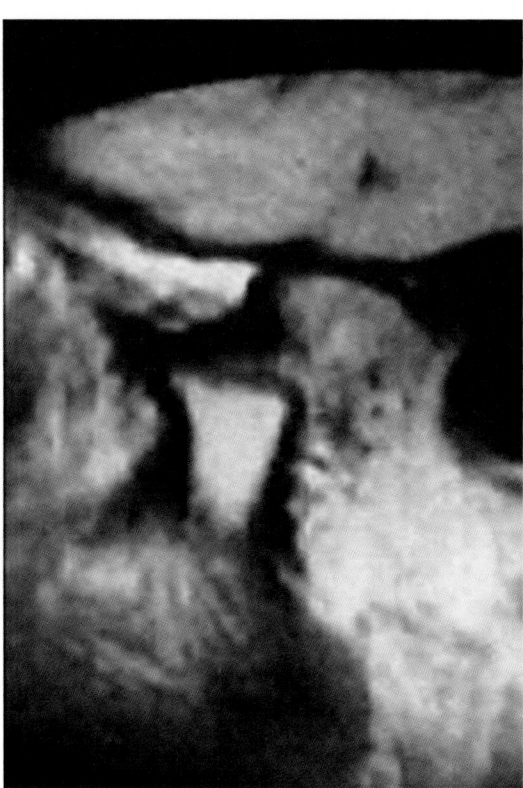

FIGURE 67.4 Sagittal view MRI of osteoarthritis of the temporomandibular joint.

Fracture. Trauma to the chin, mandible, or any part of the face may result in bony fractures of the condylar neck, condylar head, bodies of the mandible and maxilla, and temporal fossa. Untreated, these fractures will generally result in reduced range of jaw motion, pain, and fibrosis or bony ankylosis. If the fracture is uncomplicated and results in a nondisplaced fracture fragment, immediate treatment may not be necessary, as long as function is not compromised (Fig. 67.6).[115]

Muscular Disorders

Muscular pain and dysfunction are the most common symptoms of a patient with TMD. The muscles of the masticatory system are affected in the same way as other striated skeletal muscles of the body. Ligaments, nerves, and muscles all function as a complex system to stabilize the head on the shoulders, maintain a functional airway space, and allow three-dimensional movement of the mandible. This system is called the craniocervical-mandibular or the stomatognathic system. Breakdown in this complex and finely tuned system ultimately affects the musculoskeletal system, most commonly in the form of muscular disorders leading to pain in the head, face, and neck.

Myalgia due to Trauma. Masticatory muscles can be injured by acute muscle strain or by direct trauma. It is difficult to completely eliminate movement in the masticatory muscles because of the need for speech, swallowing, and chewing. If this is further compounded by dental parafunctional activities, the healing process takes longer.

Soft tissue injury results in bleeding, inflammation, and swelling, causing the muscle to respond with myalgia, muscle spasm, muscle splinting, or myositis.[116] Myofascial trigger points occur in various combinations in the muscle and are considered by Travell[117] to be the primary source of muscular pain.

Injury results in a deep, sharp ache on contraction of the

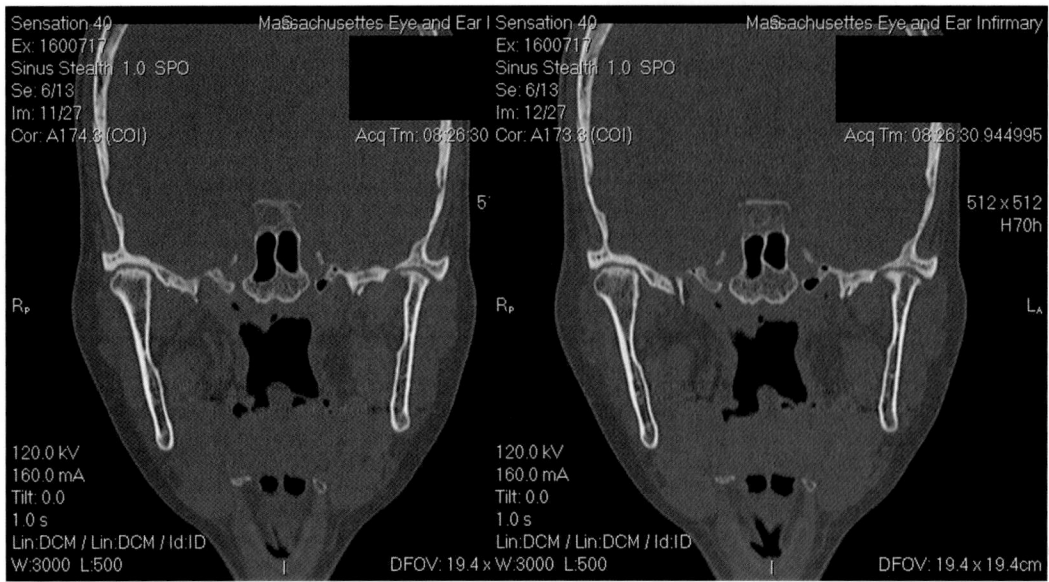

FIGURE 67.5 Coronal view CT scan of osteoarthritis of the temporomandibular joint.

muscle. Depending on the area of injury, the pain may emanate from the tendon attachments (tendonitis), the fascial component (myofascitis), or the body of the muscle (myospasm and myositis). The temporalis tendon attachment to the coronoid process is the most frequent site of masticatory tendonitis.

In acute or chronic internal derangement of the TMJ complex, the muscles that support and move the joints can be secondarily affected. Protective muscle splinting helps prevent further injury to the joint. The injured joint is often immobilized by anterior disc displacement without reduction (closed lock). Splinting of the masticatory elevator muscles is maintained until the joint is healed.

If the internal derangement is not adequately treated, the muscles remain chronically shortened and may eventually undergo contracture.[118–120] The combination of acute trauma, loss of posterior teeth, and moderate to severe parafunction may bring about an anterior disc displacement with intermittent locking of the TMJ. Patients will often report histories of trauma that are followed by a variable period of clicking, progressively increasing in frequency and culminating in an abrupt disappearance and an inability to open the mouth. Differential diagnosis of a patient who has limited mouth opening must include internal derangement as well as muscle trismus.

Myalgia secondary to injury of the cervical spine can cause headaches, facial pain, and masticatory muscle pain. Affected masticatory muscles then affect mandibular position. Mandibu-

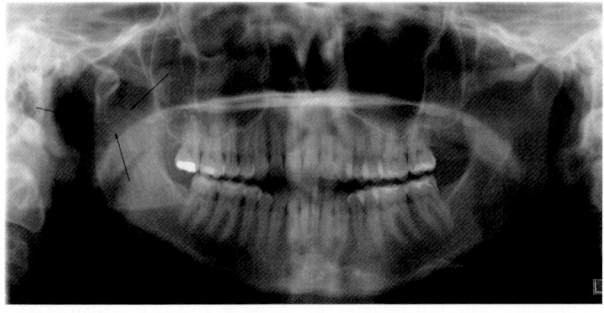

FIGURE 67.6 Fracture of the left condyle (arrows) shown on panoramic radiograph.

lar dysfunction results in tightening the muscles of the cervical spine, thereby perpetuating the cycle. This interaction is the reason that a substantial proportion of TMD patients also present with a history of cervical injury. This craniofacial and cervical syndrome requires multidisciplinary treatment of both the jaw and the neck.[121]

Disc herniations can affect the cervical muscles through protective splinting, which can eventually lead to chronic postural changes. Nerve impingement and nerve root injuries can also affect muscle function. Cervical problems are frequently comorbidities in TMD patients.[121,122]

A reduction in the space between the posterior spine of the atlas and the base of the occiput as reported by Rocabado[123] may cause pain by compression of the suboccipital tissues. The pain will be perceived as a headache starting from the back of the head.[124]

Acute or chronic trauma can shift the occiput-atlas relationship and may lead to chronic tension in the suboccipital muscles with resulting fixation and irritation of nerves C1 and C2. The pain will be referred from the back of the head to the eye, along the side of the head, along the skin over the TMJ, and down along the angle of the mandible, radiating into the neck.

Rotation of the atlas is commonly seen in patients with TMDs and may be linked to changes in occlusal contact patterns and instability of mandibular position.[125] Osteoarthritic degeneration and ligament and muscle injury also occur at this level in acceleration-deceleration injuries.

Hypermobility caused by a disruption of the C1-C2 articulation also may result in excessive stretching or kinking of the vertebral artery and may lead to temporary vertebrobasilar syndrome with symptoms of vertigo, nausea, tinnitus, and visual disturbances.[125]

The patient with a combined craniofacial-cervical syndrome will have a history of direct or indirect injury to the head and neck. The injury is usually not a direct trauma to the part, but rather a low-grade impact to the body that suddenly twists, flexes, or extends the neck.

Symptoms may range from headache, nausea, visual disturbances, neck weakness, and pain, to stiffness accompanied by noises on rotation, flexion, and extension of the head. Depending on the level of the initial injury, branches of the cervical and brachial plexus and the areas they supply can also be affected.

Secondary muscles affected can cause superimposed acute or chronic pain, requiring a specific cervical evaluation.

Depending on how the cervical problem affects the masticatory system or vice versa, occlusal appliances may reduce muscle tension.[125]

Myalgia Secondary to Parafunction. Oral parafunction includes bruxism, clenching, lip biting, thumb sucking, and any other oral habit not associated with chewing, swallowing, or speaking. Bruxism and clenching are the most common activities, with a prevalence of up to 90% in the general population.[126–130]

In most patients, parafunction is mild and intermittent and does not require treatment. Moderate or severe bruxism and clenching can damage oral structures, causing wear of the teeth, breakdown of the periodontium in the presence of inflammation, and internal derangement and muscular dysfunction.[130]

Bruxism and clenching can create excessive force for extended periods, whereas normal tooth contact during chewing and swallowing over a 24-hour period is about 20 minutes.[131] Parafunctional forces exceed normal masticatory forces, and the resultant force vector is primarily horizontal. Under such conditions, the teeth and periodontium are likely to be damaged. Ironically, most treatments are designed to protect the occlusion in function rather than in parafunction.

If the teeth, periodontium, TMJ, and muscles are considered to be "links in a chain" working together for proper function, the parafunction usually disrupts the weakest of these structures. The other structures remain relatively healthy or become secondarily affected. For example, parafunctional wear of the canines may shift force to the other teeth. If these teeth are strong enough to withstand the excessive force, the pathology may shift to the TMJ. The patient can therefore present with both tooth and joint pathology.[132–134]

Patients may present with pain in the cervical muscles as a result of chronic bruxism and clenching. Cervical muscle activity is related to occlusal contact. The patient may report restless sleep, waking up with limited mandibular range of motion, headache, facial pain, and neck pain. The pain and stiffness usually improve as the day progresses.

If a patient reports that stiffness and pain increase as the day progresses, diurnal activity should be suspected. The patient may report marked stress and depression. Palpable muscle soreness will primarily affect the elevators and the lateral pterygoid. Clenching on the wear facets by moving the mandible laterally—a provocation test—will increase the pain.

A testing device known as a Bruxcore can quantify nocturnal activity (Fig. 67.7).[135] A portable electromyographic biofeedback instrument has also been used to monitor bruxism.[136]

Repeated monitoring on different nights at a sleep laboratory is the most accurate assessment of parafunction; however, it is rarely necessary. Electromyographic analysis may show a higher resting tension level than normal, but tension depends on the specific type of muscle disorder and the specific muscle being analyzed.

Treating the parafunctional activity includes reducing the stress leading to parafunctional activity through biofeedback, stress management, medication, and counseling. The goal is to decrease the parafunction to within the adaptive capacity of the individual.

Oral structures are best protected with occlusal appliances worn at night, during the day, or both, to reduce loading on the TMJ, stress on the dentition and periodontium, and muscle activity (Fig. 67.8).[137]

Myalgia Secondary to Postural Hypertonicity. As stated above, the stability and function of the cervical region affects the position of the mandible relative to the maxilla and depends on the position of the head on the shoulders. This position is affected by gravity and the functional adaptation of the individual.[69]

A healthy craniocervical complex stabilizes head position through a series of learned and complex antagonistic muscle interactions. Forward head posture (FHP) leads to shortening and greater tension of the posterior cervical muscles.[138] The trapezius, sternocleidomastoid, and deeper muscles contract to prevent the head from tipping forward, leading to hyperactivity and chronic tension.

Chronic hyperactivity, such as working on a computer or in an office, can cause the shortened muscles to develop trigger points and the accompanying symptoms. The cervical spine is forced to adapt to the forces applied by strong cervical muscles, which may affect normal cervical lordosis.[138]

The body adapts to FHP by rounding the shoulders, leading to chronic shortening of the pectoral muscles, which further maintains FHP. Pectoral muscle tension along with FHP leads to upper thoracic breathing and tighter intercostal muscles. The anterior and middle scalenes may entrap the brachial plexus at the thoracic outlet, or the first rib can be pulled up to the clavicle, resulting in costoclavicular entrapment.[138]

Mehta and Forgione[139] have discussed the effect of chronic FHP and the relative position of the occiput, atlas, and axis with respect to each other and the craniomandibular complex. FHP and cervical muscle tension can lead to changes in occlusal contacts. Analyzing occlusal contact in maximum intercuspation with the patient in a supine position does not allow an accurate evaluation of occlusion in function. Likewise, measures to improve posture and cervical stability should be considered before definitive occlusal therapy is instituted.

Proper positioning during sleep is important for resting the postural muscles. A patient who habitually sleeps prone with the neck twisted at 90 degrees experiences the same effects as someone whose head is turned to one side all day long. In people who sleep on their sides with the lower arm outstretched under the pillow and head, the brachial plexus tends to become entrapped at the costoclavicular level. This side position can be stressful to the cervical muscles and can result in acute torticollis of the sternocleidomastoid muscle. Neck stiffness and trigger points are observed in patients with sleep habits that involve strained head positions.

Standing posture may be affected by leg-length discrepancies, hip rotation, and flat feet. Individuals who lean over machinery are likely have cervical and low-back symptoms. Shoes that are unevenly worn or that have extremely high heels affect balance and tend to cause a secondary protective adjustment of the postural muscles. This adjustment may result in chronic muscular shortening, trigger points, and spasm. Shifts in body posture and compensatory cervical changes affect mandibular position and tooth contact patterns.[69]

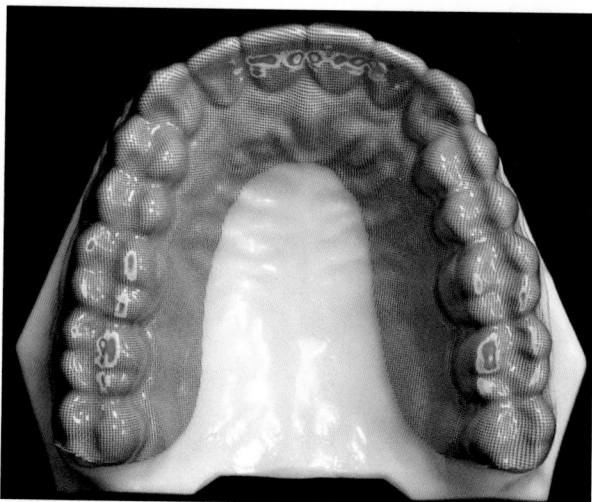

FIGURE 67.7 Bruxcore tooth grinding indicator.

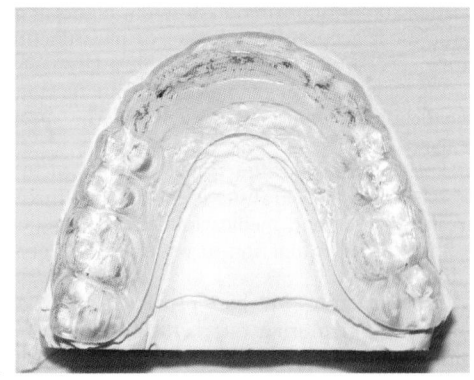
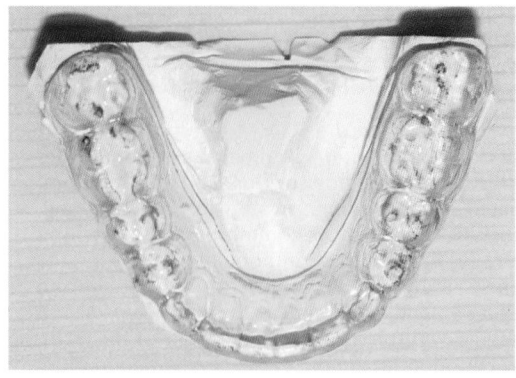

A   B

FIGURE 67.8 A,B. Oral orthosis appliance for the jaws.

Radiographs CT scans or MRI scans may be needed to evaluate spinal curvature and to rule out other pathologies.

Short-term exercise can increase range of motion and improve posture, muscle re-education can strengthen the muscles in the therapeutic postural position, and home exercise programs can maintain therapeutic postural position.[115]

Myofascial Pain and Trigger Points. In 1952, Travell and Rinzler[116] introduced the concept of myofascial pain and trigger points. They defined a myofascial trigger point as a hyperirritable locus within a taut band of skeletal muscle located in a muscle or in its associated fascia or tendon. The spot is painful on compression and can evoke characteristic referred pain and autonomic phenomena.[116]

Trigger points may be active or latent. Active trigger points may cause pain spontaneously or during movement. Latent trigger points afflict nearly half of the population by early adulthood.[140] Latent trigger points are usually not painful, but create weakness and restrict movement. Trigger points can be activated by a sudden overloading contraction, viral infection, cold temperatures, fatigue, and increased emotional stress.

The complex nature of myofascial trigger points and their common presence in acute and chronic muscle dysfunction require an understanding of their clinical features. According to Travell and Simons,[140] there are seven such features:

- local tenderness over the trigger point
- referred pain, tenderness, and autonomic phenomena
- a palpable taut band associated with the trigger points
- a local twitch response of a trigger point in a palpable taut band
- perpetuation of trigger points
- a therapeutic effect when stretching the muscle containing the trigger points
- weakness and fatigability of muscles afflicted with trigger points relative to unafflicted muscles

Myofascial pain often refers to pain at the head and neck and is considered by some to constitute tension-type headaches. Myofascial pain and trigger points of the masticatory muscles can send pain to the eyes, ears, TMJ, and teeth, depending on the specific muscles. The pain is usually a dull or intense ache that varies daily and is strongly related to posture and muscle activity. The pain can usually be localized by the patient and can be indicated on a diagram of the body. Trigger points commonly affect the muscles of posture and mastication, and pain may occur in the same dermatome, myotome, or sclerotome. Satellite trigger points may occur within the pain reference zone. Clinically, movement is restricted, passive stretching is painful, and strong contractions markedly increase the pain. Resistive testing reveals weakness from protective splinting.

Trigger points are palpated by rubbing the fingertip lightly along the long axis of the muscle. If present, a taut band will be located first, and then the more sensitive trigger point. Applying pressure on a trigger point elicits a grimace or an involuntary sound from the patient called the "jump sign." A snapping palpation of the taut band will produce a latent trigger response confirming the presence of the trigger point. Final confirmation comes on reproducing the patient's pain by digital pressure on the point.[139]

Pressure algometers quantify the amount of pressure applied to the trigger point, which allows the clinician to document the severity of the trigger point. It may also be used to objectively record the efficacy of treatment.

Treating myofascial trigger points includes spray-and-stretch techniques with ethyl chloride or fluoromethane for its cooling effects, followed by stretching, hot compresses, and range-of-motion exercises. Trigger point injections of procaine (0.5% solution in saline) or lidocaine (2% without epinephrine) have also been the standard in pain management programs (Fig. 67.9). More recently, botulinum toxin (Botox) has been added to this arsenal.[140–144]

Other techniques involve ischemic compression for 30 to 60 seconds, acupressure, and pharmacologic therapy, including analgesics, muscle relaxants, antidepressants, and NSAIDs. Physical therapy modalities such as myofascial release and craniosacral techniques, including postural correction and exercise, have also

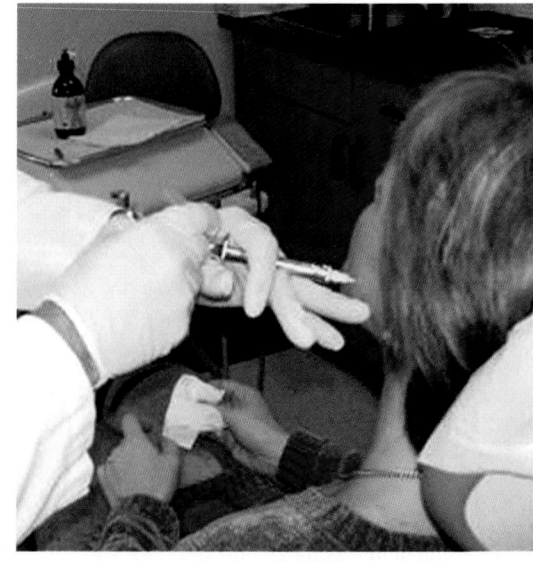

FIGURE 67.9 Trigger point injection of the masseter muscle.

been effective in managing myofascial trigger points. Stress and nutritional and hormonal factors should also be addressed.[137]

In case of the masticatory muscles, occlusal appliances may be used.[138] Dental appliances are effective in reducing muscle symptoms and trigger points in mandibular elevators. These appliances are usually flat plane and fully cover either the upper or lower teeth, depending on when they are to be worn.

Muscle Splinting.
Muscle splinting is a reflex by which skeletal muscles stabilize an injured area to protect it from further injury. The involved muscles become hypertonic and painful. The associated feeling of weakness, although alarming to the patient, is a normal protective reaction to discourage moving the affected part.

Muscle splinting is often a sequela to muscle injury and follows myositis. If splinting is protracted, muscle spasm may follow with or without trigger points, leading to a chronic cycle of myofascial pain and dysfunction.[140]

Initially, injections are not indicated; ice, rest, and relaxation are the basis of acute therapy. Stretching, ultrasound, or light massage can be used in the initial stages. Once the muscles have started to heal, splinting decreases, at which point therapy to regain mobility can begin. Mobilization techniques, gentle stretching, and range-of-motion exercises are required to prevent ongoing myospasm, contracture, and atrophy.

Muscle Spasm (Sustained).
A muscle spasm is the painful contraction of a striated muscle caused by trauma, tension, or disease.[113,125] The spasm manifests as pain and interference in function. Muscular fiber contractions occur in response to increased excitability of alpha motoneurons.

Prolonged muscle spasm is thought to be caused by the ischemia induced in a skeletal muscle by its continued contraction. The muscle fatigues and lactic acid builds up, leading to the release of bradykinin, causing pain.

In the masticatory musculature, spasm of the masseter or temporalis muscle limits range of motion, which in turn causes the jaw to deflect to the ipsilateral side on mouth opening. If a spasm is isometric, the muscle will be rigid and resistant to stretch. Condylar position can be affected in true spasm of the elevator muscles and may predispose a patient to internal derangement. As with all chronic pain, the severe pain and inability to function can bring about psychosocial problems.[113]

Spastic muscles must be differentiated by palpation from: the painful soft muscle of myositis; relatively normal, albeit painful, muscle splinting; and localized taut bands and areas of myofascial trigger points. In contrast, a muscle in spasm has a stiff hard surface that is painfully resistant to stretch.

Electromyographic recordings show high standing tension in the affected muscle but lower electromyographic activity relative to the unaffected side. Pressure threshold meters and tissue compliance measurements may help identify the muscles in spasm. Thermography is also being investigated for routine diagnostic use.[145–146]

Initial treatment should be directed to eliminating the cycling spasm. The patient should restrict movement to within painless limits, but some function is necessary to regain a normal stretch reflex, which helps relax the muscle. In spasm of a masticatory muscle, the teeth can be disengaged with a stabilization (flat plane) appliance if the mouth can open enough to insert a temporary emergency splint. Splints are thought to work by shutting off proprioceptive input from the teeth that may help maintain spastic activity.

Muscle relaxants administered judiciously can help reduce dysfunction and spasm and can be adjuncts to other therapy, such as injection of spastic muscles. Spray-and-stretch techniques and massage and acupressure techniques may also be effective.

As the muscle starts to respond to treatment, stretching and range-of-motion exercises will help prevent contractures and bring the muscle back to full function. Ongoing passive jaw motion exercises will help maintain range of motion. In the masticatory system, structural factors, such as the bite, should be corrected only after the muscle is pain-free and fully functional.[138]

Myositis.
A direct blow to a muscle can trigger a localized inflammatory response accompanied by swelling, pain, and immobilization.[138] The main presenting symptoms will be localized soreness, swelling, and pain, along with weakness and immobilization of the affected structure. Pain is generally dull, deep, boring, and constant. Episodes of sharp pain related to movement of the affected structure may also be reported.

Injury to the head and neck muscles will result in an accompanying reduction in neck movement and changes in shoulder height and head posture as a means of protecting against further trauma. The pain may be perceived by the patient as a headache. An accompanying feeling of weakness in the neck may be experienced.

Patients with myositis of the masticatory muscles may report pain in the face or jaw accompanied by a change in the bite with the inability to chew, swallow, and speak comfortably. Locally, the area may appear swollen and discolored because of extravasations of inflammatory products. An inflamed muscle will present as a soft, painful mass on palpation. Pain will be associated with active as well as passive movement of the affected structure. The skin may be warmer to the touch than the surrounding area. The patient may present with low-grade fever if secondary infection is involved. Pressure threshold measurements with a threshold meter will indicate that discomfort occurs at a lower threshold than before the injury. Proximal to the injury, there may be a cold spot caused by vasoconstriction, which may affect healing.

Initial therapy of the acute symptoms of myositis includes immediately applying ice to the affected structure to reduce swelling, limiting movement to within painless boundaries, and resting the affected part. In injured mandibular muscles, restricting mouth opening during function and using a dental intraoral bite guard to control closure should be supported by NSADIs. In a severe case, immediately applying a methylprednisolone dose pack can control the amount of the immediate swelling. Antibiotics can be used if secondary infection is possible.

After the acute symptoms have subsided, treatment should include increased heat and mobilization of the affected structure, then an exercise program to regain full range of motion, and finally a muscle strengthening program.

Fibrosis and Contracture.
Myotatic contracture occurs in muscles that are not allowed to function within their full range of motion. The muscle will lose its stretch reflex capabilities and will gradually shorten. Prolonged pain or immobilization can lead to myotatic contracture.[113]

Contracture can occur in the masticatory muscles if patients are unwilling or unable to open their mouths fully. Patients often report avoiding opening wide for fear of hearing clicking or crepitus, and others may not open wide because of past or present pain. Over time, this practice leads to the development of a habituated protective pattern, causing myotatic contracture. Likewise, restricted movement of the cervical region results in myotatic contracture.

Myofibrotic contracture often occurs as a result of infection that leads to fibrous changes in the muscle or its sheath. Trauma to a muscle and the resultant inflammation and splinting may lead to fibrosis—an irreversible condition. Radiation therapy, incision through a muscle with fibrotic healing, and disuse for long periods (more than 6 weeks) can also result in myofibrotic contracture.

In patients with masticatory muscle involvement, myotatic or myofibrotic contracture will appear with limited interincisal opening. If the elevator muscles are involved, deviation will occur on opening but not on protrusion. Lateral movement will be normal. Pain will not be present without sudden and forceful stretching or biting.

The treatment for myotatic contracture is to gradually stretch the involved muscle. Ultrasound with 5% to 10% hydrocortisone cream can be used as adjunct therapy. Massage and myofascial release along with daily stretching and exercise will bring the muscle slowly back to function. Myofibrotic contracture is irreversible and requires surgical intervention for a patient whose function is severely impaired.

Muscle Disorders Secondary to Internal Derangement. In the presence of acute or chronic internal derangement, the muscles that support and move the joints can be secondarily affected. Splinting helps prevent further injury to the joint. In cases of anterior disc displacement without reduction (closed lock), the joint will often be immobile. The masticatory elevator muscles should be splinted until the joint is healed.

The clinical finding of elevator spasm often causes the physician or dentist unfamiliar with TMD to prescribe muscle relaxants. These medications override the body's defense mechanisms and so may do more harm than good. If the internal derangement is not adequately treated, the muscles remain chronically shortened and may eventually undergo contracture. A patient with acute closed lock often presents with a history of joint clicking. The patient may or may not be able to pinpoint an eliciting event. Sometimes the patient wakes up with the jaw locked. Other times, it locks during chewing. The patient will often have loss of posterior support through tooth wear, tooth breakdown, or missing or poorly restored posterior teeth.

Closed lock may be accompanied by a change in occlusion resulting from disc displacement, accompanying spasm of the lateral pterygoid, or both. The occlusion may shift to the contralateral side with a corresponding posterior open bite developing on the ipsilateral side. The patient may attempt to position the posterior teeth into contact but is hampered by joint pain and the lateral pterygoid, which pulls the mandible in the opposite side.

After acute trauma, the occlusion settles back to its preinjured state once the TMJ inflammation has subsided. However, if the patient has a parafunctional habit or has lost vertical dimension, the joint will continue to be unevenly loaded, and healing will be delayed. In such instances, the joint may become chronically inflamed and the muscles of mastication may continue to be in a state of protective splinting, spasm, or both.

If a patient has a combination of acute trauma, loss of posterior teeth, and moderate-to-severe parafunction, anterior disc displacement with intermittent locking of the TMJ is likely. Patients often report histories of trauma that are followed by a variable period of clicking, progressively increasing in frequency and culminating in an abrupt disappearance and an inability to open the mouth. Differential diagnosis of a patient who has limited mouth opening must include internal derangement, as well as muscle trauma.

Muscle Disorders Secondary to Cervical Spinal Dysfunction. Muscle disorders may occur secondary to rotations, fixations, fusions, or injury or locking of the facets of the cervical, thoracic, lumbar, and sacral vertebrae. The history, physical examination, and radiographic evaluation, often done in conjunction with a physiatrist or orthopedist, will reflect the acuteness and severity of the vertebral problem.

Disc herniations can secondarily affect the cervical muscles through protective splinting, which can eventually lead to chronic postural changes. Nerve impingement and nerve root injuries can also affect muscle function. Commonly seen cervical problems in relation to TMDs occur at the following cervical levels.

Occiput-Atlas. A reduction in the space between the posterior spine of the atlas and the base of the occiput, as reported by Rocabado,[147] may cause pain by compressing the suboccipital tissues. The pain will be perceived as a headache starting from the back of the head.

Acute or long-standing trauma can shift the occiput-atlas relationship and may lead to chronic tension in the suboccipital muscles with resulting fixation and irritation of the C1 and C2 nerves. The pain will be referred from the back of the head to the eye, along the side of the head, along the skin over the TMJ, and down along the angle of the mandible, radiating into the neck.

Rotation of the atlas is commonly seen in patients with TMDs and may be linked to changes in occlusal patterns and instability of mandibular position.[139,147] Osteoarthritic degeneration and ligament and muscle injury also occur at this level in acceleration-deceleration injuries.

Atlas/Axis Level. Trauma to this level may disrupt the transverse ligament holding the odontoid process of the axis against the anterior arch of the atlas, allowing forward subluxation or dislocation of the atlas on the axis. A disruption of the C1-C2 articulation may also result in excessive stretching or kinking of the vertebral artery secondary to hypermobility. This may lead to temporary vertebrobasilar syndrome with symptoms of vertigo, nausea, tinnitus, and visual disturbances.

Cervical rotation will be reduced because 40% to 50% of rotation occurs at the atlas-axis articulation.[147] Pain also limits movement. Fractures are always to be considered in trauma to this region.

C4, C5, and C6. The level of greatest instability against acceleration-deceleration forces appears to be in the C4 to C6 region, with C4-C5 being primarily affected in hyperextension and C5-C6 in hyperflexion. Trauma may be to the ligaments, discs, and vertebral bodies, depending on the direction and magnitude of the force.

The cervical curve can be affected, and the patient will often have a compensatory forward head posture, further perpetuating the problem.

Cranial Neuralgias

Trigeminal Neuralgia

The cranial neuralgias, particularly trigeminal neuralgia, affect the face and have specific diagnostic criteria and treatment modalities. These disorders are covered in Chapter 66.

Neuropathic Facial Pain (see Table 67.13)

The International Association for the Study of Pain (IASP) defines neuropathic pain as "Pain initiated or caused by a primary lesion or dysfunction in the nervous system."[148] Thus, neuropathic pain results from pathology in the peripheral or central nervous system.[148] These disorders are particularly common in the head and neck, probably as a result of the dense and specialized sensory innervation of this region. Unfortunately, these disorders greatly affect the patient's life by interfering with important functions, such as feeding and speech.

In the past, any facial pain disorder without a definable cause was considered to be an idiopathic, "atypical" facial pain syndrome. Over the years, many inappropriate "descriptive" diagnoses were given to these disorders (atypical trigeminal neuralgia, atypical facial pain, atypical odontalgia, phantom tooth syndrome, and so on.) Under the current IHS classification[1] (see Tables 67.5 and 67.6), these disorders are considered "central" causes for headache and facial pain and are classified as "persistent idiopathic facial pain" (category 13.18).[1]

Complex regional pain syndrome (CRPS), a form of neuropathic pain can occur in the face.[149] CRPS is covered in detail in Chapter 25. Likewise, postherpetic neuralgia commonly affects the face and is covered in detail in Chapter 27.

PSYCHOSOCIAL CONSIDERATIONS

Assessment

As with other chronic pain conditions, psychosocial factors explain much of the variance in the outcome of persistent facial pain disorders. Affective and anxiety symptoms, especially emotional trauma, have been implicated in precipitating and maintaining chronic orofacial pain.[150] Marked somatic overconcern or somatization disorder can also compromise treatment in these disorders. Similarly, chronic disability behavior further compromises the patient's status.

It has become a minimum standard of care to address critical psychosocial factors within the diagnostic interview, as underscored by the IASP Curricula on Pain for Dental Schools.[151,152] Consistent with this attention, the Research Diagnostic Criteria includes a 31-item questionnaire addressing psychosocial and physical domains of chronic TMD. Other validated self-report facial pain scales also address psychosocial issues, and their use within multidisciplinary facial pain facilities is common.[153-155]

Treatment

As in other areas of chronic pain management, behavioral interventions have been a mainstay of treatment for persistent facial pain. Time-limited, structured relaxation training is as effective as conventional occlusal splint therapy for temporal joint dysfunction and related chronic myofascial facial pain disorders. Combined treatment is even more effective and provides longer lasting effects.[156] Similarly, improving cognitive coping skills reduces pain and improves function.[157] Behavioral interventions target reducing anxiety and improving perceived control over pain. Biofeedback-assisted relaxation can also be effective, perhaps more so in limited subpopulations.[158-160] More intensive, interdisciplinary treatment is often indicated for patients with a constellation of severe psychosocial and disability behaviors.

Cost-effective behavioral group programs have also been used in the early stages of facial pain syndromes and have reduced pain and improved coping skills. Most recently, Stowell et al.[161] compared a brief behavioral treatment program emphasizing early intervention to a standard approach in patients with "acute TMD" (pain of less than 6 months duration). One-year follow-up data revealed clinical improvement and substantially fewer jaw-related health care dollars for the early intervention program. Overall, conservative interdisciplinary treatment appears to have the most promising results. Ideally, these programs will be implemented before the chronic concomitants of facial pain develop.

CONCLUSION

Craniocervical pain is a common clinical problem and often a diagnostic challenge. Given the complex anatomy of the region and the numerous discrete syndromes, a multidisciplinary approach is frequently indicated for evaluating difficult or refractory cases.

References

1. Headache Classification Subcommittee of the International Headache Society. The International Classification of Headache Disorders: 2nd edition. *Cephalalgia* 2004;24(suppl 1):9–160.
2. Maciewicz R, Mason P, Strassman A, et al. Organization of the trigeminal nociceptive pathways. *Semin Neurol* 1988;8:255–264.
3. Mason P, Strassman A, Maciewicz R. Is the jaw-opening reflex a valid model of pain? *Brain Res* 1985;357:137–146.
4. Bell WE. Orofacial pains: classification, diagnosis and management. In: Okeson JP, ed. *Pains of Dental Origin*. 3rd ed. Hanover Park, IL: Quintessence Publishing Co.; 1985:116–143.
5. Berman LH. Contemporary concepts in endodontics: 2003 and beyond. *Gen Dent* 2003;51:224–230.
6. Silberstein SD, Lipton RB, Dalessio DJ. Wolff's headache and other headache pain. In: Graff-Radford SB, Newman A, eds. *Disorders of the Mouth and Teeth*. 8th ed. New York: Oxford University Press; 2008.
7. Ratcliff S, Becker IM, Quin L. Type and incidence of cracks in posterior teeth. *J Prosthet Dent* 2001;86(2):168–172.
8. Offenbacher S. Periodontal diseases: pathogenesis. *Ann Periodontol* 1996;1: 821–878.
9. Newman MG, Takci HH, Carranza FA. *Carranza's Clinical Periodontology*. 9th ed. Philadelphia: WB Saunders; 2002:297–313.
10. Horning GM, Cohen ME. Necrotizing ulcerative gingivitis, periodontitis and stomatitis: clinical staging and predisposing factors. *J Periodontal* 1995;66: 990–998.
11. Bartoshuk LM, Duffy VB, Reed D, et al. Supertasting, earaches and head injury: genetics and pathology alter our taste worlds. *Neurosci Biobehav Rev* 1996;20:79–87.
12. Grushka M, Sessle BJ. Burning mouth syndrome. *Dent Clin North Am* 1991; 35:171–184.
13. Mott AE, Grushka M, Sessle BJ. Diagnosis and management of taste disorders and burning mouth syndrome. *Dent Clin North Am* 1993;37:33–71.
14. Ship JA, Grushka M, Lipton JA, et al. Burning mouth syndrome: an update. *J Am Dent Assoc* 1995;126:842–853.
15. Forssell H, Jaaskelainen S, Tenovuo O, et al. Sensory dysfunction in burning mouth syndrome. *Pain* 2002;99:41–47.
16. Lee AG, Beaver HA, Brazis PW. Painful ophthalmologic disorders and eye pain for the neurologist. *Neurol Clin N Am* 2004;22:75–97.
17. Olesen J, Tfelt-Hansen P, Welch KM. The headache. In: Gobeltt H, Martin TJ, eds. *Ocular Disorders*. 2nd ed. Philadelphia: Lippincott Williams & Wilkins; 2002:899–904.
18. Sherwood MB, Garcia-Siekavizzo A, Meltzer MI, et al. Glaucoma's impact on quality of life and its relation to clinical indicators: a pilot study. *Ophthalmology* 1998;105:561–566.
19. Klein BE, Klein R, Meuer SM, et al. Migraine headache and its association with open angle glaucoma: the beaver dam eye study. *Invest Ophthalmol Vis Sci* 1993;34:3024–3027.
20. Silberstein SD, Lipton RB, Dodick DW. *Wolff's Headache and Other Headache Pain: The Eye and Headache*. 8th ed. New York: Oxford University Press; 2008:459–474.
21. Joseph A. A tooth for an eye: dental procedures in unrecognized glaucoma. *J R Soc Med* 1999;92:249.
22. Dayan MB, Turner B, McGhee C. Acute-angle closure glaucoma masquerading as systemic illness. *BMJ* 1996;313:413–415.
23. Kasper DL, Braunwald E, Fauci AS, et al. Disorders of the eye. In: Braunwald E, Fauci AS, Kasper DL, et al, eds. *Harrison's Principles of Internal Medicine*. New York: The McGraw-Hill Companies; 2005.
24. Cates CA, Newman DK. Transient monocular visual loss due to uveitis-glaucoma-hyphema (UGH) syndrome. *J Neurol Neurosurg Psychiatry* 1998; 65:131–132.
25. Folberg R, Bernardino VB, Aguilar GL, et al. Amputation neuroma mistaken for recurrent melanoma in the orbit. *Ophthalmic Surg* 1981;12:275–278.
26. Lanzino G, Andreoli A, Tognetti F, et al. Orbital pain and unruptured carotid-posterior communicating artery aneurysms: the role of sensory fibers of the third cranial nerve. *Acta Neurochir* 1993;120:7–11.
27. Hannerz J. Recurrent Tolosa-Hunt syndrome: a report of ten new cases. *Cephalalgia* 1999;19(suppl 25):33–35.
28. Hannerz J. A case of parasellar meningioma mimicking cluster headache. *Cephalalgia* 1989;9:265–269.
29. Del Catillo F, Corretger JM, Medina J, et al. Acute otitis media in childhood: a study of 20,532 cases. *Infection* 1995;23(suppl 2):70–73.
30. Woollons AC, Morton RP. When does middle ear effusion signify nasopharyngeal cancer? *N Z Med J* 1994;107:507–509.
31. Shah RK, Blevins NH. Otalgia. *Otolaryngol Clin N Am* 2003;36:1137–1151.
32. Powers WH, Britton BH. Nonotogenic otalgia: diagnosis and treatment plan. *Am J Otology* 1980;2:97–104.
33. Scarbrough TJ, Day TA, Williams TE, et al. Referred otalgia in head and neck cancer: a unifying schema. *Am J Clin Oncology* 2003;26:157–162.
34. Olesen J, Tfelt-Hansen P, Welch KM. The headache. In: Gobel H, Balioh RW, eds. *Disorders of the Ear, Nose, and Sinus*. 2nd ed. Philadelphia: Lippincott Williams & Wilkins; 2000:905–912.
35. Doherty GM, Way LW. Current surgical diagnosis and treatment. In: Baily BJ, et al, eds. *Otolaryngology—Head & Neck Surgery*. New York: The McGraw-Hill Companies; 2006.
36. Stewart MH, Siff JE, Cydulka RK. Evaluation of the patient with sore throat, earache, and sinusitis: an evidence based approach. *Emerg Med Clin North Am* 1999;17(1):153–178.
37. Henderson DH, Cooper JC, Bryan GW, et al. Otologic complaints in temporomandibular joint syndrome. *Arch Otolaryngol Head Neck Surg* 1992;118: 1208–1213.

38. Prasad KC, Kamath MP, Reddy KJM, et al. Elongated styloid process (Eagle's syndrome): a clinical study. *J Oral Maxillofac Surg* 2002;60:171–175.
39. Gibson WS Jr, Cochran W. Otalgia in infants and children—a manifestation of gastroesophageal reflux. *Int J Pediatr Otorhinolaryngol* 1994;28:213–218.
40. Poelmans J, Tack J, Feenstra L. Prospective study on the incidence of chronic ear complaints related to gastroesophageal reflux and on the outcome of antireflux therapy. *Ann Otol Rhinol Laryngol* 2002;111:933–937.
41. Evans RW, Mathew NT. Headaches & neoplasms, high & low pressure and HEENT disorders. In: Evans RW, Mathew N, eds. *Handbook of Headache*. 2nd ed. Philadelphia: Lippincott Williams & Wilkins; 2005:269–305.
42. Benninger MS, Anon J, Mabry RL. The medical management of rhinosinusitis. *Otolaryngol Head Neck Surg* 1997;117:S41–S49.
43. Cady RK, Schreiber CP. Sinus headache: a clinical conundrum. *Otolaryngol Clin N Am* 2004;37:267–288.
44. West B, Jones NS. Endoscopy-negative, computed tomography-negative facial pain in a nasal clinic. *Laryngoscope* 2001;111:581–586.
45. Fahy C, Jones NS. Nasal polyposis and facial pain. *Clin Otolaryngol* 2001; 26:510–513.
46. Tarabichi M. Characteristics of sinus-related pain. *Otolaryngol Head Neck Surg* 2000;122:84–87.
47. Jones NS, Cooney TR. Facial pain and sinonasal surgery. *Rhinology* 2003; 41:193–200.
48. Lew D, Southwick FS, Montgomery WW, et al. Sphenoid sinusitis: a review of 30 cases. *N Engl J Med* 1983;19:1149–1154.
49. Lau J, Zucker D, Engels EA, et al. *Diagnosis and treatment of acute bacterial rhinosinusitis. Evidence report/technology assessment no. 9. Contract 290-97-0019 to the New England Medical Center*. Rockville, MD: Agency for Health Care Policy and Research; March 1999.
50. Silberstein SD. Headaches due to nasal and paranasal sinus disease. *Neurol Clin N Am* 2004;22:1–19.
51. Lanza DC, Kennedy DW. Adult rhinosinusitis defined. *Otolaryngol Head Neck Surg* 1997;117:S1–S7.
52. Williams JW, Simel DL, Roberts L, et al. Clinical evaluation of sinusitis. *Ann Intern Med* 1992;117:705–710.
53. Jones NS. Sinogenic facial pain: diagnosis and treatment. *Otolaryngol Clin N Am* 2005;38:1311–1325.
54. Sofferman RA. Cavernous sinus thrombophlebitis secondary to sphenoid sinusitis. *Laryngoscope* 1983;93:797–800.
55. Tepper SJ. New thoughts on sinus headache. *Allergy Asthma Proc* 2004;25: 95–96.
56. Levine HL, Setzen M, Cady RK, et al. An otolaryngology, neurology, allergy and primary care consensus on diagnosis and treatment of sinus headache. *Otolaryngol Head Neck Surg* 2006;134:516–523.
57. Bhattacharyya N, Fried MP. The accuracy of computed tomography in the diagnosis of chronic rhinosinusitis. *Laryngoscope* 2003;113:125–129.
58. McCaffrey TV. Functional endoscopic sinus surgery: an overview. *Mayo Clin Proc* 1993;68:675–677.
59. Acquadro MA, Salman SD, Joseph MP. Analysis of pain and endoscopic sinus surgery for sinusitis. *Ann Otol Rhinol Laryngol* 1997;106:305–309.
60. Mortimore S, Wormald PJ, Oliver S. Antibiotic choice in acute and complicated sinusitis. *J Laryngol Otol* 1998;112:264–268.
61. Chow JM. Rhinologic headaches. *Otolaryngol Head Neck Surg* 1994;111(3): 211–218.
62. de Leeuw R. *Orofacial Pain: Guidelines for Assessment, Diagnosis, and Management*. 4th ed. Chicago: The American Academy of Orofacial Pain; 2008.
63. Solberg WK. Epidemiology, incidence and prevalence of temporomandibular disorders: a review. In: *The President's Conference on the Examination, Diagnosis and Management of Temporomandibular Disorders*. Chicago: American Dental Association; 1983:30–39.
64. Schiffman E, Fricton JR. Epidemiology of TMJ and craniofacial pains. In: Fricton JR, Kroening RJ, Hathaway KM, eds. *TMJ and Craniofacial Pain*. St. Louis: Ishiro Euro America; 1988:1–10.
65. Dworkin SF, Huggins KH, LeResche L, et al. Epidemiology of signs and symptoms of temporomandibular disorders: clinical signs in cases and controls. *J Am Dent Assoc* 1990;120:273–281.
66. Wabeke KB, Spruijt RJ. *On Temporomandibular Joint Sounds: Dental and Psychological Studies* [Thesis]. Amsterdam: University of Amsterdam; 1994: 91–103.
67. Huber NU, Hall EH. A comparison of the signs of temporomandibular joint dysfunction and occlusal discrepancies in a symptom-free population of men and women. *Oral Surg Oral Med Oral Pathol* 1990;70:180–183.
68. Levitt SR, McKinney MW. Validating the TMJ scale in a national sample of 10,000 patients: demographic and epidemiologic characteristics. *J Orofac Pain* 1994;8:25–34.
69. Mehta NR, Forgione AG, Rosenbaum RS, et al. Temporomandibular disorders: a triad of dysfunctions. *J Mass Dent Soc* 1984;33(4):212–213.
70. Bonjardim LR, Gaviao MB, Pereira LJ, et al. Signs and symptoms of temporomandibular disorders in adolescents. *Pesqui Odontol Bras* 2005;19:93–98.
71. Kapur N, Kamel IR, Herlich A. Oral and craniofacial pain: diagnosis, pathophysiology, and treatment. *Int Anesthesiol Clin* 2003;41:115–150.
72. Egermark I, Magnusson T, Carlsson GE. A 20-year follow-up of signs and symptoms of temporomandibular disorders and malocclusions in subjects with and without orthodontic treatment in childhood. *Angle Orthod* 2003; 73:109–115.
73. Sipila K, Zitting P, Siira P, et al. Temporomandibular disorders, occlusion,

74. Nassif NJ, Talic YF. Classic symptoms in temporomandibular disorder patients: a comparative study. *Cranio* 2001;19:33-41.
75. Johansson A, Unell L, Carlsson GE, et al. Gender difference in symptoms related to temporomandibular disorders in a population of 50-year-old subjects. *J Orofac Pain* 2003;17:29–35.
76. Macfarlane TV, Blinkhorn AS, Davies RM, et al. Oro-facial pain in the community: prevalence and associated impact. *Community Dent Oral Epidemiol* 2002;30:52–60.
77. Rasmussen P. Facial pain. IV. A prospective study of 1052 patients with a view of: precipitating factors, associated symptoms, objective psychiatric and neurological symptoms. *Acta Neurochir (Wien)* 1991;108:100–109.
78. de las Penas CF, Cuadrado ML, Gerwin RD, et al. Referred pain from the trochlear region in tension-type headache: a myofascial trigger point from the superior oblique muscle. *Headache* 2005;45:731–737.
79. Kalina R, Orcutt J. Ocular and periocular pain. In: Bonica JJ, ed. *The Management of Pain*. Philadelphia: Lee and Ferbiger; 1990:759–768.
80. Curtis AW. Myofascial pain-dysfunction syndrome: the role of nonmasticatory muscles in 91 patients. *Otolaryngol Head Neck Surg* 1980;88:361–367.
81. Alvarez DJ, Rockwell PG. Trigger points: diagnosis and management. *Am Fam Physician* 2002;65:653–660.
82. Kuttila S, Kuttila M, Le BY, et al. Characteristics of subjects with secondary otalgia. *J Orofac Pain* 2004;18:226–234.
83. Kuttila M, Le BY, Savolainen-Niemi E, et al. Efficiency of occlusal appliance therapy in secondary otalgia and temporomandibular disorders. *Acta Odontol Scand* 2002;60:248–254.
84. Kuttila SJ, Kuttila MH, Niemi PM, et al. Secondary otalgia in an adult population. *Arch Otolaryngol Head Neck Surg* 2001;127:401–405.
85. Wright EF, Syms CA III, Bifano SL. Tinnitus, dizziness, and nonotologic otalgia improvement through temporomandibular disorder therapy. *Mil Med* 2000;165:733–736.
86. Bush FM, Harkins SW, Harrington WG. Otalgia and aversive symptoms in temporomandibular disorders. *Ann Otol Rhinol Laryngol* 1999;108:884–892.
87. Wazen JJ. Referred otalgia. *Otolaryngol Clin North Am* 1989;1205–1215.
88. Egermark I, Carlsson GE, Magnusson T. A 20-year longitudinal study of subjective symptoms of temporomandibular disorders from childhood to adulthood. *Acta Odontol Scand* 2001;59:40–48.
89. Matsumoto MA, Matsumoto W, Bolognese AM. Study of the signs and symptoms of temporomandibular dysfunction in individuals with normal occlusion and malocclusion. *Cranio* 2002;20:274–281.
90. Simmons HC III, Gibbs SJ. Anterior repositioning appliance therapy for TMJ disorders: specific symptoms relieved and relationship to disk status on MRI. *Cranio* 2005;23:89–99.
91. Fink M, Wahling K, Stiesch-Scholz M, et al. The functional relationship between the craniomandibular system, cervical spine, and the sacroiliac joint: a preliminary investigation. *Cranio* 2003;21:202–208.
92. Ciancaglini R, Testa M, Radaelli G. Association of neck pain with symptoms of temporomandibular dysfunction in the general adult population. *Scand J Rehabil Med* 1999;31:17–22.
93. Svensson P, Wang K, Sessle BJ, et al. Associations between pain and neuromuscular activity in the human jaw and neck muscles. *Pain* 2004;109: 225–232.
94. Kushida CA, Morgenthaler TI, Littner MR, et al. Practice parameters for the treatment of snoring and obstructive sleep apnea with oral appliances: an update for 2005. *Sleep* 2006;29:240–243.
95. Chakfa AM, Mehta NR, Forgione AG. The effect of stepwise increases in vertical dimension of occlusion on isometric strength of cervical flexors and deltoid muscles in nonsymptomatic females. *Cranio* 2002;20:264–273.
96. Abduljabbar T, Mehta NR, Forgione AG, et al. Effect of increased maxillomandibular relationship on isometric strength in TMD patients with loss of vertical dimension of occlusion. *Cranio* 1997;15:57–67.
97. Dibbets JM, van der Weele LT. Prevalence of structural bony change in the mandibular condyle. *J Craniomandib Disord* 1992;6:254–259.
98. Buchbinder D, Kaplan A. Biology. In: Kaplan A, Assael LA, eds. *Temporomandibular Disorders: Diagnosis and Treatment*. Philadelphia: WB Saunders; 1991:11–23.
99. Pullinger AG, Bibb CA, Ding X, et al. Contour mapping of the TMJ temporal component and the relationship to articular soft tissue thickness and disk displacement. *Oral Surg Oral Med Oral Pathol* 1993;76:636–646.
100. Pullinger AG, Bibb CA, Ding X, et al. Relationship of articular soft tissue contour and shape to the underlying eminence and slope profile in young adult temporomandibular joints. *Oral Surg Oral Med Oral Pathol* 1993;76: 647–654.
101. Ward DM, Behrents RG, Goldberg JS. Temporomandibular synovial fluid pressure response to altered mandibular positions. *Am J Orthod Dentofacial Orthop* 1990;98:22–28.
102. Axelsson S, Holmlund A, Hjerpe A. Glycosaminoglycans in normal and osteoarthrotic human temporomandibular joint disks. *Acta Odontol Scand* 1992;50:113–119.
103. Wongwatana S, Kronman JH, Clark RE, et al. Anatomic basis for disk displacement in temporomandibular joint (TMJ) dysfunction. *Am J Orthod Dentofacial Orthop* 1994;105:257–264.
104. Brecht K, Johnson CM III. Complete mandibular agenesis. Report of a case. *Arch Otolaryngol* 1985;111:132–134.

105. Warner BF, Luna MA, Robert NT. Temporomandibular joint neoplasms and pseudotumors. *Adv Anat Pathol* 2000;7:365–381.
106. Elfving L, Helkimo M, Magnusson T. Prevalence of different temporomandibular joint sounds, with emphasis on disc-displacement, in patients with temporomandibular disorders and controls. *Swed Dent J* 2002;26:9–19.
107. Wright EF, Clark EG, Paunovich ED, et al. Headache improvement through TMD stabilization appliance and self-management therapies. *Cranio* 2006; 24:104–111.
108. Al-Ani Z, Gray RJ, Davies SJ, et al. Stabilization splint therapy for the treatment of temporomandibular myofascial pain: a systematic review. *J Dent Educ* 2005;69:1242–1250.
109. Castroflorio T, Talpone F, Deregibus A, et al. Effects of a functional appliance on masticatory muscles of young adults suffering from muscle-related temporomandibular disorders. *J Oral Rehabil* 2004;31:524–529.
110. Miller VJ, Karic VV, Myers SL, et al. The temporomandibular opening index (TOI) in patients with closed lock and a control group with no temporomandibular disorders (TMD): an initial study. *J Oral Rehabil* 2000;27:815–816.
111. Placios E, Volvasoni G, Shannon M, et al. *Magnetic Resonance of the Temporomandibular Joint: Clinical Consideration Radiography Management.* New York: George Thieme Publishing; 1990.
112. Okeson J. Orofacial pain: guidelines for assessment diagnosis and management. In: *The American Academy of Orofacial Pain.* Lombard, IL: Quintessence; 1996.
113. Stegenga B, de Bont LG, Boering G, et al. Tissue responses to degenerative changes in the temporomandibular joint: a review. *J Oral Maxillofac Surg* 1991;49:1079–1088.
114. Kraus H. *Diagnosis and Treatment of Muscle Pain.* Lombard, IL: Quintessence; 1988.
115. Travell J, Rinzler SH. The myofascial genesis of pain. *Postgrad Med* 1952; 11:425–434.
116. Bell D. *Clinical Management of Temporomandibular Disorders.* Chicago: Yearbook Medical Publishing; 1982;404–454.
117. De Boever JA, Carlsson GE, Klineberg IJ. Need for occlusal therapy and prosthodontic treatment in the management of temporomandibular disorders. Part II: tooth loss and prosthodontic treatment. *J Oral Rehabil* 2000;27: 647–659.
118. De Boever JA, Carlsson GE, Klineberg IJ. Need for occlusal therapy and prosthodontic treatment in the management of temporomandibular disorders. Part I. Occlusal interferences and occlusal adjustment. *J Oral Rehabil* 2000; 27:367–379.
119. Wenneberg B, Nystrom T, Carlsson GE. Occlusal equilibration and other stomatognathic treatment in patients with mandibular dysfunction and headache. *J Prosthet Dent* 1988;59:478–483.
120. Padamsee M, Mehta N, Forgione A, et al. Incidence of cervical disorders in a TMD population. *J Dent Res* 1994;73.
121. Fitz-Ritzon D. Neuroanatomy and neurophysiology of the upper cervical spine. In: Vernon H, ed. *Upper Cervical Spine.* Baltimore: Williams and Wilkins; 1988.
122. Rocabado M. Biomechanical relationship of the cranial, cervical, and hyoid regions. *J Craniomandibular Pract* 1983;1:61–66.
123. Rocabado M. Biomechanical relationship of the cranial, cervical, and hyoid regions. *J Craniomandibular Pract* 1983;1:61–66.
124. Grace A. Pathomechanics of the upper cervical spine. In: Vernone H, ed. *Upper Cervical Syndrome.* Baltimore: Williams and Wilkins; 1988.
125. Wruble MK, Lumley MA, McGlynn FD. Sleep-related bruxism and sleep variables: a critical review. *J Craniomandib Disord* 1989;3:152–158.
126. Glaros AG, Rao SM. Bruxism: a critical review. *Psychol Bull* 1977;84: 767–781.
127. Mehta NR, Forgione AG, Maloney G, et al. Different effects of nocturnal parafunction on the masticatory system: the Weak Link Theory. *Cranio* 2000; 18:280–286.
128. Graf H. Bruxism. *Dent Clin North Am* 1969;13:659–665.
129. Reding GR, Rubright WC, Zimmerman SO. Incidence of bruxism. *J Dent Res* 1966;45:1198–1204.
130. Jorgic-Srdjak K, Ivezic S, Cekic-Arambasin A, et al. Bruxism and psychobiological model of personality. *Coll Antropol* 1998;22 Suppl:205–212.
131. Glickman I, Haddad AW, Martignoni M, et al. Telemetric comparison of centric relation and centric occlusion reconstructions. *J Prosthet Dent* 1974; 31:527–536.
132. Mehta NR, Roeber FW, Haddad AW, et al. Photoelastic model for occlusal force analysis. *J Dent Res* 1975;54:1243.

133. Mehta NR, Roeber FW, Haddad AW, et al. Stresses created by occlusal prematurities in a new photoelastic model system. *J Am Dent Assoc* 1976;93: 334–341.
134. Forgione A. A simple but effective method quantifying bruxism behavior. *J Dent Res* 1974;53:127.
135. Mejias JE, Mehta NR. Subjective and objective evaluation of bruxing patients undergoing short-term splint therapy. *J Oral Rehabil* 1982;9:279–289.
136. Rugh J. Behavioral therapy. In: Mohl G, Zarb G, Carlsson G, et al, eds. *A Textbook of Occlusion.* Lombard, IL: Quintessence; 1988.
137. Mehta N. Muscular disorders. In: Kaplan A, Assael L, eds. *Temporomandibular Disorder: Diagnosis and Treatment.* Philadelphia: WB Saunders; 1991.
138. Mehta N, Forgione A. The effect of macroposture and body mechanics on dental occlusion. In: Gelb H, ed. *New Concepts in Craniomandibular and Chronic Pain Management.* Chicago: Mosby-Yearbook; 1994.
139. Travell JG, Simons DG. *Myofascial Pain and Dysfunction: The Trigger Point Manual: The Upper Extremities.* Vol.1. Baltimore: Williams & Wilkins; 1983.
140. Blitzer A, Brin MF, Greene PE, et al. Botulinum toxin injections for the treatment of oromandibular dystonia. *Ann Oto Rhino Laryngol* 1989;98:93–97.
141. Freund BJ, Schwartz M. Treatment of whiplash-associated neck pain with botulinum toxin: a pilot study. *Headache* 2000;40:231–236.
142. Reilich P, Kern U, Menses S, et al. Consensus statement: botulinum toxin in myofascial pain. *J Neurol* 2004;251(Suppl):36–38.
143. Freund BJ, Schwartz M, Symington JM. The use of botulinum toxin for the treatment of temporomandibular disorders: preliminary findings. *JOMS* 1999;57:916–920.
144. Nixdorf DR, Heo G, Major PW. Randomized controlled trial of botulinum toxin A in chronic myogenous orofacial pain. *Pain* 2002;99:465–473.
145. Fikackova H, Ekberg E. Can infrared thermography be a diagnostic tool for arthralgia of the temporomandibular joint? *Oral Surg Oral Med Oral Pathol Oral Radiol Endod* 2004;98:643–650.
146. McBeth SB, Gratt BM. Thermographic assessment of temporomandibular disorders symptomology during orthodontic treatment. *Am J Orthod Dentofacial Orthop* 1996;109:481–488.
147. Rocabado M. Biomechanical relationship of the cranial, cervical, and hyoid regions. *J Craniomandibular Pract* 1983;1:61–66.
148. Merskey H, Bogduk N. *Classification of Chronic Pain: Descriptions of Chronic Pain Syndromes and Definitions of Pain Terms.* Seattle, WA: IASP Press; 1994.
149. Mellis M, Zawawi K, Badawi E, et al. Complex regional pain syndrome in the head and neck: a review of the literature. *J Orofacial Pain* 2002;16:93–104.
150. de Leeuw R. Prevalence of traumatic stressors in patients with temporomandibular disorders. *J Oral Maxilofac Surg* 2005;63(1):42–50.
151. Charlton JE, ed. *Core Curriculum for Professional Education in Pain. Committee on Education for the International Association for the Study of Pain.* Seattle, WA: IASP Press; 2005.
152. International Association for the Study of Pain. *Proposed Outline Curricula on Pain for Dental Schools (Predoctoral and Postdoctoral).* Seattle, WA: International Association for the Study of Pain Secretariat; 1993.
153. Kafas P, Leeson R. Assessment of pain in temporomandibular disorders: the bio-psychosocial complexity. *J Oral Maxilofac Surg* 2006;35(2):145–149.
154. Levitt SR, McKinney MW. Validating the TMJ scale in a national sample of 10,000 patients: demographic and epidemiologic characteristics. *J Orofac Pain* 1994;8(1):25–35.
155. Widmer CG, Huggins KH, Fricton J. Research diagnostic criteria for temporomandibular disorders: review, criteria, examinations and specifications critique. Part III: examination and history data collection. *J Craniomandib Disord* 1992;6:335–355.
156. Madland G, Feinman C. Chronic facial pain: a multidisciplinary problem. *J Neurol Neurosurg Psychiatry* 2001;71:716–719.
157. Gatchel RJ, Stowell AW, Wildenstein L, et al. Efficacy of an early intervention for patients with acute temporomandibular disorders-related pain: a one-year outcome stud. *JADA* 2006;137(3):339–347.
158. Crider AB, Glaros AG. A meta-analysis of EMG biofeedback treatment of temporomandibular disorders. *J Orofac Pain* 1999;13:29–37.
159. Crider A, Glaros A, Gevirtz RN. Efficacy of biofeedback-based treatments for temporomandibular disorders. *J Oral Maxilofac Surg* 2005;63(10):42–50.
160. Glaros AG. Special topics: EMG biofeedback as an experimental tool for studying pain. *Biofeedback* 2007;35(2):50–53.
161. Stowell AW, Gatchel RJ, Wildenstein L. Cost-effectiveness of treatments for temporomandibular disorders: biopsychosocial intervention versus treatment as usual. *J Am Dent Assoc* 2007;138(2):202–208.

CHAPTER 68 ■ NECK AND ARM PAIN

ANITA H. HICKEY AND ZAHID H. BAJWA

INTRODUCTION

The unique anatomy of the cervical spine and upper extremity balances the attributes of strength and stability with those of flexibility and range of motion. The biomechanical properties which allow for these combined properties are associated with a high incidence of degenerative change which increases with aging and is associated with episodic or chronic pain. Although the origin of pain in the neck is often divided into axial versus radicular pain and musculoskeletal pain versus neuropathic pain, the patient presenting for treatment in the clinical setting may not always be representative of these categorical descriptions.

An understanding of the normal anatomy of the neck and upper extremity, pathophysiology of common disorders of the cervical spine, diversity of clinical presentations of neck and arm pain, and the potential contribution of systemic and psychologic factors is critical in forming a differential diagnosis, referring the patient for appropriate diagnostic tests and evaluations, and instituting timely and appropriate treatment. This chapter will focus on the anatomy of the cervical spine and upper extremity, recent data regarding the epidemiology of neck and arm pain, the critical role of the clinician in performing a thorough and targeted history and physical examination, and finally a discussion of the etiology and treatment of neck and arm pain.

The common causes of mechanical neck and arm pain, including cervical spondylosis and myelopathy, cervical radiculopathy, cervicogenic headache, brachial plexopathy, peripheral nerve entrapment syndromes of the upper extremity, and thoracic outlet syndrome, will be discussed in this chapter. Myofascial pain syndromes, fibromyalgia, and acute musculoskeletal disorders can involve the neck and upper extremities and are covered in detail elsewhere in this text. Neck and arm pain may also be secondary to primary or metastatic disease. Cancer pain is discussed more thoroughly elsewhere as well. Therapeutic modalities are covered more extensively in Part V: Methods for Symptomatic Control.

ANATOMY OF THE NECK AND ARM

Cervical Spine

The anatomy of the cervical spine is complex in order to allow for support of the weight of the cranium, to provide protection and support of the neurovascular elements of the cervical spine, and to simultaneously permit functional mobility in relationship to the surrounding structures. It is composed of 7 vertebrae, 5 intervertebral disks, 12 joints of Luschka, and 14 zygapophyseal joints, uniquely bound and connected to numerous ligaments and muscles which both limit and permit varying degrees of motion of the cervical spine.[1]

With the exception of the first two cervical vertebrae, which have unique characteristics, each of the seven cervical vertebrae is comprised of a segmental unit, which includes a vertebral body, an intervertebral disc, four uncovertebral joints of Luschka, two pedicles, two lamina, two inferior, and two superior zygapophyseal (articular facet) joints. Between each vertebral segment, a spinal nerve, radicular blood vessels, and the sinuvertebral (recurrent meningeal) nerves pass through neural openings or foramina on each side of the cervical spine (Fig. 68.1).[1]

The upper two segments of the cervical spine have unique anatomic and biomechanic characteristics when compared with the lower five segments of the cervical spine. The atlas, or C1 vertebra, is a ring shaped vertebra with paired lateral pillars which function as articulating joints or facets. The upper ellipsoid facets articulate superiorly with the occipital condyles to form the atlantooccipital joints, while the round and concave inferior facets articulate inferiorly with the axis to form the atlantoaxial joints. The anterior arch of the atlas incorporates an articular surface which contacts the anterior surface of the dens or odontoid process of the axis. The atlas is the widest of the cervical vertebrae, allowing for the spinal cord, dens, and a surrounding cushion of spinal fluid. It has a mean internal, anteroposterior dimension of approximately 31.7 mm and an internal width of 32.2 mm. The atlas is the only cervical vertebra not associated with an intervertebral disk. Its transverse process is longer than the other cervical vertebrae to support the attachments of the muscles that rotate the head, and its transverse foramen contains the vertebral artery, veins, and sympathetic nerves (Fig. 68.2).

The axis, or C2 vertebra, has a small body anteriorly from which the odontoid process arises and projects upward. Its oval shaped anterior face articulates with that on the anterior arch of the atlas. The posterior surface of the odontoid process articulates with the transverse ligament. The facets on the upper and lower surfaces of the lateral masses of the axis articulate with the atlas above and the C3 facet joints below. The atlas also has a large palpable bifid spinous process and small transverse processes with transverse openings or foramina through which the vertebral artery, veins, and the vertebral sympathetic plexuses pass. Because both the atlas and the axis lack pedicles and intervertebral foramen, the nerve roots of the first and second spinal nerves pass above and posterior to the articulating lateral masses of each vertebrae. The hypoglossal nerves traverse the occipital condyles anterolaterally through the hypoglossal foramen a mean of 12.2 mm from the posterior margin of the occipital condyle (see Fig. 68.2).[1]

The five lower cervical vertebrae share common characteristics in that they are composed of a vertebral body, an intervening intervertebral disc, two pedicles, two laminae, two vertebral arches, and a spinous process. The upper and lower surfaces of the pedicles form the articulating facets of the cervical zygapophyseal joints. The transverse processes are situated anterolaterally to the facet joints. Their trough-shaped surfaces contain the roots of the cervical spinal nerves and a foramen through which the vertebral artery, veins, and vertebral sympathetic nerve pass.[1]

The anterior portions of the C2 through C7 vertebral bodies, like those of the thoracic and lumbar spine, are connected at their upper and lower surfaces by intervertebral disks which make up the main joints of the spinal column. Each disk is made up of a central nucleus pulposis surrounded by a thick ring of fibrous cartilage called the annulus fibrosis. The disk is connected to the vertebral body above and below by a hyaline cartilage endplate whose fibers interface with the disc and the vertebral body.[1]

The nucleus pulposis contains collagen and elastin fibers embedded in a colloidal proteoglycan gel which is osmotically

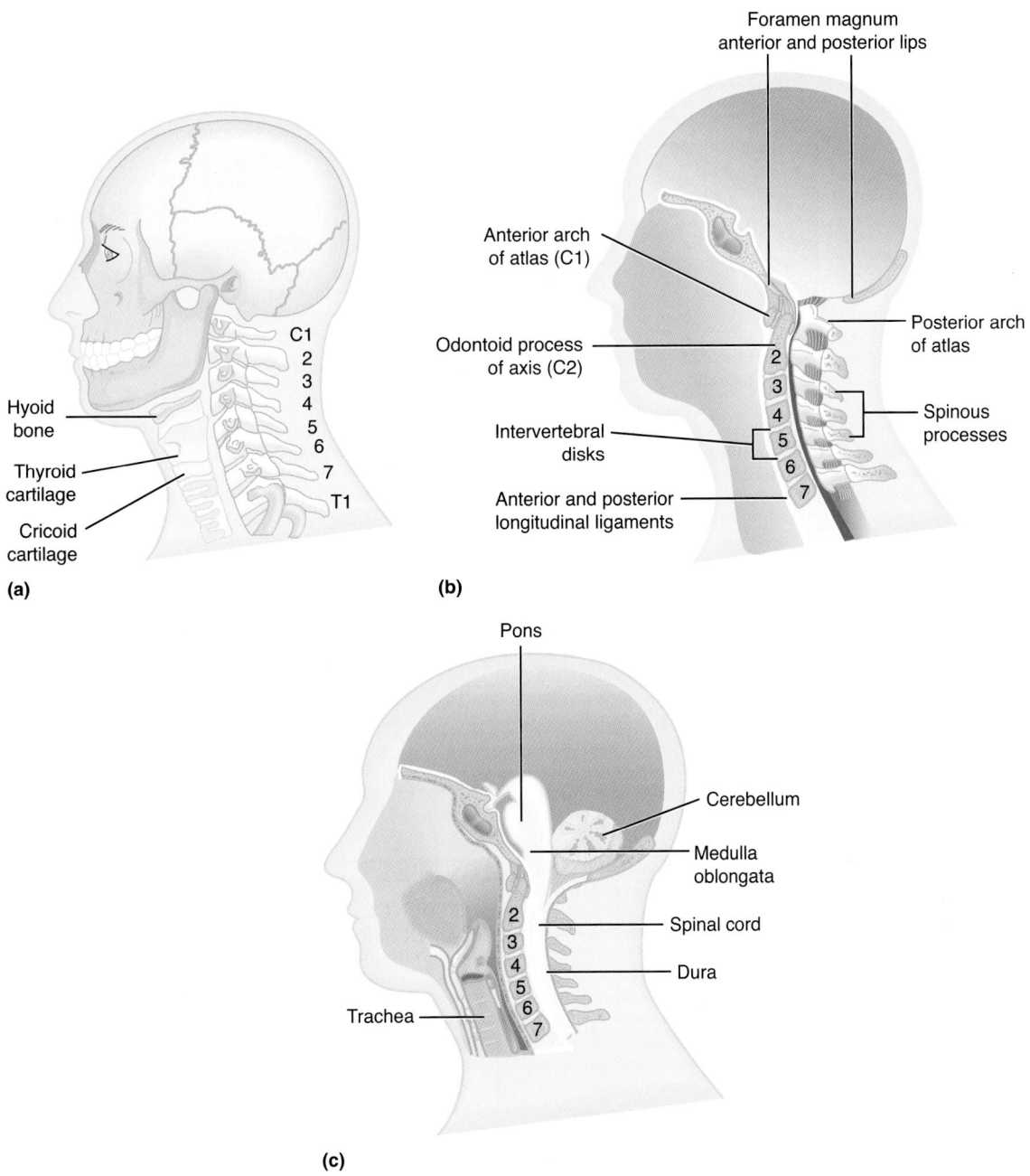

FIGURE 68.1 Anatomy of the cervical spine. **A.** Lateral view, showing landmarks of the spine, including the hyoid bone, thyroid, and cricoid cartilages, and transverse and spinous processes. **B.** View of the skeletal portion of the lower skull and cervical spine. The skull and spinous processes are shown in sagittal section, whereas the vertebral bodies are shown as normal. **C.** Sagittal view of the cervical spine showing the relationship of the brainstem, medulla oblongata, foramen magnum, and spinal canal, containing the spinal cord. Normally, the lower portion of the medulla is outside and below the foramen magnum so that subluxation of the atlas on the axis, and compression of the lower brainstem, can occur by compression from the odontoid process, which moves posteriorly against the neuraxis. (Modified from Bland JH. *Disorders of the cervical spine: diagnosis and medical management.* Philadelphia: Saunders; 1987.)

active in healthy discs with an approximately 80% water content. The annulus is made up of 15–25 concentric rings or lamellae made up of collagen fibers oriented in an alternating criss-cross oblique fashion with elastin fibers layered between the lamellae. The annulus attaches around the entire circumference of the upper and lower endplates and, together with the nucleus pulposis, forms a fluid elastic system. These properties allow the disk to absorb and more evenly distribute the mechanical stress of high impact activity. By the third decade of life, the disk has

become avascular and must rely on diffusion of nutrients and water through the endplates and lymph. The properties of the healthy disc permit disk hydration by way of compression and relaxation of the viscoelastic system, similar to the action of squeezing a sponge. With aging, atherosclerosis, and trauma, degenerative changes occur within the disk. A decrease in protein polysaccharide content and thus its water composition leads to loss of its viscoelastic properties. Degeneration of the disk increases the axial load and shear on the zygapophyseal joints and

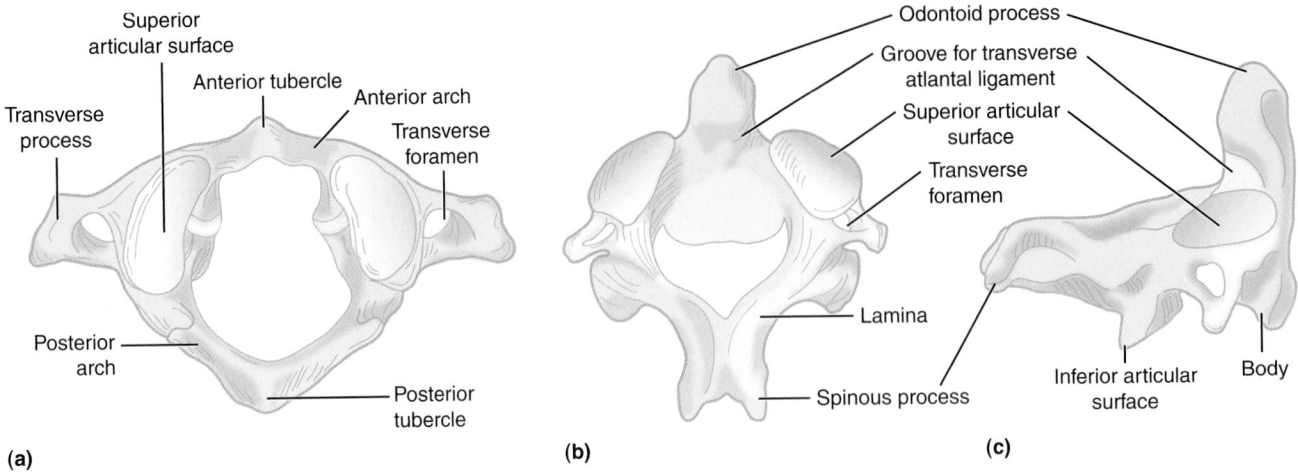

FIGURE 68.2 Anatomy of the atlas and axis. **A.** Superior view of the atlas. **B.** The axis viewed from a superior and posteroanterior aspect. **C.** Lateral view of the axis.

contributes to simultaneous degenerative changes of these posterior spinal elements (Fig. 68.3).[1]

The posterior elements of the lower segments of the cervical spine consist of two vertebral arches, a central posterior spinous process, two transverse processes, and a paired articulation. The transverse processes and posterior spinous processes serve as sites for attachment of supporting ligaments and neck muscles. The zygapophyseal facet joints are true joints with cartilaginous surfaces lined with synovium, containing synovial fluid and surrounded with a ligamentous joint capsule. As such, they are subject to the same inflammatory and degenerative diseases found in other synovial joints. The cervical zygapophyseal joints provide a guiding and gliding movement between the adjacent cervical vertebrae. The movements allowed at the atlantooccipital and atlantoaxial joint are much different than those allowed at the

C2-C3 through C7-T1 joints. Differences between the cervical and lumbar spine are summarized in Table 68.1 and Figure 68.4.[1]

Ligaments of the Cervical Spine

The ligaments of the cervical spine provide essential protection to the spinal cord and nerves during various stresses which occur owing to a top-heavy and eccentrically balanced head atop a relatively narrow elastic cervical spine. The greatest range and amplitude of movement in the cervical spine occurs between the occiput and the C3 vertebra, whereas nodding in an up and down

FIGURE 68.3 Schematic depiction of the hydraulic mechanism of the intervertebral disk. **A.** Normal disk at rest. The internal pressure is exerted in all directions, and the fibers of the annulus are taut. **B.** When the disk is compressed the fluid within the nucleus pulposus cannot compress, so the annulus must bulge. **C.** With flexion of the spine, the fluid shifts within the intervertebral disk; the cubic contents remain the same but the fluid shift causes fibers of the anterior annulus to shorten and those of the posterior annulus to elongate (*W, weight*). (From Cailliet R. *Neck and arm pain.* 2nd ed. Philadelphia: FA Davis; 1981.)

TABLE 68.1

DIFFERENCES BETWEEN THE CERVICAL AND LUMBAR SPINE

Characteristic	Cervical	Lumbar
Disk to vertebral body height ratio	1:2	1:3
Vertical height of disk	Anterior height 2× that of posterior height/ wedge shaped	Anterior height slightly greater anterior
Vertebral endplates	Convex and concave, nucleus in anterior portion of disk	Flat and parallel, nucleus centrally located
Joints of von Luschka	False joints or pseudoarthrosis, appear at 10–20 years of age	Not present in lumbar or thoracic spine
Posterior longitudinal ligament	Double layered between vertebrae Broad, thick, and complete across postvertebra	Incomplete posteriorly from L3–S1
Movement between vertebrae	Forward and backward gliding motion	Rocking movement

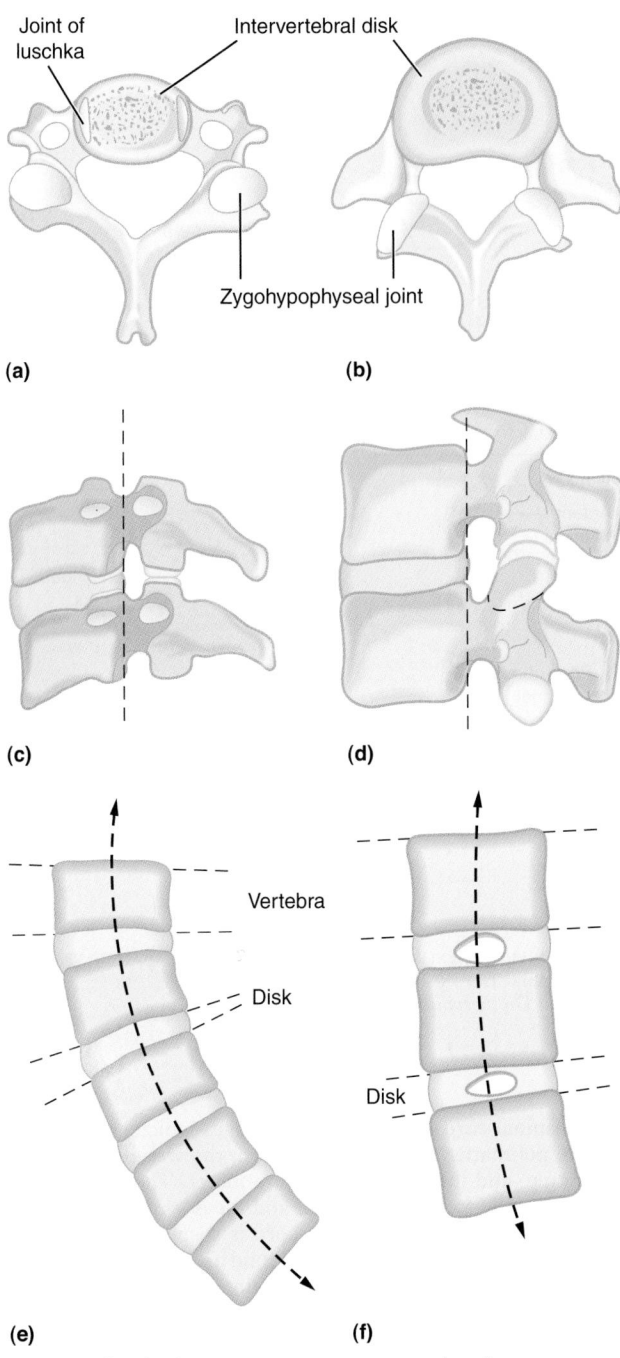

Joint of luschka

Intervertebral disk

Zygohypophyseal joint

(a)   **(b)**

(c)   **(d)**

Vertebra

Disk

Disk

(e)   **(f)**

Cervical   **Lumbar**

FIGURE 68.4 Comparative views of the cervical and lumbar functional units. **A.** Cross-section of the five joints of the cervical spine, which include an intervertebral disk, the paired uncovertebral (Luschka) joints, and the paired posterior articulations. **B.** Cross-section of the three joints of the lumbar spine, which include an intervertebral disk and the paired posterior articulations. **C,D.** Lateral views of the same vertebrae shown in **A** and **B.** The dashed lines divide the anterior supporting portion from the posterior gliding portion of each functional unit. **E,F.** Lateral views of the bodies of the vertebrae of the cervical and lumbar spines, depicting particularly the shapes of the intervertebral disks. Note that in the cervical region the anterior portion of the disk is larger (higher) than the posterior portion, whereas in the lumbar region the difference between the anterior and posterior portions is much less. (Modified from Cailliet R. *Neck and arm pain*. 2nd ed. Philadelphia: FA Davis; 1981.)

movement in the sagittal plane occurs between the atlas and the axis.[1]

Atlantooccipital Unit. Flexion and extension at the occiput to C1 level is limited to 23–24.5 degrees by impingement of the tip of the dens on the foramen magnum in flexion and the tectorial membrane in extension. The tectorial membrane is a fan-shaped continuation of the posterior longitudinal ligament to the base of the occiput where its fibers connect with the dura mater. Lateral bending is resisted by the anatomy of the occipital-C1 articulation and the alar ligaments, and averages 3.4 to 5.5 degrees per side. The alar ligaments are enclosed in a synovial membrane and extend to the margin of the foramen magnum from each side of the odontoid process. Axial rotation is also limited by the atlantooccipital joint and the alar ligament to 2.4 to 7.2 degrees per side. Lateral translation, stretch and compression, and sagittal plane translation is restricted by the tectorial membrane, the alar, and the apical ligaments, as well as the occiput-C1 articulation. The apical ligament is a vestigial remnant of the notochord and attaches from the peak of the odontoid process to the anterior foramen magnum. Other ligaments at this level include the posterior atlantooccipital membrane, which forms the connection between the anterior margin of the foramen magnum and the anterior arch of the atlas and the posterior atlantooccipital membrane, which extends posteriorly over the vertebral artery.[1]

Atlantoaxial Unit. Axial rotation is the primary movement of the C1-C2 segment. The average 23.3–38.9 degree per side rotation is limited by the atlantoaxial joints, the transverse ligament of the ipsilateral side, the alar ligaments of the contralateral side, and capsular ligaments. Flexion-rotation is 10.1–22.4 degrees and is resisted by the transverse ligament during flexion, the tectorial membrane and joint anatomy. Lateral bending is limited to 6.7 degrees mostly by the alar ligament. Posterior movement or translation at this level is resisted by abutment of the dens on the arch of C-1. The transverse ligament extends posteriorly to the odontoid process between the lateral pillars of the atlas. The destabilizing effect of a tear of the transverse ligament is equal to that of a fracture of the odontoid process.[1,2]

Other Cervical Ligaments. The posterior longitudinal ligament and the anterior longitudinal ligaments limit the degree of flexion, extension, and transverse sliding of the C2 to C7 vertebrae. The anterior longitudinal ligament blends with the annulus as it crosses the disk spaces and adheres to the front of the vertebral bodies. The posterior longitudinal ligament is a double-layered structure which is firmly bound to the posterior surface of the cervical disks and loosely bound to the posterior cervical vertebrae. It reinforces the capsular ligaments and the anterior border of the cervical spinal canal.[1]

The ligamentum flavum are paired structures forming the posterior border of the epidural space. Collectively referred to as ligament flava, they extend between the anterior inferior surface of the lamina above and to the posterior superior surface of the lamina below. Posterior to the ligamentum flavum, the interspinous ligaments extend between and connect each spinous process. The ligamentum nuchae is the superior continuation of the supraspinous ligaments of the thoracic and lumbar vertebrae. It is a strong fibrous posterior ligament which extends from the base of the skull to the tips of the posterior cervical spinous process and vertebra (Fig. 68.5).[1]

Musculature of the Neck

The capital movers are the muscles of the neck that flex and extend the head. The capital extensors include the posterior rectus capitis minor and major and the obliquus capitis superior and inferior. The groups of longer muscles that act as capital extensors while working together bilaterally include the longissimus capitis, semispinalis capitis, and splenius capitis. The capital flexors are

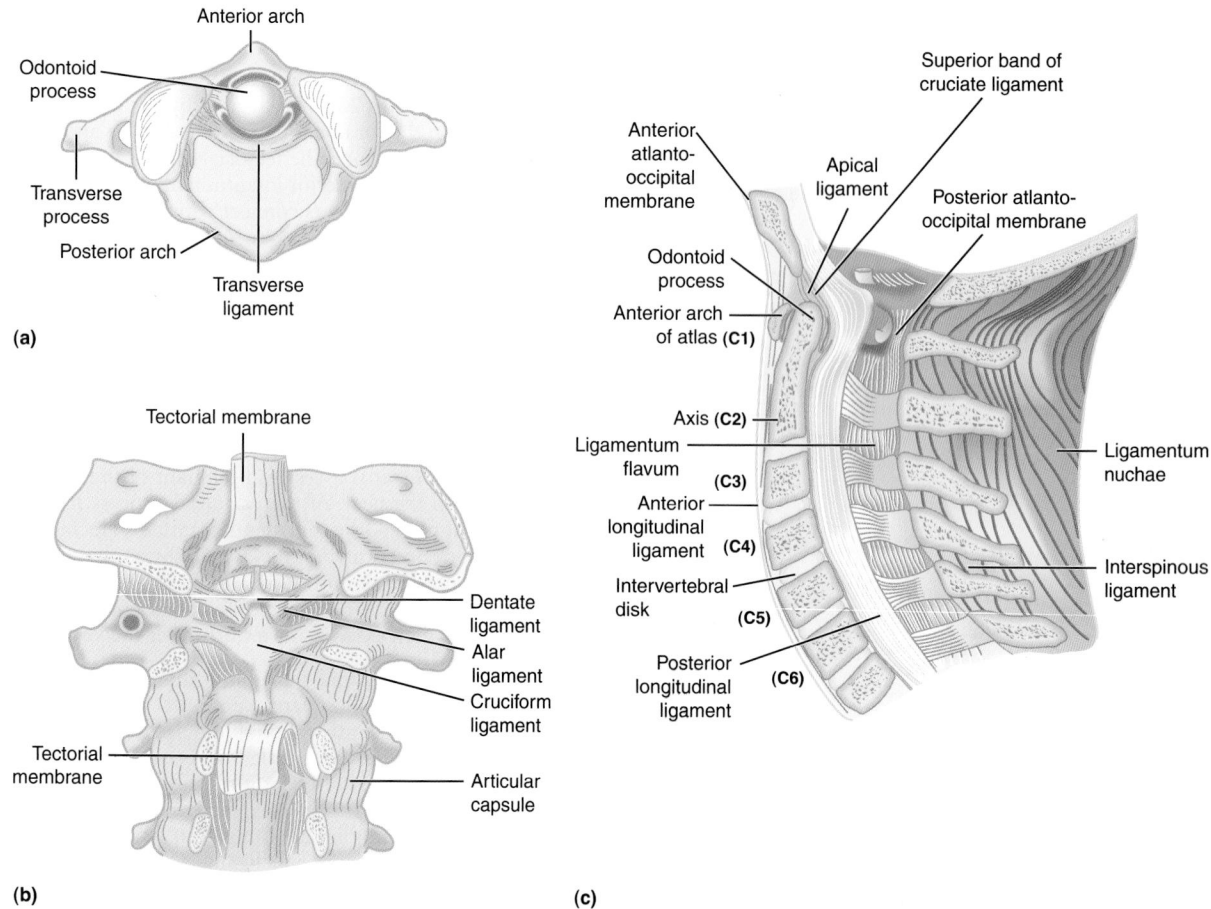

(a)

Anterior arch

Odontoid process

Transverse process

Posterior arch

Transverse ligament

Anterior atlanto-occipital membrane

Apical ligament

Superior band of cruciate ligament

Posterior atlanto-occipital membrane

Odontoid process

Anterior arch of atlas **(C1)**

Axis **(C2)**

Ligamentum flavum   **(C3)**

Anterior longitudinal ligament   **(C4)**

Intervertebral disk   **(C5)**

Posterior longitudinal ligament   **(C6)**

Ligamentum nuchae

Interspinous ligament

Tectorial membrane

Dentate ligament

Alar ligament

Cruciform ligament

Tectorial membrane

Articular capsule

(b)

(c)

FIGURE 68.5 A–C. Ligaments of various parts of the cervical spine (see text for details). (Modified from Clemente CD, ed. *Gray's anatomy of the human body.* Philadelphia: Lea & Febiger; 1985:343–344; and from Netter FH. *CIBA collection of medical illustrations. Vol 1. The nervous system.* Summit, NJ: CIBA Pharmaceutical Products; 1983.)

the short recti and the longus capitis muscles. The most extension and extensor musculature is at the atlantoaxial and C6 through T1 joints. The cervical extensors include the splenius cervicis, longissimus cervicis, and semispinalis cervicis. Maximum flexion of the cervical spine and maximum cervical lordosis occurs at C4-C5. The flexors of the cervical spine consist of the scalenus anterior, medius, and posterior. Unilateral rotators of the head include the splenius cervicis, splenius capitis, longissimus capitis, and sternocleidomastoid. The erector muscles of the vertebral column are also involved in movement of the neck (Fig. 68.6).[1]

The Vertebral Canal

A transverse cut through the cervical vertebral canal reveals its triangular shape with the base or anterior wall made of the vertebra, disk, posterior longitudinal ligament, pedicle, and neural foramina. The lateral and dorsolateral aspects of the other two sides of the triangle include the zygapophyseal joints, laminae, and ligament flava. The canal has its largest sagittal diameter, a range of 16–30 mm, at the C1-C2 level and its smallest sagittal diameter, a range of 14–23 mm, at the C5-C6 level. The cervical canal lengthens and the intervertebral foramina enlarge during flexion, whereas shortening of the cord and a decrease in the size of the foramen occurs with extension. Lateral flexion or rotation causes the ipsilateral foramina to decrease in size and the contralateral foramina to enlarge. These changes in size of the foramen become significant in the degenerative spine (Fig. 68.7).[1]

The spinal cord is covered by meninges which consist of the delicate pia matter attached to the cord, the web-like arachnoid membrane, and the strong outer dura mater. The dura mater is attached to the foramen magnum and the dorsal surfaces of the C2 and C3 vertebra. The spinal cord is suspended in and protected by surrounding cerebrospinal fluid and is attached laterally to the dural sheath by the dentate ligaments, which are thickenings of the pia mater between and anterior and posterior roots. The anterior and posterior rootlets join the anterior and posterior roots respectively at the inner aspect of the intervertebral foramina (Fig. 68.8). An enlargement of the cervical cord occurs from the C3 to T1 levels. It is larger than the lumbar enlargement as it contains the ascending and descending long tracts for the trunk as well as the upper and lower limbs. The transverse diameter of the cervical spinal cord is greater than its sagittal diameter, and the cervical cord occupies approximately 40% of the canal. With neck extension, the dura relaxes to form a corrugated appearance and the vertebra above approximates the arch of the vertebra below causing encroachment into the cervical canal. These factors, together with shortening of the cord during extension, increase the risk of impingement of the cord during neck extension.[1]

Vertebral Arteries

The vertebral arteries are the first branches from the subclavian trunk and pass cephalad as they course through the transverse foramina of C6 to C2 anterior to the cervical nerves. They are

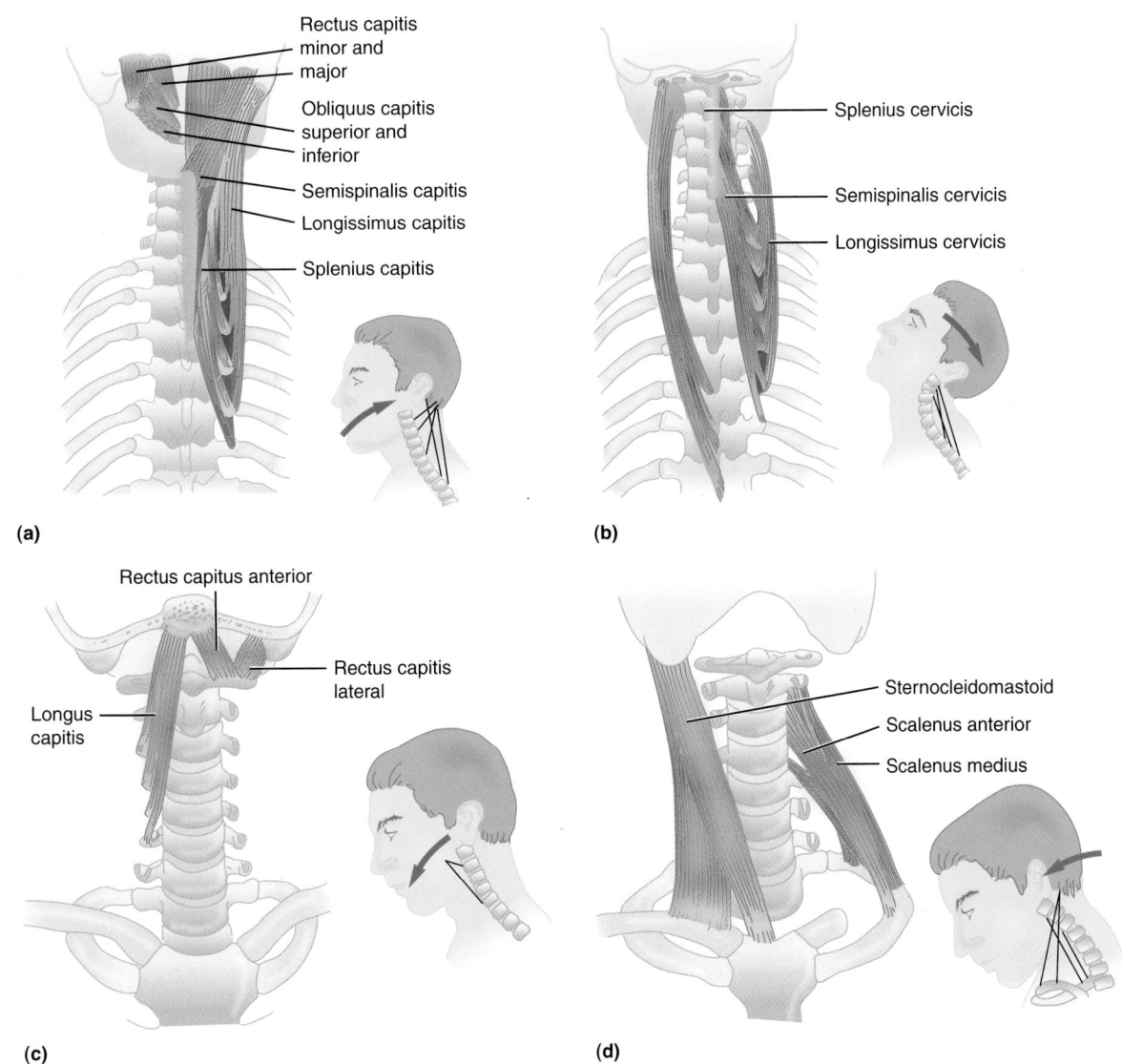

FIGURE 68.6 Musculature of the head and neck. **A.** The capital extensors attach on the skull and move the head on the neck. **B.** The cervical extensors originate from and attach on the cervical spine and alter the curvature of the spine. **C.** The capital flexors flex the head on the neck. **D.** The cervical flexors attach occlusively on the cervical vertebrae and have no significant functional attachment to the skull. (Modified from Clemente CD, ed. *Gray's anatomy of the human body.* Philadelphia: Lea & Febiger; 1985; and from Cailliet R. *Neck and arm pain.* 2nd ed. Philadelphia: FA Davis; 1981.)

accompanied by the vertebral venous plexus and the vertebral nerve and sympathetic plexus, whose fibers originate from neurons in the stellate and intermediate cervical sympathetic ganglia. Branches from the vertebral artery pass through the intervertebral foramina where they supply ligaments, dura, and bone and communicate with the posterior and anterior spinal arteries, which are also branches of the vertebral arteries. The vertebral arteries are supplied by fibers from the vertebral sympathetic plexus as are the basilar artery, circle of Willis, superior cerebellar, and posterior cerebellar artery (Fig. 68.9).[1]

Cervical Nerves

A more detailed discussion of peripheral and spinal pain mechanisms and applied anatomy relevant to pain can be found in earlier chapters of this text. The spinal nerve roots are composed

of a dorsal sensory root and a ventral motor root. The posterior root breaks into 12 or more rootlets which attach in series to the dorsolateral sulcus of the cord near Lissauer's tract and then project into the dorsal and ventral horns. Peripherally, the sensory rootlets converge into the fascicule radiculae which unite to form the dorsal root ganglion. A smaller number of rootlets make up the anterior root which arises from the ventrolateral sulcus of the cord. Each rootlet is covered by pia mater and, as they coalesce to form dorsal and ventral roots, they become separately covered in arachnoid-dural sleeves which are attached to the bony margin of the intervertebral foramen. The anterior roots are in contact with Luschka's joint, and the disk annulus and the dorsal root approximates the articular process and zygapophyseal joint capsule as they pass through the cervical intervertebral foramen. The dorsal and anterior roots join slightly beyond the dorsal root ganglion to form the composite spinal nerve.[1]

The figure eight-shaped intervertebral foramina are largest at

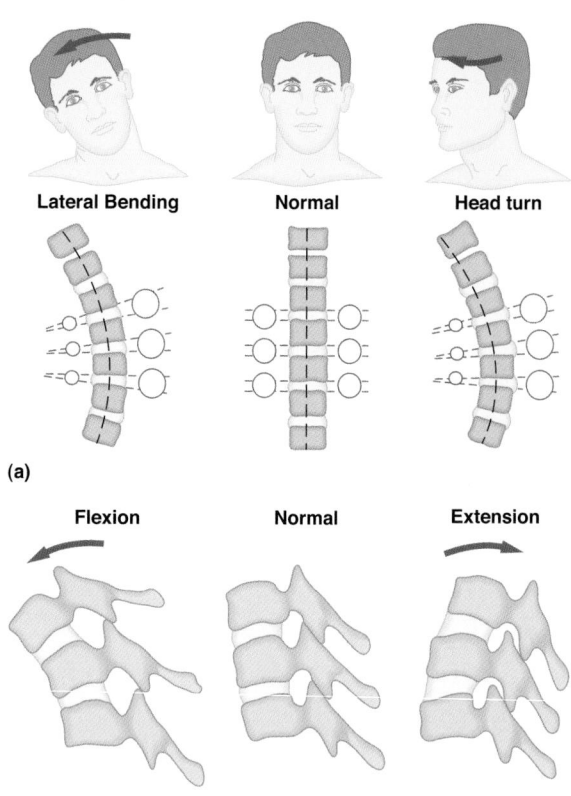

Lateral Bending   **Normal**   **Head turn**

(a)

Flexion   **Normal**   **Extension**

(b)

FIGURE 68.7 Changes in the size of the intervertebral foramina with movement of the neck. **A.** With lateral flexion and rotation of the head the foramina become smaller on the side of the head to which the head flexes laterally or rotates, and they are open on the opposite side. **B.** With forward flexion the intervertebral foramina become larger, whereas with extension they become smaller. (Modified from Cailliet R. *Neck and arm pain.* 2nd ed. Philadelphia: FA Davis; 1981.)

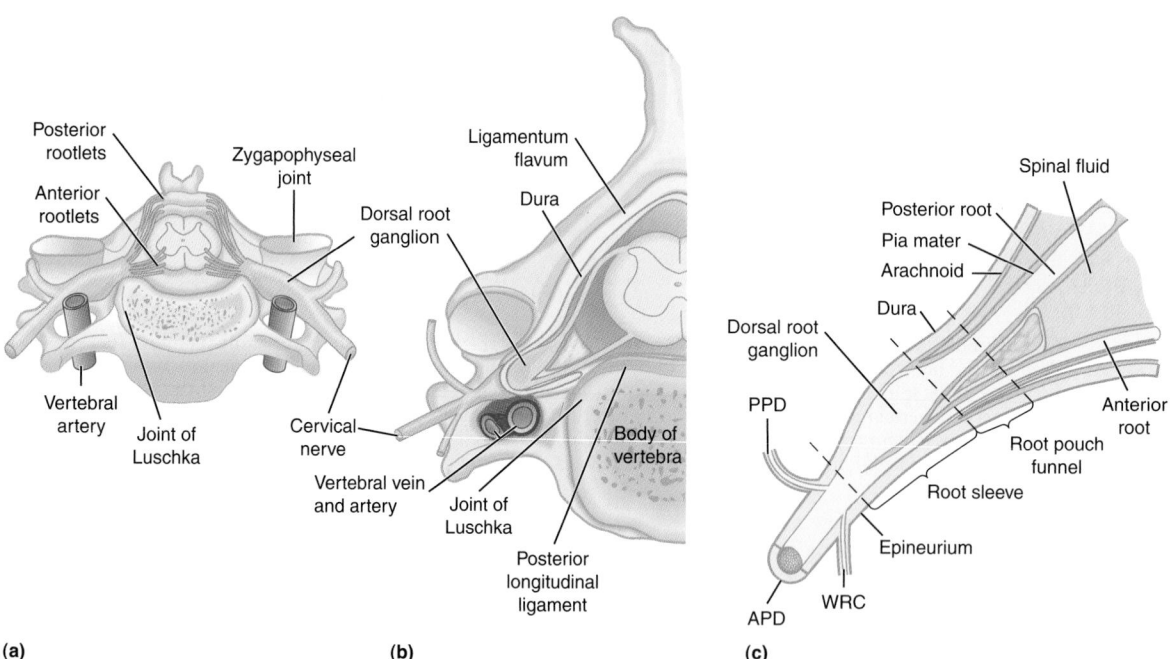

(a)   **(b)**   **(c)**

FIGURE 68.8 Transverse sections of the cervical spine. **A.** The spinal cord and anterior and posterior rootlets join to form the spinal nerve. Note the relationship of the nerves to the Luschka and zygapophyseal joints and the two vertebral arteries, which pass through the transverse foramina and are located just anterior to the nerve. **B.** Cross-section of a cervical vertebra showing some details of the relationship of the posterior root to the lateral aspect of the ligamentum flavum, which covers the zygapophyseal joint just posterior to it. The anterior root and its dural covering are close to the lateral part of the posterior longitudinal ligaments and to the capsules of the joint of Luschka. The proximal portion of the dorsal root ganglion is in the outer portion of the intervertebral foramen, whereas the remainder is in the gutter of the transverse process. **C.** Detailed anatomy of a nerve root and its meningeal covering. Note the extent of the root pouch and root sleeve. Just distal to the joining of the anterior and posterior roots is the short spinal nerve covered by epineurium (the continuation of the dura), which promptly divides into the anterior primary division (*APD*) and posterior primary division (*PPD*) and gives off a white ramus communicantes (*WRC*). (**A** modified from Bland JH. *Disorders of the cervical spine: diagnosis and medical management.* Philadelphia: Saunders; 1987; **B,C** modified from Cailliet R. *Neck and arm pain.* 2nd ed. Philadelphia: FA Davis; 1981.)

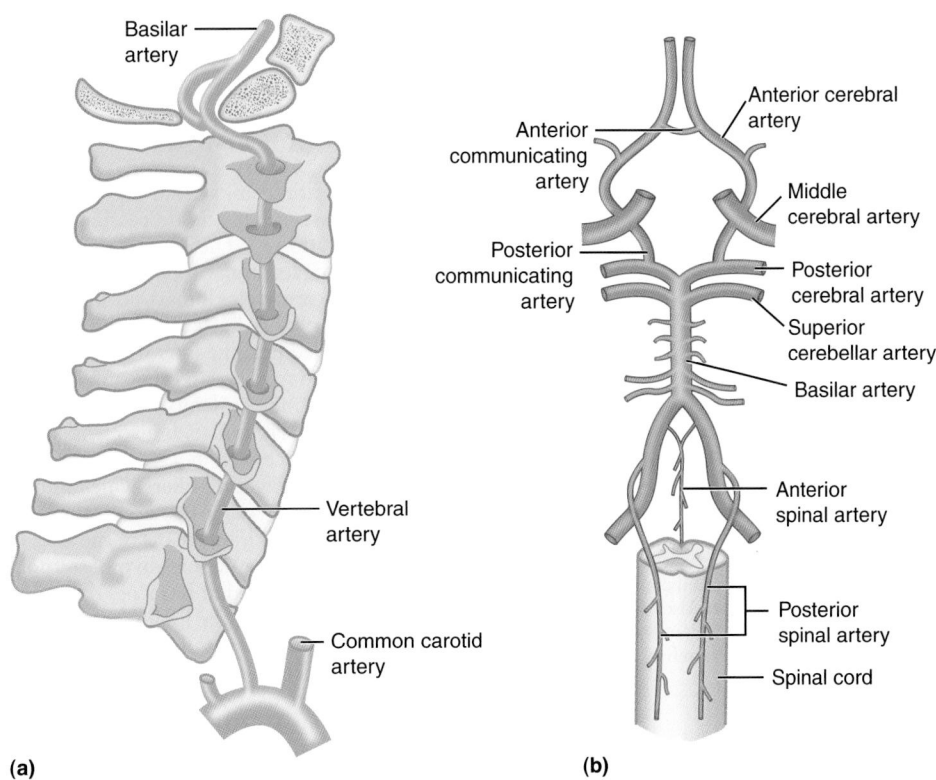

FIGURE 68.9 A. Lateral view of the cervical vertebrae depicting the course of the vertebral artery from C6 to C1 through boney ridges of the foramina transversaria. Note the double U-turn the artery makes from C2 to C1 in its posterior course around the lateral mass of the atlas. **B.** The two vertebral arteries join to form the basal arteries. Also shown is the circle of Willis. Note the origin of the anterior spinal artery and the two posterior spinal arteries from the two vertebral arteries.

the C2 to C3 level and progressively narrow and shorten to the C6 to C7 level with an average vertical diameter of 10 mm and transverse diameter of 5 mm. The first and second cervical nerves are unique in that they do not pass through an intervertebral foramen. The first cervical nerve passes between the occiput and C1 lateral to the occipital condyle and the second between C1 and C2 posterior to the lateral pillars.[1]

In addition to the nerve roots, the foramina contain the spinal radicular arteries, intervertebral veins, and venous plexuses together with loose areolar tissue and fat from the adjoining extension of the epidural space. These provide a protective cushion in the healthy spine. Each spinal nerve receives one or more gray rami communicantes from the cervical sympathetic ganglia after exiting the spinal canal. Spinal nerves one through four receive fibers from the superior cervical sympathetic ganglion, spinal nerves five and six from the intermediate ganglia, spinal nerves seven and eight from the inferior cervical ganglion, and spinal cervical nerve eight and thoracic one from the first thoracic ganglion. The meninges are supplied from a branch of the cervical spinal nerve at each level (see Figs. 68.8 and 68.10).[1]

Lateral to the intervertebral foramen, posterior to the vertebral artery, the spinal nerves separate into posterior and anterior primary divisions with the anterior motor divisions being much larger than the posterior divisions, with the exception of C1. Each spinal nerve supplies muscles (myotomes), skin (dermatomes), as well as ligamentous and boney structures (sclerotomes). The posterior primary division passes over the posterior portion of the transverse process around the articular pillar and divides into the medial sensory and lateral muscular branches, with the exception of the C1 nerve.[1]

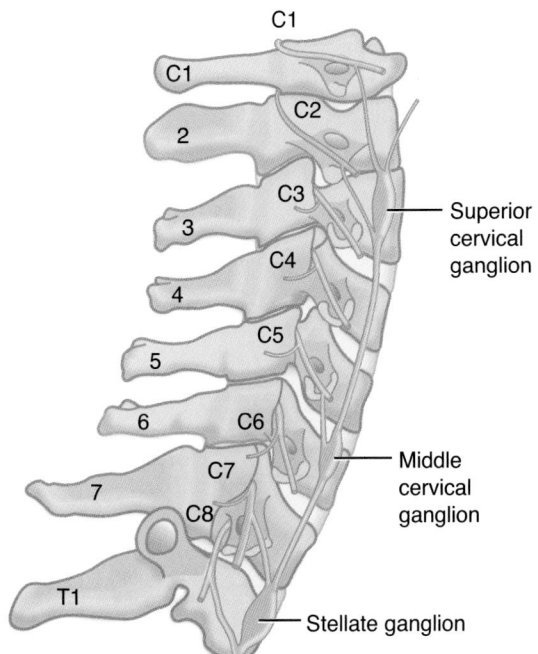

FIGURE 68.10 Lateral view showing the course and relation of the cervical nerves and the cervical sympathetic chain. (From Cooper G, Bailey B, Bogduk N. Cervical zygapophysial joint pain maps. *Pain Medicine* 2007;8[4]:344–853, with permission.)

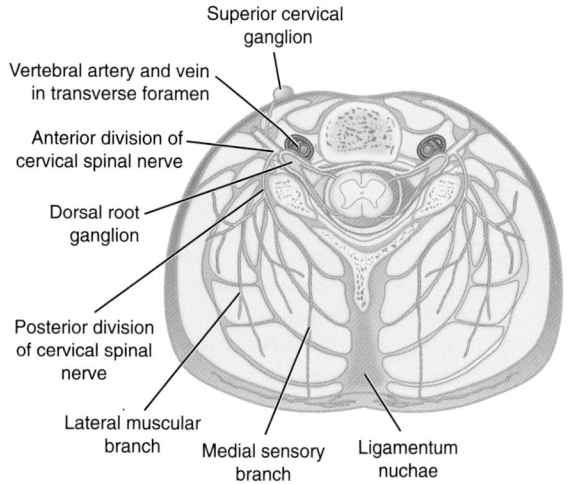

FIGURE 68.11 Cross-section of the third cervical segment showing the course and distribution of the posterior primary division, with its medial branch passing posteriorly to supply the skin and subcutaneous structures and the lateral branch supplying the muscles. Also shown is a cross-section of the superior cervical ganglion and its connection to the nerve by the white ramus communicantes. Note the vertebral vessels just anterior to the nerve.

The first cervical nerve or suboccipital nerve remains as one trunk and supplies the muscles of the suboccipital triangle. Sensory fibers from the C1 nerve supply the periosteum and body of the atlas and occiput, the atlantooccipital and atlantoaxial joints, and ligaments around these joints. It may occasionally supply skin of the scalp and communicate with the greater and lesser occipital nerves. The posterior primary divisions of the other cervical spinal nerves supply the muscles of the posterior neck (lateral branches) and skin of the neck (medial branches).[1]

The greater occipital nerve is the medial or sensory branch of the posterior division of the second cervical nerve. It communicates with the third cervical nerve to supply the scalp over the vertex and top of the head and gives muscular branches to the semispinalis capitis. The third or least occipital nerve arises from the medial sensory branch of the posterior division of the third cervical nerve (Figs. 68.11 and 68.12).[1]

The Cervical and Brachial Plexus

The cervical plexus is made up of the anterior primary divisions of the upper four cervical nerves. The brachial plexus is formed from the lower four cervical nerves, C5 through C8, together with T1 (Fig. 68.13).[1]

The anterior trunks from cervical nerves two through four divide into ascending and descending branches which form a series of three loops. These are located lateral to the vertebrae, anterior to the levator scapulae and scalenus medius muscles, and beneath the sternocleidomastoid muscle. The deep branches of the cervical plexus lie beneath the sternocleidomastoid muscle and are divided into the lateral or external group and the medial or internal group. The lateral group of branches supplies muscular branches to the scalenus medius, sternocleidomastoid, trapezius, and levator scapulae. It also sends communicating branches to the spinal accessory nerve. The medial or internal branches send off communicating fibers which join the vagus, hypoglossal and descendens hypoglossi nerves, the superior cervical sympathetic ganglion, and, by means of the ansa hypoglossi, supply the thyrohyoid, geniohyoid, omohyoid, sternothyroid, and sternohyoid muscles. The medial branches also supply the rectus capitis, lateralis, and anticus, the longus capitis and longus colli muscles, as well as the diaphragm by way of the phrenic nerve.[1]

The superficial or cutaneous branches of the cervical plexus are often referred to as the superficial cervical plexus and include the lesser occipital nerve, the great auricular nerve, the anterior cutaneous nerve, and the supraclavicular nerve. The lesser occipital nerve joins with the greater occipital and greater auricular nerves to supply the posterior scalp. Its auricular branch supplies the upper and posterior auricula and communicates with the mastoid branch of the great auricular nerve. The great auricular nerve supplies the skin of the face over the parotid gland and communicates with the facial nerve via its anterior or facial branch. Another branch supplies the lobule and lower part of the concha of the ear and communicates with the lesser occipital nerve, the auricular branch of the vagus, and the posterior auricular branch of the facial nerve. The anterior cutaneous nerve supplies the cranial, ventral, and lateral aspects of the neck as far as the sternum.[1]

Finally, the supraclavicular nerve supplies the skin and superficial fascia of the clavicular region as well as the periosteum and bone of the clavicle. Via its medial or supraclavicular branches known also as the suprasternal nerves, it supplies the skin of the infraclavicular region medially as far as the midline and laterally

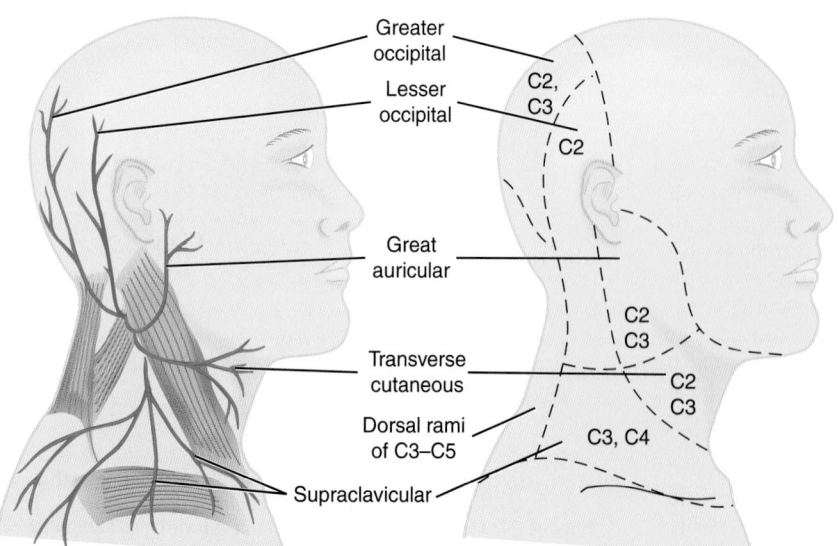

FIGURE 68.12 Cutaneous nerves derived from the cervical plexus (see text for details).

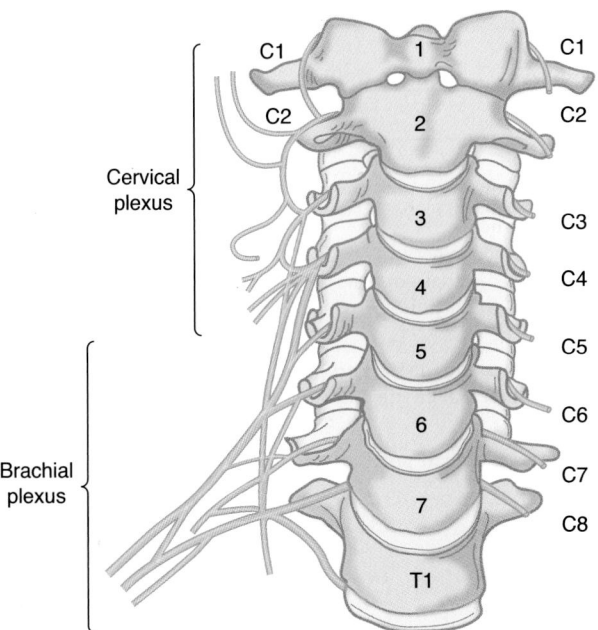

FIGURE 68.13 Anterior view showing the formation of the cervical and brachial plexuses.

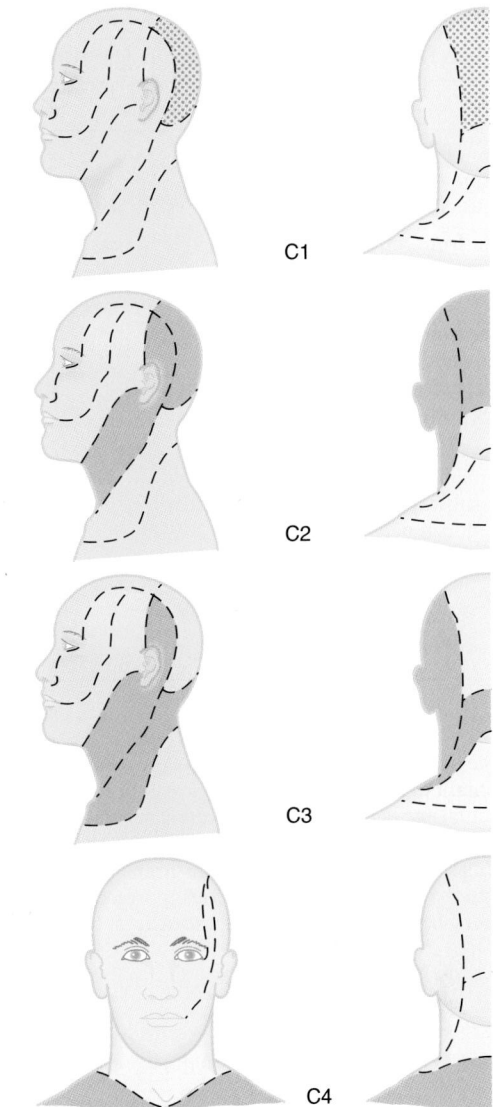

FIGURE 68.15 Dermatomes of the neck and head derived from the upper four cervical nerves.

to the junction of the medial and middle third of the clavicle. The intermediate supraclavicular nerve supplies the skin over the pectoralis major as far as the second or third rib and communicates with the cutaneous branches of the second and third intercostals nerves. The lateral supraclavicular nerves or supraacromial nerves supply the skin of the top and dorsal parts of the shoulder (Figs. 68.14 and 68.15).[1]

The brachial plexus is formed from the primary anterior divisions of the fifth through eighth cervical nerves and the first thoracic nerve with occasional contributing branches from the anterior primary divisions of the fourth cervical and second thoracic nerves. These combine to form three trunks which include: (1) the upper trunk, formed from the primary divisions of the fifth and sixth cervical nerves; (2) the middle trunk, formed from the

seventh primary division; and (3) the lower trunk formed from the eighth cervical and first thoracic primary divisions.[1] The upper trunk gives off the suprascapular nerve which supplies the shoulder joint, the supraspinatus and infraspinatus muscles, and the subclavius nerve, which supplies the subclavius muscle.

The three trunks continue from the interscalenus space in an anterolateral and inferior direction toward the first rib. These further divide into anterior and posterior divisions which pass beneath the midclavicular region to enter the apex of the axilla. Within the axilla, the anterior and posterior divisions form the lateral, medial, and posterior cords. The anterior divisions of the upper and middle trunks, containing fibers from the fifth, sixth, and seventh cervical nerves, form the lateral cord. The anterior division of the lower trunk continues as the medial cord and contains fibers from the eighth cervical and first thoracic nerves. The union of all the posterior divisions makes up the posterior cord, which thus contains fibers from all nerves of the brachial plexus. The three cords divide to give rise to the peripheral nerves of the upper extremity at the lateral border of the pectoralis minor. The lateral aspect of the median nerve and the musculocutaneous nerves derive from the lateral cord. The medial cord divides into the medial

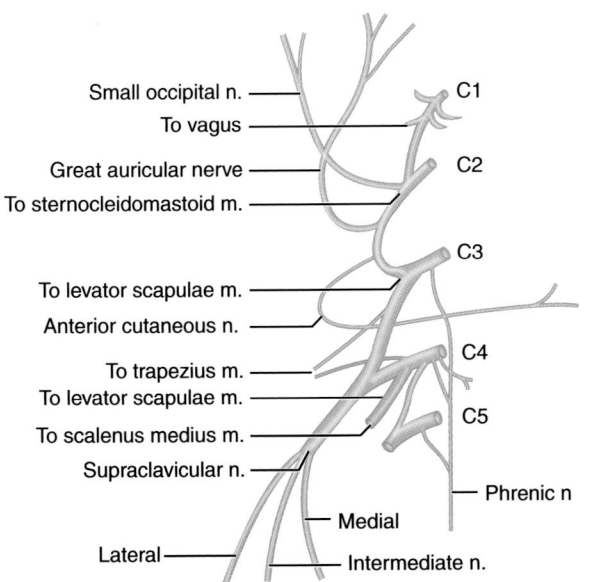

FIGURE 68.14 Origin and composition of the cervical plexus.

TABLE 68.2

ORGANIZATION AND BRANCHES OF THE BRACHIAL PLEXUS

Structure	Neurotome	Structure	Neurotome
Branches of cervical nerves		**Branches**	
To phrenic nerve	C5	Anterior pectoral	C5 to C7
To longus colli and scaleni muscles	C5 to C7	**Terminal branches**	
Branches from roots		Musculocutaneous nerve	C5 to C7
Dorsal scapular nerve	(C4), C5	Median nerve, lateral portion	C6, C7
Long thoracic nerve	C5 to C7	Medial cord origin (inferior trunk)	C8 to T1
Branches from trunks (superior trunk)		**Branches**	
Nerve to subclavius	C5, C6	Medial brachial cutaneous nerve	C8 to T1
Suprascapular nerve	C5, C6	Medial antibrachial cutaneous nerve	C8 to T1
Posterior cord origin (from all trunks)	C5 to C8, T1	**Terminal branches**	
Branches		Median nerve (medial portion)	C8 to T1
Superior subscapular nerve	C5, C6	Ulnar nerve	C8 to T1
Inferior subscapular nerve	C5, C6		
Thoracodorsal nerve	C6 to C8		
Terminal branches			
Axillary	C5, C6		
Radial	C5 to C8, T1		
Lateral cord origin (superior and middle trunk)	C5 to C7		

head of the median nerve, the ulnar nerve, the medial antebrachial and brachial cutaneous nerves, as well as a branch to the intercostobrachial nerve. The axillary and radial nerves are terminating branches from the posterior cord.[1]

In addition to supplying terminal branches to the upper extremity, the brachial plexus carries postganglionic sympathetic fibers from the cervical and thoracic sympathetic chain to the upper limbs. The brachial plexus also supplies branches to the longus colli muscle and the scalene muscles. The fifth cervical nerve sends fibers to the phrenic nerve, the rhomboid muscles, and the levator scapulae muscles via the dorsal scapular nerve. Fibers from the anterior divisions of the fifth, sixth, and seventh cervical nerves supply the serratus anterior muscle via the long thoracic nerve (Table 68.2, Figs. 68.16 and 68.17).

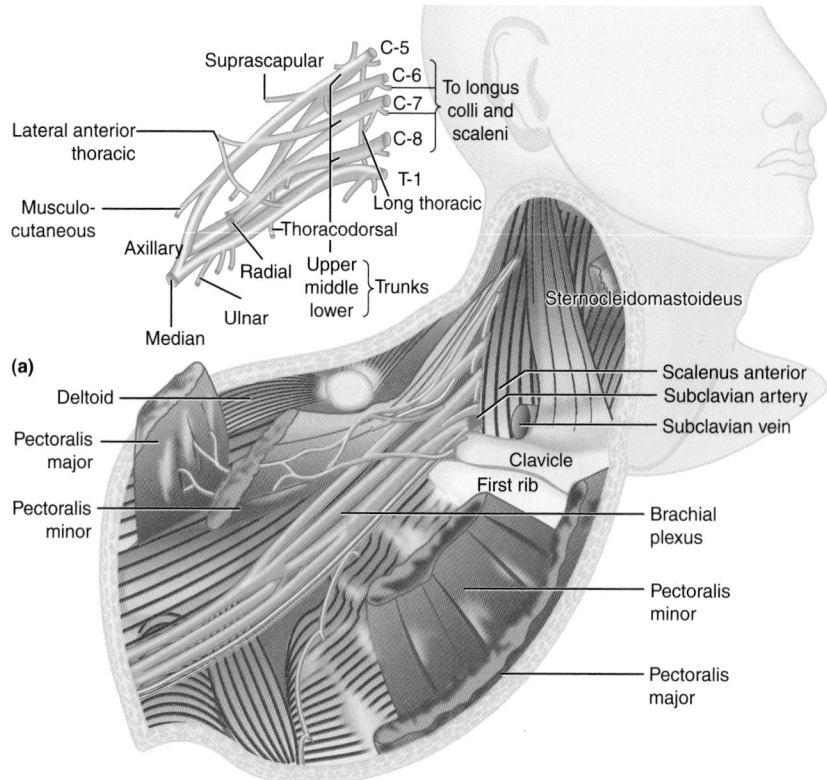

FIGURE 68.16 Anatomy of the brachial plexus. **A.** Schematic depiction of the brachial plexus. **B.** Relation of the roots of the brachial plexus to the scalene muscles showing the position of the plexus over the first rib and its course into the axilla.

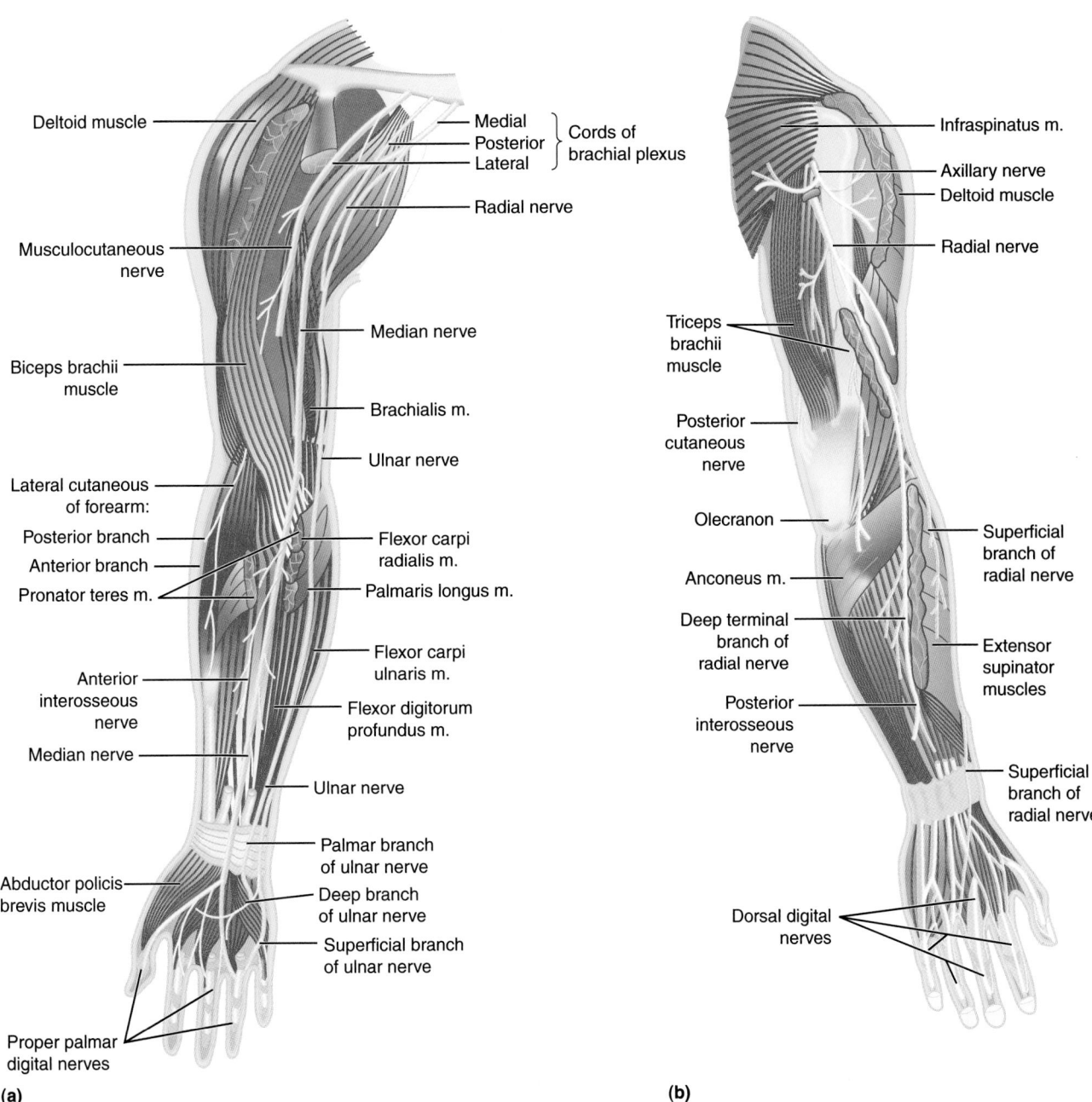

FIGURE 68.17 Anatomy of the median, ulnar, and radial nerves. Anterior view (**A**) and posterior view (**B**) of the upper limb showing the course of the three nerves and some of the muscles (m.) they supply.

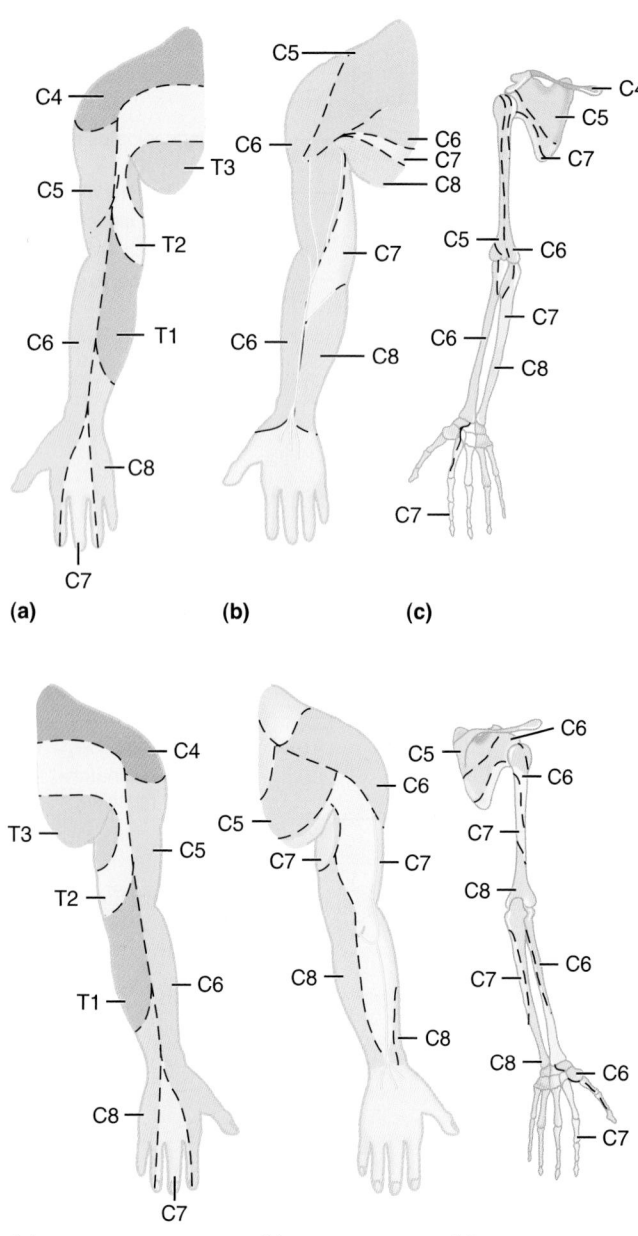

(a)   **(b)**   **(c)**

(a)   **(b)**   **(c)**

FIGURE 68.18 Segmental nerve supply to the upper limb showing the anterior view (*above*) and posterior view (*below*). **A.** Dermatomes. **B.** Myotomes. **C.** Sclerotomes.

The segmental and peripheral nerve supply of the neck and arm is summarized in Figures 68.18 and 68.19 as well as Tables 68.3, 68.4, and 68.5. Sympathetic nervous system contributions to the upper extremity from the cervical and thoracic preganglionic neurons are illustrated and described in Figure 68.20. Contributions from the anterolateral and posterolateral subclavian sympathetic nerves, which supply the subclavian artery and its branches distal to the scalene muscles, contain both sympathetic and sensory fibers.[1]

Pectoral Girdle and Shoulder Anatomy

The differential diagnosis of neck and arm pain includes many disorders of the pectoral girdle and shoulder which can result not only in shoulder pain, but also in radiation of pain to the neck and/or arm. Common disorders involving the shoulder and pectoral girdle include rotator cuff tears, tendonitis, impingement syndromes, and arthritis (Figs. 68.21 and 68.22). An understand-

ing of the complex anatomy and biomechanics of pectoral girdle and shoulder is essential for the diagnosis and treatment of pain in this region.[1]

The pectoral girdle is made up of the scapula and clavicle, the sternoclavicular and acromioclavicular joints, and the scapulothoracic and humeroacromial interfaces. Unlike the lower limb, which is built for weight-bearing as well as locomotion, the upper limb function is primarily to allow mobility and a wide range of motion for the arm and hand. The girdle does not articulate with the vertebral column, as does the pelvic girdle, but with the thoracic cage at the saddle-shaped sternoclavicular joint. The sternoclavicular joint is divided into two spaces by an articular disk and is surrounded by a strong, lax capsule. In addition to the capsule, the joint is stabilized by the interclavicular ligament superiorly, inferiorly by the costoclavicular ligament (which limits elevation and rotation of the clavicle and serves as the fulcrum of movements at the sternoclavicular joint), and the posterior sternoclavicular ligament. Dislocation of the costoclavicular joint is rare, but tends to occur

(text continues on page 1017)

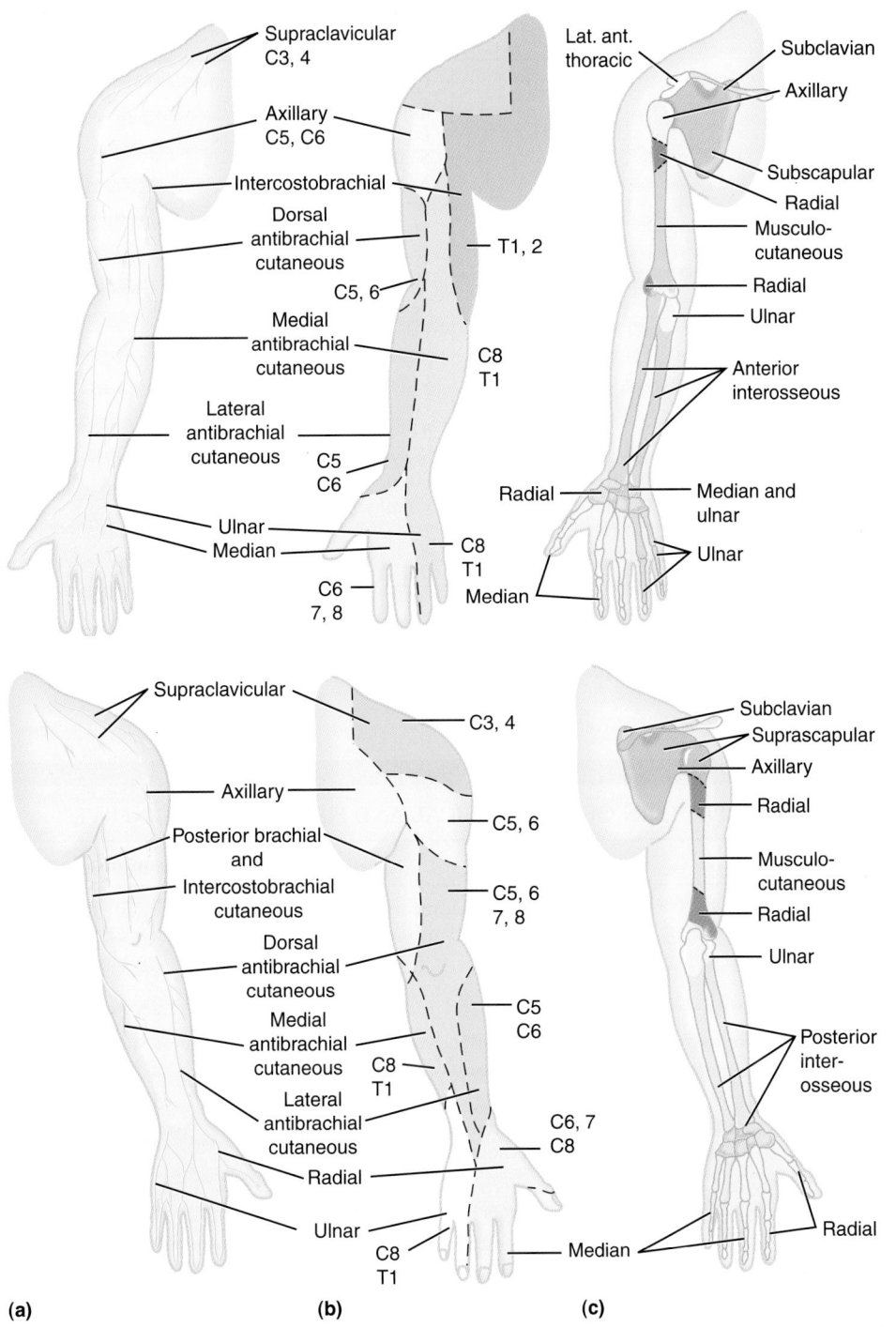

(a)   **(b)**   **(c)**

FIGURE 68.19 Peripheral nerve supply to the upper limb showing the anterior view (*above*) and posterior view (*below*). **A.** Various cutaneous nerves and their territories (**B**). **C.** Nerve supply to the bones and joints.

TABLE 68.3

NERVE SUPPLY OF MUSCLES OF THE NECK

Muscle	Nerve Supply	Muscle	Nerve Supply
Capital flexors		**Cervical spine extensors**	
Rectus capitis anterior	C1, C2	Splenius cervicis	C2 to C7
Rectus capitis lateralis	C1, C2	Longissimus cervicis	C1 to C8*
Longus capitis	C1 to C4	Semispinalis cervicis	C1 to C8*
		Multifidus	C3 to T1
Capital extensors			
Rectus capitis posterior major	C1	**Head rotators†**	
Rectus capitis posterior minor	C1	Sternocleidomastoid	See above
Oblique capitis superior	C1	Splenius cervicis	
Oblique capitis inferior	C1	Semispinalis cervicis	
Longus capitis	C1 to C4	Longissimus cervicis	
Splenius capitis	C3 to C5		
Semispinalis capitis	C3 to C5	**Other neck muscles**	
		Geniohyoid	C1
Cervical spine flexors		Thyrohyoid	C1
Scalenus anterior	C4 to C7	Sternohyoid	C1 to C3
Scalenus medius	C3 to C8	Sternothyroid	C1 to C3
Scalenus posterior	C5 to C8	Omohyoid	C1 to C3
Longus colli	C2 to C8		
Sternocleidomastoid	Cranial nerve XI; C2, C3*		

*When muscles of both sides contract.
†When the muscle of one side contracts.

TABLE 68.4

SCLEROTOMAL DISTRIBUTION PATTERN OF THE CERVICAL AND FIRST THORACIC NERVES

Segment	Sclerotome	Joints	Ligaments
C1	Periosteum and body of atlas	Atlantoaxial, medial, atlantoaxial, lateral, atlantoaxial	Alar, cruciform, apical dental, accessory atlantoaxial, articular capsules, nuchal, anterior atlanto-occipital membrane, posterior atlanto-occipital membrane
C2	Periosteum and body of axis	Medial atlantoaxial, lateral atlantoaxial, intervertebral	Anterior longitudinal, atlantoaxial membrane, atlantoaxial, capsular, cruciform, nuchal
C3	Periosteum and body of C3 vertebra and clavicle	Intervertebral, Luschka, sternoclavicular, zygapophyseal	Anterior longitudinal, posterior longitudinal, capsular, nuchal
C4	Periosteum and body of C4 vertebra and clavicle	Intervertebral, Luschka, sternoclavicular, zygapophyseal	Anterior longitudinal, posterior longitudinal, capsular, ligamentum flavum, nuchal
C5	Periosteum and body of C5 vertebra and portions of humerus, scapula, and proximal ulna	Acromioclavicular, glenohumeral Luschka, intervertebral, elbow, zygapophyseal, sternoclavicular	Anterior longitudinal, posterior longitudinal, capsular, nuchal, ligamentum flavum
C6	Periosteum and body of C6 vertebra and portions of humerus, radius, scapula, and first metacarpal bone	Glenohumeral, intervertebral, Luschka, elbow, zygapophyseal	Anterior longitudinal, posterior longitudinal, capsular, nuchal, ligamentum flavum
C7	Periosteum and body of C7 vertebra and portions of humerus, scapula, radius, and ulna	Elbow, Luschka, intervertebral, zygapophyseal	Anterior longitudinal, posterior longitudinal, nuchal, ligamentum flavum
C8	Periosteum and body of C8 vertebra and portions of humerus, ulna, carpal bones, and bones of fourth and fifth fingers	Intervertebral, Luschka, zygapophyseal, elbow, wrist, hand	Supraspinous, interspinous, anterior longitudinal, posterior longitudinal
T1	Periosteum and body of T1 vertebra	Intervertebral, zygapophyseal, costovertebral, elbows, wrist, hand	Anterior longitudinal, posterior longitudinal, supraspinous, interspinous, ligamentum flavum

TABLE 68.5

NERVE SUPPLY OF THE MUSCLES OF THE UPPER LIMBS

Region/Muscle Group/Function*	Peripheral Nerve Supply	Segmental Nerve Supply†
Shoulder rotator cuff		
Supraspinatus	Suprascapular	C5, C6
Infraspinatus	Suprascapular	C5, C6
Subscapularis	Nerve to subscapularis	C5, C6
Teres minor	Axillary	C5, C6
Scapular motion		
Elevation		
Levator scapulae	Dorsal scapular	C4, C5
Rhomboideus	Dorsal scapular	C4, C5
Trapezius (superior fibers)	Spinal accessory	CN XI
Depression		
Trapezius (inferior fibers)	Spinal accessory	CN XI
Pectoralis major	Medial/lateral pectorals	C5, C6, C7, C8, T1
Subclavius	Nerve to subclavius	C5, C6
Upward rotation		
Serratus anterior	Long thoracic	C5, C6, C7
Trapezius (upper/lower fibers)	Spinal accessory	CN XI
Downward rotation		
Levator scapulae	Dorsal scapular	C4, C5
Rhomboideus	Dorsal scapular	C4, C5
Pectoralis major and minor	Lateral/medial pectorals	C5, C6, C7, C8, T1
Latissimus dorsi	Thoracodorsal	C6, C7, C8
Abduction (protraction)		
Serratus anterior	Long thoracic	C5, C6, C7
Pectoralis major	Medial/lateral pectorals	C5, C6, C7, C8, T1
Adduction (retraction)		
Trapezius (middle fibers)	Spinal accessory	CN XI
Rhomboideus	Dorsal scapular	C4, C5
Latissimus dorsi	Thoracodorsal	C6, C7, C8
Arm motion		
Flexion		
Pectoralis major (clavicular head)	Medial/lateral pectorals	C5, C6, C7, C8, T1u
Deltoid (anterior fibers)	Axillary	C5, C6
Coracobrachialis	Musculocutaneous	C6, C7
Biceps brachii	Musculocutaneous	C5, C6
Extension		
Latissimus dorsi	Thoracodorsal	C6, C7, C8
Teres major	Subscapular	C5, C6
Deltoid (posterior fibers)	Axillary	C5, C6
Triceps brachii	Radical	C7, C8
Abduction		
Deltoid (middle fibers)	Axillary	C5, C6
Supraspinatus	Suprascapular	C5, C6
Infraspinatus	Suprascapular	C5, C6
Teres minor	Axillary	C5, C6
Adduction		
Pectoralis major and minor	Medial/lateral pectorals	C5, C6, C7, C8, T1
Latissimus dorsi	Thoracodorsal	C6, C7, C8
Teres major	Subscapular	C5, C6
Medial rotation		
Subscapularis	Nerve to subscapularis	C5, C6
Latissimus dorsi	Thoracodorsal	C6, C7, C8
Pectoralis major and minor	Medial/lateral pectorals	C5, C6, C7, C8, T1
Lateral rotation		
Infraspinatus	Suprascapular	C5, C6
Teres minor	Axillary	C5, C6

(continued)

TABLE 68.5

CONTINUED

Region/Muscle Group/Function*	Peripheral Nerve Supply	Segmental Nerve Supply†
Elbow/forearm motion		
Extension		
Triceps brachii	Radial	C6, <u>C7</u>, C8
Anconeus	Radial	<u>C7</u>, C8
Flexion		
Biceps brachii	Musculocutaneous	<u>C5</u>, C6
Brachialis	Musculocutaneous	<u>C5</u>, C6
Brachioradialis	Radial	<u>C5</u>, C6
Wrist motion		
Flexion		
Flexor carpi radialis	Median	C6, <u>C7</u>
Flexor carpi ulnaris	Ulnar	C7, <u>C8</u>
Palmaris longus	Median	<u>C7</u>, C8
Extension		
Extensor carpi radialis longus/brevis	Radial	<u>C6</u>, C7
Extensor carpi ulnaris	Radial (posterior interosseus)	<u>C7</u>, C8
Radial deviation		
Flexor carpi radialis	Median	<u>C6</u>, C7
Extensor carpi radialis longus/brevis	Radial	<u>C6</u>, C7
Ulnar deviation		
Flexor carpi ulnaris	Ulnar	C7, <u>C8</u>
Extensor carpi ulnaris	Radial (posterior interosseus)	<u>C7</u>, C8
Digits (2–5)		
Flexion		
Flexor digit superficialis	Median	C7, <u>C8</u>, T1
Flexor digit profundus	Median (anterior interosseus)	C7, <u>C8</u>, T1
Extension		
Extensor digit communis	Radial (posterior interosseus)	<u>C7</u>, C8
Extensor digit minimi	Radial (posterior interosseus)	<u>C7</u>, C8
Extensor indicis	Radial (posterior interosseus)	<u>C7</u>, C8
Abduction		
Dorsal interossei	Ulnar	C8, <u>T1</u>
Adduction		
Palmar interossei	Ulnar	C8, <u>T1</u>
Motion of thumb		
Flexion		
Flexor pollicis longus	Median (anterior interosseus)	C7, <u>C8</u>
Extension		
Extensor pollicis longus	Radial (posterior interosseus)	C7, <u>C8</u>
Extensor pollicis brevis	Radial (posterior interosseus)	C7, <u>C8</u>
Abductor pollicis longus	Radial (posterior interosseus)	C7, <u>C8</u>
Adduction		
Adductor pollicis	Ulnar	C8, <u>T1</u>
Abduction		
Abduction pollis brevis	Median	C8, <u>T1</u>
Opponens pollicis	Median	C8, <u>T1</u>
Opposition		
Opponens pollicis	Median	C8, <u>T1</u>
Hypothenar group (motion of fifth finger)		
Abduction digiti minimi	Ulnar	C8, <u>T1</u>
Flexor digiti brevis	Ulnar	C8, <u>T1</u>
Opponens digiti minimi	Ulnar	C8, <u>T1</u>

CN, cranial nerve.
*Only the primary muscle nerves are included.
†Main root is underlined.

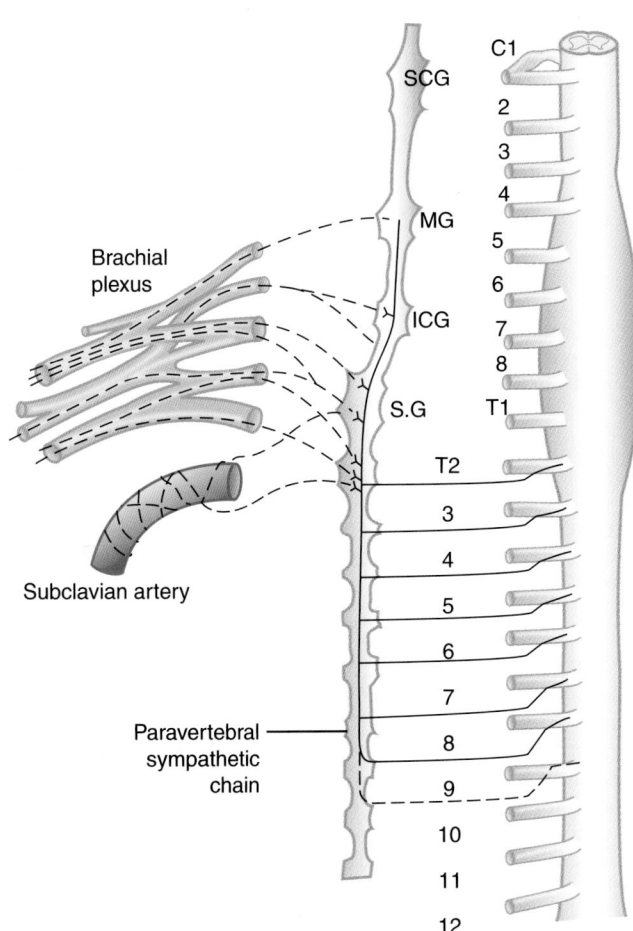

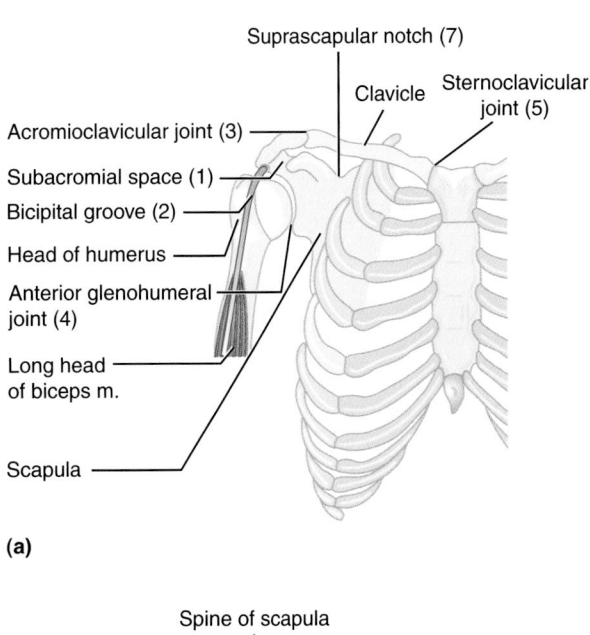

(a)

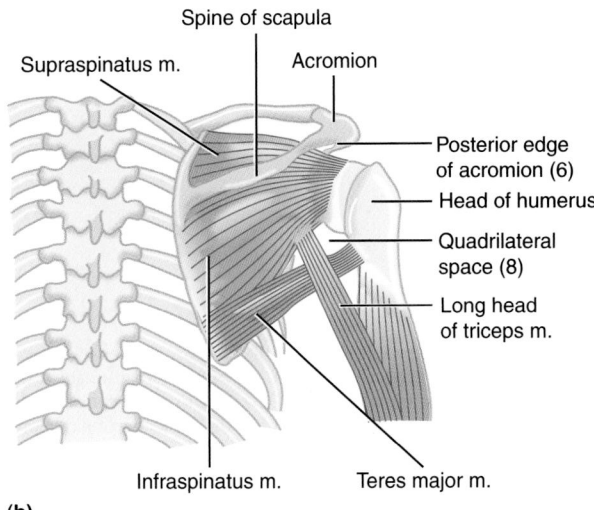

(b)

FIGURE 68.20 Schematic depiction of the origins and courses of pre-ganglionic sympathetic neurons destined to supply the upper limbs. Note that the axons of the preganglionic neurons, which are located in spinal segments T2 to T8 (and occasionally T9), pass through the anterior root as white rami communicantes and from there to the paravertebral sympathetic chain, where they ascend and synapse with postganglionic fibers primarily in the second thoracic, stellate, and intermediate and middle cervical ganglia, and occasionally in the third cervical ganglion (not shown). Some of the postganglionic fibers pass directly to the subclavian artery, but most pass as gray rami communicantes to the roots of the brachial plexus. (From Bonica JJ. *Clinical application of diagnostic and therapeutic nerve blocks.* Springfield, IL: Charles C Thomas; 1959.)

FIGURE 68.21 Anterior (**A**) and posterior (**B**) views of the shoulder identifying the various bones and joints and also the sites of pathologic processes that produce pain and tenderness. (1) Subacromial space, which can be involved with calcific tendinitis, rotator cuff tendinitis and impingement syndrome, and rotator cuff tear; (2) bicipital groove, which can be involved in bicipital tendinitis and biceps tendon subluxation and tear; (3) acromioclavicular joint, which can be involved with degenerative and infectious processes; (4) anterior glenohumeral joint, which can be the site of glenohumeral arthritis, osteonecrosis, glenoid labial tears, and adhesive capsulitis; (5) sternoclavicular joint, which can be the site of pain caused by infection, degenerative changes, or trauma; (6) posterior edge of the acromion, which can contribute to rotator cuff tendinitis, calcific tendinitis, and rotator cuff tear; (7) suprascapular notch, which can be the site of suprascapular nerve entrapment; and (8) quadrilateral space, which can be the site of axillary nerve entrapment.

anteriorly where the joint is weakest when it does occur (Fig. 68.23).

The acromioclavicular joint of the pectoral girdle is surrounded by a weak and lax capsule. It is stabilized by the acromioclavicular ligament superiorly, the fan-shaped coracoclavicular ligament, which serves as a vertical axis for scapular rotation, and the trapezoid ligament which serves as a hinge for scapular motion about the horizontal axis. A partial or complete disruption of the coracoclavicular ligament, resulting in separation of the acromioclavicular joint, may occur with a fall on the shoulder.

The scapulothoracic interface allows a gliding movement between the ventral surface of the scapula and the thorax overlying the second through the seventh ribs. The scapula is held in close approximation to the thorax by the serratus anterior, the trapezius, and the rhomboid muscles. For full abduction and forward flexion of the shoulder to occur, the scapula must undergo upward rotation. Movements of the pectoral girdle consist of upward-downward rotation, protrac-

tion-retraction, and elevation-depression (Table 68.6, Figs. 68.24 and 68.25).

The glenohumeral joint is a synovial joint which consists of the interface of the head of the humerus with the pear-shaped glenoid cavity and ring of fibrocartilage known as the glenoid labrum. These deepen the socket of the scapula and assist with stability of the glenohumeral joint. The supraglenoid and infraglenoid tubercles above and below the glenoid cavity are attachment sites for the long head of the biceps and triceps, respectively.

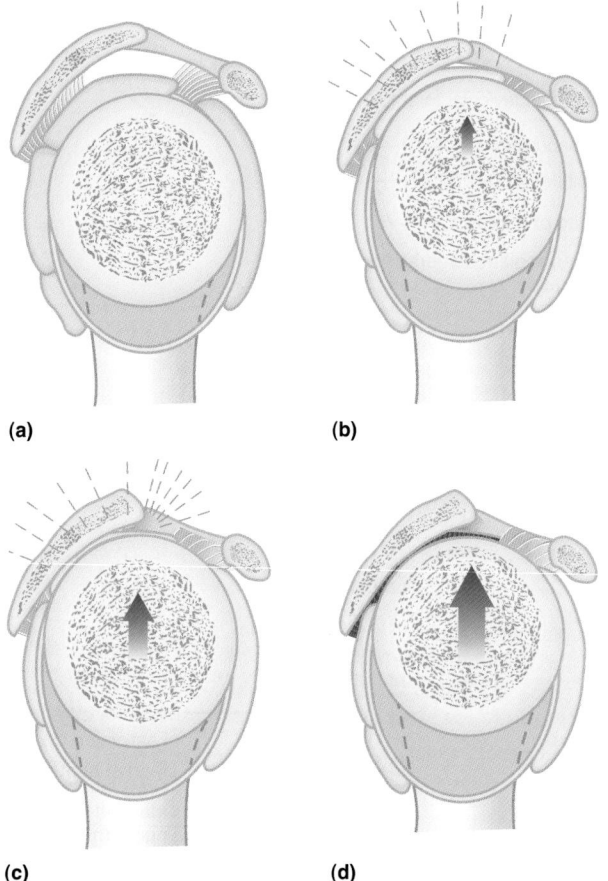

(a)   **(b)**

(c)   **(d)**

FIGURE 68.22 With progressive cuff fiber failure, the head moves upward against the coracoacromial arch. **A.** Normal relationships of the cuff and the coracoacromial arch. **B.** Upward displacement of the head, squeezing the cuff against the acromion and the coracoacromial ligament. **C.** Greater contact and abrasion, giving rise to a traction spur in the coracoacromial ligament. **D.** Still greater upward displacement, resulting in abrasion of the humeral articular cartilage and cuff tear arthropathy. (From Matsen FA. *Practical evaluation and management of the shoulder.* Philadelphia: Saunders; 1994:123, with permission.)

The joint capsule is strong but lax, to allow for mobility, and attaches to the scapula proximally and distally to the articular margins of the head of the humerus superiorly and the surgical neck of the humerus inferiorly. The ligaments of the glenohumeral joint consist of the superior, middle, and inferior glenohumeral ligaments (thickenings of the anterior capsule), the coracohumeral ligament (which attaches to the greater and lesser tuberosities and limits flexion and extension), and the coracoacromial ligament (which extends from the undersurface of the acromion to the coracoid process and acts as an articulating surface for the head of the humerus). The subacromial and subdeltoid bursae lie between the coracoacromial arch and the rotator cuff tendons and have been implicated in shoulder impingement (see Fig. 68.24).

Movement at the shoulder requires the combined motion of the glenohumeral joint and the pectoral girdle for flexion or abduction greater than 90 degrees. For example, the abduction or elevation of the arm to 180 degrees requires 60 degrees of scapular rotation to alter the angle of the glenoid fossa during its articulation with the head of the humerus (Figs. 68.26 and 68.27). Prime movers of the pectoral girdle and glenohumeral joint are listed in Tables 68.6 and 68.7.[1]

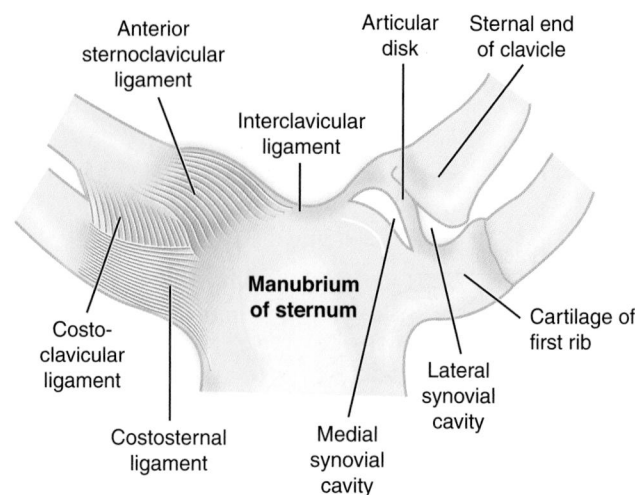

FIGURE 68.23 Anatomy of the sternoclavicular joints viewed from the front. (Adapted from Clement CD. *Gray's anatomy of the human body.* 30th ed. Philadelphia: Lea & Febiger; 1985:366–367.)

EPIDEMIOLOGY OF NECK AND ARM PAIN

Methodology and definition of neck pain varies significantly in epidemiologic studies of neck and arm pain. A critical review of the literature on the incidence of neck complaints between 1980 and 2006 was published by the Bone and Joint Decade 2000–2010 Task Force on Neck Pain and its Associated Disorders. They found that the incidence of neck complaints per 1000 patient years in the general population ranged from 0.037, when defined as patients presenting as inpatients or to hospital emergency rooms for soft tissue injuries (not from motor vehicle collisions), to 213 initially pain-free adolescents reporting pain onset over the last 3 months via questionnaire. An average of 30% to 50% 12-month prevalence among adults and 21% to 42% among children and adolescence was found. Neck pain which limited activities was less common at 2% to 11%.[3]

Other associated conditions identified with neck and arm pain include poor psychologic health, exposure to secondhand smoke in childhood, current smoking, and genetics. Associated poor

---

TABLE 68.6

PRIME MOVERS OF THE PECTORAL GIRDLE

Elevation	Trapezius (upper fibers) Rhomboids Levator scapulae
Depression	Latissimus dorsi Pectoralis major (costal fibers) Trapezius (lower fibers)
Protraction	Serratus anterior Pectoralis minor Pectoralis major
Retraction	Trapezius Rhomboids
Upward rotation	Trapezius Serratus anterior
Downward rotation	Rhomboids

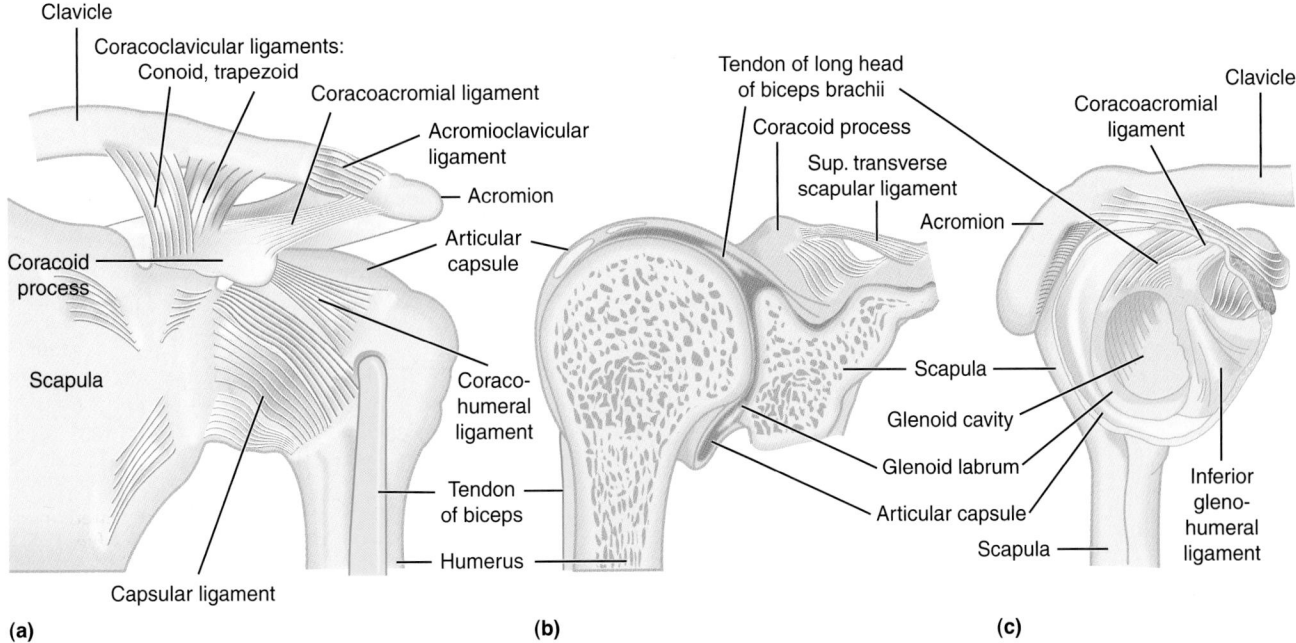

FIGURE 68.24 Anatomy of the shoulder joint. **A.** Anterior view of ligaments of the left shoulder. **B.** Coronal section through the head of the left humerus and shoulder joint, anterior half viewed from behind. **C.** Interior of the right shoulder viewed from its lateral aspect. (Adapted from Clement CD. *Gray's anatomy of the human body.* 30th ed. Philadelphia: Lea & Febiger; 1985:368–372.)

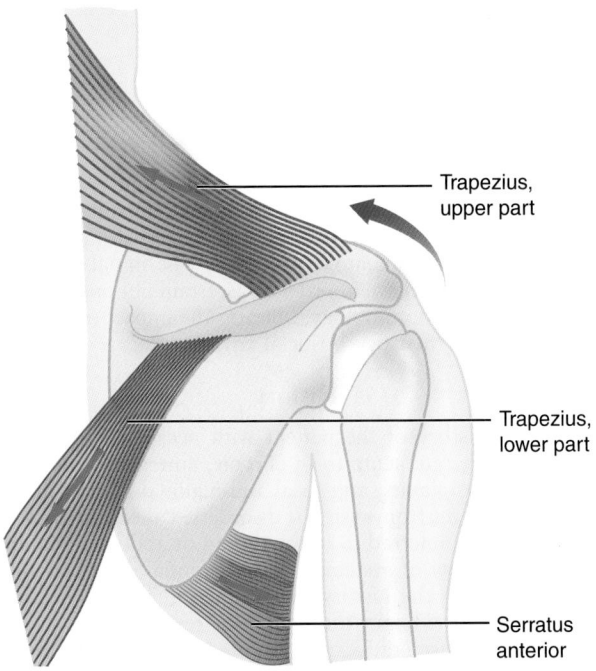

FIGURE 68.25 The muscles that rotate the scapula upward during abduction of the arm. Note that the upper part of the trapezius, which is attached to the outer part of the scapular spine, pulls upward, and that the lower part of the serratus anterior, attached to the lower part of the scapula, pulls the inferior angle laterally, while the lower portion of the trapezius, attached to the medial part of the scapular spine, pulls downward. (From Rosse C, Gaddum-Rosse P. *Hollinshead's textbook of anatomy.* 5th ed. Philadelphia: Lippincott–Raven; 1997:235, with permission.)

health, as well as musculoskeletal and psychologic health complaints, were prognostic for poor outcome. Prevalence was found to be overall higher in females with prevalence peaking in middle age. Neck pain prevalence associated with previous trauma to the neck via exposure to a motor vehicle collision was associated with subsequent neck pain prevalence at 7-year follow-up only when there had been a report of whiplash-associated disorder or pain following the collision.[3]

Controversy exists regarding the relationship between radiologic evidence of cervical spine degeneration and neck pain. One recent study reported no significant difference in the degree of neck pain in patients with or without radiographic evidence of cervical spine degenerative changes,[4] whereas another study correlated neck pain with increasing grade of disc degeneration.[5] Zlapetal et al.[6] showed increasing evidence of neck pain with increasing prevalence of atlanto-odontoid degenerative changes.

Up to 78% of asymptomatic subjects have been found to have degenerative changes on magnetic resonance imaging (MRI) accompanied by positive findings such as disc bulging and protrusion, foraminal stenosis, and abnormal spinal cord contour. This evidence suggests that degenerative findings are common in both asymptomatic and symptomatic individuals, increase linearly with age, and cannot be assumed to be the definitive cause of neck pain in symptomatic individuals.[7–9] One study comparing cervical spine MRIs of fighter pilots to age-matched controls showed premature cervical disc degeneration among pilots exposed frequently to high $+Gz$ forces.[10]

Neck pain following whiplash-associated disorders is common with more than 300 persons per 100,000 population evaluated for this complaint each year according to recent data.[11] Increased symptom severity and presence of neurologic signs is predictive of poor prognosis. Postinjury feelings of helplessness in controlling the consequences of pain, fear of movement, catastrophizing, and postinjury anxiety have also been found to be associated with higher risk of long-term disability,[12] as has changing the insurance system from a no-fault to a tort system of compensation.[13] Studies from hospital populations report that at an

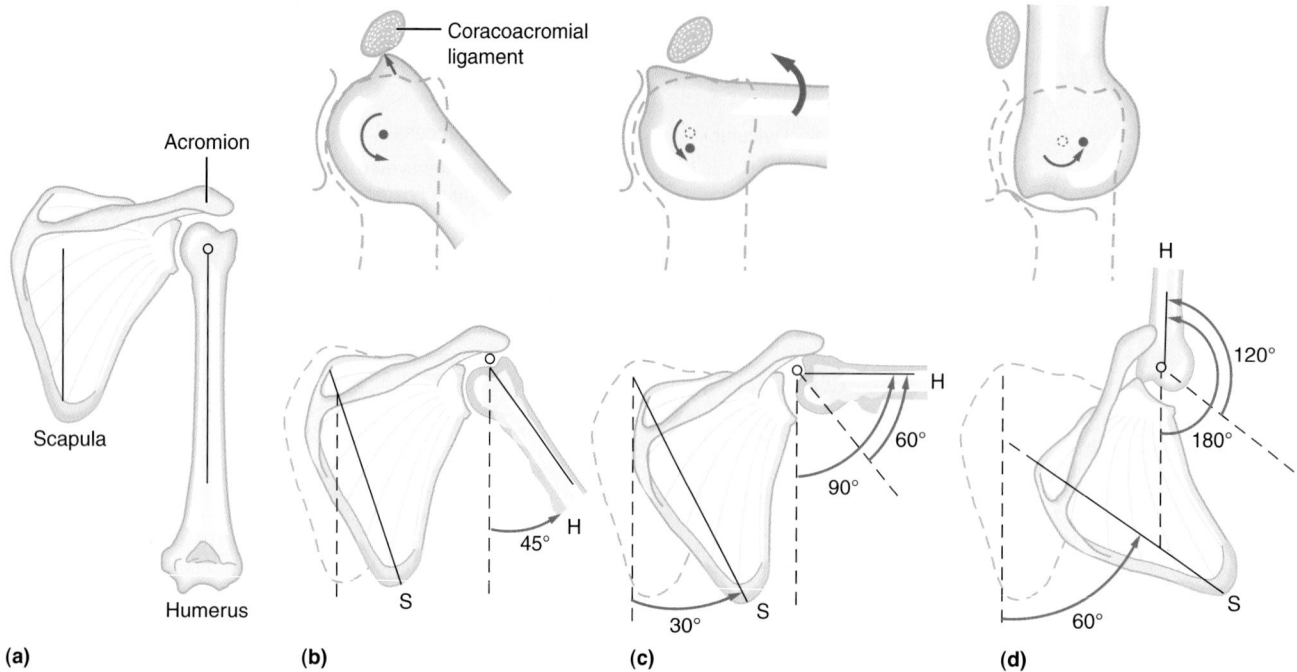

FIGURE 68.26 Biomechanics of the glenohumeral movements of arm abduction. **A.** Normal position of the head and shaft of the humerus (H). The circle in the head of the humerus indicates the center of rotation. **B.** Humerus abducted 45 degrees and the scapula (S) beginning upward rotation. The upper panel shows that the incongruity of the articulating surface of the head of the humerus, and the surface of the glenoid cavity causes the greater tuberosity of the humerus to impinge on the coracoacromial ligament. The upper panel in (C) shows that to allow the greater tuberosity to pass under the coracoacromial hood during arm abduction, the humeral head is depressed (depicted by downward movement of the center of rotation) and the humeral head rotated (*thin arrow*). The abduction movement of the arm is accomplished in a smooth coordinated movement during which for each 15 degrees of arm abduction, 10 degrees of motion occurs at the glenohumeral joint, and 5 degrees occurs because of scapular rotation on the thorax. Thus, as noted in (C), abduction of the arm to 90 degrees is accomplished by 60 degrees rotation of the humerus and 30 degrees rotation of the scapula. Full abduction of the arm, as shown in (D), is accomplished by 120 degrees of rotation at the glenohumeral joint and 60 degrees rotation of the scapula. (Modified from Cailliet R. *Shoulder pain*. 2nd ed. Philadelphia: FA Davis; 1981.)

average follow-up of 2 years, 20% to 45% of patients with soft tissue neck injuries following whiplash reported discomfort sufficient enough to interfere with their capacity to work.[14]

Onset of neck and arm pain in the workplace varies widely across various occupations. Highly repetitive work, low job satisfaction and a high level of fear avoidance are associated with development of neck and arm pain as are jobs which require prolonged bending or flexion of the neck such as computer work.[15–18]

EVALUATION OF THE PATIENT

History and Physical Examination

The patient in pain is prompted to seek help, not only to alleviate the suffering which accompanies their condition, but to address the accompanying condition of impairment or disability. The psychologic, physical, or functional handicap which coexists with pain results in loss of ability to perform normal activities and fulfill roles that are fundamental to personal identity. Ultimately, the goal of a successful evaluation should be the ability to answer the patient's three fundamental questions: (1) "What's happening to me?"; (2) "What's going to happen to me?"; and (3) "What can be done to improve what happens to me?"[19]

The differential diagnosis of neck and arm pain is broad and encompasses acute pain from work-related injury, motor vehicle

trauma and infection, emerging symptoms from enlarging tumors, vascular abnormalities or infections, manifestations of complex systemic disease processes, and exacerbation of chronic degenerative or inflammatory processes. The initial evaluation should be comprehensive in order to ascertain not only the etiology of physical symptomology, but also the impact the patient's disability has on their psychosocial environment.

History

A thorough history of the patient with neck and arm pain is essential to separate acute from chronic, emergent from urgent and routine complaints, and focal and regional injuries and degenerative changes from systemic disorders. Pain in the neck and arm may also be referred from the thorax or abdomen requiring a thorough review of systems. The differential diagnosis is frequently based on the history, which then guides further focus during the physical exam and diagnostic testing.

Immediate consideration must be made regarding the severity and urgency of the complaint. Emergent conditions can often be discerned at the time of phone request for urgent evaluation or by nurses when the patient is screened at check-in. Severe neck pain accompanied by progressive disturbance of gait, progressive motor or sensory deficits, or urinary and fecal incontinence requires prompt physician evaluation. Enlarging tumor, acute infection, and unstable inflammatory spondyloarthropathy can progress to respiratory failure and death if not treated promptly and requires immediate surgical and medical intervention. Acute

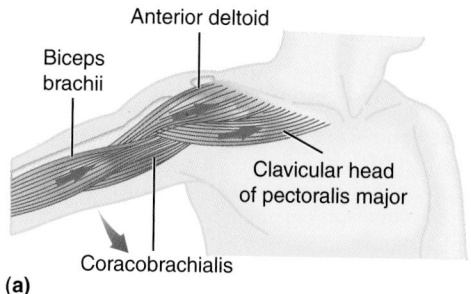

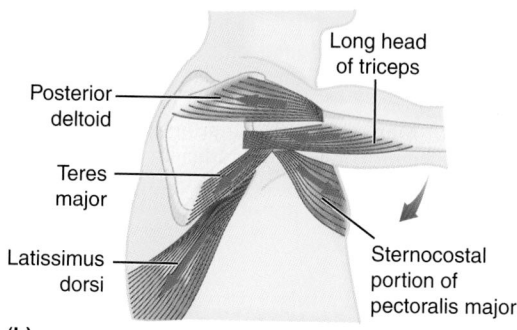

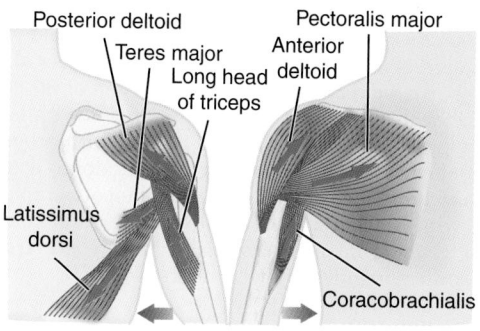

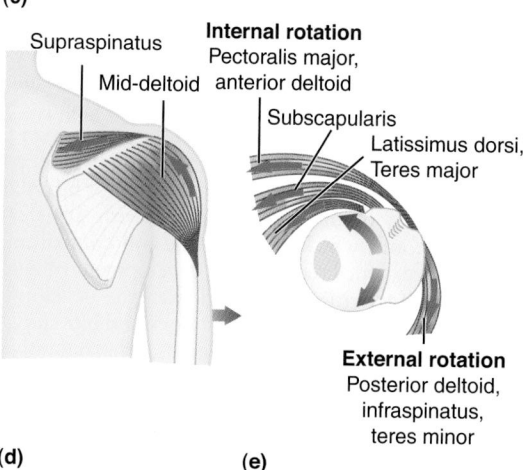

FIGURE 68.27 Muscles that move the shoulder and arm: flexors (**A**), extensors (**B**), adductors (**C**), abductors (**D**), and rotators (**E**). (Adapted from Hollinshead WH. *Anatomy for surgeons. Vol 3: The back and limbs.* 3rd ed. New York: Harper & Row; 1982:325–330.)

TABLE 68.7

PRIME MOVERS OF THE GLENOHUMERAL JOINT

Flexion	Pectoralis major (clavicular head)
	Deltoid (anterior fibers)
Extension	Latissimus dorsi
	Deltoid (posterior fibers)
Internal rotation	Pectoralis major
	Latissimus dorsi
	Teres major
	Subscapularis
External rotation	Infraspinatus
	Teres minor
	Deltoid (posterior fibers)
Abduction	Deltoid
	Supraspinatus
Adduction	Pectoralis major
	Latissimus dorsi
	Teres major
	Subscapularis

Location/Radiation

Pain in the neck and arm may be skeletal, myofascial, or neuropathic. Neuropathic pain can be further divided into peripheral or segmental nerve pathology versus autonomic and central nervous system pathology or sensitization. Cohen[22] suggests the diagnostic construct of mechanical versus nonmechanical pain. Mechanical pain is exacerbated by movement and occurs in the essentially well patient. Nonmechanical pain is often related to a medical source such as infection, neoplasm, or an inflammatory process generally seen in patients with systemic manifestations of their disease process.[22]

The purpose of a thorough history with determination of the location, pattern, and distribution of the patient's pain is to establish an initial differential diagnosis which can subsequently be confirmed or ruled out by physical examination, diagnostic laboratory, radiologic, and electrophysiologic testing. Localized pain is usually caused by disorders of joints and muscles. Segmental pain conforming to dermatomal distributions may implicate lesions of nerve roots. Pain conforming to a peripheral dermatomal and/or myotomal distribution suggests lesions of the cervical or brachial plexus or their branches. Knowledge of dermatomal, myotomal, sclerotomal, and zygapophyseal referral patterns as well as distribution of peripheral nerves of the cervical and brachial plexus are essential for determining a rational differential diagnosis (see Figs. 68.11 through 68.19 and Tables 68.3 through 68.5).

In addition to cervical nerve root inflammation or impingement, cervical and brachial referral patterns may be secondary to myofascial trigger points or referred pain from cervical zygapophyseal joints. Widespread pain may implicate fibromyalgia syndrome, rheumatologic disease such as mild systemic lupus erythematosus, polyarticular osteoarthritis, rheumatoid arthritis, polymyalgia rheumatica, hypermobility syndromes, and even osteomalacia. Nonrheumatologic syndromes must also be considered in patients presenting with widespread pain. These include neoplastic and neurologic diseases, hypothyroidism, and other endocrine disorders, chronic infections, and a variety of psychiatric conditions.[23]

Location of the patient's pain cannot in isolation lead to a correct diagnosis. All aspects of the history of present illness, past medical and surgical history, family history of hereditary illness, social, occupational, behavioral, psychologic, and demographic information are necessary to identify predisposing factors or

progressive neurologic and cognitive deficits accompanied by hemodynamic instability may also present with dissecting vertebral and extracranial carotid artery aneurysms.[20,21] Other red flags include significant head trauma in the presence of a neurologic deficit. Night pain or unrelenting pain with associated weight loss is suggestive of a neoplastic or infectious process.

mechanisms of injury. A review of systems and detailed physical exam are essential to rule out manifestations of systemic disease and presence or absence of significant neurologic deficits. Even then, further diagnostic tests as well as pharmacologic and interventional trials may be required in complex cases to confirm or rule out etiologic hypothesis.

Onset

Acute onset of pain may occur after trauma, injury, or following an unaccustomed increase in activity in a deconditioned patient; however, an acute exacerbation of a chronic condition cannot be excluded. More gradual or insidious onset is common in progressive degenerative, inflammatory, or malignant process. It is important to elicit the time at which the pain first occurred, characteristics of the pain during the interval between onset, and evaluation of precipitating events or factors.

Intensity and Pattern of Severity With Time. A cardinal principle of diagnosis is assessment of the intensity of pain both at baseline and in response to time, activities, and treatment. Although the visual analogue or numerical rating pain score system is subjective and may be influenced by psychologic, social, and occupational factors, it is essential to evaluate the trend of each patient's pain over time in order to assess the effects of pharmacologic, psychologic, behavioral, physical, and interventional therapies. Patterns of pain severity over time are often associated with certain diseases. Chronic unrelenting pain may be due to inflammatory disease or a more centralized pain syndrome. Pain due to cervical spondylosis and stenosis may be severe with activities requiring neck flexion and rotation and absent or significantly reduced when the patient's neck is held in a neutral position. Patient complaint of night pain or pain of spontaneous onset which is constant and not relieved by rest or modified by movement may raise suspicion for an infectious or neoplastic process.

Quality. Electrical, shooting, stabbing, lancinating, burning, tingling, and pins and needles are common terms used to describe neuropathic pain. Dull, aching, cramping, or throbbing pain is more often associated with pain of a musculoskeletal nature. Stiffness is often described in association with degenerative arthritis or diffuse idiopathic skeletal hyperostosis (DISH). It is not unusual for the patient to include sensory changes (numbness, pins and needles, or burning) as well as cramping and aching pain in their description of cervical radiculopathy. This is most likely due to both the cutaneous or dermatomal and muscular or myotomal distribution of the cervical nerve roots. Burning pain associated with allodynia and thermohyperesthesia suggests Complex Regional Pain Syndrome (CRPS). The more chronic the pain condition, the more likely the patient will report a poorly localized, widespread, nondermatomal pain pattern due to changes in central pain processing known to occur following persistent painful peripheral input.[24]

Modifying Factors and Drug History

Asking the patient the question, "What makes your pain better or worse?" will assist in further narrowing of the differential diagnosis. Coughing or sneezing and lateral head rotation and extension may cause exacerbation of cervical radicular pain. Chronic inflammatory pain is often worse after a period of inactivity and improves with exercise. Degenerative arthritis is often exacerbated by exercise and improves with rest. In patients with multiple pain complaints, response to medication may help guide diagnosis. In patients who have failed multiple medication trials, it is important to elicit specific reactions to medications, duration of use, dosages reached, and titration schedules implemented. An elderly patient, for example, who gives a history of intolerable sedation with an antiepileptic medication, may have been started at a standard adult dose and subsequently titrated upward using an aggressive titra-

tion schedule. This patient may be able to benefit from this same medication if it is titrated more gradually from a low dose.

Associated Symptoms

A history of neck and arm pain associated with frequently dropping objects, difficulty with writing, or other fine motor skills is useful in separating motor weakness from guarding secondary to pain. Associated symptoms may help to broaden or further refine the differential diagnosis. A patient with neck and arm pain which occurs with increased activity and is associated with diaphoresis and shortness of breath may broaden the differential diagnosis to include coronary artery disease. Indeed, the first clinical description of cervical radiculopathy by Semmes and Murphy in 1943 was titled, "The syndrome of unilateral rupture of the sixth cervical vertebral disc with compression of the seventh cervical root: a report of four cases with symptoms simulating coronary disease."[25] Association of neck and radicular arm pain with positional headaches accompanied with nausea, photophobia, and blurred vision may lead the physician to rule out low pressure headache.[26]

Family History

In addition to more common hereditary arthritides such as rheumatoid arthritis (more common in females), ankylosing spondylitis (predominantly seen in males), psoriatic arthritis, and Reiter's syndrome, there are also more uncommon hereditary diseases which can involve the cervical spine. Compression of the cervical cord from cervical root neurofibromas in patients with neurofibromatosis type 1 has been reported to present with progressive neurologic deficit.[27] Tophaceous gout of the odontoid process and larynx, epidural, mediastinal, and subcutaneous emphysema in a patient with Marfan's disease following forceful coughing, and cervical dystonia in spinocerebellar ataxia type 2 are other inherited disorders manifesting with neck pain.[28–31]

Age and Psychosocial History

The patient's age, sex, occupational, and social history is important in determining risk factors known to be associated with the development of persistent neck and upper limb pain. While sports or trauma injury and congenital defects such as Chiari I malformations are common causes of neck pain in pediatric or adolescent patients, degenerative changes are common in older patients. Jobs or activities which require repeated lifting of heavy objects, prolonged bending of the neck, working with arms at/above shoulder height, and which involve little job control and little social support are associated with the development of neck pain. Specific jobs and activities associated with the development of neck pain include prolonged computer work and bicycling.[16,17,32] Extensive neck and upper extremity pain is independently associated with psychologic ill-health, female sex, unemployed status, and smoking.[18]

Questions regarding use of pillows at night and bifocals as well as any other activities which put the patient's neck under prolonged flexion strain should be included in the social and occupational history. In some cases, simple correction of repetitive strain with postural reeducation may result in relief of symptoms.

Depression and anxiety may occur as a reaction to persistent pain and are also independent risk factors for the development of chronic pain. The depressed individual may lack the psychologic and social capabilities to cope with the complex physical, emotional, cognitive, and behavioral components of the pain experience.[33] Patients with coexisting histories of depression and anxiety may benefit from referral to a psychopharmachologist and from psychologic consultation for cognitive and behavioral therapies to assist the patient with coping strategies.

Past Medical History and Review of Systems

The past medical history, past surgical history, and review of systems may provide essential clues tying the patient's symptoms to an associated disease process. Table 68.8 lists a few coexisting diseases which may present with neck pain and radiculopathy, while Table 68.9 lists a review of systems checklist which may identify systemic involvement or an urgent, rapidly progressing process.

Surgical History

A past surgical history of neck fusion may signal risk of pseudoarthrosis or increased risk of recurrent disk disease above or below the level of fusion. Poststernotomy lesions following cardiac surgery with the clinical appearance of a C8 radiculopathy have been described. The causal mechanism is thought to be related to an occult fracture of the first thoracic rib. These are often mistaken for ulnar neuropathy at the elbow thought to be associated with surgical positioning.[34]

Physical Examination

General Observations. Many important observations can be made during the initial interview and even as the patient travels from the waiting area to the exam room. The general health and independence of the patient can be surmised from skin and muscle tone, posture, gait, and use of assistive devices. Cachexia may be a sign of debilitation due to cancer or long-standing depression. Mood, affect, and cognitive state can be ascertained during questioning as well as during the physical exam. Other important general observations include symmetry of the shoulders, abnormal head positions including lateral flexion, rotation or protrusion and evidence of muscle wasting or deformity of the neck, shoulders, or upper limbs.

A complete physical exam is paramount in the patient with neck, shoulder, and arm pain. Inspection of the skin for lesions may reveal psoriasis which may be associated with psoriatic arthritis. Vesicles typifying herpes zoster may be found in a patient complaining of radicular symptoms. Lesions typical of erythema nodosum may be indicative of inflammatory disease or cancer, and needle marks (intravenous drug abuse) may raise suspicion for vertebral column infections. Acute pain from viscera sharing the same embryologic segmental derivation as the cervical spine can present as neck, shoulder, or arm pain. These include the submandibular glands, lymph nodes, thyroid, esophagus, heart, lungs, stomach, gallbladder, pancreas, and diaphragm, necessitating a general inspection and palpation of these areas.[35] In general, a systematic approach which includes a neurologic exam, inspection, palpation of bony and soft tissue structures, followed by range of motion and special tests used in the diagnosis of

TABLE 68.8

NONCOMPRESSIVE INFECTIOUS, INFLAMMATORY, AND NEOPLASTIC CAUSES OF NECK PAIN AND RADICULOPATHY

Infection (most common in immune suppressed patients)
  Herpes Zoster, human immunodeficiency virus, Cytomegalovirus, Tuberculosis, Borrelia burgdorferi (Lyme disease)

Inflammatory
  Systemic lupis Erythematosus, Sarcoidosis, Bruns-Garland syndrome (diabetic radiculopathy), Parsonage-Turner syndrome (Neuralgic amyotrophy), Multiple Sclerosis "pseudopolyneuropathy," Gout

TABLE 68.9

A COMPREHENSIVE CHECKLIST OF ASSOCIATED FEATURES OF NECK PAIN THAT MIGHT INDICATE A RED FLAG CONDITION

System	Past History	Symptoms of	Feature or Condition
Nervous	Yes / No	Yes / No	Weakness
	Yes / No	Yes / No	Numbness
	Yes / No	Yes / No	Bladder dysfunction
	Yes / No	Yes / No	Impaired balance
	Yes / No	Yes / No	Impaired vision
	Yes / No	Yes / No	Altered Speech
	Yes / No	Yes / No	Disorientation
	Yes / No	Yes / No	Altered
	Yes / No	Yes / No	consciousness
Cardiovascular	Yes / No	Yes / No	Risk factors
	Yes / No	Yes / No	Chest pain
	Yes / No	Yes / No	Anticoagulants
	Yes / No	Yes / No	Transient ischemic attacks
Respiratory	Yes / No	Yes / No	Carcinoma
	Yes / No	Yes / No	Tuberculosis
	Yes / No	Yes / No	Cough
	Yes / No	Yes / No	Weight loss
Alimentary	Yes / No	Yes / No	Carcinoma
	Yes / No	Yes / No	Weight loss
	Yes / No	Yes / No	Loss of appetite
	Yes / No	Yes / No	Dysphagia
	Yes / No	Yes / No	Diarrhea
	Yes / No	Yes / No	Altered bowel habits
Urinary	Yes / No	Yes / No	Incontinence
	Yes / No	Yes / No	Obstruction
Reproductive	Yes / No	Yes / No	Breast lump
	Yes / No	Yes / No	Uterine dysfunction
Endocrine	Yes / No	Yes / No	Thyroid cancer
	Yes / No	Yes / No	Hyperparathyroidism
Reticulo-endothelial	Yes / No	Yes / No	Lymph nodes
Skin	Yes / No	Yes / No	Rash
Musculoskeletal	Yes / No	Yes / No	Other joint pain
Age	Yes / No	Yes / No	Other muscle pain
	Yes / No	Yes / No	Risk of Paget's disease
	Yes / No	Yes / No	Risk of myeloma

From Bogduk N. The neck. *Baillieres Clin Rheumatol* 1999;13(2):261–262, with permission.

neck pain should supplement, but not replace, the full physical examination.

Exam of the Neck.

Neurologic exam. Examination of the neck must include a neurologic exam. Tumors, infections, and carotid dissections which present as neck pain are also associated with cranial nerve palsies and sensory deficits. Delay in recognition of neurologic deficits in these cases can lead to progression of tumor or infection with poor surgical or medical outcome and prognosis.[36–38] A summary of the motor, sensory, and autonomic functions of the cranial nerves is found in Table 68.10.

In addition to examination of the cranial nerves, general head,

TABLE 68.10

SUMMARY OF THE MOTOR, SENSORY, AND AUTONOMIC FUNCTIONS OF THE CRANIAL NERVES

Cranial Nerve (CN)	Cranial Point Exit	Peripheral Innervation of Head	Function	Symptom/Sign of Damage
Olfactory (CNI)	Cribiform plate	Mucosa of nasal cavity	Smell	Anosmia
Optic (CNII)	Optic foramen	Retina of eye	Vision	Blindness
Occulomotor (CNIII)	Superior orbital fissure	All extraocular eye muscles except superior oblique and lateral rectus	Eye movement (elevation, adduction)	Eye deviates down and out Loss of papillary accommodation reflexes
Trochlear (CNVI)	Superior orbital fissure	Superior oblique (extraocular eye muscle)	Eye movement (depression of adducted eye)	Diplopia, lateral deviation of eye
Trigeminal (CNV)	V1-Superior orbital fissure V2-Foramen rotundum V3-foramen ovale	V1-Cutaneous sensation of nose, eyes, and scalp V2-Sensation of face: maxilla, nasal mucosa, upper lip, and teeth V3-Cutaneous sensation of lower face: mouth mucosa, lower jaw teeth, TMJ, anterior two-thirds of tongue Motor supply to muscles of mastication	Facial sensation mastication	Facial anesthesia Loss of pain sensation Weakness/loss of mastication
Abducent (CNVI)	Superior orbital fissure	Lateral rectus (extraocular eye muscle)	Eye movement (abduction)	Medial eye deviation
Facial (CNVII)	Entry: Internal acoustic meatus Exit: stylomastoid foramen	Motor: muscles of facial expression and scalp	Facial expression Taste Salivation, lacrimation	Paralysis of facial muscles Loss of taste (anterior two-thirds of tongue) Dry mouth, loss of lacrymation
Vestibulocochlear (CNVIII)	Internal acoustic meatus	Inner ear labyrinth structures (semicircular canal and cochlear apparatus)	Balance hearing	Vertigo, disequilibrium, Nystagmus, hearing loss
Glossopharyngeal (CNIX)	Jugular Foramen	Posterior one-third of tongue Parotid gland Mucosa and elevator muscles of pharynx	Taste salivation Innervation of pharynx	Loss of taste (Posterior one-third of tongue) Loss of gag reflex
Vagus (CNX)	Jugular foramen	Palatal muscles, pharyngeal constrictors, vocal cords Taste and sensation to epiglottis	Swallowing and talking Cardiac, gastrointestinal tract Respiration Taste	Dysphagia and hoarseness Loss of cough reflex, loss of taste
Cranial accessory	Jugular foramen	Motor supply to larynx and pharynx	Pharynx/larynx muscles	Head turning
Spinal accessory (CNXI)		Head rotation and shoulder shrugging	Trapezius, Sternocleidomastoid	Shoulder shrug weakness
Hypoglossal (Xii)	Hypoglossal canal	Intrinsic and some extrinsic tongue muscles	Tongue movement	Atrophy of tongue muscles, deviation on protrusion, Fasciculations

neck, and upper extremity sensory, motor and deep tendon exam, sensory, motor, and deep tendon exam of the lower extremities is essential. Exam findings signaling a possible cervical myelopathy include unilateral or bilateral spastic, ataxic, spastic-ataxic or Trendelenberg gait, hyperreflexia of lower extremity deep tendon reflexes and Babinsky sign, and decreased sphincter tone or loss of the anal "wink."

Sensory exam. The sensory exam is particularly useful in the patient with neuropathic pain. Sensory testing should include brush touch for allodynia, light pressure for tenderness and hyperalgesia, palpation for painful areas, as well as vibration, hot, cold, and sharp versus dull discrimination. Positive sensations, stimulus-evoked hypersensitivities such as allodynia to innocuous stimulation including light touch and cold, and hyperalgesia to noxious stimulation such as pinprick, occur focally in mononeuropathies and distally and symmetrically in polyneuropathies. In neuropathic pain syndromes such as CRPS, allodynia, and hyperalgesia may spread outside the area of the original injury or to homologous sites in the opposite limb. These sensory findings are often associated with focal autonomic abnormalities such as sweating, skin temperature and color changes, and edema are also present in CRPS. In central pain and anesthesia dolorosa, allodynia, hyperalgesia, and aftersensation (persistence of pain after the stimulus has ceased) can occur in areas demonstrated to have loss of sensation. In small fiber neuropathies, loss of thermal, pain, and sometimes touch perception with sparing of large-fiber functions such as muscle strength, deep tendon reflexes, and vibratory and proprioceptive perception is seen. These functions are all compromised in combined large- and small-fiber polyneuropathies.[39] The sensory exam should include evaluation for dermatomal patterns of sensory abnormality and for altered sensation in peripheral nerve distributions in patients with suspected peripheral nerve injury or entrapment syndromes. A "cord" level of sensory disturbance may be confined to the upper extremities due to "central cord syndrome" with involvement of decussating anterior sensory fibers.[40]

Motor exam. Motor exam is tested using the standard muscle strength scale from 0–5 (Table 68.11).

In addition to testing of motor function of the cranial nerves, myotomal or segmental nerve root motor supply should be systematically evaluated (Table 68.12).

Deficits consistent with peripheral nerve lesions or injury should also be ruled out (Table 68.13).

Reflex testing should include upper and lower extremities since lesions of the cervical spine may manifest with hypoactive reflexes at the level of the lesion, hyperactive reflexes below the lesion, and pathologic reflexes. Cutaneous reflexes will also be lost below the lesion. Reflexes are tested using the following standard scale:

- 0: absent reflex
- 1+: trace or seen only with reinforcement
- 2+: normal

TABLE 68.11

MUSCLE STRENGTH GRADING

Grade 0: Total paralysis
Grade 1: Palpable or visible contraction
Grade 2: Full range of motion with gravity eliminated
Grade 3: Full range of motion against gravity
Grade 4: Full range of motion with decreased strength
Grade 5: Normal strength
NT: Not testable

TABLE 68.12

SEGMENTAL MOTOR FUNCTION EVALUATION

C2: Breathing
C3-C4: Spontaneous breathing, trapezius function
C4–C6: Shoulder flexion, extension
Upper Extremity Strength
C5: Deltoid abduction at shoulder
C6: Biceps flexion at forearm
C6: Wrist extension (extensor carpi radialis)
C7: Wrist flexion
C7: Elbow extension (triceps)
C7: Finger extension
C8: Fingers flexion middle finger (flex dig profundus)
T1: Small finger abductors (abductor digiti minimi)
T1: Interossei (spread fingers)

- 3+: brisk
- 4+: nonsustained clonus (i.e., repetitive vibratory movements)
- 5+: sustained clonus

1+, 2+, or 3+ reflex are considered normal unless there is a significant difference between sides. 0, 4+, and 5+ are considered abnormal.

Upper extremity normal and pathologic reflexes are outlined in Table 68.14.

Inspection and palpation. After observation for abnormal posture such as abnormal loss of cervical lordosis, torticollis, and obvious atrophic musculature of the neck or upper extremity, the patient should be asked to lay supine to relax the musculature of the neck. This allows optimal examination of the boney structures of the neck.[35] While standing at the patient's side, one hand supports the neck from behind while the other is used to palpate the anterior neck structures.

The most superior boney structure of the anterior neck is the hyoid bone. It is the only bone in the skeletal structure not articulated to any other bone. It supports the root of the tongue and in turn is supported by the muscles of the neck and suspended by the stylohyoid ligaments from the styloid processes of the temporal bones. The body of the hyoid bone is palpated in the midline while the lesser and greater cornu are palpated laterally to each side of the body forming a horseshoe-like structure. The hyoid bone lies at the lower level of C3 or at the intervertebral disk between C3 and C4. Although injuries of the hyoid bone are rare outside of strangulation, fractures of the hyoid due to trauma, cardiopulmonary resuscitation, and sports injuries have been reported with complications including carotid pseudoaneurysm, pharyngeal laceration, and airway compromise.[41–44] Insertion tendonitis of the hyoid bone has also been reported as an unrecognized source of neck pain with recognizable radiologic features.[45] Below the hyoid bone, at the level of C4 to C5, is the thyroid cartilage. The first cricoid ring forms the upper border of the trachea. It lies at the level of C6. The carotid tubercle, also known as Chassaignac's tubercle, is the anterior tubercle of the C6 trans-

TABLE 68.13

MANIFESTATIONS OF PERIPHERAL NERVE INJURIES OF UPPER EXTREMITIES

Ulnar nerve: Claw hand
Radial nerve: Wrist drop
Median nerve: Cannot make "OK" sign

TABLE 68.14

UPPER EXTREMITY DEEP TENDON REFLEXES AND PATHOLOGIC REFLEXES

Reflex	Nerve Root or Function Tested	Location	Response
Scapulohumeral reflex	Tests integrity of cord segments from C4-C6	Lower aspect of medial border of scapula	Adduction and lateral rotation of the arm
Biceps reflex	C5, C6	Tap thumb placed over biceps tendon in antecubital fossa	Flexion of forearm
Brachioradialis reflex	C6	Proximal to radial aspect of wrist	Radial and dorsiflexion at wrist
Triceps reflex	C7	Tendon of triceps muscle as it crosses olecranon fossa	Extension at elbow
Hoffman's sign (pathologic if positive; upper extremity equivalent of Babinsky sign)	Test for upper motor neuron lesion	Patient's long finger in slight extension. DIP flicked downward by examiner's thumb	Involuntary flexion of thumb and little finger to make "OK" sign
Jaw reflex	Upper motor neuron lesions	Tap finger placed over mental area of chin	Jaw closing (abnormal if hyperactive)
Chvosteck's sign (pathologic if positive)	Hypocalcemia or other metabolic abnormality	Tap over facial nerve anterior to ear	Hyperactive response

DIP, Distal interphalangeal joint.

verse process and can be palpated approximately 3 cm lateral to the first cricoids ring. The carotid arteries overlie the tubercles. Caution should be taken to examine the carotid pulses individually to prevent bradycardia and/or syncope.

Soft tissues of the anterior neck include the H-shaped thyroid gland which extends from the thyroid cartilage cranially to the fourth to sixth tracheal rings inferiorly. This area should be inspected to preclude generalized enlargement of the gland and palpated to exclude thyroid masses. The exam should include inspection for palpable lymph nodes which may be due to infection or metastatic disease. Unknown primary carcinoma presents as painless enlarged cervical lymph nodes and accounts for approximately 5% of all head and neck malignancies. If malignancy is suspected, the patient should be referred for more advanced imaging and diagnostic testing.[46] By having the patient turn their head to the opposite side, the sternocleidomastoid muscle may be examined from the origins on the sternum and clavicle to its insertion on the mastoid process of the temporal bone. The anterior border of this muscle from origin to insertion defines the lateral limit of the anterior triangle of the neck and the posterior border, the anterior limit of the posterior triangle of the neck. The exam should include palpation for painful or painless masses, trigger points with associated referral patterns, and pain associated with swallowing.

Palpation of the boney landmarks of the posterior cervical spine includes the inion or external occipital protuberance in the midline, which makes the midpoint of the superior nuchal line extending laterally from the inion bilaterally. The occipital nerves run medial to the occipital arteries over the occiput approximately 3 cm from the midline. Tenderness or pain with examination of this area may be seen with occipital neuralgia. Palpation of the cervical spine is performed in a systematic way, starting with the spinous processes, and followed by the zygapophyseal joints. Pain over the midline structures may indicate a structural problem of the cervical spine. The zygapophyseal joints are located 2–3 cm from the midline. Palpation of the lateral atlantoaxial joint of C1-C2 is undertaken by rotating the patient's head to the ipsilateral side. C2, C3, C4, and C5 are usually difficult to palpate because of the normal cervical lordosis but can be easily identified if it is remembered that the C3-C4 joint is at the level of the hyoid bone and the C4-C5 joint is at the superior

aspect of the thyroid cartilage. The C6 spinous process can be easily identified as it is usually easily palpable and disappears under the examining finger on extension of the neck. The level of the C6-C7 joint can also be confirmed by its location at the level of the cricoid ring. The largest "fixed" prominence is the spinous process of C7. Referral patterns from the zygapophyseal joints have recently been studied in patients with neck, head, and shoulder pain with the most common referral patterns based on areas in which patients are relieved of pain by controlled blocks are depicted in Figures 68.28 through 68.33.[47]

Examination of the soft tissues of the posterior neck includes palpation of the suboccipital muscles and trapezius which, like the sternocleidomastoid, may be a source of cervicogenic headache. The trapezius extends from the external occipital protuberance, the medial third of the superior nuchal line of the

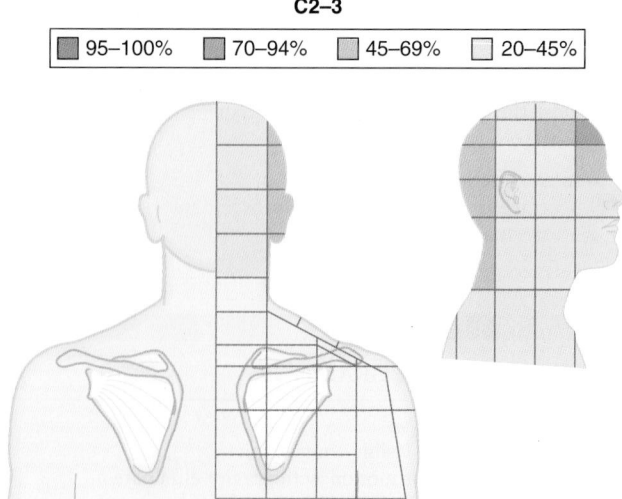

FIGURE 68.28 Distribution of pain and pain frequency in each grid area as reported by patients with pain originating from C2-C3. (From Cooper G, Bailey B, Bogduk N. Cervical zygapophysial joint pain maps. *Pain Medicine* 2007;8[4]:344–853, with permission.)

C3–4

| ■ 95–100% | ■ 70–94% | ☐ 45–69% | ☐ 20–45% |

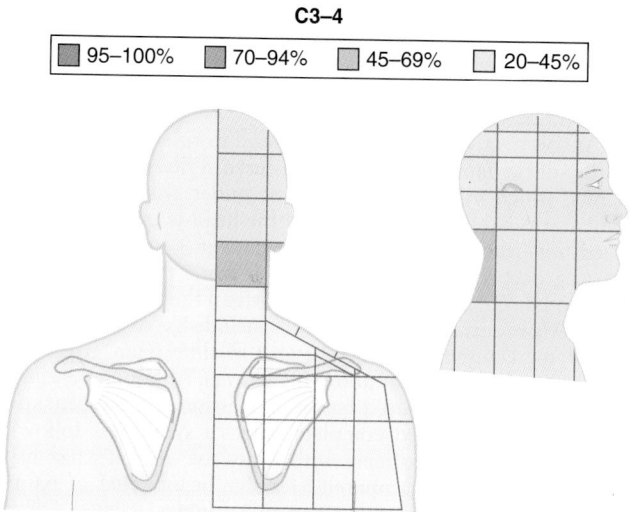

FIGURE 68.29 Distribution of pain and pain frequency in each grid area as reported by patients with pain originating from C3-C4. (From Cooper G, Bailey B, Bogduk N. Cervical zygapophysial joint pain maps. *Pain Medicine* 2007;8[4]:344–853, with permission.)

C5–6

| ■ 95–100% | ■ 70–94% | ☐ 45–69% | ☐ 20–45% |

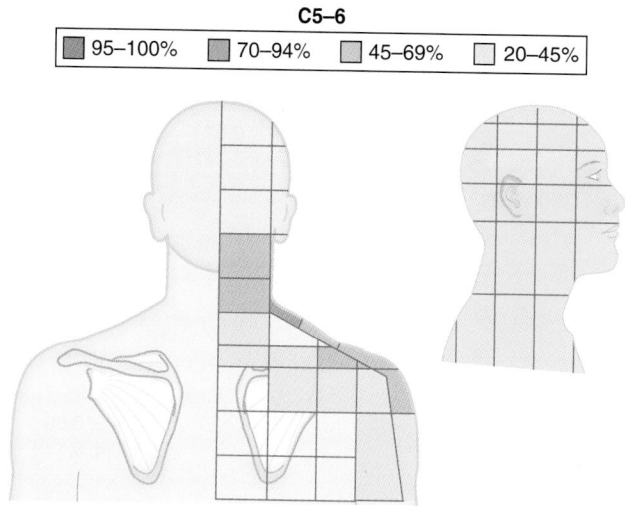

FIGURE 68.31 Distribution of pain and pain frequency in each grid area as reported by patients with pain originating from C5-C6. (From Cooper G, Bailey B, Bogduk N. Cervical zygapophysial joint pain maps. *Pain Medicine* 2007;8[4]:344–853, with permission.)

occipital bone, the ligamentum nuchae, spinous processes of the seventh cervical, and all thoracic vertebrae to the posterior border of the lateral third of the clavicle, the medial margin of the acromion, and the posterior border of the scapular spine. The scalene muscles should be not be neglected in patients with neck, arm, and head ache. Neck pain, occipital headache, extremity paresthesia, pain, and weakness may occur from scarring of the scalene muscles secondary to neck trauma such as whiplash injuries.[48] As with examination of the anterior neck, a chain of lymphnodes lies along the anterolateral border of the trapezius. Enlargement or tenderness of these may indicate infection or metastatic disease.

Special tests for neck and upper extremity
SPURLING'S MANEUVER. This maneuver is used to confirm the presence of a cervical radiculopathy. It is performed by extending

and rotating the head to the right or left. This narrows the intervertebral foramen by 20% to 30%. It has been shown to have a sensitivity of 30% and a specificity of 93% on 235 individuals referred for electrodiagnosis of upper extremity nerve pain.[49] It also increases pressure on the cervical facet joints and may intensify facet mediated pain.

VALSALVA TEST. This test is performed by having the patient place their thumb in their mouth and blow, as if to push the thumb out of their mouth. This maneuver increases the intraspinal pressure and may reveal the presence of space-occupying lesions of the cervical spine such as large intervertebral disk herniations, tumors, and stenosis due to spondylosis or osteophytes. If the mass involves the area of the spine adjacent to nerve roots, radicular pain may be reproduced.

DISTRACTION TEST. This test reduces pressure on the intervertebral disk and exiting nerve roots and simulates the effect that traction may have on treatment of neck and radicular symptoms.

C4–5

| ■ 95–100% | ■ 70–94% | ☐ 45–69% | ☐ 20–45% |

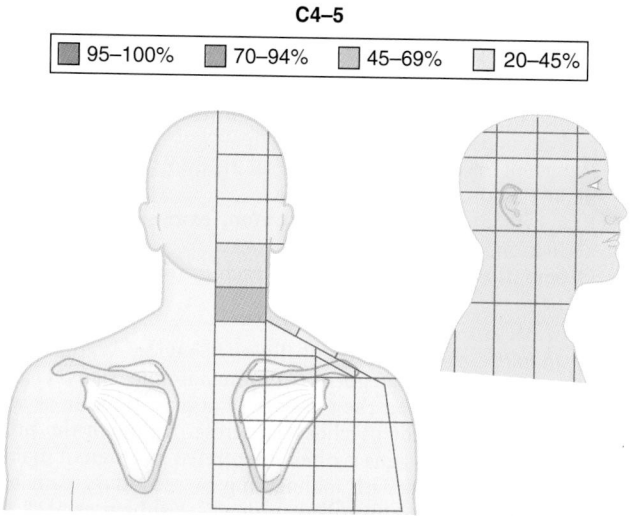

FIGURE 68.30 Distribution of pain and pain frequency in each grid area as reported by patients with pain originating from C4-C5. (From Cooper G, Bailey B, Bogduk N. Cervical zygapophysial joint pain maps. *Pain Medicine* 2007;8[4]:344–853, with permission.)

C6–7

| ■ 95–100% | ■ 70–94% | ☐ 45–69% | ☐ 20–45% |

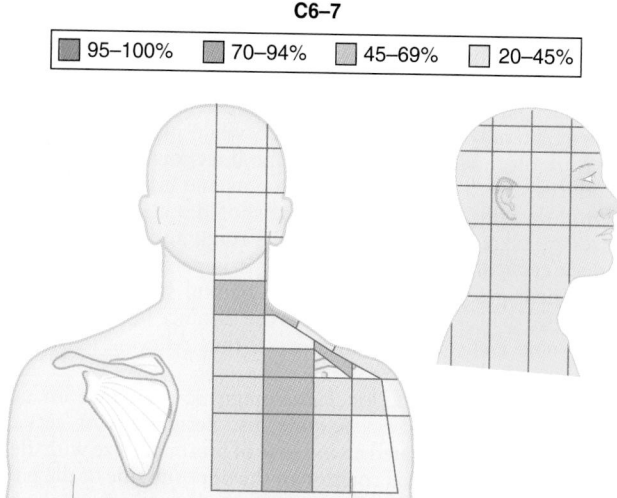

FIGURE 68.32 Distribution of pain and pain frequency in each grid area as reported by patients with pain originating from C6-C7. (From Cooper G, Bailey B, Bogduk N. Cervical zygapophysial joint pain maps. *Pain Medicine* 2007;8[4]:344–853, with permission.)

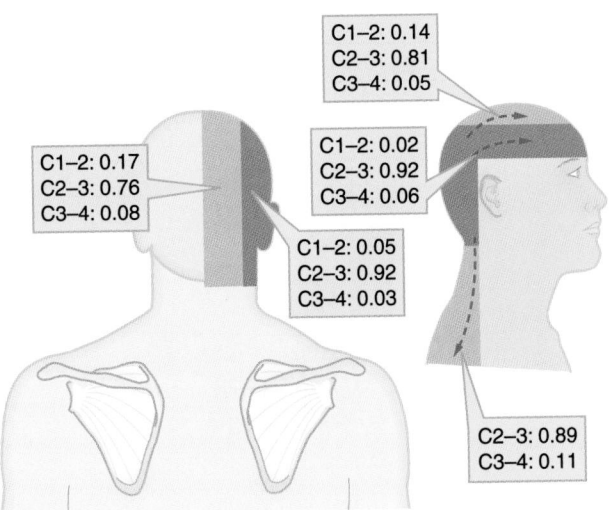

C1–2: 0.14
C2–3: 0.81
C3–4: 0.05

C1–2: 0.17
C2–3: 0.76
C3–4: 0.08

C1–2: 0.02
C2–3: 0.92
C3–4: 0.06

C1–2: 0.05
C2–3: 0.92
C3–4: 0.03

C2–3: 0.89
C3–4: 0.11

FIGURE 68.33 The probability of neck and head pain in areas depicted being secondary to C1-C2, C2-C3 and C3-C4 segments. (From Cooper G, Bailey B, Bogduk N. Cervical zygapophysial joint pain maps. *Pain Medicine* 2007;8[4]:344–853, with permission.)

It is performed by placing one hand underneath the jaws, the other beneath the occiput, and applying gentle upward pressure over 30–60 seconds. Increased pain with this maneuver may be due to inflammatory or degenerative disease, or muscle or ligamentous pathology.

JACKSON'S COMPRESSION TEST. As with Spurling's Maneuver, this test places increased pressure on the cervical facet joints and causes narrowing of the neural foramen. It may reproduce neck pain due to facet arthropathy and/or upper extremity radicular pain due to nerve root compression. To perform this test, the patient is instructed to rotate his or her head first to the right and then to the left. The examiner exerts gentle pressure to the top of the patient's head after each movement.

LHERMITTE'S SIGN. Lhermitte's sign is the production of a sensation of lightening-like paresthesias or dysesthesias in the arms or legs upon flexion of the cervical spine. It may be caused by a large disc herniation or boney compression of the anterior cord in patients with a narrowed central canal. It may also occur in patients with rheumatoid arthritis with associated instability or in patients with multiple sclerosis affecting the cervical spinal cord, tumors, and syringomyelia.[50]

SHOULDER DEPRESSION AND ABDUCTION TESTS. The shoulder depression and abduction tests are useful for evaluation of radicular pain. The shoulder depression test is performed by having the patient laterally flex his or her neck while placing downward pressure on the shoulder opposite the direction of flexion. This produces stretch on irritated nerve roots and may accentuate or reproduce radicular symptoms. The shoulder abduction test relieves pressure on the cervical nerve roots and may relieve or reduce cervical radicular symptoms. It is performed by having the patient place the hand from the painful side on the top of their head. This maneuver shortens the distance between the cervical spine and the coracoid process, thus relieving tension on the nerve root.

In vivo studies using kinematic magnetic resonance imaging of 21 patients with cervical spine disc herniations or cervical spondylosis demonstrated an increase of foraminal size with flexion combined with axial rotation to the opposite side of the pain. Foraminal size decreased at extension combined with axial rotation to the side of the pain. A decrease or no change of foraminal size was observed at either extension or axial rotation to the side of the pain alone. Cervical cord rotation or displacement was noted with axial rotation in 24% of these patients.[51] Active versus

passive range-of-motion testing is advised in patients with neurologic symptoms or those at risk of instability of the cervical spine (i.e., patients with progressive rheumatoid arthritis involving the cervical spine). In these patients, limitation of active range of motion due to pain may be protective.

ADSON'S MANEUVER. This test is used to rule out compression of the subclavian artery by an extra cervical rib or scalene muscle bands, which may result in thoracic outlet syndrome. The patient's arm hangs at their side and the head is extended and rotated toward the affected side. The patient is then instructed to breathe deeply and hold their breath while the radial pulse is monitored. The test is considered positive if the radial pulse disappears. More current testing methods include use of doppler ultrasound to record significant changes in subclavian artery flow characteristics during the above maneuvers. Although the clinical validity of the Adson's test has been questioned,[52] a recent study of 16 patients showed complete relief of symptoms following surgery in 87% of patients with a positive Adson's test using doppler ultrasound compared to a significant relief of pain in only 50% of patients with a negative doppler-assisted Adson's test.[53]

HALSTED MANEUVER (EXAGGERATED MILITARY POSITION). The Halsted maneuver is a test of neurovascular compression at the costoclavicular space. The patient assumes a military posture with the shoulders rolled backward and downward so to narrow the costoclavicular space. The radial pulse is monitored. The maneuver is considered positive if the radial pulse disappears.

Further diagnostic tests for shoulder pathology are outlined in Table 68.15.

Examination of the Shoulder and Arm. Detailed anatomy of the neck, shoulder, and upper extremities, including normal range-of-motion, is covered in the initial part of this chapter and is essential to understanding the anatomic and functional correlates of this portion of the physical exam. Physical examination of the shoulder, arm, elbow, forearm, wrist, and hand should include:

- Blood pressure
- Inspection of position, shape, muscle atrophy, swelling
- Inspection of skin for allodynia, changes in color, temperature, or trophic changes
- Palpation of muscles and tendon for tenderness, pain, trigger points, dysesthesias, and radiation patterns
- Palpation over joints during range of motion testing for crepitus, popping, or locking
- Active and passive range of motion at shoulder: abduction, adduction, internal and external rotation, flexion, and extension at shoulder
- Other tests for shoulder, see Table 68.15
- Range of motion at forearm: flexion, extension, pronation, and supination
- Range of motion at wrist: dorsal flexion, palmar flexion, ulnar flexion, and radial flexion
- Range of motion of fingers: flexion, extension, adduction, abduction, opponens, and grip
- Observation of effect on pain of each movement

Waddell signs. In their study of illness behavior, Waddell and Main[54] described 5 categories of nonanatomic signs (Table 68.16) and reported that the presence of at least three signs was indicative of significant psychosocial stress. Although the presence of three or more signs is often interpreted as a sign of malingering, no association with malingering or secondary gain has been demonstrated in controlled studies.[55] Fishbain et al.[56] reported that Waddell's signs decreased following comprehensive pain management. Pain behaviors are known to be a means for patients to communicate pain and distress. They can be positively reinforced by attention from family members or by being excused

TABLE 68.15

TESTS USED IN SHOULDER PAIN DIAGNOSIS AND SIGNIFICANCE OF POSITIVE FINDINGS

Test	Maneuver/Description	Diagnosis Suggested by Positive Result
1. Apley scratch test	1. Patient touches superior and inferior aspects of opposite scapula	1. Loss of range of water: rotator cuff problem
2. Neers sign	2. Arm in full flexion	2. Impingement syndrome
3. Hawkin's test	3. Flexion at shoulder to 90 degrees and internal rotation—arm lowered slowly to waist	3. Impingement syndrome
4. Drop-arm test	4. Supraspinatus isolated against resistance	4. Rotator cuff tear
5. Empty can test	5. Hand against back of waist with 90 degrees flexion of elbow	5. Rotator cuff tear
6. Lift-off test	6. Forward elevation to 90 degrees and active adduction	6. Rotator cuff tear (subscapularis)
7. Cross-arm test	6. Shoulder flexion to 90 degrees and 20 degrees adduction, resisting downward force exerted by examiner	7. Acromioclavicular joint
8. O'Brian's test (active compression test)	7. Anterior pressure on humerus with exterior rotation	8. Pain with thumb up may indicate acromioclavicular
9. Apprehension test	8. Post force on humerus with external rotation	9. joint arthritis or injury and thumb down a SLAP lesion
10. Relocation test	9. Pulling downward on elbow or wrist	10. Anterior glenohumeral instability
11. Sulcus sign	10. Elbow flexed to 90 degrees with forearm pronated	11. Anterior glenohumeral instability
12. Yergason's test	11. Elbow flexed to 20–30 degrees with forearm pronated	12. Inferior glenohumeral instability
13. Speed's maneuver	12. Rotation of loaded shoulder from extension to forward flexion	13. Biceps tendon instability or tendonitis
14. Clunk sign	13. Arm elevated to 160 degrees in scapular plane, loaded axially along humerus with maximal internal and external rotation	14. Biceps tendon instability or tendonitis
15. Crank test		15. Labral disorder
		16. Labral tear

from undesirable obligations. Pain behaviors may also be "unlearned," using cognitive and behavioral therapies.[57,58]

Laboratory Evaluation

Pain must be seen as a diagnosis of exclusion, for the consequences of treating pain symptomatically in the face of progressive systemic disease can result in a tragic delay of diagnosis and treatment. In general, laboratory testing is guided by the patient's history of present illness, past medical history, and physical exam. A patient who is systemically ill requires more extensive testing guided by affected organs and systems. For example, patients who are febrile or those with weight loss, anorexia, and other signs suggesting infection or neoplasm would benefit from complete blood count and differential analysis. Those with a history of hepatitis or other risk factors for liver disease would benefit from a liver enzyme panel. Patients with cold intolerance, weight gain, and lethargy should undergo thyroid function test analysis.

Morning stiffness, polyarticular involvement, rigidity, or cutaneous manifestations suggest an inflammatory arthritic component requiring a more extensive rheumatologic evaluation. Patients with a diagnosis of fibromyalgia should undergo testing of both thyroid function and vitamin D levels since hypothyroidism and vitamin D deficiency can both result in diffuse pain syndromes which mimic fibromyalgia.

Laboratory analysis of the erythrocyte sedimentation rate and C-reactive protein may also assist in evaluating inflammatory phenomena such as an autoimmune disease, infection, or neoplasm. These may be significantly elevated with an upward trend in patients who are afebrile, who have a normal white blood cell count, and who culture negative (even in the face of sepsis).[59,60]

Other laboratory tests which may be useful in ruling out systemic disease in select patients include serum calcium, which amongst other diagnoses may be elevated in patients with malignancy, and serum alkaline phosphatase, which is elevated in metastatic spine tumors and Paget's disease.[1]

TABLE 68.16

WADDELL'S SIGNS

1. Superficial and widespread tenderness or nonanatomic tenderness (it's "one" sign).
2. Stimulation tests: Axial loading and pain on simulated rotation (it's another "one" sign).
3. Distracted straight leg raise.
4. Nonanatomic sensory changes: Regional sensory changes and regional weakness (it's another "one" sign).
5. Overreaction.

Radiographic Studies

Diagnostic and functional imaging is covered in detail in Chapters 18 and 19. In general, imaging of the neck and arm should be performed in patients with a history of trauma, persistent or progressive pain, and in patients with neurologic deficits involving the neck and/or upper extremities in order to confirm or rule out treatable organic causes of pain or neurologic deficits and to guide therapeutic decision making.

Although the clinical usefulness of cervical spine radiographs for evaluation of neck pain has been questioned,[61,62] cervical spine fractures occur frequently following relatively minor trauma in the elderly patient[63] with a relative risk of up to three

TABLE 68.17

NEXUS CRITERIA FOR RADIOLOGIC EVALUATION OF THE NECK IN PATIENTS STATUS POST TRAUMA

- No midline cervical tenderness
- No focal neurologic deficit
- Normal alertness
- No intoxication
- No painful, distracting injury

times more fractures in elderly versus younger adults evaluated in the emergency room.[64] Though significant cervical spine injury is infrequent in younger patients, diagnosis is often delayed following motor vehicle and sports trauma. In published series, missed cervical spine injuries following trauma have been reported to occur in 4.6% to 33% of patients.[65,66] C2 and C5-C6 level fractures are the most commonly seen injuries.[67-69] In a recent report of 100 consecutive patients who underwent operative fixation or halo stabilization for cervical spine injuries, 10% of injuries were missed due to failure to perform plain cervical films versus failure of interpretation or failure to utilize more advanced imaging techniques.[68] A recent prospective, multicenter U.S. study designed to validate clinical criteria developed to evaluate patients with neck pain following blunt trauma[70-73] confirmed sensitivity of the set of five criteria (Table 68.17) approaching 100% for clinically important injuries.[74]

Even fewer injuries were missed in a more recent multicenter study, when the Canadian C-spine rule was applied (Fig. 68.34).[75] Anteroposterior, neutral lateral, and odontoid plain film views are recommended. A patient with persistent neck pain or tenderness despite normal plain film radiology or suspected ligamentous injury may benefit from flexion-extension views to evaluate for listhesis or instability. These views may also be helpful in determining the amount of motion occurring with flexion and extension in patients with degenerative spondylolisthesis. Prior to flexion-extension imaging, the patient should perform active range-of-motion in the presence of a physician to confirm that no significant neurologic deficit occurs during these maneuvers.

In patients with chronic neck pain, plain film views can reveal degenerative changes such as loss of disc height, bone spurs, endplate irregularity, and endplate sclerosis. In patients with prior cervical spine fusion, instability secondary to pseudoarthrosis can be appreciated.

Computerized tomography (CT) is recommended for patients with acute or chronic neck pain who have normal plain films and clinically suspected cervical spine pathology or to further define abnormalities seen on plain films.[76] It is also useful for evaluating the size and shape of the spinal canal, facet and uncovertebral joints, and transverse foramina.[77,78] When possible, patients with neurologic deficits or pain due to suspected neurologic or soft tissue injury or pathology should undergo MRI. According to a

systematic analysis and multicenter study comparing CT to MRI for assessment of cervical spine injuries following trauma to the cervical spine, midsagittal T1- and T2-weighted MRI provides an objective, quantifiable, and reliable assessment of spinal cord compression that cannot be adequately assessed by CT alone.[79] MRI and magnetic resonance myelography are comparable to CT myelography in assessing spinal stenosis and spinal nerve roots. Although CT is superior in imaging canal foraminal osteophytes, MRI is superior to CT in assessment of spinal cord gray matter and nerve root signal changes and well as ligamentous and intervertebral disk changes.[80] Use of gadolinium-enhanced MRI in symptomatic patients who have undergone surgery of the cervical spine is valuable in identifying changes consistent with postoperative infection in the acute postoperative period and in defining the extent of epidural scar formation versus reherniation of intervertebral discs in patients with recurrent neck and radicular pain.[81]

If MRI is contraindicated (i.e., due to a pacemaker or spinal cord stimulator), CT using 45-degree oblique reconstruction is superior to sagittal reconstructions oriented at 90 degrees for evaluation of the foramen for bony spurs.[82]

In regard to imaging of the shoulder, a standard series of shoulder radiographs excludes or confirms arthritis, bursitis, tendonitis, calcification, dislocation, tumor, and old or new fractures.[83] CT is useful for diagnosing bony lesions, subtle dislocation, labral tears, and full rotator cuff tears. MRI is more expensive, time consuming, less readily available in some areas, and certain pathologies such as the glenoid labrum and the surrounding ligaments may be difficult to evaluate with MRI. MRI is able to evaluate partial or full rotator cuff tears and has the advantages of noninvasive nature, lack of contrast exposure, non-ionizing radiation, high degree of resolution, and ability to evaluate multiple pathologies.

Ultrasound is used to diagnose rotator cuff tears, is noninvasive, rapid, and relatively inexpensive; however, it has been shown to have more interoperator variability in performance and interpretation of imaging.[83-87]

Advanced imaging as well as electromyography and nerve conduction velocity testing should be performed as needed for the purpose of guiding treatment decision making. Electrodiagnostic evaluation of acute and chronic pain is discussed in Chapter 16.

Multiple plain radiographic views are often needed to visualize the elbow, forearm, wrist, and hand and can also be used to confirm or rule out fractures, tendonitis, and dislocations. Minimal evaluation of the elbow should include anteroposterior views for the distal humerus and proximal forearm, as well as lateral views in maximal flexion and extension. Additional views such as radiocapitellar, cubital tunnel, oblique, and stress views may be utilized based on history or mechanism of injury and physical exam findings.[1]

COMMON CAUSES OF NECK AND ARM PAIN

Mechanical Neck Pain and Cervicogenic Headache

Neck pain from similar mechanisms may be axial, associated with radicular pain, headache, and/or symptoms suggesting spinal cord compression. The complex and highly interdependent structures of the neck may preclude identification of a single pain generator in patients with advanced disease. Muscle and ligamentous injury or pain may result from factors related to posture, poor ergonomics, stress, injury, and/or chronic muscle fatigue. Pain may also result from degenerative changes of the cervical facet joints and discs and atlantooccipital and atlantoaxial joints and irritation, inflammation, and mechanical distortion of the

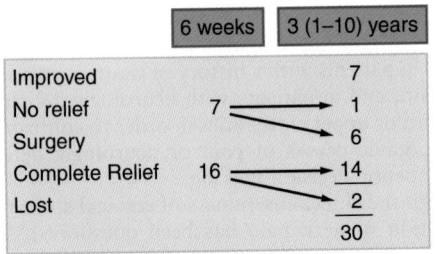

FIGURE 68.34 Canadian C-Spine rule.

cervical nerve roots and spinal cord. These processes may occur independently or concurrently and require a careful history and physical examination together with the judicial use of diagnostic tests to rule out systemic disease and rapidly progressive processes. Recent data reports a 12-month prevalence of 30% to 50% for neck pain and associated disorders in adults.[3] A knowledge and application of recent prospective studies, systemic reviews, and meta-analysis proposing guidelines for evaluation and treatment of these patients may assist with assessing the risk versus benefit for effective conservative versus interventional and surgical therapies in this large and heterogeneous population.

Cervical Spondylosis and Radiculopathy

Degenerative changes of the cervical spine reach a prevalence of nearly 95% by age 65. These changes are associated with positive changes such as disc protrusion, neural foraminal narrowing, and spinal cord contour changes in up to 78% of asymptomatic individuals.[7-9,88] In symptomatic individuals, the risk versus benefit of surgery and other interventional therapy[89] mandates an understanding of the natural course of symptomatic patients with cervical spondylosis and radiculopathy. Although the outcome of these patients when treated conservatively versus surgically is controversial,[90,91] recent investigations reveal clinical and radiographic correlates with outcome in this population, which may be of assistance in timely surgical referral when symptoms continue to progress following conservative treatment.[92-94]

Cervical spondylosis was first distinguished from acute cervical disc protrusion by Brain in 1948.[95] The latter occurs more commonly in individuals younger than age 55, is often traumatic in origin, and most frequently compresses the nerve roots versus the spinal cord. The former is a chronic degenerative condition of the cervical spine associated with formation of osteophytes. It is a universal finding associated with aging and is associated with compression of the spinal cord in most symptomatic cases. Patients older than age 55 are more likely to have central canal or neural foraminal stenosis due to spondylosis.[96] In a population-based study conducted from 1976 to 1990 in Rochester, Minnesota, a confirmed disc herniation was found to account for approximately 20% of all cervical radiculopathies and approximately 70% of all spondylosis. The average age-adjusted incidence rate per 100,000 population was 107.3 for males, 63.5 for females, and reached a peak of 202.9 for the age group between ages 50 to 54.[97,98]

Spondylosis refers to degenerative changes of the spine involving the intervertebral discs, uncovertebral joints of Lushcka, zygapophyseal joints, ligaments, and connective tissue of the cervical vertebrae. Degenerative changes of the cervical spine are seen in approximately 10% of individuals by age 25 and in 95% by age 65. The process is believed to begin with fibrosis and loss of elasticity of the disc which occurs with loss of water, protein, and mucopolysaccharides from the nucleus pulposis. Loss of disc space height initially occurs ventrally and leads to loss of cervical lordosis. This shift of biomechanical forces results in ventral vertebral body compression with resultant pathologic cervical spine kyphosis, dissection of the annulus fibrosus, posterior longitudinal ligament, and Sharpy's fibers away from the edges of the posterior vertebral body, formation of reactive bone on the edges of exposed dorsal vertebral bodies, and increased axial load-bearing by the uncovertebral and zygapophyseal joints, with resultant hypertrophy and osteophytic formation ventral and posterior to the neural foramen.

Spondylotic spurs may eventually span the width of the vertebral canal in some patients. Because the osteophytes form in response to increased motion or segmental instability, the levels most commonly affected, both by disc herniation and chronic spondylosis are C6-C7 followed by C5-C6 since these are the cervical segments at which the most extension and flexion occur.

The reduction in sagittal spinal canal diameter in cervical spondylosis results from a combination of static and dynamic factors. Static reduction of the sagittal diameter of the spinal canal occurs from disc herniation or bulging, vertebral body osteophyte growth into the anterior spinal canal, degenerative hypertrophy of the uncovertebral joints, facet joints, and ligamentum flavum combined with calcification of the posterior longitudinal ligament. The addition of dynamic factors such as flexion, extension, or subluxation can further increase the risk for compression and injury to the contents of the spinal canal and neural foramen including the spinal cord, nerve roots, arteries, and veins. These combined pathologic features are thought to be responsible for the production of the wide spectrum of clinical symptoms associated with cervical spondylosis including neck and shoulder pain, occipital pain and headaches, radicular symptoms, and cervical radiculopathies and cervical spondylotic myelopathy. Compression of the spinal cord may occur from spondylotic bars and calcified posterior longitudinal ligament ventrally or from the hypertrophic ligamentum flavum dorsally. Cumulative repetitive injury to the spinal cord is thought to occur with flexion, due to a "bowstring effect" over the ventral spondylotic bars and kyphotic spine, and compression dorsally by buckling of the ligamentum flavum. MRI flexion and extension studies observed increased cervical stenosis in twice as many patients during extension versus flexion. Risk for compression of the spinal cord is increased in individuals with congenital narrowing of the spinal canal.

Cervical spondylotic myelopathy (CSM) refers to clinically evident spinal cord dysfunction with the presence of long-tract signs due to compression of the spinal cord. Weakness or stiffness in the legs with unsteady gait together with weakness or clumsiness of the hands is pathognomonic of cervical spondylotic myelopathy. Progression of weakness may be gradual in some patients or sudden in others following minor trauma. In a prospective study at a U.K. regional neuroscience center, 23.6% of 585 patients admitted with tetraparesis or paraparesis were found to have cervical spondylotic myelopathy. Some patients may complain of hesitancy on urination; however, loss of sphincter control or urinary incontinence is rare and considered a late sign of myelopathy.

Patients with CSM generally present with neck and shoulder pain and stiffness. The patient may also present with pain in the arm, elbow, wrist, or fingers described as combined or isolated sensations of stabbing, dull, or aching pain. Arm pain may be nondermatomal in distribution and accompanied by numbness or tingling in the hands. Pain which conforms to a dermatomal distribution with associated motor and sensory deficits is referred to a radiculopathy rather than myelopathy. Some patients may present with both myelopathy and radiculopathy.

Signs of CSM on physical exam include an electrical sensation radiating down the back to the legs with flexion of the neck (Lhermitte's sign), atrophy of the intrinsic musculature of the hands, and variable sensory, vibratory, or proprioceptive loss in the extremities. Deep tendon reflexes may be reduced or absent at the level of compression with hyperreflexia below the level of the lesion together with upper motor signs such as clonus, Hoffmann's, and Babinski's sign.[95,99-101]

There are two commonly used classification systems for CSM. The classification of Crandall and Batzdorf[102] divides CSM patients into five groups of spinal cord dysfunction. These include the transverse lesion syndrome, the motor system syndrome, the central cord syndrome, the Brown-Séquard syndrome, and the brachalgia cord syndrome. These are summarized in Table 68.18. Ferguson and Caplan[103] categorize CSM into four overlapping syndromes, which are summarized in Table 68.19.

The differential diagnosis of CSM includes amyotrophic lateral sclerosis, multiple sclerosis, hereditary spastic paraplegia, spinal cord tumors, and subacute combined degeneration of the spinal cord associated with vitamin B12 deficiency.

MRI is the imaging technique of choice for evaluating the

TABLE 68.18

CRANDALL AND BATZDORF[102] CLASSIFICATION OF CLINICAL SYNDROMES IN CERVICAL SPONDYLOTIC MYELOPATHY

Transverse lesion syndrome	Most common lesion. Involves posterior column, spinothalamic and corticospinal tracts, and often anterior horn cells. Posterior column involvement uncommon and late.
Motor system syndrome	Involves anterior horn cells and corticospinal tracts primarily. Little sensory involvement. Upper and lower extremity weakness, gait disturbance, and spasticity.
Central cord syndrome	Upper extremities weaker than lower extremities. Profound hand weakness. Posterior column involved often presenting as painful paresthesias of hands.
Brown-Séquard syndrome	Unilateral spinal cord dysfunction. Involvement of corticospinal tract. Posterior column sensory loss (position, vibration) and long tract motor signs (hemiplegia) are found ipsilateral to the lesion, whereas pain and temperature are lost contralaterally. One or two levels below highest level of motor involvement.
Brachalgia cord syndrome	Upper extremity nerve root compression combined with long tract signs (analogous to Ferguson and Caplan's[103] combined medial and lateral syndrome).

patient with CSM. T2- and T1-weighted signals on MRI have been found to correlate with various degrees of injury to the spinal cord on histologic studies. Edema is seen as a high-intensity T2-weighted image. Necrotic changes in the gray matter correspond to low signals on T1-weighted studies but high signals on T2-weighted studies. T1-weighted hypointensity is an expression of irreversible damage and, therefore, the worst prognosis.[94,104] A less favorable surgical outcome is predicted by the presence of a T1-weighted hypointense signal and the presence of clonus or spasticity. A high intramedullary T2-weighted signal without clonus or spasticity is associated with a more favorable surgical outcome with a greater likelihood of reversal of MRI signal changes.[105] A recent investigation reported multiple regression analysis of various risk factors associated with surgical outcome.

TABLE 68.19

FERGUSON AND CAPLAN[103] CLASSIFICATION OF CLINICAL SYNDROMES IN CERVICAL SPONDYLOTIC MYELOPATHY

Lateral syndrome	Represents a spondylotic radiculopathy. Absence of long tract signs.
Medial syndrome	Upper motor neuron symptoms. Variable weakness of all extremities, gait abnormalities, spasticity below level of compression.
Combined medial and lateral syndrome	Most common clinical presentation.
Vascular syndrome	Acute onset and rapid progression of myelopathy. Thought to represent insufficiency or compression of anterior spinal artery and its branches to the spinal cord.

According to this analysis, the most significant prognostic factor was the transverse area of the spinal cord, followed by the duration of symptoms and the presence of multisegmental areas of high signal intensity on T2-weighted MRI. The latter was associated with upper extremity muscle atrophy and less favorable surgical recovery of neurologic function.[93]

Controversy exists regarding optimal treatment for patients with cervical spondylotic myelopathy, and many authors recommend conservative treatment due to significant risks associated with surgery and lack of data supporting long-term improved outcome in patients undergoing surgery versus conservative care.[106–109] A recent prospective 3-year follow-up study did not show, on average, that the effects of surgery in the treatment of mild and moderate forms of CSM were better than the conservative approach. Nevertheless, there was a slight but statistically significant increase in the number of patients with a negative trend in the score for daily activities in the conservatively treated group. The authors of this study recommend conservative treatment for patients with mild SCM along with careful follow-up evaluation and reassessment 3 months after the start of conservative treatment. Decompression surgery is recommended for patients who experience neurologic deterioration during this period.[90] A prospective, multicenter study with independent clinical review evaluating conservative versus surgical treatment for patients with moderate to severe CSM found that although surgical treatment was not found to improve neurologic outcome, overall pain and functional status improved significantly. When medical and surgical treatments were compared, surgically treated patients appeared to have better outcomes, despite exhibiting a greater number of neurologic and nonneurologic symptoms and greater functional disability before treatment.[91]

Conservative treatment for CSM consists of intermittent cervical immobilization with a soft collar, the use of anti-inflammatory medications, active discouragement of high-risk activities, and avoidance of risky environments involving physical overloading, excess cold, movement on slippery surfaces, manipulation therapies, or vigorous or prolonged flexion of the head. Additional conservative measures include physiotherapy with institution of a rehabilitation program and referral to a multidisciplinary pain team. Patients with moderate to severe symptoms on presentation and progressive neurologic symptoms should be referred for surgical evaluation. The aim of the surgery in these patients is to stop the progression of neurologic deterioration and prevent sudden deterioration after minor injury or in particular situations such as swimming, cycling, and physical overloading.[90,91]

Cervicogenic Headache

The term cervicogenic headache (CEH) was coined by Sjaastad in 1983.[110] He later organized the Cervicogenic Headache International Study Group (CHISG), and diagnostic criteria for CEH were published by the CHISG in 1990.[111] A revision of criteria for CEH was published by the CHISG in 1998.[112]

CEH was recognized as a unique category of headaches by the International Association for the Study of Pain in 1994, using criteria similar to that published by Sjaastad et al.[113] Revised criteria for CEH were published by the International Headache Society (IHS) in 2004.[114]

Although controversy exists regarding the defining characteristics and prevalence of CEH, there is emerging evidence of valid clinical, diagnostic, and therapeutic criteria which differentiates this syndrome from migraine headache, tension-type headache, hemicrania continua, and chronic paroxysmal hemicrania.[115,116]

CEH is defined as unilateral head or face pain which starts in the neck and is triggered by neck movement or sustained awkward neck posture. Although pain begins in the neck or occipital region, it may spread to the retroorbital, temporal, and frontal areas of the head and face where maximum pain may be perceived. Pain may occur to a lesser degree on the contralateral side; however, profound unilateral dominance should exist. Cervicogenic headache is typically described as deep and nonthrobbing with intermittent attacks lasting hours to days. In time, headaches may become constant with superimposed attacks of more intense pain. Pain in CEH should be reproducible upon palpation or stimulation of cervical spine or neck structures. It is accompanied by reduced range of motion of the neck and ipsilateral nonradicular neck, shoulder, or arm pain. Nausea, vomiting, photophobia, dizziness, blurred vision, lacrymation, and conjunctival injection may occur.

The new IHS criteria requires clinical, laboratory, or imaging evidence of a lesion or disorder within the neck or cervical spine known to be associated with the causation of headache. This should be validated by reproducible clinical signs or by controlled diagnostic blockade (Tables 68.20 and 68.21 show comparison of IHS and CHISG criteria for CEH).

TABLE 68.20

INTERNATIONAL HEADACHE SOCIETY DIAGNOSTIC CRITERIA FOR CERVICOGENIC HEADACHE

A. Pain referred from a source in the neck and perceived in one or more regions of the head and/or face fulfilling criteria C and D.
B. Clinical, laboratory, and/or imaging evidence of a disorder or lesion within the cervical spine or soft tissues of the neck known to be, or generally accepted as, a valid cause of headache.
C. Evidence that the pain can be attributed to the neck disorder or lesion based on at least one of the following:
　1. Demonstration of clinical signs that implicate a source of pain in the neck.
　2. Abolition of headache following diagnostic blockade of a cervical structure or its nerve supply using placebo or other adequate controls.
D. Pain resolves within 3 months after successful treatment of the causative disorder or lesion.

TABLE 68.21

CERVICOGENIC HEADACHE INTERNATIONAL STUDY GROUP CERVICOGENIC HEADACHE DIAGNOSTIC CRITERIA[112]

Major Criteria
A. Symptoms and signs of neck involvement; it is obligatory that one or more of the phenomena 1 to 3 are present.
　1) Precipitation of head pain, similar to the usually occurring one:
　　a) By neck movement and/or sustained, awkward head positioning, and/or
　　b) By external pressure over the upper cervical or occipital region on the symptomatic side.
　2) Restriction of the range-of-motion in the neck.
　3) Ipsilateral neck, shoulder, or arm pain of a rather vague, nonradicular nature, or, occasionally, arm pain of a radicular nature.
B. Confirmatory evidence by diagnostic anesthetic blockages.
C. Unilaterality of the head pain, without side shift.

Head Pain Characteristics
D. Moderate–severe, nonthrobbing pain, usually starting in the neck
　Episodes of varying duration, or
　Fluctuating, continuous pain.

Other Characteristics of Some Importance
E. Only marginal effect or lack of effect of indomethacin.
　Only marginal effect or lack of effect of ergotamine and sumatriptan.
　Female sex.
　Not infrequent occurrence of head or indirect neck trauma by history, usually of more than only medium severity.

Other Features of Lesser Importance
F. Various attack-related phenomena, only occasionally present and/or moderately expressed when present.
　1) Nausea
　2) Phono- and photophobia
　3) Dizziness
　4) Ipsilateral "blurred vision"
　5) Difficulties on swallowing
　6) Ipsilateral edema, mostly in the periocular area

The prevalence of CEH in the literature varies widely from 0% to 80%, depending on the population of patients studied, diagnostic criteria, and methodology.[115] A recent Norwegian study reported that 75% of tractor drivers suffered from moderate to severe generalized headache only when working on their tractor because of consecutively turning or twisting their neck for many hours daily.[117] In a series of 100 consecutive patients with neck pain following whiplash, Lord et al.[118] reported a prevalence of associated headache in 88%. Of those patients with headache as the dominant symptom, 54% were found to have neck pain originating from a C2-C3 cervical zygapophyseal joint following diagnostic blocks. This was associated with tenderness over the affected joint on physical examination.[118] In a study of 34 patients with the complaint of headache emanating from the occipital region, tenderness to exam over the tip of the transverse process of C1 and worsening of their usual headache with passive rotation of the C1 vertebra, 60% were found to have complete relief of their pain following diagnostic blockade of the atlantoaxial joint.[119] Pain maps based on regions of the head and neck in which patients were relieved of pain following controlled blocks revealed radiation of pain from the C1-C2 through the C3-C4 facet joints to the suboccipital and occipital regions as well as the vertex, frontal, orbital, and temporoparietal region of the head.[47]

The anatomic basis by which pain from the cervical spine and neck can be perceived in the face and head derives from the convergence of afferents from the trigeminal nerve with those of the first three spinal nerves in the caudal aspect of the trigeminal nucleus in the brainstem.[120,121] Musculoskeletal structures innervated by the first three cervical nerves are outlined in Table 68.22. Convergence with the spinal trigeminal nucleus and the extradural convergence of the first three cervical nerves may account for the difficulty encountered in localizing the pain in patients with CEHs.

The anatomy of the sinuvertebral nerve may also contribute to the variation of pain patterns among patients and the presence of diffuse neck and head pain in the presence of discrete injuries. The sinuvertebral nerves supply structures within the spinal canal. They arise from the rami communicantes and enter the spinal canal by way of the intervertebral foramina. Branches ascend and descend one or more levels, interconnecting with the sinuvertebral nerves from other levels and innervating the anterior and posterior longitudinal ligaments dura mater and blood vessels, as well as sending nociceptive fibers to degenerative intervertebral discs.[122,123] Neurogenic inflammation from compression ischemia of the cervical nerve and inflammatory response following exposure of spinal tissues to proinflammatory mediators such as phosholipase A2 from extruded nucleus pulposis may also contribute to neck pain and CEH.

In addition to the evidence of atlantoaxial and zygapophyseal joint evidence discussed above, there is evidence that CEH may arise from a discogenic origin. Reproduction of patient's usual headache by cervical provocation discography has been reported, as has relief of headache following decompressive surgery of the upper and lower cervical spine.[124,125] The mechanisms by which headaches are provoked by levels below C3 have caused speculation regarding the possibility of convergence of afferents from lower spinal nerves with trigeminal afferents in the spinal trigeminal nucleus. An alternate explanation could lie in the anatomy of the sinuvertebral nerves, which descend from higher levels in the cervical spine to communicate with those at lower levels. An inflammatory response could also be causative with proinflammatory mediators resulting from disc degeneration at lower cervical spinal segments precipitating a nociceptive response at adjacent spinal segments.[122]

Greater and lesser occipital nerve injections using local anesthetic and/or steroid have been reported as useful for diagnosis and short-term relief of CEH. Many authors consider entrapment of the greater occipital nerve to be one of the major underlying causes of CEH.[126-128] A recent controlled trial of nerve stimulator-guided greater and lesser occipital nerve blocks with adjuvant agents provided greater than 50% relief versus placebo with significant reduction of associated headache features and medica-

tion use in the treatment group.[129] A case report of pulsed radiofrequency for the treatment of intractable occipital headache reported 70% relief for 4 months followed by an additional 5 months of 70% relief with repeat pulsed radiofrequency.[130]

Percutaneous radiofrequency cervical medial branch neurotomy has been shown, in a rigorous double blind controlled trial, to provide relief in 70% of patients diagnosed with cervical zygapophyseal joint pain following whiplash injuries. Other therapies found to have efficacy in the treatment of CEH include the physical therapy modalities of manipulation and/or mobilization in conjunction with exercise and intramuscular lidocaine injections. In chronic neck disorders associated with a radicular component, epidural injection of methylprednisolone and lidocaine improved pain greater than cervical intramuscular injections with the same solution at 1 year follow-up.[131-133]

Diffuse Idiopathic Skeletal Hyperostosis

DISH is a form of osteoarthritis which is characterized by the calcification and ossification of soft tissues including ligaments and tendons. It may involve both the peripheral joints and the axial skeletal structures in 25% and 15% of men and women, respectively, who are older than 50 years of age. Its prevalence increases to 35% and 26%, respectively, in individuals older than 70 years. Classical axial involvement results in calcification of the ligamentum flavum in the lumbar spine, the anterior longitudinal ligament in the thoracic spine, and the posterior longitudinal ligament in the cervical spine. It is distinguished from degenerative spondylosis of the spine by earlier onset, sparing of the intervertebral disc, and its association with a number of risk factors including diabetes mellitus, obesity, hyperuricemia, dyslipidemia, hypertension, coronary artery disease, and prolonged use of isoretinal (vitamin A supplementation).

The patient with DISH typically presents with stiffness and decreased range-of-motion. Older patients with cervical spine involvement may complain of dysphagia due to pharyngeal encroachment from large anterior osteophytes. Other potential sequelae include cervical myelopathy and cervical spine fractures following relatively trivial trauma. The diagnosis of cervical spine fractures is often delayed due to the presence of baseline neck and spine pain.

The diagnosis of diffuse idiopathic skeletal hyperostosis is radiographic and is based on the criteria established by Resnick and Niwayama. These include the presence of "flowing" ossification along anterolateral margins of at least four contiguous vertebrae and the absence of changes associated with degenerative spondylosis. Treatment consists of conservative measures similar to cervical degenerative spondylosis. Operative treatment is reserved for those patients who fail to respond to conservative measures.[134]

Cervical Radiculopathies

The classical definition and clinical manifestation of cervical radiculopathies is pain, sensory loss, and motor weakness in the distribution of the affected nerve root. Although the cause of radicular symptoms has been presumed to be secondary to compression of the nerve root because of adjacent soft disc herniation or progressive degenerative changes of the cervical spine, the poor correlation between radiologic evidence of degenerative change and incidence of painful symptoms in the cervical spine has been well documented.[136-140] Other factors thought to contribute to the pathogenesis of radiculopathic symptoms include vascular insufficiency, venous engorgement, nerve root fibrosis, and inflammation. Type C cell distortion in dorsal root ganglion of cervical nerve roots has been proposed as a mechanism of accentuated neuropeptide production and increased hypersensitivity in pa-

---

TABLE 68.22

MUSCULOSKELETAL STRUCTURES OF THE NECK INNERVATED BY C1 THROUGH C3

- Muscles: Capital flexors and extensors, cervical spine flexors including the scalenus medius, scalenus posterior, longus colli and sternocleidomastoid, cervical spine extensors, head rotators and other neck muscles including the hyoid muscles, the sternothyroid, and diaphragm.
- Periosteum and body of the atlas, axis and C3 vertebra and clavicle, atlanto-occipital, atlantoaxial, intervertebral, Luschka, sternoclavicular and zygapophyseal joints associated with the C1 to C3 spinal segments, associated ligaments.

tients with acute and chronic neural foraminal compression or edema.[141]

The patient with cervical radiculopathy typically complains of burning, aching, cramping, electrical, or sharp pain which radiates to the neck and head, shoulder, arm, or chest depending on the involved nerve root(s). In acute radiculopathy, pain classically presents in a myotomal distribution versus a distal dermatomal distribution. The pain is generally accompanied by numbness and paresthesias. Motor weakness and diminution or loss of deep tendon reflexes may also be seen. Spurling's maneuver, Valsalva, coughing, and sneezing will often provoke or aggravate the patient's symptoms while the shoulder abduction sign (having the patient abduct the shoulder and place their hand on top of their head) will generally relieve their pain.

The C1 nerve passes between the occiput and C1. It is also known as the suboccipital nerve and supplies sensory fibers to the periosteum and body of the atlas, occiput, atlanto-occipital joint, and atlantoaxial joint. It is also distributed to the muscles of the suboccipital triangle. The C2 nerve passes between C1 and C2. The medial or sensory branch of C2 is also known as the greater occipital nerve. It supplies the scalp over the vertex and top of the head and supplies muscular branches to the semispinalis.

C3 arises between C2 and C3. The medial sensory branch of the posterior division of the third cervical nerve forms the third or least occipital nerve. The anterior rami of the upper four cervical nerves communicate to form the cervical plexus. Pathologic processes which affect the C1 through C3 nerves cause pain radiating to the head and neck. Pain of the upper cervical spine was covered in more detail in the section on CEHs.[142,143] The greater auricular nerve and the anterior cutaneous nerve are also derived from the second and third cervical nerves. Processes affecting these nerves can also result in pain involving the mastoid process, the lobule and concha of the ear, the skin of the face over the parotid gland, and the skin of the anterolateral aspect of the neck as far as the sternum. Via the deep cervical plexus, the second and third cervical nerves also communicate with the vagus, the hypoglossal nerve, the superior cervical sympathetic ganglion, and the diaphragm by way of the phrenic nerve (see Table 68.3).

Radiculopathy of the fourth cervical nerve root results from pathologic changes between the C3 and C4 vertebrae and is more common than a C3 radiculopathy. The supraclavicular nerve arises mainly from the fourth cervical nerve and supplies the skin and superficial fascia of the clavicular region, the periosteum, and boney structure of the clavicle as far as the midline and the skin over the pectoralis major as far as the second or third rib. It additionally communicates with the cutaneous branches of the second and third rib. The lateral supraclavicular nerve supplies the skin of the top and dorsal parts of the shoulder. Involvement of the C3 nerve may be a cause of unexplained pain along the base of the neck that radiates to the superior aspect of the shoulder and posteriorly to the scapula. Pain in the distribution of the supraclavicular nerve may also be a cause of chronic breast pain in women.

The rhomboid, trapezius, and levator scapulae muscles are supplied in part by the fourth cervical nerve root, but a motor deficit may be difficult to detect. A sensory deficit may be present over the anterolateral aspect of the neck, along the distribution of the transverse cervical and supraclavicular nerves. Because the C3, C4, and C5 nerve roots innervate the diaphragm, involvement of these three nerve roots may lead to diaphragmatic weakness.

The brachial plexus is formed by the fifth, sixth, seventh, and eighth cervical nerves together with the first thoracic nerve and frequently contributing branches from the anterior division of the fourth cervical and second thoracic nerve. The variation of brachial plexus and extradural cervical nerve connections may contribute to variations in radicular patterns among patients.

Pathologic changes at the C4-C5 level result in a C5 radiculopathy. The principal motor deficit seen in classical C5 radiculopa-

thy is supraspinatus and deltoid muscle weakness with impaired shoulder abduction. Weakness of the clavicular head of the pectoralis major, biceps, and infraspinatus muscles can also occur. The pectoralis reflex and the biceps reflex, which are innervated by the fifth and sixth cervical nerve roots, may be decreased or absent. The numbness follows the C5 sensory distribution, which is located over the top of the shoulder along its midportion, and extends laterally to the midportion of the arm. The component fibers of the suprascapular nerve are derived primarily from the fifth and sixth cervical nerves. It supplies sensory, motor, and sympathetic fibers which supply the supraspinatus and infraspinatus muscles, the shoulder joint, and periarticular structures as well as an area of skin at the apex of the shoulder. Patients often present with numbness and localized shoulder pain that can be confused with a pathologic shoulder condition. The absence of pain with a range-of-motion of the shoulder and the absence of impingement signs at the shoulder help to differentiate radiculopathy of the fifth cervical nerve root from a pathologic shoulder condition.

The sixth cervical nerve root is the second most commonly involved in cervical radiculopathy. Patients with pathology at this level typically present with pain radiating from the neck to the lateral aspect of the biceps, lateral aspect of the forearm, dorsal aspect of the web space between the thumb and index finger, and into the tips of those digits. Numbness occurs in the same distribution. Motor deficits are best elicited in the wrist extensors, but weakness of the biceps, supinator, pronator, teres, and triceps muscles may be present. The brachioradialis and biceps reflexes may be decreased or absent. The pain and paresthesias of C6 radiculopathy may mimic carpal tunnel syndrome, which is caused by median nerve entrapment at the transverse carpal ligament.

The seventh cervical nerve root is most frequently involved by cervical radiculopathy according to many clinical studies. The patient with C7 radiculopathy complains of pain radiating along the back of the shoulder, often extending into the scapular region, down along the triceps, along the dorsum of the forearm and into the dorsum of the long finger. Motor weakness is most often appreciated in the latissimus dorsi muscle, the triceps, wrist flexors, and finger extensors. The triceps reflex may be lost or diminished. Entrapment of the posterior interosseus nerve may be mistaken for the motor component of seventh cervical radiculopathy and presents with weakness in the extensor digitorum communis, extensor pollicis longus, and extensor carpi ulnaris. With entrapment of the interosseus nerve, sensory changes are absent and the triceps and wrist flexors show normal strength.

Pathology at the C7-T1 level results in radiculopathy of the eighth cervical nerve root. Patients with a C8 radiculopathy generally present with sensory changes extending over the medial aspect of the arm and forearm and into the medial hand and the fourth and fifth digits. Numbness usually involves both the dorsal and volar aspects of the digits and hand and may extend proximal to the wrist over the medial aspect of the forearm. Weakness may involve the small muscles of the hand, particularly the interossei, and the flexors and extensors of the wrist and fingers (with the exception of the flexor carpi radialis and extensor carpi radialis muscles). This may cause patients to complain of difficulty using their hands for routine tasks such as buttoning shirts and grasping objects. Compression of the C8 nerve root may initially be difficult to differentiate from ulnar entrapment at the elbow. C8 nerve root compression may affect the function of the flexor digitorum profundus in the index and long fingers, the flexor pollicis longus in the thumb, and the pronator quadratus, but these muscles are not affected by entrapment of the ulnar nerve. Also, the short thenar muscles, except for the adductor pollicis, may be involved with C8 or T1 compression but are spared with ulnar nerve involvement. Furthermore, sensory changes seen with ulnar neuropathies include numbness, tingling, and/or pain in the fourth and fifth fingers and the hand just below these fingers, but not proximal to the wrist (medial antebrachial cutaneous nerve distribution), as may be seen with C8 radiculopathy. Anterior interosseus nerve entrapment may also mimic C8 or T1 radiculopathy but lacks sensory changes, and thenar muscle involvement is absent.

Though uncommon, occurrence of T1-T2 disc herniations or other pathology at this level may result in a T1 radiculopathy. The T1 nerve is the main contributor to the adductor pollicis, the thenar muscles, the interossei, and the first two lumbricals. Classic T1 radiculopathy results in intrinsic hand weakness. Numbness occurs in the axilla, and Horner's syndrome can occur ipsilaterally.[1,101,144]

Epidemiologic data suggest that up to 90% of patients with cervical radiculopathy improve with conservative medical treatment alone.[97,98,145–147] However, due to lack of standardized diagnostic criteria and comparative randomized controlled trials comparing conservative with surgical treatment, evidence-based guidelines have been difficult to establish.

Conservative therapy in patients with cervical radiculopathy includes activity modification, education, and physical therapy with progressive passive and active modalities. Pharmacologic therapy requires a large armentarium of medications due to the heterogeneity in this patient population and the various mechanisms involved in the production of neuropathic pain. Options include over-the-counter analgesics, anticonvulsants, tricyclic antidepressants, and selective serotonin-norepinephrine reuptake inhibitors, topical anesthetic agents, nonsteroidal anti-inflammatory drugs, antiarrhythmics, muscle relaxants, nonnarcotic analgesics, and opioids.[148,149] Multiple studies suggest that epidural steroid injections may be beneficial with decreased short-term and long-term pain reported in greater than 60% of patients.[150,151] Use of flouroscopic guidance in interlaminar epidural steroid injections and use of nonparticulate steroid in transforaminal injections may significantly reduce the risk of complications.[152–154]

Outcome in patients with cervical radiculopathy following medical versus operative treatment was recently reported following a prospective, multicenter study with independent clinical review. Comparison of results of patients undergoing medical versus surgical treatments showed that, although both medically and surgically treated patients reported statistically significant improvement in their overall pain, more improvement was observed in the surgery group. Improvement in worst pain and average pain was also statistically significant in both groups. Surgically-treated patients had more neurologic and nonneurologic symptoms and more functional disability before treatment. However, despite high satisfaction in surgically-treated patients, a significant number of patients continued to report horrible or excruciating pain, multiple neurologic symptoms, and minimal or no work activity. These results are similar to those in patients with CSM in that the majority of patients improve with conservative therapy while those with persistent severe pain and progressive neurologic symptoms are generally referred for operative management, which attempts to improve pain and arrest the progression of neurologic symptoms.[91,147]

Upper Extremity Peripheral Nerve Entrapment Syndromes and Brachial Plexus Neuropathy

Acute trauma with resultant fibrosis and scar tissue, chronic trauma from overuse injuries, or space-occupying lesions can result in entrapment of peripheral nerves. Peripheral nerve entrapment syndromes typically present with pain at the site of entrapment. Pain can radiate both distally and proximally to this point. Sensory, motor, or sympathetic changes can occur in the nerve distribution distal to the site of entrapment.

The diagnosis of nerve compression or nerve entrapment is based on a careful history of the mechanism of injury or repetitive

use and a thorough physical exam together with neurologic and electrodiagnostic examinations. MRI is helpful in identifying the cause of the neuropathy, identifying the site of entrapment based on muscle denervation patterns, and detecting unsuspected space-occupying lesions.[155,156] Nerve entrapment and radiculopathies may infrequently exist simultaneously. In a retrospective analysis of 12,736 cases of carpal tunnel syndrome and ulnar neuropathy at the elbow 435 (3.4%) of these cases were found to have a coexisting cervical root lesion. However, lesions were on the same nerve in only 98 (0.8%) of these cases.[157] Upper extremity nerve entrapment syndromes are characterized in Table 68.23.

Early recognition is essential for timely diagnosis and treatment of nerve entrapment syndromes involving the upper extremity as they are thought to affect the function of many individuals, including musicians, athletes, and as many as 1 in 4 office workers.[158] Most patients respond to conservative treatment including rehabilitative exercises, passive physical therapy modalities, relative rest, and correction of training and equipment use errors. Other measures may include anti-inflammatory medications, protective padding or bracing, and injections with local anesthetic and steroids. In patients with severe or progressive neurologic deficit or intractable pain, surgical decompression may be necessary.[159]

Lesions of the Brachial Plexus

Injury to the brachial plexus resulting in functional impairment of the upper extremity can occur secondary to penetrating or blunt trauma, severe traction, or acceleration-deceleration injuries. Other etiologies include congenital, developmental or exogenous compression, vascular or infectious disease, and neoplastic disease. The relative incidence of these lesions of the brachial plexus is presented in Table 68.24.

Brachial plexus injury (BPI) can be classified into preganglionic lesions, postganglionic lesions, and a combination of preganglionic and postganglionic lesions. In a preganglionic lesion, the nerve root is avulsed. A postganglionic lesion involves the nerve distal to the sensory ganglion and is further divided into nerve ruptures or lesions in continuity.

Clinical exam and electrodiagnostic and imaging studies may help in determining the location and severity of injury, which is essential in therapeutic decisions regarding these injuries. CT myelography is considered most reliable in detecting avulsion injuries. MRI, as well as new techniques such as MR myelography, diffusion-weighted neurography, and Bezier surface reformation, provides additional useful data in the evaluation and management of brachial plexus injury.[160,161]

Treatment of traumatic BPI is conservative versus surgical and is based on various factors such as the degree of damage, the site and type of injury, the time interval between injury and surgery, and the patient's age and occupation. Surgical treatment includes neurolysis, nerve grafting, nerve transfer, and other reconstructive procedures.[162–164] Physical therapy and pain control is essential for recovery of function following operative cases and for optimization of function and palliation of pain in nonoperative cases. In addition to pharmacologic treatment options, successful treatment of pain related to brachial plexus lesions has been reported following implantation of spinal cord and deep brain stimulator systems.[165,166]

Acute Brachial Plexus Neuritis

Acute brachial plexus neuritis is an uncommon disorder of unknown etiology which is commonly misdiagnosed as cervical spondylosis or cervical radiculopathy. It was first described by Spillane[167] in 1943 and is also known as Parsonage Turner syndrome or neuralgic amyotrophy due to the case series of this condition by Parsonage and Turner[168] in 1948. Other names by

TABLE 68.23

UPPER EXTREMITY ENTRAPMENT SYNDROMES

Nerve	Usual Cause	Location of Pain	Sensory Changes	Weakness
Dorsal scapular	Scalenus medius hypertrophy	Medial scapula, lateral arm	None	Rhomboids, levator scapulae
Suprascapular	Band in supraspinatus notch	Posterolateral, shoulder, lateral arm; tender at suprascapular notch	None	Supraspinatus, infraspinatus
Long thoracic	Downward pressure on shoulder	Not usually painful; can have diffuse ache in shoulder or scapula	None	Serratus anterior
Musculocutaneous	Entrapment by coracobrachialis	Anterior arm, proximal lateral forearm	Anterolateral forearm	Biceps, brachialis
Posterior interosseous	Entrapment at proximal forearm	Proximal radial forearm	None	Wrist and finger extensors and abductors
Ulnar (at elbow)	Entrapment at cubital tunnel	Elbow, ulnar forearm, and hand	Ulnar hand, fourth and fifth digits	Flexor carpi ulnaris and intrinsics
Ulnar (at wrist)	Entrapment at Guyon's canal	Ulnar side of hand, fourth and fifth digits	Ulnar hand, fourth and fifth digits	Adductor pollicis, interossei, hypothenar muscles
Median (at elbow)	Entrapment at ligament of Struthers or pronator teres	Elbow, volar forearm	Radial hand, first, second, and third digits	Pronator teres, flexor carpi radialis, flexor digitorum superior
Median (at wrist)	Entrapment at carpal tunnel	Wrist, radial hand, first, second, and third digits	Radial hand, first, second, and third digits	Thenar muscles, first and second lumbricals
Anterior interosseous	Entrapment at pronator teres or flexor digitorum superior	Elbow, volar forearm	None	Pronator quadratus, flexor pollicis longus, first and second flexor digitorum profundus
Digital nerve	Entrapment at intermetacarpal tunnel	Finger	Half of finger	None

TABLE 68.24

CAUSES OF BRACHIAL PLEXUS LESIONS

Cause	Example(s)	Incidence (% of cases)
Trauma	Penetrating injuries (e.g., gunshot, knife); closed injuries: obstetric (newborn), mechanical distortion	70
Compression	Exogenous (knapsack paralysis); congenital abnormality; developmental abnormality	10
Vascular	Local disease of major vessels; generalized vasculopathy (lupus erythematosus, arteritis); secondary to radiation therapy	5
Infectious	Viral; bacterial (local sepsis, abscess, or cellulitis)	3
Neoplastic	Primary tumors of brachial plexus; secondary involvement of plexus by tumors of surrounding tissues (Pancoast's tumor)	10
Miscellaneous causes	Electric shock; parainfectious; following serum therapy; unknown	2

which it is referred include brachial plexus neuropathy, paralytic neuritis, and acute shoulder neuritis.

The classical presentation of the patient with acute brachial plexus neuritis is the acute onset of severe burning pain in the neck, shoulder, and upper arm not associated with a precipitating injury or trauma. The pain may or may not be associated with sensory deficit and generally subsides over the following days to weeks. It is followed by a profound weakness, sometimes to the extent of flaccidity, involving the supraspinatus, infraspinatus, and deltoid and/or biceps muscles. Involvement of the sternomastoid or diaphragm has also been described, as has isolated or single nerve involvement. Bilateral brachial plexus involvement is not uncommon. Gradual recovery of muscle strength over 3 to 4 months is the usual course of brachial neuritis; however, some patients may experience several years of permanent muscle weakness. Chronic scapulocostal pain syndromes may occur due to dysfunctional mechanics following profound weakness.

Although a viral etiology has been proposed, various infections have been reported as preceding the onset of this disorder in up to 25% of cases. Onset following influenza, hepatitis B, or other vaccinations in up to 15% of cases suggests an immunologic etiology. Familial and recurrent cases are encountered. Other reported precipitating factors include childbirth, trauma, and surgery. Pathologic studies favor an immune mediated demyelinating pathogenesis over an axon-loss mechanism.[169,170]

The annual incidence of acute brachial plexus neuritis is reported to be 1.64 cases per 100,000, athough this figure is presumed to be low because of misdiagnosis. It occurs most often between age 20 and 60 years with a reported male predominance of 2:1 to 11.5:1.[169]

Diagnosis of brachial neuritis requires a high level of suspicion. A case series report of electrodiagnostic results reports no evidence of prolongation of F-latencies and no reduction of conduction velocity or conduction block in conventional peripheral ulnar and median nerve motor studies. Proximal nerve stimulation of the cervical roots and brachial plexus revealed axonal degeneration in most cases as well as evidence of proximal conduction block consistent with demyelination. MRI is useful in evaluating muscle denervation, muscle signal intensity changes, and muscle volume loss.[171]

Treatment of brachial neuritis is primarily supportive with use of analgesic medications followed by range-of-motion exercises. An arm sling may be helpful in preventing injury and strain from the weight of the arm distracting the humeral head from the glenoid fossa.[59] Full functional recovery is expected in 80% to 90% of patients, though the course may be protracted. Ten percent to 20% of patients may continue to have significant residual muscle weakness. In cases of profound and early weakness, intravenous immunoglobulin treatment has been proposed due to its usefulness in treating other focal demyelinating peripheral nerve diseases.[172,173] Acupuncture many also be effective in treating pain and improving function.[174,175]

Thoracic Outlet Syndrome

The definition, diagnosis, and treatment of thoracic outlet syndrome (TOS) are among the most disputed of any clinical entity. The syndrome generally refers to a variety of symptoms in the upper extremity due to compression of the brachial plexus, subclavian artery, and subclavian vein. Compression of the neurovascular bundle can occur as it passes through the interscalene triangle, the costoclavicular triangle, and subcoracoid space during its passage from the base of the neck to the proximal aspect of the arm. Structural compressive etiologies include fibrous bands, scar tissue, hypertrophied or fibrous muscles, anomalous soft tissue, and cervical ribs. Previous to the coining of the term TOS in 1956 by Peet,[176] the name of this syndrome was assigned according to the etiologies of compression including: scalenus anticus syndrome, costoclavicular syndrome, hyperabduction, cer-

vical rib syndrome, or first rib syndrome. The lower trunk of the brachial plexus (C8 and T1) is most often affected. Other factors associated with the development of TOS include repetitive trauma to the brachial plexus, median sternotomy, or traumatic events such as motor vehicle accidents.[177]

TOS is variably divided into arterial, venous, or neurogenic. Alternatively, it has been classified as vascular, neurogenic, and nonspecific. The latter classification system reflects both diagnostic criteria and therapeutic recommendations and outcome.

Vascular TOS occurs in only 2% to 5% of thoracic outlet cases and is described most frequently in young individuals following vigorous arm activity or strenuous work. Patients with subclavian artery compression frequently present with pallor, pulselessness, and coolness of the affected upper extremity, transient ischemic attack, or infarcts of the hand and fingers. Decreased blood pressure in the affected arm when compared with the opposite arm of more than 20 mm Hg may also be present. Claudication may occur only with arm hyperabduction in some patients. Injury may include thrombosis, aneurysm, and/or stenosis.

Subclavian vein compression typically presents with edema and cyanosis of the upper limb with hyperabduction of the upper extremity. Thrombosis of the axillary-subclavian vein, (also known as Paget-von Schoetter syndrome), occurs in association with vigorous shoulder activity.

Doppler and duplex ultrasonography, magnetic resonance arteriography, CT angiography, and arteriography are used to confirm the diagnosis of vascular TOS. Decompression procedures or vessel reconstruction may be indicated in urgent cases and in cases not responsive to conservative therapy.[177–180]

Neurogenic and nonspecific categories of TOS comprise 95% to 98% of cases. A syndrome of painless atrophy of the hand primarily involving the abductor pollicis brevis with lesser atrophy of the interossei and hypothenar muscles known as Gilliatt-Sumner hand is the classic presentation of the true neurogenic type of TOS. This is associated with positive neurologic and electrodiagnostic findings. Sensory loss typically involves the ulnar aspect of the forearm and hand consistent with lower trunk compression, though upper trunk compression has also been reported. Pain is not the primary symptom of true neurogenic TOS; however, the patient may complain of diffuse, dull pain in the neck, shoulder, axillary region, and arm which may worsen with overhead activities and repetitive use of the arm.

The most common form of TOS is the nonspecific type. Patients generally present with the primary complaint of pain, often following a motor vehicle or work-related injury. Kelly's test and Adson's tests may be positive, but are not reliable as they have been shown to be positive in many asymptomatic individuals. Physical examination findings are often inconclusive and nonspecific and are not supported by electrodiagnostic or imaging results.[180–182] The differential diagnosis of TOS includes cervical radiculopathy or myelopathy, acute brachial neuritis, Reynaud's disease, multiple sclerosis, ulnar or median nerve entrapment syndromes, acute coronary syndrome, and CRPS.

The diagnosis of nonspecific TOS requires a detailed history and physical exam to rule out other causes of neck and upper extremity pain. Electrodiagnostic testing may help localize and quantify a brachial plexus lesion in true neurogenic TOS and rule out other segmental or systemic neuropathies.[183,184] Radiographic studies used in evaluation with the patient with suspected TOS include cervical spine and chest radiographs to rule out boney abnormalities and MRI and CT to evaluate the cervical spine for soft tissue anomalies, tumors, or degenerative disease of the cervical spine.[185]

Conservative treatment of TOS is indicated in the majority of cases and consists of activity modification education with instructions to avoid provocative positions and activities. Physical therapy programs to restore normal posture and strengthen the muscles of the pectoral girdle have also been successful in alleviating symptoms in greater than 50% of cases.[186] Surgical approaches to treatment are undertaken in intractable or urgent cases. Surgery in the nonspecific type of TOS is associated with the least favorable outcome and is generally discouraged due to the significant risks associated with surgeries in this region. New minimally invasive techniques are now being investigated and may offer reduced risk of complications.[187,188]

SPONTANEOUS LOW PRESSURE HEADACHE

Intracranial hypotension or low pressure headache is classified as by the IHS into three categories: (1) postdural puncture headache; (2) cerebrospinal fluid (CSF) fistula headache; and (3) headache attributed to low CSF pressure.[114] Alternately, intracranial hypotension is described as primary, spontaneous, intracranial hypotension or secondary, iatrogenic, intracranial hypotension. The most common causes of secondary intracranial hypotension include diagnostic lumbar puncture, inadvertent dural puncture following surgical procedures, or epidural catheter placement and CT myelography. In the hospital setting, the symptoms associated with low pressure headache are rapidly recognized due to the associated risk factors such as iatrogenic dural puncture, postsurgical dural tear, or inadvertent overdrainage of CSF shunts.

Spontaneous intracranial hypotension (SIH) has an estimated prevalence of 5 in 100,000 individuals. It is thought to result from rupture of a spinal arachnoid membrane which allows CSF to pass into the subdural or epidural space. It may be associated with a history of minor trauma such as sports activities or severe coughing, degenerative discs or osteophytes, and patient morphology consistent with Marfan's or other connective tissue disorders. The patient with SIH is often misdiagnosed or is diagnosed following a delay due to variation in clinical presentation and diagnostic test results.[189,190]

Patients with SIH present with headaches which generally begin in the occipital region and radiate to the frontal and retroorbital area. The headaches typically worsen with sitting or standing and improve with recumbency. Patients may report nausea, emesis, diplopia, neck pain, vertigo, photophobia, and hearing disturbances. In severe cases, patients may develop cranial nerve palsy, gait imbalances, mental status changes, and obtundation due to herniation of the cerebellar tonsil. Cervical epidural venous engorgement has been reported to produce radicular symptoms and neck pain in addition to headache in some patients. A cervical myelopathy secondary to severe compression from cervical epidural venous varicosities has also been reported and Lhermitte's sign may be present. Some patients report fluctuating headaches of many months duration.[26,191]

MRI with gadolinium of most, but not all, patients with SIH reveals diffuse pachymeningeal enhancement. Subdural fluid collections and brain descent may also be seen. Pituitary enlargement is typical in the symptomatic stage. In some case reports, epidural fluid collections and pachymeningeal enhancement is seen. Downward displacement or "sagging" of the brain may mimic a Chiari I malformation. Chronic subdural hematoma and subarachnoid hemorrhage has been reported in patients with SIH. Diagnostic tests may be inconclusive. Opening pressure may be normal, low, or even high. CSF analysis is nondiagnostic and may be normal, reveal xanthochromia, increased protein, and/or lymphocytic pleocytosis. In the case of normal CSF pressure, CSF hypovolemic syndrome rather than SIH syndrome has been proposed as a more accurate classification.[192,193]

Conservative treatment consists of bedrest, analgesics, and intravenous fluid administration together with intravenous or oral caffeine. For patients with neurologic deficit and intractable symptoms, an epidural blood patch at the lumbar level is recommended regardless of the level of the leak. Systemic or local infection, anticoagulants, or coagulopathy should be excluded prior to neuraxial procedures. The lumbar blood patch can be repeated if the patient does not respond.[194] For patients not responding to lumbar epidural blood patch, a blood patch at the level of the leak is recommended. Most CSF leaks have been found to be located at the cervicothoracic junction or in the thoracic spine. Spinal MRI with and without gadolinium appears to be more sensitive than radionuclide cisternography for detecting CSF leaks. To avoid the area of venous engorgement, the epidural blood patch may be delivered to the site of the leak via a catheter inserted from the lower cervical spine under flouroscopic or CT guidance.[193,195,196] Intrathecal saline infusion for emergent management of progressive obtundation prior to definitive treatment has been reported to reverse deteriorating mental status and neurologic deficits.[197] Surgical repair is recommended for patients failing treatment with epidural blood patch.[198]

References

1. Loeser JD. *Bonica's Management of Pain*. 3rd ed. Philidelphia, PA: Lippincott Williams & Wilkins; 2001:1008.
2. Wolfla CE. Anatomical, biomechanical, and practical considerations in posterior occipitocervical instrumentation. *Spine J* 2006;6(6 suppl):225S–232S.
3. Hogg-Johnson S, van der Velde G, Carroll LJ, et al. The burden and determinants of neck pain in the general population: results of the Bone and Joint Decade 2000–2010 Task Force on Neck Pain and its Associated Disorders. *Spine* 2008;33(4S):S39–S51.
4. Peterson C, Bolton J, Wood AR, et al. A cross-sectional study correlating degeneration of the cervical spine with disability and pain in United Kingdom patients. *Spine* 2003;28(2):129–133.
5. van der Donk J, Schouten JS, Passchier J, et al. The associations of neck pain with radiological abnormalities of the cervical spine and personality traitsin a general population. *J Rheumatol* 1991;18(12):1884–1889.
6. Zapletal J, Hekster RE, Straver JS, et al. Relationship between atlantoodontoid osteoarthritis and idiopathic suboccipital neck pain. *Neuroradiology* 1996;38(1):62–65.
7. Matsumoto M, Fujimura Y, Suzuki N, et al. MRI of cervical intervertebral discs in asymptomatic subjects. *J Bone Joint Surg Br* 1998;80(1):19–24.
8. Boden SD, McCowin PR, Davis DO, et al. Abnormal magnetic-resonance scans of the cervical spine in asymptomatic subjects. A prospective investigation. *J Bone Joint Surg Am* 1990;72(8):1178–1184.
9. Siivloa SM, Levoska S, Tervonen O, et al. MRI changes of cervical spine in asymptomatic and symptomatic young adults. *Eur Spine J* 2002;11(4):358–363.
10. Hamalained O, Vanharanta H, Kuusela T. Degeneration of cervical intervertebral disks in fighter pilots frequently exposed to high + Gz forces. *Aviat Space Environ Med* 1993;64(8):692–696.
11. Quinlan KP, Annest JL, Myers B, et al. Neck strains and sprains among motor vehicle occupants—United States, 2000. *Accid Anal Prev* 2004;36(1):21–27.
12. Carroll LJ, Holm LW, Hogg-Johnson S, et al. Course and prognostic factors for neck pain in whiplash-associated disorders (WAD): results of the Bone and Joint Decade 2000–2010 Task Force on Neck Pain and Its Associated Disorders. *J Manipulative Physiol Ther* 2009;32(2 suppl):S97–S107.
13. Berglund A, Alfredsson L, Jensen I, et al. Occupant- and crash-related factors associated with risk of whiplash injury. *Ann Epidemiol* 2003;13(1):66–72.
14. Merskey H, Teasell RW. Problems with insurance-based research on chronic pain. *Med Clin North Am* 2007;91(1):31–43.
15. Andersen JH, Haahr JP, Frost P. Risk factors for more severe regional musculoskeletal symptoms: a two year prospective study of a general working population. *Arthritis Rheum* 2007;56(4):1355–1364.
16. Ostegren PO, Hanson BS, Balogh I, et al. Incidence of shoulder and neck pain in a working population: effect modification between mechanical and pshychosocial exposures at work? Results from a one year follow-up of the Malmo shoulder and neck study cohort. *J Epidemiol Community Health* 2005;59(9):721–728.
17. Hannan LM, Monteilh CP, Gerr F, et al. Job strain and risk of musculoskeletal symptoms among a prospective cohort of occupational computer users. *Scand J Work Environ Health* 2005;31(5):375–386.
18. Walker-Bone K, Reading I, Coggon D, et al. The anatomical pattern and determinants of pain in the upper limbs: an epidemiologic study. *Pain* 2004;109(1–2):45–51.
19. Cohen JJ. Remembering the real questions. *Ann Intern Med* 1998;128(7):563–566.
20. Arnold M, Cumurciuc R, Stapf C, et al. Pain as the symptom of cervical artery dissection. *J Neurol Neurosurg Psychiatry* 2006;77(9):1021–1024.
21. Bassi P, Lattuada P, Gomitoni A. Cervical cerebral artery dissection: a multicenter prospective study (preliminary report). *Neurol Sci* 2003;24(suppl 1):S4–S7.
22. Cohen ML. Cervical and lumbar pain. *Med J Aust* 1996;165(9):504–508.
23. McBeth J, Macfarlane GJ, Benjamin S, et al. Features of somatization predict

the onset of chronic widespread pain: results of a large population-based study. *Arthritis Rheum* 2001;44(4):940–946.

24. Navarro X, Vivó M, Valero-Cabré A. Neural plasticity after peripheral nerve injury and regeneration. *Prog Neurobiol* 2007;82(4):163–201.

25. Semmes RE, Murphy F. The syndrome of unilateral rupture of the sixth cervical vertebral disc with compression of the seventh cervical root: a report of four cases with symptoms simulating coronary disease. *JAMA* 1943;121(15):1209–1214.

26. Albayram S, Wasserman BA, Yousem DM, et al. Intracranial hypotension as a cause of radiculopathy from cervical epidural venous engorgement: case report. *AJNR Am J Neuroradiol* 2002;23(4):618–621.

27. Leonard JR, Ferner RE, Thomas N, et al. Cervical cord compression from plexiform neurofibromas in neurofibromatosis 1. *J Neurol Neurosurg Psychiatry* 2007;78(12):1404–1406.

28. Fraser JF, Anand VK, Schwartz TH. Endoscopic biopsy sampling of Tophaceous gout of the odontoid process. Case report and review of the literature. *J Neurosurg Spine* 2007;7(1):61–64.

29. Tsikoudas A, Coateswortth AP, Martin-Hirsch DP. Laryngeal gout. *J Laryngol Otol* 2002;116(2):140–142.

30. Fujimoto K, Matsunaga R, Yamamoto F, et al. Epidural, mediastinal and subcutaneous emphysema in a patient with suspected torm frusta of Marfan's syndrome [in Japanese]. *Nihon Kokyuki Gakkai Zasshi* 2004;42(10):909–913.

31. Boesch SM, Muller J, Wenning GK, et al. Cervical dystonia in spinocerebellar ataxia type 2: clinical and polymyographic findings. *J Neurol Neurosurg Psychiatry* 2007;78(5):520–522.

32. Asplund S, Webb C, Barkdull T. Neck and back pain in bicycling. *Curr Sports Med Rep* 2005;4(5):271–274.

33. Leino P, Magni G. Depressive and distress symptoms as predictors of low back pain, neck shoulder pain, and other musculoskeletal morbidity: a 10-year follow-up of metal industry employees. *Pain* 1993;53(1):89–94.

34. Wilbourn AJ. Brachial plexus lesions. In: Dyck PJ, Thomas PK, eds. *Peripheral Neuropathy.* 4th ed. Philadelphia: Elsevier Saunders; 2005:1339–1373.

35. Bland JH. *Disorders of the cervical spine. Diagnosis and medical management.* Philadelphia: Saunders; 1994.

36. Baumgartner RW, Bogousslavsky J. Clinical manifestations of carotid dissection. *Front Neurol Neurosci* 2005;20:70–76.

37. Chennupati SK, Norris R, Dunham B, et al. Osteosarcoma of the skull base: case report and review of literature. *Int J Pediatr Otorhinolaryngol* 2008;72(1):115–119.

38. Kumandas S, Per H, Gumus H, et al. Torticollis secondary to posterior fossa and cervical spine tumors: report of five cases and literaature review. *Neurosurg Rev* 2006;29(4):333–338.

39. Horowitz SH. The diagnostic workup of patients with neuropathis pain. *Med Clin North Am* 2007;91(1):21–30.

40. Voskuhl RR, Hinton RC. Sensory impairment in the hands secondary to spondolytic compression of the cervical spinal cord. *Arch Neurol* 1990;47(3):309–311.

41. Levine E, Taub PJ. Hyoid bone fractures. *Mt Sinai J Med* 2006;73(7):1015–1018.

42. Wang W, Kong L, Dong R, et al. Fracture of the hyoid bone associated with atlantoaxial subluxation: a case report and review of the literature. *Am J Forensic Med Pathol* 2007;28(4):345–347.

43. Hashimoto Y, Moriya F, Furumiya J. Forensic aspects of complications resulting from cardiopulmonary resuscitation. *Leg Med (Tokyo)* 2007;9(2):94–99.

44. Sethi A, Sareen D, Chopra S, et al. Pharyngeal perforation with deep neck abscess secondary to isolated hyoid bone fracture. *J Laryngol Otol* 2005;119(12):1007–1009.

45. Aydil U, Ekinci O, Köybaşioğlu A, et al. Hyoid bone insertion tendinitis: clinicopathologic correlation. *Eur Arch Otorhinolaryngol* 2007;264(5):557–560.

46. Schmalbach CE, Miller FR. Occult primary head and neck carcinoma. *Curr Oncol Rep* 2007;9(2):139–146.

47. Cooper G, Bailey B, Bogduk N. Cervical zygapophysial joint pain maps. *Pain Medicine* 2007;8(4):344–853.

48. Sanders RJ, Hammond SL, Rao NM. Diagnosis of thoracic outlet syndrome. *J Vasc Surg* 2007;46(3):601–604.

49. Tong HC, Haig AJ, Yamakawa K. The Spurling test and cervical radiculopathy. *Spine* 2002;27(2):156–159.

50. Ventafridda V, Caraceni A, Martini C, et al. On the significance of Lhermitte's sign in oncology. *J Neurooncol* 1991;10(2):133–137.

51. Muhle C, Bischoff L, Weinert D, et al. Exacerbated pain in cervical radiculopathy at axial rotation, flexion, extension, and coupled motions of the cervical spine: evaluation by kinematic magnetic resonance imaging. *Invest Radio* 1998;33(5):279–288.

52. Malanga GA, Landes P, Nadler SF. Provocative tests in cervical spine examination: historical basis and scientific analyses. *Pain Physician* 2003;6(2):199–205.

53. Ledd AD, Agarwal S, Sadhu D. Doppler Adson's test: predictor of outcome of surgery in non-specific thoracic outlet syndrome. *World J Surg* 2006;30(3):291–292.

54. Waddell G, McCulloch HA, Kummel E, et al. Non-organic physical signs in low-back pain. *Spine* 1980;5:117–125.

55. Fishbain DA, Rosomoff HL, Cutler RB, et al. Secondary gain concept: a review of the scientific evidence. *Clin J Pain* 1995;11(1):6–21.

56. Fishbain DA, Cutler RB, Rosomoff HL, et al. Is there a relationship between nonorganic physical findings (Waddell signs) and secondary gain/malingering? *Clin J Pain* 2004;20(6):399–408.

57. Turk DC, Wack JT, Derns RD. An empirical examination of the "pain-behavior" construct. *J Behav Med* 1985;8(2):119–130.

58. McCahon S, Strong J, Sharry R, et al. Self-report and pain behavior among patients with chronic pain. *Clin J Pain* 2005;21(3):223–231.

59. Lossos IS, Yossepowitch O, Kandel L, et al. Septic arthritis of the glenohumeral joint. A report of 11 cases and review of the literature. *Medicine (Baltimore)* 1998;77(3):177–187.

60. Unkila-Kallio L, Kallio MJ, Peltola H. The usefulness of C-reactive protein levels in the identification of concurrent septic arthritis in children who have acute hematogenous osteomyelitis. A comparison with the usefulness of the erythrocyte sedimentation rate and the white blood-cell count. *J Bone Joint Surg Am* 1994;76(6):848–853.

61. Heller CA, Stanley P, Lewis-Jones B, et al. Value of x ray examinations of the cervical spine. *Br Med J* 1983;287(6401):1276–1278.

62. Johnson MJ, Lucas GL. Value of cervical spine radiographs as a screening tool. *Clinl Orthop Relat Res* 1997;340:102–108.

63. Malik SA, Murphy M, Connolly P, et al. Evaluation of morbidity, mortality and outcome following cervical spine injuries in elderly patients. *Eur Spine J* 2008;17(4):585–591.

64. Touger M, Gennis P, Nathanson N, et al. Validity of a decision rule to reduce cervical spine radiography in elderly patients with blunt trauma. *Ann Emerg Med* 2002;40(3):287–293.

65. Davis JW, Phreaner DL, Hoyt DB, et al. The etiology of missed cervical spine injuries. *J Trauma* 1993;34(3):342–346.

66. Bohlman HH. Acute fractures and dislocations of the cervical spine. An analysis of three hundred hospitalized patients and review of the literature. *J Bone Joint Surg Am* 1979;61(8):1119–1140.

67. Davis JW, Phreaner DL, Hoyt DB, et al. The etiology of missed cervical spine injuries. *J Trauma* 1993;34(3):342–346.

68. MacDonald RL, Schwartz MD, Mirich MD, et al. Diagnosis of cervical spine injury in motor vehicle crash victims: how many x-rays are enough. *J Trauma* 1990;30(4):392–397.

69. Brohi K, Wilson-Macdonald J. Evaluation of unstable cervical spine injury: a 6-year experience. *J Trauma* 2000;49(1):76–80.

70. Hoffman JR, Schriger DL, Mower WR, et al. Low-risk criteria for cervical-spine radiography in blunt trauma: a prospective study. *Ann Emerg Med* 1992;21(12):1454–1460.

71. Hoffman JR, Wolfson AB, Todd KH, et al. Selective cervical spine radiography in blunt trauma: methodology of the National Emergency X-Radiography Utilization Study (NEXUS). *Ann Emerg Med* 1998;32(4):461–469.

72. Hoffman JR, Wolfson AB, Todd K, et al. Selective cervical spine radiography in blunt trauma: methodology of the National Emergency X-Radiography Utilization Study (NEXUS). *Ann Emerg Med* 1998;32(4):461–469.

73. Mahadevan S, Mower WR, Hoffman JR, et al. Interrater reliability of cervical spine injury criteria in patients with blunt trauma. *Ann Emerg Med* 1998;31(2):197–201.

74. Hoffman JR, Mower WR, Wolfson B, et al. Validity of a set of clinical criteria to rule out injury to the cervical spine in patients with blunt trauma. *N Engl J Med* 2000;343(2):94–99.

75. Stiell IG, Clement CM, McKnight RD, et al. The Canadian C-spine rule versus the NEXUS low-risk criteria in patients with trauma. *N Engl J Med* 2003;349(26):2510–2518.

76. Klein GR, Vaccaro AR, Albert TJ, et al. Efficacy of magnetic resonance imaging in the evaluation of posterior cervical spine fractures. *Spine* 1999;24(8):771–774.

77. Sanchez B, Waxman K, Jones T, et al. Cervical spine clearance in blunt trauma: evaluation of a computed tomography-based protocol. *J Trauma* 2005;59(1):179–183.

78. Shedid D, Benzel EC. Cervical spondylosis anatomy: pathophysiology and biomechanics. *Neurosurgery* 2007;60(1 Suppl 1):S7–S13.

79. Fehlings MG, Rao SC, Tator CH, et al. The optimal radiologic method for assessing spinal canal compromise and cord compression in patients with cervical spinal cord injury. Part II: results of a multicernter study. *Spine* 1999;24(6):605–613.

80. Maus TP. Imaging of the spine and nerve roots. *Phys Med Rehabil Clin N Am* 2002;13(3);487–544,vi.

81. Babar S, Saifuddin A. MRI of the post-discectomy lumbar spine. *Clinical Radiology* 2002;57(11):969–981.

82. Dorenbeck U, Schreyer AG, Schlaier J, et al. Degenerative diseases of the cervical spine: comparison of a multiecho data image combination sequence with a magnetization transfer saturation pulse and cervical myelotraphy and CT. *Neuroradiology* 2004;46(4):306–309.

83. Stevenson JH, Trojian T. Evaluation of shoulder pain. *J Fam Pract* 2002;51(7):605–611.

84. Woodward TW, Best TM. The painful shoulder: part II—acute and chronic disorders. *Am Fam Physician* 2000;61(11):3291–3300.

85. Uri DS. MR imaging of shoulder impingement and rotator cuff disease. *Radiol Clin North Am* 1997;35(1):77–96.

86. Ertl JP, Kovacs G, Burger RS. Magnetic resonance imaging of the shoulder in the primary care setting. *Med Sci Sports Exerc* 1998;30(4 suppl):S7–S11.

87. Stiles RG, Otte MT. Imaging of the shoulder. *Radiology* 1993;188(3):603–613.

88. Garfin SR. Cervical degenerative disorders: etiology, presentation, and imaging studies. *Instru Course Lect* 2000;49:335–338.

89. Carragee EJ, Hurwitz EL, Cheng I, et al. Treatment of neck pain: injections and surgical interventions: results of the Bone and Joint Decade 2000–2010 Task Force on Neck Pain and Its Associated Disorders. *Spine* 2008;33 (4 suppl):S153–S169.

90. Kadanka Z, Mares M, Bednarik J, et al. Approaches to spondylotic cervical myelopathy: conservative versus surgical results in a 3 year follow-up study. *Spine* 2002;27(20):2205–2210; discussion 2210–2211.

91. Sampath P, Bendebba M, Davis JD. Outcome of patients treated for cervical myelopathy. A prospective, multicenter study with independent clinical review. *Spine* 2000;25(6):670–676.

92. Alafifi T, Kern R, Fehlings M. Clinical and MRI predictors of outcome after surgical intervention for cervical spondylotic myelopathy. *J Neuroimaging* 2007;17(4):315–322.

93. Wada E, Yonenobu K, Suzuki S, et al. Can intramedullary signal change on magnetic resonance imaging predict surgical outcome in cervical spondolytic myelopathy? *Spine* 1999;24(5):455–461.

94. Mastronardi L, Elsawaf A, Roperto R, et al. Prognostic relevance of the postoperative evolution of intramedullary spinal cord changes in signal intensity on magnetic resonance imaging after anterior decompression for cervical spondylotic myelopathy. *J Neurosurg Spine* 2007;7(6):615–622.

95. Brain RW, Northfield D, Wilkinson M. The neurological manifestations of cervical spondylosis. *Brain* 1952;75(2):187–225.

96. Truumees E, Herkowitz HN. Cervical spondylotic myelopathy and radiculopathy. *Instr Course Lect* 2000;49:339–360.

97. Malanga GA. The diagnosis and treatment of cervical radiculopathy. *Med Sci Sports Exerc* 1997;29(7 suppl):S236–S245.

98. Radhakrishnan K, Litchy WJ, O'Fallon WM, et al. Epidemiology of cervical radiculopathy. A population-based study from Rochester, Minnesota, 1976 through 1990. *Brain* 1994;117(Pt 2):325–335.

99. Malcolm GP. Surgical disorders of the cervical spine: presentation and management of common disorders. *J Neurosurg Psychiatry* 2002;73(suppl 1); i33–i41.

100. Shedid D, Benzel EC. Cervical spondylosis anatomy: pathophysiology and biomechanics. *Neurosurgery* 2007;60(1 Suppl 1):S7–S13.

101. Polston DW. Cervical radiculopathy. *Neurol Clin* 2007;25(2):373–385

102. Crandall PH, Batzdorf U. Cervical spondylotic myelopathy. *J Neurosurg* 1966;25(1):57–66.

103. Ferguson RJL, Caplan LR. Cervical spondylotic myelopathy. *Neurol Clin* 1985;3(2):373–382.

104. Ito T, Oyanagi K, Takahashi H, et al. Cervical spondylotic myelopathy: clinicopathologic study on the progression pattern and thin myelinated fibers of the lesions of seven patients examined during complete autopsy. *Spine* 1996; 21(7):827–833.

105. Fujii H, Yone K, Sakou T. Magnetic resonance imaging study of experimental acute spinal cord injury. *Spine* 1993;18(14):2030–2034.

106. Hunt WE. Cervical spondylosis: natural history and rare indications for surgical decompression. *Clin Neurosurg* 1980;27:466–480.

107. Long DM. Lumbar and cervical spondylosis and spondylotic myelopathy. *Curr Opin Neurol Neurosurg* 1993;6(4):576–580.

108. Lunsford LD, Bissonette DJ, Zorub DS. Anterior surgery for cervical disc disease. Part 2: treatment of cervical spondylotic myelopathy in 32 cases. *J Neurosurg* 1980;53(1):1–11.

109. Rowland LP. Surgical treatment of cervical spondylotic myelopathy: time for a controlled trial. *Neurology* 1992;42(1):5–13.

110. Sjaastad O, Saunte C, Hovdal H, et al. "Cervicogenic" headache. An hypothesis. *Cephalalgia* 1983;3(4):249–256.

111. Sjaastad O, Fredriksen TA, Pfaffenrath V. Cervicogenic headache: diagnostic criteria. The Cervicogenic Headache International Study Group. *Headache* 1990;30:725–726.

112. Sjaastad O, Fredriksen TA, Pfaffenrath V. Cervicogenic headache: diagnostic criteria. The Cervicogenic Headache International Study Group. *Headache* 1998;38(6):442–445.

113. Merskey H, Bogduk N, eds. *Classification of Chronic Pain: Description of Chronic Pain Syndromes and Definition of Pain Terms.* Seattle, WA: IASP Press; 1994.

114. Headache Classification Subcommittee of the International Headache Society. The international classification of headache disorders: second edition. *Cephalalgia* 2004;24(suppl 1):1–155.

115. Haldeman S, Dagenais S. Cervicogenic headaches: a critical review. *Spine J* 2001;1(1):31–46.

116. Antonaci F, Bono G, Chimento P. Diagnosing cervicogenic headache. *J Headache Pain* 2006;7(3):145–148.

117. Sjaastad O, Bakketeig LS. Tractor drivers' head and neckache: Vågå study of headache epidemiology. *Cephalalgia* 2002;22(6):462–467.

118. Lord SM, Barnsley L, Wallis BJ, et al. Third occipital nerve headache: a prevalence study. *J Neurol Neurosurg Psychiatry* 1994;57(10):1187–1190.

119. Aprill C, Axinn MJ, Bogduk N. Occipital headaches stemming from the lateral atlanto-axial (C1-2) joint. *Cephalalgia* 2002;22(1):15–22.

120. Kerr FWL. Central relationships of trigeminal and cervical primary afferents in the spinal cord and medulla. *Brain Res* 1972;43(2):561–572.

121. Busch V, Jakob W, Juergens T, et al. Functional connectivity between trigeminal and oxxipital nerves revealed by occipital nerve blockade and nociceptive blink reflexes. *Cephalalgia* 2005;26(1):50–55.

122. Groen GJ, Baljet B, Drukker J. Nerves and nerve plexuses of the juman vertebral column. *Am J Anat* 1990;188(3):282–296.

123. Schellhas KP, Garvey TA, Johnson BA, et al. Cervical diskography: analysis of provoked responses at C2-C3, C3-C4, and C4-C5. *AJNR Am J Neuroradiol* 2000;21(2):269–275.

124. Ahn Y, Lee SH, Chung SE, et al. Percutaneous endoscopic cervical discectomy for discogenic cervical headache due to soft disc herniation. *Neuroradiology* 2005;47(12):924–930.

125. Diener HC, Kaminski M, Stappert G, et al. Lower cervical disc proloapse may cause cervicogenic headache: prospective study in patients undergoing surgery. *Cephalalgia* 2007;27(9):1050–1054.

126. Biondi DM. Cervicogenic headache: a review of diagnostic and treatment strategies. *J Am Osteopath Assoc* 2005;105(4 Suppl 2):16S–22S.

127. Leone M, D'Amico D, Grazzi L, et al. Cervicogenic headache: a critical review of the current diagnostic criteria. *Pain* 1998;78(1):1–5.

128. Bovim G, Sand T. Cervicogenic headache, migraine without aura and tension-type headache. Diagnostic blockade of the greater occipital and supra-orbital nerves. *Pain* 1992;51(1):43–48.

129. Naja ZM, El-Rajab M, Al-Tannir MA, et al. Occipital nerve blockade for cervicogenic headache: A double-blind randomized controlled clinical trial. *Pain Pract* 2006;6(2):89–95.

130. Navani A, Mahajan G, Kreis P, et al. A case of pulsed radiofrequency lesioning for occipital neuralgia. *Pain Med* 2006;7(5):453–456.

131. Lord SM, Barnsley L, Wallis BJ, et al. Percutaneous radio-frequency neurotomy for chronic cervical zygapophyseal-joint pain. *New Engl J Med* 1996; 335(23):1721–1726.

132. Gross AR, Hoving JL, Haines TA, et al. Manipulation and mobilization for mechanical neck disorders. *Chochrane Database Syst Rev* 2004;1:CD004249.

133. Peloso P, Gross A, Haines T, et al. Medicinal and injection therapies for mechanical neck disorderes. *Cochrane Database Syst Rev* 2007;18(3): CD00319.

134. Sarzi-Puttine P, Atzeni F. New developments in our understanding of DISH (diffuse idiopathic skeletal hyperostosis). *Curr Opin Rheum* 2004;16(3): 287–292.

135. Childs SG. Diffuse idiopathic skeletal hyperostosis: Forestier's disease. *Orthoped Nurs* 2004;23(6):375–382.

136. Marshall LL, Trethewie ER, Curtain CC. Chemical radiculitis. A clinical, physiological and immunological study. *Clin Orthop* 1977;129:61–67.

137. Hoyland JA, Freemont AJ, Jayson MI V. Intervertebral foramen venous obstruction. A cause of periradicular fibrosis? *Spine* 1989;14(6):558–568.

138. Jayson MI. The role of vascular damage and fibrosis in the pathogenesis of nerve root damage. *Clin Orthop* 1992;279:40–48.

139. Hasue M. Pain and the nerve root. An interdisciplinary approach. *Spine* 1993; 18(14):2053–2058.

140. Garfin SR, Rydevik B, Bengt L, et al. Spinal nerve root compression. *Spine* 1995;20(16):1810–1820.

141. Boyd-Clark LC, Briggs CA, Galea MP. Segmental degeneration in the cervical spine and associated changes in dorsal root ganglia. *Clin Anat* 2004;17(6): 468–477.

142. Kouwenhoven JW, Wuisman PI, Ploegmakers JF. Headache due to an osteochondroma of the axis. *Eur Spine J* 2004;13(8):746–749.

143. Bogduk N. Cervicogenic headache: anatomic basis and pathophysiologic mechanisms. *Curr Pain Headache Rep* 2001;5(4):382–386.

144. Harrop JS, Hanna A, Silva MT, et al. Neurological manifestations of cervical spondylosis: an overview of signs, symptoms and pathophysiology. *Neurosurgery* 2007;60(1 Suppl 1):S14–S20.

145. Wainner RS, Gill H. Diagnosis and nonoperative management of cervical radiculopathy. *J Orthop Sports Phys Ther* 2000;30(12):728–744.

146. Wolff MW, Levine LA. Cervical radiculopathies: conservative approaches to management. *Phys Med Rehabil Clin N Am* 2002;13(3):589–608.

147. Sampath P, Bendebba M, Davis JD, et al. Outcome in patients with cervical radiculopathy: prospective, multicenter study with independent clinical review. *Spine* 1999;24(6):591–597.

148. Galluzze KE. Managing neuropathic pain. *J AM Osteopath Assoc* 2007; 107(10 suppl 6):ES39–ES48.

149. Chen H, Lamer TJ, Rho RH, et al. Contemporary management of neuropathic pain for the primary care physician. *Mayo Clin Proc* 2004;79(12):1533–1545.

150. Peloso P, Gross A, Haines T, et al. Medicinal and injection therapies for mechanical neck disorders. *Cochrane Database Syst Rev* 2007;18(3): CD000319.

151. Abdi S, Datta S, Trescot AM, et al. Epidural steroids in the management of chronic spinal pain: a systematic review. *Pain Physician* 2007;10:185–212.

152. Scanlan GC, Moeller-Bertram T, Romanowsky SM, et al. Cervical transforaminal epidural steroid injections more dangerous than we think? *Spine* 2007;32(11):1249–1256.

153. Manchikanti L, Bakhit CE, Pakanati RR, et al. Flouroscopy is medically necessary for the performance of epidurla steroids. *Anesth Analg* 1999;89(5): 1330–1331.

154. Hessiion WG, Stanczak JD, Davis KW, et al. Epidural steroid injections. *Semin Roentgenol* 2004;39(1):7–23.

155. Bencardino JT, Rosenberg ZS. Entrapment neuropathies of the shoulder and elbow in the athlete. *Clin Sports Med* 2006;25(3):465–487.

156. Corwin HM. Compression neuropathies of the upper extremity. *Clin Occup Environ Med* 2006;5(2):333–352, viii.

157. Morgan G, Wilbourn A. Cervical radiculopathy and coexisting distal entrapment.neuropathies: double-crush syndromes? *Neurology* 1998;50(1):78–83.

158. Wellik GM. Nerve entrapments of the wrist: early treatment preserves function. *JAAPA* 2005;18(4):18–23.

159. Dimeff RJ. Entrapment neuropathies of the upper extremity. *Curr Sports Med Rep* 2003;2(5):255–261.
160. Yoshikawa T, Hayashi N, Yamamoto S, et al. Brachial plexus injury: clinical manifestations, conventional imaging findings and the latest imaging techniques. *Radiographics* 2006;26(suppl 1):S133–S143.
161. Bertelli JA, Ghizoni MF. Use of clinical signs and computed tomography myelography findings in detecting and excluding nerve root avulsion in complete brachial plexus palsy. *J Neurosurg* 2006;105(6):835–842.
162. Kawabata H, Shibata T, Matsui Y, et al. Use of intercostals nerves for neurotization of the Musculocutaneous nerve in infants with birth-related brachial plexus palsy. *J Neurosurg* 2001;94(3):386–391.
163. Samii A, Carvalho GA, Samii M. Brachial plexus injury: factors affecting functional outcome in spinal accessory nerve transfer for the restoration of elbow flexion. *J Neurosurg* 2003;98(2):307–312.
164. Norkus T, Norkus M, Pranchevicius S, et al. Early and late reconstruction in brachial plexus palsy: a preliminary report. *Medicina (Kaunas)* 2006;42(6):484–491.
165. Owen SL, Green AL, Nandi DD, et al. Deep brain stimulation for neuropathic pain. *Acta Neurochir Suppl* 2007;97(Pt 2):111–116.
166. Verdolin MH, Stedje-Larsen ET, Hickey AH. Ten consecutive cases of complex regional pain syndrome of less than 12 months duration in active duty United States minitary personnel treated with spinal cord stimulation. *Anesth Analg* 2007;104(6):1557–1560.
167. Spillane JD. Localized neuritis of the shoulder girdle. A report of 46 patients in the MEF. *Lancet* 1943;2:532–5.
168. Parsonage M, Turner J. Neuralgic amyotrophy: the shoulder-girdle syndrome. *Lancet* 1948;1:973–8.
169. Miller JD, Pruitt S, Mcdonald TJ. Acute brachial plexus neuritis: an uncommon cause of shoulder pain. *Am Fam Phys* 2000;62(9):2067–2072.
170. Sierra A, Prat J, Bas J, et al. Blood lymphocytes are sensitized to brachial plexus nerves in patients with neuralgic amyotrophy. *Acta Neurol Scand* 1991;83(3):183–186.
171. Lo YJ, Mills KR. Motor root conduction in neuralgic amyotrophy: evidence of proximal conduction block. *J Neurol Neurosurg Psychiatry* 1999;66(5):586–590.
172. Tsairis P, Dyck PJ, Mulder DW. Natural history of brachial neuritis. *Arch Neurol* 1972;27:109–117.
173. Jaspert A, Claus D, Grehl H, et al. Multifocal motor neuropathy: clinical and electrophysiologic findings. *J Neurol* 1996;243(10):684–692.
174. Inoue M, Hojo T, Yano T, et al. The effects of electroacupuncture on peripheral nerve regeneration in rats. *Acupunct Med* 2003;21(1–2):9–17.
175. Patel G, Euler D, Audette JF. Complementary and alternative medicine for noncancer pain. *Med Clin North Am* 2007;91(1):141–167.
176. Peet RM, Hendriksen JD, Anderson TP, et al. Thoracic outlet syndrome: evaluation of a therapeutic exercise program. *Proc Staff Meet Mayo Clin* 1956;31(9):281–287.
177. Urschel HC, Kourlis H. Thoracic outlet syndrome: a 50 year experience at Baylor Univesity Medial Center. *Proc (Bay Univ Med Cent)* 2007;20(2):125–135.
178. Durham JR, Yao JS, Pearce WH, et al. Arterial injuries in the thoracic outlet syndromes. *J Vasc Surg* 1995;21(1):57–69.
179. Huang JH, Zager EL. Thoracic outlet syndrome. *Neurosurg* 2004;55(4):897–902.
180. Davidovic LB, Kostic DM, Jakovljevic NS, et al. Vascular thoracic outlet syndrome. *World J Surg* 2003;27(5):545–550.
181. Sanders RJ, Hammond SL, Rao NM. Diagnosis of thoracic outlet syndrome. *J Vasc Surg* 2007;46(3):601–604.
182. Gergoudis R, Barnes RW. Thoracic outlet arterial compression: prevalence in normal persons. *Angiology* 1980;31(8):538–541.
183. Cruz-Martinez A, Arpa J. Electrophysiological assessment in neurogenic thoracic outlet syndrome. *Electromyogr Clin Neurophysiol* 2001;41(4):253–256.
184. Rousseff R, Tzvetanov P, Valkov I. Utility (or futility?) of electrodiagnosis in thoracic outlet syndrome. *Electromyogr Clin Neurophysiol* 2005;45(3):131–133.
185. Demondion X, Herbinet P, Van Sint Jan S, et al. Imaging assessment of thoracic outlet syndrome. *Radiographics* 2006;26(6):1735–1750.
186. Mackinnon SE, Patterson GA, Navak CB. Thoracic outlet syndrome: a current overview. *Semin Thorac Cardiovasc Surg* 1996;8(2):176–182.
187. Degeorges R, Reynaud C, Becquemin JP. Thoracic outlet syndrome surgery: long-term functional results. *Ann Vasc Surg* 2004;18(5):558–565.
188. Rockind S, Shemesh M, Patish H, et al. Thoracic outlet syndrome: a multidisciplinary problem with a perspective for microsurgical management without rib resection. *Acta Neurochir Suppl* 2007;100:145–147.
189. Inamasu J, Guiot BH. Intracranial hypotension with spinal pathology. *Spine J* 2006;6(5):591–599.
190. Joo WI, Lee KJ, Rha HK, et al. Delayed diagnosis, due to the associated radiological abnormalities of spontaneous intracranial hypotension caused by cerebrospinal fluid leakage at C1-2. *Br J Neurosurg* 2008;22(2):292–294.
191. Schienvink WI. Sontaneous spinal cerebrospinal fluid leaks and intracranial hypotension. *JAMA* 2006;295(19):2286–2296.
192. Paldino M, Mogilner Ay, Tenner MS. Intracranial hypotension syndrome: a comprehensive review. *Neurosurg Focus* 2003;15(6):ECP2.
193. Miyazawa K, Shiga Y, Hasegawa T, et al. CSF hypovolemia vs intracranial hypotension in "spontaneous intracranial hypotension syndrome." *Neurology* 2003;60(6):941–947.
194. Ferrante E, Arpino I, Citterio A. Is it a rational choice to treat with lumbar epidural blood patch headache caused by spontaneous cervical CSF leak? *Cephalalgia* 2006;26(10):1245–1246.
195. Inamasu J, Nakatsukasa M. Blood patch for spontaneous intracranial hypotension caused by cerebrospinal fluid leak at C1-2. *Clin Neurol Neurosurg* 2007;109:716–719.
196. Kantor D, Silberstein SD. Cervical epidural blood patch for low CSF pressure headaches. *Neurology* 2005;65(7):1138.
197. Binder DK, Dillon WP, Fishman RA, et al. Intrathecal saline infusion in the treatment of obtundation associated with spontaneous intracranial hypotension: technical case report. *Neurosurgery* 2002;51(3):830–836.
198. Inamasu J, Guiot BH. Intracranial hypotension with spinal pathology. *Spine J* 2006;6(5):591–599.

CHAPTER 69 ■ CHEST WALL PAIN

NARASIMHA R. GUNDAMRAJ AND STEVEN RICHEIMER

GENERAL CONSIDERATIONS

The chest wall is one of the common sites of pain encountered in clinical practice. The origin of pain can be from various structures of the chest wall. These include pain from skeletal components including the spine, muscles, and nerves, or pain that is referred from outside the chest wall (Table 69.1). For instance, visceral pain from the chest can be perceived as chest wall pain. It is important to distinguish the origin of pain as arising from the chest wall or from the viscera inside. Focusing on some key points in the history and physical examination can assist in diagnosing the origin of pain. A thorough knowledge of the anatomy and physiology of the chest wall and its relationship to the vital organs enclosed inside is essential for any clinician involved in treatment of chest wall pain.

ANATOMY OF THE CHEST WALL

The chest wall is made up of skeletal structures, muscular elements, and neurovascular components. The skeletal structures of the chest wall include the ribs, vertebrae, and the sternum. From a functional standpoint, the skeletal components of the chest wall provide protection for the specialized organs that support the vital functions of the human body.

Skeletal Structures of the Chest Wall

The chest wall is made up of the vertebrae posteriorly, ribs and costal cartilages laterally, and the sternum anteriorly. The superior boundary of the thorax includes the T1 vertebra posteriorly,

CHEST PAIN CAUSED BY NEUROPATHIC, MUSCULOSKELETAL, AND OTHER DISORDERS

I. Pain primarily of neuropathic origin
  A. Disease of the spinal cord (myelopathy)
  B. Lesions of the rootlets or roots of thoracic spinal nerves (radiculopathy)
  C. Lesions of the formed spinal nerves (neuropathy)
  D. Lesions of the intercostal nerves (intercostal neuropathy)
  E. Disorders of the peripheral branches of spinal nerves (peripheral neuropathy)

II. Pain primarily of musculoskeletal origin
  A. Lesions or disease of bones
    1. Disease or lesions of the thoracic vertebrae
    2. Disease or lesions of the ribs
    3. Diseases or disorders of the costal cartilages
    4. Disease or disorders of the sternum
    5. Disease of the sternoclavicular joint
  B. Disorders of muscles
    1. Myofascial pain syndromes
    2. Chest pain caused by other disorders of muscles

III. Diseases of the skin
  A. Burns and other trauma
  B. Cicatrices
  C. Postoperative pain syndromes
  D. Mastodynia
  E. Deep axillary abscess
  F. Adiposis dolorosa
  G. Phlebitis of the anterolateral chest
  H. Other dermatologic painful disorders

IV. Chest pain caused by extrathoracic diseases
  A. Disorders of the cervical spine and shoulder
    1. Intervertebral disk disease
    2. Thoracic outlet syndromes
  B. Abdominal diseases
    1. Gas entrapment syndromes
    2. Disorders of the gastrointestinal tract
    3. Disease of the biliary tract
    4. Disease of the pancreas
    5. Other abdominal visceral disease
  C. Diseases of the diaphragm
    1. Acute primary diaphragmatitis
    2. Subphrenic abscess
    3. Diaphragmatic flutter

V. Chest pain primarily of psychological origin
  A. Abnormal emotional reactions to visceral disease
  B. Anxiety syndrome
  C. Depression syndrome
  D. Conversion reaction
  E. Hypochondriasis
  F. Psychiatric syndromes

first rib laterally, and superior margin of the sternum (Fig. 69.1). Inferiorly the thorax is bounded by the T12 vertebra and the twelfth rib posteriorly, seventh to tenth ribs and their cartilages laterally joining anteriorly to the xiphisternum.[1,2] The anteroposterior and lateral diameter of the thorax is smaller at the top compared to the inferior portion. A compromise in the space at the thoracic inlet due to pathology of the skeletal structures or thoracic viscera can compromise the neurovascular structures and also result in chest wall pain.[3,4]

Thoracic Spine

The thoracic spine is made up of 12 thoracic vertebrae (Fig. 69.2). Each thoracic vertebra is heart shaped with long and inclined spinous processes (Fig. 69.3). Costal facets are present laterally on either side of the body for articulation with the ribs. Costal facets are also present on the transverse processes (except T11 and T12) for articulation with the tubercles of the ribs.

Ribs

There are 12 pairs of ribs attached posteriorly to the spine. The upper seven pairs of ribs are attached anteriorly to the sternum by costal cartilages and are called true ribs (Fig. 69.4). The eighth, ninth, and tenth ribs are attached to each other and the seventh rib by their costal cartilages forming small synovial joints. These ribs are called false ribs. The eleventh and twelfth ribs have no anterior attachments and are called floating ribs. A typical rib is a long, curved, flat bone. The superior border is smooth and rounded. The inferior border is sharp and thin and it overhangs the costal groove which encloses the intercostals vessels and the nerves. The head of the rib has two facets for articulation with the corresponding vertebral body and the one above it. The neck is a constricted portion of the rib after the head. A prominence on the outer surface of the rib at the junction of the shaft and the neck is called the tubercle. It also has a facet for articulation with the transverse process of the corresponding vertebra. A cervical rib arising from the transverse process of the seventh cervical vertebra is seen in 0.5% of humans. It can cause pressure on the adjacent neurovascular structures—the brachial plexus and the subclavian artery.

Sternum

The sternum is a flat bone in the middle of the anterior chest wall. It is divided into three parts: manubrium, body, and xiphoid process. The manubrium is the upper portion of the sternum that articulates with the body of the sternum at the manubriosternal joint. It also articulates at the clavicles, the first costal cartilage, and the upper portion of the second costal cartilage. The body of the sternum on each side articulates with the second to seventh costal cartilages. The xiphoid process is a roughly triangular cartilaginous structure that becomes ossified in adulthood. The angle of Louis or sternal angle is the junction between the manubrium and the body of the sternum. This useful anatomic landmark is palpated by feeling for a transverse ridge on the anterior aspect of the sternum. It correlates to the second costal cartilage anteriorly and the intervertebral disc between the fourth and fifth thoracic vertebrae posteriorly.

Joints of the Chest Wall

The chest wall includes many joints. The manubriosternal joint and xiphisternal joints are fixed joints. The costochondral connections of ribs with costal cartilages are also nonsynovial joints. These costochondral joints can become the source of painful irritation. The costal cartilages often calcify with age, reducing the flexibility of the chest wall. The joints of the heads of the ribs with the vertebral bodies, and the joints of the tubercles with the transverse processes of the ribs are synovial joints that allow for the expansion movements of the chest wall. The joints of the costal cartilages with the sternum are synovial (with the exception of the first rib), but these joints allow for only slight motion and they tend to disappear with age.

Intercostal Spaces

The intercostal space between the ribs is covered with three muscles: the external intercostals, internal intercostals, and the inner-

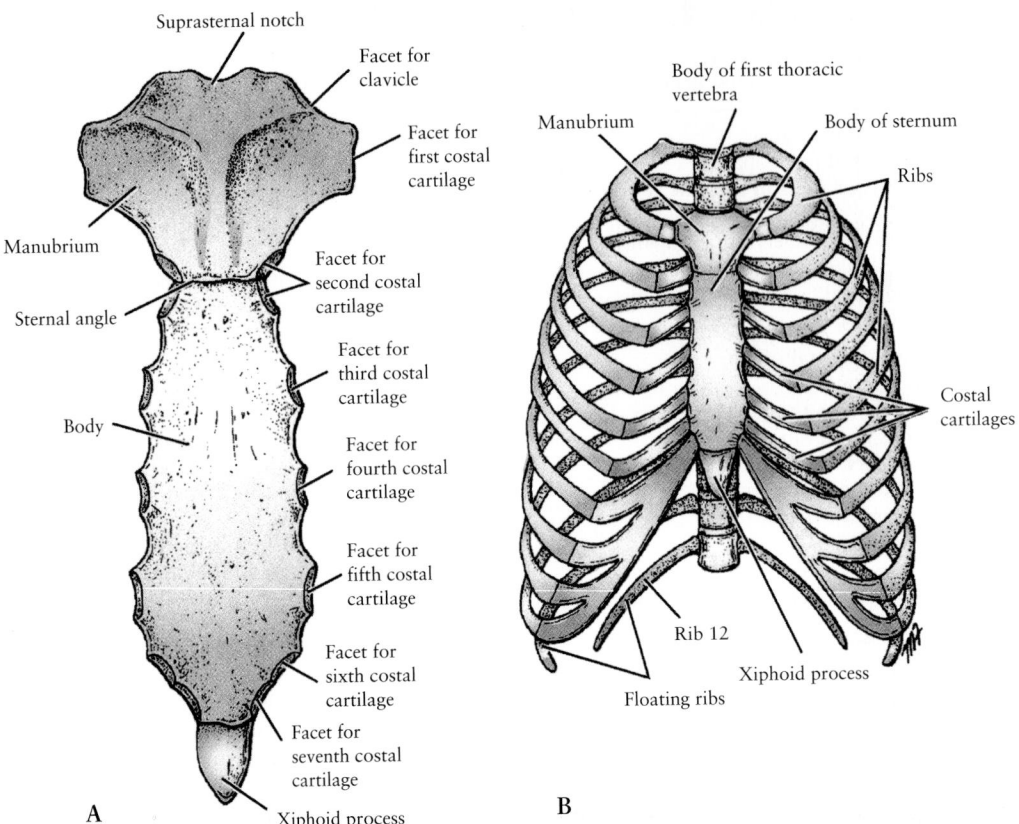

FIGURE 69.1 **A.** Anterior view of the sternum. **B.** Sternum, ribs and costal cartilages forming the thoracic skeleton. From Snell RS. *Clinical Anatomy by Regions*, 8th ed. Philadelphia: Lippincott Williams & Wilkins, 2007.

most intercostals muscle (Fig. 69.5). The innermost intercostal muscle is lined by the endothoracic fascia, which in turn covers the parietal pleura. The intercostal nerves and blood vessels run between the internal and the innermost intercostals muscles in the intercostals groove. The intercostal muscles play an important role in the mechanics of respiration. They are supplied by the corresponding intercostal nerves. The neurovascular structures in the intercostal groove are arranged from above downward as vein, artery, and nerve.

Intercostal Nerves

The anterior rami of the first 11 thoracic spinal nerves form the intercostals nerves. The anterior ramus of the twelfth nerve lies in the abdominal wall as the subcostal nerve. The rami communicantes connect the intercostals nerve to the sympathetic trunk. The collateral branch runs forward inferiorly to the intercostal nerve on the upper border of the rib below. The lateral cutaneous branch runs in the skin on the side of the chest and divides in to the anterior and posterior branches. The anterior cutaneous branch is the terminal portion of the intercostal nerves and reaches the skin near the midline anteriorly (Fig. 69.6). Muscular branches are given out to the intercostals muscles. Pleural sensory branches go to the pleura. Peritoneal sensory branches from the seventh to eleventh intercostal nerves run to the parietal peritoneum. The first intercostal nerve has a branch joining the brachial plexus. The second intercostals nerve joins the medial cutaneous nerve of the arm by the intercostobrachial nerve. In coronary artery disease, referred pain to the arm might be through this nerve.[5]

NEOPLASTIC CHEST WALL PAIN

A thorough history and physical examination is necessary to rule out pain caused by neoplasms of the thorax. Associated symptoms of cough, dyspnea, brachial plexopathy, and hoarseness due to recurrent laryngeal nerve involvement or Horner syndrome should arouse the suspicion of possible neoplastic disease. Diagnostic radiologic tests can confirm the diagnosis and the extent of involvement. If there is a high level of suspicion for neoplastic disease in a patient presenting with chest wall pain, diagnosis of the condition should be undertaken prior to any interventional procedures. Pain due to neoplastic disease is treated with a comprehensive or multimodal approach with opioid and nonopioid analgesics, physical therapy, interventional treatment with intercostal nerve blocks or epidural injections, and psychotherapy. In patients with refractory cancer pain, neuraxial delivery of opioid and local anesthetics by continuous infusion pumps or neurolytic ablation may be necessary for pain control.

Lung and breast cancers account for the majority of the thoracic neoplasms. Other neoplasms include metastatic lesions of the lung and the skeletal structures. Neoplasms of the lung present with symptoms of cough, dyspnea, hemoptysis, or obstructive symptoms due to compression of the neurovascular structures. Pain is not a common symptom with lung cancers except when there is pleural involvement. Nociceptive pain is usually localized, constant, or associated with chest wall movement and is caused by the invasion of the pleura, vertebrae, or other soft tissues of the chest wall. Deafferentation or neuropathic pain is caused by compression, infiltration, or damage to the involved spinal nerves and produces allodynia, hyperalgesia, dysesthesia, or hyperesthesia in a segmental fashion.[6] Involvement of the superior pulmonary sulcus produces Pancoast syndrome. It is characterized by pain in the shoulder and arm, motor weakness and wasting of muscles of the hand, as well as Horner syndrome.[7] The mass in the superior sulcus of the lung can cause compression of the lower trunk of the brachial plexus. Pain and motor symptoms are most commonly seen in the distribution of the ulnar nerve. Brachial plexopathy can also result from other causes such as metastatic tumors, radiation, or thoracic surgery.[8,9]

Epidural Spinal Cord Compression

Epidural spinal cord compression is the second most common central neurologic complication of systemic cancer. Pain is the initial symptom before the development of other neurologic signs and symptoms. The pain can be misdiagnosed as musculoskeletal in origin. Appropriate imaging studies can aid in the diagnosis. Treatment includes corticosteroids and radiation. Surgical decompression with laminectomy or vertebral body resection is recommended in patients who are relatively healthy.[10,11]

Superior Vena Cava Syndrome

Obstruction of the blood flow through the superior vena cava results in superior vena cava syndrome. The obstruction can be due to external compression from pathology of the lung, lymph nodes, or mediastinum. It can also result from internal obstruction. There can be coexistent thrombosis along with the external compression. Chest wall pain, cough, dyspnea along with venous engorgement of the chest wall and neck, and facial edema are the common signs and symptoms. Dyspnea is the most common symptom. Lung cancer is the most common cause followed by lymphoma. Malignancy accounts for 60% to 85% of all cases of superior vena cava syndrome with small cell lung cancer serving as the most common type of lung malignancy causing this syndrome.[12] Non–Hodgkin lymphoma is the most common type of lymphoma resulting in obstruction of the superior vena cava. Diagnosis is made based upon clinical symptoms and the findings of abnormal lesions in the chest radiograph. Confirmatory studies include contrast enhanced computed tomography (CT) scan and venous angiography. Current treatment strategies include chemotherapy, radiation, or endovascular stenting.[13] Radiation treatment is indicated for emergency relief of airway obstruction.

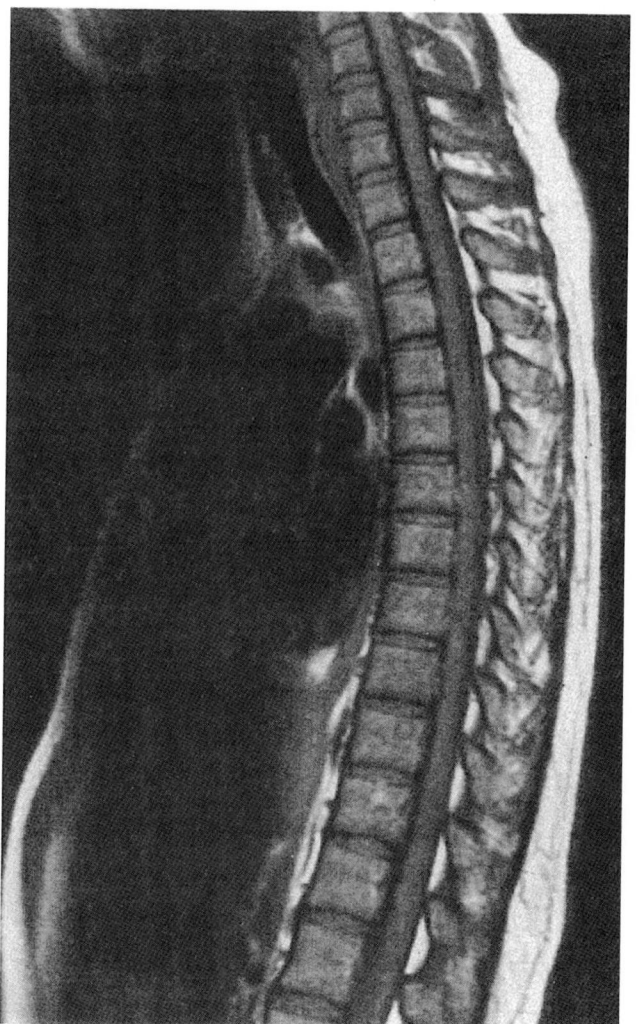

FIGURE 69.2 MRI Normal thoracic spine, midsaggittal T1-weighted image. Lee JKT, Sagel SS, Stanley RJ, et al. *Computerized Body Tomography with MRI Correlation*, 4th ed. Philadelphia: Lippincott Williams & Wilkins; 2006.

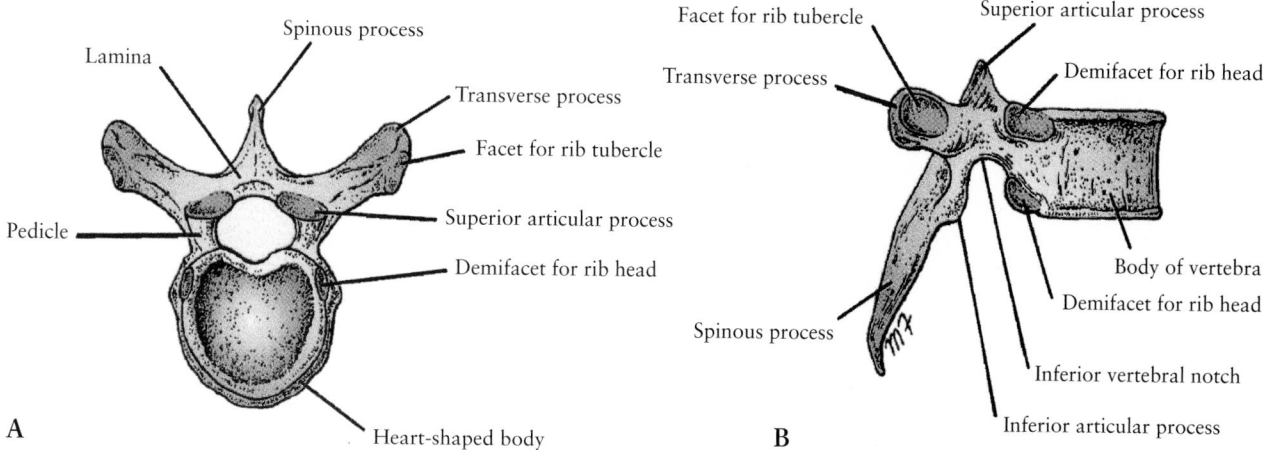

FIGURE 69.3 Thoracic vertebra **A.** Superior surface **B.** Lateral surface. From Snell RS. *Clinical Anatomy by Regions*, 8th ed. Philadelphia: Lippincott Williams & Wilkins; 2007.

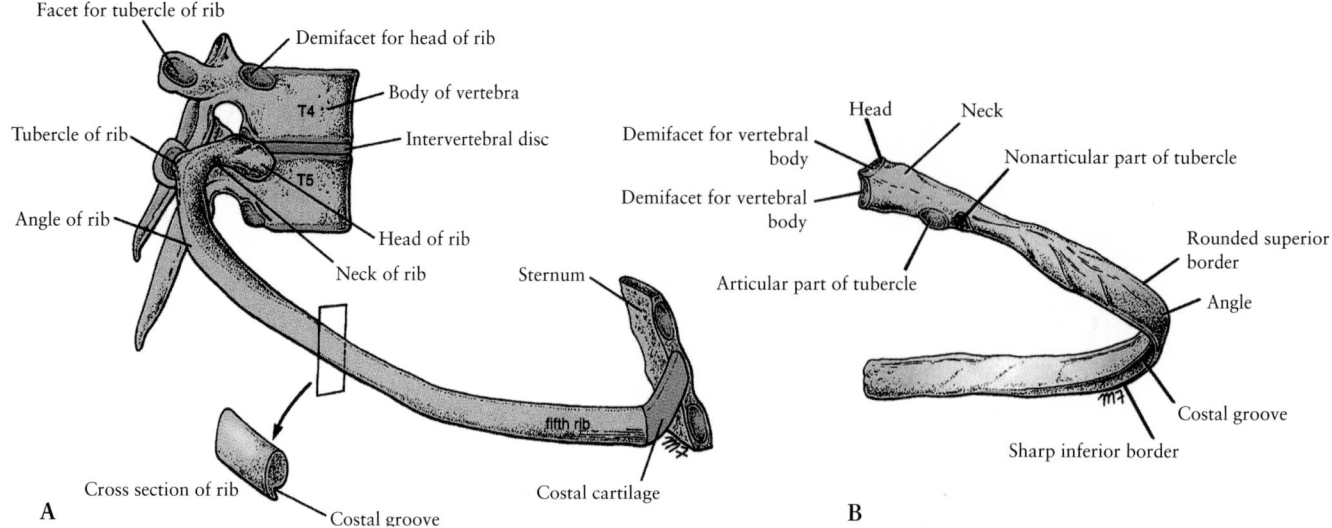

FIGURE 69.4 Fifth rib as it articulates with the vertebral column posteriorly and the sternum anteriorly. From Snell RS. *Clinical Anatomy by Regions*, 8th ed. Philadelphia: Lippincott Williams & Wilkins; 2007.

Costopleural Syndrome

Tumor invasion of the pleura, ribs, and soft tissues of the chest wall with or without involvement of the intercostals nerves can result in sharp, aching, or burning pain (Fig. 69.7). Pain is exacerbated by movements of the chest wall, deep breathing, and coughing. Lesions of the pleura closer to the diaphragm can cause localized pain in the shoulder region or referred dull aching pain in the back or upper abdomen. Mediastinal pleural involvement causes pain deep in the central portion of the chest or the shoulder region. This type of pain is often potently responsive to steroidal or nonsteroidal anti-inflammatory analgesics.

NONNEOPLASTIC CHEST WALL PAIN

Chest wall pain from other than neoplasms and visceral pain will be discussed in this section. This section includes a discussion of chest wall pain due to neuropathy including neuraxial pain, myofascial, skeletal, and joint pain.

Neuropathic Pain

Pain due to neuropathy can arise anywhere along the nervous system supplying the chest wall. The pain can be neuraxial involv-

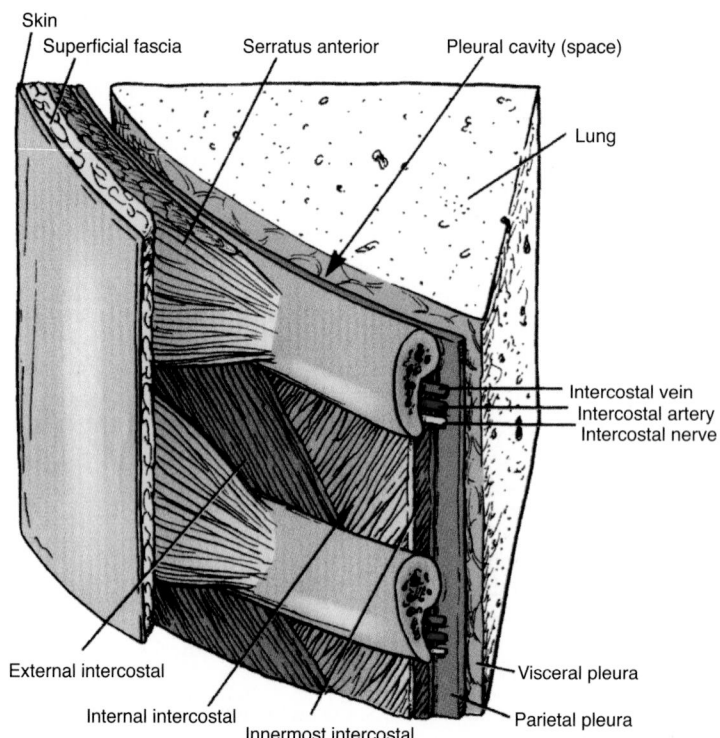

FIGURE 69.5 Intercostal space, its boundaries and contents. From Snell RS. *Clinical Anatomy by Regions*, 8th ed. Philadelphia: Lippincott Williams & Wilkins; 2007.

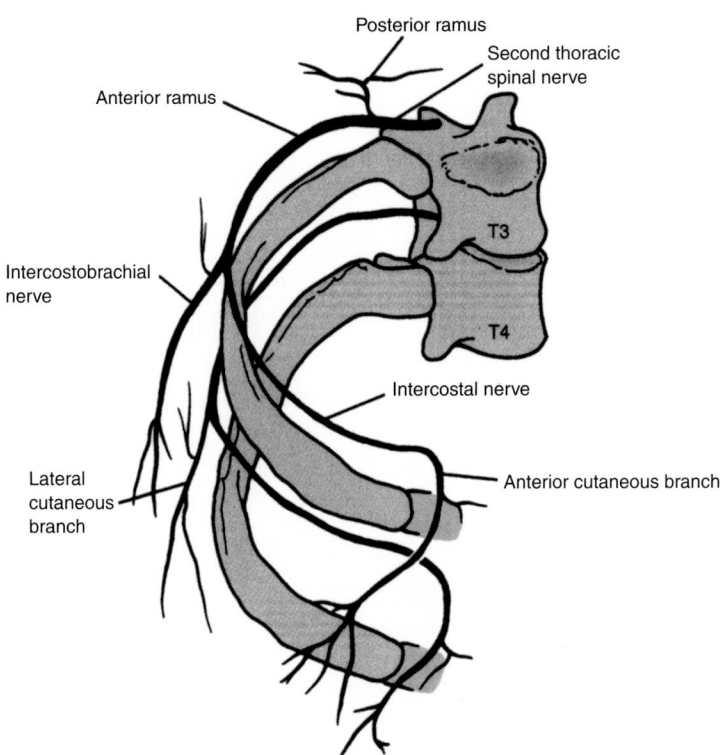

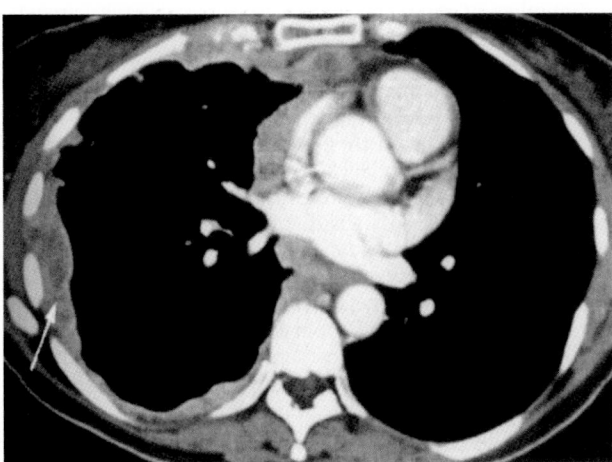

FIGURE 69.6 The distribution of two intercostals nerves to the rib cage. From Snell RS. *Clinical Anatomy by Regions*, 8th ed. Philadelphia: Lippincott Williams & Wilkins; 2007.

ing the spinal cord and nerve roots or related to peripheral nerves (Table 69.2).

Neuropathic Pain of Central Origin

Thoracic myelopathy can cause chest wall pain, back pain, or abdominal pain. Lesions can be present within the spinal cord or extramedullary or epidural spaces. Thoracic disc herniation can also result in chest wall pain (Fig. 69.8). Pain is usually the initial symptom before other neurologic symptoms. Pain is worsened in the recumbent position. If pain is the only symptom, it is often confused as myofascial or skeletal pain. Prompt diagnosis is important in light of potentially evolving cord compression. Pain that is progressive and not relieved by conventional therapy

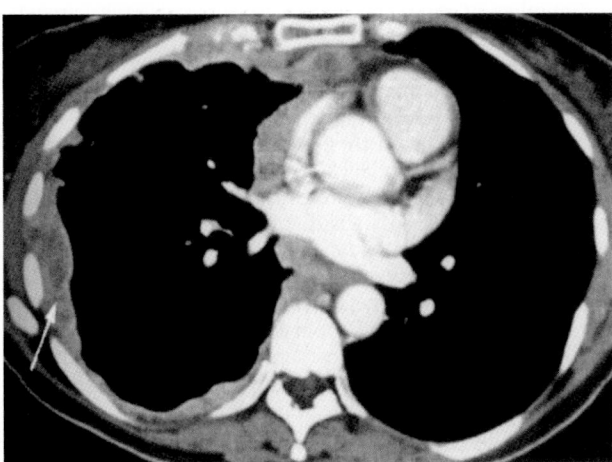

FIGURE 69.7 CT image showing right pleural thickening due to mesothelioma. Lee JKT, Sagel SS, Stanley RJ, et al. *Computerized Body Tomography with MRI Correlation*, 4th edition. Philadelphia: Lippincott Williams & Wilkins, 2006.

for musculoskeletal pain requires prompt attention to rule out neoplasm. Acute neurologic symptoms are initially treated with corticosteroids and radiation therapy.[14] Surgical decompression with laminectomy may be necessary if the symptoms are not relieved by nonsurgical methods. Lower cervical disc herniation can also present as neuropathic chest wall pain.[15,16] A relatively rare cause of thoracic neuropathic pain is seen in the form of an extramedullary granuloma in patients with neuraxial infusion pumps. Stopping the implanted infusion pump and radiographic exam with contrast through the catheter, CT myelography or magnetic resonance imaging can help make the diagnosis. Stopping the infusion may decrease the size of the mass. Surgical removal of the symptomatic granuloma is rarely necessary.[17]

Peripheral Neuropathic Chest Wall Pain

Herpes Zoster and Postherpetic Neuralgia. Acute herpes zoster, also called shingles, is caused by the deoxyribonucleic acid (DNA) virus, varicella zoster. The incidence of herpes zoster is higher in older and immunocompromised patients. Factors that decrease immune function such as chronic corticosteroid use, human immunodeficiency virus infection, cancer, and chemotherapy can increase the risk of developing herpes zoster.[18,19] Following a primary varicella infection, the virus remains dormant in the dorsal root ganglia. Acute herpes zoster is characterized by the reactivation of the latent virus in the dorsal root ganglion. It typically presents as a mononeuropathy involving the intercostal nerves. Clinically the presentation begins with burning pain, hyperesthesia or tingling followed by the characteristic vesicular rash. The prodromal sensory symptoms may be present for 1 to 2 weeks prior to the appearance of the rash.[20] The characteristic rash is initially maculopapular and progresses into vesicles with erythematous bases. The rash of herpes zoster is commonly seen involving one or two contiguous thoracic dermatomes, almost always unilateral. T5 and T6 dermatomes are most commonly affected.[21] Pain is sharp, burning, and superficial in nature. Pain can be worsened with ulceration and secondary infection of the vesicles. Associated muscle spasms can worsen the pain.

TABLE 69.2

CHEST PAIN PRIMARILY OF NEUROPATHIC ORIGIN

I. Diseases of the spinal cord (myelopathy)
   A. Intrinsic spinal cord diseases: primary tumors, metastatic tumors, syringomyelia, trauma, multiple sclerosis, infarction, abscess
   B. Extramedullary intrathecal disorders
      1. Primary tumors: meningioma, neurofibroma
      2. Metastatic tumors
   C. Epidural spinal cord compression
      1. Primarily caused by vertebral pathology
      2. Metastatic neoplasm from breast, lung, prostate
      3. Epidural abscess
      4. Hematoma
      5. Adhesive arachnoiditis

II. Diseases of the rootlets and roots of spinal nerves (radiculopathy)
   A. Infection and inflammation
      1. Herpes zoster
      2. Syphilis (tabes dorsalis)
      3. Meningitis
      4. Systemic infection
      5. Tuberculosis
      6. Other infectious diseases
   B. Mechanical compression or injury
      1. Osteoarthritis
      2. Other arthritides
      3. Ruptured intervertebral disk
      4. Fracture of vertebra
      5. Abscess or tumor of the vertebra
      6. Paget disease of the spine

III. Diseases of the formed thoracic spinal nerves (neuropathy)
   A. Vertebral compression (same as IIB)
   B. Paravertebral compression
      1. Paravertebral adenopathy
      2. Mediastinal tumors
      3. Paravertebral abscess
      4. Aortic aneurysm
   C. Primary nerve tumors
      1. Neurofibroma
      2. Schwannoma
   D. Systemic infection, neuropathy
   E. Other neuritides
      1. Alcoholism
      2. Avitaminosis
      3. Intoxication by heavy metals, food, amoebae
      4. Vitamin metabolic disorders and others

IV. Disorders of the intercostal nerves (intercostal neuralgia)
   A. Compression or injury secondary to fracture or tumors of ribs
   B. External trauma (e.g., stab wounds)
   C. Postinfectious intercostal neuropathy
   D. Postoperative neuropathy
      1. Postmastectomy syndrome
      2. Postthoracotomy syndrome

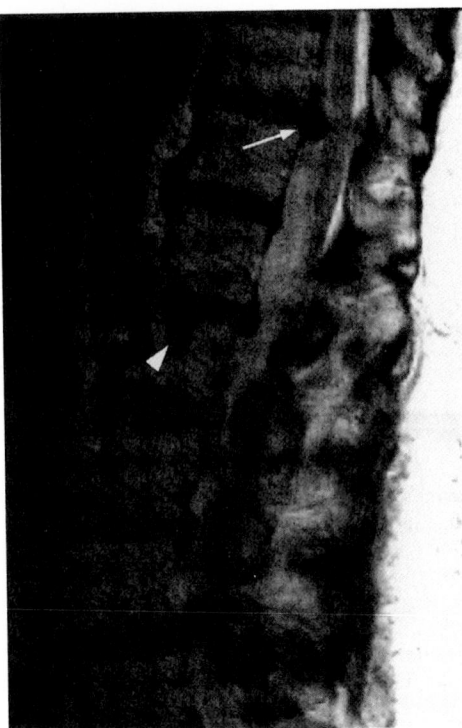

FIGURE 69.8 Sagittal T2-weighted MRI image showing a central thoracic disc herniation at T11–T12 (*arrow*). The cord is displaced posteriorly. The arrow head shows a Schmorl nodule. Lee JKT, Sagel SS, Stanley RJ, et al. *Computerized Body Tomography with MRI Correlation*, 4th edition. Philadelphia: Lippincott Williams & Wilkins; 2006.

recommended. Pharmacologic therapy involves initiating treatment with oral antiviral agents as soon as the diagnosis has been made. Studies have shown efficacy of antiviral agents if started within 72 hours.[22,23] Interventional treatments include segmental epidural blockade with dilute local anesthetic solutions, intercostal nerve blocks, and sympathetic blockade of the cervicothoracic chain with stellate ganglion blocks are recommended. If the elderly patient is suffering with a very painful bout of acute zoster, then aggressive interventional treatment can reduce the severity of the condition and reduce the risk of postherpetic neuralgia. Use of systemic corticosteroids for treatment is controversial. However it has not been associated any worsening of the disease. The number of interventional treatments can range anywhere from three to four in a 2-week period. Continuous segmental epidural blockade with thoracic epidural catheter is also recommended however it may require hospitalization of the patient. Continuous blockade of the intercostal nerves can be achieved by placing a catheter in the intercostals space connected to an isomeric infusion pump. Such therapy can be used effectively on an outpatient basis. Use of dilute local anesthetics with less toxicity can reduce complications due to local anesthetic toxicity in older patients.

Postherpetic neuralgia presents with persistence of severe sharp, burning pain in the affected dermatomes after the disappearance of the acute rash. About 20% percent of elderly patients with herpes zoster develop postherpetic neuralgia. The pain may persist for months to years without treatment. Hyperalgesia and allodynia of the effected dermatome is seen. The chronicity of the pain can result in behavioral changes affecting sleep and mood. Psychosocial symptoms and depression can worsen the pain. Treatment of postherpetic neuralgia includes symptomatic treatment of pain with medications and interventions. Medical management involves the use of neuropathic analgesics which are discussed extensively elsewhere in this text. These may include

Diagnosis of the condition is made by the clinical presentation of the characteristic rash.

The main goal of treatment of acute herpes zoster infection is not only to treat the acute condition but also to prevent central sensitization and postherpetic neuralgia. Treatment of the acute condition is initially pharmacologic. Elderly patients are more susceptible to developing postherpetic neuralgia; therefore, more aggressive treatment with additional interventional modalities is

tricyclic antidepressants, duloxetine, and anticonvulsants.[24–26] Topical treatment with local anesthetic patches, local anesthetic ointments, preparations with capsaicin, and compounded creams can be used to achieve symptomatic treatment of the condition.[27,28] Transcutaneous electrical nerve stimulation (TENS) can also be helpful.[29] Interventional treatment with intercostal nerve blocks or epidural injections may be required. Permanent implants like dorsal column spinal cord stimulators and peripheral intercostals nerve stimulators offer a novel approach to pain control in patients who require repeated interventional treatments. A trial of such a stimulator is recommended before permanent implantation. Along with the interventional treatments aggressive behavioral therapy is highly recommended. Chronic opioid therapy may be needed. A comprehensive approach using pharmacologic, interventional, rehabilitative, and behavioral treatments will help achieve pain relief and improve functional capacity of the patient.

Intercostal and Peripheral Neuropathy. Chronic intercostal neuralgia can result from trauma or compression of the intercostals nerves. Due to the proximity of the nerves to the inferior aspect of the ribs, any abnormalities of the ribs such as fractures and metastatic lesions can result in intercostal neuralgia. Prior thoracic or breast surgery and surgical lesion of the nerves can result in chronic intercostal neuralgia. Other causes include trauma or infection. Pain is characterized as sharp, superficial, burning, or lancinating in the distribution of the affected nerve. Pain is worsened by respirations and movements of the chest wall similar to the clinical presentation of pleuritic lesions. Localized tenderness to palpation may be appreciated in the intercostal space. A thorough history looking for previous trauma or surgeries can assist in the diagnosis.

Medical management of intercostal neuralgia consists of treatment with nonsteroidal anti-inflammatory agents, tricyclic antidepressants, and anticonvulsants. Intercostal nerve blocks with long-acting local anesthetics and corticosteroids can be effective (Fig. 69.9). Cryoablation or radiofrequency neurolysis of the intercostal nerves can provide longer pain relief.[30–32] We avoid chemolysis of the intercostals nerves because of concerns of postlysis neuralgia and neuritis. Long-term relief can also be achieved by implantable peripheral nerve stimulators.

Chest Wall Pain of Skeletal Origin

Skeletal chest wall pain can originate from the thoracic spine, ribs, costal cartilages, or sternum.

Abnormalities of the Thoracic Spine. Localized pain in the back can result from abnormalities of the thoracic spine. Pain is caused by stimulation of nociceptive fibers in the periosteum, joints, and ligaments. Reflex muscle spasms of the paraspinal muscles are also associated with pain. Deep palpation of the thoracic spinous processes, the paravertebral region, and movement of the spine can elicit pain.

Congenital abnormalities of the spinal curvature resulting in scoliosis can cause chest wall pain as the patient ages. Structural changes in the thoracic spine due to postural kyphosis, trauma, or disease can result in pain. Correction of lateral scoliosis with surgical or nonsurgical interventions can help alleviate the pain. Posture training with strengthening exercises and relief of muscle spasms is helpful.

Vertebral Fractures. Fractures of the vertebral body can be very painful. The pain can be particularly severe and may radiate into the chest wall. Vertebral fractures are the result of trauma, metastatic disease, or osteoporosis. Compression fractures in younger patients are mostly due to trauma. However, corticosteroid use can also result in compression fractures in younger patients. Osteoporosis is a major public health concern in the modern world. It is estimated that by the eighth decade 50% of all women will develop vertebral fractures.[33] There is significant impact on the patient with an osteoporotic vertebral fracture resulting in pain, deformity, dependence, and fear of falling. More than 200,000 people per year with osteoporotic fractures require opioid pain medications.[34,35] Radiologic diagnosis with plain films, CT scan, or magnetic resonance imaging (MRI) can assist in the diagnosis of a patient who presents with acute onset posterior axial pain with or without radicular symptoms (Fig. 69.10).

Physical examination may reveal deformity of the spine. A prominent spinous process can sometimes be palpated above or below the level of the compression fracture. Pain may not be present initially and about 50% of the patients present at a later time with the onset of pain. Most of the fractures are due to a combination of flexion with axial compression resulting in collapse of the anterior portions of the vertebral body. With osteoporosis, as the load bearing capacity of the vertebral bodies decreases, minor movements such as bending or lifting can result in a fracture in older patients. Crushed fracture of the anterior and middle columns of the vertebral body, the so-called burst fractures, can result in neurological compromise. The main goal of therapy is prevention. Treatment options for pain due to vertebral compression fractures include analgesics, bracing, and interventional treatments. Surgical treatment is indicated if there is neurological compromise. However, surgery can be invasive and result in failure of fixation in the osteoporotic spine.

Vertebral body augmentations with vertebroplasty or balloon kyphoplasty have had promising results. It involves mechanical augmentation of the compressed vertebral body by injecting acrylic bone cement material. Use of polymethylmethacrylate for

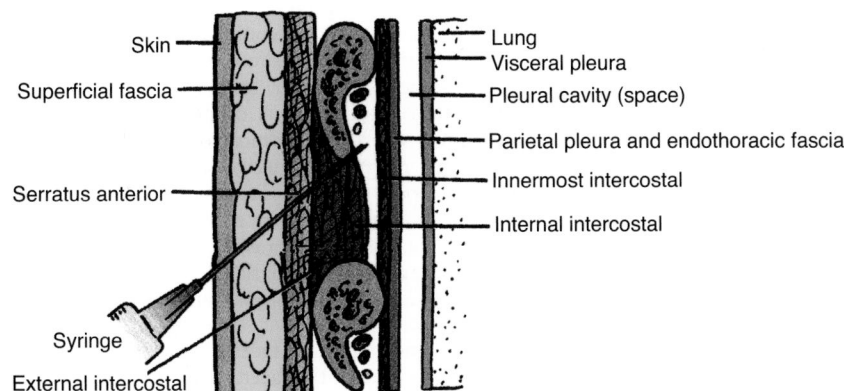

FIGURE 69.9 Intercostal nerve block. Modified from Snell RS. *Clinical Anatomy by Regions*, 8th ed. Philadelphia: Lippincott Williams & Wilkins; 2007.

FIGURE 69.10 Thoracic spine compression fracture. **A.** Axial CT shows compression fracture involving mainly the anterior aspect of T7 vertebral body. **B.** Midsaggittal T1- weighted image shows the wedged T7 vertebral body (arrow). The posterior margin is displaced into the spinal canal, producing spinal cord compression. Lee JKT, Sagel SS, Stanley RJ, et al. *Computerized Body Tomography with MRI Correlation*, 4th edition. Philadelphia: Lippincott Williams & Wilkins; 2006.

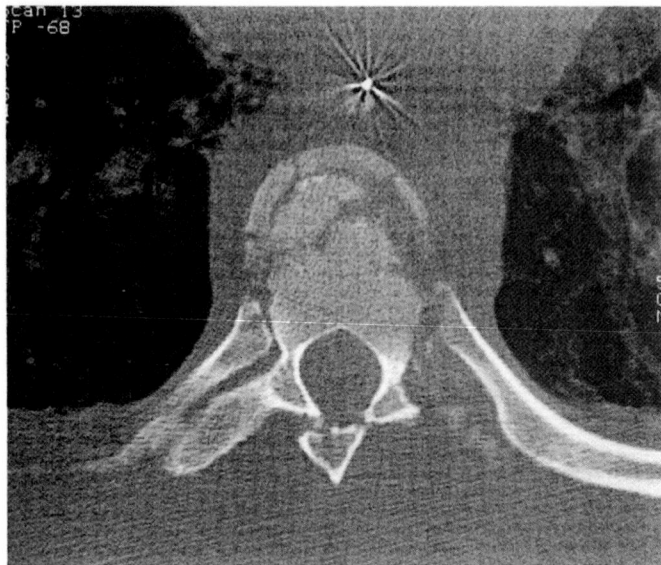

A

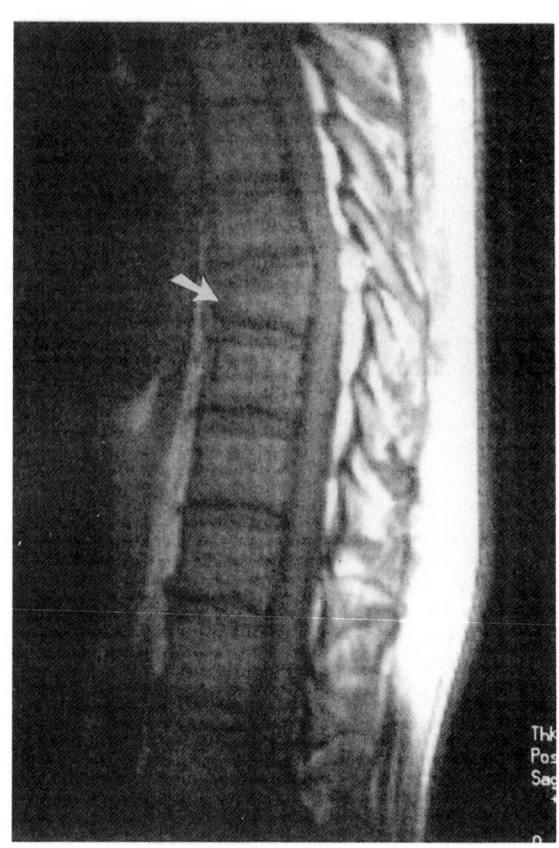

B

vertebral compression fractures was reported in France in 1991 with good results of pain relief. Polymethylmethacrylate is injected into the vertebral body via a posterolateral approach. The posterior cortex of the vertebral body must be intact prior to injection. Studies have recognized the best timing of interventional procedures to be within 6 weeks of the fracture.[36,37]

Ankylosing Spondylitis. Ankylosing spondylitis results in a stiff spine due to arthritic changes in the intervertebral joints including the costovertebral, costotransverse, and apophyseal joints. The sternoclavicular joints can also be involved.[38] Patients can present with mild to moderate pain in the posterior chest wall. Physical examination demonstrates limited movements of the spine with contracted tender paraspinal muscles. Diagnosis is made by plain films that show characteristic fused spine or "bamboo spine." Occasionally, involvement of the nerve roots due to arthritic changes in the joints can result in radicular pain. Secondary contracture of the paraspinal muscles can worsen the pain. Effective treatment involves physical therapy, trigger point muscle injections, and muscle relaxants. Progression of the arthropathy should be addressed with the expertise of a rheumatologist. Paravertebral blocks can provide relief from radicular pain. Thoracic facet joint injections with corticosteroid and local anesthetics can provide significant relief of pain. If good results are encountered with facet joint injections, longer-term relief of pain can be obtained with radiofrequency ablation of the nerve supply of the facet joint. The radiofrequency technique is generally considered to be safer than chemical ablation, because there are additional risks associated with the potential unwanted spread of the chemolysis agent.

Costovertebral Arthritis. Arthritis of the costovertebral and costotransverse joints can cause posterior chest wall pain. Pain is localized, aching, and deep in character. Pain can be increased with deep breathing, coughing, or lateral compression of the

chest. Physical examination may reveal localized deep tenderness that may be hard to distinguish from thoracic facet syndrome. Characteristics of pain and radiologic examination can delineate the pathology.[39,40] Treatment is provided with nonsteroidal antiinflammatory agents and physical therapy. Interventional treatment with injection of the joints with local anesthetic, corticosteroid mixture with fluoroscopic confirmation can alleviate the pain. It can also be diagnostic. Low dose opioid medications may be needed for treatment of chronic pain from the arthritis.[41] Rarely, resection of the joints is considered for refractory pain from isolated costovertebral joint arthritis.[42]

Diffuse Idiopathic Skeletal Hyperostosis. Another cause of posterior chest wall pain in elderly patients can be due to diffuse idiopathic skeletal hyperostosis (DISH), also called Forestier disease. Patients present with dull aching thoracic back pain, posterior chest wall pain, dysphagia, myelopathy due to involvement of the posterior longitudinal ligaments, fractures, subluxation, and, rarely, intercostal neuralgia. Physical findings include slight increase in dorsal kyphosis, minimal reduction in motion, and localized tenderness. Diagnosis is confirmed with radiologic exams with plain films and CT scans showing spinal hyperostosis resulting in linear ossification and bridging osteophytosis along the anterior and anterolateral aspects of the vertebral bodies. DISH most commonly affects the thoracic spine. Absence of sacroiliitis, true syndesmophytes, and ankylosing apophyseal joints distinguishes this syndrome from ankylosing spondylitis.[43,44] The syndrome of synovitis, pustulosis, hyperostosis, and osteitis (SAPHO syndrome) can also be a cause of anterior chest wall hyperostosis.[45] Treatment is symptomatic with nonsteroidal antiinflammatory drugs (NSAIDs) and physical therapy.

Thoracic Facet Syndrome. Thoracic facet syndrome results from abnormal locking or binding of the facet joints. Sudden or rapid turning movements of the trunk, working with hands over the head, or lifting with the trunk in a twisted position can result in this syndrome. Symptoms include moderate to severe pain on the side of the spine or anterolateral chest wall.[46,47] The pain is worsened with extension of the spine and relieved with flexion. Localized deep tenderness can be elicited to deep palpation over the facet joint. Tenderness and spasms of the erector spinae muscles can exacerbate the pain. It can mimic the pain from costovertebral arthropathy. Injection of the joint can assist in making the correct diagnosis. Treatment includes NSAIDs, physical therapy, and injection of the facet joints and medial branches with corticosteroid and local anesthetics. Radiofrequency denervation offers long term pain relief.[48,49]

Chest Wall Pain Arising from the Ribs.

Rib fractures account for one of the most common causes of acute chest wall pain of skeletal origin. Blunt trauma to the ribs is the usual cause of fractures. Other causes include severe paroxysmal coughing (tussive fracture), metastatic disease, osteoporosis, osteomalacia, and Paget disease of the bone (Fig. 69.11). Elder or child abuse should be sought in unexplained rib fractures after all other etiologies are eliminated.

Fractures may involve several ribs or multiple fractures of the same rib. Acute pain from rib fractures is usually aching, sharp, and worsened with respirations. Pain from multiple fractures can restrict breathing leading to additional pulmonary complications. Acute pain from rib fractures is treated with NSAIDs, low-dose opioids, or continuous intercostal nerve blocks. Chest wall pain from multiple rib fractures in trauma patients, in which serious consequences might occur from hypoventilation due to pain-related splinting, are candidates for a thoracic epidural catheter with a continuous epidural infusion.[50–52] Multiple studies in selected trauma patients have shown better outcomes of pain relief and reduction in pulmonary complications with thoracic epidural infusion compared to systemic opioids or intrapleural catheters.[53–56]

Occasionally, rib trauma without radiographically apparent fracture can cause localized pain and swelling with point tenderness in the area. If these are related to hypoventilation due to splinting from pain, they may be considered the same as rib fractures potentially requiring neuroaxial analgesia. Local injections with local anesthetics, intercostals nerve blocks, and NSAIDs can help relieve the pain. Topical local anesthetic patches with 5% Lidocaine may be helpful for some with pain from single rib fractures or rib injuries without a fracture. Metastatic disease from the breast, lungs, and prostate can cause isolated rib tenderness. Plain radiographs and nuclear medicine bone scans can aid in the diagnosis.

Slipping Rib Syndrome.

Slipping rib syndrome was described first in 1922 by Davies-Colley.[57] It is characterized by chest wall or abdominal pain due to irritation of the intercostal nerves. The etiology is thought to be due to trauma. There is increased mobility of the costal cartilages of eighth to tenth ribs near the sternum. The syndrome is also referred to as clicking rib, gliding rib, or displaced ribs.[58] It is also seen in children.[59,60] The cause for pain is due to anatomic variation of the eighth to tenth ribs, which, instead of articulating directly with the sternum, articulate with the costal cartilages of the upper rib. As such the sternal ends of these ribs are more prone to trauma. Injury can cause separation of the cartilages causing slipping movements of the ribs with respiration. A characteristic click can be felt with the movement of the ribs over the border of the upper cartilage. Diagnosis of the condition can be accomplished by the "hooking maneuver." The examiners curled fingers are placed over the inferior border of the rib and the rib is pulled up anteriorly. A positive test produces a clicking noise and increases the pain.[61] Slipping rib syndrome is treated conservatively with reassurance and nonopioid analgesics. Injection of the painful site (between the detached cartilage and the rib) with local anesthetic steroid combination medications may relieve pain for a longer period. Surgical excision of the involved rib and costal cartilages has also been suggested for refractory cases.

Teitze Syndrome.

Teitze syndrome is characterized by a benign, nonsuppurative, painful swelling of the second or third costal cartilages.[62] It was first described in 1921 by Teitze. Straining, severe cough, heavy manual work, nutritional deficiencies, and arthritic conditions have all been implicated as the possible causes. In 80% of the patients the condition is unilateral.[63] Pain is usually localized, but occasionally can radiate over the anterior chest wall, to the shoulder or neck. Pain is characterized as heaviness, tightness, or soreness. Pain is exacerbated by coughing and deep breathing. There is localized tenderness and swelling over the involved cartilage.[64,65] The overlying skin is normal. Radiologic diagnosis by bone scans is nonspecific. Treatment includes use of nonopioid anti-inflammatory medications. The condition usually is self limited with occasional exacerbations and remissions.

Costochondritis.

Costochondritis is one of the most common causes of anterior chest wall pain often confusing or coexisting with the pain due to coronary artery disease.[66–68] Pain is characterized as aching, sharp, or tightness in the anterior chest wall. Unlike Teitze syndrome it involves multiple sites. No swelling is palpated. There is localized tenderness involving multiple costochondral regions of the anterior chest wall. Second to fifth costal cartilages are frequently involved. Pain is aggravated with movement of the chest. Pain can radiate anteriorly or to the back. In adolescents it can cause chest wall or abdominal pain. Firm steady pressure applied over the sternum, intercostal spaces, costochondral junctions, and the ribs can reproduce the pain. The horizontal flexion test consists of having the arm flexed across the anterior chest wall and applying steady traction in a horizontal direction, while the patient's head is rotated toward the ipsilateral shoulder. The crowing rooster maneuver involves having the patient extend the neck as much as possible by looking toward the

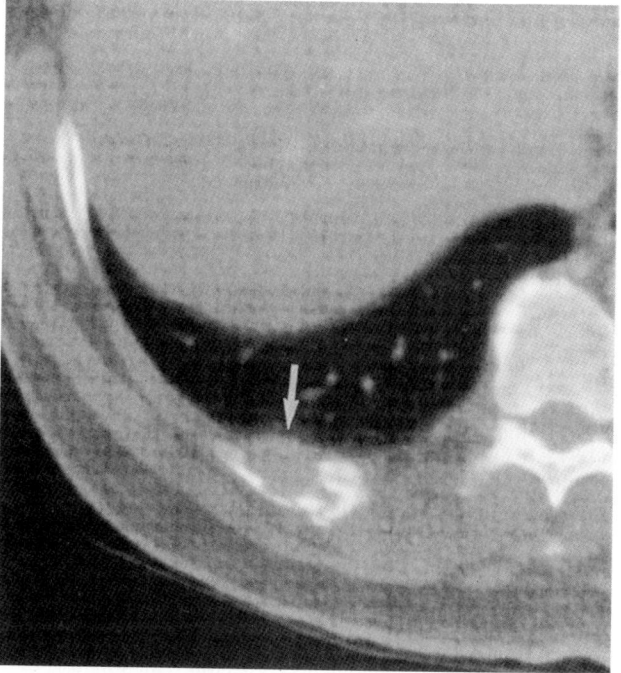

FIGURE 69.11 CT showing Rib destruction from multiple myeloma. Lee JKT, Sagel SS, Stanley RJ, et a. *Computerized Body Tomography with MRI Correlation*, 4th edition. Philadelphia: Lippincott Williams & Wilkins; 2006.

ceiling while the clinician, standing behind the patient, exerts traction on the posteriorly extended arms.

It is important to distinguish pain due to costochondritis (especially left-sided) from that because of coronary artery disease or abdominal pathology.[69] Pain due to costochondritis is usually located to the lateral side of the sternum unlike the substernal cardiac pain.[70] Pain can radiate to the left arm or shoulder. The patient gives a history of pain with movement and postural changes. Localized tenderness can be palpated. Pain usually lasts for a few minutes to hours, distinguishing it from pain of acute cardiac origin. Intercostal nerve blocks and injection of the tender costochondral areas with local anesthetic have been used for diagnostic purposes. Rarely, emergency room physicians experience a patient with both costochondritis and coronary artery disease. Careful history and physical exam along with treatment with sublingual nitroglycerin can aid in prompt diagnosis of the cardiac pain, which is relieved with the nitroglycerin.

Treatment of costochondritis is initiated with NSAIDs, physical therapy, heat application, and low-dose opioids. Once the diagnosis has been made, reassuring the patent about the benign nature of the condition can prevent patient anxiety and avoid unnecessary expensive diagnostic workup. Localized injection of the costochondral junction with local anesthetics and corticosteroids can help relieve the pain.

Costochondral Dislocation

Costochondral dislocation is commonly seen after trauma in young patients.[71] It is also encountered after thoracic surgery with rib retraction. The pain is typically dull, aching, or burning, and is usually continuous. Localized tenderness is present. Sometimes a mass is felt due to cartilaginous excess from the injury. Treatment is similar to other conditions as described above with oral analgesics and intercostals nerve blocks. Manipulation and reduction of the dislocation after adequate analgesia can correct the condition.

Chest Wall Pain of Sternal Origin

Sternoclavicular joint arthritis can be caused due to various arthritic conditions (osteoarthritis, rheumatoid arthritis, psoriatic) and rarely infections due to central venous catheters.[72–74] Infections are also seen in intravenous drug users. Traumatic subluxation and dislocation can also cause pain. Apart from trauma, such conditions are also seen after cardiac surgery when the sternum is retracted. Pain is localized to the affected joint. Localized tenderness of the joint is seen with palpation along with pain from shrugging the shoulders. Treatment consists of oral NSAIDs and injection of the joints with local anesthetic and corticosteroid. Such intervention must be avoided in infectious joints which are treated with antibiotics and analgesics.

Blunt injuries to the sternum can cause subluxation of the manubriosternal joint.[75] Manubriosternal arthritis can occur due to various arthritic conditions.[76–78] Septic arthritis of the joint is also seen.[79,80] Pain is localized to the anterior sternum or angle of Louis with occasional radiation parasternally. Pain is characterized as sharp aggravated with deep breathing, coughing or yawning. Pain may mimic anginal pain. Diagnosis is made by physical examination. Bone scans can be positive.[81] Treatment consists of systemic analgesics, topical lidocaine patches, heat, infiltration of the joint with local anesthetics, and corticosteroids. Rarely, surgical intervention to correct the manubriosternal displacement is necessary.

Xiphoidalgia. (Painful xiphoid syndrome, xiphoid cartilage syndrome, hypersensitive xiphoid)

Intermittent, inferior substernal or epigastric pain associated with tenderness of the xiphoid to palpation is characteristic of xiphoidalgia.[82,83] Pain is spontaneous without any obvious precipitating cause. It is sometimes seen along with coronary artery disease, intestinal disease, and metabolic disorders. Movements of the xiphoid with bending, stooping or turning, precipitates or

exacerbates the pain more commonly after a full meal. Along with NSAIDs, local injection of the xiphisternal joint with local anesthetic and corticosteroid can alleviate the pain.

Chest Wall Pain of Myofascial Origin

Myofascial strain can be caused by excessive muscular activity. Repeated stress due to exercise, coughing, straining, or repetitive movements (chopping wood, painting a ceiling) can result in generalized tenderness over the anterior chest wall. Pain in the intercostals or accessory thoracic muscles is usually due to trauma. Pain from the pectoralis muscles can be exacerbated with adduction movements of the shoulder. Pain between the scapula and spine from an injured rhomboid is increased with bracing of the shoulders backward. Treatment consists of reassurance, local heat or cold, NSAIDs, topical lidocaine patches, physical therapy, and avoiding precipitating activities. Infiltration of the muscle with local anesthetic can be undertaken if there is localized tenderness. Caution regarding the risk of pneumothorax is necessary for all chest wall injections.

Precordial Catch Syndrome (Chest Wall Twinge Syndrome). This is characterized by episodes of sudden, brief, sharp precordial or periapical pain. This is a benign, self-limited condition.[84,85] Sharp pains, stitches, or catches are felt in the chest wall in the left parasternal on or near the cardiac apex. Some patients report pain from assuming a slouching or bent position. Pain may last for a few seconds to up to 3 minutes. Deep breathing exacerbates the pain while shallow breathing relieves it. There is no localized tenderness. The cause is unknown. Intercostal muscle spasms and pain from the pleura have been postulated as possible causes. Treatment consists of reassurance and correction of posture. Due to the unpredictability and the benign short duration of pain, analgesics are not necessary.

Epidemic Myalgia (Bornholm Disease, Epidemic Pleurodynia, Devil's Grip). This condition is characterized by paroxysms of intense sharp chest wall and upper abdominal pain due to viral infection with coxsackie or echoviruses.[86] The paroxysms of pain are separated by pain-free intervals. Frequently there is associated fever, headache, and pharyngitis. The condition is self-limited.

Breast Pain

Pain arising from the breast is a common and nonspecific symptom in women.[87,88] Usual causes include benign cysts, fibrocystic change, or cyclical pain due to hormonal cycle changes of the menstrual cycle. Other causes of breast pain include malignancy, mastitis, ductal ectasia, breast abscess, hormone replacement therapy, or large breasts. Careful clinical evaluation and mammography to rule out malignancy should be undertaken. Pain due to malignant breast lesions does not usually present until the tumor is large (greater than 2 centimeters in diameter). Axillary lymph node involvement can present as either localized or sharp pain in the arm with involvement of the intercostobrachial nerves. Extramammary sources of breast pain should be evaluated if no other etiology is suggestive. Causes include skeletal and myofascial pain from the chest wall, radicular pain, or pain from peripheral nerves.

Chronic severe breast pain that persists for years without any obvious cause characterizes idiopathic mastalgia. Pain can be unilateral or bilateral, cyclical, or noncyclical which is usually seen in the third or early fourth decades of life. Without any organic diagnosis, the etiology is often misdiagnosed as psychologic.[89] Cyclical mastalgia responds to Danazol, Bromocriptine, or Tamoxifen. Hormonal events such as pregnancy, menopause, or use of oral contraceptives may lead to relief.[90,91]

Breast pain is treated with NSAIDs and acetaminophen. Warm compresses, ice packs, or gentle massage can relieve pain. Pain arising from the cervical or thoracic spine requires appropriate treatment of the cause as discussed elsewhere in this text. Peripheral myofascial and skeletal pain, also discussed elsewhere in this text, can be treated with injection of local anesthetic and corticosteroid.[92,93]

Adiposis Dolorosa (Dercum Disease). This syndrome is characterized by painful subcutaneous fatty tumors in various parts of the body, including the breast.[94] This can result in chronic pain in the breast. Treatment with intravenous lidocaine and resection of the fatty lesions is helpful.

Mondor Disease. Thrombosis of the superficial veins of the thoracic wall can cause pain in the anterolateral chest wall.[95] This is seen occasionally in patients who abuse intravenous drugs.[96] The disease is mostly seen in middle aged women with pendulous breasts and can cause pain in the breast.[97] Presence of a palpable tender cord is characteristic. The disease can cause anxiety in the patient. Mondor disease is self-limited. Treatment involves management of pain with NSAIDs.

Postsurgical Chest Wall Pain

Pain can persist for several months to years after surgery. It is often troublesome for the patient to live with pain after the original pathology has been corrected with surgery.

Chronic postsurgical pain is most commonly seen after thoracotomy, mastectomy, and cardiac surgery. Other rare causes of chronic postsurgical chest wall pain include video-assisted thoracoscopy, mediastinoscopy, breast reconstruction, and surgery of the cervical or thoracic spine.

Postsurgical Breast Pain and Postmastectomy Pain Syndrome. Persistent pain in the anterior chest wall, axilla, and the arm can be seen in a few patients after mastectomy.[98–100] It can also occur after minor breast surgeries, such as lumpectomy. Breast reconstruction or other cosmetic breast surgeries can be also associated with such pain. Submuscular implants and capsule formation around the implant can cause injury or impinge on the thoracodorsal, long thoracic, lateral, or medial pectoral nerves. Postsurgical complications such as wound infection, fluid or hematoma retention, and re-exploration can frequently result in pain. Although previous studies describe pain in less than 10% of patients, more recent studies report pain, paresthesias, and phantom sensations in about half of the patients.[101,102] In about half of the cases pain resolves with time. Pain is described as burning, sharp, or tight constriction of the axilla. Pain can be associated with surgical scar sensitivity. There can be associated dysesthesia or hyperesthesia of the anterior chest wall. It is presumed that injury to the intercostobrachial nerves and, rarely, the intercostals nerves is the cause. Patients are at risk for developing upper extremity problems due to restricted movement of the arm secondary to pain. Treatment consists of analgesic and neuropathic medications, physical therapy, reassurance, intercostal or paravertebral nerve blocks, or epidural analgesia.[103,104] Intraoperative infiltration of botulinum toxin into the chest wall musculature has also been suggested.[105] Persistent pain should arouse suspicion for recurrent breast disease.

Phantom breast syndrome has been a common occurrence after a mastectomy in the past.[106–108] The incidence has decreased with adequate psychosocial supportive therapy.[109,110] It can present as painful or nonpainful sensations in the region of the missing breast as if it is still present. It can develop within 3 months after the surgery. Risk factors for development of the syndrome include psychosocial factors, damaged body image, and impaired sexual function. Affected women are usually younger, premenopausal with children. Predisposing factors for phantom breast pain are similar to phantom limb syndrome and include pain in the involved breast prior to surgery.[111] Preoperative analgesia may be effective in preventing this syndrome; however, it has not been significantly studied.

Postthoracotomy Pain. Chronic chest wall pain after thoracotomy can be disabling to the patient.[112,113] Characteristics of postthoracotomy pain can be burning, aching, hyperesthesia, or allodynia along the surgical incision and the involved dermatome. Women experience more pain than men after major thoracotomy.[114] No difference has been seen in the incidence of acute or chronic pain with different types of thoracotomy incisions.[115] Adequate management of acute postsurgical pain can prevent the chronicity of pain.[116] Management of acute pain with thoracic epidural placed prior to surgery has been shown to decrease the severity of perioperative pain and decrease the incidence of chronic pain. Other causes of radicular chest wall pain and recurrent cancer have to be excluded, especially in postthoracotomy patients who experience onset of severe pain several months after the thoracotomy. Management is similar to treatment for intercostal neuralgia.[117,118] Thoracic paravertebral blocks are also helpful to control acute and chronic pain.[119,120] Pulsed radiofrequency of dorsal root ganglia or intercostal nerves is recommended for refractory pain.[121] Prior to any injections of the surgical scar site, a careful examination is necessary to avoid injury to herniated lung tissue in rare cases.[122,123] A multimodal approach to pain management provides higher success in controlling chronic postthoracotomy pain.

Postcardiac Surgery Pain. Persistent anterior chest wall pain has been reported in about 28% of patients after cardiac surgery.[124,125] Myocardial ischemia, infection, sternal or costosternal instability, sternal wires, and intercostal neuralgia (especially after dissection of the internal mammary artery from the chest wall), can be possible causes.[126] Pain can persist up to 2 years postoperatively. Initial attempts at treatment should be focused on eliminating obvious serious causes. Treatment consists of analgesic and neuropathic medications, costosternal joint injections, and surgical removal of sternal wires.[127]

Chest Pain and Psychological Factors

Patients with sudden acute chest pain, regardless of the cause, experience varying degrees of anxiety, apprehension, and fear, depending on their interpretation of the cause of pain. Those who believe they are experiencing a heart attack become extremely frightened of possible impending death. Patients with persistent angina develop reactive depression, which, if untreated, produces progressive physical and psychological deterioration.[128] Musculoskeletal chest pain can cause a great deal of anxiety and apprehension until the patients are reassured about the benign nature of the condition.[129,130] Adolescents can often present with chest pain that is mostly myofascial or psychogenic in origin.

Chest pain can also result from psychological mechanisms. Because of the potential seriousness of a physical cause of chest pain, thorough history, physical examination, and diagnostic work up is essential. Some of the features of psychological chest pain include pain at the apex of the heart, patients describing the character of pain dramatically, development of pain unrelated to physiologic events, and possible presence of an emotional precipitating event prior to the pain. Once the diagnosis of psychological chest pain has been made, reassurance, relaxation techniques, anxiolytic drugs, sedatives, tranquilizers, and time can reduce the anxiety.

Patients with chronic anxiety can present with chest pain and other symptoms. This syndrome has been called Da Cossta syndrome, neurocirculatory asthenia, vasoregulatory asthenia, effort syndrome, and soldier's heart.[131,132] Patients can present with symptoms of apical chest pain, shortness of breath, nervousness, anxiety, fatigue, generalized weakness, and low energy level. Treatment consists of reassurance, behavioral therapy, and treatment of underlying psychiatric disorders, if any. Other psychiatric disorders, such as depression, conversion reactions, hypochondriasis, and learned behavior can manifest as chest pain.

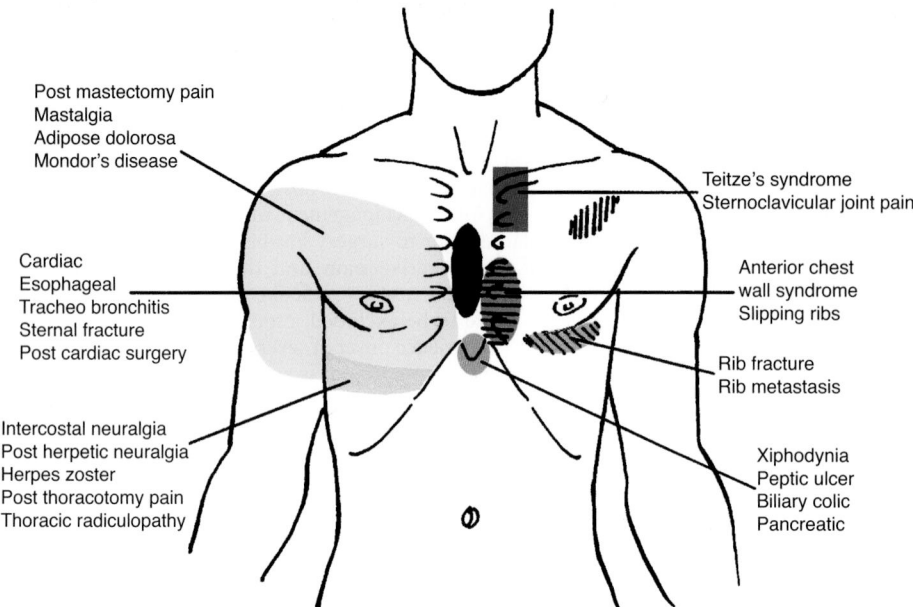

Post mastectomy pain
Mastalgia
Adipose dolorosa
Mondor's disease

Teitze's syndrome
Sternoclavicular joint pain

Cardiac
Esophageal
Tracheo bronchitis
Sternal fracture
Post cardiac surgery

Anterior chest
wall syndrome
Slipping ribs

Rib fracture
Rib metastasis

Intercostal neuralgia
Post herpetic neuralgia
Herpes zoster
Post thoracotomy pain
Thoracic radiculopathy

Xiphodynia
Peptic ulcer
Biliary colic
Pancreatic

FIGURE 69.12 Common sites of anterior chest wall pain due to chest wall structures or referred pain.

Chest Wall Pain of Cardiac Origin

In any patient who presents with chest pain the differential diagnosis must include chest pain of cardiac origin. Angina presents as substernal chest pain or tightness. However, atypical presentations of chest pain or gastric symptoms can be seen from cardiac disease. Evaluation of risk factors may help assist in making the diagnosis in atypical presentations. Chronic refractory angina pectoris is a condition where patients present with chronic and disabling chest pain despite optimal medical treatment. In such patients who are not candidates for invasive cardiac procedures, spinal cord stimulation (SCS) offers adequate pain control and improvement in the quality of life.[133,134] SCS is also mentioned as an available adjunct by the task force on the management of

stable angina pectoris of the European Society of Cardiology.[135] Angina due to acute myocardial infarction is not masked by spinal cord stimulation.[136]

CONCLUSION

Chest wall pain can result from lesions within the chest wall or referred pain from the thoracic viscera (Figs. 69.12 and 69.13). A comprehensive assessment and examination is needed to differentiate these and to further determine if the lesion involves skeletal, muscular, or neurological components of the chest wall or thoracic and abdominal viscera (Table 69.3).

(text continues on page 1067)

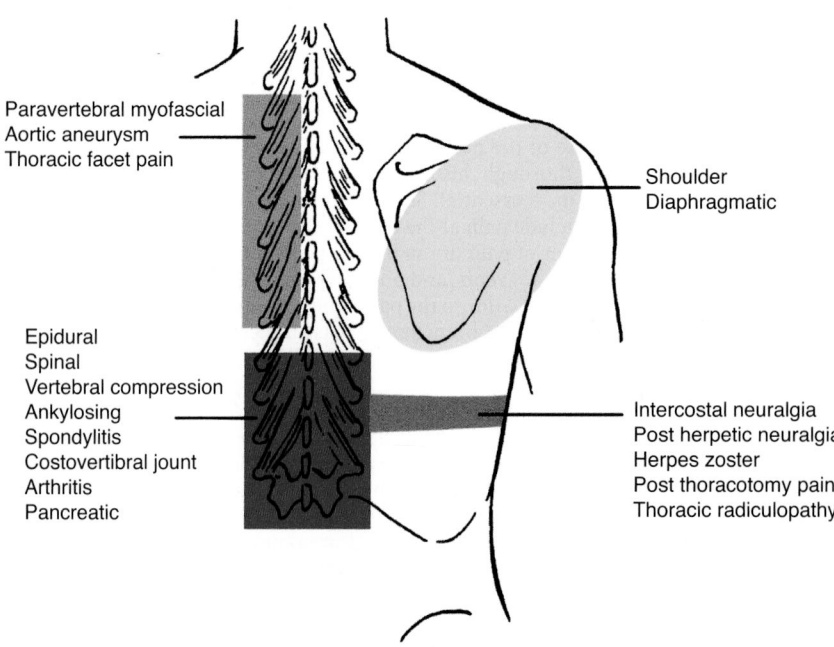

Paravertebral myofascial
Aortic aneurysm
Thoracic facet pain

Shoulder
Diaphragmatic

Epidural
Spinal
Vertebral compression
Ankylosing
Spondylitis
Costovertibral jcount
Arthritis
Pancreatic

Intercostal neuralgia
Post herpetic neuralgia
Herpes zoster
Post thoracotomy pain
Thoracic radiculopathy

FIGURE 69.13 Common sites of posterior chest wall pain due to chest wall structures or referred pain.

TABLE 69.3

PAIN IN THE CHEST: SUMMARY OF DIFFERENTIAL DIAGNOSIS

Etiology (disease)	IASP code reference†	Important diagnostic features	
		Characteristics of the pain	Associated symptoms and signs
I. Pain caused by disease of the heart and aorta			
A. Angina pectoris (stable angina, unstable angina, variant angina)	XVII-4	Mild, moderate, severe, or excruciating anterior chest pain felt predominantly retrosternally with radiation to parasternal region, left arm or right arm or both, epigastrium, and, less frequently, to the interscapular region, neck, and lower jaw; discomfort felt as severe oppression or heaviness on the chest, a sense of constriction or bandlike pressure, or a feeling of choking, strangling, or tight pressure on the neck; pain provoked by physical effort, severe emotional stress, or a large meal (except unstable angina, which occurs at rest or with little or no provocation); lasts 2–5 minutes with stable angina, 15–30 minutes or longer with unstable angina and variant angina; promptly relieved with nitroglycerin or discontinuation of effort	History of previous anginal attacks; can have normal ECG at rest, but ST depression and other ECG changes during stress test; positive evidence with radionuclide stress testing and coronary arteriography; demonstration of coronary artery spasm in variant angina
B. Acute myocardial infarction	XVII-5	Pain of same character, location, and reference as angina but of sudden onset, much more severe, and of longer duration (1–8 hours or more); little or no relief with nitroglycerin; intense pain often accompanied by strong alarm reaction and feeling of impending death	Frequently nausea, vomiting, and profuse sweating; many patients develop tenderness in pectoral muscle and deep muscle of interscapular region; some develop bradycardia and hypotension and others tachycardia and hypertension; ECG changes include Q-wave and ST-segment elevation and increased creatine kinase and other serum enzyme levels
C. Aortic stenosis	—	Dyspnea first symptom but angina occurs with severe aortic stenosis; chest pain occurs during physical exertion as a result of increased oxygen demand from increased myocardial mass and high ventricular systolic pressure	With severe disease exertional syncope is caused by decline in arterial pressure; left ventricular failure, palpitation, fatigue, weakness, peripheral cyanosis, narrow pulse pressure, and palpable systolic murmur; increased QRS complex and ST- and T-wave alterations
D. Aortic regurgitation	—	Asymptomatic early in disease; dyspnea on exertion; pain late symptom of severe disease that can occur at rest as well as with exertion and persists longer than angina of coronary artery disease; some patients have neck and abdominal pain	Dyspnea on exertion, flushing, sweating, palpitation; increased fatigue progresses to orthopnea and eventually to paroxysmal nocturnal dyspnea; high-pitched crescendo diastolic murmur along left sternal border
E. Mitral valve prolapse	—	Sharp, stabbing chest pain not provoked by exertion and unresponsive to nitroglycerin; more frequent in female subjects	Cardiac arrhythmia produces palpitation and rarely dizziness, syncope, or even sudden death; midsystolic click and late systolic murmur
F. Hypertrophic cardiomyopathy	—	Most patients asymptomatic; symptomatic patients have dyspnea on exertion because of increased stiffness of left ventricular walls; typical angina pectoris with exertion	Atrial and ventricular arrhythmias produce palpitation, dizziness, and syncope; ECG shows QRS changes of left ventricular hypertrophy and abnormal Q wave

(continued)

TABLE 69.3

CONTINUED

Etiology (disease)	IASP code reference†	Important diagnostic features	
		Characteristics of the pain	Associated symptoms and signs
G. Acute pericarditis	XVII-6	Severe, sharp chest pain; worse in supine position, partially relieved by sitting; markedly aggravated by deep breathing; pain usually retrosternal (central), radiates to the neck and trapezius ridge but not to the arms	Dyspnea occurs because of marked increase in pain with normal respiration; triphasic pericardial friction rub occurs with atrial systole, ventricular systole, and ventricular diastole, occasionally only biphasic; ECG initially shows ST-segment elevation and later T-wave flattening
H. Diseases of the thoracic aorta			
1. Dissecting aneurysm	—	Sudden, severe excruciating pain with maximal intensity at its onset; location of pain helps to localize dissection: ascending aortic dissection produces anterior chest pain in 65% of patients and posterior chest pain in 50%; dissection in descending thoracic aorta produces back pain in nearly all patients; radiation to the neck, throat, jaw, and abdomen in a small percentage of patients	Nausea, vomiting, diaphoresis, bradycardia, and hypotension or tachycardia and hypertension; loss of one or more arterial pulses; sense of impending death, apprehension
2. Nondissecting aneurysm	XVII-7	Mild to severe continuous burning, aching pain with bouts of lancinating pain; radiation to the chest, shoulder, and back caused by mechanical compression or injury of thoracic spinal nerves; erosion of bone causes boring, agonizing, intractable back pain	Dyspnea, cough, dysphagia, hoarseness; Horner syndrome; pulsating mass; radiographic evidence
II. Diseases of the respiratory system			
A. Diseases of the tracheobronchial tree			
1. Acute tracheobronchitis (infectious, irritative, thermal injury)	—	Mild to moderate burning, aching pain in the retrosternal and parasternal regions; pain severe with thermal injury; associated with sore throat	Preceded by upper respiratory infection: coryza, malaise, chilliness, slight fever, back and muscle pain; with bronchitis, initially dry and nonproductive cough but later mucoid or mucopurulent, dyspnea might be present
2. Bronchiectasis	—	Mild to moderate aching pain in retrosternal and parasternal regions	Chronic cough and sputum production; with progression, cough becomes more productive, hemoptysis common, recurrent pneumonia frequent; wheezing, dyspnea in severe cases
B. Diseases of the pulmonary circulation			
1. Acute pulmonary hypertension	—	Severe crushing, gripping pain in the center of the chest simulating that of acute myocardial infarction, but does not radiate to arms or jaw and seldom to back	Usually decrease in arterial P_{O_2} can have dyspnea, cyanosis, sweating
2. Chronic pulmonary hypertension (primary, secondary)	—	Pain in anterior chest, primarily retrosternal; radiation to neck; some patients have typical angina pectoris complicated by myocardial ischemia	Primary hypertension usually in female subjects; dyspnea, easy fatigue, less frequently syncope; right ventricular hypertrophy can progress to failure

(continued)

TABLE 69.3

CONTINUED

Etiology (disease)	IASP code reference†	Important diagnostic features	
		Characteristics of the pain	Associated symptoms and signs
3. Pulmonary embolism	—	With large embolus pain is sudden, severe, crushing, and of a visceral central type; simulates pain of myocardial infarction but does not radiate to the jaw or arms; lasts for minutes to several hours; small embolus produces localized severe pleuritic pain that is persistent and lasts a week or longer; aggravated by deep breathing or coughing	Feeling of impending death (*angor animi*), pressure on throat, desire to defecate; history of thrombi in leg, pelvis, occasionally in upper extremity; rarely, embolic fluid or fat emboli; initially the large embolus usually produces pulmonary hypertension from increased pulmonary vascular resistance, leading to decreased cardiac output, hypotension that can progress to shock, with sweating, tachypnea, dyspnea, arterial hypoxemia; hemoptysis, pleural friction rub with small embolus; radiography reveals wedge-shaped shadow
C. Diseases of the lungs			
1. Pneumonia	—	With lobar pneumonia patient develops pleuritis with moderate to severe pain in lateral chest or shoulder aggravated by deep breathing and coughing (because of involvement of central diaphragmatic pleura); little or no pain with bronchopneumonia	Systemic symptoms and signs of infection: fever, cough, occasionally nausea, vomiting, malaise, and muscle pain; blood-streaked sputum, occasionally hemoptysis; rhonchi; percussion reveals dullness; radiographic evidence
2. Lung abscess	—	Typical pleuritic chest pain if abscess produces pleuritis; characteristics similar to those of lobar pneumonia (see above)	Malaise, anorexia, sputum-producing cough, sweats, severe prostration, and fever; putrid odor (anaerobic infection); fine moist rales
3. Atelectasis	—	Rapid occlusion with massive lung collapse causes moderate to severe pain on the affected side	Rapid collapse causes dyspnea, cyanosis, hypotension, tachycardia, fever, and shock; percussion, dullness, or flatness; diminished or absent breath sounds; decreased chest excursion of affected side
D. Disorders of the pleura			
1. Pneumothorax (spontaneous)	—	Sudden moderate to severe stabbing, sharp pain felt across the chest or over abdomen or corresponding shoulder, can simulate pain of acute myocardial infarction or acute abdomen	Dyspnea, absent breath sounds; with large or tension pneumothorax tympany on percussion; decreased excursion of affected side; cardiac dullness and apex felt away from affected side; radiographic evidence
2. Pleuritis (pneumonitis, pulmonary infarct, pleural tumors, lung abscess, actinomycosis, coccidiomycosis, other infectious processes)	—	Localized, sharp, knifelike stabbing, piercing pain in various regions of the chest depending on the site of pathology (side, shoulder, epigastrium); markedly aggravated by deep breathing, coughing, laughing, movement of the chest; pain can be continuous with pleural carcinoma	Diagnostic pleural friction rub; history and systemic symptoms and signs of infection; chest signs (rales, rhonchi); radiographic evidence
3. Epidemic pleurodynia (Bornholm disease)	—	Severe paroxysmal sharp pain in side of chest wall, epigastrium, costovertebral region, and abdomen	Fever, headache; occasionally orchitis, encephalitis, and pericarditis occur during epidemic pleurodynia

(continued)

TABLE 69.3

CONTINUED

Etiology (disease)	IASP code reference†	Important diagnostic features	
		Characteristics of the pain	Associated symptoms and signs
E. Bronchogenic and metastatic carcinoma of the lung, bronchial pleura (squamous cell carcinoma, undifferentiated small or large cell adenocarcinoma, bronchoalveolar carcinoma)	—	Location, quality, and severity of pain depend on location and type of spread: a. Endobronchial carcinoma ∅ sternal and parasternal pain b. Intrapulmonary carcinoma ∅ vague central (visceral) pain c. Pleural spread ∅ sharp, stabbing, chest wall pain markedly aggravated by breathing, coughing, movement d. Mediastinal spread ∅ neuropathy with segmental pain e. Pancoast syndrome (brachial plexopathy) ∅ pain in shoulder, scapula, medial arm	Weight loss; paraneoplastic syndromes; other signs and symptoms: a. Cough, hemoptysis b. Hypoxia, dyspnea, atelectasis c. Signs and symptoms of pleuritis (see above) d. Compression of superior vena cava ∅ superior vena cava syndrome e. Horner syndrome, hoarseness, weakness of all muscles supplied by the ulnar nerve

III. Diseases of the esophagus
  A. Esophagitis
    1. Gastroesophageal reflux disease
	XIX-4	Retrosternal pain extends from suprasternal notch to xiphoid process; radiation to epigastrium, neck and back, and, rarely, arms; simulates pain of myocardial ischemia; lasts seconds to many hours; aggravated by stooping or lifting, recumbency, citrus juices, exercise, heavy meal, coffee, alcohol, aspirin, tobacco, and obesity; relieved by antacids	Dysphagia, odynophagia, regurgitation, and occasionally aspiration; diagnosis helped by pH monitoring, acid perfusion test, and esophagoscopy

2. Acute and chronic esophagitis caused by infection or chemical agents	XIX-4	Corrosive agents: immediate, severe, burning pain in throat and behind the whole length of the sternum down to epigastrium, pain is constant with periodic increases in intensity produced by esophageal spasm; infection: pain appears gradually over a period of hours or days and is constant, mild to moderate, and burning in character; both are markedly aggravated by swallowing (odynophagia) and by citrus juices and other factors listed previously for gastroesophageal reflux disease	Infection: signs and symptoms of inflammation (e.g., fever, chills); chemical esophagitis: pharyngeal erythema; moniliasis: typical soft white patches in tongue, tonsil, and buccal mucosa; other associated symptoms as above (e.g., dysphagia, odynophagia)
B. Esophageal motor disorders (achalasia; diffuse spasm unclassified motor disorders)	XIX-3	Moderate to severe retrosternal pain; radiation to epigastrium and back, neck, jaw, teeth, left arm, or both arms; aggravated by cold liquids, solids, and emotional stress; partially relieved by nitroglycerin; lasts seconds to many hours and can awaken patient from sleep; simulates pain of myocardial infarction	Dysphagia, odynophagia; diagnosis aided by manometry, scintigraphy, provocative tests (e.g., edrophonium or methacholine-induced esophageal spasm)
C. Esophageal laceration and rupture (Mallory-Weiss syndrome, Boerhaave syndrome)	—	Mallory-Weiss syndrome: laceration of distal esophagus and proximal stomach during retching, vomiting, or hiccup causes pain in lower sternum and epigastrium; Boerhaave syndrome: spontaneous rupture occurs during intense vomiting following a large meal and causes sudden, severe, excruciating crushing or tearing pain in lower retrosternal region and epigastrium, with radiation to the back	Dysphagia, odynophagia; rupture ∅ mediastinitis ∅ acute illness, epigastric tenderness, and later subcutaneous emphysema and left pleural effusion

(continued)

TABLE 69.3

CONTINUED

Etiology (disease)	IASP code reference†	Important diagnostic features	
		Characteristics of the pain	Associated symptoms and signs
D. Carcinoma	—	Moderate to severe retrosternal pain; radiation to epigastrium with lower lesions and to upper sternum with upper lesions; radiation to neck, interscapular region; pain continuous and aggravated by food ingestion	Dysphagia, odynophagia, weight loss; esophageal obstruction; radiographic, CT, and esophagoscopic evidence
E. Paraesophageal hiatal hernia	XIX-2	Generally asymptomatic; might be feeling of epigastric fullness and lower retrosternal discomfort; with incarceration and strangulation severe, excruciating epigastric and retrosternal pain	Possible massive gastrointestinal hemorrhage; radiographic and esophagoscopic evidence
IV. Diseases of the mediastinum and diaphragm			
A. Mediastinal disorders			
1. Spontaneous mediastinal emphysema	—	Sudden intense, violent, agonizing retrosternal or precordial pain; radiation to nape of neck and shoulder associated with pleural pain; persists for hours	Signs of emphysema: crunching sound in area of pain, decreased or obliterated cardiac dullness, pneumothorax, subcutaneous emphysema (crepitus); radiographic evidence
2. Acute or chronic mediastinitis	—	Continuous; mild to moderate; retrosternal, central; oppressive or burning, aching sensation; can be severe	Systemic signs of infection; history of esophageal rupture or other trauma
3. Neoplasms (anterior compartment, superior compartment, middle compartment, posterior compartment)	—	One-third of patients asymptomatic: remainder have chest pain, cough, dyspnea, and symptoms caused by compression or invasion of structures in mediastinum	Middle compartment: dysphagia, hoarseness; anterior compartment, superior compartment: retrosternal and suprasternal discomfort, local chest pain from pressure on sternum; posterior compartment: neurogenic tumors, vague chest pain, cough, radicular pain from neuropathy, superior vena cava syndrome
B. Diseases of the diaphragm			
1. Diaphragmatic pleuritis	—	Sharp, stabbing *pleuritic* pain along the nape and shoulder or in the posterior and lateral parts of the lower chest and upper abdomen, or both; aggravated by diaphragmatic motion	Signs and symptoms of pneumonitis or infectious processes with inflammation of diaphragmatic pleura
2. Acute primary diaphragmatitis (Hedblom syndrome)	—	Moderate to severe pain in lower chest, upper abdomen, and shoulder	Chills and fever; muscle spasm of abdomen; decreased lung expansion on inspiration; radiographic evidence of flattened diaphragm
3. Diaphragmatic spasm	—	Precordial pain; radiation to shoulder	Dyspnea during sustained spasm of the diaphragm can cause occlusion of esophagus; some patients develop progressive dyspnea, pallor, sweating, hypotension, and angor animi simulating that of acute myocardial infarction; occlusion of the esophagus causes dysphagia and odynophagia
4. Diaphragmatic flutter	—	Lower chest pain felt along the diaphragmatic attachment in the epigastrium, precordium; radiation to the shoulder and occasionally to the neck and arm	Dyspnea, palpitation; symptoms and signs of various causative factors (e.g., encephalitis, intoxication)

(continued)

TABLE 69.3

CONTINUED

Etiology (disease)	IASP code reference†	Important diagnostic features	
		Characteristics of the pain	Associated symptoms and signs
V. Pain of neuropathic origin			
A. Lesions or diseases of the spinal cord (myelopathy)			
1. Intramedullary lesion (tumor, syringomyelia, trauma, multiple sclerosis, abscess, hemorrhage)	I-6	Spontaneous, burning, diffuse, poorly localized pain; bouts of explosive pain; later radicular pain involving several segments, depending on the size of the lesion	Dissociation of sensation, loss of pain and temperature sensation, but little effect on proprioception; sensory changes often "spotty"; lower motor neuron signs; with multiple sclerosis spotty paresthesia, pain, symptoms and signs of other involved parts of CNS
2. Extramedullary lesion (primary or metastatic tumor; abscess; hemorrhage)	I-6	Initially localized back pain but subsequently pain is radicular; aggravated by increase in CSF pressure, such as that caused by straining, sneezing, coughing	Paravertebral tenderness, paresthesia, followed by sensory loss, muscular weakness; lower motor neuron signs at level of lesion; increased deep reflexes; CSF changes early and marked; spinal cord compression with large lesion
3. Epidural spinal cord compression (primary or metastatic tumor, hemorrhage, posterior disk protrusion, abscess, hemorrhage)	—	Localized back pain at level of site of lesion in 95% of patients; bilateral radicular pain in segments affected by lesion in 55%; aggravated by neck flexion, straight leg raising, coughing, sneezing, Valsalva maneuver	Back tenderness on deep palpation, fist pounding; no other early signs, but later muscle weakness ranging from mild degree to paraplegia; numbness and paresthesia in 50%; bladder and bowel dysfunction with low thoracic epidural spinal cord compression
B. Lesions of rootlets or roots of T-1 to T-12 (radiculopathy)			
1. Herpes zoster	I-1	Continuous aching, itching, or burning pain, often with superimposed bouts of severe lancinating pain; hyperalgesia; aggravated by trunk motion, palpation of vesicles; persists until healing of rash (1–4 weeks)	Appearance of rash, later vesicles form and then crust; hyperalgesia and hyperesthesia of skin in affected segments; occasionally systemic symptoms of infection; mood and behavioral changes with unrelieved pain
2. Postherpetic neuralgia	I-1	Severe, continuous, unrelenting burning pain, itching; accompanied by severe paroxysms of stabbing, lancinating pain that persist long after acute phase	Hyperalgesia, hypesthesia, hyperpathia; scar in area of vesicles; reactive depression, sleep disturbances, anorexia, lassitude, constipation, decreased libido; high suicide rate among those with unrelieved postherpetic neuralgia
3. Tabes dorsalis	I-6	Severe, sharp, lancinating, girdlelike (segmental) pain of brief duration with intervals of remission	History of syphilis; CSF evidence; other symptoms of CNS syphilis
4. Mechanical compression (tumor, disk protrusion, vertebral fracture, osteophyte, adhesive arachnoiditis)	—	Segmental sharp, burning pain; aggravated by cough, sneezing, straining, and movement of trunk	Hyperalgesia, hyperesthesia, hypesthesia, dysesthesia; radiographic evidence of pathology
C. Diseases of formed thoracic spinal nerves (neuropathy)			
1. Vertebral compression (arthritis, metastatic or traumatic fracture, tumor of vertebrae, osteomyelitis)	—	Segmental neuralgia usually present: continuous burning or sharp pain affecting part or entire segment of nerve, associated with paroxysms of stabbing pain; compression of anterior root produces dull, aching, occasionally stabbing pain in part of affected segment; both aggravated by movement of thoracic spine; often worse at night	Paravertebral tenderness and segmental hyperalgesia, hyperesthesia, hypesthesia; radiographic evidence (CT scan)

(continued)

TABLE 69.3

CONTINUED

Etiology (disease)	IASP code reference†	Important diagnostic features	
		Characteristics of the pain	Associated symptoms and signs
2. Paravertebral compression (mediastinal tumors, aortic aneurysm, paravertebral abscess or adenopathy)	—	Continuous moderate to severe burning, aching segmental pain; aggravated by movement of spine; occasional bouts of lancinating pain	Paravertebral tenderness; segmental hyperalgesia, hypesthesia; radiographic evidence
3. Primary neurogenic tumors (neurofibroma, schwannoma, ganglioneuroma, neuroblastoma)	—	Possibly localized back pain and tenderness but usually continuous burning, aching pain; associated with lancinating pain in distribution of affected nerve	Sensory deficit (hypesthesia), paresthesia, dysesthesia; CT scan and radiographic evidence
4. Other neuropathies (systemic infection, alcoholism, avitaminosis, diabetes, metals)	—	Continuous or intermittent mild to moderate burning pain; associated with paroxysms of stabbing pain in one or more dermatomes	History of infection, alcoholism, nutrition deficiency, exposure to ingestion of metals; hyperesthesia, hyperalgesia, hypesthesia, paresthesia, dysesthesia; other signs and symptoms of primary disorder
D. Lesion or disease of the intercostal nerves—intercostal neuropathy (compression or irritation secondary to rib fracture; trauma; primary or metastatic tumor of ribs; pleuritis)	—	Superficial continuous burning pain in distribution of affected intercostal nerve; also, local pain with rib fracture or tumor, pleuritic pain with pleuritis	History of trauma or infection; paresthesia, hyperesthesia, dysesthesia, hypesthesia; superficial and deep tenderness; radiographic evidence; palpable tumor or fracture
VI. Pain of musculoskeletal origin			
A. Lesions of the thoracic spine			
1. Fracture (trauma, neoplasm, osteoporosis, subluxation, dislocation)	—	Initially localized dull, aching pain, often referred to anterior part of chest; aggravated by motion, worse and throbbing at night; segmental pain with root compression	History of trauma; radiographic evidence; localized tenderness paravertebrally and over spinous processes; possibly segmental hyperalgesia, paresthesia
2. Metastatic or primary tumors	—	Intense aching, boring circumscribed pain; aggravated by motion and local pressure	Local tenderness or segmental hyperalgesia and hyperesthesia; CT scan and radiographic evidence
3. Arthritis or deformity of spine	—	Usually circumscribed aching pain in back and side; segmental pain with neuropathy	Signs of arthritis in other areas; deformity of spine evident; local tenderness; reflex muscle spasm; radiographic evidence
4. Ankylosing spondylitis	—	Usually circumscribed dull aching pain in back; later paraspinal contractures develop with compression of nerve root, which causes segmental pain	Tenderness on deep palpation; radiographic evidence
5. Diffuse idiopathic skeletal hyperostosis	—	Mild to moderate localized, dull, aching pain; aggravated by inactivity and cold	Tenderness and stiffness in thoracic spine; dorsal kyphosis; reduction of range of movement and in chest expansion; characteristic radiographic evidence
6. Inflammatory disease of vertebrae (osteomyelitis, actinomycosis, tuberculosis, syphilis, subperiosteal hematoma)	—	Circumscribed, continuous, aching pain; moderate to severe; aggravated by pressure, often worse at night	Local and systemic symptoms and signs of inflammation; localized tenderness paravertebrally and over spinous process

(continued)

TABLE 69.3

CONTINUED

Etiology (disease)	IASP code reference†	Important diagnostic features	
		Characteristics of the pain	Associated symptoms and signs
7. Costovertebral joint arthritis	—	Localized deep aching pain similar to that arising from vertebral pathology; aggravated by movement; relieved by local infiltration of joint	Tenderness on deep palpation; radiographic evidence
8. Apophyseal facet syndrome	—	Moderate to severe, dull, aching, localized pain and tenderness; aggravated by hyperextension; relieved by flexion of the spine	Tenderness; limitation of motion, flattening of normal kyphotic thoracic curve; paraspinal muscle spasm
B. Rib lesions			
1. Fracture or trauma (severe cough, osteoporosis, metastatic tumor)	—	Localized sharp pain at site of lesion; widespread chest pain with multiple rib fractures; pain aggravated by deep breathing, coughing, movement of thorax	History of accidental trauma or severe coughing; evidence of osteoporosis; exquisite tenderness on palpation of fracture site; radiographic evidence; with compound fracture can have pneumothorax and damage to lung, with respiratory symptoms and signs
2. Primary metastatic rib tumor (myeloma, chondrosarcoma, granuloma)	—	Mild to moderate or severe continuous unilateral dull, aching, chest pain; relatively localized but can also produce intercostal neuralgia	Palpable mass and tenderness to pressure; radiographic evidence
3. Other bone diseases (osteitis deformans, acromegaly, Paget disease, osteoporosis, hyperostosis)	—	Localized continuous aching pain; intercostal neuralgia if lesion irritates nerve	Evidence of disease elsewhere; tenderness on palpation; radiographic evidence
C. Disorders of the costal cartilages			
1. Costochondritis (anterior chest wall syndrome)	—	Unilateral or bilateral aching pain in lower anterior chest wall usually in region of cartilages of third, sixth to seventh ribs; aggravated by deep breathing, coughing, palpation	No swelling of costochondral region; more frequent in younger than older people; development of anxiety and concern about heart disease if pain is on left side
2. Tietze syndrome	—	Localized moderate dull, aching pain in upper anterior chest in region of second and perhaps third costochondral junction; aggravated by palpation, movement of chest wall, coughing, respiratory infection; worse when lying down; recurs between intervals of remission	Palpable tender tumorlike swelling at site of costochondral joint; occurs mostly in people older than 50 years; radiography not diagnostic; development of anxiety, fatigue, concern about heart disease
3. Slipping rib syndrome (rib tip syndrome, slipped cartilage)	XVII-10	Unilateral lower chest and upper abdominal localized aching or sharp pain; aggravated by hyperextension and raising of arms; relieved by forward bending to the affected side	Palpation produces tenderness and reveals upward curling of loosened end of cartilages of eighth, ninth, and tenth ribs; hooking flexed finger under costal cartilage and exerting pressure anteriorly produces clicking noise
4. Fracture of cartilage or dislocation of costochondral joint	—	Sudden sharp pain from fracture or dislocation followed by continuous dull aching, burning discomfort in area of costal margin; reference to back	History of injury; tenderness on palpation; displaced cartilage is palpable and feels like lump
D. Lesions or disorders of the sternum			
1. Fracture of sternum	—	Localized pain in region of sternum, usually sharp initially but then continuous and aching; aggravated by deep breathing or palpation	History of blunt trauma to anterior chest; tenderness to palpation; leads to manubriosternal arthralgia

(continued)

TABLE 69.3

CONTINUED

Etiology (disease)	IASP code reference†	Important diagnostic features	
		Characteristics of the pain	Associated symptoms and signs
2. Rheumatoid arthritis or osteoarthritis	—	Continuous or intermittent pain localized to the angle of Louis; aggravated by deep breathing, coughing, sneezing, and yawning	Mild swelling of joint; exquisite tenderness to palpation; systemic arthritis present; radiographic evidence of arthropathy
3. Xiphoidalgia (hypersensitive xiphoid syndrome, xiphodynia)	—	Spontaneous deep aching or sharp pain varying in intensity from a slight to agonizing discomfort that simulates pain of myocardial infarction; aggravated by movements that act on xiphoid process (e.g., bending, stooping, turning) and by increase in intragastric pressure caused by a large meal; can be constant or recurs several times a day; lasts for minutes to several hours	Pressure on xiphoid process produces spontaneous pain that can radiate deep retrosternally and to the precordium, epigastrium, and across shoulder and back; persists for weeks or months but usually disappears spontaneously
4. Arthritis of sternoclavicular joint	—	Localized sharp or aching pain in region of joint; radiation to shoulder and upper chest	Joint swollen, tender on palpation; radiographic evidence
F. Muscle disorders			
1. Myofascial pain syndromes with trigger points			
a. Anterior chest (major and minor, pectoralis; scaleni; sternalis; intercostals)	—	Frequent cause of pain in anterior chest; pain is deep and aching; aggravated by activity; sternalis and pectoralis pain can simulate pain of angina pectoris; pain relieved by injection of trigger points with local anesthetic	History of severe strain by heavy lifting; local tenderness, trigger points present; unaffected body activity
b. Lateral chest (serratus anterior; intercostals)	—	Deep aching pain on the lateral aspect of the chest extending from the lower axilla to about the seventh to the sixth ribs; pain also in area near the inferior angle of the scapula; with intercostal syndrome site of pain varies with site of trigger points; relief with trigger point injection	Localized tenderness and trigger point about the level of the sixth rib; pressure on trigger points produces spontaneous pain
c. Posterior chest (rhomboidei, latissimus dorsi multifidi, serratus posterior superior, iliocostalis thoracis)	—	Deep aching pain in different parts of the back depending on the site of the trigger point and the muscles involved; aggravated by activity of muscles, unaffected by bodily activity	Localized tenderness and trigger points
2. Acute muscle spasm	—	Sharp localized pain in area of the spastic muscle; some radiation to anterior and posterior chest; complete relief with infiltration of muscle	Palpation of spastic muscle; generalized tenderness
3. Muscle contractures	—	Constant deep aching pain, often associated with early spondylosis	Possible localized tenderness of affected muscle or in an area of reference
4. Dermatomyositis and polymyositis	—	Rarely a cause of chest pain; when present, pain aching and aggravated by palpation	Generalized weakness; elevated serum levels of skeletal muscle enzyme
VII. Pain of tegumentary origin (including the breast)			
A. Acute disorders			
1. Burns and other trauma	—	Sharp burning pain following burns, aching pain with trauma	History of injury or burn; emotional reactions

(continued)

TABLE 69.3

CONTINUED

Etiology (disease)	IASP code reference†	Important diagnostic features	
		Characteristics of the pain	Associated symptoms and signs
2. Postoperative pain	—	Fairly localized sharp, burning, aching pain primarily at the site of incision; can radiate to involve adjacent segments	Reflex muscle spasm, tenderness; hyperalgesia; tachycardia response; signs of neuroendocrine stress
3. Acute mastodynia (inflammatory)		Sharp, aching, burning pain in chest; radiation to axilla and inner arm; aggravated by movement of the breast	Extreme tenderness, tumefaction; evidence of infection
4. Deep axillary abscess		Sharp localized, diffuse dull, aching pain in axilla; radiation to anterior chest and medial arm	Tenderness, fluctuating mass; signs of infection
5. Acute dermatologic disorders (vesicles, furuncles, bullae, pustules, ulcers, erythema, cellulitis)	—	Aching, burning, itching pain localized to lesion	Possible evidence of local or systemic disease
B. Chronic disorders			
1. Postmastectomy syndrome 2. Postthoracotomy syndrome		Sharp, burning, aching pain; accompanied by bouts of lancinating pain in distribution of the dermatomes supplied by the injured nerve or in part of the segment; aggravated by light touch of skin, palpation of neuroma, and emotional stress	Hyperesthesia, hyperalgesia, hypesthesia, paresthesia; neuroma often palpable; evidence of recurrent cancer by use of CT scan or other diagnostic procedures
3. Adiposis dolorosa (Dercum disease)	—	Enlarged painful fatty subcutaneous nodule most commonly in the chest and arms but can affect any part except the face; usually darting, shooting, or stabbing pain; occurs spontaneously or provoked by palpation	Usually occurs in obese women; weakness, fatigue, emotional instability, occasional dementia
4. Chronic mastalgia	—	Chronic persistent pain; cyclic in two-thirds of patients and continuous in the other third; deep, aching, diffuse pain over entire breast without palpable evidence of pathology; about 20% have spontaneous intermittent relief while others have relief at menopause or pregnancy or with use of oral contraceptives; those with noncyclic pain have pain that can persist for 2–3 years or for as long as 30 years	Psychological tests usually reveal no abnormality; positive response to hormonal manipulation suggests a hormonal basis to the condition
5. Scleroderma (dermatomyositis, disseminating lupus erythematosus, polyarteritis nodosa)	—	Dull, aching, occasionally burning pain in the chest wall, usually in the area of the lesion; with scleroderma, chest pain can arise from skin, thoracic wall, or myocardial or esophageal lesions	Symptoms and signs of systemic disease; many types produce widespread visceral involvement
6. Other chronic dermatologic diseases	—	(See Chapter 31 for detailed discussion)	
7. Mondor disease (phlebitis of anterolateral chest)	—	Rare condition manifested by thrombosis of superficial vein of thoracic wall that produces palpable painful cord within the skin; usually sharp and persistent; intensified by deep inspiration or flexion of the trunk	Presence of painful, tender, subcutaneous cord running obliquely across thorax in distribution of one or more superficial veins; lesion indolent after several weeks

(*continued*)

TABLE 69.3

CONTINUED

Etiology (disease)	IASP code reference†	Important diagnostic features	
		Characteristics of the pain	Associated symptoms and signs
C. Cancer of the breast	—	Early breast cancer not painful; in far advanced disease skin nodule eventually breaks down and formation also causes localized breast pain; metastasis to the pleura produces pleuritic pain; metastasis to the ribs causes localized pain and can be associated with segmental neuralgia; metastasis to the spine produces back pain and later can cause epidural spinal cord compression or plexopathy	Early: retracted nipple, bleeding, distorted areola or breast contour, skin dimpling (*peau d'orange*); later: axillary supraclavicular adenopathy; metastatic lesion demonstrated by radiography and CT scan
VIII. Chest pain referred from extrathoracic disorders			
A. Disorders of the cervical spine that cause neuropathy			
1. Posterolateral protrusion of intervertebral disk (C-7, C-8) 2. Arthritis, osteophyte, fracture or other lesion that compresses root or nerve		Pain in the neck, shoulder, medial aspect of the arm, and pectoral region of the chest; with left-sided lesion, pain can simulate that of myocardial ischemia but is differentiated by aggravation by lateral flexion and the Spurling test (see Chapter 54); unaffected by activity if neck and arms not moved	Paravertebral and pectoral muscle tenderness; hyperalgesia, hyperesthesia, and paresthesia of the arm; decrease in reflexes and some muscle weakness in the upper limbs
3. Thoracic inlet syndromes (scalenus anticus syndrome; cervical rib or abnormal first rib; costoclavicular compression)	—	Pain most prominent in the shoulder and upper limbs; radiation to the upper pectoral region; aggravated by severe arm abduction and walking with swinging arms; unaffected by activity if arms not moved	Supraclavicular (scaleni) tenderness and fullness; neurovascular signs and symptoms in the upper extremities; radiographic evidence of abnormal cervical rib
4. Pancoast syndrome	—	Pain in shoulder, scapula, medial aspect of arm, and superior anterior chest; aggravated by extreme abduction of the arm and paravertebral pressure; unaffected by activity if neck and limbs are not moved	Signs and symptoms of plexopathy with paresthesia, dysesthesia, numbness in the medial aspects of the forearm and fourth and fifth fingers, also medial aspect of arm; marked weakness of muscles supplied by ulnar nerve; radiographic and CT scan evidence of lesion
B. Diseases of the abdominal viscera			
1. Gas entrapment syndromes (e.g., caused by aerophagia, excess production of gas in bowel)	—	Bloated sensation associated with pain in the epigastrium and central lower chest; if diaphragm irritated, pain also in shoulder; dull, aching pain worsens as day progresses; transiently relieved by belching; gas entrapment in hepatic flexure of colon produces discomfort in right upper quadrant and lower part of right chest, gas in splenic flexure causes pain in left upper quadrant and left lower chest	History of aerophagia, abdominal tympany; radiographic evidence

(*continued*)

TABLE 69.3

CONTINUED

Etiology (disease)	IASP code reference†	Important diagnostic features	
		Characteristics of the pain	Associated symptoms and signs
2. Peptic ulcer disease	—	Ulcer in cardia of stomach produces pain in the epigastrium and central lower anterior chest, ulcer in other locations not associated with chest pain; duodenal ulcer causes pain that radiates to xiphoid process but not higher	Peptic ulcer confirmed by radiography and endoscopy
3. Perforated ulcer	—	Sudden severe epigastric pain that can radiate to lower chest with severe hypotension; myocardial ischemia; anginal pain	History, physical signs (e.g., muscle spasm, shock, diaphoresis, hematemesis)
4. Biliary colic	—	Sudden moderate to severe epigastric pain; radiation to back; right subcostal region, and low central portion of right chest; rarely, pain confined only to chest mimicking that of myocardial infarction, but no radiation to arm or jaw	Patient can have nausea but no vomiting; in distress but no fever; subcostal tenderness
5. Acute cholecystitis	—	Pain usually localized to right upper quadrant; lasts few days rather than a few hours; chest pain rare except in patients with coexisting coronary artery disease: in these patients, biliary pain provokes angina pectoris and ECG changes (low amplitude and inversion of T wave)	Nausea, vomiting, fever, jaundice, and tender right upper quadrant mass; abdominal muscle spasm
6. Acute pancreatitis	—	Sudden severe epigastric pain associated with retrosternal oppression; radiation to lower part of left side of chest; unaffected by effort; often provokes ECG changes similar to those of myocardial ischemia and infarction	Severe abdominal muscle spasm; often hypotension, hypoventilation, elevated blood amylase level
7. Subphrenic abscess	—	Pus from perforated viscus produces subdiaphragmatic abscess with inflammation of the diaphragm; pleuritic pain in the lower chest and often the shoulder; intrapleural rupture of amebic liver abscess; sudden severe chest pain	Dyspnea, fever, pleural effusion and, occasionally, hepatomegaly
IX. Chest pain primarily of psychological origin			
A. Acute anxiety state	—	Sudden acute diffuse pain in chest in the precordial region near cardiac apex (not retrosternal); severe, sharp, stabbing pain or dull, heavy pressure experienced after effort, not during	Dyspnea (air hunger) leading to hyperventilation, tachycardia, dizziness, palpitations, perspiration, tremor, weakness, chest tightness; psychological evaluation and testing reveal evidence of anxiety
B. Chronic anxiety (cardiac neurosis, soldier's heart, neurocirculatory asthenia, irritable heart, effort syndrome)	—	Pain usually at apex of the heart; felt as dull ache with or without attacks of sharp pain over same area; either of brief duration or continuous for hours and days; associated with fatigue rather than effort; responds poorly to all medication	Chronic anxiety and apprehension; severe dyspnea; respiratory distress both at rest and with exertion, sighing respirations; possible ECG changes; low energy level; psychological evaluation and testing reveal psychopathology

(continued)

TABLE 69.3

CONTINUED

Etiology (disease)	IASP code reference†	Important diagnostic features	
		Characteristics of the pain	Associated symptoms and signs
C. Depression	—	Endogenous depression can cause atypical chest pain described as a heavy feeling or deep ache or tightness; possible radiation to left arm; usually worse in the morning, lessens as the day goes on	Feeling of overconcern with the heart; in primary affective disorder patient complains of feelings of depression, guilt, worthlessness, withdrawal, disinterest; occasional suicidal preoccupation, anorexia, weight loss, fatigue, low energy level, malaise, insomnia; psychological evaluation and testing reveal psychopathology
D. Hypochondriasis	—	Precordial or apical pain; pain described by patient in minute detail regarding location, quality, and duration but does not fit pattern of any *organic* disease, and description of the pain changes from one visit to another	Feeling of overconcern with the heart; many other complaints (e.g., dysfunction of gastrointestinal tract); may present different complaints at different visits; psychological evaluation and testing produces evidence of psychopathology
E. Operant pain (learned pain)	—	Initially patient has chest pain from disease of the heart or lungs that persists after healing because of reinforcing environmental factors; develops chronic pain behavior and abnormal illness behavior	Progressive physical deterioration over time because of inactivity, muscle weakness, and other factors that cause pain and reinforce the behavior; psychological evaluation and testing reveal psychopathology

†See Table 2-2.

Our growing treatment armamentarium includes analgesic and neuropathic medications, nerve blocks and ablations, joint injections, implanted pumps, transcutaneous or implanted electrical stimulators, as well as behavioral medicine approaches. In many cases of chest wall pain, conservative, multidisciplinary approaches are initially preferred, saving invasive treatments for the refractive cases.

References

1. Snell RS, ed. *Clinical Anatomy by Regions.* 8th ed. Philadelphia: Lippincott Williams & Wilkins; 2007:45–73.
2. Standring S, ed. *Gray's Anatomy: The Anatomical Basis of Clinical Practice.* 39th ed. London: Elsevier, Churchill Livingstone; 2005: 951–968.
3. Sanders RJ. *Thoracic Outlet Syndrome.* Philadelphia: JB Lippincott Co.; 1991.
4. Schaumburg HH, Berger AR, Thomas PK. *Disorders of Peripheral Nerves.* 2nd ed. Philadelphia: FA Davis Co.; 1992.
5. White JC. Cardiac pain: anatomic pathways and physiologic mechanisms. *Circulation* 1957;16:644–655.
6. Watson PN, Evans RJ. Intractable pain with lung cancer. *Pain* 1987;29: 163–173.
7. Pancoast HK. Superior pulmonary sulcus tumor. *JAMA* 1932;99:1391–1394.
8. Hepper NGG. Thoracic inlet tumors. *Ann Int Med* 1966;64:979–989.
9. Watson PN, Evans RJ. Intractable pain with lung cancer. *Pain* 1987;29: 163–173.
10. Kori S, Foley KM, Posner JB. Brachial plexus lesions in patients with cancer: clinical findings in 100 cases. *Neurology* 1981;31:45–50.
11. Gilbert RW, Kim JH, Posner JB. Epidural spinal cord compression from metastatic tumor. *Ann Neurol* 1978;3:40–51.
12. Posner JB. Back pain and epidural spinal cord compression. *Med Clin North Am* 1987;71:185–205.
13. Rusch V, Ginsberg RJ. Chest wall, pleura, lung, and mediastinum. In: Schwartz SI, Shires GT, eds. *Principles of Surgery.* New York: McGraw–Hill; 1999:667–790.
14. Gucalp R, Dutcher J. Oncologic emergencies. In: Fauci AS, Harrison TR, eds. *Harrisons Principles of Internal Medicine.* New York: McGraw–Hill; 1998: 627–634.
15. Yeung MC, Hagen NA. Cervical disc herniation presenting with chest wall pain. *Can J Neurol Sci* 1993;20:59–61.
16. O'Connor Rc, Andary MT, Russo RB, et al. Thoracic radiculopathy. *Phys Med Rehabil Clin N Am* 2002;13:623.
17. Hassenbusch S, Burchiel K, Coffey RJ, et al. Management of intrathecal catheter tip inflammatory masses: a consensus statement. *Pain Med* 2002;3: 313–323.
18. Donahue JG, Choo PW, Manson JE, et al. The incidence of herpes zoster. *Arch Intern Med* 1995;155:1605–1609.
19. Choo PW, Galil K, Donahue JG, et al. Risk factors for postherpetic neuralgia. *Arch Intern Med* 1997;157:1217–1224.
20. Bowsher D. Pathophysiology of postherpetic neuralgia. *Neurology* 1995;45: S58–S60.
21. Wu JJ, Huang DB, Tyring SK. Dermatologic virology. In: Hall JC, ed. *Sauer's Manual of Skin Diseases.* 9th ed. Philadelphia: Lippincott Williams & Wilkins; 2006:228–229.
22. Schmader K. Management of herpes zoster in elderly patients. *Infect Dis Clin Pract* 1995;4:293–299.
23. Dworkin RH, Perkins FM, Nagasako E. Prospects for the prevention of post herpetic neuralgia in herpes zoster patient. *Clin J Pain* 2000;16:S90–100.
24. Rowbotham M, Harden N, Stacey B, et al. Gabapentin for the treatment of postherpetic neuralgia. *JAMA* 1998;280:1837–1842.
25. Dworkin RH, Corbin AE, Young JP Jr, et al. Pre gabalin for the treatment of post herpetic neuralgia. *Neurology* 2003;60:1274–1283.
26. Argoff C, Katz N, Backonja M. Treatment of postherpetic neuralgia: a review of therapeutic options. *J Pain Symptom Manage* 2004;28:396–411.
27. Rowbatham M, Davies PS, Verkempinck C, et al. Lidocaine patch: double-blind controlled study of a new treatment method for postherpetic neuralgia. *Pain* 1996;65: 39–44.
28. Watson CP, Tyler KL, Bickers DR, et al. A randomized vehicle controlled trial of topical capsaicin in the treatment of post herpetic neuralgia. *Clin Ther* 1993;15:510–526.
29. Nathan PW, Wall PD. Treatment of post-herpetic neuralgia by prolonged electrical stimulation. *BMJ* 1974;3:645–647.
30. Trescot AM. Cryoanalgesia in interventional pain management. *Pain Physician* 2003;6:345–360.
31. Bogduk NB. Assessing a new procedure: thoracic radiofrequency dorsal root ganglion lesions. *Clin J Pain* 1996;12:76–77.
32. Stolker RJ, Vervest AC, Groen GJ. The treatment of chronic thoracic segmental pain by radiofrequency percutaneous partial rhizotomy. *J Neurosurg* 1994; 80:986–992.
33. Kostuik JP. Osteoporotic fractures of the spine. In: Vaccaro AR, ed. *Fractures*

of the Cervical, Thoracic and Lumbar Spine. New York: Marcel Dekker, Inc; 2003:635–653.

34. Cohen MS, Blair B, Garfin SR. Thoracolumbar compression fractures. In: Levine AM, Eismont FJ, Garfin SR, et al, ed. *Spine Trauma.* Philadelphia: WB Saunders Co; 1998:388–401.
35. Schwartz ED, Flanders AE. Spinal trauma. Philadelphia: Lippincott Williams & Wilkins; 2007.
36. Barr J, Barr M, Lemley T, et al. Percutaneous vertebroplasty for pain relief and spinal stabilization. *Spine* 2000;25:923–928.
37. Mathis JM, Barr JD, Belkoff M. Percutaneous vertebroplasty: a developing standard of care for vertebral compression fractures. *Am J Neuroradiol* 2001; 22:373–381.
38. Reuler JB, Girard DE, Nardone DA. Sternoclavicular joint involvement in ankylosing spondylitis. *South Med J* 1978;71:1480–1481.
39. Nathan H, Weinberg H, Robin GC. The costovertebral joints: anatomical-clinical observations in arthritis. *Arthritis Rheum* 1964;7:228–240.
40. Sanzhang C, Rothschild BM. Zygapophyseal and costovertebral/costotransverse joints: an anatomic assessment of arthritis impact. *Br J Rheumatol* 1993; 32:1066–1071.
41. Roth SH. A new role for opioids in the treatment of arthritis. *Drugs* 2002; 62:255–263.
42. Sales JR, Beals RK, Hart RA. Osteoarthritis of the costovertebral joints: the results of resection arthroplasty. *J Bone Joint Surg Br* 2007;89(10): 1336–1339.
43. Resnick D, Niwayama G. Radiographic and pathologic feature of spinal involvement in diffuse skeletal hyperostosis. *Radiology* 1976;119:559–568.
44. Forestier, Rotes–Querol. Senile ankylosing hyperostosis of the spine. *Ann Rheum Dis* 1950;9:321–330.
45. Amital H, Applbaum YH, Aamar DS, et al. SAPHO syndrome treated with pamidronate: an open-label study of 10 patients. *Rheumatology* 2005;44: 137–138.
46. Fukui S, Ohseto K, Shiotani M. Patterns of pain induced by distending the thoracic zygapophyseal joints. *Reg Anesth* 1997;22:332–336.
47. Dreyfuss P, Tibiletti C, Dreyer S. Thoracic zygopophyseal joint pain patterns. *Spine* 1994;19:807–811.
48. Stolkre RJ, Vervest ACM, Groen GJ. Percutaneous facet denervation in chronic thoracic spinal pain. *Acta Neurochir* 1993;122:82–90.
49. Chua WH, Bogduk N. The surgical anatomy of thoracic facet denervation. *Acta Neurochir* 1995;136: 40–144.
50. Cicala RS, Voeller GR, Fox T, et al. Epidural analgesia in thoracic trauma: effects of lumbar morphine and thoracic bupivacaine on pulmonary function. *Crit Care Med* 1990;18:229–231.
51. Mackersie RC, Karagianes TG, Hoyt DB, et al. Prospective evaluation of epidural and intravenous administration of fentanyl for pain control and restoration of ventilatory function following multiple rib fractures. *J Trauma* 1991;31:443–449.
52. Ullman DA, Fortune JB, Greenhouse BB, et al. The treatment of patients with multiple rib fractures using continuous thoracic epidural narcotic infusion. *Reg Anesth* 1989;14:43–47.
53. Haenel JB, Moore FA, Moore EE, et al. Extrapleural bupivacaine for amelioration of multiple rib fracture pain. *J Trauma* 1995;38:22–27.
54. Luchette FA, Radafshar SM, Kaiser R, et al. Prospective evaluation of epidural versus intrapleural catheters for analgesia in chest wall trauma. *J Trauma* 1994;36:865–870.
55. Moon MR, Luchette FA, Gibson SW, et al. Prospective randomized comparison of epidural vs parenteral opioid analgesia in thoracic trauma. *Ann Surg* 1999;229:684.
56. Shinora K, Iwama H, Akama Y, et al. Interpleural block for patients with multiple rib fractures: comparison with epidural block. *J Emerg Med* 1994; 12:441–446.
57. Davies–Colley R. Slipping rib. *BMJ* 1922;1:432.
58. Wright JT. Slipping rib syndrome. *Lancet* 1980;2:632–634.
59. Mooney DP, Shortner NA. Slipping rib syndrome in childhood. *J Pediatr Surg* 1997;32:1081–1082.
60. Porter GE. Slipping rib syndrome: an infrequently recognized entity in children: a report of three cases and review of literature. *Pediatrics* 1985;76: 810–813.
61. Heinz GJ, Zavala DC. Slipping rib syndrome. *JAMA* 1977;237:794–795.
62. Motulsky A, Rohn RJ. Teitze's syndrome: cause of chest pain and chest wall swelling. *JAMA* 1953;152:504–506.
63. Sain AK. Bone scan in Teitze's syndrome. *Clin Nucl Med* 1978;3:470–471.
64. Gill GV. Epidemic of Teitze's syndrome. *BMJ* 1977;2:499.
65. Kayser HL. Teitze's syndrome: a review of literature. *Am J Med* 1956;21: 982–989.
66. Fossgreen OFJ, Sondergaard–Petersen J, Hede J. Musculo-skeletal pathology in patients with angina pectoris and normal coronary angiograms. *J Int Med* 1999;245:237–246.
67. Scobie BA. Costochondral pain in gastroenterologic practice (letter). *N Engl J Med* 1976;295:1261.
68. Peyton FW. Unexpected frequency of idiopathic costochondral pain. *Obstet Gynecol* 1983;62:605–608.
69. Wolf E, Stern S. Costosternal syndrome: its frequency and importance in differential diagnosis of coronary heart disease. *Arch Intern Med* 1976;136: 189–191.
70. Epstein SE, Gerber LH, Borer JS. Chest wall syndrome: a common cause of unexplained cardiac pain. *JAMA* 1979;241:2793–2797.

71. Brown RT. Costochondritis in adolescents. *J Adolesc Health Care* 1981;1: 198–201.
72. Aglas F, Gretler J, Rainer F, et al. Sternoclavicular septic arthritis: a rare but serious complication of subclavian venous catheterization. *Clin Rheumatol* 1994;13:507–512.
73. Prevo RL, Rasker JJ, Kruijsen MW. Sternocostoclavicular hyperostosis or pustulotic arthrosteitis. *J Rheumatol* 1989;16:1602–1605.
74. Resnick CS, Ammann AM. Cervical spine involvement in sternoclavicular hyperostosis. *Spine* 1985;10:846–848.
75. Dastgeer GM, Mikolich DJ. Fracture- dislocation of manubriosternal joint: an unusual complication of seizures. *J Trauma* 1987;27:91–93.
76. Doube A, Clarke AK. Symptomatic manubriosternal joint involvement in rheumatoid arthritis. *Ann Rheum Dis* 1989;48:516–517.
77. Kernodle GW Jr, Allen NB. Acute gout presenting in the manubriosternal joint. *Arthritis Rheum* 1986;29:570–572.
78. Sebes JI, Salazar JE. The manubriosternal joint in rheumatoid disease. *Am J Roentgenol* 1983;140:117–121.
79. Gruber BL, Kaufman LD, Gorevic PD. Septic arthritis involving manubriosternal joint. *J Rheumatol* 1985;12:803–804.
80. Van Linthoudt D, De Torrente A, Humair L, et al. Septic manubriosternal arthritis in a patient with Reiter's disease. *Clin Rheumatol* 1987;6:293–295.
81. Parker VS, Malhotra CM, Ho G Jr, et al. Radiographic appearance of the sternomanubrial joint in arthritis and related conditions. *Radiology* 1984; 153:343–347.
82. Lipkin M, Fulton LA, Wolfson EA. Xiphoidalgia syndrome. *N Engl J Med* 1955;253:591–597.
83. Howell JM. Xiphodynia. *J Emerg Med* 1992;10:435–438.
84. Miller AJ, Texidor TA. Precordial catch: a neglected syndrome of precordial pain. *JAMA* 1955;159:1364–1365.
85. Reynolds JL. Precordial catch syndrome in children. *South Med J* 1989;82: 1228–1230.
86. Hopkins JHS. Bornholm disease. *Br Med J* 1950;27:1230–1232.
87. Preece PE, Mansel RE, Bolton PM etal. Clinical syndromes of mastalgia. *Lancet* 1976;2:670–673.
88. Wisbey JR, Kumar S, Mansel RE, et al. natural history of breast pain. *Lancet* 1983;2:672–674.
89. Preece PE, Mansel RE, Hughes LE. Mastalgia: psychoneurosis or organic disease? *BMJ* 1978;1:29–30.
90. Mansel RE, Preece PE, Hughes LE. A double blind trial of prolactin inhibitor bromocriptine in painful benign breast disease. *Br J Surg* 1978;65:724–727.
91. Mansel RE, Wisbey JR, Hughes LE. Controlled trial of the antigonadotropin danazol in painful nodular benign breast disease. *Lancet* 1982;1:928–930.
92. Gately, CA, Maddox PR, Mansel RE, et al. Mastalgia refractory to drug treatment. *Br J Surg* 1990;77:1110–1112.
93. Khan HN, Rampaul R, Blamey RW. Local anesthetic and steroid combined injection therapy in the management of non-cyclical mastalgia. *Breast* 2004; 13:129–132.
94. Petersen P, Kastrup J. Dercum's disease (adiposis dolorosa). Treatment of severe pain with intravenous lidocaine. *Pain* 1987;28:77–80.
95. Lunn GM, Potter JM. Mondor's disease. *BMJ* 1954;1:1074–1076.
96. Cooper RA. Mondor's disease secondary to intravenous drug abuse. *Arch Surg* 1990;125:807–808.
97. Camiel MR. Mondor's disease in the breast. *Am J Obstet Gynecol* 1985;152: 879–881.
98. Stevens PE, Dibble SL, Miaskowski C. Prevalence, characteristics and impact of postmastectomy pain syndrome; an investigation of women's experiences. *Pain* 1995;61:61–68.
99. Carpenter JS, Andrykowski MA, Sloan P, et al. Post mastectomy and post lumpectomy pain in breast cancer survivors. *J Clin Epedemiol* 1998;51:1285.
100. Vecht CJ, Vande Brand HJ, Wajer OJ. Post-axillary dissection pain in breast cancer due to a lesion of the intercostobrachial nerve. *Pain* 1989;38:171–176.
101. Wallace SW, Wallace AM, Lee J, et al. Pain after breast surgery: a survey of 282 women. *Pain* 1996;66:195–205.
102. Smith WC, Bourne D, Squair J, et al. A retrospective cohort study of post mastectomy pain syndrome. *Pain* 1999;83:91–95.
103. Reuben SS, Makari–Judson G, Lurie SD. Evaluation of efficacy of the perioperative administration of Venlafaxine XR in the prevention of postmastectomy pain syndrome. *J Pain Symptom Manage* 2004;27:133–139.
104. Crawford JS, Simpson J, Crawford P. Myofascial release provides symptomatic relief from chest wall tenderness occasionally seen following lumpectomy and radiation in breast cancer patients. *Int J Radiat Oncol Biol Phys* 1996; 15:1188–1199.
105. Layeeque R, Hochberg J, Siegel, et al. Botulinum toxin infiltration for pain control after mastectomy and expander reconstruction. *Ann Surg* 2004;240: 608–614.
106. Jamison K, Wellisch DK, Katz RL, et al. Phantom breast syndrome. *Arch Surg* 1979;114:93–95.
107. Kroner K, Knudsen UB, Lundby L, et al. Long term phantom breast syndrome after mastectomy. *Clin J Pain* 1992;8:346–350.
108. Staps T, Hoogenhout J, Wobbes T. Phantom breast sensations following mastectomy. *Cancer* 1985;56:2898–2901.
109. Gottrup H, Andersen J, Arendt- Nielsen L, et al. Psychophysical examination in patients with post mastectomy pain. *Pain* 2000;87:275–284.
110. Tasmuth T, Von Smitten K, Kalso E. Effect of present pain and mood on the memory of past postoperative pain in women treated surgically for breast cancer. *Pain* 1996;68:343–345.

111. Kroner K, Krebs B, Skov J, et al. Immediate and long-term phantom breast syndrome after mastectomy: incidence, clinical characteristics and relationship to pre-mastectomy breast pain. *Pain* 1989;36:327–334.

112. Keller SM, Carp NZ, Levy MN, et al. Chronic post thoracotomy pain. *J Cardiovasc Surg* 1994;35:161–164.

113. Daczman E, Gordon A, Kreisman H, et al. Long-term postthoracotomy pain. *Chest* 1991;99:270–274.

114. Ochroch EA, Gottschalk A, Troxel AB, et al. Women suffer more short and long term pain than men after major thoracotomy. *Clin J Pain* 2006;22: 491–498.

115. Athanassiadi K, Kakaris S, Theakos N, et al. Muscle-sparing versus posterolateral thoracotomy: a prospective study. *Eur J Cardiothorac Surg* 2007;31: 496–500.

116. Katz J, Jackson M, Kavanaugh BP, et al. Acute pain after thoracic surgery predicts long term postthoracotomy pain. *Clin J Pain* 1996;12:50–55.

117. Sihoe ADL, Lee TW, Wan IYP, et al. The use of gabapentin for post-operative and posttraumatic pain in thoracic surgery patients. *Eur J Cardiothorac Surg* 2006;26:795–799.

118. Senturk M, Ozcan PE, Talu GK, et al. The effects of three different analgesia techniques on long term postthoracotomy pain. *Anesth Analg* 2002;94:11.

119. Kirvela O, Antila H. Thoracic paravertebral block in chronic postoperative pain. *Reg Anesth* 1992;17:348–350.

120. Kamakar MK. Thoracic paravertebral block. *Anesthesiology* 2001;95: 771–780.

121. Cohen SP, Sireci A, Wu CL, et al. Pulsed radiofrequency of the dorsal root ganglia is superior to pharmacotherapy or pulsed radiofrequency of the intercostal nerves in the treatment of chronic postsurgical thoracic pain. *Pain Physician* 2006;9:227–236.

122. Meek JC, Bollen E, Koudstaal J, et al. Pain in scar as an early symptom of acquired thoracic lung hernia. *Eur Respir J* 1991;4:505–507.

123. Fitzpatrick C, Coppola CP, Eichelberger. Intercostal hernia and spontaneous pneumothorax in a liver transplant recipient: a case report. *J Pediatr Surg* 2007;42:5–8.

124. Eisenberg E, Pultorak Y, Pud D, et al. Prevalence and characteristics of post coronary artery bypass graft surgery pain (PCP). *Pain* 2001;92:11–17.

125. Bruce J, Drury N, Poobalan AS, et al. The prevalence of chronic chest and leg pain following cardiac surgery: a historical cohort study. *Pain* 2003;104: 265–273.

126. Mailis A, Umana M, Feindel CM. Anterior intercostal nerve damage after coronary artery bypass graft surgery with use of internal thoracic artery graft. *Ann Thorac Surg* 2000;69:1455–1488.

127. Norgaard MA, Andersen TC, Lavrsen MJ, et al. The outcome of sternal wire removal on persistent anterior chest wall pain after median sternotomy. *Eur J Cardiothorac Surg* 2006; 29: 920–924.

128. Billings RF. Chest pain related to emotional disorders. In: Levine DL, Billings RF, eds. *Chest Pain: An Integrated Diagnostic Approach*. Philadelphia: Lea and Febiger; 1977:133–150.

129. Mukerji B, Mukerji V, Alpert MA, et al. The prevalence of rheumatologic disorders in patients with chest pain and angiographically normal coronary arteries. *Angiology* 1995;46:425–430.

130. Wise CM, Semble EL, Dalton CB. Musculoskeletal chest wall syndromes in patients with noncardiac chest pain: a study of 100 patients. *Arch Phys Med Rehabil* 1992;73:147–149.

131. Vaisrub S. Editorial: Da costa syndrome revisited. *JAMA* 1975;232:164.

132. Wheeler EO, White PD, Reed EW, et al. Neurocirculatory asthenia (anxiety, neurosis, effort syndrome, neurasthenia): a 20-year follow-up study of 173 patients. *JAMA* 1950;142:878–889.

133. Borjesson M, Andrell P, Lundberg D, et al. Spinal cord stimulation in severe angina pectoris: a systematic review based on the Swedish council on technology assessment in health care report on long standing pain. *Pain* 2008;140: 501–508.

134. Di Pede F, Lanza GA, Zuin G, et al. Immediate and long term clinical outcome after spinal cord stimulation for refractory stable angina pectoris. *Am J Cardiol* 2003;91:951–955.

135. Fox K, Garcia MAA, Ardissino D, et al. Guidelines on the management of stable angina pectoris: the Task Force on the Management of Stable Angina Pectoris of the European Society of Cardiology. *Eur Heart J* 2006;27(11): 1341–1381.

136. Anderson C, Hole P, OXhoj H. Does pain relief with spinal cord stimulation for angina conceal myocardial infarction. *Br Heart J* 1994;71:419–421.

CHAPTER 70 ■ LOWER EXTREMITY PAIN

GAGAN MAHAJAN AND DAVE LOOMBA

The information in this chapter is presented in three major sections detailing: (1) specific causes of lumbosacral plexopathy; (2) specific lower extremity peripheral nerve lesions; and (3) specific causes of foot pain.

LUMBOSACRAL PLEXOPATHY

Although the lumbar and sacral plexi are separate structures, they are often referred to as a single structure—the lumbosacral plexus—that provides motor and sensory innervation to the pelvis and leg (Fig. 70.1). The lumbar plexus, which is made up of the ventral rami of the T12–L3 and a portion of the L4 nerve roots, is contained within the psoas muscle and lies anterior to the L2–L5 vertebral bodies.[1-3] The anterior and posterior divisions of the ventral rami form the terminal branches of the lumbar plexus and include the iliohypogastric (T12,L1), ilioinguinal (L1), genitofemoral (L1,L2), lateral femoral cutaneous (L2,L3), obturator nerves (L2,L3,L4), and femoral (L2,L3,L4) nerves.[3] The saphenous nerve is a branch of the femoral nerve.

The sacral plexus (Fig. 70.2), which is made up of the ventral rami of the S1–S5 nerve roots, connects with the lumbar plexus via the lumbosacral trunk. It is made up of the ventral rami of the L4–L5 nerve roots and lies just anterior to the piriformis muscle, posterior to the internal iliac vessels, and in close proximity to the hypogastric arteries and veins, lateral rectum, pelvic colon, and ureters.[2,3] Similar to the lumbar plexus, terminal branches arise from the anterior and posterior divisions of the ventral rami of the sacral plexus. The tibial nerve (made up of the anterior divisions of the ventral rami) and the common fibular (peroneal) nerve (made up of the posterior divisions) form the terminal branches of the sciatic nerve upon bifurcating from their common epineural sheath.[3] Additional terminal branches of the sacral plexus include the superior gluteal (L4,L5,S1) inferior gluteal (L5,S1,S2), posterior femoral cutaneous (S1,S2,S3), and pudendal (S2,S3,S4) nerves.[3]

There are multiple causes of lumbosacral plexopathy. These include space-occupying masses (invasive neoplasm, compression by retroperitoneal or pelvic mass), vascular/metabolic diseases (diabetes, chronic idiopathic peripheral polyneuoropathy, vasculitis, aneurysmal dilation), trauma (pelvic fractures, complications from surgery or radiation therapy), and idiopathic causes.[4] Nontraumatic lesions are the most common, as evidenced by one report of 86 cases revealing a neoplastic etiology in more than 50% and trauma in only 6%.[3] Patellar reflex impairment along with hip flexion, knee extension, and/or dorsiflexion weakness suggests lumbar plexopathy; whereas, ankle reflex impairment

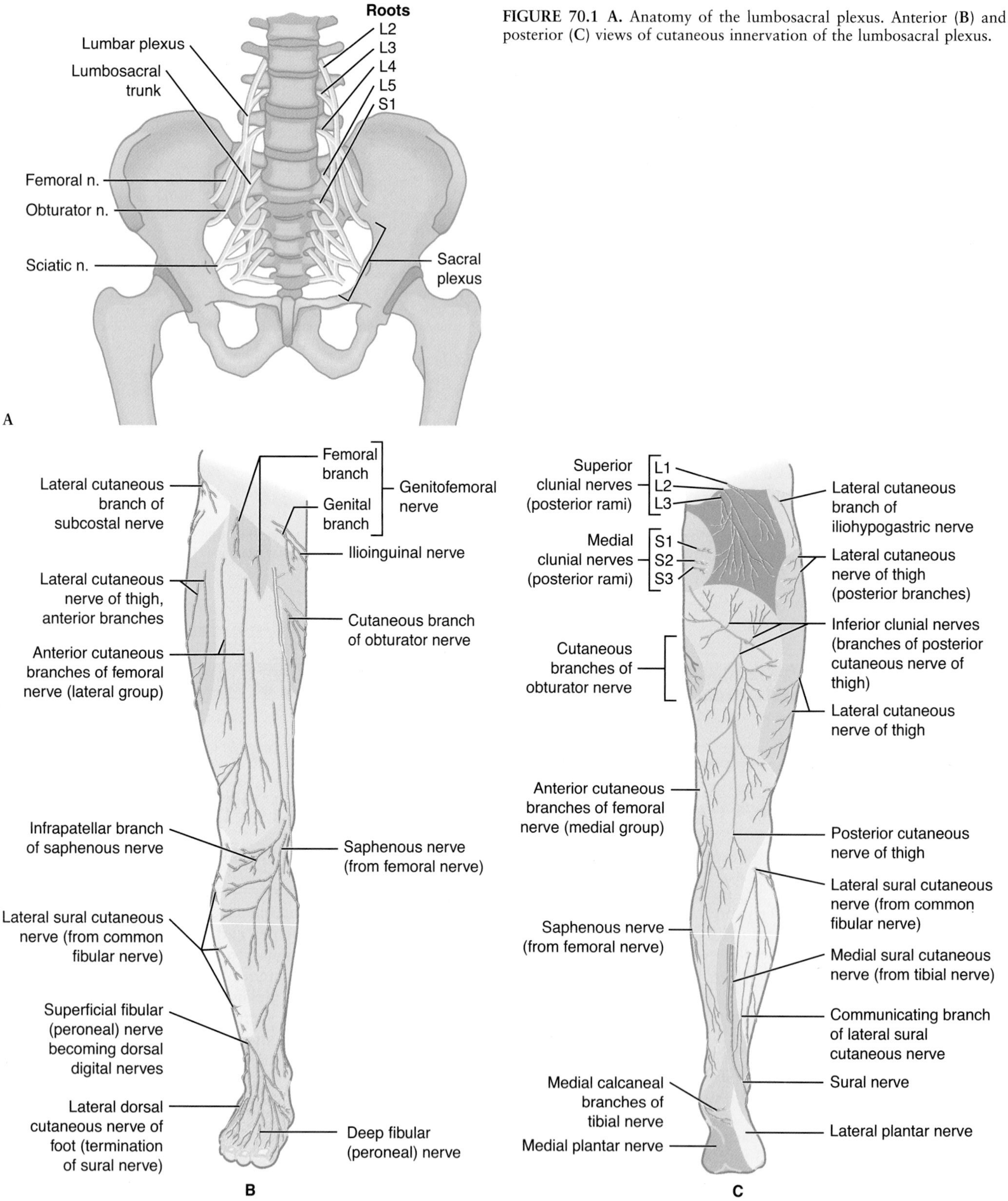

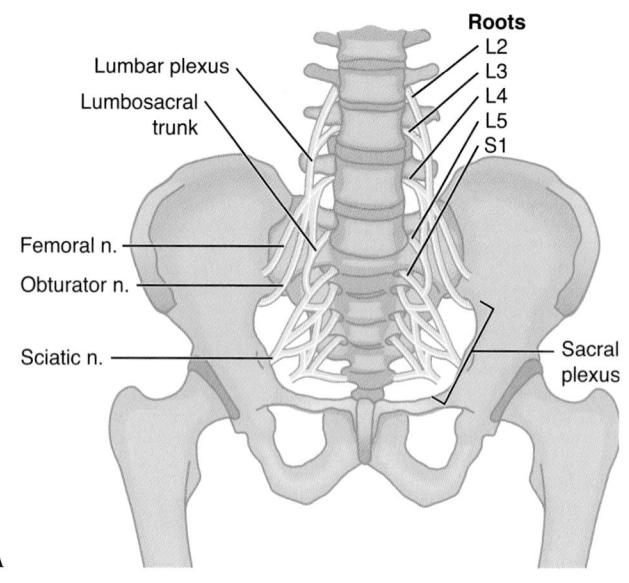

FIGURE 70.1 A. Anatomy of the lumbosacral plexus. Anterior (**B**) and posterior (**C**) views of cutaneous innervation of the lumbosacral plexus.

A (anterior pelvis diagram)

Roots
L2
L3
L4
L5
S1

Lumbar plexus
Lumbosacral trunk
Femoral n.
Obturator n.
Sciatic n.
Sacral plexus

B (anterior limb)

Lateral cutaneous branch of subcostal nerve
Lateral cutaneous nerve of thigh, anterior branches
Anterior cutaneous branches of femoral nerve (lateral group)
Infrapatellar branch of saphenous nerve
Lateral sural cutaneous nerve (from common fibular nerve)
Superficial fibular (peroneal) nerve becoming dorsal digital nerves
Lateral dorsal cutaneous nerve of foot (termination of sural nerve)
Femoral branch
Genital branch
Genitofemoral nerve
Ilioinguinal nerve
Cutaneous branch of obturator nerve
Saphenous nerve (from femoral nerve)
Deep fibular (peroneal) nerve

C (posterior limb)

Superior clunial nerves (posterior rami)
L1
L2
L3
Medial clunial nerves (posterior rami)
S1
S2
S3
Cutaneous branches of obturator nerve
Anterior cutaneous branches of femoral nerve (medial group)
Saphenous nerve (from femoral nerve)
Medial calcaneal branches of tibial nerve
Medial plantar nerve
Lateral cutaneous branch of iliohypogastric nerve
Lateral cutaneous nerve of thigh (posterior branches)
Inferior clunial nerves (branches of posterior cutaneous nerve of thigh)
Lateral cutaneous nerve of thigh
Posterior cutaneous nerve of thigh
Lateral sural cutaneous nerve (from common fibular nerve)
Medial sural cutaneous nerve (from tibial nerve)
Communicating branch of lateral sural cutaneous nerve
Sural nerve
Lateral plantar nerve

along with hip extension, knee flexion, and/or plantarflexion weakness suggests sacral plexopathy.

Depending on the cause, diagnostic workup for plexopathy can include plain film x-ray imaging, detailed neuroimaging (computed tomography [CT] and magnetic resonance imaging [MRI]), angiography, ultrasonography, electrodiagnostic studies (electromyography [EMG] and nerve conduction study [NCS]),

and laboratory studies. Diagnostic studies in isolation of the patient's medical history and physical exam findings, however, have limitations. For example, neuroimaging may not be able to differentiate between benign tumor versus malignant tumor versus radiation-induced plexopathy. Likewise, electrodiagnostic studies may not be able to differentiate between peripheral neuropathy versus plexopathy.[3] Electrodiagnostic studies, however, may be

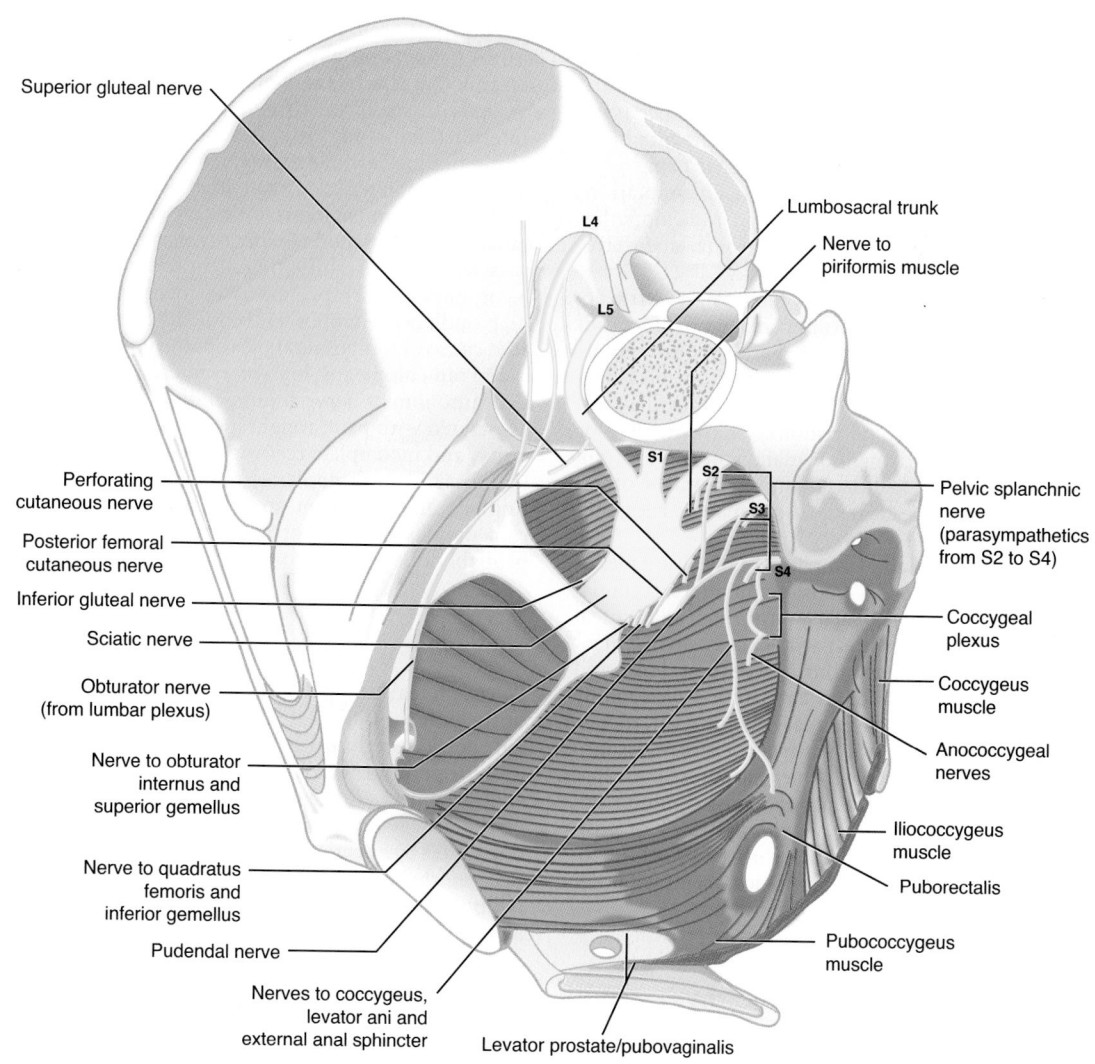

Superior gluteal nerve

L4

L5

Lumbosacral trunk

Nerve to
piriformis muscle

S1

S2

S3

S4

Pelvic splanchnic
nerve
(parasympathetics
from S2 to S4)

Perforating
cutaneous nerve

Posterior femoral
cutaneous nerve

Inferior gluteal nerve

Sciatic nerve

Obturator nerve
(from lumbar plexus)

Nerve to obturator
internus and
superior gemellus

Nerve to quadratus
femoris and
inferior gemellus

Pudendal nerve

Nerves to coccygeus,
levator ani and
external anal sphincter

Levator prostate/pubovaginalis

Coccygeal
plexus

Coccygeus
muscle

Anococcygeal
nerves

Iliococcygeus
muscle

Puborectalis

Pubococcygeus
muscle

FIGURE 70.2 Oblique sagittal view of the sacral plexus.

able to provide information on the extent of motor axon loss or on the presence of muscle denervation when clinical assessment is limited by the cause of injury.

Treatment options depend on the cause, location, severity, and duration of the plexopathy.[3] In certain situations, surgery may be the initial treatment of choice, whereas in other circumstances observation and symptom management may be the preferred approach. Conservative therapy for symptomatic relief includes medications (corticosteroids, acetaminophen, nonsteroidal anti-inflammatory drugs, anticonvulsants, tricyclic antidepressants, opioids, topical analgesics, and lidocaine patch) and injections. Spinal cord stimulation or intrathecal therapies may be considered for those who have a suboptimal response to the aforementioned and/or those who are not surgical candidates. Physical therapy is important for those with evidence of motor weakness in order to minimize muscle atrophy, prevent muscle contractures, and maintain ambulatory status. Assessment for orthotic devices (e.g., ankle-foot orthosis [AFO], etc.) and gait assistive devices (e.g., crutches, cane, walker, etc.) also may be necessary in order to prevent falls.

Neoplasms

In comparison to neoplastic involvement of the lumbosacral spinal nerves, cauda equina, or conus medullaris, lumbosacral plexus involvement is relatively uncommon and has a reported incidence of 0.71%.[5,6] Neoplastic plexopathies can involve the sacral plexus (50%), lumbar plexus (33%), or lumbosacral plexus (17%).[3,7] Most are of malignant origin, with 75% occurring by direct extension (most commonly from gastrointestinal tumors, genitourinary tumors lymphomas, sarcomas), or metastasis.[3,5] Breast cancer is the most common primary source and rarely is the diagnosis of neoplastic plexopathy made before discovery of the primary neoplasm.

Neoplastic plexus involvement portends a poor prognosis, with death often occurring within 6 months of diagnosis.[5] Insidious onset of low back pain (lumbar plexus) and/or leg pain (sacral plexus) are often the primary heralding features and can precede other neurologic symptoms.[1,3,5,7] At initial onset, unilateral leg pain is present in 90% of patients and tends to be more prominent than low back pain.[8] The pain can have both nociceptive and neuropathic features and is worse with recumbency, movement, and Valsalva maneuvers.[1] Lumbar plexus involvement is also suggested by localization of pain over the costovertebral angle, anterior abdominal wall, groin, or thigh, and by painful fixed flexion of the hip worsened by passive or active hip extension (also known as malignant psoas syndrome).[1,9,10] Within 13 months of pain onset, many patients develop additional neurologic symptoms: weakness (86%), gait dysfunction, sensory loss (73%), reflex impairment (64%), and paroxysmal or continuous paresthesias or dysesthesias.[1,3,5,6,8] Additional physical exam findings may include: (a) lower extremity edema (seen in 50%); (b) warm and dry foot (seen with sympathetic nerve involvement); (c) palpable rectal mass and perineal pain (seen in more than one third with sacral involvement); (d) incontinence and impotence (seen in 10%, usually implying extensive sacral involvement with bilateral sacral plexopathy); and (e) abdominal and pelvic pain.[1,3,6,11] The differential diagnosis, however, must also include radiation-induced plexopathy, peripheral neuropathy, radiculopathy, cauda equina syndrome, retroperitoneal hematoma, and vertebral compression fracture.[1]

In general, tumors can be classified as intrinsic or extrinsic. Intrinsic tumors can be benign (neurofibromas and plexiform lesions) or malignant (i.e., schwannoma or neurogenic sarcoma).[1] Neurofibromas, which are common in patients with neurofibromatosis type 1, are commonly seen in the paraspinal, sacral plexus, sciatic notch, and perirectal regions.[12] Patients may or may not have symptoms with benign or malignant tumors, and MRI alone may be insufficient to differentiate one from the other. Symptomatic relief with analgesic medications may be necessary until the tumor can be excised.

Extrinsic tumors are malignant. Lymphoma can cause a plexopathy due to enlarged lymph nodes (most common), extranodal disease in the muscle (e.g., psoas, iliacus, piriformis, and gluteal muscles) or subcutaneous fat, or direct sciatic nerve involvement (rare).[2] Carcinomas (colorectal, genitourinary, breast, lung, and prostate) and retroperitoneal sarcomas can cause a plexopathy by encasement of the plexus by the primary tumor itself, metastasis into the surrounding soft and bony tissue, or metastasis into the plexus itself.[1,2] Sacral chordomas, which can cause constipation, urinary frequency, and sciatica, are the most common primary malignant sacral tumors.[2] Imaging with MRI, CT or positron emission tomography-CT may help with the work-up of these extrinsic tumors. Chemotherapy, radiation therapy, and/or surgical resection of the tumor is usually indicated.

Radiation-Induced Plexopathy

Pelvic radiation therapy to treat urological cancers, gynecological cancers, and lymphomas can result in radiation-induced lumbar, sacral, or lumbosacral plexopathy. Unlike neoplastic plexopathy which is often associated with significant pain and weakness, radiation plexopathy is primarily associated with weakness, with significant pain being present in fewer than 25% of patients.[8] Weakness is noted predominantly in the distal L5-S1 innervated muscles and may be accompanied by reflex and sensory impairment, skin changes, and lymphedema; bowel or bladder disturbance is rare.[8,11] The mean duration of symptom onset is 5 years but can vary from a few months to more than three decades.[3,11] Skin changes and lymphedema are commonly seen.[8] Because of obvious therapeutic implications, neuroimaging studies are critically important in order to discriminate between tumor recurrence, radiation fibrosis, and surgical scar tissue. Electrodiagnostic studies should be included to help establish the diagnosis when neuroimaging findings are nonspecific. Characteristic electrodiagnostic findings include demyelinating conduction block and myokimia.[3] If electrodiagnostic findings are also nonspecific, the diagnosis usually needs to be confirmed by biopsy or surgical exploration. For those with only radiation-induced plexopathy, treatment is nonsurgical and involves symptom management.[3]

Diabetic and Nondiabetic Lumbosacral Radiculoplexus

Diabetic lumbosacral radiculoplexus (diabetic amyotrophy) involves microvasculitic ischemic nerve injury. It most commonly

occurs in elderly patients with chronic type 2 diabetes mellitus and does not occur in isolation of diabetic peripheral polyneuropathy.[3] Patients usually report weight loss and low back and/or leg pain that is worse at night. These symptoms are often followed by signs of weakness, atrophy, and sensory deficits involving the anterior thigh along with an absent patellar reflex. Electrodiagnostic findings include axonal loss, demyelination, and denervation changes in muscles innervated by the obturator and femoral nerves.[3] Neuroimaging is necessary to rule out other potential causes of lumbosacral plexopathy. Because the plexopathy is due to ischemic nerve injury, treatment focuses on symptom management, physical therapy, and assessment for a gait assistive device.

Nondiabetic lumbosacral radiculoplexus is an underappreciated cause of lumbosacral plexopathy. Similar to diabetic lumbosacral radiculoplexus, it involves microvasculitic (motor, sensory, and autonomic) nerve injury, initially involves the legs, and is associated with pain, weight loss, prolonged morbidity and mortality, and incomplete recovery.[13] Both nondiabetic and diabetic lumbosacral radiculoplexus also share similar electrodiagnostic findings and treatment strategies. Unlike diabetic lumbosacral radiculoplexus, it is not associated with hyperglycemia and is probably due to an autoimmune phenomenon.[13]

Abscess

Psoas, gluteal, and pelvic abscesses can present acutely or insidiously with painful fixed flexion of the hip or pain in the abdominal, pelvic, or gluteal regions. In their retrospective analysis of 23 retroperitoneal collections related to the psoas muscle, Paley et al.[14] confirmed 5 were hematomas and 18 were abscesses; and of the abscesses, 3 were caused by primary infections and the remainder by infections of spinal, renal, or gastrointestinal origin. Because their appearance on MRI and CT can be confused with lymphoma or tumor deposits, image-guided percutaneous drainage can be of diagnostic and therapeutic value.[2]

Retroperitoneal Hematoma

Retroperitoneal hematomas can occur from anticoagulant therapy, hemophilia, ruptured aortic aneurysms, idiopathically, or iatrogenically (e.g., cardiac catheterization).[2,15] The degree of neurologic deficit depends on the size of the hematoma: (a) a small hematoma compresses the intrapelvic portion of the femoral nerve within the iliacus muscle; (b) a large hematoma compresses the lumbar plexus within the psoas muscle, affecting both the obturator and femoral nerves; and (c) a widespread hematoma affects the lumbosacral plexus.[2] Signs and symptoms may include ecchymosis (flank, low back, and/or thigh) and acute or subacute onset of lower abdominal or groin pain radiating to the anterior thigh. Neuroimaging facilitates the diagnosis. Electrodiagnostic findings include axonal loss in the distribution of the femoral nerve or lumbar plexus (though involvement of the lumbosacral plexus can also occur) and EMG abnormalities in the adductor muscle.[3] Even though retroperitoneal hematomas are considered compartment syndromes, treatment is nonsurgical.[3]

Aneurysms

Aneurysms of the distal aorta, iliac arteries, intrapelvic arteries, and hypogastric arteries and arteriovenous malformations can injure the lumbosacral plexus via direct compression or ischemia from embolism of feeding vessels.[2,3] Symptoms may include low back pain with or without radicular symptoms, sensory loss, and weakness. The diagnostic work-up initially includes an abdominal and pelvic ultrasound, followed by neuroimaging and angiography. The electrodiagnostic finding includes axonal loss, but pinpointing the location is often challenging.[3] Treatment involves surgical repair of the aneurysm.

Trauma

Traumatic injuries to the lumbosacral plexus, in comparison to the brachial plexus, occur infrequently because the neural structures are (a) relatively distant to highly mobile structures and (b) well protected by muscle and bone.[3] Therefore, trauma-induced lumbosacral plexopathy typically results from penetrating or violent injuries—gunshot blast, high-speed motor vehicle or motorcycle accident, pedestrian versus motor vehicle accident, or fall from a tall height—and is often associated with pelvic bony fractures. Isolated fractures involving the nonweight-bearing anterior one third of the pelvic ring are often stable and do not result in neurovascular injury. Conversely, because the posterolateral two thirds of the pelvic ring is involved with weight bearing and lays in close proximity to neurovascular structures, fractures in this area lead to instability and neurovascular compromise.[3] Symptoms can include variable degrees of pain, sensory and reflex impairment, muscle weakness, atrophy, and gait abnormality. Treatment involves identifying the extent of neurovascular injury. Since most nerve traumatic injuries spontaneously improve (to a certain degree) and surgical repair can be technically challenging, surgery is not recommend as the initial treatment of choice.[3] Of those who do require surgery, outcomes are relatively better with repair of the lumbar instead of sacral plexus.[3] Neuropathic pain persisting beyond the anticipated healing process suggests the presence of a neuroma or scar tissue. Treatment may involve additional surgery to remove the neuroma or scar tissue, medication management, or implantation of a spinal cord or peripheral nerve stimulator.

Obstetric-Related Plexopathy

Compression of the lumbosacral plexus between the pelvic rim and fetal head can occur during the latter stages of pregnancy or during delivery (Fig. 70.3).[3] Katirji et al.[16] described seven patients with intrapartum maternal lumbosacral plexopathy who shared common features: short maternal stature, prolonged labor, pain and demyelination in an L5 nerve root distribution, foot drop, and complete resolution of symptoms within 5 months. A large fetal head or the use of forceps can also cause compression of the lumbosacral plexus. Neuroimaging may be of limited benefit when the fetus is present. Electrodiagnostic abnormalities include a demyelinating conduction block of nerves supplying the

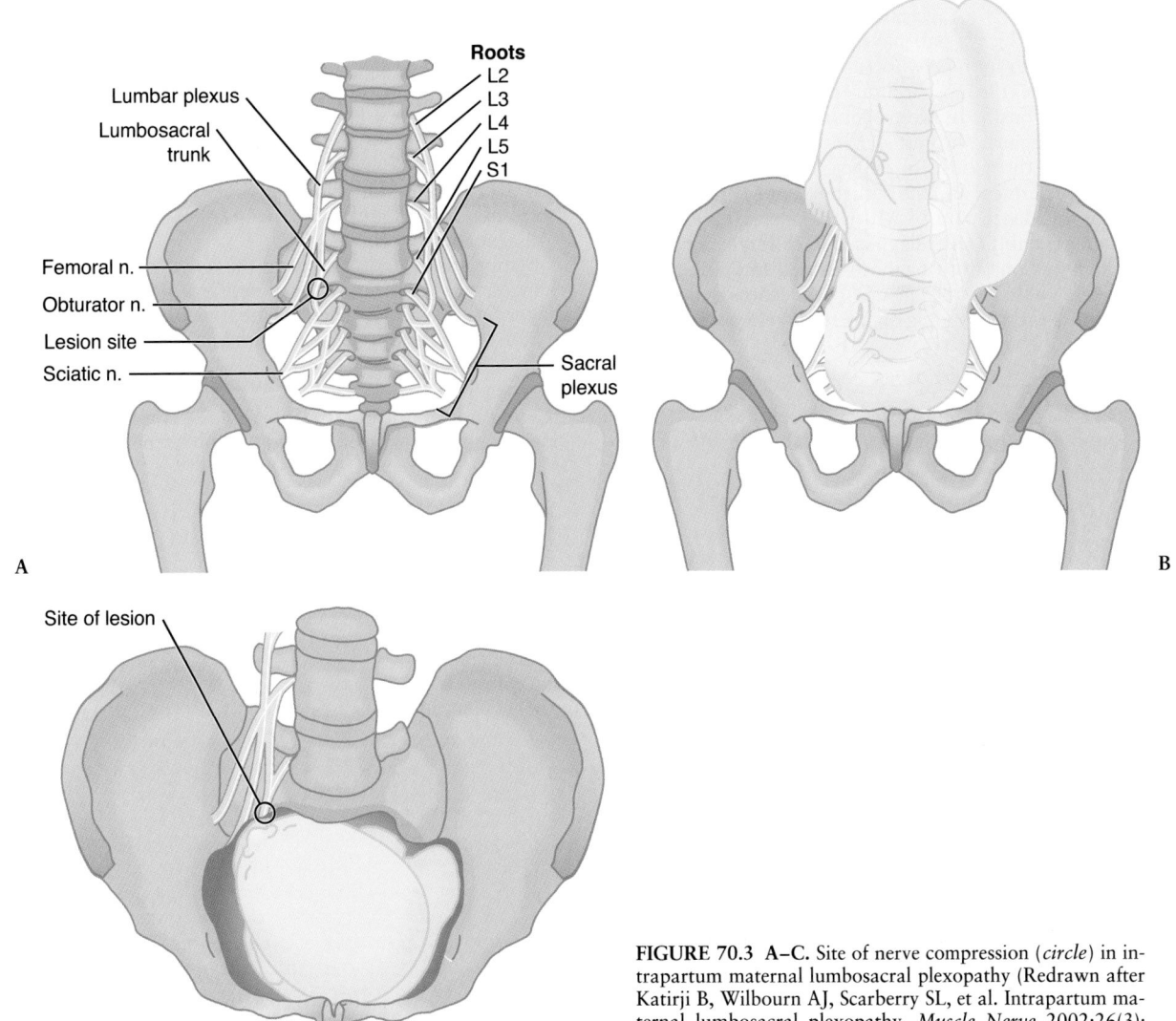

FIGURE 70.3 A–C. Site of nerve compression (*circle*) in intrapartum maternal lumbosacral plexopathy (Redrawn after Katirji B, Wilbourn AJ, Scarberry SL, et al. Intrapartum maternal lumbosacral plexopathy. *Muscle Nerve* 2002;26(3): 340–347.)

muscles of the anterolateral leg and EMG abnormalities in muscles innervated by the L5 nerve root.[3] Aside from delivery of the fetus, treatment is nonsurgical.[3]

SPECIFIC NERVE ENTRAPMENT SYNDROMES

Lateral Femoral Cutaneous Nerve Entrapment

The lateral femoral cutaneous nerve (LFCN), a purely sensory nerve, originates from the lumbar plexus and conveys fibers from posterior divisions of the ventral rami of the L2 and L3 nerve roots (Fig 70.4). Near the anterior superior iliac spine (ASIS), the LFCN divides into anterior and posterior branches and conveys sensory information from the anterolateral and lateral surfaces of the thigh, respectively. Compression of the LFCN most commonly occurs as the nerve exits the pelvis and pierces or crosses the inguinal ligament and attaches to the ASIS.[17] Entrapment of the lateral femoral cutaneous nerve (LFCN), also know as lateral femoral cutaneous neuralgia, was first characterized by Bernhard in 1878. In 1895, Roth coined the name meralgia paresthetica (MP), which is derived from the Greek words *meros* (meaning thigh) and *algos* (meaning pain).[18,19]

While MP is not rare, its exact prevalence remains unknown. It can occur at any age but is most commonly seen in patients 30 to 60 years of age.[19,20] A recent retrospective study analyzing registered patients (173,375 patient years from 1990–1998) from a computerized registration network of Dutch general practitioners probably provides the most accurate incidence of MP.[20] After looking at the relationship between comorbidity (e.g., carpal tunnel syndrome, pregnancy, hip osteoarthritis, obesity, symptoms of the pubic bone, thrombosis of the leg, diabetes mellitus, and the use of corticosteroids) and the occurrence of MP, the authors concluded the incidence rate of MP is 4.3 per 10,000 person years. Though probably underdiagnosed in children, it has been seen in as many as one third of those treated for osteoid osteoma.[19] Whether there is a true gender predilection remains unknown, as results vary depending on the study referenced.[17,20–23]

Etiology

Causes of MP have been categorized as spontaneous or iatrogenic.[21] Spontaneous causes result from entrapment due to intrapelvic (pregnancy, pelvic or abdominal tumors, uterine fibroids, degenerative pubic symphysis, diverticulitis, and appendicitis), extrapelvic (seatbelt trauma, tight garments or belts, and obesity), or mechanical (prolonged sitting, prolonged standing, and leg length discrepancy) factors; or from metabolic derangements (diabetes mellitus, hypothyroidism, alcoholism, and lead poisoning).[24,19] Rossi et al.[25] noted that obese patients (body mass index ≥30 kg/m²), but not overweight patients (body mass index 25–29.9 kg/m²),[25] showed two-fold greater risk for developing MP.[23] Interestingly, some have even reported cases of MP in patients who have lost weight.[26,27] Postulated mechanisms may include the presence of other compressive factors, lack of nutritional factors, or underlying systemic disease.[23] Iatrogenic causes of MP result from orthopaedic procedures (pelvic osteotomy, iliac crest bone graft harvest, spine surgery, and total hip replacement) and nonorthopaedic procedures (gastric bypass surgery, laparoscopic inguinal herniorrhaphy, laparoscopic cholecystectomy, laparoscopic myomectomy, coronary artery bypass grafting, aortic valve surgery, and renal transplant).[19,28]

Signs and Symptoms

While the majority of patients usually complain of unilateral sensory loss, paresthesias, or dysesthesias, the incidence of bilateral symptoms can be as high as 20%.[17] The symptoms rarely radiate proximally toward the spine.[19] Hair loss over the anterolateral thigh due to constant rubbing may be present.[19] Prolonged standing, walking, or hip extension may worsen the symptoms. Hip flexion may alleviate or worsen the symptoms. A Tinel's sign (paresthesias radiating to the anterolateral thigh) sometimes can be elicited by percussing medial to the ASIS.[23] For those patients in whom inguinal ligament LFCN entrapment is suspected, the pelvic compression test should be performed (Fig. 70.5). With the patient lying in a lateral decubitus position on the unaffected limb, the examiner maintains downward pressure on the pelvis for 45 seconds. Transient improvement of symptoms is considered a positive result. Nouraei et al.[29] showed this test had a sensitivity of 95% and a specificity of 93.3% in those with electrodiagnostically proven MP.

Symptoms extending beyond the territory of the nerve, reflex changes, muscle weakness, or muscle atrophy suggest an alternate diagnosis, such as a lumbar plexopathy, high lumbar radiculopathy, or other peripheral neuropathy.

Diagnosis

Imaging and laboratory studies should be considered when a clear cause cannot be identified: radiograph or neuroimaging of the

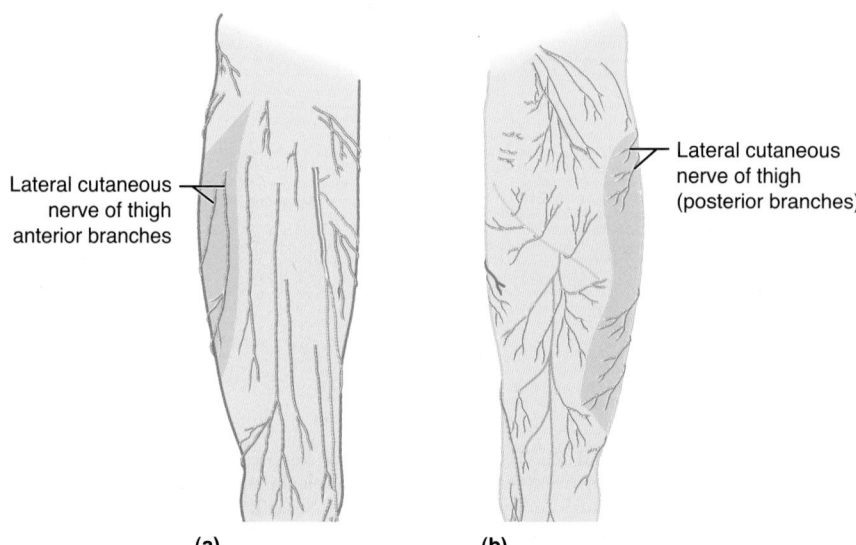

(a)   **(b)**

Lateral cutaneous nerve of thigh anterior branches

Lateral cutaneous nerve of thigh (posterior branches)

FIGURE 70.4 Cutaneous branches of the lateral femoral cutaneous nerve. Anterior (**A**) view and posterior (**B**) view.

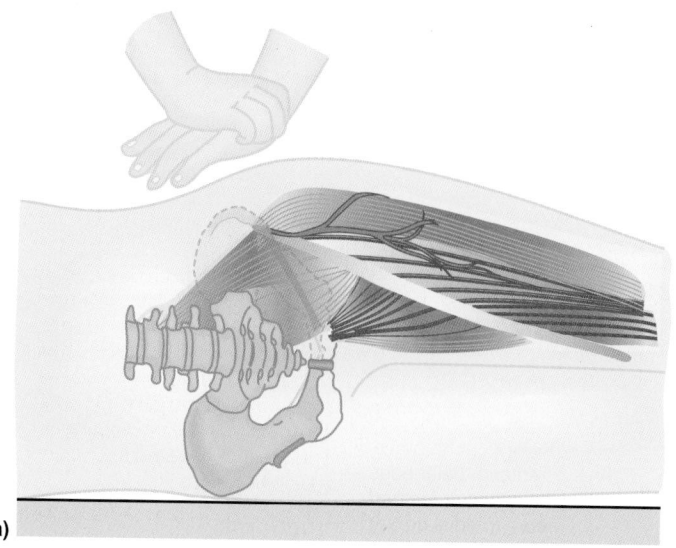
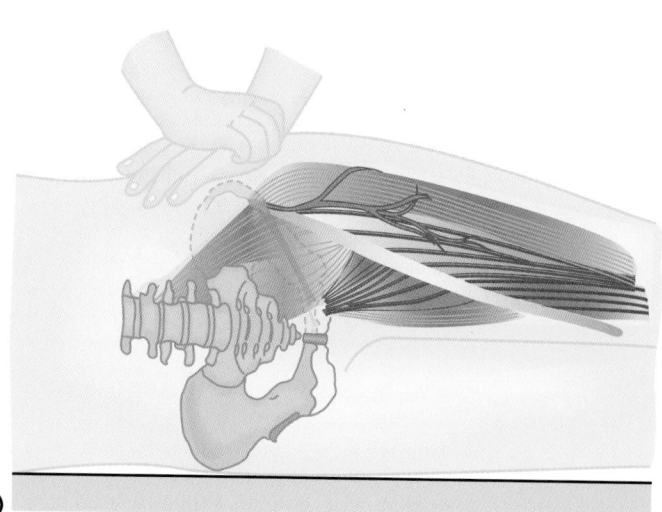

(a)   (b)

FIGURE 70.5 Pelvic compression test. Place the patient in a lateral decubitus position (**A**) and apply downward pressure on the pelvis for 45 seconds (**B**). Transient improvement of symptoms is a positive test.

pelvis to rule out pelvic tumor or fracture and neuroimaging of the lumbosacral spine to rule out disc herniation.[19] While electrodiagnostic studies can play a role in the diagnosis of MP, some argue its utility may be hampered by inherent technical difficulty, challenges in obtaining a response in obese patients, and small recordable sensory responses (absent in 71% and prolonged in 24%).[24] Furthermore, in order to obtain the best recordings one must use needle electrodes instead of surface electrodes. Others, however, claim that electrodiagnostics should play a central role in diagnosing MP. Instead of strictly looking at the absolute value of the sensory nerve action potential (SNAP) amplitude, Seror and Seror[22] demonstrated a specificity of 98.75% in their study of 120 patients when the side-to-side amplitude ratio was greater than 2.3 and the amplitude was less than 3 microvolts. Since the nerve is purely sensory, EMG testing of muscles should be normal. The value of somatosensory-evoked potentials (SSEPs) in making the diagnosis is debatable.[19] Ultimately, the greatest benefit of performing an electrodiagnostic is to rule out other entities—high lumbar radiculopathy, lumbar plexopathy, or other peripheral neuropathy—that can cause similar symptoms.

Treatment

Nonsurgical treatment for MP is typically successful, as symptoms are often mild and self-limited. In their study of 277 patients, Williams and Trzil[30] reported conservative management was successful in 91% of patients. Initial recommendations include advising patients to avoid wearing tight-fitting garments or belts, advising obese patients to lose weight, and correcting leg-length discrepancies. If symptoms persist, other treatment options include: ice, transcutaneous electrical stimulation unit, and analgesic medications and injections. Because no controlled studies have been performed, the long-term efficacy of a local anesthetic LFCN block (with or without corticosteroids) is unclear. Furthermore, whether temporary relief of symptoms alters the long-term prognosis is unknown. Using a standard treatment algorithm in 79 patients, Haim et al.[17] showed symptomatic improvement in 21 patients requiring conservative therapy and medical management, 48 patients requiring LFCN blocks using corticosteroid and local anesthetic, and 10 patients requiring surgery. At 1-year follow-up, the authors reported none of the patients had recurrence of MP symptoms.

Traditionally, the target site of injection is identified based on anatomic landmarks (1 cm medial and 1 cm inferior to the ASIS),

with a large volume of medication being injected using a fanning technique. While large volumes may increase the success rate of blocking the LFCN to obtain useful diagnostic information, it can also come at the risk of inadvertently blocking the femoral and/or obturator nerves. However, absence of immediate analgesia does not necessarily rule out the diagnosis of MP given the LCFN's anatomic variability and given failure rate of this technique being as high as 60%.[31] In a prospective, randomized, crossover study involving 20 patients, the same authors demonstrated a 100% versus 40% success rate with blocking the LFCN using a stimulating needle versus a fanning technique, respectively.[31] Use of a stimulating needle or ultrasound guidance, however, can improve the success rate of identifying the correct nerve. In their study of 10 patients, 5 of whom were obese, Hurdle et al.[32] successfully blocked the LFCN in 100%. The authors concluded that ultrasound-guided LFCN blocks offered the advantage of visualizing the adjacent structures, of using lower volumes of injectate, and of avoiding the inadvertent blockage of the femoral and/or obturator nerves.

For those who do not obtain long-term benefit from corticosteroid injections, other treatments that have been tried include cryoanalgesia of the peripheral nerve, pulsed or continuous radiofrequency (RF) of the peripheral nerve, peripheral nerve stimulation, and spinal cord stimulation. The successful outcomes reported in some of these studies need to be interpreted with caution, though, as they tend to be case reports, case series, or retrospective studies.[33–36] For those patients whose symptoms are refractory to analgesic medications, LFCN blocks, and neurostimulation, operative interventions may include surgical decompression, neurolysis, or transection of the LFCN.[30] Which of these surgical techniques is most successful remains unclear.[30,37,38] As with any neurodestructive procedure, there is a risk of nerve injury or neuroma formation.

Femoral Nerve Entrapment

The femoral nerve is a sensory (Fig. 70.6) and motor nerve and is the largest nerve of the lumbar plexus. It originates within the psoas muscle and arises from the posterior divisions of the ventral rami of the L2, L3, and L4 nerve roots (see Fig. 70.1A).[39] (The anterior divisions of the same nerve roots form the obturator nerve.) In the abdomen, the femoral nerve gives off branches to

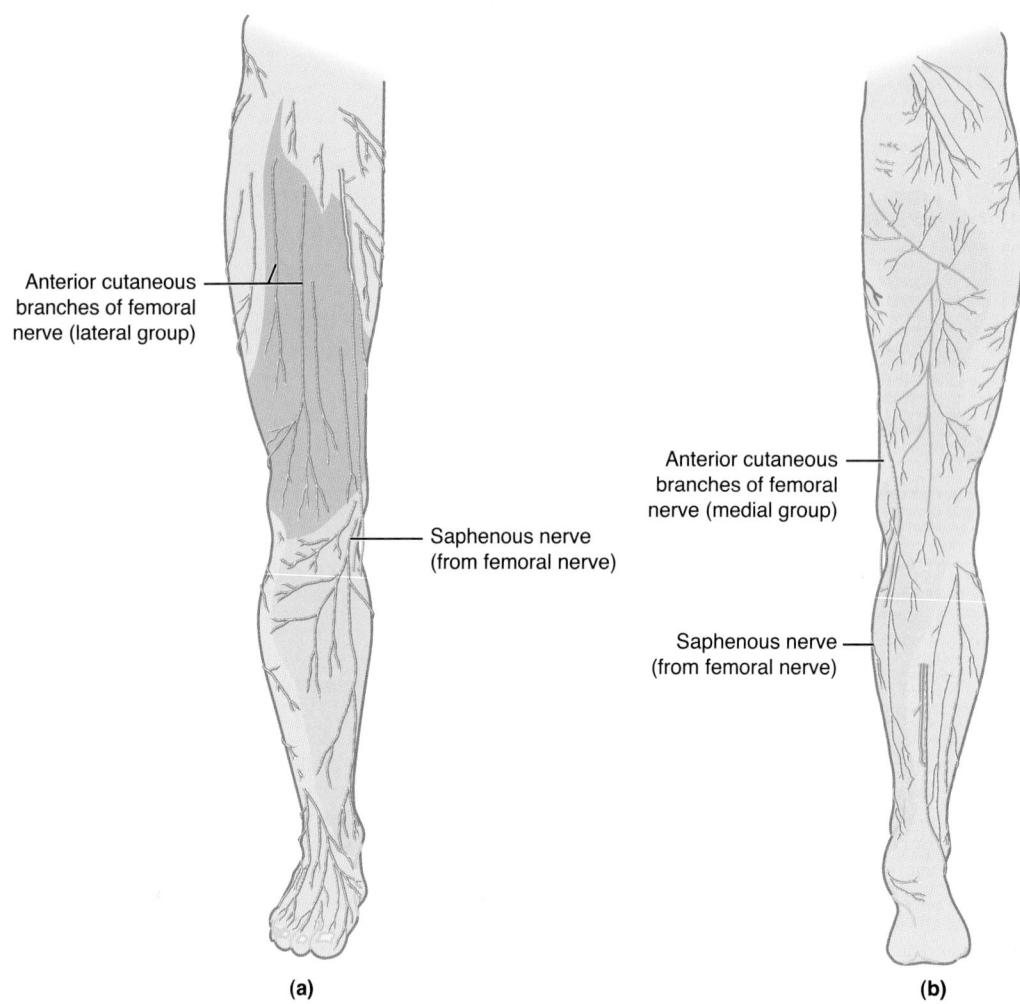

Anterior cutaneous branches of femoral nerve (lateral group)

Saphenous nerve (from femoral nerve)

Anterior cutaneous branches of femoral nerve (medial group)

Saphenous nerve (from femoral nerve)

(a)   (b)

FIGURE 70.6 Cutaneous branches of the femoral nerve. Anterior (**A**) view and posterior (**B**) view.

the iliacus and psoas muscles, and as it passes under the inguinal ligament it gives off a branch to the pectineus muscle. The nerve then enters the femoral triangle lateral to the femoral artery, and upon exiting the triangle it splits into an anterior and posterior division. The anterior division provides motor innervation to the sartorius muscle and sensory innervation (via the medial and intermediate femoral cutaneous nerves) to the anterior thigh as far distally as the knee. The posterior division provides motor innervation to the quadriceps muscles (rectus femoris, vastus lateralis, vastus intermedius, and vastus medialis) and sensory innervation (via the saphenous nerve) to the anteromedial aspect of the knee, medial calf, medial malleolus, and part of the medial arch of the foot and great toe.[39,40]

Isolated femoral neuropathy, originally known as anterior crural neuritis, was first reported in 1822 in a thesis by Descot. While most lesions are unilateral, bilateral involvement has been observed.[28] Because an isolated unilateral femoral neuropathy is uncommon, its true incidence remains unknown. Kuntzer et al.[41] reported that of 7252 electrodiagnostic examinations performed at their institution between 1988 to 1994, femoral neuropathy accounted for the diagnosis is only 32 patients (0.5%). Femoral neuropathies can cause either motor and sensory disturbances or sensory disturbances only. The latter occurs when the saphenous nerve, which is the distal sensory continuation of the femoral nerve, is involved.

Etiology

The causes of femoral neuropathy may be divided into the following categories: (a) direct nerve trauma (gunshot or knife wound, hip or pelvic fracture, hip replacement, hip prosthesis displacement, thermal energy from methylmethacrylate, inguinal herniorrhaphy, or femoral nerve block); (b) nerve ischemia due to interrupted vascularization at the intrapelvic level (common iliac artery occlusion, vascular or aortic surgery, or renal transplant with graft in the iliac fossa); (c) nerve compression (femoral artery injury in the femoral triangle, retroperitoneal hematoma, retroperitoneal mass, lithotomy positioning, prolonged hyperextension of the hip, or entrapment under the inguinal ligament with hip flexion); (d) metabolic (diabetes or pelvic radiation therapy); and (e) idiopathic.[39,41–43]

Because of a somewhat differential blood supply, the left femoral nerve is more susceptible to ischemic injury than the right.[44] The most vulnerable site of injury is located 4–6 cm above the inguinal ligament, which is where the nerve exits from the psoas muscle.[28] Because most pelvic surgical maneuvers occur proximal to the psoas muscle and out of the direct path of the nerve, neuropathy due to a compressive injury from retractors is more likely than that due to nerve transection and is independent of the type of incision (horizontal, midline, or lateral).

Most surgery-related causes of femoral neuropathy are preventable as long as retractors are used with care and positional factors are taken into account.[43] In their analysis of 32 patients with electrodiagnostically confirmed femoral neuropathy, Kuntzer et al.[41] identified an iatrogenic cause in 65% of the cases, and of these 87% were related the hip surgeries. The incidence of femoral neuropathy after total hip arthroplasty is estimated to be as high as 3%.[45] A significant number of cases of femoral neuropathy occur with gynecologic, urologic, orthopaedic, and vascular surgeries.[28,41,45] The incidence of neuropathy after abdominal hysterectomy, for example, ranges from 7% to 12%.[45] Based on their prospective study looking at femoral neuropathy subsequent to abdominal hysterectomy, Goldman et al.[46] reported the incidence of femoral neuropathy decreased from 7.45% to 0.7% when self-retaining retractors were eliminated. The compression is often indirect, as the nerve becomes entrapped between the pelvic wall and the psoas muscle upon which the retractor rests.[28] In those instances where a compressive neuropathy has occurred, direct ischemia of vasa nervorum due to deficient vascularization is the most likely mechanism of action. Urological procedures (renal transplant, radical cystectomy, transurethral resection of the bladder with exploration and biopsy of a tumor mass, percutaneous nephrolithotomy of a pelvic kidney, radical cystoprostatectomy and continent urinary diversion, and psoas hitch vesicopexy) can also be a cause of femoral nerve injury.[39] For patients undergoing renal transplant with graft in the iliac fossa, the occurrence of femoral neuropathy ranges from 0.5% to 2.2%.[28,45] Possible explanations for the cause include nerve compression combined with potential hematoma in the iliac space and prolonged vascular anastomosis or arterial clamping time.

Signs and Symptoms

Unilateral sensory loss, paresthesias, or dysesthesias in the distribution of the femoral nerve and its branches, an impaired patellar reflex, and/or hip flexion and knee extension weakness may be present. Quadriceps atrophy may be noted in chronic and severe cases. Patients with hip flexion and knee extension weakness describe frequent buckling of the knee and/or falls while ambulating.[39] Navigating stairs is often difficult, requiring patients to ascend by leading with the unaffected leg and to descend by leading with the affected leg. Kuntzer et al.[41] reported weakness and dysesthesias in 88% and 44%, respectively. Pain, if present, can be at the site of the causative lesion (iliac fossa and inguinal region) or in the distribution of the nerve itself (anterior thigh or medial calf). Inguinal pain suggests a retroperitoneal mass.[39] Pain may be exacerbated by hip extension and partially relieved with hip flexion and external rotation.[24]

Diagnosis

If femoral neuropathy is noted in the immediate postoperative period, appropriate neuroimaging and radiographic studies should be ordered to determine the cause. Because motor weakness and reflex changes can also be seen with lumbar plexopathies or radiculopathies, these diagnoses must be included in the differential. Electrodiagnostic testing can help isolate the location and extent of nerve injury. While the presence of EMG abnormalities in the vastus medialis muscle was not predictive of prognosis, the presence of NCS abnormalities, especially percentage of axonal loss, was predictive of prognosis.[47] Axonal loss, which is indicative of axonotmesis, portends a slower and possibly incomplete recovery. Kuntzer et al.[41] concluded that all patients with less than 50% axonal loss showed improvement within 1 year, whereas less than half the patients with greater than 50% axonal loss improved with conservative management alone. Furthermore, the authors found that irrespective of cause of injury, no improvement occurs after 2 years. Prognosis of recovery is greater if testing reveals only demyelinating abnormalities.[43] Abnormal EMG findings in the lumbar paraspinal muscles, however, suggest a lumbar radiculopathy or plexopathy and not a peripheral neuropathy.

Treatment

If imaging studies identify a treatable cause, then the appropriate surgery should be performed as soon as possible to minimize the extent of neurologic deficit. Based on their retrospective series (1967–2000) of 119 surgically treated patients with intrapelvic or thigh-level femoral nerve lesions (89 traumatic injuries and 30 tumors), Kim et al.[48] recommended surgery in the absence of improvement at 3 to 4 months: neurolysis if intraoperative nerve action potentials across the nerve lesion are present and resection with grafting if intraoperative nerve action potentials are absent. Though fewer patients underwent neurolysis compared to resection with grafting, the extent of recovery was greater in the former group, consistent with the severity of nerve injury. If there is no evidence of clinical or electrodiagnostic improvement after 3 to 6 months in those with iatrogenic or idiopathic femoral neuropathy, then surgical exploration with neurolysis should be considered.[43]

Assuming the femoral neuropathy is not due to traumatic injury or mass effect that necessitates surgery, recovery is typically the rule and conservative treatment is usually sufficient. The retrospective analysis, by Fanelli et al.,[49] of 2175 patients undergoing a combined sciatic-femoral nerve block showed that 45 patients (2%) experienced transient neurologic dysfunction and all but one improved within 4 to 12 weeks.[49] Extent of recovery (none, partial, or complete) and time to recovery after abdominal surgery is much more variable, the latter ranging from 2 weeks to 1 year.[43] Nonoperative treatment options include rest, analgesic medications, injections, and physical therapy. Whether temporary relief of symptoms with medications or injections alters the long-term prognosis is unknown, as the extent of recovery depends on the causative factor, extent of nerve damage, and location of injury. Longer recovery times should be anticipated when nerve damage is extensive and/or more proximal. Recovery is excellent if the etiology is due to lithotomy positioning, but is less than satisfactory when due to hip surgery or inguinal procedures.[47,50] Kuntzer et al.,[41] however, reported no association between etiology and outcome. Physical therapy is important for those with evidence of motor weakness in order to prevent muscle contractures, minimize muscle atrophy, and maintain ambulatory status. For those with significant quadriceps weakness and knee instability, orthotic and/or gait assistive devices should be considered.

Saphenous Nerve Entrapment

The saphenous nerve is the terminal sensory branch of the posterior division of the femoral nerve and is the longest cutaneous branch of the femoral nerve (Fig. 70.7). It originates near the inguinal ligament and descends within the quadriceps muscles in the subsartorial (Hunter's) canal and emerges from the canal to become subcutaneous approximately 10 cm proximal to the medial femoral condyle. The canal, which is located in the middle third of the medial thigh, also contains the femoral artery and vein. The saphenous nerve along with its two main divisions, the sartorial and infrapatellar nerves, supplies cutaneous sensation from the anteromedial aspect of the knee, medial calf, medial malleolus, and part of the medial arch of the foot.[39,40]

Etiology

Saphenous nerve injury can occur anywhere along the course of the nerve. Most saphenous neuropathies are iatrogenic or related to surgical procedures, though spontaneous neuropathies with unidentified causes can also occur.[39,51] Saphenous nerve trauma during femoral vascular surgeries and from saphenous vein harvesting for coronary artery bypass graft surgery can result in saphenous neuropathy.[52–58] After undergoing vascular reconstructions below the inguinal ligament, Adar et al.[52] reported variable

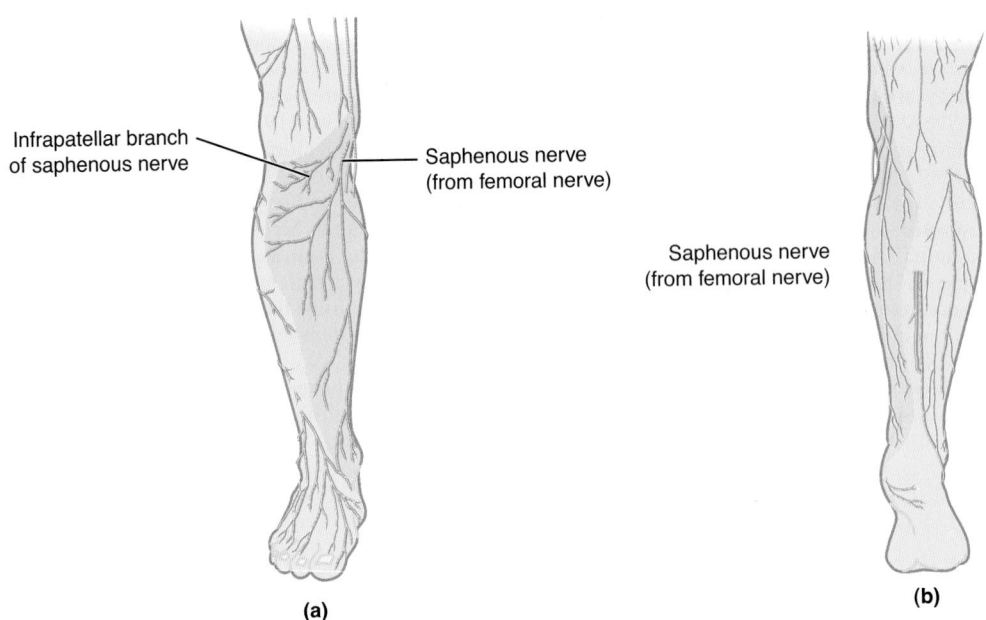

Infrapatellar branch
of saphenous nerve

Saphenous nerve
(from femoral nerve)

Saphenous nerve
(from femoral nerve)

(a)   (b)

FIGURE 70.7 Cutaneous branches of the saphenous nerve. Anterior (**A**) view and posterior (**B**) view.

degrees of saphenous neuropathy in 27 of 55 (49%) of patients, which were unrelated to surgical technical flaws. Inadvertent transection of the infrapatellar or sartorial nerves, such as during knee surgery (medial arthrotomy, medial meniscectomy, patellar realignment, total knee arthroplasty, and secondary repair for medial instability with pes transfer) can occur.[40,51,59,60] Schwabegger et al.[61] reported how a retained hemostatic clip on the infrapatellar nerve after a gracilis muscle flap resulted in neuralgia due to neuroma formation and moderate fibrosis within the subsartorial (Hunter's) canal. Resection of the neuroma resolved the pain, but sensory impairment remained. Another case report describes nerve damage resulting following a medial knee joint injection.[62]

Saphenous nerve entrapment can occur as it travels through the subsartorial (Hunter's) canal.[39,51] One case report documents distal tibial pain mimicking a tibial stress fracture from entrapment of the saphenous nerve caused by pes anserine bursitis.[63] Compression or thrombosis of the superficial femoral artery within the adductor canal can cause claudication pain in the lower leg.[56] Neural compression from the femoral vessels and adductor magnus tendons, which is more proximal to the subsartorial (Hunter's) canal, has also been reported.[64] Other case reports describe compression of the nerve due to an osteochondroma and from sitting astride and gripping a surfboard between the knees.[65,66]

Symptoms and Signs

Knee pain is the main complaint, occurring in 90% of patients in one study, and tends to be worst with walking or any exercise involving active knee extension.[52,56,66] In another study involving 15 cases of saphenous nerve entrapment, patients most commonly reported medial knee and leg pain after prolonged walking (87%) and standing (47%).[51] Additional symptoms reported by these same patients included hypoesthesia (47%), no change in sensation (47%), and hyperesthesia (6%). Point tenderness over the subsartorial canal may be elicited in some of those with a suspected entrapment neuropathy, but it is unlikely to be present in those with a traumatic nerve injury.[51,52,66] Because it is a purely sensory nerve, motor strength is unaffected. Therefore, sensory abnormalities or pain beyond the territory of the nerve, reflex changes, muscle atrophy, or muscle weakness suggests a lumbar

plexopathy, lumbar radiculopathy, or other peripheral neuropathy.

Diagnosis

Electrodiagnostic studies can be helpful, but performing a saphenous nerve conduction study can be challenging. Instead of strictly looking at the absolute value of the SNAP amplitude or latency in the affected limb, it is more important to compare the side-to-side SNAP amplitudes.[39] A SNAP amplitude of less than 50% of the unaffected limb suggests the lesion is at or distal to the dorsal root ganglion.[39] Since the nerve is purely sensory, the EMG result should be normal. The clinical utility of saphenous nerve SSEPs is low. A pelvic MRI or CT should be considered if one suspects a mass lesion in the subsartorial canal.

Treatment

Nonsurgical treatment options include rest, analgesic medications, and injections. For those with a suspected entrapment neuropathy, a saphenous nerve block (with or without corticosteroid) over the subsartorial canal can be tried. While the long-term efficacy remains unclear, the nerve block might yield a diagnostic answer. A local anesthetic saphenous nerve block provided relief in 12 of 32 (38%) cases described by Mozes et al.[67] but they did not provide lasting relief in any of the 15 cases described by Worth et al.[51] With corticosteroid added to the local anesthetic in 30 patients undergoing a series of saphenous nerve blocks, "favorable outcomes, no change and increased pain" were reported in 80%, 13%, and 7%, respectively.[56] Whether temporary relief of symptoms alters the long-term prognosis is unknown. Because ultrasound of the nerves around the knee has been described, an ultrasound-guided saphenous nerve block may improve chances of obtaining a successful block.[68] However, this has yet to be shown in a study. For those with unremitting symptoms, neurolysis or neurectomy may be indicated, though which surgical approach offers the best outcome with the fewest complications is debatable.[51,67]

Obturator Nerve Entrapment

The obturator nerve, which is a sensory and motor nerve, originates from the anterior divisions of the ventral rami of the L2,

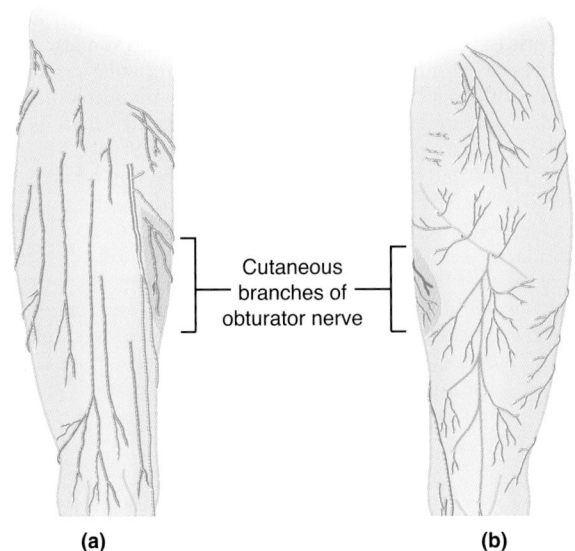

(a)   **(b)**

FIGURE 70.8 Cutaneous branches of the obturator nerve. Anterior (**A**) view and posterior (**B**) view.

L3, and L4 nerve roots (Fig. 70.8; see Fig. 70.1a). (The posterior divisions of the same nerve roots form the femoral nerve.) The obturator nerve emerges from the medial surface of the psoas major muscle at the pelvic brim and descends along the lateral pelvic wall where it passes through the fibro-osseous obturator foramen. Within the foramen, the obturator nerve splits into an anterior and posterior branch, finally emerging through the obturator foramen and entering the thigh. At the point of origin, the anterior branch supplies an articular branch to the hip joint followed by motor branches to the adductor longus and brevis, gracilis, and pectineus muscles. The sensory fibers of the anterior branch convey cutaneous information from the distal two thirds of the medial thigh. The posterior branch supplies motor branches to the obturator externus and adductor magnus muscles and sensory branches to the articular capsule, cruciate ligaments, and synovial membrane of the knee joint. A normal variant in approximately 8% to 13% of the population, the accessory obturator nerve supplies the pectineal muscles and hip joint.[69]

Etiology

An isolated obturator neuropathy is uncommon because the nerve is well-protected within the pelvis and medial thigh.[70,71] Causes of obturator neuropathy include entrapment (obturator hernia or local infection); compression (pelvic trauma, pelvic hematoma, pelvic tumor, retroperitoneal mass, fetal head or forceps in the pelvic canal during delivery, trauma or hematoma caused by cesarean section, acetabular labral cyst, extrapelvic synovial cyst, prolonged tourniquet use, or myositis ossificans); surgery (orthopaedic, gynecological, or pelvic laparoscopy); lithotomy positioning; and diabetes.[39,69–77] Of 22 patients with electrodiagnostic evidence of obturator neuropathy, Sorenson et al.[70] found perioperative complications or pelvic trauma were the most common causes. Because laparoscopic pelvic procedures could result in inadvertent electrocautery of the wrong nerve, careful visualization of the adjacent neurovascular structures should be undertaken.[39,71] The mechanism of entrapment is unclear, but Bradshaw et al.[69] concluded from their study of 32 athletes that electrodiagnostic and surgical findings (nerve entrapment by fascia and vessels over the obturator externus and adductor brevis muscles) suggest entrapment occurs at the level of the obturator foramen and proximal thigh, instead of within the obturator tunnel. Gender differences in the bony pelvic anatomy also play a

role. Higher iliac bones, a smaller transverse pelvic inlet diameter, and a narrower subpubic angle, which all contribute to a greater bend in the obturator nerve within the obturator canal, probably accounts for the higher incidence of obturator neuropathy in men.[69]

Symptoms and Signs

Symptoms of obturator neuropathy include weakness, paresthesias, sensory loss, and/or pain along the medial thigh with extension as far distally as the knee. Sorenson et al.[70] reported that patients most commonly complained of medial thigh or groin pain (73%) followed by muscle weakness (27%) and sensory impairment (27%). Unfortunately, the complaints of pain can make it challenging to differentiate whether it is due to obturator neuropathy versus a traumatic or surgical procedure. Similar to Sorenson et al.,[70] Bradshaw et al.[69] found that self-reports of numbness or paresthesia among their 32 athletes were uncommon except in those with chronic obturator neuropathy. Additional symptoms included referred pain to the ASIS, exercise-induced exacerbation of pain with radiation from the medial thigh to knee, resolution of pain with rest, exercise-induced adductor muscle weakness and spasm, and wide-based gait. Because the femoral and sciatic nerves provide partial innervation to the adductor longus and magnus, respectively, muscle weakness may be difficult to appreciate on physical exam. With chronic and severe obturator neuropathy, though, medial thigh atrophy may occur. The adductor tendon reflex may even be diminished, but since this reflex can be absent in those without neuropathy, it must be obtainable in the unaffected limb.[39] A positive Howship-Romberg's sign—pain provocation along the medial thigh to the knee with passive abduction and extension of the affected hip or passive internal rotation of the hip—suggests the diagnosis.[78] This neural tension maneuver is felt to be pathognomonic of an obturator hernia, occurring in 15% to 50% of cases.[78,79]

Diagnosis

Because motor weakness and reflex changes can also be seen with lumbar plexopathies or radiculopathies, these diagnoses must be included in the differential. When the physical exam is nonspecific, sensory and motor findings can be confirmed with electrodiagnostic testing. Sorenson et al.[70] were able to diagnose a different disorder in 15 of 38 (39%) of patients who carried a presumptive diagnosis of obturator neuropathy.[70] Radiographs of the pelvis are typically normal, unless osteitis pubis is present, and bone scans may show increased uptake in the pubic ramus on the affected side that presumably represents an inflammatory reaction that tracks along the fascia to entrap the nerve.[69] Alternatively, the periosteal changes may represent adductor insertion avulsion syndrome ("thigh splints"). If an intrapelvic or extrapelvic lesion is suspected, neuroimaging should be obtained.

Treatment

Recovery after sustaining an obturator nerve insult appears good in those with an acute neuropathy and poor in those with a chronic neuropathy. Conservative treatment measures include rest, physical therapy to stretch the groin muscles and to strengthen the adductor and pelvic muscles, soft tissue massage, and analgesic medications. Physical therapy is important for those with evidence of motor weakness in order to prevent muscle contractures, minimize muscle atrophy, and maintain ambulatory status. Among patient with acute onset neuropathy, 14 of 15 patients improved with conservative treatment or surgical exploration, whereas none of the 4 patients with chronic obturator neuropathy improved.[70] Controversy exists as to whether severity of nerve injury affects long-term prognosis. Bradshaw et al.[69] noted failure with conservative treatment in those with electrodiagnostic evidence of denervation, instead preferring definitive surgical neurolysis. Conversely, Sorenson et al.[70] found 3 of 4 patients with electrodiagnostic evidence of a complete lesion improved without surgical exploration. For those who have limited benefit with noninjection therapies, a fluoroscopically-guided obturator nerve block at the obturator foramen can be attempted.[69] Successful treatment of groin pain, medial and lateral thigh pain, and hip joint pain with continuous RF and pulsed RF of the articular branches of the obturator and femoral nerves has also been described in various case reports.[80–82] For those with persistent symptoms or severe injuries (pelvic trauma, intraoperative nerve laceration, or tumor) surgery is advocated.[39]

Sciatic Nerve Entrapment

The sciatic nerve arises from the lumbosacral plexus and is composed of the L4, L5, S1, S2, and S3 nerve roots (Fig. 70.9). It enters the lower extremity by exiting the pelvis through the sciatic notch. Variability exists, however, in the course the sciatic nerve takes as it exits the pelvis through the greater sciatic notch near the piriformis muscle. Beaton and Anson[83] found that among 1510 cadaveric extremities, in 88% the sciatic nerve exited below the piriformis muscle, in 11% the piriformis muscle was divided in two parts such that the fibular division of the sciatic nerve passed in between both parts of the piriformis muscle and the tibial division passed below the bottom-most part of the muscle, in 0.86% the fibular and tibial division of the nerve either passed above and below the muscle, respectively, and in 0.13% the entire

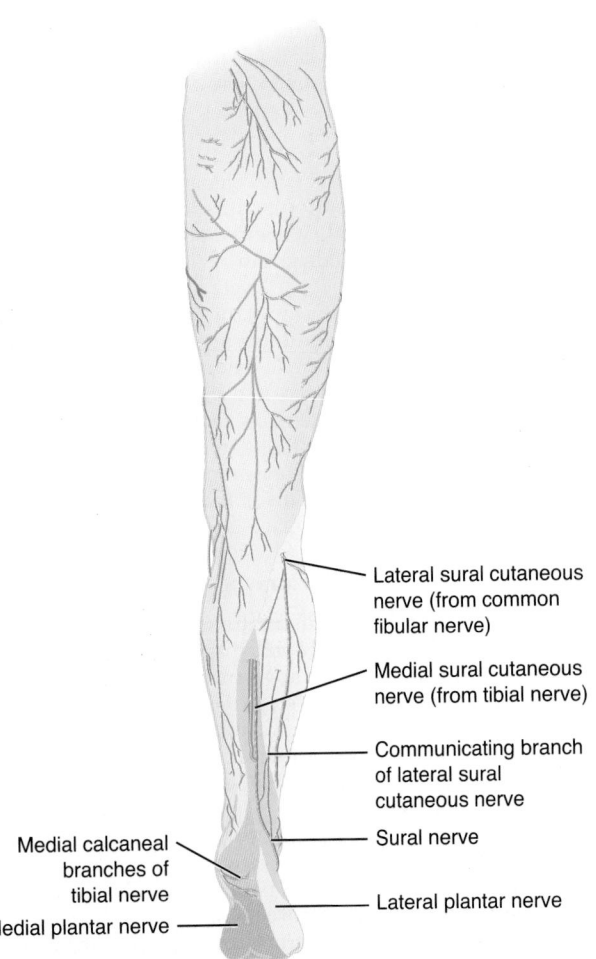

Lateral sural cutaneous nerve (from common fibular nerve)

Medial sural cutaneous nerve (from tibial nerve)

Communicating branch of lateral sural cutaneous nerve

Sural nerve

Medial calcaneal branches of tibial nerve

Lateral plantar nerve

Medial plantar nerve

FIGURE 70.9 Cutaneous branches of the sciatic nerve.

sciatic nerve pierced an undivided piriformis muscle (Fig. 70.10). The two anatomic variations where the sciatic nerve or its divisions pass in between the nerves lead to the nontraumatic variant of piriformis syndrome. Upon leaving the gluteal region, the sciatic nerve travels posterior and medial to the hip joint.

Commonly perceived of as a single nerve, the sciatic nerve is composed of lateral (fibular division) and medial (tibial division) trunks that actually lay adjacent to each other. Around the middle to distal aspect of the posterior thigh, the divisions diverge to form the common fibular and tibial nerves. Prior to diverging, the fibular division innervates the short-head of the biceps femoris muscle, with tibial nerve branches innervating the remaining hamstring (semitendinosus, semimembranosus, and long-head of the biceps femoris) muscles. With the exception of the saphenous nerve, branches of the sciatic nerve supply the sensory innervation below the knee, and branches of the sciatic nerve supply the entire motor innervation below the knee.

Etiology

After fibular neuropathy, sciatic neuropathy is the second most common lower extremity peripheral neuropathy.[84] Injury can occur anywhere along the course of the nerve from the gluteal region to the posterior thigh. Causes of sciatic neuropathy include compression (hematoma, abscess, piriformis syndrome, benign or malignant tumor, myositis ossificans, endometriosis, prolonged sitting or supine positioning without adequate pressure relief, lithotomy position, vaginal delivery due to nerve compression from the fetus's head, or pneumatic thigh tourniquet); contusion (fall from a height without fracture or dislocation); trauma (gunshot wound, laceration, femur fracture, intramuscular injection of medication into the gluteal region); stretch injury (hip arthroplasty, hip dislocation, hip or femur fracture); nerve ischemia (vasculitis, arterial thrombosis, arterial bypass surgery, diabetes mellitus, postradiation therapy); and idiopathic.[47,85–87] Based on 492 reported cases of sciatic neuropathy in the English literature from 1967–1997, Plewnia et al.[87] found that the five most common causes were: hip arthroplasty (34%), intramuscular injection of medication into the gluteal region (28%), hip fracture or dislocation (9%), benign or malignant tumor (8%), and external compression (8%).

Sciatic nerve injury is the most common neurologic complication of total hip arthroplasty—with an estimated incidence of 0.6% to 6.7% of all arthroplasties—and can be caused by stretch injury, direct trauma from retractors or fixation screws, infarction, intraneural hemorrhage, hip dislocation, thermal injury from methylmethacrylate extravasation, or compression from the prosthesis or a bony prominence.[85] In their study of 100 patients with electrodiagnostically confirmed sciatic neuropathy, Yuen et al.[84] reported that hip arthroplasty occurred in 22% and accounted for the most common cause of sciatic nerve injury. Kline et al.,[85] however, discovered that of 380 patients seen from 1967 to 1991, hip arthroplasty only accounted for a minority (3%) of cases and that injection injury from intramuscular drug administration accounted for the majority (36%) of cases. While most cases of hip arthroplasty-related sciatic neuropathy occur in the perioperative setting, delayed onset can also be seen.[88]

Sciatic nerve entrapment by the piriformis muscle, also known as piriformis syndrome, can be another cause of sciatica. Though its diagnosis remains controversial, it is reported to occur with a 6:1 female-to-male predominance.[89] It is less commonly due to sciatic nerve entrapment by the piriformis muscle, and instead is more commonly associated with direct trauma to the sciatic notch and the gluteal regions; prolonged sitting; prolonged combined hip flexion, adduction and internal rotation; and certain athletes (cyclists who ride for prolonged periods of time, tennis players who constantly internally rotate their hip with an overhead serve, and ballet dancers who constantly externally rotate their hip while dancing).[83,90–93] While the mechanism of injury may be

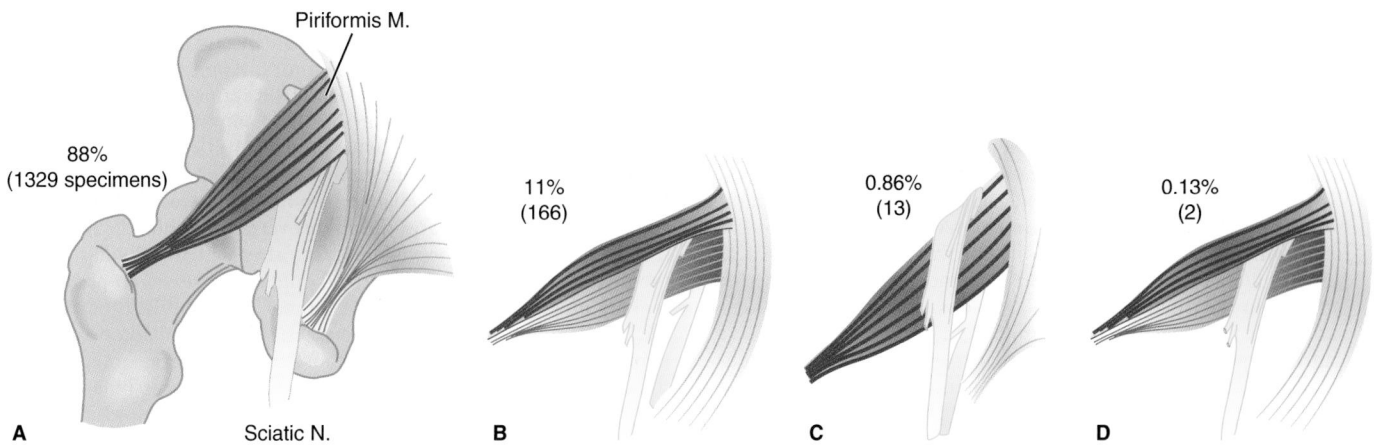

Piriformis M.

88%
(1329 specimens)

11%
(166)

0.86%
(13)

0.13%
(2)

A   Sciatic N.   B   C   D

FIGURE 70.10 A–D. Relationship of the sciatic nerve to the piriformis muscle in 1510 extremities studied.[83]

postulated, the etiology of the signs and symptoms remains less clear. Traumatic injury to the piriformis muscle may generate inflammatory and edematous changes to the muscle and surrounding fascia, subsequently compressing the sciatic nerve against the wall of the pelvis and leading to a compression neuropathy.[93] The trauma itself may induce focal hyperirritability in the piriformis muscle, which can be further exacerbated by muscle spasm or hypertrophy.

Symptoms and Signs

Signs and symptoms of sciatic neuropathy include weakness, impaired ankle reflex, paresthesias, sensory loss, and/or pain in the distribution of the nerve. Weakness of toe extension and flexion, ankle dorsiflexion and plantarflexion, and ankle eversion and inversion are the most prominent signs.[86] Clinically, absence of complete weakness of ankle dorsiflexion and plantarflexion predicts earlier or better recovery.[88] Of the two nerve trunks, weakness more commonly affects fibular- versus tibial-innervated muscles.[85,86] This is especially true in sciatic neuropathy after hip replacement.[84] While it is not entirely understood why the fibular division is more selectively injured compared to the tibial division, various reasons have been postulated: (a) superficial and lateral position, thereby placing the fibular division in closer proximity to the hip joint and exposing it to injury from hip joint trauma or surgery; (b) smaller blood supply; (c) fewer and larger fascicles; (d) less supportive endoneurium and perineurium between fascicles; and (e) relative tethering of the nerve at the sciatic notch and fibular head, thereby making it vulnerable to stretch injuries.[85,94] The exception to this rule appears to be femur fractures or gunshot wounds to the thigh, in which case the tibial division can be involved to an equal or greater extent.[84] Because of preferential fibular involvement, knee flexion weakness is commonly insignificant, and isolated injury to the fibular division can masquerade as a fibular neuropathy at the knee or fibular head.

The most common presenting symptoms with piriformis syndrome are a deep, aching buttock pain that is often associated with a limp and sitting intolerance on the affected side.[93] Squatting, climbing stairs, walking, and prolonged sitting (especially on hard surfaces) typically worsen the pain. In addition, the piriformis muscle's compression of the pudendal nerve and blood vessels may cause labial pain and dyspareunia in females and scrotal pain and impotence in males. Painful bowel movements have also been reported, presumably due to the close proximity of the piriformis muscle and the rectum.[95] The two most consistent physical exam findings are tenderness to palpation in the greater sciatic notch and reproduction of pain with maximum flexion, adduction, and internal rotation of the hip.[93] Various physical

exam maneuvers can be tried in an attempt to reproduce these findings: Freiberg's sign (buttock pain with passive, forced internal rotation of the hip), Lasègue's sign (pain and tenderness to palpation in the greater sciatic notch with the hip passively flexed to 90 degrees and the knee passively extended 180 degrees), Pace's maneuver (buttock pain with resisted abduction of the affected leg while in the seated position), and Beatty's maneuver (while laying in a lateral decubitus position on the unaffected side, buttock pain is elicited in the affected extremity when the patient actively abducts the affected hip and holds the knee several inches off the table).[89,96,97]

Diagnosis

Because the differential diagnosis can include radiculopathy, plexopathy, or fibular neuropathy, neuroimaging of the pelvis and/or lumbosacral spine may be necessary to help establish the cause of nerve damage based on the mechanism of injury. Electrodiagnostic testing can be performed to confirm the location of the lesion and to offer prognostic information based on the chronicity and severity of nerve damage. Because muscles innervated by the nerve roots are uninvolved, the lumbar paraspinal muscles are unaffected. In their retrospective analysis of 100 patients, Yuen et al.[84] noted greater severity of injury of the fibular division (64%), significant axonal loss (93%), tibialis anterior muscle EMG abnormality (92%), and low or absent extensor digitorum brevis (EDB) compound muscle action potential (CMAP) amplitude (80%). A more favorable prognosis—earlier or better recovery—was noted in those with a recordable EDB, CMAP, and presence of demyelination instead of axonal loss. Because normal sural and superficial fibular SNAP amplitudes were obtained in 29% and 9% of patients, respectively, the authors concluded that sparing of the tibial division does not necessarily exclude the diagnosis of sciatic neuropathy.

To diagnose piriformis syndrome, the symptoms and clinical exam findings must be correlated with neuroimaging of the pelvis (asymmetry of the piriformis muscle, mass effect, or anatomic variation consistent with entrapment) and electrodiagnostic studies (evidence consistent with extrapelvic compression of the sciatic nerve at the level of the piriformis muscle).[95,98,99]

Treatment

Conservative therapy for symptomatic relief includes analgesic medications, injections, and physical therapy. Physical therapy is important for those with evidence of motor weakness in order to prevent muscle contractures, minimize muscle atrophy, and maintain ambulatory status. An AFO should be considered for those with significant ankle dorsiflexion and plantarflexion weakness. Spinal cord stimulation or intrathecal therapies should be considered for those who have a suboptimal response to the aforementioned and/or those who are not surgical candidates.

Surgical treatment of sciatic neuropathy is directed at identifying the cause of nerve injury. Surgery should be considered for cases of compression due to obvious mass effect or traumatic neuropathy that fails to improve with time. Surgical exploration for trauma-induced injuries, however, requires careful deliberation. Kline et al.[85] found that medical management in those patients with a partial deficit and/or improvement in function and pain resulted in an 80% and 60% chance of useful return of function in the tibial and fibular divisions, respectively. In those patients in whom surgery (neurolysis, suture repair, or nerve graft) was performed because of evidence of a nerve action potential distal to the lesion, good-to-excellent outcomes were common for the tibial division but not so common for the fibular division. Some have suggested that the paucity of successful functional outcomes with fibular division surgeries may be related to uncoordinated muscle reinnervation (as opposed to insufficient nerve regeneration), further calling into question the practicality of fibular division surgery.[85]

If the diagnosis of piriformis syndrome is confirmed and conservative management with physical therapy and medication fails to adequately relieve symptoms, intramuscular piriformis injection of corticosteroid and local anesthetic under CT guidance, fluoroscopic guidance, or combined fluoroscopic and EMG guidance can be performed.[92,100] Because the duration of analgesia with corticosteroid can be short-lived, some have even advocated the use of botulinum toxin for prolonged analgesia in those that at least respond diagnostically to the local anesthetic.[101–103] Surgical consultation for evaluation of piriformis tendon release and sciatic neurolysis should be considered as a last resort.[93,104]

Fibular (Peroneal) Nerve Entrapment

The fibular nerve is derived from the L4, L5, S1, and S2 nerve roots as a part of the sciatic nerve (Fig. 70.11). The fibular nerve, along with the tibial nerve, is a division of the sciatic nerve. Approximately 8 cm proximal to the popliteal fossa, the fibular nerve separates from the tibial nerve and forms the common fibular nerve. As it descends into the popliteal fossa, it innervates the short head of the biceps femoris muscle. Proximal to the fibular head, the common fibular nerves gives off two branches: the sural communicating branch and the lateral cutaneous branch. The sural communicating branch becomes part of the sural nerve after receiving a branch from the tibial nerve. The lateral cutaneous branch conveys sensory information from the proximal and lateral aspect of the leg. As it winds around the fibular head, covered only by skin and a thin layer of subcutaneous tissue, the common fibular nerve is most vulnerable to injury. Approximately 1 to 2 centimeters distal to the fibular head, the common fibular nerve dives into the fibular tunnel which is made up of the aponeurosis of the soleus muscle and a wide, thick, and inflexible fibrous arch.[105] Distal to the fibular tunnel, the common fibular nerve separates into the superficial and deep fibular nerves. The superficial fibular nerve innervates the ankle everters and plantar flexors (peroneus longus and brevis muscles), after which it divides into the medial and intermediate dorsal cutaneous nerves to provide sensory innervation to most of the dorsal aspect of the foot, with the exception of the web space between the first and second toes. (Ankle inversion is unaffected because the tibial nerve innervates the tibialis posterior muscle.) The deep fibular nerve innervates the ankle and toe dorsiflexors (tibialis anterior, extensor hallucis longus, extensor digitorum longus, and peroneus tertius muscles). Distal to the ankle mortise, the deep fibular nerve gives off lateral and medial branches. The former innervates the extensor digitorum brevis and extensor hallucis brevis, and the latter supplies cutaneous sensation to the web space between the first and second toes.

Etiology

Fibular neuropathy is the most common lower extremity mononeuropathy, but its exact gender or age prevalence is unknown.[106] In a retrospective analysis looking at 5777 trauma patients, Noble et al.[107] noted 79 lower extremity peripheral nerve injuries involving the fibular,[39] sciatic,[28] tibial,[8] and femoral[4] nerves. While fibular nerve trauma most commonly occurs at the fibular head where it is superficially protected only by the skin and thin underlying fascia, injury to the fibular nerve and its branches can occur anywhere along the course of the nerve. Aprile et al.[106] demonstrated that most (83%) causes of fibular neuropathy are identifiable, with the majority (31%) being due to perioperative issues. Various causes of fibular nerve injury include entrapment, compression (improperly applied casts or braces, tight stockings, vascular abnormality, osteophytes, and intraneural or extraneural tumor); traction (leg-crossing, prolonged squatting or kneeling, prolonged ankle plantarflexion, surgical positioning, high-heeled shoes,); trauma (fracture of the proximal fibular head, knee dislocation, ankle sprain or fracture, nerve laceration, and gunshot injury); metabolic (rapid weight loss, hyperthyroidism, diabetes mellitus, vasculitic disorders, and leprosy); surgery (orthopaedic surgery, vascular surgery, and plastic surgery); or idiopathic.[24,105,107–122] In their study of 146 fibular nerve injuries requiring surgery, Piton et al.[123] classified the causes as: fibular tunnel syndrome,[62] external compression,[16] trauma,[33] iatrogenic injury,[16] tumor,[9] wound injury,[7] contusion[2] and burn injury.[1] In a larger and more recent study involving 318 fibular nerve injuries requiring surgery, Kim et al.[124] classified the causes as: stretch or contusion without fracture or dislocation,[125] tumor,[40] laceration,[39] entrapment,[30] stretch or contusion with fracture or dislocation,[22] external compression,[21] iatrogenic,[13] and gun shot.[12] Looking at 60 patients who only had entrapment, Fabre et al.[105] classified the causes as idiopathic,[53] postural,[5] and dynamic.[2] True entrapment can be classified as postural (which is associated with kneeling, crouching, squatting, or ankle plantarflexion) or dynamic (which is associated with activities such as running).[24,126–128] For those with entrapment, it is postulated that chronic nerve irritation within the fibrous arch of the fibular tunnel causes edema, which subsequently causes scar tissue formation as the nerve glides in the narrow tunnel during knee flexion and extension.[105]

Superficial fibular nerve entrapment is relatively uncommon and usually is due to compression of the nerve as it exits the anterolateral compartment 10 cm proximal to the ankle.[129–131] While deep fibular nerve entrapment can occur anywhere along

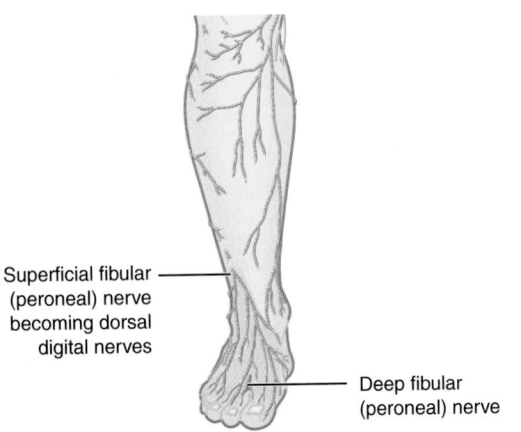

Superficial fibular (peroneal) nerve becoming dorsal digital nerves

Deep fibular (peroneal) nerve

FIGURE 70.11 Cutaneous branches of the fibular nerve.

its course, it is known as "anterior tarsal tunnel syndrome" when it becomes compressed beneath the inferior extensor retinaculum.[131–133] Postural causes of deep fibular entrapment include prolonged plantarflexion, such as with wearing high-heeled shoes.[24]

Symptoms and Signs

Symptoms of fibular neuropathy may include weakness, paresthesias, sensory loss, and/or pain in the distribution of the fibular nerve and its various branches. Patients with dynamic entrapment report activity-related leg pain with or without sensory impairment.[24] The degree and extent of neuromuscular deficit and atrophy depends on the location (common versus superficial versus deep fibular), severity, and chronicity of nerve injury. Common fibular injury typically causes dorsiflexion (ankle and toes) and eversion (ankle) weakness, leading to tripping due to dragging of toes, excessive hip and knee flexion in an attempt to clear the foot (steppage gait), and foot slap.[131] When the injury is proximal to the knee, knee flexion weakness also occurs because the biceps femoris muscle is affected. A positive Tinel's sign at the fibular head, 10 cm proximal to the ankle, or over the dorsal aspect of the ankle suggests a common fibular, superficial fibular, or deep fibular neuropathy, respectively. Fabre et al.[105] noted a positive Tinel's sign at the fibular head in 60 of the 62 (97%) cases of common fibular entrapment.[105] Sensory abnormalities, motor weakness, or pain beyond the territory of the nerve suggest an alternate diagnosis, such as a lumbar plexopathy, a lumbar radiculopathy, or other peripheral neuropathy.

Diagnosis

Electrodiagnostic studies can be performed to confirm the diagnosis, location, and extent of fibular neuropathy. Without axonal loss, the NCS reveals slowing of the nerve conduction velocity. However, when long-standing compression or direct nerve injury results in axonal loss, a decreased SNAP amplitude, a decreased compound muscle action potential amplitude, and a conduction block can be seen on NCS. The EMG portion of the study not only helps confirm axonal loss, but the extent of muscle involvement can aid in determining whether the lesion involves the common fibular, superficial fibular, or deep fibular nerve. For those with exercise-induced (dynamic) fibular neuropathy, electrodiagnostic studies may need to be done before and after exercising.[24] Once a fibular neuropathy has been confirmed electrodiagnostically, additional imaging (radiograph, CT, and MRI) or laboratory studies may be needed to isolate the cause of nerve injury.

Treatment

Nonsurgical treatment options include rest, modification of footwear or garments, analgesic medications, injections, and physical therapy. Physical therapy is important for those with evidence of motor weakness in order to prevent muscle contractures, minimize muscle atrophy, and maintain ambulatory status. Whether temporary relief of symptoms with medications or injections alters the long-term prognosis is unknown, as the extent of recovery depends on the causative factor, extent of nerve damage, and location of injury. The degree of pain relief after doing a fibular nerve block at the fibular head can provide diagnostic information. Significant fibular nerve damage resulting in ankle and foot weakness may necessitate an AFO and customized orthopaedic shoes to correct any gait disturbance.

Depending on the etiology of fibular nerve injury, surgery is advocated within 2 to 4 months if there is lack of clinical and electrophysiologic improvement.[105,123,124] In their retrospective analysis of 318 patients with preoperatively confirmed EMG evidence of knee-level common fibular nerve lesions, Kim et al.[124] reported recovery of useful function in 88% and 84% of those undergoing neurolysis and end-to-end suture repair, respectively;

recovery of useful function in 75%, 38%, and 16% for those requiring nerve grafting less than 6 cm, 6 to 12 cm, and 13 to 24 cm, respectively; and preservation of preoperative clinical function in 80% of those requiring tumor resection. For patients with idiopathic entrapment, Fabre et al.[105] advocated operative decompression if symptoms fail to resolve within 3 to 4 months because they found the surgery was safe and the time needed for recovery was shorter than that associated with conservative management.

FOOT PAIN

Pes Planus

Etiology

Pes planus, a condition also known as flatfoot, refers to the loss of the normal longitudinal arch of the medial foot (Fig. 70.12). The most common cause of pes planus is insufficiency or dysfunction of the posterior tibial tendon.[134] Congenital flatfoot is used to describe a flatfoot present since birth. Trauma, such as Lisfranc joint injuries and calcaneal fractures, can also lead to pes planus due to joint subluxation. Degenerative changes secondary to arthritis can also lead to pes planus. Tarsal coalition—a congenital fibrous union or fusion between the bones of the hindfoot and midfoot—has also been implicated as a cause of flatfoot.[135]

Symptoms and Signs

Symptoms of pes planus can vary among patients with different forms of anatomic pathology and biomechanics leading to the condition. Examination of the feet should begin with the patient in standing position. Typically, the longitudinal arch flattens upon standing and appears when the foot is not bearing weight. Heel eversion often accompanies pes planus. Severe pes planus may result in significant pain, particularly along the course of the posterior tibial tendon, which may be tender upon palpation.[136]

Diagnosis and Treatment

Radiographic imaging should be performed of the foot and ankle in three weight-bearing views—anteroposterior, oblique, and lateral. Loss of the longitudinal arch is best visualized on the weight-bearing lateral radiographs.[137] MRI can also be useful in assessing this condition, particularly in evaluation of the posterior tibial tendon. Treatment is often conservative through the use of arch supports and plantar inserts. Surgical treatment may involve posterior tibial advancement, subtalar fusion, or osteotomies, depending on the initial cause of the condition.

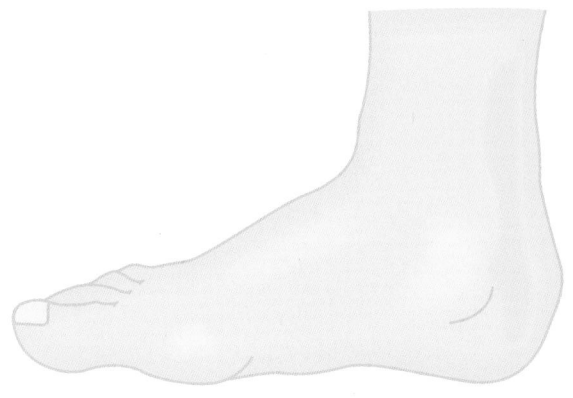

FIGURE 70.12 Pes planus.

Pes Cavus

Etiology

Cavus foot deformity is an abnormal elevation of the longitudinal arch (Fig. 70.13). This results in increased stress forces on the metatarsal heads and decreased weight bearing by the plantar region of the foot.[138] Causes of pes cavus include neuromuscular disease (such as muscular dystrophy, cerebral palsy, and spinal tumors), residual clubfoot, malunion of calcaneal or talar fractures, and burns.[138]

Symptoms and Signs

Symptomatology varies based on the extent of the deformity. Lateral foot pain can develop as a result of increased weight bearing by the lateral foot. Metatarsalgia is frequently associated with pes cavus. Intractable plantar keratosis is often seen as well. Clawing of the toes—hyperextension at the metatarsophalangeal joints and flexion of the proximal and distal interphalangeal joints—may also be present.[138] Patients may experience generalized stiffness of the joint, leading to disuse of the affected foot.

Diagnosis and Treatment

Physical examination should elucidate if the deformity is flexible or rigid. This can be determined by performance of the Coleman block test.[137] A 1-inch wood block is placed beneath the heel and lateral foot while the first, second, and third metatarsals are allowed to hang freely into plantarflexion and pronation. If heel varus corrects in this stance, the deformity is flexible. If the hindfoot does not correct, the deformity is rigid. Weight-bearing radiographs of the ankle and foot aid in the diagnosis through demonstration of hindfoot varus. MRI of the spine may be necessary to evaluate for possible spinal tumor presence if the deformity is unilateral and no inciting traumatic event is noted. In addition, neurologic consultation, electromyography, and NCS can be obtained to evaluate for polio, Charcot-Marie-Tooth disease, and other neurologic causes of pes cavus. Conservative therapy for pes cavus includes the use of orthotic shoe inserts to offset increased weight-bearing forces on the metatarsal heads. Surgical intervention is warranted if the condition is severe and is aimed at construction of a plantigrade foot. This may be accomplished through tendon transfers, osteotomies, and arthrodesis.[137]

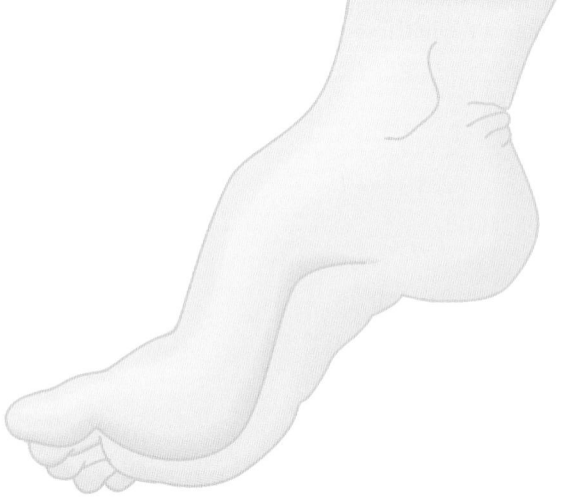

FIGURE 70.13 Pes cavus.

Plantar Fasciitis

Etiology

Plantar fasciitis is a painful inflammatory condition involving the insertion of the plantar fascia on the medial process of the calcaneal tuberosity. Pes planus, pes cavus, leg-length discrepancy, overpronation, and running all involve increased stress forces placed on the plantar fascia, and thus can lead to plantar fasciitis.[139]

Symptoms and Signs

Patients typically complain of intense sharp heel pain after the first few steps in the morning or after a period of rest. The pain is usually located along the anterior portion of the heel, with radiation into the sole of the foot.[140] The pain is exacerbated by weight-bearing activities and relieved by rest. Patients may also experience generalized stiffness of the foot and swelling of the heel.

Diagnosis and Treatment

Pain can be reproduced on palpation of the anteromedial aspect of the calcaneus as well as the proximal plantar fascia. Passive dorsiflexion of the toes and toe-walking can also reproduce pain secondary to plantar fasciitis.[140] Radiographic imaging can reveal soft tissue calcifications in the heel and may be more useful to investigate for bony tumor or fractures as an underlying cause. Ultrasound may reveal a thicker heel aponeurosis, which can be associated with plantar fasciitis. MRI can demonstrate thickening of the plantar fascia. Because of the poor sensitivity and specificity of these imaging techniques, diagnosis of plantar fasciitis is usually made through the history and physical examination. Conservative treatment involves the use of medial arch support inserts in footwear, as well as stretching exercises focusing on the plantar fascia, ice therapy, and NSAIDs.[140] Night splints can be worn to allow the plantar fascia to heal in an elongated position as opposed to the natural plantarflexed position of the foot during sleep.[141] Extracorporeal shock wave therapy for plantar fasciitis may be beneficial, but limited evidence supports it use. Case reports have demonstrated that corticosteroid injections and botulinum toxin injections can also be useful in treating plantar fasciitis. Injection of either substance is performed with a medial or lateral approach into the site of maximal tenderness. Complications include plantar fascia rupture and corticosteroid-induced fat pad atrophy.[125] Surgical release of the plantar fascia may be indicated when these treatment modalities are unsuccessful.

Heel Pad Deficiency

Etiology

The fat pad of the heel is made of individual fibrous septa containing fat and elastic fibrous tissue. The fat pad absorbs shock and distributes mechanical forces to the calcaneus. The fat pad atrophies with age, multiple glucocorticoid injections, and trauma.[142]

Symptoms and Signs

Patients typically experience deep, diffuse plantar heel pain that is exacerbated upon standing and walking/running on hard surfaces. Direct palpation of this area reproduces this pain. There is palpable atrophy of the heel pad and underlying bone may be palpated. Scar tissue and calcification can be observed.

Diagnosis and Treatment

Diagnosis is usually made through history and physical examination. NSAIDs can provide significant analgesia. Long-acting local anesthetics, such as bupivacaine, can be infiltrated into the affected area for severe, painful crises. Corticosteroids are contraindicated, as they can worsen the condition.[125] Shock-absorbing footwear inserts can be helpful by providing cushion and absorbing shock.

Tarsal Tunnel Syndrome

Anatomy

The tarsal tunnel is bounded by the flexor retinaculum, a strong fibrous band that extends from the medial malleolus to the margin of the calcaneus, and the medial surfaces of both the calcaneus and talus.[143] The posterior tibial nerve courses beneath the flexor retinaculum through this tunnel and divides into the medial and lateral plantar nerves, which innervate the small muscles of the foot and the skin on the plantar aspect of the foot and toes (Fig. 70.14).

Etiology

Compression of the posterior tibial nerve as it passes behind the medial malleolus in the tarsal tunnel may lead to tarsal tunnel syndrome, a painful condition of the ankle and plantar aspect of the foot. The branches of the posterior tibial nerve are vulnerable to compressive injury (restrictive footwear), entrapment from space-occupying lesions (i.e., ganglion cysts, osteophytes, and tumors), direct trauma, overuse injuries, and inflammation within the tarsal tunnel.[144] Hindfoot valgus deformities can further exacerbate tarsal tunnel syndrome symptoms due to increased neural tension that is secondary to an increase in eversion and dorsiflexion foot positioning. All of these conditions can lead to edema and scar tissue formation, which further limit the vascular supply and cause increased traction of the nerve between joint movements. This ultimately can result in axonal and Wallerian degeneration.

Symptoms and Signs

Pain or paresthesias in the heel, medial malleolus, or plantar surface of the foot may occur, depending on which nerve branch is compressed and the severity of the compression. When both plantar nerves are affected, symptoms extend from the posterior malleolus to the plantar aspect of the foot and dorsal surfaces of the distal aspect of the toes. Pain can be experienced in both the standing and reclining positions and may be worse at night.[143] Simultaneous dorsiflexion and eversion of the ankle exacerbates the pain due to increased nerve tension. Advanced disease leads to weakness of the intrinsic muscles of the foot and of the toe plantar flexor muscles. Physical examination typically reveals tenderness to palpation of the tibial nerve. Percussion at the medial malleolus (Tinel's sign) causes radiation of pain and paresthesias along the path of the posterior tibial nerve and its branches.[143] In addition, symptoms may be reproduced through continuous compression of the nerve for 30 seconds (Phalen's sign).[143] Sensory deficits are uncommon, but can affect the sole of the foot if present.

Diagnosis

Electromyography and nerve conduction velocity studies often reveal prolonged motor terminal latency of the medial or plantar nerves to the abductor hallucis and abductor digiti quinti muscles. In addition, they display abnormalities in sensory nerve conduction including absent nerve potentials or slow nerve conduction velocity.[145] While electrodiagnostic testing can aid in the diagnosis of tibial neuropathy, neuroimaging may still be necessary to demonstrate whether a space-occupying lesion within the tarsal tunnel is the source of the symptoms.[146] MRI demonstrates the anatomy of the tarsal tunnel and its contents and can prove useful in planning for surgical decompression.

Treatment

Nonsurgical treatment options include rest, medications (corticosteroids, acetaminophen [APAP], NSAIDs, antiseizure medications, opioids, tricyclic antidepressants, topical analgesics, lidocaine patch), injections, and physical therapy. Initial treatment includes nonsurgical measures such as avoidance of exacerbating activities, medications (corticosteroids, APAP, NSAIDs, antiseizure medications, opioids, tricyclic antidepressants, topical analgesics, lidocaine patch), TENS, physical therapy, shoe inserts, and utilization of night splints with the foot in plantarflexion. An injection of local anesthetic and steroid into the tarsal tunnel may provide analgesia.[145] Surgical decompression with release of the flexor retinaculum is employed if nonoperative measures fail. If present, space-occupying lesions of the tarsal tunnel, such as varicose veins and ganglions, are removed along with release of the flexor retinaculum. Decompression may also be accomplished through division of the proximal ridge of the abductor hallucis.[144]

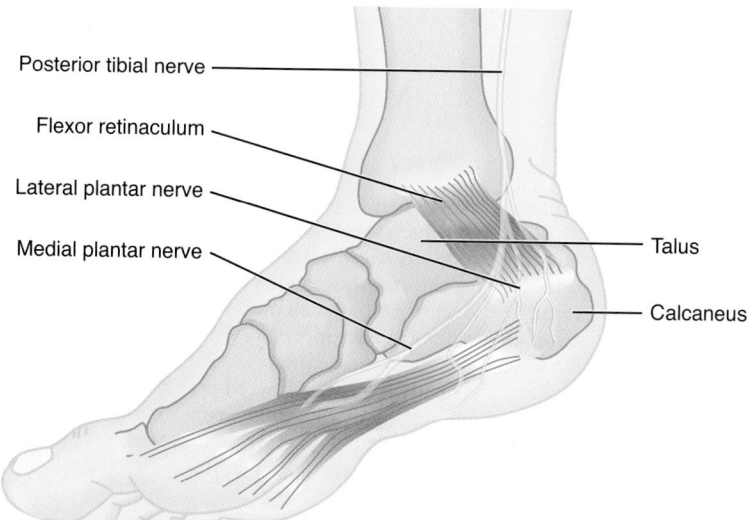

Posterior tibial nerve

Flexor retinaculum

Lateral plantar nerve

Medial plantar nerve

Talus

Calcaneus

FIGURE 70.14 Anatomy of the tarsal tunnel and posterior tibial nerve.

Surgical complications primarily involve incomplete release of the flexor retinaculum, resulting in persistent pain.[144]

Lisfranc's Joint Instability

Etiology

The Lisfranc joint (tarsometatarsal joint or metatarsal cuneiform joint) is a six-bone complex that connects the forefoot and the midfoot. It is made up of the articulation of the bases of the first three metatarsals with the cuneiforms and the fourth and fifth metatarsals with the cuboid. The joint aids in pronation and supination of the foot.[147] The great majority of Lisfranc joint injuries are associated with fractures, especially the metatarsals. While injury to the joint is generally associated with high-energy mechanisms (e.g., falls or motor vehicle collisions), resulting in severe inversion or plantarflexion, low impact mechanisms (e.g., direct trauma in sports-related injuries) are also known to cause injury.[148] The Lisfranc injury may be classified by the direction of the dislocation.

Symptoms and Signs

Lisfranc's joint instability is characterized by severe midfoot pain and the inability to bear weight. Point tenderness over the midfoot is noted on exam. Bruising on the plantar surface of the midfoot represents an occult sign of an injury. Depending on the mechanism of injury, there may be soft-tissue damage, such as edema, a wound, or vascular impairment. Pain or edema that persists after soft tissue healing is expected to have occurred should raise the index of suspicion for a Lisfranc joint injury.[148]

Diagnosis and Treatment

Radiographs will reveal fractures of the joint and displacement of the metatarsals. Because sprains are more difficult to detect, weight-bearing plain radiographs and stress radiographs taken with the foot plantarflexed and inverted have been suggested to establish the diagnosis.[149] Recently, CT scanning is becoming the imaging modality of choice in diagnosing Lisfranc injuries.[150]

Treatment depends on the type and severity of the injury, as well as the length of time between injury and diagnosis. Ligamentous injury can benefit from casting or a fitted boot. If these conservative treatments fail, surgical open reduction or joint fusion may be required.

Posterior Tibial Tendon Insufficiency

Etiology

Posterior tibial tendon insufficiency is the most common cause of acquired adult flatfoot deformity.[151] Flatfoot deformities result from flattening of the medial longitudinal arch of the foot with failing of the supporting soft tissue structures of the ankle and hindfoot. The posterior tibial tendon is the principle supporting mechanism of this arch, though ligament involvement is extensive.[134] Dysfunction of the posterior tibial tendon leads to the collapse of the arch and the formation of a pes planovalgus deformity. Arthritis may develop secondary to the foot deformity. Insufficiency of the posterior tibial tendon may result from a variety of insults, including trauma and arthritic damage. Patients are most often middle-aged females and are often obese.[152]

Symptoms and Signs

Initially, patients report pain along the medial aspect of the foot and ankle due to stretching of medial ligaments and soft tissues. On physical exam, erythema, edema, and tenderness to palpation along the course of the posterior tibial tendon can be appreciated. Later, as the arch begins to collapse, the ankle starts to roll inward, resulting in pain along the lateral aspect of the foot.[152] There may be difficulty in performing a single leg heel rise. Persistent dull aching pain due to destruction of the midfoot may culminate in difficulty with standing and ambulation.

Diagnosis and Treatment

Radiographic imaging should include weight-bearing anteroposterior and lateral radiographs of the foot to evaluate the biomechanical relationships and detect secondary arthritic changes.[152] MRI is utilized to assess the integrity of the posterior tibial tendon.

Initial treatment is supportive and involves immobilization, analgesic medications, and orthotic devices to correct pronation. Steroid injections have not been proven to be efficacious and remain controversial. When supportive measures fail, treatment consists of surgical augmentation of the posterior tibial tendon, alone, or in combination with osteotomy or arthrodesis.[152]

Ganglion

Etiology

Ganglions are mucin-filled cysts that typically arise from a joint or tendon sheath. Although the etiology is uncertain, it may represent degenerative changes or reaction to inflammation or trauma.[153]

Symptoms and Signs

Ganglion cysts are generally asymptomatic. However, pain can occur as a result of inflammatory pressure points created while walking or from wearing tight-fitting footwear.

Diagnosis and Treatment

Ganglions are commonly found along the anterolateral aspect of the ankle and are usually solitary and less than 2 cm in diameter.[154] Upon palpation, they are firm and well-circumscribed. Nonsurgical treatment options include fine needle aspiration or injection of corticosteroids into the ganglion.[154] When these measures fail, surgical excision of the cyst and stalk from its origin on the ligament or joint capsule and capsular excision should be performed. The most common surgical complication is ganglion recurrence.[154]

Metatarsalgia

Etiology

Metatarsalgia refers to pain involving one or more of the metatarsal heads and distal metatarsal shafts, secondary to chronically elevated stress forces as the total body weight is transferred to the forefoot during the mid-stance and push-off phases of walking and running.[155] Abnormal biomechanics resulting from excessive pronation, cavus deformities, foot surgeries (e.g., osteotomies), and high-heeled shoes can further increase the weight distribution on the metatarsal heads.[153] The increased prevalence of metatarsalgia among women is likely due to wearing high-heeled shoes. Other causes of metatarsalgia include intermetatarsal bursitis/neuritis, metatarsal stress fracture, metatarsophalangeal joint stress syndrome, sesamoiditis, inflammatory arthritis, interdigital neuroma, and aseptic necrosis of the second metatarsal head (Freiberg disease).[153]

Symptoms and Signs

Pain severity is gradual in nature and is aggravated with walking and running activities. Over time, calluses can form over the second and third metatarsal heads and can further increase weight bearing on the metatarsal heads. On physical examination, palpable point tenderness is elicited at the distal end of the plantar metatarsal fat pad and also can be reproduced by squeezing the metatarsal head between the thumb and index finger.[153] Interdigital neuromas can lead to metatarsalgia and should be considered when pain is present in the interdigital web spaces. Over time, the pain may progress to diffuse forefoot and midfoot pain.

Diagnosis and Treatment

Radiographic imaging (weight-bearing anteroposterior, lateral, and oblique views) of the affected foot should be obtained to exclude metatarsal stress fractures, which may also lead to forefoot pain. Ultrasound and MRI may be necessary if a neuroma, cyst, bursitis, or other soft-tissue anomaly is suspected. A serum C-reactive protein, uric acid level, and erythrocyte sedimentation rate should be obtained to exclude gout, which often presents as metatarsal pain at the base of the great toe.

Conservative treatment includes the use of analgesic medications and semi-rigid orthotic inserts to reduce pressure on the metatarsal heads. Kang et al.[156] showed that the use of metatarsal pads resulted in decreased maximal peak pressures and pressure time intervals during exercise, which translated to improved function and analgesia. Athletes can achieve significant pain reduction through the use of metatarsal bar appliances that can be placed in footwear. Surgical procedures are aimed at equalizing weight-bearing forces on the metatarsal heads and may include metatarsal shaft osteotomy or metatarsal head condyle excision.[157]

Hallux Valgus

Etiology

Hallux valgus, also known as bunion deformity, is the most common deformity of the metatarsophalangeal joint.[158] Subluxation results in lateral deviation of the proximal phalanx of the great toe and the formation of a medial prominence by the first metatarsal head (Fig. 70.15). The deformity can be congenital or can result from biomechanical instability. Use of improper footwear, such as high-heeled shoes with tight-fitting and small toe boxes, may explain the higher prevalence hallux valgus among women.[158]

Symptoms and Signs

Pain occurs in the first metatarsophalangeal joint and can be described as deep, aching, and/or lancinating. Pain is worsened with ambulation and relieved upon shoe removal. Physical examination reveals a prominence on the medial aspect of the first metatarsal head and valgus deformity of the great toe. Adventitial bursa formation over the prominent medial metatarsal head can also be observed.[159] Bursitis and overlying skin inflammation may be present. Osteoarthritic changes that occur over time may result in significant reduction in joint range of motion associated with pain.

Diagnosis and Treatment

Radiographic imaging (weight-bearing anteroposterior, lateral, and oblique views) should be obtained in order to measure the angular degree of deformity, which provides diagnostic and prognostic information.[159]

Conservative treatment involves wearing footwear with wide toe boxes and placement of pads in the first web space and over the median prominence to relieve pressure-induced pain. Oral

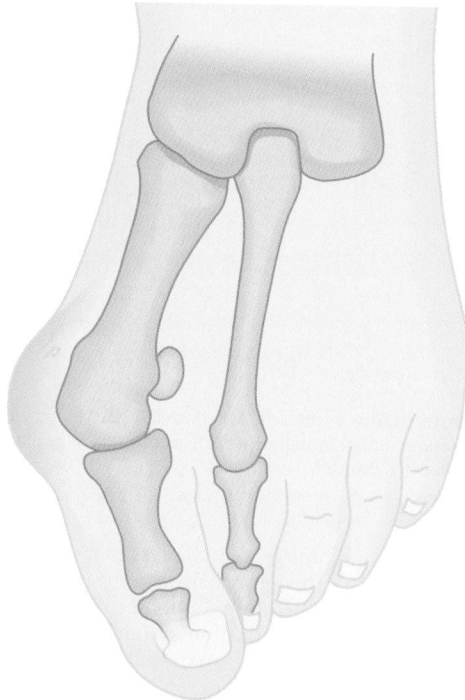

FIGURE 70.15 Hallux valgus. See text for details.

analgesic medications and corticosteroid injections into the first metatarsophalangeal joint can be used to address acute, painful inflammatory states. Surgical treatment is indicated for intractable pain associated with significant functional impairment. Surgical options include osteotomy, exostectomy, resectional arthroplasty, resectional arthroplasty with implant, capsulotendon balancing, first metatarsophalangeal joint arthrodesis, and first metatarsocuneiform joint arthrodesis.[159] A majority of these techniques involve excision of the medial prominence of the metatarsal head (bunionectomy), adductor hallucis tendon release, and occasional excision of the lateral sesamoid bone. Major surgical complications include overcorrection and recurrence.[159]

Hallux Rigidus

Etiology

Hallux rigidus is osteoarthritis of the first metatarsophalangeal joint and is associated with restricted range of motion and pain (Fig. 70.16). This results from cartilage degeneration, altered joint mechanics, and osteophyte formation. Impingement of the dorsal osteophytes results in inflammation and pressure point pain.[160] Athletic activities involving running have been associated with development of hallux rigidus.

Symptoms and Signs

Patients describe a dull, aching pain on the dorsal surface of the first metatarsophalangeal joint that occurs during weight-bearing activities involving the forefoot and often results in an antalgic gait. Unlike hallux valgus, pain from hallux rigidus is associated with or without wearing shoes. Neuropathic pain can result from first dorsal digital nerve entrapment. Physical examination reveals an osteophyte formation on the dorsal surface of the first metatarsophalangeal joint and extremely limited range of motion.

Diagnosis and Treatment

Radiographic imaging reveals degenerative changes of the first metatarsophalangeal joint. Early changes include dorsal and mar-

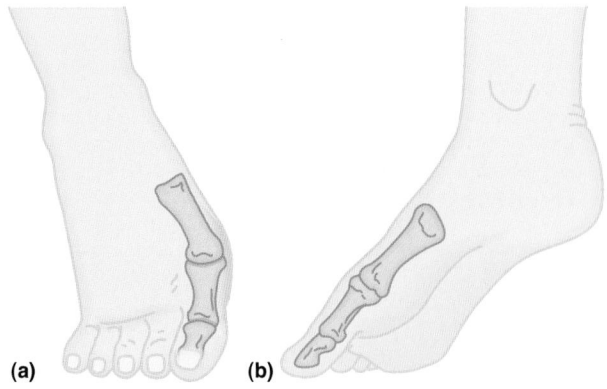

FIGURE 70.16 Hallux rigidus. **A.** Anterior view. **B.** Medial view. Arthritis of the metatarsophalangeal joint reduces motion, especially in dorsiflexion. Push-off is painful.

ginal osteophyte formation. Severe changes that can be visualized include joint space narrowing, sclerosis, joint irregularities, and sesamoid and cystic degeneration. Coughlin and Shurnas[161] proposed a Grade 0 to 4 classification system based on range of motion, physical exam findings, and radiographic results.

Conservative treatment includes rest, customized foot orthotics, and wearing low-heeled, rigid rocker bottom soled shoes with soft surfaces lining the dorsum of the foot. Corticosteroids can be injected in to the first metatarsal interspace lateral to the joint, along with local anesthetic application in the region of the first dorsal digital nerve. Several surgical treatments can be attempted to correct the condition. The least invasive, a cheilectomy, involves the excision of all irregular bony spurs contributing to decreased range of motion. This can provide significant pain relief and gain in function, although a successful outcome is inversely proportional to the degree of arthritic changes. A resection arthroplasty (Keller procedure), which involves excision of the base of the proximal phalanx, is usually reserved for patients with low functional demands.[160] A proximal phalanx and metatarsal osteotomy can also be performed. Complications, such as flaccidity and motor weakness of the hallux, are quite high.[160] Although a joint arthrodesis can provide analgesia, it results in loss of joint motion. Despite this, patients can continue to remain physically active.

Intractable Keratosis

Etiology

Intractable keratosis is characterized by hard callus formation that develops underneath the metatarsal heads due to plantar flexion.[162] Callus formation results in point pressure on the plantar fat pad.

Symptoms and Signs

Intractable keratosis presents as a painful discrete lesion that is aggravated by weight-bearing activities and causes an antalgic gait. Physical examination reveals a 1 cm focal, whitish colored lesion with circumferential erythema found on the plantar aspect of the forefoot.[161]

Diagnosis and Treatment

Radiographic imaging should be performed to exclude other pathology, including fractures, metatarsal avascular necrosis.

Conservative treatment involves wearing shoes with wide toe boxes and placing a pad underneath the uninvolved metatarsal heads in order to offload weight from the involved metatarsal

head. Pumice stones and prescription creams containing lactic acid can be used to reduce the mass of the keratosis and thereby provide symptomatic relief. Analgesic medications can provide minor relief. Corticosteroid injections are controversial as the can create fat-pad atrophy and further exacerbate the condition.[163] Surgical options can include callus tissue reduction and core removal, a variety of distal metatarsal osteotomies, and segmental resection of the proximal metatarsal.[161]

Sesamoiditis

Etiology and Pathophysiology

Sesamoiditis refers to inflammation of the two sesamoid bones on the plantar of the first metatarsophalangeal joint. This state of inflammation can occur as a result of increased stress forces on the sesamoid bones. This is exhibited in lateral displacement of the sesamoid bones seen in hallux valgus.

Symptoms and Signs

Pain is localized on the plantar aspect of the foot and is aggravated by weight-bearing activities. Postural abnormalities may contribute to this condition. Physical examination reveals pain upon dorsiflexion of the metatarsophalangeal joint.[153] In addition, direct palpation of the sesamoid bones causes significant pain.

Diagnosis and Treatment

Radiographic studies should be performed to exclude fractures and other anatomic abnormalities. If plain film radiographs are nondiagnostic, a bone scan can prove useful.

Treatment includes reducing loading forces on the sesamoid bones through the use of a walking cast. In addition, NSAIDs can provide significant analgesia and decrease inflammation. Surgical resection of the sesamoids may be considered after failure to respond to conservative treatment. The major surgical complication is hallux varus.[153]

Gout

Etiology

Elevated systemic uric acid levels cause gout. It typically occurs in association with serum uric acid concentrations greater than 7.0 mg/dL, at which uric acid crystal precipitation occurs.[164] This typically occurs due to increased uric acid production, decreased renal excretion of uric acid, or both.[165] Gout typically manifests in men with a peak age of onset in the fifth decade of life and in women in the sixth decade of life.[164]

Symptoms and Signs

The natural history of gout can be divided into three distinct stages: asymptomatic hyperuricemia, acute and intermittent gout, and chronic tophaceous gout.[165] Asymptomatic hyperuricemia can last for 10 to 30 years before an acute gouty arthritis event occurs. This event is characterized by severe pain in conjunction with edema, erythema, and rubor of the affected joint, after which resolution occurs within 1 to 2 weeks. Gout typically involves only one joint in the early course of the disease, and it is usually the first metatarsophalangeal joint. The acute and intermittent phase involves asymptomatic periods interrupted by acute attacks. These intervals can vary from months to years, but over time the frequency and duration of attacks and number of joints involved increases. Although it remains uncertain, the attacks may be associated with rapid fluctuations of serum uric acid levels. Chronic gouty arthritis typically develops after more than

10 years of acute intermittent gout. There are no pain-free intervals in this stage.

Diagnosis and Treatment

Patients report multiple painful, stiff, edematous joints, particularly in the toes, ankles, and knees. Although elevated serum uric acid levels (greater than 7.0 mg/dL) are commonly seen in gout, there may be periods of time when serum uric acid levels are normal.[165] In addition to hyperuricemia, leukocytosis, elevated erythrocyte sedimentation rates, and elevated C-reactive protein levels may be present in acute attacks. The criterion standard of diagnosis, however, remains aspiration and examination of synovial fluid from an actively affected joint. Under polarized microscopy, monosodium uric acid crystals are seen as negatively birefringent needle-like structures engulfed by polymorphonuclear neutrophils.

Treatment of acute gouty arthritis focuses on decreasing the inflammation within the joints. This is best accomplished through NSAIDs. In patients who cannot take NSAIDs, corticosteroids can be given via the oral, intravenous, or intra-articular routes. If taken within the first 12 hours of an acute gouty attack, oral colchicine can have an anti-inflammatory effect and can prevent uric acid crystal deposition. While colchicine does not lower the uric acid levels, in low doses it can be used to prevent or reduce the severity of future attacks. Patients however, may not be able to tolerate the side effects of nausea, vomiting, and diarrhea. Chronic therapy to prevent recurrence of gouty arthritic attacks is aimed at normalizing serum uric acid levels. Uricosuric agents, such as probenecid, work by increasing uric acid secretion into the urine. Xanthine oxidase inhibitors, such as allopurinol, work by inhibiting uric acid synthesis. Surgical resection of large nodular deposits of uric acid crystals, also known as tophi, can offer improvement in terms of mechanical function.[166]

Interdigital (Morton's) Neuroma

Etiology

An interdigital neuroma is characterized by a well-localized area of pain on the plantar aspect of the forefoot that radiates into the web space. It typically involves the third interspace of the foot. Although this condition is termed interdigital neuroma, it is not a true neuroma. The histopathologic changes include the degeneration of nerve fibers associated with deposition of amorphous eosinophilic material that is more congruent with neuropathy secondary to an entrapment phenomenon.[167] What causes an interdigital neuroma is unclear, although it has been hypothesized that it arises from constant traction of nerve fibers against the transverse metatarsal ligament during dorsiflexion of the toes.[168] Interdigital neuromas occur approximately 10 times more frequently in women than men. This may be explained by the state of continuous dorsiflexion of the feet when wearing high-heeled shoes.[168]

Symptoms and Signs

Patients typically complain of localized pain in the region of the metatarsal head. The third interspace is more frequently involved than the second interspace, but it rarely involves the first or fourth interspace.[169] The pain is aggravated by wearing tight-fitting shoes and walking and is alleviated by rest and removal of shoes. Upon palpation of the involved interspace, patients report a sharp pain that radiates into the toes. Often, a mass located in the interspace can be palpated. Palpating the affected interspace with one hand and squeezing the entire foot at the same time with the other hand, resulting in narrowing of the intermetatarsal space and compression of the mass can often reproduce symptoms. This can elicit an audible click, known as Mulder's sign.[161] The

differential diagnosis of interdigital neuroma should include stress fracture, tendon sheath ganglion, foreign-body reaction, nerve-sheath tumor, strain of the plantar capsule, and capsulitis or bursitis at the level of the plantar metatarsal-phalangeal joint. In many of these conditions, inflammation of the adjacent nerve also may be present, causing the neuritic sensation of an interdigital neuroma, thus complicating proper diagnosis. It is also important to distinguish interdigital pain from metatarsalgia, which gives rise to a host of other possible pathologies including avascular necrosis, synovial cysts, and tarsal tunnel compression.

Diagnosis and Treatment

Although interdigital neuromas are often diagnosed based solely on clinical findings, MRI, CT, and ultrasound have all been utilized for diagnostic purposes as well. MRI has emerged as the preferred imaging modality due to superior contrast resolution and precision. Interdigital neuromas are best visualized on short-axis (transverse) T1-weighted images through the metatarsal heads. Due to their highly vascular nature, intravenous contrast agents typically result in visual enhancement. They appear as bulbous masses arising between the metatarsal heads (Fig. 70.17).[170] Recent literature has demonstrated that despite being less costly and more portable, use of ultrasound involves a high learning curve and is quite heavily dependent on operator skill. Radiographs may reveal pathology at the metatarsophalangeal joint; however, they are not useful in the diagnosis of interdigital neuromas.

Conservative management of interdigital neuromas includes wearing shoes with wider toe boxes, adequate cushioning, and heels no higher than 1 in. Neuroma pads—soft support inserts that are placed proximal to the affected metatarsal head—are designed to separate the metatarsal heads and prevent rubbing or irritating the affected neuroma when stepping down. NSAIDs and corticosteroid injections into the affected interspace can be tried.[168] However, corticosteroids can result in local fat atrophy and metatarsalgia. Phenol neurolysis of the common interdigital nerve has also been reported to be effective.[171] When conservative management fails, surgical intervention may be indicated. This

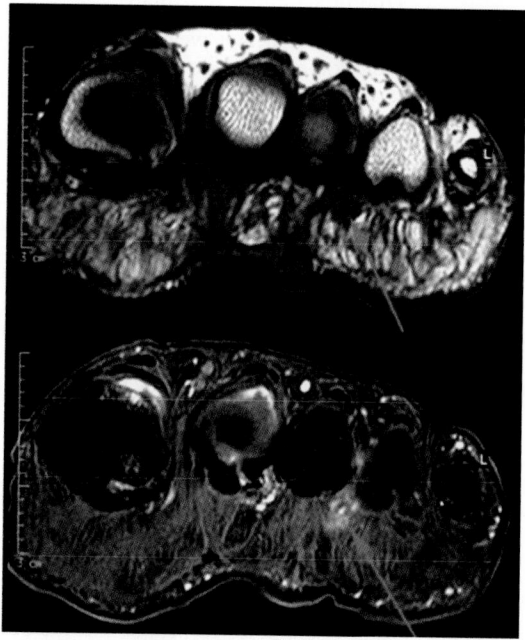

FIGURE 70.17 Interdigital neuroma. Transverse T1-weighted (top) and contrast-enhanced fat-suppressed T1-weighted (bottom). MRIs show the bulbous morphology of the perineural mass with plantar extension. The administration of contrast material reveals enhancement of the lesion.

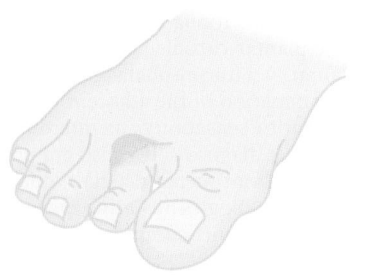
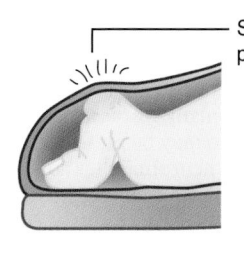

FIGURE 70.18 Hammertoe deformity, a typical small toe deformity, often causes corns and calluses with standard footwear. Extra deep shoes avoid these problems.

involves a dorsal incision in the midline of the affected interdigital space in order to release the transverse metatarsal ligament, as the nerve typically lies beneath this ligament. Postoperative recovery includes a compression dressing worn for several weeks after wound closure. Ambulation is permitted in a postoperative boot.[172] It is important to note that patients may experience decreased sensation in the interdigital web space.

Hammertoes

Etiology

Hammertoe deformities are primarily flexible or fixed plantarflexion deformities of the proximal interphalangeal (PIP) joint, with hyperextension of the metatarsophalangeal (MTP) joint and extension deformities of the distal interphalangeal joint (Fig. 70.18).[173] This results in a dorsal prominence on the PIP, which can cause pain secondary to compression and inflammation from footwear. Physical examination must include determining if the deformity is fixed or flexible. Other deformities may be present, such as hallux valgus or cavus foot deformities. Examination of the extensor surface of the PIP joint may reveal callus or ulcer formation. Intractable keratosis can develop underneath the metatarsal head of the involved toe.[153]

Diagnosis and Treatment

Radiographic imaging should include weight-bearing anteroposterior and lateral radiographs of the involved foot.

Conservative management involves the use of metatarsal pads and shoes with wide toe boxes. Surgical treatment involves MTP joint correction, but the type of surgery is influenced by whether the deformity is fixed or flexible. Fixed hammertoe deformities are corrected through resection arthroplasty of the PIP joint, with the aim of reducing soft tissue contraction forces through toe shortening. Additional procedures such as flexor/extensor tenotomies, MTP joint release, or arthroplasty may be necessary. Weil osteotomies, which primarily involve metatarsal shortening, have also been used to correct the deformity.[174] Flexible hammertoe deformities are surgically corrected with a Girdlestone flexor tendon transfer. This involves harvesting the long flexor tendon from

the plantar aspect of the foot and surgically affixing this into the extensor hood. Thus, the tendon functions as both an extensor of the interphalangeal joints and a flexor the MTP joint.[169] The major complication of Girdlestone flexor tendon transfer is a failure to identify a contracture of the flexor digitorum longus tendon during surgery, resulting in inadequate correction.[173]

Clawtoe Deformity

Etiology

Clawtoe deformity results from dorsiflexion of the proximal phalanx on the lesser MTP joint and concurrent flexion of the PIP and distal interphalangeal joints (Fig. 70.19).[173] Pain results from friction between the interphalangeal joints and the shoe. In addition, patients experience pain underneath the metatarsal heads from being in plantarflexion.[169] As with hammertoes, clawtoe deformities may be flexible or fixed. They typically involve all four of the lesser toes. The clinical evaluation is similar to that of hammertoe deformities, including inspection for possible callus and ulcer formation along the extensor surface of the proximal interphalangeal joints.

Diagnosis and Treatment

Radiographic imaging should include weight-bearing anteroposterior and lateral radiographs of the involved foot.

Conservative management includes wearing shoes that have increased depth to reduce pressure on the lesser toes and placement of arch supports underneath the metatarsal heads. Shoe inserts can be positioned proximal to the MTP joints in flexible deformities that are mild. The flexible deformity is corrected with a Girdlestone flexor tendon transfer. The fixed deformity requires a DuVries proximal phalangeal condylectomy in conjunction with the Girdlestone tendon transfer procedure.[169] As with hammertoe surgical correction, the major complication is inadequate correction and subsequent recurrence of the deformity.[173]

Hard Corn (Clavus Durum)

Corns are painful, hyperkeratotic skin lesions located over bony prominences that result from excessive pressure on the skin. Histologic specimens reveal hyperplasia of the epidermis, especially

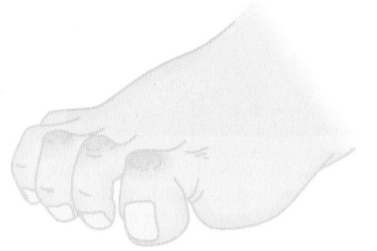
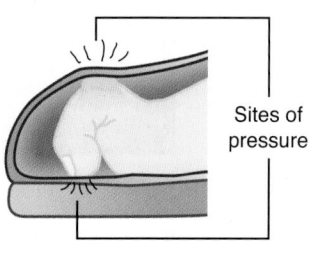

FIGURE 70.19 Clawtoe deformity, a typical small toe deformity, often causes corns and calluses with standard footwear. Extra deep shoes avoid these problems.

proliferation of the stratum corneum.[175] Hard corns are notable for their dry, horny appearance that develops over the dorsal and lateral surfaces of the fifth toe—on the lateral condyle of the proximal phalanx.

Conservative treatment is aimed at reducing pressure on the bony prominences by wearing shoes with large toe boxes. Surgical correction involves débridement of the lesion and occasionally necessitates removal of the distal portion of the proximal phalanx. The most common complication of the latter surgical procedure is excessive bone removal, resulting in a flaccid fifth toe.[176]

Soft Corn (Clavus Mollum)

Soft corns are macerated lesions that frequently occur in the fourth web space between the base of the proximal of the fourth toe and the medial condyle of the head of the proximal phalanx of the fifth toe.[169] These typically develop as a result of small bony protrusion anomalies that cause pressure points, which can then result in ulceration.[176]

As with hard corns, management first focuses on reducing pressure on the bony prominences through utilization of footwear with large toe boxes. Other treatment modalities include the use of keratolytics such as salicylic acid.[177] Surgical treatment involves removal of the bony protrusion.

Ingrown Toenail (Onychocryptosis)

An ingrown toenail is a painful condition resulting from nail plate penetration upon the medial or lateral nail fold epithelium (Fig. 70.20). This typically involves the great toe. It is associated with trauma, tight-fitting footwear, and improperly trimming the nails at the nail margins.[154] Aberrant nail curvature predisposes one to developing an ingrown toenail.

If no infection is present, initial treatment includes elevation of the nail by placing cotton between the nail plate and the skin. This can be aided by daily foot soaks and removal of any pressure points on the nail. Additional treatment involves trimming an oblique portion of the affected nail toward the posterior nail fold under a digital block.[154] The nail groove is then débrided and dressed. If infection or granulation occurs, treatment is focused on partial removal of the nail plate. This involves performing a digital nerve block, followed by a longitudinal incision from the base to the tip of the affected region of the nail plate, including the nail beneath the cuticle. The nail is then grasped with a hemo-

stat and removed from the nail groove using a rocking motion. The nail groove is then débrided and dressed.[154]

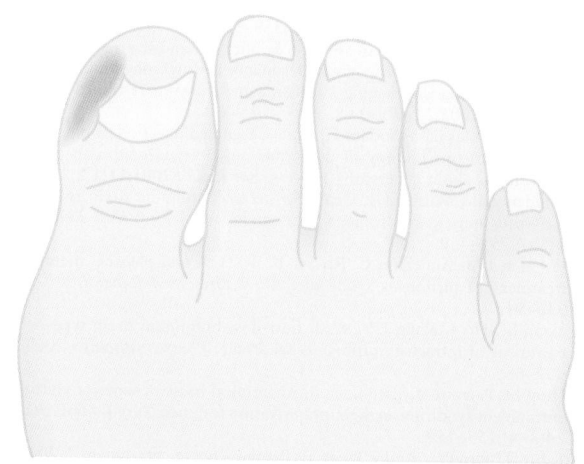

FIGURE 70.20 Ingrown toenail is often caused by improper nail cutting techniques or by wearing ill-fitting footwear that creates pressure against the lateral nail fold producing exquisite pain and tenderness.

References

1. Ramchandren S, Dalmau J. Metastases to the peripheral nervous system. *J Neurooncol* 2005;75(1):101–10.
2. Planner AC, Donaghy M, Moore NR. Causes of lumbosacral plexopathy. *Clin Radiol* 2006;61(12):987–995.
3. Wilbourn AJ. Plexopathies. *Neurol Clin* 2007;25(1):139–171.
4. Yee T. Recurrent idiopathic lumbosacral plexopathy. *Muscle & Nerve* 2000; 23(9):1439–1442.
5. Taylor BV, Kimmel DW, Krecke KN, et al. Magnetic resonance imaging in cancer-related lumbosacral plexopathy. *Mayo Clinic Proc* 1997;72(9):823–829.
6. Yadav R. Neoplastic lumbosacral plexopathy. Available at: http://emedicine.medscape.com/article/316390-overview. Accessed 8/26/2009.
7. Jaeckle KA. Neurological manifestations of neoplastic and radiation-induced plexopathies. *Semin Neurol* 2004;24(4):385–393.
8. Portenoy RK. Cancer pain. Epidemiology and syndromes. *Cancer* 1989;63(11 Suppl):2298–2307.
9. Stevens MJ, Gonet YM. Malignant psoas syndrome: recognition of an oncologic entity. *Australas Radiol* 1990;34(2):150–154.
10. Agar M, Broadbent A, Chye R. The management of malignant psoas syndrome: case reports and literature review. *J Pain Symptom Manage* 2004; 28(3):282–293.
11. Falah M, Schiff D, Burns TM. Neuromuscular complications of cancer diagnosis and treatment. *J Support Oncol* 2005;3(4):271–282.
12. Tonsgard JH, Kwak SM, Short MP, et al. CT imaging in adults with neurofibromatosis-1: frequent asymptomatic plexiform lesions. *Neurology* 1998; 50(6):1755–1760.
13. Dyck PJ, Windebank AJ. Diabetic and nondiabetic lumbosacral radiculoplexus neuropathies: new insights into pathophysiology and treatment. *Muscle Nerve* 2002;25(4):477–491.
14. Paley M, Sidhu PS, Evans RA, Karani JB. Retroperitoneal collections—aetiology and radiological implications. *Clin Radiol* 1997;52(4):290–294.
15. Ozcakar L, Sivri A, Aydinli M, et al. Lumbosacral plexopathy as the harbinger of a silent retroperitoneal hematoma. *South Med J* 2003;96(1):109–110.
16. Katirji B, Wilbourn AJ, Scarberry SL, et al. Intrapartum maternal lumbosacral plexopathy. *Muscle Nerve* 2002;26(3):340–347.
17. Haim A, Pritsch T, Ben-Galim P, et al. Meralgia paresthetica: a retrospective analysis of 79 patients evaluated and treated according to a standard algorithm. *Acta Orthop* 2006;77(3):482–486.
18. Roth V. [Meralgia Paresthetica]. *Med Obozr* 1895;43(678).
19. Harney D, Patijn J. Meralgia paresthetica: diagnosis and management strategies. *Pain Med (Malden, Mass)* 2007;8(8):669–677.
20. van Slobbe AM, Bohnen AM, Bernsen RM, et al. Incidence rates and determinants in meralgia paresthetica in general practice. *J Neurol* 2004;251(3):294–297.
21. Grossman MG, Ducey SA, Nadler SS, et al. Meralgia paresthetica: diagnosis and treatment. *J Am Acad Orthop Surg* 2001;9(5):336–344.
22. Seror P, Seror R. Meralgia paresthetica: clinical and electrophysiological diagnosis in 120 cases. *Muscle Nerve* 2006;33(5):650–654.
23. Mondelli M, Rossi S, Romano C. Body mass index in meralgia paresthetica: a case-control study. *Acta Neurol Scand* 2007;116(2):118–123.
24. Hollis MH, Lemay DE, Jensen RP. Nerve entrapment sydromes of the lower extremity. Available at: http://emedicine.medscape.com/article/1234809-overview. Accessed 8/26/2009.
25. World Health Organization. Obesity: preventing and managing the global epidemic. Report of a WHO consultation. *World Health Organization Technical Report Series* 2000;894:i–xii,1–253.
26. Kitchen C, Simpson J. Meralgia paresthetica. A review of 67 patients. *Acta Neurol Scand* 1972;48(5):547–555.
27. Baldini M, Raimondi PL, Princi L. Meralgia paraesthetica following weight loss. Case report. *Neurosurg Rev* 1982;5(2):45–47.
28. Pastor Guzman JM, Pastor Navarro H, Donate Moreno MJ, et al. [Femoral neuropathy in urological surgery]. *Actas Urol Esp* 2007;31(8):885–894.
29. Nouraei SA, Anand B, Spink G, et al. A novel approach to the diagnosis and management of meralgia paresthetica. *Neurosurgery* 2007;60(4):696–700; discussion 700.
30. Williams PH, Trzil KP. Management of meralgia paresthetica. *J Neurosurg* 1991;74(1):76–80.
31. Shannon J, Lang SA, Yip RW, et al. Lateral femoral cutaneous nerve block revisited. A nerve stimulator technique. *Reg Anesth* 1995;20(2):100–104.
32. Hurdle MF, Weingarten TN, Crisostomo RA, et al. Ultrasound-guided blockade of the lateral femoral cutaneous nerve: technical description and review of 10 cases. *Arch Phys Med Rehabil* 2007;88(10):1362–1364.
33. Shah RV, Racz GB. Pulsed mode radiofrequency lesioning of the suprascapular nerve for the treatment of chronic shoulder pain. *Pain Phys* 2003;6(4):503–506.
34. Trescot AM. Cryoanalgesia in interventional pain management. *Pain Phys* 2003;6(3):345–360.

35. Barna SA, Hu MM, Buxo C, et al. Spinal cord stimulation for treatment of meralgia paresthetica. *Pain Phys* 2005;8(3):315–318.

36. Rozen D, Ahn J. Pulsed radiofrequency for the treatment of ilioinguinal neuralgia after inguinal herniorrhaphy. *Mt Sinai J Med (New York)* 2006;73(4): 716–718.

37. Nahabedian MY, Dellon AL. Meralgia paresthetica: etiology, diagnosis, and outcome of surgical decompression. *Ann Plast Surg* 1995;35(6):590–594.

38. van Eerten PV, Polder TW, Broere CA. Operative treatment of meralgia paresthetica: transection versus neurolysis. *Neurosurgery* 1995;37(1):63–65.

39. Busis NA. Femoral and obturator neuropathies. *Neurol Clin* 199917(3): 633–653, vii.

40. Hunter LY, Louis DS, Ricciardi JR, et al. The saphenous nerve: its course and importance in medial arthrotomy. *Am J Sports Med* 1979;7(4):227–230.

41. Kuntzer T, van Melle G, Regli F. Clinical and prognostic features in unilateral femoral neuropathies. *Muscle Nerve* 1997;20(2):205–211.

42. Carter GT, McDonald CM, Chan TT, et al. Isolated femoral mononeuropathy to the vastus lateralis: EMG and MRI findings. *Muscle Nerve* 1995;18(3): 341–344.

43. Ducic I, Dellon L, Larson EE. Treatment concepts for idiopathic and iatrogenic femoral nerve mononeuropathy. *Ann Plast Surg* 2005;55(4):397–401.

44. Boontje AH, Haaxma R. Femoral neuropathy as a complication of aortic surgery. *J Cardiovasc Surg* 1987;28(3):286–289.

45. Brasch RC, Bufo AJ, Kreienberg PF, et al. Femoral neuropathy secondary to the use of a self-retaining retractor. Report of three cases and review of the literature. *Dis Colon Rectum* 1995;38(10):1115–1118.

46. Goldman JA, Feldberg D, Dicker D, et al. Femoral neuropathy subsequent to abdominal hysterectomy. A comparative study. *Eur J Obstet Gynecol Reprod Biol* 1985;20(6):385–392.

47. Schmalzried TP, Noordin S, Amstutz HC. Update on nerve palsy associated with total hip replacement. *Clin Orthop Relat Res* 1997;344:188–206.

48. Kim DH, Murovic JA, Tiel RL, et al. Intrapelvic and thigh-level femoral nerve lesions: management and outcomes in 119 surgically treated cases. *J Neurosurg* 2004;100(6):989–996.

49. Fanelli G, Casati A, Garancini P, et al. Nerve stimulator and multiple injection technique for upper and lower limb blockade: failure rate, patient acceptance, and neurologic complications. Study Group on Regional Anesthesia. *Anesth Analg* 1999;88(4):847–852.

50. Walsh C, Walsh A. Postoperative femoral neuropathy. *Surg Gynecol Obstet* 1992;174(3):255–263.

51. Worth RM, Kettelkamp DB, Defalque RJ, et al. Saphenous nerve entrapment. A cause of medial knee pain. *Am J Sports Med* 1984;12(1):80–81.

52. Adar R, Meyer E, Zweig A. Saphenous neuralgia: a complication of vascular reconstructions below the inguinal ligament. *Ann Surg* 1979;190(5):609–613.

53. Chauhan BM, Kim DJ, Wainapel SF. Saphenous neuropathy: following coronary artery bypass surgery. *New York State J Med* 1981;81(2):222–223.

54. Lederman RJ, Breuer AC, Hanson MR, et al. Peripheral nervous system complications of coronary artery bypass graft surgery. *Ann Neurolog* 1982;12(3): 297–301.

55. Roder OC, Kamper A, Jorgensen SJ. Incidence of saphenous neuralgia in arterial surgery. *Acta Chir Scand* 1984;150(1):23–24.

56. Romanoff ME, Cory PC Jr, Kalenak A, et al. Saphenous nerve entrapment at the adductor canal. *American J Sports Med* 1989;17(4):478–481.

57. Lavee J, Schneiderman J, Yorav S, et al. Complications of saphenous vein harvesting following coronary artery bypass surgery. *J Cardiovasc Surg* 1989; 30(6):989–991.

58. Senegor M. Iatrogenic saphenous neuralgia: successful therapy with neuroma resection. *Neurosurgery* 1991;28(2):295–298.

59. Miller DB Jr. Arthroscopic meniscus repair. *Am J Sports Med* 1988;16(4): 315–320.

60. Tennent TD, Birch NC, Holmes MJ, et al. Knee pain and the infrapatellar branch of the saphenous nerve. *J Roy Soc Med* 1998;91(11):573–575.

61. Schwabegger AH, Rhomberg M, Ninkovic MM, et al. Saphenous nerve neuralgia after gracilis muscle flap harvest. *Br J Plast Surg* 1998;51(5):410.

62. Iizuka M, Yao R, Wainapel S. Saphenous nerve injury following medial knee joint injection: a case report. *Arch Phys Med Rehabil* 2005;86(10): 2062–2065.

63. Hemler DE, Ward WK, Karstetter KW, et al. Saphenous nerve entrapment caused by pes anserine bursitis mimicking stress fracture of the tibia. *Arch Phys Med Rehabil* 1991;72(5):336–337.

64. Murayama K, Takeuchi T, Yuyama T. Entrapment of the saphenous nerve by branches of the femoral vessels. A report of two cases. *J Bone Joint Surg* 1991;73(5):770–772.

65. Fabian RH, Norcross KA, Hancock MB. Surfer's neuropathy. *New Engl J Med* 1987;316(9):555.

66. Hattori H, Asagai Y, Yamamoto K. Sudden onset of saphenous neuropathy associated with hereditary multiple exostoses. *J Orthop Sci* 2006;11(4): 405–408.

67. Mozes M, Ouaknine G, Nathan H. Saphenous nerve entrapment simulating vascular disorder. *Surgery* 1975;77(2):299–303.

68. Bianchi S. Ultrasound of the nerves of the knee region. Technique of examination and normal US appearance. *J Ultrasound* 2006:1–15.

69. Bradshaw C, McCrory P, Bell S, et al. Obturator nerve entrapment. A cause of groin pain in athletes. *Am J Sports Med* 1997;25(3):402–408.

70. Sorenson EJ, Chen JJ, Daube JR. Obturator neuropathy: causes and outcome. *Muscle Nerve* 2002;25(4):605–607.

71. Jirsch JD, Chalk CH. Obturator neuropathy complicating elective laparoscopic tubal occlusion. *Muscle Nerve* 2007;36(1):104–106.

72. Kleiner JB, Thorne RP. Obturator neuropathy caused by an aneurysm of the hypogastric artery. A case report. *J Bone Joint Surg* 1989;71(9):1408–1409.

73. Redwine DB, Sharpe DR. Endometriosis of the obturator nerve. A case report. *J Reprod Med* 1990;35(4):434–435.

74. Rogers LR, Borkowski GP, Albers JW, et al. Obturator mononeuropathy caused by pelvic cancer: six cases. *Neurology* 1993;43(8):1489–2592.

75. Nakayama T, Kobayashi S, Shiraishi K, et al. Diagnosis and treatment of obturator hernia. *Keio J Med* 2002;51(3):129–132.

76. Yamashita K, Hayashi J, Tsunoda T. Howship-Romberg sign caused by an obturator granuloma. *Am J Surg* 2004;187(6):775–776.

77. Stuplich M, Hottinger AF, Stoupis C, et al. Combined femoral and obturator neuropathy caused by synovial cyst of the hip. *Muscle Nerve* 2005;32(4): 552–554.

78. Yokoyama Y, Yamaguchi A, Isogai M, et al. Thirty-six cases of obturator hernia: does computed tomography contribute to postoperative outcome? *World J Surg* 1999;23(2):214–216; discussion 217.

79. Kammori M, Mafune K, Hirashima T, et al. Forty-three cases of obturator hernia. American journal of surgery. 2004;187(4):549–552.

80. Kawaguchi M, Hashizume K, Iwata T, et al. Percutaneous radiofrequency lesioning of sensory branches of the obturator and femoral nerves for the treatment of hip joint pain. *Reg Anesth Pain Med* 2001;26(6):576–581.

81. Malik A, Simopolous T, Elkersh M, et al. Percutaneous radiofrequency lesioning of sensory branches of the obturator and femoral nerves for the treatment of non-operable hip pain. *Pain Phys* 2003;6(4):499–502.

82. Wu H, Groner J. Pulsed radiofrequency treatment of articular branches of the obturator and femoral nerves for management of hip joint pain. *Pain Pract* 2007;7(4):341–344.

83. Beaton LE, Anson BJ. The Relation of the sciatic nerve and its subdivisions to the piriformis muscle. *Anat Rec* 1938;70:1–5.

84. Yuen EC, So YT, Olney RK. The electrophysiologic features of sciatic neuropathy in 100 patients. *Muscle Nerve* 1995;18(4):414–420.

85. Kline DG, Kim D, Midha R, et al. Management and results of sciatic nerve injuries: a 24-year experience. *J Neurosurg* 1998;89(1):13–23.

86. Yuen EC, So YT. Sciatic neuropathy. *Neurol Clin* 1999;17(3):617–631, viii.

87. Plewnia C, Wallace C, Zochodne D. Traumatic sciatic neuropathy: a novel cause, local experience, and a review of the literature. *J Trauma* 1999;47(5): 986–991.

88. Yuen EC, Olney RK, So YT. Sciatic neuropathy: clinical and prognostic features in 73 patients. *Neurology* 1994;44(9):1669–1674.

89. Pace JB, Nagle D. Piriform syndrome. *Western J Med* 1976;124(6):435–439.

90. Thiele GH. Coccygodynia and pain in the superior gluteal region. *JAMA* 1937;109:1271–1275.

91. Travell JG, Simons DG. *Myofascial Pain and Dysfunction: The Trigger Point Manual.* Baltimore: Williams & Wilkins; 1992.

92. Fishman SM, Caneris OA, Bandman TB, et al. Injection of the piriformis muscle by fluoroscopic and electromyographic guidance. *Reg Anesth Pain Med* 1998;23(6):554–559.

93. Benson ER, Schutzer SF. Posttraumatic piriformis syndrome: diagnosis and results of operative treatment. *J Bone Joint Surg* 1999;81(7):941–949.

94. Feinberg J, Sethi S. Sciatic neuropathy: case report and discussion of the literature on postoperative sciatic neuropathy and sciatic nerve tumors. *HSS J* 2006; 2:181–187.

95. Wallace MS, Staats P. *Pain Medicine and Management: Just the Facts.* New York: McGraw-Hill, Health Professions Division; 2004.

96. Freiburg AH. Sciatic pain and its relief by operations on muscle and fascia. *Arch Surg* 1937;34:337–350.

97. Beatty RA. The piriformis muscle syndrome: a simple diagnostic maneuver. *Neurosurgery* 1994;34(3):512–514; discussion 514.

98. Fishman LM, Zybert PA. Electrophysiologic evidence of piriformis syndrome. *Arch Phys Med Rehabil* 1992;73(4):359–364.

99. Filler AG, Haynes J, Jordan SE, et al. Sciatica of nondisc origin and piriformis syndrome: diagnosis by magnetic resonance neurography and interventional magnetic resonance imaging with outcome study of resulting treatment. *J Neurosurg* 2005;2(2):99–115.

100. Fanucci E, Masala S, Sodani G, et al. CT-guided injection of botulinic toxin for percutaneous therapy of piriformis muscle syndrome with preliminary MRI results about denervative process. *Eur Radiol* 2001;11(12):2543–2548.

101. Childers MK, Wilson DJ, Gnatz SM, et al. Botulinum toxin type A use in piriformis muscle syndrome: a pilot study. *Am J Phys Med Rehabil* 2002; 81(10):751–759.

102. Fishman LM, Anderson C, Rosner B. BOTOX and physical therapy in the treatment of piriformis syndrome. *Am J Phys Med Rehabil* 2002;81(12): 936–942.

103. Yoon SJ, Ho J, Kang HY, et al. Low-dose botulinum toxin type A for the treatment of refractory piriformis syndrome. *Pharmacotherapy* 2007;27(5): 657–665.

104. Diop M, Parratte B, Tatu L, et al. Anatomical bases of superior gluteal nerve entrapment syndrome in the suprapiriformis foramen. *Surg Radiol Anat* 2002; 24(3–4):155–159.

105. Fabre T, Piton C, Andre D, et al. Peroneal nerve entrapment. *J Bone Joint Surg Am* 1998;80(1):47–53.

106. Aprile I, Padua L, Padua R, et al. Peroneal mononeuropathy: predisposing factors, and clinical and neurophysiological relationships. *Neurol Sci* 2000; 21(6):367–371.

107. Noble J, Munro CA, Prasad VS, et al. Analysis of upper and lower extremity peripheral nerve injuries in a population of patients with multiple injuries. *J Trauma* 1998;45(1):116–122.

108. Takao M, Ochi M, Shu N, et al. A case of superficial peroneal nerve injury during ankle arthroscopy. *Arthroscopy* 2001;17(4):403–404.

109. Yilmaz S, Altinbas H, Senol U, et al. Common peroneal nerve palsy after retrograde popliteal artery puncture. *Eur J Vasc Endovasc Surg* 2002;23(5):467–469.

110. Yilmaz E, Karakurt L, Serin E, et al. [Peroneal nerve palsy due to rare reasons: a report of three cases]. *Acta Orthop Traumatol Turc* 2004;38(1):75–78.

111. Flores LP, Koerbel A, Tatagiba M. Peroneal nerve compression resulting from fibular head osteophyte-like lesions. *Surg Neurol* 2005;64(3):249–252; discussion 252.

112. Hems TE, Jones BG. Peroneal nerve damage associated with the proximal locking screws of the AIM tibial nail. *Injury* 2005;36(5):651–654; discussion 655.

113. Niall DM, Nutton RW, Keating JF. Palsy of the common peroneal nerve after traumatic dislocation of the knee. *J Bone Joint Surg Br* 2005;87(5):664–667.

114. Giannas J, Bayat A, Watson SJ. Common peroneal nerve injury during varicose vein operation. *Eur J Vasc Endovasc Surg* 2006;31(4):443–445.

115. Atkin GK, Round T, Vattipally VR, et al. Common peroneal nerve injury as a complication of short saphenous vein surgery. *Phlebology* 2007;22(1):3–7.

116. Drosos GI, Stavropoulos NI, Kazakos KI. Peroneal nerve damage by oblique proximal locking screw in tibial fracture nailing: a new emerging complication? *Arch Orthop Trauma Surg* 2007;127(6):449–451.

117. Ersozlu S, Ozulku M, Yildirim E, et al. Common peroneal nerve palsy from an untreated popliteal pseudoaneurysm after penetrating injury. *J Vasc Surg* 2007;45(2):408–410.

118. Prasad AR, Steck JK, Dellon AL. Zone of traction injury of the common peroneal nerve. *Ann Plast Surg* 2007;59(3):302–306.

119. O'Neill PJ, Parks BG, Walsh R, et al. Excursion and strain of the superficial peroneal nerve during inversion ankle sprain. *J Bone Joint Surg Am* 2007;89(5):979–986.

120. Hamdan FB, Jaffar AA, Ossi RG. The propensity of common peroneal nerve in thigh-level injury. *J Trauma* 2008;64(2):300–303.

121. Sanger JR, Kao DS, Hackbarth DA. Peroneal nerve compression by lateral gastrocnemius flap. *J Plast Reconstr Aesthet Surg* 2008 Jan 25 (Epub ahead of print).

122. Jowett AJ, Johnston JF, Gaillard F, et al. Lateral meniscal cyst causing common peroneal palsy. *Skeletal Radiol* 2008;37(4):351–355.

123. Piton C, Fabre T, Lasseur E, et al. [Common fibular nerve lesions. Etiology and treatment. Apropos of 146 cases with surgical treatment]. *Rev Chir Orthop Reparatrice Appar Mot* 1997;83(6):515–521.

124. Kim DH, Murovic JA, Tiel RL, et al. Management and outcomes in 318 operative common peroneal nerve lesions at the Louisiana State University Health Sciences Center. *Neurosurgery* 2004;54(6):1421–1428; discussion 1428–1429.

125. Young C, Rutherford D, Niedfeldt M. Treatment of plantar fasciitis. *Am Fam Phys* 2001;63(3):467–474.

126. Marwah V. Compression of the lateral popliteal (common peroneal) nerve. *Lancet* 1964;2:1367–1369.

127. Moller BN, Kadin S. Entrapment of the common peroneal nerve. *Am J Sports Med* 1987;15(1):90–91.

128. Leach RE, Purnell MB, Saito A. Peroneal nerve entrapment in runners. *Am J Sports Med* 1989;17(2):287–291.

129. McAuliffe TB, Fiddian NJ, Browett JP. Entrapment neuropathy of the superficial peroneal nerve. A bilateral case. *J Bone Joint Surg Br* 1985;67(1):62–63.

130. Styf J, Morberg P. The superficial peroneal tunnel syndrome. Results of treatment by decompression. *J Bone Joint Surg Br* 1997;79(5):801–803.

131. Fernandez E, Pallini R, Lauretti L, et al. Neurosurgery of the peripheral nervous system: entrapment syndromes of the lower extremity. *Surg Neurol* 1999;52(5):449–452.

132. Krause KH, Witt T, Ross A. The anterior tarsal tunnel syndrome. *J Neurol* 1977;217(1):67–74.

133. Miller S. In: Hetherington V, ed. *Textbook of Hallux Valgus and Forefoot Surgery*. Entrapment neuropathies. Cleveland: Vincent J. Hetherington: 2000 401–428.

134. Deland J, de Asla R, Sung I, et al. Posterior tibial tendon insufficiency: which ligaments are involved? *Foot Ankle Int* 2005;26(6):427–435.

135. Lemley F, Berlet G, Hill K, et al. Current concepts review: tarsal coalition. *Foot Ankle Int* 2006;27(12):1163–1169.

136. Pomeroy G, Pike R, Beals T, et al. Acquired flatfoot in adults due to dysfunction of the posterior tibial tendon. *J Bone Joint Surg (American)* 1999;81(8):1173–1182.

137. Younger A, Hansen S. Adult cavovarus foot. *J Am Acad Orthop Surg* 2005;13(5):302–315.

138. Wapner K, Myerson M, eds. *Pes Cavus*. Philadelphia: WB Saunders; 2000.

139. Buchbinder R. Clinical practice plantar fasciitis. *New Engl J Med* 2004;350(21):2159–2166.

140. Cole C, Seto C, Gazewood J. Plantar fasciitis: evidenced-based review of diagnosis and therapy. *Am Fam Phys* 2005;72(11):2237–2242.

141. Crawford F, Thomson C. Interventions for treating plantar heel pain. *Cochrane Database Syst Rev* 2003;3:CD000416.

142. Aldridge T. Diagnosing heel pain in adults. *Am Fam Phys* 2004;70(2):332–338.

143. ÜrgÜden M, Bilbaşar H, Özdemir H, et al. Tarsal tunnel syndrome—the effect of the associated features on outcome of surgery. *Intl Orthop* 2002;26(4):253–256.

144. DiDomenico L, Masternick E. Anterior tarsal tunnel syndrome. *Clin Podiatr Med Surg* 2006;23(3):611–620.

145. Franson J, Baravarian B. Tarsal tunnel syndrome: a compression neuropathy involving four distinct tunnels. *Clin Podiatr Med Surg* 2006;23(3):597–609.

146. Franson J, Baravarian B. Tarsal tunnel syndrome: a compression neuropathy involving four distinct tunnels. *Clin Podiatr Med Surg* 2006;23(3):597–609.

147. Englanoff G, Anglin D, Hutson H. Lisfranc fracture-dislocation: a frequently missed diagnosis in the emergency department. *Ann Emerg Med* 1995;26(2):229–233.

148. Ross G, Cronin R, Hauzenblaus J, et al. Plantar ecchymosis sign: a clinical aid to diagnosis of occult Lisfranc tarsometatarsal injuries. *J Orthop Trauma* 1996;10(2):119–122.

149. Faciszewski T, Burks R, Manaster B. Subtle injuries of the Lisfranc joint. *J Bone Joint Surg* 1990;72(10):1519–1522.

150. Early J, Bucholz R. Lisfranc injuries and their management. *Curr Orthop* 1996;10(3):169–173.

151. Beals T, Pomeroy G, Manoli A. Posterior tendon insufficiency: diagnosis and treatment. *J Am Acad Orthop Surg* 1999;7(3):112–118.

152. Kohls-Gatzoulis J, Angel J, Singh D, et al. Tibialis posterior dysfunction: a common and treatable cause of adult acquired flatfoot. *Br Med J* 2004;329(7478):1328–1333.

153. Loeser J, ed. *Bonica's Management of Pain*. 3rd ed. Philadelphia: Lippincott Williams & Wilkins; 2001.

154. Tintinalli J, ed. *Tintinalli's Emergency Medicine: A Comprehensive Study Guide*. 6th ed. Philadelphia: McGraw-Hill; 2004.

155. Hockenbury R. Forefoot problems in athletes. *Med Sci Sports Exercise* 1999;31(7S):448–458.

156. Kang J, Chen M, Chen S, et al. Correlations between subjective treatment responses and plantar pressure parameters of metatarsal pad treatment in metatarsalgia patients: a prospective study. *BMC Musculoskel Disord* 2006;7(95):1471–2474.

157. O'Kane C, Kilmartin T. The surgical management of central metatarsalgia. *Foot Ankle Int* 2002;23(5):415–419.

158. Mann R, Coughlin M. Hallux valgus: etiology, anatomy, treatment and surgical considerations. *Clin Orthop Relat Res* 1981;157:31–41.

159. Ajis A. Tailor's bunion: a review. *J Foot Ankle Surg* 2005;44(3):236–245.

160. Beertema W, Draijer W, van Os J, Pilot P. A retrospective analysis of surgical treatment in patients with symptomatic hallux rigidus: long-term follow-up. *J Foot Ankle Surg* 2006;45(4):244–251.

161. Coughlin M. Common causes of pain in the forefoot in adults. *J Bone Joint Surg* 2000;82(6):781–790.

162. Kitaoka H, Patzer G. Chevron osteotomy of lesser metatarsals for intractable plantar callosities. *J Bone Joint Surg Br* 1998;80(3):516–518.

163. Tsai W. Treatment of proximal plantar fasciitis with ultrasound-guided steroid injection. *Arch Phys Med Rehabil* 2000;81(10):1416–1421.

164. Ruddy S, Harris EJ, Harris C, eds. *Kelly's Textbook of Rheumatology*. 7th ed. Philadelphia: Elsevier; 2001.

165. Eggebeen A. Gout: an update. *Am Fam Phys* 2007;76(6):801–808.

166. Lee S, Sun I, Lu Y, et al. Surgical treatment of the chronic tophaceous deformity in upper extremities: the shaving technique. *J Plast Reconstruct Aesthetic Surg* 2008.

167. Graham C, Graham D. Morton's neuroma: a microscopic evaluation. *Foot Ankle* 1984;5(150):150–153.

168. Hassouna H. Morton's metatarsalgia: pathogenesis, aetiology and current management. *Acta Orthop Belg* 2005;71(6):646–655.

169. Skinner H, ed. *Current Diagnosis and Treatment in Orthopedics*. 4th ed. Philadelphia: McGraw-Hill; 2006.

170. George VA, Khan AM, Hutchinson CE, et al. Morton's neuroma: the role of MR scanning in diagnostic assistance. *The Foot* 2005;15(1):14–6.

171. Magnan B, Marangon A, Frigo A, et al. Local phenol injection in the treatment of interdigital neuritis of the foot (Morton's neuroma). *La Chirurgia Degli Organi di Movimento* 2005;90(4):371–377.

172. Klenerman L. Morton's neuroma. *Curr Orthop* 1997;11(1):15–18.

173. Kirchner J, Wagner E. Girdlestone-Taylor flexor extensor tendon transfer techniques. *Foot Ankle Surg* 2004;3(2):91–99.

174. Trnka H, Gebhard C, Muhlbauer M. The Weil osteotomy for treatment of dislocated lesser metatarsophalangeal joints: good outcome in 21 patients with 42 osteotomies. *Acta Orthop Scand* 2002;73(2):190–194.

175. Wolff K, ed. *Fitzpatrick's Dermatology in General Medicine*. 7th ed. New York: McGraw-Hill; 2008.

176. Canale T, ed. *Campbell's Operative Orthopaedics*. 10th ed. St. Louis: Mosby; 2003.

177. Cordoro K, Ganz J. Training room management of medical conditions: sports dermatology. *Clin Sports Med* 2005;24(3):565–598.

CHAPTER 71 ■ ACUTE LOW BACK PAIN

BRIAN E. McGUIRK AND NIKOLAI BOGDUK

Evidence has revolutionized what might be described as the traditional approach to acute low back pain. The paradigm of making a diagnosis and then prescribing a treatment for that diagnosis has been overturned. For most patients, a diagnosis cannot be made, but nor is it required. The natural history of acute low back pain is fundamentally favorable, provided that it is managed well and not dismissed, neglected, or overmedicalized. Serious causes of acute low back pain are rare and can be identified largely on the basis of history. Investigations to establish a diagnosis or to rule out serious causes are not required. Meanwhile, many conventional interventions have proven ineffective, or no more effective than sham treatment.

These facts promote an innovative approach to acute low back pain for which there is evidence of efficacy. It requires iteration through four principal phases: triage, initial management, review, and reinforcement (Fig. 71.1).

TRIAGE

The cardinal tool for triage is taking a history. A fundamental consideration is whether the patient is describing back pain and not a different, but topographically related, complaint. If the patient does have back pain, triage involves assessing the patient, with the priority being to determine if they have a serious cause of pain.

HISTORY

A comprehensive history can be taken systematically by pursuing an inquiry strategy in several domains that, generically, are pertinent to any pain problem (Table 71.1). For acute low back pain, some of these domains are rarely relevant, but several are pivotal.

Site

The International Association for the Study of Pain[1] defines lumbar spinal pain as pain perceived anywhere within a region bounded by the last thoracic spinous process, the first sacral spinous process, and the lateral borders of the erectors spinae (Figs. 71.2A,B). They define sacral spinal pain as pain perceived anywhere in a region bounded by the first sacral spinous process, the posterior sacrococcygeal joints, and the posterior superior iliac spines.

In the light of these definitions, back pain can be defined as lumbar spinal pain or sacral spinal pain or any combination of the two (Fig. 71.2B). The significance of this definition is not so much to establish what low back pain is, but to establish what it is not (Fig. 71.2).

Pain over the posterior thorax is not low back pain, but thoracic spinal pain (Fig. 71.2C). For thoracic spinal pain, the differential diagnosis is different from that for low back pain, and a different evidence base applies.[2]

Pain over the gluteal region, not encompassing the lumbar spine or sacrum, does not constitute low back pain (Fig. 71.2C). It invites a consideration of sources in the hip joint and surrounding structures. Pain over the loin is not back pain, and invites a consideration of pain emanating from the urinary tract or other viscera (Fig. 71.2D).

If the patient has pain in any of these other regions, their management should be according to algorithms for those regions. The approach being developed in this chapter applies only to patients with low back pain.

Length of Illness

The adjectives acute, subacute, and chronic are often used to describe the period over which back pain has been perceived. Definitions vary, but largely with respect to defining chronic low back pain (see Chapter 72). Acute low back pain means pain of recent onset. In conventional usage, this means pain that has not persisted for longer than 3 months. Most of the evidence on low back pain conforms to this convention. The subcategory subacute low back pain usually means pain that has lasted longer than 5 to 7 weeks, but not longer than 12 weeks.[3] If that category is applied, acute low back pain is pain that has not persisted longer than 5 to 7 weeks.

Establishing the length of illness is both relevant and important if management is to be guided by evidence. The evidence for the causes and management of acute low back pain differs considerably from that for chronic low back pain. The evidence for subacute low back pain is more closely related to that for acute low back pain, but differs in certain respects.

Spread

Low back pain need not be restricted to the lumbar or sacral regions. From various sources in the lumbar spine and sacrum, pain can be referred into the lower limb. This type of pain is classified as somatic referred pain. It is pain perceived in a region innervated by nerves other than the nerves that innervate the actual source of pain.[1] As an approximate rule, somatic referred pain is perceived in structures that share the same segmental innervation as the source of pain.

Experiments in normal volunteers and patients have shown that pain from the lumbar zygapophyseal joints, the lumbar intervertebral discs, lumbar ligaments, posterior lumbar muscles, and from the sacroiliac joint can spread across the gluteal region, into the thigh, and even into the leg and foot (Fig. 71.3).[4-9]

The location and distribution does not help in the diagnosis of the source of pain, for they are related to the segmental innervation of the source but not to the specific source itself. However, the distribution of pain is one factor that helps distinguish somatic referred pain from radicular pain. Of all things that have been revealed by research over the last 70 years, this distinction has still failed to permeate education on back pain.

Somatic referred pain tends to spread over broad areas. The patient usually finds it difficult to identify the boundaries of where it is felt, but they can indicate its centroid. Once established, somatic referred pain is sessile in nature; although the area in which it is felt may fluctuate in size with the intensity of the pain, its location tends to be fixed. In contrast, radicular pain is typically perceived along a narrow band (Fig. 71.4). Furthermore, radicular pain travels longitudinally into the lower limb. Other distinguishing features relate to the quality of pain.

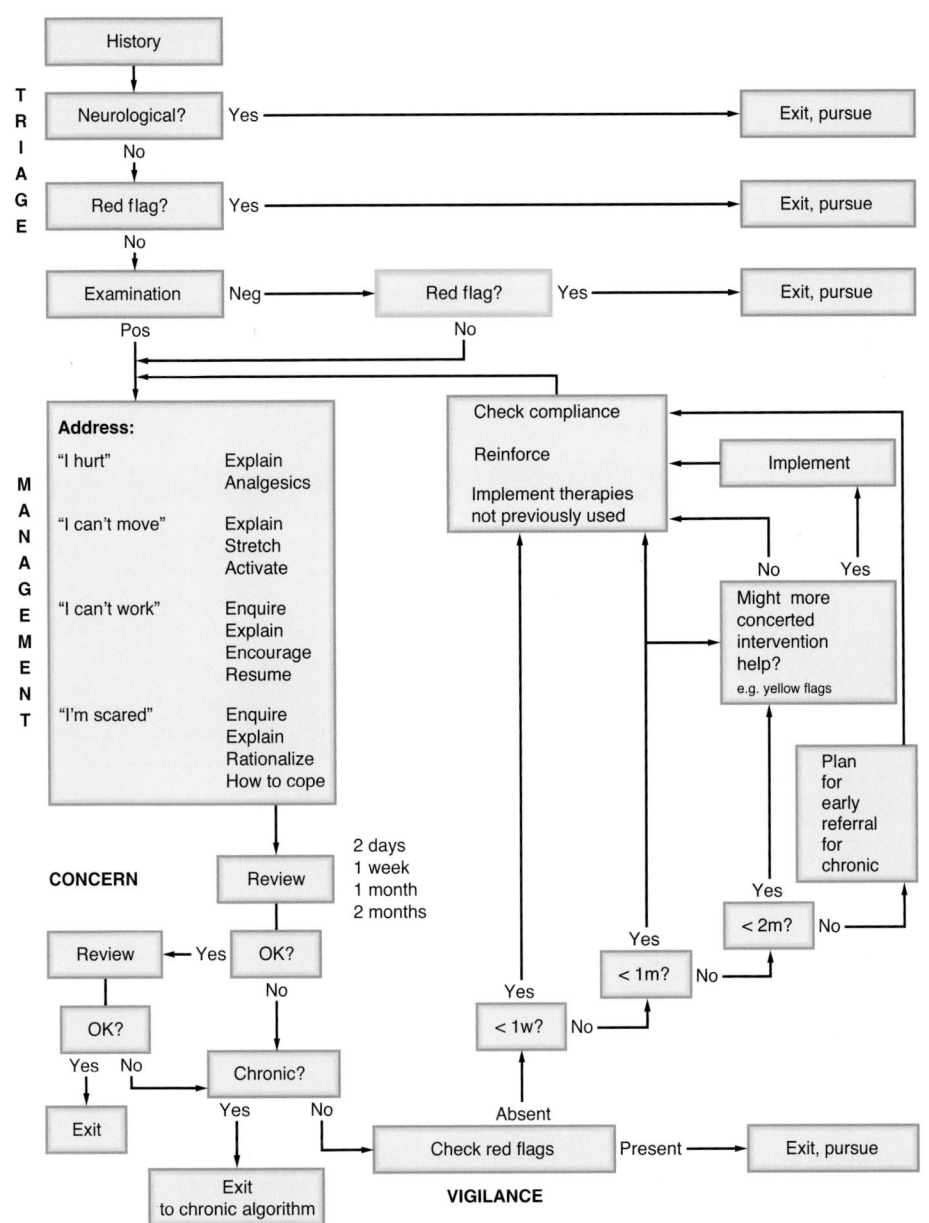

FIGURE 71.1 An algorithm for the management of acute low back pain.

TABLE 71.1

DOMAINS OF INQUIRY FOR THE SYSTEMIC HISTORY OF ANY PAIN PROBLEM

Site
Length of Illness
Spread
Quality
Intensity
Frequency
Duration
Time of onset
Mode of onset
Precipitating factors
Aggravating factors
Relieving factors
Associated features

Quality

Low back pain and somatic referred pain tend to be dull and aching in quality. In some instances, the pain feels like an expanding pressure. Although not diagnostic of the source or cause of pain, these features distinguish somatic referred pain from radicular pain. Radicular pain is lancinating, shooting, or electric in quality.

Making the distinction between somatic referred pain and radicular pain—on the basis of its distribution and quality—is a significant and important step in the assessment of patients. The investigation and subsequent management of lumbar radicular pain are distinctly different from those for somatic referred pain.[9,10] Whereas neurological examination and medical imaging are indicated for radicular pain, they are neither invited nor required for somatic referred pain. Failure to make this distinction has confounded much of the past literature on these entities. It is not evident the extent to which patients described in the past as having had radicular pain—or sciatica—actually had somatic referred pain. Consequently, the extent to which the efficacy of

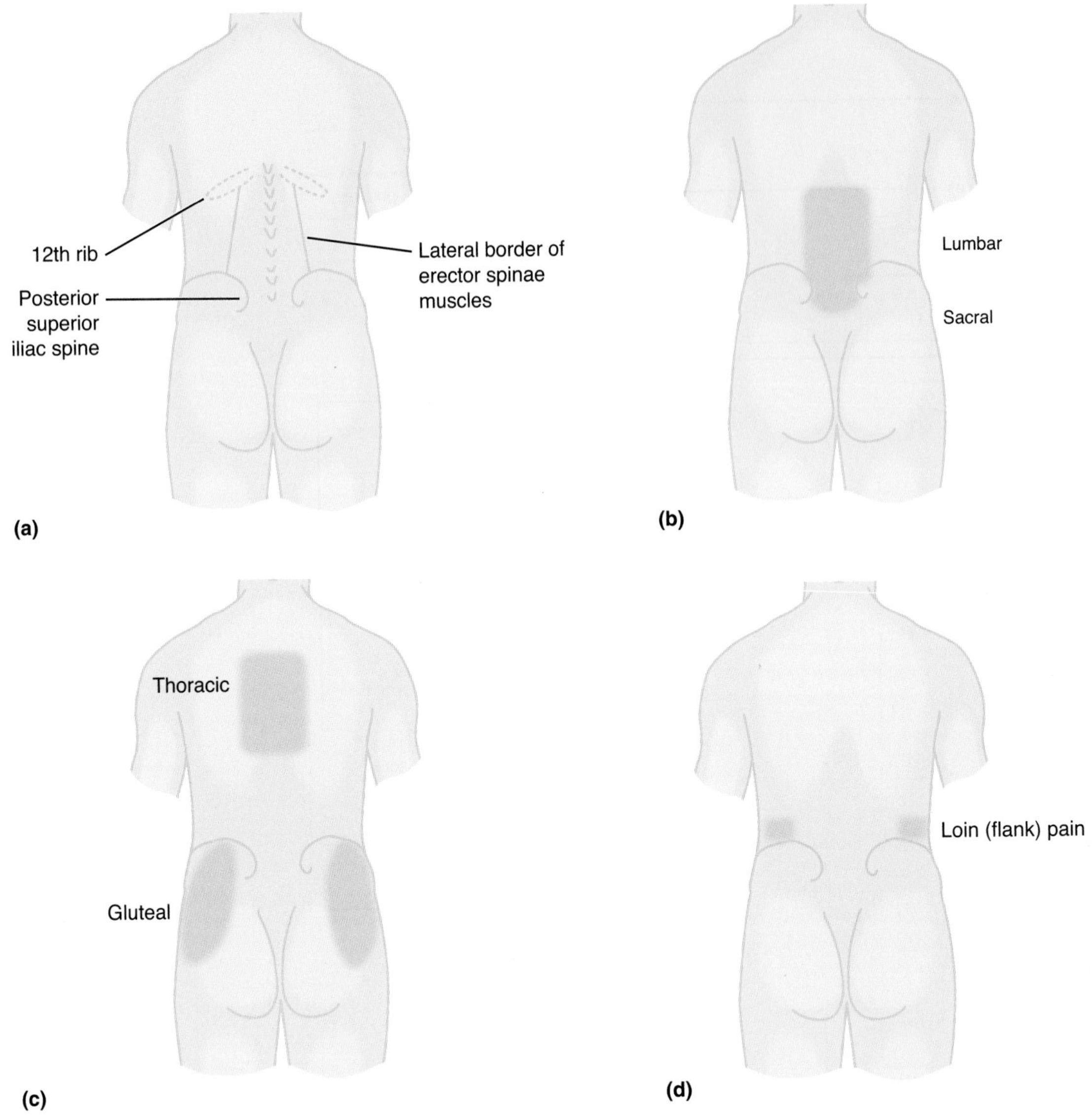

(a)

12th rib

Posterior superior iliac spine

Lateral border of erector spinae muscles

(b)

Lumbar

Sacral

(c)

Thoracic

Gluteal

(d)

Loin (flank) pain

FIGURE 71.2 The definition of what is back pain and what is not. **A.** Landmarks for the definition of lumbar spinal pain. **B.** The topographical location of lumbar spinal pain and sacral spinal pain, any combination of which amounts to low back pain. **C.** Thoracic spinal pain and gluteal pain. **D.** Loin pain.

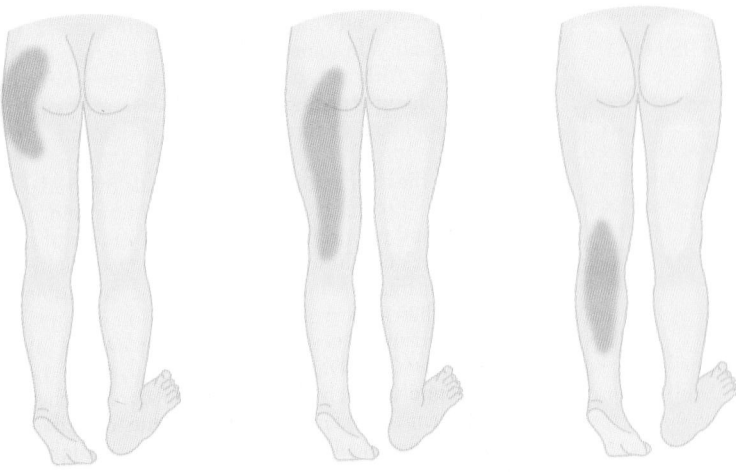

FIGURE 71.3 Various patterns of distribution of somatic referred pain from the lumbar spine.

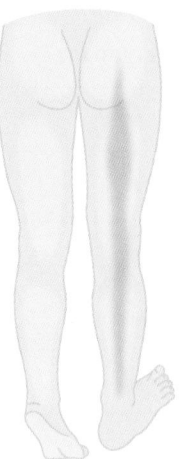

FIGURE 71.4 The pattern of radicular pain. Radicular pain is felt along a narrow band traveling into the lower limb.

treatments have been compromised for the distinction having not been made is not evident. A different base of evidence, and a different algorithm, applies for the management of acute lumbar radicular pain.[9,10]

Intensity

A patient can provide a measure of the intensity of their pain by completing a visual analog scale[12,13] or a numerical pain rating scale.[13,14] High scores, however, are difficult to interpret in a valid manner. Although they might indicate severe pain because of serious pathology, high scores may be no more than an indication that the patient feels that they are suffering, even though the cause of their pain may not be serious. Other features help to indicate if the patient has a serious cause for severe pain.

Frequency and Duration

Variables such as the frequency of episodes of pain and their duration are of greater relevance to other forms of pain, such as headache and visceral pain. In the context of low back pain, they are not critical for diagnosis. For patients whose pain is constant they are, by definition, irrelevant. For patients with intermittent pain they are of value only for gauging the patient's overall disability.

Time of Onset

Temporal variables are of greater relevance for other types of pain that are distinctly periodic in nature. The occurrence of back pain at particular times of the day, particular days of the week, or particular weeks of the month may indicate an association with particular precipitating factors or visceral disorders, but is otherwise not material to diagnosis.

Mode of Onset

When the onset of back pain has been gradual or otherwise unremarkable, there is little relevance to this variable. A sudden onset of severe pain for no obvious reason is not diagnostic of any cause, but constitutes an alerting feature to possible serious causes. Those are distinguished by associated features.

Precipitating Factors

In the sense of pathology, there are no causes of acute low back pain that bear a relationship to particular precipitating factors. However, inquiry into precipitating factors may reveal risk factors in the way the patient undertakes work, domestic, or other physical activities.

Aggravating Factors

Back pain of virtually any cause is likely to be aggravated by movement. Thus, this variable is of little diagnostic significance when positive. More informative—and alerting—is back pain that is not aggravated by movements or particular activity. It suggests a source that is not subject to compression loading in the lumbar spine or tension in its joints and ligaments. Visceral and vascular disorders have this property, as can malignancy until it starts to affect spinal joints.

Relieving Factors

Relieving factors are the complement to aggravating factors. Pain that is not relieved by rest should invite a concerted consideration of possible sinister causes.

Associated Features

The domain of associated features is the most critical and revealing domain of inquiry about low back pain. Serious causes of pain will usually be evident through the features, other than pain, that they produce. Conversely, case reports that describe missed diagnoses often reveal elements in the history that would have revealed the cause had a thorough inquiry about associated features been conducted earlier.

Associated features encompass a variety of historical and social features as well as a review of symptoms in other body systems. A checklist of these features has been developed[15] (Fig. 71.5), and found effective in field trials.[16] The checklist serves as a reminder to ask about features that constitute so-called red flag indicators. A positive response to any of the items does not necessarily implicate a serious cause of pain; that requires other evidence. However, negative responses to all of the items render vanishingly small the probability of a serious cause for back pain.

The first column of the checklist reminds the user to check for elements in the history that constitute risk factors for fracture, infection, or cancer as the cause of pain. It also prompts consideration of what might be considered rare, or exotic, causes of pain; for example, helminthic diseases in patients who are farmers or who have been exposed to animals, fungal diseases in patients exposed to birds or caves, or other infections in patients who have traveled to undeveloped countries or regions. A particularly exotic example is exposure to spear grass (a plant found in Northern Australia), whose seed can burrow into tissues using an osmotically driven corkscrew action.

The second and third columns prompt a review of body systems, diseases of which may produce back pain or are associated with it. The cardiovascular system should be assessed to look for risk factors for peripheral vascular disease. The urinary system and skin should be assessed as possible sites of infection. The endocrine system should be assessed to look for risk factors for infection (e.g., diabetes mellitus, use of corticosteroids). As well, hyperparathy-

Name:					LOW BACK PAIN		
Date of birth:			Medical Record No.				
History of:			Cardiovascular			Endocrine		
Trauma	Y	N	Risk factors?	Y	N	Diabetes?	Y	N
Sports injury	Y	N	Respiratory			Corticosteroids?	Y	N
Fever, night sweats	Y	N	Cough?	Y	N	Parathyroid	Y	N
Recent surgery	Y	N	Urinary			Musculoskeletal		
Catheterization	Y	N	Infection?	Y	N	Pain elsewhere?	Y	N
Venipuncture	Y	N	Hematuria?	Y	N	Neurological		
Illicit drug use	Y	N	Retention?	Y	N	Symptoms/signs?	Y	N
Weight loss	Y	N	Stream problems?	Y	N	Skin		
Past history of cancer	Y	N	Reproductive			Infection?	Y	N
Occupational exposure	Y	N	Menstrual?	Y	N	Rashes?	Y	N
Hobby exposure	Y	N	Hemopoietic			GIT		
(Overseas) travel	Y	N	Problems?	Y	N	Diarrhea?	Y	N
Comments:					Signature		
					Date:		

FIGURE 71.5 A checklist for red flag clinical indicators, suitable for inclusion in medical records used in general practice.[15]

roidism can present with spinal pain. The urinary, reproductive, respiratory, and hemopoietic systems should be assessed for neoplastic diseases. The musculoskeletal and gastrointestinal systems and skin should be assessed for features of spondylarthropathies. The neurological system should be assessed for features of intrinsic or extrinsic lesions of the spinal cord or nerve roots.

Fractures are an uncommon cause of acute low back pain, and when they are there should be a reason for a fracture to have occurred. Fractures may occur in patients exposed to severe trauma, but in the absence of trauma, fractures will not be the cause of back pain unless the patient has a reason for pathological fracture. The risk factors for pathological fracture are osteoporosis, prolonged use of corticosteroids (causing osteoporosis), and a past history of cancer.

Stress fractures of the pars interarticularis are a distinctive entity. In the general population their prevalence is no greater in patients with back pain than in subjects with no pain.[17] Therefore, they cannot be invoked as causes of pain in that population. However, their prevalence is far greater among athletes, particu-larly those who perform extension, rotation, or combinations of extension and rotation of their lumbar spine. In such individuals the challenge lies in identifying stress reactions before they fracture, for then the fracture can be avoided. Inquiring about a patient's sporting activities is, therefore, pertinent in the triage of patients presenting with acute low back pain.

Although infection can be a cause of back pain, accurate figures on its prevalence are not available. One estimate puts the figure at less than 0.01%,[18] but this may be an underestimate. The alerting features for infection as a possible cause are factors that explain why a patient should have a spinal infection. These include a history of body penetration (by illicit drug use, tattooing, recent surgery, catheterization, venipuncture, or a known site of infection) or compromised resistance to infection (immunosuppression, diabetes, alcohol abuse). Overt indicators are fever and night sweats.[19]

Cancer is responsible for acute low back pain in less than 0.7% of patients, and is four times more likely in patients over 50.[20] The cardinal indicators for cancer as a cause are past history of cancer, unexplained weight loss, age over 50, and symptoms of visceral dysfunction, particularly the lungs, thyroid gland, prostate, and kidney, which are the most common sources of metastases to the spine.

The significance of aortic aneurysm as a cause of back pain has possibly been understated in the past. In many cases of deaths from ruptured aortic aneurysms, the presenting feature was back pain, and the condition was overlooked.[21] In terms of history, the cardinal features are risk factors for peripheral vascular disease.

Because serious causes of acute low back pain are uncommon, the likelihood of a patient having a serious cause is very low. Moreover, the likelihood is virtually zero if the patient has no other feature of the serious disorder. Serious disorders, therefore, can effectively be ruled out if the responses to the checklist are all negative.

Positive responses do not mean that a serious cause is present. They serve only to raise suspicion. The actual diagnosis is confirmed or excluded by other actions. The clinical features that should raise suspicion about particular serious causes are listed in Table 71.2. This table also lists the appropriate confirmatory investigations (see Investigations, below).

Physical Examination

Examination of the lumbar spine has traditionally involved palpation for tenderness, and assessing active and passive ranges of movement. Some craft groups contend that passive intervertebral motion can and should be tested. The evidence from the available literature indicates that conventional physical examination procedures lack reliability, validity, or both.[22] Nothing found by various maneuvers or tests reliably implicates any source of cause of pain with any validity.

The exception to this may be spinal assessment by the McKenzie method. Two studies have shown that careful, specialized examination can identify patients with sacroiliac joint pain[23] and patients with internal disc disruption.[24] These studies, however, were based on patients with chronic low back pain, in whom these two conditions are common. Their prevalence in patients with acute low back pain is not known and, therefore, the validity of the McKenzie assessment in these patients has not been established.

Nevertheless, there are two reasons for conducting a physical examination. In the first instance, patients expect to be examined, and performing an examination is an indication that the physician is interested in the patient and concerned about them. The fact that nothing found on examination is diagnostic is immaterial in this context. The second reason is ironic. Of greater significance than finding positive features on examination is finding no physical features in the lumbar spine. Absence of somatic signs prompts a serious consideration of visceral and vascular causes of low back pain. A pertinent aphorism is: if the patient has no signs in their back, turn them over and examine their abdomen and pelvis.

Although classical teaching prescribes a neurological examination for patients with low back pain it is neither warranted nor justified. If a patient reports a history of neurological symptoms, such as weakness or numbness, a neurological examination becomes mandatory, but in that context the indication for neurological examination is the neurological symptoms—not the back pain. Neurological diseases do not present with back pain as the only feature. In patients with back pain as the sole feature, physicians might elect to perform a neurological examination in order to appear thorough, but they should be under no illusion that it serves to establish a diagnosis. This guideline should not be confused with neurological examination in a patient with radicular pain. Neurological examination is indicated if the patient has radiculopathy, but in that context, it is pain in the leg—not pain in the back—that is the indication for neurological examination.

TABLE 71.2

CLINICAL INDICATORS AND PREFERRED INVESTIGATIONS FOR POSSIBLE SERIOUS CAUSES OF SPINAL PAIN

Suspected Pathology	Clinical indicators	Preferred test	
Fracture	Severe trauma	1st line	X-ray
Stress fracture	Sporting activity involving spinal extension, rotation, or both	1st line 2nd line	Bone scan or MRI X-ray
Pathological fracture	Osteoporosis Prolonged use of corticosteroids Past history of cancer	1st line 2nd line	X-ray MRI
Infection	Fever, sweating Risk factors for infection: (invasive medical procedure, injection, illicit drug use, trauma to skin or mucous membrane, immunosuppression, diabetes mellitus, alcoholism)	1st line 2nd line	ESR, FBC, CRP MRI
Tumor	Past history of malignancy Age greater than 50 Failure to improve Weight loss Pain not relieved by rest	All cases 1st line 2nd line Prostate Myeloma	 1: ESR, CRP 2: MRI PSA IEPG, serum protein electrophoresis
Aortic aneurysm	Cardiovascular risk factors Anticoagulants No musculoskeletal signs	1st line	Ultrasound

CRP, C-reactive protein; ESR, erythrocyte sedimentation rate; FBC, full blood count; IEPG, immuno-electrophoretogram; MRI, magnetic resonance imaging; PSA, prostate specific antigen.

A component of physical examination that has not been formally studied pertains to the demeanor of the patient. This can be helpful in identifying patients with serious causes of pain. Patients with infections and cancer are typically serious, subdued, or quietly guarded in their presentation. They avoid movement, and are apprehensive about being examined. Their general demeanor is grim—as if, intuitively, they know that something serious is wrong. That appearance is distinctly not histrionic. Although they may rate their pain as severe, they do not incessantly draw attention to it. Beware the quiet patient with severe pain.

Investigations

Much research has overturned past habits of routine investigations for acute low back pain. Investigations, such as plain radiography, CT scanning, or magnetic resonance imaging (MRI), are not justified either "just in case" or to reveal something that is not evident on history. In the absence of specific clinical indicators, the yield of these investigations is next to zero.

Plain radiography lacks sensitivity and specificity for any cause of back pain other than fractures. It is indicated only for those patients who have risk factors for fracture (Table 71.2).

Neither CT nor MRI has ever been shown to demonstrate a cause of back pain in patients with no clinical indicators of fracture, infection, or cancer, or in the absence of neurological signs. In that regard, the use of CT or MRI in patients with back pain should not be confused with its use in patients with radicular pain or neurological signs. In those conditions it is the neurological features that are the indication for investigation—not the back pain.

Apart from not being diagnostic, medical imaging has the liability of needlessly alarming patients. To the uninformed patient, the vocabulary of radiology reports sounds serious and significant. Terms such as "spondylosis," "spondylolisthesis," and "degenerative changes" sound like the patient has a disease that both explains their pain and requires treatment. However, the evidence shows that these conditions are not related to pain.[25]

Nor is it an argument that patients expect imaging. They do so only when they remain uninformed. A controlled study has shown that 5 minutes of explanation deters most patients from wanting unnecessary radiographs.[26] The arguments against imaging include their lack of sensitivity and specificity, the very low likelihood of finding anything, the possibility of false-positive findings and the distress that they can cause, the possible false sense of security from a negative result, and the health hazards of radiation exposure.

Investigations are indicated only if the patient has features on history of a possible serious cause of pain (Table 71.2). In that event, imaging is not the default investigation. Laboratory tests take precedence for the assessment of infection and tumor.

Studies have shown that imaging did not detect an occult cancer if patients were under 50, had no history of cancer, no weight loss, and no signs of systemic illness.[20,27] In patients over the age of 50, or with unexplained weight loss or signs of systemic illness, imaging did not detect cancer if their erythrocyte sedimentation rate (ESR) was less than 20 mm/hour. Therefore, for suspected cancer, the indications for imaging are either a past history of cancer or a raised ESR. The appropriate imaging is either bone scan or MRI. Both are equally sensitive, but MRI has greater specificity.

In athletes in whom a stress fracture is suspected, the imperative is to detect a stress reaction before actual fracture. Doing so allows the pars interarticularis to be protected from further stress and allowed to heal. Once fractures occur, there is no guarantee that they will unite. Bone scan has been the traditional investigation, but it lacks specificity; it cannot distinguish between a stress

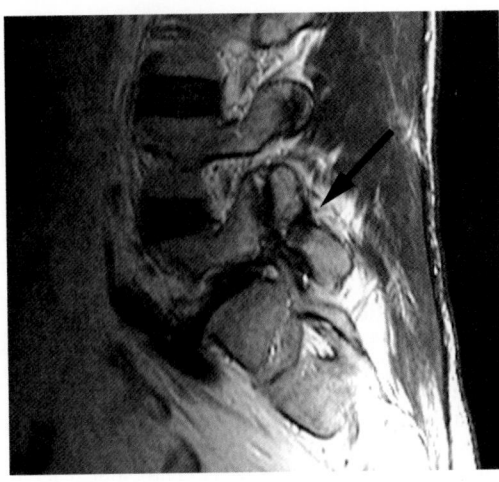

FIGURE 71.6 An MRI scan clearly showing a fracture (arrowed) of the pars interarticularis of L5 fracture. (Courtesy of Dr. Time Maus of the Mayo Clinic, Rochester, MN.)

reaction and an actual fracture. MRI can detect and distinguish both, and should be the preferred investigation (Fig. 71.6).

Formulation

The role of triage is to identify serious conditions or exclude them. If a patient has a neurological condition, possible cancer, or infection, they should be managed in a manner appropriate for the condition suspected or diagnosed. Their further management is dictated by the condition causing their pain, not by their back pain.

Mercifully, serious causes of acute low back pain are rare. Therefore, for the majority of patients, triage will not provide a diagnosis. There is no evidence as to what the causes of acute low back pain are. History alone does not provide a diagnosis, nor does physical examination or imaging in the absence of red flag indicators.

Although this may feel disheartening or contrary to the expectations of both physicians and patients, a diagnosis is not required. The natural history of acute low back pain is favorable, and successful management can be instituted without a formal, patho-anatomic diagnosis.

Physicians should also not feel obliged to make a diagnosis on the occasion of the first consultation. Indeed, it might not be possible to do so. Even serious conditions may be early in their evolution and will escape detection if investigations are undertaken too early. The protection that physicians have is vigilance. Reviewing the patient allows them to check for the evolution of new features. For that reason, review and vigilance become critical components of management.

INITIAL MANAGEMENT

The precepts of good medical management of a patient with acute low back pain can be encapsulated by the patient's cardinal complaints: "I hurt; I can't move; I can't work; and I'm scared."[28,29]

Pain

The foremost tool for the management of acute low back pain is **explanation**. That explanation has two aspects: what the patient does not have, and what the patient does have.

The practitioner should explain to the patient that the chances of a serious cause are extremely low, and are even lower because of their negative responses to the red flag checklist. If pressed, the practitioner can explain why there is no need for any special investigations. If patients ask about x-rays, the practitioner should take the time to explain why they are not indicated.

Once the red flag issues have been covered, the practitioner should provide an explanation of why the patient does have pain. It does not matter if this explanation is not academically valid; it simply has to indicate to the patient that the practitioner does know what is going on. In this regard it is not so much what the practitioner says that is important, but the manner in which they say it. Providing an explanation is the opposite of appearing uncertain or alarmed about what the problem might be. Providing an explanation is the opposite of panicking and pursuing unnecessary investigations that alarm the patient and reinforce their fears that something serious is wrong.

Individual practitioners may develop their own pattern of offering an explanation. One that has been tested[30,31] is to explain to patients, in simple terms, that they have internal disc disruption: a small injury that is presently inflamed and sore, but which will settle.[30] Depending on the situation, practitioners might prefer an alternative model. They might care to explain to the patient that they have strained their back muscles, or that their muscles are sore because they have been undertaking activities in an inefficient manner.

Whatever the model used, the art of explanation can be encapsulated by the six C's (Table 71.3). The explanation should be **credible**: It should fit the patient's circumstances and be intelligible to them. The practitioner should present the explanation in a **confident** manner; uncertainty in the explanation breeds doubts in the patient. The practitioner should be **convincing**, which requires monitoring the patient's response to the explanation and addressing any uncertainties. **Concerted** means that the practitioner should show that they are trying hard to help the patient. Throughout the explanation the practitioner should show that they **care** about the patient and their complaint. **Concern** does not mean alarm about possible serious causes of pain; it is related to caring and means taking the patient seriously. All of these attributes amount to the opposite of being fast, perfunctory, and dismissive.

The second tool at the disposal of the practitioner is the evidence on the natural history of acute low back pain. Provided that patients are managed properly, the natural history is very favorable. About 80% can be expected to fully recover.[16] Explaining this fact constitutes evidence-based practice. The practitioner should explain to the patient, in terms that they will understand, that the odds are in their favor; that there is every chance of recovering (even regardless of treatment), but that it may take time. During that time, there are certain measures that both the practitioner and the patient can take to ease the situation while this recovery takes place.

For medical practitioners, the traditional intervention for acute low back pain has been to prescribe analgesics. It is conspicuous, however, that the evidence base for this action is markedly weak.

Multiple guidelines recommend paracetamol (acetaminophen), on a time-contingent basis, as the first-line drug if analgesics are required.[2,32-35] These recommendations, however, are based on the reputation of this drug as an analgesic, and its relative lack of side effects when used in appropriate doses. Explicit evidence of its efficacy for acute low back pain is lacking. At best, its efficacy is evident only from studies in which it has been used as a control treatment. It has not been shown to be more effective than placebo.[2,36,37]

Some guidelines permit or recommend nonsteroidal anti-inflammatory drugs (NSAIDs) as a second-line drug if paracetamol proves ineffective or patients require greater analgesia. This recommendation is based on the assumption that NSAIDs are effective, or in some way more effective than paracetamol, for acute low back pain. Evidence of this is lacking. An earlier review found NSAIDs to be more effective than placebo for the outcome measure global perceived effect, but for the outcome measure relief of pain, they were not more effective than placebo.[37] A later review[38] reported that NSAIDs were more effective than placebo, but of the four studies used for the meta-analysis, two used intramuscular injections rather than oral medication. Of the remaining two studies one found no superiority over placebo,[39] but the other did find superiority.[40] The margin in favor of placebo, however, amounted to only 8 points on a 100-point pain scale, and was measured only at 7 days.

Instead of drugs, an expedient and effective alternative for the short-term relief of acute low back pain is superficial heat, in the form of low-level heatwrap therapy. Applying heat to the back has been shown to be more effective than placebo, both in general patients[41-44] and in workers with back pain,[45] and is more effective than either ibuprofen or acetaminophen.[46] It has been rated as a cost-effective intervention.[47]

Other interventions commonly used in the past for the relief of pain in patients with acute low back pain either lack formal evidence of efficacy or have been shown to be ineffective. They should be avoided, not only because they are ineffective, but also because they conflict with the precept of empowering the patient to become responsible for their own rehabilitation.

Bed rest is ineffective for acute low back pain.[48] Its use denies patients the proven benefits of staying active (see Movement, below). Although antidepressants are used to relieve pain, there is no evidence that they are effective for acute low back pain.[36] Although systematic reviews have concluded that muscle relaxants may be effective,[49] the source literature speaks otherwise. Orphenadrine, diazepam, and tizanidine are not more effective than placebo.[36] Dantrolene is more effective than placebo but only for reducing pain upon maximum voluntary contraction.[36] Methocarbamol is no more effective than the tranquilizer chlormezanone, which itself is no more effective than mefenamic acid.[36] Carisoprodol reduces pain to a greater extent than placebo but has been tested only at 4 days.[36] Baclofen reduces pain more than placebo, but only by 20%.[36] The reduction of pain by cyclobenzaprine (by 5.5 points on a 10-point scale) is barely greater than the reduction achieved by placebo (4 points), but cyclobenzaprine is not more effective than NSAIDs.[36]

For the relief of pain in patients with acute low back pain, exercises have been shown to be no more effective than other conservative interventions, including no intervention.[50,51] The role of exercises lies in restoring movement, rather than in relieving pain (see Movement, below).

For acute low back pain, belts or corsets,[52,53] traction,[54] and transcutaneous electrical nerve stimulation[55] are not effective; back school has been shown to be ineffective[55]; and there is no evidence for acupuncture.[56] Multidisciplinary pain management has explicitly been shown to be ineffective for acute low back pain.[57] It is not indicated early in the course of management. It becomes a valid option if pain persists into the subacute phase.[57]

TABLE 71.3

THE SIX C'S THAT DEFINE THE ATTRIBUTES OF GOOD EXPLANATION OF A PATIENT'S ACUTE LOW BACK PAIN

Credible
Confident
Convincing
Concerted
Caring
Concern

There is no evidence that formal behavioral therapy is effective.[54] Such evidence as might support behavioral therapy pertains to regularly reviewing the patient's progress, acknowledging any difficulties the patient has in maintaining activities of daily living and being encouraging and helpful in this regard, and promoting self-management.

Various guidelines recommend issuing patients with an educational booklet about back pain. This might serve to standardize information provided, and practitioners might consider it an aid in their endeavors, but booklets achieve little effect when used alone.[58,59] They are not a substitute for explanation, support, and encouragement provided personally by the caring practitioner.

Perhaps the most contentious intervention is manual therapy. Conclusions from systematic reviews about the evidence are mixed, and seem to reflect the inclinations or preferences of authors rather than the strength of the evidence. Whereas some reviewers accepted that there is moderate evidence that spinal manipulative therapy provides greater relief of pain in the short-term than other interventions,[60] other reviewers found that there is no evidence that spinal manipulative therapy is superior to other standard treatments for acute low back pain.[61] Moreover, manual therapy contravenes the recommendations of guidelines to avoid passive treatment.

A protocol commonly practiced in primary care is to supplement advice with either an NSAID or spinal manipulative therapy. However, when this protocol was tested, it emerged that neither adding an NSAID nor adding manipulative therapy conferred any greater benefit to patients.[62]

Movement

Multiple studies and reviews have consistently shown that maintaining activity is a crucial component in the management of acute low back pain.[16,30,48] The emphasis lies not in treating a particular pathology but in resuming or maintaining activity, in a holistic sense, in order to prevent the patient being disabled by their pain. The intervention is coupled with explanation, encouragement, and empowering the patient to take responsibility for their own management.

The practitioner should explain to the patient that the evidence shows that those who resume activities have a much more favorable prognosis and recover more quickly and more thoroughly than patients who resort to rest and avoid activities.[48] A model of explanation that has successfully been used is to explain that muscle tightness is a normal reaction to pain but one that can be deleterious; allowing the back to seize up or become stiff not only interferes with movement but can add to the pain.[30] The objective of treatment, therefore, is to prevent and overcome stiffness.

This can be achieved by teaching the patient a set of simple stretching exercises.[63] These are not exercises that require supervision or attendance at a facility, such as a physiotherapy practice or gymnasium. They are exercises that can, and should, be executed virtually anywhere that the patient needs them. In order to reduce stiffness and keep the patient mobile, the patient should perform the exercises at strategic or ceremonial times of the day, such as upon rising, before going to work, at coffee breaks, or lunchtime. In the sense of a "warm-up," they can be applied as a preparatory and preventive measure prior to undertaking a major activity, such as commencing chores. As a first-aid measure, they can be applied to ease exacerbations of pain after sustained activity or prolonged sitting. Providing a first-aid measure is one of the crucial steps in empowering the patient to be able to look after themselves. Exercises that the patient can do by themselves, and for themselves, are crucial to avoiding passive interventions and becoming dependent on them.

Work

All guidelines on occupational low back pain emphasize the benefits of returning to work or remaining at work.[64–66] Patients who do so inherit a better prognosis than those who do not.

The obstructing factor in this context lies not in the patient but in the attitude of the treating practitioner. It is easier, and faster, to write a certificate for time off work than to explain to the patient why they do not need one.[67] The attitudes of practitioners are difficult to change. Changing patients is far less of a problem.

The practitioner should share with the worker the evidence of the benefits of returning to work. They should inquire as to why the patient feels or believes that they cannot return to work.

Fears of aggravating the pain will already have been partly addressed by confidently providing a credible explanation for the pain, coupled with an explanation that activity will not do harm. That message is reinforced by helping the patient resume movements, and empowering them to do so (see Movement, above). Those movements include work.

Some patients may have pain of high intensity that temporarily impedes their ability and capacity to resume their accustomed work. For such patients modified work duties may be required. Unfortunately, there is no evidence in the form of controlled trials that vindicate the prescription of modified duties. Their reputation rests on anecdotal and observational data. The strongest evidence lies in a cohort study, which found that keeping patients at work, with modified duties as required, resulted in a greater proportion of patients fully recovered, and fewer recurrences, than did usual care.[67]

Prescribing modified duties imposes a responsibility. The practitioner should not forget the patient. The objective of modified duties is to have the patient remain at work but progressively restore their capacity for former duties. During this period, the patient and their progress need to be monitored. As soon as they are able, the patient should return to full work. A certificate and its expiration date do not magically achieve this; it is the continued involvement of the practitioner that does so.

Inquiry into the patient's beliefs about work may reveal extraneous but pertinent issues. They may resent their work environment or their supervisor. They may harbor fears about recurrences of accidents in which they were injured. Such issues raise agendas that are separate and additional to the back pain. Those agendas need to be pursued and managed parallel to the back pain itself.

In the first instance, the practitioner needs to elicit from the worker the beliefs and concerns that they have. Mistaken beliefs can be discussed and corrected. Misplaced concerns can be allayed. Otherwise, workplace intervention may be required. If the practitioner cannot exercise this, the services of a skilled practitioner in occupational medicine should be recruited.

The evidence strongly supports the efficacy of workplace intervention. Whether as an isolated intervention, or adding it to medical management, workplace intervention improves outcomes.[68] It is conspicuous, however, that the contents of the workplace intervention are immaterial. The effective ingredient does not lie in the specifics of ergonomic or related changes. What counts is that the worker has an advocate who acts on their behalf and in their interests. This is done in the context of solving problems with the participation of supervisors and management. Solutions may lie in modifying the physical work environment, social work environment, work flow, or work demands. The solution should be cast in a manner such as to benefit all parties. The worker returns to an improved environment. The employer avoids the problem of additional injuries and claims, and the burden of increased insurance premiums. Advocacy is paramount in these negotiations. Workers typically do not have access to management, whom they regard as intransigent and uncaring. The occupational physician has the appropriate "social rank" to appear before management and to explain the circumstances to them.

Workplace intervention takes time and requires a particular, skilled aptitude. General practitioners and others may not have this time or aptitude. That, however, is not a pretext for overlooking or neglecting workplace intervention. Persisting problems with return to work, in a practice or in a region, are an indication that specialist skills need to be recruited.

Fear

Fear is the most damaging characteristic that a patient with acute low back pain can harbor. Their fears might pertain to what is wrong biologically, what is going to be done medically, or what is going to happen socially. Such fears inhibit the patient's recovery. It is important, therefore, that any such fears be discovered and addressed.

It is not necessary or expected for a practitioner to address the fears that a patient might have at the first consultation. However, the possibility of fears should be noted and their exploration resumed at follow-up visits.

The practitioner can explore possible fears in the course of a normal consultation, either by being alert to what the patient might mention or allude to spontaneously, or checking for fears through simple questions, such as "What do you think is the cause of pain? What do you think needs to be done? What do you think is going to happen?"

Fears about the biology of back pain are covered by providing a credible, convincing explanation, reinforced by repetition if necessary. Fears about prognosis and consequences are covered by explaining to the patient the favorable natural history of acute low back pain. Fears about management are covered by providing the patient with a concerted plan that empowers them and does not leave them abandoned. Fears about work, employment, and future are encompassed by the workplace intervention.

REVIEW

In the past, physicians believed that if the patient does not return, they must be all right. This myth has been dispelled. A longitudinal study in British primary care followed patients after they presented to general practitioners with acute low back pain.[69] They did not return to the general practitioners, who (naturally) assumed that they had recovered. Research nurses found that only 25% of patients had recovered; the remainder continued to suffer; but they did not return to their general practitioner because they felt that they were not being helped.

Patients with acute low back pain should not be abandoned, and they should not feel abandoned. The risk of doing so is that patients will exaggerate and prolong their disability, if left to fend for themselves. The singular measure against this eventuality is planned concern. The treating practitioner should schedule a follow-up with the patient. This might be a conventional consultation, or it might be no more than a telephone follow-up. If patients have recovered, and report that they do not need further care, no more need be done; however, if patients have not recovered, face-to-face follow-up is indicated.

An algorithm with scheduled follow-up allows busy practitioners to divide their management into initial triage at the first consultation, and further exploration at the subsequent consultation. This deflates the perceived burden of having to get everything done on the first occasion.

If the patient is progressing well, further follow-up can be decreased or dispensed with. If they are not progressing, the review consultation provides the opportunity for the succeeding steps in the algorithm.

VIGILANCE

A review consultation allows the practitioner to exercise vigilance. Serious disorders may not be evident at the first consultation. Repeating the checklist for red flags serves to detect the emergence of any new features, which may require changes to the management plan. Relying on clinical monitoring, in this way, obviates the need for precipitous and inappropriate use of investigations at the first consultation.

If red flag features emerge, management appropriate for those features can be pursued. If red flag features do not emerge, the previous management can continue.

REINFORCEMENT

During the review consultation, the practitioner should assess the progress of the patient. If previous management appears to be working, no change is required. If progress to recovery seems to be slow, the practitioner should assess why this might be the case. The practitioner should check if the patient understood the previous plan of management and if they are complying with it. The review consultation provides the opportunity to reinforce previous explanations, if they were not understood, and to check, for example, if the patient has been able to execute any exercises correctly. If the patient is not complying, the reasons for that need to be elicited. Misunderstandings can be corrected. If unjustified resistance is the reason, that raises an agenda in the management plan that is not back pain.

If progress is not occurring despite adequate compliance, consideration needs to be given to implementing interventions not previously used. If exercises were not prescribed at the first consultation, they can be introduced now. If the patient is having difficulties restoring movement, a supervised exercise program conducted in a cognitive–behavioral milieu can be effective.[70]

Yellow Flags

Slow progress to recovery may be due to undetected, or unrevealed, psychosocial factors, referred to as yellow flag indicators.[71] These pertain to the patient's beliefs and behaviors concerning physical activity and domestic, social, and vocational responsibilities.

When patients believe that physical activity might harm their back, and that they should not undertake activities that make their pain worse, they avoid activities. For most patients with acute low back pain, these beliefs are not justified. Explanation, reassurance, and encouragement to resume activities are the cardinal tools for overcoming these mistaken beliefs. If required, a graded plan of resuming activities can be developed and followed. Some patients may take longer to regain activities. The guiding principle is that increments should be pursued, even if they are small.

Patients may seek to avoid domestic activities and responsibilities, such as cooking, cleaning, maintenance, shopping, and housework, for fear of pain. Avoiding such activities amplifies their disability. Encouragement to resume these activities may be not enough to convince some patients. The accustomed manner in which they do things may not be efficient. They may need help to analyze how else they might acquit the required activity, in a manner that does not aggravate their pain. The guiding principle is not to abandon the activity but to find alternative means to achieve its purpose. In this regard, the practitioner provides their own intellect to help solve the patient's problem.

Patients may avoid social activities, claiming that their back pain prevents them from doing so. But back pain does not directly preclude social activity. The mediating factor is fear that social activity will aggravate their pain. If the patient can regain movement at home, they can apply the same principles away from home. They should be helped to understand that becoming a recluse will not improve their prognosis; if anything, it will hinder their recovery. Encouragement should be coupled with suggestions of what to do if their pain threatens to be aggravated when they are "out." Instead of being an embarrassment, doing the stretching exercises can be turned into an asset (see Movement, above).

Perhaps the most destructive of the yellow flags is the aversion to work. Patients may believe that work caused their pain, work aggravates their pain, that work is too heavy for them, and that they should not work. Such beliefs require patient analysis and discussion. In the majority of cases they will not be true. The practitioner cannot afford to be dismissive and assertive. They need to understand the patient's work, and in a compassionate manner be able to indicate how work can be resumed in a safe manner. If required, the services can be engaged of an occupational physician who is familiar with the patient's industry, and can develop a return to work plan in the context of a workplace intervention.

DISCUSSION

The majority of patients with acute low back pain will not have a serious cause of pain or a serious injury. If treated well, they can expect to recover. They do not need special treatment. The measures outlined in this chapter will suffice. It has been demonstrated that following these evidence-based principles secures recovery in some 70% of patients, sustained at 12 months, with recurrence rates as low as 16%.[16] Moreover, when evidence-based care is provided in a confident, caring manner, patients overwhelmingly find it attractive.[16]

However, evidence-based care will not be universally successful. Among patients who present with acute low back pain will be two subgroups: those with serious psychosocial problems and those with undetected injuries. There are no features by which to identify these patients early in their course. They emerge by elution. As those destined to recover do so, those with difficulties remain.

The time to identify psychosocial problems is during the acute phase. If recognition and intervention are delayed until the problems become chronic, they may become too entrenched to be remediable. Confident and competent primary care practitioners should be able to address and manage psychosocial factors. They require extra time in consultations, but most are not insurmountable.[67] Early referral is required if they do prove insurmountable. Trained psychologists are more likely to achieve better outcomes if they can see patients early in the development of problems.

Patients with injuries that do not resolve with the passage of time are destined to develop chronic pain. If reiteration and reinforcement of simple interventions does not result in progress and resolution, patients at risk of becoming chronic should be identified before they do so. Appointments to pain clinics or spine specialists may take time to obtain, and they are easier to cancel than to get. Therefore, for patients with persistent pain, steps for early referral to appropriate resources become part of the closing phases of the algorithm for acute low back pain. The management of these patients follows a different algorithm, with a different evidence base (see chapter 72).

References

1. Merskey H, Bogduk N, eds. *Classification of Chronic Pain: Descriptions of Chronic Pain Syndromes and Definitions of Pain Terms.* 2nd edition. Seattle: IASP Press; 1994.
2. Australian Acute Musculoskeletal Pain Guidelines Group. *Evidence-Based Management of Acute Musculoskeletal Pain.* Brisbane: Australian Academic Press; 2003 [Online. Available at http://www.nhmrc.gov.au]
3. van Tulder MW, Koes BW, Bouter LM. Conservative treatment of acute and chronic nonspecific low back pain. A systematic review of randomized controlled trials of the most common interventions. *Spine* 1997;22:2128–2156.
4. Mooney V, Robertson J. The facet syndrome. *Clin Orthop* 1976;115:149–156.
5. Bogduk N. Lumbar dorsal ramus syndrome. *Med J Aust* 1980;2:537–541.
6. Fairbank JCT, Park WM, McCall IW, et al. Apophyseal injections of local anesthetic as a diagnostic aid in primary low-back pain syndromes. *Spine* 1981; 6:598–605.
7. Fortin JD, Dwyer AP, West S, et al. Sacroiliac joint: pain referral maps upon applying a new injection/arthrography technique. Part I: asymptomatic volunteers. *Spine* 1994;19:1475–1482.
8. Fukui S, Ohseto K, Shiotani M, et al. Distribution of referred pain from the lumbar zygapophyseal joints and dorsal rami. *Clin J Pain* 1997;13:303–307.
9. O'Neill CW, Kurgansky ME, Derby R, et al. Disc stimulation and patterns of referred pain. *Spine* 2002;27:2776–2281.
10. Bogduk N, Govind J. *Medical Management of Acute Lumbar Radicular Pain: An Evidence-Based Approach.* Newcastle: Newcastle Bone and Joint Institute; 1999.
11. Govind J. Radicular pain, diagnosis. In: Schmidt RR, Willis WD, eds. *Encyclopedia of Pain.* Vol 3. Berlin: Springer; 2007:2081–2083.
12. Strong J, Ashton R, Chant D. Pain intensity measurement in chronic low back pain. *Clin J Pain* 1991;7:209–218.
13. Briggs M, Closs JS. A descriptive study of the use of visual analogue scales and verbal rating scales for the assessment of postoperative pain in orthopedic patients. *J Pain Symptom Manage* 1999;18:438–446.
14. Farrar JT, Young JP Jr, LaMoreaux L, et al. Clinical importance of changes in chronic pain intensity measured on an 11-point numerical pain rating scale. *Pain* 2001;94:149–158.
15. Bogduk N, McGuirk B. *Medical Management of Acute and Chronic Low Back Pain. An Evidence-Based Approach.* Amsterdam: Elsevier; 2002:27–40.
16. McGuirk B, King W, Govind J, et al. Safety, efficacy, and cost-effectiveness of evidence-based guidelines for the management of acute low back pain in primary care. *Spine* 2001;26:2615–2622.
17. Bogduk N, McGuirk B. *Medical Management of Acute and Chronic Low Back Pain. An Evidence-Based Approach.* Amsterdam: Elsevier; 2002:49–63.
18. Deyo RA, Rainville J, Kent DL. What can the history and physical examination tell us about low back pain? *JAMA* 1992;268:760–765.
19. van den Hoogen HM, Koes BW, Eijk JTM, et al. On the accuracy of history, physical examination, and erythrocyte sedimentation rate in diagnosing low back pain in general practice. A criteria-based review of the literature. *Spine* 1995;20:318–327.
20. Deyo RA, Diehl AK. Cancer as a cause of back pain: frequency, clinical presentation, and diagnostic strategies. *J Gen Intern Med* 1988;3:230–238.
21. El-Farhan N, Busuttil A. Sudden unexpected deaths from ruptured abdominal aortic aneurysms. *J Clin Forensic Med* 1997;4:111–116.
22. Bogduk N, McGuirk B. *Medical Management of Acute and Chronic Low Back Pain. An Evidence-Based Approach.* Amsterdam: Elsevier; 2002:41–47.
23. Laslett M, Young SB, Aprill CN, et al. Diagnosing painful sacroiliac joints: a validity study of a McKenzie evaluation and sacroiliac provocation tests. *Aust J Physiother* 2003;49:89–97.
24. Laslett M, Oberg B, Aprill CN, et al. Centralization as a predictor of provocation discography results in chronic low back pain, and the influence of disability and distress on diagnostic power. *Spine J* 2005;5:370–380.
25. van Tulder MW, Assendelft WJ, Koes BW, et al. Spinal radiographic findings and nonspecific low back pain. A systematic review of observational studies. *Spine* 1997;22:427–434.
26. Deyo RA, Diehl AK, Rosenthal M. Reducing roentgenography use. Can patient expectations be altered? *Arch Intern Med* 1987;147:141–145.
27. Joines JD, McNutt RA, Carey TS, et al. Finding cancer in primary care outpatients with low back pain: a comparison of diagnostic strategies. *J Gen Intern Med* 2001;16:14–23.
28. Bogduk N, McGuirk B. *Medical Management of Acute and Chronic Low Back Pain. An Evidence-Based Approach.* Amsterdam: Elsevier; 2002:73–81.
29. Watson P. The MSM quartet. *Australian Musculoskeletal Medicine* 1999;4(2): 8–9.
30. Indahl A, Velund L, Reikeraas O. Good prognosis for low back pain when left untampered. A randomized clinical trial. *Spine* 1995;20:473–477.
31. Indahl A, Haldorsen EH, Holm S, et al. Five-year follow-up study of a controlled clinical trial using light mobilization and an informative approach to low back pain. *Spine* 1998;23:2625–2630.
32. Royal College of General Practitioners, Chartered Society of Physiotherapy, Osteopathic Association of Great Britain, et al. *Clinical Guidelines for the Management of Acute Low Back Pain.* London: Royal College of General Practitioners; 1996.
33. National Advisory Committee on Core Health and Disability Services, Accident Rehabilitation and Compensation Insurance Corporation. *Clinical Practice Guidelines. Acute Low Back Problems in Adults: Assessment and Treatment.* Wellington: Core Services Committee, Ministry of Health (New Zealand); 1995.
34. Agency for Health Care Policy and Research. *Acute Low Back Pain in Adults: Assessment and Treatment.* Rockville: U.S. Department of Health and Human Services; 1994.
35. van Tulder, Becker A, Bekkering T, et al. European guidelines for the manage-

ment of acute nonspecific low back pain in primary care. *Eur Spine J* 2006; 15:S169–S191.

36. Bogduk N, McGuirk B. *Medical Management of Acute and Chronic Low Back Pain. An Evidence-Based Approach.* Amsterdam: Elsevier; 2002:83–112.

37. van Tulder MW, Scholten RJ, Koes BW, et al. Nonsteroidal anti-inflammatory drugs for low back pain: a systematic review within the framework of the Cochrane Collaboration Back Review Group. *Spine* 2000;25:2501–2513.

38. Roelofs PD, Deyo RA, Koes BW, et al. Non-steroidal anti-inflammatory drugs for low back pain. *Cochrane Database Syst Rev* 2008;23;(1):CD000396.

39. Amlie E, Weber H, Holme I. Treatment of acute low-back pain with piroxicam: results of a double-blind placebo-controlled trial. *Spine* 1987;12:473–476.

40. Dreiser RL, Marty M, Ionescu E, et al. Relief of acute low back pain with diclofenac-K 12.5 mg tablets: a flexible dose, ibuprofen 200 mg and placebo-controlled clinical trial. *Int J Clin Pharmacol Ther* 2003;41:375–385.

41. French SD, Cameron M, Walker BF, et al. A Cochrane review of superficial heat or cold for low back pain. *Spine* 2006;31:998–1006.

42. Mayer JM, Ralph L, Look M, et al. Treating acute low back pain with continuous low-level heat wrap therapy and/or exercise: a randomized controlled trial. *Spine J* 2005;5:395–403.

43. Nadler SF, Steiner DJ, Erasala GN, et al. Continuous low-level heatwrap therapy for treating acute nonspecific low back pain. *Arch Phys Med Rehabil* 2003; 84:329–334.

44. Nadler SF, Steiner DJ, Petty SR, et al. Overnight use of continuous low-level heatwrap therapy for relief of low back pain. *Arch Phys Med Rehabil* 2003; 84:335–342.

45. Tao XG, Bernacki EJ. A randomized clinical trial of continuous low-level heat therapy for acute muscular low back pain in the workplace. *J Occup Environ Med* 2005;47:1298–1306.

46. Nadler SF, Steiner DJ, Erasala GN, et al. Continuous low-level heatwrap therapy provides more efficacy than ibuprofen and acetaminophen for acute low back pain. *Spine* 2002;27:1012–1017.

47. Lloyd A, Scott DA, Akehurst RL, et al. Cost-effectiveness of low-level heatwrap therapy for low back pain. *Value Health* 2004;7:413–422.

48. Waddell G, Feder G, Lewis M. Systematic reviews of bed rest and advice to stay active for acute low back pain. *Brit J Gen Pract* 1997;47:647–652.

49. van Tulder MW, Touray T, Furlan AD, et al. Muscle relaxants for nonspecific low back pain: a systematic review within the framework of the Cochrane collaboration. *Spine* 2003;28:1978–1992.

50. Hayden JA, van Tulder MW, Malmivaara A, et al. Exercise therapy for treatment of non-specific low back pain. *Cochrane Database Syst Rev* 2005 Jul 20; (3):CD000335.

51. Hayden JA, van Tulder MW, Malmivaara AV, et al. Meta-analysis: exercise therapy for nonspecific low back pain. *Ann Intern Med* 2005;142:765–775.

52. Doran DM, Newel DJ. Manipulation in treatment of low-back pain: a multi-centre study. *Br Med J* 1975;2:161–164.

53. Hsieh CY, Phillips RB, Adams AH, et al. Functional outcomes of low back pain: comparison of four treatment groups in a randomized controlled trial. *J Manipulative Physiol Ther* 1992;15:4–9.

54. van Tulder MW, Waddell G. Conservative treatment of acute and subacute low back pain. In: Nachemson A, Jonsson E, eds. *Neck and Back Pain: The Scientific Evidence of Causes, Diagnosis, and Treatment.* Philadelphia: Lippincott Williams & Wilkins; 2000:241–269.

55. van Tulder MW, Koes BW, Bouter LM. Conservative treatment of acute and chronic nonspecific low back pain. A systematic review of randomized controlled trials of the most common interventions. *Spine* 1997;22:2128–2156.

56. van Tulder MW, Cherkin DC, Berman B, et al. The effectiveness of acupuncture in the management of acute and chronic low back pain. A systematic review within the framework of the Cochrane Collaboration Back Review Group. *Spine* 1999;24:1113–1123.

57. Sinclair SJ, Hogg–Johnson SH, Mondloch MV, et al. The effectiveness of an early active intervention program for workers with soft-tissue injuries. The Early Claimant Cohort Study. *Spine* 1997;22:2919–2931.

58. Roland M. Dixon M. Randomized controlled trial of an educational booklet for patients presenting with back pain in general practice. *J Roy Coll Gen Pract* 1989; 39:244–246.

59. Little P, Roberts L, Blowers H, et al. Should we give detailed advice and information booklets to patients with back pain? A randomized controlled factorial trial of a self-management booklet and doctor advice to take exercise for back pain. *Spine* 2001;26:2065–2072.

60. Bronfort G, Haas M, Evans RL, et al. Efficacy of spinal manipulation and mobilization for low back pain and neck pain: a systematic review and best evidence synthesis. *Spine J* 2004;4:335–356.

61. Assendelft WJ, Morton SC, Yu EI, et al. Spinal manipulative therapy for low back pain. A meta-analysis of effectiveness relative to other therapies. *Ann Intern Med* 2003;138:871–881.

62. Hancock MJ, Maher CG, Latimer J, et al. Assessment of diclofenac or spinal manipulative therapy, or both, in addition to recommended first-line treatment for acute low back pain: a randomized controlled trial. *Lancet* 2007;370: 1638–1643.

63. Bogduk N, McGuirk B. The "Indahl" exercises for low back pain. *Australian Musculoskeletal Medicine* 2008;13(1):8–14.

64. Carter JT, Birrell LN, eds. *Occupational Health Guidelines for the Management of Low Back Pain at Work–Principal Recommendations.* London: Faculty of Occupational Medicine; 2000.

65. Waddell G, Burton AK. Occupational health guidelines for the management of low back pain at work: evidence review. *Occup Med (Lond)* 2001;51:124–135.

66. Staal JB, Hlobil H, van Tulder MW, et al. Occupational health guidelines for the management of low back pain: an international comparison. *Occup Environ Med* 2003; 60:618–626.

67. McGuirk B, Bogduk N. Evidence-based care for low back pain in workers eligible for compensation. *Occup Med (Lond)* 2007;57:36–42.

68. Loisel P, Abenhaim L, Durand P, et al. A population-based, randomized clinical trial on back pain management. *Spine* 1997;22:2911–2918.

69. Croft PR, Macfarlane GJ, Papageorgiou AC, et al. Outcome of low back pain in general practice: a prospective study. *Brit Med J* 1998;316:1356–1359.

70. Moffett JK, Torgerson D, Bell–Syer S, et al. Randomised controlled trial of exercise for low back pain: clinical outcomes, costs, and preferences. *Brit Med J* 1999;319:279–283.

71. Kendall NAS, Linton SJ, Main CJ. *Guide to Assessing Psychosocial Yellow Flags in Acute Low Back Pain: Risk Factors for Long-term Disability and Work Loss.* Wellington, NZ: Accident Rehabilitation and Compensation Insurance Corporation of New Zealand and the National Health Committee; 1997.

CHAPTER 72 ■ CHRONIC LOW BACK PAIN

BRIAN E. MCGUIRK AND NIKOLAI BOGDUK

By convention, chronic low back pain is defined as back pain that has persisted for longer than 3 months[1,2]; however, some authorities believe that this rubric can be applied earlier if the pain shows no signs of improving.[3] Irrespective of how it is defined, chronic low back pain is a major social problem in developed societies and, despite an abundance of research, many questions remain unresolved. There is evidence of what might be the sources of pain, but little evidence of its causes. Some entities have been refuted as causes; others remain putative but contested. Traditional approaches to assessment and investigation have been found wanting, but alternatives have not found favor. Various treatments are advocated but few have been vindicated by convincing evidence.

SOURCES

Experiments in normal volunteers have shown that noxious stimulation of the muscles of the back,[4,5] interspinous ligaments,[5,6,7] zygapophyseal joints,[8,9,10] sacroiliac joint(s),[11] and intervertebral discs[12–15] can each evoke pain in the back. Back pain can also be evoked by mechanical[15] or chemical irritation of the dura mater.[16] These structures, therefore, become the possible sources of pain in patients.

Pain evoked from these structures can also be referred to the lower limb (see Fig. 71.3). The distance to which the pain radiates seems to be proportional to the intensity of the stimulus in the back.[8] This referred pain is not produced by irritation of the lumbar spinal nerves or their roots; it is evoked from somatic structures in the lumbar spine. Consequently, it is an example of somatic referred pain.

Somatic referred pain is not synonymous with radicular pain or sciatica, even though all are felt in the lower limb. Somatic referred pain arises because of convergence in the central nervous system between nociceptive afferents from the back and from the lower limb. Since its mechanism and sources are different from those of radicular pain, somatic referred pain needs to be distinguished from radicular pain. In that regard, somatic referred pain is typically dull, aching in quality, and tends to occur in a fixed location. Although its boundaries may be difficult to establish, the subject is well aware of its centroid. In contrast, radicular pain is lancinating in quality, and travels into the limb along a narrow band[17,18] (see Fig. 71.4).

CAUSES

Although the possible sources of back pain have been demonstrated, its causes have been more elusive. Conventional methods of assessment and investigation typically fail to identify the cause of chronic low back pain in the majority of patients. This has fostered belief in the claim that a cause cannot be found in over 80% of patients with chronic low back pain.

The source of this figure is difficult to track down, but it was endorsed and enshrined by the report of the Quebec Task Force on Low Back Pain, published in 1987.[19] An earlier source is a study, published in 1966, in which British general practitioners claimed that a diagnosis was not possible in 80% of cases.[20]

These claims were correct at the time that they were made. In 1987—and more so in 1966—the investigation of low back pain was limited to plain radiography and perhaps computerized tomography. These modalities are now known to lack the sensitivity and resolution to detect lesions that might commonly cause back pain. That restriction does not apply to modern imaging and other procedures. Whereas in the past it might not have been possible to find a cause of back pain, the situation is now different.

Refuted Causes

Research has shown that many conditions traditionally considered to be possible causes of chronic low back pain are actually not causes. Multiple studies have shown that spondylolysis or spondylolisthesis cannot be held as causes of back pain in adults. These conditions occur with equal prevalence in subjects with no symptoms and in patients with back pain.[21,22] Similarly, so-called degenerative changes (spondylosis) occur only slightly more frequently in patients with back pain than they do in asymptomatic individuals.[21,22] The difference in prevalence is so small as to render degenerative changes not diagnostic. They represent no more than normal age changes.

Accepted Causes

There is no dispute that tumors and infections can cause low back pain, but these conditions are rare. Although specialist practitioners may be accustomed to greater prevalences because they are in referral practice, the prevalence of serious causes of back pain in primary care amounts to no more than 5%.[23]

Untested Causes

In its Classification of Chronic Pain, the International Association for the Study of Pain (IASP) recognizes, in principle, certain causes

of chronic low back pain that are promoted by some practitioners.[1] These include muscle sprain, ligament sprain, segmental dysfunction, and trigger points. However, the IASP requires that for the diagnosis of these conditions techniques be used that are of known reliability and validity. But no technique has been shown to be both reliable and valid for the diagnosis of these entities. Therefore, they remain only theoretical or imaginary constructs.

Known Source, Unknown Cause

It is possible to establish a source of low back pain by selectively anesthetizing structures believed to be the source[24,25] (see also Chapter 99, Diagnostic and Therapeutic Nerve Blocks). If performed under controlled conditions, using validated techniques, diagnostic blocks can identify the source of back pain in a substantial proportion of patients.

The rationale (concept validity) of diagnostic blocks is that if a particular structure is the source of pain then whenever it is anesthetized the pain should stop. Controls, however, are required to maximize construct validity. Anatomical controls involve anesthetizing the target structure on one occasion but an adjacent structure, which is not painful, on another occasion, under single-blind conditions. Physiological controls require that the patient respond in a manner consistent with the duration of action of the agent used to anesthetize the structure, which can include placebo agents.[24,25]

Sacroiliac Joint(s)

Using anatomical[26] or physiological controls,[27] studies have shown that the source of chronic low back pain can be traced to the sacroiliac joints(s) in about 20% of patients. These patients obtain complete relief of their pain when the joint is anesthetized. The actual cause, however, has not been determined. It may involve loosening of the joint following injury or pregnancy, but no method of investigation has yet been developed by which to detect such an entity reliably.

Zygapophyseal Joints

Using physiological controls, multiple studies have purported to trace the source of chronic low back pain to the lumbar zygapophyseal joints. Prevalence rates of 15%,[28] 40%,[29] and 45%[30-32] have been reported. What is contentious about these figures, however, is that complete relief of pain was not a diagnostic criterion. Rather, the investigators accepted 50% relief or 80% relief. They assumed that any pain not relieved stemmed from another concurrent source, but that source was not identified. Meanwhile, other studies have shown that patients with chronic low back pain rarely have concurrent sources of pain from the zygapophyseal joints, the sacroiliac joint, or the intervertebral discs.[26,33] Therefore, insofar as concurrent sources of pain have not been identified, partial relief of pain must be viewed as a spurious diagnostic criterion. Placebo responses have not been excluded.

When studies looked for complete relief of pain following blocks of the lumbar zygapophyseal joints, substantially lesser prevalence has been encountered. In general populations, the prevalence of complete relief of pain is about 5% or less.[34-37] Therefore, lumbar zygapophyseal joint pain may not be as common as has been held to date.

However, one study using placebo controls did find that 34% of an elderly population obtained at least 90% relief of pain.[28] Therefore, the prevalence of lumbar zygapophyseal joint pain may be population-dependent and more common in the elderly than in younger, injured workers.

The cause of zygapophyseal joint pain is not known. In patients with a history of injury upon exertion, it is conceivable that they may have suffered an articular fracture. Laboratory studies have shown that the lumbar zygapophyseal joints are sus-

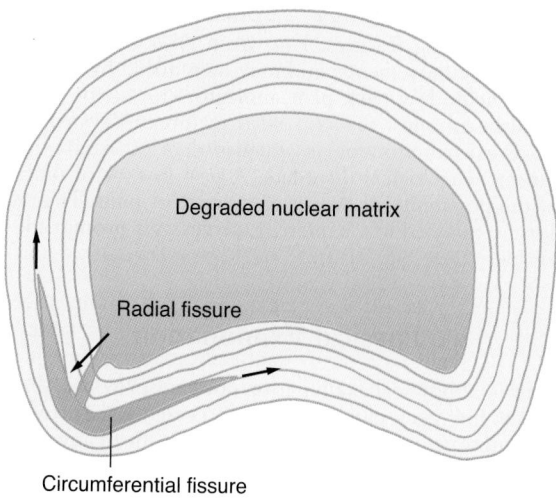

FIGURE 72.1 The features of internal disc disruption.

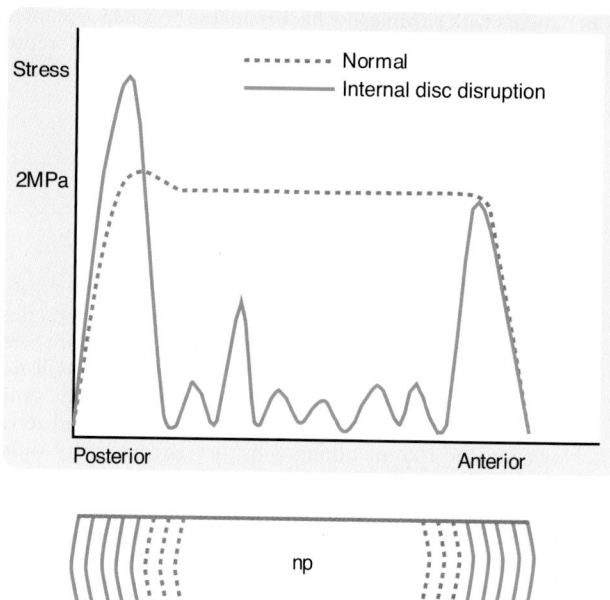

FIGURE 72.3 The biophysical features of internal disc disruption. The graph shows the stresses recorded across the diameter of normal discs and a disc with internal disruption.

ceptible to small fractures, or avulsions of the capsule, when subjected to excessive torsion. However, no studies have validated this injury (e.g., by high resolution CT scan). In elderly patients, it is tempting to attribute their pain to osteoarthrosis, but there is no correlation between the radiologic features of osteoarthrosis on CT scan and the joint being painful.[38] An emerging proposition is that painful lumbar zygapophyseal joints express inflammatory changes evident on magnetic resonance imaging (MRI) using a fat-saturation setting.[39] This has yet to be corroborated by other studies.

Internal Disc Disruption

Internal disc disruption is a condition characterized by a set of chemical, morphological, and biophysical features. It is precipitated by a small fracture of the vertebral endplate, as a result of severe compression injury or fatigue failure under compression.[40] This results in progressive degradation of the nuclear matrix, and the development of radial fissures into the annulus fibrosus (Fig. 72.1). The degree of disruption can be graded according to the extent that fissures penetrate the annulus[41,42] (Fig. 72.2). In grade I disruption, fissures reach the inner third of the annulus. In grade II disruption fissures reach the middle third of the annulus. Grade

III disruption arises when the fissure reaches the outer third, and becomes grade IV if the fissure then extends circumferentially. These chemical and morphological changes affect the biophysical properties of the disc.

Degradation of the nucleus compromises its ability to sustain compression loads. Stresses in the nucleus become irregular and reduced across the profile of the nucleus, becoming zero in some locations in some discs[40,43] (Fig. 72.3). This results in the annulus fibrosus having to bear more of the compression load. In particular, stress in the posterior annulus is increased greatly above normal levels.[40,43]

These various features correlate with the affected disc being painful on discography. Some 70% of discs with grade III or IV fissures are painful, and 70% of painful discs exhibit grade III or IV fissures.[44] Moreover, this relationship is independent of age changes in the disc.[45] Decreased nuclear stress and increased stress in the posterior annulus each, separately, correlate strongly with the disc being painful.[46]

Animal studies have shown that experimental injury to the vertebral endplate precipitates the biochemical degradation of the nuclear matrix.[47–49] Laboratory studies have shown that nuclear depressurization and increased posterior annulus stress appear immediately after fatigue failure of the vertebral endplate.[40] Endplate fractures can occur in response to as few as 100 repetitions of compression loads amounting to between 50% and 80% of the ultimate tensile stress of the endplate.[50,51] Such stresses are within the range experienced during normal, moderate to heavy lifting activities.[51]

The disc becomes painful as a result of two mechanisms acting in combination. Inflammatory chemicals, such as phospholipase, tumor necrosis factor, and nitric oxide, produced within the nucleus in response to injury, provide a basis for chemical nociception. They could stimulate nerve endings that occur normally in the outer third of the annulus, if the chemicals reach the outer annulus through radial fissures. Alternatively, or additionally, they could stimulate endings of nerves that grow into injured discs.[52,53] Meanwhile, the increased stresses in the posterior annulus constitute a stimulus for mechanical nociception in the outer annulus. Chemicals that reach the outer annulus could sensitize the nerve endings located there to mechanical stimulation.

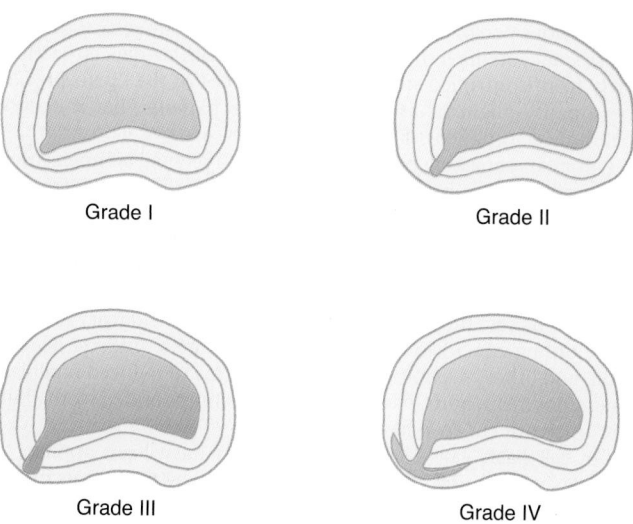

FIGURE 72.2 The grading of internal disc disruption.

In patients with chronic low back pain, the prevalence of internal disc disruption is 39%,[33] which is a worst-case figure. It represents the proportion of patients with single-level disease, and does not include patients with two-level disease.

ASSESSMENT

History

Taking a history is a conventional component of pain practice. However, in patients with chronic low back pain it is more ceremonial than diagnostic. For most patients, the history will not provide a diagnosis. Most patients will relate basically the same story of unremitting pain with limitation of movements and activity. However, the role of taking a history is to identify those patients who are not typical.

Determining the length of illness establishes that the pain is chronic, and is largely reassuring with respect to pathology. Patients are unlikely to have a serious cause if their condition has not deteriorated over several months. Nevertheless, practitioners need to be mindful of chronic infection. Spinal infections can remain indolent, and not produce additional features for a long time. In one study, delays of 1 to 8 years were encountered in 47% of patients.[54]

Confirming the site of pain is important to confirm that the patient has lumbar spinal pain, and not loin pain or gluteal pain[1] (see Chapter 71, Acute Low Back Pain). Loin (flank) pain indicates a visceral source, and primary gluteal pain suggests a hip disorder rather than spinal pain. Pain located in the lumbar or sacral spinal region can arise from many sources, but there is a partial rule concerning sacroiliac joint pain. Pain from the sacroiliac joint tends to be located over the joint, and radiates distally. Rarely, if ever, has it been found to extend above the L5 level. Therefore, pain located exclusively below L5 increases the likelihood of the sacroiliac joint being the source.

The radiation of pain needs to be carefully interpreted. Somatic referred pain in the buttock or lower limb can be expected with any source of pain in the lumbar spine. It should not be confused with radicular pain. The cardinal distinctions lie in the quality of pain and its behavior. Somatic referred pain is dull and aching in quality; it tends to occupy a broad area with boundaries that are hard to define but whose center the patient can readily indicate, and although the pain may extend further into the lower limb when severe, the pain is relatively fixed in location (see Fig. 71.3). In contrast, radicular pain is lancinating in quality, and travels along the length of the lower limb (see Fig. 71.4). Making this distinction is pivotal because the causes of somatic referred pain and radicular pain are quite different, and invite different investigations and treatment. Some authorities maintain that somatic referred pain does not extend below the knee and that, therefore, pain below the knee must be radicular in origin. This is not correct, for it has been shown that pain from the lumbar zygapophyseal joints and intervertebral discs can be referred beyond the knee, even into the foot.[8,9,10,15]

The frequency and duration of pain are not helpful discriminating variables in the assessment of chronic low back pain. Patients will typically complain of constant pain.

Neither is the intensity of pain discriminating. Whereas severe pain is an alerting feature in patients with acute low back pain (see Chapter 71, Acute Low Back Pain), it does not carry the same connotation in patients with chronic low back pain. Serious causes of pain should already have manifested other features apart from severe pain. That is not to say that conditions such as internal disc disruption do not produce severe pain—just that severe pain, in the absence of other features, does not indicate a serious cause.

Precipitating, aggravating, and relieving factors are usually not discriminating features. Pain from all sources tends to be aggravated by movements, and may be reduced by rest.

As for acute low back pain, indicators for serious causes of pain will lie amongst the associated features. A systems review should reveal symptoms of visceral disorders if these are the cause of pain or neurological disorders. A past history of illness will reveal the possibility of cancer as a cause of pain. The red flag checklist, explained in Chapter 71, serves as a prompt for what to consider[55] (see Fig. 71.5).

Physical Examination

Conventional physical examination does not provide a diagnosis of chronic low back pain. There is no evidence that tenderness, range of motion, or other features are diagnostic of any particular source or cause of pain. Some practitioners use physical features to guide treatment (e.g., improving range of motion, or where to inject therapeutic agents), but these applications are not diagnostic in a patho-anatomic sense. Some practitioners use physical features to monitor progress, or to classify patients, but, again, this does not amount to diagnosis.

Neurological examination is neither necessary nor productive in the assessment of patients with chronic low back pain. Neurological examination is indicated if the patient has neurological symptoms, but in that event their presenting feature is the neurology, not back pain. In the absence of neurological symptoms, neurological examination serves only to satisfy the examiner that features that should not be present are actually not present.

In one arena, developments have occurred. A specialized protocol of examination, based on detecting centralization of pain and other features, has been tested. It has been shown to be valid for the detection of sacroiliac joint pain[56] and of internal disc disruption.[57] It does not detect zygapophyseal joint pain.[36,37] This protocol, however, requires special training.[58]

As for acute low back pain (see Chapter 71) physical examination is perhaps most relevant when the patient exhibits no signs in the lumbar region. In that event, consideration needs to be given to a visceral or vascular cause of pain.

Psychological Assessment

About 30 years ago, several authorities promoted the psychoanalytic concept that intractable pain is a defense against unconscious psychic conflict.[59] Chronic pain was attributed to repressed hostility and aggression, guilt, resentment, loss, masked depression, and various personality disorders. Although eloquently espoused, these concepts have not found support from evidence, particularly from controlled studies.[59] The concept of the "pain-prone" personality might be applicable to some patients, but it cannot be applied to patients at large.[59]

Nor can persisting pain be attributed to seeking compensation or to pre-existing psychological disorders. Studies purporting to show this have not controlled for selection biases, overinterpretation being an inappropriate use of psychometric tests.[60] The concept of "secondary gain" is poorly substantiated by the literature.[61]

On balance, the existing data fit a more conciliatory and understanding conclusion: Chronic pain produces anxiety, depression, and other psychological distress, all due to reduced function, unemployment, and financial insecurity, compounded by the failure of treatment to relieve the pain.[60]

In the past, various psychiatric labels have been applied to patients with chronic low back pain, usually by physicians rather than psychiatrists. Patients are now protected from such incorrect practices by the *Diagnostic and Statistical Manual of Mental Disorders (DSM-IV-TR)* of the American Psychiatric Association,[62] which prescribes specific criteria that must be satisfied before particular rubrics can be applied.

The criteria for "conversion disorder" stipulate loss of sensory or motor function. This rubric is expressly precluded if pain is the sole symptom.[62]

The criteria for "hypochondriasis" stipulate that the patient has a preoccupation with fears of having a serious disease.[62] Although patients with chronic low back pain may appear preoccupied with their pain to the extent of seeking relief, this differs from having a preoccupation with a fear of having pain, or fear of a serious disorder.

Somatization disorder is a rubric that might seem to be a euphemism for psychogenic pain, but the diagnostic criteria for this condition stipulate that the patient must have pain in at least four different sites, as well as two gastrointestinal symptoms, one sexual symptom, and one pseudoneurological symptom, the latter not limited to pain.[62] Furthermore, the symptoms are not intentional. These criteria specify a complex disorder that some patients with chronic pain may have, but by definition the criteria do not apply to patients with pain in a single region, such as back pain.

The diagnostic criteria for "undifferentiated somatoform disorder" are more liberal than those for somatization disorder, and some physicians might be attracted to applying this rubric to patients with chronic low back pain. The notes for this disorder, however, specify fatigue, loss of appetite, or gastrointestinal or urinary symptoms.[62] Pain is conspicuously not mentioned, which suggests that this rubric was not designed to accommodate patients with pain for which there is no explanation.

"Factitious disorder" is characterized by the intentional production or feigning of physical or psychological signs or symptoms, in order to assume a sick role, but external incentives for the behavior are absent.[62] A further qualification is that individuals with factitious disorder present their history with dramatic flair but are extremely vague and inconsistent when questioned in greater detail. Pain may be the symptom produced, and distinction between a genuine and fabricated complaint may be difficult. Lack of external incentives distinguishes factitious disorder from malingering, and a patient who is consistent and lacks dramatic flair when describing their symptoms is unlikely to qualify as having a factitious disorder.

"Malingering" is not a formal psychiatric diagnosis, and the *DSM* does not provide diagnostic criteria for it. It states only that malingering should be strongly suspected if any combination is noted of medicolegal context of presentation, marked discrepancy between the person's claimed distress or disability and the objective findings, lack of cooperation during the diagnostic evaluation and in complying with the prescribed treatment regimen, and the presence of antisocial personality disorder.[62] For many patients with chronic low back pain, some of these features must be carefully interpreted lest they be unjustly incriminating. The criterion for medicolegal context pertains to overt, and deliberate, compensation-seeking behavior. It does not apply to injured patients covered by workers' compensation who cannot avoid a medicolegal context. Some causes of pain may lack objective findings. In other instances, physical findings on physical examination lack reliability and validity. Therefore, physicians will naturally fail to find a correlation between findings and symptoms. They should not misrepresent this natural feature of the disorder as malingering. A systematic review found little scientific evidence to justify malingering as a diagnosis in patients with chronic pain.[63] Expert opinion considers it to be a rare condition.[63]

The essential feature for "adjustment disorder" is a psychological response to an identifiable stressor that results in the development of clinically significant emotional or behavioral symptoms. Examples of stressors include termination of a relationship, business difficulties, living in a crime-ridden neighborhood, and natural disasters. Although pain is listed as a symptom by the handbook that accompanies the *DSM*,[64] it is conspicuously not

mentioned by the manual itself.[62] Rather, the manual emphasizes behavioral symptoms such as anxiety and depression. The use of this rubric may not be valid if the physician attributes pain to a stressor because superficially it is convenient to do so, instead of pursuing a diagnosis in a more rigorous manner.

The *DSM* provides an entry that explicitly accommodates patients with chronic pain. It provides three subtypes:

- *307.80 Pain Disorder Associated with Psychological Factors*
- *307.89 Pain Disorder Associated with Both Psychological Factors and a General Medical Condition*
- *Pain Disorder Associated with a General Medical Condition*

For the first two subtypes, the critical criterion is that "psychological factors are judged to have an important role in the onset, severity, exacerbation, or maintenance of the pain." What the *DSM* does not provide are guidelines by which this judgment is to be made. Therefore, the judgment becomes a matter of the physician's opinion. For these rubrics to apply, psychological factors must overtly be responsible for onset, severity, exacerbation, or maintenance of the pain. This is not the same as finding that patients have psychological features that are secondary to the persistence of pain.

The third subtype is specified as not a mental disorder. Having pain, for which psychological factors are judged not to be important, is no more than a medical condition. Unless there is explicit evidence to the contrary, most patients with chronic pain should fall into this category, especially if it is deemed that any psychological factors are secondary to the persistence of pain. It is this category that would accommodate patients with psychological features that are caused by the pain, not vice versa.

When assessed for psychological distress using the SCL-90R, patients with chronic low back pain typically show elevated scores on the scales for somatization, depression, obsessive-compulsive behavior, and psychoticism.[65,66] Respectively, these scales reflect attentional focus on physical sensations, depression, pain-related rumination and frustration, and feelings of isolation as well as loss of control.[66] These features compound the problems already faced by these patients in terms of pain and physical disability.

It is, therefore, important to identify in patients the nature and extent of their psychological distress. These features invite, and warrant, treatment or help in their own right. Moreover, if the pain genuinely cannot be diagnosed, and genuinely cannot be relieved, the psychological domain may be the only one in which treatment might be implemented.

Various instruments are available for the psychological assessment of patients with chronic pain (see Chapter 21, Psychological and Psychosocial Evaluation). Some are more suited for research purposes than for conventional practice. Others are best administered by specialist psychologists. However, in primary care, and even in specialist care, instruments may not be required.

In the first instance, a practitioner alert to the importance of psychological factors would look for these, or elicit them, in the course of a normal consultation. Formal instruments are not required to identify fear, depression, frustration, and isolation. If required, practitioners can be prompted to explore psychological factors using the Distress Risk Assessment Method (DRAM)[67] or a checklist that summarizes the features explored by that method[68] (Table 72.1).

Having identified psychological factors, the practitioner can decide if they are able to help the patient with their distress, or if they need to engage the expertise of a psychologist. Engaging a psychologist, however, should not be a dismissive behavior. Dismissing a patient to a psychologist is tantamount to blaming the pain on a psychological disorder, or the patient might so infer. Engaging a psychologist requires that the patient understand that they have psychological problems parallel to their pain problems, and that a cooperative, interdisciplinary plan of management is required.

TABLE 72.1

ELEMENTS ASSESSED BY THE DISTRESS AND RISK ASSESSMENT METHOD[67]

Somatic perception	Depression
Heart rate increase	Feels downhearted
Feeling hot all over	Feels best in morning
Sweating all over	Has crying spells or feels like it
Sweating in a particular part of the body	Has trouble getting to sleep at night
Pulse in neck	Feels that nobody cares
Pounding in head	Eats as much as used to
Dizziness	Still enjoys sex
Blurring of vision	Losing weight
Feeling faint	Has trouble with constipation
Everything appearing unreal	Heart beats faster than usual
Nausea	Gets tired for no reason
Butterflies in stomach	Mind is as clear as it used to be
Pain or ache in stomach	Tends to wake up too early
Stomach churning	Finds it easy to do the things they used to
Desire to pass water	Is restless and can't keep still
Mouth becoming dry	Is hopeful about the future
Difficulty swallowing	Is more irritable than usual
Muscles in neck aching	Finds it easy to make a decision
Legs feeling weak	Feels quite guilty
Muscles twitching or jumping	Feels that I am useful and needed
Tense feeling across forehead	Life is pretty full
Tense feeling in jaw muscles	Feels that would be better off if dead
	Still able to enjoy the things they used to

INVESTIGATIONS

Investigations that might be used in a patient with chronic low back pain are predicated by their indications and purpose. Some investigations are indicated by clinical cues in the presenting features of possible red flag conditions. Others are designed to determine the source of pain in patients who do not have red flag conditions. There are also investigations that have no place in the management of chronic low back pain but which are nevertheless commonly used.

Red Flag Conditions

In the context of chronic low back pain, the indications and tests for red flag conditions are the same as those for acute low back pain (see Chapter 71, Acute Low Back Pain). They are designed either to rule in or rule out a serious cause of pain (see Table 71.2). The prompt for these investigations is not that they have not been done but whether or not the patient has the appropriate clinical indicator. If the patient does not express an indicator, the test is not warranted or justified.

If the patient has been well managed during their acute phase they will already have been assessed and monitored for red flag conditions. Traumatic and pathological fractures will already have been considered and investigated; tumors should have progressed and manifested new features. Indolent infections are perhaps the only condition that can persist for long periods without expressing new features. However, if a patient has not been managed well in the past, it is appropriate to follow the red flag checklist (see Fig. 71.5) to determine if specific investigations are indicated.

Screening Test

Notwithstanding the security that following the red flag checklist should provide, practitioners may still be concerned lest they have overlooked a serious condition. Conversely, they may want to "clear" the patient of serious disorders before embarking upon a pursuit of the cause of pain. For this purpose, MRI is the investigation of choice.

MRI has a high sensitivity and high specificity for all manner of possibly occult or overlooked disorders. It is, therefore, the appropriate screening test. There is no justification for progressing through plain radiography, bone scan, and CT before considering MRI. Each of those other investigations has little or limited ability to detect cryptic disorders. For screening purposes, MRI can detect fractures, which would be seen on plain radiographs (see Fig. 71.6), but MRI will also detect soft-tissue lesions, which plain radiography cannot do. The increased vascular uptake that bone scan demonstrates will be evident on MRI with greater specificity. Although CT provides better resolution of bone, bony lesions will not escape detection by MRI.

Not Indicated

Foremost amongst investigations not indicated for chronic low back pain is electrophysiological testing. There is no lesion that causes low back pain that produces a conduction block in the nerves of the lower limb. Therefore, there is nothing that nerve-conduction studies can show about back pain. Some practitioners are accustomed to using conduction studies because they confuse somatic referred pain with radicular pain, and explain that they are testing for radiculopathy. However, even that practice is without foundation. It has been demonstrated that even in patients with radicular pain, conduction studies are not diagnostic.[69,70] Conduction studies are indicated only if peripheral neuropathy is in the differential diagnosis of radiculopathy. Back pain is not radiculopathy, and peripheral neuropathy is not a differential diagnosis for chronic low back pain.

Similarly, CT is not an appropriate investigation for chronic low back pain. Its use is based on the confusion between radicular pain and somatic referred pain. CT is very useful for the detection of disc herniations in patients with radicular pain, but somatic referred pain is not caused by disc herniations. Therefore, CT is not indicated. The only role for CT would be as a substitute when MRI is not available as a screening test. In that regard CT is not an alternative to MRI, for there are conditions that MRI can detect that CT cannot detect. CT is an alternative to MRI for social or economic reasons, not for medical ones.

Plain radiography is not indicated in patients with chronic low back pain. The lesions that it can detect are limited fractures and gross lesions of bone. Yet these are rare causes of chronic low back pain and are better detected by MRI, or CT if there must be an alternative.

Diagnostic Tests

Certain diagnostic tests can pinpoint the source of pain, and sometimes its cause, in patients with chronic low back pain in whom serious causes have been excluded. These encompass MRI and various invasive tests.

MRI

Irrelevant to the diagnosis of chronic low back pain are age-changes—so called degenerative changes—that may be evident on MRI or CT of the lumbar spine. Osteophytes, disc bulges, and even disc herniations occur commonly in subjects with no back pain and exhibit no relationship to pain.[70,72] However, there are certain features that can appear on MRI scans that are pertinent to establishing the cause of pain.

High-Intensity Zone. High-intensity zones (HIZs) are very bright signals that occur in the posterior annulus of lumbar intervertebral discs[42] (Fig. 72.4). They are distinguished from simple fissures in the annulus in that their intensity rivals that of cerebrospinal fluid on heavily T-2 weighted MRI images. In contrast, simple fissures appear grey. Biopsy has revealed that they represent sites of highly vascularized granulation tissue in anular tears.[73]

HIZs are not common. They occur in about 30% of patients with chronic low back pain. In these patients the presence of an HIZ correlates strongly with the affected disc being the source of the patient's pain. Multiple studies have investigated this rela-

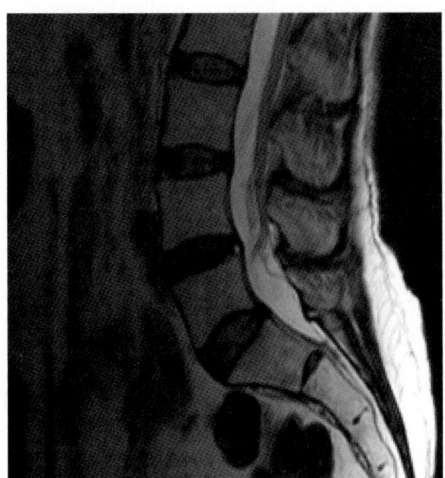

FIGURE 72.4 A sagittal MRI scan that shows a high-intensity zone in the L4–L5 intervertebral disc. (Courtesy of Dr Peter Lau, John Hunter Hospital, Newcastle, Australia.)

TABLE 72.2

THE SENSITIVITY, SPECIFICITY, AND POSITIVE LIKELIHOOD RATIO OF HIGH-INTENSITY ZONES (HIZS) AS PREDICTORS OF THE AFFECTED DISC BEING PAINFUL, AS REPORTED BY THE STUDIES CITED

Sensitivity	Specificity	Likelihood ratio	Source
0.71	0.89	6.5	42
0.27	0.95	5.4	74
0.52	0.90	5.2	75
0.81	0.79	3.9	76
0.78	0.74	3.0	77
0.31	0.90	3.1	78
0.45	0.84	2.8	79
0.27	0.85	1.8	80
0.09	0.93	1.3	81

tionship (Table 72.2). The studies differ in the sensitivities that they encountered. This indicates that not all painful discs necessarily exhibit an HIZ, which may be a function of the pathology suffered by the patient or a function of the scanning technique used. However, all studies agree on a high specificity, which generates substantial positive likelihood ratios. This means that if an HIZ is evident then the affected disc is very likely to be painful. Even the study that sought to refute the validity of the HIZ produced data consonant with this conclusion.[79] That study argued that that HIZ could not be held as a cause of pain on the grounds that it could occur in asymptomatic individuals.[79] However, the data provided nevertheless showed that the prevalence of an HIZ in patients with back pain (60%; 95% CI: 45% to 75%) was significantly greater than in asymptomatic subjects (24%; 95% CI: 11% to 37%). Moreover, in the original literature,[42] HIZs were not promoted as a cause of pain, but as an indicator that, in patients with back pain, the affected disc was likely to be the source. In that regard, the HIZ is a valid sign (see Table 72.2).

Modic Changes. Another feature that can occur on MR scans are signal changes in the bone marrow adjacent to a vertebral endplate. They are known as Modic changes, after the radiologist who first described them.[81] Modic type-I changes represent edema in the marrow, and are evident on both T1-weighted and T2-weighted images (Figs. 72.5A,B). Modic type-2 changes represent fatty infiltration in the marrow, and are best seen on T1-weighted images (Figs. 72.5C,D). Sequentially in time, these changes imply an acute and then chronic inflammatory response to an injury to the disc. These changes are strongly related to the affected disc being painful (Table 72.3). In that regard, Modic changes have only a low sensitivity, reflecting that only a minority of painful discs exhibit Modic changes, but their specificity and likelihood ratios are very high, which indicates that if Modic changes are evident the affected disc is very likely to be painful. This correlation is reinforced by pathology studies that show that endplates affected by Modic changes have a higher density of nerve fibers and cells that stain for tumor necrosis factor α.[53]

Medial Branch Blocks

The medial branches of the lumbar dorsal rami innervate the lumbar zygapophyseal joints. Each joint is supplied by the nerve above and the nerve below. Blocking these nerves with local anesthetic serves as a diagnostic test for pain stemming from these joints. The technique is described in Chapter 97 (Diagnostic and Therapeutic Nerve Blocks).

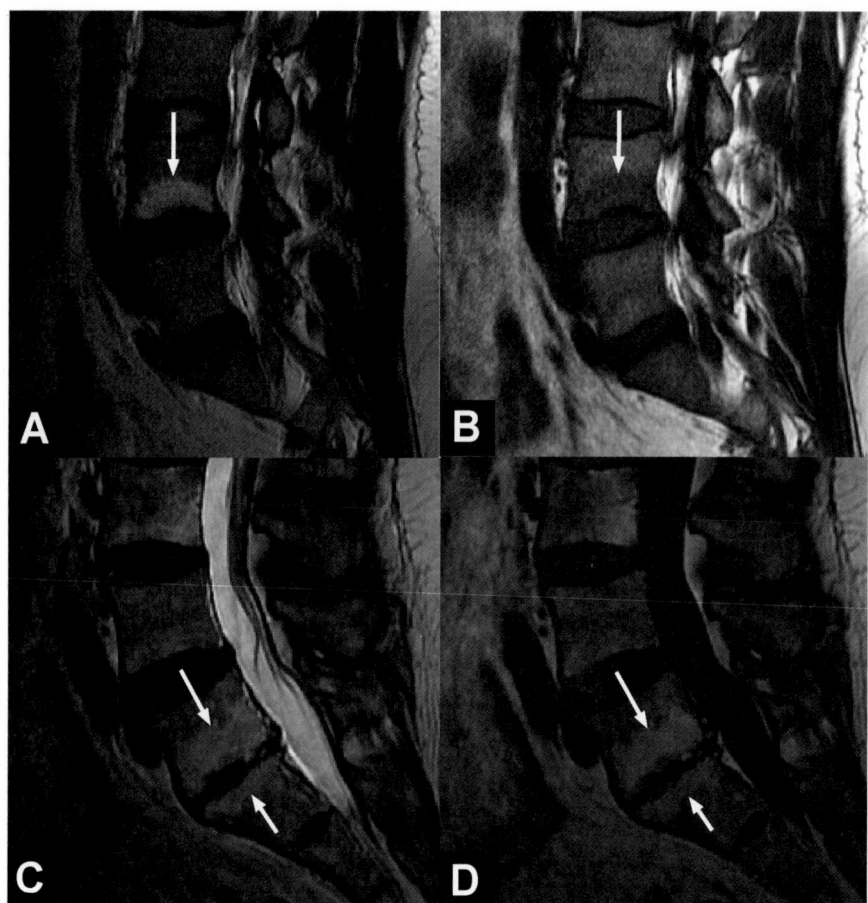

FIGURE 72.5 Magnetic resonance scans showing Modic changes around an intervertebral disc. (A) L4–L5 disc; Type 1 lesion, T2-weighted image. (B) L4–L5 disc; Type 1 lesion, T1-weighted image. (C) L5–S1 disc; Type 2 lesion, T2-weighted image. (D) L5–S1 disc; Type 2 lesion, T1-weighted image. (Courtesy of Dr Tim Maus Lau, of the Mayo Clinic, Rochester, MN.)

Lumbar medial branch blocks have been validated. They protect normal volunteers from experimentally induced pain from the joint anesthetized.[84] They do not anaesthetize other structures that might be an alternative source of pain.[85] Single, diagnostic blocks, however, carry a high false-positive rate.[30,86,87] Therefore, in order to be valid, lumbar medial branch blocks have to be controlled. Comparative local anesthetic blocks have been used in the past, but doubts have been raised about their validity (see Chapter 97, Diagnostic and Therapeutic Nerve Blocks). Because of the low prevalence of lumbar zygapophyseal joint pain, even comparative blocks still have substantial false-positive rates (see Chapter 97, Diagnostic and Therapeutic Nerve Blocks). Consequently, operators who use comparative blocks need to appreciate that some of their positive responses will be doubtful. The only way to reduce this doubt is to perform placebo-controlled blocks.

TABLE 72.3

THE SENSITIVITY, SPECIFICITY, AND POSITIVE LIKELIHOOD RATIO OF MODIC LESIONS AS PREDICTORS OF THE AFFECTED DISC BEING PAINFUL, AS REPORTED BY THE STUDIES CITED

Sensitivity	Specificity	Likelihood ratio	Source
0.38	1.00	∞	80
0.23	0.97	7.7	83
0.22	0.95	4.4	75

With these reservations in mind, it is possible to use lumbar medial branch blocks to determine if a patient has back pain stemming from one or more lumbar zygapophyseal joints. Algorithms for the efficient use of blocks have been described.[88] They recommend multilevel screening blocks in the first instance, in order to identify patients who do not have zygapophyseal joint pain, which is the most common response. Patients who report relief of the pain from screening blocks can then be subjected to repeat testing with controlled blocks, in order to identify the joint or joints that are the source of pain.

Because of the vicissitudes of controlled blocks and the criteria for a positive response (see Chapter 97, Diagnostic and Therapeutic Nerve Blocks), the prevalence of lumbar zygapophyseal joint pain is uncertain. In the general population of patients with chronic low back pain it may be 5% or less.[89] In older populations, with no history of trauma, it may be around 40%.[29]

Irrespective of the actual prevalence, lumbar zygapophyseal joint pain is worth investigating because, if diagnosed, it can be treated. The pain can be relieved by lumbar medial branch radiofrequency neurotomy[89] (see Chapter 101, Neurolytic Blockade).

Sacroiliac Joint Blocks

Pain from a sacroiliac joint can be diagnosed using controlled blocks of the joint. These blocks involve injecting local anesthetic into the cavity of the joint (see Chapter 97, Diagnostic and Therapeutic Nerve Blocks).

In 15% to 20% of patients with chronic low back pain the source of pain can be traced to a sacroiliac joint if controlled blocks are used.[26,27] Doing so has diagnostic utility. Establishing a diagnosis confirms for the patient that they do have a genuine source of pain, and that the pain is not imagined. Establishing a diagnosis protects the patient from a futile pursuit of other diagnoses by bringing about closure. It protects them from undergoing treatments that do not target the sacroiliac joint and which are, therefore, doomed to failure. Knowing that the sacroiliac joint is the source of pain allows treatments to be applied that are specific for that source.

Sacroiliac Ligaments

The dorsal sacroiliac ligaments are a potential source of pain. These ligaments are not anesthetized by intra-articular blocks of the sacroiliac joint. They can, however, be anesthetized by blocking the lateral branches of the sacral dorsal rami, which innervate them.

Conventional techniques for sacral lateral branch blocks, however, have been shown to be unreliable.[90] The nerves run at variable locations and at variable depths. For blocks to be reliable they have to be performed at multiple sites and at multiple depths within the posterior ligamentous complex. Such blocks have been shown to protect normal volunteers from experimentally induced pain from the posterior sacroiliac ligaments.[91] They can be used to identify patients who might be treated with radiofrequency neurotomy of the sacral lateral branches.

Discography

Lumbar discography is a procedure designed to determine if a lumbar intervertebral disc is the source of back pain. If supplemented by postdiscography CT, it allows a diagnosis of internal disc disruption to be established.

The procedure involves introducing fine needles into the center of the disc suspected of being the source of pain, and into adjacent discs.[92] A small volume of contrast medium is injected through the needles in order to stress the disc by pressurizing it internally. The principle is that when a symptomatic disc is stressed, the patient's accustomed pain should be reproduced, but pain should not be reproduced if asymptomatic discs are stressed.

Because discography is a provocation test, certain precautions need to be observed in order to maximize its validity. Specifically, anatomic controls and a manometric control combined with pain intensity need to be exercised.

For discography to be valid, stressing one disc should be painful but stressing discs at adjacent levels should not be painful. This criterion guards against false-positive responses owing to hyperalgesia. Validity is compromised, to an unknown degree, if two discs appear symptomatic, for in that event the number of apparently positive discs typically outnumbers the number of control discs. If no disc is asymptomatic the test cannot be regarded as positive.

Manometric controls are required because, in principle, any disc might be rendered painful if stressed with sufficient intensity. In practice, some discs withstand an excess of 100 psi internal pressure without becoming painful; others become mildly painful at high pressures up to 100 psi.[93] Conversely, normal discs are rarely painful, if at all, at low pressures of stimulation, and are minimally or only mildly painful. A sensitivity analysis allows for operational criteria to be defined.

If discography is painful at less than 50 psi and evokes pain at an intensity greater than 4 on a 10-point numerical pain rating scale, the probability of the response being false-positive should be less than 0.10.[93,94] However, the probability of a false-positive rate reduces to zero if the required pain score is held at 4 and the threshold pressure of injection is lowered to 30 psi; or if the required pressure is held at 50 psi and the pain score required is raised to 6.[93,94] Two sets of operational criteria are offered because the low-pressure criterion has high specificity but detects

fewer patients as positive, whereas the more liberal, 50 psi threshold detects more patients with only a marginal reduction in specificity.

Postdiscography CT scanning allows the demonstration of the distribution of contrast medium with the discs tested. Radial fissures are the hallmark of internal disc disruption (see Internal Disc Disruption, above). Demonstrating radial fissures upgrades the diagnosis from discogenic pain to internal disc disruption.

Warnings have been raised about possible false-positive responses to lumbar discography. In studies of normal volunteers, patients with chronic pain, and patients reportedly with "somatization," the reported false-positive rates have been 10%, 40%, and 75%, respectively.[95] However, if the operational criteria for anatomical and manometric controls are satisfied, these false-positive rates reduce to 0%, 0%, and 25% respectively.[92–94,96] Consequently, operators who adhere to the operational criteria need to be concerned about false-positive responses only in patients with somatization.

The virtue of lumbar discography lies in its diagnostic utility, both in a positive and a negative sense. Establishing a diagnosis of discogenic pain or internal disc disruption protects the patient from further pursuit of diagnosis, and from treatments that are unlikely to work because they do not stop discogenic pain. Conversely, finding discography to be negative should protect the patient from surgery to the disc based only on assumptions that the disc is the source of pain.

The therapeutic utility of lumbar discography still remains unproven. No studies have yet shown that any treatment can reliably and consistently relieve pain if directed at the disc found to be symptomatic by discography. There is some evidence that outcomes of arthrodesis are better if planned on the basis of discography than if planned on imaging alone,[97] but this has not been confirmed by other studies. Most studies of arthrodesis have not used discography to select patients. Otherwise, discography is used to select patients for a variety of intradiscal therapies that are still being evaluated (see Intradiscal Therapies, below).

TREATMENT

Metaphorically, the treatment of chronic low back pain is a political minefield. It is occupied by several schools of thought. Each school believes that its treatment is the correct one, each tries to produce evidence of its efficacy, and each zealously defends itself against any criticism from other schools. The major schools represent multidisciplinary pain management or functional restoration, interventional pain medicine, surgery, individual therapies, and salvage or palliative care.

The plight of patients with chronic low back pain can be encapsulated, in cartoon form, as a journey through a five ring circus (Fig. 72.6). The patient may start with individual therapies, trying one then another. They may be referred for multidisciplinary pain management or functional restoration. They may find their way to interventional pain medicine, where they may be treated, or subjected to diagnostic tests that lead to surgery. When surgery or other interventions fail, the patient resorts to salvage treatment or what might be called palliative care. The patient may remain for a while in a particular cycle, before passing to one or more others. They may revisit cycles.

The various schools differ in certain key characteristics. Those who promote multidisciplinary pain management or functional restoration believe that a diagnosis is not possible; some even abjure pursuing a diagnosis.[98] Their objective is to help patients improve their function and cope with their pain. Relief of pain is not a primary objective. Proponents of individual therapies do not necessarily make a diagnosis. They apply a treatment that they believe works and that they believe the patient requires or should have. Surgeons believe that particular operations will relieve the patient's pain. A valid diagnosis may or may not be

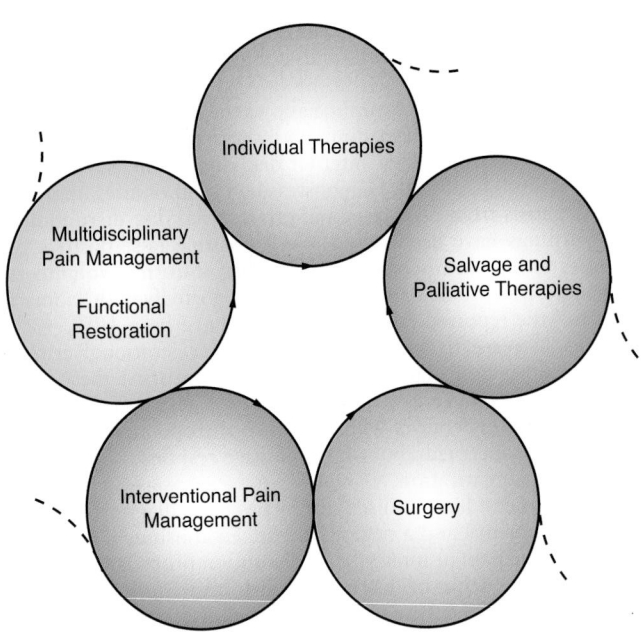

FIGURE 72.6 The-five ring circus of chronic low back pain. Patients cycle within or between various schools of treatment.

made. Interventional pain management strives to pinpoint a source of pain, and direct treatment to that source with the aim of stopping the pain. Those who undertake salvage and palliative care seek to relieve pain by interfering with nociception rather than treating its source.

Individual Therapies

Many individual therapies are available for patients with chronic low back pain. These include, but are not limited to drug therapy, exercise, manual therapy, massage, transcutaneous electrical nerve stimulation (TENS), acupuncture, back school, traction, and injections. Some practitioners may offer more than one. They may be tried serially; sometimes they are used in combination.

Most individual therapies are offered without the need for a diagnosis. For example, exercise does not require a patho-anatomical diagnosis; nor does drug therapy, TENS, or back school. Other therapies may be preceded by a diagnosis, but these diagnoses lack reliability, validity, or both. For example, acupuncture may be prescribed on the basis of pulse diagnosis or disturbed flows of energy along meridians, but these concepts have not been validated. Similarly, manual therapy may be predicated by purportedly diagnostic abnormalities of segmental motion, but these lack reliability and validity.[99,100]

The evidence supporting individual therapies is meager. At best it attests to small effect-sizes or effects for limited durations only.

Drugs

The drugs most often prescribed for chronic low back pain are simple analgesics, nonsteroidal anti-inflammatory drugs (NSAIDs), muscle relaxants, antidepressants, and tramadol. Opioids might also be used, but usually not as a first-line agent. The use of opioids is covered below under Salvage Therapy.

No studies have established the efficacy of paracetamol (acetaminophen) for chronic low back pain. Its use for this condition is based on the reputation of this agent as a relatively safe, simple analgesic. One study found that fewer patients had reduction of pain when taking paracetamol than when taking diflunisal,[101] but the difference was not statistically significant.

Systematic[102–104] and other reviews[105] of the literature indicate that NSAIDs are statistically more effective than placebo for relieving pain, but the effect-sizes have been modest or small.[106] Moreover, many studies followed patients for only 2, 4, or 6 weeks, and none beyond 12 weeks. No studies have indicated what proportion of patients achieved satisfying relief for sustained periods, and required no other treatment. NSAIDs, therefore, may have a role for the short-term relief of chronic low back pain, but there is no evidence that they are effective as a long-term alternative to other treatment.

The efficacy of muscle relaxants has been studied only for 1, 2, or 3 weeks.[105,107] Over such short periods agents such as tetrazepam and flupirtin have been found to be more effective than placebo in reducing pain, but the difference is small. For example, patients taking tetrazepam had an average reduction in pain of 50%, whereas those taking placebo had a reduction of 30%.[108] Other agents, such as diazepam and tolperisone, have not proved more effective than placebo in reducing pain.[105,107] There are no long-term data on the effectiveness of muscle relaxants.

Although antidepressants are promoted as a co-analgesic for chronic low back pain, evidence of their efficacy is limited.[109,110] They have not been studied for longer than 8 weeks. Some tricyclic antidepressants, but not others, are slightly more effective than placebo for reducing pain. Serotonin selective reuptake inhibitors are conspicuously ineffective for chronic low back pain.[110]

The available data on tramadol for chronic low back pain are curious. A compound analgesic, consisting of tramadol and acetaminophen, has been shown to be more effective than placebo in studies lasting 3 months.[111,112] The agent improves pain as well as function. What is not evident is the extent to which the improvements are due to the tramadol component or the acetaminophen component. The one study that assessed tramadol alone selected patients who tolerated tramadol and benefited from it during an open-label screening phase.[113] In those patients, tramadol was found to be more effective than placebo for relief of pain and improvement in function. Fewer patients (20.7%) discontinued tramadol for lack of adequate pain relief than did patients (51.3%) who took placebo. This effect was demonstrated in a 4-week study. Longer term data are not available.

What is evident from these data on drug therapy is that the evidence is not commensurate with the way drugs are used for chronic low back pain. Short-term data are extrapolated to imply long term efficacy, but this has not been shown. Long-term data are not available to justify long-term use. Unknown is the proportion of patients who are satisfied with the relief that they obtain and who do require other treatment.

Physiotherapy

Although medical practitioners are accustomed to referring patients with chronic low back pain for "physiotherapy" it is difficult to define exactly what this treatment constitutes. Individual physiotherapists may differ in exactly what they offer to patients. For some interventions that physiotherapists may offer, data on efficacy are available, and these are covered separately below (see Exercises, Manual Therapy, and TENS). For what might be called "routine physiotherapy" the data are fewer. A British study found that "routine physiotherapy" was neither more effective nor more cost-effective than providing advice for patients with chronic low back pain.[114]

Exercise

The European Guidelines for the Management of Chronic Non-Specific Low Back Pain recommend exercise as a first-line treatment.[103] However, exercise is not a powerful treatment. A systematic review found that exercise for chronic low back pain is more effective than no treatment and at least as effective as treatments such as usual care by a general practitioner, massage, and home exercises.[115,116] The effect-size of exercise, however, is quite small, measuring 0.57 when expressed as a standardized mean difference.[106] This amounts to a mean difference of 10 points (on a 100-point scale), when compared to no treatment, and 7.3 points when compared with other treatments.[115,116]

Proponents of high-intensity strengthening exercises have sought evidence of efficacy within the general literature on exercise for chronic low back pain, but found no clear evidence of benefit over other exercises or other interventions such as physiotherapy and massage.[117] Others likewise found trunk-strengthening exercises to be more effective than no exercises but not more effective than aerobics or McKenzie treatment.[118]

Proponents of core stabilization exercises found moderate evidence that this form of exercise is effective in improving pain and function, but strong evidence that it was not more effective than physiotherapy, manual therapy, general exercises, and minimal care.[119] Another review found that stabilization exercises were superior to usual medical care and education but not to manipulative therapy, and no additional effect was found when stabilization exercises were added to a conventional physiotherapy program.[120]

McKenzie Therapy

Systematic reviews found limited evidence concerning the efficacy of McKenzie therapy for chronic low back pain.[121,122] Advocates of the treatment cite a study that showed no superiority over stabilization exercises, and a study that showed slightly better outcomes than those of strengthening exercise at 2 months after treatment but not at 8 months.[123]

Massage

A systematic review lists several studies of massage for chronic low back pain,[124] but many are flawed by limitations such as lack of blinding and lack of follow-up after treatment. Those studies with long-term follow-up indicate that massage may be slightly more effective than acupuncture, education, or self-care at 10 weeks, but not after 52 weeks.[124]

Manipulative Therapy

Spinal manipulative therapy is perhaps the most hotly contested intervention for chronic low back pain, and the most extensively studied and most often subjected to systematic reviews. Individual studies have differed in their design and rigor. Reviews have differed in what they consider evidence of efficacy. A synthesis of the literature ventured limited and specific conclusions[125]:

> "Spinal manipulative therapy combined with strengthening exercises is as effective as prescription NSAIDs combined with exercises; flexion-distraction mobilization is more effective than exercises, for the relief of pain although not for improving disability."

In other respects, manipulative therapy appears more effective than some other interventions in the short-term, but evidence for long-term differences is either inconclusive or lacking.[125] In studies that enrolled mixed populations, with some patients having chronic low back pain, the evidence is conflicting as to whether the efficacy of spinal manipulative therapy is superior or similar to that of medical care or physiotherapy.[125] The calculated effect-size of manipulative therapy is small (0.35).[106]

Electrical Therapies

Systematic reviews of the literature have found several studies of the efficacy of transcutaneous electrical nerve stimulation (TENS) for chronic low back pain, but most assessed outcomes only immediately after treatment.[126-128] Even then, the effect size of TENS is small (0.22).[106] Only one study provided long-term follow-up (3 and 6 months) and found no significant difference from

placebo.[129] An attempted systematic review found no studies suitable for review of interferential therapy, electrical muscle stimulation, or ultrasound therapy.[126]

Traction

Multiple studies have shown that sustained traction is no more effective than sham treatment for chronic low back pain.[130] The evidence on intermittent traction is limited to two studies with opposing results.[130]

Trigger Point Injection

Despite the popularity of trigger point injection as a treatment, there are few studies of its efficacy, and even fewer of its efficacy specifically in patients with chronic low back pain.[131] Studies limited to immediate and short-term outcomes (7 days) report conflicting results. No studies have provided long-term data.

Prolotherapy

Multiple reviews have found no evidence of efficacy for prolotherapy.[132-134] Studies that used co-interventions have found positive results, but studies in which prolotherapy alone was tested found negative results.[132]

Acupuncture

Many studies have explored the efficacy of acupuncture for chronic low back pain. They vary in quality and conclusions. The pattern in the evidence is that acupuncture is better than no treatment; it may be better than TENS, but it is not more effective than sham acupuncture, massage, or self-care education.[135]

Epidural Injections

Epidural injections, by the caudal or interlaminar route, are used for the treatment of chronic low back pain, but there is no evidence of their efficacy for this condition. Epidural injections have been tested for radicular pain (see Chapter 100, Epidural Steroid Injections), but not in patients with back pain but no radicular pain. Despite this lack of evidence, some authorities curiously still recommend their use.[136]

Back School

As a stand-alone intervention, outside the context of multidisciplinary pain management (see below), back school is not an effective intervention for chronic low back pain.[137] It is not more effective than no treatment or placebo treatment.[137]

Brief Education

Brief education involves contact with a health care professional in sessions of short duration to encourage self-management, provide advice to stay active, and reduce potential concerns about back pain.[137] It is more effective than usual care in promoting return to work, but not for reducing pain or disability, although it is more effective than no treatment or massage in reducing disability.[137]

Fear-Avoidance Training

Fear-avoidance training is an intervention that has started to be assessed in recent years. It involves a physician or a psychologist encouraging patients to return to normal activities and physical exercise in order to overcome fears of aggravating pain and to reduce avoidance of activity. It has been shown to reduce pain and disability better than does usual care, and is no less effective than spinal surgery.[137]

MULTIDISCIPLINARY PAIN MANAGEMENT

In its original forms, multidisciplinary pain management involved the collaboration of various disciplines in the management of patients with chronic pain. Physicians would attend to the medical assessment of the patient and provide pharmacological interventions and perhaps other interventions. Physiotherapists would assess the patient's musculoskeletal disabilities, and provide interventions in that realm. A psychologist or psychiatrist would address the patient's psychological distress. Others, such as occupational therapists and social workers, would address the patient's vocational, social, and financial problems. If required, additional specialists, such as neurologists or surgeons, could be consulted.

Functional restoration had a separate, and later, origin. Although it, too, was multidisciplinary in nature, it was more prompted by sports medicine. In the way that athletes were known to overcome musculoskeletal injuries by concerted training and perseverance, it was proposed that injured workers could rehabilitate by work hardening. The objective was to restore function, virtually regardless of the pain.

It has now become difficult to disentangle multidisciplinary pain management from functional restoration, particularly when it comes to analyzing the literature on efficacy. Multidisciplinary pain management has adopted some of the principles and practices of functional restoration, particularly those of intensive training, whereas functional restoration adopted behavioral therapy from multidisciplinary pain management.

It is unclear the extent to which behavioral therapy is a critical component of functional restoration. As evidence of behavioral therapy for chronic low back pain, advocates cite reviews of behavioral therapy for chronic pain in general.[138] Those reviews are weighted by evidence pertaining to the treatment of temporomandibular pain, fibromyalgia, and arthritis. The literature specifically on chronic back pain is less compelling. For chronic low back pain, behavioral therapy has a moderate positive effect on pain, and a small positive effect on functional status when compared with no treatment, placebo treatment, or being put on a waiting list; however, adding behavioral therapy to usual care has no short-term or long-term effect on pain, functional status, or behavior.[139,140] Nor is behavioral therapy more effective than exercise.[141] More recent studies have shown that a group program of exercise or education using a cognitive behavioral approach is not significantly more effective than providing an educational booklet[142]; and that active physical treatment is as effective as cognitive behavioral treatment or a combination of active physical treatment and cognitive behavioral treatment.[143]

The critical component of multidisciplinary rehabilitation would appear to be the intensity of the program, particularly its physical component. A systematic review found strong evidence that intensive, multidisciplinary rehabilitation with functional restoration improves function when compared with inpatient or outpatient rehabilitation that was not multidisciplinary, and moderate evidence that it reduces pain.[144,145] It also found that less intensive multidisciplinary rehabilitation did not provide improvements in pain, function, or vocational outcomes when compared with nonmultidisciplinary rehabilitation or usual care.

Although the conclusions about intensive multidisciplinary rehabilitation are favorable, it is conspicuous that it is not a treatment that effects a cure. The outcomes are cast in terms of reductions in pain and improvements in disability. When the original literature is consulted, the magnitudes of improvement are from 6.1 to 5.7 for pain, 16.9 to 12.1 for function in one study,[146] and a 17-point reduction on a 100-point scale for pain, in another study.[147] Despite these limitations, the European Guidelines recommend multidisciplinary rehabilitation for chronic low back pain.[103]

SURGERY

Surgeons offer a variety of operations for the treatment of chronic low back pain. They include various ways of fusing the lumbar spine and various forms of disc replacement. Some surgeons select the segmental level to be treated on the basis of discography. For others, the indication for surgery seems to be persistent pain and evidence on medical imaging of disc degeneration.

Surgery has not avoided scientific scrutiny; there have been many studies of surgery for back pain, but most have only compared one technique with another. Few studies have addressed critical issues such as clinical outcome in comparison with other less invasive, less destructive, and less irreversible interventions. Only three randomized, controlled trials have done this.

One study found spine fusion to be more effective than physiotherapy, but only marginally so.[148] The continuous outcome data for pain show a distinct improvement in the surgery group at 6 and 12 months, which did not occur in the nonsurgical group; however, at 24 months there was decay in outcomes of the surgery group, such that considerable overlap occurred in the outcomes of the two groups (Fig. 72.7). The categorical outcome data are more revealing. No patient was reported to have been cured of their pain, by either intervention. The advantages of surgical treatment were only that a greater proportion of patients reported feeling much better or better (Table 72.4). Reciprocally, a greater proportion of patients who had nonsurgical treatment were unchanged. The success rate of surgery for making patients "better" was 63%. For a major intervention, this is a disappointing figure,

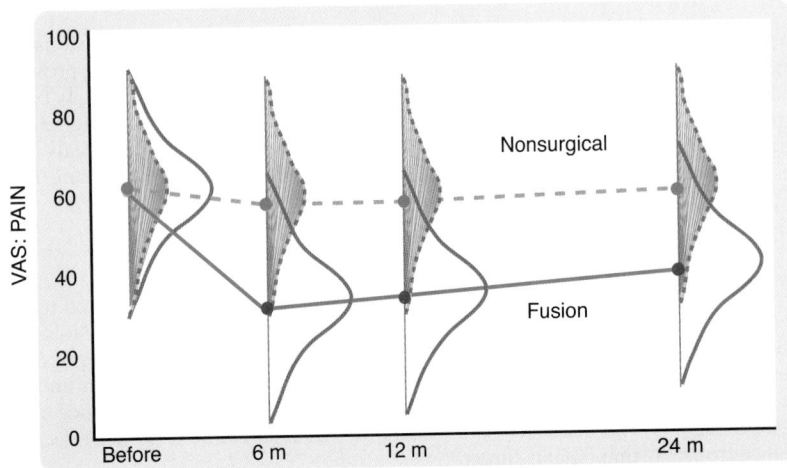

FIGURE 72.7 The outcomes at 6 months, 12 months, and 24 months of the study by Fritzell et al,[148] which compared fusion with nonsurgical therapy for chronic low back pain. Depicted are the mean visual analog scores (VAS) for pain, and their distributions based on the standard deviations reported in the study.

TABLE 72.4

THE CATEGORICAL OUTCOMES OF THE STUDY OF FRITZELL ET AL,[148] OF SURGERY COMPARED WITH NONSURGICAL CARE FOR CHRONIC LOW BACK PAIN

	Treatment group	
	Surgery	Nonsurgical
Much better	29%	14%
Better	34%	15%
Unchanged	24%	45%
Worse	14%	26%

and is dissonant with the public expectation that surgery "fixes" problems. Other conservative interventions might be just as effective if making patients "better" is the only objective. This is borne out by other studies.

A second study compared surgery with an intervention consisting of exercises and a cognitive-behavioral rehabilitation program.[149] In terms of pain and disability, the outcomes were indistinguishable statistically (Fig. 72.8). A third study also found no differences in outcomes between surgery and cognitive therapy coupled with intensive rehabilitation.[150]

Surgical treatments other than fusion have not yet been studied in this way.

INTERVENTIONAL PAIN MANAGEMENT

The objectives of interventional pain management are to pinpoint the source of a patient's pain and to direct treatment specifically to that source. If the lesion responsible for the pain cannot itself be treated, then interventions can target the nerves that mediate the pain in order to block nociception.

In terms of volume of publications, interventional pain management has attracted substantially less research than more conventional and traditional interventions for chronic low back pain, for several reasons. Interventional pain management requires expensive, specialized facilities, a license to practice invasive procedures, and the training to do so. Consequently, the procedures cannot be practiced anywhere or by anyone. As well, the number of individuals with skills in this field, who also hold academic appointments and might undertake the necessary research, num-

ber barely a handful worldwide. As a result, the literature is meager compared with that of other disciplines in chronic low back pain, but not without merit.

Zygapophyseal Joint Pain

A diagnosis of lumbar zygapophyseal joint pain can be established using controlled, diagnostic blocks of the medial branches that innervate the painful joint (see Chapter 97, Diagnostic and Therapeutic Nerve Blocks). This pain can be treated by percutaneous lumbar medial branch radiofrequency neurotomy (see Chapter 101, Neurolytic Blockade). In this procedure, electrodes are used to coagulate the nerves in order to provide long-lasting relief of pain.

The benchmark for outcomes was established in a small observational study.[151] Patients were selected on the basis of positive responses to controlled diagnostic blocks. Anatomically correct technique was meticulously executed. At 1-year follow-up, some 60% of patients maintained at least 80% relief of their pain, and 80% maintained at least 60% relief.

Two controlled trials have established that lumbar medial branch neurotomy is not a placebo.[152,153] Patients treated with the active procedure achieved superior outcomes, in terms of relief of pain and improvement in function, than did patients who underwent sham treatment.

Outcome studies have shown that, when the operation is successful, good relief is maintained.[154] If pain recurs and requires treatment, relief can be successfully reinstated by repeating the neurotomy.[155]

Patient selection is critical to a successful outcome. The patient must be shown to have zygapophyseal joint pain. Long-term outcomes are substantially and significantly better when a diagnosis is correctly established than when it is assumed.[156] Correct technique must be used.[157,158] Studies purporting to discredit medial branch neurotomy have not used anatomically accurate techniques.[157]

Sacroiliac Joint Pain

Although pain can be traced to the sacroiliac joint by using controlled diagnostic blocks, a successful treatment has proved elusive. A variety of conservative therapies are advocated,[159] but none has been validated in controlled trials. Arthrodesis of the joint is advocated and appears successful in small observational studies,[160] but has not been tested in controlled trials.

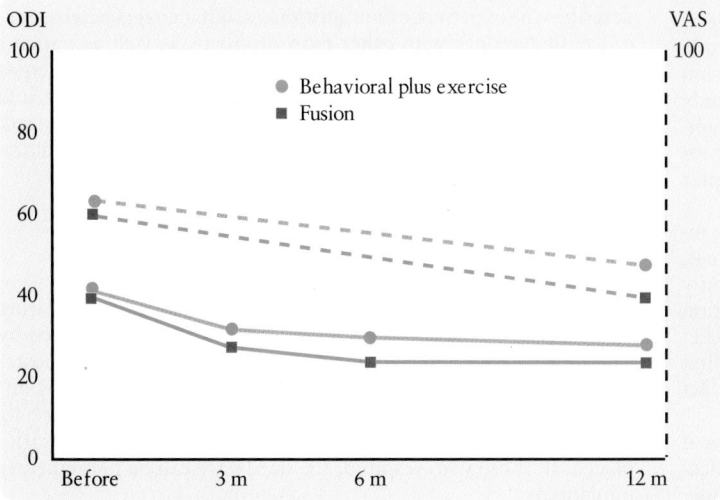

FIGURE 72.8 Outcomes of the study of Brox et al[149] that compared fusion with behavioral therapy and exercises.

Practitioners of interventional pain medicine have explored methods of denervating painful sacroiliac joints (see Chapter 101, Neurolytic Blockade). The target nerves are the lateral branches of the sacral dorsal rami. These can be coagulated using radiofrequency neurotomy.

A controlled trial has shown that sacral lateral branch radiofrequency neurotomy is undoubtedly more effective than sham treatment.[161] The duration of effect, however, is limited. Whereas 80% of patients achieved at least 50% relief of their pain at 1 month, this proportion had dropped to 60% at 6 months and 10% at 12 months.[161]

Discogenic Pain

A variety of interventions are being explored for the selective treatment of lumbar discogenic pain (see Chapter 100, Interventions for Vertebral Body and Disc Pain). Variously these target the pathology of internal disc disruption at a macroscopic or molecular level, or the nerves that transduce the pain. To date, however, only one intervention has been subject to controlled trials.

Intradiscal electrothermal anuloplasty (IDET) involves inserting a flexible electrode circumferentially into the posterior annulus of the painful disc. The electrode is heated to around 85° to 90°C, ostensibly to seal radial fissures, coagulate algogenic material within those fissures, or to coagulate the nerve endings around them.[162] The indications for the procedure are positive responses to discography, demonstration of a radial fissure on postdiscography CT scan, and preservation of sufficient disc height to enable introduction of the electrode to a suitable location.[162]

The first controlled study of IDET was conducted at a time when the efficacy of the procedure was still unknown.[163,164] It was not randomized, but instead used a convenience sample of patients denied permission to have the procedure by their insurer. These patients underwent conventional functional restoration. IDET proved significantly more effective at 1-year and 2-year follow-up. Of those treated with IDET, 54% achieved at least 50% reduction in pain, returned to work, and no longer required opioids. The corresponding figure for those who underwent rehabilitation was 10%. Furthermore, 20% of patients treated with IDET had complete relief of pain, returned to work, and did not require opioids. In the rehabilitation group, none achieved this outcome. The complement of these figures, however, is that some 50% of patients obtain no benefit from IDET. This fact affects the utility of the procedure, which emerged in latter studies.

A randomized, placebo controlled study reported an intriguing result.[165] No patient benefited from IDET, and no patient benefited from sham treatment. The placebo response rate was zero. This is curious, for it is rare for any control treatment of pain to have absolutely no effect. Failure to respond suggests substantial nocebo effects. The authors concluded that their study showed that IDET was no better than a placebo. This is somewhat egregious because no placebo effect was encountered. The study would have been more convincing if the investigators had encountered even a small response rate, commensurate with that reported in observational studies of the procedure (see Chapter 102, Interventions for Vertebral Body and Disc Pain).

The second placebo-controlled trial yielded more realistic results.[166] Patients responded both to IDET and to sham treatment, but the magnitude of improvement in pain was significantly greater in those who had active treatment. A greater proportion of patients treated with IDET (8/32) achieved at least 75% relief of pain than did patients who had sham treatment (1/24). What prevents these differences being convincing statistically is the fact that IDET fails to relieve pain in 50% of patients.

It is the failure rate that limits the utility of IDET. Even if patients are stringently selected, half will not benefit. Cynical observers might use that failure to discredit IDET as an inadequate procedure. However, for the patients who do benefit, IDET is an attractive alternative to other interventions that are recommended to them but for which there is little or no evidence of efficacy. In that regard, reviewers[167] and investigators[168] have argued that IDET is an entertainable option before embarking on surgical treatment.

The limited efficacy of IDET has been attributed to the small radius of the lesion produced by the electrodes used.[169] With such a small field of influence, the electrodes cannot be guaranteed to capture fissures within the annulus in their entirety, or to capture all the nerves that mediate the pain. This concept has prompted the development of techniques by which to produce larger thermal lesions within the annulus.

One such technique is biacuplasty, in which a broad thermal lesion is produced across the posterior annulus between a pair of water-cooled electrodes. An observational study has produced somewhat encouraging results,[170] and a controlled trial is being conducted.

SALVAGE AND PALLIATIVE CARE

Salvage or palliative care is what patients turn to when other interventions have failed. In the past, it was typically the care to which patients resorted when surgery failed to relieve their pain (see Chapter 74, Failed Back Surgery Syndrome). Nowadays it includes patients who fail interventional pain management, or even functional restoration.

The notion of "salvage" pertains to salvaging patients from the failure and complications of other interventions. The notion of "palliative care" means providing some degree of relief when a definitive cure is not possible. Three main interventions fall into this domain: intrathecal opioids, spinal cord stimulation, and oral opioids.

Intrathecal Opioids

If applied to the spinal cord, opioids can exert analgesic effects at doses substantially less than those required if they are administered by the oral route. They can be delivered from a subcutaneous reservoir connected to a catheter inserted into the intrathecal space (see Chapter 99, Neuraxial Drug Delivery).

Intrathecal opioids are provided by practitioners who have the skills to implant the devices required and who are prepared to monitor patients—to deal with obstructions and infections in the delivery system, to replenish agents in the reservoir, and to minimize dose escalation.

The efficacy of intrathecal opioids for chronic low back pain rests on reputation and experience. There is some literature that describes the experience of practitioners, but it covers heterogeneous patients: ones with other pain problems as well as patients with low back pain. No studies have described the effectiveness of intrathecal opioids exclusively in patients with chronic low back pain. Moreover, no controlled studies have been reported. The practice of intrathecal opioids is sustained by position statements.[171]

Spinal Cord Stimulation

Nociception can be reduced or blocked by electrically stimulating the posterior surface of the spinal cord. This can be achieved by electrodes placed in the epidural space or implanted in the posterior dural sac. The electrodes are driven by a battery that is implanted into a subcutaneous pocket, like a pacemaker. Patients suitable for treatment are screened using electrodes temporarily placed. In those who respond, the hardware can be permanently implanted.

Spinal cord stimulation is the mainstay of treatment for failed back surgery syndrome (see Chapter 74, Failed Back Surgery Syndrome) particularly when patients have neuropathic pain rather than somatic pain. In the past, the use of spinal cord stimulation was based exclusively on observational studies and reputation. Of late, the challenge for controlled studies has been answered.

For patients with persistent or recurrent radicular pain after spine surgery, spinal cord stimulation is more often successful than reoperation[172] and is more cost effective.[173] Adding spinal cord stimulation to conventional medical management is more effective than conventional medical management alone, in terms of achieving 50% relief of pain, and improving quality of life and functional capacity.[174]

Spinal cord stimulation is not a cure for chronic back pain. It is an option for patients who have exhausted other options. Moreover, the cardinal indication is leg pain rather than back pain, although both types of pain benefit. However, success is limited. Only about 50% of patients achieve greater than 50% relief of pain,[174] and only about 15% are able to return to work.[175]

Oral Opioids

As pain medicine matured as a specialty, previous fears and restrictions about the long-term use of opioids in patients with pain not due to cancer were gradually overcome. Patients with chronic low back pain became eligible for treatment with long-term opioids. This has become the cardinal resort for patients in whom a diagnosis cannot be made or who have not responded to interventional pain management, for whom surgery is not indicated, in whom surgery has failed, or who have not benefited from functional restoration or individual therapies.

Opioids were used for such patients in the expectation that they would relieve their pain. Indeed, in lay circles, opioids are referred to as "pain-killers," which implies eradication of pain. This has proved not the case.

There is conspicuously little evidence for the use of opioids for chronic low back pain. One review[176] identified one study of dextropropoxyphene, one of tramadol, one pertaining to topical morphine, and one of oxycodone published only in abstract form. For classical opioids, it only found one study of oxymorphone[177] and one of oxycodone.[178] The former study found oxymorphone to be more effective than placebo, but the follow-up period was only 18 days. The latter study reported oxycodone to be more effective than naproxen, but a Cochrane review[179] recalculated the differences and found them to be not statistically significant.

A third review[180] identified two additional studies. Both from the same institution, these studies found oxymorphone to be superior to placebo for relief of pain during a 12-week period of assessment.[181,182] Other studies identified by this review only compared different opioids or different formulations of the same drug.

This paucity of data has led reviewers to conclude that opioids may be efficacious for short-term relief of pain, but their long-term efficacy is not clear,[176,180] or that the benefits for the long-term management of chronic low back pain remain questionable.[179]

It is also evident from the literature that opioids are not universally effective. During the titration phase of some studies, 37%,[181] 15%,[177] or 43%[182] of patients discontinued treatment because of adverse side effects. Once the dose was stabilized, a further 17%,[181] 14%,[182] 20%,[178] or 30%[177] ceased treatment because of side effects or for lack of efficacy.

Of increasing concern are the problems of opioid-induced hyperalgesia, tolerance, and abuse.[183] In studies that have reported abuse, its prevalence ranges between 3% and 43%.[176] The literature on opioids for chronic pain in general helps little to support their use for chronic low back pain. The controlled studies have

all had short periods of follow-up.[183] Open-label follow-up studies indicate that up to 56% of patients abandon the treatment because of lack of analgesic efficacy or side effects.[183,184] The one consolation is that those patients who stay on treatment seem to maintain their analgesia.[183,184]

Despite these limitations and problems, guidelines still allow opioids for chronic low back pain[103]—perhaps reluctantly, perhaps in recognition that there is no alternative.

DISCUSSION

In light of the available evidence, it should not be surprising that patients with chronic low back pain get lost in a five-ring circus (see Fig. 72.6). None of the treatments, in any of the rings, are properly—let alone perfectly—effective. Many treatments are no more effective than sham treatment or placebo. Some are more effective than no treatment. Others are more effective than usual care, but some are not. Most offer partial reduction in pain, if any, and perhaps improvement in function or psychological state. Few treatments approach what patients seek—elimination of pain.[185]

The objective of any treatment should be to reduce the burden of illness: Once treated, patients should not need to seek other care. This is not evident in the treatment of back pain. Treatment with drugs and physical, electrical, and like therapies has not been shown to be successful. Once patients exhaust those options they seek other avenues. Multidisciplinary rehabilitation helps some patients, but does not eliminate their problem. Surgery offers the promise of a cure, but succeeds in making only some patients better.

It is only in interventional pain management that the objective has been to eliminate pain, or at least substantially reduce it. This is possible with lumbar medial branch neurotomy, but ironically this treatment appears suitable for only a minority of patients with chronic low back pain. Treatments for more common causes of pain, such as IDET, are not universally effective.

Salvage treatment and palliative care are portrayed as last resorts or ports of final call, but even they are incompletely effective. While opioids can palliate some patients, others are intolerant of them.

The reasons for this parlous state have not been explored or revealed. It is perhaps that the treatment of chronic low back pain is practice-driven, not problem-driven. Practitioners of various disciplines have been taught to treat patients by particular methods. They have chosen, or have been taught, to believe that their treatment should and does work. When the evidence proves otherwise, a dilemma arises. Established practitioners are reluctant to abandon their craft. They must persevere or face oblivion. Surgeons are not likely to stop operating just because an outsider writes that surgery does not work. Nor are physiotherapists or chiropractors going to cease prescribing exercises or manipulation. It is easier to find faults in hostile studies or reviews, and thereby deflect the burden of self-effacement and responsibility.

Research has been conducted into back pain and continues to be conducted; however, the bulk of that research is not the sort that is required. Studies focus on defending or proving contentious interventions that have been traditional, or which sounded like a good idea. What are needed are not so much answers but the right questions. Why do these patients continue to suffer, and can we fix it? The answers should not come in the forms of opinions, conjectures, or so-called theories, but with objective tests that decide the answer free of personal bias.

References

1. Merskey H, Bogduk N. *Classification of Chronic Pain. Descriptions of Chronic Pain Syndromes and Definition of Pain Terms.* 2nd edition. Seattle: IASP Press, 1994.

2. Van Tulder MW, Koes BW, Bouter LM. Conservative treatment of acute and chronic nonspecific low back pain: a systematic review of randomized controlled trials of the most common interventions. *Spine* 1997;22: 2128–2156.

3. Waddell G. *The Back Pain Revolution*. Edinburgh: Churchill Livingstone, 1998;33.

4. Kellgren JH. Observations on referred pain arising from muscle. *Clin Sci* 1938; 3:175–190.

5. Bogduk N. Lumbar dorsal ramus syndrome. *Med J Aust* 1980;2:537–541.

6. Kellgren JH. On the distribution of pain arising from deep somatic structures with charts of segmental pain areas. *Clin Sci* 1939;4:35–46.

7. Feinstein B, Langton JNK, Jameson RM, et al. Experiments on pain referred from deep structures. *J Bone Joint Surg* 1954;36A:981–997.

8. Mooney V, Robertson J. The facet syndrome. *Clin Orthop* 1976;115: 149–156.

9. McCall IW, Park WM, O'Brien JP. Induced pain referred from posterior lumbar elements in normal subjects. *Spine* 1979;4:441–446.

10. Fukui S, Ohseto K, Shiotani M, et al. Distribution of referred pain from the lumbar zygapophyseal joints and dorsal rami. *Clin J Pain* 1997;13:303–307.

11. Fortin JD, Dwyer AP, West S, et al. Sacroiliac joint: pain referral maps upon applying a new injection/arthrography technique. Part I: asymptomatic volunteers. *Spine* 1994;19:1475–1482.

12. Wiberg G. Back pain in relation to the nerve supply of the intervertebral disc. *Acta Orthop Scand* 1947;19:211–221.

13. Falconer MA, McGeorge M, Begg AC. Observations on the cause and mechanism of symptom-production in sciatica and low-back pain. *J Neurol Neurosurg Psychiatry* 1948;11:13–26.

14. Kuslich SD, Ulstrom CL, Michael CJ. The tissue origin of low back pain and sciatica: a report of pain response to tissue stimulation during operations on the lumbar spine using local anesthesia. *Orthop Clin North Am* 1991;22: 181–187.

15. O'Neill CW, Kurgansky ME, Derby R, et al. Disc stimulation and patterns of referred pain. *Spine* 2002;27:2776–2781.

16. El-Mahdi MA, Abdel Latif FY, Janko M. The spinal nerve root "innervation," and a new concept of the clinicopathological interrelations in back pain and sciatica. *Neurochirurgia* 1981;24:137–141.

17. Smyth MJ, Wright V. Sciatica and the intervertebral disc: an experimental study. J *Bone Joint Surg* 1959;40A:1401–1418.

18. Norlen G. On the value of the neurological symptoms in sciatica for the localization of a lumbar disc herniation. *Acta Chir Scand* 1944;95 (suppl): 1–96.

19. Quebec Task Force on Spinal Disorders. Scientific approach to the assessment and management of activity-related spinal disorders: a monograph for clinicians. *Spine* 1987;12 (suppl 7):S1–S59.

20. Dillane JB, Fry J, Kalton G. Acute back syndrome—a study from general practice. *Brit Med J* 1966;2:82–84.

21. van Tulder MW, Assendelft WJJ, Koes BW, et al. Spinal radiographic findings and nonspecific low back pain: a systematic review of observational studies. *Spine* 1997;22:427–434.

22. Bogduk N, McGuirk B. *Medical Management of Acute and Chronic Low Back Pain. An Evidence-Based Approach*. Amsterdam, Netherlands: Elsevier, 2002:49–63.

23. Bogduk N, McGuirk B. *Medical Management of Acute and Chronic Low Back Pain. An Evidence-Based Approach*. Amsterdam, Netherlands: Elsevier, 2002:115–125.

24. Bogduk N. Diagnostic nerve blocks in chronic pain. Best practice. *Res Clin Anaesth* 2002;16:565–578.

25. Bogduk N. Diagnostic blocks: a truth serum for malingering. *Clin J Pain* 2004;20:409–414.

26. Schwarzer AC, Aprill CN, Bogduk N. The sacroiliac joint in chronic low back pain. *Spine* 1995;20:31–37.

27. Maigne JY, Aivaliklis A, Pfefer F. Results of sacroiliac joint double block and value of sacroiliac pain provocation tests in 54 patients with low-back pain. *Spine* 1996;21:1889–1892.

28. Schwarzer AC, Aprill CN, Derby R, et al. Clinical features of patients with pain stemming from the lumbar zygapophyseal joints: is the lumbar facet syndrome a clinical entity? *Spine* 1994;19:1132–1137.

29. Schwarzer AC, Wang SC, Bogduk N, et al. Prevalence and clinical features of lumbar zygapophyseal joint pain: a study in an Australian population with chronic low back pain. *Ann Rheum Dis* 1995;54:100–106.

30. Manchikanti L, Pampati V, Fellows B, et al. Prevalence of lumbar facet joint pain in chronic low back pain. *Pain Physician* 1999;2:59–64.

31. Manchikanti L, Pampati V, Fellows B, et al. The inability of the clinical picture to characterize pain from facet joints. *Pain Physician* 2000;3:158–166.

32. Manchikanti L, Pampati V, Fellows B, et al. The diagnostic validity and therapeutic value of lumbar facet joint nerve blocks with or without adjuvant agents. *Curr Rev Pain* 2000;4:337–344.

33. Schwarzer AC, Aprill CN, Derby R, et al. The prevalence and clinical features of internal disc disruption in patients with chronic low back pain. *Spine* 1995; 20:1878–1883.

34. Carette S, Marcoux S, Truchon R, et al. A controlled trial of corticosteroid injections into facet joints for chronic low back pain. *New Engl J Med* 1991; 325:1002–1007.

35. Jackson RP, Jacobs RR, Montesano PX. Facet joint injection in low back pain: a prospective study. *Spine* 1988;13:966–971.

36. Laslett M, Oberg B, Aprill CN, et al. Zygapophysial joint blocks in chronic low back pain: a test of Revel's model as a screening test. *BMC Musculoskelet Disord* 2004;5:43.

37. Laslett M, McDonald B, Aprill CN, et al. Clinical predictors of screening lumbar zygapophyseal joint blocks: development of clinical prediction rules. *Spine J* 2006;6:370–379.

38. Schwarzer AC, Wang S, O'Driscoll D, et al. The ability of computed tomography to identify a painful zygapophyseal joint in patients with chronic low back pain. *Spine* 1995;20:907–912.

39. Czervionke LF, Fenton DS. Fat-saturated MR imaging in the detection of inflammatory facet arthropathy (facet synovitis) in the lumbar spine. *Pain Med* 2008;9:400–406.

40. Adams MA, McNally DS, Wagstaff J, et al. Abnormal stress concentrations in lumbar intervertebral discs following damage to the vertebral bodies: cause of disc failure? *Eur Spine J* 1993;1:214–221.

41. Sachs BL, Vanharanta H, Spivey MA, et al. Dallas discogram description: a new classification of CT/discography in low-back disorders. *Spine* 1987;12: 287–294.

42. Aprill C, Bogduk N. High-intensity zone: a diagnostic sign of painful lumbar disc on magnetic resonance imaging. *Br J Radiol* 1992;65:361–369.

43. McNally DS, Adams MA. Intervertebral disc mechanics as revealed by stress profilometry. *Spine* 1992;17:66–73.

44. Vanharanta H, Sachs BL, Spivey MA, et al. The relationship of pain provocation to lumbar disc deterioration as seen by CT/discography. *Spine* 1987;12: 295–298.

45. Moneta GB, Videman T, Kaivanto K, et al. Reported pain during lumbar discography as a function of anular ruptures and disc degeneration: a re-analysis of 833 discograms. *Spine* 1994;17:1968–1974.

46. McNally DS, Shackleford IM, Goodship AE, et al. In vivo stress measurement can predict pain on discography. *Spine* 1996;21:2500–2587.

47. Holm S, Holm AK, Ekstrom L, et al. Experimental disc degeneration due to endplate injury. *J Spinal Disord Tech* 2004;17:64–71.

48. Cinotti G, Della Rocca C, Romeo S, et al. Degenerative changes of porcine intervertebral disc induced by vertebral endplate injury. *Spine* 2005;15:30: 174–180.

49. Haschtmann D, Stoyanov JV, Gédet P, et al. Vertebral endplate trauma induces disc cell apoptosis and promotes organ degeneration in vitro. *Eur Spin L* 2008;17:289–299.

50. Hansson TH, Keller TS, Spengler DM. Mechanical behaviour of the human lumbar spine. II. Fatigue strength during dynamic compressive loading. *J Orthop Res* 1987;5:479–487.

51. Brinckmann P, Biggemann M, Hilweg D. Fatigue fracture of human lumbar vertebrae. *Clin Biomech* 1988;3(suppl 1):S1–S23.

52. Holm S, Baranto A, Kaigle Holm A, et al. Reactive changes in the adolescent porcine spine with disc degeneration due to endplate injury. *Vet Comp Orthop Traumatol* 2007;20:12–17.

53. Ohtori S, Inoue G, Ito T, et al. Tumor necrosis factor-immunoreactive cells and PGP 9.5-immunoreactive nerve fibres in vertebral endplates of patients with discogenic low back pain and Modic Type 1 or Type 2 changes on MRI. *Spine* 2006;31:1026–1031.

54. Malawski SK, Lukawski S. Pyogenic infection of the spine. *Clin Orthop* 1991; 272:58–66.

55. Bogduk N, McGuirk B. History. In: Bogduk N, McGuirk B, (eds). *Medical Management of Acute and Chronic Low Back Pain. An Evidence-Based Approach*. Amsterdam, Netherlands: Elsevier, 2002:27–40.

56. Laslett M, Young SB, Aprill CN, et al. Diagnosing painful sacroiliac joints: a validity study of a McKenzie evaluation and sacroiliac provocation tests. *Aust J Physiother* 2003;49:89–97.

57. Laslett M, Oberg B, Aprill CN, et al. Centralization as a predictor of provocation discography results in chronic low back pain, and the influence of disability and distress on diagnostic power. *Spine J* 2005;5:370–380.

58. Aina A, May S, Clare H. The centralization phenomenon of spinal symptoms—a systematic review. *Man Ther* 2004;9:134–143.

59. Gamsa A. The role of psychological factors in chronic pain. I. A half century of study. *Pain* 1994;57:5–15.

60. Gamsa A. The role of psychological factors in chronic pain. II. A critical appraisal. *Pain* 1994;57:17–29.

61. Fishbain DA, Rosomoff HL, Cutler R, et al. Secondary gain concept: a review of the scientific literature. *Clin J Pain* 1995;11:6–21.

62. DSM-IV-TR. *Diagnostic and Statistical Manual of Mental Disorders*. 4th edition. Text Revision. Washington DC: American Psychiatric Association, 2000.

63. Fishbain DA, Cutler R, Rosomoff HL, et al. Chronic pain disability exaggeration/malingering and submaximal effort research. *Clin J Pain* 1999; 5:244–274.

64. First MB, Frances A, Pincus HA. *DSM-IV-TR Handbook of Differential Diagnosis*. Washington, DC: American Psychiatric Association, 2002.

65. Kinney RK, Gatchel RJ, Mayer TG. The SCL-90R evaluated as an alternative to the MMPI for psychological screening of chronic low-back pain patients. *Spine* 1991;16:940–942.

66. Peebles JE, McWilliams LA, MacLennan R. A comparison of symptom checklist 90—revised from patients with chronic pain from whiplash and patients with other musculoskeletal injuries. *Spine* 2001;26:766–770.

67. Main CJ, Wood PLR, Hollis S, et al. The distress and risk assessment method: a simple patient classification to identify distress and evaluate the risk of poor outcome. *Spine* 1992;17:42–52.

68. Bogduk N, McGuirk B. Assessment. In: Bogduk N, McGuirk B, (eds). *Medical*

Management of Acute and Chronic Low Back Pain. An Evidence-Based Approach. Amsterdam, Netherlands: Elsevier, 2002;127–138.

69. Dvorak J. Neurophysiologic tests in diagnosis of nerve root compression caused by disc herniation. *Spine* 1996;21(suppl 24):39S–44S.

70. Andersson GBJ, Brown MD, Dvorak J, et al. Consensus summary on the diagnosis and treatment of lumbar disc herniation. *Spine* 1996;21 (suppl 24):75S–78S.

71. Jensen MC, Brant-Zawadzki MN, Obuchowski N, et al. Magnetic resonance imaging of the lumbar spine in people without back pain. *N Engl J Med* 1994;331:69–73.

72. Boden SD, Davis DO, Dina TS, et al. Abnormal magnetic resonance scans of the lumbar spine in asymptomatic subjects: a prospective investigation. *J Bone Joint Surg* 1990;72A:403–408.

73. Peng B, Hou S, Wu W, et al. The pathogenesis and clinical significance of a high-intensity zone (HIZ) of lumbar intervertebral disc on MR imaging in the patient with discogenic low back pain. *Eur Spine J* 2006;15:583–587.

74. Saifuddin A, Braithwaite I, White J, et al. The value of lumbar spine magnetic resonance imaging in the demonstration of anular tears. *Spine* 1998;23:453–457.

75. Ito M, Incorvaia KM, Yu SF, et al. Predictive signs of discogenic lumbar pain on magnetic resonance imaging with discography correlation. *Spine* 1998;23:1252–1260.

76. Lam KS, Carlin D, Mulhollad RC. Lumbar disc high-intensity zone: the value and significance of provocative discography in the determination of the discogenic pain source. *Eur Spine J* 2000;9:36–41.

77. Schellhas KP, Pollei SR, Gundry CR, et al. Lumbar disc high-intensity zone: correlation of magnetic resonance imaging and discography. *Spine* 1996;21:79–86.

78. Smith BMT, Hurwitz EL, Solsberg D, et al. Interobserver reliability of detecting lumbar intervertebral disc high-intensity zone on magnetic resonance imaging and association of high intensity zone with pain and anular disruption. *Spine* 1998;23:2074–2080.

79. Carragee EJ, Paragoudakis SJ, Khurana S. Lumbar high-intensity zone and discography in subjects without low back problems. *Spine* 2000;25:2987–2992.

80. Weishaupt D, Zanetti M, Hodler J, et al. Painful lumbar disk derangement: relevance of endplate abnormalities at MR imaging. *Radiology* 2001;218:420–427.

81. Ricketson R, Simmons JW, Hauser BO. The prolapsed intervertebral disc. The high-intensity zone with discography correlation. *Spine* 1996;21:2758–2762.

82. Modic MT, Steindberg PM, Ross JS, et al. Degenerative disc disease: assessment of changes in vertebral body marrow with MR imaging. *Radiology* 1988;166:193–199.

83. Braithwaite I, White J, Saifuddin A, et al. Vertebral endplate (Modic) changes on lumbar spine MRI: correlation with pain reproduction at lumbar discography. *Eur Spine J* 1998;7:363–368.

84. Kaplan M, Dreyfuss P, Halbrook B, et al. The ability of lumbar medial branch blocks to anesthetize the zygapophyseal joint. *Spine* 1998;23:1847–1852.

85. Dreyfuss P, Schwarzer AC, Lau P, et al. Specificity of lumbar medial branch and L5 dorsal ramus blocks: a computed tomographic study. *Spine* 1997;22:895–902.

86. Schwarzer AC, April CN, Derby R, et al. The false-positive rate of uncontrolled diagnostic blocks of the lumbar zygapophyseal joints. *Pain* 1994;58:195–200.

87. Manchikanti L, Pampati V, Fellows B, et al. The diagnostic validity and therapeutic value of lumbar facet joint nerve blocks with or without adjuvant agents. *Curr Rev Pain* 2000;4:337–344.

88. International Spine Intervention Society. An algorithm for the investigation of low back pain. In: Bogduk N, (ed). *Practice Guidelines for Spinal Diagnostic and Treatment Procedures.* San Francisco, CA: International Spine Intervention Society, 2004:87–94.

89. Bogduk N. Evidence-informed management of chronic back pain with facet injections and radiofrequency neurotomy. *Spine J* 2008;8:56–64.

90. Dreyfuss P, Snyder BD, Park K, et al. The ability of single site, single depth sacral lateral branch blocks to anesthetize the sacroiliac joint complex. *Pain Med* 2008;9:844–850.

91. Dreyfuss P, Henning T, Malladi M, et al.The ability of multi-site, multi-depth sacral lateral branch blocks to anesthetize the sacroiliac joint complex: a physiologic study. *Pain Med.* In press.

92. International Spinal Intervention Society. Lumbar disc stimulation. In: Bogduk N (ed). *Practice Guidelines for Spinal Diagnostic and Treatment Procedures.* San Francisco, CA: Spinal Intervention Society, 2004:20–46.

93. Derby R, Lee SH, Kim BJ, et al. Pressure-controlled lumbar discography in volunteers without low back symptoms. *Pain Med* 2005;6:213–221.

94. Wolffer et al. Pain Physician, in press.

95. Carragee EJ, Tanner CM, Khurana S, et al. The rates of false-positive lumbar discography in select patients without low back symptoms. *Spine* 2000;25:1373–1381.

96. Bogduk N, McGuirk B. Precision diagnosis. In: Bogduk N, McGuirk B, (eds). *Medical Management of Acute and Chronic Low Back Pain. An Evidence-Based Approach.* Amsterdam, Netherlands: Elsevier, 2002;169–176.

97. Colhoun E, McCall IW, Williams L, et al. Provocation discography as a guide to planning operations on the spine. *J Bone Joint Surg* 1988;70B:267–271.

98. loeser*

99. Phillips DR, Twomey LT. A comparison of manual diagnosis with a diagnosis established by a uni-level lumbar spinal block procedure. *Man Ther* 1996;2:82–87.

100. Bogduk N, McGuirk B. *Medical Management of Acute and Chronic Low Back Pain. An Evidence-Based Approach.* Amsterdam, Netherlands: Elsevier, 2002:41–47.

101. Hickey RF. Chronic low back pain: a comparison of diflunisal with paracetamol. *NZ Med J* 1982;95:312–314.

102. Van Tulder MW, Scholten RJ, Koes B, et al. Nonsteroidal anti-inflammatory drugs for low back pain: a systematic review within the framework of the Cochrane Collaboration Back Review Group. *Spine* 2000;25:2501–2513.

103. Airaksinen O, Brox JI, Cedraschi C, et al. European guidelines for the management of chronic nonspecific low back pain. *Eur Spine J* 2006;15:S192–S300.

104. Van Tam V, Becker A, Bekkering T, et al. European guidelines for the management of acute nonspecific low back pain in primary care. *Eur Spine J* 2006;15:S169–S191.

105. Malanga G, Wolff E. Evidence-informed management of chronic low back pain with nonsteroidal anti-inflammatory drugs, muscle relaxants and simple analgesics. *Spine J* 2008;8:173–184.

106. Keller A, Hayden J, Bombardier C, et al. Effect sizes of nonsurgical treatments of nonspecific low-back pain. *Eur Spine J* 2007;16:1776–1788.

107. van Tulder MW, Touray T, Furlan AD, et al. Muscle relaxants for nonspecific low back pain: a systematic review within the framework of the Cochrane collaboration. *Spine* 2003;28:1978–1992.

108. Arbus L, Fajadet B, Aubert D, et al. Activity of tetrazepam (myolastan) in low back pain: a double-blind trial vs placebo. *Clin Trials J* 1990;27:258–267.

109. Staiger TO, Gasler B, Sullivan MD, et al. Systematic review of antidepressants in the treatment of chronic low back pain. *Spine* 2003;28:2540–2545.

110. Chang V, Gonazalez P, Akuthota V. Evidence-informed management of chronic low back pain with adjunctive analgesics. *Spine J* 2008;8:21–27.

111. Ruoff GE, Resenthal N, Jordan D, et al. Tramadol/acetaminophen combination tablets for the treatment of chronic low back pain: a multicenter, randomized, double-blind, placebo-controlled outpatient study. *Clin Ther* 2003;25:1123–1141.

112. Peloso PM, Fortin L, Beaulieu A, et al. Analgesic efficacy and safety of tramadol/acetaminophen combination tablets (ultracet) in treatment of chronic low back pain: a mutlicenter, outpatient, randomized, double blind, placebo controlled trial. *J Rheumatol* 2004;31:2454–2463.

113. Schnitzer TJ, Gray WL, Paster RZ, et al. Efficacy of tramadol in treatment of chronic low back pain. *J Rheumatol* 2000;27:772–778.

114. Rivero-Arisa O, Gray A, Frost H, et al. Cost-utility analysis of physiotherapy treatment compared physiotherapy advice in low back pain. *Spine* 2006;31:1381–1387.

115. Hayden JA, van Tulder MW, Malmivaara A, et al. Exercise therapy for treatment of nonspecific low back pain. *Cochrane Database Syst Rev* 2005, Issue 3. Art. No.: CD000335,pub2. DOI: 10.1002/14651858.CD000335.pub2.

116. Hayden JA, van Tulder MW, Malmivaara AV, Koes BW. Meta-analysis: exercise therapy for nonspecific low back pain. *Ann Intern Med* 2005;142:765–775.

117. Mayer J, Mooney V, Dagenais S. Evidence-informed management of chronic low back pain with lumbar extensor strengthening exercises. *Spine J* 2008;8:96–113.

118. Slade SC, Keating JL. Trunk-strengthening exercises for chronic low back pain: a systematic review. *J Manip Physiol Ther* 2006;29:163–173.

119. Standaert CJ, Weinstein SM, Rumpeltes J. Evidence-informed management of chronic low back pain with lumbar stabilization exercises. *Spine J* 2008;8:114–120.

120. Ferreira PH, Ferreira ML, Maher CG, et al. Specific stabilization exercise for spinal and pelvic pain: a systematic review. *Aust J Physiother* 2006;52:79–88.

121. Clare HA, Adams R, Maher CG. A systematic review of efficacy of McKenzie method for low back pain. *Aust J Physiother* 2004;50:209–216.

122. Machado LA, de Souza MS, Ferreira PH, et al. The McKenzie method for low back pain: a systematic review of the literature with a meta-analysis approach. *Spine* 2006;31:E254–E262.

123. May S, Donelson R. Evidence-informed management of chronic low back pain with the McKenzie method. *Spine J* 2008;8:134–141.

124. Imamura M, Furlan AD, Dryden T, Irvin E. Evidence-informed management of chronic low back pain with massage. *Spine J* 2008;8:121–133.

125. Bronfort G, Haas M, Evans R, et al. Evidence-informed management of chronic low back pain with spinal manipulation and mobilization. *Spine J* 2008;8:213–225.

126. Poitras S, Brosseau L. Evidence-informed management of chronic low back pain with transcutaneous electrical nerve stimulation, interferential current, electrical muscle stimulation, ultrasound, and thermotherapy. *Spine J* 2008;8:226–233.

127. Brosseau L, Milne S, Robinson V, et al. Efficacy of the transcutaneous electrical nerve stimulation for the treatment of chronic low back pain: a meta-analysis. *Spine* 2002;27:596–603.

128. Khadilkar A, Milne S, Brosseau L, et al. Transcutaneous electrical nerve stimulation for the treatment of chronic low back pain: a systematic review. *Spine* 2005;30:2657–2666.

129. Deyo RA, Walsh NE, Martin DC, et al. A controlled trial of transcutaneous electrical stimulation (TENS) and exercise for chronic low back pain. *E Engl J Med* 1990;322:1627–1634.

130. Gay RE, Brault JS. Evidence-informed management of chronic low back pain with traction therapy. *Spine J* 2008;8:234–242.

131. Malanga G, Wolff E. Evidence-informed management of chronic low back pain with trigger point injections. *Spine J* 2008;8:243–252.

132. Dagenais S, Mayer J, Haldeman S, et al. Evidence-informed management of chronic low back pain with prolotherapy. *Spine J* 2008;8:203–212.

133. Yelland MJ, Del Mar C, Pirozzo S, et al. Prolotherapy injections for chronic low-back pain. *Cochrane Database Syst Rev* 2004. CD 004059.

134. Dagenais S, Yelland MJ, Del Mar C, et al. Prolotherapy injections for chronic low-back pain. *Cochrane Database Syst Rev* 2007. CD 004059.

135. Ammendolia C, Furlan AD, Imamura M, et al. Evidence-informed management of chronic low back pain with needle acupuncture. *Spine J* 2008;8:160–172.

136. DePalma MJ, Slipman CW. Evidence-informed management of chronic low back pain with epidural steroid injection. *Spine J* 2008;8:45–55.

137. Brox JI, Storheim K, Grotle M, et al. Evidence-informed management of chronic low back pain with back schools, brief education, and fear-avoidance training. *Spine J* 2008;8:28–39.

138. Gatchel RJ, Rollings KH. Evidence-informed management of chronic low back pain with cognitive behavioural therapy. *Spine J* 2008;8:40–44.

139. van Tulder MW, Ostelo R, Vlaeyen JWS, et al. Behavioral treatment for chronic back pain: a systematic review within the framework of the Cochrane Back Review Group. *Spine* 2000;25:2688–2699.

140. Ostelo RW, van Tulder MW, Vlaeyen JW, et al. Behavioural treatment for chronic low back pain. *Cochrane Database Syst Rev* 2005: CD002014.

141. Turner JA, Clancy S, McQuade KJ, et al. Effectiveness of behavioral therapy for chronic low back pain: a component analysis. *J Consult Clin Psychol* 1990;58:573–579.

142. Johnson RE, Jones GT, Wiles NJ, et al. Active exercise, education, and cognitive behavioral therapy for persistent disabling low back pain: a randomized controlled trial. *Spine* 2007;32:1578–1585.

143. Smeets RJ, Vlaeyen JW, Hidding A, et al. Active rehabilitation for chronic low back pain: cognitive-behavioural, physical, or both? First direct post-treatment results from a randomized controlled trial [ISRCTN22714229]. *BMC Musculoskeletal Disord* 2006;7:5.

144. Guzman J, Esmail R, Karjalainen K, et al. Multidisciplinary biopsychosocial rehabilitation for chronic low back pain. *Cochrane Database Syst Rev* 2002: CD000963.

145. Guzman J, Esmail R, Karjalainen K, et al. Multidisciplinary rehabilitation for chronic back pain: systematic review. *Brit Med J* 2001;322:1511–1516.

146. Bendix AF, Bendix T, Ostenfeld S, et al. Active treatment programs for patients with chronic low back pain: a prospective, randomized, observer-blinded study. *Eur Spine* 1995;4:148–152.

147. Alaranta H, Rytokoski U, Rissanen A, et al. Intensive physical and psychosocial training program for patients with chronic low back pain: a controlled clinical trial. *Spine* 1994;19:1339–1349.

148. Fritzell P, Hagg O, Wessberg P, et al. Lumbar fusion versus nonsurgical treatment for chronic low back pain: a multicenter randomized controlled trial from the Swedish Lumbar Spine Study Group. *Spine* 2001;26:2521–2534.

149. Brox JI, Sorensen R, Friis A, et al. Randomized clinical trial of lumbar instrumented fusion and cognitive intervention and exercises in patients with chronic low back pain and disc degeneration. *Spine* 2003;28:1913–1921.

150. Fairbank J, Frost H, Wilson-MacDonald J, et al. Randomised controlled trial to compare surgical stabilisation of the lumbar spine with an intensive rehabilitation programme for patients with chronic low back pain: the MRC spine stabilisation trial. *BMJ* 2005;330:1233.

151. Dreyfuss P, Halbrook B, Pauza K, et al. Efficacy and validity of radiofrequency neurotomy for chronic lumbar zygapophyseal joint pain. *Spine* 2000;25:1270–1277.

152. van Kleef M, Barendse GAM, Kessels A, et al. Randomized trial of radiofrequency lumbar facet denervation for chronic low back pain. *Spine* 1999;24:1937–1942.

153. Nath S, Nath CA, Pettersson K. Percutaneous lumbar zygapophyseal (facet) joint neurotomy using radiofrequency current in the management of chronic low back pain: a randomized double-blind trial. *Spine* 2008;33:1291–1298.

154. Gofeld M, Jitendra J, Faclier G. Radiofrequency denervation of the lumbar zygapophyseal joints: 10-year prospective clinical audit. *Pain Physician* 2007;10:291–300.

155. Schofferman J, Kine G. Effectiveness of repeated radiofrequency neurotomy for lumbar facet pain. *Spine* 2004;29:2471–2473.

156. Park J, Park JY, Kim SH, et al. Long term results from percutaneous radiofrequency neurotomy on posterior primary ramus in patients with chronic low back pain. *Acta Neurochir Suppl* 2006;99:81–83.

157. Hooten WM, Martin DP, Huntoon MA. Radiofrequency neurotomy for low back pain: evidence-based procedural guidelines. *Pain Med* 2005;6:129–138.

158. Gofeld M, Faclier G. Radiofrequency denervation of the lumbar zygapophysial joints—targeting the best practice. *Pain Med* 2008;9:204–211.

159. Zelle BA, Gruen GS, Brown S, et al. Sacroiliac joint dysfunction: evaluation and management. *Clin J Pain* 2005;21:446–455.

160. Buchowski JM, Kebaish KM, Sinkov V, et al. Functional and radiographic outcome of sacroiliac arthrodesis for the disorders of the sacroiliac joint. *Spine J* 2005;5:520–528.

161. Cohen SP, Hurley RW, Buyckenmaier CC 3rd, et al. Randomized placebo-controlled study evaluating lateral branch radiofrequency denervation for sacroiliac joint pain. *Anesthesiology* 2008;109:279–288.

162. Karasek M, Bogduk N. Intradiscal electrothermal annuloplasty: percutaneous treatment of chronic discogenic low back pain. *Tech Reg Anesth Pain Manag* 2001;5:130–135.

163. Karasek M, Bogduk N. Twelve-month follow-up of a controlled trial of intradiscal thermal anuloplasty for back pain due to internal disc disruption. *Spine* 2000;25:2601–2607.

164. Bogduk N, Karasek M. Two-year follow-up of a controlled trial of intradiscal electrothermal anuloplasty for chronic low back pain resulting from internal disc disruption. *Spine J* 2002;2:343–350.

165. Freeman BJ, Fraser RD, Cain CM, et al. A randomized, double-blind, controlled trial: intradiscal electrothermal therapy versus placebo for the treatment of chronic discogenic low back pain. *Spine* 2005;30:2369–2377.

166. Pauza KJ, Howell S, Dreyfuss P, et al. A randomised, placebo-controlled trial of intradiscal electrothermal therapy for the treatment of discogenic low back pain. *Spine J.* 2004;4:27–35.

167. Freedman BA, Cohen SP, Kuklo TR, et al. Intradiscal electrothermal therapy (IDET) for chronic low back pain in active-duty soldiers: 2-year follow-up. *Spine J* 2003;3:502–509.

168. Anderson GB, Mekhail NA, Block JE. Treatment of intractable discogenic low back pain: a systematic review of spinal fusion and intradiscal electrothermal therapy (IDET). *Pain Physician* 2006;9:237–248.

169. Bogduk N, Lau P, Govind J, et al. Intradiscal electrothermal therapy. *Tech Reg Anesth Pain Manag* 2005;9:25–34.

170. Kapural L, Ng A, Dalton J, et al. Intervertebral disc biacuplasty for the treatment of lumbar discogenic pain: results of a six-month follow-up. *Pain Med* 2008;9:60–67.

171. Deer T, Chapple I, Classen A, et al. Intrathecal drug delivery for treatment of chronic low back pain: report from the National Outcomes Registry for Low Back Pain. *Pain Med* 2004;5:6–13.

172. North RB, Kidd DH, Farrokhi F, et al. Spinal cord stimulation versus repeated lumbosacral spine surgery for chronic pain: a randomized, controlled trial. *Neurosurgery* 2005;56:98–106.

173. North RB, Kidd D, Shipley J, et al. Spinal cord stimulation versus reoperation for failed back surgery syndrome: a cost-effectiveness and cost utility analysis based on a randomized, controlled trial. *Neurosurgery* 2007;61:361–368.

174. Kumar K, Taylor RS, Jacques L, et al. Spinal cord stimulation versus conventional medical management for neuropathic pain: a mulitcentre randomised controlled trial in patients with failed back surgery syndrome. *Pain* 2007;132:179–188.

175. Kumar K, Malik S, Demeria D. Treatment of chronic pain with spinal cord stimulation verus alternative therapies: cost-effectiveness analysis. *Neurosurgery* 2002;51:106–115.

176. Martell BA, O'Connor PG, Kerns RD, et al. Systematic review: opioid treatment for chronic back pain: prevalence, efficacy, and association with addiction. *Ann Intern Med* 2007;146:116–127.

177. Hale ME, Dvergsten C, Gimbel J. Efficacy and safety of oxymorphone extended release in chronic low back pain: results of a randomized, double-blind, placebo- and active-controlled phase III study. *J Pain* 2005;6:21–28.

178. Jamison RN, Raymond SA, Slawsby EA, et al. Opioid therapy for chronic noncancer back pain: a randomized prospective study. *Spine* 1998;23:2591–2600.

179. Deshpande A, Furlan A, Mallis-Gagnon A, et al. Opioids for chronic low-back pain. *Cochrane Database Syst Rev* 2007 Jul 18;(3):CD004959.

180. Schofferman J, Mazanec D. Evidence-informed management of chronic low back pain with opioid analgesics. *Spine J* 2008;8:185–194.

181. Katz N, Rauck R, Ahdieh H, et al. A 12-week, randomized, placebo-controlled trial assessing the safety and efficacy of oxymorphone extended release for opioid-naive patients with chronic low back pain. *Curr Med Res Opin* 2007;23:117–128.

182. Hale ME, Ahdieh H, Ma T, et al. Efficacy and safety of OPANA ER (oxymorphone extended release) for relief of moderate to severe chronic low back pain in opioid-experienced patients: a 12-week randomized, double-blind, placebo-controlled study. *J Pain* 2007;8:175–184.

183. Ballantyne JC, Spin NS. Efficacy of opioids for chronic pain: a review of the evidence. *Clin J Pain* 2008;24:469–478.

184. Noble M, Tregear SJ, Treadwell JR, et al. Long-term opioid therapy for chronic noncancer pain: a systematic review and meta-analysis of efficacy and safety. *J Pain Symptom Manage* 2008;35:214–228.

185. Yelland MJ, Schulter PJ. Defining worthwhile and desired responses to treatment of chronic low back pain. *Pain Med* 2006;7:38–45.

CHAPTER 73 ■ SURGERY FOR LOW BACK PAIN

YOUSSEF GHABRIAL AND NIKOLAI BOGDUK

Surgery is a distinctive form of therapeutic intervention. It is characterized by identifying a lesion or abnormality that is then resected, repaired, reconstructed, reinforced, or replaced. In other fields of medicine, surgery has an esteemed history. Injured viscera can be repaired; tumors can be resected; blood vessels can be reconstructed or replaced. In orthopedics, fractures can be immobilized, externally or internally, and painful joints can be replaced or fused.

For the treatment of low back pain, the history of surgery is less esteemed. Whereas individual surgeons have developed and promoted various surgical techniques by which to treat back pain, the evidence of effectiveness has often been less than convincing. Failures are common, and pain clinics are familiar with patients whose pain persists despite surgical intervention (see Chapter 74).

HISTORICAL PERSPECTIVE

The origin of spine surgery is attributed[1,2] to Hibbs[3] and Albee[4] who devised techniques by which to fuse the spine to control the progressive deformity that occurred in patients with spinal tuberculosis. The technique involved applying bone grafts to the spinous processes and laminae in order to fuse the posterior elements of the spine.

Progressively, posterior fusion was modified in various ways, with respect to the source of the bone graft, and the supplemental use of wires, rods, screws, and plates to reinforce the fusion.[1,2] A particular modification was to place the graft posterolaterally, between the transverse processes.[5–7] Known as posterolateral (PL) fusion, this has become one of the standard techniques of lumbar spinal fusion (Figs. 73.1 and 73.2).

Anterior lumbar interbody fusion (ALIF) also arose for the treatment of spinal tuberculosis.[8] Idiomatically, ALIF was not simply the surgical fixation of a joint, ultimately resulting in bone fusion (arthrodesis). Rather, the critical component of the procedure was excision of the tuberculous lesion in the disc and vertebral bodies. Bone graft and fusion was then a necessary supplement to replace the missing parts and to secure spinal integrity and stability.

Progressively, these various techniques and their modifications were applied to correct deformity, such as scoliosis, and to secure stability of the spine in patients with destructive lesions. Unlike its predecessors, posterior lumbar interbody fusion (PLIF) lacked a connection with tuberculous lesions. It was developed as a supplement to removal of herniated intervertebral discs,[2,9,10] in order to secure stability.

The history of fusion for low back pain is difficult to trace. Three streams of consciousness seem to apply.

In one stream, surgery was undertaken to treat radicular pain, caused by disc herniation or by spondylolisthesis. Decompression was the cardinal component of the surgery. Posterior elements of the spine had to be removed in order to gain access to the nerve roots. Fusion was not an active component of the intervention, but was undertaken in the interests of stabilizing the spine when too much of the posterior elements had to be sacrificed in order to gain access to the vertebral canal. The apparently good results achieved for the treatment of radicular pain predisposed surgeons to believe that fusion might also work for low back pain.

In the second stream, the logic was that if back pain was aggravated by movement it should be relieved by eliminating movement. The techniques available for securing stability and correcting deformity could, therefore, be applied to treat back pain.

According to the third stream, if an intervertebral disc is the

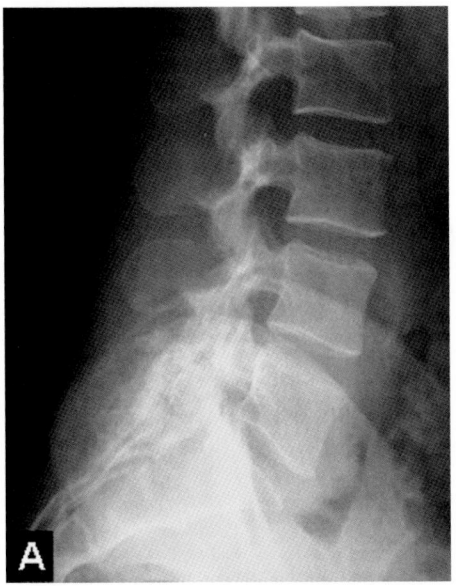
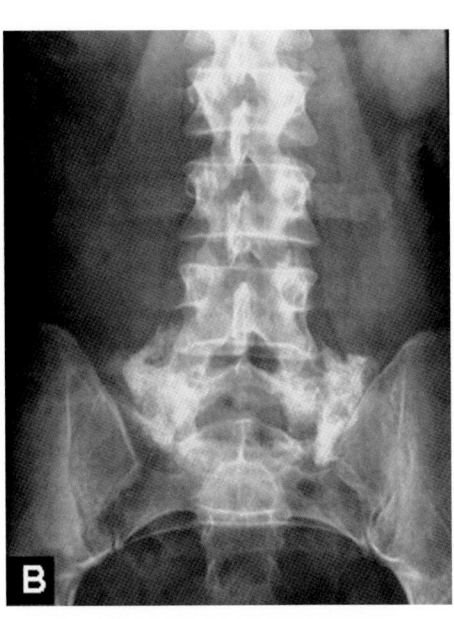

FIGURE 73.1 Radiographs of a posterolateral (intertransverse) fusion (PLF) at L5-S1, using bone graft alone. **(A)** Lateral view. **(B)** Anteroposterior view.

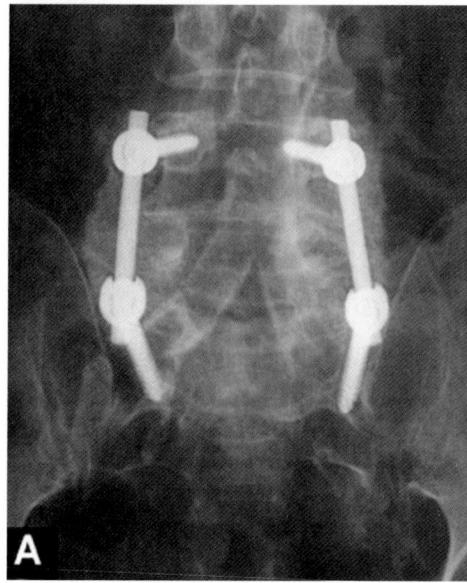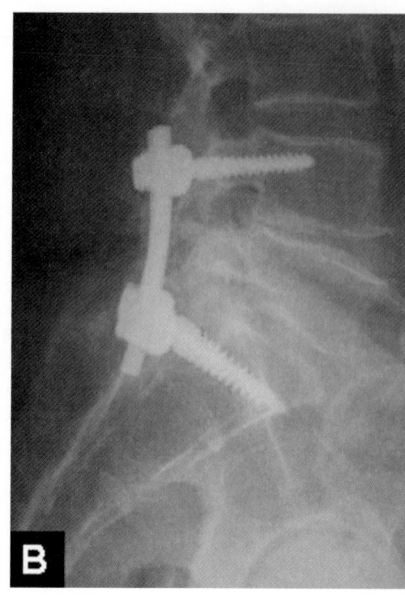

FIGURE 73.2 Radiographs of a posterolateral (intertransverse) fusion (PLF) from L4 to the sacrum, supplemented by instrumentation in the form of pedicle screws and rods. (**A**) Anteroposterior view. (**B**) Lateral view.

source of pain, excision of that disc should relieve the pain. Excision, therefore, is a cardinal component of the intervention. Fusion was required to fill that defect and restore spinal stability.

Of late, the third stream has evolved into disc replacement. Instead of fusing the spine after excision of the painful disc, the disc is replaced with a prosthesis, in the interests of retaining spinal movement. No doubt, this approach has been inspired by the success of total hip replacement for the treatment of hip pain.

TECHNIQUES

A variety of techniques has evolved for the surgical treatment of low back pain. They differ with respect to whether the surgery is performed from the front, from the back, or both; whether or not discs are excised; whether bone grafts, instruments, or both are used; and where they are placed (Fig. 73.3).

Fusion to eliminate motion has been the traditional approach for treating back pain. The opposing school of thought is that movements should be retained, in which case the offending disc should be replaced with a prosthesis.

Some surgeons believe that fusion is all that is required. The offending source of pain can be left in situ because elimination of motion should relieve the pain. Others believe that the source of pain should be removed. If a disc is perceived to be the source of pain, that disc is removed. The space it vacates can be filled with a bone graft or a prosthesis.

Noninstrumented fusion involves introducing a bone graft,

FUSION	NO FUSION

| RETAIN DISC | Posterolateral (intertransverse) |
| | Transarticular (facet) |

EXCISE DISC	Anterior interbody	Disc arthroplasty
	Posterior interbody
	Circumferential (360°)

| NON-INSTRUMENTED | INSTRUMENTED |

FIGURE 73.3 A classification of types of surgery used for low back pain.

which may be autologous bone or an allograft from a bone bank. If discs are retained, the graft is placed between transverse processes, in order to eliminate segmental motion. If discs are removed, the graft is placed in the intervertebral space. The bone graft alone can be placed between the vertebral bodies, or a metal cage or other device can be placed in order to hold the graft in place.

Fusion by bone grafting can be supplemented by instrumentation, in the form of screws and rods or plates, designed to hold the fused segments in place in order to prevent instability and to optimize the strength of fusion.

APPLICATIONS

The lumbar spine can be affected by tumors, infections, and fractures. In these cases, the lesion is identifiable by imaging and is remediable by surgery. However, back pain is not the indication for surgery. Surgery is indicated by the lesion demonstrated. For such conditions, the use of surgery is not contentious. Indeed, it is often the only option.

Surgery becomes a contentious treatment when back pain is the only feature, and no lesion is evident, or when the validity of the purported lesion is disputed. The contentious issues are the indications for surgery and its outcomes. The available evidence centers around three principal conditions or indications: spondylolisthesis, idiopathic back pain, and discogenic back pain.

SPONDYLOLISTHESIS

Spondylolisthesis is defined by forward subluxation of one vertebra on the next. Typically, the L5 vertebra subluxates on the sacrum. Less commonly, the L4 or L3 vertebra may be the one affected.

Spondylolisthesis has attracted surgical treatment for various reasons: it is an obvious deformity, it appears to be unstable, and it appears to be associated with pain. Surgery is invited in order to correct the deformity, or to stabilize it, and to relieve pain. However, the available evidence confounds this rationale.

Other than in severe cases, the deformity of spondylolisthesis does not cause disability. In lesser grades, the condition is not noticeable clinically; it becomes evident only when detected on radiographs. In children and adolescents, severe grades of spondylolisthesis may be evident if they cause gibbus deformity, which becomes a cosmetic issue. Other than correcting this cosmetic appearance, the deformity of spondylolisthesis alone neither attracts nor warrants surgery.

By some, spondylolisthesis is perceived to be an unstable state. However, in adults, instability has not been detected radiographically.[11-14] Indeed, some investigators have commented that the affected segment appears paradoxically more stable than its neighbors.[14] Therefore, the simple presence of spondylolisthesis is not evidence of instability, and should not attract surgical intervention for the purposes of securing stability. Arthrodesis might be indicated if instability was demonstrated preoperatively, but this has seldom been done in the literature on surgical treatment of spondylolisthesis.

Some patients with back pain have spondylolisthesis. This has been interpreted by some surgeons as meaning that the spondylolisthesis is the cause of back pain. The epidemiologic data speak otherwise. Spondylolisthesis is equally prevalent in subjects with no pain as in subjects with back pain.[15] Consequently, in patients with back pain, spondylolisthesis assumes the status of no more than an incidental finding and back pain is not a valid indication for surgery.

The cardinal feature of spondylolisthesis, and the only one that justifies surgery, is the onset of radicular pain. In such cases, nerve roots can be compressed or stretched by the axial and forward subluxation that the affected vertebra undergoes, or by a concurrent disc herniation; and this nerve root impairment can be demonstrated on computed tomography (CT) or magnetic resonance imaging (MRI). The objective of surgery in such cases is to decompress the affected nerve or nerves.

The cardinal component of surgery for spondylolisthesis is, therefore, decompression. However, decompression may require extensive removal of the posterior elements, including the laminae, spinous process, and even the zygapophyseal joints, in order to fully decompress the nerves. Removal of these posterior elements threatens introduction of iatrogenic instability. Fusion is, therefore, added to the intervention in order to stabilize the spine. In this regard, it has been clearly demonstrated that clinical outcomes are distinctly better in patients who undergo supplementary fusion than in those who undergo decompression alone.[16-18]

Against this background, a consideration of spondylolisthesis should be irrelevant in the context of surgery for low back pain. Since spondylolisthesis does not cause back pain, it is not an indication for the surgical treatment of back pain. However, the reputation of surgery as a successful treatment for spondylolisthesis is part of the foundation of surgery for back pain.

Many studies have not always been clear about their indications. In patients with spondylolisthesis, the clinical indications have variously been: neurogenic claudication alone, back pain or neurogenic claudication, radicular pain alone, back pain or radicular pain, back pain without or without sciatica, and back pain or leg pain. Some studies have not stated their clinical indications. Other studies have included spondylolisthesis as one of several indications for surgery, but did not report results separately for spondylolisthesis.

A literature review summarized the success rates of surgery for spondylolisthesis as reported in 34 original studies.[19] For posterior fusion alone, the success rates ranged between 37.5% and 98%, with an average of 74.8%. For anterior fusion, the success rates ranged between 80% and 95%. These data, however, were based on irregular and sometimes ill-defined criteria for clinical success. Some studies measured success in terms of patients achieving complete relief of symptoms, whereas others reported only the proportion of patients achieving some degree of improvement. Few studies, however, reported the degree of impairment before surgery and rarely have outcomes been corroborated by quantitative measures of pain, disability, return to work, and use of other health care.

Two controlled studies provide accurate and interpretable data. Both initially compared surgical treatment with conservative care, but one also compared different forms of fusion. Both provide data on the effectiveness of surgery.

The study of Weinstein et al.[20] showed a small advantage of surgery over conservative care, with respect to relief of pain, improvement of physical function, and reduction of disability. These advantages, however, were modest, amounting to 18 points difference for bodily pain and physical functioning on the SF-36, and 16.7 points on the Oswestry Disability Index (ODI). Differences in favor of surgery were evident at 3 months and at 1 year after treatment, and diminished only slightly at 2 years. Notwithstanding the comparative data, the outcomes for surgery were not great. Scores for bodily pain improved from 30 to 60, as did scores for physical functioning, but remained below normal levels. Disability reduced from 40 to 20.

The study of Moller et al.[21] showed that surgery was more effective than exercise at 2 years after treatment, but it also revealed the same curious outcomes. Although 55% of patients who underwent surgery were "much better" and 19% were "better," mean pain scores fell from 63 before treatment to only 37 at 2 years after treatment, with a range of 0 to 96.

Among the patients treated surgically, no significant differences in outcomes arose when patients were treated with instrumented or noninstrumented fusion[22]; but the same perplexing issues arose. About 50% of patients were "much better" at 2 years after treatment, and a further 20% or so were "better." The pain scores, however, showed little change. The mean pain score was 63 before treatment and 40 at 2 years after treatment. (No ranges of these scores were reported.) These data reflect clinical improvement, but do not portray resolution of the pain.

A long-term follow-up[23] of the original study[21] found that, 5 to 13 years after treatment, pain scores improved in the exercise group but not functional disability; but in the surgery group functional disability deteriorated. Pain and disability were no longer significantly different between the exercise and surgery groups. Of the patients treated surgically, 33% of the instrumented patients and 44% of the noninstrumented patients rated themselves as "much better." Mean pain scores had stabilized at 40/100.

These results, from controlled studies with good follow-up and assessment, are dissonant with the claims from descriptive studies of success rates of 80% and 90%. Either some surgeons achieve better results than others, or the success rates reported in descriptive studies have been inflated because of less rigorous assessment.

IDIOPATHIC BACK PAIN

Lumbar spinal fusion has been used extensively to treat idiopathic low back pain, that is, lumbar spinal pain of unknown origin.[24] The indications for surgery have been ambiguous or contentious, as have been the outcomes.

The indications have variously been "degenerative disc disease" or simply persisting back pain. The fact that degenerative disc disease is equally prevalent in patients with no pain, or barely more prevalent in patients with back pain,[15] has not deterred surgeons from attributing back pain to disc degeneration. The absence of any significant correlation between disc degeneration and pain renders it no more than a normal age change and an incidental finding on CT or MRI.

Another perception is that back pain arises because of instability of the lumbar spine, but no form of instability has been objectively demonstrated, using validated measures, in patients with idiopathic low back pain, which might attract spinal fusion. That rationale for spinal fusion in patients with undiagnosed low back pain appears to be little more than if movement aggravates pain then elimination of movement should relieve it. On balance, the available evidence contradicts this rationale more than it supports it.

The first systematic review of spinal fusion[25] provided little information about its efficacy for low back pain. It provided data separately and specifically on fusion for herniated discs and for spondylolisthesis. For low back pain as the indication for surgery, it found only six eligible studies, which reported successful outcomes in between 47% and 90% of patients, with an average success rate of 61%.

A later review, which limited its search to controlled studies, found no adequate scientific evidence about the efficacy or long-term effects of fusion. That absence of evidence has since been corrected. Three controlled trials have appeared, each of which compared surgery to some form of conservative care, and each of which provided outcome data for fusion.

The Fritzell study[27] showed that fusion was more effective than nonsurgical therapy. For patients treated surgically, pain scores fell from 64 at inception to 30 at 6 months, but then regressed to 43 at 2 years, with a standard deviation of 25. The ODI improved only from 47 to 36. Beforehand, the authors defined an excellent outcome as no pain, no functional restrictions, and no analgesics; and a good outcome as sporadic pain, slight restriction of function, and occasional analgesics. However, when reporting their results, these two categories were grouped together: 45% of patients achieved an excellent or good outcome. The proportion of patients with complete relief was not stated. Some 29% of patients rated themselves as "much better" and a

further 34% rated themselves as "better," with neither of these terms being defined. For a major invasive intervention, these are not particularly flattering outcomes.

The Brox study[28] found fusion to be no more effective than cognitive behavioral therapy coupled with exercises. In the fusion group, scores for back pain improved from 62 at inception to 39 at 1 year; the ODI improved from 42 to 26. For both outcome measures, these outcomes are less than modest.

The Fairbank study[29] found surgery to be minimally more effective than an intensive rehabilitation program. Pain scores were not reported, but ODI scores improved from 46.7 ± 14.5 (mean $\pm$ standard deviation) at inception to only 33.3 ± 20.8 at 24 months.

In reviewing these controlled trials, Mirza and Deyo[30] noted that, other than low back pain lasting longer than 12 months, a diagnosis was not made in any of the studies. Other observations pertained to outcomes. The improvements in ODI ranged from 8.9 to 15.6. This exceeds the threshold of 4 which is regarded by some authorities as the minimal clinically important difference, but the U.S. Food and Drug Administration (FDA) regards a change of 15 points as the threshold. This was exceeded only in the Brox study,[28] by 0.6 of a point.

For back pain, the minimal clinically important change is at least 20, according to some,[31] but 25 according to others,[32,33] and as high as 5.5 for initially intense low back pain.[33] Improvements of 21[27] and 23[28] barely exceed the minimal threshold.

These data bespeak only a modest efficacy of fusion for undiagnosed low back pain. Although some patients benefit, they are rendered only "better"; few, if any, are totally relieved of their presenting problem.

Data from another source corroborate this impression. Thomsen et al.[34] conducted a controlled trial designed to compare the effectiveness of fusion with and without pedicle screw instrumentation. The clinical indications for treatment were chronic, motion-induced back pain. The study enrolled 35 patients with isthmic spondylolisthesis, but the majority (94) were diagnosed as having instability. Outcomes at 2[34] and 5[35] years were reported. Improvements in scores on the Dallas Pain Questionnaire were modest to small, amounting to improvements from 65 to 40 for work, 60 to 50 for daily activities, 40 to 25 for anxiety and depression, and 35 to 15 for social concerns. Pain scores at inception were not reported, but at 5 years mean scores were 2 for leg pain and 4 for back pain, each with a range of 0 to 10.[35] Fusion did not achieve return to work, and some 50% of patients received a pension because of continuing back pain.

DISCOGENIC BACK PAIN

Some surgeons undertake surgical treatment for low back pain only in patients in whom a diagnosis of discogenic pain has been established. The diagnostic test is provocation discography (see Chapter 102). Various forms of treatment apply. The affected segment can be treated by leaving the symptomatic disc in situ, but fusing that segment using a posterolateral fusion. The affected disc can be resected and the disc space filled with a graft, using anterior lumbar interbody fusion or posterior lumbar interbody fusion, with either fusion being with or without instrumentation.

No controlled trials have been reported, apart from a few in which different types of fusion have been compared. The reputation of fusion for diagnosed discogenic pain rests on a small collection of descriptive studies (Table 73.1).

Although impressive outcomes are claimed by many of these studies, few were rigorously conducted and reported. Inception data were not reported, surgeons performed their own assessments, and outcomes were not corroborated by quantitative outcome measures.

Of this collection of studies, only those of Penta et al.[43] and Greenough[44] provided interpretable outcome data. Both studies

TABLE 73.1

OUTCOMES REPORTED BY VARIOUS STUDIES THAT USED DISCOGRAPHY TO SELECT SEGMENTS FOR TREATMENT BY FUSION

Source	Criteria	Success rate
Blumenthal 1988[36]	Normal activities and no medications or NSAIDs only	74%
Kozak 1990[37]	At least 75% relief of pain and return to work, or Slight restriction of activities and no analgesics	74%
Kostuik 1990[38]	Absence of significant back or leg pain Occasional use of non-narcotic analgesics	31%
Gill 1992[39]	At least 75% relief of pain and return to work, or Return to normal activities and no opioids	66%
Lee 1995[40]	No pain	26%
	Mild pain	61%
	No medications	59%
	No opioids	30%
	No restricted activities	50%
	Mild or moderate restriction	30%
	Return to full work	81%
	Return to restricted work	11%
Wetzel 1994[41]	Minimal symptoms and no analgesics, or Marked improvement, and rare use of analgesics	46%
Parker 1996[42]	Pain less than 4/10 No medications other than NSAIDs Return to at least 75% previous work capacity	39%
Penta 1997[43]	Complete relief or Good deal of relief	39% 39%
Greenough 1998[44]	Complete or almost complete relief A good deal of relief	17% 23%

came from the same center. Outcomes were assessed by an independent observer. In one study the follow-up was at least 2 years[44] while in the other it was at a minimum of 10 years.[43]

Fusion had a modest success rate at 2 years. Only 39% had complete relief, but a further 39% had what the patients called a good deal of relief.[44] These figures attenuated to 17% and 23%, respectively, in the 10 year study.[43] However, the investigators highlighted an enigma or paradox. Although 78% of patients reported a successful result, only 34% fell into the categories of "excellent" or "good" outcomes, as defined for the Low Back Outcome Score.[43] Nevertheless, these data—on patients diagnosed by discography—suggest outcomes superior to those achieved in patients in whom no diagnosis was made. An outcome of 39% with complete relief of pain[44] outweighs 29% feeling just "much better."[27]

DISC ARTHROPLASTY

Commentators have heralded intervertebral disc arthroplasty as offering the potential of restoring joint mechanics and, thereby, reducing pain and improving function; preserving motion appears to lessen adverse loading and changes in range of motion at adjacent segments.[45] Preliminary results from descriptive studies are good in some studies[46] and have yielded outcomes comparable to those of fusion for low back pain.[45] Recovery time seems to be less than for fusion.[46]

Because the advent of arthroplasty has been subjected to strong scrutiny, controlled trials and good descriptive studies have appeared early in the evolution of this technology. The available studies provide sobering insights.

Blumenthal et al.[47] compared disc arthroplasty, using a particular device, with a form of anterior lumbar interbody fusion. Zigler et al.[48] compared arthroplasty, using a different device, with circumferential fusion. These studies provide outcome data not only on disc arthroplasty but also on the conventional fusion procedures with which it was compared.

Although the Blumenthal study[47] found disc arthroplasty to be not inferior to fusion, the outcomes of both arthroplasty and ALIF were modest. Mean pain scores improved from 70 to 30, which exceeds the minimal clinically important change (MCIC) of 20 points and ODI improved from 50 to 25; but 64% of patients treated by surgery still took opioids and, although 64% returned to work, 53% had been working before surgery. These latter figures do not attest to any substantial decrease in the burden of illness; surgery did not seem to alter the patients' use of other health care or their ability to work. The proportion of patients who were completely relieved of pain was not reported. One reviewer recommended that these data argue for caution by patients and surgeons.[49]

The Zigler study[48] found disc arthroplasty to be slightly more effective, on average, than circumferential fusion, but it too reported only modest results for both surgical treatments. For arthroplasty, ODI improved from 63.4 at inception to 34.5 at 24 months, but with a standard deviation of 24.8. This latter figure indicates that a substantial proportion of patients were still substantially disabled. Pain scores improved from just above 70 to 37 with a standard deviation of 30.1. This study judged outcomes as a success if the ODI improved by 15 points, which is the MCIC required by the FDA.[30] On this basis, a 72% success rate was claimed. But this misrepresents MCIC. The MCIC does not amount to the least value at which success occurs. It is no more than the least value that patients equate with a detectable level of improvement. The study did not report the proportion of patients rendered substantially better, or free of pain. Of patients considered to have a successful outcome, 39% still took opioids, which seems contradictory. Reviewers concluded that this study lacked sufficient detail for the interested reader to perform an independent evaluation of the data to confirm or reject the authors' conclusions.[50]

These results from controlled trials of arthroplasty are starkly inferior to those of a well-reported descriptive study. In the study of Bertagnoli et al.,[51] mean pain scores improved from 7.5 to 3, and ODI improved from 54 to 29. At 2 years, 32% of patients had no back pain and a further 59% had only occasional pain, 90% took no opioids, and only 41% required NSAIDs for pain.

DYNAMIC STABILIZATION

A number of devices have been invented that can be inserted between lumbar spinous processes in order to reduce lordosis and to limit extension, without affecting flexion and other movements of the lumbar spine. Their application has been described, generically, as dynamic stabilization.

These devices were developed originally as a treatment for neurogenic intermittent claudication caused by spinal stenosis. For that indication, they have been shown to be more effective than conservative care.[52] Outcomes have been reasonable in some hands,[53] but less satisfying in others.[54,55] Others have warned against their use in spondylolisthesis.[56]

Some surgeons have taken to using these devices to treat idiopathic low back pain, but there is no published evidence of efficacy or effectiveness for that indication.

CONCLUSION

Patients look to surgery as an ultimate cure for their back pain. For them, surgery has concept validity. They are familiar with surgery being the cure for abdominal pain caused by appendicitis or cholecystitis. They are familiar with the wondrous success of hip arthroplasty for osteoarthritis of the hip. Because of such comparators, patients could be forgiven for having the same expectations of spine surgery for back pain. They are not to know that back pain is not caused by infection, or that the ball and socket joint of the hip is biomechanically simpler than a spinal motion segment.

Surgeons also are subject to concept validity. The history of spinal surgery is riven with examples of a surgeon who thinks of a good idea. The idea sounds sensible. Movement aggravates pain; therefore, eradication of movement should stop pain. The disc hurts, so removing the disc should stop pain. Motion should be preserved, so arthroplasty should replace fusion.

These concepts, however, are only superficially valid. Techniques have not been developed and validated that might test if temporarily eradicating movements succeeds in relieving pain; or that show that temporarily anesthetizing a disc completely relieves a patient's pain. Fusing or replacing a disc is a large, irreversible step. Taking this step amounts to subjecting patients to a trial by treatment. The empirical data indicate that these trials fail. An insufficient proportion of patients is completely relieved of pain to vindicate the rationale for surgery and too many patients remain unchanged or worse.

In an editorial, Fritzell[57] posed the question, "Is surgical treatment consistent with evidence-based medicine?" and answered it with, "Yes, in selected patients." But surgeons have not yet articulated the definition of the correctly selected patient and tested it prospectively. The reputation of surgery rests on the observation, after treatment, that some patients sometimes do well with some procedures. That is little solace to the majority of patients who do not do well, who suffer complications, or who are rendered worse by surgery.

There is a major mismatch between what surgeons report as their outcomes and what epidemiologists count in communities. Descriptive studies, some controlled studies, claim success rates of 60% or more. Such claims predict that, on the average, large proportions of patients should do well after surgery and that the burden of back pain should be decreasing. In contrast, epidemiologists report observations such as 67.7% of patients' back pain was worse, and in 55.8% quality of life was not better or worse.[58] Others report that surgery for back pain is palpably less effective than surgery for spinal stenosis or disc herniation, and nowhere near as effective as hip replacement.[59] Indeed, whereas patients undergoing the other orthopedic operations improve on average, those who have surgery for back pain tend to deteriorate.[59]

One explanation for this pattern might be that spine surgery for back pain is highly demanding technically and that only expert surgeons can achieve good outcomes while average surgeons do not publish but are responsible for the poorer results seen in community studies. If that is the case, then surgeons—or someone else—have a responsibility to accredit surgeons, both in the interests of patients and in the interests of optimizing outcomes and, therefore, the reputation of surgery.

The other explanation is a recurrent one. It is that patients need to be carefully and properly selected before undertaking surgery. Yet, little has been done in this regard despite repeated proclamations of the need.

The seductive feature of surgery for back pain is that, perhaps more than occasionally, patients do very well. This phenomenon reinforces faith in the concept validity of surgery for back pain. But it is a false inference statistically. It amounts to remembering the few good cases, but ignoring those who do not benefit and those who do worse.

Two reforms are necessary to change the course of spine surgery significantly. One is for surgeons to abandon their traditional style of reporting results. The quality of the literature needs improving. Quoting percentages of patients who, reportedly, had "excellent or good" outcomes might attract surgeons, but no longer convinces their critics. A convincing set a data would describe the state of the patients before treatment in terms of pain, function, and use of health care, using validated instruments. After treatment, the data should show not just the mean scores in these variables, but the proportions of patients who achieve not just the MCIC but also endpoints of value, such as complete relief of pain and minimal pain, normal function, return to work by those previously not working, and reduction of use of other health care.

The second reform is abstract and intellectual. It is a call for surgeons to reflect. Perhaps fusion or arthroplasty is a valid concept, but the means by which they are secured confounds successful implementation of the treatment. It might be that the tissue destruction required to implement these treatments interferes with the outcome. Evidence on this contention is likely to arise as more surgeons adopt minimally invasive techniques of spinal surgery.

Conversely, however, there is a conjecture that surgeons have not yet faced. It is a paradox that fusion, or arthroplasty, does not consistently work or does not last. That paradox might have an answer. An explanation that fits the enigmatic and variable outcomes of spine surgery is that arthrodesis per se, or arthroplasty per se, is not the active component of spine surgery for back pain. Rather, what relieves pain is the extensive debridement of the lumbar spine that occurs during these procedures. Denervation, not fixation or replacement, is what relieves the pain; and pain recurs as the spine is reinnervated. This conjecture, rather than ill-defined placebo effects, is what surgeons will need to consider into the 21st century.

References

1. Fraser RD. Interbody, posterior, and combined lumbar fusions. *Spine* 1995; 20(Suppl 24):167S–177S.
2. Bick EM. An essay on the history of spine fusion operations. *Clin Orthop Relat Res* 1964:35:9–15.
3. Hibbs RA. An operation for progressive spinal deformities. *New York Med J* 1991;93:1013–1016.
4. Albee FH. Transplantation of a portion of the tibia into the spine for Pott's disease: a preliminary report. *JAMA* 1991;57:885–886.
5. Watkins MB. Posterolateral fusion of the lumbar lumbosacral spine. *J Bone Joint Surg [Am]* 1953;35A:1014–1019.
6. Wiltse LL, Bateman JG, Duey R. Experiences with transverse process fusions in the lumbar spine. *J Bone Joint Surg [Am]* 1962;44A:1013.
7. Wiltse LL, Hutchinson RH. Surgical treatment of spondylolisthesis. *Clin Orthop Relat Res* 1964;35:116–135.
8. Hodgson AR, Stock FE. Anterior spine fusion for the treatment of tuberculosis of the spine. *J Bone Joint Surg* 1960;42A:295–310.
9. Jaslow IA. Intercorporal bone graft in spinal fusion after disc removal. *Surg Gynecol Obstet* 1946;82:215–218.
10. Wiltberger DR. The dowel intervertebral body fusion as used in lumbar disc surgery. *J Bone Joint Surg [Am]* 1957;39A:284–291.
11. Olsson TH, Selvik G, Willner S. Vertebral motion in spondylolisthesis. *Acta Radiol Diagn (Stockh)* 1976;17:861–868.
12. Penning L, Blickman JR. Instability in lumbar spondylolisthesis: a radiographic study of several concepts. *AJR* 1980;134:293–301.
13. Wood KB, Popp CA, Transfeldt EE, et al. Radiographic evaluation of instability in spondylolisthesis. *Spine* 1994;19:1697–1703.
14. Pearcy M, Shepherd J. Is there instability in spondylolisthesis? *Spine* 1985;10:175–177.
15. van Tulder MW, Assendelft WJJ, Koes BW, et al. Spinal radiographic findings and nonspecific low back pain: a systematic review of observational studies. *Spine* 1997;22:427–434.
16. Resnick DK, Choudhri TF, Dailey AT, et al. Guidelines for the performance of fusion procedures for degenerative disease of the lumbar spine. Part 9: fusion in patients with stenosis and spondylolisthesis. *J Neurosurg Spine* 2005;2:679–685.
17. Mardjetko SM, Connolly PJ, Shott S. Degenerative lumbar spondylolisthesis: a meta-analysis of literature 1970–1993. *Spine* 1994;19:2256S–2265S.
18. Vaccaro AR, Garfin SR. Internal fixation (pedicle screw fixation) for fusions of the lumbar spine. *Spine* 1995(Suppl 24);20:157S–165S.
19. Kwon BK, Hilibrand AS, Malloy K, et al. A critical analysis of the literature regarding surgical approach and outcome for adult low-grade isthmic spondylolisthesis. *J Spinal Disord Tech* 2005;18:S30–S40.
20. Weinstein JN, Lurie JD, Tosteson TD, et al. Surgical versus nonsurgical treatment for lumbar degenerative spondylolisthesis. *N Engl J Med* 2007;356:2257–2270.
21. Moller H, Hedlund R. Surgery versus conservative management in adult isthmic spondylolisthesis: a prospective randomized study: Part 1. *Spine* 2000;25:1711–1715.
22. Moller H, Hedlund R. Instrumented and noninstrumented posterolateral fusion in adult spondylolisthesis: a prospective randomized study: Part 2. *Spine* 2000;25:1716–1721.
23. Ekman P, Moller H, Hedlund R. The long-term effect of posterolateral fusion in adult isthmic spondylolisthesis: a randomized controlled study. *Spine J* 2005;5:36–44.
24. Deyo RA, Nachemson A, Mirza SK. Spinal-fusion surgery—the case for restraint. *N Engl J Med* 2004;350:722–726.
25. Turner JA, Herron L, Haselkorn J, et al. Patient outcomes after lumbar spine fusions. *JAMA* 1992;268:907–911.
26. Gibson JNA, Grant IC, Waddell G. The Cochrane review of surgery for lumbar disc prolapse and degenerative lumbar spondylosis. *Spine* 1999;24:1820–1832.
27. Fritzell P, Hagg O, Wessberg P, et al. 2001 Volvo Award Winner in Clinical Studies: lumbar fusion versus nonsurgical treatment for chronic low back pain: a multicenter randomized controlled trial from the Swedish Lumbar Spine Study Group. *Spine* 2001;26:2521–2532.
28. Brox JI, Sorensen R, Friis A, et al. Randomized clinical trial of lumbar instrumented fusion and cognitive intervention and exercises in patients with chronic low back pain and disc degeneration. *Spine* 2003;28:1913–1921.
29. Fairbank J, Frost H, Wilson–MacDonald J, et al. Randomised controlled trial to compare surgical stabilisation of the lumbar spine with an intensive rehabilitation programme for patients with chronic low back pain: the MRC spine stabilisation trial. *BMJ* 2005;330:1233.
30. Mirza SK, Deyo RA. Systematic review of randomized trials comparing lumbar fusion surgery to nonoperative care for treatment of chronic back pain. *Spine* 2007;32:816–823.
31. Ostelo RWJG, de Vet HCW. Clinically important outcomes in low back pain. *Best Pract Res Clin Rheumatol* 2005;19:593–607.
32. Kovacs FM, Abraira V, Royuela A, et al. Minimal clinically important change for pain intensity and disability in patients with nonspecific low back pain. *Spine* 2007;32:2915–2920.
33. van der Roer N, Ostelo RW, Bekkering GE, et al. Minimal clinically important change for pain intensity, functional status, and general health status in patients with nonspecific low back pain. *Spine* 2006;31:578–582.
34. Thomsen K, Christensen FB, Eiskjaer SP, et al. 1997 Volvo Award winner in clinical studies. The effect of pedicle screw instrumentation on functional outcome and fusion rates in posterolateral lumbar spinal fusion: a prospective randomized clinical study. *Spine* 1997;22:2813–2822.
35. Christensen FB, Hansen ES, Laursen M, et al. Long-term functional outcome of pedicle screw instrumentation as a support for posterolateral spinal fusion. Randomized clinical study with a 5-year follow-up. *Spine* 2002;27:1269–1277.
36. Blumenthal SL, Baker J, Dossett A, et al. The role of anterior lumbar fusion for internal disc disruption. *Spine* 1988;13:566–569.
37. Kozak JA, O'Brien JP. Simultaneous combined anterior and posterior fusion. An independent analysis of a treatment for the disabled low-back pain patient. *Spine* 1990;15:322–328.
38. Kostuik JP, Errico TJ, Gleason TF. Luque instrumentation in degenerative conditions of the lumbar spine. *Spine* 1990;15:318–321.
39. Gill K, Blumenthal SL. Functional results after anterior lumbar fusion at L5–S1 in patients with normal and abnormal MRI scans. *Spine* 1992;17:940–942.
40. Lee CK, Vessa P, Lee JK. Chronic disabling low back pain syndrome caused by internal disc derangements. The results of disc excision and posterior lumbar interbody fusion. *Spine* 1995;20:356–361.
41. Wetzel FT, La Rocca SH, Lowery GL, et al. The treatment of lumbar spinal pain syndromes diagnosed by discography: lumbar arthrodesis. *Spine* 1994;19:792–800.
42. Parker LM, Murrell SE, Boden SD, et al. The outcome of posterolateral fusion in highly selected patients with discogenic low back pain. *Spine* 1996;21:1909–1917.
43. Penta M, Fraser RD. Anterior lumbar interbody fusion. A minimum 10-year follow-up. *Spine* 1997;22:2429–2434.
44. Greenough CG, Peterson MD, Hadlow S, et al. Instrumented posterolateral lumbar fusion. Results and comparison with anterior interbody fusion. *Spine* 1998;23:479–486.
45. Anderson PA, Rouleau JP. Intervertebral disc arthroplasty. *Spine* 2004;29:2779–2786.
46. Gamradt SC, Wang JC. Lumbar disc arthroplasty. *Spine J* 2005;5:95–103.
47. Blumenthal S, McAfee PC, Guyer RD, et al. A prospective, randomized, multicenter Food and Drug Administration investigational device exemptions study of lumbar total disc replacement with the CHARITÉ™ artificial disc versus lumbar fusion. Part I: evaluation of clinical outcomes. *Spine* 2005;30:1565–1575.
48. Zigler J, Delamarter R, Spivak JM, et al. Results of the prospective, randomized, multicenter Food and Drug Administration investigational device exemption study of the ProDisc®-L total disc replacement versus circumferential fusion for the treatment of 1-level degenerative disc disease. *Spine* 2007;32:1155–1162.
49. Mirza SK. Point of view: commentary on the research reports that led to Food and Drug Administration approval of an artificial disc. *Spine* 2005;30:1561–1564.
50. Zindrick MR, Spratt KF. Point of view. *Spine* 2007;32:1163.
51. Bertagnoli R, Yue JJ, Shah R, et al. The treatment of disabling single-level lumbar discogenic low back pain with total disc arthroplasty utilizing the Prodisc prosthesis: a prospective study with 2-year minimum follow-up. *Spine* 2005;30:2230–2236.
52. Zucherman JF, Hsu KY, Hartjen CA, et al. A multicenter, prospective, randomized trial evaluating the X STOP interspinous process decompression system for the treatment of neurogenic intermittent claudication: two-year follow-up results. *Spine* 2005;30:1351–1358.
53. Kondrashov DG, Hannibal M, Hsu KY, et al. Interspinous process decompression with the X-STOP device for lumbar spinal stenosis: a 4-year follow-up study. *J Spinal Disord Tech* 2006;19:323–327.
54. Siddiqui M, Smith FW, Wardlaw D. One-year results of X Stop interspinous implant for the treatment of lumbar spinal stenosis. *Spine* 2007;32:1345–1348.
55. Brussee P, Hauth J, Donk RD, et al. Self-rated evaluation of outcome of the implantation of interspinous process distraction (X-Stop) for neurogenic claudication. *Eur Spine J* 2008;17:200–203.
56. Verhoof OJ, Bron JL, Wapstra FH, et al. High failure rate of the interspinous distraction device (X-Stop) for the treatment of lumbar spinal stenosis caused by degenerative spondylolisthesis. *Eur Spine J* 2008;17:188–192.
57. Fritzell P. Fusion as treatment for chronic low back pain—existing evidence, the scientific frontier and research strategies. *Eur Spine J* 2005;14:519–520.
58. Franklin GM, Haug J, Heyer NJ, et al. Outcome of lumbar fusion in Washington State Workers' Compensation. *Spine* 1994;19:1897–1904.
59. Hannson T, Hansson E, Malchau H. Utility of surgery: a comparison of common elective orthopaedic surgical procedures. *Spine* 2008;33:2819–2830.

CHAPTER 74 ■ FAILED BACK SURGERY SYNDROME

JEROME SCHOFFERMAN

Failed back surgery syndrome (FBSS) is a nonspecific term that implies the final outcome of surgery did not meet the expectations, which were established *before* surgery, of *both* the patient and the surgeon.[1] It does not and should not mean that the patient failed to get total pain relief or did not return to full function. A surgeon's expectations for the outcome in a specific patient should be based on published medical evidence, the structural problem, the number and types of prior surgeries the patient has had, the psychological health of the patient, and the skills and experience of the surgeon. The patient must also have realistic expectations and must rely to some degree on the surgeon's input regarding possible outcomes and reasonable expectations from surgery.

In the subjective realm of pain for which there is no objective test, we must rely on the patient's report to judge whether the surgery resulted in a clinically important difference.[2,3] In patients with subacute nonspecific low back pain (LBP), the minimal clinically important difference (MCID) on a 0 to 10 numerical rating scale (NRS) is about 2.5 to 4.5 units.[3] In chronic LBP, results vary according to the research methods. If baseline NRS was <7 the MCID was 1.5 to 3.2. If the baseline pain was ≥9, the MCID was 2.5 to 6.8.[4] In chronic neuropathic pain, an improvement in NRS of 1.8 units is equivalent to a change of about 30%, an improvement that most patients will consider a "somewhat satisfactory result."[2] An improvement in NRS of 3 units or more is equivalent to a change in pain of about 50%, which most patients consider an "extremely satisfactory result."

There are many options for the treatment of patients with FBSS. The patient should receive the treatment with the highest level of evidence consistent with his or her specific structural pathology while considering that person's individual values and circumstances. To achieve this, cross referrals back and forth among pain specialists, surgeons, and other providers are often necessary. For some patients, the best and most conservative treatment for FBSS is repeat surgery. At other times, surgery is a poor option and medical management, a functional restoration program, neuroaugmentation, or neuroablation might be the best treatment. Collaborative care and consultation should result in the best outcomes and the resultant cross-fertilization will provide mutual education.

In order to be prepared to treat these challenging patients, physicians should know the reasons spine surgery might fail, the structural causes of FBSS, and the best treatment options for each situation.

CAUSES OF FBSS

It has been said that the best surgical outcome occurs when the right surgeon does the right surgery on the right patient at the right time. There is a significant risk for FBSS when any of these rights goes wrong. There are several models for classifying patients with FBSS.[1,5] One valuable method is to determine whether there is a structural cause for the pain. Residual or recurrent structural pathology may be due to inadequate evaluation before surgery or mismatch of the surgery needed versus the surgery performed, unrecognized complications, or technical failure. New structural problems may have developed after surgery. Another model is based on the time course of the residual or recurrent pain after surgery. Patients who never improve or who deteriorate in the first 4 weeks after surgery are more likely to have residual pathology, a complication, or a technical failure. Patients who get somewhat better initially but then deteriorate may have developed instability, instrument failure, recurrent disc herniation, or delayed infection. Those who get better but then deteriorate after 6 months may have new pathology at the same or adjacent segment or pseudarthrosis. This first section of this chapter discusses some of the more common issues that may result in FBSS using each model.

Mismatch of the Surgery Needed versus the Surgery Performed ("Wrong Surgery")

It is axiomatic that the best results of a spine surgery require the surgeon to perform the surgery indicated for the clinical condition ("right surgery"). When a surgeon chooses an operation that is not appropriate for the structural problem, the operation is likely to fail.

There is a paradigm that I have found to be quite useful. There are surgeries aimed at improving leg pain (e.g., decompression of a nerve root or discectomy for radicular symptoms) and surgeries that are directed toward improving axial low back pain (e.g., fusion for discogenic pain or instability). It follows that if a patient had predominantly axial LBP, but had a decompression or discectomy without fusion, it was not the best surgery for the clinical problem and there is a high likelihood the surgery will fail. In other words, there was a mismatch between the clinical problem and the surgery. The surgeon performed a "leg pain operation" for low back pain.

A second type of mismatch occurs when the surgery does not address all of the patient's pathology. For example, there are patients who have pathology such as disc degeneration, disc herniations, spinal stenosis, or combinations at multiple motion segments. The surgeon may have elected to operate on only the worst segment or segments, which leaves the patient with residual problems at the adjacent segments. This type of patient required multilevel surgery or, if the number of levels is excessive, perhaps no surgery at all. Another example is the patient with both central and foraminal stenosis. The surgeon does a good decompression of the central canal but inadequate decompression of the lateral canal. The patient may be left with leg pain due to remaining foraminal stenosis, which may be incorrectly thought to be neuropathic pain. Yet another example is the patient with severe foraminal stenosis. A surgeon may decide to perform a limited decompression for fear of causing instability, which might necessitate fusion. As a result, there is inadequate decompression and the patient does not get better. The patient needed decompression and fusion, but only had decompression. This is another mismatch between the surgery needed and the surgery performed.

Another example of a mismatch between the surgery needed and the surgery performed occurs when the surgeon fails to fully consider the effect of surgery on the motion segment. For example, consider a patient with spinal stenosis and very slight spondylolisthesis who has leg pain. If the surgeon chooses decompression without fusion, many times the spondylolisthesis progresses and the patient develops progressive LBP.

Incomplete Evaluation and/or Diagnosis ("Residual Pathology")

If a patient has not been fully or correctly evaluated, it is again likely that the surgery will fail. One of the reasons for the mismatches discussed in the previous section is incomplete evaluation. Surgery performed after an incomplete evaluation may leave significant structural pathology unattended. Incomplete evaluation is often due to overreliance on imaging studies, particularly magnetic resonance imaging (MRI). Many spine specialists depend on confirmatory diagnostic spinal injections to complement the history, physical examination, and MRI scan, particularly in the complex patient. A simple study, plain radiographs done standing with flexion and extension views, is too frequently not performed before surgery. These x-rays may disclose spondylolisthesis or deformity that was not seen on supine MRI. Pain relief after transforaminal epidural injection would suggest any foraminal stenosis seen on MRI is in fact the pain generator.[7-9] Discography can be useful to identify a painful disc.[10-14] It is certainly not a good test when used in isolation, but can add additional information when used in conjunction with other testing.

Psychological health is one of the most important variables with respect to the outcome of surgery.[15] Therefore, psychological evaluation is especially important for patients ("right patient") with longstanding pain and impairment or when the surgeon has any inkling that there may be a psychological problem. It is very likely that any psychological problems present after surgery were in fact present before, but overlooked or underestimated. Most patients with chronic LBP have some psychological illness, most commonly depression, anxiety disorder, and substance abuse disorder.[16,17] Although these disorders may not cause surgery to be cancelled, treatment before surgery and psychological follow-up afterward might prove useful to increase the chances of a good result. In addition to these familiar illnesses, there is growing evidence that a patient's coping abilities, fear and fear-avoidance behavior, and past history of sexual or physical abuse may play important roles in continuing pain, impairment, and disability.[18-22]

Complications

Many of the complications of spinal surgery occur early in the postoperative period and will be recognized by the surgeon. Infection usually occurs early, but occasionally does not appear for weeks or months. Incidental durotomy, if not recognized, can lead to late pseudomeningocoele. Misplaced pedicle screws can cause new leg pain, usually in a single dermatome, and is often present immediately after surgery. Neural injury during surgery has similar symptoms and early appearance after surgery. Complications that usually occur later include facet or pedicle fractures; problems with pedicle screws; and bone graft collapse, resorption, or dislocation (after interbody fusion). Another complication is surgery performed at the wrong level. Even now with extra care being paid to marking the operative level and more, this complication still occurs. It may not be noted until a plain radiograph or CT scan is obtained during the evaluation for FBSS.

Pedicle screws can cause LBP by any of several mechanisms. There can be loosening of screws, which can result in a "wind-shield wiper effect" at the bone–screw interface and be painful. There can be pain over the screws, sometimes attributed to chronic irritation of overlying soft tissues and bursa formation. As mentioned previously, pedicle screw misplacement can cause leg pain if a screw breaches a pedicle and irritates or injures a nerve. This can be mistaken for neural injury due to surgical trauma. Therefore, if there is leg pain in a single dermatome, it is necessary to obtain a CT scan to see if there has been even slight breach of the pedicle. Removal of the internal fixation may be helpful.[24] Pseudarthrosis is a failure of fusion. Some patients with nonunions have pain, but others do not. Therefore, one cannot assume that the nonunion is the cause of the pain. Plain radiographs are not reliable to show if a fusion is solid. However, if standing films with sagittal flexion and extension views show motion, it would indicate nonunion. The most useful test is a CT scan that includes reformatted curved coronal sections that are taken out to the tips of the transverse processes in addition to the usual sagittal and axial images.[25] CT also allows visualization of the anterior column to look for lucency surrounding an interbody fusion (bone or cages).

Some patients that have undergone surgery develop instability defined as greater than 3 mm translation on standing flexion/extension x-rays. We frequently see patients who had very slight spondylolisthesis before surgery for disc herniation or spinal stenosis in whom no fusion was done because the slip was so slight. Then, some months after surgery, the back pain worsens and plain x-rays reveal progression of the slip.

Technical Failure

Despite the fact that the surgery was appropriate for the symptoms and pathology, the surgeon may not have been able to accomplish the technical goals. Technical failure is usually apparent on good quality imaging studies. There may be inadequate decompression of a foramen even though stenosis was recognized and the surgeon attempted decompression. There may be incomplete removal of a disc herniation, especially if it was a far lateral herniation. There may be misplacement of screws or incorrect connection of internal fixation.

Residual Pathology

Spinal Pathology

Residual pathology implies that the surgery did not correct all of the structural problems that were painful. There are many explanations why pathology might have been left behind. These are discussed previously.

Extra-Spinal Pathology

Residual pathology might also be due to extra-spinal disorders that can mimic spinal problems. Most likely, when an extra-spinal disorder is the cause of pain, it was present prior to surgery but not recognized. Some of the common problems that can mimic spine pain are shown in Table 74.1 and include primary hip disorders (especially osteoarthritis and osteonecrosis), greater trochanteric pain syndromes (GTPS), peripheral nerve injury or entrapment, and perhaps pirifomis syndrome.[26-30]

Painful disorders of the hip region most often are independent of spinal pathology, but at times they can coexist with a spinal disorder, especially in older patients. This is a challenging problem because there is considerable overlap between their respective symptoms and signs. Osteoarthritis of the hip is common in elderly patients with spinal stenosis. Brown et al. studied a referral population with leg pain to determine if there were signs or symptoms that might differentiate between osteoarthritis of the hip

TABLE 74.1

DIFFERENTIAL DIAGNOSIS OF SOME OF THE MORE COMMON EXTRA-SPINAL CAUSES OF FBSS BY SYMPTOMS, SIGNS, RADIOLOGY, AND INJECTIONS

Diagnosis	Symptoms	Signs	Radiology	Injections
Hip osteoarthritis	Groin pain	Limp and limited IR	Standing x-rays of pelvis and hips	Relief with intra-articular
Non-OA intra-articular hip pathology	Groin pain	Limp and limited or painful IR	If standard x-rays nondiagnostic, MRI of hip	+/− relief with intra-articular
Trochanteric bursitis	Lateral thigh pain	Tender over GT	Not generally helpful	Relief with injection of GT
Tendonitis	Pain at tendon insertion	Pain with resistance	MRI may show tendonopathy	+/− relief with injection
Nerve entrapment or neuroma	Pain in peripheral nerve distribution	Allodynia, hypoalgesia Tinel's sign	MRI	Relief with anesthesia of affected nerve
Peripheral arterial insufficiency	Arterial claudication	Poor pulses? Pain with bicycling test and treadmill	Positive arterial studies	N/A

CT, computed axial tomography; GT, greater trochanter; IR, internal rotation; MRI, magnetic resonance imaging; SIJ, sacroiliac joint pain; +/−, may be helpful.

and a spinal disorder.[27] Unfortunately the types of spinal disorders were not detailed and there was no special attention paid to the sacroiliac joint (SIJ), a condition that might easily be confused with a hip disorder. The factors that were strongly suggestive of primary hip pathology were the presence of a limp, groin pain, or limited internal rotation of the hip. Factors more suggestive of spinal stenosis were lateral thigh pain, buttock pain, and pain below the knee, particularly in the absence of groin pain.

There may be clues to hip disease in the history and examination. Groin pain with each step is highly indicative of intrinsic hip pathology. Patients at risk for osteonecrosis of the hip may have a history of dislocation, alcohol abuse, or corticosteroid use. Patients with hip pathology will often present with a limp or Trendelenburg gait as opposed to patients with spinal stenosis who usually walk in lumbar flexion. However, osteoarthritic patients with hip flexion contractures also walk bent at the waist. Limitation of or pain during hip range of motion testing, particularly internal rotation, are excellent indicators of intrinsic hip disease.[27] Weight-bearing radiographs of the hip are the standard for diagnosing hip pathology. A single, weight-bearing antero-posterior pelvis view can serve as a screening tool in patients felt to be a risk for hip osteoarthritis.

Disorders of the structures near the hip that can mimic spine pain include greater trochanteric pain syndromes (GTPS), subtle sacral fractures, piriformis syndrome, gluteal tendonitis, hamstring syndrome, ischial bursitis, or tendonitis. Most have been described in patients with FBSS.[30,32,33] Patients with GTPS typically complain of pain in the proximal lateral thigh, often with radiation to the distal thigh and occasionally below the knee.[30,32,33] Pain is usually increased by lying on the affected side, climbing stairs, and transition from sitting to standing.[33] Pain may arise from the bursa itself or from the gluteal and short external rotator tendons or iliotibial band.[32] On exam, there is tenderness over the greater trochanter but, in the variants of GTPS, there may be tenderness at other sites. Diagnosis is confirmed by relief of pain with the injection of local anesthetic and steroids into the bursa or other tender structure. Some authors feel it is necessary to use fluoroscopy to accurately inject the greater trochanteric bursa.[34]

There is controversy regarding piriformis syndrome.[31,35] On the one hand are those who feel it is a diagnosis that occurs in two-thirds of patients with sciatica of unclear etiology.[31] Others feel that, at least based on cadaver studies, anatomical causes for piriformis syndrome are rare.[35] It must be considered that the pain is actually referred from the sacroiliac or facet joints. Signs that might be suggestive of piriformis syndrome include gluteal pain and tenderness in the sciatic notch, and buttock pain with flexion, adduction, and internal rotation of the hip (FADIR). Imaging modalities are rarely helpful, although MR neurography has been suggested as useful.[31,36] After more common problems are eliminated, injection of the muscle has been reported to provide intermediate and long-term relief in many patients.[31]

Peripheral nerve trauma or entrapment can mimic radiculopathy.[28] In the patient with FBSS, the most relevant problems are lateral femoral cutaneous nerve entrapment or injury (meralgia paresthetica), which presents with pain in the lateral or anterolateral thigh; peroneal nerve entrapment; and sciatic nerve entrapment.[28,29] With entrapments, pain will be in the distribution of the peripheral nerve involved, not in a true lumbar dermatome. There may be a positive Tinel sign over the area of pathology. Diagnosis can often be confirmed by nerve conduction studies, and there will be temporary relief of pain after injection with local anesthetic in the area of presumed entrapment.

Recurrent Pathology

Pathology can recur even after perfect surgery. Disc herniations recur in up to 15% of patients after discectomy. Foraminal stenosis can recur if there is progressive degeneration of the same motion segment.

New Pathology

Pain after prior spine surgery may be totally unrelated to the index surgery. The usual structural causes of LBP can be seen in these patients.

STRUCTURAL ETIOLOGIES OF FAILED BACK SURGERY

Despite the many reasons for failed spine surgery, there are a limited number of structural etiologies for the residual or recur-

TABLE 74.2

MOST COMMON SPINAL CAUSES OF FAILED BACK SURGERY IN THREE REPORTED STUDIES[37–39]

Diagnosis	Burton (1981)	Waguespack (2002)	Slipman (2002)
Lateral stenosis	58	29	25
HNP	12–16	7	12
Painful discs	N/A	20	22
Neuropathic pain	6–16	10	10
Total %	76 to 90	66	69

All numbers are %; HNP, herniated disc.

rent pain. The three studies that looked at the most common structural causes of FBSS had very similar findings (Table 74.2).[37–39] The most common structural causes of FBSS are lateral canal stenosis (foraminal stenosis), recurrent or residual disc herniation, one or more painful degenerated discs, neuropathic pain, facet joint pain, and SIJ pain.

In 1981, Burton et al. reported an analysis of several hundred patients with FBSS.[37] About 58% had foraminal stenosis, 7% to 14% had central canal stenosis, 12% to 16% had recurrent (or residual) disc herniations, 6% to 16% had arachnoiditis, and 6% to 8% had epidural fibrosis. Other less common causes in their series included neuropathic pain, chronic mechanical pain, painful disc above a fusion, pseudarthrosis, foreign body, and surgery performed at the wrong level. They were not able to establish a diagnosis in less than 5% of their patients despite the fact that their patients were evaluated early in the CT scan era and well before MRI scans. They did use discography.

There have been major advances in diagnostic testing since the Burton paper. In 2002, Waguespack et al. and Slipman et al. reported the results of their evaluations of patients with FBSS.[38,39] In a retrospective review of 187 patients with FBSS seen at a tertiary care spine center, the authors were able to make a diagnosis in 95%. Slipman et al. were also able to make a diagnosis in more than 90% of patients.

Several authors have presented their unquantified opinions and experiences regarding the structural causes of FBSS.[40,41]

Fritsch reviewed 136 patients who had revision surgeries after clinical failure of an initial laminectomy and discectomy and found a high prevalence of recurrent disc herniations and instability.[40] Kostuik discussed some of the potential causes of failure of decompression, but provided no quantitative data.[41]

In the following section, I have used functional definitions of structural abnormalities that are a composite of those proposed by the North American Spine Society[42] and the International Association for the Study of Pain[43] modified by my clinical experiences. The differential diagnosis of some of the more common causes of FBSS along with some helpful symptoms, signs, radiological findings, and response to injections are shown in Table 74.3.

Lateral Canal Stenosis

Lateral canal stenosis (foraminal stenosis) was found in 2% to 29% of FBSS patients in the Waguespack and Slipman studies, half of what was seen 25 years ago.[37–39] The lower prevalence may be due to increased awareness of the problem, improved imaging studies, and/or better understanding of the need for meticulous decompression. Patients with lateral stenosis have pain that is predominantly in the leg or buttock region, often in the distribution of a single dermatome. Pain is usually worsened by standing and walking and relieved by sitting. MRI or CT scan shows narrowing of the canal at the index level or an adjacent segment. Stenosis can be subclassified as "up-down stenosis" due to loss of disc space height or "front-back stenosis" due to facet hypertrophy and osteophyte formation. Potential confirmation that the visualized stenosis is the cause of pain is at least temporary relief of leg pain after transforaminal epidural blockade of the suspected nerve root.[6–8] There may be longer relief if corticosteroids are administered.[9]

Lateral canal stenosis must be differentiated from neuropathic pain and mixed pain syndrome, which have similar presentations, because the treatments are different. Spinal stenosis is treated with flexion-biased body mechanics, medications, transforaminal corticosteroid injections, and/or decompression. Neuropathic pain is treated with medications or spinal cord stimulation (SCS). Mixed pain syndromes may require multiple treatments including decompression followed by medications and SCS.

TABLE 74.3

DIFFERENTIAL DIAGNOSIS OF COMMON CAUSES OF FBSS BY SYMPTOMS, SIGNS, RADIOLOGY, AND INJECTIONS

Diagnosis	Symptoms	Signs	Radiology	Injections
Lateral canal stenosis	Leg pain > LBP; relief with sitting	Loss of lumbar lordosis	MRI: foraminal stenosis	Relief with transforaminal epidural
Painful disc	LBP; ? worse with sitting	Restricted flexion in standing	MRI: degenerated disc(s)	Not indicated
Neuropathic pain	Leg pain Burning dysesthesia	Hypoalgesia Allodynia	No alternative diagnosis	Not indicated
Facet pain	Left or right LBP	?Facet tenderness	Not specific	Medial branch block relieves pain
Recurrent HNP	Vary with location. Leg pain > LBP	Variable	HNP on MRI	Epidural may provide temporary relief
SI joint pain	Gluteal pain with referral to leg and groin	May have + provocative testing	Not helpful	SI joint injection relieves pain

HNP, herniated nucleus pulposus; LBP, low back pain; MRI, magnetic resonance imaging; SIJ, sacroiliac joint pain.

Painful Disc (Discogenic Pain)

Pain that arises from within a disc without extrinsic neural compression is often referred to as discogenic pain.[42,43] One or more painful discs were the cause of FBSS in about 21% of patients.[37–39] Painful discs can occur at the index level of prior surgery, at an adjacent segment, or rarely at the index level, even in the presence of prior posterolateral fusion.[44–47] When there is a residual painful disc at the index surgical level, it is likely that it was not treated adequately by performing a fusion. When there is a painful disc at an adjacent segment, it was either present prior to surgery and not addressed or the disc degenerated after surgery.

It is clear that discs have the neural substrate to be painful.[48–50] In the normal disc the superficial layers of the annulus have sensory nerve endings that are potentially nociceptive.[50] In degenerated discs nerve fibers may extend deeper and even reach the inner third of the annulus in 50% of painful degenerated discs.[48,50] It is theorized that, in painful discs, these nerve endings become sensitized and thereby respond to innocuous stimuli with pain. In addition, recent evidence suggests that the sensory nerve supply of the disc resembles the innervation of certain enteric structures and may represent a variant of visceral pain. This may partly explain why discogenic pain seems to "behave" differently from other musculoskeletal pain.[50]

Several authors have tried to correlate symptoms and signs to identify with the presence of discogenic pain.[51–53] However, the correlations are neither sufficiently sensitive nor specific to be relied upon. Schwarzer et al. found no symptoms or signs to be specific for discogenic pain.[51] Young et al. found factors that increased the likelihood of a positive discogram were centralization of pain during mechanical (McKenzie) evaluation, pain provoked or increased when rising from sitting to standing, and midline pain.[52] In a systematic review, Hancock et al. found centralization of pain was predictive of a discogenic source.[53] Hancock et al. also found that MRI findings of high intensity zone, endplate changes, and disc degeneration correlated with discogenic pain using provocation disc injection as the reference standard.[53] Absence of degeneration on MRI was the only test that reduced the likelihood of discogenic pain being present.

An MRI scan is a picture of anatomy, not of pain. It is well established that patients without LBP might have an abnormal MRI.[54,55] Therefore, there have been efforts to find a means to determine if an abnormal disc visualized on MRI is in fact a pain generator in a particular patient.[11] Discography, perhaps more properly called provocation disc injection, can be quite useful to distinguish between discs that are and are not painful. Discography is not a definitive or perfect test, but when interpreted cautiously and in light of the history, physical examination, psychological status, imaging studies, and other diagnostic injections, it can prove very helpful.[10–14] The value of discography in patients with FBSS, especially with respect to a disc that has been operated on, has not been well examined. In this setting provocation disc injection might prove most useful when painless to exclude a disc as source of pain. When the diagnosis of discogenic pain is suggested by history and examination, MRI shows a single degenerated disc, and other potential causes of chronic LBP have been excluded, there is little need to perform discography.

Although there is no perfect reference standard, based on published reports and my personal experience, there may be a typical clinical presentation for discogenic LBP. Patients usually have dominant midline LBP that frequently radiates to the left and right of the midline, the gluteal regions, and often to the leg in a nondermatomal fashion. Pain is usually worse sitting and during transition from sitting to standing. It may improve with standing or walking. Physical examination is not specific. There may be decreased flexion in standing because of pain. There may be ten-

derness over the spinous processes, but not over the facet joints. Centralization of pain with mechanical examination is common.

Disc Herniation

Recurrent or residual disc herniation was seen in 7% to 12% of patients with FBSS.[37–39] There are two common presentations of pain from a disc herniation: radicular and axial. The topography of the pain is primarily due to the location of the herniation. A posterolateral herniation is more likely to compress or irritate a nerve root and therefore present with predominant leg pain. A midline herniation, unless very large, does not compress neural elements and presents with predominant LBP. A disc that is degenerated with a herniation can cause both leg and LBP. In the presence of epidural or perineural fibrosis, a disc herniation may cause more leg pain than expected than if there were no fibrosis.

Diagnosis of recurrent or residual disc herniation is inferred from the history and physical examination, and confirmed by MRI. There is no advantage to using gadopentate with modern scanners 6 months or more after surgery.

Facet Joint Pain

The facet joints are the cause of pain in 15% to 30% of patients with chronic LBP, and the cause of residual or recurrent pain in 3% to 16% of patients with FBSS.[39,56–58] The facet joint (FJ) is a diarthrodial joint with chondral surfaces, synovium, and meniscoid tissue. FJs are susceptible to chondral damage, inflammation, and degeneration. Injury may occur during surgery, as a result of progressive degeneration of the motion segment at the surgical level, or degeneration due to the mechanical stresses of fusion at an adjacent segment.

Shah et al. and Moshirfar et al. described a 33% and 24% incidence respectively of FJ violation in patients undergoing lumbar fusion with pedicle screw fixation.[59,60] Neither study reported the clinical status of the patients. There has been increased interest in the role of FJs since the introduction of total disc arthroplasty (TDR). Van Ooij et al. reported that FJ arthrosis was responsible for clinical failure in 11 of 27 patients.[61] Shim et al. reported radiological degradation of the facets in 32% to 36% of 61 patients after TDR.[62]

Facet arthrosis has been suggested as a relative contraindication to TDR.[63]

Although there are no reports that correlated symptoms and signs of FJ pain in patients with FBSS, several investigators and expert panels have tried to define the clinical pattern of FJ pain in chronic LBP.[52,56,64,65] Schwarzer et al. found no specific symptoms or signs that correlated positively with FJ pain, but noted that the presence of midline LBP had a negative association.[56] Young found that patients with FJ pain did not have increased pain when rising from sit to stand.[52] Laslett found symptoms and signs of facet joint pain "to be elusive."[64] A panel of physical therapist and physician experts arrived at consensus regarding features of symptoms and signs that were suggestive of FJ pain.[64] These included localized unilateral back pain, replication or aggravation of pain by unilateral pressure over the FJ or transverse process, lack of pain below the knee, pain eased in flexion (sitting), pain in extension, and pain in extension plus side bending or rotation to the ipsilateral side. Imaging studies were not felt to be helpful.

Given the ambiguities in the literature and lack of data in patients with FBSS, it is reasonable to perform medial branch blocks on most patients as part of the routine evaluation of predominant LBP unless there is another obvious cause for the problem. Features of the history that increase the likelihood of FJ pain being present are age greater that 65 and improvement in pain by lying supine. Other features include pain that is not worse with forward flexion including sitting, not worse when rising from sitting to standing, and not worse with coughing. Features from the examination include tenderness to palpation over the FJs or transverse processes. The diagnosis of FJ pain is made when there is excellent relief of the target pain on two occasions after medial branch block (MBB), or less definitively pain relief after intra-articular injection of local anesthetic into the joint.[66]

Sacroiliac Joint Pain

There is sufficient and consistent evidence that shows that the SIJ can be a cause of pain in up to 15% to 30% of patients with chronic LBP.[67,68] The prevalence of SIJ pain is at least 2% to 3% in patients with FBSS, and may be higher in patients who have had fusion to the sacrum.[39,69] The SIJ can be injured during graft harvesting, but more likely the joint becomes painful owing to transfer of stress after fusion.[70] Finally, SIJ pain could have been present before surgery due to acute or cumulative trauma, but not recognized.[71]

Again, there are no specific signs or symptoms specific for SIJ pain, but there are definite clues to the diagnosis.[52,53,68,72] Virtually all patients have pain distal to the posterior iliac crest and lateral to the midline spine. Some patients will point directly over the SIJ when asked to show where the pain is centered. Pain is frequently referred to the groin, thigh, calf, and occasionally the foot—patterns that might otherwise suggest radiculopathy or even hip joint pathology. The patient may report pain is worsened during transition from sitting to standing.[52] Pain may increase with single leg weight bearing. Most often there is tenderness directly over the SIJ. Although signs are not specific, diagnosis is probable when tenderness and three or four other provocative tests are present.[53] Plain radiographs, MRI, and CT are not definitive. The confirmation of SIJ pain requires relief of the target pain after fluoroscopically guided local anesthetic SIJ injection.[73]

Spinal Stenosis and Axial Low Back Pain

The classic symptom of central spinal stenosis is leg pain with walking (neurogenic claudication) or standing. In addition, many if not most patients with spinal stenosis also report LBP.[74–77] However, it has not been established that patients with central spinal stenosis can have primarily LBP and gluteal pain with little or no leg pain. I believe this clinical presentation is not rare, but there are no data to support this observation. In my experience, the characteristic pain pattern is LBP, especially gluteal pain, with standing or walking, and complete or near complete relief of pain sitting. This symptom complex is quite the opposite of discogenic pain, but similar to FJ pain. Patients usually experience at least temporary relief of pain after epidural steroid injection and no relief after MBB, just the opposite of FJ pain. The patients with FBSS and predominant LBP might have spinal stenosis at the index level or an adjacent segment that developed after surgery or was not addressed at surgery.

Neuropathic Pain

Neuropathic pain is defined as pain due to injury or physiological dysfunction of the peripheral or central nervous system (CNS). Neuropathic pain was the predominant problem in 5% to 9% of FBSS patients.[37,38] It is likely that there is an increased awareness and, therefore, recognition of neuropathic pain rather than an increased prevalence.

There are several potential mechanisms for neuropathic pain after spine surgery. A nerve root could have been damaged prior to surgery because of either sudden injury (acute disc herniation) or prolonged compression from foraminal stenosis or disc hernia-

tion. In this instance, radicular type pain continues despite technically successful surgery. Alternatively, a nerve could be damaged during the surgery itself, which is sometimes referred to as a "battered nerve." The incidence of new cases of arachnoiditis has probably decreased, perhaps because oil-based myelography is no longer performed, but it still occurs. There can be peripheral nerve injuries such as cluneal neuroma owing to nerve injury at an iliac crest donor site and meralgia paresthetica.[29,78,79] In theory at least, it is also possible that total or near total discectomy alters the nervous system in a model akin to phantom pain.

Neural injury or dysfunction can be responsible for both amplification and persistence of pain.[80,81] Neuropathic pain of spinal origin usually presents with a predominance of leg pain in one or two adjacent dermatomes or along the path of a peripheral nerve. In classic presentations, the pain is described as burning, dysesthetic, or electrical, but in neuropathic disorders after spine surgery, pain is more frequently described as aching and stabbing. Pain may be constant or intermittent. It is often precipitated or aggravated by simple activities because the damaged nerves are hyperexcitable and respond abnormally to even minor biomechanical changes.

By definition, in pure and uncomplicated neuropathic pain, there is no evidence of nerve root compression on imaging studies. It is important to distinguish neuropathic pain from what I'll call neurogenic pain. Neurogenic pain implies that a nerve is being compressed or irritated rather than its being permanently damaged. To further complicate matters, some patients have both neuropathic pain plus ongoing neural compression (neurogenic), which is referred to as a mixed pain syndrome.

Neuropathic pain can also be due to physiological dysfunction in the peripheral or central nervous systems without structural nerve damage. As a result of prolonged or repeated chemical or mechanical damage to afferent nerves, these nociceptors may become sensitized and hyperexcitable (peripheral sensitization). There is lowering of their activation thresholds and subsequent increased responsiveness to all stimuli.[80] In this physiologically altered setting, innocuous stimuli may be perceived as painful (allodynia), minimally noxious stimuli may be perceived as very painful (hyperalgesia), and thereby be stimulus-independent pain as well.

A similar sensitization can develop in the CNS as a result of "constant bombardment" by painful afferent stimuli (central sensitization). The site of dysfunction is thought to be primarily at the dorsal horn of the spinal cord and brainstem. Once again, normal or minimally painful stimuli are perceived as very painful. In patients with persistent axial LBP (rather than the more typical extremity pain) despite perfect surgery and no other explanation for pain, one might be able to hypothesize that this represents central sensitization and a variant of neuropathic pain.

Epidural Fibrosis

Epidural fibrosis occurs after most, if not all, posterior lumbar surgeries. There is a school of thought that fibrosis is responsible for many or most of the failures of lumbar spine surgery. The other point of view is that in most instances fibrosis is an innocent and incidental finding that does not cause pain, but has the potential to make other problems worse, such as radiculopathy due to disc herniation or spinal stenosis.

Coskun et al. performed a prospective analysis of 29 patients with FBSS to determine the relationships among the severity of epidural fibrosis, psychological factors, LBP, and disability.[82] They found that neither the postoperative pain scores nor the postoperative Oswestry Disability Index scores differed significantly with relationship to the severity of the epidural fibrosis. Moreover, postoperative pain scores were positively correlated with the scores of the mini-Minnesota Multiphasic Personality Inventory (MMPI). They concluded that epidural fibrosis was an incidental radiological finding that did not correlate with patients' complaints. Annertz et al. compared the MRI scans of eight patients with and eight patients without sciatica after lumbar discectomy.[83] Fourteen patients had focal or diffuse epidural fibrosis. There were no differences between the symptomatic and nonsymptomatic groups with respect to the presence or extent of epidural or perineural fibrosis.

Trescot et al. performed a systematic review of the effectiveness of adhesiolysis in patients with chronic spinal pain.[84] They concluded that there was strong evidence for short-term relief (>50%) and moderate evidence for relief lasting greater than 3 months of both LBP and leg pain. Some studies included patients with no prior back surgery.

Deconditioning

Deconditioning has long been considered to be at least partially responsible for the persistent pain and pain-related impairment and disability in many patients with FBSS.[85–89] There are three models for this so-called deconditioning syndrome. The pure physical deconditioning model holds that loss of muscle strength and endurance is responsible for reduced activity, impairment, and disability.[88] The cognitive-behavioral model emphasizes the fear-avoidance paradigm, which holds that some patients with LBP avoid activities out of pain-related catastrophic thinking and fear.[88] They believe that attempts to increase their function will result in increased pain and progressive structural damage and, as a result, they markedly curtail their activity. A third model is a combination of the two in which patients have both the maladaptive fear-avoidance and true physical deconditioning. As a result of the fear-avoidant decreased activity, there is disuse (perhaps better termed underuse) with progressive loss of muscle strength and endurance.[88,89]

In patients with chronic LBP and deconditioning, the paraspinal musculature is most affected.[90] There is MRI, CT scan, and ultrasound evidence that after spine surgery, many patients have decreased cross-sectional area (CSA) of their lumbar muscles.[91,92] Gejo et al. showed both decreased CSA and decreased muscle strength in 20 patients after posterior lumbar surgery.[92] In addition, four of eight patients with longer retraction times during surgery had LBP at 6 months versus none in 12 patients with shorter retraction times. Motosuneya et al. looked at the changes in muscle CSA after 5 different types of spine surgery and surprisingly found some loss of muscle strength even in those patients who had anterior spine surgery. They opined that rigid fixation and resultant protection of the paraspinal muscles was at least partly responsible.[94]

Weber et al. found that posterior spine surgery caused changes in muscle histology, but found no correlation between pain and these changes.[93] Airaksinen et al. compared muscle density by CT scan in patients after decompression for spinal stenosis.[95] There was a marked decrease in lumbar extensor muscle density that the authors felt could be explained by disuse or inactivity. The density of the lumbar flexors was higher in the group with excellent results than those with poor outcomes. Sihvonen et al. studied a select subgroup of 14 patients with good results and 21 with poor results 2 to 5 years after laminectomy.[96] They concluded that disturbed back muscle innervation and loss of muscular support leads to increased biomechanical strain and might be one important cause of the failed back syndrome.

In summary, there is consistent evidence that posterior spine surgery (and possibly anterior as well) often causes loss of muscle density, histologic changes, and probably decreased strength. There is a trend in the evidence that suggests a correlation between greater muscle changes and LBP after surgery.

Multiple studies have shown decreased muscle strength and endurance in patients with chronic LBP and no prior surgery.[85,86,95,97] Recently, some investigators have questioned the idea that patients with chronic LBP have meaningful losses of muscle strength and endurance, feeling that the evidence for the physical deconditioning model is inconclusive.[98] Bousema et al. measured the muscle strength, muscle endurance, and aerobic capacity in 124 patients with subacute LBP at presentation and at 1 year.[99] Patients who had persisting pain did not show signs of physical deconditioning. Interestingly, most patients did not show evidence of decreased physical activities either. Their study did not validate and, in fact, partially contradicted the deconditioning paradigm.

That said, virtually all investigators agree there is clear evidence that exercise is effective in reducing impairment and disability.[88,90,97,98,100,101] Many, but not all, studies also show decreases in LBP. It is suggested that the improvements are more likely due to reduction of fear, fear-avoidance, and pain catastrophizing rather than increases in strength and endurance.[102,103]

PSYCHOLOGICAL FACTORS IN FAILED BACK SURGERY ("RIGHT PATIENT")

Most patients with FBSS have some form of psychological response. In some, their psyche can be helpful; in others it can be harmful. The most common psychological illnesses in patients with chronic LBP are depression, anxiety disorder, and substance abuse disorder (although current definitions and better understanding of opioid use might change the prevalence of the latter).[17] It is most likely that these psychological illnesses make pain and function worse rather than being the underlying cause of pain. In most chronic LBP patients, psychological disorders developed after the back injury. Accordingly, they would have been present prior to surgery, and either not recognized or not considered important.[15,16] Patients with more severe psychological illnesses such as thought disorders, bipolar disorder, antisocial personality, or active addictive disease have illness that is usually very apparent. These patients are less likely to have had spine surgery.

Fear-Avoidance

In addition to the more classic psychological illnesses mentioned briefly previously, there is increasing recognition of the importance of cognitive-behavioral factors in patients with chronic LBP. The most important of these are catastrophic thinking, pain-related fear, and fear-avoidance.[18] Although not always the case, these cognitive-behavioral factors often correlate more strongly with impairment and disability than does pain severity.[14,18,19]

Fear-avoidance is the avoidance of movements or activities because of fear of one or more aspects of pain. The fears reported most often are the fear that pain will get worse due to activity, the fear that activity will lead to further structural damage, and the fear that residual pain means that something seriously wrong has been overlooked.[89,105] Any or all of these fears may lead to avoidance of normal activity and subsequent disuse (underuse), deconditioning, impairment, and disability. Physicians may contribute to its development and perpetuation by advising patients to avoid certain activities.[106]

Catastrophic thinking is an exaggerated negative orientation toward pain.[102] Patients dwell on the most negative conceivable consequences.[18] Every flare is a crisis. Every good day is just the calm before the proverbial disaster. Pain-related catastrophic thinking is the cognitive aspect of fear-avoidance behavior. In patients with acute LBP, pain catastrophizing is a powerful predictor of chronicity. Pain-related catastrophic thinking may lead to avoiding activities that might increase pain, which results in progressive limitations of function with impairment and disability. The progressive downhill spiral of catastrophic thinking, fear, fear-avoidance, and physical deconditioning is appealing as an explanation for progressive impairment and disability.[107]

Coping Abilities

Another model that is useful and correlates well with the fear-avoidance model is based on coping abilities. Coping has been defined as the purposeful strategies used to manage internal and external stressful events—in this case, pain.[108] Coping can be broadly characterized as either active or passive. Patients with active coping strategies take personal responsibility for their pain and believe they can control it. They work to maximize their function despite pain. They accept their problem and have realistic expectations. On the other hand, patients with passive coping resort to strategies that are not useful such as prayer and hoping, wishful thinking, guarding, and resting excessively.[109] Some may blame others for their pain and give responsibility for managing their pain to an outside source. They reduce their activities to avoid increasing their pain, and may develop a fear-avoidance lifestyle. Passive coping is a significant risk factor for chronicity in patients with subacute LBP and for persons in the general population who develop acute LBP.[20]

Kerns et al. described three types of patients based on their mechanism of coping: adaptive copers, interpersonally distressed, and dysfunctional.[110] For practical clinical purposes the latter two might be combined. It is sometimes useful in understanding these issues to consider adaptive copers as "persons with chronic pain" and the dysfunctional patients as "chronic pain patients." Adaptive copers have active coping strategies. Their pain seems appropriate for the peripheral stimulus, function is appropriate for the pain, and mood is consistent with the pain and impairment. They tend to stay with one physician and have reasonable expectations. They are generally easy to care for and respond to most treatments as might be expected based on the evidence.

On the other hand, dysfunctional patients are much more difficult to treat. Their pain is typically far greater than expected for the peripheral stimulus, their disability and impairment seem out of proportion to the peripheral stimulus, their mood is depressed, their expectations are not reasonable, and their behavior is demanding. They tend to go from doctor to doctor seeking an almost magical cure. In general they tend to respond poorly to most treatments—medications, rehabilitation, interventional pain techniques, and surgery.

Childhood Abuse

Persons who had a very dysfunctional childhood and subsequent LBP may be at special and higher risk for chronic pain, impairment, disability, and failed back surgery.[111,112] One explanation lies in the realm of attachment theory. As children they suffered severe disruption of parental attachments. Identified disruptions include childhood physical or sexual abuse, abandonment, or parents who had addictive disease, chronic pain syndromes, or severe psychological illness.

ESTABLISHING THE DIAGNOSIS

Role of the History

The history is the most important part of the evaluation of a patient with FBSS. It establishes the foundation for the remainder of the evaluation as well as the information necessary to interpret other diagnostic elements. The most important elements of the history include a thorough description of the current pain, a com-parison of the pain before and after surgery, the time course of the reappearance of the pain, and the response of the pain to specific activities. It is also very valuable to analyze whether the type of surgery performed was appropriate for the preoperative symptoms and condition. The history should lead to a limited differential diagnosis, suggest the emphasis for the physical examination, and provide guidelines for selecting appropriate imaging studies and diagnostic injections. It is important to remember there may be more than one diagnosis present.

Preoperative Versus Current Pain

Pain that is essentially the same before and after surgery in terms of severity, location, quality, and response to mechanical maneuvers suggests that the original problem was not corrected. There may have been an error in diagnosis, an error selecting the correct surgery, or an incomplete surgery. On the other hand, when symptoms have changed significantly, it is most likely that there is new pathology, either a complication of surgery, technical failure, or progression of the underlying disease.

Location of Pain (Especially LBP vs. Leg Pain)

It is useful to divide FBSS patients into those with predominantly LBP and those with predominantly leg pain. In general, when LBP is greater than leg pain, the most common causes are discogenic pain at the level of the index surgery or at adjacent levels, FJ pain, SIJ pain, or instability (spondylolisthesis). If fusion was attempted, there may be a pseudarthrosis, although pseudarthrosis itself may not be the cause of pain. When leg pain predominates, the more common causes include residual foraminal stenosis, recurrent or residual disc herniation, neuropathic pain, or less likely hip disease or peripheral nerve injury.

Response to Mechanical Changes

There are no studies that document the changes in pain in response to common activities in patients with FBSS. Therefore, these correlations are based on personal experience and the studies in patients with chronic LBP and no prior surgery. These responses to biomechanical stresses are clues, but obviously cannot be considered definitive.

Response to Sitting. LBP or leg pain that increases with sitting and with flexion in standing is more likely due to one or more painful discs or instability (spondylolisthesis). Leg pain that improves with sitting is usually due to spinal stenosis.

Transition from Sitting to Standing. LBP that worsens during the transition from sit to stand suggests disc pain or SIJ and speaks against FJ pain.[17] LBP that increases with standing suggests posterior element pathology such as FJ pain. Leg pain that increases with standing or walking suggests spinal stenosis.

Quality of Pain

The word the patient uses to describe the pain is occasionally helpful. Burning, electric shock-like pain, dysesthesia, or superficial (skin) tenderness to light touch (allodynia) suggests neuropathic pain. However, neuropathic pain after spine surgery may not fit these classical descriptors.

Time Course of Appearance of Pain

Preoperative LBP or Leg Pain Never Improves or Early Onset of Old Symptoms

When LBP never improves or recurs within days to a month or so after surgery, it is most likely that the symptomatic structural pathology was not adequately addressed by surgery, there was a complication such as wrong level surgery, or the wrong procedure for this particular patient was done.[5] Partial pain relief implies correction of only part of the structural problem.[5] This outcome falls in the category of residual pathology, and the differential diagnosis has already been outlined.

New Leg Pain Soon After Surgery

The early appearance of new leg pain suggests direct neural injury during surgery, misplacement of a pedicle screw, or venous thrombosis.[5,78]

Pain Improves but Recurs One to Six Months After Surgery

Pain that improved initially but recurred in 1 to 6 months may be due to residual, recurrent, or new pathology. If pain location and description resemble preoperative symptoms, residual or recurrent pathology is likely. Pain that has new characteristics is more likely due to new pathology. There may be recurrent disc herniation, failure (loosening of pedicle screws) of internal fixation, instability, and late infection.

Pain Improves but Recurs and Is Different

Pain that recurs late and has a different location or quality compared to the preoperative pain is more likely due to new pathology. Examples include painful disc at an adjacent segment, disc herniation, or FJ pain. SIJ pain from donor site injury or stress from fusion to the sacrum also can occur at this stage.

Role of Radiological Evaluation of FBSS

Herzog discussed the requirements for imaging patients with FBSS and much of the following section is a summary of his work.[1,25] Radiological examination usually includes x-rays and either MRI or CT scan. There are only rare indications for nuclear imaging studies (infection, possible malignancy, possible rheumatological illness), myelography (pseudomeningocele), or CT myelography in the setting of FBSS.

Standard radiographs with standing flexion and extension lateral views are used to assess alignment, extent of disc space narrowing, spondylolisthesis, and, when fusion has been attempted, perhaps pseudarthrosis.[25,111] MRI is the optimal exam for most FBSS patients unless the issue is pseudarthrosis, in which case plain radiographs with flexion-extension views and CT scan with multiplanar reformations is much better.[1,25,111] With MRI it is necessary that the study visualizes the left and right extraforaminal zones so as to avoid missing foraminal or extraforaminal pathology. Angled T2-weighted sections from T12-L1 to L5-S1 through the disc spaces are done to evaluate the cross-sectional area of the thecal sac, to evaluate the central canal, and to define the exact relationship of the structural changes to all the neural elements.

In evaluating patients who had surgery for disc herniation, contrast enhanced MRI became the standard, but with newer equipment and imaging sequences, nonenhanced MRI imaging is usually adequate if the radiologist monitors the study and administers contrast only if the routine sequences are not definitive. MRI is an excellent study for spinal stenosis and can detect hypertrophy of facet joints and ligamenta flava, synovial cysts, or prominence of epidural fat. It will show if decompression was adequate to decompress the nerve root. Arachnoiditis can easily be detected with MRI. In patients with spinal instrumentation using titanium alloys, there should be no significant distortion with a high field-strength MRI if the sequences are optimized for the presence of metal using fast spin echo T2-weighted sequences without fat saturation to reduce artifacts. The central canal and

neural foramina can be adequately assessed even with the presence of pedicle screws.

Role of Diagnostic Injections

Anesthetic Injections

Diagnostic anesthetic injections are the reference standard for the diagnosis of FJ and SIJ pain.[66,73] A transforaminal epidural (TFE) injection is sometimes used to determine if a nerve that appears compressed on MRI or CT scan is in fact the pain generator.[6,8] A positive TFE may be defined as relief of the target pain after anesthetizing a specific spinal nerve. In addition, pain relief during the corticosteroid phase is reported to predict a good outcome for surgery.[9]

Provocation Disc Injections (Discography)

MRI scan demonstrates disc anatomy. Findings such as hydration status, disc height, changes in adjacent vertebral body or endplates, the presence of high intensity zones, and disc herniations are all visible on MRI. However, perhaps except for high intensity zones, findings on MRI do not reliably indicate whether a disc is a source of pain. Many investigators and clinicians believe there is sufficient published evidence to suggest that discography can help identify a painful disc.[11-13] However, others feel discography is unreliable and extremely difficult to interpret.[14] It is clear that discography must be interpreted in light of the history, physical examination, psychological evaluation and status of the patient, radiological testing, and other diagnostic injections.

Provocation disc injection is based on the theory that during disc injection, a disc that is causing a patient's pain should reproduce concordant pain and, if it does not, that disc is not the pain generator. In addition, injection of adjacent discs should not be painful. In addition, in order to improve diagnostic accuracy, pressure manometry has been suggested. A disc that is painful at low pressure is more likely to be a true pain generator. The results of discography in patients with FBSS may be particularly hard to interpret because patients frequently have conditions that have been associated with false positives such as longstanding pain, psychological distress, and dorsal horn sensitization. Discography is described in detail elsewhere in this text.

TREATMENTS

There is a spectrum of treatments for FBSS that ranges from manual therapy, exercise, and medication through interventional pain management and repeat surgery (Table 74.4). Treatment of an individual patient should be based on the published evidence integrated with the physician's clinical expertise and each patient's values and circumstances. It must be recognized that just as pain management is not necessarily a failure of spine surgery, neither is corrective spine surgery a failure of pain management. Some patients with FBSS are most appropriately treated with medications, radiofrequency neurotomy (RFN), or spinal cord stimulation, but for others the best treatment might be a properly performed repeat surgery.

Nonspecific Treatments

Rehabilitation

Rehabilitation is often the first line of treatment for patients with FBSS. In most publications, the specific spinal disorders have not been reported but, interestingly, that does not seem to matter. There is a wide variety of program type, intensity, and duration.

TABLE 74.4

TREATMENT OPTIONS FOR THE STRUCTURAL CAUSES OF FBSS

Problem	Preferred treatment	Other options	Comment
Foraminal stenosis	• Decompression	• TFE • ? gabapentin	
Recurrent HNP	• Discectomy for radiculopathy	• Functional restoration may equal surgery	• Fusion if surgery needed for primary axial LBP
Painful disc	• Severe pain: fusion; • Moderate pain: rehab = fusion	• Opioid analgesics	• Intradiscal RX not studied in FBSS
Facet joint pain	• RFN		
SIJ pain	• Corticosteroid injections	• Rehabilitation • RFN • Rarely SIJ fusion	• Research re: SIJ RFN not conclusive
Spondylolisthesis	• Fusion	• RFN if facets are source of pain	
Neuropathic pain	• Medications	• SCS	
Psychological	• Cognitive-behavioral functional restoration	• Psychotherapy • Medications	

HNP, disc herniation; RFN, radiofrequency neurotomy; SIJ, sacroiliac joint; SCS, spinal cord stimulation; TFE, transforaminal epidural.

Kernan and Rainville used a 6-week, two sessions per week plus independent exercise physical therapy only program and demonstrated clinically important improvements in pain, OSI, and kinesiophobia.[112] Patients were only modestly impaired at entry. LBP (0–10) improved from 5.8 to 3.7 at discharge and 3.0 at 1 year. OSI improved from 38 to 23 to 19. At the other end of the intensity spectrum, Brox reported outcomes in patients treated for FBSS after discectomy.[100] The program was 25 hours per week for 3 weeks and included cognitive-behavioral therapy and lectures by physicians. At 1 year, LBP (0–100) improved from 65 to 51 and OSI improved from 45 to 32. Smeets et al. compared active physical therapy, cognitive-behavioral therapy without specific exercise but with graduated increases in tasks, a combined program, and waiting list.[88] There were no significant differences among the three treatment groups and all were better than waiting list.

The Cochrane review of randomized controlled studies on the effect of exercise therapy for chronic LBP concluded that "exercises may be helpful for patients with chronic LBP to increase return to normal daily activities and work."[113] Rainville et al. did a narrative review of exercise as treatment for chronic LBP and included case series and cohort studies.[114] There was no literature to suggest exercise increased LBP or caused harm. The large body of evidence they reviewed demonstrated strength training and exercise can improve LBP-related endurance performance and disability in a large proportion of patients. They found reductions in pain of 10% to 50% in most studies. Their work and the work of others confirms that, although there were improvements in strength and endurance, it may be that much of the gains occurred through desensitization of fear, altering attitudes and beliefs about pain, and improving depression.[115] Smeets et al., after their literature review, opined that it is the reactivation caused by the active treatment that is most important, not the physical reconditioning itself.[90] Miller et al. compared the outcomes of chronic LBP and FBSS patients in an interdisciplinary functional restoration program.[116] Both groups did well. The no surgery chronic LBP patients had greater reductions in pain and disability, but the FBSS patients were significantly more improved in strength and endurance measures, activities of daily living, and fear of exercise.

There can be no doubt that exercise is effective treatment that serves both to improve physical impairments and, perhaps equally important, help overcome the catastrophic thinking and fear-avoidance. In patients who have physical and cognitive-behavioral impairments that are mild to moderate, active exercise alone is sufficient. In patients who are more severely disabled, programs that include an educational program that targets negative attitudes and beliefs may be more effective than exercise alone. It may be that the necessary intensity and duration of treatment depend on the degree of impairment and maladaptive cognitive-behavioral factors.

Medications

Medication management of chronic pain is discussed in detail elsewhere in this text. There are no specific studies of the efficacy of medications for patients with FBSS. However, there are multiple studies with high levels of evidence that have demonstrated the efficacy of opioid analgesics for moderate to severe refractory chronic LBP.[117] Many of these studies did contain patients with FBSS.

There has been a systematic review and a meta-analysis on the effect of antidepressants in the treatment of chronic LBP.[118,119] Both concluded that noradrenergic, but not serotonergic, antidepressants provided modest relief of pain, but there was no evidence of improvement in function. Yaksi et al. did a randomized controlled trial of gabapentin in 55 patients with neurogenic claudication due to spinal stenosis. The gabapentin group had improved walking distance, pain, and sensory findings compared to placebo.[120] The anticonvulsant topiramate has been studied in patients with axial LBP and leg pain.[121,122] In a randomized placebo-controlled study of patients with lumbar radiculopathy, topiramate reduced the mean leg score by 19% compared to placebo, which indicated a trend but did not quite reach statistical significance.[121] However, reductions in average back pain score, worst leg pain, and others did reach statistical significance. The number needed to treat was 5.3. In a 10-week randomized controlled trial of topiramate in 96 patients with chronic LBP, Muelbacher et al. found significant improvements in pain, function, and health-related quality of life for topiramate compared to placebo.[122]

Specific Treatments

Discogenic Pain

Discogenic pain, especially in the setting of FBSS, may prove the most difficult to treat among the structural causes of chronic LBP. Only rehabilitation and fusion surgery have been thoroughly evaluated in this setting. For patients with mild to moderate pain after discectomy, a 3-week interdisciplinary functional rehabilitation program has been shown to be equal to fusion surgery.[100] This is consistent with several studies comparing intensive rehabilitation with fusion in mixed populations of idiopathic chronic LBP that included some patients with prior back surgery.[123,124] It appears that most of these studies excluded patients with severe pain and severe functional impairment. Medication management can be useful, but most studies showing efficacy evaluated nonspecific LBP, and were not limited to discogenic pain.

Facet Joint Pain

There is high quality evidence to support the efficacy of properly performed RFN for FJ pain.[125,126] Successful RFN relieves pain to a meaningful degree for about 9 to 12 months.[125] When pain recurs, RFN can be repeated. Repeat RFN is usually successful unless there has been disease progression or technical failure.[127]

Sacroiliac Joint Pain

There are no treatment options that are supported by high levels of evidence, and most of the recommendations are expert opinion or at best case series. Treatment usually begins with rehabilitation, anti-inflammatory drugs and transdermal lidocaine, support belts, and perhaps spinal manipulative therapy. If there is no meaningful improvement, best available evidence would suggest SIJ corticosteroid injection is the next step.[129] The duration of relief after steroid injection varies greatly. Some patients achieve long-lasting relief after one to three injections, but others require several injections each year.[129,130] For patients who do not respond to these treatments, SIJ RFN has been useful in a limited number of patients.[131,132] Finally, for patients with severe and refractory pain, SIJ fusion has been reported to be helpful.[133]

Spinal Stenosis

As previously noted, spinal stenosis may involve the central, lateral, or both canals. Although there are multiple nonrandomized and randomized studies comparing operative with nonoperative care, most of the data regards central stenosis or the type of stenosis was not defined. Lateral canal or foraminal stenosis is far more common than central stenosis in patients with FBSS. Central stenosis can be treated initially with medications, rehabilitation, and epidural corticosteroid injections.[134] Patients who fail with medications and rehabilitation usually do well with surgery.[135–137] The same paradigm seems appropriate for foraminal stenosis. If stenosis is severe and extensive decompression is needed, fusion may be required. For mixed pain syndromes, if decompression is not sufficient, medications and/or spinal cord stimulation may be useful.

Neuropathic Pain

Neuropathic pain is best treated sequentially. Most often medications (anticonvulsants, noradrenergic antidepressants, opioid analgesics) are used first. If there is limited success, spinal cord stimulation (SCS) is often useful. Kumar et al. randomized 100 patients with FBSS and predominant leg pain to receive either SCS plus conventional medical management to medical management alone.[138] The primary outcome measure was 50% reduction in leg pain, which was achieved in 48% of the SCS plus medication group versus only 9% of the medication only group. In addition, the SCS plus medication group had improved low back pain, quality of life, and function as well as greater treatment satisfaction. There were 32% who experienced device-related side effects. There are case series regarding the treatment of cluneal nerve injuries with injections of corticosteroids and with alcohol.[139,140]

Psychological Issues

Psychological illness is treated according to its severity and type. Patients with depression and anxiety disorders may benefit from individual psychotherapy, groups, and medications. Active addictive disease should prompt consultation by a specialist in addiction medicine.

As previously noted, cognitive-behavioral factors can be dominant, especially in the perpetuation of impairment and disability. Treatment of these problems has been discussed as well. It bears repeating that there can be significant improvements in catastrophic thinking, fear, fear-avoidance, and depression by virtue of an active supervised exercise program. The addition of an educational program and directed cognitive-behavior treatment and graduated exposure to those activities perceived by the patient as noxious may improve the outcomes in moderately or severely impaired patients, but may not be necessary in those with lesser degrees of illness.

References

1. Schofferman J, Reynolds J, Dreyfuss P, et al. Failed back surgery: etiology and diagnostic evaluation. *Spine J* 2003;3:400–403.
2. Farrar JT, Young JP, LaMoreaux L, et al. Clinical importance of changes in chronic pain intensity measured on an 11-point numerical pain rating scale. *Pain* 2001;94:149–158.
3. van der Roer N, Ostelo R, Bekkering G, et al. Minimal clinically important change for pain intensity, functional status, and general health status in patient with nonspecific low back pain. *Spine* 2006;31:578–585.
4. Kovacs F, Abraira V, Royuela A, et al. Minimal clinically important change for pain intensity and disability in patients with nonspecific low back pain. *Spine* 2007;32:2915–2920.
5. Guyer R, Patterson M, Ohnmeiss D. Failed back surgery syndrome: diagnostic evaluation. *J Am Acad Orthop Surg* 2006;14:534–543.
6. Bogduk N. Lumbar spinal nerve blocks. In: Bogduk N, ed. *International Spine Intervention Society: Practice Guidelines for Spinal Diagnostic and Treatment Procedures.* San Francisco, CA; 2004:3–19.
7. Slosar P, White A, Wetzel F. The use of selective nerve root blocks: diagnostic, therapeutic, or placebo? *Spine* 1998;20:2253–2256.
8. van Akkerveeken P. The diagnostic value of nerve root sheath infiltration. *Acta Orthop Scand* 1993;64:61–63.
9. Derby R, Kine G, Saal JA, et al. Response to steroid and duration of radicular pain as predictors of surgical outcome. *Spine* 1992;17:S176–183.
10. Derby R, Howard MW, Grant JM, et al. The ability of pressure-controlled discography to predict surgical and nonsurgical outcomes. *Spine* 1999;24:364–372.
11. Bogduk N. Lumbar disc stimulation (provocation discography). In: Bogduk N, ed. *International Spine Intervention Society: Practice Guidelines for Spinal Diagnostic and Treatment Procedures.* San Francisco, CA; 2004:20–46.
12. Bartynski W, Rothfus W. Pain improvement after intradiskal lidocaine administration in provocation lumbar discography: association with diskographic contrast leakage. *Am J Neuroradiol* 2007;28:1259–1265.
13. Wetzel FT, LaRocca H, Lowery GL, et al. The treatment of lumbar spinal pain syndromes diagnosed by discography. Lumbar arthrodesis. *Spine* 1994;19:792–800.
14. Carragee EJ, Alamin TF. Discography: a review. *Spine J* 2001;1:364–372.
15. Block AR, Ohnmeiss DD, Guyer RD, et al. The use of presurgical psychological screening to predict the outcome of spine surgery. *Spine J* 200;1(4):274–282.
16. Dersh J, Mayer T, Theodore B, et al. Do psychiatric disorders first appear preinjury or postinjury in chronic disabling occupational spinal disorders? *Spine* 2007;32:1045–1051.
17. Dersh J, Gatchel R, Mayer T, et al. Prevalence of psychiatric disorders in patients with chronic disabling occupational spinal disorders. *Spine* 2006;31:56–62.

18. Leeuw M, Goossens ME, Linton SJ, et al. The fear-avoidance model of musculoskeletal pain: current state of scientific evidence. *J Behav Med* 2007;30:77–94.
19. Crombez G, Vlaeyen J, Heuts P, et al. Pain-related fear is more disabling than pain itself: evidence on the role of pain-related fear in chronic back pain disability. *Pain* 1999;80:329–339.
20. Mercado A, Carroll L, Cassidy J, et al. Passive coping is a risk factor for disabling neck or low back pain. *Pain* 2005;117:51–57.
21. Hasenbring M, Plaas H, Bischbein B, et al. The relationship between activity and pain in patients 6 months after lumbar disc surgery: do pain-related coping modes act as moderator variables. *Eur J Pain* 2006;10:701–709.
22. Schofferman J, Anderson D, Hines R, et al. Childhood psychological trauma correlates with unsuccessful spine surgery. *Spine* 1992;17:S138–S144.
23. Schofferman J, Hines R, Anderson D, et al. Childhood psychological trauma and chronic refractory low back pain. *Clin J Pain* 1993;9:260–265.
24. Alanay A, Vyas R, Shamie AN, et al. Safety and efficacy of implant removal for patients with recurrent back pain after a failed degenerative lumbar spine surgery. *J Spinal Disord Tech* 2007;271–277.
25. Herzog RJ, Marcotte PJ. Assessment of spinal fusion. Critical evaluation of imaging techniques. *Spine* 1996;21:1114–1118.
26. Bolt P, Wahl M, Schofferman J. The roles of the hip, spine, sacroiliac joint and other structures in patients with persistent pain after back surgery. *Semin Spine Surg*. In press
27. Brown MD, Gomez–Marin O, Brookfield KF, et al. Differential diagnosis of hip disease versus spine disease. *Clin Orthop Relat Res* 2004;419:280–284.
28. Saal J, Dillingham M, Gamburd R, et al. The pseudoradicular syndrome. Lower extremity peripheral nerve entrapment masquerading as lumbar radiculopathy. *Spine* 1988;13:926–930.
29. Harney D, Patijn J. Meralgia paresthetica: diagnosis and management strategies. *Pain Med* 2007;8:669–677.
30. Tortolani P, Carbone J, Quartararo L. Greater trochanteric pain syndrome in patients referred to orthopedic spine specialists. *Spine J* 2002;2:251–254.
31. Filler A, Haynes J, Jordan S, et al. Sciatica of nondisc origin and piriformis syndrome: diagnosis by magnetic resonance neurography and interventional magnetic resonance imaging with outcome study of resulting treatment. *J Neurosurg Spine* 2005;2:99–115.
32. Fardon D. Letter to the editor. *Spine J* 2003;3:251.
33. Tortolani P, Carbone J, Quartararo L. Response to letter to the editor. *Spine J* 2003;3:251–252.
34. Cohen S, Narvaez J, Lebovigts A, et al. Corticosteroid injections for trochanteric bursitis: is fluoroscopy necessary? A pilot study. *Br J Anaesth* 2005;94:100–106.
35. Windisch G, Braun E, Anderhuber F. Piriformis muscle: clinical anatomy and consideration of the piriformis syndrome. *Surg Radiol Anat* 2007;29:37–45.
36. Lewis A, Layzer R, Engstrom J, et al. Magnetic resonance neurography in extraspinal sciatica. *Arch Neurol* 2006;63:1469–1472.
37. Burton C, Kirkaldy–Willis W, Yong–Hing K, et al. Causes of failure of surgery on the lumbar spine. *Clin Orthop* 1981;157:191–199.
38. Etiology of long-term failures of lumbar spine surgery. *Pain Medicine* 2002;3:18–22.
39. Slipman CW, Shin CH, Patel RK, et al. Etiologies of failed back surgery syndrome. *Pain Medicine* 2002;200–214.
40. Fritsch EW, Heisel J, Rupp S. The failed back surgery syndrome. Reasons, intraoperative findings, and long-term results: a report of 182 operative treatments. *Spine* 1996;21:626–633.
41. Kostuik JP. The surgical treatment of failures of laminectomy. *Spine* 1997;11:509–538.
42. Fardon DF, Herzog RJ, Mink JH, et al. Contemporary concepts in spine care. Nomenclature of lumbar disc disorders. North American Spine Society; 1995.
43. Merskey H, Bogduk N. *Classification of Chronic Pain*. 2nd ed. Seattle: IASP Press; 1994.
44. Park P, Garton HJ, Gala VC, et al. Adjacent segment disease after lumbar or lumbosacral fusion: review of the literature. *Spine* 2004;29(17):1938–1944.
45. Hilibrand AS, Robbins M. Adjacent segment degeneration and adjacent segment the consequences of spinal fusion? *Spine J* 2004;4(suppl):190–194.
46. Weatherly CR, Prickett CF, O'Brien JP. Discogenic pain persisting despite solid posterior fusion. *J Bone Joint Surg Br* 1986;668:142–143.
47. Barrick W, Schofferman J, Reynolds J, et al. Anterior fusion improves discogenic pain at levels of prior posterolateral fusion. *Spine* 2000;25:853–857.
48. Freemont A, Peacock T, Goupille P, Hoyland J, et al. Nerve ingrowth into diseased intervertebral discs in chronic low back pain. *Lancet* 1997;350:178–181.
49. Coppes M, Marani E, Thomeer R, et al. Innervation of "painful" lumbar discs. *Spine* 1997;22:2342–2350.
50. Edgar M. The nerve supply of the lumbar intervertebral disc. *J Bone Joint Surg [Br]*. 2007;1135–1139.
51. Schwarzer A, Aprill C, Derby R, et al. The prevalence and clinical features of internal disc disruption in patients with chronic low back pain. *Spine* 1995;20:1878–1883.
52. Young S, Aprill C, Laslett M. Correlation of clinical examination characteristics with three sources of chronic low back pain. *Spine J* 2003;3:460–465.
53. Hancock M, Maher C, Latimer J, et al. Systematic review of tests to identify the disc, SIJ or facet joint as the source of low back pain. *Eur Spine J* 2007;16:1539–1550.
54. Boden S, Davis D, Dina T, et al. Abnormal magnetic-resonance scans of the lumbar spine in asymptomatic subjects. *J Bone Joint Surg* 1990;72:403–408.

55. Jensen M, Brant–Zawadzki, Obuchowski N, et al. Magnetic resonance imaging of the lumbar spine in people without back pain. *N Engl J Med* 1994;331:69–73.
56. Schwarzer AC, Aprill CN, Derby R, et al. Clinical features of patients with pain stemming from the lumbar zygapophysial joints. Is the lumbar facet syndrome a clinical entity? *Spine* 1994;19:1132–1137.
57. Manchikanti L, Manchukonda R, Pampati V, et al. Prevalence of facet joint pain in chronic low back pain in postsurgical patients by controlled comparative local anesthetic blocks. *Arch Phys Med Rehabil* 2007;88:449–455.
58. Manchukonda R, Manchikanti K, Cash I, et al. Facet joint pain in chronic spinal pain: an evaluation of prevalence and false-positive rate of diagnostic blocks. *J Spinal Disord Tech* 2007;20:539–545.
59. Shah RR, Mohammed S, Saifuddin A, et al. Radiologic evaluation of adjacent superior segment facet joint violation following transpedicular instrumentation of the lumbar spine. *Spine* 2003;28:272–275.
60. Moshirfar A, Jenis LG, Spector LR, et al. Computed tomography evaluation of superior-segment facet-joint violation after pedicle instrumentation of the lumbar spine with a midline surgical approach. *Spine* 2006;31(22):2624–2629.
61. van Ooij A, Oner F, Verbout A. Complications of artificial disc replacement. *J Spinal Dis Tech* 2003;16:369–383.
62. Shim C, Lee S, Shin H, et al. Charite versus ProDisc. A comparative study of a minimum 3-year follow-up. *Spine* 2007;32:1012–1018.
63. Wong D, Annesser B, Birney T, et al. Incidence of contraindications to total disc arthroplasty: a retrospective review of 100 consecutive fusion patients with a specific analysis of facet arthrosis. *Spine J* 2007;7:5–11.
64. Laslett M, McDonald D, Aprill CN, et al. Clinical predictors of screening lumbar zygapophyseal joint blocks: development of clinical prediction rules. *Spine J* 2006;6(4):370–379.
65. Wilde V, Ford J, McMeeken J. Indicators of lumbar zygapophyseal joint pain: survey of an expert panel with the Delphi technique. *Phys Ther* 2007;87:1348–1361.
66. Bogduk N. Lumbar medial branch blocks. In: Bogduk N, ed. *International Spine Intervention Society: Practice Guidelines for Spinal Diagnostic and Treatment Procedures*. San Francisco, CA; 2004:47–64.
67. Schwarzer A, Aprill C, Bogduk N. The sacroiliac joint in chronic low back pain. *Spine* 1995;20:31–37.
68. Dreyfuss P, Dreyer S, Cole A, et al. Sacroiliac joint pain. *J Am Acad Orthop Surg* 2004;12:255–265.
69. Katz V, Schofferman J, Reynolds J. The sacroiliac joint: a potential cause of pain after lumbar fusion. *J Spinal Disord Tech* 2003;16:96–99.
70. Ebraheim NA, Elgafy H, Semaan HB. Computed tomographic findings in patients with persistent sacroiliac pain after posterior iliac graft harvesting. *Spine* 2000;25:2047–2051.
71. Chou L, Slipman CW, Bhagia SM, et al. Inciting events initiating injection-proven sacroiliac joint syndrome. *Pain Med* 2004;5:26–32.
72. Slipman C, Sterenfeld E, Chou L, et al. The predictive value of provocative sacroiliac joint stress maneuvers in the diagnosis of sacroiliac joint syndrome. *Arch Phys Med Rehab* 1998;79:288–292.
73. Bogduk N. Sacroiliac joint blocks. In: Bogduk N, ed. *International Spine Intervention Society: Practice Guidelines for Spinal Diagnostic and Treatment Procedures*. San Francisco, CA; 2004:66–86.
74. Yamashita K, Ohzono K, Hiroshima K. Five-year outcomes of surgical treatment for degenerative lumbar spinal stenosis. *Spine* 2006;31:1484–1490.
75. Atlas S, Keller R, Wu Y, et al. Long-term outcomes of surgical and nonsurgical management of lumbar spinal stenosis: 8 to 10 year results from the Maine Lumbar spine study. *Spine* 2005;30:936–943.
76. Simotas A, Dorey F, Hansraj K, et al. Nonoperative treatment for lumbar spinal stenosis. *Spine* 2000;25:197–204.
77. Malmivaara A, Statis P, Heliovaaara M, et al. Surgical or nonoperative treatment for lumbar spinal stenosis. A randomized controlled trial. *Spine* 2007;32:1–8.
78. Antonacci M, Eismont F. Neurologic complications after lumbar spine surgery. *J Am Acad Orthop Surg* 2001;9:137–145.
79. Ahlmann E, Patzakis M, Roidis N, et al. Comparison of anterior and posterior iliac crest bone grafts in terms of harvest-site morbidity and functional outcomes. *J Bone Joint Surg* 2002;84:716–720.
80. Campbell J, Meyer R. Mechanisms of neuropathic pain. *Neuron* 2006;52:77–92.
81. Sessle B. Peripheral and central mechanisms of orofacial pain and their clinical correlates. *Minerva Anesthiol* 2005;71:117–136.
82. Coskun E, Süzer T, Topuz O, et al. Relationships between epidural fibrosis, pain, disability, and psychological factors after lumbar disc surgery. *Eur Spine J* 2000;9:218–223.
83. Annertz M, Jonsson B, Stromquist B, et al. No relationship between epidural fibrosis and sciatica in lumbar postdiscectomy syndrome. A study with contrast-enhanced MRI in symptomaic and asymptomatic individuals. *Spine* 1995;20:449–453.
84. Trescot A, Chopra P, Abdi S, et al. Systematic review of effectiveness and complications of adhesiolysis in the management of chronic spinal pain: an update. *Pain Physician* 2007;10:129–146.
85. Verbunt J, Seelen H, Vlaeyen J, et al. Disuse and deconditioning in chronic low back pain: concepts and hypotheses on contributing mechanisms. *Eur J Pain* 2003;7:9–21.
86. Mayer T, Mooney V, Gatchel R, et al. Quantifying postoperative deficits of

physical function following spinal surgery. *Clin Orthop Relat Res* 1989;244: 147–157.

87. Mayer T, Polatin P, Gatchel R. Functional restoration and other rehabilitation approaches to chronic musculoskeletal pain disability syndromes. *Crit Rev Phys Rehabil Med* 1998;10:209–221.

88. Smeets R, Vlaeyen J, Hidding A, et al. Active rehabilitation for chronic low back pain: cognitive-behavioral, physical, or both? First direct post-treatment results from a randomized controlled trial. *BMC Musculoskel Disord* 2006; 7:1–16.

89. Peters M, Vlaeyen J, Weber W. The joint contribution of physical pathology, pain-related fear and catastrophizing to chronic back pain disability. *Pain* 2005;113:45–50.

90. Smeets R, Wade D, Hidding A, et al. The association of physical deconditioning and chronic low back pain: a hypothesis-oriented systematic review. *Disabil Rehabil* 2006;28:673–693.

91. Gille O, Jolivet E, Dousset V, et al. Erector spinae muscle changes on magnetic resonance imaging following lumbar surgery through a posterior approach. *Spine* 2007;32:1236–1241.

92. Gejo R, Matsui H, Kawaguchi Y, et al. Serial changes in trunk muscle performance after posterior lumbar surgery. *Spine* 1999;24:1023–1028.

93. Weber B, Grob D, Dvorak J, et al. Posterior surgical approach to the lumbar spine and its effect on the multifidus muscle. *Spine* 1997;22:1765–1772.

94. Motosuneya T, Asazuma T, Tsuji T, et al. Postoperative change of the cross-sectional area of back musculature after 5 surgical procedures as assessed by magnetic resonance imaging. *J Spinal Disord Tech* 2006;19:318–322.

95. Airaksinen O, Herno A, Kaukanen E, et al. Density of lumbar muscles 4 years after decompressive spinal surgery. *Eur Spine J* 1996;5:193–197.

96. Sihvonen T, Herno A, Paljarvi L, et al. Local denervation atrophy of paraspinal muscles in postoperative failed back syndrome. *Spine* 1993;18:575–581.

97. Hernan T, Rainville J. Observed outcomes associated with a quota-based exercise approach on measures of kinesiophobia in patients with chronic low back pain. *J Orthop Sports Phys Ther* 2007;37:679–687.

98. Smeets R, Wittink H. The deconditioning paradigm for chronic low back pain unmasked? *Pain* 2007:130:201–202.

99. Bousema E, Verbunt J, Seelen H, et al. Disuse and physical deconditioning in the first year after the onset of back pain. *Pain* 2007;130:279–286.

100. Brox J, Reikeras O, Nygaard, et al. Lumbar instrumented fusion compared with a cognitive intervention and exercises in patients with chronic low back pain after previous surgery for disc herniation: a prospective randomized controlled study. *Pain* 2006;122:145–155.

101. Miller B, Gatchel R, Lou L, et al. Interdisciplinary treatment of failed back surgery syndrome (FBSS): A comparison of FBSS and non-FBSS patients. *Pain Pract* 2005;5:190–202.

102. Smeets R, Viaeyen J, Kester A, et al. Reduction of pain catastrophizing mediates the outcome of both physical and cognitive-behavioral treatment in chronic low back pain. *J Pain* 2006;7(4):261–271.

103. Rainville J, Ahern D, Phalen L. Altering beliefs about pain and impairment in a functionally oriented treatment program for chronic low back pain. *Clin J Pain* 1993;9:196–201.

104. Grotle M, Vollestad N, Veirod M, et al. Fear-avoidance beliefs and distress in relation to disability in acute and chronic low back pain. *Pain* 2004;112: 343–352.

105. Heuts P, Vlaeyen J, Roelofs J, et al. Pain-related fear and daily functioning in patients with osteoarthritis. *Pain* 2004;110:228–235.

106. Rainville J, Pransky G, Indahl A, et al. The physician as disability advisor for patients with musculoskeletal complaints. *Spine* 2005;30:2579–2584.

107. Swinkels–Meewisse I, Roelofs J, Verbeek A, et al. Fear of movement/(re)injury, disability and participation in acute low back pain. *Pain* 2003;105: 371–379.

108. Jensen M, Keefe F, Lefebvre J, et al. One- and two-item measures of pain beliefs and coping strategies. *Pain* 2003;104:453–469.

109. Jensen M, Turner J, Romano J. Changes after multidisciplinary pain treatment in patient pain beliefs and coping are associated with concurrent changes in patient functioning. *Pain* 2007;131:38–47.

110. Kearns R, Turk D, Rudy T. The West Haven–Yale Multidimensional pain inventory. *Pain* 1985;23:345–356.

111. Kizilkilic O, Yalcin O, Sen O, et al. The role of standing flexion-extension radiographs for spondylolisthesis following single level disk surgery. *Neurol Res* 2007;29:540–543.

112. Kernan T, Rainville J. Observed outcomes associated with a quota-based exercise approach on measures of kinesiophobia in patients with chronic low back pain. *J Orthop Sports Phys Ther* 2007;11:679–687.

113. Van Tulder M, Malmivaara A, Esmail R, et al. Exercise therapy for low back pain. *Spine* 2000;25:2784–2796.

114. Rainville J, Hartigan C, Martinez E, et al. Exercise as a treatment for chronic low back pain. *Spine J* 2004;4:106–115.

115 ainville J, Hartigan C, Jouve C, et al. The influence of intense exercise-based physical therapy program on back pain anticipated before and induced by physical activities. *Spine J* 2004;4:176–183.

116. Miller B, Gatchel R, Lou L, et al. Interdisciplinary treatment of failed back surgery syndrome (FBSS): a comparison of FBSS and non-FBSS patients. *Pain Pract* 2005;5:190–202.

117. Schofferman J, Mazanec D. Evidence-informed management of chronic low back pain with opioid analgesics. *Spine J* 2008;8:185–194.

118. Staiger T, Gaster B, Sullivan M, et al. Systematic review of antidepressants in the treatment of chronic low back pain. *Spine* 2003;28:2540–2545.

119. Salerno S, Browning R, Jackson J. The effect of antidepressant treatment on chronic back pain. *Arch Intern Med* 2002;162:19–24.

120. Yaksi A, Ozgonenel L, Ozgonenel B. The efficacy of gabapentin therapy in patients with lumbar spinal stenosis. *Spine* 2007;32:939–942.

121. Khoromi S, Patsalides A, Parada S, et al. Topiramate in chronic lumbar radicular pain. *J Pain* 2005;6:829–836.

122. Muehlbacher M, Nickel M, Kettler C, et al. Topiramate in treatment of painters with chronic low back pain. A randomized, double-blind, placebo-controlled study. *Clin J Pain* 2006;22:526–531.

123. Mirza S, Deyo R. Systematic review of randomized trials comparing lumbar fusion surgery to nonoperative care for the treatment of chronic low back pain. *Spine* 2007;32:816–823.

124. Fairbank J, Frost H, Wilson–MacDonald J, et al. Randomised controlled trial to compare surgical stabilization of the lumbar spine with an intensive rehabilitation programme for patients with chronic low back pain: the MRC spine stabilization trial. *BMJ* 2005;330:1233–1239.

125. Bogduk N. Percutaneous radiofrequency lumbar medial branch neurotomy. In: Bogduk N, ed. *International Spine Intervention Society: Practice Guidelines for Spinal Diagnostic and Treatment Procedures.* San Francisco, CA; 2004:188–218.

126. Dreyfuss P, Halbrook B, Pauza K, et al. Efficacy and validity of radiofrequency neurotomy for chronic lumbar zygapophysial joint pain. *Spine* 2000;25: 1270–1277.

127. Schofferman J, Kine G. The effectiveness of repeated radiofrequency neurotomy for lumbar facet pain. *Spine* 2004;29:2471–2473.

128. Foley B, Buschbacher R. Sacroiliac joint pain: anatomy, biomechanics, diagnosis and treatment. *Am J Phys Med Rehabil* 2006;85:997–1006.

129. Slipman CW, Lipetz JS, Vresilovic EJ, et al. Fluoroscopically guided therapeutic sacroiliac joint injections for sacroiliac joint syndrome. *Am J Physical Medicine and Rehab* 2001;80:425–432.

130. Hawkins J, Schofferman J. Serial therapeutic sacroiliac joint injections: a practice audit. *Pain Med*. In press.

131. Yin W, Willard F, Carreiro J, Dreyfuss P. Sensory stimulation-guided sacroiliac joint radiofrequency neurotomy: technique based on neuroanatomy of the dorsal sacral plexus. *Spine* 2003;28:2419–2425.

132. Burnham R, Yasui Y. An alternative method of radiofreqency neurotomy of the sacroiliac joint: a pilot study of the effect on pain, function, and satisfaction. *Reg Anesth Pain Med* 2007;32:12–19.

133. Buchowski J, Kebaish K, Sinkov V, et al. Functional and radiographic outcome of sacroiliac arthrodesis for the disorders of the sacroiliac joint. *Spine J* 2005;5:520–528.

134. Simotas A, Dorey F, Hansraj K, et al. Nonoperative treatment for lumbar spinal stenosis. *Spine* 2000;25:197–204.

135. Athiviraham A, Yen D. Is spinal stenosis better treated surgically or nonsurgically? *Clin Orthop Rel Res* 2007;458:90–93.

136. Malmivaara A, Slatis P, Heliovaara M, et al. Surgical or nonoperative treatment for lumbar spinal stenosis. A randomized controlled trial. *Spine* 2007; 32:1–8.

137. Atlas S, Keller R, Wu Y, et al. Long-term outcomes of surgical and nonsurgical management of lumbar spinal stenosis: 8 to 10 year results from the Maine lumbar spine study. *Spine* 2005;30:936–943.

138. Kumar K, Taylor R, Eidabe S, et al. Spinal cord stimulation versus conventional medical management for neuropathic pain: a multicentre randomised controlled trial in patients with failed back surgery syndrome. *Pain* 2007; 132:179–188.

139. Jeong Y, Ahn K, Kim H, et al. The effects of the local steroid injection in the patients with medial superior cluneal nerve entrapments. *J Korean Acad Rehabil Med* 2005;29:276–280.

140. Mahli A, Coskun D, Altun N, et al. Alcohol neurolysis for persistent pain caused by superior cluneal nerves injury after iliac crest bone graft harvesting in orthopedic surgery: report of four cases and review of the literature. *Spine* 2002;27:E478–E481.

CHAPTER 75 ■ PSYCHOLOGICAL SCREENING OF SPINE SURGERY CANDIDATES

ANDREW R. BLOCK

INTRODUCTION

Spine surgery is being used with increasing frequency in the United States. A recent study by the Center for Evaluative Clinical Sciences of Medicare enrollees indicates that the rate of lumbar fusion has increased from 0.3 per 100,000 to 1.1 per 100,000 during the period from 1992 to 2003.[1] By 2003, spending on lumbar fusion equaled $482 million, accounting for 47% of total spine surgery spending. However frequent its use, the outcome of spine surgery is quite variable. Deyo and Mirza,[2] for example, found that 2 years after the surgery there was no significant difference between back pain patients of similar diagnosis who were treated surgically or nonsurgically. This lack of uniform positive response to spine surgery echoes other earlier data. Turner et al., reviewing all published research on spinal fusion, found that only approximately 65% to 75% of all patients achieved satisfactory clinical outcomes.[3] In these studies, poorer outcome was associated with a number of factors, including greater numbers of fused levels and the use of instrumentation.[3] Similarly, Hoffman and colleagues, in a literature review on laminectomy and discectomy, found that the mean success rate of this procedure for relief of spine pain was 67%.[4] The popular media have pounced on these and similar results, which appear to provide support for declarations such as that of *Consumer Reports*[5] identifying back surgery as the number one item in their list of "overused medical tests and treatments."

Such pessimistic appraisals of spine surgeries are contradicted by other data demonstrating that some of these procedures can lead to dramatic improvements in the patients' experience of pain and functional abilities. For example, Malter and colleagues, examining the effectiveness of laminectomy and discectomy in the treatment of spine pain, found that those patients receiving such surgery had significantly greater quality of life at 5 years postoperation than did patients provided conservative care alone.[6] The results of this study also showed that the cost-effectiveness of laminectomy and discectomy exceeded that of the medical treatment for hypertension, as well as that of single artery bypass grafting in coronary heart disease. In similar fashion, the Spine Patient Outcomes Research Trail (SPORT: 7) found that patients who underwent discectomy had significantly less pain, and greater reported functional ability than did patients receiving conservative treatment, at a 2-year follow-up. Hence, a balanced view of spine surgery is that it can be effective, although not universally so.

Failed spine surgery significantly impacts the patient, the physician, the employer, and the third-party payer. The patient, of course, continues to remain disabled, with perhaps even greater pain, increased medication dependence, and more emotional difficulty than prior to the surgery. The pain may be so great, or the surgery so unsuccessful, that reoperation is required, as is the case in 10% of those who undergo laminectomy and discectomy,[4] and 23% of those who undergo spinal fusion.[3]

The patient after failed surgery places many demands on the health care system, often requiring increasing medications and expensive multiple treatments. Patients often feel frustrated and discouraged. The physician may become angry with the patient for not responding to treatment, and the employer is always concerned about his or her obligation to pay compensation to a permanently disabled worker.

Given that spine surgery can be quite effective, and that the implications of failed spine surgeries can be so profound, it becomes critical to determine factors that may lead to poor results from such procedures. Certainly, surgical results can be less than optimal if appropriate diagnostics are not performed, or if less-than-expert surgical techniques are utilized. Improper pre- and postoperative information and treatments may also decrease surgery results. However, a growing body of research indicates that psychosocial factors are among the most significant influences on spine surgery results. For example, DeBerard et al.[8] compared the outcomes of spinal fusion in patients who had been referred for preoperative psychological evaluation (based on surgeon recognition of the presence of psychosocial concerns) versus those who were not referred for such evaluations. The referred patients had much higher medical treatment costs than those who were not referred. Similarly, Trief et al.[9] found that good emotional health, as assessed by the Mental Component Score of the SF-36, was associated with higher levels of physical functioning at 12 months and 24 months post fusion.

The purpose of this chapter is to review the major psychosocial variables that have been shown to be associated with reduced surgery outcomes. These studies demonstrate that *even when surgery is performed correctly, and is based on appropriate diagnostics, patients may fail to achieve satisfactory results due to psychosocial issues.* For a much more comprehensive review see Block et al.[10]

PERSONALITY AND EMOTIONAL FACTORS

Most spine surgery aims to correct an underlying pathological physical condition that would appear to be the source of the pain. Pain, however, is a subjective experience, one which can be assessed only indirectly, through patient self reports, behavioral changes, and utilization of pain medication. As a subjective experience, pain influences and is, in turn, influenced by psychological process such as perception, emotion, and communication. Thus, the pathophysiology underlying pain becomes only the point of initiation for a complex process, the end result of which is the presentation of the patient in the surgeon's office, desperately seeking pain relief.

There are many psychosocial factors tied to pain perception and response, but the largest research focus has been centered on issues of "personality." The American Psychiatric Association defines *personality* as "deeply ingrained patterns of behaviors, which include the way one relates to, perceives and thinks about, the environment and oneself."[1] According to this description, personality can exert wide-ranging influences over both thoughts and actions. These characteristics can determine, for example, whether people typically become depressed, anxious, or angry in response to stress. Personality may also influence one's need to maintain control, to draw attention to himself or herself, or to withdraw and become sullen. More germane to presurgical psychological screening (PPS), personality factors can exert strong influences on perception of the pain, the emotional impact of pain, and the actions one takes to achieve pain relief.

Personality factors can be reliably identified through the use of *objective* psychological tests, such as the Minnesota Multiphasic Personality Inventory, version 2 (MMPI-2). The MMPI-2 has been frequently used in studies attempting to predict outcome following spine surgery. Table 75.1 lists the major studies that have used the MMPI-2 (and its predecessor, the MMPI) with spine surgery patients. The results demonstrate that elevations on several MMPI-2 scales have been found to be associated with poorer surgical outcomes. In examining this table we must recognize that the MMPI-2 not only assesses enduring personality traits, but also more acute emotional reactions. For example, depression, as assessed by the MMPI, may be a reaction to the pain and lifestyle changes engendered by the spine injury or may be more of a chronic feeling state. The results of the MMPI-2 cannot be used to make such a differentiation. However, as is discussed in the following section, the relatively enduring nature of many of the traits displayed on the MMPI-2 may significantly influence the outcome of spine surgery. A number of other more brief, more focused, and less complicated psychometric measures have been studied in connection with spine surgery outcome, and these are reviewed below, in the context of the MMPI-2 scales with which they have some overlap.

Pain Sensitivity

Pain is a sensation primarily arising from the stimulation of nociceptors, specialized sensory neurons indicating tissue damage, or the potential for damage. However, if the subjective experience of pain was directly tied to tissue damage, then there would be a perfect correlation between nociceptor output and pain experience. Obviously, this is not the case, and there is a large body of research demonstrating that certain chronic pain patients report higher levels of pain than expected on the basis of identifiable physical pathology, a phenomenon termed excessive *pain sensitivity*. For example, patients with functional gastrointestinal pain syndromes may be hypersensitive to pain signals arising from the gut. Using balloon distension of the esophagus in patients with noncardiac chest pain, Barish and colleagues found that distension caused pain in 56% of patients compared with 20% of normal controls.[12] Similarly, Coffin and colleagues reported that patients with nonulcer dyspepsia showed greater sensitivity to balloon distension of the stomach than did normal subjects.[13] Fibromyalgia patients, too, have been shown to be more pain sensitive than normal subjects to pressure, noxious heat, and electrical impulses.[14] Finally, Schmidt and Brands reported that

TABLE 75.1

STUDIES EXAMINING THE RELATIONSHIP OF MINNESOTA MULTIPHASIC PERSONALITY INVENTORY TO SPINE SURGERY OUTCOME

Authors	Subjects	Evaluation interval	Minnesota Multiphasic Personality Inventory results
Cashion and Lynch (1979)	78 laminectomy patients, no previous surgery	1 yr	Significant differences between good and bad outcome scales Hs, D, K, F, Es
Doxey et al. (1982), Dzioba and Doxey (1984)	116 workers' compensation patients, no previous surgery; 74 received surgery, 43 not	1 yr	Hs, Ma, Pt higher in poor outcome patients
Kuperman et al. (1979)	37 discectomy patients, no previous surgery	1 yr	Hs, Hy, D, significant r^2 with outcome; r^2 of Hs + Hy + D with outcome = .58
Long (1981)	44 surgery patients, referred because of suspected nonorganic factors	6–18 mo postoperatively	Hy, Hs, Pd higher in poor outcome group
Pheasant et al. (1979)	90 patients, various procedures	6 mo, 1 yr	Hs, Hy higher in poor outcome group
Riley et al. (1996)	71 fusion patients, 30% previous surgery, 37% workers' compensation	Average 20 mo postoperatively	Cluster analysis: poorest outcome in patients with high Hs + Hy, and "depressed-pathological"
Smith and Duerksen (1979)	31 patients, various procedures, 3 previous surgery	Unclear	Hs, Hy, D significant r^2 with outcome
Sorenson and Mors (1988)	57 discectomy patients, no previous surgery	6, 24 mo postoperatively	r^2 with poor outcome: Hs = .37, D = 0.37, Hy = 0.47; also Sc, Ma
Spengler et al. (1990)	84 discectomy patients, no previous surgery	1 yr or more	Hs + Hy significantly associated with poor outcome; also Pd, Sc
Turner et al. (1986); Uomoto et al. (1988)	106 discectomy patients, 25 previous surgery	1 yr	Discriminative function using Minnesota Multiphasic Personality Inventory predicted 69.7% of outcome, function including Hs, K, L
Wiltse and Rocchio (1975)	130 chemonucleolysis patients, no previous surgery	1 yr	Success predicted by Hs + Hy, not predicted by physical findings

D, depression; Es, ego strength; Hs, hypochondriasis; Hy, hysteria; L, lie; Ma, hypomania; Pd, psychopathic deviate; Pt, psychasthenia; Sc, schizophrenia.

chronic low back pain patients were extremely sensitive to a cold pressor test (immersion of the forearm into an ice water bath), reporting higher pain levels and tolerating the ice water for a shorter period of time than did a control, nonpatient group.[15]

These studies by Barrish et al. and Coffin et al. demonstrate that patients with various clinical syndromes can display heightened pain sensitivity to controlled stimulation of tissues associated with their pain syndromes. In the field of spine pain it is much more difficult to stimulate nociceptors in a controlled fashion. There is, however, one medical test frequently used in diagnosing intervertebral disc problems that does provide for such a demonstration. This procedure, termed discography, involves injection of radiographic dye into the nucleus of a putatively disrupted disc. The injection, performed under fluoroscopy and combined with postdiscogram CT, gives evidence of the presence and extent of disc disruption. The most interesting feature of this test, as far as the present discussion is concerned, is that the injection of a disrupted disc has been demonstrated to act as a stimulus that provokes pain, often with a pattern and intensity similar to the patient's normally occurring pain. For example, Vanharanta et al.[16] found that injection of moderately to severely disrupted discs provoked pain which was similar or an exact reproduction of normally occurring pain in approximately 65% of cases. On the other hand, injection into normal-appearing discs provoked exact or similar reproduction of pain in only 18% of cases. Even stronger results along the same lines were obtained by Walsh et al.[17] Thus, discography may provide a laboratory for providing controlled stimulation of the disc in order to assess whether certain patients with low back pain display heightened pain sensitivity.

We[18] have administered the MMPI-2 to low back pain surgical candidates undergoing three-level lumbar discography, a procedure which frequently provides for a "control level," that is, injection into a nondisrupted disc. Such a test should lead to pain reproduction upon injection of disrupted discs and no pain response on injection of a normal disc, in the same subject. However, we found that many patients had at least one "false positive" pain report—that is, reproduction of pain upon injection of a normal disc level. Results showed that hypochondriasis (Hs) and hysteria (Hy) elevations were associated with false-positive reports of pain. In fact, 75% of patients with elevated Hs scores displayed at least one level with such a false positive (compared to a false-positive rate of 30% in patients no having elevated Hs scores). Interestingly, the majority of patients who had such false-positive pain reports at one disc level also had concordant pain reports (i.e., pain reproduction on injection of an abnormal or disrupted disc) at another level. Thus, these results demonstrate that excessive pain sensitivity significantly influences pain perception even in patients with objectively identifiable pathophysiology.

Pain sensitivity, as a personality factor, can be assessed by the MMPI-2 Hs and Hy scales.[19] These scales are the ones most commonly elevated in general chronic pain syndromes and in spine surgery candidates.[20] The major difference between the two scales is that Hy, in addition to pain sensitivity, measures a tendency to deny psychological and emotional problems, as well as to minimize discomfort experienced in social situations. There is a strong correlation ($r = .53$) between the two scales, and thus they are often both elevated at about the same level. Most studies examining the value of the MMPI-2 in predicting spine surgery outcome have found at least one, if not both, of the scales Hs and Hy to strongly predict poor surgical outcome (see Table 76.1). In some studies, the predictive value of these two scales far exceeds that of medical diagnostic tests, such as radiography, CT scans, or neurologic signs.[22] Such results parallel those in other chronic pain syndromes, finding that Hs and Hy elevations predict poor treatment outcome for syndromes as diverse as temporomandibular joint dysfunction, gastrointestinal disorder, and nonsurgical back pain.[23–25]

Anger

Patients with chronic pain are often filled with anger. They are frequently mad about past medical treatment, the ways they have been treated by employers, and the fact they people they considered friends now avoid them. Anger is often seen by the physician, and is frequently the impetus for a referral for PPS. A study by Fernandez and Milburn demonstrates just how frequently patients experience this emotion. These researchers asked chronic pain patients to endorse the intensity of 10 different emotions they were experiencing and found that anger was given the highest ratings of all emotions assessed.[26]

Anger as a personality trait is assessed by the psychopathic deviate (Pd) scale of the MMPI, which also evaluates rebelliousness toward authority and aggressiveness.[19] Elevations on the Pd scale have been found in at least five studies to be associated with poor surgical outcome.[21,27–30] There are numerous reasons why anger may have a negative impact on reduction of pain. First, anger may lead to maladaptive lifestyle changes, such as poor health habits, lack of physical exercise, or excessive use of drugs or alcohol.[31] Such maladaptive behaviors may have a negative impact on the patient's commitment to postoperative rehabilitation. Furthermore, anger has been shown to have an adverse effect on many health conditions, such as cardiovascular disease, headaches, asthma, and many others.[32,33] Such adverse effects may be mediated by excessive activation of sympathetic nervous system efferents or changes in the immune system, perhaps influencing the healing process.[32] Finally, a fascinating series of studies by Burns[34] demonstrates that anger may increase pain sensitivity in chronic low back pain patients, by increasing muscle tension near the site of the injury.

Of course, anger may have effects not just on the experience of pain, but also on its meaning and expression. Anger often leads to the desire for vindication or revenge, and certainly this can influence treatment results. DeGood and Kiernan have found chronic pain patients who are angry and blame their employer for their injuries report high levels of emotional distress and have poorer response to treatment.[35] It may be that for patients who experience intense anger, continued postsurgical pain reports may be tied more closely to the feelings that they have toward those they perceived have wronged them than to any improvement in the pathophysiological basis of the pain.

Clinical Depression

Many chronic pain patients experience some level of depression. For up to 85%, the intensity of this emotional experience is sufficient to meet the diagnostic criteria for clinical depression.[30] Depressive symptoms include depressed mood, diminished interest in almost all activities, weight loss or gain, insomnia or hypersomnia, agitation or psychomotor retardation, fatigue or energy loss, feelings of worthlessness or guilt, impaired concentration, and recurrent thoughts of death.[11] Depression can be assessed by scale D of the MMPI. Elevations on scale D are found in most studies to be associated with poor outcome of elective spine surgery,[27,28,30] although in several studies no relationship was reported.[21,36–38]

Several other studies have assessed depression using different instruments and found that it can be predictive of reduced spine surgery results. Kjelby-Wendt, Styf, and Carlsson[39] examining discectomy results found that patient satisfaction with surgery was strongly related to elevated scores on the Beck Depression Inventory—in fact, elevated scores were found in 55% of dissatisfied patients but in only 18% of satisfied patients. Schade et al.[40] found that depression, as assessed on a simple Likert-type scale, had strong negative correlations with return to work and overall recovery. Trief et al.[41] found that high scores on the Zung depression inventory were associated with little reduction in back pain and elevated work disability after spine surgery. Finally, DeBerard et al.[42] found that depression, assessed using the DSM-IV criteria, was strongly related to total medical costs in workers' compensation patients undergoing spinal fusion.

Chronic pain patients who are depressed may fail to respond well to spine surgery for a number of reasons. First, individuals with depression have been found to be more likely to focus on negative rather than positive events.[43] Kremer and colleagues[44] demonstrated that such tendencies can affect the chronic pain patient's perception of the improvements in function that result from treatment. In this study, activity levels of patients undergoing interdisciplinary rehabilitation were unobtrusively observed by trained staff members. Patients also recorded their own activity levels on an hourly basis. Although all patients demonstrated objective improvement in activity levels as a result of treatment, those who were depressed tended to underreport their improvements. Thus, depressed patients who undergo spine surgery may also fail to see the gains they have made.

Depression may affect the patient's viewpoint about the surgery. It is clear from research that chronic pain patients tend to have negative cognitions about their health.[45] It is not a great leap, therefore, to assume that depressed patients might experience pessimism about any treatment, including surgery. This is of great significance as den Boer et al.[46] found that negative outcome expectations for lumbar disc surgery were associated with elevated disability and elevated pain at 6 weeks and 6 months postoperatively.

Finally, depression has also been shown to be associated with a low threshold for induced pain.[47] Perhaps the depressed surgical patient may be focused on the body and hypervigilant for pain even if its pathophysiological basis has been corrected and the nociceptive stimulation greatly reduced.

In examining depression, one must consider whether the symptoms predate the back injury or are of relatively recent onset. For many patients, depression may be a personality style or a chronic emotional condition (i.e., dysthymia). For others, depressive symptoms, such as decreased concentration, sleep disturbance, and weight change, may be a direct result of the experience of protracted pain or disability.[48] Chronically depressed patients may respond more poorly to any surgical procedure aimed at pain relief compared with those patients whose depression is reactive to their medical condition and symptoms. Surgical recovery in more acutely depressed patients may actually be facilitated if clinical depression is adequately treated, through a combination of antidepressant medication and short-term psychotherapy. The improvement in depressive symptoms, including a likely decrease in pain sensitivity, may lead the patient to feel relieved by surgery beyond the correction of pathological changes in the spine.

Anxiety and Fear

Chronic back pain engenders many difficulties for the patient. Often patients are quite anxious, worrying about paying their bills and fearing that they will lose their jobs. They may be concerned about the many changes in family interaction caused by pain and limitations. Most of all, the spine surgery candidate has to face uncertainty about improvement in pain and functional ability. Such fears and worries, combined with more chronic tendencies toward emotional distress, obsessions, and compulsions, are assessed by the MMPI-2 psychasthenia (Pt) scale. Patients with Pt elevations tend to be stubborn, rigid, and self-critical.[11] In four studies, Pt elevations have been found to be associated with adverse outcomes of spine surgery (see Table 76.1).

As with the other major emotional/personality issues, the relationship of anxiety to surgical outcome has been assessed using devices other than the MMPI. Trief et al.[49] found that patients with elevated state anxiety scores on the State Trait Anxiety Inventory (STAI) achieved less pain relief and lower return to work

rates after surgery than did patients with lower anxiety. One particularly troublesome type of anxiety centers on the belief that increasing function and activity may increase the likelihood of re-injury. This type of fear measure has been assessed by several questionnaires including the Tampa Scale of Kinesophobia.[50] Den Boer et al.[51] found that elevated scores on the Tampa scale were associated with delayed return to work after lumbar disc surgery. One plausible explanation for this result is that patients with a heightened fear of movement might be less likely to engage in aggressive postoperative rehabilitation.

Anxiety may influence spine surgery outcome for any number of other reasons. First, anxiety may increase awareness of pain, as experimental pain studies have shown that anxiety can reduce the threshold for pain perception as well as pain tolerance. Kiecolt-Glaser et al.[52] have suggested that anxiety/fear may diminish surgical results by slowing healing perhaps through reduced production of pro-inflammatory cytokines, such as a interleukin 1. Recently, Starkweather et al.[53] expanded on this notion, finding that patients about to undergo spine surgery, whether discectomy or fusion, are highly stressed and have reduced Natural Killer Cell activity (NCKA). Kiecolt-Glaser et al.[52] also suggest that anxiety may increase postoperative pain, and such increased noxious sensations could then down-regulate immune function, further compromising the surgery healing process. In summary, then, anxiety may reduce surgical outcome by increasing pain sensitivity, slowing the healing process and/or reducing postoperative activity levels.

COGNITIVE FACTORS

A growing body of research is examining the ways in which patients' thoughts and beliefs concerning their pain, independent of personality or emotional factors, can strongly affect treatment outcome.[54,55] Such cognitions and coping strategies have been demonstrated to influence the level of pain experienced by the patient, level of functional ability, and adjustment to the pain and efforts to overcome it.[56-58]

Coping Strategies

Coping strategies may be defined as specific thoughts and behaviors individuals use to manage their pain or their emotional reactions to pain.[57] Coping strategies may affect the patient's level of attentiveness to pain, the ability to persist in the face of pain, and the extent to which the patient feels entitled to be taken care of as a result of the pain. There are a number of questionnaires available to assess pain-related coping strategies, including the Vanderbilt Pain Management Inventory.[57] However, the largest body of research on coping in chronic pain (and the only research directly applied to surgical screening) has used the Coping Strategies Questionnaire (CSQ).[58]

Gross administered the CSQ preoperatively to 50 lumbar laminectomy candidates.[59] Patients who obtained good results from surgery indicated on the CSQ that they felt better able to control the pain and also indicated they were more self-reliant. Other coping strategies assessed by the CSQ, such as hoping and praying and catastrophizing, were associated with poor surgical outcomes. These results are consistent with several other studies demonstrating that more passive coping strategies and perceived lack of pain control tend to be associated with greater pain levels, higher opioid consumption, greater levels of depression, and poorer treatment outcome.[58,60,61] Additional studies on cognitive aspects of pain, using questionnaires other than the CSQ, have identified similar findings. Worse subjective symptoms and poorer treatment outcome are found in chronic pain patients who tend to have negative self-statements, tend to catastrophize (e.g., greatly overestimate the impact of minor negative events), and have strong beliefs that all pain should be avoided.[55,56,62]

Recent research by den Boer et al.[51] provides further support for the strong influence of coping strategies on surgical outcome. In these studies, 336 patients undergoing spine surgery for lumbar radicular syndrome were examined. "Passive Pain Coping" was assessed preoperatively using the Pain-Coping Inventory.[63] Results indicated that passive pain coping, along with negative surgical outcome expectancy, predicted more severe disability and reduced work capacity at 6 months postsurgery. Taken together with the just-cited study by Gross, these results demonstrate that the effectiveness of surgery may be partially mediated by the manner in which the patient thinks about the experience of pain and the strategies he or she has available to cope with the pain.

BEHAVIORAL FACTORS

All the psychosocial factors discussed up to this point are internal to the patient—thoughts, feelings, and personality. Factors external to the patient can also exert profound influences upon recovery from spine surgery. Especially powerful in this regard are the responses of others to the patient's pain. Pain behavior almost always occurs in a social context, communicating to observers that the patient is in distress. Observers, in turn, may react to such behavior with attempts to relieve the patient's pain, help him or her to avoid further problems, or be supportive of limitations in activity. Employers, and even the insurance system, may also inadvertently support pain behaviors through provision of disability benefits or time off of work. Unfortunately, such solicitous responses from others, while well-intentioned, may serve to reinforce or reward pain behaviors, increasing the likelihood that patients will continue to show and experience pain.[64] Failure to alter reinforcement of pain behavior may contribute to prolonged disability after spine surgery and noninvasive treatment of spine injury.

Litigation

Chronic pain often arises from a specific injury—a motor vehicle accident, a fall, lifting an excessively heavy object, etc. In our litigious society the party injured in such situations will often consider suing the person or company perceived as being partially or fully responsible for the injury. The settlement received in such litigation has the potential to act as a reinforcer for the patient's pain complaints and behaviors, as (correctly or incorrectly) the patient may receive advice that greater disability will lead to larger sums received. Kennedy, in a frequently cited quotation about patients involved in litigation, coined the term *compensation neurosis*, "a state of mind born out of fear, kept alive by avarice, stimulated by lawyers, and cured by verdict."[65] Studies of chronic pain patients provide only limited support for the concept of compensation neurosis. Yet, it is clear that cultural and social factors can influence chronic pain behaviors. In countries other than the United States, where litigation for accidents is uncommon, continuing pain from injuries is less common. In Lithuania, where few drivers are covered by insurance, virtually no individuals involved in car accidents report disabling *whiplash* type pain at 1 to 3 years postaccident.[66] In New Zealand, which has a no-fault system for work-related injuries, workers experience less intense pain and have fewer emotional and behavioral difficulties than do injured workers in the United States.[67] Thus, patients who are in litigation do appear to have greater pain complaints and levels of disability than do nonlitigating patients.

However, when an examination is made of the effects of litigation on treatment outcome, the results are complex. Schofferman and Wasserman found that low back and neck pain patients improved despite litigation.[68] Norris and Watt found no statistically significant changes in the symptoms of litigating patients after their claims were settled.[69] For conservative pain management it appears that, while litigating patients may have significantly increased pain complaints, for most claimants, disability from injury does not resolve following the settlement of litigation.[70]

Despite the previously mentioned results, it appears that litigation surrounding an injury can exert greater influence on spine surgery outcome than on the conservative treatment of pain. LaCaille et al.[71] found that total compensation costs for lumbar fusion patients who had attorneys averaged $41,657 versus $24,837 for those without lawyers, even though there was no correlation between total compensation cost and the likelihood of achieving successful fusion. Finneson and Cooper[72] found that both "history of law suits for medicolegal problems" and "secondary gain" predicted negative results of disc surgery, a result corroborated by Manniche et al.[73] Junge et al. found that Swiss patients who were applying for disability pensions had poorer discectomy outcomes than did nonapplicants.[74] Such results do not mean that litigation patients are making up their symptoms (i.e., malingering), because surgical candidates do have a pathophysiological basis for the pain. Furthermore, an often-cited survey of orthopedic and neurosurgeons by Leavitt and Sweet found that malingering occurred in less than 5% of patients.[75] However, the results with litigating surgical patients imply that, in some cases, reinforcement of pain in the form of anticipated financial gains may increase sensitivity to pain, making patients "somatically hypervigilant"[76] and less responsive to treatment.

Workers' Compensation and Disability Payments

Another source of potential reinforcement for pain comes in the form of workers' compensation and other disability payments to those injured on the job. Such payments often begin at the time of injury and continue until the patient has been declared to have reached *maximum medical improvement*. A number of studies have shown that spine surgery outcome is reduced in patients receiving workers' compensation payments.[77–79] Hudgins, for example, examining patients 1 year postlaminectomy, found that those receiving workers' compensation were the least likely to be working and to report pain relief.[80] Klekamp, McCartty, and Spengler[81] found that 81% of patients obtained a good result from lumbar discectomy, compared to a success rate of 29% of litigating workers' compensation patients. Similarly, Trief et al.[82] found that receiving disability funds was negatively associated with return to work and improvement in work-leisure functions at 12 months postoperatively.

Poor treatment results among workers' compensation patients may not arise solely from economic considerations. Rather, workers' compensation patients have a number of additional issues that may lead to reports of high pain levels and poor treatment outcome. First, these patients have frequently been unable to work for extended periods at the time of surgery. Research on chronic pain has clearly shown that the length of time a patient has been nonfunctional strongly influences treatment outcome. Dworkin et al., using multiple regression to examine the relationships among compensation, litigation, and employment status (time off work) in 454 patients undergoing treatment for chronic pain, found that only time off work (and not workers' compensation or litigation) predicted treatment outcome.[83] In similar and even more dramatic fashion Anderson et al.[84] found that patients who were working up to the time that they went in for anterior lumbar interbody fusion were 10.5 times more likely to have returned to work by 1 year postoperative than were individuals who had not been working prior to surgery. Interestingly, this association was independent of workers' compensation status, and number of levels treated.

Responses to treatment by patients receiving workers' compensation may be influenced by a number of other job and workplace factors such as job dissatisfaction,[85] heavy physical job demands,[51,74,77] and high levels of anger or blame toward the employer.[35] Regardless of the cause, workers' compensation is so widely recognized as a risk factor that Frymoyer and Cats-Baril have proposed that *compensability* is one of the strongest predictors of excessive disability among back injury patients.[86] Thus, compensation status should be noted as a strong potential risk factor for poor outcome following surgery, especially if the patient is not working up to the date of the surgery. We should be cautious, however, in noting that compensation is a *relative risk* factor and may not be predictive of treatment response in any particular case. Rather, it should be included as one factor along with others described throughout this chapter (see Table 76.3).

Spousal Reinforcement of Pain Behavior

Chronic pain has a profound effect on those closest to the patient. Family income and family roles often change as a result of the pain. Spouses may become confused or depressed themselves in response to all these lifestyle alterations. A number of studies have shown that pain-reinforcing responses by the spouse can exert a strong influence on patients' pain behaviors. Such reinforcing actions might include taking over the patient's jobs or responsibilities, giving the patient medication, and encouraging rest while discouraging activity. Family members may be more likely to pay attention to the patient when the pain appears greatest and to ignore the patient at other times, such as when Block and colleagues, for example, found that patients who receive a high level of attention or solicitous responses from their spouses were more likely to report high pain levels in the spouses' presence than were patients with nonsolicitous spouses.[87] Lousberg and colleagues extended this result, finding that patients with solicitous spouses showed decreased physical exertion on treadmill performance in the presence of the spouse.[88] Similar results have been obtained in a number of other studies.[89,90] By extension, it would appear that spousal solicitousness may have a negative impact on surgical recovery and should be assessed prior to surgery, by measures such as the West Haven-Yale Multidimensional Pain Inventory.[91]

Why should some spouses, who profoundly desire that the patient get better, provide reinforcement for pain complaints and pain behavior? The explanation may rest on the finding that certain spouses experience strong empathy with the patient, experiencing an increase in their own arousal level when the patient appears to be experiencing pain.[92,93] Such physiological and cognitive responses to pain displays may motivate the spouse to behave toward the patient in a solicitous fashion, unwittingly reinforcing pain behavior.

Family members may provide emotional disincentives for improvement in another way. Numerous studies have demonstrated that marital distress is high among chronic pain patients.[94,95] We have shown that dissatisfied spouses have more negative outcome expectations for the patient and tend to attribute the patient's pain to psychological causes.[96] It is likely that spouses who are dissatisfied would be less supportive of the patient. Social support, particularly from the spouse, has been found to be an important influence on compliance with medical treatment recommendations[97] and recovery from invasive surgery, such as hip replacement.[98] Thus, patients who report high levels of marital distress, or have unstable or unsupportive marital relationships, may have a poorer surgical prognosis. Marital dissatisfaction should be assessed in the surgical candidate, using measures such as the Locke-Wallace Marital Adjustment Inventory, which focuses on marital satisfaction.[99]

HISTORIC FACTORS

The ways in which individuals respond to and cope with painful spine injuries are strongly influenced by their previous life experiences. Research has demonstrated a number of historic elements in the background of the spine surgery candidate that can negatively impact surgical recovery.

Abandonment and Physical and Sexual Abuse

A disproportionately high number of chronic back pain patients have been the victims of abuse or abandonment as either adults or as children. In one study, more than half of the patients evaluated at a multidisciplinary pain clinic had a history of at least one form of such abuse. In 90% of the cases the abuse occurred during adulthood.[100] These figures are substantially higher than the base rate in the U.S. population.

One unfortunate consequence associated with victimization is that such patients respond poorly to spine surgery. Schofferman and colleagues[101] found an 85% failure rate from spine surgery among patients with a significant history of childhood abuse and abandonment, compared with a 5% failure rate among patients lacking such a traumatic history. A study by Linton[102] suggests that experiences of sexual and physical abuse may predispose individuals, especially women, toward chronic pain, thereby reducing overall spine surgery results. This study surveyed a sample of the general population in Sweden, as well as chronic pain patients, about their history of physical and sexual abuse. All subjects, whether patients or not, were also questioned about any chronic pain symptoms they might have had. Among the female chronic pain patients, 35% had an abuse history. Many of the nonpatient women also reported experiencing chronic pain. For nonpatient women reporting "pronounced pain," frequency of physical abuse was 8% and frequency of sexual abuse was 46%. For the nonpatient women reporting no pain, frequency of physical abuse was 2% and frequency of sexual abuse was 23%. Further analyses of the results determined that the chances of developing chronic pain were increased fivefold by physical abuse and fourfold by sexual abuse. In this study there appeared to be little association of abuse with pain for the men. The above results suggest that for some patients, while surgery may eliminate the physical cause of pain, a history of abuse and the patterns of self-esteem and pain coping such an abhorrent situation engenders may confound the outcomes of surgery.

Premorbid Psychiatric Diagnosis and Emotional Distress

Many chronic pain patients have diagnosable mental health problems. Kinney et al.,[103] for example, found that among those reporting low back pain, 100% with chronic pain and 61% with acute pain had diagnosable psychological conditions. Lower incidence rates were reported by Coste and colleagues.[104] As noted previously in the discussion of depression, psychological problems may predate the injury. For example, Fishbain and colleagues found that 58.4% of the chronic pain patients they studied had diagnosable long-term personality disorders, while Reich and colleagues reported a 37% incidence of such disorders.[105,106] Preexisting psychological problems, whether emotional or personality based, have been found by a number of authors to be associated with poor results from spine surgery.[107,108] It would seem likely that patients with preexisting psychological problems, especially those who have had prior psychiatric treatment, might be less well equipped to deal with the stress and difficulties involved in recovering and rehabilitation following spinal surgery.

Previous Medical Use

Not only is a history of previous psychological treatment associated with poor outcome, but a preinjury history of multiple physical problems also does not bode well for surgical outcome. A number of authors have found that patients who report many illnesses and physical symptoms do not respond well. Frymoyer et al.,[109] for example, found that a history of multiple physical complaints was associated with high levels of back-related disability. Ciol and colleagues[110] reported that higher numbers of previous hospitalizations were associated with greater risk of lumbar spine re-operations in a Medicare population. Wiltse and Rocchio[38] determined that high scores on the Cornell Medical Index, a measure of past illnesses and current bodily symptoms, were associated with poor outcome of chemonucleolysis.

The influence of previous medical problems on surgical outcome appears to parallel results reported earlier in this section noting that excessive pain sensitivity, as assessed by the MMPI-2 Hs and Hy scales, is also a predictor of poor surgical outcome. It appears that patients whose personality and medical history predispose them toward reporting many physical symptoms may have more difficulty experiencing a reduction in back pain and disability as a result of spine surgery, perhaps related to their preoccupation with bodily processes and hypervigilance to noxious sensations.

Substance Abuse

Excessive use and abuse of opioid medication and alcohol appear to be red flags for poor surgical outcome. To the extent that patients depend on such substances, their responsibility for pain relief and improvements in functional ability through participation in postoperative rehabilitation may be diminished. It is clear that many chronic pain patients use excessive amounts of opioids. For example, Polatin and colleagues[108] found that 19% of spine pain patients entering a work-hardening program had a substance abuse history, and even higher rates were reported in other studies. Unfortunately, there is little research addressing the relationship of substance abuse and spine surgery outcome. The only study to directly report such results is that of Spengler and colleagues,[111] who examined 30 of their spine surgery failures and found that 25 were "continually abusing medication and alcohol."

Determining when a patient is abusing drugs or alcohol is not as easy as it might seem. In recent years there has been an increasing acceptance of the use of analgesic substances, including opioids, in patients with chronic pain. A number of studies have demonstrated that chronic opioids provide significant pain relief in chronic pain patients.[112,113] Thus, some surgical candidates may be taking doses of opioids at the time of evaluation, which, just a few years ago, would have been considered unacceptable. One could argue that patients who are denied opioids by their physicians are not necessarily abusing substances when they seek pain relief through street drugs or alcohol. However, the argument is complex, as is exemplified in a research extensive review by Martell et al.[114] This study found that the efficacy of long-term opioid use in reducing chronic pain was no more effective than placebo. Further, the prevalence of lifetime substance abuse in chronic pain patients taking opioid therapy was 36% to 56%, and the current level of substance abuse disorders was 43%. In sum, these studies indicate that substance abuse should only be considered a risk factor if the patient meets DSM-IV criteria for substance abuse, and especially when these medications or alcohol provide inadequate pain relief and do not help to maintain the patients' functional ability.[11]

CONCLUSION

A growing body of research reviewed in this chapter indicates that psychosocial factors can strongly influence spine surgery outcome. These results suggest that PPS should be included as a component of the diagnostic process in many spine surgery candidates. Table 75.2 provides a set of general referral guidelines that a physician can keep in mind when considering the need for PPS. When the surgeon, comparing a patient with other spine surgery candidates he or she has evaluated, judges that the patient displays four or more of these points listed in Table 75.2, a referral for PPS should be initiated. Such a referral is especially critical to the extent that the planned surgery is highly invasive (involving multiple levels, instrumentation, and so forth), is exploratory, involves a reoperation, or when the pain is particularly protracted (greater than 1 year in duration).

The major psychosocial factors contributing to poor surgical outcome are listed in Table 75.3. PPS surgical prognosis is based on the number of these risk factors identified. Research from our laboratory[115] has found that patients with nine or more risk factors are at risk for poor surgical outcome. In our study, 204 spine surgery candidates underwent PPS, using a semistructured interview and psychological testing including the MMPI. Outcome of spine surgery was assessed at approximately 6 months postoperatively. Poor outcome (measured in terms of continued pain greater than 4 on a 10-point scale, continued use of opioid medications, and severe activity restrictions) was obtained in 83% of patients having nine or more risk factors. Poor results were obtained in only approximately 18% of patients with fewer than nine risk factors. Such findings parallel those of other researchers who found, using a similar *scorecard* approach to identifying risk factors, that patients with a high level of overall risk respond poorly to spine surgery.[21,72,74] For a more complete discussion of determination of prognosis, as well as psychological intervention in surgical candidates, see Block.[10]

The results reviewed in this chapter demonstrate that spine surgery may not be very effective when applied to patients having a high level of psychosocial risk. For such patients, more conservative intervention appears more appropriate and effective. Fortunately, a cost-effective alternative to spine surgery exists—the multidisciplinary chronic pain management program (CPMP).

TABLE 75.2

REFERRAL GUIDELINES FOR PRESURGICAL PSYCHOLOGICAL SCREENING

Excessive pain behavior
Symptoms inconsistent with identified pathology
High levels of depression or anxiety
Sleep disturbance: insomnia or hypersomnia
Excessively high or low expectations about surgical outcome
Marital distress or sexual difficulties
Negative attitude toward work or employer
Emotional lability or mood swings
Inability to work or greatly decreased functional ability (<3 mo)
Escalating or large doses of narcotics or anxiolytics
Litigation or continuing disability benefits resulting from spine injury
Referral considerations
   0–1 items: not necessary to refer unless desired by patient
   2–3 items: consider referral for presurgical psychological screening
   4+ items: strongly consider referral for presurgical psychological screening

TABLE 75.3

PRESURGICAL PSYCHOLOGICAL SCREENING RISK FACTORS FOR POOR SURGICAL OUTCOME

Personality Factors (assessed by objective tests, such as the MMPI-2)
  Pain sensitivity
  Anger
  Depression
  Anxiety and obsessions

Poor Coping Strategies (assessed by objective tests)
  Catastrophizing
  Low self-efficacy or pain control

Behavioral Factors
  Spousal reinforcement of pain (West Haven-Yale Multidimensional Pain Inventory)
  Litigation pending
  Workers' compensation
  Blaming employer for injury

Historic Factors
  Abuse and abandonment
  Past psychological treatment
  Multiple previous medical problems
  Substance abuse

Presurgical Psychological Screening Prognosis
  Good: 0–4 risk factors
  Fair: 5–8 risk factors
  Poor: 9–14 risk factors

Such programs teach patients to manage and cope with pain and its impacts, through a combination of physical conditioning, education, psychological treatment, relaxation training, and vocational counseling. Several recent studies have shown that the CPMP approach can be as effective in treating spine pain patients as is spine surgery. Brox et al.[116] studied 64 Swedish patients with evidence of severe disc degeneration lasting more than 1 year. These patients were randomly assigned to undergo either: (1) lumbar fusion with posterior transpedicular screws and postoperative physical therapy; or (2) a modified CPMP involving cognitive-behavioral intervention with three daily physical exercise sessions for 3 weeks. At 1-year follow-up, both groups had significant improvements in function, as measured by the Oswestry Disability Index (ODI), but there was no significant difference in functional improvement between those treated surgically and those treated nonsurgically. In addition, there were no significant differences in pain, use of analgesics, emotional distress, and return to work. Fear-avoidance beliefs were reduced significantly more in the non-surgically treated group.[117] The early complication rate for the surgically treated group was 18%.

Additional support for the use of CPMP has been obtained by Fairbank et al.[118] who examined 349 patients who were uncertain if they should undergo spine surgery. These patients were randomly assigned to spinal fusion or to "intensive rehabilitation"—a CPMP. The surgical group underwent spine stabilization procedures. Subjects were followed for 24 months. The patients treated with spine surgery showed a slightly greater improvement in function as measured by the ODI, but no other comparisons between the two groups reached significance. Intraoperative complications occurred in 19 patients who underwent surgery. An additional study of these same patients[119] found that the cost of CPMP was far less than that for surgery (£4256 vs. £7830), while the percentage of patients returning to work at 2 years' was equivalent.[17] Thus, CPMP was much more cost-effective than spinal fusion. Turk and Burwinkle,[120] in a separate

review of the literature, confirm and extend such findings.[18] They found that the CPMP approach is approximately 26 times more cost-effective in returning patients to work than is spine surgery. The studies comparing CPMPs to spine surgery suggest that, even when medical diagnostics reveal spinal pathology potentially amenable to surgery, many patients may achieve comparable results, with less long-term risk, by undergoing treatment at a CPMP.

In summary, through the use of PPS the surgeon can reduce the costs arising from futile procedures and can help the high-risk patient avoid a downward slide into increasing pain and disability. Based on the PPS, surgeons may decide to (1) refer the patient for treatment at a CPMP; (2) postpone elective surgery until psychosocial factors are addressed; (3) avoid surgery and other treatment altogether; or (4) proceed with surgery but involve psychologists early during rehabilitation. PPS, thus, offers the potential to sharpen patient selection for spine surgery, and tailor treatments to both the patient's physical and psychological needs.

References

1. Weinstein JN, Lurie JD, Olson PR, et al. United States' trends and regional variations in lumbar spine surgery. *Spine* 2006;31:2707–2714.
2. Deyo RA, Mirza SK. Trends and variations in the use of spine surgery. *Clin Orthop Relat Res* 2006;443:139–146.
3. Turner JA, Ersek M, Herron L, et al. Patient outcomes after lumbar spinal fusions. *JAMA* 1992;268:907–911.
4. Hoffman RM, Wheeler KJ, Deyo RA. Surgery for herniated lumbar discs: a literature synthesis. *J Gen Intern Med* 1993;8:487–496.
5. Treatment traps to avoid. *Consumer Reports* November, 2007. Available online at http://www.consumerreports.org/health/doctors-hospitals/medical-ripoffs/overview/medical-ripoffs-ov_1.htm. Accessed March 26, 2009.
6. Malter AD, Larson EB, Urban N, et al. Cost-effectiveness of lumbar discectomy for the treatment of herniated intervertebral disc. *Spine* 1996;21:1048–1055.
7. Weinstein JN, Lurie JD, Tosteson TD, et al. Surgical vs. nonoperative treatment for lumbar disk herniation: the spine patient outcomes research trial (SPORT) observational cohort. *JAMA* 2006;296:2451–2459.
8. DeBerard MS, Masters KS, Colledge AL, et al. Outcomes of posterolateral lumbar fusion in Utah patients receiving worker's compensation. *Spine* 2001;26:738–747.
9. Trief PM, Ploutz-Snyder R, Fredrickson BE. Emotional health predicts pain and function after fusion: a prospective multicenter study. *Spine* 2006;31:823–830.
10. Block AR, Gatchell RJ, Deardorff WW, et al. *The Psychology of Spine Surgery*. Washington, DC: American Psychological Association; 2003.
11. American Psychiatric Association. *Diagnostic and Statistical Manual of Mental Disorders*, 4th ed. Washington, DC: American Psychiatric Association; 1994.
12. Barish CF, Castell DO, Richter JE. Graded esophageal balloon distention: a new provocative test for noncardiac chest pain. *Dig Dis Sci* 1986;31:1292–1298.
13. Coffin B, Azpiroz F, Guarner F, et al. Selective gastric hypersensitivity and reflux hyporeactivity in functional dyspepsia. *Gastroenterology* 1994;107:1345–1351.
14. Lautenbacher S, Rollman GB, McCain GA. Multimethod assessment of experimental and clinical pain in patients with fibromyalgia. *Pain* 1994;59:45–53.
15. Schmidt AJ, Brands AM. Persistence behavior of chronic low back pain patients in an acute pain situation. *J Psychosom Res* 1986;30:339–346.
16. Vanharanta H, Sachs BL, Spivey MA, et al. The relationship of pain provocation to lumbar disc deterioration as seen by CT/Discography. *Spine* 1987;12:295–298.
17. Walsh TR, Weinstein JN, Spratt KF, et al. Lumbar discography in normal subjects. *J Bone Joint Surg* 1990;72:1081–1088.
18. Block AR, Vanharanta H, Ohnmeiss DD, et al. Discographic pain report. Influence of psychological factors. *Spine* 1996;21:334–338.
19. Graham JR. *The MMPI-2: assessing personality and psychopathology*. New York: Oxford University Press; 1990.
20. Keller LS, Butcher JN. *Assessment of Chronic Pain Patients with the MMPI-2 [MMPI-2 Monographs]*. Vol 2. Minneapolis: University of Minnesota Press; 1991.
21. Spengler DM, Ouelette EA, Battié M, et al. Elective discectomy for herniation of a lumbar disc. *J Bone Joint Surg Am* 1990;72:230–237.
22. Schwartz RA, Greene CS, Laskin DM. Personality characteristics of patients with myofascial pain-dysfunction (MPD) syndrome unresponsive to conventional therapy. *J Dent Res* 1979;58:1435–1439.
23. Millstein-Prentky S, Olson R. Predictability of treatment outcome in patients

with myofascial pain-dysfunction (MPD) syndrome. *J Dent Res* 1979;58: 1341–1346.

24. Whitehead WE. Behavioral medicine approaches to gastrointestinal disorders. *J Consult Clin Psychol* 1992;60:605–612.

25. Kleinke CL, Spangler AS Jr. Predicting treatment outcome of chronic back pain patients in a multidisciplinary pain clinic: methodological issues and treatment implications. *Pain* 1988;33:41–48.

26. Fernandez E, Milburn TW. Sensory and affective predictors of overall pain and emotions associated with affective pain. *Clin J Pain* 1994;10:3–9.

27. Herron L, Turner JA, Ersek M, et al. Does the Millon Behavioral Health Inventory (MBHI) predict lumbar laminectomy outcome? A comparison with the Minnesota Multiphasic Personality Inventory (MMPI). *J Spinal Disord* 1992;5:188–192.

28. Dvorak J, Valach L, Fuhrimann P, et al. The outcome of surgery for lumbar disc herniation. II. A 4–17 years' follow-up with emphasis on psychosocial aspects. *Spine* 1988;13:1423–1427.

29. Long CJ. The relationship between surgical outcome and MMPI profiles in chronic pain patients. *J Clin Psychol* 1981;37:744–749.

30. Sørenson LV, Mors O. Presentation of a new MMPI scale to predict outcome after first lumbar diskectomy. *Pain* 1988;34:191–194.

31. Leiker M, Hailey BJ. A link between hostility and disease: poor health habits? *Behav Med* 1988;14:129–133.

32. Williams R, Williams V. *Anger Kills*. New York: HarperCollins; 1994.

33. Friedman HS. *Hostility, Coping, and Health*. Washington, DC: American Psychological Association; 1992.

34. Burns JW. Arousal of negative emotions and symptom-specific reactivity in chronic low back pain patients. *Emotion* 2006;6:309–319.

35. DeGood DE, Kiernan B. Perception of fault in patient with chronic pain. *Pain* 1996;64:153–159.

36. Doxey NC, Dzioba RB, Mitson GL, et al. Predictors of outcome in back surgery candidates. *J Clin Psychol* 1988;44:611–622.

37. Turner JA, Herron L, Weiner P. Utility of the MMPI pain assessment index in predicting outcome after lumbar surgery. *J Clin Psychol* 1986;42:764–769.

38. Wiltse LL, Rocchio PD. Preoperative psychological tests as predictors of success of chemonucleolysis in the treatment of low-back syndrome. *J Bone Joint Surg Am* 1975;75:478–483.

39. Kjelby-Wendt G, Styf J, Carlsson SG. The predictive value of psychometric analysis in patients treated by extirpation of lumbar intervertebral disc herniation. *J Spinal Disord* 1999;12:375–379.

40. Schade V, Semmer N, Main CJ, et al. The impact of clinical, morphological, psychosocial, and work-related factors on the outcome of lumbar discectomy. *Pain* 1999;80:239–249.

41. Trief PM, Ploutz-Snyder R, Fredrickson BE. Emotional health predicts pain and function after fusion: a prospective multicenter study. *Spine* 2006;31: 823–830.

42. DeBerard MS, Masters KS, Colledge AL, Holmes EB. Presurgical biopsychosocial variables predict medical and compensation costs of lumbar fusion in Utah workers' compensation patients. *Spine J* 2003;3:420–429.

43. Seligman MEP. *Helplessness: On Depression, Development, and Death*. San Francisco: WH Freeman; 1975.

44. Kremer EF, Block AR, Atkinson JJ. Assessment of pain behavior: factors that distort self-report. In: Melzack R, ed. *Pain Management and Assessment*. New York: Raven; 1983:165–171.

45. Pincus T, Santos R, Morley S. Depressed cognitions in chronic pain patients are focused on health: evidence from a sentence completion task. *Pain* 2007; 130:84–92.

46. den Boer JJ, Oostendorp RA, Beems T, et al. Continued disability and pain after lumbar disc surgery: the role of cognitive-behavioral factors. *Pain* 2006; 123:45–52.

47. Merskey H. The effect of chronic pain upon the response to noxious stimuli by psychiatric patients. *J Psychosom Res* 1965;9:291–298.

48. Cavanaugh S, Clark DC, Gibbons RD. Diagnosing depression in the hospitalized medically ill. *Psychosomatics* 1983;24:809–815.

49. Trief PM, Ploutz-Snyder R, Fredrickson BE. Emotional health predicts pain and function after fusion: a prospective multicenter study. *Spine* 2006;31: 823–830.

50. Roelofs J, Goubert L, Peters ML, et al. The Tampa Scale for Kinesiophobia: further examination of psychometric properties in patients with chronic low back pain and fibromyalgia. *Eur J Pain* 2004;8:495–502.

51. den Boer JJ, Oostendorp RA, Beems T, et al. Reduced work capacity after lumbar disc surgery: the role of cognitive-behavioral and work-related risk factors. *Pain* 2006;126:72–78.

52. Kiecolt-Glaser JK, Page GG, Marucha PT, et al. Psychological influences on surgical recovery. Perspectives from psychoneuroimmunology. *Am Psychol* 1998;53:1209–1218.

53. Starkweather AR, Witek-Janusek L, Nockels RP, et al. Immune function, pain, and psychological stress in patients undergoing spinal surgery. *Spine* 2006;31:E641–E647.

54. Jensen MP, Turner JA, Romano JM. Self-efficacy and outcome expectancies: relationship to chronic pain coping strategies and adjustment. *Pain* 1991;44: 263–269.

55. Keefe FJ, Brown GK, Wallston KA, et al. Coping with rheumatoid arthritis pain: catastrophizing as a maladaptive strategy. *Pain* 1989;37:51–56.

56. Waddell G, Newton M, Henderson I, et al. A Fear-Avoidance Beliefs Questionnaire (FABQ) and the role of fear-avoidance beliefs in chronic low back pain and disability. *Pain* 1993;52:157–168.

57. Brown GK, Nicassio PM. Development of a questionnaire for the assessment of active and passive coping strategies in chronic pain patients. *Pain* 1987; 31:53–64.

58. Rosensteil AK, Keefe FJ. The use of coping strategies in chronic low back pain patients: relationship to patient characteristics and current adjustment. *Pain* 1983;17:33–44.

59. Gross AR. The effect of coping strategies on the relief of pain following surgical intervention for lower back pain. *Psychosom Med* 1986;48:229–241.

60. Keefe FJ, Dolan E. Pain behavior and pain coping strategies in low back pain and myofascial pain dysfunction syndrome patients. *Pain* 1986;24:49–56.

61. Turner JA, Clancy S. Strategies for coping with chronic low back pain: relationship to pain and disability. *Pain* 1986;24:355–364.

62. Gil KM, Abrams MR, Phillips G, et al. Sickle cell disease pain: relation of coping strategies to adjustment. *J Consult Clin Psychol* 1990;57:725–731.

63. Kraaimaat FW, Evers AW. Pain-coping strategies in chronic pain patients: psychometric characteristics of the pain-coping inventory (PCI). *Int J Behav Med* 2003;10(4);343–363.

64. Fordyce WE. *Behavioral Methods for Chronic Pain and Illness*. St. Louis: Mosby; 1976.

65. Kennedy F. The mind of the injured worker: its affect on disability periods. *Compensation Medicine* 1946;1:19–24.

66. Schrader H, Obelieniene D, Bovim G, et al. Natural evolution of late whiplash syndrome outside the medicolegal context. *Lancet* 1996;347:1207–1211.

67. Carron H, DeGood DE, Tait R. A comparison of low back pain patients in the United States and New Zealand: psychosocial and economic factors affecting severity of disability. *Pain* 1985;21:77–89.

68. Shofferman J, Wasserman S. Successful treatment of low back pain and neck pain after a motor vehicle accident despite litigation. *Spine* 1994;19: 1007–1010.

69. Norris SH, Watt I. The prognosis of neck injuries resulting from rear-end vehicle collisions. *J Bone Joint Surg Br* 1983;65:608–611.

70. Hadjistavropoulos T. Chronic pain on trial: the influence of litigation and compensation on chronic pain syndromes. In: Block AR, Kremer EF, Fernandez E, eds. *Handbook of Pain Syndromes: Biopsychosocial Perspectives*. Mahwah, NJ: Lawrence Erlbaum Associates; 1998.

71. LaCaille RA, DeBerard MS, LaCaille LJ, et al. Obesity and litigation predict workers' compensation costs associated with interbody cage fusion. *Spine J* 2007;7:266–272.

72. Finneson BE, Cooper VR. A lumbar disc surgery predictive score card: a retrospective evaluation. *Spine* 1979;4:141–144.

73. Manniche C, Asmussen KH, Vinterberg H, et al. Analysis of preoperative prognostic factors in first-time surgery for lumbar disc herniation, including Finneson's and modified Spengler's score systems. *Dan Med Bull* 1994;41: 110–115.

74. Junge A, Dvorak J, Ahrens S. Predictors of bad and good outcomes of lumbar disc surgery: a prospective clinical study with recommendations for screening to avoid bad outcomes. *Spine* 1995;20:460–468.

75. Leavitt F, Sweet JJ. Characteristics and frequency of malingering among patients with low back pain. *Pain* 1986;25:357–364.

76. Chapman CR. Pain: the perception of noxious events. In: Sternbach RA, ed. *The Psychology of Pain*. New York: Raven; 1978:169–202.

77. Davis RA. A long-term outcome analysis of 984 surgically treated herniated lumbar discs. *J Neurosurg* 1994;80:414–421.

78. Greenough CG, Fraser RD. The effects of compensation on recovery from low-back injury. *Spine* 1989;14:947–955.

79. Haddad GH. Analysis of 2932 workers' compensation back injury cases. The impact of the cost to the system. *Spine* 1987;12:765–769.

80. Hudgins WR. Laminectomy for treatment of lumbar disc disease. *Tex Med* 1976;72:65–69. *Spine* 1987;12:765–771.

81. Klekamp J, McCarty E, Spengler DM. Results of elective lumbar discectomy for patients involved in the workers' compensation system. *J Spinal Disord* 1998;11;277–282.

82. Trief PM, Grant W, Fredrickson B. A prospective study of psychological predictors of lumbar surgery outcome. *Spine* 2000;25:2626–2631.

83. Dworkin RH, Handlin DS, Richlin DM, et al. Unraveling the effects of compensation, litigation and employment on treatment response in chronic pain. *Pain* 1985;23:49–59.

84. Anderson PA, Schwaegler PE, Cizek D, Leverson G. Work status as a predictor of surgical outcome of discogenic low back pain. *Spine* 2006;31:2510–2515.

85. Bigos SJ, Battié MC, Spengler DM, et al. A prospective study of work perceptions and psychosocial factors affecting the report of back injury. *Spine* 1991; 16:1–6.

86. Frymoyer JW, Cats-Baril WL. An overview of the incidences and cost of low back pain. *Orthop Clin North Am* 1991;22:263–271.

87. Block AR, Kremer EF, Gaylor M. Behavioral treatment of chronic pain: the spouse as a discriminative cue for pain behavior. *Pain* 1980;9:243–252.

88. Lousberg R, Schmidt AJ, Groenman NH. The relationship between spouse solicitousness and pain behavior: searching for more evidence. *Pain* 1992;51: 75–79.

89. Kerns RD, Southwick S, Giller E, et al. The relationship between reports of pain-related social interactions and expressions of pain and affective distress. *Behav Ther* 1991;22:101–111.

90. Romano JM, Turner JA, Jensen MP, et al. Chronic pain patient-spouse interactions predict pain behavior. *Pain* 1995;63:353–360.

91. Kerns RD, Turk DC, Rudy EE. The West Haven-Yale Multidimensional Pain Inventory (WHYMPI). *Pain* 1985;23:345–356.

92. Block AR, Boyer SL. The spouse's adjustment to chronic pain: cognitive and emotional factors. *So Sci Med* 1984;19:1313–1317.

93. Block AR. Investigation of the response of the spouse to chronic pain behavior. *Psychosom Med* 1981;43:415–422.

94. Romano JM, Turner JA, Clancy SL. Sex differences in the relationship of pain patient dysfunction to spouse adjustment. *Pain* 1989;39:289–295.

95. Schwartz L, Slater MA, Birchler GR, et al. Depression in spouses of chronic pain patients: the role of patient pain and anger, and marital satisfaction. *Pain* 1991;44:61–67.

96. Block AR, Boyer SL, Silbert RV. Spouse's perception of the chronic pain patient: estimates of exercise tolerance. In: Fields HL, Dubner R, Cervero F, eds. *Advances in Pain Research and Therapy*. Vol 9. New York: Raven; 1985: 897–904.

97. O'Brien ME. Effective social environment and hemodialysis adaptation: a panel analysis. *J Health Soc Behav* 1980;21:360–370.

98. Mutran EJ, Reitzes DC, Mossey J, et al. Social support, depression, and recovery of walking ability following hip fracture surgery. *J Gerontol B Psychol Sci Soc Sci* 1995;50:S354–S361.

99. Locke JJ, Wallace KM. Short-term marital adjustment and prediction tests: their ability and validity. *J Marriage Fam Ther* 1959;21:251–255.

100. Haber J, Roos C. Effects of spouse abuse and/or sexual abuse in the development and maintenance of chronic pain in women. *Adv Pain Res Ther* 1985; 9:889–895.

101. Schofferman J, Anderson D, Hines R, et al. Childhood psychological trauma correlates with unsuccessful lumbar spine surgery. *Spine* 1992;17(suppl 6): S138–S144.

102. Linton SJ. A population-based study of the relationship between sexual abuse and back pain: establishing a link. *Pain* 1997;73:47–53.

103. Kinney RK, Gatchel RJ, Mayer TG. The SCL-90R evaluated as an alternative to the MMPI for psychological screening of chronic low-back pain patients. *Spine* 1991;16:940–942.

104. Coste J, Paolaggi JB, Spira A. Classification of nonspecific low back pain. I. Psychological involvement in low back pain: a clinical, descriptive approach. *Spine* 1992;17:1028–1037.

105. Fishbain DA, Goldberg M, Meagher BR, et al. Male and female chronic pain patients categorized by DSM-III psychiatric diagnostic criteria. *Pain* 1986;26: 181–197.

106. Reich J, Tupen JP, Abramowitz SI. Psychiatric diagnosis of chronic pain patients. *Am J Psychiatry* 1987;150:471–475.

107. Keel PJ. Psychosocial criteria for patient selection: review of studies and concepts for understanding chronic back pain. *Neurosurgery* 1984;15:935–941.

108. Polatin PB, Kinney RK, Gatchel RJ, et al. Psychiatric illness and chronic low-back pain. The mind and the spine—which goes first? *Spine* 1993;18:66–71.

109. Frymoyer JW, Pope HJ, Clements JH, et al. Risk factors in low back pain. An epidemiological survey. *J Bone Joint Surg Am* 1983;65:213–218.

110. Ciol MA, Deyo RA, Kreuter W, et al. Characteristics in Medicare beneficiaries associated with reoperation after lumbar spine surgery. *Spine* 1994;19: 1329–1334.

111. Spengler DM, Freeman C, Westbrook R, et al. Low-back pain following multiple lumbar spine procedures. Failure of initial selection? *Spine* 1980;5: 356–360.

112. Arkinstall W, Sandler A, Goughnour B, et al. Efficacy of controlled-release codeine in chronic non-malignant pain: a randomized, placebo-controlled clinical trial. *Pain* 1995;62:169–178.

113. Moulin DE, Iezzi A, Amireh R, et al. Randomized trial of oral morphine for chronic non-cancer pain. *Lancet* 1996;347:143–147.

114. Martell BA, O'Connor PG, Kerns RD, et al. Systematic review: opioid treatment for chronic back pain: prevalence, efficacy, and association with addiction. *Ann Intern Med* 2007;146:116–127.

115. Block AR, Ohnmeiss DD, Guyer RD, et al. The use of presurgical psychological screening to predict the outcome of spine surgery. *Spine J* 2001;1:274–282.

116. Brox JI, Sørensen R, Friis A, et al. Randomized clinical trial of lumbar instrumented fusion and cognitive intervention and exercises in patients with chronic low back pain and disc degeneration. *Spine* 2003;28(17):1913–1921.

117. Brox JI, Reikeras O, Nygaard Ø, et al. Lumbar instrumented fusion compared with cognitive intervention and exercises in patients with chronic back pain after previous surgery for disc herniation: a prospective randomized controlled study. *Pain.* 2006;122(1–2):145–155.

118. Fairbank J, Frost H, Wilson-MacDonald J, et al. Randomised controlled trial to compare surgical stabilisation of the lumbar spine with an intensive rehabilitation programme for patients with chronic low back pain: the MRC spine stabilisation trial. *BMJ* 2005;330:1233.

119. Rivero-Arias O, Campbell H, Gray A, et al. Surgical stabilisation of the spine compared with a programme of intensive rehabilitation for the management of patients with chronic low back pain: cost utility analysis based on a randomised controlled trial. *BMJ* 2005;330:1239.

120. Turk DC, Burwinkle TM. Assessment of chronic pain in rehabilitation: Outcomes measures in clinical trials and clinical practice *Rehab Psych* 2005;50: 56–64.

CHAPTER 76 ■ RATIONAL PHARMACOTHERAPY FOR PAIN

ARTHUR G. LIPMAN

Pharmacology is the science that deals with the origin, nature, chemistry, effects, and uses of drugs. Commonly, pharmacology is subdivided into pharmacodynamics (how drugs work; mechanisms of action) and pharmacokinetics (how drugs are absorbed, distributed, biotransformed [metabolized], and eliminated) in the body. Pharmacology is laboratory (nonclinical) nonclinical science done largely in animal and in vitro models in the laboratory setting. Clinical pharmacology, often termed therapeutics in the UK and some other countries, is the discipline intended to translate finding from the laboratory bench to the patient bedside. Despite attempts in the U.S. to develop clinical pharmacology as a subspecialty of internal medicine, and subsequently pediatrics and psychiatry, very few clinical pharmacologists are in practice and fewer still are in training programs today. By definition, the term pharmacology and even clinical pharmacology are somewhat restrictive.

Pharmacotherapy is, simply put, the treatment of disease by medicines. This is now a recognized health science discipline and describes the practice of clinicians including many physicians, pharmacists, advanced practice nurses, pharmacologically oriented psychologists, and others. Pharmacotherapy encompasses what those who attempted to develop clinical pharmacology envisioned without restricting practice to subspecialty-certified physicians. It is an academic discipline and numerous respected journals and an increasing number of health science textbooks now have pharmacotherapy in their titles. This more inclusive term includes those aspects of pharmacology and findings from clinical pharmacology that apply directly to the use of pharmacologically active substances in patient care.

Clinicians must have access to contemporary information on how drugs work to use them optimally in managing pain. Pharmacology is the science of how the drugs work, not their application in treating patients. Thus this section of *Bonica's Management of Pain* has been redesignated Pharmacotherapy.

Pharmacotherapy is a potent tool in pain management. However, we must use drugs wisely to provide optimal patient benefit. Several core concepts in rational pharmacotherapy are introduced in this chapter as a prelude to the four subsequent chapters on specific pharmacotherapy for pain management.

DRUGS ARE BOTH UNDERUSED AND OVERUSED IN PAIN MANAGEMENT

There is a broad consensus among pain clinicians that pain, especially chronic nonmalignant pain, often is undertreated.[1] One of the reasons for this is concern about medication misuse. Increasing reports of adverse events and even fatalities associated with analgesic use indicate that some practitioners may use analgesic pharmacotherapy unwisely or excessively. It is important to view drugs as tools that can be used well or poorly. Adverse events are not due to the drugs, per se, they are due to the way the drugs are used. Clinicians are encouraged to not label any class of drugs as "good" or "bad," but to recognize that they only become so designated because of the way they are used. However, there are some drugs within various classes that one should consider suboptimal, for example, meperidine,[2] as discussed in more detail in the opioids chapter. This section will attempt to identify medication use that is more apt to have positive than adverse outcomes.

PHARMACOTHERAPY ALONE IS RARELY OPTIMAL THERAPY FOR CHRONIC PAIN

Analgesic pharmacotherapy often is appropriate alone for acute pain. However, chronic malignant and nonmalignant pain usually responds better to multimodal treatment.[3] Many adverse events due to medications might not occur if lower drug doses are used, and concurrent nonpharmacological therapy often reduces drug dose requirements (Table 76.1). Using multiple drugs to address symptoms of other drugs sometimes leads to complex regimens with adverse events, that is, polypharmacy.[4] Although it is usually wise to simplify drug regimens, use of more than one drug in combination may reduce the risk of adverse events when the drugs are additive or synergistic and the adverse events are commonly dose related. A common example is concurrent use

TABLE 76.1

EXAMPLES OF PAIN INTERVENTION ALTERNATIVES TO INCREASING OPIOID DOSE

Etiology	Treatment
Bony pain	NSAID with opioid
Neuropathic pain	TCAs, anticonvulsants, local anesthetics, topical capsaicin, nerve blocks
Infectious damage	Incision and drainage, anti-infectives
GI spasm	Anticholinergic agents
Constipation	Stimulating laxatives
Lymphedema	Physical therapy, compression

From Lipman AG. Efficacy of opioids in cancer pain syndromes. *Pain* 1995; 63:135–136.

of an opioid and a nonsteroidal antiinflammatory drug (NSAID) because these two drug classes are mutually dose sparing. One might consider such use of multiple drugs for pharmacotherapy as "rational polypharmacy."

It often is useful to consider medications for chronic nonmalignant pain as temporary interventions to facilitate the patient's adapting self-management techniques such as physical activation, cognitive restructuring, or responding to medical procedures such as serial nerve blocks.

Every Use of Medication for Pain is an Experiment

It is axiomatic that every drug has the potential to do harm. We should only use pharmacotherapy when the potential benefit outweighs the potential harm; that is, there is a favorable risk to benefit ratio. Clinicians should consider pain pharmacotherapy a trial to determine outcome before committing to ongoing pharmacotherapy. All medication orders should expire at a predetermined time and only be continued after it is clear that the benefits outweigh the risks. It is helpful in most cases to tell patients that new medications are being ordered for a limited time to determine if they should be continued. This practice would eliminate many adverse outcomes from ongoing drug therapy. This practice might also lessen inappropriate patient expectations about their drug therapy for pain. It is usually unwise to continue any medication without a clear determination that it is more helpful than harmful.

In addition to risk to benefit considerations, clinicians should always consider cost to benefit issues. Frequently, new drugs and dosage forms offer incremental advantages over previously available agents, but the new agents do so at a markedly greater cost. The pharmaceutical industry often aggressively markets new and patent-protected drugs and dosage forms while there is rarely a financial incentive for a pharmaceutical manufacturer or distributor to promote generic drugs because pharmacists can legally substitute generic equivalent drugs unless the prescriber specifies otherwise. At the extreme, entire older classes of drugs, which may still be agents of choice, have been largely replaced by newer, far more expensive agents. For example, tricyclic antidepressants still are drugs of choice for neuropathic pain, but no company promotes them. Aggressive marketing of various antiepileptic and serotonin-norepinephrine reuptake-inhibiting drugs that are as effective or nearly as effective as the tricyclic antidepressants for this indication has resulted in the newer, more expensive drugs being considered by many clinicians as the only drugs for neuropathic pain.

Patient Preference: Symptom Control versus Side Effects

Patients vary both in their desire to take medications to manage their pain and in their response to the medications. Many patients are highly averse to taking medications, especially opioids, even when those medications can greatly reduce the pain. This aversion may be due to fears or misconceptions about the medications, and clinicians should inquire about their patients' beliefs and preferences when considering pharmacotherapy. When a patient with allergies indicates a preference for a particular antihistamine, we normally provide that medication. However, when a chronic pain patient expresses a preference for a particular opioid, many clinicians become suspect that there is an ulterior motive for specifying a drug of choice. The perceived preference may be due to prior experience, observation of other patients' good or bad response to opioids, or misconceptions. We should ascertain the basis for our patients' expressed preferences when feasi-

ble rather than draw our own—often inaccurate—conclusions. Obviously, we should correct wrong information on which patients express preferences.

Some chronic pain patients prefer to be more alert even though the trade-off may be more intense pain. Others prefer as much pain relief as possible with the accompanying dulling of their senses. Neither preference is right or wrong. It is very reasonable to counsel patients about the side effects of the analgesics and adjuvants we are considering and ask them their preferences regarding comfort versus alertness. One of the most problematic misconceptions among chronic pain patients is that medication will "cure" their pain. It is important to determine if the patient harbors such beliefs and to correct them when possible.

There is great interpatient variability in response to analgesics. We see this commonly with NSAIDs but cannot explain the mechanism. With opioids, it also is common and we know several sources of genetic polymorphism that cause interpatient variability[5] as described in more detail in Chapter 78. Clinicians should actively counsel patients about the need to adjust medications and doses to optimize response: one size does not fit all.

Whenever Possible Treat the Cause of the Pain

A commonly espoused concept in opioid pharmacotherapy is to increase the medication dose until the patient experiences either adequate pain relief or unacceptable side effects. While there may be some wisdom in this approach, it also has two major problems.[6] One is that opioids are not the therapy of choice for all types of pain. For example, bone pain in which there is inflammation often responds better to NSAIDs than to opioids, and nearly always responds better to a combination of these two drug classes than to opioids alone. Likewise, neuropathic pain nearly always responds better to a combination of opioids and tricyclic antidepressants or anticonvulsant medications with fewer side effects than will be seen with one class alone. Again, a combination of both a neuropathic pain-specific agent with an opioid is usually synergistic. Opioids can actually blunt pain from constipation, but would probably exacerbate the constipation. It is far better to identify the cause of the pain and to treat it with specific modalities than to simply use opioids and increase the dose to response. Examples of painful conditions that are indications for such alternate modalities include incision and drainage with anti-infectives for painful infected cysts, physical therapy for myofascial pain, and massage with pressure for pain due to painful lymphatic drainage blockade.

The second limitation is that several opioid dosage forms, most notably the newer long acting ones, are very expensive. The great interpatient variability in response to opioids supports changing drugs when a patient does not respond as expected after two or three dose increments. Such patients may well respond better to other opioids to which they are rotated in such cases. Thus, serial trials of different opioids to find the optimal drug are sometimes indicated.

Synergism and Potentiation

Additive effects may occur when we use two pharmacological agents concurrently and the combined effect equals the sum of the two agents' effects. Unless doing so provides a specific benefit, for example, dose sparing with drugs that have problematic dose-related adverse effects, additive pharmacotherapy usually is not warranted. It simply complicates the regimen reducing patient adherence (compliance) and often increases cost. Synergism occurs when two drugs act together to produce a supradditive action. This often is desirable. An example is using an NSAID with an opioid for their mutually synergistic effects. Synergism occurs because of the two different mechanisms and the NSAID being anti-inflammatory with the opioid acting largely centrally while NSAID provides peripheral anti-inflammatory activity. Potentiation is an effect in which one drug enhances the action of another. An example is the concurrent use of acetaminophen and morphine, which has been demonstrated in rat model.[7] Both drugs are simple analgesics, that is, they have no anti-inflammatory activity. The opioid is far more active than the acetaminophen but the latter increases the effectiveness of the former by acting at the serotonergic system in the brain. Although the concurrent use of acetaminophen can be clinically useful, the net clinical advantage of combination therapy is less than occurs when an opioid is used with an NSAID producing the two-way advantage of synergism.

Outcomes Analyses of Pain Pharmacotherapy

Clinical studies of analgesics have traditionally focused largely, if not exclusively, on efficacy. Efficacy is defined simply as the ability of an agent to have a desired effect. Studies of analgesic efficacy for chronic pain typically last only 3 to 6 weeks. Commonly, reduction in pain intensity is the measured outcome. Every pain clinician knows that long-term effectiveness is the outcome measure needed to determine the usefulness of a drug for chronic pain and that patients' ability to function, to carry out activities of daily living, is often more important than pain intensity, per se. These should be the criteria for effectiveness.

The pharmaceutical industry is beginning to conduct true effectiveness studies in support of their products. When more clinicians insist upon such evidence before adopting new drugs that are supported only by the short-term efficacy studies needed for the drugs to be approved for human use, we will see more true effectiveness studies.

Clinical outcomes studies comprise only one of the three types of studies needed to assess the place of drugs in pain management. Health-related quality of life (HRQoL) research is a relatively new discipline that provides important information for such subjective complaints as pain.[8] The gold standard for HRQoL is the Medical Outcomes Study Short Form 36 (MOS SF-36).[9] While this instrument provides useful population data, it lacks the specificity and sensitivity needed for utility as a clinical monitoring tool in chronic pain management. The Treatment Outcomes of Pain Survey (TOPS) is a pain-enhanced SF-36 that is useful for monitoring outcomes of chronic pain patients.[10] HRQoL studies provide valuable clinical information on how interventions affect patients' ability to function, not just their subjective pain intensity report.

The third type of study that is becoming increasingly important is pharmacoeconomic (PE) analyses. Pain management has become more complex, more invasive, and more expensive in recent years. Five types of PE studies that help define which interventions are apt to provide the most benefit are listed in Table 76.2.[11]

TABLE 76.2

TYPES OF PHARMACOECONOMIC ANALYSES

Cost-effectiveness
Cost-utility
Cost benefit
Cost-minimization
Cost-consequence

Adapted from Asche CV, Seal B, Jackson KC 2nd, Oderda GM. Economic evaluations in pain management: principles and methods. *J Pain Palliat Care Pharmacother* 2006;20(3):15–23.

Approved Drugs and Drugs for Nonapproved Uses

For a drug to be available for routine clinical use in the United States, the manufacturer or distributor (sponsor) must hold an approved new drug application (NDA) from the U.S. Food and Drug Administration (FDA). The FDA can legally issue an NDA only after the sponsor has completed three phases of clinical studies under a license for those studies called an investigational new drug exemption (IND). The IND specifies exactly how and in whom the investigators can use the drug and use outside of those restrictions can lead to criminal penalties. Only clinicians explicitly named on the IND or persons under their direct supervision can legally participate in the studies. Once the FDA licenses a new drug for human use, any licensed prescriber can legally use it for any human use. However, the sponsor cannot legally advertise or market the newly approved drug for indications outside of the labeling even when good scientific evidence supports such use. This includes any continuing professional education activities directly supported by the sponsor. Furthermore, the indications that are listed in the labeling (package insert) for the newly approved drug can, by law, only include those indications approved by the FDA based on clinical studies submitted by the sponsor in support of the NDA.

If the sponsor provides an unrestricted educational grant to a professional society, hospital, or other such uninterested party, that organization can sponsor continuing professional education in which presenters can discuss nonapproved uses of the drug based on scientific and professional publications and findings. Thus, for example, a sponsor cannot legally promote an antiepileptic drug that is not FDA approved for neuropathic pain management for that indication even if there is good scientific evidence of the efficacy of the drugs for that indication. Neither can professionals paid directly by the sponsor make continuing education presentations in which they discuss "off-label" use in any program. That would be defined as marketing the drug for an unapproved use. However, this in no way constrains licensed prescribers from prescribing the medication for off-label use as long as an NDA has been issued for another human use.

If a patient suffers an adverse event from a drug prescribed off label, the harmed parties can initiate civil (malpractice) litigation against the prescriber and the health care facility where this occurred. There normally are no grounds for criminal action against the practitioner for prescribing an approved drug even though it was for an unapproved indication. Published scientific evidence supporting the use of the drug as prescribed is normally a good defense in such actions. The lack of such evidence greatly increases the prescribers' exposure to civil litigation.

Pain patients often have comorbid mood disorders and sometimes they are already involved in litigation relating to the cause of their pain. These factors may increase the risk of litigation against pain clinicians if the patients are dissatisfied with the care they receive. Therefore, pain clinicians should remain aware of legal issues when planning an implementing pharmacotherapy for such patients. Opioids and other such potent medications are essential in pain management, however, and clinicians should not hesitate to use such pharmacotherapy when indicated. Clinicians should always carefully document what they are doing as recommended by the Federation of State Medical Boards of the United States. In its 2004 Model Policy for the Use of Controlled Substances for the Treatment of Pain (http://www.fsmb.org/pdf/2004_grpol _Controlled_Substances.pdf) the Federation explicitly states that quality medical practice dictates pain relief and that inadequate care results from lack of knowledge. The Model Policy further states that (state medical) boards should define boundaries of practice. Criteria for evaluating the use of con-

TABLE 76.3

GUIDELINES FOR EVALUATING THE USE OF
CONTROLLED SUBSTANCES FOR PAIN CONTROL

- Evaluation of the patient
- Written treatment plan with stated objectives
- Informed consent and agreement for treatment
- Periodic review at reasonable intervals
- Consultation as necessary for additional evaluation
- Accurate and complete medical records to include
  —The medical history and physical examination
  —Diagnostic, therapeutic, and laboratory results
  —Evaluations and consultations
  —Treatment objectives
  —Discussion of risks and benefits
  —Treatments
  —Medications (including date, type, dosage, and quantity prescribed)
  —Instructions and agreements
  —Periodic reviews
- Compliance with controlled substance laws and regulations

Federation of State Medical Boards of the United States, Inc. Model policy for the use of controlled substances for the treatment of pain. Available online at: http://www.fsmb.org/pdf/2004_grpol_Controlled_Substances.pdf. Accessed June 25, 2009.

trolled substances and information to document in the medical record when doing so are listed in Table 76.3.

Rational Pharmacotherapy

The criteria for rational pharmacotherapy are simple. The drug must be legal, that is, there must be an NDA for at least one human use. If the drug is used for a nonapproved use, the clinician should assure that there is good evidence supporting that use. The clinician must be confident that the potential benefit for use of the drug in that specific patient in the regimen prescribed presents potential benefits that outweigh the potential risks. To make that determination, the clinician must understand both the pharmacodynamics and pharmacokinetics of the drug. The recent increase in deaths due to methadone is attributable in part to the prescribers not understanding the long elimination half-life of the opioid. When any opioid dose is increased before the drug has reached steady-state serum levels, there is risk of accumulation toxicity. Due to the relatively high cost of commercially available long acting opioids, several third party payers encouraged primary care clinicians to change their patients from the more expensive analgesics to methadone. However, methadone, a pharmacologically long acting opioid, has a much longer half-life than pharmaceutically long acting opioids such as sustained-acting oxycodone. That difference in half-life without necessary changes in the opioid regimen when initiating methadone appears to be at least one factor in the increased number of methadone deaths observed in the last decade.[12]

CONCLUSION

Pharmacotherapy is essential in the management of nearly all acute pain and the majority of chronic pain patients. Safe and

rational use requires attention to the risk to benefit ratio in each clinical situation. It is not logical to provide analgesics for every patient in pain, nor is it reasonable to deny analgesic medication when it is needed.

Pharmacotherapy is the most common modality used to treat pain. Too often pharmacotherapy is used as a sole intervention. Most patients with moderate to severe acute pain or any chronic pain would benefit more from multimodal therapy.

Recent statements and publications emphasizing the risks of pharmacotherapy without providing a balanced discussion of the benefits of these drugs have discouraged some clinicians from using needed medications for pain. The U.S. Drug Enforcement Administration (DEA) has taken positions that discourage opioid pharmacotherapy [13] and the American Heart Association has discouraged NSAID use due to cardiovascular risk without addressing the major improvement in quality of life that millions of patients receive from these medications.[14] The DEA posits that reducing opioid use will reduce opioid abuse. While that may be true, it would occur at the cost of countless pain patients suffering unnecessarily. The American Heart Association position looks at the cardiovascular risks associated with NSAIDs. However, it does not consider the impact of painful inflammatory diseases such as osteoarthritis, which erode the quality of life of millions of patients.

Pain clinicians must be effective advocates for rational pharmacotherapy for their patients. To do so, we must be knowledgeable about the drugs we use. We also must assure that our patients and their families have accurate information to help them use the medications correctly. The following four chapters provide a scientific basis for that advocacy and use.

References

1. The Undertreatment of Pain – Legal, Regulatory, and Research Perspectives and Solutions. *J Law Med Ethics* 2001:29(1).
2. Cohen MJ, Schecter WP. Perioperative pain control: a strategy for management. *Surg Clin North Am* 2005;85(6):1243–1257.
3. White PF. Multimodal pain management—the future is now! *Curr Opin Investig Drugs* 2007;8(7):517–518.
4. Nogueras C, Miralles R, Roig A, et al. Polypharmacy as part of comprehensive geriatric assessment: disclosure of false diagnosis of atrial fibrillation by drug revision. *J Am Geriatr Soc* 2007;55(9):1476–1478.
5. Somogyi AA, Barratt DT, Coller JK. Pharmacogenetics of opioids. *Clin Pharmacol Ther* 2007;81(3):429–444.
6. Lipman AG. Efficacy of opioids in cancer pain syndromes. *Pain* 1995;63:135.
7. Sandrini M, Vitale G, Ottani A, et al. The potential of analgesic activity of paracetamol plus morphine involves the serotonergic system in rat brain. *Inflam Res* 1999 48(3):120–127.
8. Moinpour CM, Donaldson GW, Redman MW. Do general dimensions of quality of life add clinical value to symptom data? *J Natl Cancer Inst Monogr* 2007;(37):31–38.
9. Ware JE Jr, Sherbourne CD. The MOS 36-item short-form health survey (SF-36). I. Conceptual framework and item selection. *Med Care* 1992;30(6):473–483.
10. Wittink HM, Rogers WH, Lipman AG, et al. Older and younger adults in pain management programs in the United States: differences and similarities. *Pain Med* 2006;7(2):151–163.
11. Asche CV, Seal B, Jackson KC II, et al. Economic evaluations in pain management: principles and methods. *J Pain Palliat Care Pharmacother* 2006;20(3):15–23.
12. Centers for Disease Control and Prevention (CDC). Increase in poisoning deaths due to non-illicit drugs—Utah, 1991–2003. *MMWR Morb Mortal Wkly Rep* 2005;54:33–36.
13. Lipman AG. Does the DEA truly seek balance in pain medicine? A chronology of confusion that impedes good patient care. *J Pain Palliat Care Pharmacother* 2005:19 (1):7–9.
14. Antman EM, Bennett JS, Daugherty A, et al. Use of nonsteroidal anti-inflammatory drugs: an update for clinicians: a scientific statement from the American Heart Association. *Circulation* 2007;115:1634–1642.

CHAPTER 77 ■ NONSTEROIDAL ANTI-INFLAMMATORY DRUGS AND ACETAMINOPHEN

ASOKUMAR BUVANENDRAN AND ARTHUR G. LIPMAN

INTRODUCTION

Nonsteroidal anti-inflammatory drugs (NSAIDs) are a diverse group of compounds with analgesic, antipyretic, and anti-inflammatory activity. The prototypical NSAID, aspirin, has been largely replaced by newer NSAIDs which often are better tolerated and which do not present the aspirin-associated risk of Reye's syndrome in children who are exposed to influenza viruses.[1] Today, NSAIDs are the most widely prescribed drugs in the world, with sales greater than 2 billion dollars in the United States and 6 to 8 billion dollars worldwide. They are valuable in the management of both acute and chronic painful and inflammatory conditions and are administered by both systemic and local (topical) routes.

The earliest agent in this class, which has been used in folk medicine for millennia, is willow bark. Hippocrates wrote about the use of powdered willow bark for pains and fever in the fifth century BCE. Edward Stone formally reported salicylic acid extracted from the bark and leaves of willow, myrtle, and a number of other plants, as a medication for fever in 1763. Felix Hoffmann, a chemist at Bayer Pharmaceuticals in Germany, rediscovered the acetylsalicylic acid formulation which Bayer then named Aspirin and began marketing it for pain, fever, and inflammation early in the twentieth century. Only in the mid-twentieth century did aspirin become the generic name for that compound.

The newer NSAIDs were introduced in the 1960s, the first being indomethacin which was soon followed by ibuprofen. Numerous other NSAIDs promptly followed, most of which claimed better efficacy and safety than earlier compounds. In the past two decades, several NSAIDs have been removed from commercial availability due to potentially lethal side effects after they were in general use. Phenylbutazone and oxyphenbutazone lost popularity and were withdrawn due to blood dyscrasias. Suprofen caused nephrotoxicity. Benoxaprofen, bromfenac, and ibufenac (which was marketed in the United Kingdom, not the United States) caused serious hepatotoxicity. Two of the three cyclooxygenase-2 (COX-2) selective NSAIDs approved in the United States in the 1990s were subsequently withdrawn from the market as noted below in the discussion of the COX-2 selective agents. Today, over two dozen NSAIDs are commercially available in the United States for clinical use (Table 77.1) and several others are available in other countries as well.

MECHANISM OF ACTION

Prostaglandin Synthesis and Pharmacology

NSAIDs act by inhibiting prostaglandin synthesis in vivo. Prostaglandins (PGs) are derived from arachidonic acid and other polyunsaturated fatty acids; the 20-carbon polyunsaturated essential fatty acid (arachidonic acid) is the major source in mammalian tissues. PGs derived from arachidonic acid contain two double bonds. These are PGE_2, thromboxane and prostacyclin. Analogous compounds synthesized from eicosatrienoic (linoleic) and eicosapentaenoic acids contain one fewer or one more double-bond in the side chains (PGE_1, PGE_3, respectively).[2] The PGs, thromboxanes, hydroxy acids, and leukotrienes which retain the 20-carbon unsaturated fatty acid backbone are collectively known as eicosanoids.[3] Their release, usually as a result of trauma, is the major stimulus for eicosanoid production, as PGs cannot be stored and are released as soon as they are synthesized.[4] Cell membrane disruption causes phospholipid release, which is converted to arachidonic acid by the action of phospholipase A_2. Arachidonic acid then acts as a substrate for the COX enzyme.

PGs also are involved in the pyretic response. After injection of pyrogens, cerebrospinal fluid (CSF) PG levels rise. That effect can be prevented by pretreatment with aspirin.[5] Acetaminophen (paracetamol) is analgesic and antipyretic but lacks clinically useful peripheral anti-inflammatory activity. Acetaminophen blocks PG synthetase within the blood brain barrier, but not peripherally in a clinically meaningful way. Therefore, it is not an NSAID, per se, although it is commonly used for many of the same indications as NSAIDs. Acetaminophen is discussed in more detail later in the chapter.

Prostanoids do not generally activate nociceptors directly; they sensitize them to mechanical stimuli and chemical mediators of nociception such as bradykinin.[6] PGE_2 is the predominant eicosanoid released from endothelial cells of small blood vessels[7] and is a key mediator of both peripheral and central pain sensitization.[3] Because it is the prostanoid most associated with inflammatory responses, the formation of PGE_2 at inflammatory sites is often considered an indicator of local COX activity and suppression of PGE_2 is an indicator of a decreased inflammatory process.[8] The production of PGE_2 is slow in onset and of long duration in response to inflammation.[9]

COX is encoded by 2 genes.[10] Although the isomerization of PGH_2 into PGE_2 has been well-characterized biochemically and pharmacologically, the enzyme responsible, PGE synthase (PGES), was only recently purified and cloned.[11,12]

COX-1 and COX-2 Selectivity

The existence of more than one COX isoform, and specifically one that is positively regulated by cytokines and negatively regulated by glucocorticoids, was long suspected. In the early 1990s, an inducible COX isoenzyme was cloned.[13] The recognition of two COX isoforms, then designated COX-1 and COX-2, generated intense efforts to characterize the relative contribution of each isoform to prostanoid production in specific situations (Fig. 77.1).

COX-1 and COX-2 are membrane-associated enzymes with a 60% amino acid sequence homology.[14] In spite of their structural similarity, the two COX isoforms have different gene expression profiles, distinct kinetic properties, and different interactions with PLA_2s and synthases.[15] COX-1 is expressed constitutively and produces prostanoids that fine-tune physiologic processes requiring instantaneous or continuous regulation such as hemos-

TABLE 77.1

ACETAMINOPHEN AND NONSTEROIDAL ANTI-INFLAMMATORY DRUGS (NSAIDS) AVAILABLE IN THE UNITED STATES

Medication	Proprietary (trade) name	Half-life (H)*	Percent protein bound	Usual 24-hour adult dose range	Adult daily dose and frequency		Usual daily pediatric dose mg/kg/per 24 hours
					Dosage	Schedule	
Para-aminophenol derivative							
Acetaminophen	Tylenol, others	2	20–50	2–4 g	325–650 mg	Q4H	Dose varies with body weight and age
					650 mg–1 g	QID	
Salicylates							
Aspirin	Multiple	2–3	~90	2.4–6 g	600–1500 mg	QID	80–100 mg/kg/24h
buffered aspirin	Ascriptin, Bufferin, others			2.4–6 g	600–1500 mg	QID	80–100 mg/kg/24h
enteric-coated aspirin	Ecotrin, others			2.4–6 g	600–1500 mg	QID	80–100 mg/kg/24h
Choline magnesium trisalicylate	Trilisate Tricosal	2–3	90	1.5–3 g	500–1000 mg 750–1500 mg	TID BID	50–65 mg/kg/24h
Diflunisal	Dolobid	8–12	99	1–1.5 g	500–750 mg	BID	NA
Salsalate	Disalcid	1	90	1.5–3 g	750–1500 mg	BID	NA
Propionic acid derivatives							
Fenoprofen	Nalfon	2	99	1.2–2.4 g	300–600 mg	QID	900 mg–1.8 g per body surface area meter[2]
Flurbiprofen	Ansaid	2	99	200 mg	100 mg	BID	NA
Ibuprofen	Motrin, Advil, others	6	99	1.2–2.4 g (pain) 2.4–3.2g (inflammation)	OTC: 200–400 mg Rx: 400, 600; 800 mg Maximum: 3200 mg	QID QID	30–40 mg/kg/day as 3–4 doses
Ketoprofen	Orudis	2–4	99	225 mg	75 mg	TID	NA
Naproxen	Naprosyn, others	14	99	750 mg–1 g	250, 375, 500 mg	BID	10–20 mg/kg/24h as 2 doses
Naproxen Sodium	Aleve, Anaprox	14	99	550–1100 mg	275–550 mg	BID	10–20 mg/kg/24h as 2 doses
Oxaprozin	Daypro	40–60	99	1.2 g	1.2 g	Once daily	1 = 20 mg. kg/d

Fenamates						
Meclofenamate	Meclomen	2–3	99	50–100 mg	150–400 mg	TID, QID	NA
Diclofenac	Voltaren, in Arthrotec	1–2	99	50 mg, 75 mg	150–200 mg	TID, BID	2–3 mg/kg/24h
Tolmetin	Tolectin	5	99	400, 600, 800 mg	800–2400 mg	TID, QID	20–30 mg/kg/24h as 3–4 doses
Ketorolac	Toradol	4–6	99	Oral: 10 mg Q6H for not >5 days total	Oral: not >60 mg/day; Parenteral 30–60 mg, then 15–30 mg	QID	IV: 0.5 mg/kg/day single dose only; IM: 1 mg/kg/day single dose only
Mefenamic acid	Ponstel	3–4	99	250 mg	1.0–4.0 g	QID	NA
Enolic acid derivatives (oxicams)							
Meloxicam	Mobic	15–20	99	7.5 mg (OA), 15 mg (RA)	7.5–15 mg	Once daily, Once daily	NA
Piroxicam	Feldene	40–50	99	10, 20 mg	20 mg	Once daily	NA
Nabumetone	Relafen	24	99	500–750 mg	1.0–1.5 g	BID	NA
Acetic acid derivatives							
Etodolac	Lodine	7	99	200–300 mg maximum: 1200 mg	400–1200 mg	BID, TID, QID	15–20 mg/kg/24h
Indomethacin	Indocin, Indocin SR, others	2.–4.5	90	25–50 mg; SR: 75 mg; rarely >150 mg	<200 mg	TID or QID, BID	2–4 mg/kg/24h
Sulindac	Clinoril	8–16	99	150, 200 mg	400 mg	BID to TID	NA
COX-2 selective NSAID (coxib)							
Celecoxib	Celebrex	6–12	97	100–200 mg, 400 mg acute pain	200 mg	1–2 times daily	3 mg/kg BID

NA, not applicable; OTC, over-the-counter; Q4H, every 4 hours; QID, four times/day; TID, three times/day; Rx, prescription; SR, sustained release.

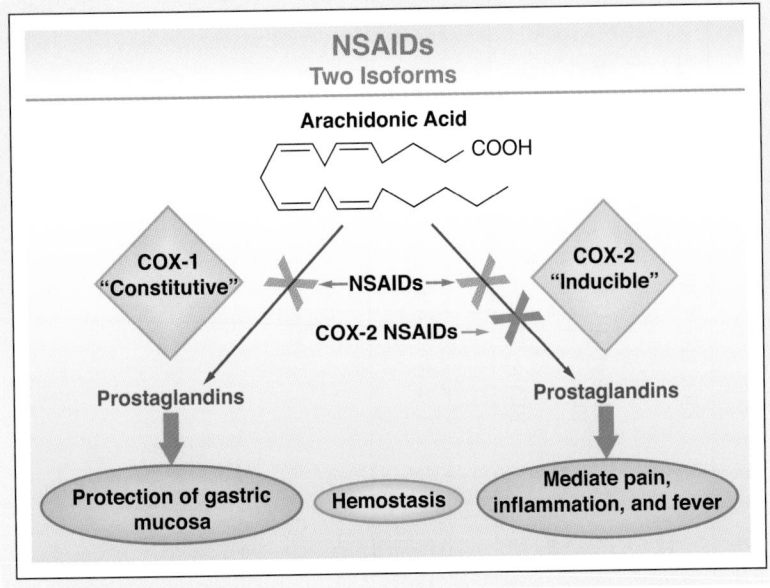

FIGURE 77.1 Simplified arachidonic acid pathway differentiating COX-1 and COX-2 effects.

tasis.[14] COX-2 expression is usually low but can be induced by numerous factors including neurotransmitters, growth factors, proinflammatory cytokines, lipopolysaccharide, calcium, phorbol esters, and small peptide hormones.[16] However, there are exceptions to the original constitutive versus inducible theory of COX expression. COX-1 expression can be induced in some stress conditions, such as nerve injury, and many tissues, including the central nervous system (CNS) and the kidney, constitutively express COX-2.[16] In the spinal cord, there are detectable basal levels of both COX-1 and COX-2 that might enable immediate reactions to transmitter release that result in prostanoid production.[17] A third isoform designated COX-3, that was identified in dogs, is formed as a splice variant of COX-1.[18] Because canine COX-3 can be inhibited by therapeutic concentrations of acetaminophen, initial reports postulated that COX-3 inhibition was the mechanism of action of acetaminophen. However, this does not appear to be true; more recent evidence indicates that COX-3 is not expressed in humans.[19]

Peripheral and Central Induction of COX-2

The original hypothesis formulated by John Vane in his Nobel Prize-winning work on the mechanism of action of NSAIDs was that these compounds inhibited prostanoid production in the periphery preventing a sensitizing action of PGE_2 on the peripheral terminals of sensory fibers.[20] Peripheral inflammation induces an increase in COX-2[21] and PGES expression in the CNS. The proinflammatory cytokine interleukin 1β (IL-1β) is up-regulated at the site of inflammation and plays a major role in inducing COX-2 in local inflammatory cells by activating the transcription factor NF-$_k$B.[22] IL-1β is also responsible for the induction of COX-2 in the CNS in response to peripheral inflammation. However, this is not the consequence either of neural activity arising from the sensory fibers innervating the inflamed tissue or of systemic IL-1β in the plasma. Rather, peripheral inflammation produces some other signal molecule that enters the circulation, crosses the blood-brain barrier, and acts to elevate IL-1β, leading to COX-2 expression in neurons and nonneuronal cells in many different areas of the spinal cord.[3,23] An elevation of COX-2 also occurs at many levels in the brain and spinal cord, mainly in the endothelial cells of the brain vasculature.[24] Thus, there appear to be two forms of input from peripheral inflamed tissue to the CNS. The first is mediated by electrical activity in sensitized nerve fibers innervating the inflamed area, which signals the location

of the inflamed tissue as well as the onset, duration, and nature of any stimuli applied to this tissue.[21] This input is sensitive to peripherally acting COX-2 inhibitors and to neural blockade with local anesthetics, as with epidural anesthesia.[25] The second is a humoral signal originating from the inflamed tissue, which acts to produce a widespread induction of COX-2 in the CNS. Regional anesthesia does not affect this[23,26]; it only is blocked by centrally acting COX-2 inhibitors.[23,25] One implication of this is that patients who receive neuraxial anesthesia for surgery might also need a centrally acting COX-2 inhibitor to optimally reduce postoperative pain and the postoperative stress response.[25] Therefore, the permeability of the blood-brain barrier to both nonselective and COX-2 selective NSAIDs is important.[27,28] Inhibitors of COX-2 that better penetrate the blood-brain barrier might represent more efficient analgesics and could also act to reduce many of the more diffuse aspects of inflammatory pain, such as generalized aches and pains, depression, and loss of appetite, which are key aspects in determining the "quality of life" response to treatment.[29] The main process by which a drug passes from the circulation into the CNS is passive diffusion. Lipophilicity and ionization are critical determinants of this transfer.[30] The CSF represents a convenient sampling point for drugs that enter the CNS; however, there are very few NSAIDs for which the CSF pharmacokinetics have been defined.[31] The high lipid solubility of indomethacin allows it to rapidly cross into the CSF and equilibrate with the free plasma concentration.[32] Similar results are seen with ketoprofen.[33]

PHARMACOKINETICS

NSAIDs are weak acids with pK_a values typically lower than 5. Since weak acids will be 99% ionized two pH units above their pK_a, these anti-inflammatory agents are present in the body mostly in the ionized form. Although NSAIDs differ in their individual pharmacokinetic properties, some general factors affecting NSAID pharmacokinetics can enable clinicians to select among the different agents available.

Absorption

Most NSAIDs are rapidly absorbed following oral administration, with peak plasma concentrations generally reached within

2 to 3 hours, though slow-release dosage forms have been developed to maintain active plasma levels for prolonged times. Factors affecting gastric emptying may profoundly affect the time course of the clinical effect of an NSAID. The extent of drug absorption from the gastrointestinal (GI) tract is more important than the rate.[34] Rectal and topical administration minimize GI side effects that are common with these agents. In general, the rate and extent of NSAID absorption is comparable for the rectal and oral routes.[35] Rectal NSAIDs have been used effectively, primarily for short-term postoperative analgesia[36] in some European countries. They are not commonly used in the United States largely due to cultural preferences.

There is good evidence that topical NSAIDs can be safe and effective and that they produce less GI toxicity than systemic forms of the same drugs.[37,38] These topical forms can be effective for inflammation of the knee and surface tissues; they generally are not effective for deeper structures. Topical NSAIDs must be properly formulated. Although extemporaneously compounded topical NSAIDs have been used, these are often ineffective. The vehicle and formulation can profoundly influence the efficacy of the topical dosage form.[39] In the United States, both a diclofenac topical patch (Flector, King Pharmaceuticals, Inc., Bristol, TN) and gel (Voltaren Gel, Novartis Consumer Health, Inc., Parsippany, NJ) were commercially available at the time of this writing. A Canadian topical solution formulation (Pennsaid, Nuvo Research Inc., Mississauga, Ontario, Canada) that is not yet available in the United States at the time of this writing is also supported by good clinical studies.[40] Topical NSAID dosage forms available in several countries are listed in Table 77.2.

Intravenous and intramuscular NSAIDs forms are available in several countries. Ketorolac is the only parenteral NSAID available in the United States. Parecoxib, an injectable analog for the COX-2 selective NSAID valdecoxib was under study, but those trials ceased when valdecoxib was withdrawn. Parenteral administration may be advantageous in renal colic due to a more rapid onset than oral administration, but has demonstrated no advantage over oral forms for any other indication.[41] Several injectable NSAID dosage forms, such as diclofenac and ibuprofen, were in phase II and III trials at the time this chapter was written.

Distribution

NSAIDs other than aspirin are generally lipid soluble, weakly acidic, and highly bound to plasma proteins, primarily albumin. In most cases, less than 1% of the total plasma concentration exists in the unbound form. Hypoalbuminemia increases the free fraction of NSAIDs in the plasma, thus affecting the distribution and elimination of these agents.[42] The high degree of serum protein binding increases interaction risk with other highly serum protein bound drugs. Most NSAIDs have distribution volumes between 0.1–0.15 L/kg.

In inflammatory joint disease, NSAID effectiveness corresponds to the affected joint synovial fluid drug levels. Those correlate closely with the drug concentration at the active site, since there is simple transport of drugs across the synovial membrane.[43,44] The amount of drug in synovial fluid is dependent on the amount of albumin in the joint, which is lower than in plasma.[45]

Elimination

Hepatic biotransformation is the major elimination pathways for most NSAIDs[46] which are metabolized by cytochrome P-450-mediated oxidation and/or glucuronide conjugation. Renal excretion of unmetabolized drug is a minor elimination pathway for most NSAIDs, accounting for less than 10% of the administered dose. Some NSAID metabolites are excreted to a significant extent via the bile.

Pathophysiologic Conditions Affecting the Kinetics of Nonsteroidal Anti-Inflammatory Drugs

Renal Failure

Renal failure influences NSAID kinetics by reducing renal excretion of the drugs and metabolites normally eliminated in the urine and by affecting the distribution and biotransformation of drugs.

Absorption and Distribution. The absorption of NSAIDs is not impaired in renal failure patients. However, the plasma protein binding of many acidic compounds such as the NSAIDs is impaired in renal failure patients.[47] The result is an increase in the volume of distribution of the unbound fraction of the drug in plasma.

Elimination. An increase in the unbound fraction of the drug in plasma may lead to an increase in total plasma clearance of the NSAID. The clearance of those NSAIDs for which formation of acyl glucuronides is a major elimination pathway is significantly reduced in patients with renal failure.[48] The acyl glucuronide forming NSAIDs (diflunisal, ketoprofen, naproxen, indoprofen, benoxaprofen, tiaprofenic acid) are usually rapidly excreted in urine, but accumulate in plasma of patients with renal failure. The effect of renal failure on the oral clearance of several NSAIDs (e.g., ibuprofen, fenbufen, isoxicam, and piroxicam) is small.[49] Most of these compounds are metabolized by oxidative pathways. All NSAIDs are very highly bound to plasma proteins, and hemodialysis will not likely result in increased elimination of these agents. No dosage adjustments are therefore necessary for hemodialysis patients receiving NSAIDs.[48]

Hepatic Disease

Absorption and Distribution. Because the majority of NSAIDs are low clearance drugs, mild to moderate liver disease should theoretically not interfere with their oral bioavailability. Since the liver is the major organ for the synthesis of albumin, the major binding protein for NSAID in plasma, hepatic dysfunction would be expected to cause alterations in the unbound drug fraction in plasma.

Elimination. Since most NSAIDs have a small total intrinsic clearance (oral clearance) relative to blood flow, hepatic clearance is essentially independent of flow and reflects drug metabolizing capacity. The elimination of ibuprofen does not seem to be affected in patients with mild to moderate liver disease.[50]

SPECIFIC DRUGS

All NSAIDs are analgesic, anti-inflammatory, and antipyretic. Differences among the drugs in their approved label indications reflect the studies submitted for approval rather than the actual indications for which the drugs are effective. Characteristics and available dosage forms of commercially available NSAIDs in the United States and much of the world are listed in Table 77.1. Initial selection of an NSAID for a specific patient should be based on the patient's past experience, dosing frequency compatibility with the patient's lifestyle, and cost. No population studies suggest that any one NSAID is more effective than another, but interpatient variability in response does occur. Because patients respond differently to various NSAIDs for reasons that are not

TABLE 77.2

APPROVED TOPICAL NSAIDS IN THE UNITED STATES, CANADA, NEW ZEALAND, IRELAND, FINLAND, FRANCE, AND ISRAEL*

Country (database)	Diclofenac	Ketoprofen	Ibuprofen	Piroxicam
United States (FDA, www.fda.gov)	Flector patch (diclofenac epolamine 1.3% patch, King Pharmaceuticals, Inc., Bristol, TN) Voltaren Gel (diclofenac sodium 1% gel, Novartis Consumer Health, Inc., Parsippany, NJ)	NA	NA	NA
Canada (Health Canada Drug Product Database, http://www.hc-sc.gc.ca/dhp-mps/prodpharma/databasdon/index-eng.php)	Pennsaid (diclofenac sodium 1.5% topical solution, Nuvo Research Inc., Mississauga, Ontario, Canada) Voltaren Emulgel (diclofenac 1% topical gel, Novartis Consumer Health, Inc., Parsippany, NJ)	NA	NA	NA
New Zealand (MEDSAFE, http://www.medsafe.govt.nz/profs/Datasheet/DSForm.asp)	NA	Oruvail topical gel (ketoprofen 2.5%, Sanofi-Aventis, Surrey, England)	NA	NA
Ireland Irish Medicines Board, http://www.imb.ie/EN/Medicines/HumanMedicines/HumanMedicinesListing.aspx)	Diclac 1% Gel (diclofenac sodium 1%, Rowex Ltd., Cork, Ireland) Difene Gel (diclofenac sodium 1%, Astellas Pharma Co., Ltd, Dublin, Ireland) Difene Spray Gel (diclofenac sodium 4%, Astellas Pharma Co., Ltd., Dublin, Ireland) Flector Tissugel 1% Medicated Plaster (diclofenac epolamine 1%, Novartis Consumer Health, Inc., Parsippany, NJ) Voltarol Emulgel (diclofenac diethylamine 1%, Novartis Consumer Health, Inc., Parsippany, NJ)	Fastum 2.5 gel (ketoprofen 2.5% gel, Menarini, Florence, Italy) Oruvail (ketoprofen 2.5% gel, Sanofi-Aventis, Surrey, England)	Ibugel 5% (ibuprofen 5% gel, Dermal Laboratories Ltd., Herts, United Kingdom) Nurofen Gel (ibuprofen 5% gel, Reckitt Benckiser Ireland Ltd., Dublin, Ireland) Phorpain (ibuprofen 5% gel, Goldshield Pharmaceuticals Ltd., Surrey, England)	Feldene Gel (piroxicam 0.5% gel, Pfizer, New York, NY)

Country (Regulatory agency)	Diclofenac	Ketoprofen	Ibuprofen	Piroxicam
Finland (National Agency for Medicines, http://namweb.nam.fi/namweb/do/haku/view?locale = en)	EEZE Spray (diclofenac 4% spray, Antula Healthcare, Stockholm, Sweden) Flector (diclofenac epolamine 1% plaster IBSA, Farmaceutici Italia Srl, Lodi, Italy) Voltaren emulgel (diclofenac diethylamine 1%, Novartis Consumer Health, Inc., Parsippany, NJ)	Ketorin 2.5% Gel (ketoprofen 2.5% gel, Orion Oyj, Epsoo, Finland) Orudis Gel (ketoprofen 2.5% gel, Sanofi-Aventis, Surrey, England)	NA	Feldene Gel (piroxicam 0.5%, Pfizer, New York, NY)
France (French Health Products Safety Agency, http://agmed.sante.gouv.fr/htm/1/amm/amm0.htm)	Flector (1% diclofenac epolamine plaster (Laboratoires Genevrier SA, Antibes, France) Voltaren emulgel (diclofenac diethylamine 1% gel, Novartis Consumer Health, Inc., Parsippany, NJ) Diclofenac 1% Gel (diclofenac diethylamine 1% gel, Merck, Whitehouse Station, NJ)	Ketoprofen 2.5% Gel (multiple manufacturers)	Ibuprofen 5% Gel, Solution (multiple manufacturers)	Piroxicam Gel (piroxicam 0.5% gel, Pfizer, New York, NY)
Israel (The Israel Drug Registry, http://www.health.gov.il/units/pharmacy/trufot/index.asp?safa = e)	Dicloplast (diclofenac sodium patch 140 mg, CTS Chemical Industries, Tel Aviv, Israel) Voltaren Emulgel (diclofenac diethylamine 1% gel, Novartis Consumer Health, Inc., Parsippany, NJ) Diclofenac Sodium 1% (diclofenac sodium 1% gel, Vitamed, Benyamina, Israel) Dicloren Gel (diclofenac sodium 1%, Trima, Kibbutz Maabarot, Israel)	Fastum Gel (ketoprofen 2.5% gel, Menarini, Florence, Italy)	Deep Relief (ibuprofen 5% and levomenthol 3%, Mentholatum Company, Hertfordshire, England) Nurofen Gel (5% ibuprofen gel, Reckitt Benckiser Healthcare Ltd., Hull, England)	Exipan (Piroxicam 0.5% gel, Perrigo Israel Pharmaceuticals, Bnei Brak, Israel) Feldene Gel (piroxicam 0.5% gel, Pfizer, New York, NY)

NA, not available.
*Websites accessed in December 2008.

well understood, it is appropriate to try an NSAID at full dose for about 3 weeks and then to rotate to another NSAID if the desired effect does not occur. There is no evidence that a patient who does not respond to an NSAID in one chemical subclass (e.g., propionic acid derivatives) will respond any better to an NSAID from another chemical subclass class than to a different propionic acid derivative NSAID.

Salicylates

Aspirin

The aspirin elimination half-life increases from 2.5 hours at low doses to 19 hours at high doses. It is well absorbed from the stomach and small intestine, with peak blood levels achieved 1 hour after an oral dose. There is then rapid conversion of aspirin to salicylates from a high first-pass effect, which occurs in the wall of the small intestine and the liver. The metabolic pathways follow first-order and zero-order kinetics.[51]

Aspirin inhibits the biosynthesis of prostaglandins through irreversible acetylation and consequent inactivation of COX. This differs from the newer NSAIDs, which are reversible COX inhibitors.[52] Most cells can synthesize COX; platelets cannot. Thus, the acetylation of their microsomal enzyme lasts for the life of the platelet (10–14 days). The ability of aspirin to acetylate proteins helps explain its anti-inflammatory superiority over most other salicylates. Aspirin is the only NSAID that has been associated with Reye's syndrome, a potentially lethal disorder that produces seizures and coma. It has occurred with the use of aspirin during a viral illness in children,[53] and aspirin is now rarely, if ever, used in pediatrics.

Diflunisal

Diflunisal has potentially better GI tolerability than aspirin because diflunisal is not metabolized to salicylic acid in plasma according to the results of a study comparing it at 250 mg and 500 mg twice a day to aspirin at 600 mg four times a day.[54] Diflunisal has a shorter half-life and causes less inhibition of platelet aggregation than aspirin.

Acetic Acid Derivatives

Indomethacin

Indomethacin is well absorbed following oral and rectal administration, but the extent of absorption varies widely among patients. There is also a large interpatient variability in elimination half-life caused by extensive enterohepatic recirculation of the drug. It is highly bound to serum albumin. Metabolism involves demethylation and deacetylation in the liver with subsequent excretion of inactive metabolites and unchanged drug in the bile and urine.[55] Its clinical application is somewhat limited by a relatively high incidence of gastritis and renal dysfunction. It is used in patients with acute gouty arthritis and osteoarthritis. Indomethacin is often used in neonatology to facilitate closure of patent ductus arteriosus.

Sulindac

Sulindac resulted from the search for a drug similar to indomethacin but with less toxicity. Sulindac is an inactive prodrug that is converted after absorption by liver microsomal enzymes to sulindac disulfide, the active metabolite.[56] As few as 25% of patients on sulindac have GI problems, primarily constipation.[57] Sulindac was considered in early studies to be the least nephrotoxic of the NSAIDs, but subsequent studies failed to support this contention.[58]

Tolmetin and Etodolac

These two NSAIDs claim fewer side effects than others in the class. Tolmetin is excreted in the urine partly unchanged, partly conjugated, and as an inactive dicarboxylic acid metabolite.[59] Tolmetin can cause edema due to sodium retention and abnormal liver function, both of which are reversible upon discontinuation of this NSAID.

Etodolac is an acidic compound with a pK$_a$ of 4.65 and is available as tablets and capsules with a dosage of up to 1 gram daily, and maximum of 1.0 gram/day. Clinical doses of 200 to 300 mg twice a day for the relief of low back or shoulder pain have been equated to analgesia with naproxen 500 mg twice a day.[60] Large clinical trials demonstrated a similar incidence of abdominal pain and dyspepsia is similar to several other NSAIDs, and gastrointestinal ulceration occurs in less than 0.3% of patients.[61] Dyspepsia occurs with etodolac in 10% of patients with a somewhat lower incidence of abdominal pain.

Ketorolac

Ketorolac is currently the only parenteral NSAID available for clinical analgesic use in the United States. It is almost entirely bound to plasma proteins (>99%). This results in a small apparent volume of distribution with extensive metabolism by conjugation and excreted renally.[62] The analgesic effect occurs within 30 minutes with maximum effect between 1–2 hours and duration of 4–6 hours (FDA-approved labeling).[63] It has antipyretic effects 20 times that of aspirin and thus can mask febrile response when given routinely to patients postoperatively. Several studies have demonstrated efficacy comparable to or exceeding that of morphine for treatment of moderate postoperative pain treatment but with fewer side effects.[64] Although ketorolac prolongs bleeding time, it does not do so excessively; however, postoperative bleeding associated with intraoperative ketorolac use has been reported.[65] There is evidence that ketorolac may act at the CNS in addition to the peripheral mode of action.[32] Dental surgery studies with ketorolac also indicate that ketorolac acts centrally[66]; however, measurements of the drug in CSF demonstrate poor penetration of the compound from plasma.[67]

When first used postoperatively at an initial dose of 60 mg followed by 30 mg doses every 4 hours, ketorolac was associated with acute tubular necrosis, especially in patients who had undergone fluid-restricted procedures. Some deaths resulted. Subsequently, to minimize this risk, doses were commonly reduced by 50% to 75%, but concerns about nephrotoxicity continue. The appropriate analgesic dose of parenteral ketorolac is controversial. There have been reports of death due to GI and operative site bleeding[69] resulting in the drug being recalled in Germany and France. In a response to these adverse events, the drug's manufacturer recommended reducing the dose of ketorolac from 150 to 120 mg per day.[63] The European Committee for Proprietary Medicinal Products recommended a further reduction of the maximum daily dose to 60 mg for the elderly and to 90 mg for the nonelderly.[70] Currently, there is consensus that the dose should be as low as 7.5–10 mg every 6 hours.[71,72] The intranasal route of administration may often produce higher levels of the drug in the CNS and CSF[73] with minimal GI side effects. Studies are underway to determine the efficacy of this drug when administered intranasally.[74]

Oral ketorolac was approved for use in the United States approximately 3 years after the parenteral form and has an efficacy similar to that of naproxen and ibuprofen.[68] The parenteral form can be administered at single doses of 30 to 60 mg or as 30 mg intramuscularly or intravenously every 6 hours, whereas the oral dose is limited to 10 to 20 mg every 4 to 6 hours for no more than 5 days because of toxicity.

Diclofenac

Oral diclofenac is a carboxylic acid functional group with rapid and complete absorption. Substantial concentrations of drug are attained in synovial fluid, which may be one of the sites of action of diclofenac.[75] Concentration-effect relationships have been established for total bound, unbound, and synovial fluid diclofenac concentrations.[76] Diclofenac is eliminated following biotransformation to glucuronidated and sulphated metabolites that are excreted in urine with very little drug eliminated unchanged. Diclofenac has a greater high effect than other NSAIDs producing less systemic availability. Diclofenac may also have a significantly higher incidence of hepatotoxicity than other NSAIDs. The excretion of conjugates may be related to renal function. Conjugate accumulation occurs in end-stage renal disease; however, no accumulation is apparent upon comparison of young and elderly individuals.[77] Dosage adjustments for the elderly, children, or for patients with certain comorbidities (e.g., hepatic disease or rheumatoid arthritis) may not be required. Significant drug interactions occur with aspirin, lithium, digoxin, methotrexate, cyclosporin, cholestyramine, and colestipol.[78]

Parenteral diclofenac is used in Europe, and there is evidence that it reduces opioid dose requirements and pain after thoracotomy.[79] Experimental diclofenac sodium topical gel has produced effective pain relief for superficial burns.[80] Commercially available transdermal diclofenac patches provide pain relief from minor sports injuries[81] and have recently been demonstrated to be effective for postoperative pain relief.[82]

Propionic Acid Derivatives

This class of NSAIDs includes ibuprofen, fenoprofen, ketoprofen, flurbiprofen, and naproxen. A newer drug in this class is oxaprozin, which permits a once-daily dose regimen, but no other advantage over other NSAIDs.[83]

Ibuprofen

Ibuprofen was the first NSAID to become available without prescription in the United States. It is well absorbed; peak plasma levels of 15–20 µg/mL are achieved about 1 to 2 hours after a single dose. The half-life is about 3.5 hours. The drug is primarily hepatically metabolized with less than 10% excreted unchanged in the urine and bile.[84] Ibuprofen at a dose of 1200 mg/day has a predominately analgesic effect in arthritis patients. Normally, a minimum dose of 1600 mg a day is needed for clinically useful anti-inflammatory activity. At 2400 mg per day, it produces GI side effects of which nausea and dyspepsia are predominant. Renal side effects of ibuprofen appear to be dose-dependent and were not reported at the recommended dosage as over-the-counter drug (200 to 800 mg per day). Even at anti-inflammatory doses of more than 1600 mg per day, renal side effects are almost exclusively encountered in patients with low intravascular volume and low cardiac output, particularly in the elderly.[85]

Concomitant administration of ibuprofen and aspirin antagonizes the irreversible platelet inhibition induced by aspirin. Therefore, the treatment with ibuprofen in patients with increased cardiovascular risk may limit the cardioprotective effects of aspirin.[86] Other routes of administration of this drug are under study.

Ketoprofen

Oral ketoprofen reaches peak plasma levels in 1.5 to 2 hours. The half-life is 2.4 hours with an analgesic duration of 4 to 6 hours.[87] The maximum recommended dose is 300 mg. An investigational topical patch contains 100 mg of the drug. Pharmacokinetic data indicate that the plasma levels of ketoprofen 100 mg administered orally are higher than when applied by patch. Because the patch facilitates ketoprofen delivery over a full day, the drug remains continually present in the tissue adjacent to the site of application. High tissue but low plasma ketoprofen concentra-

tions produce a therapeutic effect while plasma concentrations remain low enough to minimize systemic adverse events.[88]

Fenoprofen

The calcium salt of fenoprofen is more common; it is well absorbed and achieves a peak plasma level of 20–30 µg/mL two hours after a single oral dose with a plasma half-life of 2 to 3 hours.[89] Steady state plasma levels are reached within the first 24 hours of therapy. Fenoprofen is well tolerated compared to aspirin and causes minimal occult GI bleeding; nevertheless, dyspepsia remains the most common side effect. Most of the drug is excreted as glucuronide in the urine.

Naproxen

Naproxen sodium is also available without a prescription in the United States. Naproxen is well absorbed from the upper GI tract. Its long half-life of 13 hours makes it suitable for twice-daily administration,[90] and it takes more than 2 days to reach steady state serum levels. Excretion is almost entirely renal, primarily as an inactive glucuronide metabolite.

Naproxen has been used for the treatment of arthritis and other inflammatory diseases with superior efficacy to aspirin.[91] It causes less GI irritation than aspirin. Naproxen increases bleeding time by inhibiting platelet aggregation. When given during pregnancy, it can cross the placenta in 20 minutes and cause neonatal jaundice. Naproxen appears to have one of the safest cardiovascular profiles of all NSAIDs.

Oxaprozin

Oxaprozin is approved for the management of adult rheumatoid arthritis, osteoarthritis, ankylosing spondylitis, soft tissue disorders, and postoperative dental pain. Oxaprozin has a high oral bioavailability (95%), with peak plasma concentrations at 3 to 5 hours after dosing.[92] It is metabolized in the liver by oxidative and conjugative pathways and is readily eliminated by the renal and fecal routes. Oxaprozin inhibits nuclear translocation of NF-kappa B and metalloproteases and modulates the endogenous cannabinoid system.[93] In a randomized study of patients with refractory shoulder pain, oxaprozin (1200 mg) once a day was superior to three doses/day of diclofenac (50 mg) in reducing pain and improving quality of life.[94]

Oxaprozin diffuses readily into inflamed synovial tissues after oral administration.[95] Although discovered more than 20 years ago, it is now under intensive investigation because of its unusual pharmacodynamic properties. Other than being a nonselective COX inhibitor, the drug is capable of inhibiting both anandamide hydrolase in neurons, with consequent potent analgesic activity, and NF-kappaB activation in inflammatory cells.[93] Moreover, oxaprozin induces apoptosis of activated monocytes in a dose-dependent manner. As monocyte-macrophages and NF-kappaB pathways are crucial for synthesis of proinflammatory and histotoxic mediators in inflamed joints, oxaprozin appears to have pharmacodynamic properties exceeding those presently assumed as markers of classical NSAIDs.[96]

Oxicam Derivatives

Piroxicam, the first drug in this class, provides peak serum concentration following oral dosing slowly and has a long elimination half-life of 48.5 hours. This allows once daily dosing, but piroxicam may take up to 1 week to achieve steady state blood concentrations.[97]

Meloxicam

Meloxicam is approved for the treatment of osteoarthritis in the United States. It has also been evaluated for the treatment of rheumatoid arthritis, ankylosing spondylitis, and acute rheumatic pain.[98] Meloxicam is a nonselective COX inhibitor that has been shown to be somewhat COX-2 preferential at low therapeutic dose. It is unclear that this is clinically meaningful at normal therapeutic doses. Therefore, meloxicam should be considered a nonselective NSAID.

In clinical trials at a low dose, meloxicam was as effective as piroxicam, diclofenac, and naproxen with less GI toxicity,[99] but this may not hold true at the commonly required higher dose. Meloxicam's half-life of approximately 20 hours makes it appropriate for once daily dosing.[99] Meloxicam has not been reported to cause deterioration in renal function in patients with moderate renal failure, and there is no evidence of drug accumulation with continued use. However, the FDA-approved labeling recommends that only the 7.5 mg dose be used in patients with renal insufficiency. Dose adjustment is not required in the elderly. Meloxicam interacts with some medications, including cholestyramine, lithium, and some inhibitors of cytochrome P450 -2C9 and -3A4. Consequently, increased clinical vigilance is indicated when using it concurrently with other medications metabolized by those enzymes. Concentration-dependent therapeutic and toxicological effects have yet to be extensively elucidated for meloxicam.[100] Its pharmacokinetic profile is characterized by a prolonged, almost complete absorption, and the drug is more than 99.5% bound to plasma proteins. Meloxicam is metabolized primarily to four biologically inactive metabolites, which are excreted in both urine and feces. Steady state plasma concentrations are achieved within 3–5 days. The pharmacokinetic parameters of meloxicam are linear over the dose range 7.5–30 mg, and bioequivalence has been shown for a number of different formulations.

COX-2 Selective Nonsteroidal Anti-Inflammatory Drugs

COX-2 selective NSAIDs were developed to reduce the incidence of serious GI adverse effects associated with the administration of traditional NSAIDs on the assumption that these side effects were COX-1 mediated. Marketing efforts to differentiate these drugs from nonselective NSAIDs led to the term COX-2 specific inhibitors. That is misleading because these drugs are selective, not specific, in their COX-2 affinity. The initial COX-2 selective NSAIDs approved by Food and Drug Administration (FDA) were celecoxib and rofecoxib.

Celecoxib

Celecoxib, the first COX-2 selective NSAID, was approved by the FDA on December 31, 1998. It now has approval for the relief of pain from osteoarthritis, rheumatoid arthritis, acute pain, dysmenorrhea, and for familial adenomatous polyposis. It has good selectivity for the COX-2 enzyme. Peak plasma levels occur 3 hours after oral administration, and the drug crosses into the CSF.[27] Celecoxib is 97% serum protein bound with an apparent volume of distribution of 400 L. It is metabolized via cytochrome P450 -2C9 and is eliminated predominantly by the liver. It is not indicated for pediatric use and is a category C drug for pregnancy. The drug has a half-life of about 11 hours.[101] Adverse events noted in the various clinical trials include headache, edema, dyspepsia, diarrhea, nausea, and sinusitis. It is contraindicated in patients who have a sulfonamide allergy or a known hypersensitivity to aspirin or other NSAIDs.

Because celecoxib does not interfere with platelet function[102] (there is no COX-2 in human platelets), it can be administered perioperatively as a multimodal analgesic without increased risk of bleeding.

The efficacy and upper GI safety of celecoxib compared with nonselective NSAIDs was evaluated in 13,274 patients with os-

teoarthritis (SUCCESS-I study).[103] Patients were randomly assigned to receive either celecoxib 100 or 200 mg twice daily or nonselective NSAID therapy (diclofenac 50 mg twice daily or naproxen 500 mg twice daily) for 12 weeks. Both celecoxib doses were as effective as the nonselective NSAIDs in treating osteoarthritis and significantly more gastric ulcer-related complications occurred in the nonselective NSAID patients (0.8/100 patient-years) compared with the celecoxib group (0.1/100 patient-years) (odds ratio $= 7.02$; $p = 0.008$). The number of cardiovascular thromboembolic events was low and not different between the groups. The results of the SUCCESS-I study are different from the "CLASS" trial.[104] which did not demonstrate an advantage of celecoxib in reducing the incidence of upper GI ulcer complications, which is attributed by the SUCCESS-I study authors to the low dropout rate and design of the newer study.

Rofecoxib

Rofecoxib is a selective COX-2 inhibitor that was originally indicated for use in osteoarthritis, rheumatoid arthritis, dysmenorrhea, and acute pain following its approval in 1999. Rofecoxib was withdrawn from the worldwide market voluntarily by its manufacturer after data indicated an increased incidence of myocardial infarctions associated with its use. Subsequent studies suggest that the cardiovascular toxicity was due, at least in part, to dose-related blood pressure elevations. Had lower doses of rofecoxib been used more frequently, the recall may not have been necessary. Consistent clinical reports indicate that some patients who responded well to rofecoxib do not benefit as much from celecoxib, and vice versa.

Valdecoxib and Parecoxib

Valdecoxib is a derivative of isoxazole, and binds noncovalently to COX-2, forming a tight and relatively stable enzyme-inhibitor complex. It is a potent inhibitor of PGE_2 production in humans.[105] Valdecoxib has good oral bioavailability (83%) and a minimal first-pass effect. It achieves maximal plasma concentration in 3 hours with an elimination half-life of about 8–11 hours.[106] Valdecoxib was approved for use in osteoarthritis (10 mg), rheumatoid arthritis (10 mg),[107] and acute pain (up to 40 mg). Clinical studies in high-risk cardiac patients demonstrated a significant increased incidence of major cardiovascular adverse events, and the identification of increased risk for serious skin reactions (toxic epidermal necrolysis, Stevens-Johnson syndrome, erythema multiforme) led the FDA to recommend the withdrawal of this COX-2 inhibitor from the U.S. market in 2003. Parecoxib is a parenteral derivative of valdecoxib that has not been approved for marketing in the United States largely because of cardiovascular toxicity concerns.

Use in Postoperative Care. A meta-analysis of clinical studies evaluating these drugs compared to nonselective NSAIDs (which do not differentiate between COX-1 and COX-2 effects) for postoperative pain showed that the analgesic efficacy of COX-2 inhibitors in the 6 hours after surgery was similar to or better than ibuprofen.[108] A meta-analysis examined whether there is any advantage of multimodal analgesia with acetaminophen, nonselective NSAIDs, or COX-2 selective NSAIDs when added to morphine patient-controlled analgesia.[109] The results suggested that all of the analgesic agents provided an opioid dose-sparing effect (25%–55%) and the addition of NSAIDs to morphine was associated with a decrease in the incidence of postoperative nausea and vomiting and sedation. Clinical trials of COX-2 selective NSAIDs used preoperatively and into the postoperative period (2 weeks) for patients undergoing both major surgery[110] and minimally invasive surgery[111] demonstrated improved clinical outcomes. Preoperative administration of oral COX-2 selective NSAIDs can reduce the CSF PGE_2 levels in humans during the perioperative period resulting in improved outcomes following hip replacement surgery.[25] In addition to the reducing CSF PGE_2 levels, the COX-2 selective NSAIDs were able to modulate the CSF interleukin-6. The exact mechanism responsible for the reduction in the interleukins has yet to be determined, but is probably related to the PGE_2 pathway.[25]

Other COX-2 Selective Nonsteroidal Anti-Inflammatory Drugs. Additional drugs in the class have been formulated and shown efficacy in clinical trials. None has been approved by the FDA, although etoricoxib is commonly used in several other countries. Clinical experience consistently shows that some patients respond to one NSAID better than another and that applies to the COX-2 selective NSAIDs as well. It is unfortunate that celecoxib is the only such drug currently available in the United States.

Nonsteroidal Anti-Inflammatory Drug Controversies

NSAIDs are indicated in a multimodal analgesic approach. Recent practice guidelines for acute pain management in the perioperative setting specifically state "unless contraindicated, all patients should receive around-the-clock regimen of NSAIDs, COX-2 inhibitors, or acetaminophen."[112] The routine perioperative use of nonselective NSAIDs may predispose patients to an increased risk of bleeding.[113] In contrast, the COX-2 selective agents can be administered preemptively to surgical patients without the added risk of increased perioperative bleeding reported with nonselective NSAIDs.[114] The lack of perioperative bleeding with COX-2 selective NSAIDs offers a significant advantage compared to nonselective NSAIDs for a variety of orthopaedic surgical procedures. Although some animal studies with high dose NSAIDs suggest inhibition of bony in-growth postoperatively, there is no clinical evidence at normal doses to support that. As a result, many orthopaedic surgeons resist postoperative NSAID analgesia while others embrace it.

For chronic pain management, the concurrent use of an NSAID with an opioid or another analgesic with a different mechanism of action than the NSAIDs represents a rational combination in most cases. NSAIDs and opioids are mutually dose-sparing, and nearly all opioid and NSAID adverse effects are dose related.

Cardiovascular Effects

A more recent concern about the perioperative administration of NSAIDs, especially the COX-2 selective agents for short-term use, has been their possible role in increasing cardiovascular morbidity.[115] A joint meeting of the FDA Arthritis Advisory Committee and the Drug Safety and Risk Management Advisory Committee was convened in February 2005 to discuss the safety of COX-2 selective and nonselective NSAIDs. These committees jointly reaffirmed that COX-2 selective agents are important treatment options for pain management and that the preponderance of data demonstrate that the cardiovascular risk associated with celecoxib is similar to that associated with commonly used, older nonselective NSAIDs. Their rationale was that COX-2 selective NSAIDs collectively increased cardiovascular risk compared with placebo but not when compared with nonselective NSAIDs. The Committee concluded that short-term use of NSAIDs does not appear to increase cardiovascular risk and that rigorous scientific studies are needed to characterize the longer-term cardiovascular risks of these analgesics. Subsequently, on April 7, 2005, the FDA announced a series of labeling changes for all NSAIDs, including nonprescription forms. These included a FDA boxed warning for the potential increased risk of cardiovascular events and GI bleeding associated with all prescription NSAIDs, including celecoxib. The manufacturers were asked to revise their labeling to include a medication guide for patients to help make them aware of the potential for cardiovascular and GI adverse events. In addition, the FDA asked manufacturers of all over-the-counter NSAIDs to revise their labels to include more specific information about potential cardiovascular and GI risks and information to assist consumers in the safe use of these drugs.

Allergy and Hypersensitivity

All NSAIDs, including aspirin, may induce hypersensitivity reactions of two general types. Both may be related to the inhibition of PG synthesis. The two types of hypersensitivity are the syndrome of asthmatic attacks in patients with vasomotor rhinitis, nasal polyposis, and bronchial asthma and the syndrome of urticaria and angioedema. Prostaglandin E_2 is a bronchodilator. It stabilizes histamine stores in mastocytes and thus helps to inhibit the inflammatory response.[116] In a susceptible person, the result of the inhibition of PG biosynthesis may be spontaneous degranulation of mastocytes with release of histamine in the respiratory tract and skin, leading to bronchoconstriction and asthma as well as urticaria syndrome called Samter's triad which is COX-1 mediated. Therefore, COX-2 selective NSAIDs may be safely administered to these patients. The general recommendation is to use any NSAID for the shortest time and at the lowest dose that is clinically appropriate. For many patients with chronic, painful, inflammatory disorders, chronic NSAID therapy continues to present a favorable risk to benefit ratio. Those patients should be monitored, especially for blood pressure elevation and renal function.

Gastrointestinal Toxicity

The first evidence that aspirin could damage the stomach was reported in 1938 based on gastroscopic observations.[117] In the 1950s and 1960s, case control studies demonstrated NSAID-associated melena. NSAIDs cause hemorrhagic gastric erosions in the corpus and antrum. The mortality rate attributed to NSAID-related GI toxicity is 0.22%/year with an annual relative risk of 4.21. An estimated 16,500 NSAID-related deaths occur due to gastric complications, which is similar to the number from acquired immunodeficiency syndrome (16,685) and exceeds the number of deaths due to multiple myeloma and asthma. Risk factors identified for the development of NSAID-induced ulcers include advanced age, history of ulcer, concomitant use of corticosteroids, higher doses of NSAIDs, including the use of more than one NSAID, concomitant administration of anticoagulation, serious systemic disorder, cigarette smoking, consumption of alcohol, and concomitant infection with *Helicobacter pylori*.

The mechanisms by which NSAIDs cause ulceration in the stomach are contact irritation of the epithelium and suppression of PG synthesis.[118] NSAID-induced gastropathy correlates with the time and dose for gastric PG suppression.[119] Inhibition of PG synthesis reduces the gastric mucosa ability to defend itself against luminal irritants because bicarbonate secretions, blood flow, and epithelial cell turnover are influenced by PG. Gastric bleeding from pre-existing ulcers can also occur due to NSAID suppression of platelet aggregation.[120] Mediators in the pathway by which decreased PG levels cause gastric irritation and damage have been extensively studied. These include leukotrienes,[121] TNF-α,[122] and neutrophil adherence substances.[122]

NSAID-induced enteropathy has been documented in the small intestine and colon, although the exact mechanism is not fully understood. Various strategies can reduce NSAID gastroenteropathy.[123] Agents used to prevent NSAID-induced ulcers include sucralfate (efficacy controversial), H_2-receptor antagonists (famotidine), proton-pump inhibitors (omeprazole), and prostaglandins (misoprostol). Enteric-coated and slow-release NSAID dosage forms have not reduced ulcer risk.

NSAID-induced gastric complications prompted development of COX-2 selective agents. Preferential use of those selective agents to minimize gastropathy resulted in increased cardiovascular toxicity culminating in the withdrawal of two of the three. But cardiovascular toxicity is not specifically related to the selective NSAIDs. Celecoxib appears to have one of the safer cardiovascular profiles of all NSAIDs.

For patients with no cardiovascular risk factors and who have low risk for GI complications, monotherapy with nonselective NSAIDs is appropriate. For patients who do not require aspirin prophylaxis and are at risk for NSAID-induced GI complications, an initial approach would be to prescribe either a COX-2 selective NSAID or a traditional NSAID and a proton-pump inhibitor.

Hematologic and Cardiovascular Effects

All NSAIDs, not just the COX-2 selective agents, may increase risk of serious cardiovascular thrombotic events, myocardial infarction, and stroke. As noted above, NSAIDs inhibit prostaglandin formation. But different prostaglandins have different, sometimes opposing, functions. Thromboxane$_{A2}$ (TX_{A2}) is a platelet activator and vasoconstrictor, whereas prostacyclin (PGI_2) is a platelet inhibitor and vasodilator. Furthermore, activated platelets divert some of their endoperoxides to vascular cells ("endoperoxide steal") to further provide substrate for PGI_2 formation.[124] Platelet activity results from a balance between PGI_2 effects on endothelium and TX_{A2} effects on platelets. Platelets are especially vulnerable to COX inhibition because, unlike most other cells, platelets cannot regenerate this enzyme. Aspirin irreversibly acetylates the COX enzyme and that inhibits platelet aggregation for the 10 to 14 day lifespan of the platelet.[124] Other nonselective NSAIDs reversibly inhibit COX causing only a transient reduction in TX_{A2} formation. As a result, platelet activation inhibition resolves after most of the drug is eliminated.[124] A single 300 to 900 mg dose of ibuprofen can inhibit platelet aggregation for 2 hours after administration, and the effect is largely dissipated by 24 hours.[125] Similarly, both sulindac and diclofenac also inhibit platelet aggregation for less than 24 hours. The antiplatelet effects of long-acting NSAIDs such as piroxicam can last for several days after the drug is discontinued.[126] Overall nonaspirin NSAIDs cause "transient, dose-dependent, and modest bleeding time abnormalities," which often do not exceed normal limits.[124]

While in vitro studies examining the effect of NSAIDs on platelet function provide useful information, the clinical effect in patients is more important. The test primarily used to assess platelet function is bleeding time, but this test is highly operator-dependent and is subject to technical artifact. In addition, its clinical utility as a preoperative tool for predicting intraoperative bleeding remains controversial. Studies show variable effects of NSAIDs on bleeding. In one total hip arthroplasty study, 140 patients taking NSAIDs had more intraoperative and postoperative blood loss than those who did not.[127] In addition to potentially increasing perioperative bleeding, NSAIDs may increase myocardial infarction and stroke. An unbalanced biosynthesis of PGI_2 and TX_{A2} may play a role in atherogenesis and thrombosis. Prolonged administration of COX-2 selective NSAIDs may cause adverse events through inhibition of PGI_2. These include a blood pressure elevation, initiating and early development of atherosclerosis, and the architectural and functional response of blood vessels to stress. All of these effects may predispose individuals to an exaggerated thrombotic response upon rupture of an atherosclerotic plaque.[128] Aspirin and nonselective NSAIDs suppress both COX-1 and COX-2 and therefore reduce both TX_{A2}, and PGI_2. In contrast, COX-2 selective NSAIDs suppress PGI_2 production without affecting TX_{A2} synthesis.[129] Some authors posit that this may increase acute myocardial infarction risk that has been observed with prolonged use of some of the COX-2 selective agents. However, the fact that this outcome has not been associated with celecoxib suggests that it is not a coxib-specific effect. A more probable mechanism that others posit is that the risk of

myocardial infarction with all NSAIDs results more from modest, renally-mediated systolic blood pressure elevations over time.[130]

Renal Toxicity

Aspirin and all other NSAIDs can transiently decrease renal function. This effect may occur more often in patients with underlying renal disease.[129] The postulated mechanism is the inhibition of the renal PG synthesis, which may be important in the autoregulation of renal blood flow. Aspirin may also block the diuretic effect of spironolactone by inhibiting its binding to the tubular-cell receptor.

The renal profile of NSAIDs appears related to sodium retention, which is COX-2 inhibition mediated, and glomerular filtration rate changes due to inhibition of COX-1/COX-2. All NSAIDs are associated with hypertension and edema. Most of these events are of minor clinical significance with discontinuation rates due to hypertension and edema when used for short term.[130] Most cases resolve with discontinuation of therapy, which is generally seen over 1 to 8 weeks. The risk factors for NSAID-induced renal toxicity include the following: chronic NSAID use, multiple NSAID use, dehydration, volume depletion, congestive heart failure, vascular disease, hyperreninemia, shock, sepsis, systemic lupus erythematosus, hepatic disease, sodium depletion, nephrotic syndrome, diuresis, concomitant drug therapy (diuretics, angiotensin-converting enzyme inhibitors, beta blockers, potassium supplements), and age 60 years or older.[129]

Hepatic Toxicity

Aspirin is hepatotoxic in certain situations and this effect is non–dose-dependent. The effect is reversible when the drug is discontinued.[131] As noted above, diclofenac appears to be the most potentially hepatotoxic agent of the newer NSAIDs.

Central Nervous System Effects

Direct toxic reactions are of several types. Tinnitus or deafness are usually early warning signs of toxicity. Toxic manifestations are directly related to free drug levels, and those vary inversely with albumin levels. The adverse event is typically reversed when the dose is reduced or discontinued. NSAIDs are the most frequently implicated drugs in hypersensitivity-induced aseptic meningitis. Ibuprofen, sulindac, tolmetin, and naproxen have been implicated in causing drug-induced aseptic meningitis. Patients typically complain of fever, headache, and stiff neck that generally commences within weeks of beginning therapy.[132]

Acetaminophen

Acetaminophen is a para aminophenol derivative with analgesic and antipyretic properties similar to aspirin. Antipyresis is likely from direct action on the hypothalamic heat-regulating centers via inhibiting action of endogenous pyrogen.[133] Recent reports suggest that acetaminophen may act via the serotonergic pathway to provide analgesia.[134] Although equipotent to aspirin in inhibiting central PG synthesis, acetaminophen has no significant peripheral PG synthetase inhibition. Therefore, it lacks clinically useful peripheral anti-inflammatory activity, which makes it less desirable than NSAIDs for painful, inflammatory disorders. Doses of 600 to 650 mg are more effective than doses of 300 to 325 mg, but little additional benefit is seen at doses above 1000 mg, indicating a possible ceiling effect.[135]

Acetaminophen has few side effects in the usual dosage range; no significant GI toxicity or platelet functional changes occur. However, recent studies demonstrate that acetaminophen can cause blood pressure elevations. It is not clear if this presents risk of cardiovascular side effects similar to NSAIDs in light of the finding that NSAID-induced blood pressure elevation over time is associated with cardiovascular thrombotic effects.[136]

Nephrotoxicity also can occur with acetaminophen but less frequently than it occurs with NSAIDs. Acetaminophen is almost entirely metabolized in the liver, and the minor metabolites are responsible for the hepatotoxicity seen in overdose.[137] Inducers of the P-450 enzyme system in the liver (such as alcohol) increase the formation of metabolites and therefore increase hepatotoxicity. In certain patients (chronic ethanol users, malnutrition, and fasting patients), repeating therapeutic or slightly excessive doses may precipitate hepatotoxicity. A dose of 2600 to 3200 mg per day may represent a safer chronic daily dose, and acetaminophen dosing should not exceed 4 g/day.[138] Toxic doses appear to be a function of baseline glutathione levels and other dose-related factors. Genetically-determined glutathione is an important factor in overdose toxicity. Patients with high glutathione stores may tolerate much higher doses, but the 4 gram limit is important for safety because many patients lack sufficient glutathione stores to safely tolerate higher daily doses. Clinicians should carefully inquire and educate patients about other over-the-counter symptom-control products that patients may be taking which also contain acetaminophen.

Acetaminophen is completely and rapidly absorbed following oral administration. Peak serum concentrations are achieved within 2 hours and therapeutic serum concentrations are 10–20 mcg/mL.[139] About 90% of acetaminophen is hepatically metabolized to sulfate and glucuronide conjugates for renal excretion with a small amount secreted unchanged in the urine.[140]

The bioavailability of rectal acetaminophen is variable and is approximately 80% of that following oral administration. The rectal rate of absorption is slower, with maximum plasma concentration occurring 2 to 3 hours after administration.[141] Doses of 40–60 mg/kg of rectal acetaminophen have been shown to have opioid-sparing effect in postoperative pain models.[142] Propacetamol, an injectable prodrug of paracetamol, is completely hydrolyzed within 6 minutes of administration and 1 gram of propacetamol yields 0.5 grams of paracetamol. Injectable paracetamol has been shown to reduce opioid consumption by about 35%–45%[143] in postoperative pain studies,[143,144] including after cardiac surgery.[145] There is widespread use of the intravenous form in many other countries, but it was not available in the United States at the time of this writing. Acetaminophen has been reported to produce a dose ceiling effect at intravenous doses of 5 mg/kg, which resulted in a serum concentration of 14 mg/mL.[146]

CONCLUSION

The NSAIDs are important drugs which provide excellent analgesic, antipyretic, and anti-inflammatory effects as monotherapy and can be especially useful in combination with opioids for more severe pain. Acetaminophen provides comparable analgesic and antipyretic activity but lacks clinically useful anti-inflammatory activity. Like NSAIDs, acetaminophen administered concurrently with opioids often is opioid dose-sparing due to synergistic analgesic activity. Acetaminophen often is better tolerated than NSAIDs, most notably due to its lack of GI distress and chronic use-associated blood pressure elevations, ulcerogenicity, and nephrotoxicity. However, acetaminophen, like all drugs, does have toxicities, and chronic use requires monitoring for blood pressure and renal effects.

References

1. Flowers R, Moncada S, Vane J. Analgesic-anti-pyretics and anti-inflammatory agents: drugs employed in the treatment of gout. In: Gilman A, Goodman L, Rall T, et al, eds. *The Pharmacological Basis of Therapeutics.* 7th ed. New York: Macmillan; 1985.
2. Park JY, Pillinger MH, Abramson SB. Prostaglandin E2 synthesis and secretion: the role of PGE2 synthases. *Clin Immunol* 2006;119(3):229–240.
3. Samad TA, Sapirstein A, Woolf CJ. Prostanoids and pain: unraveling mechanisms and revealing therapeutic targets. *Trends Mol Med* 2002;8(8):390–396.
4. Cashman J, McAnulty G. Nonsteroidal anti-inflammatory drugs in perisurgical pain management: mechanisms of action and rationale for optimum use. *Drugs* 1995;49(1):51–70.
5. Ferreira SH, Vane JR. New aspects of the mode of action of non-steroidal anti-inflammatory drugs. *Annu Rev Pharmacol* 1974;14:57–73.
6. Ferreira SH. Prostaglandins, aspirin-like drugs and analgesia. *Nat New Biol* 1972;240(102):200–203.
7. Gerritsen ME, Cheli CD. Arachidonic acid and prostaglandin endoperoxide metabolism in isolated rabbit and coronary microvessels and isolated and cultivated coronary microvessel endothelial cells. *J Clin Invest* 1983;72(5):1658–1671.
8. Giuliano F, Warner TD. Origins of prostaglandins E2: involvement of cyclooxygenase (COX)-1 and COX-2 in human and rat systems. *J Pharmacol Ther* 2002;303(3):1001–1006.
9. Higgs GA. Arachidonic acid metabolism, pain and hyperalgesia: the mode of action of non-steroid mild analgesics. *Br J Pharmacol* 1980;10(Suppl 2):233S–235S.
10. Dray A, Bevan S. Inflammation and hyperalgesia: the team effort. *Trends Pharm Sci* 1993;14(8):287–290.
11. Mancini JA, Blood K, Guay J, et al. Cloning, expression, and up-regulation of inducible rat prostaglandin E synthase during lipopolysaccharide-induced pyresis and adjuvant-induced arthritis. *J Biol Chem* 2001;276(6):4469–4475.
12. Jakobsson PJ, Morgenstern R, Mancini J, et al. Common structural features of MAPEG—a widespread superfamily of membrane associated proteins with highly divergent functions in eicosanoid and glutathione metabolism. *Protein Sci* 1999;8(3):689–692.
13. O'Banion MK, Sadowski HB, Winn V, et al. A serum and glucocorticoid-regulated 4-kilobase mRNA encodes a cyclooxygenase-related protein. *J Biol Chem* 1991;266(34):23261–23267.
14. Smith WL, DeWitt DL, Garavito RM, et al. Cyclooxygenases: structural, cellular, and molecular biology. *Annu Rev Biochem* 2000;69:145–182.
15. Kraemer SA, Meade EA, DeWitte DL. Prostaglandin endoperoxide synthase gene structure: identification of the transcriptional start site and 5' flanking regulatory sequences. *Arch Biochem Biophys* 1992;293(3):391–400.
16. O'Banion MK. Cyclooxygenase-2: molecular biology, pharmacology and neurobiology. *Crit Rev Neurobiol* 1999;13(1):45–82.
17. Yaksh TL, Dirig DM, Conway CM, et al. The acute antihyperalgesic action of nonsteroidal, anti-inflammatory drugs and release of spinal prostaglandin E2 is mediated by the inhibition of constitutive spinal cyclooxygenase-2 (COX-2) but not COX-1. *J Neurosci* 2001;21(16):5847–5853.
18. Chandrasekharan NV, Dai H, Roos KL, et al. COX-3, a cyclooxygenase-1 variant inhibited by acetaminophen and other analgesic/antipyretic drugs: cloning, structure and expression. *Proc Natl Acad Sci U S A* 2002;99(21):13926–13931.
19. Qin N, Zhang SP, Reitz TL, et al. Cloning, expression and functional characterization of human cyclooxygenase-1 splicing variants: evidence for intron 1 retention. *J Pharmacol Exp Ther* 2005;315(3):1298–1305.
20. Vane JR. The mode of action of aspirin and similar compounds. *J Allergy Clin Immunol* 1976;58(6):691–712.
21. Kroin JS, Buvanendran A, McCarthy RJ, et al. Cyclooyxgenase-2 (COX-2) inhibitor potentiates morphine antinociception at the spinal level in a postoperative pain model. *Reg Anesth Pain Med* 2002;27(5):451–455.
22. Dai YQ, Jin DZ, Zhu XZ et al. Triptolide inhibits COX-2 expression via NF-kappa B pathway in astrocytes. *Neurosci Res* 2006;55(2):154–160.
23. Samad TA, Moore KA, Sapirstein A, et al. Interleukin-1beta mediated induction of COX-2 in the CNS contributes inflammatory pain hypersensitivity. *Nature* 2001;410(6827):471–475.
24. Laflamme N, Lacroix S, Rivest S. An essential role of interleukin-1beta in mediating NF-kappaB activity and COX-2 transcription in cells of the blood-brain barrier in response to a systemic and localized inflammation but not during endotoxemia. *J Neurosci* 1999;19(24):10923–10930.
25. Buvanendran A, Kroin JS, Berger RA, et al. Up-regulation of prostaglandin E2 and interleukins in the central nervous system and peripheral tissue during and after surgery in humans. *Anesthesiology* 2006;104(3):403–410.
26. Kroin JS, Ling ZD, Buvanendran A, et al. Upregulation of spinal cyclooxygenase-2 in rats after surgical incision. *Anesthesiology* 2004;100(2):364–369.
27. Dembo G, Park SB, Kharasch ED. Central nervous system concentration of cyclooxygenase-2 inhibitors in humans. *Anesthesiology* 2005;102(2):409–415.
28. Buvanendran A, Kroin JS, Tuman KJ, et al. Cerebrospinal fluid and plasma pharmacokinetics of the cyclooxygenase 2 inhibitor rofecoxib in humans: single and multiple oral drug administration. *Anesth Analg* 2005;100(5):1320–1324.
29. Bartfai T. Immunology telling the brain about pain. *Nature* 2001;410(6827):425–427.
30. Bonati M, Kanto J, Tognoni G. Clinical pharmacokinetics of cerebrospinal fluid. *Clin Pharmacokinet* 1982;7(4):312.
31. Gaucher A, Netter P, Faure G, et al. Diffusion of oxyphenbutazone into synovial fluid, synovial tissue, joint cartilage and cerebrospinal fluid. *J Clin Pharmacol* 1982;25(1):107–112.
32. Bannwarth B, Netter P, Pourel J, et al. Clinical pharmacokinetics of nonsteroidal anti-inflammatory drugs in the cerebrospinal fluid. *Biomed Pharmacother* 1989;43(2):121–126.

33. Netter P, Lapicque F, Bannwarth B, et al. Diffusion of intramuscular ketoprofen into the cerebrospinal fluid. *Eur J Clin Pharmacol* 1985;29(3):319–321.

34. Cooke AR, Hunt JN. Relationship between pH and absorption of acetylsalicylic acid from the stomach. *Gut* 1969;10(1):77–78.

35. Eller MG, Wright C 3rd, Della-Coletta AA. Absorption kinetics of rectally and orally administered ibuprofen. *Biopharm Drug Dispos* 1989;10(3):269–278.

36. Montané E, Vallano A, Aguilera C. Analgesics for pain after traumatic or orthopaedic surgery: what is the evidence—a systematic review. *Eur J Clin Pharmacol* 2006;62(11):971–988.

37. Moore RA. Topical nonsteroidal anti-inflammatory drugs are effective in osteoarthritis of the knee. *J Rheumatol* 2004;31(10):1893–1895.

38. Lin J, Zhang W, Jones A, et al. Efficacy of topical nonsteroidal anti-inflammatory drugs in the treatment of osteoarthritis: meta-analysis of randomised controlled trials. *BMJ* 2004;329(7461):324.

39. Galer BS. Topical NSAIDs not created equal—understanding topical analgesic drug formulations. *Pain* 2008;139(1):237–238.

40. Tugwell PS, Wells GA, Shainhouse JZ. Equivalence study of a topical diclofenac solution (Pennsaid) compared with oral diclofenac in symptomatic treatment of osteoarthritis of the knee: a randomized controlled trial. *J Rheumatol* 2004;31(10):2002–2012.

41. Tramèr M, Williams J, Carroll D, et al. Comparing analgesic efficacy of non-steroidal anti-inflammatory drugs given by different routes for acute and chronic pain. *Acta Anaesth Scand* 1998;42(1):71–79.

42. Evans AM, Hussein Z, Rowland M. Influence of albumin on the distribution and elimination kinetics of diclofenac in the isolated perfused rat liver: analysis by the impulse-response technique and the dispersion model. *J Pharm Sci* 1993;82(4):421–428.

43. Soren A. Kinetics of salicylates in blood and joint fluid. *J Clin Pharmacol* 1957;15(2–3):173–177.

44. Mäkelä AL, Lempiäinen M, Ylijoki H. Ibuprofen levels in serum and synovial fluid. *Scand J Rheumatol Suppl* 1981;39:15–17.

45. Fowler PD, Shadforth MF, Crook PR, et al. Plasma and synovial fluid concentrations of diclofenac sodium and its major hydroxylated metabolites during long-term treatment of rheumatoid arthritis. *Eur J Clin Pharmacol* 1983;25(3):389–394.

46. Davies NM, Skjodt NM. Choosing the right nonsteroidal anti-inflammatory drug for the right patient: a pharmacokinetic approach. *Clin Pharmacokinet* 2000;38(5):377–392.

47. Gibaldi M. Drug distribution in renal failure. *Am J Med* 1977;62(4):471–474.

48. Verbeeck RK. Pathophysiologic factors affecting the pharmacokinetics of nonsteroidal anti-inflammatory drugs. *J Rheumatol Suppl* 1988;17:44–57.

49. Cook ME, Wallin JD, Thakur VD. Comparative effects of nabumetone, sulindac, and ibuprofen on renal function. *J Rheumatol* 1997;24(6):1137–1144.

50. Menkes CJ. Renal and hepatic effects of NSAIDs in the elderly. *Scand J Rheumatol Suppl* 1989;83:11–13.

51. Levy G. Clinical pharmacokinetics of aspirin. *Pediatrics* 1978;62(5 Pt 2 Suppl):867–872.

52. Flower RJ. Drugs which inhibit prostaglandin biosynthesis. *Pharmacol Rev* 1974;26(1):33–67.

53. Farrell SJ, ed. Liver disease produced by nonsteroidal anti-inflammatory drugs. In: *Drug-Induced Liver Disease*. Edinburgh: Churchill Livingstone; 1994:371.

54. Huskisson EC, Williams TN, Shaw LD, et al. Difunisal in general practice. *Curr Med Res Opin* 1978;5(7):589–592.

55. Duggan DE, Hogans AF, Kwan KC, et al. The metabolism of indomethacin in man. *J Pharmacol Exp Ther* 1972;181(3):563–575.

56. Wood LJ, Mundo F, Searle J, et al. Sulindac hepatotoxicity: effects of acute and chronic exposure. *Aust N Z J Med* 1985;15(4):397–401.

57. Huskisson EC, Franchimont P, eds. Clinoril in the treatment of rheumatic disorders. In: *Proceedings of a symposium held at the 8th European Rheumatology Congress, Helsinki, Finland, 1–7 June 1975*. New York: Raven Press; 1976.

58. Quintero E, Ginés P, Arroyo V, et al. Sulindac reduces the urinary excretion of prostaglandins and impairs renal function in cirrhosis with ascites. *Nephron* 1986;42(4):298–303.

59. Grindel JM, Migdalof BH, Plostnieks J. Absorption and excretion of tolmetin in arthritic patient. *Clin Pharmacol Ther* 1979;26(1):122–128.

60. Pena M. Etodolac analgesic effects in musculoskeletal and postoperative pain. *Rheumatol Int* 1990;10 Suppl:9–16.

61. Schattenkirchner M. An updated safety profile of etodolac in several thousand patients. *Eur J Rheumatol Inflamm* 1990;10(1):56–65.

62. Gills JC, Brogden RN. Ketorolac. A reappraisal of its pharmacodynamics and pharmacokinetic properties and therapeutic use in pain management. *Drugs* 1997;53(1):139–188.

63. Toradol IV/IM [Package insert]. Nutley, NJ: Roche Laboratories; 1994.

64. Stouten E, Armbruster S, Houmes RJ, et al. Comparison of ketorolac and morphine for postoperative pain after major surgery. *Acta Anaesthesiol Scand* 1992;36(7):716–721.

65. Greer I. Effects of ketorolac tromethamine on hemostasis. *Pharmacotherapy* 1990;10(6[Pt 2]):71S–76S.

66. Gordon SM, Brahim JS, Rowan J et al. Peripheral prostanoid levels and non-steroidal anti-inflammatory drug analgesia: replicate clinical trials in a tissue injury model. *Clin Pharmacol Ther* 2002;72(2):175–183.

67. Rice AS, Lloyd J, Bullingham RE, et al. Ketorolac penetration into the cerebrospinal fluid of humans. *J Clin Anesth* 1993;5(6):459–462.

68. Forbes JA, Kehm CJ, Grodin CD, et al. Evaluation of ketorolac, ibuprofen,

69. Strom BL, Berlin JA, Kinman JL, et al. Parenteral ketorolac and risk of gastrointestinal and operating site bleeding. A postmarketing surveillance study. *JAMA* 1996;275(5):376–382.

70. Choo V, Lewis S. Ketorolac doses reduced. *Lancet* 1993;342(8863):109.

71. Sevarino FB, Sinatra RS, Paige D, et al. The efficacy of intramuscular ketorolac in combination with intravenous PCA morphine for postoperative pain relief. *J Clin Anesth* 1992;4(4):285–288.

72. Reuben SS, Connelly NR, Lurie S, et al. Dose-response of ketorolac as an adjunct to patient-controlled analgesia morphine in patients after spinal fusion surgery. *Anesth Analg* 1998;87(1):98–102.

73. Quadir M, Zia H, Needham TE. Development and evaluation of nasal formulation of ketorolac. *Drug Deliv* 2000;7(4):223–229.

74. Vyas TK, Shahiwala A, Marathe S, et al. Intranasal drug delivery for brain targeting. *Curr Drug Deliv* 2005;2(2):165–175.

75. Elmquist WF, Chan KK, Sawchuk RJ. Transsynovial drug distribution: synovial mean transit time of diclofenac and other nonsteroidal antiinflammatory drugs. *Pharm Res* 1994;11(12):1689–1697.

76. Chan KK, Vyas KH, Brandt KD. In vitro protein binding of diclofenac sodium in plasma and synovial fluid. *J Pharm Sci* 1987;76(2):105–108.

77. Morgan GJ, Poland M, DeLapp RE. Efficacy and safety of nabumetone versus diclofenac, naproxen, ibuprofen, and piroxicam in the elderly. *Am J Med* 1993;95(2A):19S–27S.

78. Davies NM, Anderson KE. Clinical pharmacokinetics of diclofenac. Therapeutic insights and pitfalls. *Clin Pharmacokinet* 1997;33(3):184–213.

79. Rhodes M, Conacher I, Morritt G, et al. Nonsteroidal anti-inflammatory drugs for postthoracotomy pain. A prospective controlled trial after lateral thoracotomy. *J Thorac Cardiovasc Surg* 1992;103(1):17–20.

80. Magnette J, Kienzler JL, Alekxandrova I, et al. The efficacy and safety of low dose diclofenac sodium 0.1% gel for the symptomatic relief of pain and erythema associated with superficial natural sunburn. *Eur J Dermatol* 2004; 14(4):46–48.

81. Galer BS, Rowbotham M, Perander J, et al. Topical diclofenac patch relieves minor sports injury pain: results of a multicenter controlled clinical trial. *J Pain Symptom Manage* 2000;19(4):287–294.

82. Alessandri F, Lijoi D, Mistrangelo E, et al. Topical diclofenac patch for postoperative would pain in laparoscopic gynecologic surgery: a randomized study. *J Min Invas Surg* 2006;13(3):195–200.

83. Miller L. Oxaprozin: a once-daily nonsteroidal anti-inflammatory drug. *Clin Pharm* 1992;11(7):591–603.

84. Brooks CD, Schlagel CA, Sekhar NC, et al. Tolerance and pharmacology of ibuprofen. *Curr Ther Res* 1973;15(4):180–181.

85. Mann JF, Goerig M, Brune K, et al. Ibuprofen as an over-the-counter drug: is there a risk for renal injury? *Clin Nephrol* 1993;39(1):1–6.

86. Catella-Lawson F, Reilly MP, Kapoor SC, et al. Cyclooxygenase inhibitors and the antiplatelet effect of aspirin. *N Engl J Med* 2001;345(25):1809–1817.

87. Geisslinger G, Menzel S, Wissel K, et al. Pharmacokinetics of ketoprofen enantiomers after different doses of the racemate. *Br J Clin Pharmacol* 1995; 40(1):73–75.

88. Mazieres B. Topical ketoprofen patch. *Drugs* 2005;6(6):337–344.

89. Gruber CM Jr. Clinical pharmacology of fenoprofen: a review. *J Rheumatol* 1976;2:8–17.

90. Ryley NJ, Lingam G. A pharmacokinetic comparison of controlled-release and standard naproxen tablets. *Curr Med Res Opin* 1988;11(1):10–15.

91. Sevelius H, Segre E, Bursick K. Comparative analgesic effects of naproxen sodium, aspirin, and placebo. *J Clin Pharmacol* 1980;20(7):480–485.

92. Davies NM. Clinical pharmacokinetics of oxaprozin. *Clin Pharmacokinet* 1998;35(6):425–436.

93. Kean WF. Oxaprozin: kinetic and dynamic profile in the treatment of pain. *Curr Med Res Opin* 2004;20(8):1275–1277.

94. Heller B, Tarricone R. Oxaprozin versus diclofenac in NSAID-refractory periarthritis of the shoulder. *Curr Med Res Opin* 2004;20:1279–1290.

95. Kurowski M, Thabe H. The transsynovial distribution of oxaprozin. *Agents Actions* 1989;27(3–4):458–460.

96. Dallegri F, Bertolotto M, Ottonello L, et al. A review of the emerging profile of the anti-inflammatory drug oxaprozin. *Expert Opin Pharmacother* 2005; 6(5):777–785.

97. Caldwell JR. Comparison of the efficacy, safety, and pharmacokinetic profiles of extended-release ketoprofen and piroxicam in patients with rheumatoid arthritis. *Clin Ther* 1994;16(2):222–235.

98. Fleischmann R, Iqbal I, Slobodin G. Meloxicam. *Expert Opin Pharmacother* 2003;3(10):1501–1512.

99. Vidal L, Kneer W, Baturone M, et al. Meloxicam in acute episodes of soft tissue rheumatism of the shoulder. *Inflamm Res* 2001;50 Suppl 1:S24–29.

100. Gates BJ, Nguyen TT, Setter SM, et al. Meloxicam: a reappraisal of pharmacokinetics, efficacy and safety. *Expert Opin Pharmacother* 2005;6(12): 2117–2140.

101. Kessenich C. Cyclooxygenase 2 inhibitors: an important new drug classification. *Pain Manag Nurs* 2001;2(1):13–18.

102. Leese PT, Hubbard RC, Karim A, et al. Effects of celecoxib, a novel cyclooxygenase-2 inhibitor, on platelet function in healthy adults: a randomized, controlled trial. *J Clin Pharmacol* 2000;40(2):124–132.

103. Singh G, Fort JG, Goldstein JL, et al. Celecoxib versus naproxen and diclofenac in osteoarthritis patients: SUCCESS-I study. *Am J Med* 2006;119(3): 255–266.

acetaminophen, and an acetaminophen-codeine combination in postoperative oral surgery pain. *Pharmacotherapy* 1990;10(6[Pt 2]):94S–105S.

104. Silverstein FE, Faich G, Goldstein JL et al. Gastrointestinal toxicity with cele-coxib vs nonsteroidal anti-inflammatory drugs for osteoarthritis and rheuma-toid arthritis: the CLASS study: a randomized controlled trial. Celecoxib Long-term Arthritis Safety Study. *JAMA* 2000;284(10):1247–1255.

105. Alsalameh S, Burian M, Mahr G, et al. Review article: the pharmacological properties and clinical use of valdecoxib, a new cyclo-oxygenase-2 selective inhibitor. *Aliment Pharmacol Ther* 2003;17(4):489–501.

106. Jain KK. Evaluation of intravenous parecoxib for the relief of acute post-surgical pain. *Expert Opin Invest Drugs* 2000;9(11):2717–2723.

107. Fenton C, Keating GM, Wagstaff AJ, et al. Valdecoxib: a review of its use in the management of osteoarthritis, rheumatoid arthritis, dysmenorrhoea and acute pain. *Drugs* 2004;64(11):1231–1261.

108. Rømsing J, Møniche S. A systemic review of COX-2 inhibitors compared with traditional NSAIDs, or different COX-2 inhibitors for postoperative pain. *Acta Anaesthesiol Scand* 2004;48(5):525–546.

109. Elia N, Lysakowski C, Tramèr M. Does multimodal analgesia with acetamino-phen, nonsteroidal antiinflammatory drugs, or selective cyclooxygenase-2 in-hibitors and patient controlled analgesia morphine offer advantages over mor-phine alone? Meta-analysis of randomized trials. *Anesthesiology* 2005; 103(6):1296–1304.

110. Buvenandran A, Kroin JS, Tuman KJ, et al. Effects of perioperative administra-tion of a selective cyclooxygenase 2 inhibitor on pain management and recovery of function after knee replacement. *JAMA* 2003;290(18):2411–2418.

111. Buvanendran A, Tuman KJ, McCoy DD et al. Anesthetic techniques for mini-mally invasive total knee arthroplasty. *J Knee Surg* 2006;19(2);133–136.

112. American Society of Anesthesiologists Task Force on Acute Pain Manage-ment. Practice guidelines for acute pain management in the perioperative set-ting: an updated report by the American Society of Anesthesiologists Task Force on Acute Pain Management. *Anesthesiology* 2004;100(6):1573–1581.

113. Connelly C, Panush R. Should nonsteroidal anti-inflammatory drugs be stopped before elective surgery? *Arch Intern Med* 1991;151(10):1963–1966.

114. Souter AJ, Fredman B, White PF. Controversies in the perioperative use of nonsteroidal antiinflammatory drugs. *Anesth Analg* 1994;79(6):1178–1190.

115. Bhattacharyya T, Smith RM. Cardiovascular risks of coxibs: the orthopaedic perspective. *J Bone Joint Surg Am* 2005;87(2):245–246.

116. Szczklik A, Gryglewski RJ, Czerniawska-Mysik G. Clinical patterns of hyper-sensitivity to nonsteroidal anti-inflammatory drugs and their pathogenesis. *J Allergy Clin Immunol* 1977;60(5):276–284.

117. Douthwaite AH, Lintott SAM. Gastroscopic observation of the effect of aspi-rin and certain other substances on the stomach. *Lancet* 1938;2:1222–1225.

118. Wallace JL, McCafferty DM, Carter L, et al. Tissue-selective inhibition of prostaglandin synthesis in rat by tepoxalin: anti-inflammatory without gastro-pathy. *Gastroenterology* 1993;105(6):1630–1636.

119. Lanza FL. A review of gastric ulcer and gastroduodenal injury in normal volunteers receiving aspirin and other nonsteroidal anti-inflammatory drugs. *Scand J Gastroenterol Suppl* 1989;163:24–31.

120. Hawkey CJ, Hawthrone AB, Hudson N, et al. Separation of the impairment of haemostasis by aspirin from mucosal injury in the human stomach. *Clin Sci* 1991;81(4):565–573.

121. Vaananen PM, Keenan CM, Grisham MB, et al. A pharmacological investiga-tion of the role of leukotrienes in the pathogenesis of experimental NSAID-gastropathy. *Inflammation* 1992;16(3):227–240.

122. Santucci L, Fiorucci S, Giansanti M, et al. Pentoxifylline prevents indometha-cin induced acute gastric mucosal damage in rats: role of tumour necrosis factor alpha. *Gut* 1994;35(7):909–915.

123. Wallace JL. Nonsteroidal anti-inflammatory drugs and gastroenteropathy: the second hundred years. *Gastroenterology* 1997;112(3):1000–1016.

124. Schafer A. Effects of nonsteroidal anti-inflammatory drugs on platelet func-tion and systemic hemostasis. *J Clin Pharmacol* 1995;35(3):209–219.

125. Lind S. The bleeding time does not predict surgical bleeding. *Blood* 1991; 77(12):2547–2552.

126. Weintraub M, Case K, Kroening B. Effects of piroxicam on platelet aggrega-tion. *Clin Pharmacol Ther* 1978;23:134–135.

127. An HS, Mikhail WE, Jackson WT, et al. Effects of hypotensive anesthesia, nonsteroidal anti-inflammatory drugs, and polymethylmethacrylate on bleed-ing in total hip arthroplasty patients. *J Arthroplasty* 1991;6(3):245–250.

128. Egan KM, Wang M, Fries S, et al. Cyclooxygenases, thromboxane, and ath-erosclerosis: plaque destabilization by cyclooxygenase-2 inhibition combined with thromboxane receptor antagonism. *Circulation* 2005;111(3):334–342.

129. Taber SS, Mueller BA. Drug-associated renal dysfunction. *Crit Care Clin* 2006;22(2):357–374.

130. Whelten A. COX-2 specific inhibitors and the kidney: effect on hypertension and oedema. *J Hypertens Suppl* 2002;20:S31–S35.

131. O'Connor N, Dargan PI, Jones AL. Hepatocellular damage from nonsteroidal anti-inflammatory drugs. *QJM* 2003;96(11):787–791.

132. Marinac J. Drug and chemical-induced aseptic meningitis: a review of the literature. *Ann Pharmacolother* 1992;26(6):813–822.

133. Lipton JM, Rosenstein J. Thermoregulatory disorders after removal of a cra-niopharyngioma from the third cerebral ventricle. *Brain Res Bull* 1981;7(4): 369–673.

134. Pickering G, Loriot MA, Libert F, et al. Analgesic effect of acetaminophen in humans: first evidence of central serotonergic mechanism. *Clin Pharmacol Ther* 2006;79(4):371–378.

135. Skoglund LA, Skjelbred P, Fyllingen G. Analgesic efficacy of acetaminophen 1000 mg, acetaminophen 2000 mg, and the combination of acetaminophen 1000 mg and codeine phosphate 60 mg versus placebo in acute postoperative pain. *Pharmacotherapy* 1991;11(5):364–369.

136. Gaziano JM. Nonnarcotic analgesics and hypertension. *Am J Cardiol* 2006; 97(9A):10–16.

137. Stewart DM, Dillman RO, Kim HS, et al. Acetaminophen overdose: a growing health care hazard. *Clin Toxicol* 1979;14(5):507–513.

138. Bertin P, Keddad K, Jolivet-Landreau I. Acetaminophen as symptomatic treat-ment of pain from osteoarthritis. *Joint Bone Spine* 2004;71(4):266–274.

139. Douglas DR, Sholar JB, Smilkstein MJ. A pharmacokinetic comparison of acetaminophen products (Tylenol Extended Relief vs regular Tylenol). *Acad Emerg Med* 1996;3(8):740–744.

140. Steventon GB, Mitchell SC, Waring RH. Human metabolism of paracetamol (acetaminophen) at different dose levels. *Drug Metabol Drug Interact* 1996; 13(2):111–117.

141. Cobby TF, Crighton IM, Kyriakides K, et al. Rectal paracetamol has a signifi-cant morphine-sparing effect after hysterectomy. *Br J Anaesth* 1999;83(2): 253–256.

142. Peduto VA, Ballabio M, Stefanini S. Efficacy of propacetamol in the treatment of postoperative pain. Morphine-sparing effect in orthopedic surgery. *Acta Anaesthesiol Scand* 1998;42(3):293–298.

143. Delbos A, Boccard E. The morphine-sparing effect of propacetamol in or-thopedic postoperative pain. *J Pain Symptom Manage* 1995;10(4):279–286.

144. Sinatra RS, Jahr JS, Reynolds LW, et al. Efficacy and safety of single and repeated administration of 1 gram intravenous acetaminophen injection (par-acetamol) for pain management after major orthopedic surgery. *Anesthesiol-ogy* 2005;102(4):822–831.

145. Cattabriga L, Pacini D, Lamazza G, et al. Intravenous paracetamol as adjuvant treatment for postoperative pain after cardiac surgery: a double blind random-ized controlled trial. *Eur J Cardiothorac Surg* 2007;32(3):527–531.

146. Hahn TW, Mogensen T, Lund C, et al. Analgesic effect of i.v. paracetamol: possible ceiling effect of paracetamol in postoperative pain. *Acta Anaesthesiol Scand* 2003;47(2):138–145.

CHAPTER 78 ■ OPIOID ANALGESICS

CHARLES E. INTURRISI AND ARTHUR G. LIPMAN

Opioid analgesics remain the most effective and commonly used treatment modality for moderate to severe pain.[1] Not every pain patient will benefit from opioid therapy, and more patients benefit from these strong analgesics when the drugs are used as one component of multimodal therapy.

During the past 20 years there has been a dramatic increase in our knowledge of the sites and mechanisms of action of opioids.[2] The development of analytical methods has also been of great importance by facilitating pharmacokinetic (PK) studies of the disposition and fate of opioids in patients. These PK studies and recent discoveries about pain and opioid receptor-related genetic polymorphisms have begun to provide a better understanding of some of the sources of interindividual variation in the response to opioids and suggest ways to minimize some of their adverse effects.[1,3] Although major gaps remain in our knowledge of opioid pharmacology, ultimately, the rational and appropriate clinical use of these drugs is based on the knowledge of their pharmacological properties derived from well-controlled clinical trials.

The term *analgesic* (from the Greek an-, without + algesis, sense of pain) refers to a drug that relieves pain without a significant loss of other sensations. *Opioid* (the preferred term) is any compound that binds to an opioid receptor. Opioids include the exogenous opioid receptor agonists and antagonists as well as the endogenous opioid peptides. The term *opiate* originally referred to any drug derived from opium but now includes the natural opium products (e.g., morphine), the semisynthetic derivatives (e.g., hydromorphone), or completely synthetic congeners (e.g., methadone). The term *narcotic* was originally associated with the opioids. It is now used in a legal context to refer to any drug considered to possess abuse or addictive potential. Because it is a value-laden word, avoidance of the term narcotic when discussing opioids with patients is often advisable.

CLASSIFICATION BASED ON INTERACTIONS WITH AN OPIOID RECEPTOR

Opioid analgesics can be classified based on their interactions with opioid receptors, namely mu (μ), delta (δ), and kappa (κ). Mu opioid receptor agonists (agents that occupy and activate the receptor) are the major source of clinically used opioid agonist and antagonist drugs. Kappa opioid receptor ligands provide a few drugs; however, their clinical pharmacology is complicated by concurrent mu opioid receptor antagonist activity (see later). Delta opioid receptor ligands were in clinical investigation at the time of this writing; none was yet available for clinical use.

Each of the opioid receptors is a G protein-coupled receptor (GPCR) and signals via a second messenger, cyclic adenosine monophosphate (cAMP), or an ion channel.[2] Alterations in the levels of cAMP and the transcription factor, CREB (cAMP response element binding protein) during chronic morphine treatment are associated with numerous cellular changes, some of which can lead to the development of tolerance and physical dependence.[4] Molecular genetic approaches have used gene-target-

ing (knockout) technology to disrupt the gene that codes for each of the three opioid receptors. Mice that lack the mu opioid receptor (MOR-deficient mice) do not respond to morphine with analgesia, respiratory depression, constipation, physical dependence, reward behaviors, or immunosuppression.[5] These results confirm and extend previous pharmacologic and receptor binding studies and demonstrate that the mu receptor mediates the analgesic and adverse effects of morphine. Pharmacologic evaluation of the effects of the microinjection of morphine and other opioids has been combined with anatomic characterization of the distribution of opioid receptors to provide insight into the sites of action of morphine and other clinically used mu opioids. Thus, mu opioid receptors (MORs) are found in the periphery (following inflammation), at pre- and postsynaptic sites in the spinal cord dorsal horn, and in the brainstem, thalamus, and cortex, in what constitutes the ascending pain transmission system.[6] In addition, MORs are found in the midbrain periaqueductal grey, the nucleus raphe magnus, and the rostral vental medulla where they comprise a descending inhibitory system that modulates spinal cord pain transmission.[6] Activation of the high density of mu opioid receptors in the human colon appears to be the major mechanism of opioid-induced constipation.[7] At a cellular level, opioids decrease calcium ion entry resulting in a decrease in presynaptic neurotransmitter release (e.g., substance P release from primary afferents in the spinal cord dorsal horn). They also enhance potassium ion efflux resulting in the hyperpolarization of postsynaptic neurons and a decrease in synaptic transmission. A third mode of opioid action is to inhibit GABAergic transmission in a local circuit, for example, in the brainstem, where GABA acts to inhibit a pain inhibitory neuron. This disinhibitory action of the opioid has the net effect of exciting a descending inhibitory circuit.

The opioid receptors are part of an endogenous system that includes a large number of endogenous opioid peptide ligands. Based on cloning, three distinct families of classical opioid peptides, the enkephalins, endorphins, and dynorphins, have been identified.[2] The physiologic roles of the endogenous opioid peptides are not completely understood. They appear to function as neurotransmitters, neuromodulators, and, in some cases, as neurohormones.[5] They play a role in some forms of stress-induced analgesia and in the analgesia produced by electrical stimulation of discrete brain areas such as the periaqueductal grey.[2,6]

Animal studies suggest that the reinforcing and rewarding properties of opioids (e.g., euphoria) that are associated with opioid abuse involve the mesolimbic dopamine system, not the supraspinal systems most prominently involved in the production of analgesia and physical dependence.[8]

CLASSIFICATION BASED ON OPIOID AGONIST OR ANTAGONIST ACTIVITY

The expression of agonist or antagonist activity is an important pharmacodynamic property used to classify opioids. The morphine-like agonist drugs represent one end of the pharmacodynamic spectrum. They bind predominately or exclusively to MORs and produce analgesia and the other mu opioid receptor-mediated effects described later. The opioid antagonists, such as naloxone, represent the other end of the spectrum since their binding to an opioid receptor does not trigger the signaling cascade that leads to the pharmacodynamic effects seen with opioid agonists. Rather, receptor occupancy by a sufficient concentration of an opioid antagonist prevents or reverses opioid receptor-mediated agonist effects.

Between these two types of pharmacodynamic actions fall the effects of the mixed agonist-antagonist drugs. These opioid drugs (see Table 78.1) can demonstrate agonist (at the kappa receptor) or antagonist (at the mu receptor) activity. What occurs clinically depends on whether the patient is opioid-naïve or has prior exposure to a mu opioid agonist. Buprenorphine is a partial agonist opioid. This classification derives principally from its pharmacodynamic activity observed in preclinical test systems wherein the difference in efficacy between a full agonist and a partial agonist can be more readily measured. Clinically, the consequences of buprenorphine's partial agonism can be observed as its ability to precipitate opioid withdrawal in some patients who have been receiving repeated doses of a mu agonist.

OPIOID PHARMACODYNAMICS

Receptor-Mediated Cellular, Synaptic, and Circuit Level Events Inhibit Pain Transmission

At the cellular level, activation of an opioid receptor (mu, kappa, or delta) by an opioid inhibits voltage gated (VG) calcium (Ca++) channels and the opening of certain potassium (K+) channels. The presynaptic block of VG Ca++ channels reduces transmitter release, while the increase in outward K+ currents hyperpolarizes postsynaptic neurons (increasing an inhibitory postsynaptic potential). These effects on transmitter release are believed to decrease synaptic transmission of pain signals in the spinal cord dorsal horn.

At the neuronal circuit level, opioids can disinhibit an inhibitory interneuron. This is the basis of descending modulation of pain transmission as discussed below.

Functional Localization of Opioid Receptors

Each of the three types of opioid receptors is expressed in defined patterns throughout the central nervous system (CNS). The MORs exist in peripheral tissues following activation by injury or inflammation, then in the spinal cord dorsal horn, the thalamus, limbic system, and in the somatosensory cortex (Fig. 78.1A). This distribution provides an anatomic basis for the modulation of ascending pain transmission by mu opioids. MORs also are located in the midbrain periaqueductal grey, the nucleus raphe magnus, and rostral ventral medulla (Fig. 78.1B). Opioids inhibit GABAergic neurons and remove the tonic *inhibition* of the pain inhibitory neurons (PIN) that project from the rostral ventral medulla to the spinal cord dorsal horn. Thus, opioids produce a disinhibition of the PIN, which results in the *activation* of descending inhibition and the descending modulation of pain transmission (Fig. 78.1C).

Mu opioid receptors are also located peripherally and the development of peripheral mu opioid antagonists has provided a new class of drugs to manage opioid bowel dysfunction. See Peripheral effects of opioids later.

THE PHARMACODYNAMIC EFFECTS OF OPIOIDS

The pharmacodynamic effects of opioids are discussed using the prototype morphine and the morphine-like opioids. In some cases

the term *opioids* refers to properties common to both morphine-like and mixed agonist–antagonist opioids. Later individual opioids are discussed in the context of how they compare to and differ from morphine and other morphine-like opioids.

The desirable and undesirable effects of morphine can be divided into those that may occur with a single dose and those that occur with repeated administration including tolerance, physical dependence, and addiction (Table 78.2).

CENTRAL NERVOUS SYSTEM OPIOID EFFECTS

Analgesia

The relief of pain by morphine is relatively selective in that other sensory modalities are not affected. While continuous dull pain has been relieved more effectively than sharp intermittent pain, morphine-like opioids can relieve severe, acute pain associated with renal or biliary colic. Some patients report that they still perceive pain, but that it is no longer as distressing as it was prior to morphine. Recent reports and long-standing clinical observations support the concept that pain includes both sensory-discriminative aspects (e.g., perception of the location, type, and intensity) and reactive or affective meaning of the pain experience (e.g., its unpleasantness). Under experimental conditions, positron emission tomography (PET) imaging studies localized and separated these two dimensions of pain. The sensory-discriminative aspects are processed in the somatosensory cortex (SSC) while the affective component is processed in the anterior cingulate cortex (ACC).[9] The presence of MORs in both of these brain areas is consistent with the ability of morphine-like opioids to alter both dimensions of pain.

In contrast to nonopioid analgesics, there is no easily measurable ceiling to the dose-dependent analgesic effects of morphine-like opioids. Nevertheless, there is often a practical ceiling imposed by the dose-dependent adverse effects including sedation, mental clouding, nausea and vomiting, or respiratory depression (Table 78.2). The actual dose required for analgesia can vary greatly depending on the type or source of pain and a variety of patient factors. The most important principle that derives from these properties of the morphine-like opioids is to titrate the dose for each patient to an acceptable level of analgesia that balances the degree of pain relief with the limits that are imposed by concomitant adverse effects.

Mood Effects

The morphine-like opioids can produce alterations in mood including the relief of anxiety, euphoria (pleasant feelings), as well as dysphoria (unpleasant feelings). Chronic pain patients receiving opioids often report initial relief of depression (a common concomitant of chronic pain), but this usually proceeds to exacerbation of depression after a few days to weeks. Thus, the mood effects appear as both desirable and undesirable effects in Table 78.2. Reports of euphoria or dysphoria usually depend on the individual and the circumstances of the morphine experience. Most "normals" not in pain as well as many patients in pain, report some dysphoria after receiving morphine. That is associated with difficulty in mental activities, dizziness, and decrease in physical activity.

The reinforcing and rewarding properties of these drugs that are associated with opioid abuse involve the mesolimbic dopamine system and appear to be distinct from those systems involved in analgesia and the production of physical dependence.[8]

TABLE 78.1

OPIOID ANALGESICS COMMONLY USED FOR SEVERE PAIN

Name	Equianalgesic parenteral dose[a]	Parenteral/ oral potency	Starting oral dose range (mg)	Comments	Precautions
			Mu (morphine-like) Agonist Opioids		
Morphine	10	6[b]	30–60[b]	Standard of comparison for opioid analgesics. Extended-release preparations (MS Contin[R], OramorphSR[R], and Kadian[R]).	Those with impaired ventilation, bronchial asthma, increased intracranial pressure and liver failure. Lower doses for elderly.
Hydromorphone (Dilaudid[R])	1.5	5	4–8	Slightly shorter acting. High potency parenteral dosage form for tolerant patients.	Like morphine.
Methadone (Dolophine[R])	10	2	5–10	Good oral potency. Long but variable plasma half-life. Rotation dose depends on prior opioid dosage. See text.	Like morphine. May accumulate with repetitive dosing causing excessive sedation.
Levorphanol (Levo-Dromoran[R])	2	2	2–4	Like methadone.	Like methadone.
Oxymorphone (Opana[R])	1	6[b]	5–10	Immediate-release (Opana[R]) and extended-release (Opana ER[R]) oral dosage. Also available as a rectal suppository.	Like morphine. Do not take with food or alcohol.
Oxycodone	15	2	5–20	Immediate- release (Roxicodone[R] and OxyIR[R]) and extended-release (Oxy-Contin[R]) oral dosage. Also in combination with nonopioids for less severe pain.	Like morphine.
Fentanyl	0.1	—	—	Transdermal fentanyl (Duragesic[R]). Also as Oral Transmucosal Fentanyl Citrate (Actiq[R]) for breakthrough pain.	Transdermal creates skin reservoir of drug and 12-hr delay in onset and offset. Fever increases absorption.

Drug				Comments (oral use)	Comments
Meperidine, pethidine (Demerol[R])	75	4	not recommended	Slightly shorter acting than morphine. Used orally for less severe pain.	Normeperidine metabolite accumulates with repetitive dosing causing CNS excitation. Not for patients with impaired renal function or receiving monoamine oxidase inhibitors.[c]
Codeine	130	1.5	30–60	Used orally in combination with nonopioids for less severe pain.	Like morphine.
Hydrocodone	—	30	2.5–10	Used orally in combination with nonopioids for less severe pain (Vicodin[R], Lorcet[R], Lortab[R], and many others).	
Mixed agonist-antagonist opioids					
Pentazocine (Talwin[R])	60	3	- see comments -	Used orally for less severe pain. A mixed agonist-antagonist—see precautions.	May cause psychotomimetic effects. May precipitate withdrawal in opioid dependent patients. Not for myocardial infarction pain.
Nalbuphine (Nubain[R])	10	- see comments -	- see comments -	Not available orally. Like IM pentazocine but not Scheduled.	Incidence of psychotomimetic effects lower than with pentazocine.
Butorphanol (Stadol[R])	2	- see comments -	- see comments -	Not available orally. Like IM nalbuphine.	Like nalbuphine.
Partial mu agonist opioid					
Buprenorphine (Buprenex[R])	0.3	- see comments -	- see comments -	Not available orally. Only parenteral form approved in U.S. for pain. Does not produce psychotomimetic effects.	May precipitate withdrawal in opioid-dependent patients. Not readily reversed by naloxone. Avoid in labor.

For these equianalgesic parenteral doses (based on intramuscular administration studies, also see comments) the time of peak analgesia in nontolerant patients ranges from one-half to one hour and the duration from four to six hours. The peak analgesic effect is delayed and the duration prolonged after oral administration.

[a]These doses are recommended starting parenteral doses from which the optimal dose for each patient is determined by titration and the maximal dose limited by adverse effects. For single IV bolus doses use half the parenteral dose.

[b]A value of 3 is used when calculating an oral dosage regimen of every 4 hrs around-the-clock.

[c]Irritating to tissues on repeated administration.

IM, intramuscular; IV, intravenous.

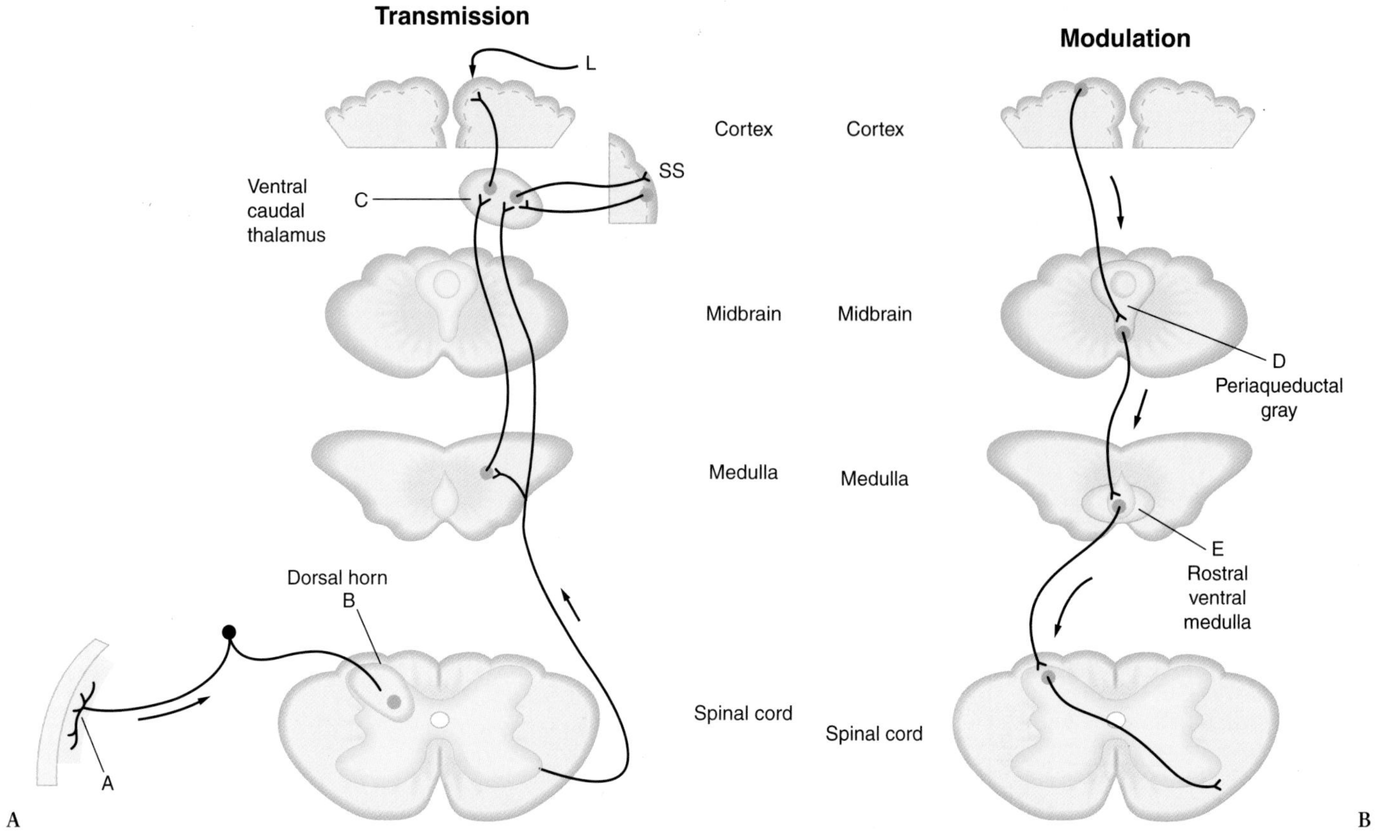

Transmission

Modulation

Cortex

Cortex

Ventral
caudal
thalamus

C

L

SS

Midbrain

Midbrain

D
Periaqueductal
gray

Medulla

Medulla

E
Rostral
ventral
medulla

Dorsal horn
B

Spinal cord

Spinal cord

A

B

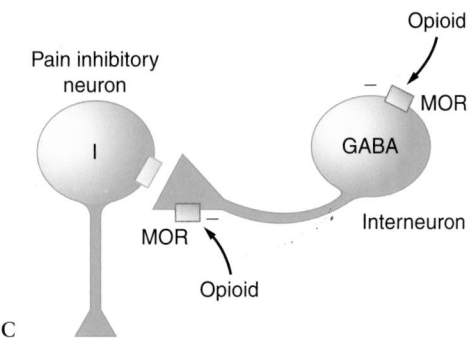

Pain inhibitory
neuron

I

MOR

Opioid

Opioid

MOR

GABA

Interneuron

C

FIGURE 78.1 (**A**) Sites of action common to all mu opiods; the location of mu opioid receptor (MORs). Modulation of ascending pain transmission pathways. MORs are found (**A**) in the periphery following inflammation (**B**) at pre- and postsynaptic sites in spinal cord dorsal horn (**C**) in the thalamus and in the limbic (**L**) and somatosensory (**SS**) cortex. (**B**) Descending modulation of pain transmission; the location of MORs. MORs are found in (**D**) the midbrain periaqueductal grey, the nucleus raphe magnus and (**E**) the rostral ventral medulla. Mu opioids activate a descending inhibitory system that modulates spinal cord dorsal horn pain transmission. (**C**) Descending modulation of pain transmission; GABAergic neurons and descending inhibition. A brainstem pain inhibitory neuron (**I**) is tonically inhibited by a GABAergic neuron. Opioids inhibit GABAergic neurons and remove the inhibition of the pain inhibitory neurons (PIN) that project from the rostral ventral medulla to the spinal cord dorsal horn. Thus, opioids produce a disinhibition of the PIN which results in the activation for descending inhibition. (Redrawn after: In Katzung B, ed., *Basic and Clinical Pharmacology*, 9th ed. New York: McGraw-Hill, 2004.)

Sedation

Morphine-like opioids produce drowsiness and sedation, which may be useful in certain clinical situations (e.g., pre-anesthesia) but usually are not desirable concomitants of analgesia, particularly in ambulatory patients. The CNS depressant actions of these drugs are at least additive to the sedative and respiratory depressant effects of sedative-hypnotics such as alcohol, barbiturates, and benzodiazepines.

Reducing the dose and interval, that is, giving a lower dose more frequently, produces a lower peak opioid serum concentration, which may counteract excessive sedation. In addition, other CNS depressants including sedative-hypnotics and antianxiety agents that add to or potentiate the sedative effects of opioids should be discontinued if possible. Concurrent administration of a central stimulant (e.g., dextroamphetamine, methylphenidate) twice daily helps counteract the sedative effects of opioids. Tolerance usually develops to the sedative effects of opioid analgesics within the first several days of repeated administration.

Nausea and Vomiting

The morphine-like analgesics produce nausea and vomiting by stimulating the chemoreceptor trigger zone (CTZ) in the area postrema of the medulla. The incidence of nausea and vomiting is markedly greater in ambulatory patients suggesting that these drugs also alter vestibular sensitivity. The ability of opioid analgesics to produce nausea and vomiting appears to vary with drug and among patients; some advantage may result from opioid rotation. Alternately, a centrally acting antiemetic such as a phenothiazine (e.g., prochlorperazine), a gastric prokinetic agent (e.g., metoclopramide), or a $5HT_3$ receptor antagonist (e.g., ondansetron) may be used in combination with the opioid. For some patients initiating treatment by the parenteral route and then switching to the oral route may reduce the emetic symptoms.[10]

Respiratory Depression

Respiratory depression is potentially the most serious adverse opioid effect. The morphine-like agonists act on brainstem respi-

TABLE 78.2

THE DESIRABLE AND UNDESIRABLE PROPERTIES OF MORPHINE AS AN ANALGESIC

Desirable	Undesirable
Analgesic	Sedation
Mood effects	Mental clouding
Sedation	Dizziness
	Mood effects
	Dysphoria
	Nausea and vomiting
	Respiratory depression
	Suppression of the cough reflex
Tolerance (to respiratory depression)	Tolerance (to analgesia)
	Physical dependence
	Substance dependence or addiction
	Spasmogenic
	Constipation

ratory centers to produce dose-related respiratory depression to the point of apnea. In humans, death due to overdose of a morphine-like agonist is nearly always due to respiratory arrest. Therapeutic doses of morphine may depress all phases of respiratory activity (rate, minute volume, and tidal exchange). However, as CO_2 accumulates, it stimulates central chemoreceptors, resulting in a compensatory increase in respiratory rate, which masks the degree of respiratory depression. At equianalgesic doses, the morphine-like agonists produce an equivalent degree of respiratory depression. Therefore, individuals with impaired respiratory function or bronchial asthma are at greater risk of experiencing clinically significant respiratory depression in response to usual doses of these drugs. Respiratory depression and CO_2 retention produces cerebral vasodilation and increased cerebrospinal fluid pressure unless the PCO_2 is normalized by artificial ventilation. Respiratory depression occurs most commonly in opioid-naïve patients following acute opioid administration and it is associated with other signs of CNS depression including sedation and mental clouding. Tolerance develops rapidly to this effect with repeated drug administration, often allowing use of opioids in the management of chronic pain without significant risk of respiratory depression. Obstructive sleep apnea is common in overweight chronic pain patients and it presents risk for opioid-induced respiratory depression, especially when the patients are sleeping. Recent reports suggest that opioids, and perhaps more so methadone, may induce potentially life-threatening central sleep apnea.[11,12] Respiratory depression can be reversed by timely administration of the opioid antagonist naloxone. In patients chronically receiving opioids who develop respiratory depression, naloxone diluted 1:10 should be titrated carefully to prevent the precipitation of severe withdrawal symptoms while reversing the respiratory depression. An endotracheal tube should be placed in the comatose patient before administering naloxone to prevent aspiration associated respiratory compromise with excessive salivation and bronchial spasm. In patients receiving meperidine chronically, naloxone may precipitate seizures by blocking the depressant action of meperidine and allowing the convulsant activity of the active metabolite, normeperidine, to be manifest.

The mixed agonist-antagonists, pentazocine, nalbuphine, butorphanol, and the partial agonist buprenorphine have different dose-response characteristics for their respiratory depression curves from the morphine-like opioids. While therapeutic doses of pentazocine produce respiratory depression equivalent to that of morphine, increasing the dose does not ordinarily produce a proportional increase in respiratory depression. Whether this apparent ceiling to respiratory depression offers any significant clinical advantage has not been determined. Also, naloxone reversal of the respiratory depression produced by buprenorphine requires relatively large doses (5–10 mg) and is delayed in onset.[13]

Constriction of the Pupil

Opioids stimulate the Edinger-Wesphal (parasympathetic) nucleus of the oculomotor nerve to produce miosis. Pinpoint pupils (along with respiratory depression and loss of consciousness) are the three pathognomonic signs of opioid overdose. These effects are antagonized by the opioid antagonist, naloxone. However, severe anoxia results in mydriasis.

Antitussive Effect

Opioids depress the cough centers in the medulla and, in turn, depress the cough reflex. However, the receptor mechanisms involved with cough differ from those involved with other opioid effects such as analgesia. Therefore, the dextrorotatory isomers of opioids (e.g., dextromethorphan), which do not bind to opioid receptors, are nevertheless effective antitussives.

Hypothalamic Effects

Morphine affects both body temperature and circulating neuroendocrine hormone levels by actions on the hypothalamus. Morphine alters hypothalamic heat-regulating resulting in a slightly lower body temperature. The release of corticotrophin-releasing hormone (CRH) and gonadotropin-releasing hormone (GnRH) are inhibited resulting in a decrease in luteinizing hormone (LH), follicle stimulating hormone (FSH), and adrenocorticotropic hormone (ACTH). Prolactin and antidiuretic hormone (ADH) release are increased. Based on observations in methadone maintenance patients, tolerance develops to the effects of morphine on these hypothalamic releasing factors.

The term *opioid-induced androgen deficiency* (OPIAD) describes clinically meaningful decrease in testosterone levels that occurs in the majority of men receiving ongoing morphine or other potent mu agonist opioid pharmacotherapy for chronic nonmalignant pain.[14] Worsening of pain, depressed mood, and refractoriness to treatment are common in such patients. Trials of androgen supplements have been helpful and this phenomenon also appears to occur in women, presumably due to progesterone suppression.

Central Nervous System Excitation

In contrast to the obvious opioid CNS depressant effects, there are excitatory effects. Dose-dependent convulsions occur in rodents but are rare in humans. However, normeperidine, a principal metabolite of meperidine, causes anxiety, tremors, myoclonus, and generalized seizures when it accumulates with repetitive dosing.[15] Naloxone does not reverse, and may even exacerbate, this hyperexcitability. The morphine-like opioids can produce multifocal myoclonus when administered in high doses to opioid-tolerant patients.

Opioid Tolerance, Dependence, and Addiction

The properties of the opioid analgesics that are most likely to lead to their being misused, or the patient mistreated, are effects mediated in the CNS that are seen following chronic administration. These include tolerance, physical dependence, and psychological dependence (addiction) (Table 78.2). It must be emphasized that while the development of tolerance and physical dependence are predictable pharmacologic effects seen in humans and laboratory animals in response to repeated administration of an opioid, these effects are distinct from the behavioral pattern seen in some individuals and described by the terms *substance dependence* (DSM IV) or *addiction*.[16] See Chapters 21 and 32 for more on addiction and dependence.

The Opioid Tolerant Patient and Opioid-Induced Hyperalgesia

Clinically Observable Tolerance

Tolerance to opioid effects occurs, but it is widely misunderstood by many. It is useful to subdivide tolerance into three dimensions: (1) tolerance to analgesia, (2) tolerance to other CNS-depressing effects and nausea, and (3) tolerance to opioid-induced constipation. Effective ongoing opioid therapy for chronic pain often requires increasing the dose numerous times in the first days to weeks of therapy until a consistently effective dose is found. This may be initial tolerance or simply reflect a dose-finding period. Once an effective dose is found which keeps the patient reasonably comfortable for a few days, it is relatively uncommon to have to increase the dose further unless the painful pathology increases or a new painful disorder occurs, the patient skips doses, the dosage form is changed, a drug interaction occurs or some other nonpharmacological event such as diversion occurs. These types of events probably account for the majority of patient requests for increasing opioid doses. This phenomenon has been termed "pseudotolerance." Clinically meaningful tolerance to analgesia occurs unpredictably in a minority of patients receiving opioids chronically for management of pain with a physiological basis. Many chronic cancer and noncancer pain patients remain comfortable without increasing pain complaints for months or even years without an increase in opioid dose. A minority require escalating opioid doses for reasons that remain unclear. When a patient no longer responds to increasing doses of a particular opioid that was previously effective, consider rotation to another opioid.

Conversely, nearly everyone develops some meaningful degree of tolerance to opioid-induced sedation, respiratory depression, nausea, and inhibition of coordination after 5 to 7 days of ongoing (around the clock) opioid pharmacotherapy. At the initiation of opioid therapy, an antiemetic may be needed, but commonly it is not needed after a few days of therapy. Many patients cannot drive a motor vehicle or operate machinery safely in the first days of opioid treatment. However, after a week of regularly scheduled opioid, most people can drive safely. When the dose is increased or if the patient abstains from the medication for a few days, another week may be required to reacquire tolerance to impaired eye-foot-hand coordination.

Tolerance to opioid-induced constipation does not appear to occur. Management of this common and sometimes debilitating side effect is discussed later.

Proposed Mechanisms of Tolerance

Opioid tolerance may be classified as associative or pharmacologic. Associative or contextual tolerance refers to changes in response that result when an opioid is administered in the presence of specific environmental cues that can induce tolerance specific to that setting.[17] Pharmacologic (nonassociative) tolerance is divided into pharmacodynamic tolerance, which is the result of neuronal adaptations that reduce the sensitivity of the system to the drug, and pharmacokinetic tolerance wherein the disposition of the drug is increased so that the effective concentra-

tion is reduced. Generally, pharmacodynamic mechanisms are thought to be most responsible for in vivo opioid tolerance. However, a contribution by associative tolerance cannot be excluded.

In the clinical setting, pharmacodynamic tolerance (hereafter simply tolerance) develops when a given dose of an opioid produces a decreasing effect, or when a larger dose is required to maintain the original effect. Some reports suggest that a degree of tolerance to analgesia appears to develop in most patients receiving opioid analgesics chronically.[18] Although tolerance to opioid analgesia appears to develop rapidly in animal models, it does so much more slowly in humans. Other reports however document that many patients do not experience tolerance to analgesia, that is, the same dose of opioid continues to provide effective analgesia over days to years unless there is increasing pathology.[19]

An early sign of the development of tolerance is the patient's complaint of a decrease in the duration of effective analgesia. The rate of tolerance development varies greatly among cancer patients; some demonstrate tolerance within days of initiating opioid therapy while others will remain well-controlled for many months on the same dose.[20] Unfortunately, pharmacodynamic tolerance cannot be adequately evaluated in the clinical situation. Factors described previously as causing "pseudotolerance" should be considered and addressed before concluding that pharmacodynamic tolerance has occurred. Both an increase in pain and the development of tolerance often respond to an increase in the opioid dose. Since the analgesic effect is a logarithmic function of the dose of opioid, a doubling of the dose may be required to restore full analgesia. Although controversial, the experience with cancer patients suggests that there appears to be no limit to the development of tolerance and with appropriate adjustment of dose, many, but not all patients can continue to obtain pain relief without intolerable adverse effects. Titration to effect remains the hallmark of effective opioid therapy.

Preclinical studies suggest that apparent opioid tolerance may result from excitatory CNS changes that facilitate transmission of and increase sensitivity to pain.[21] This condition is termed opioid-induced hyperalgesia (OIH). The basic phenomenon appears to result from the up-regulation of pronociceptive systems. The neuroanatomic substrates and signaling pathways involved in OIH are emerging.[21] However, the magnitude of the contribution of OIH to clinical opioid tolerance and its consequences for continued opioid therapy remain controversial. There is general agreement that during opioid withdrawal, OIH may occur and contribute to an exacerbation of pain.[22] Therefore, avoid acute withdrawal. Switching from a morphine-like opioid to a mixed agonist-antagonist (pentazocine, nalbuphine, and butorphanol) or the partial agonist buprenorphine must be avoided because of those drugs' ability to induce abrupt opioid withdrawal and cause concomitant hyperalgesia in opioid-dependent individuals.[1] Using a combination of an opioid with a nonopioid can enhance analgesia and reduce the rate of tolerance development since tolerance does not develop to the nonopioid component of the mixture. Opioid dose-sparing strategies can be used at the initiation of opioid therapy. Rotation to an alternative mu opioid agonist usually results in a relative reduction of opioid dosage due to incomplete cross-tolerance (see later) among this class of opioids.[23] The use of bolus or continuous epidural local anesthetics in patients with localized pain, for example, perineal pain, can dramatically reduce the need for systemic opioids and thus diminish opioid tolerance.

Animal study data on tolerance do not translate well to humans. The rates of development and loss of tolerance are not well defined in patients. The rate and extent of tolerance can vary greatly among different opioids and among patients receiving the same doses of a single opioid.

Cross-tolerance refers to the effects of one drug that confers tolerance to another drug, usually of the same class. While some cross-tolerance appears to occur among mu opioid agonists, the more relevant observation is that this cross-tolerance is incomplete. Therefore, when rotating from one opioid to another, this phenomenon must be taken into account in dosage calculations by initiating dosage with 25% to 50% of the calculated equianalgesic dose and titrating as required for pain relief.

The Opioid Dependent Patient

Physical dependence is the term used to describe an altered physiological state produced by repeated administration of an opioid which requires the continued administration of an opioid to prevent the emergence of a stereotypical withdrawal or abstinence syndrome that is characteristic for the particular opioid. The signs and symptoms of opioid withdrawal are described elsewhere.[24] The administration of an opioid antagonist to a physically dependent individual produces an immediate withdrawal syndrome. Patients who have received repeated doses of a morphine-like agonist, to the point at which they are physically dependent, may experience an opioid withdrawal reaction when given a mixed agonist-antagonist. Prior exposure to a morphine-like drug can greatly increase a patient's sensitivity to the antagonist component of a mixed agonist-antagonist. The severity of withdrawal is a function of the dose and duration of administration of the opioid just discontinued, that is, the patient's prior opioid exposure. The time course of the withdrawal syndrome is a function of the elimination half-life of the opioid to which the patient has become dependent (Table 78.3). Abstinence symptoms will appear within 6 to 12 hours and reach a peak at 24 to 72 hours, following cessation of a short half-life drug such as morphine, while onset may be delayed for 36 to 48 hours with methadone, a long half-life drug. Therefore, even for a patient in whom pain has been relieved by a procedure or treatment, it is necessary to slowly decrease the opioid dose to prevent withdrawal.

There is not one best method to taper opioids. Several different approaches have worked well. For patients who are anxious about tapering an opioid and those who may be especially sensitive to mild withdrawal effects, a slower taper may be indicated. A tapering rate of 10% to 20% per day is usually well tolerated.[25]

PLASMA HALF-LIFE VALUES FOR OPIOIDS AND THEIR ACTIVE METABOLITES

1. Shorter half-life opioids	Plasma half-life (hours)
Morphine	2 to 3.5
Morphine-6-glucuronide	2
Hydromorphone	2 to 3
Oxycodone	2 to 4
Fentanyl	3.7
Codeine	3
Meperidine	3 to 4
Pentazocine	2 to 3
Butorphanol	2.5 to 3.5
Buprenorphine	3 to 5
Nalbuphine	5
Longer half-life opioids	
Oxymorphone	7.5 to 9.5
Levorphanol	12 to 16
Propoxyphene	12
Normeperidine	14 to 21
Methadone	13 to 50
Norpropoxyphene	30 to 40

Experience indicates that the usual daily dose required to prevent withdrawal is approximately one-fourth of the previous daily dose. This dose is called, for want of a better term, the detoxification dose and is typically given in four divided parts. Commonly, the initial detoxification dose is given for 2 days and then decreased by one-half (administered in four divided doses) for 2 days until a total daily dose of 10 to 15 mg per day (in morphine equivalents) is reached. After 2 days on this dose, the opioid can be discontinued. Thus, a patient who had been receiving 240 mg per day of morphine equivalent for pain would require an initial detoxification dose of 60 mg given as 15 mg every 6 hours. This dose is decreased by 50% per day over the next 3 to 5 days.

Cross-dependence refers to the ability of one opioid to substitute for another in preventing the withdrawal syndrome. Cross dependence among the opioids allows rotation as described previously, and allows detoxification with an alternate opioid. For example, methadone can be substituted for morphine in the previous example by switching the patient to oral methadone at one-fourth to one-eighth of the patient's morphine dose and decreasing the dosage as described above.

The Opioid Addicted Patient With Pain

The terms *substance dependence* (DSM IV) and *addiction* describe a pattern of drug use characterized by a continued craving for an opioid that is manifested as compulsive drug seeking behavior leading to an overwhelming involvement with the use and procurement of the drug. Within these definitions most, but not all individuals, who are addicted to opioids will have acquired some degree of physical dependence. However, the converse is not true, so that an individual can be physically dependent on an opioid analgesic without being addicted. Fear of addition is a major concern limiting the use of appropriate doses of opioids. Recent national surveys indicate a significant increase in nonmedical use of prescription opioids. Increased reports of this problem coincided with attempts to make opioids more widely available to patients in pain. It is important to recognize the responsibility of clinicians to assess and monitor patients who are receiving long-term opioid treatment for pain to limit the abuse of these drugs.

Peripheral Effects of Opioids

In addition to the central effects, opioids have several important peripheral effects. The colon contains a large population of mu opioid receptors, and opioid-induced constipation can be a difficult clinical problem. Occupation and activation of those receptors by mu opioid agonists inhibits peristalsis. Stimulating laxatives are the most appropriate type of laxative to manage this and they often, but not always, are effective. Stool softeners alone usually are not.

Peripherally acting mu opioid antagonists are a new class of drugs useful in managing opioid-induced constipation that is not responsive to laxatives.[26] Methylnaltrexone, the first such drug in the class, was approved to manage opioid-induced constipation in advanced illness in 2008 as a subcutaneous injection.[27] At the time of this writing, an oral formulation was under study. Alvimopan, an oral peripheral mu opioid receptor antagonist, is the second drug in the class. It was approved soon after methylnaltrexone, but only for limited term use under strict controls for the management of postoperative ileus.[28]

Itching has been associated with morphine, presumably due to morphine-induced release of histamine from mast cells.[29] This phenomenon has not been well studied, but clinical reports suggest that it is more common with morphine than with other opioids. This is not indicative of an immune reaction that presents risk of anaphylactoid events. Systemic antipruritic agents have been used empirically. Rotation to another opioid is the most common management strategy.

Other peripheral opioid effects are associated with muscle relaxation. These include the cardiovascular system and cardiac rhythm, and relaxation of the ureter and bladder.

Opioid Effects in Pregnancy and on the Neonate

Pregnant women taking opioids may deliver an opioid-dependent infant. An estimated 1% to 2% of pregnant women take opioids.[30] A recent retrospective study[31] found that women on methadone maintenance had better outcomes than those who underwent methadone-assisted withdrawal and remained off methadone during pregnancy.

Routes for Opioid Administration

The oral (PO) route is generally the preferred route for opioid administration in ambulatory care due to convenience and relatively low cost. Immediate release oral opioid dosage forms include solutions, compressed tablets, and gelatin capsules. Although solutions are absorbed more promptly, it is not clear that this offers a clinically important advantage for most patients. The risk of patients incorrectly measuring the volume producing inconsistent and sometimes excessive doses is real.

Opioids can be administered systemically by oral, parenteral, rectal, sublingual, transdermal, and transmucosal routes. The mu agonists can be categorized as short-acting, long-acting, and ultra-short acting. Short half-life morphine-type opioids require frequent administration to maintain analgesia. Immediate-release morphine products provide about 4 hours of pain relief, and need to be dosed accordingly. Pharmaceutically formulated long-acting formulations (e.g., Avinza, Kadian, MS Contin, Opana ER, Oramorph-SR, OxyContin orally, and Duragesic transdermally) provide alternatives to frequent opioid administration of inherently short-acting drugs. Pharmacologically long-acting opioids, methadone and levorphanol, that have longer half-lives (Table 78.3) provide analgesia for 6 to 12 hours. Although methadone protects against opioid withdrawal for 24 or more hours, an oral dose only provides effective analgesia for about 8 hours. Pharmaceutically long-acting opioid dosage forms are generally relatively expensive, although generic forms of the original 8-hour formulations are now reasonably priced. The pharmacologically long-acting opioids, methadone and levorphanol, are relatively inexpensive.

Clinicians should be cautious about using extemporaneously compounded sustained release opioids. Although there are franchised compounding pharmacies that prepare these—and some market them aggressively—most inconsistently and unreliably release the active ingredient over time. Uneven pain control, exacerbation of pain and even overdose may result. The rapid onset of action of fentanyl mu agonists favors their use as a preoperative adjunct and their high lipophilicity facilitates transdermal and subcutaneous administration. When these highly lipophilic opioids are absorbed through or injected under the skin, they create a depot in subcutaneous fat from which the drug is slowly released. This depot effect also makes them very difficult to titrate to response.[32] However, when these medications are administered transmucosally or sublingually they are rapidly absorbed due to the lack of the buccal and sublingual fat. This prompt onset makes those routes useful in managing breakthrough pain.

Buprenorphine also has been formulated as a long-acting transdermal patch which was available in some countries, but not in the United States at the time of this writing.

The intravenous (IV) route of administration is generally preferred in immediate postoperative and intensive care settings. Intramuscular (IM) injection is painful and may produce uneven absorption. The subcutaneous (SC) route is preferred for injection when the intravenous route is impractical. The pharmacokinetics of SC administered opioids result in levels comparable to the IM route with the advantages that the SC route is far simpler to use and more comfortable for the patient. There is little or no rationale for IM opioid injections.

Table 78.1 lists relative equianalgesic doses and durations of action for commonly used opioids.

Alternative Noninvasive Routes

When oral administration is not possible, consider alternative noninvasive routes before resorting to injections, infusions, or the placement of epidural or intrathecal catheters.

Sublingual Administration

Transmucosal absorption occurs following sublingual administration of a reasonably lipophilic opioid. Oral transmucosal dosing may provide less consistent absorption than oral administration due to anatomical and physiological variability in the mucosa, for example, thickening due to pathology, pH. This route generally should not be considered when patients can take medications orally because oral administration is simpler and oral solid dosage forms provide more exact doses than liquid doses that must be measured before administration.

Sublingual administration entails placing of a small volume of concentrated liquid or a readily dissolvable solid dosage form under the tongue. Other locations in the mouth that can be used are the cheek pouch (buccal administration) and the anterior lip pouch. Clinical experience supports these routes but they have not been systematically studied. Patients should not eat or drink anything for about 15 minutes after taking an oral transmucosal dose. Doing so may increase the amount of drug that is swallowed, causing inconsistent interdose absorption.

Because opioids often cause dry mouth, it is important to counsel patients about this restriction. Some of an oral transmucosal dose tends to trickle down the throat or be actively swallowed, in which case that portion will undergo normal gastrointestinal absorption. Factors that influence the percentage of the dose that is swallowed include the volume of liquid and the condition of the oral mucosa. In general, no more than 1 mL of liquid should be placed under the tongue or in a mucosal pouch. Larger volumes tend to increase the amount of drug that is swallowed. Additional doses can be administered in a few minutes if necessary. It is necessary to moisten the mouth before dosing if it is dry as the result of disease or therapy. Stomatitis and excessive keratinization of the oral mucosa may make absorption inconsistent. The oral pH can influence absorption across the oral mucosa. Whereas normal mouth pH is 6.5, for many cancer patients receiving therapy it is above 7. The percentage of sublingual opioid absorbed increases with higher pH.[33] Because recently ingested foods and liquids can influence oral cavity pH, it is advisable to rinse the mouth with water before taking or administering an oral transmucosal dose, and to not eat or drink anything for the next 15 to 20 minutes.

The rectal route of administration is an alternative for patients unable to take drugs orally.

Table 78.4 lists rectal opioid times to peak and duration of action. This route of administration is generally acceptable for short-term use, but some patients find it esthetically objectionable.

This route is most commonly considered for short-term use and in care of terminal patients. The advantages of the rectal route include ease of use, lack of equipment, and low cost. Rectal

TABLE 78.4

RECTAL OPIOID TIMES TO PEAK AND DURATION OF ACTION

Morphine immediate release oral tablets	
peak	1.1 hour
duration	<6 hours
Morphine controlled release oral tablets	
peak	5.4 hours
duration	8–12 hours
Morphine oral solution	
peak	0.5 hours
duration	4–6 hours
Morphine rectal suppositories	
peak	1.1 hours
duration	<6 hours
Hydromorphone rectal suppositories	
peak	1 hour
duration	4–6 hours
Methadone oral tablets	
peak	2 hours
duration	6–8 hours
Oxycodone oral tablets and solution	
peak	3.1 hours
duration	8–12 hours

Table adapted from Warren D. Practical use of rectal medications in palliative care. *Pain Symptom Manage* 11:378–387, 1996.

administration is contraindicated for patients with painful anal lesions.[34]

Several opioid rectal suppository dosage forms are commercially available, some of which contain doses that are too low to be practical in advanced disease and palliative care. Therefore, extemporaneously compounded dosage forms are often needed. For such extemporaneously prepared forms, the rate and consistency of release of active ingredient from the dosage form and the risk of dose dumping resulting in toxicity are concerns.[35]

Rectally and orally administered morphine provides similar analgesic effect and serum levels. Although there is far less absorption following a rectal dose, a significant portion of an orally administered dose undergoes first-pass metabolism which is avoided with rectal administration. This effect may be unique to morphine and may not apply to other opioids. Immediate-release oral tablets, liquids, and suppositories of morphine have been used rectally with good effect.[36] Do not assume dose equivalency for other oral opioid dosage forms given rectally because of differences in physicochemical and pharmacokinetic properties. Controlled-release dosage forms do not necessarily have the same effects and duration of action when administered orally and rectally. Lower peak serum levels and more interpatient variability occur with all controlled-release dosage forms when they are given rectally rather than orally. MS Contin administered rectally produces clinical effects similar to those obtained with the same dose taken orally, and may produce less rectal irritation than commercially available rectal morphine suppositories.[37] Some palliative care nurses administer tablets rectally in a small mass of butter or an empty gelatin capsule. This is unnecessary and may delay absorption of the opioid. Simply ensure that the rectum is empty before inserting the tablets.

Oxycodone produces similar areas under the curve (AUCs) when administered rectally and orally.[38] Although rectal oxycodone suppositories are available in some countries, only oral solid and liquid forms are marketed in the United States. The commer-

cially available oral liquid could be used rectally, but administration would be required every 3 to 4 hours for continual analgesia.

Informal, anecdotal reports of both immediate-release and controlled-release oral solid dosage forms administered via the vagina and through colostomy and ileostomy stomas also have been mentioned, but no data to support such use have been published. A comparative study of morphine administered rectally and through a colostomy led the investigators to conclude that the opioid should not be given through a colostomy due to poor and inconsistent absorption.[39] Animal studies of methadone administered vaginally indicate possible usefulness of that route.[40] But clinical data to support that hypothesis were not identified in a comprehensive literature search.

Nebulized opioids have been used and may provide good pain relief. However, that is not a cost-effective administration method for analgesia. Nebulized opioids are sometimes used as an alternative to sublingual administration to treat dyspnea (air hunger) in advanced disease.[41] Very small particles are needed to deliver drug to the alveoli. Use of an administration method other than a high quality small particle nebulizer can result in drug deposition on the palate with little clinical effect. Hand-held, squeeze bulb devices are not useful. Nebulized opioid administration requires sterile solutions, which increase expense as compared to oral and sublingual routes.

Epidural, Intrathecal, and Intraventricular Administration

The term spinal administration is sometimes unclear due to inconsistent differentiation between epidural and intrathecal administration. It is therefore better to avoid the term spinal and specify either epidural or intrathecal (subarachnoid). Both of these routes are being used increasingly, the former commonly for postoperative pain control and the latter more for chronic administration. In obstetrical analgesia, a single intrathecal dose followed by continuous or intermittent epidural administration often is used. Epidural patient-controlled analgesia also is used in some settings.[42]

The epidural space is a fat-filled potential space that contains blood vessels (Fig. 78.2). Therefore, epidural opioid administra-

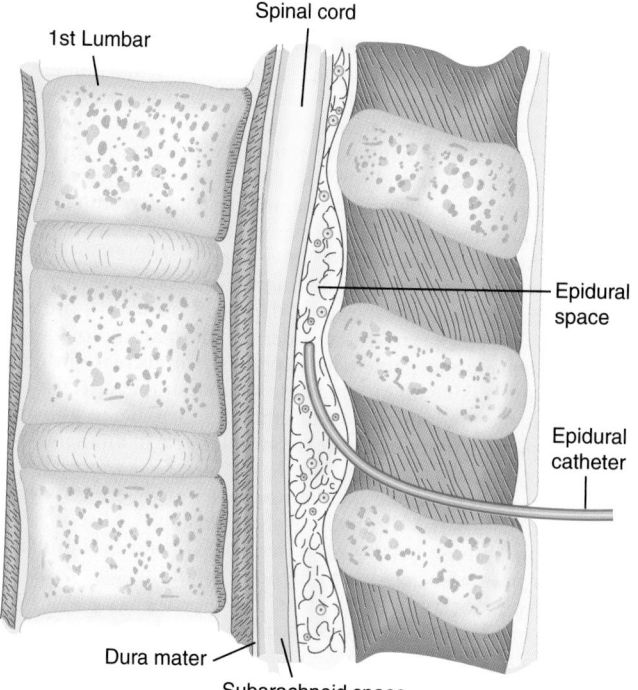

FIGURE 78.2 Drug delivery catheter in the epidural space.

tion can cause systemic effects albeit much more slowly and less than with intravenous and other systemic routes. The intrathecal route avoids some of the supraspinally mediated toxicity associated with the systemic delivery of these medications. The epidural and intrathecal routes each have advantages and disadvantages. Epidural administration allows opioid placement at any dermatomal level and does not require puncturing of the dura. However, larger doses are required and systemic effects may occur with epidural administration, increasing the risk of adverse effects. For morphine, intrathecal doses are typically one-tenth of those needed for an equianalgesic epidural dose. Intrathecal administration requires puncturing the dura, which delivers drug closer to the spinal cord receptors. Disadvantages of intrathecal use include increased potential for meningitis and risk of postdural puncture headaches. Dose-related problems associated with spinal analgesia include pruritus, urinary retention, and delayed respiratory depression.

Intraventricular administration has been used in cancer patients unresponsive to opioids administered by other routes.[43] The Ommaya reservoir has been used for this method of drug delivery.

With any direct central administration method, the pharmacokinetics of the opioids can vary greatly from systemic administration. Physicochemical drug characteristics, especially lipophilicity, become very important with these routes.

SOME SPECIFIC OPIOID CHARACTERISTICS

Morphine

The oral bioavailability of morphine varies from 35% to 75%, which helps to explain some of the interpatient variability in response. Its average plasma half-life of 3 hours is somewhat shorter than its 4- to 6-hour duration of analgesia; this limits accumulation. With repetitive administration, its pharmacokinetics remain linear and there does not appear to be autoinduction of biotransformation even following large chronic doses.[44] These pharmacokinetic properties contribute to the safe use of morphine over time. The two major morphine metabolites are morphine-3 glucuronide (M3G) and morphine-6 glucuronide (M6G). M6G appears to contribute to the analgesic activity of morphine.[45,46] M6G is eliminated by the kidney and, because it has a somewhat longer half-life than the parent compound, will accumulate relative to morphine in patients with renal insufficiency. A survey of steady-state morphine and M6G levels and adverse effects in 109 cancer patients indicated that myoclonus or cognitive impairment was not associated with M6G accumulation.[47] For a subset of the 20 patients with the highest M6G levels (>2000 ug/mL), the M6G level and concurrent organ failure was associated with the most severe toxicity (respiratory depression and/or obtundation).[47] It is appropriate to consider an alternate opioid for a patient receiving morphine who experiences a decrease in renal function and a concomitant increase in undesirable effects.

M3G is the predominant metabolite of morphine in humans. It lacks opioid activity but has excitatory effects in animals after direct injection into the CNS. This has led to the suggestion that M3G may be responsible for the neuroexcitatory effects sometimes seen with large chronic morphine dosing.[48] M3G has an elimination half-life even longer than M6G, and accumulated M3G has been associated with myoclonus and hyperalgesia although that association is not clear.[49]

Based on single dose studies in patients with either acute or chronic pain, the relative potency of intramuscular to oral morphine is 1:6. However, with repeated administration, when patients are dosed on a regular schedule (around the clock), the parenteral to oral dose ratio is reduced to 1:2 or 1:3 (Table 78.1).

This presumably is due to accumulation of the M6G metabolite, which is active and has a longer half-life than the parent drug.

The sustained-release morphine preparations provide analgesia with a duration of 8 to 12 hours (MS Contin, Roxanol-SR) or 12 to 24 hours (Kadian, Avinza) and allow patients greater freedom from repetitive dosing, especially during the night. Patients may be titrated using the immediate release morphine and, once stabilized, converted to the sustained-release preparation according to a schedule appropriate for the form used. To manage acute "breakthrough" pain, "rescue" medication (immediate release morphine) should be made available to the patient receiving delayed-release preparations.

Allergy to morphine has historically been associated more with trace plant protein in morphine derived from natural sources (opium). Today, most morphine formulations are very pure and contain so little plant protein that this problem is relatively uncommon. When it does occur, a synthetic opioid is indicated. True allergy to the morphine molecule is rare.

Hydromorphone

Hydromorphone is a short half-life opioid used as an alternative to morphine by the oral and parenteral routes. It is a semisynthetic compound. It is more soluble than morphine and is available in a concentrated parenteral dosage form at 10 mg/mL which can be advantageous for opioid tolerant patients and cachectic patients in whom the volume of the opioid solution must be limited.

Methadone

Methadone use in pain management has dramatically increased in recent years with mixed effects. The original interest in methadone was based on its high (1:2) oral to parenteral potency ratio, which is a reflection of its high oral bioavailability that averages 85%. It was found to be useful in opioid rotation, because its incomplete cross-tolerance with opioids like morphine allow a significant reduction in dose when switching from morphine to methadone. Methadone is relatively inexpensive and its metabolites do not have opioid activity or apparent toxicity. As with other opioids, it may provide a larger therapeutic window in a particular patient although this cannot be determined prior to a therapeutic trial. Preclinical studies demonstrated the NMDA receptor antagonist activity of both isomers of methadone. In animals this NMDA receptor antagonist activity included antihyperalgesic activity and the ability to prevent the development of morphine tolerance.[1,50] However, it remains to be determined whether effects occur in humans at the doses of methadone used clinically.

A major limitation on the use of methadone as a first-line opioid for pain management relates to its safety. Its population pharmacokinetics are variable with a plasma half-life that averages 24 hours but may range from 13 to 50 hours. Since initially the duration of analgesia is often only 4 to 8 hours, repetitive analgesic dosing of methadone can lead to drug accumulation, because of this discrepancy between its plasma half-life and the duration of analgesia during initial dosing. Sedation, confusion, and even death can occur when patients are not carefully monitored and dosage adjusted during the accumulation period that can last from 5 to 10 days. More recently a second safety issue relates to concerns about the potential for methadone to prolong the QTc interval and predispose patients to torsade de pointes (TdP), a life-threatening arrhythmia.

Finally, there is the stigma among pain patients and the public attached to the use of methadone for the treatment of opioid addiction.

Oxycodone

Oxycodone is a mu opioid agonist that also may have kappa agonist activity. The latter may be advantageous in visceral pain such as occurs in gallbladder and pancreatic disease.[51]

Oxymorphone

Oxymorphone, a congener of morphine, is parenterally approximately 10 times more potent than morphine. Immediate- and extended-release oral formulations (Opana and Opana ER) have recently been released. The extended release dosage is indicated for every 12 hour dosing. As with other extended release dosage forms, it should not be used on an-as-need (PRN) schedule or used in opioid naive patients. It is contraindicated in patients with severe hepatic impairment. Opana ER is available in 5 to 40 mg tablets. The usual starting dose oral dose is 5 mg. Food enhances the bioavailability, so Opana ER should be taken 1 hour prior to a meal or 2 hours after a meal. Coingestion of alcohol with Opana ER may also increase plasma levels of oxymorphone. Oxymorphone remains available for parenteral and rectal (suppository) administration.

Levorphanol

Levorphanol is a longer half-life opioid (Table 78.3) that sometimes can be a useful alternative to morphine, but it must be used cautiously to prevent accumulation. For patients who are unable to tolerate morphine and methadone, levorphanol represents a useful medication with a good oral to parenteral potency ratio of 1:2.

Meperidine

The primary metabolite of meperidine (pethidine), normeperidine, has a unique neurotoxicity, which can lead to symptoms ranging from irritability to grand mal seizures. Because the metabolite half-life is much longer than the parent compound, the metabolite accumulates rapidly. Therefore, meperidine should not be used for longer than 24 to 48 hours. Many hospitals and health centers have removed it from their formularies for this reason.

Meperidine may have a relatively unique usefulness in managing rigors associated with anesthetics and amphotericin.[52] Other opioids and benzodiazepines have been suggested as alternatives for managing rigors, but controlled trials to document that are lacking.

Codeine

Codeine is an analgesic of limited usefulness because it is actually a prodrug that must be metabolized to morphine for effect. Because over 10% of the population lacks the cytochrome P-450 hepatic enzyme isoform needed for that metabolism, many patients get poor or no analgesia from codeine. Toxicity has occurred in nursing infants whose mothers ingested relatively low dose codeine when the mothers were rapid metabolizers, a more rare polymorphism than the poor metabolism phenotype, causing morphine levels that can be lethal to the infants.[53] Codeine is observed to produce more nausea and undesired central effects per unit of analgesia than equianalgesic morphine doses. While many clinicians believe that codeine is safer than other opioids, data do not support that contention. Codeine's usefulness is more as an antitussive and antidiarrheal agent than as an analgesic.

Codeine abuse is common. This may be due in part to its availability in antitussive formulations, for example, elixir terpin hydrate with codeine, which are only Schedule V controlled substances that can be purchased without a prescription in many jurisdictions.

Hydrocodone

Hydrocodone is a pure mu agonist much like morphine or oxycodone. Despite its name, hydrocodone is far more similar to morphine than codeine. Hydrocodone is the only opioid that is scheduled in the United States Federal Controlled Substances Act, which specifies it is to be a Schedule III controlled substance when formulated as a combination dosage form, for example, hydrocodone plus acetaminophen. Single ingredient hydrocodone dosage forms would be Schedule II. As such, the combinations are the most widely prescribed and, therefore, most widely abused opioids in the United States. There is no scientific rationale for hydrocodone being scheduled differently than oxycodone. The dose limit on hydrocodone-acetaminophen tablets and capsules is due to the acetaminophen, not the opioid.

Propoxyphene

Propoxyphene is a weak analgesic which also has a toxic metabolite resulting in being included on the Beer's List of inappropriate medications for elderly patients.[54] Studies have long supported the position that most of the efficacy of the commonly used propoxyphene-acetaminophen combination is due to the acetaminophen.[55]

Propoxyphene has been removed from many leading hospital formularies.

Tramadol

Tramadol is a weak mu agonist and weak norepinephrine-serotonin reuptake inhibitor. Neither mechanism alone explains its analgesic efficacy. The probable mechanism is synergism between these two weak effects. Tramadol at a dose of 100 mg four times daily may produce analgesia similar to that of oral morphine 5 to 10 mg, four times daily. Higher doses of tramadol offer no advantage and produce greater toxicity. Due to its mechanism, tramadol is more useful in neuropathic than nociceptive pain and it appears more appropriate as a chronic than acute use analgesic because the dose must be titrated up slowly to minimize risk of lowering seizure threshold.[56] A combination of tramadol 75% with acetaminophen 25% appears to be as effective as the single ingredient analgesic. Tramadol is not a controlled substance but it does have abuse potential and can be highly toxic when misused.[57]

Table 78.5 lists metabolites of commonly used opioids.

SELECTING AMONG THE OPIOIDS FOR CLINICAL USE

Table 78.1 lists other morphine-like agonists that may be substituted for morphine. An alternative opioid to morphine may be selected based on the need with a particular patient to overcome an adverse effect of morphine (e.g., vomiting or sedation). Other reasons include the cost, a patient's favorable prior experience with another opioid or even local availability of other morphine-like opioids. There is no evidence to suggest that any other opioid has greater analgesic efficacy than morphine in the population as a whole but interpatient variability does exist. Only clinical

TABLE 78.5

OPIOID METABOLITES

Parent drug (% eliminated unchanged)	Duration of analgesia	Metabolites (% if known)	Metabolite half-lives (hours)	Primary metabolite elimination	Comments
Morphine (~7.2% IV, ~3.7% PO)	4–6				In renal failure, Vd may be smaller producing increased plasma levels; enterohepatic circulation of parent drug and glucuronide metabolites
		morphine-3-glucuronide (57–74) morphine-6-glucuronide (4.7–12)	2.8–4	Renal	T½ ~41–141 hours in renal failure, contributes to dose dependent myoclonus and seizures; T½ ~89–136 hours in renal failure; may cause narcosis in renal failure; Intrathecally ~100 times more potent than morphine; accumulates with chronic dosing
		morphine-3-ethereal sulfate (5–10) normorphine (3.5) morphine-N-oxide	Duration 2 × longer than parent drug		
Codeine 11.1%[5]	4–6	codeine-6-glucuronide norcodeine morphine (10)		Renal	primary elimination form; profound narcosis has occurred in chronic renal failure equipotent to codeine in analgesic activity formation dependent on CYP 450 2D6; genetic polymorphism impacts effectiveness and toxicity
Fentanyl (<10%)	1–2	norfentanyl		renal, hepatic	may be extensively liver metabolized metabolized to despropionyl fentanyl may cause neurotoxic side effects structurally similar to normeperidine
		4-N-anilinopiperidine			
Hydromorphone (5.6%)		hydromorphone-3-glucuronide hydromorphone-6-glucuronide nor-metabolites		Renal	clearance dependent on hepatic blood flow; shown to accumulate in renal failure in one patient formed from intermediate metabolites, dihydroisomorphine, and dihydromorphine
Levorphanol	6–8	levorphanol glucuronide		Renal	liver metabolized by glucuronide conjugation
Meperidine 5% (uncontrolled urine pH)	2.5–3.5	normeperidine (5–30)	15–30	Renal, hepatic	bioavailability increases from 50% to 80% in cirrhosis; T½ of meperidine and normeperidine prolonged in cirrhosis; urinary pH affects elimination of unchanged meperidine in urine; 25% in acidic urine vs. 1% to 2% in alkaline urine; T½ prolonged in renal failure(>30 hr); double the CNS excitatory effects and half the analgesic effect of meperidine; urinary elimination is pH dependent: uncontrolled pH f_e = 0.05–0.06, acidic urine f_e = 0.30, alkaline urine f_e <0.031
		meperidinic acid			inactive metabolite

Drug (f_e)	Half-life (h)	Metabolites	Route of elimination	Comments
Methadone 21% (acidic urine increases the fraction of elimination [f_e])	4–6 initially; 6–8 after steady state (1–2 days)		renal, biliary	in an anephric patient, 98% of methadone was found in feces as metabolite, suggesting a shift in metabolism from renal to fecal urinary excretion of methadone and metabolites is dose dependent and is the major route of elimination in doses >55 mg/day; 10% to 45% of methadone is eliminated in feces as metabolites
		1,5-demethyl-2-ethyl-3,3-diphenyl-1-pyrroline 2-ethyl-5-methyl-3,3-diphenyl-1-pyrroline		unpredictable T½ with chronic dosing long term analgesia is 10 times morphine; major metabolite $f_e = 0.30$
		methadone-N-oxide		minor metabolite
Oxycodone	3–6	noroxymorphone	hepatic, renal	minor metabolite
		oxymorphone		renally excreted, primarily as metabolites
		noroxycodone		active metabolite; renally excreted as oxymorphone-glucuronide
Propoxyphene 1.5%	4–6			may depress cardiac conduction secondary to anesthetic properties; half-life not altered in renal failure
		norpropoxyphene (25)	renal	local anesthetic properties; cardiac conduction abnormalities can result with accumulation (not reversed by naloxone); not hemodialyzable
	22.9–36.6			
Buprenorphine	6–8			one source says it is almost completely metabolized in the liver, but another source says the majority is excreted unchanged in feces and undergoes enterohepatic circulation with metabolites
		glucuronidation products	renal	may have weak analgesic properties
		norbuprenorphine	renal	primary route of elimination is renal; hepatic, biliary, and fecal routes also involved
Butorphanol 5%	3–4			extensively liver metabolized; Cl_{Cr} <30 mL/min half-life increased from 5.75 to 10.5 hours in single-dose, intranasal administration
		norbutorphanol	biliary	no analgesic activity
		hydroxybutorphanol	renal	analgesic activity; major metabolite; 60% to 80% renally excreted
Nalbuphine 7%	3–6			hepatic metabolism; metabolites and parent compound excreted in urine and feces
				major route of elimination is biliary secretion
Pentazocine 4.9%	3–6			(l) isomer responsible for analgesic activity; large interpatient variability in metabolism and oral bioavailability
				bioavailability in cirrhotic patients increased to 60% to 70%
		alcoholic and carboxylic acid metabolites	renal	inactive metabolites
		pentazocine glucuronide	renal	inactive metabolite

Table adapted from the following references: McEvoy G, ed. AHFS Drug Information 2008. Bethesda: American Society of Health-System Pharmacists, 2008; Babul N, Darke A. Putative role of hydromorphone metabolites in myoclonus. *Pain* 1993;52:123; Chan G, Matzke G. Effects of renal insufficiency on the pharmacokinetics and pharmacodynamics of opioid analgesics. *Drug Intell Clin Pharm* 1987;21:773–783; Lötsch J, Stockmann A, Brune K, et al. Pharmacokinetics of morphine and its glucuronides after intravenous infusion of morphine and morphine-6-glucuronide in healthy volunteers. *Clin Pharmacol Ther* 1996;60:316–325; Mulvana D, Duncan G, Shyu W, et al. Quantitative determination of butorphanol and its metabolites in human plasma by gas chromatography-electron capture negative-ion chemical ionization mass spectrometry. *J Chromatogr B Biomed Appl* 1996;682:289–300; Gutstein HB, Akil H. Opioid Analgesics. In: Bruton LL, Lazo JS, Parker KL, eds. *Goodman and Gilman's The Pharmacological Basis of Therapeutics.* New York: McGraw-Hill, 2006:547–590; Shyu W, Morgenthien E, Barbhaiya R. Pharmacokinetics of butorphanol nasal spray in patients with renal impairment. *Br J Clin Pharmacol* 1996;41:397–402; Steinberg R, Gilman D, Johnson F. Acute toxic delirium in a patient using transdermal fentanyl. *Anesth Analg* 1992;75:1014–1016.

trial can adequately determine the opioid that is the best choice for a specific patient.

CONCLUSION

Opioids are essential analgesics for the management of severe pain. The risk to benefit ratio can be favorable when they are used properly. Respiratory depression is a risk particularly in the opioid naïve while the chronic toxicity may be related to endocrinopathy, especially androgen deficiency.

Titration to response remains the only effective way to determine the optimal opioid and dose for a specific patient. The initial opioid to be used should be based on past patient experience, dosing schedule compatibility with the patient's life style and probable adherence to the regimen, and cost. Regular observation for adverse effects is essential. When adverse events occur, consider whether changing to a different opioid may be preferable to additional drugs to treat the adverse effect. If opioid efficacy wanes, consider whether nonopioid therapy might then suffice and if androgen deficiency is a contributor. Opioid rotation also should be considered. Because of the comorbidities that occur with chronic pain, opioid monotherapy is seldom indicated; rather, additional pharmacotherapies, concurrent physical therapy, and psychotherapy are often required for appropriate pain management.

Opioid pharmacokinetics and pharmacodynamics are well characterized at all stages of life. Caution is indicated in elderly and renally impaired patients due to possible opioid accumulation. Additive and synergistic effects with other central nervous system depressant medications are common. All opioid regimens should be reevaluated at regular intervals and the medication should be tapered off if it is no longer needed or is no longer providing more benefits than adverse effects.

Pain remains a major public health problem and opioids are an important part of the analgesic armamentarium. Used wisely, opioids have great value.

References

1. Inturrisi CE. Clinical pharmacology of opioids for pain. *Clin J Pain* 2000;18: S3–S13.
2. Gutstein HB, Akil H. Opioid Analgesics. In: Bruton LL, Lazo JS, Parker KL, eds. *Goodman & Gilman's The Pharmacological Basis of Therapeutics*. New York: McGraw-Hill, 2006:547–590.
3. Lötsch J, Geisslinger G. Current evidence for a genetic modulation of the response to analgesics. *Pain* 2006;121:1–5.
4. Angst MS, Clark JD. Opioid-induced hyperalgesia: a qualitative systematic review. *Anesthesiology* 2006;104:570–587.
5. Nestler EJ. Molecular mechanisms of drug addiction. *Neuropharmacology* 2004;47 suppl 1:24–32.
6. Kieffer BL, Gavériaux-Ruff C. Exploring the opioid system by gene knockout. *Prog Neurobiol* 2002;66:285–306.
7. Terman GW, Bonica JJ. Spinal Mechanisms and Their Modulation. In: Loeser JD, Butler SH, Chapman CR, Turk DC, eds. *Bonica's Management of Pain*. Philadelphia: Lippincott Williams and Wilkins, 2001:73–152.
8. Fakata KL, Lipman AG. Gastrointestinal Opioid Physiology and Pharmacology. In: Yuan SH, ed. *Opioid Bowel Dysfunction*. Binghamton, NY: Haworth Medical Press, 2005.
9. O'Brien CP, Gardner EL. Critical assessment of how to study addiction and its treatment: human and non-human animal models. *Pharmacol Ther* 2005; 108:18–58.
10. Rainville P, Duncan GH, Price DD, et al. Pain affect encoded in human anterior cingulate but not somatosensory cortex. *Science* 1997;277:968–971.
11. Foley KM. Problems of overarching importance which transcend organ systems. In: Bennett JC, Plum F, eds. *Cecil's Textbook of Medicine*. Philadelphia: WB Saunders, 1996.
12. Walker JM, Farney RJ, Rhondeau SM, et al. Chronic opioid use is a risk factor for the development of central sleep apnea and ataxic breathing. *J Clin Sleep Med* 2007;3(5):455–461.
13. Webster LR, Choi Y, Desai H, et al. Sleep-disordered breathing and chronic opioid therapy. *Pain Med* 2008;9(4):425–432.
14. Gal TJ. Naloxone reversal of buprenorphine-induced respiratory depression. *Clin Pharmacol Ther* 1989;45:66–71.
15. Daniell HW. Hypogonadism in men consuming sustained-action oral opioids. *J Pain* 2002;3(5):377–384.
16. Kaiko RF, Foley KM, Grabinski PY, et al. Central nervous system excitatory effects of meperidine in cancer patients. *Ann Neurol* 1983;13:180–185.
17. O'Brien C. Drug Addiction and Drug Abuse. In: Bruton LL, Lazo JS, Parker KL, eds. *Goodman & Gilman's The Pharmacological Basis of Therapeutics*. New York: McGraw-Hill, 2006:607–627.
18. Mitchell JM, Basbaum AI, Fields HL. A locus and mechanism of action for associative morphine tolerance. *Nat Neurosci* 2000;3:47–53.
19. McQuay H. Opioids in pain management. *Lancet* 1999;353:2229–2232.
20. Lipman AG, Jackson KC. Opioids. In: Warfield C, Bajwa Z, eds. *Principles and Practice of Pain Management*, 2nd ed. New York: McGraw-Hill, 2003.
21. Kanner RM, Foley KM. Patterns of narcotic drug use in a cancer pain clinic. *Ann N Y Acad Sci* 1981;362:161–172.
22. Carroll IR, Angst MS, Clark JD. Management of perioperative pain in patients chronically consuming opioids. *Reg Anesth Pain Med* 2004;29:576–591.
23. Inturrisi CE. Opioid Rotation. In: Schmidt RF, Willis WD, eds. *Encyclopedia of Pain*. Berlin, Heidelberg, New York: Springer, 2007:1561–1564.
24. O'Brien C. Drug addiction and drug abuse. In: Hardman JG, Limbird LE, eds. *Goodman & Gilman's The Pharmacological Basis of Therapeutics*. New York: McGraw-Hill, 2001:621–642.
25. Hare BD, Lipman AG. Uses and Misuses of Medication in the Treatment of Chronic Pain. In: Hare BD, Fine P, eds. *Chronic Pain, Problems in Anesthesia*. Philadelphia: JB Lippincott Co., 1990.
26. Yuan CS, ed. *Handbook of Opioid Bowel Syndrome*. Binghamton NY: Haworth Medical Press, 2005.
27. Thomas J, Lipman AG, Slatkin N, et al. *J Pain Symptom Manage* 2008;35: 103–113.
28. Curran MP, Robyns GW, Scott LJ, et al. Alvimopan. *Drugs* 2008;68(14): 2011–2019.
29. Barke KE, Hough LB. Opiates, mast cells and histamine release. *Life Sci* 1993; 53(18):1391–1399.
30. Minozzi S, Amato L, Vecchi S, et al. Maintenance agonist treatments for opiate dependent pregnant women. *Cochrane Database Syst Rev* 2008 Apr 16;(2): CD006318.
31. Jones HE, O'Grady KE, Malfi D, et al. Methadone maintenance vs. methadone taper during pregnancy: maternal and neonatal outcomes. *Am J Addict* 2008; 17(5):372–386.
32. Ashburn MA, Lipman AG. Management of pain in the cancer patient. *Anesth Analg* 1993;76:402–416.
33. Weinberg DS, Inturrisi CE, Reidenberg B, et al. Sublingual absorption of selected opioid analgesics. *Clin Pharmacol Ther* 1988;44:335–342.
34. Jacox A, Carr DB, Payne R, et al. Management of Cancer Pain. Clinical Practice Guideline. AHCPR Publication Number 94-0592. Rockville, MD: Agency for Health Care Policy and Research, US Department of Health and Human Services, Public Health Service, 1994.
35. Allen L. Suppositories as drug delivery systems. *J Pharm Care Pain Symptom Control* 1997;5:17–26.
36. Maloney CM, Kesner RK, Klein G, et al. The rectal administration of MS Contin: clinical implications of use in end stage cancer. *Am J Hospice Care* 1989;6:34–35.
37. Kaiko RF, Fitzmartin RD, Thomas GB, et al. The bioavailability of morphine in controlled release 30 mg tablets. *Pharmacotherapy* 1992;12:107–113.
38. Leow KP, Smith MT, Watt JA, et al. Comparative oxycodone pharmacokinetics in humans after intravenous, oral and rectal administration. *Ther Drug Monit* 1992;14:479–484.
39. Højsted J, Rubeck-Petersen K, Rask H, et al. Comparative bioavailability of morphine suppository given rectally and in a colostomy. *Eur J Clin Pharmacol* 1990;39:49–50.
40. Swanson BN, Gordon WP, Lynn RK, et al. Seminal excretion, vaginal absorption, distribution and whole blood kinetics of d-methadone in the rabbit. *J Pharmacol Exp Ther* 1978;206:507–514.
41. Viola R, Kiteley C, Lloyd NS, et al. The management of dyspnea in cancer patients; a systematic review. *Support Care Cancer* 2008;16(4):329–337.
42. Cata JP, Noguera EM, Parke E, et al. Patient-controlled epidural analgesia (PCEA) for postoperative pain control after lumbar spinal surgery. *J Neurosurg Anesthesiol* 2008;20:256–260.
43. Karavelis A, Foroglou G, Selviaridis P, et al. Intraventricular administration of morphine for control of intractable cancer pain in 90 patients. *Neurosurgery* 1996;39(1):57–61.
44. Inturrisi CE, Hanks GWC. Opioid Analgesic Therapy. In: Doyle D, Hanks GWC, MacDonald N, eds. *Oxford Textbook of Palliative Medicine*. Oxford: Oxford University Press, 1993:166–182.
45. Portenoy RK, Thaler HT, Inturrisi CE, et al. The metabolite morphine-6-glucuronide contributes to the analgesia produced by morphine infusion in patients with pain and normal renal function. *Clin Pharmacol Ther* 1992;51:422–431.
46. Lotsch J. Opioid metabolites. *J Pain Symptom Manage* 2005;29(5 suppl): S10–S24.
47. Tiseo PJ, Thaler HT, Lapin J, et al. Morphine-6-glucuronide concentrations and opioid-related side effects: a survey in cancer patients. *Pain* 1995;61: 47–54.
48. Smith MT. Neuroexcitatory effects of morphine and hydromorphone: evidence implicating the 3-glucuronide metabolites. *Clin Exp Pharmacol Physiol* 2000; 27:524–528.

49. McNicol E, Horowicz-Mehler N, Fisk RA, et al. Management of opioid side effects in cancer-related and chronic noncancer pain: a systematic review. *J Pain* 2003;4(5):231–256.

50. Davis AM, Inturrisi CE. d-Methadone blocks morphine tolerance and N-methyl-D-aspartate-induced hyperalgesia. *J Pharmacol Exp Ther* 1999;289:1048–1053.

51. Staahl C, Dimcevski G, Andersen SD, et al. Differential effect of opioids in patients with chronic pancreatitis: an experimental pain study. *Scand J Gastroenterol* 2007;42(3):383–390.

52. Holtzclaw BJ. Control of febrile shivering during amphotericin B therapy. *Oncol Nurs Forum* 1990;17(4):521–524.

53. Ferner RE. Did the drug cause death? Codeine and breastfeeding. *Lancet* 2008;372(9639):606–608.

54. Sloane PD, Zimmerman S, Brown LC, et al. Inappropriate medication prescribing in residential care/assisted living facilities. *J Am Geriatr Soc* 2002;50(6):1001–1011.

55. Miller RR, Feingold A, Paxinos J. Propoxyphene hydrochloride. A critical review. *JAMA* 1970;213(6):996–1006.

56. Christoph T, Kögel B, Strassburger W, et al. Tramadol has a better potency ratio relative to morphine in neuropathic than in nociceptive pain models. *Drugs* 2007;8(1):51–57.

57. Shadnia S, Soltaninejad K, Heydari K, et al. Tramadol intoxication: a review of 114 cases. *Hum Exp Toxicol* 2008;27:201–205.

CHAPTER 79 ■ SKELETAL MUSCLE RELAXANTS AND ANALGESIC BALMS

KENNETH C. JACKSON AND CHARLES E. ARGOFF

SKELETAL MUSCLE RELAXANTS

The class of medications commonly termed skeletal muscle relaxants remains an ill-defined and confusing enigma to many clinicians and scientists. To some extent, this results from the assumption that these medications act in a similar fashion and that this mechanism produces reliable production of skeletal muscle relaxation. Neither is true. These medications produce a range of effects that remain poorly defined for clinicians (Table 79.1).[1-4] The class includes carisoprodol, chlorzoxazone, cyclobenzaprine, metaxalone, methocarbamol, and orphenadrine.[5] These agents are approved by the U.S. Food and Drug Administration (FDA) for the relief of discomfort associated with an acute, painful musculoskeletal conditions. Baclofen and tizanidine have FDA-approved indication of the treatment of spasticity due to multiple sclerosis, spinal cord disease, or injury. Benzodiazepines, principally diazepam, also are commonly used for adjunctive relief of skeletal muscle spasm. Chief among the challenges to clinicians using these drugs is discerning the role of the agents across the continuum of painful disorders.

Historically, skeletal muscle relaxants have been prescribed for acute and chronic conditions associated with muscle-related pain. The majority of these agents are indicated for use during the initial presentation of acute low back pain (LBP), which often results from soft-tissue mechanical injury and normally occurs in the muscles, ligaments, and/or tendon structures around the lumbar spine. Acute pain may include local pain and tenderness, muscle spasm, and limited range of motion, but what actually constitutes painful muscle spasm remains controversial.[6] Muscle spasm may be a variant of the myofascial pain presentation and, as such, not really a spasm.[7]

To better understand the potential pharmacologic benefit of these agents, consider the regulation of muscle activity in both the peripheral tissues and central nervous system (CNS). At the level of the peripheral muscle, tissues are comprised of intrafusal fibers that signal changes in muscle length. These lie in parallel with extrafusal muscle fibers that normally serve to contract or stabilize joints. When muscle tissue is stretched, the intrafusal fibers stretch resulting in an increase in neural discharges carried by afferent nerve fibers. This signal is transmitted to the dorsal horn and synapses with alpha-motoneurons in the ventral horn,

producing excitatory postsynaptic potentials. The result is a type of negative feedback, with muscle contraction of the intrafusal muscle fibers where the original stretch signal originated. These muscle fibers also maintain an efferent component, facilitated by small gamma-motoneurons that originate in the ventral horn of the spinal cord and travel together with the alpha-motoneurons that innervate extrafusal muscle fibers. The gamma-motoneurons adjust the sensitivity of the muscle fibers and regulate muscle tension over a wide range of muscle lengths. This complex system of afferent and efferent signaling through the motoneurons when at homeostasis leads to stabilization of muscle structures (Fig. 79.1).

In the dorsal horn, a complex network of excitatory and inhibitory interneurons mediates motor reflexes in response to deep and cutaneous stimulation. Such reflexes mediate ipsilateral flexion and contralateral extension in response to noxious stimuli to coordinate a protective or escape response. Impulses from cutaneous afferents travel through the dorsal horn of the spinal cord and terminate on excitatory interneurons, which in turn terminate on presynaptic terminals of the intrafusal fibers further promoting excitation at the ventral horn alpha-motoneuron. Inhibitory centers in the bulbar reticular formation and facilitatory centers from several brain regions further regulate both corticospinal and reflex muscle activity.[8,9]

Excitatory neurotransmitters in the CNS play a major role in the modulation of movement in the spinal cord and include substances like glutamate, aspartate, and substance P. These neurotransmitters are released from the terminals of primary afferent fibers to mediate reflexes that enhance motor tone at the spinal level.[10] Gamma-aminobutyric acid (GABA) is a major inhibitory CNS neurotransmitter that emanates from supraspinal and interneuronal inputs. GABA is believed to play a major role in presynaptic inhibition of motoneurons in the dorsal horn.[10]

Any change in the homeostasis of the peripheral or CNS components related to maintaining proper muscle tone can lead to production of an acute reflex muscle spasm. When this occurs, there are two main potential issues. Either a reflex increase in muscle tone activates polysynaptic reflexes and produces hyperexcitability of alpha and/or gamma motoneurons, or there is supraspinal activation of descending facilitatory systems.[11] In settings of chronic muscle spasticity, the processes appear to be more involved, with pathology from supraspinal CNS descending path-

TABLE 79.1

PHARMACOTHERAPIES COMMONLY USED FOR MUSCLE SPASM

Drug	Onset	Duration	Common dosing	Side effects	Important drug interactions
Sedative Carisoprodol (Soma, Meda Pharmaceuticals, Somerset, NJ)	30 min	4–6 hours	350 PO QID	Ataxia, dizziness, drowsiness, N/V, withdrawal potential	Additive effects with alcohol and other CNS depressants
Chlorzoxazone (Parafon Forte)	~1 hour	3–4 hours	250–750 mg PO TID-QID	Dizziness, drowsiness, headache, N/V	
Metaxalone (Skelaxin, King Pharmaceuticals Inc., Bristol, TN)	1 hour	4–6 hours	400–800 mg PO TID	Dizziness, drowsiness, headache, N/V, rash	
Methocarbamol (Robaxin)	30 min (PO)	N/A	750–1000 mg PO QID	Blurred vision, dizziness, drowsiness	
TCA-Like Cyclobenzaprine (Flexeril)	~1 hour	12–24 hours	5–10 mg PO TID	Drowsiness, dizziness, dry mouth	Additive effects with alcohol and other CNS depressants; seizures with tramadol and MAOIs; additive effects with TCAs
Antihistamine Orphenadrine (Norflex)	1 hour (PO)	4–6 hours	100 mg PO BID	Tachycardia, lightheadedness, N/V, dry mouth	Additive effects with alcohol and other CNS depressants; coadministration with propoxyphene can lead to confusion, anxiety, and/or tremors
GABA-Type Diazepam (Valium)	30 minutes (PO)	Variable, depending on elimination	2–10 mg PO TID	Sedation, fatigue, hypotension, ataxia, respiratory depression	Potentiation of effects when taken with phenothiazines, opioids, barbiturates, MAOIs
Baclofen (Lioresal)	3–4 days (PO) 30 min (IT)	Variable (PO) 4–6 hours (IT)	5 mg PO TID titrated up to 40–80 mg/day	Drowsiness, slurred speech, hypotension, constipation, urinary retention	Antidepressants (short-term memory loss); additive effects with imipramine
Central Alpha-2 Agonists Tizanidine (Zanaflex)	2 weeks	Variable	2–8 mg PO TID–QID	Drowsiness, dry mouth, dizziness, hypotension, increased spasm/tone	Additive effects with alcohol and other CNS depressants; reduced clearance with oral contraceptives

IT, intrathecal; MAOIs, monoamine oxidase inhibitors; N/A, not applicable; N/V, nausea/vomiting; PO, oral; QID, four times daily; TID, three times daily.

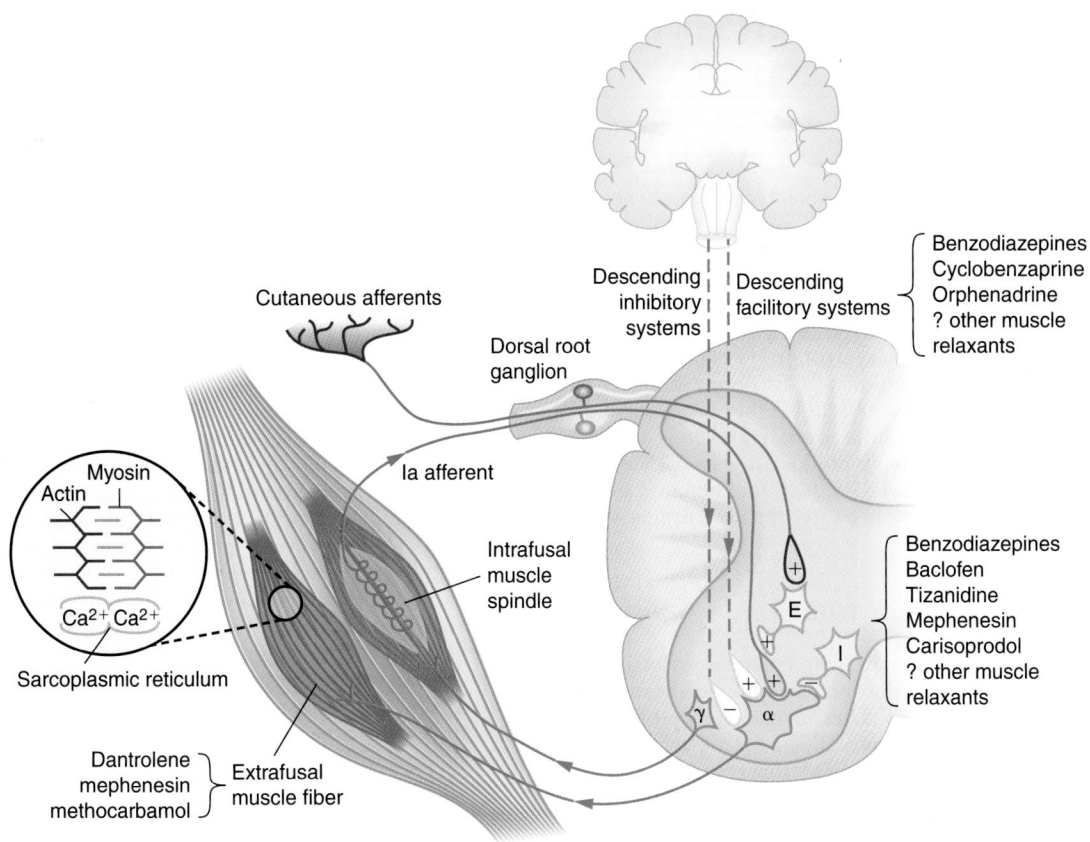

FIGURE 79.1 Neural regulation of muscle tone: possible sites of action of skeletal muscle relaxants. See text for details. (+, excitatory effect; −, inhibitory effect; α, alpha-motoneuron; Ca^{2+}, calcium ion; E, excitatory interneuron; γ, gamma-motoneuron; I, inhibitory interneuron.)

ways that produce excessive excitation or diminished inhibition of alpha-motoneurons in the dorsal horn.[12]

Mechanism of Action

In animal studies, skeletal muscle relaxants act at various CNS sites that are important in muscle activity regulation. The exact mechanism of action for these various agents is not clear. A variety of mechanisms appear to be associated with the activity of this diverse group of agents (Table 79.2). Animal models have

TABLE 79.2

AGENTS BY PROPOSED MECHANISM OF ACTION

CNS depressants
- **Antihistamine**
  orphenadrine
- **Sedatives**
  carisoprodol, chlorzoxazone, metaxalone, methocarbamol
- **TCA-like**
  cyclobenzaprine

Central alpha-2 agonists
tizanidine

GABA-agonists
baclofen
benzodiazepines

historically shown that muscle relaxants exert their activity by blocking polysynaptic neurons in the spinal cord and inhibiting interneuronal activity within the descending reticular formation.[1] Mephenesin, an early predecessor to today's muscle relaxants, in animal models affected monosynaptic and polysynaptic reflexes.[13,14] Subsequent animal data showed that mephenesin and methocarbamol prolonged the refractory period of skeletal muscle by a direct action on skeletal muscle fibers.[15] Very little has been described about the effects of skeletal muscle relaxants such as cyclobenzaprine, methocarbamol, carisoprodol, and chlorzoxazone on neurotransmission. These medications are also known to have a significant sedative profile. This was a quality that was exploited when older treatment paradigms included significant bedrest. Interestingly, other medications with sedative properties are also known to depress polysynaptic reflexes. This situation certainly sheds some degree of confusion as to the specific utility of skeletal muscle relaxants, especially in relation to the purported effects versus nonspecific sedation.

The pharmacologic capacity of other commonly used drugs is less well characterized in specific relation to muscle spasm. Diazepam, a benzodiazepine, suppressed polysynaptic reflexes in cats, but required doses higher than would be used clinically.[16] Benzodiazepines act by potentiating the postsynaptic effects of GABA within the CNS.[12] Baclofen (parachlorophenyl GABA) is a lipophilic derivative of GABA that binds to $GABA_B$ but not to $GABA_A$ receptors and may exert its effect, in part, by inhibiting the evoked release of excitatory amino acids (e.g., glutamate) and substance P.[10] Tizanidine, a newer antispasticity agent, is an α_2-adrenergic receptor agonist that may also act by decreasing spinal excitatory amino acid release.[16]

CENTRALLY-ACTING SEDATIVE-HYPNOTIC MUSCLE RELAXANTS

Carisoprodol

Carisoprodol is converted in the liver to meprobamate, a schedule IV controlled substance. Meprobamate produces physical and psychologic dependence.[18–23] Substance abuse appears to be problematic with carisoprodol, probably due to meprobamate formation. In recent years, several states have begun treating carisoprodol as a controlled substance within their state formularies. Due to the dependence potential, carisoprodol should be cautiously tapered as opposed to immediately discontinued following long-term use. At the end of November 2007, the European Medicines Agency recommended the suspension of marketing authorization for carisoprodol-containing products for its 12 member states. Its Committee for Medicinal Products for Human Use concluded that the risk of their use is greater than the benefits.[24]

Chlorzoxazone

Chlorzoxazone may be less effective than the other skeletal muscle relaxants.[25] Chlorzoxazone does not have any significant drug interactions, but does have a significant adverse effect profile that includes a rare idiosyncratic hepatocellular reaction.[26] The use of this agent may be questionable considering the potential lack of efficacy and significant toxicity profile.[27]

Metaxalone

Metaxalone does not have any significant drug interactions and appears to have a fairly benign side effect profile. Hemolytic anemia and impaired liver function may occur but are uncommon. Fatalities attributed to the use of metaxalone have been reported.[28,29] Metaxalone is contraindicated in patients with severe renal or hepatic impairment. Because this drug was FDA-approved over 30 years ago, there are few published placebo-controlled studies of metaxalone for musculoskeletal pain.[30]

Methocarbamol

Methocarbamol is available in an oral form and a parenteral form for IV or intramuscular use. Complications with the injectable form include pain, skin sloughing, and thrombophlebitis. This drug also was FDA-approved over 30 years ago, and as a result, there are few published studies comparing it to placebo for the treatment of musculoskeletal pain.[31]

ANTIHISTAMINE MUSCLE RELAXANT

Orphenadrine Citrate

Orphenadrine is a derivative of diphenhydramine and accordingly exhibits antihistaminic and anticholinergic properties. There have been reports of severe adverse reactions with parenteral use (e.g., anaphylactoid reaction). Orphenadrine use with propoxyphene may cause confusion, anxiety, and tremors, perhaps because of additive effects. Anticholinergic actions of orphenadrine have been noted to produce significant adverse effects at high dosages (e.g., tachycardia, palpitations, urinary retention, blurred vision).[32]

TRYCYCLIC ANTIDEPRESSANT-LIKE MUSCLE RELAXANT

Cyclobenzaprine

Cyclobenzaprine is more structurally and pharmacologically similar to the tricyclic antidepressants (TCAs) than it is to the centrally acting sedative-hypnotic skeletal muscle relaxants. As with the other skeletal muscle relaxants, cyclobenzaprine does not act directly on muscle tissue. Animal data suggest cyclobenzaprine acts primarily at the level of brainstem, reducing tonic somatic motor activity.[33] While no evidence exists in humans to support this mechanism, it is interesting to note that the newer 5 mg dose has yielded similar clinical efficacy with less sedation than the 10 mg dose.[34] This may prove to be an important distinction from the centrally acting sedative-hypnotic muscle relaxants.

The value of muscle relaxant monotherapy remains the subject of some skepticism; these agents may be used as adjuncts to other therapies. This appears to apply to cyclobenzaprine as well. In an open-label study of patients with acute neck or low back pain associated with muscle spasm who were randomized to be treated for 7 days with either cyclobenzaprine 5 mg orally three times daily alone or with cyclobenzaprine 5 mg orally three times daily in combination with ibuprofen at doses of 400 mg orally three times daily or 800 mg three times daily, no significant treatment differences were found among these groups.[35]

Cyclobenzaprine has a similar adverse event profile as the TCAs. Thus, one might want to avoid using cyclobenzaprine and a TCA concurrently unless the combination is truly clinically indicated. Anticholinergic side effects, including dry mouth, urinary retention, and constipation, occur with cyclobenzaprine. Use of cyclobenzaprine is contraindicated in the setting of arrhythmias, congestive heart failure, hyperthyroidism, or during the acute recovery phase of a myocardial infarction. Concurrent use with proserotonergic agents such as selective serotonin reuptake inhibitors may predispose patients to life-threatening serotonin syndrome.[36]

Cyclobenzaprine labeling suggests that concomitant use with tramadol may place patients at higher risk for developing seizures.[33] Concomitant use of cyclobenzaprine with monoamine oxidase inhibitors or use within 14 days after their discontinuation is contraindicated. Cyclobenzaprine can enhance the effects of agents with CNS-depressant activity. Older patients appear to have a higher risk for CNS-related adverse reactions, such as hallucinations and confusion, when using cyclobenzaprine. Withdrawal symptoms have been noted with the discontinuation of chronic cyclobenzaprine use. Use of a medication taper may be warranted for patients with chronic use.

GABA-AGONIST MUSCLE RELAXANTS

Diazepam

Diazepam is the most commonly prescribed and referenced benzodiazepine in the treatment of muscle spasms.[37] It has hypnotic, anxiolytic, antiepileptic, and antispasmodic properties. Sedation and abuse potential are the main concerns with this agent and class. It is important to slowly taper this agent after long-term use to avoid any withdrawal symptoms.

Baclofen

Studies have shown baclofen to have superior efficacy than diazepam.[2] Baclofen is unique in that it can be administered intrathecally in cases of severe spasticity and for patients who do not tolerate or have failed oral therapy. Baclofen should be tapered slowly after long-term use to avoid a withdrawal reaction and rebound phenomena. It should be used with caution in the elderly and for patients with renal impairment.

CENTRAL ALPHA-2 AGONIST MUSCLE RELAXANTS

Tizanidine

Tizanidine is related chemically to clonidine, but has significantly less antihypertensive effect.[38] The main adverse effect for most patients with this agent is sedation.[39] Currently, tizanidine is FDA-approved for the management of increased muscle tone associated with spasticity resulting from CNS disorders, such as multiple sclerosis or spinal cord injury. Two studies report use of tizanidine in back pain or muscle spasm, either alone or in combination with ibuprofen, and another reports effectiveness in myofascial pain.[40-42] A multicenter, placebo-controlled study evaluated the efficacy and safety of tizanidine in the treatment of low back pain; tizanidine was found to provide pain relief and less restriction of movement than placebo. Drowsiness was the most common side effect but, for acute LBP patients, this effect may actually be desired, especially at night.[40] A study of 105 patients with acute LBP received tizanidine 4 mg orally three times daily with ibuprofen 400 mg orally three times daily or ibuprofen 400 mg orally three times daily compared to placebo. The results suggested that the tizanidine/ibuprofen combination was more effective for moderate or severe acute LBP than ibuprofen only.[41] Use tizanidine with caution in renal impairment; clearance is decreased by 50% in patients with creatinine clearance <25 mL/minute. Coadministration with alcohol can increase the AUC of tizanidine by approximately 20% and increase C_{max} by approximately 15%. Use with oral contraceptives can decrease the clearance of tizanidine and place patients at higher risk for sedating adverse effects.

ACUTE LOW BACK PAIN

Available data indicate that skeletal muscle relaxants are more effective than placebo to relieve acute LBP.[25] Unfortunately, most of the data are dated and are derived from studies for which the designs and analyses would not be acceptable today. No data clearly show that any one agent is more efficacious than another. Some data suggest that chlorzoxazone may be less effective than other drugs and, as such, puts into question the use of this agent.[25,43]

Most clinical guidelines list skeletal muscle relaxants as optional agents for use individually or in combination with a nonsteroidal anti-inflammatory agent (NSAID). The federal clinical practice guideline published in 1995 specifically noted that skeletal muscle relaxants alone or in combination with an NSAID were no more effective than using an NSAID alone.[44] This conclusion has been supported in systematic reviews by van Tulder and colleagues.[25,43] Skeletal muscle relaxants have been shown to more effective than placebo for patients with acute LBP with respect to outcomes such as short-term pain relief, global efficacy, and improvement of physical outcomes.[45-48] No quality evidence allows a direct comparison of skeletal muscle relaxants to NSAIDs. Most clinicians and researchers agree that skeletal muscle relaxants may benefit patients with acute LBP by reducing the duration of their discomfort and accelerating recovery. A meta-analysis of cyclobenzaprine studies for acute LBP concluded that, despite limitations in the available evidence, the combination of a NSAID with cyclobenzaprine appears to be warranted.[49] It is probably best to consider the use of skeletal muscle relaxants as an adjunct or alternative to NSAIDs, especially in cases where NSAID toxicity is a concern or when NSAID monotherapy proves suboptimal.

Various systematic reviews have been published reviewing the randomized controlled trials of muscle relaxants in the treatment of LBP.[25,43,50] These analyses concur that there is strong evidence that muscle relaxants are more effective than placebo for acute LBP, but do not indicate superiority of a specific type of muscle relaxant. Muscle relaxants also appear to be useful in acute cervical pain presentations.[51-53]

Baclofen and tizanidine are well established for the treatment of spasticity secondary to upper motor neuron or spinal disorders.[12,17,54] Limited clinical evidence exists for the treatment of acute muscle spasm with baclofen. As noted previously, tizanidine has some evidence but can be extremely sedating, especially at doses that prove analgesic for acute back pain.

CHRONIC LOW BACK PAIN

Despite the common use of skeletal muscle relaxants, relatively few data clarify their appropriateness in the treatment of chronic back pain.[25,50] No skeletal muscle relaxant has an indication for use in chronic back pain. Despite this lack of evidence, muscle relaxants are often prescribed on a long-term basis.[55] Only baclofen and tizanidine have FDA-approved indications for spasticity. When used in acute back pain, skeletal muscle relaxants are used to treat muscle spasms and associated pain during the normal recovery period of 1 to 3 weeks. Since this correlates with the time course that most patients recover from their acute injury, it is difficult to discern the exact nature of the utility for these medications. As a group, these agents may provide some global palliative quality, but probably do not affect the course of the underlying morbidity, per se.

Skeletal muscle relaxants have CNS-depressant effects and should be used with caution, particularly for patients with concomitant use of alcohol, anxiolytics, opioid analgesics, or other sedating medications. There is strong evidence that skeletal muscle relaxants are associated with increased risk for total adverse effects, especially those related to the CNS.[25,43,50] Many chronic pain patients appear to benefit from less pharmacotherapy, especially substances that may cloud cognitive and functional capacities.[56] Pill tapers can be used where patients who are appropriate candidates for streamlining can have their muscle relaxant therapy slowly discontinued over a relatively short time (e.g., 2 weeks). In some situations, patients may require more interventions (e.g., behavioral medicine support). These patients are probably best managed by interdisciplinary pain programs or by a psychiatrist.

TOPICAL ANALGESIC BALMS

Applying medicines topically is an ancient practice that, while often perceived as pragmatic, can become quite problematic. Many ancient cultures utilized a variety of natural substances (e.g., herbs and plants) for a variety of medicinal uses, including analgesia. Today, a variety of topical remedies is available to patients with painful conditions, primarily as over-the-counter (OTC) analgesic balm, many of which have been available for decades. The majority of these preparations contain counterirritants such as camphor, menthol, and salicylates either alone or in combination with each other or a variety of other medicinal

TABLE 79.3

BENEFITS AND LIMITATIONS OF TOPICAL ANALGESICS

Benefits	Limitations
• Avoid need for oral absorption • Avoid metabolic complications and systemic adverse effects • Ease of dose termination in the event of untoward side effects • Direct access to the target site • Convenient administration • Improved patient acceptance and adherence • Alternative route when oral not viable (e.g., patient with emesis)	• Absorption pharmacokinetic issues due to molecular size, lipophilicity, and skin permeability • Topical enzymatic activity may occur and reduce efficacy. • Localized skin irritation, such as erythema, can occur.

(Adapted from Hare BD, Lipman AG. Uses and Misuses of Medication in the Treatment of Chronic Pain. In Hare BD, Fine P, eds. *Chronic pain, problems in anesthesia.* Philadelphia: JB Lippincott Co.; 1990.)

ingredients. Capsaicin, a counterirritant, and nonsalicylate NSAIDs are also available in prescription and OTC topical formulations. Lidocaine and a variety of other substances used topically are discussed elsewhere in this book.

Topical drug administration would appear to maintain many potential benefits, especially in pain presentations that have a defined local and peripheral component.[57] The most obvious benefit is avoiding potential negative sequelae common with systemic administration of analgesics (e.g., adverse effects, drug interactions, need for an effective serum concentration). At the same time, topical administration can be prone to a variety of limitations, often inversely related to the benefits of topical application. Benefits and limitations are summarized in Table 79.3. Direct topical drug application appears to avoid numerous problems that occur with systemic administration of medications. This is especially true for NSAIDs, where toxicity with systemic administration can be very difficult for many patients. As described below, topical NSAIDs appear to be useful for some acute pain presentations (e.g., soft tissue injuries and postsurgical pain).

NSAIDs have the most evidence base among the topical analgesics. Moore and colleagues[58] conducted a meta-analysis reviewing analgesic efficacy for acute pain related to soft tissue trauma, sprains, and strains. They also analyzed pain relief for chronic pain conditions, such as osteoarthritis and tendonitis. The number needed to treat (NNT) was 3.9 for the acute pain conditions and 3.1 for the chronic pain conditions. The authors noted that local skin reactions were uncommon (3.6% of patients) in the studies. As could be expected, systemic adverse effects were extremely uncommon at less than 0.5% of patients exposed to this drug class. The evidence is not as compelling for the role of topical NSAIDs when compared to oral administration.[59] While topical administration does not appear to afford the same therapeutic profile, this route of administration is also better tolerated and may be of benefit in patients who would not otherwise be able to use an NSAID orally.

Topical Counterirritants

Topical counterirritants comprise a group of substances primarily for use by patients in a variety of OTC analgesic compounds.

These include capsaicin, camphor, menthol, and salicylates which appear to provide analgesic benefit by desensitizing peripheral nociceptive receptors. Galeotti and colleagues[60] suggested that menthol's analgesic properties may be mediated through selective activation of kappa-opioid receptors.

Capsaicin appears to have the best evidence for use among the topical analgesics, primarily in osteoarthritis. Analgesic activity for capsaicin is attributed to depletion of substance P from peripheral nerve terminals. This requires both time and consistent dosing. A recent systematic review of topical capsaicin for musculoskeletal pain found an NNT of 8.1 for pain relief.[61] A variety of guidelines list capsaicin as a useful adjunct for use in patients with osteoarthritis. The European League Against Rheumatism and the American College of Rheumatology both recommend capsaicin for the treatment of pain in osteoarthritis.[62,63] The main issue related to capsaicin use is the adverse effect profile, which occurs to some extent with all patients and is an expected consequence of the mechanism of action. In the aforementioned systematic review, side effects were problematic in approximately one-third of the patients.[61] Typical experiences include local adverse reactions such as pain upon application, burning, stinging, and redness at the site of application. This adverse effect profile is probably the biggest disadvantage for this medication, causing either early discontinuation or reduced patient compliance, leading to absence of efficacy.[64,65]

The other counterirritants can be classified as rubefacients, including salicylates. There are few good efficacy data for these medications, probably in part because these substances have been used for so long. The benefit of these agents may also be due to the actual administration process (i.e., rubbing), causing increased stimulation in the area.

While salicylates may also have activity similar to other NSAIDs, their topical mechanism remains poorly elucidated. Mason and colleagues[66] reviewed the use of topical salicylates for acute musculoskeletal pain. These authors noted that topical salicylates produced a significant reduction in pain compared to placebo, with a NNT of 2.1. The benefit of this medication class for chronic use is limited by both lack of efficacy data and the potential for adverse effects with continued administration.

CONCLUSION

Skeletal muscle relaxants and topical analgesic balms comprise a cadre of substances that are commonly used for a variety of pain conditions. Skeletal muscle relaxants have value for acute back pain, mainly as adjunctive agents with other forms of analgesia and physical therapy. The use of these agents in chronic pain conditions remains controversial. This is in part due to the lack of efficacy data available for the use of these substances in chronic back pain conditions. Moreover, these agents maintain a substantial adverse effect profile that often is counterproductive for patients with chronic pain.

Topical analgesic balms are commonly used for self-care in acute painful conditions. Capsaicin is the one substance within this group with potential value in osteoarthritis. The main challenge with this substance is managing expectations and adverse effects.

References

1. Elenbaas JK. Centrally acting oral skeletal muscle relaxants. *Am J Hosp Pharm* 1980;37(10):1313–1323.
2. Waldman HJ. Centrally acting skeletal muscle relaxants and associated drugs. *J Pain Symptom Manage* 1994;9(7):434–441.
3. Balano KB. Anti-inflammatory drugs and myorelaxants. Pharmacology and clinical use in musculoskeletal disease. *Primary Care* 1996;23(2):329–334.
4. Patel AT, Ogle AA. Diagnosis and management of acute low back pain. *Am Fam Physician* 2000;61:1779–1786, 1789–1790.

5. Jackson KC. Evaluation of skeletal muscle relaxant use for acute musculoskeletal pain and injury in ambulatory care. *J Pain* 2003;4(2 suppl 1):84(934).

6. Johnson EW. The myth of skeletal muscle spasm. *Am J Phys Med Rehabil* 1989;68(1):1.

7. Rivner MH. The neurophysiology of myofascial pain syndrome. *Curr Pain Headache Rep* 2001;5(5):432–440.

8. Magoun HW, Rhines R. An inhibitory mechanism in the bulbar reticular formation. *J Neurophysiol* 1946;9:165–171.

9. Schreiner LH, Lindsley DB, Magoun HW. Role of brain stem facilitatory systems in maintenance of spasticity. *J Neurophysiol* 1949;12(3):207–216.

10. Davidoff RA. Antispasticity drugs: mechanisms of action. *Ann Neurol* 1985; 17(2):107–116.

11. Stanko JR. A review of oral skeletal muscle relaxants for the craniomandibular disorder (CMD) practitioner. *Cranio* 1990;8(3):234–243.

12. Young RR, Delwaide PJ. Drug therapy: spasticity (first of two parts). *N Engl J Med* 1981;304(1):28–33.

13. Henneman E, Kaplan A, Unna K. A neuropharmacological study on the effect of myanesin (Tolserol) on motor systems. *J Pharmacol Exp Ther* 1949;97(3): 331–341.

14. Latimer CN. Action of mephenesin upon three monosynaptic pathways of cat. *J Pharmacol Exp Ther* 1956;118(3):309–317.

15. Crankshaw DP, Raper C. Some studies on peripheral actions of mephenesin, methocarbamol and diazepam. *Br J Pharmacol* 1968;34(3):579–590.

16. Ngai SH, Tseng DTC, Wang SC. Effect of diazepam and other central nervous system depressants on spinal reflexes in cats: a study of site of action. *J Pharmacol Exp Ther* 1966;153(2):344–351.

17. Wagstaff AJ, Bryson HM. Tizanidine: a review of its pharmacology, clinical efficacy and tolerability in the management of spasticity associated with cerebral and spinal disorders. *Drugs* 1997;53(3):435–452.

18. Littrell RA, Hayes LR, Stillner V. Carisoprodol (Soma): A new and cautious perspective on an old agent. *South Med J* 1993;86(7):753–756.

19. Bailey DN, Briggs JR. Carisoprodol: an unrecognized drug of abuse. *Am J Clin Pathol* 2002;117(3):396–400.

20. Reeves RR, Carter OS, Pinkofsky HB, et al. Carisoprodol (Soma): abuse potential and physician unawareness. *J Addict Dis* 1999;18(2):51–56.

21. Reeves RR, Carter OS, Pinkofsky HB. Use of carisoprodol by substance abusers to modify the effects of illicit drugs. *South Med J* 1999;92(4):441.

22. Rust GS, Hatch R, Gums JG. Carisoprodol as a drug of abuse. *Arch Fam Med* 1993;2(4):429–432.

23. Elder NC. Abuse of skeletal muscle relaxants. *Am Fam Physician* 1991;44(4): 1223–1226.

24. European Medicines Agency Press Release. European Medicines Agency recommends suspension of marketing authorizations for Carisoprodol-containing medicinal products. Doc ref. EMEA/520463/2007. Available at: http://www.emea.europa.eu.Accessed

25. van Tulder MW, Touray T, Furlan AD, et al. Muscle relaxants for non-specific low back pain. *Cochrane Database Syst Rev* 2003;2:CD004252.

26. Powers BJ, Cattau EL Jr, Zimmerman HJ. Chlorzoxazone hepatotoxic reactions. An analysis of 21 identified or presumed cases. *Arch Intern Med* 1986; 146(6):1183–1186.

27. Jackson KC II. Pharmacotherapy in lower back pain. *Drugs Today (Barc)* 2004; 40(9):765–772.

28. Moore KA, Levine B, Fowler D. A fatality involving metaxalone. *Forensic Sci Int* 2005;149(2–3):249–251.

29. Poklis JL, Ropero-Miller JD, Garside D, et al. Metaxalone (Skelaxin)-related death. *J Anal Toxicol* 2004;28(6):537–541.

30. Dent RW Jr, Ervin DK. A study of metaxalone (Skelaxin) vs. placebo in acute musculoskeletal disorders: a cooperative study. *Curr Ther Res Clin Exp* 1075; 18(3):433–440.

31. Tisdale SA Jr, Ervin DK. A controlled study of methocarbamol (Robaxin) in acute painful musculoskeletal conditions. *Curr Ther Res Clin Exp* 1975;17(6): 525–530.

32. Gareri P, De Fazio P, Cotroneo A, et al. Anticholinergic drug-induced delirium in an elderly Alzheimer's dementia patient. *Arch Gerontol Geriatr* 2007; 44(suppl 1):199–206.

33. Flexeril [package insert]. Fort Washington, PA: McNeil Consumer & Specialty Pharmaceuticals; 2003.

34. Borenstein DG, Korn S. Efficacy of a low-dose regimen of cyclobenzaprine hydrochloride in acute skeletal muscle spasm: results of two placebo-controlled trials. *Clin Ther* 2003;25(4):1056–1073.

35. Childers MK, Borenstein D, Brown RL, et al. Low-dose cyclobenzaprine versus combination therapy with ibuprofen for acute neck or back pain with muscle spasm: a randomized trial. *Curr Med Res Opin* 2005;21(9):1485–1493.

36. Keegan MT, Brown DR, Rabinstein AA. Serotonin syndrome from the interaction of cyclobenzaprine with other serotoninergic drugs. *Anesth Analg* 2006; 103(6):1466–1468.

37. Cherkin DC, Wheeler KJ, Barlow W, et al. Medication use for low back pain in primary care. *Spine* 1998;23(5):607–614.

38. Coward DM. Tizanidine: neuropharmacology and mechanism of action. *Neurology* 1994;44(11 suppl 9):S6–S10.

39. Smith HS, Barton AE. Tizanidine in the management of spasticity and musculoskeletal complaints in the palliative care population. *Am J Hosp Palliat Care* 2000;17(1):50–58.

40. Berry H, Hutchinson DR. A multicentre placebo-controlled study in general practice to evaluate the efficacy and safety of tizanidine in acute low back pain. *J Int Med Res* 1988;16(2):75–82.

41. Berry H, Hutchinson DR. Tizanidine and ibuprofen in acute low back pain: results of a double-blind multicentre study in general practice. *J Int Med Res* 1988;16(2):83–91.

42. Malanga GA, Gwynn MW, Smith R, et al. Tizanidine is effective in the treatment of myofascial pain syndrome. *Pain Physician* 2002;5(4):422–432.

43. van Tulder MW, Koes BW, Bouter LM. Conservative treatment of acute and chronic nonspecific low back pain. A systematic review of randomized controlled trials of the most common interventions. *Spine* 1997;22(18):2128–2156.

44. Bigos SJ, Bowyer OR, Braen GR, et al. *Clinical Practice Guideline Number 14: Acute Low Back Problems in Adults.* Rockville, MD: U.S. Department of Health and Human Services, Agency for Health Care Policy and Research; 1994. Publication 95-0642.

45. Barrata R. A double-blind study of cyclobenzaprine and placebo in the treatment of acute musculoskeletal conditions of the low back. *Curr Ther Res* 1982; 32(5):646–652.

46. Berry H, Hutchinson D. A multicentre placebo-controlled study in general practice to evaluate the efficacy and safety of tizanidine in acute low-back pain. *J Int Med Res* 1988;16(2):75–82.

47. Lepisto P. A comparative trial of DS 103-282 and placebo in the treatment of acute skeletal muscle spasms due to disorders of the back. *Curr Ther Res* 1979; 26(4):454–459.

48. Gold RH. Orphenadrine citrate: sedative or muscle relaxant? *Clin Ther* 1978; 1(6):451–453.

49. Browning R, Jackson JL, O'Malley PG. Cyclobenzaprine and back pain. A meta-analysis. *Arch Intern Med* 2001;161:1613–1620.

50. Chou R, Peterson K, Helfand M. Comparative efficacy and safety of skeletal muscle relaxants for spasticity and musculoskeletal conditions: a systematic review. *J Pain Symptom Manage* 2004;28(2):140–175.

51. Dillin W, Uppal GS. Analysis of medications used in the treatment of cervical disk degeneration. *Orthop Clin North Am* 1992;23(3):421–433.

52. Basmajian JV. Cyclobenzaprine hydrochloride effect on skeletal muscle spasm in the lumbar region and neck: two double-blind controlled clinical and laboratory studies. *Arch Phys Med Rehabil* 1978;59(2):58–63.

53. Basmajian JV. Reflex cervical muscle spasm: treatment by diazepam, phenobarbital or placebo. *Arch Phys Med Rehabil* 1983;64(3):121–124.

54. Davidoff RA. Antispasticity drugs: mechanisms of action. *Ann Neurol* 1985; 17(2):107–116.

55. Dillon C, Paulose-Ram R, Hirsch R, et al. Skeletal muscle relaxant use in the United States: data from the Third National Health and Nutrition Examination Survey (NHANES III). *Spine* 2004;29(8):892–896.

56. Hare BD, Lipman AG. Uses and misuses of medication in the treatment of chronic pain. In: Hare BD, Fine P, eds. *Chronic Pain, Problems in Anesthesia.* Philadelphia: JB Lippincott & Co; 1990.

57. Stanos SP. Topical agents for the management of musculoskeletal pain. *J Pain Symptom Manage* 2007;33(3):342–355.

58. Moore RA, Tramèr MR, Carroll D, et al. Quantitative systematic review of topically applied non-steroidal anti-inflammatory drugs. *BMJ* 1998;316(7128): 333–338.

59. Lin J, Zhang LW, Jones A, et al. Efficacy of topical non-steroidal anti-inflammatory drugs in the treatment of osteoarthritis: meta-analysis of randomised controlled trials. *BMJ* 2004;329(7461):324.

60. Galeotti N, Di Cesare Mannelli L, Mazzanti G, et al. Menthol: a natural analgesic compound. *Neuruosci Lett* 2002;322(3):145–148.

61. Mason L, Moore RA, Derry S, et al. Systematic review of topical capsaicin for the treatment of chronic pain. *BMJ* 2004;328(7446):991.

62. Jordan KM, Arden NK, Doherty M, et al. EULAR recommendations 2003: an evidence based approach to the management of knee osteoarthritis. Report of a Task Force of the Standing Committee for International Clinical Studies Including Therapeutic Trials (ESCISIT). *Ann Rheum Dis* 2003;62(12): 1145–1155.

63. Recommendations for the medical management of osteoarthritis of the hip and knee: 2000 update. American College of Rheumatology Subcommittee on Osteoarthritis Guidelines. *Arthritis Rheum* 2000;43(9):1905–1915.

64. Bley KR. Recent developments in transient receptor potential vanilloid receptor 1 agonist-based therapies. *Expert Opin Investig Drugs* 2004;13(11):1445–1456.

65. Szallasi A. Vanilloid (capsaicin) receptors in health and disease. *Am J Clin Pathol* 2002;118(1):110–121.

66. Mason L, Moore RA, Edwards JE, et al. Systematic review of efficacy of topical rubefacients containing salicylates for the treatment of acute and chronic pain. *BMJ* 2004;328(7446):995–997.

CHAPTER 80 ■ NEUROPATHIC PAIN PHARMACOTHERAPY

ELON EISENBERG AND DAVID PETERSON

INTRODUCTION

Neuropathic pain is chronic pain due to direct central or peripheral nerve damage. While all pain may be considered neurogenic, neuropathic pain results from damage to the nervous system, per se. An estimated 1.5% to 8% of the general population suffer from neuropathic pain.[1,2] Neuropathic pain may result from a large variety of insults, examples of which are listed in Table 80.1. Common examples of peripheral neuropathic pain include lumbar or cervical radiculopathy, painful diabetic neuropathy (PDN), and postherpetic neuralgia (PHN). Neuropathic pain of central origin includes central poststroke pain, pain due to multiple sclerosis, and postspinal cord injury pain.

Neuropathic pain may be continuous or intermittent, and is typically described as burning, aching, or paresthetic. It may or may or may not be lancinating. Allodynia, an abnormal sensitivity of the painful site to normally innocuous stimuli such as running water or cold air, is commonly associated with neuropathic pain.[3] Neuropathic pain has negative effects on multiple domains of life; the quality of life of patients with neuropathic pain is comparable to that experienced by patients suffering from cancer or chronic heart failure. This is further aggravated by the fact that neuropathic pain is often undiagnosed and undertreated.[4] Various types of neuropathic pain are discussed in more detail in Part I of this book.

Many different drugs are used to manage neuropathic pain due to the lack of specific medications that effectively treat it. Pharmacotherapy for neuropathic pain involves a wide variety of agents including, but not limited to, antidepressants, anticonvulsants, opioids, and topical agents. Even with the newest of these drugs, effective pain relief occurs in less than half of chronic neuropathic pain patients.[5,6] In patients with refractory neuropathic pain, combination therapy with two or more agents possessing different mechanisms is often indicated.[7] Additional approaches for the management of intractable neuropathic pain,

for example, implantation of neuromodulation devices such as spinal cord stimulators, intrathecal drug delivery pumps, are discussed in Chapter 95.

Most pharmacological studies of neuropathic pain management have focused on a few subtypes of peripheral neuropathic pain, notably PDN, PHN, and, to some degree, trigeminal neuralgia. Thus, while evidence of treatment efficacy in these indications clearly exists, the effectiveness of these treatments in other forms of neuropathic pain is less clear.

This chapter reviews pharmacotherapy for neuropathic pain and emphasizes the strengths and the limitations of different treatments. It also addresses unresolved issues related to pharmacological treatment of neuropathic pain.

ANTIDEPRESSANTS

Four classes of antidepressant medications have been studied in neuropathic pain treatment: tricyclic antidepressants (TCAs), selective serotonin and norepinephrine reuptake inhibitors (SNRIs), selective serotonin reuptake inhibitors (SSRIs), and monoamine oxidase inhibitors (MAOIs). Certain drugs in the first two classes are commonly considered first line recommended treatments for neuropathic pain.[5,6,8] Table 80.2 lists major properties of common antidepressants.

Tricyclic Antidepressants (TCAs)

Table 80.3 summarizes the placebo-controlled trials of various drugs for neuropathic pain and shows efficacy for amitriptyline, imipramine, nortriptyline, desipramine, clomipramine, and maprotiline at daily doses ranging from 30 to 200 mg for PHN, PDN, postmastectomy pain, central poststroke pain, and mixed types neuropathies. These results are commonly extrapolated to all types of neuropathic pain and clinical experience suggests some broad utility for the drugs. A systematic literature review presenting numbers needed to treat (NNTs) found TCAs the most efficacious antidepressants for neuropathic pain with an overall NNT of 3.1 (95% confidence interval [CI] 2.7–3.7).[5] However, a few trials failed to demonstrate TCA efficacy for spinal cord injury pain,[18] cisplatin-induced neuropathy,[19] HIV neuropathy,[20,21] phantom limb pain,[22] lumbar radiculopathy,[23] and neuropathic cancer pain.[24] Inability to demonstrate effectiveness of the TCAs in these neuropathic pain types may represent a true lack of therapeutic benefit, or it may be due to study design weaknesses or other factors. More studies are needed to clarify the value of specific TCAs in different types of neuropathic pain.

In many countries, TCAs may be overlooked as first line neuropathic pain drugs because they are generic and are not actively marketed. Newer, more expensive drugs for neuropathic pain may be selected despite comparatively lower effectiveness (higher NNTs), in part because of aggressive marketing by the pharmaceutical industry. The analgesic efficacy of the TCAs is likely to

TABLE 80.1

CAUSES OF NEUROPATHIC PAIN PERIPHERAL OR CENTRAL SOMATOSENSORY NERVOUS SYSTEM (EXAMPLES)

Trauma (surgery, frostbite, amputation)
Inflammation (Guillain Barré syndrome)
Infection (AIDS neuropathy, postherpetic neuralgia)
Degenerative spine disease
Ischemic disorders
Metabolic disorders (diabetes mellitus)
Neoplastic disorders
Congenital disorders (Fabry's disease)
Toxicity (chemotherapy)
Immunologic disorders

TABLE 80.2

COMPARISON OF ANTIDEPRESSANTS IN NEUROPATHIC PAIN[9-17]

Agent	Normal adult daily dose in psychiatric disorders[a]	Usual number of doses per day	Elimination half-life ($t_{1/2}$)	Dosing adjustments	Serotonin: norepinephrine selectivity ratio[b]
Selective Serotonin Receptor Inhibitors (SSRIs)					
Citalopram	20–40 mg	1	35 hours	20 mg/day in hepatic impairment or elderly.	3500–3900
Escitalopram	10–20 mg	1	27–32 hours	10 mg/day in hepatic impairment or elderly.	7100
Fluoxetine	20–80 mg	1	24–72 hours (acute), 96–144 hours (chronic), Norfluoxetine 96–384 hours	Decrease dose in hepatic impairment	300–545
Fluvoxamine	100–300 mg	1–2	16 hours	Decrease dose in hepatic impairment and elderly.	580–620
Paroxetine HCL	20–60 mg	IR: 1 XR: 1	21 hours	Maximum dose = 40 mg/day in hepatic impairment or elderly.	300–450
Paroxetine mesylate	20–60 mg	1	33 hours	Maximum dose = 40 mg/day in renal or hepatic impairment, or elderly.	300–450
Sertraline	50–200 mg	1	62–104 hours	Decrease dose in hepatic impairment and elderly.	1400–2750
Serotonin and norepinephrine reuptake inhibitors (SNRIs)					
Desvenlafaxine	50–100 mg	1	11 hours	Decrease dose in moderate or severe renal disease.	85
Duloxetine	40–120 mg	1–2	8–17 hours	Do not give to patients with hepatic impairment. Decrease dose in severe renal disease.	9
Venlafaxine	75–375 mg	IR: 2–3 XR: 1	3–7 hours, ODV 9–13 hours	Decrease dose in hepatic or renal impairment.	115–120
Tricyclic antidepressants (TCAs)[c]					
Amitriptyline	100–300 mg	1–4	9–27 hours	Lower doses in elderly and hepatic impairment.	8
Clomipramine	100–300 mg	1–3	15–60 hours	Lower doses in elderly and hepatic impairment.	130
Desipramine	75–300 mg	1–3	10–30 hours	Lower doses in elderly and hepatic impairment.	0.05
Imipramine	100–300 mg	1–4	5–30 hours	Lower doses in elderly and hepatic impairment.	27
Maprotiline	100–225 mg	1–3	25–50 hours	Lower doses in elderly and hepatic impairment.	0.002
Nortriptyline	50–150 mg	1–4	20–55 hours	Lower doses in elderly and hepatic impairment.	0.24

IR, immediate release; ODV, O-desmethylvenlafaxine; XR, extended release.

[a]Dosing is per product U.S. approved dosing; dosing in pain syndromes may vary from that listed.

[b]These are estimates of selectivity ratio; actual selectivity ratios are concentration dependent; numbers <1 indicate greater affinity for norepinephrine than serotonin.

[c]TCAs may be safely administered once daily; some practitioners prefer to dose them more frequently.

TABLE 80.3

SUMMARY OF RANDOMIZED CONTROLLED TRIALS OF ANTIDEPRESSANTS IN TREATMENT OF NEUROPATHIC PAIN PUBLISHED AS PEER-REVIEWED ARTICLES

Study	Drug	Diagnosis	Design	Number of patients treated with active drug	Maximal dosage (mg)	Treatment duration (weeks)	Results
Leijon[147] 1989	Amitriptyline	CPSP	crossover	15	75	4	A>P
Cardenas[18] 2002	Amitriptyline	SCI	parallel	44	125	6	A=P
Max[25] 1987	Amitriptyline	DPN	crossover	29	150	6	A>P
Vrethem[148] 1997	Amitriptyline	DPN and other polyneuropathies	crossover	33	75	4	A>P
Watson[149] 1982	Amitriptyline	PHN	crossover	24	137.5	3	A>P
Max[150] 1988	Amitriptyline	DPN	crossover	34	150	6	A>P
Robinson[22] 2004	Amitriptyline	Phantom limb	parallel	39	125	6	A=P
Kalso[151] 1995	Amitriptyline	Postmastectomy	crossover	15	100	4	A>P
Kieburtz[20] 1998	Amitriptyline	HIV neuropathy	parallel	46	100	10	A=P
Shlay[21] 1998	Amitriptyline	HIV neuropathy	parallel	58	75	14	A=P
Kvinesdal[152] 1984	Imipramine	DPN	crossover	12	100	5	A>P
Sindrup[153] 1992	Imipramine	DPN	crossover	18	150	2	A>P
Sindrup[31] 2003	Imipramine	DPN	crossover	29	150	4	A>P
Gomez–Perez[74] 1985	Nortriptyline	DPN	crossover	18	60	4	A>P
Raja[101] 2002	Nortriptyline	PHN	crossover	46	140	8	A>P
Panerai[154] 1990	Nortriptyline	Mixed neuropathies	crossover	24	100	3	A>P
Khoromi[23] 2007	Nortriptyline	Radiculopathy	crossover	34	100	9	A=P
Sindrup[155] 1990	Clomipramine	DPN	crossover	19	75	2	A>P
Panerai[154] 1990	Clomipramine	Mixed neuropathies	crossover	24	100	3	A>P
Sindrup[155] 1990	Desipramine	DPN	crossover	19	200	2	A>P
Max[156] 1991	Desipramine	DPN	crossover	20	250	6	A>P
Kishore-Kumar[157] 1990	Desipramine	PHN	crossover	19	250	6	A>P
Raja[101] 2002	Desipramine	PHN	crossover	13	160	8	A>P
Vrethem[148] 1997	Maprotiline	DPN and other polyneuropathies	crossover	33	75	4	A>P
Goldstein[34] 2005	Duloxetine	DPN	parallel	342	120	12	A>P
Raskin[35] 2005	Duloxetine	DPN	parallel	232	120	12	A>P
Wernicke[36] 2006	Duloxetine	DPN	parallel	226	120	12	A>P
Sindrup[31] 2003	Venlafaxine	Mixed neuropathies	crossover	30	225	4	A>P
Rowbotham[30] 2004	Venlafaxine	DPN	crossover	163	225	6	A>P
Tasmuth[33] 2002	Venlafaxine	Post mastectomy	crossover	13	75	4	A=P
Yucel[158] 2005	Venlafaxine	Mixed neuropathies	parallel	8	150	8	A=P[a]
Sindrup[41] 1990	Paroxetine	DPN	crossover	20	40	2	A>P
Sindrup[40] 1992	Citalopram	DPN	crossover	20	40	3	A>P
Max[27] 1992	Fluoxetine	DPN	crossover	46	40	6	A>P

CPSP, central poststroke pain; DPN, diabetic peripheral neuropathy; PHN, postherpetic neuralgia; SCI, spinal cord injury.
[a]The study showed significant effect of venlafaxine in the manifestations of hyperalgesia and temporal summation, but not on the ongoing pain intensity.

be independent of their antidepressant effect.[25] Over one-fifth (21%) of the patients with chronic pain have been diagnosed with depression associated with their pain.[26] Concomitant chronic pain and depression favor the use of an antidepressant (TCA or another) over other medication classes. TCAs are associated with dose-dependent adverse events, the most common being sedation, constipation, dry mouth, urinary retention, and orthostatic hypotension. Tricyclic antidepressants can be administered once daily, usually at bedtime, exploiting their sedating properties. The dose used for neuropathic pain, typically 100 mg a day or less, is below the antidepressant dose for most patients, lowering the risk of side effects. Secondary amine TCAs (e.g., desipramine, nortriptyline) are better tolerated than tertiary amine TCAs (e.g., amitriptyline, imipramine), but are equally effective.[27,28] Nonetheless, TCAs may not be tolerated by many patients. The anticholinergic effects of TCAs are a relative contraindication in patients with benign prostatic hyperplasia, cardiac conduction defects, and other morbidities sensitive to parasympatholytic action. Desipramine has only one-quarter of the anticholinergic and sedative activity of amitriptyline at comparable doses, making desipramine a TCA of choice.[29]

Use of a low initial dose and slow dose titration of all TCAs is important to minimize patients stopping the medication prematurely due to side effects. Dry mouth is the most common adverse event and it is often best managed with sugarless candies or chewing gum, especially sugarless lemon candy to stimulate serous saliva flow. Sips of water provide only transient relief. The most common starting dose for TCAs is 25 mg, but frail elderly and other highly sensitive patients may tolerate an initial 10 mg dose better. Increase the dose by the same number of mg as the starting dose every 3 to 5 days until some diminution of pain complaints occurs or the daily dose totals 100 mg. The maximal effect often occurs within 3 weeks at that dose, generally before antidepressant effects peak.

The anticholinergic effects of TCAs can cause cardiac toxicity including ventricular ectopic activity, myocardial infarction, and sudden death. A screening electrocardiogram (EKG) might be considered in patients over 40 years of age or who have other risk factors prior to initiating a TCA. According to recent recommendations, these drugs should not be used in patients who have ischemic heart disease or increased risk of sudden cardiac death.[8]

Selective Serotonin and Norepinephrine Reuptake Inhibitors

The SNRIs duloxetine and venlafaxine are newer antidepressants with effectiveness for neuropathic pain. Results with venlafaxine for neuropathic pain have been inconsistent. Venlafaxine was effective for PDN and for various forms of polyneuropathy at daily doses of 150 to 225 mg.[30,31] In one placebo-controlled trial, perioperative venlafaxine at a daily dose of 75 mg prevented the development of postmastectomy pain syndrome,[32] but in other trials on patients with postmastectomy pain[33] syndrome and mixed type neuropathies, efficacy at dose range of 75 to 150 mg could not be demonstrated.

Three large randomized controlled trials[34–36] and one open-label 52-week extension trial[37] showed that duloxetine was effective for PDN at daily doses of 60 to 120 mg. Duloxetine 60 mg per day has similar efficacy to duloxetine 120 mg per day and the lower dose but is far more tolerable. It can be administered once daily. At that dose the drug significantly improved sleep and quality of life. The most common adverse effects reported in these clinical trials were nausea, somnolence, dizziness, and constipation—all of which tended to decrease over time. Initiating treatment at a daily dose of 30 mg for one week followed by an increase to 60 mg per day during the second week is likely to improve tolerability.[38] Duloxetine has not been associated with cardiac toxicity. Do not use it concomitantly with MAOIs or in patients with markedly impaired liver function.

The relative efficacy (NNTs) of the SNRIs in the treatment of PDN have been calculated as 4.6 (CI 2.9–10.6) for venlafaxine and 5.2 (CI 3.7–8.5) for duloxetine[6] indicating that they are less effective than the far less expensive TCAs.[39]

Selective Serotonin Reuptake Inhibitors

Reports of the effectiveness of SSRIs in neuropathic pain management are inconsistent. Some reports may not have separated analgesic effect from the effects of mood elevation on pain perception. One well controlled trial documented that fluoxetine was no more effective than placebo[27] while both amitriptyline and desipramine were efficacious. Two other trials support efficacy of citalopram[40] and paroxetine[41] (both at 40 mg per day) in PDN. Although SSRIs show a favorable safety profile compared to TCAs and are generally well tolerated, they are far less efficacious in the treatment of neuropathic pain, with NNT of 6.8 (CI 4.4–441), and therefore should not be regarded as first-line agents.[5]

ANTICONVULSANTS

Some systematic reviews and evidence-based guidelines for the treatment of neuropathic pain regard selected anticonvulsants as first line therapy. Drugs include the calcium channel α2-δ ligands gabapentin and pregabalin for PHN and PDN, and carbamazepine for trigeminal neuralgia. Additionally, lamotrigine, oxcarbazepine, and, to a lesser extent, other anticonvulsants have been reported as effective in neuropathic pain in randomized controlled trials. Table 80.4 summarizes these trials.

Pregabalin

Perhaps the most extensively studied drug in this class is pregabalin, which is believed to exert its analgesic effect by binding to the α2-δ subunit of voltage-gated calcium channels on primary afferent neurons, reducing the release of neurotransmitters from their central terminals.[42] Pregabalin was effective for PHN and PDN in numerous multicenter, randomized, controlled trials.[43–51] A recent trial demonstrated better pain relief with pregabalin than placebo in patients with spinal cord injury pain.[52] It has not been studied in other types of neuropathic pain. The effective daily dose of 300 to 600 mg reduces pain and improves sleep, functioning, and quality of life. Pregabalin has several advantages compared to other anticonvulsants: it is usually administered twice daily, can be rapidly titrated, has early onset of analgesic effect, and linear pharmacokinetics. No drug interactions have been reported with pregabalin. The most commonly reported adverse events were dose-dependent and included dizziness, somnolence, dry mouth, and edema.[12,13]

Gabapentin

There is also strong evidence of gabapentin's efficacy for PHN and PDN at doses of 900 to 3600 mg per day. Although less broadly studied than pregabalin in these syndromes, gabapentin has shown efficacy in HIV-associated painful neuropathy, pain in Guillain Barré syndrome, phantom limb pain, spinal cord injury pain, and cancer-related neuropathic pain.[7,53–64] In contrast, three trials did not support the efficacy of gabapentin in various forms of neuropathic pain. In a small trial comparing gabapentin and placebo for phantom pain, the authors concluded that "gabapentin did not substantially affect pain."[65] In another study, gabapentin had only a mild effect on pain in patients with complex regional pain syndrome type I (CRPS I).[66] A more recent and larger trial did not demonstrate any benefit for gabapentin over placebo in chemotherapy-induced painful peripheral neuropathy.[67] Gabapentin is believed to have similar mechanism of analgesia to pregabalin. However, unlike pregabalin it requires thrice daily dosing, has nonlinear pharmacokinetics, and may take days or weeks to reach an effective dose. Gabapentin is relatively safe, with no clinically relevant drug interactions. The main adverse effects are somnolence, dizziness, and peripheral edema.[12,13] Clinically, some clinicians report that some patients who fail to respond to gabapentin may respond to pregabalin and vice versa.

Carbamazepine

Carbamazepine is commonly used to treat trigeminal neuralgia. Most carbamazepine studies in trigeminal neuralgia were conducted in the 1960s and 1970s using small samples sizes. In these studies pain relief was superior with carbamazepine compared to placebo.[68–71] Carbamazepine was also one of the first anticonvulsants used in PDN, and was superior to placebo in two small trials.[72,73] Pain reduction was similar between carbamazepine and the tricyclic antidepressant nortriptyline in a more recent trial.[74] Carbamazepine was more effective than placebo in patients with mixed types of neuropathic pain in one controlled trial.[75] NNT to achieve 50% pain relief with carbamazepine in trigeminal neuralgia and painful diabetic neuropathy were 2.6 (range 2.2–3.3) and 3.3 (range 2–9.4), respectively, in systematic reviews.[76,77] However, these figures are based primarily on old trials, most of which were conducted in small patient groups for relatively short treatment periods. Nonetheless, study-quality

TABLE 80.4

SUMMARY OF THE RANDOMIZED CONTROLLED TRIALS OF ANTIEPILEPTIC DRUGS IN TREATMENT OF NEUROPATHIC PAIN PUBLISHED AS PEER-REVIEWED ARTICLES

Study	Drug	Diagnosis	Design	Number of patients treated with active drug	Maximal dosage (mg)	Treatment duration (weeks)	Results
Nicol[70] 1969	Carbamazepine	TN	crossover	20	2400	2	A>P
Campbell[68] 1966	Carbamazepine	TN	crossover	77	800	2	A>P
Killian[69] 1968	Carbamazepine	TN	crossover	27	1000	5 days	A>P
Vilming[159] 1986	Carbamazepine	TN	parallel	6	900	3	A>tizanidine
Lechin[160] 1989	Carbamazepine	TN	crossover	48	1200	8	A<pimozide
Lindstrom[79] 1987	Carbamazepine	TN	crossover	12	Maximal tolerated	2	A = tocinide
Rull[72] 1965	Carbamazepine	DPN	crossover	30	400	2	A>P
Wilton[73] 1974	Carbamazepine	DPN	crossover	40	400	2	A>P
Gomez-Perez[74] 1996	Carbamazepine	DPN	crossover	16	200	4	A = nortriptyline
Harke[75] 2001	Carbamazepine	Mixed types	parallel	43	600	8 days	A>P
Dogra[80] 2005	Oxcarbazepine	DPN	parallel	69	1800	16	A>P
Grosskopf[161] 2006	Oxcarbazepine	DPN	parallel	71	1200	16	A = P
Thienel[94] 2004	Topiramate	DPN	parallel	878	400	22	A = P[a]
Raskin[93] 2004	Topiramate	DPN	parallel	214	400	12	A>P
Khoromi[95] 2005	Topiramate	LR	crossover	42	400	8	A = P; A>P[b]
Hahn[56] 2004	Gabapentin	HIV neuropathy	parallel	15	2400	4	A>P
Rice[61] 2001	Gabapentin	PHN	parallel	223	2400	7	A>P
Rowbotham[62] 1998	Gabapentin	PHN	parallel	113	3600	8	A>P
Pandey[59] 2002	Gabapentin	GBS	crossover	18	15mg/kg	1	A>P
Pandey[60] 2005	Gabapentin	GBS	parallel	12	900	1	A>P
Caraceni[55] 2004	Gabapentin	Neuropathic cancer pain	parallel	79	1800	8 days	A>P
Backonja[53] 1998	Gabapentin	DPN	parallel	84	3600	8	A>P
Morello[58] 1999	Gabapentin	DPN	crossover	26	1800	6	A = amitriptyline
Gilron[7] 2005	Gabapentin	DPN + PHN	crossover	57	3200	5	A>P; A<morphine A<A + morphine[c]
van de Vusse[66] 2004	Gabapentin	CRPS	crossover	58	1800	3	A>P
Bone[54] 2002	Gabapentin	Phantom limb	crossover	19	2400	6	A>P
Levendoglu[57] 2004	Gabapentin	SCI	crossover	20	3600	8	A>P
Tai[64] 2002	Gabapentin	SCI	crossover	7	1800	4	A>P[d]
Serpel[63] 2002	Gabapentin	Mixed types	parallel	153	2400	8	A>P
Eisenberg[82] 2001	Lamotrigine	DPN	parallel	29	400	8	A>P
Simpson[84] 2000	Lamotrigine	HIV-N	parallel	20	300	14	A>P
Simpson[83] 2003	Lamotrigine	HIV-N	parallel	150	600	11	A = P; A>P[e]
Finnerup[85] 2002	Lamotrigine	SCI	crossover	22	400	8	A = P; A>P[f]
Vestergaard[86] 2001	Lamotrigine	CPSP	crossover	30	200	8	A>P
Zakrzewska[87] 1997	Lamotrigine	TN	crossover	14	400	2	A>P
McCleane[89] 1999	Lamotrigine	Mixed types	parallel	50	200	8	A = P
Richter[48] 2005	Pregabalin	DPN	parallel	161	600	6	A>P
Lesser[47] 2004	Pregabalin	DPN	parallel	240	600	5	A>P
Rosenstock[49] 2004	Pregabalin	DPN	parallel	76	300	8	A>P
Freynhagen[39] 2005	Pregabalin	DPN + PHN	parallel	273	600	12	A>P
Sabatowski[50] 2004	Pregabalin	PHN	parallel	157	300	8	A>P
Dworkin[45] 2003	Pregabalin	PHN	parallel	89	600	8	A>P
van Seventer[51] 2006	Pregabalin	PHN	parallel	273	600	13	A>P
Atli[162] 2005	Zonisamide	DPN	parallel	13	600	12	A = P
Atli[162] 2005	Zonisamide	DPN	parallel	13		12	A = P
Otto[92] 2004	Valproic acid	Mixed types	crossover	31	1500	4	A = P
Kochar[91] 2005	Valproic acid + sodium valproate	PHN	parallel	48	1000	9	A>P
Vilholm[97] 2008	Levetiracetam	Postmastectomy	crossover	26	3000	4	A = P

CPSP, central poststroke pain; DPN, diabetic polyneuropathy; GBS, Guillain-Barré syndrome; HIV-N, HIV neuropathy; LR, lumbar radiculopathy; SCI, spinal cord injury; TN, trigeminal neuralgia.

A, active drug; P, placebo; > indicates that active drug was superior to the comparator in terms of pain reduction; < indicates that active drug was superior to the comparator in terms of pain reduction; = indicates that active drug was equal to the comparator in terms of pain reduction.

[a]findings from three double-blind placebo-controlled trials.

[b]No significant difference between topiramate and placebo in pain score (primary outcome measure), but significant difference in global pain relief score.

[c]In this four-arm study, gabapentin was superior to placebo but less effective than morphine and the combination of gabapentin plus morphine.

[d]A significant decrease of "unpleasant feeling" and a trend toward a decrease in both the "pain intensity" and "burning sensation."

[e]Lamotrigine was superior to placebo in patients who received antiviral neurotoxic therapy, but not in patients who did not receive this therapy.

[f]Lamotrigine was superior to placebo in patients with incomplete spinal cord injury and evoked pain, but equal to placebo in patients with complete injury and without evoked pain.

rating for carbamazepine in trigeminal neuralgia is regarded as level 1 (good quality evidence), and only level 3 (no good evidence) for diabetic neuropathy and other forms of neuropathic pain.[76,77] The analgesic mechanism of carbamazepine is related to voltage-dependent sodium channel blocking, which results in decreased ectopic nerve discharges and neural membranes stabilization.[78] Adverse events are common and include dizziness, nausea, drowsiness, blurred vision, and ataxia.[73] Rare, but serious, side effects include leukopenia, impairment of liver function, and reduction of sodium plasma levels. A limitation of using carbamazepine is its association with Stevens-Johnson syndrome.[12,13]

Oxcarbazepine

Oxcarbazepine is believed to have a similar analgesic mechanism to carbamazepine. Randomized, controlled trials[79] demonstrated its effectiveness for trigeminal neuralgia at daily doses of 600 to 1200 mg; patients with intractable trigeminal neuralgia may need doses as high as 2400 mg per day. Oxcarbazepine was more effective than placebo in reducing pain associated with diabetic neuropathy in one randomized trial.[80] In several open-label trials oxcarbazepine improved mixed types of neuropathic pain from baseline.[81] In summary, oxcarbazepine seems similar to carbamazepine for trigeminal neuralgia, but there are only limited data regarding its efficacy and safety for other types of neuropathic pain. Hyponatremia has occurred with this drug; sodium levels should be monitored.

Lamotrigine

Lamotrigine has shown efficacy in some randomized, controlled trials for painful diabetic neuropathy,[82] HIV-related neuropathy,[83,84] spinal cord injury pain,[85] central poststroke pain,[86] and trigeminal neuralgia.[87] At the same time, equivocal or negative (active therapy not superior to placebo) results were reported from studies with lamotrigine for HIV-related neuropathy,[83] pain related to complete spinal cord injury,[85] diabetic polyneuropathy,[88] and mixed neuropathies.[89] The overall safety profile for lamotrigine is dose-related. Common side effects include nausea, vomiting, sedation, drowsiness, dizziness, headaches, malaise, visual disturbances, and ataxia. Skin rash that may deteriorate to dangerous or life-threatening Stevens-Johnson syndrome or toxic epidermal necrolysis is the most serious adverse event of lamotrigine. Slow titration may reduce the risk of developing these syndromes. The appearance of skin rash requires discontinuation of lamotrigine.[90]

Other Anticonvulsants

Valproic acid and sodium valproate at a daily dose of 1000 mg were superior to placebo in reducing postherpetic neuralgia.[91] In contrast, 1500 mg of valproic acid failed to show superiority to placebo for mixed types of neuropathic pain in another randomized, controlled trial.[92] Topiramate was effective for PDN in one controlled trial,[93] but not in another, much larger trial.[94] Topiramate also yielded equivocal results in one randomized, controlled trial in patients with painful lumbar radiculopathy.[95] Topiramate was titrated up to a daily dose of 400 mg in all three trials. Several new anticonvulsants such as levetiracetam, zonisamide, tiagabine, and lacosamide have been used in open label studies or small-scale randomized, controlled trials, but currently available data are too limited to confidently assess the efficacy of any of these newer drugs. One example is levetiracetam, which initially showed some indication of efficacy for painful neoplastic plexopathies in an open-label case series report,[96] but more recently

failed to relieve postmastectomy pain syndrome when compared to placebo in a randomized controlled trial.[97]

OPIOIDS

Nine randomized controlled trials tested the efficacy of oral opioids for PDN, PHN, phantom pain, nerve root pain, and neuropathic pain of diverse etiologies (Table 80.5). Eight trials demonstrated effectiveness of morphine, oxycodone, methadone, or levorphanol in reducing spontaneous neuropathic pain.[75,98–104] Efficacy was demonstrated by either superiority over placebo or a dose-dependent analgesic response. The only negative study is a recent trial in which morphine showed no superiority over placebo in patients with chronic lumbar radicular pain.[23] Six studies[98–101,103,104] were recently pooled in a meta-analysis[105] resulting in a mean pain intensity to be 14 points lower in opioid treated patients than in those treated with placebo (95% C.I. -18 to -10; $p < .001$). From a different standpoint, the overall NNT of opioids for reducing neuropathic pain by 50% is 2.5 (95% CI 2.0–3.2).[5] A systematic review of seven short-term (less than 24 hours) and two intermediate-term (4 weeks) randomized, controlled trials concluded that according to these trials opioids can reduce the intensity of dynamic mechanical allodynia and perhaps of cold allodynia in peripheral neuropathic pain. These findings are clinically relevant because dynamic mechanical allodynia and cold allodynia are the most prevalent types of evoked pain in neuropathic pain.[106]

Although opioids clearly reduce neuropathic pain, several questions related to chronic opioid use in neuropathic pain remain unanswered. Secondary outcome parameters such as physical and mental health, sleep, disability, and quality of life, which were measured in some of these trials, yielded inconsistent results. Data are limited regarding efficacy of opioids for central neuropathic pain. Opioid studies were limited to 8 weeks or less. Therefore, no data on long-term safety and efficacy of opioids in the treatment of neuropathic pain are available. This is particularly important because of emerging information regarding long-term complications of opioid use such as hypogonadism,[107,108] increased risk of bone fractures in the elderly,[109,110] immunological changes,[111] and the potential for opioid-induced hyperalgesia.[112,113] Available trials do not clearly address the issues of addiction and abuse which have major medical, legal, and social implications. These unanswered questions about opioid treatment of neuropathic pain require further assessment.

TRAMADOL

Tramadol is a unique agent with a dual mechanism of analgesia: it has a weak affinity for mu-opioid receptors and it weakly inhibits serotonin and norepinephrine reuptake.[12,13] Randomized controlled trials show that tramadol can reduce pain in patients with PHN,[114] PDN,[115] mixed forms of painful polyneuropathy[116] and postamputation pain (Table 80.5).[117] Its efficacy for PDN and PHN seems somewhat reduced as compared to that of other opioids with NNT of 3.9 (CI 2.7–6.7).[5] Due to dose-dependent adverse effects, a gradual titration from 50 mg two to three times daily to a maximal dose of 200 mg twice daily is generally required. Common adverse events include drowsiness, nausea, constipation, dizziness, and potential for abuse. Concomitant use of serotonin reuptake inhibitors may increase the risk for serotonergic syndrome.

NMDA RECEPTOR ANTAGONISTS

In spite of numerous animal studies in which N-methyl-D-aspartic acid (NMDA) receptor antagonists yielded promising results,

TABLE 80.5

SUMMARY OF RANDOMIZED CONTROLLED TRIALS OF OPIOIDS AND TRAMADOL IN TREATMENT OF
NEUROPATHIC PAIN PUBLISHED AS PEER-REVIEWED ARTICLES

Study	Drug	Diagnosis	Design	Number of patients treated with active drug	Maximal dosage (mg)	Treatment duration (weeks)	Results
Watson[103] 1998	Oxycodone	PHN	crossover	50	60	4	A>P
Huse[99] 2001	Morphine	Phantom limb	crossover	12	300	4	A>P
Harke[75] 2001	Morphine	Mixed peripheral	parallel	21	90	8 days	A=P
Raja[101] 2002	Morphine	PHN	crossover	38	225	8	A>P
Raja[101] 2002	Methadone	PHN	crossover	26	80	8	A>P
Gimbel[98] 2003	Oxycodone	DPN	parallel	82	120	6	A>P
Watson[104] 2003	Oxycodone	DPN	crossover	45	80	4	A>P
Morley[100] 2003	1. Methadone low-dose	Mixed neuropathic	crossover	19	low dose 10	20 days	AL=P
	2. Methadone high-dose		crossover	17	high dose 20		AH>P
Rowbotham[102] 2003	Levorphanol low-dose vs. levorphanol high-dose	mixed neuropathic	parallel	38 43	low dose 3.15 high dose 15.75	8	AH>AL
Khoromi[23] 2007	Morphine	Radiculopathy	crossover	41	90	9	A=P
Boureau[114] 2003	Tramadol	PHN	parallel	63	400	6	A>P
Harati[115] 1998	Tramadol	DPN	parallel	65	400	6	A>P
Sindrup[116] 1999	Tramadol	Mixed neuropathic	crossover	43	400	4	A>P
Wilder-Smith[117] 2005	Tramadol	Postamputation	parallel	33	594	1 month	A>P

AH, active drug at high dose; AL, active drug at low dose.

clinical trials with oral drugs were generally negative (Table 80.6). Two small trials showed efficacy of the NMDA receptor antagonist dextromethorphan for PDN but not for PHN or neuropathies of mixed etiologies. Memantine, which also has NMDA receptor blocking properties, was not effective in diabetic polyneuropathy, postherpetic neuralgia, or phantom limb pain.[5] In contrast, intravenous administration of subanesthetic doses of ketamine produced short-term analgesia (lasting for hours) in multiple forms of neuropathic pain.[118] Regardless of the difference in outcomes between short- and long-term studies, a recent trial showed that short-term intravenous administration of ketamine may be useful in predicting long-term response to oral dextromethorphan.[119]

SODIUM CHANNEL BLOCKERS

Carbamazepine, oxcarbazepine, mexiletine, intravenous lidocaine, and topical lidocaine are all sodium channel blockers. The first two have already been reviewed earlier in this chapter.

Mexiletine, an orally available analog of lidocaine with antiarrhythmic properties,[12] was evaluated in several randomized, controlled trials for the treatment of painful diabetic polyneuropathy. These trials are summarized in Table 80.6. With the exception of one trial in which a relatively high dose of the drug produced modest effect, no significant pain relief was demonstrated.[120–122]

High doses of mexiletine are commonly associated with adverse effects such as chest pain, dizziness, gastrointestinal disturbances, palpitations, tremor, and potential for worsening of existing arrhythmia.[12,13]

A meta-analysis of randomized, controlled trials demonstrated the effectiveness of intravenous lidocaine for various types of peripheral neuropathic pain syndromes. Pain was reduced by about 10 mm more (on a 100 mm scale) with lidocaine than with placebo.[123] Major drawbacks of this therapy are the lack of data on long-term efficacy and the apparent necessity for repeated infusions for sustained pain relief. This may therefore be an impractical approach for many patients. Interestingly, a positive correlation between the response to a single lidocaine infusion and long-term response to oral mexiletine has been reported.[124] Topical lidocaine is reviewed later in this chapter.

NONSTEROIDAL ANTI-INFLAMMATORY AGENTS

Although evidence for the role of inflammation in neuropathic pain is emerging and it is estimated that half of all clinical cases of neuropathic pain are associated with inflammation of the peripheral nerves,[125] no controlled clinical trials that tested the effectiveness of nonsteroidal anti-inflammatory agents (NSAIDs) for neuropathic pain exist. Only a pilot, randomized, open-label

TABLE 80.6

SUMMARY OF RANDOMIZED CONTROLLED TRIALS OF OTHER DRUGS IN TREATMENT OF NEUROPATHIC PAIN PUBLISHED AS PEER-REVIEWED ARTICLES

Study	Drug	Diagnosis	Design	Number of patients treated with active drug	Maximal dosage (mg)	Treatment duration (weeks)	Results
			Topical agent				
Chad[163] 1990	Capsaicin cream	DPN	parallel	28	0.075% × 4/day	4	A = P
Scheffler[164] 1991	Capsaicin cream	DPN	parallel	19	0.075% × 4/day	8	A > P
Capsaicin study group[165] 1991	Capsaicin cream	DPN	parallel	138	0.075% × 4/day	8	A > P
Tandan[166] 1992	Capsaicin cream	DPN	parallel	11	0.075% × 4/day	8	A > P
Low[167] 1995	Capsaicin cream	DPN	parallel	40	0.075% × 4/day	12	A = P
Bernstein[168] 1989	Capsaicin cream	PHN	parallel	16	0.075% × 3–4/day	6	A > P
Watson[169] 1993	Capsaicin cream	PHN	parallel	74	0.075% × 4/day	6	A > P
Watson[170] 1992	Capsaicin cream	Postmastectomy	parallel	14	0.075% × 4/day	6	A = P
Ellison[171] 1997	Capsaicin cream	Postsurgical	parallel	49	0.075% × 4/day	8	A > P
Paice[172] 2000	Capsaicin cream	HIV neuropathy	parallel	15	0.075% × 4/day	8	A = P
McCleane[173] 2000	Capsaicin cream	Mixed neuropathic	parallel	33	0.025% × 4/day	4	A > P
Rowbotham[134] 1995	Lidocaine gel	PHN	crossover	39	5%	4	A > P
Rowbotham[135] 1996	Lidocaine patch	PHN	crossover	35	5%	24 hours	A > P
Galer[133] 1999	Lidocaine patch	PHN	crossover	32	5%	2–14	A > P
Galer[174] 2002	Lidocaine patch	Focal neuropathies	crossover	96	5%	3	A > P
Estanislao[175] 2004	Lidocaine gel	HIV neuropathy	crossover	61	5%	2	A = P
Meier[136] 2003	Lidocaine patch	Focal neuropathies	crossover	39	5%	1	A > P
Lynch[137, 146] 2005	Ketamine cream	Mixed neuropathies	parallel	22	1%	3	A = P
			NMDA receptor antagonists				
Nelson[176] 1997	Dextromethorphan	DPN	crossover	13	960	6	A > P
Sang[177] 2002	Dextromethorphan	DPN	crossover	19	400	9	A > P
Sang[177] 2002	Memantine	DPN	crossover	19	55	9	A = P
Nelson[176] 1997	Dextromethorphan	PHN	crossover	13	960	6	A = P
Sang[177] 2002	Dextromethorphan	PHN	crossover	17	400	9	A = P
Sang[177] 2002	Memantine	PHN	parallel	17	35	9	A = P
Eisenberg[178] 1998	Memantine	Phantom limb	crossover	12	20	5	A = P
Nikolajsen[179] 2000	Memantine	Phantom limb	parallel	15	20	5	A = P
Maier[180] 2003	Dextromethorphan	Mixed neuropathies	crossover	18	30	4	A = P
McQuay[181] 1994	Riluzole	Mixed neuropathies	crossover	17	81	20 days	A = P
Galer[182] 2000	Riluzole	Mixed neuropathies	crossover	12	100	2	A = P
Galer[182] 2000	Mexiletine	DPN	crossover	21	200	2	A = P
Dejgard[183] 1988	Mexiletine	DPN	crossover	16	10 mg/kg	26	A > P
Stracke[121] 1992	Mexiletine	DPN	parallel	47	675	5	A = P
Oskarsson[120] 1997	Mexiletine	DPN	parallel	95	675	3	A = P
Wright[122] 1997	Mexiletine	DPN	parallel	14	600	3	A = P

(continued)

TABLE 80.6

CONTINUED

Study	Drug	Diagnosis	Design	Number of patients treated with active drug	Maximal dosage (mg)	Treatment duration (weeks)	Results
NMDA receptor antagonists (continued)							
Kiebyrtz[20] 1998	Mexiletine	HIV neuropathy	parallel	48	600	10	A=P
Kemper[184] 1998	Mexiletine	HIV neuropathy	crossover	16	600	6	A=P
Chabal[185] 1992	Mexiletine	Peripheral nerve injury	crossover	11	750	9	A>P
Wallace[186] 2000	Mexiletine	Mixed neuropathies	crossover	20	900	10 days	A=P
Chiou-Tan[187] 1996	Mexiletine	Spinal cord injury	crossover	11	450	4	A=P
Drug combinations							
Gilron[7] 2005	Gabapentin + morphine vs. gabapentin vs. morphine	Mixed neuropathies	crossover	49 / 48 / 49	60+2400 / 3600 / 120	5	C>M = G>P[a]
Khoromi[23] 2007	Morphine + nortriptyline v. morphine vs. nortriptyline	radiculopathy	crossover	34 / 41 / 34	90+100 / 90 / 100	9	C = M = N = P[b]
Hanna[144] 2006	Gabapentin + oxycodone vs. gabapentin + placebo	DPN	parallel	163 / 165	3600+80 / 4800	12	G+O>G+P[c]
Lynch[137,146] 2005	Ketamine + amitriptyline vs. ketamine vs. amitriptyline	Mixed neuropathies	parallel	23 / 22 / 22	2%+1% cream / 1% cream / 2% cream	3	C = K = A = P[d]
Cannabinoids							
Karst[140] 2003	1',1'dimethylheptyl-Delta8-tetrahydrocannabinol-11-oic acid (CT3)	Mixed neuropathies	crossover	19	80	7 days	A>P
Abrams[139] 2007	Cannabis	HIV neuropathy	parallel	27	3.65 mg smoked X3/day	5 days	A>P
Berman[141] 2004	Tetrahydrocannabinol ± cannabidiol	Brachial plexus avulsion	parallel	93	129.6 ± 120	14 days	A>P
Svendsen[188] 2004	Dronabinol	Central pain (multiple sclerosis)	crossover	24	10	3	A>P
Rog[142] 2005	Tetrahydrocannabinol + cannabidiol	Central pain (multiple sclerosis)	parallel	34	67.5+62.5	4	A>P

[a]Combination therapy superior to each drug alone; all are superior to placebo.
[b]Combination, each drug alone, and placebo showed similar efficacy.
[c]Combination of gabapentin + oxycodone was superior to the combination of gabapentin + placebo.
[d]Combination of ketamine + amitriptyline cream, each drug alone and their combination showed similar efficacy.

clinical trial which showed comparable effectiveness of lidocaine patch 5% to that of naproxen 500 mg twice daily for the treatment of neuropathic pain associated with carpal tunnel syndrome is available.[126]

ZICONOTIDE

Ziconotide, the first N-type calcium channel blocker, is a synthetic formulation of *Conus magus* cone snail venom.[127] It produces analgesia by selectively and reversibly blocking N-type calcium channels in the CNS.[128,129] Intrathecal administration via an implanted pump or catheter is necessary because systemic ziconotide produces profound hypotension.[128] Intrathecal ziconotide resulted in significantly greater visual analogue scale (VAS) pain score reductions than placebo in chronic malignant and nonmalignant pain during clinical trials ($p < .001$).[127,130] Common adverse events include dizziness (47%), nausea (41%), nystagmus (27%), confusion (25%), somnolence (22%), gait abnormalities (18%), blurred vision (14%), headache (13%), memory impairment (13%), and vomiting (13%).[127,130] Ziconotide's narrow therapeutic index commonly results in toxicity, particularly with aggressive initial dosing and titration.[128,129] The U.S. labeling for ziconotide recommends an initial continuous infusion of 2.4 mcg/day, with dose titrations 2 or 3 times weekly.[130] Later, an expert consensus statement recommended an initial dose of only 0.5 mcg/day, with weekly dose increases of no more than 0.5 mcg/day as needed for pain control.[131] Lower starting doses and slower titration reduce the risk of serious adverse events and premature drug discontinuation.[130,131] Risks inherent with intrathecal drug delivery include infection, subarachnoid hemorrhage, catheter-tip inflammatory masses, and pump failure.[132] Ongoing studies offer promise that new N-type calcium channel blockers will provide effective and well tolerated analgesia with less invasive routes of administration.[128]

TOPICAL AGENTS

Capsaicin

Topical capsaicin cream 0.075% applied 3 to 4 times daily was effective in three of five published randomized controlled trials in painful diabetic neuropathy, in two postherpetic neuralgia trials, one trial in postsurgical pain, and one in patients with mixed neuropathies. Topical capsaicin was not superior to placebo in randomized controlled trials for postmastectomy pain syndrome and for HIV neuropathy. The NNT with topical capsaicin to reach 50% pain reduction is therefore 6.7 (95% CI 4.6–12).[5] The proposed mechanism of action is depletion of vanilloid receptors, but neurolysis may also be responsible for the activity of topical capsaicin. Capsaicin application is associated with burning sensation, particularly during the first weeks of treatment, an adverse event that may often limit its use. Therefore, therapy should begin with the lower 0.025% concentration and the higher 0.075% concentration should be used only after a full container of the weaker formulation has been used up. Patients should be instructed to avoid touching eyes and mucous membranes with the drug or fingers that have been exposed to it. Counsel patients that within a week most people become reasonably tolerant to the burning on application that is common when starting therapy especially since up to a month is required for maximal analgesic effect. Experienced clinicians consider topical capsaicin more of an adjunctive than primary therapy for neuropathic pain.

Topical Lidocaine Patches

Application of topical lidocaine 5% patches was effective for PHN in three short-term, randomized, controlled trials,[133–135] and also in patients with other focal peripheral neuropathies.[126,136] The maximal recommended daily dose is three patches applied simultaneously every 12 hours. With the exception of mild skin reactions, lidocaine patches are not associated with adverse reactions, although caution is required in patients receiving oral Class I antiarrhythmic medications (e.g., mexiletine) and in patients with severe hepatic dysfunction.[8]

Topical Ketamine

One short-term, randomized, controlled trial evaluated the analgesic effect of topical ketamine 1% as compared to topical amitriptyline 2%, a combination of both, or placebo in patients with mixed types of neuropathic pain. No difference in pain reduction between treatments was found.[137]

CANNABINOIDS

Although cannabinoids are not formally approved for the treatment of neuropathic pain by drug regulatory agencies, many patients use cannabis for pain relief.[138] A recent double-blind, placebo-controlled, crossover study showed that smoking a single high-dose (7%) or low-dose (3.5%) cannabis cigarette produced better analgesia for a few hours than placebo in 38 patients with central and peripheral neuropathic pain. No effect on evoked pain was seen. Modest cognitive effects, particularly memory, at higher doses were noted.[138] Cannabis (3.56% tetrahydrocannabinol) or identical placebo cigarettes, smoked three times daily for 5 days also was tested in patients with HIV-induced painful neuropathy.[139] The first cannabis cigarette reduced pain by a median of 72% versus 15% with placebo. Smoked cannabis produced a daily median pain reduction of 34% compared to 17% with placebo. In contrast to the aforementioned study, cannabis reduced experimentally induced mechanical hyperalgesia. All these results were statistically significant. The agent 1′,1′dimethylheptyl-Delta8-tetrahydrocannabinol-11-oic acid (CT-3), a potent analgesic cannabinoid in animals, was tested in a randomized, placebo-controlled, double-blind crossover trial in 21 patients with mixed forms of chronic neuropathic pain. The two tested doses (40 and 80 mg/day) of CT-3 produced more analgesia that placebo, but no dose response analgesic effect was observed. No major adverse effects were observed.[140] In another study, 48 patients with intractable pain related to brachial plexus avulsion were treated for 2 weeks with two different oromucosal spray preparations of whole plant extracts of delta (9) tetrahydrocannabinol (THC) with or without cannabidiol (CBD) or placebo. The active compounds, but not the placebo, significantly improved pain and sleep. The study medications were generally well tolerated.[141] The THC-CBD oromucosal spray was also tested in 66 patients with central pain due to multiple sclerosis and was superior to placebo in reducing pain and sleep disturbances. The active drug was, again, well tolerated.[142] Another study on patients with multiple sclerosis compared the efficacy of orally administered 10 dronabinol at a maximum daily dose of 10 mg versus placebo. Median spontaneous pain intensity and median pain relief score were significantly superior during dronabinol treatment than during placebo treatment. A recent meta-analysis concluded that cannabinoids are effective for neuropathic pain in multiple sclerosis, although small number of trials and patients were notable limitations of the review.[143] While the reports on cannabis efficacy in neuropathic pain management are inconsistent, it is reasonable to conclude at this time that the cannabinoids have shown effectiveness for neuropathic pain in a few recent controlled trials, and seem to be well tolerated. However, their long-term efficacy and safety have not been tested yet.

DRUG COMBINATIONS

Not uncommonly, administration of a single drug does not produce adequate analgesia. Pharmacologically, it seems reasonable to coadminister drugs with different mechanisms of action. While combination therapy is commonly used in clinical practice, limited data are available regarding the efficacy and safety of this practice. Most trials produced positive results. One trial found that concomitant use of gabapentin and morphine in patients with mixed forms of neuropathic pain produced superior efficacy and safety than each drug alone.[7] Similar results were reported for the combination of gabapentin with oxycodone[144] and for gabapentin with venlafaxine.[145] These trials imply that combination therapy could enhance analgesia while decreasing side effects. In contrast, Khoromi et al.[23] could not demonstrate superiority of morphine, nortriptyline, or their combination over placebo in patients with chronic lumbar root pain. One randomized controlled trial compared the efficacy of topical amitriptyline 2%, ketamine 1%, and a combination of both in patients with mixed types of neuropathic pain. Although reduction in pain scores was observed in all groups, there was no difference in efficacy between the groups.[137] Interestingly, an open-label trial demonstrated that topical amitriptyline 2%/ketamine 1%, given over 6 to 12 months, was associated with long-term analgesic effectiveness in treating neuropathic pain.[146]

References

1. Torrance N, Smith BH, Bennett MI, et al. The epidemiology of chronic pain of predominantly neuropathic origin. Results from a general population survey. *J Pain* 2006;7(4):281–289.
2. Hall GC, Carroll D, Parry D, et al. Epidemiology and treatment of neuropathic pain: the UK primary care perspective. *Pain* 2006;122(1–2):156–162.
3. Yarnitsky D, Eisenberg E. Neuropathic pain: between positive and negative ends. *Pain Forum* 1998;7:241–242.
4. Taylor RS. Epidemiology of refractory neuropathic pain. *Pain Pract* 2006; 6(1):22–26.
5. Finnerup NB, Otto M, McQuay HJ, et al. Algorithm for neuropathic pain treatment: an evidence based proposal. *Pain* 2005;118(3):289–305.
6. Attal N, Cruccu G, Haanpää M, et al. EFNS guidelines on pharmacological treatment of neuropathic pain. *Eur J Neurol* 2006;13(11):1153–1169.
7. Gilron I, Bailey JM, Tu D, et al. Morphine, gabapentin, or their combination for neuropathic pain. *N Engl J Med* 2005;352(13):1324–1334.
8. Dworkin RH, O'Connor AB, Backonja M, et al. Pharmacologic management of neuropathic pain: evidence-based recommendations. *Pain* 2007;132(3): 237–251.
9. Tatsumi M, Groshan K, Blakely RD, et al. Pharmacological profile of antidepressants and related compounds at human monoamine transporters. *Eur J Pharmacol* 1997;340(2–3):249–258.
10. Owens MJ. Selectivity of antidepressants: from the monoamine hypothesis of depression to the SSRI revolution and beyond. *J Clin Psychiatry* 2004;65 suppl 4:5–10.
11. Maheswaran AM, ed. *Mosby's Drug Consult.* 16th ed. St. Louis, MO: Elsevier Mosby; 2006.
12. McEvoy GK, Snow EK, Miller J, et al., eds. *AHFS 2008 Drug Information.* Bethesda, Md: American Society of Health-System Pharmacists; 2008.
13. Brungon LL, Lazo JS, Parker KL, eds. *Goodman and Gilman's The Pharmacological Basis of Therapeutics.* 11th ed. New York: McGraw-Hill; 2006.
14. Hardman JG, Limbird LE, eds. *Goodman and Gilman's The Pharmacological Basis of Therapeutics.* 10th ed. New York: McGraw-Hill; 2001.
15. Bymaster FP, Dreshfield-Ahmad LJ, Threlkeld PG, et al. Comparative affinity of duloxetine and venlafaxine for serotonin and norepinephrine transporters in vitro and in vivo, human serotonin receptor subtypes, and other neuronal receptors. *Neuropsychopharmacology* 2001;25(6):871–880.
16. Deecher DC, Beyer CE, Johnston G, et al. Desvenlafaxine succinate: A new serotonin and norepinephrine reuptake inhibitor. *J Pharmacol Exp Ther* Aug 2006;318(2):657-665.
17. Desvenlafaxine (Pristiq) package insert. Philadelphia: Wyeth Pharmaceuticals, Inc.; 2008.
18. Cardenas DD, Warms CA, Turner JA, et al. Efficacy of amitriptyline for relief of pain in spinal cord injury: results of a randomized controlled trial. *Pain* 2002;96(3):365–373.
19. Hammack JE, Michalak JC, Loprinzi CL, et al. Phase III evaluation of nortriptyline for alleviation of symptoms of cis-platinum-induced peripheral neuropathy. *Pain* 2002;98(1–2):195–203.
20. Kieburtz K, Simpson D, Yiannoutsos C, et al. A randomized trial of amitripty-

line and mexiletine for painful neuropathy in HIV infection. AIDS Clinical Trial Group 242 Protocol Team. *Neurology* 1998;51(6):1682–1688.
21. Shlay JC, Chaloner K, Max MB, et al. Acupuncture and amitriptyline for pain due to HIV-related peripheral neuropathy: a randomized controlled trial. Terry Beirn Community Programs for Clinical Research on AIDS. *JAMA* 1998;280(18):1590–1595.
22. Robinson LR, Czerniecki JM, Ehde DM, et al. Trial of amitriptyline for relief of pain in amputees: results of a randomized controlled study. *Arch Phys Med Rehabil* 2004;85(1):1–6.
23. Khoromi S, Cui L, Nackers L, Max MB. Morphine, nortriptyline, and their combination vs. placebo in patients with chronic lumbar root pain. *Pain* Jul 2007;130(1–2):66–75.
24. Mercadante S, Arcuri E, Tirelli W, et al. Amitriptyline in neuropathic cancer pain in patients on morphine therapy: a randomized placebo-controlled, double-blind crossover study. *Tumori* 2002;88(3):239–242.
25. Max MB, Culnane M, Schafer SC, et al. Amitriptyline relieves diabetic neuropathy pain in patients with normal or depressed mood. *Neurology* 1987; 37(4):589–596.
26. Breivik H, Collett B, Ventafridda V, et al. Survey of chronic pain in Europe: prevalence, impact on daily life, and treatment. *Eur J Pain* 2006;10(4): 287–333.
27. Max MB, Lynch SA, Muir J, et al. Effects of desipramine, amitriptyline, and fluoxetine on pain in diabetic neuropathy. *N Engl J Med* 1992;326(19): 1250–1256.
28. Rowbotham MC, Reisner LA, Davies PS, et al. Treatment response in antidepressant-naive postherpetic neuralgia patients: double-blind, randomized trial. *J Pain* 2005;6(11):741–746.
29. Lipman AG. Analgesic drugs for neuropathic and sympathetically maintained pain. *Clin Geriatr Med* 1996;12(3):501–515.
30. Rowbotham MC, Goli V, Kunz NR, et al. Venlafaxine extended release in the treatment of painful diabetic neuropathy: a double-blind, placebo-controlled study. *Pain* 2004;110(3):697–706.
31. Sindrup SH, Bach FW, Madsen C, et al. Venlafaxine versus imipramine in painful polyneuropathy: a randomized, controlled trial. *Neurology* 2003; 60(8):1284–1289.
32. Reuben SS, Makari-Judson G, Lurie SD. Evaluation of efficacy of the perioperative administration of venlafaxine XR in the prevention of postmastectomy pain syndrome. *J Pain Symptom Manage* 2004;27(2):133–139.
33. Tasmuth T, Härtel B, Kalso E. Venlafaxine in neuropathic pain following treatment of breast cancer. *Eur J Pain* 2002;6(1):17–24.
34. Goldstein DJ, Lu Y, Detke MJ, et al. Duloxetine vs. placebo in patients with painful diabetic neuropathy. *Pain* 2005;116(1–2):109–118.
35. Raskin J, Pritchett YL, Wang F, et al. A double-blind, randomized multicenter trial comparing duloxetine with placebo in the management of diabetic peripheral neuropathic pain. *Pain Med* 2005;6(5):346–356.
36. Wernicke JF, Pritchett YL, D'Souza DN, et al. A randomized controlled trial of duloxetine in diabetic peripheral neuropathic pain. *Neurology* 2006;67(8): 1411–1420.
37. Raskin J, Smith TR, Wong K, et al. Duloxetine versus routine care in the long-term management of diabetic peripheral neuropathic pain. *J Palliat Med* 2006;9(1):29–40.
38. Dunner DL, Wohlreich MM, Mallinckrodt CH, et al. Clinical consequences of initial duloxetine dosing strategies: comparison of 30 and 60 mg QD starting doses. *Curr Ther Res* 2005;66(6):522–540.
39. Cruccu G. Treatment of painful neuropathy. *Curr Opin Neurol* 2007;20(5): 531–535.
40. Sindrup SH, Bjerre U, Dejgaard A, et al. The selective serotonin reuptake inhibitor citalopram relieves the symptoms of diabetic neuropathy. *Clin Pharmacol Ther* 1992;52(5):547–552.
41. Sindrup SH, Gram LF, Brøsen K, et al. The selective serotonin reuptake inhibitor paroxetine is effective in the treatment of diabetic neuropathy symptoms. *Pain* 1990;42(2):135–144.
42. Dooley DJ, Donovan CM, Meder WP, et al. Preferential action of gabapentin and pregabalin at P/Q-type voltage-sensitive calcium channels: inhibition of K+-evoked [3H]-norepinephrine release from rat neocortical slices. *Synapse* 2002;45(3):171–190.
43. Sharma U, Allen R, Glessner C, et al. Pregabalin effectively relieves pain in patients with diabetic polyneuropathy: study 1008-914 [abstract 686-p]. *Diabetes* 2000;40(suppl 1):167.
44. Strojek K, Floter T, Balkenohl M, et al. Pregabalin in the management of chronic neuropathic pain (NeP): a novel evaluation of flexible and fixed dosing [abstract 804]. *Diabetes* 2004;53(suppl 2):59.
45. Dworkin RH, Corbin AE, Young JP Jr, et al. Pregabalin for the treatment of postherpetic neuralgia: a randomized, placebo-controlled trial. *Neurology* 2003;60(8):1274–1283.
46. Freynhagen R, Strojek K, Griesing T, et al. Efficacy of pregabalin in neuropathic pain evaluated in a 12-week, randomised, double-blind, multicentre, placebo-controlled trial of flexible- and fixed-dose regimens. *Pain* 2005; 115(3):254–263.
47. Lesser H, Sharma U, LaMoreaux L, et al. Pregabalin relieves symptoms of painful diabetic neuropathy: a randomized controlled trial. *Neurology* 2004; 63(11):2104–2110.
48. Richter RW, Portenoy R, Sharma U, et al. Relief of painful diabetic peripheral neuropathy with pregabalin: a randomized, placebo-controlled trial. *J Pain* 2005;6(4):253–260.
49. Rosenstock J, Tuchman M, LaMoreaux L, et al. Pregabalin for the treatment

of painful diabetic peripheral neuropathy: a double-blind, placebo-controlled trial. *Pain* 2004;110(3):628–638.

50. Sabatowski R, Gálvez R, Cherry DA, et al. Pregabalin reduces pain and improves sleep and mood disturbances in patients with post-herpetic neuralgia: results of a randomised, placebo-controlled clinical trial. *Pain* 2004;109(1–2):26–35.

51. van Seventer R, Feister HA, Young JP Jr, et al. Efficacy and tolerability of twice-daily pregabalin for treating pain and related sleep interference in post-herpetic neuralgia: a 13-week, randomized trial. *Curr Med Res Opin* 2006;22(2):375–384.

52. Siddall PJ, Cousins MJ, Otte A, et al. Pregabalin in central neuropathic pain associated with spinal cord injury: a placebo-controlled trial. *Neurology* 2006;67(10):1792–1800.

53. Backonja M, Beydoun A, Edwards KR, et al. Gabapentin for the symptomatic treatment of painful neuropathy in patients with diabetes mellitus: a randomized controlled trial. *JAMA* 1998;280(21):1831–1836.

54. Bone M, Critchley P, Buggy DJ. Gabapentin in postamputation phantom limb pain: a randomized, double-blind, placebo-controlled, cross-over study. *Reg Anesth Pain Med* 2002;27(5):481–486.

55. Caraceni A, Zecca E, Bonezzi C, et al. Gabapentin for neuropathic cancer pain: a randomized controlled trial from the Gabapentin Cancer Pain Study Group. *J Clin Oncol* 2004;22(14):2909–2917.

56. Hahn K, Arendt G, Braun JS, et al. A placebo-controlled trial of gabapentin for painful HIV-associated sensory neuropathies. *J Neurol* 2004;251(10):1260–1266.

57. Levendoglu F, Ogun CO, Ozerbil O, et al. Gabapentin is a first line drug for the treatment of neuropathic pain in spinal cord injury. *Spine* 2004;29(7):743–751.

58. Morello CM, Leckband SG, Stoner CP, et al. Randomized double-blind study comparing the efficacy of gabapentin with amitriptyline on diabetic peripheral neuropathy pain. *Arch Intern Med* 1999;159(16):1931–1937.

59. Pandey CK, Bose N, Garg G, et al. Gabapentin for the treatment of pain in Guillain-Barré syndrome: a double-blinded, placebo-controlled, crossover study. *Anesth Analg* 2002;95(6):1719–1723.

60. Pandey CK, Raza M, Tripathi M, et al. The comparative evaluation of gabapentin and carbamazepine for pain management in Guillain-Barré syndrome patients in the intensive care unit. *Anesth Analg* 2005;101(1):220–225.

61. Rice AS, Maton S. Gabapentin in postherpetic neuralgia: a randomised, double blind, placebo controlled study. *Pain* 2001;94(2):215–224.

62. Rowbotham M, Harden N, Stacey B, et al. Gabapentin for the treatment of postherpetic neuralgia: a randomized controlled trial. *JAMA* 1998;280(21):1837–1842.

63. Serpell MG. Gabapentin in neuropathic pain syndromes: a randomised, double-blind, placebo-controlled trial. *Pain* 2002;99(3):557–566.

64. Tai Q, Kirshblum S, Chen B, et al. Gabapentin in the treatment of neuropathic pain after spinal cord injury: a prospective, randomized, double-blind, cross-over trial. *J Spinal Cord Med* 2002;25(2):100–105.

65. Smith DG, Ehde DM, Hanley MA, et al. Efficacy of gabapentin in treating chronic phantom limb and residual limb pain. *J Rehabil Res Dev* 2005;42(5):645–654.

66. van de Vusse AC, Stomp-van den Berg SG, Kessels AH, et al. Randomised controlled trial of gabapentin in Complex Regional Pain Syndrome type 1 [ISRCTN84121379]. *BMC Neurol* 2004;4:13.

67. Rao RD, Michalak JC, Sloan JA, et al. Efficacy of gabapentin in the management of chemotherapy-induced peripheral neuropathy: a phase 3 randomized, double-blind, placebo-controlled, crossover trial (N00C3). *Cancer* 2007;110(9):2110–2118.

68. Campbell FG, Graham JG, Zilkha KJ. Clinical trial of carbazepine (tegretol) in trigeminal neuralgia. *J Neurol Neurosurg Psychiatry* 1966;29(3):265–267.

69. Killian JM, Fromm GH. Carbamazepine in the treatment of neuralgia. Use of side effects. *Arch Neurol* 1968;19(2):129–136.

70. Nicol CF. A four year double-blind study of tegretol in facial pain. *Headache* 1969;9(1):54–57.

71. Rockliff BW, Davis EH. Controlled sequential trials of carbamazepine in trigeminal neuralgia. *Arch Neurol* 1966;15(2):129–136.

72. Rull JA, Quibrera R, González-Millán H, et al. Symptomatic treatment of peripheral diabetic neuropathy with carbamazepine (Tegretol): double blind crossover trial. *Diabetologia* 1969;5(4):215–218.

73. Wilton TD. Tegretol in the treatment of diabetic neuropathy. *S Afr Med J* 1974;48(20):869–872.

74. Gómez-Pérez FJ, Choza R, Ríos JM, et al. Nortriptyline-fluphenazine vs. carbamazepine in the symptomatic treatment of diabetic neuropathy. *Arch Med Res* 1996;27(4):525–529.

75. Harke H, Gretenkort P, Ladleif HU, et al. The response of neuropathic pain and pain in complex regional pain syndrome I to carbamazepine and sustained-release morphine in patients pretreated with spinal cord stimulation: a double-blinded randomized study. *Anesth Analg* 2001;92(2):488–495.

76. Maizels M, McCarberg B. Antidepressants and antiepileptic drugs for chronic non-cancer pain. *Am Fam Physician* 2005;71(3):483–490.

77. McQuay H, Carroll D, Jadad AR, Wiffen P, Moore A. Anticonvulsant drugs for management of pain: a systematic review. *BMJ* 1995;311(7012):1047–1052.

78. Burchiel KJ. Carbamazepine inhibits spontaneous activity in experimental neuromas. *Exp Neurol* 1988;102(2):249–253.

79. Lindstrom P. The analgesic effect of carbamazepine in patients with new onset trigeminal neuralgia. *Pain* 1987;4:S85.

80. Dogra S, Beydoun S, Mazzola J, et al. Oxcarbazepine in painful diabetic neuropathy: a randomized, placebo-controlled study. *Eur J Pain* 2005;9(5):543–554.

81. Magenta P, Arghetti S, Di Palma F, et al. Oxcarbazepine is effective and safe in the treatment of neuropathic pain: pooled analysis of seven clinical studies. *Neurol Sci* 2005;26(4):218–226.

82. Eisenberg E, Lurie Y, Braker C, et al. Lamotrigine reduces painful diabetic neuropathy: a randomized, controlled study. *Neurology* 2001;57(3):505–509.

83. Simpson DM, McArthur JC, Olney R, et al. Lamotrigine for HIV-associated painful sensory neuropathies: a placebo-controlled trial. *Neurology* 2003;60(9):1508–1514.

84. Simpson DM, Olney R, McArthur JC, et al. A placebo-controlled trial of lamotrigine for painful HIV-associated neuropathy. *Neurology* 2000;54(11):2115–2119.

85. Finnerup NB, Sindrup SH, Bach FW, et al. Lamotrigine in spinal cord injury pain: a randomized controlled trial. *Pain* 2002;96(3):375–383.

86. Vestergaard K, Andersen G, Gottrup H, et al. Lamotrigine for central poststroke pain: a randomized controlled trial. *Neurology* 2001;56(2):184–190.

87. Zakrzewska JM, Chaudhry Z, Nurmikko TJ, etc. Lamotrigine (lamictal) in refractory trigeminal neuralgia: results from a double-blind placebo controlled crossover trial. *Pain* 1997;73(2):223–230.

88. Vinik AI, Tuchman M, Safirstein B, et al. Lamotrigine for treatment of pain associated with diabetic neuropathy: results of two randomized, double-blind, placebo-controlled studies. *Pain* 2007;128(1–2):169–179.

89. McCleane G. 200 mg daily of lamotrigine has no analgesic effect in neuropathic pain: a randomised, double-blind, placebo controlled trial. *Pain* 1999;83(1):105–107.

90. Mockenhaupt M, Messenheimer J, Tennis P, et al. Risk of Stevens-Johnson syndrome and toxic epidermal necrolysis in new users of antiepileptics. *Neurology* 2005;64(7):1134–1138.

91. Kochar DK, Garg P, Bumb RA, et al. Divalproex sodium in the management of post-herpetic neuralgia: a randomized double-blind placebo-controlled study. *QJM* 2005;98(1):29–34.

92. Otto M, Bach FW, Jensen TS, et al. Valproic acid has no effect on pain in polyneuropathy: a randomized, controlled trial. *Neurology* 2004;62(2):285–288.

93. Raskin P, Donofrio PD, Rosenthal NR, et al. Topiramate vs placebo in painful diabetic neuropathy: analgesic and metabolic effects. *Neurology* 2004;63(5):865–873.

94. Thienel U, Neto W, Schwabe SK, et al. Topiramate in painful diabetic polyneuropathy: findings from three double-blind placebo-controlled trials. *Acta Neurol Scand* 2004;110(4):221–231.

95. Khoromi S, Patsalides A, Parada S, et al. Topiramate in chronic lumbar radicular pain. *J Pain* 2005;6(12):829–836.

96. Dunteman ED. Levetiracetam as an adjunctive analgesic in neoplastic plexopathies: case series and commentary. *J Pain Palliat Care Pharmacother* 2005;19(1):35–43.

97. Vilholm OJ, Cold S, Rasmussen L, et al. Effect of levetiracetam on the postmastectomy pain syndrome. *Eur J Neurol* 2008;15:851–857.

98. Gimbel JS, Richards P, Portenoy RK. Controlled-release oxycodone for pain in diabetic neuropathy: a randomized controlled trial. *Neurology* 2003;60(6):927–934.

99. Huse E, Larbig W, Flor H, et al. The effect of opioids on phantom limb pain and cortical reorganization. *Pain* 2001;90(1–2):47–55.

100. Morley JS, Bridson J, Nash TP, et al. Low-dose methadone has an analgesic effect in neuropathic pain: a double-blind randomized controlled crossover trial. *Palliat Med* 2003;17(7):576–587.

101. Raja SN, Haythornthwaite JA, Pappagallo M, et al. Opioids versus antidepressants in postherpetic neuralgia: a randomized, placebo-controlled trial. *Neurology* 2002;59(7):1015–1021.

102. Rowbotham MC, Twilling L, Davies PS, et al. Oral opioid therapy for chronic peripheral and central neuropathic pain. *N Engl J Med* 2003;348(13):1223–1232.

103. Watson CP, Babul N. Efficacy of oxycodone in neuropathic pain: a randomized trial in postherpetic neuralgia. *Neurology* 1998;50(6):1837–1841.

104. Watson CP, Moulin D, Watt-Watson J, et al. Controlled-release oxycodone relieves neuropathic pain: a randomized controlled trial in painful diabetic neuropathy. *Pain* 2003;105(1–2):71–78.

105. Eisenberg E, McNicol ED, Carr DB. Efficacy and safety of opioid agonists in the treatment of neuropathic pain of nonmalignant origin: systematic review and meta-analysis of randomized controlled trials. *JAMA* 2005;293(24):3043–3052.

106. Eisenberg E, McNicol ED, Carr DB. Efficacy of mu-opioid agonists in the treatment of evoked neuropathic pain: systematic review of randomized controlled trials. *Eur J Pain* 2006;10(8):667–676.

107. Daniell HW. Hypogonadism in men consuming sustained-action oral opioids. *J Pain* 2002;3(5):377–384.

108. Rajagopal A, Vassilopoulou-Sellin R, Palmer JL, et al. Symptomatic hypogonadism in male survivors of cancer with chronic exposure to opioids. *Cancer* 2004;100(4):851–858.

109. Takkouche B, Montes-Martínez A, Gill SS, et al. Psychotropic medications and the risk of fracture: a meta-analysis. *Drug Saf* 2007;30(2):171–184.

110. Vestergaard P, Rejnmark L, Mosekilde L. Fracture risk associated with the use of morphine and opiates. *J Intern Med* 2006;260(1):76–87.

111. Vallejo R, de Leon-Casasola O, Benyamin R. Opioid therapy and immunosuppression: a review. *Am J Ther* 2004;11(5):354–365.
112. Chang G, Chen L, Mao J. Opioid tolerance and hyperalgesia. *Med Clin North Am* 2007;91(2):199–211.
113. Chu LF, Clark DJ, Angst MS. Opioid tolerance and hyperalgesia in chronic pain patients after one month of oral morphine therapy: a preliminary prospective study. *J Pain* 2006;7(1):43–48.
114. Boureau F, Legallicier P, Kabir-Ahmadi M. Tramadol in post-herpetic neuralgia: a randomized, double-blind, placebo-controlled trial. *Pain* 2003; 104(1–2):323–331.
115. Harati Y, Gooch C, Swenson M, et al. Double-blind randomized trial of tramadol for the treatment of the pain of diabetic neuropathy. *Neurology* 1998;50(6):1842–1846.
116. Sindrup SH, Andersen G, Madsen C, et al. Tramadol relieves pain and allodynia in polyneuropathy: a randomised, double-blind, controlled trial. *Pain* 1999;83(1):85–90.
117. Wilder-Smith CH, Hill LT, Laurent S. Postamputation pain and sensory changes in treatment-naive patients: characteristics and responses to treatment with tramadol, amitriptyline, and placebo. *Anesthesiology* 2005;103(3): 619–628.
118. Hocking G, Visser EJ, Schug SA, et al. Ketamine: Does life begin at 40? *Pain Clin Updates* 2007;XV(1).
119. Cohen SP, Chang AS, Larkin T, et al. The intravenous ketamine test: a predictive response tool for oral dextromethorphan treatment in neuropathic pain. *Anesth Analg* 2004;99(6):1753–1759.
120. Oskarsson P, Ljunggren JG, Lins PE. Efficacy and safety of mexiletine in the treatment of painful diabetic neuropathy. The Mexiletine Study Group. *Diabetes Care* 1997;20(10):1594–1597.
121. Stracke H, Meyer UE, Schumacher HE, et al. Mexiletine in the treatment of diabetic neuropathy. *Diabetes Care* 1992;15(11):1550–1555.
122. Wright JM, Oki JC, Graves L III. Mexiletine in the symptomatic treatment of diabetic peripheral neuropathy. *Ann Pharmacother* 1997;31(1):29–34.
123. Tremont-Lukats IW, Challapalli V, McNicol ED, et al. Systemic administration of local anesthetics to relieve neuropathic pain: a systematic review and meta-analysis. *Anesth Analg* 2005;101(6):1738–1749.
124. Galer BS, Harle J, Rowbotham MC. Response to intravenous lidocaine infusion predicts subsequent response to oral mexiletine: a prospective study. *J Pain Symptom Manage* 1996;12(3):161–167.
125. Watkins LR, Maier SF. Neuropathic pain: the immune connection. *Pain Clin Updates* 2004;XII(1).
126. Nalamachu S, Crockett RS, Gammaitoni AR, et al. A comparison of the lidocaine patch 5% vs naproxen 500 mg twice daily for the relief of pain associated with carpal tunnel syndrome: a 6-week, randomized, parallel-group study. *MedGenMed* 2006;8(3):33.
127. Klotz U. Ziconotide—a novel neuron-specific calcium channel blocker for the intrathecal treatment of severe chronic pain—a short review. *Int J Clin Pharmacol Ther* 2006;44(10):478–483.
128. Snutch TP. Targeting chronic and neuropathic pain: the N-type calcium channel comes of age. *NeuroRx* 2005;2(4):662–670.
129. Wermeling DP. Ziconotide, an intrathecally administered N-type calcium channel antagonist for the treatment of chronic pain. *Pharmacotherapy* 2005; 25(8):1084–1094.
130. Lynch SS, Cheng CM, Yee JL. Intrathecal ziconotide for refractory chronic pain. *Ann Pharmacother* 2006;40(7–8):1293–1300.
131. Fisher R, Hassenbusch S, Krames E, et al. A consensus statement regarding the present suggested titration for Prialt (ziconotide). *Neuromodulation* 2005; 8(3):153–154.
132. Ghafoor VL, Epshteyn M, Carlson GH, et al. Intrathecal drug therapy for long-term pain management. *Am J Health Syst Pharm* 2007;64(23): 2447–2461.
133. Galer BS, Rowbotham MC, Perander J, etc. Topical lidocaine patch relieves postherpetic neuralgia more effectively than a vehicle topical patch: results of an enriched enrollment study. *Pain* 1999;80(3):533–538.
134. Rowbotham MC, Davies PS, Fields HL. Topical lidocaine gel relieves postherpetic neuralgia. *Ann Neurol* 1995;37(2):246–253.
135. Rowbotham MC, Davies PS, Verkempinck C, et al. Lidocaine patch: double-blind controlled study of a new treatment method for post-herpetic neuralgia. *Pain* 1996;65(1):39–44.
136. Meier T, Wasner G, Faust M, et al. Efficacy of lidocaine patch 5% in the treatment of focal peripheral neuropathic pain syndromes: a randomized, double-blind, placebo-controlled study. *Pain* 2003;106(1–2):151–158.
137. Lynch ME, Clark AJ, Sawynok J, et al. Topical 2% amitriptyline and 1% ketamine in neuropathic pain syndromes: a randomized, double-blind, placebo-controlled trial. *Anesthesiology* 2005;103(1):140–146.
138. Wilsey B, Marcotte T, Tsodikov A, et al. A randomized, placebo-controlled, crossover trial of cannabis cigarettes in neuropathic pain. *J Pain* 2008;9(6): 506–521.
139. Abrams DI, Jay CA, Shade SB, et al. Cannabis in painful HIV-associated sensory neuropathy: a randomized placebo-controlled trial. *Neurology* 2007; 68(7):515–521.
140. Karst M, Salim K, Burstein S, et al. Analgesic effect of the synthetic cannabinoid CT-3 on chronic neuropathic pain: a randomized controlled trial. *JAMA* 2003;290(13):1757–1762.
141. Berman JS, Symonds C, Birch R. Efficacy of two cannabis based medicinal extracts for relief of central neuropathic pain from brachial plexus avulsion: results of a randomised controlled trial. *Pain* 2004;112(3):299–306.
142. Rog DJ, Nurmikko TJ, Friede T, et al. Randomized, controlled trial of cannabis-based medicine in central pain in multiple sclerosis. *Neurology* 2005; 65(6):812–819.
143. Iskedjian M, Bereza B, Gordon A, et al. Meta-analysis of cannabis based treatments for neuropathic and multiple sclerosis-related pain. *Curr Med Res Opin* 2007;23(1):17–24.
144. Hanna M, Wilson MC, O'Brien C. Neuropathic pain: optimising patient outcome with combination therapy. Abstract from 5th Congress of the European Federation of IASP Chapters (EFIC) *Eur J Pain* 2006 10(Suppl 1):s120.
145. Simpson DM. Gabapentin and venlafaxine for the treatment of painful diabetic neuropathy. *J Clin Neuromusc Dis* 2001;3:53–62.
146. Lynch ME, Clark AJ, Sawynok J, et al. Topical amitriptyline and ketamine in neuropathic pain syndromes: an open-label study. *J Pain* 2005;6(10): 644–649.
147. Leijon G, Boivie J. Central post-stroke pain—a controlled trial of amitriptyline and carbamazepine. *Pain* 1989;36(1):27–36.
148. Vrethem M, Boivie J, Arnqvist H, et al. A comparison of amitriptyline and maprotiline in the treatment of painful polyneuropathy in diabetics and non-diabetics. *Clin J Pain* 1997;13(4):313–323.
149. Watson CP, Evans RJ, Reed K, et al. Amitriptyline versus placebo in postherpetic neuralgia. *Neurology* 1982;32(6):671–673.
150. Max MB, Schafer SC, Culnane M, et al. Amitriptyline, but not lorazepam, relieves postherpetic neuralgia. *Neurology* 1988;38(9):1427–1432.
151. Kalso E, Tasmuth T, Neuvonen PJ. Amitriptyline effectively relieves neuropathic pain following treatment of breast cancer. *Pain* 1996;64(2):293–302.
152. Kvinesdal B, Molin J, Frøland A, et al. Imipramine treatment of painful diabetic neuropathy. *JAMA* 1984;251(13):1727–1730.
153. Sindrup SH, Bach FW, Gram LF. Plasma beta-endorphin is not affected by treatment with imipramine or paroxetine in patients with diabetic neuropathy symptoms. *Clin J Pain* 1992;8(2):145–148.
154. Panerai AE, Monza G, Movilia P, et al. A randomized, within-patient, crossover, placebo-controlled trial on the efficacy and tolerability of the tricyclic antidepressants chlorimipramine and nortriptyline in central pain. *Acta Neurol Scand* 1990;82(1):34–38.
155. Sindrup SH, Gram LF, Skjold T, et al. Clomipramine vs desipramine vs placebo in the treatment of diabetic neuropathy symptoms. A double-blind crossover study. *Br J Clin Pharmacol* 1990;30(5):683–691.
156. Max MB, Kishore-Kumar R, Schafer SC, et al. Efficacy of desipramine in painful diabetic neuropathy: a placebo-controlled trial. *Pain* 1991;45(1):3–9; discussion 1–2.
157. Kishore-Kumar R, Max MB, Schafer SC, et al. Desipramine relieves postherpetic neuralgia. *Clin Pharmacol Ther* 1990;47(3):305–312.
158. Yucel A, Ozyalcin S, Koknel Talu G, et al. The effect of venlafaxine on ongoing and experimentally induced pain in neuropathic pain patients: a double blind, placebo controlled study. *Eur J Pain* 2005;9(4):407–416.
159. Vilming ST, Lyberg T, Lataste X. Tizanidine in the management of trigeminal neuralgia. *Cephalalgia* 1986;6(3):181–182.
160. Lechin F, van der Dijs B, Lechin ME, et al. Pimozide therapy for trigeminal neuralgia. *Arch Neurol* 1989;46(9):960–963.
161. Grosskopf J, Mazzola J, Wan Y, et al. A randomized, placebo-controlled study of oxcarbazepine in painful diabetic neuropathy. *Acta Neurol Scand* 2006;114(3):177–180.
162. Atli A, Dogra S. Zonisamide in the treatment of painful diabetic neuropathy: a randomized, double-blind, placebo-controlled pilot study. *Pain Med* 2005; 6(3):225–234.
163. Chad DA, Aronin N, Lundstrom R, et al. Does capsaicin relieve the pain of diabetic neuropathy? *Pain* 1990;42(3):387–388.
164. Scheffler NM, Sheitel PL, Lipton MN. Treatment of painful diabetic neuropathy with capsaicin 0.075%. *J Am Podiatr Med Assoc* 1991;81(6):288–293.
165. Treatment of painful diabetic neuropathy with topical capsaicin. A multicenter, double-blind, vehicle-controlled study. The Capsaicin Study Group. *Arch Intern Med* 1991;151(11):2225–2229.
166. Tandan R, Lewis GA, Krusinski PB, et al. Topical capsaicin in painful diabetic neuropathy. Controlled study with long-term follow-up. *Diabetes Care* 1992; 15(1):8–14.
167. Low PA, Opfer-Gehrking TL, Dyck PJ, et al. Double-blind, placebo-controlled study of the application of capsaicin cream in chronic distal painful polyneuropathy. *Pain* 1995;62(2):163–168.
168. Bernstein JE, Korman NJ, Bickers DR, et al. Topical capsaicin treatment of chronic postherpetic neuralgia. *J Am Acad Dermatol* 1989;21(2 pt 1): 265–270.
169. Watson CP, Tyler KL, Bickers DR, et al. A randomized vehicle-controlled trial of topical capsaicin in the treatment of postherpetic neuralgia. *Clin Ther* 1993;15(3):510–526.
170. Watson CP, Evans RJ. The postmastectomy pain syndrome and topical capsaicin: a randomized trial. *Pain* 1992;51(3):375–379.
171. Ellison N, Loprinzi CL, Kugler J, et al. Phase III placebo-controlled trial of capsaicin cream in the management of surgical neuropathic pain in cancer patients. *J Clin Oncol* 1997;15(8):2974–2980.
172. Paice JA, Ferrans CE, Lashley FR, et al. Topical capsaicin in the management of HIV-associated peripheral neuropathy. *J Pain Symptom Manage* 2000; 19(1):45–52.
173. McCleane G. Topical application of doxepin hydrochloride, capsaicin, and a combination of both produces analgesia in chronic human neuropathic pain: a randomized, double-blind, placebo-controlled study. *Br J Clin Pharmacol* 2000;49(6):574–579.

174. Galer BS, Jensen MP, Ma T, et al. The lidocaine patch 5% effectively treats all neuropathic pain qualities: results of a randomized, double-blind, vehicle-controlled, 3-week efficacy study with use of the neuropathic pain scale. *Clin J Pain* 2002;18(5):297–301.

175. Estanislao L, Carter K, McArthur J, et al. A randomized controlled trial of 5% lidocaine gel for HIV-associated distal symmetric polyneuropathy. *J Acquir Immune Defic Syndr* 2004;37(5):1584–1586.

176. Nelson KA, Park KM, Robinovitz E, et al. High-dose oral dextromethorphan versus placebo in painful diabetic neuropathy and postherpetic neuralgia. *Neurology* 1997;48(5):1212–1218.

177. Sang CN, Booher S, Gilron I, et al. Dextromethorphan and memantine in painful diabetic neuropathy and postherpetic neuralgia: efficacy and dose-response trials. *Anesthesiology* 2002;96(5):1053–1061.

178. Eisenberg E, Kleiser A, Dortort A, et al. The NMDA (N-methyl-D-aspartate) receptor antagonist memantine in the treatment of postherpetic neuralgia: a double-blind, placebo-controlled study. *Eur J Pain* 1998;2(4):321–327.

179. Nikolajsen L, Gottrup H, Kristensen AG, et al. Memantine (a N-methyl-D-aspartate receptor antagonist) in the treatment of neuropathic pain after amputation or surgery: a randomized, double-blinded, cross-over study. *Anesth Analg* 2000;91(4):960–966.

180. Maier C, Dertwinkel R, Mansourian N, et al. Efficacy of the NMDA-receptor antagonist memantine in patients with chronic phantom limb pain—results of a randomized double-blinded, placebo-controlled trial. *Pain* 2003;103(3):277–283.

181. McQuay HJ, Carroll D, Jadad AR, et al. Dextromethorphan for the treatment of neuropathic pain: a double-blind randomised controlled crossover trial with integral n-of-1 design. *Pain* 1994;59(1):127–133.

182. Galer BS, Twilling LL, Harle J, et al. Lack of efficacy of riluzole in the treatment of peripheral neuropathic pain conditions. *Neurology* 2000;55(7):971–975.

183. Dejgard A, Petersen P, Kastrup J. Mexiletine for treatment of chronic painful diabetic neuropathy. *Lancet* 1988;1(8575–8576):9–11.

184. Kemper CA, Kent G, Burton S, et al. Mexiletine for HIV-infected patients with painful peripheral neuropathy: a double-blind, placebo-controlled, crossover treatment trial. *J Acquir Immune Defic Syndr Hum Retrovirol* 1998;19(4):367–372.

185. Chabal C, Jacobson L, Mariano A, et al. The use of oral mexiletine for the treatment of pain after peripheral nerve injury. *Anesthesiology* 1992;76(4):513–517.

186. Wallace MS, Magnuson S, Ridgeway B. Efficacy of oral mexiletine for neuropathic pain with allodynia: a double-blind, placebo-controlled, crossover study. *Reg Anesth Pain Med* 2000;25(5):459–467.

187. Chiou-Tan FY, Tuel SM, Johnson JC, et al. Effect of mexiletine on spinal cord injury dysesthetic pain. *Am J Phys Med Rehabil* 1996;75(2):84–87.

188. Svendsen KB, Jensen TS, Bach FW. Does the cannabinoid dronabinol reduce central pain in multiple sclerosis? Randomised double blind placebo controlled crossover trial. *BMJ* 2004;329(7460):253.

CHAPTER 81 ■ ANGER AND PAIN

JOSHUA WOOTTON

CULTURAL BACKGROUND

Aristotle, referencing Homer's *Iliad*, suggested that "Anger may be defined as an impulse, accompanied by pain, to a conspicuous revenge for a conspicuous slight,"[1,p54] emphasizing that "the angry man feels pain."[1,p63] There was no suggestion of the separation of emotional distress from its physical consequences. Unlike many of his contemporaries, Aristotle undertook a reasoned approach to the understanding of anger but nevertheless placed it clearly in the context of emotional and physical pain. In his essay *On Anger*, Seneca urged his elder brother Novatus to eschew anger and agreed that he was "right to have a particular dread of this most hideous and frenzied of all emotions,"[2,p17] even likening the emotional experience to "a brief insanity."[2,p17] It was a common thematic thread to philosophers and physicians in ancient Greece and Rome that anger tended to reveal itself as a form of madness and that attempts to control it reflected strength of character and spirit.[3] Attempts to control anger in antiquity, however, were usually concerned with altering its often dramatic appearance, not with regulating its impact on the body. The possible harmful effects of managing the expression of anger were paid little consideration.

Scripture, too, characterizes anger as being at the heart of sin or separation from God and admonishes against the dangers of its excesses. In Hebrew, Christian, and Islamic religious writings, God is often portrayed as angry toward those who oppose his will,[2] but the faithful are taught to suppress their angry impulses "for the anger of man does not work the righteousness of God" (Jas. 1:20). The Qur'an teaches that "Allah loves those who restrain anger" ('Al-'Imran 3:134), while the Psalms caution us to "Be angry, but sin not" (Pss. 4:4). In other passages, we are encouraged not only to avoid expressions of anger, but to resist even the emotion itself. In the Gospel of Matthew, we find that "everyone who is angry with his brother shall be liable to judgment" (Matt. 5:22), while elsewhere in the Psalms, we are exhorted to "Refrain from anger; and forsake wrath!" (Pss. 37:8), and in the Sunnah of Islam, the Prophet advises, again and again, "Do not become angry and furious" (Hadith-Sahih Al-Bukhari 8.137).

This deeply ingrained cultural awareness—that not only are angry actions dangerous, but the emotion of anger itself can be harmful—led to the inclusion of anger as one of the "seven deadly sins" in the religious West,[4] a theme popularized and later woven into the fabric of Western cultures through literature, drama, and art, including in European cultures the enduring and influential classics of Dante's *Divine Comedy* and Chaucer's *Canterbury Tales*.

PSYCHOANALYTIC BACKGROUND

One important difference between historical and more contemporary discussions of anger is that the former, while often concerned with the negative consequences of expressing anger, were seldom concerned with the possible harmful effects of its inhibition.[3] Anger in psychoanalytic theory does not carry the metaphysical weight of sin, but its expression through hostility and aggressive impulses often lies at the core of conflict, competing drives, and the formation of pathological symptoms, including pain. Although Freud was an atheist, his frequent excursions into the fields of religion, religious experience, and anthropology are testi-

mony to his respect for the conscious and unconscious impact of culture upon the individual; he was the first to emphasize the idea that the individual and culture are linked dynamically and that disturbances may occur in the developmental interaction between the two, leaving behind a disposition to future neuroses.[5] He was also an astute observer of the phenomenon of pain from organic origins being maintained for intrapsychic reasons, long past the point of expectable physical healing and recovery.[6,7]

Early in his work, Freud arrived at the idea that pain is a common symptom of *conversion* and that, although there is usually an organic basis for the onset of pain, it can later be influenced and extended in duration and scope by a process through which mental conflict is displaced onto the body, resulting in the somatic expression of symptoms. Conversion, in this context, is closer to the contemporary term *somatization*, referring both to conversion and psychophysiological disorders. The repression of negative affects, such as anger, resentment, and guilt, is transmuted into the expression of physical symptoms. The defensive process of somatization continues until relief from the intrapsychic burden of intolerable affect is no longer necessary or desomatization takes place through support—often psychotherapeutic—of the individual's more mature defenses and coping strategies.

Freud's later work was focused more on patients whose pain was less directly associated with an original organic insult and more configured with mood disturbance. In *Mourning and Melancholia*, he delineated the intrapsychic origins of depression as a process through which aggression, originally directed toward the lost object, is turned against the self[8]—somewhat oversimplified in the popular formula "anger turned inward." According to this template, pain and mourning may be seen as affective responses to separation and as unconscious defenses against aggression.[8,9,10] Freud's successors related pain to aggression and hostility more directly, and the idea that the symptom of physical pain can be an unconscious defense against anger and aggression became a widely shared interpretation in psychoanalytic theory; however, as Merskey points out, the evidence has been largely anecdotal, with the relationship between anger and pain often being made more plausible by retrospective analysis.[7]

Like Freud, Engel acknowledged that pain may originate with actual physical injury, but his study of the "pain-prone patient" gave the most enduring and widely influential psychoanalytic expression of chronic pain as a symbolic displacement of anger and aggression.[11] He also suggested that patients are frequently unwilling or unable to acknowledge the hostility and aggressive impulses behind their pain, leaving them with the difficult task of attempting to adjust to symptoms that are borne of conflicts that they can neither recognize nor accept. The presence of chronic pain, then, may reflect underlying conflicts—in turn, giving rise to intolerable affects, which, when repressed, are given dynamic expression through the body. Szasz, as well, held that repression of emotional distress is often the principal mechanism underlying chronic pain and suggested that, by focusing their attention on their pain, many patients are coping with their distress symbolically and through a more socially acceptable expression of their conflicts.[12]

Burns summarizes the evidence supporting this view that repression of affect is the mechanism at the heart of chronic pain.[13,14] First, he cites the phenomenon of the "conversion-V" profile on the Minnesota Multiphasic Personality Inventory (MMPI-2), depicted by clinical elevations on Scales 1 and 3, Hypochodriasis and Hysteria, with a comparatively lower score on Scale 2, Depression. The resulting V-configuration suggests the presence of somatic preoccupation and a hysterical constellation of defenses, deployed in the service of relieving depressed affect. Second, he further reports evidence of the link between the tendency to suppress anger and aggression and the symptomatic expression of chronic pain and disability. Finally, he points to the persistent observation that inhibition of emotion, particularly emotions arising in the context of traumatic events, has physiological consequences.

Where the first of these three lines of evidence is concerned, the conversion-V configuration of scores on the MMPI and MMPI-2 has been studied extensively, and applied to chronic pain, for more than 30 years.[13,15] The first scale of this "neurotic triad" of scores is Hypochondriasis (Hs). High scores on Hypochondriasis tend to reflect patterns of neurotic concern over physical health.[16,17] The third scale, Hysteria (Hy), was developed specifically as an aid to measuring the predisposition to develop symptoms of conversion or somatization and reflects a high degree of reliance upon hysterical defenses.[16,17] When these two scales are clinically elevated and the second scale, Depression (D), which reflects both mood and neurovegetative aspects of depression, is comparatively lower, the indication of the resulting V-configuration is that intolerable affect is being displaced onto somatic concerns, principally through the mechanism of repression.[14,15,16,17,18,19]

Where the second line of evidence is concerned, Burns' observations of trends in the scientific literature suggesting the link between chronic pain and the inhibition of anger[14] have been replicated and amplified by numerous subsequent studies, although not always with psychoanalytic theory in the foreground.[20,21,22,23,24,25] The suggestion is that patients with chronic pain are more likely to experience anger than those without pain and more likely also to inhibit their anger.[24] Burns' third source of evidence concerns the physiological response, both conscious and unconscious, to efforts at inhibition.[13] Suppression reflects the more obvious example of physiological cost; however, repression also has a dynamic element that must be balanced in the psychosomatic economy of mind and body interrelationship.[20,21,22,24] Within the framework of psychoanalytic theory, the physiological exertion demanded by inhibition was often seen as related to the persistence of conversion, as well as the intensity and duration of somatization.[8,10,26]

The following case of a young woman referred for evaluation of her chronic abdominal pain will serve to illustrate the psychoanalytic perspective on inhibition and its relation to anger and pain.

Case 1: Ms. Ostrakova was a 20-year-old single library aide and part-time student at a nearby community college, who presented with a 2-year history of chronic abdominal pain. She had undergone two separate, complete gastroenterological work-ups at two different medical centers, without any positive findings. She associated the beginning of her difficulties with a chicken sandwich, prepared by her elder sister, in which the meat was apparently undercooked. She explained that she had become quite ill within a short time, with fever, nausea, and vomiting. These symptoms resolved after a few days, but her abdominal pain persisted and became progressively more debilitating until, by the time she arrived in clinic, she had taken a leave of absence from both college and her job and was attempting to manage her pain with a medication regimen that included short-acting opioids. Ms. Ostrakova was fit and slender and her demeanor, while somewhat subdued, was affable and cooperative. She had no psychiatric history or history of substance abuse, and her medical history was notable only for robust health prior to the onset of her abdominal pain. Her psychosocial history, however, was remarkable for early childhood trauma and abuse and a childhood household of domestic turmoil and violence. She described a history of fighting in school and finally being remanded at age 17 by the juvenile court system to a residential treatment facility for "anger management" in another state. When asked about the therapeutic aspect of her 1-year treatment program, she replied, "They just taught us how to keep our anger inside, not to let it out, so we wouldn't always get into fights. We had to avoid fighting to prove we had learned how to manage our anger."

As the interview progressed, it became clear that the patient had learned much about recognizing anger when she experienced it, and suppressing it in the moment, but little about the potential cost to herself and her body. A psychometric assessment reflected little endorsement of depressive symptoms on the Beck Depression Inventory or the MMPI-2 but clinically elevated scores on Hs and Hy, and her history reflected many of the psychosocial factors depicted by Engel as disposing toward "pain-proneness." The latter included parents who were abusive toward each other and toward their children, a father who was alcoholic and emotionally and physically domineering, and a mother who was often debilitated by pain of uncertain etiology.[11,27]

In her treatment program, the patient appeared to have gotten the message, right or wrong, that, if she showed no outward signs of anger, she would be considered successfully rehabilitated. The experience of anger, therefore, became an obstacle between her court-mandated residential treatment and her successful return home. Over time, the experience of anger was transformed by a developing awareness of intolerable affect—displaced onto her body in the more acceptable symptomatic expression of physical pain. When Ms. Ostrakova's elder sister provided the organic insult of an undercooked chicken sandwich, resulting in gastroenterological distress, the patient, who might previously have responded with anger leading to physical confrontation, began instead to experience the pain associated with simple repression of her affect—unconsciously "keeping her anger inside." This is the classic picture of somatization, depicted in psychoanalytic theory, which continues to be influential in our assessment of patients with chronic pain.

CURRENT RESEARCH IN ANGER AND ITS RELATION TO PAIN

The role of anger in exacerbating pain and in disposing toward the development of chronic pain is, in some respects, similar to that of other negative emotions or distressed affective states, such as anxiety and depression.[28] According to the prevailing gate control and neuromatrix theories of pain, negative emotions can increase the intensity and duration of pain by altering or dysregulating the descending and central pain modulation systems.[29,30,31,32] Precisely how this takes place remains an open question for further research, but an integrated neurobiological model is beginning to emerge with implications for treatment of both chronic pain and disorders of anger.

Physiological Mechanisms in Anger and Pain Research

Merskey noted that pain can make individuals aggressive for purely biological reasons, associated with the activation of the fight-or-flight mechanisms and high autonomic arousal.[7] He added that we may not need to look much further in our attempts to explain why patients with chronic pain become angry. Whereas angry responses can be adaptive, especially when they prompt the search for constructive solutions to problems within the medical setting, chronically angry reactions of the sort observed in some patients with chronic pain are often seen as maladaptive and disruptive—indicative not of discrete situations of fight-or-flight, but of sustained and simmering autonomic arousal.[32] Parsing the relationship here has proven challenging because of two related questions: Does chronic pain induce sustained sympathetic arousal and therefore lead to continual expressions of anger? Does the situation of chronic pain arise more easily among individuals who are disposed to express anger and aggression?

Robinson and Riley outlined four models or mechanisms through which the relationship between pain and negative emotion has been usefully described, both from a clinical perspective and as a template for empirical design[28]:

- Negative emotion increases sensitivity;
- Pain is caused by negative emotion;
- Negative affect occurs as a result of chronic pain;
- Pain and negative emotion are concomitant.

The first of these is simply the observation that negative emotion increases somatic sensitivity. In other words, negative emotions increase awareness and recognition of pain. Evidence in support of this mechanism comes from studies in which induced changes in mood have been correlated with increased reports of pain and decreased tolerance for experimentally induced pain, as well as in the clinical observation that depressed patients tend to interpret sensations negatively, experiencing them more often as painful.[28]

The second mechanism—that pain is caused by negative emotion—is most closely allied with the psychoanalytic view of pain as a symptom of underlying or repressed conflict, but inhibition of negative emotion and affect can also result in elevations of autonomic and central nervous system activity, raising serum cortisol levels and leading to neurovegetative dysfunction and increased pain. Cacioppo et al.'s meta-analytic study of the physiological correlates of negative emotions concluded that the experience of anger, whether expressed or suppressed, tends to be accompanied by increased diastolic blood pressure, skin conductance, stroke volume, cardiac output, peripheral resistance, finger pulse, and heart rate, all suggesting a high sympathetic response.[33] Considering the impact of sustained autonomic arousal, negative emotions, not surprisingly, may also be seen as causal in the expression of stress-related illness and pain in which somatic reactivity can lead to musculoskeletal disorder.[28,34,35] Robinson and Riley's third mechanism echoes Merskey's suggestion that negative affect may be seen simply as a reaction to the situation of chronic pain, arising within a stress-diathesis framework,[7,28,36] whereas their fourth proposed mechanism posits that pain and negative emotion arise concomitantly from shared neurobiological pathways.[28]

Taken together, these four mechanisms are broadly consistent with the gate control and neuromatrix theories of pain; however, the last—that anger, anxiety, depression, and pain share neurobiological pathways—suggests a physiological context in which negative emotions can alter the descending and central pain modulation processes.[37] Serotonin, norepinephrine, and dopamine all play roles in the modulation of pain, as well as in the development of negative emotions. That pain and depression both respond to certain antidepressant medications has long been cited as evidence of common neurobiological pathways.[28,38,39] Relative cortisol levels and dopaminergic transfer and regulation have also been implicated in the relationship between anger and pain,[28,40,41,42,43] but the key neurotransmitter implicated in the modulation of anger is dopamine, with the focus of activity in the nucleus accumbens.[43,44,45,46]

From an evolutionary perspective, the emotion of anger is clearly primitive and derived from ancient limbic regions of the brain, as opposed to the cortex and prefrontal cortex, which assume a more modulatory role in its experience and expression.[44] The regions of primary activity for anger—along with its conceptual counterparts, appetitive impulsivity, drive, motivation, pleasure, and psychoticism—appear to be associated with the core regions of temperament: the amygdala and nucleus accumbens or ventral striatum, as well as the cingulate cortex.[44,45] Lara and Akiskal suggest that anger is influenced by dopaminergic transfer and regulation in these regions, with high anger being associated with either enhanced postsynaptic response to dopamine or increased synaptic dopamine concentration or both.[44] Wood outlines evidence to suggest that the inhibition of tonic pain is mediated by activation of mesolimbic dopamine neurons, arising from the ventral tegmental area and projecting to the nucleus accumbens.[43]

Ironically, anger may be associated both with an increase or a decrease in the experience of pain.[37,47,48,49] Acute stress may activate mechanisms of pain-suppression through the release of endogenous opioids and substance P within the ventral tegmental area, but prolonged exposure to stress—as in the case of sustained anger or proneness to anger—tends to result in a reduction of dopaminergic output in the nucleus accumbens, potentiating the subsequent development of hyperalgesia.[43] The outcome appears to be that inhibition of pain may occur initially when a painful stimulus is first perceived but that, upon further exposure and evaluation, sensitization may occur.[37] The experience of anger appears to undergo change over time, leading to associations with both traits and temperament—factors related to the thematic and serial evaluation of stimuli—an observation that has led to the study of anger-related features of both mood and personality disorders.[50,51,52] The influence of anger on the changes involved in mood states suggests a dynamic relationship associated with the tonic and phasic balance of dopaminergic activity.[43,44] In this case, the inhibition of pain may be principally related to physiological changes occurring in the initial or situational experience of anger, such as changes in cardiovascular reactivity and autonomic arousal that have been shown to modulate the experience of pain.[47] Pain sensitization, on the other hand, appears more associated with the ability to regulate anger and the emotional evaluation of the experience—individual differences that influence dopaminergic output.[37,44] This, in turn, suggests that the experience of anger, relative to personality and temperament, as well as how we manage anger, are important variables in the modulation of pain.[37,44,46,47,48,49,50,51,52]

Other physiological mechanisms under study include the effects of anger on muscle reactivity, the immune system, and endogenous opioid dysfunction.[32] Consideration of the last of these will be deferred to discussion of the related work on anger management, later in this chapter. Where the first is concerned, studies on muscle reactivity have suggested that anger may increase musculoskeletal tension in specific sites that contribute to pain.[53,54] The experience of anger, whether inhibited or expressed, and the trait of hostility have been associated with increased likelihood of reporting high levels of tension near the site of pain and injury.[55] A further mechanism through which anger may influence pain is distress-related immune dysregulation.[56] While brief, situational stressors involving activation of the fight-or-flight mechanisms have been shown to result in potentially beneficial changes to the immune system, exposure to prolonged stress and negative emotion, such as sustained anger and hostility, have been associated with deleterious effects in a broad range of health concerns, immunological suppression, and generalized inflammatory processes associated with chronic pain.[57,58,59,60] Because immunological changes must be observed longitudinally, this work has tended to emphasize the impact of sustained anger and hostility associated with enduring personality traits and temperament.[59,60]

Psychological Constructs in Anger and Pain Research

The etymology of "anger" is not the same for every modern language, but it appears to have come into modern English usage via Old Norse, angra, "to grieve, vex," later angr, "distress, grief," Old English, enge, "narrow, painful," influenced by the Proto-Indo-European root, angh-, "painfully constricted," and finally into Middle English, where its associations with pain endured.[61] The relative importance of the term in ordinary discourse can be illustrated through the frequency of its use: Of the roughly 700,000 words in common English usage, "anger" is ranked 3,253rd in frequency of appearance in spoken and written communication.[62] Focusing on the logic underpinning the ordinary language use of the word "anger," Smedslund offered a contemporary definition of anger that depicts the psycholinguistic core of the construct, rather than emphasizing the characteristic features of its expression: "a feeling involving a *belief* that a person one cares for has, intentionally or through neglect, been treated without respect, and a *want* to have that respect re-established."[34,35,63] In Smedslund's conceptual framework, the "person one cares for," particularly in the context of pain, is ordinarily the self.

Fernandez emphasizes the dimensions of *action tendency* and *cognitive appraisal* in the study of the relationship between anger and pain.[34,35] The former concerns the behavioral tendencies associated with anger, including aggression and impulses directed toward the restoration of control, the removal of obstacles, and the seeking of redress. This becomes an important consideration in the context of whether action is expressed or suppressed and, if expressed, how adaptively. The latter suggests a framework within which the individual seeks to explain otherwise ambiguous interior experiences or changes in arousal. Both of these dimensions are anticipated by and subsumed under Smedslund's ordinary language definition of anger, and both have proven critical to the study of the relationship between anger and pain.

The cognitive appraisal theory of emotion—perhaps most elegantly and economically portrayed in Lazarus's cognitive-motivational-relational theory[64]—suggests that the experience of an emotion, like anger, is the joint effect of (1) the event of physiological arousal in response to incoming stimuli and (2) the cognitive appraisal of its meaning with respect to the particular setting in which the event occurs (Table 81.1). Cognitive appraisal, then, is the process through which physiological states, such as arousal, are interpreted in light of the perceived situation. This becomes critical in the management of anger and, by extension, to the psychotherapeutic treatment of patients with chronic pain, because how events are appraised tends to influence selection and deployment of coping strategies.[65,66] Lazarus further distinguished between primary and secondary appraisals, with the former referring to the interpretation of how a particular situation affects considerations of well-being and the latter, referring to considerations of how to cope with the situation.[64] Secondary appraisals, he suggests, can actually shape the experience of an emotion through the selection of a particular coping strategy.[64,67]

Anger Management Style

Much of the research on anger and its relationship to pain has highlighted the related constructs of hostility, aggression, and anger management style.[32] *Anger* is the term denoting the emotion, characterized by physiological arousal and accompanying conscious and unconscious impulses toward aggression. *Aggression* typically refers to the behavioral expression of the emotion, ordinarily through acts of vindication, punishment, and destruction, directed toward others or objects.[68] Freud's focus was ultimately less on anger than on aggression, as one of the two primary instinctual drives.[6,69] In psychoanalytic theory, aggression in its stimulation of defensive functions and coping strategies plays an important role in the development of personality. This distinction between anger and aggression suggests that, while anger is usually conceived as a transient state, aggression is a more durable and endogenously derived motivational force. The word *anger* can be used in this manner—to denote a more dispositional quality—but, frequently, the term *hostility* is used in reference to the tendency to make consistently negative cognitive appraisals regarding the motivations of others.[35]

Conceptual links with aggression and hostility further raise the distinction between state anger and trait anger, a critical consideration in researching the influence of anger upon chronic pain. A good starting point for the distinction is offered by Spielberger, who characterizes state anger as a transitory emotional episode, whereas trait anger is described as a more stable pattern of personality attributes, similar to hostility.[68] One way of representing this is that trait anger reflects a relatively stable dimension of proneness to anger in which individual differences are reflected in the frequency, intensity, and duration with which state anger is experienced over time.[70] This, in turn, suggests that characteristic defensive patterns and reliance upon particular coping strategies tend to result in what may be described as more enduring styles of anger management.

Anger management style is a term denoting the relative tendencies of individuals either (1) to suppress or internalize their anger or (2) to express or externalize their anger. The construct of anger management style is often represented in research as anger-in, anger-out, and anger-control.[32] *Anger-in* characterizes the tendency to inhibit the expression of angry thoughts and feelings, whereas *anger-out* describes the tendency to express angry thoughts and feelings directly, whether verbally, physically, or both. High trait anger, according to Deffenbacher, is more associated with the tendency to express anger negatively, less constructively, and with less control than with the tendency to suppress anger; he further notes that there is a stronger connection between the suppressed anger and anxiety than between suppressed anger and forms of expressed anger.[70] *Anger-control* refers to an individual's perceived control over the experience and expression of anger and is usually interpreted as positive, unless too much control approaches no expression at all.[32]

Although the International Association for the Study of Pain (IASP) appears to separate the sensory and emotional dimensions of the experience of pain, when it defines pain as an "unpleasant sensory and emotional experience associated with actual or potential tissue damage,"[71] several studies point to the simultaneous processing of pain in the somatosensory cortex and emotion-related cerebral systems.[37,72] Mollett and Harrison summarize the case for the application of emotional theories to the study of pain and propose that emotion may influence the processing of pain in several ways[37]:

- Negative emotion increases pain intensity and decreases threshold and tolerance;
- Positive emotion decreases pain intensity and increases threshold and tolerance;
- Pain may produce negative emotion or increase the memory for negative emotion.

This template emphasizes the relationship between anger and pain and strongly implicates anger in the development and maintenance of chronic pain. It further highlights the role of anger management style as a critical influence in how pain is experienced.

Anger-In

In his study of emotion regulation, Gross utilized a process model to illustrate two features of trait anger-in: First that, while the mechanism of suppression tends to decrease negative emotional expression, it also decreases positive emotional expression and second that, while suppression has little impact on the experience of negative emotion, it tends to decrease the experience of positive emotion.[73] In his analysis of emotion regulation, he concluded that, as a means of regulating negative emotion, cognitive appraisal is more adaptive than suppression and tends to decrease both the experience and expression of negative emotion, while increasing the experience and expression of positive emotion. He added that there may be times when cognitive appraisal cannot adequately be mobilized and suppression may be, in the moment, the best available means of regulating negative emotion, but such instances are more likely to involve evaluation in the moment of

TABLE 81.1

RS LAZARUS'S COGNITIVE-MOTIVATIONAL-RELATIONAL THEORY OF EMOTION*

Event (stimulus)	Physiological response	Setting/circumstances	Cognitive appraisal	Emotion	Secondary appraisal
Feeling oneself being pushed or shoved	Autonomic arousal, pain	A cashier's line in a busy store where customers are jostling for position	"A stranger has pushed me aside! *This is unfair!*"	Anger (increased pain associated with the unfair slight to one's identity or ego)	The setting may suggest that an angry outburst will prove less effective than a sympathetic, reasoned appeal to civility.
Feeling oneself being pushed or shoved	Autonomic arousal, pain	A pedestrian crosswalk at a busy urban traffic intersection	"A stranger has pushed me out of harm's way! *I was nearly struck by that automobile!*"	Relief, gratitude (reduced pain); if anger is experienced, it is likely directed toward the impatient motorist or toward oneself for being careless	The setting may suggest that a personal expression of gratitude toward one's protector is more appropriate than an angry outburst directed toward the fleeing motorist.

*The same or similar events and physiological responses may be interpreted or appraised differently, depending upon the setting or circumstances, resulting in different emotional responses.

state anger. The overarching conclusion is that suppression as a trait mechanism for modulating intolerable affect is problematic.

Engel noted that inhibition of anger, whether through repression or suppression, is a common attribute among pain-prone patients, but psychoanalytic theory offered little insight into the causal relationship or cognitive, emotional, and physiological mechanisms through which inhibited anger can affect pain.[11,24,25] More recent studies of anger-in as a form of emotional regulation confirm that suppression is a prevalent style of management among patients with chronic pain but also point to applications of Wegner's ironic process theory as a means of delineating the mechanisms involved.[24,25,74] According to this template, suppression of negative emotion requires the coordination of two distinct cognitive processes: the first represents a resource-dependent operating process that serves to eliminate awareness of unwanted thoughts and feelings, whereas the second represents a monitoring process that remains vigilant to the awareness of unwanted thoughts and feelings to be suppressed (Table 81.2). Under ordinary conditions, the monitor works to identify material to be suppressed, while the operating process performs the suppression; however, when under stress or high demand, the operating process may not have sufficient resources to perform its task. Stress, in this context, may be reflected in both cognitive and somatic symptomatology, with cognitive dissonance thwarting both suppression and cognitive appraisal and the corresponding demands on the body being expressed through cardiovascular and musculoskeletal symptoms. Burns et al. reported that patients with chronic low back pain who reflect an anger-in style of management are more likely than other groups to experience high levels of muscle tension at the site of pain and injury when experiencing anger and to show relatively high systolic and diastolic blood pressure.[55]

The irony implicit in Wegner's theory of mental processing is that, under such conditions, the monitor may be serving to bring unwanted thoughts and feelings into conscious awareness without sufficient resources for suppression to take place. The result is that unsuccessful efforts to suppress anger can paradoxically lead to heightened awareness of the cognitive and emotional experience of anger, thereby increasing sensitivity to pain and influencing subsequent perceptions and interpretations of pain according to the unsuccessfully suppressed, unwanted cognitions and intolerable affect.[24,25] Carson et al. conducted studies on

constructs related to anger-in, including the construct of ambivalence of emotional expression (AEE) and the construct of forgiveness.[75,76] Their findings suggest that those who are ambivalent about expressing their emotions and those who cannot forgive others for perceived wrongs and insults may experience higher levels of low back pain and psychological distress, mediated by higher levels of anger. Where treatment is concerned, it is possible that psychotherapeutic interventions designed to resolve patients' ambivalence toward expressing their emotions and to encourage the development of cognitive reappraisals supportive of conciliation and forgiveness may facilitate the management of pain.

Anger-Out

Like anger-in, the emotional regulatory strategy of anger-out—managing anger directly with physical or verbal expression—has been shown repeatedly to be associated with increased responsiveness to pain and higher levels of chronic pain intensity and disability.[32,77,78] It must be noted, here, that anger-out, in this context, usually refers to the trait of immediately responding to the emotional experience of anger with expression of anger—not the same as the considered, constructive expression of anger signifying the mobilization of more mature defensive processes. Hostility and tendencies toward aggression are hallmarks of trait anger-out. Bruehl et al. have done the most complete review of anger-out studies to date and conclude that elevated trait anger-out is associated with heightened chronic pain intensity and low levels of improvement in individuals suffering from a broad range of medical conditions associated with chronic pain.[77] They examine a number of proposed mechanisms underlying the effects of trait anger-out upon acute experimental, acute clinical, and chronic pain, but the emphasis here will be upon chronic pain.

The authors submit that there is little evidence for the influence of either neuroticism or the psychoanalytic construct of repression.[77] The former—a willingness to over-endorse a broad spectrum of symptoms—has sometimes led to spurious correlations between elevated pain and indicators of an anger-out style of management, but the available evidence tends to suggest that the relationship of anger-out to pain is independent of the broader palette of negative affect, including depression and anxiety. Where the latter is concerned, one might expect that trait anger-

---

TABLE 81.2

DM WEGNER'S IRONIC PROCESSES THEORY OF MENTAL CONTROL*

Monitoring cognitive processes	Setting/circumstances	Operating cognitive processes	Mental control outcome
Vigilance toward unwanted thoughts or reminders of previous events leading to overwhelming anger	*Stress-free* or low-stress circumstances evoking occasional or random thoughts or reminders of previous events leading to anger *Stress-laden* or high-stress circumstances evoking frequent thoughts or reminders of previous events associated with harm or an unfair slight to one's ego or identity leading to anger	Effortful, conscious attempts at suppression of or distraction from unwanted thoughts and reminders	*Successful* suppression of or distraction from monitored thoughts and reminders *Failed* suppression of or distraction from monitored thoughts and reminders leading to preoccupation and rumination

*Note that when the operating processes are under high stress, the monitoring processes, which ordinarily serve to identify thoughts to be suppressed, can become the source of continual unwanted reminders of events leading to overwhelming anger.

out would be negatively associated with the classic psychoanalytic constructs of conversion and somatization and therefore consistently lead to an amelioration of pain. As previously noted, however, the hostility and aggression embodied in trait anger-out do not promote the mature and adaptive expressions of anger reflecting successful management that might lead to reduced pain intensity and sensitivity. Other behavioral mechanisms have been considered, including the observation that individuals whose scores are elevated on measures of anger-out show decreased cardiovascular reactivity when encouraged to express their anger versus suppress it and, among a high anger-out group of women, verbal expression of anger during provocation was associated with improved blood pressure recovery, following the stressful event. Although there are some indications that these findings are related to improvement in situations involving acute pain, Bruehl et al. point out that implications for the effect of behavioral anger expression upon chronic pain have yet to be fully delineated.

Although not specifically applied to the variable of management style, Greenwood et al. suggest several behavioral mechanisms that may influence the relationship between anger and pain.[32] First, anger may foster the development of pain behaviors associated with the negative consequences of expressing anger. The high correlation between hostility and absenteeism from work, for example, suggests that anger may contribute to the maintenance of pain-related illness. Second, the effects of anger upon marital functioning may lead to spousal responses that exacerbate and maintain pain and pain behaviors. Finally, anger can impact pain by contributing to conflicts and mistrust in relationships between patients and their medical providers. Studies by Burns et al. concluded that high scorers on anger-out and hostility were correlated with patients' reports of weaker alliances with their physicians and with interference in their abilities to improve with pain management.[79,80]

Proposed mechanisms underlying the relationship of anger-out and pain have also included a number of physiologically-based models.[77] Anger-out has been associated with greater visceral adipose tissue is some studies, a potential source of impact on lower spine mechanics. Like anger-in, anger-out has also been found to be correlated with increases in stress-induced muscle tension among patients with low back pain. Neither of these models, however, can account for the effects of anger-out on acute pain responsiveness and sensitivity. Genetic mechanisms have been suggested as well, but Bruehl et al. assert that none has been adequately investigated, to date, despite promising connections with genetic factors related to personality traits, emotional reactivity, and endogenous opioid system functioning. A related mechanism, referred to as "trait X," suggests that high anger-outs express their anger because they believe it is beneficial and it feels better to discharge it than the alternative. The idea is that behaviorally expressing anger for high anger-outs actually reduces arousal and restores emotional and physiological homeostasis more efficiently. The authors comment that trait X state interactions may well reflect some degree of functional regulatory benefit, especially in the immediate aftermath of expressing anger, but the more enduring trait anger dimension has yet to be sufficiently investigated.

Opioid Deficit Hypothesis

Bruehl, in collaboration with others, has also called attention to the role of endogenous opioid dysfunction in the relationship between anger-out and pain.[21,23,77,78,81,82] The essential premise is that mechanisms associated with anger-out may impose an excessive burden or strain on the body's ability to produce endogenous opioids, inhibiting the natural management of chronic pain. Bruehl et al. conducted studies in which subjects with low scores in anger-out reported increased acute pain intensity following opioid blockade with naloxone, versus following placebo

blockade, whereas subjects high in anger-out reported smaller naloxone blockade effects.[21,23] The implication is that there is less effective endogenous opioid response among those who score high in anger-out, with opioid dysfunction partially mediating the positive correlation between anger-out and chronic pain intensity.[78]

Burns et al. further established that the use of exogenous opioid analgesics remediates opioid deficits such that anger-out is related to chronic pain severity only among patients not taking opioid medications.[82] The results suggest that regular use of opioid medications among those who are high in anger expression may compensate for overtaxed endogenous opioid mechanisms. In another, related study, Bruehl et al. investigated whether impaired central opioid inhibitory functioning, assessed via changes in plasma beta-endorphin release, could explain exaggerated pain responsiveness and anger expression in high anger-out subjects.[78] As with the opioid blockade studies and the study of the mediating effects of exogenous opioids, the results of this pain-induced endogenous opioid release study support the opioid deficit hypothesis and demonstrate that greater trait anger-out is associated with higher perceived pain intensity and less endogenous opioid release.

Taken together, these studies provide strong evidence for the idea that patients whose anger management style involves physical and verbal expression show comparative deficits in opioid analgesia because of endogenous opioid dysfunction. Bruehl et al. have taken this one step further with the opioid triggering hypothesis, suggesting that, for individuals high in anger-out, the dramatic expression of anger serves to activate endogenous opioid response that would otherwise remain quiescent when anger associated with pain and stress is either not expressed or only moderately expressed.[77] Those who are low in anger-out appear to elicit a sufficient endogenous opioid response without expressing their anger, but the expression of anger among high anger-outs may actually represent an adaptive mechanism designed to trigger the release of endogenous opioids. Patients high in anger-out may therefore have a higher threshold for the activation of endogenous opioid response, with the increased arousal of dramatic anger expression serving as a triggering mechanism.

MEASUREMENT OF ANGER

Anger, both state and trait, as well as the related constructs of aggression, hostility, and anger management style have been assessed for research purposes with a broad spectrum of tools, ranging from projective tests, like the Rorschach and TAT, to physiological measures principally associated with autonomic arousal.[35] Self-report questionnaires and inventories tend to predominate in anger-related research, however, both for their ease of administration and for their more readily documented validity and reliability. Several of the self-report instruments measuring anger that are more widely utilized in pain research are reviewed below. Extensive commentary on each, as well as critical reviews of many more instruments designed to measure some aspect of anger, are available in *Tests in Print VII*[83] and the *Mental Measurements Yearbook, 19th ed.*[84] The instruments discussed below are summarized in Table 81.3.

State-Trait Anger Expression Inventory-2 (STAXI-2)

The STAXI-2 was developed by Spielberger and is widely regarded as the most psychometrically sound and comprehensive tool in the assessment of anger and hostility.[35,68] It represents the integration and culmination of several precursors developed by Spielberger, including the State-Trait Anger Scale (STAS), the

TABLE 81.3

INSTRUMENTS DESIGNED TO ASSESS ANGER

Instrument	Format	Administration	Availability
State-Trait Anger Expression Inventory (STAXI-2)	57 items distributed across 6 scales, 5 subscales, and an anger expression index; ages 16 years and up	5–10 minutes; scored by hand	**PAR** Psychological Assessment Resources, Inc. (http://www3.parinc.com)
Targets and Reasons for Anger and Pain Sufferers (TRAPS)	10-point Likert scale assessing degree or intensity of anger toward 10 common objects of anger (e.g., self, significant others, employer, physician) and 10 common reasons for anger	10–20 minutes for an interactive administration; has been adapted for briefer self-administration; scored by hand	Fernandez E, Salinas N, Swift P, et al. Psychosocial factors that predict anger in chronic pain sufferers. *Annals of Beh Med* 1995; 17(Suppl.)S164. Fernandez E, Salinas N, Swift P, et al. Psychosocial factors that predict anger in chronic pain sufferers. Sixteenth Annual Scientific Meeting of the Society of Behavioral Medicine, San Diego, 1995. (Use by permission of primary author.)
Multidimensional Anger Inventory (MAI)	30-item instrument, with multiple variations, assessing the duration, frequency, and magnitude of anger, including differentiation between anger-in and anger-out expression and common situations leading to anger	10–20 minutes; scored by hand	Siegel JM. The multidimensional anger inventory. *J Pers Soc Psychol* 1986;51:191–200. (Use by permission of author.)
Novaco Anger Scale and Provocation Inventory (NAS-PI)	60 items distributed across 3 subscales (cognitive, arousal, behavioral) plus a 25-item inventory eliciting responses to specific situations	25 minutes; scored by hand	**WPS** Western Psychological Services (http://portal.wpspublish.com)
Anger Disorders Scale (ADS)	70 items distributed over 5 categories (provocations, cognitions, arousal, motives, behaviors)	short form, 5–10 minutes; long form, 10–20 minutes; scored by hand or software	**MHS** Multi-Health Systems, Inc. (http://www.mhs.com/mhs)
Minnesota Multiphasic Personality Inventory (MMPI-2)	567 true-false items distributed across multiple validity and clinical scales, with 6 assessing some aspect of anger, hostility, or aggression	60–90 minutes with a short form available; scored by hand or software	**Pearson** Education, Inc., Pearson Assessments for Educational, Clinical, and Psychological Use (http://www.pearsonassessments.com)

Anger Expression Scale (AES), and the first version of the STAXI-2. The instrument consists of six scales: Trait Anger, Anger Expression-Out, Anger Expression-In, Anger Control-Out, Anger Control-In, and State Anger, as well as five subscales and an Anger Expression Index. It can be administered in 5 to 10 minutes and is scored by hand, making it practical for clinical applications as well as research. The STAXI-2 purports to measure tendencies toward angry action, as well as more dispositional or trait-based hostility, along with tendencies to suppress or express the experience of anger. This makes the inventory well-suited for research in anger management styles and clinically well-adapted to assess the needs of patients for psychotherapeutic applications of anger management. Normative data are published for adolescents, adults, and psychiatric patients, and evidence for high reliability and validity are detailed in the testing manual.

The Targets and Reasons for Anger in Pain Sufferers (TRAPS)

Although the STAXI-2 is applied to the study of pain more frequently than other inventories of anger, it was not designed for use with chronic pain patients and does not assess specifically pain-related dimensions of anger. Fernandez developed a structured inventory, the TRAPS, later adapted for self-administration by Okifuji et al., that allows chronic pain patients to rate their levels of anger on a Likert-type scale toward 10 common objects or targets of their anger: whole world, self, God/destiny, significant other, employer, insurance company, attorney or legal system, health care providers, person who caused the accident.[35,85] Patients may also be instructed to identify and rank their reasons for being angry toward these targets. The results, especially when the TRAPS is administered in a structured interview, allow clinicians and patients to explore together the relative importance of specific targets of and reasons for anger, suggesting interventions and strategies for reducing the impact of anger on pain. Normative data and information on reliability and validity are not yet available.

Multidimensional Anger Inventory (MAI)

Siegel developed the MAI as a brief instrument designed to assess responses to anger-eliciting situations in an attempt to increase sensitivity to the multidimensional nature of the construct.[35,86] Factor analytic solutions arrived at the following dimensions or factors: anger-arousal, hostile outlook, range of anger-eliciting situations, and anger expression, the last being divided into anger-in and anger-out. Although it was developed specifically to assess anger in cardiovascular patients, factor analytic replications in more heterogeneous populations suggest its utility on a broader scope, especially with other health-related groups. Reliability and scale validity information are available through the author's report.[86]

Novaco Anger Scale and Provocation Inventory (NAS-PI)

This inventory, developed by Novaco, consists of two principal sections: The Novaco Anger Scale (NAS) purports to measure the general inclination toward reacting with anger, whereas the Provocation Inventory (PI) asks patients to respond to descriptions of specific situations that tend to elicit anger.[87] The NAS contains 60 items divided equally over three subscales: (1) a cognitive subscale, measuring anger justification, rumination, hostile attitude, and suspicion; (2) an arousal subscale, measuring anger intensity, duration, somatic tension, and irritability; and (3) a behavior subscale, measuring impulsive reaction, verbal aggression, physical confrontation, and direct expression. The PI contains 25 items, each describing a situation that tends to elicit anger, with subjects being instructed to rate their degree of anger or annoyance on a 5-point Likert-type scale. The situations include scenarios such as "getting your car stuck in the mud or sand" and "being joked about or teased." The items are grouped into five subscales summarizing the theme of the provocation: disrespectful treatment, unfairness, frustration, annoying traits of others, and irritations. The NAS-PI attempts to characterize how an individual experiences anger and what sorts of situations provoke it. The instrument has been widely used to evaluate the role of anger in diverse environments, from community-based to correctional settings, and may prove useful in evaluating the role of anger in healthcare settings. Normative data, reliability, and validity are well-documented in the testing manual.[87]

Anger Disorders Scale (ADS)

The ADS is a self-report instrument consisting of 70 items distributed over five categories characterizing human emotion: provocations, cognitions, arousal, motives, and behaviors.[88] A short-form consisting of only 18 items may be used as a screening tool to obtain scores on three factors: reactivity/expression, anger-in, and vengeance.[89] The ADS is designed to assess and identify dimensions of anger that are associated with dysfunction and impairment in clinical populations. It yields information concerning the duration that an individual stays angry, the breadth of stimuli that may serve as triggers for an individual's anger, and the frequency of angry episodes. Information on reliability and concurrent and discriminative validity are available in the testing manual.

Minnesota Multiphasic Personality Inventory-2 (MMPI-2)

The MMPI-2 is a 576-item, true–false, self-report instrument designed to assess a broad range of psychopathology and personality traits and characteristics.[16,17] It is arguably the best known and most widely used psychometric assessment tool available, and it has been applied to the investigation of pain in hundreds of empirical studies.[15] Several MMPI-2 scales are relevant to the study of anger and its relationship to pain, including the Psychopathic Deviate (Pd) clinical scale, as well as the supplementary scales of Hostility (Ho) and Overcontrolled-Hostility (O-H) and the content scales of Anger (ANG), Cynicism (CYN), and Aggression (AGG). All of these scales are well-validated and are designed to reflect some aspect of trait anger, and some, like the O-H and Ho scales, have been distributed separately for convenience and shortened time of administration.

PSYCHOTHERAPEUTIC MANAGEMENT

When anger and problems with the management of anger are aspects of a patient's presentation with chronic pain, ignoring the indication for psychotherapeutic intervention may well jeopardize any chance of successfully treating or managing his or her pain.[90] As we have seen, trait anger and certain styles of anger management are fertile ground for the development of chronic pain, but anger may emerge as a critical factor in response to chronic pain, as well. The following case of a middle-aged patient with chronic headaches will serve to illustrate the mutually influential roles of anger and pain in the context of treatment:

Case 2: Mr. Alvarez was a 45-year-old single man, referred to the Pain Center by his new primary care physician and his new neurologist for the treatment of longstanding chronic daily headaches with tension-type and migrainous features. He arrived for his initial evaluation more than an hour late but loudly insisted upon being seen, saying that the traffic was not his fault and that he had a severe headache requiring immediate attention. He was irritable in his exchanges with support staff and paced back and forth in the waiting area, to the discomfiture and consternation of other patients. When he was finally escorted to an examination room, he informed the nurse that he hoped he did not have to wait long to see the physician. Once his pain physician joined him for the evaluation, he seemed deferential and cooperative, as he related his medical history and the history of his headaches. His physician noted, however, that he expressed considerable anger toward previous providers, toward his wife and children, and toward his employer, none of whom, according to the patient, responded with adequate sympathy to his distress or provided any respite from his pain. As his physician rose to conclude the interview, the patient looked at the prescriptions he had been given as a first line of intervention and, tossing them onto the desk, said, "I didn't come here for more pills. I told you, I came for Botox injections, and I'm not leaving here without them." When it was explained that authorization from his insurance carrier had to be obtained and that he might well respond favorably to a less invasive procedure, the patient's anger became increasingly confrontational. When it became clear that he was not going to get what he wished, he vociferously decried "the incompetence of doctors" and stormed from the examining room, upsetting a chair and waste bin in the process.

In the succeeding days, as the patient's stricken pain physician consulted with Mr. Alvarez's referring providers and assembled his medical records, several points became clear. This was not the patient's only reported angry exchange in healthcare settings and, indeed, it appeared that Mr. Alvarez frequently changed primary care physicians and specialists, whether by his own decision or mutual agreement.

It was a surprise when Mr. Alvarez made and kept a follow-up appointment, but less surprising when the outcome was much the same, with the patient discharging his anger and frustration toward staff and his pain physician. It was at the conclusion of his second appointment that he was referred to the pain psychologist to do biofeedback and learn relaxation techniques. This puzzled but did not threaten him, because the physiological benefit of treatment was emphasized, and he was affable enough during the initial visit and anamnesis, which revealed much about the relationship between his anger and his pain. He exhibited many of the behavioral mechanisms, previously mentioned, through which anger can exercise influence over pain.[32] His anger toward his employer led to frequent arguments and resulting exacerbations of his headaches, in turn resulting in high absenteeism, which led to further conflicts at work. His anger toward his wife frequently led to retaliation in various forms on her part, which, again, resulted in exacerbations of his pain and the development of pain behaviors designed both to justify his disability and to elicit sympathy. Finally, his anger in the medical setting led to inconsistent and poorly planned care that, in turn, thwarted his attempts to gain relief, allowing his headache and associated behavioral patterns to become firmly entrenched.

It was nevertheless an unexpected development to Mr. Alvarez when the pain psychologist suggested that his anger may be exerting a dramatic impact on his headaches. The patient characterized himself as "quick to anger but quick to get over it" and cited trends within his family of origin, especially his own parents, to be dramatically expressive of anger. He added with irony, "I thought that's what you psychologists were always saying—'to get it off my chest and not hold it in.'" He portrayed himself honestly and clearly as a high anger-out individual, a style of anger management shown repeatedly to be associated with increased responsiveness to pain and higher levels of pain intensity and disability.[32,77,78] In addition to doing biofeedback training and learning relaxation techniques, the goal of psychotherapy in this second case was to encourage the patient to adopt and practice more adaptive strategies for anger management. Neither Mr. Alvarez's anger-out style nor Ms. Ostrakova's anger-in style, depicted in the first case, was conducive to the successful management of their chronic pain.

Considerations in the Selection of Psychotherapy

Where the special practice of pain psychology is concerned, supportive and psychoanalytically-informed psychotherapies have been viewed as useful in the management of pain, primarily when behavioral and cognitive-behavioral treatments have failed to bring relief.[91,92] The psychodynamic approach may be a logical starting point, however, for patients whose anger, pain, and disability are sustained by intrapsychic conflicts or unconscious motives associated with childhood trauma or primary or secondary gain.[90,93] The drawbacks associated with pursuing such a course of treatment can be manifold, but there may be times when patients are unable to move forward until they are satisfied that their conflicts and motives are revealed and understood. A problem for the successful management of pain, however, is that psychotherapies focusing on the primacy of the experience of emotion are typically long-term and may require many months, if not years, to result in meaningful insight and progress. Such treatments, at least near their outset, can also lead patients to an uncritical acceptance of their feelings, further validating the experience of negative emotions such as anger; therefore, the selection of appro-

priate psychotherapy and the skill of the psychotherapist are perhaps most critical in cases where a psychodynamic or supportive approach is indicated.

If the principal obstacles to successful adjustment to chronic pain are factors such as anger management style and negative cognitions underlying anger and hostility, then a more direct approach to treatment would be to challenge the behaviors reflecting and maintaining anger, as well as the negative cognitions driving it. Challenging established behaviors with new, more adaptive ones is the goal of behavioral therapy, whereas identifying, examining, and restructuring the negative cognitions behind negative emotions is the work of cognitive therapy. Both are well established as offering greater efficacy in the implementation of change and the modulation of the effects of anger upon chronic pain, but both depend upon the patient's willingness to collaborate with treatment and his or her readiness for and motivation to change.[90,94]

The influence of any psychosocial risk factor, such as trait anger and hostility, may signal reluctance on the part of the patient to give up his or her pain and suffering or relinquish the refuge of disability.[90] In the first case study, Ms. Ostrakova complained of pain, but her symptoms were driven by powerful and enduring unconscious conflicts associated with her history of childhood trauma and abuse. The high correlations between histories of abuse and the subsequent development of difficulties with both anger and chronic pain are well documented in the psychoanalytic and scientific literatures.[11,27,95–99] For patients who have suffered abuse as children or who have been exposed as adults to situations involving catastrophic loss or harm, chronic pain may come to represent a means of psychologically symbolizing and organizing unbearable memories and intolerable affects.[90] In Ms. Ostrakova's case, coming to an understanding of the relationship between her history and the development of her symptoms may well represent an essential step toward taking an active role in her treatment, and the selection of treatment to facilitate this step is likely to involve a form of supportive and psychodynamic psychotherapy. Ironically, a year of inpatient treatment with behavioral and cognitive-behavioral interventions appears only to have altered the patient's style of anger management from anger-out to anger-in.

Investigators have found that patients vary widely regarding how prepared they are to collaborate in their own treatment and make the changes necessary to manage their anger and their pain more effectively. Assessing a patient's *readiness for change* is frequently a critical prelude to effective psychotherapeutic intervention and may shed insight into why some patients never seem to improve. Cognitive therapy often begins with the patient's response to two questions: What do you want (to change)? What are you willing to do to get it?[90,99] The first question is easy for most patients with chronic pain, but the second implies work and sacrifice and is not so easy when patients are prone to anger and preoccupied with their own suffering and deprivation. Assessing a patient's readiness for change is one way of answering the second question.

Kerns et al. applied Prochaska's transtheoretical model of the stages of change to the situation of chronic pain and arrived at four successive levels in patients' willingness to collaborate with treatment and undertake the behavioral changes necessary to manage their pain more effectively[100,101,102]:

- *Precontemplation*: patients who have no intention of changing their current patterns of behavior—"You're the doctor. Fix my pain!"
- *Contemplation*: patients who have begun to recognize the necessity of making changes in their behavior but have not yet committed to doing so—"I know it's up to me. I just don't know how to do it."

■ *Action*: patients who have committed to a plan of action and are engaged in making changes—"I'm doing something about my pain."

■ *Maintenance*: patients who are attempting to sustain the changes they have undertaken—"I'm using what I've learned in treatment to manage my pain better."

Angry and hostile patients, in particular, may be stuck in the precontemplative stage of readiness for change, and their often unrealistic expectations of their physicians may lead them to feel that effective treatment is being withheld. This was the case with Mr. Alvarez, whose anger was driven by his disappointment in providers who never seemed willing to do enough to help him manage his pain. Unlike Ms. Ostrakova, however, his style of managing anger did not reflect defensive inhibition of affect, and his chronic pain was not associated with unconscious conflicts. His anger, although more volatile, also proved more tractable to the psychoeducational component of cognitive therapy, and he was ultimately able to make the transition more easily from the precontemplative to the contemplative stage of readiness for change.

Behavioral and Cognitive-Behavioral Therapies

Templates for behavioral and cognitive-behavioral intervention in cases of chronic pain are offered in succeeding chapters. Here, their specific relevance to the treatment of anger will be explored. Behavioral approaches to the treatment of anger have tended to revolve around relaxation training and applications of relaxation techniques to reducing autonomic arousal and uncomfortable musculoskeletal tension. Suinn's template for anxiety/anger management training (AMT) represents one of the more enduring expressions of this form of treatment.[103,104] He proposes a brief, structured therapy involving six to eight sessions in which guided imagery directed toward arousing anger is subsequently and serially paired with relaxation techniques designed to deactivate arousal. Patients are first instructed in the elicitation of the body's natural relaxation response—which can be accomplished using meditation, progressive muscle relaxation, body scans or other forms of autogenic training, or diaphragmatic breathing techniques—and, once they have mastered this, the psychotherapist offers structured practice in the use of the technique to contain or defuse sympathetic nervous system reactivity cued by suggestions and visualizations of stressful images. The use of biofeedback technology in the assessment of progress can frequently hasten mastery of this strategy by presenting the patient with tangible evidence of progress.

Recall that in Lazarus's cognitive appraisal theory of emotion, the experience of anger is the joint effect of (1) the event of physiological arousal and (2) the cognitive appraisal of its meaning.[64] While much of behavioral therapy directed toward the management of anger is concerned with the former, cognitive therapy is directed toward the latter. As we have seen, anger, by Smedslund's definition, involves the appraisal by the subject that he or she—or a person for whom he or she cares—has been treated without respect.[63] This, of course, may actually be the case in a given situation, and therein lies the foundation of the biological basis for anger[43,44,73]; but anger, as our Greco-Roman and Judeo-Christian roots attest, does not necessarily conform to logic. The experience of anger can quickly and easily become associated with irrational, automatic thoughts and beliefs concerning the motives of others and the sources of threat to our well-being.

The approach of cognitive therapy is to offer a corrective process to the development and maintenance of errors in our thinking and beliefs.[35,90,105,106,107,108] Through the process of cognitive restructuring or reappraisal, patients are led to examine whether, in the process of trying to make sense of their anger and pain, they may be making fundamental errors in their thinking and relying upon mistaken beliefs. Patients are encouraged to challenge their automatic thoughts and uncritically held beliefs regarding their experiences of anger through the template of cognitive appraisal theory—that is, that situations are ordinarily neutral until we assign meaning to them. We are often unaware of this step of assigning meaning because we do not usually stop to examine the thoughts and beliefs that influence our emotional responses to certain situations and, even when we do, we may not consider the accuracy of these thoughts and beliefs. The essence of the cognitive model of treatment suggests that much of our emotional distress and self-defeating behavior is based simply upon inaccurate and irrational thinking and that, once our attention is drawn to these upsetting cognitions, we can test their veracity and value to see whether they form an appropriate basis for our emotions and behavior.

As they learn to identify negative cognitions, patients begin to monitor their cognitive appraisals more rigorously and critically, cognitively restructuring their primary and secondary appraisals of situations resulting in anger. Common reappraisals of the experience of anger might include reexamining the intention of the one toward whom our anger is directed, reconsidering the harm done by the perceived slight or insult, or reinterpreting the outcome of a situation to determine whether a perceived breach of respect actually resulted in harm or injury.[35] In the case of Mr. Alvarez, several negative cognitions were identified as being based on dysfunctional family-of-origin models and over-rehearsed expression. His primary negative cognition—"Everyone is out to take advantage of me"—may have reflected some degree of utility in the gang-controlled streets of his childhood barrio, but was dysfunctional and even harmful in the medical setting, where his physicians and other providers were genuinely concerned to help him. Their response to his anger was to defend themselves by disengaging and retreating, often to the detriment of his care. A corollary negative cognition—"No one will help you voluntarily; you have to demand what you need from people"—was equally destructive of the medical alliance. Through cognitive reappraisal and the opportunity to test different interpretations, the patient ultimately proved to himself that people, especially people whose job is to take care of him, really are often willing to help and that consistently making demands of others tends to result in less return than welcoming their responses to reasonable requests. Mr. Alvarez's anger-out style, once a barrier to his receiving the best from his medical care, receded and was replaced by a more genuinely collaborative attitude toward his physicians.

SUMMARY

The cultural background of anger lays the groundwork for understanding its role both as an emotion and as a trait, as well as its relationship to pain. Psychoanalytic theory emphasized the harmful effects of inhibiting the experience and expression of anger, placing it at the core of conflicts between competing drives and the formation of pathological symptoms. More recent research has brought additional clarity to the relationship between anger and pain, suggesting a number of possible mechanisms through which state and trait anger can influence sensitivity to pain and the development and maintenance of chronic pain. This trend, in turn, has led to improved objective psychological measures of anger and the observation that style of anger management may be a principal modulating factor in the relationship between anger and pain. Anger management style has become a critical consideration in the development of effective psychotherapeutic treatments for anger-related psychopathology, with behavioral and cognitive therapies for anger often resulting in improved management of chronic pain.

References

1. Aristotle. *Rhetoric*. Roberts WR, trans. Whitefish, MT: Kessinger Press; 2004: 54–63.

2. Seneca. *Moral and Political Essays*. Procope JF, ed. Cooper JM, trans. Cambridge, UK: Cambridge University Press; 1995:17.

3. Kemp S, Strongman KT. Anger theory and management: a historical analysis. *Am J Psychol* 1995;108:397–417.

4. Thurman RAF. *Anger*. New York: Oxford University Press; 2005.

5. Freud S. On psycho-analysis. In: Strachey J, ed, trans. *Complete Psychological Works*. Vol 12. standard ed. London: Hogarth Press; 1958:209. (Original work published 1913.)

6. Breuer J, Freud S. Studies on hysteria. In: Strachey J, ed, trans. *Complete Psychological Works*. Vol 2. standard ed. London: Hogarth Press; 1955. (Original work published 1893–1895.)

7. Merskey H. History of psychoanalytic ideas concerning pain. In: Gatchel RJ, Weisberg JN, eds. *Personality Characteristics of Patients with Pain*. Washington, DC: American Psychological Association; 2000:25–35.

8. Freud S. Mourning and melancholia. In: Strachey J, ed, trans. *Complete Psychological Works*. Vol 14. standard ed. London: Hogarth Press; 1957. (Original work published 1917.)

9. Freud S. Beyond the pleasure principle. In: Strachey J, ed, trans. *Complete Psychological Works*. Vol 18. standard ed. London: Hogarth Press; 1955. (Original work published 1920.)

10. Freud S. Inhibitions, symptoms, and anxiety. In: Strachey J, ed, trans. *Complete Psychological Works*. Vol 20. standard ed. London: Hogarth Press; 1959. (Original work published 1926.)

11. Engel GL. "Psychogenic" pain and the pain-prone patient. *Am J Med* 1959; 26:899–918.

12. Szasz TS. *Pain and Pleasure: A Study of Bodily Feelings*. London: Tavistock; 1957.

13. Burns JW. Repression predicts outcome following multidisciplinary treatment of chronic pain. *Health Psychol* 2000;19:75–84.

14. Burns JW. Repression in chronic pain: an idea worth recovering. *Appl Prev Psychol* 2000;9:173–190.

15. Keller LS, Butcher JN. *Assessment of Chronic Pain Patients with the MMPI-2*. Minneapolis, MN: University of Minnesota Press; 1991.

16. Butcher JN. *MMPI-2: A Practitioner's Guide*. Washington, DC: American Psychological Association; 2005.

17. Graham JR. *MMPI-2: Assessing Personality and Psychopathology*. New York: Oxford University Press; 2005.

18. Vendrig AA. The Minnesota multiphasic personality inventory and chronic pain: a conceptual analysis of a longstanding but complicated relationship. *Clin Psychol Rev* 2000;20:533–559.

19. Schlessinger D. MMPI-2 characteristics in a chronic pain population. *Assessment* 2002;9:406–414.

20. Jansen SJ, Spinhoven P, Brosschot JF. Experimentally induced anger, cardiovascular reactivity, and pain sensitivity. *J Psychosom Res* 2001;51:479–485.

21. Bruehl S, Burns JW, Chung OY, et al. Anger and pain-sensitivity in chronic low back pain patients and pain-free controls: the role of endogenous opioids. *Pain* 2002;99:223–233.

22. Bruehl S, Chung OY, Burns JW. Differential effects of expressive anger regulation on chronic pain intensity in CRPS and non-CRPS limb pain patients. *Pain* 2003;104:647–654.

23. Bruehl S, Chung OY, Burns JW, et al. The association between anger expression and chronic pain intensity: evidence for partial mediation by endogenous opioid dysfunction. *Pain* 2003;106:317–324.

24. Quartana PJ, Burns JW. Painful consequences of anger suppression. *Emotion* 2007;7:400–414.

25. Quartana PJ, Yoon KL, Burns JW. Anger suppression, ironic processes, and pain. *J Behav Med* 2007;30:455–469.

26. Engel GL. The psychoanalytic approach to psychsomatic medicine. In: Marmor J, ed. *Modern Psychoanalysis: New Directions and Perspectives*. 1995:251–273. (Original work published 1968.)

27. Adler RH, Zlot S, Hurny C, et al. Engel's "psychogenic pain and the pain-prone patient": a retrospective, controlled clinical study. *Psychosom Med* 1989;51:87–101.

28. Robinson ME, Riley JL. The role of emotion in pain. In: Gatchel RJ, Turk DC, eds. *Psychosocial Factors in Pain: Critical Perspectives*. New York: Guilford Press; 1999:74–88.

29. Melzack R. From the gate to the neuromatrix. *Pain* 1999;(suppl 6): S121–S126.

30. Melzack R. Pain and the neuromatrix in the brain. *J Dent Educ* 2001; 65:1378–1382.

31. Melzack R. Evolution of the neuromatrix theory of pain. *Pain Pract* 2005;5: 85–94.

32. Greenwood KA, Thurston R, Rumble M, et al. Anger and persistent pain: current status and future directions. *Pain* 2003;103:1–5.

33. Cacioppo JT, Bernston GG, Klein DJ, et al. The psychophysiology of emotion across the lifespan. *Annu Rev Gerontol Geriatr* 1997;17:27–74.

34. Fernandez E, Turk DC. The scope and significance of anger in the experience of chronic pain. *Pain* 1995;61:165–175.

35. Fernandez E. *Anxiety, Depression, and Anger in Pain: Research Findings and Clinical Options*. Dallas, TX: Advanced Psychological Resources; 2002.

36. Banks SM, Kerns RD. Explaining high rates of depression in chronic pain: a diathesis-stress framework. *Psychol Bull* 1996;119:95–110.

37. Mollet GA, Harrison DW. Emotion and pain: a functional cerebral systems integration. *Neuropsychol Rev* 2006;16:99–121.

38. Mico JA, Ardid D, Berrocoso E, et al. Antidepressants and pain. *Trends Pharmacol Sci* 2006;27:348–354.

39. Maizels M, McCarberg B. Antidepressants and antiepileptic drugs for chronic pain. *Am Fam Physician* 2005;71:483–490.

40. Hagelberg N, Forssell H, Aalto S, et al. Altered dopamine D2 receptor binding in atypical facial pain. *Pain* 2003;106:43–48.

41. Hagelberg N, Jaaskelainen SK, Martikainen IK, et al. Striatal dopamine D2 receptors in modulation of pain in humans: a review. *Eur J Pharmacol* 2004; 500:187–192.

42. Field T, Hernandez—Reif M, Diego M, et al. Cortisol decreases and serotonin and dopamine increase following massage therapy. *Intern J Neuroscience* 2005;115:1397–1413.

43. Wood PB. Stress and dopamine: Implications for the pathophysiology of chronic widespread pain. *Med Hypotheses* 2004;62:420–424.

44. Lara DR, Akiskal HS. Toward an integrative model of the spectrum of mood, behavioral, and personality disorders based on fear and anger traits: II. Implications for neurobiology, genetics and psychopharmacological treatment. *J Affect Disord* 2006;94:89–103.

45. Salamone JD, Correa M, Mingote SM, et al. Beyond the reward hypothesis: alternative functions of nucleus accumbens dopamine. *Curr Opin Pharmacol* 2005;5:34–41.

46. Svrakic DM, Cloninger R. Classification of personality disorders: implications for treatment and research. In: Soares JC, Gershon S. eds. *Handbook of Medical Psychiatry*. New York: Marcel Dekker, Inc.; 2003:117–148.

47. Janssen SA, Spinhoven P, Brisschot JF. Experimentally induced anger, cardiovascular reactivity, and pain sensitivity. *J Psychosom Res* 2001;51:479–485.

48. Janssen SA. Negative affect and sensitization to pain. *Scand J Psychol* 2002; 43:131–137.

49. Burns JW, Bruehl S, Caceres C. Anger management style, blood pressure reactivity, and acute pain sensitivity: evidence for "trait x situation" models. *Ann Behav Med* 2004;27:195–204.

50. Cloninger CR. Antisocial personality disorder: a review. In: Maj M, Akiskal HS, Messich JE, eds. *Personality Disorders*. New York, NY: Wiley; 2005: 125–169.

51. Serretti A, Mandelli L, Lorenzi C, et al. Temperament and character in mood disorders: influence of DRD4, SERTPR, TPH, and MAO-A polymorphisms. *Neuropsychobiology* 2006;53:9–16.

52. Dersh J, Polatin PB, Gatchel RJ. Chronic pain and psychopathology: Research findings and theoretical considerations. *Psychosom Med* 2002;64:773–786.

53. Turk DC, Monarch ES. Biopsychosocial perspective on chronic pain. In: Turk DC, Gatchel RJ, eds. *Psychological Approaches to Pain Management: A Practitioner's Handbook*. New York, NY: Guilford Press; 2002:3–29.

54. Burns JW. Arousal of negative emotion and symptom-specific reactivity in chronic low back pain patients. *Emotion* 2006;6:309–319.

55. Burns JW, Bruehl S, Quartana PJ. Anger management style and hostility among patients with chronic pain: effects upon symptom-specific physiological reactivity during anger- and sadness-recall interviews. *Psychosom Med* 2006;68:786–793.

56. Kiecolt-Glaser JK, McGuire L, Robles TF, et al. Emotions, morbidity, and mortality. *Annu Rev Psychol* 2002;53:83–107.

57. Segerstrom SC, Miller GE. Psychological stress and the human immune system: a meta-analytic study of 30 years of inquiry. *Psychol Bull* 2004;130: 601–630.

58. Kop WJ. The integration of cardiovascular behavioral medicine and psychoneuroimmunology. *Brain Behav Immun* 2003;17:233–237.

59. Graham JE, Robles TF, Kiecolt-Glaser JK, et al. Hostility and pain are related to inflammation in older adults. *Brain Behav Immun* 2006;20:389–400.

60. Boyle SH, Jackson WG, Suarez EC. Hostility, anger, and depression predict increases in C3 over a 10-year period. *Brain Behav Immun* 2007;21:816–823.

61. Harper D, ed. Anger. Dictionary.com. *Online Etymology Dictionary*. 2001. Available at: http://dictionary.reference.com/browse/anger. Accessed January 8, 2008.

62. Parker PM, ed. Anger. *Webster's Online Dictionary*. 2004. Available at: http://websters-online-dictionary.org/definition/anger Accessed: February 8, 2008.

63. Smedslund J. How shall the concept of anger be defined? *Theory Psychol* 1993;3:5–33.

64. Lazarus RS. Cognitive-motivational-relational theory of emotion. In: Hanin YL, ed. *Emotions in Sport*. Champaign, IL: Human Kinetics; 2000:39–64.

65. Anshel MH, Jamison J, Raviv S. Cognitive appraisals and coping strategies following acute stress among skilled competitive male and female athletes. *J Sport Behav* 2001;24:128–143.

66. Grant LD, Long BC, Willms JD. Women's adaptation to chronic back pain: daily appraisals and coping strategies, personal characteristics, and perceived spousal responses. *J Health Psychol* 2002;7:545–563.

67. Cheng C, Cheung MWL. Cognitive processes underlying coping flexibility: differentiation and integration. *J Pers* 2005;73:859–886.

68. Spielberger CD. *The State-Trait Anger Expression Inventory-2*. Odessa, FL: Psychological Assessment Resource; 1999.

69. Freud S. New introductory lectures on psychoanalysis. In: *Complete Psycho-*

logical Works. Vol 22. standard ed. London: Hogarth Press; 1964. (Original work published 1933.)

70. Deffenbacher JL. Trait anger: theory, findings, and implications. In: Spielberger CD, Butcher JN, eds. *Advances in Personality Assessment.* Hillsdale, NJ: Lawrence Erlbaum; Vol 9. 1990:177–202.

71. International Association for the Study of Pain. IASP Task Force on Taxonomy. In: Merskey H, Bogduk N, eds. *Classification of Chronic Pain: Description of Chronic Pain Syndromes and Definition of Pain Terms.* Seattle, WA: IASP Press; 1994.

72. Chapman CR, Nakamura Y, Donaldson G, et al. Sensory and affective dimensions of phasic pain are indistinguishable in the self-report and psychophysiology of normal laboratory subjects. *J Pain* 2001;2:279–294.

73. Gross JJ. Emotion regulation: affective, cognitive, and social consequences. *Psychophysiology* 2002;39:281–291.

74. Wegner DM. Ironic processes of mental control. *Psychol Rev* 1994;101:34–52.

75. Carson JW, Keefe FJ, Goli V, et al. Forgiveness and chronic low back pain: a preliminary study examining the relationship of forgiveness to pain, anger, and psychological distress. *J Pain* 2005;6:84–91.

76. Carson JW, Keefe FJ, Lowry KP, et al. Conflict about expressing emotions and chronic low back pain. *J Pain* 2007;8:405–411.

77. Bruehl S, Chung OY, Burns JW. Anger expression and pain: an overview of findings and possible mechanisms. *J Behav Med* 2006;29:593–606.

78. Bruehl S, Chung OY, Burns JW, et al. Trait anger expressiveness and pain-induced beta-endorphin release: support for the opioid dysfunction hypothesis. *Pain* 2007;130:208–215.

79. Burns J, Higdon L, Mullen J, et al. Relationships among patient hostility, anger expression, depression, and the working alliance in a work hardening program. *Ann Behav Med* 1999;21:77–82.

80. Burns JW, Johnson BJ, Devine J, et al. Anger management style and the prediction of treatment outcome among male and female chronic pain patients. *Behav Res Ther* 1998;36:1051–1062.

81. Bruehl S, McCubbin J, Hardin R. Theoretical review: altered pain regulatory systems in chronic pain. *Neurosci Biobehav Rev* 1999;23:877–890.

82. Burns JW, Bruehl S. Anger management style, opioid analgesic use, and chronic pain severity: a test of the opioid-deficit hypothesis. *J Behav Med* 2005;28:555–563.

83. Murphy LL, Plake BS, Spies RA, eds. *Tests in Print VII: An Index to Tests, Test Reviews, and the Literature on Specific Tests.* Vol 7. Lincoln, NE: Buros Institute of Mental Measurements; 2006.

84. Buros Institute. *The Seventeenth Mental Measurements Yearbook.* Spies RA, Plake BS, Geisinger KF, et al., eds. Lincoln, NE: Buros Institute of Mental Measurements; 2007.

85. Okifuji A, Turk DC, Curran SL. Anger in chronic pain: Investigations of anger targets and intensity. *J Psychosom Res* 1999;47:1–12.

86. Siegel JM. The multidimensional anger inventory. *J Pers Soc Psychol* 1986;51:191–200.

87. Novaco RW. *Novaco Anger Scale and Provocation Inventory (NAS-PI).* Los Angeles, CA: Western Psychological Services; 2003.

88. DiGiuseppe R, Tafrate R. *Understanding Anger and Anger Disorders.* New York, NY: Oxford University Press; 2004.

89. DiGiuseppe R, Tafrate RC. *Anger Disorders Scale: Short (ADS:S).* North Tonawanda, NY: Multi-Health Systems, Inc.; 2004.

90. Wootton RJ, Caudill-Slosberg MA, Frank JB. Psychotherapeutic management of chronic pain. In: Warfield CA, Bajwa ZH, eds. *Principles and Practice of Pain Medicine.* 2nd ed. New York, NY: McGraw-Hill; 2004:157–169.

91. Grzesiak RC, Ury GM, Dworkin RH. Psychodynamic psychotherapy with chronic pain patients. In: Gatchel RJ, Turk DC, eds. *Psychological Approaches to Pain Management: A Practitioner's Handbook.* New York, NY: Guilford Press; 1996;148–178.

92. Postone N. Psychotherapy with cancer patients. *Am J Psychother* 1998;52:412–424.

93. Wootton RJ. Supportive dynamic and existential therapy. *J Cancer Pain Symptom Palliation* 2005;1:73–78.

94. Howells K, Day A. Readiness for anger management: clinical and theoretical issues. *Clin Psychol Rev* 2003;23:319–337.

95. Linton SJ, Larden M, Gillow AM. Sexual abuse and chronic musculoskeletal pain: prevalence and psychological factors. *Clin J Pain* 1996;12:215–221.

96. Goldberg RT. Childhood abuse, depression, and chronic pain. *Clin J Pain* 1994;10:277–281.

97. Whitehead WE, Crowell MD, Davidoff AL, et al. Pain from rectal distention in women with irritable bowel syndrome: relationship to sexual abuse. *Dig Dis Sci* 1997;42:796–804.

98. Nickel R, Egle UT, Hardt J. Are childhood adversities relevant in patients with low back pain? *Eur J Pain* 2002;6:221–228.

99. Wessler R, Hankin S, Stern J. *Succeeding with Difficult Clients: Applications of Cognitive Appraisal Therapy.* San Diego, CA: Academic Press; 2001.

100. Prochaska JO, DiClemente CC. The transtheoretical approach. In: Norcross JC, Goldfried MR, eds. *Handbook of Psychotherapy Integration.* New York, NY: Basic Books; 1992:300–334.

101. Prochaska JO, Velicer WF. The transtheoretical model of health behavior change. *Am J Health Promotion* 1997;12:38–48.

102. Kerns RD, Rosenberg R, Jamison RN, et al. Readiness to adopt a self-management approach to chronic pain: the pain stages of change questionnaire (PSOCQ). *Pain* 1997;72:227–234.

103. Suinn R. *Anxiety Management Training: A Behavior Therapy.* New York, NY: Plenum Press; 1990.

104. Suinn RM. Anxiety/anger management training. In: Koocher GP, Norcross JC, eds. *Psychologists' Desk Reference.* New York: Oxford University Press; 2005:271–273.

105. Turk DS. Cognitive behavioral approach to the treatment of chronic pain patients. *Reg Anesth Pain Med* 2003;28:573–579.

106. Winterowd C, Beck AT, Gruener D. *Cognitive Therapy with Chronic Pain Patients.* New York: Springer; 2003.

107. Thorn BE. *Cognitive Therapy for Chronic Pain.* New York: Guilford Press; 2004.

108. Vlayen JWS, Morley S. Cognitive behavioral treatments for chronic pain: what works for whom? *Clin J Pain* 2005;21:1–8.

CHAPTER 82 ■ COGNITIVE BEHAVIORAL THERAPY FOR CHRONIC PAIN

LUIS F. BUENAVER, CLAUDIA M. CAMPBELL, AND JENNIFER A. HAYTHORNTHWAITE

INTRODUCTION

The early foundations of modern cognitive–behavioral therapy for chronic pain derive from a rich history of scientific work in the behavioral and social sciences. In the 1960s and 1970s, Fordyce, working in a rehabilitation setting, applied established behavioral principles to the study of pain and pain-related behavior and demonstrated that patients' reports of pain and their daily activities could be changed using social consequences (the reader is referred to[1,2] for an excellent example of the application of behavioral principles for the management of pain). About the same time, the field of behavioral medicine formed and promoted a multifactorial conceptualization of physical health and illness in which psychological and behavioral factors reciprocally interact with biological factors. This approach was particularly suited to the study of pain, as cognitive and emotional processes had long been established as influencing pain (e.g., Beecher's work with soldiers returning from war[3] and Melzack and Wall's Gate Control Theory of Pain[4]). Albert Ellis'[5] work on irrational thoughts and Aaron Beck's[6–7] work on cognitive factors influencing depression had already gained prominence by the 1970s, and Turk et al.'s[8] influential book expanded these perspectives to include social learning principles and pain-specific cognitive processes, synthesizing a cognitive–behavioral perspective on pain. These key developments and the concurrent explosion of research in the behavioral sciences changed treatment approaches for chronic pain, which had previously employed a largely biomedical approach, focusing on specific anatomy, physiology, and neurochemistry in order to modify nociceptive input.

Often, persistently painful clinical conditions require multidimensional treatment that targets pain reduction and a return to daily functioning. Cognitive–behavioral treatments (CBT) began receiving empirical support in the early 1980s,[8–10] and have become the most frequently used behavioral medicine approach for pain management, focusing on pain-related cognitions and behaviors. CBT for pain management is based on empirical work indicating that a person's beliefs about pain are associated with various functional outcomes[11–13] and that changes in patients' beliefs about pain are related to changes in functioning.[14,15] A substantial body of literature strongly supports the assertion that multifaceted pain treatment approaches incorporating cognitive-behavioral interventions are beneficial,[16,17] although not for every patient.[18] Specific underlying assumptions characterize CBT interventions for chronic pain.[19] People are viewed as actively (versus passively) engaged with their environment, processing both external and internal stimuli. Cognitive schemas are mental frameworks that represent an individual's understanding of the world. They develop from social and cultural experiences and are shaped by learning. Cognitive schemas are used to process external and internal stimuli from people's environments and guide behavior; therefore, these schemas become important targets for CBT. CBT for chronic pain also assumes that cognitions influence affective and physiological arousal, and these associations are viewed as reciprocal with affect, physiology, and behavior similarly influencing cognitions. The patient's active engagement with the environment includes changing his or her own behavior, manipulating the environment, and attempting to change others' behavior. Fundamental to this perspective is the tenet that people with pain are not helpless; they can and should replace maladaptive cognitions and behaviors (that precipitate, maintain, and exacerbate pain) to more adaptive ones. The concept of replacement is integral to a behavioral approach, in which consequences control behavior; in order for the behavior (or cognition) to change with any durability, it should be replaced with an alternative that is reinforced.

Cognitive, affective, and behavioral responses to pain are significant features of the pain experience because they influence long-term pain-related outcomes and therefore serve as key targets for psychosocial interventions directed at improving pain-related quality of life.[13,20,21] Thus, CBT for pain management involves the integration of cognitive, affective, and behavioral factors into the case conceptualization and treatment of patients. Psychological variables such as catastrophizing, negative thinking, maladaptive coping, pain behaviors (e.g., learned responses), and mood are of particular interest. Within the cognitive–behavioral framework of pain, patient perceptions and expectations of their circumstances significantly contribute to pain-related outcomes (e.g., health status, disability). Therefore, learning new cognitive and behavioral responses to pain and the factors that shape the pain experience (e.g., stress, social interactions) can enhance patient perceptions of control over pain, improve mood via changes in negative thinking, and replace maladaptive behaviors with adaptive ones, thereby decreasing pain and pain-related disability.

Cognitive–behavioral techniques have been applied and tested with a broad range of chronic pain conditions. Similar to pharmacological management of pain, the actual nature of the therapy is individually determined based on the clinical presentation. For example, some patients present with high levels of catastrophizing and an array of maladaptive beliefs about their pain and current life circumstances. For this patient, CBT may emphasize cognitive therapy more so than behavioral therapy. For another

patient, inactivity and deconditioning may be primary, so goal setting and behavioral activation may receive more emphasis. The actual CBT intervention is specifically tailored to the patient's needs identified during a careful assessment of the presenting problem and clinical picture.

Some people are not good candidates for CBT, particularly because a significant level of motivation and commitment is required of patients.[22] For this reason, patients who are not interested in CBT are less likely to benefit since CBT requires the person to practice skills outside of therapy and attend treatment consistently. Sometimes these patients become more engaged after exposure to relaxation (see below) or use of biofeedback, but motivation (see discussion of readiness to change) and openness to considering the treatment are crucial. Patients who expect a "quick fix" or conceptualize their condition as purely "organic" and unaffected by psychosocial factors are unlikely candidates for CBT. Comorbid conditions, such as a personality disorder or substance abuse/dependence or a serious mental illness, may necessitate alternate mental health care and stabilization prior to initiating CBT for pain. Finally, the patient's social environment must be considered and incorporated into treatment whenever possible. The family, disability system, and other social forces can strongly influence the patient's ability to make behavioral, cognitive, and emotional changes. If not properly supportive of treatment goals, the social environment can undermine treatment efforts.

The typical modes of treatment delivery for CBT have historically been individual therapy or group treatment. Individual sessions are composed of one-on-one meetings in private and confidential settings where treatment is tailored to the patient. CBT approaches typically are structured according to individual need and are relatively short-term. Given the considerable practitioner time and often prohibitive cost associated with individual treatment, group therapy (see Chapter 86) has become an increasingly viable option.

The qualifications and training of the therapist providing cognitive-behavioral interventions for pain have not been studied or standardized to meet the standards used for the treatment of anxiety or depression.[23] In addition to basic skills in psychotherapy, the personal attributes of the competent clinician include placing a high priority on helping patients reduce symptoms quickly and valuing a collaborative working relationship in which both the practitioner and the patient collaborate in guiding the change process. A substantial period of theoretical training and supervised clinical experience is required for effective application of skills. Some essentials for the CBT practitioner include making case formulations/conceptualizations based on presenting problems and the factors that maintain them; developing a strong, active, collaborative therapeutic alliance; planning treatment sessions according to the conceptualization, continually monitoring progress and altering the course if appropriate; working toward patient goals; guiding the patient in identifying and modifying maladaptive cognitions; facilitating behavior change; working on treatment adherence; and strategizing with the patient for relapse prevention.

Unfortunately, few clinical trials of CBT in the pain literature adequately describe the expertise of CBT interventionists or document that they meet a minimal standard of expertise in administering these specialized interventions.[17,24] In many trials and most clinical settings, these interventionists are generally doctorate-level clinical psychologists with additional postdoctoral training in pain management. According to the American Psychological Association (APA), the doctoral degree in psychology with at least 1 year of supervised postgraduate work and completion of a state licensure exam is considered entry level for an independent professional and additional specialty certification in CBT is available to licensed psychologists through the American Board of Professional Psychology (ABPP). However, other countries (e.g., Australia) have outlined competencies for the non–doctoral-level

CBT practitioner in a number of disciplines including nursing and social work. While few CBT practitioners have additional specialized training in working with pain patients, a notoriously difficult population, training opportunities with experts in the field exist. For example, the International Association for the Study of Pain lists specific educational opportunities on their Web site.

TYPES OF CBT AND SPECIFIC TECHNIQUES

In this section we discuss traditional types of CBT, including coping skills training, cognitive restructuring, and some innovative modalities for treatment delivery (e.g., telephone and Web-based treatments). For a discussion of the application of contextual cognitive behavior therapy and exposure-based therapies, the reader is referred to Chapter 83. Although CBT therapist techniques and delivery systems vary by provider and/or program, the approaches are similar because they include some common ingredients: educational content; setting personalized treatment goals and identifying targets for intervention; refinement of existing pain coping skills and development of new skills; behavioral skill rehearsal during and between sessions; use of goal setting and homework; identifying and changing maladaptive beliefs and thoughts; and involvement of family or other sources of social support. Treatment sessions are structured (e.g., sessions often follow the same sequence: review of homework, new topic introduction and skill rehearsal, goal setting, and new homework assignment) yet personalized and substantial time in early sessions is devoted to education, as well as setting expectations for active participation on the part of the patient both during and between sessions.

Coping Skills Training

The objective of coping skills training is to shape the patient's conceptualization of chronic pain as a chronic illness, similar to diabetes, which requires self-management on a daily basis. Through education and skill development, patients develop an effective arsenal of pain coping skills. These skills typically include relaxation, cognitive restructuring, distraction, problem solving, behavioral activation and pacing, goal setting, and stress management, briefly renewed here.

Education and Rationale

Providing patients with education and information about the nature and course of an illness, available treatment plans, and the process and outcomes of diagnostic and therapeutic procedures is an essential aspect of CBT treatment. One of the goals of providing patients with information is to enhance their cognitive control over an aversive event by promoting control-enhancing reappraisals of the particular situation.[25] Preparatory information provided to patients facing stressful and painful invasive medical procedures reduces negative affect and pain.[26] Thus, education and information can increase self-management and feelings of control over pain.[27]

An integral educational component in coping skills interventions involves teaching patients about the gate control theory of pain.[4,28] Many patients find it helpful to know that experts conceptualize pain as a multidimensional experience consisting of sensory, affective, and evaluative components, and not simply a sensory event that signals tissue damage. This lays the groundwork for discussing the processing of pain as a dynamic sequence in which the cognitive and affective centers of the brain influence the transmission of nociceptive signals by activating descending systems that block pain through a gating mechanism located in the spinal cord. When described in everyday language, the concept of a gating mechanism in the spinal cord that modulates the experience of pain can be appealing to many patients. Some useful real-life examples that can be incorporated into the discussion of the gate control model include the common example of athletes performing while injured, the experience of phantom pain following an amputation, or the often experienced exacerbation of pain perceived during/following stressful events.

Early in treatment for many patients, it is important to establish a plausible rationale for the use of psychological interventions (i.e., CBT) to manage chronic pain because many patients are skeptical and quick to reject psychological approaches to pain management. The gate control theory of pain can be quite helpful in explaining the idea that in addition to biological factors, psychological factors play a role in shaping their pain experience. If pain is acknowledged as a personal/subjective experience influenced by thoughts, behaviors, and feelings, then the therapist can help the patient identify factors that maintain, aggravate, or alleviate their pain.

Relaxation and Imagery Techniques

Relaxation training is often one of the first skills taught in CBT for pain. There are a number of different relaxation techniques available for use in pain management (see Chapter 85 for more detail), including progressive muscle relaxation, imagery, deep breathing, hypnosis, yoga, and meditation. The common dimension of these various techniques is a neurophysiologic response referred to as the "relaxation response."[29] This response involves a reduction in the tone of the sympathetic nervous system that produces muscle relaxation along with attenuated neuroendocrine response to adverse external conditions, culminating with a general sense of well-being and decreased anxiety. Progressive muscle relaxation,[30,31] which involves systematically and progressively contracting and relaxing various muscle groups, imagery,[8] and deep breathing,[8] are methods frequently used in the treatment of chronic pain.

Relaxation methods are designed to enhance patients' stress-management skills by giving them different strategies to regulate cognitive–affective processes and autonomic responses associated with persistent pain. However, in order to achieve maximum benefit, relaxation exercises require a commitment from the patient to set aside time to practice consistently and ultimately implement the techniques. Relaxation strategies, particularly imagery techniques, can also serve to redirect the patients' focus away from their pain and onto the relaxation task at hand. Patients who become proficient at effectively implementing relaxation strategies can increase their perception of control over their pain. Once the general principles and exercises have been explained to the patient, the procedures can also be tailored to reflect the components that are most effective and most relaxing for the patient.

Though relaxation exercises can be time consuming and require motivation on the part of the patient, research supports the efficacy of relaxation therapy in augmenting improvement and minimizing or preventing potential relapses associated with conventional therapy alone.[32] Though some reviews find a lack of evidence supporting the analgesic effectiveness of relaxation exercises in chronic pain,[33] other reviews find evidence supporting the benefits of relaxation,[34] particularly with children and adolescents.[35] In general, there is very good evidence supporting the efficacy of relaxation in reducing the frequency of and pain associated with chronic headache, with outcomes comparable to those obtained with pharmacological treatments.[36,37] Furthermore, moderate to large effect sizes have been demonstrated with relaxation in the treatment of chronic back pain.[34]

Goal Setting

Goal setting is typically initiated in the first therapy session and goals are individualized to the patient based on their baseline level of functioning. Often the first goal in CBT treatment pertains to the practice of relaxation because the first session typically includes both educational information about the gate control theory and then the rationale and demonstration of relaxation. In setting a goal, patients are guided in identifying realistic, attainable goals that are measurable. For example, an appropriate goal for the patient who has just been taught relaxation might be to practice for a set period (e.g., 15 minutes) once each day until the next treatment session. For the unusual patient who already meditates daily, the goal might focus on monitoring pain before, during, and after meditation. Or the goal might include practicing new relaxation strategies as an "experiment" to see if different types of relaxation have different effects on pain. As the patient becomes more accustomed to and adept in the behaviors that promote goal attainment and as their level of functioning improves, goals can gradually become more challenging. However, the difficulty level of a goal should not be increased until the patient has demonstrated an appropriate level of skill and/or proficiency in the attainment of previous goals regardless of their level of pain. The sense of accomplishment derived from achieving one's goals can be quite rewarding for many people, though the social reinforcement received from family members, friends, and health care providers can also be very helpful. Furthermore, engaging in similar goal setting activities with other patients that share the experience of chronic pain can be very effective in motivating patients and reinforcing their behavior. This may be one of the advantages of participating in a group multidisciplinary pain management intervention relative to individual treatment.

Pacing

Pacing refers to the method of finding a manageable and realistic or optimal pace when engaging in specific behaviors and/or activities in order to not exhaust or deplete one's self or precipitate or aggravate pain. Due to the nature of chronic pain, it is often difficult for patients to predict when pain will flare up or, conversely, when they will have a relatively pain-free day. As a result, many chronic pain sufferers exert themselves and are overly active on days when pain is low to manageable. This is in contrast to alternating periods of under-activity during periods of high intensity pain. Unfortunately, periods of over-activity can potentially precipitate and/or aggravate a pain episode. This is particularly the case in low back pain, osteoarthritis, and many cases of complex regional pain syndrome. The patient engages in an activity until the pain prevents them from continuing and they are consequently forced into a period of rest and potential analgesic use secondary to the pain. This frequently repeated pattern often results in feelings of frustration, distress, and demoralization. Not surprisingly, patients may become avoidant and engage in maladaptive forms of coping, which leads to further decreased activity and resulting physical deconditioning accompanied by a loss of flexibility and strength.[38] Often, periods of increased activity tend to become shorter while periods of inactivity become longer. Behavioral techniques that can help with these alternating cycles of over- and under-activity include goal setting and pacing.[39]

Through proper planning and prioritizing tasks by importance, patients will be able to find an optimal pace at which to engage in identified activities and maintain a consistent level of activity over time as compared to cycling between periods of over- and under-activity. Once patients identify a desired activity, they establish a baseline level or rate of that activity which they are able to maintain daily regardless of other circumstances. Once a baseline is established, a goal is set to slightly increase the activity and, initially, the difficulty level of the goal should be minimal so that it is attainable regardless of whether the patient is in pain or not. Thus, the increase in activity early in the process should be easily managed and is expected to have minimal impact on pain. During this process, it is important for the patient to maintain the activity despite the level of pain; this way, activities are not contingent upon the patient's level of pain and goals are set and achieved regardless of the patient's pain level. Proceeding in a stepwise and systematic fashion will increase the patient's activity level and improve their self confidence.

Distraction

Distraction procedures, one of the many cognitive coping skills often promoted and refined during CBT, focus attention away from pain, allowing for a filtering process where some information reaches conscious attention and other information (in this case, pain) is suppressed.[40] Techniques using mental imagery, counting or even virtual reality are often used to distract.[41,42] Attention diversion can produce analgesia in laboratory settings,[43] during medical procedures,[44] and in the context of ongoing chronic pain.[45] These procedures may increase pain tolerance and decrease perceived pain intensity, as pain ceases to be the focus of attention potentially due to competing demands on the attentional system and/or other physiological processes. While these adjunctive treatments have been shown to be effective, when the distraction stops, pain often returns as the central focus of awareness and may subsequently be accompanied by greater pain.[40,45]

Distraction techniques may work best when pain intensity is constant or increases slowly[46] and may be more difficult to apply when pain intensity is high and accompanied by high somatic awareness.[47] However, distraction may be an effective strategy when pain is less intense. Nurses often use distraction to help patients manage painful or distressing procedures. Distraction is a very promising analgesic for brief medical interventions such as wound debridement for burn patients,[48] dislocations from fractures,[49] and for venous cannulation pain, which is often necessary prior to more invasive procedures.[50] The widespread clinical utility of distraction is an inexpensive, simple to apply method for reducing acute pain during medical procedures that has no known side effects, and which can reduce distress and be of great benefit to chronic pain patients when practiced regularly.

Cognitive Restructuring

Cognitive restructuring illustrates the essence of cognitive therapy[6] in which patterns of dysfunctional or negative thinking that can precipitate feelings of emotional distress (e.g., anxiety, depression, anger), physiological arousal, and maladaptive behaviors are identified. Patients are taught to identify and subsequently replace distorted cognitions in order to change negative mood states, lower and regulate physiological arousal, and replace maladaptive behaviors with behaviors that are likely to be associated with or result in positive outcomes. Hence, adaptive coping is encouraged through realistic appraisal of events. The basic premise behind cognitive restructuring is that patients' emotions and behavior can be greatly influenced by their thoughts. If people can actively change their "self-talk" or what they say to themselves along with the mental images they bring to mind, then they can change the way they feel. An extensive literature indicates that the thoughts and interpretations that people have in response to pain significantly influence their experience of pain (e.g., see Chapters 7 and 21). When these thoughts are negative, they may exacerbate the overall experience of pain, thereby increasing pain-related suffering; conversely, balanced, rational, and realistic thoughts can serve to attenuate the pain experience and improve both psychological and physical function.

Cognitive restructuring is a vital component of chronic pain treatment. The first step in identifying distorted thinking involves developing awareness of these thoughts. Teaching the concept of automatic thoughts, which are the words and images that "automatically" pop into our heads throughout the day or when we are engaged in particular activities, lays the foundation for increasing awareness of negative thinking. It is then often helpful to illustrate for patients how thoughts can impact mood and behavior. One method of accomplishing this entails introducing the ABCD model, based on the work of Ellis[51] and Beck,[6] in which patients are taught to identify a precipitating event (A) when they notice that they are experiencing a negative mood (C). It is often challenging for many patients to distinguish the difference between thoughts (B) and feelings (C). Once a patient has identified thoughts, treatment focuses on identifying distorted thoughts (B) and accompanying maladaptive assumptions and beliefs (B) evoked by the event. Next, after identifying the negative thoughts and erroneous assumptions, several techniques are used to restructure or replace the distorted or irrational thoughts with more realistic and balanced thoughts. A commonly used approach is reality checking or hypothesis testing in which patients are taught to regard a distorted thought as a hypothesis (versus reality) that needs to be tested empirically. Patients are taught to challenge faulty thinking by examining the evidence supporting or refuting the negative thought. Following this, balanced and realistic thoughts that do not ignore the negative aspects of the situation but rather also include other aspects (i.e., neutral, positive) of the situation are developed in order to produce more balanced thinking (D) to replace the distorted thinking. Typically, these concepts are introduced in a therapy session and the patient is given a negative thought log to take home and use to identify precipitating events, distorted thoughts, emotional/behavioral consequences, evidence for and against their negative thoughts, and the resulting balanced thoughts generated to replace the negative thinking. The goal of cognitive restructuring is to recognize and modify negative thoughts in order to regulate emotional distress, physiological arousal, and/or maladaptive behavior.

Homework Adherence

Participation in homework assignments is one of the guiding principles inherent to CBT and has been repeatedly shown to have significant clinical importance in a variety of conditions.[52] While few studies examining the role of CBT homework in chronic pain populations exist, the use of homework in biofeedback treatment showed a trend toward greater improvement.[53] Homework facilitates the learning of new adaptive behaviors that can be generalized to the patient's natural environment. The more the patient practices the skills taught in treatment, the more proficient he or she becomes in successfully implementing these behaviors, which results in greater derived benefits. Successful implementation of the new adaptive behaviors reinforces the continued use of these skills for pain management. Consequently, it is crucial to emphasize to patients that homework is integral to their treatment success, because it facilitates the generalization and maintenance of these skills to situations outside the clinic setting. Many chronic pain patients take a passive approach to managing their pain, especially patients who seek care in tertiary pain care settings. As a result, it is important that homework assignments initially be a collaborative experience to help patients work toward taking responsibility for their pain management. Providing a rationale for homework, assigning specific (versus general) tasks, having a homework difficulty level that is reasonable and appropriate to the client, and reviewing homework completion and progress can help enhance patient compliance and improve long-term outcomes.[54] The reader is referred to a helpful resource for the practi-

tioner by Johnson and Kazantzis[54] that discusses obstacles to the use of homework in chronic pain populations and provides strategies to promote homework compliance and overcoming/problem solving obstacles.

Relapse Prevention, Developing a Maintenance Plan, and Managing Flare-Ups

As previously noted, any intervention involving a cognitive shift or behavior change requires substantial dedication and work on the part of the patient. Continued dedication to maintenance of behavior change can be quite difficult for a patient without the weekly guidance and support of the interventionist. However, an important aspect of CBT includes discussion of relapse prevention and plans for any difficulty in maintaining treatment gains. The goals of relapse prevention include working to anticipate potential triggers of pain exacerbation, mood deterioration, or loss of physical function, identifying obstacles to maintaining behavior change, and noting any high-risk situations which may prompt relapse, as well as developing a plan for unanticipated challenges. The basic relapse prevention model includes components of behavioral skills training, cognitive interventions, and lifestyle change.[55] Identification of challenging situations and events (flare-up, new pain episode, re-injury, stress, psychological strain, etc.) and problem solving approaches to help the patient get back on track is essential. Little empirical literature exists on the best way to approach relapse prevention in chronic pain patients,[56] though suggestions are offered and discussed in CBT manuals for pain (see Table 82.1). Patients are encouraged to set realistic expectations about treatment, realize that setbacks both during and after treatment are expected, and create opportunities to practice new skills. It is also useful to have the patient keep track of situations that have exacerbated pain in the past in order

TABLE 82.1

USEFUL BOOKS AND SELF-HELP WORKBOOKS FOR PAIN MANAGEMENT

Workbooks
Pain
Managing Pain before It Manages You—Revised Edition (Caudill, 2001)
Chronic Pain Control Workbook (Catalano & Hardin, 1997)
Cognitive Therapy for Chronic Pain: A Step-by-Step Guide (Thorn, 2004)
Living a Healthy Life with Chronic Conditions: Self-Management of Heart Disease, Arthritis, Diabetes, Asthma, Bronchitis, Emphysema & Others—2nd Edition (Lorig, Holman, Sobel, Laurent, González, & Minor, 2000)

Related topics
The Relaxation & Stress Reduction Workbook—5th Edition (Davis, McKay, & Eshelman, 2000)
Mind Over Mood: Change How You Feel by Changing the Way You Think (Greenberger & Padesky, 1995)

Books
Getting Off the Pain Roller Coaster: Psychological Aspects of Pain & Pain Management (Weiss & Weiss, 1995)
Taking Control of Your Headaches: How to Get the Treatment You Need—Revised Edition (Duckro, Richardson, & Marshall, 1999)

(*Adapted from* Buenaver LF, McGuire L, Haythornthwaite JA. Cognitive-Behavioral self-help for chronic pain. *J Clin Psychol* 2006 Nov;62[11]:1389–1396, with permission.)

to anticipate and effectively plan for those situations in the future. Brainstorming between the therapist and patient can facilitate better management and implementation of appropriate skills in future situations.

Although relapse rates following CBT for psychiatric conditions are quite low compared to pharmacological therapies,[57,130] the examination of maintenance programs and relapse rates has been relatively neglected in the literature on CBT for pain, an omission that was noted in the early 1990s[56] and has not been adequately addressed since. A very recent editorial[131] emphasized the dearth of information on this important topic, which has not received increased attention since the original calls for action. While treatment gains following CBT generally maintain over 6 and 12 months following the end of treatment[132] and even improve (although some decline), efficacy is also seen over long periods of follow-up.[133] In a recent and innovative posttreatment relapse study, Naylor and colleagues[121] developed and assessed the effects of a Therapeutic Interactive Voice Response (TIVR) system (an automated, telephone-based tool they created for maintenance enhancement) in chronic musculoskeletal pain patients. Following 11 weeks of group CBT, patients received either standard care or TIVR, which included components of daily self-monitoring, review of coping skills, behavioral rehearsal of coping skills, and personalized feedback messages based on the patient's daily reported pain. Compared to standard care following CBT, the TIVR group showed continued gains at 4 months and reported reduced typical pain level, catastrophizing, and increased physical functioning/activity.[121] This innovative approach to maintaining and even enhancing treatment gains shows tremendous promise for CBT interventions.

OUTCOMES AND PREDICTORS OF OUTCOMES

Outcomes

Hundreds of studies demonstrate the effectiveness of CBT[57] and several meta-analyses specifically support the efficacy of CBT for chronic pain. One of the earliest meta-analyses found that CBT interventions for chronic pain reduced pain intensity, improved coping and reduced behavioral expressions of pain, compared with other active treatments.[17] Other reviews summarize positive outcomes for specific pain conditions including arthritis,[58] migraine/chronic headache,[59] chronic musculoskeletal pain,[60] chronic cancer pain,[61] rheumatoid arthritis and osteoarthritis,[62] myofascial temporomandibular disorders,[63,64] chronic low back pain,[21] carpal tunnel syndrome pain,[65] and chronic pelvic pain.[66] CBT benefits patients with chronic fatigue syndrome, irritable bowel syndrome[67] and works in children.[68–70] The outcomes appear more variable in fibromyalgia.[71] In an interesting review, Bradley and colleagues[72] compared patients with a "well understood" chronic pain condition (RA, osteoarthritis) to those without a specific origin (fibromyalgia, chronic fatigue syndrome, irritable bowel syndrome), finding that CBT produced positive outcomes for all patients except those with fibromyalgia.

In a recent meta-analysis, Hoffman and colleagues[21] concluded that CBT for chronic low back pain produces dramatic improvements in pain (see section I) with additional benefits in pain-related interference, health-related quality of life, and depression. In another meta-analysis, CBT in arthritis patients was compared to a number of other treatment approaches (e.g., biofeedback, stress management, emotional disclosure, hypnosis, psychodynamic therapy) for improving outcomes related to arthritis pain.[58] This examination included 18 studies of CBT in arthritis patients and found that CBT produced a significant decrease in pain; however, the strongest findings were for quality of life related variables such as self-efficacy, mood, and pain coping.

Unfortunately, the lack of studies examining interventions other than CBT precluded these authors from making meaningful comparisons between the effectiveness of CBT to other treatments.[58]

New studies are now being published addressing the cortical changes that occur following cognitive–behavioral interventions. For example, imaging studies have revealed changes in specific brain areas following CBT for a variety of psychiatric disorders.[73] More relevantly, in a positron emission tomography (PET) study in irritable bowel syndrome patients, Lackner et al.[74] found changes in cortical–limbic region neural activity subserving hypervigilance and emotion regulation after a brief course of cognitive therapy. Several authors have noted that changes in brain activity following psychological interventions often parallel those of pharmacological studies.[73]

Predictors of Treatment Outcomes

Not all patients complete treatment,[75] and among those who do respond there are differences in the degree of benefit experienced.[18,76] Understanding the factors that predict positive (or negative) treatment outcomes is important for programs to help tailor approaches or match patients to the most appropriate treatment,[13,76] control costs by funding the treatments most likely to be effective, and improve mechanisms that contribute to treatment efficacy.[77] Most studies have not found an association between response to CBT and age, sex, race, education, and pain duration,[15,77] suggesting that all patients potentially may be helped by this therapy. Similarly, multidisciplinary treatment for chronic back pain reduces pain intensity and improves return to work regardless of medical background, medical diagnosis, and physical impairment.[33,78,79] However, specific outcomes vary widely across patients exposed to CBT, yielding effect sizes in the small to moderate range.[17,18] Patients who are emotionally distressed engage in a high degree of negative thinking about their pain, or lack faith in their ability to effectively manage their pain; they may experience less favorable outcomes. For example, depression has been associated with poorer treatment outcomes.[80–83] On the other hand, stronger belief in one's ability to control pain[15,84–86] and less catastrophizing or negative thinking in response to pain[15,87,88] are associated with favorable treatment outcomes. Research examining associations between physical/ sexual abuse history and pain-related treatment outcomes has been inconsistent, demonstrating both poor outcomes[89] and outcomes comparable to patients with no prior abuse history.[90]

In an interesting review article focused on back pain, McCracken and Turk[77] concluded that low expectations for returning to work, greater somatic focus, or greater perceived pain and disability predicted poorer outcomes and in some cases poor program compliance or early discharge from programs. More controlling, less organized, less cohesive, and less supportive family circumstances also were associated with less treatment benefit.[77] Secondary gain or when treatment has financial implications for the patient is a complicated concept that remains important to consider,[91] but a simplistic approach is clearly not validated.[92] The Minnesota Multiphasic Personality Inventory (MMPI) has frequently been used to predict who will benefit most from treatment; however, these studies also have mixed and confounding conclusions.[93]

Readiness to Change

The Transtheoretical Model of Behavior Change integrates theoretical models to explain how people may be more or less successful in treatments focusing on behavior change. One of the key constructs in this model, stage of change, speaks to the "readiness" of a person to modify a certain problem behavior. Five stages include (1) precontemplation: the person has no intention of making a behavioral change in the near future; (2) contemplation: the person thinks about the possibility of making a change, but has not yet fully committed to action; (3) preparation: the person is considering making a change soon (within a month); (4) action: the person is actively working on changing behavior and modifying their environment to help implement change; and (5) maintenance: the person is working to maintain changes and using relapse prevention. These stages are thought to be important in treatment settings, as practitioners may be more successful if they tailor their intervention to the prominent stage of a given patient (thus helping catalyze movement and aiding the patient in progressing from one stage to the next). This model has been applied to pain and particularly the patient's readiness to adopt self-management therapies.[94] The Pain Stages of Change Questionnaire (PSOCQ) was developed to assess readiness to change in pain patients, which assesses both stage of readiness and acceptance of being personally responsible for pain control.[94] The validity[94,95] and clinical utility of the PSOCQ have been demonstrated.[75,96,97] The PSOCQ has been shown to predict treatment dropout,[75,96] and positive increases in attitudes regarding self-management as well as predict subsequent improvements in outcomes.[97] The interested reader is referred to reviews of this literature.[98,99] Noting limitations to the PSOCQ, the Multidimensional Pain Readiness to Change Questionnaire (MPRCQ[100]), and a more recent revised version, the MPRCQ2,[101] was developed to examine readiness to change a wider range of behaviors in multidisciplinary chronic pain management settings. These questionnaires have also been adapted for specific pain conditions, including osteoarthritis[102] and fibromyalgia (in a Dutch population[103]).

The assessment of these stages in pain patients has paved the way for additional research on motivating patients to engage in treatment and improving outcomes by tailoring treatment to the patient's level of readiness. Motivating pain patients in the early stages of readiness (precontemplation, contemplation) can be quite challenging. Jensen and colleagues[22] set forth a motivational model for pain self-management and others have found that motivation and adherence mediate the relationship between readiness to change and goal attainment.[104] Motivational interventions are discussed in detail in Chapter 87.

ALTERNATIVE APPROACHES TO TRADITIONAL CBT

Self-Help

Recent developments in technology, as well as an interest in the broader dissemination of CBT treatments, have encouraged the use of alternative modes of delivering treatment. Self-help interventions organized via group formats, workbooks, books, audiotapes, minimal contact formats, and telephone- and Internet-based delivery systems have been found to reduce pain, pain-related disability, depression, and anxiety in arthritis, low back pain, headache, and temporomandibular joint disorder.[105] Much self-help is provided through groups, and the use of lay leaders to facilitate such support/educational groups has contributed to the widespread application of the *Arthritis Self Management Program* (ASMP) through the Arthritis Foundation.[106] This program provides the strongest outcome data on the benefits of skill development as compared to disease education in order to enhance self-management. Self-management incorporates techniques designed to increase patients' confidence and skills in daily management of their arthritis. The ASMP has been found to be cost efficient in reducing pain and improving patient functioning in such areas as exercise, anxiety, depression, decision-making, and problem-solving.[106] Some of the latest work by Lorig and her colleagues[107] extends the use of written self help materials

to include a tailored, written intervention based on the ASMP. Following completion of a one-page assessment, rheumatoid arthritis and osteoarthritis patients receive a tailored summary report with recommendations for developing a personal plan, as well as a variety of supportive materials including *The Arthritis Helpbook* and relaxation tapes. Quarterly written contacts included personalized feedback, encouragement about changes made, and recommendations for further changes. Participants receiving this personalized intervention reported increased self-efficacy and reductions in physician visits as well as reductions in global disease severity ratings. Compared to the ASMP, these participants also reported significant reductions in disability and greater increases in self-efficacy.[107] Overall, such self-help programs appear to achieve reductions in pain and disability primarily through increases in self-efficacy, and these changes can maintain over long periods.

The benefits of self-help may vary according to the structure of the program or the pain condition. Four group sessions of self-management led by trained laypersons supplemented with an educational book and video helped patients with chronic low back pain reduce worry or concern about back pain, increase confidence in self-care, and lower disability scores up to 12 months posttreatment.[108] On the other hand, when support groups are not well attended or sessions are spread over fairly long periods, little differential benefit of lay- or professionally-led support groups over treatment as usual has been observed.[109] Self-help has less clear benefits for patients suffering from irritable bowel syndrome (IBS), where self help was no better than a waiting list control group in reducing gastrointestinal symptoms and distress and both had less impact than CBT.[110] Even without symptom reduction, however, there is some indication that a comprehensive self-help guidebook can reduce IBS patient costs by as much as 40%.[111]

Limitations to self-help techniques are, as of yet, largely unknown, but include the potential for greater rates of attrition. Studies assessing the efficacy of self-help techniques often use highly controlled research settings for investigating treatments, and are selective in obtaining participant groups; these factors may further limit the generalizability to patients who are more medically or psychologically/psychiatrically complicated.[105] However, it appears clear that self-help may be particularly useful for patients with limited resources, who travel a long distance for specialty care, or are resistant to seeking mental health care. Thus, the development of brief, self-help-oriented interventions have the potential to vastly increase the number of patients who can successfully access and benefit from psychological interventions. Self-help workbooks for chronic pain are currently available, although none has been empirically examined to our knowledge, although the workbook by Lorig and her colleagues listed in Table 82.1 is based on their extensive research using similar materials. For patients seeking self-help, the workbooks and/or books listed in Table 82.1 can be recommended.

Home-Based and Minimal Contact CBT Treatments

The headache literature has a long history of demonstrating the cost-efficiency of minimal contact CBT interventions for managing chronic tension and migraine headache. An early meta-analysis concluded that home-based behavioral treatment for headache sufferers yields equivalent or superior benefits when compared to clinic-based treatments.[112] In minimal-contact therapy (MCT), CBT and self-management skills are introduced in the clinic typically by a specially trained professional, and training and practice occur primarily at home using written materials and audiotapes. Meta-analyses of the self-help literature suggest that some degree of therapist contact may have incremental benefits,[113] and in MCT the therapist contact can be delivered by diverse methods, including infrequent meetings, telephone calls, and/or mailings and use of electronic contacts such as electronic mail. Issues of confidentiality need to be discussed and ground rules established before using electronic communication strategies. MCT may be more affordable for many patients seeking care and have been shown to be more cost-effective in the treatment of headaches.[114] MCT gains can be equally well maintained as intensive individual protocols.[115]

MCT has been examined in greatest detail within the headache and facial pain literatures. A meta-analysis of headache clinical trials indicated that home-based behavioral treatment yields treatment effects that are equivalent or superior to clinic-based treatments.[112] As a viable, cost-effective alternative for many chronic headache sufferers, minimal contact interventions for headache average a five-fold increment in cost-effectiveness.[112] The use of MCT in dental/facial pain is limited to two studies, both of which provide encouraging results. Following two group sessions supplemented with written materials and individualized therapist feedback temporomandibular joint disorder (TMD) patients reported reduced pain and interference in daily activities as compared to usual care.[116] Using MCT to teach principles of habit reversal, a small group of 10 TMD patients reported reductions in pain, pain interference, and life stress that were maintained 8 months posttreatment.[117]

The extension of home-based interventions to Web-based designs raises the potential for improving pain and other outcomes while being cost/time effective and broadly dispersed. Increasingly, CBT interventions are enhanced through use of advanced communication technology in order to expand access and reduce costs. For example, telephone psychotherapy has been successfully used as a supplement to antidepressant treatment in primary care[118] and is being tested for the treatment of depression in patients with multiple sclerosis.[119] Automated telephone contact that includes personalized messages enhances outcomes following group CBT,[120] possibly due to encouraging consistent use of skills or enhancing self-monitoring.[121] Work on Internet-based cognitive behavioral self-help treatment for pain management is just developing and early studies show good outcomes despite high rates of attrition.[122] The addition of telephone support does not seem to enhance outcomes,[123] but may substantially reduce dropout.[124]

Spousal/Caregiver Involvement in Treatment

The involvement of family members in CBT can be critical in helping the patient with chronic pain make substantial and enduring changes. A recent meta-analysis documents the beneficial impact of family involvement in CBT treatments for chronic illness, concluding that the involvement of family members in psychosocial treatment increased treatment effects on depression and, in some cases, reduced mortality.[125] While little research has focused on spousal/caregiver involvement in CBT for pain, there are undoubtedly bidirectional interactions between intractable pain and the psychosocial environment/familial relationships. For example, a strong concordance between the patient's perceived pain level and the spouse's rating of that pain may lead to improved outcomes.[126] Keefe and colleagues have extensively studied patient and caregiver interactions as well as novel interventions involving a spouse or other caregiver in treatment.[13] Spouse-assisted coping skills training shows a trend to reduce pain, pain behaviors, and psychological disability when compared to individualized coping skills training,[127] and these gains are generally maintained at 6 and 12 months.[128] The addition of exercise to spouse-assisted coping skills training improves physical fitness, strength, pain coping, and self-efficacy.[129] Keefe and colleagues[129] interpret these caregiver-assisted interventions as shaping the social context that influences pain and further suggest that the most appropriate patients for these interventions may

be those who prefer a "communal style of coping" with pain, whereas those with a poor relationship or communication skills may benefit less from these treatments.[13]

NEW DIRECTIONS AND CONCLUSIONS

Prevention and/or Early Intervention

A significant body of literature documents the efficacy of CBT in the treatment of a wide range of chronically painful conditions. CBT reduces pain and improves pain-related psychological and physical function both alone and as an adjunct to other treatments. While potentially any patient can benefit from CBT, effect sizes are moderate at best and many people do not show substantial improvement. Continued research needs to identify treatment nonresponders and how to best address their health care needs. Most often, CBT is a treatment that is offered late in the course of chronic pain, often after the patient has experienced multiple treatment failures and continues to experience substantial pain, pain-related disability, and distress. As our knowledge of risk factors increases, a logical direction for clinical care and research is to identify which patients may benefit most from early CBT interventions. By capturing people early in their transition from acute to chronic pain, it may be possible to reduce or even stop the development of a clinical pain condition in part through the use of prevention strategies. An excellent example of this potential is provided by a study of CBT for patients with rheumatoid arthritis for less than 2 years.[134] As compared to medical management, the CBT group showed immediate reductions in depressive symptoms that sustained for 18 months, when additional improvements in disability and anxiety were also observed. Thus, CBT effectively altered the 18-month course of early rheumatoid arthritis. Linton found that a CBT group intervention prevented long-term sick leave and reduced health care use in at-risk people with subacute or recurrent spine pain.[135] A similar study with neck and back pain community residents with little disability showed similar positive outcomes in the CBT group, particularly with long-term sick leave.[136] Of note, these studies by Linton and his colleagues recruited patients from the community and early in the pain trajectory. Since studies of irritable bowel,[137] fibromyalgia,[138] and headache[139] indicate substantial differences in personality, mood, and psychiatric comorbidity between patients and community residing nonpatients, the recruitment processes used in existing studies of CBT likely influenced the strength of findings (i.e., small to moderate effect sizes). Prevention holds the potential to reduce the skyrocketing costs of health care and the significant suffering and disability associated with chronic pain. The cognitive behavioral conceptualization of chronic pain suggests that capturing patients at the primary care level, when a patient enters the health care system, may provide the best opportunity to improve coping skills and correct misperceptions about pain that contribute to persistent pain and pain-related disability.

Tailoring Treatment

Tailored treatment or treatment matching involves determining *a priori* which patients are most likely to benefit from a particular treatment. Although the heterogeneity of patient groups likely accounts for at least some of the limitations of CBT,[76] few studies have systematically evaluated treatment tailoring or matching prospectively. One of the more promising approaches to treatment tailoring utilizes profiles derived from the Multidimensional Pain Inventory,[140,141] which has been shown to predict differential response to CBT in some studies.[76]

The challenges of providing these specialized services in the context of escalating medical costs suggest a need to develop a more sophisticated, stepped care approach to providing CBT interventions, especially if these interventions are to be made available early in the transition from acute to chronic pain. A stepped care approach has been proposed for the management of back pain,[142] which might have broad applicability to many types of pain. Level 1 care recommends self-help via groups, workbooks, or the Internet; Level 2 care provides minimal contact CBT with a trained specialist; and Level 3 care provides intensive individual or group CBT with a trained specialist. Steps 2 and 3 are generally beyond the scope of current medical practice, but could be integrated into physical therapy or case management interventions.[142]

CONCLUSIONS

Chronic pain results from a complex interaction of biological, psychological, and social variables, and responses to pain are shaped not only by the pathophysiology of the underlying disease, but also by their inherent cultural and psychosocial contexts. CBT is an effective treatment for many patients who experience chronic pain, producing reductions in pain and pain-related interference, improvements in mood and coping, and reductions in negative beliefs and cognitions such as catastrophizing. Since we know so little about the characteristics of nonresponders and continue to face challenges in the health care system around access to these specialized services, studies that identify patient characteristics that enable treatment matching or test a stepped care approach to treatment are warranted. Whether the development of the next generation of CBT interventions and established exposure-based treatments (see Chapter 83) are differentially effective for subtypes of patients will need to be determined, as will new avenues for treating CBT nonresponders.

References

1. Fordyce WE, Fowler RS Jr, Lehmann JF, et al. Some implications of learning in problems of chronic pain. J Chronic Dis 1968;21(3):179–190.
2. Fordyce WE, Fowler RS, DeLateur B. An application of behavior modification technique to a problem of chronic pain. Behav Res Ther 1968;6(1):105–107.
3. Beecher HK. Pain in men wounded in battle. Ann Surg 1946;123(1):96–105.
4. Melzack R, Wall PD. Pain mechanisms: a new theory. Science 1965;150(699):971–979.
5. Ellis A. Reason and Emotion in Psychotherapy. Oxford, England: Lyle Stuart, 1962.
6. Beck AT. Cognitive Therapy and the Emotional Disorders. Oxford, England: International Universities Press, 1976.
7. Beck A, Rush AJ, Shaw BF, et al. Cognitive Therapy of Depression. New York: Guilford Press, 1979.
8. Turk DC, Meichenbaum D, Genest M. Pain and Behavioral Medicine: A Cognitive-Behavioral Perspective. New York: Guilford Press, 1983.
9. Turner JA, Chapman CR. Psychological interventions for chronic pain: a critical review. I. Relaxation training and biofeedback. Pain 1982;12(1):1–21.
10. Turner JA, Chapman CR. Psychological interventions for chronic pain: a critical review. II. Operant conditioning, hypnosis, and cognitive-behavioral therapy. Pain 1982;12(1):23–46.
11. Jensen MP, Turner JA, Romano JM, et al. Coping with chronic pain: a critical review of the literature. Pain 1991;47(3):249–283.
12. Gatchel RJ, Peng YB, Peters ML, et al. The biopsychosocial approach to chronic pain: Scientific advances and future directions. Psychol Bull 2007;133(4):581–624.
13. Keefe FJ, Rumble ME, Scipio CD, et al. Psychological aspects of persistent pain: current state of the science. J Pain 2004;5(4):195–211.
14. Burns JW, Kubilus A, Bruehl S, et al. Do changes in cognitive factors influence outcome following multidisciplinary treatment for chronic pain? A cross-lagged panel analysis. J Consult Clin Psychol 2003 Feb;71(1):81–91.
15. Turner JA, Holtzman S, Mancl L. Mediators, moderators, and predictors of therapeutic change in cognitive-behavioral therapy for chronic pain. Pain 2007;127(3):276–286.
16. Astin JA, Beckner W, Soeken K, et al. Psychological interventions for rheumatoid arthritis: a meta-analysis of randomized controlled trials. Arthritis Rheum 2002;47(3):291–302.
17. Morley S, Eccleston C, Williams A. Systematic review and meta-analysis of randomized controlled trials of cognitive behaviour therapy and behaviour therapy for chronic pain in adults, excluding headache. Pain 1999;80(1–2):1–13.
18. Vlaeyen JW, Morley S. Cognitive-behavioral treatments for chronic pain: what works for whom? Clin J Pain 2005;21(1):1–8.
19. Okifuji A, Ackerlind S. Behavioral medicine approaches to pain. Anesthesiology Clin 2007 Dec;25(4):709–719.
20. Turk DC, Okifuji A. Psychological factors in chronic pain: evolution and revolution. J Consult Clin Psychol 2002;70(3):678–690.
21. Hoffman BM, Papas RK, Chatkoff DK, et al. Meta-analysis of psychological interventions for chronic low back pain. Health Psychol 2007;26(1):1–9.
22. Jensen MP, Nielson WR, Kerns RD. Toward a motivational model of pain self-management. J Pain 2003;4(9):477–492.
23. Sudak DM, Beck JS, Wright J. Cognitive behavioral therapy: a blueprint for attaining and assessing psychiatry resident competency. Acad Psychiatry 2003;27(3):154–159.
24. Yates SL, Morley S, Eccleston C, et al. A scale for rating the quality of psychological trials for pain. Pain 2005;117(3):314–325.
25. Averill JR. Personal control over aversive stimuli and its relationship to stress. Psychol Bull 1973;80(4):286–303.
26. Suls J, Wan CK. Effects of sensory and procedural information on coping with stressful medical procedures and pain: a meta-analysis. J Consult Clin Psychol 1989;57(3):372–379.
27. Foster G, Taylor SJ, Eldridge SE, et al. Self-management education programmes by lay leaders for people with chronic conditions. Cochrane Database Syst Rev 2007;(4):CD005108.
28. Melzack R, Casey KL. Sensory, motivational, and central control determinants of pain: a new conceptual model. In: Kenshalo DR, ed. The Skin Senses Springfield, IL: Charles C Thomas, 1968;423–443.
29. Hoffman JW, Benson H, Arns PA, et al. Reduced sympathetic nervous system responsivity associated with the relaxation response. Science 1982;215:190–192.
30. Bernstein DA, Borkovec TD. Progressive relaxation training: a manual for the helping professions. Champaign, IL: Research Press, 1973.
31. Bernstein DA, Carlson CR, Schmidt JE. Progressive relaxation: abbreviated methods. In: Lehrer PM, Woolfolk RL, Sime WE, eds. Principles and Practice of Stress Management. 3rd ed. New York, NY: Guilford Press, 2007;88–122.
32. Orlando B, Manfredini D, Salvetti G, et al. Evaluation of the effectiveness of biobehavioral therapy in the treatment of temporomandibular disorders: a literature review. Behav Med 2007;33(3):101–118.
33. McQuay HJ, Moore RA, Eccleston C, et al. Systematic review of outpatient services for chronic pain control. Health Technol Assess 1997;1(6):i–iv, 1–135.
34. Ostelo RW, van Tulder MW, Vlaeyen JW, et al. Behavioural treatment for chronic low-back pain. Cochrane Database Syst Rev 2005;(1):CD002014.
35. Eccleston C, Yorke L, Morley S, et al. Psychological therapies for the management of chronic and recurrent pain in children and adolescents. Cochrane Database Syst Rev 2003;(1):CD003968.
36. Holroyd KA, Drew JB. Behavioral approaches to the treatment of migraine. Semin Neurol 2006;26(2):199–207.
37. Andrasik F. What does the evidence show? Efficacy of behavioural treatments for recurrent headaches in adults. Neurol Sci 2007;28(0):S70–S77.
38. Leeuw M, Goossens MI, Linton S, et al. The fear-avoidance model of musculoskeletal pain: current state of scientific evidence. J Behav Med 2007;30(1):77–94.
39. Kole-Snijders AM, Vlaeyen JW, Goossens ME, et al. Chronic low-back pain: what does cognitive coping skills training add to operant behavioral treatment? Results of a randomized clinical trial. J Consult Clin Psychol 1999 Dec;67(6):931–944.
40. Johnson MH. How does distraction work in the management of pain? Curr Pain Headache Rep 2005;9(2):90–95.
41. Hoffman HG, Patterson DR, Carrougher GJ, et al. Effectiveness of virtual reality-based pain control with multiple treatments. Clin J Pain 2001;17(3):229–235.
42. Wismeijer AA, Vingerhoets AJ. The use of virtual reality and audiovisual eyeglass systems as adjunct analgesic techniques: a review of the literature. Ann Behav Med 2005;30(3):268–278.
43. McCaul KD, Malott JM. Distraction and coping with pain. Psychol Bull 1984;95(3):516–533.
44. Uman LS, Chambers CT, McGrath PJ, et al. A systematic review of randomized controlled trials examining psychological interventions for needle-related procedural pain and distress in children and adolescents: an abbreviated Cochrane Review. J Pediatr Psychol 2008;33(8):842–854.
45. Anderson KO, Cohen MZ, Mendoza TR, et al. Brief cognitive-behavioral audiotape interventions for cancer-related pain: immediate but not long-term effectiveness. Cancer 2006;107(1):207–214.
46. Melzack R, Guite S, Gonshor A. Relief of dental pain by ice massage of the hand. Can Med Assoc J 1980;122(2):189–191.
47. Eccleston C, Crombez G, Aldrich S, et al. Attention and somatic awareness in chronic pain. Pain 1997;72(1–2):209–215.
48. Hoffman HG, Patterson DR, Seibel E, et al. Virtual reality pain control during burn wound debridement in the hydrotank. Clin J Pain 2008;24(4):299–304.
49. Ruland RT, Hogan CJ, Cannon DL, et al. Use of dynamic distraction external fixation for unstable fracture-dislocations of the proximal interphalangeal joint. J Hand Surg [Am] 2008;33(1):19–25.

50. Agarwal A, Yadav G, Gupta D, et al. The role of a flash of light for attenuation of venous cannulation pain: a prospective, randomized, placebo-controlled study. *Anesth Analg* 2008;106(3):814–816.

51. Ellis A. *Rational-Emotive Therapy and Cognitive Behavior Therapy* New York: Springer, 1984.

52. Kazantzis N, Deane FP, Ronan KR. Homework assignments in cognitive and behavioral therapy: a meta-analysis. *Clin Psychol: Sci Pract* 2000;7(2): 189–202.

53. Blanchard EB, Nicholson NL, Radnitz CL, et al. The role of home practice in thermal biofeedback. *J Consult Clin Psychol* 1991;59(4):507–512.

54. Johnson MH, Kazantzis N. Cognitive behavioral therapy for chronic pain: strategies for the successful use of homework assignments. *J Ration Emo Cog Behav Ther* 2004 Sep;22(3):189–218.

55. Marlatt GA. Relapse prevention: theoretical rationale and overview of the model. In: Marlatt GA, Gordon JR, eds. *Relapse Prevention.* New York: Guilford Press; 1985;3–70.

56. Turk DC, Rudy TE. Neglected topics in the treatment of chronic pain patients—relapse, noncompliance, and adherence enhancement. *Pain* 1991; 44(1):5–28.

57. Butler AC, Chapman JE, Forman EM, et al. The empirical status of cognitive-behavioral therapy: a review of meta-analyses. *Clin Psychol Rev* 2006;26(1): 17–31.

58. Dixon KE, Keefe FJ, Scipio CD, et al. Psychological interventions for arthritis pain management in adults: a meta-analysis. *Health Psychol* 2007;26(3): 241–250.

59. Lake AE 3rd. Behavioral and nonpharmacologic treatments of headache. *Med Clin North Am* 2001;85(4):1055–1075.

60. Haigh R, Clarke AK. Effectiveness of rehabilitation for spinal pain. *Clin Rehabil* 1999;13(suppl 1):63–81.

61. Thomas EM, Weiss SM. Nonpharmacological interventions with chronic cancer pain in adults. *Cancer Control* 2000;7(2):157–164.

62. Bradley LA, McKendree-Smith NL. Central nervous system mechanisms of pain in fibromyalgia and other musculoskeletal disorders: behavioral and psychologic treatment approaches. *Curr Opin Rheumatol* 2002;14(1):45–51.

63. Turner JA, Mancl L, Aaron LA. Brief cognitive-behavioral therapy for temporomandibular disorder pain: Effects on daily electronic outcome and process measures. *Pain* 2005;117(3):377–387.

64. Sherman JJ, Turk DC. Nonpharmacologic approaches to the management of myofascial temporomandibular disorders. *Curr Pain Headache Rep* 2001; 5(5):421–431.

65. Feuerstein M, Burrell LM, Miller VI, et al. Clinical management of carpal tunnel syndrome: a 12-year review of outcomes. *Am J Ind Med* 1999;35(3): 232–245.

66. Reiter RC. Evidence-based management of chronic pelvic pain. *Clin Obstet Gynecol* 1998;41(2):422–435.

67. Kroenke K, Swindle R. Cognitive-behavioral therapy for somatization and symptom syndromes: a critical review of controlled clinical trials. *Psychother Psychosom* 2000;69(4):205–215.

68. Chen E, Joseph MH, Zeltzer LK. Behavioral and cognitive interventions in the treatment of pain in children. *Pediatr Clin North Am* 2000;47(3):513–525.

69. Christie D, Wilson C. CBT in paediatric and adolescent health settings: a review of practice-based evidence. *Pediatr Rehabil* 2005;8(4):241–247.

70. Eccleston C, Morley S, Williams A, et al. Systematic review of randomised controlled trials of psychological therapy for chronic pain in children and adolescents, with a subset meta-analysis of pain relief. *Pain* 2002;99(1–2): 157.

71. Bennett R, Nelson D. Cognitive behavioral therapy for fibromyalgia. *Nat Clin Pract Rheumatol* 2006;2(8):416–424.

72. Bradley LA, McKendree-Smith NL, Cianfrini LR. Cognitive-behavioral therapy interventions for pain associated with chronic illnesses. *Semin Pain Med* 2003:1:44–54.

73. Roffman JL, Marci CD, Glick DM, et al. Neuroimaging and the functional neuroanatomy of psychotherapy. *Psychol Med* 2005;35(10):1385–1398.

74. Lackner JM, Lou CM, Mertz HR, et al. Cognitive therapy for irritable bowel syndrome is associated with reduced limbic activity, GI symptoms, and anxiety. *Behav Res Ther* 2006;44(5):621–638.

75. Kerns RD, Rosenberg R. Predicting responses to self-management treatments for chronic pain: application of the pain stages of change model. *Pain* 2000; 84(1):49–55.

76. Turk DC. The potential of treatment matching for subgroups of patients with chronic pain: lumping versus splitting. *Clin J Pain* 2005;21(1):44–55.

77. McCracken LM, Turk DC. Behavioral and cognitive-behavioral treatment for chronic pain: outcome, predictors of outcome, and treatment process. *Spine* 2002;27(22):2564–2573.

78. Flor H, Fydrich T, Turk DC. Efficacy of multidisciplinary pain treatment centers: a meta-analytic review. *Pain* 1992;49(2):221–230.

79. Gatchel RJ, Okifuji A. Evidence-based scientific data documenting the treatment and cost-effectiveness of comprehensive pain programs for chronic nonmalignant pain. *J Pain* 2006;7(11):779–793.

80. Gatchel RJ, Gardea MA. Psychosocial issues: their importance in predicting disability, response to treatment, and search for compensation. *Neurol Clin* 1999;17(1):149–166.

81. Feuerstein M, Beattie P. Biobehavioral factors affecting pain and disability in low back pain: mechanisms and assessment. *Phys Ther* 1995;75(4):267–280.

82. Hansen JS, Bendtsen L, Jensen R. Predictors of treatment outcome in headache patients with the Millon Clinical Multiaxial Inventory III (MCMI-III). *J Headache Pain* 2007;8(1):28–34.

83. Vowles KE, Gross RT, Sorrell JT. Predicting work status following interdisciplinary treatment for chronic pain. *Eur J Pain* 2004;8(4):351–358.

84. Jensen MP, Turner JA, Romano JM. Changes after multidisciplinary pain treatment in patient pain beliefs and coping are associated with concurrent changes in patient functioning. *Pain* 2007;131(1–2):38–47.

85. Harkapaa K, Jarvikoski A, Mellin G, et al. Health locus of control beliefs and psychological distress as predictors for treatment outcome in low-back pain patients: results of a 3-month follow-up of a controlled intervention study. *Pain* 1991;46(1):35–41.

86. Spinhoven P, Linssen AC. Behavioral treatment of chronic low back pain. I. Relation of coping strategy use to outcome. *Pain* 1991;45(1):29–34.

87. Sullivan MJ, Thorn B, Haythornthwaite JA, et al. Theoretical perspectives on the relation between catastrophizing and pain. *Clin J Pain* 2001;17(1):52–64.

88. Tota-Faucette ME, Gil KM, Williams DA, et al. Predictors of response to pain management treatment. The role of family environment and changes in cognitive processes. *Clin J Pain* 1993;9(2):115–123.

89. McMahon MJ, Gatchel RJ, Polatin PB, et al. Early childhood abuse in chronic spinal disorder patients: a major barrier to treatment success. *Spine* 1997; 22(20):2408–2415.

90. Bailey BE, Freedenfeld RN, Kiser RS, et al. Lifetime physical and sexual abuse in chronic pain patients: psychosocial correlates and treatment outcomes. *Disabil Rehabil* 2003;25(7):331–342.

91. Fishbain DA, Rosomoff HL, Cutler RB, et al. Secondary gain concept: a review of the scientific evidence. *Clin J Pain* 1995;11(1):6–21.

92. Fishbain DA, Cutler RB, Rosomoff HL, et al. Is there a relationship between nonorganic physical findings (Waddell signs) and secondary gain/malingering? *Clin J Pain* 2004;20(6):399–408.

93. Bradley LA, McKendree-Smith NL. Assessment of psychological status using interviews and self-report instruments. In: Turk DC, Melzack R, eds. *Handbook of Pain Assessment.* 2nd ed. New York: Guilford; 2001;292–319.

94. Kerns RD, Rosenberg R, Jamison RN, et al. Readiness to adopt a self-management approach to chronic pain: the Pain Stages of Change Questionnaire (PSOCQ). *Pain* 1997;72(1–2):227–234.

95. Jensen MP, Nielson WR, Romano JM, et al. Further evaluation of the pain stages of change questionnaire: is the transtheoretical model of change useful for patients with chronic pain? *Pain* 2000;86(3):255–264.

96. Biller N, Arnstein P, Caudill MA, et al. Predicting completion of a cognitive-behavioral pain management program by initial measures of a chronic pain patient's readiness for change. *Clin J Pain* 2000;16(4):352–359.

97. Glenn B, Burns JW. Pain self-management in the process and outcome of multidisciplinary treatment of chronic pain: evaluation of a stage of change model. *J Behav Med* 2003;26(5):417–433.

98. Kerns RD, Habib S. A critical review of the pain readiness to change model. *J Pain* 2004;5(7):357–367.

99. Dijkstra A. The validity of the stages of change model in the adoption of the self-management approach in chronic pain. *Clin J Pain* 2005;21(1):27–37.

100. Nielson WR, Jensen MP, Kerns RD. Initial development and validation of a multidimensional pain readiness to change questionnaire. *J Pain* 2003;4(3): 148–158.

101. Nielson WR, Jensen MP, Ehde DM, et al. Further development of the Multidimensional Pain Readiness to Change Questionnaire: The MPRCQ2. *J Pain* 2008;9(6):552–565.

102. Heuts PH, de Bie R, Drietelaar M, et al. Self-management in osteoarthritis of hip or knee: a randomized clinical trial in a primary healthcare setting. *J Rheumatol* 2005;32(3):543–549.

103. Dijkstra A, Vlaeyen JW, Rijnen H, et al. Readiness to adopt the self-management approach to cope with chronic pain in fibromyalgic patients. *Pain* 2001; 90(1–2):37–45.

104. Heapy A, Otis J, Marcus KS, et al. Intersession coping skill practice mediates the relationship between readiness for self-management treatment and goal accomplishment. *Pain* 2005;118(3):360–368.

105. Buenaver LF, McGuire L, Haythornthwaite JA. Cognitive-behavioral self-help for chronic pain. *J Clin Psychol* 2006;62(11):1389–1396.

106. Lorig K, Holman H. Arthritis self-management studies: A twelve-year review. *Health Educ Q* 1993;20(1):17–28.

107. Lorig KR, Ritter PL, Laurent DD, et al. Long-term randomized controlled trials of tailored-print and small-group arthritis self-management interventions. *Med Care* 2004;42(4):346–354.

108. Von Korff M, Moore JE, Lorig K, et al. A randomized trial of a lay person-led self-management group intervention for back pain patients in primary care. *Spine* 1998;23(23):2608–2615.

109. Linton SJ, Hellsing AL, Larsson I. Bridging the gap: support groups do not enhance long-term outcome in chronic back pain. *Clin J Pain* 1997;13(3): 221–228.

110. Payne A, Blanchard EB. A controlled comparison of cognitive therapy and self-help support groups in the treatment of irritable bowel syndrome. *J Consult Clin Psychol* 1995;63(5):779–786.

111. Robinson A, Lee V, Kennedy A, et al. A randomised controlled trial of self-help interventions in patients with a primary care diagnosis of IBS. *Gut* 2006.

112. Haddock CK, Rowan AB, Andrasik F, et al. Home-based behavioral treatments for chronic benign headache: a meta-analysis of controlled trials. *Cephalalgia* 1997;17(2):113–118.

113. Gould RA, Clum GA. A meta-analysis of self-help treatment approaches. *Clin Psychol Rev* 1993;13:169–186.

114. Rowan AB, Andrasik F. Efficacy and cost-effectiveness of minimal therapist contact treatments of chronic headaches: a review. *Behav Ther* 1996;27: 207–234.

115. Blanchard EB, Appelbaum KA, Guarnieri P, et al. Two studies of the long-term follow-up of minimal therapist contact treatments of vascular and tension headache. *J Consult Clin Psychol* 1988;56(3):427–432.

116. Dworkin SF, Turner JA, Wilson L, et al. Brief group cognitive-behavioral intervention for temporomandibular disorders. *Pain* 1994;59(2):175–187.

117. Townsend D, Nicholson RA, Buenaver L, et al. Use of a habit reversal treatment for temporomandibular pain in a minimal therapist contact format. *J Behav Ther Exp Psychiatry* 2001;32(4):221–239.

118. Simon GE, Ludman EJ, Tutty S, et al. Telephone psychotherapy and telephone care management for primary care patients starting antidepressant treatment: a randomized controlled trial. *JAMA* 2004;292(8):935–942.

119. Mohr DC, Burke H, Beckner V, et al. A preliminary report on a skills-based telephone-administered peer support programme for patients with multiple sclerosis. *Mult Scler* 2005;11(2):222–226.

120. Naylor MR, Helzer JE, Naud S, et al. Automated telephone as an adjunct for the treatment of chronic pain: a pilot study. *J Pain* 2002;3(6):429–438.

121. Naylor MR, Keefe FJ, Brigidi B, et al. Therapeutic interactive voice response for chronic pain reduction and relapse prevention. *Pain* 2008;134(3): 335–345.

122. Strom L, Pettersson R, Andersson G. A controlled trial of self-help treatment of recurrent headache conducted via the Internet. *J Consult Clin Psychol* 2000; 68(4):722–727.

123. Andersson G, Lundstrom P, Strom L. Internet-based treatment of headache: does telephone contact add anything? *Headache* 2003;43(4):353–361.

124. Buhrman M, Faltenhag S, Strom L, et al. Controlled trial of Internet-based treatment with telephone support for chronic back pain. *Pain* 2004;111(3): 368–377.

125. Martire LM, Lustig AP, Schulz R, et al. Is it beneficial to involve a family member? A meta-analysis of psychosocial interventions for chronic illness. *Health Psychol* 2004;23(6):599–611.

126. Martire LM, Keefe FJ, Schulz R, et al. Older spouses' perceptions of partners' chronic arthritis pain: implications for spousal responses, support provision, and caregiving experiences. *Psychol Aging* 2006;21(2):222–230.

127. Keefe FJ, Caldwell DS, Baucom D, et al. Spouse-assisted coping skills training in the management of osteoarthritic knee pain. *Arthritis Care Res* 1996;9(4): 279–291.

128. Keefe FJ, Caldwell DS, Baucom D, et al. Spouse-assisted coping skills training

129. Keefe FJ, Blumenthal J, Baucom D, et al. Effects of spouse-assisted coping skills training and exercise training in patients with osteoarthritic knee pain: a randomized controlled study. *Pain* 2004;110(3):539–549.

130. Hollon SD, Stewart MO, Strunk D. Enduring effects for cognitive behavior therapy in the treatment of depression and anxiety. *Annu Rev Psychol* 2006; 57:285–315.

131. Morley S. Relapse prevention: still neglected after all these years. *Pain* 2008; 134(3):239–240.

132. Turner JA, Mancl L, Aaron LA. Short- and long-term efficacy of brief cognitive-behavioral therapy for patients with chronic temporomandibular disorder pain: a randomized, controlled trial. *Pain* 2006;121(3):181–194.

133. Keefe FJ, Caldwell DS, Williams DA, et al. Pain coping skills training in the management of osteoarthritic knee pain II: follow-up results. *Behav Ther* 1990;21:435–447.

134. Sharpe L, Sensky T, Timberlake N, et al. Long-term efficacy of a cognitive behavioural treatment from a randomized controlled trial for patients recently diagnosed with rheumatoid arthritis. *Rheumatology* 2003;42(3):435–441.

135. Linton SJ, Andersson T. Can chronic disability be prevented? A randomized trial of a cognitive-behavior intervention and two forms of information for patients with spinal pain. *Spine* 2000;25(21):2825–2831.

136. Linton SJ, Ryberg M. A cognitive-behavioral group intervention as prevention for persistent neck and back pain in a non-patient population: a randomized controlled trial. *Pain* 2001;90(1–2):83–90.

137. Drossman DA, McKee DC, Sandler RS, et al. Psychosocial factors in the irritable bowel syndrome: a multivariate study of patients and nonpatients with irritable bowel syndrome. *Gastroenterology* 1988;95(3):701–708.

138. Aaron LA, Bradley LA, Alarcon GS, et al. Psychiatric diagnoses in patients with fibromyalgia are related to health care-seeking behavior rather than to illness. *Arthritis Rheum* 1996;39(3):436–445.

139. Ziegler DK, Paolo AM. Headache symptoms and psychological profile of headache-prone individuals: a comparison of clinic patients and controls. *Arch Neurol* 1995;52(6):602–606.

140. Kerns RD, Turk DC, Rudy TE. The West Haven-Yale Multidimensional Pain Inventory (WHYMPI). *Pain* 1985;23(4):345–356.

141. Turk DC, Rudy TE. Toward an empirically derived taxonomy of chronic pain patients: integration of psychological assessment data. *J Consult Clin Psychol* 1988;56:233–238.

142. Von KM, Moore JC. Stepped care for back pain: activating approaches for primary care. *Ann Intern Med* 2001;134(9 Pt 2):911–917.

CHAPTER 83 ■ PAIN AND ANXIETY AND DEPRESSION

LANCE M. MCCRACKEN

INTRODUCTION

Chronic pain upsets, frightens, discourages, and demoralizes those who experience it. Chronic pain imposes limits on daily functioning and creates conflicts between what the individual and society expect and what the individual finds him or herself able to do. It presents diagnostic ambiguities and apparent contradictions, such as the oft-quoted notion that "hurt does not equal harm." It is essentially impossible to fully predict or control in many circumstances. As chronic pain continues, these experiences can create an accumulating sense of uncertainty, threat, loss, and helplessness, and can lead to the experience of significant anxiety and depression, among other emotions.

The purpose of this chapter is to describe and examine anxiety and depression in the context of chronic pain. It will briefly review the extent of these emotional experiences, the impacts they impose on patients, and processes by which they interact with other experiences of chronic pain to adversely influence patient

behavior and overall functioning. It will also detail the nature of cognitive behavioral treatment approaches to anxiety and depression and describe new developments that may improve management of these conditions for chronic pain sufferers in the future.

PREVALENCE OF ANXIETY AND DEPRESSIVE DISORDERS IN CHRONIC PAIN

Identified rates of significant anxiety and depressive disorders in chronic pain sufferers depend entirely on the particular population under study, the methods used to collect the data, and the criteria used for defining cases (Table 83.1). Nonetheless, anxiety and depression appear significantly more among persons with chronic pain than those without. A recent national survey in the United States (N = 5877) found that among chronic pain sufferers, 35.1% experienced anxiety disorders and 20.2% experienced

TABLE 83.1

SELECTED PREVALENCE FIGURES FOR ANXIETY AND DEPRESSIVE DISORDER IN COMMUNITY AND CLINICAL SAMPLES WITH AND WITHOUT CHRONIC PAIN

Study	Sample	Diagnostic method	Prevalence anxiety	Prevalence depression
McWilliams et al.[1]	U.S. general population sample with chronic arthritis, bone, joint pain N = 5877	Composite International Diagnostic Interview—Short Form for Major Depression (CIDI)	35.1%	20.2%
Currie and Wang[6]	Canadian household survey N = 118,533 total (N = 10,600 with chronic pain)	CIDI		5.9% for those without pain 19.8% for those with pain
Von Korff et al.[2]	U.S. general population sample with chronic spinal pain N = 5692	CIDI	26.5%	17.5%
Kroenke et al.[17]	U.S. primary care clinic sample N = 965	Structured Clinical Interview for *The Diagnostic and Statistical Manual of Mental Disorders*, 4th edition	19.5% at least one anxiety disorder 8.6% Posttraumatic Stress 7.6% Generalized Anxiety 6.8% Panic 6.2% Social Anxiety	
Moussavi et al.[14]	Nationally representative samples from 60 countries N = 245,404 (4.5% diagnosed with angina, 4.1% with arthritis)	CIDI		3.2% overall 15.0% of those with angina 10.7% of those with arthritis 23.0% of those with two or more chronic medical conditions

depressive disorders in the past year.[1] In this study, chronic pain was defined as "severe arthritis, rheumatism, or another bone or joint disease."[1] A more recent study found similar rates of anxiety and depressive disorders in persons with "chronic spinal pain" at 26.5% and 17.5%, respectively.[2] They defined chronic pain as "chronic back or neck problems" in the prior 12 months. Both of these studies were based on data from a general population survey, the National Comorbidity Study,[3] and employed a standard diagnostic interview, the Composite International Diagnostic Interview (CIDI) from the World Health Organization (WHO).[4] For comparison purposes, the results from a nationally representative household survey in the United States (N = 9282), relying on precisely the same methods as those producing the data above, demonstrated 12-month prevalence estimates of 18.1% for anxiety disorders and 9.5% for mood disorders, regardless of the presence of pain.[5] Hence, from these data collected in the United States, rates of anxiety and depressive disorders in those with chronic pain in the community are roughly 1.5 to 2.0 times as great as those in the community in general.

Results from a large household survey in Canada show that depression is more than three times more prevalent in individuals with chronic pain compared to those without.[6]

A recent survey of community-dwelling adults carried out in 17 countries in Europe, America, the Middle East, Africa, Asia, and the South Pacific (N = 85,088), found that "mental disorders" are more common among persons with chronic back or neck pain than in those without. The pooled odds ratios were 2.3 (95% CI = 2.1, 2.5) for major depression, 2.8 (95% CI = 2.5, 3.2) for dysthymia, 2.7 (95% CI = 2.4, 3.1) for generalized anxiety disorder, 2.1 (95% CI = 1.9, 2.4) for agoraphobia or panic, 1.9 (95% CI = 1.7, 2.2) for social phobia, and 2.6 (95% CI = 2.3, 3.0) for posttraumatic stress disorder.[7] Other results from the same data showed that rates of depression and anxiety increase substantially as the extent of pain increases, nearly doubling in persons with pain in multiple areas of the body.[8]

Perhaps not surprisingly, data from chronic pain sufferers who present in clinic populations show generally higher rates of depression and anxiety disorders compared with those with chronic pain in the general population. Overall, current prevalence estimates in clinical samples range from 7.0% to 62.5% for anxiety disorders,[9,10] and from 30.0% to 54.0% for major depression.[10,11] In particular, the rate of current depression among individuals with chronic pain in clinical settings is at least six times the rate in the general population.

IMPACT OF ANXIETY AND DEPRESSIVE DISORDERS ON PATIENT FUNCTIONING

The high rates of anxiety and depressive disorders in chronic pain are worrying, particularly given the well-documented impacts of these disorders on health, impacts that are reflected clearly in the WHO slogan that there can be "no health without mental health."[12] Mental health problems are generally known to increase risk for other diseases and injury and to impede access to health services for comorbid conditions.[12] This situation is more troubling still for the worldwide shortage of appropriate services for such conditions, most dramatically in the less developed countries, but also in Europe and the United States.[13] Even in developed countries, only about half of those with severe mental health disorders receive even minimal services.[13]

Out of the two sets of psychiatric conditions, it appears that depressive disorders have by far the largest impact on general "disease burden" worldwide. A recent WHO survey including observations from 245,404 participants in 60 countries[14] found a 12-month prevalence of 3.2% for ICD-10 depressive episode. In this survey, between 9.3% and 23.0% of participants with one or more chronic medical conditions also had depression. In comparison to persons with chronic asthma, angina, arthritis, and diabetes alone, those with depression had the lowest rated health. Those with depression comorbid with another chronic medical condition had much lower rated health than those with the chronic medical conditions alone. And, finally, those with two or more chronic medical conditions and comorbid depression had the lowest mean health scores overall.

Based on a recent large-scale study, persons without chronic spinal pain were estimated to function at an average of 93.5% of full role performance, compared to an average of 76.5% for persons with chronic spinal pain.[2] About one-third of this difference in role performance was associated with a combination of physical comorbidities and, importantly, anxiety and depressive disorders. Results from a large, representative, population-based survey in Europe (N = 21,425) showed that the presence of pain and depression was associated with more than twice as many days per month of decreased work productivity as in either condition alone, and more than five times as many days as in the absence of either condition.[15] Other data from primary care clinics in the United States similarly showed that "disabling chronic pain" is four times more prevalent in those with major depression compared to those without.[16] These data further showed that the presence of major depression brought with it a significant risk of alcohol abuse or dependence and six times the risk of significant anxiety-related problems.

Just as depressive disorders clearly add to the impact of chronic pain, anxiety disorders, based on somewhat fewer studies, appear to do the same. A study of 965 randomly sampled patients in primary care in the United States showed that 19.5% had at least one anxiety disorder.[17] Compared to the patients without anxiety disorders, the 188 patients with at least one anxiety disorder reported two to three times as many days in the past three months when their symptoms interfered with their usual activities and more then one and one half times as many physician visits.[17] The implication of these data is that those with chronic pain and significant anxiety-related problems would be expected to carry the added burden of anxiety-related interference with functioning and additional health care use.

The presence of anxiety and depression places patients with chronic pain at risk for a wide range of unwanted health-related outcomes in addition to the general effects on functioning detailed above. These include sleep disturbance,[18] complaints of cognitive dysfunction,[19] opioid abuse (OR = 1.46),[20] delayed seeking of treatment,[15] reduced treatment effects,[21] and dissatisfaction with treatment.[22] Suicide is relatively rare in chronic pain sufferers but appears to occur at twice or three times the rate of the general population.[23] It is nonetheless important as it is arguably the most limiting of all possible outcomes in chronic pain management. Here too, clear features of anxiety and depression, such as helpless, hopeless, or catastrophic thinking, and desire for escape or avoidance, are identified as key psychological processes that increase a patient's risk.[23]

For its part, the adverse effect of depression on pain treatment appears mutual in that, just as depression negatively impacts on treatment of pain, pain negatively impacts on treatment for depression.[24] Also, effective treatment for depression can reduce pain, reduce interference with daily activities due to pain, and improve overall health status, such as in older adults with arthritis.[25]

PROCESSES IN THE INTERACTION OF ANXIETY, DEPRESSION, AND CHRONIC PAIN

In the past, there was often debate about which came first: pain or the types of psychopathology associated with anxiety and depression. For some, this type of linear thinking may be beside the point, such as in clinical situations and treatment planning. It also belies the fact that the terms "chronic pain," "anxiety," and "depression" represent merely ways of speaking about conglomerations of underlying experiences, behavior, and circumstances that interact complexly. Certainly, the temporal order of these events can occur in any direction in any individual case. Most frequently, however, experiences of chronic pain are regarded as antecedent to the emergence of later anxious and depressive behavior. This is somewhat better demonstrated in the case of depression than anxiety.[10]

According to the commonly applied "diathesis-stress" model, individuals who later develop patterns of significant anxiety and depression do so, in part, as a result of particular pre-existing susceptibilities. The occurrence of chronic pain then "activates" these patterns by bringing with it stressors and emotionally pertinent circumstances.[10,11] As mentioned, experiences of uncertainty or threat are commonly associated with chronic pain and are typical occasions for anxiety and fear. Likewise, experiences of loss, broadly speaking, also are commonly associated with chronic pain and are typical occasions for depression.

Attempting to answer the question of which came first, pain or patterns of emotional suffering, may serve no practical clinical purposes. Patients may be better served by an understanding of how experiences of anxiety and depression maintain or worsen a pattern of suffering and disability associated with chronic pain, lend complications to the process of treatment, or contribute to excess health care use, for example. Perhaps the most useful task is to identify the key elements among the patient's problems that are most manipulable and most likely to yield large and durable improvements in health and functioning. In fact, the most manipulable circumstances in those with chronic pain may include the circumstances that give rise to anxious and depressive behavior patterns more so than the circumstances directly underlying the pain experience itself.

The Fear-Avoidance Model and Processes of Depression and Pain

For its part, anxiety has been incorporated into a well-integrated model of chronic pain and disability, the so-called "fear-avoidance model," a model that has garnered a moderate degree of empirical support.[26,27] According to this model, when persons with chronic pain experience fear or anxiety related to their pain and act accordingly by avoiding their pain and related situations, the result is increasing emotional impact overall and greater disability. This pattern of behavior has been reliably demonstrated in a range of chronic pain conditions including both acute and chronic low back pain,[28,29] general musculoskeletal pain,[30] rheumatoid arthritis,[31] osteoarthritis,[32] and fibromyalgia.[33] Other studies have shown that reduction in fear and avoidance plays an important role in the process of successful multidisciplinary treatment for chronic pain.[34,35]

The proposed processes behind the fear-avoidance model include respondent and operant-based learning in tandem with processes of physical deconditioning (loss of physical capacity) or disuse (reduced activity), hypervigilance, and possibly muscular reactivity. Cognitive processes, including catastrophizing, also figure importantly in the cyclical process of mutually reinforcing behavioral, cognitive, emotional, and musculoskeletal influences on reduced functioning.[26] However, the proposed processes of disuse and deconditioning in this model have so far evaded clear empirical demonstration.[36]

Anxious or fearful behavior patterns can vary greatly in terms of the nature of the specific situations that occasion the behavior, how many different situations there are that do so, or how generalized these are. The fear-avoidance model concerns fear and anxiety directly related to pain and activity or movement. Fear of pain from the particular pain problem and fear of movement (kinesophobia) represent the specific end of the continuum, health anxiety and fear of general pain perhaps represent points midway in the continuum, and generalized worry or "trait anxiety" represent the more general end. Studies suggest that measures of more specific, pain-related, movement-related, and possibly health-related forms of anxious behavior are most useful for understanding adjustment to chronic pain, while measures of non-specific, trait-like, or general anxiety appear less useful.[37,38]

The case for how depression contributes to the behavior disturbance of chronic pain is less formalized, as it has not been incorporated into a specific model of distress and disability, as has anxiety or fear. Clearly, the extent to which chronic pain sufferers also suffer with symptoms of depression is correlated with their level of disability or quality of life, both in the general population samples,[1,6] and in clinic samples.[30,39–42] The role of depression in the overall impact of chronic pain may include processes as negative automatic thoughts or attributional styles,[43] relations between depression and passive coping or avoidance,[44,45] or a mediating role of depression in relation to effects of insomnia on pain-related disability.[46]

Practically, by definition, persons with depression and chronic pain have a greater burden of discouraging, ruminative, and distressing thinking (e.g., "I am a worthless person," "My situation is hopeless," "My pain is unbearable") and will therefore experience greater overall emotional distress and greater limitations in functioning as a result, presumably, as they "believe" their thinking, feel the emotions provoked by the circumstances described in their thoughts, or act as if they were true. In addition, their negative thoughts may occasion behavior patterns that are punishing to others, such as complaining, crying, or irritable behavior. These may produce maladaptive social interactions, either alienating others, or gaining ultimately unhelpful forms of social support, an effect suggested in a number of studies on catastrophizing.[47] Behavior patterns of avoidance, which are implicated in the effects of depression, are well documented in their adverse affects on functioning.[45] These adverse effects arise quite straightforwardly because unnecessary or overgeneralized avoidance of unwanted experiences prevents participation in productive, satisfying, or healthy activities at least some of the time.[48] Finally, the effects of sleep-related behavior in relation to depression may be complex. These may include disabling effects of fatigue and other bodily symptoms from actual impaired sleep,[49] or perceptions of a need to rest or reduce activities based solely on the belief that sleep was inadequate,[18,50] or a combination of both.

Confounded Content in Anxiety, Depression, and Pain

Clearly anxiety, depression, and chronic pain have considerable overlap in their psychological and behavioral features. In the case of depression and chronic pain, for example, there is controversy over whether the "somatic features" of each might lead standard depressive inventories to overestimate the presence of depression.[51,52] Anxiety, chronic pain, and depression are each aversive

psychological experiences. Each experience includes: (a) unpleasant feelings in the body and in emotions; (b) patterns in thinking that include a mixture of attempts to solve the problem, unproductive rumination, as well as the presence of distressing or discouraging content; and (c) behavior patterns acquired in the past because they limit contact with, or avoid, the experiences, even though the long-term workability of these patterns appears extremely limited. These behavior patterns will include the avoidance, escape, or corrective rituals associated with anxiety; the generally low activity and persistent treatment seeking of chronic pain; and the withdrawal, excessive sleep, and even the complaints, irritable behavior, or emotional blunting, of depression. These are patterns of behavior that are both topographically and functionally similar, and, again, predominantly avoidant. They may differ more in their originating circumstances than in the psychological processes that maintain them.

TREATMENT OF ANXIETY AND DEPRESSION

In a recent high quality review, it was reported that there are now over 325 published outcome studies on cognitive-behavioral therapy (CBT) and at least 16 "methodologically rigorous" meta-analyses of these studies.[53] There were several general conclusions from this review: large effect sizes were found for CBT for depression, generalized anxiety disorder, panic disorder, social phobia, and posttraumatic stress disorder, with an overall mean effect size of 0.95 (Cohen's d: >20 = small, >05 = medium, >0.08 = large). It was also concluded that CBT was "somewhat superior" to antidepressant medication in treatment of depression.

CBT is sometimes faulted for having limited evidence for the durability of its treatment effects. In the extreme, it is sometimes suggested that effects of CBT are short-term only. The research literature shows that this is not true, and that CBT produces relapse rates, in conditions such as depression and panic, that are half as large as those from pharmacological therapies.[53,54] Twelve-month follow-up data after treatment for depression showed that CBT responders were significantly less likely to relapse than medication responders who were subsequently withdrawn from medication (31.0% versus 76.0%) and no more likely to relapse than patients continuing on medication (31.0% versus 47.0%).[55] Data like these have led experts to conclude that "as effective as medications are for many psychiatric disorders, there is no evidence that they are anything more than palliative; that is, they suppress symptoms so long as they are taken, but often do little to alter the course of the underlying disorder or to reduce subsequent risk once their use is discontinued."[54]

More and more, it appears that antidepressant medications may have significant limitations. A Cochrane review of nine studies including active placebos (which mimic some of the side effects of antidepressants and may prevent "unblinding" effects) versus antidepressants revealed that just two of these showed statistically significant effects in favor of the active drug in terms of improvement in mood.[56] The nine trials produced a pooled effect size of 0.39. One positive trial result contributed to significant heterogeneity in the combined result. Removing this one trial led to a reduced effect size of 0.17. These trials were all relatively short duration, just 6 weeks on average and 12 weeks in the longest case, and, hence, tell us little about longer term results of interest in clinical practice. Recent analyses of published and unpublished trials, available through the Food and Drug Administration in the United States, suggest that the published literature on antidepressants may present an unrealistically high effect size, perhaps one third higher, compared to results that include unpublished trials.[57]

Results of studies with pharmacological therapies for anxiety disorders tend to reveal a similarly sobering pattern as with recent studies of depression. For example, benzodiazepines appear inferior to CBT, particularly in the longer run (6 or 12 months after treatment), for generalized anxiety disorder[58] and for panic disorder.[59] From these results, CBT shows the lowest rate of referral for further psychological or psychiatric treatment in comparison to medication alone for patients with generalized anxiety disorders,[58] and benzodiazepines alone are not recommended for those who have access to appropriate forms of CBT for panic disorder.[59] Currently, serotonin reuptake inhibitor (SSRI) medications are considered the first line pharmacological therapy for anxiety disorders such as panic. There are data that show CBT and SSRI each used alone are about equivalent in efficacy 9 months following the start of treatment, but combined CBT plus SSRI therapy appears marginally better.[60] On the other hand, naturalistic SSRI use during CBT for panic disorder is associated at pretreatment with greater agoraphobia and at posttreatment with delayed reductions in panic severity.[61] Results from cost-efficacy analyses following a randomized trial of three monotherapies (CBT, imipramine, and paroxetine) and two combination therapies (each medication combined with CBT) for panic disorder demonstrated that CBT alone was the most cost-effective both at the end of the maintenance phase and 6 months after the termination of treatment.[62] Trials of SSRIs for panic disorder show relatively high dropout rates (i.e., low tolerability) of between 25% to 50% during 12 months.[63] Relapse of symptoms is relatively high following treatment with medications and especially so after discontinuation of medication, an effect that is reduced with the addition of CBT.[64]

Clearly the efficacy of CBT for anxiety and depression is well-supported by research. On top of this success, particular methods within CBT may be in a process of refinement. For example, there has been a gradual revolution afoot in the analysis of treatment components and treatment process. More than 10 years ago, a component analysis of CBT for depression (N = 150) showed that both the behavioral activation component of CBT (an approach to increasing behavior that yields a sense of pleasure and mastery) and combined components of behavioral activation and skills training for modifying automatic thoughts were as effective as the entire package of these components plus a component that focused on changing core cognitive schemas.[65] These results held both immediately posttreatment and at 6-month follow-up. Additional results showed that the behavioral activation condition was as effective as the full set of components at altering negative thinking and dysfunctional attributional styles. These results run contrary to the popularly accepted cognitive model of depression, as this model proposes that the modification of negative schemata is necessary for treatment effects in CBT. It appears that a relatively simple treatment for depression aimed at direct behavior change and not on changing the way people think can be as effective as a more complicated form of treatment that emphasizes cognitive change.

A recent randomized trial comparing behavioral activation to cognitive therapy and antidepressant medication (N = 241) found that, in severely depressed patients, behavioral activation produced similar positive effects as did antidepressant medication, and both of these treatments produced better results than cognitive therapy.[66] This version of behavioral activation was an updated version that highlights the role of avoidance and withdrawal in depression, seeks to promote engagement with activities consistent with long-term goals, and to redirect attention away from the content of rumination and onto direct experience. In a follow-up study, the research group found a subgroup of patients they deemed as experiencing an "extreme nonresponse" to cognitive therapy.[67] Through the use of logistic regression, they found that the extreme nonresponders to cognitive therapy were characterized by high baseline depression severity, functional impairment, and problems with their primary social support. These patients reported major life stressors or interpersonal problems and regarded themselves as having long-standing difficulties with depression. When patients with these same characteristics were identified among those treated in the behavioral activation condition, they did not evidence nonresponses to this treatment. Perhaps cognitive therapy is more complicated to deliver because of its focus on patient behavior, beliefs, and attitudes, as opposed to the smaller number of straightforward overt behavioral strategies included in behavioral activation. Perhaps a more limited focus is an advantage when the length of treatment is constrained.[67]

More than 16 years ago, Sullivan and colleagues[68] called for increased recognition of depression in chronic pain and for treatments specifically targeting depressive symptoms in chronic pain. Although we do know that CBT is effective for anxiety and depression and that treatments for chronic pain based on cognitive behavioral principles can result in decreased depression and anxiety,[69] this leaves the question still unanswered about how to most effectively treat anxiety and depression in the context of chronic pain or whether to do so will result in significantly better overall treatment results. The current literature leads one to assume this would be the case.

COGNITIVE BEHAVIORAL TREATMENT OF PAIN-RELATED FEAR AND AVOIDANCE

Unlike depression, the model connecting fear and anxiety-related processes to chronic pain has spawned specific treatment methods, primarily including exposure-based methods. Exposure-based treatments essentially include having the patient make contact with particular situations, involving movements and pain, that provoke fear and avoidance, but having them do so in a way that does not include avoidance and so that they do not attempt to control their fearful feelings by avoidance or escape. Exposure trials are typically performed along a graded hierarchy of fear-eliciting situations, from low levels of threat to higher levels. These treatments for pain-related fear and avoidance have typically also included a component called "behavioral experiments," which include methods to identify and challenge irrational expectations during exposure.[70] Repeated trials using these methods together are presumed to reduce fearful feelings and correct mistaken fearful beliefs or expectations.

In what was apparently the first published demonstration of exposure for treatment of pain-related fear and avoidance, Vlaeyen et al.[70] conducted a replicated, single-case, cross-over experimental design comparing in vivo exposure with methods designed to increase activity in a graded fashion. The participants in this study (N = 4) were selected for their high levels of fear of movement. Based on graphical and time series analyses of daily ratings of pain-related cognitions and fears, improvements only occurred during the graded exposure and not during the graded activity condition. These investigators also found that reductions in fear of pain correlated with reductions in catastrophizing and disability. These results from the Netherlands were essentially replicated by a group in Sweden.[71] In a subsequent study, the actual exposure component, and not educational sessions included with exposure, appeared responsible for improvements in daily activity, and that improvements from treatment maintained at a 6-month follow-up.[72] The results of graded exposure in vivo for fearful patients with chronic pain have been extended to patients with complex regional pain syndrome (CRPS).[73] Again, relative to baseline phases of randomly determined durations across patients, an exposure condition was associated with decreased fear, disability, and pain. Interestingly, the exposure condition also appeared to reduce patients' signs and symptoms of CRPS.

Until recently, all of the investigations of graded exposure for chronic pain utilized single subject design methods and therefore small sample sizes. In what appears to be the first randomized controlled trial in this area, including 44 patients with chronic low back pain, Woods and Asmundson[74] showed that, relative to a graded activity condition, patients in the graded exposure condition had greater improvements in measures of fear of pain and movement, pain-related anxiety, catastrophizing, pain, anxiety, and depression. Improvements in disability, however, did not reach statistical significance. Improvements were maintained at a 1-month follow-up.

In a more recently reported trial including patients with "at least moderate pain-related fear" (N = 85), it was demonstrated that exposure-based treatment appeared roughly equal in efficacy to graded activity in terms of improvements in functional disability and physical activity-related complaints, immediately and 6 months following treatment.[75] On the other hand, the exposure treatment demonstrated clear superiority in reducing pain, catastrophizing, and perceived harmfulness of activities. Effects of the exposure condition on disability and physical activity-related complaints were mediated by decreases in pain, catastrophizing, and perceived harmfulness of activities. Although the results from both randomized trials are certainly not discouraging, they seem less definitive in asserting the specific efficacy of exposure-based methods than were results from the studies relying on single subject designs.

DEVELOPMENTS IN CONTEXTUAL COGNITIVE BEHAVIORAL THERAPY

Developments in the cognitive and behavioral therapies have been described as a series of "waves."[76] The first consisted of the application of laboratory-based principles to human behavior problems in what was simply called Behavior Therapy, or, in the field of chronic pain management, the "operant approach."[77] The second wave included the addition of cognitive therapy methods to behavior therapy to define what is now understood as CBT.[78] The "third wave" includes a number of approaches that integrate the behavioral and cognitive elements of the first two waves, but also expands these within a conceptual framework that is less mechanistic and more contextual. The methods that emerge within this wave include notions like acceptance, mindfulness, and values. Examples of these "third wave" approaches include Mindfulness-based Stress Reduction,[79] Dialectical Behavior Therapy,[80] Mindfulness-based Cognitive Therapy,[81] Acceptance and Commitment Therapy (ACT),[82] and an approach to chronic pain based on ACT called Contextual Cognitive Behavioral Therapy (CCBT).[83]

The therapeutic model underlying ACT and CCBT includes six core processes. These include acceptance, contact with the present moment (a feature of mindfulness), cognitive defusion (a loosening of the general role of verbal/cognitive processes in their influence on behavior and their blocking of nonverbal influences), committed action, self-as-context (as distinct from a verbally constructed sense of self), and value-based action.[83] In turn, these six processes entail an overall process referred to as "psychological flexibility," which is a quality of behavior that allows it to change or persist in line with long-term goals and values relatively free from restrictions on behavior based on interactions between verbally-based and direct (nonverbally-based) influences on that behavior.

Research supports the role of the core therapeutic processes described here in relation to the functioning of patients with chronic pain. For example, acceptance of pain is associated with emotional, physical, and social functioning, health care use in both retrospective[84,85] and prospective[86] studies in patients with heterogeneous pain problems, and in patients with rheumatoid arthritis[87] and low back pain.[88] Mindfulness,[41] values-based action,[89] and general psychological flexibility[90] are, likewise, significantly and generally related to key aspects of patient functioning. In relation to focus of this chapter, more than 20 studies of these contextual processes in chronic pain demonstrate that these processes are particularly strong in their correlations with anxiety (range r = -0.29 to -0.72) and depression (range r = -0.45 to -0.59).

There are at least seven treatment outcome studies that demonstrate the benefits of treatment methods for chronic pain related to the ACT and CCBT model. In these studies, both mindfulness-based methods alone[91-93] and broader packages of methods (including exposure, mindfulness, values-based methods, and other methods to increase psychological flexibility)[94,95] yield significant results across a range of domains, including results with clear clinical significance.[96] These latter results, for example, include effect sizes of 1.2 immediately post treatment (N = 171) and above 0.90 at a 3-month follow-up (N = 114) for both pain-related anxiety and depression, following a 3 or 4 week course of interdisciplinary residential treatment in the United Kingdom. Whereas the mindfulness-based methods for chronic pain have been analyzed in fully randomized controlled trials, the results regarding the comprehensive multicomponent packages of methods await a high quality, fully randomized, controlled trial. To date, published studies have included a small randomized trial of participants "at risk" for work loss due to pain or stress,[97] and a nonrandomized trial with a waiting phase comparison.[94]

The particular value in acceptance-based, contextual, and mindfulness-based methods for anxiety and depression in chronic pain sufferers appears to arise from their specific focus on processes for addressing rumination,[98] undermining avoidance, and reducing the impact of distressing and restricting influences in patterns of emotional thinking.[82]

SUMMARY

The suffering that comes with chronic pain is undeniable in the community and even more so in the clinic. This suffering takes many forms but commonly includes the experiences of anxiety and depression. Between 1 out of 5 and 1 out of every 2 individuals with chronic pain will meet criteria for an anxiety or depressive disorder or both. The added burden of anxiety or depressive conditions on top of chronic pain is important because this constitutes real human suffering, and because it significantly impacts on general health, work, and health care use. Despite the quite large burden imposed by anxiety and depression on individuals, the community, and national resources, these problems are not adequately addressed, even among the most advantaged countries around the world, where less than half of those in need receive even minimal services.

Talk of individuals in categories like chronic pain, anxiety, and depression is just a way of speaking, a way of organizing events in the world. This way of speaking has uses as well as limitations.[99] A more adequate analysis of the medical, psychological, and social processes responsible for the suffering and disability of chronic pain will require looking underneath these categories to the interrelated experiences and behavior patterns that constitute the problem and to the situations and history that determine and maintain these patterns. It is not an adequate technical analysis to say that depression "makes pain worse," or even to say that fear causes avoidance and that this avoidance causes disability and further distress.

What is remarkable about the categories of chronic pain, anxiety, and depression is all the psychological features they share in common. Each of these includes contact with aversive experiences particularly in the body and in the mind. Each of these includes thoughts and beliefs that, if taken literally, add considerably to emotional suffering, and, if followed, lead to behavior patterns that restrict the individual's functioning further still. Each of these includes prominent patterns of avoidance, including both decreases in healthy overt activity and processes of struggling to control or limit contact with the many related, collateral, aversive experiences. While the particular history that gave rise to the chronic pain, anxiety, or depression may have unique features, such as the experiences of threat or uncertainty that lead to anxiety, or the experiences of loss that lead to depression, the psychological processes that maintain the suffering and life disruption they occasion appear largely overlapping. One day, treatments may focus not on symptoms of chronic pain, anxiety, or depression, but on underlying psychological dimensions of avoidance, loss of contact with reality, and general psychological inflexibility.[82]

Cognitive behavioral approaches to anxiety and depression are highly effective for reducing the symptoms of these conditions and for improving patient functioning. There is also evidence that cognitive behavioral approaches for chronic pain can generally effectively reduce the impacts of anxiety and depression. Still, cognitive behavioral methods develop and evolve. These developments emerge from theoretical advances and from research results. Among the particularly intriguing results, for example, it was recently concluded that perhaps it is *not* necessary to challenge irrational thoughts in CBT,[100] and that a modern version of behavioral activation, a method for changing behavior without first changing thoughts and feelings, can be more effective in treating depression than a more comprehensive cognitive behavioral approach that places a greater emphasis on changing thoughts.[66]

A short time ago, the remark was made that "these are interesting times to be doing depression research,"[101] by this it was meant that this is a time of potential controversy and a time for questioning notions, such as the notion that depression is primarily a function of altered brain chemistry, some personality-based vulnerability, or an irrational response. One might equally say that it is an interesting time to be doing anxiety or chronic pain research for the same controversies that emerge. Recent analyses suggest that the human suffering and lost vitality that arise with chronic pain, anxiety, and depression emerge not from a defect in the individual but from a somewhat arbitrary extreme within normal human functioning. Newer developments in the cognitive behavioral therapies that emerge from this way of thinking include processes like acceptance, mindfulness, and values, where in the past the key processes may have been "control," "coping," and "cognitive restructuring." As research results continue to accumulate, methods that derive from these processes may be shown to significantly expand the range and adequacy of our treatment methods for individuals suffering with chronic pain.

References

1. McWilliams LA, Cox BJ, Enns MW. Mood and anxiety disorders associated with chronic pain: an examination in a nationally representative sample. *Pain* 2003;106(1-2):127–133.
2. Von Korff M, Crane P, Lane M, et al. Chronic spinal pain and physical–mental comorbidity in the United States: results from the national comorbidity survey replication. *Pain* 2005;113(3):331–339.
3. Kessler RC, McGonagle KA, Zhao S, et al. Lifetime and 12-month prevalence of DSM-III-R psychiatric disorders in the United States: results from the National Comorbidity Survey. *Arch Gen Psychiatry* 1994;51(1):8–19.
4. World Health Organization. *Composite International Diagnostic Interview.* Geneva, Switzerland: World Health Organization; 1990.
5. Kessler RC, Chiu WT, Demler O, et al. Prevalence, severity, and comorbidity of 12-month DSM-IV disorders in the National Comorbidity Survey Replication. *Arch Gen Psychiatry* 2005;62(6):617–627.
6. Currie SR, Wang J. Chronic back pain and major depression in the general Canadian population. *Pain* 2004;107(1-2):54–60.
7. Demyttenaere K, Bruffaerts R, Lee S, et al. Mental disorders among persons with chronic back or neck pain: results from the world mental health surveys. *Pain* 2007;129(3):332–342.
8. Gureye O, Von Korff M, Kloa L, et al. The relation between multiple pains

and mental disorders: results from the World Mental Health Surveys. *Pain* 2008;135(1-2):82–91.
9. Fishbain DA, Cutler BR, Rosomoff HL, et al. Comorbidity between psychiatric disorders and chronic pain. *Current Review of Pain* 1998;2(1):1–10.
10. Dersh J, Polatin PB, Gatchel RJ. Chronic pain and psychopathology: research findings and theoretical considerations. *Psychosom Med* 2002;64(5):773–786.
11. Banks SM, Kerns R D. Explaining high rates of depression in chronic pain: a diathesis–stress framework. *Psychol Bull* 1996;119(1):95–110.
12. Prince M, Patel V, Saxena S, et al. Global mental health 1: no health without mental health. *Lancet* 2007;370(9590):859–877.
13. Wang PS, Aguilar–Gaxiola S, Alonso J, et al. Use of mental health services for anxiety, mood, and substance disorders in 17 countries in the WHO world mental health surveys. *Lancet* 2007;370(9590):841–850.
14. Moussavi S, Chatterji S, Verdes E, et al. Depression, chronic diseases, and decrements in health: results from the World Health Surveys. *Lancet* 2007;370(9590):851–858.
15. Demyttenaere K, Bonnewyn A, Bruffaerts, et al. Comorbid painful physical symptoms and depression: prevalence, work loss, and help seeking. *J Affective Disord* 2006;92(2–3):185–193.
16. Arnow BA, Humkeler EM, Blasey CM, et al. Comorbid depression, chronic pain, and disability in primary care. *Psychosom Med* 2006;68(2):262–268.
17. Kroenke K, Spitzer RL, Williams JBW, et al. Anxiety disorders in primary care: prevalence, impairment, comorbidity, and detection. *Ann Intern Med* 2007;146(5):317–325.
18. Tang NKY, Wright KJ, Salkovskis PM. Prevalence and correlates of clinical insomnia co-occurring with chronic back pain. *J Sleep Res* 2007;16(1):85–95.
19. Roth RS, Geisser ME, Theisen–Goodvich M, et al. Cognitive complaints are associated with depression, fatigue, female sex, and pain catastrophizing in patients with chronic pain. *Arch Phys Med Rehabil* 2005;86(6):1147–1154.
20. Edlund MJ, Steffick D, Hudson T, et al. Risk factors for clinically recognized opioid abuse and dependence among veterans using opioids for chronic non-cancer pain. *Pain* 2007;129(3):355–362.
21. Finset A, Wigers SH, Gotestam G. Depressed mood impedes pain treatment response in patients with fibromyalgia. *J Rheumatol* 2004;31(5):976–980.
22. Bair MJ, Kroenke K, Sutherland JM, et al. Effects of depression and pain severity on satisfaction in medical outpatients: analysis of the Medical Outcomes Study. *J Rehabil Res Dev* 2007;44(2):143–152.
23. Tang NKY, Crane C. Suicidality in chronic pain: a review of the prevalence, risk factors, and psychological links. *Psychol Med* 2006;36(5):575–586.
24. Kroenke K, Shen J, Oxman TE, et al. Impact of pain on the outcomes of depression treatment: results from the RESPECT trial. *Pain* 2008;134(1–2):209–215.
25. Lin EH, Katon W, Von Korff M, et al. Effect of improving depression care on pain and functional outcomes among older adults with arthritis. *JAMA* 2003;290(18):2428–2434.
26. Vlaeyen JWS, Linton SJ. Fear-avoidance and its consequences in chronic musculoskeletal pain: a state of the art. *Pain* 2000;85(3):317–332.
27. Leeuw M, Goossens MEJB, Linton SJ, et al. The fear-avoidance model of musculoskeletal pain: current state of the scientific evidence. *J Behav Med* 2007;30(1):77–93.
28. Crombez G, Vlaeyen JWS, Heuts PHTG, et al. Pain-related fear is more disabling then the pain itself: evidence on the role of pain-related fear in chronic back pain disability. *Pain* 1999;80(1–2):329–339.
29. Grotle M, Vollestad NK, Brox, JI. Clinical course and impact of fear-avoidance beliefs in low back pain. *Spine* 2006;31(9):1038–1046.
30. McCracken LM, Spertus IL, Janeck AS, et al. Behavioral dimensions of adjustment in persons with chronic pain: pain-related anxiety and acceptance. *Pain* 1999;80(1–2):283–289.
31. Strahl C, Kleinknecht RA, Dinnel DL. The role of pain anxiety, coping, and pain self-efficacy in rheumatoid arthritis patient functioning. *Behav Res Ther* 2000;38(9):863–873.
32. Heuts PHTG, Vlaeyen JWS, Roelofs J, et al. Pain-related fear and daily functioning in patients with osteoarthritis. *Pain* 2004;110(1–2):228–235.
33. Turk DC, Robinson JP, Burwinkle T. Prevalence of fear of pain and activity in patients with fibromyalgia syndrome. *J Pain* 2004;5(9):483–490.
34. McCracken LM, Gross RT, Eccleston C. Multimethod assessment of treatment process in chronic low back pain: comparison of reported pain-related anxiety with directly measured physical capacity. *Behav Res Ther* 2002;40(5):585–594.
35. Woby SR, Watson PJ, Roach NK, et al. Are changes in fear-avoidance beliefs, catastrophizing, and appraisals of control, predictive of changes in chronic low back pain and disability? *Eur J Pain* 2004;8(3):201–210.
36. Smeets RJEM, Wade D, Hiddings A, et al. The association of physical deconditioning and chronic low back pain: a hypothesis-oriented systematic review. *Disabil Rehabil* 2006;28(11):673–693.
37. McCracken LM, Gross RT, Aikens J, et al. The assessment of anxiety and fear in persons with chronic pain: a comparison of instruments. *Behav Res Ther* 1996;34(11–12):927–933.
38. Hadjistavropoulos HD, Asmundson GJG, Kowalyk KM. Measures of anxiety: is there a difference in their ability to predict functioning at three-month follow-up among pain patients? *Eur J Pain* 2004;8(1):1–11.
39. Haythornthwaite JA, Sieber WJ, Kerns RD. Depression and the chronic pain experience. *Pain* 1991;46(2):177–184.
40. Romano JM, Turner JA, Jensen MP. The Chronic Illness Problem Inventory as a measure of dysfunction in chronic pain patients. *Pain* 1992;49(1):71–75.

41. McCracken, LM, Gauntlett-Gilbert J, Vowles KE. The role of mindfulness in a contextual cognitive-behavioral analysis of chronic pain-related suffering and disability. *Pain* 2007;131(1–2):63–69.

42. Keeley P, Creed F, Tomenson B, et al. Psychosocial predictors of health-related quality of life and health service utilization in people with chronic low back pain. *Pain* 2008;135(1–2):142–150.

43. Ingram RE, Atkinson JH, Slater MA, et al. Negative and positive cognition in depressed and nondepressed chronic-pain patients. *Health Psychol* 1990;9(3):300–314.

44. Carroll LJ, Cassidy JD, Cote P. The role of pain coping strategies in prognosis after whiplash injury: passive coping predicts slow recovery. *Pain* 2006;124(1):18–26.

45. McCracken LM, Samuel VM. The role of avoidance, pacing, and other activity patterns in chronic pain. *Pain* 2007;130(1–2):119–125.

46. Naughton F, Ashworth P, Skevington SM. Does sleep quality predict pain-related disability in chronic pain patients? The mediating role of depression and pain severity. *Pain* 2007;127(3):243–252.

47. Sullivan MJL, Thorn B, Haythornthwaite JA, et al. Theoretical perspectives on the relation between catastrophizing and pain. *Clin J Pain* 2001;17(1):52–64.

48. Hayes SC, Wilson KG, Gifford EV, et al. Experiential avoidance and behavioral disorders: a functional dimensional approach to diagnosis and treatment. *J Consult Clin Psychol* 1996;64(6):1152–1168.

49. Haack M, Mullington JM. Sustained sleep restriction reduces emotional and physical well-being. *Pain* 2005;119(1–3):56–64.

50. Semler CN, Harvey AG. Misperception of sleep can adversely affect daytime functioning in insomnia. *Behav Res Ther* 2005;43(7):843–856.

51. Williams AC, Richardson PH. What does the BDI measure in chronic pain? *Pain* 1993;55(2):259–266.

52. Geisser ME, Roth RS, Robinson ME. Assessing depression among persons with chronic pain using the Center for Epidemiological Studies-Depression Scale and the Beck Depression Inventory: a comparative analysis. *Clinical J Pain* 1997;13(2):163–170.

53. Butler AC, Chapman JE, Forman EM, et al. The empirical status of cognitive-behavioral therapy: a review of meta-analyses. *Clin Psychol Rev* 2006;26(1):17–31.

54. Hollon SD, Stewart MO, Strunk D. Enduring effects for cognitive behavior therapy in the treatment of anxiety and depression. *Ann Rev Psychol* 2006;57:285–315.

55. DeRubeis RJ, Hollon SD, Amsterdam JD, et al. Cognitive therapy vs. medications in the treatment of moderate to severe depression. *Arch Gen Psych* 2005;62(4):409–416.

56. Montcrieff J, Wessely, S, Hardy R. Active placebos versus antidepressants for depression. *Cochrane Database Syst Rev* 2004;(1):CD003012.

57. Turner EH, Matthews AM, Linardatos E, et al. Selective publication of antidepressant trials and its influence on apparent efficacy. *N Engl J Med* 2008;358(3):252–260.

58. Power KG, Simpson RJ, Swanson V, et al. Controlled comparison of pharmacological treatment of generalized anxiety disorder in primary care. *Br J Gen Prac* 1990;40(336):289–294.

59. Wantanabe N, Churchill R, Furukawa TA. Combination of psychotherapy and benzodiazepine versus either therapy alone for panic disorder: a systematic review. *BMC Psychiatry* 2007;7:18.

60. van Apeldoorn FJ, van Hout WJPJ, Mersch PPA, et al. Is a combined therapy more effective than either CBT or SSRI alone? Results of a multicenter trial on panic disorder with or without agoraphobia. *Acta Psychiatr Scand* 2008;117(4):260–270.

61. Arch JJ, Craske MG. Implications of naturalistic use of pharmacologicotherapy in CBT treatment for panic disorder. *Behav Res Ther* 2007;45(7):1435–1447.

62. McHugh RK, Otto MW, Barlow DH, et al. Cost-efficacy of individual and combined treatments for panic disorder. *J Clin Psychiatry* 2007;68(7):1038–1044.

63. Dannon PN, Iancu I, Lowengrub K, et al. A naturalistic long-term comparison study of selective serotonin reuptake inhibitors in the treatment of panic disorder. *Clin Neuropharmacol* 2007;30(6):326–334.

64. Choy Y, Peselow ED, Case BG, et al. Three-year medication prophylaxis in panic disorder: to continue or discontinue? A naturalistic study. *Compr Psychiatry* 2007;48(5):419–425.

65. Jacobson NS, Dobson KS, Traux PA, et al. A component analysis of cognitive-behavioral treatment for depression. *J Consult Clin Psychol* 1996;64(2):295–304.

66. Dimidjian S, Hollon SD, Dobson KS, et al. Randomized trial of behavioral activation, cognitive therapy, and antidepressant medication in the acute treatment of adults with major depression. *J Consult Clin Psychol* 2006;74(4):658–670.

67. Coffman SJ, Martell CR, Dimidjian S, et al. Extreme nonresponse in cognitive therapy: can behavioral activation succeed where cognitive therapy fails? *J Consult Clin Psychol* 2007;75(4):531–541.

68. Sullivan MJL, Reesor K, Mikail S, et al. The treatment of depression in chronic low back pain: review and recommendations. *Pain* 1992;50(1):5–13.

69. Hoffman BM, Papas RK, Chatkoff DK, et al. Meta-analysis of psychological interventions for chronic low back pain. *Health Psychol* 2007;26(1):1–9.

70. Vlaeyen JWS, de Jong J, Geilen M, et al. Graded exposure in vivo in the treatment of pain-related fear: a replicated single-case experimental design in four patients with chronic low back pain. *Behav Res Ther* 2001;39(2):151–166.

71. Boersma K, Linton S, Overmeer T, et al. Lowering fear-avoidance and enhancing function through exposure in vivo: a multiple baseline study across six patients with back pain. *Pain* 2004;108(1–2):8–16.

72. de Jong JR, Vlaeyen JWS, Onghena P, et al. Fear of movement/(re)injury in chronic low back pain: education or exposure in vivo as mediators to fear reduction? *Clin J Pain* 2005;21(1):9–17.

73. de Jong JR, Vlaeyen WSJ, Onghena P, et al. Reduction of pain-related fear in complex regional pain syndrome type I: the application of graded exposure in vivo. *Pain* 2005;116(3):264–275.

74. Woods MP, Asmundson GJG. Evaluating the efficacy of graded in vivo exposure for the treatment of fear in patients with chronic back pain: a randomized controlled clinical trial. *Pain* 2008;136(3):271–280.

75. Leeuw M, Goossens MEJB, van Breukelen GJP, et al. Exposure in vivo versus operant graded activity in chronic low back pain patients: results of a randomized controlled trial. *Pain* 2008;138(1):192–207.

76. Hayes SC. Acceptance and commitment therapy, relational frame theory, and the third wave of behavior therapy. *Behav Ther* 2004;35(4):639–665.

77. Fordyce, WE. *Behavioral Methods for Chronic Pain and Illness*. Saint Louis: Mosby; 1976.

78. Turk DC, Meichenbaum D, Genest M. *Pain and Behavioral Medicine: A Cognitive-Behavioral Perspective*. New York: Guilford; 1983.

79. Kabat-Zinn J. *Full Catastrophe Living: Using the Wisdom of Your Body and Mind to Face Stress, Pain, and Illness*. New York: Dell Publishing; 1990.

80. Linehan MM. *Cognitive-behavioral treatment of borderline personality disorder*. New York: Guilford; 1993.

81. Segal ZV, Williams JMG, Teasdale JD. *Mindfulness-based cognitive therapy for depression*. New York: Guilford; 2002.

82. Hayes SC, Luoma JB, Bond FW, et al. Acceptance and commitment therapy: model, process and outcome. *Behav Res Ther* 2006;44(1):1–25.

83. McCracken LM. *Contextual Cognitive-Behavioral Therapy for Chronic Pain, Progress in Pain Research and Management*. Vol 33. Seattle: IASP Press; 2005.

84. McCracken LM, Eccleston C. Coping or acceptance: what to do about chronic pain? *Pain* 2003;105(1–2):197–204.

85. Nicholas MK, Asghari A. Investigating acceptance in adjustment to chronic pain: is acceptance broader than we thought? *Pain* 2006;124(3):269–279.

86. McCracken LM, Eccleston C. A prospective study of acceptance of pain and patient functioning with chronic pain. *Pain* 2005;118(1–2):164–169.

87. Kratz AL, Davis MC, Zautra AJ. Pain acceptance moderates the relation between pain and negative affect in female osteoarthritis patients. *Ann Behav Med* 2007;33(3):291–301.

88. Mason VL, Mathias B, Skevington SM. Accepting low back pain: it is related to a good quality of life? *Clin J Pain* 2008;24(1):22–29.

89. McCracken LM, Yang SY. The role of values in a contextual cognitive-behavioral analysis of chronic pain. *Pain* 2006;123(1–2):137–145.

90. McCracken LM, Vowles KE. Psychological flexibility and traditional pain management strategies in relation to patient functioning with chronic pain: an examination of a revised instrument. *J Pain* 2007;8(9):700–707.

91. Pradhan EK, Baumgarten M, Langenberg P, et al. Effect of mindfulness-based stress reduction in rheumatoid arthritis patients. *Arth Rheum* 2007;57(7):1134–1142.

92. Sephton SE, Salmon P, Weissbecker I, et al. Mindfulness meditation alleviates depressive symptoms in women with fibromyalgia: results of a randomized clinical trial. *Arth Rheum* 2007;57(1):77–85.

93. Morone NE, Grecco CM, Weiner DK. Mindfulness meditation for the treatment of chronic low back pain in older adults: a randomized controlled pilot study. *Pain* 2008;134(3):310–319.

94. McCracken LM, Vowles KE, Eccleston C. Acceptance-based treatment for persons with complex, long standing chronic pain: a preliminary analysis of treatment outcome in comparison to a waiting phase. *Behav Res Ther* 2005;43(10):1335–1346.

95. McCracken LM, MacKichan F, Eccleston C. Contextual cognitive-behavioral therapy for severely disabled chronic pain sufferers: effectiveness and clinically significant change. *Eur J Pain* 2007;11(3):314–322.

96. Vowles KE, McCracken LM. Acceptance and values-based action in chronic pain: a study of effectiveness and treatment process. *J Consult Clin Psychol* 2008;76(3):397–407.

97. Dahl J, Wilson KG, Nilsson A. Acceptance and commitment therapy and the treatment of persons at risk for long-term disability resulting from stress and pain symptoms: a preliminary randomized trial. *Behav Ther* 2004;35:785–802.

98. Ramel W, Goldin PR, Carmona PE, et al. The effects of mindfulness meditation on cognitive processes and affect in patients with past depression. *Cognit Ther Res* 2004;28(4):433–455.

99. Brown TA, Barlow DH. Dimensional versus categorical classification of mental disorders in the fifth edition of the *Diagnostic and Statistical Manual of Mental Disorders* and beyond: comments on the special section. *J Abnorm Psychol* 2005;114:551–556.

100. Longmore RJ, Worrell M. Do we need to challenge thoughts in cognitive behavior therapy? *Clin Psychol Rev* 2007;27(2):173–187.

101. Jacobson NS, Gortner ET. Can depression be de-medicalized in the 21st century: scientific revolutions, counter-revolutions and the magnetic field of normal science. *Behav Res Ther* 2000;38(2):103–117.

CHAPTER 84 ■ HYPNOSIS

JEANNE HERNANDEZ

HISTORY OF HYPNOSIS IN PAIN AND SYMPTOM CONTROL

Hypnosis is a word derived from the Greek word meaning "sleep." The fairly ancient practice was used by the Druids, the Celts, and by the Egyptians, who frequented "sleeping temples" for relaxation and healing. In the 1770s, the Austrian physician Franz Mesmer (1734–1815) was interested in the effect of physical energy and magnetism on the body and spirit. He placed his patients in a tub of iron filings and, with wide sweeps of his arm, made "passes" up and down the patients' bodies. The success of the practice, termed mesmerism, was attributed to animal magnetism, whereas the benefits were probably due to the hypnotic effect of his arm-waving ritual. In the 1830s, practical uses of mesmerism were discussed by Oliver in the U.S. and by the French Academy of Medicine. In Scotland, James Braid (1795–1860) termed the word "hypnosis" in 1843, thinking it to be a stage of sleep that influenced the nervous system, and distinguishing it from the state of mental concentration. Braid concluded that the relaxing suggestions diverted the patients away from critical thinking and led them into trance. In the early 1900s, Pavlov also viewed hypnosis as an incomplete sleep state that allowed patients to mentally separate from what was going on around them.

John Esdaile (1808–1859)[1] began using trance inductions with surgery patients in 1845 in India, where there were not anesthetics available; he found the hypnotized patients to have increased resistance to infection, greater comfort, and quicker recovery times. In Europe, the School of Hypnotic Study was being formed in Nancy, where the view was that suggestion led to hypnotic trance states that were quite normal phenomena. Neurologist Jean-Martin Charcot (1825–1893) also noted that hysteria was effectively treated with hypnotism; while he brought hypnotism into favorable light, he viewed it as a part of the hysteria process and not a normal healthy phenomenon. Interestingly, recent brain research shows us how he was correct in his assessment and that there is a link between the propensity to hysteria and high hypnotizability.

Pierre Janet (1849–1947) saw hypnosis as dissociation or a split away from cognitive consciousness, which was sometimes normal and healthy and other times related to dissociative states or multiple personalities. In the late 1800s, Freud became interested in accessing repressed memories through hypnosis, recognizing it as a pathway to the unconscious mind. However, he was not a good hypnotist and therefore abandoned it; in doing so, he led others away as well. Fortunately he did continue his interest in the hypnotic properties of dreams and free associations.

In the mid-1840s, the introduction of chloroform and ether into surgical practice was another reason for the apparent hiatus in the use and study of hypnosis in medicine. In the 1950s, its use in understanding the workings of the mind and its application to psychotherapy began to pick back up. In the U.S., psychologist Clark Hull[2] documented its use for anesthesia, posthypnotic amnesia, and pain relief. Milton Erickson conducted many of these experiments and went on to study the mechanisms of trance practices brought to him by Jay Haley and Margaret Meade.

Erickson had an exquisite understanding of the mechanisms of the unconscious mind, and his personal understanding of its effectiveness for reducing physical pain left him well poised to research, practice, and teach hypnosis for symptom control and pain management. The American Society of Clinical Hypnosis (ASCH) was founded in 1957 as a spin off from the Society for Clinical and Experimental Hypnosis (SCEH), founded in 1949. Hypnosis was endorsed by both the American Psychological Association (APA) and the American Medical Association (AMA) in the late 1950s. The British Medical Association endorsed its use in 1958 as an anesthetic in certain surgical situations.

In a way, there is a great difference between the linear and precise thinking of modern medicine and the spiritual and imagination-rich mosaic thinking of the hypnotherapist, and yet they come together in this chapter in the discussion of pain as a psychological event, and of the role of expectancy and hope in pain management and general wellness. The early researchers and practitioners identified the spiritual and magical element of hypnosis having to do with the positive expectation noted in the early practices of Mesmer with his magnets, Freud with his dream work, and Erickson with his positive mindset of hope and respect for the patients. These men all identified the role of the unconscious mind in psychosomatic symptom formation and, in doing so, let down the Cartesian wall between the mind and the body. They also recognized that the highly hypnotizable may be more likely to develop psychosomatic symptoms but also may be more likely to benefit from hypnotic treatment. Upcoming sections will discuss pain as a psychological event that is moderately plastic and open to suggestion. Research shows that the triggered memory of pain and the expectation of future pain can be as painful as injury-induced pain.

In the 1970s there began to be an interest and upsurge in multidisciplinary pain management. Fordyce,[3] Bonica, and many others were at the forefront of the physicians, scholars, and researchers who moved the field forward in the 1980s. While the ideal was for patients to be holistically treated by all disciplines together, psychological management is still usually done separate from medical treatment. Recently, Turk[4] reviewed outcome data for patients receiving care from interdisciplinary chronic pain and rehabilitation programs (ICPRP) as opposed to other care. He found that pain reduction and activity level of patients in ICPRPs was as good as or better than that of patients receiving standard medical treatment and that iatrogenic complications, medication use, and health care use was less, with more patients returning to work. Other studies compare psychological treatment for chronic pain favorably to more invasive measures and to narcotic use. A recent systematic Cochrane review concluded that cognitive interventions combined with exercise is recommended for chronic low back pain.[5] There is also strong evidence that intensive multidisciplinary biopsychosocial rehabilitation improves function when compared with inpatient or outpatient nonmultidisciplinary treatments.[6] A recent study reconfirms the cost-effectiveness of perioperative hypnosis to patients or to their hospitals.[7] Given the evidence, we may expect that less invasive and less costly treatments may become the preferred options of patients, their providers, and insurance companies. An extensive review of the research[8] found hypnosis to meet the APA's criteria as an effective treatment for pain, and superior to medication.

Hypnotic trance will be explained as a state of mind and its use in behavioral medicine in general will be described. The discussion will include the current understanding of how hypnosis works at the unconscious level in general and for pain relief, citing recent literature on brain mechanisms of pain. Recent research will be outlined, suggesting hypnosis' application to specific types and locations of pain, and some commonly used hypnotic maneuvers to treat them. Even though some studies discuss symptom relief (tension, twitches, allergies, anxiety, rashes) as separate from pain itself, usually symptom relief leads to pain relief down the road. The chapter describes both traditional and newer practices of pain hypnosis, and provides information on certification and training. The chapter is concluded with a discussion on chronic pain, where the emotional suffering related to pain is a notable dynamic.

HYPNOSIS BY DEFINITION

Hypnosis is a process of bypassing the critical thinking cognitive mind to access the unconscious processes. Without the critical thinking filters, the hypnotized person may be more suggestible and more easily influenced by the hypnotist. During hypnotic trance, a person can focus intently on just one aspect of an experience, or dissociate from the experience to the point of losing track of their body and whereabouts. Succinctly, hypnosis is simply a programmed entrance into "trance," which is itself a perfectly normal state that we engage in whenever we are totally absorbed in a task or experience and are not reviewing the characteristics of our experience. Formally, hypnosis is "a social interaction in which one person, designated the subject, responds to suggestions offered by another person, designated the hypnotist, for experiences involving alterations in perception, memory, and voluntary action,"[9] hopefully for the sake of some change the patient desires. Professionals should be thoroughly trained in hypnosis before practicing it, and should work only in the areas of their professional expertise. ASCH and SCEH train and certify professionals in medical hypnosis; certification requires a professional degree in health or mental health and specific training that includes the ethical uses of hypnosis.

Conscious, Unconscious, and Content of Consciousness

A brief review of the conscious and unconscious minds will serve as the groundwork for discussing the mechanisms of hypnosis itself as well as the psychosomatic process of logging an emotional experience as pain.

A. *Consciousness: what you are oriented toward in the present*
   1. *Content of consciousness: perceptions and specific thoughts; what is on your mind and in your thoughts, including what is "on the back burner"*
   2. *Selective consciousness: what you choose to have in the front rather than in the back or periphery of your mind*
B. *Unconscious*
   1. *Long-term memory: which you may or may not access when necessary*
   2. *Short-term memory: which has happened recently*
   3. *Automatic functioning that usually but not always bypasses your conscious mind. This is sometimes called the primary process or body language that demonstrates when you are angry, happy, or frightened. It also includes behavior such as scratching an itch or catching yourself before you fall.*

   4. *Programmed physiology that you have little or no access to in normal thinking state, such as your heart beating, breathing, allergic responses, healing rate, etc.*
   5. *Deeper processes such as the essential self, spiritual self, soul, and body's core identity. Other parts of the self are the immune system, the neurological map, or the body and the core spiritual self.*

We might say that the conscious mind includes awareness and cognition, and the unconscious mind includes everything else, including your physical self. Cognition is a tool to help with survival and with the expression of the essential self; it is a small part of the whole self constellation, in a somewhat figure/ground relationship. The unconscious mind is adaptive and capable of profound change, potentially with both positive and negative outcomes.

When you are "associated" to a situation, you see it through your own eyes, and you are fully present to it; an example of this is the child who is involved in a task but is not monitoring himself and who needs an adult to oversee his behavior. In reflective thinking, you are of two minds at once, contemplating an idea or situation by looking into your unconscious mind to find new perspectives for viewing or approaching it. The conscious mind and the unconscious mind can operate autonomous of one another, in the condition of dissociation (dis-"associated"), occurring when ideas are split off from the normal (associated) experience and when, to some extent, you are not paying attention. When dissociated, you may take a global experience of the situation and break it down into parts, amplifying one part while diminishing concentration on the other part—when, for instance, you notice one aspect of the situation and no longer notice others. You may see the situation and also see yourself in the situation, or you may see the situation differently. This can occur during trauma or during hypnosis; for instance, during surgery, you can dissociate from pain by imagining yourself at the beach and seeing the beach at the same time, or dissociate from a body part during surgery and believe it to be having surgery or recuperating across the room. In an internally directed trance state, the patient may shut off pain and influence healing, immune functions, heart rate, blood flow, and autoimmune responses not commonly accessed in the normal conscious. Again, hypnosis is merely the programmed entrance into trance or dissociation at some level, and hypnotherapy is the programmed entrance into trance for therapeutic purposes.

Actually, the hypnotist or hypnotherapist is merely guiding the patient to self-hypnosis. Unless the state is induced with hypnotic medications or other psychoactive substances, the patient is the one to suspend vigilance, and their ability to do so is likely to depend on: (1) the relationship that they have with the hypnotist, (2) the skill of the hypnotist inducing the trance, (3) the safety of the situation and environment, (4) the patient's level of hypnotizability, (5) the patient's expectancy that they will receive benefit and relief, (6) the patient's need for the trance—pain itself can be a trance state to tap into, and (7) the patient's past experience with trance states, ranging from dissociative disorders leading from experienced trauma, to meditation and past hypnosis training.

Complementarity, the quantum physics concept of relativity, helps explain the use of hypnosis for pain control. Basically, it is impossible to be wholly in one state (fully present and focused in one perspective) and keep the other fully in mind at the same time; the difference is being *in* the moment, versus *thinking about* the moment. When you are fully locked into pain, you cannot get perspective to solve the pain problem; you need to dissociate from the pain somewhat to get a better perspective on it. Once you dissociate from it, you can no longer feel it. The hypnotherapist facilitates the process. Other examples of split consciousness or going back and forth between the conscious and the unconscious minds are the rewriting the endings of dreams (lucid dreaming), remembering that the stove is on while watching television (split concentration), and accessing memories—all of which are normal functioning, but also, in a way, related to hypnosis. These principles of trance and hypnotic states are important to understanding hypnotic pain management. The more access to the unconscious mind one can gain by self or guided hypnosis, to imagine or create another way of being or feeling, the more control of pain and physiological symptoms one may have.

CENTRAL MECHANISMS

Central Mechanisms of Hypnosis

Hypnosis has been viewed as magical, energy-related, sleep-related (Braid and Pavlov), psychosomatic, pathological (Charcot), dissociative,[10–12] and the consequence of normal suggestibility[13]—all of which are partly true. Recent brain imaging research using functional magnetic resonance imaging (fMRI) and positron emission tomography (PET) shed more light on the process. In general, the studies show that there are many brain areas involved in the hypnotic process, including simultaneous increased activities in some areas and selective shutting down of others. Some studies look at performance on certain tasks (learning, verbal, auditory) and in certain situations (pain, for example) before and during hypnosis, while others compare high and low hypnotizable patients or subjects.

Clinicians as far back as Freud have known that some people are more suggestible or susceptible to hypnosis than others. About 15% of people are highly suggestible, 65% are moderately, and 20% are not very suggestible.[11] While hypnotizability is a fairly stable trait and not related to intelligence, it can be taught and also modified according to situation, hypnotist skill, patient motivation level and expectancies, induction and trance relevance to the patient, and patient physical and psychological state. Experienced hypnotists help patients lower their vigilance by setting the appropriate conditions and by sensing and identifying the way their patients unconsciously process information.[14,15]

High and Low Hypnotizability

Over the last two decades, Gruzelier[16] has been involved in numerous experiments studying high and low hypnotizable brain responses to experimental tasks during pain episodes and other situations. His studies seemed to show that in a hypnotic state, subjects can selectively ignore what is in their perceptual field while still knowing what is there. This is important regarding pain, in that often the patient's focus is as much on misery and helplessness as it is on their physiology; the clinician may not be able to change the physical condition, but they may help the patient to selectively disregard the pain and the suffering. Gruzelier[16] found that, in general, highly hypnotizable subjects exhibit more neurophysiological and cognitive flexibility,[17] which include "superior abilities in absorption, creativity, dissociation, attention and vividness of imagery; these are all well known correlates of hypnotizability." Regarding hemisphere involvement, high hypnotizables under hypnosis demonstrate more right hemispheric frontolimbic influence. Further, there is more neuronal flexibility going from the right to left and from the left to right hemispheres, and, according to Gruzelier, "in stimulus repetitions, highs showed a shift from an initial right-sided preference, in line with the right hemisphere's role in global orienting, to a left hemisphere preference, in line with the left-sided involvement in the local orienting process,"[16,18] indicating absorption. One study found greater informational exchange in the prefrontal areas of highly hypnotizable patients during hypnosis.[18] High hypnotizables were better able to inhibit pain from their conscious awareness. fMRIs showed them to have a significantly larger rostrum area, the corpus callosum area involved in transferring problem solving information between the left and the right hemispheres. Gruzelier emphasized another difference between highs and lows during an auditory attention task: pre-hypnosis, highs increased ERP N100 activity (engaging frontal attentional circuits), while lows had little activity, indicating distraction; under hypnosis, highs had little activity, indicating disengagement of the frontal process, or distraction, while lows' activity progressively increased.[19]

Other studies involving mental tasks showed increased activity in the anterior cingulate under hypnosis in highs more than in lows (indicating that they were monitoring the task), and a decrease in the inferior frontal gyrus activity (indicating that they were disengaging from executive functioning).[16] In other words, highs under hypnosis are relatively better at actively not paying attention to what they still know is in the field; they seem to let go of attending it. This seems to represent frontolimbic inhibition on the left side and a shift to the right brain, engaging the patients' ability to feel or imagine things different than they were before. Hypnosis involves activation of the hippocampus and inhibition of the amygdala activity at the same time.[20] A fractal analysis of electroencephalographs (EEGs) in patients under hypnosis showed dissociation of centralized activity and a loss of the normal patterns of integrated physiological responses, which results in a trance state.[21]

Central Mechanisms of Hypnotic Analgesia

Price, Barber, and Hawkins[22] provided a statistical path analysis to show four necessary elements of hypnotic analgesia—relaxation; absorption; disorientation from time, space, or sense of self; and automaticity—and their relationship order. Automaticity is the condition in which the suggestion bypasses cognition and leads directly to the sensation or experience, such that the suggestion of sinking into a warm bathtub will allow you to relax your back muscles and smile, without your having to think about it or consciously relax or lower your shoulders. Studies show that imagining heat actually increases blood flow that relaxes muscles, thereby validating automaticity. The principle is similar to direct suggestion and to suggestion through expectancy and placebo.

Some suggest that hypnotic analgesia works by activating endogenous pain inhibitory systems that descend to the spinal cord, where it prevents transmission to the brain of pain coming from nociception. One study evoked experimental pain in subjects by stimulating the sural nerve, causing the nociceptive flexion reflex (NFR).[23] Hypnotic suggestion could both increase and decrease the NFR, leading the researchers to conclude that hypnotic suggestion actually controlled the response at the spinal level by activating descending antinociceptive mechanisms. However, this does not appear to stem from the opioid system alone,[24,25] in that the administration of naloxone, an opioid antagonist, does not reverse hypnotic analgesia. It would seem, then, that there are nonopiate cortical fugal or brain-to-spinal-cord descending control mechanisms.

The relationship between pain and hypnotic or dissociative faculties of the brain are made clearer in recent studies of complex regional pain syndrome (CRPS), which begins with excruciating pain and can progress to include dramatic physiological changes and neglect or dissociation from the painful limb. According to studies, within moments of an injury or absence of sensory input, there is a reorganization of the somatosensory cortex representation of the injured limb that leads the patient to behaviorally isolate or "favor" the limb. fMRI studies show that the degree of change in the somatosensory cortex is directly related to the degree of perceived pain.[26,27] Even when there is painless stimulation in the CRPS patient's uninjured counterpart limb, there is pain-related activation all through the brain, including cerebral, motor, parietal, bilateral S2, frontal lobe, and the anterior and posterior parts of the anterior cingulate cortex (aACC and pACC).[28] When the CRPS pain lessens, however, both the cortical reorganization and impaired tactile sensation return to normal.[29,30] Wobst[31] summarizes the PET, fMRI, and evoked potential studies on pain, concluding that the ACC, insular, frontal cortices, amygdala, S1 and S2, and the lateral thalamus are all involved in pain when the body processes the pain in regard to location and duration. The studies show that the affective (cognitive and evaluative) components of pain are processed in the medial thalamus and progress back to the ACC.[32–35]

At the same time, other areas of the brain work to calm and heal; following the awareness of physical or emotional pain, the right ventral prefrontal cortex is involved with soothing responses that are triggered by soothing hypnotic therapeutic suggestions and messages, which proceed to help the right parietal lobe to reorganize and to perceive the body intact and comfortable (see section later on CRPS and phantom limb pain).

In a hypnosis study of experimentally induced pain, high and low hypnotizables responded differently.[36] Under hypnosis with the low hypnotizable subjects, increased pain ratings corresponded with increased frontal gamma oscillations; however, gamma oscillations did not increase in high hypnotizable subjects as the pain ratings increased. The gamma frequencies were noted primarily in the bilateral anterior cingulum (within the limbic system), which supports the understanding of pain being tied in with a complex of emotional responses. The mid-cingulate cortex may modulate and influence sensory, affective, cognitive, and behavioral aspects of nociception at least in the hypnotic state.[37] Raij et al.[38] used fMRI to compare brain mechanistic responses to noxious stimulation perceptions versus hypnotically hallucinated pain; they found that both real and imagined pain produced similar brain responses, although perception of hallucinated pain was less than the actual induced pain. In both cases, there was activity in the rostral and perigenual ACC and in the pericingulate regions of the medial prefrontal cortex. They conclude that the medial prefrontal cortex is involved in monitoring real and hallucinated pain which then influences how noxious stimuli are experienced and processed. A study exposed subjects to pain (1) in the waking state, (2) with hypnotic relaxation, or (3) with hypnosis suggesting depersonalization (out of body experiences).[39] All the subjects showed somatosensory, insular, and cerebral activation with pain; however, the depersonalization group showed less activation in the contralateral somatosensory cortex, parietal cortex and prefrontal cortex, putamen, and ipsilateral amygdala. DePascalis, Magurano, and Bellusci[40] and others have shown somatosensory event-related increase during pain, followed by a reduction when subjects were administered hypnotic analgesia. DePascalis[41] found that highs experiencing hypnotic analgesia showed smaller total, delta, and beta amplitudes in the right hemisphere; they experienced more theta activity in the left hemisphere during pain and more in the right hemisphere with hypnotic analgesia, decreasing both the sympathetic activity and the overall experience of pain. Meier et al[42] showed that hypnotic hypalgesia decreased subjects' experimental pain; when suggestions about increasing pain were made, somatosensory evoked potentials, auditory evoked potentials, and EEGs remained unchanged from the hypalgesic state, indicating that the physical response to pain and its affective component can indeed be separated. Thus, hypnotizability level certainly appears to impact the ultimate outcome of hypnosis in general as well as for pain management.

PAIN AS A PLASTIC EXPERIENCE

Why is hypnosis particularly appropriate for acute and chronic pain management? How can it be that Jensen and Barber[43] showed hypnotic analgesia to be more effective than other analgesics, including morphine, for reducing pain? We can begin to

answer it by viewing pain as a psychosomatic event and a complex interweaving of physiological, psychological events, and the memories and expectations of like experiences, interacting on two-way streets through the body. In other words, it is a perception or conclusion derived from a real physiological signal, expectations, and memories of similar past experiences; the perception itself generates feedback to the body. Physical injury and disease cannot fully predict the amount of perceived pain a patient experiences; other determining factors are anxiety and trauma, context of the injury, depression, expectation, social support, and numerous other personality factors and cognitive styles. Interestingly, as is discussed elsewhere in this chapter, those who are highly hypnotizable are often the most likely to experience psychosomatic symptoms of the overlap of psychological interpretation and nociception, but they are also most likely to benefit by hypnosis and other well applied psychological treatment.

Chapman[44] describes nociception as an unconscious messaging about tissue damage through the nervous system, not to be equated with pain, which is the conscious awareness of that nociception. He defines pain as "a complex, compelling unpleasant bodily awareness normally associated with tissue trauma." One purpose of pain is to engage the cognitive problem solving part of the brain in a plan to resolve the tissue damage. Biologically, pain is a cascade of neurotransmitter and biochemical responses to nociception involving the hypothalamic-pituitary-adrenal (HPA)-axis and the limbic system and causing changes in blood pressure and blood sugar, serotonin, and norepinephrine levels, thereby affecting concentration, mood, behavior, healing, and sleep. Pain can interfere with psychological and physical well-being. When the nociception is not medically treated and stopped, the body's unconscious responses to it can continue on to cause permanent change and damage in other physiological and psychological systems. At the same time, psychological stress and suffering can lead to the same cascade of physiological stress responses and even lead to the construction of the sense of pain where no damage exists, which helps to explain why some events, physical or otherwise, cause pain to some people more than others.[44]

Hypnotherapy for pain aims to disengage pain from suffering and soothe both the physical and emotional stress. In the case of acute pain during surgery or procedures and after injury, the patient's focus can be directed away from the experience, or the experience can be reframed as beneficial and healing, and one not to be feared. Directing the patient's focus away from the pain and back into them is also a way to alleviate suffering, in that the pain would then be differentiated from the patient's sense of self. Whereas pain is stressful, hypnotherapy is a relaxing and comforting experience that induces brain waves and levels of autonomic functioning that soothe the sympathetic nervous system and enhance healing and resistance to disease.[45] By changing the cognitive mind's and body's responses to nociception, patients may simultaneously alleviate pain, promote healing, and learn to manage future pain better, all within the same cost-effective applications. For a detailed review of techniques according to medical problems, see Brown and Fromme[46] and Hammond.[47]

TESTING HYPNOTIZABILITY

Hypnotizability level does appear to influence hypnotic pain management and the outcome of hypnosis in general, although there are ways for the experienced hypnotist to work with it successfully. Researchers may be more likely than clinicians to use hypnotizability scales before engaging in subject or patient interactions. Some say that testing for hypnotizability may actually interfere with the research, because testing itself is hypnotic training and subjects become more hypnotizable with practice.[48] Nonetheless, when hypnotizability is very important, such as before attempting intraoperative hypnotic analgesia, it may be wise to use the Stanford Hypnotic Susceptibility Scale (SHSS), Form C,[49] which is a fairly long (over an hour) and stringent test with a broad sampling of hypnotic suggestions. The Stanford Hypnotic Clinical Scale (SHCS)[50] is a shorter version that gives scores for adults in 25 minutes; there are also versions for children. The Hypnotic Induction Profile (HIP)[51] gives scores for adults and children in 5–15 minutes; it is based upon a simple procedure (the eye roll) that goes beyond suggestibility to autonomic function. The Harvard Group Scale[52] may be read or administered by tape recording, and should be used when there is a need to maintain a pool of subjects of varying suggestibility. The Waterloo-Stanford Group Scale of Hypnotic Susceptibility (WSGC)[53] is a group version of the Stanford Hypnotic Susceptibility Scale, Form C that may best be used for measuring suggestibility. The Hypnotic State Assessment Questionnaire (HSAQ)[54] assesses patients' hypnotic state at one point in time, and may be used during clinical or experimental sessions. Weitzenhoffer[55] points out that suggestibility and hypnotizability are different and that some research has failed because subjects were not really hypnotized, but rather merely followed suggestions. To be sure of hypnotizability, he recommends administering the Stanford Profile Scales of Hypnotic Susceptibility, I and II,[49] or at least one of them, and the next best assurance that the patient is in a hypnotic state would be to use a score of 10 as a cut-off on SHSS:C.

Lynn, Council, and Green[56] outline various hypnotherapists views on assessing hypnotizability levels. Many[48] object to the use of such tests, stating that they are obtrusive, undermine the therapeutic relationship, and do not adequately measure hypnotic capacity or take into consideration change in hypnotizability over time. Other options to using tests are to assess the patient's success with the first induction[57] or to use a conversational assessment of hypnotizability.[58] A series of questions can give the clinician a good idea of how easy it will be to get a patient into a hypnotic state; for example, questions about past hypnotic states or trauma, dissociative tendencies in various realms of life, right/left brain characteristics.

A scale that may be informative to a psychologist treating pain patients is the Tellegen Absorption Scale,[59] a 34-item true-false test that correlates well with hypnotic susceptibility. Wickramasekera[60] found that patients scoring high on absorption scales or tests of hypnotic susceptibility and also scoring high on neuroticism as measured by the Marlowe-Crown[61] were more likely to develop psychosomatic pain or symptoms, by dissociating traumatic or undesirable experiences and converting them into somatic symptoms or pain, creating what Damasio termed "psychological markers." Wickram developed a 25-item scale to be used to identify patients who were more likely to somatize. He points to the neural flexibility and "ideational fluency" that Gruzeleir[16] suggested was related to a propensity to dissociate that can leave one vulnerable to schizotypy, affective distress, mood disorders, and somatic markers or memories that stay beyond conscious awareness. In simpler terms, highly hypnotizable patients are more likely to create a somatic marker for a psychological event, and are more likely to trigger a memory of previous pain when they experience a new pain.[44] A meta-analysis[62] shows classic, modern, and mixed forms of hypnosis to be effective for treating psychosomatic disorders (those which meet the criteria for somatoform disorder), which would include both hypersensitivity to pain, hyperawareness of symptoms and to body processes in general, and the transduction or conversion of emotions and memories into somatic markers. This is remarkable given the range of disorders and symptoms including: tinnitus, duodenal ulcers, asthma, irritable bowel syndrome (IBS), osteoarthritis, chronic pain, and dyspepsia. Also, DuHamel et al.[63] found that their high hypnotizable burn patients had significantly more intrusive avoidance and arousal symptoms with their injury-related trauma. Roelofs, Hoogduin, and Keijsers[64] showed that they could use hypnosis to induce catalepsy and altered perception of

the cataleptic limb in high hypnotizable subjects, suggesting the formation of conversion disorders or psychosomatic illness. Younger et al.[65] show a linear correlation between hypnotizability and somatic complaints commonly assumed to be of a psychosomatic nature.

CURRENT RESEARCH AND APPLICATIONS OF MEDICAL HYPNOSIS FOR PAIN

The applications of hypnosis to medicine are numerous and go beyond the scope of this chapter, as not all involve pain; Table 84-1 outlines common applications of hypnosis in medicine in general. Information on the effect of hypnosis on emotional pain and on physical pain, related or not to medical conditions, is undoubtedly not best found in the medical research, but rather in books, articles, and trainings offered by the clinicians who regularly use it but who are not researchers. This is in part because every effective hypnotherapy session is, in research terms, an N of 1. However, research in hypnosis and its clinical use in medicine are increasing, due to the recent surge in brain research and the increased understanding of what pain is, and due to increased attention to the number of the people in chronic pain and in health care utilization and costs. Hypnosis research is important because, without published results, it is difficult for hospitals and insurance companies to justify reimbursing and endorsing its use in medicine.

Earlier research on psychological treatment of medical conditions often compares such treatment to standard care practices with and without the addition of cognitive behavioral therapy (CBT). CBT often consists of a standardized program that is more applicable to research than hypnosis. CBT differs from hypnosis in that the therapist intends to speak directly to the patient's cognitive conscious mind, without deliberately sending any direct or indirect messages to his/her unconscious. A hypnosis session may likely include behavioral suggestions in and out of trance, and messages to the conscious and the unconscious mind at the same time. Both may include homework. Kirsch, Montgomery, and Sapirstein[57] looked at 18 studies of CBT with and without additional hypnosis. The addition of hypnosis to CBT substantially enhanced treatment outcome, such that the patients who received additional hypnosis did better than 70% of those with just CBT treatment. In most cases the authors mean CBT administered in the medium of hypnosis.

As we go on to discuss the research on medical hypnosis, there

TABLE 84.1

COMMON APPLICATIONS OF HYPNOSIS IN MEDICINE

Headaches	Smoking cessation
Muscle cramps	Eating disorders
Pain disorders such as CRPS	Perioperative preparation
Chronic diseases	Post-operative pain and
Burns	recuperation
Minor procedures – analgesic or anesthetic	Allergies
	Wound care
Colonoscopies	Hypertension
Blood drawing	Chronic disease management
Dentistry	Cancer related anxiety and
Surgery – anesthetic	depression
Cancer	Nausea and emesis
Labor and delivery	Dental and needle phobia
Bone growth and healing	Skin rashes and warts
	Immune and autoimmune disorders

are some points to bear in mind. First, we expect there to be quite a difference between the methods and benefits of hypnosis in clinical practice and the process of studying it in research. We must assume that clinicians in their office would not exactly follow a research protocol, and that they would modify even a hypnotic script to fit their patient's situation. Also, pain hypnosis is used primarily for chronic pain, less often for procedural and least for surgical pain, where hypnosis is usually used as an adjunct to medicine. Under strict standards, for hypnosis to be considered the dependent variable in research, it must deliver suggestions that could not be just as well delivered to the patient cognitive-behaviorally (as in telling the patient what to do). However, some highly hypnotizable or well-trained patients have ready access to the unconscious mind and absorb even a CBT message quite deeply or literally; a good example of this is the patient who testifies that they always gets all the side effects mentioned on the inserts of their medications. Finally, most patients in severe pain or in traumatic conditions are already in a trance and in a manner of speaking hypnotized, so that the comparison between CBT and hypnosis is muddy at best. In effect, the strict standards of the research may dilute the power of hypnosis. Fortunately, clinical success with hypnosis does not depend wholly on the results of research studies.

Efficacy and Effectiveness

To move the practice of hypnosis in medicine along, research on effectiveness (how hypnosis works in the real world, in quasi-experimental design) should be as methodical as the research on efficacy (how a technique works within the controlled research situation).[66-69] A 1982 article[70] reported skepticism about the effect of hypnosis on pain due to the lack of controlled studies comparing hypnosis with credible placebos or other treatment methods. Hawkins[71] updated that article with a review of research articles up to the year 2000, and was able to conclude that hypnosis is effective for pain related to cancer, burns, gastrointestinal problems, and for invasive medical procedures. He also noted that poor-quality reviews were not more likely to produce positive conclusions about efficacy, and that there was a paucity of good studies in the areas of obstetrics, headache, and chronic pain. Montgomery, DuHamel, and Redd[8] did a meta-analysis of pain analgesia studies using healthy subjects and patient samples and taking into consideration hypnotizability levels; they concluded hypnosis to be effective in both arenas for 75% of their population. Hypnotic analgesia compared favorably in effect to standard care and to attention.[72] Hypnosis has compared favorably to empathic attention[73] and to autogenic training (AT) for psychosomatic and medical disorders.[74] Yapko,[48] however, suggests that AT is in itself a hypnotic induction and that the comparison of the two treatments presents a problem.

The research process itself raises some concerns. One is that research studies focus on the precise content of the intervention, not how it can be flexibly adapted to the real life patient situation. Another concern is the outcome measure itself: we intend for patients to be noticing pain less, but then we ask them to tune into it and rate it at the end of the study. Also, many studies do not account for hypnotizability, which would color research results. Another issue is expectancy—the patient's expectation that hypnosis will resolve their pain—which seems to predict pain relief. Jensen and Patterson[75] suggest that most of hypnosis studies lack adequate controls for expectancy and placebo effects, even though the studies find that hypnotic analgesia is effective in treating chronic pain. Clearly, raising the patient's expectancy is a good thing, as are raising their levels of self efficacy and curiosity about finding new ways to cope, and encouraging the placebo effect. A study looking at changes in various psychological responses to pain postoperatively and after 3 months found hypnosis to be effective; the positive effect was not significantly

related to hypnotic ability, concentration of treatment (e.g., daily vs. up to weekly), or initial response pattern to treatment, but it was moderately related to the participants' expectancy ratings of treatment after the first session.[76]

All of this being said, Amundson, Aladdin, and Gill[77] point out that research probably underestimates the effectiveness of clinical hypnosis. Many are concerned about the randomized controlled trial (RCT) approach to hypnosis research that is so distinct from the patient-centered and cooperative relationship based nature of clinical hypnotherapy.[78,79] Clinical one-on-one hypnotic sessions take a patient's unique issues and personal variables into consideration, and scripted or standardized protocols cannot address the psychological and emotional issues intertwined with the pain. Spiegel and Kahn[80] discuss the difficulties inherent in using an outside hypnotherapist as the interventionist in research or therapy, which lacks the all-important therapeutic relationship; they also point out that the relationship between the hypnotherapist and the treating physician is important. It would seem that hypnotic protocols would be most effective when designed for each patient by a therapist who is interactively responsive to the patient; according to one extensive study, 30% of therapy outcome is based on the therapeutic relationship, even when the treatment is medication, while another 15% is due to expectancy.[81] Nonetheless, research showing the effectiveness of hypnosis must be stringent if it is to be widely available in medicine and adequately reimbursed by insurance companies. In fact, when comparing the delivery of hypnotic analgesia with the hypnotist present, manualized protocols, standardized audiotapes, or individualized audiotapes (as would be prepared for patients in clinical practice), a meta-analysis indicates that any delivery is better than none[82]; however, since clinicians understand the importance of being fully present and flexible in a hypnotic session, more research in this area is needed. Interesting delivery formats are now on the horizon. Patterson, Wiechman, Jensen et al.[83] have attempted to improve absorption that may be missing with audiotapes by creating virtual reality (VR) computer-based presentations that immerse patients in a three dimensional computer-generated environment, to absorb the patients' attention and divert it away from the pain experience. VR induces and sustains a hypnotic state without a therapist. Questions arise as to whether this intervention satisfies the research definitions for hypnosis, and whether the same effect could be accomplished by naturalistic absorption or with audiotapes alone.

Here is an example of a clinical application of hypnosis that is distinct from a research protocol. A female patient in her 30s had been extensively evaluated for her deep, sharp right side pelvic pain that came on for 15 to 20 minutes as often as every hour, even during the night. She rarely had pain when she was on birth control pills, other than after sexual intercourse. There was a small area of endometriosis, successfully removed, and one cyst that ruptured, but otherwise no diagnoses explained the pain. She and her husband were anxious to be off birth control pills in order to conceive, and she also exhibited generalized high vigilance. She asked a hypnotherapist to help find any unconscious motivations for the pain. She is highly hypnotic and motivated, with high expectancy. The therapist worked interactively with her on a wide range of techniques to find what worked uniquely for her in managing and accepting the nerve pain, which she practiced self hypnotically at home. Hypnosis helped with vigilance, and therapy helped other issues about trust. The therapeutic relationship supported the work on hyper vigilance, trust, and specific fears that related to pregnancy.

Clinically, and in research, even when patients do not receive pain relief with hypnotic analgesia, they seem to receive satisfaction from the sessions. Jensen et al.[84] reported that out of the benefits listed by subjects in their pain hypnosis study, 23% reported pain-related benefits as the reason for satisfaction, 58% reported other than pain benefits, 13% were neutral, and

8% reported a negative experience. Subjects cited increased sense of control and positive shifts in perspective, with no subjects reporting dissatisfaction. Dawson et al.[85] have said that pain treatment satisfaction in general has more to do with the provider–patient relationship than pain-related outcomes.

We will briefly mention two other variables. Both direct and indirect hypnotic suggestions for pain or symptom relief seem to be effective (e.g., progressively relaxing muscles versus imagining lying on a beach at a peaceful island, which would warm and relax muscles). In regards to whether hypnosis is more effective when labeled as hypnosis or introduced using other terms, Jensen and Patterson[75] concluded that in the short-term there is probably no difference, but over time, there may be a benefit for the patient in attributing improvement to hypnosis or self-hypnosis.

Review of Research Studies According to Pain Problems or Situations

Research on hypnosis has waxed and waned over the years and varied in focus. Many of the new studies are physician driven and are looking for nonmedicinal, noninvasive self-management treatments that improve medical outcome. Even though pain is common to most medical disorders and procedures, each carries its own unique cluster of symptoms and might indicate a different psychological or hypnotic approach for healing and management, differing lengths of treatment time, and varying depths of trance. Research and clinical reports show the importance of matching the appropriate protocol to the type of pain experienced.[86] The following sections will outline recent research on hypnosis when used as one of the treatment modes, grouped according to medical condition. Under each heading, research findings, primarily since the year 2000, are followed by some suggestions and techniques for use in clinical practice. Most of the articles address acute and procedural pain. Hopefully, the sections will serve as a background and a resource for hypnotherapists and clinicians, and for those planning to embark upon such medical research.

Perioperative and Procedural Uses

As described previously, hypnotic analgesia was first reported as successful in surgery before there were any chemical anesthetic alternatives. In this century, while there are sporadic reports of its successful use as the only anesthetic,[87] it is now most often used as an adjunct to chemical anesthetics or to analgesics. Studies have looked at improved well-being or enhanced healing and recovery time after surgery or procedures and reduction in hospital costs. Hypnosis successfully targets a number of surgical and postsurgical variables, such as anxiety, blood pressure, and patients' sense of control over their feelings[88]; pain, nausea, vomiting, blood loss, wound healing[89]; pain, knee strength, edema, inflammation, and postsurgical anxiety after anterior cruciate ligament (ACL) surgery[90]; both objectively and subjectively rated healing, when level of hypnotizability was controlled[91]; postoperative anxiety and pain level, even after a single session of hypnosis before surgery[92]; pain and distress, where the effects were mediated by patient expectancy[93]; shorter hospital stays; and less parenteral narcotic use.[94] A study showed hypnosis to lessen procedural pain and result in a speedier medical procedure; positive results did not correlate with hypnotizability, possibly because the hypnotist facilitated self hypnosis before and during the procedure, such that subjects received individualized treatment.[95]

Three studies used hypnosis as it might be used clinically. Enqvist and Fischer[96] aimed to reduce preoperative stress that might influence healing and recovery from a surgery, specifically to reduce medication use, inflammation, infection, postoperative pain, and edema. Using one surgeon who was blind to the grouping, patients were given a 20 minute tape containing an induction, suggestions of finding a safe place, having control of bodily responses to surgery, dissociating, and alleviating pain. Subjects were also asked to use their chosen way of relaxing for 2 minutes, and to let soft music bring them back to awareness. In a controlled study, Dyas[97] used a conversational induction containing positive language patterns and suggestions that included counting down (into trance), relaxing breathing, finding a safe place, and dissociating from the surgical procedure; reinforcing words were used during surgery, and posthypnotic suggestions addressed continued relaxation and comfort. Another controlled study used music with or without the audio taped voice of a hypnotherapist during surgery under general anesthesia[98]; the addition of hypnosis was beneficial, and the author suggests the results would be even more significant using individualized tapes and in situations where less anesthesia is used.

Obviously both physical and emotional pain during surgery can present a problem, as pain is both traumatic and stressful and relief from it can improve healing, save money, and make for happier patients and surgeons. The most important patient variable to consider for use in surgery as the sole or primary anesthesia seems to be hypnotizability. To be sure the patient is highly hypnotizable and can go into a deep state, stringent testing should be done.[49,56] The sole use of hypnosis should be reserved for the patient who is highly hypnotizable, experienced with hypnosis, and for whom the payoff is likely to be great. Preoperative preparation for surgery described by Kessler and Dane[99] is also effective and satisfying to patients. Kessler found that the most significant variable related to the anxiety in surgery that can affect the surgical outcome variables related previously was the expectation of negative surgical outcomes, coming from previous experiences of either the patient or to those close to them; he designed a short screening questionnaire to identify patients who are in most need of hypnotic preparation (Kessler, personal communication, 1996). Subsequent perioperative hypnotic treatment can be done with any level of trance, even conversational,[58] to assure that the anxiety level regarding the procedure is optimally low and that the mind set is positive; this can speed up healing and recovery and allay concerns about procedure and recovery processes. During such perioperative preparations I have twice discovered male patients who fully expected to die because they were grieving the death of fathers who died during the same procedure or at their like chronological age; we took the time to work through those issues before surgery took place.

The most important factors regarding preparation for surgery involve positive expectancy and the positive interpretation of the surgical events and sounds the patient may unconsciously notice. The optimal protocol will include some critical details of the surgery that the patient can interpret positively: "when you feel the surgeon touch your stomach with a knife, that will be an indication that he is finding the best place on your belly for the smallest opening to allow him to remove the part of your intestine that needs to come out so that he can reattach the healthy tissue and allow your intestines to work normally again" and "when you feel a little tugging, that will be an indication that he is closing the opening with a nice line of little stitches," "since you will be hungry from not eating before surgery, you can begin to look forward to your favorite food soon after surgery," and "you can let your thoughts be on that beach you love so much, and you can listen only to sentences from your own doctor and that begin with your first name." In that way, the surgeon can request the patient to lower their blood pressure, divert blood away from the surgical site, and the surgeon can prepare the patient for any changes in the surgical plan, and even imbed suggestions to lose interest in unhealthy food or cigarettes. For a review of other "patient-friendly" terms see Bennett and Disbrow.[100]

Complex Regional Pain Syndrome

Complex regional pain syndrome (CRPS) is one of two pain syndromes responsive to hypnosis that are particularly interesting because they demonstrate the brain mechanisms of pain. CRPS is a complicated condition wherein the pain is disproportionate to the injury or event leading up to it; the continuing acute-level pain has no confirmed mechanism.[101] Even when there is neuropathology, the symptoms, which can lead to muscle atrophy and bone demineralization, appear to be sympathetically driven. Treatment usually includes some psychotherapy to manage anxiety and often to disclose a series of emotional events that trigger a flight/flight or psychophysiologically defensive response. The psychological meanings attached to a nociception or to perceived pain may trigger the brain to temporarily rewrite the neurosensory map of the pain area. This in turn leads to a relative neglect syndrome of that limb, which can establish, in lay terms, a "cry for help" in the form of pain and distress symptoms.[26,102,103]

Treatment should include psychologically working through the incidents in the patient's life that led to the need for the defensiveness,[104,105] addressing anxiety and stress management, and counteracting the neglect of the injured limb in order to reintegrate it back into the body. This can be done using mental imagery,[106] desensitization training,[107] or hypnosis, which can accomplish all of the above at the same time. The process of neglect is a dissociative process beginning at a deep level. Given other work on hypnotizability and psychosomatic disorders, we can hypothesize that highly hypnotizable people may be more likely to develop CRPS under the right conditions, and also assume that hypnosis would more readily help them resolve the complex syndrome.

Phantom Limb Pain

The other pain disorder responding to psychologically addressing brain mechanisms is phantom limb pain. Pain in an amputated limb can come from damaged nerve endings that are at the stump or that connect with the neurons in the spinal cord. It can also come from a change in the somatosensory cortex map of the body that results either from lack of sensory input from the missing or paralyzed limb, or from a peripheral nerve injury that leads to lack of sensation.[108] This may lead to a neurological need or a cry out to find the missing limb that takes the form of pain sensation.[109]

Long before there were fMRI studies, Erickson said "If you can have phantom limb pain you can have phantom limb pleasure"; implying the power of the unconscious mind to change the interpretation of information from the periphery or the somatosensory cortex, from negative to positive. The patient can do this with self-hypnosis or with deep trance hypnotherapy, to resolve pain by creating a more positive mind/body messaging system (to counteract pain) and a better transfer of information between the cognitive and the unconscious areas of the brain (this may counteract neglect due to changes in the somatosensory mapping). Giraux and Sirigu[110] have patients imagine that they are still using the missing or paralyzed limb to relieve pain. This is similar to the positive rehabilitative effects found when asking patients to imagine doing the physical therapy if they are not yet ready to actually do it. Flor et al.[111] had patients touch the stump for sensory stimulation; both studies[110,111] demonstrated pain relief. This works along the same lines as having CRPS patients gently stroke and soothe (desensitize) their limbs that were previously too painful to touch, in order to restore the somatosensory map that was altered due to excruciating pain.[112] Evidence for the relationship between the somatosensory cortex and pain comes from research where the somatosensory map was reorganized back to the original somatosensory map by using an electrical prosthetic limb[113] or by use of a mirror-image of the remaining limb to "trick" the mind into thinking there were two functioning limbs.[114] Hypnosis may also be used to accomplish the end goal of resolving the need to find the missing limb. Older and more traditional hypnotic trances for phantom pain may be found in Hammond.[47]

This author used hypnosis to assist a young college student patient who had lost his leg in an automobile accident. He felt positional pain leading him to believe that his leg was bent in a painful position under his body. First, we discussed the actual cause of the pain as a somatosensory reorganization that was his mind's first attempt to help him survive that he could now revise; this mini-lecture was partly informational and partly a hypnotic confusion technique and an induction into trance. He was guided to imagine moving the leg to a more comfortable position and then soothing it so that it would recover from the bent position. This reduced some but not all the pain. In the next session, we used a technique of connecting spiritually with the limb as a valuable part of himself.[112] He was hypnotically guided to bring his attention into his leg ("go down your leg to the injury") and gently nurse and soothe the injury. He was guided to recognize that his leg was a valuable part of himself that he could always have relationship with (as he did with elders who had passed on) and he was guided to watch his leg go to a spiritual place to rest outside of his body where he knew it would be safe in the universe and would wait for the rest of his body in the future at the end of his life. He was then guided to visualize the perimeter (the map) of his body at present (without the leg), and to see and feel the body moving without the leg, and to practice this in his mind, free from pain. His guided imagery had him sensing himself going to class and doing in the future the things he had done in the past. This lengthy set of sessions helped with the majority of his pain; his keen focus on getting back to his life and on to his active career certainly helped him to take positive suggestions. The treatment is in line with the research on the brain mechanisms discussed previously and in line with trends toward success reported by Oakley et al.[115]

Burns

There is a relatively long history of using hypnosis for burn pain, which can be very intense for an extended period of time. Wound care procedures necessary for recovery from burns is painful as well, and pain medication usually does not cover all of the pain. Burn pain is often severe enough to evoke a negative trauma-related trance state in itself, if not shock, at the very same time that a positive mind set is important for recovery. As mentioned previously, distraction is a useful pain management technique for certain situations, but hypnosis appears to afford more pain relief than distraction alone during dressing changes. Frenay[116] also found it more effective for pain reduction than stress reducing strategies for decreasing pain and anxiety during wound care; in that study, the wording was individualized according to the hypnotherapist's observations and their judgment of the patient's clinical needs. One case study has experimented with immersive virtual reality (VR) (mentioned earlier in this chapter).[83] In that study, patients engaged in the VR during wound care; those who remained with the program enjoyed the experience, had no medication side effects, and their pain and anxiety significantly dropped with the VR.

Clinicians will appreciate the work of Ewin,[117–119] a teaching surgeon and psychiatrist who, in addition to using hypnosis during procedures and surgery, also used hypnotic imagery to prevent the symptom formation after skin is burned. He would immediately give suggestions to counteract the body's response to a burn (reddening and blistering) such as swimming in a cold stream in the evening, and he took advantage of the trauma-induced trance state after a burn incident. I used the technique for a hand burn resulting from picking up a frying pan that had been on the stove. I imagined moving my hand in a cool mountain stream visited during childhood, and when that cold was fully re-experienced, I imagined a sequence of events that included swimming in a pool that day, and moved through time to the very near future (watching TV in the next room), skipping the episode of the burn completely; I rehearsed the sequence a few times, letting the unconscious mind do the work of deleting the burn experience. Also, to regain my body's trust and prevent avoidance or resistance in the future, I immediately telepathically sent my hand an apology and an assurance about taking better care of the hand from then on.

For debridement and healing of burns, good techniques might include hallucinating anesthesia or numbness in the area, and displacing the limb or area of the body that is in pain to another side of the room, or to a special imaginary healing place, so that the body can rest easy and be ready for its return after trance; trance can be extended by posthypnotic suggestion to last as long as is necessary. There may be a place as well for amnesia for the more painful and traumatic events of the accident, which would have to be addressed in trance individually. Trance phenomenon will allow for the conscious and unconscious minds to work together to know that an accident occurred while conveniently forgetting about parts of it, both at the same time; it is also possible for a patient to know they are being treated for an injury and to forget the pain, both at the same time.

Dentistry

Hypnosis has been successfully resolving pain and anxiety surrounding dental work for over 80 years, and was arguably used as much for dental work as for other purposes through World War II. Kay Thompson, a dentist who was also an Ericksonian hypnotherapist, pointed out potential psychosomatic element of pain in the oral cavity, as the mouth is the first infant connection to the mother, the first source of gratification, and the first experience of getting attention to one's needs (through crying).[120,121] For whatever reasons, pain in or near the head may be more likely to result in anxiety and a loss of self-control and efficacy, and patients are relatively quick to appreciate caring support and attention.

A study comparing Ericksonian hypnosis to progressive muscle relaxation tapes, education about procedures, and a control group showed the Ericksonian hypnosis group to have less anxiety about dental procedures; in the protocol, negative thoughts were restructured (the sound of the dentist drill as a suggestion to go deeper into trance) and patients were to visualize success over pain and to use age-regression to a painless time in the past.[122] A study comparing patients' pain before and after dental work offered five hypnosis sessions which included relaxation, imagery, catalepsy, analgesia, and anesthesia, with posthypnotic suggestions to patients; they were also given self-hypnosis tapes.[123] The patients showed less pain frequency and duration and an increase in daily functioning compared to baseline, even at 6-month follow-up. A study comparing educational sessions or occlusal appliances to hypnorelaxation for temporomandibular joint (TMJ) pain showed that the hypnosis group reduced current and worst pain significantly more than the control groups did.[124] Hypnosis has been shown to be an effective adjunct in dental surgery to reduce pain, pain medication use, and anxiety,[82] and pre- and intraoperative hypnosis audiotapes used for third molar extraction with anesthesia reduced anxiety and pain medication use.[96]

For surgery and procedures, a depth of hypnosis is often used wherein the patient is responsive to the dentist's requests (to open wider, close, etc.) but does not feel the procedure itself. Hypnotic suggestions may be for relaxation, for creating numbing, for going by trance to another place while safely leaving the tooth with the dentist, and for feeling pressure rather than pain. In addition to dental procedural pain and anxiety, many dentists learn hypnosis for needle phobia, gagging, bruxism, saliva control, and TMJ, all of which will necessitate specific suggestions.

Pediatric Pain

Children are in general more hypnotizable than adults for a number of reasons. They have much richer fantasy lives, are relatively more curious, and are encouraged to use imagination in play; there are fewer parameters and fixed interpretations of the world in general, as they are still learning and are relatively trusting of adults and authority. Critical thinking develops as the brain matures, and it is only in adolescence where society demands more realistic and responsible thinking. In general, peak hypnotizability may be as late as latency (8–12 years of age), when children are the most open-minded, curious, imaginative, and willing to suspend judgment and when they are reasonably knowledgeable. Learning pain management and self control early can help children tolerate medical procedures (shots, fracture settings, etc.) and eliminate negative associations to pain that may remain with them as adults. Children are not reflective thinkers, and so they are more likely to be psychosomatic in their presentation of emotional or situational problems; the bank of literature on childhood stomach aches tells us that for them, stomach aches may be a benchmark for distress that may otherwise go unexpressed.

Training in self hypnosis improved children's functional abdominal pain 80%,[125] and self-hypnosis tapes improved the respiratory functioning of anxious children in a pulmonary center by 95%.[126] A prospective controlled trial explored the efficacy of adding self-hypnosis training to the use of analgesic cream for lumbar puncture-induced pain and anxiety in 6- to 16-year-old cancer patients[127]; the additional hypnosis led to a decrease in anticipatory and procedure-related pain and anxiety. A retrospective study found a significant decrease in self-reported pain intensity, duration, and frequency of headaches, with no adverse effects, after adolescents were taught self-hypnosis.[128] An hour of self-hypnosis training given to children, along with instructions to practice several times a day, led to less stressful and speedier urological procedures, by both parental and staff report.[129] Manual-based clinical hypnosis has been found more effective than distraction,[130] cognitive-behavioral treatments,[131] and play and distraction.[132] Hypnosis can also help children undergo acupuncture.[133] However, reviews of the research still found hypnosis to be not robust enough to fall within best practice guidelines for managing procedure-related pain in pediatric oncology;[66] several researchers call for more randomized control trials for the clear-cut benefits of hypnosis and other psychological interventions to be shown, although no studies refute the likelihood that it is beneficial and shows a better side-effect profile.[134–136]

Designing trances or trance experiences for children will of course involve taking their developmental age into consideration, as well as the degree of trauma and fear involved in what they will be experiencing. First, it is important to remember that children are highly suggestible, and are still vulnerable to trauma long before they can understand its context or verbalize their problem. On the other hand, even babies can be lulled or stroked into a soothing situation and be spoken to in reassuring words, songs, and sounds. Olness and Gardner[137] suggest framing therapeutic suggestions and stories in the context of what they know, such as bubbles, pop-up books, dolls, and stories, and utilizing story book figures as the characters of the stories. Nature, favorite pleasant places, cars, magical travel, music, and repetitive action such as ball bouncing or yo-yo tossing can be used in inductions. For adolescents and older children who are more interested in relationships, stories and images could include peer groups. All aged children may be quite intrigued with some of the classic induction techniques such as the pendulum, arm levitation, and the coin drop. It is particularly important to speak to the child in language he/she can understand, to consider play as a way to make the experience more pleasant, and to speak with a tone of voice that allows the child to feel supported and respected, and to add suggestions about self control and self-efficacy and safety. For detailed discussion of hypnosis with children, see Olness and Kohen.[138]

A case example is a 13-year-old patient who broke his nose while playing baseball; his mother brought him to a facial trauma doctor I was working with at the time. Concern for his anxiety was relatively great since the same surgeon in the same hospital had previously done surgery on the youngster's throat after a near-fatal small airplane crash. Before trance, any fears or discomfort were discussed so that he would be safe in the procedure room. As the room was being set up for him, we discussed any of his concerns and his baseball game. I hypnotically coached him to go back in his mind to complete the game as he wanted it to end, and along the way, and I suggested to him that he could forget about whatever parts of the whole afternoon that would make him more comfortable, and that he did not need to remember. I gave him permission to suggest to me how to make the experience safer and more comfortable for him. He proceeded to ask one resident to leave, because she was talking about trivial personal issues and not paying attention to his procedure. To our surprise, when the patient woke up the next morning, he removed all the bandages and packing and went down to breakfast without mentioning or questioning the bandages or the hospital experience, but he did remember some pretty girls he saw on the way there. Since that incident, the author includes suggestions to follow his doctor's instructions, so that any necessary aftercare does not also go by the wayside!

Irritable Bowel Syndrome

Most IBS patients have low thresholds of pain in their bowels, along with abnormal autonomic nervous system functioning and considerable symptom discomfort.[139] Hypnotherapy has been shown to improve pain, autonomic symptom dysfunction, and well-being,[140] even at follow-ups beyond 5 years.[141] The Manchester Model[142] hypnosis protocol has been consistently effective for treatment of bowel and other physical symptoms, depression, and anxiety[143,144]; improvement in symptom scores is associated with improvement in IBS-related thoughts.[145] When Palsson's North Carolina hypnotic protocol[146] is administered to IBS patients, their daily diary reports show an approximate 50% reduction in pain.[147] In a study comparing the North Carolina protocol[147,139] administered with the manual presentation versus with individually tailored presentation, the manualized induction group had less emotional stress after the treatment, but the individualized induction group continued to improve and did better at 10 months than the group who received the scripted trance, and showed less emotional distress.[148]

Hypnotic suggestions to improve gut symptoms and IBS pain can include those to warm hands, progressively relax, move attention away from gut symptoms, and to calm and comfort the gut, in addition to suggestions for enhanced overall well-being, self-efficacy, self management, and control. The North Carolina protocol is lengthy; it includes all the previously listed elements and also suggests dissociation away from the pain and to a carefree place. This appears to break the cycle of pain, and patients reset their perceptions of pain. The protocol includes seven scripted, therapist-guided sessions and an audiotape for home use. The Manchester Model[142] now has 12 scripted sessions and an audiotape for home use; the scripts include suggestions to warm the hands and transfer the warmth mechanically to the gut, for control and normalization of gut functions, as well as suggestions for ego-strengthening and self control in handling IBS symptoms.

Headaches

In general, migraine, tension, and mixed headaches respond to hypnosis.[149] Migraine headache frequency, duration, and severity decreased in one study when patients were given one group hypnosis session and 12 weeks of follow-up with hypnosis audiotapes.[150] Tension headache pain, vitality, and mental health improved when patients were offered guided imagery audiotapes.[151] There have been many comparisons of autogenic training (AT) to hypnosis for headache control. AT focuses specifically on relaxing muscles, which is in part what hypnosis would address,

so that similar effectiveness is expected. Studies show AT to be more effective,[152] less effective,[153] or equally effective for headache pain.[154] Both treatments seem to help patients perceive more self control of pain[155]; improvement in pain scores seems to be related to hypnotizability, and formal hypnosis with a formal induction seems to improve the chances of success.[153]

To treat a headache it is usually important to know whether the patient has tension, migraine, or cluster headaches. For tension headaches, direct suggestions could be to breathe in and out through the skin in the head and neck, to loosen the scalp, to let the hair fall naturally directly from the scalp, or to cool or warm the inside of the head (depending on the type of headache). Indirect suggestions might be to imagine being in a relaxing place or in a cold place, with cool wet rag at the neck. For migraines, Gibbons[156] suggests diving into water, as this lowers blood pressure and heart beat and may alleviate circulatory congestion in the head. Suggestions for cold (skiing, hiking in the snow) may also be helpful. Patients may also constrict blood vessels by imagining them to become tight, cool, and narrower. Tension headaches may respond to suggestions that help to open the blood vessels, such as warm climates, relaxation, or warm water. Hammond[149] finds self-hypnosis effective for tension headache management; he suggests that patients who report daily morning headaches may respond well to the use of self-hypnosis tapes at bedtime, which aim to allay tension while they are sleeping.

Cancer

Caner pain may be distinct from other long-term or chronic pain, in that changes or increases in pain may trigger end of life concerns, grief, depression, and anxiety. In addition, there are very often painful and bothersome side effects to cancer treatment, such as nausea, vomiting, tissue or nerve damage, weakness, and fatigue, many of which respond to hypnosis quite well. The feedback loop between diseases such as cancer, negative cognitions, and suffering are discussed elsewhere, as is the effect of stress and distress on immunosuppression, which can compromise patients' recovery times and resistance to secondary illnesses.

Hypnosis is particularly effective in reducing stress through direct and indirect suggestions to relax, and through enhancing patients' sense of self-efficacy and self-control. Spiegel and Bloom[157] showed positive effects with hypnosis in terminal cancer patients, possibly including giving patients a slightly longer lifespan; the latter benefit was not replicated in the recent study, possibly due to the improved medical treatments that extend the lives of all patients who were subjects.[158] This does point out the importance of alternative medicine therapists ensuring that patients are not discounting or ignoring medical care.

A number of studies compared hypnosis to cognitive behavioral therapy (CBT) for control of cancer pain. One showed bone marrow transplant patients to benefit more from hypnosis than from CBT or attentional control, as they had less pain at worst times, and for shorter durations.[159] Other studies show the benefits of hypnosis over CBT for pain, anxiety, and overall distress.[93,130,160] A prospective randomized study with advanced stage cancer patients showed that a manualized presentation of four weekly hypnosis sessions with addition audiotapes for home use significantly decreased pain; suggestions were comprehensive, including relaxation, comfort, dissociation, and more specific pain control techniques.[161]

Quality of life is particularly important with cancer because end-of-life patients may have grieving to do as well as personal, relationship, and spiritual business to tend. To address this, one study randomly assigned patients to 10 minute self-hypnosis audiotapes teaching either progressive relaxation (a passive coping strategy) or breathing exercises (an active coping strategy), to be used three times a week.[162] Positive attitudes increased and negative attitudes and anxiety decreased in both groups, with more improvement shown with the active coping strategy; this may have had to do, again, with perceived self control. Quality of life, particularly vitality, improved for metastatic breast cancer patients who were given 4 weeks of self hypnosis training, in comparison to those offered 4 weeks of training in a Japanese healing method called Johrei and to wait-list controls[163]; both treatment groups improved in mood and anxiety scores. Other studies have shown quality of life improvement for cancer patients using hypnosis.[164,165] The latter study's protocol looks similar to what might occur in a clinical setting; it offered four 30-minute sessions of hypnosis weekly, using traditional inductions and individualized suggestions for symptom management and ego strengthening. Hypnotic suggestions that foster or support existential, religious or other beliefs about life after death for patients, and for those who socially support them, might be given early in treatment.[166]

Osteoarthritis

The research literature on the use of hypnosis with arthritic pain is sparse. One study found Erickson hypnosis to compare favorably to Jacobson relaxation and control conditions for treatment of osteoarthritis pain.[69] Pain relief was directly related to imagery and hypnotic susceptibility, but not to expectancy. Hypnotic suggestions addressed relaxation, positive imagery and age regression to a more comfortable time; the authors used the words of "mental imagery" rather than "hypnosis," and the words "pain" and "analgesia" were not used.

Clinically, suggestions to alleviate arthritis pain may include warm water, warm blankets, warm sun, and stroking the area with arm hands. Also, suggestions to initiate moving arthritic parts or walking while exhaling and to keep the breath flowing, can alleviate unnecessary tensing. The patient may self-hypnotically rehearse moving the arthritic area, thereby limbering the body before actually moving, to help the mind and body work together. Patients might move around while keeping in mind the image of themselves at a much younger age and at pain-free times. They might also focus more intently on the *goal* for moving (specifically what they will do on the other side of the room once they get there) rather than on the sensation of moving. Time distortion to a pain-free time in the past or future, and getting involved with increased focus on what they are doing, may also distract them from physical feelings. Other suggestions might be to let go of the sensation of gravity in the body, and to lighten their steps.

There are references to anger as a psychosomatic link to some arthritis pain. As with other emotional links to pain, hypnotic treatment is likely to be even more successful when such psychological or emotional components are addressed. Often, defensiveness or fear underlie the anger and can lead to body tension; the extent of this would be relatively easy to discover during the very important pretreatment assessment.

MEDICAL HYPNOSIS TECHNIQUES

Principles of Preparation, Induction, and Suggestions

The traditional hypnotherapy session may be divided into four phases: induction; a period of deepening involvement of the unconscious mind while lessening involvement of the conscious mind; the therapy itself; and then a gradual transition back to conscious awareness. Beforehand a pretreatment assessment should include learning the patient's analogies or metaphors about the pain (stabbing, slicing, cold, daggers, or tingling) and learning what the pain means to the patient in terms of suffering, insult, guilt, religious beliefs, associations to past traumas, future expectations and fears, and social, cultural, or familial losses.

That information will help the therapist know the extent of the patient's fears and concerns and the nature of their suffering, and determine the appropriate therapy and support that is needed. It will also tell the therapist what specific words or metaphors to use in their messages and suggestions to the patient, and what overall approach to use. The better the therapist understands the mechanisms of the unconscious mind, particularly where pain, stress, and memories are concerned, the easier it may be to do effective pain management work.

Ethics for using hypnosis are even more stringent than when using other psychological techniques, in that trances allowing access to unconscious processes can potentially leave the patient more vulnerable. ASCH guidelines also include preparing the patient for hypnosis by dispelling myths about what hypnosis is and is not, advising them of what they might experience, and ensuring that hypnosis is not against their religious beliefs or that it will not violate safety boundaries; this protects both the patient and the clinician. They should know that the therapist will not shield them from any pain they should keep in order to protect themselves; it is sometimes best to allow patients to keep a certain small percentage of their pain, and to recognize any pain that they might need to address. Patients should be advised and comforted to know that the therapist is guiding them into a condition of self-hypnosis, and is not *doing* hypnosis *to* them. They should also be advised that everyone has their own level of susceptibility that is independent of intelligence and emotional or moral fortitude, and that can vary according to day or time. They should also be given permission to stop the session and to talk to the therapist whenever they need to do so.

One variable to consider is the level of involvement in treatment the patient desires. Some patients are proactive in their treatment and cope best by knowing everything there is to know about the process and prognosis, while others avoid knowing the clinical details. Giving the patient the amount of detail he or she wants to keep them comfortable will help in keeping good rapport. In one study, researchers found that over time, patients who attributed the pain control to themselves did better with pain.[155] For the benefit of positive expectancy, using the word hypnosis may benefit the patient outcome, because some patients prefer handing over the pain management to the clinician (as in the often heard phrases "Just hypnotize me and make me stop [smoking] or [eating] so much." That mindset signifies an external locus of control, which is not a good indicator of pain management in general or for therapeutic success; however, it may indicate success with hypnosis in that the patient may be willing to suspend vigilance with little resistance.

It is best to provide a quiet, pleasant, and emotionally safe space for the hypnosis sessions, which, of course, may be compromised in many clinical, surgical, and emergency settings. Again, the most important element is the patient/clinician relationship, and there are techniques health care providers can use to gain rapport and help anxious and traumatized patients relax in emergency rooms, operating rooms, and busy clinics (see http://www.anodyne.net). In the clinical setting, proper posture helps patients truly "let go" and relax; they may do best when sitting with both feet on the floor and with hands resting on the knees, so that they are not likely to fall asleep but they do not have to work at balancing. An emotionally safe one-on-one session would facilitate the patient's recovery of memories and hidden associations to the pain. Setting up positive expectancy, including the clinician's and the rest of the treatment staff's positive belief in success, also improves the success of hypnosis; this is the variable that confounds many research studies, according to Jensen and Patterson.[75]

Styles of hypnosis vary depending on the preferred approach of the therapist, the context, and the needs of the patient. Research indicates that all therapy techniques work more or less equally well, and that the most effective is the one the therapist feels most comfortable using, as they direct their attention toward the patient's chosen outcome and remain flexible about changing approaches as the patient's needs change.[167] In hypnosis, the patient is suspending vigilance and giving over access into his or her unconscious mind, so that the onus is on the therapist to choose words carefully and to maintain the safe therapeutic space. That being said, the inductions, certainly the messages, and the length of the sessions will necessarily differ according to the circumstance of pain—chronic, acute, surgical, or trauma-induced pain. Emergency situations are often best handled with a very direct authoritarian approach. In emergencies and where pain is suddenly acute, the patient may be anxious and may want someone to take charge, and they may need suggestions for quick relief; indeed, the pain and trauma involved may already have induced a trance state. Depth of trance is not necessarily related to outcome; the purpose of the trance is to get suggestions to the unconscious mind efficiently, and hypnosis aims to facilitate that at whatever level. Hypnotic anesthesia for surgery demands a deep trance and a longer induction. For other medical procedures where the patient is to be conversant (such as with epidural injections or spinal cord stimulator placements or brain surgery), a lighter trance may be in order. Light trances may allow patients to observe and learn self-hypnosis, while the therapist can gain information on how the work is going and even explore sensations in the pain area to gain more diagnostic information. Conversational trances can occur when the therapist establishes very good rapport with the patient, when the patient is already in an altered state of mind, and when the therapist talks directly to the unconscious mind using hypnotic language and techniques (for example, the Ericksonian techniques described later). Hypnosis may bring up unexpected memories or associations that should be addressed and resolved when they occur or when they are recognized; this might necessitate varying levels of trance during the session.

Common Induction Procedures

Inductions can be done conversationally, naturalistically, using rituals or chanting, by directing the patient inward, or by using objects such as a coin or crystal on a chain. In general the induction involves fixating or narrowing the patient's attention and deepening their involvement while at the same time suggesting dissociation from conscious awareness of the field. Good rapport-building skill and the use of hypnotic phrasing and words allow a seamless transition from induction into therapy. Therapy can begin during induction or after the patient is at the necessary level of trance.

A number of classic induction procedures are often taught in hypnosis training:

- Chiasson induction: The patient is asked to hold their hand out in front of them, and to notice their arm or hand move slowly toward their face. The therapist suggests that the patient's eyes feel so heavy that they want to close. When the hand comes closer to the face and as the fingers open, trance will also occur.
- Reversed arm levitation induction: the patient starts with their arm out in front of them, and as it slowly drops to the table (lap, chair arm) and rests there, they will go deeper into trance.
- Catalepsy induction: the patient holds the arm out in front of them and is given the suggestion that they will lose the feeling of it being there and that they will not be able to move it.
- Chevreul pendulum technique[168]: the patient holds a shiny object at eye level, and has their eyes follow the swinging movement; the therapist suggests that the arm is getting tired and will slowly sink to the table. The moment the pendulum hits the table, the patient will go deeper into trance and may close their eyes for comfort.
- Coin technique: The patient holds a coin in their fist out at arm's length. The therapist may suggest that the coin is a balloon that expands, so that the hand opens; eventually the coin drops, which the patient knows is the signal to enter into trance.
- Magnetic hands: the patient holds two hands out in front of themself, with the suggestion to watch how they slowly come together like magnets, eventually touching one another, which is the invitation into trance.
- Imagery induction: The patient is asked to go in their mind to a personally ideal, specific place or location and to hear, sense, smell, and totally be *in* the setting.
- Going down a staircase: The patient is guided to walk slowly down a flight of stairs (often 20); as the therapist talks, inducing trance, the therapist will imbed a count-down of the number of stairs until the patient gets to the bottom, when they will drop into trance. The lead out of trance will be to reverse the numbers (from 0 to 20) as the patient walks back up into the conscious mind.
- Progressive relaxation: The patient is guided to relax muscle groups progressively, starting at their feet and working upward or starting at their head and working down. The advantage of this technique is that it is easily used self-hypnotically.
- Eye fixation: The patient is asked to watch something intently until they cannot anymore, and when the eyes decide to close they may go into trance.
- Rapid eye roll[169]: The technique is also an indicator of hypnotizability. The patient is asked to take a deep breath and hold it, then to roll the eyes upward to look into the top of the eye sockets, then to close the eyes, as the patient slowly breathes out, they will relax into a trance.

When there is a sufficient level of trance, therapy can continue to help the patient feel better and give them tools to forget pain, change the perception, put it into perspective, or view the sensations constructively.

Suggestions and Imagery

The link between thoughts, feelings, behaviors, physiological state, and pain can allow any of them to change when any of the others does. Curiosity and imagination can be essential keys to change, and change can happen for the patient when they imagine that they are in the state of mind or body that will allow the change to occur. For instance, when I want to be relaxed, I can imagine being at the beach, to put me in the right frame of mind, or I can go to the beach. If I want someone to like me, I can imagine that they already do, to show them how to treat me. If I want to dance gracefully, I can imagine myself gracefully gliding across a dance floor, to access body memories. Body states, behaviors, and feelings are modified more easily in trance than out of trance. When the patient uses their own images, those images are more likely to be relevant and more likely to be successfully used in future self hypnosis sessions. To encourage dissociation away from the body, the suggestion may be a very detailed trip up in the air in a balloon, off into the clouds, on a row boat in a magical lake, on a magic carpet over a peaceful place, up on a mountain top, or down on a beach. Any of these can help move the focus out of the here and now and out of the body. Turning inward, but still dissociating away from pain, suggestions might be to take a journey from the top of the spine all the way down the back to the sit bones,[170] to go inside the organ or area of the body that has pain and do something soothing, (expand the space, add a healing potion, stroke the inside walls of the area) according to the patient's image of the pain problem,[171] or to go into (working with) the inner workings of the brain to change the interpretation or sensation of pain.[172] All these utilize the complementarity principle, to be discussed below.

For hypnosis to be effective, the message or suggestion needs to go (1) from the conscious to the unconscious mind, reflectively or by self-hypnosis; (2) directly to the unconscious mind while the conscious mind is in deep trance; or (3) indirectly to the unconscious mind by confusing the conscious mind or by some otherwise subliminal technique. Techniques to do the latter include (1) imbedded commands (If **you** are like me you **will feel** that the couch is **better** than the chair for going **in**to **trance**); (2) suggestions of dissociation ("While you are aware of the pain at a conscious level, your unconscious mind is already beginning the healing process all by itself without you having to do anything"); (3) the "yes" set, wherein the therapist says a series of truisms the patient will endorse, and then presents the therapeutic message that the patient may have otherwise doubted ("You did well last week and you did well yesterday, and you are doing well now, and you will continue to do well tonight as well"); (4) implied causatives, which assume that when the patient does **A**, **B** will follow ("Whenever you begin the healing you will probably notice the pain that leads to the automatic healing responses in your unconscious mind that know how to resolve pain all on their own"); and (5) confusion, which forces one to suspend the conscious mind so as to think through and resolve the cognitive conflict the confusion created (see Erickson section later). Direct versus indirect style of suggestion is exemplified by whether the patient is told, for instance, to "Lower your shoulders" or "Take the creases out of your forehead" as opposed to "You may remember the pleasure of a very warm shower on your back and shoulders at the end of a winter day" or "If you have ever had a soothing massage, would your shoulders remember that now?" and "Does your forehead remember how it was so smooth when you were a baby, sleeping peacefully in your cradle?" or "As your eyes slowly begin to close, it is as though you can feel the day's tension roll right down your face, from your hair and all down over your chest and onto the floor in front of you."

The unconscious operates more in machine language than the sophisticated conscious mind, so keeping language extremely simple, using metaphors and sparing words, is usually more effective, unless you are accessing the patient's unconscious mind by using a confusion technique, imbedding two conversations and hidden messages at the same time, or creating a state of boredom so that the patient will go deeper into unconsciousness. Whatever the purpose for the trance, it is usually a good idea to add in suggestions to enhance self-esteem and self-efficacy. *Convincers* can assist the effect of therapy by raising the patient's level of positive expectancy that hypnosis works. Traditional ways to do this might include glove anesthesia, wherein the therapist guides the patient to create numbness in one hand, catalepsy or the arm raise as discussed previously, or simply calling attention to the lost sense of time that occurs during trance. Finally, *fractionation* involves changing the patients' depth of trance, coming out and back into trance, which effectively deepens the trance; may make the trance more effective and may show the patient that he is an interactive partner in the process.

For surgical and procedural anesthesia or analgesia and for trauma situations, acute pain relief is the primary concern. However, the suggestions made for trust and emotional comfort during and after surgery, speedy recovery, ease with the hospital and healing processes, reduction in anesthetic and pain medications, self-confidence, amnesia for presurgical pain, and future well-being can be posthypnotic and address postsurgical issues. With chronic pain, posthypnotic suggestions can help the patient process and reframe nociception that continues to occur after the hypnotic session. The suggestions can be general or specific, suggesting that whenever the patient feels x, the patient can automatically do y ("In the future, whenever you feel tension in your head, you can automatically say your special releasing words to yourself, release and relax," or "Whenever you want relief from daily tension you can say the word 'ease' to yourself, and you will automatically feel the wave of release throughout your neck area.")

Finally, the patient can be guided out of trance with suggestions that encourage more cognitive thought and less unconscious processing. References to recognizing time, temperature of the room, the therapist's voice ("as distinct from your own"), or feeling the heart beat, as the therapist picks up the pace and volume of their speech, can all guide the patient back to conscious awareness. There may be side effects to trance which are not convenient, such as foggy thinking, lethargy, disorientation, slow heart beat, lack of vibrancy, and a temporary amnesia for what was going on before the trance. They may be erased with another brief series of suggestions so that the patient feels refreshed and in control at the end of trance.

CHRONIC PAIN MANAGEMENT

Jensen and Patterson[75] reviewed 19 studies on the efficacy of hypnosis for chronic pain, and outlined the control conditions used for comparison. Eight studies involved headache pain alone; and others included cancer, sickle cell, low back, temporomandibular, and mixed chronic pain problems. There were six types of control conditions: measuring change from baseline; hypnosis versus standard care; hypnosis added to another treatment, including physical therapy, medication, education or advice, or an occusal appliance; hypnosis versus biofeedback; an attentional control condition; and minimal effect control conditions (this allows for passage of time and patient expectancy that a change could occur). They also addressed conditions (or independent variables) that effect success with hypnosis, namely suggestibility, frequency of treatment sessions, frequency of self-hypnosis practices, patient-rated outcome expectations, initial treatment response, and diagnostic group. The overall conclusion was that hypnotic analgesia was significantly more effective than no treatment and than other standard care conditions, although other hypnotic-like treatments, such as progressive relaxation and autogenic training, produced similarly effective pain control.

We have mentioned chronic pain as distinct from acute and procedural pain throughout this chapter, although almost all the techniques mentioned also may apply to chronic pain. Chronic pain carries the expectation that it may never go away, and the extra burden of itself as a prolonged physiological stressor. In addition, its emotional suffering component may magnify with time.[172–174] To that aim, Hilgard and Hilgard[173] asked their patients to rate their suffering and pain separately so that they might learn to differentiate them. Chronic pain is of the type that the patient can well afford to disregard, forget or modify; there are hypnotic techniques for all those possibilities. Treatment may include dissociation from the nociception and from the awareness of pain; time distortion, which allows the patient to mentally "be" in the future or the past when they do not feel good; selective amnesia for the original injury that caused the pain; displacement of the pain to a place outside the body, imaginary numbing of the pain, and altered perception of the pain that recognizes nociception as just a signal and nothing more.

Brown[175] outlines group pain therapy sessions, which may be done in 8–12 week formats. The techniques are taught to the patient through personal experience during sessions, and then the patients practice them for home use. Brown classifies pain management techniques in four categories—alleviation, alteration, attenuation, and awareness.

1. Alleviating the sensations or symptoms involves making direct or indirect suggestions to make the pain go away, to substitute pain sensations for other sensations or for different ones, to create numbness, or to imagine analgesia.
2. Alteration involves changing the overall experience of pain by temporary forgetting it or losing sensation of it, by altering

the meaning of it, such as aching after winning a sports event, or changing the sensation (from pain to pressure or tingling), or by dissociating from the pain or by depersonalizing from the body.

3. Avoiding involves taking pain away using distraction, engaging in fantasy, distorting time, age regression or progression, by getting absorbed in a mental task, or by imagining the pain somewhere else in the body.

4. Awareness techniques include focusing the conscious mind on the component parts of the pain, and studying the component parts of one's pain awareness, or the component parts of the mind and body's nociception process itself.

Brown's awareness techniques also highlight complementarity, in that when a patient thinks about their thinking, they tend to go into trance and cannot pay attention to pain. Brown suggests having patients pinch the skin between the thumb and the forefinger[51] to induce just enough pain to test out each of the listed techniques and to find out which ones work best; in subsequent practice sessions, each patient will hone the techniques that worked the best for them personally. Brown suggests beginning with secondary pain areas (for instance, the leg pain that accompanies back pain, or compensatory pain) before working with the primary one. Finally, pain management training should include a section on relapse prevention, to be sure that patients know how to manage the psychological and behavioral triggers in their lives that exacerbate pain, and that they have a variety of techniques to use for different situations, types, and levels of pain.

Spira and Speigel[176] discuss practical ways hypnotherapists can work with patients' varying levels of hypnotizability, presenting a tabular outline of techniques to use according to the patients' hypnotizability (low, moderate, and high) and pain levels (mild, moderate, or severe). The table shows strategies that help low hypnotizables, who will do best learning to release tension for mild pain, differentiate pain from their responses to moderate pain, and distract themselves during severe pain bouts. Moderately hypnotic patients may best attend to their own positive coping resources to managing pain and other problems; as pain increases they may imagine themselves to be in a positively resourceful state. Patients who are highly hypnotizable can alter mild pain directly by triggering memories of past successful alterations to go directly to that state; as pain progresses, they may dissociate from the experience.

Ericksonian Naturalistic Approaches to Pain and Symptom Management

Erickson was an expert at pain management from personal and professional experience; his techniques and philosophies are taught worldwide and through the Milton H. Erickson Foundation. Neurolinguistic programming (NLP) was developed as an attempt to understand how and what Erickson knew about the unconscious minds of his patients; a good part of NLP's focus is on getting into rapport with the patient's unconscious processes, to help them make changes that other parts of their mind are resisting (see http://www.NLPU.com for more information on medical and pain related applications). Erickson believed that hypnotic trance should be cooperative and interactive and that induction should guide the patient inside him- or herself. He believed patients were unique and resourceful in resolving their own pain and suffering, if they could become "unstuck" and open up to doing so. He oriented patients toward positive change, and his rapport with patients was a study in and of itself. He spoke directly to the patient's unconscious mind (or body processes) and bypassed conscious *and* unconscious resistance by utilizing the patient's language, posture, mood, words, and thinking patterns; this requires the attentive listening and observation skills. To treat pain and symptoms, particularly psychosomatic pain,

he stressed the importance of seeing the symptom as a valid part of the patient's experience with some positive purpose that the therapist must welcome in order to work with it.

Erickson managed his own pain by absorbing himself deeply into the awareness of his pain and verbalizing his perceptions of it; this advanced technique diverted his attention away from the sensation itself. His other pain management techniques included altering or reinterpreting the signal, reframing it as a positive thing, eliciting positive early memories to replace the present feelings, or disregarding conscious awareness of pain signal. He was also a master at introducing confusion at the cognitive level, to send the patient into trance, and then confusing perception of pain signals. He disengaged the conscious mind with techniques the conscious mind could not follow. Examples of confusion techniques include:

- Including syntactical errors into conversation ("wondering how *you will* it will happen for you . . . to *go into trance*")
- Putting two opposing ideas in the same sentence ("You can use self-hypnosis or I will lead you there"), or offering like alternatives ("You can go into trance all by yourself or you can go into self-hypnotic trance".)
- Distracting with strange wording ("Isn't it always the way it is when you think you have control")
- Making blatant suggestions and negating them ("Maybe you were kind of hysterical, or that really doesn't make sense at all")
- Using double meanings (such as in a story about shattering window panes or taking them out to let air through the frame)
- Interspersing an important suggestion into a sentence ("It's apparent (*as a parent*) that *you do a good job* at work anywhere.")
- Leading the patient away from their train of thought with surprise or humor ("Wow, I just remembered . . . sorry to interrupt . . . and you were saying . . . or is there another way you wanted to feel?)
- Suggesting the obvious ("Sooner or later you will feel relaxed and drop into trance," or "You may not yet know how you will get relief, but as your pain waxes and wanes. . . .")
- Reframing the experience ("You know you are still alive when you are lucky enough to still feel your pain.")
- Paradoxical states of being, to make feeling pain inconsistent with some other state of mind the patient can remember experiencing
- Describing the pain in a sentence and saying it backward
- Reversing the perceived direction or pathway of the pain

Lankton and others use a number of Erickson's tools for treatment of pain that include metaphors, stories, and anecdotes or jokes to pull attention away and disconnect from cognitive control. Lankton and Lankton[177,178] devised the triple imbedded metaphor technique that begins with a naturalistic trance induction and then progresses deeper with the use of three concurrent stories. The technique relies on excellent rapport and the design of stories and language specific to the patient and imbeds suggestions for cognitive, behavioral, emotional, and physiological changes at deep levels. The use of metaphors fosters a shift to the right side (more hypnotic and feeling) of the brain. Lankton's hypnotic trances for treatment of physical pain highlight confusion of the pain perception, time distortion, humor for distraction and rapport, and posthypnotic suggestion.[179]

Kay Thompson,[180] an Ericksonian who was also a dentist, used distraction techniques with children, and played many word games, such as "panes" of glass that could shatter and be disposed of, seeing through a pain of glass, "untying the knots to not feel" pain, and her famous phrase to start the process of pain management, "When everything that can and should be done about the pain has already been done, you can forget about the pain now."

Obviously there is overlap in the pain management tools that practitioners use; what differs is the style of presentation, the particular suggestions for physiological healing according to the specific type and site of pain. Above all, the patient needs to know that their pain and suffering are acknowledged by the therapist; trust, rapport, safety, confidence, and expectancy are all beneficial to the outcome.

CONCLUSION

Trance is a natural phenomenon, and health care providers have been using hypnosis to guide the patients into pain relieving trances for over 200 years. Recent research on the central mechanisms of pain and of hypnosis has highlighted a role for hypnosis in many medical disciplines, concluding that patients prepared hypnotically for surgery do better than 89% of other patients, and that 75% of both healthy subjects and patients respond positively to hypnotic analgesia, even when hypnotizability is not controlled. Ongoing efficacy and effectiveness studies on hypnosis have improved techniques such that even in the wake of the improved medicines and procedures that modern pain clinics have to offer, hypnosis is still poised to take a respectable role in interdisciplinary pain medicine.

References

1. Esdaile J. *Mesmerism in India and its Practical Application in Surgery and Medicine.* London: Longman, Brown, Green & Longmans; 1846.
2. Hull CH. *Hypnosis and Suggestibility: An Experimental Approach.* Carmarthen, Wales: Crown House Publishing; 2002. (Originally published 1933).
3. Fordyce WE. *Behavioral Methods for Chronic Pain and Illness.* St. Louis, MO: Mosby; 1976.
4. Turk D. Cost Effectiveness. From: Past and current state of multidisciplinary treatment programs. Presented at: 26th Annual Scientific Meeting of the American Pain Society; May 2–5, 2007; Washington, DC.
5. Van Tulder M, Becker A, Bekkering T, et al. On behalf of the COST B13 Working Group on Guidelines for the Management of Acute Low Back Pain in Primary Care. *Eur Spine J* 2006;15(suppl 2):S169–S191.
6. Guzman J, Esmail R, Karjalainen K, et al. Multidisciplinary rehabilitation for chronic low back pain: systematic review. *BMJ* 2001;322(7301):1511–1516.
7. Montgomery GH, Bovberg DH, Schnur JB et al. A randomized clinical trial of a brief hypnosis intervention to control side effects in breast surgery patients. *J Natl Cancer Inst* 2007;99(17):1304–1312.
8. Montgomery GH, DuHamel KN, Redd WH. A meta-analysis of hypnotically induced analgesia: how effective is hypnosis? *Int J Clin Exp Hypn* 2000;48: 138–153.
9. Kihlstrom JF. Hypnosis. *Ann Rev of Psychol* 1985;36:385–418.
10. Janet P. The subconscious. In: Badger RG, ed. *Subconscious Phenomena.* Boston: Gorham Press; 1910.
11. Hilgard ER. *Hypnotic Susceptibility.* New York: Harcourt Brace Jovanovich; 1965.
12. Bowers K. Imagination and dissociation in hypnotic responding. *Int J Clin Exp Hypn* 1992;40:253–275.
13. Bernheim H. *Hypnosis and Suggestion in Psychotherapy.* 1884. New edition translated. New York: University Books; 1963.
14. Haley J. *Uncommon Therapy: The Psychiatric Techniques of Milton H. Erickson, MD.* New York: W.W. Norton & Co., Ltd.; 1986.
15. Bandler R, Grinder J. *Patterns of the Hypnotic Techniques of Milton H. Erickson, MD.* New edition. Scotts Valley, CA: Grinder DeLozier Associates; 1996.
16. Gruzelier JH. Frontal function, connectivity and neural efficiency underpinning hypnosis and hypnotic susceptibility. *Contemp Hypn* 2006;23(1): 1513–1532.
17. Evans FJ. Hypnotisability: individual differences in dissociation and the flexible control of psychological processes. In: Lynn SJ, Rhue JW, eds. *Theories of Hypnosis.* London: Guilford Press; 1991:144–168.
18. Horton JE, Crawford HJ, Harrington G, et al. Increased anterior corpus callosum size associated positively with hypnotizability and the ability to control pain. *Brain* 2004;127 (8):1741–1747.
19. Gruzelier JH, Gray M, Horn P. The involvement of frontally modulated attention in hypnosis and hypnotic susceptibility: cortical evoked potential evidence. *Contemp Hypn* 2002;19:179–189.
20. De Benedittis G, Sironi VA. Arousal effects of deep brain stimulation in hypnosis. *Int J Clin Exp Hypn* 1988;36:96–106.
21. Lee J, Spiegel D, Kim S, et al. Fractal analysis of EEG in hypnosis and its relationship with hypnotizability. *Int J Clin Exp Hypn* 2007;55(1):14–31.
22. Price DD, Barber J, Harkins S. Path analysis of the hypnotic experience, 1988.

23. Danzinger N, Fournier E, Bouhassira D, et al. Different strategies of modulation can be operative during hypnotic analgesia: a neurophysiological study. *Pain* 1998;75:85–92.
24. Barber J, Mayer D. Evaluation of the efficacy and neural mechanisms of a hypnotic analgesia procedure in experimental and clinical dental pain. *Pain* 1977;4:4–48.
25. Goldstein A, Hilgard ER. Failure of the opiate antagonist naloxone to modify hypnotic analgesia. *Proc Natl Acad Sci U S A* 1975;72:2041–2043.
26. Maihöfner C, Handwerker HO, Neundörfer B, et al. Patterns of cortical reorganization in complex regional pain syndrome. *Neurology* 2003;61(12): 1707–1715.
27. Pleger B, Ragert P, Schwenkreis P, et al. Patterns of cortical reorganization parallel impaired tactile discrimination and pain intensity in complex regional pain syndrome. *Neuroimage* 2006;32(2):503–510.
28. Maihofner C, Handwerker HO, Birklein F. Functional imaging of allodynia in complex regional pain syndrome. *Neurology* 2006;67(8):1526.
29. Maihofner C, Handwerker HO, Neundorfer B, et al. Cortical reorganization during recovery from complex regional pain syndrome. *Neurology* 2004; 63(4):693–701.
30. Pleger B, Tegenthoff M, Ragert P, et al. Sensorimotor retuning (corrected) in complex regional pain syndrome parallels pain reduction. *Ann Neurol* 2005; 57:425–429.
31. Wobst AHK. Hypnosis and surgery: past, present, and future. *Anesth Analg* 2007;104(5):1199–1208.
32. Derbyshire SW, Whalley MG, Stenger A et al. Cerebral activation during hypnotically induced and imagined pain. *Neuroimage* 2004;23(1):392–401.
33. Vogt BA, Berger, Derbeyshire SW. Structural and functional dichotomy of human midcingulate cortex. *Eur J Neurosci* 2003;18:3134–3144.
34. Vogt BA, Derbyshire S, Jones AK. Pain processing in four regions of human cingulated cortex localized with co-registered PET and MR imaging. *Eur J Neurosci* 1996;l8:1461–1473.
35. Peyaron R, Laurent B, Garcia–Larrea L. Functional imaging of brain responses to pain: a review and meta-analysis. *Neurophysiol Clin* 2000;30: 263–288.
36. Croft RJ, Williams JD, Jaenschel C, et al. Pain perception and 40 Hz oscillations: the effect of hypnotic analgesia. *Int J Psychophysiol* 2002;41:101–108.
37. Faymonville M, Roediger L, Del Fiore G, et al. Increased cerebral functional connectivity underlying the antinociceptive effects of hypnosis. *Brain Res Cogn Brain Res* 2003;17(2):255–262.
38. Raij T, Numminen J, Narvanen S, et al. Brain correlates of subjective reality of physically and psychologically induced pain. *Proc Natl Acad Sci U S A* 2005;102(6):2147–2151.
39. Röder CH, Michal M, Overbeck G, et al. Pain response in depersonalization: a functional imaging study using hypnosis in healthy subjects. *Psychother Psychosom* 2007;76(2):115–121.
40. De Pascalis V, Magurano MR, Bellusci A. Pain perception, somatosensory event-related potentials and skin conductance responses to painful stimuli in high, mid, and low hypnotizable subjects: effects of differential pain reduction strategies. *Pain* 1999;83:499–508.
41. de Pascalis V. Physiological correlates of hypnosis and hypnotic susceptibility. *Int J Clin Exp Hypn* 1999;47(2):117–142.
42. Meier W, Klucken M, Soyka D, et al. Hypnotic hypo-and hyperalgesia: divergent effects on pain ratings and pain-related cerebral potentials. *Pain* 1993; 53:175–181.
43. Jensen MP, Barber J. Hypnotic analgesia of spinal cord injury pain. *Austral J Clin Exp Hypn* 2000;28:150–168.
44. Chapman CR. Psychological aspects of pain: a consciousness studies perspective. In: Pappagallo M, ed. *The Neurological Basis of Pain.* New York: McGraw-Hill; 2005:157–167.
45. Liossi C. Hypnosis in cancer care. *Contemp Hypn* 2006;23(1):47–57.
46. Brown DP, Fromme E. *Hypnosis and Behavioral Medicine.* Hillside, NJ: Lawrence Erlbaum Associates Publishers; 1987.
47. Hammond DC. *Handbook of Hypnotic Suggestions and Metaphors.* New York: W.W. Norton & Co.; 1991.
48. Yapko MD. *Trance Work: An Introduction to the Practice of Clinical Hypnosis.* 3rd ed. New York: Bruner–Routledge; 2003.
49. Weitzenhoffer AM, Hilgard ER. *Stanford Hypnotic Susceptibility Scale: Form C.* Palo Alto, CA: Consulting Psychologists Press; 1962.
50. Morgan AH, Hilgard ER. Stanford Hypnotic clinical scale (for children and for adults). *Am J Clin Hypn* 1978–1979;21:134–147, 148–169.
51. Speigel H, Spiegel D. Trance and treatment. In: *Clinical Uses of Hypnosis.* New York: Basic Books; 1978.
52. Shor RE, Orne MT. *Harvard Group Scale of Hypnotic Susceptibility.* Palo Alto, CA: Consulting Psychologists Press; 1962.
53. Bowers K. Waterloo–Stanford Group C (WSGC) scale of hypnotic susceptibility: normative and comparative data. *Int J Clin Exp Hypn* 1993;41(1):35–46.
54. Kronenberger WG, LaClave L, Morrow C. Assessment in response to clinical hypnosis: Development of the Hypnotic State Assessment Questionnaire. *Am J Clin Hypn* 2002;44(3–4):257–272.
55. Weitzenhoffer AM. Scales, scales and more scales. *Am J Clin Hypn* 2002;44: 209–219.
56. Lynn SJ, Council JR, Green, JP. Assessing hypnotic responsiveness in clinical and research settings. *Am J Clin Hypn* 2003;44:181–183.
57. Kirsch I, Montgomery, Sapirstein G. Hypnosis as an adjunct to cognitive-

behavioral psychotherapy: a meta-analysis. *J Consult Clin Psychol* 1995; 63(2):214–220.

58. Kessler RS, Dane JR, Galper DI. Conversational assessment of hypnotic ability to promote hypnotic responsiveness. *Am J Clin Hypn* 2002;44(3–4):273–282.

59. Tellegen A, Atkinson G. Openness to absorbing and self-altering experiences ("absorption"), a trait related to hypnotic susceptibility. *J Abnorm Psychol* 1974;83:268–277.

60. Wickramasekera I. Secrets kept from the mind but not from the body or behavior: the unsolved problems identifying and treating somatization and psychophysiological disease. *Adv Mind–Body Med* 1998;14:81–132.

61. Crown DP, Marlowe D. A new scale of social desirability independent of psychopathology. *J Consult Psychol* 1960;24:349–354.

62. Flammer E, Alladin A. The efficacy of hypnotherapy in the treatment of psychosomatic disorders: meta-analytic evidence. *Int J Clin Exp Hypn* 2007; 55(3):251–274.

63. DuHamel KN, Difede J, Foley F, et al. Hypnotizability and trauma symptoms after burn injury. *Int J Clin Exp Hypn* 2002;50(1):33–50.

64. Roelofs K, Hoogduin KAL, Keijsers GPJ. Motor imagery during hypnotic arm paralysis in high and low hypnotizable subjects. *Int J Clin Exp Hypn* 2002;50(1):51–66.

65. Younger JW, Rossetti GC, Borckardt JJ, et al. Hypnotizability and somatic complaints: a gender-specific phenomenon. *Int J Clin Exp Hypn* 2007;55(1):1–13.

66. Wild MR, Espie CA. The efficacy of hypnosis in the reduction of procedural pain and distress in pediatric oncology: a systematic review. *J Dev Behav Pediatr* 2004;25(3):207–213.

67. Nash M. Salient findings: Pivotal reviews and research on hypnosis, soma, and cognition. *Int J Clin Exp Hypn* 2004;52:82–88.

68. Chaves JF, Dworkin SF. Hypnotic control of pain: historical perspectives and future prospects. *Int J Clin Exp Hypn* 1994;4:356–376.

69. Gay MC, Philippot P, Luminet O. Differential effectiveness of psychological interventions for reducing osteoarthritis pain: a comparison of Erickson hypnosis and Jacobson relaxation. *Eur J Pain* 2002;6:1–16.

70. Turner JA, Chapman CR. Psychological interventions for chronic pain: a critical review II. Operant conditioning, hypnosis, and cognitive-behavioral therapy. *Pain* 1982;12(1):23–46.

71. Hawkins RMF. A systemic meta-review of hypnosis as an empirically supported treatment for pain. *Pain Rev* 2001;8:47–73.

72. Patterson DR, Jensen M. Hypnosis and clinical pain. *Psychol Bull* 2003;128:495–521.

73. Lang EV, Berbaum KS, Faintuch S et al. Adjunctive self-hypnotic relaxation for outpatient medical procedures: a prospective randomized trial with women undergoing large core breast biopsy. *Pain* 2006;126(1–3):155–164.

74. Stetter F, Kupper S. Autogenic training: a meta-analysis of clinical outcome studies. *Appl Psychophysiol Biofeedback* 2002;27(1):45–98.

75. Jensen M, Patterson D. Control conditions in hypnotic analgesia clinical trials: challenges and recommendations. *Int J Clin Exp Hypn* 2005;63(2):170–197.

76. Jensen M, Hanley M, Engel J, et al. Hypnotic analgesia for chronic pain in persons with disabilities: a case series. *Int J Clin Exp Hypn* 2005;53(2):198–228.

77. Amundson JK, Alladin A, Gill E. Efficacy vs. effectiveness research in psychotherapy: implications for clinical hypnosis. *Am J Clin Hypn* 2003;46:11–30.

78. Iphofen R, Corrin A, Ringwood–Walker C. Design issues in hypnotherapeutic research. *Eur J Clin Hypn* 2005;6(2):30–36.

79. Roberts LM. Trial design in hypnotherapy: does the RCT have a place? *Eur J Clin Hypn* 2005;6(2):16–19.

80. Spiegel SB, Kahn S. Being "the other therapist": the varieties of adjunctive experience with hypnosis. *Int J Clin Exp Hypn* 2001;49(4):339–351.

81. Hubbe M, Duncan B, Miller S. *Heart and Soul of Change*. Washington, DC: American Psychological Association; 1999.

82. Montgomery GH, David D, Winkel G, et al. The effectiveness of adjunctive hypnosis with surgical patients a meta-analysis. *Anesth Analg* 2002;94(6):1639–1645.

83. Patterson DR, Wiechman SA, Jensen M, et al. Hypnosis delivered through immersive virtual reality for burn pain: a clinical case series. *Int J Clin Exp Hypn* 2006;54(20):130–142.

84. Jensen M, McArthur KD, Barber J, et al. Satisfaction with, and the beneficial side effects of hypnotic analgesia. *Int J Clin Exp Hypn* 2006;54(4):432–447.

85. Dawson T, Spross JA, Jablonski ES, et al. Probing the paradox of patients' satisfaction with inadequate pain management. *J Pain Symptom Manage* 2002;23:211–220.

86. Patterson DR. Treating pain with hypnosis. *Curr Dir Psychol Sci* 2004;13:252–255.

87. Wain HJ. Reflections on hypnotizability and its impact on successful surgical hypnosis: a sole anesthetic for septoplasty. *Am J Clin Hypn* 2004;46(4):313–321.

88. Hart RR. The influence of a taped hypnotic induction treatment procedure on the recovery of surgery patients. *Int J Clin Exp Hypn* 1980;28(4):234–332.

89. Gurgevich S. Clinical hypnosis and surgery. *Alternative Med Alert* 2003;6(10):109–120.

90. Cupal DD, Brewer BW. Effects of relaxation and guided imagery on knee strength, reinjury anxiety, and pain following anterior cruciate ligament reconstruction. *Rehab Psychol* 2001;46(1):28–43.

91. Ginandes C, Brooks P, Sando W, et al. Can medical hypnosis accelerate post-

92. Massarini M, Rovetto F, Tagliaferri C. A controlled study to assess the effects on anxiety and pain in the postoperative period. *Eur J Clin Hypn* 2005;6(1):8–15.

93. Montgomery GH, Weltz CR, Seltz M, et al. Brief presurgery hypnosis reduces distress and pain in excisional breast biopsy patients. *Int J Clin Exp Hypn* 2002;50(1):17–32.

94. Lobe TE. Perioperative hypnosis reduces hospitalization in patients undergoing the Nuss procedure for pectus excavatum. *J Laparoendosc Adv Surg Tech A* 2006;16(6):639–642.

95. Lang EV, Joyce JS, Spiegel D, et al. Self-hypnotic relaxation during interventional radiological procedures: Effects on pain perception and intravenous drug use. *Int J Clin Exp Hypn* XLIV 1996;(2):106–119.

96. Enqvist B, Fischer K. Preoperative hypnotic techniques reduce consumption of analgesics after surgical removal of third mandibular molars: a brief communication. *Int J Clin Exp Hypn* 1997;45(2):102–108.

97. Dyas R. Augmenting intravenous sedation with hypnosis, a controlled retrospective study. *Contemp Hypn* 2001;18(3):128–134.

98. Nilsson U, Rawal N, Uneståhl LE, et al. Improved recovery after music and therapeutic suggestions during general anesthesia: a double-blind randomized, controlled trial. *Acta Anaesthesiol Scand* 2001;45:812–817.

99. Kessler R, Dane JR. Psychological and hypnotic preparation for anesthesia and surgery: an individual differences perspective. *Int J Clin Exp Hypn* 1996; 44(3):189–207.

100. Bennett H, Disbrow EA. Preparing for surgery and medical procedures. In: Goleman D, Gurin J, eds. *Mind–Body Medicine: How to Use your Mind for Better Health*. Yonkers, NY: Consumer Reports Books; 1993:401–427.

101. Harden RN, Bruehl S, Stanton–Hicks M, et al. Proposed new diagnostic criteria for complex regional pain syndrome. *Pain Med* 2007;8(4):326–331.

102. Moseley GL. Why do people with complex regional pain syndrome take longer to recognize their affected hand? *Neurology* 2004;62:2182–2216.

103. Galer BS, Butler S, Jensen M. Case reports and hypotheses: a neglect-like syndrome may be responsible for the motor disturbance in reflex sympathetic dystrophy. *J Pain Symptom Manage* 1995;10:358–392.

104. Gainer MJ. Somatization of dissociated traumatic memories in a case of reflex sympathetic dystrophy. *Am J Clin Hypn* 1993;36(2):124–131.

105. King JH, Nuss S. Reflex sympathetic dystrophy treated by electroconvulsive therapy: intractable pain, depression, and bilateral electrode ECT. *Pain* 1993; 55:393–396.

106. Berklein F, Maihöfner C. Use your imagination: training the brain and not the body to improve chronic pain and restore function. *Neurology* 2006; 67(12):2115–2116.

107. Burton AW, Hassenbusch SJ III, Warneke C, et al. Complex regional pain syndrome (CRPS): survey of current practices. *Pain Pract* 2004;4(2):74–83.

108. Melzak R. Phantom limbs. *Sci Am* 1992;266(4):120–126.

109. Wall PD. *Pain: The Science of Suffering*. London: Weidenfeld and Nicolson; 1999.

110. Giraux P, Sirigu A. Illusory movements of the paralyzed limb restore motor cortex activity. *Neuroimage* 2003;20:S107–111.

111. Flor H, Denke C, Schaefer M, et al. Effect of sensory discrimination training on cortical reorganization and phantom limb pain. *Lancet* 2001;357:1763–1764.

112. Hernandez J. Psychological treatment for CRPS symptoms that addresses its central mechanisms. Submitted to *J Pain Med*, 2008.

113. Lotze M, Flor H, Grodd W, et al. Phantom movements and pain: an fMRI study in upper limb amputees. *Brain* 2001;124:2268–2277.

114. Ramachandran VS, Rogers–Ramachandran D. Synaesthesia in phantom limbs induced with mirrors. *Proc Biol Sci* 1996;263:377–386.

115. Oakley DA, Whitman LG, Halligan PW. Hypnotic imagery as a treatment for phantom limb pain: two case reports and a review. *Clin Rehabil* 2002; 16(4):368–377.

116. Frenay MC, Faymonville ME, Devlieger S, et al. Psychological approaches during dressing changes of burned patients: a prospective randomized study comparing hypnosis against stress reducing strategy. *Burns* 2001;27(8):793–799.

117. Ewin D. The effect of hypnosis and mental set on major surgery and burns. *Am J Clin Hypn* 1986;26:5–8.

118. Ewin D. Emergency room hypnosis for the burned patient. *Am J Clin Hypn* 1986;29:7–12.

119. Ewin D. The use of hypnosis in the treatment of burn patients. *Psychiatr Med* 1992;10(4):79–87.

120. Thompson K. *The Use of Hypnosis for Pain*. Phoenix, AZ: Milton H. Erickson Congress; 1992.

121. Kane S, Olness K, eds. *The Art of Therapeutic Communication: The Collected Works of Kay Thompson*. Conn: Crown House Publishers; 2004.

122. Moore R, Bordgaard I, Abrahamsen R. A 3-year comparison of dental anxiety treatment outcomes: hypnosis, group therapy, and individual desensitization vs. no specialist treatment. *Eur J Oral Sci* 2002;110:287–295.

123. Simon EP, Lewis DM. Medical hypnosis for temporomandibular disorders: treatment efficacy and medical utilization outcome. *Oral Surg Oral Med Oral Pathol Oral Radiol Endod* 2000;90:54–63.

124. Winocur E, Gavish A, Emodi–Perlman A, et al. Hypnorelaxation as treatment for myofascial pain disorder: a comparative study. *Oral Surg Oral Med Oral Pathol Oral Radiol Endod* 2002;93:429–434.

surgical wound healing? Results of a clinical trial. *Am J Clin Hypn* 2003;45:333–351.

125. Anbar RD. Self-hypnosis for the treatment of functional abdominal pain in childhood. *Clin Pediatr (Phila)* 2001;40:447–451.
126. Anbar R, Giesler S. Identification of children who may benefit from self-hypnosis at a pediatric pulmonary center. *BMC Pediatr* 2005;5(1):6.
127. Liossi C, White P, Hatira P. Randomized clinical trial of local anesthetic versus a combination of local anesthetic with self-hypnosis in the management of pediatric procedure-related pain. *Health Psychol* 2006;25(3):307–315.
128. Kohen DP, Zajac R. Self-hypnosis training for headaches in children and adolescents. *J Pediatr* 2007;150(6):635–639.
129. Butler LD, Symons BK, Henderson SL, et al. Hypnosis reduces distress and duration of an invasive medical procedure for children. *Pediatry* 2005;115: e77–85.
130. Liossi C, Hatira P. Clinical hypnosis versus cognitive-behavioral training for pain management with pediatric cancer patients undergoing bone marrow aspirations. *Int J Clin Exp Hypn* 1999;47:104–116.
131. Zeltzer L, Lebaron S. Hypnosis and nonhypnotic techniques for reduction of pain and anxiety during painful procedures in children and adolescents with cancer. *J Pediatr* 1982;101(6):1032–1035.
132. Wall VJ, Womack W. Hypnotic versus active cognitive strategies for alleviation of procedural distress in pediatric oncology patients. *Am J Clin Hypn* 1989;31(3):181–191.
133. Zeltzer LK, et al. A phase I study on the feasibility and acceptability of an acupuncture/hypnosis intervention for chronic pediatric pain. *J Pain Symptom Manage* 2002;24(4):437–446.
134. Ladas EJ, Post–White J, Hawks R, et al. Evidence for symptoms management in the child with cancer. *J Pediatr Hematol Oncol* 2006;28(9):601–615.
135. Lassetter JH. The effectiveness of complementary therapies on the pain experience of hospitalized children. *Holist Nurs* 2006;24(3):196–208.
136. Uman LS, Chambers CT, McGrath PJ, et al. Psychological interventions for needle-related procedural pain and distress in children and adolescents. *Cochrane Database Syst Rev* 2006;18(4):CD005179.
137. Olness K, Gardner GG. *Hypnosis and Hypnotherapy with Children*. 2nd ed. New York: Grune and Stratton; 1988.
138. Olness K, Kohen DP. *Hypnosis and Hypnotherapy with Children*. 3rd ed. New York: Guilford Press; 1996.
139. Palsson OS. Standardized hypnosis treatment for irritable bowel syndrome: the North Carolina protocol. *Int J Clin Exp Hypn* 2006;54(1):51–64.
140. Simren M, Ringstron G, Bjornsson ES, et al. Treatment with hypnotherapy reduces the sensory and motor component of the gastrocolonic response in irritable bowel syndrome. *Psychosom Med* 2004;66(2):233–238.
141. Gonsalkorale WM, Miller V, Afzal A, et al. Long-term benefits of hypnotherapy for irritable bowel syndrome. *Gut* 2003;52:1623–1629.
142. Whorwell PJ, Prior A, Faragher EB. Controlled trial of hypnotherapy in the treatment of severe refractory irritable bowel syndrome. *Lancet* 1984;2: 1232–1234.
143. Gonsalkorale WM, Houghton LA, Whorwell PJ. Hypnotherapy in irritable bowel syndrome: a large-scale audit of a clinical service with examination of factors influencing responsiveness. *Am J Gastroenterol* 2002;97:954–961.
144. Lea R, Houghton LA, Calvert EL, et al. Gut-focused hypnotherapy normalizes disordered rectal sensitivity in patients with irritable bowel syndrome. *Aliment Pharmacol Ther* 2003;17:635–642.
145. Gonsalkorale WM, Toner BB, Whorwell PJ. Cognitive change in patients undergoing hypnotherapy for irritable bowel syndrome. *J Psychosom Res* 2004;56(3):271–278.
146. Palsson OS. Standardized hypnosis treatment protocol for irritable bowel syndrome. Copyright 1998. Available at http://www.ibshypnosis.com. Accessed April 15, 2009.
147. Palsson OS, Turner MJ, Johnson DA, et al. Hypnosis treatment for severe irritable bowel syndrome: investigation of mechanism and effects on symptoms. *Dig Dis Sci* 2002;47(11):2605–2614.
148. Barabasz A, Barabasz M. Effects of tailored and manualized hypnotic inductions for complicated irritable bowel syndrome patients. *Int J Clin Exp Hypn* 2006;54(1):100–102.
149. Hammond DC. Review of the efficacy of clinical hypnosis with headaches and migraines. *Int J Clin Exp Hypn* 2007;55(2):207–219.
150. Emmerson GH, Trexler G. A hypnotic intervention for migraine control. *Aust J Clin Exp Hypn* 1999;27:54–61.
151. Mannix LK, Chandurkar RS, Rybicvki LA, et al. Effect of guided imagery on quality of life for patients with chronic tension-type headache. *Headache* 1999;29:326–334.
152. Ter Kuile. High hypnotizables showed more improvement than lows. AT was slightly more effective for headache pain. *Headache* 1995;35:630–636.
153. Zitman FG, Van Dyck, Spinhoven P, et al. Hypnosis and autogenic training in the treatment of tension headaches: a two-phase constructive design study with follow-up. *Psychosom Res* 1992;36(3):219–228.
154. Van Dyck R, Zitman FG, Linssen ACG, et al. Autogenic training and future oriented hypnotic imagery in the treatment of tension headache: outcome and process. *Int J Clin Exp Hypn* 1991;39:6–23.
155. Spinhoven P, Linssen ACG, Van Dyck R et al. Autogenic training and self-hypnosis in the control of tension headaches. *Gen Hosp Psychiatry* 1992;14: 408–415.
156. Gibbons DE Suggestions for pain control. In: Hammond DC, ed. Handbook of *Hypnotic Suggestions and Metaphors*. New York: W.W. Norton & Co; 1990.
157. Spiegel D, Bloom JR. Group therapy and hypnosis reduce metastatic breast carcinoma pain. *Psychosom Med* 1983;45:333–339.
158. Spiegel D, Butler LD, Giese–David J, et al. Effects of supportive-expressive group therapy on survival of patients with metastatic breast cancer: a randomized prospective trial. *Cancer* 2007;110:1130–1138.
159. Syrjala KL, Cummings C, Donaldson GW. Hypnosis or cognitive behavioral training for the reduction of pain and nausea during cancer treatment: a controlled clinical trial. *Pain* 1992;48(2):137–146.
160. Mundy EA, DuHamel KN, Montgomery GH. The efficacy of behavioral interventions for cancer treatment–related side effects. *Semin Clin Neuropsychiatry* 2003;8(4):253–275.
161. Elkins GR, Cheung A, Marcus J, et al. Hypnosis to reduce pain in cancer survivors with advanced disease: a prospective study. *J Cancer Integ Med* 2004; 2:167–172.
162. Laidlaw TM, Willett MJ. Self-hypnosis tapes for anxious cancer patients: an evaluation using personalized emotional index (PEI) diary data. *Contemp Hypn* 2002;19(1):25–33.
163. Laidlaw T, Bennett, BM, Dwivedl P, et al. Quality of life and mood changes in metastatic breast cancer after training in self hypnosis or Johrei: a short report. *Contemp Hypn* 2005;22(2):84–93.
164. Classon C, Butler LD, Koopman C, et al. Supportive-expressive group therapy and distress in patients with metastatic breast cancer: a randomized clinical intervention trial. *Arch Gen Psychiatry* 2001;58:494–501.
165. Liossi C, White P. Efficacy of clinical hypnosis in the enhancement of quality of life of terminally ill cancer patients. *Contemp Hypn* 2001;18(3):145–160.
166. Spira JL. *Group Therapy for Medically Ill Patients*. New York: Guilford Press; 1997.
167. Duncan BL, Miller SD, Sparks JA. *The Heroic Client: Revolutionary Way to Improve Effectiveness Through Client-Directed Outcome-Informed Therapy*. San Francisco: Jossey–Bass; 2004.
168. Easton RD, Shor RE. Information processing analysis of the Chevreul pendulum illusion. *J Exp Psychol: Hum Percept Perform* 1975;1(3):231–236.
169. Ewin DM. Rapid eye roll induction. In: Hammond DC (Ed.). Hypnotic induction and suggestion: an introductory manual. Des Moines: American Society of Clinical Hypnosis; 1998:49–50.
170. Lankton S. *Ericksonian Approach to Hypnotherapy*. Advanced Training Workshops. Pensacola, FL; April 27–29, 1994.
171. Hernandez J. The use of self-relations therapy in pain management. In: *Walking in Two Worlds: The Relational Self in Theory, Practice and Community*. Phoenix: Zeig, Tucker & Theisen, Inc.; 2002.
172. Hernandez J. *Dialogues With Pain: Internal Body Conversations that Resolve Suffering*. Carmarthen, UK: Crown House Publishing; 2008.
173. Hilgard ER, Hilgard J, Barber J. *Hypnosis in the Relief of Pain* (Rev. ed.). New York: Brunner–Mazel; 1994.
174. Chapman CR, Gavrin J. Suffering: the contribution of persistent pain. *Lancet* 1999;353(9171):2233–2237.
175. Brown DP, Fromme E. *Hypnosis and Behavioral Medicine*. Hillside, NJ: Lawrence Erlbaum Associates; 1987.
176. Spira JL, Spiegel D. Hypnosis and related techniques in pain management. *Hosp J* 1992;8:89–119.
177. Lankton S, Lankton C. *The Answer Within: A Clinical Framework of Ericksonian Hypnotherapy*. New York: Brunner–Mazel Publishers; 1983.
178. Lankton C, Lankton S. *Tales of Enchantment: Goal-Oriented Metaphors for Adults and Children*. New York: Brunner–Mazel Publishers; 1989.
179. Lankton S. *Pain Management*. Milton H. Erickson. Congress, Phoenix, AZ; 2007.
180. Thompson K. The curiosity of Milton H. Erickson, MD In: Zeig JK, ed. *Ericksonian Approaches to Hypnosis and Psychotherapy*. New York: Brunner–Mazel; 1982:413–421.

CHAPTER 85 ■ RELAXATION AND IMAGERY TECHNIQUES

KAREN L. SYRJALA AND JEAN C. YI

Relaxation with imagery (R&I) is one of the most widely used methods for nonpharmacologic relief of pain, with strong empirical support.[1,2] A form of R&I is nearly always a component of multidimensional chronic pain treatment and is typically part of broader cognitive behavioral treatment programs for chronic pain. In addition, R&I is effective with acute and cancer pain problems. Beyond efficacy in reducing reports of pain, R&I can be beneficial in limiting the impact of pain on function.[3]

Numerous techniques and terms are used within the rubric of R&I, including progressive muscle (tense–release) relaxation, autogenic relaxation, imagery, visualization, and meditation. Although it is possible to separately describe relaxation methods versus imagery methods in practice, nearly all relaxation incorporates a form of imaging, whereas nearly all imagery begins with a form of relaxation. Consequently, clinicians need to understand and be able to use both components. Relaxation is used to pull focus away from pain and to induce a physical state of decreased muscle tension, as well as decreased autonomic and affective arousal. In theory, this state is inconsistent with the pain experience and, in itself, may reduce pain perception. Imagery provides a directly competing cognitive focus, which can block perception of pain during total concentration on imagery. After imagery is completed, pain reduction may continue through a shift in cognitive interpretation of nociceptive signals or through more direct neurochemical mechanisms. Both relaxation and imagery disrupt the pain–dysfunction feedback loop by increasing patient focus on feelings of well-being, thereby decreasing the focus on pain, as well as the tension, anxiety, depression, and inactivity related to pain.

As described in this chapter, R&I has been shown to be effective in the treatment of chronic low back pain, cancer pain, rheumatoid arthritis, childbirth, and acutely painful procedures. Headache and temporomandibular disorder (TMD) pain have been treated successfully with relaxation alone or combined with imagery. In this chapter we first consider some basic information, including a historical perspective of R&I techniques, theoretical bases including physiologic effects, and advantages and disadvantages of the methods. We then detail clinical methods and efficacy, as well as possible complications that a clinician should be prepared to manage. For further details on the application of specific approaches, the reader is referred to several books with useful information for professionals.[4–8] In addition, Bernstein and Borkovec[9] have a widely used manual for training professionals in progressive relaxation. For reviews of research or practice of R&I, see articles by Fernandez and Turk,[10] Keefe and Caldwell,[11] McCaffery and Beebe,[12] the NIH Technology Assessment Panel,[13] Syrjala and Abrams,[14] Syrjala and Roth-Roemer,[15] Turner and Romano,[16] Vessey and Carlson,[17] and Wallace.[18]

With the increased public attention to self-help and alternative therapies, bookstores are full of books and audiotapes instructing patients how to use imagery on their own. Clinicians will find several that they can recommend for patient use, along with professional care, in treatment of specific pain problems. *Books and audiotapes should not be considered adequate treatment alone. Most patients require initial professional assistance to* *adapt methods to their individual needs.[19,20] Tapes alone can bias patients against trying R&I with a professional, because they believe "it doesn't work for me."*

BASIC INFORMATION

History

Relaxation was in use by the 1930s as a technique for reducing tension and anxiety. Progressive muscle relaxation (PMR) was introduced by Jacobson,[4] who found that by extensive practice with systematic tensing and releasing of muscle groups, anxious patients could learn to discriminate the resulting sensations and produce an experience of deep relaxation. Wolpe[21] modified the procedure into a program that could be completed in six 20-minute training sessions with twice-daily home practice. He then incorporated relaxation into his systematic desensitization therapy for phobias, reasoning that relaxation would provide a response incompatible with fear. The relaxed state was paired with gradual exposure to the feared stimulus. The patient first imagined the exposure while relaxing and then actually confronted the feared object in real life. This method of treatment for phobias is still used today.

Autogenic training (AT) originated with a Berlin psychiatrist, Johannes H. Schultz, and was popularized in North America by Luthe.[22] AT does not require tensing of muscles but instead consists of turning attention to each muscle group in turn, suggesting sensations of heaviness and warmth. After progression through the muscle groups, attention is turned to slowing the heart rate, developing a regular respiration pattern, and regulating the viscera and cooling the forehead. The objective of AT is autonomic regulation as well as muscle relaxation. In its passive concentration, AT resembles meditation. In its content it incorporates the use of imagery, although these images are limited and intentionally repetitive.

Benson[5] has described the relaxation response as a form of meditation without the religious or lifestyle connotations of transcendental meditation, Zen, or yoga. In the two most tested meditation strategies for pain, the relaxation response and mindfulness meditation, patients are taught awareness in the moment, without judgment. Procedures vary, but awareness can focus on breathing, a phrase, or on a detached observation.[6,8,23]

Although relaxation began as a treatment for anxiety, since the time that behavioral psychologists began working with pain patients, R&I techniques have been a key element of standard treatment.[7] A sequential combination of PMR and AT is most frequently taught, with deep breathing and guided imagery often incorporated. Although not technically included in any of the original versions of relaxation already mentioned, deep breathing can be the first step toward helping patients focus attention before proceeding with further relaxation. Guided imagery serves as a distraction technique and, more important, as an effective means of introducing alternative thoughts, images, or ways to perceive pain. As such, the imagery component can be critical to the success of relaxation as a pain relief tool.[10]

Theoretical Bases

The mechanisms through which R&I reduces pain are still under debate, except for consensus on the obvious mechanisms of tension relief and altered sympathetic arousal.[13] Little is known about brain physiologic changes in response to relaxation, but more is known about peripheral physiologic change. Even brief PMR training has produced significant reductions in heart rate, respiratory rate, and electromyographic (EMG) forearm muscle tension.[24] Furthermore, during relaxation, physiologic changes have been greater than those observed during hypnosis for systems not under voluntary control (e.g., heart rate and tonic muscle tension). Other documented physiologic responses to relaxation include decreases in oxygen consumption, blood pressure, and serum lactic acid levels; increases in skin resistance; and alterations in blood flow.[25] Investigators have found that plasma norepinephrine levels either increase or do not change after relaxation.[26] It has been hypothesized that these peripheral changes, which indicate a decreased arousal of the sympathetic nervous system, are related to decreased end-organ responsiveness to norepinephrine.[25]

Reduced sympathetic activity after relaxation does not fully explain the pain reductions found in a substantial number of conditions.[16,27-29] In tension headaches and TMD pain, the reduction in reported pain may be due, at least in part, to muscle relaxation effects[30] and decreased sympathetic arousal, although not all studies have supported this finding. Altered blood flow may account for some of the effect with migraine headache. Other physiologic and cortical processes almost certainly are involved in accomplishing the pain relief reported with imagery in some acute and chronic pain conditions.

Measured brain responses to relaxation include increased electroencephalogram alpha and theta waves,[25] but research has confirmed few other brain activity changes. Theorists have speculated that relaxation and meditation shift areas of brain activation or that pain relief is a function of changes in catecholamines, endorphins, or other neurochemical systems.[13,25] Some data suggest that a spinal–thalamic–frontal cortex–anterior cingulate pathway influences subjective response to pain, whereas a spinal–thalamic–somatosensory cortex pathway influences pain sensation. Noxious signaling may be modulated through a descending pathway that involves the periaqueductal grey. At the dorsal spinal cord, serotonin and norepinephrine appear to play important roles in sensory modulation.[3] Although these mechanisms have been hypothesized for some time, they remain difficult to test. Another area of the brain that has been implicated in pain has been the rostral anterior cingulate cortex (rACC).[31] Using imagery strategies, deCharms and colleagues were able to demonstrate that teaching healthy volunteers or chronic pain patients to control activation of the rACC, as monitored with real-time functional MRI, led to a decrease in pain perception.[31]

Advantages

R&I has three primary advantages over the similar but more complex technique of hypnosis (see Chapter 84): (1) Patients can be trained in the use of the skills with relative ease; (2) no special equipment or extensive training of the therapist is required; and (3) patients readily accept R&I techniques, whereas they are more likely to reject hypnosis.[32]

Although it can be difficult to predict who will benefit from R&I, the lack of serious complications and the relative ease and low cost with which it can be tried make this a method with minimal risks.[33] Unlike the practice of hypnosis, R&I is essentially a skill that can be learned. It also does not depend to any extent on the "susceptibility" of the patient, although it does require willingness to practice. If a patient is unable to visualize images, PMR can be taught with potential benefit, and methods can be adapted to the particular capabilities and preferences of a patient. Thus, the flexibility within the method leaves room for adaptation to a wide variety of styles or needs. Expectations of patients tend to be more realistic than for hypnosis. While hypnosis may benefit from positive expectations and wishes for a "magic cure," higher levels of fear of loss of control can work against patient receptiveness, whereas fear is rarely aroused by R&I utilization.

Disadvantages

R&I requires the participation of the patient. To optimize benefit, patients must practice outside the trainer's office. Although self-control is one of its appeals to patients, lack of practice is one of the greatest problems in its use.[30] Further disadvantages follow as corollaries to R&I's advantages. These include the lack of implied "magic cure" that can be hoped for with either a medical intervention or hypnosis. Ease of use and lack of cost can be associated in patients' minds with lower expected efficacy. The effects of R&I may not be immediately apparent but can accumulate over time, as will be discussed in the studies to follow, thus requiring not only practice but also patience. R&I is a subjective experience not unlike pain; as such, its effects can be difficult to measure and confidence in their benefits may be low. In addition, imaging ability may be a moderator of reduction in pain when using guided imagery.[2] Finally, for most conditions, R&I is not an adequate stand-alone treatment for pain, but must be considered a complementary method used in combination with appropriate medical treatment.

CLINICAL INFORMATION

Indications

Indications for treating pain vary with the type of pain and the condition of the patient. Relaxation is recommended for any patient for whom tension is a significant cause of pain or for whom tension and fear may be augmenting the pain problem. In acute pain situations such as childbirth, trauma, or procedural pain, R&I may be combined with meditation and other distraction strategies that decrease the focus on discomfort and speed the passage of time. Relaxation is clearly indicated in the treatment of tension, migraine, and cluster headaches and in TMD pain. In other chronic conditions and in cancer pain, clinical trials have indicated that R&I and meditation reduce pain.[14,20,28,34] With the limitations of time in the current medical practice environment, R&I is most strongly recommended for patients who have chronic conditions that cannot be adequately relieved with medical intervention alone. In addition, patients will benefit from R&I training if they must regularly repeat acutely painful procedures because fear and phobias can increase over time with exposure to these stimuli.

Contraindications

Contraindications are few and usually relate more to the mental status and characteristics of the patient than to the pain condition itself. Pain or sedation that prevents a patient from focusing attention, or a delirium that disrupts cognition, needs to be treated with other methods until concentration is possible. Then, briefer images with a short relaxation component can permit participation by a patient who otherwise could not sustain the mental effort needed for more extended training. Sometimes these patients feel ease of intense discomfort by combining images with physical massage or pressure on a part of the body (shoulder, hand, lower arm, or calf muscles) that is not in pain. Of course, clinicians must be cautious and should consider having someone else in the room if they decide that physical touch with imagery is needed to help a patient with pain that cannot be relieved with medical methods alone.

Certainly religious objections,[14] intense fear of loss of control, or resistance to trying the method for any reason should be respected. Skepticism is not a reason to withhold treatment if the patient is willing to give the technique a valid try—clinicians can encourage a healthy skepticism and empirical testing attitude. Similarly, patients who ask for biological explanations for why mental strategies might work usually respond well to information about physiologic mechanisms behind R&I. These patients also may do best with PMR in the beginning because this helps to enhance awareness of physical changes that occur as the body relaxes. The same is true for patients who seem out of touch with their bodies and unaware of tension or for patients who are action-oriented "doers not thinkers."

Intense anxiety or preoccupation that prohibits focus on imagery must be attended to pharmacologically or with discussion before beginning R&I. Because anxiety can increase during imagery, the clinician should assess a highly anxious patient and ensure that emotional expression is tolerable. Usually a patient presenting with extreme anxiety needs to express thoughts and feelings first. Then the clinician can re-evaluate the patient's ability to focus. Ability to engage in a discussion of places that the patient enjoys should indicate adequate ability to participate in imagery.

Two additional circumstances can complicate the use of R&I: One is the patient who is feeling very out of control; the other is the patient who has a strong need to be in control. For patients who feel completely out of control of their experience and environment, a clinician can appropriately take charge of the situation and let patients know the clinician is going to ensure their safety during the process. Clinicians need to convey to patients that the situation is manageable and the pain can be relieved. If these messages seem to reassure and calm the patient, the clinician should be able to move into imagery. For patients who give indications that they must be in control, clinicians will want to assess whether these patients might respond best to permissive, indirect imagery versus more structured PMR methods. PMR helps in this situation because patients can be told exactly what steps the clinician will take. Generally, patients feel safest with PMR because it is clear that patients control their own responses. Alternatively, if imagery is used, the clinician can encourage patients to select as many features of the imagery as possible and can incorporate options and permission to have other thoughts or experiences during the imagery. Another strategy is to have patients tell the clinician what they see, feel, hear, and do in their imagery, with the clinician asking questions rather than leading the imagery process.

Techniques

Preparation of the Patient

Relaxation may be learned and practiced by virtually anyone. The techniques can be taught by those who have had relatively limited training, but clinicians should be aware of and prepared to handle possible complications. Before relaxation training begins, the clinician should explain to pain patients the rationale for the particular procedure being used. Also, the clinician should assess for treatment expectancy as these are related to outcome measures of pain management.[35] In a recent study, pretreatment negative expectancies predicted negative affect and poorer health-related quality of life a full year after R&I plus cognitive–behavioral treatment.[35] Many patients view relaxation as irrelevant to their pain problem, or even as an indication that their doctors think the pain is "just tension" or "all in my head." Most patients are helped in their disbelief by a brief discussion of the physiologic pathways of pain perception, hypothesized neuroendocrine effects, and the feedback loop between pain and tension or fear. Patients can also be told that relaxation training is harmless and, if nothing else, will leave the patient feeling relaxed. The clinician can then suggest that the procedure be tried as an "experiment," with nothing to lose. This approach is preferable to promising patients dramatic pain relief because this rarely occurs initially. Patients also need to understand that R&I is a skill, like learning to read. Benefits take time to reach their peak, and daily home practice is necessary to become adept at the procedure and to maintain benefits. Audiotapes can be helpful in supporting home practice.

To prevent surprises and help patients feel secure, clinicians should describe the basic steps involved in the technique and estimate the length of time required to complete the procedure. Although increased comfort can be achieved in as little as 5 minutes, deep relaxation requires at least 20 minutes for new practitioners and may continue for up to 45 minutes. Patients can be advised that they will likely be most comfortable with their eyes closed, although this is not mandatory, and that they are free to move at any time to make themselves more comfortable. Use of a reclining chair with a headrest is desirable, or patients can sit on the floor or a regular chair. They should not lie on a bed, unless the goal is rest for a sleep-deprived patient in pain. Lying on a bed tends to evoke falling asleep rather than completing the imagery. When using imagery, it is critical to assess for images that would be helpful as what one patient considers relaxing might not be so for another patient.[14] Unplugging the phone and minimizing other noises or disruptions are helpful. In hospital rooms this is not always possible. Therefore it is helpful to add a statement such as "and just allow any sounds around you to fade to the distance, part of the background that adds to your feeling of being in a different place, a place all your own right now." Surprisingly, after imagery, patients often indicate that they were unaware of any sounds or disruptions even though they may seem intrusive to the clinician.

Training Procedures

Deep breathing is the most rapidly learned of the relaxation techniques. Very little training is needed to obtain benefits. Controlled breathing also can be quite effective in capturing and holding a very distressed patient's attention and may be the first step toward using imagery to further distract the patient from the distress. One component that is often not stressed but can be quite valuable in relieving pain is making a sound while breathing, usually just emphasizing the sound of air leaving the lungs and mouth. Another component of deep breathing that can improve effectiveness when panic is a component of acute pain, is to remind the patient to exhale first, not inhale. Shallow breathing is a feature of panic, reducing available oxygen volume. Exhaling first allows oxygen to be inhaled more fully. Variations on this method are commonly used in childbirth preparation.[34] Typical instructions for deep breathing are given in Table 85.1.

PMR is the most routine of the techniques. Because it requires the patient to tense and release muscle groups, it provides feedback to the clinician (as well as the patient) on the participation of the patient. The tense–release format provides momentum from which the patient can achieve relaxation well below usual levels of tension relief. Before implementing this technique with a patient, clinicians are urged to read the manual by Bernstein and Borkovec[9] or another in-depth "how-to" for this method.

Autogenic relaxation is similar to PMR in that it progresses through the body, focusing attention on relaxing each area of

TABLE 85.1

INSTRUCTIONS FOR DEEP BREATHING[a]

> I. Perform the following steps in sequence:
>   A. Deep breathing may be done in any position. If possible, sit, lie, or stand comfortably, with a straight spine.
>   B. Exhale the air in your lungs.
>   C. Inhale through your nose while counting slowly to four as you:
>   1. First fill the lower section of your lungs. Your diaphragm will push your abdomen outward to make room for the air.
>   2. Second, fill the middle part of your lungs as your lower ribs and chest move forward to accommodate the air.
>   3. Third, fill the upper part of your lungs as you raise your chest and shoulders slightly and draw your abdomen in a little to support your lungs.
>   4. With practice, these three steps can be performed in one smooth, continuous inhalation.
>   D. Hold your breath for a slow count of three.
>   E. Exhale through your mouth, making a relaxing, whooshing sound like the wind as you blow out to a slow count of 4.
>   F. As you exhale, follow the same order as the inhalation:
>   1. First, pull your abdomen in.
>   2. Next, exhale from your middle chest.
>   3. Finally, exhale from your upper chest as you allow your shoulders to sink and relax and your abdomen to puff out again slightly.
>
> II. As the pattern becomes automatic, scan your body for other areas of tension, then return to the sound and feeling of breathing as you become more and more relaxed.
>
> III. Imagine all the tension from your body being pulled into your lungs and being exhaled with your breath.
>
> IV. Continue deep breathing for 5–10 minutes at a time. If you become lightheaded at any point, alternate six regular breaths with six deep breaths.
>
> V. As you continue deep breathing, scan your body for any area that may remain tense, focus on this place and imagine breathing directly through this area.
>
> VI. When you have learned to relax yourself using deep breathing, practice it whenever and wherever you feel yourself getting tense.

[a]Following the instructions provided results in the most complete relaxation, but the steps can be shortened or adapted depending on the clinical situation.
Adapted from Davis M, Eshelman EF, McKay M. *The Relaxation and Stress Reduction Workbook*. Oakland, CA: New Harbinger Publications, 1982.

the body in turn. Autogenics, however, does not require tensing muscles first. The focus is on imagining a feeling of warmth and heaviness in each area. Imagery may be inserted after completion of the relaxation phase or may be combined with the relaxation phrases. This technique is useful with patients who are quite fatigued and uncomfortable. The imagery component may relate only to feelings of warmth, heaviness, and sensations that accompany relaxation or may be augmented at length depending on the will and interest of patient and clinician.

Incorporating imagery into relaxation can greatly enhance efficacy as a pain relief tool.[10,20,36] Imagery also increases the enjoyment of patients and therefore the likelihood that they will use the technique. Activating all the senses in the mind can create distraction as well as hypnotic-like experiences of comfort, wellbeing, and mastery of a problem. For instance, patients can be asked to choose a place where they have felt most at ease or joyful. As patients recapture the familiar experience of a place with sight, sound, taste, smell, and touch, they also recapture the feelings of comfort. Clinicians can then suggest to patients that by imagining themselves in that place, patients can once again be comfortable and in control of how they feel. The content of images can vary greatly, from going to pleasant places to modifying the pain experience directly.[14,37] Patients without these abilities may respond more to the relaxation component of R&I. Choice of images may be the most important factor in the success

of imagery. Pleasantness may be more important to encouraging use of the imagery than in enhancing its effect on pain.[40] Pain reduction is greater when patients can choose their images and when they make statements to themselves in the imagery that they are able to tolerate or modify the pain.[39] More success in using imagery may be achieved by patients with greater ability to generate images and those who have a capacity to experience images as if they are real.[38,39]

An alternative imagery strategy is more akin to meditation. This approach involves focusing on the pain rather than away from it and picturing details of the pain location.[41] There is some indication that for more extreme, unremitting types of pain such as with terminal cancer, focusing on the pain rather than away from it is more effective in achieving pain reduction.[42] Table 85.2 lists some of the more commonly used imagery strategies for pain control. These can be incorporated into imagery of going to a favorite place or can be combined with deep breathing.

In execution, meditation most resembles deep breathing. Instead of focusing sequentially on each part of the body, meditation requires a cultivated "detached observation."[6,8] Two similar approaches to meditation have been useful in medical settings. One involves repeating a phrase or word to oneself and is referred to as the *relaxation response*[5]; the other is called *mindfulness meditation*.[8,23] Mindfulness meditation is similar to the imagery approaches that transform painful sensation.[41] Attention is fo-

TABLE 85.2

IMAGERY OPTIONS FOR PAIN CONTROL—STRATEGIES

I. **Escape or distraction by having the patient go to a favorite place**
  A. Use multisensory imagery: color, shades of light, texture of objects, sensations against the skin (e.g., air temperature), smells, taste, sounds, physical sensations
  B. To increase absorption, change the surroundings, have the patient move deeper into the place or on to another location that moves the person further away from the pain, and find something unexpected.
  C. Introduce another person or object with a "message" the patient most needs to hear right now; have the patient connect with that person in a caring way (look into the other person's eyes, touch hands, hear the words that are most helpful right now).
  D. For pain relief through distraction, include physical action in the imagery; have the patient walk, run, feel the strength and power of his or her muscles, how well the body works, how healthy and comfortable it feels to move.
  E. Use positive suggestions—what is felt.
    1. Pain or discomfort is not mentioned.
    2. Talk about "moving attention to that area of the body that you would like to feel more comfortable, more at ease."

Advantages
Most enjoyable so patients are more likely to practice
Takes less effort from the patient

Disadvantages
Provides distraction, but without analgesic suggestions it may not extend pain relief past the period of the imagery

II. **Block pain with images of analgesia or anesthesia.**
  A. Numbness via ice or anesthetic
  B. Flip switches to change the channel so the pain message cannot connect to the brain.
  C. Turn down the signal of the pain message to the brain; count down the numbers (using the 0 to 10 point scale for pain) to a pain number that is acceptable to the patient.

Advantages
Provides direct analgesic suggestions
Gives patients control over the pain and the use of imagery at any time, thus extending relief past the period of imagery

Disadvantages
Takes more active participation by the patient
Patients may feel they have failed if it "doesn't work"
May be easier for more suggestible patients

III. **Sensory transformations**
  A. After relaxing, go to the pain location with the mind; as a neutral observer, explore the pain and watch as it changes. Have patients notice what the pain says to them and how they can respond to ease the pain.
  B. Use images that can change as the pain changes and have the patient observe these changes in color, shape, density, texture, size.
  C. Use images that compete with the pain description.
    1. Blow cold arctic air through a burning pain.
    2. Take a knotted cramping pain, gather the knot into a fist and throw it away, or loosen the knot, watch as it softens, smoothes, eases.

Advantages
Takes less energy than blocking pain
Goes with the patient's focus rather than fighting against it
Can be done quickly without lengthy relaxation for patients in acute pain
Can be very successful in easing pain and greatly reducing tendency to tighten around pain

Disadvantages
Less likely to eradicate pain; instead teaches the patient to modify and work with the pain
Pain may initially seem worse because of the focus on it, scaring the patient

IV. **Additional strategies can be used with hypnotic trance (see Chapter 84)**

cused not on changing pain perception but on insight developed from distinguishing all sensations as they occur moment by moment. Thoughts about pain are observed from the position of a neutral observer. Although relaxation response training is easy to implement, data do not clearly document its effectiveness as a pain reduction method. Mindfulness meditation, on the other hand, has been shown to reduce pain in chronically ill patients.[23,28] In a feasibility study comparing mindfulness, massage, and control groups of patients recruited from an internal medicine practice, the two treatment groups did not differ, and both groups had reductions in pain compared with controls.[43] Differences appeared at the 12-week follow-up when the massage group was unable to maintain gains whereas the mindfulness group was able to do so.[43] In another study using pain-free volunteers, pain tolerance increased after mindfulness practice.[44] For meditation, an experienced clinician is recommended as a trainer. Instructions for using the relaxation response and instructions for mindfulness meditation are detailed thoroughly in the Kabat-Zinn book.[8]

Related to mindfulness-based approaches, McCracken and colleagues have promoted using acceptance to treat chronic pain.[45–48] The utility of acceptance is that people are taught to acknowledge the pain they are experiencing while continuing to live their lives rather than avoiding activities because of fear of re-injury or worsening pain.[45] In one study of this method, participants were less depressed and reduced the amount of time resting due to pain.[46] Caution should be used in interpreting these findings as a randomized controlled trial has yet to be done testing acceptance. However, it may be a promising new approach in pain management.

Effectiveness

Comparisons have been made between R&I strategies and hypnosis or biofeedback, as well as between different relaxation techniques. Numerous studies have also tested packages of cognitive–behavioral skills training that have included a form of R&I. Each of these interventions, including hypnosis, biofeedback, and cognitive–behavioral packages, elicits similar physiologic responses and subjective reductions in pain when compared with no treatment.[1,16,20,25,27,29,36,49,50] In general, research results indicate that R&I demonstrates greater effect size than other strategies alone and that packages of cognitive–behavioral skills are not always superior to R&I alone.[10,11,49] Hypnosis, biofeedback, and audiotaped relaxation are less effective than live PMR in achieving reductions in sympathetic arousal.[24,51] However, a taped version of guided imagery has been found to be effective.[52] An exception may be frontalis EMG levels, which have shown greater reductions with autogenic relaxation than with tense–release relaxation, although both approaches produce some decrease in EMG.[53] This finding may interest clinicians choosing between relaxation techniques for the treatment of tension headache.

Much of the research on the effectiveness of relaxation alone for pain reduction has been conducted with tension headache patients. In general, the results of these studies suggest that relaxation is effective and that benefits are maintained at follow-up.[16] Relaxation training alone appears to be a reasonable first step for headache sufferers, with the addition of biofeedback for those patients who are unsuccessful with relaxation alone.[54] Similarly, research with TMD pain patients suggests that many can be treated successfully with relaxation alone, although some patients may benefit from the addition of biofeedback.[55] With other conditions, relaxation is best implemented in combination with imagery.

Pain reduction is not the only goal of many treatments. R&I may target health-related quality of life and not just pain.[56] R&I has achieved superior results in return to work rates when compared with medication alone.[50] Health care visits also have decreased in the year following R&I interventions.[50] The next sections discuss efficacy of a single method of R&I within specific medical conditions, as this is how most clinical trials of R&I methods are tested.

Chronic Conditions

R&I is usually one element in a set of cognitive–behavioral treatments for chronic pain, rather than an independent pain control technique. Research indicates that R&I can contribute to reduced pain levels, reduced medication use in a number of chronic conditions, and reduced disability, although the role of R&I versus other cognitive methods is not yet clear.[29,49,50] The evidence for sustained improved function is less consistent but more often than not supports improvement in disability after treatment.[29,49,57–59] Chapter 82 presents a thorough review of the effectiveness of cognitive–behavioral strategies that usually include R&I.

Kabat-Zinn and colleagues[8,23,28] have used mindfulness meditation to successfully treat a variety of chronic problems, including pain located in the low back, neck, shoulder, arm, leg, face, head, chest, peripheral nerves, and multiple sites. About 10% to 20% of patients refuse to use this strategy for pain control. A majority (72%) who are willing to try are able to reduce their pain by 33% or more. In addition, improvement has been noted in body image, activity, mood disturbance, and medication use. Compliance both during and after participation in the program has been high. These results support the contention that meditation may have a generalized beneficial effect for chronic pain patients.

Headache. Tension headache research dominates the literature and generally reveals relaxation to be as effective or more effective than biofeedback.[16,27,60,61] The same results have been found with migraine headache, although fewer studies are available. The most careful explorations into the relative roles of relaxation and biofeedback in relieving headache have been reported by Blanchard et al.[54,60,62] and Andrasik et al.[63] (see Chapter 61). In terms of both cost-effectiveness and success, the optimal therapy for tension, migraine, or mixed tension and migraine pain appears to be a two-step treatment beginning with PMR. For those patients who do not show substantial reduction in headache activity with PMR, the second step is instituted. For vascular headache patients, the second step is thermal biofeedback; for tension headache patients, frontalis EMG biofeedback is the second step. Blanchard et al.[64] found that with this two-step therapy 73% of tension headache patients and 52% of vascular headache patients were much improved. While all groups improved with relaxation, tension headache patients improved the most.

Philips and Hunter[65] tested the effects of PMR versus PMR with calming imagery for tension headache patients. The two groups showed similar improvements in pain. The authors suggested that the addition of imagery produced a larger improvement in pain based on several outcome measures even though no individual measure showed significantly superior effects.

The superiority or equivalence of relaxation and biofeedback has not been consistent across studies. LaCroix et al.,[66] for instance, found that thermal biofeedback was superior to frontalis EMG feedback and relaxation for migraine patients, although all groups improved. However, Vasudeva et al.[67] conducted a randomized control trial with people who had migraines with aura using biofeedback and relaxation and found that those in the biofeedback condition had significant reductions in pain, anxiety, and depression compared to the control group that was told to relax without any further instruction.

With regard to home practice, Andrasik et al.[63] reported that posttreatment practice was unrelated to maintenance of effects. It should be noted, however, that all patients in this study were provided with regular therapist visits.

Low Back Pain. Studies comparing relaxation with other techniques for low back pain indicate that relaxation is an effective treatment[68,69] but that combining relaxation with other cognitive–behavioral strategies may be advantageous (see Chapter 82). Turner[70] compared PMR treatment with PMR plus additional cognitive-behavioral therapy or no treatment. The two treatment groups both reported reduced pain intensity and disability immediately after treatment and at 1.5- and 2-year follow-up. The cognitive–behavioral group, however, showed some superiority in maintaining treatment gains and in hours worked per week. A number of other studies by Turner et al. support the use of relaxation as one component of effective cognitive–behavioral treatment for chronic pain.[16,29,49,70,71] McCauley et al.[72] compared PMR with hypnosis in the treatment of low back pain and found that both treatments were similarly effective and superior to a placebo EMG treatment.[73]

Though studies indicate that relaxation contributes to the efficacy of combination treatments for low back pain, the value of adding specific components to treatment packages remains unclear. In particular, the usefulness of combining imagery with relaxation training for treatment of chronic conditions needs to be examined. Furthermore, outcome variables other than symptom relief, such as employment status, medication, and health care use need to be evaluated when considering the utility of R&I for low back pain.[68]

Temporomandibular Disorder Pain. The research on relaxation and cognitive–behavioral packages that include PMR for TMD pain supports the conclusion that relaxation is effective in reducing pain and is at least as successful as biofeedback, the most commonly compared treatment.[71] Funch and Gale[55] reported that biofeedback and audiotaped relaxation training were equally effective in reducing TMD pain. Patients who were more successful using relaxation were generally younger, had experienced TMD pain for a shorter period of time, and reported other psychophysiologic disorders. The differential effect of relaxation and biofeedback with different patients also was found in a single-subject, multiple-baseline study by Moss et al.[74] In this study, relaxation with EMG feedback was most effective for three out of four patients tested. In a large, randomized, controlled clinical treatment, Dworkin et al.[71] compared patients receiving usual treatment for TMD with patients receiving usual treatment plus a package of cognitive–behavioral skills that included relaxation training. The skills-trained group reported continued improvement over 12 months of follow-up and overall lower pain scores. Researchers also found a strong trend toward reduced pain interference with function. Turner et al.[59] compared PMR to self-care, consisting of dispensing general health information but no advice or treatment, and found that participants in the PMR condition made clinically significant changes in pain level, activity interference, depression, and jaw function. These gains were maintained over a 1-year follow-up.

Arthritis and Autoimmune Diseases. The benefits of self-management strategies that include relaxation for coping with arthritis pain and dysfunction are well documented.[75–82] Educational strategies that may or may not include relaxation exercises are widely used in arthritis and are cost-effective and pain relieving over and above the efficacy of medication alone.[11,77,83] Even more so than with low back pain and other chronic conditions, arthritis and autoimmune diseases are not treated with R&I alone, but rather with R&I as a component of educational and other cognitive skills training.[11,84] Consequently, it is difficult to know to what extent R&I is an essential component of these techniques. There is no reason to believe that patients with arthritis pain or autoimmune diseases would respond differently than patients with other chronic illnesses such as low back pain or cancer, even though each disease has its own unique characteristics and therefore stressors that tax coping.

Cancer Pain. Cancer patients may experience acute treatment-related pain or chronic pain (see Chapters 41–49). Chronic pain with cancer may be stable (e.g., postmastectomy pain) or progressive (e.g., tumor invasion pain). R&I is commonly used in the management of cancer pain and is effective.[84,85] Successful treatment depends to some extent on tailoring therapy to the type of pain. In clinical reports, R&I, sometimes called *hypnosis*, is touted.[86,87] However, there are few controlled trials on the efficacy of R&I with adult cancer patients.[88] As noted by Jay et al.,[89] adult research has focused on persistent pain, whereas pediatric research has focused on procedural pain. Spiegel and Bloom[90] provided group "self-hypnosis" training to breast cancer patients and reported an additive analgesic effect of hypnosis, with smaller increases in pain and suffering over time. Syrjala et al.[36] provided three groups of bone marrow transplant patients with training in "hypnosis," cognitive–behavioral training including PMR, or support with no training. The group receiving hypnosis reported lower average levels of oral pain after chemoradiotherapy than the other two groups. In a follow-up study, Syrjala and colleagues[20] tested R&I against three other groups: a standard treatment control, a supportive psychotherapy intervention, and a cognitive–behavioral package, which included R&I. Again, in this clinical trial R&I was the most effective treatment for pain, with cognitive–behavioral methods showing no mean additive effect over and above the R&I alone. There was an indication that some patients who may not have benefited from the R&I alone benefited from the cognitive–behavioral package. However, power was not adequate to test this hypothesis. These data indicate a valuable role for imagery in helping cancer patients cope with pain. Results also suggest a need to individualize patient treatments.

Relaxation with EMG was found to be an effective means of pain reduction in a sample of Taiwanese patients with advanced cancer.[91] EMG data indicate that relaxation not only decreased pain but also anxiety and physiological arousal. This study also demonstrates cross-cultural validity for the use of relaxation techniques.

Acute Conditions

Childbirth. Preparation for childbirth usually includes breathing exercises with a visual focus and sometimes includes formal relaxation training (see Chapter 56). As Tan[34] noted in his review, studies on the effectiveness of these strategies in reducing pain in childbirth are supportive but equivocal. Many studies do not include actual measures of pain level in reporting favorable outcomes. Despite the equivocal data on pain reduction associated with childbirth preparation, the reduced distress resulting from such programs probably supports their continued use.

Acute Traumatic, Procedural, and Postoperative Pain. A number of sources confirm the benefits of relaxation training before various procedures and surgery.[92] Only anecdotal evidence was found for the use of deep breathing, relaxation, and imagery during acute trauma, although hypnosis has been demonstrated effective during burn debridement.[93] In a review of nonpharmacological interventions for burn patients, relaxation was found to be effective in reducing pain.[94] This is a difficult area to research because of the unpredictable availability of patients and the wide variety of possible injuries. By and large, support for the use of R&I strategies in trauma situations must be extrapolated from research on other acute pain conditions.

Relaxation training before stressful procedures has been shown to be effective in reducing a number of measures of pain and distress. For example, patients trained in PMR and deep breathing before sigmoidoscopy rated themselves as less anxious and made fewer requests to stop the procedure than patients who were not trained in relaxation.[95] Both relaxation and information have been reported to reduce heart rate and observer ratings of distress during endoscopy. Only relaxation also increased positive mood.[96] Even greater effect size was seen in a study of imagery and self-hypnosis during radiologic procedures. In this randomized controlled trial, patients receiving the R&I and hypnosis treatment reported less pain, used less analgesic medication, reported less anxiety, and had fewer procedural interruptions due to hemodynamic instability.[97] In a departure from using specialists to provide R&I to patients, Lang and colleagues[97,98] have trained radiology nurses and technicians to provide R&I during painful procedures. Patients receiving R&I reported lower pain scores, with a strong trend toward less drug use.[98]

Laboratory and clinical studies have found that the effectiveness of relaxation training in acute situations may depend on the coping style of the patient. In the laboratory, it has been reported that patients who were more external in their "locus of control" were better able to use relaxation training than were patients who were more internal—that is, saw themselves as the agent of control.[99] During procedural discomfort, patients who reported that they preferred to avoid thinking about unpleasant things were helped more by relaxation than by information, whereas the reverse was true of the nonavoiders.[96] In addition, patients who indicated that they were less independent benefited from both relaxation and information, whereas those who were more independent benefited from neither. Relaxation and information were not demonstrated to be harmful to patients who were not matched on intervention and coping style. Finally, with postoperative patients, Scott and Clum[100] found that brief relaxation training was profitable for those who had "sensitizing" coping styles that focus on problems, but not for those who were avoiders. In sum, avoiders and "external locus of control" patients may do particularly well with escape-oriented pleasant imagery, whereas other patients may respond well to all types of R&I.

Pediatric Applications

Research on the use of relaxation techniques with children is less extensive and well controlled than the research with adults. Lavigne et al.,[101] Vessey and Carlson,[17] Rheingans,[102] and Eccleston et al.[103] provide reviews of painful pediatric conditions and the interventions that have been successful. The terminology used in much of the published research is inconsistent. For example, treatments are interchangeably defined as active fantasy, guided imagery, breathing, hypnosis, relaxation, or imagery.

Children are generally able to participate in imagining as a distraction from pain or fantasy to modify the pain experience from approximately 5 years of age.[17] Initially, imagery differs from play or active fantasy and storytelling only in its intention. We have found it particularly effective to use stuffed animals or soft puppets onto which the child can transfer the pain, fear, or anger that accompany pain. When left with the child, these toys become an object with which the child can repeat the imagery when the clinician is not present. As children mature to adolescence, imagery and relaxation methods increasingly resemble those used with adults. However, adolescents and children are closer to fantasy than many adults and therefore require little or no time in relaxation and need to move to fantasy imagery more quickly. Adolescents respond well to imagery with themselves as heroes and the agents of change and success. Pain transformations can be included in these images of mastery.

In research with pediatric cancer patients, interventions have focused on procedure-related pain and distress.[89,104–106] Effective treatments have included breathing and imagery, sometimes incorporated into a cognitive–behavioral package. Although numerous studies demonstrate that R&I can reduce distress related to procedures, and sometimes pain, light sedation has largely supplanted a need for R&I with repeated invasive procedures such as lumbar punctures and bone marrow aspirations.

A small number of case studies suggest that relaxation, particularly if coupled with imagery, can be effective in treating other pediatric pain problems. Distraction and breathing exercises have received some support as useful techniques for relieving pain during debridement for pediatric burn patients.[101] Weydert et al.[107] compared guided imagery with PMR to deep breathing for treating recurrent abdominal pain in children. Participants in this study improved more in the guided imagery with PMR condition than in the breathing condition. In addition, participants were able to maintain their gains over a 2-month follow-up. Unlike relaxation research with adults, which has focused on tension headache, pediatric research has focused on autogenic relaxation for migraine. This research clearly supports the use of autogenics for relief of migraine in children.[101]

Because children are easily engaged in active imagery, this component can be successfully introduced into most interventions with children in pain. Clinicians interested in the use of imagery are also referred to the literature on hypnosis, as many researchers using imagery with children have termed their interventions "hypnosis."

Complications

Minor Problems. One of the advantages of relaxation techniques in comparison with more invasive therapies is the lack of lasting adverse effects. Most complications are rare, harmless, and can be quickly resolved. Muscle cramps can develop with PMR, in which case the patient can be asked to generate less tension in problem areas for shorter periods of time. If necessary, a pause can be taken while the patient massages cramped muscles. Unless the patient comments or appears uncomfortable, spasms should simply be ignored. Patients can be reassured that muscle spasms are common when people relax and occur in many people when they fall asleep. Movements are common and not disruptive. They can be normalized by the clinician including suggestions for shifting to a more comfortable position at any time. Talking and laughter usually stop if they are ignored. Alternatively, they can be casually acknowledged, such as "and just notice that different thoughts or feelings may come up and that's fine, just a part of letting things flow through your mind and away, feeling even more at ease."

Because some patients experience intrusive thoughts as disruptive, they should be told ahead of time that such thoughts are to be expected. Suggest that as thoughts arise, they can be allowed to "float through the mind, knowing that anything important will still remain later, but that right now there are no other things to focus on or to do but to let these normal thoughts just drift away."

If a patient falls asleep, the therapist might need to speak in a progressively louder voice until the patient is again awake. Patients who report falling asleep regularly during home practice should be instructed to practice earlier in the day and in a sitting position, not lying down.

Problems Requiring Attention. Problems requiring the therapist to be more careful and attentive are infrequent. The more common difficulties and some solutions are described in Table 85.3. For certain patients, tension or pain can be localized in an area not sufficiently covered by the standard relaxation of body parts. TMD pain, as an example, benefits from exercises and relaxation targeted to the jaw area.[71] If residual tension remains, it is helpful to develop a tension or relaxation strategy that specifically targets the localized area. This might involve taking time after relaxing to go to any place in the body that continues to feel tight or uncomfortable, going to that place with the mind and watching while imagining breathing through that place and noticing the changes in sensations. Sensory transformation imagery may be used to expand on this experience.

Pain patients commonly have an initially greater awareness of the pain as attention is focused on internal states. In this case, patients can be instructed to observe the pain in a detached man-

TABLE 85.3

PROBLEMS AND SOLUTIONS ENCOUNTERED IN CLINICAL PRACTICE

Problem	Solutions

Fatigued or in severe pain	First
	   Use medications for better pain control.
	   Consider medication options for fatigue or depression.
	Then
	   Use brief images; little induction is needed.
	   As appropriate, use touch on the hand, foot, or shoulder to help the patient focus, to anchor the patient away from the location of the pain, and to provide a competing sensation to the pain.
	   Begin simply, do only what is possible (e.g., breathing with an image of pain changing).

Lack of concentration	Use brief images.
	   If preoccupied, talk about preoccupations.
	   Perhaps try at a later time.

Highly distressed	Need to talk out feelings first. If feeling out of control, need signs that you are in control and believe the situation is manageable. Patients can relax because you are in control and will make sure they are okay.
Unsupportive family	Talk to the family. Involve the family in helping the patient. Help the patient solve the problem.
Not practicing	Review what gets in the way. Problem solve barriers. Try to remove guilt or "homework" associations so patient will claim the activity, not see it as externally imposed.
Skeptical patients	Encourage an experimenting attitude—"see what happens."
Religious patients	Explore whether faith and help of God can be incorporated as a focus of imagery. Discuss but defer if patient thinks imagery violates beliefs. Ensure that patient is always in control, can stop any time. Offer an option to observe or listen to a tape first.
Crying, increased anxiety, or other negative effects	Ask if patient is okay and wants to stop or continue. Talk about it; start again if patient is comfortable. Open eyes if feel safer.
Falling asleep	For patients in severe pain with sleep deprivation, encourage to continue with a deep, restful sleep. Raise the tone of voice and incorporate suggestions for more active imagery. If patients complain of falling asleep during home practice, suggest practice sitting up and at a time of day when more alert.
Unresponsive patients	Explore whether the patient has control fears or other barriers. Discuss what was experienced. Decide if worth trying again or if change in method is indicated. Reassure the patient that it often takes practice and gets easier with practice or that you may need to try several approaches to find the one that works best for him or her.

Reprinted from Syrjala KL, Abrams JR. Hypnosis and imagery in the treatment of pain. In: Turk DC, Gatchel RJ (eds.) *Psychosocial Approaches to Pain Management: A Practitioner's Guide*, 2nd ed. New York: Guilford Press, 2002:187–208, with permission.

ner (as described for meditation). Usually the intensity will lessen. Alternatively, the clinician can move the patient's attention to another part of the body or to images away from the body.

Patients who have been particularly out of touch with body sensations can suddenly become aware of any number of strange, unfamiliar sensations while relaxing and focusing on the body. Patients might feel as though they are floating and disoriented to such an extent that they must open their eyes until they once again feel comfortable. If this sensation or others are frightening, the clinician will need to respond with reassurance. Other discomforting sensations can include tingling, nausea, lightheadedness, or a sense of losing control.

Patients who fear losing control require perhaps the greatest care in designing an appropriate intervention. These patients often respond initially to PMR because the procedure feels most in their control. Explaining the steps of the procedure also helps to ease their fears. Another strategy is to offer choices for what they would like to try. With these patients, it is particularly important to include statements that they are in complete control of their experiences and what they choose to do, that at any time they can choose to change their experience or even to stop.

An increase in anxiety has been reported in some patients learning relaxation.[108] In our experience, this occurs in approximately 2% of patients. Switching to a different relaxation (e.g., PMR) that more fully occupies the patient's attention may help reduce such anxiety. Discussion of the nature of the anxiety may reveal an alternative set of thoughts or images that can provide a more neutral focal point for the patient. Often patients feel some relief from expressing pent-up feelings. However, other patients may feel embarrassed or reluctant to try imagery again. This circumstance requires the use of clinical skill in deciding the best approach for each individual.

Sexual arousal can occur from the relaxation and rarely from perceived seductiveness in the setting. If treated matter-of-factly as similar to other normal intrusive thoughts, this usually resolves on its own.[9]

Failure to practice relaxation strategies is by far the most common problem encountered. Clinicians can remind patients of other learning experiences, such as reading or biking, in which practice led to mastery. Discussion of changes in the home environment that would assist practice may also be helpful. Above all, clinicians must emphasize that practice is an important element of learning and using any relaxation technique successfully.

CONCLUSIONS

R&I techniques—including PMR, AT, deep breathing, imagery, and meditation—can be valuable in the treatment of both acute and chronic pain syndromes. The number of randomized controlled trials that demonstrate efficacy of R&I for many types of pain are sufficient to conclude that this is an effective strategy for pain treatment. The advantages of R&I include its relative cost-effectiveness and lack of lasting adverse effects. Although the specific physiologic mechanisms through which R&I reduces pain have not been proven, relaxation reduces muscle tension, quiets the sympathetic nervous system, and provides a cognitive distraction from distress and pain sensations. R&I may also lead to neuroendocrine changes that inhibit pain perception.

For headache and TMD pain, relaxation appears to be the treatment of choice, with biofeedback instituted for those patients who do not benefit from relaxation. For other chronic conditions, R&I may be as effective as biofeedback or any other packages of cognitive–behavioral skills. Furthermore, R&I is difficult to distinguish from hypnosis either in procedure or in effect. Similarly, with acute pain, R&I is as effective as other cognitive-behavioral approaches that have been studied.

There are no populations that should be excluded from using R&I, except for those with religious or other firm objections.

Children and adults equally benefit from the methods. Older adults also benefit.[109] Although R&I would rarely be used for painful conditions without considering appropriate medical treatments as well, R&I helps patients to be active participants in their health and should be considered whenever medical care alone is not adequate to alleviate pain.

Continuing challenges are to make this method less dependent on people with highly specialized expertise and to facilitate the incorporation of R&I into routine practice through training of nurses, technicians, and physicians providing front-line care. Other strategies are being tested that would combine video, printed, and audiotaped materials to patients who do not have access to experts or to provide these same types of materials through World Wide Web treatment groups. Matching patient characteristics to specific R&I techniques may also improve use. The survival of R&I as a pain strategy to combine with medical treatment may depend on these efforts to make R&I widely accessible.

Acknowledgment

The authors are supported by grants from the National Cancer Institute (CA63030, CA78990, and CA112631).

References

1. Morley S, Eccleston C, Williams A. Systematic review and meta-analysis of randomized controlled trials of cognitive behavior therapy and behavior therapy for chronic pain in adults, excluding headache. *Pain* 1999;80:1–13.
2. Kwekkeboom K, Huseby-Moore K, Ward S. Imaging ability and effective use of guided imagery. *Res Nurs Health* 1998;21:189–198.
3. Gatchel RJ, Peng YB, Peters ML, et al. The biopsychosocial approach to chronic pain: scientific advances and future directions. *Psychol Bull* 2007;133:581–624.
4. Jacobson E. *Progressive Relaxation*. Chicago: University of Chicago Press, 1974.
5. Benson H. *The Relaxation Response*. New York: Academic Press, 1975.
6. Benson H, Proctor W. *Beyond the Relaxation Response: How to Harness the Healing Power of Your Personal Beliefs*. New York: New York Times Book Co, 1984.
7. Turk DC, Meichenbaum D, Genest M. *Pain and Behavioral Medicine: A Cognitive Behavioral Perspective*. New York: Guilford Press, 1983.
8. Kabat-Zinn J. *Full Catastrophe Living: Using the Wisdom of Your Body and Mind to Face Stress, Pain, and Illness*. New York: Dell Publishing, 1990.
9. Bernstein DA, Borkovec TD. *Progressive Relaxation Training: A Manual for the Helping Professions*. Champaign, IL: Research Press, 1973.
10. Fernandez E, Turk DC. The utility of cognitive coping strategies for altering pain perception: a meta-analysis. *Pain* 1989;38:123–135.
11. Keefe FJ, Caldwell DS. Cognitive behavioral control of arthritis pain. *Adv Rheumatol* 1997;81:277–290.
12. McCaffery M, Beebe A. *Pain: Clinical Manual for Nursing Practice*. St. Louis: Mosby, 1989.
13. NIH panel, assessment. Integration of behavioral and relaxation approaches into the treatment of chronic pain and insomnia: NIH Technology Assessment Panel on integration of behavioral and relaxation approaches into the treatment of chronic pain and insomnia. *JAMA* 1996;276:313–318.
14. Syrjala KL, Abrams JR. Hypnosis and imagery in the treatment of pain. In: Gatchel RJ, Turk DC, eds. *Psychological Approaches to Pain Management: A Practitioner's Handbook*. New York: The Guilford Press, 1996:231–258.
15. Syrjala KL, Roth-Roemer SL. Nonpharmacologic approaches to pain. In: Berger A, ed. *Principles and Practices of Supportive Oncology*. Philadelphia, Pennsylvania: Lippincott–Raven, 1998:79–93.
16. Turner JA, Romano JM. Evaluating psychological interventions for chronic pain: issues and recent developments. In: Benedetti C, Chapman CR, Moricca G, eds. *Advances in Pain Research and Therapy*. New York: Raven Press, 1984:257–296.
17. Vessey JA, Carlson KL. Nonpharmacological interventions to use with children in pain. *Pediatr Nurs* 1996;19:169–182.
18. Wallace KG. Analysis of recent literature concerning relaxation and imagery interventions for cancer pain. *Cancer Nurs* 1997;20:79–87.
19. Ferrell BR, Ferrell BA, Ahn C, et al. Pain management for elderly patients with cancer at home. *Cancer* 1994;74:2139–2146.
20. Syrjala KL, Donaldson GW, Davis MW, et al. Relaxation and imagery and cognitive behavioral training reduce pain during cancer treatment: a controlled clinical trial. *Pain* 1995;63:189–198.
21. Wolpe J. *The practice of behavior therapy*. New York: Pergamon, 1969.

22. Luthe W. Autogenic training: method, research, and application in medicine. *Am J Psychother* 1963;17:174–195.

23. Kabat-Zinn J. An outpatient program in behavioral medicine for chronic pain patients based on the practice of mindfulness meditation: theoretical considerations and preliminary results. *Gen Hospl Psychiatry* 1982;4:33–47.

24. Paul GL. Physiological effects of relaxation training and hypnotic suggestion. *J Abnorm Psychol* 1969;74:425–437.

25. Kutz I, Borysenko JZ, Benson H. Meditation and psychotherapy: a rationale for the integration of dynamic psychotherapy, the relaxation response, and mindfulness meditation. *Am J Psychiatry* 1985;142:1–8.

26. Lehmann JW, Goodale IL, Benson H. Reduced pupillary sensitivity to topical phenylephrine associated with the relaxation response. *J Human Stress* 1986; 12:101–104.

27. Turner JA, Chapman CR. Psychological interventions for chronic pain: a critical review (I.) relaxation training and biofeedback. *Pain* 1982;12:1–21.

28. Kabat-Zinn J, Lipworth L, Burney R. The clinical use of mindfulness meditation for the self-regulation of chronic pain. *J Behav Med* 1985;8:163–190.

29. Turner JA, Jensen MP. Efficacy of cognitive therapy for chronic low back pain. *Pain* 1993;52:169–177.

30. Adams N, Poole H, Richardson C. Psychological approaches to chronic pain management: part 1. *J Clin Nurs* 2006;15:290–300.

31. deCharms RC, Maeda F, Glover GH, et al. Control over brain activation and pain learned by using real-time functional MRI. *Proc Natl Acad Sci U S A* 2005;102:18626–18631.

32. Hendler CS, Redd WH. Fear of hypnosis: the role of labeling in patients' acceptance of behavioral interventions. *Behav Ther* 1986;17:2–13.

33. Lin YC, Lee AC, Kemper KJ, Berde CB. Use of complementary and alternative medicine in pediatric pain management service: a survey. *Pain Med* 2005;6: 452–458.

34. Tan S-Y. Cognitive and cognitive behavioral methods for pain control: a selective review. *Pain* 1982;12:201–228.

35. Goossens ME, Vlaeyen JW, Hidding A, et al. Treatment expectancy affects the outcome of cognitive-behavioral interventions in chronic pain. *Clin J Pain* 2005;21:18–26.

36. Syrjala KL, Cummings C, Donaldson GW. Hypnosis or cognitive behavioral training for the reduction of pain and nausea during cancer treatment: a controlled clinical trial. *Pain* 1992;48:137–146.

37. Spiegel D, Moore R. Imagery and hypnosis in the treatment of cancer patients. *Oncology* 1997;11:1179–1189.

38. Kwekkeboom K, Huseby-Moore K, Ward S. Imaging ability and effective use of guided imagery. *Res Nurs Health* 1998;21:189–198.

39. Worthington EL. The effects of imagery content, choice of imagery content, and self-verbalization on the self-control of pain. *Cognit Ther Res* 1978;2: 225–240.

40. Syrjala K, Danis B, Abrams J, et al. *Coping Skills for Bone Marrow Transplantation.* Seattle: Fred Hutchinson Cancer Research Center, 1992;1–16.

41. Levine S. *Who Dies? An Investigation of Conscious Living and Conscious Dying.* Garden City, NY: Anchor Press, 1982.

42. McCaul KD, Malott JM. Distraction and coping with pain. *Psychol Bull* 1984; 95:516–533.

43. Plews-Ogan M, Owens JE, Goodman M, et al. A pilot study evaluating mindfulness-based stress reduction and massage for the management of chronic pain. *J Gen Intern Med* 2005;20:1136–1138.

44. Kingston J, Chadwick P, Meron D, et al. A pilot randomized control trial investigating the effect of mindfulness practice on pain tolerance, psychological well-being, and physiological activity. *J Psychosom Res* 2007;62:297–300.

45. McCracken LM, Eccleston C. A prospective study of acceptance of pain and patient functioning with chronic pain. *Pain* 2005;118:164–169.

46. McCracken LM, Vowles KE, Eccleston C. Acceptance-based treatment for persons with complex, long standing chronic pain: a preliminary analysis of treatment outcome in comparison to a waiting phase. *Behav Res Ther* 2005; 43:1335–1346.

47. McCracken LM, Gauntlett-Gilbert J, Vowles KE. The role of mindfulness in a contextual cognitive-behavioral analysis of chronic pain-related suffering and disability. *Pain* 2007;131:63–69.

48. McCracken LM, Vowles KE, Gauntlett-Gilbert J. A prospective investigation of acceptance and control-oriented coping with chronic pain. *J Behav Med* 2007;30:339–349.

49. Turner JA, Clancy S. Comparison of operant behavioral and cognitive behavioral group treatment for chronic low back pain. *J Consult Clin Psychol* 1988; 56:261–266.

50. Gatchel RJ, Okifuji A. Evidence-based scientific data documenting the treatment and cost effectiveness of comprehensive pain programs for chronic nonmalignant pain. *J Pain* 2006;7:779–793.

51. Lehrer PM. How to relax and how not to relax: a reevaluation of the work of Edmund Jacobson-I. *Behav Res Ther* 1982;20:417–428.

52. Lewandowski W, Good M, Draucker CB. Changes in the meaning of pain with the use of guided imagery. *Pain Manag Nurs* 2005;6:58–67.

53. Haynes SN, Moseley D, McGowan WT. Relaxation training and biofeedback in the reduction of frontalis muscle tension. *Psychophysiology* 1975;12: 547–552.

54. Blanchard EB, Andrasik F, Neff DF, et al. Sequential comparisons of: relaxation, training, and biofeedback in the treatment of three kinds of chronic headache or the machines may be necessary some of the time. *Behav Res Ther* 1982;20:469–481.

55. Funch DP, Gale EN. Biofeedback and relaxation therapy for chronic temporomandibular joint pain: predicting successful outcomes. *J Consult Clin Psychol* 1984;52:928–935.

56. Baird CL, Sands LP. Effect of guided imagery with relaxation on health-related quality of life in older women with osteoarthritis. *Res Nurs Health* 2006;29: 442–451.

57. Nicholas MK, Wilson PH, Goyen J. Comparison of cognitive behavioral group treatment and an alternative non-psychological treatment for chronic low back pain. *Pain* 1992;48:339–347.

58. Spence SH, Sharpe L, Newton-John T, et al. Effect of EMG biofeedback compared to applied relaxation training with chronic, upper extremity cumulative trauma disorders. *Pain* 1995;63:199–206.

59. Turner JA, Mancl L, Aaron LA. Short- and long-term efficacy of brief cognitive behavioral therapy for patients with chronic temporomandibular disorder pain: a randomized, controlled trial. *Pain* 2006;121:181–194.

60. Blanchard EB, Andrasik F, Silver BV. Biofeedback and relaxation in the treatment of tension headaches: a reply to Belar. *J Behav Med* 1980;3:322–232.

61. Blanchard EB, Andrasik F. Psychological assessment and treatment of headache: recent developments and emerging issues. *J Consult Clin Psychol* 1982; 50:859–879.

62. Blanchard EB, Andrasik F, Ahles TA, et al. Migraine and tension headache: a meta-analytic review. *Behav Ther* 1980;11:613–631.

63. Andrasik F, Blanchard EB, Neff DF, et al. Biofeedback and relaxation training for chronic headache: a controlled comparison of booster treatments and regular contacts for long-term maintenance. *J Consult Clin Psychol* 1984;52: 609–615.

64. Blanchard EB, Andrasik F, Neff DF, et al. Biofeedback and relaxation training with three kinds of headache: treatment effects and their prediction. *J Consult Clin Psychol* 1982;50:562–575.

65. Philips C, Hunter M. The treatment of tension headache II. EMG normality and relaxation. *Behav Res Ther* 1981;19:499–507.

66. Lacroix JM, Clarke MA, Bock JC, et al. Biofeedback and relaxation in the treatment of migraine headaches: comparative effectiveness and physiological correlates. *J Neurol Neurosurg Psychiatry* 1983;46:525–532.

67. Vasudeva S, Claggett AL, Tietjen GE, et al. Biofeedback-assisted relaxation in migraine headache: relationship to cerebral blood flow velocity in the middle cerebral artery. *Headache* 2003;43:245–250.

68. McCracken LM, Turk DC. Behavioral and cognitive behavioral treatment for chronic pain: outcome, predictors of outcome, and treatment process. *Spine* 2002;27:2564–2573.

69. Chou R, Huffman LH, American Pain Society, et al. Nonpharmacologic therapies for acute and chronic low back pain: a review of the evidence for an American Pain Society/American College of Physicians clinical practice guideline. *Ann Intern Med* 2007;147:492–504.

70. Turner JA. Comparison of group progressive-relaxation training and cognitive-behavioral group therapy for chronic low back pain. *J Consult Clin Psychol* 1982;50:757–765.

71. Dworkin SF, Turner JA, Wilson L, et al. Brief group cognitive-behavioral intervention for temporomandibular disorders. *Pain* 1994;59:175–187.

72. McCauley JD, Frank RG, Callen KE, et al. Hypnosis compared to relaxation in the outpatient management of chronic low back pain. *Arch Phys Med Rehabil* 1983;64:548–552.

73. Sanders SH. A component analysis of behavioral methods used in the treatment of chronic pain patients. Poster session presented at: Annual Meeting of Association of Advanced Behavioral Therapy, 1982; Los Angeles.

74. Moss RA, Wedding D, Sanders SH. The comparative efficacy of relaxation training and masseter EMG feedback in the treatment of TMJ dysfunction. *J Oral Rehabil* 1983;10:9–17.

75. Appelbaum KA, Blanchard EB, Hickling EJ, et al. Cognitive behavioral treatment of a veteran population with moderate to severe rheumatoid arthritis. *Behav Ther* 1988;19:489–502.

76. Keefe FJ, Caldwell DS, Williams DA, et al. Pain coping skills training in the management of osteoarthritic knee pain: a comparative study. *Behav Ther* 1990;21:49–62.

77. Lorig KR, Mazonson PD, Holman HR. Evidence suggesting that health education for self-management in patients with chronic arthritis has sustained health benefits while reducing health care costs. *Arthritis Rheum* 1993;36: 439–446.

78. O'Leary A, Shoor S, Lorig K, et al. A cognitive-behavioral treatment for rheumatoid arthritis. *Health Psychol* 1988;7:527–544.

79. Parker JC, Smarr KL, Buckelew SP, et al. Effects of stress management on clinical outcomes in rheumatoid arthritis. *Arthritis Rheum* 1995;38: 1807–1818.

80. Radojevic V, Nicassio PM, Weisman MH. Behavioral intervention with and without family support for rheumatoid arthritis. *Behav Ther* 1992;23:13–30.

81. Baird CL, Sands L. A pilot study of the effectiveness of guided imagery with progressive muscle relaxation to reduce chronic pain and mobility difficulties of osteoarthritis. *Pain Manag Nurs* 2004;5:97–104.

82. Astin JA, Beckner W, Soeken K, et al. Psychological interventions for rheumatoid arthritis: a meta-analysis of randomized controlled trials. *Arthritis Rheum* 2002;47:291–302.

83. Superio-Cabuslay E, Ward MM, Lorig KR. Patient education interventions in osteoarthritis and rheumatoid arthritis: a meta-analytic comparison with nonsteroidal anti-inflammatory drug treatment. *Arthritis Care Res* 1996;9: 292–301.

84. Keefe FJ, Abernethy AP, Campbell C. Psychological approaches to under-

standing and treating disease-related pain. *Annu Rev Psychol* 2005;56: 601–630.

85. Redd WH, Montgomery GH, DuHamel KN. Behavioral intervention for cancer treatment side effects. *J Natl Cancer Inst* 2001;93:810–823.
86. Margolis CG. Hypnotic imagery with cancer patients. *Am J Clin Hypn* 1982; 25:128–134.
87. Donovan MI. Relaxation with guided imagery: a useful technique. *Cancer Nurs* 1980;3:27–32.
88. Bardia A, Barton DL, Prokop LJ, et al. Efficacy of complementary and alternative medicine therapies in relieving cancer pain: a systematic review. *J Clin Oncol* 2006;24:5457–5464.
89. Jay SM, Varni JW, Elliott C. Acute and chronic pain in adults and children with cancer. *J Consult Clin Psychol* 1986;54:601–607.
90. Spiegel D, Bloom JR. Group therapy and hypnosis reduce metastatic breast carcinoma pain. *Psychosom Med* 1983;45:333–339.
91. Tsai PS, Chen PL, Lai YL, et al. Effects of electromyography biofeedback-assisted relaxation on pain in patients with advanced cancer in a palliative care unit. *Cancer Nurs* 2007;30:347–353.
92. Seers K, Carroll D. Relaxation techniques for acute pain management: a systematic review. *J Adv Nurs* 1998;27:466–475.
93. Patterson DR, Everett JJ, Burns GL, et al. Hypnosis for the treatment of burn pain. *J Consult Clin Psychol* 1992;60:713–717.
94. de Jong AE, Middelkoop E, Faber AW, et al. Nonpharmacological nursing interventions for procedural pain relief in adults with burns: a systematic literature review. *Burns* 2007;33:811–827.
95. Kaplan RM, Atkins CJ, Lenhard L. Coping with a stressful sigmoidoscopy: evaluation of cognitive and relaxation preparations. *J Behav Med* 1982;5: 67–82.
96. Wilson JF. Behavioral preparation for surgery: benefit or harm. *J Behav Med* 1981;4:79–102.
97. Lang EV, Joyce JS, Spiegal D, et al. Self-hypnotic relaxation during interventional radiological procedures: effects on pain perception and intravenous drug use. *Int J Clin Exp Hypn* 1996;44:106–119.

98. Lang EV, Berbaum KS. Educating interventional radiology personnel in non-pharmacologic analgesia. *Acad Radiol* 1997;4:753–757.
99. Clum GA, Luscomb RL, Scott L. Relaxation training and cognitive redirection strategies in the treatment of acute pain. *Pain* 1982;12:175–183.
100. Scott LE, Clum GA. Examining the interaction effects of coping style and brief interventions in the treatment of postsurgical pain. *Pain* 1984;20:279–291.
101. Lavigne JV, Schulein MJ, Hahn YS. Psychological aspects of painful medical conditions in children. II. personality factors, family characteristics and treatment. *Pain* 1986;27:147–169.
102. Rheingans JI. A systematic review of nonpharmacologic adjunctive therapies for symptom management in children with cancer. *J Pediatr Oncol Nurs* 2007; 24:81–94.
103. Eccleston C, Morley S, Williams A, et al. Systematic review of randomised controlled trials of psychological therapy for chronic pain in children and adolescents, with a subset meta-analysis of pain relief. *Pain* 2002;99:157–165.
104. Broome ME, Lillis PP, McGahee TW, et al. The use of distraction and imagery with children during painful procedures. *Oncol Nurs Forum* 1992;19: 499–502.
105. Broome ME, Rehwaldt M, Fogg L. Relationships between cognitive behavioral techniques, temperament, observed distress, and pain reports in children and adolescents during lumbar puncture. *J Pediatr Nurs* 1998;13:48–54.
106. Jay SM, Elliott CH, Katz E, et al. Cognitive behavioral and pharmacologic interventions for childrens' distress during painful medical procedures. *J Consult Clin Psychol* 1987;55:860–865.
107. Weydert JA, Shapiro DE, Acra SA, et al. Evaluation of guided imagery as treatment for recurrent abdominal pain in children: a randomized controlled trial. *BMC Pediatr* 2006;6:29.
108. Heide FJ, Borkovec TD. Relaxation-induced anxiety: paradoxical anxiety enhancement due to relaxation training. *J Consult Clin Psychol* 1983;51: 171–182.
109. Morone NE, Greco CM. Mind–body interventions for chronic pain in older adults: a structured review. *Pain Med* 2007;8:359–375.

CHAPTER 86 ■ GROUP THERAPY FOR CHRONIC PAIN

BEVERLY E. THORN, REGINA MCCONLEY, AND BARBARA B. WALKER

Group treatment has become a common method of helping patients manage chronic pain.[1] First appearing in the pain management literature in the early 1980s, case reports[2] and open clinical trials[3,4] focused on adapting individual treatments for small-group formats and exploring the acceptability of a group format to patients. Since that time, numerous controlled research trials have established the efficacy of group treatment for helping patients manage chronic painful conditions.

Although case reports and open clinical trials continue to accumulate in the literature and provide valuable information, in an evidence-based practice, randomized controlled trials (RCTs) provide stronger support.[5] As a result, findings presented in this chapter are based on searches of the scientific literature that were performed as recommended within the practice of evidence-based medicine.[6] Specifically, Medline, PsycINFO, and the Cochrane Collaboration Databases were searched dating back to 1980 using combinations of controlled vocabulary terms, keywords, and methodological filters in an effort to identify the highest level of evidence currently available on group treatment of chronic pain. Details of these searches may be found in Appendix A.

These literature searches revealed that controlled trials have primarily centered around four different types of groups: (a) cognitive-behavioral therapy (CBT) groups that focus on teaching pain self-management skills; (b) mindfulness-based pain reduction groups that are sometimes included as part of CBT but often

delivered separately; (c) education groups; and (d) supportive/expressive groups. The vast majority of well-controlled trials have found that group CBT is efficacious for treatment of chronic pain; as a result, the focus of this chapter is on group CBT for the management of chronic pain conditions.

BASIC CONSIDERATIONS OF GROUP TREATMENT FOR PAIN MANAGEMENT

Rationale for Group Treatment

Evidence for Efficacy of Group Treatment for Chronic Pain

To find the best available evidence in an evidence-based practice, one searches specifically for meta-analyses and systematic reviews that synthesize the evidence quantitatively. To our knowledge, no meta-analyses or systematic reviews of group cognitive–behavioral treatments (CBT) as a treatment for chronic pain have been published to date. Our literature search did reveal numerous controlled studies (both randomized controlled trials [RCTs] and nonrandomized controlled trials) that have compared (1) group treatment to individual treatment and (2) group treatment to wait-list controls, to treatment as usual, and to other kinds of group treatment (e.g., relaxation or education/support groups) and (3) behavioral group treatments to group exercise and physical therapy treatments. These are reviewed below.

Group vs. Individual Treatment. Table 86.1 summarizes the controlled studies that have directly compared the efficacy of group-administered treatment to individually-administered treatment for chronic pain.[7–12] Although relatively few studies have compared group to individual treatment, they have consistently demonstrated few meaningful differences in outcome between the two treatment modalities.

One of the earliest RCTs comparing group to individual treatment[8] found no differences in outcome between the two modes of treatment for headache patients with the exception that at the 6-month follow-up, participants in the group condition showed less of a tendency to drift back toward baseline levels of pain ratings. Since participants knew prior to treatment that they would be randomly assigned to group or individual treatment formats, posttreatment interviews queried their perceptions regarding the treatment modality to which they were ultimately assigned. Patients in group treatment highlighted the benefit of being able to share openly with other headache sufferers and to discuss their progress with others in the group. Patients in individual treatment valued the personalized attention given via the dyadic therapeutic relationship and expressed concern that group treatment would not have offered sufficient therapist time for each individual. Thus, participants who participated in each treatment modality seemed to highlight the positive aspects of the treatment modality to which they were assigned as the reasons why this would be the preferred mode of treatment.

Another early RCT focusing on patients with pain in the upper extremities also demonstrated minimal overall differences between individual and group treatment.[10] At 6-months and 2-year follow-up, those who received the group treatment reported less pain-related interference than those who were treated individually, and treatment outcome was otherwise equally efficacious.[10,11] It is interesting to note that posttreatment satisfaction ratings were higher for individually-treated patients, and individual treatment was more effective than group treatment on the outcome measure of self-reported coping strategies. One limitation of these early RCTs, however, was the relatively low number of participants in each condition, which limited the statistical power. A benefit of the studies was the collection of patient satisfaction data.

Several more recent trials have confirmed these general findings. In patients with chronic low back pain, Rose et al.[9] reported few differences in an RCT comparing patients treated individually and those treated in groups. In a sample of patients with mixed chronic pain, Frettloh et al.[7] also found few statistically significant differences in treatment outcome between individual and group modalities, although the effect sizes in improvement at follow-up suggested that group treatment may have been superior to individual treatment.[7] In another RCT of mixed chronic pain patients, Turner-Stokes et al.[12] compared outpatient group and individual therapies and found that both treatments resulted in improvements on measures of depression, anxiety, medication consumption, general activity, and pain severity. Those treated in a group showed greater initial gains than those treated individually, but these treatment differences were not sustained over time. Patients treated individually showed slower initial gains, but evidenced the same benefits as those who had been treated in a group at the end of treatment. These authors also reported less of a tendency for the treatment gains made by individually-treated patients to drift back toward baseline over time. In this study, however, group treatment was delivered for more hours at a time and over a shorter duration (8 weeks) than individual

treatment (spread over 16 weeks), and this difference could explain the slower treatment gains witnessed with the individually-treated patients. These few distinctions notwithstanding, these authors and others have generally concluded that there are very few meaningful differences between outcomes resulting from group and individually administered treatments for chronic pain.

Group CBT vs. Wait-List, Treatment as Usual, or Other Group Treatments. Table 86.2 summarizes the controlled studies that have compared group-administered CBT to wait-list control conditions, treatment as usual conditions, or other group treatments such as relaxation, education, or supportive/expressive group therapy.[13–47] There are an impressive number of controlled trials that have been carried out by different research groups focusing on different populations of pain patients that together establish the efficacy of CBT for chronic pain. In most cases, RCTs that compared group CBT to other types of group treatments also included a wait-list condition to control for the natural progression of the chronic pain disorder. Below we highlight findings from studies comparing group CBT to other types of group treatment because they have played an important role in identifying specific mechanisms responsible for treatment efficacy.

CBT is a generic term used to describe a complex and multifaceted treatment. Although the general principles associated with CBT are likely consistent across studies (i.e., teaching pain self-management strategies and that one's thoughts and feelings influence one's ability to cope with pain), the specific treatment components vary across studies. CBT almost always includes one or more modules on recognizing and modifying maladaptive or distorted pain-related cognitions and beliefs, enhancing cognitive coping, learning relaxation strategies (including one or more types of relaxation techniques such as biofeedback, autogenic relaxation, progressive or passive muscle relaxation, meditation, and/or self-hypnosis), and completing regular homework assignments for skills acquisition. Frequently, but less consistently, CBT includes modules focusing on stress management (sometimes referred to as stress inoculation), paced physical activity, assertive communication, pleasant activity scheduling, and coping self-statements.

Because of the varied approaches that have all been subsumed under the label of CBT in the literature, it has been difficult to identify the specific treatment components that account for treatment efficacy. Controlling for nonspecific treatment effects (e.g., attention from therapist, expectations of health care provider and patient) is an important step toward determining the specific components of treatment efficacy. Comparing patients receiving group treatment for chronic pain to those on a wait-list does not allow for this type of analysis although wait-lists do control for the natural progression of the disorder over time and potential reactivity associated with self-monitoring or keeping pain diaries (if included as part of the study). The social context in which the treatment is administered is of particular relevance for the study of the active components of group treatment approaches. Therefore, studies comparing one type of group treatment to another type of group treatment provide better evidence for the nonspecific treatment effects of group treatment (e.g., social support from group members, group problem solving).

There are a limited number of studies in which one group treatment for pain has been compared to another. One study in patients with mixed chronic pain, for example, compared group education plus CBT to group education plus group discussion to control for attention.[27] These authors found that both groups showed equal improvements in pain coping and knowledge, and both were superior to a wait-list control condition. An economic evaluation of the treatments resulted in the authors' suggestion that the extra health care costs associated with the addition of the CBT modules were not warranted based on the outcomes.[27,48] It is important to note that the education modules that were offered to all participants included structured physical fitness

(text continues on page 1275)

TABLE 86.1
INDIVIDUAL VS. GROUP THERAPY

Authors	N	Study	Treatment type	Treatment components	Duration	Outcome measures	Results	Limitations	Follow-up (f/u)
Frettlöh & Kröner-Herwig, 1999	102 mixed chronic pain	Non-randomized Controlled Trial*	Group CBT (N = 34) vs. Individual CBT (= 34) vs. control (TAU = 34)	Education, relaxation, imagery, cognitive restructuring	12 weeks	Subjective disability, catastrophizing (katastrophisierende Kognitionen), depression (Depressivität), coping (kognitives Coping), pain diary	Group & individual >control for majority of outcomes. Group = individual for depression and most other measures. Larger effect sizes for group compared to individual at f/u	Session duration not specified *Information obtained from English abstract only	6 mos.
Johnson & Thorn, 1989	22 Headache	RCT	Group CBT(N = 7) vs. Individual CBT (N = 7) vs. Wait-list Control (WLC) (N = 8)	Psychoeducation, Cognitive Coping Strategies, Relaxation	5 weekly 90 minute sessions	McGill Pain Questionnaire MPQ, Brief Symptom Inventory (BSI), Self-monitoring cards (for pain intensity, no. of prescribed medications, no. of OTC medications, no. of prescribed pills consumed, no. of OTC pills consumed)	Improvement in pain ratings and decrease in anxiety across groups from Times 1 to 2. Decreases in number of times individuals took medication and in number of different medications taken. GCBT = ICBT overall	Small sample size, limited power	1, 3, & 6 mos.
Rose et al., 1997	84 chronic low back pain	RCT	Part 1: Group CBT (N = 26) vs. Individual CBT (N = 24) Part 2: compared 15-hr (N = 22), 30-hr (N = 22), or 60-hr duration treatments	Education, Cognitive therapy, graded aerobic exercise, relaxation	15, 30, or 60 hours duration	VAS pain severity scale (0 to 100), Roland & Morris Disability Questionnaire, Modified Somatic Perception Questionnaire (MSPQ), Modified Zung Depression Inventory, Pain Locus of Control Scale, Pain self-efficacy Questionnaire	Individual = group treatments on outcome measures. Individual tx more strongly associated with changes in disability and on MSPQ. No differences in program duration on outcome.	No control for baseline differences on some variables	6 mos.
Spence, 1989, & Spence, 1991 (2-yr follow-up)	45 Chronic work-related pain of the upper extremity (19 followed at 2 yrs)	RCT	Group CBT (GCBT) (N = 13) vs. Individual CBT (ICBT) (N = 14) vs. WLC (N = 15)	Goal setting, cognitive restructuring, relaxation, cognitive skills training, dealing with sleep problems, assertiveness training	9 weekly sessions at 1.5 hours	BDI Spielberger State-Trait Anxiety Inventory (STAI) Coping Strategies Questionnaire (CSQ) McGill Pain Rating Index (PRI) Sickness Impact Profile (self-report & other-report) Daily Self-Monitoring	GCBT & ICBT> WLC for reductions on all outcome measures. Improvements maintained at f/u GCBT = ICBT 2 yr f/u: Less relapse for GCBT for pain ratings and interference, GCBT = ICBT for other outcomes	Small sample size, Limited power	6 mos, 2 years
Turner-Stokes et al., 2003	113 mixed chronic pain	RCT	Group cognitive-behavioral therapy (CBT)(N = 66) vs. Individual CBT (N = 47)	Group and individual: relaxation, cognitive coping strategies, activity pacing, encouraged to exercise by building up with achievable goals	Group: 1 full afternoon per week for 8 weeks Individual: 1 hour sessions every other week for 8 weeks	West-Haven Yale Multi-dimensional Pain Inventory (WHYMPI), State-Trait Anxiety Inventory (STAI), Beck Depression Inventory (BDI), General activities, analgesic medication consumption, and pain severity	Both groups: significant improvements in pain interference, control over pain, and depression. Group = individual at follow-up. Rapid improvements in Group, slower improvements in individual. Differences leveled off at f/u Group = individual overall	Treatment intervals differ according to group or individual assignment	6–12 mos.

TABLE 86.2

GROUP COGNITIVE AND BEHAVIORAL THERAPY STUDIES

Authors	N	Study	Treatment type	Treatment components	Duration	Outcome measures	Results	Limitations	Follow-up (f/u)
Thorn et al., (2007)	34 Headache	RCT compared order of treatment modules	Cognitive-behavioral therapy (CBT) (N = 22) vs. WLC (N = 11)	Cognitive restructuring, cognitive coping, relaxation, assertiveness, behavioral pacing, homework	10 90-minute group sessions	Pain Catastrophizing Scale (PCS), Pain Anxiety Symptoms Scale (PASS), Beck Depression Inventory – II (BDI-II), Headache Management Self-Efficacy Scale(HMSE), Pain and Medication via pain diaries	CBT>WLC for improvements in catastrophizing, anxiety, headache management self-efficacy. 50% treated patients showed clinically significant reductions in h.a. frequency, medication use no difference in outcome based on order of treatment	Small sample size rendered limited power to detect potential differences in order of treatment modules	6 mos, 12 mos.
Li et al., 2006	64 with work-related injuries	RCT	Training on Work Readiness (T) (N = 34) vs. Control (C) (N = 30)	T: individual vocational counseling (3 sessions), CBT, pain and stress management, relaxation, stages of change assessment, job acquisition, pre-employment training	T: 3 weekly group sessions at 2–3 hours, 3 one hour individual sessions	Spinal Function Sort (SFS), Loma Linda University Medical Centre Activity Sort (LLUMC), Chinese Lam Assessment of Stages of Employment Readiness (C-LASER), Chinese State Trait and Anxiety Inventory (C-STAI), Short form Health Survey (SF-36)	T>C for improvements in anxiety, work readiness, readiness to change, and perceived health status T: within-group improvements from baseline for most SF-36 subscales & physical capacity	Lack of f/u, stages of change may require longer time period for assessment	None specified
Linton et al., 2005	185 workers with back/neck pain	RCT	CBT (N = 69) vs. CBT and physical therapy (CBT + PT) (N = 69), vs. Minimal treatment (N = 47)	CBT: problem solving, homework, skills training, stress management, relaxation CBT + PT: CBT plus personalized exercise program Minimal: medical visit and advice, educational booklet	6 weekly 2 hour sessions	Sick absenteeism, health care visits, Outcome Evaluation Questionnaire, VAS pain ratings, HAD, Pain Catastrophizing Scale (PCS), Tampa Scale of Kinesophobia (TSK), ADLs, Roland Morris Disability Questionnaire (RMDQ)	CBT + PT = CBT for most measures. CBT + PT >Minimal for reductions in health care visits. At f/u: CBT + PT fewest sick days, followed by CBT and Minimal. Both treatment groups 5 times less likely to be on long term sick leave than Minimal.	Different intervention lengths	1 year
Gold et al., 2004	185 women with vertebral fracture	RCT	Part 1: Intervention (I)(N = 94) vs. Education control (EC) (N = 91) Part 2: Crossover: EC becomes I group after 6 mos. Initial I group self maintenance	I: exercise, coping skills (relaxation, stress reduction) EC: education of health issues for women	Part 1: I: 5 weekly exercise & coping sessions (22.5 min) EC: 1 weekly session at 45 min Part 2: I: self-maintain EC = I group	Trunk extension strength, Functional Status Index (FSI), Global Severity Index of Hopkins Symptom Checklist-Revised	Part 1: I: I >EC for improvement in trunk extension & psychological symptoms EC: worse for all three outcomes Part 2: EC showed within-group improvements in trunk extension & psychological symptoms after intervention I: decrease in back strength from post-tx, improvement in psychological state maintained	Different session lengths for I & EC, no control group at F/U. I group did not receive education in cross-over design	6 mos.

(continues)

TABLE 86.2

CONTINUED

Authors	N	Study	Treatment type	Treatment components	Duration	Outcome measures	Results	Limitations	Follow-up (f/u)
Van Lankveld et al., 2004	59 rheumatoid arthritis	RCT compared couples to patient only group	Couples (C) (N = 31) vs. Patient only (P) (N = 28)	Education, cognitive restructuring, encouragement to use active coping skills	C: 2 weekly 1.5 hour sessions for 4 weeks	Disease Activity Score (DAS): swollen joint count Impact of Rheumatic Diseases on General Health & Lifestyle (IRGL), Coping with Rheumatoid Stressors Questionnaire (CORS), Maudsley Marital Questionnaire (MMQ)	Sample improvements in disease activity, cognitions, coping, physical & psychological function (C = P). At f/u: C >P for improvements in disease related communication with spouse	Possible selection bias of highly invested couples because of study design	6 mos.
Ersek et al., 2003	45 elderly with chronic pain	RCT	Self Management (SM) (N = 17) vs. Educational booklet Control (EB) (N = 23)	SM: education, self-monitoring, communication, relaxation, individualized goals, homework EB: booklet with information about pain, medications, instructions for self-management, and pain resources	SM: 7 group sessions at 90 min	SF-36, Graded Chronic Pain Scale, Geriatric Depression Scale, Survey of Pain Attitudes (SOPA), survey assessing use of pain management strategies, treatment usefulness scales	SM>EB for improvements in pain intensity and physical role function (pre-post change); Clinically significant improvement in 43% SM & 13% EB; SM = EB at f/u.	Brief follow-up	3 mos.
Tkachuk, 2003	28 Irritable Bowel Syndrome (IBS)	RCT	CBT (n = 14) vs. Home based symptom monitoring with weekly telephone contact (SMTC) (n = 14)	CBT: Education, relaxation, cognitive restructuring, assertiveness training SMTC: daily symptom monitoring, discussion of symptom patterns	10 90 min sessions for 9 weeks	Daily monitoring IBS scores, BDI II, cognitive emotional distress (CSFBD), trait anxiety (STAI-T), discomfort with assertion (AQ), quality of life (SF-36)	CBT >SMTC for pain relief ratings, improvement in GI Symptoms, quality of life. Maintained at f/u. 1/3 treated patients experienced clinically significant improvement	Brief f/u	3 mos.
Leibing et al., 1999	55 rheumatoid arthritis	RCT	CBT (N = 19) vs. Treatment as Usual (TAU) (N = 36), change in medication matched control group (CN) (N = 20)	CBT: Education, relaxation, cognitive restructuring, pain management, pleasant activity scheduling	CBT: 12 weekly sessions at 90 min	C-reactive protein (CRP), blood sedimentation rate (Westergren), swollen joint count, Hannover Functional Ability Questionnaire (HFAQ), Medication types, VAS pain intensity, Affective pain score, pain diary, STAI, Depression Scale (DS), Arthritis Helplessness Scale (AHI), Bernese Coping Modes	Overall increase in disease activity across sample. CBT less progressive inflammation than TAU. CBT >CN for pain reduction, improvements in depression, anxiety, helplessness. CBT: improved depression, helplessness, positive coping from baseline	Potential Type I error from multiple significance tests. Lack of f/u	None specified

Study	Population	Design	Conditions	Treatment	Duration	Measures	Results	Limitations	Follow-up
Potts et al., 1999	60 non-cardiac chest pain	RCT	CBT (N = 34) vs. WLC (N = 26)	CBT: Education, relaxation, biofeedback, graded exercise, challenging automatic thoughts, homework WLC: delayed treatment	6 sessions at 2 hours	HADS, Nijmegen hyperventilation scale, Sickness Impact Profile (SIP), Nottingham Health Profile (NHP), Chest pain diaries, Hyperventilation: portable carbon dioxide monitor, Exercise electrocardiography (ECG)	CBT >WLC for improvements in chest pain frequency, pain free days, anxiety, and depression, disability, and exercise tolerance. Similar results for delayed treatment group once treated. Overall, 76% had improvements in chest pain. Maintained at f/u	Lack of control group at f/u	6 mos.
Cole, 1998	113 mixed chronic pain	Non-randomized controlled trial	CBT (N = 88) vs. TAU (N = 25)	Coping skills pain self-management, adjustment, stress management, relaxation, self-esteem, positive thinking	75 min, 1 per week for 16 weeks	Multidimensional Pain Inventory (MPI), Minnesota Multiphasic Personality Inventory-2 (MMPI-2), Beck Depression Inventory (BDI) Reported narcotic medication usage, health care visits, work status	CBT: decreases in BDI and MPI scores, & health care visits from baseline, increase in return to work F/U: medication decreased from 75% at baseline to 44%, health care visits decreased from 5 per month to 1 per month. Work status increased from 10% to 31%	Patients not randomly assigned. No direct comparison between CBT and control groups	1 year
Keel et al., 1998	27 Fibromyalgia (FM)	RCT	CBT (N = 14) vs. Autogenic (N = 13)	CBT: stress inoculation, cognitive restructuring, activities for pain diversion, information, relaxation, group discussion, stretching, aerobic exercise Autogenic: practice relaxation	15 weekly sessions lasting 1–2 hours.	Feiburg Personality Inventory Locus of Control Scale Rosenzweig Picture-Frustration Diary (of active hours, resting hours, sleep index, pain intensity, and medication consumption) General Symptom Checklist	2 CBT clients vs. 1 autogenic had clinically significant improvement in medication consumption, physical therapies, sleep, pain scores, general symptoms At f/u: CBT >autogenic for improvement in pain ratings. 4 CBT vs. 0 autogenic had clinically significant improvements at f/u	Small sample size; Statistical analyses not described	3 mos.
Keel et al., 1998	411 low back pain	Non-randomized controlled trial	Experimental (E) (N = 243) vs. Standard physiotherapy (S)(N = 168)	E: coping strategies, stress management, relaxation, simulated work situations fitness training, education and group activity, individual physiotherapy or psychotherapy for acute pain, S: mostly individual physiotherapy	E: 4 week (27 day) inpatient program S: 3 week (20 day) inpatient program	Work situation, physical activities, pain history, pain drawing, VAS pain rating, RMDQ, Psychological General Well-being Index (PGWB), health costs, quality of life, impairment	E = S for improvements in functional ability, limitations in daily life, health care visits E: higher proportion of individuals in work rehabilitation (23% work incapacity decrease), E >S daily hours worked, decrease in professional handicaps. At f/u: larger proportion of S worsened	Pre-existing differences between groups on demographic variables. Different predominant treatment modalities in each condition (E = group, S = individual)	3 mos., 1 year
Basler et al, 1997	94 low back pain	RCT	CBT (N = 36) vs. TAU (N = 40)	Education, relaxation, modifying thoughts and feelings, pleasant activity scheduling, postural training	12 weekly sessions at 150 minutes	Pain diary (pain intensity, control over pain, medication consumption), Heidelberg Coping Scale (HCS), Dusseldorf Disability Scale (DDS)	CBT: decreases in pain intensity, improvements in coping with pain, mental performance, and disability Gains maintained at 6 month f/u TAU: Little or no change	High attrition rate at f/u	6 mos.

(continued)

TABLE 86.2

CONTINUED

Authors	N	Study	Treatment type	Treatment components	Duration	Outcome measures	Results	Limitations	Follow-up (f/u)
van Dulmen et al., 1996	45 IBS	Non-randomized controlled trial	CBT (N = 25) vs. WLC (N = 20)	Patient education (e.g., roles of cognitions, behaviors, in IBS), homework, discussion, progressive muscle relaxation	8 weekly sessions lasting for 2 hours	Diary (duration of pain, daily avoidance behavior, GI complaints), Abdominal Complaint Inventory, Symptom Checklist 90 (SCL-90)	CBT >WLC for improvement in Daily Abdominal Complaint Score (DAC), duration, avoidance, and number of successful coping strategies delayed treatment group: decreases in DAC, Improvements maintained at f/u	No WLC at f/u, wide range of f/u assessment times (6 mos. to 4 years)	Mean = 2.25 years
Vlaeyen et al., 1996	131 FM	RCT	Cognitive educational intervention (ECO = 47) vs. Attention control condition of education & discussion (EDI = 39) vs. WLC (N = 40)	ECO: imaginative transformation of pain, relaxation & biofeedback, homework EDI: education, sharing thoughts with group members, listening to music, homework	ECO & EDI = 12 90 minute sessions conducted in 6 weeks	Pain cognition list, Coping Strategies Questionnaire (CSQ), Behavioral Approach Test, Pain Behavior Scale, McGill Pain Questionnaire (MPQ) Multidimensional Pain Locus of Control Scale, Checklist for Interpersonal Pain Behavior, Fear Survey Schedule, BDI	ECO = EDI for improvements in pain coping and knowledge EDI >WLC on knowledge and pain control. At 12 month f/u, ECO = EDI, although ECO had an increase in pain intensity	Potential confounding of treatment (EDI group shared thoughts, completed homework). Low education level of participants may have made ECO difficult	12 months
Newton-John et al., 1995	44 chronic back pain	RCT	CBT (= 16) vs. Electro-myographic Feedback (EMGBF = 16) vs. WLC (= 12)	CBT: education, goal setting, relaxation, cognitive restructuring, homework EMGBF: education, diaphragmatic breathing, adaptation, homework	8 sessions at 1 hour (2 sessions per week)	BDI, STAI, (CSQ), Pain Disability Index, Pain Beliefs Questionnaire (PBQ)	CBT & EMGBF >WLC for improvements in intensity, disability, adaptive beliefs, & depression. Improvements maintained at f/u, along with improvements in anxiety and active coping	Small sample size per group	6 mos.
James et al., 1993	33 headache	RCT	CBT with Goals (Goal Group) (N = 13) vs. CBT with no goals (Open Group) (N = 13) vs. WLC (N = 7)	Both CBT groups: education, coping, developing appropriate self-talk, generalization of skills, relaxation Goal: specific time goals for coping with pain/stress Open: instructions to cope as long as possible	6 weekly sessions at 90 minutes	Goal specificity: coping with daily stressors and pain, daily self monitoring, pain index, medication intake, downtime, Pain Behavior Questionnaire, SCL-90, SIP, BDI, STAI, Cognitive Coping Index	Goal & Open groups >WLC for improvements in pain coping skills, Goal group >Open & WLC group for reduction of headache and non-narcotic medication use	Lack of f/u period	None specified

Author, Year	Sample	Design	Conditions (N)	Treatment components	Measures	Sessions	Results	Comments/Limitations	Follow-up
Turner & Jensen, 1993	102 low back pain	RCT	Relaxation (R) (N = 17) vs. cognitive therapy (C) (N = 21) vs. cognitive therapy & relaxation (CR) (N = 16) vs. WLC (N = 18)	R: imagery, progressive muscle relaxation (PMR); C: identify negative thoughts, counter negative automatic thoughts; CR: combined treatment	VAS pain ratings, SIP, BDI, Observed Pain Behaviors, Cognitive Errors Questionnaire, BDI	6 weekly sessions at 2 hours	R, C, & CR >WLC for improvements in pain ratings, and disability. At f/u: all three patient groups improved. At both f/u, patients in all groups improved R = C = CR	No comparison to control group at f/u, attrition rates for control condition	6, 12 mos.
Kneebone & Martin, 1992	35 headache	Non-randomized controlled trial. Compared couples to standard non-couple and control groups	Partners involved (PI)(N = 12) vs. No partners (NPI)(N = 10) vs. No treatment control (NTC)(N = 13)	PI & NPI: self-monitoring relaxation, cognitive restructuring, assertiveness, group process (e.g., support), homework PI: partners educated in reinforcement principles	Headache activity, intensity, medication usage, relaxation practice, Partner Involvement Questionnaire, Dyadic Adjustment Scale (DAS), self-monitoring forms	10 weekly sessions at 1.5–2 hours	PI = NPI for relaxation time, PI >NPI for partner involvement: spouse assisted with relaxation. PI: decrease headache activity from baseline NPI: decreased medication usage from baseline. NTC increased medication usage. At f/u, NPI >NTC for reductions in medication. Other measures: PI = NPI at f/u	Potential for Type 1 inflation. Low motivation across treatment groups to practice relaxation	2 mos., 12 mos.
Nicholas et al., 1991	58 low back pain	RCT	Cognitive Therapy (CT) + relaxation (N = 8) or CT (N = 10) vs. Behavior Therapy + relaxation (N = 9) or BT (N = 10) vs. attention (ATC N = 10) & no attention control (N = 11)	All groups: physiotherapy, education, exercise CT: cognitive restructuring, distraction, imagery, self-monitoring BT: activity pacing, medication reduction, reinforcement Relaxation: PMR ATC: group discussion about back pain	Pain Rating Chart STAI, PBQ, CSQ, SIP, SIP-Others (SIP-O), Medication intake, report of alternative treatments, visits to health care facilities	5 1.5–2 hour sessions twice per week	Sample improved on affective distress, functional impairment, medication use, and active coping. Both CBT groups & both BT groups >ATC & control for improvements in pain intensity, self-reported disability, pain beliefs, and active coping. BT >CBT for improvements in impairment. Improvements somewhat maintained at f/u	Physiotherapy included as part of all treatments Small sample size	6, 12 mos.
Subramanian, 1991 & Subramanian, 1994	39 mixed chronic pain Long term F/U = 22	RCT	Structured group therapy (N = 19) vs. WLC (N = 20)	Therapy: stress management, relaxation cognitive restructuring (coping thoughts, self-defeating, self-enhancing thoughts), assertiveness training	SIP, Pain level (0–10 scale) used a control variable Profile of Mood States (POMS), social support questionnaire	8 weekly 2 hour sessions	Therapy >WLC for improvements in physical and psychosocial dysfunction, negative mood states. Within-group improvements also apparent. Long term f/u: Improvements maintained, improvement in pain severity observed, 77% improved from post to f/u, 36% reduction in prescription medication usage	No comparison group at long term f/u	6 mos. Long-term: 18–22 mos.

(*continued*)

TABLE 86.2

CONTINUED

Authors	N	Study	Treatment type	Treatment components	Duration	Outcome measures	Results	Limitations	Follow-up (f/u)
Peters & Large, 1990	68 chronic pain	RCT	Group inpatient program (IPMP)(N = 29) vs. Group outpatient program (OPMP)(N = 23) vs. control (C)(N = 16)	IPMP: education, pain management, relaxation, cognitive restructuring, exercise, vocational counseling, reinforcement OPMP: education, activity goal setting, exercise, medication & stress management, relaxation	Inpatient: 4 weeks Outpatient: 9 weekly sessions at 2 hours	BDI, MPQ, General Health Questionnaire (GHQ), SIP, Pain Behaviour Checklist, pain drawings, VAS ratings, VAS stair climbing test, physiological measures, physical endurance	Sample improvements in disability, GHQ scores, BDI, & MPQ scores IPMP & OPMP >control for improvements in disability, VAS pain ratings, and pain behavior	Results may have been influenced by timing of the assessments, lack of f/u	None specified
Turner et al., 1990	96 chronic low back pain patients	RCT	Group behavioral and aerobic exercise (BE) (N = 18) vs. Behavioral Therapy only (B)(N = 18) Aerobic exercise only (E)(N = 21) vs. WLC (N = 23)	BE: behavioral intervention followed by exercise in each session B: reinforcement role-playing, discussion, homework, communication E: Exercises 5 times per week	BE & B: 8 weekly 2 hour sessions E: 5 weekly sessions	McGill Pain Questionnaire (MPQ), SIP, Pain Behavior Checklist (PBC), PBC-spouse ratings, Physical Work Capacity (PWC), Center for Epidemiological Studies Depression Scale (CES-D), recorded pain behaviors	All 3 groups improved more than the WLC from pre to post treatment (tx), BE >WLC from pre to post tx on self-report and observer rated pain behavior measures, BE >E on PBC Spouse ratings Follow-up: all tx groups improved over time	Interaction with therapists varied by condition	6, 12 mos.
Linton et al., 1989	66 nurses with back pain	RCT	Physical and behavioral preventive intervention (PBI)(N = 36) vs. WLC (N = 30)	PBI: physical therapy, "low back school", relaxation, pain control instruction, goal-setting, problem-solving, coping, identifying high-risk situations	PBI: 8 hours per day for 5 weeks	Daily pain diaries, VAS intensity, fatigue, anxiety, sleep, pain behavior, activities of daily living (ADLs), BDI, AHI, marital satisfaction, absenteeism, medication intake	PBI >WLC for improvements in pain intensity, fatigue, pain behavior, sleep, ADLs, helplessness Most differences maintained at f/u	Use of non-standardized measures of sleep quality, ADLs, marital satisfaction	6 mos.
Puder, 1988	69 mixed chronic pain	RCT	Stress inoculation training (SIT) (N = 31) vs. WLC (N = 38)	SIT: explaining treatment, reviewing progress, problem solving	10 weekly 2 hour group sessions	Daily pain diary, non treatment technique usage: psychological support, exercise, heat/cold, massage, TENS, injections	SIT >WLC for improvements in pain interference, coping, decreased analgesic intake, discontinuation of heat/cold, and home traction technique. No diff. according to age Improvements maintained at f/u	Use of non-standardized measures	1, 6 mos.

Study	N / Population	Design	Conditions	Treatment	Sessions	Measures	Results	Limitations	Follow-up
Bradley et al., 1987	53 rheumatoid arthritis	RCT	Biofeedback assisted CBT (N = 17) vs. Structured group social support therapy (SGT) (N = 18), No adjunct treatment (NAT) (N = 18)	CBT: thermal biofeedback, education, relaxation, behavioral goal setting, self-reward SGT: education, discussion of coping strategies, encouragement to develop improved strategies	CBT: 5 thermal sessions, 10 family/friend meetings SGT: 15 sessions family/friends	STAI, Depression Adjective Checklist (DACL), Health Locus of Control Scale (HLCS), AHI, pain behaviors, rheumatologist ratings of disease activity level, rheumatoid factor titers, sedimentation rate (Westergren)	CBT >SGT & NAT for decreases in pain behavior, pain ratings, rheumatoid activity (RAI), NAT: lower RAI scores than SGT SGT & NAT increased in depression and rheumatoid factor titer across assessments, CBT & SGT >NAT for improvement in anxiety CBT maintained improvement at f/u	Session duration not specified	6 mos.
Larsson et al., 1987	36 high school students with tension/migraine headaches	RCT	Self Help Relaxation (SHR) (N = 12) vs. Problem Discussion Condition (PDC) (N = 10) vs. Untreated Self Monitoring Condition (SM) (N = 12)	SHR: relaxation programs, rapid cue controlled strategy, homework, help solving problems during relaxation PDC: discussion of conflicts in everyday life, role-play, identifying stressors, assertiveness	5 weekly sessions SHR = 3 hours PDC = 7 hours	Headache Diary: frequency, duration headache free days, peak intensity, modified Depression Scale for Female adolescents, Children's Manifest Anxiety Scale, Social Relationship-Competence Questionnaire (SRCQ)	Headache Activity: Greatest reductions for SHR group, SHR >SM and PDC Headache sum and peak intensity: SHR >PDC during pre-follow-up interval Headache duration and headache free days: SHR >SM and PDC	Small sample size, different therapist interaction for two interventions.	5 mos.
Bradley et al., 1985	33 rheumatoid arthritis (RA)	RCT	Thermal Biofeedback and group cognitive behavioral (CB = 11) vs. Social support (SS = 10) vs. NAT (= 12)	CB: thermal biofeedback, education, skills acquisition, self-instructional training, application SS: education, support, encouragement to develop own coping strategies, NAT = control	CB: 5 individual thermal sessions, 10 family meetings SS: 15 family meetings	STAI, DACL, VAS ratings of pain intensity, unpleasantness, severity of morning stiffness, pain behaviors, HLCS, rheumatoid factor titers, Westergren, rheumatologist ratings of disease activity.	CB >NAT group for significant decreases in pain intensity, Pre to Post: CB less pain behavior from pre to post, less rheumatoid activity, and rheumatoid factor titer. CB & SS less anxiety and depression. SS increase in sedimentation rate NAT: sig. reduction in morning stiffness	Small sample size, lack of f/u	None specified
Linton et al., 1985 & Melin & Linton, 1988	28 chronic pain	RCT Long-term f/u	Regular treatment (RT) vs. Applied Relaxation and operant activities (RT + BT) vs. WLC	RT: prescribed treatment plan RT+BT: plan and relaxation training, operant training, reinforcement of well behaviors, decrease in medication	12 sessions	BDI, Activities of Daily Living questionnaire, self-monitoring of pain, medication consumption, sleep f/u measures also included pain, health, activity, level, sleep, occupation	RT + BT >RT & WLC for improvements in pain level and leisure activity. Improvements maintained at f/u	Small sample size Long term f/u: WLC group received individual treatment prior to assessment	14–16 mos.

(continued)

TABLE 86.2

CONTINUED

1276

Authors	N	Study	Treatment type	Treatment components	Duration	Outcome measures	Results	Limitations	Follow-up (f/u)
Moore & Chaney, 1985	43 mixed chronic pain	RCT	Couples group therapy (CBT)(N = 17) vs. Patient only group Therapy vs. (N = 14) WLC(N = 12)	Couples & patient only: education, goal-setting, problem solving, relaxation and controlled breathing, direct pain reduction method, coping strategies, homework.	16 hour program, Couples: 8 bi-weekly 2 hour sessions	VAS pain severity (patient and spouse) MMPI Hs, D, & Hy scales only, SIP, PARS IV Community Adjustment Scale (spouses) Locke Marital Adjustment Test (LMAT) Utilization of medical resources medication usage	Couples and patient only groups >WLC for improvements in VAS ratings, pain severity & pain behavior ratings, somatization, & PARS (spouse rating) Patient only groups >controls on LMAT & SIP scores Treatment gains maintained at f/u Couples = patient only therapy	Small sample sizes for each condition	3, 7 mos.
Cohen et al., 1983	25 Chronic Low Back Pain	RCT	Behavioral Intervention (BT)(N = 13) vs. Physical Therapy (PT) (N = 12)	PT: pain control strategies, relaxation, exercise, pool therapy, use of body mechanics, BT: goal setting, activity pacing, problem-solving, assertiveness	10 weekly 2 hour sessions	Physical Abilities & Walking Abilities testing, Knowledge and Functional Measure of Body Mechanics, CES-D, Psychological Adjustment to Role Scale (PARS-V)	PT: Greater low back control and decreases in CES-D score. BT & PT: Lower anxiety and depression per patients and sig. others on PARS-V, others. Decreases in physical and activity limitations for both groups.	Small sample size, validity data for some instruments not provided	None specified
Figueroa, 1982	15 tension headache patients	RCT	Behavior therapy (BT)(N = 5), psychotherapy (P)(N = 5), self-monitoring (SM = 5)	BT: problem solving, relaxation, anxiety management training, stress inoculation P: discussion, conflict resolution, discussion of stressful events	BT: 7 ninety minute sessions P: 7 ninety minute sessions (twice weekly)	Headache questionnaire, Headache checklist (e.g., level of relaxation, number of headaches, duration, severity, medication usage, disability), self monitoring forms	Pre to f/u: BT >P and SM for improvements in perceived disability. BT >SM for reductions in headache frequency and duration, medication usage, level of relaxation, and pain severity.	Small sample size, use of non-standardized measures	Time not specified
Turner, 1982	36 Chronic low back pain patients	RCT	CBT (N = 13), vs. Relaxation (N = 14) training, WLC/attention conditions (N = 9)	CBT: stress inoculation, behavioral goals, cognitive and affective responses to pain, coping self-statements, relaxation Wait list/attention: gave daily pain ratings to therapist in weekly phone calls	5 weekly 90 minute sessions	SIP, SIP Significant Other (SIP-O), VAS ratings, Self-ratings of improvement, Beck Depression Inventory, Work hours, health care usage	CBT and Relaxation groups >WLC for improvements in pain, depression, disability, and spousal ratings of physical and psychosocial function At f/u: CBT improved on SIP, SIP Significant Other, pain severity, Relaxation: worse pain severity 1.5–2 year f/u: both groups retain improvements, CBT >in hours worked per week	Small sample size	1 month, 1.5–2 years

training after each of 12 sessions, and this behavioral component may have served to increase the overall outcome efficacy of both groups. Furthermore, the discussion modules (attention control) included weekly homework assignments, which is typical of CBT groups but atypical of control conditions. The authors suggest that the homework assignments may have served as a form of graded exposure for the fearful participants, thereby resulting in treatment gains in the control group. It is also important to mention that both treatment groups in the above study used limited therapist time in an effort to reduce treatment costs. It may be that the principles associated with cognitive–behavioral change require some threshold amount of therapeutic intervention in order to be successfully implemented. These findings and others led Vlaeyen and colleagues to raise the important point that the active components of group treatment need further careful study.

Another study assessed the efficacy of group CBT for pain using education booklets as the control condition[18] and found significant pre- to posttreatment differences in favor of the CBT self-management groups. Although the use of education booklets do not control for the nonspecific treatment effects of group interaction or support, this study suggests that merely offering facts about pain and pain management outside a therapeutic context does not appear to be efficacious.

Several other studies have compared group CBT to relaxation training or another group condition. In one study of patients with low back pain, patients receiving group CBT and those receiving relaxation training improved compared to wait-list controls, although at follow-up, those who received CBT showed greater treatment gains than those receiving relaxation training.[47] In a similar study with fibromyalgia patients, those who received group CBT showed greater improvement in pain ratings than those who received autogenic relaxation training.[23] Focusing on high school students with migraine and tension-type headaches, Larsson et al.[40] compared self-help relaxation groups to problem discussion groups and untreated self-monitoring groups and found self-help relaxation to be superior to the other two conditions. Together, these studies suggest that CBT groups are superior to relaxation-only groups and that relaxation groups alone are superior to groups offering only education or discussion.

A specialized subset of studies comparing one type of group treatment to another are those that have compared group CBT offered only to the patient to group CBT offered to both the patient and his or her partner. Moore and Chaney[44] found that among patients with mixed chronic pain syndromes, couples group therapy and patient only group therapy were both superior to a wait-list control group, but the patient-only groups showed significant improvement on more outcome variables than did the couples groups. Another study found similar improvements in physical and psychological functioning, cognitions, and coping among both couples groups and patient-only groups, although at 6-month follow-up, patients in the couples groups reported greater improvement in communication with their spouse than did patients in the patient-only groups.[17] Patients with chronic headache differ in some ways from those with other chronic pain syndromes, and therefore it is interesting to note that one study found that partner involvement in chronic headache management groups actually reduced efficacy compared to nonpartner involvement.[31] Further research is necessary to determine whether this finding is unique to chronic headache patients or if other variables are associated with this outcome.

Behavioral Group Treatment vs. Exercise and Physical Therapy Group Treatments. Physical therapy has long been considered an essential component of chronic pain management, and as a result it is important to consider its role in treatment groups for chronic pain. Although most studies have focused on the efficacy of physical therapy and exercise in individual chronic pain patients, we located two RCTs specifically comparing group behavioral approaches to group physical therapy. In one study, chronic low back pain patients who received group behavioral treatment and those who received group physical therapy both showed significant decreases in activity limitations, anxiety, and depression.[45] In another study, Turner et al.[36] examined the differential efficacy of group behavioral therapy alone, group aerobic exercise training alone, group behavioral therapy plus group aerobic exercise, and a wait-list control group. The three treatment groups showed greater improvement than the wait-list control group, and all groups showed increasing improvement over the 6- and 12-month follow-ups. It is important to note that in this study, the combined behavioral plus exercise group treatment showed the greatest improvement overall, suggesting that physical activity may be an important component to incorporate into group treatment for chronic pain.

Although it did not compare *group-administered* physical therapy (PT) to group CBT, the results of one additional study may shed light on this issue because it explored the incremental benefits of adding individual PT training to 6 sessions of group CBT in recently injured patients with low back pain.[15] Random assignments were made to a minimal treatment condition (physical examination, reassurance and encouragement to stay active, informational brochure), CBT alone, or CBT plus PT. The treatment gains were similar between those patients who received CBT alone and those who received CBT plus PT although the CBT plus PT group incurred fewer health care visits after treatment. Both treatment groups showed large reductions in risk for developing long-term sick disability leave compared to the minimal treatment group.

To summarize, converging lines of evidence described above and in Table 86.2 provide strong evidence that chronic pain patients benefit significantly more from group CBT than from being on a waiting list or receiving medical treatment as usual. The specific mechanisms of treatment efficacy have yet to be clearly identified, but studies to date have shed some light on these mechanisms. As efficacy research moves from open trials to RCTs designed specifically to compare group CBT to other active group treatments, future studies are likely to emerge that will help identify the active components of efficacious treatment.

Mindfulness-Based Approaches to Pain Management. There is a small but growing literature of controlled trials on mindfulness-based pain and stress-reduction or other meditative therapies for chronic pain. A meta-analysis of controlled studies of mindfulness for a wide range of clinical populations (including, but not limited to chronic pain) reported significant, moderate effect size improvement on standardized measures of physical and mental well-being.[49] Regarding group meditation treatments specific to chronic pain, we were able to locate two RCTs[50,51] and three non-randomized controlled trials.[52,53,54] (See Table 86.3 for a summary.) Most of these studies compared group meditation to standard care and found meditation to be more beneficial with respect to pain perception, pain coping and measures of affect immediately post-treatment and also at follow-up.

The studies cited above studied mindfulness as a stand-alone treatment, but mindfulness-based pain and stress reduction groups are also sometimes included as part of an integrated CBT package. In an open clinical trial comparing a group of highly disabled patients with pain (n = 53) to a group of less-disabled patients (n = 234), McCracken and colleagues[55] found that mindfulness training plus CBT (referred to as "Contextual Cognitive-Behavioral Therapy"- CCBT) resulted in large decreases in psychosocial disability and depression, and large increases in acceptance of pain in both groups, with treatment gains maintained at 3-month follow-up. Even in highly disabled patients, CCBT resulted in statistically significant and clinically meaningful treatment gains. Clearly, well-controlled trials with adequately powered samples are needed, but the literature to date suggests that group meditation treatments may prove to be efficacious for chronic pain management.

TABLE 86.3

MINDFULNESS BASED GROUP INTERVENTIONS

Authors	N	Study	Treatment type	Treatment components	Duration	Outcome measures	Results	Limitations	Follow-up (f/u)
Carson et al., 2005	43 low back pain	RCT	Loving-kindness meditation (Medi)(N = 18) vs. standard care (TAU) (N = 25)	Medi: silent mental phrases to direct positive feelings toward others attend to feelings of love instead of anger/ resentment, discussion, practice	8 weekly 90 min sessions	McGill Pain Questionnaire (MPQ), Brief Pain Inventory (BPI), State-Trait Anger Expression Inventory (STAI), Anger Expression & Control, Brief Symptom Inventory (BSI), diary, VAS ratings of pain & anger, affect, pain, & fatigue	Medi: improvement in pain intensity, usual pain, psychological distress, and anxiety from baseline. TAU: little change Pre to f/u: Medi improved in usual pain, anxiety, psychological distress, and the phobia scale of the BSI	No direct comparison between intervention and TAU group.	3 mos.
Plews-Ogan et al., 2005	30 musculo-skeletal pain	RCT	Mindfulness Based Stress Reduction (MBSR)(N = 10) vs. Massage (N = 10) vs. standard care (TAU)(N = 10)	MBSR: meditation and yoga, nonjudgmental awareness, practice Massage: Swedish, deep tissue, neuromuscular, pressure point	MBSR: 8 weekly 2.5 hour sessions Massage: 8 weekly 1 hour sessions	Pain intensity, pain unpleasantness, Short-Form Health Survey 12 (SF-12)	Post treatment (tx): Massage >TAU for improvements in unpleasantness & mental status. MBSR = TAU At f/u: MBSR >TAU for improvement in mental health score	Small sample size limits statistical power	4 weeks
Grossman et al., 2007	58 females with Fibromyalgia (FM)	Non-randomized controlled trial	Mindfulness-based stress reduction (MBSR = 39) vs. Active Social Support (= 13)	MBSR: mindfulness practice, awareness during yoga, stressful situations, social interactions, homework Support: social support, relaxation training, stretching exercises, discussion, homework	8 weekly 2.5 hour sessions plus one all day session	Quality of Life Profile for the Chronically Ill (QoL), Hospital Anxiety and Depression Scale (HADS), Pain Perception Scale (PPS), Inventory of Pain Regulation (IPR), Visual analog ratings (VAS)	MBSR >support for improvements in VAS pain, QoL subscales, pain coping, depression, and somatic complaints Improvements maintained at f/u	Unequal n limits statistical power	3 yrs
Sagula & Rice, 2004	57 mixed chronic pain	Non-randomized controlled trial	Mindfulness meditation (MM)(N = 39) vs. Control (C)(N = 18)	MM: 20 min daily meditation (body scan, mindfulness on breath, hatha yoga), meditation log, development of resources for self-healing	8 weekly 90 min sessions	Response to Loss Scale (RTL)(e.g., Growth, Cope/ Awareness), Beck Depression Inventory (BDI), STAI	MM >C for reductions in depression, state anxiety, and intensity of grief from loss associated with pain. Growth: MM = C	Unequal sample sizes limits statistical power lack of f/u	None specified
Kabat-Zinn et al., 1985	90 mixed chronic pain	Non-randomized controlled trial	Stress Reduction and Relaxation (SR & RP)(N = 69) vs. Pain Clinic control group (PC)(N = 21)	SR & RP: meditation training, Hatha yoga, homework, 45 min daily meditation	10 weekly 2 hour sessions	McGill-Melzack Pain Rating Index (PRI), Body Parts Problem Assessment (BPPA) scale, medically oriented symptom checklist (MSCL), Profile of Mood States (POMS), revised Hopkins Symptom Checklist (SCL-90R)	Sample improvements in pain indices, mood, and psychological symptoms. SR & RP >PC for improvements in anxiety, hostility and somatization. SR & RP: Larger proportion of individuals with clinically significant improvements. Maintenance at f/u	Wide range in f/u assessments	2.5–15 mos.

Advantages of Group Treatment

Efficiency and Cost-Effectiveness

Given the general lack of difference in treatment outcomes between group and individual CBT, it could reasonably be argued that group treatment is a more efficient modality of therapy for chronic pain disorders. Certainly, group treatment is more cost-effective in terms of practitioner time and patient expense.

Social Proximity and Support

There are several other advantages to using a group modality with patients who have chronic pain-related conditions: A group approach provides social interaction and support from others who share common distressing experiences including the pain itself as well as secondary stressors associated with the pain such as frustrating interactions with the healthcare system, economic hardship, and deteriorating family relationships. Individuals struggling with chronic pain often feel isolated and misunderstood. Disclosing thoughts and feelings to others who share similar concerns offers patients a greater sense of legitimacy than might be experienced by sharing thoughts and feelings with a therapist or significant other who does not experience pain. A qualitative study of previously treated group members confirmed that being listened to, understood, accepted, tolerated, and affirmed were highly valued perceived benefits of the group approach for pain management.[56]

Beyond the social support provided by others who share similar concerns (which is considered a non-specific treatment factor), group CBT seems to offer additional benefits. Studies have shown group CBT to be superior to group relaxation sessions[47] and to group discussion sessions,[40] both of which offer the type of social support received in group CBT. Maunder and Esplen[57] reported that a supportive-expressive group for patients with inflammatory bowel disease did not improve symptoms of GI distress/pain, patient quality of life, anxiety, or depression, and they concluded that, at least for this population, supportive-expressive group therapy alone is not efficacious.

Vicarious Learning and Modeling of Collaborative Approach

Group treatment provides clinicians with multiple scenarios to choose from and build upon during group discussions, which is helpful when illustrating a particular teaching point. Taking advantage of a salient example and using it for the benefit of the entire group maximizes the likelihood that patients will understand the intervention through vicarious learning (i.e., other group members observing a therapeutic interaction between an individual patient and the therapist).

Moreover, group treatment provides a fertile venue for modeling a collaborative approach to treatment between the patient and the practitioner. Early in the group process, the leader establishes the expectation that patients will actively participate in group discussions, self-monitor their activities, and complete homework assignments. Through selective reinforcement of patients who actively engage in their treatment by participating in the group and completing the homework assignments, the leader can strive to increase active coping in all of its members. A qualitative study of group CBT treatment with women suffering from chronic pelvic pain revealed that this collaborative approach facilitates a therapeutic progression beginning with developing self-knowledge, followed by assuming responsibility for self-management, and ending with increasing self-control and personal mastery of emotions.[58]

Interpersonal Group Process

A final potential advantage of group treatment is the use of group process to facilitate treatment gains (i.e., utilizing the interpersonal exchange between group members in addition to the exchange between therapist and the patient). A group of patients provides an opportunity to capitalize on the moment-by-moment interchanges among group members as well as the interpersonal relationships that develop over time. It is noteworthy that group members will often accept positive feedback, negative feedback, and confrontation from other group members better than from the group leader. This may be due in part to feeling more understood by a fellow patient (someone who has "walked in my shoes"), but may also be due to the power of the interpersonal process that occurs in group settings.

Practical Issues

Open vs. Closed Groups

Most controlled studies in the literature have focused on time-limited, closed groups. In research, this is a necessity to control for a number of confounding variables that ongoing, open groups would introduce into a research design. There are also clinical advantages to running a closed group where all members start and end group treatment at the same time. From a practical perspective, however, running closed groups can prove difficult in some clinical settings because new patients would be required to wait until a new group starts to begin treatment. In response to this, some clinics have begun experimenting with a hybrid model which involves running revolving closed, time-limited groups but allowing new members to enter the group once each month so no patient has to wait longer than 3–4 weeks to start treatment. The effectiveness and feasibility of this model for treating chronic pain patients in groups is currently being explored by the third author of this chapter (BBW) as part of a collaborative effort between Indiana University and Volunteers in Medicine of Monroe County (www.vimmonroecounty.org). If both effective and feasible, this group model for helping patients manage chronic pain will hopefully be adopted by other clinics in addition to other members of the Volunteers in Medicine Alliance (www.vimi.org) across the country.

Length of Group

The length of the groups varied in the RCTs reviewed for this chapter, ranging from 5 to 12 sessions, with a modal number of 10 sessions. Most RCTs reported meeting weekly for 90-minute sessions. Time-limited groups are the accepted standard in research trials because treatment manuals are usually highly structured, and demonstrating fidelity of treatment through therapist adherence to the protocol is an important component of treatment implementation.[59] Furthermore, treatment groups of varying lengths would introduce variance that would reduce the statistical power required to detect real differences between treatment and control groups. On the other hand, clinical realities often necessitate varying the length of a particular treatment component based upon whether or not the intervention has been understood by the group members. In clinical settings, there may indeed be some situations in which it would be well advised to repeat a particular unit, continue coverage of a particular topic, or adapt the treatment protocol in some other way. As an example of this, when faced with an opportunity to treat pain patients with very little education, the first author of this chapter (BET) recognized the need to adapt the written materials used in group CBT for this population. An RCT is currently being conducted to test the efficacy of this adapted protocol in this subset of chronic pain patients with low literacy. If shown to be efficacious, the adapted materials could then be used in other clinical trials and in clinical settings with similar populations.

Number of Participants

A group composed of approximately five members is of sufficient size to facilitate interaction among group members, accommodate the absence of a member without jeopardizing group cohesiveness, and provide enough time to attend to each patient during the individual sessions. Most CBT groups will have more women than men, since women have more chronic pain problems, present more frequently for pain treatment than men,[60] and may be more receptive to group interventions based on their tendency to cope via a communal support process.[61] Differences in age, ethnicity, and cultural background do not appear to jeopardize the group process, perhaps because chronic pain serves as a unifying factor, making other potentially divisive issues less important. We were unable to identify any studies addressing the issue of whether it is important to racially match group leaders with participants. In an unpublished follow-up qualitative study using post-treatment key informant interviews with African American members of a CBT headache management group two years after the RCT had been completed,[13] those interviewed thought that including therapists of different racial and ethnic backgrounds as group leaders would enhance the comfort level of participants and thus increase both their willingness to participate and their chances of treatment completion. In mixed race groups, it is probably preferable to have at least one of the co-therapists be a person of different racial and/or ethnic background.

Individuals Who May be Inappropriate for Groups

Almost anyone deemed appropriate for individual CBT for pain management is appropriate for group treatment, but there are a few exceptions. Patients with moderate to severe dementia or other cognitive impairment, psychosis, or chronic interpersonal relationship problems are inappropriate for group treatment. In addition, it is not unusual for chronic pain patients to have problems managing anger, and in some cases the degree of anger and hostility may be a contraindication for group treatment. In these cases, however, it is often possible to help the patient learn to regulate their anger and hostility in individual treatment and then invite them to participate in a group at a later date. Keefe et al.[1] noted that they sometimes use a "time-out" strategy for group members whose anger is disruptive or in other ways countertherapeutic, in which patients meet individually with group leaders while continuing to attend the group but remaining silent for two to three sessions. Clearly, if a patient expresses a strong preference for individual treatment or if his or her schedule prohibits involvement at the prescribed group time, an individual approach will need to be employed.

CORE COMPONENTS OF GROUP CBT FOR CHRONIC PAIN

As mentioned earlier, CBT is an umbrella term for a variety of treatment components. The core principles behind CBT involve the conceptualization that one's thoughts, feelings, and behaviors are critically important components in helping a patient engage in appropriate pain self-management. Common treatment components frequently include training in cognitive restructuring, cognitive coping, relaxation, paced physical activity, and assertive communication.

Overview of CBT Rationale and Components

The purpose of group CBT, like individual CBT, is to teach non-medication based methods of reducing pain and distress and to increase overall level of functioning despite the presence of pain. During the cognitive modules of CBT, patients are taught to iden-tify the habitual thought patterns that exacerbate their pain and related distress. These thought patterns take the form of situation-specific automatic thoughts (e.g., "I might as well quit my job because I'm missing so much work."), more global attitudes and beliefs about their pain and the way they think it should be treated (e.g., "If I have back pain, I should lie down and rest as much as possible to let it heal."), and deep-seated core beliefs about the self (e.g., "I am basically useless now."). These distortions in thinking are associated with negative emotions (anxiety, depression, anger) and maladaptive coping behaviors (e.g., inappropriate reliance on pain medications). Cognitive coping techniques often include training in positive coping self-statements and cognitive distraction techniques. The behavioral modules of CBT teach patients specific stress management techniques such as relaxation, assertiveness, and pacing oneself instead of doing too much or too little in response to pain cues. Sometimes expressive writing is also included to help the patient process strong negative emotions. Behavioral approaches teach patients how to manage stressful events that cause pain, exacerbate pain, and/or are caused by pain. The distinction between "cognitive" and "behavioral" modules is somewhat artificial, since both cognition and behavior are involved in each component of treatment.

Example of a Typical CBT Group Program

Since there is considerable variability in the number and content of group CBT modules, no one treatment description captures all CBT programs. In general, however, each session consists of a review of what was learned the previous week, an introduction to a new skill or concept, and a homework assignment designed to reinforce the use of new techniques and promote understanding of new ideas.

The first session is designed to provide the rationale for a CBT approach and introduce the ground rules, including those regarding confidentiality. The second through the ninth sessions typically involve teaching specific cognitive and behavioral skills. The tenth session is used to promote a sense of closure and help patients begin to generalize what they have learned in past sessions. This is achieved by discussing how all of the techniques and concepts taught in the group can be integrated and maintained over time. See Table 86.4 for an outline of a 10-week CBT program. See also Haythornthwaite (Chapter 82) for a discussion of CBT for chronic pain not necessarily focused on group treatment.

Example of Cognitively-Focused Group CBT

Below we offer a more specific discussion of the cognitive aspects of our group CBT program. The manual covering the basic structure and detailing the cognitive components of treatment is available in Thorn.[62] Since the emphasis on cognitions is greater in this program than many other CBT programs for pain management, the four core components of the cognitive focus are featured below and the distinctive aspects associated with group treatment are highlighted when relevant.

Stress-Appraisal-Pain Connection

The first core component in cognitively-focused group CBT introduces the group to the importance of understanding the Stress-Appraisal-Coping Model of Pain. Group leaders help patients understand that pain produces stress, stress increases pain, and managing stress reduces the negative impact of pain on one's life. Moreover, stress itself can trigger and/or exacerbate pain. Thus, it is crucial that patients with chronic pain learn about stress and how to manage stress more effectively.

After reviewing the physiological mechanisms of the stress

TABLE 86.4

MAJOR OBJECTIVES OF TEN GROUP CBT SESSIONS

Session number	Major objectives
1	Establish rapport, explain therapy rationale, goals, format and rules, introduce the connection between stress and pain, and introduce the concept of stress appraisal
2	Introduce the stress-appraisal-coping model of pain, begin identification of automatic thoughts or images, recognize connection between automatic thoughts and emotional/physical shifts
3	Evaluate automatic thoughts for accuracy, identify sources of distorted thoughts, challenge negative, distorted automatic thoughts, construct realistic alternative responses
4	Identify underlying beliefs about the cause, treatment, and control over pain, challenge negative distorted beliefs, construct new beliefs
5	Identify core beliefs, challenge negative, distorted core beliefs, construct new, more adaptive beliefs
6	Introduce passive muscle relaxation techniques; construct and use positive coping self-statements; incorporate coping self-statements into relaxation
7	Introduce the principles of behavioral pacing (i.e., planned use of discrete periods of time engaging in productive, but potentially stressful, activities ["uptime"], alternating with periods of restful, relaxing activities ["downtime"], and the benefits associated with use of pacing)
8	Learn and practice expressive writing or verbal narration of expressive writing exercise
9	Introduce the principles of assertiveness (e.g., making direct, simple, nonapologetic requests; saying no to a request without hostility or guilt); plan an assertive communication
10	Review concepts and skills learned, provide feedback about helpful and challenging aspects of the treatment, continue to practice and use skills in everyday life

response, group leaders introduce the concept that judgments about and reactions to situations are more important than the actual situations themselves and that stressors are typically appraised as threats, losses, or challenges. The concept of "appraisal" is introduced as a determinant of "coping," which is comprised of thoughts, feelings, and behavior. As part of the session, group members are asked to generate a list of stressors that are both pain-related and non-pain-related and then share them with the group.

As homework, group members are asked to add to their list of pain-related and non-pain-related stressful situations daily throughout the week. Beside each stressor, they are asked to record the type of appraisal (threat, loss, or challenge), and then to note how their appraisal of those stressors influenced their coping (thoughts, images, feelings, behaviors, and pain).

Recognizing, Evaluating, and Changing Automatic Pain-Related Thoughts

The second core component in cognitively-focused group CBT teaches patients to recognize, challenge, and then reconstruct

maladaptive automatic thoughts. Group members are taught that automatic thoughts are the ongoing, internal stream-of-consciousness dialogue that often occurs just below one's immediate level of awareness. Patients must first learn to recognize their own automatic, pain-related thoughts, especially those that are negative and/or irrational. To accomplish this, group members are asked to consider thoughts or images that run through their mind when their mood or sense of well-being worsens. For example, in response to a worsening of pain while standing at work, a patient might have the automatic thought: "I might as well apply for disability since I can't work the way I used to." Patients are often surprised by the large number of negative and irrational thoughts that occur just outside of their immediate awareness. Group leaders explain that these thoughts have a powerful impact on their emotions, behaviors, and other thoughts whether the individual is aware of them or not. Bringing these thoughts into one's awareness provides greater control over the thoughts because once one is aware of a thought, one can evaluate it. It is emphasized that all thoughts contain at least a grain of truth and some are completely true, but many thoughts are distorted. These distorted thoughts, especially negative ones, coincide with negative emotions and can lead to or exacerbate feelings of helplessness and hopelessness. Once group members learn to identify common cognitive distortions, they can begin to recognize how their own negative, distorted automatic thoughts influence their moods, behavior, and pain. Next, group members are guided through a process of Socratic questioning to help determine whether their distorted thoughts are completely true, partially true, or not at all true. Socratic questioning is a "tell me more" technique where patients are taught to ask themselves a series of questions that will ultimately guide them to the answer. In the case of automatic thoughts, patients ask themselves, "what are the facts that support this thought?" and "what are the facts that do not support this thought?" Evaluating the rationality of their distorted automatic thoughts provides a segue into learning to construct alternative thoughts that are more realistic and adaptive. The purpose of focusing on distorted thoughts is not so much to change the *content* of the thought as it is to uncouple the emotion from the thought. The thought becomes "just a thought" by removing the power of "truth" from it.

Identifying and Evaluating Intermediate Pain-Related Beliefs

The third core component of cognitively-focused group CBT teaches group members to recognize thought processes such as underlying beliefs that are more deeply ingrained than situation-specific automatic thoughts. With intermediate beliefs, the focus is on those beliefs that are pain-related. Patients are taught that their pain-related intermediate beliefs are beliefs related to the cause of pain (e.g., "My pain is bad because I have collapsed discs in my spine."), beliefs about appropriate treatment of their pain (e.g., "When I'm in pain my family should take better care of me."), and beliefs about their ability to influence their pain (e.g., "The only thing that can help my pain is strong pain medication."). Intermediate beliefs are often represented by rules and assumptions that patients make about the way things "should," "must," or "ought to be" in the situations in which they find themselves. It is thought that intermediate beliefs give rise to automatic thoughts.[63]

In order to help patients recognize these attitudes and beliefs about pain and the way it should be treated, group leaders first ask patients to identify key automatic thoughts (ones that come up repeatedly), explaining that they may be linked to underlying beliefs. Using a "downward arrow" technique described by Burns,[64] patients are asked to consider: "if that (automatic) thought is true, what does it mean to you?" Patients often need help identifying the underlying belief systems that are driving the irrational automatic thoughts. Intermediate beliefs may be harder to identify because they are not as easily recognized as irrational by the patient. For example, the automatic thought "I might as well apply for disability, because I can't work the way I used to" could be driven by the belief that "I should be able to lift the same amount of freight that I could before the accident, in the same way, in the same amount of time." The self-expectation held by the patient giving the above example feels completely true to the patient when he first identifies his belief. Using a process of Socratic questioning similar to that used to examine automatic thoughts (e.g., "What are the facts supporting this belief?" "What are the facts not supporting this belief?"), group leaders can help patients begin to question these attitudes and assumptions about the way they (and the world) "should" be.

In many cases, patients' intermediate beliefs promote the attitude of a passive patient receiving a diagnosis, treatment, and cure. Here, the group leader can take advantage of the group process to help patients understand how their attitudes and beliefs about the cause and treatment of their pain impact what they choose to do (or not do) to help themselves. For example, with very little therapist intervention, one group member can open the door to considering alternative beliefs by saying something like, "So . . . none of these surgeries and none of the medicines have worked to cure our pain, and we've been trying it for years. Maybe it's time to try something else." As the group leaders help patients realize that beliefs and attitudes, like automatic thoughts, are also *just thoughts* and not necessarily absolute truths, they become more receptive to the idea of taking more responsibility for pain self-management behaviors rather than relying on the belief of a cure and the attitude that their health and well-being are in the hands of physicians.

Identifying and Evaluating Core Pain-Related Beliefs

In the fourth core component of cognitively-focused group CBT, group members learn that core beliefs are rigid, long-held beliefs about one's basic worth or lovability as a human being. For most people, most of the time, negative core beliefs do not predominate over positive core beliefs. However, it is thought that during times of significant stress (e.g., a pain flare-up), underlying beliefs often become negatively distorted, which in turn negatively impacts thoughts, feelings, and behavior.[63] Core pain-related beliefs reflect the patient's sense of self as an individual in pain. Unfortunately, with increasing pain duration and mounting associated problems, patients with chronic pain often adopt the core pain-related belief that "I am a disabled chronic pain patient" and assume the role commensurate with such an identity.

Core beliefs are probably the most difficult to change because they are so deeply ingrained and often thought to be indisputable facts. However, building on previous sessions and patient success with mastering automatic thoughts and intermediate beliefs, group leaders teach that core beliefs are not absolute truths; rather, they are ideas that can be altered. Again utilizing the Downward Arrow Technique[64] patients are asked to identify a frequently occurring automatic thought, perhaps stemming from a previously identified intermediate belief. They are then asked to consider, "If that automatic thought is true, what does it mean *about* me?" Building from a previous example, the automatic thought "I might as well apply for disability," driven by the belief "I should be able to work the same as I used to," might in turn be driven by the pain-related core belief "I am a worthless chronic pain patient." It is also sometimes useful to get at pain-related core beliefs by having patients ask the "Why me?" question. Often patients feel that they are in pain because they deserve some sort of punishment, are basically unlovable anyway, or have always felt unworthy.

Challenging and changing patients' negative core pain-related beliefs are a formidable challenge. Here the group process is invaluable as patients will more readily accept confrontation about the belief "I am unlovable because I have chronic pain" from a

fellow pain patient than from a group leader. It is also useful to help patients examine the disadvantages as well as the advantages to holding on to negative core pain-related beliefs. With help, patients often recognize that adopting their negative core beliefs gives them permission to give up and no longer try to cope. Patients are often motivated to challenge their beliefs when they come to this recognition. Another tool used to help patients challenge their core pain-related beliefs is to experiment with the "acting as if" exercise.[63] In this exercise, group members are asked to consider what specific things they would do differently if they did not hold their core pain-related belief. Ideally, the treatment component examining core pain-related beliefs will ultimately help the patient dissociate pain from both disability and suffering, allowing the patient to adopt a new identity that "I am a well person with pain."

FACTORS AFFECTING PSYCHOTHERAPEUTIC OUTCOME

Although there are many potential factors affecting group treatment outcome for pain management, we have chosen to highlight four: the importance of changing cognitions, the importance of practicing skills to maintain treatment gains, the need for sufficient therapist contact to promote change, and the role of the group process itself.

The Importance of Cognitive Change

The CBT approach is based upon strong evidence that thoughts influence emotions and behavior, and this has been found to be particularly true with regard to the experience of pain. Highly negative cognitions regarding a patient's pain and its sequelae are predictive of poor patient coping with chronic pain.[65] For example, negative pain-related cognitions have been shown to be a robust predictor of higher perceived pain intensity, lower tolerance of painful procedures, greater psychological distress and psychosocial dysfunction, higher analgesic use, and greater pain interference, disability, and inability to work.[66–68] In addition, negative cognitions are a better predictor of poor coping (and therefore, poor adaptive outcome) than disease severity, perceived pain intensity ratings, age, sex, depression or anxiety.[66,67,69–75] Given this evidence, the basis of cognitively-focused CBT for pain is on helping patients become aware of, examine, and gain control over the thoughts that influence their feelings, coping behavior and physiology. Furthermore, with CBT, early changes in pain catastrophizing and perceived helplessness are related to later treatment changes in pain severity and functioning.[76,77]

Compliance with Homework and Skills Practice to Maintain Treatment Gains

When considering whether a valid clinical trial has been conducted, there must be some demonstration that adequate levels of independent treatment components have actually been given.[60] Treatment enactment refers to the extent that clients actually apply what they have learned out of the treatment session. Homework or practice of skills learned in treatment is one way to measure treatment enactment. Scharff and Marcus[78] found that headache participants who practiced the skills taught in treatment (which included physical therapy, headache-free diets, and relaxation) were more likely to maintain their treatment gains when measured at follow-up. Likewise, completion of homework assignments were significantly related to treatment outcome in IBS patients participating in group CBT.[19] Vlaeyen et al.,[27] comparing group education plus CBT to group education plus attention control (group discussion), noted that in the CBT group, compliance with completion of homework assignments was quite low. The researchers noted that the education level of their participants was low and that the homework assignments might have been too difficult for them to complete. Ironically, failure to understand or complete the homework may result in an unintended decrease in self-efficacy, which would certainly limit the efficacy of the intended treatment.

Importance of Therapist Skill and Adequate Time with Therapist

Vlaeyen et al.[27] also noted that the treatment in their clinical trial was designed to be low-cost and therefore included minimal therapist interventions. It is quite possible that the complex cognitive and behavioral skills that must be acquired by patients prior to treatment gains require a threshold level of therapist intervention in order to be comprehended by the client. Thus, without a skilled therapist guiding the acquisition of cognitive-behavioral change in the CBT group, subsequent lack of understanding may have resulted in unintended frustration and reduced overall efficacy.

Importance of Group Process

In our review of the group pain management literature, we located one open clinical trial that offered interesting qualitative information regarding the importance of group process. Moore, Berk, and Nypaver[79] studied 51 patients completing multidisciplinary inpatient pain management programs in small groups (3–4 individuals). Overall, patients showed a decrease in pain, disability, and hypochondriasis after treatment, and at 6-month follow-up, treatment gains were maintained and more patients were employed. Failure to improve depended in part on whether other members of the same treatment group also failed to respond. The authors noted that each group seemed to quickly acquire a temperament unique to that group, with some evolving toward positive cooperation and some being more adversarial or negative in nature. Examination of the group data showed that if one individual failed to benefit from treatment (or left the program prematurely due to dissatisfaction) others in the group were also more likely to have not improved. This study highlights the importance of social factors in chronic pain and underscores the caveat that group treatment should be designed to capitalize on these social influences.

SUMMARY AND CONCLUSIONS

Group treatment approaches for pain management have been clearly established as efficacious, and the vast majority of controlled research studies have focused on CBT group approaches. The available research suggests that there are few differences in treatment outcome between group and individual CBT for chronic pain. Thus, since group treatment is more efficient in terms of therapist time and more economical for patients, we suggest that group treatment is generally the favored modality. Certainly, not all patients are appropriate for group pain management, and logistical difficulties in organizing and running a group prevent the universal adoption of group treatment as the only method of appropriate treatment. Relatedly, some patients may need more intensive psychotherapy than what the typical group approach has to offer. It is therefore quite appropriate to refer certain patients for individual treatment after the completion of group treatment.

FUTURE DIRECTIONS

It is important to note that although the extant research literature has established the efficacy of group CBT for pain management, the external validity of research-based efficacy trials has yet to be studied (i.e., effectiveness studies). Since the efficacy studies cover a wide range of pain problems and come from a variety of research laboratories both inside and outside the United States, we may feel more confident in the generalizability of the results. Future research exploring appropriate adaptations for local populations with special needs will help establish the effectiveness of group (GBT) approaches for real-world settings.

Two other areas in need of more research are cost-effectiveness studies and research examining the specific mechanisms associated with treatment efficacy. Regarding cost-effectiveness, such research is particularly difficult to carry out in health care settings without readily available (electronic and universal) health care utilization information. Regarding the identification of specific treatment factors responsible as the agent of change, the research conducted up to this point offers a promising start that efficacious group CBT is more than simply therapeutic and social support.

Finally, there is a clear need for a systematic review and meta-analysis of group treatments for chronic pain. As health care practitioners of all disciplines become more and more reliant upon systematic reviews to support evidence-based practice, a thorough systematic review and meta-analysis of group treatments for chronic pain would represent a certain contribution to the literature.

APPENDIX A

Search Strategies

Medline and Cochrane Database searches were performed in March 2007 using OVID as an interface to search for group treatments for (1) gastrointestinal disorders, (2) back, facial, neck, neuralgia and intractable pain, (3) pelvic pain, dysmenorrheal and vulvar diseases, and (4) headache disorders.

1. Database: Ovid MEDLINE(R) <1950 to March Week 2 2007> Search Strategy:
   1 exp psychotherapy, group/ (18366)
   2 exp Colonic Diseases, Functional/ (5158)
   3 1 and 2 (12)
   4 limit 3 to (humans and english language) (10)
2. Database: Ovid MEDLINE(R) <1950 to March Week 2 2007> Search Strategy:
   1 exp psychotherapy, group/ (18366)
   2 back pain/ or facial pain/ or neck pain/ or neuralgia/ or pain, intractable/(24526)
   3 1 and 2 (22)
   4 limit 3 to (humans and english language) (20)
   5 limit 4 to case reports (1)
   6 4 not 5 (19)
3. Database: Ovid MEDLINE(R) <1950 to March Week 2 2007> Search Strategy:
   1 exp Psychotherapy, Group/ (18366)
   2 exp pelvic pain/ or exp dysmenorrhea/ (3924)
   3 exp Vulvar Diseases/ (10719)
   4 2 or 3 (14610)
   5 1 and 4 (3)
4. Database: Ovid MEDLINE(R) <1950 to March Week 2 2007> Search Strategy:
   1 exp group psychotherapy/ (18366)
   2 exp Headache Disorders/ (17650)
   3 1 and 2 (17)
   4 limit 3 to (humans and english language) (12)

5 limit 4 to case reports (3)
6 4 not 5 (9)
7 from 6 keep 1–9 (9)

PsycINFO was also searched in March 2007 using CSA Illumina as an interface, and this search yielded 40 records focusing on group treatment for pain:

Database: PsycINFO/ CSA Illumina
  Query: DE=("pain" or "aphagia" or "back pain" or "chronic pain" or "headache" or "migraine headache" or "muscle contraction headache" or "myofascial pain" or "neuralgia" or "trigeminal neuralgia" or "somatoform pain disorder")AND DE=("group psychotherapy" or "encounter group therapy" or "marathon group therapy" or "therapeutic community") NOT DE= ("neoplasms")

In November 2007, these searches were repeated and broader, more sensitive searches were also performed by incorporating keywords in addition to controlled vocabulary to minimize the possibility of missing relevant studies and to include studies on mindfulness. These broader searches in both Medline and PsycINFO are detailed below.

Database: Ovid MEDLINE(R) <1950 to November Week 2 2007>
  1 pain.mp. or exp Pain/ (353317)
  2 headache.mp. or exp Headache Disorders/ (49645)
  3 1 or 2 (379062)
  4 "group treatment".mp. (1467)
  5 "group psychotherapy".mp. or exp Psychotherapy, Group/ (19229)
  6 4 or 5 (20189)
  7 3 and 6 (318)
  8 cancer.mp. or exp Neoplasms/ (1982859)
  9 7 not 8 (281)
  10 limit 9 to (humans and english language) (224)
  11 limit 10 to yr = "1980–2008" (195)
  12 limit 11 to "therapy (sensitivity)" (88)

Database: Ovid MEDLINE(R) <1950 to November Week 2 2007>
  1 pain.mp. or exp Pain/ (353317)
  2 exp Meditation/ or mindfulness.mp. (696)
  3 1 and 2 (52)
  4 limit 3 to (humans and english language) (51)
  5 limit 4 to "therapy (sensitivity)" (19)
  6 limit 3 to evidence based medicine reviews (1)
  7 limit 3 to "review articles" (15)

Database: PsycINFO / CSA Illumina
  Query: DE = ("pain" or "aphagia" or "back pain" or "chronic pain" or "headache" or "migraine headache" or "muscle contraction headache" or "myofascial pain" or "neuralgia" or "trigeminal neuralgia" or "somatoform pain disorder") and DE = ("mindfulness")
  Records retrieved = 14.

References

1. Keefe FJ, Beupre PM, Gil KM. Group therapy for patients with chronic pain. In: Turk DC, Gatchel RJ, eds. *Psychological Approaches to Pain Management: A Practitioner's Handbook.* 2nd ed. New York: The Guilford Press; 2002: 234–256.
2. Gamsa A, Braha RE, Catchlove RF. The use of structured group therapy sessions in the treatment of chronic pain patients. *Pain* 1985;22(1):91–96.
3. Blanchard EB, Schwarz SP. Adaptation of a multicomponent treatment for irritable bowel syndrome to a small-group format. *Biofeedback Self Regul* 1987;12(1):63–69.
4. Herman E, Baptiste S. Pain control: mastery through group experience. *Pain* 1981;10(1):79–86.
5. Straus SE, Richardson WS, Glasziou P, et al. *Evidence-Based Medicine: How*
to Practice and Teach EBM. 3rd ed. London: Elsevier Churchill Livingstone; 2005.
6. McKibbon A. *PDQ: Evidence-Based Principles and Practice.* Hamilton: B.C. Decker; 1999.
7. Frettloh J, Kroner-Herwig B. Individual versus group training in the treatment of chronic pain: which is more efficacious? *J Clin Psychol (Ger.)* 1999;28: 256–266.
8. Johnson PR, Thorn BE. Cognitive behavioral treatment of chronic headache: group versus individual treatment format. *Headache* 1989;29(6):358–365.
9. Rose MJ, Reilly JP, Pennie B, et al. Chronic low back pain rehabilitation programs: a study of the optimum duration of treatment and a comparison of group and individual therapy. *Spine* 1997;22(19):2246–2251.
10. Spence SH. Cognitive-behavior therapy in the management of chronic, occupational pain of the upper limbs. *Behav Res Ther* 1989;27(4):435–446.
11. Spence SH. Cognitive-behaviour therapy in the treatment of chronic, occupational pain of the upper limbs: a 2 yr follow-up. *Behav Res Ther* 1991;29(5): 503–509.
12. Turner-Stokes L, Erkeller-Yuksel F, Miles A, et al. Outpatient cognitive behavioral pain management programs: a randomized comparison of a group-based multidisciplinary versus an individual therapy model. *Arch Phys Med Rehabil* 2003;84(6):781–788.
13. Thorn BE, Pence LB, Ward LC, et al. A randomized clinical trial of targeted cognitive behavioral treatment to reduce catastrophizing in chronic headache sufferers. *J Pain* 2007;8(12):938–949.
14. Li EJ, Li-Tsang CW, Lam CS, et al. The effect of a "training on work readiness" program for workers with musculoskeletal injuries: a randomized control trial (RCT) study. *J Occup Rehabil* 2006;16(4):529–541.
15. Linton SJ, Boersma K, Jansson M, et al. The effects of cognitive-behavioral and physical therapy preventive interventions on pain-related sick leave: a randomized controlled trial. *Clin J Pain* 2005;21(2):109–119.
16. Gold DT, Shipp KM, Pieper CF, et al. Group treatment improves trunk strength and psychological status in older women with vertebral fractures: results of a randomized, clinical trial. *J Am Geriatr Soc* 2004;52(9):1471–1478.
17. Van Lankveld W, van Helmond T, Näring G, et al. Partner participation in cognitive-behavioral self management group treatment for patients with rheumatoid arthritis. *J Rheumatol* 2004;31(9):1738–1745.
18. Ersek M, Turner JA, McCurry SM, et al. Efficacy of a self-management group intervention for elderly persons with chronic pain. *Clin J Pain* 2003;19(3): 156–167.
19. Tkachuk G, Graff LA, Martin GL, et al. Randomized controlled trial of cognitive-behavioral group therapy for irritable bowel syndrome in a medical setting. *J Clin Psychol Med Settings* 2003;10(1):57–69.
20. Leibing E, Pfingsten M, Bartmann U, et al. Cognitive-behavioral treatment in unselected rheumatoid arthritis outpatients. *Clin J Pain* 1999;15(1):58–66.
21. Potts SG, Lewin R, Fox KA, et al. Group psychological treatment for chest pain with normal coronary arteries. *QJM* 1999;92(2):81–86.
22. Cole JD. Psychotherapy with the chronic pain patient using coping skills development: outcome study. *J Occup Health Psychol* 1998;3(3):217–226.
23. Keel PJ, Bodoky C, Gerhard U, et al. Comparison of integrated group therapy and group relaxation training for fibromyalgia. *Clin J Pain* 1998;14(3):232–328.
24. Keel PJ, Wittig R, Deutschmann R, et al. Effectiveness of in-patient rehabilitation for sub-chronic and chronic low back pain by an integrative group treatment program (Swiss Multicentre Study). *Scand J Rehabil Med* 1998;30(4): 211–219.
25. Basler HD, Jäkle C, Kröner-Herwig B. Incorporation of cognitive-behavioral treatment into the medical care of chronic low back patients: a controlled randomized study in German pain treatment centers. *Patient Educ Couns* 1997; 31(2):113–124.
26. van Dulmen AM, Fennis JF, Bleijenberg G. Cognitive-behavioral group therapy for irritable bowel syndrome: effects and long-term follow-up. *Psychosom Med* 1996;58(5):508–514.
27. Vlaeyen JW, Teeken-Gruben NJ, Goossens ME, et al. Cognitive-educational treatment of fibromyalgia:a randomized clinical trial. I. Clinical effects. *J Rheumatol* 1996;23(7):237–245.
28. Newton-John TR, Spence SH, Schotte D. Cognitive-behavioural therapy versus EMG biofeedback in the treatment of chronic low back pain. *Behav Res Ther* 1995;33(6):691–697.
29. James LD, Thorn BE, Williams DA. Goal specification in cognitive-behavioral therapy for chronic headache pain. *Behav Ther* 1993;24:305–320.
30. Turner JA, Jensen MP. Efficacy of cognitive therapy for chronic low back pain. *Pain* 1993;52(2):169–177.
31. Kneebone II, Martin PR. Partner involvement in the treatment of chronic headaches. *Behav Change* 1992;94:201–215.
32. Nicholas MK, Wilson PH, Goyen J. Operant-behavioural and cognitive-behavioural treatment for chronic low back pain. *Behav Res Ther* 1991;29(3): 225–238.
33. Subramanian K. Structured group work for the management of chronic pain: an experimental investigation. *Res Soc Work Pract* 1991;1:32–45.
34. Subramanian K. Long-term follow up of a structured treatment for the management of chronic pain. *Res Soc Work Pract* 1994;4(2):32–45.
35. Peters JL, Large RG. A randomised control trial evaluating in- and outpatient pain management programmes. *Pain* 1990;41(3):283–293.
36. Turner JA, Clancy S, McQuade KJ, et al. Effectiveness of behavioral therapy for chronic low back pain: a component analysis. *J Consult Clin Psychol* 1990; 58(5):573–579.

37. Linton SJ, Bradley LA, Jensen I, et al. The secondary prevention of low back pain: a controlled study with follow-up. *Pain* 1989;36(2):197–207.

38. Puder RS. Age analysis of cognitive-behavioral group therapy for chronic pain outpatients. *Psychol Aging* 1988;3(2):204–207.

39. Bradley LA, Young LD, Anderson KO, et al. Effects of psychological therapy on pain behavior of rheumatoid arthritis patients. Treatment outcome and six-month followup. *Arthritis Rheum* 1987;30(10):1105–1114.

40. Larsson B, Melin L, Lamminen M, et al. A school-based treatment of chronic headaches in adolescents. *J Pediatr Psychol* 1987;12(4):553–566.

41. Bradley LA, Turner RA, Young LD, et al. Effects of cognitive-behavioral therapy on pain behavior of rheumatoid arthritis (RA) patients: preliminary outcomes. *Scand J Behav Ther* 1985;14: 51–64.

42. Linton SJ, Melin L, Stjernlöf K. The effects of applied relaxation and operant activity training on chronic pain. *Behavioral Psychotherapy* 1985;13:87–100.

43. Melin L, Linton SJ. A follow-up study of a comprehensive behavioural treatment programme. *Behav Psychother* 1988;16(4):313–321.

44. Moore JE, Chaney EF. Outpatient group treatment of chronic pain: effects of spouse involvement. *J Consult Clin Psychol* 1985;53(3):326–334.

45. Cohen MJ, Heinrich RL, Naliboff BD, et al. Group outpatient physical and behavioral therapy for chronic low back pain. *J Clin Psychol* 1983;39(3): 326–333.

46. Figueroa J. Group treatment of chronic tension headaches: a comparative treatment study. *Behav Modif* 1982;6:229–239.

47. Turner JA, Comparison of group progressive-relaxation training and cognitive-behavioral group therapy for chronic low back pain. *J Consult Clin Psychol* 1982;50(5):757–765.

48. Goossens ME, Rutten-van Mölken MP, et al. Cognitive-educational treatment of fibromyalgia: a randomized clinical trial. II. Economic evaluation. *J Rheumatol* 1996;23(7):1246–1254.

49. Grossman P, Niemann L, Schmidt S, et al. Mindfulness-based stress reduction and health benefits. A meta-analysis. *J Psychosom Res* 2004;57(1):35–43.

50. Carson JW, Keefe FJ, Lynch TR, et al. Loving-kindness meditation for chronic low back pain: results from a pilot trial. *J Holist Nurs* 2005;23(3):287–304.

51. Plews-Ogan M, Owens JE, Goodman M, et al. A pilot study evaluating mindfulness-based stress reduction and massage for the management of chronic pain. *J Gen Intern Med* 2005;20(12):1136–1138.

52. Grossman P, Tiefenthaler-Gilmer U, Raysz A, et al. Mindfulness training as an intervention for fibromyalgia: evidence of postintervention and 3-year follow-up benefits in well-being. *Psychother Psychosom* 2007;76(4):226–233.

53. Kabat-Zinn J. The clinical use of mindfulness meditation for the self regulation of chronic pain. *J Behav Med* 1985;8(2):163–190.

54. Sagula D, Rice KG. The effectiveness of mindfulness training on the grieving process and emotional well-being of chronic pain patients. *J Clin Psychol Med Settings* 2004;11(4):333–342.

55. McCracken LM, MacKichan F, Eccleston C. Contextual cognitive-behavioral therapy for severely disabled chronic pain sufferers: Effectiveness and clinically significant change. *Eur J Pain* 2007;11(3):314–322.

56. Steihaug S, Ahlsen B, Malterud K. "I am allowed to be myself": women with chronic muscular pain being recognized. *Scand J Public Health* 2002;30(4): 281–287.

57. Maunder RG, Esplen MJ. Supportive-expressive group psychotherapy for persons with inflammatory bowel disease. *Can J Psychiatry* 2001;46(7):622–626.

58. Albert H. Psychosomatic group treatment helps women with chronic pelvic pain. *J Psychosom Obstet Gynaecol* 1999;20(4):216–225.

59. Lichstein KL, Riedel BW, Grieve R. Fair tests of clinical trials: A treatment implementation model. *Adv Behav Res Ther* 1994;16:1–29.

60. Unruh A. Gender variations in clinical pain experience. *Pain* 1996;65 (2–3)123–167.

61. Lyons RF, Mickelson KD, Sullivan MJL, et al. Coping as a communal process. *J Soc Pers Relat* 1998;15(5):579–605.

62. Thorn BE. *Cognitive Therapy for Chronic Pain: A Step by Step Guide.* New York: The Guilford Press; 2004.

63. Beck JS. *Cognitive Therapy: Basics and Beyond.* New York: The Guilford Press; 1995.

64. Burns DD. *Feeling Good: The New Mood Therapy.* New York: Avon Books; 1999.

65. Sullivan MJL, Thorn BE, Haythornthwaite J, et al. Theoretical perspectives on the relation between catastrophizing and pain. *Clin J Pain* 2001;17:52–64.

66. Jacobsen PB, Butler RW. Relation of cognitive coping and catastrophizing to acute pain and analgesic use following breast cancer surgery. *J Behav Med* 1996;19:17–29.

67. Keefe FJ, Brown GK, Wallston KA, et al. Coping with rheumatoid arthritis: catastrophizing as a maladaptive strategy. *Pain* 1989;37:51–56.

68. Sullivan MJ, Adams H, Sullivan M. Communicative dimensions of pain catastrophizing: social cueing effects on pain behavior. *Pain* 2004;107:220–226.

69. Flor H, Behle DJ, Birbaumer N. Assessment of pain-related cognitions in chronic pain patients. *Behav Res Ther* 1993;31:63–73.

70. Geisser ME, Robinson ME, Keefe FJ, et al. Catastrophizing, depression and the sensory, affective and evaluative aspects of chronic pain. *Pain* 1994;59: 79–83.

71. Gil KM, Thompson RJ Jr, Keith BR, et al. Sickle cell disease pain in children and adolescents: change in pain frequency and coping strategies over time. *J Pediatr Psychol* 1993;18:621–637.

72. Martin MY, Bradley LA, Alexander RW, et al. Coping strategies predict disability in patients with primary fibromyalgia. *Pain* 1996;46:45–53.

73. Robinson ME, Riley JL 3rd, Myers CD, et al. The Coping Strategies Questionnaire: a large sample, item level factor analysis. *Clin J Pain* 1997;13:43–49.

74. Sullivan MJL, Neish N. The effects of disclosure on pain during dental hygiene treatment: the moderating role of catastrophizing. *Pain* 1999;79:155–163.

75. Sullivan MJL, Rouse D, Bishop S, et al. Thought suppression, catastrophizing, and pain. *Cognit Ther Res* 1997;21:555–568.

76. Burns, Kubilus, Breuhl S, et al. Do changes in cognitive factors influence outcome following multidisciplinary treatment for chronic pain? A cross-lagged panel analysis. *J Consult Clin Psychol* 2003;71:81–91.

77. Burns JW, Glenn B, Bruehl S, et al. Cognitive factors influence outcome following multidisciplinary chronic pain treatment: a replication and extension of a cross-lagged panel analysis. *Behav Res Ther* 2003;41(10):1163–1182.

78. Scharff L, Marcus DA. Interdisciplinary outpatient group treatment of intractable headache. *Headache* 1994;34(2):73–78.

79. Moore ME, Berk SN, Nypaver A. Chronic pain: inpatient treatment with small group effects. *Arch Phys Med Rehabil* 1984;65(7):356–361.

CHAPTER 87 ■ MOTIVATING PAIN PATIENTS FOR BEHAVIORAL CHANGE

AKIKO OKIFUJI AND DENNIS C. TURK

INTRODUCTION

Motivation is perhaps the primary determinant of human behavior, influencing the initiation, direction, intensity, and persistence.[1] Historically, motivation has not been a central issue in the biomedical world as the modal biomedical approach to treat illness appeared to require very little active participation from patients. However, as our understanding of how patients' behaviors impacted their illness and influenced their adherence to treatment regimens increased, it has become of a significant issue and concern. This is especially true for treatment and management of chronic illnesses, such as chronic pain for which there often is no cure, since these diseases require patients to become actively involved in the self-management of their symptoms and lifestyles. Moreover, self-management and adherence to recommendations will likely be required for extended periods of time.

There is a large volume of literature indicating that even relatively simple behaviors, such as taking medication in the prescribed manner, is problematic. Studies have reported that depending on how it is defined and measured, the rates of nonadherence to medication range from 30% to 60%.[2] In general, one-third of patients can be expected to be nonadherent.[3]

For chronic pain patients, rehabilitation rather than complete cure is most realistic. One of the critical requirements for successful rehabilitation is that patients adopt an active, participatory role in their treatments. Literature consistently acknowledges that multidisciplinary pain care that includes an activating therapy is helpful for restoring functioning and improving the quality of life.[4] However, such a treatment requires patients to make significant lifestyle changes including the incorporation of various functional activities in their daily routines. Maintaining these changes over long periods of time is often difficult even for healthy individuals. For example, a report by the U.S. Surgeon General[5] noted that 50% of those who sign up with gyms at the beginning of a year drop out within the first 6 months. Thus, it is hardly surprising that pain patients find it difficult to adhere to regular physical activity regimens and ones that may actually cause some exacerbation of their symptoms. In the one study that directly examined the issue of compliance with pain rehabilitation, Lutz et al.[6] followed patients 8 months after they had been successfully treated at pain rehabilitation and found that, based on self-report, the overall rate of adherence with the recommendations of the treatment program was only 12.2%, and the rates of adherence with each of the specifically recommended behaviors (e.g., progressive ambulation and stretching exercises, regular application of ice and heat, relaxation) averaged approximately 42%.

Another dilemma for successful implementation of activating therapy is that it can be contrary to the very nature of pain where the motivating drive is to avoid or escape from any activities that might increase pain or that patients anticipate will induce pain. Yet another disincentive is that most people have learned "if something hurts, don't do it." That is, they have come to equate hurt with harm. Combined with our culture dictating the notion that we should not have to tolerate discomfort and pain, patients may perceive activating therapies as a counterintuitive approach. Certainly, pain plays a protective role; in a case of acute injury, for example, resting and inactivity facilitates the healing process but may be inappropriate when pain is persistent.

Thus, clinicians are frequently faced with the challenge of how to motivate patients to actively engage in the treatment protocols. Long-term treatment success depends on regular adherence to recommended self-care regimens for people with chronic pain conditions.[3,7,8] Historically, clinicians would invest less energy in patients who show little commitment to therapies. "You can lead a horse to water, but you can't make it drink" was a typical way of conceptualizing the issue.[9] However, as noted earlier, motivation to commit to the treatment plan and adherence with regimen are essential in successful pain rehabilitation (pharmacologic as well as rehabilitative), and this makes how we can motivate patients for behavioral change a critical clinical issue in pain management.

CONCEPT OF READINESS TO CHANGE: TRANSTHEORETICAL MODEL OF BEHAVIOR CHANGE

The transtheoretical model of behavior change was developed in an attempt to understand motivation to adhere to the health care regimens. The transtheoretical model offers an integrative framework describing the process of behavior change.[10] The transtheoretical model was originally developed to understand how people change their addictive behaviors. The model, however, has been extended to many medical problems including chronic pain.[11] The basic assumptions underlying the model are the notions that people differ in their readiness and willingness to take on behavioral change and that there are certain processes of changes that facilitate the advancement of one's readiness. The model is organized around a major construct: stages of change.

According to the model, patients attempting to change health-related behavior move from one stage to another, often in a cyclic

fashion (see Fig. 87.1; descriptions of each stage is in Table 87.1), although the movement through these stages is not necessarily linear. Some behaviors are easier to change than others; it is reasonable to assume that several attempts may be necessary to achieve significant behavioral change. A good example of the nonlinear change of stages may occur in smoking cessation where average smokers take 7–8 attempts to quit before succeeding.[12] The description of each stage as well as typical patient behavior seen at each stage point is listed in Table 87.1.

There are three critical parameters of the model that determines the likelihood of advancing one's readiness.

1. **Processes of change** are one of the dimensions of the transtheoretical model that enables understanding of *how* shifts in behavior may be achieved. Change processes involve both covert and overt activities and experiences that patients engage in when they attempt to change their behavioral patterns. Each process is a broad category and an eclectic collection of techniques, methods, and interventions can be recommended to facilitate the change process. Ten processes, cluster into two groups: the cognitive–experiential cluster of processes and the behavioral processes (Table 87.2). As can be seen, there are various strategies that come from the disparate theoretical orientations to target each process (right-hand column of Table 87.2).
2. **Self-Efficacy** is defined as personal confidence in the ability to change problem situations.[13] If people think that there is no way that they can do the prescribed activities, it is highly unlikely that the treatment will be successful.
3. **Decisional Balance** is defined as a personal "balance sheet" of gains and losses for changing and not changing their behaviors.[14] People are likely to advance their change stages when they perceive themselves to have adequate skills to cope and feel confident in executing those skills (i.e., high efficacy belief) and when they perceive more gains of changing and losses of not changing than more losses of changing and gains of not changing (decisional balance). We will discuss the decisional balance process later in the chapter as a part of reviewing the motivational enhancement techniques.

Some of the behavioral strategies such as counterconditioning and stimulus control are generally a major part of the multidisciplinary rehabilitation for chronic pain. The cognitive-behavioral self-management skill training that is generally a part of the pain rehabilitation also improve self-efficacy[15]; however, baseline levels of self-efficacy vary across patients, and there is a linear relationship between the baseline level of self-efficacy and posttreatment level of self-efficacy and subsequent treatment benefit self-management skill training.[16] Strategies targeting experiential processes are recommended as the primary approach to help people with low level of treatment readiness and self-efficacy.[17] Thus, using the concept of the change process seems a promising way to optimize the clinical outcomes of pain rehabilitation.

Motivation Enhancement Therapy

Motivation enhancement therapy (MET), developed by Miller et al.,[18] is one of the therapeutic methods to target motivation and readiness. It shares the assumption with the transtheoretical model that people vary in their readiness to adhere to treatment regimen and provides a problem-focused, patient-centered, clinician-directed approach with the aim of helping patients move through the stages of change. Although some of the techniques and approaches overlap with those of cognitive–behavior therapy (CBT), one of the most prevalent behavioral medicine approaches in treating chronic pain patients, the two therapy approaches have some distinct characteristics. The nature of the therapy course is no doubt variable depending upon the personal styles

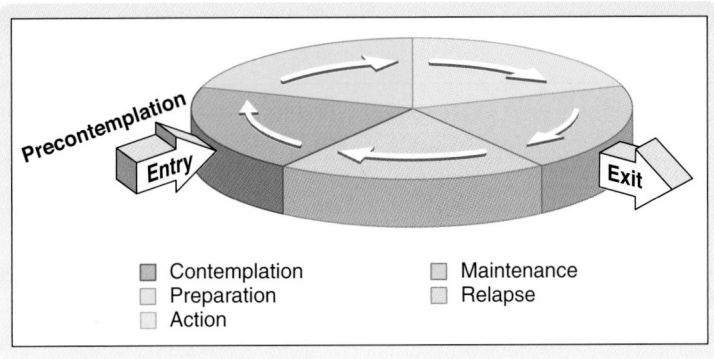

FIGURE 87.1 Stages of changes.

of the clinicians, and there is a danger of oversimplification of complex therapy modalities; however, for the sake of comparison and contrast, we summarize the characteristics of MET as compared to CBT in Table 87.3.

MET is broadly grounded in the Rogerian tradition of psychotherapy[19] in conjunction with behavioral analyses. It is nonconfrontational and patient-centered, exploring and reaching resolution of ambivalence toward behavior change. As in the Rogerian practice, a MET clinician helps patients explore their inner phenomenology that is explored without judgment or criticism. In order to facilitate this process, MET encourages a clinician to exercise empathetic listening and to ask open-ended questions.

Empathy is often confused with sympathy or agreement. In the Rogerian approach, empathy is expressed as understanding and acceptance without imposing the clinician's own perspectives. The patient's thoughts and feelings can be acknowledged through reflective comments no matter how much the clinician considers those maladaptive. Such acknowledgement is not achieved by simply repeating what the patient has just said. Rather, the clinician reflects back to the patient what the clinician "thinks" the patient meant. The term "active listening" or "reflective listening" is often used to describe the skill. Such empathetic atmosphere creates a sense of security for the patient which, in combination with a feeling of being understood and accepted, is considered critical for facilitating intrinsic motivation for behavioral change.

Asking open-ended questions helps the clinician to better understand the individualized phenomenology of the patient regarding the problem that is the target of behavior change in a nonthreatening manner. It also aids the patient to achieve a clearer view on the issue. Asking open-ended questions, however, is not time-efficient; asking questions that can be responded with a short "yes" or "no" answer can save time. As you can see in the following sections describing the MET techniques, however, asking open-ended questions is vital in successful implementation of MET. Some examples of open-ended and close-ended questions are listed in Table 87.4.

The MET offers a collection of therapeutic techniques to help patients: (1) clearly recognize their problems, (2) perform decisional balance work, and (3) produce self-motivational statements and internalize those motivational statements via improved self-efficacy. MET also provides the guidance for how to handle resistance and setbacks. In the following section, we will describe the basic MET methods, including how to deal with resistance and what not to do while engaging in MET.

TABLE 87.1

STAGES OF CHANGE

Stages	Descriptions	Patients' behaviors
Precontemplation	Patient does not perceive a need to change and actively resists change.	• Unwilling to discuss • "Who? Me?"
Contemplation	Patient begins to see a need for change and may consider making a change in the future	• Somewhat ambivalent or fearful of change • "Yes, but. . ."
Preparation	Patient feels ready to change and takes a first concrete (behavioral) change	• Sees more pros for change than cons • "I'll start this on Sunday!"
Action	Patient actively engages in behaviors consistent with regimen	• Feels more confident
Maintenance	Patient executes plans to sustain the changes made	• Feels comfortable with the change • Identifies self as the changed entity
Relapse	Some patients fail to sustain the effort	Variable

TABLE 87.2

PROCESSES OF CHANGE

Processes	Definition	Therapeutic strategies that may help targeting the process
Experiential Processes		
Consciousness raising	Increasing information about self and problem	Observations, confrontations, interpretations, bibliotherapy
Self-reevaluation	Assessing how one feels and thinks about oneself with respect to a problem	Value clarification, imagery, corrective emotional experience
Dramatic relief	Experiencing and expressing feelings about one's problem and solutions	Role playing, psychodrama, grieving losses
Environmental reevaluation	Assessing how one's problems affect the physical environment	Empathy training, documentaries
Social liberation	Increasing alternatives for nonproblem behaviors available in society	Advocating for rights of repressed, empowering, policy interventions
Behavioral Processes		
Counterconditioning	Substituting alternatives for problem and anxiety related behaviors	Relaxation, desensitization, assertion, positive self-statements
Helping relationships	Being open and trusting about problems with someone who cares	Therapeutic alliance, social support, self-help groups
Reinforcement management	Rewarding oneself or being rewarded by others for making changes	Contingency contracts, overt and covert reinforcement, self-reward
Stimulus control	Avoiding stimuli that elicit problem behaviors	Adding stimuli that encourage alternative behaviors, restructuring one's environment, avoiding high risk cues, fading techniques
Self-liberation	Choosing and committing to act or believe in ability to change	Decision-making therapy, resolution

HELP PATIENTS RECOGNIZE THE PROBLEMS AND GOALS

Patients come to clinics with various expectations and goals. Some patients expect to be pain-free, whereas some patients focus on improving the quality of life even if pain is not totally resolved. However, many patients are often unaware of what should happen to achieve their goals and what their role should be for meeting the expectation. The next step to help patients become more aware of what needs to happen is to delineate the gap between where they are now and where they want to be when they get better. For example, the discussion may start with questions such as:

- How is your life different from your life before pain began?
- How has your pain stopped you from doing what you want to do?
- What are you now doing to cope with your pain problem? How are they working for you?
- How do you think your pain and disability impact your relationship with your spouse/family?
- What do you miss most about your life before the pain began?

Then the discussion should be turned into what patients want to see happen through treatment. For example,

- What would your life look like with better pain management?
- What change would you like to see most?
- What are you doing now that is helping you to make these things happen?

TABLE 87.3

MOTIVATION ENHANCEMENT THERAPY VERSUS COGNITIVE–BEHAVIORAL THERAPY APPROACHES

	MET	CBT
Orientation	Patient-centered	Goal-oriented
Therapist–patient relationship	Collaborative	Top-down
Focus	Stage change	Action
Therapist's task	More listening	More talking
Dealing with ambivalence	Explore ambivalence	Direct persuasion
Approaches to reasons for change	Elicit reasons for change	Give reasons for change

TABLE 87.4

CLOSE-ENDED QUESTIONS VERSUS OPEN-ENDED QUESTIONS: EXAMPLES

Close-ended questions	Open-ended questions
Are you having a problem exercising?	Tell me about the problem you are having about exercising
Do you overuse your pain medications when your pain is really bad?	What do you do when your pain is really bad?
Would you be able to come to the clinic every week for trigger point injections?	How would you feel about coming to the clinic for trigger point injections?

- What other things could you do, or do more of, to help your goal come true?

This line of discussion can also help identify specific discrepancy between what a patient wants from therapy (e.g., "I want to get well") and what he or she is doing (e.g., "I can't do my exercise because I am not well"). The process facilitates the realization of the possibility that patients' own behaviors contribute to the maintenance of pain and prevent them from obtaining their goal of getting better. Such realization in turn forms a background on which motivation for behavioral change can be built.

Not only can clarification of the gap between a present state and a goal state help drive the motivation to change, but it also creates the opportunity to move to specific plans. A clinician and patient can start "brainstorming" as to what possible ways there are to make the change probable. Plans can be prioritized by patients' preference and practical concerns as well as perceived effectiveness of the actions. Possible problems and obstacles should also be thoroughly explored to better prepare the patient.

It is common to find that the patient, after years of functional impairment and other related problems, feels very helpless and convinced that there is nothing they can do to manage their plight. Such resistance can seriously arrest the process of behavioral change. We will discuss how to deal with resistance later in this chapter.

Decisional Balance

Motivation for behavioral changes is rarely linear. Often, we may understand the need for behavioral change but remain reluctant to commit ourselves to do the things needed for the change. People experiencing persistent pain are no exception. Nearly all pain patients would want to improve, and many of them may intuitively understand how behavioral changes can help their pain. Despite this, many patients may remain feeling ambivalent or conflicted about committing themselves for behavioral change. One often hears comments like "I know I need to be more active, but..."

To a large extent, activating rehabilitation and self-management pain care recommends daily practice of the learned skills and modification of lifestyle, aiming at the long-term, gradual improvement. Thus, activities required for these approaches typically do not pay off immediately despite substantial work involved. This tends to lead patients to focus more on immediate "cost" of self-management activities, such as postexercise soreness and time commitment. Decisional balance helps patients explore all sides of the story on the consequences of not only "doing" but also "not doing" activities that they think need to be done.

The decisional balance procedure involves creating a personal "balance sheet" of both advantages and disadvantages of committing to change compared to not committing. For example, suppose that a clinician would like to facilitate a more active lifestyle for a patient who has dealt with pain by staying in bed or resting for years. The patient will be asked to list what they think are good things and not so good things about maintaining the status quo; in other words, not changing and keeping doing what they have been doing. The patient will also be asked to list good and not so good things about changing their way to be more active and keep functioning despite pain. An example of a "balance sheet" is shown in Table 87.5. The clinician can help patients explore the impact of the change and no change on various life domains and the emotional and cognitive consequences of their action (or nonaction). The sheet will help facilitate the resolution of the potential "I want to, but..." conflict. The section of "not so good" things about change can also help the clinician see what areas of coping and other supportive care can be implemented to increase the sense of self-efficacy for the change.

Self-Motivational Statements

Self-motivational statements or "change-talks" by patients represent an important step toward better readiness for behavioral change. In MET, it is critical that thoughts reflecting their intention to change are discussed and help them internalize such thoughts. There are three steps in this phase. First, such thoughts should be elicited and verbalized. Then the thoughts need to be elaborated, as such thoughts, if remaining abstract, may result in perpetual wishful thinking with no actual behavioral change. And finally, elicitation and elaboration of such thoughts are reinforced. Going through this process helps patients identify problems and goals, and they then explore what it would mean to change versus not change. At this point, the patients may spontaneously come up with statements reflecting their willingness and intention to commit themselves for behavioral changes. If so, the therapy can start with the second step. However, for many chronic pain patients whose maladaptive habitual patterns are so ingrained in their lifestyles, some time may be devoted to help patients feel comfortable with change talks.

In order to guide a patient through this process, the clinician may ask questions such as:

- What encourages you that you can change if you want to?
- What do you think would work for you, if you decided to change?
- What will make (engaging in exercise program, etc.) it easier for you?

One of the supportive yet effective methods for the elicitation of self-motivational statements is to review past success. By recognizing that they were able to commit to change and were successful in doing so, it breeds the ground for optimism and improves the sense of self-efficacy. For example, in the earlier phase in treatment, the clinician may ask patient to list what and how they were able to change something in their lives, and guide the patient by asking

- What do you remember when you were able to...?
- What was it like when you changed...?
- When else in your life have you made a significant change? How did you do it?

Some patients may have a tendency to disregard past success and instead focus on past failure. It is also common to encounter the extremely negative cognitive style in which patients generalize past failure to all future actions. In a case like this, it is helpful to explore their past failure and help them reframe the experience. Provision of education regarding outcome literature and how certain behaviors increase their probability of recovery may also be beneficial.

It is extremely important for a clinician to recognize self-motivational statements. Typically, initial self-motivational statements are rather only vaguely directed toward the perceived needs

TABLE 87.5

DECISIONAL BALANCE SHEET

Staying in bed or resting every time I feel pain (status quo)		Trying to stay active (change)	
Good things	Not so good things	Good things	Not so good things
• Helps me rest • I will not get tired or sore	• Life has to come to a halt • I do not feel that good anyway • I may get even more deconditioned • I have to ask for help from others • Cannot participate in social things • More depression • May gain weight • Will never be able to go back to work	• Things can get done • Keep in touch with friends • Feel better about the day • Feel more independent • May gain physical strength • Less burden on family	• I may feel worse • I may feel stressed out

(e.g., "I know I really need to take the home exercise program more seriously," "I am wondering if I should start thinking of how I can manage my anxiety better," "It may not be a bad idea for me to go back to work"). How such statements are responded to by the clinician can determine whether they can be transformed to more concrete motivation and actual behavioral actions. Basic responses by the clinicians should clarify the issue at hand in terms of how the change can be made based upon what concerns. The statements can further be elaborated with responses like:

■ Tell me in what ways you think you can do that.
■ Sounds like you have some thoughts about it. What other concerns have you noticed about this problem?
■ What are some reasons why you want to do this?
■ How do you think you can enjoy this change?

The clinician must remain cautious during the process of elaboration. It is common to see that premature or presumptuous encouragement by the clinician can result in undue pressure for the patient. A discouraged patient is likely to become resistant to change. It is important to remember that MET is clinician-directed but patient-centered.

The attempts at self-motivational statements and subsequent elaborations should be positively reinforced. The clinician's encouraging responses can significantly impact the patient's frame of mind about the change. Simple comments such as "I think it's a wonderful idea," "I see how important this is to you," and "You have a point there" can help the process of eliciting self-motivational statements conclude in a positive and productive manner.

WHAT NOT TO DO IN MOTIVATION ENHANCEMENT THERAPY

One of the important aspects in MET is to avoid placing a patient in a passive role in the clinician–patient interaction. This is a very easy trap for the clinician to get in. For example:

Clinician: How long have you had this pain?
Patient: Seven years.
Clinician: Where does it hurt?
Patient: My back.
Clinician: Are you working now?
Patient: No.
Clinician: Are you receiving disability?
Patient: Yes.

The process like this is counterproductive for activating rehabilitation because it sets a tone of the treatment where the clinician is the expert who can tell what to do, whereas the patient is the passive recipient of the treatment.

We are not saying that a clinician should never provide advice. As an expert, a clinician can provide options and choices. What is important here is to emphasize that there are options and to help the patient achieve their own conclusion of what would work for him or her. Ultimate responsibility of behavioral change lies with the patient, and it should be communicated clearly through the MET process.

Value judgment by the clinician can also be detrimental in helping the patient increase motivation for behavioral change. Consider the following interaction:

Clinician: It seems that you are only interested in getting medications from us. You have not done anything we asked you to do such as exercise, habit change, and mood monitoring; no wonder you are not doing so well.

Patient: Well, I need my medicine because it takes some edge off my pain. I am not doing that badly. I am doing fine.

Value judgments by clinicians can elicit defensiveness, often leading patients to discount the very problem that needs to be addressed. "Oh, it's no big deal," and the change stage could return all the way back to the precontemplative stage (see Table 87.1 for the description of the stage). When the patients consider the problem "no problem," it is very hard, if not impossible, to motivate them for behavioral changes.

DEALING WITH SETBACKS AND RESISTANCE

Changes are hard to make. As noted earlier, patients are likely to hold some ambivalence about committing to change, particularly when the change involves the fundamental part of their lifestyle. Resistance is expected, can occur at any phase of MET, and may take various forms such as arguing, interrupting, denying, ignoring, challenging, minimizing, and sidetracking. Some example behaviors of these resistance forms are listed in Table 87.6. One of the hallmarks of MET is that a clinician does not fight resistance but works with it. Too often, an eager clinician gets overdriven to argue for the change, only to find that the patient backs off from the previous self-motivational stance and becomes reluctant to commit. MET requires a clinician to direct a patient to move toward the behavioral change without imposing, ordering,

TABLE 87.6

EXAMPLES OF RESISTANCE

Resistance	Behaviors
Arguing	Contests the accuracy of information or the clinician's expertise
Interrupting	Interrupts the clinician in a defensive manner
Denying	Shows unwillingness to admit/recognize problems
Ignoring	Does not follow the discussion or conversational direction
Challenging	Challenges the accuracy, effectiveness, or applicability of what the clinician says
Minimizing	Minimizes the risk of problem behaviors (or not doing something) or minimizing the benefit of change
Sidetracking	Changes the direction of the conversation away from the direction that the clinician was pursuing
Blaming	Blames others for the problem and does not acknowledge any responsibility for him/herself
Non-answering	Gives a response that is no answer to the question asked
Disagreeing	"Yes, but…"—disagrees with a suggestion without offering any constructive alternative

or arguing for it. How do we do this? The approach here is to stay on the same side with patients yet help them to argue for change. There are several specific techniques that a clinician can employ to work with resistance.

Simple Reflection

In simple reflection, clinicians express their acknowledgement of the patients' comments that reflects resistance in a nonconfrontational manner. For example, patients may argue that they are too exhausted and sore to do the home exercise program after taking care of the household chores; the clinician may respond:

- I see that you are frustrated for not being able to make the change you want.
- It is hard for you to work out after a long day.

The simple reflection method is to provide the sense that the patient is heard and understood. Notice that the reflection does not have any hint of value judgment (e.g., "It is really too bad that you cannot save any energy to exercise because we are not asking you to do that much, you know"), which would defeat the purpose of the simple reflection technique that is to be used to signal that the patient's concern was heard and taken seriously.

Amplified Reflection

Amplified reflection is an applied variation of simple reflection in which the clinician reflects back the patient's comment in an overexaggerated manner. With the example of not being able to do the home exercise above, the clinician may respond: "It is absolutely impossible for you to do the exercise."

The amplified reflection adds the core meaning or intensity of the emotion associated with the patient's statement. By doing

so, it helps patients better see the balance of their ambivalence. Facing the exaggerated form of their own statement often helps them focus more on the other side of their original comment. Consider a case where a patient complains of postexercise soreness.

Patient: I am so sore after doing those exercises that I cannot do anything but lay in bed for the rest of the day. The house is a mess and I do not feel better.
Clinician: There is absolutely no way that the exercise can help you get better.

The amplification must be done in an empathetic manner. There can be a fine line between empathetic amplification and sarcasm. The same statement above, with a slightly different tone, can be delivered as a sarcastic criticism. If the patient feels that the clinician is being sarcastic or inpatient, the reflection will likely encourage further resistance and retard the process of change.

Double-Sided Reflection

Double-sided reflection is used to highlight the ambivalent feeling that the patient has expressed. With the example above, the clinician may respond: "On the one hand, you find it very difficult to incorporate exercise in your life, and at the same time, it is frustrating because you really want to do it."

Miller and Rollnick[20] recommend the use of "and" rather than "but" to bridge the two sides of the ambivalence. It also seems advisable that one ends the reflection with the motivational side, perhaps reflecting the motivational statement the patient has previously used.

Agreement With Twist

This is another variation of the reflection in which the clinician initially reflects and then reframes the patient's statement. Initial reflection is typically presented as an empathetic agreement, affirming that the patient was well heard. Then the clinician offers a reframed perspective on the same subject in a nonthreatening manner. For example:

Patient: I know I do not do all the stuff the physical therapist wants me to do. But it is so hard, and I don't think she (the physical therapist) understands how hard it is for me to do the program everyday.
Clinician: You have a point there. It is so frustrating for you not to be able to do the exercise, even though you are so anxious to find a way to do it and move forward with your program.

This subtle change in the direction can help the patient move further toward change while maintaining the therapeutic relationship.

Personal Choice and Control

The psychotherapy literature suggests that one of the conditions in which resistance tends to arise is when a patient perceives a loss of, or a threat of losing, personal choice and control.[21] Typically, resistance is stronger when the importance of the threatened freedom is greater, often resulting in people asserting their option by doing something counteractive to the required behavior. In MET, it is essential that the affirmation of personal choice and control be reminded throughout the course of treatment that it is ultimately their choice to follow through the treatment recommendation. For example:

Patient: All of you keep telling me to do the home program, even though I keep telling you I do not want to do it.

Clinician: It is your choice, of course. It is your health after all. We can only make the recommendations and the rest is up to you.

Such an interaction can help the patient understand that the choice is theirs; at the same time, it fosters a sense of responsibility for the patient to commit to the treatment regimen.

Shifting Focus

Some patients, particularly those with tendency to "catastrophize" (i.e., a cognitive and emotional process that involves magnification of pain related-stimuli, feelings of helplessness, and a negative orientation toward pain) and use the black–white cognitive styles, tend to get trapped into the mode of "cannot do because. . ."; there is always a reason why they cannot do what they need or want to do. For them, obstacles and barriers to advance behavioral changes can become so great that those could be the only thing they would focus. A clinician can defuse such intense focus and help the patient move out of the trap and onto the step necessary to make the desired change. For example:

> *Patient*: There is absolutely no way I can do those exercises. You do not know how much it hurts for me to even lift my 2-year-old. I have not been able to do anything I want for years, and how can I possibly do what they want me to do?
>
> *Clinician*: I see your frustration. It sounds like pain really influences your life. Tell me more the kind of things you would like to do in your life.

Shifting focus can help defuse the resistance and instead focus on something that can be workable and supportive for behavioral change.

RESEARCH OUTCOMES

A growing body of research supports the conclusion that MET is effective in promoting healthful behaviors. Past research has shown that MET has been effective for facilitating change to reduce problem behaviors, such as smoking,[22–24] alcohol abuse,[25,26] problem gambling,[27] behaviors related to eating disorders,[28] and high-risk sexual behaviors.[29,30] MET has also been shown to increase wellness behaviors such as promoting exercise in myocardial infarction patients[31] and cancer survivors,[32] adherence with glucose control regimen in diabetics,[33] and attendance for mammography screening.[34] MET has become a popular method to address obesity and research shows its efficacy for children[35] as well as adult diabetic patients.[36] MET has been shown to help normalize the lipid profiles of hyperlipidemic individuals via increased fitness.[37]

MET can easily be integrated in various clinical settings. Brief MET counseling in a primary care setting may reduce substance use among high-risk adolescents.[38] In a busy clinical setting, clinicians may regard a full course of MET impossible to implement. There is some evidence, however, that implementing even a small part of MET can be efficacious in promoting behavioral change. A recent study has reported that a brief decisional balance session can promote safer sexual practice and reduce problem drinking among high-risk college men.[39] MET can also be implemented through phone counseling. Phone MET has been shown to help adherence for osteoporosis medication[40] and reduce alcohol abuse.[41]

Unfortunately, MET has not been extensively tested for pain patients, although there are some excellent chapters describing MET,[42–44] reflecting the growing awareness of the importance of motivation in pain treatment. Available evidence strongly suggests that the state of motivation for change is critical in better treatment outcomes for pain patients.[45,46] Furthermore, a recent study suggests that implementing MET prior to the initiation of the CBT-based self-management skill training for pain patients may enhance the treatment attendance,[47] and similar results have been shown with cocaine users.[48] A recent pilot, single-group

study also shows significant symptom reduction in fibromyalgia patients undergoing a brief exercise program with phone-based MET.[49] They found a dose-response trend with those who received more than four MET calls showing greater symptom reduction than those who received less than four calls.

CONSIDERATIONS FOR AND POTENTIAL PITFALLS OF MOTIVATIONAL ENHANCEMENT THERAPY

Although research consistently shows the effectiveness of MET for promoting behavioral change in various clinical settings, it is important to remind ourselves that it certainly is not a panacea for pain patients. MET primarily places a focus upon specific changes to either increase or decrease certain types of behaviors to further the effectiveness of pain treatments. If the treatment itself is too complicated or too difficult for the patient, behavioral change would not yield satisfactory outcomes, therefore de-reinforcing the behavioral change itself. Once discouraged, it is reasonable to assume that resistance to another type of behavioral change would become greater. The effectiveness of MET, therefore, partially depends upon the reasonableness of the pain treatment itself. The MET clinician needs to be actively involved in the pain treatment team to assure the successful interaction of MET and the pain regimens recommended by the team.

As some MET experts have pointed out,[42,50] MET is neither for every patient nor for every clinician. For example, MET assumes a fairly equal balance of power between a clinician and a patient (i.e., clinician ≠ expert), and some patients may be uncomfortable or feel even threatened by such relationship with the health care provider. In a case like this, MET may prove to be detrimental rather than helpful, and the clinician may do better with the traditional top-down approaches to aim at behavioral change. Similarly, although MET is certainly a learnable skill, it may not be so for some clinicians. Some may feel more at home with more directive, confrontational style and find it more effective for their practice. Like any other behavioral modalities, the goodness of fit between a patient and clinician is critical for successful execution of MET for pain patients.

Finally, the outcome literature of MET for pain patients is scarce at this time. In addition, MET is a flexible approach with various techniques; how different parameters influence patients' behaviors is not well understood. MET also involves different formats (e.g., individual, group, phone, mail) as well as intensity of the program (e.g., number of sessions). The effectiveness of MET may depend upon various other factors such as target behaviors, clinical context, and overall pain treatment plan. Future research needs to take these factors in consideration to further our understanding of how we can optimize the effectiveness of MET for pain patients to achieve behavior change for more adaptive lifestyles.

Perhaps the most effective way to help people change is to encourage and assist them in accomplishing improvements based on their own efforts. Coercing and encouraging by themselves may be ineffective, whereas behavioral experience and success will have the greatest likelihood on increasing a sense of self-efficacy.[13] The emphasis is on the "self." Obtaining "evidence" demonstrating that one can actually bring about changes, especially changes that are important to patients, will provide the greatest incentive and motivation to continue to engage in necessary self-management behaviors.

CONCLUSION

In this chapter, we have noted the importance of motivation for behavior change, particularly for patients who have chronic pain. For these individuals, self-management and adherence to prescribed regimens over long periods of time are essential. We reviewed the theoretical basis of behavioral change and the basics of the therapeutic approaches to enhance motivation for change, MET. There are multiple areas of treatments that require significant behavioral, cognitive, and emotional changes for pain patients. Pain clinicians, across disciplines, often face behavioral issues, such as maladaptive behaviors related to medication use and resistance and nonadherence to exercise and other self-management behaviors, all of which become a significant hindrance for optimal treatment implementation. MET is one approach that has been designed specifically to target motivation and to help clinicians help patients commit to behavioral change that should facilitate the overall pain therapies. Although there is limited empirical evidence for MET in pain medicine, there are a growing number of studies in other areas demonstrating the efficacy of MET in reducing maladaptive behaviors and increasing wellness behaviors, suggesting that MET can be a powerful tool for pain clinicians as well.

Acknowledgment

Support for preparation of this manuscript was provided by grants from the National Institutes of Health, National Institute of Arthritis Musculoskeletal Diseases and Skin Diseases (R01AR4888) to the first author and (R01AR44724) to the second author.

References

1. Geen R. *Human Motivation: A Social Psychological Approach*. Pacific Grove: Brooks/Cole; 1995.
2. Masek BJ. Compliance and medication. In: Doleys DN, Meredith RL, Ciminero AR, eds. *Behavioral Medicine: Assessment and Treatment Strategies*. New York, NY: Plenum Press; 1982.
3. Turk DC, Rudy TE. Neglected topics in the treatment of chronic pain patients—relapse, noncompliance, and adherence enhancement. *Pain* 1991; 44(1):5–28.
4. Okifuji A. Interdisciplinary pain management with pain patients: evidence for its effectiveness. *Semin Pain Med* 2003;1(2):110–119.
5. U.S. Department of Health and Human Services. *Physical activity and health: a report of the Surgeon General*. Atlanta, GA: Centers for Disease Control and Prevention, National Center for Chronic Disease Prevention; 1996.
6. Lutz RW, Silbret M, Olshan N. Treatment outcome and compliance with therapeutic regimens: long-term follow-up of a multidisciplinary pain program. *Pain* 1983;17(3):301–308.
7. Hayden JA, van Tulder MW, Malmivaara A, et al. Exercise therapy for treatment of non-specific low back pain. *Cochrane Database Syst Rev* 2005;3: CD000335.
8. Oliver K, Cronan T. Predictors of exercise behaviors among fibromyalgia patients. *Prev Med* 2002;35(4):383–389.
9. Meichenbaum DH, Turk DC. *Facilitating Treatment Adherence: A Practitioner's Guidebook*. New York, NY: Plenum Press; 1987.
10. Prochaska J, DiClemente C. The transtheoretical approach: toward a systematic eclectic framework. In: Norcross JC, ed. *Handbook of Eclectic Psychotherapy*. New York: Brunner/Mazel; 1986:163–200.
11. Kerns RD, Rosenberg R, Jamison RN, et al. Readiness to adopt a self-management approach to chronic pain: the Pain Stages of Change Questionnaire (PSOCQ). *Pain* 1997;72(1–2):227–234.
12. Crane R. The most addictive drug, the most deadly substance: smoking cessation tactics for the busy clinician. *Prim Care* 2007;34(1):117–135.
13. Bandura A. Self-efficacy: toward a unifying theory of behavioral change. *Psychol Rev* 1977;84(2):191–215.
14. Mann L. Use of a "balance sheet" procedure to improve quality of personal decision making: a field experiment with college applicants. *J Vocat Behav* 1972;2(3):291–300.
15. Gowans SE, deHueck A, Voss S, et al. A randomized, controlled trial of exercise and education for individuals with fibromyalgia. *Arthritis Care Res* 1999;12(2): 120–128.
16. Buckelew SP, Huyser B, Hewett JE, et al. Self-efficacy predicting outcome among fibromyalgia subjects. *Arthritis Care Res* 1996;9(2):97–104.
17. Prochaska J, Velicer W, DiClemente C, et al. Patterns of change: dynamic typology applied to smoking cessation. *Multivariate Behav Res* 1991;26(1): 83–107.
18. Miller W. Motivational interviewing with problem drinkers. *Behav Psychother* 1983;11:147–172.
19. Rogers C, Dymond R. *Psychotherapy and Personality Change*. Chicago, IL: University of Chicago Press; 1954.
20. Miller W, Rollnick S. *Motivational Interviewing: Preparing People for Change*. 2nd ed. New York, NY: Guilford Press; 2002.

21. Brehm SS, Brehm JW. *Psychological Reactance: A Theory of Freedom and Control*. New York: Academic Press; 1981.
22. Town GI, Fraser P, Graham S, et al. Establishment of a smoking cessation programme in primary and secondary care in Canterbury. *N Z Med J* 2000; 113(1107):117–119.
23. Velasquez MM, Hecht J, Quinn VP, et al. Application of motivational interviewing to prenatal smoking cessation: training and implementation issues. *Tob Control* 2000;9(suppl 3):III36–III40.
24. Ruger JP, Weinstein MC, Hammond SK, et al. Cost-effectiveness of motivational interviewing for smoking cessation and relapse prevention among low-income pregnant women: a randomized controlled trial. *Value Health* 2008; 11(2):191–198.
25. Brown RL, Saunders LA, Bobula JA, et al. Remission of alcohol disorders in primary care patients. Does diagnosis matter? *J Fam Pract* 2000;49(6): 522–528.
26. Handmaker NS, Miller WR, Manicke M. Findings of a pilot study of motivational interviewing with pregnant drinkers. *J Stud Alcohol* 1999;60(2): 285–287.
27. Hodgins DC, Currie SR, el-Guebaly N. Motivational enhancement and self-help treatments for problem gambling. *J Consult Clin Psychol* 2001;69(1): 50–57.
28. Feld R, Woodside DB, Kaplan AS, et al. Pretreatment motivational enhancement therapy for eating disorders: a pilot study. *Int J Eat Disord* 2001;29(4): 393–400.
29. Carey MP, Braaten LS, Maisto SA, et al. Using information, motivational enhancement, and skills training to reduce the risk of HIV infection for low-income urban women: a second randomized clinical trial. *Health Psychol* 2000; 19(1):3–11.
30. Kalichman SC, Cherry C, Browne-Sperling F. Effectiveness of a video-based motivational skills-building HIV risk-reduction intervention for inner-city African American men. *J Consult Clin Psychol* 1999;67(6):959–966.
31. Song R, Lee H. Managing health habits for myocardial infarction (MI) patients. *Int J Nurs Stud* 2001;38(4):375–380.
32. Bennett JA, Lyons KS, Winters-Stone K, et al. Motivational interviewing to increase physical activity in long-term cancer survivors: a randomized controlled trial. *Nurs Res* 2007;56(1):18–27.
33. Smith DE, Heckemeyer CM, Kratt PP, et al. Motivational interviewing to improve adherence to a behavioral weight-control program for older obese women with NIDDM. A pilot study. *Diabetes Care* 1997;20(1):52–54.
34. Bernstein J, Mutschler P, Bernstein E. Keeping mammography referral appointments: motivation, health beliefs, and access barriers experienced by older minority women. *J Midwifery Womens Health* 2000;45(4):308–313.
35. Schwartz RP, Hamre R, Dietz WH, et al. Office-based motivational interviewing to prevent childhood obesity: a feasibility study. *Arch Pediatr Adolesc Med* 2007;161(5):495–501.
36. West DS, DiLillo V, Bursac Z, et al. Motivational interviewing improves weight loss in women with type 2 diabetes. *Diabetes Care* 2007;30(5):1081–1087.
37. Kreman R, Yates BC, Agrawal S, et al. The effects of motivational interviewing on physiological outcomes. *Appl Nurs Res* 2006;19(3):167–170.
38. Stern SA, Meredith LS, Gholson J, et al. Project CHAT: a brief motivational substance abuse intervention for teens in primary care. *J Subst Abuse Treat* 2007;32(2):153–165.
39. LaBrie JW, Pedersen ER, Thompson AD, et al. A brief decisional balance intervention increases motivation and behavior regarding condom use in high-risk heterosexual college men. *Arch Sex Behav* 2008;37(2):330–339.
40. Cook PF, Emiliozzi S, McCabe MM. Telephone counseling to improve osteoporosis treatment adherence: an effectiveness study in community practice settings. *Am J Med Qual* 2007;22(6):445–456.
41. Brown RL, Saunders LA, Bobula JA, et al. Randomized-controlled trial of a telephone and mail intervention for alcohol use disorders: three-month drinking outcomes. *Alcohol Clin Exp Res* 2007;31(8):1372–1379.
42. Jensen M. Enhancing motivation to change in pain treatment. In: Gatchel R, Turk D, eds. *Psychological Approaches to Pain Management*. New York, NY: Guilford; 1996:78–111.
43. Turk D, Okifuji A, Sherman J. Psychologic aspects of back pain: implications for physical therapists. In: Twomey L, Taylor J, eds. *Physical Therapy of the Low Back*. New York, NY: Churchill Livingstone;2000:351–384.
44. Jones KD, Burckhardt CS, Bennett JA. Motivational interviewing may encourage exercise in persons with fibromyalgia by enhancing self efficacy. *Arthritis Rheum* 2004;51(5):864–867.
45. Kerns RD, Rosenberg R. Predicting responses to self-management treatments for chronic pain: application of the pain stages of change model. *Pain* 2000; 84(1):49–55.
46. Heapy A, Otis J, Marcus KS, et al. Intersession coping skill practice mediates the relationship between readiness for self-management treatment and goal accomplishment. *Pain* 2005;118(3):360–368.
47. Habib S, Morrissey S, Helmes E. Preparing for pain management: a pilot study to enhance engagement. *J Pain* 2005;6(1):48–54.
48. McKee SA, Carroll KM, Sinha R, et al. Enhancing brief cognitive-behavioral therapy with motivational enhancement techniques in cocaine users. *Drug Alcohol Depend* 2007;91(1):97–101.
49. Ang D, Kesavalu R, Lydon JR, et al. Exercise-based motivational interviewing for female patients with fibromyalgia: a case series. *Clin Rheumatol* 2007; 26(11):1843–1849.
50. Squires DD, Moyers TB. *Motivational Interviewing: a Guideline Developed for the Behavioral Health Recovery Management Project*. Albuquerque, NM: University of New Mexico, Center on Alcoholism, Substance Abuse and Addictions; 2001.

CHAPTER 88 ■ BASIC CONCEPTS IN BIOMECHANICS AND MUSCULOSKELETAL REHABILITATION

JAMES P. MCLEAN, GARY P. CHIMES, JOEL M. PRESS, MICHAEL L. HEARNDON, STUART E. WILLICK, AND STANLEY A. HERRING

INTRODUCTION

For the clinician treating patients with painful conditions, it is common practice to focus attention on the anatomic region of a patient's chief complaint (e.g., they present with right shoulder pain). Oftentimes, however, while they may complain of pain in a certain region, the underlying cause of the pain may lie elsewhere. For example, for many patients who present with shoulder pain related to rotator cuff tendonopathy, it would be unusual for the main cause of the rotator cuff to be because of some underlying pathology with the rotator cuff (although this certainly can occur with some conditions, such as a proximal myopathy). Rather, more commonly, the rotator cuff is the victim of suboptimal biomechanics elsewhere along the kinetic chain (whether that be at the scapula, thoracic spine, or hips), and therefore has been asked to perform in a manner for which it had never been designed.

The goal of this chapter is to provide an overview of the biomechanical approach to assessing and managing patients with musculoskeletal pain generators. The initial section will focus on the principles of biomechanical analysis, including assessment of range of motion, strength, and endurance. Further, we will explore more biomechanical function with a discussion of neuromuscular control, muscle balance, neural tension, and kinetic chain theory. We will also review the distinction between prehabilitation and posthabilitation, as well as detailing the nature of a patient-therapist relationship.

The second section will focus on the clinical application of these basic principles. These include therapeutic exercise, flexibility training, and strength training. We will also discuss manipulation, spinal traction, and the physical modalities. In the final section, we provide three clinical cases to demonstrate how the biomechanical assessment of peripheral musculoskeletal pain complaints can be used to better manage and treat our patients. It is our hope that these sections will help the pain physician to include a functional biomechanical assessment as part of their comprehensive pain management regimen.

By emphasizing biomechanical principles, the contents of this chapter represent a fundamental change from the customary emphasis on the use of physical therapy and physical modalities in treating musculoskeletal pain. Patients are often treated for musculoskeletal disorders with passive modalities such as hot packs, cold packs, massage, electrical stimulation, and deep heat. Unfortunately, these passive therapies are overused. While they certainly can play an important role in providing symptomatic relief of musculoskeletal pain, passive modalities should be used only as methods to facilitate *active* rehabilitation. The patient most needs to become actively involved in a therapeutic exercise program specifically designed to improve musculoskeletal functioning.

Musculoskeletal rehabilitation is a process whereby poor posture, muscle imbalances, and other biomechanical deficits are corrected using specific exercises to gain better static and dynamic control of the musculoskeletal system. The physical restoration process may involve passive therapeutic modalities to facilitate the exercise program. Clinicians treating musculoskeletal pain and dysfunction must identify and work to correct deficits in the patient's biomechanics.

This chapter introduces general concepts in clinical biomechanics that are crucial to the understanding of musculoskeletal rehabilitation. The first section, Basic Considerations, presents an overview of these biomechanical concepts. In the second section, Clinical Considerations, specific techniques used to treat musculoskeletal pain are reviewed. In keeping with the philosophy that lasting improvements in biomechanical functioning are due to exercise programs prescribed specifically for each patient's pain symptoms and biomechanical deficits, therapeutic exercise is emphasized; passive therapeutic modalities are given less attention. The concepts presented here can be applied to soft tissue injuries throughout the body. The diagnosis and treatment of specific injuries are covered in the final section of this chapter.

BASIC CONSIDERATIONS

This section introduces basic concepts in musculoskeletal rehabilitation. Using specific examples, we review the importance of optimizing range of motion, strength, endurance, and neuromuscular control. The role of muscle agonist/antagonist interactions and adverse neural tension (ANT) is included. There is a certain degree of overlap between the various biomechanical concepts that are presented. For example, although strength and endurance are related, they are presented separately because clinical pain syndromes related to deficits in strength differ from those related to deficits in endurance.

Range of Motion

Lack of adequate range of motion is probably the most common biomechanical deficit seen and one of the easiest to address. Deficits in range of motion can cause pain directly or may lead to pain elsewhere. An example of a range-of-motion deficit that causes pain directly occurs when electricians experience shoulder pain while doing overhead work because of limitations in glenohumeral forward flexion. An example of a range-of-motion deficit that leads to pain in a distant body segment occurs when electricians with limited glenohumeral forward flexion experience low back pain while performing overhead activities because they must increase their lumbar lordosis to compensate for the lack of shoulder elevation (Fig. 88.1). The compensatory increase in lumbar lordosis is an example of a maladaptive substitution pattern due to a biomechanical deficit (e.g., decreased latissimus dorsi length).

The musculoskeletal clinician must have adequate examination skills to identify all range-of-motion limitations, decide which of these contribute most significantly to patients' symptoms, and implement appropriate therapies to correct the deficits.

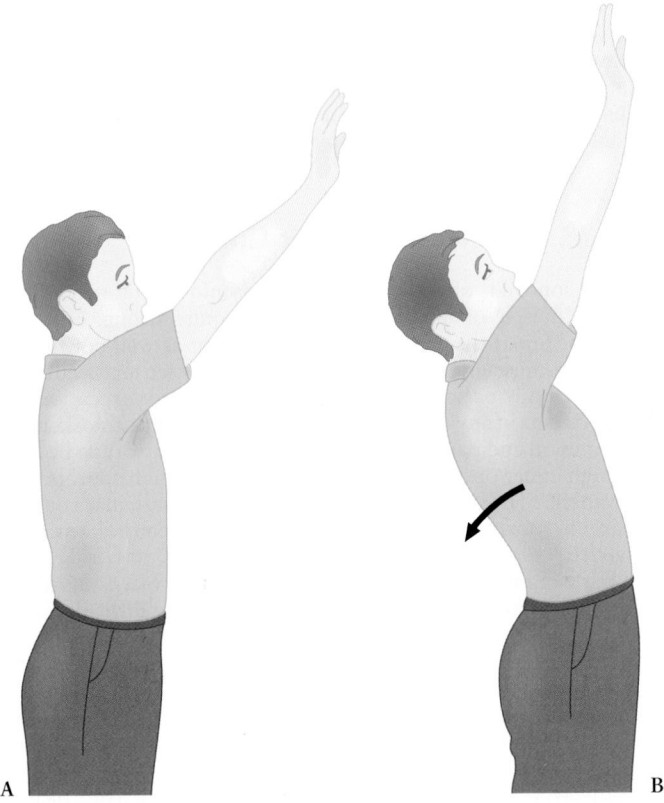

FIGURE 88.1 The individual with limited glenohumeral forward flexion (**A**) compensates with exaggerated lumbar lordosis during overhead activities (**B**). This maladaptive substitution pattern can lead to low back pain.

Range-of-motion restrictions can be due to shortening of muscle-tendon units, restrictions in joint capsule distensibility, ANT, or bone-on-bone contact at joint interfaces. The first three conditions are almost always amenable to specific stretching techniques. These are discussed later in this chapter under Clinical Considerations. Range-of-motion deficits due to bone-on-bone contact are not improved with therapeutic exercise or physical modalities.

Strength

Strength assessment is part of the comprehensive examination of the patient, whether it is through manual muscle testing (MMT), or a more formal dynamometric assessment. As a general rule, the patient should be examined in muscles surrounding the region that is painful. In addition, assess strength in the regions immediately proximal and distal to the painful region. For example, in a patient with elbow pain, the clinician should evaluate strength in the shoulder, elbow, and wrist.

Additionally, since many pain complaints may have an underlying spine etiology (e.g., a radiculopathy), it is often useful to examine the key myotomes in the affected region. Using the same example of elbow pain, the clinician would evaluate muscle strength of the C5-T1 myotomes bilaterally to assess for focal weakness. A useful set of muscles for assessing specific myotomes are those that are used as part of the comprehensive assessment for spinal cord injury, as per the American Spinal Injury Association guidelines, as these key muscles have been tested to assure their reliability in assessing specific myotomes (Table 88.1).

If the clinician finds that a patient has what appears to be weakness, the next delineation is whether the weakness is a "true" weakness or is pain-limited. While this is obviously challenging,

TABLE 88.1

AMERICAN SPINAL INJURY ASSOCIATION MYOTOMES

Mytome	Movement tested
C5	Elbow flexion
C6	Wrist extension
C7	Elbow extension
C8	Finger flexion (at the DIP joint)
T1	Fifth digit abduction
L2	Hip flexion
L3	Knee extension
L4	Ankle dorsiflexion
L5	Long toe (hallux) extension
S1	Ankle plantarflexion

there are a few clues that may help the clinician determine whether a patient is limiting their effort secondary to pain. First, the clinician is able to elicit a more vigorous effort if the patient knows that maximum effort will only be required for a moment. Second, it is unusual for patients to be able to exert a submaximal effort in a smooth manner; instead, they will often exert an initial effort and then stop further exertion (i.e., "give-way" weakness, or "catch-and-release"). If the patient has pain-limited weakness, this is of course clinically important, because it demarcates a painful range of forceful motion. However, it is important to distinguish pain-limited weakness from a true focal weakness, which may be a harbinger of a potentially serious neurologic cause.

Two primary factors contribute to relative strength deficits in ambulatory patients without major nerve or muscle injury. The first might be considered a relative disuse weakness. In relative disuse, the body part is not immobilized but is infrequently used in a manner that develops strength. Triceps weakness in sedentary office workers is a good example of this. Although these individuals may be "pushing papers" all day long, they may go for decades without ever performing elbow extensions against enough resistance to prevent gradual weakness from developing. On MMT, they will likely earn an elbow extension grade of 4/5 to 5/5. This relative weakness may never be symptomatic unless the workload required in that individual's triceps muscle suddenly increases. This would occur, for example, if the person decided to build a deck onto the back of the house and began hammering for long periods.

Similarly, many of us do not maintain full strength in our hip extensors (especially for extension past the neutral position) or the muscles that help elevate the upper limbs, especially those that upwardly rotate the scapula. These simply are not movements that we do against resistance very often during routine activities of daily living. Mild strength deficits due to relative inactivity are frequently asymptomatic. They become symptomatic if the individual has a rapid increase in activity or if age-related changes such as loss of motor units or decreasing activity level further weaken muscle groups that already have mild strength deficits. Mild or relative weakness of the hip extensors and abductors has particular relevance in the setting of low back pain due to the functioning of the hip extensors and abductors as lumbopelvic stabilizers. Mild weakness of the scapular rotators has particular relevance in the setting of shoulder pain, due to the role of these muscles in overhead activities.

The second primary factor that contributes to relative strength deficits in ambulatory patients without major nerve or muscle injury is a process sometimes referred to as muscle de-education.[1] This is a process in which the individual fails to activate, or abnormally activates, a given muscle because of pain, fatigue, maladaptive biomechanics, or psychologic reasons. Over time, the normal neuromuscular engram for the intended movement becomes harder to retrieve, and the neuromuscular control system has essentially "forgotten" the normal pattern of use for that muscle. Most often, muscle de-education involves the patient losing the ability to fire a muscle with the correct timing, or strongly enough, for the movement intended. The patient adopts a maladaptive neuromuscular firing pattern and substitutes other muscles to perform the task. Sometimes the muscle de-education process consists of the patient firing a muscle too strongly or losing the ability to relax the muscle appropriately.

An example of a patient substituting one muscle for another is the individual who preferentially fires hamstrings to perform hip extension, rather than using the strongest hip extensor, the gluteus maximus. If this maladaptive firing pattern continues over time, the gluteus maximus becomes de-educated and weak. This can result in poor pelvic control and secondary low back pain. The concept of muscle de-education emphasizes the close interaction between neural control mechanisms and musculoskeletal function in the development of musculoskeletal pain.

A classic example of a patient losing the ability to appropriately relax a muscle is the individual who presents with unilateral upper back and posterior neck pain. This is often due to the patient holding the scapula in an elevated position. The levator scapulae and upper trapezius are short and tight, and there are pain and tenderness in these muscles. This hiked-shoulder posture is assumed when people work hunched over a desk or when they are tense. Some individuals do not bring the scapula back down to its normal position, and over time they "forget" how to relax the scapular elevators, and forget where their scapula should be normally positioned.

The clinician treating musculoskeletal pain must identify all strength deficits, decide which ones are clinically relevant to the patient's symptoms, and implement an appropriate rehabilitation plan to correct those deficits and re-educate muscles that have lost their normal patterns of firing.

Endurance

Endurance refers to the capacity to continue to functionally exert oneself. While patients with pain complaints may occasionally be limited by cardiovascular endurance, the more common context for assessing endurance in a pain patient is muscular endurance.

As an individual bears weight during a functional activity, the forces of their activity (e.g., the ground reaction force while walking) have to be borne by the different structures throughout the kinetic chain. These include bone, joints, articular cartilage, ligaments, and muscles. Ideally, muscles bear a substantial amount of these reactive forces, which reduces the forces transmitted across other structures. However, with repetitive iterations, muscles may fatigue, and therefore, while muscles may be able to bear reactive forces initially, with each repetition, forces are then transmitted to other structures.

The phenomenon of muscle fatigue has important implications both diagnostically and therapeutically. Oftentimes, patients will complain of pain presentations that are initially mild, but worsen with increased activity. They may initially appear normal on physical examination. Therefore, it may be necessary during examination to exercise a patient to fatigue to simulate those circumstances when the patient is having pain. For example, if a patient complains of knee pain that worsens with walking long distances or climbing stairs, a component of the pain complaint may be poor muscular endurance in the quadriceps muscle. When testing knee extension by MMT, the strength may appear normal, since the patient's limitation is muscular endurance rather than peak torque production (which is what one tests with MMT). Therefore, the patient may be better assessed by performing repetitive single leg squats, which can fatigue the quadriceps

relatively quickly within the time frame of the examination, and allow the clinician to assess whether poor muscular endurance is contributing to the patient's pain complaint. Similarly, if the clinician assesses that poor muscular endurance is contributing to a patient's pain complaint, then improving muscular endurance should be a focus in the patient's physical therapy protocol.

Neuromuscular Control

Motor control is often overlooked in musculoskeletal rehabilitation. A muscle or muscle group may be quite strong, but if it does not fire at the appropriate time, it might as well not fire at all. Neuromuscular control is a combination of sensory feedback from the body part, premotor planning, and motor execution.[2,3] Impairments in any of these pathways can lead to musculoskeletal dysfunction and pain. Normal neuromuscular control can be lost through injury or disuse and can be regained through appropriate retraining.[4] For some movements, proper neuromuscular control is an easy task. For other movements, motor control requires practice.

For example, if you ask patients to fire their biceps muscles, they will be able to flex their elbows without any difficulty. But if you ask patients to fire their multifidus or lower trapezius muscles, they may not be able to do so even if you show them pictures of those muscles in an anatomy text and explain their actions.[5,6] Multifidus and lower trapezius are under voluntary control just like biceps, but our ability to consciously use them to gain fine control over segmental spine motion and scapular rotation, respectively, is far less than our ability to consciously activate biceps to precisely flex the elbow. Specialized exercises can improve one's ability to execute fine control of the neuromusculoskeletal system.

When trying to gain fine motor control, one needs to maximize control of individual muscles and smoothly integrate the actions of different muscle groups in succession during dynamic activities.[7-9] For example, when lifting an object, a person must first fire the foot and ankle muscles to stabilize the feet on the ground. Then one must fire the thigh muscles to stabilize the knee. Next, the hip girdle muscles must stabilize the pelvis before the spine extensors can elevate the torso. If the gluteus maximus fails to kick in before the erector spinae fires, the pelvis will remain anteriorly tilted and abnormal motion will occur in the lumbar spine.

Normal motor sequencing is a highly synchronized process that can easily break down. Several causes of deficits exist in neuromuscular control. One is a lesion in the motor pathways, either centrally or peripherally. This can be dramatic in obvious cases such as cerebellar lesions or cerebral palsy. Subtle nerve injury, however, can cause subtle loss of neuromuscular control. For example, mild irritation of the C5 nerve root can cause abnormal firing patterns of the shoulder girdle muscles and result in upper back and shoulder pain.[10] Mild irritation of the L5 nerve root can cause abnormal firing patterns of ankle and lumbopelvic stabilizers and lead to ankle or lumbopelvic instability and pain. For optimal success, a comprehensive rehabilitation program addresses biomechanical deficits in both the musculoskeletal and neuromuscular systems.

Another cause of impairment in neuromuscular control is loss of sensory feedback from a body part. This can be dramatic in obvious cases such as occur with a lesion of the sensory portion of the internal capsule or severe vitamin B_{12} deficiency. More subtle loss of sensory feedback can also alter normal neuromuscular firing patterns, however. A common example of this is the inversion ankle sprain. One can strengthen the foot and ankle indefinitely, but if proprioception retraining is not added to the rehabilitation plan, the patient may have persistent ankle pain due to poor fine motor control of the ankle stabilizers.[11,12] Proprioception and fine motor control training is crucial for many injuries involving the spine, knee, and shoulder, as well as the ankle.[2,13–18]

The clinician must recognize deficits in neuromuscular control that may be contributing to the patient's musculoskeletal pain and implement a rehabilitation plan that includes correction of those deficits.

Muscle Balance and Agonist/Antagonist Interactions

When a patient has a pain complaint in a specific peripheral structure (e.g., the shoulder), pain in that region can be a function of suboptimal biomechanics at that joint. One cause of suboptimal positioning is an imbalance between agonist and antagonist muscle groups.

One of the most common examples of agonist and antagonist muscle groups occurs about the shoulder. For various postulated reasons, the flexor/adductor/internal rotator muscles of the shoulder girdle are often more active than the corresponding extensor/abductor/external rotator muscles. When this is the case, the glenohumeral joint sits in a plane that is suboptimal for many functional activities, particularly overhead activities.[19,20]

There are several mechanisms for the relative imbalance of agonist and antagonist groups. First, some activities, such as sitting at a desk using a laptop computer, will emphasize positioning that activates one agonist group (in this case, a slumped posture that internally rotates, adducts, and flexes the shoulder girdle) and de-emphasizes the corresponding antagonist group. Second, muscle balance theory states that a strong, tight muscle group will reflexively inhibit the antagonist group.[1,21] The clinical implications of such agonist/antagonist interactions are important. If a patient is having trouble strengthening a muscle group during a physical therapy program, simultaneous stretching of the antagonist muscle group may be necessary to facilitate strengthening of the target muscle group. Similarly, if the patient is not progressing with correcting range-of-motion deficits in a particular muscle group, the rehabilitation plan may need to include strengthening of the antagonist muscle group.[22] This concept is best illustrated by the following common examples of muscle imbalance that are clinically associated with painful musculoskeletal dysfunction.

The first example is that of the patient with subacute or chronic posterior neck pain. This patient often presents with cervical hyperlordosis due to tightness of the long cervical extensors and weakness of the cervical flexors.[23] Both of these biomechanical deficits need to be addressed to restore proper cervicothoracic posture and movement. Similarly, one contributor to abnormal motion at the patellofemoral joint, with subsequent patellofemoral arthralgia, is muscle imbalance in the structures that control the patella. Typical biomechanical deficits in this case are tightness of the laterally situated iliotibial band (ITB) and weakness of the medial thigh muscles, including hip adductors and vastus medialis obliques.[24] In treatment, it is necessary to stretch the lateral patellar stabilizers and strengthen the medial patellar stabilizers to improve patellofemoral tracking.

Another common area of muscle imbalance is the shoulder girdle, where one frequently finds tightness of the strong anterior shoulder muscles, including pectoralis minor, pectoralis major, and latissimus dorsi, with associated inhibition and weakness of the posterior shoulder muscles, including middle and lower trapezius and rhomboids.[25] This forward-rounded shoulder posture (Fig. 88.2) can be a cause of interscapular pain, rotator cuff pain secondary to abnormal scapular movement (Fig. 88.3), and upper limb pain due to ANT in the brachial plexus.

Similar symptoms can be seen with imbalance between tight scapular elevators, principally levator scapulae and upper trapezius, and inhibited, weak scapular depressors, including lower trapezius and serratus anterior. This pattern of muscle imbalance causes the patient to have a shoulder-elevated posture and is also

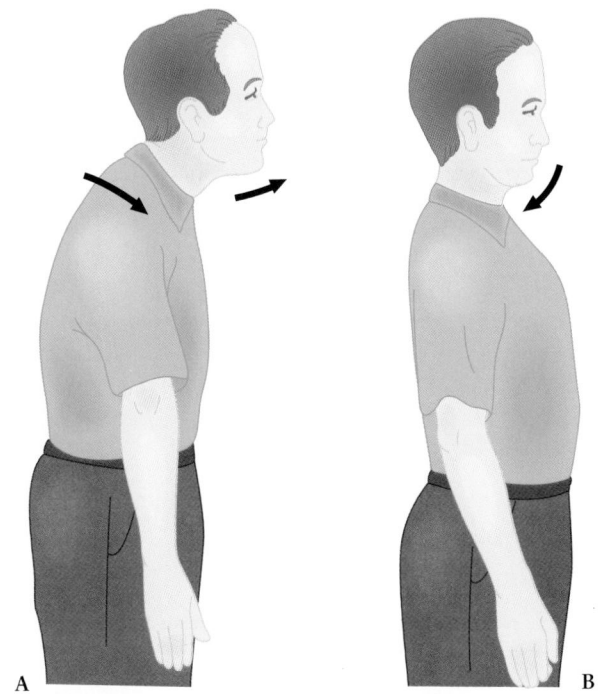

FIGURE 88.2 The forward-rounded shoulders posture offers a prime example of muscle imbalance that can lead to musculoskeletal dysfunction. The anterior shoulder muscles are tight and the neck and posterior shoulder muscles are put at mechanical disadvantage. **A.** Excessive cervicothoracic kyphosis necessitates a compensatory cervico-occipital extension to keep the eyes level. **B.** Posture rehabilitation includes stretching the anterior shoulder girdle, strengthening the scapular retractors, and chin tucks to improve cervicothoracic alignment.

often seen in patients presenting with posterior neck and shoulder pain. The rehabilitation plan should include stretching of the tight muscle groups with simultaneous strengthening of their antagonists to restore normal muscle balance.

A fourth common site of muscle imbalance is the hip girdle, where tight hip flexors are often seen clinically with inhibited, weak hip extensors.[1] Perhaps the most important clinical sequela of this type of muscle imbalance is not hip dysfunction per se. Instead, poor pelvic control by gluteus maximus results in an increase in anterior pelvic tilt, which leads to lumbar hyperlordosis and low back pain.[26] The rehabilitation of low back pain almost always includes restoration of neutral lumbar posture. In this case, that would necessitate restoring full range of motion of the hip flexors as well as full strength of the hip extensors.[27]

A few instances of agonist/antagonist interactions pose particularly troublesome problems for the neuromuscular control system. Consider again the relationship between the upper and lower trapezius. Working together, they couple forces to stabilize the scapula in a retracted and upwardly rotated position, a function crucial for all overhead activities. Yet, they also have antagonistic roles in that the upper trapezius is a scapular elevator while the lower trapezius is a scapular depressor. Such a complex relationship between two different parts of the same muscle, innervated by a single nerve, cannot always be accommodated by the neuromuscular control system and can result in scapulothoracic dyskinesis. In this case, the lower trapezius tends to become inhibited and weak.

An equally complex relationship exists between the tensor fascia lata and gluteus maximus, the two muscles that insert into and control the ITB. Working as agonists, the two muscles serve as hip abductors. Yet they are also antagonists in that the tensor fascia lata is a hip flexor and internal rotator, whereas the gluteus maximus is a hip extensor and external rotator. As in the above

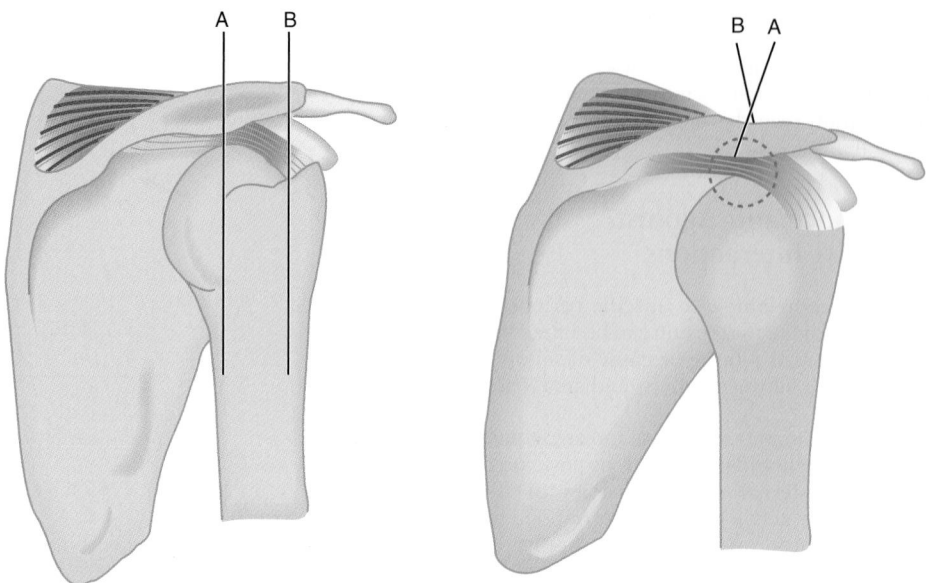

FIGURE 88.3 Line A represents a vertical line drawn through the angle of the acromion and Line B represents a line through the long axis of the humerus. The left figure represents the positioning of the humerus and scapula in anatomical position, whereas the right figure represents the same system with the scapula malpositioning from tightness/overdevelopment of the anterior muscles (pectoralis minor). As a result, the scapula is placed into a position of protraction and anterior rotation. In the right figure, the scapula (line A) is rotated, while the humerus (line B) due to effects of gravity, remains fixed in place, therefore resulting in an angle between the scapula and humerus. This angle creates a new dynamic for the supraspinatus tendon. The insertion of the supraspinatus tendon on the superior-anterior aspect of the greater tubercle of the humerus is now more closely approximated to inferior aspect of the acromion. The aberrant positioning of the scapula will predispose the supraspinatus tendon to impingement.

example, this can tax the resources of the neuromuscular control mechanisms that dictate appropriate firing patterns. In this example, the tensor fascia lata usually dominates, with the gluteus maximus becoming inhibited. If fine control of the ITB is lost, hip pain (trochanteric bursopathy) or knee pain (ITB insertionopathy) can result.

Other examples exist where muscles serve paradoxic functions. The tibialis anterior and tibialis posterior (TP) muscles work together to invert the foot and support the arch of the foot. Yet they are also antagonists in that the latter is an ankle plantar flexor, whereas the former is a dorsiflexor. At times, during normal walking gait, running gait, and going up or down stairs, both muscles must be active for dynamic arch support, but we need one or the other to stop firing because we need the action of its antagonist. Abnormal firing patterns of TP can lead to TP tendinopathy. Inhibition of either the tibialis anterior or TP can lead to arch collapse, plantar fasciitis, or foot pain.

Similarly, the extensor carpi radialis brevis (ECRB) and longus cooperate with the extensor carpi ulnaris to extend the wrist. But the ECRB is left in a quandary during wrist extension movements that require radial deviation, such as hitting a backhand in tennis, or repeatedly loading luggage onto a conveyer belt. At these moments, ECRB must fire to produce wrist extension and radial deviation. But the extensor carpi ulnaris, an ulnar deviator of the wrist, abandons its partner in wrist extension to allow radial deviation of the wrist to occur. This neuromuscular predicament impedes the ability of the wrist extensors to adequately concentrically generate or eccentrically absorb forces, and leads to ECRB overload (called lateral epicondylopathy or tennis elbow).

In each of the above examples of contradictory agonist/antagonist interactions, there exists a common, associated overuse injury such as rotator cuff tendinopathy due to scapulothoracic dyskinesis, ITB friction syndrome, posterior tibial tendinopathy, or forearm extensor tendinopathy.

The clinician must recognize muscle imbalances that contrib-

ute to the patient's musculoskeletal pain and implement a rehabilitation plan that restores proper balance by treating both the agonist and antagonist muscle groups involved. Neuromuscular control must be optimized through specific muscle education and training.

Neural Tension

Neural structures in the central nervous system (CNS) and peripheral nervous system (PNS) move when body parts move. Like muscles, tendons, and joint capsules, the connective tissue associated with the nervous system can lose its normal elasticity and range of motion. If symptomatic, this condition is called ANT. Alternative names include adverse neurodynamic tension or, sometimes, dural tension. ANT can be defined as abnormal physiologic or mechanical responses of the nervous system as its tissues are taken through a range of motion.[28]

ANT is most commonly recognized as the condition that produces a positive straight-leg raise test. It is also commonly recognized as the entity that produces a positive Kernig's sign in a patient with meningitis. Less commonly recognized, however, is that ANT can exist in areas other than the lumbosacral roots that contribute to the sciatic nerve. Even in the absence of meningitis, it can exist in the spinal cord and the surrounding connective tissue, the cervical roots, brachial plexus, and peripheral nerves. ANT can cause range of motion restriction, pain with movement, paresthesias in the distribution of the nerves affected, and diminished neuromuscular control.

Normal and abnormal movement of neural structures during movement of the musculoskeletal system has been partly characterized. The posterior part of the human spinal canal increases between 5 and 9 cm in length as the spine goes from full extension to full flexion.[29–31] Thus, trunk and neck movement is associated with gliding movements of the spinal cord within the canal. The dura is connected to the bony and ligamentous structures of the spinal canal via the ligaments of Hoffman.[32] Abnormal adhesions between the dura and surrounding structures may form, however, and have been implicated in enhancing pain consequent to disc herniations.[33] Upper and lower limb movements also have mechanical consequences for the spinal cord and its roots.[34] The median nerve elongates 20% as the upper limb moves from elbow and wrist flexion to full elbow and wrist extension.[35] Further stretching of the nerve fibers in the brachial plexus is obtained by adding ipsilateral shoulder depression and contralateral cervical flexion.[36]

The nervous system is linked to the musculoskeletal system in several ways. First, neural movement is mechanically coupled with musculoskeletal movement. Second, the nervous system is physiologically connected to the musculoskeletal system at the neuromuscular junction. Third, the nervous system itself can be considered to be in part a connective tissue. Myelin possesses elastic features that allow the myelin sheath to change conformation as nerves stretch, with opening of the clefts of Schmidt-Lantermann.[37-40] The endoneurium, perineurium, and epineurium surrounding peripheral nerves all contain collagen,[41] the common substrate of all connective tissue.

The connective tissues within peripheral nerves allow for the necessary gliding of adjacent fascicles against each other during limb movements, especially when the limb goes through its full range of motion. Also built into the neurodynamic system is an allowance for a considerable amount of motion between the peripheral nerve and the surrounding tissues in which it lies.[35,42] Tunturi[43] demonstrated the presence of elastin in the dura mater of dogs, suggesting that dura possesses the capability of distensibility.

Certain regions of the body exist in which the connective tissue of the nervous system is more abundant. For example, the fibular nerve (also called the peroneal nerve) has 17% more connective tissue associated with it as it passes around the fibular head than as it courses through the popliteal fossa.[44] The amount of connective tissue in peripheral nerves ranges from 21% to 81%, with greater amounts present when the nerve passes a joint.[45] The connective tissue elements associated with the CNS and PNS protect neural tissue from injury during gliding movements and compressive events.

The spinal nerve roots lie at the junction of the CNS and PNS and are at particular risk for mechanical stress and ANT for three reasons. The first is that the connective tissue covering the roots is at a transition between the CNS and PNS and is not as well developed as its more proximal or distal counterparts.[46] Second, the spinal nerve roots are more tightly adherent to the walls of the intervertebral foramen than in other places.[47,48] Third, stenosis of the intervertebral foramen, which can cause abnormal neural gliding, is a common occurrence.

Often, a close association exists between ANT and muscle tightness. A prime example of this is patients with lumbosacral nerve root tension who also have marked hamstring tightness. Both the nerve root and the muscle must be mobilized if normal biomechanics in the region are to be restored.[49,50] ANT and muscle tightness often coexist and can easily be mistaken for one another. Careful physical examination is required to distinguish between the two.

Several special physical examination maneuvers that test for ANT in the spine and limbs are described later in the chapter. The clinician treating pain syndromes must be able to identify when ANT is contributing to the patient's symptoms and then implement an appropriate neural mobilization program.

Kinetic Chain Theory

Kinetic chain theory states that biomechanical deficits in one region can be responsible for symptoms in a distant body part. A corollary to kinetic chain theory is the concept of force distribution. A biomechanical system functions optimally when all its parts are able to absorb and generate forces appropriately. Loss of optimal function in one region of the kinetic chain may predispose to overload in another region. The following two examples illustrate this idea. First, if a volleyball player is generating inadequate hip extension or ankle plantarflexion moments during jumping, the athlete's quadriceps can become overloaded and patellar tendinopathy may result as the quadriceps is forced to compensate for the deficiencies of its kinetic chain partners. Second, if a golfer lacks adequate hip rotation, there will be a compensatory increase in lumbar axial rotation during the driving swing that may result in low back pain. Thus, the clinician must assess function in parts along the kinetic chain both proximal and distal to the painful area.

Kibler and colleagues[51-53] have eloquently synthesized a grand unifying theory of kinetic chain functioning. They describe how for any injury, there are five separate elements that make up the musculoskeletal injury complex that may be identified as contributing to the production or continuation of symptoms (Fig. 88.4). These elements include (1) the tissue injury complex—the actual area of anatomic disruption; (2) the clinical symptom complex—the group of symptoms the patient experiences, such as pain, stiffness, and impaired performance; (3) the functional biomechanical deficit—the set of muscle inflexibilities, weakness,

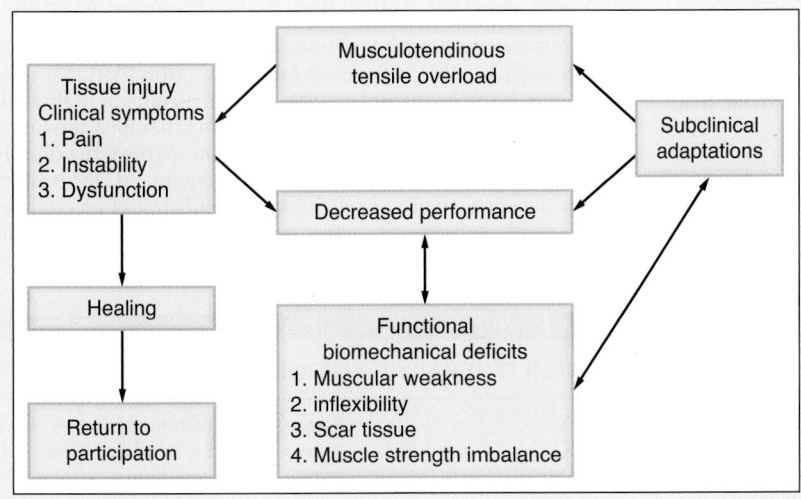

FIGURE 88.4 The vicious cycle: Tissue injury can lead to maladaptive biomechanical alterations, which in turn can lead to further tissue injury.

and imbalance that cause inefficient mechanics; (4) the functional adaptation complex—the set of functional substitutions that the patient uses in an attempt to reduce pain and maintain performance; and (5) the tissue overload complex—the group of muscles and other soft tissue structures that are subject to overload injury secondary to the initial injury or maladaptive biomechanics, thus causing or prolonging symptoms. These five elements are often interactive and additive, setting up a vicious cycle of continuing musculoskeletal problems.

Prehabilitation and Posthabilitation

The focus of the management of a patient with an acute pain complaint is typically targeted on resolving their current symptoms. However, given that pain complaints are often caused by suboptimal biomechanics, it is important for the clinician to rehabilitate beyond the resolution of the symptoms. This is termed posthabilitation. If the suboptimal biomechanics that led to the pain presentation are still present, then it is likely that the patient may have another exacerbation of the same pain complaint in the future. Indeed, for many common peripheral musculoskeletal pain complaints (e.g., ankle sprains), the best predictor of a future pain episode is a prior episode of the same condition.[11,54–57]

While it is certainly valuable to address a patient's pain complaints at the time of injury through rehabilitation and to prevent recurrences afterward via posthabilitation, the ideal scenario would be to prevent injuries from occurring. Prehabilitation is a focus on preventing injuries before they occur, primarily focusing on optimizing biomechanics to prevent those injuries associated with identifiable biomechanical deficits.

For example, Frank Noyes and his colleagues[58,59] have developed the Sportsmetric program as a systematic training program designed to reduce the incidence of ACL tears in female athletes. This is based on the biomechanical studies of Mary Lloyd Ireland and others who have demonstrated a clear causality between suboptimal biomechanics and increased incidence of ACL tears in female athletes.[60–66] It is important to remember that the absence of symptoms does not imply absence of pathology in the musculoskeletal system. The pain accompanying overuse injuries presents well after there are pathologic changes in the tissues and disappears before those tissues have fully healed. Therefore, the rehabilitation process must be comprehensive and continue after pain resolution. The goal of posthabilitation is prevention of injury recurrence.

Identifying Predisposing Factors

The astute musculoskeletal clinician searches for the reasons the patient developed an injury. In the case of acute trauma, the cause is obvious. In the case of soft tissue overload injuries, however, the clinician will need to look further. If the underlying precipitants of tissue overload are not addressed, the patient is at risk for recurrence.

Patient-Therapist Relationship

The relationship that the patient and therapist develop from their first session together and throughout treatment is crucial to the outcome of the rehabilitation process. The therapist must gain the trust of the patient and develop an exercise program that fits his or her musculoskeletal, cognitive, and psychologic needs. Some patients require more information or more reassurance. Other self-motivated patients may simply need to be shown how to do their home exercise program correctly and require less attention from the therapist.

Regardless of the specific needs of the patient, the therapist and physician must empower the patient to become an active participant in the rehabilitation process. This is done by educating the patient about his or her particular musculoskeletal pathomechanics and ensuring that the patient is involved in a home exercise program designed to make lasting biomechanical improvements. It is the additional responsibility of the therapist to help motivate the patient to be conscientious about performing the exercises (see Chapter 87). Should the patient-therapist relationship hinder the rehabilitation process at any time, consideration should be given to having the therapist adopt different strategies for that particular patient or to changing therapists.

CLINICAL CONSIDERATIONS

Therapeutic Exercise

The musculoskeletal rehabilitation clinician uses therapeutic exercise like the cardiologist prescribes antihypertensive medication or the surgeon uses a scalpel. The goal of therapeutic exercise is to correct biomechanical deficits that are contributing to the patient's injury and restore and maintain normal structure-function relationships in the musculoskeletal system. Although it is appropriate for the exercise program to be overseen by a physician and therapist, patients should do the majority of exercises independently, either at home or in a gym setting. The importance of promoting patient independence in a home exercise program, with regular reevaluation and advancement of the rehabilitation program, is critical in our changing health care environment. The principal components of therapeutic exercise are flexibility, strength, and neuromuscular control training.

Flexibility Training

An individual's flexibility results from a combination of genetic factors (primarily collagen type) as well as musculoskeletal usage patterns. Injury and lack of use predispose to contracture of soft tissues. Potential benefits of flexibility training include increased range of motion, decreased risk of musculotendinous injuries, decreased soreness, and improved musculoskeletal performance.[54,55] Several methods exist to improve flexibility. They include static stretching, ballistic stretching, contract-relax stretching, neural stretching, and manual mobilization. Each of these techniques is reviewed. Which technique to choose depends on the tissue to be stretched and the preferences of the physician, therapist, and patient.

Passive, Assisted Active, and Active Range of Motion

The terms passive range of motion (PROM), active assisted range of motion (AAROM), and active range of motion (AROM) refer to different levels of therapist and patient involvement in flexibility exercises (Table 88.2). PROM entails the therapist moving a joint through its range of motion with the patient maximally relaxed. The patient does not actively participate. PROM is often used in the early stages of rehabilitation and should be complemented with subsequent active participation by the patient.

TABLE 88.2

PHYSICAL THERAPY CATEGORIES

PROM	Passive range of motion
AAROM	Active assisted range of motion
AROM	Active range of motion

PROM is also used when the patient is unable to actively participate, for example, when trying to improve range of motion in a plegic limb. In AAROM, the patient actively moves the joint through its available range of motion as much as he or she is able, and then the therapist assists with overpressure at the end range of motion to make further gains in flexibility. AAROM is used when the patient is able to move the body part being targeted but not well enough at the end range of motion to improve flexibility. The goal of a progressive flexibility program is to enable the patient to perform the exercises independently. When possible, therefore, the patient should be advanced to AROM exercises without hands-on assistance from the therapist.

In static stretching, the length of the muscle-tendon unit is slowly increased until the patient feels a mild to moderate pulling sensation in the belly of the muscle being targeted. Sometimes the pulling sensation is felt at the musculotendinous junction or at the tendon-bone junction if there is overuse soreness or other pathology in these areas. If the patient feels pain or a severe pulling sensation, then the muscle-tendon unit is being over-stretched and is at risk for injury. Severe discomfort during stretching is a signal that either the muscle should be relaxed by a few centimeters or a different stretch should be tried. During the course of a sustained static muscle stretch, the inverse myotatic stretch reflex is initiated, resulting in relaxation of the muscle.[67,68] It is important to take advantage of this phenomenon by extending the stretch by a few degrees or centimeters every 10 seconds. Thus, "static" stretching is not truly static when appropriately performed. This slow, controlled method of stretching is generally considered the safest way to improve flexibility of muscle-tendon units.

Some debate exists over the optimum amount of time that a muscle should be placed on stretch to effect lasting elongation of the tissue. Most clinicians advocate that a stretch should be held for a minimum of 30 seconds[69]; others prefer 120 seconds.[70] Also, no clear guidelines exist on the frequency with which a muscle should be stretched to effect lasting elongation of the tissue. Generally, two or more stretches per day, each held for at least 30 seconds, are required to improve range of motion. Some prescriptions might call for stretching a muscle every 2 to 3 hours.

Ballistic Stretching

Ballistic stretching is a higher-level technique used to increase the length of the muscle-tendon unit. In ballistic stretching, the muscle is positioned near the end of its range of motion and then repetitively brought just past the point where it provides natural resistance. These repetitive "bouncing" motions can be low or high amplitude and low or high velocity. Repetitive low-velocity movements up to and just past the muscle's end range of motion are called on-off stretching. The primary advantage of ballistic stretching is that, when performed correctly, rapid and significant gains in flexibility can be achieved.[71] The primary disadvantage is that it often requires the assistance of a qualified therapist or trainer. Another disadvantage is that the risk of over-stretching is greater than with static stretching. A session of ballistic stretching should be followed by static stretching of the target muscles.

Contract-Relax Technique

Contract-relax stretching is also considered a higher level stretching technique. Like ballistic stretching, the contract-relax technique has the potential to provide rapid gains in flexibility and it also often requires the intervention of a qualified therapist or trainer. This technique takes advantage of a period of muscle relaxation that follows muscle contraction. The patient firmly contracts the target muscle isometrically against resistance for approximately 5 seconds. Immediately following the contraction, the muscle is stretched. This contract-relax cycle can be repeated several times. Contract-relax stretching is sometimes referred to by the less descriptive term proprioceptive neuromuscular facilitation and is a form of the so-called muscle-energy stretching techniques.

Neural Tension Assessment and Mobilization

Restricted motion of neural elements can coexist and be interrelated with other soft tissue biomechanical deficits. Several reasons exist for this interrelationship. First, motion restrictions in the musculoskeletal system can cause secondary motion restrictions in the anatomically-related neural elements. One example of this includes tight, hypertrophied scalene muscles that restrict normal gliding of the brachial plexus as they pass out of the neck. Second, soft tissue edema or hematoma from acute trauma or chronic overuse can cause irritation of a nerve passing through the injured area. For example, sciatic ANT has been associated with repetitive hamstring strain.[49,72] Third, primary nerve irritation, for example, from a discogenic inflammatory process, can cause abnormal neuromuscular control that leads to secondary biomechanical deficits in the muscles served by that nerve root. Thus, ANT is rarely seen in isolation and should not be treated in isolation from other biomechanical deficits.

Before adding neural mobilization to the rehabilitation program, the clinician must determine whether ANT is present and, if so, whether it is relevant to the patient's symptom complex. Several physical examination maneuvers can be performed that assess for ANT in the lower and upper limbs.

The best technique for assessing ANT in the lower limbs is the slump test (Fig. 88.5). The starting position for this test has the patient seated with hands placed behind the buttocks, palms up on the examination table. The patient then places the chin on his or her chest and slumps the torso forward. This motion draws the spinal cord cephalad.[73] The examiner then sequentially extends the knee and dorsiflexes the ankle. These steps pull the lumbosacral nerve roots caudad.[74,75] At each stage, the examiner asks the patient what he or she feels. If the maneuver reproduces the patient's usual leg pain, and having the patient extend the neck relieves symptoms, the test is considered positive for ANT. It is crucial that the geometric relationship between the thighs, pelvis, and thoracolumbar spine remains constant so as to avoid tensing and relaxing myofascial structures and thus better isolate movement in the neuraxis. A crossed slump test occurs when extending the asymptomatic leg reproduces pain in the patient's symptomatic leg. This is analogous to a crossed straight-leg test.

The slump test is preferred over the better known straight-leg raise test for several reasons. First, the slump test is more sensitive because it adds cephalad gliding of the spinal cord, while the straight-leg raise maneuver only offers caudad gliding of the nerve roots. Second, the slump test adds specificity because neck flexion and extension help distinguish motion restrictions in neural tissue from other soft tissue inflexibilities. Using the standard straight-leg raise test, it is often difficult to distinguish between ANT and hamstring or gastrocnemius tightness. Both the straight-leg raise and the slump test can be modified to preferentially test tension in the peroneal/L5 nerve fibers versus the tibial/S1 fibers by inversion and plantarflexion of the foot.[74]

The brachial plexus tension test is the upper limb homologue to the slump test. First, the cervical roots are pulled distally by sequential shoulder depression, shoulder abduction, and external rotation, forearm supination, and elbow, wrist, and finger extension. The examiner asks the patient what he or she feels at each stage. Reproduction of pain or paresthesias in the limb is considered a positive test. If the neck is side bent to the contralateral side, thus drawing the cervical cord away from the limb being tested, symptoms should be exacerbated. If the neck is side bent toward the ipsilateral side, symptoms should be alleviated (Fig. 88.6). Side-to-side comparisons should be done. The brachial plexus tension test was first described by Elvey[76] and has been subject to cadaveric and clinical verification.[77]

Brachial plexus tension testing maneuvers with median, ulnar,

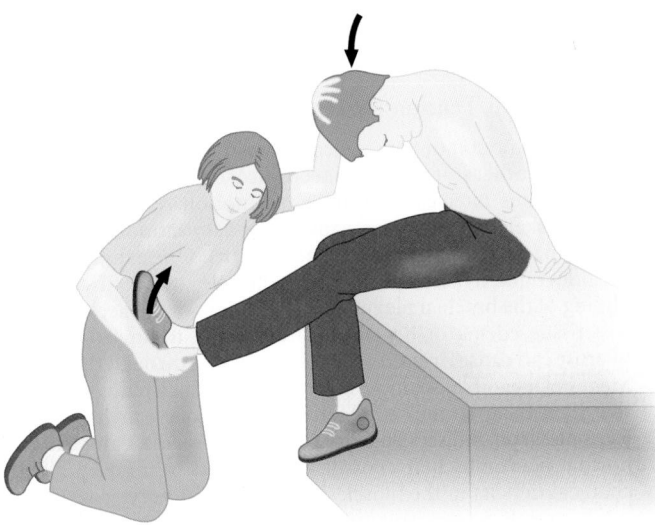

FIGURE 88.5 The slump test for adverse neural tension. Full spine flexion causes cephalad gliding of the spinal cord. Sequential knee extension and ankle dorsiflexion cause caudad gliding of the lumbosacral nerve roots. The examiner checks for reproduction of symptoms, side-to-side differences, and alleviation of symptoms with cervical extension.

and radial nerve bias have been described.[28] Because it can be difficult to differentiate between tightness in neural elements versus inflexibilities of myofascial structures along the kinetic chain, some clinicians refer to these physical examination maneuvers by the more generic term upper limb tension tests rather than brachial plexus tension tests. If the maneuvers reproduce neurologic symptoms, then the clinician can feel more confident that ANT is present.

The results of the neural tension maneuvers guide the initial neural mobilization maneuvers. The therapist instructs the patient to place the limb in the position where neural tension is first noted. Then the patient is instructed to slowly relax the limb a few degrees to a more comfortable position and then stretch a few degrees back toward the position of symptom reproduction. By gently repeating this maneuver with ever larger amplitudes, the connective tissues associated with the nerve gradually regain normal gliding motion.

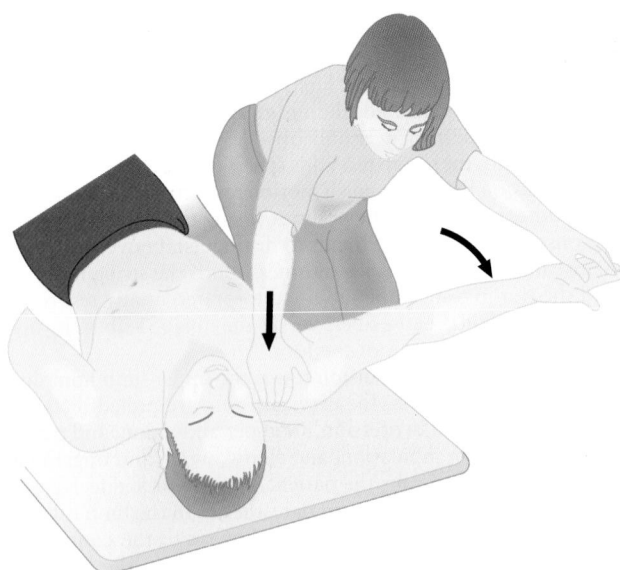

FIGURE 88.6 The brachial plexus tension test: The examiner sequentially performs shoulder depression and abduction, forearm supination, wrist and finger extension, and elbow extension. After each movement, the patient is asked about symptom production. Contralateral cervical lateral flexion should increase limb symptoms, and ipsilateral cervical lateral flexion should alleviate limb symptoms.

Manual Joint Mobilization

Joint mobilization is a technique applied by a therapist to a spinal or peripheral joint in which an oscillatory movement is performed to restore full range of motion in the joint. Manual joint mobilizations differ fundamentally from the previous types of range-of-motion techniques discussed. Mobilizations are aimed at improving accessory movements rather than voluntary movements. Voluntary movements are movements that individuals can perform themselves, such as glenohumeral joint flexion, interphalangeal joint flexion, and lumbar flexion. In contrast, accessory movements are joint movements that individuals have no ability to perform and only occur passively. Examples of accessory joint movements include anterior-posterior gliding of the glenohumeral joint, interphalangeal joints, and individual vertebral segments. Accessory movements can be gliding, rolling, spinning, or compression/distraction motions of the joint. Joint mobilization maneuvers target range-of-motion restrictions in the joint and joint capsule itself, rather than the muscles that span the joint. Joint mobilizations can be diagnostic as well as therapeutic: They can help distinguish capsular versus muscular patterns of tightness.

Joint mobilizations are classified into four categories of increasing aggressiveness. Grade I mobilizations are small-amplitude movements performed in the middle of a joint's normal range of movement. Grade II mobilizations are large-amplitude movements performed within the free range of the joint but not moving into any resistance or stiffness. Grade I and II mobilizations can prevent further loss of joint range of motion but do not increase range of motion. They almost always precede grade III and IV maneuvers during a therapy session. Grade III joint mobilizations are large-amplitude movements performed up to the limit of the available joint range of motion. Grade IV mobilizations are small-amplitude movements performed at and just beyond the limit of the joint's range of motion. Manual joint mobilizations should only be performed by a therapist or clinician with advanced training in these techniques. Experienced manual therapists can mobilize virtually any joint in the body.

Common Stretching Errors

Probably the most common cause of ineffective stretching is not holding the stretch long enough or not performing it frequently enough. Improper technique is another common cause of ineffective stretching. Often, individuals will fail to make gains in flexibility because the stretches target the single joint muscles in a muscle group, rather than the more important biarthrodial muscles. A

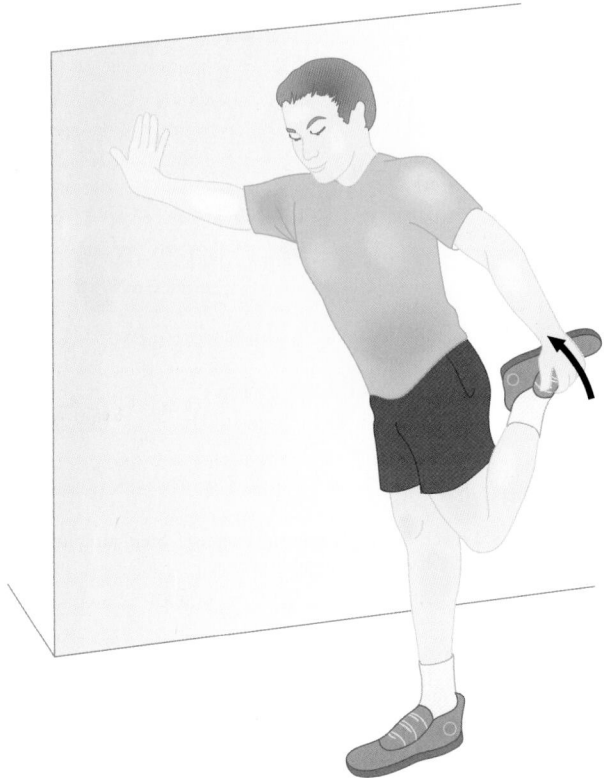

FIGURE 88.7 A common error in quadriceps stretching is failure of the patient to stabilize the pelvis. The position shown here provides pelvic stabilization and greater stretch to all four of the quadriceps muscles.

prime example of this is the classic standing quadriceps stretch, which might address the vastus lateralis, vastus intermedius, and vastus medialis but neglects the rectus femoris, which crosses the hip joint as well as the knee joint (Fig. 88.7). Sometimes a stretching position inadvertently stretches tissues other than the target tissue. Finally, the flexibility program must address all the relevant structures contributing to the inflexibility. Joint capsule mobilization maneuvers alone will not be successful if the muscles crossing that joint are also tight. Similarly, muscle stretching alone will not be successful if an underlying motion restriction exists in neural structures. Carefully documenting an exercise history will help determine whether the exercises are being performed correctly.

Strength Training

Strength deficits often contribute to musculoskeletal pain. Strength deficits can cause pain in one of two main ways. First, a muscle can be a primary pain generator if it lacks adequate strength or endurance to perform a given task and therefore fatigues. Second, a muscle group lacking sufficient strength to properly control a joint may cause abnormal, painful motion in that joint. Many ways exist to improve muscle strength.

Exercise Prescription

A strength training prescription should include the patient's diagnosis, the muscles to be worked, the modality of strength training, the frequency, the number of repetitions per set and number of sets per workout, the intensity of the exercise, and precautions. Exercise prescriptions should be flexible. The clinician must reevaluate the patient at appropriate intervals and modify the program as necessary.

Specificity of Training Effects

Training effects tend to be very specific to the type of exercise performed. For example, strengthening the biceps in isolation does not increase triceps strength. Training for quick, explosive power does not improve endurance, and vice versa. Training muscle groups to generate force does not necessarily increase their ability to absorb force. Strength training for the lower limb does not improve balance unless it is done in a manner that challenges balance. Therefore, the goals of the rehabilitation program must be clear, and the prescription must be written to fulfill those goals.

Neural Versus Muscular Mechanisms of Strength Gains

Physiologically, strength gains come about through neural and muscular mechanisms. It is well established that neural mechanisms play a significant role in strength gains during training. As early as 1967, researchers showed that rats on a training program improved muscle strength without a concomitant increase in muscle bulk.[78] The ability of muscle to undergo strength gains without hypertrophy has been confirmed in humans.[79,80] The mechanism of strength gains without muscle hypertrophy has been shown to be improved synchronization of motor unit firing. Neural mechanisms are more important than muscular mechanisms in the early stages of training, before muscle hypertrophy has had a chance to occur.[79-82] Later in the course of a training program, muscular mechanisms predominate. The quantitative electrodiagnostic techniques used to investigate changes in neural synchronization during strength training have been shown to be reliable and sensitive[83-85] and continue to be used to investigate training effects on the neuromuscular system.[86-88]

Static Versus Dynamic Strength Training

Static Strength Training. Strength training can be broadly classified into static or dynamic exercises. Static strength training is more commonly referred to as isometric exercise. In isometric exercise, a muscle or group of muscles works against a resistance without any change in muscle length or joint angle. Isometric exercise is the strength training method of choice in the earliest stages of rehabilitating injured muscle, tendon, ligament, or joints. Isometric exercise offers the primary advantage of avoiding movement in painful or frail structures, while allowing strength gains to occur. Isometric exercise is used in patients with osteoarthritis, if putting joints through a range of motion may be painful or impossible. Isometric exercise is also used in the initial stages of the rehabilitation of strains and sprains and advanced tendinosis, when movement of the injured structure puts it at risk for further injury.

Isometric exercise of any given muscle or muscle group should be varied in several ways. First, the joint angle should be varied. For example, in the earliest stages of rehabilitation for forearm extensor tendinopathy, the patient should be given a light hand weight to hold for a set amount of time with the wrist in a neutral position. Then the patient should statically hold the weight with the wrist in varying degrees of flexion and extension. The exercise should be gradually advanced by adding weight and by increasing the length of time of each repetition. The position should be held until mild to moderate fatigue develops in the target muscles.

Isometric exercises can be performed to either isolate a single muscle or work several segments of the kinetic chain simultaneously. In the rehabilitation of forearm extensor tendinopathy, for example, the wrist extensor strengthening can be done with the entire upper limb supported except for the hand. Alternatively, the upper limb can be unsupported to simultaneously work the shoulder girdle. The latter method offers the advantage of working proximal parts of the kinetic chain, where relative weakness may have predisposed to distal overload. At appropriate times during the rehabilitation course, the patient's program should be advanced to short arc and then longer arc dynamic strengthening exercises.

Dynamic Strength Training. Dynamic exercises have various classifications. One can speak of concentric versus eccentric exercise, isokinetic versus isotonic exercise, closed kinetic chain versus open kinetic chain exercise, and plyometric exercise.

Concentric and eccentric exercise. Concentric muscular contraction refers to an action in which the muscle shortens to move a body segment. An example of concentric movement is shortening of the quadriceps muscle as one extends the knee while ascending stairs. An eccentric muscle contraction is one in which the muscle lengthens while resisting a force. An example of an eccentric movement is controlled lengthening of the quadriceps muscle as the knee flexes while descending stairs. The muscle has to lengthen to accommodate the normal mechanics of descent and also has to fire to prevent the knee from buckling. Eccentric exercise works muscles harder and is more likely to cause muscle overload than concentric exercise.[89-93]

Frequently, strength training regimens include both concentric and eccentric exercise. When rehabilitating a particular injury, however, one should emphasize the movement that overloaded the structure in the first place. For example, if a furniture mover suddenly overloaded his elbow flexors by trying to stop a falling couch with his forearm, the initial strength retraining program should progress from gentle isometric exercises to slow, gentle eccentric elbow flexor exercises. In normal human movements, one often finds an eccentric contraction preceding a concentric contraction in the same muscle. This sequence of eccentric and concentric contractions forms a natural pattern called the stretch-shortening cycle.[94]

Isokinetic and isotonic exercise. In isokinetic exercise, the target muscle moves a joint through a range of motion at fixed angular velocity, but the torque generated by the movement may vary. This is accomplished with the use of specialized equipment that can be programmed to provide resistance to joint movement at any predetermined fixed rate, usually measured in degrees per second. Although isokinetic exercise is useful for quantifying strength for research purposes, or quantifying a patient's progress during the course of rehabilitation, it is a type of movement that is rarely performed during real-life activities.[95] The applicability of isokinetic movements performed in the laboratory is further limited because of the dissociation between joint angular velocities and muscle shortening.[96,97] Therefore, rehabilitation protocols should emphasize more functionally relevant exercises.

Isotonic muscle contraction refers to a muscle contracting through a range of motion while maintaining either a constant tension within the muscle or a constant torque applied against a resistance. Like isokinetic movements, isotonic movement is rarely reproduced during daily activities and is therefore more of an academic concept than a practical one.

Closed and open kinetic chain exercise. Closed kinetic chain exercise refers to work done with the distal end of the limb fixed in space. Open kinetic chain exercise refers to work done with the distal end of the limb free in space. When a person does push-ups, for example, the hands are fixed on the floor, and the upper limbs function in a closed kinetic chain situation. When someone throws a baseball, however, the hand moves through space and the upper limb functions in an open chain fashion.

Advantages and disadvantages exist to both open and closed kinetic chain exercise. In general, if the movement to be trained is an open chain movement, such as lifting boxes, then the clinician should prescribe open kinetic chain exercises. Closed kinetic chain work is preferred when the patient needs to strengthen muscles that are primarily used in closed kinetic chain situations, for example, when strengthening knee and hip extensors in a

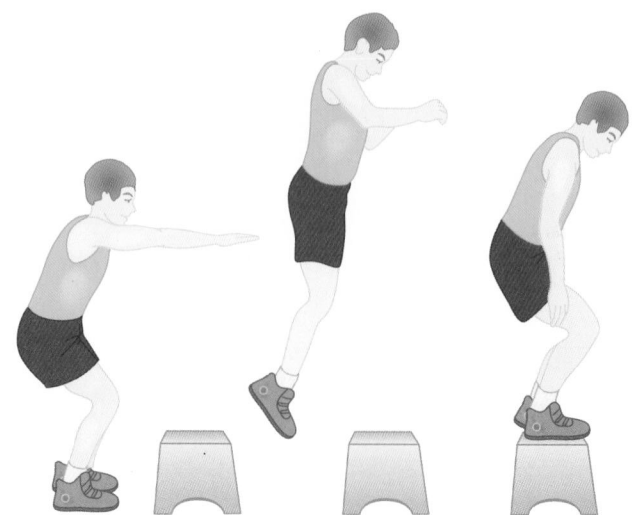

FIGURE 88.8 Lower body plyometric exercise: Step jumping builds strength, endurance, balance, and agility.

post-polio patient who is having difficulty arising from a chair. Closed kinetic chain work offers several additional advantages over open kinetic chain exercise. Closed kinetic chain exercise promotes cocontraction of multiple muscles that cross a joint, thus providing greater joint stability. It also tends to work more segments of the kinetic chain, thus providing a more complete workout while also promoting improved sequencing of movements. Finally, closed kinetic chain work generally demands greater proprioceptive feedback than open kinetic chain exercise, thus improving this important sensory modality.

Combination strengthening exercises. A current trend exists to simultaneously work multiple muscle groups throughout the kinetic chain, rather than strengthen individual muscles in isolation. Two primary advantages exist to exercising multiple body parts at once. First, it is more time efficient. Second, most normal activities involve activating multiple muscle groups simultaneously or in sequence. Therefore, combination exercises are considered more functional than exercises that isolate individual muscles. An advanced form of combination exercise is plyometric exercise.

Plyometric exercise is a higher level dynamic form of exercise that can combine strength, endurance, power, balance, and agility training. Plyometric maneuvers simultaneously bring multiple muscle groups through a rapid stretch-shorten cycle. A simple example of lower body plyometric training is step jumping (Fig. 88.8). In this exercise, the hip extensors, knee extensors, and ankle plantar flexors rapidly fire concentrically. On landing, they fire eccentrically while lengthening. An example of upper body plyometric exercise could be throwing a basketball at a target while balancing on one leg. To avoid injury, an individual must attain an adequate baseline level of strength and flexibility before starting a plyometric training program.

Manipulation

Manual manipulation of the musculoskeletal system dates back at least to the times of Hippocrates and Galen.[98,99] After a long period of obscurity, manipulation reemerged at the end of the last century with the founding of osteopathy in 1874[100] and chiropractic medicine in 1895.[99] Manipulation enjoys widespread popularity today, with an estimated 12 million Americans undergoing 90 to 120 million manipulations per year.[101-103] Joint manipulation differs from joint mobilization in that manipulation employs low-amplitude high-velocity thrusts, while mobilization employs higher-amplitude, low-velocity movements. Theoretically, if a manual therapist or chiropractor can improve a patient's joint alignment through manipulation, then biomechanics will also be improved.[104–106]

Despite its popularity, the exact mechanism of action whereby manipulation alleviates pain remains unclear. Manipulation of the musculoskeletal system is postulated to have several beneficial effects. First, it is believed to help restore joint symmetry, particularly in reference to the spine.[107–109] Second, it may aid in mechanical restoration of muscular and fascial range and ease of motion.[110,111] Third, manipulative techniques have been theorized to induce sensory afference, which may diminish pain through a gate theory effect.[111–113] Fourth, some authors have postulated that manipulation increases endorphin release.[104,109,111] These theories have not been subjected to rigorous scientific testing, however. Many believe that manipulation benefits patients primarily through a placebo effect.[114]

In the past, many practitioners of manipulation have extended the benefits of this modality to areas beyond the musculoskeletal system, such as the endocrine, immune, and digestive systems.[99] Such leaps in logic have led those in conventional medicine to question the practice of manipulation. Fortunately, a greater percentage of practitioners of manipulation now rely on this technique to restore structure-function relationships only in the musculoskeletal system.

Clearly, no current consensus exists on the mechanism whereby manipulation improves musculoskeletal function. Furthermore, there is no consensus on whether manipulation is beneficial at all, due to a lack of well-designed randomized controlled studies. One meta-analysis,[115] two reviews,[116,117] and two controlled clinical trials[118,119] indicate that manipulation decreases spine pain in selected populations, at least for short periods (e.g., less than 1 month). A review of randomized controlled trials found limited evidence that manipulation is better than placebo but not superior to other conservative measures for acute low back pain.[120] The same review found strong evidence that manipulation is better than placebo and moderate evidence that it is better than analgesics, rest, and massage for chronic low back pain.[120] Further study is needed to determine whether and how manipulation is effective.

Contraindications to high-velocity thrust manipulation include progressive neurologic impairment, unstable vertebral segments, severe osteoporosis, rheumatoid arthritis, bone or spinal cord tumors, spondyloarthropathy, bleeding diathesis, and poor manipulative skills. Risks are greater with cervical spine manipulations and include injury to nerve root, spinal cord, vertebral artery, and other soft tissue and osseous structures.[102,121]

Spinal Traction

Like manipulation, spinal traction techniques date back to ancient times[122] and are widely used today but are not universally accepted in conventional medicine circles. Also like manipulation, the literature on spinal traction is fraught with inconsistencies and methodologic flaws.[120] Reviews of randomized clinical trials have failed to find proof of efficacy for spinal traction,[120,123–126] particularly for lumbar traction. However, numerous reports of positive results of traction exist,[127–133] primarily in uncontrolled and/or nonrandomized clinical trials.

Proponents argue that if correctly performed, spinal traction can aid by widening the intervertebral foramina, decreasing intradisc pressure, allowing migration of herniated disc material back into place, decreasing facet joint friction, stretching paraspinal musculature, and straightening spinal curves, both in the lumbar[134–136] and cervical[137–139] regions. Three studies, two using epidurography[130,140] and one using computed tomography[133] to visualize disc herniations, have demonstrated reduction in disc prolapse following traction. Long-term maintenance of the reduction has not been demonstrated, however. In fact, disc material has been observed to return to its prolapsed state following traction therapy.[140] It has been speculated, but not proven, that traction improves nutrition of the disc by decreasing intradisc pressure and facilitating imbibition.[141] Traction has been advocated in the treatment of facet arthralgia and muscle spasm.[142] Some argue that the primary benefit of traction is from immobilization rather than the traction itself.[143]

Many ways exist to apply traction to the axial skeleton. Devices can be accommodated for use in a regular bed or hospital bed. There are also specially constructed, mechanical, single piece, and split traction tables.[110] Motorized and hydraulic traction tables are also available.[143] A therapist can manually apply traction,[100,107,144] although duration and force are more difficult to control when compared to mechanical or motorized traction. Some degree of traction can be obtained simply with positioning—for example, right side-lying on several pillows to provide left axial distraction. Autotraction is a technique that relies on patients' pulling their torsos cephalad with their arms, while the pelvis is fixed. Autotraction can be inexpensive and provides built-in protection against overdistraction because the patient controls the force applied. The patient's upper limb strength may be inadequate to generate the force necessary for distraction, however, and the time frame is limited by the patient's endurance.[145,146] Furthermore, autotraction puts the patient at risk for shoulder injury. Some prefer gravity traction, in which the patient is suspended from a crossbar either in a fully inverted position or in an upright position. Both orientations provide distraction forces of approximately 50% body weight through the axial skeleton.[147]

Traction devices can apply longitudinal, rotational, and side-bending forces. In addition to specifying the type of traction device used, traction prescriptions differ in terms of frequency of application, time per session, and force applied. No standardization of these parameters exists and prescriptions vary widely among practitioners.

Contraindications to traction are similar to those for high-velocity manipulation and include fracture, spine instability, osteoporosis, tumor, infection, pregnancy, hiatal hernia, and claustrophobia.[148]

Physical Modalities

Physical modalities such as heat, cold, and electrical stimulation can be useful adjuncts to the physical restoration program. The primary goals of physical modalities are to decrease pain and inflammation to facilitate the exercise program. They should rarely, if ever, be used in isolation without an appropriate exercise program.

Heat

General Physiologic Effects of Heating Modalities. Many different heating modalities are available to raise the temperature in superficial and deep tissues. The physiologic effects of tissue heating can be broadly classified into hemodynamic, neuromuscular, joint and connective tissue, and analgesic effects.

The hemodynamic effects of tissue heating are related to increased blood flow. Forearm blood flow increases two- to three-fold following application of heat.[149] Vasodilation is postulated to speed healing of nonacute soft tissue injuries by increasing local metabolism and ingress of nutrients, leukocytes, and antibodies and increasing egress of breakdown products.[150,151] Heat also increases nerve conduction velocities in most peripheral nerves.[149,152] The clinical significance of this effect in musculoskeletal rehabilitation is unclear. A more relevant neuromuscular effect of tissue heating is the inhibition of group II muscle spindle fibers.[153] Inhibition of spindle fibers can relax muscle and facilitate stretching.

Tissue heating facilitates stretching of muscle-tendon units by direct effects on connective tissue as well as by indirect effects via the muscle spindles. Lehmann and colleagues[154] showed that tendon distensibility increases with increasing temperature. They further showed that heat combined with stretching produced greater gains in tendon distensibility than heat or stretching alone. Heating superficial joints such as metacarpophalangeal joints can decrease stiffness in these structures and facilitate a stretching program.[155]

Although heat is often used for its analgesic effect, the mechanism whereby heat reduces pain has not been clarified. Possible mechanisms include general relaxation effect, endorphin release, vasodilation causing washout of pain mediators, and vasodilation leading to a decrease in ischemic pain.[156-158]

General Precautions for the Use of Heat. Heat use should be avoided in patients who are unable to provide feedback about their tissue temperature. This includes insensate patients and those whose cognitive condition impairs their ability to accurately warn the therapist of adverse effects—principally burns. Heat should also be avoided in patients with arterial insufficiency. The vasodilation produced can cause metabolic activity to exceed the ability of the arterial system to deliver oxygen to the area, resulting in tissue ischemia.[150,159] Vasodilation can also result in increased bleeding in patients with a bleeding diathesis. Heat is contraindicated in acute musculoskeletal injury because it can increase acute hemorrhage and edema. Theoretical objections have been raised against the use of heat near tumors due to the fear of increased rate of tumor growth or hematogenous spread.[158]

Superficial Heat. Heat may be transferred to body tissues by means of conduction, convection, or conversion. The first two are forms of superficial heat, while the last is used to heat deeper tissues. Superficial heat modalities are most useful for facilitating range of motion exercises in the hands and feet, where the target tendons and joints are superficial and not well protected by an insulating subcutaneous fat layer.

Hydrocollator packs, which transfer heat by conduction, are a commonly used modality to heat superficial tissues. They are made of silicon dioxide enclosed in canvas. These packs are heated to 65° C to 90° C and are applied to the skin over insulating towels for 20 to 30 minutes.[160] Hydrocollator packs have been shown to raise tissue temperatures up to 3° C at a depth of 1 cm below the skin.[161] The ability of hydrocollator packs to significantly elevate the temperature of tissue deeper than 1 cm is questionable.[161,162] Hot water packs, electrical heating pads, and chemical packs heat by convection. Hydrocollator packs have the advantage of offering greater temperature control than most of the convection modalities. Whirlpool and Hubbard tanks, however, provide superficial heat by convection and offer very good temperature control. Heated water tanks should not exceed 40° C.

Perhaps the most common misapplication of superficial heating modalities occurs when it is used in an attempt to heat deep structures. Studies have shown that the modalities listed in this section do not raise the temperature in tissues deeper than the subcutaneous fat, which serves as an excellent insulator against heat.[161,162]

Deep Heat.
Ultrasound. Ultrasound is the safest and most commonly used of the deep heating modalities. Ultrasound employs sound waves above the frequency threshold of human hearing to heat deep tissues. The ultrasound frequencies used range from 0.8 to 1.0 MHz. Although ultrasound produces some nonthermal effects on biological tissues, such as streaming, microstreaming, cavitation,

and standing waves, the effects of the nonthermal effects are not thought to be clinically significant.[163-166] It is the thermal effects that are important.

The literature on the clinical benefits of ultrasound remains mixed. One group found no difference between exercise plus ultrasound and exercise plus sham ultrasound in a randomized, double-blind study in patients with lateral epicondylalgia, although both groups showed improvement over time.[167] Similarly, ultrasound plus exercise showed no benefit over exercise alone in a randomized, double-blind, placebo-controlled study on patients with painful knee osteoarthritis.[157] A review of the ultrasound literature concluded that most positive studies lacked adequate controls and that additional research was required to determine efficacy.[157]

Shortwave and microwave diathermy. Ultrasound has largely replaced shortwave and microwave diathermy as the deep heating modality of choice. They are included here largely for historical reasons only.

Shortwave diathermy employs radio waves to heat deep tissues. The Federal Communications Commission has restricted medical use to specific frequencies and most shortwave diathermy machines in the United States operate at 27.12 MHz.[160] Temperature elevations of 4° C to 6° C can be attained in muscle.[168] Thermal effects tend to be greatest in water-poor tissues, however, and subcutaneous fat may be heated up to 15° C.[169] Shortwave diathermy has been used to heat connective tissue in nearly every part of the body, including pelvic floor structures via transvaginal and transrectal application.[170] Pulsed shortwave diathermy has produced statistically significant pain relief in patients with rotator cuff tendinopathy,[171] neck pain,[172] and other soft tissue injuries.[173]

In addition to the general precautions of heat mentioned above, shortwave diathermy is also contraindicated in the setting of implants such as pacemakers, stimulators, surgical implants, contact lenses, and metallic intrauterine devices. Such devices can cause excessive heating to occur in the tissues immediately surrounding the implant. Additionally, shortwave diathermy can cause excessive bleeding if applied to the menstruating uterus. The safety of shortwave diathermy has not been established in those with immature skeletons and therefore is not recommended in the pediatric population.

Microwave diathermy differs from shortwave diathermy in that it employs electromagnetic radiation of much greater frequency. The Federal Communications Commission has approved microwave frequencies between 915 and 2456 MHz for medical use. Lower frequencies penetrate to deep tissues better than higher frequencies.[174,175] At 915 MHz, subcutaneous fat temperature may be increased 10° C to 15° C, with deep muscle temperature elevations of 3° C to 4° C at 2 to 4 cm below the skin.[176]

The contraindications for other forms of deep heat application hold for microwave diathermy as well (see Fig. 88.1). Microwaves can produce cataracts, so both patients and therapists should wear protective goggles.[177] Although human fetuses have been exposed to microwave diathermy without deleterious effects, the overall safety in fetuses and children has not been established and its use is therefore discouraged in pregnant women and young children. Because tissues with a high water content are selectively heated, application of microwave over fluid-filled cavities, cysts, or blisters can produce unacceptable local heating.[178] The use of microwave diathermy has, however, been used to speed resolution of hematomas.[179] Most clinicians feel that the presence of an acute inflammatory condition such as inflammatory arthritis is a contraindication to microwave diathermy.[180] There are some reports, however, of improved patient comfort after application of microwave to rheumatoid joints.[181,182]

Cryotherapy

Cryotherapy has several benefits in the treatment of musculoskeletal pain. Its ability to slow nerve conduction[149,183-185] and produce local analgesia[186] is well known. It has also been shown to improve tendon distensibility[154] and modify muscle stretch reflexes.[187-191] In combination, these effects can greatly facilitate a stretching program aimed at restoring full range of motion. Chilling a body part initially stimulates local reflexes to enhance sympathetic tone and produce vasoconstriction.[192,193] Vasoconstriction reduces blood flow, slows local metabolism, and lessens swelling.[194]

Technique. Ice packs, iced compression wraps, iced whirlpools, frozen steaks, and frozen bags of peas all work equally well in cooling body parts. The preferences of the therapist and patient usually determine the specific method of cryotherapy. Iced compression wraps offer a few advantages. Compression wraps help reduce swelling and can also add proprioceptive feedback for the individual who is exercising while icing (cryokinetics) or stretching while icing (cryostretching). Commercial products are available that are specifically designed for different body parts and that allow the individual to apply ice and compression simultaneously. These usually allow people to participate in other activities such as working or doing household chores because they do not have to fumble with a clumsy plastic bag of ice cubes. The recommended duration of cryotherapy is 20 to 30 minutes. This can be repeated up to once per hour. Longer periods of application increase the risk of local tissue damage and reactive hyperemia.[195]

Precautions. The most common adverse reaction of cryotherapy is local tissue damage from overzealous icing. Skin burns, frostbite, and nerve injury can occur.[196] Delayed tissue healing may occur if cryotherapy is used for extended periods because of reduction in blood flow and slowing of local metabolism.[197] Cryotherapy should be used judiciously or not at all in the extremities of patients with Raynaud's disease, cold urticaria, cryoglobulinemia, and atherosclerotic disease, because of the risk of inducing limb ischemia. As is true with heat therapy, cryotherapy is contraindicated in insensate patients who are unable to provide feedback on the status of the treated area. Properly applied ice treatments of less than 30 minutes in healthy individuals will not cause injury.[186,191]

Functional Electrical Stimulation and Surface Electromyography

Transcutaneous electrical stimulation for the treatment of pain is discussed in Chapter 91. In the rehabilitation of muscle dysfunction, functional neuromuscular electrical stimulation (NMES) and surface electromyography (SEMG) are sometimes used to aid the muscle reeducation process. Muscles can become de-educated or lose their normal firing patterns for several reasons, including partial denervation, disuse from prolonged immobilization or bed rest, and maladaptive substitution patterns. Specialized muscle reeducation techniques are often useful after tendon transfers as well, when the muscle is being asked to fire in a new pattern.[198] Electrical stimulation of muscle can help maintain muscle bulk during a period of disuse. It can also assist in the early stages of a muscle reeducation process, by giving the muscle a "jump start."[199-201] Once the patient feels the muscle firing with electrical stimulation, it is easier to start voluntarily firing the muscle. Feedback from the muscle can be transmitted to the patient using SEMG recordings. The patient can see the EMG signal recorded from the muscle undergoing reeducation and try to improve the firing pattern to make those tracings match a set of normal tracings.

The use of functional NMES/SEMG to help patients self-regulate the activity of motor units started in the 1960s.[202-204] It has been used fairly extensively in the functional rehabilitation of stroke patients.[205-208] In the nonstroke population, it has been used to reeducate muscles around the shoulder,[209,210] forearm

and hand,[211-213] lumbar spine,[214,215] and knee.[216-221] As the benefits of functional NMES/SEMG become more widely appreciated, there will be greater elucidation of normal and abnormal firing patterns of muscle groups during dynamic activities. Functional NMES is contraindicated in patients with pacemakers, local infection or malignancy, recent fracture or serious muscle/tendon disruption, local skin lesions, seizure disorder, and pregnancy.[198]

Miscellaneous Physical Modalities

Numerous other physical modalities have been used through the millennia in the treatment of musculoskeletal pain ranging from aromatherapy to snake venom to healing touch. The majority of these alternative modalities are not discussed here due to a lack of scientific literature about their efficacy. Two less mainstream modalities that are becoming popular, vibration and low-energy laser therapy, warrant brief mention, however.

Vibration. A wide variety of vibration therapy products are commercially available. Physical therapists prefer models that operate with frequencies around 150 Hz and amplitudes around 1.5 mm.[222-224] In uncontrolled studies, vibration therapy has been reported to be 70% successful in the treatment of sinusitis and musculoskeletal pain.[225-227] These effects were not reversed by naloxone, suggesting that the mechanism of action did not involve stimulation of the natural opiate system.[228]

French investigators have also reported success with vibratory stimulation in the treatment of chronic pain.[229,230] In a prospective controlled study, Guieu and colleagues[230] found vibration to be more effective than sham treatment for short-term relief of chronic pain. Another arm of the same study found the combination of transcutaneous electrical nerve stimulation plus vibration to have additive effects for short-term relief of chronic pain.[230] In a series of experiments, the same group of investigators has explored possible roles of vibratory stimulation in modulating the Met-enkephalin and substance P pathways via activation of large afferent nerve fibers.[231-235] The definitive mechanism of action whereby vibration therapy reduces pain remains under investigation.

Low-Energy Laser. While low-energy laser treatments are available outside the United States for treating pain from osteoarthritis, back pain, headache, and neuritis, they are not yet approved for clinical use in this country. Energy levels used are usually in the range of 1 to 100 mW.[236,237] Pain relief has been reported to be as high as 60% to 80% of subjects, although other investigators have found no benefit.[237]

One double-blind controlled trial of low-energy laser versus sham treatment found it to be associated with decreased pain and improved grip strength in patients with lateral epicondylitis 4 weeks after treatment.[238] Other randomized, placebo-controlled studies failed to find benefit from low-energy laser treatments in this condition[239,240] and in ankle sprains.[241] A randomized, double-blind study evaluated the effect of low-energy laser versus sham treatment on chronic low back pain. Both treatment groups were also placed on an exercise program. Both groups had a decrease in pain, but there was no difference between those who received laser treatments and those who received sham treatments.[242]

The mechanism of action of low-energy laser remains unproven. Proponents of this modality report that it accelerates wound healing by stimulating DNA synthesis and collagen production and improves the function of damaged neurologic tissue.[236] Further research is needed to definitively assess its efficacy and indications.

CASE STUDY

We examined a 26-year-old runner with left anterior knee pain. She complained that she had developed the pain over the past several months as she had been increasing her mileage and intensity in anticipation for a 10k road race. The pain tends to worsen as she progresses in her runs, bothers her when climbing up and especially down stairs, and is also bothersome when she sits for prolonged periods, such as when she drives or sits in a lecture hall or movie theater.

Her history is classic for patellofemoral syndrome, the most common cause of anterior knee pain in young, female runners. In working through her assessment, we used a kinetic chain evaluation to assess her biomechanics and help her develop a treatment plan. The starting point of the kinetic chain evaluation was to determine whether the location of her pain (in this case, the knee) was the culprit of her pain, or merely a victim of suboptimal biomechanics. Given that most young females do not have primary problems related to the patellofemoral articulation, most cases of patellofemoral syndrome are related to asking the patellofemoral articulation to do more than it is anatomically designed to do. The most common kinetic chain deficits are asking a relatively small structure to absorb forces that are better absorbed by a larger, more powerful structure, or asking an anatomic structure to range beyond its normal arc of motion to compensate for lack of range of motion at another joint. Therefore, our investigation focused on determining which structures above or below her knee were inadequately absorbing forces or were limited in their range of motion.

Upon further history, she noted that she did all of her training along the left side of a local crowned road (so as to be running against traffic). Because she is running on a sloped surface, this predisposes her to muscle imbalances about the hip, both in terms of the forces exerted and the amount of ranging at each joint. Interestingly, she did note that she had fewer symptoms when running on flat surfaces.

On physical examination, she also exhibited relative muscle imbalances. When examining her performing squatting maneuvers and single-leg squatting maneuvers, she initially performed without any lapses in form. However, after sufficient repetitions to fatigue the muscles, she started to have alterations in her biomechanics. What was most noticeable was that when she was viewed from the front, her knee appeared to track medially.

This is a common phenomenon in patellofemoral syndrome, namely that the femur was medially rotating and adducting her thigh relative to her patella. If one were to look at the patellofemoral articulation in isolation, it may appear that the patella was tracking laterally relative to the femur. This is sometimes compared to a train falling off a track. However, the motion of the patella relative to the femur is an illusion largely created by focusing only on the site of pain (the patella), and not focusing on the larger biomechanical system. The patella itself remains relatively fixed, but because the femur is displacing medially (from internal rotation and adduction at the hip), a better analogy would be the track slipping out beneath the train (Fig. 88.9).

One explanation for the malpositioning of the femur is relative disuse of the gluteus maximus, which is an external rotator, abductor, and extender of the femur at the hip joint. Therefore, if one performs a closed kinetic chain activity such as a single leg-squat or running (which is a series of successive and coordinated single leg squats), relative disuse of the gluteus maximus will result in the opposite motion of the thigh, namely internal rotation, adduction, and flexion. This is indeed what we saw with our patient (Fig. 88.10).

Armed with this insight, we were able to develop a treatment plan aimed at correcting her biomechanical deficit, particularly focusing on activation of her gluteus maximus during closed kinetic chain activities. These exercises included lunges and squatting activities. One exercise that we have found particularly helpful in helping cue the patient to activate her gluteus maximus is the "belt squat." We placed a belt just above the knee of the patient while she performed squatting maneuvers. The belt serves as a reminder to maintain the thigh in a position of abduction and external rotation throughout the range of motion. If the thigh were to slip into internal rotation or adduction, the tension in the belt would ease, and may even drop to the floor. In addition to the physical therapy program, we worked on her running hygiene, particularly focusing on having her run on flat surfaces to minimize her developing muscle imbalances about her pelvic girdle.

This case highlights several key points that were addressed elsewhere in this chapter. First, when a physician interacts with a patient who has a pain complaint, one has to consider whether the site of pain is the culprit or merely the victim of suboptimal biomechanics at another region within the kinetic chain. Second, if there is a kinetic chain deficit, one should look for a body part being asked to compensate for force absorption or range of motion that is inadequately addressed at another body part. Finally, once the kinetic chain deficit is identified, a targeted physical therapy program should be designed to compensate for

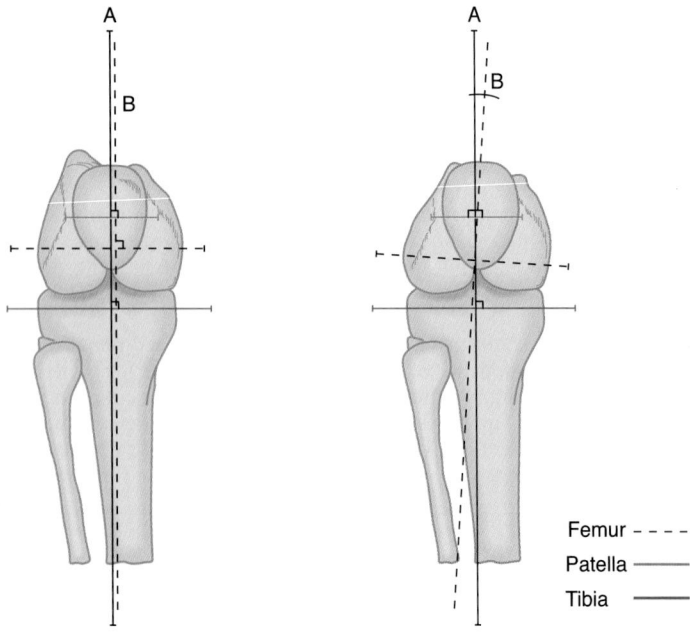

Femur - - - -
Patella ——————
Tibia ——————

FIGURE 88.9 Line A is a line connecting the midpoint of the patella and the tibial tuberosity. Because of the strong attachment of the patella to the tibia via the patellar ligament, this line remains relatively fixed in place in both open kinetic chain and closed kinetic chain biomechanics. Line B represents long axis through the patellar groove of the femur. In open kinetic chain biomechanics, because the distal limb segment is not fixed, any motion of the femur (line B), will be matched by a corresponding motion in the patella and tibia, and therefore Lines A and B will remain parallel, as seen in the left panel. In closed kinetic chain biomechanics, the distal limb segment is fixed, and therefore the tibia and patella (line A) are not free to rotate with the femur (line B). Therefore, any motion of the femur will not necessarily be reflected in the position of the tibia and patella, and therefore an angle will develop between lines A and B. More specifically, when the femur internally rotates or adducts (as is seen when the gluteus maximus is not sufficiently activated), the patellar groove of the femur tracks medially relative to the patella and tibia, and it will appear that the patella is tracking laterally relative to the femur.

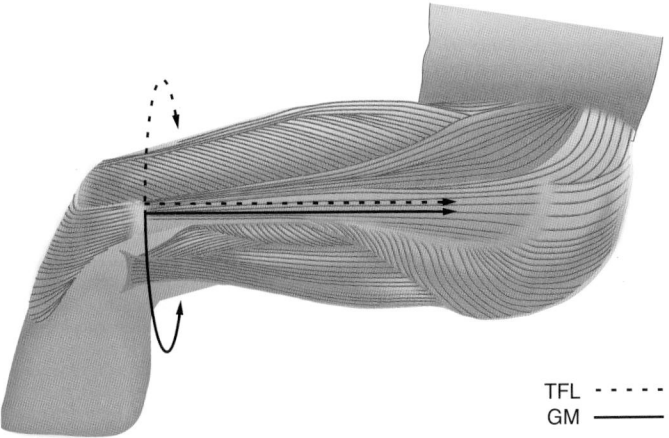

TFL - - - - -
GM ————

FIGURE 88.10 The ITB and the muscles attaching to it proximally, namely the tensor fascia lata anteriorly and gluteus maximus posteriorly. The tensor fascia lata acts on the femur to induce internal rotation (dotted arc), whereas the gluteus maximus induces external rotation (solid arc). When both muscles act together, the rotational forces cancel out, and their combined moment applies traction to ITB, resulting in pure hip abduction (solid and broken lines).

the kinetic chain deficit, which will allow the patient to resume their prior activities without re-exacerbating their initial pain complaint.

CONCLUSION

The goal of physical rehabilitation is to maximize the functioning of the patient's neuromusculoskeletal system. Therapies are directed at correcting pertinent biomechanical deficits by restoring full, pain-free range of motion, adequate strength and endurance for the patient's desired activity levels, and proper neuromuscular control. The mainstay of treatment is therapeutic exercise. Most exercises can be done by the patient in a home exercise program after careful instruction by a therapist. Manual techniques by a specially trained therapist can be very helpful, especially in the early stages of the rehabilitation program. The patient's progress should be reevaluated at appropriate intervals, and his or her therapeutic exercise programs should be upgraded as needed. Therapeutic modalities such as ice and ultrasound can be helpful to facilitate the exercise program. The majority of the work in most successful programs is done by the patient, not the therapist.

References

1. Janda V. Muscle weakness and inhibition (psuedoparesis). In: Grieve GP, ed. *Back Pain Syndrome in Modern Manual Therapy of the Vertebral Column.* New York: Churchill Livingstone; 1986:197–201.
2. Rutherford OM, Jones DA. The role of learning and coordination in strength training. *Eur J Appl Physiol Occup Physiol* 1986;55(1):100–105.
3. Schaible HG, Grubb BD. Afferent and spinal mechanisms of joint pain. *Pain* 1993;55(1):5–54.
4. O'Sullivan P, Twomey L, Allison G. Dysfunction of the neuromuscular system in the presence of low back pain—implications for physical therapy management. *J Manual Manipulative Ther* 1997;5:20–26.
5. Cooper RG, Stokes MJ, Sweet C, et al. Increased central drive during fatiguing contractions of the paraspinal muscles in patients with chronic low back pain. *Spine* 1993;18(5):610–616.
6. Hides JA, Stokes MJ, Saide M, et al. Evidence of lumbar multifidus muscle wasting ipsilateral to symptoms in patients with acute/subacute low back pain. *Spine* 1994;19(2):165–172.
7. Nygren Pierce M, Lee WA. Muscle firing order during active prone hip extension. *J Orthop Sports Phys Ther* 1990;12(1):2–9.
8. Janda V. Muscles, central motor regulation and back problems. In: Korr I, ed. *The Neurologic Mechanisms of Manipulative Therapy.* New York: Plenum Press; 1977:27–41.
9. Jull V, Janda V. Muscles, and motor control in low back pain: assessment and management. In: Twomey L, Taylor J, eds. *Physical Therapy for the Low Back (Clinics in Physical Therapy).* New York: Churchill Livingstone; 1987: 253–278.
10. Davidson RI, Dunn EJ, Metzmaker JN. The shoulder abduction test in the diagnosis of radicular pain in cervical extradural compressive monoradiculopathies. *Spine* 1981;6(5):441–446.
11. Tropp H, Askling C, Gillquist J. Prevention of ankle sprains. *Am J Sports Med* 1985;13(4):259–262.
12. Tropp H, Ekstrand J, Gillquist J. Stabilometry in functional instability of the ankle and its value in predicting injury. *Med Sci Sports Exerc* 1984;16(1): 64–66.
13. Wyke B. Articular neurology—a review. *Physiotherapy* 1972;58(3):94–99.
14. Spencer JD, Hayes KC, Alexander IJ. Knee joint effusion and quadriceps reflex inhibition in man. *Arch Phys Med Rehabil* 1984;65(4):171–177.
15. Solomonow M, Baratta R, Zhou BH, et al. The synergistic action of the anterior cruciate ligament and thigh muscles in maintaining joint stability. *Am J Sports Med* 1987;15(3):207–213.
16. Proske U, Schaible HG, Schmidt RF. Joint receptors and kinaesthesia. *Exp Brain Res* 1988;72(2):219–224.
17. Knapik JJ, Bauman CL, Jones BH, et al. Preseason strength and flexibility imbalances associated with athletic injuries in female collegiate athletes. *Am J Sports Med* 1991;19(1):76–81.
18. Pitman MI, Nainzadeh N, Menche D, et al. The intraoperative evaluation of the neurosensory function of the anterior cruciate ligament in humans using somatosensory evoked potentials. *Arthroscopy* 1992;8(4):442–447.
19. Burkhart SS, Morgan CD, Kibler WB. The disabled throwing shoulder: spectrum of pathology Part III: The SICK scapula, scapular dyskinesis, the kinetic chain, and rehabilitation. *Arthroscopy* 2003;19(6):641–661.
20. Kibler WB. The role of the scapula in athletic shoulder function. *Am J Sports Med* 1998;26(2):325–337.
21. Máčková J, Janda V, Máček M, et al. Impaired muscle function in children and adolescents. *J Manual Medicine* 1989;4:157–160.
22. Janda V. Muscle strength in relation to muscle length, pain and muscle imbalance. In: Harris-Rindahl K, ed. *Muscle Strength.* New York: Churchill Livingstone; 1993:83–91.
23. Watson DH, Trott PH. Cervical headache: an investigation of natural head posture and upper cervical flexor muscle performance. *Cephalalgia* 1993; 13(4):272–284; discussion 32.
24. Sommer HM. Patellar chondropathy and apicitis, and muscle imbalances of the lower extremities in competitive sports. *Sports Med* 1988;5(6):386–394.
25. Kamkar A, Irrgang JJ, Whitney SL. Nonoperative management of secondary shoulder impingement syndrome. *J Orthop Sports Phys Ther* 1993;17(5): 212–224.
26. Adams MA, Dolan P. Recent advances in lumbar spinal mechanics and their clinical significance. *Clin Biomech (Bristol, Avon)* 1995;10(1):3–19.
27. Bullock-Saxton JE, Janda V, Bullock MI. Reflex activation of gluteal muscles in walking. An approach to restoration of muscle function for patients with low-back pain. *Spine* 1993;18(6):704–708.
28. Butler D, Gifford L. The concept of adverse mechanical tension in the nervous system. *Physiotherapy* 1989;75:622–626.
29. Inman V, Saunders J. The clinico-anatomical aspects of the lumbosacral region. *Radiology* 1942;38:669–678.
30. Breig A. *Adverse Mechanical Tension in the Central Nervous System.* Stockholm, Sweden: Williams & Wilkins; 1978.
31. Louis R. Vertebroradicular and vertebromedullar dynamics. *Anat Clin* 1981; 3:1–11.
32. Spencer DL, Irwin GS, Miller JA. Anatomy and significance of fixation of the lumbosacral nerve roots in sciatica. *Spine* 1983;8(6):672–679.
33. Parke WW, Watanabe R. Adhesions of the ventral lumbar dura. An adjunct source of discogenic pain? *Spine* 1990;15(4):300–303.
34. Bowsher D. *Introduction to the Anatomy and Physiology of the Nervous System.* 5th ed. Oxford, UK: Blackwell; 1988.
35. McLellan DL, Swash M. Longitudinal sliding of the median nerve during movements of the upper limb. *J Neurol Neurosurg Psychiatry* 1976;39(6): 566–570.
36. Millesi H. The nerve gap. Theory and clinical practice. *Hand Clin* 1986;2(4): 651–663.

37. Renyi GSD. The structure of cells in tissues as revealed by microdissection. *J Comp Neurol* 1929;47:405–425.

38. Glees P. Observations on the structure of the connective tissue sheaths of cutaneous nerves. *J Anat* 1943;77(Pt 2):153–159.

39. Robertson JD. The ultrastructure of Schmidt-Lanterman clefts and related shearing defects of the myelin sheath. *J Biophys Biochem Cytol* 1958;4(1):39–46.

40. Singer M, Bryant SV. Movements in the myelin Schwann sheath of the vertebrate axon. *Nature* 1969;221(5186):1148–1150.

41. Thomas P, Olsson Y. Microscopic anatomy and function of the connective tissue components of peripheral nerves. In: Dyck P, ed. *Peripheral Neuropathy*. 2nd ed. Philadelphia: Saunders; 1984.

42. Wilgis EF, Murphy R. The significance of longitudinal excursion in peripheral nerves. *Hand Clin* 1986;2(4):761–766.

43. Tunituri AR. Elasticity of the spinal cord dura in the dog. *J Neurosurg* 1977;47(3):391–396.

44. Sunderland S, Bradley KC. The cross-sectional area of peripheral nerve trunks devoted to nerve fibers. *Brain* 1949;72(3):428–449.

45. Sunderland S. *Nerve and Nerve Injuries*. 2nd ed. Edinburgh, UK: Churchill Livingstone; 1978.

46. Parke WW, Watanabe R. The intrinsic vasculature of the lumbosacral spinal nerve roots. *Spine* 1985;10(6):508–515.

47. Blikra G. Intradural herniated lumbar disc. *J Neurosurg* 1969;31(6):676–679.

48. Savolaine ER, Pandya JB, Greenblatt SH, et al. Anatomy of the human lumbar epidural space: new insights using CT-epidurography. *Anesthesiology* 1988;68(2):217–220.

49. Turl SE, George KP. Adverse neural tension: a factor in repetitive hamstring strain? *J Orthop Sports Phys Ther* 1998;27(1):16–21.

50. Jönhagen S, Németh G, Eriksson E. Hamstring injuries in sprinters. The role of concentric and eccentric hamstring muscle strength and flexibility. *Am J Sports Med* 1994;22(2):262–266.

51. Kibler WB. Clinical aspects of muscle injury. *Med Sci Sports Exerc* 1990;22(4):450–452.

52. Kibler WB, Chandler TJ, Pace BK. Principles of rehabilitation after chronic tendon injuries. *Clin Sports Med* 1992;11(3):661–671.

53. Kibler WB, Chandler TJ, Stracener ES. Musculoskeletal adaptations and injuries due to overtraining. *Exerc Sport Sci Rev* 1992;20:99–126.

54. McHugh MP, Tyler TF, Tetro DT, et al. Risk factors for noncontact ankle sprains in high school athletes: the role of hip strength and balance ability. *Am J Sports Med* 2006;34(3):464–470.

55. Thacker SB, Stroup DF, Branche CM, et al. The prevention of ankle sprains in sports. A systematic review of the literature. *Am J Sports Med* 1999;27(6):753–760.

56. Bullock-Saxton JE, Janda V, Bullock MI. The influence of ankle sprain injury on muscle activation during hip extension. *Int J Sports Med* 1994;15(6):330–334.

57. Gross MT, Liu HY. The role of ankle bracing for prevention of ankle sprain injuries. *J Orthop Sports Phys Ther* 2003;33(10):572–577.

58. Hewett TE, Stroupe AL, Nance TA, et al. Plyometric training in female athletes. Decreased impact forces and increased hamstring torques. *Am J Sports Med* 1996;24(6):765–773.

59. Noyes FR, Dunworth LA, Andriacchi TP, et al. Knee hyperextension gait abnormalities in unstable knees. Recognition and preoperative gait retraining. *Am J Sports Med* 1996;24(1):35–45.

60. Ireland ML. The female ACL: why is it more prone to injury? *Orthop Clin North Am* 2002;33(4):637–651.

61. Ireland ML, Ott SM. Special concerns of the female athlete. *Clin Sports Med* 2004;23(2):281–298, vii.

62. Leetun DT, Ireland ML, Willson JD, et al. Core stability measures as risk factors for lower extremity injury in athletes. *Med Sci Sports Exerc* 2004;36(6):926–934.

63. Willson JD, Ireland ML, Davis I. Core strength and lower extremity alignment during single leg squats. *Med Sci Sports Exerc* 2006;38(5):945–952.

64. Krosshaug T, Nakamae A, Boden BP, et al. Mechanisms of anterior cruciate ligament injury in basketball: video analysis of 39 cases. *Am J Sports Med* 2007;35(3):359–367.

65. Grindstaff TL, Hammill RR, Tuzson AE, et al. Neuromuscular control training programs and noncontact anterior cruciate ligament injury rates in female athletes: a numbers-needed-to-treat analysis. *J Athl Train* 2006;41(4):450–456.

66. Fagenbaum R, Darling WG. Jump landing strategies in male and female college athletes and the implications of such strategies for anterior cruciate ligament injury. *Am J Sports Med* 2003;31(2):233–240.

67. Brukner P, Khan K. *Clinical Sports Medicine*. Sydney, Australia: McGraw-Hill; 1995.

68. Moore MA, Hutton RS. Electromyographic investigation of muscle stretching techniques. *Med Sci Sports Exerc* 1980;12(5):322–329.

69. Bandy WD, Irion JM. The effect of time on static stretch on the flexibility of the hamstring muscles. *Phys Ther* 1994;74(9):845–850; discussion 50–52.

70. De Lateur BJ. Flexibility. *Phys Med Rehabil Clin N Am* 1994;5(2):295–307.

71. Sady SP, Wortman M, Blanke D. Flexibility training: ballistic, static or proprioceptive neuromuscular facilitation? *Arch Phys Med Rehabil* 1982;63(6):261–263.

72. Kornberg C, Lew P. The effect of stretching neural structures on grade one hamstring injuries. *J Orthop Sports Phys Ther* 1989;10(12):481–487.

73. Reid JD. Effects of flexion-extension movements of the head and spine upon the spinal cord and nerve roots. *J Neurol Neurosurg Psychiatry* 1960;23:214–221.

74. Breig A, Troup JD. Biomechanical considerations in the straight-leg-raising test. Cadaveric and clinical studies of the effects of medial hip rotation. *Spine* 1979;4(3):242–250.

75. Supik LF, Broom MJ. Sciatic tension signs and lumbar disc herniation. *Spine* 1994;19(9):1066–1069.

76. Elvey R, ed. Brachial plexus tension test and pathoanatomic origin of arm pain. Multidisciplinary International Conference on Manipulative Therapy; Melbourne, Australia; 1979.

77. Selvaratnam PJ, Matyas TA, Glasgow EF. Noninvasive discrimination of brachial plexus involvement in upper limb pain. *Spine* 1994;19(1):26–33.

78. Gordon EE, Kowalski K, Fritts M. Protein changes in quadriceps muscle of rat with repetitive exercises. *Arch Phys Med Rehabil* 1967;48(6):296–303.

79. Milner-Brown HS, Stein RB, Lee RG. Synchronization of human motor units: possible roles of exercise and supraspinal reflexes. *Electroencephalogr Clin Neurophysiol* 1975;38(3):245–254.

80. Moritani T, DeVries HA. Neural factors versus hypertrophy in the time course of muscle strength gain. *Am J Phys Med* 1979;58(3):115–130.

81. Moritani T, deVries HA. Potential for gross muscle hypertrophy in older men. *J Gerontol* 1980;35(5):672–682.

82. Komi PV. Training of muscle strength and power: interaction of neuromotoric, hypertrophic, and mechanical factors. *Int J Sports Med* 1986;7(Suppl 1):10–15.

83. DeVries HA. "Efficiency of electrical activity" as a physiological measure of the functional state of muscle tissue. *Am J Phys Med* 1968;47(1):10–22.

84. Petrofsky JS. Frequency and amplitude analysis of the EMG during exercise on the bicycle ergometer. *Eur J Appl Physiol Occup Physiol* 1979;41(1):1–15.

85. Moritani T, Nagata A, deVries HA, et al. Critical power as a measure of physical work capacity and anaerobic threshold. *Ergonomics* 1981;24(5):339–350.

86. deVries HA, Tichy MW, Housh TJ, et al. A method for estimating physical working capacity at the fatigue threshold (PWCFT). *Ergonomics* 1987;30(8):1195–1204.

87. Ng A, Dao H, Lee A. Altered EMG/force relationship in older humans. *Med Sci Sports Exerc* 1998;30(5 Suppl):S255.

88. Yao W, Fuglevand RJ, Enoka RM. Motor-unit synchronization increases EMG amplitude and decreases force steadiness of simulated contractions. *J Neurophysiol* 2000;83(1):441–452.

89. Komi P. Relationship between muscle tension, EMG and velocity of contraction under concentric and eccentric work. In: Deswmedt J, ed. *New Developments in Electromyography and Clinical Neurophysiology*. Basel, Switzerland: S Karger; 1973:730–735.

90. Ingemann-Hansen T, Halkjaer-Kristensen J. Force-velocity relationships in the human quadriceps muscle. *Scand J Rehabil Med* 1979;11:85–89.

91. Fugl-Meyer AR, Mild KH, Hornsten J. Output of skeletal muscle contractions. a study of isokinetic plantar flexion in athletes. *Acta Physiol Scand* 1982;115(2):193–199.

92. Westing SH, Seger JY. Eccentric and concentric torque-velocity characteristics, torque output comparisons, and gravity effect torque corrections for the quadriceps and hamstring muscles in females. *Int J Sports Med* 1989;10(3):175–180.

93. Westing SH, Seger JY, Karlson E, et al. Eccentric and concentric torque-velocity characteristics of the quadriceps femoris in man. *Eur J Appl Physiol Occup Physiol* 1988;58(1–2):100–104.

94. Komi P. The stretch-shortening cycle and human power output. In: Jones N, ed. *Human Muscle Power*. Champaign, IL: Human Kinetics Publishers; 1986:27–38.

95. Winters D. *The Biomechanics and Motor Control of Human Gait*. Waterloo, Canada: University of Waterloo Press; 1987.

96. Herzog W, ter Keurs HE. Force-length relation of in-vivo human rectus femoris muscles. *Pflugers Arch* 1988;411(6):642–647.

97. Herzog W, ter Keurs HE. A method for the determination of the force-length relation of selected in-vivo human skeletal muscles. *Pflugers Arch* 1988;411(6):637–641.

98. Halderman S. Spinal manipulative therapy in the management of low back pain. In: Finneson B, ed. *Low Back Pain*. Philadelphia: JB Lippincott Company; 1980:245–275.

99. Harris J. History and development of manipulation and mobilization. In: Basmajian J, ed. *Manipulation, Traction and Massage*. Baltimore: Williams & Wilkins; 1985:3–21.

100. Greenman PE. *Principles of Manual Medicine*. Baltimore: Williams & Wilkins; 1989.

101. Haldeman S. Spinal manipulative therapy. A status report. *Clin Orthop Relat Res* 1983;(179):62–70.

102. Powell FC, Hanigan WC, Olivero WC. A risk/benefit analysis of spinal manipulation therapy for relief of lumbar or cervical pain. *Neurosurgery* 1993;33(1):73–78; discussion 8–9.

103. Eisenberg DM, Kessler RC, Foster C, et al. Unconventional medicine in the United States. Prevalence, costs, and patterns of use. *N Engl J Med* 1993;328(4):246–252.

104. Greenman PE. Models and mechanisms of osteopathic manipulative medicine. *Osteopath Med News* 1987;4:1–20.

105. Neumann H. *Introduction to Manual Medicine*. Heidelberg, Germany: Springer-Verlag; 1989.

106. Dvorak J, Dvorak V. *Manual Medicine—Diagnostics*. Sttugart, Germany: Thieme Medical Publishers; 1990.

107. Cyriax J, Russel G. *Textbook of Orthopaedic Medicine: Treatment by Manipulation, Massage and Injection*. London: Bailliere Tindall; 1980.

108. Heilig D. The thrust technique. *J Am Osteopath Assoc* 1981;81(4):244–248.

109. Hruby R. Pathophysiological models and the selction of osteopathic manipulative technique. *J Osteopath Med* 1992;6:25–30.

110. Hinterbruchner C. Traction. In: Basmajian JV, ed. *Manipulation, Traction, and Massage*. 3rd ed. Baltimore: Williams & Wilkins; 1985:172–201.

111. Korr IM. Somatic dysfunction, osteopathic manipulative treatment, and the nervous system: a few facts, some theories, many questions. *J Am Osteopath Assoc* 1986;86(2):109–114.

112. Korr IM. Proprioceptors and somatic dysfunction. *J Am Osteopath Assoc* 1975;74(7):638–650.

113. Kimberly PE. Formulating a prescription for osteopathic manipulative treatment. *J Am Osteopath Assoc* 1980;79(8):506–513.

114. Fisk JW. *Medical Treatment of Neck and Back Pain*. Springfield, IL: Thomas; 1987.

115. Ottenbacher K, DiFabio RP. Efficacy of spinal manipulation/mobilization therapy. A meta-analysis. *Spine* 1985;10(9):833–837.

116. Shekelle PG. Spinal manipulation. *Spine* 1994;19(7):858–861.

117. Shekelle PG, Adams AH, Chassin MR, et al. Spinal manipulation for low-back pain. *Ann Intern Med* 1992;117(7):590–598.

118. Hadler NM, Curtis P, Gillings DB, et al. A benefit of spinal manipulation as adjunctive therapy for acute low-back pain: a stratified controlled trial. *Spine* 1987;12(7):702–706.

119. MacDonald RS, Bell CM. An open controlled assessment of osteopathic manipulation in nonspecific low-back pain. *Spine* 1990;15(5):364–370.

120. van Tulder MW, Koes BW, Bouter LM. Conservative treatment of acute and chronic nonspecific low back pain. A systematic review of randomized controlled trials of the most common interventions. *Spine* 1997;22(18):2128–2156.

121. Raskind R, North CM. Vertebral artery injuries following chiropractic cervical spine manipulation–case reports. *Angiology* 1990;41(6):445–452.

122. Hoehler FK, Tobis JS, Buerger AA. Spinal manipulation for low back pain. *JAMA* 1981;245(18):1835–1838.

123. Scientific approach to the assessment and management of activity-related spinal disorders. A monograph for clinicians. Report of the Quebec Task Force on Spinal Disorders. *Spine* 1987;12(7 Suppl):S1–S59.

124. Bigos SJ. Acute low back problems in adults. In: Services USDoHaH, ed. *Clinical Practice Guidelines 14*. Washington, DC: Government Printing Office; 1994.

125. van der Heijden GJ, Beurskens AJ, Dirx M. Efficacy of lumbar traction: a randomized clinical trial. *Physiotherapy* 1995;81:29–35.

126. Beurskens AJ, de Vet HC, Koke AJ, et al. Efficacy of traction for non-specific low back pain: a randomised clinical trial. *Lancet* 1995;346(8990):1596–1600.

127. Cyriax J. The treatment of lumbar disc lesions. *BMJ* 1950;2:14–34.

128. Harris PR. Cervical traction. Review of literature and treatment guidelines. *Phys Ther* 1977;57(8):910–914.

129. Mathews JA. The effects of spinal traction. *Physiotherapy* 1972;58(2):64–66.

130. Gupta RC, Ramarao SV. Epidurography in reduction of lumbar disc prolapse by traction. *Arch Phys Med Rehabil* 1978;59(7):322–327.

131. Oudenhoven RC. Gravitational lumbar traction. *Arch Phys Med Rehabil* 1978;59(11):510–512.

132. Saunders HD. Use of spinal traction in the treatment of neck and back conditions. *Clin Orthop Relat Res* 1983;(179):31–38.

133. Onel D, Tuzlaci M, Sari H, et al. Computed tomographic investigation of the effect of traction on lumbar disc herniations. *Spine* 1989;14(1):82–90.

134. Cyriax J. Conservative treatment of lumbar disc lesions. *Physiotherapy* 1964;50:300–303.

135. Hood LB, Chrisman D. Intermittent pelvic traction in the treatment of the ruptured intervertebral disk. *Phys Ther* 1968;48(1):21–30.

136. Gillstrom P, Ericson K, Hindmarsh T. Autotraction in lumbar disc herniation. A myelographic study before and after treatment. *Arch Orthop Trauma Surg* 1985;104(4):207–210.

137. Judovich BD. Herniated cervical disc; a new form of traction therapy. *Am J Surg* 1952;84(6):646–656.

138. Colachis SC Jr, Strohm BR. A study of tractive forces and angle of pull on vertebral interspaces in the cervical spine. *Arch Phys Med Rehabil* 1965;46(12):820–830.

139. Nayak N. Cervical traction: prescription patterns. *Arch Phys Med Rehabil* 1993;74:1268.

140. Mathews JA, Hickling J. Lumbar traction: a double-blind controlled study for sciatica. *Rheumatol Rehabil* 1975;14(4):222–225.

141. Goldfish G. Lumbar traction. In: Tollison CD, Kriegel ML, eds. *Interdisciplinary Rehabilitation of Low Back Pain*. Baltimore: Williams & Wilkins; 1989: xviii, 365.

142. Saunders HD, Saunders R. *Evaluation, Treatment, and Prevention of Musculoskeletal Disorders*. Chaska, MN: Saunders Group; 1993.

143. Rogoff J. Motorized intermittent traction. In: Basmajian JV, ed. *Manipulation, Traction, and Massage*. 3rd ed. Baltimore: Williams & Wilkins; 1985: 201–207.

144. Grieve GP. *Mobilisation of the Spine: A Primary Handbook of Clinical Method*. 5th ed. Edinburgh: Churchill Livingstone; 1991.

145. Larsson U, Choler U, Lidstrom A, et al. Auto-traction for treatment of lumbago-sciatica. A multicentre controlled investigation. *Acta Orthop Scand* 1980;51(5):791–798.

146. Tesio L, Merlo A. Autotraction versus passive traction: an open controlled study in lumbar disc herniation. *Arch Phys Med Rehabil* 1993;74(8):871–876.

147. Nosse LJ. Inverted spinal traction. *Arch Phys Med Rehabil* 1978;59(8):367–370.

148. Yates DA. Indications and contra-indications for spinal traction. *Physiotherapy* 1972;58(2):55–57.

149. Abramson DI, Chu LS, Tuck S Jr, et al. Effect of tissue temperatures and blood flow on motor nerve conduction velocity. *JAMA* 1966;198(10):1082–1088.

150. Schmidt KL, Ott VR, Rocher G, et al. Heat, cold and inflammation. *Z Rheumatol* 1979;38(11–12):391–404.

151. Weber D, Brown A. Physical therapeutic modalities. In: Braddom RL, ed. *Physical Medicine & Rehabilitation*. Philadelphia: Saunders; 1996.

152. Denys EH. AAEM minimonograph #14: The influence of temperature in clinical neurophysiology. *Muscle Nerve* 1991;14(9):795–811.

153. Mense S. Effects of temperature on the discharges of muscle spindles and tendon organs. *Pflugers Arch* 1978;374(2):159–166.

154. Lehmann JF, Masock AJ, Warren CG, et al. Effect of therapeutic temperatures on tendon extensibility. *Arch Phys Med Rehabil* 1970;51(8):481–487.

155. Weinberger A, Fadilah R, Lev A, et al. Intra-articular temperature measurements after superficial heating. *Scand J Rehabil Med* 1989;21(1):55–57.

156. Lehmann JF, Brunner GD, Stow R. Pain threshold measurements after therapeutic application of ultrasound, microwave, and infrared. *Arch Phys Med Rehabil* 1958;39:560–565.

157. Falconer J, Hayes KW, Chang RW. Therapeutic ultrasound in the treatment of musculoskeletal conditions. *Arthritis Care Res* 1990;3(2):85–91.

158. Lehmann JF. *Therapeutic Heat and Cold*. 4th ed. Baltimore: Williams & Wilkins; 1990.

159. Michlovitz SL, Wolf SL. *Thermal Agents in Rehabilitation*. 2nd ed. Philadelphia: Davis; 1990.

160. Prentice WE. *Therapeutic Modalities in Sports Medicine*. 2nd ed. St. Louis: Times Mirror/Mosby College Pub; 1990.

161. Lehmann JF, Silverman DR, Baum BA, et al. Temperature distributions in the human thigh, produced by infrared, hot pack and microwave applications. *Arch Phys Med Rehabil* 1966;47(5):291–299.

162. Abramson DI, Tuck S Jr, Chu LS, et al. Effect of paraffin bath and hot fomentations on local tissue temperatures. *Arch Phys Med Rehabil* 1964;45:87–94.

163. Coakley WT. Biophysical effects of ultrasound at therapeutic intensities. *Physiotherapy* 1978;64(6):166–169.

164. Miller DL, Nyborg WL, Whitcomb CC. Platelet aggregation induced by ultrasound under specialized conditions in vitro. *Science* 1979;205(4405):505–507.

165. Webster DF, Harvey W, Dyson M, et al. The role of ultrasound-induced cavitation in the 'in vitro' stimulation of collagen synthesis in human fibroblasts. *Ultrasonics* 1980;18(1):33–37.

166. ter Haar GR, Stratford IJ. Evidence for a non-thermal effect of ultrasound. *Br J Cancer Suppl* 1982;5:172–175.

167. Haker E, Lundeberg T. Pulsed ultrasound treatment in lateral epicondylalgia. *Scand J Rehabil Med* 1991;23(3):115–118.

168. Lehmann JF, DeLateur BJ, Stonebridge JB. Selective muscle heating by short-wave diathermy with a helical coil. *Arch Phys Med Rehabil* 1969;50(3):117–223.

169. Kantor G. Evaluation and survey of microwave and radiofrequency applicators. *J Microw Power* 1981;16(2):135–150.

170. Zanetić F, Marković B, Starcević L. Short-wave therapy as a complementary treatment for chronic prostatitis [in Croatian]. *Med Arh* 1981;35(3):157–159.

171. Binder A, Parr G, Hazleman B, et al. Pulsed electromagnetic field therapy of persistent rotator cuff tendinitis. A double-blind controlled assessment. *Lancet* 1984;1(8379):695–698.

172. Foley-Nolan D, Barry C, Coughlan RJ, et al. Pulsed high frequency (27MHz) electromagnetic therapy for persistent neck pain. A double blind, placebo-controlled study of 20 patients. *Orthopedics* 1990;(4):445–451.

173. Wilson DH. Treatment of soft-tissue injuries by pulsed electrical energy. *Br Med J* 1972;2(5808):269–270.

174. Witters DM, Kantor G. An evaluation of microwave diathermy applicators using free space electric field mapping. *Phys Med Biol* 1981;26(6):1099–1114.

175. Dutreix J, Cosset JM, Salama A, et al. Experimental studies of various heating procedures for clinical application of localized hyperthermia. *Prog Clin Biol Res* 1982;107:585–596.

176. DeLateur BJ, Lehmann JF, Stonebrid JB, et al. Muscle heating in human subjects with 915 MHz. Microwave contact applicator. *Arch Phys Med Rehabil* 1970;51(3):147–151.

177. Richardson WA, Duane TD, Hines HM. Experimental lenticular opacities produced by microwave irradiations. *Arch Phys Med Rehabil* 1948;29(12):765–769.

178. Worden R, Herrick J, Wakim K. The heating effects of microwave with and without ischemia. *Arch Phys Med Rehabil* 1948;29(29):763–769.

179. Lehmann JF, Dundore DE, Esselman PC, et al. Microwave diathermy: effects on experimental muscle hematoma resolution. *Arch Phys Med Rehabil* 1983;64(3):127–129.

180. Basford J. Physical agents. In: DeLisa JA, ed. *Rehabilitation Medicine: Principles and Practice*. 2nd ed. Philadelphia: Lippincott; 1993:404–424.

181. Weinberger A, Fadilah R, Lev A, et al. Treatment of articular effusions with local deep microwave hyperthermia. *Clin Rheumatol* 1989;8(4):461–466.

182. Lehmann JF, McMillan JA, Brunner GD, et al. Comparative study of the efficiency of short-wave, microwave and ultrasonic diathermy in heating the hip joint. *Arch Phys Med Rehabil* 1959;40:510–512.

183. Hodgkin AL, Katz B. The effect of temperature on the electrical activity of the giant axon of the squid. *J Physiol* 1949;109(1–2):240–249.

184. Stalberg E, Ekstedt J, Broman A. The electromyographic jitter in normal human muscles. *Electroencephalogr Clin Neurophysiol* 1971;31(5):429–438.

185. Bolton CF, Sawa GM, Carter K. The effects of temperature on human compound action potentials. *J Neurol Neurosurg Psychiatry* 1981;44(5):407–413.

186. Knight K. *Cryotherapy: Theory, Technique and Physiology.* Chattanooga, TN: Chattanooga Corporation; 1985.

187. Eldred E, Lindsley DF, Buchwald JS. The effect of cooling on mammalian muscle spindles. *Exp Neurol* 1960;2:144–157.

188. Petajan JH, Watts N. Effects of cooling on the triceps surae reflex. *Am J Phys Med* 1962;41:240–251.

189. Knutsson E, Mattsson E. Effects of local cooling on monosynaptic reflexes in man. *Scand J Rehabil Med* 1969;1(3):126–132.

190. Miglietta O. Action of cold on spasticity. *Am J Phys Med* 1973;52(4):198–205.

191. Hartviksen K. Ice therapy in spasticity. *Acta Neurol Scand* 1962;38:79–84.

192. Franchimont P, Juchmes J, Lecomte J. Hydrotherapy—mechanisms and indications. *Pharmacol Ther* 1983;20(1):79–93.

193. Guyton AC. *Textbook of Medical Physiology.* 7th ed. Philadelphia: Saunders; 1986.

194. Berne RM, Levy MN. *Physiology.* 2nd ed. St. Louis: Mosby; 1988.

195. Taber C, Contryman K, Fahrenbruch J, et al. Measurement of reactive vasodilation during cold gel pack application to nontraumatized ankles. *Phys Ther* 1992;72(4):294–299.

196. Tsairis P. Peripheral nerve injuries in athletes. In: Jordan BD, Tsairis P, Warren RF, eds. *Sports Neurology.* Rockville, MD: Aspen Publishers; 1989:180–192.

197. Lundgren C, Muren A, Zederfeldt B. Effect of cold-vasoconstriction on wound healing in the rabbit. *Acta Chir Scand* 1959;118:1–4.

198. Kasman G. *Clinical Applications in Surface Electromyography.* Gaithersburg, MD: Aspen Publishers; 1998.

199. Graupe D, Kohn KH. A critical review of EMG-controlled electrical stimulation in paraplegics. *Crit Rev Biomed Eng* 1987;15(3):187–210.

200. Hefftner G, Jaros GG. The electromyogram (EMG) as a control signal for functional neuromuscular stimulation–Part II: practical demonstration of the EMG signature discrimination system. *IEEE Trans Biomed Eng* 1988;35(4):238–242.

201. Hefftner G, Zucchini W, Jaros GG. The electromyogram (EMG) as a control signal for functional neuromuscular stimulation–Part I: Autoregressive modeling as a means of EMG signature discrimination. *IEEE Trans Biomed Eng* 1988;35(4):230–237.

202. Marinacci AA, Horande M. Electromyogram in neuromuscular re-education. *Bull Los Angel Neuro Soc* 1960;25:57–71.

203. Andrews JM. Neuromuscular re-education of the hemiplegic with the aid of the electromyograph. *Arch Phys Med Rehabil* 1964;45:530–532.

204. Johnson HE, Garton WH. Muscle re-education in hemiplegia by use of electromyographic device. *Arch Phys Med Rehabil* 1973;54(7):320–322 passim.

205. Winchester P, Montgomery J, Bowman B, et al. Effects of feedback stimulation training and cyclical electrical stimulation on knee extension in hemiparetic patients. *Phys Ther* 1983;63(7):1096–1103.

206. Fields RW. Electromyographically triggered electric muscle stimulation for chronic hemiplegia. *Arch Phys Med Rehabil* 1987;68(7):407–414.

207. Cozean CD, Pease WS, Hubbell SL. Biofeedback and functional electric stimulation in stroke rehabilitation. *Arch Phys Med Rehabil* 1988;69(6):401–405.

208. Kraft GH, Fitts SS, Hammond MC. Techniques to improve function of the arm and hand in chronic hemiplegia. *Arch Phys Med Rehabil* 1992;73(3):220–227.

209. Taylor W. Dynamic EMG biofeedback in assessment and treatment using a neuromuscular re-education model. In: Cram J, ed. *Clinical EMG for Surface Recordings.* Nevada City, CA: Clinical Resources; 1990:175-196.

210. Reid D, Saboe L, Chepeha J. Anterior shoulder instability in athletes: comparison of isokinetic resistance exercise and an electromyographic biofeedback re-education program—a pilot program. *Physiother Can* 1996:251–256.

211. Grieco A, Occhipinti E, Colombini D, et al. Muscular effort and musculoskeletal disorders in piano students: electromyographic, clinical and preventive aspects. *Ergonomics* 1989;32(7):697–716.

212. Montes R, Bedmar M, Sol Martin M. EMG biofeedback of the abductor pollicis brevis in piano performance. *Biofeedback Self Regul* 1993;18(2):67–77.

213. Reynolds C. Electromyographic biofeedback evaluation of a computer keyboard operator with cumulative trauma disorder. *J Hand Ther* 1994;7(1):25–27.

214. Asfour SS, Khalil TM, Waly SM, et al. Biofeedback in back muscle strengthening. *Spine* 1990;15(6):510–513.

215. Lofland KR, Mumby PB, Cassisi JE, et al. Assessment of lumbar EMG during static and dynamic activity in pain-free normals: implications for muscle scanning protocols. *Biofeedback Self Regul* 1995;20(1):3–18.

216. LeVeau BF, Rogers C. Selective training of the vastus medialis muscle using EMG biofeedback. *Phys Ther* 1980;60(11):1410–1415.

217. Wise HH, Fiebert I, Kates JL. EMG biofeedback as treatment for patellofemoral pain syndrome. *J Orthop Sports Phys Ther* 1984;6(2):95–103.

218. Draper V. Electromyographic biofeedback and recovery of quadriceps femoris muscle function following anterior cruciate ligament reconstruction. *Phys Ther* 1990;70(1):11–17.

219. Draper V, Ballard L. Electrical stimulation versus electromyographic biofeedback in the recovery of quadriceps femoris muscle function following anterior cruciate ligament surgery. *Phys Ther* 1991;71(6):455–461; discussion 61–64.

220. Shelton GL, Thigpen LK. Rehabilitation of patellofemoral dysfunction: a review of literature. *J Orthop Sports Phys Ther* 1991;14(6):243–249.

221. Ingersoll CD, Knight KL. Patellar location changes following EMG biofeedback or progressive resistive exercises. *Med Sci Sports Exerc* 1991;23(10):1122–1127.

222. Bishop B. Vibratory stimulation. Part I. Neurophysiology of motor responses evoked by vibratory stimulation. *Phys Ther* 1975;54:1273–1282.

223. Bishop B. Vibratory stimulation. Part III. Possible applications of vibration in treatment of motor dysfunctions. *Phys Ther* 1975;55(2):139–143.

224. Bishop B. Vibratory stimulation. Part II. Vibratory stimulation as an evaluation tool. *Phys Ther* 1975;55(1):28–34.

225. Lundeberg T. The pain suppressive effect of vibratory stimulation and transcutaneous electrical nerve stimulation (TENS) as compared to aspirin. *Brain Res* 1984;294(2):201–209.

226. Lundeberg T, Ekblom A, Hansson P. Relief of sinus pain by vibratory stimulation. *Ear Nose Throat J* 1985;64(4):163–167.

227. Lundeberg T, Nordemar R, Ottoson D. Pain alleviation by vibratory stimulation. *Pain* 1984;20(1):25–44.

228. Lundeberg T. Naloxone does not reverse the pain-reducing effect of vibratory stimulation. *Acta Anaesthesiol Scand* 1985;29(2):212–216.

229. Guieu R, Tardy-Gervet MF, Blin O, et al. Pain relief achieved by transcutaneous electrical nerve stimulation and/or vibratory stimulation in a case of painful legs and moving toes. *Pain* 1990;42(1):43–48.

230. Guieu R, Tardy-Gervet MF, Roll JP. Analgesic effects of vibration and transcutaneous electrical nerve stimulation applied separately and simultaneously to patients with chronic pain. *Can J Neurol Sci* 1991;18(2):113–119.

231. Guieu R, Dano P, Tardy-Gervet MF, et al. Effects of naloxone on the analgesia induced by vibratory stimulation [in French]. *Presse Med* 1989;18(24):1207–1208.

232. Guieu R, Tardy-Gervet MF, Giraud P. Met-enkephalin and beta-endorphin are not involved in the analgesic action of transcutaneous vibratory stimulation. *Pain* 1992;48(1):83–88.

233. Guieu R, Tardy-Gervet MF, Giraud P. Substance P-like immunoreactivity and analgesic effects of vibratory stimulation on patients suffering from chronic pain. *Can J Neurol Sci* 1993;20(2):138–141.

234. Guieu R, Tardy-Gervet MF, Giraud P, et al. Met-enkephalin and substance P. Comparison of CSF levels in patients with chronic pain based on a sampling procedure [in French]. *Rev Neurol (Paris)* 1993;149(6–7):398–401.

235. Tardy-Gervet MF, Guieu R, Ribot-Ciscar E, et al. Transcutaneous mechanical vibrations: analgesic effect and antinociceptive mechanisms [in French]. *Rev Neurol (Paris)* 1993;149(3):177–185.

236. Basford JR. Low-energy laser therapy: controversies and new research findings. *Lasers Surg Med* 1989;9(1):1–5.

237. Basford JR, Hallman HO, Sheffield CG, et al. Comparison of cold-quartz ultraviolet, low-energy laser, and occlusion in wound healing in a swine model. *Arch Phys Med Rehabil* 1986;67(3):151–154.

238. Vasseljen O Jr, Hoeg N, Kjeldstad B, et al. Low level laser versus placebo in the treatment of tennis elbow. *Scand J Rehabil Med* 1992;24(1):37–42.

239. Haker E, Lundeberg T. Is low-energy laser treatment effective in lateral epicondylalgia? *J Pain Symptom Manage* 1991;6(4):241–246.

240. Haker EH, Lundeberg TC. Lateral epicondylalgia: report of noneffective midlaser treatment. *Arch Phys Med Rehabil* 1991;72(12):984–988.

241. de Bie RA, de Vet HC, Lenssen TF, et al. Low-level laser therapy in ankle sprains: a randomized clinical trial. *Arch Phys Med Rehabil* 1998;79(11):1415–1420.

242. Klein RG, Eek BC. Low-energy laser treatment and exercise for chronic low back pain: double-blind controlled trial. *Arch Phys Med Rehabil* 1990;71(1):34–37.

CHAPTER 89 ■ PAIN REHABILITATION

STEVEN STANOS

"Rehabilitation is a continuous process."[1]

Rehabilitation may be described as a "return to ability . . . the return to the fullest physical, mental, social, vocational, and economic usefulness that is possible for the individual."[2] The focus is placed more on one's abilities rather than their disabilities.[2]

HISTORICAL OVERVIEW: PAIN REHABILITATION AND FUNCTIONAL RESTORATION

History of Pain Rehabilitation

Early evidence of a rehabilitation approach to the injured person or worker dates back to the Egyptians under Ramses II in 1500 BC where organized treatments of injured workers, fees for treatment, and compensation for injury were established.[3] The development of more expertise and a more rational treatment and management approach of pain was delayed until the birth of the field of anesthesia in the 1840s and the isolation and synthesis of morphine by Serturner in 1806 and salicylates from willow bark in the late 1800s.[4] The modern development of a rehabilitation model evolved only after World War I and World War II with the birth of the fields of physical and occupational therapy as a means to "rehabilitate" injured returning soldiers.[5] Pain rehabilitation developed in the context of evolution of the medical specialties of physical medicine and rehabilitation, anesthesia, psychiatry, and occupational medicine during the twentieth century. John Bonica championed a more comprehensive "multidisciplinary" approach in the United States in 1947 and later at the University of Washington in 1960.[6] Wilbert Fordyce, a psychologist and collaborator of Bonica, incorporated operant

conditioning and other behavioral approaches with more specialized 8-week inpatient programs in the late 1960s. In 1982, John Loeser formalized a more "structured program" at the University of Washington, a 3-week daily program, which has become a model for "interdisciplinary" treatment. A more biopsychosocial approach to pain rehabilitation has also been facilitated by the merging of behavioral and cognitive fields and the subsequent cognitive-behavioral approach to the assessment and treatment of pain in the 1980s and 1990s.[7–9] A proliferation of pain treatment facilities was seen between 1980 and 1995 and included the advancement of interventional procedures.[10] A more recent conceptualization of pain focuses on behaviors within the pain system, a biopsychomotor model of pain, which incorporates three interdependent behavioral subsystems: (1) communicative, (2) protective, and (3) social response behaviors.[11] This model assumes that a pain system can only be adaptive if the sensory component of the pain system is accompanied by behaviors designed to act on the source or cause of injury or illness. This may help to explain the wide variability observed in pain behaviors seen across different patients despite relatively similar levels of reported pain intensity and objective tissue pathology. The biopsychomotor model of pain can be extended to include behavioral factors such as communicative behavior (grimacing), protective behaviors (i.e., withdrawing a limb from the fire), and behaviors designed to elicit social responses (i.e., empathy and solicitous behavior from others). This model, like the biopsychosocial one, emphasizes that dysfunction may develop in behavioral systems separate from pain sensation, and subsequent treatments targeting pain behavior would more likely lead to greater clinical outcomes and provide a more pragmatic and inclusive model for the spectrum of pain rehabilitation (Fig. 89.1).

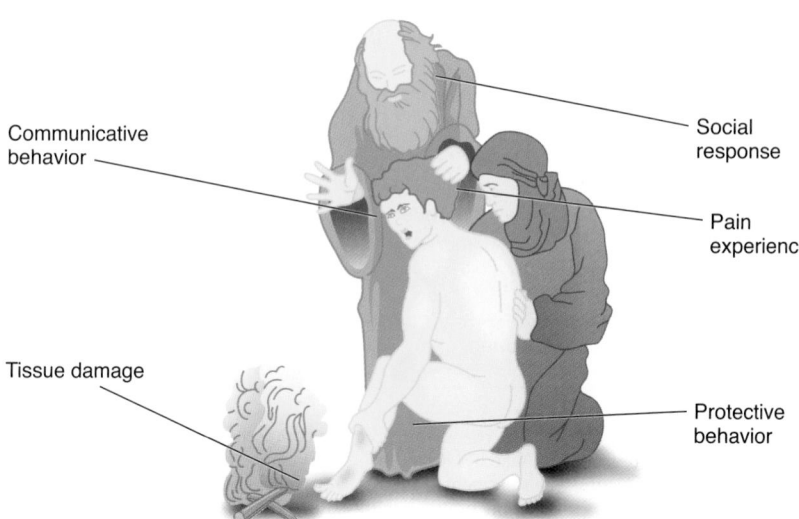

Communicative behavior

Tissue damage

Social response

Pain experience

Protective behavior

FIGURE 89.1 Biopsychomotor response to pain. (Redrawn from Sullivan MJ. Toward a biopsychomotor conceptualization of pain. *Clin J Pain* 2008;24:281–290, with permission.)

History of Functional Restoration and Work Rehabilitation

Functional restoration (FR) programs, based on a return-to-work model, evolved along with advancements in occupational medicine beginning in the 1970s. Prior to this, programs of "habit training" focused on restoring workers affected by disease or injury in the 1920s and later by the incorporation of vocational rehabilitation mandated at the federal level in 1923 and the Vocational Rehabilitation Act. In the 1950s, more objective measures were used to track progress and measure outcomes and served as the starting point for more formal work conditioning and work hardening programs championed by Lillian Wegg and Florence Cromwell.[12,13] In the 1970s, work hardening emerged as a formal industrial management service[14] and adopted a similar multidisciplinary approach used in the management of chronic pain and disability. Standardized work stimulation equipment, assessment, and treatment protocols were incorporated into standard practice in the 1980s and led to formal accreditation by the Commission on Accreditation of Rehabilitation Facilities (CARF) in the late 1980s and early 1990s.[15–17]

Gatchel et al.[18] described eight classic critical elements of a functional restoration approach which serves as the foundation for most multi- and interdisciplinary rehabilitation based programs. Elements include quantification of physical deficits on an ongoing basis, psychosocial and socioeconomic assessment used to individualize and monitor progress, and an emphasis on reconditioning of the injured area or body part. The team-centered FR approach also includes generic simulation of work or activity, disability management with cognitive-behavioral approaches, psychopharmacologic management focusing on improving analgesia, sleep, and affective distress, many times detoxifying patients from medications (i.e., opioids or benzodiazepines).[18]

What Is Pain Rehabilitation?

A pain rehabilitation model can be applied to the entire spectrum of pain conditions, from acute musculoskeletal injuries, to subacute and recurrent injuries aggravated by poor ergonomics and/or physical impairments, to more complex chronic pain conditions where interplay of biologic, psychologic, and social influences is more apparent. Pain rehabilitation is based on a structured, individualized approach. The formal assessment identifies specific problems and needs most relevant to the patient and relates the problem to impairments and psychosocial factors, selecting appropriate measures to monitor progress and treatment. The rehabilitation program includes planning and coordinating various interventions with a focus on treating the specific impairments by restoring function and identifying compensatory strategies. Additionally, addressing activity limitations by addressing environmental and personal factors may help in restoring patients to previous levels of functioning and preventing or limiting disability.[1]

A traditional definition of rehabilitation, based on a biomedical model, places the concept of rehabilitation as a secondary intervention, used to restore patients to their previous level of (residual) physical, psychologic, and social functioning, and if possible, return them to (modified) work.[19] Waddell and Burton[20] question this assumption in that the biomedical definition assumes that disability is a "matter of permanent impairment," that sickness and disability imply an incapacity to work, that rehabilitation focuses on "irremediable permanent impairment," and that rehabilitation is a second-stage process following acute medical management and only is carried out after treatment ceases. Waddell and Burton[20] have implied this may be inappropriate in that in many chronic pain conditions (i.e., low back pain) objective factors (pathology and impairment) accounts for

a small part of the incapacity. These chronic conditions are characterized more by "symptoms and distress" than tissue abnormality.[20] A number of biopsychosocial risk factors (i.e., lower level of education, higher preoperative pain, low work satisfaction, longer duration of sick leave, somatic complaints, and passive avoidance coping) have been identified as predictors of poor outcomes after surgical interventions contributing to loss of function, increased disability, and persistent elevated levels of subjective reports of pain.[21,22] These biopsychosocial risk factors may serve as important and potential targets for pain rehabilitation.

Stakeholders in Rehabilitation

Pain rehabilitation also involves the coordination of a number of important stakeholders involved in the care of the individual patient or worker. Stakeholders may include various health care providers, managed care organizations and insurers, the workers' compensation carrier, society, the individual patient, and family members. This complex health care process and related list of stakeholders involved may sometimes add, as described by Shultz and Gatchel,[23] a political dimension to the individual patient's assessment and treatment process. Success in treatment may vary depending on stakeholder and may indirectly lead to antagonistic, confrontational, and misinterpreted feelings by the patient suffering with pain. Criteria of success may vary significantly depending on whether it is assessed by the patient or by society in general (Fig. 89.2). Many times, contrary to what is seen in other areas of clinical medicine, the pain rehabilitation clinician may find himself or herself in a potentially conflicting role in the treatment of patients with chronic pain (Table 89.1). The focus of care should remain on providing appropriate clinical services, serving as a patient advocate or adjudicator, without crossing ethical boundaries resulting in harm to the client.[24]

This chapter will focus on an overview of assessment and treatment strategies included in a pain rehabilitation-based approach to acute and chronic pain conditions. As part of the clinical continuum, the more comprehensive and integrated treatment approaches commonly referred to as multidisciplinary, interdisciplinary, and/or FR[25] will be examined. Important psychologic factors related to chronic pain and disability, the continuum of treatment models from more acute to integrative approaches,

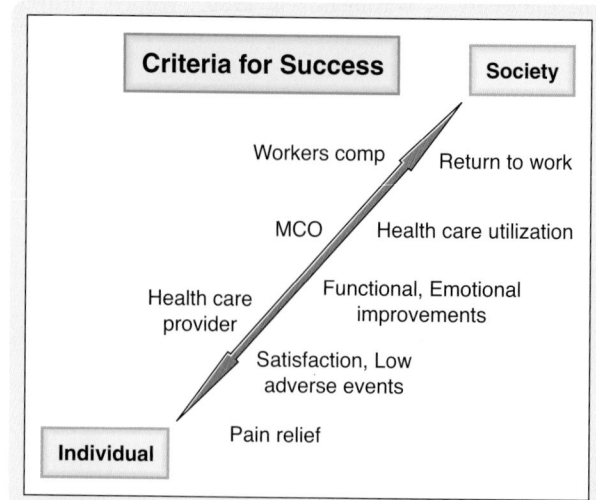

FIGURE 89.2 Criteria for success in comprehensive pain programs. (Redrawn from Gatchel RJ, Okifuji A. Evidence-based scientific data documenting the treatment and cost-effectiveness of comprehensive pain programs for chronic nonmalignant pain. *J Pain* 2006;7(11):779–793, with permission.)

TABLE 89.1

CONFLICTING ROLES OF REHABILITATION SPECIALIST

1. Clinical service provider working to reduce the client's suffering
2. Client's advocate working to protect the client in conflicts with an insurer
3. An adjudicator working to help the insurer detect evidence of client's fraudulent behavior

From Sullivan JM, Main C. Service, advocacy and adjudication: balancing the ethical challenges of multiple stakeholder agendas in the rehabilitation of chronic pain. *Dis Rehab* 2007;29:1596–1603, with permission.

specific responsibilities of members of a pain rehabilitation team (i.e., physical and occupational therapist, psychologist, relaxation therapist, and vocational specialist), and an overview of more specific work rehabilitation approaches including work conditioning, work hardening, and functional capacity testing will be reviewed.

MODELS OF REHABILITATION

Conceptual models of pain rehabilitation are based on historical advances that initially described pain as a purely sensory phenomenon evolving to include a more mind body approach to understanding disability and function (Table 89.2). Hippocrates and Galez (c. 150 AD) described an imbalance of bodily "humors" as a means of developing chronic pain and distress as a model for understanding suffering.[26] In the 1600s, a dualistic mechanistic model emerged. René Descartes (1596–1650) theorized damage to the body would stimulate specific neural pathways, giving rise to the sensation of pain.[26] Through the mid nineteenth century, medicine focused on the individual's unique manifestations of the disease process. In the mid 1800s, the expanding understanding of pathologic anatomy shifted the focus to a more biomedical model. In 1965, Melzack and Wall[27] proposed the gate control theory of pain which proposed that pain experience was determined by physical, motivational, cognitive, and emotional factors, and transmission of nerve impulses could be modulated by spinal gating mechanisms at the level of the dorsal horn. Melzack[28] elaborated on this more dynamic role of pain networks further with the "neuromatrix" model, arguing that the brain and central nervous system play a dominant role in the pain experience.

Biopsychosocial Approach Versus Biomedical Model for Pain Management

The biomedical model assumes a causal relationship between a specific physical pathology and the presence or intensity of pain

TABLE 89.2

HISTORICAL OVERVIEW: MODELS OF PAIN

Hippocrates and Galen[26]	Bodily humors
Descartes[26]	Dualistic theory
Melzack and Wall 1964[27]	Gate control theory
Engel 1977[28]	Biopsychosocial approach in medicine
Melzack and Wall 1990s[28]	Neuromatrix model
Turk, Gatchel[7]	Biopsychosocial approach
Sullivan[11]	Biopsychomotor approach

symptoms. It emphasizes the importance of eliminating pain by restoring normal function in the organ or body part from which pain is thought to emanate. Although the more disease-based biomedical model enabled the medical sciences to flourish and improved our ability to treat infection and other disease processes, its fundamentally limited scope led to less profound success and relative treatment resistance in the treatment of many chronic pain states. A biomedical model may be more advantageous in treating more acute pain states, where interventional procedures, pharmacotherapy, and surgical interventions may lead to recovery of pain or hasten time to recovery. But the biomedical model poorly addresses related mental health issues and frequently relies on dualistic decision pattern whereby if the patient does not respond to an intervention, then the pain may be not be "real" or just "in their heads."[29] Many more complex pain conditions remain resistant to a purely biomedical approach (i.e., chronic low back pain, neuropathic pain, and fibromyalgia).[30] George Engel helped to shift the thinking from a purely biomedical model of disease management to a more comprehensive biopsychosocial model of illness.[31] Recently, the World Health Organization has embraced a biopsychosocial model of disability (Fig. 89.3) which incorporates a dynamic interaction between the individual health condition and contextual factors.[32]

The pain rehabilitation approach is based on a fundamental understanding of the individual's unique condition as it relates to (1) impairment, (2) disability, and (3) functional limitation. Impairment is the loss of normality psychologically, physically, or functionally at the level of the organs and body systems.[33] Examples of physiologic impairments include muscle weakness, loss of range of motion, and pain. Disablity is a restriction or lack of ability to perform activities due to related impairments such as inability to function in a specific vocation, as a spouse, student, or parent. Functioning has been described as an umbrella term for body functions, body structures, activities, and participation, denoting a positive interaction between the individual or patient and contextual factors (i.e., background of the individual's life and current situation). Functional limitation is a deviation from the normal behavior of performing activities of daily living (ADLs) and may include problems with transfers, standing, ambulation, running, and stair climbing.[33] A formal model proposed by the International Classification of Functioning, Disability, and Health integrates the individual components into a biopsychosocial based model where a "health condition" is substituted by

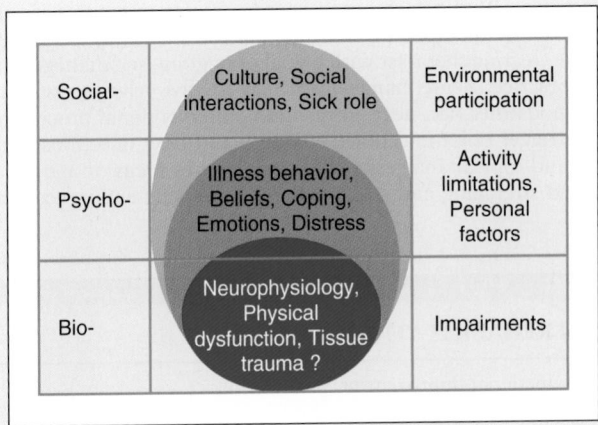

FIGURE 89.3 Domains of the biopsychosocial approach to pain rehabilitation. (Redrawn from Waddell G, Burton AK. Concepts of rehabilitation for the management of low back pain. *Best Pract Res Clin Rheum* 2005; 19:655–670, with permission.)

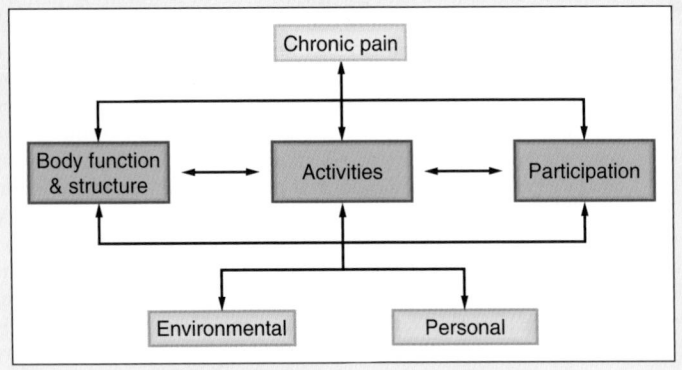

FIGURE 89.4 A formal model demonstrating the relationship among individual components that affect an individual's function was proposed by the International Classification of Functioning, Disability and Health. This model was proposed for any "health condition," and here we have substituted "chronic pain" for the more generic term. (Redrawn from Weigl M, Cieza C, Cantista P, Stucki G. Physical disability due to musculoskeletal conditions. *Best Pract Res Clin Rheum* 2007;21:167–190, with permission.)

"chronic pain" (Fig. 89.4). Chronic pain is affected by body function, activities, and participation as well as influences from the environment and personal factors.

A patient-centered approach is necessary if one is to effectively address these important individual concepts. A team-centered approach focuses on helping patients to achieve individual goals which enable them to improve physical and psychosocial function, decrease pain, and improve quality of life. By working together, the rehabilitation team is able to help patients achieve better outcomes than could be achieved by an individual practitioner or intervention (i.e., surgical procedure, injection, pharmacotherapy). Basic treatment goals of both acute and chronic pain rehabilitation programs focus on functional improvement, improved abilities to perform ADLs, return to leisure, sport, or vocational activities, and improved pharmacologic management of pain and related affective distress (Table 89.3).

Treatment Approaches: Pain Rehabilitation

A pain rehabilitation approach encompasses a wide range of treatment options including more directed therapies for acute pain conditions to more comprehensive and collaborative multi- and interdisciplinary approaches (Table 89.4).

Acute Rehabilitation

An approach to managing acute pain conditions relies on a more focused understanding of causative and aggravating factors, changes to affected tissues and related overload stresses, and includes three important phases: (1) acute, (2) recovery, and (3) functional. Within each phase, specific treatment focuses are applied by the therapist or clinician and tools or skills are taught by the treating therapist with a goal of ongoing self management and practice. Acute management may involve relative rest, passive modalities (ice, heat, ultrasound), interventional procedures (i.e., trigger point injections, epidural, and facet injections), and oral and topical analgesics. Recovery phases focus on more advanced stretching and strengthening, increasing endurance, and

assessing and treating postural changes that may be contributing to chronic pain.[34]

More Comprehensive Team Models: A Pain Continuum

Rehabilitation treatment models include a continuum of care based on patient severity and needs with increasing complexity of treatment philosophies, a need for greater communication, and decreasing individual team member autonomy.[35] Each of these models occupies a position along a continuum of care based on increasing levels of coordination, diversity of philosophies, and decreased hierarchical structure and practitioner autonomy. The left side of the treatment continuum (Fig. 89.5) shows the least collaborative model, parallel practice, where health care providers function quite independently. As one moves to the right, services become more coordinated with decreasing level of autonomy and increasing diversity of philosophies. From a structure standpoint, moving left to right increases the complexity of care while reliance on hierarchy and clearly defined roles decreases. Complexity and diversity of outcomes increases while from a process perspective, communication, participants, synergy, and importance of consensus building increases. Multi- and interdisciplinary treatment is even more structured, usually involving a number of specialties with less evidence of practitioner autonomy.

With parallel practice, independent health care practitioners are working within their defined scope of practice such as in an emergency room setting or an acute cardiac unit (i.e., nurse, phlebotomist, physician, radiology technician) where the goal is rapid assessment and treatment in the most efficient manner. Consultation may include a pain physician referring a patient to an addiction specialist or surgeon for recommendations and shared treatment responsibilities. Collaborative practice may include the use of a case manager to help coordinate treatment between the patient and physical therapist. In a collaborative approach, information is shared on an ad-hoc basis; practitioners normally practice independently sharing information regarding

TABLE 89.3

PAIN REHABILITATION GOALS

1. Functional improvement
2. Improvement in ADLs
3. Relevant psychosocial improvement
4. Rational pharmacologic management (analgesia, mood, and sleep)
5. Return to leisure, sport, work, or other productive activity

TABLE 89.4

PAIN REHABILITATION LEVELS OF CARE

Unimodal (acute)
Collaborative
Coordinated
Multidisciplinary
  Work conditioning
  Work hardening
Interdisciplinary
Integrative

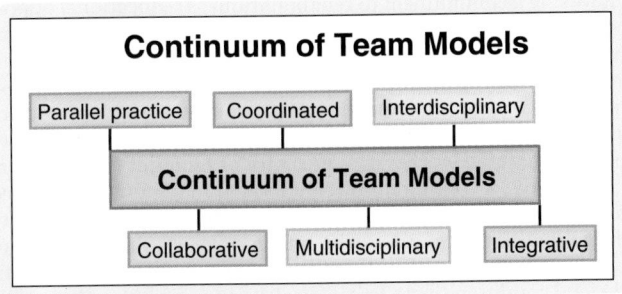

FIGURE 89.5 Continuum of team models. The most common practice model is parallel practice in which each practitioner oversees only the problems within their isolated discipline with little or no interaction with other practitioners caring for the same patient. The most effective models for caring for those with chronic pain involve programs designed to allow for frequent, direct, and repeated interactions among the providers caring for each patient in the form of multidisciplinary and interdisciplinary treatment programs. (Redrawn from Boon H, Verhoef M, O'Hara D, et al. From parallel practice to integrative health care: a conceptual framework. *BMC Health Service Research* 2004;4:15, with permission.)

a particular patient. In coordinated treatment, patient records are shared among clinicians providing treatment for a specific therapy where the case coordinator or case manager is responsible for ensuring information is transferred to all team members. Differentiating between multi- and interdisciplinary treatment will be reviewed in greater detail below. Although commonly used interchangeably, the terms inter- and multidisciplinary have important distinguishing features.

Multidisciplinary Treatment

Focused treatment programs for acute conditions may involve individual physical therapy directed by the pain physician, followed by a coordinated program including ongoing communication with the patient's case manager and therapist. With chronic pain conditions, more diverse assessment and treatment teams include multi- and interdisciplinary programs. In the multidisciplinary model, patient care is planned and managed by a team leader, usually a pain specialist (anesthesiologist, physiatrist, neurologist, psychiatrist, or primary care provider) or a psychologist, and is often hierarchical with one or two individuals directing the services of a range of team members, many with individual goals. Treatment may be delivered at different facilities or centers where individual patient progress is not regularly shared between distinct disciplines. The growth of multidisciplinary pain treatment centers in the 1980s led to the need for development of standards and formal accreditation processes. A committee on standards for Pain Treatment Facilities was established by the American Pain Society in the early 1980s and a process was subsequently developed to accredit multidisciplinary pain centers (MPCs) by the Commission on Accreditation of Rehabilitation Facilities (CARF). Non-CARF accredited programs also exist. Further, the International Association for the Study of Pain delineated four levels of pain programs[36]: multidisciplinary pain centers, multidisciplinary pain clinics, pain clinics, and modality-oriented clinics. Multidisciplinary pain clinics and centers, many of which include an even more integrated comprehensive interdisciplinary approach, include similar basic treatment disciplines; however, the MPC centers are usually associated with major health science institutions with an additional focus on pain-related research and outcomes.

Interdisciplinary Treatment

Even more collaborative, the interdisciplinary model involves team members working together toward a common goal. Team members are able to communicate and consult with other team members on an ongoing basis, facilitated by regular face-to-face meetings. Incorporation of the cognitive and behavioral psychologic approaches along with the development and emergence of the field of health psychology led to the development of more interdisciplinary models under the more general "multidisciplinary" umbrella. Interdisciplinary pain programs may also be referred to as functional restoration programs, which provide outcome-focused, coordinated, goal-oriented services. FR as an approach implies an emphasis on quantification and graded increases in function versus pain reduction, cognitive-behavioral therapy, occupational therapy, and work conditioning. FR programs were developed in the mid-1980s by Mayer et al.[37] in the United States and have been incorporated with the basic program structure of interdisciplinary programs. The basic treatment model is based on Fordyce's classic contingency management techniques and graded activity related to operant learning processes. FR aims at decreasing or eliminating learned pain behaviors.[38]

The interdisciplinary model provides practical strategies for assessing and treating pain-related deconditioning, psychosocial distress, and socioeconomic factors related to disability. An interdisciplinary team model is characterized by team members working together for a common goal, making collective therapeutic decisions, and having face-to-face meetings and patient team conferences to facilitate communication and consultation. Importantly, in this model, team members possess a combination of skills that no single individual demonstrates alone. Interdisciplinary teams may be led by a physician (medical director), psychologist, or nurse and include comprehensive assessment including pain medicine, pain psychology, and vocational rehabilitation. In some institutions, physical and occupational therapy assessments are also included in the formal assessment. Interdisciplinary programs are usually housed in one facility with periodic interdisciplinary team meetings to assess and adjust treatment progress, program coordination, and discharge planning. Programs primarily focus on restoring joint mobility, muscle strength, endurance, and conditioning and cardiovascular fitness. Coordinated vocational and therapeutic recreation services are also important aspects of care and focus on aiding patients in returning to work, improving behavioral factors (i.e., coping, catastrophizing, and problem solving) in the workplace, clarifying return to work level of functioning, and many times, individual occupational therapy.

In general, formal interdisciplinary programs vary in intensity, and may include 3–8 weeks of 4 to 8 hours per day programs with tailored group and individual therapies usually provided in an outpatient or, less often, in an inpatient hospital setting. Long-term follow-up studies of interdisciplinary treatment programs have demonstrated improved return to work rates, pain reduction, and quality of life.[39,40] The reader is referred to the chapter on Interdisciplinary Pain Treatment (Chapter 105).

Outcomes of Multi- and Interdisciplinary Treatment Programs

An early prospective trial documented high rates of return to work versus control subjects with improved physical capacities, self-reported disability, depression, and pain scores.[41] Maintained posttreatment improvements in pain, perceived health, and psychological and physical function have been demonstrated in long-term studies (6 months and 5 years).[42,43] The interdisciplinary treatment approach is supported by evidence suggesting these programs are more cost-effective and provide at least equal or greater efficacy than other pain treatments (i.e., spinal cord stimulation and implantable devices, conservative care, and surgery).[44] Additional evidence-based studies have demonstrated outcomes and treatment cost-effectiveness data supporting FR treatment which included multidisciplinary and interdisciplinary treatment programs.[45–47] A recent analysis examined the cost utility of interdisciplinary treatment of chronic spinal pain.[48] Cost utility involved the calculation of cost of the specific treatment relative to desired treatment goal (increased functioning and decreased pain) relative to pharmacologic treatment with or without anesthetic interventions. Interdisciplinary treatment was associated with better cost utility supporting interdisciplinary treatment as both less costly and more effective.[48] Although early intervention and referral for pain rehabilitation treatment should intuitively favor greater outcomes as compared to referrals late in the treatment process, studies have demonstrated that patients with long-term disability, many of whom have a greater incidence of pretreatment surgery, may still benefit from comprehensive treatment with similar improved return to work rates and decreased lost time rates.[49] Rehabilitation-based multidisciplinary treatment has demonstrated high cost-benefit with regards to decreasing treatment costs and increasing workplace return to work.[50,51]

TEAM BUILDING AND STAKEHOLDER COORDINATION

Case Management

Case management involvement is an important resource in the management of work-related injuries. Case management has been conceptualized as a system-based approach based on Bronfenbrenner's systems theory[52] which incorporates an interaction of microsystems (worker factors), mesosystems (workplace, health care utilization, insurance system factors), and macrosystems (economic, social, and legislative). Case managers are primarily assigned to injured workers' cases to help facilitate communication between stakeholders and medical providers and coordinate and clarify issues related to return to work and job description, respectively. A practical problem-based approach in rehabilitation management process is the rehabilitation cycle and includes four important interdependent steps: assessment, assignment, intervention, and evaluation (Fig. 89.6).[53] Case management assessment includes identification of patient problems and modification and adjustment of goals. The assignment step involves the assignment to specific health care professionals who understand intervention principles and goals. Intervention more specifically refers to treatment disciplines and interventions with specific goals and milestones. Finally, evaluation refers to the evaluation of goals and level of achievement.[54]

Tate et al.[55] suggested success of any collaborative workplace rehabilitation relationship is contingent upon (1) company policy endorsing a commitment to rehabilitation, (2) educational opportunities offered or available for the injured worker by the employer, and (3) identification of key decision-making points involved in the ongoing relationship. Training the nurse case mangers in basic fundamentals led to improved work placement as compared to untrained case managers who were more likely to place the injured worker in a sedentary or light duty job position.

Applying a continuum of care model, many times facilitated by strong case management presence, includes a coordination of disciplines, services, providers, and care levels. A continuum of care model developed in Canada for the treatment of musculoskeletal conditions included medical management, active physical therapy, chiropractic management, and multidisciplinary assessment and rehabilitation. Implementation of the program resulted in more rapid and sustained recovery, greater patient satisfaction, and dramatic cost savings as compared to usual care.[56]

Applying Team Values

Decision-making in pain rehabilitation has been found to incorporate common decision values shared by the team members, worker, and stakeholders. Shared "general values," as described by Loisel et al.,[57] are those that stress work is therapeutic, pain is multidimensional, and interventions should be graded. These values should in turn be shared by the team members, the worker, and stakeholders facilitated by reassurance and the delivering of a single message as a way of more successfully returning a patient to work or previous level of function.[57] Theses same values can be applied to the many barriers presented to the individual patient and stakeholder (Table 89.5).

ASSESSMENT, GOAL SETTING, AND PROGRESSION THROUGH TREATMENT

Pain Rehabilitation Principles

Assessment of patients prior to entering a rehabilitation program is based on a comprehensive examination of physical, psychologic, and social or relevant vocational factors. Also, the evaluating clinician must work to develop trust and rapport with the patient in order to understand barriers to recovery (i.e., contentious relationships involving family, employer, case manager, and/or the legal system) that may potentially lead to a delay or reduction of clinical improvement. Many times, the success of developing that relationship starts at the initial evaluation. Understandably, patients undergoing a rehabilitation program are

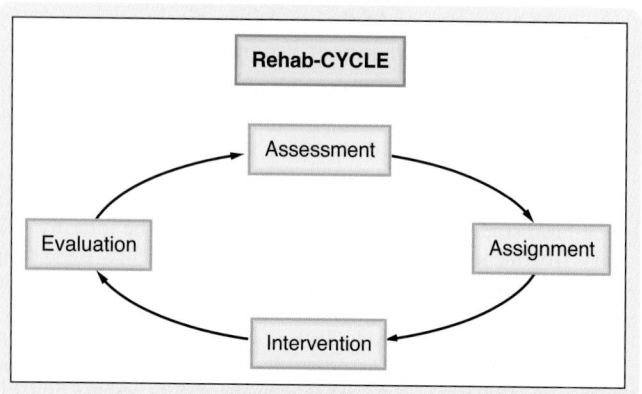

FIGURE 89.6 The rehabilitation cycle. (Redrawn from Stucki G, International Classification of Functioning, Disability, and Health (ICF): a promising framework and classification for rehabilitation medicine. *Am J Phys Med Rehab* 2005;84(10):733–740, with permission.)

TABLE 89.5

STRATEGIES APPLIED BY THE REHABILITATION TO OVERCOME BARRIERS TO COLLABORATION

Stakeholders	Strategies applied
Worker	Pain management
	Relaxation
	Education
	Confrontation
	Rational polypharmacy: analgesia, sleep, mood
Employer	Education
	Asking for employer's opinion on the TRW setting
	Sensitize the employer to its support role in relation to the worker
	Asking the insurer to use its authority to exert influence on the employer
Insurer	Education
	Sensitize to the issues involved in the intervention
	Clarification of the roles and objectives
	Meeting with the insurer's case worker before meeting the worker or the employer to ensure consistency in information delivered
	Acting without interfering
	Choosing convincing information
	Asking for the case worker's support for the intervention
Physician	Inform the physician about the rehabilitation process
	Convincing him/her to take action to facilitate return to work
	Recommendation that worker find another physician if too great a hindrance to the TRW process

TRW, therapeutic return to work.
Adapted from Loisel P, Durand M, Baril J, et al. Interorganizational collaboration in occupational rehabilitation: perceptions of an interdisciplinary rehabilitation team. *J Occup Rehab* 2005;15(4):581–590.

often asked to make significant changes in the ways they cope with pain and function. Readiness to make such important changes has been found to be associated with treatment success[58,59] and readiness to self-manage pain increases from pre- to post-MPC treatment.[60] Based on the transtheoretical model of behavior change, individuals are seen to progress through a number of stages involving decisions about change and include precontemplation, contemplation, action, maintenance, and acceptance phases.[61] These basic concepts are important for the physician to explore during the evaluation and often become a focus of discussion between other potential treatment disciplines (i.e., pain psychologist, physician, and vocational counselor) when deciding whether the patient is an appropriate candidate for treatment. The pain rehabilitation clinician must be consistent and clear in promoting exercise and activity as essential, safe, and effective for the correction of functional impairments. The clinician must also be aware of various fears, negative attitudes, financial and vocational stressors many chronic pain working and nonworking patients are sometimes struggling with, and be able to confront the patients on these issues in an open and understanding manner (Table 89.6).[62]

REHABILITATION SPECIALISTS: ACTIVITIES AND CONCEPTUAL MODELS

A pain rehabilitation team may include a pain physician (i.e., anesthesiologist, physiatrist, psychiatrist, neurologist, and/or primary care physician), physical and/or occupational therapist, a pain psychologist, relaxation (biofeedback) therapist, vocational and therapeutic recreational therapists, social workers, and nurses. Ongoing communication between treating disciplines, including monitoring of progress and adjustment of patient goals, is coordinated by the pain physician. A rehabilitation model is based on a clear, concise, and consistent therapeutic message which focuses on the patient assuming a more active role in self management, flare up management, and exercise progression. Goals of treatment remain somewhat consistent across all disciplines and focus on improving function and decreasing pain. More specialized roles of individual therapists (i.e., physical and occupational therapy, pain psychology, and vocational rehabilitation) and treatment goals will be reviewed below based on a FR approach.

The Therapist's Role: Building an Effective Therapeutic Relationship

Besides obvious clinical skills and application of therapies by specific disciplines, the relationship between treating therapist (i.e., physical therapist, occupational therapist, psychologist, etc.) and patient is based on an ability to establish a mutually effective relationship based on ongoing respect, collaboration, and exchange of ideas. A successfully established working alliance will only help to improve outcomes. A process model for patient-practitioner collaboration includes a four-component model based on initially developing a therapeutic relationship, followed by mutual inquiry, problem solving, and negotiation.[63] The therapist must also be cognizant of the patient's beliefs, skills, emotional state, and expectations in effectively developing and adjusting a specific treatment plan and subsequent interventions.[64] A therapeutic relationship involves the establishment of clear and attainable short- and long-term goals, the therapy intervention and training, and discharge planning (i.e., home exercise program). Therapists involved in pain rehabilitation treatment must be adept in their ability to assess initial levels of functional ability and then monitor and progressively increase the individual patient's level and complexity of therapeutic exercises. Therapists assess secondary impairments in addition to their primary pain-related diagnoses (i.e., general inflexibility, deconditioning, regional myofascial pain and dysfunction, and other related postural abnormalities), which expands the area of treatment. Physical and occupational therapists apply a more functional cognitive and behaviorally mediated therapeutic approach and help the patient slowly integrate other aspects of the program into his or her home program.

The basic principles of cognitive-behavioral therapy are also introduced and facilitated by the physical and occupational therapy team members and may include goal setting, education, monitoring and documenting exercise and conditioning progress, and ongoing challenging and redirecting of maladaptive thoughts and behaviors.[65–67] The integration of these approaches may help foster patient optimism, decreases the fear of reinjury, and maximizes patient compliance. Common cognitive-behavioral objectives may be applied across disciplines as well as by pain psychology professionals in helping the pain rehabilitation patient change maladaptive thoughts and behaviors and include helping patients to combat demoralization, view pain as more manageable, alter

TABLE 89.6

PATIENT PERCEPTIONS

Pathways to becoming injured	Seeking treatment	Seeking return to adequate work	Living as an injured worker
Work, workplace, and degree of unsafe practices lead to injury	Desperate for a diagnosis; difficulty accessing appropriate and timely treatment	Returned to modified work yet disillusioned to find accommodations short-lived or nonexistent	Financial hardships; loss of marriages; change in family structure
Fear of unemployment; continued hazardous job	Negative attitudes by doctors and other health practitioners toward the injured worker	Lack of choice and control over vocational issues	Legal action with compensation system drained of financial resources, adding to distress
Lack of knowledge about reporting injuries	Medical uncertainty led to different diagnoses from different specialists; uncertainty led to more doctor shopping and inconsistent message regarding level of activity and restrictions	Workers believed employer-based actions on the need of company rather than the workers	Psychological deterioration; limitation in self-care activities led to feelings of dependency and social isolation

From Beardwood BA, Kirsh B, Clark NJ. Victims twice over: perceptions and experiences of injured workers. *Qual Health Res* 2005;15:30–48, with permission.

or unlearn maladaptive thoughts or behaviors, bolster confidence, and improve problem solving (Table 89.7).

Incorporating Behavioral Approaches in Pain Rehabilitation

Pain rehabilitation approaches rely heavily on incorporating behavioral principles and approaches (i.e., operant, cognitive, and respondent) into active therapies. The cornerstone of operant therapy is graded activity. The basic premise of a graded activity program is based on Fordyce's combined use of graded activity

TABLE 89.7

PAIN TEAM SHARED PRIMARY OBJECTIVES OF A COGNITIVE-BEHAVIORAL APPROACH FOR PAIN PATIENTS

1. To combat demoralization by assisting patients to change their view of their pain from overwhelming to manageable
2. To teach patients the coping strategies and techniques to help them to adapt and respond to pain and the resultant problems
3. To assist patients to reconceptualize themselves as active, resourceful, and competent
4. To learn the associations between thoughts, feelings, and behavior and subsequently to identify and alter automatic, maladaptive patterns
5. To utilize more adaptive ways of thinking, feeling, and behaving
6. To bolster self-confidence and patients' attribution of successful outcomes to their own efforts
7. To help patients anticipate problems proactively and generate solutions, thereby facilitating maintenance and generalization

Adapted from Main CJ, Sullivan JM, Watson PJ. *Pain Management: Practical Application of the Biopsychosocial Perspective in Clinical and Occupational Settings.* 2nd ed. Edinburgh: Churchill Livingstone; 2007 and Turk DC, Okifuji A. A cognitive-behavioral approach to pain management. In: Melzack R, Wall PD, eds. *Handbook of Pain Management: A Clinical Companion to Wall and Melzack's Textbook of Pain.* Edinburgh: Churchill Livingstone; 2003:533–541.

progression and contingency management techniques. This treatment targets helping patients to increase healthy behaviors with positive reinforcement while at the same time decreasing maladaptive pain behaviors and beliefs and increasing tolerance for activity.[68,69] Often, graded activity programs are also incorporated with exercise therapy and problem-solving training.[70]

Physical Therapy

Physical therapists specialize in gait training, locomotion, core strengthening and stability, joint deficiencies, and proper biomechanics. Active treatments include instruction in strengthening, postural re-education, and related therapeutic exercise (see Chapter 92). Passive treatment modalities (i.e., local application of heat, cold modalities) may be more efficacious for acute injuries; they are used more judiciously with chronic pain conditions. The use of modalities with chronic pain rehabilitation should shift to an emphasis on facilitating increased activity before or after formal treatment sessions or exercise and as a means of managing pain flare-ups more independently.

Manual therapy, the manipulation of soft tissues, continues to occupy a large part of the modern physical therapist's scope of practice. Not necessarily new to medicine, manual techniques were described by Hippocrates (460 BC) with traction and immobilization as a means of reducing fractures.[71] Galen[72] later recommended techniques to treat "outwardly dislocated" vertebrae. Modern physical therapy's use of manual techniques is based on principles of osteopathic medicine introduced by Andrew T. Still in 1871 and chiropractic treatment pioneered by Daniel Palmer in the late 1800s. Today, many therapists receive special training and certification from a number of "schools" of manual therapy including Maitland, Paris, Kaltenborn, and McKenzie (Table 89.8).[73,74]

Therapeutic Exercise

Therapeutic exercises targets muscle and joint deficiencies (i.e., weakness, decreased conditioning, and contracture) and serves as the basis for rehabilitation of patients with acute or chronic musculoskeletal, postoperative, and posttraumatic rehabilitation

TABLE 89.8

MANUAL THERAPY

Manual Therapy school	Basic principles	Key terminology
Maitland (Australian)	Graded oscillatory movements to evaluate and treat joint stiffness and restore lost mobility	"S.I.N.S." algorithm *Severity, Irritability Nature of the complaint Stage of the pathology*
Paris, Stanley B. (New Zealand)	Focus on examination of spine, facet joint primary source for dysfunction in spine	Incorporates Maitland and Kaltenborn principles
Kaltenborn (Norwegian)	Arthrokinematics principles (e.g., concave-convex, closed-loosely packed positions), treat hypomobility even if asymptomatic	
McKenzie, R (Australia)	Directional preference • "centralization" vs. "peripheralization" of symptoms • Over pressure	
Cyriax, James (England)	Identify "lesion" Heat and friction massage for contractile structures and forceful manipulation with manual distraction to treat intra-articular displacement	

protocols (Table 89.9). The pain clinician must be cognizant of basic principles of physiology and guiding a patient through an individualized active strengthening program. This section will review important definitions and concepts related to therapeutic exercise. With rehabilitation of any injury, strength and endurance are important targets for assessment and treatment. Muscular strength is the ability of a muscle to generate force against resistance. Maintenance of strength of one's muscle or, more importantly, muscle groups, will help to improve function and prevent new or reinjury. Strength training also incorporates balance and coordination of movement. Muscular endurance is the ability to perform repetitive muscular contractions against some resistance over time. Endurance will tend to increase with strength. Improvements in muscular endurance may be more advantageous with regards to improving daily function.

In general, skeletal muscular contraction can be divided into three types of contractions: isometric, concentric, and eccentric.[75] Isometric contraction occurs when the muscle contracts without changing length. Isometric or static strength is necessary for performing many ADLs and in functional tasks or sports activities where a stable base of support is necessary for effective and efficient movement of joints. In pain rehabilitation, isometrics may be useful when joint motion is painful, a joint or joints are immobilized, or muscle or muscle groups are weak. In concentric contraction, the muscle shortens in length while tension increases to overcome or move some resistance. With eccentric contraction, resistance is greater than the muscular force being produced, lengthening the muscle while producing tension. This type of muscle activation may be associated with a higher incidence of delayed onset muscle soreness after exercise.[76] Thus, concentric exercises may be the focus of the program prior to progressing to more eccentric, unloaded ones.

Strength and muscular endurance are dependent on size of muscle or muscle groups, number of muscle fibers, neuromuscular function and efficiency, and biomechanical factors. Neuromuscular training (NT) is a growing area of practice with most work in rehabilitation of musculoskeletal injuries including anterior cruciate ligament reconstruction. NT can include balance exercises, plyometrics, agility training, and joint mobility exercises. Plyometric exercise, initially used to enhance sports performance, may also be used in later stages of an active therapy program as a means of returning the patient to previous levels of sport or work. Plyometric exercise causes a lengthening of the muscle-tendon unit followed immediately by shortening, hence called the stretch-shortening cycle. Plyometrics are used with various demands placed on the musculoskeletal system, usually initiated at lower intensity and progressed to more difficult and physically challenging higher intensity levels. The higher intensity levels may serve to resolve postinjury neuromuscular impairment and prepare the body to respond more effectively and safely to rapid changes in position and movement as well as greater levels of force seen in higher intensity exercise and physically demanding work tasks.[77]

Exercise Prescription

Exercise prescription for the patient with pain should include four basic goals[34,78]:

1. Changing sedentary behaviors to more active ones
2. Modifying risk factors for disability (e.g., obesity, hypertension, deconditioning)
3. Maintaining or improving exercise capacity as it relates to strength, aerobic capacity, balance, and flexibility
4. Enhance psychosocial function

Exercise prescription and focus may vary depending on the patient's age, medical comorbidities, and individual pain-related impairments (i.e., muscle strength, joint pain, joint contracture). Endurance exercise may help to reverse the cycle of deconditioning and weakness commonly seen with chronic pain patients and is an important part of the pain rehabilitation program. The phys-

TABLE 89.9

COMMON THERAPEUTIC EXERCISES

Exercise type	Description	Therapeutic uses
Closed kinetic chain	Proximal segment of the extremity moves on a fixed distal segment (e.g., leg press, squats, elliptical walker)	Shoulder and knee rehabilitation, dynamic stability
Concentric	Muscle contracts as it shortens (e.g., flexion phase of a biceps or hamstring curl)	Increase muscle mass and strength
Core stability	Targets low back, trunk, and abdominal muscles (e.g., sit up, back extension, abdominal crunch, Pilates)	Relief of low back pain or pregnancy-related pelvic pain
Eccentric	Muscle contracts as it lengthens (e.g., extension phase of biceps or hamstring curl)	Sport-specific strengthening to prevent injury
Isometric	Muscle contracts, but its length stays the same (e.g., holding a weight in a stationary position for a few seconds)	Muscle toning and strengthening when joint mobility is not advised; quadriceps exercises to treat patellofemoral pain syndrome
Isotonic	Constant resistance applied to a muscle through a joint range of motion (e.g., free-weight lifting)	General muscle conditioning
Open kinetic chain	Distal segment of the extremity moves about the proximal segments (e.g., long arc quadriceps extension, most weight-lifting exercises using the arms)	Functional improvement in ADLs

From Rand, SE, Goerlich C, Marchand K, et al. The physical therapy prescription. *Am Fam Physician* 2007; 76:1661–1666, with permission.

iologic effects of exercise have been shown to have analgesic effects, enhance mood, and improve self-efficacy. Circuit exercise programs, popular with the elderly population, have been shown to provide significant improvements in cardiorespiratory fitness, muscular strength, body composition, and serum cholesterol levels.[79]

Occupational Therapy

Activities of Daily Living

Occupational therapy focuses primarily on functional mobility and ADLs, as well as activity tolerance and ergonomic retraining. Occupational therapists typically concentrate on educating patients regarding proper posture and ergonomics related to upper limb functional activities such as lifting and computer usage as well as proper standing, sitting, carrying, and lifting postures. In general, occupational therapists address upper extremity related ADLs including feeding, hygiene, grooming, bathing, and dressing. Occupational therapists spend considerable time with the patient, educating them on the potential for increases in pain with reinitiation of movement early in the treatment process. Focus may later change to lifting training and tolerance building. Coaching on proper body mechanics could include a basic assess-

ment of maladaptive movement patterns, restriction in joint and soft tissue structures, as well as abnormal postures and bending or lifting techniques which may exacerbate and/or be the cause of ongoing pain and dysfunction. Occupational therapists are also responsible for managing and directing more individualized work conditioning and work hardening programs as well as administering functional capacity evaluations many times in coordination with the vocational rehabilitation team and employer.

Pacing

Another important concept occupational therapists are primarily responsible for is directing and instructing patients on activity, work, and leisure pacing. Pacing may be either an appropriate or a maladaptive behavior. Good pacing may include activity scheduling, taking breaks to complete a pain-inducing activity as compared to over-doing activities, and the "crashing and burning" approach with prolonged periods of rest and "down time" in order to recover from activity related flare-ups (Table 89.10).

The therapist is then able to work with the patients in improving their daily routines, incorporating pacing, taking appropriate breaks, and prioritizing activities while incorporating self-management skills learned in other disciplines such as relaxation techniques and stretching into the patient's daily routine at work, at home, and in leisure activities. Occupational therapists may also provide job site interventions which include assessing ergo-

TABLE 89.10

PACING: USEFUL VERSUS MALADAPTIVE RESPONSES

Useful	Maladaptive
1. Gradual increase in activity	Overdo activities
2. Increase on a quota system	Increase activity until "intolerable" pain
3. Varies mixed activities and rest	"Crash and burn": take extended periods of rest or prolonged down time after an activity or pain flare up
4. Realistic and manageable	Too busy to incorporate

Adapted from Harding VR, Williams AC. Extending physiotherapy skills using a psychological approach: cognitive-behavioral management of chronic pain. *Physiotherapy* 1995;81(11):681–688.

nomics and monitoring for job site safety issues. Services may also include job site training where a trained occupational or physical therapist accompanies the injured worker.

Pain Psychology

Psychologic interventions as part of a pain rehabilitation program have been shown to enhance recovery, decrease disability, and enhance psychosocial functioning.[80–83] Psychologic interventions focus on addressing maladaptive cognitions, passive avoidance, depression, anger, and pain-related anxiety. Initial focus of psychologic treatment includes challenging patients to change maladaptive thoughts and behaviors. As stated earlier, an individual's readiness to make important changes has been hypothesized to be an important factor in treatment success and serves as an important initial clinical question posed by the treating psychologist.[84–86] Over time, patients are also challenged to consider taking a more active role in management and incorporating nonpharmacologic and pharmacologic therapies into their individualized program. Problem solving training may help to teach patients to choose more effective responses to pain and improve function.[87] Incorporating group pain psychology interventions with an active physical therapy program has been shown to enhance posttreatment outcomes as compared to physical therapy alone on measures of functional impairment, employment of active coping strategies, medication use, and self-efficacy beliefs.[88]

Combining group cognitive-behavioral therapy and relaxation therapy with an individually based multidisciplinary treatment (cognitive-behavioral therapy, physical and occupational therapy, and social work) program demonstrated an additive effect with greater improvement on measures of pain, sleep, activity levels, and medication use.[89,89a]

Relaxation Training

Further, incorporating relaxation techniques (i.e., deep breathing, progressive muscle relaxation) with therapeutic stretching can help the patient progress in the exercise program and improve activity tolerance. Biofeedback is a treatment that has been shown to be quite effective in the management of pain.[90] The treatment serves to help a patient become more aware of their physiologic responses to pain or other stressors. In general, relaxation training focuses on helping the patient to acquire self-management tools for reducing tension and decreasing pain. Initial treatment involves basic education explaining how biofeedback-assisted

therapies work and helping the patient to understand they are able to control or modulate physiologic functioning of their own bodies by "seeing" or "hearing" their own physiologic function (i.e., breathing, limb temperature, and sweat).

Skills training includes training with basic biofeedback technologies such as respiratory biofeedback, surface electromyography, and/or thermal biofeedback. Techniques include diaphragmatic breathing, progressive muscle relaxation, and autogenic techniques. Patients are encouraged to log their practice sessions in their relaxation practice log. Relaxation training is provided in one-on-one and in group settings usually provided by a health psychologist, biofeedback specialist, or physical or occupational therapist. At the conclusion of formal treatment, patients should be independent with relaxation self-management techniques and be able to incorporate practice and technique integration with normal daily activities and during times of symptom flare-up or elevated levels of distress.

WORK REHABILITATION: WORK CONDITIOING AND WORK HARDENING

Work conditioning and work hardening are an important core component of work therapy in the field of industrial and pain rehabilitation. This field of modern occupational therapy developed after World War II with a focus of FR in wounded veterans as a means of securing employment in the civilian world after returning from duty. Work therapy also includes acute treatment, job analysis and placement, and functional capacity evaluation. Multidisciplinary principles were applied to occupational therapy based work rehabilitation in the 1950s with the development of improved assessment tools and systems and the addition of vocational counseling, medical management, and industrial engineering. In the 1970s, work hardening and conditioning programs were combined with behavioral medicine approaches that focused on reducing abnormal illness behaviors in a more comprehensive treatment of injured workers primarily with low back pain. Eventually, standards were established and subsequently updated by CARF in the late 1989s and early 1990s, respectively. Work rehabilitation usually begins once a patient has reached a treatment plateau in active physical therapy and is unable to return to work due to pain-related impairments (Table 89.11).

TABLE 89.11

WORK REHABILITATION

Musculoskeletal exercise	Stability–mobility Strength–endurance Balance–coordination
Aerobic training	Equipment based Aerobic classes Functional activities
Education	Principles Technique training Problem solving
Work activity	Simulated activity Actual equipment Actual work

From Isernhagen SJ. Work Hardening. In: Demeter SL, Andersson GB, eds. *Disability Evaluation.* 2nd ed. St. Louis: Mosby; 2003:769–780, with permission.

TABLE 89.12

COMPONENTS IN A TYPICAL WORK HARDENING PROGRAM

Step I Job analysis	Step II Establishing work tolerance baseline	Step III Individual work hardening plan/goals
Understand worker's specific job require- ments Critical Job Tasks Physical Job Demands Psychosocial Demands High-risk Job Factors *If job analysis available: review and vali- date primary job functions *If job analysis not available: on site job task analysis	Medical History Worker Interview Job Description with Critical Job Demands Pain Assessment Physical Assessment Work Posture and Mobility Strength, Sensation, Coordination, Lifting, Reaching, Carrying, Pushing and Pulling, Stooping, Bending, Kneeling, Sitting and Standing, Work Task Stimulation	1. Increase duration of daily participation 2. Increase physical tolerances to the level of critical job demands 3. Improve body mechanics and postures 4. Develop pain management strategies 5. Develop problem-solving skills for self- management at the work site 6. Facilitate appropriate worker behaviors

Work conditioning is usually concentrated on the physical components of flexibility, strength, coordination, and endurance and involves one discipline of treatment (i.e., physical or occupational therapy). A more multidisciplinary approach is seen with work hardening, which incorporates behavioral and vocational components with a formal focus on return to job-specific tasks or positions. Work conditioning is routinely coordinated with acute medical management as compared to work hardening, which is usually provided later in therapy within the rehabilitation phase of treatment.

Work hardening programs were initially described by Matheson at Rancho Los Amigos Hospital[91] as a work-oriented program focused on improvement in the client's productivity versus symptom reduction or increased physical capacity. A "client" can be described as an injured worker with impairments that do not match their job position, a worker with disease-based impairments with diminishing physical capacity, a job applicant who may not have the physical abilities to perform the intended job, or a currently employed worker in transition to a job requiring higher physical function.[92]

Work hardening is an individualized, work specific, multi- and interdisciplinary program centered primarily on returning patients (i.e., the injured worker) to their previous level of work or work demands. Work hardening uses real or simulated work tasks and progressively increasing conditioning, flexibility, neuromuscular control, and tolerances (Tables 89.12 and 89.13). Goals of work hardening include (1) attaining optimal physical tolerances and abilities, (2) maximizing cognitive and psychosocial functioning, (3) developing appropriate worker behaviors, (4) reducing fear and increasing confidence for the resumption of productive work, and (5) identifying problems that may necessitate placement in an alternative job.[93,94]

An individualized work hardening program incorporates a three step process which includes an initial formal job analysis to determine specific duties, completion of a baseline work tolerance evaluation, and establishment of the individual work hardening plan. Work hardening standards have been established by a number of groups and may vary depending on the state or the federal governing body.[95]

Occupational therapy manages most work conditioning and work hardening treatments as part of the pain rehabilitation program. Assessment of the injured worker is more comprehensive than the assessment done during standard occupational therapist evaluations. Patients are placed in programs of a set number of days, usually 4 to 5 days per week over a 4 to 8 week period. Both programs are highly based on objective measures obtained during the program evaluation which includes tolerances and ca-

pacities for lifting, pulling, standing, sitting, reaching, climbing, kneeling, and/or crawling. The treatment program is based on the individual patient's own job demands and work level (sedentary, light, medium, heavy) and developing improved conditioning and tolerances for activities (Table 89.14). Although formal psychologic counseling is not a core discipline, these programs are based on helping patients work through and unlearn fear avoidance beliefs and movement patterns, pain-related fear, catastrophizing, and pain-related anxiety.

TABLE 89.13

WORK HARDENING PROGRAM STANDARDS

1. Improve strength and endurance in relation to return to work goal
2. Simulation of critical work demands, tasks, and environment of the job worker will return to
3. Education: body mechanics, pacing, safety, and injury prevention, promoting worker responsibility and self-management
4. Assess for need for job modifications (i.e., equipment changes or additions, ergonomic modification). Availability for on site job modification assessments
5. Individualized written plan which includes observable and measurable goals
6. Safe work or therapy environment that is appropriate for reaching vocational goals
7. Quality assurance system, outcomes based on program and worker goals
8. Documentation or reporting system that includes initial plan, regularly scheduled team conference notes with monitoring of progress, record of attendance, and compliance
9. Evaluation and modification of work behaviors (i.e., timeliness, attendance, interpersonal relationships)
10. Criteria for admission includes physical recovery sufficient to allow for progressive reactivation and participation for a minimum of 4 hours a day for 3 to 5 days a week along with a defined work goal
11. Criteria for discharge clearly stated (i.e., patient met goal stated in plan, patient did not participate according to program plan, goals not feasible to attain)

Adapted from State of Washington Department of Labor and Industries. Work Hardening Program Standards. Available at: http://www.lni.wa.gov/ClaimsIns/Files/ReturnToWork/WhStds.pdf. Accessed October 12, 2008.

TABLE 89.14

PHYSICAL DEMAND AND LEVEL OF JOB DUTY

Physical demand	Occasionally	Frequently	Constantly
Sedentary duty	Lift or carry up to 10 lbs	Negligible	Negligible
	Sit 6–8 h	—	—
	Stand or walk 0–2 h	—	—
Light duty	Lift or carry up to 20 lbs	Up to 10 lbs	Negligible
	Stand 4–8 h	—	—
	Walk 0–4 h	—	—
Medium duty	Lift or carry up to 50 lbs	Up to 20 lbs	Up to 10 lbs
	Stand or walk 8 h	—	—
Heavy duty	Lift or carry up to 100 lbs	Up to 50 lbs	Up to 20 lbs
	Stand or walk 8 h	—	—
Very heavy duty	Lift or carry over 100 lbs	Over 50 lbs	Over 20 lbs
		—	—

From U.S. Department of Labor. *Dictionary of Occupational Titles.* Washington, DC: U.S. Government Printing Office; 1986.

Outcomes of Work Conditioning and Work Hardening Programs

Reviews of work conditioning and work hardening programs have found evidence of improved return to work rates and fewer work days off in treated patients versus controls.[96–98]

MEASURING PHYSICAL CAPACITY

Functional capacity testing provides a means of measuring function by obtaining objective and subjective data with performance-based testing. Testing can be divided into two groups of tests including examining isolated parts of the body or "functional units" (i.e., lumbar spine, shoulder) and the ability of the functional unit to interact with other bodily functional units or activities such as lifting capacity. Lifting capacity many times involves the interplay of the biomechanical chain of a number of systems. A common example of the biomechanical chain includes transferring forces from a simple lifting task from the ground. Here, forces of the biomechanical chain include transferring forces from the hands through the elbow and shoulder (upper extremity functional unit) to the lumbar spine and hips (lower extremity functional unit) to placing the object and transmitting forces to the floor.

Functional Capacity Testing

Functional capacity evaluation (FCE) is a process where the individual's ability to perform a specific task or physical demands of a job is assessed, bridging the gap between observed physical impairment and work capacity. Matheson[99] describes the FCE as "a systematic method of measuring an individual's ability to perform meaningful tasks in a safe and dependable basis." FCEs have three specific purposes: (1) to improve the likelihood that the patient will be safe in a job task, (2) to assist in improving role performance through assessing and identifying functional decrements as a means of providing appropriate treatment or therapy, and (3) to determine presence of disability for bureaucratic or legal entities that may assign a quantifiable level of impairment or apportionment or deny monetary or medical disability benefits.[100]

The FCE is a valuable tool for the physician, vocational counselor, therapist, or employer to establish a specific attainable work goal based on objective data. In theory, by comparing performance demonstrated on the FCE to the required physical job demands of the individual worker, meeting or exceeding all job requirements simulated during testing will help to determine if the patient is safe to return to work.[101] Better performance on a FCE, many times defined by lower number of failed tasks during testing, may be associated with lower risk of recurrence after return to work.[102,103]

Various types of FCEs can be performed as a means of obtaining specific vocational goals including establishing functional goal setting, disability rating, job and occupation matching, and work capacity evaluation.[104] In general, the FCE can be done before treatment and usually once a patient has reached a treatment plateau or has completed a formal acute or subacute therapy program. As a means of determining impairment of disability, a FCE may compare measured functional capacity either to the patient's preinjury baseline abilities or population norms. Accurate measurements of a worker's preinjury capacities rarely exist, and health care providers are many times inaccurate in estimating the worker's preinjury functional level or physical capabilities.[105]

The FCE is used to establish a final level of functioning and includes a statement regarding validity, effort, and pain behaviors. A number of validated FCE tests and programs are available from a number of vendors and are individually designed for specific disorders such as low back pain or upper extremity conditions. These tests can be incorporated into a larger battery of tests used in the formal FCE.

Strength testing may include assessing lifting, carrying, pushing and pulling, work stimulation, and circuit testing (Table 89.15).

Common assessment and job simulation devices include the Purdue Pegboard Test, the Crawford Small Parts Dexterity Test, and the Jebsen Hand Dexterity Test. Testing usually lasts between 2 to 6 hours and may also be performed over a number of days to observe for fluctuations in performance depending on change in pain or to make sure the patient meets the demands of more continuous work-related physical activity.

Performance reliability is used to determine performance credibility based on the assumption an individual will produce similar outcomes in a series of trials.[106] Additional objective measures may also be assessed including increase in heart rate during and immediately following performance of a strenuous task. Perfor-

FUNCTIONAL CAPACITY EVALUATION LIFTING PROTOCOLS

Test	Test of	Specific tests	Progression	
Isoinsertional Lifting Evaluation	Occasional lifting tolerance	4 lifts: floor to knuckle, 12 inch to knuckle, waist to shoulder, shoulder to overhead carry	Weight increased in 10 lb increments, if too much pain, decrease by 5 lb	
Dynamic Carrying, Pushing and Pulling Tests		1. Carrying 2. Pushing (sled) 3. Pulling (Sled)	Resistance increased in 10 lb increments	
Progressive Isoinertial Lifting Evaluation (PILE)	Frequent lifting capacity	Lumbar PILE: (floor to 30 inch high shelf) Cervical PILE: (30 inch shelf to 54 inch shelf)	Starting weight 13 lb (male), 8 lb (female)	End Points: 85% of max predicted age adjusted heart rate, 55% to 60% body weight

mance credibility can be subjectively determined by assessing for consistency and incongruity between specific tasks and tests. Reports of pain and pain behavior should be specific to the body part and correlate with the level or area of injury.[107] Performances that do not follow normal or expected patterns may also be indicative of less than sincere effort.

Subjective credibility measures may include the individual's perceived physical strain or effort and may be rated on a number of Ratings of Perceived Exertion scales. In one example scores range from 6 to 19 (e.g., 6 [no exertion], 7 ["very, very light"], 15 ["hard"] to 19 ["very, very hard"]) and increase linearly with exercise intensity. Values of the scale correlate to heart rate (0.8–0.9), ranging from 60–200 beats per minute.[108]

Grip strength assessment in the FCE serves two important purposes: to assess hand grip strength and to document performance of maximum voluntary efforts. A common test used in many clinics and mentioned in FCE reports is the Jamar hand dynamometer (Sammons Preston Rolyan, Bolingbrook, IL), a calibrated hydraulic hand dynamometer, which measures static grip strength at five grip spans. The therapist is able to produce a graphical representation of the forces produced at five grip positions, revealing a classic "biomechanical curve," with the lowest force values occurring in positions one and five and the highest at positions two, three, or four. Inability to produce this bell-shaped curve could cast doubt on the individual's sincerity of full maximal effort. Force variability of multiple trials can be applied to normative data and can also be used to indicate noncredible performance.[109]

Functional Capacity Testing Utility

An important and controversial area of FCE results lies in its ability to demonstrate validity, reliability, and accuracy.[110,111] Lemstra et al.[112] examined the tester's ability to judge maximal effort in a standard lifting protocol. They found high specificity but low sensitivity (62%) with only a small number of commonly used maximal lifting tests (5 of 17) able to differentiate between maximal and submaximal effort.[112] Results of a functional capacity test can be used in conjunction with a more detailed understanding of the individual's job description as a means of establishing return to work restrictions and formal levels of work (see Table 89.14).[112,113]

What Does an "Invalid" Test Mean?

In clinical practice, "invalid" test results may be related to the patient demonstrating less than full effort in performance. Although not always consistent with malingering, a number of other causes (i.e., physical ability, disability, pain intensity, and fear of reinjury) have been identified and should be considered when interpreting and making clinical decisions based on an invalid test or test with evidence of less than "full" or "maximal effort" (Table 89.16).[114–118]

The result of an FCE can have far reaching consequences including injured workers having compensation terminated or losing their job or seeing a reduced medico-legal settlement in patients believed to be exhibiting submaximal effort.[119] In order to establish one's functional capacity, the injured worker must perform at his or her maximal ability or effort. A number of tests have been used as a means of validating effort. Methods used to assess sincerity of effort include Waddell nonorganic signs, pain behavior description, symptom magnification, coefficients of variation, correlations between physical evaluation and function, grip measurements, and temporal relationship between heart rate and increased levels of pain with activity.[119]

CAUSES OF INVALID FUNCTIONAL CAPACITY EVALUATION TESTS/LESS THAN FULL EFFORT

1. Malingering syndrome
2. Factitious disorder
3. Learned illness behavior
4. Conversion disorder, pain disorder, or other somatoform disorders
5. Depressive disorders
6. Test anxiety
7. Fear of symptom exacerbation or injury
8. Fatigue
9. Medication and psychoactive substance effects
10. Lowered self-efficacy expectations
11. Need to gain recognition of symptoms

From American Institutes for Research. *Synthesis of research and development of prototypes for a new disability determination methodology: measurement concepts and issues relevant to the Social security Administration's disability determination process.* Washington, DC: American Institutes for Research; 1999.

ROLE OF OPIOID MANAGEMENT IN PAIN REHABILITATION

The role of chronic opioid management in pain rehabilitation remains a controversial topic. Pain rehabilitation programs as early as the 1960s focused primarily in reducing and or eliminating opioids secondary to fears of tolerance and development of iatrogenic addiction. This approach still characterizes many interdisciplinary programs today. However, the shift to more liberal use of opioids for chronic noncancer-related pain in the1990s and the assumption that risk for addiction was minimal led to increased use of opioids in the treatment of chronic pain.[120–123] The more recent reappraisal of the benefits and potential harms of chronic opioid use has also led to more questions regarding the accuracy of predicting aberrant behavior, and quantifying rates of addiction[124–127] use has been complicated by an appreciation for not only the potential risk for developing aberrant behaviors and addiction in a small percentage of patients but also for the development of other potential opioid-induced adverse effects, including cognitive impairment, endocrine function (sexual dysfunction and opioid induced hypogonadism), and mood.[128–131]

Risk stratification for determining potential risk for abuse and misuse and more comprehensive screening prior to initiating an opioid trial is finding greater acceptance in the evolving field of pain management.[132] Unfortunately, many patients referred for pain rehabilitation treatment may include a greater number of opioid treatment "failures" and/or patients additionally managed with other controlled substances (i.e., benzodiazepines and hypnotics). A number of reasons for "failing" should be considered during the evaluation and subsequent treatment planning and include ruling out improper or maladaptive opioid or controlled substance use, poorly designed opioid and/or pharmacologic regimen, poor or limited analgesic response with adverse effects, opioid induced pain sensitivity, or a combination of these factors (Table 89.17).

A pain rehabilitation approach may also offer a patient self-management treatment tools with potentially similar or even greater clinical outcomes than those achieved by his or her opioids. Concurrent pharmacologic management may include a structured taper off the currently used opioid, conversion to methadone, or conversion to buprenorphine products. Use of U.S. Food and Drug Administration-approved buprenorphine products for opioid dependence (i.e., buprenorphine and buprenorphine and naloxone) requires specialized licensure by clinicians. Treatment of withdrawal signs and symptoms primarily includes the use of oral or transdermal clonidine, an α_2-adrenergic ago-

nist,[133] and adjuvants for withdrawal-related myalgias, insomnia, anxiety, and gastrointestinal distress.[134]

The advantage of a structured and relatively controlled environment of most multidisciplinary and interdisciplinary treatment programs is that it offers an opportunity for patients with limited or maximized improvement on chronic opioids to reduce or eliminate opioids while at the same time learning to apply new nonpharmacologic approaches to management of their pain. This structured environment is ideal for more successfully integrating a more rational polypharmacy approach.

Behavioral medicine treatments can be effectively incorporated into a structured multi- or interdisciplinary rehabilitation based program. Treatment of the chemically dependent patient can include two types of therapies: (1) psychotherapeutic strategies and (2) mind-body therapies.[135] Psychotherapeutic strategies include supportive-expressive psychotherapy, drug counseling, family therapy, and motivational enhancement therapy. Mind-body therapies, in general, include cognitive-behavioral therapy, group support and education therapy, and relaxation therapy (i.e., deep breathing, imagery, hypnosis, and biofeedback) (Table 89.18).

Patients can be successfully weaned or have their opioid dose decreased during a FR rehabilitation-based approach. Active opioid withdrawal did not adversely impact short-term outcomes following a 3-week outpatient pain program,[136] and physical and emotional functioning were favorable in a fibromyalgia cohort that completed an interdisciplinary pain rehabilitation program which included withdrawal of opioids, nonsteroidal anti-inflammatory drugs, benzodiazepines, and muscle relaxants.[137]

TABLE 89.17

POTENTIAL SCOPE AND SPECTRUM OF USE OF OPIOIDS IN PAIN REHABILITATION

1. Rule out improper or maladaptive use of opioids for their non-analgesic reasons (i.e., depression, psychologic tolerance, anxiety)
2. Adjust regimen, limit short-acting, limit total daily dose while patient learns additional nonpharmacologic skills to manage pain and pain-related disability
3. Detoxification secondary to failed analgesia, poor functional outcomes related to use
4. Slow taper down in total daily dose while monitoring for changes in mood, cognition
5. Detoxification secondary to development of possible opioid induced hyperalgesia
6. Detoxification secondary to pain condition not fully or partially responsive to opioid analgesics

TABLE 89.18

BEHAVIORAL TREATMENT TECHNIQUES FOR THE CHEMICALLY DEPENDENT PATIENT

Psychotherapeutic Strategies
  Supportive-Expressive Psychotherapy
  Multidimensional Family Therapy
  Motivational Enhancement Therapy

Mind-body Therapies
  Cognitive-Behavioral Therapy
  Relaxation Techniques
    Meditation, guided, or self-guided imagery, progressive muscle relaxation, deep breathing

Adapted from Wooten J. Behavioral Medicine Treatment in the Management of the Chemically Dependent Patient. In Smith HS, Passik SD, eds. *Pain and Chemical Dependency*. New York: Oxford University Press; 2008:253–258.

CONCLUSION

Rehabilitation is a continuous process, relying on a comprehensive, pragmatic approach that focuses on an individual's physical impairments and function-related disability. The field of modern pain rehabilitation developed along with the growth of a number of medical specialties (i.e., anesthesia, rehabilitation medicine, psychiatry, neurology, and occupational medicine), physical and occupational therapy, and health psychology. Pain rehabilitation assessment and treatment is based on a biopsychosocial model. A narrower dualistic biomedical model may fail to adequately assess and help patients to manage the complexities of ongoing pain, affective distress, and environmental and social issues. Treatment goals in pain rehabilitation programs include improving psychosocial functioning, decreasing pain, improving aerobic conditioning, and facilitating safe and successful return to work status, return to leisure pursuits, and activities at home and in the community.

A pain rehabilitation approach includes planning and coordinating various medical interventions (i.e., pharmacologic and nonpharmacologic), educational activities, and coordinating a patient's participation with specific rehabilitation-based disciplines (i.e., physical and occupational therapy, pain psychology, relaxation and other mind body therapies). Vocational rehabilitation can serve as an additional treatment option and may be coordinated in patient-specific work-based therapies such as work conditioning and work hardening programs. Work conditioning and work hardening may be more specific levels of treatment for the injured worker as a bridge to progress patients after completing acute rehabilitation and more closely simulating work activities, respectively, prior to returning to previous levels of sport, function, or work. Functional capacity testing may be used as a more objective means of establishing a baseline level of function, establish treatment and work goals, or finalize return to work level of functioning. Validity measures may also help to identify physical and psychosocial factors that are contributing to the injured worker's level of functioning and clarify discrepancies in tolerances and effort.

The pain rehabilitation clinician must work with the patient in conjunction with various stakeholders (i.e., case managers, insurance providers and adjustors, legal personnel, and family members). The clinician's role may include additional responsibilities beyond only working to help patients decrease pain and increase function, but also as an advocate for the patient with insurers, employers, and rare circumstances as adjudicator, helping the insurer or employer to decrease or identify inconsistent or fraudulent patient behavior. Optimal patient outcomes are facilitated by the clinician and team members establishing a therapeutic environment with the patient characterized by ongoing coordination of care, communication between treatment team members and the patient, providing consistency of message, and collaboration between team members.

References

1. Weigl M, Cieza C, Cantista P, et al. Physical disability due to musculoskeletal conditions. *Best Pract Res Clin Rheumatol* 2007;21:167–190.
2. Hopkins HL, Smith HD, Tiffany EG. Rehabilitation. In: Hopkins HL, Smith HD, eds. *Willard and Spackman's Occupational Therapy*. 6th ed. Philadelphia: JB Lippincott; 1983.
3. Foley BS, Buschbacher RM. Occupational rehabilitaiton. In: Braddom RL, ed. *Physical Medicine and Rehabilitation*. 3rd ed. Philadelphia: Saunders Elsevier; 2007:1047–1054.
4. Zimmermann M. The history of pain concepts and treatment before IASP. In: Merskey H, Loeser J, Dubner R, eds. *The Paths of Pain. 1975–2005*. Seattle: IASP Press; 2005.
5. Murphy W. *Healing the Generations: A History of Physical Therapy and the American Physical Therapy Association*. Alexandria, VA: American Physical Therapy Association; 1995.
6. Bonica JJ. Organization and function of a pain clinic. *Northwest Med* 1950; 49:593–596.
7. Turk DC. Biopsychosocial perspective on chronic pain. In: Gatchel RJ, Turk DC, eds. *Psychological Approaches to Pain Management: A Practitioner's Handbook*. New York: Guilford Press; 1996:33–52.
8. Keefe FJ, Dunsmore J, Burnett R. Behavioral and cognitive-behavioral approaches to chronic pain: recent advances and future directions. *J Consult Clin Psychol* 1002;60:528–536.
9. Weiner BK. The biopsychosocial model and spine care. *Spine* 2008;33: 219–223.
10. Brena SF. Pain control facilities: patterns of operation and problems of organization in the USA. *Clin Anesth* 1985;3.
11. Sullivan MJ. Toward a biopsychomotor concpetualization of pain. *Clin J Pain* 2008;24:281–290.
12. Curry R. Understanding patients with chronic pain in work hardening programs. Work programs special interest section newsletter (American Occupational Therapy Association). 1989;3:3.
13. Wegg L. Role of occupational therapist in vocational rehabilitation. *Am J Occup Ther* 1957;11:4.
14. Wegg L. Essentials of work evaluation. *Am J Occup Ther* 1960;14:65.
15. Commission on Accreditation of Rehabilitation Facilities. *Standards Manual*

for Organizations Serving People with Disabilities. Tucson, AZ: Author; 1989.
16. Commission on Practice. *Occupational Therapy Services in Work Practice: Official Statement*. Bethesda, MD: American Occupational Therapy Association; 1992.
17. Matheson LN. Work hardening for patients with back pain. *J Musculoskel Med* 1993;10:53–63.
18. Gatchel RG, Mayer TG, Hazard RG, et al. Editorial: functional restoration. Pitfalls in evaluating efficacy. *Spine* 1992;17:988–994.
19. Nocon A, Baldwin S. *Trends in Rehabilitation Policy. A Review of the Literature*. London: Kings Fund; 1998.
20. Waddell G, Burton AK. Concepts of rehabilitation for the management of low back pain. *Best Pract Research Clin Rheum* 2005;19:655–670.
21. den Boer JJ, Oostendorp RA, Beems T, et al. Reduced work capacity after lumbar disc surgery: role of cognitive-behavioral related risk factors. *Pain* 2006;126(1–3):72–78.
22. Donceel P, DuBois M. Predictors of work incapacity continuing after disc surgery. *Scand J Work Environ Health* 1999;25:264–271.
23. Schultz IZ, Stowell AW, Feurstein M, et al. Models of return to work for musculoskeletal disorders. *J Occup Rehabil* 2007;17:327–352.
24. Sullivan JM, Main C. Service, advocacy and adjudication: balancing the ethical challenges of multiple stakeholder agendas in the rehabilitation of chronic pain. *Dis Rehab* 2007;29:1596–1603.
25. Mayer T, Gatchel R, Kishino N, et al. Objective assessment of spine function following industrial injury. A prospective study with comparison group and one year follow-up. *Spine* 1985;10:482–493.
26. Descartes R. *De Homine*. Leyden: Moyardus and Leffen; 1662.
27. Melzack R, Wall P. Pain mechanisms: a new theory. *Science* 1965;150: 971–979.
28. Melzack R. From the gate to the neuromatrix. *Pain* 1999;6:S121–S126.
29. Pransky G, Shaw WS, Franche R, et al. Disability prevention and communication among workers, physicians, employers, and insurers: current models and opportunities for improvement. *Disabil Rehabil* 2004;26:625–634.
30. Carragee EJ. Persistent low back pain. *N Engl J Med* 2005;352:1891–1898.
31. Engel GL. The need for a new medical model: a challenge for biomedicine. *Science* 1977;196:129–136.
32. World Health Organization. *International Classification of Functioning, Disability and Health*. Geneva: World Health Organization:2001. Available at: http://www3.who.int/icf/icftemplate/cfm. Accessed August 28, 2009.
33. American Physical Therapy Association. The guide to physical therapist practice, 2nd ed. *Phys Ther* 81(1):9–738.
34. Fiatarone MA. Exercise to prevent and treat functional disability. *Clin Geriatr Med* 2002;18:431–462.
35. Boon H, Verhoef M, O'Hara D, et al. From parallel practice to integrative health care: a conceptual framework. *BMC Health Serv Res* 2004;4:15.
36. Loeser 1991. Desirable characteristics for pain management facilities. In: Bond MJ, ed. *Pain Research and Management*. Amsterdam: Elsevier; 1991. 411–416.
37. Mayer T, Gatchel R, Kishino N. Objective assessment of spine function following industrial injury: A prospective study with comparison groups and one-year follow up. *Spine* 1985;B:82–93.
38. Fordyce WE. *Behavioral Methods for Chronic Pain and Illness*. St. Louis: Mosby; 1976.
39. Norrefalk JR, Linder J, Ekholm J, et al. A 6-year follow-up study of 122 patients attending a multiprofessional rehabilitation programme for persistent musculoskeletal-related pain. *Int J Rehabil Res* 2007;30(1):9–18.
40. Angst F, Brioschi R, Main CJ, et al. Interdisciplinary rehabilitation in fibromyalgia and chronic back pain: a prospective outcome study. *J Pain* 2006;7: 807–815.
41. Mayer TG, Gatchel RJ, Mayer H, et al. A prospective two-year study of functional restoration in industrial low back injury. An objective assessment procedure. *JAMA* 1987;258:1763–1767.
42. Westman A, Linton S, Theorell T, et al. Quality of life and maintenance of improvements after early multimodal rehabilitation: a 5-year follow-up. *Disab Rehab* 2006;28:437–446.
43. Grahn B, Ekdahl C, Borgquist L. Effects of a multidisciplinary rehabilitation programme on health-related quality of life in patients with prolonged musculoskeletal disorders: a 6-month follow-up of a prospective controlled study. *Disabil Rehabil* 1998;20:285–297.
44. Turk DC. Clinical effectiveness and cost effectiveness of treatment for patients with chronic pain. *Clin J Pain* 2002;18:355–365.
45. Chou R, Qaseem A, Snow V, et al. Diagnosis and treatment of low back pain: a joint clinical practice guideline from the American College of Physicians and the American Pain Society. *Ann Intern Med* 2007;147(7):478–491.
46. Gatchel RJ, Okifuji A. Evidence-based scientific data documenting the treatment and cost-effectiveness of comprehensive pain programs for chronic nonmalignant pain. *J Pain* 2006;7(11):779–793.
47. Guzman J, Esmail R, Karjalaninen K. Multidisciplinary rehabilitation for chronic low back pain: systematic review. *BMJ* 2001;322:1511–1516.
48. Hatten A, Gatchel R, Polatin P, et al. A cost-utility analysis of chronic spinal pain treatment outcomes: converting SF-36 data into quality-adjusted life years. *Clin J Pain* 2006;22:700–711.
49. Jordan K, Mayer TG, Gatchel RJ. Should extended disability be an exclusion criterion for tertiary rehabilitation? Socioeconomic outcomes of early versus late functional restoration in compensation spinal disorders. *Spine* 1998;23: 2110–2116.

50. Ekto-Andersen J, Ingvarsson E, Kullendorff M, et al. High cost-benefit of early team-based biomedical and cognitive-behavior intervention for long-term pain-related sickness absence. *J Rehabil Med* 2008;40:1–9.

51. Norrefalk JR, Ekholm K, Linder J, et al. Evaluation of a multiprofessional rehabilitation programme for persistent musculoskeletal-related pain: economic benefits of return to work. *J Rehabil Med* 2008;40:15–22.

52. Bronfenbrenner U. *The Ecology of Human Development: Experiments by Nature and Design.* Cambridge, MA: Harvard University Press; 1979.

53. Stucki G. International Classification of Functioning, Disability, and Health (ICF): a promising framework and classification for rehabilitation medicine. *Am J Phys Med Rehab* 2005;84(10):733–740.

54. Steiner WQ, Ryser L, Huber E, et al. Use of the ICF model as a clinical problem-solving tool in physical therapy and rehabilitation medicine. *Phys Ther* 2002;82:(11):1098–1107.

55. Tate DG, Habeck RV, Schwartz G. Disability management: a comprehensive framework for prevention and rehabilitation in the workplace. *Rehabil Lit* 1986;47:230–235.

56. Stephens B, Gross DP. The influence of a continuum of care model on the rehabilitation of compensation claimants with soft tissue disorders. *Spine* 2007;32:2898–2904.

57. Loisel P, Falardeau M, Baril R, et al. The values underlying team decision-making in work rehabilitation for musculoskeletal disorders. *Disab Rehab* 2005;27:561–569.

58. Jensen MP. Enhancing motivation to change in pain treatment. In: Turk DC, Gatchel RJ, eds. *Psychological Approaches to Pain Management: A Practitioner's Handbook.* New York: Guilford Press; 1996:78–111.

59. Kearns RD, Rosenberg R, Jamison RN, et al. Readiness to adopt a self-management approach to chronic pain: the Pain Stages of Change Questionnaire (PSCOQ). *Pain* 1997;72:227–234.

60. Jensen MP, Nielson WR, Turner JA, et al. Changes in readiness to self-manage pain are associated with improvement in multidisciplinary pain treatment and pain coping. *Pain* 2004;111:84–95.

61. Prochaska J, DiClemente C. *The Transtheoretical Approach: Crossing Traditional Boundaries of Therapy.* Homewood, IL: Dow Jones Irwin; 1984.

62. Beardwood BA, Kirsh B, Clark NJ. Victims twice over: perceptions and experiences of injured workers. *Qual Health Res* 2005;15:30–48.

63. Jensen GM, Lorish CD. Promoting patient cooperation with exercise programs: linking research, theory, and practice. *Arthritis Care Res* 1994;4: 181–189.

64. Meichenbaum D, Turk DC. *Facilitation Treatment Adherence: A Practitioner's Guidebook.* New York: Plenum; 1987.

65. Harding V, Williams AC. Extending physiotherapy skills using a psychological approach: cognitive-behavioral management of chronic pain. *Physiotherapy* 1996;81:681–688.

66. Main CJ, Sullivan JM, Watson PJ. *Pain Management: Practical Application of the Biopshcyosocial Perspective in Clinical and Occupational Settings* 2nd ed. Edinburgh: Churchill Livingstone; 2007.

67. Turk DC, Okifuji A. A cognitive-behavioral approach to pain management. In: Melzack R, Wall PD, eds. *Handbook of Pain Management: A Clinical Companion to Wall and Melzack's Textbook of Pain.* Edinburgh: Churchill Livingstone; 2003:533–541.

68. Fordyce WE. *Behavioral Methods for Chronic Pain and Illness.* St. Louis: Mosby; 1976.

69. Fordyce WE, Fowler RS, Lehmann JF, et al. Operant conditioning in the treatment of chronic pain. *Arch Phys Med Rehabil* 5:399–408.

70. van den Hout JH, Vlaeyen JW, Heuts PH, et al. Secondary prevention of work-related disability in nonspecific low back pain: does problem-solving therapy help? A randomized clinical trial. *Clin J Pain* 2003;29:87–96.

71. Ackerknecht EH. *A Short History of Medicine.* New York: Ronald Press; 1975.

72. Schiotz EH, Cyriax J. *Manipulation: Past and Present.* London: William Heinemann; 1978.

73. Hall RC, Nitz AJ. Basic concepts of orthopedic manual therapy. In: Malone T, McPoil T, Nitz A, eds. *Orthopedic and Sports Physical Therapy.* 3rd ed. St Louis: Mosby; 1997:191–209.

74. Maitland GD. *Vertebral Manipulation.* 4th ed. Boston: MA: Butterworth; 1984. McKenzie R. *The Lumbar Spine: Mechanical Diagnosis and Therapy.* Waikane, New Zealand: Spinal Publications; 1981:95–106.

75. Prentice WE. Impaired muscle performance: regaining muscular strength and endurance. In: Voight M, Hoogenboom B, Prentice WE, eds. *Musculoskeletal Interventions. Techniques for Therapeutic Exercise.* New York: McGraw-Hill Medical; 2007.

76. Gabriel D, Kamen G, Frost G. Neural adaptations to resistive exercise: mechanisms and recommendations from training practices. *Sports Med* 2006;36: 133–149.

77. Chmielewski TL, Myer GD, Kauffman D, et al. Plyometric exercise in the rehabilitation of athletes: physiological responses and clinical application. *J Orthop Sports Phys Ther* 2006;36(5):308–319.

78. Rand SE, Goerlich C, Marchand K, et al. The physical therapy prescription. *Am Fam Physician* 2007;76:1661–1666.

79. Takeshima N, Rogers ME, Islam MM, et al. Effect of concurrent aerobic and resistance circuit exercise training on fitness in older adults. *Eur J Appl Physiol* 2004;93:173–182.

80. Evers QW, Kraaimaat FW, van Riel PL, et al. Tailored cognitive-behavioral therapy in early rheumatoid arthritis for patients at risk: a randomized controlled trial. *Pain* 2002;100:141–153.

81. Morley S, Williams A. A systematic review and meta-analysis of randomized clinical trials of cognitive behavior therapy and behavior therapy for chronic pain in adults, excluding headache. *Pain* 1990;80:1–13.

82. Tulder can MW, Ostelo RW, Vlayen JW, et al. Behavioral treatment for chronic low back pain: a systematic review within the framework of the Cochrane back review group. *Spine* 2001;26:270–281.

83. Ostelo RW, Tulder M, Vlaeyen J, et al. Behavioral treatment for chronic low-back pain. *Cochrane Database Syst Rev* [Online Update Software] 2005;1: CD002014.

84. Jensen MP. Enhancing motivation to change in pain treatment. In: Turk DC, Gatchel RJ, eds. *Psychological Approaches to Pain Management: A Practitioner's Handbook.* New York: Guilford Press; 1996:78:111.

85. Kerns RD, Rosenberg R, Jamison RN. Readiness to adopt a self-management approach to chronic pain: the Pain Stages of Change Questionnaire (PSCOZ). *Pain* 1997;72:227–234.

86. Jensen MP, Nielson WR, Turner JA, et al. Changes in readiness to self-manage pain are associated with improvement in multidisciplinary pain treatment and pain coping. *Pain* 2004;111:84–95.

87. van den Hout JH, Vlaeyen JW, Heuts PH, et al. Secondary prevention of work-related disability in nonspecific low back pain: does problem-solving therapy help? A randomized clinical trial. *Clin J Pain* 2003;19:87–96.

88. Nichoal MK, Wilson PH, Goyen J. Comparison of cognitive-behavioral group treatment and an alternative non-psychological treatment for chronic low back pain. *Pain* 1992;48:339–347.

89. Linton SJ, Melin L, Stjernlof K. The effects of applied relaxation and operant activity training on chronic pain. *Behav Psychother* 1985;13:87–100.

89a. Nicholas MK, Wilson PH, Goyen J. Comparison of cognitive-behavioral group treatment and an alternative non-psychological treatment for chronic low back pain. *Pain* 1992;48:339–347.

90. Astin JA. Mind-body therapies for the management of pain. *Clin J Pain* 2004; 20:27–32.

91. Matheson LN. Work hardening for patients with back pain. *J Musculoskel Med* 1993;10:53–63.

92. Isernhagen S. Work hardening. In: Demeter SL, Andersson GB, eds. *Disability Evaluation.* 2nd ed. St. Louis: Mosby; 2003.

93. Maultsy Burt C. Work evaluation and work hardening. In: Pedretti LC, Early MB, eds. *Occupational Therapy.* 5th ed. St Louis: Mosby; 2001.

94. Lindstrom I, Ohlund C, Eek C, Wallin L, et al. The effect of graded activity on patients with subacute low back pain: a randomized prospective clinical study with an operant-conditioning behavioral approach. *Phys Ther* 1002; 72:279–290.

95. State of Washington Department of Labor and Industries. Work Hardening Program Standards. Available at: http://www.lni.wa.gov/ClaimsIns/Files/ReturnToWork/WhStds.pdf. Accessed October 12, 2008.

96. Bendix AF, Bendix T, Baegter K, et al. Comparison of three intensive programs for chronic low back pain patients: a prospective, randomized, observer-blinded study with one year follow-up. *Scand J Rehab Med* 1997;29:81–89.

97. Schonstein E, Kenny D, Keating J, et al. Physical conditioning programs for workers with back and neck pain: a Cochrane systematic review. *Spine* 2003; 28:E391–395.

98. Schonstein E, Kenny DT, Keating J, et al. Work conditioning, work hardening and functional restoration for workers with back and neck pain. *Cochrane Database Syst Rev* 2003;1:CD001822.

99. Matheson L. Functional capacity evaluation. In: Andersson G, Demeter S, Smith G, eds. *Disability Evaluation.* Chicago: Mosby Yearbook; 1996.

100. Matheson LN, Mooney V, Grant JE, et al. Standardized evaluation of work capacity. *J Back Musculoskel Rehabil* 1996;6:249–264.

101. Innes E, Straker L. A clinician's guide to work-related assessments: 1-purposes and problems. *Work* 1998;11:183–189.

102. Isernhagen SJ. *The Comprehensive Guide to Work Injury Management.* Gaithersburg, MD: Aspen Publishers; 1995:821.

103. Gross DP, Battié MC. The prognostic value of functional capacity evaluation in patients with chronic low back pain: part 2. *Spine* 2004;29:920–924.

104. Matheson LN. The functional capacity evaluation. In: Demeter SL, Andersson GB, eds. *Disability Evaluation.* 2nd ed. St. Louis: Mosby; 2003.

105. Fishbain D, Khalil T, Abdel-Moty E, et al. Physician limitations when assessing work capacity: a review. *J Back Musculoskel Rehabil* 1995;5:107–113.

106. Matheson LN. How do you know that he tried his best? The reliability crisis in industrial rehabilitation. *Industrial Rehab Quart* 1988;1:10–12.

107. Owens KA, Buchholz RL. Functional capacity assessment, worker evaluation strategies, and the disability management process. In: Shrey DE, Lacerte M, eds. *Principles and Practices of Disability Management in Industry.* Boca Raton, FL: CRC Press; 1995:269–299.

108. Borg GA. Psychophysical bases of perceived exertion. *Med Sci Sports Exerc* 1982;14:377–381.

109. Matheson L, Carlton R, Niemeyer L. Grip strength in the disabled sample: reliability and normative standards. *Industrial Rehab Quart* 1988;1(3):9.

110. Vasudevan SV. Role of functional capacity assessment in disability evaluation. *J Back Musculoskel Rehabil* 1996;6:265–276.

111. Vlozo CA. Work evaluations: critique of the state of the art of functional assessment of work. *Am J Occup Ther* 1993;47:203–209.

112. Lemstra M, Olszynski WP, Enright W. The sensitivity and specificity of functional capacity evaluations in determining maximum effort. *Spine* 2004;29: 953–959.

113. U.S. Department of Labor. *Dictionary of Occupational Titles.* Washington, DC: US Government Printing Office; 1986.

114. Gross DP, Battié MC. Factors influencing results of functional capacity evaluations in workers' compensation claimants with low back pain. *Phys Ther* 2005;85:315–322.

115. Gross DP, Battié MC. The construct validity of a functional capacity evaluation administered within a workers' compensation environment. *J Occup Rehab* 2003;13:287–295.

116. Cutler RB, Fishbain DA, Steele-Rosomoff R, et al. Relationships between functional capacity measures and baseline psychological measures in chronic pain patients. *J Occup Rehab* 2003;13:249–258.

117. Lackner JM, Carosella AM. The relative influence of perceived pain control, anxiety, and functional self efficacy on spinal function among patients with chronic low back pain. *Spine* 1999;24:2254–2260.

118. Geisser ME, Robinson ME, Miller QL, et al. Psychosocial factors and functional capacity evaluation among persons with chronic pain. *J Occup Rehab* 2003;13:259–276.

119. Lechner DE, Bradbury SF, Bradley LA. Detecting sincerity of effort: a summary of methods and approaches. *Phys Ther* 1998;78:867–888.

120. Moulin DE, Iezzi A, Amireh R, et al. Randomised trial of oral morphine for chronic non-cancer pain. *Lancet* 1996;347:143–147.

121. Tennant FS, Uelmen GF. Narcotic maintenance for chronic pain. Medical and legal guidelines. *Postgrad Med* 1983;73:81–94.

122. Portenoy RK. Chronic opioid therapy in nonmalignant pain. *J Pain Symptom Manage* 1990;5:46–62.

123. Porter J, Jick HN. Addiction rare in patients treated with narcotics. *N Engl J Med* 1980;302:123.

124. Kalso E, Edwards JE, Moore RA, et al. Opioids in chronic non-cancer pain: systematic review of efficacy and safety. *Pain* 2004;112:372–380.

125. Eisenberg E, McNicol ED, Carr DB. Efficacy and safety of opioid agonists in the treatment of neuropthic pain of nonmalignant origin: systematic review and meta-analysis of randomized controlled trials. *JAMA* 2005;293:3043–3052.

126. Fishbain DA, Bole B, Lewis J, et al. What percentage of chronic nonmalignant pain patients exposed to chronic opioid analgesic therapy develop abuse/addiction and/or aberrant drug-related behavior? A structured evidence-based review. *Pain Med* 2008;9:444–459.

127. Furlan A, Sandoval J, Mailis-Gagnon A, et al. Opioids for chronic noncancer pain: a meta-analysis of effectiveness and side effects. *CMAJ* 2006;174:1589–1594.

128. Ballantyne JC, Mao J. Opioid therapy for chronic pain. *N Engl J Med* 2003;349:1943–1953.

129. Mao J. Opioid-induced abnormal pain sensitivity: implications in clinical opioid therapy. *Pain* 2002;100:213–217.

130. Angst MS, Clark JD. Opioid-induced hyperalgesia: a qualitative systematic review. *Anesthesiology* 2006;104(3):570–587.

131. Daniell HW. Hypogonadism in men consuming sustained-action oral opioids. *J Pain* 2002;3:377–384.

132. Michna E, Ross EL, Hynes WL, et al. Predicting aberrant drug behavior in patients treated for chronic pain: importance of abuse history. *J Pain Symptom Manage* 2004;28:250–258.

133. Charney DS, Heninger GR, Kleber HD. The combined use of clonidine and naltrexone as a rapid, safe, and effective treatment of abrupt withdrawal from methadone. *Am J Psychiatry* 1986;143:831–837.

134. Collins ED. Pharmacologic approaches to opioid dependence and withdrawal. In: Smith HS, Passik SD, eds. *Pain and Chemical Dependency*. New York: Oxford University Press; 2008:247–251.

135. Wooten J. Behavioral medicine treatment in the management of the chemically dependent patient. In: Smith HS, Passik SD, eds. *Pain and Chemical Dependency*. New York: Oxford University Press; 2008:253–258.

136. Rome JD, Townsend CO, Bruce BK, et al. Chronic noncancer pain rehabilitation with opioid withdrawal: comparison of treatment outcomes based on opioid use status at admission. *Mayo Clin Proc* 2004;79:759–768.

137. Hooten WM, Townsend CO, Sletten CD, et al. Treatment outcomes after multidisciplinary pain rehabilitation with analgesic medication withdrawal for patients with fibromyalgia. *Pain Med* 2007;8:8–16.

CHAPTER 90 ■ ASSESSMENT AND TREATMENT OF CHEMICAL DEPENDENCY

ANDREW J. SAXON, JAMES P. ROBINSON, AND MARK D. SULLIVAN

INTRODUCTION

This chapter on assessment and treatment of chemical dependency provides guidance, particularly for practitioners interested in pain medicine, on how various forms of substance dependence are diagnosed and managed clinically. Since detection and management of opioid addiction pose a major concern for physicians using opioids to treat patients, and since diagnosis of opioid addiction in this context is often confounded by pain issues, the chapter focuses special attention on this complex clinical conundrum. More specifically, the chapter focuses on patients with chronic nonmalignant pain (CNMP) because issues related to opioid addiction are more vexing in these patients than in patients with cancer or other life-threatening illnesses.

Various surveys indicate that individuals with chronic pain disorders are more likely to have substance use disorders than are individuals in the general population,[1,2] and individuals with substance use disorders also have high rates of pain disorders.[3] Therefore, practitioners treating pain disorders are likely to encounter patients with substance use disorders and will need to know how to screen for and recognize these disorders, diagnose these disorders, make appropriate referrals for and/or treat these disorders, monitor for these disorders during ongoing pain treatment, and how to manage therapy for chronic pain in the context of these disorders.

The first section of the chapter presents the assessment and treatment of all major forms of chemical dependency from the perspective of addiction medicine. The second section focuses on assessment and treatment of opioid addiction from the perspective of the pain specialist.

ASSESSMENT AND TREATMENT OF CHEMICAL DEPENDENCY—ADDICTION MEDICINE PERSPECTIVE

The panoply of substance use disorders includes intoxication, withdrawal, abuse, dependence, and substance-induced psychiatric disorders (for example psychosis, mood disturbance, or anxiety caused directly by the use of the substance). Substance use disorders occur with a variety of commonly used substances such as alcohol, cannabis, cocaine, opioids, sedative/hypnotics, stimulants like amphetamines and methylphenidate, inhalants, psychedelic agents, and nicotine. A standardized set of criteria characterizing these disorders is provided in the *Diagnostic and Statistical Manual of Mental Disorders* (*DSM-IV TR*).[4] Intoxication and withdrawal differ by substance and can generally be diagnosed through history and physical examination. The criteria for abuse and dependence, which will be covered in greater detail below, are identical across substances.

The use of the term "dependence" has generated some confusion and controversy. In contrast to a commonly held conception of "dependence" as notating purely physiologic changes that occur in response to repeated exposure to a substance, in *DSM-IV TR*, "dependence" refers to a syndrome of physiologic signs and symptoms combined with an array of behavioral disturbances. Some have suggested that the phrase "substance dependence," referring to the *DSM-IV TR* syndrome, be replaced with the term "addiction" to avoid confusion between purely physiologic dependence and the syndrome of substance dependence.[5] Others feel that the term "addiction" has negative connotations leading to stigmatization. In any event, it should be understood that the terms "addiction" and "substance dependence" are essentially synonymous and interchangeable.

Screening and Recognition

Some initial evidence must arise through screening to suggest that a patient has a substance use disorder to trigger a thorough diagnostic assessment. In many cases, screening and diagnostic evaluation may overlap. Recently, the idea of "universal precautions" in pain medicine has been advanced to detect potential substance use problems in all pain patients so there may be some value in routine use of some or all of these screening procedures.[6]

History

Generally, a thorough history of substance use obtained through a matter-of-fact, nonjudgmental interviewing style will provide a great deal of information or even a formal diagnosis. Most patients are not aware of guidelines for safe quantities of alcohol consumption and will readily divulge the amount of their drinking. Many patients are more reluctant to discuss use of illicit substances, but some will freely admit to such use if they do not fear sanctions or punishment. Oftentimes, this openness is more likely to occur during initial intake. Patients may be less forthright during the course of treatment if they believe they have something to lose by admitting to use. If time allows, it is worth asking explicitly about frequency and quantity of use for each class of substance along with route of administration. It is also quite important to ask about any history of current and past problematic substance use as such problematic use is known to increase the risk of recurrence in the context of pain management. It is useful to know what types of substance use disorder treatments have been useful for the patient in the past.

Recommended safe quantities of alcohol use consist of no more than 4 standard drinks per day (or more than 14 total per week) for men and 3 standard drinks (or more than 7 total per week) for women.[7] The recommended quantities are less for women because women tend to have less total body water and thus a lower volume of distribution for alcohol.[8] Quantities of different forms of alcohol that define a standard drink are listed in Table 90.1. If patients acknowledge regularly consuming more than the recommended amounts or describe heavy drinking such as 5 or more drinks on one occasion for men or 4 or more for women, a more thorough diagnostic evaluation for alcohol abuse or dependence should be pursued.

For illicit substances, any suggestion of more than occasional recreational use of marijuana should prompt a more thorough diagnostic evaluation. It is also important to look for nicotine dependence, as this has been associated with increased risk of opioid misuse in a number of studies.[1,9]

Physical Examination

Signs of possible substance use problems evident on physical exam include hypertension (common with excessive alcohol use),

TABLE 90.1

QUANTITIES OF ALCOHOL THAT DEFINE A STANDARD DRINK (14 GRAMS PURE ALCOHOL)

Beverage	Percent alcohol	Quantity in standard drink (in fluid ounces)
Beer	5%	12
Malt Liquor	7%	8.5
Table Wine	12%	5
Fortified Wine	17%	3.5
Liqueur	24%	2.5
Brandy	40%	1.5
Spirits (gin, vodka, whiskey)	40%	1.5

track marks indicative of recent or past injection drug use, pupillary constriction or dilation, inflamed nasal turbinates from intranasal substance insufflation, wheezes or rhonchi on lung exam from substance smoking, enlarged, tender liver from excessive alcohol use, other substance toxicity or hepatitis, or any stigmata of excessive alcohol use such as flushed facies, spider angiomas, palmar erythema, etc. Any of these findings should trigger further screening and a possible thorough diagnostic evaluation.

Laboratory

Routine blood work can provide an indication of excessive alcohol use. Suggestive findings include elevations in liver transaminases or macrocytic, hyperchromic red blood cells related to alcohol's interference with folate absorption and subsequent folate deficiency. Positive serologies for past or current hepatitis B or C infection or human immunodeficiency virus infection would raise concerns about a substance use related mode of transmission.

In addition, specific laboratory testing to detect presence of substances in body fluids offers a convenient component of screening. Typically urine is tested,[10] though tests can also be readily performed in oral fluid or blood.[11,12] Substances that have been used are likely to remain present in urine for a longer period than they will in other body fluids (Table 90.2). For urine testing, a screening test is typically performed via immunoassay. When needed, confirmatory tests using gas chromatography/mass spectrometry can be ordered. It is important to note that the routine urine assay for opioids does not detect oxycodone, which requires a specific screening test. Likewise methadone is not detected by the opiate assay and necessitates a specific screening test. Heroin can only be detected shortly after use if its intermediate metabolite, 6-monoacetyl morphine, is present. Subsequently, 6-monoacetyl morphine is rapidly metabolized to morphine. If morphine appears in a urine toxicology specimen, it could represent either pharmaceutical morphine use or heroin use. It is difficult to detect alcohol in urine, blood, oral fluid, or breath unless the use has been quite recent.

Self-Report Questionnaires

A number of self-report questionnaires have been designed to help in screening for substance use disorders, and these can be utilized prior to, concurrent with, or subsequent to the history, physical, and laboratory evaluation to help determine whether a patient warrants more thorough diagnostic evaluation. Although the instruments described below have definite utility in primary care and general populations as well as selected samples such as psychiatric patients, they have not been tested in pain patients.

In screening for alcohol use disorders, the most frequently

TABLE 90.2

DRUG DETECTION TIMES IN URINE AND DRUG PLASMA HALF-LIVES

Drug	Detection time in urine (based on standard cut-off values)	Plasma half-life
Amphetamine	2–3 days	12 hours
Cocaine Metabolite (Benzoylecgonine)	2–3 days	7.5 hours
Opioids		
Morphine Glucuronide	2 days	7.5 hours
Codeine Glucuronide	3 days	12 hours
Heroin Metabolite (6-mono acetyl morphine)	2–4 hours	20 minutes
Methadone	3 days single use 7–9 days maintenance dosing	24 hours
Oxycodone	2 days	5 hours
Hydromorphone	1–2 days	2.5 hours
Hydrocodone	1–2 days	4 hours
Barbiturates		
Short-Acting	1 day	25 hours
Intermediate-Acting	2–3 days	38 hours
Long-Acting	≥16 days	100 hours
Benzodiazepines		
Short-Acting	1 day	1.5 hours
Intermediate-Acting	2–4 days	10 hours
Long-Acting	≥7 days	48 hours
Cannabis single use	3 days	20 hours
Cannabis chronic use	≥30 days	20 hours

used instruments are the Alcohol Use Disorders Identification Tests (AUDIT)[13] and the Michigan Alcohol Screening Test (MAST).[14] The AUDIT has 10 items related to quantity and frequency of alcohol consumption and to maladaptive behaviors associated with alcohol use and can be completed in about 5 minutes. Each item is scored 0 to 4. A score of 8 or more for men under age 60 or 4 or more for women or men over age 60 are considered positive screens indicative of need for further assessment. The MAST contains 25 questions and focuses more on problem behaviors associated with alcohol use. Each item counts for 1 point, and a score of 6 or more indicates a positive screen with need for further assessment. There are shorter versions of the MAST which also appear to function as adequate screening instruments.

In the context of managing pain patients where urine toxicology should be readily available, self-report instruments to screen for drug use problems are probably less useful than a positive urine toxicology. However, if use of a self-report screening instrument is desired, the most commonly used instrument is the Drug Abuse Screening Test (DAST).[15] The DAST is based on the MAST and has 28 items concerning both intensity and frequency of drug use and problematic behaviors associated with drug use. As with the MAST, each item counts for 1 point, and a score of 6 or more points to the needs for further assessment. Shorter versions of the DAST also exist.

Diagnostic Assessment

As noted above, criteria provided in *DSM-IV TR* represent the most standard way to make a diagnosis of a substance use disorder. Substance abuse is considered a less serious disorder and substance dependence more serious. Abuse and dependence are mutually exclusive. Once a patient has progressed to dependence, the patient can no longer be diagnosed with abuse, even if the substance use has become less problematic. In that circumstance, a diagnosis of dependence in partial remission would be made. At times, it proves fruitful to interview family members if the patient is not forthcoming.

Substance Abuse

Table 90.3 contains *DSM-IV TR* criteria for substance abuse. The presence of one or more of four possible criteria is needed

TABLE 90.3

DSM-IV TR CRITERIA FOR SUBSTANCE ABUSE

A. A maladaptive pattern of substance use leading to clinically significant impairment or distress as manifested by one (or more) of the following, occurring within a 12-month period
  (1) Recurrent substance use resulting in a failure to fulfill major role obligations at work, school, or home
  (2) Recurrent substance use in situations in which it is physically hazardous
  (3) Recurrent substance-related legal problems
  (4) Continued substance use despite having persistent or recurrent social or interpersonal problems caused or exacerbated by the effects of the substance
B. The symptoms have never met the criteria for substance dependence for this class of substances

Reprinted with permission from American Psychiatric Association. *Diagnostic and Statistical Manual of Mental Disorders*. 4th ed, text revision. Arlington, VA: American Psychiatric Publishing Incorporated; 2000.

to make the diagnosis. The essence of substance abuse involves the repeated use of the substance in risky situations or in situations in which the use results in legal problems or interferes with social or occupational functioning. The use need not be frequent, and withdrawal usually does not occur. Individuals usually begin with substance abuse and may then progress to dependence. To determine the presence or absence of the diagnosis, the interviewer should focus one by one in turn on each substance of potential relevance and systematically go over each of the criteria with the patient for each substance.

Substance Dependence

Table 90.4 displays the *DSM-IV TR* criteria for substance dependence. There are two physiologic criteria, tolerance and withdrawal, and five behavioral criteria. Three or more of the seven criteria must be present at any one time over a 12-month period to make the diagnosis. Thus, an individual could meet both physiologic criteria but would not be diagnosed with dependence unless she or he met at least one behavioral criterion. This situation could occur, for example, with a pain patient treated chronically with opioids who might display tolerance to the effects of opioids and withdrawal signs and symptoms if the medication is stopped but has no behavioral evidence of dependence, with an attention deficit hyperactivity disorder patient treated chronically with stimulants, or with an anxiety disorder patient treated chronically with benzodiazepines. Conversely, an individual might not have either tolerance or withdrawal but could have the *DSM-IV TR* defined substance dependence if she or he meets at least three of the behavioral criteria, although this scenario occurs rarely in clinical practice. As with diagnosing abuse, the interviewer should go systematically through each of the criteria with the patient and cover each substance separately. Inspection of the criteria reveals that questions about each criterion are unlikely to be interpreted by patients as critical or threatening and unlikely to engender resistance or deception, particularly if posed in a matter of fact, nonjudgmental fashion. Although this procedure sounds time consuming, it frequently can be accomplished in a matter of minutes for each substance of concern. As mentioned at the outset, the diagnosis of opioid dependence in a patient with CNMP being treated with opioids may not be as straightforward as simple application of the *DSM-IV TR* criteria and will be discussed in detail below.

Diagnosis of a substance use disorder certainly should not preclude appropriate interventions for a pain problem and, in many instances, with appropriate monitoring and safeguards may not preclude opioid treatment of chronic pain.

Co-Occurring Psychiatric Disorders

Mental health disorders frequently co-occur with substance use disorders.[16,17] It is likely that chronic pain patients who have substance dependence will have another nonsubstance related co-occurring psychiatric disorder.[18] Oftentimes co-occurring psychiatric and substance use disorders interact with negative synergy so that exacerbation of one disorder in turn exacerbates the other.[19] Thus, if a pain patient does have a substance use disorder, it is imperative to evaluate that patient for other co-occurring psychiatric disorders and provide appropriate clinical intervention (including pharmacotherapy and/or psychotherapy) for any that are diagnosed.

Monitoring During Ongoing Pain Treatment

Even if a patient does not manifest a substance use disorder at the onset of chronic pain treatment, a disorder can certainly arise during the course of treatment. Maintaining vigilance for the development of a disorder involves both observation of the patient for behavioral evidence and routine monitoring techniques.[6] Be-

haviors that may increase the index of suspicion include missing appointments, having medication shortages, failure to pay bills, or a markedly changed affect during appointments.

Depending on the setting and resources available, it may prove worthwhile to establish routine monitoring procedures for all pain patients even in the absence of concern. This approach normalizes these procedures, allows patients to expect them, and creates structure that may actually help the patient to feel supported while removing any sense of stigma or accusation that may supervene if the procedures are applied only for cause. The procedures that will be utilized should be specified at the outset of treatment in a written treatment agreement. One routine monitoring procedure to consider is urine toxicology testing as described above.[20]

Another potential procedure is unscheduled medication call backs. For this procedure, patients are telephoned and asked to return to the office within 24 hours with all their outstanding medication. When the patients come in, pill counts are performed to insure that all expected outstanding medication is accounted for. It is also possible to obtain a urine toxicology specimen at that time.

Treatment and/or Referral

Some general comments about treatment and referral will be made and then specific interventions for dependence on each particular class of substances will be outlined. Most physicians get virtually no training or experience in treatment of substance use disorders and, therefore, often feel helpless or hopeless in the face of these disorders. Although most patients with these disorders who do get treatment get it in specialized settings that operate in parallel to and oftentimes outside of mainstream medicine, many patients will refuse a referral to such settings, and a growing body of literature supports the efficacy of brief physician intervention as a reasonable first attempt at treating these disorders.

Brief Interventions

Brief office interventions conducted by physicians have demonstrated efficacy in reducing alcohol consumption for patients with problematic alcohol use that does not rise to the level of alcohol abuse or dependence and may also have some benefit in these latter disorders.[21,22] Motivational interventions (see below) which can be incorporated into brief office interventions have demonstrated modest efficacy in drug dependence.[23]

Brief interventions should be delivered in a manner that is matter-of-fact, nonjudgmental, supportive, and empathic and definitely not in a manner that is confrontational. The first step consists of stating concern about the patient's level of alcohol use (or any level of illicit drug use). It is helpful to give the patient direct examples from his or her medical record including bothersome symptoms, physical findings, specific diseases, or lab abnormalities. The next step involves giving direct advice to cut down (or quit) the substance use along with an offer to help. If the patient is not receptive to this advice and the situation is not emergent, the physician can encourage her or him to consider it carefully and reflect on why she or he considers ongoing use to be a reasonable course of action. A follow-up can be arranged for further discussion.

If the patient appears receptive to advice to cut down or quit, the physician can help the patient to establish a specific goal to cut down or abstain (for abuse or dependence). Also, the physician can provide explicit behavioral suggestions such as avoiding acquaintances who use, avoiding places where use has previously occurred, or seeking social support for quitting, including attending mutual-help groups such as Alcoholics Anonymous or Narcotics Anonymous. A follow-up appointment should be scheduled to monitor progress.

TABLE 90.4

PROBLEMS IN THE APPLICATION OF *DSM-IV TR* CRITERIA OPIOID DEPENDENCE TO PATIENTS WITH CHRONIC NONMALIGNANT PAIN

DSM-IV TR criterion for drug dependence	Problem in application to CNMP patients
1. Tolerance	Pain specialists expect their patients to develop some tolerance to opioids and do not consider opioid tolerance to be an indicator of addiction or inappropriate use. Many believe that there is no inherent limit to opioid dosing, so that it is easy to compensate for tolerance by increasing a patient's opioid dose.
2. Withdrawal	Pain specialists expect their patients to be at risk for withdrawal reactions in response to abrupt opioid tapers and do not consider such reactions to be an indicator of addiction or inappropriate opioid use.
3. Substance taken in larger amounts or over a longer period of time than was intended	The "amount" criterion is ambiguous because many pain physicians maintain that there is no definable ceiling for opioid dosing, and, therefore, no definite way to determine that a patient is taking too much of a drug. The "duration" criterion is ambiguous, because CNMP can last indefinitely.
4. There is a persistent desire or unsuccessful efforts to cut down or control substance use	CNMP patients express a desire for opioids and explain this by maintaining that the opioids are needed to control their pain. Similarly, patients attribute difficulties in tapering opioids to pain increases during tapers, rather than to addiction. It is difficult for the treating physician to know whether these explanations represent rationalizations for addictive behavior or are accurate portrayals.
5. A great deal of time is spent in activities necessary to obtain the substance, use the substance, or recover from its effects	This is ambiguous in two ways. First, CNMP patients often do not have to go to great lengths to get opioids because their physicians prescribe them at office visits. Second, if a CNMP patient does engage in drug-seeking behavior, his or her behavior might be construed as evidence of pseudoaddiction. This term implies that the patient's behavior is attributable to inappropriate prescribing on the part of the treating physician, rather than to addiction on the part of the patient.
6. Important social, occupational, or recreational activities are given up or reduced because of substance use	CNMP patients often give up these activities but routinely report that they are forced to do so because of their pain, rather than because of opioid addiction. Treating physicians generally do not have reliable methods to determine why the patients fail to engage in work and social activities.
7. Substance use is continued despite knowledge of having a persistent or recurrent physical or psychological problem that is likely to have been caused or exacerbated by the substance use	CNMP patients routinely downplay adverse consequences of their opioid use. If they do acknowledge adverse consequences, they express the view that they would suffer even more if they did not have opioids to control their pain. Treating physicians generally do not have reliable methods to determine the validity of patients' attributions.

Criteria reprinted with permission from American Psychiatric Association. *Diagnostic and Statistical Manual of Mental Disorders*. 4th ed, text revision. Arlington, VA: American Psychiatric Publishing Incorporated; 2000.

If the patient has alcohol dependence and is willing to try for abstinence, the brief intervention could be combined with prescription of an appropriate alcohol treatment medication as described below. If the patient has developed opioid dependence, the brief intervention could be combined with a recommendation to try buprenorphine, also described below. If the pain physician treating the patient has a federal waiver to prescribe buprenorphine, arrangements could be made to stop the opioid analgesic the patient is currently taking and make a switch to buprenorphine.

Specialty Substance Use Disorders Treatment

If a referral to a specialized substance dependence treatment provider is needed, the referral could be made to an individual practitioner, another physician, psychologist, social worker, or chemical dependency counselor who specializes in substance dependence treatment and could work with the patient in a private office setting using one or more of the psychotherapeutic or behavioral interventions detailed below. Frequently, the referral will be made to an addiction treatment or chemical dependency program or agency. The American Society of Addiction Medicine publishes Patient Placement Criteria that can aid in determining what level of addiction treatment is appropriate for a given patient. These criteria have not, however, been fully scientifically validated and are based largely on expert opinion.[24,25]

Medically Supervised Withdrawal

Some patients who manifest withdrawal when stopping their substance use may need medically supervised withdrawal (also known as detoxification) to stop the substance safely and engage in treatment. The most common substances which require supervised withdrawal are alcohol, sedative-hypnotics, and opioids, although occasionally patients may have very unpleasant withdrawal symptoms from cocaine or amphetamines and need some support and monitoring. Medically supervised withdrawal can be accomplished on an outpatient or inpatient basis depending upon the severity of the withdrawal. Alcohol or sedative-hypnotic withdrawal can be so severe as to be life-threatening. Usually, benzodiazepines are prescribed over several days in tapering doses.[26] Supervised opioid withdrawal for opioid dependence can be accomplished using methadone in a licensed treatment program[27] (see below) or with buprenorphine[28] by appropriately qualified physicians. Alternatively, the α_2 adrenergic agonist, clonidine, can be prescribed to attenuate opioid withdrawal signs and symptoms and tapered over several days.[29] Some paradigms, known as ultrarapid opioid withdrawal, have been developed whereby opioid withdrawal is precipitated with an opioid antagonist such as naloxone or naltrexone under sedation or general anesthesia to complete the withdrawal in a brief period of time. These rapid procedures have no better outcomes than more gradual withdrawal but do have more adverse events such as pulmonary problems and psychiatric instability so they are not recommended.[30] It is very important to understand that medically supervised withdrawal (detoxification) alone does not constitute treatment. If medically supervised withdrawal is not immediately followed by more definitive chemical dependency treatment, relapse is almost universal.

Opioid Agonist Treatment

Many patients with primary opioid dependence do not want to undergo withdrawal or have tried it previously with subsequent relapse. These patients might be referred to a federally licensed opioid treatment program.[31] These programs provide opioid agonist therapy with either methadone or buprenorphine. Because these medications have long half-lives, they can prevent the emergence of opioid withdrawal when taken on a once a day basis. (More detail on the clinical use of these medications for the treatment of opioid dependence is provided below.) The structure of the program is largely dictated by federal and state regulations. Patients must have a minimum of a 1 year history of opioid dependence. In the early stages of treatment, patients must come to the clinic daily for observed doses of medication with take home doses of medication for weekend days when the clinic is closed. The maximum allowed first dose of methadone is 30 mg with subsequent gradual dose escalation to an optimally therapeutic dosage. A physical examination and basic laboratory tests are required, as is periodic urine toxicology testing. Regular counseling visits are also mandated. As patients stabilize in treatment, as evidenced by regular attendance at dosing visits and other appointments, remaining on a stable dose of medication, and ceasing illicit substance use as demonstrated by drug free toxicology specimens, take home doses of medication become available so that patients do not have to attend clinic every day. After 2 years of continuous treatment, stable patients may receive up to a maximum of 1 month's take home doses. Opioid agonist treatment has exceptionally good outcomes not only in terms of reducing illicit opioid use but also in terms of reducing other substance use, in reducing mortality and morbidity, reducing criminal justice involvement, and improving employment.[32,33] It is considered to be as cost effective as other potential life-saving treatments such as coronary bypass surgery or renal dialysis.[34] All physicians are permitted to prescribe methadone for pain management, but only specially licensed facilities can prescribe methadone for opioid dependence. Prescription of methadone for pain in patients with signs of opioid dependence has obvious inherent risks and should be undertaken with careful monitoring precautions in place.

Intensive Outpatient Treatment

For patients who do not have opioid dependence or who have opioid dependence but do not want agonist therapy and have completed withdrawal, intensive outpatient treatment is often employed. This type of treatment is generally abstinence based; that is, it emphasizes the goal of total abstinence from alcohol and all illicit substances. Some programs would accept pain patients on prescribed opioid therapy if the patient has a goal of abstinence from other substance use. Intensive outpatient treatment involves behavioral interventions usually via a group format with several meetings per week over a 4 to 12 week period so that patients receive up to 72 or more hours of total treatment.[35] Frequent urine toxicology testing is also typically performed. The therapeutic content of the group sessions varies but often includes one or more of the types of behavioral interventions described below. Attendance at mutual help groups such as Alcoholics Anonymous is strongly encouraged. Not surprisingly, patients who complete these programs have better outcomes than those who drop out. Depending upon the setting and patient characteristics, the dropout rate can be substantial.

Inpatient Treatment

For patients who fail outpatient treatment or for those who can obtain funding for it, inpatient treatment is an option. Inpatient treatment could be as brief as a few days[36] but frequently lasts 28 days, and can be extended for many months in a model known as a therapeutic community[37] for patients who have severe, intractable substance use disorders that do not respond to any other interventions. Ongoing outpatient treatment subsequent to completion of inpatient treatment is often recommended. Inpatient treatment, like intensive outpatient treatment, is almost always abstinence based. Many short-term inpatient programs would accept pain patients on opioid therapy if the patients committed to abstinence from other substances. Most therapeutic communities would not accept patients receiving opioid therapy even for pain. The content of the care in inpatient treatment does not differ substantially from the content delivered in intensive outpatient treatment, but inpatient treatment provides a controlled environment that minimizes the risk of relapse and can compress more hours of actual treatment into a shorter overall time frame.[38] In the aggregate, it appears that the quantity or "dose" of behavioral treatment received, rather than the setting in which it occurs, serves as the key mediator of outcome.

Specific Behavioral Treatments

Numerous types of behavioral interventions are used to treat substance dependence and many have been empirically validated. Mastery of specific techniques often requires considerable training and practice. Most studies comparing various behavioral intervention techniques find, as with setting, that the specific technique is less important than the total amount of behavioral intervention received. Many practitioners do not deliver the specific interventions in their pure form. In addition to the amount of intervention received, other important mediators of success are the skill of the specific therapist and the therapeutic alliance achieved between the therapist and patient regardless of what technique is used.[39] To impart at least passing knowledge of the names and basic philosophies of the more common techniques, brief descriptions are provided.

Motivational Interviewing. Motivational interviewing is a directive, patient-centered counseling style for eliciting behavior change by helping patients to explore and resolve ambivalence. Compared with nondirective counseling, it is more focused and goal-directed. The examination and resolution of ambivalence is its central purpose, and the counselor is intentionally directive in pursuing this goal using the following techniques[40]:

- Seeking to understand the person's frame of reference, particularly via reflective listening
- Expressing acceptance and affirmation
- Eliciting and selectively reinforcing the client's own self-motivational statements, expressions of problem recognition, concern, desire, and intention to change, and ability to change
- Monitoring the client's degree of readiness to change, and ensuring that resistance is not generated by jumping ahead of the client
- Affirming the client's freedom of choice and self-direction

Relapse Prevention Therapy. Relapse prevention is a cognitive-behavioral intervention based upon the notion that learning processes play an important role in the development of maladaptive behavior patterns. As applied to substance dependence, relapse prevention explores the positive and negative consequences of continued substance use, encourages self-monitoring to recognize substance cravings early on and identify high-risk situations for use, and develops strategies for coping with and avoiding high-risk situations and the desire to use.[41] A central element of this treatment is anticipating the problems that patients are likely to meet and helping them develop effective coping strategies. The skills that patients learn through relapse prevention therapy remain after the completion of treatment, and many maintain the gains they made in treatment throughout the year following treatment.

Drug Counseling. Drug counseling focuses directly on reducing or stopping the patient's substance use. It also addresses related areas of impaired functioning such as employment status, illegal activity, family/social relationships, as well as the content and structure of the patient's recovery program. Through its emphasis on short-term behavioral goals, drug counseling helps the patient develop coping strategies and tools for abstaining from substance use and then maintaining abstinence. The addiction counselor encourages 12-step participation and makes referrals for needed supplemental medical, psychiatric, employment, and other services. Individuals are encouraged to attend sessions 1 or 2 times per week.[42]

Twelve-Step Facilitation Therapy. Twelve-step facilitation consists of a structured and manual-driven approach to facilitating early recovery from substance dependence. It is intended to be implemented on an individual basis in 12 to 15 sessions and is based on behavioral, spiritual, and cognitive principles that form the core of 12-step fellowships such as Alcoholics Anonymous and Narcotics Anonymous. Twelve-step facilitation seeks to achieve two general goals in patients with substance dependence: acceptance of the need for abstinence from substances and surrender, or the willingness to participate actively in 12-step fellowships as a means of sustaining sobriety. These goals are in turn broken down into a series of cognitive, emotional, relationship, behavioral, social, and spiritual objectives.[43] Twelve-step facilitation has shown excellent results for patients with alcohol dependence but has not yet been thoroughly tested for patients with drug dependence.

Contingency Management. Contingency management treatments are based upon operant conditioning principles as elucidated by B. F. Skinner: if a behavior is reinforced or rewarded, it is more likely to occur in the future.[44] In many contingency management treatments, patients leave urine specimens multiple times each week and receive explicit reward for each specimen that tests negative for drugs. These rewards often consist of vouchers that have a monetary value and can be exchanged for retail goods. However, contingencies that lack monetary value can also be used. For example, in opioid treatment programs or office-based buprenorphine treatment, the frequency of attendance can be contingent on drug free urine specimens. Patients who provide drug-negative urine specimens get more take home medication or larger prescriptions, and those who provide drug-positive specimens have their take home privileges reduced or have to pick up a prescription more frequently. Contingency management has been demonstrated to reduce substance use significantly in numerous studies, but its implementation in clinical practice has lagged.[45]

Pharmacotherapies

Currently there are four U.S. Food and Drug Administration (FDA)-approved medications for the treatment of alcohol dependence (disulfiram, acamprosate, oral naltrexone, and injectable naltrexone) and 3 available FDA-approved medications for the treatment of opioid dependence (methadone, buprenorphine, and naltrexone). All of the alcohol treatment medications can be used by all physicians, including pain specialists if desired, within the scope of their own practice. Although methadone can be prescribed for the treatment of opioid dependence only within licensed clinics, buprenorphine can be prescribed by appropriately qualified physicians (as described below) outside of licensed clinics. Naltrexone for either alcohol or opioid dependence is not likely to have much utility in pain patients because of its antagonism of μ-opioid receptors and its tendency either to precipitate opioid withdrawal in patients on opioids or block the effects of opioid analgesics. Nevertheless, it may rarely have potential benefit in selected pain patients not currently on opioids. There are currently no FDA approved pharmacotherapies for dependence on other substances such as cocaine, methamphetamine, sedative-hypnotics, or cannabis, so these disorders must be treated with behavioral interventions alone.

Disulfiram. By inhibiting aldehyde dehydrogenase, a key enzyme in the major metabolic pathway for ethanol, disulfiram causes accumulation of acetaldehyde after alcohol ingestion. The buildup of acetaldehyde usually causes an "alcohol-disulfiram reaction" that typically ensues within minutes of alcohol ingestion.[46] Different individuals exhibit varying degrees of the reaction which may last for several hours. Signs and symptoms of the alcohol-disulfiram reaction include diaphoresis, flushing, tachycardia, hypotension, nausea, vomiting, and headache. The concept behind the idea of disulfiram is that patients taking disulfiram will fear getting an uncomfortable reaction and thus will be deterred from drinking alcohol. To some extent, change occurs during the informed consent discussion between physician and patient at the time the patient agrees to take disulfiram. During that discussion, the patient may, by agreeing to try disulfiram, be arriving at a decisive interest in achieving abstinence from alcohol.

Patients must have achieved some time of abstinence before starting disulfiram to avoid provoking the alcohol-disulfiram reaction. Typically, 48 hours of abstinence proves sufficient. The usual starting dose of disulfiram is 250 mg/day. Genetic variability may determine sensitivity to the medication, and patients with high levels of aldehyde dehydrogenase may be less sensitive to the effects of disulfiram and require higher doses of medication up to 500 mg/day. Some patients may not tolerate 250 mg/day and should have the dose reduced to 125 mg/day.

Disulfiram is associated with a number of mild side effects such as headache, metallic aftertaste, erectile dysfunction, mild fatigue or sedation, and rash. Such side effects frequently dissipate spontaneously or with a dosage decrease. Much more serious adverse events such as optic neuritis, peripheral neuropathy, hepatic injury, or psychotic symptoms or delirium, though rare, necessitate immediate disulfiram discontinuation. Disulfiram-induced hepatic injury can occur idiosyncratically at an estimated rate of 1/25,000 to 1/30,000 patient treatment years.[47] Disulfiram-induced hepatic injury can rapidly proceed to total liver failure. It most usually occurs within the first 6 months of treatment. Symptoms include extreme fatigue, malaise, anorexia, fever, jaundice, scleral icterus, nausea, vomiting, and bilirubinuria. Baseline liver function tests should be obtained prior to initiation of disulfiram treatment and then at 1–2 month intervals during the first 6 months of treatment. With the decreased risk of disulfiram-induced hepatic injury after the first 6 months of treatment, liver monitoring can subsequently be done every 3–6 months if treatment continues. Many patients who might be considered for disulfiram therapy present with moderately elevated transaminases related to alcohol use (particularly in the context of hepatitis C). These modest transaminase elevations do not represent a total contraindication to disulfiram therapy. Very rapid rises in bilirubin and transaminases occur in disulfiram-induced hepatic injury and indicate the need to stop disulfiram at once. If the medication is discontinued promptly, the signs and symptoms of liver injury typically fully resolve. If the medication is not stopped, total hepatic failure and death can supervene unless a liver transplant is performed.

Patients with pre-existing cirrhosis or other serious liver disease generally are not good candidates for disulfiram. Other contraindications include pregnancy or lactation, history of prior hypersensitivity to disulfiram, or significant coronary artery disease. The latter group could experience myocardial ischemia during a severe alcohol-disulfiram reaction.

Disulfiram has greater benefit with monitoring of medication administration. Although the largest study to date demonstrated that disulfiram dosed at 250 mg per day over 1 year did not lead to increased abstinence rates or longer time to first drink compared to placebo, it did lead to significantly fewer drinking days over the study year.[48]

Acamprosate. Acamprosate, which has seen widespread use in Europe for many years, received FDA approval for the treatment of alcohol dependence in 2004. Acamprosate is believed to modulate both the major excitatory system in the brain, the glutamate system, and the major inhibitory system, the gamma amino butyric acid (GABA) system. Alcohol interacts with these systems as well, but when alcohol is stopped after chronic exposure, glutamatergic hyperactivity and GABA hypoactivity contribute substantially to the alcohol withdrawal syndrome. Acamprosate theoretically acts to counteract these imbalances and so may attenuate symptoms associated with subsyndromal, prolonged alcohol withdrawal such as insomnia, anxiety, and restlessness which could provoke alcohol cravings and relapse.[49,50] Acamprosate also may diminish reinforcement derived from alcohol ingestion[49] and the amount of alcohol consumed by patients in treatment who do experience relapse.[51] Numerous controlled studies of acamprosate demonstrated higher total abstinence rates and longer time to relapse for acamprosate compared to placebo.[52] For reasons that remain incompletely understood, acamprosate failed to show efficacy in two large clinical trials conducted in the United States.[53,54] It has been proposed that subjects in the U.S. studies may not have experienced sufficient prolonged subsyndromal withdrawal to benefit from acamprosate.[55]

Acamprosate has very limited oral bioavailability. It achieves steady state after 5 days and is not metabolized by the liver but is excreted unchanged in the urine. The usual dose is 666 mg (two 333 mg tablets) three times daily. The labeling indicates that acamprosate should be started after a modicum of abstinence has been achieved, but there are no safety issues if acamprosate is taken concomitantly with alcohol and abstinence is not essential. In fact, acamprosate should be continued if a patient relapses to alcohol use.

It is recommended that a serum creatinine level to evaluate kidney function be obtained prior to initiation of therapy since the dose should be lowered in patients with impaired kidney function. Acamprosate is FDA category C, so women of childbearing age must use an effective method of birth control when on acamprosate. All patients should be monitored for suicidal thoughts since such thoughts occurred more frequently among acamprosate-treated patients than among placebo-treated patients in clinical trials. Diarrhea is the only common side effect noted with acamprosate.

It is recommended that acamprosate treatment be continued for 12 months, and follow-up studies show increased abstinence rates that persist 1 year after cessation of treatment.[56] Advantages of acamprosate include its lack of drug-drug interactions and the fact that it is not contraindicated in patients with serious liver disease.

Naltrexone. The μ-opioid antagonist, naltrexone, originally developed to treat opioid dependence (see below), was subsequently approved to treat alcohol dependence in 1994 and is now available in generic form. An involvement of the endogenous opioid systems in the reinforcing effects of alcohol seems likely based on the fact that opioid antagonists block the alcohol-induced release of dopamine into the nucleus accumbens.[57] The ability of alcohol to promote the release of endogenous opioids[58,59] or to affect opioid receptor binding[60] may account for dopamine release engendered by alcohol and for the blockade of this event by opioid antagonists. Naltrexone changes the subjective experience of alcohol consumption in humans, rendering it less reinforcing and more sedating.[61] Naltrexone has demonstrated efficacy in delaying and preventing relapse to heavy drinking and reducing the percentage of drinking days, but not in promoting total abstinence in numerous (but not all) clinical trials.[62]

Naltrexone is rapidly and almost fully absorbed after oral administration, achieves its peak effect after 1 hour, and has a half-life of approximately 4 hours (metabolite half-life = 12 hours). The usual dose is 50 mg per day, which is sufficient to occupy the majority of μ-opioid receptors.[63] Many clinicians begin naltrexone at 25 mg per day for a few days to minimize side effects and then titrate up to 50 mg per day. Though data are sparse, some clinicians will also increase naltrexone to 100 mg per day if a suboptimal response occurs at 50 mg per day, and the 100 mg per day dose demonstrated modest efficacy in the COMBINE Study.[53]

Common side effects of naltrexone include nausea, headache, dizziness, fatigue, sedation, and anxiety and typically resolve with continued treatment. Naltrexone does have a black box label warning for acute hepatitis, although most of these events occurred at doses of 300 mg per day in clinical trials for obesity, and there is little evidence of hepatotoxity at currently recommended doses for alcohol dependence. Nevertheless, given the black box warning, it is judicious to obtain liver function tests prior to initiation and then at 1, 3, 6 and 12 months during therapy.

Because naltrexone blocks μ-opioid receptors, opioid medications will be much less effective in the situation in which an injury or serious medical condition calls for acute pain control. If given in adequate doses (usually higher than would otherwise be required), opioids can generally overcome the blockade, but close monitoring of the patient in an inpatient setting to observe for and manage respiratory depression is advised.

Long-Acting Injectable Naltrexone. Although oral naltrexone generally appears efficacious compared to placebo in reducing relapse to heavy drinking, it has not performed well in some studies. However, when patients found to be nonadherent for oral naltrexone are factored out in several other studies, naltrexone demonstrates efficacy for treatment of alcohol dependence compared to placebo.[64,65] Consequently, long-acting intramuscular naltrexone, FDA approved in 2006 for treatment of alcohol dependence, may eliminate concerns about adherence and has been shown to be effective compared to placebo in reducing heavy drinking.[66] An additional advantage of long-acting intramuscular naltrexone includes lower rates of first-pass hepatic metabolism, exposing the liver to significantly lower peak dosages than daily oral dosing. The reduced first-pass metabolism of intramuscular naltrexone leads to lower levels of the active metabolite 6β-naltrexol, which has been correlated with side effects such as nausea. Lower levels of this metabolite may lead to better tolerability of the intramuscular form of naltrexone. Long-acting injectable naltrexone is indicated for patients who have achieved some period of abstinence which could be as brief as several hours. The dosage is one 360 mg gluteal injection every 4 weeks. Patients can be started directly on the injection without a trial on oral medication.

Naltrexone for Opioid Dependence. For opioid dependent patients who have withdrawn from opioids and who do not wish to continue opioid therapy, oral naltrexone offers, from a theoretical standpoint, an ideal pharmacotherapy. Once a state of full withdrawal is achieved as verified by a naloxone challenge test, naltrexone can be started. With naltrexone on board, the effect of exogenously administered opioids will be blocked so that no euphoria is experienced and physiologic dependence cannot be reestablished. Unfortunately, very few opioid dependent patients remain on naltrexone for an extended period, so it performs only slightly better than placebo.[67] Some populations such as individuals with legal mandates or impaired professionals may do better on naltrexone. As noted above, naltrexone represents a poor choice of pharmacotherapy for most pain patients since it prevents the use of opioid analgesics. If it is prescribed, the typical dose is 50 mg per day.

Methadone. As noted above, methadone can only be prescribed for the treatment of opioid dependence through federally licensed and regulated clinics. Thus, in most cases, pain patients who need methadone treatment must be referred to one of these clinics. Such clinics are not available in many geographic regions and at times also have waiting lists.

Methadone is prescribed quite differently when used to treat opioid dependence than when prescribed for pain. Typically, for treatment of opioid dependence, a single daily dose is provided in liquid form. The maximum initial dose is 30 mg. The lowest effective dose of methadone for treatment of opioid dependence is approximately 50 mg, with an optimum average dose for most patients of approximately 80 mg (± 20 mg), although some patients require a dose higher than this range. The daily dose should be sufficient to prevent emergence of withdrawal symptoms at least through the 24-hour dosing period. The dose should be sufficient to greatly diminish or eliminate opioid cravings and opioid use (as determined by both self-report and urine toxicology testing). The dose should create sufficient tolerance such that illicit opioid use does not cause euphoria. The dose should not be so high that side effects such as sedation, constipation, or loss of libido occur.[31]

Patients who do not stabilize within a few weeks should be evaluated both at the end of the 24-hour dosing cycle just prior to the next scheduled dose to assess the presence of withdrawal signs and symptoms and at 4 hours postdose to observe the patient for any evidence of intoxication or excessive opioid effect at the time of peak plasma levels.[31] If the patient does have withdrawal signs prior to the dose and no intoxication postdose, an upward adjustment in dose is probably warranted. When patients fail to stabilize after successive dose increases, consideration could be given to obtaining a trough (predose) serum methadone level. Levels below 100 ng/mL are associated with withdrawal symptoms and inadequate dosage.[68] There are rare ultra rapid metabolizers of methadone who will not become stable on a single daily dose and will exhibit low trough serum levels of methadone. For this small group of patients, splitting the dose by giving them half of the dose observed and the other half as a take-home for the evening generally promotes stabilization.

For patients on methadone maintenance, their daily dose of methadone will rarely be fully, if at all, efficacious in managing acute or chronic pain. These patients will typically need opioid analgesics, either methadone tablets or another opioid of choice, given throughout the day in appropriately divided doses given in addition to the daily dose of methadone. For acute pain, these additional opioids can be discontinued when the pain subsides. For chronic pain, the additional opioids will need to be ongoing in most cases.

Buprenorphine. Although buprenorphine can be prescribed through licensed clinics, its pharmacologic characteristics make it a very attractive medication for office-based therapy. Its partial agonist action means that it has a ceiling effect for central nervous system and respiratory depressive effects, making it far safer in overdose than methadone and other full μ-opioid agonists.[69] This partial agonist property also makes it easier to withdraw from this medication than from methadone. Withdrawing from methadone can take months or years and be difficult for patients.

In addition, buprenorphine has slow onset when administered sublingually (1.5 to 3 hours to peak plasma levels), a long half-life, and high affinity plus slow dissociation from the receptor.[70,71] Thus, it prevents the emergence of withdrawal symptoms for 24 hours or longer, and, by occupying the majority of receptors, it makes very few receptors available for binding of full agonists. Buprenorphine's long half-life allows for once daily or even thrice weekly dosing. Buprenorphine is poorly absorbed by the oral route and undergoes extensive first pass hepatic metabolism, so for treatment of opioid dependence, it is administered sublingually.

Buprenorphine prescription in the office setting was made possible in the United States by the Drug Addiction Treatment Act of 2000 (DATA).[72] DATA allows for office-based opioid maintenance therapy for opioid dependence using schedule III, IV, or V medications approved for this use by the FDA. In 2002, the FDA approved buprenorphine and buprenorphine/naloxone for this purpose, and they are the only medications at this time with this indication. In order to prescribe buprenorphine, physicians must obtain a waiver from the Drug Enforcement Agency which requires specialty training in addictions or completion of 8 hours of training in management of opioid dependence provided by an approved association, and physicians must be able to refer patients to appropriate counseling and ancillary services. The waiver allows physicians to prescribe buprenorphine to up to 100 patients at a given time.

Buprenorphine is available for sublingual administration as a single agent or as a combination buprenorphine-naloxone preparation with a ratio of 4 mg buprenorphine to 1 mg of naloxone. The advantage of the combination buprenorphine-naloxone preparation is the prevention of abuse. Buprenorphine has adequate bioavailability sublingually, while naloxone is minimally bioavailable sublingually, so the naloxone has no effect on patients when administered as intended. If the combination medication is dissolved in an attempt to inject buprenorphine, however, naloxone, which also has a high affinity for the μ receptor, will exert its antagonist properties resulting in withdrawal instead of euphoria. The single agent should be reserved for use only in situations where there is no concern for potential abuse, such as in an inpatient setting or in individuals who are at greater risk to potential withdrawal symptoms if exposed to naloxone, such as pregnant women or those transitioning from methadone. Due to the partial agonist properties of buprenorphine, patients need to be clearly educated that they should not take this medication soon after taking other opioid drugs because buprenorphine in that situation may precipitate withdrawal.

An important component of the clinical skill in using buprenorphine involves the induction procedures. Patients who have been taking full agonist opioids must abstain from their full agonist opioids long enough to evidence signs of mild opioid withdrawal. If patients take the first dose of buprenorphine when not in active opioid withdrawal, there is a risk that buprenorphine as a partial agonist will precipitate more severe opioid withdrawal. Patients often require a fair amount of empathic emotional support to assure them that they can handle a period of several hours without opioids and can tolerate a brief episode of mild withdrawal prior to starting buprenorphine. Usually, it is not the mild withdrawal symptoms themselves that are troublesome, so much as the anxiety about more severe withdrawal. If patients are in mild to moderate withdrawal at the time of starting buprenorphine, the first dose usually alleviates much of the withdrawal within 30–60 minutes.

Induction of buprenorphine should thus begin approximately 12–24 hours after last use of a short-acting opioid drug or 24–48 hours after last use of a long-acting opioid drug, and patients should be showing objective signs of withdrawal at the time of initiation of therapy. On the first day of induction, the maximum dose should not exceed 8 mg to 12 mg. Because the transition from methadone to buprenorphine is more difficult than the transition from short-acting opioids, patients who are receiving methadone for pain and wish to transition can be first switched from methadone to a short-acting opioid, then inducted onto buprenorphine. For patients receiving methadone in a licensed clinic for the treatment of opioid dependence, this switch to a short-acting opioid is not legally permissible, and such patients must be inducted directly from methadone to buprenorphine.

If, after beginning buprenorphine, patients still have withdrawal symptoms after receiving the maximum first day dose, they should be treated symptomatically with adjunctive agents such as clonidine, antiemetics, antidiarrheals, and benzodiazepines for specific withdrawal symptoms. Over the course of the next 2 to 6 days, patients should be assessed for signs and symptoms of withdrawal with increases in buprenorphine given for persistent symptoms up to a total of 16 mg on the second day and a maximum of 32 mg per day by the end of the first week. Withdrawal symptoms beyond this time typically indicate persisting illicit opioid abuse.

Following induction, patients will stabilize on a dose over the following 1 to 2 months, and the dose should be adjusted to the lowest effective dose to prevent withdrawal symptoms, prevent craving of opioids, and suppress illicit opioid abuse. Once this dose is established, patients can be maintained on this medication indefinitely or may choose to taper off.[73]

Numerous studies have found buprenorphine to be effective in retaining patients in treatment and reducing illicit opioid abuse. A systematic review of studies, which compared 13 studies involving 2544 subjects in trials of buprenorphine versus either placebo or methadone, found buprenorphine to be effective as a maintenance therapy for opioid dependence when compared to placebo.[74] Compared with methadone, however, especially at higher doses of methadone, buprenorphine may not be quite as effective at maintaining patients in treatment or reducing illicit opioid use. Nevertheless, since buprenorphine is a safer medication than methadone, it often makes clinical sense to use buprenorphine as a first line agent. If a patient fails buprenorphine treatment, the patient can be transitioned to methadone maintenance in a licensed clinic.[75] Transition from methadone to buprenorphine is clinically more difficult than transition from buprenorphine to methadone.

As a partial agonist, buprenorphine has analgesic properties, but its analgesic effects may not always be as powerful as those of a full agonist. However, recent evidence suggests that buprenorphine produces less hyperalgesia than full agonist opioids[76] and so may have some benefit for pain control in patients not responding well to full agonists. Also, while buprenorphine has a ceiling on its respiratory depressant action, it does not appear to have a ceiling on its analgesic activity, so higher doses should continue to elicit greater analgesia.[77] Thus, buprenorphine has tremendous potential for management of patients who have combined chronic pain and opioid dependence. It allows the physician treating such a patient to continue to manage the patient in his or her own office for both disorders along with referral for ancillary counseling if needed rather than terminating such a patient or sending the patient to an addiction treatment provider or facility with the risk of a failure to follow through. As noted, some clinical skill is required to support the patient in abstaining from full agonist opioids long enough to evidence signs of opioid withdrawal such that buprenorphine induction can take place. Patients being treated with buprenorphine for combined pain and opioid dependence may get better analgesia by taking the buprenorphine in divided doses throughout the day rather than as a single daily dose. Although more data on the treatment of combined pain and opioid dependence are needed, preliminary reports indicate a positive response for many patients.[78]

THE PAIN MEDICINE PERSPECTIVE ON ADDICTION IN CHRONIC PAIN PATIENTS

For specialists in pain medicine, addiction to opioids looms over addiction to any other kind of substance as an issue of concern. Since pain specialists frequently prescribe opioids for patients with CNMP, they must be concerned about whether their opioid prescriptions are being misused by patients with pre-existing opioid addiction, and whether the prescriptions are creating addiction to opioids.

Historic and Regulatory Issues

Challenges associated with opioid therapy in CNMP occur against the backdrop of an uneasy relationship between physicians who prescribe opioids and the regulatory and law enforcement agencies that are charged with the prevention and prosecution of illegal uses of opioids. Interactions with these agencies have almost certainly affected the opinions that physicians have expressed in publications about opioid therapy.

Historically, attitudes about prescribing opioids to patients with CNMP have gone through a succession of well-known shifts. When pain medicine emerged as a specialty in the mid-1970s, there was a reasonable consensus, based only on expert opinion and not on data, that long-term opioid therapy was problematic because of the risks of tolerance, physical dependence, and addiction.[79] Starting in the 1970s, researchers began to report that cancer patients treated with long-term opioid therapy did not show progressive tolerance, and, more generally, that opioid therapy for these patients was a reasonable therapeutic option.[80,81] During the 1980s, insights gleaned during the 1970s about cancer patients began to be applied to CNMP patients. For example, an influential paper by Portenoy and Foley[82] on a case series of 38 patients showed that it was possible to achieve long-term effective pain control for CNMP patients with opioids.

Several factors converged to lead to significant changes in the regulatory climate during the 1990s. With accumulating data demonstrating that opioids can be effective in the treatment of CNMP,[83] both physician pain specialists and patients insisted that long-term opioid therapy can benefit CNMP patients and that regulatory and legislative barriers to treatment that might relieve their suffering should be removed. Regulators and legislators responded by making opioid therapy for CNMP more accessible and acceptable.[84,85]

Pain physicians were not unanimously enthusiastic about opioid therapy during the 1990s. For example, physicians associated with multidisciplinary pain rehabilitation programs generally maintained a less sanguine view toward opioids.[86] However, pain physicians who favored opioid therapy combined forces with patient advocate groups to promote five assertions:

1. Long-term opioid therapy is an effective tool in the management of CNMP.
2. The concept of addiction as used by psychiatrists and addiction medicine specialists may not universally or easily apply to patients receiving opioid therapy for CNMP.
3. The likelihood that CNMP patients will develop addiction to prescription opioids is low.
4. There is no inherent ceiling to opioid therapy, so that it is appropriate for physicians to titrate doses upward until a patient either experiences satisfactory analgesia or develops side effects that preclude further dose escalations.
5. Patients have a right to pain relief and to receive opioids for that purpose in the absence of specific contraindications.

There is ample evidence that consumption of prescription opioids has increased markedly during the past 15 years.[87,88] Along with this increase in availability, large scale data have emerged indicating that misuse of prescription opioids has become more frequent over time and represents a significant public health problem.[84,89] Also, there has been a rise in opioid-related deaths.[90] On a smaller scale, several researchers have reported data on small cohorts of pain patients indicating that inappropriate/aberrant use of prescription opioids is far more common than physicians during the 1980s and 1990s supposed.[91–93] Finally, accumulating evidence from randomized controlled trials suggests that opioids are only modestly beneficial for patients with CNMP and appear to have limited efficacy at best for some common conditions such as chronic low back pain.[94,95] In the face of these new data, at least some pain specialists have recently urged greater restraint in the use of opioids for CNMP.[96]

Conceptions of Opioid Dependence and Opioid Abuse—The Pain Medicine Perspective

The *DSM-IV TR* criteria for identifying opioid dependence provide an appropriate starting point for the identification of

such dependence among CNMP patients. However, when these criteria are applied to CNMP patients, important ambiguities arise.[97,98] One key issue is whether patients have a legitimate need for opioids. *DSM-IV TR* states, "Opioid Dependence includes signs and symptoms that reflect compulsive, prolonged self-administration of opioid substances that are used for no legitimate medical purpose."[4] But many CNMP patients report that they **do** have a legitimate medical purpose for consuming opioids, and most pain specialists would agree (at least in principle) with such an assertion. In fact, if one accepts the premises (1) that pain has such strong motivational consequences that it "forces" people to engage in whatever activities are needed to obtain pain relief and (2) that relief of pain represents a legitimate goal for patients, many of the behaviors of CNMP patients in relation to opioids would be construed as understandable and legitimate, even though comparable behaviors by individuals who are not in pain would be construed as strong evidence for opioid dependence. Thus, acceptance of these premises challenges the relevance of several of the *DSM-IV TR* criteria to CNMP patients.

Another problem in applying *DSM-IV TR* criteria for opioid dependence to pain patients is that withdrawal and tolerance are two of the criteria. An individual who demonstrates both physical dependence and tolerance to an opioid would meet *DSM-IV TR* criteria for the diagnosis of opioid dependence if he/she met any one of the other five criteria. Pain specialists assume that patients who receive long-term opioid therapy will develop opioid tolerance and physical dependence but maintain that such predictable changes should not be accepted as indicators of addiction in these patients. For example, Portenoy[99] states: "Although physical dependence, like tolerance, has been suggested to be a component of addiction. . ., the clinical experience gained in the population with chronic pain strongly affirms that addiction should be defined in a manner that fully distinguishes it from physical dependence. . . . The fundamental distinction between addiction and physical dependence implies that clinicians should never label patients who are presumed to be at risk for an abstinence syndrome (that is, physically dependent) as *addicted*."[99] Because of the conviction among pain specialists that physical dependence is not an indicator of abnormal behavior on the part of a patient, most prefer the term "addiction" to the term "dependence" when discussing opioid-related behavior that is abnormal. Trescot et al.[100] describe addiction as follows: "Addiction is a dysfunctional use behavior that includes one or more of the following: impaired control over drug use, compulsive use, continued use despite harm, and craving." This definition emphasizes inappropriate behavior in relation to opioids and omits any reference to physical dependence or tolerance.

A third issue that complicates the application of the *DSM-IV TR* definition of opioid dependence to patients with CNMP is that pain specialists[101,102] have often accepted the premise from cancer pain management[103] that there is no inherent ceiling to opioid dosing. Also, it is not unusual for patients to receive opioids for several years. Consequently, it is difficult to apply the *DSM-IV TR* criterion "Substance taken in larger amounts or over a longer period of time that was intended."[4]

Finally, the social context within which opioid therapy for CNMP occurs also complicates any discussion of opioid addiction in CNMP patients. In contrast to heroin or methamphetamine, prescription opioids are substances that can be obtained and used legally. But in contrast to alcohol, prescription opioids are not freely available to pain patients. Physicians act as gate keepers who control the access of patients to the medications. Since decisions about opioid use emerge out of a dialog between patients and physicians, patients' opioid usage patterns are influenced by some combination of their perceptions of their opioid needs, their ability to communicate their preferences to treating physicians, and the beliefs and preferences of treating physicians regarding opioid therapy. As one example of the complexities introduced by these social factors, a patient who is in fact addicted to opioids but has a very accommodating physician might not display behaviors indicative of addiction because his or her habit is routinely "fed" by the prescribing physician. At the opposite extreme, a patient under the care of a physician who refuses to prescribe any opioids might engage in drug seeking behaviors and seem preoccupied with getting opioids.[104]

Given the above complications, it is difficult to say exactly what *DSM-IV TR* opioid dependence means when the term is applied to a patient with CNMP. The fact that the patient takes an opioid on a regular basis does not prove addiction, even if his or her daily dose is high. The patient may appear preoccupied with obtaining opioids, but this phenomenon could be construed as evidence of the "irresistible force" of persistent uncontrolled pain. In principle, a physician could conclude that a patient was addicted if the patient took opioids when he or she was not experiencing pain, or took them in order to get "high" rather than to get relief from pain. But physicians essentially never have this kind of detailed information about the experiences of patients just before or just after they take opioids. The problems of applying *DSM-IV TR* criteria to pain patients are summarized in Table 90.4.

In practice, pain physicians typically rely on indirect indicators when they make inferences about opioid dependence in CNMP patients.[93,98] For example, they are likely to suspect such dependence when patients engage in aberrant behaviors (Table 90.5), demonstrate poor judgment in relation to opioids (e.g., drive while heavily sedated), or insist on increasing doses of opioids despite demonstrating behaviors that suggest drug toxicity.

The term "pseudoaddiction," introduced by Weissman and Haddox[104] in 1989, pulls together many of the concepts which have been developed by pain specialists and which distinguish their perspective on opioid use and abuse from that of addiction medicine physicians. Weissman and Haddox[104] said: "We have termed this syndrome pseudoaddiction because of the strikingly similar behavioral pattern seen in patients such as the one reported here to patients with idiopathic opioid psychologic dependence, namely, an overwhelming and compulsive interest in the acquisition and use of opioid analgesics. However, unlike true opioid psychologic dependence where the underlying cause is unknown, pseudoaddiction is an iatrogenic syndrome caused by the undermedication of pain."[104] They indicate that the appropriate treatment for pseudoaddiction is an increase in the opioid dose prescribed for a patient.

The concept of pseudoaddiction implies that patients may be driven to seek opioids compulsively because of the severity of their pain. Thus, as the term pseudoaddiction reveals, behaviors that are normally taken as indicators of addiction are now construed as indicators of the overwhelming "force" of untreated pain. Also, the concept is at least compatible with the idea that true opioid abuse is uncommon among CNMP patients being treated with opioids. In essence, it implies that even when a patient behaves in a manner that suggests drug addiction, the problem rests with the treatment program rather than with the patient. Finally, the recommended physician response to pseudoaddiction—to increase a patient's opioid dose—is at least compatible with the idea that there is no inherent limit to opioid dosing.

Clinical Management of Opioid Addiction Within Specialty Pain Clinics

Pain specialists who prescribe opioids regularly for CNMP have to develop strategies for managing opioid addiction. However, there is no simple or uniform set of management procedures. Several factors contribute to difficulties in describing the behavior of pain specialists in relation to opioid addiction. First, a pain specialist's decisions about opioids for a patient depend on his or her assessment about whether opioids will benefit the patient, as well as his or her judgments about whether the patient is engaging in aberrant behaviors in relation to opioids. Second, there is significant variation across pain specialists with regard to use of opioids and management of opioid addiction. Finally, the procedures used by pain physicians to manage opioid addiction are generally not evidence-based. Fortunately, there are now consensus-based guidelines for managing opioid therapy[100]; the present discussion relies on these guidelines.

The management of issues related to opioid addiction can be divided into six areas: (1) initial screening and decision to use opioids; (2) establishing ground rules; (3) monitoring opioid therapy; (4) taking other steps to reduce the likelihood of aberrant behavior; (5) tapering opioids; and (6) referrals to other specialists.

1. Initial Screening: There is widespread agreement among experts that pain specialists should inquire about whether patients have present or past drug abuse problems and should be attentive to signs that patients might be prone to flout rules established by physicians. For example, if a patient reports being "fired" by other physicians because of disagreements regarding opioid therapy, this should be a red flag. In addition to interviewing CNMP patients about their past histories regarding drugs and alcohol, pain specialists can ask them to fill out a questionnaire designed to determine the risk that they will engage in aberrant behavior if they are treated with opioids. Several such questionnaires have been developed during the past several years.[9,93,105] These instruments are backed by some empirical data that support their validity. At this point, there is no instrument that is clearly superior to the others.[106] Finally, it is prudent for pain physicians to insist on an initial screening urine toxicology specimen before deciding whether to treat a CNMP patient with opioids.[6]

2. Establishing Ground Rules: There is agreement among experts that patients should sign a treatment agreement before opioid

---

TABLE 90.5

EXAMPLES OF ABERRANT BEHAVIORS RELATED TO OPIOID USE

1. Used additional opioids than those prescribed
2. Used additional opioids than those prescribed more than once
3. Forged prescription
4. Sold prescription
5. Admitted to seeking euphoria from opioids
6. Admitted to wanting opioids for anxiety
7. Overdose
8. Injected drug
9. Abnormal urine/blood screen
10. Abnormal urine/blood screen positive for two or more substances
11. Solicited opioids from other providers
12. Unauthorized emergency room visits
13. Concurrent abuse of alcohol
14. Unauthorized dose escalation
15. Resisted therapy changes/alternative therapy
16. Reported lost or stolen prescriptions
17. Canceled clinic visit
18. Requested early refills
19. Requested refills instead of clinic visit
20. Abused prescribed drug
21. Was discharged from practice (because of aberrant behavior)
22. No show or no follow-up
23. Third party required to manage patient's medications

Modified from Webster LR, Webster RM. Predicting aberrant behaviors in opioid-treated patients: preliminary validation of the Opioid Risk Tool. *Pain Med* 2005;6(6):432–442.

therapy is instituted.[100,107] A pain specialist can choose from several prototypes that are in the medical literature[108] or can create his or her own. The treatment agreement should delineate behaviors that are considered appropriate or inappropriate by the prescribing physician. Agreed upon treatment goals and criteria for treatment success are crucial.

3. Monitoring Opioid Therapy: Pain physicians should monitor the therapeutic responses of patients who have been started on opioids and should determine whether they are experiencing side effects such as constipation. As far as monitoring for aberrant use is concerned, physicians should certainly keep careful track of their opioid prescriptions, so they know whether patients are exceeding their allotments. In some instances, information sharing among pharmacies alerts prescribing physicians to situations in which a patient obtains opioids from more than one physician. Also, physicians may insist on random urine toxicology screens and pill counts. There is no consensus among pain specialists about how to orchestrate these management tools.

4. Other Steps to Reduce the Likelihood of Aberrant Behavior: Traditionally, pain specialists have advocated for the use of long-acting opioids taken on a time contingent basis, rather than short-acting opioids that patients take on an as needed basis. One rationale for this recommendation is that experience with cancer pain suggests that a continuous background level of an opioid reduces the likelihood that a patient will experience severe spikes in pain that are very hard to control pharmacologically. Another rationale is behavioral. Some experts[109,110] have argued that if opioids are taken on an as needed basis, they end up reinforcing a patient's experience of pain and set the stage for excessive drug consumption by the patient. The strategy of having CNMP patients use long-acting opioids on a time contingent basis was originally promulgated by physicians working in multidisciplinary pain rehabilitation programs (see below). Although the appropriateness of this strategy is supported by animal research demonstrating a reduced risk of opioid-induced hyperalgesia when rats are maintained on steady levels of an opioid than when they are repeatedly subjected to opioid withdrawal,[111,112] the empirical evidence to support the efficacy of the strategy among CNMP patients is at best modest.[113] In the absence of definitive data, we believe it is prudent for a physician to consider the use of long-acting, time contingent opioid therapy, especially when he or she is treating a patient who has demonstrated poor judgment with respect to opioid consumption in the past. Another strategy is to use a "pain cocktail" in order to keep a patient blinded to his or her opioid regimen.[114] Thirdly, the treating physician might reduce the likelihood of aberrant behavior by prescribing opioids thought to have a relatively low abuse potential (e.g., methadone), rather than ones that historically have been associated with high abuse potential (e.g., oxycodone).[115] Fourth, the physician should give careful consideration to the issue of dose escalations. One of us (James P. Robinson) has found it useful to titrate a patient's dose until there appears to be reasonable pain control but to also make it clear to the patient that once a stable dose has been reached, it will not be increased. Finally, the physician should consider a range of adjuvant therapies that might help patients maintain control over their opioid consumption by contributing to pain relief and functional improvement. These include antidepressant or anticonvulsant medication, exercise therapy, and psychologic counseling.

5. Tapering Opioids: A pain physician might decide to taper a patient's opioids either because opioid therapy was judged to be ineffective or because the patient engaged in aberrant behavior in relation to opioids. However, if the aberrant behavior is an indicator of opioid dependence, a taper might well be ineffective, even if the patient stops receiving opioids from the pain physician. The problem in this setting is that the patient might resume opioid consumption either by getting prescriptions from another physician or by obtaining opioids illicitly. In this regard, anecdotal reports from outpatient clinics and numerous case series from pain rehabilitation programs indicate that CNMP patients can usually go through opioid tapers uneventfully.[110,116] However, follow-up of patients who go through such tapers is woefully deficient and informal observation by one of us (James P. Robinson) suggests that after patients complete treatment at a pain rehabilitation program, it is not at all uncommon for them to be restarted on opioid medications by their community physicians. It is also sobering to note that data from addiction medicine research indicate a high probability of relapse when opioid-dependent individuals undergo medically supervised withdrawal in the absence of further treatment.[27,30] Thus, it is entirely possible that pain specialists have generally been lulled into a false sense that opioid tapers are relatively easy to perform. If the aberrant behaviors actually do represent opioid dependence, in most cases it makes more sense to begin office-based buprenorphine treatment or to refer the patient for opioid agonist therapy elsewhere to reduce risk of relapse to problematic opioid use.

6. Referrals to Other Specialists: There is no consensus among pain specialists about the circumstances under which CNMP patients should be referred for specialty services regarding the opioids. The decision is easy in extreme situations (e.g., when a patient who is receiving opioids for CNMP shows up with new needle tracks and admits to using heroin). But pain specialists routinely encounter patients who insist on receiving high doses of opioids and ones who engage in at least low level aberrant behaviors, such as "losing" opioid prescriptions or requesting early refills. Most pain specialists treat at least some of these patients without assistance. As noted above, they typically cannot assess the effectiveness of their treatments, since they rarely get follow-up data on the patients. If a pain specialist does decide that he or she needs help, there are at least three choices. One is to refer the patient to an addiction medicine specialist, especially one who works closely with facilities that can provide supervised detoxification and rehabilitative services for people with drug dependence as described earlier in the chapter. A second option is to refer the patient to a pain rehabilitation program. This type of referral has the advantage of potentially managing the patient's opioid problem in the context of an overall pain management program. However, the down side of such a referral is that most pain rehabilitation programs are not well suited to addressing the needs of patients with significant addiction problems. The deficiencies of pain programs in this regard are so magnified now that virtually all such programs are carried out on an outpatient basis, in contrast to the inpatient treatment that was the norm when multidisciplinary pain rehabilitation was first introduced.[117]

Practitioners at pain programs have only one option for more specialized care for patients with drug dependence: referral to an addiction medicine specialist. We are not aware of any detailed published data on the frequency with which such referrals are made. Informal observation indicates that when staff at pain centers identify potential drug problems among patients undergoing screening for possible program admission, they triage them into three groups: (1) patients who are taking modest opioid doses and have no red flags for aberrant behaviors are typically admitted to the pain rehabilitation program, with the expectation that they can be tapered while going through the program; (2) ones who have no red flags for aberrant behaviors but are on high opioid doses are often started on opioid tapers prior to program admission, with the expectation that the taper could be completed as they go through their program; (3) ones with red flags for substance abuse are typically referred to addiction medicine specialists.

With the advent of buprenorphine, a third choice has emerged for a pain specialist who has a patient exhibiting aberrant behaviors which ultimately lead to a diagnosis of opioid dependence. Pain specialists can now attempt to treat combined CNMP and opioid dependence in their offices using buprenorphine and referral to counseling or other ancillary services as needed.

CONCLUSION: AREAS WHERE IMPROVED COMMUNICATION BETWEEN PAIN SPECIALISTS AND ADDICTION MEDICINE SPECIALISTS IS NEEDED

From the foregoing discussion, it is apparent that addiction specialists and pain specialists have considerable overlap in their patient populations, but that their work with these patients has developed in two separate parallel tracks largely devoid of mutual interaction. The schism between the two fields is highlighted by the fact that attorneys have pitted addiction specialists and pain specialists against each other in legal proceedings involving alleged inappropriate prescribing of opioids.[118] Pain specialists, like most physicians, do not believe they have the knowledge or skill to treat addiction. Increasing evidence shows that in mild to moderate cases of addiction to nonopioid substances, particularly alcohol, physician intervention can control or ameliorate the problem. In cases of opioid dependence, physicians, including pain specialists, can manage these patients in their offices using buprenorphine. In fact, many pain specialists are in a unique position to do so because they already have a therapeutic relationship with the patient, and they have extensive expertise in opioid pharmacology. Addiction specialists should work to educate and empower pain specialists to manage cases of addiction when possible.

From the opposite perspective, pain problems are highly prevalent among patients seeing addiction specialists for acknowledged substance dependence.[3,119,120] Oftentimes, the pain problem goes untreated, exacerbating the addiction problem and creating a situation analogous but not identical to the pseudo-addiction described above. Pain specialists could help addiction specialists by educating them about prescribing opioids for pain when appropriate and monitoring functional outcomes to determine if the opioids are effective as well as by training addiction specialists in nonpharmacologic interventions for pain.

Of the many possible issues on which pain specialists and addiction medicine specialists might fruitfully collaborate, we note the following:

1. The conceptualization of drug dependence/addiction. Addiction specialists are accustomed to applying *DSM-IV TR* criteria, but pain specialists understandably lack confidence in these criteria, at least for the diagnosis of opioid dependence, in the context of a CNMP patient being treated with opioids. Although it would be difficult to accomplish, rigorous study of the application of *DSM-IV TR* criteria to this population might help to eliminate some of this uncertainty.
2. Identification of outcome variables. Whether treatment is directed at pain, addiction, or the combination of the two, it is important for physicians to identify criteria for determining when treatment has been successful. Pain specialists certainly consider pain reduction as an important outcome of treatment but also focus on patients' ability to function and the overall quality of their lives. Informal observation suggests that addiction medicine specialists have a perspective on criteria for successful treatment that is similar to that of pain specialists, but

we are not aware of any collaborative efforts between the two specialties to identify these criteria.
3. Follow-up data on CNMP patients who receive opioid therapy, with attention to long-term opioid dependence. As noted above, it is possible that pain specialists have grossly underestimated the difficulties of tapering opioids in CNMP patients because they have not systematically followed the patients. The experiences and research methods of addiction medicine might help pain specialists fill this important gap.
4. Rules of thumb regarding when pain specialists should refer CNMP patients to addiction medicine specialists.
5. Strategies for optimal management of dual diagnosis patients (i.e., ones with CNMP and addiction).
6. Consideration of what is actually being treated when CNMP patients receive opioid therapy—especially at high doses. This chapter has focused on the possibility that when pain specialists try to alleviate patients' pain by prescribing opioids, they might inadvertently maintain opioid addiction or cause opioid addiction. Another possibility is that the opioids prescribed by pain physicians may function as psychotropic drugs rather than analgesics. This reflects the fact that CNMP patients may seek opioids in large part because the opioids blunt emotional distress associated with anxiety or depressive disorders.[121] These possibilities highlight the complexities of opioid therapy and of the patients who seek such therapy. Dialog among pain specialists, addiction medicine specialists, and other specialists (such as psychiatrists) might lead to more rational methods for evaluating and treating these challenging patients.

References

1. Michna E, Ross EL, Hynes WL, et al. Predicting aberrant drug behavior in patients treated for chronic pain: importance of abuse history. *J Pain Symptom Manage* 2004;28(3):250–258.
2. Manchikanti L, Cash KA, Damron KS, et al. Controlled substance abuse and illicit drug use in chronic pain patients: An evaluation of multiple variables. *Pain Physician* 2006;9(3):215–225.
3. Rosenblum A, Joseph H, Fong C, et al. Prevalence and characteristics of chronic pain among chemically dependent patients in methadone maintenance and residential treatment facilities. *JAMA* 2003;289(18):2370–2378.
4. American Psychiatric Association. *Diagnostic and Statistical Manual of Mental Disorders.* 4th ed, text revision. Arlington, VA: American Psychiatric Publishing Incorporated; 2000.
5. O'Brien CP, Volkow N, Li TK. What's in a word? Addiction versus dependence in DSM-V. *Am J Psychiatry* 2006;163(5):764–765.
6. Gourlay DL, Heit HA, Almahrezi A. Universal precautions in pain medicine: a rational approach to the treatment of chronic pain. *Pain Med* 2005;6(2):107–112.
7. Dawson DA, Grant BF, Li TK. Quantifying the risks associated with exceeding recommended drinking limits. *Alcohol Clin Exp Res* 2005;29(5):902–908.
8. Swift R. Direct measurement of alcohol and its metabolites. *Addiction* 2003;98(Suppl 2):73–80.
9. Butler SF, Budman SH, Fernandez K, et al. Validation of a screener and opioid assessment measure for patients with chronic pain. *Pain* 2004;112(1–2):65–75.
10. Heit HA, Gourlay DL. Urine drug testing in pain medicine. *J Pain Symptom Manage* 2004;27(3):260–267.
11. Dolan K, Rouen D, Kimber J. An overview of the use of urine, hair, sweat and saliva to detect drug use. *Drug Alcohol Rev* 2004;23(2):213–217.
12. Wolff K, Farrell M, Marsden J, et al. A review of biological indicators of illicit drug use, practical considerations and clinical usefulness. *Addiction* 1999;94(9):1279–1298.
13. Berner MM, Kriston L, Bentele M, et al. The alcohol use disorders identification test for detecting at-risk drinking: a systematic review and meta-analysis. *J Stud Alcohol Drugs* 2007;68(3):461–473.
14. Selzer ML. The Michigan alcoholism screening test: the quest for a new diagnostic instrument. *Am J Psychiatry* 1971;127(12):1653–1658.
15. Gavin DR, Ross HE, Skinner HA. Diagnostic validity of the drug abuse screening test in the assessment of DSM-III drug disorders. *Br J Addict* 1989;84(3):301–307.
16. Tiet QQ, Mausbach B. Treatments for patients with dual diagnosis: a review. *Alcohol Clin Exp Res* 2007;31(4):513–536.
17. Brooner RK, King VL, Kidorf M, et al. Psychiatric and substance use comorbidity among treatment-seeking opioid abusers. *Arch Gen Psychiatry* 1997;54(1):71–80.
18. Manchikanti L, Giordano J, Boswell MV, et al. Psychological factors as pre-

dictors of opioid abuse and illicit drug use in chronic pain patients. *J Opioid Manag* 2007;3(2):89–100.

19. Brady KT, Sinha R. Co-occurring mental and substance use disorders: the neurobiological effects of chronic stress [see comment]. *Am J Psychiatry* 2005; 162(8):1483–1493.

20. Manchikanti L, Manchukonda R, Pampati V, et al. Does random urine drug testing reduce illicit drug use in chronic pain patients receiving opioids? *Pain Physician* 2006;9(2):123–129.

21. Moyer A, Finney JW, Swearingen CE, et al. Brief interventions for alcohol problems: a meta-analytic review of controlled investigations in treatment-seeking and non-treatment-seeking populations. *Addiction* 2002;97(3):279–292.

22. Kaner EF, Beyer F, Dickinson HO, et al. Effectiveness of brief alcohol interventions in primary care populations. *Cochrane Database Syst Rev* 2007;2: CD004148.

23. Carroll KM, Ball SA, Nich C, et al. Motivational interviewing to improve treatment engagement and outcome in individuals seeking treatment for substance abuse: a multisite effectiveness study. *Drug Alcohol Depend* 2006; 81(3):301–312.

24. Staines G, Kosanke N, Magura S, et al. Convergent validity of the ASAM Patient Placement Criteria using a standardized computer algorithm. *J Addict Dis* 2003;22(Suppl 1):61–77.

25. Magura S, Staines G, Kosanke N, et al. Predictive validity of the ASAM Patient Placement Criteria for naturalistically matched vs. mismatched alcoholism patients. *Am J Addict* 2003;12(5):386–397.

26. Mayo-Smith MF. Pharmacological management of alcohol withdrawal. A meta-analysis and evidence-based practice guideline. American Society of Addiction Medicine Working Group on Pharmacological Management of Alcohol Withdrawal. *JAMA* 1997;278(2):144–151.

27. Sees KL, Delucchi KL, Masson C, et al. Methadone maintenance vs 180-day psychosocially enriched detoxification for treatment of opioid dependence: a randomized controlled trial. *JAMA* 2000;283(10):1303–1310.

28. Oreskovich MR, Saxon AJ, Ellis ML, et al. A double-blind, double-dummy, randomized, prospective pilot study of the partial mu opiate agonist, buprenorphine, for acute detoxification from heroin. *Drug Alcohol Depend* 2005; 77(1):71–79.

29. Gold MS, Redmond DE Jr, Kleber HD. Clonidine blocks acute opiate-withdrawal symptoms. *Lancet* 1978;2(8090):599–602.

30. Collins ED, Kleber HD, Whittington RA. Anesthesia-assisted vs buprenorphine- or clonidine-assisted heroin detoxification and naltrexone induction: a randomized trial. *JAMA* 2005;294(8):903–913.

31. Center for Substance Abuse Treatment. *Medication-Assisted Treatment for Opioid Addiction in Opioid Treatment Programs. Treatment Improvement Protocol (TIP) Series 43.* Rockville, MD: Substance Abuse and Mental Health Services Administration; 2005. DHHS Publication No. (SMA) 05-4048.

32. Gunne LM, Gronbladh L. The Swedish methadone maintenance program: a controlled study. *Drug Alcohol Depend* 1981;7(3):249–256.

33. Kakko J, Svanborg KD, Kreek MJ, et al. 1-year retention and social function after buprenorphine-assisted relapse prevention treatment for heroin dependence in Sweden: a randomised, placebo-controlled trial.[comment] *Lancet* 2003;361(9358):662–668.

34. Barnett PG. The cost-effectiveness of methadone maintenance as a health care intervention. *Addiction* 1999;94(4):479–488.

35. McLellan AT, Hagan TA, Meyers K, et al. "Intensive" outpatient substance abuse treatment: comparisons with "traditional" outpatient treatment. *J Addict Dis* 1997;16(2):57–84.

36. Broome KM, Simpson DD, Joe GW. The role of social support following short-term inpatient treatment. *Am J Addict* 2002;11(1):57–65.

37. Smith LA, Gates S, Foxcroft D. Therapeutic communities for substance related disorder. *Cochrane Database Syst Rev* 2006;1:CD005338.

38. McKay JR, Donovan DM, McLellan T, et al. Evaluation of full vs. partial continuum of care in the treatment of publicly funded substance abusers in Washington State. *Am J Drug Alcohol Abuse* 2002;28(2):307–338.

39. Meier PS, Barrowclough C, Donmall MC. The role of the therapeutic alliance in the treatment of substance misuse: a critical review of the literature. *Addiction* 2005;100(3):304–316.

40. Miller WR, Rollnick, S. *Motivational Interviewing: Preparing People for Change.* 2nd ed. New York: Guilford Press; 2002.

41. Marlatt GA, Donovan DM, eds. *Relapse Prevention: Maintenance Strategies in the Treatment of Addictive Behaviors.* 2nd ed. Guilford Press: New York; 2005.

42. Mercer DE, Woody GE. *An Individual Drug Counseling Approach to Treat Cocaine Addiction: The Collaborative Cocaine Treatment Study Model.* Washington, DC: U.S. Government Printing Office; 1999.

43. Nowinski J, Baker S, Carroll KM. *Twelve-Step Facilitation Therapy Manual: A Clinical Research Guide for Therapists Treating Individuals with Alcohol Abuse and Dependence.* Rockville, MD: U.S. Department of Health and Human Services, Public Health Service, National Institutes of Health, National Institute on Alcohol Abuse and Alcoholism; 1995.

44. Skinner BF. *The Behavior of Organisms: An Experimental Analysis.* New York: D. Appleton-Century Company; 1938.

45. Petry NM. Contingency management treatments. *Br J Psychiatry* 2006;189: 97–98.

46. Wright C, Moore RD. Disulfiram treatment of alcoholism. *Am J Med* 1990; 88(6):647–655.

47. Björnsson E, Nordlinder H, Olsson R. Clinical characteristics and prognostic markers in disulfiram-induced liver injury. *J Hepatol* 2006;44(4):791–797.

48. Fuller RK, Branchey L, Brightwell DR, et al. Disulfiram treatment of alcoholism. A Veterans Administration cooperative study. *JAMA* 1986;256(11): 1449–1455.

49. Myrick H, Anton R. Recent advances in the pharmacotherapy of alcoholism. *Curr Psychiatry Rep* 2004;6(5):332–338.

50. Litten RZ, Fertig J, Mattson M, et al. Development of medications for alcohol use disorders: recent advances and ongoing challenges. *Expert Opin Emerg Drugs* 2005;10(2):323–343.

51. Chick J, Lehert P, Landron F, et al. Does acamprosate improve reduction of drinking as well as aiding abstinence? *J Psychopharmacol* 2003;17(4): 397–402.

52. Mann K, Lehert P, Morgan MY. The efficacy of acamprosate in the maintenance of abstinence in alcohol-dependent individuals: results of a meta-analysis. *Alcohol Clin Exp Res* 2004;28(1):51–63.

53. Anton RF, O'Malley SS, Ciraulo DA, et al. and the COMBINE Study Research Group. Combined pharmacotherapies and behavioral interventions for alcohol dependence: the COMBINE study: a randomized controlled trial. *JAMA* 2006;295(17):2003–2017.

54. Mason BJ, Goodman AM, Chabac S, et al. Effect of oral acamprosate on abstinence in patients with alcohol dependence in a double-blind, placebo-controlled trial: the role of patient motivation. *J Psychiatr Res* 2006;40(5): 383–393.

55. Kiefer F, Mann K. Pharmacotherapy and behavioral intervention for alcohol dependence. *JAMA* 2006;296(14):1727–1728; author reply 1728–1729.

56. Sass H, Soyka M, Mann K, et al. Relapse prevention by acamprosate. Results from a placebo-controlled study on alcohol dependence. *Arch Gen Psychiatry* 1996;53(8):673–680.

57. Benjamin D, Grant ER, Pohorecky LA. Naltrexone reverses ethanol-induced dopamine release in the nucleus accumbens in awake, freely moving rats. *Brain Res* 1993;621(1):137–140.

58. De Waele JP, Gianoulakis C. Enhanced activity of the brain beta-endorphin system by free-choice ethanol drinking in C57BL/6 but not DBA/2 mice. *Eur J Pharmacol* 1994;258(1–2):119–129.

59. Olive MF, Koenig HN, Nannini MA, et al. Stimulation of endorphin neurotransmission in the nucleus accumbens by ethanol, cocaine, and amphetamine. *J Neurosci* 2001;21(23):RC184.

60. Tabakoff B, Hoffman PL. Alcohol interactions with brain opiate receptors. *Life Sci* 1983;32(3):197–204.

61. McCaul ME, Wand GS, Eissenberg T, et al. Naltrexone alters subjective and psychomotor responses to alcohol in heavy drinking subjects. *Neuropsychopharmacology* 2000;22(5):480–492.

62. Srisurapanont M, Jarusuraisin N. Opioid antagonists for alcohol dependence. *Cochrane Database Syst Rev* 2002;2:CD001867.

63. Lee MC, Wagner HN Jr, Tanada S, et al. Duration of occupancy of opiate receptors by naltrexone. *J Nucl Med* 1988;29(7):1207–1211.

64. Volpicelli JR, Rhines KC, Rhines JS, et al. Naltrexone and alcohol dependence. Role of subject compliance. *Arch Gen Psychiatry* 1997;54(8):737–742.

65. Chick J, Anton R, Checinski K, et al. A multicentre, randomized, double-blind, placebo-controlled trial of naltrexone in the treatment of alcohol dependence or abuse. *Alcohol* 2000;35(6):587–593.

66. Garbutt JC, Kranzler HR, O'Malley SS, et al. Efficacy and tolerability of long-acting injectable naltrexone for alcohol dependence: a randomized controlled trial. *JAMA* 2005;293(13):1617–1625.

67. Minozzi S, Amato L, Vecchi S, et al. Oral naltrexone maintenance treatment for opioid dependence. *Cochrane Database Syst Rev* 2006;1:CD001333.

68. Bell J, Seres V, Bowron P, et al. The use of serum methadone levels in patients receiving methadone maintenance. *Clin Pharmacol Ther* 1988;43(6):623–629.

69. Walsh SL, Preston KL, Stitzer ML, et al. Clinical pharmacology of buprenorphine: ceiling effects at high doses. *Clin Pharmacol Ther* 1994;55(5):569–580.

70. Greenwald MK, Johanson CE, Moody DE, et al. Effects of buprenorphine maintenance dose on mu-opioid receptor availability, plasma concentrations, and antagonist blockade in heroin-dependent volunteers. *Neuropsychopharmacology* 2003;28(11):2000–2009.

71. Johnson RE, McCagh JC. Buprenorphine and naloxone for heroin dependence. *Curr Psychiatry Rep* 2000;2(6):519–526.

72. Drug Addiction Treatment Act of 2000 (DATA). Public Law 106–310, 106th Congress, October 17, 2000, Title XXXV.

73. Center for Substance Abuse Treatment. *Clinical Guidelines for the Use of Buprenorphine in the Treatment of Opioid Addiction. Treatment Improvement Protocol (TIP) Series 40.* Rockville, MD: Substance Abuse and Mental Health Services Administration; 2004.

74. Mattick RP, Breen C, Kimber J, et al. Buprenorphine maintenance versus placebo or methadone maintenance for opioid dependence. *Cochrane Database Syst Rev* 2002;4:CD002207.

75. Kakko J, Grönbladh L, Svanborg KD, et al. A stepped care strategy using buprenorphine and methadone versus conventional methadone maintenance in heroin dependence: a randomized controlled trial. *Am J Psychiatry* 2007; 164(5):797–803.

76. Koppert W, Ihmsen H, Körber N, et al. Different profiles of buprenorphine-induced analgesia and antihyperalgesia in a human pain model. *Pain* 2005; 118(1–2):15–22.

77. Cowan A. Buprenorphine: new pharmacological aspects. *Int J Clin Pract Suppl* 2003;(133):3–8; discussion 23–24.

78. Malinoff HL, Barkin RL, Wilson G. Sublingual buprenorphine is effective in the treatment of chronic pain syndrome. *Am J Ther* 2005;12(5):379–384.

79. Halpern LM, Robinson J. Prescribing practices for pain in drug dependence: a lesson in ignorance. *Adv Alcohol Subst Abuse* 1985–1986;5(1–2):135–162.

80. Twycross RG, Wald SJ. Long-term use of diamorphine in advanced cancer. In: Bonica JJ, Albe-Fessard D, eds. *Advances in Pain Research and Therapy.* Vol 1. New York: Raven Press; 1976.

81. Kanner RM, Foley KM. Patterns of narcotic drug use in a cancer pain clinic. *Ann N Y Acad Sci* 1981;362:161–172.

82. Portenoy RK, Foley KM. Chronic use of opioid analgesics in non-malignant pain: report of 38 cases. *Pain* 1986;25(2):171–186.

83. Kalso E, Edwards JE, Moore RA, et al. Opioids in chronic non-cancer pain: systematic review of efficacy and safety. *Pain* 2004;112(3):372–380.

84. Gilson AM, Maurer MA, Joranson DE. State policy affecting pain management: recent improvements and the positive impact of regulatory health policies. *Health Policy* 2005;74(2):192–204.

85. Joranson DE, Gilson AM, Dahl JL, et al. Pain management, controlled substances, and state medical board policy: a decade of change. *J Pain Symptom Manage* 2002;23(2):138–147.

86. Butler SH, Murphy TM. Use and abuse of drugs in chronic noncancerous pain states. In: Loeser JD, Egan KJ, eds. *Managing the Chronic Pain Patients.* New York: Raven Press; 1989:129–142.

87. Reid MC, Engles-Horton LL, Weber MB, et al. Use of opioid medications for chronic noncancer pain syndromes in primary care. *J Gen Intern Med* 2002;17(3):173–179.

88. Gilson AM, Ryan KM, Joranson DE, et al. A reassessment of trends in the medical use and abuse of opioid analgesics and implications for diversion control: 1997–2002. *J Pain Symptom Manage* 2004;28(2):176–188.

89. Soderstrom CA, Dischinger PC, Kerns TJ, et al. Epidemic increases in cocaine and opiate use by trauma center patients: documentation with a large clinical toxicology database. *J Trauma* 2001;51(3):557–564.

90. Franklin GM, Mai J, Wickizer T, et al. Opioid dosing trends and mortality in Washington State workers' compensation, 1996–2002. *Am J Ind Med* 2005; 48(2):91–99.

91. Chabal C, Erjavec MK, Jacobson L, et al. Prescription opiate abuse in chronic pain patients: clinical criteria, incidence, and predictors. *Clin J Pain* 1997; 13(2):150–155.

92. Passik SD, Kirsh KL. Opioid therapy in patients with a history of substance abuse. *CNS Drugs* 2004;18(1):13–25.

93. Webster LR, Webster RM. Predicting aberrant behaviors in opioid-treated patients: preliminary validation of the Opioid Risk Tool. *Pain Med* 2005; 6(6):432–442.

94. Martell BA, O'Connor PG, Kerns RD, et al. Systematic review: opioid treatment for chronic back pain: prevalence, efficacy, and association with addiction. *Ann Intern Med* 2007;146(2):116–127.

95. Ballantyne JC. Opioid analgesia: perspectives on right use and utility. *Pain Physician* 2007;10(3):479–491.

96. Washington State Agency Medical Directors' Group. *Interagency guideline on opioid dosing for chronic non-cancer pain: an educational pilot to improve care and safety with opioid treatment.* Olympia, WA: Washington State Department of Labor and Industries; 2007.

97. Savage SR, Joranson DE, Covington EC, et al. Definitions related to the medical use of opioids: evolution towards universal agreement. *J Pain Symptom Manage* 2003;26(1):655–667.

98. Ballantyne JC, LaForge KS. Opioid dependence and addiction during opioid treatment of chronic pain. *Pain* 2007;129(3):235–255.

99. Portenoy RK. Opioid therapy for chronic nonmalignant pain: clinician's perspective. *J Law Med Ethics* 1996;24(4):296–309.

100. Trescot AM, Boswell MV, Atluri SL, et al. Opioid guidelines in the management of chronic non-cancer pain. *Pain Physician* 2006;9(1):1–39.

101. Glajchen M. Chronic pain: treatment barriers and strategies for clinical practice. *J Am Board Fam Pract* 2001;14(3):211–218.

102. Passik SD, Kirsh KL. Will the number of milligrams of an opioid dose ever re-achieve the truly meaningless status it deserves? *J Pain Palliat Care Pharmacother* 2007;21(1):39–41.

103. Portenoy RK. Opioid therapy for chronic nonmalignant pain: a review of the critical issues. *J Pain Symptom Manage* 1996;11(4):203–217.

104. Weissman DE, Haddox JD. Opioid pseudoaddiction—an iatrogenic syndrome. *Pain* 1989;36(3):363–366.

105. Holmes CP, Gatchel RJ, Adams LL, et al. An opioid screening instrument: long-term evaluation of the utility of the Pain Medication Questionnaire. *Pain Pract* 2006;6(2):74–88.

106. Passik SD, Kirsh KL. An opioid screening instrument: long-term evaluation of the utility of the pain medication questionnaire by Holmes et al. *Pain Pract* 2006;6(2):69–71.

107. Coluzzi F, Pappagallo M, The National Initiative on Pain Control. Opioid therapy for chronic noncancer pain: practice guidelines for initiation and maintenance of therapy. *Minerva Anestesiol* 2005;71(7–8):425–433.

108. Burchman SL, Pagel PS. Implementation of a formal treatment agreement for outpatient management of chronic nonmalignant pain with opioid analgesics. *J Pain Symptom Manage* 1995;10(7):556–563.

109. Fordyce W. *Behavioral Methods for Chronic Pain and Illness.* Saint Louis, MO: Mosby; 1976.

110. Sizemore WA. Behavioral aspects of managing medications for chronic pain not caused by cancer. In: Loeser JD, Egan KJ, eds. *Managing the Chronic Pain Patient.* New York: Raven Press; 1989:117–127.

111. Ibuki T, Marsala M, Masuyama T, et al. Spinal amino acid release and repeated withdrawal in spinal morphine tolerant rats. *Br J Pharmacol* 2003; 138(4):689–697.

112. Dunbar SA, Karamian I, Yeatman A, et al. Effects of recurrent withdrawal on spinal GABA release during chronic morphine infusion in the rat. *Eur J Pharmacol* 2006;535(1–3):152–156.

113. McCarberg BH, Barkin RL. Long-acting opioids for chronic pain: pharmacotherapeutic opportunities to enhance compliance, quality of life, and analgesia. *Am J Ther* 2001;8(3):181–186.

114. Loeser J, Egan KJ. Inpatient pain treatment program. In: Loeser JD, Egan KJ, eds. *Managing the Chronic Pain Patient.* New York: Raven Press; 1989: 37–49.

115. Maruta T, Swanson DW. Problems with the use of oxycodone compound in patients with chronic pain. *Pain* 1981;11(3):389–396.

116. Addison R. Treatment of chronic pain: the Center for Pain Studies, Rehabilitation Institute of Chicago. In: Ng LK, ed. *New Approaches to Treatment of Chronic Pain: A Review of Multidisciplinary Pain Clinics and Pain Centers.* Washington, DC: U.S. Government Printing Office; 1981:12–32.

117. Fordyce WE, Fowler RS Jr, Lehmann JF, et al. Operant conditioning in the treatment of chronic pain. *Arch Phys Med Rehabil* 1973;54(9):399–408.

118. Acker CJ. Take as directed: the dilemmas of regulating addictive analgesics and other psychoactive drugs. In: Meldrum ML, ed. *Opioids and Pain Relief: A Historical Perspective.* Seattle, WA: IASP Press; 2003:35–55.

119. Trafton JA, Oliva EM, Horst DA, et al. Treatment needs associated with pain in substance use disorder patients: implications for concurrent treatment. *Drug Alcohol Depend* 2004;73(1):23–31.

120. Larson MJ, Paasche-Orlow M, Cheng DM, et al. Persistent pain is associated with substance use after detoxification: a prospective cohort analysis. *Addiction* 2007;102(5):752–760.

121. Sullivan MD, Edlund MJ, Zhang L, et al. Association between mental health disorders, problem drug use, and regular prescription opioid use. *Arch Intern Med* 2006;166(19):2087–2093.

CHAPTER 91 ■ PHYSICAL THERAPY AGENTS

ROGER J. ALLEN AND ANN M. WILSON

INTRODUCTION

In the management of pain, physical therapists are available to aid in facilitating the patient's functional restoration via the prescription and pacing of therapeutic exercise and activities.[1–4] In concert with the functional physical restoration focus, physical therapy may also utilize therapeutic physical agents (frequently referred to as physical "modalities") for pain attenuation.[5–7] The philosophies and approaches to pain management may vary by clinical facility, yet the use of physical agents is widespread. While the application of physical agents may facilitate tissue repair, inflammation control, or temporary palliative relief, the use of a passive modality as a sole treatment approach is unlikely to lead to long-term improvement in a patient's functional status. In treatment planning for pain management, thoughtful use of physical agents coordinates their application with physical restoration activities.

The physical agents used for pain management typically involve application of some form of heat, cold, light, electromagnetic, or acoustic energy to the body tissue involved in generating pain.[5,6,8] In the context of pain management, delivery of such energy to the tissues may assist in modifying the underlying process generating the pain or altering the transmission or perception of the pain message.[6] Physical agents may influence pain by a number of mechanisms such as causing temporary analgesia,[4,8] resolving inflammation and facilitating tissue repair,[5,6] modifying axonal conduction,[6] generating a counterirritant,[6] or altering muscle activation or increasing extensibility.[6] In addition, physical agents may also curb the development of maladaptive central neuropathic changes that could precipitate secondary chronic pain generators[9-11] or provide other means of palliative relief from pain perception.[7]

The utilization and selection of specific physical agents for pain management should be done on a case-by-case basis predicated on clinical impressions regarding the loci and underlying pathophysiologic processes of pain generation.[12] For a particular agent to be therapeutically useful, its effects must either address the pathophysiologic changes occurring at the tissue level or alter neural pain transmission or central processing.[12] If the origin of nociceptive pain is due to damaged and/or inflamed tissue, then locally operating agents are indicated. However, if pain is being generated by peripheral neuropathic factors or a central neuroplastic remodeling component, then potentially effective agents should be chosen from those capable of influencing neural transmission or central processing.

While pathophysiology is the primary consideration in the selection of physical agents for acute or subacute pain, additional factors must be addressed when considering physical agents for use in treating patients with chronic pain. For example, as distal subacute lesions evolve into chronic pain syndromes, the loci of pain generation may migrate.[10,12-17] Central pain generators may develop from neuroplastic remodeling of the dorsal horn, thalamus, or cerebral cortex.[10,15] Restrictions in activity and mobility in response to initial pain from the inciting lesion may lead to connective tissue changes and alterations in vascular physiology that develop into secondary pain generation sites.[13,14,16,17] Following resolution of the original lesion, secondary structural and pathophysiologic changes associated with lack of active motion may be perpetuating the pain from multiple and elusive locations.[14,18] The application of physical agents to the original lesion site may prove ineffective if the sources of the chronic pain are secondary generation sites or neural remodeling.

Another consideration related to the use of physical agents for the treatment of chronic pain is that while physical agents may influence pain processes in a number of ways, they are frequently used to provide temporary analgesia.[9,12,19] Thoughtful case-by-case consideration should be given to providing patients with chronic pain an external source of passive palliative relief.[2,12] Temporary pain relief via the use of physical agents may create a therapeutic window for the therapist to mobilize tissue or address movement impairments.[2] For some patients, however, a maladaptive cycle of pain behavior may develop from psychologic dependence on passive external palliative agents. Ultimately, this may reduce progress toward functional restoration by hindering the motivation to also actively engage in therapeutic physical activity.[2,12] Passive application of an agent that temporarily reduces pain may not only provide disincentives for the patient to approach pain management from an active or functional perspective but may also reinforce an external locus of control, whereby the patient attributes pain relief to procedures unrelated to his or her own activity or pacing.[2]

The various agents used by physical therapists in the manage-ment of pain include superficial heat and cold, light (such as low-level laser or monochromatic infrared energy), therapeutic ultrasound, shortwave diathermy, electrical currents (such as transcutaneous electrical nerve stimulation [TENS] and interferential current), and materials used to facilitate multimodal somatosensory desensitization.[12]

SUPERFICIAL THERMAL AGENTS

Thermotherapy

Thermotherapy, or the application of superficial heat, is used to increase circulation, enhance healing, increase soft tissue extensibility, and/or control pain. Heat may be delivered to superficial tissues via conduction with agents such as hot packs, paraffin wax dips, microwavable rice-filled cloth bags, electric heating pads, or air-activated wearable heat wraps. Superficial heat can also be delivered via convection using agents such as hydrotherapy or fluidotherapy. In the twentieth century, heat from infrared lamps was another popular way to deliver superficial heat. These lamps have largely been replaced by other agents due to safety concerns and are no longer in use in clinical practice.[20] In the context of pain management, potential therapeutic benefits of superficial heat are due to its effects on various metabolic, neuromuscular, and hemodynamic processes.

While the physiologic effects of superficial heat primarily influence tissue healing and acute nociceptive pain generation, thoughtfully applied thermotherapy may have utility in the comprehensive management of chronic pain. The oxygen-hemoglobin dissociation curve shifts to the right with mild increases in tissue temperature, making more oxygen available for tissue repair. Increases in enzymatic activity increase oxygen uptake by the cell, thus enhancing healing.[6] Increased skeletal muscle temperature (to 42° C) has been reported to decrease firing rates of gamma and type II muscle spindle efferents, while increasing Golgi tendon organ type Ib fiber firing rates.[21-23] This may reflexively reduce skeletal muscle tone and spasm by lowering alpha motor neuron firing rates.[24] Superficial thermal agents will not likely elevate muscle temperatures to the levels required to alter type II or type Ib activity due to their limited depth of penetration. Instead, heating the skin may lead to a decrease in gamma efferent activity, which in turn may lead to a decrease in muscle spindle activity and a reduction in muscle spasm.[6] Reducing skeletal muscle activity may also assist in breaking the pain-spasm-pain exacerbation cycle.[6,25]

Elevations in nociceptive threshold have been reported due to superficial heat.[26] By increasing activity of afferent thermoreceptive fibers, superficial heat may produce inhibitory modulation of dorsal horn pain gates.[6] Indirectly, pain may be influenced via local vasomotor effects and increased blood flow. Skin surface thermoreception directly releases bradykinins, leading to local vasodilation of the heated area.[27] Dorsal horn synapses from first order thermal receptor afferents inhibit sympathetic vasomotor efferents in the intermediolateral grey area, thus decreasing vasoconstriction neurogenically.[6] While sympathetic vasomotor outflow is decreased, local vasodilation and increased vascular perfusion may influence pain further by decreasing tissue ischemia,[28] returning nociceptors to normal firing thresholds by helping to resolve hyperalgesia, and clearing exacerbating metabolites such as prostaglandins from the region. Blood flow increases of as much as 30 mL per 100 g of tissue have been reported.[21] However, these effects influence superficial blood vessels and the tissues they supply. There is less evident vasodilation in deep muscle vasculature because of the limited ability of superficial agents to increase temperature in deeper structures.[6]

When applied in forms such as hot packs, paraffin, hydrotherapy, and fluidotherapy, superficial heat has been broadly evaluated for effectiveness in the treatment of rheumatoid arthritis. Five well controlled studies have found it a beneficial adjunct,[29–33] while two found it ineffective[34,35] and possibly harmful by increasing collagenase activity which may have damaged compromised articular cartilage.[35] Uncontrolled, comparative studies report beneficial effects of superficial heat for trigger point pain in the neck and back,[36] neck and shoulder pain,[37] and chronic low back pain.[38–42]

Thermotherapy is contraindicated for the following conditions: applying heat over hemorrhagic areas; regions of acute injury, inflammation, malignancy, impaired sensation, or thrombophlebitis; the abdomens of pregnant women; or with patients with relevant cognitive impairments.[5,6,43] Caution should be used when applying heat over areas of impaired circulation, edema, superficial metal implants or open wounds, with patients manifesting poor thermal regulation, cardiac insufficiency, or acute inflammatory disorders, or with hypotensive patients or anyone prone to syncope when heating large body surface areas.[5,6,12,35,43]

Cryotherapy

Cryotherapy, or the therapeutic use of cold, can be used to control pain, minimize edema, reduce inflammation, enhance movement, and attenuate spasticity.[6] Cryotherapy can be administered with conductive agents such as ice bags or cold compression units. Cryotherapy can also be administered with convective agents such as cold whirlpool immersion, contrast baths, in which alternating heat and cold are used, or by evaporation using vapocoolant sprays. The therapeutic effects of cold result from its actions on metabolic, neuromuscular, and hemodynamic processes.[6]

A primary indication for cryotherapy is to minimize secondary hypoxic injury to adjacent tissue areas immediately following acute trauma.[5] By lowering metabolism of damaged and surrounding cells, they become more resistant to hypoxia resulting from disrupted blood supply to the region, making this the primary reason that cold is the agent of choice for the first 24–48 hours after injury.[44] This mechanism of minimizing the extent of tissue damage is dependent on immediate application of cold following trauma and is not a mechanism likely to be utilized in the management of chronic pain states.

Decreases in nociceptive input and pain perception via application of cold may occur because of influences in both local and central nervous system mechanisms. Vasoconstrictive response to cold decreases local release of vasodilating substances and chemical mediators, which in turn decreases nociceptor sensitization.[6,25] For every 1° C drop in interstitial temperature, nerve conduction velocity of somatosensory afferent fibers drops approximately 2 m/sec due to metabolic changes in the axon. A-delta fibers display the most sensitivity to cold mediated velocity attenuation.[21] The effects of application of a cryotherapy agent for 10–15 minutes may transcend immediate changes and produce pain reductions for more than an hour.[6] Prolonged analgesia may be the result of A-delta nociceptive fiber conduction block and the maintenance of subnormal deep tissue temperature for 1–2 hours following cold exposure.[6,45] Extended cold application has been shown to produce reversible neurapraxia.[46] Theoretically, by interrupting the pain-spasm-pain cycle, cold application may reduce muscle spasm, thus continuing pain relief after tissue temperature has recovered to precryotherapy levels.[6] Finally, by applying vapocoolant sprays over skeletal muscle and combining it with stretch, evaporative cooling may reduce muscle spasm and allow muscle with excess neurogenic tone to be stretched for increased range of motion.[6,47,48] The vapocoolant spray has been hypothesized to be effective in this capacity by providing a counterirritation to cutaneous afferents, which in turn leads to a reflex decrease in motor neuron activity and resistance to stretch.[6]

Existing literature is clear in support of the efficacy of cryo-

therapy in acute trauma management. It may also play a role in treating chronic pain. Uncontrolled comparative studies[47,49] and case studies[50,51] have reported that in the treatment of muscle spasms and myofascial pain, cryotherapy may be a beneficial adjunct. Additional comparative studies have reported it to be a useful clinical tool in managing chronic headache,[52,53] trigeminal neuralgia,[54] chronic osteoarthritis,[55] and low back pain.[42,56]

Cryotherapy is contraindicated for patients with Raynaud's disease or phenomenon; cryoglobulinemia or paroxysmal cold hemoglobinuria; those prone to cold urticaria, cold intolerance, or hypersensitivity; or over skin areas of impaired somatosensory discrimination, deep open wounds, areas of circulatory compromise or peripheral vascular disease, and regenerating peripheral nerves.[5,6,43] Cryotherapy should be used with caution over the main branch of a superficial nerve, on individuals with unstable hypertension, in patients with poor sensation, or those with poor thermoregulation.[5,6,43]

LIGHT THERAPY: LASER AND MONOCHROMATIC INFRARED ENERGY

Laser therapy utilizes light energy that has the unique properties of monochromaticity, coherence, and collimation.[6,57] These properties allow laser light to deliver electromagnetic light energy to tissue depths slightly below the dermis. Indirect physiologic effects occur at deeper levels due to the promotion of chemical reactions that mediate processes at greater tissue depths.[6,57–59]

Low level laser therapy (LLLT) used in rehabilitation settings to promote healing and manage pain utilizes lasers with power outputs less than 500 mW at a power density of 50mW/cm², and wavelengths ranging from 600–1300 nm.[5] This affords a depth of tissue penetration between 1–4 mm.[6,59]

The type of laser most frequently utilized for LLLT are semiconductor diode lasers that produce light in the red and near infrared portions of the electromagnetic spectrum. Diode lasers are usually hand-held probes that allow for treatment of small, localized areas. Superluminous diodes (SLDs) also produce light in the red and near infrared portions of the electromagnetic spectrum. They are brighter but less powerful than diode lasers. The advantage of SLDs is to allow hands-free operation and the ability to treat larger surface areas.[59,60]

While the mechanisms by which low-level lasers may modulate pain are not well established, there is consensus in the literature that LLLT can induce photomodulation effects of chromophores within affected tissue.[5,6,59,61,62] Cellular chromophores (light absorbing molecules) absorb photons from laser light as it penetrates the skin. Via influence over respiratory chain enzymes, chromophores may then undergo photobiomodulation in the form of either photobiostimulation or photobioinhibition.[5,63] A dose-response interaction effect occurs based on the Arndt-Schultz law of photobiologic activation.[5,63] Low doses of laser light activate photobiostimulation responses that are potentially efficacious for wound healing, whereas higher doses of laser light initiate a photobioinhibition response that may be beneficial for pain management.[5,63]

With possible application to temporary pain relief, LLLT has been hypothesized to influence nerve conduction velocity. There are reports in the literature indicating both slight increases and decreases in peripheral nerve conduction velocity due to low-level laser application with resulting changes in distal latencies.[64–67] Other studies report no effect on nerve conduction velocity following LLLT.[68,69] The influence of LLLT on clinically significant changes in nerve conduction velocity appears uncertain at this time. Other mechanisms by which LLLT may influence perceived pain remain to be explored.

Numerous studies have addressed the effects of LLLT with

respect to treating a wide array of pain generating conditions. Findings and applications cited here were derived only from controlled studies on human volunteers. For most disorders, the literature is split between studies showing some clinically significant beneficial effect over controls and those that do not. Trigger point stimulation with LLLT has been reported to relieve pain in two studies.[70,71] However, findings regarding myofascial pain treatment via laser have largely shown no significant effect over controls.[72–74] One of five controlled studies found a positive therapeutic response for epicondylitis.[75–79] The use of laser for rheumatoid arthritis pain has been found beneficial in four studies[80–83] and to have no clinical effect over controls in three.[84–86] Five studies found LLLT useful in the treatment of osteoarthritic pain, while two found no benefit.[87–93]

Controlled human studies reporting benefits from LLLT have been published that address pain conditions originating from specific loci including postherpetic pain,[94] perioral herpes pain,[95] postsurgical abdominal pain,[96] and trigeminal pain.[97,98] Laser therapy did not demonstrate significant benefits in controlled human studies reviewed regarding effects on muscle soreness,[99,100] plantar fasciitis,[101] chondromalacia,[102] orofacial pain,[103] temporomandibular joint disorder,[104] ankle pain,[105] or tendinopathies.[106–108]

Contraindications to LLLT include exposing any of the following to laser light: photosensitive skin areas; hemorrhagic areas; any area within 4–6 months after radiation therapy[6]; neoplastic lesions; unclosed fontanelles in children; the abdomens of pregnant women; over the heart, vagus nerve, or sympathetic innervation routes to the heart of cardiac patients; or locally to endocrine glands.[5,6,43,57] In addition, exposure of the cornea of the eye is also contraindicated. Therefore, both patient and therapist must utilize protective eye wear. LLLT should be used with caution over areas with compromised somatosensation, epiphyseal regions of long bones in children, gonads, infected areas, and with patients displaying fever, epilepsy, or mental confusion.[5,6,43]

Infrared radiation, once widely used as a superficial heating agent, has recently emerged as another form of light therapy that may have effects on processes leading to pain relief, tissue repair, and restoration of protective sensation. The new infrared devices produce monochromatic infrared energy (MIRE) from the near-infrared portion of the electromagnetic spectrum at a wavelength of 890 nm through a series of 60 gallium aluminum arsenide diodes in a flexible pad.[20]

The physiologic effects of MIRE on biologic tissues are thought to be due to photochemical reactions in the skin similar to LLLT rather than thermal reactions. Light energy from MIRE devices causes an increase in plasma nitric oxide (NO) from red blood cells, leading to vasodilation and increased circulation. NO is thought to facilitate vascular perfusion, resulting in improved tissue oxygenation, delivery of nutrients, and removal of waste products of metabolism.[109] The vascular effects and increased oxygenation to the tissues may facilitate wound healing and may explain the promotion of nerve growth and resultant improvement in sensation that has been observed in individuals with peripheral neuropathy.[20,110,111]

The precautions and contraindications to MIRE include avoiding placement over the low back or pelvic regions of pregnant women or over cancerous lesions. Goggles are not required during treatment because the diode arrays block the infrared radiation from the eyes. However, the pads should not be placed over the eyes.[20]

The small volume of literature available on MIRE suggests that it has potential for the treatment of pain and spasm associated with temporomandibular joint dysfunction, healing of chronic wounds, and restoration of sensation in individuals with peripheral neuropathy.[20]

THERAPEUTIC ULTRASOUND

Ultrasound is one of the most commonly used thermal agents in rehabilitation medicine[5,112,113] and is widely used as an adjunct to the management of pain and inflammation by physical therapists.[4,114–116] It is capable of producing elevations in temperature at tissue depths of up to 5 cm through the conversion of acoustic energy into heat within body tissue.[6,117] Therapeutic ultrasound can be used as a thermal agent to increase deep tissue temperature or increase pain threshold or as a nonthermal agent to facilitate tissue repair.[6] Ultrasound can also be used to facilitate the passage of medication, such as hydrocortisone preparations, into the tissues.[6]

Therapeutic ultrasound utilizes a reverse piezoelectric effect. Acoustic waves are generated by a crystal sound head at frequencies of either 1 or 3 MHz.[12] Amplitude densities are typically between 0.1 and 3 watts/cm^2.[12] Frequency and depth of penetration of the therapeutic ultrasound beam are inversely related. That is, 3 MHz ultrasound is capable of producing heat in tissues up to 2 cm from the skin surface, while ultrasound delivered at 1 MHz can reach depths of up to 5 cm.[6,118] These parameters are in contrast to ultrasound sources used for diagnostic imaging whose purpose is not to generate heat. Diagnostic ultrasound beams carry higher frequencies and lower wattage.[12]

Molecules within soft tissue vibrate due to rarefaction and compression as acoustic waves pass through them. Heat is generated, and thus increased tissue temperature, from the microfriction caused by this increased vibratory movement of molecules.[5] Sonic impedance variations within body tissue also facilitate heat generation in the presence of acoustic waves. In general, tissues with high absorption coefficients (i.e., those with low water content or collagen-rich structures such as tendon, cartilage, and bone) will attenuate more ultrasound energy than tissues with low absorption coefficients such as fat or muscle.[6,118] The thermal effects of ultrasound, which include acceleration of metabolic rate, increased circulation, reduction of pain and muscle spasm, changes in nerve conduction velocity, and increases in collagen tissue extensibility, are essentially the same as those of superficial thermal agents except that the structures heated are different.

The nonthermal effects of ultrasound are thought to be caused by the processes of cavitation, microstreaming, and acoustic streaming.[6,118] As oscillating acoustic waves pass through soft tissue, microscopic bubbles, or cavities, are formed from the effect of cyclic drops in pressure on normally present minute gas pockets. Ultrasound produces a state of stable cavitation such that the microscopic bubbles formed pulsate without imploding. A flow of fluid is then established around the pulsating microbubbles, which is referred to as microstreaming, along with acoustic streaming which is the circular flow of cellular fluids.[5,6,117] These processes have been reported to alter vascular wall permeability, cell membrane activity, and facilitate soft tissue healing.[5,117–119] In order to produce the beneficial nonthermal effects of ultrasound without causing an appreciable rise in tissue temperature, a pulsed mode with a duty cycle of 20% or less is used.[6]

The primary clinical indications for continuous (thermal) ultrasound are soft tissue shortening due to decreased collagen tissue extensibility in structures within 5 cm of the skin surface or pain. Via alterations in tertiary molecular bonding, heating collagen increases its extensibility. This property allows therapists to utilize ultrasound in treating structural contributors to chronic pain[13,14] such as maladaptive shortening of connective tissue, joint contractures, scar tissue, and tissue adhesions.[5,6,117]

Increased nociceptive thresholds may occur with exposure to continuous thermal ultrasound, thus giving the agent the potential to reduce perceived pain by influencing peripheral nociceptive activation and transmission.[5,6,12,21,117] Hypothesized mechanisms for increased nociceptive threshold include heat activation of large diameter afferent fibers, alteration of nociceptor receptor sensitivity, and counterirritation.[117]

Ultrasound has been reported in the literature to be effective in helping manage pain originating from a variety of sources and sites. Some examples of these include myofascial trigger points,[117] muscle spasms,[120] epicondylitis,[121] carpal tunnel syndrome,[122] tendonitis,[123] back pain,[124] complex regional pain syndrome (CRPS),[125] phantom limb pain,[126] and soft tissue lesions.[127]

Nonthermal (pulsed) ultrasound is used to stimulate cellular activity during acute inflammation and repair.[6] This phenomenon has been studied extensively in vitro and with animal models.[5] The majority of human trials have been limited to individuals with chronic wounds that may not, however, respond to the ultrasonic energy in the same way.[118]

Another application of nonthermal ultrasound is for treating pain and inflammation via phonophoresis. Steroid preparations such as dexamethasone or hydrocortisone or an analgesic such as lidocaine is used between the sound head and the skin surface as a coupling medium.[6,117] Ultrasound alters the permeability of the stratum corneum which facilitates the passage of the medication transdermally into the tissues.[6,128] While the purpose of this mode of medication delivery is to facilitate local tissue effects, drugs administered via phonophoresis do enter general circulation and systemic contraindications must be taken into account.[6]

In controlled human studies, ultrasound has been reported to be an effective clinical tool in the management of shoulder pain,[129] adhesive capsulitis,[130] pain associated with prolapsed intervertebral discs,[124] and soft tissue lesions.[127] Mixed results have been reported in controlled studies for its effectiveness in the management of carpal tunnel syndrome,[122,131] elbow epicondylitis, shoulder calcific tendonitis,[123,132] and osteoarthritis.[133,134] No significant benefit over controls has been reported in controlled studies reviewed assessing the effectiveness of ultrasound for treating subacromial bursitis,[135] shoulder peritendonitis,[136] postextraction dental pain,[137,138] and perineal postlabor pain.[139,140]

The potential influences of therapeutic ultrasound on pain mechanisms primarily occur at the tissue level. It is therefore of little potential value for treating central pain states or chronic pain conditions perpetuated by neuroplastic remodeling.[12] Consideration of utilizing this physical agent with patients experiencing chronic pain should be based on individual evidence that the patient's pain generation has a nociceptive component due to an active peripheral lesion or inflammation.[12]

Contraindications include the direction of ultrasonic acoustic energy over gonads; pregnant abdomens; orbits of the eyes; epiphyseal growth plates in skeletally immature patients; fractures; malignant lesions; hemorrhagic, ischemic, thrombotic, insensate, or infected regions; plastic implants or cemented areas of prosthetic joints; areas exposed to radiotherapy within 6 months; spinal cord region postlaminectomy; and electronic implants and neurostimulators.[5,6,12]

DIATHERMY

Diathermy is the therapeutic application of short wave (10–100 MHz) or microwave (300 MHz–300 GHz) electromagnetic radiation that is converted to heat within body tissue.[5,12] The only type of diathermy in clinical use today is shortwave diathermy (SWD). SWD devices use high frequency alternating currents that oscillate as specified radio frequencies between 10 and 50 MHz. The radio frequency most commonly used for the shortwave devices used in therapy is 27.12 MHz.[6] Diathermy can be delivered continuously (continuous SWD [CSWD]) or pulsed, in which the electromagnetic radiation is interrupted at intervals (pulsed SWD [PSWD]). Thermal effects are present with CSWD, while PSWD can be delivered in such a way that the thermal effects are either minimized or negligible. (For the purposes of this chapter, the term PSWD will be used to describe only nonthermal pulsed SWD.)

SWD has potential advantages over other agents. It is capable of delivering heat to deeper tissue levels than superficial agents such as hot packs.[6] Larger areas can be heated than with other penetrating agents such as ultrasound.[6] Finally, a transmission impedance change does not occur with shortwave radiation while passing from soft tissue to bone. As a result, unlike ultrasound, shortwave energy is not reflected by bone and does not produce differential heating at tissue interfaces or present risk of burning at the periosteum.[6]

Heating of soft tissue may be accomplished by CSWD, whereas PSWD may be used to induce nonthermal physiologic effects.[5,6] When shortwave radiation is delivered to the tissue via CSWD, molecular kinetic energy increases physiologically lead to thermal effects such as increased rate of nerve conduction, increased collagen extensibility, vasodilation, increased nociceptive threshold, and acceleration of enzymatic activity.[6] Superficial heating produces physiologic heating effects within a few millimeters of the dermis, whereas CSWD may be used to produce these effects in tissues up to 3 cm from the surface.[6]

Short duration, low amplitude pulses of electromagnetic energy at a low duty cycle does not generate sustained increases in tissue temperature because of vascular perfusion and resultant dissipation of transient heat.[6] However, the application of pulsed energy produces a number of subthermal physiologic changes.[141] While nonthermal physiologic mechanisms are not fully understood, the result may be modification of cellular protein synthesis and adenosine triphosphate production via modified ion binding.[5,142–144] Electromagnetic field influences on ion binding produce a cascade of physiologic responses, including alterations in myosin phosphorylation, growth factor activation in fibroblasts and neurons, and macrophage activation.[6,145]

Most of the recent literature on the clinical efficacy of SWD is focused on the promotion of healing. Application of PSWD for 40–45 minutes is reported to increase microvascular perfusion of local tissue in normal subjects and at sites adjacent to ulcers in patients with diabetes.[6,146,147] By increasing local perfusion, PSWD has the capability to enhance nutrient availability, increase oxygenation of deep tissue, decrease anaerobic metabolism, and assist phagocytosis.[6] While CSWD and PSWD produce different ratios of thermal to nonthermal effects, both modes of application appear to result in increased cellular metabolism and functioning.[5]

The potential indications for clinical application of CSWD include decreased joint and stiffness of large muscular areas. When combined with stretching, CSWD increases joint range of motion.[6] Clinical indications for nonthermal PSWD may include pain control secondary to edema reduction and enhanced healing of soft tissue injuries, peripheral nerve lesions, and fractures.[6]

Recent studies on the clinical efficacy of SWD have addressed its nonthermal effects and evaluated its potential to augment tissue healing, with a few studies addressing SWD application in the management of chronic pain. Pulsed electromagnetic fields, which is another term used in the literature for PSWD, have been reported useful for nonunion fractures,[148,149] failed arthrodeses,[150] and osteonecrosis.[151] Significant reductions in neck pain and increase in range of motion in patients with cervical spine injuries after using PSWD have been reported in two controlled studies.[152,153] Early controlled investigations reported beneficial results from SWD treatment of osteoarthritis, while more recent studies have not found diathermy to produce reductions in osteoarthritic pain intensity over controls.[133,154,155] In reviewed studies, diathermy has failed to manifest significant benefits over controls in treating ankle sprains.[156–158] Single uncontrolled studies are available with positive outcomes using PSWD in the treatment of posttraumatic algoneurodystrophy[159] and low back pain.[160]

The manner in which electromagnetic energy from SWD increases tissue temperature gives rise to noteworthy contraindications and precautions. Materials such as metals, fat, and tissues with high free water concentrations tend to absorb disproportionate amounts of electromagnetic energy.[6] Therefore, CSWD is contraindicated in the presence of metal implants, pacemakers, neurostimulators, malignancy, pregnancy, or over the eyes, testes, or open growth plates.[5,6,12] PSWD is contraindicated in the presence of pacemakers, neurostimulators, or copper-bearing intrauterine contraceptive devices.[6,43] SWD selectively heats liquid and adipose tissue, so precautions must be taken with obese patients, when a patient begins perspiring,[6] and over moist wound dressings.[5]

In addition to the contraindications listed for other thermal agents previously mentioned in this chapter, further contraindications to SWD include malignancy, pregnancy, and over insensate skin regions. CSWD should also not be applied over the eyes or epiphyseal growth plates in skeletally immature patients due to potential damage from heat generation.[5,12]

SWD has good tissue penetration properties and the ability to heat deep structures, yet its use in the treatment of pain is now very rare. This is primarily due to the potential hazards associated with its use. Its therapeutic index is uncomfortably low. The shortwave devices in use today have the capability of delivering PSWD at either a thermal or nonthermal level in order to help address and minimize some of the hazards listed above. In general, therapists typically use superficial agents or ultrasound rather than SWD for pain management. Nonthermal PSWD is most often used to facilitate wound healing.

ELECTRICAL CURRENT

The use of electrical stimulation for pain modulation has traditionally been referred to as TENS or electroanalgesia.[161] While the tissue level is the primary site of action for managing pain for most physical agents, TENS is thought to operate by interrupting the neural propagation of pain.[162] TENS can be delivered in different ways to modulate various types of pain. For example, sensory or motor-level stimulation is used to modulate peripheral nociceptive pain or peripheral neurogenic pain while noxious level stimulation may be used if the pain is centrally mediated or in the management of CRPS.[6,163]

There are four different modes of TENS currently in clinical use that may produce electroanalgesia: sensory level stimulation, motor level stimulation, brief-intense stimulation, and noxious level stimulation.[6,161] Sensory level stimulation is used for immediate temporary relief of acute, chronic, or postoperative pain. This type of stimulation, which is also known as high frequency or "conventional" TENS, delivers high frequency (30–150 pps), short duration (50–150 μseconds) pulses at an amplitude just below the motor threshold that causes comfortable paresthesia in the area of the electrodes.[161] Conventional TENS affects primarily large diameter afferent fibers and is thought to work via the "gate control" theory proposed by Melzack and Wall.[6,161,164] This type of TENS is appropriate for use during exercise, work, or functional activities. It should be noted that for a given patient, determination of an effective TENS electrode placement site typically requires some time and experimentation.[12]

Motor level stimulation is used for the management of chronic pain or in instances where longer duration pain relief is desired. This type of TENS, which is also known as "acupuncture-like" TENS, delivers low frequency (2–4 pps), long duration (100–200 μseconds) pulses at an amplitude that causes muscle twitches. This type of TENS is proposed to control pain by stimulating the production and release of endogenous opiates such as enkephalins and endorphins.[6,161] Acupuncture-like TENS is usually applied over a trigger point, motor point, or acupuncture point related to the painful region. It is not recommended for use during activities of daily living or exercise because of interference from muscle twitching.[161]

Brief-intense TENS combines the stimulus parameters that cause both sensory level and motor level stimulation, which is then delivered at the highest tolerable intensity. It is most often recommended for use during painful procedures such as wound débridement or joint mobilization.[161] Brief-intense TENS is high frequency (60–200 pps), long duration (150–500 μseconds) pulses at an amplitude that will cause strong paresthesia and a motor response under or between the electrodes.[161]

Noxious, or painful, level stimulation, which is sometimes called "hyperstimulation," is thought to lead to analgesia via activation of the descending pain suppression system mediated by the release of endogenous opiates.[161] This type of TENS is usually only attempted if other types of stimulation have not been effective. Noxious level stimulation requires low or high frequency, long duration (250 μseconds–1 second) pulses at an amplitude that causes a painful stimulus that is maintained for 30–60 seconds. This type of TENS is typically applied over acupuncture, motor, or trigger points. It is generally quite uncomfortable and should only be used with patients who are fully aware of the expected discomfort and who agree to its application.[161]

Although TENS is usually delivered via small battery-operated monophasic or biphasic pulsed current devices, two other types of current can also have similar effects on pain modulation. The parameters that are available on interferential current (IFC) units and high voltage pulsed current (HVPC) devices can be manipulated to create sensory level conventional TENS parameters. IFC is a waveform produced by the intersection of two circuits of medium frequency alternating current of slightly different frequencies. When the two circuits intersect, there is a summation or amplitude modulation that is equal to the difference in frequency between the two circuits.[6] This amplitude modulation is called a "beat frequency" and can be adjusted to coincide with conventional TENS parameters. It has been suggested that IFC may be more comfortable than other waveforms because it offers less skin impedance and penetrates more deeply than other types of current.[6] These claims are controversial, and there is not clinical data at this time to suggest that IFC is superior to conventional TENS parameters delivered by low voltage devices.[165]

HVPC is a type of current in which monophasic pulses of short duration (usually <100 μseconds) are used. The combination of the short pulse duration and high peak current generated by HVPS devices allows for comfortable stimulation.[165] HVPC can be easily adjusted to mimic conventional TENS. Its comfort makes it an ideal alternative to conventional TENS delivered by a low voltage device.[165]

While the primary indication for TENS is attenuation of acute and subacute pain, it has theoretical utility for chronic pain conditions where peripheral nociception is not the primary mechanism of pain generation. Foley[10] has suggested TENS as a treatment option used to reduce painful input to the spine as early as possible in order to fight central pain generation via dorsal horn remodeling of N-methyl-D-aspartate. It has also been hypothesized to use early sensory-level TENS to body regions other than the painful locus, thus providing a competing attentional stimulus to decrease the probability of long-term cortical remodeling.[12]

Significant clinical effectiveness has been reported in controlled human studies for TENS in the management of pain associated with osteoarthritis,[166–171] neck pain,[172] trigeminal neuralgia,[173] migraine headache,[174] postamputation and phantom limb pain,[175,176] peripheral neuropathy pain,[177,178] and shoulder pain secondary to stroke.[179] There is less consistency in the clinical efficacy literature for the use of TENS to help manage low back pain,[180–186] myofascial pain,[187,188] and pain associated with rheumatoid arthritis.[189–191]

In addition to the use of TENS for direct pain attenuation, electrical currents can also be utilized to resolve inflammation, enhance healing, and facilitate delivery of topical medication transdermally.[6,192,193]

Iontophoresis is the utilization of direct current to facilitate transdermal delivery of local ionizable anesthetics and anti-inflammatories.[192,193] Ionic medications carrying a positive electrical charge are drawn to cathode electrodes and repelled by anode electrodes, while negatively charged medication compounds display the reverse behavior.[194] Iontophoresis was originally thought to drive the ions through the skin and into deeper tissues. Recent work suggests that iontophoresis may promote transdermal penetration by increasing the permeability of the stratum corneum.[6]

For managing chronic pain conditions via iontophoresis, several ionic compounds are in use. Negatively charged medications include dexamethasone for inflammation and salicylates for both acute and chronic muscle and joint pain.[192,194] Positively charged medications include hydrocortisone for inflammation, lidocaine for soft tissue pain and inflammation, and magnesium sulfate for skeletal muscle spasms.[192,194] Physical therapy clinics are typically equipped to administer medication via iontophoresis. However, the patient must bring the ionic medication preparation prescribed by the referring physician to the clinic.[12]

Given its reliance on direct current, sustained application of iontophoresis will produce a hydrochloric acid concentration beneath the anode and a hydroxide alkaline reaction beneath the cathode.[193] When used to excess, the accumulated pH changes may result in electrochemical skin burns. These subdermal pH changes also have the potential to affect drug ionization and stability.[12] However, iontophoresis has been demonstrated to effectively deliver select medications to the site of interest.[195-197] The actual depth of penetration of drug delivery with iontophoresis is uncertain. Several studies have found diffusion of various drugs at tissue depths ranging from 3-20 mm.[6]

Although there are few controlled studies in the literature addressing the use of iontophoresis for managing chronic pain, there are reports of significant clinical effectiveness for dexamethasone delivered using this method in treating postherpetic neuralgia,[195] plantar fasciitis,[196] and myofascial pain of the shoulder (applied in combination with lidocaine).[197]

Contraindications to the use of electrical current include its use in individuals with either a demand-type pacemaker or known cardiac arrhythmias; over the anterior cervical region or carotid sinuses; over the abdomen, pelvis, or low back during pregnancy; in the presence of an implanted defibrillator, or any other implanted electrical device; and for individuals with venous or arterial thrombosis or thrombophlebitis.[6,43] The use of iontophoresis is contraindicated for patients with sensitivity to ionic medications and over open skin lesions.[5]

Precautions should be exercised when using electrical stimulation in the presence of skin irritation or open wounds, malignancies, osteoporosis (with motor-level TENS), or cardiomyopathies; over tissues susceptible to hemorrhage or hematoma, on patients with movement control disorders or impaired cognition, on craniofacial regions for patients with a history of stroke or seizures, and on patients who are driving or operating heavy machinery.[6,43] With the use of adhesive electrodes, precautions should be taken to prevent skin damage due to adhesive irritants and pH changes under electrodes when using direct current for iontophoresis or for prolonged applications such at TENS.[6,12]

SOMATOSENSORY DESENSITIZATION

Desensitization therapy involves exposing a patient's painful skin region to direct physical contact with a progression of materials that have the potential to trigger somatosensory irritation.[12,198-200] The indication for this therapeutic tool is treatment of allodynia associated with chronic pain conditions such as CRPS.[2,199-201]

Allodynia is a painful response to non-noxious somatosensory

stimulation.[2,202] One of the hallmarks of CRPS, allodynia is not the same phenomenon as the normal hyperalgesia that follows tissue damage.[2,203,204] Patients experiencing allodynia may avoid the most seemingly innocuous tactile contact, sometimes refraining from wearing even delicate clothing over the affected area.[202,205,206] Allodynia treatment via desensitization aims at attenuating this abnormal chronic pain response and helping the patient return the affected area (frequently a limb) to normal somatosensory exposure and functional usage.[2,199-201,207,208] Somatosensory desensitization is also used in the treatment and prevention of postamputation phantom limb pain.[200,209,210]

Typical desensitization protocols involve having the patient rub the painful skin field with a progressive series of coarse or irritating materials.[200,201] Early desensitization therapy for CRPS used the chemical irritant capsaicin as the desensitizing agent.[211] In current practice, materials may progress from soft fabrics to items such as small pebbles or dry pasta.[201,205] Twice daily, the patient rubs the material over the affected area for approximately 2 minutes, then rests for 2-3 minutes, and finally rubs again for 2 more minutes.[12,201,205] Each week, the patient advances to a coarser or potentially more irritating material. Treatment course may span 2 to 4 months and includes home application and in-clinic checks at least weekly.[12,206,212]

Attenuation of allodynia via desensitization may be due to multifaceted mechanisms. These have been hypothesized to involve somatosensory habituation,[203] reintroduction of large fiber diameter afferent pain inhibition,[12,201] altered central processing of somatosensory input either at the dorsal horn or parietal lobe,[201,203] prevention of the development of new permanent neuroplastic pain pathways in the neuromatrix,[213] and normalization of exposure to the distal environment.[210] During the course of desensitization, the patient is encouraged to begin reintroduction of the limb or body area into normalized functional usage. With direction from the therapist, this reintroduced usage may facilitate a positive spiral of ascending exogenous analgesia and activity. Normal activities of daily living then become a continuation of the desensitization therapy and its ongoing effectiveness.[12,201,205]

Light touch somatosensory input is not the only tactile allodynia trigger. Some patients who have undergone successful desensitization to light touch or who never manifested light touch allodynia may still find non-noxious levels of pressure, vibration, or thermal variation to be painfully intolerable.[201,205,206,212,214,215] Desensitization therapy may therefore be specific to a given somatosensory modality. Therapeutic desensitizing agents must be matched to the type of somatosensory stimulation triggering the allodynia.[201,206,215] Therapeutic somatosensory desensitization may be performed using light touch,[199,200,205] thermal,[215] pressure,[206,212] or vibratory[213,216] stimuli.

While efficacy evidence from controlled studies is lacking, case studies have reported success in managing tactile,[205] thermal,[215] vibratory,[214] and pressure-related allodynia.[206,212] In one case study on the effects of pressure desensitization, the patient increased usage of analgesic medication during the desensitization trial.[206] Significant reductions in subsequent pain medication usage and pain intensity, combined with improved functional usage, suggested that use of analgesics to tolerate the desensitization therapy may not interfere with the treatment's effectiveness.[206]

Somatosensory desensitization is contraindicated over an active lesion that may be harmed by contact with physically irritating materials or mechanical pressure.[12]

CONCLUSION

There is a broad spectrum of therapeutic physical agents available to aid in the management of both acute and chronic pain conditions (Table 91.1). Determination of the suitability of physical agents and selection of the appropriate modality should be made

TABLE 91.1

CLINICAL APPLICATIONS AND EVIDENCE LEVELS FOR PHYSICAL THERAPY AGENTS

Agent	Uses	Clinical evidence level* and references
Thermotherapy Hot packs Paraffin wax Fluidotherapy Electric heating pads Air-activated wraps Rice-filled cloth bags	• increase circulation • increase soft tissue extensibility (up to 0.5 cm from surface) • reduce pain-spasm-pain cycle • decrease stiffness • pain control	Grade I[26,29-35]
Cryotherapy Ice bags Ice massage Cold compression units Vapocoolant sprays	• minimize inflammation • minimize edema • attenuate spasticity • pain control	Grade II[42,45-56]
Light Therapy Laser Monochromatic infrared	• increase microvessel circulation • tissue repair • pain control	Grade I[61,64-108]
Ultrasound Continuous (thermal) Pulsed (nonthermal) Phonophoresis	• increase circulation • increase soft tissue extensibility (up to 5 cm from surface) • facilitate tissue repair (nonthermal) • pain control	Grade I[119-140]
SWD CSWD (thermal) PSWD (nonthermal)	• increase circulation • increase soft tissue extensibility (up to 3 cm from surface) • facilitate tissue repair (pulsed nonthermal SWD) • pain control	Grade I[146-160]
TENS Interferential current Iontophoresis	• minimize inflammation • pain control	Grade I[166-193,195-197]
Somatosensory Desensitization	• allodynia attenuation	Grade III[206,212,215,216]

*The rating of clinical evidence level for pain management appearing in this table utilizes a hierarchy of three grades (I–III) describing the strength and quality of evidence that was developed by Canadian task force groups.[5,12] All three grades refer only to peer-reviewed studies published in refereed journals.
Grade I—Controlled studies conducted on human volunteers, regardless of blindness or level of randomization.
Grade II—Noncontrolled studies conducted on human volunteers.
Grade III—Human case studies.
Clinical evidence level should not be equated with a rating of clinical efficacy. For several indications of specific agents, separate Grade I studies may have yielded contradictory results.

with careful consideration of the mechanism of pain generation and pursued with careful treatment response monitoring.[12] It should be re-emphasized that while the use of physical agents for treating pain is common in physical therapy settings, their use should be viewed as adjunctive.[19,217] Effective pain management involves not just the attenuation of pain perception, but also restoration of compromised or lost function. Appropriate, comprehensive treatment integrates the application of physical agents with other indicated therapeutic activities to address the mechanisms of pain generation and facilitate functional restoration.

References

1. Loeser JD. Multidisciplinary pain programs. In: Loeser JD, ed. *Bonica's Management of Pain*. 3rd ed. Baltimore, MD: Lippincott Williams & Wilkins; 2001:255–264.

2. Galer BS, Schwartz L, Allen RJ. The complex regional pain syndromes: type I / reflex sympathetic dystrophy and type II causalgia. In: Loeser JD, ed. *Bonica's Management of Pain*. 3rd ed. Baltimore, MD: Lippincott Williams & Wilkins, 2001:388–411.
3. Witttink H, Michel TH. *Chronic Pain Management for Physical Therapists*. Boston: Butterworth Heinemann; 2002.
4. Strong J, Unrugh AM, Wright A, et al, eds. *Pain: A Textbook for Therapists*. Edinburgh: Churchill Livingstone; 2002.
5. Belanger AY. *Evidence-Based Guide to Therapeutic Physical Agents*. Philadelphia: Lippincott Williams & Wilkins; 2002.
6. Cameron MH. *Physical Agents in Rehabilitation: From Research to Practice*. Philadelphia: WB Saunders; 2003.
7. Wells PE, Frampton V, Bowsher D. *Pain Management in Physical Therapy*. Norwalk, CT: Appleton & Lange; 1988.
8. Robinson AJ, Snyder-Mackler L. *Clinical Electrophysiology: Electrotherapy and Electrophysiological Testing*. Baltimore: Williams & Wilkins; 1995.
9. Berger JM, Katz RL. Sympathetically maintained pain. In: Ashburn MA, Rice LJ, eds. *The Management of Pain*. Philadelphia: Churchill Livingstone; 1998: 335–349.
10. Foley R. Neuroplasticity of pain and the psychology of pain. Preconference

course presented at: Combined Sections Meeting of the American Physical Therapy Association; February 12, 2003; Tampa, FL.

11. Allen RJ, Hulten JM. Effects of tactile desensitization on allodynia and somatosensation in a patient with quadrilateral complex regional pain syndrome. *Neuro Rep* 2001;25(4):132–133.

12. Allen RJ. Physical agents used in the management of chronic pain by physical therapists. *Phys Med Rehabil Clin N Am* 2006;17:315–345.

13. Allen RJ. Deactivation pain: developmental sequelae of secondary pain generation sites resulting from reduced mobility. Paper presented at: Annual Conference & Exposition of the American Physical Therapy Association; June 21, 2001; Anaheim, CA.

14. Allen RJ, Koshi LR. Development of chronic pain secondary to excessive limb immobilization following orthopaedic trauma. *J Ortho Sports Phys Ther* 2005;35(1):A63–A64.

15. Chandler EH, Bonica JJ. Supraspinal mechanisms of pain & nociception. In: Loeser JD, ed. *Bonica's Management of Pain.* 3rd ed. Baltimore, MD: Lippincott Williams & Wilkins; 2001:388–411.

16. Butler SH, Galer BS, Bernirshka S. Disuse as a cause of signs and symptoms of CRPS-1. Paper presented at: Annual Meeting of the International Association for the Study of Pain; 1996; Vancouver, WA.

17. Butler SH, Nyman M, Gordh T. Immobility in volunteers transiently produces signs and symptoms of complex regional pain syndrome. In: Devor M, Rowbotham MC, Wiesenfield-Hallin Z, eds. Proceedings of the 9th World Congress on Pain. *Progress in Pain Research and Management.* Vol 16. Seattle: IASP Press; 2000:657–660.

18. Allen RJ. Deactivation pain and dosing therapeutic exercise for patients with chronic pain. Paper presented at: Combined Sections Meeting of the American Physical Therapy Association; February 6, 2004; Nashville, TN.

19. American Physical Therapy Association. *Guide to Physical Therapy Practice.* Fairfax, VA: American Physical Therapy Association; 2001.

20. Nolan TP, Michlovitz SL. Emerging modalities: is there evidence? In: Michlovitz SL, Nolan TP. *Modalities for Therapeutic Intervention.* 4th ed. Philadelphia, PA: FA Davis; 2006:285–291.

21. Lehmann JF, DeLateur BJ. Therapeutic heat. In: Lehmann JF, ed. *Therapeutic Heat and Cold.* Baltimore: Williams & Wilkins; 1990:429–432.

22. Mense S. Effects of temperature on the discharges of muscle spindles and tendon organs. *Pflugers Arch* 1978;374:159–166.

23. Rennie GA, Michlovitz SL. Biophysical principles of heating and superficial heating agents. In: Michlovitz SL, ed. *Thermal Agents in Rehabilitation.* Philadelphia: FA Davis; 1996.

24. Fountain FP, Gersten JW, Senger O. Decrease in muscle spasm produced by ultrasound, hot packs, and IR. *Arch Phys Med Rehabil* 1960;41:293–299.

25. Newton RA. Contemporary views on pain and the role played by thermal agents in managing pain symptoms. In: Michlovitz SL, ed. *Thermal Agents in Rehabilitation.* Philadelphia: FA Davis; 1990:18–42.

26. Benson TB, Copp EP. The effects of therapeutic forms of heat and ice on the pain threshold of the normal shoulder. *Rheumatol Rehabil* 1974;13:101–104.

27. Fox RH, Hilton SM. Bradykinin formation in human skin as a factor in heat vasodilation. *J Physiol* 1958;142:219–232.

28. Kramer JF. Ultrasound: evaluation of its mechanical and thermal effects. *Arch Phys Med Rehabil* 1984;65:223–227.

29. Ayling J, Marks R. Efficacy of paraffin wax baths for rheumatoid arthritic hands. *Physiotherapy* 2000;86:190–201.

30. Mainardi CL, Walter JM, Spiegel PK, et al. Rheumatoid arthritis: failure of daily heat therapy to affect its progression. *Arch Phys Med Rehab* 1979;60: 390–393.

31. Sukenik S, Buskila D, Neumann L, et al. Mud pack therapy in rheumatoid arthritis. *Clin Rheumatol* 1992;11:243–247.

32. Sukenik S, Buskila D, Neumann L, et al. Sulfur bath and mud pack treatment for rheumatoid arthritis in the Dead Sea area. *Ann Rheum Dis* 1990;49: 99–102.

33. Sukenik S, Newmann L, Flusser D, et al. Balneotherapy for rheumatoid arthritis at the Dead Sea. *Isr J Med Sci* 1995;31:210–214.

34. Dellhag B. Wollersjö I, Bjelle A. Effect of hand exercise and wax bath treatment in rheumatoid arthritis patients. *Arthritis Care Res* 1992;5:87–92.

35. Harris ED Jr, McCroskery PA. The influence of temperature and fibril stability on degradation of cartilage collagen by rheumatoid synovial collagenase. *N Engl J Med* 1974;290:1–6.

36. McCray RE, Patton NJ. Pain relief at trigger points: a comparison of moist heat and shortwave diathermy. *J Othop Sports Phys Ther* 1984;5:175–178.

37. Cordray YM, Krusen EM Jr. Use of hydrocollator packs in the treatment of neck and shoulder pains. *Arch Phys Med Rehab* 1959;40:105–108.

38. Constant F, Collin JF, Guillemin F, et al. Effectiveness of spa therapy in chronic low back pain: a randomized clinical trial. *J Rheumatol* 1995;22: 1315–1320.

39. Constant F, Guillemin F, Collin JF, et al. Use of spa therapy to improve the quality of life of chronic low back pain patients. *Med Care* 1998;36: 1309–1314.

40. Guillemin F, Constant F, Collin JF, et al. Short and long-term effect of spa therapy in chronic low back pain. *Br J Rheumatol* 1994;33:148–151.

41. Konrad K, Tatrai T, Hunka A, et al. Controlled trial of balneotherapy in treatment of low back pain. *Ann Rheum Dis* 1992;51:820–822.

42. Landen BR. Hear or cold for the relief of low back pain? *Phys Ther* 1967; 47:1126–1128.

43. Batavia M. *Contraindications in Physical Rehabilitation: Doing No Harm.* St. Louis, MO: Saunders; 2006.

44. Knight KL. *Cryotherapy in Sports Injury Management.* Champaign: Human Kinetics; 1995.

45. Douglas WW, Malcolm JL. The effect of localized cooling on cat nerves. *J Physiol* 1955;130:53–54.

46. Bassett FH III, Kirkpatrick JS, Engelhardt DL. Cryotherapy-induced nerve injury. *Am J Sport Med* 1992;22:516–518.

47. Travell J. Ethyl chloride for painful muscle spasm. *Arch Phys Med Rehabil* 1952;33:291–298.

48. Prentice WE. An electromyographic analysis of the effectiveness of heat or cold and stretching for inducing relaxation in injured muscle. *J Orthop Sports Phys Ther* 1982;3:133–140.

49. Mennel J. Spray-stretch for the relief of pain from muscle spasm and myofascial trigger points. *J Am Podiatr Assoc* 1976;66:873–876.

50. Nielson AJ. Spray and stretch for myofascial pain. *Phys Ther* 1978;58: 567–569.

51. Nielson AJ. Case study: myofascial pain of the posterior shoulder relieved by spray and stretch. *J Orthop Sports Phys Ther* 1981;3:21–26.

52. Robbins LD. Cryotherapy for headache. *Headache* 1989;29:598–600.

53. Diamond S, Freitag FG. Cold as an adjunctive therapy for headache. *Postgrad Med* 1986;79:305–309.

54. De Coster D, Bossuyt M, Fossion E. The value of cryotherapy in the management of trigeminal neuralgia. *Acta Stomatol Belg* 1993;90:87–93.

55. Halliday SM, Littler TR, Littler EN. A trial of ice therapy and exercise in chronic arthritis. *Physiotherapy* 1969;55:51–56.

56. Melzack R, Jeans ME, Stratford JG, et al. Ice massage and transcutaneous electrical stimulation: Comparison of treatment for low-back pain. *Pain* 1980; 9:209–217.

57. Bukowski EL, Dellagata EM. Electromagnetic radiation: laser, ultraviolet and diathermy. In: Michlovitz SL, Nolan TP, eds. *Modalities for Therapeutic Intervention.* 4th ed. Philadelphia, PA: FA Davis; 2006:141–164.

58. Anderson RR, Parrish JA. The optics of the skin. *J Invest Dermatol* 1981; 77:13–19.

59. Enwemeka CS. Therapeutic light. *Rehab Manag* 2004;17(1):20–25.

60. Enwemeka CS. Light is light. *Photomed Laser Surg* 2005;23(2):159–160.

61. Schindl A, Schindl M, Pernerstorfer-Schön H, et al. Low intensity laser therapy: a review. *J Investig Med* 2000;48:312–326.

62. Calderhead RG. Basics. In: Ohshiro T, Calderhead RG, eds. *Low-level Laser Therapy: A Practical Introduction.* New York: John Wiley & Sons; 1988: 1–18.

63. Baxter GD. *Therapeutic Lasers: Theory and Practice.* New York: Churchill Livingstone; 1994.

64. Baxter GD, Walsh DM, Allen JM, et al. Effects of low-intensity infrared laser irradiation upon conduction in the human median nerve in vivo. *Exp Physiol* 1994;79:227–234.

65. Snyder-Mackler L, Bork CE. Effect of helium-neon laser irradiation on peripheral sensory nerve latency. *Phys Ther* 1988;68:223–225.

66. Basford JR, Hallman HO, Matsumoto JY, et al. Effects of 830 nm continuous laser diode irradiation on median nerve function in normal subjects. *Lasers Surg Med* 1993;13:597–604.

67. Lowe AS, Baxter GD, Walsh DM, et al. Effect of low-intensity laser (830 nm) irradiation on skin temperature and antidromic conduction latencies in the human median nerve: relevance of radiant exposure. *Lasers Surg Med* 1994; 14:40–46.

68. Basford JR, Daube JR, Hallman HO, et al. Does low-intensity helium-neon laser irradiation alter sensory nerve action potentials or distal latencies? *Lasers Surg Med* 1990;10:35–39.

69. Greathouse DG, Currier DP, Gilmore RL. Effects of clinical infrared laser on superficial radial nerve conduction. *Phys Ther* 1985;65:1184–1187.

70. Snyder-Mackler L, Barry AJ, Perkins AI, et al. Effects of helium-neon laser irradiation on skin resistance and pain in patients with trigger points in the neck or back. *Phys Ther* 1989:69:336–341.

71. Olavi A, Pekka R, Pertti K, et al. Effects of the infrared laser therapy at treated and non-treated trigger points. *Acupunct Electrother Res* 1989;14:9–14.

72. Thorsen H, Gam AN, Jensen H, et al. Low-energy laser treatment – effect in localized fibromyalgia in the neck and shoulder regions. *Ugeskr Laeger* 1991; 153:1801–1804.

73. Thorsen H, Gam AN, Svensson BH, et al. Low-level laser therapy for myofascial pain in the neck and shoulder girdle. A double-blind, cross-over study. *Scand J Rheumatol* 1992;21:139–141.

74. Waylonis GW, Wilke S, O'Toole D, et al. Chronic myofascial pain: management by low-output helium-neon laser therapy. *Arch Phys Med Rehabil* 1988; 69:1017–1020.

75. Vasseljen O Jr, Høeg N, Kjelstad B, et al. Low-level laser versus placebo in the treatment of tennis elbow. *Scand J Rehab Med* 1992;24:37–42.

76. Lundeberg T, Haker E, Thomas M. Effect of laser versus placebo in tennis elbow. *Scand J Rehabil Med* 1987;19:135–148.

77. Krasheninnikoff M, Ellitsgaard N, Rogvi-Hansen B, et al. No effect of low-power laser in lateral epicondylitis. *Scand J Rheumatol* 1994;23:260–263.

78. Haker E, Lundeberg T. Laser treatment applied to acupuncture points in lateral humeral epicondylalgia. A double-blind study. *Pain* 1990;43:243–247.

79. Haker EH, Lundeberg TC. Lateral epicondylalgia: report of noneffective mid-laser treatment. *Arch Phys Med Rehab* 1991;72:984–988.

80. Palmgren N, Jensen GF, Kaa K, et al. Low-power laser therapy in rheumatoid arthritis. *Laser Med Sci* 1989;4:193–196.

81. Goats GC, Flett E, Hunter JA, et al. Low-intensity laser and phototherapy for rheumatoid arthritis. *Physiotherapy* 1996;82:311–320.

82. Walker JB, Akhanjee LK, Cooney MM, et al. Laser therapy for pain of rheumatoid arthritis. *Clin J Pain* 1987;3:54–59.

83. Goldman JA, Chiapella J, Casey H, et al. Laser therapy in rheumatoid arthritis. *Laser Surg Med* 1980;1:93–101.

84. Johannsen F, Hauschild B, Remvig L, et al. Low-energy laser therapy in rheumatoid arthritis. *Scand J Rheumatol* 1994;23:145–147.

85. Hall J, Clarke AK, Elvins DM, et al. Low-level laser therapy is ineffective in the management of rheumatoid arthritic finger joints. *Br J Rheumatol* 1994;33:142–147.

86. Bliddal H, Hellesen C, Ditlevsen P, et al. Soft-laser therapy of rheumatoid arthritis. *Scand J Rheumatol* 1987;16:225–228.

87. Willner R, Abeles M, Myerson G, et al. Low-power infrared laser biostimulation of chronic osteoarthritis in hand. *Laser Surg Med* 1985;5:149–150.

88. Jensen H, Harreby M, Kjer J. Infrared laser—effect in painful arthrosis of the knee? *Ugeskr Laeger* 1987;149:3104–3106.

89. Walker J. Relief from chronic pain by low-power laser irradiation. *Neurosci Lett* 1983;43:339–344.

90. Stelian J, Gil I, Habot B. Improvement of pain and disability in elderly patients with degenerative osteoarthritis of the knee treated with narrow-band light therapy. *J Am Geriat Soc* 1992;S40:23–26.

91. Bülow PM, Jensen H, Danneskiold-Samsøe B. Low-power Ga-Al-As laser treatment of painful osteoarthritis of the knee. *Scand J Rehab Med* 1994;26:155–159.

92. Basford JR, Sheffield CG, Mair SD, et al. Low energy helium-neon laser of thumb osteoarthritis. *Arch Phys Med Rehab* 1987;68:794–797.

93. Lonauer G. Controlled double-blind study on the efficacy of HeNe laser beams versus HeNe infrared laser beams in the therapy of activated osteoarthritis of finger joints. *Lasers Surg Med* 1986;6:172–175.

94. Moore KC, Hira N, Kumar PS, et al. A double-blind crossover trial of low-level laser therapy in the treatment of post herpetic neuralgia. *Laser Ther* 1988;1:7–9.

95. Schindl A Neumann R. Low-intensity laser therapy is an effective treatment for recurrent herpes simplex infection. Results from a randomized, double-blind, placebo-controlled trial. *J Invest Dermatol* 1999;113:221–223.

96. Moore KC, Hira N, Broome IJ, et al. The effect of infrared diode laser irradiation on the duration and severity of postoperative pain. A double-blind trial. *Laser Ther* 1992;4:145–150.

97. Eckerdal A, Bastian HL. Can low reactive-level laser therapy be used in the treatment of neurogenic facial pain? A double-blind, placebo-controlled investigation of patients with trigeminal neuralgia. *Laser Ther* 1996;8:247–252.

98. Walker JB, Akhanjee LK, Cooney MM. Laser therapy for pain of trigeminal neuralgia. *Clin J Pain* 1987;3:183–187.

99. Craig JA, Barlas P, Baxter GD, et al. Delayed-onset of muscle soreness: lack of effect of combined phototherapy/low-intensity laser therapy at low pulse repetition rates. *J Clin Laser Med Surg* 1996;14:375–380.

100. Craig JA, Barron J, Walsh DM, et al. Lack of effect of combined low-intensity laser therapy/phototherapy (CLILT) on delayed onset muscle soreness in humans. *Lasers Surg Med* 1999;24:223–230.

101. Basford JR, Melanga GA, Krause DA, et al. A randomized controlled evaluation of low-intensity laser therapy: plantar fasciitis. *Arch Phys Med Rehab* 1998;79:249–254.

102. Rogvi-Hansen B, Ellitsgaard N, Funch M, et al. Low-level laser treatment of chondromalacia patellae. *Int Orthop* 1991;15:359–361.

103. Hansen HJ, Thorøe U. Low-power laser biostimulation of chronic oro-facial pain. A double-blind, placebo controlled cross-over study in 40 patients. *Pain* 1990;43:169–179.

104. Conti PC. Low-level laser therapy in the treatment of temporomandibular disorders (TMD): a double-blind pilot study. *Cranio* 1997;15:144–149.

105. de Bie RA, de Vet HC, Lenssen TF, et al. Low-level laser therapy in ankle sprains: a randomized clinical trial. *Arch Phys Med Rehab* 1998;79:1415–1420.

106. Siebert W, Seichert N, Seibert B, et al. What is the efficacy of "soft" and "mild" lasers in therapy of tendinopathies? A double-blind study. *Arch Orthop Trauma Surg* 1987;106:358–363.

107. Vecchio P, Cave M, King V, et al. A double-blind study of the effectiveness of low-level laser treatment of rotator cuff tendonitis. *Br J Rheumatol* 1993;32:740–742.

108. Darre EM, Klokker M, Lund P, et al. Laser therapy of Achilles tendonitis. *Ugeskr Laeger* 1994;156:6680–6683.

109. Leonard DR, Farooqi MH, Myers S. Restoration of sensation, reduced pain, and improved balance in subjects with diabetic peripheral neuropathy: a double-blind, randomized, placebo-controlled study with monochromatic near-infrared treatment. *Diabetes Care* 2004;27:168–172.

110. Kochman AB, Carnegie DH, Burke TJ. Symptomatic reversal of peripheral neuropathy in patients with diabetes. *J Am Podiatr Assoc* 2002;92:125–130.

111. Kochman A. Restoration of sensation, improved balance and gait reduction in falls in elderly patients with use of monochromatic infrared photo energy and physical therapy. *J Geriatr Phys Ther* 2004;27:16–19.

112. Robertson VJ, Spurritt D. Electrophysical agents: implications of EPA availability and use in private practices. *Physiotherapy* 1998;84:335–344.

113. Reobroeck ME, Dekker J, Oostendorp RA. The use of therapeutic ultrasound by physical therapists in Dutch primary health care. *Phys Ther* 1998;78:470–478.

114. ter Haar G, Dyson M, Oakley EM. The use of ultrasound by physiotherapists in Britain, 1985. *Ultrasound Med Bio* 1987;13:659–663.

115. Young S. Ultrasound therapy. In: Kitchen S, Bazin S, eds. *Clayton's Electrotherapy*. 10th ed. London: WB Saunders; 1996:243–267.

116. Robertson VJ, Baker KG. A review of therapeutic ultrasound: effectiveness studies. *Phys Ther* 2001;81:1339–1350.

117. Ziskin MC, McDiarmid T, Michlovitz SL. Therapeutic ultrasound. In: Micklovitz SL, ed. *Thermal Agents in Rehabilitation*. Philadelphia, PA: FA Davis; 1990:134–169.

118. Sparrow KJ. Therapeutic ultrasound. In: Michlovitz SL, Nolan TP, eds. *Modalities for Therapeutic Intervention*. 4th ed. Philadelphia, PA: FA Davis; 2006:79–96.

119. Michlovitz SL, Lynch PR, Tuma RJ. Therapeutic ultrasound: its effects on vascular permeability. *Fed Proc* 1982;41:1761.

120. Fountain FP, Gersten JW, Sengu O. Decrease in muscle spasm produced by ultrasound, hot packs, and IR. *Arch Phys Med Rehab* 1960;41:293.

121. Binder A. Hodge G, Greenwood AM, et al. Is therapeutic ultrasound effective in treating soft tissue lesions? *Br Med J* 1985;290:512–514.

122. Ebenbichler GR, Resch KL, Nicolakis P, et al. Ultrasound treatment for treating the carpal tunnel syndrome: randomized "sham" controlled trial. *BMJ* 1998;316:731–735.

123. Ebenbichler GR, Erdogmus CB, Resh KL, et al. Ultrasound therapy for calcific tendinitis of the shoulder. *N Engl J Med* 1999;340:1533–1538.

124. Nwunga VC. Ultrasound in treatment of back pain resulting from prolapsed intervertebral disc. *Arch Phys Med Rehab* 1983;64:88–89.

125. Portwood MM, Lieberman JS, Taylor RG. Ultrasound treatment of reflex sympathetic dystrophy. *Arch Phys Med Rehab* 1987;68:116–118.

126. Tepperberg I, Marjey EJ. Ultrasound therapy of painful postoperative neurofibromas. *Am J Phys Med* 1953;32:27–30.

127. Van der Heijden GJ, Leffers P, Wolters PJ, et al. No effect of bipolar interferential electrotherapy and pulsed ultrasound for soft tissue shoulder disorders: a randomised controlled trial. *Ann Rheum Dis* 1999;58:530–540.

128. Bommannan D, Okuyama H, Stauffer P, et al. The use of high frequency ultrasound to enhance transdermal drug delivery. *Pharm Res* 1992;9:559–564.

129. Munting E. Ultrasonic therapy for painful shoulders. *Physiotherapy* 1978;64:180–181.

130. Roden D. Ultrasonic waves in the treatment of chronic adhesive subacromial bursitis. *J Irish Med Assoc* 1952;30:85–88.

131. Oztas O, Turan B, Bora I, et al. Ultrasound therapy effect in carpal tunnel syndrome. *Arch Phys Med Rehab* 1998;79:1540–1544.

132. Perron M. Malouin F. Acetic acid iontophoresis and ultrasound for the treatment of calcifying tendonitis of the shoulder: a randomized control trial. *Arch Phys Med Rehab* 1997;78:379–384.

133. Svarcová J, Trnavský K, Zvárová J. The influence of ultrasound, galvanic currents, and shortwave diathermy on pain intensity with osteoarthritis. *Scand J Rheumatol Suppl* 1987;67:83–85.

134. Falconer J, Hayes KW, Chang RW. Effect of ultrasound on mobility in osteoarthritis of the knee. *Arthritis Car Res* 1992;5:29–35.

135. Downing DS, Weinstein A. Ultrasound therapy of subacromial bursitis. A double blind trial. *Phys Ther* 1986;66:194–199.

136. Flax HJ. Ultrasound treatment of peritendinitis calcarea of the shoulder. *Am J Phys Med* 1964;43:117–124.

137. Hasish I, Hai HK, Harvey W, et al. Reduction of postoperative pain and swelling by ultrasound treatment: a placebo effect. *Pain* 1988;33:303–311.

138. Hashish I, Harvey W, Harris M. Anti-inflammatory effects of ultrasound therapy: evidence for a major placebo effect. *Br J Rheumatol* 1986;25:77–81.

139. Everett T, McIntosh J, Grant A. Ultrasound therapy for persistent post-natal perineal pain and dyspareunia: a randomized placebo-controlled trial. *Physiotherapy* 1992;78:263–267.

140. Creates V. Study of ultrasound treatment to the painful perineum after childbirth. *Physiotherapy* 1987;73:162–165.

141. Hayne CR. Pulsed high frequency energy—its place in physiotherapy. *Physiotherapy* 1984;70(12):459–466.

142. Markov MS. Electric current electromagnetic field effects on soft tissue: implications for wound healing. *Wounds* 1995;7(3):94–110.

143. Markov MS, Pilla AA. Electromagnetic field stimulation of soft tissues: pulsed radio frequency treatment of post-operative pain and edema. *Wounds* 1995;7(4):143–151.

144. Pilla AA, Markov MS. Bioeffects of weak electromagnetic fields. *Rev Environ Health* 1994;10(3–4):155–169.

145. Canaday DJ, Lee RC. Scientific basis for clinical application of electric fields in soft tissue repair. In: Brighton CT, Pollack SR, eds. *Electromagnetics in biological medicine*. San Francisco: San Francisco Press; 1991:275–291.

146. Mayrovitz HN, Larsen PB. A preliminary study to evaluate the effect of pulsed radio frequency field treatment on lower extremity peri-ulcer skin microcirculation of diabetic patients. *Wounds* 1995;7(3):90–93.

147. Mayrovitz HN, Larsen PB. Effects of pulsed electromagnetic fields on skin microvascular blood perfusion. *Wounds* 1992;4(5):197–202.

148. Bassett CA. Fundamental and practical aspects of therapeutic uses of pulsed electromagnetic fields (PEMFs). *Crit Rev Biomed Eng* 1989;17:451–529.

149. Bassett CA, Mitchell SN, Schink MM. Treatment of therapeutically resistant nonunions with bone grafts and pulsing electromagnetic fields. *J Bone Joint Surg Am* 1982;24:1214–1220.

150. Konrad K, Sevcic K, Földes K, et al. Therapy with pulsed electromagnetic fields in aseptic loosening of total hip prostheses: a prospective study. *Clin Rheumatol* 1997;15:325–328.

151. Ryaby JT. Clinical effects of electromagnetic and electric fields on fracture healing. *Clin Ortho Relat Res* 1998;355 suppl:S205–S215.

152. Foley-Nolan D, Barry C, Coughlan RJ, et al. Pulsed high frequency (27MHz) electromagnetic therapy for persistent neck pain: a double-blind placebo-controlled study of 20 patients. *Orthopedics* 1990;13:445–451.

153. Foley-Nolan D, Moore K, Codd M, et al. Low energy high frequency pulsed electromagnetic therapy for acute whiplash injuries. *Scand J Rehabil Med* 1992;24:51–59.

154. Moffett JA, Richardson PH, Frost H, Osborn A. A placebo controlled double-blind trial to evaluate the effectiveness of pulsed shortwave therapy for osteoarthritic hip and knee pain. *Pain* 1996;67:121–127.

155. Clarke GR, Willis LA, Stenners L, et al. Evaluation of physiotherapy in the treatment of osteoarthrosis of the knee. *Rheumatol Rehab* 1974;13:190–197.

156. Pasila M, Visuri T, Sundholm A. Pulsating shortwave diathermy: value in the treatment of recent ankle and foot sprains. *Arch Phys Med Rehabil* 1978;59:383–386.

157. Barker AT, Barlow PS, Porter J, et al. A double-blind clinical trial of low-power pulsed shortwave therapy in the treatment of a soft tissue injury. *Physiotherapy* 1985;71:500–504.

158. McGill SN. The effect of pulsed shortwave therapy on lateral ligament sprain of the ankle. *N Z J Physiother* 1988;10:21–24.

159. Comorosan S, Pana I, Pop L, et al. The influence of pulsed high peak power electromagnetic energy (Diapulse) treatment on posttraumatic algoneurodystrophies. *Rev Roum Physiol* 1991;28:77–81.

160. Wagstaff P, Wagstaff S, Downey M. A pilot study to compare the efficacy of continuous and pulsed magnetic energy (shortwave diathermy) on the relief of low back pain. *Physiotherapy* 1986;72:563–566.

161. Nolan TP. Electrotherapeutic modalities: electrotherapy and iontophoresis. In: Michlovitz SL, Nolan TP, eds. *Modalities for Therapeutic Intervention*. 4th ed. Philadelphia, PA: FA Davis; 2006:97–121.

162. Snyder-Mackler L. Electrical stimulation for pain modulation. In: Robinson AJ, Snyder-Mackler L, eds. *Clinical Electrophysiology: Electrotherapy and Electrophysiologic Testing*. 2nd ed. Baltimore: Williams & Wilkins; 1995:333–358.

163. Fedorczyk JM, Michlovitz SL. Pain and limited motion. In: Michlovitz SL, Nolan TP, eds. *Modalities for Therapeutic Intervention*. 4th ed. Philadelphia, PA: FA Davis; 2006:185–206.

164. Melzack R, Wall PD. Pain mechanisms: a new theory. *Science* 1965;150:971.

165. Alon G. Principles of electrical stimulation. In: Nelson RM, Hayes KW, Currier DP, eds. *Clinical Electrotherapy*. 3rd ed. Stamford, CT: Appleton & Lange; 1999:55–139.

166. Taylor P, Hallett M, Flaherty L. Treatment of osteoarthritis of the knee with transcutaneous electrical nerve stimulation. *Pain* 1981;11:233–240.

167. Fargas-Babjak A, Rooney P, Gerecz E. Randomized trial of Codetron for pain control in osteoarthritis of the hip/knee. *Clin J Pain* 1989;5:137–141.

168. Smith CR, Lewith GT, Machin D. TNS and osteoarthritis. Preliminary study to establish a controlled method of assessing transcutaneous electrical nerve stimulation as a treatment for pain caused by osteoarthritis of the knee. *Physiotherapy* 1983;69:266–268.

169. Grimmer K. A controlled double-blind study comparing the effects of strong burst mode TENS and high rate TENS on painful osteoarthritic knees. *Austr J Physiother* 1992;38:49–56.

170. Lewis D, Lewis B, Sturrock RD. Transcutaneous electrical nerve stimulation in osteoarthritis: a therapeutic alternative? *Ann Rheum Dis* 1984;43;47–49.

171. Zizic TM, Hoffman KC, Holt PA, et al. The treatment of osteoarthritis of the knee with pulsed electrical stimulation. *J Rheumatol* 1995;22:1757–1761.

172. Nordemar R. Thörner C. Treatment of acute cervical pain–a comparative group study. *Pain* 1981;10:93–101.

173. Taylor DN, Katims JJ, Ng LK. Sine-wave auricular TENS produces frequency-dependent hypoesthesia in the trigeminal nerve. *Clin J Pain* 1993;9:216–219.

174. Solomon S, Guglielmo KM. Treatment of headache by transcutaneous electrical stimulation. *Headache* 1985;25:12–15.

175. Finsen V, Persen L, Løvlien M, et al. Transcutaneous electrical nerve stimulation after major amputation. *J Bone Joint Surg* 1988;70:109–112.

176. Katz J, Melzack R. Auricular transcutaneous electrical nerve stimulation (TENS) reduces phantom limb pain. *J Pain Symptom Manage* 1991;6:73–83.

177. Kumar D, Marshall HJ. Diabetic peripheral neuropathy: amelioration of pain with transcutaneous electrical nerve stimulation. *Diabetes Care* 1997;20:1702–1705.

178. Thorsteinsson G, Stonnington HH, Stillwell GK, et al. Transcutaneous electrical stimulation: a double-blind trial of its efficacy for pain. *Arch Phys Med Rehabil* 1977;58:8–13.

179. Leandri M, Parodi CI, Corrieri N, et al. Comparison of TENS treatments in hemiplegic shoulder pain. *Scand J Rehab Med* 1990;22:69–72.

180. Melzack R, Jeans ME, Stratford JG, et al. Ice massage and transcutaneous electrical stimulation: Comparison of treatment for low-back pain. *Pain* 1981;9:209–217.

181. Melzack R, Vetere P, Finch L. Transcutaneous electrical nerve stimulation for low back pain. A comparison of TENS and massage for pain and range of motion. *Phys Ther* 1983;63:489–493.

182. Cheing GL, Hui-Chan CW. Transcutaneous electrical nerve stimulation: nonparalleled antinociceptive effects on chronic pain and acute experimental pain. *Arch Phys Med Rehabil* 1999;80:305–312.

183. Lehmann TR, Russel DW, Spratt KF, et al. Efficacy of electroacupuncture and TENS in the rehabilitation of chronic low back pain patients. *Pain* 1986;26:277–290.

184. Deyo RA, Walsh NE, Martin DC, et al. A controlled trial of transcutaneous electrical nerve stimulation (TENS) and exercise for chronic low back pain. *N Engl J Med* 1990;322:1627–1634.

185. Marchand S, Charest J, Li J, et al. Is TENS purely a placebo effect? A controlled study on chronic low back pain. *Pain* 1993;54:99–106.

186. Herman E, Williams R, Stratford P, et al. A randomized controlled trial of transcutaneous electrical nerve stimulation (CODETRON) to determine its benefits in a rehabilitation program for acute occupational low back pain. *Spine* 1994;19:561–568.

187. Graff-Radford SB, Reeves JL, Baker RL, et al. Effects of transcutaneous electrical nerve stimulation on myofascial pain and trigger point sensitivity. *Pain* 1989;37:1–5.

188. Kruger LR, van der Linden WJ, Cleaton-Jones PE. Transcutaneous electrical nerve stimulation in the treatment of myofascial pain dysfunction. *S Afr J Surg* 1998;36:35–38.

189. Abelson K, Langley GB, Sheppeard H, et al. Transcutaneous electrical nerve stimulation in rheumatoid arthritis. *N Z Med J* 1983;96:156–158.

190. Langley GB, Sheppeard H, Johnson M, et al. The analgesic effects of transcutaneous electrical nerve stimulation and placebo in chronic pain patients: a double-blind non-crossover comparison. *Rheumatol Int* 1984;4:119–123.

191. Møystad A, Krogstad BS, Larheim TA. Transcutaneous electrical nerve stimulation in a group of patients with rheumatic disease involving the temporomandibular joint. *J Prosthet Dent* 1990;64:596–600.

192. Ciccone CD. *Pharmacology in Rehabilitation*. 4th ed. Philadelphia: FA Davis; 2007.

193. Ciccone CD. Iontophoresis. In: Robinson AJ, Snyder-Mackler L, eds. *Clinical Electrophysiology: Electrotherapy and Electrophysiologic Testing*. 2nd ed. Baltimore: Williams & Wilkins; 1995:277–310.

194. Henley EJ. Transcutaneous drug delivery: iontophoresis and phonophoresis. *Crit Rev Phys Rehabil Med* 1991;2:139–151.

195. Ozawa A, Haruki Y, Iwashita K, et al. Follow-up of clinical efficacy of iontophoresis therapy for postherpetic neuralgia (PHN). *J Dermatol* 1999;26:1–10.

196. Gudeman SD, Eisele SA, Heidt RS, et al. Treatment of plantar fascitis by iontophoresis of 0.4% dexamethazone. A randomized, double-blind, placebo-controlled study. *Am J Sports Med* 1997;25:312–316.

197. Delacerda FG. A comparative study of three methods of treatment for shoulder girdle myofascial syndrome. *J Orthop Sports Phys Ther* 1982;4:51–54.

198. Cheshire WP, Snider CR. Treatment of reflex sympathetic dystrophy with topical capsaicin: case report. *Pain* 1990;42(3):307–311.

199. Walsh MT, Muntzer E. Therapist's management of complex regional pain syndrome (reflex sympathetic dystrophy). In: Macklin EJ, ed. *Rehabilitation of the Hand and Upper Extremity*. 5th ed. St. Louis, MO: Mosby; 2002.

200. Waylett-Rendall J. Desensitization of the hand. In: Hunter JM, Macklin EJ, Callahan AD, eds. *Rehabilitation of the Hand*. 4th ed. St. Louis, MO: Mosby; 1995:693–700.

201. Allen RJ, Wu C. Multimodal somatosensory desensitization therapy for patients with chronic pain. Paper Presented at: Annual Conference of the Occupational Therapy Association; October 2, 2004; Ocean Shores, WA.

202. Turk DC, Okifuji A. Pain terms and taxonomies of pain. In: Loeser JD, ed. *Bonica's Management of Pain*. 3rd ed. Baltimore, MD: Lippincott Williams & Wilkins; 2001:17–25.

203. Harden RN. Complex regional pain syndrome. *Br J Anaes* 2001;87(1):99–106.

204. Harden RN, Bruehl S, Galer BS, et al. Complex regional pain syndrome: are the IASP diagnostic criteria valid and sufficiently comprehensive? *Pain* 1999;83:211–219.

205. Allen RJ, Hulten JM. Effects of tactile desensitization on allodynia and somatosensation in a patient with quadralateral complex regional pain syndrome. Paper presented at: Combined Sections Meeting of the American Physical Therapy Association; February 23, 2002; Boston, Mass.

206. Allen RJ, Wu C, Horiuchi GM, et al. Pressure desensitization effects on pressure tolerance and function in patients with complex regional pain syndrome. *Ortho Phys Ther Prac* 2004;16(4):13–16.

207. Robinson JL. Complex regional pain syndrome. Bulletin: State of Washington Department of Labor and Industries 1997;PB97–051:1–9.

208. Hardy MA, Hardy SG. Reflex sympathetic dystrophy: the clinician's perspective. *J Hand Ther* 1997;10(2):137–150.

209. Loeser JD. Pain after amputation: phantom limb and stump pain. In: Loeser JD, ed. *Bonica's Management of Pain*. 3rd ed. Baltimore, MD: Lippincott Williams & Wilkins; 2001:412–423.

210. Melzack R. From the gate to the neuromatrix. *Pain* 1999;6 suppl:S121–S126.

211. Cheshire WP, Snyder CR. Treatment of reflex sympathetic dystrophy with topical capsaicin: case report. *Pain* 1990;42(3):307–311.

212. Allen RJ, Wu C, Horiuchi G, et al. Somatosensory specific desensitization in the treatment of patients with complex regional pain syndrome: effects of pressure desensitization. *J Ortho Sports Phys Ther* 2005;35(1):A27.
213. Fisher GT, Boswick JA Jr. Neuroma formation following digital amputations. *J Trauma* 1983;23(2):136–142.
214. Bin G, Cruccu G, Hagbarth KE, et al. Analgesic effect of vibrations and cooling on pain induced by intraneural electrical stimulation. *Pain* 1984;18: 239–248.

215. Allen RJ, Stephenson KM, Sundahl BT, et al. Thermal desensitization for treatment of severe thermal sensitivity and associated functional deficits secondary to complex regional pain syndrome of the upper limb. *Phys Ther Case Reports* 2001;4(2):59–66.
216. Lundeberg T, Nordemar R, Ottoson D. Pain alleviation by vibratory stimulation. *Pain* 1984;20(1):25–44.
217. American Physical Therapy Association. Position on exclusive use of physical agents modalities. House of Delegates Reference Committee 1995;25–95.

CHAPTER 92 ■ EXERCISE THERAPY FOR LOW BACK PAIN

ELLEN MCGOUGH AND JOYCE M. ENGEL

Exercise is the most frequently administered intervention used by physical therapists to treat low back pain (LBP) and prevent its recurrence.[1] Exercise for therapeutic purposes is defined as the systematic, planned performance of bodily movements, postures, or physical activities.[1] Regular exercise improves general fitness, results in a sense of well-being, and is associated with lower incidence and severity of comorbid conditions such as depression, fatigue, and insomnia, which are often associated with persistent pain.[2] There is support for the efficacy of exercise interventions for LBP; however, there is not yet a clear understanding concerning which components of exercise account for its benefits. There is also support for individualized exercise programs for patients with LBP across the spectrum of acute to persistent LBP.[3,4] The purpose of this chapter is (1) to describe the physical therapy (PT) evaluation and decision-making process for the development of individualized exercise programs for LBP, (2) to discuss physical and psychosocial aspects of exercise programs that may affect patient outcomes, and (3) to present available evidence for exercise approaches used for LBP.

LBP of musculoskeletal origin is a common problem and a major cause of disability. In 2006, an estimated one in four adult Americans reported that they have had a day-long pain episode in the past month with 10% stating the pain lasted a year or more.[5] Eighty percent of the population report LBP at some time during their lives,[6] and LBP is the most common cause of work-related disability in people under 45 years of age.[7] Despite the common use of pain medications, two thirds experiencing chronic or persistent pain cannot perform routine activities.[8] The annual financial cost (direct medical expenses, lost income, lost productivity) of all persistent pain syndromes is at least $100 billion.[8] Over and above the financial cost of LBP, the human cost, in terms of suffering and impact upon quality of life, cannot be estimated.

According to the American Chronic Pain Association, "persistent" pain is a more accurate description than "chronic" pain, as the former includes information on how pain can interrupt functioning, well-being, and quality of life.[9] The term persistent pain therefore will be used throughout this chapter. LBP is considered a condition, rather than a disease,[6] with multiple physical and psychosocial factors that impact the prognosis for recovery across the continuum of acute to persistent LBP conditions.[10] LBP not originating from serious spinal pathology or nerve root pain is often classified as "nonspecific LBP" due to our current inability to identify pathologic changes.[11] However, several classification systems have been developed to provide a framework for selecting PT interventions for the treatment of musculoske-

tal LBP, including approaches to exercise.[12–15] Despite the fact that the majority of patients with isolated LBP cannot be given a precise pathoanatomic diagnosis, exercise interventions hold promise for reduction of pain and disability.[3,16,17]

Exercise for musculoskeletal LBP is just one component of a multimodal PT treatment program which often includes education of anatomy and pathomechanics, postural modification, body mechanics training, manual therapy, functional training, and physical modalities (e.g., thermotherapy, cryotherapy, electrical stimulation). Due to the complex nature of persistent pain, multidisciplinary interventions are often indicated which typically include exercise, relaxation training, cognitive restructuring, vocational counseling, and medication management.[18–20]

Designing an individualized exercise program is a dynamic process initially based on the patient's impairments and exercise tolerance and then adapted to address the patient's goals of restoring function and returning to activity and participation. Specific exercises are used for the purpose of reducing LBP symptoms and addressing physical impairments, such as muscle weakness, loss of range of motion (ROM), or decreased motor control. Specific exercise approaches are often selected based on different theories of underlying pathophysiology (e.g., disc pathology,[21] lack of segmental motor control,[22–25] or dysfunction in joint mechanics caused by factors such as hypermobility or hypomobility[26,27]). Exercise interventions designed to address body region impairments are often based on theories of movement dysfunction and muscle imbalance. This type of exercise program focuses on the correction of postural alignment, modification of faulty movement patterns, and improvement of neuromuscular control imbalances between agonist and antagonist muscle groups.[15,28]

Over the course of LBP management, patients should transition from specific exercises to a more global exercise program focused on conditioning and prevention of relapse. Global exercise programs encompass exercises for general conditioning, including aerobic, flexibility, strengthening, and endurance exercises, and should be incorporated as soon as the patient demonstrates adequate tolerance and movement control. The purposes of global exercises are to enhance fitness, promote well-being, prevent injury, and improve activity and social participation. The ultimate goal is to integrate this type of exercise program into the patient's daily routine.

The overall goal of rehabilitation programs for individuals with LBP is to restore function, assist patients in returning to activity and social participation, and prevent relapse or recurrence. Functional restoration involves not only improving performance of physical skills, but it comprises the integration of skills into the individual's social and physical environments. When designing an individualized exercise program, there are multiple dimensions of physical function to consider including balance, cardiopulmonary fitness, flexibility, mobility, muscle performance, neuromuscular control, postural control, postural stability, and equilibrium.[1,29] In addition to physical factors, psychosocial, environmental, and personal factors should be taken into consideration when designing an individualized exercise program.[30,31]

There is broad agreement that LBP and disability should be managed according to a biopsychosocial model which includes health-related, personal, psychologic, and social dimensions and the interactions between them.[10,19,31] While the origin of LBP and disability may be caused by a biologic condition, the development of persistent LBP and incapacity are subject to dominant psychosocial influences.[10] The International Classification of Functioning Disability and Health Model is a biopsychosocial model designed to measure health and disability at the individual and population levels.[31]

Disability is an umbrella term for impairments, activity limitations, and participation restrictions.[31] Three dimensions related to functioning and disability include (1) body functions and structures, (2) activities at the individual level, and (3) participation in society. Impairments of body functions and structures are defined as problems with physiologic functions and/or anatomic parts, such as loss of joint ROM or reduced muscle strength. Activity restrictions are problems with executing a task or action and reduced participation includes lessened involvement in lived situations such as work, recreation, or social activities. Contextual factors include aspects of the human-built, social, and attitudinal environments that create the lived experience of functioning and disability as well as personal factors such as sex, age, coping styles, social background, education, and overall behavior patterns that may influence how disablement is experienced by the individual.[32] Environmental factors may include physical or social barriers or facilitators to activity and participation.[31,33]

Changes in attitudes and beliefs may have as much impact as physiologic changes, resulting from exercise, on the activity and participation of individuals.[10,34–36] This indicates that physical, psychosocial, environmental, and personal factors should all be considered when designing individualized exercise programs. The physical therapy examination and decision-making process is described in Figure 92.1.

INDIVIDUALIZED EXERCISE PROGRAMS

Physical Therapy Musculoskeletal Examination

Individualizing the exercise program by mutual goal setting to meet both physical and psychosocial needs is essential in maximizing exercise adherence and achieving patient satisfaction.[37] Individually designed exercise programs with higher dosage and regular practitioner follow-up are associated with improvement in pain and function, especially in patients with persistent pain.[3] Supervision and adequate compliance are common aspects of randomized clinical trials that have demonstrated positive outcomes for exercise interventions for persistent LBP.[4]

Exercise programs designed by physical therapists should be individualized to the unique needs and abilities of the patient,[1] many of which can be identified in a comprehensive musculoskeletal examination. The goals of a PT musculoskeletal examination for patients with LBP include (1) to identify impairments contributing to LBP, (2) to screen for potential contraindications and precautions to exercise, (3) to screen for coexisting conditions (e.g., cardiopulmonary), (4) to record baseline measurements of impairments and activity restriction, (5) to identify barriers to

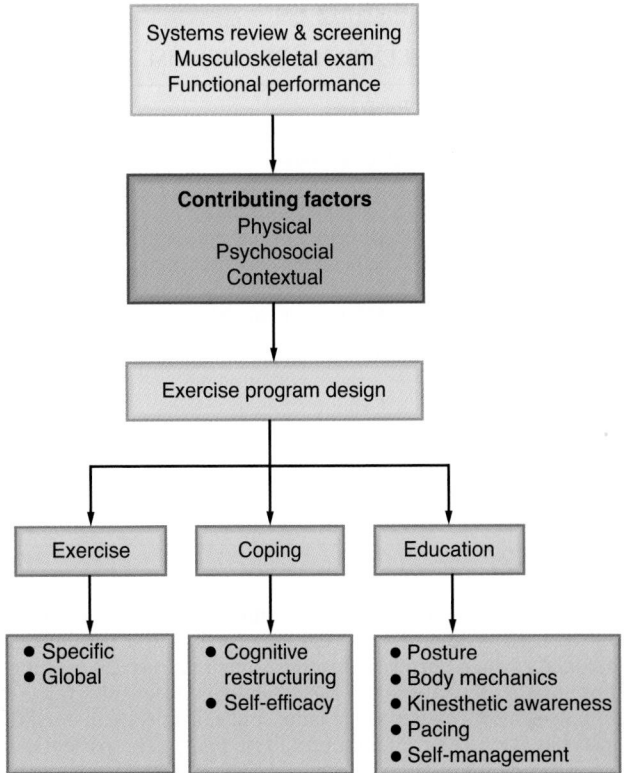

FIGURE 92.1 Physical therapy evaluation.

activity and participation, (6) to establish baseline exercise tolerance, and (7) to understand the patient's goals, preferences, and resources for carrying out an exercise program. A PT evaluation also involves learning about the patient's understanding and beliefs about his or her back problem. In addition, the obligation to manage pain and relieve one's suffering is now recognized by governing bodies as fundamental to health care.[38]

A systematic musculoskeletal examination involves the patient's history, a systems review, special tests, and measurements.[39] In addition to questions regarding pain patterns and the nature of the back problems, the examination should include inquiry related to medical history (including previous musculoskeletal problems and interventions used), psychosocial issues, and environmental barriers to activities and participation. A systems review is conducted to screen for red flags and to identify potential problem areas. Screening of the neurologic system through testing of key muscles, sensation, and reflexes is an essential component of a LBP evaluation. Current guidelines also emphasize attention to psychosocial factors, such as the patient's attitudes, beliefs, concerns, and expectations about their back pain.[11] Screening of psychosocial factors is recommended to provide indicators for chronic conditions, referred to as yellow flags,[40] which may identify patients at risk for developing persistent pain.

Anatomical structures that may contribute to pain should be tested with a systematic approach to the examination including tests of active and passive movement, tissue palpation, end range testing, repeated movements, and sustained postures.[21,39,41] Examination of a patient's postural alignment, willingness to move, body mechanics, and movement patterns should also be incorporated to gain an understanding of problems related to posture and general mobility.[39] Functional performance tests and task analysis provide information related to the ability to perform activities needed to return to activity and participation, including employment.[1,39,41]

TABLE 92.1

ELEMENTS OF EXERCISE PROGRAMS

Exercises	Coping	Education
Specific exercises	Cognitive restructuring	Anatomy
Movement control	Reduce fear of moving	Pathomechanics
Spinal stabilization	Clarify misconceptions	Body mechanics
Direction of movement	Self management	Postural alignment
Submaximal strengthening	Self-efficacy	Exercise technique
Specific mobility/flexibility		Kinesthetic awareness
Symptom reduction		Exercise progression
Global exercises		Activity modification
Aerobic conditioning		Pacing
General strength training		
Endurance training		
General stretching		
Coordination and agility		
Balance		

The results of a comprehensive musculoskeletal examination will be used to identify physical impairments and psychosocial factors for which purposeful exercise interventions can be aimed. A comprehensive approach for an individualized program, including elements of exercise, coping, and education, can be developed based on the examination (Table 92.1). The patient's response and ability to perform specific exercises serve as an additional source of feedback for both the patient and physical therapist. During the acute stage of management, the selection of specific exercises is based on the patient's responses to the exercise direction and intensity and is modified according to the patient's symptoms and movement patterns. Advancing the exercises and functional activities is facilitated when the physical therapist re-evaluates and modifies the exercise program to maximize patient progress and fit the appropriate stage of management.

Designing Individualized Exercise Programs

When considering exercises for LBP, it is important to consider the purpose of the exercises and the stage of management. The purpose refers to the patient's and clinician's goals for the exercise intervention: (1) specific exercises designed for symptom reduction or addressing physical impairment (e.g., impaired muscle performance, joint mobility, flexibility, or kinesthetic awareness) and (2) global exercises for improving overall strength, flexibility, and endurance. The stage of management refers to a time frame or the physiologic status of the tissue.[42] Acute pain is often defined on the basis of the duration of an episode of LBP (i.e., one that persists less than 4–6 weeks[11,43]), as well as the suspicion of inflammation, since signs and symptoms including pain, muscle guarding, and tissue irritability are typically present. Subacute pain is defined as LBP persisting 4–12 weeks[11,43] and/or reduced tissue irritability and increased tolerance for movement. Depending on the stage of management, an exercise program for LBP may comprise specific exercises alone, specific and global exercises, or primarily global exercises. At any stage of management, matching the patient's baseline exercise and pain tolerance is essential to facilitate program adherence.[37]

Exercise Interventions for the Acute and Subacute Stages of Management

Acute Lower Back Pain

Designing an exercise program for a patient with acute or subacute LBP includes recommendations about body position, move-

ment direction, exercise intensity, and activity level.[1,14,23] Common impairments and functional limitations associated with acute LBP include constant pain and muscle guarding, increased pain upon muscle contraction and stretching, and interference with activities of daily living (ADLs).[1] Although the timeline for recovery from an acute episode of LBP is generally considered to be within 4–6 weeks, relapse or recurrence is common.

During acute episodes of LBP, advice to stay active is recommended over bedrest since inactivity does not promote recovery and may even be detrimental to recovery.[10,11,44] Early advice to stay active has been associated with faster recovery, slightly less pain, greater functional recovery, less chronic disability, and less time off work.[11,43–45] Advice to continue typical activities and participation including work (when reasonable) is also recommended for the management of acute LBP.[11] Job modifications might need to be considered to facilitate continued participation in work activities.

Low intensity and specific exercises are recommended for patients with acute LBP[11,43] including direction specific and submaximal isometric muscle contractions performed in a neutral spine position or within the pain-free ROM.[24,25,46] Moderate-to-strong intensity muscle contractions are poorly tolerated during the acute phase of management.[11,43] Gentle active or passive exercises specific for symptom reduction are beneficial in reducing acute LBP,[47,48] but stretching is not recommended for acute injuries.[49] Additional treatments, such as manual therapy, cryotherapy, and transcutaneous electrical nerve stimulation (TENS), may assist with pain modulation and tolerance for movement during the acute stage of management.[25,42,43] Thermotherapy is generally contraindicated during the acute stage of management.[50]

Subacute Lower Back Pain

Pain intensity and tolerance for movement differ during the acute versus subacute stages of management indicating that exercises should be adjusted specifically for the stage of management.[51] As acute pain and muscle guarding subside, impairment may persist in muscle function, motor control, postural awareness, and functional activities during the subacute and persistent stages of management. The subacute stage of management involves a focus on postural and kinesthetic awareness, with the incorporation of submaximal strengthening and gentle stretching. Exercises should be completed in the pain-free ROM with emphasis to avoid further tissue irritation. Education in body mechanics, ergonomics, and relaxation are incorporated into the exercise program at this stage of management.[1] In addition, education on relapse prevention and self-management of acute pain episodes is important.[1] The application of treatments such as manual therapy, electrotherapy, cryotherapy, and thermotherapy may be indicated to address soft tissue impairments and facilitate improved exercise tolerance.[50]

Persistent Lower Back Pain Stage of Management

The international guidelines for persistent LBP place less emphasis on advice for positioning, posture, and biomechanics than the guidelines for acute and subacute LBP. Instead, emphasis is placed on promoting activity and participation, improving coping strategies, and assisting patients in changing beliefs and attitudes about their pain.[11] Persistent pain and disability are associated with physical deactivation and deconditioning, influenced by both physical and psychosocial factors.[52]

In patients with persistent LBP, individualized exercise programs with regular clinician follow-up and a higher exercise dosage are associated with clinically significant improvement in pain and function.[3] Some experts have recommended that exercise programs be guided not by the patient's pain complaints, but instead by a predetermined step-wise system for exercise and activity progression. Fordyce[53] outlined such an approach when he applied operant conditioning principles to a graded exercise program for persons with persistent pain. An individual's tolerance to activity is achieved through the use of a quota system.

Quota Programs for Exercise Dosage

A quota system is a practical approach to making baseline exercise recommendations and progressively increasing the patient's tolerance for activity. Intervention should begin with a series of baseline trials in which the patient is asked to perform a demonstrated exercise to their tolerance. Tolerance is defined as the point at which a patient stops exercising due to pain or fatigue. The physical therapist then establishes a quota for each prescribed exercise or activity to be performed daily. Typically, initial quotas are slightly lower than baseline trials (e.g., approximately 75% of baseline mean) and are increased by predetermined small increments (e.g., about 10% every few days). The patient is praised for meeting his or her goal. Unlike traditional exercise programs in which the patient exercises to his or her perceived tolerance, the patient instead achieves a quota. The quota system eliminates the linking of pain with function that might result in overdoing on "good days" and avoiding exercise or activity on "bad days." Rest breaks are scheduled instead of according to the patient's perceived need. Resting at the time of the individual's reported pain onset or exacerbation is avoided as it reinforces pain behaviors.[53,54] A gradual increase in activity also lessens the likelihood of an exacerbation of pain. Quota programs have been effective in increasing functional performance in persons with LBP.[55–57] Modalities (heat or cold) may be applied to prepare the patient for therapeutic exercise or to initiate activities.[58]

Relapse Management

Frequently, patients with persistent pain experience an acute pain episode or a significant exacerbation of their pain resulting from increased activity. Until the patient has recovered from the acute incident, the intensity of strength, flexibility, and aerobic conditioning exercises should be reduced, but the patient should be encouraged to maintain a tolerable level of exercise to avoid dehabilitation from inactivity. The patient may return to specific exercises to manage symptoms and regain mobility. An incremental, gradual increase in conditioning exercises can then be implemented.[58]

The Application of Common Exercise Approaches for Lower Back Pain

Specific Exercise

Through one-on-one evaluation and specific exercise instruction, the patient will ideally develop an understanding of principles for movement control and activity progression that will lay the foundation for progressing to a global exercise program and facilitate return to activity and participation. Specific exercise such as spinal stabilization or direction specific exercise may play a mediating role in reactivation through mechanisms involving early symptom management, improved kinesthetic awareness, and spinal region motor control.[25,59]

Spinal Stabilization Exercise Application. Spinal region motor control during functional activities can be enhanced through specific exercises, such as spinal stabilization exercises.[22,59] Submaximal training of deep lumbar musculature for the purpose of spinal segmental stabilization and movement control has also been referred to as motor control exercises for the lumbar region.[25] Research suggests that local impairments in the muscle system may be a problem of motor control rather than a problem of strength.[22,59] Spinal stabilization is a specific exercise approach designed to enhance the control of spinal orientation and intervertebral movement via training of deep trunk muscles, specifically the lumbar multifidus and transversus abdominis,[23] and sometimes also the rectus abdominis, quadratus lumborum, internal oblique abdominals, and erector spinae.[60] Spinal stabilization training is aimed at controlling pain and protecting the spinal segment from reinjury by reestablishing and enhancing motor control.[22] Restoring controlled segmental movement during static and dynamic functional activities is the ultimate goal of spinal stabilization exercises.[22]

Spinal stabilization (or motor control) exercises should be administered with direct one-on-one supervision, sometimes using ultrasound imaging, surface electromyography, or pressure monitoring devices to provide feedback to the physical therapist and patient about desired muscle recruitment.[24,25] Spinal stabilization exercises are low intensity and designed to be completed frequently throughout the day and integrated into daily activities.[23] Usually starting in the supine position with the hips and knees flexed, the therapist assists the patient in finding a neutral lumbo-pelvic position defined by anatomic landmarks and patient comfort. The patient is then asked to perform submaximal muscle contractions of the deep abdominal or multifidi muscles. Exercise progression proceeds from static (isometric) exercise in a supported position (supine or prone) to static exercise in less supported positions (e.g., 4-point, kneeling, or standing). Dynamic exercises through a controlled ROM are integrated into functional activities. The application of spinal stabilization during functional activities is emphasized across all stages of management, such as transitions from supine to sitting, sitting to standing, and ultimately to activities addressing the patient's participation goals. To facilitate improved functional mobility, the patient is instructed to perform submaximal muscle contractions during functional activities, especially when anticipating positions of potential mechanical stress.[60] The rate of a patient's progress toward performing higher functioning activities is dependent on their ability to develop controlled movement of the lumbo-pelvic region. The ultimate goal of spinal stabilization exercises is to integrate local motor control into functional movement, especially to prevent potential mechanical stress or pain.[60]

Directional Preference Exercise. Another form of specific exercise is the McKenzie approach to LBP. Exercises based on directional preference (DP) are at the foundation of the McKenzie approach.[14] DP is identified as a posture or repeated end-range movement in a single direction (flexion, extension, or side-glide/rotation) that immediately decreases lumbar midline pain or reduces the extent of referred symptoms to the extremities.[14] Exercises effective for symptom reduction are selected following a systematic examination in which the patient performs a series of repeated and sustained movements.[21] The position and direction of spinal movement that produces an immediate improvement in symptoms is selected for the patient to perform at home.[14] Patients are instructed to perform specific exercises that reduce peripheralization of symptoms and minimize LBP.[14] Peripheralization of symptoms occurs when movements or positions cause symptoms to radiate away from the midline of the back, into the buttock, or into the lower extremity. This applies to axial LBP as well as symptoms associated with sciatica. Centralization of symptoms occurs when symptoms move toward the midline of the spine, away from the periphery.[14,61] The patient is instructed that if centralization occurs during exercise, they are performing the exercise correctly. Conversely, exercises that cause symptoms to radiate away from the midline of the back, and perhaps into the buttock or low extremity, involve the wrong movement direction and/or incorrect position.[61]

In conjunction with DP exercises, postural correction and body mechanics instruction are a major component of an intervention using the McKenzie approach. For example, a common condition of mechanical LBP presents when pain increases during flexed postures and movements.[14,61] In this case, the patient would be assisted in an exercise progression that facilitates lumbar extension. Education to maintain posture with a bias toward lumbar extension with the use of lumbar rolls or back supports would be emphasized. Instruction would also be provided to maintain lumbar lordosis during all functional movements.

In summary, specific exercises such as DP and spinal stabilization are typically used for symptom relief, early mobility, and local motor control. Specific exercises are not only beneficial during the acute phase of management, but also in addressing specific impairments at any stage of recovery. For example, a patient with persistent pain may benefit from spinal stabilization exercises along with a general strengthening and conditioning for impaired spinal region motor control.[25,62] Similarly, a patient with persistent pain may address a local impairment, through symptom reduction and improving mobility, with the use of DP exercise.[47,48] While maintaining a focus on increasing activity and participation, an individual with persistent LBP may be able to manage local impairments through the use of specific exercises.

Global Exercise

The purpose of a global exercise program is to improve overall strength, endurance, mobility, and aerobic capacity. With the resolution of acute symptoms, a gradual progression of global exercise is indicated to improve strength and endurance of large muscle groups, optimize general flexibility, and increase aerobic capacity. Muscle strength and endurance training of the upper and lower extremities, with an emphasis on neutral spine mechanics and motor control, is important for promoting general muscle strength and endurance while avoiding excessive end-range forces of joints in the lumbar region.[63] The emphasis on neutral spine mechanics and motor control is also recommended when performing exercises for flexibility and aerobic conditioning.[63] During supervised exercise sessions, the physical therapist is able to provide feedback about motor control and body mechanics during functional activities. In addition, the patient is encouraged to integrate principles of motor control and body mechanics into the performance of daily functional activities.[63]

The overall goal of a global exercise program is to develop a regular exercise routine that is integrated into one's daily life and promotes well-being, prevention of injury, and enhanced activity and social participation. Matching the patient's goals and personal preferences for exercise is essential for maximizing exercise program adherence. In addition, considering physical and psychosocial barriers and facilitators to exercise is critical.[30]

Through recommendations for the type of exercise, progression, and individual modifications (e.g., postural alignment, exercise tolerance), satisfaction and adherence are likely to be enhanced.

Types of aerobic exercises may include brisk walking, running, swimming, or biking. Exercise that allows partial unloading of joints such as aquatic exercises, use of an elliptical trainer, or biking are often better tolerated by those with arthritic changes or difficulty with high-impact weight-bearing exercise (especially spinal stenosis or lower extremity osteoarthritis). Postural alignment as well as impact forces should be considered for all patients with LBP including education about shock absorbing footwear and exercise surfaces. Walking typically results in extension movements of the spine[15]; therefore, patients who have no change in symptoms or reduced symptoms with extension may benefit from walking, if impact force is controlled (footwear, angle of the treadmill platform, quality of the platform used). In contrast, patients demonstrating increased pain with extension movements of the spine may do better with aerobic exercises in which the spine is neutral or slightly flexed (e.g., stationary bike).[64]

For the average healthy adult to maintain health and reduce the risk of chronic disease, aerobic exercise 30 minutes/day, 5 days/week at moderate intensity (or 20 minutes/day, 3 days/week at vigorous intensity) is recommended by the American College of Sports Medicine (ACSM) and the American Heart Association (AHA). Moderate intensity is defined as physical activity that involves exercising with enough intensity to raise one's heart rate and break a sweat, but still be able to carry on a conversation.[65] Muscle strengthening activities may include resistance exercises to strengthen major muscle groups, such as upper and lower extremity progressive weight training, or weight-bearing exercises such as squats and lunges. A minimal strength training intensity of 8–12 repetitions, 2 days/weeks is recommended by the ACSM and AHA.[65]

Recommendations regarding exercise dosage are similar for adults of all age groups, but older adults will need more attention to balance and safety issues for exercise.[65] As patients become more active, their general health improves, but the risk of musculoskeletal injury increases.[65] Therefore, guidance in pacing of activity, self-management of symptoms, postural alignment, and safe body mechanics are critical in facilitating continued activity and participation. It is essential that guidelines for exercise performance and progression be provided to each patient (Table 92.2).

Educational and Psychosocial Approaches

Positive outcomes of exercise interventions for persistent LBP may occur as a result of modified pain perception, improved mood, improved physical fitness, and a sense of well-being.[34] Cognitive-behavioral strategies are most often considered in cases of persistent pain, but may also be beneficial in preventing disability if initiated during the acute or subacute stages of management.[66] In conjunction with exercise interventions, cognitive-behavioral strategies to minimize fears and misconceptions around activity and LBP may contribute to improved function and reduced disability.[11,36,66] Persons experiencing acute pain may learn to avoid activities and participation due to a fear of continued pain and (re)injury. This cycle of fear of pain resulting in reduced activity and participation becomes well established and may result in decreased strength, mobility, endurance, and suffering.[36] Psychosocial factors associated with LBP outcomes include coping strategies, emotional reactions, attitudes, and belief systems.[35,67]

Cognitive-behavioral strategies focus on changing patients' self-perceived efficacy to cope with pain (e.g., reduction of catastrophizing or exaggerated negative thoughts) and pain interference (decreased activity and participation) in persons with chronic LBP.[68,69] Vlaeyen and Linton[70] proposed that a gradual modification and introduction of activities and participation, despite pain, would ultimately lead to fear reduction and increased

TABLE 92.2

EXERCISE GUIDELINES

Exercise guidelines for patients
Starting and ending position
Exercise dosage
Intensity
Frequency
Duration
Quality of movement
Speed
Accuracy
ROM
Movement control
System for progression
Guide by symptoms and/or impairments (acute and subacute LBP)
Quota (persistent LBP)
Physiological (e.g., heart rate)
Formula for progression
Strategies to overcome barriers
Physical environment
Psychosocial environment
Integration into daily routine

function. Results demonstrate improvements in self-reports of pain-related fear, catastrophizing, and disability.[71] Self-efficacy is defined as the sense of control that comes from patients' own beliefs in their ability to perform specific behaviors and coping skills.[72] Even brief educational interventions using an educational booklet have positive effects on patients' beliefs about LBP and have shown improved physical outcomes.[73]

EVIDENCE FOR THE EFFICACY OF EXERCISE FOR LOWER BACK PAIN

There is support for the efficacy of exercise interventions for LBP; however, there is not yet a clear understanding concerning which components of exercise account for its benefits. Several possible reasons exist for the lack of clarity around the efficacy of various exercise interventions, including (1) research study design and methodology problems,[3,74] (2) unclear definitions for acute, subacute, and persistent (or chronic) LBP,[51] (3) the inclusion of heterogeneous study populations in many studies,[75,76] (4) multimodal treatment interventions in addition to exercise,[3,17] and (5) the main effect of exercise programs may be a result of factors other than physiologic changes (i.e., psychosocial factors).[34]

Evidence for the Efficacy of Specific Exercise Approaches

Efficacy of Spinal Stabilization Exercises

In a study by Hides et al.,[24] fewer recurrences of LBP occurred following spinal stabilization exercises for first-episode LBP patients when compared to no exercise intervention. In patients with persistent LBP, supervised trunk strengthening or stabilization exercise programs incorporating flexibility and body mechanics instruction have been shown to be more effective than a waiting list, TENS, advice to take regular walks, or to independently complete a home program.[4] The greatest benefits of spinal stabilization occur during the initial phases of the rehabilitation pro-

cess,[62] whether the stage of management is considered acute, subacute, or persistent.[19]

Recent studies have shown immediate or short-term benefits of incorporating spinal stabilization exercises, but limited long-term benefits beyond those of a general exercise program. In a randomized clinical trial involving patients with LBP, patients who participated in a spinal stabilization exercise program or manipulation treatment reported higher function and global perceived effects at 8 weeks versus patients participating in general exercise groups (aerobic, strengthening, and stretching). The stabilization and manipulation groups, however, were no different in their pain and disability from the general exercise group at 6- and 12-months follow-up.[25] Therefore, spinal stabilization exercises may be more beneficial than general exercises alone during the initial phases of the rehabilitation process.

Spinal stabilization exercises have not demonstrated long-term efficacy beyond that of general exercise programs. Two randomized clinical trials compared general exercise alone versus general exercises plus spinal stabilization exercises.[77,78] The groups performing spinal stabilization exercises in addition to more global exercises had similar long-term outcomes to those performing group exercises or participating in a conventional PT program (i.e., exercise, manual therapy, education, modalities).[77,78] In addition, general (or global) exercises reduced disability in the short-term to a greater extent than a stabilization-enhanced exercise approach in patients with recurrent LBP.[77] Another randomized controlled trial demonstrated no additional benefit, in terms of pain, function, or disability, of adding specific stabilization exercises to conventional PT treatment.[79]

Improved trunk ROM, muscle endurance, and decreased pain were reported in women with persistent LBP after completing a 4-week program of proprioceptive neuromuscular facilitation (PNF) exercises.[80] PNF exercises applied to the lumbar region would be considered a form of specific exercise for local motor control and strengthening. Improvement was reported after 4 weeks of training with dynamic resistance exercises, demonstrating better outcomes than the static (isometric) exercises.[80]

Efficacy of Directional Preference Exercises

The application of specific exercises based on DP shows potential benefit for patients early in the rehabilitation process during the acute, subacute, or persistent stages of management.[47,48] Pooled results of four trials comparing passive therapy with McKenzie exercises for acute LBP showed a statistically significant decrease in pain and disability favoring the McKenzie approach at 1-week follow-up. At 4 weeks, however, no difference in disability levels was noted between treatments.[46] At 12-weeks follow-up, patients advised to stay active produced superior results over the McKenzie exercises. One of the few studies including patients with persistent LBP (85% had symptoms >12 weeks), to evaluate the effect of 8 weeks of the McKenzie exercise approach versus intensive dynamic strengthening, showed a greater reduction in pain at 2 weeks in the McKenzie exercise group. At the 8-week and 8-month follow-up, however, there were no significant differences between groups in self-reported disability, global change of back-related quality of life, over-the-counter pain medications, or the number of visits to a general practitioner.[48]

Evidence for the Efficacy of Using Classification Systems for Exercise Selection

Matching the Exercise Program to the Patient

Treatment-based classification systems for LBP that match exercise approaches to patient baseline characteristics and impairments have recently been studied.[12,26,76] Long et al.[47] reported significantly greater short-term (2 weeks) improvement in pain and function when patients were matched to a specific exercise direction based on symptom relief, compared to those matched with the opposite direction or multidirectional exercises. Since 46% of patients were considered to have chronic complaints, it appears that exercises based on DP have the potential to produce at least short-term improvement during all stages of LBP (acute, subacute, or persistent stages of management).[19,47]

A preliminary clinical prediction rule for identifying patients likely to respond to spinal stabilization exercises was developed by Hicks et al.[26] For patients completing a spinal stabilization program, a higher likelihood for improvement at 8 weeks (>50%) on the Oswestry Disability Questionnaire[81] was associated with 4 characteristics: (1) age of no more than 40 years, (2) straight leg raise greater than 91 degrees, (3) positive prone instability test, and (4) aberrant movement patterns. Fritz et al.[27] reported lower disability scores among patients receiving stabilization exercises who were classified with segmental hypermobility versus those classified with segmental hypomobility. A history of recurrent episodes of LBP is also an important indicator supporting the implementation of a spinal stabilization approach.[26]

In an attempt to study the impact of identifying LBP subgroups within acute and subacute LBP, Brennan et al.[62] compared the outcomes of patients with LBP receiving treatment (manipulation, spinal stabilization exercises, or DP exercises) matched and unmatched to their baseline subgrouping. Patients who received specific exercise interventions matched to their baseline impairments showed a significantly greater improvement on the Oswestry Disability Scale[81] after 4 weeks of treatment than those randomly assigned to a treatment group. This study provides support for individualized exercise programs based on LBP subgroups during the acute and subacute stages of management; however, these subgroups do not appear to hold up for persistent LBP.[62]

Selecting specific exercises based on baseline physical impairments may be most beneficial during the acute and subacute stages of management, but persistent pain appears to be more closely associated with psychosocial factors.[62] Elevated baseline scores on the Fear-Avoidance Beliefs Questionnaire[82] (indicating fear of movement) during the acute stage of LBP have been associated with altered movement patterns, activity limitations, and reduced participation at later stages of management.[36,83] A psychosocial approach to fear-avoidance beliefs involves a de-emphasis on anatomic findings, encourages the patient to take an active role in his or her rehabilitation, and educates the patient to view back pain as a condition, not a serious disease and that pain does not equal harm.[66] George et al.[66] randomly assigned patients (<8 weeks of symptoms) to receive fear-avoidance-based PT (psychosocial approach + standard care PT) or standard care PT for a 4-week intervention period. Scores on the Oswestry Disability Questionnaire[81] at 4 weeks and 6 months were found to be dependent on an interaction between the type of PT (PT + fear avoidance approach versus standard PT) and the initial level on the Fear-Avoidance Beliefs Questionnaire.[82] Therefore, baseline fear-avoidance beliefs remained a significant predictor of disability at 4-weeks and 6-months follow-up.

Investigating the extent to which patients' adjustment to persistent LBP was influenced by their fear-avoidance beliefs, their

---

TABLE 92.3

THE BENEFITS OF EXERCISE FOR LOWER BACK PAIN

- Reduce risk for musculoskeletal injury
- Reduce risk of comorbidity
- Improve mood
- Increase sense of well-being
- Improve activity and participation
- Reduce the risk of reoccurrence or relapse of LBP

TABLE 92.4

THE PURPOSE OF SPECIFIC VERSUS GLOBAL EXERCISES

- Specific exercises are used for the purpose of reducing symptoms, improving mobility, and enhancing motor control. This creates the foundation for the performance of global exercises and functional activities.
- Global exercise programs encompass exercises for general conditioning including aerobic, flexibility, strengthening, and endurance exercises for the purpose of promoting well-being, preventing injury, and enhancing activity and social participation. The ultimate goal is to integrate a global exercise program into one's daily routine.

---

tendency to catastrophize (excessive negative thoughts), and their appraisals of control, Woby et al.[36] explored the relative predictive utility of these factors. Fear-avoidance beliefs about activity were the only significant predictor of patients' disability, even after adjusting for age, sex, and pain intensity. It follows that patients with elevated levels of fear-avoidance beliefs related to their back pain may be more successful when cognitive restructuring interventions are incorporated into the delivery of the exercise programs.

Evidence for the Efficacy of Global Exercise

Aerobic conditioning, muscle strengthening, stretching, and skill-training exercises (e.g., work tasks, sport specific activities) are associated with decreased pain, improved function, and reduced disability in patients with LBP.[16,17] Improved aerobic fitness and decreased trigger point tenderness following a program of moderate-to-high intensity aerobic exercise have been demonstrated in patients with fibromyalgia.[84] Moderate-to-low intensity exercise is effective for more sedentary individuals. In addition, adequate loads during strength training appear to improve strength and may decrease symptom severity in patients with fibromyalgia.[84] It is likely that these benefits of exercise also apply to patients with persistent LBP.

In general, there is strong evidence that global exercise is effective for improving pain, function, and disability levels when compared to no treatment in patients with subacute and chronic low back pain.[3,16,17,34] In individuals with persistent LBP, exercise

---

TABLE 92.5

INDIVIDUALIZED EXERCISE PROGRAMS

- Individually designed exercise programs with a higher dose (intensity, frequency, duration) and regular follow-up are associated with improved pain, function, and disability in patients with persistent pain.
- Individualizing the exercise program by mutual goal setting to meet both physical and psychosocial needs is essential in maximizing exercise adherence and achieving patient satisfaction.
- Exercise program delivery should be adjusted to meet the patient's psychosocial needs and goals.
- Adherence and satisfaction are likely to be enhanced by considering the patient's goals, environmental barriers, interests, and preferences.
- Cognitive-behavioral strategies integrated into an exercise program may improve mood, enhance participation, and reduce disability.

TABLE 92.6

EFFICACY OF EXERCISE INTERVENTIONS FOR LBP

Classification systems
- Developing subgroups or classification systems may aid in specific exercise selection.
- Physical impairments may be most important when designing exercise programs for patients during the acute and subacute stages of management.
- Psychosocial factors become more important than physical impairments in the management of chronic or persistent pain. For example, fear-avoidance beliefs need to be addressed.

Specific exercises
- Specific exercises demonstrate efficacy for short-term improvement in pain and function during the acute, subacute, and persistent stages of management.
- Spinal stabilization exercises have not demonstrated long-term efficacy beyond that of global or general exercise programs. However, there may be clinical value at all stages of management that is not easily measured.
- Spinal stabilization exercises have demonstrated short-term benefits in all stages of management and in preventing recurrence of LBP.
- Exercises based on directional preference (e.g., McKenzie approach) show potential benefit for symptom reduction during the first few weeks of the acute, subacute, or persistent stages of management.

Global exercises
- There is strong evidence that global exercise programs are effective for improving pain, function, and disability in patients with musculoskeletal LBP, especially persistent LBP.
- Aerobic conditioning, muscle strengthening, stretching, and skill-training exercises are associated with decreased pain, improved function, and reduced disability.
- Attention to program progression, self-management of symptoms, postural alignment, and body mechanics are important for enhancing long-term activity and participation in global exercise programs.

alone is as effective for improving pain, function, and disability as a multimodal PT program that includes manual therapy and modalities in addition to exercise.[34] Global exercise programs are generally accepted as an effective intervention for subacute and chronic LBP, particularly when patients have been advised in program progression, self-management of symptoms, postural alignment, and safe body mechanics. Program design, exercise intensity, delivery type, and individualization of exercise interventions have been identified as elements that impact pain levels and function in adults with persistent LBP.[3]

CONCLUSION

The four core topics of the chapter are summarized in Tables 92.3 through 92.6.

References

1. Kisner C, Colby LA. *Therapeutic Exercise.* 5th ed. Philadelphia: F.A. Davis Company; 2007.
2. Engel JM. Relaxation and related techniques. In: Hertling D, Kessler RM, eds. *Management of Common Musculoskeletal Disorders: Physical Therapy Principles and Methods.* 4th ed. Philadelphia: Lippincott Williams & Wilkins; 2006: 261–266.
3. Hayden JA, van Tulder MW, Tomlinson G. Systematic review: strategies for using exercise therapy to improve outcomes in chronic low back pain. *Ann Intern Med* 2005;142(9):776–785.
4. Liddle SD, Baxter GD, Gracey JH. Exercise and chronic low back pain: what works? *Pain* 2004;107:176–190.
5. Centers for Disease Control and Prevention. New report finds pain affects millions of Americans. Available at http://www.cdc.gov/nchs/pressroom/06 facts/hus06.htm. Accessed March 20, 2008.
6. Cieza A, Stucki G. New approaches to understanding the impact of musculoskeletal conditions. *Best Pract Res Clin Rheumatol* 2004;18(2):141–154.
7. Deyo RA, Weinstein JN. Low back pain. *N Engl J Med* 2001;344:363–370.
8. American Pain Foundation. Pain facts & figures. Available at http://www.painfoundation.org/print.asp?file=Newsroom/PainFacts.htm. Accessed March 12, 2008.
9. Asher A. Persistent pain. Available at http://backandneck.about.com/od/p/g/persistentpain.htm Accessed March 20, 2008.
10. Waddell G, Burton AK. Concepts of rehabilitation for the management of low back pain. *Best Pract Res Clin Rheumatol* 2005;19:655–670.
11. Van Tulder M, Becker A, Bekkering T, et al. European guidelines for the management of acute nonspecific low back pain in primary care. *Eur Spine J* 2006; 15(suppl 2):S169–S191.
12. Fritz JM, Cleland JA, Childs JD. Subgrouping patients with low back pain: evolution of a classification approach to physical therapy. *J Orthop Sports Phys Ther* 2007;37:290–302.
13. Fritz JM, Delitto A, Erhard RE. Comparison of classification-based physical therapy with therapy based on clinical practice guidelines for patients with acute low back pain: a randomized clinical trial. *Spine* 2003;28:1363–1371.
14. McKenzie R, May S. *The Lumbar Spine Mechanical Diagnosis & Therapy.* Vol 1. Raumati Beach, Australia: Spinal Publications New Zealand Ltd.; 2003.
15. Sahrmann SA. *Diagnosis and Treatment of Movement Impairment Syndromes.* St. Louis: Mosby; 2002.
16. Taylor NF, Dodd KJ, Shields N, et al. Therapeutic exercise in physiotherapy practice is beneficial: a summary of systematic reviews 2002–2005. *Aust J Physiother* 2007;53:7–16.
17. Hayden JA, van Tulder MW, Malmivaara A, et al. Exercise therapy for treatment of non-specific low back pain. *Cochrane Database Syst Rev* 2005;3: CD000335.
18. Jousset N, Fanello S, Bontoux L, et al. Effects of functional restoration versus 3 hours per week physical therapy: a randomized controlled study. *Spine* 2004; 29:487–493.
19. Klaber Moffet JK, Mannion AF. What is the value of physical therapies for back pain? *Best Pract Res Clin Rheumatol* 2005;19:623–638.
20. Molton IR, Graham C, Stoelb BL, et al. Current psychological approaches to chronic pain. *Curr Opin Anesthesiol* 2007;20:485–489.
21. Donelson RG, McKenzie RA. Mechanical assessment and treatment of spinal pain. In: Frymoyer JW, ed. *The Adult Spine: Principles and Practice.* 2nd ed. Philadelphia: Lippincott-Raven Publishers; 1997:1821–1835.
22. Jull GA, Richardson CA. Motor control problems in patients with spinal pain: a new direction for therapeutic exercise. *J Manipulative Physiol Ther* 2000; 23:115–111.
23. Richardson A, Jull GA. Muscle control-pain control. What exercises would you prescribe? *Man Ther* 1995;1:2–10.
24. Hides JA, Jull GA, Richardson CA. Long-term effects of specific stabilizing exercises for first-episode low back pain. *Spine* 2001;26:E243–E248.
25. Ferreira ML, Ferreira PH, Latimer J, et al. Comparison of general exercise, motor control exercise and spinal manipulative therapy for chronic low back pain: a randomized trial. *Pain* 2007;131:31–37.
26. Hicks GE, Fritz JM, Delitto A, et al. Preliminary development of a clinical prediction rule for determining which patients with low back pain will respond to a stabilization exercise program. *Arch Phys Med Rehabil* 2005;86:1753–1762.
27. Fritz JM, Whitman JM, Childs JD. Lumbar spine segmental mobility assessment: an examination of validity for determining intervention strategies in patients with low back pain. *Arch Phys Med Rehabil* 2005;86:1745–1752.
28. Maluf KS, Sahrmann SA, Van Dillen LR. Use of a classification system to guide nonsurgical management of a patient with chronic low back pain. *Phys Ther* 2000;80:1097–1111.
29. Liemohn W. Aerobic conditioning and low back function. In: Liemohm W, ed. *Exercise Prescription and the Back.* New York McGraw-Hill; 2001:89–97.
30. Rimmer JH. Use of the ICF in identifying factors that impact participation in physical activity/rehabilitation among people with disabilities. *Disabil Rehabil* 2006;28:1087–1095.
31. World Health Organization. *International Classification of Functioning, Disability and Health.* Geneva: World Health Organization; 2001.
32. Jette AM. Toward a common language for function, disability, and health. *Phys Ther* 2006;86:726–734.
33. Üstün TB, Chatter S, Bickenback J, et al. The International Classification of Functioning, Disability and Health: a new tool for understanding disability and health. *Disabil Rehabil* 2003;25:565–571.
34. Mannion AF, Müntener M, Taimela S, et al. A randomized clinical trial of three active therapies for chronic low back pain. *Spine* 1999;24:2435–2448.
35. Woby SR, Watson PJ, Roach NK, et al. Are changes in fear-avoidance, catastrophizing, and appraisals of control, predictive of changes in chronic low back pain and disability. *Eur J Pain* 2004;8:201–210.
36. Woby SR, Watson PJ, Roach NK, et al. Adjustment to chronic low back

pain—the relative influence of fear-avoidance beliefs, catastrophizing, and appraisals of control. *Behav Res Ther* 2004;42:761–774.

37. Bergman S. Management of musculoskeletal pain. *Best Pract Res Clin Rheumatol* 2007;21:153–166.

38. Fishman SM. Pain question & answer. Available at http://www.painfoundation.org/page.asp?file = QandA/FifthVitalSign.htm. Accessed March 7, 2008.

39. Magee DE. *Orthopedic Physical Assessment*. 4th ed. Philadelphia: Saunders; 2002.

40. Waddell G. Objective clinical evaluation of physical impairment in chronic low back pain. *Spine* 1992;17:617–628.

41. Hertling D. Lumbar spine. In: Hertling D, Kessler RM, eds. *Management of Common Musculoskeletal Disorders: Physical Therapy Principles and Methods*. 4th ed. Philadelphia: Lippincott Williams & Wilkins; 2006:843–934.

42. Hall CM. Patient Management. In: Hall CM, Thein Brody L, eds. *Therapeutic Exercise: Moving Toward Function*. 2nd ed. Philadelphia: Lippincott Williams & Wilkins; 2005:10–34.

43. Philadelphia Panel. Philadelphia Panel evidence-based clinical practice guidelines on selected rehabilitation interventions for low back pain. *Phys Ther* 2001; 81:1641–1674.

44. Hagen KB, Jamtvedt G, Hilde G, et al. The updated Cochrane review of bed rest for low back pain and sciatica. *Spine* 2005;30:542–546.

45. Underwood M. Exercise and the prevention of back pain disability. *Br J Sports Med* 2000;34:5.

46. Machado LA, de Souza MS, Ferreira PH, et al. The McKenzie method for low back pain: a systematic review of the literature with a meta-analysis approach. *Spine* 2006;31:E2540262.

47. Long A, Donelson R, Fung T. Does it matter which exercise? A randomized control trial of exercise for low back pain. *Spine* 2004;29:2593–2602.

48. Peterson T, Kryger P, Ekdahl C, et al. The effect of McKenzie therapy as compared with that of intensive strengthening training for treatment of patients with subacute or chronic low back pain: a randomized controlled trial. *Spine* 2002;27:1702–1709.

49. Prentice WE, Voight MI. *Techniques in Musculoskeletal Rehabilitation*. New York: McGraw-Hill; 2001.

50. Prentice WE. *Therapeutic Modalities in Rehabilitation*. 3rd ed. New York: McGraw-Hill; 2005.

51. Pengel HM, Maher CG, Refshauge KM. Systematic review of conservative interventions for subacute low back pain. *Clin Rehabil* 2002;16:811–820.

52. Verbunt J, Seelen HA, Vlaeyen JW, et al. Disuse and deconditioning in chronic low back pain: concepts and hypotheses on contributing mechanisms. *Eur J Pain* 2003;7:9–21.

53. Fordyce WE. *Behavioral Methods for Chronic Pain and Illness*. St. Louis: C. V. Mosby; 1976.

54. Turner J, Romano J. Psychological and psychosocial evaluation. In: Loeser J, Butler S, Chapman C, et al., eds. *Bonica's Management of Pain*. 3rd ed. Philadelphia: Lippincott Williams & Wilkins; 2001:329–341.

55. Ostelo RWJG, van Tulder MW, Vlaeyen JWS, et al. Behavioral treatment for chronic low-back pain. *Cochrane Database Syst Rev* 2005;1:CD002014.

56. Schwartz L, Engel JM, Jensen MP. Pain in persons with cerebral palsy. *Arch Med Rehabil* 1999;80(10):1243–1246.

57. Keefe FJ, Williams DA, Smith SJ. Assessment of pain behaviors. In: Turk DC, Melzack R, eds. *Handbook of Pain Assessment*. 2nd ed. New York: Guilford Press; 2001:170–187.

58. Engel JM. Chronic pain management in the adult. In: Hertling D, Kessler RM, eds. *Management of Common Musculoskeletal Disorders: Physical Therapy Principles and Methods*. Philadelphia: Lippincott Williams & Wilkins; 2006: 53–59.

59. Hodges PW, Richardson CA. Inefficient muscular stabilization of the lumbar spine associated with low back pain: a motor control evaluation of transverses abdominis. *Spine* 1996;21:2640–2650.

60. McGill SM. Lumbar spine stability: mechanisms of injury and restabilization. In: Liebenson C, ed. *Rehabilitation of the Spine: A Practitioner's Manual*. Baltimore: Lippincott Williams & Wilkins; 2007:93–111.

61. McKenzie R. *Treat Your Own Back*. Waikanae, New Zealand: Spinal Publications Ltd.; 1985.

62. Brennan GP, Fritz JM, Hunter SJ, et al. Identifying subgroups of patients with acute/subacute "nonspecific" low back pain: results of a randomized clinical trial. *Spine* 2006;31:623–631.

63. Hall CM. Therapeutic exercise for the lumbopelvic region. In: Hall CA, Thein Brody L, eds. 2nd ed. *Therapeutic Exercise: Moving Toward Function*. Baltimore: Lippincott Williams & Wilkins; 2005:349–401.

64. Bennett K, Belza B. Therapeutic exercise for arthritis. In: Hall CM, Thein Brody L, eds. *Therapeutic Exercise: Moving Toward Function*. 2nd ed. Baltimore: Lippincott Williams & Wilkins; 2005:229–243.

65. Haskell WL, Lee I, Pate PR, et al. Physical activity and public health: updated recommendations for adults from the American College of Sports Medicine and the American Heart Association. *Circulation* 2007;116:1081–1093.

66. George SZ, Fritz JM, Bialosky JE, et al. The effect of a fear-avoidance-based physical therapy intervention for patients with acute low back pain: results of a randomized clinical trial. *Spine* 2003;28:2551–2560.

67. Skargren EI, Öberg BE. Predictive factors for 1-year outcome of low-back pain and neck pain in patients treated in primary care: comparison between the treatment strategies of chiropractic and physiotherapy. *Pain* 1998;77:201–207.

68. Compas BE, Haaga DA, Keefe FJ, et al. Sampling of empirically supported psychological treatments from health psychology: smoking, chronic pain, cancer, and bulimia nervosa. *J Consult Clin Psychol* 1998;66:89–112.

69. Turner JA, Jensen MP. Efficacy of cognitive therapy for chronic low back pain. *Pain* 1993;52:169–177.

70. Vlaeyen JWS, Linton SJS. Fear-avoidance and its consequences in chronic musculoskeletal pain: a state of the art. *Pain* 2000;85:317–332.

71. Vlaeyen J, de Jong J, Sieben J. Graded exposure in vivo for pain-related fear. In: Turk D, Gatchel R, eds. *Psychological Approaches to Pain Management: A Practitioner's Handbook*. New York: Guilford Press; 2002:210–333.

72. Burckhardt CS. Educating patients: self-management approaches. *Disabil Rehabil* 2005;27:703–709.

73. Burton AK, Waddell G, Tillotson KM, et al. Information and advice to patients with back pain can have a positive effect. A randomized controlled trial of a novel educational booklet in primary care. *Spine* 1999;24:2484–2491.

74. van Tulder M, Malmivaara A, Hayden J, et al. Statistical significance versus clinical importance: trials on exercise therapy for chronic low back pain as example. *Spine* 2007;32:1785–1790.

75. Koes BW, Assendelft WJ, van der Heijden GJ, et al. Spinal manipulation for low back pain. An updated systematic review of randomized clinical trials. *Spine* 1996;21:2860–2871.

76. Fritz JM, Cleland JA, Childs JD. Subgrouping patients with low back pain: evolution of classification approach to physical therapy. *J Orthop Sports Phys Ther* 2007;37:290–302.

77. Koumantakis GA, Watson PJ, Oldham JA. Trunk muscle stabilization training plus general exercise versus general exercise only: randomized controlled trial of patients with recurrent low back pain. *Phys Ther* 2005;85:209–225.

78. Critchley DJ, Ratcliffe J, Noonan S, et al. Effectiveness and cost-effectiveness of three types of physiotherapy used to reduce chronic low back pain disability: a pragmatic randomized trial with economic evaluation. *Spine* 2007;32: 1474–1481.

79. Cairns MC, Foster NE, Wright C. Randomized controlled trial of specific spinal stabilization exercises and conventional physiotherapy for recurrent low back pain. *Spine* 2006;31:E670–E681.

80. Kofotolis N, Kellis E. Effects of two 4-week proprioceptive neuromuscular facilitation programs on muscle endurance, flexibility, and functional performance in women with chronic low back pain. *Phys Ther* 2006;86:1001–1012.

81. Fairbank JCT, Pynsent PB. The Oswestry Disability Index. *Spine* 2000;25: 2940–2953.

82. Waddell G, Newton M, Henderson I, et al. A Fear-Avoidance Beliefs Questionnaire (FABQ) and the role of fear-avoidance beliefs in chronic low back pain and disability. *Pain* 1993;52:157–168.

83. Thomas J, France C. Pain-related fear is associated with avoidance of spinal motion during recovery from low back pain. *Spine* 2007;16:E460–E466.

84. Mannerkorpi K. Non-pharmacological treatment of chronic widespread musculoskeletal pain. *Best Pract Res Clin Rheumatol* 2007:513–534.

CHAPTER 93 ■ COMPLEMENTARY AND ALTERNATIVE MEDICINE

CHARLES A. SIMPSON

INTRODUCTION

This chapter will look at therapies that are often classified as being "complementary" and/or "alternative" to conventional medical interventions for pain. A contemporary definition of complementary and alternative medicine (CAM) will be considered in the context of the complex and clinically challenging field of evidence-based pain medicine. A rationale for studying unorthodox treatments of pain is presented. The challenges of an evidence-based approach to incorporating complementary therapies into integrated pain management are explored. And finally, a brief survey of several commonly available complementary medicine therapies and the evidence regarding their utility are provided.

WHAT IS COMPLEMENTARY AND ALTERNATIVE MEDICINE?

Identifying and defining alternative approaches to health and healing have been problematic for decades. How these various professions, therapies, and approaches to healing have been characterized by the dominant, conventional medical mainstream is emblematic of the history, antagonisms, and misunderstandings between the two camps. How the alternative medicine disciplines have defined themselves is also instructive of the differences. Drawing meaningful distinctions between conventional biomedicine and the array of alternative methods may be useful to illuminate how each can contribute to better care for patients in pain.

THE DIVIDE

The emergence of organized medicine early in the last century marginalized a large number of existing healing disciplines, some of which enjoyed long and successful traditions treating the public. As Cohen points out,

> Although American colonies began with pluralistic notions of health care, the poor state of science, paltry qualifications of many would-be physicians, general lack of medical standards, and a cornucopia of charlatans eventually led to state regulation of healers—largely through the mechanism of licensure—and thereby to the triumph of biomedicine over competing communities of healers such as naturopathic and homeopathic physicians. Legally, state statutes made unlawful practice of medicine a crime and defined medicine in broad terms, encompassing any activity that potentially could be construed as diagnosis and treatment.[1]

As a result, Western, scientific, reductionistic biomedicine became the "real" medicine in legal terms. The resulting cultural authority of conventional medicine (CM) discounted traditional healers. The hegemony of this dominant paradigm was not seriously challenged until the last few decades of the twentieth century.

Fringe Medicine and Quackery

In the early 1960s British author Brian Inglis developed a model in his book titled *Fringe Medicine*.[2] This title consigned nonstandard approaches to healing to the periphery of science and the health care system.[2] Inglis considered such professions as homeopathy, bone setting, herbalists, and psychotherapy as fringe medicine. Being on the fringe implied that healers of this stripe were so far removed from the mainstream so as to pose no threat to the public or to the dominance of biomedicine.

In the succeeding 30 years, many of these fringe approaches to healing persisted and grew despite persistent opposition from the dominant medical establishment. In the 1950s, the American Medical Association (AMA), for example, developed ethics policies that forbade physicians from interacting with "unscientific, cult practitioners" such as chiropractors. The AMA Committee on Quackery was formed in 1963 targeting vitamins, homeopathy, chiropractic, naturopathy, all alternative cancer treatments, and other practices which compete with the drug sales of pharmaceutical companies.[3] In the case of *Wilk v. American Medical Association*, the AMA was found to have engaged in an unlawful restraint of trade under the Sherman Antitrust Act. And while the AMA's Committee on Quackery was disbanded, other groups have taken up the charge (see http://www.quackwatch.com).

Unorthodox Medicine

This unhappy stand-off persisted until Eisenberg's seminal study in 1993[4] revealed the depth and breadth to which these fringe practices have penetrated health care delivery. This paper reported a survey of respondents' use of a variety of unorthodox medical practices. These were defined by Eisenberg in exclusionary terms, that is, in terms of what these therapies are *not*. Unorthodox medicine in Eisenberg's view was *not* taught in medical schools, *not* available in hospitals, and *not* generally considered real medicine.[4]

Today, neither of these perspectives, fringe or unorthodox, provides meaningful distinctions between mainstream conventional biomedicine and those forms of healing that are different. Neither perspective bears up to careful scrutiny of the current state of complementary and alternative medicine. Eisenberg et al.[4] amply demonstrated that the volume of visits for health care delivered outside of the orthodox mainstream exceeds that of conventional care provided in physician offices—hardly an image of a fringe factor in the overall picture of the health care delivery system.

The popularity of complementary medicine with the public has not gone unnoticed by conventional medical institutions either. Health insurance plans, hospitals, and academic medical centers have integrated, to one extent or another, nontraditional health care providers and therapies into their programs. A survey of regional health plans in the northeast United States[5] found nearly universal coverage for chiropractic, with just under half of insurers covering acupuncture (usually for chronic pain) and massage therapy.[5] A 2005 American Hospital Association survey revealed that 370 of 1394 respondent institutions (26.5%) offer some form of complementary health care.[6] Complementary medicine topics are being integrated into the curricula of up to 64% of U.S. medical schools.[7] The American Medical Student Association has developed the Educational Development for Complementary and Alternative Medicine program to promote medical school education on alternative medicine topics. The Consortium of Academic Health Centers for Integrative Medicine includes 38 highly esteemed academic medical centers including Harvard, Duke, Thomas Jefferson, and Yale. The stated mission of this consortium is "to help transform medicine and health care through rigorous scientific studies, new models of clinical care, and innovative educational programs that integrate biomedicine, the complexity of human beings, the intrinsic nature of healing, and the rich diversity of therapeutic systems."[8]

Complementary and Alternative Medicine

The fringe and unorthodox labels are a carry-over from more contentious times. Other labels have included nontraditional medicine as opposed to traditional medical care. Considering that most of these nontraditional therapies pre-date most conventional interventions, for example, in the case of acupuncture, by 3000 years, traditional versus nontraditional seems irrational. Integrative and integrated medicine have some currency as well. Integrative medicine often refers to alternative medicine therapies delivered by CM practitioners or at least in conventional medical settings. Integrated medicine implies the thoughtful collaboration of conventional and alternative medicine providers in the treatment of patients. Alternative medicine suggests that the therapies are used in place of conventional medicine. Complementary medicine is supported by evidence showing that most patients use both conventional and complementary interventions, seeking to integrate their own care. The favored terminology by the National Institutes of Health has been "complementary and alternative medicine (CAM)." This chapter will use the distinction of CM to refer to Western biomedicine and CAM to cover those professions, practitioners, and therapies that lie outside of conventional medicine. These definitions too will likely lose currency over time.

Complementary medicine practitioners tend to consider their approaches as holistic and in contrast to a reductionistic approach that is ascribed to modern, specialty-driven biomedicine. Holistic practitioners use,

> [r]ather than focusing on illness or specific parts of the body, this ancient approach to health considers the whole person and how he or she interacts with his or her environment. It emphasizes the connection of mind, body, and spirit. The goal is to achieve maximum well-being, where everything is functioning the very best that is possible. With Holistic Health people accept responsibility for their own level of well-being, and everyday choices are used to take charge of one's own health.[9]

In contrast, the reductionistic approach of CM adheres to the theory that every complex phenomenon in medicine can be explained by analyzing simple, basic, physical mechanisms.

Bridging the Divide: One Kind of Medicine

The current trend toward evidence-based medicine (EBM) may eventually point the way to a reconception and resolution of the distinction between CM and CAM. CAM is frequently dismissed by critics as being unscientific and without evidence of its safety, efficacy, and effectiveness. However, over the last decade the emergence of complementary medicine on the national research agenda through the National Institutes of Health National Center for Complementary and Alternative Medicine (NCCAM) promises to develop the academic and intellectual infrastructure that

can explore the evidence that demonstrates the utility of complementary therapies. Originally formed as the Office of Complementary Medicine, the Federal budget for NCCAM grew from $2 million in fiscal year 1992 to $121.4 million in fiscal year 2007. The body of research is growing. There are currently more than 1200 randomized controlled trials (RCTs) and 150 Cochrane Collaboration reviews of alternative therapies.

Angell and Kassirer noted several years ago in a *New England Journal of Medicine* editorial[10] that in the future, medicine will be divided into those approaches to health and healing that are backed by scientific evidence and those that are not. "There cannot be two kinds of medicine—conventional and alternative. There is only medicine that has been adequately tested and medicine that has not, medicine that works and medicine that may or may not work. Once a treatment has been tested rigorously, it no longer matters whether it was considered alternative at the outset."[10] This perspective may well put to rest the arbitrary and, at times antagonistic, differentiation between CAM and conventional medicine.

A recent Institute of Medicine report on complementary medicine emphasizes, "The committee recommends that the same principles and standards of evidence of treatment effectiveness apply to all treatments, whether currently labeled as CM or CAM."[11] This evidence-based perspective will erode the barriers between health care that is provided in the tradition of Western scientific medicine and the healing disciplines that, in some instances, predate modern medicine by 3000 years.

Yet, there clearly are differences between health care available in physician offices, clinics, and hospitals and that provided by CAM practitioners. There are three features of CAM that tend to distinguish it from CM. CAM therapies are individualized to each patient. CAM almost universally incorporates a philosophy of health that emphasizes and leverages the innate capacity for healing in every individual. And finally, CAM tends to acknowledge the existence of properties of living systems that are resistant to understanding by contemporary reductionistic scientific methods of inquiry.

What Is Different About Complementary and Alternative Medicine?

These distinguishing features present significant challenges to research and assembling meaningful evidence. They also create opportunities to develop more effective, efficient, and humanizing care for a very difficult population of patients—those with pain. A recent observation by Cicerone on evidence-based practice and the limits of rational rehabilitation points out that, "we need to acknowledge the subjective meanings of illness and disability to the patients we serve. Any efforts to build our practice based on the best available systematic evidence are unlikely to succeed unless we include patients' values and beliefs and incorporate this perspective into our rehabilitation research. This aspect of evidence-based rehabilitation raises important questions about our fundamental roles and how we will choose to practice and define our field in the future."[12]

Individualized treatment is a hallmark of most CAM therapies. For example, an acupuncture practitioner may evaluate 2 patients, both with the same CM diagnosis, but develop two radically different treatment plans based on the Oriental Medicine (OM) examination findings and assessment. This approach seems to work well for patients. Studies of patients who obtain care from CAM practitioners reveal high levels of satisfaction with the practitioners and the outcome of the therapies. CAM providers spend time with their patients, and they are successful in explaining to patients the nature of their health problems. Treatment planning tends to be collaboration between therapist and patient. Interventions are developed that are consistent with each patient's own needs and preferences.

Philosophy of care is not something that most CM practitioners ponder extensively. However, philosophical discourse underlies many CAM therapies. Chiropractic, for example, contains an extensive literature that can only be described as philosophy. Beginning with the founder, D. D. Palmer, chiropractic thinkers have historically focused on not so much the rational scientific underpinnings of this healing art, but on the art itself. Innate intelligence is posited by Palmer and his successors as a fundamental life force that, when fully expressed without interference, the ultimate expression of health occurs, naturally and without need of intrusion from outside agents. In this chiropractic philosophical world view, the aim of the chiropractor is to locate and correct interferences with this natural expression of the life force. Identified as "qi" in OM, "prana" in yoga, "doshas" in Ayurvedic medicine, and "vix medica naturae" in naturopathic medicine, each discipline has elaborated some measure of a conceptual life force that guides and propels healing and health.

CM, with its intellectual traditions anchored in Western scientific thought, is understandably skeptical of notions of innate intelligence, qi, or other conceptualization of a putative life force. Finding no testable hypotheses to investigate a possible life force, CM has largely dismissed such philosophical musing. Oschman[13] provides a comprehensive review of this seeming impenetrable intellectual barrier between CAM and CM world views.

Who Uses Complementary and Alternative Medicine?

The research on CAM utilization is often confusing and contradictory. Research is complicated by a number of factors, including a lack of consensus on what therapies, interventions, and practitioner types constitute CAM, varying methodologies for collecting data, the variety of populations and settings in which data are gathered, and the different countries being studied in which the availability of CAM may vary considerably due to tradition, licensure, and cultural acceptance.

However, despite the inconsistent nature of the research efforts, it is certain that CAM use is widespread across populations, clinical conditions, settings, and sociodemographic groups. In 1993, Eisenberg and colleagues' paper[4] alerted the CM community to the magnitude of CAM utilization. This discovery revealed an ongoing phenomenon in the general population that has been verified and replicated in many subpopulations. A search of CAM on PubMed[14] with search terms "CAM utilization" returned over 500 citations. These include abstracts referring to various clinical populations (cancer, inflammatory bowel disease, autoimmune deficiency syndrome, diabetes, hypertension, allergies, rheumatic conditions, chronic fatigue, fibromyalgia, emergency department patients) and sociodemographic populations (veterans, racial and ethnic groups, geriatrics, women, children, athletes). In short, no matter what population is examined, CAM use is prevalent.

CAM use is particularly widespread among patients with chronic pain conditions. Nayak et al.[15] reported on a small sample of spinal cord injury patients with chronic pain. About 40% of respondents had used some form of CAM during the preceding year. Forty-four percent of chronic pain patients being treated with opioids reported concomitant CAM use.[16] Twenty-seven percent of veterans with cancer or chronic pain reported CAM use.[17] More veterans would have used CAM had it been covered by insurance. Tsao et al.[18] found that, given a choice of several CAM interventions, over 60% of pediatric patients (and their parents) opted to try at least one CAM approach in addition to CM treatments.

Categorizing Complementary and Alternative Medicine Therapies

There is considerable diversity in CAM practices and deciding which discipline to include under the rubric CAM and which to

exclude can be problematic and markedly affects the study results of CAM utilization. Eisenberg,[4] for example, limited his survey inquiries to 16 commonly used interventions but included "relaxation therapy . . . lifestyle diets, spiritual or religious healing by others." Eisenberg does note a categorical difference, however, between CAM therapies that are delivered by a professional, such as massage and acupuncture, and those that are largely self-administered without the involvement of a trained and licensed provider, such as lifestyle diets and intercessory prayer. Hospitals reporting the integration of CAM most frequently identify massage, body movement therapies (qi-gong, yoga, tai chi), relaxation, acupuncture, guided imagery, and therapeutic touch as the CAM modalities of choice.[6] Conspicuous by their absence from the hospitals are some of the most frequently encountered CAM modalities, such as chiropractic, nutraceutical, and herbal therapies. NCCAM has categorized CAM in 5 domains: alternative medical systems, mind–body interventions, biologically-based treatments, manipulative and body-based methods, and energy therapies.[19]

For purposes of the discussion in this chapter, CAM therapies will be limited to those commonly accessible in the community to chronic pain patients and, for the most part, administered under the guidance of licensed health care professionals. While this approach may exclude some valuable and frequently used therapies, it does encompass CAM therapies that are in regular use by chronic pain patients, are at least somewhat institutionalized, have been used or referred to by conventional medicine providers, and are capable of being integrated clinically and administratively into the CM care of chronic pain patients.

The array of CAM therapies are categorized further here by their intellectual and philosophical nature as being either essentially biologically-based or energy-based. Biologically-based therapies are explained and practiced fundamentally in ways that are familiar to practitioners trained in the CM model of Western scientific inquiry. Clinical conditions are mostly described in terms of disturbed anatomy and physiology. Treatment interventions are categorized by their physiologic effects. Outcomes are measured in objective clinical terms. These disciplines, such as chiropractic and natural medicine, often view themselves as being within the context of orthodox scientific thought. Many of these therapies have been rigorously scrutinized through the lens of Western medical scientific investigation. The disciplines themselves are developing intellectual, administrative, and physical infrastructure to conduct research as part of a commitment to evidence-based practices.

In contrast, energy-based therapies are most often founded on putative notions of natural systems of "invisible energetic relations and connections that govern living form and function."[13] While some of these energy-based therapies have undergone scientific inquiry, most notably acupuncture, the fundamental world view of energy-based healers has not been altered to conform to the understandings offered by rational reductionistic methods. For example, science has attempted to understand the physiologic basis of acupuncture in terms of its neuroendocrine effects. However, few acupuncture practitioners endorse or, more importantly, practice within this intellectual context. Most acupuncture practitioners prefer instead to explain what they do in the language of OM, such as the flow of chi.

WHY CONSIDER COMPLEMENTARY AND ALTERNATIVE MEDICINE THERAPIES IN PAIN MANAGEMENT?

There is a compelling case for why CM physicians, especially in the challenging field of pain medicine, should better understand

CAM therapies. Based on the study results of CAM utilization, it is quite likely that a pain patient is using at least one CAM therapy concurrently with CM treatments. There are potential complications that arise with the combination of CAM and CM therapies, and awareness of these enhances safety and quality of care. Users often fail to reveal their use of CAM therapies to their CM providers. Understanding the rationale for and evidence that supports CAM use in pain conditions places the clinician in a helpful role of providing objective information to pain patients. And, perhaps most significantly, CAM therapies can be effective and improve the quality of care for chronic pain patients.

Over 60 million Americans suffer from chronic pain. It is estimated that 40% of them fail to achieve adequate relief.[20] Surveys of CAM users note a high prevalence of chronic conditions, including chronic pain. Observers of the CAM scene note that "consumers will continue to use CAM, particularly in chronic conditions, in which patients struggle to find any treatment that may cure their condition or improve their quality of life."[21]

Most CAM interventions are "low-tech, high-touch" in nature. They are often perceived as inherently safe and natural by patients and practitioners. However, there is a growing body of evidence that illuminates adverse reactions to commonly used CAM therapies either by themselves or when combined with CM. Drug–herb interactions, for example, present potential challenges to patient safety and compromises of therapeutic intent. Eisenberg[4] noted that patients use CAM and CM concurrently for the same condition upward of 83% of the time. What is potentially more troublesome is that CAM users failed to disclose CAM use to CM physicians.[4] Subsequent investigation indicates that this failure to disclose has not improved over time.[7] Better understanding by both CM and CAM practitioners of risks can modify the potential for adverse outcomes.

Avoiding adverse CM–CAM interactions can obviously improve patient care. Asking patients about their use of CAM, especially from an objective and evidence-based perspective, can enhance patient communication. The cultural competency of being able to provide nonjudgmental acknowledgment of CAM use, particularly when supported by objective evidence of safety and effectiveness, can reinforce a productive therapeutic relationship between patient and CM physician.

It is well recognized that effective physician–patient communication is a critical element in predicting better patient satisfaction and compliance.[22] Moreover, as reliable evidence of CAM effectiveness emerges, CM physicians may be in a position to integrate evidence-based CAM approaches in an active manner rather than passively accepting what chronic pain patients may already be attempting to integrate on their own.

Challenges of Evidence-Based Complementary and Alternative Medicine Therapies

Assessing the evidence about CAM therapies for chronic pain is problematic from a number of perspectives. CAM therapies are often inherently resistant to analysis by commonly used clinical research methods. For example, in the hierarchy of evidence, the RCT is considered to be the criterion standard. Yet many argue that this methodology, while well suited to the study of drugs, may not be the best research design to study complex, individualized treatments routinely offered by CAM practitioners.[23,24]

For instance, trials of manipulative therapy have been plagued by the difficulty in developing a "sham" manipulation and concurrently controlling for the nonspecific effects of the hands-on practitioner–patient interaction with the theoretically inert sham treatment. Similarly, acupuncture research using sham acupuncture points irritate acupuncture practitioners who note that any needling at any point on the body affects the flow of chi, and therefore cannot be considered an inert intervention in the same way that a placebo pill is used in a clinical trial of drug therapy.

Functional magnetic resonance imagine and positron emission tomography imaging studies have demonstrated changes when sham acupuncture procedures are delivered.[25]

Further, evidence about treatment interventions for chronic pain is confounded by the complex nature of the condition itself. Patient selection is often a significant challenge to study validity. Aggregating patients with low back pain, for example, into a conceptually uniform study group ignores the wide variety of conditions that may fall into this pain population. It is no wonder that trials with this fundamental design flaw frequently come up with equivocal results for almost any intervention, whether conventional or complementary, and fail to reveal significant differences in effectiveness between treatments.

The challenges of applying evidence of this nature to the practical realities of treating patients have been increasingly recognized.[12] Fortunately, the research community, particularly in the CAM fields, is actively developing research strategies that are more appropriate both for the individualized nature of CAM interventions and the complex, multifactorial nature of chronic conditions such as chronic pain.

Finally, publication and indexing biases are obstacles to assembling reliable evidence about CAM therapies.[26] As in CM, studies with positive results are more likely to be submitted for publication. Many studies of CAM are in foreign language journals, thus limiting their exposure to English-speaking audiences. A more subtle bias also is observed in CM-published research on CAM. As one CAM researcher put it, "A negative study of acupuncture concludes that 'acupuncture doesn't work.' The analogue would be a negative drug trial that concluded 'medicine does not work.' "[27]

Despite these challenges in developing an evidence-based approach to the use of CAM therapies in chronic pain conditions, clinical evidence is accumulating. Many formerly unproven and unscientific therapies have, in fact, been shown to be safe and effective. Achieving the goal of Angell and Kassirer's[10] "one kind of medicine" is becoming a reality in health care and in the treatment of chronic pain.

THE COMPLEMENTARY AND ALTERNATIVE MEDICINE THERAPIES

Biophysiologic Therapies

These therapies are based mainly on concepts of biology and physiology commonly accepted in conventional biomedicine. These therapies rely on clinical theories, therapeutic approaches, and rationales that are couched in terms consistent with current scientific understanding of biology and physiology familiar to conventional medicine.

Manipulation

Manipulation is the most widely used CAM therapy.[4] It is widely practiced by a variety of specialties including Doctors of Chiropractic (DC), Osteopathic Physicians (DO), Medical Doctors (MD), physical therapists, and some lay practitioners. It is estimated that DCs deliver over 90% of all manipulative therapy.[28] Chiropractic training in manipulative techniques is arguably the most extensive among manipulation practitioners.

Manipulation is thought to improve pain by locating and treating disturbed joint and muscle function described as dysfunction, subluxation, fixation, and other terminology that may vary by discipline, training, and technique. Of the CAM therapies, manipulation has been studied the most extensively. NCCAM has identified 537 clinical trials of manipulative and other body work therapies such as massage. While the results are often and predictably inconclusive, there is clear evidence that manipulation is superior to sham treatment and equivalent to other conservative interventions for acute spinal pain.[29] More recent investigations show long-term benefit for neck pain,[30] headaches,[31] and chronic mechanical spine pain.[32] A recent clinical practice guideline from the American Pain Society and the American College of Physicians recommends manipulation, among other CAM treatments, for both acute and chronic low back pain.[33]

Natural Medicine Therapies

A number of CAM practices use nutritional supplements and herbs (known collectively as nutraceuticals) in the treatment of chronic pain. While these natural medicine approaches are most commonly identified with Naturopathic Physicians (ND), herbs and supplements are frequently used by acupuncture/OM and chiropractic providers as well.

Natural medicine can be used directly for analgesia (white willow bark, for example), anti-inflammatories (Omega-3 fatty acids), and antispasmodics (valerian and passiflora are examples). Nutritional and herbal interventions are most commonly applied to modify perceived underlying physiologic disturbances such as fibromyalgia, depression, osteoarthritis, and rheumatoid arthritis. Of commonly used nutritional approaches, glucosamine and chondroitin sulfate have been most extensively studied. Glucosamine has been shown to slow cartilage deterioration and relieve pain in knee osteoarthritis.[34,35]

Many nutraceutical interventions are thought to modify disturbed metabolism that underlie chronic pain conditions such as fibromyalgia.[36] While much nutraceutical information on the Internet is proprietary and commercial in nature, there are evidence-based sources of information for a number of painful conditions.[36]

Body Awareness Therapy

A number of approaches to chronic pain treatment involve the idea of improving postural coordination by using conscious processes to alter automatic postural coordination and ongoing muscular activity. These body awareness therapies (BAT) may be practiced by physical and occupational therapists, massage therapists, as well as nonlicensed body-work professionals. Two common BAT have been described: Alexander technique (AT) and Feldenkrais.

AT is described as "a method that works to change (movement) habits in our everyday activities. It is a simple and practical method for improving ease and freedom of movement, balance, support, and coordination. The technique teaches the use of the appropriate amount of effort for a particular activity, giving you more energy for all your activities. It is not a series of treatments or exercises, but rather a reeducation of the mind and body."[37]

A systematic review of AT[38] revealed few high-quality RCTs but noted promising results with Parkinson's disease and back pain.

Feldenkrais is a technique said to improve function by "expanding the self-image through movement sequences that bring attention to the parts of the self that are out of awareness and uninvolved in functional actions. Better function is evoked by establishing an improved dynamic relationship between the individual, gravity, and society."[39] Jain and colleagues[40] provide a recent review of the method, its use and the relevant research, and research gaps concerning this BAT.

Therapeutic Massage

Massage therapy encompasses more than 150 named body work systems and perhaps thousands of variations and individual techniques. Therapeutic, clinical, or medical massage is engaged to treat specific clinical conditions. The physiologic effects of massage are well documented, including muscular relaxation, improved blood and lymph circulation, and neurohormonalimmu-

nologic effects. There are more than 20 clinical trials of massage for pain. Physical Medicine and Rehabilitation Clinics of North America reviewed therapeutic massage in 1999.[41] A recent Cochrane review of massage for low back pain concluded that, "Massage might be beneficial for patients with subacute and chronic nonspecific low-back pain, especially when combined with exercises and education."[42] A more recent review concluded that there is robust evidence in favor of massage therapy for chronic low back pain and more modest support for massage in the treatment of chronic headache, shoulder pain, mixed pain conditions, fibromyalgia, and carpal tunnel syndrome.[43]

Breath Pattern Retraining

In 1975, Lum[44] introduced the concept of disordered breathing patterns as the underlying cause of "a collection of bizarre and unrelated symptoms" including cardiovascular, neurologic, respiratory, gastrointestinal, musculoskeletal, psychologic, and other syndromes. More recently, Chaitow[45] has emphasized disturbed breathing patterns as the cause of chronic pain. Proposed mechanisms are summarized as "respiratory alkalosis, leading to reduced oxygenation of tissues (including the brain), smooth muscle constriction, heightened pain perception, speeding up of spinal reflexes, increased excitability of the corticospinal system, hyperirritability of motor and sensory axons, changes in serum calcium and magnesium levels, and encouragement of myofascial trigger points." Breath pattern retraining therapists note that the respiratory mechanism is the only physiologic function that is under both autonomic and voluntary control.

A recent RCT involving chronic low back pain patients revealed equivalent improvement from 12 sessions of breath therapy as measured on a visual analogue scale (VAS), Roland-Morris Scale, and short form 36 health questionnaire (SF-36) when compared to high-quality, extended physical therapy.[46] Breath therapy was found to be safe.

Prolotherapy

The use of proliferation therapy (prolotherapy) has waxed and waned for nearly a century. Often provided by CM practitioners, prolotherapy is also frequently in the therapeutic armamentarium of ND. Following an injury, failure of adequate tendon or ligament healing is thought to result in instability, connective tissue insufficiency, or lack of tensile strength. Normal use of these compromised structures causes pain. Prolotherapy consists of injections of an array of substances intended to trigger growth factors in local connective tissue and restart the repair sequence that results in more normal and functional tissue.

A recent critical review of prolotherapy[47] retrieved over 30 studies of prolotherapy for spinal pain. These reflected wide variation in treatment protocols and concluded that, "clinical studies published to date indicate that it may be effective at reducing spinal pain." A Cochrane review concluded that, "If used alone, prolotherapy injections do not have a role in the treatment of chronic low-back pain. When combined with other treatments, they may give prolonged partial relief of pain and disability."[48]

Trigger Point Manipulation

Travell and Simons offered an early treatise on myofascial trigger points (TrP) which were defined originally as "a hyperirritable spot in skeletal muscle that is associated with a hypersensitive palpable nodule in a taut band. The spot is tender when pressed and can give rise to characteristic referred pain, motor dysfunction, and autonomic phenomena."[49]

The understanding of the etiology of TrPs has evolved. Current thinking has been summarized as, "TrPs are evoked by the abnormal depolarization of motor end plates . . . presynaptic, synaptic, and postsynaptic mechanisms of abnormal depolarization (i.e., excessive release of acetylcholine [ACh], defects of acetylcholinesterase, and upregulation of nicotinic ACh-receptor activity, respectively)."[50]

No objective diagnostic tests for TrPs are available. TrPs are diagnosed by manual palpation to identify a tender nodule, often at characteristic locations in muscle that, when stimulated, produce characteristic radiating pain as reported by the patient. Despite this low-tech diagnostic method, TrP detection has good test-retest reliability.[51] Various approaches to treating TrPs have been elaborated including manual compression, "spray and stretch," injection, dry needling, and modalities (ultrasound, electric stimulation, low-level laser). TrP treatment is often rendered by certain CM physical medicine practitioners, but most frequently by chiropractors, acupuncturists, massage practitioners, and other CAM providers.

The Tensegrity Model

Tensegrity (or biotensegrity) is not a therapy in itself, but rather a concept of how biologic systems function, from the ultrastructure of the cell to the organism. The concept is attributed to sculptor Kenneth Snelson and the term was coined by Buckminster Fuller to represent "tensional integrity."[52] Snelson noted, "Tensegrity describes a closed structural system composed of a set of three or more elongate compression struts within a network of tension tendons, the combined parts mutually supportive in such a way that the struts do not touch one another, but press outwardly against nodal points in the tension network to form a firm, triangulated, prestressed, tension and compression unit."[52] Donald E. Ingber of Harvard Medical School and Stephen M. Levin,[53] an orthopedic surgeon, have applied tensegrity concepts to biology and medicine. Ingber has postulated that cell function is regulated mechanically via tensegrity. Levin contends that the integrity of the musculoskeletal system "is a function of continuous tension, discontinuous compression, so that the skeleton, rather than being a frame of support to which the muscles and ligaments and tendons attach, has to be considered as compression components suspended within a continuous tension network."[53] Many body work practitioners including physical therapists, chiropractors, massage therapists, martial artists, and others have incorporated the tensegrity model into evaluation and treatment approaches.

Energy-Based Therapies

Energy medicine is a domain in CAM that deals with energy fields of two types: veritable, which can be measured, and putative, which have yet to be measured.

The veritable energies include mechanical vibrations (such as sound) and electromagnetic forces, including visible light, magnetism, monochromatic radiation (such as laser beams), and rays from other parts of the electromagnetic spectrum. These veritable energy-based therapies involve the use of specific, measurable wavelengths and frequencies to treat patients.

In contrast, putative energy fields are based on the concept that human beings are infused with a subtle form of energy. This vital energy or life force is known under different names in different cultures and traditions, such as "qi" in traditional Chinese medicine (TCM), "ki" in the Japanese Kampo system, "doshas" in Ayurvedic medicine, and elsewhere as "prana," "etheric energy," "fohat," "orgone," "odic force," "mana," and "homeopathic resonance." Vital energy is believed to flow throughout the material human body, but it has not been unequivocally measured by means of conventional instrumentation. Nonetheless, therapists claim that they can work with this subtle energy, see it with their own eyes, and otherwise sense its presence and quality and then use it to effect changes in another's physical body to influence health.

Veritable Energy Therapies

Magnetic Therapy

Magnetic therapy has a long and controversial history in medicine. It has recently regained popularity in the marketplace. Application is by way of electromagnetic coils in connection with acupuncture treatment and by way of static magnets. Magnetic therapy is typically applied to the skin overlying the affected area. The popular press indicates the use of magnets for treating a wide variety of chronic pain problems such as migraine, osteoarthritis, and injury to muscles, ligaments, and tendons. Contraindications are few but do include pregnancy, pediatric age, and presence of implantable electronic devices.

Contemporary clinical trials of magnet therapy have produced conflicting results. A study of carpal tunnel syndrome in 2002 found no statistically significant difference between magnets and placebo.[54] But the authors did note, "Although this study did not show magnets to be more effective than the placebo, the reduction in pain with this simple intervention was remarkable."[54] In a double blind, placebo-controlled trial, static magnets produced statistically significant ($p < 0.05$) short term pain relief in osteoarthritis of the knee.[55] Systematic reviews of magnet therapy are scarce and EBM reviews are lacking.

Microcurrent Stimulation

Microcurrent has been used in CM for the treatment of nonunion fracture and delayed healing. The exact mechanism of action is unknown but may involve intracellular regulation of calcium. Microcurrent has found application in the treatment of soft tissue disorders as well.

McMakin[56-58] has published three studies of this modality, which is termed frequency-specific microcurrent (FSM), in chronic pain patients. The studies are case series reports involving head, neck, and facial pain,[56] chronic low back pain,[57] and fibromyalgia associated with cervical spine trauma.[58] In the most recent study, McMakin and colleagues[58] began to explore the mechanisms of FSM. Their subjects revealed reductions in inflammatory cytokines, increase in beta-endorphins as well as subjective reports of pain relief in fibromyalgia.

Low-Level Laser Therapy

Low-level laser therapy (LLLT) is a form of phototherapy that involves the application of low power laser light to areas of the body in order to stimulate healing. It is also known as cold laser, soft laser, or low-intensity laser. It is hypothesized that photons are absorbed in the mitochondria. The light energy is converted to chemical energy within the cell affecting the permeability of the cell membrane, which in turn produces various physiologic effects. These physiologic changes affect a variety of cell types including macrophages, fibroblasts, endothelial cells, and mast cells.

LLLT is widely used in physical therapy, chiropractic, and other physical medicine practice. While reportedly safe, the modality is relatively new and is still controversial with respect to its effectiveness. A MEDLINE search retrieved over 500 citations. A recent systematic review of LLLT for acute and chronic neck pain concluded, "Significant positive effects were reported in four of five trials."[59] Cochrane reviews of LLLT used in osteoarthritis and rheumatoid arthritis revealed "conflicting evidence of benefit . . . for the treatment of osteoarthritis."[60] LLLT for rheumatoid arthritis is somewhat more positive about the therapy, "provides short-term pain relief for patients with rheumatoid arthritis."[61] Significantly, both reviews noted positive therapeutic results and called for more high quality research on LLLT.

Putative Energy Therapies

Acupuncture and Oriental Medicine

Among the putative energy therapies, none has received more notice and scrutiny than acupuncture. Acupuncture, the use of fine wire needles inserted into various points along meridians, is but one therapy within OM. The practice of OM itself includes a range of systems, interventions, schools of thought, and techniques. One such system, TCM, is widely taught and practiced in the United States. TCM encompasses herbs, massage, qigong, and acupuncture.

In the TCM view, the body is a delicate balance of two opposing and inseparable forces: yin and yang. Yin represents the cold, slow, or passive principle, while yang represents the hot, excited, or active principle. Among the major assumptions in TCM are that health is achieved by maintaining the body in a "balanced state" and that disease is due to an internal imbalance of yin and yang. This imbalance leads to blockage in the flow of qi (or vital energy) and of blood along pathways known as meridians. TCM practitioners typically use herbs, acupuncture, and massage to help unblock qi and blood in patients in an attempt to bring the body back into harmony and wellness.[62] These therapies are intended to balance the flow of qi rather than to produce a specific physiologic effect.

While not synonymous with TCM, needle acupuncture has received the most attention in the research and clinical communities. It is the most common OM therapy received by patients. Acupuncture describes a family of procedures involving stimulation of anatomic locations on the skin by a variety of techniques. There are a number of approaches to diagnosis and treatment in American acupuncture that incorporate medical traditions from China, Japan, Korea, and other countries. The most studied mechanism of stimulation of acupuncture points employs penetration of the skin by thin, solid, metallic needles, which are manipulated manually or by electrical stimulation.[63]

The body of research literature on acupuncture is robust. A search on PubMed for "acupuncture" returned more than 9000 citations. Limiting the search terms to "acupuncture and chronic pain" returned 500 articles. The Cochrane Collaboration lists 123 reviews for "acupuncture" and 18 EBM reviews specifically for "acupuncture and chronic pain." A comprehensive review of this literature base is well beyond the scope of this chapter, but it is apparent that there is conclusive evidence of the effectiveness and safety of this therapy for pain and other clinical conditions.

It is clear that acupuncture is widely used by chronic pain patients. A telephone survey reported by Breivik et al.[64] found 13% of chronic pain patients in Europe to be using acupuncture. Research methodology challenges in the investigation of acupuncture stubbornly persist. Meta-analyses frequently conclude that while acupuncture can be shown to be effective for pain relief, the therapy itself has not been shown to be superior to other therapies.[65]

Craniosacral Therapy

Craniosacral therapy (CST) developed from the work of an American osteopath, William Sutherland, in the early 1900s. It is founded on the notion of the primary respiratory mechanism that involves intrinsic motions of the cranial bones, the dura, and the flow of cerebrospinal fluid. Rhythmic motions are said to be measurable with instruments, but in clinical practice, it is by palpation that a CST practitioner identifies disturbed cranial rhythms and applies corrective gentle manipulations. Restricted motion of the cranial bones at the sutures is thought to impede CSF flow and lead to disordered function and disease.

CST is known in the osteopathic profession preferentially as cranial osteopathy. The chiropractic profession has a technique that encompasses much of CST and others as well, known as sacro-occipital technique. CST is also practiced by a variety of other hands-on practitioners including physical therapists, massage therapists, dentists, and lay practitioners.

CST is included under the putative energy category in that the motions of the primary respiratory mechanism have not been irrefutably demonstrated. Skeptics and critics have challenged the existence of these subtle rhythms.[66] Reliability studies of the manual diagnosis of disturbed cranial rhythms have been disappointing.[67] The Cochrane Collaboration contains no EBM reviews of CST. A systematic review of CST "found insufficient evidence to support craniosacral therapy."[68]

Homeopathy

Homeopathy is a system of diagnosis and treatment founded by Samuel C. Hahnemann in Germany in the late eighteenth century. Homeopathy is currently practiced widely in Europe and Great Britain and by many practitioner types in the United States including MD, DO, DC, ND, and lay providers. Clinical evaluations include detailed history interviews that lead to individualized treatment regimens depending on a host of physical, emotional, and psychologic factors. The therapies include the use of homeopathic remedies which are derived from plant, mineral, and other extracts that have been serially diluted, often to the point where, statistically at least, no physical molecules of the original substance remain.

This fact challenges fundamentally the notions of science and the physical universe that underlie CM. Most CM practitioners simply cannot accept the idea that a substance that has nothing physically "there" can have any real effect beyond that attributable to placebo. Nonetheless, a number of studies in reliable scientific journals report the apparent effectiveness of the medicine.

There is an extensive literature on homeopathy. A MEDLINE search covering 1996–2005 for "homeopathy" returned over 1300 citations. Many of these are foreign-language publications. A strictly nonscientific sampling of these abstracts indicates that pain and chronic pain conditions have not typically been studied. A search of the British journal *Homeopathy* for "pain" retrieved only 14 abstracts. As with natural medicine approaches to pain treatment, a homeopathic practitioner is more likely to be evaluating and treating underlying causes of pain rather than treating pain itself.

Ayurvedic Medicine

Ayurveda, which literally means "the science of life," is a natural healing system developed in India. Ayurvedic texts claim that the sages who developed India's original systems of meditation and yoga developed the foundations of this medical system. It is a comprehensive system of medicine that places equal emphasis on the body, mind, and spirit, and strives to restore the innate harmony of the individual. Some of the primary Ayurvedic treatments include diet, exercise, meditation, herbs, massage, exposure to sunlight, and controlled breathing. In India, Ayurvedic treatments have been developed for various diseases (e.g., diabetes, cardiovascular conditions, and neurological disorders). However, a survey of the Indian medical literature indicates that the quality of the published clinical trials generally falls short of contemporary methodological standards with regard to criteria for randomization, sample size, and adequate controls.[69]

In the pre-biblical Ayurvedic origins, every creation, inclusive of a human being, is a model of the universe. In this model, the basic matter and the dynamic forces (Dosha) of nature determine health and disease, and the medicinal value of any substance (plant and mineral). The Ayurvedic practices (chiefly that of diet, life style, and the Panchkarama) aim to maintain the Dosha equilibrium. Despite a holistic approach aimed to cure disease, therapy is customized to the individual's constitution (Prakruti). Numerous Ayurvedic medicines (plant-derived in particular) have been tested for their biological (especially immunomodulation) and clinical potential using modern ethnovalidation, and thereby setting an interface with modern medicine.[69]

A MEDLINE search for "Ayurvedic medicine" returned 66 results. A systematic review of Ayurvedic medicine for treatment of rheumatoid arthritis concluded that, "There is a paucity of RCTs of Ayurvedic medicines for rheumatoid arthritis. The existing RCTs fail to show convincingly that such treatments are effective therapeutic options for rheumatoid arthritis."[70] However, as with many other CAM therapies, especially the energy-based modalities, the issues raised by double-blind methodologies and placebo effects have not been thoroughly accounted for. The spiritual strength of the Ayurvedic healer and the utility of the placebo effect are both acknowledged and considered significant in many non-Western healing traditions.[71]

Touch Therapies

Touch is a fundamental human sense. The skin is arguably the largest sensory organ of the body. The power of human touch has been recognized throughout the history of medicine. Therapeutic touch (TT) and its derivatives are energy-based therapies that have become common in some hospitals and other clinical settings.

From the TT web site:

> Therapeutic Touch is a contemporary healing modality drawn from ancient practices and developed by Dora Kunz and Dolores Krieger. The practice is based on the assumptions that human beings are complex fields of energy, and that the ability to enhance healing in another is a natural potential.
> Therapeutic Touch (TT) is used to balance and promote the flow of human energy. It is taught in colleges around the world and has a substantial base of formal and clinical research. This research has shown that TT is useful in reducing pain, improving wound healing, aiding relaxation, and easing the dying process. It can be learned by anyone with a sincere interest and motivation toward helping others.[72]

A MEDLINE search for "therapeutic touch and pain" returned three citations. A Cochrane Review found insufficient evidence that TT enhances wound healing.[73] However, a pilot trial of TT in a cognitive–behavioral therapy (CBT) program found chronic pain patients who received TT in addition to relaxation and CBT fared better in terms of enhanced self-efficacy and unitary power, as well as having lower attrition rates than patients who only received relaxation training and CBT.

A study at the University of Wisconsin-Eau Claire studied another touch therapy (Tellington touch) in patients about to undergo venipuncture.[74] The intervention is described as "gentle physical touch and consisting of four components: a mental attitude of openness, use of the hands and fingers, breath awareness, and moderate finger/hand pressure." Analysis of qualitative descriptions by patients and the phlebotomist-nurse demonstrated that this massage-like, caring touch promoted relaxation and produced a helpful distraction in patients about to undergo a potentially painful procedure. While further study is warranted, the implications for physicians and others who have hands-on contact with patients of any sort, and chronic pain patients in particular, seem obvious. Human-to-human contact can have powerful effects in relieving anxiety and pain. The development of these skills by physicians and other caregivers may be of significant benefit to patients.

Reiki and Energy Healing Therapies

Reiki (pronounced RAY-kee) is Japanese for universal life energy. It is derived from rei, meaning "free passage" or "transcendental spirit" and ki, meaning "vital life force energy" or "universal life energy." Reiki is based on the belief that when spiritual energy is channeled through a reiki practitioner, the patient's spirit is healed, which in turn heals the physical body.[75] Reiki practice usually involves no direct physical contact between practitioner and recipient. By the practitioner holding his or her hands over the patient's body, the recipient is said to draw energy from the universal life force through the practitioner.

In the late 1800s, Mikao Usui developed modern Reiki from ancient Asian healing traditions said to be thousands of years old. Introduced to the West in the 1970s, Reiki has become a popular CAM therapy in the United States.[76] Reiki and other energy healing (EH) therapies have also attracted the attention of conventional medicine practitioners and researchers. A recent review noted,

> The National Institutes of Health is funding numerous EH studies that are examining its effects on a variety of conditions, including temporomandibular joint disorders, wrist fractures, cardiovascular health, cancer, wound healing, neonatal stress, pain, fibromyalgia, and AIDS. Several well-designed studies to date show significant outcomes for such conditions as wound healing and advanced AIDS, and positive results for pain and anxiety, among others. It is also suggested that EH may have positive effects on various orthopaedic conditions, including fracture healing, arthritis, and muscle and connective tissue. Because negative outcomes risk is at or near zero throughout the literature, EH is a candidate for use on many medical conditions.[77]

Reiki is practiced by a variety of licensed health care practitioners including CM and CAM physicians, allied health care providers, psychotherapists, massage practitioners, as well as nonlicensed Reiki masters. Although Reiki and other EH therapies are not without their critics[78] these high-touch, low-tech interventions are being adopted by hospitals, clinics, and physician offices as useful adjuncts to patient care.[79,80] Higher patient satisfaction, improved clinical outcomes, and lower costs are ascribed to implementing Reiki and other EH therapies.

CONCLUSION

Far from being on the fringes of modern health care, many CAM therapies have been in regular and frequent use by many chronic pain patients. Patients may seek out these therapies on their own from CAM practitioners, but they are increasingly provided in conventional health care settings as well.

Many of these unconventional therapies are being subjected to the same rigorous investigation that is expected of all contemporary evidence-based medical practices. Arguably, many CAM therapies hold up very well to this scrutiny and do so certainly as well as many commonly prescribed CM treatments.

The fact that CAM therapies are in common use by chronic pain patients suggests the need to better understand them. The emerging evidence that they are safe, clinically effective, and cost-effective when appropriately rendered further recommends them. That CAM therapies explicitly incorporate the power of intention, awareness, and healing in the human interaction of the therapeutic encounter may well be the key to achieving a more individualized, sensitive, and humanized approach to the treatment of a most difficult and challenging patient population—those with chronic pain.

References

1. Cohen M. *Healing at the Borderland of Medicine and Religion*. Chapel Hill: University of North Carolina Press; 2006;16.
2. Inglis B. *Fringe Medicine*. London: Faber and Faber; 1964.
3. Kent M. False cry of quackery. *Health Freedom Issues*. Available at: http://askwaltstollmd.com/body_quackery.html. Accessed May 15, 2007.
4. Eisenberg D, Kessler RD, Foster C, et al. Unconventional medicine in the United States—prevalence, cost, and patterns of use. *N Engl J Med* 1993;328(4):426–525.
5. Cleary-Guida M, Okvat HA, Oz MC, et al. A regional survey of health insurance coverage for complementary and alternative medicine: current status and future ramifications. *J Altern Complement Med* 2001;7(3):269–273.
6. Ananth S, Martin W. Health Forum 2005 Complementary and Alternative

Medicine Survey. Chicago, IL: Health Forum–American Hospital Association; 2006.

7. Eisenberg DM, Davis RB, Ettner SL, et al. Unconventional medicine in the U.S.: prevalence, costs, and patterns of use. *JAMA* 1998;290:1569–1575.

8. Consortium of Academic Health Centers for Integrative Medicine (CAHCIM). March 16, 2008. Consortium of Academic Health Centers for Integrative Medicine (CAHCIM). June 12, 2007. Available at: http://www.imconsortium.org/cahcim/home.html. Accessed August 27, 2009.

9. Walter S. *The Illustrated Encyclopedia of Body–Mind Disciplines*. New York, NY: The Rosen Publishing Group; 1999.

10. Angell M, Kassirer JP. Alternative medicine—the risks of untested and unregulated remedies. *N Engl J Med* 1998;339(12):839–841.

11. Board on Health Promotion and Disease Prevention Institute of Medicine of the National Academies. *Complementary and Alternative Medicine in the United States. Committee on the Use of Complementary and Alternative Medicine by the American Public.* Washington, DC: The National Academies Press; 2005.

12. Cicerone KD. Evidence-based practice and the limits of rational rehabilitation. *Arch Phys Med Rehabil* 2005;86(6):1073–1074.

13. Oschman J. *Energy Medicine in Therapeutics and Human Performance.* Edinburgh, Scotland: Butterworth-Heinemann; 2003.

14. NCCAM. About CAM on PubMed. Available at: http://nccam.nih.gov/camonpubmed/. Accessed June 18, 2007.

15. Nayak S, Matheis RJ, Agostinelli S, et al. The use of complementary and alternative therapies for chronic pain following spinal cord injury: a pilot survey. *J Spinal Cord Med* 2001;24(1):54–62.

16. Fleming S, Rabago DP, Mundt MP, et al. CAM therapies among primary care patients using opioid therapy. *BMC Complement Altern Med* 2007;7:15.

17. McEachrane-Gross F, Liebschutz JM, Berlowitz D. Use of selected complementary and alternative medicine (CAM) treatments in veterans with cancer or chronic pain: a cross-sectional survey. *BMC Complement Altern Med* 2006;6:34.

18. Tsao J, Meldrum M, Kim S, et al. Treatment preferences for CAM in children with chronic pain. *Evid Based Complement Alternat Med* 2007;4(3):367–374.

19. NCCAM. Home page. Available at: http://nccam.nih.gov. Accessed August 27, 2009.

20. Whitten CE, Evans CM, Cristobal K. Pain management doesn't have to be a pain: working and communicating effectively with patients who have chronic pain. *Perm J* 2005;9(2):41–48.

21. Lundgren J, Ugalde V. The demographics and economics of complementary alternative medicine. *Phys Med Rehabil Clin N Am* 2004;15(4):955–961.

22. Hirsh AT, Atchison JW, Berger JJ, et al. Patient satisfaction with treatment for chronic pain: predictors and relationship to compliance. *Clin J Pain* 2005; 21(4):302–310.

23. Paterson C, Dieppe P. Characteristic and incidental (placebo) effects in complex interventions such as acupuncture. *BMJ* 2005;330(7501):1202–1205.

24. Sullivan MD. Placebo controls and epistemic control in orthodox medicine. *J Med Philos* 1993;18(2):213–231.

25. Langevin H, Hammerschlag R, Lao L, et al. Controversies in acupuncture research: selection of controls and outcome measures in acupuncture clinical trials. *J Altern Complement Med* 2006;12(10):943–953.

26. Shekell P, Morton SC, Suttorp MJ, et al. Challenges in systematic reviews of complementary and alternative medicine topics. *Ann Intern Med* 2005; 142(12 Pt 2):1042–1047.

27. Hammerschlag R. Personal communication, February 20, 2005.

28. Shekelle PG, Adams AH, Chassin MR, et al. Spinal manipulation for low-back pain. *Ann Intern Med* 1992;117(7):590–598.

29. Koes B, van Tulder M. Low back pain (acute). *Clin Evid* 2006;15:1619–1633.

30. Bronfort G. The effectiveness of cervical adjustment for acute and chronic neck pain: excerpts from a systematic review and best evidence synthesis. *Journal of the American Chiropractic Association* 2003;40:42.

31. McCrory DC, Penzien DB, Hasselblad V, et al. *Evidence Report: Behavioral and Physical Treatments for Tension-Type and Cervicogenic Headache.* Des Moines, IA: Foundation for Chiropractic Education and Research; 2001.

32. Muller R, Giles LGF. Long-term follow-up of a randomized clinical trial assessing the efficacy of medication, acupuncture, and spinal manipulation for chronic mechanical spinal pain syndromes. *J Manipulative Physiol Ther* 2005; 28(1):3–11.

33. Chou R, Huffman LH, American Pain Society, et al. Nonpharmacologic therapies for acute and chronic low back pain: a review of the evidence for an American Pain Society/American College of Physicians clinical practice guideline. *Anna Intern Med* 2007;147(7):492–504.

34. Clegg DO, Reda DJ, Harris CL, et al. Glucosamine, chondroitin sulfate, and the two in combination for painful knee osteoarthritis. *N Engl J Med* 2006; 354(8):795–808.

35. Hochberg MC, Zhan M, Langenberg P. The rate of decline of joint space width in patients with osteoarthritis of the knee: a systematic review and meta-analysis of randomized placebo-controlled trials of chondroitin sulfate. *Curr Med Res Opin* 2008. [Epub ahead of print].

36. Holdcraft LC, Assefi N, Buchwald D. Complementary and alternative medicine in fibromyalgia and related syndromes. *Best Pract Res Clin Rheumatol* 2003; 17:667-83.

37. Rickover R. The complete guide to the Alexander technique. Available at: http://www.alexandertechnique.com/at.htm. Accessed August 27, 2009.

38. Erntst E, Canter PH. The Alexander technique: a systematic review of controlled clinical trials. *Forsch Komplementarmed Klass Naturheilkd* 2003;10(6):325–329.

39. The Feldenkrais Educational Foundation of North America and the Feldenkrais Guild of North America. The Feldenkrais method of somatic education. Available at: http://www.feldenkrais.com/method/standards/index.html#what. Accessed

40. Jain S, Janssen K, DeCelle S. Alexander technique and Feldenkrais method: a critical overview. *Phys Med Rehabil Clin N Am* 2004;15(4):811–825, vi.

41. Braverman DL, Schulman RA. Massage techniques in rehabilitation medicine. *Phys Med Rehabil Clin N Am* 1999;10(3):631–649, ix.

42. Furlan AD, Imamura M, Dryden T, et al. Massage for low-back pain. Available at: http://www.cochrane.org/reviews/en/ab001929.html. Accessed

43. Tsao J. Effectiveness of massage therapy for chronic, non-malignant pain: a review. *Evid Based Complement Alternat Med* 2007;4(2):165–179.

44. Lum LC. Hyperventilation: the tip of the iceberg. *J Psychosom Res* 1975; 19(5-6):375–383.

45. Chaitow L. Breathing pattern disorders, motor control, and low back pain. *J Osteopath Med* 2004;7(1):34–41.

46. Mehling WE, Hamel KA, Acree M, et al. Randomized, controlled trial of breath therapy for patients with chronic low back pain. *Altern Ther Health Med* 2005; 11(4):44–52.

47. Dagenais S, Haldeman S, Wooley JR. Intraligamentous injection of sclerosing solutions (prolotherapy) for spinal pain: a critical review of the literature. *Spine J* 2005;5(3):310–328.

48. Dagenais S, Yelland MJ, Del Mar C, et al. Prolotherapy injections for chronic low-back pain. Available at: http://www.cochrane.org/reviews/en/ab004059.html. Accessed

49. Travell JG, Simons DG. *Myofascial Pain and Dysfunction: The Trigger Point Manual: The Upper Extremities.* Vol 1. Baltimore, MD: Williams & Wilkins; 1983.

50. McPartland J. Travell trigger points—molecular and osteopathic perspectives. *J Am Osteopath Assoc* 2004;104(6):244–249.

51. Al-Shenqiti AM, Oldham JA. Test-retest reliability of myofascial trigger point detection in patients with rotator cuff tendonitis. *Clin Rehabil* 2005;19(5):482–487.

52. Snelson K. Weaving, mother of tensegrity. Available at: http://www.kennethsnelson.net/icons/struc.htm. Accessed

53. Levin S. Continuous tension, discontinuous compression: a model for biomechanical support of the body. A presentation to the North American Academy of Manipulative Medicine in 1980. Available at: http://www.biotensegrity.com/index.php?option=com_content&task=view&id=14&Itemid=29. Accessed October 18, 2007.

54. Carter R, Hall T, Aspy CB, et al. The effectiveness of magnet therapy for treatment of wrist pain attributed to carpal tunnel syndrome. *J Fam Pract* 2002; 51(1);38–40.

55. Wolsko PM, Eisenberg DM, Simon LS, et al. Double-blind placebo-controlled trial of static magnets for the treatment of osteoarthritis of the knee: results of a pilot study. *Altern Ther Health Med* 2004;10(2):36–43.

56. McMakin C. Microcurrent treatment of myofascial pain in the head, neck, and face. *Top Clin Chiropr* 1998;5:29–35.

57. McMakin C. Microcurrent therapy: a novel treatment for chronic low back myofascial pain. *J Bodywork Movement Ther* 2004;8(2):143–153.

58. McMakin C, Gregory WM, Phillips TM. Cytokine changes with microcurrent treatment of fibromyalgia associated with cervical spine trauma. 2005;9(3):169–176.

59. Chow RT, Barnsley L. Systematic review of the literature of low-level laser therapy (LLLT) in the management of neck pain. *Lasers Surg Med* 2005;37(1):46–52.

60. Brosseau L, Welch V, Wells GA, et al. Low level laser therapy for treating rheumatoid arthritis. Cochrane Database of Reviews. Available at: *http://www.cochrane.org/reviews/en/ab002046.html,* Accessed August 27, 2009.

61. Brosseau L, Welch V, Wells GA, et al. Low level laser therapy (Classes I, II and III) for treating rheumatoid arthritis. Available at: www.cochrane.org/reviews/en/ab002049.html. Accessed

62. National Center for Complementary and Alternative Medicine. Traditional Chinese Medicine: An introduction. Available at: *http://nccam.nih.gov/health/whatiscam/D428.pdf,* Accessed August 27, 2009.

63. Acupuncture. NIH Consensus Statement Online 1997 Nov 3–5. 1997;15(5):1-34. Available at: http://consensus.nih.gov/1997/1997Acupuncture107html.htm. Accessed

64. Breivik H, Collett B, Ventafridda V, et al. Survey of chronic pain in Europe: prevalence, impact on daily life, and treatment. *Eur J Pain* 2006;10(4):287-333.

65. Manheimer E, White A, Berman B, et al. Meta-analysis: acupuncture for low back pain. *Ann Intern Med* 2005;142(8):651–663.

66. Bledsoe BE, Licciardone JC. The elephant in the room: does OMT have proved benefit? *J Am Osteopath Assoc.* 2004;104(10):405–406.

67. Moran RW, Gibbons P. Intraexaminer and interexaminer reliability for palpation of the cranial rhythmic impulse at the head and sacrum. *J Manipulative Physiol Ther* 2001;24(3):183–190.

68. Green C, Martin CW, Bassett K, et al. A systematic review of craniosacral therapy: biological plausibility, assessment reliability and clinical effectiveness. *Comp Ther Med* 1999;7(4):199–270.

69. Chopra A, Doiphole VV. Ayurvedic medicine. Core concept, therapeutic principles, and current relevance. *Med Clin North Am* 2002;86(1):75–89, vii.

70. Park J, Ernst E. Ayurvedic medicine for rheumatoid arthritis: a systematic review. *Semin Arthritis Rheum* 2005;34(5):705–713.

71. Jonas WB, Levin JS. *Essentials of Complementary and Alternative Medicine.* Baltimore MD: Lippincott Williams & Wilkins; 1999;210.

72. Therapeutic Touch. Home page. Available at: http://www.therapeutic touch.org/. Accessed August 27, 2009.

73. O'Mathuna DP, Ashford RL. Therapeutic touch for healing acute wounds. *Cochrane Database Syst Rev* 2003;4:CD002766.

74. Wendler MC. Effects of Tellington touch in healthy adults awaiting venipuncture. *Res Nurs Health* 2003;26:40–52.

75. Holisitconline.com. Reiki infocenter. Available at: http://www.holistic-online.com/Reiki/hol_reiki_introduction.htm. Accessed August 27, 2009.

76. Chu DA. Tai Chi, Qi Gong and Reiki. *Phys Med Rehabil Clin N Am* 2004; 15(4):773–781, vi.

77. Dinucci EM. Energy healing: a complementary treatment for orthopaedic and other conditions. *Orthop Nurs* 2005;24(4):259–269.

78. Jarvis WT. Reiki. Available at: http://www.ncahf.org/articles/o-r/reiki.html. Accessed August 27, 2009.

79. Sawyer J. The first Reiki practitioner in our OR. *AORN J* 1998;67:674–677.

80. The International Center for Reiki Training. Reiki in hospitals. Available at: http://www.reiki.org/reikinews/reiki_in_hospitals.html. Accessed August 27, 2009.

CHAPTER 94 ■ PERIPHERAL NERVE STIMULATION

MICHAEL J. DORSI AND ALLAN J. BELZBERG

INTRODUCTION

Over the past 40 years peripheral nerve stimulation (PNS) has been established as a treatment option for refractory neuropathic pain. Since the first reports of pain relief following implantation of PNS in the 1960s, several authors have published their results with PNS for intractable painful mononeuropathy, complex regional pain syndrome, postherpetic neuralgia, trigeminal neuralgia, occipital neuralgia, and supraorbital neuralgia. This chapter will focus on PNS for painful mononeuropathy and occipital neuralgia.

MECHANISMS OF PAIN RELIEF

The exact mechanism of pain relief following PNS is not clearly understood. The original scientific basis for the use of electrical stimulation for the treatment of pain was provided in 1965 by Melzack and Wall's "gate control theory of pain."[1] They proposed that the transmission of pain from the periphery to the brain is regulated by a "gate" in the dorsal horn of the spinal cord. The gate may be opened by input from c- and Aδ-fiber nociceptive neurons and closed by nonnocieptive large fiber input. According to this theory, electrical stimulation increases large fiber input enough to "close" the gate and override the input from nociceptors. Wall and Sweet were the first to report a clinical correlation to this theory by placing temporary electrodes on sensory peripheral nerves or spinal roots in eight patients with intense chronic cutaneous pain, providing symptomatic relief.[2]

Several lines of evidence question the validity of the gate control theory: (1) normal pain thresholds are not affected by coactivation of large fibers, (2) in neuropathic pain conditions, low frequency stimulation of large-diameter afferents evokes pain, (3) large fiber neuropathies are rarely associated with increased pain, and (4) stimulation is inefficacious for chronic and acute nociceptive pain.

Alternative explanations for the effects of PNS on pain have been brought forward. Following peripheral nerve injury, mechanical allodynia can be mediated by Aβ-fibers[3] and maintained by central sensitization of dorsal horn neurons.[4] It has been shown that repetitive electrical stimulation of a peripheral nerve may produce excitation failure in c-fiber nociceptors and suppress activity in the dorsal horn of the spinal cord.[5,6] The peripheral effects may be due to stimulation-induced blockade of cell membrane depolarization which prevents axonal conduction.[7] Additional insights have been derived from animal studies in which spinal cord stimulation has been shown to ameliorate mechanical allodynia. In nerve injury animal models, spinal cord stimulation (SCS) has been shown to decrease hyperexcitability and long-term potentiation of dorsal horn neurons and ameliorate mechanical allodynia.[8–10] In addition, stimulation may affect dorsal horn excitability by decreasing the release of excitatory amino acids (glutamate and aspartate) and increasing the release of inhibitory neurotransmitters (GABA).[11]

INDICATIONS FOR PERIPHERAL NERVE STIMULATION

The initial flurry in PNS occurred in the 1970s and was championed by Long, Nashold, Picaza, and others. PNS was tested as a novel therapy for diverse intractable pain conditions including mononeuropathy, sciatica, metastatic disease, reflex sympathetic dystrophy, causalgia, amputation stump pain, and occipital neuralgia. Despite promising results in selected patients, the procedure never gained widespread popularity. Through the 1980s and 1990s there was a lull in the use of PNS for pain and a dearth of research publications on the topic. A second flurry in PNS occurred when one of the most challenging neuropathic pain syndromes to treat, occipital neuralgia, was taken on by Weiner and Reed. They first reported their results in treating this disorder with PNS in 1999.[12] They employed a percutaneous technique of electrode insertion in the vicinity of the occipital nerves, rather than direct electrode contact with the nerve, to treat occipital neuralgia. The following year saw publication by Slavin and Burchiel of their technique of stimulation for both occipital and trigeminal pain problems.[13] There are now a variety of both open and percutaneous methods for PNS in addition to targeting numerous regions of the body. For example, percutaneously inserted PNS electrodes have been used for control on inguinal pain,[14] abdominal pain, and low back pain.[16]

Electrical stimulation of peripheral nerves is used in a variety of medical applications in addition to pain control. The most common application is testing neuromuscular conduction during anesthesia. Other applications include pacing of a paralyzed phrenic nerve and vagal nerve stimulation for treatment of epilepsy or depression.

Careful patient selection increases the success rate of utilizing PNS for neuropathic pain. PNS is often reserved for chronic, severe pain that has proven refractory to conventional medical and surgical interventions including medications, physical therapy, nerve blocks, transcutaneous electrical nerve stimulation, or surgical neurolysis. Patient selection criteria should include: (1) pain localized predominantly to one nerve, (2) relief of symptoms after peripheral nerve block with local anesthetic, (3) absence of surgically correctable lesions including entrapment syndromes and tumors, and (4) satisfactory results on psychological or psychiatric assessment (Table 94.1).

When considering the use of PNS for peripheral mononeuropathy, the pain should be concordant with the sensory distribution of a single peripheral nerve. There can be a secondary phenomenon with pain occurring outside the primary nerve distribution as seen in central sensitization with secondary hyperalgesia. Peripheral nerve block with local anesthetic of the candidate nerve should decrease both the primary pain and secondary hyperalgesia. Patients who report excellent relief of pain following blocks are considered candidates for a PNS trial.

The value of a nerve block as predictor of PNS success for occipital neuralgia is less clear. Relief of pain symptoms after

TABLE 94.1

PATIENT SELECTION CRITERIA FOR PNS

1. Pain localized to one nerve
2. Positive response to peripheral nerve block
3. Absence of surgically correctible pathology (i.e., entrapment, tumor, etc.)
4. Satisfactory mental health screening

occipital nerve block suggests that the pain is being mediated by the occipital nerve. However, relief of pain after injection may not predict therapeutic response to PNS because the method of pain relief from these two modalities differs significantly.[17]

Transcutaneous electrical nerve stimulation (TENS) has shown efficacy for pain relief in a variety of conditions including neuropathic pain. The use of TENS has not reliably predicted success or failure of PNS. TENS provides global stimulation to the painful area, but does not provide the equivalent intensity of stimulation to that of PNS. It is our experience that lack of pain relief with TENS does not predict failure of PNS, however, exacerbation of symptoms with TENS is a poor prognostic indicator.

The selection of patients becomes much broader when looking at some of the more current indications for PNS. Treatment for a posttraumatic mononeuropathy and even occipital neuralgia may give way to novel uses such as treatment for migraines[18], cluster headaches,[19] and perhaps fibromyalgia.[20] Strict patient selection criteria still need to be established for these indications. The relative ease of electrode implantation (especially using percutaneous techniques), reversibility, testability, and adjustability make PNS an enticing therapeutic option, particularly in comparison with more destructive or ablative surgical options.

Imaging plays a supplementary role in screening for PNS by helping rule out correctable pathology along the neuraxis. Plain film radiographs can identify potential sites of osseous entrapment due to fractures, callus formation, or calcified fibrous bands. Magnetic resonance imaging (MRI) plays a role in ruling out compressive masses and intrinsic lesions such as tumors. The advent of MRI neurography has been a significant improvement in the ability to image peripheral nerves. The technique is still being refined, but will undoubtedly play an increasing role in improving our understanding of peripheral nerve pathology.

Electromyography and nerve conduction studies are part of the routine evaluation of patients with nerve injury and neuropathic pain. Rarely, these studies bring to light an as yet undiagnosed nerve entrapment syndrome masquerading as complex regional pain syndrome. These studies may be intolerable for patients suffering with cutaneous hyperalgesia or allodynia. Notwithstanding, the distinct possibility of missing a potentially treatable and correctable nerve entrapment justifies pursuing complete diagnostic evaluations.

Benefit may be obtained by addressing psychosocial factors contributing to the painful condition. Patients are encouraged to undergo formal consultation with a psychiatrist or psychologist. This may alert the treating physician to factors such as mood disorders, personality disorders, drug-seeking or manipulative behaviors, or secondary gain issues that would otherwise negatively impact compliance with stimulator use and overall outcome. As with any other pain treatment modality, the presence of psychiatric illness does not preclude the use of PNS.

Our experience with PNS has been primarily for the treatment of patients with painful peripheral entrapment neuropathy or traumatic neuroma formation. The most common peripheral nerves treated with PNS include the median, radial, ulnar, posterior tibial, and common peroneal nerves. Other targeted nerves include the ilioinguinal[21] and supraorbital nerves.[22]

The initial surgical approach for most entrapment neuropathies remains neuroplasty (see Chapter 104 for more detailed discussion of surgical approaches for treatment of painful peripheral nerve disorders). Treatment of painful neuromas begins with "neuroma relocation" in which the neuroma is resected and the freshly cut end of the nerve is buried in local muscle. Inevitably, a new neuroma will form, but the new neuroma is buried deep in the extremity and is theoretically less like to be stimulated and cause pain. In many cases, revision neuroplasty or neuroma relocation successfully relieves the pain. Only after attempts with neuroplasty or neuroma relocation have failed do we consider implanting a peripheral nerve stimulator.

SCS is often an option in the same group of patients we are considering for PNS. We typically perform a trial of SCS in the majority of patients prior to considering PNS. Some advantages of SCS over PNS include ease of implantation, variety of electrode designs, avoidance of the injured nerve and scar tissue from previous surgeries, and the ability to provide broad coverage areas. Generally, SCS is more effective than PNS for chronic pain involving the lower extremities. Unlike PNS, SCS does not evoke stimulation of the motor fibers of an injured mixed motor sensory peripheral nerve. Therefore, we consider PNS for patients who have failed SCS due to coverage/electrode issues or those with injury to purely sensory nerves (no risk of motor fiber stimulation). We are quicker to go to PNS in upper extremity problems where migration of cervical SCS electrodes may be more problematic.

Contraindications for use of PNS relate mainly to surgical risk. Coagulopathy or infections at the surgical site are contraindications to an elective surgical procedure. A remote infection with the possibility of seeding an implant is considered a relative contraindication. Similar to SCS where the electrodes are in the epidural space, the presence of an electrode next to a nerve is a relative contraindication to use of MRI. Careful consideration of risk versus benefit is required in patients who are likely to require serial MRIs (e.g., presence of a malignancy). Postoperative complications may include infection, nerve ischemia or compression, scarring, electrode migration, failure to provide adequate stimulation, mechanical failure including disconnection of the stimulator hardware, tenderness at the site of the implant, and cosmetic concerns. In addition, replacement of batteries requires an additional surgical procedure approximately every 2 years.

OUTCOMES

There is limited available data regarding outcomes associated with use of PNS. In the majority of our selected patients, PNS has been successful. Although most patients do not experience complete relief of pain, they report that the stimulator reduces the pain to a tolerable level. Following PNS, most patients are able to resume activities of daily living, return to work, and reduce their use of opiate analgesics. Our experience with PNS for painful mononeuropathy is comparable with that of several published series. Despite the lack of randomized controlled trials of PNS, there is a substantial body of literature reporting favorable results with low complication rates. In a review of 23 patients, with PNS implanted for pain radiating from the lumbar spine into the lower extremities, Picaza reported 50% to 100% pain relief in 20 patients.[23] In addition most patients reported reduced drug intake and improved social performance. Campbell and Long implanted PNS on the major nerve in the painful area of 33 patients with various refractory chronic pain conditions.[24] They evaluated relief from pain produced by nerve stimulation, along with assessments of narcotic withdrawal, ability to return to work, sleep pattern, and relief from depression. They reported excellent results in eight patients and intermediate results in seven. The most impressive results occurred in patients with traumatic peripheral nerve injuries. The majority of failures were in patients with sciatica or cancer pain. Nashold placed peripheral nerve stimulators on 38 peripheral nerves in 35 patients.[25] Successful relief of pain was obtained in 52.6% of patients with upper extremity PNS and 31% of patients with stimulation of the sciatic nerve. Failures in the lower extremity were found primarily in lesions of the posterior tibial nerve at the ankle. They speculated that the stress of weight bearing may decrease the efficacy and durability of the stimulator system. In a retrospective study of 24 consecutive PNS implants in patients with chronic peripheral nerve pain, Strege reported significantly improved pain scores in 18 patients.[26] In addition, most patients reported improved sleep, reduction of narcotics analgesics, and eight were able to return to work. Of the six failures, three failed the temporary stimulator trial and never were implanted. Late equipment failure was encountered in three patients that had initial success.

Novac and Mackinnon placed peripheral nerve stimulators in the upper extremity in 12 patients and in the lower extremity in 5 patients with various peripheral nerve pathologies.[27] Eleven patients experienced good or excellent pain relief from stimulation. Unlike Strege's series, there was no difference in pain relief for those patients who received an upper extremity implant and those who received a lower extremity implant. This may reflect structural improvements in the stimulator design. In addition, of the 12 patients who were unable to work before the operation, 6 returned to work after the operation.

Eisenberg reported long-term results for PNS implanted for iatrogenic nerve injuries and entrapment neuropathies in upper and lower extremities. Forty-six patients were followed for a median of 10.8 years after PNS. Cuff or paddle electrodes were sutured directly to the affected peripheral nerves. Thirty-six patients (78%) continued to experience at least 50% pain relief without any analgesic medications. The results were similar between patients with upper extremity pain (83% good outcomes) and lower extremity pain (73% good outcomes).[28]

In the largest series to date, Mobbs et al. reviewed 38 patients with 41 nerve stimulators implanted for blunt or sharp nerve trauma, iatrogenic or injection injuries, or persistent pain after surgery for entrapment or tumor.[29] Pain relief greater than 50% was obtained for 61% of patients. Activity levels were significantly improved in 47% of patients following stimulator implant.

The earliest report of successful treatment of occipital neuralgia with a peripheral nerve stimulator was by Picaza who reported good–excellent results in three of six patients treated.[23] Waisbrod later reported in his series of PNS patients, one patient treated for occipital neuralgia with a "very good" result.[30] The use of PNS for occipital neuralgia increased following the development of a percutaneous technique for implanting cylindrical leads along the upper cervical nerve roots.[31] Using the percutaneous technique, Weiner and Reed obtained good–excellent results in 85% of 35 patients with occipital neuralgia.[12] Slavin reported that 7 of 10 patients (70%) with implanted PNS systems, followed for 5–32 months, experienced adequate pain control, continuous employment, and decreased analgesic intake.[32]

The most common reported complications of PNS for occipital stimulation have been infection and electrode migration. To decrease the rate of electrode migration, Oh et al. implemented a semi-open technique involving placement of a single subcutaneous paddle-style electrode (Resume II/Itrel III; Medtronic Inc, Minneapolis, MN.) over the distal C1-2-3 spinal nerve branches at the skull base.[33] They reported good–excellent pain relief in 7 of 10 patients followed for 6 months without electrode migration.

A recent systematic review of the literature concluded that occipital nerve stimulation was a "useful tool" in the treatment of varied types of chronic severe headaches including: occipital nerve stimulation for the treatment of chronic headache including occipital neuralgia, migraine, transformed migraine, chronic daily headache, cluster headache, hemicrania continua, and cervicogenic headache.[34] All of the articles reviewed reported positive outcomes for pain relief, severity and frequency of pain, and use of analgesics. The outcome for PNS treatment in a variety of facial pain syndromes was reported by Johnson and Burchiel.[35] They reported on 10 patients with postherpetic or traumatic neuropathic pain treated by subcutaneous stimulation in the distribution of the supraorbital or infraorbital nerves. Seven of ten (70%) reported reduction in pain of at least 50% at 24 months. Other investigators have reported similar positive results in the treatment of otherwise intractable facial pain.[36,37]

TECHNIQUE FOR IMPLANTATION OF PERIPHERAL NERVE STIMULATOR

A two-stage procedure is typically performed for placement of a peripheral nerve stimulator. The first stage consists of implantation of a temporary "trial" electrode to assess whether PNS provides pain relief. Under general anesthesia, the nerve to be stimulated is identified proximal to the area of injury. Meticulous dissection is performed proximally to distally to free the nerve of scar and adjacent tissues. Once the nerve is clearly visible, care is taken to preserve the overlying epineurium and fascia and avoid devascularization. If indicated, an internal neurolysis or neuroma relocation is performed. For mixed motor/sensory nerves, direct nerve stimulation is used to discriminate between motor and sensory fascicles. After the ideal location is identified, the stimulating electrode is placed directly on the nerve and sutured directly to adjacent fascia or muscle to prevent migration. (Fig. 94.1) A temporary extension cable is connected to the electrode, and tunneled subcutaneously to exit the skin several centimeters from the surgical incision. The cable is secured to the skin with a 3-0 nylon suture.

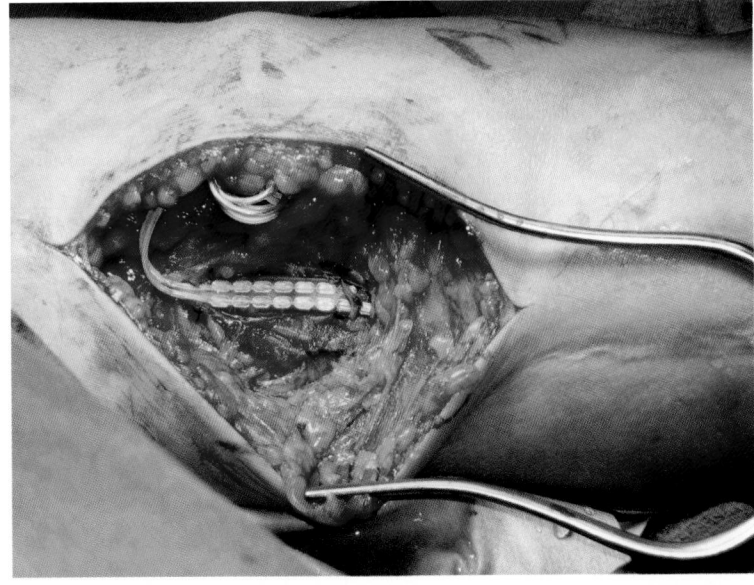

FIGURE 94.1 The stimulator electrode is placed directly on the ulnar nerve. To prevent migration, the electrode has been sutured to adjacent fascia. The wires of the electrode have been tunneled proximally via a subcutaneous track.

Over the next 2 to 7 days, a computer-based program is used to test the stimulation parameters. The patient uses the computer interface that automatically changes amplitude, rate, and pulse width of stimulation and records the patient's location and intensity of stimulation and pain relief. The goal of this trial period is to identify a set of parameters that produces a light, but not painful vibratory sensation in the distribution of the peripheral nerve. If the trial provides optimal coverage and pain relief, the patient proceeds to the second stage of surgery.

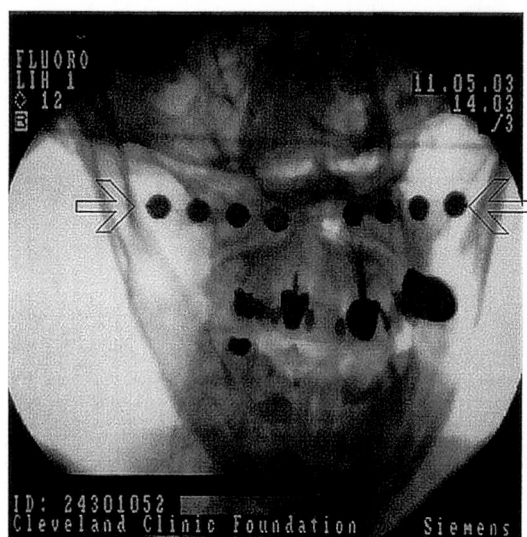

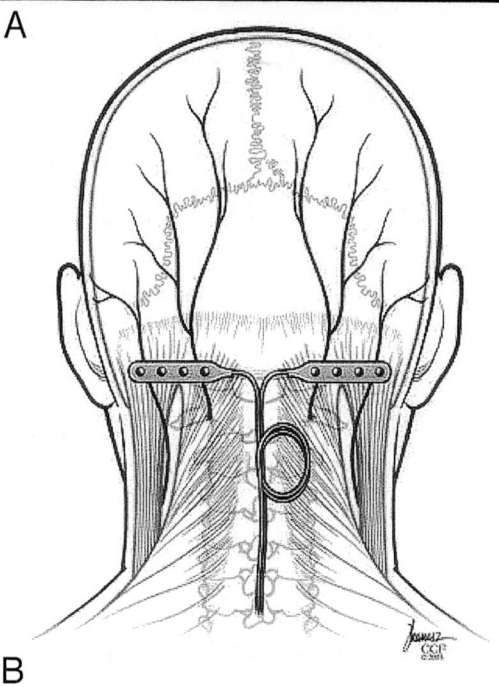

FIGURE 94.2 Radiograph (**A**) and schematics (**B**) of the midline subcutaneous approach in surgical lead positioning for electrical stimulation of the occipital nerve. (**A**) Bilateral position of subcutaneous Resume leads (*arrows*) after initial adjustment and just before intraoperative stimulation testing. Note that both leads are at the level of C1–2 dens and aimed laterally. (**B**) Schematic of the lead positioning in the subcutaneous occipital area. Note that the lead cable extensions form the loop just below the implant's position and via the same midline incision. (Reproduced with permission from Kapural L, Mekhail N, Hayek SM, et al. Occipital nerve electrical stimulation via the midline approach and subcutaneous surgical leads for treatment of severe occipital neuralgia: a pilot study. *Anesth Analg* 2005;101:171–174.)

Under general anesthesia, the original incision is opened to visualize the connection of the electrode to the temporary extension cable. The cable is then disconnected and extracted through the skin. A second incision and subcutaneous pocket must be created for the receiver/battery. In the upper extremity, the pocket is created in the deltopectoral groove; in the lower extremity it is made in the anterior thigh. A hollow, metallic tunneling device is passed subcutaneously from the pocket to the electrode. A permanent extension cable (Medtronic 7496-51) is connected to the electrode and passed through to the pocket. The cable is attached to a receiver/battery (Medtronic 3470). The receiver/battery is then internalized in the subcutaneous pocket. Both incisions are closed in multiple layers. For patients who do not obtain satisfactory results with the trial stimulation, the electrode and temporary extension cable are surgically removed. Postoperatively, the patients receive 24 hours of antibiotics. Once again the computer-based program is used to confirm the ideal stimulation parameters.

For occipital nerve stimulators, subcutaneous field stimulation is achieved by use of a percutaneous electrode inserted through a needle. The needle is placed perpendicular to the course of the nerve. There are different types of electrodes that can be placed. Although easy to place, cylindrical leads have disadvantages, including a tendency for lead migration and poor directionality of stimulation. Kapural et al. described the use of a paddle-style surgical lead introduced bilaterally via a midline approach[38] (Fig. 94.2). All six patients in this study experienced 50% or greater pain relief at 3-month follow-up. The wire type electrode, compared to the plate electrode on a nerve, is much less likely to cause perineural fibrosis.

CONCLUSION

PNS is a viable option for selected patients with a diverse array of intractable pain conditions. The best results have been obtained for treatment of painful traumatic mononeuropathy of the upper extremity and occipital neuralgia. Further research is needed to elucidate the mechanisms underlying the analgesic effects of PNS. As stimulator technology advances, new surgical techniques will arise to broaden the indications for PNS.

References

1. Melzack R, Wall PD. Pain mechanisms: a new theory. *Science* 1965;19;150(699):971–979.
2. Wall PD, Sweet WH. Temporary abolition of pain in man. *Science* 1967;6;155(758):108–109.
3. Campbell JN, Raja SN, Meyer RA, et al. Myelinated afferents signal the hyperalgesia associated with nerve injury. *Pain* 1988;32:89–94.
4. Woolf CJ, Shortland P, Sivilotti LG. Sensitization of high mechanothreshold superficial dorsal horn and flexor motor neurons following chemosensitive primary afferent activation. *Pain* 1994;58(2):141–155.
5. Torebjörk HE, Hallin RG. Responses in human A and C fibres to repeated electrical intradermal stimulation. *J Neurol Neurosurg Psychiatry* 1974;37(6):653–664.
6. Ignelzi RJ, Nyquist JK, Tighe WJ Jr. Repetitive electrical stimulation of peripheral nerve and spinal cord activity. *Neurol Res* 1981;3(2):195–209.
7. Ignelzi RJ, Nyquist JK. Excitability changes in peripheral nerve fibers after repetitive electrical stimulation. Implications in pain modulation. *J Neurosurg* 1979;51(6):824–833.
8. Yakhnitsa V, Linderoth B, Meyerson BA. Effects of spinal cord stimulation on dorsal horn neuronal activity in a rat model of mononeuropathy. *Pain* 1999;79:223–233.
9. Wallin J, Fiska A, Tjolsen A, et al. Spinal cord stimulation inhibits long-term potentiation of spinal wide dynamic range neurons. *Brain Res* 2003;973:39–43.
10. Cui JG, Linderoth B, Meyerson BA. Effects of spinal cord stimulation on touch-evoked allodynia involve GABAergic mechanisms. An experimental study in the mononeuropathic rat. *Pain* 1996;66(2–3):287–295.
11. Cui JG, O'Connor WT, Ungerstedt U, et al. Spinal cord stimulation attenuates

augmented dorsal horn release of excitatory amino acids in mononeuropathy via a GABAergic mechanism. *Pain* 1997;73:87–95.

12. Weiner RL, Reed KL. Peripheral neurostimulation for the control of intractable occipital neuralgia. *Neuromodulation* 1999;2:369–375.

13. Slavin KV, Burchiel KJ. Use of long-term nerve stimulation with implanted electrodes in the treatment of intractable craniofacial pain. *J Neurosurg* 2000; 92:576.

14. Rauchwerger JJ, Giordano J, Rozen D, et al. On the therapeutic viability of peripheral nerve stimulation for ilioinguinal neuralgia: putative mechanisms and possible utility. *Pain Pract* 2008;8(2):138–143. Epub 2008 Jan 18.

15. Paicius RM, Bernstein CA, Lempert–Cohen C. Peripheral nerve field stimulation in chronic abdominal pain. *Pain Physician* 2006;9:261–266.

16. Paicius RM, Bernstein CA, Lemper–Cohen C. Peripheral nerve field stimulation for the treatment of chronic low back pain: preliminary results of long-term follow-up: a case series. *Neuromodulation* 2007;10:279–290.

17. Schwedt TJ, Dodick DW, Trentman TL, et al. Response to occipital nerve block is not useful in predicting efficacy of occipital nerve stimulation. *Cephalalgia* 2007;27:271–274.

18. Hord ED, Evans MS, Mueed S, et al. The effect of vagus nerve stimulation on migraines. *J Pain* 2003;4(9):530–534.

19. Magis D, Allena M, Bolla M, et al. Occipital nerve stimulation for drug-resistant chronic cluster headache: a prospective pilot study. *Lancet Neurol* 2007; 6(4):314–321.

20. Thimineur M, De Ridder D. C2 area neurostimulation: a surgical treatment for fibromyalgia. *Pain Med* 2007;8(8):639–646.

21. Rauchwerger JJ, Giordan J, Rozen D, et al. On the therapeutic viability of peripheral nerve stimulation for ilioinguinal neuralgia: putative mechanisms and possible utility. *Pain Pract* 2008;8(2):138–143. Epub 2008 Jan 18.

22. Asensio–Samper JM, Villanueva VL, Pérez AV, et al. Peripheral neurostimulation in supraorbital neuralgia refractory to conventional therapy. *Pain Pract* 2008;8(2):120–124. Epub 2008 Jan 7.

23. Picaza JA, Cannon BW, Hunter SE, et al. Pain suppression by peripheral nerve stimulation. Part II. Observations with implanted devices. *Surg Neurol* 1975; 4(1):115–126.

24. Campbell JN, Long DM. Peripheral nerve stimulation in the treatment of intractable pain. *J Neurosurg* 1976;45(6):692–699.

25. Nashold BS Jr, Goldner JL, Mullen JB, et al. Long-term pain control by direct peripheral nerve stimulation. *J Bone Joint Surg Am* 1982;64(1):1–10.

26. Strege DW, Cooney WP, Wood MB, et al. Chronic peripheral nerve pain treated with direct electrical nerve stimulation. *J Hand Surg [Am]* 1994;19(6): 931–939.

27. Novak CB, Mackinnon SE. Outcome following implantation of a peripheral nerve stimulator in patients with chronic nerve pain. *Plast Reconstr Surg* 2000; 105(6):1967–1972.

28. Eisenberg E, Waisbrod H, Gerbershagen HU. Long-term peripheral nerve stimulation for painful nerve injuries. *Clin J Pain* 2004;20(3):143–146.

29. Mobbs RJ, Nair S, Blum P. Peripheral nerve stimulation for the treatment of chronic pain. *J Clin Neurosci* 2007;14(3):216–221.

30. Waisbrod H, Panhans C, Hansen D, et al. Direct nerve stimulation for painful peripheral neuropathies. *J Bone Joint Surg Br* 1985;67(3):470–472.

31. Weiner RL. Aló KM, Feler CA et al. Occipital stimulation for the treatment of chronic headache. *Abstracts of the Fourth Congress of the International Neuromodulation and Functional Electrical Neurostimulation Society*. Lucerne, Switzerland, August 1998.

32. Slavin KV, Nersesvan H, Wess C. Peripheral neurostimulation for treatment of intractable occipital neuralgia. *Neurosurgery* 2006;58(1):112–119.

33. Oh MY, Ortega J, Bellotte JB, et al. Peripheral nerve stimulation for the treatment of occipital neuralgia and transformed migraine using a C1-2-3 subcutaneous paddle style electrode: a technical report. *Neuromodulation* 2004;7: 103–112.

34. Jasper JF, Hayek SM. Implanted occipital nerve stimulators. *Pain Physician* 2008;11(2):187–200.

35. Johnson MD, Burchiel KJ. Peripheral stimulation for treatment of trigeminal postherpetic neuralgia and trigeminal posttraumatic neuropathic pain: a pilot study. *Neurosurgery* 2004;55:135–142.

36. Slavin KV, Colpan ME, Munawar N, et al. Trigeminal and occipital peripheral nerve stimulation for craniofacial pain: a single-institution experience and review of the literature. *Neurosurg Focus* 2006;21:E6.

37. Dunteman E. Peripheral nerve stimulation for unremitting ophthalmic postherpetic neuralgia. *Neuromodulation* 2002;5:32–37.

38. Kapural L, Mekhail N, Hayek SM, et al. Occipital nerve electrical stimulation via the midline approach and subcutaneous surgical leads for treatment of severe occipital neuralgia: a pilot study. *Anesth Analg* 2005;101:171–174.

CHAPTER 95 ■ SPINAL CORD STIMULATION

RICHARD B. NORTH AND BENGT LINDEROTH

HISTORY

In antiquity, some healers successfully treated pain by placing electrogenic fish on or near the painful area of the patient's body.[1] This crude form of electrotherapy enjoyed a measure of success but was limited in scope by the geographic and ecologic constraints associated with keeping the fish alive and available. Thus, electrotherapy was not widespread until creation of the Leyden jar in 1745 made it possible for physicians not only to deliver electrotherapy at will but also to exert a modicum of control over how much electrical current the patient received. This was an exciting medical advance, and by the nineteenth century, physicians were considered well-equipped only if they had a portable generator and could provide electrotherapy for a wide range of indications. The advent of empirical medicine in the twentieth century, however, caused most physicians to abandon the application of electrical shocks to treat pain. Fortunately, in the mid-1960s, neurosurgeon C. Norman Shealy[2] recognized that Melzack and Wall's newly published *Gate Control Theory of Pain*[3] provided a theoretical basis for a new form of electrotherapy that could be delivered with implanted electrodes. Shealy[2] called his innovation "dorsal column stimulation"; today, we know it as spinal cord stimulation (SCS).

Melzack and Wall's[3] Gate Control Theory proposes that the balance of activity between large and small nerve fibers in the peripheral nervous system determines whether or not pain signals are transmitted centrally. According to the theory, when small fiber input is dominant, a pain "gate" opens in the dorsal horn (DH) of the entrance segment of the spinal cord; this gate closes when large fibers dominate. Because electrical stimulation depolarizes large fibers before it affects small fibers, the theory suggests that it should be possible for stimulation to close the pain gate. This hypothesis inspired Shealy[2] to deliver current directly to a dying cancer patient's spinal cord with an implanted electrode and external pulse generator in a successful bid to relieve the patient's otherwise intractable pain. Paradoxically, although the electrical stimulation therapies inspired by the Gate Control Theory have succeeded, the theory itself remains controversial because it predicts that all types of pain will be inhibited. Instead, clinical experience and clinical studies have indicated that SCS exerts its beneficial impact on neuropathic pain, but acute and nociceptive pain signals remain relatively unaffected.[4,5] Furthermore, large fiber activity can itself signal pain (for example, the pain of sunburn).[6]

Despite the fact that the Gate Control Theory does not adequately explain all aspects of the therapies it inspired, it provides a useful description of the general concept of the transmission of pain signals and has stood the test of time to a remarkable degree.[7]

Today, SCS is a minimally invasive, reversible therapy implemented with sophisticated techniques and implanted equipment, including a variety of electrodes and multioutput pulse generators. Unlike most surgical procedures undertaken to relieve pain, SCS does not ablate pain pathways or result in anatomic change. SCS also offers its candidates the advantage of undergoing a screening trial with a temporary SCS system before proceeding (or not) to implantation.

Pain and its relief by SCS vary by condition and from patient to patient. When SCS is delivered to the right patient by the right (experienced) clinician in the right setting using the right equipment, pain relief is optimized and can be sustained for decades. It is important to remember, however, that SCS is expected to reduce, not eliminate, pain, particularly pathologic (neuropathic) pain which constitutes a state of disease. SCS is not expected or intended to relieve nociceptive or evolutionarily useful pain.

Investigators are continually improving SCS patient care by refining techniques and equipment, and as we learn more about the mechanism of action of SCS, we will be able to potentiate the impact of SCS.

MECHANISMS OF ACTION

Introduction

The work of several investigative teams in the four decades since Shealy[2] implanted the first "dorsal column stimulation" electrode has helped us identify promising avenues of research, refine experimental techniques, and develop evidence in support of hypotheses that explain aspects of the mechanisms of action of SCS. The challenge in experimental studies is to mimic the human painful condition and deliver stimulation, for example in rats, with parameters that would be clinically relevant in humans. Even in a homogeneous population of laboratory animals, however, the yield of neuropathic pain models is uncertain, and clinical studies must grapple with even greater variability among human subjects and painful pathologies. Furthermore, the clinical application of SCS elicits a discernible tingling, known as paresthesia, which confounds experimental blinding. An additional challenge is the fact that the universally agreed upon measurement of the effectiveness of SCS (reduction in pain) is subjective and depends to an uncomfortable degree on a patient's ability to remember the intensity of past pain in order to make a valid comparison with current pain. Pain assessment also relies on rather crude measurements, such as verbal rating scales and the visual analogue scale. Thus, patient assessment is assisted by measures of medication use, physical activity, well-being, etc.

Despite these obstacles, researchers have learned enough to propose distinct mechanisms of action for the therapeutic effects of SCS in the treatment of neuropathic, ischemic, and visceral pain.

Neurophysiology

SCS affects both spinal and supraspinal circuits[8-11] but does not rely solely on antidromic activation of the dorsal columns.[12,13] Some SCS effects survive disruption of supraspinal circuits by transection of the spinal cord rostral to the electrode;[14,15] others do not.[16]

Neurochemistry

SCS modulates DH and/or supraspinal neurotransmitters; thus, the beneficial effects of SCS often outlast active stimulation (see

below). SCS might[17] or might not[18] cause release of spinal opioids. Most studies indicate that endogenous opioids are not involved in the pain relieving effects of SCS; for example, the effects of SCS are not reversed by the opioid antagonist naloxone,[19] and the neuropathic pain of SCS patients is usually resistant to opioid therapy. In patients with angina, however, SCS during atrial pacing and at-rest releases the opioid peptide β-endorphin into cardiac circulation, indicating that SCS affects "local myocardial turnover of the opioid peptides leuenkephalin, β-endorphin, and calcitonin-gene-related peptide [a powerful vasodilator]."[20]

Mechanisms in Neuropathic Pain

Nerve or nervous system injury can lead to neuropathic pain, which is often radiating, generally described as "burning," and commonly involves hyperalgesia (an extreme sensitivity to pain) and allodynia (pain from normally nonpainful stimuli). In contrast, dull, aching nociceptive pain, which is mediated by receptors in skin, muscle, bone, viscera, etc., is responsive to opioids. Since SCS is not thought to cause the release of endogenous opioids,[18] the clinical expectation is that SCS will be more effective as a treatment of neuropathic, ischemic, and visceral pain than of nociceptive pain. The fact that SCS is effective in treating ischemic pain, which is considered a form of nociceptive pain, does not mean that SCS directly affects nociceptive pain. Instead, SCS exerts a beneficial effect on the underlying ischemic condition (see below).

Allodynia occurs when the activation of nerve fibers in the periphery causes hyperactivity of wide dynamic range neurons (WDRs) in the superficial laminae of corresponding DHs.[21] SCS relieves allodynia by suppressing this hyperactivity.[22] Treatment with γ-aminobutyric acid (GABA) agonists also has this effect, and SCS induces GABA release in the DH of rats[8] and activates the GABA-B receptor.[23,24] SCS also decreases DH release of the excitatory amino acids glutamate and aspartate in rats.[24]

Investigators have also proposed that electrostimulation might relieve pain by blocking conduction of primary afferents at the branch points of dorsal column fibers and collaterals.[6] This explanation is insufficient, however, because the effect of SCS extends beyond the dorsal columns, and electrical stimulation does not inhibit every type of pain.[25] Dorsal column activation, however, is more successful than ventral stimulation,[26] which might activate the spinothalamic tract fibers that evoke pain.

SCS inhibition of the pathologic response (increased firing frequency of WDRs, after-discharge in response to pressure, etc.) of DH neurons in rats exhibiting symptoms of allodynia after peripheral nerve injury continues for more than 10 minutes,[22] consistent with SCS-induced release of DH and cerebral neurotransmitters, and changes the concentration of neurotransmitters and their metabolites in cerebrospinal fluid.[26-29]

Through the use of microdialysis techniques, investigators have examined the effects of SCS on the cerebral neurotransmitter serotonin and on substance P, a polypeptide implicated in the transmission of pain impulses and in sensitizing DH neurons. In decerebrate cats, SCS invokes DH release of serotonin and substance P, but in anesthetized cats, SCS only induces a detectable DH release of substance P.[27,30]

The problem of applicability of research results from unconscious animals to conscious humans led investigators to create an experimental model using supraspinal microdialysis in conscious rats.[31,32] Application of this method revealed that a repeat 30-minute dose of SCS after a 90-minute resting period causes GABA and glutamate levels in ventrolateral periaqueductal grey matter to decrease, perhaps signaling pain inhibition (this rest/repeat scheme does not affect the concentration of serotonin or of substance P-like immunoreactivity).[8,31] Investigators also used models of painful neuropathy to explore the impact of SCS on the pain threshold in rats and found that during and after SCS, the threshold of withdrawal from innocuous mechanical stimuli increases and that SCS affects only the component of the flexor reflex mediated by A-fibers (not the late component mediated by C-fibers).[33] Thus, current thinking holds that, to a large extent, SCS acts on a segmental spinal level,[15] although additional inhibitory influences might be transmitted by descending serotonergic and noradrenergic pathways. A related study used the partial sciatic nerve ligation model to examine how SCS affects the response to innocuous stimuli in postligation rats with and without allodynia and in controls. Only in the allodynic rats did SCS significantly depress abnormal responses and spontaneous discharge of WDR neurons.[22] The same research group introduced acetylcholine (ACH) into the list of transmitters possibly involved in the beneficial effects of SCS after a microdialysis study demonstrated that ACH is released in the DHs of rats whose pain-related symptoms after nerve injury decreased in response to stimulation.[34] These effects seem to be caused by activation of muscarinic M4 and M2 receptors in the DH.[34,35] This finding might lead to new ways to enhance an otherwise inadequate effect of SCS in certain patients.

Along these lines, based on the fact that extracellular GABA levels are lower in allodynic rats than in controls but increase in allodynic rats that respond to SCS (not all rats respond),[36] investigators have attempted to potentiate the therapeutic effect of SCS in nonresponding rats with concurrent intrathecal administration of normally subtherapeutic levels of GABA or the GABA-B agonist baclofen.[23] This strategy caused a marked increase in the rats' threshold for withdrawal from innocuous mechanical stimulation. Intrathecal administration of the selective α1-adenosine receptor agonist R-phenyl isopropyl adenosine produced similar results.[24] Administration of subtherapeutic doses of these agents as adjunct therapy with SCS causes nonresponding rats to respond to SCS.[37]

In the first clinical study based on this response, however, the addition of intrathecal baclofen and/or adenosine potentiated SCS in only 2 of 5 patients.[38] This result caused investigators to increase the dose of intrathecal gabapentin and intravenous pregabalin in non-SCS-responding rats with partial sciatic nerve lesion. In these rats, the drugs reduced tactile allodynia in a dose-dependent manner and enhanced suppression of hyperexcitability of WDR neurons.[39] A similar dose-dependent effect occurred with intrathecal administration of an otherwise subtherapeutic dose of clonidine.[40] Thus, the investigators conducted a pilot study that offered intrathecal baclofen (and, in a few cases, intrathecal adenosine) to 48 patients who did not successfully respond to technically adequate SCS.[41] Although 20 patients achieved satisfactory pain relief with baclofen plus SCS or baclofen alone, only 11 continued treatment: 7 with a combination SCS system and intrathecal baclofen pump and 4 with only a baclofen pump. At mean 67 months postimplant, 2 SCS/intrathecal patients had their pumps removed and the remaining 9 in the group (5 SCS/ intrathecal, 4 intrathecal) reported continued pain relief. The baclofen dose was increased 160% from baseline, but 5 patients reduced use of other analgesics.

Among the things rats and humans have in common are that nerve injury alone sometimes causes allodynia and that SCS is not universally therapeutic. Seeking the reason for the distinctions (information that would not only shed light on the mechanisms of action of SCS but also on patient selection for the therapy), investigators used the original spared nerve injury model and variations of the model to create lesions in rats at various points on the sciatic nerve.[42] The investigators found that the location of the lesion affects both the incidence of allodynia, which varied from 50% to 73%, and responsiveness to SCS, which was only 8% with the original spared nerve model but increased to 40% to 50% after peroneal axotomy, tibial axotomy, or partial or full tibial tight ligation. The allodynia caused by these lesions was less severe than that invoked by the original model; thus, SCS

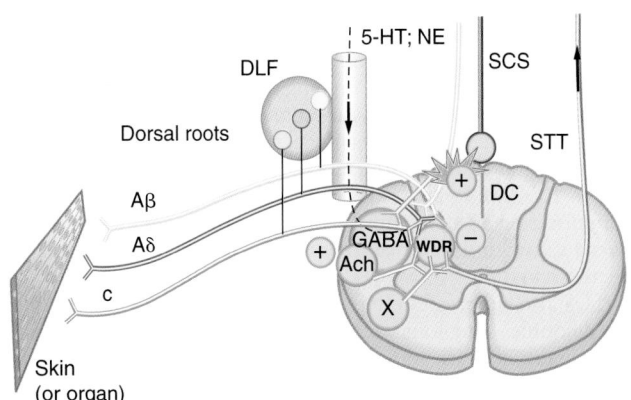

FIGURE 95.1 Schematic illustration of mechanisms and neurotransmitters possibly involved in the effects of SCS in neuropathic pain. SCS activation of dorsal column collaterals secondarily induces release of GABA from DH interneurons, activating mainly GABA-B receptors and decreasing the release of excitatory amino acids from hyperexcited second-order DH WDR neurons. SCS also causes cholinergic neurons to activate M4 and M2 muscarinic type receptors (Ach). Several other transmitters, adenosine and hitherto unknown substances are also likely involved. Furthermore, the orthodromic SCS-induced activity in the dorsal columns might—via neuronal circuitry in the brain stem (or even more rostrally)—induce descending inhibition via serotonergic (5-HT) and noradrenergic (NE) pathways in the dorsolateral funiculus (DLF), which might contribute to inhibitory influences in the DHs. DC, dorsal columns; STT, spinothalamic tract.

was more effective in rats with mild allodynia than in those with severe allodynia. This finding was confirmed by further study.[43] The mechanisms and neurotransmitters known or hypothesized to be involved in the effects of SCS in neuropathic pain are illustrated in Figure 95.1. We have yet to identify all of the neurotransmitters and neuromodulators affected by SCS, let alone to decipher their doubtless complicated interactions.[24,26,31]

Putative Mechanisms in Complex Regional Pain Syndrome

Theoretically, SCS exerts its positive effect on pain in patients with complex regional pain syndrome (CRPS) by reducing central hyperexcitability, by inhibiting sympathetic efferent activity to prevent development of abnormal contacts between peripheral sympathetic and damaged somatosensory fibers,[44] or by preventing vasoconstriction, which can excite damaged sensory afferent fibers.[44,45] In the only clinical study to investigate the impact of SCS on peripheral vasodilatation in CRPS I patients who experienced pain relief, however, SCS did not induce peripheral vasodilatation.[46]

Spinal Cord Stimulation Mechanisms in Ischemic Pain

SCS is thought to induce vasodilatation and improve microperfusion in patients with ischemic pain, which is sharp, aching, heavy, and tiring[47] and a signal of restricted blood flow. Thus, SCS has a beneficial effect on the cause, not merely the symptoms, of ischemic pain. This might explain why ischemic pain is the only type of nociceptive pain known to respond to SCS and why the mechanisms seem to be fundamentally distinct from those that provide relief of neuropathic pain.[18,26,48]

Peripheral Vascular Disease

To investigate the mechanism of SCS in the treatment of peripheral vascular disease (PVD), investigators developed a new animal model that involves applying mechanical pressure to an artery in the groin of rats.[49] Using this model, SCS delivered with clinically relevant stimulation parameters recovered normal microcirculation in 100% of treated rats versus 28% of controls. In addition, administering SCS preemptively reduced the amplitude of the invoked spasm and significantly shortened the time to recovery of microcirculation.[50]

SCS also suppresses efferent sympathetic activity (maintained by nicotinic ganglionic receptors and α-1-adrenoreceptors)[49] and might activate antidromic mechanisms at intensities far below the motor threshold,[51-55] thus causing peripheral vasodilation by stimulating release of calcitonin gene-related peptide (CGRP)[50-52] from the terminals of sensory fibers that contain transient receptor potential vanilloid-1 receptors[56,57] and the release of nitric oxide from a different location (possibly endothelial cells).[57]

The balance between these two mechanisms seems to depend on the activity level of the sympathetic nervous system, the intensity of SCS, and individual patient factors (genetic differences, diet, etc.).[54]

The fact that SCS has a powerfully beneficial effect on vasospastic conditions, such as Raynaud's Syndrome, is consistent with theories that the cause of Raynaud's Syndrome is a combination of heightened sensitivity or increased density of α-adrenergic receptors[58] and CGRP-system dysfunction.[59] A stimulation-induced "normalization" of function in each system could underlie the efficacy of SCS in treating this condition.

Because administering an autonomic ganglion blocking agent attenuates SCS-induced vasodilatation, SCS is believed to exert some of its effects by inhibiting sympathetic efferents. The outcome, however, differs among different laboratories and strains of rats. This result, for instance, did not occur on administration of a ganglionic blocking agent in North American studies.[51,52,54] Instead, these studies as well as experiments by Wu et al.[56,57] favored antidromic activation as the most important mechanism of SCS-induced peripheral vasodilatation. In fact, antidromic activation dominated at low autonomic baseline activity, while the sympatholytic effects of SCS were clear with high baseline activity.[55,60] Later studies have indicated that even small diameter fibers are involved at SCS intensities much below the motor threshold[56,57] and have pointed toward additional mechanisms.[61-63] A review of the mechanisms involved in SCS-induced vasodilation is included in a report by Wu et al.[64]

The mechanisms and neurotransmitters known or hypothesized to be involved in the effects of SCS in ischemic pain are depicted in Figure 95.2.

Angina

Investigators studying the mechanism of action of SCS in patients with otherwise refractory angina agree that SCS reduces ischemia[65] but disagree about how this occurs. Positron emission tomography has indicated that SCS causes a redistribution of coronary blood flow in patients with refractory angina[66,67] (even though experimental studies have failed to demonstrate this effect[68]). On the other hand, the decrease in the depression extending from the end of the S wave to the beginning of the T wave (ST-segment depression) that appears on electrocardiograms during SCS treatment and the observed SCS-induced reversal of lactate production to extraction might indicate an accompanying decrease in cardiac myocyte oxygen demand.[69]

The SCS-induced protective changes that increase myocardial resistance to critical ischemia[70] are manifest by the improved tolerance of patients to a deliberately paced increase in heart

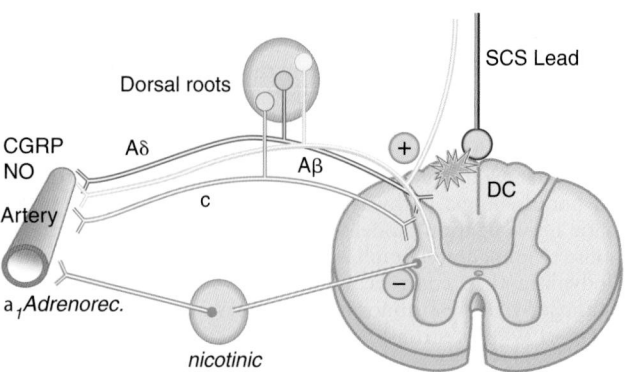

Sympathetic Efferent Fibers

FIGURE 95.2 Schematic illustration of mechanisms and neurotransmitters possibly involved in effects of SCS in ischemic pain. SCS probably indirectly exerts inhibition onto medullary neurons, thus perpetuating sympathetic efferent vasoconstriction via nicotinic ganglionic receptors, mainly α1 (α1 adrenorec = adrenoreceptors) peripheral receptors. In parallel, SCS activates an antidromic loop inducing peripheral release of CGRP, probably also involving small diameter fibers. An inhibition of nociceptive transmission has also been indicated in experimental studies but is clinically unlikely. DC, dorsal columns; NO, nitric oxide; SCS Lead, spinal cord stimulation lead.

rate,[71] and by increased time-to-angina in exercise tests.[18] This effect might signal an SCS-induced inhibition of the excitatory effect of ischemia on the intrinsic cardiac nervous system (such an excitatory effect might lead to dysrhythmia and increased ischemia).[70-72] The possibility that SCS modulates cardiac neurons is supported by the finding that transcutaneous electrical nerve stimulation increases blood flow in intact human hearts but not in transplanted, denervated hearts.[54]

Because SCS reduces total body, but not cardiac-specific, norepinephrine spillover during pacing to moderate angina,[73] part of the anti-ischemic effect of SCS might owe its potency to an overall reduction in sympathetic activity. An experimental study using induced cardiac infarcts in a rabbit model, however, indicates that the decrease in infarct size with SCS therapy shares some mechanisms with "ischemic preconditioning" but, notably, does not cause cardiac ischemia.[74] Further studies of these phenomena are on-going.

Figure 95.3 illustrates the mechanisms and neurotransmitters known or hypothesized to be involved in the effects of SCS in angina.

Mechanisms in Visceral Pain

The treatment of visceral pain is a relatively new application for SCS, and investigators have proposed that SCS might exert its positive effect on visceral pain (and dysfunction) by moderating the so-called "brain-gut" axis (the neural circuitry thought to control the interface among visceral afferent sensation, intestinal motor function, and the brain).[61,75-77]

In fact, moving an active SCS electrode along the neuroaxis demonstrates that electric activation occurs at various levels; thus, in addition to the its beneficial effects on pain and ischemia, SCS inhibits the viscero-somatic reflexes involved with the particular spinal segmental level being stimulated (Fig. 95.4).

Computer Modeling Studies

Finite element computer models of SCS electrical fields in the spinal cord[78-80] have confirmed the current and voltage distribu-

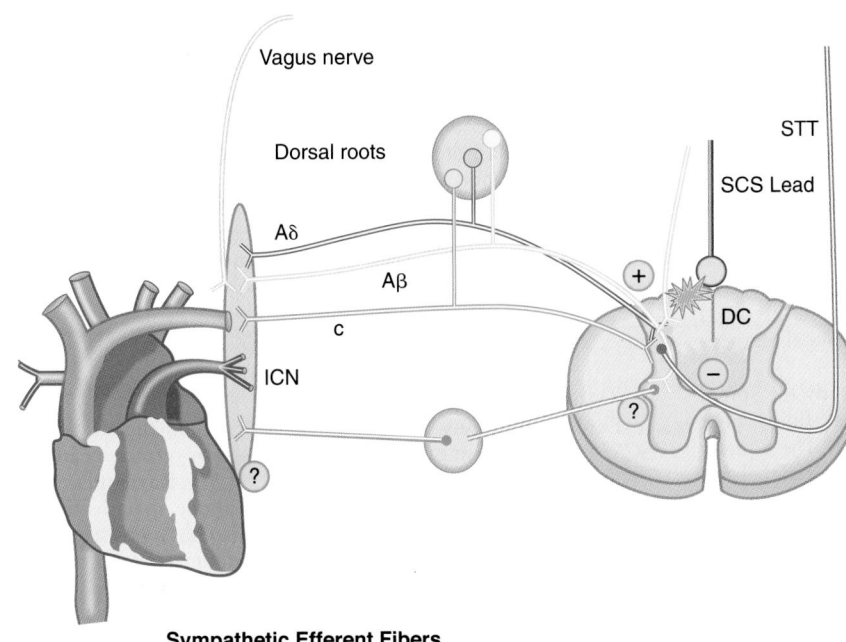

Sympathetic Efferent Fibers

FIGURE 95.3 Schematic illustration of some mechanisms possibly involved in the effects of SCS on coronary ischemic pain. SCS might exert indirect inhibitory effects on nociceptive transmission to higher centers and on the level of sympathetic activity; SCS might also have antidromically transmitted effects. Intrinsic cardiac neurons (ICN) are deeply involved in monitoring ischemic events in the heart, and this function is drastically influenced by SCS. The interplay between somatosensory and autonomic influences and the effects of SCS is presently largely unknown but is the subject of intense investigation. DC, dorsal columns; SCS Lead, spinal cord stimulation lead; STT, spinothalamic tract.

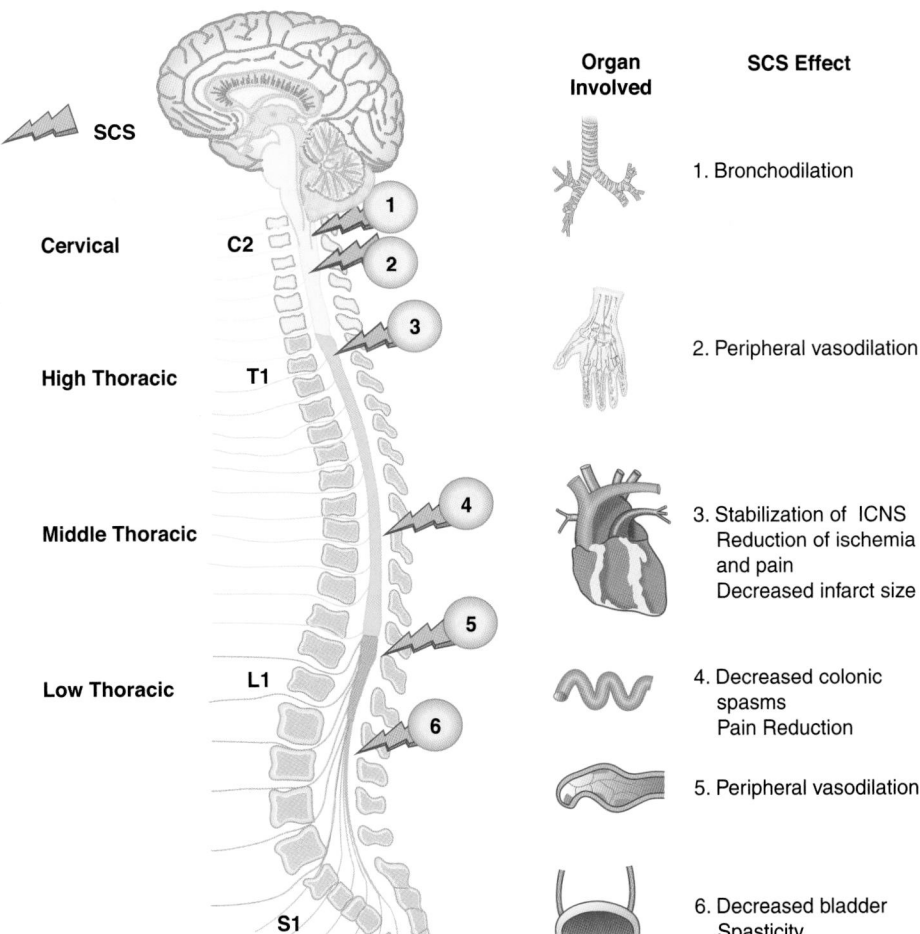

FIGURE 95.4 SCS applied at different levels of the neuroaxis might, in addition to affecting pain and peripheral blood flow, induce changes in different target organs mediated via stimulation induced changes in local autonomic activity, dorsal root reflexes, or viscero-somatic reflexes. Some of these changes in target organ function might be beneficial (redrawn after Linderoth B, Foreman RD. Mechanisms of spinal cord stimulation in painful syndromes: role of animal models. *Pain Med* 2006;7:514–526).

tion measurements previously obtained from cadavers and primates.[81] Application of these models has also led to the prediction that (1) an electrode's longitudinal position governs its segmental effect; (2) bipolar stimulation with contacts separated by 6 to 8 mm optimizes selection of midline, longitudinally-oriented fibers (a longer distance reduces therapeutic effect by favoring dorsal root stimulation); and (3) the electrical field between two cathodes placed on either side of the physiologic midline does not sum constructively in the midline. Clinical experience confirms that the correct position and spacing of SCS electrodes is essential for therapeutic success and that, instead of expanding the area of paresthesia, positioning electrodes cephalad to the involved spinal levels commonly elicits unwanted, excessive, local segmental effects.[82]

The first computerized models developed to study the spinal canal approximated the meninges, cerebrospinal fluid, fiber tracts, and grey matter with geometric shapes.[83,84] The equally simplistic, two-dimensional initial computer models of dorsal epidural stimulation[85–87] were soon replaced by a three-dimensional model that took into account fiber tracts, their branch points, and dorsal roots.[78,88]

In 1991, Holsheimer and Struijk developed a new model[89] that merged this three-dimensional construct with a McNeal-type[90] cable model of the electrical behavior of myelinated nerve fibers and data derived from mammalian myelinated fibers.[91] The resulting "University of Twente SCS Computer Model" allowed investigators to determine the impact of the location and configuration (anode/cathode, on/off) of SCS electrodes (e.g., to maximize recruitment of deep, midline, longitudinal axons rather than of the lateral, or dorsal root, fibers that can cause discomfort and motor responses) and to suggest ways to optimize SCS equipment design.

The University of Twente model was further refined when the investigators were able to apply data from human sensory fibers.[92] This improved the accuracy of predictions about the impact of various SCS threshold voltages.[93] An additional improvement streamlined the mathematical techniques used to predict stimulation effects when computing the three-dimensional action potential field.[94] Model predictions for "transverse tripole" electrode performance have been validated in part by clinical studies.[95]

INDICATIONS

Neuropathic Pain

In the United States, the major indication for SCS is the treatment of neuropathic pain arising from failed back surgery syndrome (FBSS). Two randomized controlled trials have demonstrated the superiority of treating FBSS with SCS versus reoperation[96] or optimized conventional medical management.[97] Of course, an FBSS patient with gross instability or a neurologic deficit caused by neural compression that is evident on an imaging study would undergo a corrective surgical procedure before or instead of SCS.

It is easier to achieve pain relief in the limbs than in the low back because low back pain is more likely than leg pain to have a nociceptive component, which is not expected to respond to SCS, and because pain/paresthesia overlap in the low back is generally more difficult to achieve, even with complex electrode arrays and detailed psychophysical tests. At one time, achieving low back pain relief with SCS was considered rare; however, Law's[98] research on techniques to guide paresthesia coverage kept the low back available as an SCS therapeutic target, and clinicians have built on his work to define the best electrodes[99] and contact combinations[79] for achieving pain relief in the low back.

The use of SCS to treat pain in the limbs arising from CRPS I (reflex sympathetic dystrophy) is also supported by data from a randomized controlled trial.[100,101] In that study, 5 years post-treatment, the 20 patients remaining in the group that actually received SCS reported better pain relief and superior global perceived effect than did those patients remaining in the alternate group who did not receive SCS.[102]

Other neuropathic pain indications for SCS include phantom limb/postamputation syndrome, postherpetic neuralgia, root injury pain, and pain/spasm arising from spinal cord injury or lesion.

Ischemic Pain

In Europe, clinicians have gathered evidence on the efficacy of SCS in the treatment of ischemic pain caused by refractory angina (including syndrome X),[103–106] PVD,[107,108] Raynaud's Syndrome, and diabetic neuropathy. As noted above, in patients with ischemia, SCS not only treats the pain, it also has a positive effect on the underlying ischemia. Thus, the outcome criteria used to document the impact of SCS on critical limb ischemia arising from PVD include survival, limb salvage, and measures of microcirculation,[109] as well as pain relief.

In Raynaud's Syndrome, the few published studies (all of which involve small numbers of patients) demonstrate the positive effect of SCS therapy.[110–114] This is not surprising because, compared with PVD patients, patients with vasospastic conditions are relatively young, present with relatively few obliterative vessel wall processes, and have symptoms that are often temporarily relieved by destroying or blocking the corresponding sympathetic ganglia.

Some clinicians are using cervical SCS in exploratory trials to improve cerebral blood flow in patients recovering from stroke,[115] coma,[116] or brain tumors.[117]

Visceral Pain and Dysfunction

SCS and other forms of neurostimulation are also being used to treat visceral dysfunction and pain associated with such diseases as interstitial cystitis,[118] pancreatitis,[119] motility disorders, urinary urgency and frequency,[120] pelvic pain,[121] vulvodynia,[122] and pelvic floor dysfunction.[123]

POTENTIAL BENEFICIAL OUTCOMES

Technical Goal

The technical goal of therapeutic SCS is to cover a patient's pain with a comfortable level of paresthesia. Clinicians consider this blanket of paresthesia a necessary but not sufficient condition for therapeutic success.

If an electrode migrates or if pain changes location, appropriate paresthesia coverage can be lost. Thus, contemporary SCS systems are designed to allow adjustment of stimulation parameters postimplant to steer paresthesia to a new location or to recapture coverage. Only occasionally does readjustment for these purposes require a surgical intervention.

It is possible for paresthesia to cover the painful area without providing an analgesic effect. Such clinical failure can become evident during the screening trial or can arise after a period of success. On rare occasions, a patient who experiences technical success and pain relief dislikes the sensation of paresthesia and decides not to continue the therapy.

Clinical Goal

The generally accepted clinical goal of SCS treatment for pain is a minimum of 50% pain relief, but this and other measures all have limitations.[124] Additional reported benefits of SCS include (1) reduced consumption of medication and other health care resources; (2) improved ability to engage in the activities of daily living, quality of life, neurologic function, and symptoms of emotional depression; and (3) return to work when uncontrolled chronic pain was the only impediment (and generally when the patient has been out of work for less than 2 years).[125,126]

In patients suffering from ischemic pain, SCS can improve microcirculation and tissue oxygenation. This, in turn, can promote the healing of ischemic ulcers and increase the possibility of limb salvage.

PROGNOSTIC FACTORS

Demographics provide no help in choosing the ideal SCS candidate. Age is only a factor in children, where the safety and effectiveness of SCS is not established and in the elderly, who might have difficulty dealing with the patient interface (or recharging a battery), but, as for example with driving cars, the effect of advanced age must be assessed on an individual basis.

Researchers have reported some outcome differences between men and women, but these have been minor and of little if any practical value. Thus, the only sex-related caveat is that the safety of SCS during pregnancy is not established (although pregnant women have continued to use SCS rather than suffer known and suspected adverse effects of alternative pain treatments). Even a very short life expectancy does not rule out SCS, which can be cost effective even for short-term use if an external stimulator is used.

Also, we can not reliably predict SCS outcome based on worker's compensation or litigation status, but some clinicians err on the side of caution and consider the unresolved possibility of secondary gain a relative contraindication to allowing a patient to undergo a screening trial.

For FBSS patients, it seems that the chance of success with SCS decreases as the number of relevant prior surgical procedures and the time since the last surgical procedure increases. The type of surgical procedure the patient has experienced is also important; some ablative procedures, such as rhizotomy, dorsal root ganglionectomy, or dorsal root entry zone lesioning might obliterate the neural substrate upon which SCS is thought to depend.[127]

For patients with PVD, investigators have reported that 1-year limb salvage is more likely to occur if the baseline supine $TcPO_2$ is >10 mm Hg, the baseline sitting-supine score is >17 mm Hg, and the treatment difference is >4 mm Hg.[128] Some investigators believe that a 50% improved $TcPO_2$ score during a 2-week screening period predicts limb salvage,[129] regardless of baseline score or disease stage.[130] In the case of diabetic neuropathy, however, these investigators found the stage of neuropathy to be inversely related to SCS treatment success,[131] independent of the stage of the disease.[132]

PATIENT SELECTION

One of the first things we learned about SCS was that achieving a successful outcome required the right patient. In any group of patients, the presence of seemingly identical pain syndromes was not enough to predict identical (or even any) SCS success in each individual. A major advantage of SCS, however, is that it is possible to perform a screening trial, which involves temporary (7–10 days) placement of an electrode to determine the extent of pain/

paresthesia overlap and the resulting therapeutic effect. In some European countries, a trial period of several weeks is required for reimbursement of hospital costs.

The screening trial offers the most meaningful prognostic sign of the outcome of SCS, but, of course, not all potential SCS patients proceed to a screening trial. Information to determine a patient's suitability for a screening trial is gathered from the patient's history and from the results of a physical examination and imaging studies.

Among the important aspects of the patient's history are the location, intensity, duration, and characteristics of the pain and the patient's psychologic status. Radiating pain that has an objective basis, is distributed in a manner consistent with information gleaned from a physical examination and imaging studies, and can be labeled with a specific diagnosis is the most straightforward to treat. Imaging studies that are useful for diagnostic purposes can also provide anatomic information that can be helpful or even vital during SCS implantation.

In the United States, Medicare and many health insurance companies require SCS candidates to undergo a routine psychologic evaluation. Although no psychologic test predicts the result of SCS treatment (and physicians routinely expect new patients to meet reasonable psychologic/behavioral standards), patients who have been living with chronic pain often benefit from psychologic screening with the attendant possibility of therapy. Any major psychiatric comorbidity must be addressed before a patient undergoes a SCS screening trial.

Relative contraindications include:

- Unresolved major psychiatric comorbidity
- Unresolved possibility of secondary gain
- Inappropriate dependency on pharmaceuticals
- Inconsistency among the history, pain ratings and description, physical examination, and diagnostic studies
- Abnormal pain ratings
- A predominance of nonorganic signs (e.g., Waddell's signs)
- Alternative therapies with a risk/benefit ratio comparable to that of SCS remain to be tried
- Pregnancy
- Occupational risk (e.g., of falling)
- Local or systemic infection
- Presence of a demand pacemaker or cardioverter defibrillator
- Foreseeable need for magnetic resonance imaging (MRI)
- Presence of a major comorbid chronic pain syndrome
- Anticoagulant or antiplatelet therapy

Absolute contraindications include:

- Inability to control the device
- Gross spinal instability at risk for progression or nerve compression amenable to surgery causing a serious neurologic deficit that requires immediate attention
- Coagulopathy, immunosuppression, or other condition associated with an unacceptable surgical risk
- Need for therapeutic diathermy

TECHNIQUE

A discussion of techniques used for the various types of SCS screening trials and for SCS implantations is beyond the scope of this chapter. Instead, we refer the reader to previous publications.[133–135]

SCREENING TRIAL

Before the introduction of percutaneous catheter electrodes in the 1970s, physicians used a variety of methods to screen potential SCS candidates, including transcutaneous electrical stimulation, which were found to lack prognostic value. The percutaneous electrodes developed to facilitate a screening trial were immediately adopted for chronic use as well. Today, SCS systems in the United States are generally only implanted in patients who pass a screening trial. In Europe, the screening trial is commonly bypassed in patients with typical angina pectoris, a short-cut that reflects the fact that more than 80% of these patients enjoy significant pain relief with SCS.

Beyond indicating that SCS therapy might be successful, the benefits of a screening trial include allowing a patient to experience the sensation of paresthesia before undergoing implantation of the expensive pulse generator. The trial also provides important information that will dictate the choice of a permanent electrode and pulse generator and the optimum stimulating configuration. A successful screening trial commonly is defined by at least 50% patient-reported pain relief despite appropriate (provocative) physical activity and stable or reduced analgesic consumption. Patient satisfaction is another vital outcome. Medicare and many third-party payers require a successful screening trial before implantation.

Screening Electrode Choice

A percutaneous catheter electrode placed under fluoroscopy provides easy access to multiple target spinal levels and facilitates mapping of pain/paresthesia overlap to determine the optimal longitudinal level for the electrode.

An insulated surgical plate/paddle electrode inserted by laminectomy limits access to spinal levels and mapping but is required if a percutaneous catheter electrode does not access the epidural space satisfactorily. Screening with a surgical plate/paddle electrode is also necessary in some patients to eliminate uncomfortable extraneous stimulation or provide sufficient pain/paresthesia overlap.

Electrode Positioning

Patients remain conscious during trial electrode placement in order to describe paresthesia coverage and have the opportunity to react to changes in stimulation parameters or unanticipated intraoperative events.

Parameter Adjustment

Trained professionals work with patients to adjust simulator parameters during the screening trial and after implantation to find the settings that maximize comfortable pain/paresthesia overlap, reduce or eliminate extraneous stimulation, and minimize power requirements. Patients are instructed at each stage so as to operate the device appropriately.

Procedural Risk Reduction

Implanting an electrode for a screening trial or chronic stimulation is associated with certain risks, including spinal cord or nerve injury, dural puncture, epidural hematoma, and infection. Risk can be reduced by ordering a preimplant MRI of the target spinal levels, performing the procedure under fluoroscopy with the patient conscious, maintaining a meticulously sterile environment, administering prophylactic antibiotics, and observing the patient for a reasonable of time postprocedure (e.g., overnight). Discharge instructions must indicate when and how patients should contact their physicians, the device manufacturer, and emergency care providers.

Trial Duration

A typical screening trial with a temporary percutaneous electrode lasts a week. In some circumstances, a shorter trial will be adequate, while in others, a longer trial might be beneficial.

Removal of Trial Electrode

Using the same percutaneous catheter electrode for screening and permanent stimulation would reduce the cost of the hardware, but this savings would be offset by the increased cost of anchoring the electrode, which must take place in an operating room. Anchoring a trial electrode for potential permanent stimulation also increases incisional pain, which might confound interpretation of the trial; anchoring also requires use of a percutaneous extension cable, which increases the risk of infection. On the other hand, a percutaneous catheter electrode designed solely for screening is relatively inexpensive can be inserted under sterile conditions with fluoroscopy and can be removed easily.

Using the same electrode for the screening trial and permanent stimulation might eliminate the possibility that the replacement electrode will not reproduce the pain/paresthesia overlap, but this strategy also eliminates the opportunity to improve upon the results of the screening trial—which can inform the patient as well as the physician.

Also, unless the trial electrode is routinely removed, a patient and/or clinician's expectation that the screening trial electrode will become permanent might bias the results of the screening trial.

DEVICE OPTIONS

In alphabetical order, the major manufacturers of SCS equipment are Boston Scientific (previously Advanced Bionics, Inc., Natick, MA), Medtronic, Inc. (Minneapolis, MN), and St. Jude's Medical (Previously Advanced Neuromodulation Systems, St. Paul, MN).

Choice of Electrode

Percutaneous catheter electrodes are available with up to eight contacts and can be implanted singly, creating a one-dimensional array or multiply, creating a two-dimensional array. Multiple percutaneous electrodes can be introduced one by one through a Tuohy needle to rest side by side. Use of three or more such electrodes in parallel permits programming of lateral anodes "guarding" a central cathode, which might mitigate dorsal root recruitment causing uncomfortable side effects; however, it can be difficult to achieve and maintain appropriate spacing between electrodes. Figures 95.5 and 95.6 illustrate a selection of available electrodes.

An important role, therefore, remains for plate/paddle electrodes, which cannot be introduced through a needle and thus require surgical exposure via laminectomy. These electrodes have as many as 16 contacts in one-, two-, or three-column configurations and are insulated to prevent excess stimulation of dorsal structures.[136] The spacing of the columns is fixed, precluding adjustment as well as postoperative migration of one column with respect to another.

Factors that dictate choice of electrode include the location of the pain, the amount of extraneous stimulation that must be managed, and the physician's qualifications and experience (anesthesiologists, for example, might be expected to use only percutaneous electrodes).

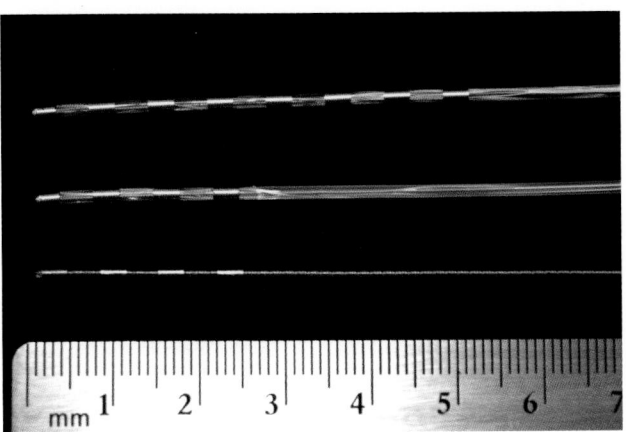

FIGURE 95.5 Percutaneous catheter electrodes have as many as eight cylindrical contacts designed for introduction through a needle.

Choice of Pulse Generator

Pulse generators are distinguished by their power sources and output configurations. The oldest style that remains in use incorporates a radiofrequency receiver and has no battery. Patients using this generator must wear an external antenna and transmitter during stimulation. In contrast, the so-called "totally implanted pulse generator" (IPG) has an implanted battery and is operated via an external remote control device. The earliest IPGs depended upon a primary cell that required surgical replacement when the battery was exhausted, but the newest generators, introduced in 2004, have rechargeable batteries. Since the 1980s, all generators have allowed noninvasive postoperative reassignment of each electrode contact (to anode, cathode, or off), and generators now support up to 16 independent contacts. The newest "multichannel" generators are capable of simultaneously or sequentially delivering pulses with different amplitudes and widths to different combinations of contacts, which of course consumes more energy compared with the simpler generators and thus motivates use of the rechargeable devices.

Factors that dictate the choice of stimulator/power generator include the patient's ability to control the device, the amount of

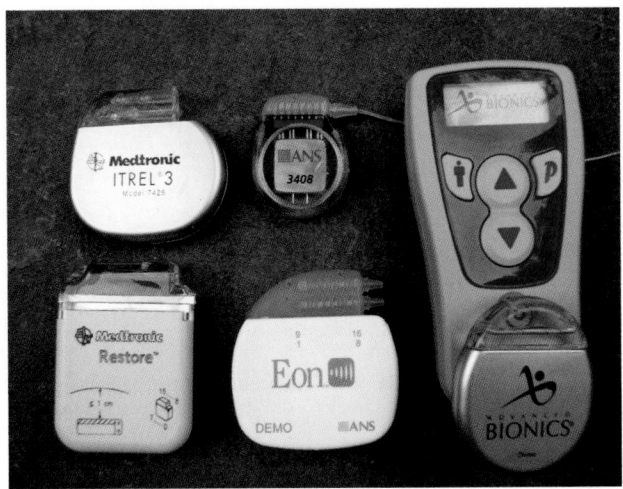

FIGURE 95.7 Contemporary implanted pulse generators support up to 16 contacts and have radiofrequency (RF) antennae for telemetry, which are visible only in generators powered by RF.

power required, and patient convenience. Figure 95.7 presents a sample of generators.

Programming a Spinal Cord Stimulation System

The number of contact combinations possible with either a surgical plate/paddle or percutaneous catheter electrode has grown markedly as the number of contacts has increased. In fact, more programming options exist than can be tested (for example, whereas a four-contact electrode offers 50 functional bipolar combinations of anodes and cathodes, an eight-contact electrode increases the choices to 6050, etc.). Thus, all three SCS manufacturers employ computerized equipment to find the best options for an individual patient and save these settings for subsequent use. Not only is initial programming important, skillful reprogramming can compensate for changes in impedance (e.g., due to postural changes or fibrosis), electrode migration, and changes in pain location or intensity.

Although each manufacturer's adjustment system is unique, each asks the patient to describe the area of pain and paresthesia and rate pain overlap and intensity at various settings (Fig. 95.8).

PATIENT MANAGEMENT

The patient should have a postoperative surgical check and SCS adjustment, and on postoperative day 7 to 14, return for suture or staple removal and any needed additional adjustment. From that point on, monthly visits should gradually taper to yearly visits.

Patients should understand that SCS is expected to reduce, not eliminate, pain. It is, therefore, important for clinicians to remember that other pain treatments remain available, especially those designed to treat nociceptive pain, which SCS is not expected to affect.

On/off time has a direct effect on battery longevity, but there are no studies of the impact of an imposed duty cycle on pain relief. In some patients, pain relief persists for a week or more after the device is turned off; others must operate the stimulator continuously. It is possible but rare for an SCS patient to achieve complete resolution of pain and request removal of the system.

Stimulation induces a subtle loss of normal sensation in SCS

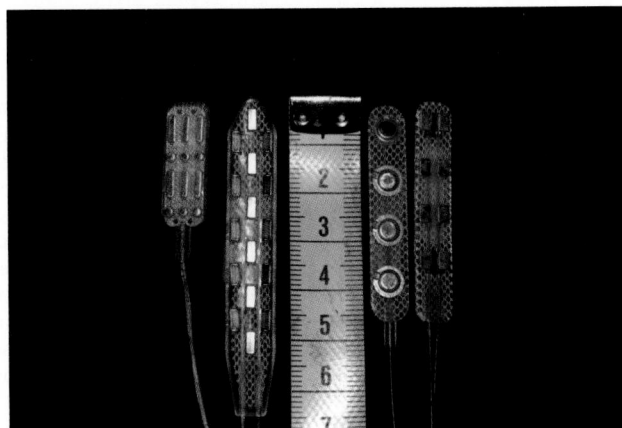

FIGURE 95.6 These laminectomy electrodes include two (on the left) with three columns of contacts; the smaller of these has a grooved dorsal surface (visible at top through the silicone elastomer) to stabilize it against lateral movement while allowing transverse flexibility. Older designs (on the right) have only one or two columns of contacts.

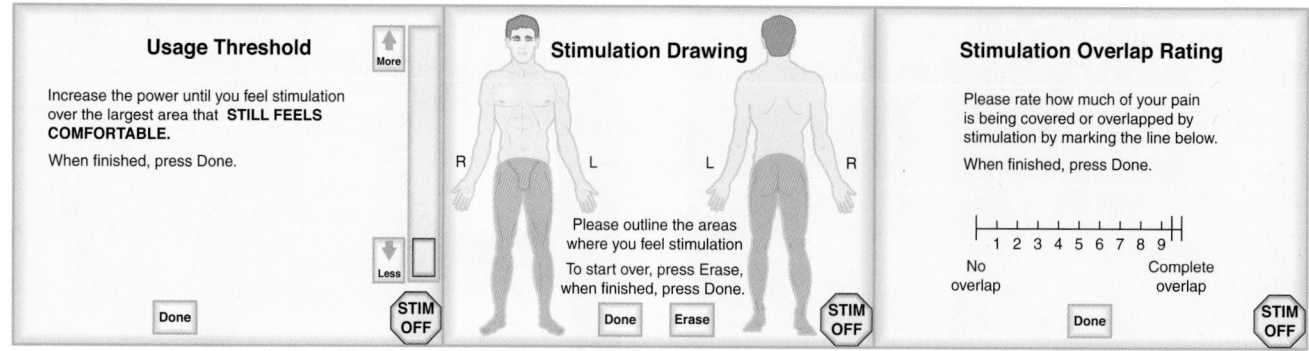

FIGURE 95.8 This computerized patient-interactive system allows the patient to (1) adjust amplitude to a specified level, (2) draw the area of paresthesia to be compared with a pain drawing and (3) rate pain/paresthesia overlap.

patients, but this loss is not sufficient to cause undesirable side effects, such as Charcot joints.[4,137] A change in paresthesia intensity corresponding to a change in posture is a normal, generally benign, side effect of SCS related to normal movement of the spinal cord with respect to the electrode(s).[138]

These side effects might, however, make certain activities hazardous; thus, we instruct patients to turn off SCS before driving a car or climbing a ladder, etc. The incidence of SCS side effects increases as stimulation amplitude and recruitment increase.[139]

As is standard practice, except in emergency cases that require immediate attention, a physician has the discretion to accept or reject any new patient who was implanted elsewhere. The device manufacturers provide all SCS patients with identification cards with the necessary contact information to facilitate appropriate emergency treatment.

Spinal Cord Stimulation Patient Precautions

SCS systems mighty affect or be affected by electromagnetic fields, and this necessitates certain precautions. MRI is generally contraindicated in SCS patients. Manufacturers generally recommend that implants be disabled before a patient enters an electromagnetic field produced by antitheft devices, a metal detector, or any other security scanning device. A patient must also refrain from scuba diving more than (typically) 10 meters deep or entering hyperbaric chambers with an absolute pressure above (typically) 2.0 atmospheres. Everyday precautions include avoiding placing excessive mechanical stress on the system.

Special steps must be taken before an SCS patient undergoes certain routine medical tests (such as cardiac monitoring) or radiation therapy with the pulse generator in the active field. Radiofrequency ablation, electrocautery, and lithotripsy also require caution. Ultrasound over the device and diathermy in any location are contraindicated in SCS patients.

SPINAL CORD STIMULATION TREATMENT CHALLENGES

Clinical Failure

The loss of pain relief despite pain/paresthesia overlap in a functioning system occurs in a minority of patients. This clinical failure might have a neurochemical basis, and it might respond to adjuvant medical therapy with baclofen or gabapentin. Clinical failure can also occur if the patient develops (1) pain in a new location that can not be covered by paresthesia unless the equip-

ment is revised surgically, (2) troublesome postural changes in paresthesia coverage, or (3) excessive pain/irritation at the implant site that is not caused by infection and cannot be treated locally.

Biological Failure

Infection, the most common biological failure, is almost always treated successfully (treatment, however, is expensive because it generally requires removal and replacement of the SCS system). The risk of infection is small, however, and is reduced by maintaining sterility and administering prophylactic intravenous antibiotics. Should an infection occur, specimen culture will guide antibiotic therapy. Unless the infection is limited to the skin over the implant, the entire SCS system should be removed until the infection resolves, when a new system can be implanted. Clinicians have reported patients with an "allergic reaction" to the implant, but this is rare and might be undiagnosed infection. A second biological failure, the development of fibrosis around implanted electrodes, can impede treatment, but this problem generally can be overcome through reprogramming.

Psychologic Failure

Psychologic problems, such as conversion disorder,[140] can require system removal.

Technical Failure

Technical failure, the inability to achieve or loss of clinically useful pain/paresthesia overlap, can result from suboptimal electrode choice or placement, from electrode migration, or from equipment malfunction. Technical failure can be mitigated by increasing clinician skill and experience, which includes adoption of the best implantation techniques; for example, the risk of percutaneous electrode migration can be nearly eliminated by applying an adhesive to the anchor/strain relief during implantation,[135] and the risk of fatigue fracture can be lessened by implanting the pulse generator in the lateral abdomen instead of the buttock and by creating strain relief coils in appropriate places.

In patients with suspected spinal stenosis or another anatomic anomaly that increases the risk of spinal cord or nerve injury, it is prudent to obtain an MRI of the target spinal areas before implantation of a surgical plate/paddle electrode. With the SCS system in place, computed tomography myelography is an alternative.

The risk of dural puncture is reduced by using an anesthetic technique that permits patient feedback during implantation of an electrode and avoiding placement in scarred areas, and the risk of epidural hematoma is reduced by preoperative review of the patient's coagulation history, medications, and blood chemistry and by monitoring the patient for a reasonable amount of time. Uncomfortable extraneous paresthesia or motor responses can be avoided by careful electrode implantation and postoperative adjustment or by use of an insulated surgical plate/paddle electrode.

Equipment Failure

Every part of an SCS system can fail. The electrode/lead/extension conductors can develop an open circuit through fatigue, fracture, or corrosion, insulation might fail, the generator battery can be depleted prematurely, or the generator itself can fail (e.g., by supplying excessive or unacceptable stimulation).[141,142]

COST EFFECTIVENESS

Although the initial expense of implanted SCS equipment creates a potential barrier to patient access, investigators have established that SCS is cost effective in the treatment of FBSS,[143–146] CRPS,[147] PVD, and angina.[104,148] Cost recovery occurs in approximately 3 years in patients with FBSS or CRPS, after 1 year in patients with angina who are not candidates for coronary artery bypass surgery, and immediately in patients with angina who would otherwise receive coronary artery bypass surgery only for symptom relief.

The cost effectiveness of SCS will be improved by the development of new equipment and techniques and can be enhanced by minimizing the incidence of complications (especially those, such as infection, that require surgical intervention and system replacement) and by careful patient selection.

The incidence of complications can be reduced if the specialist is meticulous, technically proficient, and knowledgeable (e.g., a simple technique nearly eliminates percutaneous electrode migration).[135] One improvement that has had a direct impact on cost effectiveness is the development of equipment designed to facilitate noninvasive reprogramming to optimize pain/paresthesia overlap. Another improvement, the introduction of rechargeable batteries, is intended to extend the life of expensive implanted pulse generators.[149]

SPINAL CORD STIMULATION CHALLENGES

In common with most medical therapies, we can improve patient outcomes with SCS by improving patient selection criteria, equipment design, implantation techniques, and clinician training. Continued investigation of the mechanisms of action of SCS will allow us to potentiate the benefits of the therapy, and developing refined outcome measures and appropriate research techniques will help us to optimize clinical application.

The increasing presence of magnetic fields in our environment and in the use of higher field strengths in MRI investigations motivates the development of nonmagnetic electrodes and pulse generators that will tolerate the magnetic fields.

SCS remains an underused therapy that should be considered early in the treatment continuum for a large group of patients.

References

1. Largus S. *Compositiones*. Helmreich G, ed. Leipzig: Tuebner; 1887.
2. Shealy CN, Mortimer JT, Reswick JB. Electrical inhibition of pain by stimula-

tion of the dorsal columns: preliminary clinical report. *Anesth Analg* 1967; 46(4):489–491.
3. Melzack P, Wall PD. Pain mechanisms: a new theory. *Science* 1965; 150(3699):971–978.
4. Lindblom U, Meyerson BA. Influence on touch, vibration and cutaneous pain of dorsal column stimulation in man. *Pain* 1975;1:257–270.
5. Linderoth B, Meyerson BA. Dorsal column stimulation: modulation of somatosensory and autonomic function. In: McMahon SB, Wall PD, eds. *The Neurobiology of Pain. Seminars in the Neurosciences*. London: Academic Press; 1995:263–277.
6. Campbell JN, Davis KD, Meyer RA, et al. The mechanism by which spinal cord stimulation affects pain: evidence for a new hypothesis. *Pain* 1990;5: S228.
7. Dickenson AH. Gate control theory of pain stands the test of time. *Br J Anaesth* 2002;88(6):755–757.
8. Stiller CO, Linderoth R, O'Connor WT, et al. Repeated spinal cord stimulation decreases the extracellular level of gamma-aminobutyric acid in the periaqueductal gray matter of freely moving rats. *Brain Res* 1995;699(2):231–241.
9. Hautvast RW, Ter Horst GJ, DeJong BM, et al. Relative changes in regional cerebral blood flow during spinal cord stimulation in patients with refractory angina pectoris. *Eur J Neurosci* 1997;9(6):1178–1183.
10. De Jongste MJL, Hautvast RWM, Ruiters MHJ, et al. Spinal cord stimulation and the induction of c-fos and heat shock protein in the central nervous system of rats. *Neuromodulation* 1998:2:73–85.
11. Linderoth B, Foreman RD. Physiology of spinal cord stimulation: review and update. *Neuromodulation* 1999;2(3):150–164.
12. Saadé NE, Atweh SF, Jabbur SJ, et al. Effects of lesions in the anterolateral columns and dorsolateral funiculi on self-mutilation behavior in rats. *Pain* 1990;42(3):313–321.
13. El-Khoury C, Hawwa N, Baliki M, et al. Attenuation of neuropathic pain by segmental and supraspinal activation of the dorsal column system in awake rats. *Neuroscience* 2002;112(3):541–553.
14. Foreman RD, Beall JE, Coulter JD, et al. Effects of dorsal column stimulation on primate spinothalamic tract neurons. *J Neurophysiol* 1976;39(3):534–546.
15. Ren B, Linderoth B, Meyerson BA. Effects of spinal cord stimulation on the flexor reflex and involvement of supraspinal mechanisms: an experimental study in mononeuropathic rats. *J Neurosurg* 1996;84(2):244–249.
16. Roberts MHT, Rees H. Physiological basis of spinal cord stimulation. *Pain Rev* 1994;1:184–198.
17. Tonelli L, Setti T, Falasca A, et al. Investigation on cerebrospinal fluid opioids and neurotransmitters related to spinal cord stimulation. *Appl Neurophysiol* 1988;51(6):324–332.
18. Meyerson BA, Linderoth B. Spinal cord stimulation: mechanisms of action in neuropathic and ischemic pain. In: Simpson BA, ed. *Electrical Stimulation and the Relief of Pain*. New York: Elsevier; 2003:161–182.
19. Freeman TB, Campbell JN, Long DM. Naloxone does not affect pain relief induced by electrical stimulation in man. *Pain* 1983;17:189–195.
20. Eliasson T, Mannheimer C, Waagstein F, et al. Myocardial turnover of endogenous opioids and calcitonin-gene-related peptide in the human heart and the effects of spinal cord stimulation on pacing-induced angina pectoris. *Cardiology* 1998;89(3):170–177.
21. Hanai F. C fiber responses of wide dynamic range neurons in the spinal dorsal horn. *Clin Orthop Relat Res* 1998;349:256–267.
22. Yakhnitsa V, Linderoth B, Meyerson BA. Spinal cord stimulation attenuates dorsal horn neuronal hyperexcitability in a rat model of mononeuropathy. *Pain* 1999;79(2–3):223–233.
23. Cui JG, Linderoth B, Meyerson BA. Effects of spinal cord stimulation on touch-evoked allodynia involve GABAergic mechanisms: an experimental study in the mononeuropathic rat. *Pain* 1996;66:287–295.
24. Cui JG, O'Connor WT, Ungerstedt U, et al. Spinal cord stimulation attenuates augmented dorsal horn release of excitatory amino acids in mononeuropathy via a GABAergic mechanism. *Pain* 1997;73:87–95.
25. Linderoth B, Foreman RD. Physiology of spinal cord stimulation. Review and update. *Neuromodulation* 1999;2:150–164.
26. Linderoth B. *Dorsal Column stimulation and Pain: Experimental Studies of Putative Neurochemical and Neurophsyiological Mechanisms* (doctoral thesis). Stockholm, Sweden: Karolinska Institute; 1992.
27. Linderoth B, Gazelius B, Franck J, et al. Dorsal column stimulation induces release of serotonin and substance P in the cat dorsal horn. *Neurosurgery* 1992;31:289–297.
28. Cui JG, Sollevi A, Linderoth B, et al. Adenosine receptor activation suppresses tactile hypersensitivity and potentiates spinal cord stimulation in mononeuropathic rats. *Neurosci Lett* 1997;223,173–176.
29. Meyerson BA, Brodin E, Linderoth B. Possible neurohumoral mechanisms in CNS stimulation for pain suppression. *Appl Neurophysiol* 1985;48:175–180.
30. Bonica JJ, Yaksh T, Liebeskind JC, et al. Biochemistry and modulation of nociception and pain. In: Bonica JJ, ed. *The Management of Pain*. 2nd ed. Philadelphia: Lea & Febiger; 1990:95–121.
31. Linderoth B, Stiller CO, O'Connor WT, et al. An animal model for the study of brain transmittor release in response to spinal cord stimulation in the awake, freely moving rat: preliminary results from the periaqueductal grey matter. *Acta Neurochir Suppl (Wien)* 1993;58:156–160.

32. Meyerson BA, Herregodts P, Linderoth B, et al. An experimental animal model of spinal cord stimulation for pain. *Stereotact Funct Neurosurg* 1994; 62(1–4):256–262.

33. Meyerson BA, Ren B, Herregodts P, et al. Spinal cord stimulation in animal models of mononeuropathy: effects on the withdrawal response and the flexor reflex. *Pain* 1995 61(2):229–243.

34. Schechtmann G, Song Z, Ultenius C, et al. Cholinergic mechanisms in the pain relieving effect of spinal cord stimulation in a model of neuropathy. *Pain* 2008;139(1):136–145.

35. Song Z, Meyerson BA, Linderoth B. Muscarinic receptor activation potentiates the effect of spinal cord stimulation on pain related behaviour in rats with mononeuropathy. *Neurosci Lett* 2008;436:7–12.

36. Stiller CO, Cui JG, O'Connor WT, et al. Release of gamma-aminobutyric acid in the dorsal horn and suppression of tactile allodynia by spinal cord stimulation in mononeuropathic rats. *Neurosurgery* 1996;39(2):367–374.

37. Cui JG, Meyerson BA, Sollevi A, et al. Effect of spinal cord stimulation on tactile hypersensitivity in mononeuropathic rats is potentiated by simultaneous GABA(B) and adenosine receptor activation. *Neurosci Lett* 1998;247: 183–186.

38. Meyerson BA, Cui JG, Yakhnitsa V, et al. Modulation of spinal pain mechanisms by spinal cord stimulation and the potential role of adjuvant pharmacotherapy. *Stereotact Funct Neurosurg* 1997;68(1–4 Pt 1)129–140.

39. Wallin J, Cui JG, Yakhnitsa V, et al. Gabapentin and pregabalin suppress tactile allodynia and potentiate spinal cord stimulation in a model of neuropathy. *Eur J Pain* 2002;6:261–272.

40. Schechtmann G, Wallin J, Meyerson BA, et al. Intrathecal clonidine potentiates suppression of tactile hypersensitivity by spinal cord stimulation in a model of neuropathy. *Anesth Analg* 2004;99:135–139.

41. Lind G, Schechtmann G, Winter J, et al. Baclofen–enhanced spinal cord stimulation and intrathecal baclofen alone for neuropathic pain: long-term outcome of a pilot study. *Eur J Pain* 2008;12:132–136.

42. Li D, Yang H, Meyerson BA, et al. Response to spinal cord stimulation in variants of the spared nerve injury pain model. *Neurosci Lett* 2006;400: 115–120.

43. Smits H, Ultenius C, Deumens R, et al. Effect of spinal cord stimulation in an animal model of neuropathic pain relates to degree of tactile 'allodynia.' *Neuroscience* 2006;143:541–546.

44. Baron R, Binder A, Schattschneider J, et al. Pathophysiology and treatment of complex regional pain syndromes. In: Dostrovsky JO, Carr DB, Koltzenburg M, eds. *Proceedings of the 10th World Congress on Pain.* Seattle: IASP Press; 2003:683–704.

45. Häbler H-J, Eschenfelder S, Brinker H, et al. Neurogenic vasoconstriction in the dorsal root ganglion may play a crucial role in sympathetic-afferent coupling after spinal nerve injury. In: Devor M, Rowbotham MC, Wiesenfeld-Hallin Z, eds. *Progress in Pain Research and Management.* Seattle: IASP Press; 2000:661–667.

46. Kemler MA, Barendse GA, van Kleef M, et al. Pain relief in complex regional pain syndrome due to spinal cord stimulation does not depend on vasodilation. *Anesthesiology* 2000;92(6):1653–1660.

47. Kimble LP, McGuire DB, Dunbar SB, et al. Gender differences in pain characteristics of chronic stable angina and perceived physical limitation in patients with coronary artery disease. *Pain* 2003;101:45–53.

48. Linderoth B. Spinal cord stimulation in ischemia and ischemic pain. In: Horsch S, Claeys L, eds. *Spinal Cord Stimulation III: An Innovative Method in the Treatment of PVD and Angina.* Darmstadt: Steinkopff Verlag; 1995:19–35.

49. Linderoth B, Gherardini G, Ren B, et al. Preemptive spinal cord stimulation reduces ischemia in an animal model of vasospasm. *Neurosurgery* 1995;37(2): 266–271.

50. Gherardini G, Lundeberg T, Cui JG, et al. Spinal cord stimulation improves survival in ischemic skin flaps: an experimental study of the possible mediation via the calcitonin gene-related peptide. *Plast Reconstr Surg* 1999;103(4): 1221–1228.

51. Croom JE, Foreman RD, Chandler MJ, et al. Cutaneous vasodilation during dorsal column stimulation is mediated by dorsal roots and CGRP. *Am J Physiol* 1997;272:H950–H957.

52. Croom JE, Foreman RD, Chandler MJ, et al. Reevaluation of the role of the sympathetic nervous system in cutaneous vasodilatation during dorsal spinal cord stimulation: are multiple mechanisms active? *Neuromodulation* 1998; 1:91–101.

53. Tanaka S, Barron KW, Chandler MJ, et al. Low intensity spinal cord stimulation may induce cutaneous vasodilatation via CGRP release. *Brain Res* 2001; 896:183–187.

54. Tanaka S, Barron KW, Chandler MJ, et al. Role of primary afferent in spinal cord stimulation-induced vasodilatation: characterization of fiber types. *Brain Res* 2003;959(2):191–198.

55. Tanaka S, Barron KW, Chandler MJ, et al. Local cooling alters neural mechanisms producing changes in peripheral blood flow by spinal cord stimulation. *Auton Neurosci* 2003;104(2):117–127.

56. Wu M, Komori N, Qin C, et al. Sensory fibers containing vanilloid receptor-1 (VR-1) mediate spinal cord stimulation-induced vasodilation. *Brain Res* 2006;1107:177–184.

57. Wu M, Komori N, Qin C, et al. Roles of peripheral terminals of transient receptor potential vanilloid-1 containing sensory fibers in spinal cord stimulation-induced peripheral vasodilation. *Brain Res* 2007;1156:80–92.

58. Freedman RR, Sabharwal SC, Desai N, et al. Increased α-adrenergic responsiveness in idiopathic Raynaud's disease. *Arthritis Rheum* 1989:32:61–65.

59. Bunker CB, Terenghi G, Springall DR, et al. Deficiency of calcitonin gene-related peptide in Raynaud's phenomenon. *Lancet* 1990;336:1530–1533.

60. Tanaka S, Komori N, Barron KW. Mechanisms of sustained cutaneous vasodilatation induced by spinal cord stimulation. *Auton Neurosci* 2004; 114(1–2):55–60.

61. Qin C, Farber JP, Linderoth B, et al. Neuromodulation of thoracic intraspinal visceroreceptive transmission by electrical stimulation of spinal dorsal column and somatic afferents in rats. *J Pain* 2008;9(1):71–78.

62. Wu M, Komori N, Qin C, et al. Extracellular-signal-regulated kinase (ERK) and protein kinase B (AKT) pathways involved in spinal cord stimulation (SCS)-induced vasodilation. *Brain Res* 2008;1207:73–83.

63. Yang X, Farber JP, Wu M, et al. Roles of dorsal column pathway and transient receptor potential vanilloid type 1 in augmentation of cerebral blood flow by upper cervical spinal cord stimulation in rats. *Neuroscience* 2008;152(4): 950–958.

64. Wu M, Linderoth B, Foreman RD. Putative mechanisms behind effects of spinal cord stimulation on vascular diseases: a review of experimental studies. *Auton Neurosci* 2008;1381(1–20):9–23.

65. Mannheimer C, Eliasson T, Andersson B, et al. Effects of spinal cord stimulation in angina pectoris induced by pacing and possible mechanisms of action. *BMJ* 1993;307:477–480.

66. Mobilia G, Zuin G, Zanco P, et al. Effects of spinal cord stimulation on regional myocardial blood flow in patients with refractory angina. A positron emission tomography study [in Italian]. *G Ital Cardiol* 1998;28(10):1113–1119.

67. Hautwast RW, Blanksma PK, DeJongste MJ, et al. Effect of spinal cord stimulation on myocardial blood flow assessed by positron emission tomography in patients with refractory angina pectoris. *Am H Cardiol* 1996;77:462–467.

68. Kingma JG Jr, Linderoth B, Ardell JL, et al. Neuromodulation therapy does not influence blood flow distribution or left-ventricular dynamics during acute myocardial ischemia. *Auton Neurosci* 2001;91(1–2):47–54.

69. Eliasson T, Augustinsson LE, Manneheimer C. Spinal cord stimulation in severe angina pectoris: presentation of current studies, indications and practical experience. *Pain* 1996;65:169–179.

70. Cardinal R, Ardell J, Linderoth B, et al. Spinal cord activation differentially modulates ischemic electrical responses to different stressors in canine ventricles. *Autonom Neurosci* 2004;111(1):34–47.

71. Foreman RD, Linderoth B, Ardell JL, et al. Modulation of intrinsic cardiac neuronal activity by spinal cord stimulation: Implications for its therapeutic in angina pectoris. *Cardiovasc Res* 2000;47(2):367–375.

72. Foreman RD, DeJongste MJL, Linderoth B. Integrative control of cardiac function by cervical and thoracic spinal neurons. In: Armour JA, Ardell JL, eds. *Basic and Clinical Neurocardiology.* London: Oxford University Press; 2004:153–186.

73. Norrsell H. Eliasson T, Mannheimer C, et al. Effects of pacing-induced myocardial stress and spinal cord stimulation on whole body and cardiac norepinephrine spillover. *Eur Heart J* 1997;18(12):1890–1896.

74. Southerland EM, Milhorn D, Foreman RD, et al. Preemptive, but not reactive, spinal cord stimulation mitigates transient ischemia-induced myocardial infarction via cardiac adrenergic neurons. *Am J Physiology Heart Circ Physiol* 2007;292(1):H311–317.

75. Guru K, Mailis A, Ashby P, et al. Postsynaptic potentials in motoneurons caused by spinal cord stimulation in humans. *Electroencephalogr Clin Neurophysiol* 1987;66(3):275–280.

76. Foreman, RD. Mechanisms of visceral pain: from nociception to targets. *Drug Dis Today: Dis Mech* 2004;1:457–463.

77. Greenwood-Van Meerveld B, Johnson AC, Foreman RD, et al. Attenuation by spinal cord stimulation of a nociceptive reflex generated by colorectal distention in a rat model. *Auton Neurosci* 2003;104(1):17–24.

78. Coburn B, Sin W. A theoretical study of epidural electrical stimulation of the spinal cord—Part I: Finite element analysis of stimulus fields. *IEEE Trans Biomed Eng* 1985;32:971–977.

79. Holsheimer J, Strujik JJ, Rijkhoff NJ. Contact combinations in epidural spinal cord stimulation: a comparison by computer modeling. *Stereotact Funct Neurosurg* 1991;56:220–233.

80. Holsheimer J, Wesselink WA. Effect of anode-cathode configuration on paresthesia coverage in spinal cord stimulation. *Neurosurgery* 1997;41:654–660.

81. Sances A, Swinotek TJ, Larson SJ, et al. Innovations in neurologic implant systems. *Med Instrum* 1975;9:213–216.

82. Law JD. Spinal stimulation: statistical superiority of monophasic stimulation of narrowly separated bipoles having rostral cathodes. *Appl Neurophysiol* 1983;46:129–137.

83. Ranck JB, BeMent SL. The specific impedance of the dorsal columns of the cat: An anisotropic medium. *Exp Neurol* 1965;11:451–463.

84. Geddes LA, Baker LE. The specific resistance of biological material: a compendium of data for the biomedical engineer and physiologist. *Med Biol Eng* 1967;5:271–293.

85. Coburn B. Electrical stimulation of the spinal cord: two-dimensional finite element analysis with particular reference to epidural electrodes. *Med Biol Eng Comp* 1980;18:573–584.

86. Rusinko JB, Walker CF, Sepulvedo NG. Finite element modeling of potentials within the human thoracic spinal cord due to applied electrical stimulation. In: *Frontiers of Engineering in Health Care.* Vol. 3. Houston, TX: Proceedings of the IEEE Transactions on Biomedical Engineering Conference; 1981: 76–81.

87. Sin WK, Coburn B. Electrical stimulation of the spinal cord: a further analysis relating to anatomic factors and tissue properties. *Med Biol Eng Comp* 1983; 21:264–269.

88. Coburn B. A theoretical study of epidural electrical stimulation of the spinal cord—Part II: effects on long myelinated fibers. *IEEE Trans Biomed Eng* 1985;32:978–986.

89. Holsheimer J, Struijk JJ. How do geometric factors influence epidural spinal cord stimulation? A quantitative analysis by computer modeling. *Stereotact Funct Neurosurg* 1991;56:234–249.

90. McNeal DR. Analysis of a model for excitation of myelinated nerve. *IEEE Trans Biomed Eng* 1976;23:329–337.

91. Chiu SY, Ritchie JM, Rogart RB, et al. A quantitative description of membrane currents in rabbit myelinated nerve. *J Physiol* 1979;292:149–166.

92. Wesselink WA, Holsheimer J, Boom HB. A model of the electrical behaviour of myelinated sensory nerve fibres based on human data. *Med Biol Eng Comput* 1999;37(2):228–235.

93. Struijk JJ, Holsheimer J, Barolat G, et al. Paresthesia thresholds in spinal cord stimulation: a comparison of theoretical results with clinical data. *IEEE Trans Rehab Eng* 1993;1:101–108.

94. Hoekema R, Venner K, Struijk JJ, et al. Multigrid solution of the potential field in modeling electrical nerve stimulation. *Comput Biomed Res* 1998;31: 348–362.

95. Oakley JC, Espinosa E. Bothe H, et al. Transverse tripolar spinal cord stimulation: results of an international multicenter study. *Neuromodulation* 2006; 9(3):183–191.

96. North RB, Kidd DH, Farrokhi F, et al. Spinal cord stimulation versus repeated lumbosacral spine surgery for chronic pain: a randomized, controlled trial. *Neurosurgery* 2005;56(1):98–106.

97. Kumar K, Taylor RS, Jacques L, et al. Spinal cord stimulation versus conventional medical management for neuropathic pain: a multicentre randomised controlled trial in patients with failed back surgery syndrome. *Pain* 2007; 132(1–2):179–188.

98. Law JD. Spinal stimulation in the "failed back surgery syndrome": comparison of technical criteria for palliating pain in the leg vs. in the low back. *Acta Neurochir* 1992;117:95.

99. North RB, Kidd DH, Olin J, et al. Spinal cord stimulation for axial low back pain: a prospective, controlled trial comparing dual with single percutaneous electrodes. *Spine* 2005;30(12):1412–1418.

100. Kemler MA, Barendse GA, van Kleef M, et al. Spinal cord stimulation in patients with chronic reflex sympathetic dystrophy. *N Engl J Med* 2000; 343(9):618–624.

101. Kemler MA, De Vet HC, Barendse GA, et al. The effect of spinal cord stimulation in patients with chronic reflex sympathetic dystrophy: two years' follow-up of the randomized controlled trial. *Ann Neurol* 2004;55(1):13–18.

102. Kemler MA, de Vet HC, Barendse GA, et al. Effect of spinal cord stimulation for chronic complex regional pain syndrome Type I: five-year final follow-up of patients in a randomized controlled trial. *J Neurosurg* 2008;108(2): 292–298.

103. Mannheimer C, Eliasson T, Augustinsson LE, et al. Electrical stimulation versus coronary artery bypass surgery in severe angina pectoris: the ESBY study. *Circulation* 1998;97(12):1157–1163.

104. Andréll P, Ekre O, Eliasson T, et al. Cost-effectiveness of spinal cord stimulation versus coronary artery bypass grafting in patients with severe angina pectoris—long-term results from the ESBY study. *Cardiology* 2003;99(1): 20–24.

105. Ekre O, Eliasson T, Norrsell H, et al. Long-term effects of spinal cord stimulation and coronary artery bypass grafting on quality of life and survival in the ESBY study. *Eur Heart J* 2002;23(24):1938–1945.

106. Norrsell H, Pilhall M, Eliasson T, et al. Effects of spinal cord stimulation and coronary artery bypass grafting on myocardial ischemia and heart rate variability: further results from the ESBY study. *Cardiology* 2000;94(1): 12–18.

107. Ubbink DT, Vermeulen H. Spinal cord stimulation for non-reconstructable chronic critical leg ischaemia. *Cochrane Database Syst Rev* 2005;3: CD004001.

108. Ubbink DT, Vermeulen H. Spinal cord stimulation for critical leg ischemia: a review of effectiveness and optimal patient selection. *J Pain Symptom Manage* 2006;31(4 Suppl): S30–S35.

109. Ubbink DT, Spincemaille GH, Prins MH, et al. Microcirculatory investigations to determine the effect of spinal cord stimulation for critical leg ischemia: the Dutch multicenter randomized controlled trial. *J Vasc Surg* 1999;30(2): 236–244.

110. Barolat G, Myklebust JR, Wenninger W. Effects of spinal cord stimulation on spasticity and spasms secondary to myelopathy. *Appl Neurophys* 1988; 51:29–44.

111. Augustinsson LE, Linderoth B, Mannheimer C. Spinal cord stimulation in various ischaemic conditions. In: Illis L, ed. *Spinal Cord Dysfunction. III: Functional Stimulation*. Oxford: Oxford Medical Publications; 1992:272– 295.

112. Robaina FJ, Dominguez M, Diaz M, et al. Spinal cord stimulation for relief of chronic pain in vasospastic disorders of the upper limbs. *Neurosurgery* 1989;24:63–67.

113. Ktenidis K, Claeys L, Bartels C, et al. Spinal cord stimulation in the treatment of Buerger's disease. In: Horsch S, Claeys L, eds. *Spinal Cord Stimulation: An Innovative Method in the Treatment of PVD and Angina*. Darmstadt, Germany: Springer-Verlag Telos; 1995:207–214.

114. Francaviglia N, Silvestro C, Maiello M, et al. Spinal cord stimulation for the treatment of progressive systemic sclerosis and Raynaud's syndrome. *Br J Neurosurg* 1994;8:567–571.

115. Robaina F, Clavo B. Spinal cord stimulation in the treatment of post-stroke patients: current state and future directions. *Acta Neurochir Suppl* 2007;97 (Pt 1):277–282.

116. Kuwata T. Effects of the cervical spinal cord stimulation on persistent vegetative syndrome: experimental and clinical study (in Japanese). *No Shinkei Geka* 1993;21(4):325–331.

117. Robaina F, Clavo B. The role of spinal cord stimulation in the management of patients with brain tumors. *Acta Neurochir Suppl* 2007;97(Pt 1):445–453.

118. Peters KM. Neuromodulation for the treatment of refractory interstitial cystitis. *Rev Urol* 2006;4:S121–S125.

119. Khan YN, Raza SS, Khan EA. Spinal cord stimulation in visceral pathologies. *Pain Med* 2006;7:S121–S125.

120. Elabbady AA, Hassouna MM, Elhilali MM. Neural stimulation for chronic voiding dysfunctions. *J Urol* 1994;152:2076–2080.

121. Kapural L, Narouze SN, Janicki TI, et al. Spinal cord stimulation is an effective treatment for the chronic intractable visceral pelvic pain. *Pain Med* 2006; 7(5):440–443.

122. Whiteside JL, Walters MD, Mekhail N. Spinal cord stimulation for intractable vulvar pain. A case report. *J Reprod Med* 2003;48(10):821–823.

123. Kenefick NJ. Sacral nerve neuromodulation for the treatment of lower bowel motility disorders. *Ann R Coll Surg Engl* 2006;88(7):617–623.

124. North RB. The glass is half full [commentary on the fallacy of 50% pain relief]. *Pain Forum* 1999;8:195–197.

125. Waddell G. The clinical course of low back pain. In: *The Back Pain Revolution*. Edinburgh: Churchill Livingstone; 1998:103–107.

126. Waddell G, Burton AK. Occupational health guidelines for the management of low back pain at work: evidence review. *Occup Med (Lond)* 2001;51(2): 124–135.

127. North RB, Ewend MG, Lawton MT, et al. Failed back surgery syndrome: 5-year follow-up after spinal cord stimulator implantation. *Neurosurgery* 1991;28(5):692–699.

128. Ubbink DT, Gersbach PA, Berg P, et al. The best TcPO2 parameters to predict the efficacy of spinal cord stimulation to improve limb salvage in patients with inoperable critical leg ischemia. *Int Angiol* 2003;22(4):356–363.

129. Petrakis IE, Sciacca V. Transcutaneous oxygen tension (TcPO2) in the testing period of spinal cord stimulation (SCS) in critical limb ischemia of the lower extremities. *Int Surg* 1999;84(2):122–128.

130. Petrakis IE, Sciacca V. Spinal cord stimulation in critical limb ischemia of the lower extremities: our experience. *J Neurosurg Sci* 1999;43(4):285–293.

131. Petrakis IE, Sciacca V. Spinal cord stimulation in diabetic lower limb critical ischaemia: transcutaneous oxygen measurement as predictor for treatment success. *Eur J Vasc Endovasc Surg* 2000;19(6):587–592.

132. Petrakis IE, Sciacca V. Does autonomic neuropathy influence spinal cord stimulation therapy success in diabetic patients with critical lower limb ischemia? *Surg Neurol* 2000;53(2):182–188.

133. North RB. Spinal cord stimulation. In: Connolly ES, McKhann GM, Huang J, Choudhri TF, Mocco J, eds. *Fundamentals of Operative Techniques in Neurosurgery*. 2nd ed. New York, NY: Thieme; in press.

134. North RB, Linderoth B. Spinal cord stimulation for chronic pain. In: Schmidek HH, Roberts D, eds. *Schmidek & Sweet: Operative Neurosurgical Techniques: Indications, Methods, and Results*. 5th ed. Vol. 2. Philadelphia, PA: Elsevier; 2005:2165–2186.

135. Renard VM, North RB. Prevention of percutaneous electrode migration in spinal cord stimulation by a modification of the standard implantation technique. *J Neurosurg Spine* 2006;4(4):300–303.

136. North RB, Kidd DH, Zahurak M., et al. Spinal cord stimulation for chronic, intractable pain: two decades' experience. *Neurosurgery* 1993;34:384–395.

137. Marchand S, Bushnell MC, Molina-Negro P, et al. The effects of dorsal column stimulation on measures of clinical and experimental pain in man. *Pain* 1991;45:249–257.

138. Olin JN, Kidd DH, North RB. Postural changes in spinal cord stimulation thresholds. *Neuromodulation* 1998;1(4):171–175.

139. Law JD, Kirkpatrick AF. Pain management update: spinal cord stimulation. *Am J Pain Manage* 1991;2:34–42.

140. Parisod E, Murray RF, Cousins MJ. Conversion disorder after implant of a spinal cord stimulator in a patient with a complex regional pain syndrome. *Anesth Analg* 2003;96(1):201–206.

141. Cameron T. Safety and efficacy of spinal cord stimulation for the treatment of chronic pain: a 20-year literature review. *J Neurosurg* 2004;100(3 Suppl Spine): 254–267.

142. Kumar K, Bucher E, Linderoth B, et al. Spinal cord stimulation: avoiding complications from spinal cord stimulation: practical recommendations from an international panel of experts. *Neuromodulation* 2007;10(1):24–33.

143. Bell GK, Kidd D, North RB. Cost-effectiveness analysis of spinal cord stimulation in treatment of failed back surgery syndrome. *J Pain Symptom Manage* 1997;13:286–295.

144. North RB, Kidd D, Shipley J, et al. Spinal cord stimulation versus reoperation

for failed back surgery syndrome: a cost effectiveness and cost utility analysis based on a randomized, controlled trial. *Neurosurgery* 2007;61(2):361–369.

145. Blond S, Buisset N, Dam Hieu P, et al. Cost-benefit evaluation of spinal cord stimulation treatment for failed-back surgery patients (in French). *Neurochirurgie* 2004;50(4):443–453.

146. Kumar K, Malik S, Demeria D. Treatment of chronic pain with spinal cord stimulation versus alternative therapies: cost-effectiveness analysis. *Neurosurgery* 2002;51(1):106–116.

147. Kemler MA, Furnée CA. Economic evaluation of spinal cord stimulation for chronic reflex sympathetic dystrophy. *Neurology* 2002;59:1203–1209.

148. Yu W, Maru F, Edner M, et al. Spinal cord stimulation for refractory angina pectoris: a retrospective analysis of efficacy and cost-benefit. *Corno Artery Dis* 2004;15(1):31–37.

149. Hornberger J, Kumar K, Verhulst E, et al. Rechargeable spinal cord stimulation versus nonrechargeable system for patients with failed back surgery syndrome: a cost-consequences analysis. *Clin J Pain* 2008;24(3):244–252.

CHAPTER 96 ■ MOTOR CORTEX AND DEEP BRAIN STIMULATION

MING L.CHENG AND EMAD N. ESKANDAR

INTRODUCTION

Deep brain stimulation (DBS) has been used for the last three decades for the treatment of pain. Worldwide, but particularly in the United States, the number of patients treated by DBS and the number of practitioners offering this treatment has progressively decreased. This is in part because of the development of spinal therapies that are less invasive, but also the perception of variability in its efficacy after an initial wave of optimism in the 1970s.[1] This skepticism, especially for neuropathic pain,[2,3] resulted in the reversion of DBS for pain in the United States to what is essentially experimental status, with few published reports[4] in recent years regarding its use and advancement. Yet, a review of the literature supports a clear role for DBS for specific indications, such as patients with low back pain[5] who are not helped by other forms of therapy. The use of DBS for treatment of pain continues sporadically in the United States and more frequently in Europe and Japan.

The use of DBS as a treatment for pain has evolved along two separate tracks that correspond to the effect of stimulation upon the two main targets of stimulation: the periaqueductal gray region (PAG), and the sensory thalamus, known also as the ventral posterior lateral (VPL) nucleus of the thalamus. Although there are exceptions, in general, stimulation of the former affects nociceptive pain, while stimulation of the latter is more selective for neuropathic, deafferentation pain and the allodynia and dysesthesia related to neuropathic pain of peripheral origin. Stimulation of either the VPL thalamus, PAG, or periventricular gray (PVG) is achieved by stereotactic implantation of a quadripolar DBS electrode, which is then connected to an implanted pulse generator placed just inferior to the clavicle over the chest wall.

Motor cortex stimulation (MCS) is a newer therapy that was initially performed by Tsubokawa in 1990.[6] Unlike DBS, MCS is only effective for neuropathic pain with no data to suggest efficacy for chronic nociceptive conditions such as back pain. MCS is used primarily for the treatment of two pain syndromes: central pain after stroke and painful trigeminal neuropathy. Patients may also present with evoked pain in the form of allodynia or dysesthesia that can be markedly relieved by MCS. MCS may be useful for pain from peripheral nerve injury.[7,8] MCS is achieved by placing an electrode in the epidural space directly overlying the primary motor cortex, which is then similarly connected to an implanted pulse generator.

Both forms of brain stimulation have in common the use of electrical stimulation to effect a change in the patient's perception of pain that does not depend upon destruction of neural tissue. Nonablative therapies, including electrical stimulation and intrathecal drug delivery, have become the mainstays of neurosurgical intervention for pain. Brain stimulation, while clearly in this category, is not a substantial part of the armamentarium of neurosurgeons in the United States. Greater investigation in the form of well-controlled, well-structured prospective trials is necessary to establish guidelines and clearly define the efficacy of cranial stimulation therapies. With better scientific evidence, practitioners who are currently not offering cranial stimulation are likely to more readily offer them to patients who have no other options in the treatment of their pain syndromes.

DEEP BRAIN STIMULATION

Basic Considerations

Sensory Thalamic Deep Brain Stimulation

Early attempts to relieve pain through stimulation in deep brain structures began in the late 1960s and stimulated targets in the striatum[9] and in the septal region.[10] After the introduction of dorsal column spinal cord stimulation, the intracranial target for pain moved to the sensory thalamus in the 1970s.[11–13] This move to the next higher relay in the dorsal column/medial lemniscus system was logical, and the approach produced clinical results in patients that were in many ways similar to dorsal column stimulation. This included the time course of pain relief, a preferential effect upon neuropathic pain, and the effect of paresthesias over the painful treatment area. The rationale for sensory thalamic DBS was initially quite similar to the gate control theory for spinal cord stimulation, with the earliest known trials in the 1960s[14] predicated on a 1911 theory[15] suggesting that pain results from an imbalance between nociceptive and non-nociceptive portions of the sensory pathway, with stimulation of the sensory thalamus restoring this balance.

There are multiple modern theories and experimental studies that posit mechanisms for pain relief via sensory thalamic stimulation.[16–19] Most of these appear to lack clinical relevance since they were generally performed with acute nociceptive stimuli in intact animals under general anesthesia, whereas the conditions clinicians treat are much more chronic in nature and there are well-established differences between the two mechanistically. In one such study, stimulation of sensory thalamus in the rat did not attenuate acute pain. This correlates with what we know today regarding poor efficacy with nociceptive stimuli using the sensory thalamus as the target for stimulation.[20,21] More relevant studies include one with cats that utilized a trigeminal ganglionectomy model of neuropathic pain.[22] This resulted in deafferentation hyperactivity that was inhibited in 40% of neurons with stimulation of the sensory thalamus and the internal capsule of the cats, with a long poststimulatory effect observed. In a partial sciatic injury model in rats, hind paw hypersensitivity was markedly suppressed with sensory thalamus stimulation with the effect lasting well beyond the duration of the stimulation.[23]

In humans, there is evidence that neuropathic and especially central pain leads to significant somatotopic alterations in the sensory thalamus.[24–26] As in animal studies, human microelectrode recordings taken within neuronal cells in the sensory thalamus have demonstrated substantial hyperexcitability and altered neuronal responses with spontaneous activity in patients with neuropathic pain states. In humans with deafferentation pain syndromes (e.g., phantom limb pain), an altered somatotopy as a consequence of deafferentation has been identified with areas in which receptive fields appear empty, displaced, and reorganized.[27,28] Patients report burning pain with thalamic stimulation that is referred to the painful regions of the body that is similar to the pain they experience clinically, and this elicited effect is more pronounced in patients that report allodynia and dysesthesia as part of their pain syndrome. In contrast, with stimulation in the same location in the sensory thalamus of patients without chronic pain states who are undergoing DBS for movement disorder, this group reports only sensations of nonpainful paresthesias overlaid with warmth and cold.

Stimulation of sensory fibers in the posterior limb of the internal capsule produces paresthesias that are essentially indistinguishable from sensory thalamus stimulation.[29] This suggests that similar underlying neurophysiologic mechanisms are at work. However, motor effects are common with stimulation of the internal capsule and are avoided by empirically adjusting stimulation parameters. In nonstroke patients where the thalamus is intact, there are no known benefits of using the internal capsule as the DBS target; when pain originates from a central lesion in the thalamus, however, internal capsule DBS is a clear option.[13]

Periaqueductal Gray/Periventricular Gray Deep Brain Stimulation

Stimulation of the PAG affects the experience of pain in a completely different fashion than that seen with stimulation of the thalamus. In 1969,[30] a report of powerful analgesia obtained with stimulation of the PAG in rats was followed by a series of confirmatory studies.[20,31] These studies marked a watershed in pain research by demonstrating the existence of an endogenous pain-relief mechanism in the body. Later studies demonstrated that analgesia can be produced with stimulation in an anatomically related area in the posterior wall of the third ventricle, the PVG.[32,33]

Since that time, it has been shown that rather than altering sensory pathways, the PAG is a critical player in the endogenous opioid system that extends from the arcuate to the raphe nuclei in the brain.[34] Stimulation anywhere along this system has been shown to produce analgesic effects that are reversible with naloxone.[35] Stimulation of the PAG itself has been shown to activate the endogenous opioid system[36,37] with release of met-enkephalin that coincides with pain relief[38] and to similarly increase β-endorphin levels in the cerebrospinal fluid.[39] If the opioid system is activated with PAG stimulation, then it stands to reason that tolerance to stimulation, or cross tolerance between stimulation and the analgesic effect of exogenous opioids would occur. Both

of these phenomena have indeed been described,[40] with tolerance maximizing during the first 2 years after initiation of electrical stimulation of the PAG and decreases thereafter.[41]

Much of the literature regarding PAG stimulation is not relevant to its clinical application in the setting of chronic nociceptive pain. Almost all PAG stimulation experiments have been performed using acute pain stimuli, and it is the mechanisms underlying chronic pain that appear to differ from those mediating acute pain. Nonetheless, one study in an adjuvant-induced arthritic rat model of chronic nociceptive pain demonstrated abatement of scratching and biting behaviors felt to be signs of pain through the application of periventricular stimulation.[33,42]

Indications and Target Choice

Sensory thalamic and PAG DBS are therapies that are reserved for those patients whose pain remains poorly controlled despite more conservative treatment. The low utilization of DBS for pain is in some measure due to advances in modern pain therapy and the success of spinal cord stimulators and implantable intrathecal drug delivery systems in treating chronic pain. However, even more limiting to the use of DBS is the lack of scientific evidence demonstrating safety and efficacy.

Sensory Thalamic Deep Brain Stimulation

Certain neuropathic pain conditions have been successfully treated with DBS. Among these are conditions that have a supraspinal etiology, such as refractory trigeminal pain or peripheral neuropathic conditions that are associated with extensive degeneration of dorsal column primary afferent fibers. Examples include peripheral nerve injury, postherpetic neuralgia, and phantom limb pain.[43] All of these conditions may respond to sensory thalamic stimulation. In cases where central neuropathic pain is referable to damage to the thalamus itself, the sensory limb of the internal capsule has been stimulated successfully.[12,44]

Periaqueductal Gray and Periventricular Gray Deep Brain Stimulation

There are multiple reports of PAG and PVG stimulation in patients with somatogenic or nociceptive pain. Many of these patients suffered from chronic low back pain, and relief with opiates predicted responsiveness to PAG/PVG DBS.[45–47] There have also been reports of using PAG/PVG stimulation to treat intractable pain associated with cancer and in patients with other diagnoses similarly characterized by chronic nociceptive pain, including pancreatitis, ostitis, and osteoporosis. The outcome of such studies has been variable[1,3,5,21,48] with good long-term reduction of pain ranging from 19% to 79% and treatment of nociceptive pain superior to neurogenic pain.[3] There have been more recent reports that have targeted both sensory thalamus and the PAG/PVG locations, with reportedly good results.[4]

Surgical Technique

Targeting

Ideally, the location of chronic electrodes to be implanted for DBS is determined before surgery through a combination of known coordinates relative to the anterior commissure-posterior commissure (AC-PC) line for a particular DBS target, and the use of anatomic atlases and preoperative imaging including computed tomography and magnetic resonance imaging (MRI) to directly target the structure if it can be visualized. The target for the sensory thalamus[43] is approximately 2 to 3 mm anterior to PC (y coordinate) and 12 to 13 mm from midline (x coordinate) for

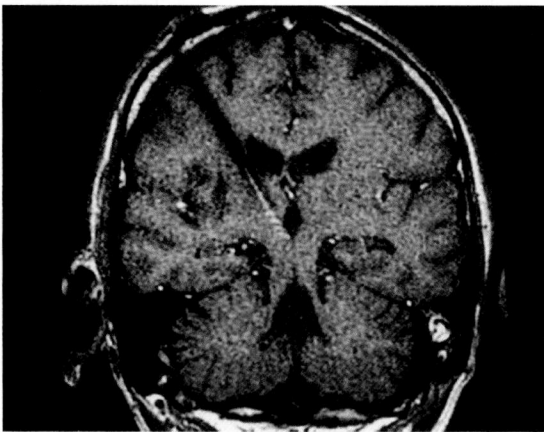

FIGURE 96.1 T1 coronal image with implanted PVG electrode. (Reproduced with permission from Owen SL, Green AL, Stein JF, et al. Deep brain stimulation for the alleviation of post-stroke neuropathic pain. *Pain* 2006;120[1–2]:202–206.)

facial pain, 14 to 15 mm for upper extremity pain, and 16 to 17 mm for lower extremity pain (Fig. 96.1). The z coordinate is approximately at the level of the AC-PC plane. The target for PVG (see Figure 96.1) is approximately 2 to 5 mm anterior to PC (y coordinate), 2 mm lateral to the medial wall of the third ventricle (x coordinate), at the level of the AC-PC plane (z coordinate).

In practice, most centers perform microelectrode recordings (MER) to confirm the trajectory and depth chosen to reach the particular target. The target is thus corroborated by the physiology of the neurons encountered during the recording pass. Some practitioners believe that MER is an absolute necessity and most practice it, but there are centers that place DBS electrodes guided solely by imaging. Such variation in practices probably reflects the fact that there is an absence of evidence that establishes the clinical superiority of microelectrode recording for the most common targets for DBS, as opposed to those used movement disorder surgery.

Potential indications and targets in DBS for pain are as indicated above: sensory VPL thalamus (or ventralis caudalis [VC] in the Hassler system), PAG, and PVG. There are many different approaches to physiologic mapping based upon MER. Single and multiunit neuronal recordings are performed at different depths along the predetermined trajectory by different surgeons with anywhere from one to five microelectrodes, and the results are typically plotted to determine the optimal trajectory and depth for chronic electrode implantation. Most practitioners use microstimulation with the microelectrode and/or macrostimulation with the chronic electrode to test for desired paresthesias in the anatomic region affected by pain and to ensure that there are no complications such as motor stimulation prior to permanent implantation. The extensiveness of the application of MER is often inversely correlated with the degree of confidence of the surgeon in the targeting accuracy, which in turn depends upon multiple factors that may include image quality and field distortion on MRI, intracranial content shift from cerebrospinal fluid loss and pneumocephalus, and change in patient position.

Microelectrode Recording

The first known report of single unit physiology was from the preparation of a muscle fiber connected to a neuron, performed over 80 years ago by a British physiologist, Lord Edgar Adrian Douglas.[49] The recording was made with an intracellular microelectrode that was created 5 years prior by a female scientist, Ida Henrietta Hyde. During the 1930s, 1940s, and 1950s, a veritable explosion in neurophysiology included such investigations as the use of the giant squid axon in elucidating the action potential, the recording of light response in the retina, and eventually to the MER mapping of the brain that is performed commonly with DBS procedures today.

The sensory thalamus is known as the VC nucleus of the thalamus in the Hassler nomenclature. Commonly used in movement disorder surgery, neurosurgeons are generally quite familiar with the ventralis intermedius (Vim) nucleus of the thalamus as a target, and VC thalamus is immediately posterior to Vim. During a typical approach, the microelectrode track starts 15 to 20 mm above the target. While the angle of approach may vary somewhat, typically the caudate is avoided by an approach just lateral to the structure. Thalamic neurons typically have large amplitude discharges without significant background spiking from more distant cells. Single unit activity is either tonic or in bursts with lower firing rates of 10–30 Hz. Recordings in VC reveal very noisy spontaneous activity and many high voltage cells. These cells generally respond to superficial light tough such as light brushing of the skin or a puff of air.[50,51] These cells respond faithfully without fatigue. The largest volume of VC is occupied by tactile cells representing the face and digits. In contrast, more anterior recordings in Vim reveal moderately active high voltage neurons that respond to contralateral passive joint movement, squeezing of muscle bellies, or pressure on deep structures such as tendons. In patients with tremor, kinesthetic cells fire rhythmically at tremor frequency.

The floor of the thalamus can be identified by the sudden loss of spontaneous neuronal activity as the microelectrode leaves the gray matter. A careful analysis of the neuronal activity of these various cell types can confirm that the appropriate target in the VC thalamus is selected. Further confirmation can be obtained with stimulation. Since Vim is thought to be the relay nucleus for kinesthetic sensation and VC the relay nucleus for superficial tactile sensation, high frequency stimulation can generally reflect this difference. The threshold (0.25–0.5 volts) for inducing paresthesias in the VC nucleus is usually much lower than that of the Vim nucleus, and in the pathologic state, the thresholds are even lower.[50] Consequently, low threshold paresthesias in the distribution of the patient's pain indicate that the electrode is correctly positioned. Neurons in the VC nucleus representing the face are found most medial, those representing the lower limbs more lateral near the internal capsule, and those representing the upper extremity and hand intermediate.

Compared to the sensory thalamus, the PVG/PAG targets are much smaller. The PVG is comprised of the nucleus endymalis and part of the nucleus parafascicularis. As a target, although it is smaller than the sensory thalamus, discrimination is easier since unlike the nuclei of the thalamus, the PVG is a discrete structure that is not surrounded by physiologically similar neurons. The trajectory of the electrode pass brings the electrode through white matter within millimeters of entry of the PVG, and due to its discrete nature the neuronal firing serves as a good confirmation marker. Intraoperative stimulation within the target produces subjective warmth that washes over the face or the torso symmetrically, even though the stimulation is unilateral. Stimulation at higher intensities may produce ocular oscillation and feelings of unease or fear.

Stimulation Regimen

For the sensory thalamus, a period of trial stimulation is performed to ensure that stimulation-induced paresthesias are present and distributed in the correct area, that they are not unpleasant or painful,[52] and that adequate pain relief is delivered. A frequency of 40 to 70 Hz is generally used, and the stimulation required to achieve this effect is typically just higher than that required to evoke paresthesias in the area of interest, and must be continued for 15 to 30 minutes. If the effect is not placebo, there is typically a poststimulation effect in patients that lasts for several hours or longer. Over the course of the first year, the pain-relief obtained may fade. In contrast to sensory thalamic stimulation, PVG stimulation is generally performed at a subthreshold intensity.

Complications

Intracranial placement of leads is associated with a small but known risk of hemorrhage that occurs in a few percent of patients. Dysesthesias and motor disturbances may occur, which can often be remedied with adjustment of stimulation parameters. Infection is a risk with any surgery, and the risk increases with the length of the surgery and the length of the trial period with externalized extension leads. Proper risk management, such as the routine use of prophylactic antibiotics and attention to sterile technique and good surgical principles, will reduce the possibility of an adverse event.

MOTOR CORTEX STIMULATION

Basic Considerations

The first motor cortex intervention for the treatment of central pain syndromes began with the observation by Penfield that stimulation of the primary motor cortex elicited sensory responses in surgical epilepsy patients. Based upon this finding, Sweet and White[53] performed pre- and postcentral gyrectomies on 3 patients with neuropathic trigeminal pain. This, while providing long-lasting pain relief, was an aggressive technique with obvious consequences, and has not been reported in the literature since.

It is not immediately obvious why stimulation of the motor cortex would relieve pain, and to date, there are conflicting theories and supporting evidence regarding the possible mechanism of MCS. Animal studies in the 1950s established that electrical stimulation of the sensorimotor cortex reduced spinal cord afferent activity.[54] Activity of spinothalamic neurons was subsequently shown to be reduced in monkeys with such stimulation.[55] The initial report of MCS was in 1990, when Tsubokawa[6] described its application in central thalamic pain with 7 patients, obtaining "excellent or good" pain relief. MCS was shown to increase cerebral blood flow, improve pain and limb movement, and decrease hemiparesis. Simultaneously, the group reported that the stimulation decreased neuronal hyperactivity in cats that were subjected to spinothalamic tractotomy; this effect occurred with motor, but not sensory, cortex stimulation. These results were in marked contrast to those of another study of cat trigeminal deafferentation pain,[22] in which stimulation of both sensory and motor cortices inhibited hyperactivity. Interestingly, activated corticofugal pathways were found to pass by both the sensory limb of the internal capsule and the sensory thalamus, both previously known stimulation targets for neuropathic pain, suggesting a similar mechanism of action. Neuronal labeling studies further demonstrated that motor cortex fibers possessed reciprocal connectivity with the sensory thalamus.[56] Recently, it was reported that the response to high intensity stimulation is selectively inhibited by MCS in rats.[57] Positron emission tomography (PET) cerebral blood flow studies performed with MCS[8,58–60] resulted in a relative decrement in thalamic blood flow with chronic pain that is ameliorated after MCS.[61–63] In a recent report, regional cerebral blood flow is increased in the thalamus, cingulate, insula, and orbitofrontal cortex following MCS (Fig. 96.2).[63] This study also suggested that decreases in subjective pain levels may be due in part to changes in mood.[63]

Indications

In clinical practice, MCS has proven useful only for neuropathic pain. Given the availability and efficacy of spinal cord stimulation

and intrathecal drug therapy, the main indications for MCS are supraspinal pain after hemorrhage and infarction,[8] postsurgical trigeminal deafferentation pain such as anesthesia dolorosa, and other forms of neuropathic facial pain such as postherpetic neuralgia. Further reports have extended the indications for surgery to include nonthalamic intracranial poststroke syndromes, including lateral brainstem infarcts,[64] phantom limb pain, multiple sclerosis, spinal cord injury, and even other neuropathic pains of the extremities.[65] In many cases, in addition to the deep, aching, and burning of central pain, these patients have shooting pain or the evoked pain of allodynia, dysesthesia, or hyperalgesia, all of which can improve markedly with MCS. For the indications described here, MCS has a better chance of success than either sensory thalamic or internal capsule stimulation.[66] For extremity neurogenic pain, it would be reasonable to perform trials for less invasive spinal cord stimulation prior to a decision regarding intracranial therapy.

Treatment efficacy for poststroke pain is variable, ranging from 45% to 75% in the overall proportion of patients reporting significant pain relief. The integrity of the corticospinal system is an important predictor of MCS efficacy; if the patient has pronounced weakness after stroke or there is difficulty in inducing motor activation with cortical stimulation during the procedure, the likelihood for a poor outcome increases dramatically.[67] There is no clear relationship between outcome and the location of the lesion that is causing central pain. Some relatively weak nonpredictive associations have been noted between MCS responsiveness and thiamylal and ketamine sensitivity and morphine resistance.[68] Success with repetitive transcranial magnetic stimulation (rTMS) may predict treatment success with MCS.[69,70] Even when the initial response is positive, however, over the course of the first year, pain relief may fade.

In contrast, outstanding results have been documented for the use of MCS in neuropathic trigeminal pain, with 75% to 100% of patients obtaining good or excellent pain relief.[7,71–73] These patients have often undergone treatment for trigeminal neuralgia and failed with one of the surgical techniques, such as glycerol, radiofrequency or balloon rhizotomy, gamma knife surgery, and even in some cases microvascular decompression. Of all brain stimulation techniques and indications, MCS for neuropathic trigeminal pain appears to be the most promising.

Surgical Technique

Anatomic identification of the motor cortex and its associated somatotopy has been a subject of multiple reports[6,8,74] going back to the classic neurophysiologic findings of Penfield in motor and sensory cortex. With modern frameless navigation equipment, image-guided intraoperative localization is becoming part of standard surgical practice. Some centers have even integrated functional MRI imaging into their localization procedure.[75] Nevertheless, localization still depends on visual identification of appropriate landmarks and therefore should be confirmed with intraoperative mapping using somatosensory evoked potentials, phase inversion, and low-frequency, high-intensity stimulation to produce peripheral muscle activity (Figs. 96.3 and 96.4). Since many patients with central pain present with severe discomfort in the distal extremities, proper somatotopic coverage may be extensive, potentially requiring wide exposure. In cases involving the distal lower extremities, exposure for electrode placement of the interhemispheric portion of the motor cortex may be necessary. In such cases, craniotomy for epidural lead placement is clearly preferable over the burr hole technique introduced by the initial practitioners of MCS.[7,72,76] In some such cases, subdural electrode placement has been used to treat distal leg pain, and it may also be performed when relief with epidural stimulation loses efficacy.[77,78]

A standard craniotomy is required for this procedure. The

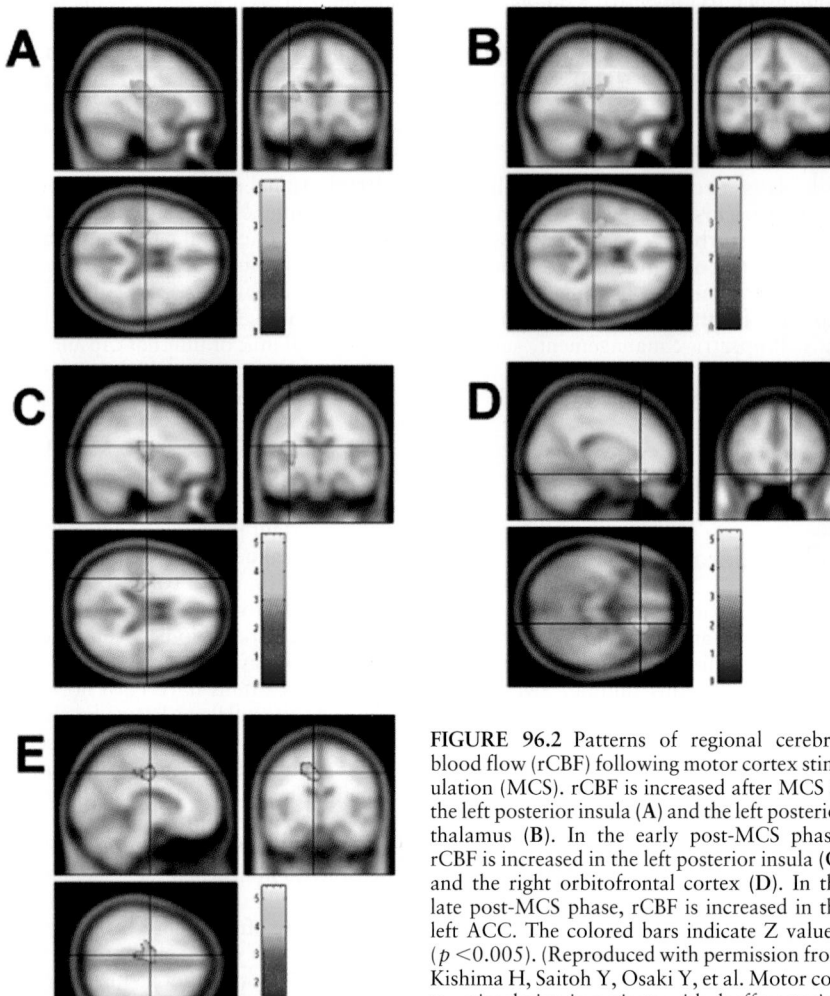

FIGURE 96.2 Patterns of regional cerebral blood flow (rCBF) following motor cortex stimulation (MCS). rCBF is increased after MCS in the left posterior insula (**A**) and the left posterior thalamus (**B**). In the early post-MCS phase, rCBF is increased in the left posterior insula (**C**) and the right orbitofrontal cortex (**D**). In the late post-MCS phase, rCBF is increased in the left ACC. The colored bars indicate Z values; ($p < 0.005$). (Reproduced with permission from Kishima H, Saitoh Y, Osaki Y, et al. Motor cortex stimulation in patients with deafferentation pain: activation of the posterior insula and thalamus. *J Neurosurg* 2007;107[1]:43–48.)

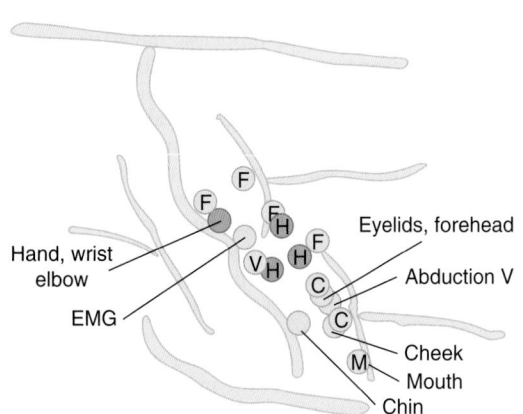

FIGURE 96.3 Blue circles correspond to position of motor cortex stimulation. Dark blue = hand, light blue = face, fingers (F), hand (H), abduction of fifth finger (V), cheek (C), mouth (M), EMG responses (EMG). (Reproduced with permission from Nguyen JP, Lefaucher JP, Le Guerinel C, et al. Motor cortex stimulation in the treatment of central and neuropathic pain. *Arch Med Res* 2000;31[3]:263–265.)

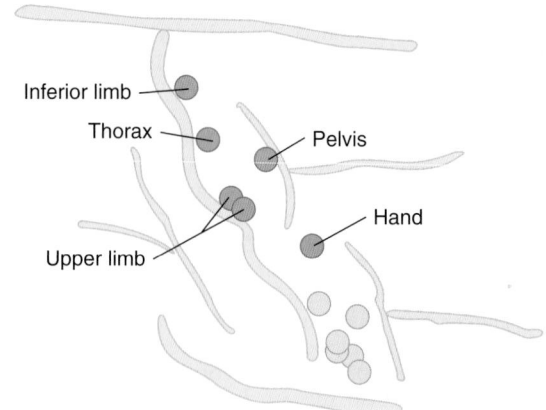

FIGURE 96.4 Circles correspond to the position of motor cortex stimulation that resulted in good or excellent pain reduction. Dark blue = hand, light blue = face. (Reproduced with permission from Nguyen JP, Lefaucher JP, Le Guerinel C, et al. Motor cortex stimulation in the treatment of central and neuropathic pain. *Arch Med Res* 2000;31[3]: 263–265.)

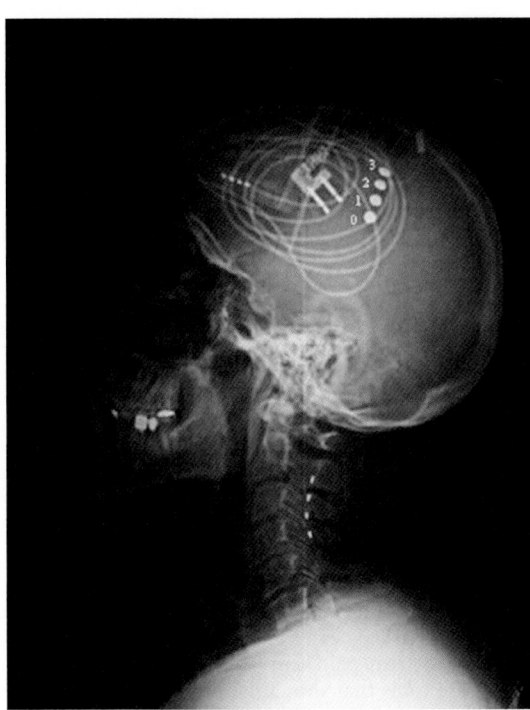

FIGURE 96.5 Skull radiograph of a patient with an epidural electrode over the right motor cortex for MCS. (Reproduced with permission from Di Lazzaro V, Oliviero A, Pilato F, et al. Comparison of descending volleys evoked by transcranial and epidural motor cortex stimulation in a conscious patient with bulbar pain. *Clin Neurophysiol* 2004;115[4]: 834–838.)

electrode is placed in the epidural position (Fig. 96.5). More than one electrode may be necessary to provide coverage of the required area for stimulation in patients with central pain. The procedure has been performed with induction of either local[7,64,66,67,71–73,76,79,80] or general anesthesia.[77,81–85] Like all surgical procedures where hardware is implanted, careful technique and strict antibiotic prophylaxis is required.

Stimulation Regimen

As in sensory thalamic DBS and spinal cord stimulation, a period of trial stimulation of 2 or more weeks is typical. Stimulation-induced paresthesias are not usually present with MCS,[7,8] but pain relief generally occurs after a few minutes of stimulation and improves over the ensuing 10 to 15 minutes. There is typically a poststimulation effect in patients that lasts for several hours or longer. Usually, a cycle mode of 5 to 30 minutes of stimulation is followed by minutes to hours with the stimulation off. A wide range of frequencies from 5 to 130 Hz and pulse durations from 60 to 450 μsec have been used with success. Intensity is often set in a range from 0.5 to 10 volts to at an appropriate subthreshold level, for example, 80% of the voltage required for muscle contraction.[86,87] Pain relief is most common at voltages around 5 volts, and amplitudes greater than 6 volts have been associated with seizures during programming, especially as the amplitude approaches 9 volts.[88] A customized empiric approach is usually utilized for each patient to adjust each of the parameters to increase pain relief while limiting side effects for each patient.

Complications

Surgical complications, including infection and epidural hematoma, have been reported with MCS. Local pain at the site of the electrode has in a few cases required dural denervation.[8] Like all previously discussed surgical procedures, the risk of infection is always present, heightened by the necessity of hardware implantation. Hardware breakage is also possible, requiring surgery for repair.

Complications due to stimulation include seizures that have been reported during the trial phase of MCS when multiple stimulation parameters are tested, but no reports have noted the progression of seizures beyond the trial phase. Other side effects from stimulation include dysesthesias[67,72,89], dysarthria, and fatigue.[82]

TRANSCRANIAL MAGNETIC STIMULATION

Basic Considerations

Repetitive TMS is a therapy was applied to psychiatric and neurodegenerative diseases prior to consideration for pain. It is reasonable that with the advent of this new technology, trials using primary motor cortex as the rTMS target would occur for pain syndromes that have benefited from MCS. The underlying rationale for the use of rTMS comes from MCS studies, with the implicit assumption that rTMS might have similar or related effects on the motor cortex as electrical stimulation. PET blood flow studies suggest that there are several brain areas that are affected by MCS (see discussion in previous MCS section). Some reports suggest that rTMS of motor cortex creates a physiologic effect that is similar, but not identical to electrical stimulation.[90] A 2006 study with rTMS showed improvement with stimulation of primary motor cortex, but not with sensory, supplementary motor, or premotor cortex stimulation.[91] This finding does correlate with what we know about the anatomic target of MCS, and indeed suggests that rTMS may have a similar physiologic basis of action.[92] In addition, as with MCS, pain relief can last beyond stimulation, but the poststimulation duration is shorter, lasting minutes to hours for rTMS compared to hours to days with MCS.

Targeting

Determination of the target area for rTMS can be performed with frameless navigation systems that are similar to the ones neurosurgeons use in the operating theater.[91] Repetitve TMS is applied through a coil that is held and positioned with an articulated coil holder, and the motor threshold is then determined with stimulation (Fig. 96.6). Single pulse TMS can be used to elicit

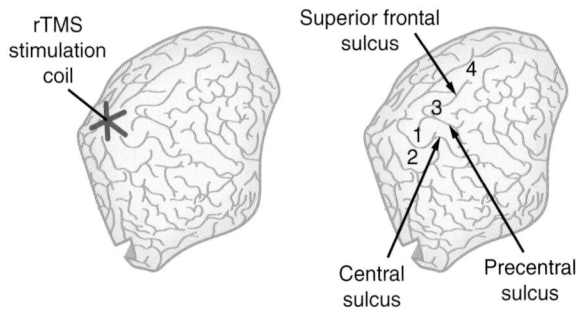

FIGURE 96.6 The use of a navigation system for rTMS. The stimulation coil (left) is centered over the motor cortex; the numbers on the right show motor cortex (1), relative to the sensory cortex (2), the premotor area (3), and the supplementary motor area (4). (Reproduced with permission from Hirayama A, Saitoh Y, Kishima H, et al. Reduction of intractable deafferentation pain by navigation-guided repetitive transcranial magnetic stimulation of the primary motor cortex. *Pain* 2006;122[1–2]: 22–27.)

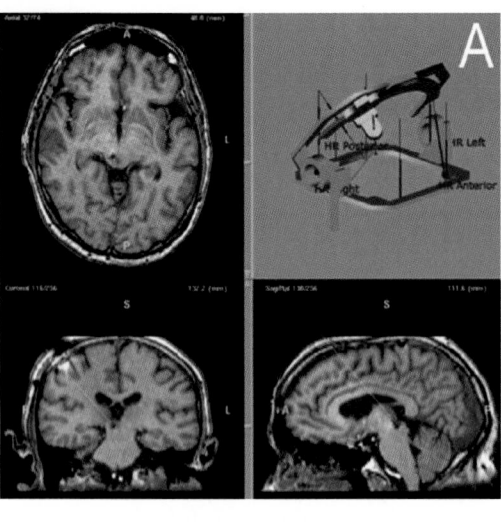
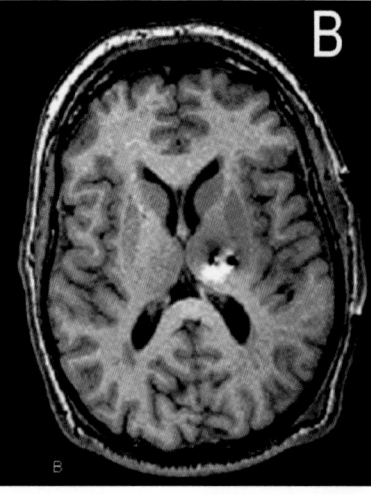

FIGURE 96.7 A. T1-weighted MRI showing planned trajectory ad target for placement of a PAG/PVG in the axial, frontal, and sagittal planes. **B.** Postoperative MRI showing VPL electrode (lateral) and the wire to the PVG electrode (medial and inferior). (Reproduced with permission from Owen SL, Green AL, Stein JF, et al. Deep brain stimulation for the alleviation of post-stroke neuropathic pain. *Pain* 2006;120[1–2]:202–206.)

muscle twitching on electromyography (EMG), so it is possible to map the area corresponding to each extremity, including the painful areas.[93–95] In areas with substantial damage to motor fibers, stimulation of up to 100 A/μs can be used, with higher stimulation intensities resulting in scalp pain.[91] In some studies, electroencephalography recordings and craniometric principles were used for target localization, but there is substantial difficulty and a lack of repeatability in freehand performance of stimulation. Thus it is recommended to utilize a frameless navigation system for localization of the primary motor cortex. The principle of combining an accurate targeting technology with neurophysiologic confirmation is utilized in the stereotactic placement of DBS electrodes with MER. Analogously, the best option for rTMS is the use of a frameless navigation system with single pulse TMS for neurophysiologic confirmation.[91]

Stimulation Parameters

After determination of the motor threshold, typically the stimulation intensity is set at 80% or 90% below the threshold level. Stimulation is then performed in trains of pulses with intervals between the trains. For example, a routine rTMS session of 500 stimulations may consist of 10 trains of 10 second TMS pulses of 5 Hz, allowing 50 second intervals between trains. High frequency rTMS enhances and low frequency inhibits neuronal firing in the cortex.[96,97] Repetitive TMS at high frequencies of 10 to 20 Hz has been reported to result in good pain control,[95,98] while rTMS at a low frequency of 1 Hz was effective only in one report in normal patients with acute nociceptive pain from capsaicin.[99] It is possible that the choice of stimulation frequency may depend upon the type of pain that is being treated. For example, poststroke central pain seems to respond better to low frequency rTMS, while trigeminal neuropathy responds to high frequencies.

CONCLUSION

Neuropathic pain is a difficult to treat effectively. It is often not responsive to drug therapy, and the only recourse becomes surgical intervention with the implantation of some form of stimulation device. While stimulation therapies may not offer complete relief, good outcomes are far from rare and offer possibilities for patients who have exhausted typical avenues of treatment. Chronic nociceptive pain, most commonly represented by patients with back pain, is similarly a problem that can be difficult to

treat with pharmacologic intervention alone. The neurosurgeon's armamentarium should include the full range of implanted intrathecal drug delivery devices and stimulation technologies for these difficult to treat pain conditions. Deep brain and cortical stimulation are tools that should be part of this armamentarium and should be among the options available to patients, especially those with supraspinal pain where spinal pain therapies are irrelevant. In extremity and back pain, these therapies should be considered when spinal therapies fail to provide pain relief.

Unfortunately, DBS for pain has suffered from a lack of high quality studies, despite anecdotal and limited observational evidence that suggest its use would appropriate in certain conditions where other therapies are not available. Prospective, well-designed studies with uniform, structured protocols for patient selection, implantation, and stimulation should be performed with MCS to ensure that this promising therapy does not suffer the same fate. Since paresthesias are not a hallmark of MCS, it is possible to prospectively study this therapy by providing stimulation to patients in a blinded fashion. Such studies are critical since, when properly applied, MCS can offer carefully selected patients the possibility of pain relief where no other therapies or recourses are available. It is possible that patients with syndromes that do not respond to MCS may respond to DBS at either the PVG/PAG or the sensory thalamic target. It is also possible that in some intractable cases where stimulation at any one site does not provide complete relief, combination stimulation therapy with leads in multiple sites (Fig. 96.7) including combinations of spinal cord and intracranial interventions, could provide pain relief.

References

1. Richardson DE. Deep brain stimulation for the relief of chronic pain. *Neurosurg Clin N Am* 1995;6(1):135–144.
2. Levy RM, Lamb S, Adams JE. Treatment of chronic pain by deep brain stimulation: long term follow-up and review of the literature. *Neurosurgery* 1987; 21(6):885–893.
3. Gybels J, Kupers R, Nuttin B. Therapeutic stereotactic procedures on the thalamus for pain. *Acta Neurochir (Wien)* 1993;124(1):19–22.
4. Owen SL, Green AL, Stein JF, et al. Deep brain stimulation for the alleviation of post-stroke neuropathic pain. *Pain* 2006;120(1–2):202–206.
5. Kumar K, Toth C, Nath RK. Deep brain stimulation for intractable pain: a 15-year experience. *Neurosurgery* 1997;40(4):736–746, discussion 746–747.
6. Tsubokawa T, Katayama Y, Yamamoto T, et al. Treatment of thalamic pain by chronic motor cortex stimulation. *Pacing Clin Electrophysiol* 1991;14(1): 131–134.
7. Meyerson BA, Lindblom U, Linderoth B, et al. Motor cortex stimulation as treatment of trigeminal neuropathic pain. *Acta Neurochir Suppl (Wien)* 1993; 58:150–153.
8. Nguyen JP, Lefaucheur JP, Decg P, et al. Chronic motor cortex stimulation in

the treatment of central and neuropathic pain. Correlations between clinical, electrophysiological and anatomical data. *Pain* 1999;82(3):245–251.

9. Ervin FR, Brown CE, Mark VH. Striatal influence on facial pain. *Confin Neurol* 1966;27(1):75–90.

10. Gol A. Relief of pain by electrical stimulation of the septal area. *J Neurol Sci* 1967;5(1):115–120.

11. Hosobuchi Y, Adams JE, Rutkin B. Chronic thalamic stimulation for the control of facial anesthesia dolorosa. *Arch Neurol* 1973;29(3):158–161.

12. Hosobuchi Y, Adams JE, Rutkin B. Chronic thalamic and internal capsule stimulation for the control of central pain. *Surg Neurol* 1975;4(1):91–92.

13. Adams JE, Hosobuchi Y, Fields HL. Stimulation of internal capsule for relief of chronic pain. *J Neurosurg* 1974;41(6):740–744.

14. Mazars GJ. Intermittent stimulation of nucleus ventralis posterolateralis for intractable pain. *Surg Neurol* 1975;4(1):93–95.

15. Head H, Holmes G. Sensory disturbances from cerebral lesions. *Brain* 1911: 34:102–254.

16. Fields HL, Adams JE. Pain after cortical injury relieved by electrical stimulation of the internal capsule. *Brain* 1974;97(1):169–178.

17. Nyquist JK, Greenhoot JH. Responses evoked from the thalamic centrum medianum by painful input: suppression by dorsal funiculus conditioning. *Exp Neurol* 1973;39(2):215–222.

18. Gerhart KD, Yezierski RP, Fang ZR, et al. Inhibition of primate spinothalamic tract neurons by stimulation in ventral posterior lateral (VPLc) thalamic nucleus: possible mechanisms. *J Neurophysiol* 1983;49(2):406–423.

19. Benabid AL, Henriksen SJ, McGinty JF, et al. Thalamic nucleus ventro-posterolateralis inhibits nucleus parafascicularis response to noxious stimuli through a non-opioid pathway. *Brain Res* 1983;280(2):217–231.

20. Mayer DJ, Liebeskind JC. Pain reduction by focal electrical stimulation of the brain: an anatomical and behavioral analysis. *Brain Res* 1974;68(1):73–93.

21. Duncan GH, Bushnell MC, Marchand S. Deep brain stimulation: a review of basic research and clinical studies. *Pain* 1991;45(1):49–59.

22. Namba S, Nishimoto A. Stimulation of internal capsule, thalamic sensory nucleus (VPM) and cerebral cortex inhibited deafferentation hyperactivity provoked after gasserian ganglionectomy in cat. *Acta Neurochir Suppl (Wien)* 1988;42:243–247.

23. Kupers RC, Gybels JM. Electrical stimulation of the ventroposterolateral thalamic nucleus (VPL) reduces mechanical allodynia in a rat model of neuropathic pain. *Neurosci Lett* 1993;150(1):95–98.

24. Tasker RR. Identification of pain processing systems by electrical stimulation of the brain. *Hum Neurobiol* 1982;1(4):261–272.

25. Tasker RR, DeCarvalho GT, Dolan EJ. Intractable pain of spinal cord origin: clinical features and implications for surgery. *J Neurosurg* 1992;77(3): 373–378.

26. Lenz FA, Seike M, Richardson RT, et al. Thermal and pain sensations evoked by microstimulation in the area of human ventrocaudal nucleus. *J Neurophysiol* 1993;70(1):200–212.

27. Lenz FA, Tasker RR, Dostrovsky JO, et al. Abnormal single-unit activity recorded in the somatosensory thalamus of a quadriplegic patient with central pain. *Pain* 1987;31(2):225–236.

28. Rinaldi PC, Young RF, Albe-Fessard D, et al. Spontaneous neuronal hyperactivity in the medial and intralaminar thalamic nuclei of patients with deafferentation pain. *J Neurosurg* 1991;74(3):415–421.

29. Namba S, Wani T, Shimizu Y, et al. Sensory and motor responses to deep brain stimulation. Correlation with anatomical structures. *J Neurosurg* 1985; 63(2):224–234.

30. Reynolds DV. Surgery in the rat during electrical analgesia induced by focal brain stimulation. *Science* 1969;164(878):444–445.

31. Mayer DJ, Wolfle TL, Akil H, et al. Analgesia from electrical stimulation in the brainstem of the rat. *Science* 1971;174(16):1351–1354.

32. Rhodes DL, Liebeskind JC. Analgesia from rostral brain stem stimulation in the rat. *Brain Res* 1978;143(3):521–532.

33. Kupers RC, Vos BP, Gybels JM. Stimulation of the nucleus paraventricularis thalami suppresses scratching and biting behaviour of arthritic rats and exerts a powerful effect on tests for acute pain. *Pain* 1988;32(1):115–125.

34. Sakata S, Shima F, Kato M, et al. Dissociated mesencephalic responses to medial and ventral thalamic nuclei stimulation in rats. Relationship to analgesic mechanisms. *J Neurosurg* 1989;70(3):446–453.

35. Akil H, Mayer DJ, Liebeskind JC. Antagonism of stimulation-produced analgesia by naloxone, a narcotic antagonist. *Science* 1976;191(4230):961–962.

36. Basbaum AI, Clanton CH, Fields HL. Opiate and stimulus-produced analgesia: functional anatomy of a medullospinal pathway. *Proc Natl Acad Sci U S A* 1976;73(12):4685–4688.

37. Yaksh TL, Yeung JC, Rudy TA. Systematic examination in the rat of brain sites sensitive to the direct application of morphine: observation of differential effects within the periaqueductal gray. *Brain Res* 1976;114(1):83–103.

38. Young RF, Bach FW, Van Norman AS. Release of beta-endorphin and methionine-enkephalin into cerebrospinal fluid during deep brain stimulation for chronic pain. Effects of stimulation locus and site of sampling. *J Neurosurg* 1993;79(6):816–825.

39. Akil H, Richardson DE, Hughes J, et al. Enkephalin-like material elevated in ventricular cerebrospinal fluid of pain patients after analgetic focal stimulation. *Science* 1978;201(4354):463–465.

40. Hosobuchi Y. Tryptophan reversal of tolerance to analgesia induced by central grey stimulation. *Lancet* 1978;2(8079):47.

41. Kumar K, Wyant GM, Nath R. Deep brain stimulation for control of intracta-

42. De Castro Costa M, De Sutter P, Gybels J, et al. Adjuvant-induced arthritis in rats: a possible animal model of chronic pain. *Pain* 1981;10(2):173–185.

43. Hamani C, Schwalb JM, Rezai AR, et al. Deep brain stimulation for chronic neuropathic pain: long-term outcome and the incidence of insertional effect. *Pain* 2006;125(1–2):188–196.

44. Namba S, Nakao Y, Matsumoto Y, et al. Electrical stimulation of the posterior limb of the internal capsule for treatment of thalamic pain. *Appl Neurophysiol* 1984;47(3):137–148.

45. Hosobuchi Y. Subcortical electrical stimulation for control of intractable pain in humans. Report of 122 cases (1970–1984). *J Neurosurg* 1986;64(4):543–553.

46. Tsubokawa T, Yamamoto T, Katayama Y, et al. Thalamic relay nucleus stimulation for relief of intractable pain. Clinical results and beta-endorphin immunoreactivity in the cerebrospinal fluid. *Pain* 1984;18(2):115–126.

47. Arnér S, Meyerson BA. Lack of analgesic effect of opioids on neuropathic and idiopathic forms of pain. *Pain* 1988;33(1):11–23.

48. Gybels J, Kupers R. Central and peripheral electrical stimulation of the nervous system in the treatment of chronic pain. *Acta Neurochir Suppl (Wien)* 1987; 38:64–75.

49. Adrian ED, Zotterman Y. The impulses produced by sensory nerve-endings: part II. The response of a single end-organ. *J Physiol* 1926;61(2):151–171.

50. Lenz FA, Dostrovsky JO, Kwan HC, et al. Methods for microstimulation and recording of single neurons and evoked potentials in the human central nervous system. *J Neurosurg* 1988;68(4):630–634.

51. Albe-Fessard D, Arfel G, Guiot G, et al. Electrophysiological studies of some deep cerebral structures in man. *J Neurol Sci* 1966;3(1):37–51.

52. Tasker RR, Vilela Filho O. Deep brain stimulation for neuropathic pain. *Stereotact Funct Neurosurg* 1995;65(1–4):122–124.

53. Lende RA, Kirsch WM, Druckman R. Relief of facial pain after combined removal of precentral and postcentral cortex. *J Neurosurg* 1971;34(4):537–543.

54. Lindblom UF, Ottosson JO. Influence of pyramidal stimulation upon the relay of coarse cutaneous afferents in the dorsal horn. *Acta Physiol Scand* 1957; 38(3–4):309–318.

55. Coulter JD, Maunz RA, Willis WD. Effects of stimulation of sensorimotor cortex on primate spinothalamic neurons. *Brain Res* 1974;65(2):351–356.

56. Rouiller EM, Tanné J, Moret V, et al. Dual morphology and topography of the corticothalamic terminals originating from the primary, supplementary motor, and dorsal premotor cortical areas in macaque monkeys. *J Comp Neurol* 1998;396(2):169–185.

57. Senapati AK, Huntington PJ, Peng YB. Spinal dorsal horn neuron response to mechanical stimuli is decreased by electrical stimulation of the primary motor cortex. *Brain Res* 2005;1036(1–2):173–179.

58. Canavero S, Bonicalzi V. Cortical stimulation for central pain. *J Neurosurg* 1995;83(6):1117.

59. Peyron R, Garcia-Larrea L, Deiber MP, et al. Electrical stimulation of precentral cortical area in the treatment of central pain: electrophysiological and PET study. *Pain* 1995;62(3):275–286.

60. Hsieh JC, Meyerson BA, Ingvar M. PET study on central processing of pain in trigeminal neuropathy. *Eur J Pain* 1999;3(1):51–65.

61. García-Larrea L, Peyron R, Mertens P, et al. Electrical stimulation of motor cortex for pain control: a combined PET-scan and electrophysiological study. *Pain* 1999;83(2):259–273.

62. Saitoh Y, Osaki Y, Nishimura H, et al. Increased regional cerebral blood flow in the contralateral thalamus after successful motor cortex stimulation in a patient with poststroke pain. *J Neurosurg* 2004;100(5):935–939.

63. Kishima H, Saitoh Y, Osaki Y, et al. Motor cortex stimulation in patients with deafferentation pain: activation of the posterior insula and thalamus. *J Neurosurg* 2007;107(1):43–48.

64. Katayama Y, Tsubokawa T, Yamamoto T. Chronic motor cortex stimulation for central deafferentation pain: experience with bulbar pain secondary to Wallenberg syndrome. *Stereotact Funct Neurosurg* 1994;62(1–4):295–299.

65. Brown JA, Barbaro NM. Motor cortex stimulation for central and neuropathic pain: current status. *Pain* 2003;104(3):431–435.

66. Tsubokawa T, Katayama Y, Yamamoto T, et al. Chronic motor cortex stimulation in patients with thalamic pain. *J Neurosurg* 1993;78(3):393–401.

67. Katayama Y, Fukaya C, Yamamoto T. Poststroke pain control by chronic motor cortex stimulation: neurological characteristics predicting a favorable response. *J Neurosurg* 1998;89(4):585–591.

68. Yamamoto T, Katayama Y, Hirayama T, et al. Pharmacological classification of central post-stroke pain: comparison with the results of chronic motor cortex stimulation therapy. *Pain* 1997;72(1–2):5–12.

69. Migita K, Uozumi T, Arita K, et al. Transcranial magnetic coil stimulation of motor cortex in patients with central pain. *Neurosurgery* 1995;36(5): 1037–1039, discussion 1039–1040.

70. Krings T, Naujokat C, von Keyserlingk DG. Representation of cortical motor function as revealed by stereotactic transcranial magnetic stimulation. *Electroencephalogr Clin Neurophysiol* 1998;109(2):85–93.

71. Ebel H, Rust D, Tronnier V, et al. Chronic precentral stimulation in trigeminal neuropathic pain. *Acta Neurochir (Wien)* 1996;138(11):1300–1306.

72. Nguyen JP, Keravel Y, Feve A, et al. Treatment of deafferentation pain by chronic stimulation of the motor cortex: report of a series of 20 cases. *Acta Neurochir Suppl* 1997;68:54–60.

73. Rainov NG, Fels C, Heidecke V, et al. Epidural electrical stimulation of the

motor cortex in patients with facial neuralgia. *Clin Neurol Neurosurg* 1997; 99(3):205–209.

74. Herregodts P, Stadnik T, De Ridder F, et al. Cortical stimulation for central neuropathic pain: 3-D surface MRI for easy determination of the motor cortex. *Acta Neurochir Suppl* 1995;64:132–135.

75. Roux FE, Ibarrola D, Tremoulet M, et al. Methodological and technical issues for integrating functional magnetic resonance imaging data in a neuronavigational system. *Neurosurgery* 2001;49(5):1145–1156; discussion 1156–1157.

76. Nguyen JP, Lefaucher JP, Le Guerinel C, et al. Motor cortex stimulation in the treatment of central and neuropathic pain. *Arch Med Res* 2000;31(3):263–265.

77. Saitoh Y, Shibata M, Hirano S, et al. Motor cortex stimulation for central and peripheral deafferentation pain. Report of eight cases. *J Neurosurg* 2000;92(1): 150–155.

78. Tani N, Saitoh Y, Hirata M, et al. Bilateral cortical stimulation for deafferentation pain after spinal cord injury. Case report. *J Neurosurg* 2004;101(4): 687–689.

79. Sharan AD, Rosenow JM, Turbay M, et al. Precentral stimulation for chronic pain. *Neurosurg Clin N Am* 2003;14(3):437–444.

80. Son UC, Kim MC, Moon DE, et al. Motor cortex stimulation in a patient with intractable complex regional pain syndrome type II with hemibody involvement. Case report. *J Neurosurg* 2003;98(1):175–179.

81. Brown JA, Pilitsis JG. Motor cortex stimulation for central and neuropathic facial pain: a prospective study of 10 patients and observations of enhanced sensory and motor function during stimulation. *Neurosurgery* 2005;56(2): 290–297, discussion 290–297.

82. Carroll D, Joint C, Maartens N, et al. Motor cortex stimulation for chronic neuropathic pain: a preliminary study of 10 cases. *Pain* 2000;84(2–3):431–437.

83. Nuti C, Peyron R, Garcia-Larrea L, et al. Motor cortex stimulation for refractory neuropathic pain: four year outcome and predictors of efficacy. *Pain* 2005; 118(1–2):43–52.

84. Roux FE, Ibarrola D, Lazorthes Y, et al. Chronic motor cortex stimulation for phantom limb pain: a functional magnetic resonance imaging study: technical case report. *Neurosurgery* 2001;48(3):681–687, discussion 687–688.

85. Velasco M, Velasco F, Brito F, et al. Motor cortex stimulation in the treatment of deafferentation pain. I. Localization of the motor cortex. *Stereotact Funct Neurosurg* 2002;79(3–4):146–67.

86. Bonicalzi V, Canavero S. Motor cortex stimulation for central and neuropathic pain (Letter regarding Topical Review by Brown and Barbaro). *Pain* 2004; 108(1–2):199–200, author reply 200.

87. Henderson JM, Lad SP. Motor cortex stimulation and neuropathic facial pain. *Neurosurg Focus* 2006;21(6):E6.

88. Henderson JM, Boongirl A, Rosenow JM, et al. Recovery of pain control by intensive reprogramming after loss of benefit from motor cortex stimulation for neuropathic pain. *Stereotact Funct Neurosurg* 2004;82(5–6):207–213.

89. Fukaya C, Katayama Y, Yamamoto T, et al. Motor cortex stimulation in patients with post-stroke pain: conscious somatosensory response and pain control. *Neurol Res* 2003;25(2):153–156.

90. Di Lazzaro V, Oliviero A, Pilato F, et al. Comparison of descending volleys evoked by transcranial and epidural motor cortex stimulation in a conscious patient with bulbar pain. *Clin Neurophysiol* 2004;115(4):834–838.

91. Hirayama A, Saitoh Y, Kishima H, et al. Reduction of intractable deafferentation pain by navigation-guided repetitive transcranial magnetic stimulation of the primary motor cortex. *Pain* 2006;122(1–2):22–27.

92. Kimbrell TA, Dunn RT, George MS, et al. Left prefrontal-repetitive transcranial magnetic stimulation (rTMS) and regional cerebral glucose metabolism in normal volunteers. *Psychiatry Res.* 2002;115(3):101–113.

93. Lefaucheur JP, Drouot X, Menard-Lefaucheur I, et al. Neurogenic pain relief by repetitive transcranial magnetic cortical stimulation depends on the origin and the site of pain. *J Neurol Neurosurg Psychiatry* 2004;75(4):612–616.

94. Lefaucheur JP, Drouot X, Keravel Y, et al. Pain relief induced by repetitive transcranial magnetic stimulation of precentral cortex. *Neuroreport* 2001; 12(13):2963–2965.

95. Pleger B, Janssen F, Schwenkreis P, et al. Repetitive transcranial magnetic stimulation of the motor cortex attenuates pain perception in complex regional pain syndrome I. *Neurosci Lett* 2004;356(2):87–90.

96. Kimbrell TA, Little JT, Dunn RT, et al. Frequency dependence of antidepressant response to left prefrontal repetitive transcranial magnetic stimulation (rTMS) as a function of baseline cerebral glucose metabolism. *Biol Psychiatry* 1999; 46(12):1603–1613.

97. Speer AM, Kimbrell TA, Wassermann EM, et al. Opposite effects of high and low frequency rTMS on regional brain activity in depressed patients. *Biol Psychiatry* 2000;48(12):1133–1141.

98. Töpper R, Foltys H, Meister IG, et al. Repetitive transcranial magnetic stimulation of the parietal cortex transiently ameliorates phantom limb pain-like syndrome. *Clin Neurophysiol.* 2003;114(8):1521–1530.

99. Tamura Y, Okabe S, Ohnishi T, et al. Effects of 1-Hz repetitive transcranial magnetic stimulation on acute pain induced by capsaicin. *Pain* 2004;107(1–2): 107–115.

CHAPTER 97 ■ DIAGNOSTIC AND THERAPEUTIC NERVE BLOCKS

MICHELE CURATOLO AND NIKOLAI BOGDUK

INTRODUCTION

Local anesthetic blocks are procedures in which a local anesthetic agent is deliberately injected onto a peripheral nerve in order to temporarily stop conduction of action potentials along it. Local anesthetic agents block conduction of action potentials by acting on the sodium channels of the nerve cell membranes. Their effect is temporary because their pharmacologic action is reversible.

Nerve blocks are an attractive tool in pain medicine because they are the only means by which to stop pain completely. Analgesics may reduce pain, but only local anesthetics stop it.

Virtually any nerve in the body can be blocked in order to relieve pain. All that is required is access to the nerve and the agent with which to anesthetize it. Many textbooks and manuals have been published that describe the techniques used to do so, but it is not the intention or purpose of this chapter to duplicate these publications. Many of the available procedures have an application in anesthesia for surgical procedures, but they are not germane to the practice of pain medicine. Some procedures have a role in securing relief of pain postoperatively; for those, the distinction between the discipline of pain medicine and the practice of anaesthesia is uncertain.

This chapter focuses on the principles of local anesthetic blocks used in pain medicine. It illustrates the more commonly used and useful procedures and reviews the evidence concerning their validity and utility. Neurolytic blocks are covered in Chapters 45, 64, 71, and 103.

APPLICATIONS

The short duration of action of local anesthetic agents limits the utility of local anesthetic blocks in pain medicine. For acute pain, their premier utility lies in providing protection from incident pain. For chronic pain, their premier use is as a diagnostic test. Otherwise, they have putative roles as a prognostic test and as palliative interventions.

COMMON PRINCIPLES

Irrespective of the purpose for which local anesthetic blocks are used, certain principles apply. These pertain to the physician, the patient, the preparation for the procedure, its contraindication, the procedure itself, and its complications.

Physician

Any physician who performs nerve blocks should be suitably trained and experienced. He or she needs to understand the pain problem being addressed and how the proposed procedure relates to the patient's management. He or she needs to be familiar with the patient, the patient's complaints, and how the patient expresses him- or herself. The physician should be able to explain to the patient the nature and significance of the procedure to be undertaken and, together with the patient, be able to assess and interpret the response. These requirements require training in more than the execution of the procedure.

The physician needs a detailed knowledge of the anatomic basis of the procedure, not only to execute it accurately but also to avoid complications. Similarly, he or she needs to be able to deal with the possible side effects and complications of local anaesthetic agents. For procedures performed under radiologic guidance, the physician needs to be able to obtain the correct views and to interpret them accurately.

More difficult to define and to achieve is technical excellence to perform the procedure expeditiously yet accurately with the minimum of stress to the patient. This includes avoiding painful structures during the insertion of the needle and keeping the number of adjustments during its course to a minimum. Acquisition of these skills requires good mentoring or forethought on the part of the practitioner and may take months or years of training.

Patient

The patient should understand the purpose of the procedure to be undertaken. This requires distinguishing between diagnostic and therapeutic procedures. Unless they are properly informed, patients may mistake a diagnostic block as a treatment and be disappointed when it appears not to have worked when the effect wears off. When a therapeutic block lacks evidence of efficacy, the patient should understand that the chances of success are unknown and that any estimate might be entirely speculative. In this regard, there is a difference between a patient consenting to a procedure and being fully informed about it.

The patient should be aware of the potential side effects and complications of the procedures, what actions are to be taken to avoid them, and what will be done in the event that they occur.

Both for diagnostic blocks and therapeutic blocks, the patient will be required to assess and report their response. Therefore, before the procedure the patient should be instructed in how to use instruments such as the visual analog scale or numerical pain-rating scale. Patients who have pain in multiple sites but who undergo blocks for only one site need to understand which pain is being tested and must be able to report the effects of the block on that particular site of pain. Relief of pain will need to be corroborated by testing activities that usually are limited by pain. For this purposes, the patient must be able to specify a set of suitable activities before the block and be able to test for their restoration after the block.

Preparation

The preparation of the patient differs according to the nature of procedure to be undertaken and the region in which the target nerve lies. For most procedures, and particularly for those that involve small doses of local anesthetic agents, standard preparations are neither indicated nor required.

Orders for "nil by mouth" are indicated only for procedures in which loss of consciousness and aspiration of gastric contents are possible complications. Examples include cervical transforaminal blocks and procedures that involve high doses of local anesthetic. In the opinion and experience of the authors, the majority of nerve blocks can be performed safely with the patient having had a light meal 2–4 hours before the procedure. Indeed, fasting may compromise the procedure if the patient is uncomfortable or distressed for not having eaten.

For most local anesthetic blocks, establishing an intravenous line is not indicated nor is continuous monitoring of respiratory and cardiovascular function required. The doses of local anesthetic typically administered do not pose hazards that require these preparations. However, appropriate precautions are indicated for procedures that are performed close to vital structures, such as the spinal cord or the vertebral artery, or when large doses of a local anesthetic agent are to be administered. In such cases, an intravenous line should be placed before the procedure in order to ensure access for the rapid administration of fluids and resuscitation drugs, should these be necessary. Vital functions should be monitored (i.e., electrocardiogram, pulse oximetry, and blood pressure). A means of ventilating the patient with 100% oxygen with a bag and mask or via endotracheal tube and suction should be available, along with drugs and equipment to manage a cardiac arrest.

Local anesthetic blocks do not require routine sedation. Proper explanation, continuous communication, and good technique will provide patient comfort without the need for systemic medication. In the case of diagnostic blocks, there is a theoretical risk that using sedation may confound the validity of response, for which reason it is best avoided. In addition, sedation may mask the onset of central nervous complications of local anesthetics and, therefore, delay early intervention.

Only occasional patients will require sedation: those who are markedly apprehensive or who have a manifest anxiety over needles or invasive procedures. In such cases, sedation can be secured by intravenous administration of modest doses of sedatives (midazolam, propofol) or short-acting opioids (fentanyl, alfentanil, remifentanil). The dose should be titrated so as to provide sufficient sedation only for the duration of the procedure; the patient should be fully awake after the procedure in order to be able to report its effects. If sedation is used, it should be complemented with monitoring of respiratory and cardiovascular function. Supplemental oxygen may be required.

Contraindications

Blocks are contraindicated in patients who are unwilling to undergo the procedure or who have attributes that compromise the safe execution of the procedure. The latter include inability to lie still, allergy to the drugs to be used, infection at the site of injection, and anatomic abnormalities.

A coagulation disorder or anticoagulation therapy is a relative contraindication. Blocks of superficial nerves in easily accessible parts of the body may be safely undertaken. Reservations apply for blocks of deep nerves in sites where hemorrhage could compromise vital structures. Patients with compromised cardiovascular function are more susceptible to either the toxic effects of local anesthetic or the effects of blockade of sympathetic nerves. Appropriate precautions should be taken with such patients if large volumes of a local anesthetic agent are to be used.

Complications

The potential complications of local anesthetic blocks can be categorized as systemic effects of the drugs injected, physiologic effects of the procedure, inadvertent damage to structures other than nerves, and damage to nerves.

Systemic Effects

Allergy to local anesthetic agents is rare. The physiologic consequences and treatment are as for any anaphylactic reaction.

Local anesthetics have direct toxic effects on the central nervous system (CNS) and cardiovascular system (CVS). These effects become increasingly pronounced as blood levels of the offending agent rise. High or rapidly rising blood levels can occur because of inadvertent intravascular injection of the local anesthetic, unusually rapid absorption from a highly vascular region, or the administration of an excessive dose of agent.

Several precautions can be taken to reduce the risk of intravascular injection. For procedures performed under fluoroscopic guidance, a test dose of contrast medium can be administered before injecting the local anesthetic agent. This will show vascular uptake. For procedures where the uptake may be to a small but vital vessel, such as a radicular artery, digital subtraction angiography serves to demonstrate the vessel more clearly. For injections undertaken without radiographic guidance, certain steps can test for intravascular injection or reduce its consequences.

The needle should be aspirated before injection and after each 2–5 mL of injectate, if such volumes are used, in order to ensure no bloody return. For blocks using large volumes, 3–4 mL of a mixture of local anaesthetic plus 1:200,000 epinephrine (15–20 μg) may be injected as an initial test dose. If injected intravascularly, such a mixture will cause, with a high degree of probability, a brief and transient (2–3 minutes) rise in the heart rate of 20–25 beats per minute, and a rise in systolic blood pressure of 20–30 points because of the beta and alpha effects of the epinephrine.[1] This precaution was originally developed to detect inadvertent intravascular injection during epidural anaesthesia, but it applies equally well for other regional techniques.

A rising, or high, blood level of local anaesthetic is typically manifest by the onset of CNS features such as anxiety, agitation, tinnitus, muscle twitching, peri-oral numbness or tingling, and dizziness. As plasma levels rise, tonic-clonic seizures can occur. At even higher plasma levels, neuronal inhibition occurs leading to respiratory arrest, coma, and cardiovascular collapse. Although most anesthetics produce signs of CNS toxicity prior to either seizure or CVS toxicity, this is not always the case. With highly lipophilic, highly protein bound agents (e.g., bupivacaine), CVS collapse may even precede CNS symptoms.[2]

If a patient manifests features of toxicity during the course of an injection, the injection should be stopped immediately and assistance should be enlisted or summoned. Oxygen (100%), via a bag and mask, should be commenced immediately. If the patient's oxygen saturation, as judged from pulse oximetry, falls below 90%, positive pressure ventilation should be instituted. A small, anticonvulsant dose of thiopental (50–100 mg) should be administered. Cardiovascular parameters should be monitored and adverse effects treated: hypotension with fluids and pressors (ephedrine 5–10 mg); hypertension with vasodilators (labetalol 5–10 mg); and tachycardia with beta blockers (esmolol 5 mg, metoprolol 2.5–5 mg).

These measures will often abort progressive local anesthetic toxicity. However, if the toxicity appears to be proceeding toward convulsions (agitation, limb jerking, loss of consciousness), further measures are necessary. Positive pressure ventilation with oxygen should be commenced in order to ensure oxygen saturation greater than 90%. If ventilation is difficult, or if the patient convulses, muscle paralysis with 50–100 mg succinylcholine should be administered to ensure adequate ventilation. Cardiovascular monitoring and treatment of adverse CVS effects should continue. Recent evidence from animal studies[3–5] and a number of case reports of successful resuscitation from cardiovascular collapse following local anesthetic toxicity suggest that intravenous administration of lipid emulsion may be a life-saving adjunct.[6–9]

Physiologic Effects

Although undertaken to relieve pain, nerve blocks will, or may, block other sensory functions, motor function, balance, and sympathetic function. When these are to be expected but pose no immediate hazard, the patient should be warned to expect them and to not be alarmed by their onset. Appropriate precautions should be taken to compensate against loss of function and to avoid injury. Examples of side effects pertinent to blocks used in pain medicine are numbness or weakness in the limb following spinal nerve blocks, ataxia following third occipital nerve blocks, and hypotension or Horner's syndrome following sympathetic nerve blocks.

Blocks targeting particular nerves may spill over to adjacent nerves and produce unwanted effects (e.g., intercostal nerve blocks may produce inadvertent epidural blockade; brachial plexus blocks may produce sympathalgia or phrenic nerve block). Patients undergoing such blocks should be closely monitored for adverse effects and treated early and vigorously in the event that they do occur.

Damage to Non-neural Structures

The needles used for local anesthetic blocks have the potential to pierce and damage structures along the course of the insertion or near the target point. Examples include pneumothorax following intercostal nerve block or thoracic spinal nerve block, piercing the esophagus during stellate ganglion blocks, piercing pelvic viscera during sacral spinal nerve blocks, and penetrating the aorta or inferior vena cava during celiac plexus blocks.

Piercing a blood vessel has the potential to produce bleeding or hematoma. In patients with normal clotting mechanisms, it is rare for such bleeding or hematoma to produce significant sequelae. In patients with abnormal coagulation, bleeding may produce hypovolemia, and hematoma may exert pressure effects on adjacent structures. For these reasons, coagulopathy is a relative contraindication for local anaesthetic blocks.

Damage to Nerves

Targeting a nerve with an injection carries the risk of nerve damage. The resultant symptoms range from minor paraesthesia to severe pain. The damage may be caused by piercing the nerve with the needle or by what is injected. Components of the injectate, such as preservative, may be neurotoxic, epinephrine may cause spasm of the vasa nervorum and result in ischemic damage, or the pressure of injection may damage the nerve physically. A prospective audit, at one institution, found that the incidence of neuropathy, encountered following 1065 blocks for surgery, was 0.22%.[10]

Procedure

In order to be valid or effective, nerve blocks need to be accurate. This involves placing the injection as close as possible to the target nerve. Several techniques are available to secure accurate placement. They differ for unaided (i.e., "blind") techniques and for image-guided techniques.

Blind Techniques

For blind techniques, the oldest method of correct needle placement is to probe the nerve gently with the tip of the needle. This maneuver produces a paraesthesia in the area of distribution of the nerve. Once paraesthesia is elicited, the needle is held steady and the local anaesthetic is injected. This technique, however, has now become almost obsolete. Probing some nerves (e.g., autonomic nerves) does not elicit paraesthesia but, more importantly, probing nerves risks damaging them.

Mixed nerves, containing sensory and motor fibers, can be located by using an insulated needle connected to a peripheral nerve stimulator. By passing an electric current through the needle, the motor fibers in the nerve are stimulated, producing a twitch in the muscles supplied by the nerve. This stimulation is usually not painful because motor fibers are activated at lower current intensity than sensory fibers. A typical setting is a frequency of 1–2 Hz and a current strength of 1 mA. At this setting, a twitch will be produced as the needle approaches the nerve but still lies some distance from it. Reducing the current to 0.4–0.5 mA allows the needle to be advanced further. A well-defined twitch at this intensity of current implies that the needle is close to the nerve.

Data from clinical anesthesia practice show a high success rate of blocks facilitated by a nerve stimulator.[11] However, large volumes of local anesthetic are typically administered for operative anesthesia, and it is unclear if these data can be extrapolated to blocks in pain medicine, in which small volumes of local anesthetic are used in order to maximize the selectivity of the block. Although rare, neurologic complications may occur when nerve stimulators are used.[12]

For some blocks, palpable landmarks can be used to secure the accuracy of the block. A classical example is the intercostal block, for which the rib is an adequate landmark for the target site.

Image-Guided Techniques

When nerves and landmarks are not palpable and precision is required, unaided techniques do not ensure accuracy and selectivity of the block. In such circumstances, image guidance can be used to secure safety, accuracy, and selectivity.

Fluoroscopy is the most commonly used form of image guidance in pain medicine. Its limitations are that fluoroscopy shows only bones. Therefore, it is suitable only for target nerves that bear a dependable relationship to a bony landmark. The accuracy of the block is achieved by directing the needle to the landmark. Safety is achieved both by choosing a course that does not incur intervening structure that should not be damaged and by having the needle not stray from the intended target. Selectivity is achieved by administering a test-dose of contrast medium to establish that the injectate will flow into the region of the target nerve and will not flow onto other structures where anesthetization might compromise the selectivity of the block. The advantages of fluoroscopy are that it demonstrates a wide field of view around the target region; with C-arm fluoroscopy, views of any orientation can be obtained in order to define the location of the needle during its course or at its target point; intermittent images are rapidly applied and continuous imaging is possible if required; and the apparatus is not excessively expensive, which keeps the cost of the procedure at acceptable levels. A particular advantage of fluoroscopy is that, in the event of intravascular injection, it will reveal rostral or caudal flow of contrast medium away from the target point. This facility is not available from devices that produce planar images.

Some operators use computed tomography (CT) guidance instead of fluoroscopy. They are attracted by the definition that CT provides of viscera and vessels that should be avoided by the needle. Ostensibly, this allows for a safer placement of the needle. For injections into narrow joint cavities or irregularly orientated joints such as the sacroiliac joint, CT offers the virtue of depicting the cavity and its orientation directly. Consequently, a path for the needle can be planned to coincide directly with the joint. The disadvantages of CT guidance are numerous. Each time the needle position is checked, the patient must be rescanned. This interrupts the procedure, prolongs it, and involves considerable radiation exposure. More critically, planar image does not reveal flow of contrast medium in vessels that run out of the plane of view. Serial reconstruction does not compensate for this because by the time the images are acquired, the contrast medium will have left the field of view. Safety with respect to inadvertent intravascular injection has not been demonstrated for CT guidance. CT is far more expensive than fluoroscopy. For these reasons, fluoroscopic guidance remains the modality of choice for pain medicine procedures. Only in selected cases would CT guidance be justified.

Ultrasound guidance is being increasingly used and explored in pain medicine.[13] It demonstrates muscles, ligaments, vessels, joints, and bones. Moreover, if high-resolution transducers are used, thin nerves can be directly visualized. Ultrasound does not involve radiation exposure, either to the patient or to the operator, and continuous screening can be used. Fluid injected is easily visualized in a real-time fashion. Ultrasound is less expensive than CT and may be less expensive than fluoroscopy. For these reasons, ultrasound guidance is emerging as an attractive alternative to other modalities of image guidance. Its limitations, at present, are the poor resolution of narrow-gauge needles (although, with experience, operators can infer the location of the needle from the movements of the soft tissues) and, in anatomically complex regions, echoes from overlying structures interfere with the image of the target area. The available data are too sparse to endorse or recommend the routine use of ultrasound for procedures in which fluoroscopy has an established role.

TEST BLOCKS

Test blocks are ones that are not therapeutic injections, prognostic tests, or diagnostic tests in the strict and correct sense of those terms. They are performed simply to test if a particular nerve is involved in the patient's symptoms. A nerve is anesthetized and the response is either that the patient's pain is relieved or not. The block is not prognostic because it is not used to predict the outcomes of any subsequent treatment. Nor is it diagnostic because the block is not used to distinguish one source of pain from another. It is used only to see if the nerve anesthetized is involved in the patient's symptoms.

Virtually any nerve in the body can be blocked in this way. Examples include supraorbital blocks for headache, suprascapular nerve blocks for pain in the shoulder, blocks of the median, ulnar, or radial nerves for pain in the hand, lateral femoral cutaneous nerves blocks for meralgia paraesthetica, ilioinguinal and iliohypogastric nerve blocks for pain after herniography, tibial nerve blocks for pain in the foot, and phrenic nerve blocks for shoulder pain or hiccups.

Proponents have typically stated that such blocks can produce "useful information," but the nature of that information, and its utility, have been poorly elaborated. In some cases, the blocks are used to "confirm" the diagnosis, but the diagnosis will already be evident from other clinical information. It may be satisfying to the operator to be able to relieve the patient's pain. The patient may find it gratifying to have their pain relieved, but any effect will be temporary because of the limited duration of action of local anaesthetic agents. The pivotal question—both clinically and philosophically—is: what then?

If the patient's response is used to predicate a subsequent treatment, the test becomes a prognostic block. In that event, however, the block and the response to it need to be valid, and the treatment needs to be effective. If those requirements are not satisfied, the blocks amount to no more than an interesting exercise.

In this context, the art of performing local anesthetic blocks has not been developed into a clinical science. Although a nerve may be blocked and although pain might be relieved, the validity and utility of this information has not been developed.

Particularly egregious in this regard is the practice of paravertebral blocks. Thoracic paravertebral blocks have been advo-

cated for pain in the chest wall, lumbar paravertebral blocks for determining specific nociceptive pathways, and transsacral blocks for back pain or pelvic pain. In the first instance, paravertebral blocks are not target-specific; they have not been shown to anesthetize particular nerves or particular nociceptive pathways specifically. In particular, they are of no diagnostic value for spinal pain, for the block is directed to ventral rami, distal to any afferents from the vertebral column. Nor have any controlled studies shown that responses to these blocks are valid. If pain pathways need to be sought, fluoroscopically-guided spinal nerve blocks have greater face validity. Individual nerves can be selectively targeted accurately, and injections can be constrained to affect only that nerve.

PROGNOSTIC BLOCKS

A prognostic block is one undertaken to test if a definitive treatment will be successful. The rationale is that if a nerve block with local anesthetic relieves the pain, then a treatment capable of interrupting conduction along the nerve should relieve the pain for a prolonged period, if not permanently.

For prognostic blocks to be valid, evidence is required to complete a table like that depicted in Table 97.1. There needs to be a strong association between a positive response to the block and a successful outcome from treatment and between a negative response to the block and failure of treatment. Such data are hard to produce and are simply not available. They would require a study in which patients undergo treatment irrespective of their response to blocks. They also require a treatment that is dependably effective. Unless that is the case, failures may be due to the failure of treatment rather than an error in the response to blocks. Few such treatments exist.

In the absence of proper evidence, practitioners who use prognostic blocks assume that a positive response to a block should be predictive of a favorable outcome to treatment. This has not always proven to be the case. In the past, prognostic blocks of peripheral somatic nerves were used to test the outcome of surgical neurectomy. This treatment proved ineffective. Neuroma formation and deafferentation pain complicated the treatment. Positive responses to sympathetic blocks have not consistently been associated with favorable or sustained outcomes from sympathectomy—either surgical or chemical. In such cases, it is not evident if the response to blocks was false or if sympathectomy is intrinsically not effective.

Spinal Nerve Blocks

In some patients with radicular pain, medical imaging is not diagnostic. CT or magnetic resonance imaging (MRI) may show more than one spinal nerve affected by a disc herniation or by foraminal

---

TABLE 97.1

A CONTINGENCY TABLE ILLUSTRATING THE NATURE OF EVIDENCE REQUIRED TO ESTABLISH THE VALIDITY OF A PROGNOSTIC BLOCK

		Response to treatment	
		Relief	No relief
Response to prognostic block	Relief	a	b
	No relief	c	d

stenosis, and the clinical features do not help to determine which nerve is the source of symptoms. Spinal nerve blocks were developed to assist surgeons to determine the symptomatic level in such cases so that surgery could be directed at the correct segmental level.

Spinal nerve blocks involve placing a needle, under fluoroscopic guidance, into the intervertebral foramen that lodges the target nerve. If anesthetizing that nerve relieves the patient's pain, then that nerve is implicated as the source of pain. If anesthetizing the nerve does not relieve the pain, that nerve is excluded as the source of pain, and investigations can be redirected to another nerve.

Cervical Spinal Nerve Blocks

Because of the proximity of the vertebral artery and the spinal cord, cervical spinal nerve blocks require consummate skill in obtaining the correct view, delivering the needle, and checking its location. Comprehensive guidelines for the safe conduct of the procedure have been published by the International Spine Intervention Society.[14]

An oblique view of the cervical spine is obtained such that the target intervertebral foramen is maximally wide. A spinal needle is inserted so that it initially touches the anterior edge of the superior articular process behind the foramen. From this position, the tip of the needle is adjusted so that it enters the foramen, tangential to the anterior surface of the superior articular process, approximately opposite the equator of the foramen (Fig. 97.1A). In an anteroposterior view, the tip of the needle is adjusted so that it lies opposite the longitudinal bisector of the articular pillar (Fig. 97.1B).

Once the needle has been placed, a test dose of contrast medium is injected to check that the injection is not intravascular (Fig. 97.1C), and a further dose is injected to show that the injectate flows medially along the nerve as far as the dural sac (Fig. 97.1D). Once flow has been shown to be safe and appropriate, between 0.5 and 1.5 mL of 1% lidocaine (or an alternative local anesthetic) is then injected.

Lumbar Spinal Nerve Blocks

Various techniques for lumbar spinal nerve blocks have been described. They differ essentially in terms of the depth to which the needle is inserted. The classical technique requires placing the needle on the anterior wall of the intervertebral foramen, just below the pedicle. Other techniques involve placing the needle above the target nerve or behind it. Explicit guidelines for each of these techniques have been prepared by the International Spine Intervention Society.[15]

The subpedicular approach aims at a target point immediately below the 6 o'clock position on the pedicle that lies above the target nerve. If this target point is obstructed by the lamina, by the superior articular process, or by a flange of the transverse process, the fluoroscope is adjusted in a manner to move the obstructing structure out of the line of view (Fig. 97.2). A spinal needle is then inserted toward the target point, taking care not to touch or injure the nerve. Its final position is checked on anteroposterior and lateral views (Fig. 97.3A,B). A test dose of contrast medium is injected to check that the injection is not intravascular and that the injectate flows along the target nerve (Fig. 97.3C,D). Once correct flow has been achieved, 1–1.5 mL of local anesthetic (0.5% bupivacaine or

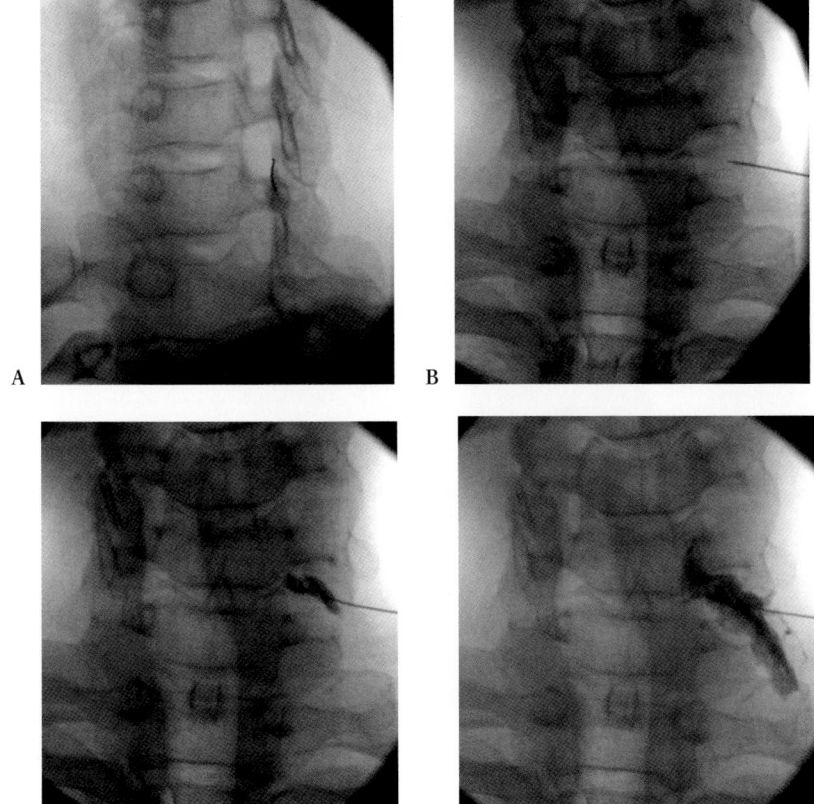

FIGURE 97.1 Steps in the execution of a C7 spinal nerve block. **A.** Oblique view showing a needle in position tangential to the superior articular process of C7. **B.** Anteroposterior view of the needle, showing its tip midway across the width of the articular pillars. **C.** Anteroposterior view of a test dose of contrast medium injected into the intervertebral foramen. **D.** Anteroposterior view after injection of sufficient contrast medium to reach the dural sac. (Radiographs provided by Dr. Paul Dreyfuss, Seattle, WA, and reproduced with permission from Bogduk N, ed. *Guidelines for Spinal Diagnostic and Treatment Procedures.* San Francisco: International Spine Intervention Society; 2004.)

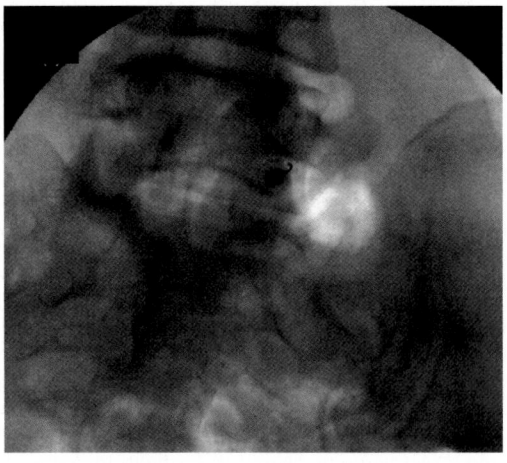

FIGURE 97.2 An oblique view of a needle passing to the subpedicular target point for an L5 spinal nerve block.

2% lidocaine) can be injected. In order to ensure adequate anesthetization of the nerve, some operators elect to deliver the local anesthetic in equal aliquots in front of, above, and behind the nerve. To do so requires withdrawing the needle slightly and monitoring its position in lateral views.

Sacral Spinal Nerve Blocks

Sacral spinal nerve blocks are a complement to lumbar spinal nerve blocks in that the S1 spinal nerve is commonly affected by lumbar spine pathology. In practice, they are effectively limited to S1 spinal nerve blocks. Techniques for other sacral spinal nerves have not been described nor has an application been described. However, the technique would be analogous to that for S1.

S1 spinal nerve blocks involve introducing a spinal needle through the S1 posterior sacral foramen and into the sacral canal (Fig. 97.4). This procedure requires familiarity and versatility with the radiographic anatomy of the posterior sacrum because the posterior sacral foramen may be hard to identify. Care needs to be taken not to insert the needle too far such that it passes through the anterior sacral foramen and into the pelvic cavity. Detailed guidelines for this procedure have been published.[15]

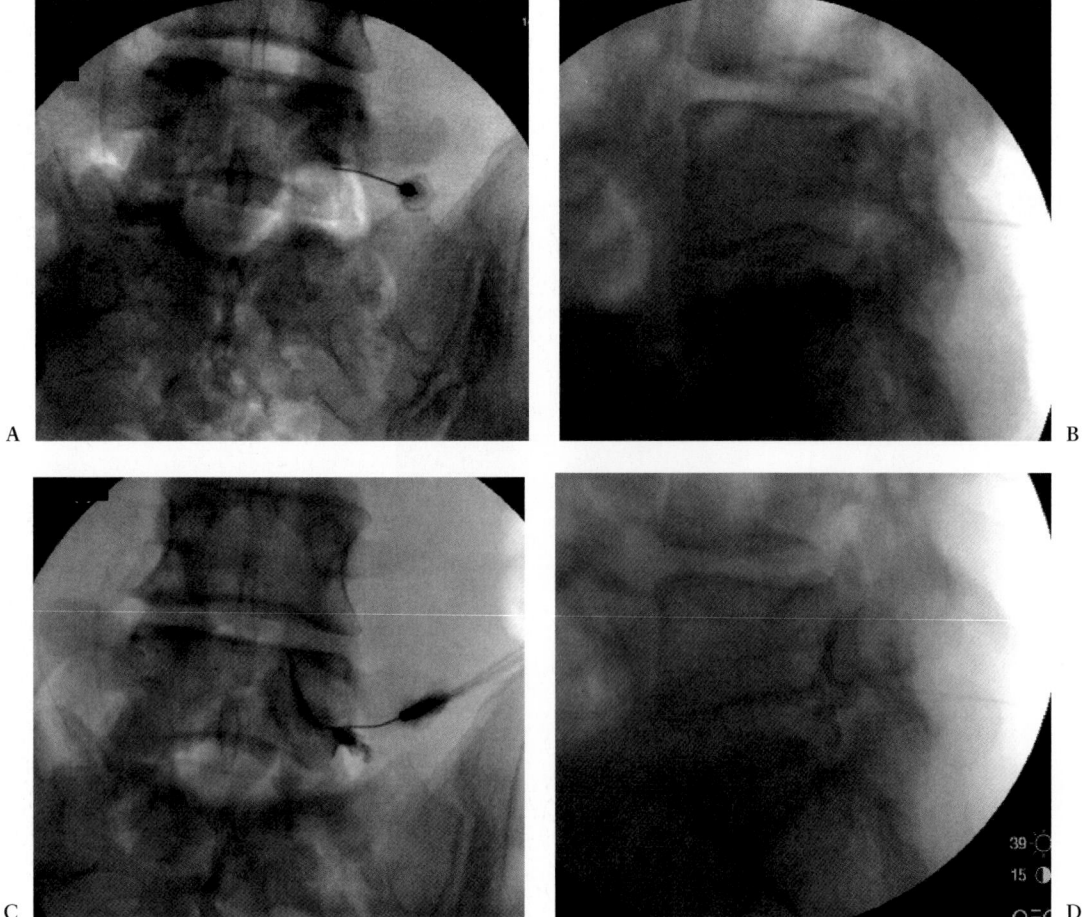

FIGURE 97.3 Steps in the execution of an L5 spinal nerve block. **A.** Anteroposterior view showing a needle delivered below the pedicle of L5. **B.** Lateral view showing the tip of the needle on the back of the vertebral body. **C.** Anteroposterior view showing contrast medium outlining the target nerve. **D.** Lateral view showing contrast medium running rostrally behind the vertebral body.

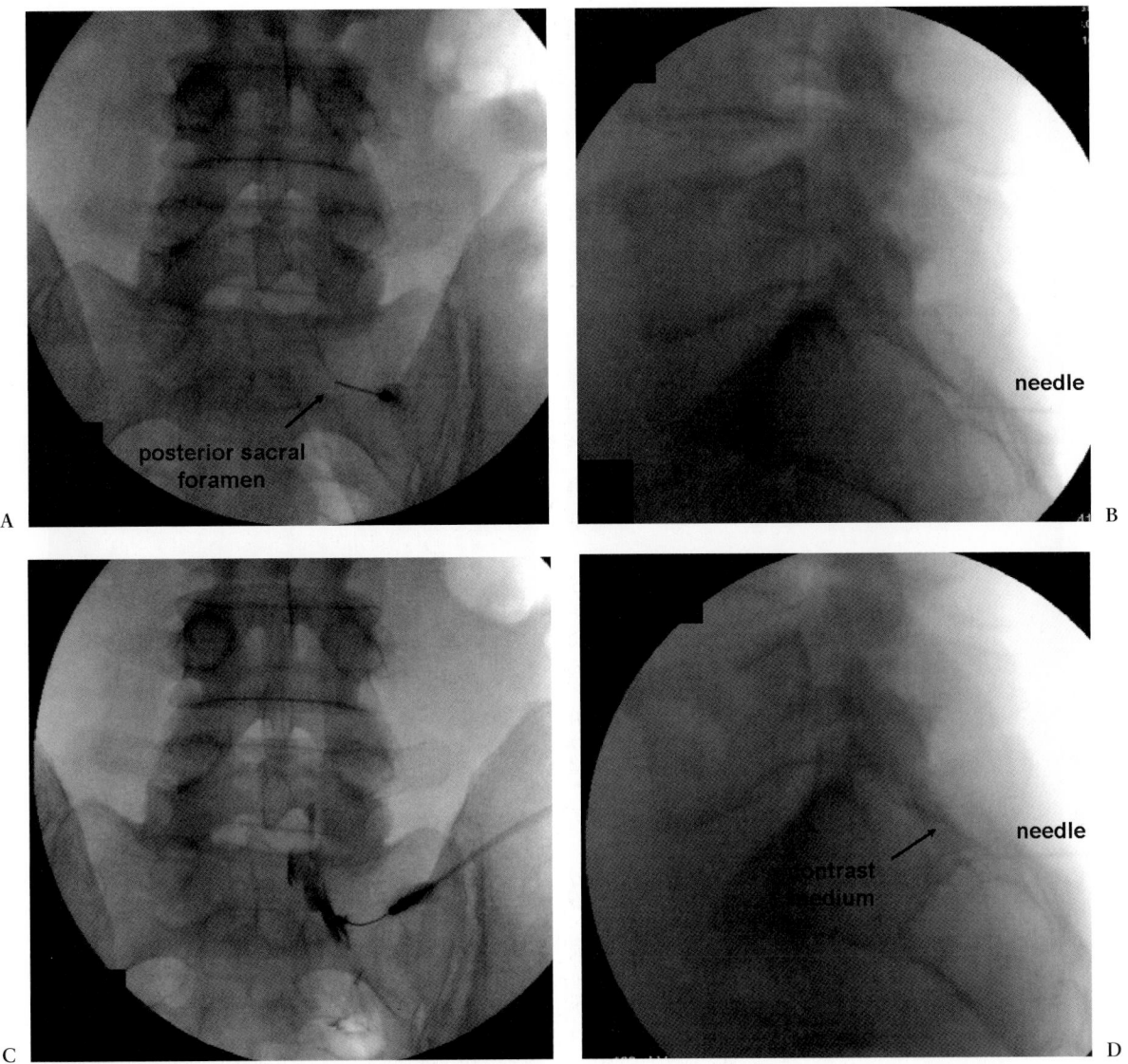

FIGURE 97.4 Steps in the execution of an S1 spinal nerve block. **A.** Anteroposterior view of a need placed through the S1 posterior sacral foramen. **B.** Lateral view showing the tip of the needle inside the sacral canal. **C.** Anteroposterior view showing contrast medium outlining the target nerve. **D.** Lateral view showing contrast medium running rostrally through the sacral canal.

Thoracic Spinal Nerve Blocks

There have been no published studies of the utility of thoracic spinal nerve blocks, but guidelines for their performance have been published.[16] In practice, they are sometimes performed to select patients for radiofrequency treatment of thoracic spinal nerves[17,18] and in the diagnosis of neuropathic pain affecting the chest wall.

The technique recommended by the International Spine Intervention Society involves placing a needle first onto the edge of the lamina overlying the target spinal nerve and then advancing the needle beyond the edge until its tip rests just behind the nerve (Fig. 97.5).[16] This maneuver is facilitated by prebending the tip of the needle slightly so that it can be rotated laterally off the lamina and subsequently medially into the intervertebral foramen. The technique requires careful adjustment of the needle in order not to injure the nerve. Once the needle has been placed, contrast medium is used to check for appropriate flow of injectate along the nerve (see Fig. 97.5) and to avoid intravascular injection.

Validity

Data on the validity of spinal nerve blocks are limited because of two factors. First, nerve blocks should be performed under controlled conditions in order to guard against false-positive responses, but only one study of spinal nerve blocks has used control blocks. Secondly, the predictive validity of blocks requires a study in which patients with positive responses to blocks and patients with negative responses both be submitted to treatment. Only such a study would provide proper data on the sensitivity and specificity of the blocks. Such studies are difficult to justify ethically and have not been conducted.

Partial data are available from studies that report the proportion of patients with positive responses to blocks in whom pathology is found at surgery. This proportion is not the sensitivity of the test, but is its positive predictive value in the sample tested. Since that value is dependent on the nature of the sample studied, it is not generalizable to other samples or to practice at large.

For lumbar spinal nerve blocks, various studies have reported positive predictive values that ranged between 80% and

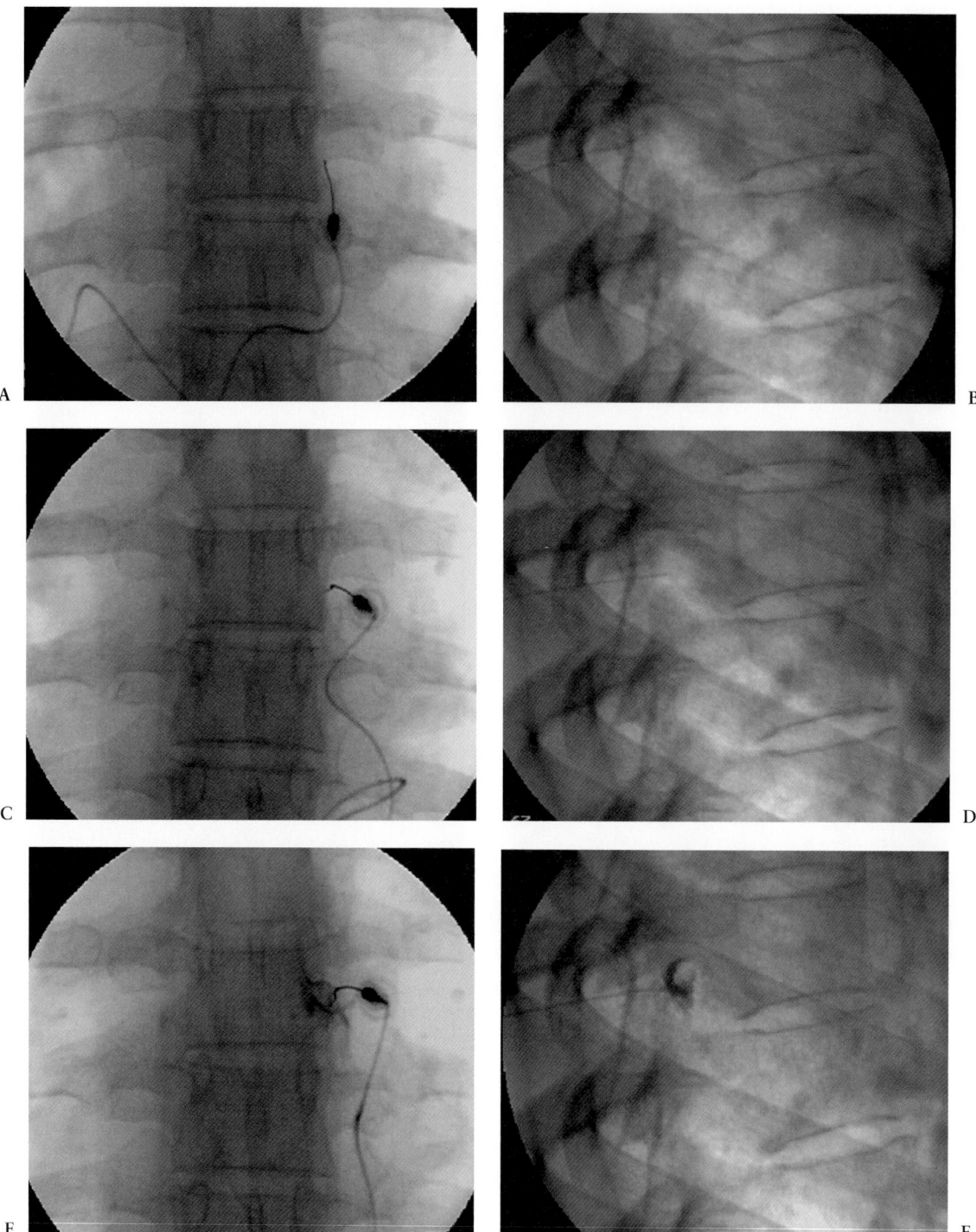

FIGURE 97.5 Steps in the execution of a thoracic spinal nerve block. **A.** Anteroposterior view of a needle placed on the edge of the dorsal surface of the lamina. **B.** Lateral view of the needle resting on the dorsal surface of the lamina. **C.** Anteroposterior view of the needle inserted slightly more deeply, lateral to the lamina, with its tip directed medially. **D.** Lateral view of the needle with its tip projecting just beyond the lamina and lying dorsal to the spinal nerve. **E.** Anteroposterior view of an injection of contrast medium that outlines the nerve. **F.** Lateral view of the injection of contrast medium. (Radiographs produced by Dr. Way Yin, Bellingham, WA, and reproduced with permission from Bogduk N, ed. *Guidelines for Spinal Diagnostic and Treatment Procedures.* San Francisco: International Spine Intervention Society; 2004.

100%.[19–22] These high values imply that the false-positive rate of lumbar spinal nerve blocks is low and, therefore, that their specificity is likely to be high. In one study, a small number of patients with negative responses to blocks nevertheless underwent surgery.[21] Pathology was found in all cases but not at the level tested; in no case did surgery find pathology at the level tested when the block had been negative. These patients proved to have multilevel disease or anomalous nerve roots. This implies that the false-negative rate of lumbar spinal nerve blocks is low and, therefore, that their sensitivity is high.

One study measured sensitivity by performing lumbar spinal nerve blocks in 46 patients with clinical and radiologic evidence of nerve root compression, subsequently confirmed at surgery.[23] The sensitivity was 100%, with 95% confidence intervals of 88% to 100%. That same study measured specificity by performing blocks in 23 patients at levels known by radiology not to be symptomatic. No false-positive responses were encountered, and the specificity of lumbar spinal nerve blocks was estimated as "around 90%."[23]

The one study that used controlled blocks enlisted 18 patients with cervical radiculopathy and 83 with lumbar radiculopathy but did not stratify the results according to region investigated.[24] Using a criterion standard of good outcome from surgery, it found a sensitivity of 93% but a specificity of only 33%. Spinal nerve blocks were no better than MRI in predicting good outcome, but the particular advantage of spinal nerve blocks demonstrated in this study was the ability of negative responses to blocks to predict poor outcome, particularly when MRI was negative or ambiguous.

No studies have explored the predictive validity of either cervical or thoracic spinal nerve blocks. When used to select patients for procedures such as dorsal root ganglion radiofrequency, these blocks have been assumed to be valid, but that validity has not been established.

SYMPATHETIC BLOCKS

Blocks of various elements of the sympathetic nervous system have a status somewhere intermediate between diagnostic and prognostic. They are not diagnostic in the strict sense of that adjective, for the cause of pain is usually evident from clinical assessment or other investigations. Fundamentally, they are used to test if the patient's clinical features are mediated by sympathetic nerves. Knowing this does not affect management unless the response to blocks is used to prognosticate the response to neurolytic treatment of the sympathetic nerves.

Cervical Sympathetic Blocks

Cervical sympathetic blocks have been used largely in the evaluation of patients with complex regional pain syndromes of the upper limb. Other applications have been for patients with pain in the face or head.

The procedure requires delivering an aliquot of local anesthetic onto the stellate ganglion. The traditional approach has been a blind technique based on surface markings and palpation. The alternative is a fluoroscopically-guided technique.

The blind technique classically involved injecting a large volume of local anesthetic in order to ensure saturation of the ganglion. Whereas this might be acceptable for therapeutic or palliative purposes, large volumes compromise the validity of cervical sympathetic blocks because structures other than the target nerve are anesthetized. Indeed, one critic has declared that very little of the injectate reaches the area of the stellate ganglion and much spreads elsewhere.[25] In a study of eight volunteers, MRI showed that injectate was not delivered to the stellate ganglion but passed

anterior to it.[26] For these reasons, a fluoroscopically-guided technique is preferred.

The lower cervical sympathetic chain runs anterolateral to the cervical vertebral column, in the trough between the scalene muscles laterally and the longus cervicis medially. The target point for blocks is the anterolateral surface of the vertebral body of C7. This can be visualized on an oblique view of the cervical spine (Fig. 97.6A). In order to avoid puncturing overlying vessels and viscera, these need to be displaced by fingers palpating above and below the target point. A needle can then be inserted toward the target point along an oblique view. Its final position should be confirmed on an anteroposterior view (Fig. 97.6B). Thereafter, an aliquot of contrast medium is injected to demonstrate flow along the gutter and not into one of the adjacent muscles (Fig. 97.6C,D).

Ultrasound guidance is an alternative to fluoroscopic guidance and offers certain advantages in this region. Ultrasound demonstrates the common carotid artery, internal jugular vein, thyroid gland, and esophagus—all of which need to be avoided during passage of the needle (Fig. 97.7). In a study that compared ultrasound guidance with the blind technique, the volume of local anesthetic required was reduced to 5 mL, the onset of block was sooner, and hematoma was avoided (but occurred in 3 out of 12 cases with the blind technique).[27] A disadvantage is that ultrasound guidance requires training and confidence in the technology and technique. The potential of ultrasound guidance to reduce complications and improve accuracy has still to be demonstrated in clinical studies.

Lumbar Sympathetic Blocks

Lumbar sympathetic blocks involve anesthetizing the lumbar sympathetic trunk, typically at the L3 level. They have traditionally been used to test if they relieve pain or other features of complex regional pain syndrome. They have also been used to test if low back pain is relieved. Although blind techniques relying on surface markings only have been used in the past, they have not shown to be valid. The preferred technique should be fluoroscopically guided in order to show that the local anesthetic is deposited accurately onto the sympathetic trunk and does not spread to other structures that might compromise the validity of the block.

The target point is the anterolateral corner of the L3 vertebral body, immediately anterior to the surface of the psoas major, which is where the lumbar sympathetic trunk runs. A target point over the lower third of the vertebral body is recommended in order to avoid the lumbar vessels which cross the middle of the vertebral body. In an oblique view of the lumbar spine, this point coincides with what appears to be the anterior margin of the vertebral body (Fig. 97.8A). In such a view, a spinal needle is directed parallel to the x-ray beam, toward the target point. Correct depth can be achieved by first directing the needle to touch the vertebral body, but then redirecting the needle so that it lies tangential to the margin of the body but at the same depth of insertion. The depth of insertion should be checked on a lateral and on an anteroposterior view (Fig. 97.8B,C). In the anteroposterior view, the tip of the needle should lie on the interpedicular line. Once the needle has been placed, an aliquot of contrast medium should be injected to check dispersal. It should flow longitudinally in the retroperitoneal space, anterior to psoas major and the lateral edge of the vertebral body (Fig. 97.8D). If the injection occurs into the psoas major, a radiate pattern of spread will appear, as the contrast medium disperses between the fascicles of the muscle. In that event, the needle needs to be relocated anterior to the muscle and outside its fascial sheath. Once appropriate flow of contrast medium has been established,

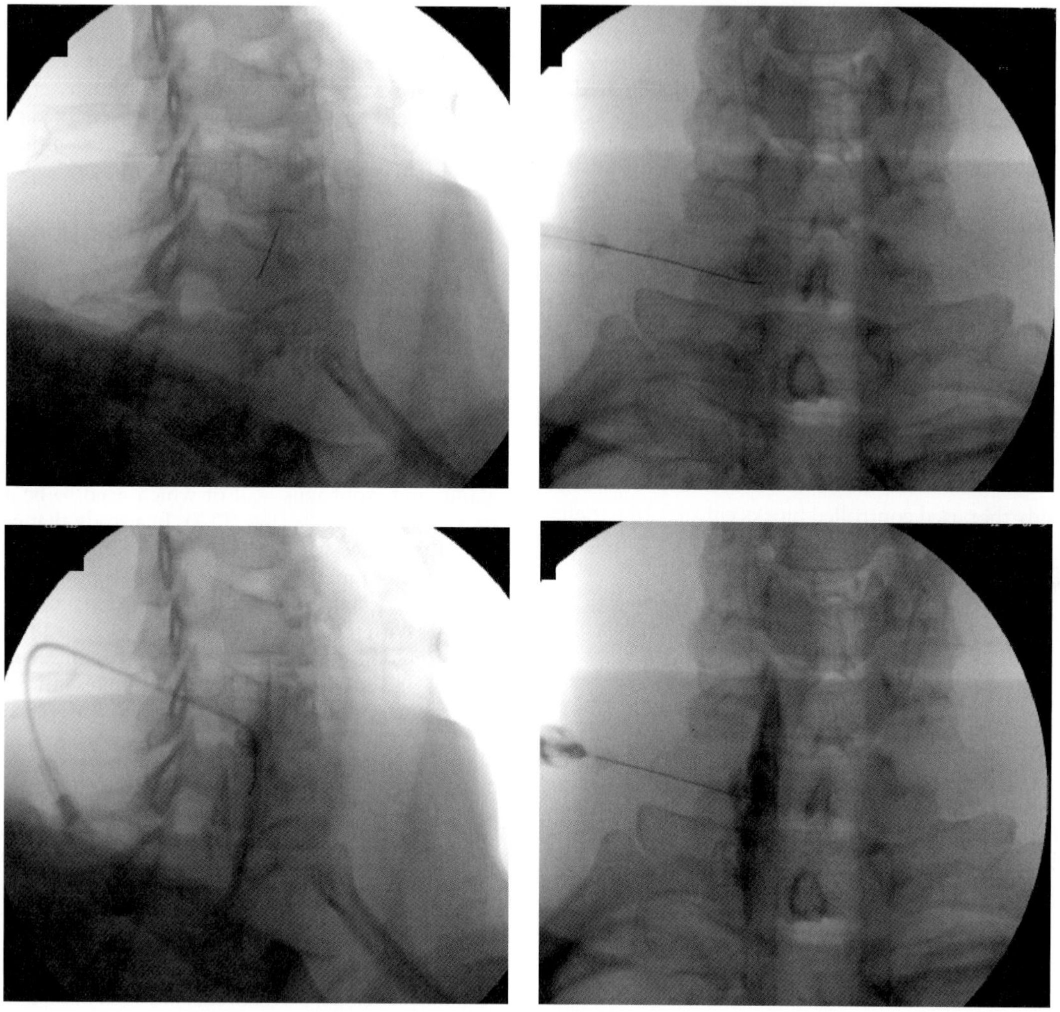

FIGURE 97.6 Stages in the execution of a lower cervical sympathetic block. **A.** In an oblique view, a needle is inserted onto the anterolateral surface of the C7 vertebral body. **B.** An anteroposterior view confirms the anterolateral location of the tip of the needle. **C.** An oblique view shows the longitudinal spread of contrast medium. **D.** An anteroposterior view shows contrast medium spread freely in the tissue plane of the sympathetic trunk, and not within the neck muscles. (Illustrations kindly provided by Dr. Milton Landers.)

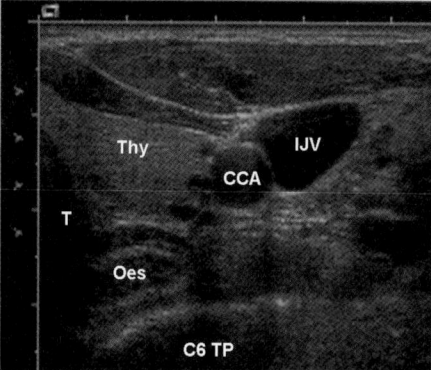

FIGURE 97.7 Ultrasound anatomy of the neck in the plane used for stellate ganglion block. Note how an anteroposterior approach, using either the traditional blind technique or fluoroscopy guidance, carries the risk of incurring the thyroid gland, common carotid artery, internal jugular vein, or esophagus. Under ultrasound guidance, an oblique approach lateral to the great vessels is possible. CCA, carotid artery; IJV, jugular vein; Oes, esophagus; T, trachea; Thy, thyroid gland; TP, transverse process of C6. (Illustration kindly provided by Dr. Urs Eichenberg, University Hospital, Berne, Switzerland.)

a similar aliquot of local anesthetic is injected to anesthetize the sympathetic trunk.

Validity

The use of fluoroscopy establishes the face validity of these blocks (i.e., the sympathetic trunk is accurately and selectively infiltrated). Face validity is confirmed physiologically by observing a rise in skin temperature in the limb of the target side, which shows that the sympathetic trunk has indeed been anesthetized.

What has not been shown is that sympathetic blocks have construct validity (i.e., that the physiologic response is due to the effects of local anesthetic and not to nonspecific factors such as placebo). This requires the execution of controlled blocks, but because of their traditional standing, sympathetic blocks have been exempt from the requirement for controls. They are assumed to be valid and, therefore, that diagnostic and prognostic inferences based on them are always correct. No research has shown this to be so. Research that has been conducted has damaged the traditional illusion.

A study showed that stellate ganglion blocks with normal saline were as effective as blocks with local anesthetic.[28] Statistically, a difference arose in that patients who received local anes-

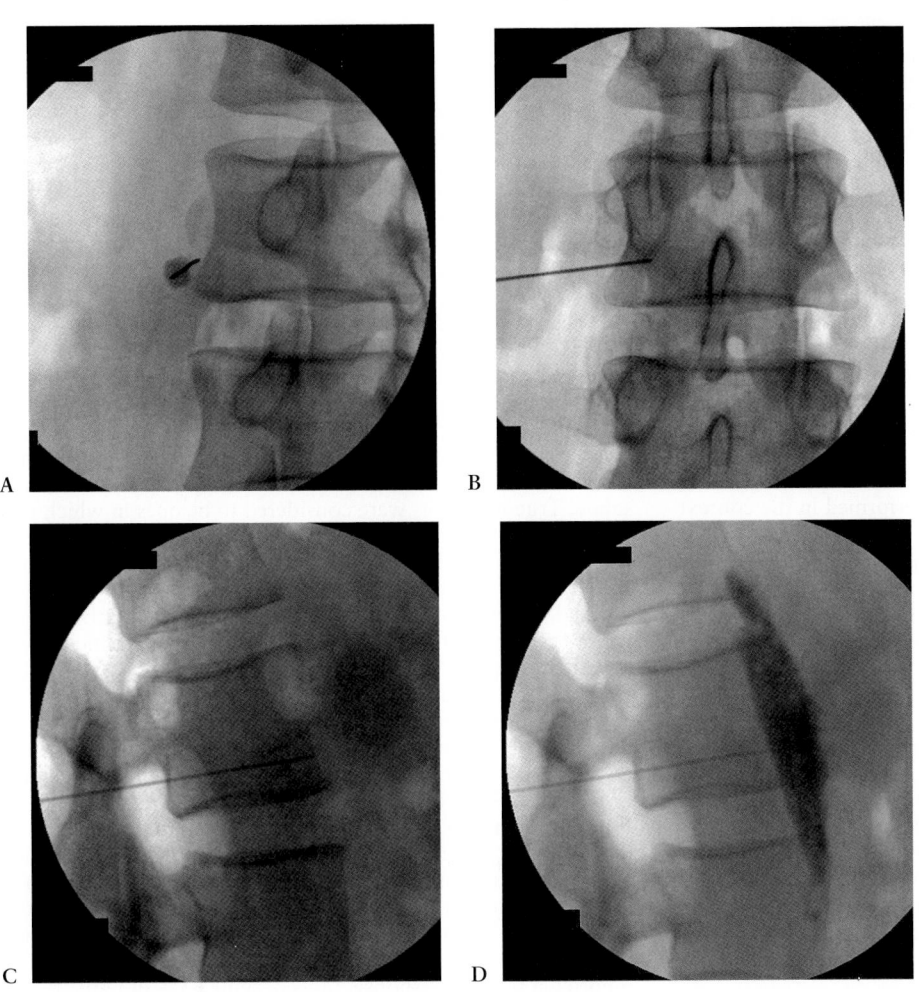

FIGURE 97.8 Stages in the conduct of a lumbar sympathetic block. **A.** An oblique view showing a needle passing tangential to the lower anterolateral surface of the L3 vertebral body. **B.** Anteroposterior view, showing the needle in place over the antero-lateral aspect of the L3 vertebral body. **C.** Lateral view showing the needle in place over the anterolateral aspect of the L3 verte-bral body. **D.** Lateral view showing contrast medium spreading longitudinal over the an-terior surface of the psoas major muscle. (Illustrations kindly provided by Dr. Milton Landers.)

thetic tended to have relief of pain lasting into the next day. Accordingly, the authors recommended that diagnostic decisions be based not on the immediate response, but on the response evident on the next day. However, this is not a secure operational criterion because some patients who received normal saline also had prolonged responses. The only way to secure the validity of stellate ganglion blocks is to perform controls in each and every patient. Unless this is done, the investigator cannot distinguish a true-positive response from a placebo response. Failing to use controlled blocks in the past may have led to overestimates of so-called sympathetic-mediated pain. Unless and until studies are conducted using controlled blocks, its true prevalence will not be known, and it remains possible that its prevalence may be zero. No studies have tested the validity of lumbar sympathetic blocks. Nor has the prognostic validity of sympathetic blocks—cervical or lumbar—been established. No one has com-pared response to blocks—either single or controlled—to out-comes of sympathectomy. Not using controlled blocks may be one reason why sympathectomy often proves ineffective.

Miscellaneous

Other blocks of the sympathetic nervous system are practiced, ostensibly widely. These include blocks of the celiac plexus, splanchnic nerves, and hypogastric plexuses, and blocks of the ganglion impar. However, there is no evidence on their validity as either diagnostic or prognostic procedures. The literature per-taining to these procedures focuses exclusively on their therapeu-tic benefits (see below).

DIAGNOSTIC BLOCKS

Many conditions associated with chronic pain have no detectable morphological correlate. The cause of pain is not evident on con-ventional medical imaging. For some such conditions, although the cause might not be evident, the source of pain can be estab-lished using diagnostic blocks.

The rationale for diagnostic, local anesthetic blocks is that if a structure is the source of pain, then anesthetizing it or its nerve supply should relieve the pain. If the suspected structure is not the source of pain, anesthetizing it should not relieve the pain.

Two types of blocks have been used to pinpoint sources of pain: intra-articular blocks and nerve blocks. Intra-articular blocks involve injecting local anesthetic into a joint suspected of being the source of pain. Diagnostic nerve blocks are restricted to small nerves that have a limited and specific distribution. Blocks of larger nerves are not diagnostic of a particular source because of their widespread distribution.

Principles

Controls

There are no objective tests for the presence of pain or for its relief. Investigators rely only on what the patient reports, but patients can report relief of pain for reasons other than the effect of a local anesthetic injected during a diagnostic block. They may have an expectation that the block will relieve their pain, particularly if they have been coached or instructed to expect a positive response. Unprompted, they might want the response to be positive so that they qualify for the resultant treatment that promises to relieve their pain permanently. Patients with medico-legal claims might choose to report relief in order to vindicate their claim.

Because of these extraneous, confounding factors, a positive response to a block cannot be summarily attributed to the effect of the local anesthetic injected. Some form of control is necessary if the response is to be valid and for the interpretation of the response to be correct. The ultimate form of control is a placebo-control in which an inactive agent is injected to test for spurious responses. However, for two reasons, placebos cannot be administered in an arbitrary manner. In the first instance, administering a placebo on a single-blind basis is considered unethical in some jurisdictions. Patients would need to be informed that they might receive an inactive agent. In the second instance, for placebo blocks to be meaningful, they must be performed in the context of at least three injections.

The first injection must be an active agent, in order to provide prima facie information that anesthetising the target structure does, in fact, relieve the patient's pain. There is no point wasting resources and effort testing with a placebo a structure that is not involved in the patient's pain. The second injection cannot routinely be the placebo, for mischievous patients would know that the second injection is always the "dummy." In order to retain the effects of chance, the second injection must be randomized to be either an active or inactive adjacent. A third injection is required to administer the complimentary agent. Under those conditions, a genuine response is one in which the patient reports complete relief of pain on each occasion that a local anaesthetic was used and no relief when the placebo was used. The validity of the response is made more secure if the injections are performed under double-blind conditions, so that the operator does not subconsciously communicate cues to the patient as to what to expect.

Whereas the triple-block, placebo paradigm satisfies scientific rigor, it is not readily implemented in clinical practice. It involves multiple procedures and additional costs. Furthermore, a positive response to placebo does not necessarily rule out that the tested joint is symptomatic. An alternative paradigm is available, but it is not as widely applicable as has hitherto been thought.

In textbooks of pain medicine, eminent authorities have advocated comparative local anesthetic blocks in order to guard against placebo responses.[29-32] These involve administering a particular agent on the occasion of the first block, but using a different agent on a second occasion. The agents advocated are lignocaine and bupivacaine. The paradigm maintains that a genuine patient will report short-lasting relief when lignocaine is used and long-lasting relief when bupivacaine is used.

An important consideration for the interpretation of responses to comparative blocks is that it is not the absolute duration of relief that is important but the relative duration. In some individuals, lignocaine lasts longer than does bupivacaine in other individuals. It is not a matter that the typical duration of action of lignocaine is 2 hours and that of bupivacaine is 4 hours. Lignocaine can last as long as 7 hours in some individuals, and bupivacaine as little as 1 hour in others. However, it has been shown that in the one individual, when both agents are injected simultaneously into symmetrical sites, bupivacaine consistently outlasts lidocaine.[33,34] Therefore, the essential criterion for a positive response to comparative blocks is that the effect of bupivacaine is longer than that of lignocaine.

The comparative block paradigm was promoted on theoretical grounds, capitalizing on the known difference in duration of action of lignocaine and bupivacaine; when promoted, however, it had not been tested empirically. For more conventional diagnostic blocks, the paradigm has still not been tested, but it has been

tested in two ways in the context of diagnostic blocks of the medial branches of the cervical dorsal rami.

In one study, Barnsley et al.[35] administered lidocaine and bupivacaine on separate occasions under double-blind conditions. They considered true-positive responses to be ones in which the patients reported longer-lasting relief of their pain when bupivacaine was used than when lignocaine was used. To establish the validity of the response, they used a statistical test involving the binomial distribution. They found that the chances that the patients had guessed the correct agents were less than 2 in 10,000, on which grounds they concluded that the comparative block paradigm was valid.

Another study used a more conventional strategy. Lord et al.[36] subjected patients to triple blocks under double-blind conditions, using lidocaine, bupivacaine, and normal saline in a randomized manner. They compared the diagnostic decision that would have been made on the basis of the responses to the two local anesthetics alone, with the decision based on the response to normal saline. True responses were considered to be ones in which pain was relieved on each occasion when a local anesthetic was used but not relieved when normal saline was used. False responses were ones in which pain was relieved when normal saline was injected. Contingency tables revealed that comparative blocks had a specificity of 88%. This means that among patients with a positive response to comparative blocks, there is only a 12% chance that it is due to placebo effects.

On the other hand, the sensitivity of comparative blocks was only 54%.[36] This means that, when strictly applied, the criteria for a positive response do not detect all patients with a genuine response. These criteria exclude some patients who do not respond to placebo blocks but who experience paradoxically longer-lasting relief following lignocaine than with bupivacaine. This type of response may be due to the different duration of action of lidocaine on open sodium channels in patients with ongoing pain. Consequently, failure to satisfy the comparative block criterion does not necessarily mean that the patient has reported a placebo-response. Indeed, some 65% of patients who report discordant responses to lignocaine and bupivacaine do not respond to placebo blocks.[36]

Accordingly, the strength of comparative blocks lies not in detecting placebo responders. It lies in identifying true-responses. If a patient has longer-lasting relief with bupivacaine, the investigator can be 88% certain that the response is true. If the criteria are relaxed to accept complete relief of pain irrespective of which agent lasted longer, the investigator can be 65% certain that the response is true.

Which type of control an investigator chooses to use and which criteria should be used to assess comparative blocks is a matter of preference depending on the circumstances. If an investigator wants to be or needs to be absolutely certain, placebo-controlled, triple blocks should be used. If a certainty of 88% is enough, comparative blocks with strict criteria can be used. If, on the other hand, the investigator can tolerate a false-positive rate of 35%, comparative blocks with relaxed criteria will suffice.

Criteria for Positive Response

For a response to a diagnostic block to be valid, certain criteria should be satisfied. On each occasion that the nerve is blocked, the patient should obtain complete relief of pain. That should be validated by recording the intensity of pain before and after the block, using either a visual analog scale or numerical rating scale. Moreover, for the block to be physiologically and pharmacologically meaningful, the pain should return as the effect of the local anesthetic wears off. Recording the return of pain, therefore, becomes part of the assessment. Prolonged relief of pain, lasting days, weeks, or months, does not constitute a valid response, for it is not compatible with the expected action and effect of administering a local anesthetic. Such prolonged responses are uninterpretable. They are not consistent with a joint or other structure being the source of nociception. A painful structure should resume being painful once the local anesthetic has ceased to operate. Prolonged responses suggest either a placebo response or some sort of modulatory effect on pain perception, the nature of which has not been determined.

A positive response to blocks should be corroborated by narrative and activity. The patient should volunteer that they feel distinctly better, and they should be able to undertake and demonstrate activities that previously were prevented or restricted by their pain. If activities are not restored, the utility of the block is questionable. If activities, ostensibly restricted by the pain, are not restored when pain is relieved, some factor other than the pain must still be responsible for the restriction.

Applications

In principle, any local anesthetic block used as a diagnostic block should be subjected to controls. Unless controls are used, the response of the patient cannot be held to be valid and diagnostic decisions based on them may be incorrect. Yet, conspicuously lacking in the literature are any data on the use of controls for traditional local anesthetic blocks. It would seem that such blocks are excused the need for controls because of their traditional standing. Data on controlled, diagnostic blocks are available only for blocks of the medial branches of the dorsal rami.

Cervical Medial Branch Blocks

The medial branches of the cervical dorsal rami supply the zygapophysial joints of the cervical spine and its medial posterior muscles (multifidus, interspinales, and semispinalis). Blocks of these nerves would relieve pain from any of these structures. However, there are no known causes of chronic neck pain that lie in the posterior neck muscles.[37] Therefore, in practice, cervical medial branch blocks are a test for pain stemming from the cervical zygapophysial joints.

At typical cervical levels, the medial branch runs across the lateral surface of the ipsisegmental articular pillar (Fig. 97.9A). The target point for blocks at these levels lies at the centroid of the articular pillar or slightly higher at the C3 and C6 levels (Fig. 97.9B).[37,38] The C7 medial branch has a variable location across the C7 superior articular process, anywhere between its apex and the root of the C7 transverse process. For blocks at this level, the target point has to be adjusted accordingly.[38]

Cervical medial branch blocks are the only means available by which either to implicate or to refute the cervical zygapophysial joints as the source of neck pain. A joint is implicated if controlled diagnostic blocks completely relieve the patient's pain.

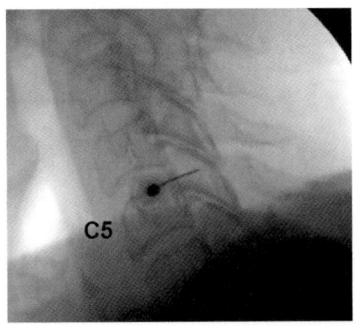

FIGURE 97.10 A lateral fluoroscopic view of the cervical spine showing a needle in place on the articular pillar of C5 for a C5 medial branch block.

In order to anesthetize a particular joint, each of the two nerves that innervate the joint must be blocked. At typical cervical levels, each joint is innervated by the medial branches that have the same segmental numbers as the joint. Thus, the C5-C6 joint is supplied by the C5 and C6 medial branches.

Cervical medial blocks require placing a needle, under fluoroscopic guidance, on to the nerve to be blocked. Explicit guidelines for the performance and evaluation of these blocks have been published by the International Spine Intervention Society.[38] For typical cervical medial branches, the needle is introduced using a lateral view. Correct depth of insertion is established once the needle reaches the articular pillar (Fig. 97.10).

For blocks of the C7 medial branch, additional measures need to be taken in order to avoid false-negative responses because of variations in the location of this nerve. Since this nerve can lie anywhere between the apex of the C7 superior articular process and the root of the transverse process, measures are required to ensure that local anesthetic covers this entire region. That might be accomplished with a single injection onto the lateral aspect of the superior articular process, provided that a test dose of contrast medium shows that the entire area is covered. Otherwise, two injections are required: one at the apex and one at the root of the transverse process (Fig. 97.11). Anteroposterior views are required to confirm the depth of insertion because, in some patients, needles that appear correctly placed in lateral views may actually be displaced laterally by a thick C7 transverse process.[38] A third placement, a few millimeters lateral to the superior articular process, is recommended in order to target C7 medial branches that sometimes are displaced off bone by a slip of the multifidus muscle.

Once the needle has been placed, some operators recommend using a test dose of contrast medium (0.1–0.2 mL) before inject-

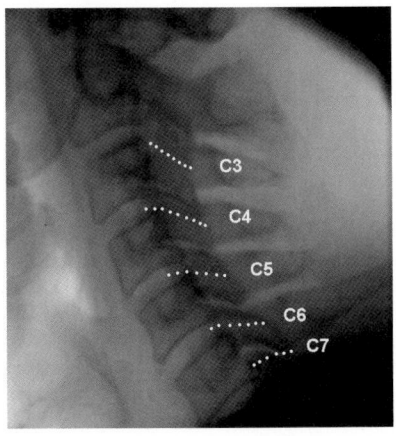

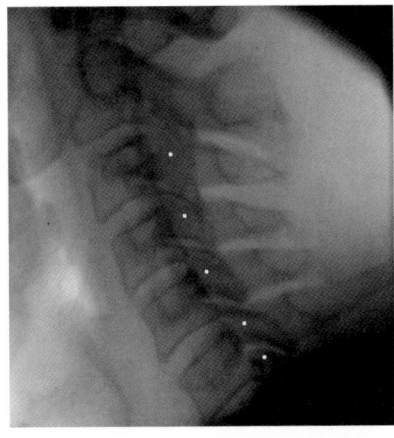

FIGURE 97.9 A lateral radiograph of the cervical spine on which the courses of the cervical medial branches and the target points for medial branch blocks have been depicted. **A.** The courses of the typical cervical medial branches are plotted by dotted lines. **B.** The dots mark the target points for medial branch blocks.

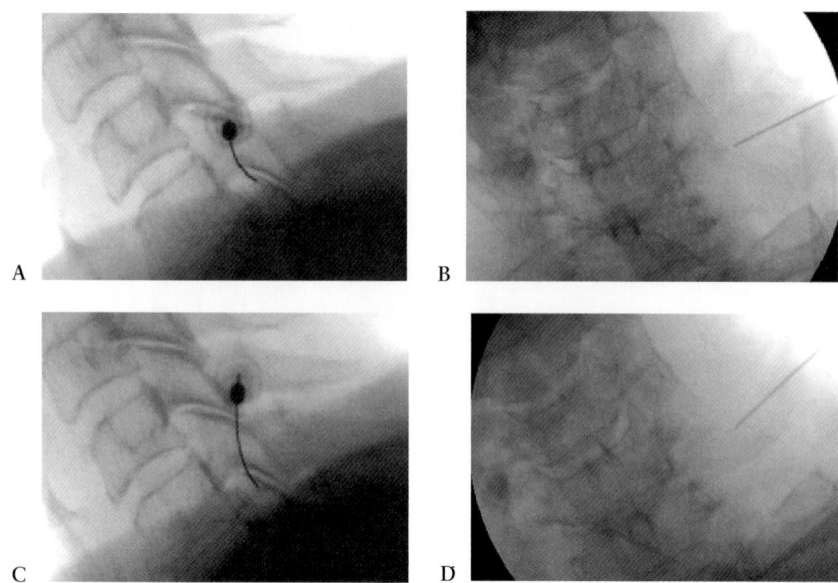

FIGURE 97.11 Fluoroscopy views of needles placed for a C7 medial branch block. **A.** Lateral view of a needle placed high on the apex of the C7 superior articular process. **B.** Anteroposterior view of the needle placed on the superior articular process. **C.** Lateral view of a needle placed at the base of the C7 transverse process. **D.** Anteroposterior view of the needle placed on the based of the transverse process. Comparison with Figure 99.11B shows that the needle lies lower and more peripherally along the transverse process.

ing local anesthetic to guard against venous uptake and, therefore, false-negative responses. For cervical medial branch blocks, the mean prevalence of vascular uptake is 3.9% (95% confidence intervals: 3.84% to 3.96%).[39] Avoiding vascular uptake avoids possible false-negative responses. Thereafter, only a tiny aliquot of local anesthetic (0.3 mL) is required to anesthetize the nerve. Greater volumes of injectate spread away from the target zone and are, therefore, superfluous and threaten the face validity of the block.

Validity

It has been shown that cervical medial branch blocks are target specific. Material injected onto the target points floods the location of the target nerve, but does not spread to adjacent nerves or the spinal nerves.[37] Nor do cervical medial branch blocks anesthetize the posterior neck muscles in a nonspecific manner. Excess injectate typically spreads across the cleavage plane between multifidus and semispinalis capitis.[38]

Single medial branch blocks are not valid. They have false-positive rates of 27%.[40] Therefore, in order to be valid, cervical medial branch blocks must be controlled in each and every case. The choice lies between placebo-controlled blocks and comparative local anesthetic blocks (see "Controls," above).

Two types of positive response to comparative blocks can occur. A concordant response is one in which pain is completely relieved for a duration concordant with the duration of action of the local anesthetic used. A discordant response is one in which pain is completely relieved but the duration of effect is longer when a short-acting agent is used. In the context of cervical medial branch blocks, both responses have been validated.

Concordant responses have a high specificity (88%) when compared with placebo-controlled blocks.[36] This means that positive responses are very unlikely to be false. However, concordant responses have a low sensitivity (54%).[36] This means that they do not detect all patients with cervical zygapophysial joint pain who do not have placebo-responses.

Discordant responses have a high sensitivity (100%). They detect all patients who have zygapophysial joint pain, but their specificity is limited (65%).[36] That means that positive responses can include some placebo responses.

For practical purposes, these different sensitivities and specificities make little difference in practice because the prevalence

of cervical zygapophysial joint pain is high (60%) (see below). Given a concordant response, a practitioner can be 88% confident that the positive response is true-positive (Table 97.2). In comparison, although a discordant response has a lower specificity, its sensitivity is high, which means that the practitioner can be 81% confident that a positive response is true-positive (see Table 97.2).[41]

Multiple and independent studies have shown that cervical zygapophysial joint pain is a common basis for chronic neck pain. In patients with chronic neck pain after whiplash, the prevalence estimates have been 54% (40% to 68%)[42] and 60% (46% to 73%).[43] In drivers who sustain a whiplash injury at high impact speeds, the prevalence has been found to be 74% (65% to 83%).[44] In patients with headache after whiplash, the prevalence of C2-C3 zygapophysial joint pain was 53% (37% to 68%).[45] In patients with neck pain, not restricted to those with whiplash, the prevalence of cervical zygapophysial joint pain has been at least 36% (27% to 45%) in a rehabilitation practice[46] and 60% (50% to 70%) in a pain clinic.[47] These data render cervical zygapophysial joint pain as the single-most common cause of chronic neck pain.

Cervical medial branch blocks have established utility. They are the only means by which to diagnose the most common cause of chronic neck pain. Moreover, patients correctly diagnosed can be treated successfully with percutaneous radiofrequency neurotomy (see Chapter 103).[48–51] Those patients who obtain complete relief from cervical medial branch blocks can expect a 70% chance of achieving complete relief of pain after cervical medial branch neurotomy.[48–51]

Third Occipital Nerve Blocks

The C2-C3 zygapophysial joint is innervated by the third occipital nerve, which is the superficial medial branch of the C3 dorsal ramus. Third occipital nerve blocks, therefore, are a particular subset of cervical medial branch blocks. They are used in patients with upper cervical pain and headache, to test if that pain stems from the C2-C3 zygapophysial joint.

The third occipital nerve runs transversely across the lateral aspect of the C2-C3 zygapophysial joint (Fig. 97.12A) and may lie at a level anywhere between opposite the apex of the C3 superior articular process to opposite the bottom of the C2-C3 intervertebral foramen. Consequently, in order to cover all possible loca-

TABLE 97.2

CONTINGENCY TABLES SHOWING THE EFFECT ON DIAGNOSTIC
CONFIDENCE OF DIFFERENT SPECIFICITIES AND SENSITIVITIES OF A
DIAGNOSTIC TEST IN DETECTING A CONDITION WITH A PREVALENCE OF 60%

Specificity	Sensitivity	Prevalence	Blocks	Condition Present	Condition Absent	Diagnostic Confidence
0.88	0.54	60%	Positive	324	48	88%
			Negative	276	352	
				600	400	
0.65	1.00	60%	Positive	600	140	81%
			Negative		260	
				600	400	

Diagnostic confidence is the measure of how confident the practitioner can be that the condition really is
present when a test is positive. It amounts to the positive predictive value that applies for a particular
prevalence, and is derived from the specificity and sensitivity of the test by the equations[41]:

$$[\text{posttest odds}] = [\text{pretest odds}] \times [\text{positive likelihood ratio}]$$
$$[\text{positive likelihood ratio}] = [\text{sensitivity}] / [1 - \text{specificity}]$$
$$[\text{pretest odds}] = [\text{prevalence}] / [1 - \text{prevalence}]$$
$$[\text{diagnostic confidence}] = [(\text{posttest odds}) / (\text{posttest odds} + 1)] \times 100\%$$

tions of this nerve, blocks are recommended at each of three
locations: over the middle of the C2-C3 zygapophysial joint,
below this point, and above it (Fig. 97.12B).[38,45]

Third occipital nerve blocks are performed using a lateral view
of the C2-C3 joint. The needle is placed at each of the three target
points required for this nerve (Fig. 97.13). They are rendered
valid by performing comparative blocks. A positive response is
complete relief of pain on each occasion that the nerve is blocked.

The utility of third occipital blocks lies in the investigation of
cervicogenic headache. In patients with posttraumatic neck pain,
in whom headache is the dominant complaint, the prevalence of
pain from the C2-C3 zygapophysial joint is 56%.[38] No other
blocks and no other diagnostic tests have established any other
source of cervicogenic headache with a prevalence that rivals this
figure.[52,53] A positive response to controlled, third occipital nerve
blocks is prognostic of an 88% success rate for completely relieving headache by third occipital radiofrequency neurotomy.[54]

A study using healthy volunteers has shown that the third
occipital nerve can be visualized by ultrasound and reliably blocked
under ultrasound guidance.[55] This technology may become an
alternative to fluoroscopic guidance in the future.

Lumbar Medial Branch Blocks

The medial branches of the lumbar dorsal rami supply the zygapophysial joints of the lumbar spine and its medial posterior muscles (multifidus, interspinales). At typical lumbar levels, each medial branch runs across the neck of the superior articular process
of the vertebra below (Fig. 97.14). At the L5 level, it is the dorsal

ramus itself that crosses the neck of the S1 superior articular
process, before giving rise to its medial branch opposite the caudal
edge of this process.

If defined strictly, lumbar medial branch blocks are a test for
pain mediated by the particular nerves anesthetized. They would
relieve pain from any of the structures innervated by these nerves.
However, there is no known pathology that affects the muscles
supplied by the lumbar medial branches, which can be a cause
of chronic pain. Therefore, in practice, medial branch blocks are
a test for pain from the zygapophysial joints, which can be a
source of pain in the same way that synovial joints of the appendicular skeleton are believed to be sources of pain.

No studies have identified the pathology responsible for zygapophysial joint pain. It may be a form of osteoarthritis or a form
of occult injury, but this pathology has not been demonstrated
on any form of medical imaging. Age changes, as seen on plain
radiographs, do not correlate with pain,[56,57] and changes as seen
on CT do not correlate with the joint being painful.[58] There are
preliminary findings that a form of synovitis, demonstrable by
MRI, might be the underlying pathology, but this pathology has
still to be correlated with relief of pain following blocks.[59]

Lumbar medial branch blocks are the only means available
by which either to implicate or to refute the lumbar zygapophysial
joints as the source of back pain. A joint is implicated if controlled
diagnostic blocks completely relieve the patient's pain.

In order to anesthetize a particular joint, each of the two
nerves that innervate the joint must be blocked. In this regard,
the numbering of the nerves is one segment less than that of the
joint that they supply. Thus, the L4,L5 medial branches supply

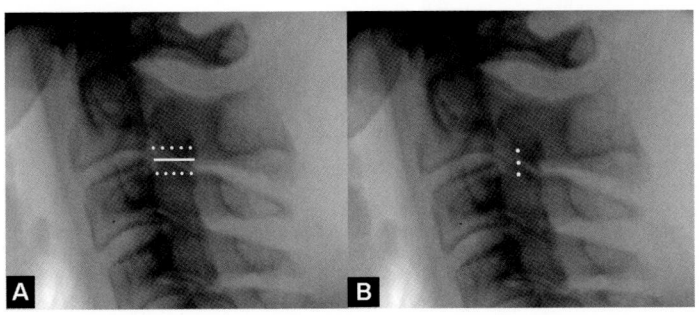

A   B

FIGURE 97.12 A lateral radiograph of the C2-C3 level of the cervical
spine showing the location of the third occipital nerve and target
points for blocks of this nerve. **A.** The bold line indicates the mean
course of the nerve, and the dotted lines mark its upper and lower
limits. **B.** The dots mark the three locations at which blocks should
be undertaken in order to cover all variants of the location of the
third occipital nerve.

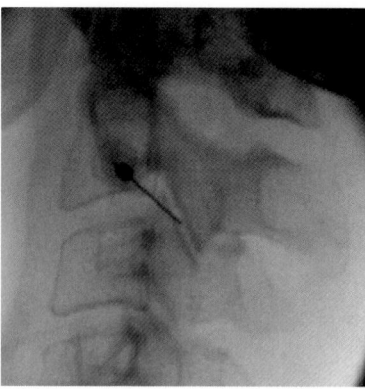

FIGURE 97.13 A lateral fluoroscopy view of the C2-C3 level showing a needle in place for the middle of three positions for blocks of the third occipital nerve.

the L5-S1 joint, and the L2,L3 nerves supply the L3-L4 joint. Since this dissonance may lead to confusion in records or communication, a recommended annotation is that sequential nerves be recorded using a comma, because they are coupled but nevertheless separate entities, whereas joints should be recorded using a hyphen, because the two segments are connected.[60]

Lumbar medial blocks require placing a needle under fluoroscopic guidance on to the nerve to be blocked. Explicit guidelines for the performance and evaluation of these blocks have been published by the International Spine Intervention Society.[60] The target point for lumbar medial branch blocks lies at the junction of the ventral and middle third of the neck of the superior articular process at each segmental level. The recommended approach to this target is along an oblique view of the target area (Fig. 97.15A). A declined view (i.e., viewing the segment from behind and below) confirms that the needle lies on the neck of the superior articular process (Fig. 97.15B). Once the needle has been placed, a test dose of contrast medium should be injected in order to exclude venous uptake, which occurs in about 3.7% of injections (95% confidence intervals: 3.3% to 4.1%).[39] The nerve can be anesthetized with as little as 0.3 mL of local anaesthetic. More than 0.5 mL is essentially wasted, because the excess injectate spreads away from the target point, between the back muscles.

The validity of lumbar medial branch blocks has been studied more than any other block in pain medicine. The blocks are target-specific. Provided that the correct target points are used and provided that small volumes are used, the injectate remains exclusively on the target nerve.[61] Placements more proximal along the nerve risk having the injectate spread into the intervertebral foramen.[61] Construct validity has been demonstrated. Medial

branch blocks protect normal volunteers from experimentally-induced zygapophysial joint pain.[62] However, in order to be valid in patients, the blocks must also be controlled.

Single blocks of the lumbar medial branches are not valid because they have false-positive rates of between 25% and 41%.[63–65] This means that if the prevalence of lumbar zygapophysial joint pain is 15% (see below), for every three blocks that appear to be positive, two will be false-positive. If the prevalence is 5%, five out of every six blocks will be false-positive. Such yields of false-positive results are unacceptable and indicate that a valid diagnosis cannot be made using a single diagnostic block. In order to reduce false-positive diagnoses, controlled blocks must be used in each and every case.

Comparative local anesthetic blocks have been advocated and used as controls for lumbar medial branch blocks on the grounds that they have been validated for the cervical spine. In the cervical spine, comparative blocks have a specificity of either 65% or 88%, depending on the stringency of the criteria for a positive response.[36] These values are acceptable for cervical medial branch blocks because cervical zygapophysial joint pain is so common. However, in the lumbar spine, where zygapophysial joint pain is far less common, comparative blocks result in inordinate numbers of false-positive results.

For a specificity of 65%, and a prevalence of 40%, the diagnostic confidence of positive comparative blocks is only 66% (Table 97.3). For a prevalence of 15%, this confidence drops to 32% and is even less for lower prevalence rates. For a specificity of 88% and a prevalence of 15%, the diagnostic confidence is only 60%, but rises to 85% if the prevalence is 40% (see Table 97.3). These calculations show that for comparative blocks to be valid in the lumbar spine, the prevalence of zygapophysial joint pain must be substantial, and the strictest criteria for a positive response must be applied (i.e., the patient must have complete relief of pain on each occasion that the nerves are blocked and must have longer-lasting relief when the long-acting agent is used). Unless these conditions apply, the false-positive rates render diagnostic confidence unacceptably low. For certainty about the response when the prevalence is low, placebo-controls are unavoidable.

The available data on the prevalence of lumbar zygapophysial joint pain is mixed and contentious and differs according to the sample studied and the criteria used to define a positive response. Using the criterion of 50% relief of pain, the prevalence has been reported as 15% (10% to 20%) among younger, injured workers.[66] Using a criterion of 75% relief of pain, the prevalence was 45% (39% to 54%) in patients attending a pain clinic,[65] and for a criterion of 90% relief, the prevalence was 40% (27% to 53%) in elderly patients with no history of trauma.[67]

The criterion of 50% relief was adopted early in the study of lumbar zygapophysial joint pain when it was believed that pain

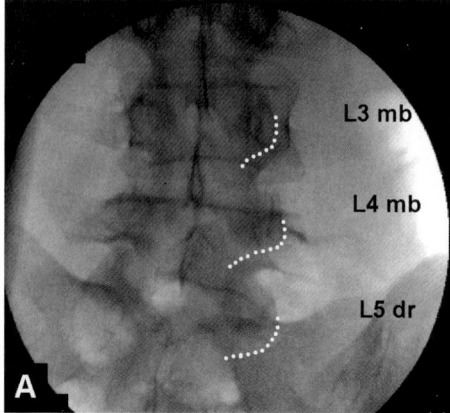

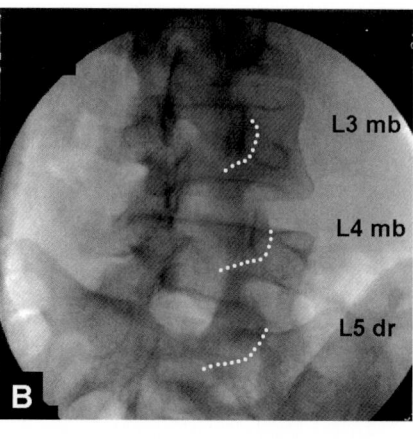

FIGURE 97.14 Radiographs of the lower lumbar spine on which the courses of the medial branches (mb) of the lower lumbar dorsal rami and the L5 dorsal ramus (dr) have been depicted. **A.** Anteroposterior view. **B.** Oblique view.

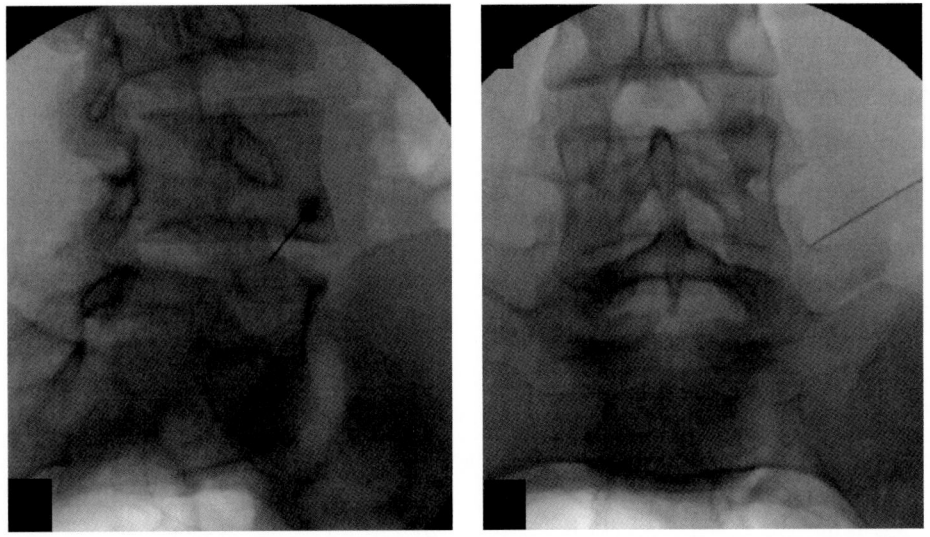

FIGURE 97.15 Radiographs of an L4 medial branch block. **A.** Oblique view showing a needle resting on the neck of the superior articular process of L5. **B.** Declined view showing the needle aiming obliquely onto the neck of the superior articular process at its junction with the transverse process.

TABLE 97.3

CONTINGENCY TABLES SHOWING THE EFFECT ON DIAGNOSTIC CONFIDENCE OF DIFFERENT SPECIFICITIES OF A DIAGNOSTIC TEST AND DECREASING PREVALENCE RATES

Specificity	Prevalence	Blocks	Condition		Diagnostic confidence
			Present	Absent	
0.88	40%	Positive	400	72	85%
		Negative		528	
			400	600	
	15%	Positive	150	102	60%
		Negative		748	
			150	850	
	5%	Positive	50	114	30%
		Negative		846	
			50	950	
0.65	40%	Positive	400	210	66%
		Negative		528	
			400	600	
	15%	Positive	150	328	32%
		Negative		748	
			150	850	
	5%	Positive	50	333	13%
		Negative		846	
			50	950	

The calculations assume a sensitivity of 100%. Diagnostic confidence is the measure of how confident the practitioner can be that the condition really is present when a test is positive. It amounts to the positive predictive value that applies for a particular prevalence and is derived from the specificity and sensitivity of the test by the equations[41]:

$$[\text{posttest odds}] = [\text{pretest odds}] \times [\text{positive likelihood ratio}]$$
$$[\text{positive likelihood ratio}] = [\text{sensitivity}] / [1 - \text{specificity}]$$
$$[\text{pretest odds}] = [\text{prevalence}] / [1 - \text{prevalence}]$$
$$[\text{diagnostic confidence}] = [(\text{posttest odds}) / (\text{posttest odds} + 1)] \times 100\%$$

from these joints could occur in patients with other sources of pain. The 50% criteria allowed for pain to persist from these other sources. However, studies subsequently showed that rarely does lumbar zygapophysial joint pain occur together with lumbar discogenic pain[68] or sacroiliac joint pain.[69] Consequently, if the zygapophysial joints are the only source of pain, patients should be completely relieved of their pain when the responsible joints are blocked. There is no provision for partial relief. However, when investigators have used a criterion of complete relief of pain, the prevalence of lumbar zygapophysial joint pain has been only 5%,[70,71] 6%,[72] or 7%.[73] But each of these studies used only single, diagnostic blocks. Therefore, the prevalence subject to controlled blocks would be expected to be even less.

These data leave the prevalence of lumbar zygapophysial joint pain in doubt. It appears to be low in injured patients, but may approach 40% in elderly patients. These data affect the utility of lumbar medial branch blocks.

Because of the low prevalence of lumbar zygapophysial joint pain, the pretest likelihood is that the patient will have a negative response to lumbar medial branch blocks. Consequently, it would be inappropriate to test each joint one at a time.[74] Doing so wastes resources. The efficient use of lumbar medial branch blocks would be initially to perform a screening block, in which the L3, L4, and L5 medial branches are blocked simultaneously. If these blocks prove negative, zygapophysial joint pain is effectively refuted. Joints are most often symptomatic at L4-L5 and L5-S1,[67] and an investigator would need good cause to test joints at higher segmental levels. If the screening blocks are positive, controlled blocks can be pursued to determine if the response is valid and to establish which particular joint is the source of pain.

Establishing a diagnosis of lumbar zygapophysial joint pain allows treatment to be offered in the form of lumbar radiofrequency medial branch neurotomy.[75] If they are selected on the basis of positive responses to controlled blocks, 60% of patients so treated can expect to obtain at least 80% relief of pain lasting 12 months, and 80% can expect at least 60% relief.[76] If pain recurs, neurotomy can be repeated in order to reinstate relief.[77]

Intra-Articular Blocks

Intra-articular injections are performed on joints of the appendicular skeleton for a variety of reasons. These include therapeutic injections and diagnostic arthrography. However, diagnostic blocks, using local anesthetic agents, are not common practice. The diagnosis of peripheral joint pain is established largely on the basis of physical examination and medical imaging, and there is no requirement for diagnostic blocks in routine practice. Some practitioners might use joint blocks in patients in whom the source of pain is ambiguous, such as hip joint blocks to distinguish hip joint pain from referred pain to the groin or buttock,

but such practices are not widely used, and their validity and utility have still to be established.

Diagnostic joint blocks have a greater application in the diagnosis of spinal pain because the joints of the spine are less accessible to physical examination, and medical imaging is typically unhelpful in pinpointing a particular joint as the source of pain.

In the past, intra-articular blocks of the zygapophysial joints were used as a means of diagnosing zygapophysial joint pain. The practice still continues in some circles. However, intra-articular blocks of the spine have never been validated and have not been shown to have therapeutic utility. They have been supplanted by medial branch blocks, which have been validated and which do have therapeutic utility.

It is unclear whether joint pain is the result of intra- or periarticular pathology or both. If periarticular lesions are involved, intra-articular blocks would not be sensitive for the diagnosis of joint pain. Periarticular infiltrations are performed in clinical practice, but their validity and therapeutic utility is unknown.

There are two spinal joints for which nerve blocks are not practical and for which intra-articular blocks remain the only means of determine if that joint is the source of pain. They are the lateral atlantoaxial joint and the sacroiliac joint.

Lateral Atlantoaxial Joint Blocks

Experimental studies in normal volunteers have shown that the lateral atlantoaxial joint (C1-C2) can produce pain in the upper cervical spine and in the head.[78] In principle, therefore, this can be a source of cervicogenic headache and neck pain.

Lateral atlantoaxial joint blocks involve delivering a needle into the cavity of the joint. The recommended technique[79] involves a posterior approach, using fluoroscopic guidance. The technique for lateral atlantoaxial joint blocks does not allow for any but minimal deviations of the needle from a straight course from skin to the target point. Therefore, these blocks should be performed only by operators who can use bevel control to restrict movements to less than a few millimeters from a straight course. The needle is inserted first to reach the lateral mass of the atlas and is then adjusted to enter the joint (Fig. 97.16A). Contrast medium is injected in order to establish that the injectate enters the joint cavity and does not escape from it (Fig. 97.16B). This establishes the face validity of the injection. Once correct placement has been confirmed, about 1 mL of local anesthetic can be injected. A positive response is one in which the injection completely relieves the patient's pain. The proximity of the target area to the dural sac, spinal cord, internal carotid artery, and vertebral artery poses significant risks during lateral atlantoaxial joint injection. Misplaced injections of local anesthetic could result in a high spinal block. Intra-arterial injection of depot corticosteroids could result in embolism and stroke.

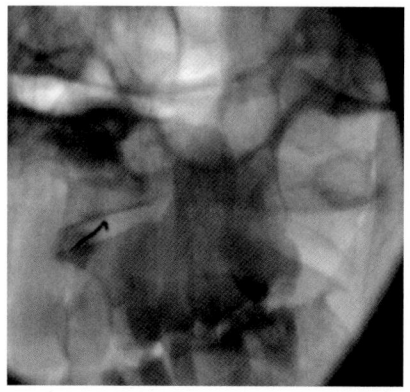 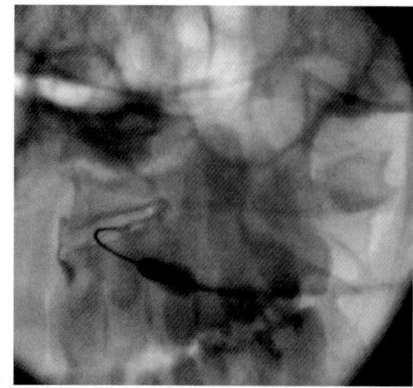

A   B

FIGURE 97.16 Anteroposterior fluoroscopy views of a lateral atlantoaxial joint injection. **A.** The needle has been advanced into the cavity of the joint. **B.** Contrast medium outlines the joint cavity and the internal surface of the lateral capsule.

The validity of lateral atlantoaxial joints has not been tested. Single diagnostic blocks may have a false-positive rate which has not yet been measured. In principle, controlled blocks are required in order to maximize validity. Controls using comparative local anesthetic blocks might be used, but the validity of comparative blocks inside joints, where blood flow is low, has not been established. Anatomic controls might be an alternative, in which the control is to block an adjacent joint (e.g., C2-C3), but the results of such controls have not yet been reported.

There are few prevalence studies of lateral atlantoaxial joint pain, but the available data indicate a nonzero prevalence. One study, using single diagnostic blocks, found that at least 16% of patients presenting with headache responded to lateral atlantoaxial joint blocks.[80] Another study found a prevalence of at least 13%.[81] Each of these may be underestimates because not all eligible patients underwent diagnostic blocks. Conversely, the figures might lower because controlled blocks were not used.

Lateral atlantoaxial joint blocks have therapeutic utility because patients can be treated by atlantoaxial arthrodesis. Follow-up studies have reported that arthrodesis succeeds in providing sustained relief of pain.[82–84] Intra-articular injections of corticosteroids are a more conservative alternative, but benefit only about 1 in 8 patients over the long-term.[81]

Sacroiliac Joint Blocks

Sacroiliac joint blocks are a test for back pain stemming from a sacroiliac joint. They involve introducing a needle under fluoroscopic control into the lower end of the cavity of the joint (Fig. 97.17).[85] A test dose of contrast medium establishes that the injectate lies within the joint cavity and does not escape from it. Subsequently, an aliquot of about 1.5 mL of local anesthetic can be injected in order to anesthetize the joint. A positive response is complete relief of the patient's pain.

Two types of controls have been used in order to maximize the validity of sacroiliac joint blocks. One study used anatomic controls by previously anesthetizing lumbar zygapophysial joints.[86] Another study used comparative local anesthetic blocks.[87] Respectively, these studies found a prevalence (95% confidence intervals) of 13% (6% to 20%) and 19% (9% to 29%). These figures indi-

cate that the sacroiliac joint is the source of pain in a substantial proportion of patients with chronic low back pain. Sacroiliac joint blocks are the only means of identifying this subgroup of patients.

The therapeutic utility of sacroiliac joint blocks is still evolving. Various studies have explored the efficacy of percutaneous radiofrequency denervation of the joint in patients who are positive to blocks. The magnitude and duration of relief from these procedures has still to be established (see Chapter 103).

Occipital Nerve Blocks

Blocks of the greater occipital nerve have been promoted in the past as a diagnostic test for headache, but they have a curious and checkered history.[53,88] Despite their popularity, there are no data on their validity or utility.

Greater occipital nerve blocks were introduced originally for the diagnosis of a particular form of occipital neuralgia. The cause of pain was described as compression of the greater occipital nerve between the posterior arch of the atlas and the lamina of C2.[89] The diagnostic test was to anesthetize the greater occipital nerve where it emerged from the posterior neck muscles onto the scalp.

Eventually, it was shown that the greater occipital nerve could not be injured in this way.[90,91] In addition, a rarely cited publication was uncovered in which one of the original authors voiced circumspection about the validity and effectiveness of greater occipital nerve blocks.[92] However, this did not stem the enthusiasm for greater occipital nerve blocks.

A belief in entrapment neuropathy developed, according to which the greater occipital nerve could be bound in scar tissue where it emerged from the posterior neck muscles. No histologic evidence of such scar has ever been produced nor has a reason for its development been articulated, let alone demonstrated. The greater occipital nerve emerges from beneath an aponeurotic sling, between the trapezius and sternocleidomastoid.[90] This fibrous sling could easily be mistaken for so-called scar tissue.

The lack of rationale for greater occipital nerve blocks as a diagnostic test is curious. Beyond the point where it is typically blocked, this nerve supplies only the skin of the posterior scalp. There is no known disease that affects this skin in order to be a cause of chronic pain. Therefore, greater occipital nerve blocks cannot be used to determine a source of pain. The same applies to lesser occipital nerve blocks. At best, therefore, greater occipital nerve blocks can only be used to establish that afferent activity in this nerve, in some way, modulates the perception of pain. The term "mediates" cannot apply for there is no source from which nociceptive afferent traffic along the nerve might arise.

Although several studies have described the use of greater occipital nerve blocks in the diagnosis of headache, none has used controlled blocks to test for placebo responses and none has articulated what diagnosis is established if the blocks are positive. Nor can greater occipital nerve blocks be held to be selective or target specific when volumes such as 5 mL[93] or 10 mL[94,95] of local anesthetic are used.[96] Under these conditions, it is hard to determine if greater occipital nerve blocks are more than a historical curiosity based on the mistaken belief that any pain in a given area must be mediated by the most obvious nerve in that area.

There is, however, a curious mystery about greater occipital nerve blocks. It has been shown that their effect on primary headache syndromes clearly outlasts the duration of local anesthetic used.[96,97] This phenomenon implies some sort of neuromodulatory effect. It would seem that this effect has been misinterpreted in the past as a diagnostic response. The mechanism of the effect and its clinical significance have not been determined.

The use of greater occipital nerve blocks as a predicate for avulsion of the greater occipital nerve has been particularly tragic. Despite seemingly widespread use in the past, this radical surgical procedure has never been shown to be effective for occipital head-

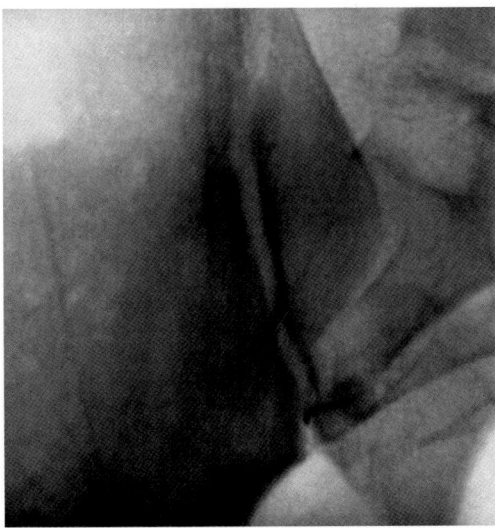

FIGURE 97.17 An anteroposterio fluoroscopy view of a needle placed for an intra-articular block of sacroiliac joint. (Radiograph provided by Dr. Paul Dreyfuss, and reproduced with permission from Bogduk N, ed. *Practice Guidelines for Spinal Diagnostic and Treatment Procedures*. San Francisco: International Spine Intervention Society; 2004.)

ache. Such data as are available indicate that any beneficial effects are temporary at best,[98] yet the treatment cannot be repeated.

PROTECTIVE PROCEDURES

Protective local anesthetic blocks are ones in which a region of the body is anesthetized in order to reduce or eliminate incident pain or to facilitate function or other treatment. Examples include femoral nerve blocks during the application of traction for a fractured femur, brachial plexus blocks to allow application of physical therapy in patients with complex regional pain syndromes of the upper limb, and intercostal blocks to permit deeper breathing in patients with painful fractures of the ribs or chest pain after thoracotomy. In these examples, it is recognized that the period of relief required is temporary and that other interventions will eventually treat the pain or spontaneous healing is anticipated. If required, the blocks can be repeated to prolong the duration of effect, but the blocks are not repeated ad infinitum.

Axillary Brachial Plexus Block

Axillary blocks of the brachial plexus involve introducing a needle through the floor of the axilla, aimed toward its apex, until it is felt to penetrate the axillary sheath. The block is increasingly performed under ultrasound guidance, which has been shown to be at least equivalent or even superior to the technique involving nerve stimulation.[99,100] Some 30 to 40 mL of local anesthetic are then injected to anesthetize the major branches of the brachial plexus that innervate the upper limb. If desired, a catheter can be introduced in the same manner in order to allow for a continuous infusion of local anesthetic.

Case reports have attested to the usefulness of continuous infusions of local anesthetic as an adjunct in the management of complex regional pain syndromes of the upper limb.[101–103] Anesthetizing the limb allows physical therapy to be applied without pain. For the manipulation of forearm fractures in children, axillary blocks are as effective as deep sedation with ketamine and midazolam.[104]

Femoral Nerve Block

The target point for femoral nerve blocks lies below the inguinal ligament, lateral to the femoral artery. While palpating the pulse of the femoral artery, a needle is introduced through the skin, about 1 cm lateral to the artery. Proper placement is established either by using a nerve stimulator or ultrasound guidance. Typically between 8 mL and 10 mL of local anesthetic is administered.

Although femoral nerve blocks may be used as an intraoperative or postoperative procedure for analgesia, their particular application as a pain medicine procedure is to relieve the pain of femoral fractures while the patient is transferred or is awaiting other interventions. Controlled trials have shown that adding a femoral nerve to intravenous analgesia block increases the reduction of pain scores by an average of 3.6 points (on a 10-point scale)[105] and that femoral nerve blocks provide superior relief of pain and anxiety than does intravenous metamizol.[106]

Intercostal Nerve Blocks

Intercostal nerve blocks can be performed opposite the angle of the rib or in the midaxillary line. They require palpating the rib above the target nerve and introducing a needle first to touch the lower edge of that rib. Thereafter, the needle is allowed to slip under the rib and a further 3–5 mm deeper. Ultrasound guidance allows the visualization of the pleura and is therefore expected to be safer than the blind technique, although no controlled trials have proven this hypothesis. Typically 3–4 mL of local anesthetic (1 mL under ultrasound guidance) is used to anesthetize the nerve. In patients with rib fractures, intercostal nerve blocks reduce pain and increase oxygen saturation.[107]

PALLIATIVE BLOCKS

There is no basis for local anesthetic blocks to be therapeutic in the conventional sense. Local anesthetics have a limited duration of action, and their effects are expected to wear off. Any relief should be temporary, under normal circumstances.

However, for some conditions for which there is no other proven treatment, some physicians administer local anesthetic blocks despite their temporary effect. Although temporary, that relief may be satisfying to patients. Using blocks in this way cannot be construed as therapeutic for there is little prospect of enduring relief. A better description is that such blocks are palliative.

Nevertheless, there is anecdotal evidence that in some patients, repeating blocks can lead to prolonged periods of relief well beyond the duration of action of the agent used. Neither the proportion of patients who respond in this way or the mechanism of this effect is known. It may be a peculiar effect of local anesthetic on open sodium channels in patients with chronic pain. It may be a placebo effect. It may be due to some settling effect on CNS pathways.

Notwithstanding this lack of information, palliative blocks are an attractive option for some practitioners and for some patients when other options are not available or impractical.

Common to all palliative blocks is a lack of formal evidence of efficacy. Patients should be informed of this lest they be under the illusion that these are in fact legitimate therapeutic procedures. Those who pay for multiple repeat blocks have grounds for concern. In some countries, where insurers are responsible for income replacement, insurers would like to see that palliative blocks improve function and allow return to work.

There is little purpose in performing palliative blocks if the effects last only for the duration of action of the agent used. This achieves nothing but a temporary illusion of therapy.

If relief is prolonged, it needs to shown to be useful. In the first instance, a visual analog scale or numeric pain rating scale (NPRS) should be used to document the magnitude of relief. Also documented should be the restoration of activities, for if function does not improve, the risk–benefit or cost–benefit ratio may be considered as unfavorable.

Palliative blocks are, therefore, a very contentious intervention. Patients enjoy the relief; physicians enjoy providing it. The exercise, however, is questionable if all that is achieved is some degree of temporary relief of pain.

A Cochrane Review searched for evidence that local anesthetic blocks were effective for complex regional pain syndromes.[108] It found only two small studies whose data were statistically equivocal about whether or not blocks achieved greater than 50% relief of pain for at least hours and no valid data on longer term effects.

Sympathetic blocks are practiced, seemingly, widely for the treatment of the pain of acute herpes zoster and for postherpetic neuralgia. Despite an abundance of descriptive studies advocating sympathetic blocks for these conditions, reviews of the literature have found that sympathetic blocks might reduce the duration of acute herpes but do not affect the intensity of pain and do not reduce the incidence of postherpetic neuralgia, nor are they effective for postherpetic neuralgia.[109,110] The evidence is stronger for epidural and intrathecal blocks for these conditions.[110]

There is substantial evidence for the efficacy of neurolytic blocks of the celiac plexus for the treatment of cancer pain and the pain of pancreatitis (see Chapters 45 and 64). Local anesthetic blocks of this plexus are substantially less effective.[111]

Blocks of the superior hypogastric plexus have been reported to be of value for intractable pain in the penis.[112] Blocks of the ganglion impar have been reported as providing at least 50% relief of pain in patients with chronic perineal pain.[112] Larger series and no controlled trials of these procedures have not been reported, possibly because of the rarity, in any one center, of the conditions for which they are used.

CONCLUSION

Anesthesiologists were prominent amongst those who founded the discipline of pain medicine. From their background and training in surgical anesthesia, they brought with them the art of local anesthetic blocks. In a new discipline, these blocks were a powerful tool: they could stop the symptom of which the patient complained. Over the last 30 years, however, the standards of science in medicine have escalated. The art of local anesthetic blocks has not kept pace with the science required of them.

Most of the publicity concerning evidence-based medicine has centered on the standards set and expected for studies of the efficacy of treatments. For such studies, rules now apply concerning randomization, blinding, controls, follow-up, outcome measures, and intention-to-treat analysis. These same rules do not apply to diagnostic tests, but others do.

The rules for operative anesthesia are straightforward and easy to apply. In operative anesthesia, the objective is to protect the patient from feeling pain once the surgery commences. Adequacy of anesthesia can be tested by a applying a noxious stimulus and asking the patient of any effect. If they are numb, the patient, the anesthetist, and the surgeon are all satisfied. At a philosophical level, it does not matter if the patient had a placebo effect. The block, nevertheless, served its purpose.

A different set of rules applies to pain medicine. The situation differs in that the objective of local anesthetic blocks is to stop ongoing pain, be that for diagnostic, prognostic, palliative, or therapeutic purposes. This is a different idiom from that of securing surgical anesthesia.

Paramount is the validity of the local anesthetic block, and placebo effects are a serious, potential, confounding influence. It does matter if the patient has a placebo response when diagnostic and therapeutic decisions are based on that response. Notwithstanding the mysteries of the placebo response and what it means, most fundamentally a placebo response is a false-positive response. It means that any decision about diagnosis may not be correct, and any decision about treatment is likely to be wrong.

Because false-positive responses can occur, sometimes commonly, practitioners cannot assume that all positive responses to blocks are true-positive. A block cannot be held to be valid unless it is subjected to some sort of control.

It is in this regard that the art of local anesthetic blocks has lagged behind the pace of contemporary science. Eminent authorities in the past have described a vast litany of the types of blocks that could be performed; some even implied that they should be done. At a scientific and clinical level, however, those recommendations pertained only to the execution of blocks. They did not address their validity and interpretation.

The assumption that single diagnostic blocks cannot be false-positive is wrong. Whenever this has been tested, substantial and sometimes prohibitive false-positive rates have been encountered. There is no reason why blocks that have not been tested for validity should be immune to false-positive response.

For prognostic blocks, the assumption has been that uncontrolled blocks will faithfully predict the outcome of treatment. This assumption may be convenient for expeditious practice, but it does not amount to evidence-based practice. Two confounding influences apply. The prediction of the blocks may be incorrect

because the response to blocks is not valid, and the treatment may not work because its efficacy has not been established.

It is for these reasons that the present chapter does not resemble its forerunners or corresponding chapters in other books. Local anesthetic blocks have not been described just because they can be done. Instead, the present chapter has focused on why blocks might be done. Some degree of evidence is required to find the answer to that question. As a result, the present chapter does not describe blocks for which there is barely anecdotal evidence. Prominence has been given to those blocks for which there is evidence and in proportion to the volume and quality of evidence available. This results in an irony.

Certain blocks, held in high esteem by anesthesiologists and widely practiced, have been accorded less prominence than in previous texts. Either evidence of their validity and utility is lacking or, in some cases, the emerging evidence has challenged their assumed validity. Sympathetic blocks are the prime example. When subjected to controls, these blocks prove not to be valid, and no studies have refuted this challenge.

Other blocks, such as transforaminal blocks, have some evidence, but it is incomplete. There is room either for these blocks still to be refuted or properly validated.

Meanwhile, it transpires that the most extensive and most rigorous evidence about local anesthetic blocks pertains to those not held to be classical and, therefore, exempt from the requirements for controls. Medial branch blocks have been tested, more so than any other form of local anesthetic blocks. Variously, they have been shown to protect healthy volunteers from experimentally induced pain; they have been shown to have target-specificity; their false-positive rates are known and are large, but can be reduced by using controls; and positive responses are associated with successful outcomes of treatment. For no other local anesthetic block have these requirements been satisfied.

The foundations of pain medicine in general and interventional pain medicine in particular depend on the validity of local anesthetic blocks. The evidence, at present, would indicate that whereas medial branch blocks are sound, all other blocks are questionable. The challenge, if not duty, of experts in this discipline is to make up the difference. It is often said that no evidence of efficacy is not evidence of no efficacy, but a retort applies. Assumption is not a substitute for evidence. Perhaps future editions of this chapter can be enriched by a greater, appropriate body of evidence.

References

1. Moore DC, Batra MS. The components of an effective test dose prior to epidural block. *Anesthesiology* 1981;55:693–696
2. Nancarrow C, Rutten AJ, Runciman WB, et al. Myocardial and cerebral concentrations and the mechanisms of death after fatal intravenous doses of lidocaine, bupivacaine, and ropivacaine in sheep. *Anesth Analg* 1998;69:276–283.
3. Weinberg GL, VadeBoncouer T, Ramaraju GA, et al. Pretreatment or resuscitation with a lipid infusion shifts the dose–response to bupivacaine-induced asystole in rats. *Anesthesiology* 1998;88:1071–1075.
4. Weinberg GL, Ripper R, Murphy P, et al. Lipid infusion accelerates removal of bupivacaine and recovery from bupivacaine toxicity in the isolated rat heart. *Reg Anesth Pain Med* 2006;31:296–303.
5. Weinberg G, Ripper R, Feinstein DL, et al. Lipid emulsion infusion rescues dogs from bupivacaine-induced cardiac toxicity. *Reg Anesth Pain Med* 2003;28:198–202.
6. Warren JA, Thoma RB, Georgescu A, et al. Intravenous lipid infusion in the successful resuscitation of local anesthetic-induced cardiovascular collapse after supraclavicular brachial plexus block. *Anesth Analg* 2008;106:1578–1580.
7. Litz RJ, Roessel T. Heller AR, et al. Reversal of central nervous system and cardiac toxicity after local anesthetic intoxication by lipid emulsion injection. *Anesth Analg* 2008;106:1575–1577.
8. Ludot H, Tharin JY, Belouadah M, et al. Successful resuscitation after ropivacaine and lidocaine-induced ventricular arrhythmia following posterior lumbar plexus block in a child. *Anesth Analg* 2008;106:1572–1574.
9. Brull SJ. Lipid emulsion for the treatment of local anesthetic toxicity: patient safety implications. *Anesth Analg* 2008;106:1337–1339.

10. Watts SA, Sharma DJ. Long-term neurological complications associated with surgery and peripheral nerve blockade: outcomes after 1065 consecutive blocks. *Anaesth Intensive Care* 2007;35:24–31.

11. Fanelli G, Casati A, Garancini P, et al. Nerve stimulator and multiple injection technique for upper and lower limb blockade: failure rate, patient acceptance, and neurologic complications. Study Group on Regional Anesthesia. *Anesth Analg* 1999;88:847–852.

12. Auroy Y, Benhamou D, Bargues L, et al. Major complications of regional anesthesia in France. The SOG Regional Anesthesia Hotline Service. *Anesthesiology* 2002;97:1274–1280.

13. Curatolo M, Eichenberger U. Ultrasound-guided blocks for the treatment of chronic pain. *Tech Reg Anesth Pain Manage* 2007;11:95–102.

14. International Spine Intervention Society. Cervical transforaminal injection of corticosteroids. In: Bogduk N, ed. *Practice Guidelines for Spinal Diagnostic and Treatment Procedures*. San Francisco: International Spine Intervention Society; 2004:237–248.

15. International Spine Intervention Society. Lumbar spinal nerve blocks. In: Bogduk N, ed. *Practice Guidelines for Spinal Diagnostic and Treatment Procedures*. San Francisco: International Spine Intervention Society; 2004:3–17.

16. International Spine Intervention Society. Thoracic transforaminal injections. In: Bogduk N, ed. *Practice Guidelines for Spinal Diagnostic and Treatment Procedures*. San Francisco: International Spine Intervention Society; 2004:295–313.

17. Stolker RJ, Vervest AC, Groen GJ. The treatment of chronic thoracic segmental pain by radiofrequency percutaneous partial rhizotomy. *J Neurosurg* 1994;80:986–992.

18. van Kleef M, Barendse GA, Dingemans WA, et al. Effects of producing a radiofrequency lesion adjacent to the dorsal root ganglion in patients with thoracic segmental pain. *Clin J Pain* 1995;11: 325–332.

19. Aspinall S, Mohammed S, Sanderson PL. The value of nerve root injection in the evaluation of sciatica in patients with normal MRI scans. *J Bone Joint Surg* 2000;82B(suppl III):279.

20. Hasueisen DC, Smith BS, Myers SR, et al. The diagnostic accuracy of spinal nerve injection studies. Their role in the evaluation of recurrent sciatica. *Clin Orthop Relat Res* 1985;198:179–183.

21. Dooley JF, McBroom RJ, Taguchi T, et al. Nerve root infiltration in the diagnosis of radicular pain. *Spine* 1988;13:79–83.

22. Castro WHM, van Akkerveeken PF. Der diagnostische Wert der selektiven lumbalen Nervenwurzelblockade. *Z Orthop Ihre Grenzgeb* 1991;129:374–379.

23. van Akkerveeken PF. The diagnostic value of nerve root sheath infiltration. *Acta Orthop Scand Suppl* 1993;251:61–63.

24. Sasso RC, Macadaeg K, Nordmann D, et al. Selective nerve root injections can predict surgical outcome for lumbar and cervical radiculopathy: comparison to magnetic resonance imaging. *J Spinal Disord Tech* 2005;18:471–478.

25. Haddox JD. A call for clarity. In: Campbell JN, ed. *Pain 1996. An updated review. Refresher course syllabus*. Seattle: IASP Press; 1996:97–99.

26. Hogan QH, Erickson SJ, Haddox JD, et al. The spread of solutions during stellate ganglion block. *Reg Anesth* 1992;17:78–83.

27. Kapral S, Krafft P, Gosch M, et al. Ultrasound imaging for stellate ganglion block: Direct visualization of puncture site and local anesthetic spread. A pilot study. *Reg Anesth* 1995;20:323–328

28. Price DD, Long S, Wilsey B, et al. Analysis of peak magnitude and duration of analgesia produced by local anesthetics injected into sympathetic ganglion of complex regional pain syndrome patients. *Clin J Pain* 1998;14:216–226.

29. Bonica JJ. Local anesthesia and regional blocks. In Wall PD, Melzak R, eds. *Textbook of Pain*. 2nd ed. Edinburgh: Churchill Livingston; 1989:724–743.

30. Bonica JJ, Buckley FP. Regional analgesia with local anesthetics. In Bonica JJ, ed. *The Management of Pain*. Vol. 2. Philadelphia: Lea & Febiger; 1990:1883–1966.

31. Boas RA. Nerve blocks in the diagnosis of low back pain. *Neurosurg Clin N Am* 1991;2:807–816.

32. Bonica JJ, Butler SH. Local anaesthesia and regional blocks. In Wall PD, Melzack R, eds. *Textbook of Pain*. 3rd ed. Edinburgh: Churchill Livingstone; 1994:997–1023.

33. Moore DC, Bridenbaugh LD, Bridenbaugh PO, et al. Bupivacaine for peripheral nerve block: a comparison with mepivacaine, lidocaine, and tetracaine. *Anesthesiology* 1970;32:460–463.

34. Moore DC, Bridenbaugh LD, Bridenbaugh PO, et al. Bupivacaine: a review of 2,077 cases. *JAMA* 1970;214:713–718.

35. Barnsley L, Lord S, Bogduk N. Comparative local anaesthetic blocks in the diagnosis of cervical zygapophysial joints pain. *Pain* 1993;55:99–106.

36. Lord SM, Barnsley L, Bogduk N. The utility of comparative local anaesthetic blocks versus placebo-controlled blocks for the diagnosis of cervical zygapophysial joint pain. *Clin J Pain* 1995;11:208–213.

37. Barnsley L, Bogduk N. Medial branch blocks are specific for the diagnosis of cervical zygapophysial joint pain. *Reg Anesth* 1993;18:343–350.

38. International Spine Intervention Society. Cervical medial branch blocks. In: Bogduk N, ed. *Practice Guidelines for Spinal Diagnostic and Treatment Procedures*. San Francisco: International Spine Intervention Society; 2004:112–137.

39. Verrils P, Mitchell B, Vivian D, et al. The incidence of intravascular penetration in medial branch blocks: cervical, thoracic, and lumbar spines. *Spine* 2008;33:E174–E177.

40. Barnsley L, Lord S, Wallis B, et al. False-positive rates of cervical zygapophysial joint blocks. *Clin J Pain* 1993;9:124–130.

41. Sackett DL, Haynes RB, Guyatt GH, et al. *Clinical Epidemiology: A Basic Science for Clinical Medicine*. 2nd ed. Boston: Little, Brown & Co.; 1991:119–139.

42. Barnsley L, Lord SM, Wallis BJ, et al. The prevalence of chronic cervical zygapophysial joint pain after whiplash. *Spine* 1995;20:20–26.

43. Lord S, Barnsley L, Wallis BJ, et al. Chronic cervical zygapophysial joint pain after whiplash. A placebo-controlled prevalence study. *Spine* 1996;21:1737–1745.

44. Gibson T, Bogduk N, Macpherson J, et al. The accident characteristics of whiplash associated chronic neck pain. *J Musculoskeletal Pain* 2000;8:87–95.

45. Lord SM, Barnsley L, Wallis BJ, et al. Third occipital nerve headache: a prevalence study. *J Neurol Neurosurg Psychiatry* 1994;57:1187–1190.

46. Speldewinde GC, Bashford GM, Davidson IR. Diagnostic cervical zygapophysial joint blocks for chronic cervical pain. *Med J Aust* 2001;174:174–176.

47. Manchikanti L, Singh V, Rivera J, et al. Prevalence of cervical facet joint pain in chronic neck pain. *Pain Physician* 2002;5:243–249.

48. Lord SM, Barnsley L, Wallis BJ, et al. Percutaneous radio-frequency neurotomy for chronic cervical zygapophyseal-joint pain. *N Engl J Med* 1996;335:1721–1726.

49. Lord SM, McDonald GJ, Bogduk N. Percutaneous radiofrequency neurotomy of the cervical medial branches: a validated treatment for cervical zygapophysial joint pain. *Neurosurgery Quarterly* 1998;8:288–308.

50. McDonald GJ, Lord SM, Bogduk N. Long-term follow-up of patients treated with cervical radiofrequency neurotomy for chronic neck pain. *Neurosurgery* 1999;45:61–68.

51. Barnsley L. Percutaneous radiofrequency neurotomy for chronic neck pain: outcomes in a series of consecutive patients. *Pain Med* 2005;6:282–286.

52. Bogduk N. The neck and headaches. *Neurol Clin* 2004;22:151–171.

53. Bogduk N, Bartsch T. Cervicogenic headache. In: Silberstein SD, Lipton RB, Dodick DW, eds. *Wolff's Headache*. 8th ed. New York: Oxford University Press; 2008:551–570.

54. Govind J, King W, Bailey B, et al. Radiofrequency neurotomy for the treatment of third occipital headache. *J Neurol Neurosurg Psychiat* 2003;74:88–93.

55. Eichenberger U, Greher M, Kapral S, et al. Sonographic visualization and ultrasound-guided block of the third occipital nerve: prospective for a new method to diagnose C2–C3 zygapophysial joint pain. *Anesthesiology* 2006;104:303–308.

56. Lawrence JS, Bremner JM, Bier F. Osteo-arthrosis. Prevalence in the population and relationship between symptoms and x-ray changes. *Ann Rheum Dis* 1966;25:1–24.

57. Magora A, Schwartz A. Relation between the low back pain syndrome and x-ray findings. *Scand J Rehabil Med* 1978;8:115–126.

58. Schwarzer AC, Wang SC, O'Driscoll D, et al. The ability of computed tomography to identify a painful zygapophysial joint in patients with chronic low back pain. *Spine* 1995; 20:907–912.

59. Czervionke LF, Fenton DS. Fat-saturated MR imaging in the detection of inflammatory facet arthropathy (facet synovitis) in the lumbar spine. *Pain Med* 2008;9(4):400–406.

60. International Spine Intervention Society. Lumbar medial branch blocks. In: Bogduk N, ed. *Practice Guidelines for Spinal Diagnostic and Treatment Procedures*. San Francisco: International Spine Intervention Society; 2004:47–65.

61. Dreyfuss P, Schwarzer AC, Lau P, et al. Specificity of lumbar medial branch and L5 dorsal ramus blocks: a computed tomographic study. *Spine* 1997;22:895–902.

62. Kaplan M, Dreyfuss P, Halbrook B, et al. The ability of lumbar medial branch blocks to anesthetize the zygapophysial joint. A physiologic challenge. *Spine* 1998;23:1847–1852.

63. Schwarzer AC, Aprill CN, Derby R, et al. The false-positive rate of uncontrolled diagnostic blocks of the lumbar zygapophysial joints. *Pain* 1994;58:195–200.

64. Manchikanti L, Pampati V, Fellows B, et al. Prevalence of lumbar facet joint pain in chronic low back pain. *Pain Physician* 1999;2:59–64.

65. Manchikanti L, Pampati V, Fellows B, et al. The diagnostic validity and therapeutic value of lumbar facet joint nerve blocks with or without adjuvant agents. *Curr Rev Pain* 2000;4:337–344.

66. Schwarzer AC, Aprill CN, Derby R, et al. Clinical features of patients with pain stemming from the lumbar zygapophysial joints. Is the lumbar facet syndrome a clinical entity? *Spine* 1994;19:1132–1137.

67. Schwarzer AC, Wang SC, Bogduk N, et al. Prevalence and clinical features of lumbar zygapophysial joint pain: a study in an Australian population with chronic low back pain. *Ann Rheum Dis* 1995;54:100–106.

68. Schwarzer AC, Aprill CN, Derby R, et al. The prevalence and clinical features of internal disc disruption in patients with chronic low back pain. *Spine* 1995; 20:1878–1883.

69. Schwarzer AC, Aprill CN, Bogduk N. The sacroiliac joint in chronic low back pain. *Spine* 1995;20:31–37.

70. Laslett M, Oberg B, Aprill CN, et al. Zygapophysial joint blocks in chronic low back pain: a test of Revel's model as a screening test. *BMC Musculoskel Disord* 2004;5:43.

71. Laslett M, McDonald B, Aprill CN, et al. Clinical predictors of screening lumbar zygapophysial joint blocks: development of clinical prediction rules. *Spine* 2006;6:370–379.

72. Carette S, Marcoux S, Truchon R, et al. controlled trial of corticosteroid injections into facet joints for chronic low back pain. *N Engl J Med* 1991;325:1002–1007.

73. Jackson RP, Jacobs RR, Montesano PX. Facet joint injection in low-back pain. A prospective statistical study. *Spine* 1988;13:966–971.
74. International Spine Intervention Society. An algorithm for the investigation of low back pain. In: Bogduk N, ed. *Practice Guidelines for Spinal Diagnostic and Treatment Procedures.* San Francisco: International Spine Intervention Society; 2004:87–94.
75. International Spine Intervention Society. Lumbar medial neurotomy. In: Bogduk N, ed. *Practice Guidelines for Spinal Diagnostic and Treatment Procedures.* San Francisco: International Spine Intervention Society; 2004:188–218.
76. Dreyfuss P, Halbrook B, Pauza K, et al. Efficacy and validity of radiofrequency neurotomy for chronic lumbar zygapophysial joint pain. *Spine* 2000;25:1270–1277.
77. Schofferman J, Kine G. Effectiveness of repeated radiofrequency neurotomy for lumbar facet pain. *Spine* 2004;29:2471–2473.
78. Dreyfuss P, Michaelsen M, Fletcher D. Atlanto-occipital and lateral atlanto-axial joint pain patterns. *Spine* 1994;19:1125–1131.
79. International Spine intervention Society. Lateral atlanto-axial joint blocks. In: Bogduk N, ed. *Practice Guidelines for Spinal Diagnostic and Treatment Procedures.* San Francisco: International Spine Intervention Society; 2004:138–151.
80. Aprill C, Axinn MJ, Bogduk N. Occipital headaches stemming from the lateral atlanto-axial (C1-2) joint. *Cephalalgia* 2002;22:15–22.
81. Narouze SN, Casanova J, Mekhail N. The longitudinal effectiveness of lateral atlantoaxial intra-articular steroid injection in the treatment of cervicogenic headache. *Pain Med* 2007;8:184–188.
82. Joseph B, Kumar B. Gallie's fusion for atlantoaxial arthrosis with occipital neuralgia. *Spine* 1994;19:454–455.
83. Ghanayem AJ, Leventhal M, Bohlman HH. Osteoarthrosis of the atlanto-axial joints. Long-term follow-up after treatment with arthrodesis. *J Bone Joint Surg* 1996;78:1300–1307.
84. Schaeren S, Jeanneret B. Atlantoaxial osteoarthritis: case series and review of the literature. *Eur Spine J* 2005;14:501–506.
85. International Spine Intervention Society. Sacroiliac joint blocks. In: Bogduk N, ed. *Practice Guidelines for Spinal Diagnostic and Treatment Procedures.* San Francisco, International Spine Intervention Society; 2004;66–85.
86. Maigne JY, Aivaliklis A, Pfefer F. Results of sacroiliac joint double block and value of sacroiliac pain provocation tests in 54 patients with low back pain. *Spine* 1996;21:1889–1892.
87. Bogduk N, Bartsch T. Headaches of cervical origin: focus on anatomy and physiology. In: Goadsby PJ, Silberstein SD, Dodick DW, eds. *Chronic Daily Headache for Clinicians.* London: BC Decker; 2005:369–381.
88. Hunter CR, Mayfield FH. Role of the upper cervical roots in the production of pain in the head. *Am J Surg* 1949;78:743–749.
89. Bogduk N. The anatomy of occipital neuralgia. *Clin Exp Neurol* 1980;17:167–184.
90. Bilge O. An anatomic and morphometric study of C2 nerve root ganglion and its corresponding foramen. *Spine* 2004;29:495–499.
91. Mayfield FH. Symposium on cervical trauma. Neurosurgical aspects. *Clin Neurosurg* 1955;2:83–90.
92. Bovim G, Fredriksen TA, Stolt-Nielsen A, et al. Neurolysis of the greater occipital nerve in cervicogenic headache. A follow up study. *Headache* 1992;32:175–179.
93. Saadah HA, Taylor FB. Sustained headache syndrome associated with tender occipital nerve zones. *Headache* 1987;27:201–205.
94. Gawel MJ, Rothbart PJ. Occipital nerve block in the management of headache and cervical pain. *Cephalalgia* 1992;12:9–13.
95. Bogduk N. Role of anesthesiologic blockade in headache management. *Curr Pain Headache Rep* 2004;8:399–403.
96. Afridi SK, Shields KG, Bhola R, et al. Greater occipital nerve injection in primary headache syndromes—prolonged effects from a single injection. *Pain* 2006;122:126–129.
97. Anthony M. headache and the greater occipital nerve. *Clin Neurol Neurosurg* 1992;94:297–301.
98. Chan VW, Perlas A, McCartney CJ, et al. Ultrasound guidance improves success rate of axillary brachial plexus block. *Can J Anaesth* 2007;54:176–182.
99. Casati A, Danelli G, Baciarello M, et al. A prospective, randomized comparison between ultrasound and nerve stimulation guidance for multiple injection axillary brachial plexus block. *Anesthesiology* 2007;106:992–996
100. Murray P, Floor K, Atkinson RE. Continuous brachial plexus blockade for reflex sympathetic dystrophy. *Anaesthesia* 1995;50:633–635.
101. Ribbers GM, Geurts AC, Rijken RA, et al. Axillary brachial plexus blockade for the reflex sympathetic dystrophy syndrome. *Int J Rehabil Res* 1997;20:371–380.
102. Wang LK, Chen HP, Chang PJ, et al. Axillary brachial plexus block with patient controlled analgesia for complex regional pain syndrome type I: a case report. *Reg Anesth Pain Med* 2001;26:68–71.
103. Kriwanek KL, Wan J, Beaty JH, et al. Axillary block for analgesia during manipulation of forearm fractures in the pediatric emergency department a prospective randomized comparative trial. *J Pediatr Orthop* 2006;26:737–740.
104. Mutty CE, Jensen EJ, Manka MA Jr, et al. Femoral nerve block for diaphyseal and distal femoral fractures in the emergency department. *J Bone Joint Surg* 2007;89:2599–2603.
105. Schifere A, Gore C, Gorove L, et al. A randomized controlled trial of femoral nerve blockade administered preclinically for pain relief in femoral trauma. *Anesth Analg* 2007;105:1852–1854.
106. Osinowo OA, Zahrani M, Softah A. Effect of intercostal nerve block with 0.5% bupivacaine on peak expiratory flow rate and arterial oxygen saturation in rib fractures. *J Trauma* 2004;56:345–347.
107. Cepeda MS, Carr DB, Lau J. Local anesthetic sympathetic blockade for complex regional pain syndrome. *Cochrane Database Syst Rev* 2005;19(4):CD00598.
108. Wu CL, Marsh A, Dworkin RH. The role of sympathetic nerve blocks in herpes zoster and postherpetic neuralgia. *Pain* 2000;87:121–129.
109. Kumar V, Krone K, Mathieu A. Neuraxial and sympathetic blocks in herpes zoster and postherpetic neuralgia: an appraisal of current evidence. *Reg Anesth Pain Med* 2004;29:454–461.
110. Levy MJ, Topazian MD, Wiersema MJ, et al. Initial evaluation of the efficacy and safety of endoscopic ultrasound-guided direct Ganglia neurolysis and block. *Am J Gastroenterol* 2008;103:98–103.
111. Rosenberg SK, Tewari R, Boswell MV, et al. Superior hypogastric plexus block successfully treats severe penile pain after transurethral resection of the prostate. *Reg Anesth Pain Med* 1998;23:619–620.
112. Toshniwal GR, Dureja GP, Prashanth SM. Transsacrococcygeal approach to ganglion impar block for manage3ment of chronic perineal pain: a prospective study. *Pain Physician* 2007;10:661–666.

CHAPTER 98 ■ EPIDURAL STEROID INJECTIONS

NIKOLAI BOGDUK

Epidural injection of steroids is one of the oldest procedures practiced in pain medicine. Reportedly, it is the most commonly performed interventional pain procedure in the United States.[1] This history and popularity, however, stand in stark contrast to the evidence of its limited efficacy.

HISTORICAL BACKGROUND

The first recorded use of epidural steroid injections dates back to 1952, when Robecchi and Capra[2] reported the relief of lumbar and sciatic pain in a woman after a periradicular injection of hydrocortisone onto the first sacral roots through the S1 posterior sacral foramen. This route of injection was popularised in the Italian[2–9] and French literature.[10–13] However, it was soon supplanted by other routes of administration. Although developments occurred worldwide, a lumbar route was promoted particularly in the United Kingdom, and a caudal route was promoted in the United States. Implicitly, these routes were based on existing techniques for obtaining epidural anaesthesia and were developed because they were easier to perform than sacral transforaminal injections and because of the desire to reach nerve roots other than the first sacral.

From the late 1950s until the close of the twentieth century, a large body of literature appeared worldwide reporting the effectiveness of injections by the lumbar[14–37] and caudal epidural[38–51] routes. This literature became responsible for the reputation of epidural steroids as an effective treatment for lumbar and sacral radicular pain (i.e., sciatica).

TECHNIQUES

Several techniques are available for the delivery of corticosteroids into the epidural space. They differ with respect to where the needle is placed and whether or not fluoroscopic guidance is used. A survey found that there is no uniformity of practice in the United States.[52] Different routes of administration and image-guidance are used to different extents within and between academic institutions and private practices.

Lumbar Epidural Steroids

The lumbar route for administering epidural steroids involves passing a needle through an interlaminar space, usually along the midline through the interspinous ligament or slightly to the side of this ligament. The procedure requires that the needle penetrates the ligamentum flavum to enter the epidural space but to fall short of piercing the dural sac. The perceived advantage of the lumbar route is that the needle is directed close to the site of pathology. There is no agreed volume or composition of the therapeutic agent. Authors have recommended various preparations of corticosteroids, either alone or mixed with local anesthetic or normal saline, in total volumes ranging from 2 mL to 43 mL,[53–55] but volumes of 2–5 mL are typical.

Caudal Epidural Steroids

The caudal route of administration involves introducing a needle into the epidural space via the sacral hiatus. The hiatus is located by palpation, and the needle is introduced through the overlying skin until it is felt to penetrate the membrane that encloses the hiatus. The purported attraction of this approach is that it is easily performed and decreases the possible risk of inadvertent dural puncture and, therefore, of inadvertent intrathecal injection.

Caudal injections require a substantial volume of fluid to be injected in order to reach the lumbar nerve roots which lie some 10 cm or more cephalad from the site of injection. Authors have recommended various preparations of corticosteroids, mixed with various local anesthetic agents or normal saline, in volumes ranging from 10 mL to 64 mL.[53–55]

Fluoroscopic Guidance

Epidural injections have traditionally been a clinical procedure. The operator relies on palpation to identify the site of injection. For depth of insertion, they rely on dexterity and various techniques such as loss of resistance[16] or the hanging drop method.[17] Some commentators, however, have argued that such reliance on manual skills leads to errors.

It has been demonstrated that caudal injections can fail to reach the epidural space in up to 35% of cases.[50,56–59] Injections can lie dorsal to the sacrum or coccyx or be intravascular (Fig. 98.1),[60] the latter despite no blood appearing on aspiration before injection. Lumbar injections can be subdural or superficial to the ligamentum flavum in some 17% of cases[50,61]; they can be

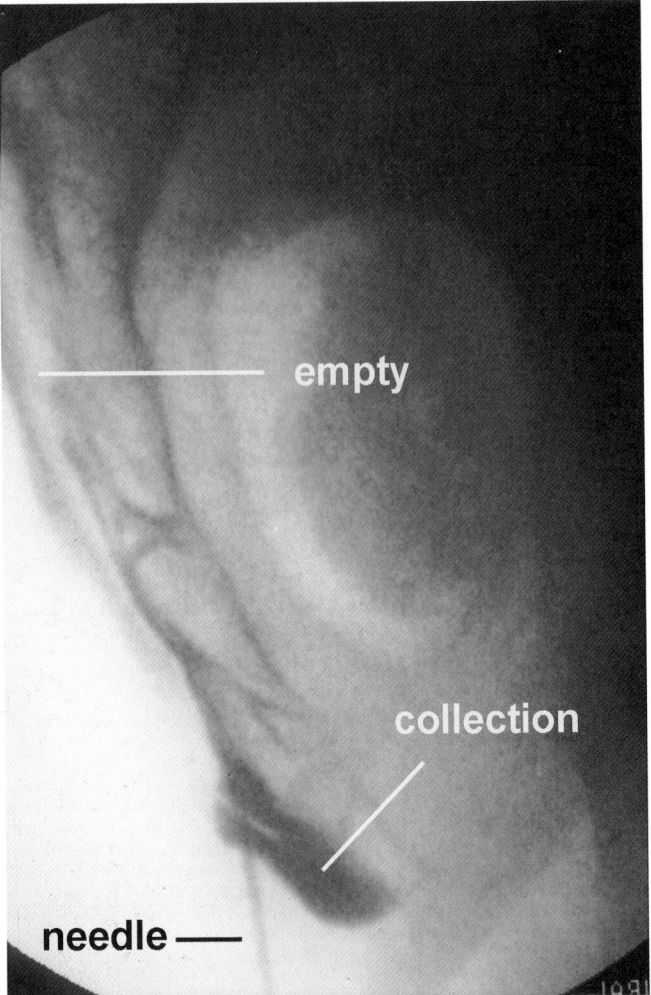

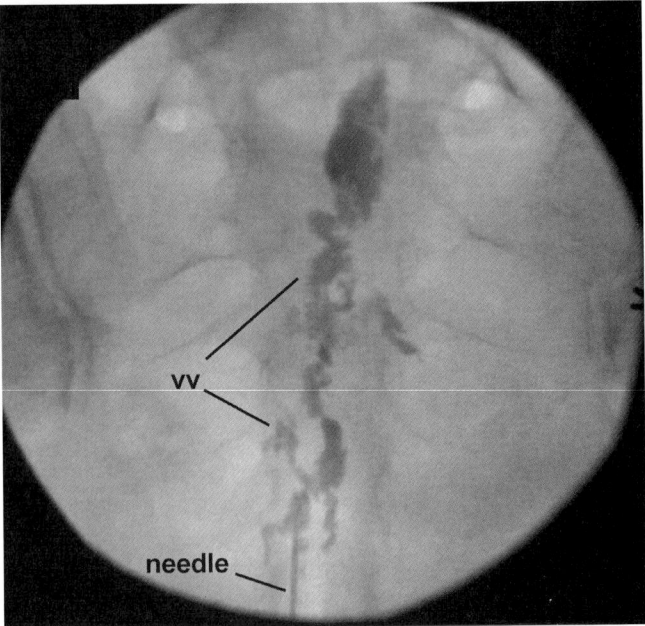

FIGURE 98.1 Aberrant caudal injections. **A.** Lateral radiograph of an attempted caudal epidural injection in which the contrast medium formed a collection dorsal to the coccyx. The sacral canal contains no contrast medium. **B.** Anteroposterior radiograph of an attempted caudal epidural injection in which the contrast medium has filled veins (vv) in the epidural space. (Kindly provided by Dr. Paul Dreyfuss, Seattle, WA.)

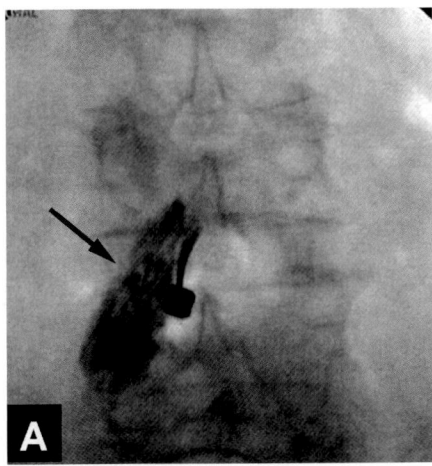
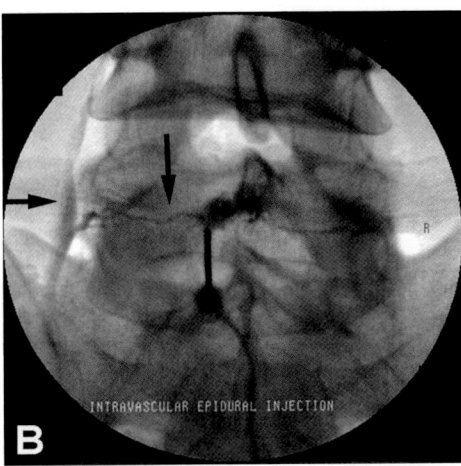

FIGURE 98.2 Aberrant lumbar interlaminar injections. **A.** Anteroposterior radiograph of an attempted interlaminar epidural injection in which the contrast medium outlined a fascicle of the lumbar multifidus muscle. **B.** Anteroposterior radiograph of an attempted interlaminar epidural injection in which the contrast medium has filled veins (*arrows*). (Kindly provided by Dr. Milton Landers, Wichita, KS.)

intravascular (Fig. 98.2). Errors are more common in patients with large body mass index,[58] when landmarks are difficult to palpate,[57] and generally in the execution of caudal injections.[58] Furthermore, even if the needle is accurately placed in the epidural space, the injectate can fail to reach the target level[62,63] or can remain in the posterior epidural space and not reach the disc-nerve root interface.[62]

Because of such errors when epidural injections are performed unaided, commentators have argued that they should be performed using fluoroscopic guidance, particularly for caudal injections.[56–58,60,64,65] Not all operators have heeded this call. Some continue to practice the procedures "blind" in a radiographic sense, but others have adopted fluoroscopic guidance.

Fluoroscopically-guided procedures differ from the classical procedures in that radiographs are used to locate the target site and to guide the needle to it (Figs. 98.3 and 98.4), and a test dose of contrast medium is injected into order to verify that the subsequent injection of therapeutic agent will be epidural and not intrathecal, subdural, or into a blood vessel. In other respects, the agents and volumes used are as for the classical procedures.

TRANSFORAMINAL INJECTIONS

Another procedure is related to epidural injections, but its taxonomic status is contentious. The procedure involves administering steroids under fluoroscopic guidance into the intervertebral foramen that lodges the affected spinal nerve. Literally and accurately, it is a transforaminal injection of steroids. Although the injectate does technically reach the epidural space, it remains around the nerve-root sleeve or on the floor of the vertebral canal. In this respect, transforaminal injections differ from classical epidural injections, in which the injectate spreads diffusely throughout the epidural space. In order to emphasise the difference, some operators use names such as "transforaminal epidural" or "selective epidural," although selectivity has never been formally established.

Transforaminal injections were developed in the belief that interlaminar or caudal injections were essentially too diffuse and that injecting directly onto the affected nerve should be more effective.[54,55] Various techniques have been described.

At lumbar levels, the variants differ only with respect to where the tip of the needle is placed.[66] In the original version,[54] the needle is directed onto the back of the vertebral body immediately opposite the lower pole of the pedicle (Fig. 98.5A,B).[66] Once the needle has been placed, a test dose of contrast medium shows that the injection is neither intrathecal nor intravascular and

flows along the target nerve (Fig. 98.5C,D). The second and third variants are designed to cope with distortions of the anatomy of the nerve, such as swelling or upward displacement, or to avoid puncturing vessels on the floor of the vertebral canal.[66] They involve placing the tip of the needle above the nerve (Fig. 98.6A) or behind it (Fig. 98.6B). In all variants, once the injection of contrast medium has demonstrated correct and safe placement of the needle, an aliquot of local anesthetic is injected (typically 1–2 mL), followed by a similar aliquot of corticosteroid preparation.

At sacral levels, the needle is delivered through the posterior sacral foramen so that its tip lies above the S1 spinal nerve and below the S1 pedicle (Fig. 98.7). Once a test dose of contrast medium establishes safe and accurate placement, local anesthetic and steroid are administered as for lumbar injections.

Number of Injections

In the published literature on interlaminar and caudal injections, most authors have used only one[17,18,22–24,27–31,50] or occasionally up to three injections.[16,25,33,36] Some have used up to six injections if they appeared to be of benefit, with the proviso of not using more than three if they did not appear to be of benefit[21]; one author describes using up to 10 injections.[20] For transforaminal injections, the literature describes using up to three injections, with an average of around two required to achieve optimal outcome.[67–69]

RATIONALE

It is conspicuous in the literature that a rationale for the epidural injection of steroids was not articulated in the early studies.[53–55] Implicitly, steroids were expected to be effective because they were believed to be effective for the treatment of other pain problems such as arthritis and tenosynovitis. Only later did authors seek a rationale. The belief that emerged was that since corticosteroids were anti-inflammatory, radicular pain must be caused by inflammation of the nerve roots. Circumstantial evidence was brought to bear in support of this belief.[53–55] More recently, animal studies have reinforced the belief by demonstrating inflammatory mediators in herniated disc material, such as phospholipase A2,[70] interleukins,[71,72] tumor necrosis factor α,[73,74] and nitric oxide.[71,75] In patients, however, evidence of inflammation has not yet been produced. Nor is demonstration of inflammation a perquisite for the use of epidural injections of steroids.

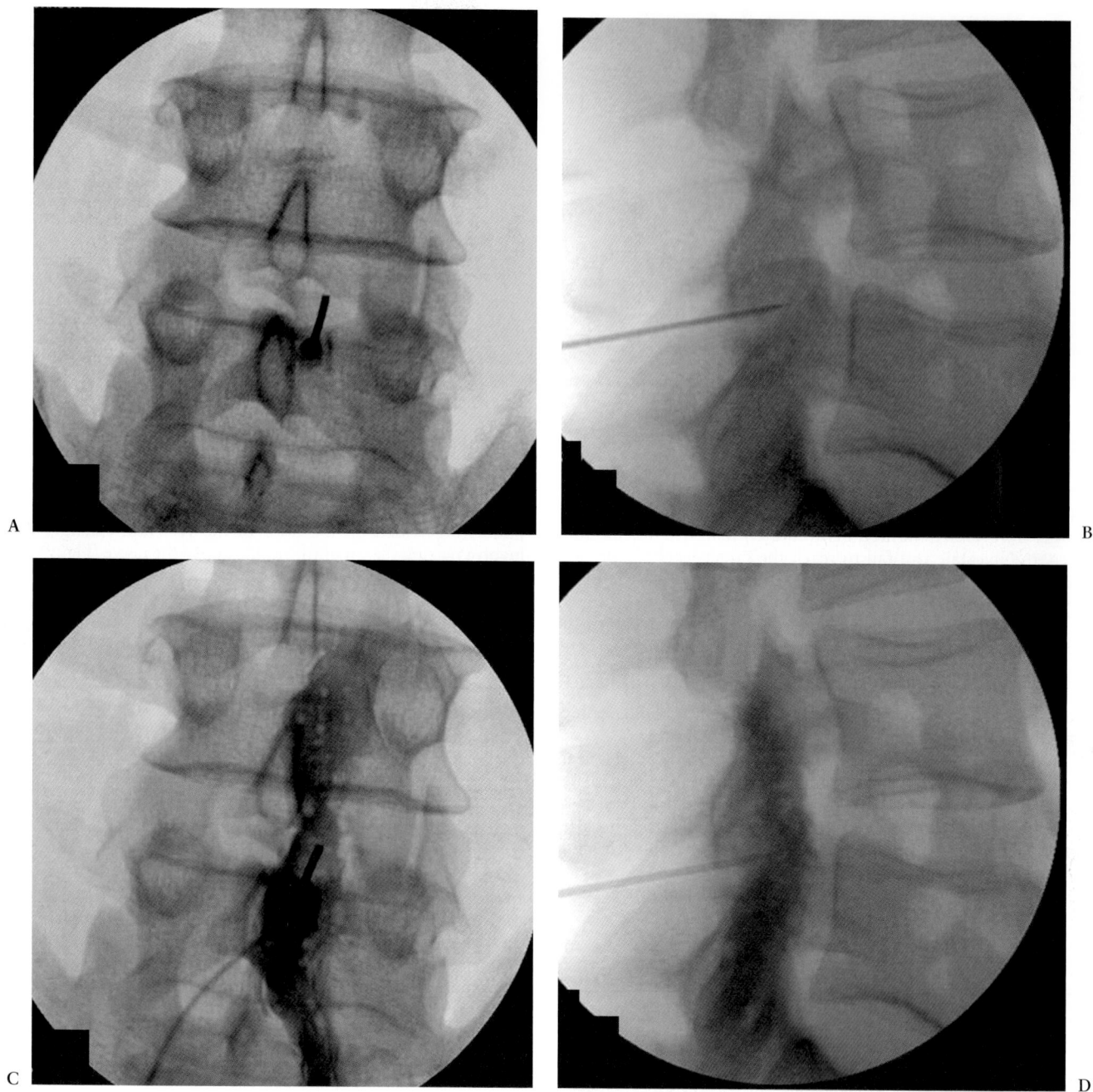

FIGURE 98.3 Images of stages of a fluoroscopically-guided, lumbar interlaminar injection of steroids. **A.** Anteroposterior view of the needle placed to the right of the midline, through the L4-L5 interlaminar space. **B.** Lateral view of needle placed. **C.** Anteroposterior view after injection of contrast medium. The contrast medium outlines the lateral epidural space and the L5 nerve root sleeves. **D.** Lateral view after injection of contrast medium. (Kindly provided by Dr. Milton Landers, Wichita, KS.)

Inflammation remains no more than a satisfying, retrospective hypothesis to rationalize the use of steroids.

INDICATIONS

For various reasons, the sole indication for epidural injection of steroids is radicular pain (i.e., sciatica). The foremost reason is that the treatment explicitly targets nerve roots, which implies a radicular origin for the pain. Secondly, whenever a rationale has

been articulated, the procedure has always been cast in terms of treating inflammation of nerve roots. Thirdly, the vast majority of the literature explicitly refers to the treatment of sciatica. However, it has not always been evident that the patients actually did have radicular pain and not somatic referred pain.

Some operators have extended the indications to include back pain without radicular pain. This application, however, is not compatible with the expressed rationale for epidural steroids, for there is no evidence that back pain is an inflammatory disorder. Nor is there any evidence that disorders of the spinal nerve, dorsal

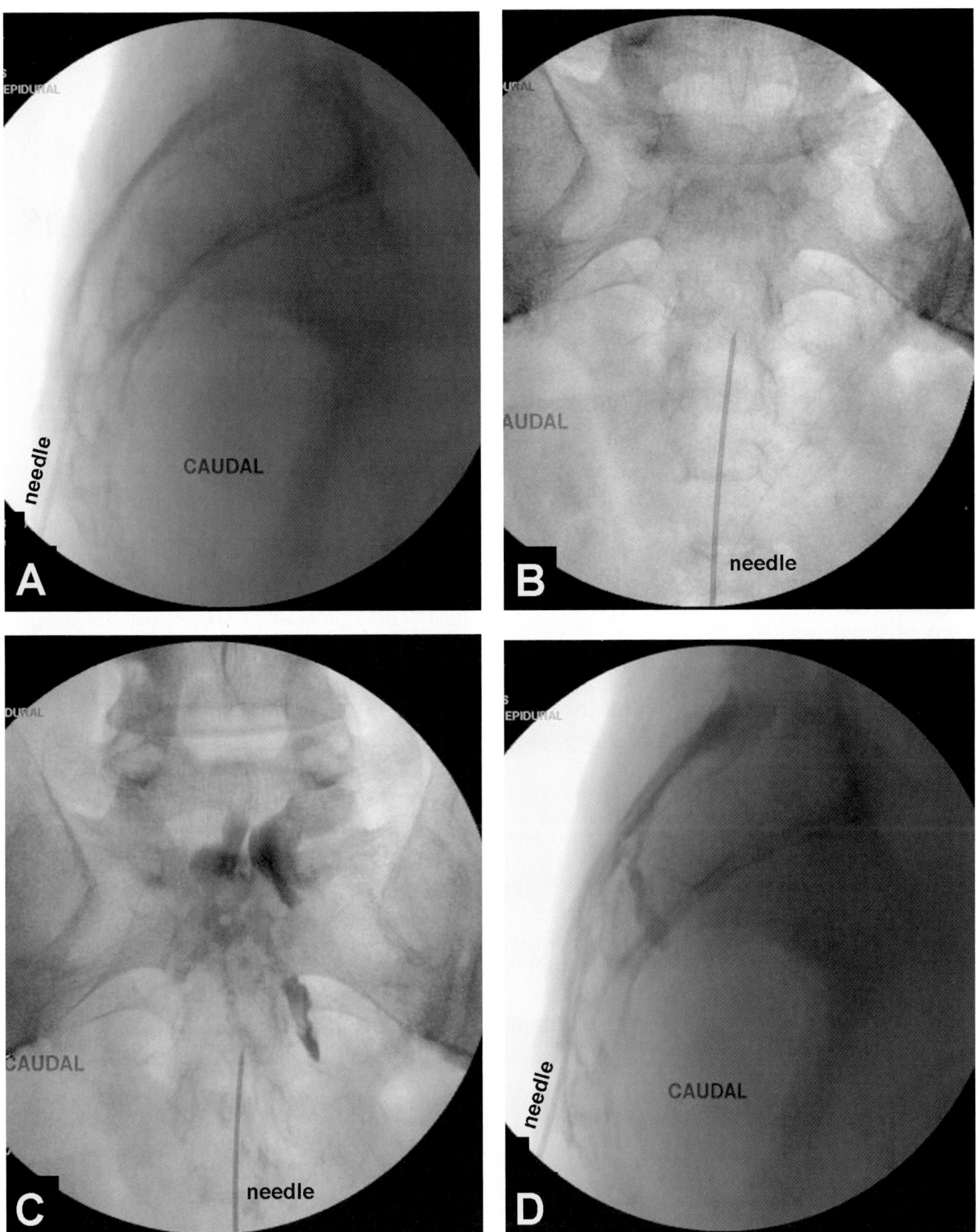

FIGURE 98.4 Images of stages of a fluoroscopically-guided caudal injection of steroids. **A.** Lateral view showing the needle passing through the sacral hiatus and into the sacral canal. **B.** Anteroposterior view of needle placed in the sacral canal. **C.** Anteroposterior view after injection of contrast medium which fills the sacral canal as far as the L5-S1 intervertebral disc. **D.** Lateral view after injection of contrast medium. (Kindly provided by Dr. Milton Landers, Wichita, KS.)

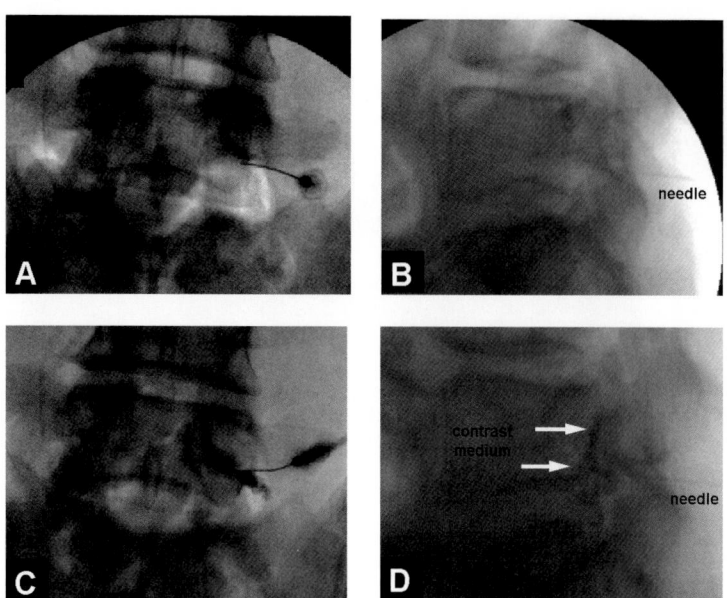

FIGURE 98.5 Fluoroscopic images of stages in the conduct of a right L5 transforaminal injection, using the subpedicular placement. **A.** Anteroposterior view; needle in place. **B.** Lateral view; needle in place. **C.** Anteroposterior view after injection of contrast medium, which outlines the sleeve of the L5 nerve roots. **D.** Lateral view after injection of contrast medium.

root, or dorsal root ganglion cause back pain without also causing radicular pain.

COMPLICATIONS

The possible complications of epidural injections of steroids can be classified according to the generic risks of all types of injections in general, those due the pharmacologic effects of steroids and local anesthetic agents, and those pertaining to the epidural site of injection. A unique, idiosyncratic complication pertains to transforaminal injections.

Generic Complications

Infection is a risk of any penetrating procedure. Following epidural injections of steroids, infection has only rarely been recorded and only in case reports.[76–79]

Pharmacologic Complications

Allergic reaction to local anesthetic[40] has been a rare complication of epidural injection of steroids. Hypotension because of sympathetic efferent blockade has been reported in about 2.5% of patients undergoing lumbar epidural injection of steroids,[18,31] but not after caudal injections.[53] Allergic reaction to steroids is a rare complication.[80] More commonly, epidural injection of steroids suppresses the secretion of glucocorticoids by the adrenal gland for about 2 to 3 weeks.[81,82] Overt, steroid side effects, such as hypercorticism or a Cushingoid syndrome, however, have been recorded only following the frequent administration, or the administration of large doses, of steroids (e.g., 120 mg of methylprednisolone).[83–86]

Site-Specific Complications

The site-specific risks of epidural injections are those that arise because of the proximity of the needle to the thecal sac. These hazards are shared with other spinal procedures such as lumbar puncture and epidural anesthesia.

Dural puncture has an incidence of 5% following lumbar epidural steroids but only 0.6% following caudal epidural steroids.[53–55] Inadvertent dural puncture does not constitute a complication in its own right, if it is recognized. The major risk of dural puncture is that, if it goes unrecognized, drugs will be deliv-

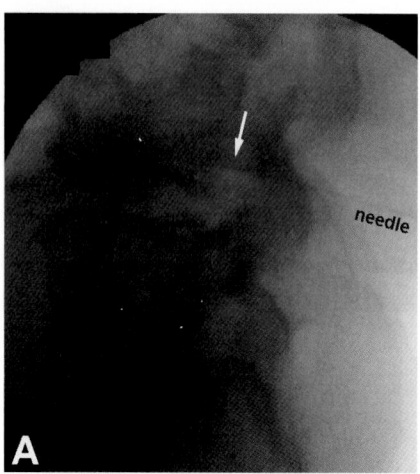

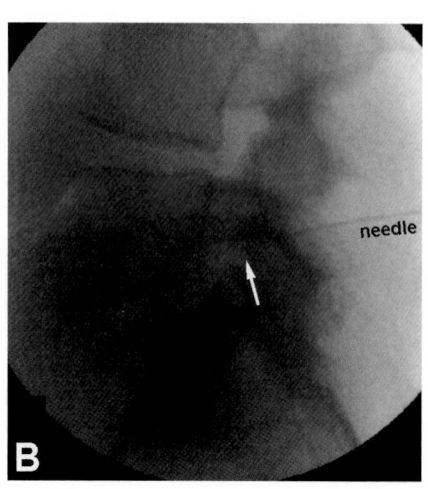

FIGURE 98.6 Lateral fluoroscopic images of alternative placements of a needle for lumbar transforaminal injections. **A.** Supraneural position, L4 nerve. **B.** Retroneural position, L5 nerve. The arrows point to the tip of the needle.

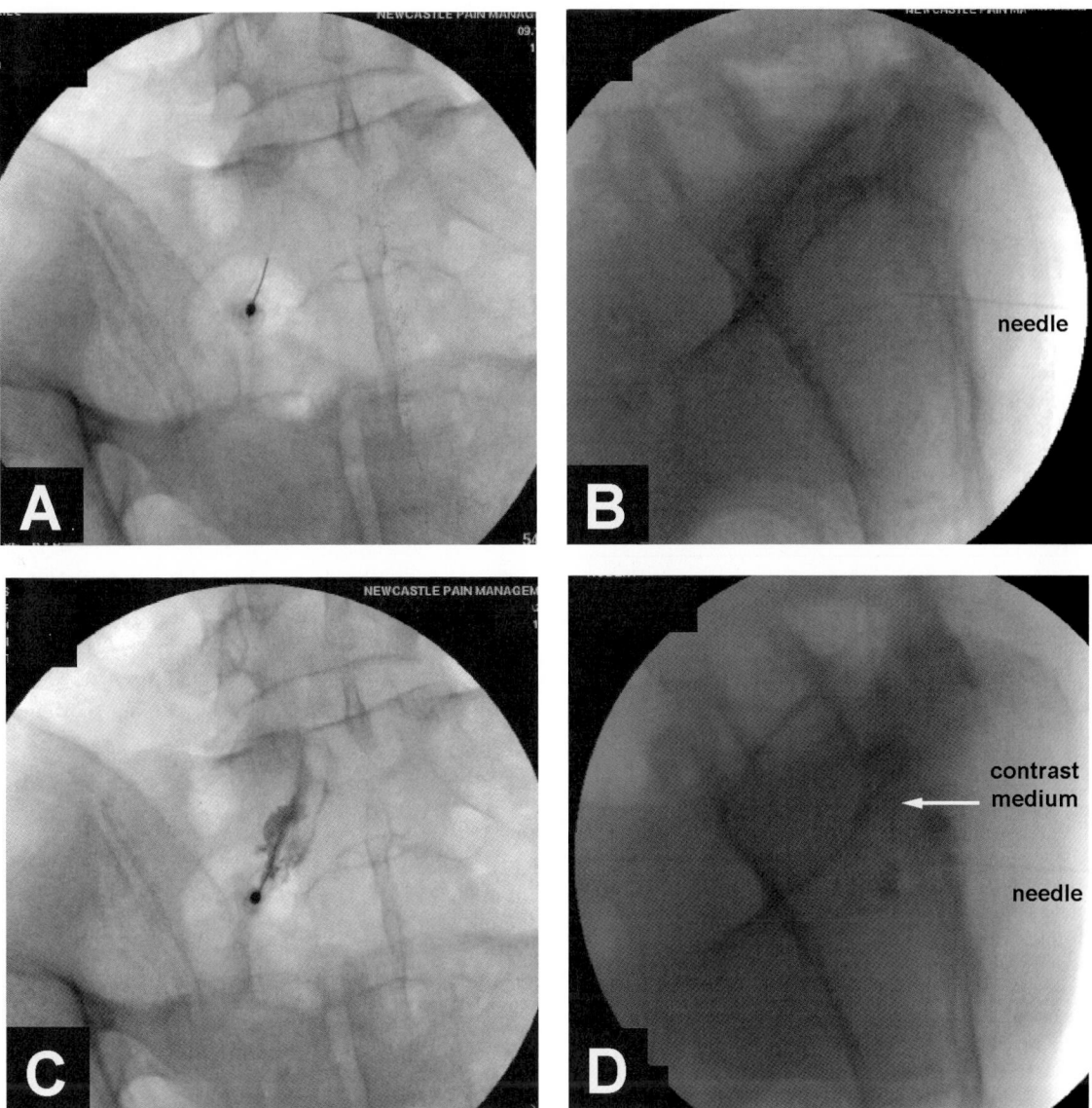

FIGURE 98.7 Fluoroscopic images of stages in the conduct of a left S1 transforaminal injection. **A.** Anteroposterior view of needle placed. **B.** Lateral view of needle placed. **C.** Anteroposterior view after injection of contrast medium, which outlines the S1 nerve root sleeve. **D.** Lateral view after injection of contrast medium, which is faintly seen within the sacral canal because only a thin film of contrast medium covers the S1 nerve root sleeve.

ered into the intrathecal space. If so injected, local anesthetics may cause spinal anesthesia,[40,44] and steroid preparations may have neurotoxic effects because of the additives that they contain.[53–55]

Exacerbation of pain is an enigmatic side effect of epidural steroid injection. Its mechanism is unknown but it is common with a weighted, mean incidence of 1%.[53,54] Analysis of the literature indicates that exacerbation of sciatic pain is related to the injection of large volumes of fluid into the epidural space, and it has been suggested that this symptom can be avoided by injecting slowly.[87]

Headache is a particularly troublesome side effect of epidural steroid injections. There are few reports of headache following caudal epidural steroids,[43] but many more for lumbar epidural steroids.[17,18,20,21,27,31] The incidence of headache is about 1% following lumbar injections.[53,54] Its mechanism has not been established. It may be due to unrecognized dural puncture with

resultant leakage of cerebrospinal fluid or inadvertent injection of air into the subarachnoid space.[88,89] Although this complaint is generally believed to be self-limiting,[90] it can persist. Headaches persisting for more than 1 year have been recorded in 0.1% of women who underwent epidural anesthesia.[91] Options for management include abdominal binders, forced fluid intake, and autologous blood patches.[92]

Transforaminal Injections

Minor and transient side effects occur in about 9% of lumbar transforaminal injections.[93] These include transient headaches (3%), increased back pain (2%), facial flushing (1%), increased leg pain (0.6%), and vaso-vagal reaction (0.3%).

More disconcerting is the complication of spinal cord injury. This has been reported in 6 patients who underwent lumbar transforaminal injections: 2 at L3–L4,[94] 1 at S1,[94] 1 at L2–L3,[95] 1 at L4–L5,[96] and 1 at T12–L1.[97] The mechanism of injury has not been explicitly demonstrated, but the prevailing view is that the injection penetrates a radicular artery that reinforces a medullary artery, and that when particulate steroids are injected they act as an embolus and infarct the conus medullaris.[98]

For this reason, investigators have studied the prevalence and size of particles in various steroid preparations. Results have differed with respect to average size of particles and the size of aggregates that they form, but as a general rule, preparations of methylprednisolone and triamcinolone tend to have large particles capable of embolizing a small artery, preparations of betamethasone may or may not have particles, and dexamethasone exhibits no particles.[99,100] These data have been published so that operators might make an informed choice about which steroid preparation to use with the view to minimising the risk of embolization, but it remains unclear that direct injection of any of these agents in to an artery supplying the spinal cord is safe.

EFFICACY

Classical Injections

Observational studies have reported successful outcomes in between 18% and 90% of patients treated with lumbar epidural steroids, and between 33% and 77% of patients treated with caudal injections.[53–55] These outcomes have been attributed to the use of steroids, but this inference has not been corroborated by controlled studies.

Systematic reviews have differed in their conclusions about the efficacy of blind epidural injections of steroids. The first systematic review concluded that epidural steroids are not effective.[101] A later review was more conciliatory.[102] An exhaustive, narrative review covered all publications then available in all languages and found no evidence of efficacy.[53] Three later reviews found no evidence of efficacy,[103–105] but a meta-analysis claimed a trend in favor of efficacy.[106] Two reviews concluded that epidural steroids might be effective.[107,108] A French review,[109] two from the Netherlands,[110,111] and a review conducted for the American Association of Neurologists found only modest evidence for accelerating resolution of radicular pain in the short-term (between 2 and 6 weeks after administration) and no evidence of longer-term efficacy.[112]

The reasons for this dissonance lie in how the available data are treated statistically and in differences in the definition of success and its duration. Some reviewers have considered a study to constitute evidence of efficacy if the study reported a $p < 0.05$ for any outcome measures, irrespective of duration. Others did not consider immediate relief or relief lasting less than 4 weeks to be of clinical significance, and only accepted responses at 3 months or longer to constitute evidence of efficacy.

The results of these reviews have done little to dissuade practitioners from using epidural steroids. It is pertinent, therefore, to examine in some detail both the studies held by some to constitute evidence of efficacy and those studies which deny efficacy. The latter include some studies that have appeared since the publication of several systematic reviews or not included by them.

Caudal Injections

An early study found no differences in the proportions of patients who were completely relieved, improved, unchanged, or worse at 1 to 3 months after epidural injections of procaine plus a combination of methylprednisolone and lidocaine or procaine alone.[43] Two later studies used injections of saline as the control treatment. Although the results in both studies showed a trend

---

TABLE 98.1

THE RESULTS OF BREIVIK ET AL.[113] IN A STUDY OF CAUDAL EPIDURAL INJECTIONS OF STEROIDS

Therapeutic agent	Response	
	Relieved	Not relieved
Steroid + Bupivacaine	9	7
Saline + Bupivacaine	5	14

Outcomes were assessed at between 3 and 18 months after treatment. Although a larger proportion of patients were relieved, the difference in outcome is not statistically significant. On chi squared analysis $p = 0.072$, and on Fisher's exact test $p = 0.07$.
Data from Breivik H, Hesla PE, Molnar I, et al. Treatment of chronic low back pain and sciatica. Comparison of caudal epidural injections of bupivacaine and methylprednisolone with bupivacaine followed by saline. In: Bonica JJ, Albe-Fessard D, eds. *Advances in Pain Research and Therapy.* Vol. 1. New York: Raven Press; 1976:927–932.

---

in favour of epidural steroids (Tables 98.1 and 98.2), neither study observed statistically significant differences between active treatment and control.

When such studies are included in a meta-analysis, they contribute toward a trend in favor of epidural steroids, but the rules of meta-analysis are that artificial pooling of studies is not a substitute for a proper study of adequate power. No such studies of caudal epidural steroids have been published.

Lumbar Interlaminar Injections

Although celebrated as the first controlled study to show that epidural steroids were effective, the study of Dilke et al.[87] found statistically significant differences only in certain, secondary outcome measures, such as return to work at 30 days. With respect to relief of pain, epidural injection of steroids was not demonstrably more effective than injection of normal saline into an interspinous ligament (Table 98.3). Differences in outcome approach statistical significance only if patients with unknown outcomes and those who required surgery are disregarded. If those who required

---

TABLE 98.2

THE RESULTS OF BUSH AND HILLIER[114] IN A CONTROLLED TRIAL OF CAUDAL INJECTIONS OF EPIDURAL STEROIDS

	Response				p Value
	No pain	Better	No change	Worse	
At 4 weeks					
Treated	2	5	4	1	0.66
Control	2	3	3	3	
At 1 year					
Treated	6	4	2	2	0.57
Control	6	1	1	3	

The treated group received saline, procaine, and triamcinolone. The control group received saline only. Chi squared analysis yields nonsignificant p values.
Data from Bush K, Hillier S. A controlled study of caudal epidural injections of triamcinolone plus procaine for the management of intractable sciatica. *Spine* 1991;16:572–575.

TABLE 98.3

THE OUTCOMES AT 3 MONTHS AFTER TREATMENT WITH EITHER A LUMBAR INTERLAMINAR INJECTION OF STEROIDS OR AN INJECTION OF SALINE INTO AN INTERSPINOUS LIGAMENT[83]

Pain	Treatment		p Value
	Steroids	Saline	
None	16	8	
Not severe	24	20	
Severe	1	6	0.05
Surgery	7	10	0.06
Unknown	3	4	0.10

On chi squared analysis, the p value is 0.05 if patients who had surgery or whose outcomes were unknown are disregarded. If patients who had surgery are classified as failures, the p value increases to 0.06. If unknown results are included, the p value becomes 0.10.
Data from Dilke TF, Burry HC, Grahame R. Extradural corticosteroid injection in management of lumbar nerve root compression. *BMJ* 1973;2: 635–637.

TABLE 98.5

THE RESULTS OF A CONTROLLED TRIAL AT 3 MONTHS AFTER TREATMENT WITH LUMBAR EPIDURAL INJECTIONS OF STEROIDS OR SALINE[116]

Outcome measure	Treatment	
	Steroid	Normal saline
Oswestry disability (0–100)	32	35
Pain (Visual Analog Score; 0–100)	39	40
Sickness Impact Profile (0–100)		
Overall	12	13
Physical	10	9
Restricted activity (days)	6	9

Data from Carette S, LeClaire R, Marcoux S, et al. Epidural corticosteroid injections for sciatica due to herniated nucleus pulposus. *N Eng J Med* 1997;336:1634–1640.

surgery are classified as failures, statistical significance is not achieved.

The only other study to report a positive result showed that epidural injection of steroids achieved greater improvements in pain than did an injection of saline into an interspinous ligament.[35] Baseline data and final outcomes, however, were not reported, and the effects attenuated after 12 weeks.

A Japanese study[20] reported that the efficacy of epidural steroids was not different from that of an epidural injection of local anesthetic alone. This observation was elaborated by another study.

Klenerman et al.[115] compared the effects of epidural injections of steroids, of local anesthetic alone, of saline alone, and of dry needling of an interspinous ligament. They categorized their outcomes as "failed" (less than 25% relief) or "not failed" (greater than 75% relief). The latter category included patients who were "improved" or "cured," but the numbers in these subcategories were too small to be subjected to statistical analysis separately. At 2 months after treatment, the outcomes in the several groups were not statistically different (Table 98.4). The fact that epidural injection of steroids was not demonstrably more effective than simply dry needling of an interspinous space is remarkable.

More recent studies also have found no attributable effect of steroids. Their outcomes were the same, irrespective of what was injected.

Carette et al.[116] found no differences in outcome at 3 months, whether patients were treated with lumbar epidural injections of

steroids or an epidural injection of normal saline (Table 98.5). In particular, the use of steroids made no difference to disability.

Using the liberal outcome measure of "relieved or not," Valat et al.[117] found no statistically significant difference in outcome after active or sham treatment. Although a slightly larger proportion of patients were relieved by steroids at day 20 after treatment, the difference was not significant. By day 35, the proportions relieved were essentially identical (Table 98.6).

For the outcome measure—any degree of relief at 35 days—the number needed to treat (NNT)[118,119] was 100.[117] This statistic means that 100 patients would need to be treated before 1 could be claimed to have obtained any degree of relief lasting 35 days expressly because of the injection of steroids. In all other patients with successful outcomes, the success is due to the nonspecific effects of having an injection and not due to the injection of steroids. This statistic describes a very ineffective and inefficient treatment.

Another study compared the outcomes of interlaminar or intramuscular injection of steroids.[120] It reported that there was no significant difference in outcome at 35 days but provided no explicit data on pain or function. The only numerical data were that the surgery rates in the two groups (31% and 41%, respectively) were not significantly different statistically.

A large and rigorous study compared interlaminar injection of steroids with injection of normal saline into an interspinous ligament.[121] With respect to relief of pain, the outcomes at 3 weeks favored interlaminar injections, but the difference was extinguished by 6 weeks. At no time, from 3 weeks to 1 year after

TABLE 98.4

THE RESULTS OF THE CONTROLLED TRIAL OF LUMBAR EPIDURAL INJECTIONS CONDUCTED BY KLENERMAN ET AL.[115]

Response	Treatment			
	Normal saline	Methylprednisolone and lidocaine	Bupivacaine	Dry needling
Failed	5	4	5	2
Not failed	11	15	11	10

Data from Klenerman L, Greenwood R, Davenport HT, et al. Lumbar epidural injections in the treatment of sciatica. *Brit J Rheumatol* 1984;23:35–38.

TABLE 98.6

THE RESULTS OF A CONTROLLED TRIAL OF LUMBAR
INTERLAMINAR EPIDURAL INJECTIONS OF STEROIDS
OR NORMAL SALINE[117]

	Proportion relieved		
	Normal saline (N = 42)	Steroids (N = 43)	NNT
Day 20	0.36	0.51	6.5
Day 35	0.48	0.49	100

NNT, number needed to treat.
Data from Valat JP, Giraudeau B, Rozenberg S, et al. Epidural
corticosteroid injections for sciatica: a randomised, double-blind, controlled
clinical trial. *Ann Rheum Dis* 2003;62:639–643.

treatment, were the proportions of patients who obtained at least 50% relief of pain different. There were no differences in disability scores or improvements in disability scores. At 3 weeks, the proportion of patients who obtained 75% improvement in disability was higher (12.5%) in those treated with interlaminar injections (3.7%), but this difference did not persist beyond 3 weeks. In this study, the NNT for 50% relief at 3 weeks was 11, but for lack of sustained benefit, no NNT was applicable at later times.

Utilization

A utilization review found that over 70% of the epidural injections of steroids performed in the United States are performed on patients with chronic pain (lasting more than 6 months).[122] No controlled studies have shown epidural steroids to be effective in this population. Most of the observational studies and all of the controlled studies of epidural steroids have been conducted on patients with acute or subacute pain or in mixed populations the majority of whom had pain for less than 3 months. Yet, even in those populations they have been shown not be effective. So, there is no evidence, direct or by extrapolation, to support the use of epidural injections of steroids for treating chronic pain, yet this is their most common use.

Back Pain

Proponents of the use of epidural steroids for back pain rely on a handful of observational studies that claim effectiveness.[123,124] In doing so, these proponents seem unperturbed that epidural steroids for sciatica were originally promoted on the basis of observational studies, only to have their efficacy eventually refuted by controlled trials. Without a rationale, and without evidence of efficacy, the use of epidural steroids for back pain appears more like a treatment looking for an application than a condition warranting an intervention. Others warn that the low success rates obtained for back pain are commensurate with placebo response rates.[125]

Fluoroscopically-Guided Injections

Those who decry "blind" injections yet advocate fluoroscopically-guided injections believe that fluoroscopically-guided lumbar or caudal injections should, in theory, be more effective because they are more accurate. But there is no evidence to this effect. As controlled studies have been published that refute the efficacy of blind injections, no contrary studies have been conducted and published that show that fluoroscopically-guided injections are, nonetheless, effective. In the absence of direct evidence, and in the absence of evidence that blind injections are effective, the effectiveness of fluoroscopically-guided injections makes rational sense, but remains no more than hearsay.

Transforaminal Injections

The introduction of fluoroscopically-guided, transforaminal injections of steroids was heralded by an observational study that used a novel outcome measure. That study enrolled 30 patients who were on a waiting list for surgery.[67] After being treated with transforaminal injections of steroids, 47% obtained complete relief of pain that was lasting and only 20% required surgery (Fig. 98.8). The efficacy of transforaminal injections was cast in terms of their ability to spare patients from having surgery.

A subsequent, observational study used more familiar outcome measures. It reported that 52 out of 69 patients obtained greater than 50% relief of the pain after treatment with transforaminal injections of steroids at follow-up times of between 28 and 144 weeks.[68] Other, observational studies echoed these outcomes.[126,127] Betamethasone and triamcinolone have been equally effective.[128]

Controlled trials soon followed. Two reported negative results, and three reported positive results. The first controlled trial[129] used avoidance of surgery as the outcome measure. It found that only 8 of 28 patients (29%) required surgery after treatment with transforaminal injections of betamethasone, compared with 18 out of 27 patients (67%) treated with transforaminal injections of bupivacaine. A later publication reported a 5-year follow-up of these patients, which showed that the outcome was enduring.[130] In neither publication were pain scores or disability reported. The second controlled trial[131] found no difference in effect on leg pain following transforaminal injections with betamethasone or with bupivacaine. A supplementary publication reported that betamethasone was more effective than bupivacaine in a subgroup of patients who had contained disc herniations, but only up to 4 weeks after treatment.[132] At longer-term follow-up, that superiority extinguished.

The third trial compared transforaminal injections of steroids with paraspinal injections of normal saline.[69] The outcomes favored transforaminal injections (Table 98.7). Mean pain scores were significantly lower in those patients treated with transforaminal steroids, and a significantly greater proportion of those patients obtained greater than 50% relief. Disability scores, however, were not appreciably different. What are conspicuous in these data are the magnitude of improvement in the control group and the proportion of patients who obtained greater than 50% relief of radicular pain simply following paraspinal injections of normal saline. There is no biologic link between the mechanism of radicular pain and either the pharmacologic properties of normal saline or the back muscles. These data underscore the powerful placebo effect of injections.

The fourth controlled trial compared the outcomes of transforaminal injection of methylprednisolone and bupivacaine with those of transforaminal injections of bupivacaine alone.[133] It found no differences at 1 day, 4 weeks, 6 weeks, or 3 months. In the two groups, pain scores dropped from 73 to 54, and from 77 to 55, respectively. One difference in this study was that patients received only one injection, whereas in previous studies they received at least one and up to three injections.

The fifth trial compared transforaminal injections of steroids

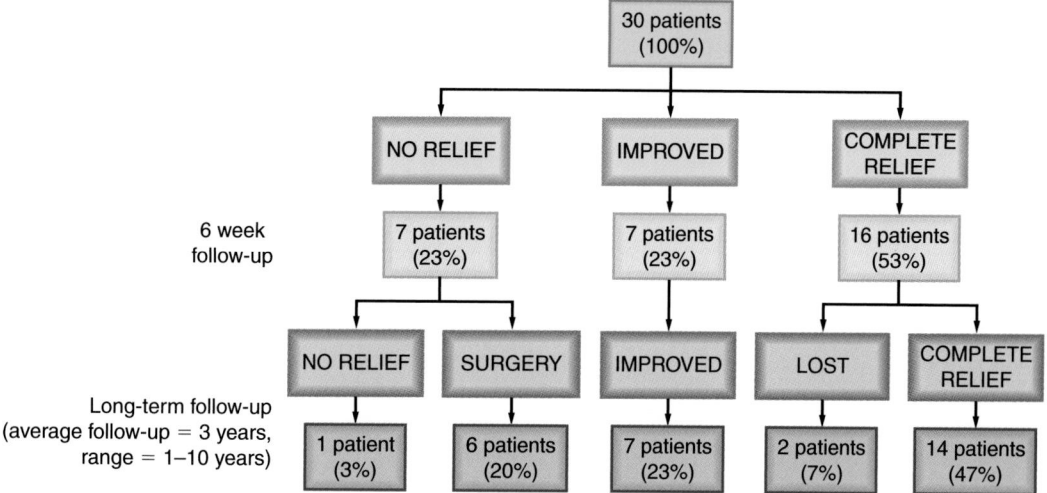

FIGURE 98.8 The results of an observational study of the efficacy of lumbar transforaminal injection of steroids. (Data from Weiner BK, Fraser RD. Foraminal injection for lateral lumbar disc herniation. *J Bone Joint Surg* 1997;79B:804–807.)

with conventional interlaminar injections.[134] No differences in outcome were evident at 6 days after treatment, but by 30 days and at 6 months after treatment, those patients treated with transforaminal injections showed statistically significant, greater improvements in pain and function relating to work and leisure.

Other studies have sought to compare the effectiveness of transforaminal injections with those of either interlaminar or caudal injections. A retrospective case-control study[135] and a practice audit[136] found in favor of transforaminal injections, as did a prospective study.[137]

Synopsis

Table 98.8 encapsulates the evidence on epidural injections of steroids. Blind caudal injections are not more effective than epidural injections of normal saline either for short-term outcomes or in the long-term.[113,114] For long-term outcomes, blind lumbar interlaminar injections are no more effective than epidural injections of normal saline or injections of normal saline into interspinous ligaments.[35,115–117,121] For short-term outcomes (i.e., less than 4 weeks), the evidence is mixed and conflicting. Whereas some have found interlaminar injections of steroids to be somewhat more effective than interlaminar injections of saline,[121] others have found no significant difference[117] or no effect greater than that from an injection of normal saline into an interspinous ligament.[87] For fluoroscopically-guided injections, there is still no evidence of efficacy. Transforaminal injections of steroids are more effective for the relief of pain than intramuscular injections of normal saline or steroids but are not more effective than transforaminal injections of local anesthetic. The only strong evidence is that transforaminal injections spare patients from surgery.

TABLE 98.7

THE RESULTS OF A CONTROLLED TRIAL THAT COMPARED THE OUTCOMES OF TREATMENT WITH TRANSFORAMINAL INJECTIONS OF STEROIDS AND PARASPINAL INJECTIONS OF NORMAL SALINE[69]

	Treatment	
Outcome	Transforaminal injection of steroids (N = 25)	Paraspinal normal saline (N = 23)
Pain (0–100) (mean ± sd)		
Baseline	88 ± 14	94 ± 14
12 months	16 ± 8	36 ± 11
Roland Morris		
Baseline	8.8	9.6
12 months	22.1	18.3
>50% relief of pain	21	11
	84%	48%

Data from Vad VB, Bhat AL, Lutz GE, et al. Transforaminal epidural steroid injections in lumbosacral radiculopathy. *Spine* 2002;27:11–16.

TABLE 98.8

A SYNOPSIS OF THE EVIDENCE ON EPIDURAL INJECTIONS OF STEROIDS BY VARIOUS ROUTES

	Route	Efficacy
Blind	Caudal	Short-term (<4 weeks) Epidural Steroids = Epidural Normal Saline Long-term (>4 weeks) Epidural Steroids = Epidural Normal Saline
	Lumbar	Short-term (<4 weeks) Epidural Steroids = Interspinous Normal Saline Epidural Steroids = Epidural Normal Saline Epidural Steroids > Epidural Normal Saline Long-term (>4 weeks) Epidural Steroids = Epidural Normal Saline Epidural Steroids = Interspinous Normal Saline
Fluroscopically-Guided	Caudal Lumbar	No evidence available
Transforaminal		Transforaminal Steroids>IM Normal Saline Transforaminal Steroids>IM Steroids Transforaminal Steroids > Interlaminar Steroids Transforaminal Steroids = Transforaminal LA Surgery Sparing

IM, intramuscular; LA, local anaesthetic.

CONCLUSION

The history of epidural injections of steroids constitutes a vivid example of a common medical misconception. Practitioners do not distinguish between observed effect and attributable effect. All treatments can seem to work to some extent or other. However, they may not work for the reasons that a treatment is believed to work. The attributable effect is the extent to which a treatment works for reasons other than the nonspecific effects of treatment and is revealed only by controlled trials.

Observational studies of epidural injections of steroids have reported success rates of various magnitudes. Therefore, they do appear to work. For short-term outcomes (i.e., 20–30 days), some studies have shown an attributable effect, but others have found none. Until a clearer picture emerges, the use of epidural injections of steroids might still be justified for providing more rapid relief of radicular pain in the short-term. For long-term relief, however, controlled studies have consistently found no attributable effect. Epidural injections of steroids work for reasons other than the injection of steroids. In the case of blind injections, injections of normal saline, even into interspinous ligaments, are as effective. This indicates that the act of injection, or the ceremony associated with it, may be the paramount therapeutic ingredient.

The same may still apply to transforaminal injections. For the relief of pain, transforaminal injections are more effective than intramuscular injections of saline or of steroids, but transforaminal injections of steroids are no more effective than transforaminal injections of local anesthetic alone. This raises two sets of possibilities.

Steroids and local anesthetic may have the same effect pharmacologically or physically when injected by the transforaminal route, both might be either analgesic or anti-inflammatory, or both might simply irrigate the target nerve.

On the other hand, transforaminal injections may have strong nonspecific effects. Performing injections in a special procedure room using sophisticated equipment has the attributes for a strong placebo effect. The technology and ceremony involved may produce a placebo effect greater than that produced by relatively banal intramuscular injections.

The study of Thomas et al.[134] took steps to control for this effect. The intramuscular injections were performed with the same facilities and ceremony as were the transforaminal injections. Although some, though not all, of the outcomes favored transforaminal injections, it was conspicuous that the outcomes of the intramuscular injections were not insubstantial. This leaves the question of whether the steroids have a systemic effect unresolved.

Epidural injections of steroids are the most enigmatic of treatments in pain medicine. It is not that the most commonly performed procedure in pain medicine lacks evidence of efficacy. Conventional injections have been shown to be no more effective than sham treatment. Yet they continued to be used. Since there is no scientific reason for their continued use, the reasons must be social, financial, or both.

Traditions and habits are hard to break. While so long as epidural steroids were believed to work, practitioners had something to offer their patients. If they are deemed not to work, these practitioners are disempowered. Unless they are given an alternative, they have nothing to offer their patients and nothing for which they might be reimbursed. For these reasons, evidence of lack of efficacy becomes threatening professionally and financially. Under those conditions, it seems preferable to ignore the evidence and to maintain tradition.

At present, transforaminal injections appear to be an alternative to conventional injections. Their reputation tenuously relies on one study that has shown that they spare patients from surgery, and one study that shows that they are just more effective than intramuscular injections of steroids. Their efficacy needs to be corroborated by confirmatory studies. However, it is possible that future studies will deny any efficacy. In that event, transforaminal injections may follow the same historical evolution as conventional injections have done. Giving the patient an injection, rather than what is injected, may be the reason why the treatment appears to work.

References

1. Manchikanti L. State of interventional pain medicine. *Pain Physician* 2000; 3:241–255.
2. Robechhi A, Capra R. L'idrocortisone (composto F). Prime esperienze cliniche in campo reumatologico. *Minerva Med* 1952;98:1259–1263.
3. Biella A, Cicognini P. L'acetato di idrocortisone nel trattamento della sindrome sciatalgica. *Minerva Med* 1954;1:1863–1865.
4. Ruggieri F, Capello A. L'idrocortisone nel trattamento della lumbosciatalgica. *Minerva Ortop* 1956;7:388–392.
5. Cappio M. Il trattamento idrocortisonico per via epidurale sacrale delle lombosciatalgie. *Reumatismo* 1957;9:60–70.
6. Cappio M, Fragasso V. Osservazioni sull'uso dell'idrocortisone per via epidurale ed endorachidea nelle lombosciatalgie. *Riforma Med* 1955;22:605–607.
7. Cappio M, Fragasso V. Il prednisolone per via epidurale sacrale nelle lombosciatalgie. *Reumatismo* 1957;5:905–908.
8. Fragasso V. Il prednisolone idrosolubile per via epidurale sacrale nelle lombosciatalgie. *Gaz Med Ital* 1959;118:358–360.
9. Canale L. Il desametazone per via epidurale sacrale nelle lombosciatalgie. *Gaz Med Ital* 1963;122:210–213.
10. Gilly R. Essai de traitement de 50 cas de sciatiques et de radiculalgies lombaires par le Celestene chronodose en infiltrations pararadiculaire. *Marseille Medicale* 1950;107:341–345.
11. Lievre JA, Bloch-Michel H, Pean G, et al. L'hydrocortisone en injection locale. *Rev Rhum* 1953;20:310–311.
12. Gerest MF. Le traitement de la nevralgie sciatique par les injections epidurales d'hydrocortisone. *J Med Lyon* 1958;261–264.
13. Renier JC. L'infitration epidurale par le premier trou sacre posterieur. *Revue du Rhumatisme et des Maladies Osteo-articulaire* 1959;26:526–532.
14. Zappala G. Iniezione peridurale segmentaria di Hydrocortone nella sindrome dolorosa da ernia discale. *Policlinico – Sez Prat* 1955;62:1229–1231.
15. Yamazaka N. Interspinal injection of hydrocortisone or prednisolone in the treatment of intervertebral disc herniation. *J Jpn Orthop Assoc* 1959;33:689.
16. Barry PJC, Kendall PH. Corticosteroid infiltration of the extradural space. *Ann Phys Med* 1962;6:267–273.
17. Harley C. Extradural corticosteroid infiltration. *Ann Phys Med* 1967;9: 22–28.
18. Burn JM, Langdon L. Lumbar epidural injection for the treatment of chronic sciatica. *Rheum Phys Med* 1970;10:368–374.
19. Swerdlow M, Sayle-Creer W. A study of extradural medication in the relief of the lumbosciatic syndrome. *Anaesthesia* 1970;25:341–345.
20. Ito R. The treatment of low back pain and sciatica with epidural corticosteroids injection and its pathophysiological basis. *J Jpn Orthop Assoc* 1971; 45:769–777.
21. Jurmand SH. Corticotherapie peridurale des lombalgies et des sciatiques d'origine discale. *Concours Medicale* 1972;94:5061–5070.
22. Winnie AP, Hartman JT, Meyers HL, et al. Pain clinic. II: intradural and extradural corticosteroids for sciatica. *Anesth Analg* 1972;51:990–1003.
23. Hartman JT, Winnie AP, Ramaurthy S, et al. Intradural and extradural corticosteroids for sciatic pain. *Orthop Rev* 1974;3:21–24.
24. D'Hoogue R, Compere A, Gribmont B, et al. Peridural injection of corticosteroids in the treatment of the low back pain-sciatica syndrome. *Acta Orthop Belg* 1976;42:157–165.
25. Brown FW. Management of diskogenic pain using epidural and intrathecal steroids. *Clin Orthop Relat Res* 1977;129:72–78.
26. Bullard JR, Houghton FM. Epidural treatment of acute herniated nucleus pulposus. *Anesth Analg* 1977;56:862–863.
27. Warr AC, Wilkinson JA, Burn JMB, et al. Chronic lumbosciatic syndrome treated by epidural injection and manipulation. *Practitioner* 1977;209:53–59.
28. Heyse-Moore GH. A rational approach to the use of epidural medication in the treatment of sciatic pain. *Acta Orthop Scand* 1978;49(4):366–370.
29. Jackson DW, Rettig A, Wiltse LL. Epidural cortisone injection in the young athletic adult. *Am J Sports Med* 1980;8:239–243.
30. Green PW, Burke AJ, Weiss CA, et al. The role of epidural cortisone injection in the treatment of diskogenic low back pain. *Clin Orthop* 1980;153: 121–125.
31. Berman AT, Garbarinbo JL, Fisher SM, et al. The effects of epidural injection of local anesthetics and corticosteroids on patients with lumbosciatic pain. *Clin Orthop* 1984;188:144–151.
32. Andersen KH, Mosdal C. Epidural application of corticosteroids in low-back pain and sciatica. *Acta Neurochir* 1987;87:52–53.
33. Hickey RF. Outpatient epidural steroid injections for low back pain and lumbosacral radiculopathy. *NZ Med J* 1987;100:594–596.
34. Matthews JA, Mills SB, Jenkins VM, et al. Back pain and sciatica: controlled trials of manipulation, traction, sclerosant and epidural injections. *Brit J Rheumatol* 1987;26:416–423.
35. Ridley MG, Kingsley GH, Gibson T, et al. Outpatient lumbar epidural corticosteroid injection in the management of sciatica. *Brit J Rheumatol* 1988;27: 905–909.
36. Rosen CD, Kahanovitz N, Bernstein R, et al. A retrospective analysis of the efficacy of epidural steroid injections. *Clin Orthop* 1988;228:270–272.
37. Mangar D, Thomas PB. Epidural steroid injections in the treatment of cervical and lumbar pain syndromes. *Regional Anesth* 1991;16:246.
38. Beyer W. Das zervikale und lumbale Bandscheiben-syndrom und seine Behandlung mit novocain-prednisolon-injektionen an die Nervenwurzeln. *Munch Med Wschr* 1960;102:1164–1165.
39. Gardner WJ, Goebert HW, Sehgal AD. Intraspinal corticosteroids in the treatment of sciatica. *Trans Am Neurol Assoc* 1961;86:214–215.
40. Goebert HW, Jallo SJ, Gardner WJ, et al. Painful radiculopathy treated with epidural injections of procaine and hydrocortisone acetate: results in 113 patients. *Anesth Analg* 1961;140:130–134.
41. Lindholm R, Salenius P. Caudal, epidural administration of anaesthetics and corticoids in the treatment of low back pain. *Acta Orthop Scand* 1964;1: 114–116.
42. Czarski Z. Leczenie rwy kulszowej wstrzykiwaniem hydrokortyzonu i nowokainy do rozworu krzyzowego. *Przeglad Lekarski* 1965;21:511–513.
43. Beliveau P. A comparison between epidural anaesthesia with and without corticosteroids in the treatment of sciatica. *Rheum Phys Med* 1971;11:40–43.
44. Mount HT. Hydrocortisone in the treatment of intervertebral disc protrusion. *Can Med Assoc J* 1971;105:1279–1280.
45. Mount HT. Epidural injection of hydrocortisone for the management of the acute lumbar disc protrusion. In: Morley TP, ed. *Current Controversies in Neurosurgery.* Philadelphia: Saunders; 1976:67–72.
46. Sharma PK. Indications, technique and results of caudal epidural injection for lumbar disc retropulsion. *Postgrad Med J* 1977;53:1–6.
47. Yates DW. A comparison of the types of epidural injection commonly used in the treatment of low back pain and sciatica. *Rheum Rehab* 1978;17:181–186.
48. Gordon J. Caudal extradural injection for the treatment of low back pain. *Anaesthesia* 1980;35:515–516.
49. Stanton-Hicks M. Therapeutic caudal or epidural block for lower back or sciatic pain. *JAMA* 1980;243:369–370.
50. White AH, Derby R, Wynne G. Epidural injections for diagnosis and treatment of low-back pain. *Spine* 1980;5:78–86.
51. Wiltse LL. Therapeutic caudal or epidural block for lower back or sciatic pain. *JAMA* 1980;243:369.
52. Cluff R, Mehio AK, Cohen SP, et al. The technical aspects of epidural steroid injections: a national survey. *Anesth Analg* 2002;95:403–408.
53. Bogduk N, Christophidis N, Cherry D, et al. *Epidural use of steroids in the management of back pain and sciatica of spinal origin. Report of the Working Party on Epidural use of Steroids in the Management of Back Pain.* Canberra: National Health and Medical Research Council; 1993.
54. Bogduk N, Aprill C, Derby R. Epidural steroid injections. In: White AH, ed *Spine Care: Diagnosis and Conservative Treatment.* Vol. 4. St Louis: Mosby; 1995:322–343.
55. Cabot W. Spine update: epidural steroids. *Spine* 1995;20:845–848.
56. el-Khoury G, Ehara S, Weinstein JN, et al. Epidural steroid injection: a procedure ideally performed with fluoroscopic control. *Radiology* 1988;168: 554–557.
57. Stitz MY, Sommer HM. Accuracy of blind versus fluoroscopically guided caudal epidural injection. *Spine* 1999;24:1371–1376.
58. Price CM, Rogers PD, Prosser AS, et al. Comparison of the caudal and lumbar approaches to the epidural space. *Ann Rheum Dis* 2000;59:879–882.
59. Bartynski WS, Grahovac SZ, Rothfus WE. Incorrect needle position during lumbar epidural steroid administration: inaccuracy of loss air pressure resistance and requirement of fluoroscopy and epidurography during needle insertion. *AJNR* 2005;26:502–505.
60. Manchikanti L, Cash KA, Pampati V, et al . Evaluation of fluoroscopically guided caudal epidural injections. *Pain Physician* 2004;7:81–92.
61. Mehta M, Salmon N. Extradural block. Confirmation of the injection site by X-ray monitoring. *Anaesthesia* 1985;40:1009–1012.
62. Whitlock EL, Bridwell KH, Gilula LA. Influence of needle tip position on injectate spread in 406 interlaminar lumbar epidural steroid injections. *Radiology* 2007;243:804–811.
63. Fredman B, Nun MB, Zohar E,et al. Epidural steroids for treating "failed back surgery syndrome": is fluoroscopy really necessary? *Anesth Analg* 1999; 88:367–372.
64. Young IA, Hyman GS, Packia-Raj LN, et al. The use of lumbar epidural/transforaminal steroids for managing spinal disease. *J Am Acad Orthop Surg* 2007;15:228–238.

65. Renfrew DL, Moore TE, Kathol MH, et al. Correct placement of epidural steroid injections: fluoroscopic guidance and contrast administration. *AJNR* 1991;12:1003–1007.

66. International Spine Intervention Society. Lumbar transforaminal injections. In: Bogduk N, ed. *Practice Guidelines for Spinal Diagnostic and Treatment Procedures*. San Francisco; International Spine Intervention Society; 2004: 163–187.

67. Weiner BK, Fraser RD. Foraminal injection for lateral lumbar disc herniation. *J Bone Joint Surg* 1997;79:804–807.

68. Lutz GE, Vad VB, Wisneski RJ. Fluoroscopic transforaminal lumbar epidural steroids: an outcome study. *Arch Phys Med Rehabil* 1998;79:1362–1366.

69. Vad VB, Bhat AL, Lutz GE, et al. Transforaminal epidural steroid injections in lumbosacral radiculopathy: a prospective randomized study. *Spine* 2002; 27:11–16.

70. Saal JS, Franson RC, Dobrow R, et al. High levels of inflammatory phospholipase A2 activity in lumbar disc herniations. *Spine* 1990;15:674–678.

71. Kang JD, Geirgescu HI, Larkin L, et al. Herniated lumbar intervertebral discs spontaneously produce matrix metalloproteinases, nitric oxide, interleukin-6, and prostaglandin E2. *Spine* 1996;21:271–277.

72. Takahashi H, Suguro T, Okazima Y, et al. Inflammatory cytokines in the herniated disc of the lumbar spine. *Spine* 1996;21:218–224.

73. Olmarker K, Larson K. Tumor necrosis factor α and nucleus-pulposus-induced nerve root injury. Spine 1998;23:2538–2544.

74. Olmarker K, Rydevik B. Selective inhibition of tumor necrosis factor-alpha prevents nucleus pulposus-induced thrombus formation, intraneural edema, and reduction of nerve conduction velocity: possible implications for future pharmacologic treatment strategies of sciatica. *Spine* 2001;26:863–869.

75. Brisby H, Byröd G, Olmarker K, et al. Nitric oxide as a mediator of nucleus pulposus-induced effects on spinal nerve roots. *J Orthop Res* 2000;18: 815–820.

76. Chan ST, Leung S. Spinal epidural abscess following steroid injection for sciatica: case report. *Spine* 1989;14:106–108.

77. Dougherty JH, Fraser RA. Complications following intraspinal injections of steroids. *J Neurosurg* 1978;48:1023–1025.

78. Goucke CR, Graziotti P. Extradural abscess following local anaesthetic and steroid injection for chronic low back pain. *Brit J Anesth* 1990;65:427–490.

79. Shealy CN. Dangers of spinal injections without proper diagnosis. *JAMA* 1966;197:1104–1106.

80. Simon DL, Kunz RD, German JD, et al. Allergic or pseudoallergic reaction following epidural steroid deposition and skin testing. *Reg Anesth* 1989;14: 253–255.

81. Burn JM, Langdon L. Duration of action of epidural methyl prednisolone. A study in patients with the lumbosciatic syndrome. *Am J Phys Med* 1974;53: 29–34.

82. Jacobs S, Pullan PT, Potter JM, et al. Adrenal suppression following extradural steroids. *Anesthesia* 1983;38:953–956.

83. Knight CL, Burnell JC. Systemic side-effects of extradural steroids. *Anaesthesia* 1980;35:593–594.

84. Simon D, Carron H, Rowlingson J. Correspondence. *J Bone Joint Surg* 1985; 67A:981.

85. Stambough JL, Booth RE Jr, Rothman RH. Transient hypercorticism after epidural steroid injection: a case report. *J Bone Joint Surg* 1984;66A: 1115–1116.

86. Tuel SM, Meythaler JM, Cross LL. Cushing's syndrome from epidural methylprednisolone. *Pain* 1990;40:81–84.

87. Dilke TF, Burry HC, Grahame R. Extradural corticosteroid injection in management of lumbar nerve root compression. *BMJ* 1973;2:635–637.

88. Abram SE, Cherwenka RW. Transient headache immediately following epidural steroid injection. *Anesthesiology* 1979;50:461–462.

89. Katz JA, Lukin R, Bridenbaugh PO, et al. Subdural intracranial air: an unusual cause of headache after epidural steroid injection. *Anesthesiology* 1991;74: 615–618.

90. Brownridge P. The management of headache following accidental dural puncture in obstetric patients. *Anaesth Intensive Care* 1983;11:4–15.

91. MacArthur C, Lewis M, Knox EG. Investigation of long term problems after obstetric epidural anaesthesia. *BMJ* 1992;304:1279–1282.

92. Bridenbaugh PO, Greene NM. Spinal (subarachnoid) neural blockade. In: Cousins MJ, Bridenbaugh PO, eds. *Neural Blockade in Clinical Anaesthesia and Management of Pain*. 2nd ed. Philadelphia: Lippincott; 1988;213–251.

93. Botwin KP, Gruber RD, Bouchlas CG, et al. Complications of fluoroscopically guided transforaminal lumbar epidural injections. *Arch Phys Med Rehabil* 2000;81:1045–1050.

94. Houten JK, Errico TJ. Paraplegia after lumbosacral nerve root block: report of three cases. *Spine J* 2002;2:70–75.

95. Somayaji HS, Saifuddin A, Casey AT. Spinal cord infarction following therapeutic computed tomography-guided left L2 nerve root injection. *Spine* 2005; 30:E106–E108.

96. Quintero N, Laffont I, Bouhmidi L, et al. Transforaminal epidural steroid injection and paraplegia: case report and bibliographic review. *Ann Readapt Med Phys* 2006;49:242–247.

97. Glaser SE, Falco F. Paraplegia following a thoracolumbar transforaminal epidural steroid injection. *Pain Physician* 2005;8:309–314.

98. Bogduk N. Complications associated with transforaminal injections. In: Neal JM, Rathmell JP, eds. *Complications in Regional Anesthesia and Pain Medicine*. Philadelphia: Saunders Elsevier; 2007:259–265.

99. Benzon HT, Chew TL, McCarthy RJ, et al. Comparison of the particle sizes of different steroids and the effect of dilution. *Anesthesiology* 2007;106: 331–338.

100. Derby R, Lee SH, Date ES, et al. Size and Aggregation of Corticosteroids used for epidural injections. *Pain Medicine* 2008;9:227–234.

101. Kepes ER, Duncalf D. Treatment of backache with spinal injections of local anesthetics, spinal and systemic steroids: a review. *Pain* 1985;22:33–47.

102. Benzon HT. Epidural steroid injections for low back pain and lumbosacral radiculopathy. *Pain* 1986;24:277–295.

103. Koes BW, Scholten RJ, Mens JM, et al. Efficacy of epidural steroid injections for low-back pain and sciatica: a systematic review of randomized clinical trials. *Pain* 1995;63:279–288.

104. Koes BW, Scholten RJ, Mens JM, et al. Epidural steroid injections for low back pain and sciatica: an updated systematic review of randomized clinical trials. *Pain Digest* 1999;9:241–9247.

105. Nelemans PJ, de Bie RA, de Vet HC, et al. Injection therapy for subacute and chronic benign low back pain. *Spine* 2001;26:501–515.

106. Watts RW, Silagy CA. A meta-analysis on the efficacy of epidural corticosteroids in the treatment of sciatica. *Anaesth Intensive Care* 1995;23:564–569.

107. Vroomen PC, de Krom MC, Slofstra PD, et al. Conservative treatment of sciatica: a systematic review. *J Spinal Dis* 2000;13:463–469.

108. McLain RF, Kapural L, Mekhail NA. Epidural steroid therapy for back and leg pain: mechanisms of action and efficacy. *Spine J* 2005;5:191–201.

109. Rozenberg S, Dubourg G, Khalifa P, et al. Efficacy of epidural steroids in low back pain and sciatica. *Rev Rhum Engl Ed* 1998;66:79–85.

110. van Tulder MW, Koes B, Seitsalo S, et al. Outcome of invasive treatment modalities on back pain and sciatica: an evidence-based review. *Eur Spine J* 2006;15(Suppl 1):S82–S92.

111. Luijsterburg PA, Verhagen AP, Ostelo RW, et al. Effectiveness of conservative treatments for the lumbosacral radicular syndrome: a systematic review. *Eur Spine J* 2007;32:1942–1948.

112. Armon CA, Argoff CE, Samuels J, et al. Assessment: use of epidural steroid injections to treat radicular lumbosacral pain: report of Therapeutics and Technology Assessment Subcommittee of the American Academy of Neurology. *Neurology* 2007;68:723–729.

113. Breivik H, Hesla PE, Molnar I, et al. Treatment of chronic low back pain and sciatica. Comparison of caudal epidural injections of bupivacaine and methylprednisolone with bupivacaine followed by saline. In: Bonica JJ, Albe-Fessard D, eds. *Advances in pain research and therapy*. Vol. 1. New York: Raven Press; 1976:927–932.

114. Bush K, Hillier S. A controlled study of caudal epidural injections of triamcinolone plus procaine for the management of intractable sciatica. *Spine* 1991; 16:572–575.

115. Klenerman L, Greenwood R, Davenport HT, et al. Lumbar epidural injections in the treatment of sciatica. *Brit J Rheumatol* 1984;23:35–38.

116. Carette S, Leclaire R, Marcoux S, et al. Epidural corticosteroid injections for sciatica due to herniated nucleus pulposus. *N Eng J Med* 1997;336: 1634–1640.

117. Valat JP, Giraudeau B, Rozenberg S, et al. Epidural corticosteroid injections for sciatica: a randomized, double-blind, controlled clinical trial. *Ann Rheum Dis* 2003;62:639–643.

118. Cook RJ, Sackett DL. The number needed to treat: a clinically useful measure of treatment effect. *BMJ* 1995;310:452–454.

119. Laupacis A, Sackett DL, Roberts RS. An assessment of clinically useful measures of the consequences of treatment. *New Engl J Med* 1988;318:1728–1733.

120. Wilson-MacDonald J, Burt G, Griffin D, et al. Epidural steroid injection for nerve root compression: a randomised, controlled trial. *J Bone Joint Surg* 2005;87B:352–355.

121. Price C, Arden N, Coglan L, et al. Cost-effectiveness and safety of epidural steroids in the management of sciatica. *Health Technology Assessment* 2005; 9(33):1–74.

122. Fanciullo GJ, Hanscom B, Seville J, et al. An observational study of the frequency and pattern of use of epidural steroid injection in 25,479 patients with spinal and radicular pain. *Reg Anesth Pain Med* 2001;26:5–11.

123. Manchikanti L, Singh V, Rivera JJ, et al. Effectiveness of caudal epidural injections in discogram positive and negative chronic low back pain. *Pain Physician* 2002;5:18–29.

124. Buttermann GR. The effect of spinal steroid injections for degenerative disc disease. *Spine J* 2004;4:495–505.

125. Southern D, Lutz GE, Cooper G, et al. Are fluoroscopic caudal epidural steroid injections effective for managing chronic low back pain? *Pain Physician* 2003;6:167–172.

126. Botwin KP, Gruber RD, Bouchlas CG, et al. Fluoroscopically guided lumbar transforaminal epidural steroid injections degenerative lumbar stenosis: an outcome study. *Am J Phys Med Rehabil* 2002;81:898–905.

127. Yang SC, Fu TS, Lai PL, et al. Transforaminal epidural steroid injection for discectomy candidates: an outcome study with a minimum of two-year follow-up. *Chang Gung Med J* 2006;29:93–99.

128. Blankenbaker DG, De Smet AA, Stanczak JD, et al. Lumbar radiculopathy: treatment with selective lumbar nerve blocks—comparison of effectiveness of triamcinolone and betamethasone injectable suspensions. *Radiology* 2005; 237:738–741.

129. Riew KD, Yin Y, Gilula L, et al. The effect of nerve-root injections on the need for operative treatment of lumbar radicular pain: a prospective, randomized, controlled, double-blind study. *J Bone Joint Surg Am* 2000;82A:1589–1593.

130. Riew KD, Park JB, Cho YS, et al. Nerve root blocks in the treatment of lumbar

radicular pain. A minimum five-year follow-up. *J Bone Joint Surg* 2006;88: 1722–1725.

131. Karppinen J, Malmivaara A, Kurunlahti M, et al. Periradicular infiltration for sciatica: a randomized controlled trial. *Spine* 2001;26:1059–1067.
132. Karppinen J, Ohinmaa A, Malmivaara A, et al. Cost-effectiveness of periradicular infiltration for sciatica: subgroup analysis of a randomized controlled trial. *Spine* 2001;26:2587–2595.
133. Ng L, Chaudhary N, Sell P. The efficacy of corticosteroids in periradicular infiltration for chronic radicular pain. *Spine* 2005;30:857–862.
134. Thomas E, Cyteval C, Abiad L, et al. Efficacy of transforaminal versus inter-

spinous corticosteroid injection in discal radicalgia—a prospective, randomized, double-blind study. *Clin Rheumatol* 2003;22:299–304.
135. Schaufele MK, Hatch L, Jones W. Interlaminar versus transforaminal epidural injections for the treatment of symptomatic lumbar intervertebral disc herniations. *Pain Physician* 2006;9:361–366.
136. Manchikanti L, Pakanati RR, Pampati V. Comparison of three routes of epidural steroid injections in low back pain. *Pain Digest* 1999;9:277–285.
137. Ackerman WE, Ahmad M. The efficacy of lumbar epidural steroid injections ion patients with lumbar disc herniations. *Anesth Analg* 2007;104: 1217–1222.

CHAPTER 99 ■ INTRATHECAL DRUG DELIVERY IN THE MANAGEMENT OF PAIN

RICHARD K. OSENBACH

INTRODUCTION

During the past 25 to 30 years, implantable drug delivery devices designed for long-term continuous infusion of medications have become an increasingly important part of the armamentarium for physicians involved in the management of patients with chronic intractable pain syndromes. Spinal drug delivery was initially indicated for and generally limited to patients with intractable pain secondary to cancer. However, over the years, the application of intrathecal (IT) drug delivery (ITDD) has expanded to include treatment of patients with chronic benign pain conditions. Indeed, the use of ITDD for nonmalignant pain syndromes has now exceeded that for patients with cancer-related pain. In addition to opiates, alternative agents have been and are currently being studied as to their safety and efficacy for IT infusion in patients with chronic pain. In addition to chronic pain conditions, IT drug delivery is also utilized for the treatment of other neurological disorders such as spinal- and cerebral-origin spasticity, Parkinson disease, and others. The purpose of this chapter is to outline the current status of neuraxial drug infusion for the treatment of chronic pain including basic concepts of intraspinal drug delivery, the various pharmacological agents either currently in use or in development, the use of ITDD devices, as well as the outcomes associated with the use of this technology for the management of chronic pain.

HISTORICAL REVIEW

The development of ITDD devices represents one of the more substantial advances of the past several decades in the field of chronic pain management. The advent of intraspinal opioid therapy is directly linked to the discovery and isolation of opioid receptors in the early 1970s and the discovery of their existence in both the brain and spinal cord. Yaksh et al. discovered that direct application of morphine to the spinal cord in experimental animals produced measurable analgesic effects and, several years later, it was shown that the intraspinal injection of morphine (epidurally or intrathecally) produced effective analgesia in humans.[1] In 1981, the first report describing the continuous infusion of IT morphine in patients with intractable pain due to underlying malignancy was published.[2] Since this initial publication, a sizeable body of literature has appeared detailing the applica-

tion, safety, and efficacy of intraspinal opiates in the management of chronic pain.[3–16]

BASIC PHARMACOLOGY OF INTRATHECAL DRUG ADMINISTRATION

The safe and effective implementation of intraspinal infusion therapy is predicated on a thorough knowledge of the pharmacology of the individual drugs and an understanding of the pharmacodynamics of intraspinal (intrathecal or epidural) drug delivery. Initial IT pharmacokinetic studies primarily focused on the use of intrathecal methotrexate (MTX); however, detailed IT pharmacodynamic profiles have now been defined for a variety of drugs, most notably the opioids, and in particular morphine.

The distribution and absorption of a drug administered intrathecally is based on multiple variables which may be divided into patient characteristics, cerebrospinal fluid (CSF) characteristics, drug characteristics, and factors associated with the injection technique[17–18] (Table 99.1). Probably the most important of these factors is the characteristic of the particular drug that is injected or infused. Following injection into the lumbar subarachnoid space, the rostral ascent of a particular drug and the ultimate cisternal concentration is determined primarily by its lipid solubility. Hydrophilic substances (e.g., morphine) do not readily cross the blood brain barrier (BBB), and infusion into the lumbar thecal space produces high lumbar CSF concentrations of the infused agent.[18] Hydrophilic drugs are distributed mainly by bulk flow of CSF such that a concentration gradient develops in a caudal-to-rostral direction. Although steady-state cisternal concentrations may not be insignificant, especially for hydrophilic compounds, lumbar drug infusion does not usually result in a significant concentration of the drug within the ventricular system. Because of the relatively small volume of CSF in the spinal canal (about 75 mL) and the relatively slow clearance of hydrophilic drugs from the CSF, infusion of even small doses of hydrophilic compounds will result in a relatively high concentration of the drug at the desired target site of action, namely the spinal cord. In contrast, drugs with significant lipid solubility will be preferentially absorbed into the substance of the spinal cord or diffuse across the subarachnoid-dural barrier into the epidural space.[18] Lipophilic drugs (e.g., fentanyl, sufentanil) usually do not reach significant cisternal concentrations. Consequently, li-

TABLE 99.1

FACTORS AFFECTING DISTRIBUTION OF INTRATHECALLY INJECTED DRUGS

Patient Factors
Age
Height
Weight
Configuration of spinal column
Patency of spinal canal
Patient position postinjection
Intraabdominal/intrathoracic pressure

CSF Factors
Specific gravity
Baricity (solution density/CSF density)
CSF flow characteristics

Drug Factors
Lipid partition coefficient (i.e., lipid solubility)
Dose
Volume of injection

Technique of Injection
Location (lumbar vs. intraventricular)
Rate of injection
Turbulence of injection

pophilic agents may be useful in producing more segmental analgesia without the supraspinal effects which occasionally occur with more hydrophilic drugs.

Continuous IT infusion of a drug using an implanted delivery system has significant theoretical and practical advantages over bolus administration through a tunneled catheter or subcutaneous reservoir. Continuous infusion assures a constant high concentration of drug in the CSF which is highly desirable since the concentration gradient represents the primary driving force for diffusion of the drug to its target site in the spinal cord. Continuous IT infusion also results in a more predictable concentration gradient and is generally associated with fewer adverse side effects than is bolus administration of the same agent.

Morphine is one of the best-studied agents in terms of IT pharmacodynamics. During the continuous IT infusion of morphine, a steady-state caudal-to-rostral concentration gradient develops with lumbar-to-cisternal ratios of morphine ranging anywhere from 4:1 to 7:1.[18] Even though cisternal levels are *relatively* low, they are not necessarily clinically insignificant, and supraspinal side effects, most notably respiratory depression, can occur. Other drugs of clinical interest for which lumbar-to-cisternal levels have been measured include baclofen (2.0–8.7:1) and the alpha-2 adrenergic agonist clonidine (3.2:1).[18]

PATIENT SELECTION FOR INTRATHECAL DRUG DELIVERY

It can be said that successes are created, not simply discovered. Indeed, this is clearly the case in selecting patients for ITDD. In many cases, treatment failure with any type of implantable device (ITDD, spinal cord stimulator, etc.) can often be attributed to suboptimal patient selection. Without question, one of the most important factors for producing a successful outcome with this type of therapy is scrupulous patient selection. It is imperative that patients with chronic pain who are considered for ITDD undergo a comprehensive multidisciplinary evaluation. It may be

prudent to involve the expertise of various specialists such as neurologists, neurosurgeons, anesthesiologists, psychiatrists, psychologists, nurses, physical and occupational therapists, social workers, and vocational rehabilitation specialists.

One must remember that experience of pain is perceptual, and each patient enters into pain management with individual beliefs, experiences, and concerns. Due to the biopsychosocial nature of chronic pain, the nature and magnitude of these influences must be assessed in order to properly evaluate the potential risks and benefits of ITDD for an individual patient. Factors such as good pain coping skills, realistic expectations, strong family support, minimal influence of psychosocial stressors, and lack of cognitive disturbances are more likely to result in a successful outcome.

Each patient should undergo a detailed pain history which includes a review of all prior pain treatments and the results of such treatments. A history of lack of benefit from all prior treatment is a poor prognostic sign. All patients should have a relatively recent spinal imaging study to exclude obvious, surgically correctable conditions such as spinal stenosis or spinal instability and make certain that there is no pathology that would otherwise preclude safe placement of an IT catheter. Absolute contraindications to pump implantation include the presence of systemic infection, local cutaneous infection near the potential surgical sites, uncorrectable coagulopathy, known allergies to components of either the pump or catheter, and active intravenous (IV) drug abuse. Relative contraindications include emaciation or patients with a body habitus that may not be conducive to an implant (e.g., inadequate subcutaneous tissue to create a pocket for the implanted pump). Careful consideration must be given to patients receiving anticoagulation therapy. Although implantation is not contraindicated in these patients, all anticoagulation must be reversed prior to any type of invasive procedure. Patients with an unfavorable psychological profile should not be considered for ITDD until any psychological concerns have been addressed and resolved. Lastly, although recovering drug addiction is not an absolute contraindication, these patients need extremely careful assessment prior to proceeding with this therapy; it is important to understand that placement of an ITDD device does not lead directly or inevitably to cessation of all oral opioids.

Chronic pain conditions for which ITDD has been utilized are outlined in Table 99.2. It is important to assess the type and

TABLE 99.2

CHRONIC PAIN STATES CURRENTLY TREATED WITH CHRONIC SPINAL DRUG INFUSION

Cancer pain
Postlaminectomy syndrome
Nerve root injury
Adhesive spinal arachnoiditis
Brachial or lumbosacral plexitis
Complex regional pain syndrome
　　Type I (reflex sympathic dystrophy)
　　Type II (causalgia)
Spinal cord injury pain
Phantom pain
Postherpetic neuralgia
Painful peripheral neuropathy
Poststroke pain
Intractable angina
HIV-related pain

topography of pain in each patient. In general, ITDD is most effective for pain located below the upper thoracic region although ITDD can be successfully applied in patients with cervical and upper extremity pain. In general, it has traditionally been thought that nociceptive pain and mixed nociceptive/neuropathic pain responds best to IT drug infusion and that patients with pure neuropathic pain are not good candidates for this therapy. However, there is evidence to suggest that neuropathic pain can respond to opioid therapy, albeit at higher doses.[19] In order to improve analgesia in patients with predominantly neuropathic pain, many clinicians have adopted the practice of polyanalgesia or combination therapy, combining IT opioids with alternative medications such as local anesthetics and clonidine.[20] Additionally, the recent approval of ziconitide by the U.S. Food and Drug Administration (FDA) has provided another alternative for treatment of neuropathic pain.[21,22]

The ideal patient for IT opioid infusion is one who has previously demonstrated a positive analgesic response to systemic opioids. This is especially true for patients who experience therapy-limiting side effects with the use of systemic agents. However, if a patient has never shown any response to adequate doses of several different systemic opiates, there is no evidence to suggest that IT delivery of opiates will produce any better analgesic response.

ROLE OF PSYCHOLOGICAL EVALUATION

Karl Marx stated that "the only antidote for mental suffering is physical pain." Indeed, the vast majority of patients with chronic pain conditions have psychosocial issues that influence their condition. This is in keeping with the accepted theory of the biopsychosocial nature of chronic pain. Many patients with chronic pain exhibit a degree of suffering and pain behavior that is out of proportion to the underlying condition. Indeed, there are individuals who possess certain behavioral and psychological factors that may "predispose" them to the development of and enhancement of the experience of pain. Moreover, many of these patients lack the requisite psychological tools to effectively cope with their condition and, as a result, develop maladaptive psychological and behavioral issues. Consequently, given the nature of chronic pain, it is recommended that all patients undergo evaluation by an experienced pain psychologist before even proceeding with a trial of IT therapy. Although psychological evaluation has never been shown to clearly result in improved outcomes, it does provide an insight into the psychosocial effects of chronic pain on an individual patient. In addition, evaluation by an experienced pain psychologist can identify risk factors that are known to be associated with poor outcomes (Table 99.3). It should be emphasized that the purpose of the psychological evaluation is not to simply "clear" or, for that matter, exclude the patient for an implant, but rather to gain an understanding of the psychological factors that might influence the outcome in a particular patient. It is also important to realize that while a given patient might initially be noted to have an unfavorable psychological profile, this does not necessarily constitute an absolute contraindication to implantation at some time in the future. Patients who are willing to work with a psychologist and/or psychiatrist can progress to the point where they are appropriate candidate for ITDD at some point in the future. Table 99.3 outlines some of the more important questions that should be addressed with the psychological evaluation and also lists a number of risks factors that may influence outcome.

TRIALING TECHNIQUES FOR INTRATHECAL DRUG DELIVERY

Prior to implantation of a permanent ITDD device, all patients, *without exception*, should undergo some type of screening trial

TABLE 99.3

PSYCHOLOGICAL RISK FACTORS ASSOCIATED WITH POOR OUTCOME OF IMPLANTABLE PAIN DEVICES

Risk Factors

Thought disorders

Personality disorders
    Borderline personality
    Anti-social personality

Mood disorders
    Major depression

Somatization disorders
    Undifferentiated somatoform disorder
    Conversion disorder
    Hypochondriasis
    Body dysmorphic disorder

Addiction disorder

Alcohol or drug abuse in primary caregiver

History of physical and/or sexual abuse

Emotional abuse or neglect in primary caregiver

Catastrophizing

Dementia or other cognitive disturbances

Excessive anxiety

High levels of psychosocial distress

Suggested Referral Questions for Psychological Evaluation

Identify any untreated or under treated major affective disorder

Axis II (personality/character) disorder
    Effects on the perception of pain, compliance, cooperation, etc.

Any untreated or under treated alcohol or drug problems (present or past)

Exceptions/attributions regarding pain and proposed therapy

Nonphysical factors and their contribution to patient's pain perception and behavior

Type and degree of social support

---

to determine effectiveness and potential drug-related side effects. Indeed, in a 2006 Canadian survey, all centers indicated that a trial injection or infusion was carried out before placement of an implanted ITDD system.[23] Even before proceeding with the trial, it is imperative that the patient and physician establish the specific goals for determining that success of the trial. Goals are not necessarily uniform across all patients, but must be individualized on a case-by-case basis, depending on the particular circumstances. Obviously, one of the goals, and probably the most important goal from the patient's point of view, is absolute pain reduction. Nearly all of the literature that has been published regarding neuromodulation procedures defines a "successful trial" as a 50% reduction in the patient's baseline pain. Although 50% pain reduction would seem to be a reasonable achievement if not arguably an excellent result in the chronic pain population, I would submit that this figure should not be used as the sole determining factor of the success or failure of an individual trial. There are certainly patients for whom a lesser reduction in pain is sufficient and results in improvement in activities, reduction in medication use, etc. On the other hand, there are clearly patients who will be disappointed with the outcome if they experience anything short of complete pain resolution, which reminds one of the philosophy that "one man's junk is another man's treasure." Indeed, some patients are simply unable to psychologically cope with the realization that they will have some degree of pain for the duration of their life. These patients often have difficulty discontinuing systemic opioids following pump implantation, demand frequent increases in their IT drug dose, and generally do not demonstrate the kind of improvement in function commensurate with their stated degree of pain reduction. These patients often pose difficult long-term management problems, which make it imperative that the implanting physician clearly outlines the *reasonable* benefits and expectations of the therapy *before* even proceeding with the trial. By establishing reasonable goals and expectations at the outset, future problems can often be avoided. Indeed, clinicians who fail to follow this basic principle will, more often than not, be left to deal with an unhappy and frustrated patient.

Although pain reduction is obviously important, perhaps the most important and revealing outcome measure is improvement in function. The type and degree of functional improvement will vary between patients. Nonetheless, it is important to establish reasonable goals for functional improvement that can be measured and confirmed after institution IT drug delivery. Physical and occupational therapists can be quite valuable in assisting the clinician in developing achievable goals and monitoring the patient during therapy. These individuals also provide an independent evaluator other than the implanting physician for whom there is always going to be some inherent bias in evaluating the outcome of treatment. Besides improvement in physical function, other important and useful measures of outcome include improvements in vocational activity (i.e., return to work), increase in social and avocational activities, improvement in sleep patterns, improvement in mood/affect, reduction in adjuvant medication use, and reduction in health care utilization. There exist a number of valuable standardized and validated measurement tools that are can be utilized to assess outcomes. These include tools such as SF-36, the Brief Pain Inventory (BPI), various mood scales, etc. These questionnaires can be administered prior to treatment and at various intervals thereafter to provide objective measurements that can then be correlated with the patient's reported degree of pain reduction.

It can not be sufficiently emphasized that careful patient selection is the key to success of not only ITDD but also of any other invasive type of therapy. It should also be remembered that a successful trial does not guarantee long-term success. Indeed, many patients with an implantable pain device (ITDD system, SCS system, etc.) who incur failure of their pump battery or pulse generator never have their power source replaced because they felt the therapy was not sufficiently effective.

Aside from the criteria that will be used to determine the success or failure of the trial, there are a number of issues including: (1) the method that will be used for screening, (2) duration of the trial, (3) which drug to use and what starting dose, (4) the potential use of a placebo, and (5) what to do with systemic opioids during the trial. There are several accepted screening methods available for IT trials including include single IT bolus injection, multiple IT boluses, continuous epidural, or IT infusion.

There is currently no clear consensus among clinicians as to the ideal trial technique. Each has it advantages and disadvantages. The single IT bolus represents the simplest, most cost-effective method of screening for IT drug delivery. However, depending on the dose injected, bolus injection may result in subanalgesic drug levels, thus producing a "false negative trial." Additionally, drug-related adverse side effects are generally more common following bolus injection than continuous infusion and these side effects may obscure the analgesic response. There is also a higher likelihood of a placebo response when using a single injection technique. Even though a single low-dose bolus of opioid produces a positive response, it is difficult to determine an accurate starting dose for the implanted pump. Finally, although single shot bolus trials are simple to perform, they do not provide the ability to evaluate the effect of the therapy on function as well as some of the other outcome measures that have been discussed. Although multiple IT boluses are more costly and time-consuming, they do provide the ability to titrate the dose and establish a dose-response curve. It is also possible with this technique to employ placebo injections for comparison with active drug administration. On the other hand, multiple boluses are often associated with an increased incidence of side effects, lack correlation with continuous infusion, and require multiple dural punctures unless a temporary IT catheter is used.

The continuous or functional trial is probably the one preferred by the majority of implanters. In fact, in a survey of implanters at academic teaching institutions conducted in 1999, 52% indicated they preferred continuous infusion for performing screening trials. Fifty-nine percent of implanters utilized the IT route, 17% used epidural infusion, and 22% employed both route at various times.[24] Intuitively, it would seem that continuous infusion would have clear advantages over bolus techniques. Continuous infusion can be performed using either the IT or epidural route. Although either is acceptable, it is important to understand the difference between IT and epidural drug delivery (Table 99.4). Regardless of the route chosen, continuous infusion allows for controlled dose titration and assessment of a reasonable starting dose once the pump is implanted. On balance there is a reduced risk of side effects with continuous infusion. There is also less chance of a placebo response since continuous infusion allows for the placebo response to dissipate over time as the trial is continued. Perhaps, most importantly, a continuous trial, particularly if continued for a sufficient period of time, allows for assessment of functional outcome which is perhaps the most important determining factor of success. Notwithstanding the advantages, there are some relative disadvantages to continuous

TABLE 99.4

COMPARISON OF EPIDURAL VS. INTRATHECAL DRUG INFUSION

Criterion	Intrathecal	Epidural
Onset of Action	Faster onset	Slower onset
Systemic Effects	Minimal systemic effects	Larger systemic effects
Duration of Effect	Long-lasting	Short-lasting
Dosage	Smaller dose (1/10 Epidural dose for morphine)	Larger dose required
Adverse Effects	Post-LP headache Risk of meningitis	More systemic side effects Risk of epidural abscess Respiratory depression

infusion. It is more complicated and requires greater expertise for placement of a tunneled catheter and is obviously more costly to perform than a bolus trial. Although it has been suggested that continuous trials are associated with increased morbidity, that has not been the author's experience. Again, as long as one adheres to strict surgical principles and is diligent in management of the patient during the trial, the morbidity is generally very low.

Anderson et al. randomized 40 patients to either IT bolus injection or continuous epidural infusion (CEI) and compared the outcome of the two groups in terms of pain reduction.[25] Twenty-seven patients had a successful trial and went on to implantation of a permanent device for long-term therapy (IT bolus = 17, CEI = 19). A "successful" response occurred in 64% and 60% of the CEI and IT bolus groups, respectively. Drug-related complications were more common in the IT bolus group (88%) compared with the CEI group (70%). The cost of CEI ($4,762) was considerably higher than that for the IT bolus group ($1,862). Follow-up data were available for 24 patients ((IT bolus = 10, CEI = 14). The patients who were trialed with a single IT bolus experienced a 57% reduction in pain scores (80 to 34) at 6 months compared to a 48% reduction in pain scores (82 to 43) in the CEI group. The authors concluded that the differences in pain and functional response to long-term IT opioids among patients selected by either trial method are not large.

The use and value of placebo administration has been raised previously. The rationale of the use of a placebo is to reduce the likelihood of a "false positive" trial. Unfortunately, normal individuals commonly exhibit a placebo response and the rate of placebo response may exceed 60% in patients with chronic pain. It may also be difficult to interpret the response, and a positive placebo response should not necessarily be taken as an equivalent to a negative trial. Once again, because a sufficiently long continuous trial will generally allow for dissipation of any placebo response, most implanters (including the author) do not utilize placebo infusion as a routine part of their screening trial.

Other issues that need to be addressed include the duration of the trial, the specific medication(s) and dosages administered, and the handling of baseline systemic opiates during the trial. There is currently no standard protocol in existence that addresses issues such as trial duration, trialing with specific medications, or how to handle baseline opioids during the trial. The author's current protocol includes slowly weaning the patient off all opioid medications and giving the patient an opioid-free drug holiday for 6 weeks prior to commencing the trial. An exception is made for the patient with pain related to cancer. This is clearly not the standard practice of most implanting physicians and could even be considered somewhat controversial. This practice is based on the fact that almost all patients referred to the author (and probably to most implanting physicians) for IT opioids have been on long-term systemic opioids, sometimes at exceedingly high doses. Under these circumstances it is likely that the patient has developed opioid tolerance and/or hyperalgesia. Under such circumstances, it is very difficult if not impossible to obtain significant pain reduction with relatively low doses of IT opioids. It has also been our experience that, even in cases where it is possible to obtain reasonable analgesia, many patients are then reluctant to taper off their systemic opioids. This practice requires extreme dedication by both the patient and clinician and an indelible trust on the part of the patient in his/her physician.

A tunneled externalized catheter is implanted and a continuous functional outpatient trial is conducted for anywhere between 2 and 4 weeks. By providing the patient a drug holiday, it is possible to begin the IT infusion at very low doses (usually around 0.25–0.5 mg per day of IT morphine) of medication. For patients with nociceptive pain or mixed nociceptive/neuropathic pain, we usually start with an opioid. If the pain is predominantly neuropathic, bupivacaine or clonidine is added to the infusion. The patient is evaluated at least three times per week to determine the analgesic response, degree of functional improvement, and the development of side effects. Incremental dose escalation is performed and if a significant degree of pain reduction or functional improvement is not realized by the time the patient reaches 2 to 4 mg of IT morphine (or its equivalent) per day, the trial is terminated and the catheter is removed. Again, the success or failure of the trial is based on the goals that have been agreed on by the clinician and patient prior to proceeding with the trial. If the trial is deemed a success, the patient is then returned to the operating room for revision of the catheter and implantation of the pump. Patients are provided short-acting opioids during the immediate postoperative period for management of surgical pain and these are weaned and discontinued over a 2-week period. Patients are routinely counseled that they may experience incident pain that will usually be transient depending on their daily activities and are provided with nonpharmacological coping strategies for managing these situations. During the past 2 years that we have been using this protocol, we have realized a higher degree of success compared with previous implants and have been able to maintain patients on a low stable dose of mediation. Interestingly, there have been occasional patients whose pain actually improves once they have been weaned off systemic opioids to such a degree that they never even proceed with the trial.

IMPLANTABLE PUMP TECHNOLOGY

Fully implantable infusion pumps were first used for the continuous delivery of heparin, insulin, and intraarterial chemotherapy and later applied to intraspinal drug infusion. There are two basic types of fully implantable devices for continuous delivery of IT medications: constant flow pumps and programmable pumps.[26,27]

The first generation pumps were constant flow devices preprogrammed to deliver medication at a single, fixed, constant rate. The initial prototype of the constant flow pump consists of a hollow titanium two-chambered device which consists of a drug reservoir and a chamber that contains a volatile two-phase fluorinated hydrocarbon (FHC) which functions as a propellant. Installation of medication into the drug reservoir results in compression of the propellant which transforms it to a liquid state. As the propellant is warmed by the patient's body temperature, the FHC is transformed from liquid to vapor which then exerts continuous pressure on a system of bellows which expand and force the drug out of the reservoir and into the IT catheter. The standard pump holds a volume just under 50 cc and is filled by puncturing a special inlet septum with a noncoring Huber needle. Flow rates designed to deliver 1.0 to 6.0 cc's per day are pre-set and calibrated at the factory. Although this pump is relatively simple and inexpensive compared to fully programmable devices, the major disadvantage is that dosage alterations require the pump to be drained and refilled with a different concentration of drug. Also, flow rates can be altered by certain physical and physiological factors and these fluctuations in drug delivery rate can result in parallel fluctuations in analgesia (Table 99.5).

The second type of fully implanted drug delivery device is a fully programmable pump such as the SynchroMed Infusion System (Medtronic Neurological, Minneapolis, MN). The current model (SynchroMed II) consists of a collapsible drug reservoir into which the drug is injected through a self-sealing septum. The pump is powered by a lithium-cadmium battery which drives an internal peristaltic pump. The pump contains an electronic module with a computer chip which allows one to program variable infusion rates, bolus injections, etc. A small radiofrequency antenna allows the pump to be noninvasively interrogated by telemetry and programmed with an external handheld programmer. The pump can be programmed for a variety of delivery modes which can be tailored to the individual circumstances. The pump

TABLE 99.5

FACTORS AFFECTING DRUG DELIVERY WITH CONSTANT FLOW INFUSION PUMPS

- Body temperature
  - calibrated for 37°C
  - 10% to 13% increase in flow per 1°C rise
- Geographical elevation
  - calibrated for elevation of implanting center
  - flow increases at higher altitudes
- Blood pressure (at site of drug discharge)
  - inversely proportional
  - 3% change for every 10 mm Hg MAP
- Drug viscosity
- Reservoir capacity
  - flow rate calibrated for 50% capacity
  - 4% variability at extremes of volume
- Pump "Dead Space"
  - 4 mL "dead volume"
  - correction factor for concentration

comes with a catheter access port (CAP) side port which is extremely valuable for trouble shooting catheter-related problems.

SURGICAL TECHNIQUE OF PUMP IMPLANTATION

Implantation of an ITDD system is usually a straightforward procedure for the properly trained and experienced implanter. However, despite the perceived simplicity of the implant procedure, there are numerous pitfalls that can lead to complications. It is clearly preferable to avoid rather than have to manage complications. In general, many complications can be avoided through attention to meticulous aseptic operative technique, gentle tissue handling, and adherence to certain technical points in terms of catheter insertion and pump implantation.[28] It should be clearly recognized that implantation of a permanent ITDD should only occur following a successful trial.

Implantation of an ITDD can be performed either under local anesthesia with IV sedation or general anesthesia, depending on the clinician's preference and the overall condition of the patient. All patients should receive a single dose of prophylactic antibiotics directed toward the normal skin flora within 30 minutes of incision. No postoperative antibiotics are prescribed as there is no literature to support their use in an otherwise clean surgical wound. The patient is positioned and secured in a lateral decubitus position. The pump can be placed on either side, either in the subcostal region or lower quadrant of the abdomen. It is important to position the pump such that it does not impinge on or sit directly over any bony prominence (e.g., iliac crest, rib cage) as this is likely to result in local pain and the need for revision of the pump pocket site. Other factors that occasionally need to be taken into account include the presence of either current or expected ostomies (e.g., percutaneous gastrostomy and/or suprapubic catheter) and body habitus (emaciation or morbid obesity). Although implantation of a pump is not absolutely contraindicated in these patients, there is likely a higher risk of infection and every effort should be made to implant the pump as far from these sites as possible.

Prior to pump implantation, all patients should undergo an appropriate imaging study of the spine (CT with IV contrast, CT-myelography, or MRI) to ensure there is no anatomical ob-

struction that might preclude safe catheter insertion. The first step is to insert and properly position the catheter in the subarachnoid space.[28] This should always be performed with the use of intraoperative C-arm fluoroscopy to verify the correct position of the catheter. A small stab incision is made in the mid-lower lumbar region based on fluoroscopic imaging. Keeping in mind that the spinal cord terminates around T12 or L1, needle entry should be caudal to this level, ideally at L2-3 or L3-4. The exact insertion site may vary depending on the spinal anatomy, the presence of spinal instrumentation, etc. A lumbar puncture is performed with a no.15 gauge Tuohy needle using a paramedian approach with a shallow insertion angle. Midline insertion should be avoided as the steep angle required makes catheter insertion more difficult. Additionally, a midline catheter will likely incur constant stress from pinching between the spinous processes and this more often than not leads to fracture of the catheter. The shallower the angle of insertion, the easier the catheter will advance and the more likely it is that the catheter will be ultimately wind up in the dorsal subarachnoid space. After obtaining good flow of CSF, the catheter is inserted through the needle and is threaded rostrally. Either a one- or two-piece catheter can be used depending on the clinical situation and the preference of the implanter. The catheter should pass easily with minimal resistance. Under no circumstances should the catheter be forced passed the point of an apparent obstruction. Doing so can lead to complications including inadvertent entry of the catheter into the substance of the spinal cord which can result in serious neurological sequelae. The tip of the catheter should generally be positioned in the upper most portion of the lumbar cistern (Fig. 99.1). For the average patient with failed back surgery syndrome and pain in the axial lumbar region and/or lower extremities, this is an ideal position given that most of these patients will be receiving a hydrophilic agent such as morphine or hydromorphone. If the pain topography is more rostral, such as the cervical spine or upper extremities, the catheter may need to be positioned more rostrally in order to get a sufficient concentration of the drug to the target area of the spinal cord. If one is using a predominantly lipophilic agent (e.g., fentanyl or sufentanil), the tip of the catheter needs to be positioned within a couple of levels of the segmental level of pain. Once the catheter has been advanced to the desired level, the guide wire is gently removed. This is best performed by straightening out the catheter and applying gentle traction to the guide wire. CSF should be observed to flow spontaneously from the end of the tubing although it is occasionally necessary and acceptable to gently aspirate the catheter to commence CSF flow. Once CSF flow is confirmed, the tubing is temporarily occluded with a smooth clamp to prevent loss of excessive amounts of CSF.

With the Tuohy needle still in place to prevent inadvertent damage to the catheter, a skin incision is made incorporating the needle and carried down to the lumbodorsal fascia. A small pocket should be fashioned to accommodate a strain relief loop of catheter and prevent kinking in the lumbar incision. The needle is then withdrawn leaving the catheter in place and the catheter is anchored at the fascial insertion site to prevent migration using one of the standard anchoring devices and permanent suture material. The author's preference is to use a butterfly-type V-wing anchor which, when sutured in placed, closes around the catheter. This technique avoids placing any suture material around the catheter itself and minimizes the risk of occlusion.

With the catheter securely in place, the next step is to create a subcutaneous pocket in the abdominal region. The pocket should be sufficiently large to easily accommodate the pump and allow closure of the wound without any significant tension. However, one should avoid making the pocket too large as this can allow the pump to rotate within the pocket in the event the anchoring sutures break. Using a tunneling rod, the catheter is then tunneled from the back to the abdominal pocket and continued

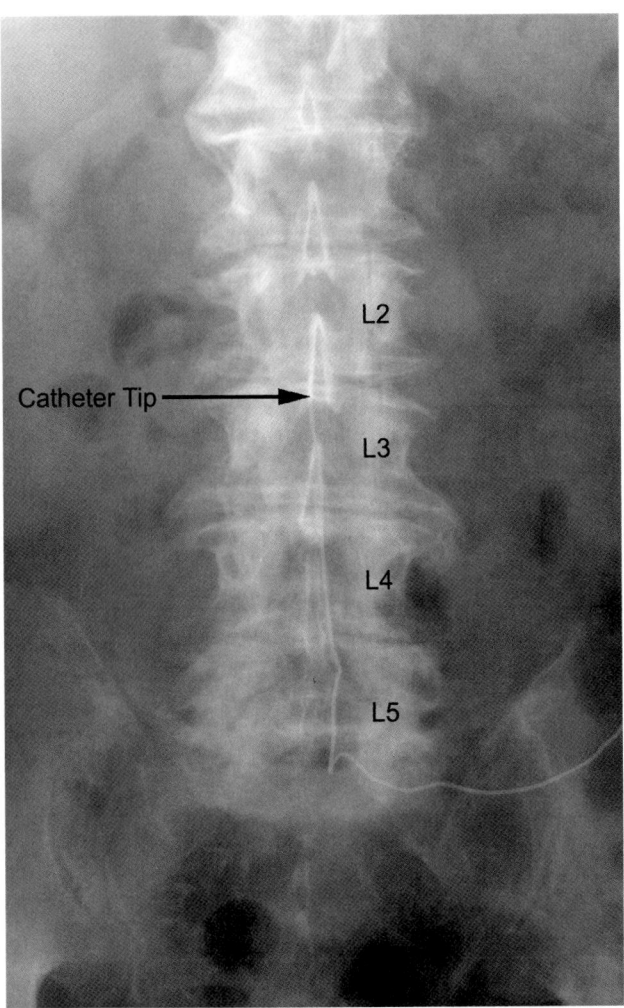

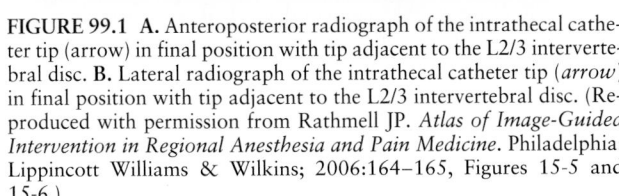

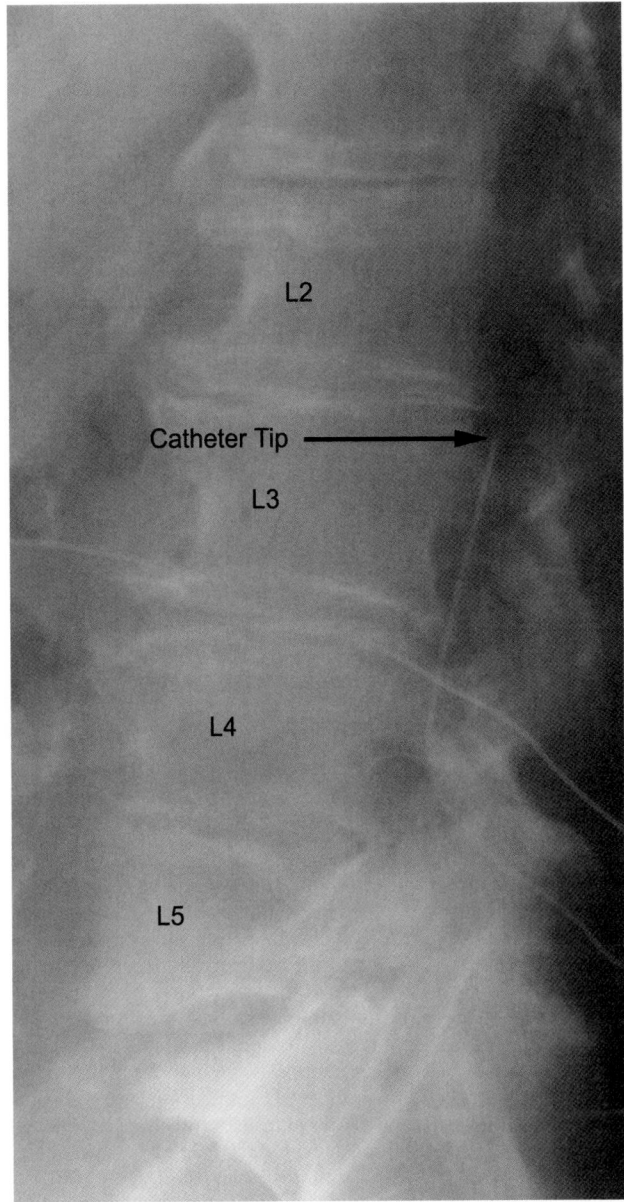

FIGURE 99.1 A. Anteroposterior radiograph of the intrathecal catheter tip (arrow) in final position with tip adjacent to the L2/3 intervertebral disc. **B.** Lateral radiograph of the intrathecal catheter tip (*arrow*) in final position with tip adjacent to the L2/3 intervertebral disc. (Reproduced with permission from Rathmell JP. *Atlas of Image-Guided Intervention in Regional Anesthesia and Pain Medicine.* Philadelphia: Lippincott Williams & Wilkins; 2006:164–165, Figures 15-5 and 15-6.)

flow of CSF is confirmed from the catheter. If a two-piece catheter is used, the distal (i.e., intrathecal) catheter is trimmed by an appropriate amount (if so desired) and then connected to the proximal catheter using a pin connector; this connection is then covered with a strain relief sleeve to prevent kinking at the connection site. This pin connector is then used as a second anchoring site, thereby creating a gentle strain relief loop between the fascial anchor and the pin connector. The amount of the distal catheter that is trimmed should be measured and recorded in order to accurately calculate the catheter volume. Once the pump has been prepared and filled with drug (this will vary depending on the type of pump), it is brought onto the surgical field and connected to the proximal catheter. The pump is then placed into the subcutaneous pocket, ensuring that the refill side is toward the skin and secured in place with permanent sutures, utilizing either the suture loops attached to the pump or by placing the pump into a Dacron pouch and securing the pouch to the fascia. This is an important maneuver to prevent the pump from flipping, thus preventing access to the refill port. Any excess proximal catheter should be gently coiled beneath the pump. It is generally recommended that a generous amount of proximal catheter be left in

the pouch since this will create an additional strain relief loop in the system. After securing the catheter and anchoring the pump, the catheter access port (if there is one) should be entered with a 24-gauge noncoring needle and CSF aspirated and reinjected to ensure patency of the system. A small amount of non-ionic preservative-free contrast can also be injected to confirm patency of the system. If contrast is used it should be flushed from the catheter using preservative-free saline. The surgical wounds are then meticulously closed in anatomical layers. The pump can then be programmed and the system primed to bring active drug to the tip of the catheter.

MEDICATIONS FOR INTRATHECAL DRUG DELIVERY

Although IT morphine often provides adequate analgesia with an acceptable side effect profile, it is ineffective or poorly tolerated in many patients. Initially, it was believed that IT delivery of opiates at fractional doses of those used systemically or even epidurally to achieve effective analgesia would eliminate many of the problems associated with systemic opiates. In retrospect, this was a rather naive assumption. As more infusion systems are implanted (particularly for noncancer pain), it has become apparent that many of the difficulties associated with the long-term administration of systemic opiates such as physiologic tolerance, hyperalgesia, and other dose-limiting side effects (e.g., nausea, constipation, pruritus, peripheral edema, respiratory depression) also occur with IT opiates. It has become more apparent that spinal opiates are either completely or relatively ineffective in treating many neuropathic pain syndromes (e.g., spinal cord injury pain, postherpetic neuralgia, and reflex sympathetic dystrophy), albeit with some exceptions. Basic research in animal models of pain shows that multiple neurotransmitters (e.g., glutamate, gamma-aminobutyric acid [GABA], substance P [SP], acetylcholine, and opioids) are intimately involved in the neurophysiology of pain transmission.[13,29] Consequently, much of the research effort in spinal drug infusion has centered around the investigation and development of alternative pharmacologic classes of agents that have antinociceptive effects when administered intrathecally in animals. These agents are discussed later. Although not currently approved by the FDA specifically for IT therapy, the use of some of these agents (e.g., clonidine, local anesthetics) is nonetheless now well accepted, and they are routinely used "off-label" as reasonable alternatives to morphine or other opiates.

Opioids

Morphine

The discovery of spinal opioid receptors in the 1970s represents the initial event that spawned interest in the IT administration of morphine. Several types of opioid receptors have been identified (mu, delta, kappa). Mu receptors are the most important subtype in so far as the major clinical effects of morphine are concerned.[13] Indeed, high concentration of mu receptors have been identified in the dorsal horn of the spinal cord, the presumed spinal site of action of morphine and other opioids used for IT infusion. Intrathecal morphine is considered to be about 10 times more potent than the same dose administered epidurally and approximately 100 times as potent as the same dose given IV. The most commonly used conversion values for morphine are: 1 mg IT morphine = 10 mg epidural morphine = 100 mg IV morphine = 300 mg oral morphine. It should be clearly understood that these figures represent estimates and that the relative potency of morphine administered by different routes may not be the same in all patients or in patients who have been receiving chronic systemic therapy.

The advantages of IT drug administration include the lack of an absorption phase and essentially 100% bioavailability. Because of the small volume of distribution (spinal CSF volume is approximately 75 mL) of morphine when injected or infused into the CSF, a dose of IT morphine yields significantly higher CSF concentration than that which occurs when given epidurally where significant vascular absorption occurs. In addition, because the rate of elimination of morphine from the CSF and plasma is similar, the duration of action of IT morphine is relatively long. Following IT administration, morphine is not detectable in serum for the first 2 hours.[30] Because morphine is a hydrophilic compound, there is slow rostral spread of the drug through bulk flow of CSF, one factor responsible for clearance of morphine from the CSF. This slow rostral spread is also thought to be responsible for the delayed respiratory depression that can occur following IT administration, particularly in opioid-naïve patients. Studies have indicated that following IT infusion of morphine in the upper lumbar region, a steady-state concentration gradient develops over a period of about 72 hours, with a lumbar: cervical concentration ration of around 7–8:1. Elimination of IT

morphine occurs through vascular absorption through the blood supply of the spinal cord. CSF elimination of opioids in general is bioexponential and dependent on the lipid solubility of the drug. With a single bolus injection of morphine, there is thought to be little metabolism of the drug. However, with chronic infusion morphine is metabolized to morphine-6-glucuronide (M-6-G) which has been shown in animal studies to have a potency 10 to 45 times that of morphine itself.[30] Preservative-free morphine is currently the only opioid that is approved for intrathecal use by the FDA.

Hydromorphone

Despite the paucity of clinical studies, the use of IT hydromorphone as an alternate opioid has steadily increased. Hydromorphone was initially utilized for ITDD in patients who manifested intolerable side effects to IT morphine or inadequate analgesia. Indeed, based on the large clinical experience with hydromorphone, this agent has been recommended as a "Line 1" agent by the most recent Polyanalgesia Consensus Conference.[31] Intrathecal hydromorphone is approximately 5 to 6 times more potent than IT morphine and is somewhat more lipophilic.[13] Perhaps its main attraction is that IT hydromorphone is generally associated with fewer side effects than is IT morphine.

Fentanyl and Sufentanil

There has been a considerable amount of both human and animal research regarding the IT use of both fentanyl and sufentanil.[13] Both fentanyl and sufentanil are highly potent mu receptor agonists which are highly lipid soluble. Both have a rapid onset (approximately 10 minutes) and relatively long duration of action (1–4 hours for fentanyl, 2–6 hours for sufentanil) following acute IT administration. Because of the lipid solubility of these agents, it is important that the tip of the delivery catheter be positioned within a few spinal segments of the segmental pain level. While this is not particularly critical for treatment of axial lumbar and/or lower extremity pain, it is important for treatment of pain at more rostral levels. In such cases, if the catheter is not located relatively close to the segmental level of pain, the drug will be absorbed into the spinal cord preventing the development of adequate concentration at the intended target site.

There have been numerous preclinical studies that have documented the analgesic efficacy of IT fentanyl or sufentanil in animals, mostly in response to acute or bolus administration. The long-term clinical use of these agents is limited to only a few studies containing small numbers of subjects.[13,32] Overall, the analgesic response to long-term infusion to either agent was favorable and relatively well-tolerated. Effective dosages have been in the microgram range: 10 to 115 µg/day for fentanyl and 12 to 77 µg/day for sufentanil.

Meperidine. There is relatively little information regarding the use of IT meperidine. There has been a single prospective study detailing the chronic IT delivery of meperidine, with or without clonidine in 10 patients with cancer-related pain.[31,33] The study showed that patients experienced a significant reduction in neuropathic pain. However, between 1 and 3 weeks into therapy, it was discovered that plasma levels of meperidine and its metabolite normeperidine rapidly increased. In fact, the concentration of normeperidine exceeded that of meperidine in one patient. These observations are important as increased levels of meperidine and/or normeperidine can lead to neurotoxicity.

Methadone. Methadone is a racemic mixture of the D- and L-isomers that produce different effects. The D-isomer has been shown to block the N-methyl-D-aspartate (NMDA) receptor in both in vitro and in vivo models. There has been a single prospective clinical trial of IT methadone for the treatment of chronic noncancer pain in patients who had failed prior IT trial with other IT analgesics.[34] Thirteen of 24 patients (54%) reported some degree of pain reduction during the course of treatment, prompting the authors to conclude that methadone might be a potentially useful neuraxial agent for treatment of chronic pain. However, there have been no stability or toxicity studies to allow one to conclude that this medication is safe for long-term use.

Local Anesthetics

Local anesthetics have played a central role in the treatment of pain for decades, although it was not until the 1990s that continuous infusion of these agents was routinely used.[6] Currently, local anesthetics such as bupivacaine are commonly given by continuous chronic IT infusion, often combined with opiates for the treatment of both cancer and nonmalignant pain. In low concentrations, local anesthetics such as bupivacaine are nontoxic and alter neurotransmission in a predictable and reversible fashion.

Bupivacaine is the most common local anesthetic used for continuous IT infusion. It appears to be most effective in patients with a neuropathic component of pain, although it may also provide some degree of benefit for patients with nociceptive pain. The utilization and dose escalation of bupivacaine is mainly limited by its side effects, which include sensorimotor blockade at higher doses, and hemodynamic instability. Usually, clinically relevant side effects do not occur with doses less than 15 mg/d, although administration of doses, as high as 118 mg/d has been reported with apparently no adverse effects. Optimal dosing is reached with progressive titration beginning with a daily dose of 3 to 5 mg/d. There has been some interest in liposomal encapsulation for local delivery by the IT route because this tends to reduce the toxicity and cardiovascular effects while increasing the anesthetic duration.

Ropivacaine is a long-acting amide type of local anesthetic that is unique in that it blocks sensory nerve fibers to a greater extent than motor fibers. It is similar to bupivacaine in onset and duration of sensory blockade. The potential advantage of ropivacaine is that it produces less motor block and has less cardiovascular toxicity than bupivacaine. As of yet there have been no clinical studies published on the long-term use of IT ropivacaine for the management of chronic pain.[31]

Tetracaine is another local anesthetic that acts through blockade of sodium channels. Unfortunately, tetracaine has been shown to have direct neurotoxicity in animals manifested by damage to both the dorsal and ventral roots, chromatolytic deterioration of motor neurons, and vacuolation of the spinal cord. Because of the potential neurotoxicity, tetracaine should not be used for long-term IT drug delivery.[31,33]

Alpha-2 Adrenergic Agonists

Alpha-2 adrenergic receptors play an important role in spinal antinociception. Alpha-2 receptor agonists in general, and clonidine in particular, are believed to produce their antinociceptive effects through inhibitory interactions with both pre- and postsynaptic primary afferent nociceptive projections onto secondary neurons in the spinal dorsal horn. Clonidine in particular has been felt to act by postsynaptic activation of descending noradrenergic inhibitory systems. It has also been suggested that the analgesic effects of this class of drugs might also be produced through the inhibition of SP release.[35] Clonidine-induced spinal analgesia is reversed by alpha-adrenergic antagonists such as yohimbine but not by naloxone, providing further evidence of it mechanism of action.

Clonidine is one of the best studied of the nonopioid substances which have been adapted for intraspinal delivery. Clonidine has been shown to have analgesic action in both cancer and nonmalignant pain syndromes when administered intraspi-

nally.[13] Clonidine is a highly lipid-soluble drug which is rapidly absorbed and eliminated from CSF. Bolus administration of IT clonidine results in dose-dependent analgesia at doses of 150, 300, and 450 μg and effective analgesia has also been shown with continuous intrathecal infusion. Intraspinal clonidine appears to be devoid of any local neurotoxicity. The rapid onset of antinociceptive action when given intrathecally provides a strong argument that the major pharmacologic effects occur at the segmental spinal level. However, delayed supraspinal analgesic effects can not be completely discounted since it has been shown that application of clonidine to the locus ceruleus results in analgesia. Since IT injection does not usually result in high cisternal concentrations of clonidine, these supraspinal effects might be explained by systemic absorption and central redistribution of the drug.

Although clonidine is the most common drug in this class to be used for spinal analgesia, other agents such as epinephrine, tizanidine, and dexmedetomidine continue to be studied for spinal infusion. Because the antinociceptive actions of the alpha-2 adrenergic agonists (and most of the other alternative agents discussed later) occur through a nonopioid mechanism, they are often effective in individuals who have become tolerant to morphine or other opiates. These agents (clonidine in particular) shift the opioid dose-response curve to the left and appear to be synergistic with opioids; in other words, the analgesia produced by the combination of clonidine with an opiate often results in a magnitude of analgesia greater than that produced by either agent alone. The major side effects of spinal clonidine include hypotension, bradycardia, and sedation. The hypotensive effects most commonly occur with lower and moderate doses and are generally counteracted at higher doses by a direct peripheral vasoconstrictive effect.[36] Unlike the opiates, clonidine does not cause respiratory depression. Clonidine has been studied in various animal models for possible neurotoxicity prior to its clinical use and has been found safe.[37] Currently, clonidine is approved for medium-term epidural infusion in patients with cancer pain.

Eisenach et al. examined the effects of both IV and IT clonidine on both nociceptive and neuropathic pain in human volunteers.[38] Nociceptive pain was produced using thermal heat stimulation; neuropathic pain was induced by an intradermal injection of capsaicin, which consistently produces sustained pain, hyperalgesia, and allodynia, hallmarks of neuropathic pain. Injection of 150 mg of IT but not IV clonidine resulted in a significant reduction in nociceptive pain from noxious thermal stimulation. The same dose of IT clonidine also resulted in significantly less pain and hyperalgesia following intradermal capsaicin injection, although development of allodynia was not affected. Both IV (150 micrograms) and IT (50 and 150 micrograms) clonidine reduced mean arterial blood pressure to a similar degree. Filos et al. examined the dose-response hemodynamic and analgesic effects of IT clonidine in humans in a prospective randomized double-blind study. Postoperative patients received 150, 300, or 450 micrograms (Groups I, II, and III, respectively) of IT clonidine by bolus lumbar injection 45 minutes after tracheal extubation.[39] Analgesia was assessed by Visual Analogue Scale (VAS) scores at standard time points for 24 hours following surgery, as was blood pressure, heart rate, sedation, and respiratory rate. Pain relief was defined as "the time to first request (in minutes) for supplemental analgesics." IT clonidine reduced pain scores in a dose-dependent fashion. Pain relief was as follows: Group I, 402 ± 75 minutes; Group II, 570 ± 76 minutes; and Group III, 864 ± 80 minutes, with significant differences ($p <0.01$ to 0.001) observed among all three groups. Only the 150-microgram dose (Group I) produced a significant reduction ($p <0.05$) in mean arterial blood pressure (21% ± 13%). Mild sedation occurred in all three groups, but respiratory rate was unaffected.

Clonidine has become a popular agent for spinal infusion in patients with reflex sympathetic dystrophy (RSD), now know as complex regional pain syndrome (CRPS) type I. Rauck et al. studied the efficacy of epidural clonidine in 26 patients with severe pain from CRPS I using a randomized, double-blind, placebo-controlled design.[40] Cervical or lumbar catheters were placed in patients with upper or lower extremity RSD, respectively. Epidural clonidine (300 or 700 micrograms) and placebo were randomly administered on 3 consecutive days and the analgesic response assessed at specified intervals for 6 hours following injection using VAS scores and the McGill Pain Questionnaire (MPQ). Patients considered positive responders were offered entry into a trial of continuous epidural clonidine infusion. Within 20 minutes of injection, both doses of clonidine but not placebo produced significant reductions in both VAS and MPQ scores that persisted for the 6-hour study period. Blood pressure was reduced by a similar amount with both clonidine doses. Nineteen patients were subsequently treated with continuous clonidine infusion (32 ± 6 µg/h; range 14 to 50 µg/h) for 43 ± 8 days (range 7 to 225 days). Their VAS scores, which were measured at weekly intervals during infusion, were significantly reduced compared with those recorded prior to clonidine therapy. Clonidine is currently approved by the FDA for continuous epidural infusion. Clonidine is not currently approved for intrathecal infusion. However, it may receive FDA approval for this application in the near future.

Although clonidine has been the most widely studied of the alpha-2 agonists, several other agents have also received attention as potential spinal analgesic agents. Tizanidine is another alpha-2 agonist that has shown promise as a potential analgesic substance. Leiphart et al. studied the effects of tizanidine in a rat model of mononeuropathic pain that is believed to mimic the hyperalgesia and allodynia typical of many neuropathic pain syndromes in humans.[41] Tizanidine increased the intensity of the mechanical stimulus required to induce paw withdrawal and reduced the duration of limb withdrawal from both normal temperature and cooled surfaces in a dose-dependent fashion. The effects of tizanidine were limited to the hyperalgesic limb and served only to normalize reactive latencies. However, morphine affected both the experimental and unaffected hind limb and increased withdrawal latencies to supernormal values. These findings suggest that IT tizanidine may be more specific for the hyperalgesia and allodynia associated with neuropathic pain states and perhaps may be valuable in managing patients that exhibit these findings.

Dexmedetomidine, another alpha-2 agonist with a higher alpha-2 receptor affinity than clonidine, has been studied experimentally for its effects on neuropathic pain.[42] A dose of 1 µg of dexmedetomidine or 10 µg of clonidine administered intrathecally following sciatic nerve section resulted in a significant reduction in autotomy behavior (self-mutilation thought to be a sign of neuropathic pain) compared with both IT morphine and saline controls. Interestingly, morphine (but not alpha-2 agonists) caused a significant reduction in autotomy behavior when given prophylactic ally or before sciatic nerve section. This finding suggests that morphine may prevent autotomy if administered prophylactic ally, whereas alpha-2 agonists may be useful for treating established pain on a chronic basis. This observation could potentially have practical implications on the prevention or treatment of certain pain states such as pain following peripheral nerve injury or phantom pain. To date there have been no studies in humans to investigate the efficacy or toxicity of this agent when given intrathecally.

Finally, catecholaminergic analgesia has been studied in animals using adrenal medullary allografts and, more recently, in humans with chromaffin cell xenografts.[43,44] When injected into the spinal subarachnoid space, catecholamines have been shown to produce profound analgesia. Catecholamine analgesia may involve an independent mechanism as well as concurrent activation of opioid systems within the spinal dorsal horn. Implantation of adrenal medullary tissue into the subarachnoid space has been shown to produce elevated levels of catecholamines and met-enkephalin, an endogenous opioid peptide. Using a model of

chronic pain in the rat, Sagen et al. have shown that adrenal medullary transplants reduce pain responses to acute noxious stimuli.[43] Furthermore, the analgesic effects are blocked by naloxone and are partially inhibited by phentolamine, providing further evidence of a strong opiate mechanism for this therapy.

Buchser et al. implanted purified bovine chromaffin cells in seven patients with terminal cancer and intractable pain.[44] Four patients suffered from neuropathic pain, and two from nociceptive pain, and the remaining patient had a mixed type of pain. The cells were introduced in a hollow fiber with a semipermeable membrane that was implanted with a minimally invasive procedure in the IT space. No pharmacologic immunosuppression was given. The implants remained in place for a mean duration of 74 days (range 41 to 172). All of the implants were retrieved and analyzed after the patients died. Opiate reduction in the four patients receiving epidural morphine at the time of the implant ranged from 30% to 100%. McGill pain ratings improved 50% to 80% in five patients. Pain reduction measured by VAS scores improved between 10% and 80% in five patients and was unchanged in two patients. Viable cells were identified after explantation in six of the seven patients. Although this study represents the first successful trial of encapsulated xenogenic cells in humans, the preliminary findings regarding analgesia probably warrant a randomized study to evaluate the efficacy of this therapy.

Calcium Channel Antagonists

Calcium is a critical element in the regulation of intracellular processes, including modulation of neuronal excitability, release of neurotransmitters, activation of second messenger systems, and gene transcription. Calcium has been found to play an important role in nociception and pain transmission. Regulation of calcium entry into cells is controlled by voltage-sensitive calcium channels (VSCCs) consisting of at least six neuronal subtypes (L, N, P, Q, R, and T). VSCCs are abundantly expressed on presynaptic nerve terminals where they regulate the calcium-dependent release of neurotransmitters that control synaptic transmission. As it turns out, N-type VSCCs are concentrated in the most superficial laminae of the dorsal horn of the spinal cord, where most primary nociceptive afferent fibers (A-delta and C fibers) terminate. Selective antagonists of N-type calcium channels such as ziconotide (also known as SNX-111), a synthetic agent derived from omega-conopeptide that selectively binds to N-type VSCC, have consistently been antinociceptive in animal models of acute, chronic, and neuropathic pain.[45,46] Based on animal studies, numerous studies of ziconotide have been conducted in humans to determine both safety and efficacy. Based on these studies ziconotide was ultimately approved by the FDA for IT use in humans.[47,48]

Staats et al. conducted a double-blind, randomized, placebo-controlled trial of the safety and efficacy of ziconotide (SNX-111) in 102 patients with chronic intractable neuropathic pain with VAS scores in excess of 50 (0 to 100 mm scale), despite the use of systemic opiate analgesics.[49] A positive response was defined as a reduction in baseline VAS score after 6 days of at least 30% without any concomitant increase in opiate requirements. Patients that received SNX-111 experienced a 37% reduction in VAS scores compared to only 3% in the placebo group ($p < 0.0002$). Adverse events included dizziness, nausea, nystagmus, abnormal gait, urinary retention, constipation, and confusion. Another study by Brose et al. reported the results of a Phase I/II open-label, dose-escalation study of IT SNX-111 in 31 patients with intractable pain that had been inadequately controlled with IT morphine.[50] Many of these patients had neuropathic or mixed neuropathic-nociceptive pain syndromes, including cancer, AIDS pain, phantom limb pain, and poststroke (thalamic) pain. SNX-111 was administered for up to 7 days with assessments performed at 4-hour intervals. Daily-dose escalation depended on the patient's response. Twenty-five patients (84%) experienced what was considered to be partial or complete pain relief that was accompanied by concomitant reductions in pain medication requirements. The most common side effects (the majority of which were reported by Staats) included mental confusion, word-finding difficulties, nystagmus, gait, and balance problems. The frequent side effects associated with intrathecal ziconotide have limited the overall use of this agent.

N-methyl-D-aspartate Receptor Antagonists

The involvement of excitatory amino acids (EAAs) and the NMDA receptor system in nociceptive transmission, along with a clearer understanding of the development of central sensitization and wind-up phenomena, have generated considerable interest in developing antagonists of this receptor for the treatment of chronic pain, particularly neuropathic pain states. NMDA receptors alter opioid receptor sensitivity in a variety of pain states and have been implicated in the development of both opioid tolerance and opioid-induced hyperalgesia. Ketamine has been the most studied and has been used both epidurally and intrathecally for the treatment of postoperative and chronic pain.

Yang et al. conducted a double-blind crossover study to evaluate the effects of ketamine on spinal morphine analgesia in 20 patients with cancer pain.[51] All patients underwent placement of an IT catheter for injection of spinal analgesics. Patients were randomly assigned to initially receive twice-daily bolus injections of either morphine alone or morphine plus 1 mg of benzethonium-preserved ketamine. The initial dose of IT morphine was 0.05 mg; this dose was escalated in daily increments that did not exceed the preceding dose until acceptable analgesia was achieved. After achieving and maintaining adequate analgesia, patients were crossed over and the titration was repeated. Although overall pain reduction was comparable in both groups, patients that received a combination of morphine and ketamine required on average less than 50% (0.17 to 0.02 mg/d) of the daily morphine dose for acceptable analgesia compared to those that received morphine alone (0.38 to 0.04 mg; $p < 0.05$). Moreover, the frequency with which patients required upward titration of their morphine dose was considerably less in those that received both morphine and ketamine. Finally, the rescue dose of morphine required for breakthrough pain was more than three times greater in the group that received morphine alone.

To date, the use of NMDA receptor antagonists has been limited due to side effects. All of the NMDA receptor antagonists to some extent produce phencyclidine-like side effects such as disinhibition, hallucinations, paranoid delusions, and rises in arterial blood pressure.[52] There is also animal data suggesting that some of the NMDA antagonists may be neurotoxic when administered intrathecally. Using a sheep model for IT infusion, Hassenbusch et al. conducted a randomized, double-blind toxicity study of three NMDA antagonists: dextrorphan, dextromethorphan, and memantine.[53] Gross and histologic examination as well as neurologic measures demonstrated that all three agents produced a dose-dependent chronic inflammatory response of the spinal cord that led to necrosis. Although these agents are not currently suited for widespread use in humans, their beneficial effects, especially on wind-up pain and hyperalgesia, suggest that further efforts should be directed toward developing an agent that retains its analgesic properties while eliminating most of the side effects.

Gamma-Aminobutyric Acid Agonists

Gamma-aminobutyric acid (GABA) and glycine are inhibitory neurotransmitters that are widely distributed throughout the nervous system. The beneficial effects of GABA agonists such as baclofen in reducing both spinal- and cerebral-origin spasticity have been well chronicled. Less well known are the potential analgesic effects of these agents. GABA can be readily found within the pain transmission system, particularly in Lissauer's tract, and in laminae I, II, and III of the dorsal horn of the spinal cord. Baclofen is a GABA-B agonist and has been shown to be analgesic when administered intrathecally in animals. The antinociceptive effects of GABA agonists are not reversed by naloxone, suggesting that GABA-aminergic analgesia is not mediated through endogenous opiates. IT baclofen diminished allodynic behavioral responses following IT administration of prostaglandin F2-alpha and reduced c-fos gene expression in an animal model of neurogenic pain.[54]

Taira et al. studied the effects of a single-bolus injection of IT baclofen (50 to 100 μg) in 14 patients with neuropathic pain syndromes (8 with poststroke pain and 6 with spinal cord injury pain).[54] Nine of the fourteen patients experienced marked pain relief within 1 to 2 hours of the injection, which lasted 10 to 24 hours. Injection of placebo produced no effect. Both spontaneous pain and allodynia and hyperalgesia were reduced whereas discriminative pain and touch were unaffected.

Herman et al. demonstrated similar analgesic effects of IT baclofen in patients with pain and spasticity following spinal cord lesions, although the two effects appeared to be temporally distinct.[55] In other words, after a bolus of IT baclofen, suppression and reappearance of the neuropathic pain occurred separate from the spasm-related pain. Not only did spinal baclofen reduce the pain associated with spasticity, it also diminished the dysesthetic pain. In contrast to this study, Loubsher et al. assessed the effects of spinal baclofen in 12 patients with spinal cord injury.[56] Six patients were determined to have neurogenic pain, three had musculoskeletal pain related to spasms, and three had both components. After 12 months, 78% of the patients with a neurogenic component to their pain were unchanged, whereas 83% of the patients experienced improvement in the musculoskeletal pain component. These authors concluded that IT baclofen does in fact reduce pain associated with spasticity but has little effect on chronic neuropathic spinal cord injury pain.

Several studies have been conducted on the effects of midazolam, a GABA-A agonist. Serrao et al. performed a prospective, double-blind, randomized, dummy-controlled trial comparing the therapeutic effects of epidural steroid injection (ESI) with IT midazolam (2 mg) in 28 patients with chronic mechanical lower back pain.[57] Pain was assessed before and 2 months after treatment using the short-form MPQ as well as VAS and verbal rating scales. Although both treatments resulted in improvement in pain, the group treated with IT midazolam was able to reduce their intake of oral analgesics to a greater extent than those who received ESI. Based on the available data, and considering that baclofen is already approved by the FDA for IT infusion using an implanted pump, the use of IT baclofen for neuropathic pain seems to warrant further investigation with a larger scale multicenter study.

Gabapentin

The use of IT gabapentin has been evaluated in a number of rodent models.[33] Injection of an IT bolus of gabapentin resulted in reduction in mechanical allodynia and thermal hyperalgesia. There was no demonstrable effect on acute nociceptive pain assessed by the formalin or hot plate test. IT gabapentin produced no deleterious hemodynamic effects but did lead to mild neurological dysfunction when dose in excess of 300 μg were used.

Somatostatin and Somatostatin Analogues

Somatostatin is a tetradecapeptide that is widely distributed throughout the central nervous system (CNS). Somatostatin was initially discovered by virtue of its ability to inhibit the secretion of growth hormone from the pituitary gland. However, its distribution is not limited to the pituitary axis. Indeed, somatostatinergic neurons can be found in the spinal cord, primarily in the substantia gelatinosa where they seem to exert inhibitory effects on nociceptive neurons.[58] Somatostatin is also present in other areas of the CNS concerned with pain transmission and modulation such as the periaqueductal grey (PAG) and both ascending and descending pain-modulating systems in the brainstem. The presence of somatostatin in primary afferent axons that terminate in lamina II of the dorsal horn of the spinal cord, spinal interneurons, descending inhibitory pathways, and PAG presents a strong circumstantial argument for an antinociceptive role of this substance. Single cell recordings have indicated that somatostatin inhibits the responses of dorsal horn neurons to noxious stimulation.[59] Somatostatin has been shown to elevate pain thresholds in experimental animals and has been reported to produce analgesia in humans when administered by either an epidural or intrathecal route.[60-63] The exact mechanism of action is unclear although it does not appear to be opioid-mediated since the antinociceptive effects of somatostatin are not antagonized by naloxone.

Mollenholt et al. administered somatostatin either epidurally or intrathecally in eight patients with terminal cancer.[63] At a mean daily dose of 1252 µg (range 250 to 3000 µg), somatostatin proved to be an effective analgesic agent in six of these patients. Although none of the patients exhibited any signs of neurologic dysfunction during treatment, autopsy findings demonstrated demyelination of the spinal roots in two patients and demyelination of the dorsal columns in another patient. Aside from concerns regarding neurotoxicity, another major problem is that somatostatin is an unstable peptide subject to rapid enzymatic degradation, making it unsuitable for long-term use.

Octreotide, a stable, nonenzymatically degraded, nontoxic analogue of somatostatin, has yielded promising results as a spinal analgesic for cancer pain. Penn et al. reported the efficacy and preclinical neurotoxicity of IT octreotide in six patients with terminal cancer.[60] At a concentration of 500 µg/mL, octreotide was found to be stable within the SynchroMed model 8611 programmable infusion pump (Medtronic Neurological, Minneapolis, MN) over a 4-week period. Insignificant concentration changes were measured at the catheter tip, and within the pump drug reservoir. Preclinical toxicity testing in dogs showed no evidence of histopathologic changes. Based on the stability and toxicity studies, six patients were treated with IT octreotide. Dosing was initiated at 2.5 to 5.0 µg/h and increased by increments of 2.5 to 5.0 µg/h to a maximum dose of 20 µg/h or 240 µg/d as necessary to achieve pain control. Treatment was continued for periods of 13 to 91 days (mean duration 45.5 days). Baseline mean VAS scores of 9.7 were significantly reduced to 1.7 after 1 week of treatment. Although VAS scores increased to 3.6 at 1 month, the improvements remained statistically significant. The same authors have reported long-term experience with octreotide in two patients with nonmalignant pain.[61] Although this experience is modest if not anecdotal, it nevertheless provides additional evidence for a sustained analgesic effect of IT octreotide in nonmalignant disease states.

There does appear to be some element of tolerance, necessitating upward titration of the dose over time. Although octreotide does in fact produce analgesia, many factors currently make this agent impractical for widespread clinical use. First, the commercially available preservative-free preparation comes at a concentration of 500 µg/mL, necessitating frequent refills. Additionally, in order to avoid damaging the infusion device, the pH must be adjusted. Perhaps the most important factor is the extreme cost—in excess of $20,000 per year—which makes this agent unsuitable. Notwithstanding the limitations of octreotide, these results should prompt further investigation into the development of other somatostatin analogues that might be equally effective but more practical for clinical development.

Tricyclic Antidepressants

Tricyclic antidepressants (TCAs) have long been known to participate in the modulation of pain transmission. The analgesic effects of TCAs are believed to be mediated through effects on monoaminergic and serotonergic pathways in the CNS, specifically, prevention of reuptake of these transmitters. In vitro testing has also shown that the TCAs bind with the NMDA receptor complex, possibly meaning that the antiallodynic and hyperalgesic effects of the TCAs are mediated via an NMDA receptor mechanism.[64] The effect of IT TCAs on pain behavior has been studied in several animal models. Presently, IT administration of TCAs in humans is not possible due to the lack of preclinical toxicity data, the observed development of motor impairment at high doses in rat experiments, and the unavailability of preservative-free preparations. However, the profound reduction in hyperalgesia and the synergistic effect with opiates provide ample reason to pursue and develop this class of agents as an effective mode of pain control.

Acetylcholinesterase Inhibitors

Acetylcholine (ACH) is a ubiquitous neurotransmitter in all parts of both the central and peripheral nervous systems. Choline acetyltransferase, the rate-limiting enzyme in the synthesis of ACH, is abundant in nerve terminals within the dorsal horn of the spinal cord. Moreover, the presence of acetylcholinesterase in certain descending raphe-spinal projections implies that ACH may be implicated in the modulation of nociception. ACH diminishes the response of dorsal horn interneurons to excitatory amino acids. Some neurons are depolarized by cholinergic substances, whereas others become hyperpolarized. IT administration of both muscarinic and nicotinic agents has indicated that analgesic effects are mediated only through muscarinic receptors. Animal studies have shown that spinal neostigmine produces analgesia (albeit transiently) and also enhances the analgesia provided by IT clonidine, but with fewer side effects.

Based on animal data, human applications of the use of IT neostigmine have been performed. Hood et al. studied the effects of IT neostigmine in 28 healthy volunteers.[65] Although IT administration of neostigmine was antinociceptive to a noxious cold stimulus, significant side effects occurred, including nausea, vomiting, reversible lower extremity weakness, and, at larger doses, tachycardia and hypertension. Although neostigmine alone is probably not suitable based on the side-effect profile, further studies may be warranted using this agent in patients who have become tolerant to opiates.

Adenosine

Although the results have been conflicting, some studies have demonstrated that adenosine, an endogenous nucleoside, and its analogues may participate in pain modulation. Belfrage et al. performed an open-label trial to determine the safety and efficacy of IT adenosine in 14 patients with neuropathic pain accompanied by tactile hyperalgesia or allodynia.[66] Patients were given IT injections of either 500 or 1000 µg of adenosine (n = 9), and areas of tactile pain were mapped. Spontaneous and evoked pain were assessed (VAS scale of 0 to 100) before and 1 hour after injection. Median VAS scores for spontaneous and evoked pain were reduced from 65 to 24 ($p < 0.01$) and 71 to 12 ($p < 0.01$), respectively. Parallel increases in tactile pain thresholds in areas of allodynia were also observed. The median reduction in the area of tactile hyperalgesia/allodynia was 90% ($p < 0.001$). Twelve of the fourteen patients experienced pain relief for a median of 24 hours. The only noted side effect was transient lumbar pain at the site of injection.

Nitric Oxide

Nitric oxide (NO) is synthesized from L-arginine by activation of NO synthase. Because NO easily penetrates cell membranes, it has been identified as a substance that may potentially act like a neurotransmitter. Because synthesis of NO is induced through an NMDA receptor mechanism, and because NMDA receptors have been implicated in the wind-up phenomenon, NO may in fact participate in the development of this pathologic state. There is evidence of increased synthesis of NO in the dorsal root ganglion animal models of neuropathic pain. Yaksh and Malmberg have injected arginine analogues that functionally inhibit NO synthesis intrathecally and found that they induce a dose-dependent reduction in the formation of the hyperalgesic state. Although there are currently no human trials to evaluate the role of NO synthesis inhibitors, this may represent fertile ground for future research.[67]

Prostaglandin Inhibitors

Prostaglandins (PGs) are another well known group of substances that participate as neurotransmitters. PGs are synthesized at the spinal cord level in the identical way to that which occurs systemically. Activation of the NMDA receptor and subsequent calcium influx are thought to lead to activation of phospholipase A_2, and ultimately to the formation of cyclooxygenase products. PGs increase calcium conductance in dorsal root ganglion cells, thereby increasing the release of SP and other peptides. Potentially, inhibition of IT PG formation might result in a reduction in neurotransmitters such as SP, thereby decreasing nociception. The effects of nonsteroidal antiinflammatory agents are mediated through inhibition of PG synthesis. In fact, recent attention has been directed toward evaluating the analgesic effects of IT nonsteroidal agents. Malmberg and Yaksh have studied the effects of IT ketorolac on nociception.[68] IT ketorolac was found to inhibit the development of hyperalgesia in a rat model of neuropathic pain, but it had minimal affect on the acute phase of pain. When administered concomitantly with morphine, ketorolac produced a synergistic analgesic effect on both the fast and slow components of pain. Further research is obviously needed to define the exact role of the various PG substances as they relate to pain transmission, as well as to study the potential for spinal toxicity.

Calcitonin Gene-Related Peptide Antagonists

Calcitonin gene-related peptide (CGRP) is another neuropeptide found in dorsal root ganglion cells, A-delta and C fibers, Lissauer's tract, and the terminals of primary afferents in laminae I, II, and V of the dorsal horn.[64] There are two types of CGRP, and perhaps as many as four receptor subtypes. A noxious thermal stimulus has been shown to result in increased levels of CGRP in lamina II or the substantia gelatinosa. Moreover, some studies have shown that IT administration of CGRP actually increases nociceptive transmission, although the data on this are conflicting. It has been suggested that CGRP may enhance the effects of SP by either inhibition of the enzyme that degrades SP or augmentation of SP release. Yu et al. showed that, although IT administration of CGRP does not produce any apparent effect on pain transmission, IT injection of CGRP 8-37, a known CGRP receptor antagonist, does induce a dose-dependent reduction in nociception.[69] Notwithstanding the work of Yu et al., the conflicting

evidence regarding CGRP indicates that the role of this substance needs to be more clearly defined before human trials of CGRP antagonists can be conducted.

Substance P Antagonists

Substance P belongs to the family of substances known as the tachykinins. It is believed to be involved in the transmission or modulation of nociceptive information. SP is stored in synaptic vesicles in primary afferents located in lamina I and II of the dorsal horn and preferentially binds to the NK-1 receptor. Based on SP's presumed role in pain transmission, studies have focused on whether antagonists of SP may be effective in producing analgesia. Again, data are conflicting regarding the effects of IT SP antagonists. Unfortunately, further studies have been hampered by the fact that these substances are neurotoxic and subject to rapid biodegradation, thus hindering application to human clinical trials.

CLINICAL STRATEGY FOR INTRATHECAL DRUG INFUSION

In order to develop a rational approach to the safe and effective use of IT medications, a panel of experts in the field of spinal drug delivery was initially convened in 2000.[70] This initial Polyanalgesic Consensus Conference provided an algorithm for the use of various agents for IT delivery. There have been two additional consensus panels convened in the past 7 years to update the information published in 2000.[31,33] The most recent update, conducted in 2007, produced a number of new recommendations regarding concentration and dosing of IT agents (Table 99.6) as well as an updated algorithm for implementation of the various agents currently in use (Table 99.7).

Line 1 contains morphine, hydromorphone, and ziconotide, all used as single agents. Morphine remains the only opioid currently approved by the FDA for chronic IT administration. Hydromorphone has been elevated to a Line 1 agent owing to it's increasing IT use and the growing body of preclinical and clinical evidence supporting it's safety and effectiveness. Ziconotide has recently been approved by the FDA and is the only nonopioid analgesic approved for long-term IT use. Both morphine and hydromorphone require close monitoring of dose and concentration

TABLE 99.6

CURRENT SUGGESTED DOSE AND CONCENTRATION LIMITATIONS FOR IT DRUG DELIVERY

Drug	Maximum concentration	Maximum daily dose
Morphine	20 mg/mL	15 mg/day
Hydromorphone	10 mg/mL	4 mg/day
Fentanyl	2 mg (2000 µg)/mL	Unknown
Sufentanil†	50 µg/mL	Unknown
Bupivicaine	40 mg/mL	30 mg/day
Clonidine	2 mg (2000 µg)/mL	1.0 mg (1000 µg)/day
Ziconitide‡	100 µg/mL	19.2 µg/day

†Sufentanil is not available for compounding
‡Maximum daily dose based on recommendations of Elan
(Adapted from Deer T, Krames EJ, Hassenbusch SJ, et al. Polyanlgesic Consensus Conference 2007: Recommendations for the Management of Pain by Intrathecal (Intraspinal) Drug Delivery: Report of an Interdisciplinary Expert Panel. *Neuromodulation* 2007;10:300–328.)

TABLE 99.7

2007 POLYANALGESIC CONSENSUS PANEL INTRATHECAL TREATMENT ALGORITHM

Line no.1	Morphine	Hydromorphone	Ziconitide
Line no.2	Fentanyl plus Ziconitide	Morphine/Hydromorphone plus Bupivicaine/Clonidine	Morphine/Hydromorphone
Line no.3	Clonidine plus Ziconitide	Morphine/Hydromorphone/Fentanyl	Bupivicaine and/or Clonidine
Line no.4	Sufentanil	Sufentanil plus Bupivicaine and/or Clonidine Plus Ziconitide	
Line no.5	Ropivicaine, Buprenorphine, Midazolam, Merperidine, Ketorolac		
Line no.6	EXPERIMENTAL AGENTS	Gabapentin, Octerotide, Conopeptide, Neostigmine, Adenosine	

(Adapted from Deer T, Krames EJ, Hassenbusch SJ, et al. Polyanlgesic Consensus Conference 2007: Recommendations for the Management of Pain by Intrathecal (Intraspinal) Drug Delivery: Report of an Interdisciplinary Expert Panel. *Neuromodulation* 2007;10:300–328.)

due to the potential of formation of a catheter tip inflammatory mass. Ziconotide has a limited use due to the relatively narrow therapeutic window associated with this medication.

Line 2 includes fentanyl which has been suggested as an alternative for patients who develop intractable supraspinal side effects to any of the Line 1 agents. It is believed that fentanyl far less likely than other opioids to result in granuloma formation so this is a reasonable alternative for patients with increased risk for this problem. Line 2 also begins to explore the use of polyanalgesic therapy when a single agent fails to provide adequate analgesia. Morphine or hydromorphone may be combined with either bupivacaine, clonidine, or ziconotide. It had previously been thought that clonidine when co-administered with opioids may provide some protective effect regarding granuloma formation; however, there have now been several reports of granuloma formation in patients receiving clonidine.

If a combination of medications on Line 2 fails to provide adequate relief, Line 3 suggests the possibility of clonidine alone or the use of opioids combined with bupivacaine and clonidine and possibly even ziconotide. This approach obviously becomes more complicated in terms of management. If Line 3 approaches are unsuccessful, one can consider switching to sufentanil, the primary Line 4 drug. Sufentanil has been safely used in humans and is thought to have granuloma-sparing effects. In Lines 2, 3, and 4, the addition of agents such as bupivacaine, clonidine, and ziconotide, may prove most beneficial for patients with pure neuropathic or mixed nociceptive/neuropathic pain. The agents listed in Line 5 of the algorithm were not considered experimental by the panel, but there is little information regarding their use in the literature. Because of the paucity of safety and efficacy data, they should only be used by highly experienced implanters and only with complete informed consent. Finally, the agents listed on Line 6 are still considered experimental and should only be used by experienced implanters with on a treatment protocol that has been approved by the local Institutional Review Board.

COMPLICATIONS OF SPINAL DRUG DELIVERY

A thorough understanding of the potential complications that might occur during the course of spinal drug infusion is essential for any clinician involved in the implantation and/or management of spinal drug delivery systems. Unfortunately complications are inevitable, even for the most seasoned clinicians. While complications are bound to occasionally occur, it is critical that they are recognized and dealt with in a timely fashion. To that end, it is imperative that anyone involved with this therapy have a fundamental knowledge of the neuroanatomy, physiology, and phar-

macological effects as these factors relate to spinal drug delivery. Complications associated with ITDD can be generally divided into surgical complications related to the implant procedure, device-related complications, and pharmacological complications (Table 99.8).[71]

Surgical Complications

Wound Hematoma/Seroma and Epidural Hematoma

Bleeding is obviously a risk of any surgical procedure. Bleeding can occur either intraoperatively or postoperative, can be superfi-

TABLE 99.8

COMPLICATIONS OF INTRATHECAL DRUG DELIVERY

Surgical Complications
- Wound hematoma or seroma
- Intraspinal hematoma
- Wound infection
- Meningitis
- Epidural abscess
- Postdural puncture headache
- Persistent cerebrospinal fluid leak
- Malposition of subcutaneous pump pocket
- Neurological injury

Device-Related Complications
- Catheter-related problems
  - Migration
  - Fracture
  - Occlusion
- Mechanical pump failure

Pharmacological Complications
- Drug-related side effects
- Tolerance
- Withdrawal and abstinence syndromes
- Opioid-induced hyperalgesia
- Inflammatory catheter tip mass (granuloma)

Complications Associated with Pump Refill
- Contamination of pump reservoir
- Accidental subcutaneous administration
- Accidental intrathecal bolus during intended refill

cial or deep, and can be related to either mechanical (surgical) or systemic factors. Fortunately, severe bleeding is rarely a problem with implantation of ITDDs. The strategy for management of bleeding problems due to systemic factors such as coagulopathies, medications, etc., is obviously prevention. Prior to proceeding with insertion of a catheter for screening or implantation of the pump system, all patients should be screened for risk factors that could cause intraoperative or postoperative bleeding. A careful medical history including family history of bleeding problems is usually the most accurate method of screening for coagulation disorders. Laboratory studies such as prothrombin and partial thromboplastin times, platelet function assays, etc., may be ordered although these studies can sometimes be normal even in the presence of a coagulopathic state, further emphasizing the importance of a thorough clinical history. If the patient is being treated with anticoagulant medications such as aspirin, clopidogrel, or Coumadin, these agents must be stopped for a sufficient period of time prior to the procedure, usually 7 to 10 days. It is important to check with the patient's primary physician or specialist to ascertain that it is indeed safe to discontinue these medications.

Intraoperative bleeding is rare since these procedures do not usually require extensive surgery, and the anatomical areas that are involved are not particularly vascular. Most of the bleeding problems associated with ITDDs involve the subcutaneous tissues, particularly the pump pocket. Failure to obtain meticulous hemostasis in the subcutaneous tissues can lead to complications such as wound hematoma/seroma and/or infection. Infiltration of the surgical sites with local anesthetic containing 1:200,000 epinephrine can be helpful in reducing superficial bleeding. The judicious use of electrocautery for the majority of the dissection will also minimize bleeding. A word of caution: extensive use of electrocautery in one location can destroy and devitalize tissue making it a perfect nidus for infection. Also, electrocautery should be avoided on the skin edges as this can lead to poor wound healing and subsequent wound breakdown and/or infection.

Clinically significant intraspinal bleeding related to needle or catheter insertion is rare. The risk of intraspinal bleeding can be minimized by keeping the number of needle passes to a minimum. Tumors can occasionally be a source of bleeding so extra caution should be exercised when implanting a pump in a patient with spinal metastases. Significant bleeding from the needle may be managed by gentle irrigation through the needle which will usually be sufficient. A small amount of epidural bleeding will not be clinically significant. However, accumulation of sufficient blood in the epidural space can lead to the development of a clinically significant epidural hematoma. This is usually heralded in the immediate postoperative period by severe escalating back pain and the onset of neurological dysfunction. An epidural hematoma sufficiently large to produce neurological dysfunction is a neurosurgical emergency. Consequently, any patient who develops neurological symptoms or signs in the immediate postoperative period should undergo an immediate imaging study (CT or MRI) of the spine and neurosurgical consultation should be obtained.

Wound hematoma and/or seroma occur more commonly than clinically significant epidural bleeding. This complication is usually due to inadequate hemostasis. A wound hematoma is usually manifest by local pain, pressure, and swelling over the surgical wound and may or may not be accompanied the serous or serosanguineous drainage. Most wound hematomas or seromas can be managed conservatively and will resolve spontaneously. However, in the event of a large collection, either surgical evacuation or percutaneous aspiration may be indicated. In the event of a wound hematoma or seroma, early pump refills should be limited since puncture of the skin may increase the risk of infection. Also, a large hematoma overlying the pump will make accessing the refill port more difficult and increase the chances of accidental subcutaneous injection of the medication.

Infectious Complications

The incidence of infection following implantation of an ITDD is relatively low since one is dealing with a clean (Class I) surgical wound. Indeed, the presence of an active systemic infection or localized soft tissue infection near the site of implantation should be a contraindication for implantation until the problem has been resolved. Most wound infections present relatively early (within 1–4 weeks) after pump implantation. The usual presentation includes pain, swelling, erythema, tenderness over the surgical incision, sometimes accompanied by purulent drainage. Although fever may be present, absence of fever should not produce any false sense of security. In the absence of systemic symptoms and/or signs of infection, some authorities have advocated a period of conservative management for several weeks including percutaneous aspiration, intravenous antibiotics, and, in some cases, instillation of antibiotics directly into the pump pocket. Although there are likely anecdotal reports of success with this strategy, the author's observations are that this almost never works and only delay the inevitable. In the author's opinion, if an infection of the pump pocket occurs, the device (including the catheter) should be removed. Occasionally, if there is absolutely no evidence of extension of the infection toward the lumbar catheter insertion site, it is sometimes possible to leave the intrathecal catheter in situ and occlude it just above the fascial insertion site such that once the infection is resolved the catheter can be revised and a new pump implanted in a site remote from the previous infection. Notwithstanding this exception, the safest and most conservative approach is to remove the entire system and start from scratch once the infection has resolved. In circumstances where the device requires removal, the clinician must have a strategy for reinstitution of systemic analgesics in order to prevent the development of withdrawal syndrome.

Meningitis is another infectious complication that, although rare, can occur following pump implantation. The clinical presentation of bacterial meningitis includes fever, chills, intractable headache, malaise, nausea/vomiting, neck/back pain, and nuchal rigidity. Most patients who develop meningitis look ill and progression of the condition can be extremely rapid. The key to treatment is early recognition of the clinical signs. If meningitis is suspected, a lumbar puncture should be performed to obtain CSF and broad spectrum antibiotics should be instituted. What to do with the device is somewhat less clear. Again, the most conservative approach is to remove the hardware. If there is absolutely no indication of infection of the surgical site and the infection appear limited to the CSF, it may be reasonable to remove the IT catheter and leave the pump in situ in which case the pump should be emptied of active drug and filled with preservative-free saline and set to run at the minimum flow rate. However, the pump can not simply be stopped and then restarted after the infection is cleared.

Epidural abscess is rare following implantation of a pump although there are numerous case reports of epidural abscess following insertion of epidural catheters. The clinical presentation of epidural abscess is similar to that of an epidural hematoma although the onset is generally more delayed and the progression of symptoms may be slower. Early diagnosis requires a high degree of suspicion and any patient who develops neurological signs or symptoms should undergo an imaging study to exclude this problem. If an epidural abscess is confirmed and the patient demonstrates signs of neurological dysfunction, neurosurgical consultation should be obtained immediately and consideration given toward surgical decompression. Although epidural abscess has traditionally been considered a neurosurgical emergency, there are increasing reports of nonoperative management of this condition. If the patient has no sign of neurological dysfunction, it may be possible to manage the problem with antibiotics combined with close clinical observation. This approach is probably most applicable to abscesses that occur in the lumbar region since the cauda equina is more resistant to compression than the spinal cord itself. Again, the most conservative approach regarding the implant is removal. Most postoperative epidural abscesses are due to *Staphylococcus aureus* and should be treated with at least 6 weeks of intravenous antibiotics.

Cerebrospinal Fluid Leak and Postdural Puncture Headache

Insertion of the IT catheter requires performing a lumbar puncture with no.15 gauge Tuohy needle. Therefore, CSF leak and postdural puncture headache (PDPH) are definite risks associated with pump implantation. This problem may occur as a result of multiple dural punctures or as a result of CSF that can leak around the catheter where it enters the dura. Some implanters try to minimize this risk by placing a purse string suture around the catheter below the fascial insertion site. If this technique is employed, one must be careful not to make the suture so tight that it occludes the catheter.

PDPH is classically described as a severe postural headache that occurs when the patient goes from the supine to upright position, although there are clearly patients who lack a significant postural component. The diagnosis is usually fairly straightforward. Initial management includes bedrest, fluids, and the use of an abdominal binder. Medications such as IV caffeine (500 mg in 1000 cc normal saline given over 1 hour) and ACTH (1.5 µg/kg in 1 liter of normal saline given over 1 hour) are sometime effective. If conservative measures fail to eliminate the problem, an epidural blood patch is indicated. This should be done using strictly aseptic conditions and fluoroscopic guidance in order to avoid damage to the IT catheter. If the leak persists after all of these measures, surgical exploration to seal the leak may be required.

Occasionally, patients will present with a CSF hygroma beneath the lumbar incision. In most cases, this will resolve spontaneously given time and patience. It is usually not necessary and generally not recommended that these collections be aspirated owing to possible introduction of infection or damage to the catheter. If the collection is large and/or the patient is symptomatic, then surgical exploration to close the leak around the catheter is required.

Neurological Injury

Neurological injury following pump implantation is most commonly associated with the development of an epidural hematoma or abscess. Although uncommon, direct neurological injury can also occur from insertion of the needle or IT catheter. Direct neurological injury should almost always be preventable providing one adheres to certain principles. First, prior to surgery, all patients should have an imaging study of the spine, preferably an MRI to ensure that the spinal canal is patent and that the catheter can be inserted safely. This is especially important in patients with cancer and spinal metastases to make certain that the tumor will not interfere with passage of the catheter. Also, an imaging study will exclude the presence of problems such as a low-lying or tethered cord. Secondly, the needle should be inserted in the lower to mid-lumbar region in order to avoid direct injury to the conus, which usually terminates around T12 or L1. The position of the conus can be seen on the MRI and therefore avoided. Once the needle has been inserted and free flow of CSF confirmed, the catheter should be inserted and positioned using fluoroscopy. The catheter should be gently advanced; under no circumstance should the catheter be forced if undue resistance is met. If this occurs, the entire catheter and needle assembly should be removed and the process repeated. The position of the catheter tip should be confirmed with fluoroscopy. Ideally, the catheter tip should be positioned in the upper portion of the lumbar cistern. By keeping the catheter caudal to the conus and spinal cord, this will minimize the risk of cord compression due to IT granu-

loma. If the catheter goes retrograde, it should also be removed and repositioned. If the catheter remains low in the lumbar region, it can potentially "knot" and damage the nerve roots of the cauda equina in the event it needs to be removed. It is not uncommon for the catheter to cause transient nerve root irritation that is usually manifest by radicular pain. This is usually self-limited and resolves over several days to weeks. However, in the event it persists, it may become necessary to remove the catheter.

Device-Related Complications

Catheter Problems

Complications related to the catheter system represent a considerable source of morbidity in patients with ITDDs. Catheter-related problems include fracture, migration, kinking, occlusion, and dislodgement. In three separate clinical trials conducted by Medtronic, catheter-related complications were reported in 20% to 25% of patients who received an implant. This included both one- and two-piece catheters. During a 1- to 2-year follow-up period, approximately 80% of the catheters remained complication-free. Correction of a catheter complication not only requires additional surgery, but also results in interruption of therapy and production of a potential withdrawal syndrome. Given that approximately 20,000 new implants are performed annually with a catheter complication rate of 25%, that means that 5,000 catheter revisions are required yearly. With an average cost of revision around $10,000, the annual revision cost is about $50,000,000.

A catheter problem is usually manifest by loss of analgesia in which case it will be necessary to troubleshoot the system to diagnose the specific problem. A sequential systematic approach will usually identify the problem. Following is the author's protocol for evaluating a potential catheter or pump-related problem. First, proper function of the pump itself can generally be confirmed through telemetry. We routinely interrogate the device and ensure that the expected information is accurate. The accuracy of the pump prescription is checked and new medication with the appropriate concentration is instilled. The residual drug volume is checked against that predicted by the telemetry and these volumes should agree. Plain radiographs that include the entire catheter and pump system are obtained to exclude disconnection of the catheter from the pump as well as fracture, migration, or kinking of the catheter. Although most catheter fractures can be seen with plain radiographs, some are subtle and can not be detected with plain x-rays. If a physical problem with the catheter is identified, the patient is scheduled for catheter revision as soon as possible. If the integrity of the system appears intact and the pump appears to be functioning properly, an MRI is obtained to exclude the presence of a catheter granuloma. If this evaluation fails to reveal the source of the problem, then a dye study is performed to further evaluate the catheter. The catheter access port (CAP, Fig 99.2) is accessed using either a no.24 or no.25 gauge needle provided in the CAP kit. Prior to injecting anything being injected, the catheter should be aspirated to confirm CSF flow and several milliliters of CSF should be removed. The removed CSF can be analyzed for drug levels, although this usually takes several weeks to obtain results. If CSF can not be removed, nothing should be injected as this could potentially push drug within the catheter directly into the CSF resulting in a drug overdose. Assuming one can easily aspirate CSF, a small amount of dye is slowly injected and observed under fluoroscopy. If the catheter is patent and there is no obstruction at the tip, dye should be observed to flow from the catheter and then dissipate quickly in the subarachnoid space. It is also possible to study the catheter by placing a radioisotope such as Indium in the drug reservoir and imaging the system over a period of 2 to 3 days which is the time that it usually takes for the tracer to appear in the CSF depending on the flow rate of the pump.

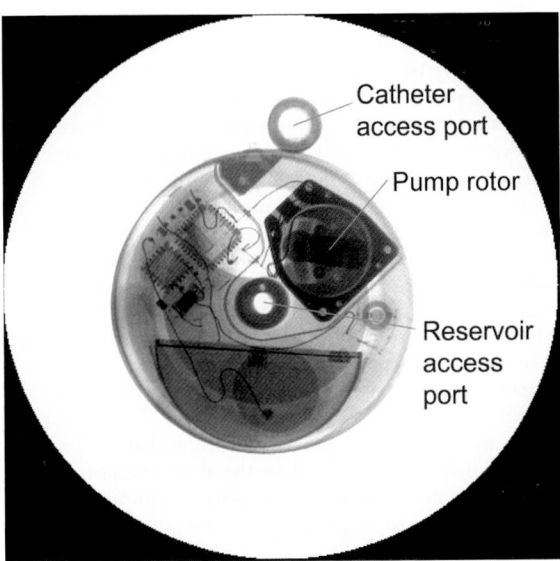

FIGURE 99.2 Plain radiograph of the Medtronic SynchroMed programmable intrathecal drug delivery pump. (Used with permission from the manufacturer. The pump shown is the most common pump in use worldwide in 2009, the SynchroMed pump manufactured by Medtronic Neurological, Minneapolis, MN.) (Reproduced with permission from Deer TR. Complications associated with intrathecal drug delivery systems. In: Neal JM, Rathmell JP, eds. *Complications in Regional Anesthesia and Pain Medicine*. Philadelphia: Saunders Elsevier; 2007:229, Figure 23-2.)

Refill Complications

Complications related to refilling a drug delivery device include inadvertent subcutaneous administration, accidental IT injection, and pump programming errors. All of these complications are avoidable by adhering to a strict protocol for pump refills. The danger during initiation of ITDD and refilling of the reservoir is apparent from a recent postmarketing study carried out by Medtronic. They reported that mortality after initiation of ITDD or device interventions (reprogramming, refilling of the drug reservoir) occurred as a result of multiple factors, including excessive intrathecal morphine dosing during initiation of ITDD, lack of close supervision of concomitant opioid or respiratory depressant drug intake, and early hospital discharge preventing monitoring for respiratory depression early after initiation of ITDD.[72] Before refilling any drug delivery device, one should check to ensure that the drug prescription matches that currently in the pump. Refills should be performed sterilely to avoid contamination of the drug reservoir. Refills should only be performed with the appropriate needles that are provided in the pump refill kit. The drug reservoir is accessed with no.22 gauge Huber needle and the catheter access port with a no.24 or no.25 gauge needle, depending on the model of the pump. The needle intended for entering the CAP should *never* be utilized for accessing the drug reservoir. In this instance, if the smaller needle is accidentally inserted into the CAP, the entire volume of medication will be directly injected into the IT space. The CAP bypasses the drug reservoir and pump and can not be accessed with a no.22 gauge needle. If there is any question that the needle is in the appropriate port, it is prudent to confirm this with fluoroscopy. The provider performing the refill should confirm that the residual volume of the reservoir matches that predicted by telemetry. Once the refill has been completed and the pump reprogrammed, the pump prescription should again be double checked for accuracy.

Inadvertent injection into the subcutaneous tissues around the pump as well as injection through the CAP directly into the IT space have both been reported. This can obviously lead to significant problems such as respiratory depression. Moreover, respira-

tory depression is likely to be delayed in onset and occur long after the patient has left the office. If subcutaneous injection occurs, treatment with an opioid antagonist may be warranted. This should be done under careful observation using small incremental doses to avoid severe complications such as hypertension, cardiac arrhythmias, and pulmonary edema. In the event that direct injection into the CSF does occur and it is recognized, the drug infusion should be stopped and the patient admitted to the hospital for observation and closely monitored for any signs of respiratory or hemodynamic problems. Again, judicious use of opioid antagonists as described is warranted. It is also possible to remove some of the drug through a high volume lumbar puncture although this will not remove all of the drug. If the patient develops signs of respiratory compromise in spite of these measures, the guiding principle should be "airway, breathing, and circulation" and there should be no hesitation in proceeding with endotracheal intubation of the patient and providing mechanical ventilatory support until the drug effects have dissipated.

Pharmacological Complications and Drug-Related Side Effects

Side Effects of Intrathecal Opioids

It is commonly believed that switching from systemic to IT delivery of opioids alleviates all of the clinically significant side effects. This is clearly a misconception, as IT opioid infusion is commonly associated with side effects. Often, these side effects are mild and well-tolerated and do not interfere with therapy. Indeed, just as patients develop tolerance to the analgesic effects of the drug (see later), they also tend to develop tolerance to the side effects. On the other hand, some patients develop side effects that may be so bothersome as to have a significant impact on the treatment. The most common side effects experienced by patients receiving ITDD include respiratory depression, gastrointestinal symptoms, urinary dysfunction, hormonal alterations, and itching.

Aside from true anaphylaxis, which is extremely rare with the use of opioids, respiratory depression is the most clinically concerning drug-related side effect. Respiratory depression results from the supraspinal interaction of the drug with mu-2 opioid receptors in the brainstem. It can occur from rostral spread of the drug and is probably more common when using hydrophilic agents which can attain significant concentrations in the cisternal CSF. It can also occur with systemic absorption into the blood and redistribution to the CNS. It is most likely to occur in patients who are opioids naïve. In fact there are relatively few reports of clinically significant respiratory depression in patients who have been exposed to opioids for even relatively short periods of time. It is also quite uncommon in patients being treated for cancer pain. Besides lack of prior exposure to opioids, additional risk factors for respiratory depression include advanced age, absence of severe pain, debilitated physical condition, preexisting pulmonary disease, sleep apnea, and, of course, additional opioids dosing by alternative routes. Respiratory depression can occur as early as 4 hours following IT dosing although it is often delayed in onset up to 24 hours. Treatment consists of support of respiration and the judicious use of a mu-receptor antagonist such as naloxone or kappa-agonist–mu-anatagonist such as nalbuphine using appropriate precautions as outlined previously in this chapter.[71]

Urinary retention is another common side effect of IT opioids, reported in 20% to 40% of patients. It is a direct spinal side effect that is caused by reduction in detrusor muscle tone and detrusor-urethral sphincter dyssynergia. It does occur with the intraventricular administration of morphine. It is believed to be mediated primarily through mu- and delta-receptors. It is more common in males and rare in women and individuals who are opioid tolerant. It is often self-limited and usually resolves within

24 to 48 hours. Treatment entails intermittent bladder catheterization until the problem resolves. One can also consider adjunct pharmacological treatment with opioids antagonists and/or phenoxybenzamine. If the problem persists, an alternative strategy involves switching to another opioid.[71]

Gastrointestinal side effects such as nausea, vomiting, and constipation are less common than with systemic delivery. However, they still occur in up to 25% to 30% of patients, especially those who are opioid naïve. Nausea and vomiting are mediated by the interaction of opioids with the chemoreceptor trigger zone. Treatment is usually symptomatic with antiemetic agents.

Pruritus occurs in about 25% of patients exposed to IT opioids and is perhaps even more common in opioid-naïve individuals. It is more common with morphine than other opioids and is believed to result from degranulation of mast cells. The problem is usually self-limited and can be managed with antihistamines albeit with mixed results. In the case of severe persistent itching, the best approach is to probably switch to an alternative opioid such as hydromorphone or fentanyl. It is important to differentiate opioid-induced pruritus from true allergy. Most patients and many clinicians not familiar with the actions of IT opioids will misconstrue itching as an allergic reaction. In fact, true allergic reactions to morphine or its congeners is very rare.[71]

Finally, there is compelling evidence that opioids can have a negative effect on neuroendocrine function.[73] Morphine has been shown to inhibit the release of gonadotropin- and corticotrophin-releasing hormones from the hypothalamus, resulting in reduced circulating levels of luteinizing hormone (LH), follicle-stimulating hormone (FSH), ACTH, and beta-endorphin. The end result is reduction in serum levels of cortisol and testosterone. Clinically, the end effect is reduction in libido and/or impotency. In men, reductions in testosterone can also result in decreased muscle mass and increased fat mass. In addition to the effects just noted, IT morphine administration can also produce significant fluid retention, possibly due to alterations in antidiuretic hormone function.

Opioid Tolerance

Tolerance can be defined as the requirement for progressively escalating doses of medication in order to achieve the same degree of clinical effect. In pharmacological terms, tolerance represents a pharmacodynamic effect manifested by a rightward shift in the dose-response curve. Two mechanisms for opioid tolerance have been proposed: desensitization (i.e., decreased activation) of opioid receptors following prolonged exposure to opioids, and opioid receptor down regulation.[74] Desensitization involves changes in opioid receptor physiology that are believed to result from alterations in G-protein receptor function. This change apparently results in an uncoupling of G-protein from the opioid or possibly a switch in coupling such that the receptor couples with a nonanalgesic G-protein. In any event, the end result is decrease in analgesia. Down regulation, the second mechanism believed to produce opioid tolerance occurs when opioid receptors are internalized from the cell membrane by endocytosis, due to substances termed arrestins.

Although tolerance is used mostly in terms of loss of analgesia, it should be noted that tolerance also occurs to other effects of a given drug. Tolerance is believed to be an important causal factor in the loss or complete failure of analgesia in patients with implanted drug delivery systems, particularly those patients primarily receiving opioid medications. Tolerance usually develops over the course of time, and the rate at which tolerance develops may vary between individuals. Moreover, tolerance does not usually develop equally to all effects of a given drug at the same rate. Before concluding that loss of analgesia is indeed related to tolerance, it is important for the clinician to exclude other reasons such as problems with the delivery system or progression of disease.

Management of tolerance depends to large degree on the baseline treatment protocol for a given patient.[71] In some cases, simple dose titration by 10% to 30% per day will overcome the problem. If indeed the problem is simply a tolerance issue, then increasing the dose should result in demonstrably improved pain control, at least for some period of time. Depending on the delivery system, dose escalation will be limited by the volume that can be safely infused. The maximum infusion rate generally recommended for an epidural infusion is around 10 to 15 mL/hour; for IT infusion, the rate should not exceed more than 10% of the patient's calculated CSF volume (typically 75 mL total, limiting the daily infusion to 7.5 mL/day). These limitations can sometimes make restoration of analgesia impossible by dose titration alone unless the infusion prescription can be prepared in a higher concentration, although there are also limits to this as well (Table 99.6).

It has been suggested that continuous drug delivery is less likely or will less rapidly lead to the development of tolerance although there are no studies that clearly demonstrate this to be the case. Switching to a more potent opioid may result in a slower development of tolerance by reducing the rate of receptor down regulation. One can also consider switching to a different opioid assuming there is incomplete cross tolerance between the two drugs. Another strategy is to add other agents such as clonidine that act through alternative spinal modulating systems and therefore might have some opiate-sparing effects. Finally, it has been suggested that a local anesthetic agent be substituted for the opioid to provide an opioid-free interval.

Opioid-Induced Hyperalgesia

Opioid-induced hyperalgesia is a condition that is manifest by a dramatically augmented sensitivity to stimuli that would be considered noxious and/or allodynia, defined as a pain that is produced by a normally nonnoxious stimulus. This phenomenon has been increasingly recognized in patients who have been treated with long-term opioid therapy and is yet another potential cause loss of analgesia with IT drug infusion. Opioid-induced hyperalgesia is not simply an escalation of the patient's original pain condition. Rather, the "abnormal" pain often originates from an area that is anatomically distinct from the original pain. In some patients, pain seems to increase and become more diffuse over time despite escalation in their opioid regimen. It has recently been shown that opioid-induced hyperalgesia may also develop in the context of short-term therapy in the absence of physical dependence or withdrawal.[74] Several mechanisms have been proposed for this phenomenon: glutamate activation of NMDA receptors as well as increases in excitatory peptide neurotransmitters such as cholecystokinin (CCK).[74]

Intrathecal Inflammatory Masses (Intrathecal Granuloma)

Inflammatory mass associated with the tip of an IT catheter is a potentially serious complication that, if not promptly recognized and managed, can result in spinal cord damage and irreversible neurological dysfunction. IT granuloma was first reported in 1991 and, over the course of time, additional case reports and small case series appeared in the literature. By 2000, 41 cases had been reported. Due to the growing concern regarding this problem, a consensus panel met and subsequently published recommendations on the management of catheter tip inflammatory masses. A similar consensus panel was reconvened in 2007 and the recommendations and guidelines of this panel were recently published.[75] The panel reviewed the pertinent literature including preclinical data, information on pathophysiology of inflammatory mass formation, and clinical data, and ultimately developed an algorithm for prevention and treatment.

An inflammatory catheter tip mass typically is comprised of both acute and chronic reactive inflammatory cells derived from

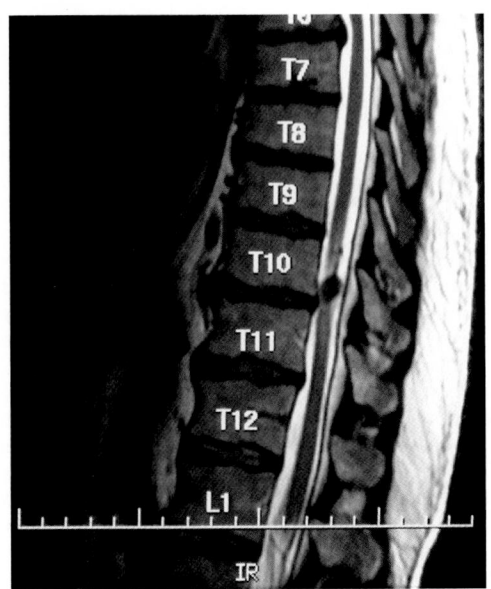
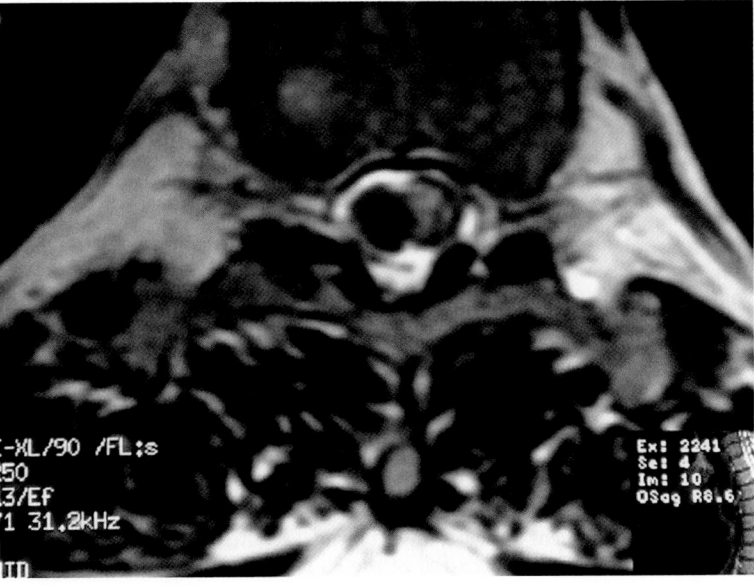

FIGURE 99.3 MRI study of a patient with an inflammatory mass surrounding the tip of an implanted intrathecal drug delivery catheter. **A.** Midline, sagittal, T2-weighted image. The inflammatory mass involves the dorsal aspect of the spinal cord at the level of the inferior end plate of T10. **B.** Axial, T2-weighted image through the inflammatory mass. The mass displaces the spinal cord toward the left. (Reproduced with permission from Deer TR. Complications associated with intrathecal drug delivery systems. In: Neal JM, Rathmell JP, eds. *Complications in Regional Anesthesia and Pain Medicine.* Philadelphia: Saunders Elsevier; 2007:229, Figure 23-1.)

the arachnoid and/or fibrosis that do not directly involve the spinal cord parenchyma. Although these masses represent a build-up of granulation tissue and have been termed "granulomas," they do not fit the classical histopathological description of a true granuloma. An infectious agent has never been associated with these inflammatory masses. There are a number of preclinical studies in both dogs and sheep that demonstrate that catheter-tip inflammatory masses occur predictably in animals receiving IT morphine infusions. Based on preclinical studies, the panel concluded that these masses likely occurred as a result of infusion of high concentrations and/or high daily doses of IT morphine.

Although most of the preclinical evidence implicated the use of morphine, more recent data indicate that other opioid infusions may be associated with inflammatory catheter tip masses. There has also been a more recent report implicating IT baclofen as a potential causative agent.

Although the occurrence of inflammatory masses in humans is less predictable than is animal models which are short-term in duration, it is believed that the incidence in humans increases with the duration of IT therapy, ranging between 0.4% after 2 years of treatment up to 1.16% after 6 years of treatment. Moreover, animal data fails to clarify whether there is even a minimal dose in humans that will not incite granuloma formation. Notwithstanding, these data do support the concept that both concentration and total dose of all opioids, with the exception of fentanyl, are important in the development of inflammatory masses. Based on the available data, the 2007 consensus panel has published recommendations for maximum dosages and concentration of the currently used IT agents (Table 99.6).

The first clinical clue to the development of an inflammatory catheter tip mass in a patient who has otherwise been doing well is often an increase in the patient's pain and the requirement for continuous dose escalation. In such cases, absent an obvious progression of disease, one should begin to consider that diagnosis of an inflammatory mass. Any patient who develops new neurological symptoms should be evaluated with spinal imaging,

preferably MRI. A catheter tip inflammatory mass can usually be detected with MRI (Fig. 99.3).

Management of the patient with an inflammatory catheter tip mass depends on the clinical situation, but is primarily related to the presence or absence of neurological signs and/or symptoms. If a mass is detected and the patient does not have neurological symptoms, it is possible to retract the catheter caudally a few centimeters out of the granuloma and reduce the drug dose and/or concentration. One additional suggestion has been to switch to a "safer" medication such as fentanyl or ziconotide. If symptoms persist despite these changes, the patient should be rapidly weaned off all IT opioids, the medication should be removed from the pump, and the pump filled with saline. One needs to pay close attention to signs of withdrawal, not only from opioids but also from adjuvant medications that may also be in the pump such as clonidine and/or baclofen. If the symptoms resolve after removing the catheter from the mass, the patient should be re-imaged in 6 months to confirm resolution of the granuloma before reinstituting the therapy. If a small granuloma is still evident, one must weight the options of further retraction of the catheter versus removal of the catheter. If neurological signs and symptoms persist or in the event that a granuloma is detected that is producing significant spinal cord compression, then the system should be removed. In patients with a large granuloma compressing the spinal cord and producing neurological dysfunction, consultation with a neurosurgeon should be obtained to determine whether removal of the granuloma itself is warranted.

Drug Withdrawal

Disruption of the IT catheter, pump battery failure, and human error during refill and reprogramming can all lead to sudden cessation of drug delivery and result in drug withdrawal. Of the medications that are currently used for IT delivery, distinct abstinence syndromes are most commonly associated with opioids, baclofen, and clonidine. There are currently no reports of withdrawal associated with the use of IT ziconotide.

The clinical symptoms and signs associated with opioid withdrawal include any or all of the following: increased lacrimation and rhinorrhea, diaphoresis, mydriasis, pilomotor erection, restlessness, irritability or agitation, gastrointestinal symptoms (nausea, vomiting, diarrhea), tremor, abdominal cramping, and, of course, increased pain levels.[71] In severe cases, acute opioid withdrawal can lead to pulmonary edema or cardiovascular collapse resulting in death. The most common causes of opioid withdrawal are catheter disruption and pump refill/programming errors. Because of the risk of opioid withdrawal, antagonist medication must be used with extreme caution in patients undergoing chronic opioid therapy. Treatment should be aimed at respiratory and hemodynamic support with restoration of the drug infusion as soon as possible.

Baclofen withdrawal is a serious complication that, if unrecognized, can be life-threatening. It is usually heralded by increase in spasticity, sometimes to the point of rigidity, pruritus, hyperthermia, drowsiness progressing to obtundation, respiratory depression, rhabdomyolysis, acute renal failure, acute multiorgan failure, and even death.[71] Early recognition is the key to treatment. The treatment of baclofen withdrawal requires urgent attention, the goal being restoration of the IT baclofen infusion as soon as possible. For patients with signs of severe baclofen withdrawal, it is not sufficient to merely provide oral medication until the problem can be fixed. In such cases, it may be prudent to place a temporary lumbar drain and restart the infusion until such time as the problem can be correctly diagnosed and treated. Abrupt cessation of clonidine can also be associated with adverse effects such as rebound hypertension, particularly in patients receiving higher doses. All patients receiving clonidine should be provided a prescription for either oral or transdermal clonidine and advised to contact the implanting physician should they develop any symptoms or signs of clonidine withdrawal.

OUTCOME OF INTRATHECAL DRUG INFUSION

Cancer Pain

Continuous IT infusion of opioids was first used for the management of cancer pain in the early 1980s and, over the next decade, remained the single most common indication for ITDD. During the past several years, it seems the use of IT opioids for cancer pain has possibly diminished, due in large measure to the development of more effective long-acting oral opioids as well as the development of less expensive drug infusion reservoirs. Nevertheless, continuous IT opiate infusion remains one of the most effective and satisfying methods of controlling cancer pain and affording patients maximal independence.

Intrathecal opioids are indicated for the management of cancer pain in two circumstances: (1) in patients whose pain is refractory to reasonable doses of oral opiates, and (2) in patients who are unable to tolerate sufficient doses of oral medications needed to adequately treat their pain due to undesirable systemic side effects, mainly sedation. Although appropriate management of the patient is the paramount goal, the current climate of health care in the United States has dictated an ever increasing recognition of the cost of care. In order to justify the cost of an implanted system, potential candidates for pump implantation should have a life expectancy of at least 3 to 6 months. Cost analysis studies comparing implanted programmable pumps to external infusion systems have shown that for patients requiring treatment more than 3 months, an IDP is the more cost effective device.[76,77]

Continuous infusion of intrathecal opiates has proven to be a highly effective and safe method for controlling cancer pain.[2,4,5,9] Adequate pain control which results in significant reduction in oral narcotic intake and increase in activity can be achieved in the majority of patients. A retrospective multicenter survey regarding intraspinal opiate therapy revealed the average reduction in pain to be just over 60% (n = 382) regardless of etiology.[9] Increase in activity was noted in nearly 82% of patients (n = 399) with 59% realizing moderate to significant increases in activities of daily living (ADL). Just over 95% of patients reported either good (42.9%) or excellent (52.4%) pain relief. There were no significant differences in the level of pain relief reported between patients with cancer and those with nonmalignant pain syndromes. Complications related to the delivery system occurred in 21.6% of patients (n = 380) and were most often related to the catheter. Adverse drug effects were reported in approximately one quarter of the patients. The most common adverse effects were nausea and vomiting (25.2%) and pruritus (13.3%).

Perhaps the best evidence for the use of ITDD in patients with cancer pain comes from the study of Smith et al..[76] The authors performed a randomized controlled trial of ITDD versus conventional medical management (CMM) in a cohort of 202 patients. Entry criteria include inadequately controlled pain of 5 or greater (0–10 VAS scale). Clinical success was defined as either a 20% reduction in baseline VAS score, or equivalent VAS score accompanied by at least a 20% reduction in toxicity following 4 full weeks of treatment. Nearly 85% (60 of 71) of patients randomized to ITDD achieved clinical success compared to 70% (51 of 72) of patients who received CMM ($p = 0.05$). Mean pain scores fell from 7.8 to 3.7 (52%) for the ITDD group compared to 7.8 to 4.8 in the CMM group ($p = 0.055$). Toxicity scores fell 50% for the ITDD group compared with only 17% for the CMM group ($p = 0.004$). Interestingly, the ITDD also showed improved survival, with 54% alive at 6 months compared with 37% in the CMM group.

Intrathecal Drug Delivery for Chronic Noncancer Pain

During the past two decades, there has been an increasing trend toward the use of chronic intrathecal opiates in the management of refractory nonmalignant pain syndromes.[6–12,14–16] Nonmalignant pain related to failed back surgery syndrome is now the most common indication for the use of ITDD. However, in spite of encouraging results in carefully selected patients with noncancer-related pain, the use of intraspinal opiates for nonmalignant pain has remained a controversial issue among clinicians, lay persons, and government regulators. Indeed, much of the fear regarding this issue has been born of the belief that the use of opiates in nonmalignant pain invariably leads to tolerance and drug abuse. However, numerous retrospective and prospective studies suggest that these previously held beliefs are for the most part erroneous. Nonmalignant pain syndromes for which IT opiates have been and might be used are outlined in Table 99.2. The treatment strategy in patients with nonmalignant pain syndromes should obey the principle that the least invasive and least costly interventions should be attempted first, reserving more invasive and expensive therapies for patients who fail the former. Unfortunately, patient selection for IT administered opiates is not as straightforward as in patients with cancer. Although there are ample reports of significant pain reduction using ITDD, translation of pain reduction into functional improvement has been more difficult to achieve.

Winkelmüller et al. reported on 120 patients with nonmalignant pain syndromes managed with long-term intrathecal opiates with an average follow-up of more than 3 years.[11] Nearly three-quarters (74.2%) of the patients derived benefit from the therapy, with a mean pain reduction of 58%. Overall, 92% of patients were satisfied with the treatment and 81% reported an improvement in their quality of life. The incidence of tolerance was low, only 5.8% (seven patients) and was successfully managed in four patients by means of "drug holidays." Anderson et al. investigated the long-term efficacy and safety of intrathecal morphine in 33 patients with non-malignant pain.[12] These investigators noted a significant reduction in pain which persisted up to 2 years. Although the daily intrathecal dose of morphine dose appeared to increase for the initial months of treatment, this tended to stabilize and remain constant after 1 year.

Roberts et al. reported their results of ITDD for noncancer pain in 84 patients who were followed on average for 3 years.[14] Nearly two thirds of their patients suffered from low back and/or radicular pain. Mean pain reduction was around 60% and 74% of patients self-reported increased activity levels as well as significant reduction in oral medication. Unfortunately, these gains were not accompanied by change in work status. Technical complications requiring an additional surgical procedure occurred in 40% of patients. These patients were initially receiving relatively high doses of morphine (9.95 mg/day) and by the end of 6 months, the mean daily dose had escalated to 15.3 mg/day.

Finally, Deer et al. reported the results of ITDD for the treatment of low back pain from the National Outcomes Registry for Low Back Pain.[15] Out of 166 patients enrolled to be trialed for an ITDD system, 136 (82%) received a permanent implant. Scores for back and leg pain scores fell by an average of 47% and 31% respectively at 12 months follow-up for those who received an implant. In additional more than 65% of patients demonstrated reduction in Oswestry scores by at least one level compared with baseline. At 1 year follow-up, 80% of patients indicated they were "satisfied" with the therapy, and 87% said they would undergo the procedure again for the same outcome.

CONCLUSION

IT drug delivery has clearly evolved and progressed since its inception nearly 30 years ago. This technique represents a viable option for patients with intractable pain conditions that can not be adequately managed with other means. Although the surgical procedure for pump implantation is relatively "simple," the management of patients with ITDD systems is far from simple. Indeed, ITDD, particularly for patients with nonmalignant pain conditions, represents an indefinite long-term commitment on the part of both the patient and clinician. Multiple issues tend to develop over the course of treatment including drug-related side effects and system complications that must be addressed. Consequently, this therapy should not be entered into lightly. In spite of the potential problems associated with this therapy, it can be useful and rewarding, so long as one adheres to the principles of judicious patient selection, meticulous surgical technique, and diligent patient management.

References

1. Yaksh T, Rudy TA Analgesia mediated by a direct spinal action of narcotics. *Science* 1976;192:1357–1358.
2. Onofrio BM, Yaksh TL, Arnold PG. Continuous low-dose intrathecal morphine administration in the treatment of chronic pain of malignant origin. *Mayo Clin Proc* 1981;56:516–520.
3. Cousins MJ, Mather LE. Intrathecal and epidural administration of opioids. *Anesthesiology* 1984;61:276–310.
4. Krames ES, Gershow J, Glassberg A, et al. Continuous infusion of spinally administered narcotics for the relief of pain due to malignant disorders. *Cancer* 1985;56:696–702.
5. Onofrio BM, Yaksh TL. Long-term pain relief produced by intrathecal morphine infusion in 53 patients. *J Neurosurg* 1990;72:200–209.
6. Krames ES, Lanning RM. Intrathecal infusion analgesia for nonmalignant pain: analgesic efficacy of intrathecal opioid with or without bupivicaine. J Pain Symptom Manage 1993;8:539–548.
7. Krames ES. Intrathecal infusional therapies for intractable pain: patient management guidelines. *J Pain Symptom Manage* 1993;8:36–46.
8. Krames ES. Intraspinal opioid therapy for chronic nonmalignant pain: current practice and clinical guidelines. *J Pain Symptom Manage* 1996;11:333–352.
9. Paice, JA, Penn RD, Shott S. Intraspinal morphine for chronic pain: a retrospective, multicenter study. *J Pain Symptom Manage* 1996;11:71–80.
10. Tutak U, Doleys DM Intrathecal infusion systems for treatment of chronic low back and leg pain of noncancer origin. *South Med J* 1996;89:295–300.
11. Winkelmüller M, Winkelmüller W. Long-term effects of continuous intrathecal opioid treatment in chronic pain of nonmalignant etiology. *J Neurosurg* 1996;85:458–467.
12. Anderson A, Burchiel KJ. A prospective study of long-term intrathecal morphine in the treatment of nonmalignant pain. *Neurosurgery* 1999;44:289–301.
13. Bennett G, Serafini M, Burchiel K, et al. Evidence-based review of the literature on intrathecal delivery of pain medications. *J Pain Symptom Manage* 2000; 20:S12–S36.
14. Roberts LJ, Finch PM, Goucke, et al. Outcome of intrathecal opioids in chronic non-cancer pain. *Eur J Pain* 2001;5:353–361.
15. Deer T, Chapple I, Classen A, et al. Intrathecal drug delivery for treatment of chronic low back pain: report from the National Outcomes Registry for Low Back Pain. *Pain Med* 2004;5:6–13.
16. Turner JA, Sears JM, Loeser J. Programmable intrathecal opioid delivery systems for chronic non-cancer pain: a systematic review of effectiveness and complications. *Clin J Pain* 2007;23:180–195.
17. Payne R. CSF distribution of opioids in animals and man. *Acta Anesthesiol Scand Suppl* 1987;1:38–46.
18. Kroin JS, Ali A, York M, et al. The distribution of medication along the spinal canal after chronic intrathecal administration. *Neurosurgery* 1993;33:226–230.
19. Hassenbusch SJ, Stanton-Hicks M, Covington E, et al. Long-term intraspinal infusion of opioids in the treatment of neuropathic pain. *J Pain Symptom manage* 1995;10:527–543.
20. Walker SM, Goudas LC, Cousins MJ, et al. Combination spinal analgesic chemotherapy: a systematic review. *Anesth Analg* 2002;95:674–715.
21. Rauck RL, Wallace MS, Leong M, et al. A randomized, double-blind, placebo-controlled study of intrathecal ziconitide in adults with severe chronic pain. *J Pain Symptom Manage* 2006;31:393–406.
22. Wallace MS, Charapata SG, Fisher R, et al. Intrathecal ziconotide in the treatment of chronic nonmalignant pain: a randomized, double-blind, placebo-controlled clinical trial. *Neuromodulation* 2006;9:75–86.
23. Peng PW, Fedoroff I, Jacques L, et al. Survey of the practice of spinal cord stimulators and intrathecal analgesic delivery implants for management of pain in Canada. *Pain Res Manag* 2007;12(4):281–285.
24. Fanciullo GJ, Rose RJ, Lunt PG, et al. The state of implantable pain therapies in the United States: a nationwide survey of academic teaching programs. *Anesth Analg* 1999;88(6):1311–1316.
25. Anderson V, Burchiel K, Cooke B. A Prospective Randomized Trial of Intrathecal Injection vs. Epidural Infusion in the Selection of Patients for Continuous Intrathecal Opioid Therapy. *Neuromodulation* 2003;6:142–152.
26. Johnston J, Reich S, Baily A, et al. Shiley INFUSAID Pump technology. *Ann N Y Acad Sci* 1988;531:57–65.
27. Synchromed Infusion System. Clinical Reference Guide for Pain Therapy. Minneapolis, Minn: Medtronic Neurological; 1998.
28. Follett KA, Burchiel KJ, Deer T, et al. Prevention of intrathecal drug delivery catheter-related complications. *Neuromodulation* 2003;6:32–41.
29. Dougherty PM, Staats PS. Intrathecal drug therapy for chronic pain. From basic science to clinical practice. *Anesthesiology* 1999;91:1891–1918.
30. Nordberg G, Hedner T, Mellstrand T, et al. Pharmacokinetic aspects of intrathecal morphine analgesia. *Anesthesiology* 1984;60:448–454.
31. Deer T, Krames EJ, Hassenbusch SJ, et al. Polyanlgesic Consensus Conference 2007: Recommendations for the Management of Pain by Intrathecal (Intraspinal) Drug Delivery: Report of an Interdisciplinary Expert Panel. *Neuromodulation* 2007;10:300–328.
32. Waara-Wolleat KL, Hildebrand KR, Stewart GR. A review of intrathecal fentanyl and sufentanil for the treatment of chronic pain. *Pain Med* 2006;7:251–259.
33. Hassenbusch SJ, Portnoy RK, Cousins M, et al. Polyanalgesic Consensus Conference 2003: An update on the management of pain by intraspinal drug delivery-report of an expert panel. *J Pain Symptom Management* 2004;27:540–563.
34. Mironer YE, Tollison CD. Methadone in the intrathecal treatment of chronic nonmalignant pain resistant to other neuron-axial agents: the first experience. *Neuromodulation* 2001;4:25–31.
35. Eisenach JC. Three novel spinal analgesics: clonidine, neostigmine, amitriptyline. *Reg Anesth* 1996;21:81–83.
36. Eisenach J, Detweiler D, Hood D. Hemodynamic and analgesic actions of epidurally administered clonidine. *Anesthesiology* 1993;78:277–287.
37. Gordh T, Post C, Olsson Y. Evaluation of the toxicity of subarachnoid clonidine, guanfacine, and a substance P-antagonist on rat spinal cord and nerve roots: light and electron microscopic observations after chronic intrathecal administration. *Anesth Analg* 1986;65:1303–1311.
38. Eisenach JC, Hood DD, Curry R. Intrathecal, but not intravenous clonidine reduces experimental thermal or capsaicin-induced pain and hyperalgesia in normal volunteers. *Anesth Analg* 1998;87:591–596.
39. Filos KS, Goudas LC, Patroni O, et al. Hemodynamic and analgesic profile after intrathecal clonidine in humans. A dose-response study. *Anesthesiology* 1994;81:591–601.
40. Rauck RL, Eisenach JC, Jackson K, et al. Epidural clonidine treatment for refractory reflex sympathetic dystrophy. *Anesthesiology* 1993;179:1163–1169.
41. Leiphart JW, Dills CV, Zikel OM, et al. A comparison of intrathecally administered narcotic and nonnarcotic analgesics for experimental chronic neuropathic pain. *J Neurosurg* 1995;92:595–599.

42. Puke MJC, Zsuzanna W: The differential effects of morphine and the alpha-2 adrenoreceptor agonists clonidine and dexmedetomidine on the prevention and treatment of experimental neuropathic pain. *Anesth Analg* 1993;77:104–109.

43. Sagen J, Wang H, Pappas GD. Adrenal medullary implants in the rat spinal cord reduce nociception in a chronic pain model. *Pain* 1990;42:69–79.

44. Buchser E, Goddard M, Heyd B, et al. Immunoisolated xenogeneic chromaffin cell therapy for chronic pain. Initial clinical experience. *Anesthesiology* 1996;85:1005–1012.

45. Bowersox S, Gadbois T, Singh T, et al. Selective N-type neuronal voltage-sensitive calcium channel blocker, SNX-111, produces spinal antinociception in rat models of acute, persistent, and neuropathic pain. *J Pharmacol Exper Ther* 1996;279:1243–1249.

46. Malmberg A, Yaksh TL. Voltage-sensitive calcium channels in spinal nociceptive processing: blockade of N- and P-type channels inhibits formalin-induced nociception. *J Neurosci* 1994;14:4882–4890.

47. Brose WG, Gutlove DP, Luther RR, et al. Use of intrathecal SNX-111, a novel, N-type, voltage-sensitive, calcium channel blocker, in the management of intractable brachial plexus avulsion. *Clin J Pain* 1997;13:256–259.

48. McGuire D, Bowersox S, Fellman JD, et al. Sympatholysis after neuron-specific, N-type, voltage-sensitive, calcium channel blockade: first demonstration of N-channel function in humans. *J Cadiovasc Pharmacol* 1997;30:400–403.

49. Staats P, Charapata S, Presley R. Chronic, intractable neuropathic pain: marked analgesic efficacy of ziconotide. 4th International Congress of the International Neuromodulation Society. Lucerne: International Neuromodulation Society; 1998

50. Brose W, Pfeifer B, Hassenbusch S. SNX-111 produces analgesia in patients with intractable pain: phase I/II results [abstract]. 11th World Congress of Anesthesiologists. Australia: World Congress of Anesthesiologists; 1996

51. Yang CH, Wong CS, Chang JY, et al. Intrathecal ketamine reduces morphine requirements in patients with terminal cancer pain. *Can J Anesth* 1996;43:379–383.

52. Muir K, Lees K. Clinical experience with excitatory amino acid antagonist drugs. *Stroke* 1995;26:503–513.

53. Hassenbusch S, Satterfield WC, Gradert TL, et al. Preclinical toxicity study of intrathecal administration of the pain-relievers dextrorphan, dextromethorphan, and memantine in the sheep model. *Neuromodulation* 1999;2:230–239.

54. Taira T, Kawamura H, Tanikawa T, et al. A new approach to control central deafferentation pain: spinal intrathecal baclofen. *Stereotact Funct Neurosurg* 1995;65:101–105.

55. Herman RM, D'Luzansky SC, Ippolito R. Intrathecal baclofen suppresses central pain in patients with spinal lesions. A pilot study. *Clin J Pain* 1992;8:338–345.

56. Loubser PG, Akman NM. Effects of intrathecal baclofen on chronic spinal cord injury pain. *J Pain Symptom Manage* 1996;12:241–247.

57. Serrao JM, Marks RL, Morley SJ, et al. Intrathecal midazolam for the treatment of chronic mechanical low back pain: a controlled comparison with epidural steroid in a pilot study. *Pain* 1992;48:5–12.

58. Terenius L. Somatostatin and ACTH are peptides with partial antagonist-like selectivity for opiate receptors. *Eur J Pharmacol* 1976;38:211–213.

59. Sandkühler J, Fu QG, Helmchen C. Spinal somatostatin superfusion in vivo affects activity of cat nociceptive dorsal horn neurons: comparison with spinal morphine. *Neuroscience* 1990;34:565–576.

60. Penn RD, Paice JA, Kroin JS. Octreotide: a potent new non-opiate analgesic for intrathecal infusion. *Pain* 1992;49:13–19.

61. Paice J, Penn RD, Kroin JS. Intrathecal octreotide for relief of intractable non-malignant pain: 5-year experience with two cases. *Neurosurgey* 1996;38:203–207.

62. Meynadier J, Chrubasik J, Dubar M, et al. Intrathecal somatostatin in terminally ill patients. A report of two cases. Pain 1985;23:9–12.

63. Mollenholt P, Rawal N, Gordh T, et al. Intrathecal and epidural somatostatin for patients with cancer. Analgesic effects and postmortem neuropathological investigations of spinal cord and nerve roots. *Anesthesiology* 1994;81:534–542.

64. Staats P, Mitchell VD. Future directions for intrathecal therapies. *Prog Anesthesiol* 1997;11:367–382.

65. Hood DD, Eisenach JC, Tuttle R. Phase I safety assessment of intrathecal neostigmine methylsulfate in humans. *Anesthesiology* 1995;82:331–343.

66. Belfrage M, Segerdahl M, Arnér S, et al. The safety and efficacy of intrathecal adenosine in patients with chronic neuropathic pain. *Anesth Analg* 1999;89:136–142.

67. Malmberg AB, Yaksh TL. Spinal nitric oxide synthesis inhibition blocks NMDA-induced thermal hyperalgesia and produces anti-nociception in the formalin test in rats. *Pain* 1993;54:291–300.

68. Malmberg AB, Yaksh TL. Pharmacology of the spinal action of ketorolac, morphine, ST-91, U50488H, and L-PIA on the formalin test and an isobiologic analysis of the NSAID interaction. *Anesthesiology* 1993;79:270–281.

69. Yu LC, Hansson P, Lundeberg T. The calcitonin gene-related peptide antagonist CGRP8-37 increases the latency to withdrawal responses in rats. *Brain Res* 1994;653:223–230.

70. Bennett G, Burchiel K, Buchser E, et al. Clinical guidelines for intraspinal infusion: report of an expert panel. *J Pain Symptom Manage* 2000;20:S37–S43.

71. Patt RB, Hassenbusch SJ. Implantable technology for pain control: identification and management of problems and complications. In: Waldman SW, ed. *Interventional Pain Management.* 2nd ed. Philadelphia, Pa: WB Saunders; 2001:654–670.

72. Coffey RJ, Divisions of Neuromodulation Clinical Research, Regulatory Vigilance, and Biostatistics, Medtronic, Inc., Minneapolis, MN. Mortality associated with implantation and management of intrathecal opioid drug infusion systems to treat non-cancer pain: Identification, analysis and mitigation of risk factors. Oral presentation during the American Society of Regional Anesthesia and Pain Medicine Annual Pain Meeting, Huntington Beach, California, November 20, 2008.

73. Cole BE. Neuroendocrine implications of opioids therapy. *Curr Pain Headache Rep* 2007;11:89–92.

74. DuPen A, Shen D, Ersek M. Mechanisms of opioid-induced tolerance and hyperalgesia. *Pain Manag Nurs* 2007;8:113–121.

75. Deer T, Krames ES, Hassenbusch SJ, et al. Management of intrathecal catheter-tip inflammatory masses: an updated 2007 consensus statement from an expert panel. *Neuromodulation* 2008;11:77–91.

76. Smith TJ, Staats PS, Deer T, et al. Randomized clinical trial of an implantable drug delivery system compared with comprehensive medical management for refractory cancer pain: impact on pain, drug-related toxicity, and survival. *J Clin Oncol* 2002;20:4040–4049.

77. Bedder MD, Burchiel KJ, Larson A. Cost analysis of two implantable narcotic delivery systems. *J Pain Symptom Management* 1991;6:368–373.

CHAPTER 100 ■ INTRADISCAL THERAPIES FOR LOW BACK PAIN

WAY YIN AND NIKOLAI BOGDUK

Intradiscal therapies are interventions in which agents—physical or chemical—are delivered into an intervertebral disc either to stop pain or to reverse or remove processes responsible for the pain. Fundamental to the use of such interventions is the belief that the lumbar intervertebral discs are a common source of chronic low back pain. This belief has a long history and is based on a variety of circumstantial and direct evidence.

DISCOGENIC PAIN

As long ago as 1940, Roofe[1] reported finding nerve fibers in lumbar discs. In 1947, authorities as eminent as Inman and Saunders[2] noted that the intervertebral discs were innervated and remarked that they might be a source of back pain. Other investigators at that time reported that probing the disc, in patients under local anesthesia, evoked back pain[3,4]; and a modern study has since reproduced these observations.[5] Also in that same era, discography was developed—initially as a diagnostic test for disc herniation—but investigators noted that stimulating the disc with injections of contrast medium reproduced the patient's low back pain.[6–9] This implied that the disc was responsible for the patient's back pain.

Resistance to the belief that lumbar intervertebral discs could be a source of pain was based initially on the assumption that discs were not innervated and, so, could not be painful, but a study in 1959 confirmed that the outer anulus fibrosus was endowed with free nerve endings and complex receptors.[10] Later studies corroborated these findings[11] and established that the innervation arose from the sinuvertebral nerves, ventral rami, and grey rami communicantes.[12,13] Using modern staining techniques, studies confirmed the presence of nociceptive nerves in the anulus fibrosus.[14–17] Furthermore, in addition to the normal innervation, damaged or degenerated discs can attract an ingrowth of new nerves, which follow blood vessels and granulation tissue.[18–20]

Once these data eliminated opposition on anatomic grounds, the opposition to belief in discogenic pain turned to the validity of how it could be diagnosed. This has remained a contentious issue.

Some practitioners rely on imaging findings of disc degeneration to implicate the disc as a source of back pain, but this lacks validity. So-called degenerative changes are as prevalent in patients with back pain as in asymptomatic subjects.[21]

Others rely on discography to detect painful discs. The validity of discography as a diagnostic test has been challenged on the grounds that disc stimulation can be painful in asymptomatic subjects,[22] but competing studies[23] and a meta-analysis[24] have shown that the false-positive rate of lumbar discography is no greater than 9% and is substantially less if strict operational criteria are followed.[25] Those criteria require that a disc be classified as symptomatic only if injecting the disc with contrast medium reproduces the patient's pain at pressures of injection less than 50 psi, preferably at less than 15 psi, and that the evoked pain is of an intensity greater than 6 out of 10 on a numerical pain rating scale.[23–25]

Magnetic resonance imaging (MRI) can help to target poten-

tially painful discs. Discs that exhibit high-intensity zones in the posterior anulus are very likely to be painful on discography.[26–32] Similarly, discs that exhibit Modic endplate changes are also likely to be painful.[29,33,34]

PATHOLOGY

Until recent years, the pathology responsible for discogenic pain has been elusive. However, it is now evident that the lumbar disc responds to a variety of nutritional, metabolic, and mechanical insults in a similar manner.[35,36] Those responses are expressed as what, to date, have been called degenerative changes.

The disc matrix is produced by chondrocytes in the nucleus pulposus (NP), and synthesis is promoted by factors such as transforming growth factor (TGF) and insulin-like growth factor (IGF), which reside in the matrix (Fig. 100.1). Under normal conditions, the matrix is continually renewed. For this to occur, old matrix has to be degraded. The chondrocyte produces enzymes, known matrix metalloproteinases (MMPs), which degrade the matrix. These enzymes are controlled by tissue inhibitors of matrix metalloproteinases (TIMMPs).[35,36]

Injury disturbs the normal balance between synthesis and degradation toward degradation (see Fig. 100.1).[35,36] Injury results in the liberation of phospholipases, which in turn act on arachidonic acid to produce prostaglandins and leukotrienes (LTs). LTs are chemotactic and attract macrophages. Macrophages release superoxide and cytokines such as tumor necrosis factor alpha (TNFα), interleukins, and interferon. These cytokines stimulate the chondrocyte to produce more MMPs and, thereby, promote matrix degradation. The cytokines also stimulate nitric oxide synthetase to produce nitric oxide (NO). NO inhibits the chondrocyte, but also combines with superoxide to produce peroxynitrite, which inhibits the TIMMPs, thereby promoting matrix degradation. Superoxide itself inhibits the chondrocyte, and directly degrades the matrix.

As the nucleus degrades it is no longer able to retain water and loses its hydrostatic properties. Pressures within the nucleus become irregular and reduced (see Fig. 73-3),[37,38] and the nucleus is less able to sustain compression loads. Meanwhile, compression loads are increasingly borne by the posterior anulus, which

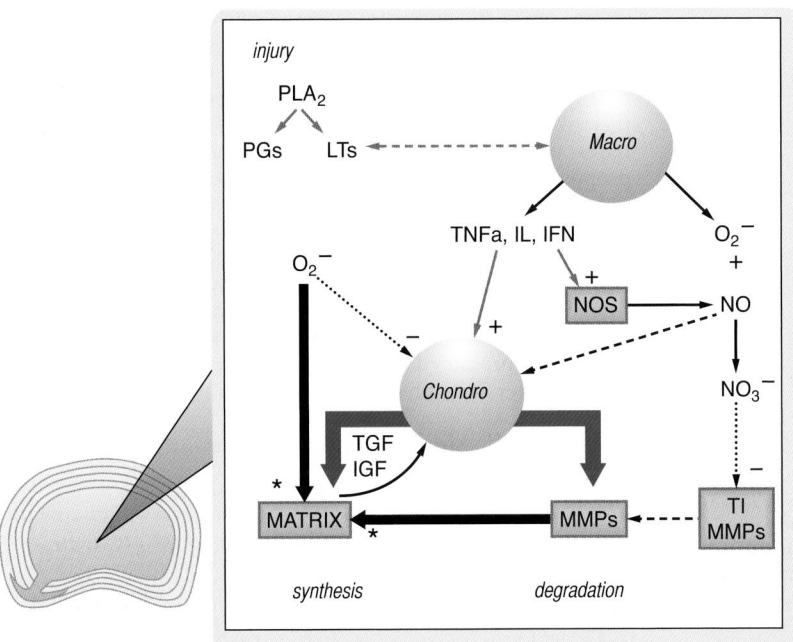

FIGURE 100.1 The molecular biology of disc degeneration and internal disc disruption. Bold arrows and plus signs (+) indicate production, promotion, or stimulation. Dashed arrows indicate attraction. Dotted arrows and minus signs (−) indicate inhibitory influences. Open arrows and asterixes (*) indicate degradative effects. Chondro, chondrocyte; IFN, interferon; IGF, insulin-like growth factor; IL, interleukins; LTs, leukotrienes; Macro, macrophage; MMPs, matrix metalloproteinases; NOS, nitric oxide synthetase; NO, nitric oxide; NO₃, peroxynitrite; O₂⁻, hyperoxide; PGs, prostaglandins; PLA₂, phospholipase A2; TFG, transforming growth factor; TIMMPs, tissue inhibitors of MMPs; TNFα, tumor necrosis factor alpha.

is subjected to loads substantially above normal (see Fig. 73-3).[37,38]

The depressurized nucleus is unable to brace the anulus internally. As a result, the inner anulus buckles and delaminates. Progressive disruption of the anulus leads to the development of radial fissures, which are characteristic of the condition known as internal disc disruption.[39–41] The severity of disruption can be graded according the extent to which fissures penetrate the anulus (see Fig. 73-2). Grade III fissures reach the outer third of the anulus, and become grade IV fissures if they extend circumferentially around the outer anulus.

Classical, macroscopic, degenerative changes, such as osteophytes, loss of disc height, or simple loss of disc signal on MRI, do not correlate with pain, but other features do. Reduced pressures in the nucleus,[42] increased pressure in the posterior anulus,[42] and grade III radial fissures[43,44] each correlate strongly with the disc being painful on discography. In particular, radial fissures are the hallmark of painful discs. They do not represent age-changes[44] and are most likely features of previous injury. Some 70% of painful discs exhibit radial fissures, and some 70% of discs with radial fissures are painful.[43]

In patients with chronic low back pain, the prevalence of internal disc disruption is at least 39%.[45] The diagnostic features are a reproduction of the patient's pain by disc stimulation at low pressures of injection, provided that stimulation of adjacent discs does not reproduce pain, and demonstration of a radial fissure on postdiscography computed tomography (CT) scan.[25]

The mechanism of pain appears to be a combination of mechanical and chemical factors. The increased pressures in the posterior anulus provide a basis for mechanical pain. The inordinate pressures in the posterior anulus would stimulate the nociceptive nerve endings in the outer anulus. Inflammatory mediators from the degraded nucleus provide a basis for chemical pain. Mediators that track through the radial fissure would reach the nerve endings in the outer anulus. They could stimulate the nerve endings to produce chemical nociception, or they could sensitize the endings and lower their threshold to mechanical stimulation. Both mechanisms could be amplified if new nerve fibers are attracted into the disc by the radial fissure.[18–20]

THERAPIES

Some intradiscal therapies target the innervation of the disc (Fig. 100.2). They seek to interrupt nociception from the affected disc

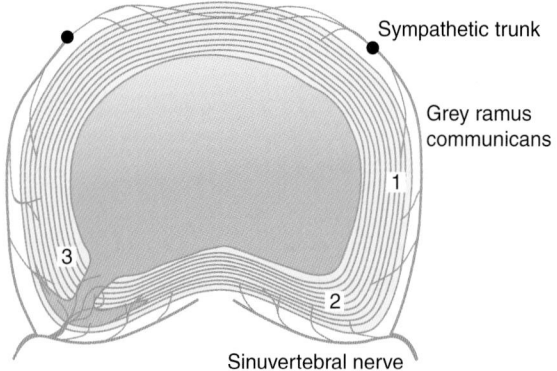

FIGURE 100.2 A sketch of a transverse section of a lumbar intervertebral disc showing the structural elements that are targets of some intradiscal therapies. The disc is innervated laterally and anteriorly by branches of the sympathetic trunk and grey rami communicantes (1), and posteriorly by the sinuvertebral nerves (2). Nerve endings are normally found within the outer third of the anulus fibrosus. Radial fissures (3) attract a neoinnervation in which nerve fibers extend deeper into the disc. Treatments can be directed at the degraded nucleus, the radial and circumferential fissures, or the nerve endings that mediate discogenic pain.

without seeking to alter its pathology. Other therapies seek to alter the macroscopic features of internal disc disruption by coagulating fissures or by removing degraded matrix from within radial fissures or the nucleus. At a molecular level, various therapies target agents involved in the degradative systems of the disc (see Fig. 100.1).

Denervation

Attempts have been made to denervate painful discs at a variety of sites using a variety of means. Most have proved unsuccessful.

Ramus Communicans Lesions

Once it was demonstrated that lumbar discs derive some of their innervation from the grey rami communicants,[12] the possibility was raised of treating discogenic pain by thermocoagulating the ramus communicans.[46] The weakness of this rationale, however, is that the grey rami constitute only one of the sources of innervation, and they innervate the anterior and lateral aspects of the disc—not the posterior anulus, which appears to be the most likely source of pain. This weakness is borne out by the only study of grey ramus communicans coagulation.

A prospective, controlled study compared the effects of thermal radiofrequency lesioning in the region of the ramus communicans with those of injections of lidocaine over the same site.[47] In terms of pain scores and SF-36 scores, significant differences arose in favor of radiofrequency treatment at 4 months following intervention. However, the degree of relief afforded by radiofrequency therapy was modest, amounting to only a 46% mean decrease in pain, and the authors did not stratify their data to demonstrate the number of patients experiencing high-grade relief (75%–100%).[47] Moreover, the study was confounded because patients who received radiofrequency therapy also received an injection of triamcinolone (40 mg) at the site treated, which the control group did not receive. It is, therefore, not evident if the modest improvements seen in the study group arose from the radiofrequency lesion created or the injection of corticosteroids.[47]

Intranuclear Radiofrequency

The NP is normally devoid of nerve endings. Therefore, placing radiofrequency lesions in the nucleus has no prospect of coagulating nerves in the immediate vicinity of the electrode. However, proponents of intranuclear radiofrequency argued that the electric field produced around the electrode would be sufficient to heat and destroy nerve fibers in the outer anulus fibrosus, and thereby provide relief of pain.[48] This belief was based on a theoretical assessment of the magnitude of the electric field and the proposition that temperatures of 45° C would be achieved in the outer anulus and would be enough to coagulate nerves.

Cadaver studies rapidly dispelled this notion.[49,50] Significant heating did not occur in the outer anulus. Nevertheless, the procedure continued to enjoy some popularity in some circles. A controlled trial eventually demonstrated that intradiscal radiofrequency achieved no greater relief of pain than sham therapy.[51] What were promoted as successful outcomes in earlier observational studies amounted to no more than placebo responses.

Sinuvertebral Nerve Lesions

Since the sinuvertebral nerves innervate the posterior anulus fibrosus, they would be a logical target for denervating a painful posterior anulus. However, because these nerves are often plexiform, they are unlikely to be selectively and completely targeted by conventional means of denervation. Although anecdotal references may be found in lectures, monographs, and texts,[52–54] no controlled or prospective studies of the efficacy of sinuvertebral nerve lesions for the treatment of lumbar disc pain are currently available.

Intradiscal Electrothermal Therapy

The use of a resistance-coil flexible heating element deployed within the fibers of the posterior anulus or along the nuclear-anular boundary was developed in the mid-1990s. Under the trade name of IDET, the technology proposed that therapeutic benefits resulted from "several heat related effects," including "destruction of pain receptors on the outer layers of the disc . . . [thermal-induced] remodeling of the collagen fibers that make up the anulus fibrosus . . . [and] cauterization and subsequent disintegration of vascular ingrowth."[55–59] None of these conceptual mechanisms have ultimately been verified by in vitro studies.[55–57] Nevertheless, IDET has been the focus of intense study and sometimes conflicting reviews.[59–63]

Eight observational studies[64–73] have demonstrated a mean reduction in pain by at least 30 points. The proportion of patients who achieve greater than 50% has ranged from 50%[66,67,74] to 70%,[64,65] and up to 20% of patients achieve complete relief.[66,67] Outcomes are maintained for 2 years.[67,71,73]

Two randomized, placebo-controlled trials have been published with differing results.[75,76] In one study, where rigorous selection criteria were applied, and both diagnostic provocation discography and subsequent IDET (or sham) was performed by highly experienced practitioners, a clear difference was demonstrated between placebo and experimental groups.[75] By the general criteria applied to many surgical studies ($\geq$50% relief), IDET was effective in 40% of patients. Furthermore, the degree of relief was stratified in this study—a courtesy seldom extended by studies of pain treatment. Twenty-two percent (7/32) of patients undergoing IDET for lumbar disc pain experienced 75% to 100% relief of pain. The duration of relief was not addressed in this study, for it was designed explicitly to test IDET against placebo. In that regard, it warned that patients undergoing intradiscal therapy could experience placebo effects, but it showed that the effects of IDET could not be wholly attributed to placebo effects.

The other controlled study[76] enrolled a similar number of patients (albeit with different demographics) with similar complaints to those of the former study.[75] Intriguingly, it found no effect, either from active treatment or from sham treatment. The lack of any placebo effect stands in marked contrast with the majority of other sham-controlled studies in clinical medicine. This lack of any demonstrable or measurable response remains unexplained. Since that study was not able to reproduce the responses seen in observational studies and since no placebo effects were demonstrated, that study does not provide evidence that those responses are due to placebo effects.

Although providing relief in a relatively small subset of patients with disc pain, IDET currently represents the most thoroughly investigated percutaneous intradiscal therapy for symptomatic internal disc disruption. The majority of prospective studies demonstrate that in well selected patients, 40% to 50% may experience greater than 50% reduction in pain with improvements in other functional outcome measures and that a small fraction (approximately 20%) may expect high-grade to complete relief which is durable.

Nucleoplasty

Application of frequency alternating current radio between two closely apposed electrodes separated by an insulator can result in the generation of a stable plasma field in conductive tissue. Moving such an electrode—and thereby the plasma field—through tissue results in vaporization of tissue in the path of the plasma field, leaving a void. Percutaneous application of this technology for the removal of disc tissue is a patented technology

marketed as "nucleoplasty," or "percutaneous plasma disc decompression." The procedure involves creation of several tunnel-like voids in the disc nucleus following multiple passes of the plasma field generated by the electrode or "nucleotome." The vaporized disc material is subsequently vented out of the disc nucleus. Vaporization of solid disc nucleus results in a reduction of mass in the disc nucleus, theoretically decreasing intradiscal pressures and thus resulting in disc decompression.

Nucleoplasty is purported to reduce pressures in the NP.[77] Although this might be of relevance for the treatment of radicular pain due to disc herniation, it is unlikely to be relevant to the treatment of discogenic pain. The pressures within a disc are not uniform (see Fig. 73-3).[37,38] Therefore, it is not evident that reducing pressure at one site affects pressure elsewhere or throughout the disc. Moreover, in painful discs, nuclear pressures are already reduced, not raised. The offending pressures are in the posterior anulus, not in the nucleus. Therefore, nucleoplasty lacks an anatomic rationale for the treatment of discogenic pain.

In vivo animal studies have demonstrated that plasma discectomy alters cytokine expression in experimentally induced disc degeneration.[78] The relevance of these changes to the effectiveness of nucleoplasty for discogenic pain remains unknown.

Clinical applications for plasma discectomy, like those for other techniques for percutaneous discectomy, have typically focused on the treatment of radicular pain associated with disc protrusion, herniation, or bulge.[79] No prospective, randomized, controlled studies are available (at this time) regarding the use of percutaneous plasma discectomy for either radicular pain or discogenic pain.

Observational studies with follow-up longer than 1 month include retrospective case series[80,81] and limited nonrandomized prospective series with varying levels of follow-up and patient selection criteria.[82,83] Two studies are available but it is not clear whether they evaluated patients prospectively or retrospectively.[84,85] All available studies grouped patients with low back pain and radicular pain together, which precludes any determination of efficacy for either specific condition. No available studies have specifically examined the efficacy of percutaneous plasma discectomy in patients with rigorously determined primary discogenic pain.

Chemical Therapies

Chemical therapies for discogenic pain target one or other of the agents involved in disc degradation. Some have proved unsuccessful; others show promise.

Intradiscal Steroids

Because phospholipase A2 (PLA2) has been implicated in disc degeneration and disc injury, intradiscal injection of corticosteroids has a rationale. By inhibiting PLA2, steroids prevent the arachidonic acid cascade and the production of prostaglandins and leukotrienes (see Fig. 100.1). However, intradiscal steroids were first used before the molecular biology of the disc was known, ostensibly because of their reputation of efficacy in treating arthritis.

Feffer[86] published the first report in 1956. He treated 60 patients with intradiscal injections of hydrocortisone, each at two levels (L4-L5 and L5-S1), using a transdural, midline approach. Patients were selected for treatment because they were "either in extreme pain and not responding to bedrest or had rapidly recurring symptoms in spite of bedrest, plaster-of-Paris jackets, back supports, and other conservative measures."[86] Seven were injected for diagnostic purposes when the etiology was in doubt.[86] Discography was performed during the treatment, but was not used as a selection criterion. Patients were maintained at strict bedrest for 2 to 3 weeks before and after injection. Responses were graded on the basis of pain, spasm, scoliosis, sciatic irritability, and neurologic findings. Feffer reported that 37 of 60 patients had "rapid remission of symptoms . . . usually . . . in four to six hours, and major discomfort had disappeared in twenty-four hours. Remissions have been permanent in thirty-three of these patients for a maximum follow-up period of eight months. . . ."[86] Nucleograms in 55 of the 60 patients were interpreted as abnormal. Five patients had "normal nucleograms," none of whom showed improvement. In 16 of the 18 failures reported, laminectomy and discectomy was performed and "all the discs . . . demonstrated irreversible changes."

Feffer[87] subsequently published a reappraisal of his original methodology with longer-term follow-up in 1969. This retrospective report described 244 patients with follow-up between 4 and 10 years, of whom 46.7% reported "permanent remission" of symptoms. Interestingly, Feffer[87] noted better responses in patients over the age of 50 with predominant back rather than radicular complaints.

These encouraging results later prompted a double-blind comparison between intradiscal injection of hydrocortisone and chymopapain injection in patients with "long-term back pain and/or sciatica."[88] The purpose of this study was to determine the effects of chymopapain, then considered a promising and relatively novel therapeutic alternative, against a reference. Intradiscal hydrocortisone was used as a control as it was felt to have "some therapeutic value," and the author felt ethically "disinclined to use a true placebo."[88] Twenty patients were randomized prospectively to receive either a single intradiscal injection of hydrocortisone or chymopapain based on diagnostic discography. Twelve of 20 patients (60%) undergoing chymopapain injection were reported to have demonstrated "good" (near complete to complete relief) or "fair" results, and as did 53% of patients who underwent hydrocortisone injection. Although detailed outcome measures were not reported, the author concluded that chymopapain injection was more effective than intradiscal hydrocortisone injection, but the differences did not reach statistical significance. The possibilities of placebo responses to injection (potentially approaching 60%–70%) were discussed, but dismissed.[88]

Following the withdrawal of chymopapain from the commercial medical market in the mid-1970s, Wilkinson and Schuman[89] published the results of a case series of 29 patients who had normal myelography and no focal neurologic symptoms. Unlike previous reports where a water-soluble steroid (hydrocortisone) was injected, these investigators used a suspension of methylprednisolone. No controls were used. Sequential injections were performed if an initial response was seen in the first 3 months following initial injection. Fifty-eight percent of initial injections were performed in patients with discogenic pain (defined as "back pain with little or no radiation into the lower extremities"), and 42% of injections were performed for predominant complaints of radicular pain. For patients with predominant "discogenic pain," 31% had "good results" with 37% reporting a good result in the radicular pain group. When the authors stratified their outcomes and excluded patients who had failed single injection or who had undergone prior lumbar spine surgery, the interpretation of respondents experiencing a "good result" increased to 54% in the low back pain group and 40% in the radicular pain group. The statistical significance of these findings was not reported.[89]

Due to the heterogeneous patient populations, methodologies, and outcome measurements from these initial studies, Simmons et al.[90] performed a more rigorous prospective double blind, controlled trial comparing intradiscal injections of 80 mg methylprednisolone suspension against 1.5 mL 0.5% bupivacaine injected at the time of diagnostic discography. More rigorous patient selection criteria and outcome measures were applied, and only those patients with discography-proven single level disc pain in the absence of disc extrusion were considered. Patients were excluded if their age was greater than 50 or if previous surgery had been performed. Outcome measures included visual analog pain scores (VAS), Oswestry pain questionnaire, and pain diagrams. The period of follow-up was extremely short (10–14 days). Only 21% of patients who were randomized to methylprednisolone suspension and 9% who received bupivacaine reported overall improvement. When individual outcome measures were compared, improvements in VAS were seen in 43% of patients who received steroid and in 36% of those who received bupivacaine. Oswestry Pain Questionnaire responses showed similar responses (36% improved with steroid, 27% with bupivacaine).

Another more recent randomized control trial was performed with 1-year follow-up.[91] Patients complaining of predominant back pain were randomized at the time of provocation discography to receive intradiscal methylprednisolone suspension (40 mg) or 1 mL normal saline. Selection criteria were fairly rigorous: only patients with single level disc concordant pain were enrolled, and postsurgical patients were excluded. It is unclear whether workers compensation patients were excluded. Discography was not manometrically-controlled. The severity of degeneration at the symptomatic level was not recorded. Of 120 patients enrolled (60 into each of the steroid and saline groups), 77% in the steroid group and 87% in the saline group completed follow-up. These authors noted no discernible improvements in Oswestry Disability Index (ODI) or VAS pain scores in either group.[91]

Others have used different selection criteria. A retrospective case series examined the effects of intradiscal prednisolone acetate (25 mg) injection in patients with painful discs associated with MRI evidence of Type I and Type II endplate changes on following provocation discography.[92] Prospective outcome data were recorded for all 74 patients whose charts were reviewed retrospectively, and included VAS, Quebec disability score, and other subjective measures. A change in VAS was recorded at 1 month following injection, with VAS and disability scores measured as secondary outcomes at 1, 3, and 6 months following injection. Compared to patients with Type II changes, moderate and statistically significant improvements in VAS were seen in patients with Type I or Type I and Type II changes at 1 month following injection. The mean reduction in VAS was 5.3 mm in patients with Type II lesions, but 30.2 mm for Type I, and 29.4 mm for combined Type I and II lesions. At 1 month, only 1 of 11 patients with Type II lesions reported greater than 50% relief of pain, whereas 18/33 patients with Type I lesions and 13/25 patients with combined lesions reported that degree of relief. However, the treatment effects between groups became indistinguishable at 6 months. Although the authors concluded that intradiscal injection of steroid in patients with chronic low back pain and predominant Type I endplate changes on MRI, significant limitations remained with regard to the relatively low number of patients demonstrating such findings and the retrospective nature of the study.

In essence, despite favorable reports from observational studies, two randomized placebo-controlled studies have indicated that intradiscal steroid injections are not effective in the management of discogenic, chronic low back pain. Whether more rigorously selected patients with internal disc disruption may benefit from intradiscal steroid injection remains unclear, but the size of such a subpopulation is likely to be small.

Etanercept

Because TNFα is involved in the degradation of lumbar discs (see Fig. 100.1), there is a rationale for using TNF-blocking agents to treat discogenic pain. One such agent is etanercept, which binds TNF receptors.

A placebo-controlled study assessed the efficacy of intradiscal injection of etanercept in doses increasing from 0.1 mg to 1.5 mg.[93] No differences were found at 1 month, either within or between patients treated with etanercept or normal saline, with respect to relief of pain or disability. Prima facie, these results deny a role for intradiscal etanercept in the treatment of discogenic pain, although the possibility remains that higher doses might still be effective.

Methylene Blue

Methylene blue, a common histologic stain, has also been used in clinical medicine for over 100 years. As a dye, it has been used to detect mucosal defects in urology and gastroenterology and to stain cement in orthopaedics. In general medicine, it has been used to treat methemoglobinemia and hepatopulmonary syndrome and pruritus ani. It has weak neurolytic effects, but its main actions appear to be inhibition of guanylate cyclase and NO synthesis. The latter property affords it a role in the treatment of discogenic pain by blocking the degradative effects of NO (see Fig. 100.1).

Investigators from China have reported a prospective pilot study in which 24 patients underwent injection of methylene blue into one (18/24) or two (6/24) discs immediately following provocative discography.[94] Patients were followed for a minimum of 12 months, with mean duration of follow-up 18 months. Outcome measures included the ODI and VAS pain ratings. The mean improvement in VAS in the single level injection group was 5.65 and 4.40 in the two-level group, with ODI improvements of 36 and 24, respectively. These changes were statistically significant. Across the entire treatment group, VAS was reduced from 7.52 ± 1.31 to 2.18 ± 1.79 (71% reduction) at 12 months, and ODI was reduced from 48.71 ± 5.28 to 15.38 ± 13.63 (68% reduction). Three of 24 patients showed no improvement or improvement less than 2 points on VAS. Of the remaining 21 patients, 11 were reported to have rated pain at less than VAS 2 at 12 months, with 5/21 (24%) apparently experiencing complete relief.

These results are extraordinary. No other intervention for chronic back pain has ever achieved such outcomes. However, the context of the study is unclear. It is not evident if the patients expected the treatment to work or if they faced fusion if the injections did not work. It is not known if patients in China respond to research studies in a manner different that of patients in the Western world. If methylene blue is as effective as reported, it urgently needs to be tested both in different populations and under controlled conditions.

Ozone

Intradiscal injections of ozone have been promoted largely in the Italian literature,[95-100] although some English-language publications have appeared.[101-104] The professed rationale is that ozone suppresses intradiscal inflammation.[105-107]

However, although back pain is mentioned in the indications, radicular pain appears to have been the primary indication. No studies have reported the effectiveness of ozone for back pain. Furthermore, although high rates of success in large numbers of patients have been enthusiastically promoted, the available literature is composed largely of case reports and retrospective case series, in which validated outcome measures have not been used.

Although touted as "safe," several cases of serious complications and death associated with intradiscal injection of O_2/O_3 have been reported.[108-110] The injection of an oxidizing gas—in relatively large volumes—in and around the disc may be especially problematic if safeguards against intra-arterial or subarachnoid injection are not rigorously maintained.

Proliferants

Some investigators have sought to ameliorate disc pain through the injection of substances purported to enhance healing of diseased disc tissue. Typically, solutions have been used that contain chondroitin sulfate, glucosamine hydrochloride, dimethylsulfoxide (DMSO), bupivacaine, and hypertonic dextrose[111,112] or hypertonic dextrose alone.[113]

An initial prospective case series involved 30 patients receiving an average of 2.5 intradiscal injections of a compounded mixture of chondroitin sulfate, glucosamine hydrochloride, DMSO, bupivacaine, hypertonic dextrose, and nonionic contrast dye.[111] The investigators reported that 57% of patients experienced greater than 50% improvement in pain sustained over a minimum follow-up of 12 months. Some 30% of patients reported reduction of pain score to 0 or 1 on a 10-point scale.

A subsequent retrospective study compared the efficacy of intradiscal injection of the aforementioned with IDET with more modest results.[113] The study was hampered by differing group sizes between IDET (74) and intradiscal injection (35), as well as mean duration of follow-up (IDET: 15.5 months; disc injection: 8 months) and uncontrolled cross-over (17% of patients undergoing intradiscal injection had previously failed IDET). The results of this study demonstrated meager improvements in both groups (mean VAS reduction from IDET: 1.27; from intradiscal injection: 2.2). No other functional outcomes were assessed, and the durability of relief in the intradiscal injection group was not with the IDET group.

In a more recent study, single and repeated intradiscal injections of hypertonic dextrose with bupivacaine were studied in 76 patients with primary complaints of leg pain, with or without back pain.[113] An average of 3.5 injections were performed into discs that were positive on provocative discography. Approximately 50% of patients were reported to experience significant improvements in pain, although the percentage experiencing complete relief was not stratified, and a strong selection bias existed for patients who reported improvements in pain while undergoing intradiscal dextrose injections. The authors also did not explain the elicitation of "concordant pain reproduction" in patients undergoing discography without low back pain and their inclusion in the study.

Whether intradiscal injections of hypertonic dextrose, with or without other agents, such as local anesthetics, chondroitin, glucosamine, or DMSO, successfully relieves pain arising from symptomatic internal disc disruption remains unclear. Since numerous pharmacologically active agents were used in these noncontrolled studies, the specific agent (or combination) that may affect a positive clinical response is difficult to ascertain. Although authors have referred to injection of these agents as "regenerative" or "proliferative" therapies, chondroitin and glucosamine have not been shown to have any specific anabolic effect on the disc, and DMSO is neurolytic. The term "regenerative" seems more appropriate for emerging intradiscal therapies that have a known positive effect on connective tissue metabolism.

Regenerative Therapies

A variety of cytokines, growth factors, and virus-mediated gene therapies are known to promote favorably the metabolism of connective tissues. Several are being explored for the restitution of degraded discs. To date, however, these agents have largely been studied only in laboratory animals or tissue cultures. Such studies as have been conducted in humans have addressed only safety. Efficacy has not been addressed.

Thompson et al.[114] were the first to examine the effects of various growth factors on mature canine intervertebral disc cell cultures. In their model, certain growth factors, especially human platelet derived transforming growth factor-β (TGF-β_1) and epidermal growth factor (EGF), resulted in marked increases in matrix synthesis and cell proliferation (EGF) or matrix synthesis alone (TGF-β_1). Increases in matrix synthesis with TGF-β_1 were dramatic. The effect of growth factors, however, was time-limited to several days. Other investigators have demonstrated that application of platelet-derived growth factor (PDF) and IGF-1 may reduce the rate and number of human anular cells undergoing apoptosis in vitro.[115]

In vivo injection of another human growth factor, osteogenic protein-1 (OP-1, also known as bone morphogenic protein-7), into rabbits resulted in mild increases (12%–15%) in disc height up to 8 weeks following injection.[116] Subsequent studies of intradiscal OP-1 in a rabbit, anular-puncture, degenerated disc model demonstrated reversal of loss of disc space height sustained at 24 weeks.[117] Sustained restoration of disc space height at 12 weeks in a chemically-induced (intradiscal injection of chondroitinase ABC) degenerative rabbit disc model has also been reported.[118]

Nishida et al.[119] pioneered the feasibility of adenovirus-mediated gene transfer to rabbit nuclear cells in vitro and in vivo. Subsequently, their group was able to demonstrate the in vivo feasibility of TGF-β_1 gene transfer utilizing an adenovirus vector (Ad/CMV-hTGFβ_1) in rabbit intervertebral discs.[120] In discs injected with Ad/CMV-hTGFβ_1 a 30-fold increase in active TGFβ_1 production 1 week after injection was seen with a 100% increase in proteoglycan synthesis over saline-injected controls. Proponents of gene therapies argue that although temporary increases in matrix synthesis or nuclear cell proliferation demonstrated with direct intradiscal injection of growth factors is promising, the relatively short biologic half-life of growth factors would require sustained delivery systems in vivo. Such technical challenges would be difficult to overcome with existing technologies. Thus, if existing intervertebral disc nuclear chondrocytes could be induced to produce growth factors endogenously, an intrinsically self-sustaining source of growth factors may be more attractive.

The feasibility of utilizing adenoviral vectors to induce genetic changes in disc nuclear cells or the direct injection of human growth factors has not yet been investigated in humans. Concerns remain regarding the regulation of growth factor effects or induced cellular synthetic activity in nontarget tissues.

Although disc cells account for only about 1% of the disc tissue by volume,[121] they play a crucial role in matrix synthesis. As cells are of crucial value to the metabolic health of the disc and its nuclear matrix, an alternative therapeutic strategy would focus on augmenting intradiscal cell populations through introduction of autogenic or allogenic cartilaginous chondrocytes, NP cells, or mesenchymal stem cells.

The effects of injection of an autogenously collected NP and NP cell cultures in an anular stab model of disc degeneration in rabbits have demonstrated that disc degeneration and formation of type II collagen can be delayed.[122] Subsequent investigation of the effects of allogenic NP demonstrated similar delays in the formation of degenerative changes without stimulating an immune response.[123] The determination of the degree of disc degeneration in both studies was performed semi-quantitatively, using histologic stains to examine changes in cell populations and type II collagen 24 weeks[122] or 16 weeks[123] after injection. Nuclear degeneration not reversed by the introduction of autologous or allogenic NP aspirates.

Other researchers have focused on autologous chondrocyte transplantation. Reintroduction of fresh or cryopreserved NP in a degenerative rat model suggested that degeneration could be delayed.[124] A detailed in vivo study of the effects of cultured autologous nuclear chondrocytes was performed in dogs. Plain film radiographs, disc height analysis, MRI imaging, and histologic analysis was performed at 3, 6, 9, and 12 months after autologous transplantation. The discs subjected to tissue harvest were examined to determine whether disc repair occurred. Transplanted cells retained viability and underwent expected morphological changes from tissue culture once reintroduced into the disc. The transplanted chondrocytes produced type I and II collagen and proteoglycans similar to normal tissue, and at longer time intervals following transplantation, disc height was better

retained. No inflammatory reactions were seen.[121] A human safety trial has been initiated with interim results suggesting that intradiscal reintroduction of autogenous chondrocytes may better disc height after lumbar discectomy.[125,126]

More recently, the effects of intradiscal transplantation of autogenic and allogenic mesenchymal stem cells (MSCs) have been investigated. MSCs possess a theoretical advantage of mature cell transplants in their pluripotency. Proponents of intradiscal MSC transplantation argue that since the causes of disc degeneration are likely multifactorial, the use of autogenic or allogenic stem cells minimizes the likelihood of host antigenic recognition and MSCs, once differentiated, may be less susceptible to genetic senescence or apoptosis. The use of allogenic MSCs may offer "off the shelf" availability—rather than requiring labor intensive autogenic cell harvesting and culture—and potentially avoid genetic predisposition to degeneration.

Several investigations have demonstrated that MSCs can be introduced into animal discs, remain viable, and differentiate into NP-like cells, produce matrix, and retard experimental disc degeneration.[127–129] In vitro experiments with human MSCs demonstrated differentiation of MSCs into NP-like chondrocytes if cocultured with human NP cells. Differentiation required direct cell-cell contact.[130] Subsequent investigations demonstrated that MSCs differentiated into chondrocytes-like cells if implanted in a three-dimensional matrix, including several hydrophilic gels. Partial depolymerization and deacetylation of chitin from crustaceans creates a hydrogel (chitosan). Combining chitosan with glycerophosphate creates a temperature sensitive hydrogel (C/Gp) which is liquid at room temperature and gels at body temperature, which would make C/Gp an ideal delivery vehicle for MSCs clinically. Bovine MSCs have been demonstrated to differentiate toward NP-like chondrocytes (as opposed to articular chondrocytes) when placed in C/Gp gel without added differentiating media in vitro.[130] The ability of MSCs to differentiate into NP-like chondrocytes (and not osteocytes or articular chondrocytes) in a gel environment without specific differentiating media is intriguing. Stem cells cultured in a three-dimensional gel matrix in a hypoxic environment tended to differentiate into NP-like cells, the addition of TGFβ-1 resulted in concert to activate genes expressed by NP cells, including those that encode matrix proteins and cell surface receptors.[131]

The identification of technically feasible delivery vehicle for MSCs (such as temperature sensitive hydrogels), their demonstrated in vivo ability to differentiate into NP-like cells in a hypoxic disc nucleus-like environment, and their ability to produce nuclear matrix aggrecans and proteoglycans once differentiated is extremely promising. The pace at which discreet mechanisms controlling MSC differentiation are being discovered is rapid. A complete understanding of the control pathways that regulate differentiation of implanted MSCs and their long-term in vivo viability remain as important questions to be answered before studies in humans can be considered.

Proponents of regenerative-, gene-, and cell-based therapies have predominantly focused on preventing or reversing disc degeneration associated with loss of nuclear matrix, cells, or restoring internal disc mechanical integrity. In experimental animal models of disc degeneration, usually incited by anular stab incisions, several approaches including direct intradiscal injection of growth factors or cell transplantation with or without a hydrogel lattice have been demonstrated to delay or partially reverse degenerative changes. However, a correlation between experimentally-induced animal disc degeneration and human disc pain has not been established.

Animal models of disc degeneration have mostly involved the creation of an anular injury (usually an incision) in young, otherwise healthy discs. It has not been the intent of these models to establish whether or not the induced degenerative changes are painful, but to mimic chemical, histologic, and radiographic changes that parallel degenerative changes in humans. No naturally occurring model of disc degeneration in commonly used laboratory mammals has been identified that closely mimics the degenerative changes seen in bipedal primates such as humans.

An important, and possibly crucial, caveat is that tissue cultures and animals may not be valid and realistic models of the human condition. In humans, the lumbar discs are persistently subjected to large compression loads during activities of daily living. What has still to be demonstrated is that intradiscal agents can exert their effects in the face of a hostile mechanical environment.

Ultimately, a focus on preventing or treating disc degeneration per se may have limited clinical relevance in man, as loss of disc height, anular bulges, protrusions, and even herniation are found in the majority of asymptomatic adults.[132–135] Progressive degeneration over 5 years in people initially asymptomatic does not correlate with the development of pain.[136] The ubiquitous nature of lumbar disc degeneration and its high prevalence in both symptomatic and asymptomatic individuals has underscored the importance of disassociating the presence of degeneration with identification of a particular symptom complex.[137] Although regenerative approaches show promise, including the possibility of creating a fully tissue engineered disc from homologous nuclear and anular cells,[138] the ultimate role of regenerative approaches in patients with disc pain remains far from clear, but technological advancements in this field may ultimately prove clinically useful once specific clinical applications and the timing of intervention becomes clear.

References

1. Roofe PG. Innervation of annulus fibrosus and posterior longitudinal ligament. *Arch Neurol* 1940;44:100–103.
2. Inman VT, Saunders JBCM. Anatomicophysiological aspects of injuries to the intervertebral disc. *J Bone Joint Surg* 1947;29:461–475.
3. Wiberg G. Back pain in relation to the nerve supply of the intervertebral disc. *Acta Orthop Scand* 1949;19:211–221.
4. Falconer MA, McGeorge M, Begg AC. Observations on the cause and mechanism of symptom-production in sciatica and low-back pain. *J Neurol Neurosurg Psychiatry* 1948;11:13–26.
5. Kuslich SD, Ulstrom CL, Michael CJ. The tissue origin of low back pain and sciatica: a report of pain response to tissue stimulation during operations on the lumbar spine using local anesthesia. *Orthop Clin North Am* 1991;22:181–187.
6. Lindblom K. Diagnostic puncture of intervertebral disks in sciatica. *Acta Orthop Scand* 1948;17:231–239.
7. Lindblom K. Technique and results in myelography and disc puncture. *Acta Radiol* 1950;34(4–5):321–330.
8. Hirsch C. An attempt to diagnose the level of a disc lesion clinically by disc puncture. *Acta Orthop Scand* 1949;18:132–140.
9. Gardner WJ, Wise RE, Hughes CR, et al. X-ray visualization of the intervertebral disk with a consideration of the morbidity of disk puncture. *Arch Surg* 1952;64(3):355–364.
10. Malinsky J. The ontogenetic development of nerve terminations in the intervertebral discs of man. (Histology of intervertebral discs, 11th communication). *Acta Anat (Basel)* 1959;38:96–113.
11. Yoshizawa H, O'Brien JP, Thomas-Smith WT, et al. The neuropathology of intervertebral discs removed for low-back pain. *J Pathol* 1980;132:95–104.
12. Bogduk N, Tynan W, Wilson AS. The nerve supply to the human lumbar intervertebral discs. *J Anat* 1981;132:39–56.
13. Groen G, Baljet B, Drukker J. The nerves and nerve plexuses of the human vertebral column. *Am J Anat* 1990;188:282–296.
14. Korkala O, Grönblad M, Liesi P, et al. Immunohistochemical demonstration of nociceptors in the ligamentous structures of the lumbar spine. *Spine* 1985;10(2):156–157.
15. Konttinen YT, Grönblad M, Antti-Poika I, et al. Neuroimmunohistochemical analysis of peridiscal nociceptive neural elements. *Spine* 1990;15:383–386.
16. Ashton IK, Walsh DA, Polak JM, et al. Substance P in intervertebral discs: binding sites on vascular endothelium of the human annulus fibrosus. *Acta Orthop Scand* 1994;65:635–639.
17. Roberts S, Eisenstein SM, Menage J, et al. Mechanoreceptors in intervertebral discs. Morphology, distribution, and neuropeptides. *Spine* 1995;20:2645–2651.
18. Freemont AJ, Peacock TE, Goupille P, et al. Nerve ingrowth into diseased intervertebral disc in chronic back pain. *Lancet* 1997;350(9072):178–181.
19. Coppes MH, Marani E, Thomeer RT, et al. Innervation of "painful" lumbar discs. *Spine* 1997;22:2342–2349.
20. Freemont AJ, Watkins A, Le Maitre C, et al. Nerve growth factor expression and innervation of the painful intervertebral disc. *J Pathol* 2002;197:286–292.
21. van Tulder MW, Assendelft WJ, Koes BW, et al. Spinal radiographic findings and nonspecific low back pain: a systematic review of observational studies. *Spine* 1997;22:427–434.
22. Carragee EJ, Tanner CM, Khurana S, et al. The rates of false-positive lumbar discography in select patients without low back symptoms. *Spine* 2000;25:1373–1381.
23. Derby R, Lee SH, Kim BJ, et al. Pressure-controlled lumbar discography in volunteers without low back symptoms. *Pain Med* 2005;6:213–221.
24. Wolffer LR, Derby R, Lee JE, et al. Systematic review of lumbar provocation discography in asymptomatic subjects with meta-analysis of false-positive rates. *Pain Physician* 2008;11:513–538.
25. International Spinal Intervention Society. Lumbar disc stimulation. In: Bogduk N, ed. *Practice Guidelines for Spinal Diagnostic and Treatment Procedures*. San Francisco, CA: International Spinal Intervention Society; 2004:20–46.
26. Aprill C, Bogduk N. High-intensity zone: a diagnostic sign of painful lumbar disc on magnetic resonance imaging. *Br J Radiol* 1992;65:361–369.
27. Schellhas KP, Pollei SR, Gundry CR, et al. Lumbar disc high-intensity zone: correlation of magnetic resonance imaging and discography. *Spine* 1996;21:79–86.
28. Saifuddin A, Braithwaite I, White J, et al. The value of lumbar spine magnetic resonance imaging in the demonstration of anular tears. *Spine* 1998;23:453–457.
29. Ito M, Incorvaia KM, Yu SF, et al. Predictive signs of discogenic lumbar pain on magnetic resonance imaging with discography correlation. *Spine* 1998;23:1252–1260.
30. Lam KS, Carlin D, Mulholland RC. Lumbar disc high-intensity zone: the value and significance of provocative discography in the determination of the discogenic pain source. *Eur Spine J* 2000;9:36–41.
31. Carragee EJ, Paragoudakis SJ, Khurana S. Lumbar high-intensity zone and discography in subjects without low back problems. *Spine* 2000;25:2987–2992.
32. Peng B, Hou S, Wu W, et al. The pathogenesis and clinical significance of a high-intensity zone (HIZ) of lumbar intervertebral disc on MR imaging in the patient with discogenic low back pain. *Eur Spine J* 2006;15:583–587.
33. Braithwaite I, White J, Saifuddin A, et al. Vertebral end-plate (Modic) changes on lumbar spine MRI: correlation with pain reproduction at lumbar discography. *Eur Spine J* 1998;7:363–368.
34. Weishaupt D, Zanetti M, Hodler J, et al. Painful lumbar disk derangement: relevance of endplate abnormalities at MR imaging. *Radiology* 2001;218:420–427.
35. Peng B, Wu W, Hou S, et al. The pathogenesis of discogenic low back pain. *J Bone Joint Surg Br* 2005;87:62–67.
36. Hadjipavlou AG, Tzermiadianos MN, Bogduk N, et al. The pathophysiology of disc degeneration: a critical review. *J Bone Joint Surg* 2008;90-B(10):1261–1270.
37. Adams MA, McNally DS, Wagstaff J, et al. Abnormal stress concentrations in lumbar intervertebral discs following damage to the vertebral bodies: cause of disc failure? *Eur Spine J* 1993;1:214–221.
38. McNally DS, Adams MA. Intervertebral disc mechanics as revealed by stress profilometry. *Spine* 1992;17:66–73.
39. Crock HV. A reappraisal of intervertebral disc lesions. *Med J Aust* 1970;1:983–989.
40. Crock HV. Internal disc disruption: a challenge to disc prolapse fifty years on. *Spine* 1986;11:650–653.
41. Bogduk N. The lumbar disc and low back pain. *Neurosurg Clin North Am* 1991;2:791–806.
42. McNally DS, Shackleford IM, Goodship AE, et al. In vivo stress measurement can predict pain on discography. *Spine* 1996;21:2580–2587.
43. Vanharanta H, Sachs BL, Spivey MA, et al. The relationship of pain provocation to lumbar disc deterioration as seen by CT/discography. *Spine* 1987;12:295–298.
44. Moneta GB, Videman T, Kaivanto K, et al. Reported pain during lumbar discography as a function of anular ruptures and disc degeneration: a reanalysis of 833 discograms. *Spine* 1994;17:1968–1974.
45. Schwarzer AC, Aprill CN, Derby R, et al. The prevalence and clinical features of internal disc disruption in patients with chronic low back pain. *Spine* 1995;20:1878–1883.
46. Sluijter ME. Radiofrequency lesions of the communicating ramus in the treatment of low back pain. In: Racz G, ed. *Techniques of Neurolysis*. Boston: Kluwer Academic Publishers; 1989:145–159.
47. Oh WS, Shim JC. A randomized controlled trial of radiofrequency denervation of the ramus communicans nerve for chronic discogenic low back pain. *Clin J Pain* 2004;20:55–60.
48. Van Kleef M, Barendse GAM, Wilmink JT. Percutaneous intradiscal radiofrequency thermocoagulation in chronic non-specific low back pain. *Pain Clin* 1996;9:259–268.
49. Troussier B, Lebas JF, Chirossel JP, et al. Percutaneous intradiscal radiofrequency thermocoagulation: a cadaveric study. *Spine* 1995;20:1713–1718.
50. Houpt JC, Conner ES, McFarland EW. Experimental study of temperature distributions and thermal transport during radiofrequency current therapy of the intervertebral disc. *Spine* 1996;21:1808–1813.
51. Barendse GA, van den Berg SG, Kessels AH, et al. Randomized controlled trial of percutaneous intradiscal radiofrequency thermocoagulation for chronic discogenic back pain: lack of effect from a 90-second 70°C lesion. *Spine* 2001;26:287–292.
52. Kline MT. Radiofrequency techniques in clinical practice. In: Waldman SD, Winnie AP, eds. *Interventional Pain Management*. 1st ed. Philadelphia: WB Saunders Company; 1996:185–217.
53. Kline MT, Yin W. Radiofrequency techniques in clinical practice. In: Waldman S, ed. *Interventional Pain Management*. 2nd ed. Philadelphia: WB Saunders Company; 2001:243–293.
54. Ruiz-Lopez R, Pichot C. Percutaneous therapeutic procedures for disc lesions. In: Raj P, Lou L, Erdine S, et al, eds. *Interventional Pain Management: Image Guided Procedures*. 2nd ed. Philadelphia: WB Saunders Company;2008:560.
55. Kleinstueck FS, Diederich CJ, Nau WH, et al. Acute biomechanical and histo-

logical effects of intradiscal electrothermal therapy on human lumbar discs. *Spine* 2001;26(20):2198–2207.

56. Kleinstueck FS, Diederich CJ, Nau WH, et al. Temperature and thermal dose distributions during intradiscal electrothermal therapy in the cadaveric lumbar spine. *Spine* 2003;28:1700–1708.

57. Freeman BJ, Walters RM, Moore RJ, et al. Does intradiscal electrothermal therapy denervate and repair experimentally induced posterolateral annular tears in an animal model? *Spine* 2003;28(23):2602–2608.

58. Karasek M, Bogduk N. Intradiscal electrothermal annuloplasty: percutaneous treatment of chronic discogenic low back pain. *Tech Reg Anesth Pain Manag* 2001;5:130–135.

59. Bogduk N, Lau P, Govind J, et al. Intradiscal electrothermal therapy. *Tech Reg Anesth Pain Manag* 2005;9:25–34.

60. Freeman BJ. IDET: a critical appraisal of the evidence. *Eur Spine J* 2006; 15(suppl 3):S448–S457.

61. Andersson GB, Mekhail NA, Block JE. Treatment of intractable discogenic low back pain. A systematic review of spinal fusion and intradiscal electrothermal therapy (IDET). *Pain Physician* 2006;9:237–248.

62. Andersson GB, Mekhail NA, Block JE. Intradiscal electrothermal therapy (IDET). *Spine* 2006;31:1402; author reply 1402–1403.

63. Appleby D, Anderson G, Totta M. Meta-analysis of the efficacy and safety of intradiscal electrothermal therapy (IDET). *Pain Med* 2006;7:308–316.

64. Kapural L, Makhail N, Korunda Z, et al. Intradiscal thermal annuloplasty for the treatment of lumbar discogenic pain in patients with multilevel degenerative disc disease. *Anesth Analg* 2004;99:472–476.

65. Kapural L, Hayek S, Malak O, et al. Intradiscal thermal annuloplasty versus intradiscal radiofrequency ablation for the treatment of discogenic pain: a prospective matched control trial. *Pain Med* 2005;6:425–431.

66. Karasek M, Bogduk N. Twelve-month follow-up of a controlled trial of intradiscal thermal anuloplasty for back pain due to internal disc disruption. *Spine* 2000;25:2601–2607.

67. Bogduk N, Karasek M. Two-year follow-up of a controlled trial of intradiscal electrothermal anuloplasty for chronic low back pain resulting from internal disc disruption. *Spine J* 2002;2:343–350.

68. Lutz C, Lutz GE, Cooke PM. Treatment of chronic lumbar diskogenic pain with intradiskal electrothermal therapy: a prospective outcome study. *Arch Phys Med Rehabil* 2003;84:23–28.

69. Maurer P, Block JE, Squillante D. Intradiscal electrothermal therapy (IDET) provides effective symptom relief in patients with discogenic low back pain. *J Spinal Disord Tech* 2008;21:55–62.

70. Nunley PD, Jawahar A, Brandao SM, et al. Intradiscal electrothermal therapy (IDET) for low back pain in worker's compensation patients: can it provide a potential answer? Long-term results. *J Spinal Disord Tech* 2008;21:11–18.

71. Lee MS, Cooper G, Lutz GE, et al. Intradiscal electrothermal therapy (IDET) for treatment of chronic lumbar discogenic pain: a minimum 2-year clinical outcome study. *Pain Physician* 2003;6:443–448.

72. Saal JA, Saal JS. Intradiscal electrothermal treatment for chronic discogenic low back pain. A prospective outcome study with minimum 1-year follow-up. *Spine* 2000;25:2622–2627.

73. Saal JA, Saal JS. Intradiscal electrothermal treatment for chronic discogenic low back pain. Prospective outcome study with a minimum 2-year follow-up. *Spine* 2002;27:966–974.

74. Cohen SP, Larkin T, Abdi S, et al. Risk factors for failure and complications of intradiscal electrothermal therapy: a pilot study. *Spine* 2003;28:1142–1147.

75. Pauza KJ, Howell S, Dreyfuss P, et al. A randomized, placebo-controlled trial of intradiscal electrothermal therapy for the treatment of discogenic low back pain. *Spine J* 2004;4:27–35.

76. Freeman BJ, Fraser RD, Cain CM, et al. A randomized, double-blind, controlled trial: intradiscal electrothermal therapy versus placebo for the treatment of chronic discogenic low back pain. *Spine* 2005;30:2369–2377; discussion 2378.

77. Chen YC, Lee SH, Chen D. Intradiscal pressure study of percutaneous disc decompression with nucleoplasty in human cadavers. *Spine* 2003;28:661–665.

78. O'Neill CW, Liu JJ, Leibenberg E, et al. Percutaneous plasma decompression alters cytokine expression in injured porcine intervertebral discs. *Spine J* 2004; 4:88–98.

79. Mirzai H, Tekin I, Yaman O, et al. The results of nucleoplasty in patients with lumbar herniated disc: a prospective clinical study of 52 consecutive patients. *Spine J* 2007;7:88–92.

80. Sharps LS, Isaac Z. Percutaneous disc decompression using nucleoplasty. *Pain Physician* 2002;5:121–126.

81. Yakovlev A, Tamimi MA, Liang H, et al. Outcomes of percutaneous disc decompression utilizing nucleoplasty for the treatment of chronic discogenic pain. *Pain Physician* 2007;10:319–328.

82. Singh V, Piryani C, Liao K, et al. Percutaneous disc decompression using coblation (Nucleoplasty) in the treatment of chronic discogenic pain. *Pain Physician* 2002;5:250–259.

83. Gerszten PC, Welch WC, King JT Jr. Quality of life assessment in patients undergoing nucleoplasty-based percutaneous discectomy. *J Neurosurg Spine* 2006;4:36–42.

84. Calisaneller T, Ozdemir O, Karadeli E, et al. Six months post-operative clinical and 24 hour post-operative MRI examinations after nucleoplasty with radiofrequency energy. *Acta Neurochir (Wien)* 2007;149:495–500.

85. Masala S, Massari F, Fabiano S, et al. Nucleoplasty in the treatment of lumbar diskogenic back pain: one year follow-up. *Cardiovasc Intervent Radiol* 2007; 30:426–432.

86. Feffer HL. Treatment of low-back and sciatic pain by the injection of hydrocortisone into degenerated intervertebral discs. *J Bone Joint Surg Am* 1956; 38-A:585–590.

87. Feffer HL. Therapeutic intradiscal hydrocortisone. A long-term study. *Clin Orthop Relat Res* 1969;67:100–104.

88. Graham CE. Chemonucleolysis: a double blind study comparing chemo-

89. nucleolysis with intra discal hydrocortisone: in the treatment of backache and sciatica. *Clin Orthop Relat Res* 1976;117:179–192.

89. Wilkinson HA, Schuman N. Intradiscal corticosteroids in the treatment of lumbar and cervical disc problems. *Spine* 1980;5:385–389.

90. Simmons JW, McMillin JN, Emery SF, et al. Intradiscal steroids. A prospective double-blind clinical trial. *Spine* 1992;17:S172–S175.

91. Khot A, Bowditch M, Powell J, et al. The use of intradiscal steroid therapy for lumbar spinal discogenic pain: a randomized controlled trial. *Spine* 2004; 29:833–836.

92. Fayad F, Lefevre-Colau MM, Rannou F, et al. Relation of inflammatory Modic changes to intradiscal steroid injection outcome in chronic low back pain. *Eur Spine J* 2007;16:925–931.

93. Cohen SP, Wenzell D, Hurley RW, et al. A double-blind, placebo-controlled, dose-response pilot study evaluating intradiscal eternacept in patients with chronic discogenic low back pain or lumbosacral radiculopathy. *Anesthesiology* 2007;107:99–105.

94. Peng B, Zhang Y, Hou S, et al. Intradiscal methylene blue injection for the treatment of chronic discogenic low back pain. *Eur Spine J* 2007;16:33–38.

95. Alexandre A, Buric J, Paradiso R, et al. Il trattamento delle ernie discali lombari con iniezione intradiscale di O2-O3. *Rivista Italiana di Ossigeno-Ozonoterapia* 2002;1(2):165–169.

96. Gjonovich A, Sattin GF, Girotto L, et al. Lombalgie ribelli: l'ossigneo-ozono terapia a confronto con altre metodiche. *Rivista di Neuroradiologia* 2001; 14(suppl 1):35–38.

97. Leonardi M, Simonetti L, Barabara C. Effetti dell'ozono sul nucleo polposo: reperti anatomo-patologici su un caso operato. *Rivista di Neuroradiologia* 2001;14(suppl 1):57–59.

98. Andreula CF. Ernie discali lombosacrali e patologia degenerativa correlata. Trattamento interventistico spinale con chemiodiscolisi con nucleoptesi con O3 e infiltrazione periradicolare e periganglionare. *Rivista di Neuroradiolgia* 2001;14(suppl 1): 81–88.

99. Andreula C, Kambas I. Il dolore lombosacrale da ernie discali lombosacrali e patologia degenerativa correlata. Trattamento interventistico spinale con chemiodiscolisi con miscela di ossigeno-ozono e infiltrazione periradicolare e periganglionare. Personale esperienza su 500 casi. *Rivista di Italiana di Ossigeno-Ozonoterapia* 2003;2:21–30.

100. Scarchilli A. Tre anni di follow-up nel trattamento delle lobalgie e lobosciatalgie con ozonoterapia intradiscale. *Rivista di Neuroradiologia* 2001;14(suppl 1):39–41.

101. Andreula CF, Simonetti L, De Santis F, et al. Minimally invasive oxygen-ozone therapy for lumbar disk herniation. *AJNR Am J Neuroradiol* 2003; 24:996–1000.

102. Muto M, Andreula C, Leonardi M. Treatment of herniated disc by intradiscal and intraforaminal oxygen-ozone (O2-O3) injection. *J Neuroradiol* 2004;31: 183–189.

103. Buric J, Molino Lova R. Ozone chemonucleolysis in non-contained lumbar disc herniations: a pilot study with 12 months follow-up. *Acta Neurochir Suppl* 2005;92:93–97.

104. Gallucci M, Limbucci N, Zugaro L, et al. Sciatica: treatment with intradiscal and intraforaminal injections of steroids and oxygen-ozone versus steroid only. *Radiology* 2007;242:907–913.

105. Richelmi P, Valdenassi L, Berte F. Basi farmacologiche dell'azione dell'ossigeno-zono terapia. *Rivista di Neuroradiologia* 2001;14(suppl 1):17–22.

106. Iliakis E, Valadakis V, Vynios DH, et al. Efetti biochimici e istoligici dell'ozono sul disco intervertebrale. *Rivista di Neuroradiologia* 2001;14(suppl 1):23–30.

107. Leonardi M, Barabara C, Agati R, et al. Trattamento percutaneo dell'ernia discale lobare con iniezione intradiscale di miscela di ozono. *Rivista di Neuroradiologia* 2001;14(suppl 1):51–53.

108. Lo Giudice G, Valdi F, Gismondi M, et al. Acute bilateral vitreo-retinal hemorrhages following oxygen-ozone therapy for lumbar disk herniation. *Am J Ophthalmol* 2004;138:175–177.

109. Ginanneschi F, Cervelli C, Milani P, et al. Ventral and dorsal root injury after oxygen-ozone therapy for lumbar disk herniation. *Surg Neurol* 2006; 66:619–20; discussion 20–21.

110. Gazzeri R, Galarza M, Neroni M, et al. Fulminating septicemia secondary to oxygen-ozone therapy for lumbar disc herniation: case report. *Spine* 2007; 32:E121–E123.

111. Klein RG, Eek BC, O'Neill CW, et al. Biochemical injection treatment for discogenic low back pain: a pilot study. *Spine J* 2003;3:220–226.

112. Derby R, Eek B, Lee SH, et al. Comparison of intradiscal restorative injections and intradiscal electrothermal treatment (IDET) in the treatment of low back pain. *Pain Physician* 2004;7:63–66.

113. Miller MR, Mathews RS, Reeves KD. Treatment of painful advanced internal lumbar disc derangement with intradiscal injection of hypertonic dextrose. *Pain Physician* 2006;9:115–121.

114. Thompson JP, Oegema TR Jr, Bradford DS. Stimulation of mature canine intervertebral disc by growth factors. *Spine* 1991;16:253–260.

115. Gruber HE, Norton HJ, Hanley EN Jr. Anti-apoptotic effects of IGF-1 and PDGF on human intervertebral disc cells in vitro. *Spine* 2000;25:2153–2157.

116. An HS, Takegami K, Kamada H, et al. Intradiscal administration of osteogenic protein-1 increases intervertebral disc height and proteoglycan content in the nucleus pulposus in normal adolescent rabbits. *Spine* 2005;30:25–31; discussion 31–32.

117. Masuda K, Imai Y, Okuma M, et al. Osteogenic protein-1 injection into a degenerated disc induces the restoration of disc height and structural changes in the rabbit anular puncture model. *Spine* 2006;31:742–754.

118. Imai Y, Okuma M, An HS, et al. Restoration of disc height loss by recombinant human osteogenic protein-1 injection into intervertebral discs undergo-

ing degeneration induced by an intradiscal injection of chondroitinase ABC. *Spine* 2007;32:1197–1205.

119. Nishida K, Kang JD, Suh JK, et al. Adenovirus-mediated gene transfer to nucleus pulposus cells. Implications for the treatment of intervertebral disc degeneration. *Spine* 1998;23:2437–2442; discussion 2443.

110. Nishida K, Kang JD, Gilbertson LG, et al. Modulation of the biologic activity of the rabbit intervertebral disc by gene therapy: an in vivo study of adenovirus-mediated transfer of the human transforming growth factor beta 1 encoding gene. *Spine* 1999;24:2419–2425.

111. Ganey T, Libera J, Moos V, et al. Disc chondrocyte transplantation in a canine model: a treatment for degenerated or damaged intervertebral disc. *Spine* 2003;28:2609–2620.

112. Okuma M, Mochida J, Nishimura K, et al. Reinsertion of stimulated nucleus pulposus cells retards intervertebral disc degeneration: an in vitro and in vivo experimental study. *J Orthop Res* 2000;18:988–997.

113. Nomura T, Mochida J, Okuma M, et al. Nucleus pulposus allograft retards intervertebral disc degeneration. *Clin Orthop Relat Res* 2001:94–101.

114. Nishimura K, Mochida J. Percutaneous reinsertion of the nucleus pulposus. An experimental study. *Spine* 1998;23:1531–1538; discussion 1539.

115. Meisel HJ, Ganey T, Hutton WC, et al. Clinical experience in cell-based therapeutics: intervention and outcome. *Eur Spine J* 2006;15(suppl 3):S397–S405.

116. Meisel HJ, Siodla V, Ganey T, et al. Clinical experience in cell-based therapeutics: disc chondrocyte transplantation. A treatment for degenerated or damaged intervertebral disc. *Biomol Eng* 2007;24:5–21.

117. Hiyama A, Mochida J, Iwashina T, et al. Transplantation of mesenchymal stem cells in a canine disc degeneration model. *J Orthop Res* 2008;26:589–600.

118. Sakai D, Mochida J, Iwashina T, et al. Regenerative effects of transplanting mesenchymal stem cells embedded in atelocollagen to the degenerated intervertebral disc. *Biomaterials* 2006;27:335–345.

119. Sakai D, Mochida J, Iwashina T, et al. Differentiation of mesenchymal stem cells transplanted to a rabbit degenerative disc model: potential and limitations for stem cell therapy in disc regeneration. *Spine* 2005;30:2379–2387.

120. Richardson SM, Walker RV, Parker S, et al. Intervertebral disc cell-mediated mesenchymal stem cell differentiation. *Stem Cells* 2006;24:707–716.

121. Risbud MV, Albert TJ, Guttapalli A, et al. Differentiation of mesenchymal stem cells toward a nucleus pulposus-like phenotype in vitro: implications for cell-based transplantation therapy. *Spine* 2004;29:2627–2632.

122. Boden SD, Davis DO, Dina TS, et al. Abnormal magnetic-resonance scans of the lumbar spine in asymptomatic subjects. A prospective investigation. *J Bone Joint Surg Am* 1990;72:403–408.

123. Jensen MC, Brant-Zawadzki MN, Obuchowski N, et al. Magnetic resonance imaging of the lumbar spine in people without back pain. *N Engl J Med* 1994;331:69–73.

124. Boos N, Rieder R, Schade V, et al. 1995 Volvo Award in clinical sciences. The diagnostic accuracy of magnetic resonance imaging, work perception, and psychosocial factors in identifying symptomatic disc herniations. *Spine* 1995;20:2613–2625.

125. Boos N, Semmer N, Elfering A, et al. Natural history of individuals with asymptomatic disc abnormalities in magnetic resonance imaging: predictors of low back pain-related medical consultation and work incapacity. *Spine* 2000;25:1484–1492.

126. Elfering A, Semmer N, Birkhofer D, et al. Risk factors for lumbar disc degeneration: a 5-year prospective MRI study in asymptomatic individuals. *Spine* 2002;27:125–134.

127. Modic MT, Ross JS. Lumbar degenerative disk disease. *Radiology* 2007;245:43–61.

128. Mizuno H, Roy AK, Vacanti CA, et al. Tissue-engineered composites of anulus fibrosus and nucleus pulposus for intervertebral disc replacement. *Spine* 2004;29:1290–1297; discussion 1297–1298.

129. Sakai D, Mochida J, Iwashina T, et al. Differentiation of mesenchymal stem cells transplanted to a rabbit degenerative disc model: potential and limitations for stem cell therapy in disc regeneration. *Spine* 2005;30:2379–2387.

130. Richardson SM, Walker RV, Parker S, et al. Intervertebral disc cell-mediated mesenchymal stem cell differentiation. *Stem Cells* 2006;24:707–716.

131. Risbud MV, Albert TJ, Guttapalli A, et al. Differentiation of mesenchymal stem cells towards a nucleus pulposus-like phenotype in vitro: implications for cell-based transplantation therapy. *Spine* 2004;29:2627–2632.

132. Boden S, Davis D, Dina T, et al. Abnormal magnetic-resonance scans of the lumbar spine in asymptomatic subjects. A prospective investigation. *J Bone Joint Surg Am* 1990;72:403–408.

133. Jensen MC, Brant-Zawadzki MN, Obuchowski N, et al. Magnetic resonance imaging of the lumbar spine in people without back pain. *N Engl J Med* 1994;331:69–73.

134. Boos N, Rieder R, Schade V, et al. 1995 Volvo Award in clinical sciences. The diagnostic accuracy of magnetic resonance imaging, work perception, and psychosocial factors in identifying symptomatic disc herniations. *Spine* 1995;20:2613–2625.

135. Boos N, Semmer N, Elfering A, et al. Natural history of individuals with asymptomatic disc abnormalities in magnetic resonance imaging: predictors of low back pain-related medical consultation and work incapacity. *Spine* 2000;25:1484–1492.

136. Elfering A, Semmer N, Birkhofer D, et al. Risk factors for lumbar disc degeneration: a 5-year prospective MRI study in asymptomatic individuals. *Spine* 2002;27:125–134.

137. Modic MT, Ross JS. Lumbar degenerative disk disease. *Radiology* 2007;245:43–61.

138. Mizuno H, Roy AK, Vacanti CA, et al. Tissue-engineered composites of anulus fibrosus and nucleus pulposus for intervertebral disc replacement. *Spine* 2004;29:1290–1297; discussion 1297–1298.

CHAPTER 101 ■ NEUROLYTIC BLOCKADE FOR NONCANCER PAIN

JAYANTILAL GOVIND† AND NIKOLAI BOGDUK

INTRODUCTION

Definition

Stedman's Medical Dictionary defines neurolysis as either the selective, iatrogenic destruction of neural tissue to secure the relief of pain, or a procedure in which the nerve is electively freed surgically from inflammatory tissue.[1] This chapter deals with the former half of this definition. It covers using chemical or physical means to damage peripheral nerves focally in order to prevent the transmission of nociceptive information along the target nerve so as to provide relief of pain. Surgical interventions are described in Chapter 104.

Etymologically, the term "neurolysis" actually means teasing apart or dissolving a nerve and "neurotomy" means opening a nerve, but no superior term has been advanced and accepted to refer to producing focal damage to a nerve while leaving it intact. In this chapter, the term "neurolytic blockade" has been adopted as a general term to refer to all procedures whose intent is to prevent the conduction of nociceptive traffic along the treated nerve. Reflecting convention, rather than good etymolog-

---

†Dr. Govind worked assiduously to compose this chapter and he considered it a great honor to be able to contribute to the Bonica text. Sadly, he did not see the culmination of his work. He passed away on the 20th of June, 2009. In Australia he is remembered as someone who strove to have interventional pain medicine accountable to the evidence. N. Bogduk.

ical practice, "neurolysis" has been retained in the context of chemical procedures and "neurotomy" in the context of physical procedures.

PRINCIPLES

Neurolytic blockade is a therapeutic option when the actual source of pain cannot be treated. The objective is to relieve the pain by blocking the nerves that transmit nociception from its source.

The primary indication for neurolytic blockade is complete relief of pain when the target is anesthetized temporarily with controlled, local anesthetics (see Chapter 97). Longer-lasting relief can then be achieved using chemical or physical agents.

Of the chemical agents, phenol and alcohol are the most commonly used, and there are no comparative data by which to choose between the two. Glycerol has a special application in the management of trigeminal neuralgia.

Of the physical modalities, heat and cold have both been used to interrupt conduction along peripheral nerves. In both instances, an electrode is placed on the nerve and used to produce a small lesion that incorporates a segment of the nerve. Cold lesions (cryoneurotomy) are produced by passing carbon dioxide through the electrode. Thermal lesion (thermal neurotomy) are produced by passing a radiofrequency (RF) current through the electrode. Variants of RF neurotomy have been developed in which the emphasis lies in the frequency and modulation of the current applied rather than the heat that it generates.

History and Trends

The earliest form of neurolytic blockade was surgical neurectomy in which the nerves from a source of pain were simply transected. This approach has largely been abandoned for several reasons: neurectomy did not achieve long-term results, and when pain returned the procedure could not be repeated; painful neuromas could develop on the proximal stump of transected nerve; and transecting large nerves could result in deafferentation pain.

Chemical and physical neurolytic blockades were developed to overcome or circumvent these problems. Neuroma-formation could be avoided by not transecting the nerve. If the nerve recovered and pain recurred, the neurolytic procedure could be repeated. Small nerves, not readily accessed surgically, could be targeted with electrodes or injections in order to avoid having to target their larger, parent nerves.

Limitations

Classical pathology teaching describes how nerves recover after they have been transected. Wallerian degeneration occurs in the distal stump and is completed within 24 hours in small nerve fibers and in 48 hours in larger nerve fibers. In the proximal stump, regeneration of axon tubules occurs within hours of the transection. The process is driven by neurotrophic agents, such as tumour necrosis factor alpha, T cells, macrophages, leukocyte inhibitory factor, and cell adhesion molecules, which are expressed in a highly coordinated fashion.[2–4] A growth cone, containing mitochondria, vesicular elements, neurofilaments, and endoplasmic reticulum, emerges from the proximal stump, and proceeds into the distal stump, if it is accessible; Schwann Cells undergo mitotic activity and form a framework for developing fibers.[2] Regeneration occurs at a rate of approximately 1 mm per day, so that reinnervation of a structure 5 cm away would take approximately 50 days. This process requires an intact dorsal

root ganglion to synthesize the regenerative proteins and other nutrients.

Neurolytic blockade involves a different pathology, much of which has not been explored and explained. The differences arise according to where in the nerve the lesion is made, the nature of the lesion, and its size.

If the dorsal root ganglion is destroyed, regeneration will not occur because the cell nucleus is not available to drive the process. Consequently, permanent relief of pain (but also permanent side effects and complications) can be expected from neurolytic procedures that target a dorsal root ganglion.

If a peripheral nerve is targeted, chemical neurolysis does not destroy it. Instead, the chemical applied denatures the components of the axons in one way or another focally. Chemicals can bind to membrane proteins or other elements, or they can exert an osmotic effect which focally desiccates the nerve. The nerve can recover from such processes. All that is required is that the damaged elements be replaced in the normal course of maintenance of the cell membrane or other constituents. The rate at which this happens, however, has not been established.

Cryoneurotomy works by freezing intracellular water; the ice expands and essentially fractures the nerve membrane, thereby preventing conduction along it. From this effect, the nerve can recover by reconstituting the damaged segment of membrane. This process appears to be relatively fast: it is measurable in weeks.

Thermal RF neurotomy denatures all the proteins in the segment of nerve incorporated in the lesion made. Nevertheless, the nerve remains macroscopically intact. Regeneration does not occur by classical processes because the nerve is sealed by the coagulated proteins, not transected and left open. Therefore, growth cones cannot emerge. Before the nerve can regenerate, the coagulated material has to be removed by endocellular repair mechanisms. The rate of this process has not been determined, but appears to be measurable in months, based on the duration of effect of thermal RF neurotomy. Critical in this regard is the length of nerve affected. It is axiomatic that if a short segment (1–2 mm) is coagulated, recovery will be faster than if a longer segment (10–15 mm) is coagulated.

CHEMICAL NEUROLYTIC BLOCKADE

Principles

Phenol, alcohol, and glycerol are locally neurotoxic in a dose-dependent manner. These dehydrating agents cause a nonselective destruction of neuronal tissues followed by necrosis, nonsegmental demyelination, Wallerian degeneration, and complete conduction block, occurring within 10 minutes of application.[5–15]

Phenol

First introduced by Lister in 1867 as an antiseptic, phenol (carbolic acid) is a neurolytic agent with local anesthetic properties. Concentrations of less than 1% produce local anesthesia without toxicity or neurolysis and may be used as a topical anesthetic. In higher doses (>8.5 g) phenol causes central nervous depression and cardiovascular collapse.[7] Phenol can be injected directly onto peripheral nerves or into the subarachnoid space in order to target dorsal root ganglia. Nonselective neuronal destruction leading to Wallerian degeneration is its principle mode of action.

Alcohol

Alcohol (absolute alcohol, ethanol, ethyl alcohol) is a clear volatile hygroscopic liquid[9] that exerts its analgesic effect by non-selective neuronal destruction.[10–12] Because of its irritant effect, alcohol may exacerbate local pain on injection and may produce dose-dependent burning and dysesthesia. Prior injection of local anesthetic may minimize this effect. Alcohol has produced variable results and some consider the risk of complications outweighs its benefits.[10]

Applications

Alcohol or phenol have been widely used to perform neurolytic blockades of various parts of the sympathetic nervous system of the abdomen. Targets have included the lumbar sympathetic trunks and the splanchnic nerves but most commonly the celiac plexus and ganglia. Indications have included pain due to carcinoma of the pancreas or chronic pancreatitis, and pain due to various types of abdominal or pelvic cancers.

Various techniques are available by which to block the celiac plexus, ranging between anterior or posterior approaches, using fluoroscopy, computed tomography, or endoscopic ultrasound for guidance.[16] For cancer pain in general, one review found that neurolytic celiac plexus blocks provided benefit for 70% to 90% of patients until death or beyond 3 months, regardless of the technique used.[17] Others, however, have warned of a narrow risk-benefit ratio.[18] Neurolytic blocks of the celiac plexus, superior hypogastric plexus, or lumbar sympathetic chain, supplemented by drug therapy, are each more effective than drug therapy alone.[19]

For patients with unresectable carcinoma of the pancreas, a review concluded that neurolytic celiac plexus blocks reduced pain and analgesic consumption, but although improvements were significant statistically, they were of minimal clinical significance.[20] A strong, controlled study found that neurolytic celiac plexus blocks reduced pain significantly more than systemic analgesic therapy and a sham injection, but did not significantly reduce opioid consumption or improve quality of life.[21] Neurolytic plexus blocks are more effective in patients with carcinoma of the head of the pancreas than in patients with carcinoma of the tail, but are not effective in patients with advanced tumour proliferation.[22]

For the pain of chronic pancreatitis, the evidence is less robust and less heartening. Response rates are low,[16] and unequivocal data on efficacy and long-term outcomes are lacking.[23]

Descriptive studies promoted neurolytic lumbar sympathetic blocks as a worthwhile treatment for rest pain in patients with peripheral vascular disease, particularly those in whom surgery could not be performed.[24,25] A controlled trial showed that neurolytic blocks were far more effective than local anesthetic blocks.[26]

Phenol or alcohol can be injected intrathecally in order to target particular nerve roots. Mixing the neurolytic agent with glycerine produces a hyperbaric solution, which can be guided under gravity to the target nerve or nerves. Adding contrast medium to the solution allows the movement of the solution to be monitored. With skillful technique, the solution can even be guided into a single nerve-root pouch by appropriately tilting the patient. As a treatment for cancer pain, such injections have been promoted in case reports and book chapters, but there have been no controlled trials.[27] The treatment provides complete relief of pain in up to half of the patients treated.[28] The duration of effect is measurable in weeks or months, which may be sufficient for patients with short life-expectancy.

For the treatment of lumbar zygapophysial joint pain, in one trial 42% of the study sample reported more than 80% pain relief over a mean period of 6.2 years (range 1–10), and litigation made no difference to the outcomes.[29] These claims have not been corroborated by any other study.

Glycerol

Propane-1,2,3-triol, or glycerol, is a colorless, hygroscopic, syrupy liquid,[13] which has a unique application in the management of trigeminal neuralgia. Percutaneous retrogasserian glycerol rhizolysis is achieved by the instilling, under fluoroscopic guidance, no more than 0.3 mL into the Gasserian cistern. Glycerol nonselectively damages both the axons and the myelin sheath,[14] and 30% to 76% of patients suffer sensory loss.[15] Some achieve good pain relief without detectable facial numbness.[30] Onset of analgesia takes about 1 to 10 days to occur, but can be delayed for up to 6 weeks.[31] It provides excellent pain relief while largely sparing trigeminal nerve function in most patients.[31] As many as 72% of patients can be totally free of pain for 3 years, and in one series, 60% remained pain free for more than 10 years after a single injection.[30] Within the first year, 10% to 53% recur,[31] while 25% to 83% recur between 2 and 5 years.[32] These long durations of effect are concordant with the trigeminal ganglion being the target of the treatment. Damaging ganglion cells prevents or impedes regeneration of the peripheral nerve fibers that they subtend.

Glycerol is preferred when pain is localized to the first division as it rarely produces corneal anaesthesia, but the overall efficacy is less than for RF neurotomy.[33] In the elderly or where microvascular decompression is contraindicated, glycerol gangliolysis is safer, more effective than stereotactic surgery, and is more cost-effective.[34]

CRYONEUROTOMY

Cryoneurotomy relieves pain by causing a variable degree of nerve injury. Freezing is achieved by a simultaneous reduction in pressure and temperature as expanding carbon dioxide is forced through a specialized probe. An ice ball averaging 3.5 to 5.5 mm in diameter rapidly forms at temperatures as low as $-50°$ C to $-70°$ C. Subzero temperatures cause nonselective but reversible conduction block, and the effect is prolonged when the intracellular contents are crystallized. There is little clinical difference provided that the temperature is maintained below $-20°$ C for 1 minute.[35,36]

Nerve injury is dose-dependent and ranges from a mild neurapraxia to changes of Wallerian degeneration, associated with very minimal inflammatory reaction. Within a few days of freezing, the lesion is seen as a dense cellular matrix of macrophages.[37] In contrast to chemical neurolysis, painful neuromas, neuritis, or dysesthesia are avoided as exact regeneration is facilitated by an intact epineurium and perineurium.[35,36] The duration of the block depends on the rate of nerve regeneration at the proximal stump, which averages 1 to 3 mm per day.[35,36] Cryolesioning is a safe, simple, and repeatable procedure: it produces a temporary block and its therapeutic effect may last for many weeks. The main disadvantage is that the relief of pain is often of short duration and is unpredictable.[38]

Cryotherapy is an effective adjunct to the pharmacologic management of trigeminal neuralgia when other more invasive treatments are contraindicated. In most patients, the relief of pain is immediate, and in one series, at least 58% remained pain free for 12 months with a mean time to recurrence of 20 months.[39]

For chronic lumbar zygapophysial joint pain, modest outcomes have been noted in two studies. One study claimed a 72% success rate 6 weeks after cryotherapy.[40] The other found that

62% of patients reported at least 50% relief of pain for 12 months, with parallel improvements in activities of daily living.[41]

Cryoneurotomy has been reported as useful for the management of postthoracotomy pain and intercostal neuralgia.[42] In these conditions, the short duration of relief obtained may be enough to render patients comfortable while natural healing occurs or other measures are implemented.

THERMAL RADIOFREQUENCY

Introduction

Thermal (continuous) percutaneous RF procedures have now evolved as one of the better and more practical neurosurgical procedures for the management of chronic disabling pain. With modern imaging and the development of sophisticated equipment, precise ablation of neural pathways is possible. When meticulously executed in correctly selected patients, the RF neurotomy with temperature monitoring has proven itself to be safer and more effective than any other procedure. The technique required principally depends on the source of nociception and the accessibility of the nerves that innervate it. Critical to its correct application is an understanding and appreciation of its limitations, the pathophysiology of the primary condition, and a valid diagnosis.

Physics

Thermal RF should not be confused with electrocautery. Tissues are not burned or oxidized. Rather, they are coagulated in situ by the application of a high-frequency, alternating electric field.[43] The objective of RF lesioning is to deliver sufficient heating power into biological tissue such that the tissue temperature is raised above the "lethal temperature" range of 45° to 50° C, since neural cells exposed to these temperatures for 20 seconds or more will be destroyed by heat.[44,45] This requires an RF generator, an insulated electrode with an exposed ("active") tip of 2 to 10 mm, and a ground or dispersive ("passive") plate with a large surface area. The electrode is placed either into (e.g., central nervous system) or onto (e.g., peripheral nerve) the target structure. The larger dispersive plate is positioned at a convenient location of the body remote from the electrode. The patient completes the electrical circuit and the generator delivers the alternating current between exposed tip of the insulated electrode and the large dispersive plate.

The passage of low-energy, high frequency alternating current (100,000–500,000 Hertz) causes intense oscillation of ions. This oscillation heats charged molecules, notably proteins.[46] The exposed, active tip of the electrode acts as an antenna around which the current concentrates into a greater density. Consequently, greater heating occurs in the tissues around the electrode, and it is the tissue about the electrode-tip, rather than the electrode itself, that becomes the source of heat. The tissues heat the electrode, and a thermocouple, built into the electrode, monitors the temperature generated. Once a certain temperature is reached, lesion formation ("coagulation") occurs.

Tissue temperature (T) is related directly to current density (I) but inversely to the fourth power of the radius (R) from the electrode (i.e., $T = IR^{-4}$). Current density is less at the distal tip of the electrode than at its sides. Therefore, the lesion extends little, if at all, in a longitudinal direction from the tip. Rather, it extends radially around the circumference of the exposed shaft and generally assumes the shape of a prolate spheroid (football).[46] However, because the tissue temperature drops rapidly

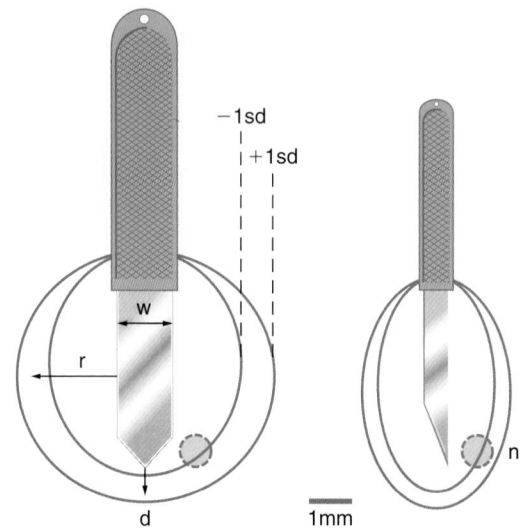

FIGURE 101.1 Longitudinal sections through thermal radiofrequency electrodes, showing the geometry of the lesions that they produce. The lesion has a transverse radius (r) that is proportional to the width (w) of the electrode. Less lesion is produced distally (d). For the same electrode on different occasions, the size of the lesion varies around a mean value in a normal distribution. Smaller electrodes generate smaller lesions. Smaller lesions may fail to incorporate a target nerve completely, even if the electrode is placed close to the nerve.

with distance from the electrode, the lesion is limited in size to 2 mm or less beyond the surface of the electrode (Fig. 101.1).

The physical variables that govern lesion size include current density, its rate of application, lesioning temperature, electrode size, the duration of heating, and impedance.[45–48] Temperature is the fundamental lesioning parameter and temperature monitoring remains central to the safety of the procedure and quantification of lesion size.[49,50] Because there is no consistent relation between temperature and voltage, temperature-controlled RF lesioning is preferred to voltage-controlled lesioning in order to create reproducible and well-defined lesion sizes.[51] The use of lower temperatures may not be acceptable in the clinical setting because it may not produce a permanent or long-term or sufficiently extensive lesion. Above 60° C,[52,53] soft tissues generally will coagulate, and if the surface temperature of the electrode is elevated to 80° to 85° C, then tissues within a short distance from the surface will be heated to 60° to 65° C or more. Once the electrode surface temperature reaches 80° C, lesion size increases with time as the temperature is maintained. Most of the increase in size occurs within 60 seconds, but an appreciable growth continues between 60 and 90 seconds.[53] After 90 seconds, further growth is prevented because the coagulated tissues present an increasing impedance (resistance) to flow of current and, therefore, the generation of any further lesion.

The lesion should be generated by increasing the temperature by about 1° C per second. This avoids cavitation, steam formation, microexplosions, and charring,[45–47] but more critically, in the event that the patient experiences adverse sensations, heating can be aborted promptly before any damage is done.

The size of the lesion is directly proportional to the diameter (width) of the electrode. Since lesions develop from the surface of the electrode, those formed by a larger electrode will reach further away from its center. Lesions made by small-diameter electrodes will extend only a short distance from their surface (see Fig. 101.1). In practice, the radius of a lesion is equal in length to between 1 and 2 times the width of the electrode used. Beyond this range, tissues may escape coagulation.[53]

Because electrodes generate lesions radially, they must be

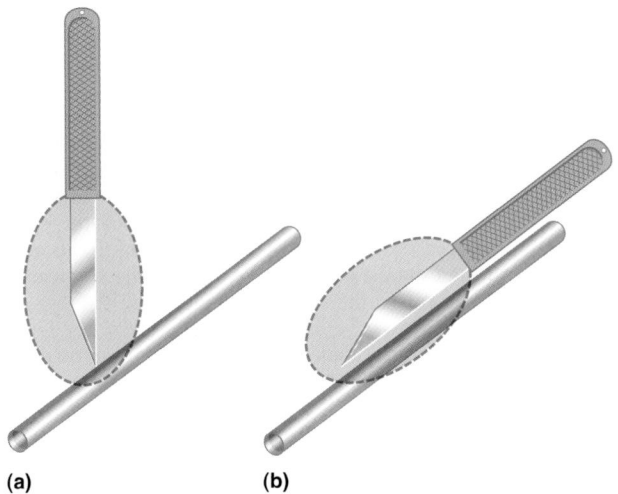

(a)   **(b)**

FIGURE 101.2 The influence of orientation on the effects of thermal radiofrequency neurotomy. **A.** If an electrode is placed perpendicular to the target nerve, it may coagulate the nerve only partially and for a short length because of the limited range over which the electrode generates a lesion distally. **B.** If an electrode is placed parallel to a nerve, it incorporates a large volume of the nerve along a greater length.

placed close and parallel to the target nerve in order for the lesion to be optimally effective.[52] If the electrode is placed perpendicular to the nerve, the lesion made may fail to incorporate the target nerve (Fig. 101.2). Throughout the lesioning process, the electrode must be held in place lest it dislodges, and its proper placement should be checked by periodic fluoroscopic monitoring.

Pathology

Heating by RF causes many cells to die rapidly at temperatures greater than 45° C. Similar effects are produced irrespective of whether the electrode is placed either inside the dorsal root ganglion or onto a peripheral nerve. Above 55° C, there is an indiscriminate destruction of both small and large myelinated fibers, focal necrosis, hemorrhages, extensive edema, and features of Wallerian degeneration.[54–59] Even with a low voltage of 0.1 V, an electrode placed inside a dorsal root ganglion and heated to 67° C causes a total loss of myelinated fibers with hemorrhage.[59]

Physiology

The study by Letcher and Goldring[60] is often misrepresented as showing that RF neurotomy selectively destroys small-diameter fibers, while preserving large-diameter fibers. Rather, what the study showed was that depression of C-fiber and A-δ fiber action potentials preceded depression of the potentials of A-β fibers, but within a short time, all fibers were ultimately and equally affected and the disappearance of action potentials was independent of fiber size. No class of fiber was exempt from the effects of heat.[60] These findings were confirmed in two independent, clinical studies which showed that RF neurotomy of the medial branches of the lumbar dorsal rami resulted in electromyographic abnormalities in over 80% of patients.[61,62] These abnormalities indicated that large-diameter, alpha motor neurons were not spared by RF neurotomy.

Applications

In general medicine, thermal RF is widely used for the treatment of supraventricular tachyarrhythmias.[63] Water-cooled electrodes

permit the generation of larger lesions to ablate thick ventricular muscle effectively.[64] In pain medicine, thermal RF has been used to treat trigeminal neuralgia, to interrupt pain pathways in the spinal cord or brainstem, and to treat various types of spinal pain and miscellaneous other types of pain.

Trigeminal Neuralgia

For the symptomatic treatment of trigeminal neuralgia, various descriptors, such as RF trigeminal neurolysis, RF thermocoagulation of the Gasserian ganglion, or retrogasserian thermorhizotomy, each refer to the generation of thermal lesions in an area between the trigeminal ganglion and its sensory root. Under fluoroscopic guidance, the electrode is introduced via the foramen ovale until the active tip sits at the posterior end of Meckel's cave, the average depth of insertion being 5 to 6 cm. Once the electrode appears to be adequately placed, a test electric stimulus is delivered to the nerve. If the electrode has been accurately placed, test stimulation will evoke pain in the area in which the patient normally experiences pain. Lesioning temperature may range between 55° and 90° C,[32,65,66] and the current may be applied either continuously for up to 300 seconds[65] or in 45 to 90 second cycles.[66]

The evidence of efficacy for trigeminal RF neurotomy consists of several large, observational studies, some encompassing over 1000 patients.[67] In one series, 41% of patients sustained relief for 20 years.[66] However, because of methodological inconsistencies, a recent systematic review[68] found only four studies on which sound conclusions could be based.[65,66,69,70] Nevertheless, collectively, these studies reaffirmed the general, favorable impression conveyed by the literature at large. Compared with other commonly used ablative techniques, RF neurotomy provided the highest rate of complete pain relief, and some 75% of patients were free of all pain for at least 6 months. At 12 months, RF provided a higher rate of complete pain relief than stereotactic radio-surgery.[68] In a later, unrelated study,[71] 90% of patients reported complete pain relief with their first RF, and a significant proportion continued to enjoy excellent relief some 15 years later. Presumably due to neuronal regeneration, the success rate diminishes and pain returns, such that just over 50% remain completely relieved at 5 years,[68] with a 14-year recurrence rate of 25% in one series.[71]

Common side effects are sensory loss sufficient to affect quality of life in more than 30% of patients, keratitis in some 10%, and dysesthesia in 4% to 10%. Although rare, reported complications include cranial nerve palsies, brain stem injury, meningitis, and vascular fistula formations (see also Chapter 106).[72–75]

Central Ablative Procedures

In conditions where pain is intractable and refractory to most forms of nonsurgical and minimally invasive intervention, relief may be secured by interrupting pathways in the spinal cord.[76] The most common target sites are the dorsal root entry zones, the spinothalamic tract, and trigeminal pathways.

Dorsal Root Entry Zone Lesions. Dorsal root entry zone (DREZ) lesioning is performed for the relief of central (deafferentation) and peripheral (neuropathic) pain caused by disease of peripheral nerves or injuries to them.[76,77] In these conditions, deafferentation results in spontaneous activity in the apical neurons of the dorsal grey column of the segments to which the affected nerves relay.[78] DREZ lesioning involves inserting a small electrode into this region in order to ablate the spontaneously active cells.[77] Multiple lesions are usually required in order to capture all the active neurons. Better outcomes are obtained when the dorsal root and the dorsal horn are primarily affected by the injury and both the pain and the pathology are topographically well-defined. Conversely, DREZ lesioning is contraindicated where pain is poorly localized because identifying the level at which the operation should be performed is difficult.[76] The ablative process includes the central portion of the dorsal root, the tract of Lissauer, and layers I–V of the dorsal horn. In this manner, the lateral portion of the dorsal horn, where C fibers predominate, is destroyed. By sparing the medial portion of the dorsal horn, tactile and proprioception senses are preserved.

Better outcomes are obtained if test electrical stimulation is used. Stimulation not only confirms the relevant segments but also identifies additional zones of dorsal horn electrical hyperactivity which would have been missed if topographical landmarks alone are used.[79,80]

Controlled trials have not been performed, but this may be understandable given the nature of the disorder and the nature of the intervention. Advocacy is based on multiple observational studies in which significant proportions of recipients report remarkable relief. DREZ lesioning has been particularly effective for the pain of brachial plexus avulsion with 66% to 87% patients affirming more than 70% relief,[81–85] and an appreciable proportion not requiring supplementary medication.[83] For traumatic spinal cord injuries, percentage relief of pain can range from at least 50% to complete relief with no limitation of activity or the need for opioids.[86,87] With respect to postamputation pain, the outcomes are better for phantom pain than for stump pain alone.[83] DREZ lesioning has not been particularly effective for postherpetic neuralgia. Some 18% to 47% report complete pain relief but such relief is not consistently maintained.[81] The close neuroanatomical relationship between the site of DREZ lesioning, the lateral corticospinal tract, and the dorsal column can lead to severe neurologic complications such as motor weakness, bladder or sexual dysfunction, and dysesthesia (see also Chapter 106).[88]

Cordotomy. Percutaneous cordotomy can be used to treat unilateral intractable pain transmitted by the lateral spinothalamic tract.[89] A lesion made in the antero-lateral segment of the spinal cord totally abolishes pain and temperature in one-half of the body below the lesion.[89] The procedure is typically performed percutaneously at the C1-C2 level, using a lateral approach to insert the electrode. Indications for these procedures have included severe neuropathic pain arising from brachial plexus root avulsion imitating phantom pain, electric burns, postherpetic neuralgia, and cancer pain.[90] In patients with cancer pain, some 70%[91] or more[92,93] initially obtain worthwhile relief. This relief wanes with time, but persists in most for the duration of remaining life (see also Chapter 104).

Trigeminal Procedures. Pain mediated by the trigeminal nerve can be treated by ablating various sites within the central nervous system, such the descending trigeminal tract (trigeminal tractotomy), the nucleus caudalis (trigeminal nucleotomy), or all of the substantia gelatinosa of the nucleus caudalis (nucleus caudalis dorsal root entry zone [NCDREZ]). Nociceptive type pain is most sensitive to NCDREZ ablation.[81]

Indications have included severe glossopharyngeal neuralgia, craniofacial dysesthesia, posttraumatic neuropathy, and anesthesia dolorosa.[90] For intractable facial pain, such as "end-stage" trigeminal neuralgia that has failed all other means of treatment including microvascular decompression,[81] NCDREZ lesioning has been successful in 60% to 70% of cases (see also Chapter 104).[94,95]

Medial Branch Neurotomy

Some forms of spinal pain are mediated by the medial branches of the dorsal rami. These nerves innervate the zygapophysial joints and certain paramedian posterior muscles of the vertebral column. Since there are no disorders known to affect, selectively, only particular segments of the back muscles, pain mediated by the medial branches is regarded as arising from the zygapophysial

joints. The actual source of pain, however, is immaterial, for the singular indication for medial branch RF neurotomy is complete relief of pain following controlled, diagnostic blocks of these nerves (see Chapter 97).[96–99]

The medial branches of the dorsal rami are small targets and can vary in location, particularly at cervical levels. Therefore, the principle of medial branch neurotomy is not so much to place the electrode on the target nerve, but to place a sufficient number of lesions in a sufficient number of locations so that the matrix of lesions produced covers all possible locations of the nerve. For this purpose, a detailed knowledge of both the surgical and radiographic anatomy of the nerves is mandatory.[100–102]

Cervical Medial Branch Neurotomy. Of the numerous techniques that have been used for cervical RF neurotomy,[103–106] only one has been validated.[103] This technique has been endorsed by the International Spine Intervention Society, and its execution has been described in detail in that society's guidelines.[107] Techniques reported by other investigators have not been tested in a similar rigorous manner, and their efficacy is not known.

Idiosyncrasies of the anatomy of the typical cervical medial branches govern the technique required to secure optimal coagulation of these nerves. The electrode must lie parallel to the target nerve. Therefore, since the nerves run obliquely across the articular pillar at the C3, C4, C5, and C6 levels, essentially parallel to the plane of the zygapophysial joints, the electrode must be inserted parallel to this plane (i.e., cephalo-ventrally). Furthermore, since the surface of the articular pillar is curved, two insertions are required in order to coagulate a maximal length of nerve. An oblique insertion is used to reach the nerve over the anterolateral sector, and a sagittal insertion is used to reach the nerve over the lateral sector of the pillar (Fig. 101.3). In both insertions, an appropriate number of lesions must be made in order to match the size of the electrode and the lesion that it produces with the possible locations of the nerve. These differ at different segments. At C5, the nerve typically crosses the central two-fourths of the articular pillar. At segments progressively further away from C5, the nerve tends to lie higher on the pillar.[53,107]

At the C7 level, the medial branch crosses the lateral aspect of the superior articular process of C7. This process is insufficiently curved to warrant an oblique insertion. The nerve can be reached with a sagittal insertion alone. Nevertheless, the nerve can lie as high as the tip of the superior articular process or as low as the base of the transverse process. Therefore, multiple lesions must be made to capture the nerve in all of its possible locations.

Once the electrode has been placed, a lesion is generated by maintaining a temperature of 80° to 85° C and maintained for 90 seconds. Throughout the lesioning process, the electrode must be held in place lest it dislodges, and its proper placement verified by periodic monitoring.

Once the first lesion has been made, the operator must judge if and how many further lesions need to be made in order to accommodate all the possible locations of the target nerve. This requires knowing the variations in location at each segmental level[53,107] and estimating the size of the lesion made by the electrode used. In general, if a large gauge electrode (16G) is used, one or two lesions may suffice, but if a small gauge electrode (22G) is used, three, four, or five lesions may be required. In both instances, patients with taller articular pillars will require a greater number of lesions than patients with short pillars.

Of all the techniques described in the literature, this is the only technique that has been tested and has consistently shown to confer sustainable and complete relief of pain.[103,108–111] Alternative techniques including the simultaneous insertion of multiple electrodes or shortening the operative time[112] have not generated comparable or better outcomes.

A placebo-controlled trial firmly demonstrated that the effects of cervical RF neurotomy, when meticulously executed in correctly selected patients, were not due to chance.[103] The treatment

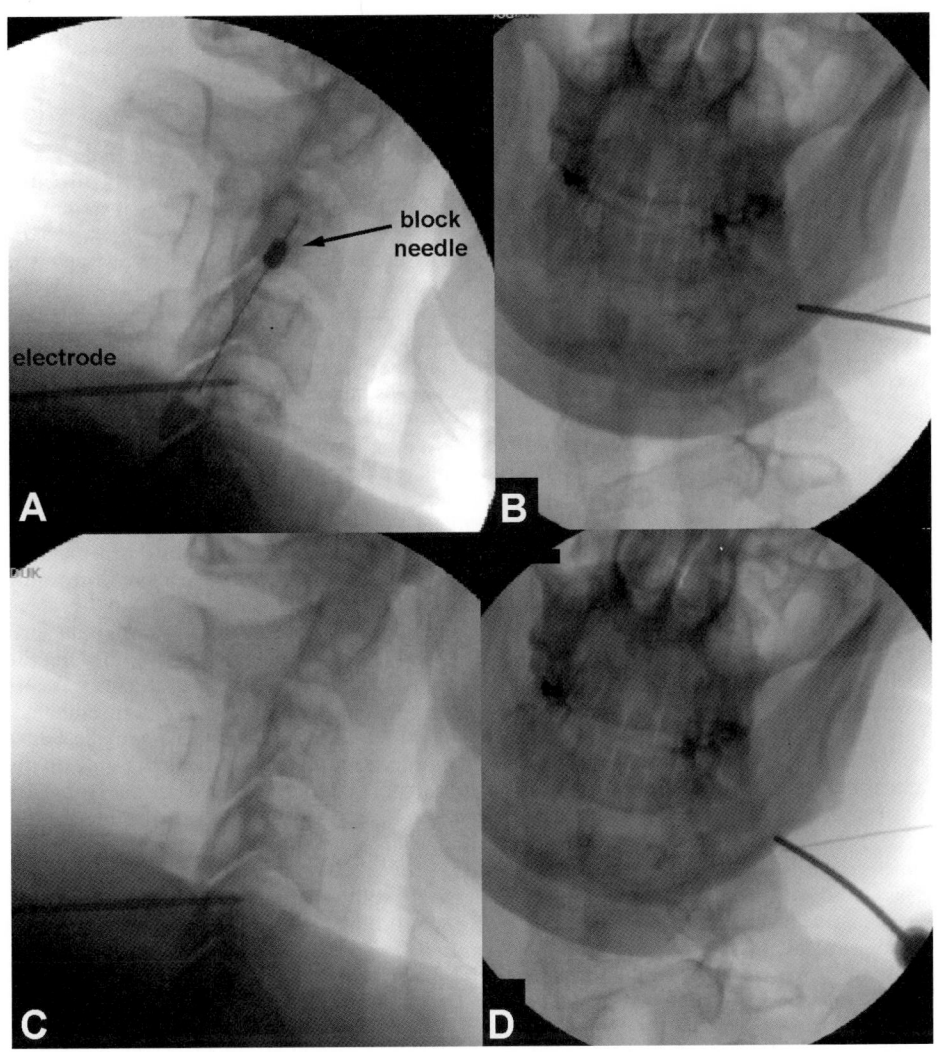

FIGURE 101.3 Fluoroscopy view of electrode placements in the execution of a C5 medial branch RF neurotomy. **A.** Lateral view of an oblique insertion. The tip of the electrode lies over the anterolateral surface of the C5 articular pillar. (A block needle remains in place over the target area, in case supplementary local anaesthesia is required). **B.** Anteroposterior view of an oblique insertion. The tip of the electrode lies just medial to lateral margin of the silhouette of the C5 articular pillar. **C.** Lateral view of a sagittal insertion. The tip of the electrode lies over the lateral surface of the C5 articular pillar. **D.** Anteroposterior view of a sagittal insertion. The tip of the electrode lies tangential to the lateral surface of the C5 articular pillar.

was so effective that a sample of 24 had 100% power for the results obtained. Patients reporting complete relief of their index pain required no other supplementary treatment, and activities of daily living previously impeded by pain were reinstated. To achieve maximal coagulation of each of the two targeted nerves, the procedure required at least 2 to 3 hours operating time. In the control group, the median time for recurrence of pain was 8 days after surgery. The median duration of relief of pain, following active treatment, was 263 days.[103]

Long-term follow-up confirmed that at least 64% of patients so treated obtained complete relief of their pain for a median duration of 422 days.[53,109] If pain recurred, relief was reinstated by repeating the procedure. Patients, who initially obtain relief for greater than 90 days, had an 82% chance of further success by a repeat procedure. If initial relief lasted less than 90 days, the chances of successful repeat treatment reduced to 33%.[109] Successful treatment led to the complete resolution of psychologic distress,[113] and treatment was equally effective in litigants and nonlitigants.[108,111,114]

No other form of treatment for neck pain has been shown to be as effective as RF medial branch neurotomy. Three independent reviews have concluded that cervical medial branch neurotomy is an efficacious treatment for proven cervical zygapophysial joint pain.[115–117]

Unlike for trigeminal neuralgia or DREZ lesioning, the relief of pain after medial branch neurotomy is not permanent. The ganglion cells of the nerve are not targeted, and the nerve regener-

ates. With optimal coagulation, the average duration of relief is about 9 months but may last for up to 12 months or longer.[53,103,109] Pain may recur once the nerve has regenerated, but the return of pain is usually gradual and may not return to its former intensity. Should pain become intolerable and interfere with the activities of daily living, relief can be reinstated by repeating the procedure. Multiple repetitions are possible without compromising the outcomes.[53,103,109] Confirmatory diagnostic blocks should always precede any repetition of the procedure lest a different or new source of pain be overlooked.[53]

At typical levels (C3-C7 inclusive), side effects of cervical medial branch neurotomy are uncommon and self-limiting (Table 101.1).

Skin burns are avoided by using a firmly applied dispersive/ground plate with a large surface area rather than a spinal needle to dissipate electrical energy. Meticulous technique and strict asepsis should guard against infection and hematoma formation. Neurologic complications are avoided by ensuring that electrodes always remain external to the vertebral column and do not reach either the vertebral artery or the intervertebral foramen.

Concerns about Charcot's joints are unfounded.[119,120] There are no published reports of Charcot's arthropathy directly attributable to RF neurotomy, nor does selective denervation of the wrist joint cause Charcot's arthropathy.[121] Contemporary pathophysiology implicates a neurovascular mechanism, diabetes has replaced tertiary syphilis as the most common cause,[122] and arthropathy can occur in advance of abnormal neurology.[123,124]

TABLE 101.1

INCIDENCE OF SIDE EFFECTS FOLLOWING
RADIOFREQUENCY AT TYPICAL CERVICAL
LEVELS[53,118]

Side effects	Incidence %
Vasovagal syncope	2
Dermoid cyst	1
Köbner's phenomenon	1
Neuritis	2
Numbness in the cutaneous territory of one of the coagulated nerves	29
Dysesthesia in the cutaneous territory of one of the nerves coagulated	19

Charcot's joints classically occur in weight-bearing joints of the lower limb in which all the surrounding muscles are insensate, resulting in instability.[125] This does not occur with spinal RF neurotomy. The medial branches innervate only the deep paramedian muscles. The superficial and lateral muscles are spared. Thus, the spinal motion segment is not rendered insensate. Meanwhile, the disc and articular processes maintain stability passively.

Catastrophic spinal cord injuries have occurred only when electrodes have been egregiously misplaced.[126] They are avoided by careful placement of electrodes in the correct target zone and monitoring of their location during the generation of lesions.

Third Occipital Headache. Pain from upper cervical segments can be referred into to the head, where it is perceived as headache. This type of headache is known as cervicogenic headache. Its mechanism is convergence in the trigeminocervical nucleus between afferents of the upper three cervical spinal nerves and trigeminal afferents.[127,128] Of the possible sources of cervicogenic headache, the strongest volume of evidence implicates the C2-C3 zygapophysial joint.[127–134] Pain stemming from the C2-C3 zygapophysial joint is mediated by a single nerve: the third occipital nerve (TON).[100] Accordingly, headache stemming from this joint have, appropriately, been called third occipital headache.[130] The TON is the superficial medial branch of the C3 dorsal ramus.[100]

In accordance with the guidelines of the International Headache Society,[135] the essential criterion for the diagnosis of third occipital headache is complete relief of pain following controlled, diagnostic blocks of the TON (see Chapter 97). Once so diagnosed, third occipital headache can be treated by third occipital RF neurotomy.

The TON crosses the C2-C3 zygapophysial joint transversely and may lie anywhere along the height of the C3 superior articular process, but more often, the nerve courses along the lower half of the convexity of the C2-C3 zygapophysial joint.[100] To ensure maximal efficiency, RF lesions must be placed along the entire height of the C3 superior articular process in order to encapsulate the nerve at all possible locations. Oblique and the sagittal insertions of electrode are standard, as for medial branches at typical cervical levels (Fig. 101.4).[107] Meticulous technique is required to ensure optimal outcomes. This involves placing the electrodes accurately and holding them in place during coagulation.[108]

Placebo-controlled trials of third occipital neurotomy have not been conducted because active neurotomy causes numbness in the cutaneous territory of the TON, and this effect cannot be masked. Observational studies are, therefore, the best possible evidence of effectiveness. They have shown that at least 85% of patients with proven third occipital headaches can be rendered

completely free of pain, provided that meticulous surgical technique is used.[108,111] The median duration of relief is at least 297 days, and when pain recurs, relief can be reinstated by repeat neurotomy. Outcomes have not been affected by litigation status.[108,111]

Third occipital neurotomy is associated with distinctive side effects (Table 101.2). Numbness is to be expected because the TON has a cutaneous distribution that is larger and more constant than that of typical cervical medial branches. Touch-evoked hypersensitivity and dysesthesia typically resolve spontaneously, usually within 2 weeks, but may last up to 6 weeks. The TON also innervates the semispinalis capitis and contributes substantially to cervical proprioception and tonic neck reflexes. Therefore, neurotomy is commonly associated with a mild ataxia. Generally, this ataxia is not disabling, for patients can rely on visual cues to locate horizontal objects, and thereby stabilize the orientation of their head. No long-term effects have been reported.

Because of possible problems with ataxia, presumptive bilateral neurotomy is not recommended in patients with bilateral third occipital headache. If bilateral neurotomy is indicated, it is recommended that one side be treated first and the other side be tested with a prognostic block to test that subsequent neurotomy on this side does not produce disabling ataxia.

Randomized, placebo-controlled studies have been published which purported to test the efficacy of RF neurotomy for the treatment of cervicogenic headache.[136–139] In all studies, patients were selected on clinical grounds which have not been validated. Therefore, there was no guarantee that patients actually had a cervical source of pain. In no study were patients selected on the basis of controlled diagnostic blocks. Therefore, the segmental source of pain was not established. In all studies, multiple segments were treated in every patient, but in no study was an anatomically validation surgical technique used. For these reasons, none of these studies constitutes a valid test of the treatment of cervicogenic by RF neurotomy.[134,140]

Lumbar Medial Branch Neurotomy. Confusion and inconsistencies have plagued the conduct and assessment of lumbar medial branch neurotomy. The crucial problem has been adherence to the surgical anatomy of the procedure. Other problems pertain to how electrodes are placed and how patients are selected.

At typical lumbar levels, the medial branches of the lumbar dorsal rami cross the neck of the superior articular process.[140] At the L5 level, it is the dorsal ramus itself that crosses the superior articular pillar before forming its medial branch, so the dorsal ramus becomes the target nerve rather than the medial branch.

At typical lumbar levels, the medial branch does not lie consistently at an exact location. Rather, it can lie somewhat higher or lower across the junction of the transverse process and superior articular process. Therefore, a single point does not constitute the target point for neurotomy. Rather, a target zone applies across which a matrix of lesions needs to be placed in order to accommodate possible variations in the exact location of the nerve.[140] These considerations are less of a problem for the L5 dorsal ramus, whose course over the ala of the sacrum is comparatively more constant.

Electrodes that are placed perpendicular to the target nerve may fail to incorporate the nerve in a lesion or may coagulate the nerve incompletely because little lesion is produced distal to the tip of the electrode. In order to coagulate the nerve adequately and reliably, electrodes must be placed parallel to the nerve. This requires an insertion in a ventro-cephalad direction at an angle of approximately 45 degrees to the transverse plane of the vertebra that the nerve crosses.[140,141] In addition, electrodes need to be angled about 15 degrees medially in order to avoid the mamillo-accessory ligament, especially when this ligament is ossified.[140,141]

At all levels, the target zone lies along the middle two-quarters of the neck of the superior articular process.[140,141] Lesions placed

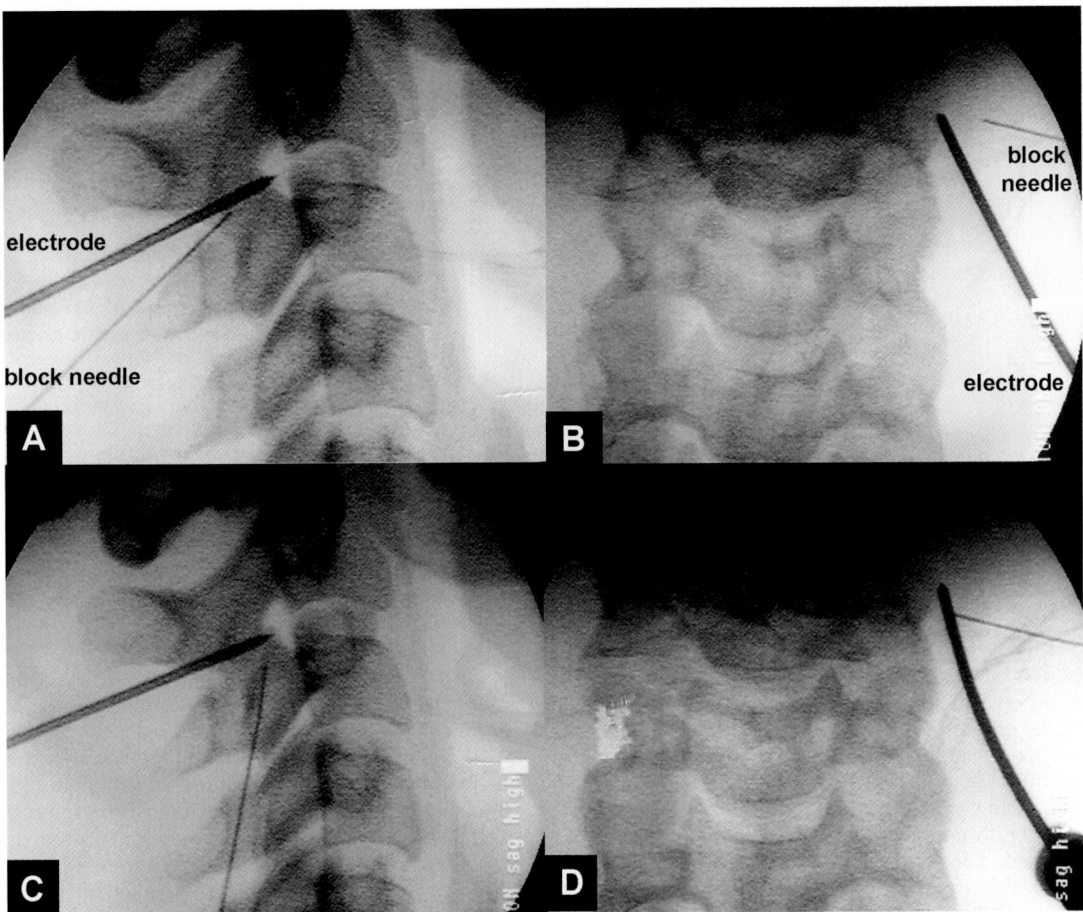

FIGURE 101.4 Fluoroscopy views of electrode placement for third occipital radiofrequency neurotomy. **A.** Lateral view of oblique insertion of electrode. The electrode tip lies over the anterolateral aspect of the C2-C3 zygapophysial joint. The electrode lies in the higher of two positions required to encompass the third occipital nerve thoroughly. (A block needle overlies the target zone in case supplementary anaesthesia is required.) **B.** Anteroposterior view of an oblique insertion. The tip of the electrode lies medial to the lateral margin of the silhouette of the C2-C3 zygapophysial joint. **C.** Lateral view of a sagittal insertion. The tip of the electrode lies over the lateral aspect of the C2-C3 zygapophysial joint. The electrode lies in the highest of three positions required to encompass the third occipital nerve thoroughly **D.** Anteroposterior view of a sagittal insertion. The electrode lies tangential to the C2-C3 zygapophysial joint.

proximal to this area risk incorporating the lateral branch of the dorsal ramus. Distal to this area, lesion will not capture the medial branch because it is covered by the mamillo-accessory ligament.[140] When correctly placed over this target zone, an electrode with a 10 cm active tip should adequately incorporate an adequate length of the target nerve. Electrodes with a 5 mm tip need to be placed proximally and then distally along the target zone in order to capture the optimal length of nerve. The matrix of

lesions produced should extend onto the root of the transverse process and slightly dorsally across the root of the superior process. Such a matrix encompasses all possible locations of the nerve.[140,141] The number of lesions required to produce this matrix depends on the size of the electrode used. With larger gauge electrodes, an adequate matrix can be produced with one or two lesions. If smaller electrodes are used, four, six, or more lesions will need to be placed lest the nerve escape coagulation.

As recommended by the International Spine Intervention Society,[141] the procedure requires obtaining a caudally declined view of the target area, such that the transverse process is viewed edge-on, coupled with a slight lateral obliquity. In this view, the electrode is inserted parallel to the x-ray beam so that it lodges against the neck of the superior articular process (Fig. 101.5A). Depth of insertion is established in other views. In an oblique view, the active tip of the electrode should cross the junction of the transverse process and superior articular process (Fig. 101.5B). In an anteroposterior view, the electrode should fit snugly against the lateral surface of the superior articular process (Fig. 101.5C). In a lateral view, the active tip should lie opposite the middle two-fourths of the neck of the superior articular process (Fig. 101.5D). In this location, a lesion is produced. Depending on the gauge of the electrode used and the length of its active tip, one or more

TABLE 101.2

THE SIDE EFFECTS OF THIRD OCCIPITAL NEUROTOMY[108]

Side effect	Incidence
Numbness	97%
Ataxia	95%
Dysesthesia	55%
Hypersensitivity	15%
Itch	10%

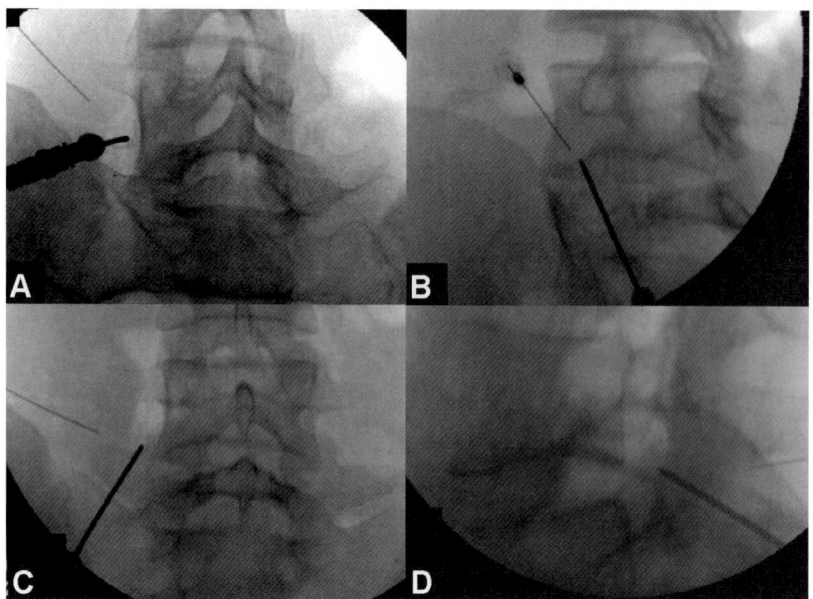

FIGURE 101.5 Fluoroscopy views of an electrode in place for an L4 medial branch radiofrequency neurotomy. **A.** Declined (pillar) view showing the tip of the electrode lodged in the notch between the superior articular process and transverse process of L5. **B.** Oblique view showing the tip of the electrode crossing the junction of the superior articular process and transverse process. **C.** Anteroposterior view showing the electrode orientated obliquely, cephalad, and medially against the lateral surface of the superior articular process. **D.** Lateral view showing the active tip of the electrode lying opposite the middle two-fourths of the neck of the superior articular process.

lesions may need to be placed in order to cover variations in the location of the nerve. If the lesion placed on the neck of the superior articular process is small, another lesion should be placed on the root of the transverse process. If a short active tip is used, a second lesion should be placed after withdrawing the electrode 5 mm from each of its deeper positions.

Techniques that do not comply with this protocol cannot be relied on to achieve adequate coagulation of the target nerve. Common flaws in this regard are placing the electrode perpendicular to the nerve, making one lesion rather than a matrix, and using small gauge electrodes which produce almost trivial lesions.[140]

Pivotal to the effectiveness of lumbar medial branch neurotomy is selection of patients. The essential indication is complete relief of pain or near complete relief following controlled diagnostic medial branch blocks (see Chapter 97). Unless this criterion is satisfied, there are no grounds for believing that the patient has pain mediated by these nerves and that neurotomy should relieve this pain.

Several controlled trials of lumbar medial branch neurotomy have been published, but none has satisfied the requirements outlined above. Patients were not selected on the basis of controlled diagnostic blocks. Electrodes were placed perpendicular to the nerve. Single lesions were made. Small gauge electrodes were used. Under those circumstances, it is not surprising that efficacy was not demonstrated in these trials. It is conspicuous, as well, that systematic reviews[142,143] of this procedure did not recognize these technical flaws of the studies, and how they affect conclusions about the efficacy of lumbar medial branch neurotomy.[144]

The benchmark for effectiveness of lumbar medial branch neurotomy was established by an observational study.[62] That study showed that, when properly executed in correctly selected patients, good outcomes can be expected. Some 80% of patients maintain at least 60% relief of their pain at 12 months, and some 60% of patients maintain at least 80% relief.

Subsequently, a larger cohort study treated 209 patients selected on the basis of positive responses to controlled diagnostic lumbar medial branch blocks.[145] Of the 174 patients who completed the audit, 68% experienced greater than 50% relief sustained for between 6 and 24 months.

Two placebo-controlled trials have established that the effects of lumbar medial branch neurotomy cannot be attributed to placebo. The first used a suboptimal technique—electrodes were placed perpendicular to the target nerves. Consequently, the du-

ration of relief of pain was limited. Nevertheless, in that context, it was clearly evident that active treatment was superior to sham treatment.[146] The second study[147] selected patients on the basis of controlled, diagnostic blocks and placed electrodes parallel to the target nerves and in multiple locations. It showed superior outcomes from active treatment than from sham treatment.

Relief from lumbar medial branch neurotomy is not permanent. Progressively, the nerve regenerates over a period determined by the accuracy and thoroughness of coagulation. If pain recurs with sufficient intensity to warrant treatment, the procedure can be repeated and the relief of pain reinstated.[148]

If correctly and carefully executed, lumbar medial branch neurotomy should have no complications. In one large series, no complications were reported barring temporary localized pain and self-limiting neuritic pain.[149] Postsurgical neuritis with dysesthesia and hypoesthesia, including exacerbation of the primary pain, has been reported.[150,151] Injuries to the spinal nerve or ventral ramus have occurred when the electrode has been incorrectly placed or has dislodged during the procedure.[126,152,153]

Damage to spinal nerves or the spinal cord should not occur. They have occurred only when operators have misinterpreted the radiographic anatomy and have grievously placed electrodes in the wrong location or when the electrode has dislodged but its position has not been monitored during the procedure.[126,152,153] Injuries have also occurred when operators have conducted the procedure under general anesthesia.[126] Under general anesthesia, patients cannot report inappropriate sensations indicative of a lesion being generated in the wrong location.

Thoracic Medial Branch Neurotomy. Some practitioners have reported performing RF neurotomy of the medial branches of the thoracic dorsal rami.[154] A dissection study, however, revealed that the target points used in that study were remote from the medial branches and, therefore, that those nerves could not have been coagulated.[155] A technique for thoracic medial branch neurotomy based on accurate anatomy has not been developed, let alone tested.

Sacroiliac Pain

Opinion and the evidence is divided as to how the sacroiliac joint is innervated.[156] Some maintain the joint receives its innervation posteriorly from the lateral branches of the L5 and S1 and S2 dorsal rami, and anteriorly from branches of the lumbar and sacral ventral rami.[157–160] Others maintain that the innervation

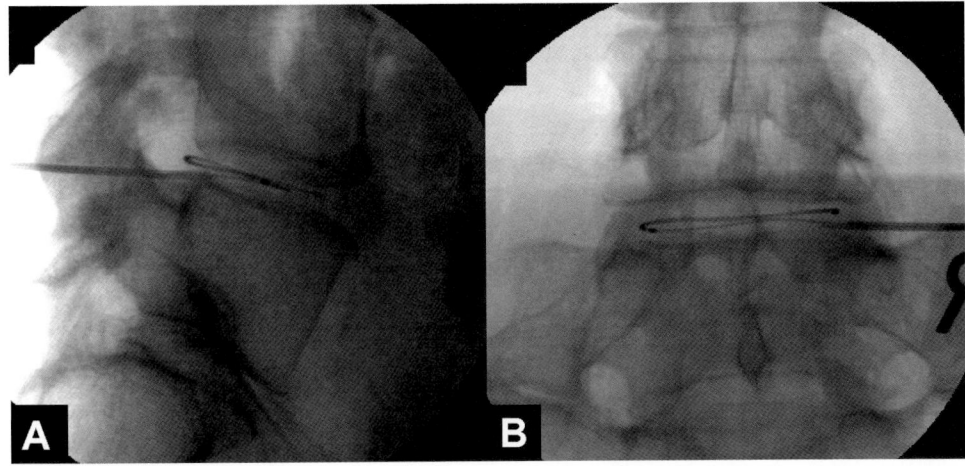

FIGURE 101.6 Electrode placement for intradiscal electrothermal anuloplasty of an L4-L5 intervertebral disc. **A.** Lateral view. **B.** Anteroposterior view. (Illustrations kindly provided by Dr. Paul Dreyfuss, Seattle, WA.)

is exclusively from the sacral dorsal rami.[161] This latter view allows for sacroiliac pain to be treated by RF neurotomy of the lateral branches of the sacral dorsal rami.

Various techniques have been developed and advocated on the basis of descriptive studies. Some placed a strip of lesions along the posterior edge of the sacroiliac joint.[162] Others have placed electrodes around the lateral perimeter of the posterior sacral foramina, using single[163,164] or multiple[165] electrodes. Some have used electrical stimulation to find the target nerves.[163]

The outcomes of sacroiliac RF treatment have been modest and short-lasting. Between 30% and 50% of patients reported at least 50% relief of their pain for 3 or 6 months. Better outcomes have been reported when nerves were targeted,[163,164] rather than when electrodes were placed in the posterior capsule and ligaments.[162] Higher success rates have been reported in studies in which patients who reported at least 70% relief of their pain following a single intra-articular block underwent stimulation-guided RF.[163]

A placebo-controlled study has shown that the outcomes of active RF neurotomy for sacroiliac pain are patently superior to sham therapy.[166] However, the duration of successful outcomes was limited, as in the observational studies. The application of RF neurotomy requires a more enduring efficacy for it to become an entertainable option for sacroiliac pain.

Discogenic Pain

Investigators have explored various applications of thermal RF or related technologies to treat back pain stemming from the lumbar intervertebral discs. Some applications have been discredited. For some, the evidence is mixed. For others, it remains encouraging. Other intradiscal therapies are covered in Chapter 100.

Intranuclear Monopolar Radiofrequency. The first application of RF treatment for discogenic pain involved placing a monopolar electrode into the center of the nucleus pulposus in order to produce a single lesion. The rationale was that such a lesion produced sufficient heat to destroy the nerve endings in the outer anulus. A clinical study reported an impressive success rate for this procedure.[167] Subsequently, a clinical study found outcomes to be short-lasting,[168] and a controlled study found no effect greater than sham treatment.[169] Laboratory studies showed that intranuclear lesions did not generate temperatures in the outer anulus capable of coagulating nerves.[170,171]

Intradiscal Electrothermal Anuloplasty. Intradiscal electrothermal anuloplasty (IDET) involves threading a flexible electrode,

in a circumferential fashion, into the anulus of a painful disc (Fig. 101.6). The electrode emits radiant heat, which produces a narrow lesion around and along the length of the electrode. The originally proposed rationale was that heating the anulus stiffened it by denaturing its collagen,[172] but histologic evidence of such an effect has not been forthcoming. Electron microscopic features of extensive collagen disorganization with shrinkage and chondrocyte damage described in one study[173] could not be confirmed in a contemporary study in which normal morphology prevailed.[174] Other conjectures have been that IDET might seal radial or circumferential fissure or coagulate nerve endings.[175,176] These conjectures require that the electrode be placed very close to such fissures or into the innervated zone of the anulus. Studies have shown that temperatures recorded 10 mm away from the tip were insufficient to denature nociceptors[177] or to affect the nerve count in laboratory animals.[178] Temperatures greater than 45° C were achievable at least 9 mm away from the active tip, but not all discs responded uniformly.[179]

Some outcome studies reported very low success rates,[180–183] but many reported notable,[184–189] or substantial,[190–196] reductions in pain. Overall, the data from descriptive studies suggest that IDET achieves an average reduction of pain of about 4 on a 0 to 10 scale, and that around 50% of patients can expect at least 50% reduction of their pain (Fig. 101.7).

A case-control study found IDET to be more effective than treatment by thermal RF anuloplasty (see below).[194] A cohort study[195,196] found IDET to be more effective than rehabilitation.

A notable feature is that IDET was not universally effective. Some 50% of patients obtain no benefit at all.[195,196] Most of the remainder obtain at least 50% relief of pain, and some obtain complete relief. Outcomes are largely stable over 1 and 2 years.[195–198]

Two randomized controlled studies have provided conflicting results. In one of these trials, the success rate for IDET was zero, but it was zero as well for placebo treatment.[199] These results raise intriguing questions. A zero success rate for active treatment is incompatible with the results of most outcome studies. This implies either a different selection of patients or a different execution of the technique. The lack of any placebo effect is quite curious. If IDET works because of placebo effects, one would expect successful outcomes in at least a proportion of patients treated with sham therapy. It seems somewhat ingenuine to conclude that IDET is a placebo when no placebo effect is encountered.

The second randomized controlled trial[200] provided more realistic results. Consistent with previous outcome studies, over 50% of patients obtained no benefit, but the remainder benefited to greater or lesser degrees. In those patients, outcomes for pain and physical function were significantly better than in patients

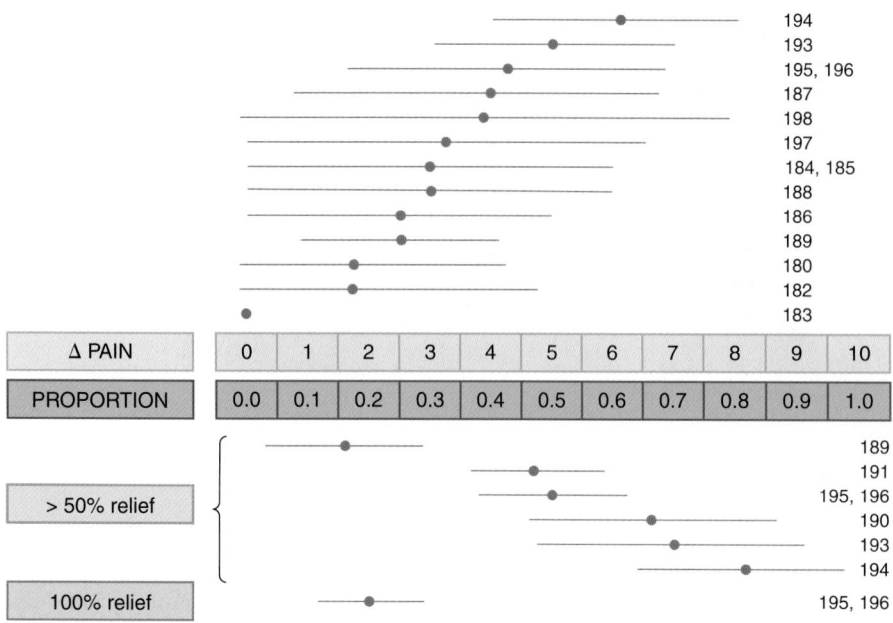

FIGURE 101.7 A graphic summary of outcomes for intradiscal electrothermal therapy reported in observational studies, a case-control study, and a cohort study. For studies that reported outcomes as reductions in pain, the mean reduction and standard deviation of each study have been depicted above the scale labeled "Δ pain" (change in pain expressed as reduction on a 0–10 analog pain scale). For studies that reported proportions of patients obtaining at least 50% relief of pain and complete relief of pain, the proportion and its 95% confidence intervals have been depicted below the scale labeled "proportion." Each datum point is accompanied by the reference number of the study.

who received sham treatment. This study provided the evidence that the effects of IDET could not be attributed wholly to placebo effects, but having encountered placebo responses, it also warned also that all intradiscal therapies should be subjected to controlled trials in order to refute placebo effects.

Despite being methodologically sound, this latter study[200] was criticized in a Cochrane Review for having a sample that representative of an "average" orthopaedic practice.[201,202] This criticism is gratuitous because it ignores the difficulties in getting patients to enroll in placebo-controlled studies of surgery and because IDET is not designed for average or all patients. It is applicable only for patients with internal disc disruption who satisfy strict indications.[175,176,203] For such patients, no form of conservative treatment, including cognitive behavioral therapy, has been shown to be as effective as IDET. Nor do these patients undergo spontaneous resolution if left untreated.[204]

Other reviews have been more charitable.[205,206] Both reaffirmed that with proper selection, IDET had the potential to reduce fusion surgery by at least 50%,[206] and hence is a valid option before undertaking spinal surgery.[205]

The reasons for the limited success rates of IDET have not been explored, but technical issues seem to apply.[176] The electrodes used have a limited field of influence. They create lesions to within only 2 mm from their surface. Fissures or nerves outside this field would escape coagulation, even if the electrode seems reasonably placed. Large fissures would not be encompassed by the small-sized lesion. For such reasons, alternative technologies have been developed and explored.

Complications associated with IDET have included injuries to the cauda equina.[207–209] This implies that electrodes were misplaced into the vertebral canal, but the techniques used in these cases were not illustrated in the reports. Neurologic complications can be avoided by careful attention to where the electrode is placed and by having the patient awake during the procedure so that they can warn of the onset of adverse symptoms. In cases where neurologic injuries have occurred, operators persisted in the procedure despite the onset of burning pain.[126] Vertebral osteonecrosis has been cited in two publications[210,211] but has not been distinguished from infection or a pre-existing intraosseous disc herniation.[126] Disc herniation,[212] discitis, infections, nerve root damage, allergic reaction, and vascular injury such as retroperitoneal bleeding have also been reported.[213]

Thermal Radiofrequency Anuloplasty. Thermal RF anuloplasty is analogous to IDET in that it requires inserting a flexible electrode into the anulus fibrosus. However, instead of applying radiant heat, the electrode operates in the manner of thermal RF to heat surrounding tissues.[214,215]

No randomized trials of this intervention have been conducted. An outcome study found reductions in pain in only a modest proportion of patients.[216,217] A case-control study found thermal RF anuloplasty to be less effective than IDET.[194]

Intradiscal Biacuplasty. Intradiscal biacuplasty is an emerging innovation for the treatment of discogenic pain. It involves placing electrodes bilaterally into the posterolateral corners of the target disc (Fig. 101.8). The innovation is that each electrode is cooled by passing water through it. For this reason, the procedure is also known as "cold RF." Cooling each electrode prevents coagulation around the active tip, which prevents the development of high impedance in the tissues.[218] As a result, current can be passed between the two electrodes over a prolonged time (15 minutes) to generate a lesion between the electrodes across the entire posterior anulus. The lesion produced is larger, both in depth and in height, than that produced by IDET. Temperatures sufficient to ablate nociceptors are confined to the anulus fibrosus.[218] In human cadaveric[219,220] and porcine discs,[218] no histopathologic changes to either osseous or neural tissues were evident following cold RF. Theoretically, these technical differences offer the promise of greater efficacy than with previous intradiscal therapies.

Transdiscal biacuplasty is still being evaluated in a multicenter trial. At one center, mean pain scores were reduced from 7.2 (1.9) to 3.4 (1.9), and 7 out of 13 patients reported at least 50% relief of pain at 6 months after treatment.[221] Improvements in pain were associated with improvements in disability and physical function, as well as decrease in use of opioids. At another center, 4 out of 8 patients had greater than 50% reduction in pain at 6 months.[222] These outcomes have still to be corroborated in larger numbers of patients. However, the procedure is easy to perform and is painless to the patients, which renders it an attractive, potential option for discogenic pain.

Radiofrequency Dorsal Root Ganglion

RF dorsal root ganglion (RF-DRG) is known by various names in which thermal RF lesions are directed at dorsal root ganglia.

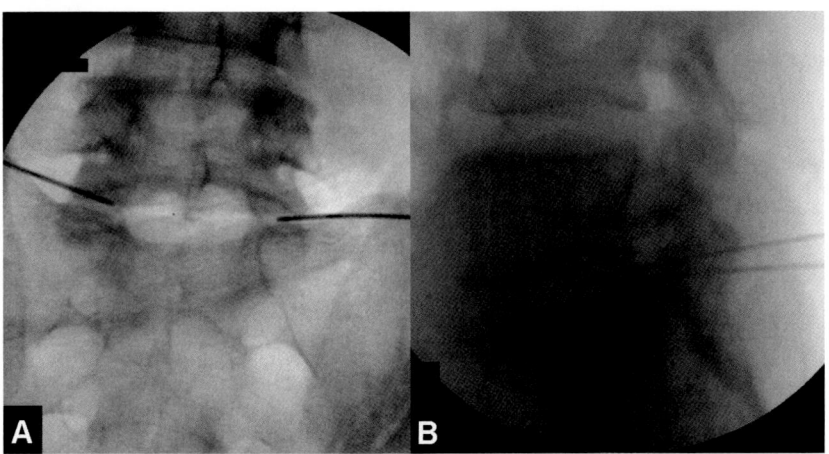

FIGURE 101.8 Fluoroscopy views of electrodes in position for intradiscal biacuplasty of an L5-S1 disc. **A.** Anteroposterior view. **B.** Lateral view.

The professed objective was not to coagulate the ganglion but to place a lesion close enough to provide relief of pain while only partially affecting the ganglion. It has been used to treat chronic pain mediated by cervical, lumbar, or thoracic dorsal root ganglia.

Descriptive studies promoted the use of RF-DRG for cervical,[223] thoracic,[224,225] and eventually lumbar,[226] pain syndromes. Outcomes were reported in terms of whether the patients were "pain-free" or had "good" (50%–100%) relief of their pain. Other outcome measures were not provided.

A descriptive study of cervical RF-DRG reported that 2/20 patients (10%) were pain free at 3 months, 4/20 were so at 6 months, and 2/17 (11%) at 12 months.[223] Eight patients had good relief at 3 months, but their numbers dropped to 2 at 6 months, and 2 at 12 months. In a controlled trial, success was defined as a reduction by 2 points or more on a 10-point VAS.[227] A significantly greater proportion of patients (8/9) had a successful outcome following active treatment than those (2/11) who underwent sham treatment. Follow-up, however, was limited to only 8 weeks. At this time the actively treated patients had reduced their mean pain scores from 6.4 to 3.3, whereas the sham-treated patients maintained the same scores (5.9, 6.0). Although this study provided data to the effect that the initial effects of cervical RF-DRG were not due to placebo, they do not attest to a successful, lasting effect. The data of the preceding observational study would predict that outcomes would attenuate substantially beyond 8 weeks.

A retrospective review of 361 patients treated by lumbar RF-DRG found 61 to be free of pain at 2 months.[226] This number became 23 at a mean follow-up of 22.9 months, but the range of that period was 2 to 70 months. A further 103 patients reported incomplete but greater than 50% relief at 2 months. This number dropped to 73 at longer-term follow-up. When tested in a placebo-controlled trial, lumbar RF-DRG was no more effective than sham treatment.[228]

The first study of thoracic RF-DRG announced that 30/45 patients (67%) were pain free and a further 11 (24%) had greater than 50% reduction in pain at 2 months.[224] At long-term follow-up, ranging from 13 to 46 months, 20 patients were pain free and 15 had greater than 50% relief of pain. The second study did not reproduce these outcomes.[225] At 8 weeks, only 8 of 43 patients (18%) had complete relief of pain, and 9 (21%) had greater than 50% relief. At follow-up beyond 36 weeks, only 5 patients (12%) were pain free, and 8 (18%) had greater than 50% relief. Patient selection may have been the reason for this dissonance. The first study had a large proportion (38%) of patients with postsurgical pain (thoracotomy, mastectomy, abdominal scar), in whom good outcomes were achieved. Such patients were absent from the second study. Conversely, the second study had a large proportion (47%) of patients with neuralgia. In the first study, patients with neuralgias had less than average outcomes. The second study did not stratify its results according to diagnosis. The efficacy of thoracic RF-DRG has not been tested in a controlled trial.

Sympathectomy

Surgical sympathectomy has a long heritage for the treatment of peripheral vascular disease and various chronic pain problems. For peripheral vascular disease, sympathectomy confers quantifiable clinical improvement. Subjectively, some 50% of patients secure complete relief of their pain with partial improvement in a further 31%.[229] Objectively, improvement in cutaneous[230,231] and muscle perfusion,[232] promote the healing of ischemic ulcers,[233] limit the spread of gangrene, and prevent amputation.[234] For chronic pain problems, the evidence is less than impressive.

Despite concerns expressed as long ago as 1942 about the efficacy of surgical sympathectomy for the management of noncancer pain,[235] the procedure was enthusiastically pursued for the management of reflex sympathetic dystrophy or complex regional pain syndrome (CRPS), migraine, dysmenorrhoea, epilepsy, chronic pancreatitis, postherpetic neuralgia of the trigeminal nerve, postdiscectomy syndrome, and phantom limb pain.[236,237] However, systematic reviews have found no tangible evidence supportive of sympathectomy for the management of neuropathic pain.[238,239] Furthermore, postsympathectomy neuralgia is a common complaint with a reported incidence between 15% to 50%.[240,241]

Despite this background, some operators have advocated thermal RF as an alternative to surgical sympathectomy.[242] Evidence, however, is limited to small case series.

For chronic abdominal pain, caused by pancreatitis or of unknown origin, one study of 10 patients reported good relief of pain lasting over 12 months following RF ablation of the splanchnic nerves.[243]

There is some evidence, from observational studies, that RF sympathetic neurotomy can improve vascular function in disorders of the upper limb, but those studies provide no data on the relief of pain.[244] For the relief of pain by RF stellate ganglion neurotomy in patients with CRPS, an attempted review found only one publication, which provided inadequate data.[245] That review offered its own outcome data, claiming that one-third of patients achieved more than 50% reduction of pain. Follow-up, however, was limited, with a drop-out rate of 69%. A later, retrospective study found that stellate ganglion neurotomy provided at least 50% relief of pain in 35 of 86 with various, unspecified pain syndromes.[242] The duration of relief was said to have an average of 52 weeks, with a range of 2 to 186 weeks, but these figures were based on a follow-up of only 27 of the patients.

TABLE 101.3

PAIN DISORDERS TREATED WITH PULSED RF[266,267]

Pain Types	Conditions Treated
Somatic	Arthritis; back, neck, shoulder, elbow, sacroiliac, temporomandibular, and hip joint pain
Visceral	Groin pain, orchialgia
Neuropathic	CRPS, trigeminal and glossopharyngeal neuralgia, radicular pain
Headaches	Posttraumatic, occipital neuralgia
Postsurgical	Tonsillectomy, postherniorrhaphy neuralgia, postlaminectomy syndrome

Miscellaneous

Thermal RF neurotomy has been used to treat miscellaneous chronic pain problems, such as cluster headache,[246,247] other oral and facial pain,[248,249] and hip pain.[250] The evidence is limited to case reports.

PULSED RADIOFREQUENCY

Pulsed RF was developed as an alternative to thermal RF. Instead of delivering a sustained current and thereby generating heat, the current is delivered in pulses, with temperature maintained at or below 42° C. Doing so avoids the production of a destructive lesion, but purportedly, the pulsed electric field exerts therapeutic effects.[251–254] Relief of pain is attributed to the electric field exerting a "central modulatory" effect ostensibly through a series of yet to be defined physiologic events.[155,252–254]

Proponents of pulsed RF attribute its antinociceptive effect to activation of transcription factors such as *c-fos*[255,256] and ATF3.[257] However, although one study reported the expression of *c-fos* in spinal neurons exposed to pulsed RF at 38° C but not to thermal RF at an equivalent temperature,[256] another study showed no difference in *c-fos* expression when exposed to either thermal RF or pulsed RF.[258] In any event, the *c-fos* is not a marker of relief of pain. Expression of *c-fos* is not associated with long-term neuronal plasticity, nor does *c-fos* exert a preferential antinociceptive effect.[259,260] It is little more than an expression of neuronal activity. Rats exposed to cat odor show greater *c-fos*

expression than controls,[261] and persistent *c-fos* expression can occur in the presence of chronic social stress.[262] The data are no different for ATF3. Elevated levels occur in cardiac ischemia, liver toxicity,[263] and seizures.[264] Like *c-fos*, ATF3 is thought to be a marker of neuronal injury,[265] but its precise physiologic significance is not known.

Whether delivered percutaneously, transcutaneously,[266] or intra-articularly,[267] pulsed RF has been widely applied for all manner of pain, irrespective of pain pathophysiology (Table 101.3). The number of publications, however, is disproportionate with the quality of published evidence. A narrative review[268] and a systematic review[266] both found the descriptive literature uncompelling for lack of diagnostic criteria, small effect-sizes, lack of follow-up, incomplete follow-up, lack of controls, and the confounding effect of cointerventions. For cervical and lumbar zygapophysial joint pain and trigeminal neuralgia, pulsed RF has neither surpassed nor equaled the published benchmark set by thermal neurotomy.[53,62,103,109] The results of two controlled trials do not dispel these conclusions.

In one randomized controlled trial, thermal RF was shown unequivocally to be superior to pulsed RF in the management of trigeminal neuralgia.[269] Within the first 3 months of commencing the trial, all patients who received pulsed RF showed no signs of improvement and all required their medications. The trial was abandoned and the entire study sample was treated with thermal RF. At the end of 6 months, all patients treated with thermal RF were pain free and none required medications.

In the second controlled trial, 23 patients with suspected cervical radicular pain were randomized into a group of 11 who were treated with pulsed RF and a group of 12 who were treated with sham RF.[270] Relief of pain by at least 50% at 3 months was obtained in 9 of those treated with pulsed RF and by 4 of those who received sham treatment. Significant differences evident at 3 months were lost by 6 months. At no stage did active treatment achieve significantly greater improvements in function or quality of life than did sham treatment. No patient was rendered pain free, and all patients still required medications.

A third study[271] showed that the results of pulsed RF for lumbar medial branch neurotomy were inferior to those achieved by thermal RF.

CONCLUSION

The field of neurolytic blockade for chronic pain provides a suitable canvas upon which to illustrate the vicissitudes of evidence-

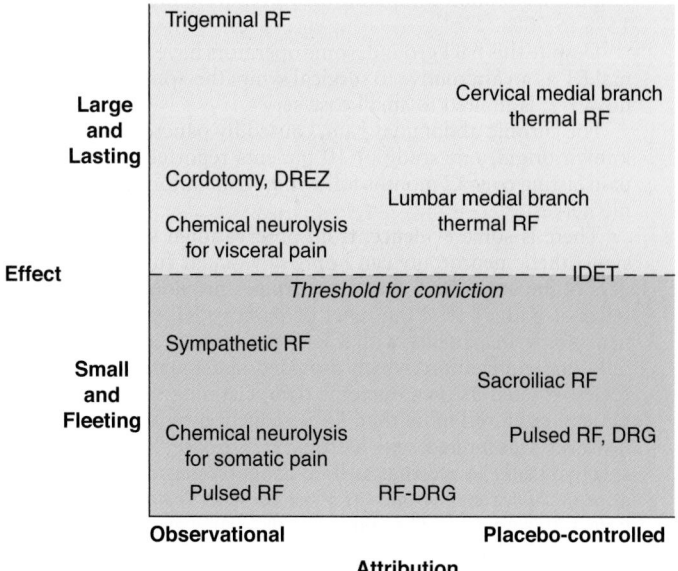

FIGURE 101.9 A graphical representation of the extent to which the evidence for various neurolytic procedures is convincing or not, according the nature of studies and the nature of the effect of treatment.

based medicine. Although it has become fashionable in some circles, to demand randomized controlled trials as the only acceptable form of evidence, this is an extreme view. Other levels of evidence can be sufficiently convincing. For neurolytic procedures, the evidence for various procedures is spread across a spectrum of credibility and conviction (Fig. 101.9).

At the heart of evidence appraisal is not whether a study is a controlled trial or not, but whether the evidence is convincing or not. In other fields of medicine, it has been shown that rarely have placebo-controlled trials overturned practices that were based on well-conducted observational studies.[272–274] This is reflected in the domain of neurolytic blockade. The issue is whether or not the evidence presented reaches some threshold of conviction (see Fig. 101.9).

There have been no placebo-controlled trials of thermal RF neurotomy for trigeminal neuralgia. Yet, no one challenges the effectiveness of this treatment for lack of controlled trials. This treatment is firmly established because of strong observational data. The effect of this treatment is strong and lasting. A large proportion of patients obtains complete or near complete relief of pain, and the duration of that relief can be measured in years, if not decades. For most practitioners, this is enough to attract conviction that thermal RF neurotomy is a worthwhile treatment for trigeminal neuralgia. Only the most ardent pundit would deny conviction, and none has done so publicly about this intervention.

In this case, the principle reflected is that conviction about effectiveness is achieved if a successful outcome can be demonstrated to occur consistently across multiple studies, consistently for a large proportion of patients, and that outcome is enduring. Moreover, the relief obtained is consistent with the known biological basis of the intervention. In the case of trigeminal thermal RF neurotomy, all these criteria have been satisfied.

Other RF interventions pale in comparison. Data to show that relief occurs in a substantial proportion of patients, that it occurs consistently across large numbers of patients, that it is enduring, or that relief means complete relief of pain are lacking. Investigators have sought recognition of their procedure on the basis of single studies with small sample sizes. What passes for success is little more than 50% relief of pain, whose duration is measured in weeks and occurs in a minor proportion of patients. No evidence is provided that this limited degree of relief reduces the burden of illness: that patients require no other form of treatment or that physical and social activities are restored by the treatment.

It is not that observational studies are an insufficient level of evidence. The issue is that most observational studies in this field provide insufficient evidence to achieve a threshold of conviction, or they provide evidence of insufficient effect to be convincing.

For sympathetic RF and for chemical neurolytic blockade for somatic pain, evidence is lacking for a substantial effect consistently across large numbers of patients that is lasting in duration. In the case of chemical neurolytic blockade for cancer pain, a worthwhile effect has been demonstrated consistently across a number of studies, although some questions still remain concerning benefits for variables other than pain. There has been no demand for controlled trials probably because of the limited life expectancy of the patients for whom these treatments are used. The same applies for treatments such as cordotomy.

For pulsed RF, outcomes are modest or poor, occur in minor proportions of patients, and are of short duration. There is not a demonstrated rationale for the procedure. When peripheral nerves have been the target of treatment, outcomes either fail to achieve the benchmarks reported for thermal RF or have been shown to be inferior to those of thermal RF.

Demands for stronger evidence are justified if there is no evident rationale or biological basis for why the treatment should work, if treatment effects are small, or if treatment effects are large but have not been shown to occur consistently across large samples. Without placebo-controlled trials, under these circumstances, consumers of information cannot determine if the reported results are no more than fortuitous but statistically accidental outcomes.

In the field of neurolytic blockade, various interventions have suffered different fates when subjected to placebo controls. Some have been vindicated but others have been shown to be no more effective than placebo, despite previous enthusiasm for them.

Despite being heralded as a successful procedure, lumbar RF-DRG proved no more effective than placebo. Pulsed RF-DRG proved more effective, statistically, than placebo in some measures, but not consistently across all measure. Nor were its effects enduring. It amounts to a procedure that produces some outcomes, in some patients, for a short time.

For thermal RF, the evidence differs for different applications. For some the evidence is convincing, or should be so, for others it has not reached the threshold of conviction.

A rigorous, placebo-controlled trial showed that cervical medial branch RF neurotomy was not a placebo. Subsequent follow-up studies showed that the effects were either enduring or can be reinstated by repeat treatment at about yearly intervals. Moreover, the validated outcomes were complete relief of pain, restoration of function, and no need for other health care.

For lumbar medial branch RF neurotomy, the evidence is also reasonable. A placebo effect has been refuted, outcome studies have shown prolonged effects, and relief can be reinstated if pain recurs. Still to be shown, however, is if treatment restores function, reduces the need for other health care, and secures return to work. A persisting problem is that not all operators perform this procedure in a manner that has been shown to be effective.

Sacroiliac RF is still in evolution. Although placebo effects have been refuted, the magnitude of relief obtained and its duration remain limited. For thoracic medial branch RF neurotomy, evidence is simply lacking.

RF cordotomy and DREZ lesioning are spared the requirement for randomized controlled trials because of the delicacy of the procedure and the target involved. Ethically, it is hard to justify placebo-controlled trials of invasive procedures on the spinal cord. Outcome studies could, perhaps, be more rigorous than they have been in order to attract greater conviction about the effectiveness of these procedures, but given the highly specialized nature of these procedures, the available evidence is probably enough.

The most curious example of evidence is IDET. Although there is an abundant literature and although placebo-controlled trials have been conducted, conviction about this procedure is marginal or contentious. The low success rate of this procedure limits its attraction. Had IDET been consistently successful in a consistently large proportion of patients, it might have attracted more widespread conviction. Proponents have gathered behind the defense that this procedure should be used only in patients who satisfy particular, stringent indications. Yet, even in such cases, the success rate remains modest. A treatment more consistently effective than IDET will readily replace it as an alternative to lumbar fusion.

References

1. *Stedman's Medical Dictionary.* 27th ed. Philadelphia: Lippincott Williams & Wilkins; 2000.
2. Stoll G, Jander S, Myers RR. Degeneration and regeneration of the peripheral nervous system: from Augustus Waller's observations to neuroinflammation. *J Peripher Nerv Syst* 2002;7:13–27.
3. Ramer MS, Priestley JV, McMahon SB. Functional regeneration of sensory axons into the adult spinal cord. *Nature* 2000;403:312–316.
4. Chen ZL, Yu WM, Strickland S. Peripheral regeneration. *Annu Rev Neurosci* 2007;30:209–233.
5. Phenol. In: Micromedex® [intranet database]. Version 5.1. Greenwood Village, Colo: Thomson Reuters (Healthcare) Inc., 2008.
6. Iggo A, Walsh EG. Selective block of small fibres in the spinal roots by phenol. *Brain* 1960;83:701–708.
7. Wood KM. The use of phenol as a neurolytic agent: a review. *Pain* 1978;5: 205–229.

8. Nathan PW, Sears TA, Smith MC. Effect of phenol solution on the nerve roots of the cat: an electrophysiological and histological study. *J Neuro Sci* 1965;2:7–29.
9. Alcohol. In: Micromedex® [intranet database]. Version 5.1. Greenwood Village, Colo: Thomson Reuters (Healthcare) Inc., 2008.
10. Gregg RV, Costantini CH, Ford DVI, et al. Electrophysiologic investigation of alcohol as a neurolytic agent. *Anesthesiology* 1985;63:A250.
11. Taylor JJ, Woolsey RM. Dilute ethyl alcohol: effect on the sciatic nerve of the mouse. *Arch Phy Med Rehabil* 1976;57:233–237.
12. Woolsey RM, Taylor JJ, Nagel JH. Acute effects of topical ethyl alcohol on the sciatic nerve of the mouse. *Arch Phy Med Rehabil* 1972;53:410–414.
13. Glycerol. In: Micromedex® [intranet database]. Version 5.1. Greenwood Village, Colo: Thomson Reuters (Healthcare) Inc., 2008.
14. Burchiel KJ, Russell LC. Glycerol neurolysis: neurophysiologic effects of topical glycerol application in a rat saphenous nerve. *J Neurosurg* 1985;63:784–788.
15. Lunsford LD. Percutaneous retrogasserian glycerol rhizotomy. In: Rovit RL, Muralie R, Jannetta PJ, eds. *Trigeminal Neuralgia*. Baltimore: Lippincott Williams & Wilkins; 1990:145–164.
16. Noble M, Gress FG. Techniques and results of neurolysis for chronic pancreatitis and pancreatic cancer pain. *Curr Gastroenterol Rep* 2006;8:99–103.
17. Eisenberg E, Carr DB, Chalmers TC. Neurolytic celiac plexus block for treatment of cancer pain: a meta-analysis. *Anesth Analg* 1995;80:290–295.
18. de Leon-Casasola OA. Critical evaluation of chemical neurolysis of the sympathetic axis for cancer pain. *Cancer Control* 2000;7:142–148.
19. de Oliveira R, dos Reis MP, Prado WA. The effects of early or late neurolytic sympathetic plexus block on the management of abdominal or pelvic cancer pain. *Pain* 2004;110:400–408.
20. Yan BM, Myers RP. Neurolytic celiac plexus block for pain control in unresectable pancreatic cancer. *Am J Gastroenterol* 2007;102:430–438.
21. Wong GY, Schroeder DR, Carns PE, et al. Effect of neurolytic celiac plexus block on pain relief, quality of life, and survival in patients with unresectable pancreatic cancer: a randomized controlled trial. *JAMA* 2004;291:1092–1099.
22. Rykowski JJ, Hilgier M. Efficacy of neurolytic celiac plexus block in varying locations of pancreatic cancer: influence on pain relief. *Anesthesiology* 2000;92:347–354.
23. Bhutani MS, Pasricha PJ. Neurolytic approaches for the treatment of pain in patients with chronic pancreatitis. *Curr Treat Options Gastroenterol* 2003;6:375–379.
24. Löfström B, Zetterquist S. Lumbar sympathetic blocks in the treatment of patients with obliterative arterial disease of the lower limb. *Int Anesthesiol Clin* 1969;7:423–438.
25. Cousins MJ, Reeve TS, Glynn CJ, et al. Neurolytic lumbar sympathetic blockade: duration of denervation and relief of rest pain. *Anaesth Intensive Care* 1979;7:121–135.
26. Cross FW, Cotton LT. Chemical lumbar sympathectomy for ischemic rest pain. A randomized prospective controlled clinical trial. *Am J Surg* 1985;150:341–345.
27. Candido K, Stevens RA. Intrathecal neurolytic blocks for the relief of cancer pain. *Best Pract Res Clin Anaesthesiol* 2003;17:407–428.
28. Ischia S, Luzzani A, Ischia A, et al. Subarachnoid neurolytic block (L5-S1) and unilateral percutaneous cervical cordotomy in the treatment of pain secondary to pelvic malignant disease. *Pain* 1984;20:139–149.
29. Silver HR. Lumbar percutaneous facet rhizotomy. *Spine* 1990;15:36–40.
30. Liu JK, Apfelbaum RI. Treatment of trigeminal neuralgia. *Neurosurg Clin N Am* 2004;15:319–334.
31. Peters G, Nurmikko TJ. Peripheral and gasserian ganglion-level procedures for the treatment of trigeminal neuralgia. *Clin J Pain* 2002;18:28–34.
32. Brown JA. Percutaneous techniques: part IV trigeminal neuralgia. In: Winn HR, ed. *Youmans Neurological Surgery*. 5th ed. New York: WB Saunders; 2004:2996–3004.
33. Molet J. Neurosurgical treatment of facial neuralgias and neuropathic pain of the face. *Pain Rev* 1999;6:35–51.
34. Pollock B, Ecker RD. A prospective cost-effectiveness study of trigeminal neuralgia surgery. *Clin J Pain* 2005;21:317–322.
35. Evans PJ, Lloyd JW, Green CJ. Cryoanalgesia: the response to alterations in the freeze cycle temperature. *Br J Anaesth* 1981;53:1121–1127.
36. Lloyd JW, Barnard JD, Glynn CJ. Cryoanalgesia: a new approach to pain relief. *Lancet* 1976;2:932–934.
37. Collins GH, West NR, Parmely JD, et al. The histopathology of freezing injury to the rat spinal cord. A light microscope study. I. Early degenerative changes. *J Neuropathol Exp Neurol* 1986;45:721–741.
38. Evans PJ. Cryoanalgesia. The application of low temperatures to nerves to produce anaesthesia or analgesia. *Anaesthesia* 1981;36:1003–1013.
39. Zakrzewska JM, Nally FF. The role of cryotherapy (cryoanalgesia) in the management of paroxysmal trigeminal neuralgia: a six-year experience. *Br J Oral Maxillofac Surg* 1988;26:18–25.
40. Bärlocher CB, Krauss JK, Seiler RW. Kryorhizotomy: an alternative technique for lumbar medial branch rhizotomy in lumbar facet syndrome. *J Neurosurg* 2003;98:14–20.
41. Birkenmaier C, Veihelmann A, Trouillier H, et al. Percutaneous cryodenervation of lumbar facet joints: a prospective clinical trial. *Int Orthop* 2007;31:525–530.
42. Wang JK. Cryoanalgesia for painful peripheral nerve lesions. *Pain* 1985;22:191–194.
43. IEEE Committee on Man and Radiation (COMAR). Medical aspects of radiofrequency radiation overexposure. *Health Phys* 2002;82:387–391.
44. Foster KR. Thermal and nonthermal mechanisms of interaction of radiofrequency energy with biological systems. *IEEE Trans Plasma Sci* 2000;28:15–23.
45. Cosman ER, Nashold BS, Ovelman-Levitt J. Theoretical aspects of radiofrequency lesions in the dorsal root entry zone. *Neurosurgery* 1984;15:945–950.
46. Organ LW. Electrophysiologic principles of radiofrequency lesion making. *Appl Neurophysiol* 1976–1977;39:69–76.
47. Alberts WW, Wright EW, Feinstein B, et al. Experimental radiofrequency brain lesion size as a function of physical parameters. *J Neurosurg* 1966;25:421–423.
48. Cosman ER, Ritman WJ, Nashold BS, et al. Radiofrequency generation and its effect on tissue impedance. *Appl Neurophysiol* 1988;51:230–242.
49. Haines DE, Watson DD. Tissue heating during radiofrequency catheter ablation: a thermodynamic model and observations in isolated perfused and superfused canine right ventricular free wall. *Pacing Clin Electrophysiol* 1989;12:962–976.
50. Jain MK, Wolf PD. Temperature-controlled and constant-power radiofrequency ablation: what affects lesion growth? *IEEE Trans Biomed Eng* 1999;46:1405–1412.
51. Buijs EJ, van Wijk RM, Geurts JW, et al. Radiofrequency lumbar facet denervation: a comparative study of the reproducibility of lesion size after 2 current radiofrequency techniques. *Reg Anesth Pain Med* 2004;29:400–407.
52. Bogduk N. Macintosh J, Marsland A. Technical limitations to the efficacy of radiofrequency neurotomy for spinal pain. *Neurosurg* 1987;20:529–535.
53. Lord SM, McDonald GJ, Bogduk N. Percutaneous radiofrequency neurotomy of the cervical medial branches: a validated treatment for cervical zygapophysial joint pain. *Neurosurg Q* 1998;8:288–308.
54. Hamann W, Hall S. Acute effect and recovery of primary afferent nerve fibres after graded radiofrequency lesions in anaesthetized rats. *Br J Anaesthesia* 1992;68:443P.
55. Zervas NT, Kuwayama A. Pathological characteristics of experimental thermal lesions. Comparison of induction heating and radiofrequency electrocoagulation. *J Neurosurg* 1972;37:418–422.
56. Kanpolat Y, Onol B. Experimental percutaneous approach to the trigeminal ganglion in dogs with histopathological evaluation of radiofrequency lesions. *Acta Neurochir Suppl (Wien)* 1980;30:363–366.
57. Podhajsky RJ, Sekiguchi Y, Kikuchi S, et al. The histologic effects of pulsed and continuous radiofrequency lesions at 42 degrees C to rat dorsal root ganglion and sciatic nerve. *Spine* 2005;30:1008–1013.
58. Smith HP, Whorter JM, Challa VR. Radiofrequency neurolysis in a clinical mode: neuropathological correlation. *J Neurosurg* 1981;55:246–253.
59. de Louw AJA, Vles HS, Freling G, et al. The morphological effects of a radiofrequency lesion adjacent to the dorsal root ganglion (RF-DRG)—an experimental study in the goat. *Eur J Pain* 2001;5:169–174.
60. Letcher FS, Goldring S. The effect of radiofrequency current and heat on peripheral nerve action potential in the cat. *J Neurosurg Sci* 1968;29:42–47.
61. Oudenhoven RC. Paraspinal electromyography following facet rhizotomy. *Spine* 1977;2:299–304.
62. Dreyfuss P, Halbrook B, Pauza K, et al. Efficacy and validity of radiofrequency neurotomy for chronic lumbar zygapophysial joint pain. *Spine* 2000;25:1270–1277.
63. Kuck KH, Akhtar M. New horizons for electrical therapy in managing ventricular and supraventricular tachyarrhythmias. *Pacing Clin Electrophysiol* 1993;16:503–505.
64. Ruffy R, Imran MA, Santel DJ, et al. Radiofrequency delivery through a cooled catheter tip allows the creation of larger endomyocardial lesions in the ovine heart. *J Cardiovasc Electrophysiol* 1995;6:1089–1096.
65. Zakrzewska JM, Jassim S, Bulman JS. A prospective longitudinal study on patient with trigeminal neuralgia who underwent radiofrequency thermocoagulation of the Gasserian ganglion. *Pain* 1999;79:51–58.
66. Kanpolat Y, Savas A, Bekar A, et al. Percutaneous controlled radiofrequency trigeminal rhizotomy for the treatment of idiopathic trigeminal neuralgia: a 25-year experience with 1,600 patients. *Neurosurgery* 2001;48:524–534.
67. Wilkins RH. Trigeminal neuralgia: historical overview, with emphasis on surgical treatment. In: Burchiel K, ed. *Surgical Management of Pain*. New York: Thieme; 2002:288–303.
68. Lopez BC, Hamlyn PJ, Zakrzewska JM. Systematic review of ablative neurosurgical techniques for the treatment of trigeminal neuralgia. *Neurosurgery* 2004;54:973–982.
69. Latchaw JP Jr, Hardy RW, Forsythe SB, et al. Trigeminal neuralgia treated by radiofrequency coagulation. *J Neurosurg* 1983;59:479–484.
70. Oturai AB, Jensen K, Eriksen J, et al. Neurosurgery for trigeminal neuralgia: comparison of alcohol block, neurectomy, and radiofrequency coagulation. *Clin J Pain* 1996;12:311–315.
71. Taha JM, Tew JM Jr, Buncher CR. A prospective 15-year follow up of 154 consecutive patients with trigeminal neuralgia treated by percutaneous stereotactic radiofrequency thermal rhizotomy. *J Neurosurg* 1995;85:189–993.
72. Harrigan M, Chandler WF. Abducens nerve palsy after radiofrequency rhizolysis for trigeminal neuralgia: case report. *Neurosurgery* 1998;43:623–625.
73. Berk C, Honey CR. Brain stem injury after radiofrequency trigeminal rhizotomy. *Acta Neurochir (Wien)* 2004;146:635–636.
74. Torroba L, Moreno S, Lorenzana L, et al. Purulent meningitis after percutaneous radiofrequency trigeminal rhizotomy. *J Neurol Neurosurg Psychiatry* 1987;50:1081–1082.
75. Kaplan M, Erol FS, Ozveren MF, et al. Review of complications due to foramen ovale puncture. *J Clin Neurosci* 2007;14:563–568.
76. Romanelli P, Ersposito V, Adler J. Ablative procedures for chronic pain. *Neurosurg Clin N Am* 2004;15:335–342.

77. Nashold JRB, Nashold BS Jr, Pearlstein RD. The DREZ operation for the relief of deafferentation pain. In: Kaye AH, Black PMcL, eds. *Operative Neurosurgery*. London: Churchill Livingstone; 2000:1521–1537.

78. Guenot M, Bullier J, Sindou M. Clinical and electrophysiological expression of deafferentation pain alleviated by dorsal root entry zone lesion in rats. *J Neurosurg* 2002;97:1402–1409.

79. Falci S, Best L, Bayles R, et al. Dorsal root entry zone micro-coagulation for spinal cord injury-related central pain: operative intramedullary electrophysiological guidance and clinical outcome. *J Neurosurg* 2002;97:193–200.

80. Tomás R, Haninec P. Dorsal root entry zone (DREZ) localization using direct spinal cord stimulation can improve results of the DREZ thermocoagulation procedure for intractable pain relief. *Pain* 2005;116:159–163.

81. Gorecki JP. Dorsal root entry zone and brainstem ablative procedures. In Winn HR ed. *Youman's Neurological Surgery*. 5th ed. Philadelphia: WB Saunders; 2004:3045–3058.

82. Sindou MP, Blondet E, Emery E, et al. Microsurgical lesioning in the dorsal root entry zone for pain due to brachial plexus avulsion: a prospective series of 55 patients. *J Neurosurg* 2005;102:1018–1028.

83. Mertens P, Sindou M. Surgery in the dorsal root entry zone for treatment of chronic pain [in French]. *Neurochirurgie* 2000;46(5):429–426.

84. Blumenkopf B. Neuropharmacology of the dorsal root entry zone. *Neurosurgery* 1984;15:900–903.

85. Parry CB. Pain in avulsion of brachial plexus. *Neurosurgery* 1984;15:960–965.

86. Sindou MP. Microsurgical DREZotomy. In: Schmidek HH, Sweet WH, eds. *Operative Neurosurgical Techniques*. 3rd ed. Philadelphia: WB Saunders; 1995:1585–1594.

87. Denkers M, Biagi HL, O'Brien AM, et al. Dorsal root entry zone lesioning used to treat central neuropathic pain with traumatic spinals cord injury: a systematic review. *Spine* 2002;27:E177–E184.

88. Sampson JH, Cashman RE, Nashold BS Jr, et al. Dorsal root entry zone lesions for intractable pain after trauma to the conus medullaris and cauda equina. *J Neurosurg* 1995;82:28–34.

89. Kanpolat Y. Cordotomy for pain. In: Winn HR, ed. *Youman's Neurological Surgery*. 5th ed. Philadelphia: WB Saunders; 2003:3059–3071.

90. Kanpolat Y. The surgical treatment of chronic pain: destructive therapies in the spinal cord. *Neurosurg Clin N Am* 2004;15:307–317.

91. Sanders M, Zuurmond W. Safety of unilateral and bilateral percutaneous cervical cordotomy in 80 terminally ill cancer patients. *J Clin Oncol* 1995;13:1509–1512.

92. Crul BJ, Blok LM, van Egmond J, et al. The present role of percutaneous cervical cordotomy for the treatment of cancer pain. *J Headache Pain* 2005;6:24–29.

93. Ischia S, Luzzani A, Ischia A, et al. Role of unilateral percutaneous cervical cordotomy in the treatment of neoplastic vertebral pain. *Pain* 1984;19:123–131.

94. Bullard DE, Nashold BS Jr. The caudalis DREZ for facial pain. *Stereotact Funct Neurosurg* 1997;68:168–174.

95. Bernard EJ Jr, Nashold BS Jr, Caputi F, et al. Nucleus caudalis DREZ lesions for facial pain. *Br J Neurosurg* 1987;1:81–91.

96. Geurts JW, Lou L, Gauci CA, et al. Radiofrequency treatments in low back pain. *Pain Pract* 2002;2:226–234.

97. Slipman CW, Bhat AL, Gilchrist RV, et al. A critical review of the evidence for the use of zygapophysial injections and radiofrequency denervation in the treatment of low back pain. *Spine J* 2003;3:310–316.

98. Hooten WM, Martin DP, Huntoon MA. Radiofrequency neurotomy for low back pain: evidence based procedural guidelines. *Pain Med* 2005;6:129–138.

99. Hall DJ. Facet joint denervation: a minimally invasive treatment for low back pain in selected patients. In: Herkowitz HN, Dvorak J, Bell GR, et al., eds. *The Lumbar Spine: Official Publication of the International Society for the Study of the Lumbar Spine*. 3rd ed. Philadelphia: Lippincott Williams & Wilkins; 2004:307–311.

100. Bogduk N. The clinical anatomy of the cervical dorsal rami. *Spine* 1982;7:319–330.

101. Bogduk N, Lord SM. Cervical zygapophysial joint pain. *Neurosurg Q* 1998;8:107–117.

102. Bogduk N, Wilson AS, Tynan W. The human lumbar dorsal rami. *J Anat* 1982;134:383–397.

103. Lord SM, Barnsley L, Wallis BJ, et al. Percutaneous radio-frequency neurotomy for chronic cervical zygapophyseal-joint pain. *N Engl J Med* 1996;335:1721–1726.

104. Hildebrandt J, Argyrakis A. Percutaneous nerve block of the cervical facets—a relatively new method in the treatment of chronic headache and neck pain. *Man Med* 1986;2:48–52.

105. Sluijter ME, Mehta M. Treatment of chronic neck and back pain by percutaneous thermal lesions. In: Lipton S, Miles J, eds. *Persistent Pain: Modern Methods of Treatment*. London: Academic Press; New York: Grune & Stratton; 1981;3:141–179.

106. Vervest ACM, Stolker RJ, Groen GJ. Radiofrequency lesioning for pain treatment: a review. *Pain Clin* 1995;8:175–189.

107. International Spine Intervention Society. Percutaneous radiofrequency cervical medial branch neurotomy. In: Bogduk N, ed. *Practice Guidelines for Spinal Diagnostic and Treatment Procedures*. San Francisco, CA: International Spine Intervention Society, 2004:249–284.

108. Govind J, King W, Bailey B, et al. Radiofrequency neurotomy for the treatment of third occipital headache. *J Neurol Neurosurg Psychiat* 2003;74:88–93.

109. McDonald GJ, Lord SM, Bogduk N. Long-term follow-up of patients treated with cervical radiofrequency neurotomy for chronic neck pain. *Neurosurgery* 1999;45:61–68.

110. Shin WR, Kim HI, Shin DG, et al. Radiofrequency neurotomy of cervical medial branches for chronic cervicobrachialgia. *J Korean Med Sci* 2006;21:119–125.

111. Barnsley L. Percutaneous radiofrequency neurotomy for chronic neck pain: outcomes in a series of consecutive patients. *Pain Med* 2005;6:282–286.

112. Geurts JWM, van Wilk RMAW, Stolker R. In defense of radiofrequency neurotomy. [author reply]. *Reg Anesth Pain Med* 2002;27:441–442.

113. Wallis BJ, Lord SM, Bogduk N. Resolution of psychological distress of whiplash patients following treatment by radiofrequency neurotomy: a randomised, double-blind, placebo-controlled trial. *Pain* 1997;73:15–22.

114. Sapir DA, Gorup JM. Radiofrequency medial branch neurotomy in litigant and nonlitigant patients with cervical whiplash: a prospective study. *Spine* 2001;26:E268–E273.

115. Centre for Health Services and Policy Branch. Percutaneous radio-frequency neurotomy treatment of chronic cervical pain following whiplash injury. Vancouver, University of British Columbia, British Columbia Office of Health Technology Assessment 01:5T;2001.

116. Cousins MJ, Walker S. Chronic pain: management strategies that work. *Anaesth Analg* 2001;92(suppl):15–25.

117. Boswell MV, Shah RV, Everett CR, et al. Interventional techniques in the management of chronic spinal pain; evidence-based practice guidelines. *Pain Physician* 2005;8:1–47.

118. Lord SM, McDonald GJ, Bogduk N. Side effects and complications of cervical percutaneous radio-frequency neurotomy—an audit of 83 procedures [abstract]. *Anaesth Intensive Care* 1998;26:322–328.

119. Merrill DG. Hoffman's glasses: evidence-based medicine and the search for quality in the literature of interventional pain medicine. *Reg Anesth Pain Med* 2003;28:547–560.

120. Drinka PJ, Jaschob K. Treatment of chronic cervical zygapophyseal-joint pain. *New Eng J Med* 1997;336:1530–1531.

121. Buck-Gramcko D. Denervation of the wrist joint. *J Hand Surg Am* 1977;2:254–261.

122. Hutton CW. Osteoarthritis. In Weatherall DJL, Wedingham JGG, Warrell DA, eds. *Oxford Textbook of Medicine*. 3rd ed. New York: Oxford University Press; 1996:3079.

123. Norman A, Robbins H, Milgram JE. The acute neuropathic arthropathy—a rapid, severely disorganising form of arthritis. *Radiology* 1968;90:1159–1164.

124. Kate I, Rabinowitz JG, Dziadiw R. Early changes in Charcot's joints. *AJR* 1961;86:965–974.

125. Lord SM, Bogduk N. Treatment of chronic zygapophyseal joint pain (letter). *N Eng J Med* 1997;336:1531.

126. Bogduk N, Dreyfuss P, Baker R, et al. Complications of spinal diagnostic and treatment procedures. *Pain Med* 2008;9, Supplement 2:S11–S34.

127. Bogduk N. Cervicogenic headaches: anatomic basis and pathophysiologic mechanisms. *Curr Pain Headache Rep* 2001;5:382–386.

128. Bogduk N. The neck and headaches. *Neurol Clin N Am* 2004;22:151–171.

129. Trevor-Jones R. Osteo-arthritis of the paravertebral joints of the second and third cervical vertebrae as a cause of occipital headaches. *S Afr Med J* 1964;38:392–394.

130. Bogduk N, Marsland A. On the concept of third occipital headache. *J Neurol Neurosurg Psychiat* 1986;49:775–780.

131. Lord SM, Barnsley L, Wallis BJ, et al. Third occipital headache: a prevalence study. *J Neurol Neurosurg Psychiatry* 1994;57:1187–1190.

132. Lord SM, Bogduk N. The cervical synovial joint as a source of post-traumatic headache. *J Musculoskeletal Pain* 1996;4:81–94.

133. Govind J, King W, Giles P, et al. Headaches and the cervical zygapophysial joints (cervicogenic/cervical headache) [abstract]. *J Bone Joint Surg* 2005;87-B(suppl 3):399.

134. Bogduk N, Bartsch T. Cervicogenic headache. In: Silberstein SD, Lipton RB, Dodick DW, eds. *Wolff's Headache and Other Head Pain*. 8th ed. New York: Oxford University Press; 2008:551–570.

135. Headache Classification Subcommittee of the International Headache Society. The International Classification of Headache Disorders: 2nd edition. *Cephalalgia* 2004;24(suppl 1)9–160.

136. van Suijlekom HA, van Kleef M, Barendse GA, et al. Radiofrequency cervical zygapophyseal joint neurotomy for cervicogenic headaches: a prospective study of 15 patients. *Funct Neurol* 1998;13:297–303.

137. Stovner LJ, Kolstad F, Helde G. Radiofrequency denervation of facet joints C2-C6 in cervicogenic headache: a randomized, double-blind, sham-controlled study. *Cephalalgia* 2004;24:821–830.

138. Haspeslagh SR, van Suijlekom HA, Lamé IE, et al. Randomised controlled trial of cervical radiofrequency lesions as a treatment for cervicogenic headache [ISRCTN07444684]. *BMC Anesthesiol* 2006;6:1.

139. Bogduk N. Cervicogenic headache. *Cephalalgia* 2004;24:819–820.

140. Lau P, Mercer S, Govind J, et al. The surgical anatomy of lumbar medial branch neurotomy (facet denervation). *Pain Med* 2004;5:289–298.

141. International Spine Intervention Society. Percutaneous radiofrequency lumbar medial branch neurotomy. In: Bogduk N, ed. *Practice Guidelines for Spinal Diagnostic and Treatment Procedures*. San Francisco, CA: International Spine Intervention Society, 2004:188–210.

142. Geurts JW, van Wijk RM, Stolker RJ, et al. Efficacy of radiofrequency procedures for the treatment of spinal pain: a systematic review of randomized clinical trials. *Reg Anesth Pain Med* 2001;26:394–400.

143. Niemistö L, Kalso E, Malmivaara A, et al. Radiofrequency denervation for neck and back pain: a systematic review within the framework of the Cochrane Collaboration Back Review Group. *Spine* 2003;28:1877–1888.
144. Hooten WM, Martin DP, Huntoon MA. Radiofrequency neurotomy for low back pain: evidence-based procedural guidelines. *Pain Med* 2005;6:129–138.
145. Gofeld M, Jitendra J, Faclier G. Radiofrequency denervation of the lumbar zygapophysial joints: 10-year prospective clinical audit. *Pain Physician* 2007;10:291–300.
146. van Kleef M, Barendse GA, Kessels A, et al. Randomized trial of radiofrequency lumbar facet denervation for chronic low back pain. *Spine* 1999;24:1937–1942.
147. Nath S, Nath CA, Pettersson K. Percutaneous lumbar zygapophysial (facet) joint neurotomy using radiofrequency current in the management of chronic low back pain: a randomized double blind trial. *Spine* 2008;33(12):1291–1297; discussion 1298.
148. Schofferman J, Kine G. Effectiveness of repeated radiofrequency neurotomy for lumbar facet pain. *Spine* 2004;29:2471–2473.
149. Kornick C, Kramarich SS, Lamer TJ, et al. Complications of lumbar facet radiofrequency denervation. *Spine* 2004;29:1352–1354.
150. Kapural L, Mekhail N. Radiofrequency ablation for chronic pain control. *Curr Pain Headache Rep* 2001;5:517–525.
151. North RB, Han M, Zahurak M, et al. Radiofrequency lumbar facet denervation: analysis of prognostic factors. *Pain* 1994;57:77–83.
152. Abbott Z, Smuck M, Haig A, et al. Irreversible spinal nerve injury from a dorsal ramus radiofrequency neurotomy: a case report. *Arch Phys Med Rehabil* 2007;88:1350–1352.
153. Coskun DJ, Gilchrist J, Dupuy D. Lumbosacral radiculopathy following radiofrequency ablation therapy. *Muscle Nerve* 2003;28:754–756.
154. Stolker RJ, Vervest AC, Groen GJ. Percutaneous facet denervation in chronic thoracic spinal pain. *Acta Neurochir (Wien)* 1993;122:82–90.
155. Chua WH, Bogduk N. The surgical anatomy of thoracic facet denervation. *Acta Neurochir* 1995;136:140–144.
156. Fortin JD, Kissling RO, O'Connor BL, et al. Sacroiliac joint innervation and pain. *Am J Orthop* 1999;28:687–690.
157. Vilensky JA, O'Connor BL, Fortin JD, et al. Histologic analysis of neural elements in the human sacroiliac joint. *Spine* 2002;27:1202–1207.
158. Ebraheim NA, Lu J, Biyani A, et al. The relationship of the lumbosacral plexus to the sacrum and the sacroiliac joint. *Am J Orthop* 1997;26:105–110.
159. Atlihan D, Tekdemir I, Ateš Y, et al. Anatomy of the anterior sacroiliac joint with reference to lumbosacral nerves. *Clin Orthop Relat Res* 2000;376:236–241.
160. Ikeda R. Innervation of the sacroiliac joint. Macroscopical and histological studies [in Japanese]. *Nippon Ika Daigaku Zasshi* 1991;58:587–596.
161. Grob K, Neuhuber W, Kissling R. Die innervation des sacroiliacalgelenkes beim menschen. *Zeitschr Rheumatol* 1995;27:117–122.
162. Ferrante FM, King LF, Roche EA, et al. Radiofrequency sacroiliac joint denervation for sacroiliac syndrome. *Reg Anesth Pain Med* 2001;26:137–142.
163. Yin W, Willard F, Careiro J, et al. Sensory stimulation-guided sacroiliac joint radiofrequency neurotomy: technique based on neuroanatomy of the dorsal sacral plexus. *Spine* 2003;28:2419–2425.
164. Buijs EJ, Kamphuis ET, Groen GJ. Radiofrequency treatment of sacroiliac joint-related pain aimed at the first three sacral dorsal rami: a minimal approach. *Pain Clin* 2004;16:139–146.
165. Burnham RS, Yasui Y. An alternate method of radiofrequency neurotomy of the sacroiliac joint: a pilot study of the effect on pain, function, and satisfaction. *Reg Anesth Pain Med* 2007;32:12–19.
166. Cohen SP, Jurhara C, Hurley RW, et al. A randomized, placebo-controlled study evaluating lumbosacral primary dorsal rami and lateral branch radiofrequency denervation for sacroiliac joint pain. *Anesthesiology* 2008;109:279–288.
167. Van Kleef M, Barendse GA, Wilmink JT, et al. Percutaneous intradiscal radiofrequency thermocoagulation in chronic non-specific low back pain. *Pain Clin* 1996;9:259–268.
168. Erçelen O, Bulutçu E, Oktenoglu T, et al. Radiofrequency lesioning using two different time modalities for the treatment of lumbar discogenic pain: a randomized trial. *Spine* 2003;28:1922–1927.
169. Barendse GAM, van Den Berg SG, Kessels AH, et al. Randomized controlled trial of percutaneous intradiscal radiofrequency thermocoagulation for chronic discogenic back pain: lack of effect from a 90-second 70 C lesion. *Spine* 2001;26:287–292.
170. Troussier B, Lebas JF, Chirossel JP, et al. Percutaneous intradiscal radiofrequency theromocoagulation. A cadaveric study. *Spine* 1995;20:1713–1718.
171. Houpt JC, Conner ES, McFarland EW. Experimental study of temperature distributions and thermal transport during radiofrequency current therapy of the intervertebral disc. *Spine* 1996;21:1808–1812.
172. Saal JS, Saal JA. Management of chronic discogenic low back pain with a thermal intradiscal catheter. A preliminary report. *Spine* 2000;25:382–388.
173. Shah RV, Lutz GE, Lee J, et al. Intradiscal electrothermal therapy: a preliminary histologic study. *Arch Phys Med Rehabil* 2001;82:1230–1237.
174. Kleinstueck FS, Diederich CJ, Nau WH, et al. Acute biomechanical and histological effects of intradiscal electrothermal therapy on human lumbar discs. *Spine* 2001;24:2198–2207.
175. Karasek M, Bogduk N. Intradiscal electrothermal annuloplasty: percutaneous treatment of chronic discogenic low back pain. *Tech Reg Anesth Pain Manag* 2001;5:130–135.
176. Bogduk N, Lau P, Govind J, et al. Intradiscal electrothermal therapy. *Tech Reg Anesth Pain Manag* 2005;9:25–34.
177. Kleinstueck FS, Diederich CJ, Nau WH, et al. Temperature and thermal dose distributions during intradiscal electrothermal therapy in the cadaveric lumbar spine. *Spine* 2003;28:1700–1709.
178. Freeman B, Walters RM, Moore RJ, et al. Does intradiscal electrothermal therapy denervate and repair experimentally induced posterolateral anular tears in an animal model? *Spine* 2003;28:2602–2608.
179. Bono CM, Iki K, Jalota A, et al Temperatures within the lumbar disc and endplates during intradiscal electrothermal therapy: formulation of a predictive temperature map in relation to distance from the catheter. *Spine* 2004;29:1124–1129.
180. Derby R, Eek B, Chen Y, et al. Intradiscal electrothermal annuloplasty (IDET): a novel approach for treating chronic discogenic back pain. *Neuromodulation* 2000;3:82–88.
181. Gerszten PC, Welch WC, McGrath PM, et al. A prospective outcomes study of patients undergoing intradiscal electrothermy (IDET) for chronic low back pain. *Pain Physician* 2002;5:360–364.
182. Spruit M, Jacobs WC. Pain and function after intradiscal electrothermal treatment (IDET) for symptomatic lumbar disc degeneration. *Eur Spine J* 2002;11:589–593.
183. Davis TT, Delamarter RB, Sra P, et al. The IDET procedure for chronic discogenic low back pain. *Spine* 2004;29:752–756.
184. Saal JA, Saal JS. Intradiscal electrothermal treatment for chronic discogenic low back pain; a prospective outcome study with minimum 1-year follow-up. *Spine* 2000;25:2622–2627.
185. Saal JA, Saal JS. Intradiscal electrothermal treatment for chronic discogenic low back pain: prospective outcome study with a minimum 2-year follow-up. *Spine* 2002;27:966–974.
186. Endres SM, Fiedler GA, Larson KL. Effectiveness of intradiscal electrothermal therapy in increasing function and reducing chronic low back pain in selected patients. *WMJ* 2002;101:31–34.
187. Lutz C, Lutz GE, Cooke PM. Treatment of chronic lumbar diskogenic pain with intradiskal electrothermal therapy: a prospective outcome study. *Arch Phys Med Rehabil* 2003;84:23–28.
188. Lee MS, Cooper G, Lutz GE, et al. Intradiscal electrothermal therapy (IDET) for treatment of chronic lumbar discogenic pain: a minimum 2-year clinical outcome study. *Pain Physician* 2003;6:443–448.
189. Freedman BA, Cohen SP, Kuklo TR, et al. Intradiscal electrothermal therapy (IDET) for chronic low back pain in active-duty soldiers: 2-year follow-up. *Spine J* 2003;3:502–509.
190. Singh V. Intradiscal electrothermal therapy: a preliminary report. *Pain Physician* 2000;3:367–373.
191. Cohen SP, Larkin T, Abdi S, et al. Risk factors for failure and complications of intradiscal electrothermal therapy: a pilot study. *Spine* 2003;28:1142–1147.
192. Mekhail N, Kapural L. Intradiscal thermal annuloplasty for discogenic pain: an outcome study. *Pain Pract* 2004;4:84–90.
193. Kapural L, Makhail N, Korunda Z, et al. Intradiscal thermal annuloplasty for the treatment of lumbar discogenic pain in patients with multilevel degenerative disc disease. *Anesth Analg* 2004;99:472–476.
194. Kapural L, Hayek S, Malak O, et al. Intradiscal thermal annuloplasty versus intradiscal radiofrequency ablation for the treatment of discogenic pain: a prospective matched control trial. *Pain Med* 2005;6:425–431.
195. Karasek M, Bogduk N. Twelve-month follow-up of a controlled trial of intradiscal thermal anuloplasty for back pain due to internal disc disruption. *Spine* 2000;25:2601–2607.
196. Bogduk N, Karasek M. Two-year follow-up of a controlled trial of intradiscal electrothermal anuloplasty for chronic low back pain resulting from internal disc disruption. *Spine J* 2002;2:343–350.
197. Maurer P, Block JE, Squillante D. Intradiscal electrothermal therapy (IDET) provides effective symptom relief in patients with discogenic low back pain. *J Spinal Disord Tech* 2008;21:55–62.
198. Nunley PD, Jawahar A, Brandao SM, et al. Intradiscal electrothermal therapy (IDET) for low back pain in worker's compensation patients: can it provide a potential answer? Long-term results. *J Spinal Disord Tech* 2008;21:11–18.
199. Freeman BJ, Fraser RD, Cain CM, et al. A randomized, double-blind, controlled trial: intradiscal electrothermal therapy versus placebo for the treatment of chronic discogenic low back pain. *Spine* 2005;30:2369–2377.
200. Pauza KJ, Howell S, Dreyfuss P, et al. A randomized, placebo-controlled trial of intradiscal electrothermal therapy for the treatment of discogenic low back pain. *Spine J* 2004;4:27–35.
201. Gibson JN, Waddell G. Surgery for degenerative lumbar spondylosis: updated Cochrane review. *Spine* 2005;30:2312–2310.
202. Gibson JA, Waddell G. Untitled. [Letter in Response]. *Spine* 2006;31:1402–1403.
203. International Spine Intervention Society. Intradiscal electrothermal therapy. In: Bogduk N, ed. *Practice Guidelines for Spinal Diagnostic and Treatment Procedures.* San Francisco, CA: International Spine Intervention Society; 2004:219–236.
204. Ryne AL, Smith SE, Wood KE, et al. Outcome of unoperated discogram-positive low back pain. *Spine* 1995;20:1997–2000.
205. Appleby D, Andersson G, Totta M. Meta-analysis of the efficacy and safety of intradiscal electrothermal therapy (IDET). *Pain Med* 2006;7:308–316.
206. Andersson GB, Mekhail NA, Block JE. Treatment of intractable discogenic low back pain. A systematic review of spinal fusion and intradiscal electrothermal therapy (IDET). *Pain Physician* 2006;9:237–248.
207. Epstein NE. Laser-assisted diskectomy performed by an internist resulting in cauda equina syndrome. *J Spinal Disord* 1999;12:77–79.

208. Hsia AW, Isaac K, Katz JS. Cauda equina syndrome from intradiscal electro-thermal therapy. *Neurology* 2000;55:320.
209. Ackerman WE III. Cauda equina syndrome after intradiscal electrothermal therapy. *Reg Anesth Pain Med* 2002;27:622.
210. Scholl BM, Theiss SM, Lopez-Ben R, et al. Vertebral osteonecrosis related to intradiscal electrothermal therapy: a case report. *Spine* 2003;28(9):E161–E164.
211. Djurasovic M, Glassman SD, Dimar JR II, et al. Vertebral osteonecrosis associated with the use of intradiscal electrothermal therapy: a case report. *Spine* 2002;27:E325–E328.
212. Cohen SP, Larkin T, Polly DW Jr. A giant herniated disc following intradiscal electrothermal therapy. *J Spinal Disord Tech* 2002;15:537–541.
213. Kapural L, Cata JP. Complications of percutaneous techniques used in the diagnosis and treatment of discogenic lower back pain. *Tech Reg Anesth Pain Manag* 2007;11:157–163.
214. Finch PM. Radiofrequency denervation of the annulus fibrosus: a rationale. *Tech Reg Anesth Pain Manag* 2004;8:41–45.
215. Wright RE, Brandt SA, Barkow SH, et al. Quantitative annular thermometry in humans and sheep during radiofrequency and electrothermal anuloplasty. *Tech Reg Anesth Pain Manag* 2001;5:136–141.
216. Erdine S, Yucel A, Celik M. Percutaneous annuloplasty in the treatment of discogenic pain: retrospective evaluation of one year follow-up. *Agri* 2004;16:41–47.
217. Finch PM, Price LM, Drummond PD. Radiofrequency heating of painful annular disruptions: one-year outcomes. *J Spinal Disord Tech* 2005;18:6–13.
218. Petersohn JD, Conquergood LR, Leung M. Acute histologic effects and thermal distribution profile of disc biacuplasty using a novel water-cooled bipolar electrode system in an in vivo porcine model. *Pain Med* 2008;9:26–32.
219. Kapural L, Mekhail N, Kapural M, et al. Histological and temperature studies of a novel transdiscal heating system in human cadaver discs. *Anesthesiology* 2006;105:A705.
220. Kapural L, Mekahil N, Hicks D, et al. Histological changes and temperature distribution studies of a novel bipolar radiofrequency heating system in degenerated and nondegenerated human cadaver lumbar discs. *Pain Med* 2008;9:68–75.
221. Kapural L, Ng A, Dalton J, et al. Intervertebral disc biacuplasty for the treatment of lumbar discogenic pain: results of a six-month follow-up. *Pain Med* 2008;9:60–67.
222. Bogduk N, Lau P, Gowaily K. A pilot audit of the effectiveness of transdiscal biacuplasty for the treatment of beck pain due to internal disc disruption. Proceedings of the Spine Society of Australia. *J Bone Joint Surg* 2009 (In press).
223. van Kleef M, Spaans F, Dingemans W, et al. Effects and side effects of a percutaneous thermal lesion of the dorsal root ganglion in patients with cervical pain syndrome. *Pain* 1993;52:49–53.
224. Stolker RJ, Vervest AC, Groen GJ. The treatment of chronic thoracic segmental pain by radiofrequency percutaneous partial rhizotomy. *J Neurosurg* 1994;80:986–992.
225. van Kleef M, Barendse GA, Dingemans WA, et al. Effects of producing a radiofrequency lesion adjacent to the dorsal root ganglion in patients with thoracic segmental pain. *Clin J Pain* 1995;11:325–332.
226. van Wijk RM, Geurts JW, Wynne HJ. Long-lasting analgesic effect of radiofrequency treatment of the lumbosacral dorsal root ganglion. *J Neurosurg* 2001;94:227–231.
227. van Kleef M, Liem L, Lousberg R, et al. Radiofrequency lesion adjacent to the dorsal root ganglion for cervicobrachial pain. a prospective double blind randomized study. *Neurosurgery* 1996;38:1127–1131.
228. Geurts JW, can Wijk RM, Wynne HJ, et al. Radiofrequency lesioning of dorsal root ganglia for chronic lumbosacral radicular pain: a randomised, double-blind, controlled trial. *Lancet* 2003;361:21–26.
229. Cousins MJ, Reeve TS, Glynn CJ, et al. Neurolytic lumbar sympathetic blockade: duration of denervation and relief of rest pain. *Anaesth Intensive Care* 1979;7:121–135.
230. Lantsberg L, Goldman M. Lower limb sympathectomy assessed by laser Doppler blood flow and transcutaneous oxygen measurements. *J Med Eng Technol* 1990;14:182–183.
231. Maga P, Kuzdzał J, Nizankowski R, et al. Long term effects of thoracic sympathectomy on microcirculation in the hands of patients with primary Raynaud disease. *J Thorac Cardiovasc Surg* 2007;133:1428–1433.
232. Walsh JA, Glynn CJ, Cousins MJ, et al. Blood flow, sympathetic activity and pain relief following lumbar sympathetic blockade or surgical sympathectomy. *Anaesth Interns Care* 1984;13:18–24.
233. Dabrowski J, Mikosiński J, Kuśmierek J. Scintigraphic and ultrasonographic assessment of the effect of lumbar sympathectomy upon chronic arteriosclerotic ischemia of lower extremities. *Nucl Med Rev Cent East Eur* 2003;6:17–22.
234. Wang WH, Lai CS, Chang KP, et al. Peripheral sympathectomy for Raynaud's phenomenon: a salvage procedure. *Kaohsiung J Med Sci* 2006;22:491–499.
235. Bates W, Judovich BD. Intractable pain. *Anesthesiology* 1942;3:663–672.
236. Dobrogowski J. Chemical sympathectomy. *Pain Clin* 1995;8:93–99.
237. Bay JW, Dohn DF. Surgical sympathectomy. In Wilkins RH, Rengachary SS eds. *Neurosurgery*. 2nd ed. New York: McGraw-Hill; 1996:3251–3256.
238. Mailis-Gagnon A, Furlan A. Sympathectomy for neuropathic pain. *Cochrane Database Syst Rev* 2002;1:CD002918.
239. Mailis-Gagnon A, Furlan A. Sympathectomy for neuropathic pain. *Cochrane Database System Rev* 2003;2:CD002918.
240. Mockus MB, Rutherford RB, Rosales C, et al. Sympathectomy for causalgia. Patient selection and long-term results. *Arch Surg* 1987;122:668–672.
241. Kramis RC, Roberts WJ, Gillette RG. Post-sympathectomy neuralgia: hypotheses on peripheral and central neuronal mechanisms. *Pain* 1996;64;1–9.
242. Forouzanfar T, van Kleef M, Weber WE. Radiofrequency lesions of the stellate ganglion in chronic pain syndromes: retrospective analysis of clinical efficacy in 86 patients. *Clin J Pain* 2000;16:164–168.
243. Garcea G, Thomasset S, Berry DP, et al. Percutaneous splanchnic nerve radiofrequency ablation for chronic abdominal pain. *ANZ J Surg* 2005;75:640–644.
244. Wilkinson HA. Percutaneous radiofrequency upper thoracic sympathectomy: technical applications. *Neurosurgery* 1996;38:715–725.
245. Geurts JWR, Stolker RJ. Percutaneous radiofrequency lesion of the stellate ganglion in the treatment of pain in the upper extremity reflex sympathetic dystrophy. *Pain Clin* 1993;6:17–25.
246. Sanders M, Zuurmond WW. Efficacy of sphenopalatine ganglion blockade in 66 patients suffering from cluster headache: a 12- to 70-month follow-up evaluation. *J Neurosurg* 1997;87:876–80.
247. Salar G, Ori C, Iob I, et al. Percutaneous thermocoagulation for sphenopalatine ganglion neuralgia. *Acta Neurochir (Wien)* 1987;84:24–28.
248. Salar G, Iob I, Ori C. Combined thermocoagulation of the 5th and 9th cranial nerves for oral pain of neoplastic aetiology. *J Maxillofac Surg* 1986;14:1–4.
249. Salar G, Ori C, Baratto V, et al. Selective percutaneous thermolesions of the ninth cranial nerve by lateral cervical approach: report of eight cases. *Surg Neurol* 1983;20:276–279.
250. Kawaguchi M, Hashizume K, Iwata T, et al. Percutaneous radiofrequency lesioning of sensory branches of the obturator or femoral nerves for the treatment of hip joint pain. *Reg Anesth Pain Med* 2001;26:576–581.
251. Sluijter ME, Cosman ER, Rittman WB III, et al. The effects of pulsed radiofrequency fields applied to the dorsal root ganglion-a preliminary report. *Pain Clin* 1998;11:109–117.
252. Munglani R. The longer term effect of pulsed radiofrequency for neuropathic pain. *Pain* 1999;80:437–439.
253. Sluijter M. Racz G. Technical aspects of radiofrequency. *Pain Pract* 2002;2:195–200.
254. Mikeladze G, Espinal R, Finnegan R, et al. Pulsed radiofrequency application in the treatment of chronic zygapophyseal joint pain. *Spine J* 2003;3:360–362.
255. Geurts JW, Lou L, Gauci CA, et al. Radiofrequency treatments in low back pain. *Pain Pract* 2002;2:226–234.
256. Higuchi Y, Nashold BS Jr, Sluijter M, et al. Exposure of dorsal root ganglion in rats to pulsed radiofrequency current activated dorsal horn lamina I and II neurons. *Neurosurgery* 2002;50:850–856.
257. Hamann W, Abou-Sherif S, Thompson S, et al. Pulsed radiofrequency applied to dorsal root ganglion causes a selective increase in ATF3 in small neurons. *Eur J Pain* 2006;10:171–176.
258. Van Zundert J, de Louw AJ, Joosten EA, et al. Pulsed and continuous radiofrequency current adjacent to the cervical dorsal root ganglion of the rat induces late cellular activity in the dorsal horn. *Anaesthesiology* 2005;102:125–131.
259. McClung CA, Nestler EJ. Neuroplasticity mediated by altered gene expression. *Neuropsychopharmacolgy* 2008;33:3–17.
260. Sandkühler J, Treier AC, Liu XG, et al. The massive expression of c-fos protein in the spinal dorsal horn neurons is not followed by long-term changes in spinal nociception. *Neuroscience* 1996;73:657–666.
261. Dielenberg RA, Hunt GE, McGregor IS. "When a rat smells a cat": the distribution of fos immunoreactivity in rat brain following exposure to a predatory odor. *Neuroscience* 2001;104:1085–1097.
262. Matsuda S, Peng H, Yoshimura H, et al. Persistent c-fos expression in the brains of mice with chronic social stress. *Neurosci Res* 1996;26:157–170.
263. Chen BP, Wolfgang CD, Hai T. Analysis of ATF3, a transcription factor induced by physiological stresses and modulated by gaddl53/Chop 10. *Mol Cell Biol* 1996;16:1157–1168.
264. Hai T, Wolfgang CD, Marsee DK, et al. ATF3 and stress responses. *Gene Expr* 1999;7:321–335.
265. Tsujino H, Kondo E, Fukuoka T, et al. Activating transcription factor 3 (ATF3) induction by axotomy in sensory and motor neurons: a novel neuronal maker of nerve injury. *Mol Cell Neurosci* 2000;15:17–182.
266. Malik K, Benzon HT. Pulsed radiofrequency: a critical review of efficacy. *Anaesth Intensive Care* 2007;35:863–873.
267. Sluijter ME, Teixeira A, Serra V, et al. Intra-articular application of pulsed radiofrequency for arthrogenic pain—report of six cases. *Pain Pract* 2008;8:57–61.
268. Bogduk N. Pulsed Radiofrequency. *Pain Med* 2006;7:396–407.
269. Erdine S, Ozyalcin NS, Cimen A, et al. Comparison of pulsed radiofrequency with conventional radiofrequency in the treatment of idiopathic trigeminal neuralgia. *Eur J Pain* 2007;11:309–311.
270. Van Zundert J, Patijn J, Kessels A, et al. Pulsed radiofrequency adjacent to the cervical dorsal root ganglion in chronic cervical radicular pain: a double blind sham controlled randomized clinical trial. *Pain* 2007;127:173–182.
271. Tekin I, Mirzai H, Ok G, et al. A comparison of conventional and pulsed radiofrequency denervation in the treatment of chronic facet joint pain. *Clin J Pain* 2007;23:524–529.
272. Hopayian K. The need for caution in interpreting high quality systematic reviews. *BMJ* 2001;323:681–684.
273. Benson K, Hartz AJ. A comparison of observational studies and randomized, controlled trials. *N Engl J Med* 2000;342:1878–1886.
274. Concato J, Shah N, Horwitz RI. Randomized, controlled trials, observational studies, and the hierarchy of research designs. *N Engl J Med* 2000;342:1887–1892.

CHAPTER 102 ■ SURGERY OF THE PERIPHERAL NERVOUS SYSTEM AS A TREATMENT FOR PAIN

ANTHONY C. WANG, JAMES N. CAMPBELL, AND PARAG G. PATIL

INTRODUCTION

In this chapter, we consider ablative and decompressive surgical approaches to pain that target the peripheral nervous system. Ablative procedures interrupt signal flow between pain generators in the periphery and brain. For example, cutting a peripheral nerve may prevent transmission of pain-encoding signals from an injured region to the spinal cord. By contrast, nonablative procedures may relieve pain due to compression of nerves by adjacent connective tissue.

There are four major categories of pain surgery involving the peripheral nervous system: peripheral neurectomy, nerve entrapment release, dorsal rhizotomy and ganglionectomy, and sympathectomy. The treatment of trigeminal neuralgia, one of the most prevalent diseases successfully treated with surgery, is presented in Chapter 103. Ablative procedures aimed at the spinal cord, such as the dorsal root entry zone operation for brachial plexus avulsion or cordotomy for cancer pain, are presented in Chapter 104.

There are two fundamental approaches to control intractable pain: attempts to palliate symptoms and attempts to eliminate pain definitively. Pharmacologic, psychologic, physiotherapeutic, neuro-modulatory, and neuro-interventional approaches each attempt to reduce the severity of pain symptoms. Surgical approaches have great appeal for their potential to eliminate pain altogether. In fact, nerve decompressions are among the most common peripheral nerve surgeries. By contrast, ablative procedures such as neurectomy and ganglionectomy are notorious for achieving only short-term benefits, a reputation that undermines their appeal. In support of such skepticism, animal research suggests that axotomy alone may be sufficient to induce pain.[1] However, regardless of the perception that inappropriate patient selection may lead to considerable morbidity, the experience of some clinicians remains that ablative procedures have the capacity to relieve pain enduringly and that ablative procedures are useful therapeutic ventures in properly selected patients.

PERIPHERAL NEURECTOMY

Basic Considerations

There are two reasons that a nerve may be cut to eliminate pain. One reason is to denervate a peripheral pain-producing structure to treat nociceptive pain. For example, facet rhizotomy denervates the facet joint as a treatment for axial spine pain. A second reason to cut a nerve is to remove an abnormal focus of nerve injury (e.g., excision of a neuroma). In this case, there is some irony in the use of neurectomy to treat pain, as transection of a somatic nerve may have been the original cause of the pain. To understand how neurectomy may relieve pain, we must consider some aspects of the pathophysiology of neuropathic pain.

Pathophysiology of Neuropathic Pain

When sensory nerve fibers are severed, the proximal axons remain in continuity with cell bodies in the dorsal root ganglion.

These axons sprout and seek Schwann-cell guides. Schwann cells are believed to up-regulate expression of neurotrophic factors, which induce axonal growth.[2–5] If the perineurium of the injured nerve has remained intact, as in the case of crush or certain thermal injuries, the sprouts may successfully reinnervate the target tissue. Successful regeneration may also occur when the transected ends of the nerve are surgically reapproximated (neurorrhaphy). However, when Schwann-cell guides are not present, the axon sprouts are unable to reach the target tissue and randomly double-back on themselves. This disordered process of growth ultimately results in a densely packed cluster of nerve sprouts known as a neuroma.

Weir Mitchell[6] brought attention to the problem of painful nerve injury after caring for wounded soldiers during the American Civil War. A century later, Denny-Brown and Kirk[2] presented one of the first studies demonstrating that axotomy can induce behavioral signs of pain in an animal model. More recent studies have suggested that axotomy of a major nerve, by itself, may induce hyperalgesia in animals. Although nontraumatic neuropathies may induce pain in diverse ways, the single nerve lesion offers a useful model through which to understand the mechanisms of neuropathic pain.

At least four pathophysiologic mechanisms appear to play a role in nerve-injury pain:

Ectopic generation of action potentials. Though normally silent, nociceptive afferents may become spontaneously active following nerve injury, producing action-potential activity in the absence of a stimulus.[3] This activity may be experienced as spontaneous pain. In addition to abnormal signaling in the nerve itself, the activity may sensitize central neurons, such that inputs from non-nociceptive, tactile afferents produce pain (allodynia).[7]

Ectopic excitability. Uninjured nerve trunks are minimally sensitive to mechanical stimuli. Gentle percussion over a nerve is not painful. Following injury, however, regenerating fibers may abnormally respond to mild, mechanical stimuli. Such ectopic mechanical excitability gives rise to Tinel's sign, an electrical sensation in the nerve's original target distribution, elicited by mechanical stimulation at the location of regenerating axons. Furthermore, ectopic excitability to mechanical stimuli may be accompanied by chemical sensitization. For example, injured nociceptive axons may become abnormally sensitive to catecholamines. As a result, the physiologic release of norepinephrine from sympathetic terminals may induce pain (sympathetically maintained pain [SMP]).[4,5]

Nervi nervorum. Nerves themselves appear to be innervated by nociceptive fibers. These nervi nervorum fibers may be sensitized to mechanical stimuli following nerve injury. Such a mechanism may explain, for example, the local tenderness and mechanical hyperalgesia of the ulnar nerve when it is entrapped at the elbow or the local tenderness of nerves entrapped by scar tissue.[8]

Ephaptic conduction. Under normal conditions, signals in adjacent afferent nerve fibers are insulated from each other. Activity in an injured nerve fiber may cross to a nearby fiber, through a direct electrical connection between the two. During such ephaptic transmission, or cross-talk, a non-noxious sensory stimulus may evoke activity in nociceptive fibers and thereby cause pain.

Some of the mechanisms of ectopic generation of action potentials and ectopic excitability have been described. When an axon is severed, the axonal transport of sodium channels and other ion channels from the neuronal cell body to the sensory terminal is interrupted. As a result, channels may be expressed ectopically in the neuroma formed at the nerve injury site. Nociceptive fibers in the neuroma thereby become sensitive to normally nonpainful stimuli, producing pain when these stimuli are present.[9,10] In addition, nerve injury may lead to profound changes in gene expression, promoting ectopic excitability.[11]

Other mechanisms may also contribute to neuropathic pain. While inflammatory and neuropathic pain syndromes are traditionally considered separately, immunologic studies have implicated several pathways through which inflammatory responses may alter nociceptive processing, resulting in neuropathic pain.[12] Evidence supports what may be termed the wallerian degeneration hypothesis.[13] According to this hypothesis, uninjured nociceptors that are adjacent to nerves undergoing wallerian degeneration may become spontaneously active and develop sensitivity to catecholamines, resulting in spontaneous pain and SMP. To the extent that neuropathic pain results from these mechanisms, peripheral neurectomy may be expected to worsen pain, since the nerve undergoes wallerian degeneration distal to the site of neurectomy.

Rationale for Neuroma Relocation Surgery

The concept of surgery to remove a neuroma as a treatment of nerve injury pain is a flawed one. Neuromas arise from nerve fibers proximal to a region of transection or severe injury which remain in continuity with their cell bodies in the dorsal root ganglia. Cutting the nerve at a location that is proximal to the site of nerve injury to remove the neuroma results in the formation of a new neuroma at the proximal location. Surgery in which neuromas are "removed" should therefore be termed neuroma relocation surgery.

Not all neuromas are painful. The tissue milieu surrounding the nerve may determine whether a neuroma becomes painful or remains painless. The use of peripheral neurectomy as a treatment for painful neuromas is therefore predicated on the hope that relocation of the neuroma may convert it from a painful one to a painless one. For example, relocating a neuroma to a nonpressure-sensitive area may alleviate pain in some patients. Relocation of neuromas into muscle was first described in 1918. Since that time, the identification of anatomic locations appropriate for nerve relocation has improved outcomes substantially.[14–22]

Thus, an important consideration in peripheral neurectomy is the role of location in the production of pain. If the location of nerve injury contributes to pain, then relocating the neuroma to a mechanically favorable area may be advantageous. However, to the extent that there is location-independent ectopic generation of action potentials in the neuroma, neuroma relocation surgery will fail. Additionally, some investigators have argued that central mechanisms may account for pain in many situations of nerve injury.[23] In this circumstance, neuroma relocation surgery may also fail. However, our observations as well as those of other experienced clinicians suggest that in patients with nerve injury pain, where anesthetic block of the injured nerve relieves pain, peripheral neurectomy may provide significant pain relief.

Clinical Considerations

Preoperative Evaluation

Clinical scenarios favoring peripheral neurectomy may be broadly divided into two circumstances: neuropathic pain resulting from nerve injury and nociceptive pain from a diseased tissue other than nerve. Nerve injury pain is characterized by numbness, burning, and allodynia. Tinel's sign may be present at the site of

a painful neuroma. Candidates for neuroma relocation surgery should respond to local anesthetic blockade.

Successful anesthetic blockade is an important prerequisite for effective neuroma relocation surgery. If blockade of the putative, pain-generating neuroma fails to relieve pain nearly entirely, the rationale for neuroma relocation surgery is precarious. The decision to operate may be made with more confidence if more than one block is done. Once candidate nerves are identified, local anesthetic blocks indicate the level of benefit that can be obtained following nerve ablation. A successfully applied block should induce anesthesia in the distribution of each target nerve, but not beyond, to indicate the specificity of the blockade. Injection of saline or injections away from the nerve may enhance blockade specificity by identifying nonspecific responses (e.g., placebo responses).

Findings associated with complex regional pain syndrome, such as edema, hyperalgesia, and trophic changes, also suggest that neurectomy will not alleviate pain. Notably in such cases, peripheral nerve blockade typically produces little relief. Patients should be additionally assessed for hyperalgesia to cooling stimuli. This finding is suggestive of SMP, discussed below. Finally, local tenderness in combination with Tinel's sign suggests nerve entrapment. In this instance, nerve decompression would be indicated rather than neurectomy. It is important to note that even subtle entrapments without significant motor or sensory loss may induce severe pain.

Even after one has identified a specific nerve as the pain generator, and one has determined that there are no contraindications to neuroma relocation surgery, a wait-and-see approach may remain most appropriate. For example, where injury is relatively recent and the nerve relatively minor, one may choose to observe. The pain may resolve spontaneously. Where there is only partial nerve injury with remaining function, neurectomy may sacrifice function without any assurance that the new neuroma will be less painful than the old one. In this circumstance, nerve repair should be considered before performing neuroma relocation surgery.

Nerve repair has potential to relocate neuromas with the advantage of restoring neurologic function. The clinician sometimes faces the ironic situation that to repair an injured nerve, a normal nerve (e.g., sural nerve) may be sacrificed to provide donor grafts. In effect, nerve repair is, in a sense, still a neuroma relocation operation—the neuroma is relocated to the donor nerve. Repair of an injured nerve, when feasible, is generally preferable to permanent transection. By contrast, if a nerve has already been completely severed, the risk of relocating the neuroma is low. Thus, in a case of a well-defined neuroma, when an anesthetic block relieves pain, surgical neurectomy may be the preferred first-line of surgical therapy.

Careful analysis may lead to rewarding outcomes. The following case presents the history, preoperative evaluation, and treatment of a patient with neuropathic pain:

> A 44-year-old woman presented with a chief complaint of right vaginal pain. This problem had been present for 3 years and originated with an excisional biopsy of a right-sided vaginal ulcer near the introitus. The pain was always present, but especially disturbing were lightning attacks of pain that occurred unpredictably several times a day. Examination disclosed a subtle sensory loss in the right vulvar area. Medication trials were minimally helpful. An anesthetic block of the right pudendal nerve led to 50% pain relief. A combined ilioinguinal and genitofemoral nerve block also led to 50% pain relief. A local anesthetic block of all three nerves together led to 100% pain relief. As treatment, the right pudendal nerve was severed distal to the sacral spinous ligament through a perivulvar approach, and the patient, predictably, had 50% of her pain relieved. At a separate surgery, the right ilioinguinal and genitofemoral nerves were severed through a retroperitoneal approach. At 3-year follow-up, the patient had complete relief. There were no adverse sequelae.

In this case, both lumbosacral neural segments provided innervation to the painful neuromas. Failure to appreciate this would have led to a less than satisfactory result. This case underscores the need for complete blockade of pain during the application of local anesthetic to ensure that all involved nerves are identified.

Operative Technique

Once peripheral neurectomy has been selected as the treatment of choice, the primary surgical issue is where to relocate the neuroma. Troublesome neuromas typically are in areas near joints, scars, and structures that may tether the nerve. The idea of surgery is to relocate the neuroma to a new location where tethering does not occur.[17] Nerves may be cut back to locations such that the ends can be placed in healthy, well-vascularized muscle. Some have also advocated that neuromas be placed in holes in bone.[23b] Placement of a cut nerve into these environments does not change the fact that the cut ends of the nerve will sprout and that a neuroma will form. However, with relocation of the neuroma into muscle or bone, chances are reduced that the new neuroma will be subject to the tension and shearing forces likely to play a role in pain generation.

Alternatives to neuroma relocation exist. The nerves may be cauterized, frozen, burned, or injected with toxic chemicals. These options have been reported to be successful, but their advantages over surgical neurectomy have not been demonstrated. A surgical procedure where the neurectomy is done sharply, with limited damage to the surrounding environment of the nerve, is most appealing from a mechanistic perspective. Damage to the surrounding tissues, such as necrosis due to phenol injection, may create a new focus for pain generation.[24]

Indications and Outcomes for Treatment of Neuropathic Pain

Ordinarily, neurectomy should be reserved for those situations in which nerve decompression is unlikely to provide a satisfactory result and nerve repair is not possible. Division of major nerves can cause significant motor deficits, sensory deficits, and pain. Ablation of such nerves as a treatment of pain should ordinarily be considered only if the nerve is already divided. Nerve graft repair should be considered as an alternative to repeat transection. Neurectomy of minor nerves has a role in pain treatment and the risk-reward ratio may be favorable.

Amputation Stump Pain

In cases of stump pain, it is worthwhile to examine the patient for tender neuromas. A prosthetic device, for example, may apply pressure to the neuroma, causing pain. Surgical relocation of neuromas to more proximal or protected locations may provide significant benefit in these cases.[25]

Intercostal and Intercostobrachial Pain

Chest trauma or thoracotomy may damage intercostal nerves. Shoulder trauma and axillary node dissection may damage the intercostobrachial nerve. Motor deficits associated with intercostal and intercostobrachial neurectomy are clinically insignificant. Hence, neurectomy is usually without significant drawbacks. This procedure can be safely accomplished through video-assisted thoracoscopy, as well as through an open procedure.[26]

Perineal and Inguinal Pain

Injuries to the pudendal, ilioinguinal, iliohypogastric, and genitofemoral nerves may result in severe pain. These injuries are often due to abdominal and pelvic surgery, episiotomy, hernia repair, entrapment, or blunt trauma. For example, the Pfannenstiel transverse incision may injure the ilioinguinal/iliohypogastric

nerves. Groin pain from inguinal herniorrhaphy is not uncommon. Stulz and Pfeiffer[27] reported relief of pain with neurectomy in 70% (16 of 23) of patients with ilioinguinal and iliohypogastric neuralgia as a complication of prior surgery. Starling and Harms[28] reported similar rates of success: 89% (17 of 19) for ilioinguinal neuralgia and 71% (12 of 17) for genitofemoral neuralgia. In the largest series to date, Amid[29] reported 95% improvement in pain among 225 patients. Our own experience supports the use of neurectomy, but the incidence of long-term favorable outcomes is much more modest.[30]

Meralgia Paresthetica

Entrapment or injury of the lateral femoral cutaneous nerve, meralgia paresthetica, may result in pain and dysesthesia in the anterolateral thigh. In cases where the diagnosis is unclear, local anesthetic blockade may be helpful. Transection should ordinarily be considered as a back-up procedure when decompression is not feasible and nonsurgical approaches, such as weight loss, have failed.[31]

Saphenous Neuralgia

Entrapment of the saphenous nerve in the subsartorial canal[32] may occur with or without a history of trauma. Damage to the saphenous nerve may occur when the saphenous vein is harvested.[33] The condition is associated with pain (with or without numbness) along the anterior and medial leg and the dorsum of the foot. Proximal neurectomy may be used if the nerve has been directly injured. Otherwise, in our experience, the nerve should be decompressed as first-line treatment.

Morton's Neuroma

This condition involves compression of the digital nerve, typically between the third and fourth tarsal bones. The compression leads to a swelling of the nerve, which is mistakenly called a neuroma. Patients present with pain in this region worsened by wearing shoes and walking. If conservative measures (e.g., orthotics) fail, neurectomy may be offered. Indeed, this operation is a common procedure for this condition. Johnson et al.[34] reported relief of pain in 67% (22 of 33) of patients, with 6 years average follow-up, following excision of the plantar interdigital neuroma. Others have reported surgical success rates of up to 90%.[35,36]

General Results for Neurectomy for Neuropathic Pain

What are the predicted results of neurectomy for nerve injury pain? The question is difficult to answer because the patients undergoing this treatment are heterogeneous. In addition, measurement of patient outcome varies greatly among studies with regard to methodological rigor, length of follow-up, and technique. As suggested by the studies cited above, success rates vary from modest to high.

Burchiel and colleagues[37] have taken a systematic approach to the treatment of nerve injury pain, moving the field toward a definition of the indications for neuroma surgery. In their study, 42 patients with nerve injury pain were divided into four treatment groups:

1. Patients with distal sensory neuromas treated by excision of the neuroma and implantation of the proximal nerve into muscle or bone marrow.
2. Patients with suspected distal sensory neuromas in which the involved nerve was sectioned proximal to the injury site and implanted.
3. Patients with proximal neuromas-in-continuity of major sensorimotor nerves treated by neuroplasty, which frees a nerve from adjacent tissue.
4. Patients with nerve injuries at points of anatomic entrapment treated by neuroplasty and transposition.

Surgical success (rated as a greater than 50% subjective improvement in pain levels, subjectively rated pain relief as "good" or "excellent," and no postoperative narcotic usage) varied between the groups. In the 40 patients who received postoperative follow-up care over 2 to 32 months (average of 11 months), 16 (40%) met these criteria. By group, successful pain relief was accomplished in 44% (8 of 18) of group 1, 40% (4 of 10) of group 2, 0% (0 of 5) of group 3, and 57% (4 of 7) of group 4.

After obtaining these results, Burchiel et al.[37] attempted to determine retrospectively the extent to which indicators of nerve injury predicted surgical success. Such indicators included Tinel's sign, hyperalgesia, a "discrete nerve syndrome," litigation, and prior procedures. Some predictors showed promise. For example, a discrete nerve syndrome, defined as a condition in which a single nerve could account for all the neurologic findings and pain distribution, tended to predict success. However, none of the relationships between preoperative diagnostic variables and treatment success achieved statistical significance at the $p < 0.05$ level.

One can only speculate why the results of this series differ substantially from those of other series. Perhaps patient selection accounts for differences, yet Burchiel and colleagues[37] appeared to discriminate patients at high risk for failure. Surgical technique could also play a role, but there is no evidence on which to base such a statement. In some cases, neuromas are innervated by more than one nerve. For example, proximal resection of the superficial radial nerve to treat dorsoradial wrist neuromas often relieves pain only temporarily. Further inspection reveals that the lateral antebrachial cutaneous nerve may also innervate these neuromas, and thus success may require sectioning this nerve as well.[38]

Another reason for failure in neuroma relocation surgery may relate to the discovery that the distal side of a severed nerve may also form a neuroma at the site of injury. Plexus formation distal to the neurectomy may allow intact nerve fibers from other nerves to sprout in retrograde fashion to innervate this distal site. This retrograde sprouting may create a potentially painful neuroma on the "wrong" side.[39] Neuroma relocation surgery should perhaps attend to neuroma formation on both sides of a severed nerve.

Indications and Outcomes for the Treatment of Nociceptive Pain

Neurectomy may be performed to interrupt the flow of pain signals through intact nerves from a diseased, pain-generating tissue to the spinal cord. In these cases, a balance is sought between elimination of input from the pain-generating tissue and the potential formation of a painful neuroma. Following neurectomy, regrowth of the transected nerve and invasion of the diseased tissue by surrounding nerves may result in a return of pain. In addition, intact and otherwise "normal" nerve fibers may be sensitized by the release of growth factors in partially denervated tissues. Progression of the underlying disease process may also enlarge the injured tissue region, producing pain beyond the region of surgery. In spite of these considerations, in the following disease processes, neurectomy may be an effective treatment of nociceptive pain.

Axial Spine Pain

The medial branches of dorsal rami innervate the paraspinal muscles, the interspinous ligament, and the zygapophyseal (facet) joints. Pain associated with movement of the lower back, which is relieved by rest and is not attributable to other spine pathology, may be relieved through bilateral, percutaneous radiofrequency or chemical ablation of these branches in the lumbar spine.[40,41] A success rate of 85% with mean duration of relief of 10.5 months was reported by Schofferman and Kine[42] through this procedure. In addition, neck pain associated with whiplash injury

may benefit from a similar procedure in the cervical spine.[43] The mechanism of pain relief is thought to relate to denervation of the facet joint. Since the dorsal ramus innervates several structures, other mechanisms are possible. Evidence is indeterminate for similar pain of thoracic origin.

Many experts suggest diagnostic anesthetic blocks of the facets prior to a facet denervation procedure. Good results are expected only in patients who get excellent benefit from the blocks. Patients who have axial pain in addition to radicular symptoms tend not to benefit from facet denervation procedures alone. Among preexisting symptoms, only paraspinal tenderness has been shown to predict treatment success, while increased pain with facet loading maneuvers predicts less favorable outcomes.[44,45]

The procedure is performed percutaneously with radiofrequency heat lesions. The advantages of this procedure are that it can be done on an outpatient basis and morbidity is low. The disadvantage is that the procedure often confers only temporary relief or often no relief at all, regardless of the temporary effects of diagnostic facet blocks. In addition to continuous, high-temperature radiofrequency medial branch ablation, pulsed radiofrequency, cryodenervation, and phenol neurolysis have also been used to provide intermediate to long-term pain relief.

In patients with no prior spine surgery, these procedures have been reported to provide initial relief for 60% to 70% of patients.[33,43,44,46] Rates are reported to be considerably lower (20% to 50%) for patients with prior spine surgery.[33,46,47] However, a history of spine surgery is associated with treatment failure not only for radiofrequency denervation, but other interventions as well, including epidural steroid injection and open surgery. Our view is that this is a low-morbidity procedure that can provide effective, albeit impermanent, pain relief for patients with axial spine pain. Recurrence of pain following denervation can be treated with repeated neurotomy with comparable efficacy. See Chapter 101 for a detailed discussion of neurolytic blocks, including radiofrequency neurolysis.

Extremity Joint Pain

Denervation procedures aim to eliminate pain arising from degenerative processes in the joint, while preserving functions that may be lost after other forms of joint surgery. Buck-Gramcko[48] reported retention of wrist mobility with substantial reduction of pain in 69% (135 of 195) of patients following wrist denervation surgery. Wilhelm[49] reported success in 90% of patients with tennis elbow treated by denervation. Dellon et al.[50] reported satisfaction in 86% (60 of 70) of patients following partial denervation surgery for persistent, postoperative knee pain. Pulsed radiofrequency denervation has also been used to provide relief, though generally with shorter effect when compared to conventional radiofrequency ablation, and limited evidence to support the efficacy of this approach.[51]

Pelvic Pain

Neurectomy of the superior hypogastric (presacral) plexus has been advocated as a treatment for medically refractory pelvic pain. In 1948, Ingersoll and Meigs[52] reported complete relief of primary dysmenorrhea in 81% (72 of 89) of women treated with neurectomy. More recently, with the development of more effective analgesics, ablative approaches to pelvic pain have been largely limited to patients with secondary dysmenorrhea associated with endometriosis. Nezhat et al.[53] reported at least 50% relief from pain in 70% to 85% of patients with various stages of endometriosis with 1-year follow-up, following presacral neurectomy combined with excision and vaporization of endometriotic lesions. Debate over the proper role of presacral neurectomy has been ongoing for well over 50 years. Introduction of the biopsychosocial model of chronic pain has potential to spare many women from surgery.

Cancer Pain

Peripheral neurectomy is infrequently used in the treatment of pain due to cancer. This is due to the availability of alternative strategies with low morbidity and higher success rates, such as spinal opiates. Transecting a peripheral nerve may fail to relieve pain because of overlapping receptive fields of adjacent nerves or central plasticity. Sectioning major peripheral nerves results not only in numbness but also in unacceptable motor loss. Peripheral neurectomies are rarely indicated in the extremities. However, localized chest or abdominal wall pain can successfully be treated with intercostal neurectomies. Alcohol injection, cryoprobe, or radiofrequency lesions provide similar success to open surgery and lowered morbidity for the treatment of cancer pain.

NERVE ENTRAPMENT RELEASE

Basic Considerations

Pathophysiology of Nerve Entrapment Pain

Nerve entrapment syndromes result from pressure applied directly to a nerve, causing pain, paresthesias, or weakness in the sensory distribution of the nerve.[38,54,55] Entrapment commonly develops where peripheral nerves traverse confined anatomic spaces, rest in superficial locations or in proximity to joints, or become tethered to adjacent tissues. Structural factors such as anomalous nerves, cervical ribs, muscles, or connective tissue bands also may contribute. Repetitive motion, nerve traction due to joint position, chronic vibration, and high force constitute physical stressors that increase the risk of symptomatic entrapment.

While the degree of compression required to cause nerve injury may vary, axonal degeneration follows pressure in a dose-dependent relationship.[56] Symptoms can arise following a few significant events or after a longer period of repetitive mild insults. The time course and force of injury are just two of the prognostic considerations. The length of the affected nerve region, as well as the presence and severity of nerve ischemia are important factors in the development of symptomatic nerve entrapment. Finally, nerves become more vulnerable to injury in the presence of concurrent systemic metabolic disease, and nerves lose their regenerative capacity with age.

Several pathophysiologic mechanisms have been proposed to explain pain associated with peripheral nerve entrapment at the cellular level. Evidence for these mechanisms arises from studies of animal models.[56-58] Following local nerve compression, internodes along myelinated fibers distort in shape. Demyelination appears earliest in the segment nearest to the point of compression.[59,60] Eventually, segmental demyelination leads to diffuse demyelination and, ultimately, axonal degradation. Compressive injury usually affects larger, more peripherally located myelinated nerves as opposed to smaller or unmyelinated fibers.

Nerve ischemia may also play an important role in nerve entrapment pain syndromes. Focal pressures of 20 to 30 mm Hg may impede venous blood flow, while higher pressures may reduce arterial supply.[61,62] Within 4 hours of extraneural compression, increasing permeability of the blood-nerve barrier leads to development of subperineurial edema.[63-66] As there is no lymphatic drainage of the endoneurial space, sustained intraneural pressure elevations persist for at least 24 hours after compressive forces are removed. Following such injury, reactive inflammation, fibrin deposition, and proliferation of endoneurial fibroblasts and capillary endothelial cells lead to intraneural fibrosis of perineurial and epineurial tissues.

Ischemia does not appear to play a role in the initial demyelination associated with acute compressive injury.[67,68] Rather, nodes of Ranvier adjacent to the point of compression are out-wardly displaced and disrupt the myelin sheath. Segmental demyelination follows, stemming from these sites of myelin invagination.[69,70] Disruption of anterograde axoplasmic flow of vital nutrient proteins reduces terminal membrane excitability. Long-standing ischemia thereby results in replacement of funicular contents with fibrotic tissue, producing derangements in electrical conductivity.[71]

Nerve Entrapment and Systemic Disease

Several endocrine and rheumatologic diseases show an association with increased risk for nerve entrapment. Approximately 15% of upper extremity nerve entrapment patients have diabetes. This may result from an increased association of peripheral neuropathies with entrapment. Both hypo- and hyperthyroidism have been shown to pose an increased risk for nerve entrapment, which is thought to result from glycogen deposition in Schwann cells.[72] Up to 30% of acromegalics are diagnosed with nerve entrapment syndromes, which often resolve with treatment of the underlying acromegaly.[73,74] Obesity and pregnancy have well-documented associations with entrapment syndromes, with as many as two thirds of pregnant women experiencing temporary symptoms.[75] Rheumatoid arthritis is also thought to contribute to entrapment in anatomic locations where synovial overgrowth can produce compression of a nerve. There is an estimated 45% incidence of entrapment neuropathy in rheumatoid arthritis patients.[76,77] Amyloidosis, carcinomatosis, gout, mucopolysaccharide storage diseases, and polymyalgia rheumatica are all suspected to pose an increased risk for exacerbation of nerve entrapment.

Clinical Considerations

Preoperative Evaluation

Clinical Findings. Patients suffering from nerve entrapment syndromes present with pain, paresthesias, or motor weakness along a specific nerve distribution. Nocturnal pain, either sharp or burning, classically develops before the onset of daytime or persistent symptoms. Muscular changes, such as atrophy or fasciculation, as well as sensory alterations, such as altered two-point discrimination or temperature sensation, can occur in advanced cases. Specific symptoms result from the location and severity of compression.

On physical examination, Tinel's sign may be present. Tinel's sign is an electric radiating sensation in the distribution of the nerve, produced by percussion over the nerve. Tinel's sign represents ectopic excitability, a hallmark of nerve entrapment, and may be accompanied by local tenderness. Provocative maneuvers may reproduce or exacerbate symptoms and have significantly positive predictive value in the diagnosis of entrapment syndromes.

In many cases, diagnosis of a specific entrapment syndrome may be difficult to make. Compensation of one muscle group by another may create uncertainty in identifying etiology of the entrapment. Furthermore, entrapment syndromes may be accompanied by concurrent radiculopathy, producing synergistic pain, thereby adding to the diagnostic challenge.[78] In addition, pain associated with entrapment syndromes may not be well-localized. For example, radial nerve entrapment may present with global arm pain. Finally, results of electrodiagnostic studies may be normal in some cases, further increasing the diagnostic dilemma.

Electrodiagnostic Studies. Physical findings may be supported by electrodiagnostic studies. Nerve conduction studies (NCS) measure action potentials along axons while electromyography studies (EMG) measure muscle fiber activity. In sensory NCS, a stimulus is applied to the nerve and a sensory nerve action potential

(SNAP) is measured at various distal points along the nerve. Alterations in axon number, diameter, myelination, or temperature all affect the magnitude and temporal profile of the SNAP. In motor NCS, a stimulus is applied to the nerve and a compound motor action potential (CMAP) is measured from the innervated muscle. Changes in conduction velocity, amplitude of CMAP, and distal motor latency suggest that conduction inhibition exists between the point of initial stimulation and the site of recording. Needle EMG examines the spontaneous electrical activity of individual muscle fibers resulting from denervation, reinnervation, or acute muscle injury.

These studies aid in the differentiation of peripheral nerve entrapments from brachial plexopathy and radiculopathy by defining the nature and extent of neurologic dysfunction. For example, although NCS cannot be performed in structures like the brachial plexus due to an inability to record and stimulate across the region of compression, a plexus lesion would be expected to affect the function of multiple peripheral nerves. In entrapment neuropathy, large myelinated sensory fibers are typically affected before motor fibers. Hence, NCS are most often effective earlier in the disease than motor conduction studies (ulnar compression at the elbow is a notable exception to this rule). Entrapment is represented by abnormal recordings of evoked SNAPs along a short nerve segment. Prolonged latency or reduced motor conduction velocity are also indicative of injury, although they are less sensitive measures. Fibrillation seen on EMG occurs as a result of wallerian degeneration of distal nerve segments and suggests advanced entrapment. In general, a combination of studies and measurement points yields the best information with which to form a diagnosis.

Comparison among the nerves of interest and a nearby unaffected nerve is often more accurate than comparison of a nerve with normal reference values. Cooler temperature, increasing age, and patient size all serve to prolong sensory latencies, confounding reference values. As a result, and to avoid such confounding factors, it is common to perform sensory latency comparisons at as many as three sites (median-ulnar midpalmar, median-ulnar ring finger, and median-radial thumb) in the diagnosis of carpal tunnel syndrome (CTS).[79] While the greater number of studies increases the likelihood of false-positive results,[80] summation of the latencies of these three studies has proven to be the most sensitive and specific test for CTS.[81]

Following entrapment release, it is notable that clinical improvement may not correlate reliably with electrodiagnostic studies. However, in patients with persistent symptoms following treatment, comparison with pretreatment studies may be helpful. If earlier studies are unavailable, a series of postoperative studies over several months should be obtained.

Imaging Studies. Developments in ultrasonography and magnetic resonance imaging (MRI) have resulted in a potentially expanded role for imaging in the diagnosis of entrapment neuropathies. Ultrasonography now offers the highest available resolution for visualizing the location of entrapment (Fig. 102.1). However, ultrasound is unable to show pathologic changes within nerves. In contrast, signal and configuration characteristics seen in chronically compressed or tethered peripheral nerves have been well-characterized by MRI (Fig. 102.2). On MRI, indicators for nerve abnormality include focal enlargement, T2 hyperintensity, and an indistinguishable or nonuniform fascicular pattern. In addition, MRI simultaneously visualizes muscular alterations due to atrophy and neurogenic edema.

Specific MRI findings have been correlated with clinical findings, electrodiagnostic findings, and postoperative outcomes for several nerve entrapment syndromes.[82–85] With current technology, MRI may be a useful adjunct in the diagnosis of entrapment. Specific indications for MRI may include ulnar entrapment, entrapment in the presence of superimposed neuropathy, entrapment where other tests are equivocal, and postoperative evalua-

tion of entrapment.[86] The value of MRI imaging in the setting of uncommon entrapments is less clear.

Operative Technique

Substantial experimental evidence supports three treatments of peripheral nerve entrapment: splinting, local corticosteroid injection, and surgical release. Splinting reduces the offending stimulus through postural correction and reduction of repetitive injury, thereby decreasing reactive inflammation. Local corticosteroid injections have been shown to be helpful in mild cases. Surgical release of anatomic compression is the mainstay of treatment in more advanced cases of peripheral nerve entrapment.[87]

In general, operative release of entrapment can be quite rewarding, as the risks of surgery are typically low and pain improvement is often dramatic. Avoidance of additional trauma to the compressed nerve is of great importance to surgical outcome. Occasionally, unexpected sources of entrapment may be found during surgical exposure, such as cysts, soft tissue masses, and bony prominences. Choices of surgical approach and operative technique are based largely upon individual surgeon preferences.[88] Rates of success and complications vary with the location of entrapment and the etiology of pain.

Specific Indications

Entrapments of the Median Nerve

Carpal Tunnel Syndrome. CTS results from compression of the median nerve between bones of the wrist and the flexor retinaculum. CTS is the most common nerve compression syndrome, with an annual incidence of 150 per 100,000 population and a 2:1 female predominance.[89,90] Patients with CTS present with pain along the radial half of the hand, particularly at night, and weakness of median innervated muscles. Phalen's sign—recreation of pain through complete wrist flexion for 30 to 60 seconds—is a sensitive and specific marker of mild to moderate CTS.[91,92] Electrodiagnostic studies typically demonstrate decreased median-nerve conduction velocity at the wrist. Imaging findings on MRI, when performed, may demonstrate increased signal intensity in the nerve, volar bowing of the flexor retinaculum, and flattening of the median nerve at the level of the hamate.[93]

Initial therapy includes splinting, activity modification, and nonsteroidal anti-inflammatory medications for mild disease. Corticosteroid injections offer nearly a 70% positive response initially, although eventual recurrence of symptoms is high.[94]

Surgical decompression of the carpal tunnel is indicated in cases that have failed conservative management or in cases with severe or rapid onset of symptoms. Some 80% of patients achieve excellent pain relief with surgery, while another 10% achieve partial relief; less than 1% of patients experience worsening of their pain symptoms. For patients with motor weakness, similar results have been reported with 84% of patients returning to baseline function and another 9% experiencing some improvement.[92,95–97] Early surgery in patients with ongoing pain has been associated with improved resolution of symptoms.

Incomplete decompression of the nerve is seen in the majority of cases in which pain relief is incomplete, absent, or transient. Another cause of recurrent pain includes postoperative fibrosis. Failure to appreciate the path of the recurrent motor (thenar) branch of the nerve can result in postoperative weakness following release. Injury to the palmar cutaneous branch can result in postoperative pain in the wrist and proximal thenar eminence.[98,99]

Anterior Interosseus Syndrome. Anterior interosseus syndrome results from isolated injury or entrapment of this largely motor branch of the median nerve.[100] The nerve arises distal to the

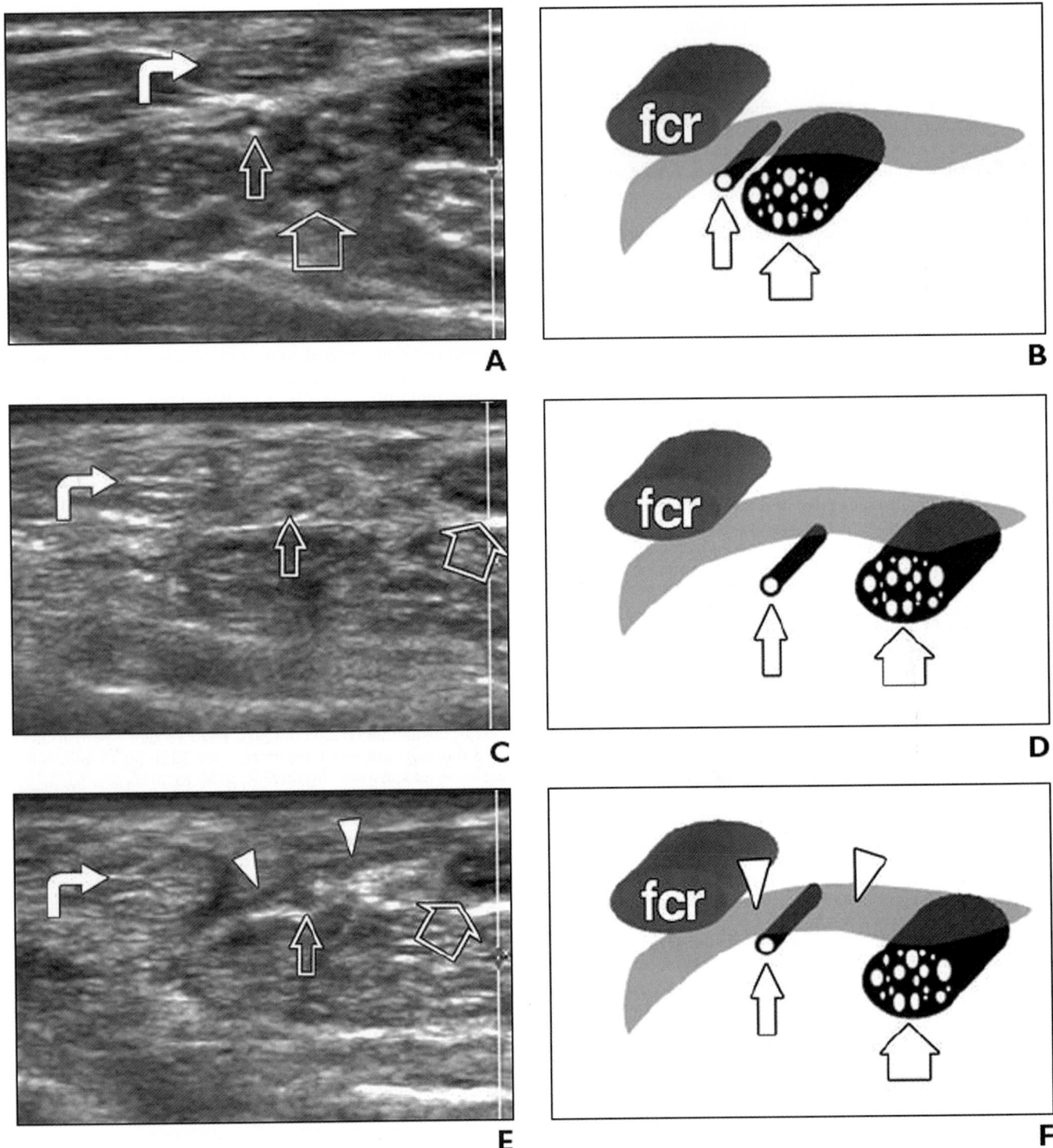

FIGURE 102.1 Series of transverse 17-5–MHz sonography images obtained from proximal to distal over palmar cutaneous branch of median nerve (MN) in 35-year-old healthy man with corresponding diagrams. Relationships of palmar cutaneous branch of MN (thin open arrows) with MN (*thick open arrows*), flexor carpi radialis tendon (*curved arrow* in **A,C,E,G**; *fcr* in **B,D,F,H**), and antebrachial fascia (*arrowheads*, **E–H**) are shown. **A,B.** Palmar cutaneous branch of MN detaches from MN as one of its most radial fascicles. **C,D.** Palmar cutaneous branch of MN gradually deflects to approach flexor carpi radialis tendon. **E,F.** Palmar cutaneous branch of MN runs slightly deep in relation to antebrachial fascia.   (*continued*)

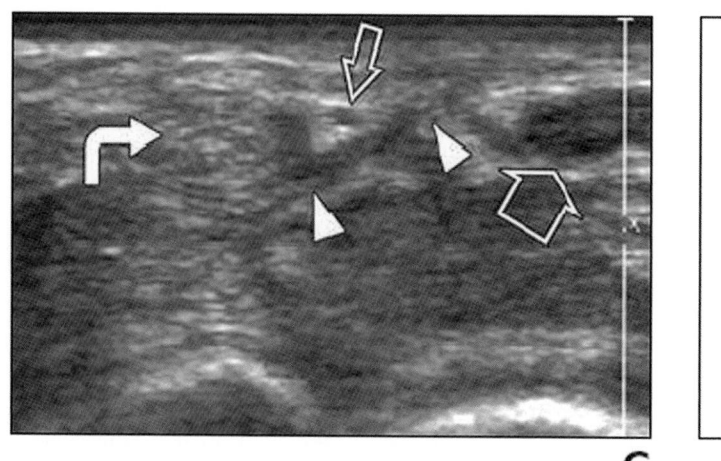

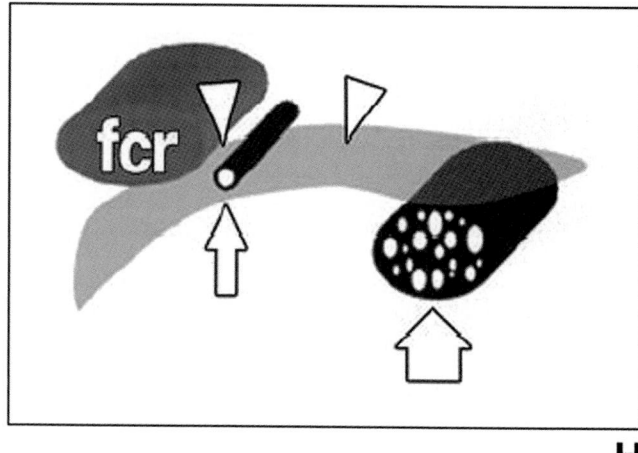

FIGURE 102.1 (*Continues*) **G,H.** Palmar cutaneous branch of MN lies adjacent to flexor carpi radialis tendon after piercing fascia. (Reproduced with permission from Tagliafico A, Pugliese F, Bianchi S, et al. High-resolution sonography of the palmar cutaneous branch of the median nerve. *Am J Roentgen* 2008;191:107–114.)

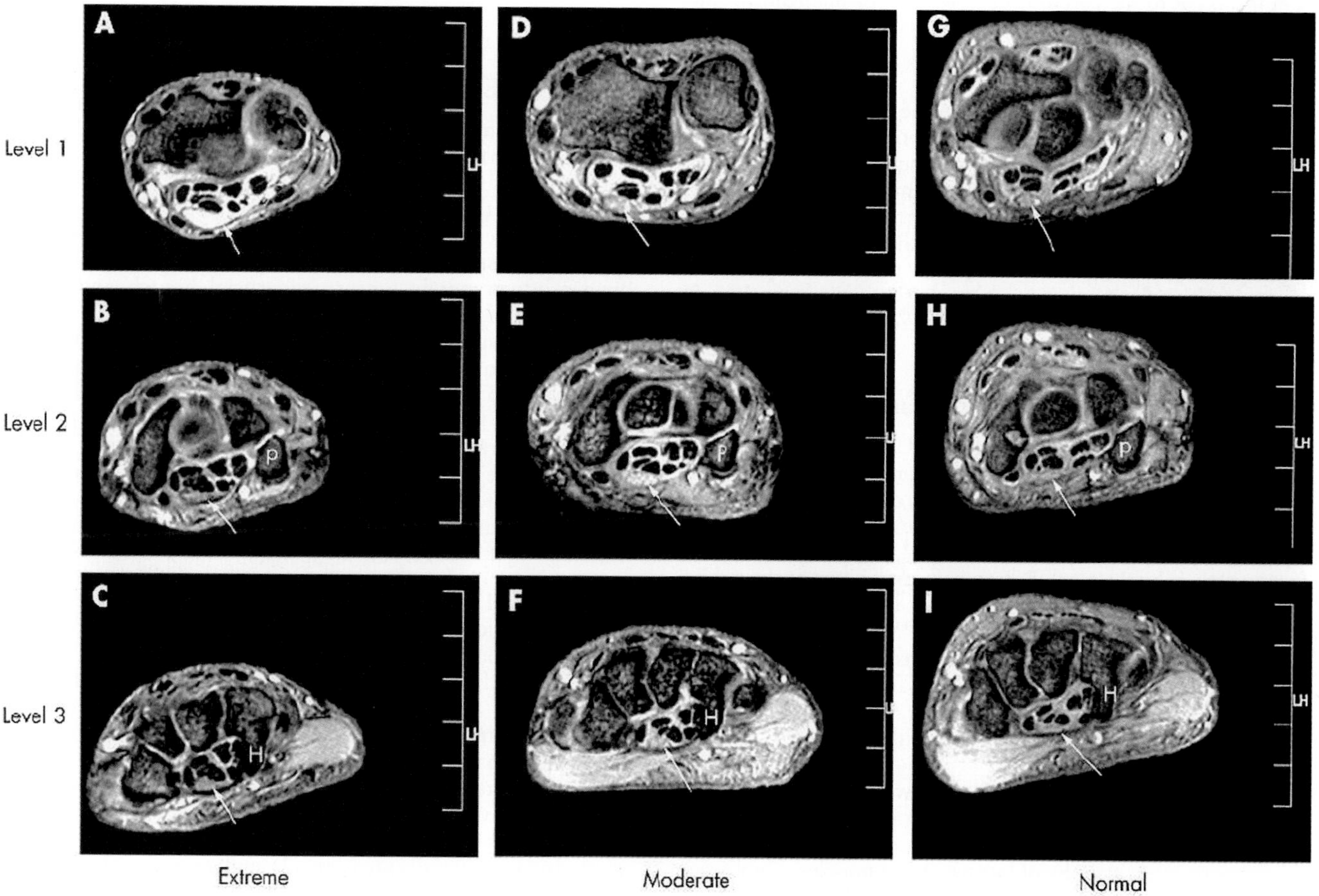

	Extreme	Moderate	Normal
Level 1	A	D	G
Level 2	B	E	H
Level 3	C	F	I

FIGURE 102.2 T2-weighted gradient echo images at the distal part of the distal radioulnar joint level (DRUJ) (1), at the level of the pisiform (2), and at the level of the hook of the hamate (3) in three different stages of idiopathic carpal tunnel syndrome. Solid arrow indicates the cross section of the median nerve. Upper part represents the dorsal side, and the righthand side represents the ulnar side. H, hook of the hamate; P, pisiform bone. **A–C.** Extreme stage. Enlargement and high signal intensity of the flattened median nerve are seen at level 1, and enlargement of the median nerve at levels 2 and 3. Palmar bowing of the TCL is evident. **D–F.** Moderate stage. Enlargement and high signal intensity of the median nerve are seen at level 2. They are slightly appreciated at level 3, and still not seen at level 1. Palmar bowing of the TCL is well appreciated. **G–I.** Normal wrist. Enlargement of the median nerve is not seen at any level. Isointensity of the nerve to the hypothenar muscle is seen throughout the cross sections. Palmar bowing of the TCL is not seen. (Reproduced with permission from Uchiyama S, Itsubo T, Yasutomi T, et al. Quantitative MRI of the wrist and nerve conduction studies in patients with idiopathic carpal tunnel syndrome. *J Neurol Neurosurg Psych* 2005;76:1103–1108.)

medial epicondyle, and is vulnerable to injury in supracondylar and forearm fractures.[101-103] In severe cases, there may be weakness of flexor pollicis longus, flexor digitorum profundus to the index finger, and pronator quadratus.

Patients with anterior interosseus syndrome may present with a characteristic pinch as compensation for weakness in the long flexors of the index finger and thumb. The condition may also present with pain in the forearm associated with tenderness in the proximal volar forearm. EMG may confirm changes associated with muscular denervation. Surgical exploration with neuroplasty is most commonly performed for patients whose pain does not respond to anti-inflammatory medications or avoidance of repetitive pronation/supination activity.[104-108]

Entrapment by the Ligament of Struthers. Struthers' ligament can cause compression of the median nerve, brachial artery, or brachial vein as they pass beneath it, proximal to the medial epicondyle. A variant bony spicule (supracondylar process) arising from the humerus at this level can place the nerve at risk for entrapment.[109] A rare disorder, this pathology can potentially be mistaken for CTS.[110] Motor weakness of the pronator teres, flexor carpi radialis, and flexor digitorum profundus (to the first two digits), while not always present, indicate a point of compression proximal to the carpal tunnel. Release of the ligament and excision of the supracondylar process typically provides pain relief.

Pronator Syndrome. Pronator syndrome presents as a vague, aching pain in the volar aspect of the elbow and forearm that is exacerbated by activities involving grasping or pronation of the forearm.[111] On physical examination, tenderness can usually be elicited by deep palpation over the pronator teres. Compression occurs at the lacertus fibrosus, within the muscle between the two heads of pronator teres, or beneath the flexor superficialis tendon at its origin. Avoiding maneuvers that exacerbate the pain and intra-muscular injection of corticosteroids may be attempted prior to surgical release.

Entrapments of the Ulnar Nerve

Ulnar Nerve Entrapment at the Elbow. Ulnar nerve entrapment at the elbow (UNEE) is the second most common peripheral nerve entrapment syndrome after CTS. At the elbow, the ulnar nerve is bounded medially and anteriorly by the medial epicondyle and laterally by the olecranon. A dense fascial layer overlies this space, forming the cubital tunnel. Entrapment may occur at the cubital tunnel, in the epicondylar groove, beneath the arcade of Struthers, or at the medial intermuscular septum.[112] Antecedent trauma, inflammatory change, and mass lesions increase the risk of UNEE. Subluxation of a hypermobile ulnar nerve over the medial epicondyle may lead to traumatic injury. An anomalous and potentially compressive anconeus epitrochlearis muscle may be found in up to 30% of patients.[113-115]

UNEE typically presents insidiously with paresthesias in the ulnar distribution of the forearm, wrist, and hand. Muscle weakness leads to impaired grip and clumsiness in the hand, and in more severe cases, atrophy of intrinsic hand muscles. Tinel's sign and the elbow flexion-pressure test, which is done with manual compression of the ulnar nerve just proximal to the cubital tunnel for 30 seconds, offer significant sensitivity and specificity for UNEE.[116,117] Electrodiagnostic studies may demonstrate reduced sensory and motor conduction velocity across the elbow.

The optimal surgical technique for entrapment release in UNEE has not been established. Options include transposition of the nerve and in situ decompression. For transposition, the ulnar nerve is displaced anterolaterally in order to shorten its course around the medial epicondyle. Transposition may be subcutaneous, intramuscular, or submuscular, with respect to the flexor-pronator muscle mass.[118-126] Among the larger case series,

successful surgical results of 90% have been reported, regardless of technique.[127-131] Many surgeons favor in situ decompression as an initial surgical treatment, particularly when patients have milder symptoms and isolated compression at only one site.[132-136]

Traumatic etiology, chronic symptoms, absence of sensory potentials, and severe muscular weakness are among the indicators of poor prognosis for surgical outcome. Pain symptoms more often resolve, while motor symptoms may only partially improve, after surgery. Persistent pain following ulnar nerve decompression at the elbow may be due to injury of the medial antebrachial cutaneous nerve.

Ulnar Nerve Entrapment at the Wrist. The ulnar nerve and artery course through Guyon's canal and may become entrapped there.[137] This canal is bounded by the volar and transverse carpal ligaments and palmaris brevis muscle, with the pisiform bone proximally and medially, and the hook of the hamate laterally and distally. Common causes of entrapment include local masses, such as ganglion formation, lipomas, and uremic tumoral calcinosis, or anatomic variants, such as the presence of abductor digit minimi within the canal.[138] Evaluation is typically based on physical examination and electrodiagnostic studies. MRI, when a dedicated wrist coil is utilized, offers noninvasive visualization of Guyon's canal.[139] Surgical decompression involves unroofing of the canal and removal of any masses.[140,141]

Entrapments of the Radial Nerve

Compression neuropathy of the radial nerve occurs at the radial tunnel, a 5-cm space extending from the capitulum of the humerus to the distal edge of the supinator muscle. It is bounded anteromedially by the brachialis muscle, anterolaterally by brachioradialis and extensor carpi radialis brevis, and posteriorly by the capitulum. Just distal to the lateral epicondyle, the radial nerve divides into a purely sensory superficial branch and a deep branch, the posterior interosseous nerve.

While the superficial branch passes superior to the supinator muscle, the posterior interosseous nerve courses in a plane between the two heads of the supinator muscle as they both continue into the forearm. Potential sources of compression at this level include the fibrous bands that anchor the radial nerve to the elbow, the recurrent radial artery and its associated vessels and branches (collectively known as the leash of Henry), and the arcade of Frohse at the fibrous origin of the supinator and other muscles.[140,142-144]

Radial Tunnel Syndrome and Posterior Interosseous Nerve Syndrome. Classically, there are two distinct clinical syndromes involving this pathology—one primarily involving pain and the other, motor dysfunction. Radial tunnel syndrome itself is a frequently-cited, yet somewhat controversial diagnosis, as some argue against its existence. It consists of pain symptoms including deep aching pain, often worse at night, in the extensor muscle mass at the lateral elbow. On physical examination, several particular maneuvers are suggestive of this diagnosis: (1) reproduction of pain by resisting extension of the third digit, with the elbow and wrist in full extension; (2) tenderness to palpation over the entry of the posterior interosseous nerve into the supinator muscle, approximately 5 cm distal to the radial head; and (3) reproduction of pain with the application of a tourniquet at this level.[145-148]

In contrast to radial tunnel syndrome, posterior interosseous nerve syndrome is defined primarily by motor symptoms, including progressive weakness of the wrist and digit extensor muscle group. Due to the relatively distal point of compression, innervation to the brachioradialis, extensor carpi radialis muscles, and supinator are typically unaffected. Weakness in wrist extension is incomplete, such that there is radial deviation. Pain, when present, is secondary in this constellation of symptoms.

Development of this entrapment syndrome is associated with repetitive forceful movements involving elbow extension and forearm pronation and supination.[149] Mass lesions, elbow dislocation, vascular malformations, and synovial inflammation are other potential etiologies of compression, and MRI or ultrasound may useful in the identification of compression. Electrodiagnostic studies are of limited utility for most patients. Hence, the diagnosis is typically clinical.

Operative release of entrapment includes an exploration of all the branches of the radial nerve, such that the posterior interosseous branch can be fully liberated.[150] Few large case series have been analyzed, and reported outcomes vary in the region of 70%. In some series, however, improved functional outcomes have been reported in over 90% of treated patients.[151-153]

Superficial Sensory Branch Entrapment. Entrapment of the superficial sensory branch of the radial nerve can occur through externally compressive apparel such as watch bands. Chronic intermittent compression tends to cause numbness and dysesthesias over the dorsal surface of the hand, whereas blunt injury at this location typically causes highly refractory pain. Operative neuroplasty has yielded significant improvement of symptoms in 74% to 86% of patients.[154-156] Of note, superficial sensory branch entrapment may be associated with De Quervain's tenosynovitis, and release of the extensor compartment is sometimes performed in combination with neuroplasty.

Entrapment of the Suprascapular Nerve

Suprascapular nerve entrapment presents with shoulder pain along the border of the trapezius muscle, and often denervation of the associated musculature.[157-160] On physical examination, it is exacerbated with abduction and external rotation of the arm. The suprascapular nerve passes through the suprascapular notch and beneath the suprascapular ligament before entering the supraspinatus fossa.[161] Compression at the suprascapular ligament is common, and thus, a palsy involving both supraspinatus and infraspinatus is more frequently seen than an isolated infraspinatus denervation on EMG. History of trauma such as shoulder dislocation or scapular fracture is usually present. When this is absent, suprascapular ligament compression, tumor, ganglion, or Parsonage-Turner neuritis should be considered. Reported pain relief and strength increase after surgery have been excellent, with improvement in over 90% of patients.[159,160,162-165] Early surgical treatment appears to yield better results than a delayed operation.[166]

Thoracic Outlet Syndrome

The term "thoracic outlet syndrome" (TOS) was coined by Peet to describe compression at the thoracic inlet of the neurovascular bundle comprised of the brachial plexus, subclavian vein, and subclavian artery.[166b] TOS is most commonly neurogenic in origin. In TOS, unlike other upper extremity entrapments, nerve conduction studies across the putative entrapment site are not feasible. The diagnosis is therefore typically based upon clinical criteria.

TOS has been subdivided into three syndromic zones, according to likelihood of entrapment of the brachial plexus, subclavian artery, and subclavian veins. Anterior scalene syndrome occurs with brachial plexus or subclavian artery compression in the interscalene triangle. Costoclavicular syndrome occurs with compression of any nearby structures in the space between the clavicle and the first rib. Retropectoralis minor syndrome can involve any adjacent structure as well, and compression occurs at the attachment site of pectoralis minor at the coracoid process (the subcoracoid tunnel).[167-170]

In cases of pure peripheral nerve compression, insidious onset of pain and paresthesias in the neck, shoulder, arm, or hand is typical, whereas motor weakness occurs in just 10% of patients.

Nearly 90% of cases involve the ulnar nerve distribution.[171] Symptoms may be reproduced when assuming a spear-throwing position or with downward pressure on the shoulder. Tenderness (with or without Tinel's sign) over the anterior scalene muscle in the supraclavicular fossa may also be present.[172]

Diagnosis can be aided by imaging and electrodiagnostic studies. In particular, a radiograph demonstrating anomalous bony findings, such as a cervical rib, in the presence of corresponding symptoms is highly predictive of good surgical outcome. Comparing MRIs of the thoracic outlet in the standard anatomic position and following hyperabduction and external rotation of the arm may reveal significant narrowing of the costoclavicular space in patients with TOS compared to normal healthy subjects.[168]

With careful attention to patient selection and surgical technique, good results have been reported with surgical management. Surgery can involve first rib resection, anterior scalenectomy, resection of the costoclavicular ligament, or neuroplasty, depending upon suspected pathology.[172] The majority of surgeons employ a transaxillary or supraclavicular approach.

In general, immediate pain relief with surgery is good, although results often deteriorate over time. Numerous outcome studies for the transaxillary approach report greater than 90% of patients enjoy initial symptomatic relief. However, long-term follow-up has revealed that less than 50% of patients sustain relief at 5 years, and less than 10% of patients have relief persisting at 20 years.[170,171,173] While reported in fewer numbers and with shorter follow-up, outcomes for the supraclavicular approach appear to be equally good in terms of initial results.[174,175] Complications of surgery for TOS are unfortunately common and include vascular injury, brachial plexus injury, and thoracic wall injury.[176] The pathophysiology, diagnosis, and management of TOS is discussed in more detail in Chapter 39.

Entrapments of Lower Extremities

Of the entrapment syndromes seen in the lower extremities, meralgia paresthetica (symptoms along the lateral femoral cutaneous nerve) is the most common. Inciting factors are many, including trauma, weight gain, and clothing. Indeed, trauma is the foremost cause of peripheral nerve injury in the lower extremities, particularly around the pelvic, inguinal, and ankle regions, often involving the femoral, obturator, ilioinguinal, iliohypogastric, genitofemoral, and posterior tibial nerves. Described chronic compressive syndromes include entrapment of the lateral femoral cutaneous, sciatic, saphenous, posterior tibial, common peroneal, deep peroneal, and plantar digital nerves. Results from surgical management of meralgia paresthetica and Morton's neuroma (of a plantar digital nerve) are discussed with other pathologies treated by neurectomy, and will be omitted here.

Sciatic Nerve Entrapment. The posterior L4 to S3 sacral plexus nerve roots typically give rise to the sciatic nerve, which travels anterior to the piriformis muscle before passing beneath its inferior border to exit the pelvis through the greater sciatic foramen posterior to the piriformis muscle, along with the superior and inferior gluteal vessels and nerves. When the sciatic nerve instead travels above or even through the piriformis muscle, a syndrome of gluteal region pain, weakness in hip abduction resulting in a lurching gait, and tenderness to palpation just lateral to the greater sciatic notch can be induced.[177] Weakness in knee flexion in the absence of paraspinous muscle weakness can be suggestive of this peripheral injury as well, and there is often discrete tenderness between the greater trochanter and ischium.

This entrapment syndrome is six times more common in women than in men and often associated with repetitive trauma such as horseback riding, muscular hypertrophy or ossification, or with iatrogenic injury to the sciatic nerve.[178] It can closely mimic the sciatica caused by lumbar disc herniation or spinal stenosis, and MRI is particularly helpful in determining the likelihood of a peripheral nerve entrapment in relation to the far more common spinal etiologies. Electrodiagnostic tests are very difficult to perform reliably in this region, and are generally of little utility. Focal tenderness directly over the piriformis muscle, together with normal MRI of lumbar spine, is suggestive of sciatic nerve entrapment.

Surgical management involves sectioning of the overlying piriformis muscle and has provided excellent relief in a limited number of reported cases.[179,180] A feared complication of this procedure is complete sectioning of one of the associated gluteal vessels, which can retract into the pelvis, necessitating laparotomy for hemostasis.[181] There have been case reports of spontaneous entrapment neuropathies involving the distal portions of the sciatic nerve in the thigh.[182,183]

Saphenous Nerve Entrapment. Iatrogenic saphenous nerve injury is commonly a result of saphenous vein harvesting. A similar syndrome that also presents as dysesthesias and pain involving the medial aspect of the knee and anterior tibial region has been treated successfully with surgical release in the subsartorial (Hunter's) canal.[32,184] A fascial band between the abductor magnus and vastus medialis muscles is the offending factor, and pain can typically be elicited on examination with palpation over the canal.

Tibial Nerve Entrapment. Tibial nerve entrapment at the popliteal fossa results from compression by the tendinous arch of the origin of the soleus muscle, as well as from nerve tumors, Baker's cyst, and trauma. As it crosses medially in the popliteal fossa, the tibial nerve travels superficially to the popliteus muscle, while passing under the tendinous arch of the soleus muscle before entering the space between the heads of the gastrocnemius and plantaris muscles.[185,186]

Symptoms of tarsal tunnel syndrome result from compression of the posterior tibial nerve at the medial malleolus. The tarsal tunnel itself refers to the deep posterior compartments of the distal leg as they pass beneath the flexor retinaculum, which is formed from the superficial and deep aponeuroses of the leg.[187] Symptoms typically include pain and dysesthesias involving the plantar surface of the foot and sometimes the heel, depending on whether the posterior tibial nerve trifurcates and gives rise to the medial calcaneus sensory branch proximal to the point of compression. Tinel's sign over the flexor retinaculum is quite sensitive and specific in the diagnosis of entrapment, particularly when combined with the dorsiflexion-eversion maneuver.[188] Both MRI and electrodiagnostic studies are extremely helpful in confirming and assessing severity of the pathology, particularly in recurrent cases and in those rare instances refractory to conservative management.[189-192] The differential diagnosis is wide and includes such common etiologies as complex regional pain syndrome, plantar fasciitis, and Achilles tendonitis.

Surgical sectioning of the flexor retinaculum and release of the nerve has demonstrated only moderate success, perhaps in part due to the success of conservative management in such a large proportion of cases.[193-195] Pfeiffer and Cracchiolo[196] reported 44% of patients received significant improvement after decompression, and two subsequent studies showed similar overall benefit. Sammarco and Chang[197] later reported significantly better surgical outcomes in patients with duration of symptoms lasting less than 1 year, compared with disease present for greater than 1 year. Still, Turan et al.[198] demonstrated that surgical management is still of benefit in those with longstanding symptoms, providing excellent results in 61% of patients who experienced symptoms for more than 5 years.

Peroneal Nerve Entrapments. Once the sciatic nerve reaches the popliteal fossa, it gives rise to the common peroneal nerve, which then wraps around the fibular head and passes into the peroneal tunnel alongside the peroneus longus tendon. There, it trifurcates, giving off superficial and deep peroneal nerve branches, as well as a sensory branch to the tibiofibular joint and knee.[199] Entrapment syndromes typically arise due to compression in the knee (due to fatty tissue deposition or Baker's cyst) or at the peroneal tunnel, but the superficial and deep branches can be compressed at the fascial exit of the superficial branch over the anterolateral aspect of the lower shin,[200] and at the anterior tarsal tunnel bounded by the fascial layers over the talus and the inferior extensor retinaculum, respectively. Several small series of patients undergoing decompression of the superficial and deep branches have shown the efficacy of surgical treatment, but large reports guiding decision-making in surgical decompression are lacking.[201-205]

The common peroneal nerve rests in a particularly superficial position at the fibular neck, and thus is susceptible to external compression as well as to traction injury. It is also a common site of intraneural ganglia.[199] Neuropathy is commonly found in women who habitually sit in a cross-legged position. Similarly, prolonged squatting or kneeling can cause compressive symptoms. Repetitive plantarflexion and inversion of the foot is often the mechanism of traction upon the nerve, and a constricting band at the level of the fibular head is often found at the time of operation. Symptoms most commonly include foot drop, weakness of ankle, dorsiflexion and eversion, and pain in the peroneal nerve dermatome along the lateral leg. The pain symptoms can be easily confused with such common ailments as shin splints or tibial stress fracture, as well as with an L5 radiculopathy or compartment syndrome. Electrodiagnostic studies are helpful in isolating the region of entrapment.[206]

Surgical decompression must not be delayed, although conservative management is successful in approximately one third of cases.[207] In one analysis, 87% of patients with motor dysfunction obtained good improvement, whereas only 54% of patients with purely sensory deficits experienced long-term relief.[208] However, the average time between onset of symptoms and operation was 14 months in this study. In another series, surgical intervention was shown to yield a 97% immediate success rate when performed within 2 months of onset of injury, whereas in cases lasting 4 to 8 months, only a 38% benefit was found.[209]

DORSAL RHIZOTOMY AND GANGLIONECTOMY

Basic Considerations

The Bell-Magendie model describes a dorsal root comprised solely of primary afferent fibers, while the ventral root contains only efferent fibers. Dorsal rhizotomy and ganglionectomy procedures seek to take advantage of this apparent physiologic segregation to halt the inflow of nociceptive signals to the spinal cord at particular levels, while sparing motor outputs. Injury to motor fibers in the ventral root is avoided (Fig. 102.3). No neuroma forms at the cut ends of the rootlets, as nerve fibers that enter the spinal cord are deprived of their cell body and hence degenerate.[210]

Theoretically an appealing treatment option for pain, rhizotomy in practice often fails to confer the lasting benefit that one might expect. Early surgeons performed dorsal rhizotomy for a broad range of conditions including stump pain, intercostal neuralgia, angina, visceral pain, and spastic hemiplegia. After comparing operative results for pain with those for spasticity in 1911, Groves remarked, "Strangely enough, the division of the posterior spinal roots has given the least satisfactory results in those very cases where we should have expected it to be the most efficient . . . the relief of pain."[211]

An important problem with rhizotomy is that the sensory afferents that arise from a region of the body may provide contributions to multiple spinal nerves. Conversely, fibers from a single

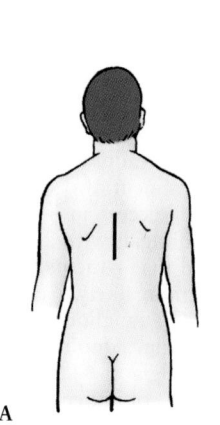

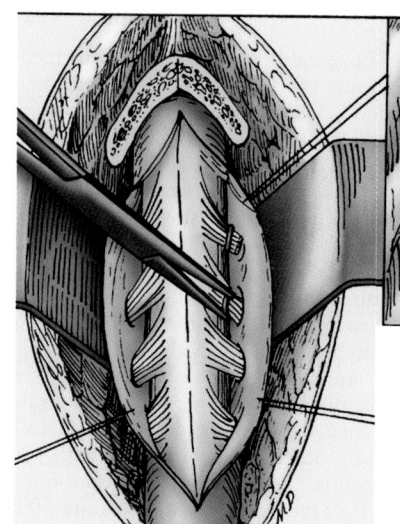

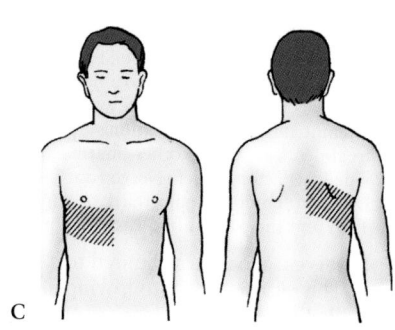

FIGURE 102.3 Dorsal rhizotomy. **A.** Location of midline dorsal incision for T4 to T7 dorsal rhizotomy. **B.** Intradural dorsal rhizotomy with application of metal clip on the rootlets of a root already transected above and being applied to the rootlets of a root below just prior to sectioning them. Inset on the right depicts extradural dorsal rhizotomy showing division of the dorsal root central to the ganglion prior to extirpation of the ganglion by a lesion that will be made just distal to the ganglion. **C.** Expected area of sensory loss following right T4 to T7 dorsal rhizotomy.

spinal nerve may innervate multiple segments of the spinal cord. As a result, sensory dermatomes overlap considerably, so that ablation of a single dorsal root produces little sensory deficit.[212] The earliest studies[213,214] of the dermatomes appreciated this complexity, and early surgeons performed rhizotomy at two to three levels or more to achieve pain control.[211] Extensive remodeling of sensory dermatomes, attributed to intraspinal sprouting of dorsal root axons,[215] functional reorganization of existing sensory pathways,[216] and other mechanisms, has since been described.

A second potential explanation of surgical failure involves the presence of unmyelinated sensory fibers in the ventral roots. In 1894, Sherrington[217] noted degeneration of fibers on the cord side of a transected ventral root.[218] He suggested that these fibers, which he presumed would double back and reenter the cord through the dorsal root, might provide a physiologic basis for the observation that stimulation of the ventral root results in pain. Microscopy has demonstrated that some fibers do, in fact, enter the cord through ventral roots, cross the ventral horn, and synapse within the dorsal horn or enter the dorsal columns.[219] Thus, dorsal rhizotomy may fail ultimately because of the presence of afferents that reach the spinal cord via the ventral root. However, the actual frequency of ventral root sensory nerves is not known.

To obviate this problem, consideration may be given to performance of a sensory ganglionectomy. The cell body for all primary afferents is believed to reside in the dorsal root ganglion, regardless of whether the fibers reach the spinal cord via the dorsal or ventral roots. One report cites a patient with recurrent pain following dorsal rhizotomy that experienced enduring pain relief following removal of the dorsal root ganglia at the same level,[220] providing further evidence that afferents concerned with pain may enter the spinal cord through ventral roots. Ganglionectomy has gained acceptance in the treatment of certain pain disorders.[221] However, including ganglionectomy in a dorsal rhizotomy has not been demonstrated to yield better long-term results, though late recurrence with ganglionectomy is also common.

Clinical Considerations

Preoperative Evaluation

Dorsal rhizotomy or sensory ganglionectomy may be attempted for treatment of both nociceptive and neuropathic pain, although in our experience, pain often recurs within a few years. Prediction

of the potential effect of an operation can be fairly simple, if only a single level is affected. A number of confounding anatomic situations, such as root-to-root anastomosis or overlap of root innervation, must be considered.[222] Identification of the appropriate spinal level and roots or ganglia for ablation is accomplished through paravertebral local anesthetic nerve blocks. Spinal epidural or subarachnoid blocks can be used for screening purposes when considering sacral rhizotomy. For greater accuracy in diagnosis, these blocks should be performed at multiple levels, with placebo controls. There is a tendency for the anesthetic to leak into the epidural space, and this may lead to a false positive result.

Although rhizotomies are now done infrequently for pain, some patients do gain enduring pain relief from rhizotomy or ganglionectomy, with acceptable morbidity. The challenge is to select the patients most likely to benefit. Feasibility dictates the appropriate procedures, to some extent. If the clinical problem is limited to one root, ganglionectomy has appeal in order to avoid the problem of ventral root afferents. Unfortunately, surgical ganglionectomy involves destruction of a substantial portion of the facet, and therefore may not be practical if two or more roots are involved. Rhizotomy may be preferable in this instance; however, the problem of pain recurrence may be higher. No clinical studies directly compare rhizotomy and ganglionectomy, and differences in outcome between the two procedures are not well understood.

Dorsal rhizotomy and sensory ganglionectomy spare motor efferents and do not lead to the formation of neuromas. However, careful attention must be given to the potential complications of dorsal root surgery. Ablations of the dorsal roots attenuate not only pain, but also vibratory, temperature, and proprioceptive inputs. Loss of these sensory functions may be troublesome, particularly in the extremities. In addition, with the ablation of the highly vascularized dorsal roots, blood supply to the spinal cord can be jeopardized. Ablation of more than six dorsal roots increases this risk considerably.[212] Finally, dorsal rhizotomy and ganglionectomy, if unsuccessful, preclude the use of dorsal column stimulation as a means of pain treatment, because the primary afferents on which the stimulator acts undergo wallerian degeneration.

The following case presents evaluation and treatment of a patient with neuropathic pain, in an ideal setting for performance of a ganglionectomy, although with eventual pain recurrence:

A 42-year-old woman underwent an anterior cervical discectomy and fusion with harvesting of a bone graft from the left iliac crest. An anterior abdominal wall hernia developed at the site of bone harvest.

This defect was repaired with mesh, and the patient developed severe pain at the repair site. Eventually the repair site was explored, and injury to the subcostal nerve (T12) was noted. The neuroma was resected back and relocated to a healthy muscular bed away from scar. Pain was relieved for several weeks and then returned. An additional attempt at neuroma relocation surgery met with the same fate. Opioid treatments as well as other pharmacologic approaches failed to provide satisfactory relief. Nerve root blocks of T12 but not of T11 or L1 led to complete pain relief. A ganglionectomy was performed at T12, and the patient had sustained pain relief for 2 years.

In this case, pain was limited to a single, clearly defined spinal level. The return of pain following neurectomy demonstrated the high likelihood of reformation of a painful neuroma. A single ganglionectomy both eliminated the pain and precluded the reformation of a painful neuroma. However, the pain recurred after 2 years. In our experience, peripheral nerve stimulation, spinal cord stimulation, and intrathecal pain pumps may be preferable and nondestructive first-line therapies for radicular pain prior to performance of sensory rhizotomy or ganglionectomy.

Operative Technique

Dorsal rhizotomy is performed using either an intradural or extradural approach, while ganglionectomy is by extradural approach. For intradural rhizotomy, a laminectomy is performed at the levels of interest and the dura is opened, where sensory rootlets are then identified at the intervertebral foramina, followed proximally, and divided. For extradural rhizotomy, the lateral facet is removed and the appropriate nerve roots are exposed laterally. The proximal spinal root is dissected free, and the dorsal rootlet is identified and divided. For ganglionectomy, the dorsal root ganglion is also dissected free and removed. In some cases, separation of the ganglion from the motor root is difficult and there may be resections of this structure as well, a factor to be borne in mind when selecting the ablative approach. Ganglionectomy can also be performed from a foraminal approach with minor disruption of the facet. Sacral rhizotomy may be accomplished though sacral laminectomy and division of the thecal sac between the S1 and S2 roots.[223]

Specific Indications and Outcomes

Indications for dorsal rhizotomy or ganglionectomy may be broadly divided into procedures for cancer and noncancer pain,[224] and are outlined by the Joint Section on Pain in its 1994 recommendations. In addition,[224b] dorsal rhizotomy can be a useful therapy in treatment of certain spasticity disorders, including spastic cerebral palsy. Barrash and Leavens[225] reported success in 70% (50 of 71) of patients with cancer, with 10.5-month average follow-up. By contrast, Onofrio and Campa[226] reported an overall success rate of 41% (46 of 112) in patients with localized idiopathic pain. Wilkinson[227] reported excellent pain reduction in 74% of patients with dorsal root ganglionectomy alone, with no adverse complications, for pain refractory to other treatments. The differences in success rate between cancer and noncancer pain could potentially result from earlier mortality among patients with cancer-related pain, given the significant incidence of late-recurring pain.

Cranial and Cervical Pain

Rhizotomy of C1 to C4 in combination with cranial nerves V, IX, and X may provide effective pain relief from extensive head and neck cancers.[228] In considering such a procedure, one would have to consider the morbidity of such an extensive operation in terms of sensory loss. In some cancer victims, however, sensory loss is already extensive. Dorsal cervical rhizotomy may also be combined with trigeminal tractotomy. Cancers of the lung or breast with brachial plexus involvement, with loss of function in the upper limb, may also benefit from cervical rhizotomy.

Occipital Neuralgia

The greater occipital nerve, formed by the posterior primary ramus of C2, and the lesser occipital nerve, formed by the C2 and C3 roots in the cervical plexus, jointly innervate the occipital region of the scalp. Occipital neuralgia is headache characterized by severe paroxysmal lancinating or continuous pain, localized to this innervated region.[229] Occipital neuralgia may be due to migraine, compression of the C2 root, entrapment of greater occipital nerve at the superior nuchal line, or nerve injury.[230]

C2 or C3 ganglionectomy, as well as upper intradural cervical rhizotomy, have been used successfully in treatment of occipital neuralgia. Stechison and Mullin[231] reported success in 4 of 4 patients with idiopathic greater occipital neuralgia, with 2-year average follow-up. Lozano et al.[232] reported that patients with occipital neuropathic pain due to trauma are more likely to experience significant pain reduction following C2 ganglionectomy than other patient groups with occipital pain. Onofrio and Campa[226] reported relief from occipital neuralgia in 64% (9 of 14) of patients immediately, and 50% (7 of 14) of patients after months to years following ablation of 1 to 3 cervical roots. Dubuisson[233] reported success in 71% (10 of 14) of patients, with 33-month average follow-up, following partial posterior rhizotomy at C1 to C3. Cervical nerve block has been shown to be useful for confirmation of occipital neuralgia, and possibly as a patient selection tool for rhizotomy.[234] In a recent study, Burchiel and colleagues[235] reported the return of pain within a year in 65% (13 of 20) of patients undergoing C2 or C3 ganglionectomy. Occipital nerve stimulation may be considered a favorable alternative to C2 or C3 ganglionectomy.[236]

Thoracic Pain

Pain associated with chest wall invasion of pleural-based or chest wall malignancies, as well as localized thoracic pain secondary to nerve invasion or compression, can be an indication for dorsal rhizotomy or ganglionectomy. Arbit et al.[237] reported complete pain relief in 64% (9 of 14) and 50% to 100% pain relief in an additional 29% (4 of 14) of patients with cancer pain, with 22-month median follow-up, following thoracic dorsal and ventral rhizotomy. Smith[238] reported success in 10 of 10 patients with intercostal pain due to thoracotomy,[7] herpes zoster,[2] and cancer,[1] following thoracic ganglionectomy.

Postsurgical Truncal Pain

Persistent pain following thoracotomy or laparotomy may be responsive to dorsal rhizotomy. White and Kjellberg[212] reported successful treatment of intercostal neuralgia in three of four patients, with 8-month median follow-up, following thoracic rhizotomy. Loeser[224] reported success in 33% (1 of 3) of patients at more than 3 months. By contrast, Onofrio and Campa[226] reported on 18 patients with postthoracotomy pain and 5 patients with postlaparotomy pain, none of whom obtained benefit. White and Kjellberg[212] also reported successful treatment of postherniorrhaphy neuralgia in 3 of 4 patients, with 2-year median follow-up, following thoracolumbar rhizotomy. There are no large series of patients upon which to base management decisions.

Sacral Pain

Cancers of the colon, rectum, urinary tract, cervix, and prostate may result in pain attributable to sacral roots. Unfortunately, ablation of the second and third sacral roots may affect bladder, sphincter, and sexual function. Thus, sacral root division is indicated in cases of pelvic cancer pain, where patients have already lost bladder and bowel function. It is a simple procedure that may confer striking benefit. Saris et al.[239] reported success in 47% (7 of 15) of patients with colorectal cancer presenting with perianal pain, with 1-year median follow-up, following bilateral S3 to S5 rhizotomy. Felsoory and Crue[223] reported satisfactory

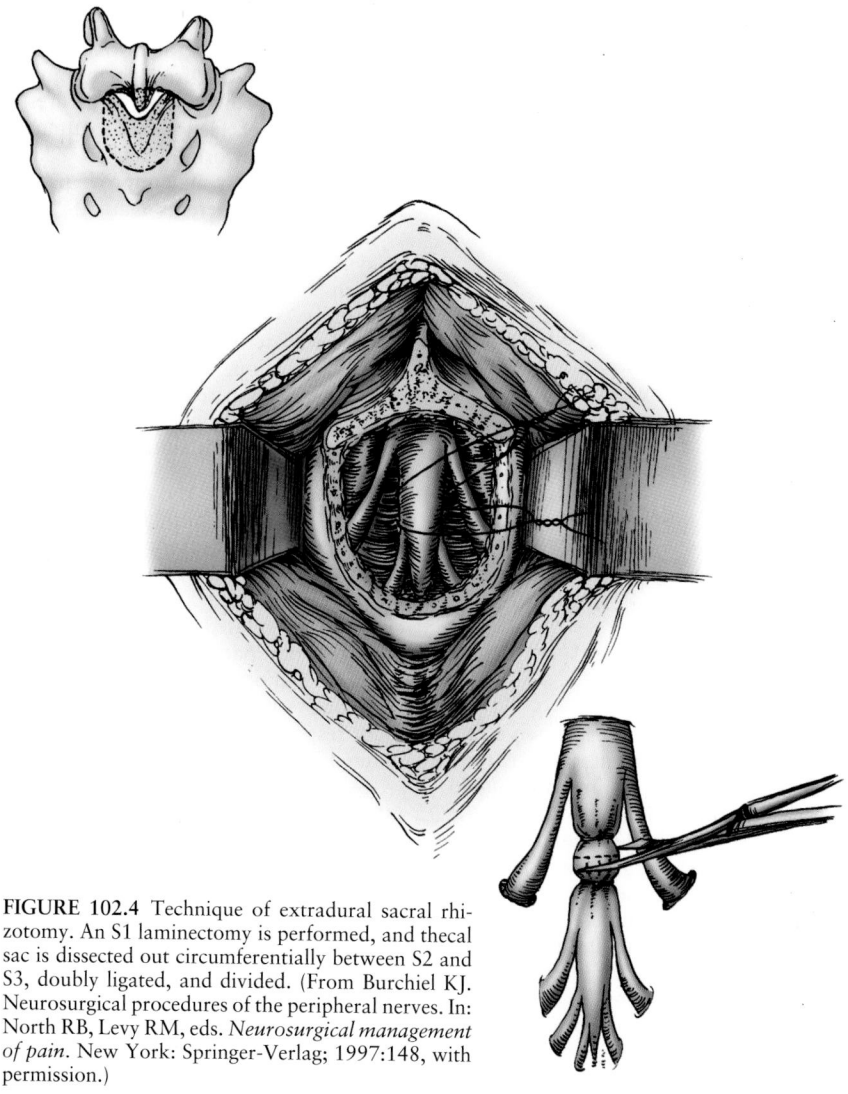

FIGURE 102.4 Technique of extradural sacral rhizotomy. An S1 laminectomy is performed, and thecal sac is dissected out circumferentially between S2 and S3, doubly ligated, and divided. (From Burchiel KJ. Neurosurgical procedures of the peripheral nerves. In: North RB, Levy RM, eds. *Neurosurgical management of pain*. New York: Springer-Verlag; 1997:148, with permission.)

results in 69% (20 of 28) of patients with colorectal,[17] cervical,[5] anal,[3] and other[3] cancers, with unstated follow-up duration, following transection of the cauda equina at L5-S1. The surgical anatomy is depicted in Figure 102.4.

Extremity Pain

Rhizotomy or ganglionectomy are indicated for denervation of a functionally useless limb. There are few other indications in the treatment of extremity pain. That multiple roots may be involved, the morbidity of sensory loss, and the problem of frequent pain recurrence, lead to infrequent use of these procedures for extremity pain. Ganglionectomy for monoradicular extremity pain has been proposed, but remains unproven.[240] North et al.[241] reported greater than 50% relief from failed back surgery syndrome in none of the 13 patients they studied, with 5.5-year average follow-up. By contrast, Taub et al.[242] reported success in 59% (36 of 61) of patients with intractable monoradicular sciatica following dorsal root ganglionectomy, with 5 to 9 years median follow-up. This unusually high rate of success likely reflects very careful patient selection.

The choice of rhizotomy or ganglionectomy for treatment of extremity pain requires a balance between compromise of function due to elimination of sensation and the elimination of pain. For the upper extremity, White and Kjellberg[212] reported success-ful treatment of diffuse upper extremity pain in 50% (7 of 14) of patients, with 3-year median follow-up, following rhizotomy at various levels. Following the procedure, none of the patients complained of unpleasant numbness or clumsiness of the hand, perhaps reflecting the seriousness of the preoperative condition. In the lower extremity, they reported successful treatment of lateral femoral cutaneous neuralgia in 67% (4 of 6) of patients, with 3-year median follow-up, following L2 to L3 rhizotomy. Spinal cord stimulation may offer a nondestructive alternative to rhizotomy or ganglionectomy for the treatment of extremity pain.[243]

Visceral Pain

Though rarely used today due to the advent of other techniques, dorsal rhizotomy has been reported to be highly effective in controlling visceral pain. White and Kjellberg[212] reported successful treatment of medically intractable angina in 75% (3 of 4) of patients, with 14-month median follow-up, following T1 to T4 rhizotomy. Success was 50% (3 of 6) for treatment of other forms of visceral pain.

Axial Spine Pain

Lumbar median branch rhizotomy via percutaneous radiofrequency ablation is indicated for treatment of facet arthropathy pain and is discussed in detail in Chapter 101. Local and radicular pain due to lumbar spine disease is largely unresponsive, in the longer term, to dorsal rhizotomy. Loeser[224] reported success in 75% (12 of 16) at up to 3 months, but only 14% (2 of 14) at more than 3 months for patients with disk disease. Onofrio and Campa[226] reported improvement in 17% (11 of 64) of patients with lumbosacral pain following rhizotomy, with unstated follow-up. Wetzel et al.[244] reported success in 55% (28 of 51) at up to 6 months and 19% (7 of 37) at 2 years for patients with lumbar radiculopathy after lumbar surgery.

Postherpetic Neuralgia

Dermatomal pain following herpetic infection responds poorly to dorsal rhizotomy. Loeser[224] reported failure in two of two patients. Onofrio and Campa[226] reported success in only 20% (one of five) of patients, with 5-year follow up, following unilateral rhizotomy. The treatment of postherpetic neuralgia is discussed in Chapter 27.

SYMPATHECTOMY

Basic Considerations

Sympathetic Efferents

Sympathetic efferents reach their target structures in two steps. Preganglionic sympathetic efferents arise in the intermediolateral cell column of the spinal cord at T1 to L3. Thinly myelinated fibers emerge in the ventral roots and transit briefly through the spinal nerve before exiting to form the white rami communicantes, leading to the paravertebral sympathetic ganglia. Some preganglionic fibers form synapses in the sympathetic chain with postganglionic neurons, from which unmyelinated fibers return to the spinal nerves, forming the gray rami communicantes. These postganglionic efferents provide sympathetic innervation to blood vessels, sweat glands, and other structures. Other preganglionic fibers pass through the paravertebral sympathetic chain without forming synapses and continue to the prevertebral ganglia. In the prevertebral ganglia, these efferents synapse with postganglionic effector neurons. From the prevertebral ganglia, unmyelinated fibers innervate the abdominal and pelvic viscera. Sympathectomy has been used in the treatment of pain from the limbs, the heart, and abdominal viscera. Presacral neurectomy and thoracic sympathectomy for cardiac pain are discussed earlier in this chapter and are not further addressed here.

Sympathetically Maintained Pain

In some patients with chronic pain syndromes, the pain depends on the activity of sympathetic efferents in the painful area. This pain, termed SMP, is defined as that aspect of pain that is relieved by blockade of sympathetic efferents.[245] Pain that is unaffected by the activity of sympathetic efferents is termed sympathetically independent pain. The diagnosis of SMP is empiric; that is, it is made based on response to treatment. In any pain syndrome, a portion may be sympathetically maintained, while another part is sympathetically independent. Notably, complex regional pain syndrome and other neuropathic conditions may or may not be associated with SMP.

Traditionally, three distinct mechanisms have been considered as ways through which ablation of sympathetic nerves or ganglia may lead to pain relief:

1. The sympathetic efferents in T1 to L3 that pass through paravertebral sympathetic ganglia to abdominal and pelvic viscera do not travel alone. They are accompanied by afferents, with cell bodies in the dorsal root ganglia of T1 to L3, which convey sensory information about distension and inflammation of visceral organs to the central nervous system. As a result of this colocalization, ablation of prevertebral ganglia (or the nerves originating from them) interrupts the flow of nociceptive signals from visceral structures to brain, thereby producing pain relief. Hence, as a treatment for visceral pain, sympathectomy is a form of sensory neurectomy.

2. Sympathectomy may improve pain associated with ischemia. Sympathetic efferents maintain arterial tone. In vasospastic and vasoocclusive conditions, the vasodilation consequent to sympathectomy may ameliorate ischemia, thereby decreasing pain.[246]

3. Finally, sympathectomy may eliminate norepinephrine-mediated activation of nociceptors and thereby relieve SMP. In this section, we concentrate on this latter mechanism and extremity pain related to complex regional pain syndromes in which a component of pain has been demonstrated to be sympathetically maintained.

Understanding of the pathophysiologic mechanisms underlying SMP continues to increase. The involvement of both A and polymodal C nociceptors is evident, though incompletely elucidated.[247,248] Immunologically-mediated mechanisms involving prostaglandin, bradykinin, substance P, neuropeptide Y, and calcitonin gene-related peptide, have also been proposed in treatment-resistant patients.[249,250] Increased expression of class I and II human leukocyte antigen in patients diagnosed with reflex sympathetic dystrophy suggests a genetic predisposition to poor treatment response,[251] although a relationship to SMP has not been defined.

By definition, SMP is eliminated by blockade of sympathetic efferent innervation of the painful area. Thus, anesthetic blockade of the relevant sympathetic ganglia relieves pain in patients with SMP. Stimulation of the sympathetic chain evokes pain in patients with SMP but not in those without SMP.[25] Moreover, Walker and Nulson[252] noted that stimulation of the severed distal end of the sympathetic chain evokes pain in those diagnosed with SMP but not in other patients. Thus, the central connections of sympathetic efferent fibers are not required for stimulation of the sympathetic system to evoke pain. These observations establish that efferent sympathetic fibers, rather than afferent sensory fibers that may travel with sympathetic fibers, account for SMP in nonvisceral pain syndromes.

Several independent lines of pharmacologic evidence support the claim that norepinephrine released from sympathetic fibers is critical in SMP. First, regional infusion of guanethidine, which acts to deplete norepinephrine from sympathetic terminals, relieves pain in patients with SMP.[253] Second, in patients whose pain had been relieved by either sympathetic block or sympathectomy, a cutaneous injection of norepinephrine into the previously painful area rekindles the pain and hyperalgesia. However, norepinephrine injected intracutaneously into normal subjects induces less pain and less hyperalgesia.[254,255] Finally, administration of sympathetic β-adrenergic antagonists, such as prazosin, phenoxybenzamine, or phentolamine, relieves SMP.[256–259]

Following nerve injury, neuromas that form may acquire sensitivity to norepinephrine. Injection of pH-balanced norepinephrine solution into normal subcutaneous tissues causes little pain. However, injection of norepinephrine onto painful neuromas does induce pain.[260] Thus, nerve injury may be associated with the induction of SMP.

These observations suggest that an abnormal increase in the amount of norepinephrine released from sympathetic terminals is not likely to be the mechanism of SMP. Rather, it is the response to norepinephrine that appears to be critical. Studies continue to support this theory, demonstrating the benefit of perioperative pharmacologic sympathetic block in reducing recurrence.[261,262] Whether this change is due to an up-regulation of β-adrenergic receptors or increased receptor sensitivity is unknown.

Clinical Considerations

Preoperative Evaluation

SMP cannot be diagnosed purely from history and physical examination of the patient.[263] However, it must be differentiated from similar-appearing chronic pain syndromes, particularly peripheral nerve injury. A number of clinical features are helpful: (1) In general, SMP does not occur in places other than the extremities or face. As a rule, the likelihood of developing SMP parallels the density of sympathetic innervation of the skin. Hence, truncal pain is far less likely to be due to SMP than is extremity pain. (2) Signs that may be inferred to represent increased sympathetic activity in the painful area do not necessarily denote the presence of SMP.[264] For example, limbs associated with SMP may be warmer, cooler, or the same temperature as unaffected limbs. Similarly, differences in sweating, nail growth, and muscle tone do not reliably contribute to the diagnosis of SMP. Nonetheless, sweating abnormalities in particular, as well as temperature alterations in general, may have some diagnostic utility.[265] We have found that among patients with traumatic nerve or soft tissue injury with touch-evoked pain, all patients with SMP and 50% of patients with sympathetically independent pain have striking sensitivity to mild cooling stimuli.[7,266]

Due to adverse effects and lack of definitive supporting evidence, surgical sympathectomy is typically reserved for medically-refractory SMP. Careful patient selection is critical to success. Thus, preoperative evaluation is of great importance. Mechanical allodynia with temperature change and cooling hyperalgesia together form an indication for sympathetic blockade.[264] The effect of sympathetic blockade via regional blockade or systemic infusion, in turn, plays an important role in identifying patients who might benefit from sympathectomy. High rates of recurrence, either due to sympathetic chain regeneration or new-onset complex regional pain syndrome, as well as significant adverse effects of the operation, serve to further highlight the need for discriminating patient selection. Finally, early intervention is important to optimize patient outcomes.

Quantitative Sensory Testing. Essentially all patients with SMP have cooling hyperalgesia.[263,266] In fact, patients with SMP often spontaneously volunteer that the one stimulus that they most dread is cooling of the painful area. Cooling hyperalgesia occurs less frequently in patients with sympathetically independent pain. This suggests that cooling hyperalgesia is a highly sensitive, though not specific, indicator of SMP.

Local Anesthetic Sympathetic Ganglion Blocks. The traditional procedure to diagnose SMP is percutaneous injection of local anesthetic onto the sympathetic ganglia serving the painful region. In local anesthetic sympathetic ganglion blocks (LASB), ganglia are localized through anatomic landmarks, ideally under fluoroscopic guidance, and local anesthetic is injected into the region. The presence of local anesthetic at the ganglia prevents norepinephrine from being released into peripheral tissues. While frequently used to diagnose SMP, LASB results must be interpreted with care: (1) Incomplete block of individual ganglia may falsely underestimate the contribution of SMP to a painful condition. The extent of sympathetic block must be evaluated by assaying for effects of sympathetic block, such as changes in skin temperature; (2) Spread of local anesthetic onto somatic afferents in the nerve roots, or blockade of sensory afferents that accompany sympathetic efferents, may induce pain relief by way of somatic block rather than sympathetic block. Careful sensory examination must be performed to ensure that somatic afferents are not affected by injection of local anesthetic; (3) LASB may evoke a placebo response, causing overestimation of pain relief. In addition to these interpretive issues, LASB has some risk. Complica-

tions reported with LASB include pneumothorax, phrenic and laryngeal nerve block, cardiac arrhythmia, kidney injury, hemorrhage, and inadvertent intravascular or epidural injections (see Chapter 97 for a detailed discussion of the role of local anesthetic blocks in the diagnosis of SMP).

Systemic Phentolamine Infusion. An alternative strategy to assess the potential efficacy of sympathectomy involves intravenous infusion of phentolamine, a short-acting antagonist of β-adrenergic receptors.[257,259] There is good correlation between pain relief with LASB and that with systemic phentolamine infusion (SPI).[259,263] As a systemic infusion, phentolamine does not provide any information about anatomic localization, as is available with LASB. However, SPI has a number of advantages over LASB: (1) the test is painless in that the phentolamine is delivered systemically and does not require fluoroscopy or needles to be placed in the paravertebral space; (2) with SPI, a significant observation period can be used prior to the administration of the drug, and the patient can be blinded to the time of drug administration, allowing a placebo-control period in every trial; (3) SPI appears to be safer than LASB, with only nasal stuffiness and peripheral vasodilation reported as side effects.[267] Furthermore, because the activity of nearby sensory afferents is preserved, SPI appears to be a more specific diagnostic test for SMP.[259,263]

Intravenous Regional Block. A third method to detect SMP involves regional intravenous infusion of an agent that impedes peripheral release of norepinephrine,[253] known as a Bier block. Sympatholytic agents studied include bretylium, reserpine, and guanethidine.[266] To avoid systemic circulation of the sympatholytic agent, a tourniquet is applied to the limb during the test. The central advantage of intravenous regional block (IRB) is localization of sympathetic block to the limb of interest. However, there are shortcomings: (1) some patients poorly tolerate the required tourniquet application; (2) the dramatic release of sympathetic neurotransmitter accompanying infusion of guanethidine in SMP patients may be severely painful; (3) the blocking agent may leak beyond the tourniquet, in some instances with significant hemodynamic effects; (4) the need for a tourniquet makes IRB difficult to perform either in the trunk or in the lower extremity; (5) it is difficult to evaluate placebo responses with IRB. Though frequently mentioned as a means to diagnose and to treat SMP, we believe that IRB has few advantages. The same degree of β-receptor blockade can be achieved with systemic phentolamine.

Medical Treatment of SMP. Once the diagnosis of SMP is made, the mainstay of treatment is medical sympatholysis, with surgical intervention reserved for refractory cases. A remarkable feature of SMP is that extended sympathetic blockade may lead to long-term or permanent relief from the disorder. When the goal of blockade is diagnosis, the diagnostic technique should be specific to the sympathetic nervous system. By contrast, when the goal is treatment, there need not be specificity. There are several medical and interventional means by which to achieve sympatholysis. The choice of technique should be based on considerations of safety, comfort, and efficacy.

Multiple sympathetic ganglion blocks with local anesthetics have, in the past, served as the criterion standard for treatment. However, local anesthetic treatment of peripheral nerves may work as well by inducing similar blockade of the distal sympathetic fibers. For example, SMP in the upper extremity could be treated either by LASB of thoracic sympathetic ganglia or by local anesthetic application to the appropriate nerves.

Alternatively, while epidural administration of anesthetic may lack specificity as a means to diagnose SMP, it may provide an effective treatment regimen. Epidural clonidine, though limited by hemodynamic effects, provides extensive analgesia.[268] SPI has been used successfully to treat SMP in a patient with pain in all extremities due to Sjögren's associated polyneuropathy.[269]

When episodic treatments fail to provide adequate relief, chronic treatment with oral sympatholytics may reduce SMP. Both phenoxybenzamine and prazosin have been used in this manner.[256,258] However, the systemic hypotension that frequently accompanies the use of these agents may preclude adequate sympathetic blockade. Finally, topical clonidine, which is likely to inhibit local norepinephrine release, may be a low-morbidity treatment of SMP in some patients, albeit locally.[254,270] If well tolerated, this and other medical techniques could substantially reduce the need for surgical sympathectomy; indeed the role for surgical sympathectomy remains in question.

Operative Techniques

To achieve sympathectomy of the upper extremity, it is necessary to resect the T2, T3, and T4 sympathetic ganglia. Removal of less than all three ganglia risks inadequate sympathectomy for pain. One of our patients required extension of the sympathectomy to T5. This is best achieved through a thoracoendoscopic technique, although the data on this operation have been acquired through open supraclavicular transaxillary or posterior costotransversectomy approaches. By contrast, the lumbar sympathetic chain, most commonly involving L2 and L3 ganglia, is generally accessed through an anterolateral retroperitoneal surgical approach. Percutaneous approaches have been suggested, but these procedures often do not achieve enduring results. In addition, the scarring produced by these approaches makes later surgical treatment more difficult.

Many clinicians have reported limited success in the treatment of pain by surgical sympathectomy.[271,272] Failure of sympathectomy may reflect inadequacies either of the preoperative evaluation, as discussed above, or of the extent of the sympathectomy. For example, sympathetic outflow to the arm derives predominantly from the T2 and T3 ganglia and not from the stellate ganglion. Failure to remove the T2 ganglion, at a minimum, will result in continued sympathetic innervation of the hand. An important feature in the lower extremity is that sympathetic innervation is often bilateral. Bilateral lumbar sympathectomy of L2 to L4 is typically necessary (Fig. 102.5). A typical patient history is one of impressive relief of pain lasting several weeks following an ipsilateral lumbar sympathectomy. The pain then returns, and at that time the pain may be relieved by a contralateral block of the lumbar sympathetic ganglia. Patients will typically have enduring relief of pain following contralateral lumbar sympathectomy.[273,274] As in the upper extremity, complete sympathectomy is required for pain relief; the partial denervation that is successful for vascular diseases is not adequate as a treatment for pain.

Specific Indications and Outcomes

Ulmer and Mayfield[275] reported successful treatment of 96% (67 of 70) of soldiers with burning pain due to nerve injury by surgical sympathectomy of appropriate ganglia. In studies of a civilian population, Manart et al.[276] reported a "good" response to thoracic sympathectomy in 59% (13 of 22) of patients with burning posttraumatic pain, even when diagnostic blockades were not typically performed. For patients selected for preoperative diagnostic sympathetic block, Mockus et al.[277] reported improvement in 94% (29 of 31) of patients, with 3.4 years average follow-up. AbuRahma[278] reported 1-year satisfactory improvement of pain in 20 of 21 patients. Overall success rates of 90% or greater with surgical sympathectomy have been reported by several groups.[279] Thompson[280] reported successful surgical treatment in 46% (55 of 120) of patients with SMP following minor trauma, who were unresponsive to medical therapy. Overall, long-term successful outcomes in 70% to 85% of cases of thoracic, and slightly less in lumbar sympathectomy, can be expected.

As noted, results of sympathectomy largely depend upon careful patient selection.[258] Our experience has been that patients do extremely well if the pain responds dramatically to sympathetic ganglion block and systemic infusion of phentolamine, and there is provocation of pain with injection of norepinephrine when the patient is under the influence of a LASB. While our conclusions are preliminary, it appears that if one or more of these elements are missing, the patient does not fare as well. The modest response rates to sympathectomy in earlier series may reflect improper patient selection and inadequate sympathectomy (e.g., bilateral sympathectomy required for lower extremity pain) or more extensive unilateral ganglionectomy for total denervation of an extremity.

Postoperative Complications

Surgical sympathectomy may be associated with idiosyncratic complications. One frequent complication, affecting up to 20%

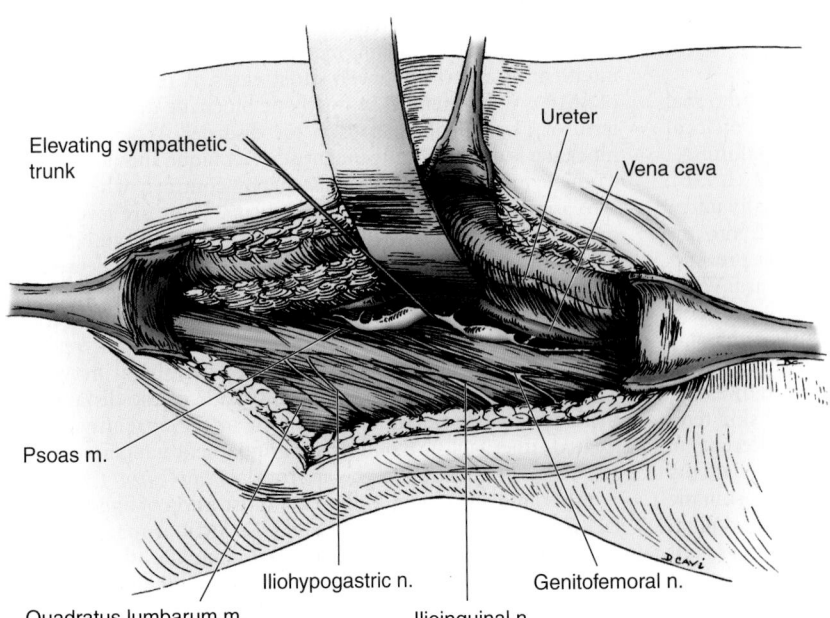

FIGURE 102.5 Open lumbar sympathectomy is done through retroperitoneal exposure of the sympathetic chain. (From Wilkinson HA. Neurosurgical procedures of the sympathetic nervous system. In: North RB, Levy RM, eds. *Neurosurgical management of pain.* New York: Springer-Verlag; 1997:170, with permission.)

to 50% of patients, is postsympathectomy pain.[277,281,282] This condition is characterized by the sudden onset, a few weeks after the procedure, of superficial burning pain, deep aching pain, and cutaneous hyperalgesia.[283] The pain arises in the proximal regions of limbs and the trunk, despite surgical ablation of sympathetic innervation to the distal limbs. Fortunately for the majority of patients, postsympathectomy pain resolves spontaneously in several weeks to a few months and no further surgical intervention is warranted.[281]

Ablation of sympathetic input to a region of skin results in sudomotor paralysis. In the upper extremity, the resultant dryness can be uncomfortable. In the lower extremity, dryness is better tolerated. Postural hypotension also can be a transient problem. However, even in patients with sympathectomy of all four extremities, this problem is usually not enduring. Compensatory hyperhidrosis, as well as pathologic gustatory sweating, may be found in patients following sympathectomy.[284] Two additional complications of sympathectomy include paradoxical vasoconstriction and ileus. Sympathetic fibers arising from the celiac and mesenteric ganglia modulate gastrointestinal motility. Both complications are generally transient.

CONCLUSION

The peripheral nervous system offers a number of attractive strategies for treatment of pain. Peripheral nerves may be transected or released from regions of entrapment. Where regional pain control is required, sensory roots or ganglia may be the targets of therapy. In cases where pain has a significant sympathetically maintained component, sympathectomy may offer significant and long-lasting pain relief.

As for all surgical procedures, careful patient selection and clear establishment of the etiology of the painful condition is critical to ensure successful analgesia. Enthusiasm for these surgical procedures must be tempered by a keen appreciation of potential complications.

Nerve transection may either produce or eliminate pain. This leaves the clinician with the sometimes daunting task of deciding if, when, and how to perform neurectomy. Each patient must be carefully evaluated. In the case of minor nerves previously transected, the clinician should not labor over the decision to relocate the neuroma to a protected, unscarred site. In this instance there is little to lose.

Pain due to mechanical compression may be relieved through release of nerve root entrapments. Carpal tunnel release and release of ulnar nerve entrapment at the elbow are among the most commonly performed peripheral nerve procedures. However, many less common forms of nerve root entrapment may be overlooked or misdiagnosed. A systematic understanding of peripheral neuroanatomy on the part of the pain clinician is essential to accurate diagnosis and treatment of these pain syndromes.

Dorsal rhizotomy is seldom used in modern practice, but a survey of the existing literature reveals that patients certainly exist in whom rhizotomy conferred long-term benefit. Today's pain clinician does well to keep this option in mind in properly selected cases. Ganglionectomy has certain theoretical advantages over rhizotomy and neurectomy and is still another technique that should be considered in certain cases. However, recurrence of pain several years after surgery may be quite common.

Sympathectomy is helpful in patients with persistent SMP who are refractory to medical management. Recognition of the clinical symptoms of SMP, such as cold allodynia, and appropriate selection of sympathetic blockade modalities are required to make the diagnosis and to provide a successful treatment strategy. Hence, the key to success with this procedure, as with most surgery, is meticulous patient selection and proper execution of the operation.

References

1. Kim KJ, Yoon YW, Chung JM. Comparison of three rodent neuropathic pain models. *Exp Brain Res* 1997;113:200–206.
2. Denny-Brown D, Kirk E. Hyperesthesia from spinal and root lesions. *Trans Am Neurol Assoc* 1968;93:116–120.
3. Wall PD, Gutnick M. Properties of afferent nerve impulses originating from a neuroma. *Nature* 1974;248:740–743.
4. Wall PD, Gutnick M. Ongoing activity in peripheral nerves: the physiology and pharmacology of impulses originating from a neuroma. *Exp Neurol* 1974;43:580–593.
5. Wall PD, Waxman S, Basbaum AI. Ongoing activity in peripheral nerve: injury discharge. *Exp Neurol* 1974;45:576–589.
6. Mitchell SW. *Injuries of Nerves and Their Consequences*. Philadelphhia: J. B. Lippincott; 1872.
7. Frost SA, Raja SN, Campbell JN, et al. Does hyperalgesia to cooling stimuli characterize patients with sympathetically maintained pain (reflex sympathetic dystrophy)? In: Dubnar R, Gebhart GF, Bond MR, eds. *Proceedings of the Vth World Congress on Pain*. New York: Elsevier; 1988.
8. Lang E, Spitzer A, Pfannmüller D, et al. Function of thick and thin nerve fibers in carpal tunnel syndrome before and after surgical treatment. *Muscle Nerve* 1995;18:207–215.
9. Koschorke GM, Meyer RA, Campbell JN. Cellular components necessary for mechanoelectrical transduction are conveyed to primary afferent terminals by fast axonal transport. *Brain Res* 1994;641:99–104.
10. Koschorke GM, Meyer RA, Tillman DB, et al. Ectopic excitability of injured nerves in monkey: entrained responses to vibratory stimuli. *J Neurophysiol* 1991;65:693–701.
11. Xiao Y, Segal MR, Rabert D, et al. Assessment of differential gene expression in human peripheral nerve injury. *BMC Genomics* 2002;3:28.
12. Thacker MA, Clark AK, Marchand F, et al. Pathophysiology of peripheral neuropathic pain: immune cells and molecules. *Anesth Analg* 2007;105:838–847.
13. Campbell JN, Meyer RA. Mechanisms of neuropathic pain. *Neuron* 2006;52:77–92.
14. Atherton DD, Elliot D. Relocation of neuromas of the lateral antebrachial cutaneous nerve of the forearm into the brachialis muscle. *J Hand Surg Eur Vol* 2007;32:311–315.
15. Atherton DD, Leong JC, Anand P, et al. Relocation of painful end neuromas and scarred nerves from the zone II territory of the hand. *J Hand Surg Eur Vol* 2007;32:38–44.
16. Dellon AL, Kim J, Ducic I. Painful neuroma of the posterior cutaneous nerve of the forearm after surgery for lateral humeral epicondylitis. *J Hand Surg Am* 2004;29:387–390.
17. Dellon AL, Mackinnon SE. Treatment of the painful neuroma by neuroma resection and muscle implantation. *Plast Reconstr Surg* 1986;77:427–438.
18. Hazari A, Elliot D. Treatment of end-neuromas, neuromas-in-continuity and scarred nerves of the digits by proximal relocation. *J Hand Surg Br* 2004;29:338–350.
19. Novak CB, van Vliet D, Mackinnon SE. Subjective outcome following surgical management of lower-extremity neuromas. *J Reconstr Microsurg* 1995;11:175–177.
20. Novak CB, van Vliet D, Mackinnon SE. Subjective outcome following surgical management of upper extremity neuromas. *J Hand Surg Am* 1995;20:221–226.
21. Sood MK, Elliot D. Treatment of painful neuromas of the hand and wrist by relocation into the pronator quadratus muscle. *J Hand Surg Br* 1998;23:214–219.
22. Stahl S, Rosenberg N. Surgical treatment of painful neuroma in medial antebrachial cutaneous nerve. *Ann Plast Surg* 2002;48:154–158; discussion 158–160.
23. D'Mello R, Dickenson AH. Spinal cord mechanisms of pain. *Br J Anaesth* 2008;101:8–16.
23b. Boldrey E. Amputation neuroma in nerves implanted in bone. *Ann Surg* 1943;188:1052–1057.
24. Kirvelä O, Nieminen S. Treatment of painful neuromas with neurolytic blockade. *Pain* 1990;41:161–165.
25. White JC, Sweet WH. *Pain and the Neurosurgeon: A Forty-Year Experience*. Springfield: Charles C. Thomas; 1969.
26. Lai YY, Chen SC, Chien NC. Video-assisted thoracoscopic neurectomy of intercostal nerves in a patient with intractable cancer pain. *Am J Hosp Palliat Care* 2006;23:475–478.
27. Stulz P, Pfeiffer KM. Peripheral nerve injuries resulting from common surgical procedures in the lower portion of the abdomen. *Arch Surg* 1982;117:324–327.
28. Starling JR, Harms BA. Diagnosis and treatment of genitofemoral and ilioinguinal neuralgia. *World J Surg* 1989;13:586–591.
29. Amid PK. Causes, prevention, and surgical treatment of postherniorrhaphy neuropathic inguinodynia: triple neurectomy with proximal end implantation. *Hernia* 2004;8:343–349.
30. Aasvang E, Kehlet H. Surgical management of chronic pain after inguinal hernia repair. *Br J Surg* 2005;92:795–801.
31. Williams PH, Trzil KP. Management of meralgia paresthetica. *J Neurosurg* 1991;74:76–80.
32. Luerssen TG, Campbell RL, Defalque RJ, et al. Spontaneous saphenous neuralgia. *Neurosurgery* 1983;13:238–241.

33. Lora J, Long D. So-called facet denervation in the management of intractable back pain. *Spine* 1976;1:121–126.

34. Johnson JE, Johnson KA, Unni KK. Persistent pain after excision of an interdigital neuroma. Results of reoperation. *J Bone Joint Surg Am* 1988;70:651–657.

35. Dereymaeker G, Schroven I, Steenwerckx A, et al. Results of excision of the interdigital nerve in the treatment of Morton's metatarsalgia. *Acta Orthop Belg* 1996;62:22–25.

36. Gauthier G. Thomas Morton's disease: a nerve entrapment syndrome. A new surgical technique. *Clin Orthop Relat Res* 1979:90–92.

37. Burchiel KJ, Johans TJ, Ochoa J. The surgical treatment of painful traumatic neuromas. *J Neurosurg* 1993;78:714–719.

38. Mackinnon SE, Dellon AL. *Surgery of the Peripheral Nerve.* New York: Thieme Medical Publishers; 1988.

39. Belzberg AJ, Campbell JN. Evidence for end-to-side sensory nerve regeneration in a human. Case report. *J Neurosurg* 1998;89:1055–1057.

40. Bogduk N, Long DM. The anatomy of the so-called "articular nerves" and their relationship to facet denervation in the treatment of low-back pain. *J Neurosurg* 1979;51:172–177.

41. Shealy CN. Percutaneous radiofrequency denervation of spinal facets. Treatment for chronic back pain and sciatica. *J Neurosurg* 1975;43:448–451.

42. Schofferman J, Kine G. Effectiveness of repeated radiofrequency neurotomy for lumbar facet pain. *Spine* 2004;29:2471–2473.

43. Lord SM, Barnsley L, Wallis BJ, et al. Percutaneous radio-frequency neurotomy for chronic cervical zygapophyseal-joint pain. *N Engl J Med* 1996;335:1721–1726.

44. Cohen SP, Bajwa ZH, Kraemer JJ, et al. Factors predicting success and failure for cervical facet radiofrequency denervation: a multi-center analysis. *Reg Anesth Pain Med* 2007;32:495–503.

45. Cohen SP, Hurley RW, Christo PJ, et al. Clinical predictors of success and failure for lumbar facet radiofrequency denervation. *Clin J Pain* 2007;23:45–52.

46. Silvers HR. Lumbar percutaneous facet rhizotomy. *Spine* 1990;15:36–40.

47. Oudenhoven RC. Paraspinal electromyography following facet rhizotomy. *Spine* 1977;2:299–304.

48. Buck-Gramcko D. Denervation of the wrist joint. *J Hand Surg Am* 1977;2:54–61.

49. Wilhelm A. Tennis elbow: treatment of resistant cases by denervation. *J Hand Surg Br* 1996;21:523–533.

50. Dellon AL, Mont MA, Mullick T, et al. Partial denervation for persistent neuroma pain around the knee. *Clin Orthop Relat Res* 1996:216–222.

51. Tekin I, Mirzai H, Ok G, et al. A comparison of conventional and pulsed radiofrequency denervation in the treatment of chronic facet joint pain. *Clin J Pain* 2007;23:524–529.

52. Ingersoll FM, Meigs JV. Presacral neurectomy for dysmenorrhea. *N Engl J Med* 1948;238:357–360.

53. Nezhat CH, Seidman DS, Nezhat FR, et al. Long-term outcome of laparoscopic presacral neurectomy for the treatment of central pelvic pain attributed to endometriosis. *Obstet Gynecol* 1998;91:701–704.

54. Omer GE, Spinner M, Van Beek AL. *Management of Peripheral Nerve Problems.* 2nd ed. Philadelphia: WB Saunders; 1998.

55. Pečina MM, Krmpotić-Nemanić J, Markiewitz AD. *Tunnel Syndromes: Peripheral Nerve Compression Syndromes.* 3rd ed. Boca Raton, FL: CRC Press; 2001.

56. Rempel D, Dahlin L, Lundborg G. Pathophysiology of nerve compression syndromes: response of peripheral nerves to loading. *J Bone Joint Surg Am* 1999;81:1600–1610.

57. Mackinnon SE, Dellon AL, Hudson AR, et al. A primate model for chronic nerve compression. *J Reconstr Microsurg* 1985;1:185–195.

58. Novak CB, Mackinnon SE. Nerve injury in repetitive motion disorders. *Clin Orthop Relat Res* 1998:10–20.

59. Ochoa J, Fowler TJ, Gilliatt RW. Anatomical changes in peripheral nerves compressed by a pneumatic tourniquet. *J Anat* 1972;113:433–455.

60. Ochoa J, Marotte L. The nature of the nerve lesion caused by chronic entrapment in the guinea-pig. *J Neurol Sci* 1973;19:491–495.

61. Dahlin LB, Lundborg G. The neurone and its response to peripheral nerve compression. *J Hand Surg Br* 1990;15:5–10.

62. Rydevik B, Lundborg G, Bagge U. Effects of graded compression on intraneural blood blow. An in vivo study on rabbit tibial nerve. *J Hand Surg Am* 1981;6:3–12.

63. Dyck PJ, Lais AC, Giannini C, et al. Structural alterations of nerve during cuff compression. *Proc Natl Acad Sci U S A* 1990;87:9828–9832.

64. Lundborg G. Structure and function of the intraneural microvessels as related to trauma, edema formation, and nerve function. *J Bone Joint Surg Am* 1975;57:938–948.

65. Lundborg G, Myers R, Powell H. Nerve compression injury and increased endoneurial fluid pressure: a "miniature compartment syndrome." *J Neurol Neurosurg Psychiatry* 1983;46:1119–1124.

66. Powell HC, Myers RR. Pathology of experimental nerve compression. *Lab Invest* 1986;55:91–100.

67. Abramowitz J, Dion JE, Jensen ME, et al. Angiographic diagnosis and management of head and neck schwannomas. *AJNR Am J Neuroradiol* 1991;12:977–984.

68. Rudge P, Ochoa J, Gilliatt RW. Acute peripheral nerve compression in the baboon. *J Neurol Sci* 1974;23:403–420.

69. Drake CG. Diagnosis and treatment of lesions of the brachial plexus and adjacent structures. *Clin Neurosurg* 1964;11:110–127.

70. Stull MA, Moser RP Jr, Kransdorf MJ, et al. Magnetic resonance appearance of peripheral nerve sheath tumors. *Skeletal Radiol* 1991;20:9–14.

71. Fullerton PM. The effect of ischaemia on nerve conduction in the carpal tunnel syndrome. *J Neurol Neurosurg Psychiatry* 1963;26:385–397.

72. Beard L, Kumar A, Estep HL. Bilateral carpal tunnel syndrome caused by Graves' disease. *Arch Intern Med* 1985;145:345–346.

73. O'Duffy JD, Randall RV, MacCarty CS. Median neuropathy (carpal-tunnel syndrome) in acromegaly. A sign of endocrine overactivity. *Ann Intern Med* 1973;78:379–383.

74. Schiller F, Kolb FO. Carpal tunnel syndrome in acromegaly. *Neurology* 1954;4:271–282.

75. Weimer LH, Yin J, Lovelace RE, et al. Serial studies of carpal tunnel syndrome during and after pregnancy. *Muscle Nerve* 2002;25:914–917.

76. Kline DG, Hudson AR. *Nerve Injuries: Operative Results for Major Nerve Injuries, Entrapments, and Tumors.* 1st ed. Philadelphia: WB Saunders; 1995.

77. Neary D, Ochoa J, Gilliatt RW. Sub-clinical entrapment neuropathy in man. *J Neurol Sci* 1975;24:283–298.

78. Dellon AL, Mackinnon SE. Chronic nerve compression model for the double crush hypothesis. *Ann Plast Surg* 1991;26:259–264.

79. Jablecki CK, Andary MT, So YT, et al. Literature review of the usefulness of nerve conduction studies and electromyography for the evaluation of patients with carpal tunnel syndrome. AAEM Quality Assurance Committee. *Muscle Nerve* 1993;16:1392–1414.

80. Rivner MH. Statistical errors and their effect on electrodiagnostic medicine. *Muscle Nerve* 1994;17:811–814.

81. Robinson LR, Micklesen PJ, Wang L. Strategies for analyzing nerve conduction data: superiority of a summary index over single tests. *Muscle Nerve* 1998;21:1166–1171.

82. Britz GW, Haynor DR, Kuntz C, et al. Carpal tunnel syndrome: correlation of magnetic resonance imaging, clinical, electrodiagnostic, and intraoperative findings. *Neurosurgery* 1995;37:1097–1103.

83. Hochman MG, Zilberfarb JL. Nerves in a pinch: imaging of nerve compression syndromes. *Radiol Clin North Am* 2004;42:221–245.

84. Jarvik JG, Yuen E, Kliot M. Diagnosis of carpal tunnel syndrome: electrodiagnostic and MR imaging evaluation. *Neuroimaging Clin N Am* 2004;14:93–102.

85. Mäurer J, Bleschkowski A, Tempka A, et al. High-resolution MR imaging of the carpal tunnel and the wrist. Application of a 5-cm surface coil. *Acta Radiol* 2000;41:78–83.

86. Grant GA, Britz GW, Goodkin R, et al. The utility of magnetic resonance imaging in evaluating peripheral nerve disorders. *Muscle Nerve* 2002;25:314–331.

87. Hughes R. Treatment of peripheral nerve disorders. *Curr Opin Neurol* 2005;18:554–556.

88. Arle JE, Zager EL. Surgical treatment of common entrapment neuropathies in the upper limbs. *Muscle Nerve* 2000;23(8):1160–1174.

89. Martin BI, Levenson LM, Hollingworth W, et al. Randomized clinical trial of surgery versus conservative therapy for carpal tunnel syndrome [ISRCTN84286481]. *BMC Musculoskelet Disord* 2005;6:2.

90. Stevens JC, Sun S, Beard CM, et al. Carpal tunnel syndrome in Rochester, Minnesota, 1961 to 1980. *Neurology* 1988;38:134–138.

91. Jarvik JG, Yuen E, Haynor DR, et al. MR nerve imaging in a prospective cohort of patients with suspected carpal tunnel syndrome. *Neurology* 2002;58:1597–1602.

92. Phalen GS. The carpal-tunnel syndrome. Clinical evaluation of 598 hands. *Clin Orthop Relat Res* 1972;83:29–40.

93. Mackinnon SE, Novak CB, Landau WM. Clinical diagnosis of carpal tunnel syndrome. *JAMA* 2000;284:1924–1926.

94. O'Connor D, Marshall S, Massy-Westropp N. Non-surgical treatment (other than steroid injection) for carpal tunnel syndrome. *Cochrane Database Syst Rev* 2003;1:CD003219.

95. Cseuz KA, Thomas JE, Lambert EH, et al. Long-term results of operation for carpal tunnel syndrome. *Mayo Clin Proc* 1966;41:232–241.

96. Gainer JV Jr, Nugent GR. Carpal tunnel syndrome: report of 430 operations. *South Med J* 1977;70:325–328.

97. Gerritsen AA, de Vet HC, Scholten RJ, et al. Splinting vs surgery in the treatment of carpal tunnel syndrome: a randomized controlled trial. *JAMA* 2002;288:1245–1251.

98. Lanz U. Anatomical variations of the median nerve in the carpal tunnel. *J Hand Surg Am* 1977;2:44–53.

99. Werner RA, Andary M. Carpal tunnel syndrome: pathophysiology and clinical neurophysiology. *Clin Neurophysiol* 2002;113:1373–1381.

100. Kiloh LG, Nevin S. Isolated neuritis of the anterior interosseous nerve. *Br Med J* 1952;1:850–851.

101. Collins DN, Weber ER. Anterior interosseous nerve syndrome. *South Med J* 1983;76:1533–1537.

102. Spinner M, Schreiber SN. Anterior interosseous-nerve paralysis as a complication of supracondylar fractures of the humerus in children. *J Bone Joint Surg Am* 1969;51:1584–1590.

103. Warren JD. Anterior interosseous nerve palsy as a complication of forearm fractures. *J Bone Joint Surg Br* 1963;45:511–512.

104. Lake PA. Anterior interosseous nerve syndrome. *J Neurosurg* 1974;41:306–309.

105. Spinner M. The anterior interosseous-nerve syndrome, with special attention to its variations. *J Bone Joint Surg Am* 1970;52:84–94.

106. Yasunaga H, Shiroishi T, Ohta K, et al. Fascicular torsion in the median nerve within the distal third of the upper arm: three cases of nontraumatic anterior interosseous nerve palsy. *J Hand Surg Am* 2003;28:206–211.

107. Kim DH, Murovic JA, Kim YY, et al. Surgical treatment and outcomes in 15 patients with anterior interosseous nerve entrapments and injuries. *J Neurosurg* 2006;104:757–765.

108. Joist A, Joosten U, Wetterkamp D, et al. Anterior interosseous nerve compression after supracondylar fracture of the humerus: a metaanalysis. *J Neurosurg* 1999;90:1053–1056.

109. Laha RK, Dujovny M, DeCastro SC. Entrapment of median nerve by supracondylar process of the humerus. Case report. *J Neurosurg* 1977;46:252–255.

110. Aydinlioglu A, Cirak B, Akpinar F, et al. Bilateral median nerve compression at the level of Struthers' ligament. Case report. *J Neurosurg* 2000;92:693–696.

111. Werner CO, Rosén I, Thorngren KG. Clinical and neurophysiologic characteristics of the pronator syndrome. *Clin Orthop Relat Res* 1985:231–236.

112. Spinner M, Spencer PS. Nerve compression lesions of the upper extremity. A clinical and experimental review. *Clin Orthop Relat Res* 1974;104:46–67.

113. Clark CB. Cubital tunnel syndrome. *JAMA* 1979;241:801–802.

114. Hirasawa Y, Sawamura H, Sakakida K. Entrapment neuropathy due to bilateral epitrochleoanconeus muscles: a case report. *J Hand Surg Am* 1979;4:181–184.

115. Matev B. Cubital tunnel syndrome. *Hand Surg* 2003;8:127–131.

116. Novak CB, Lee GW, Mackinnon SE, et al. Provocative testing for cubital tunnel syndrome. *J Hand Surg Am* 1994;19:817–820.

117. Greenwald D, Blum LC III, Adams D, et al. Effective surgical treatment of cubital tunnel syndrome based on provocative clinical testing without electrodiagnostics. *Plast Reconstr Surg* 2006;117:87e–91e.

118. Dellon AL. Operative techniques for submuscular transposition of the ulnar nerve. *Contemp Orthop* 1988;16:17–24.

119. Harrison MJ, Nurick S. Results of anterior transposition of the ulnar nerve for ulnar neuritis. *Br Med J* 1970;1:27–29.

120. Kleinman WB, Bishop AT. Anterior intramuscular transposition of the ulnar nerve. *J Hand Surg Am* 1989;14:972–979.

121. Learmonth JR. A technique for transplanting the ulnar nerve. *Surg Gynec Obstet* 1942;75:792–793.

122. Lowe JB III, Novak CB, Mackinnon SE. Current approach to cubital tunnel syndrome. *Neurosurg Clin N Am* 2001;12:267–284.

123. Nouhan R, Kleinert JM. Ulnar nerve decompression by transposing the nerve and Z-lengthening the flexor-pronator mass: clinical outcome. *J Hand Surg Am* 1997;22:127–131.

124. Pasque CB, Rayan GM. Anterior submuscular transposition of the ulnar nerve for cubital tunnel syndrome. *J Hand Surg Br* 1995;20:447–453.

125. Richmond JC, Southmayd WW. Superficial anterior transposition of the ulnar nerve at the elbow for ulnar neuritis. *Clin Orthop Relat Res* 1982:42–44.

126. Siegel DB. Submuscular transposition of the ulnar nerve. *Hand Clin* 1996;12:445–448.

127. Bartels RH, Menovsky T, Van Overbeeke JJ, et al. Surgical management of ulnar nerve compression at the elbow: an analysis of the literature. *J Neurosurg* 1998;89:722–727.

128. Bartels RH, Verhagen WI, van der Wilt GJ, et al. Prospective randomized controlled study comparing simple decompression versus anterior subcutaneous transposition for idiopathic neuropathy of the ulnar nerve at the elbow: Part 1. *Neurosurgery* 2005;56:522–530.

129. Dellon AL. Review of treatment results for ulnar nerve entrapment at the elbow. *J Hand Surg Am* 1989;14:688–700.

130. Dellon AL. Techniques for successful management of ulnar nerve entrapment at the elbow. *Neurosurg Clin N Am* 1991;2:57–73.

131. Kim DH, Han K, Tiel RL, et al. Surgical outcomes of 654 ulnar nerve lesions. *J Neurosurg* 2003;98:993–1004.

132. Amadio PC. Anatomical basis for a technique of ulnar nerve transposition. *Surg Radiol Anat* 1986;8:155–161.

133. Chan RC, Paine KW, Varughese G. Ulnar neuropathy at the elbow: comparison of simple decompression and anterior transposition. *Neurosurgery* 1980;7:545–550.

134. Heithoff SJ. Cubital tunnel syndrome does not require transposition of the ulnar nerve. *J Hand Surg Am* 1999;24:898–905.

135. LeRoux PD, Ensign TD, Burchiel KJ. Surgical decompression without transposition for ulnar neuropathy: factors determining outcome. *Neurosurgery* 1990;27:709–714.

136. Miller RG. The cubital tunnel syndrome: diagnosis and precise localization. *Ann Neurol* 1979;6:56–59.

137. Grantham SA. Ulnar compression in the loge de Guyon. *JAMA* 1966;197:509–510.

138. Moneim MS. Ulnar nerve compression at the wrist. Ulnar tunnel syndrome. *Hand Clin* 1992;8:337–344.

139. Zeiss J, Jakab E, Khimji T, et al. The ulnar tunnel at the wrist (Guyon's canal): normal MR anatomy and variants. *AJR Am J Roentgenol* 1992;158:1081–1085.

140. Kleinert JM, Mehta S. Radial nerve entrapment. *Orthop Clin North Am* 1996;27:305–315.

141. Uriburu IJ, Morchio FJ, Marin JC. Compression syndrome of the deep motor branch of the ulnar nerve. (Piso-Hamate Hiatus syndrome). *J Bone Joint Surg Am* 1976;58:145–147.

142. Chien AJ, Jamadar DA, Jacobson JA, et al. Sonography and MR imaging of posterior interosseous nerve syndrome with surgical correlation. *AJR Am J Roentgenol* 2003;181:219–221.

143. Konjengbam M, Elangbam J. Radial nerve in the radial tunnel: anatomic sites of entrapment neuropathy. *Clin Anat* 2004;17:21–25.

144. Spinner M. The arcade of Frohse and its relationship to posterior interosseous nerve paralysis. *J Bone Joint Surg Br* 1968;50:809–812.

145. Lister GD, Belsole RB, Kleinert HE. The radial tunnel syndrome. *J Hand Surg Am* 1979;4:52–59.

146. Moss SH, Switzer HE. Radial tunnel syndrome: a spectrum of clinical presentations. *J Hand Surg Am* 1983;8:414–420.

147. Rinker B, Effron CR, Beasley RW. Proximal radial compression neuropathy. *Ann Plast Surg* 2004;52:174–180; discussion 181–183.

148. Verhaar J, Spaans F. Radial tunnel syndrome. An investigation of compression neuropathy as a possible cause. *J Bone Joint Surg Am* 1991;73:539–544.

149. Roquelaure Y, Raimbeau G, Dano C, et al. Occupational risk factors for radial tunnel syndrome in industrial workers. *Scand J Work Environ Health* 2000;26:507–513.

150. Mayer JH, Mayfield FH. Surgery of the posterior interosseous branch of the radial nerve. *Surg Gynecol Obstet* 1947;84:(5):979–982.

151. Atroshi I, Johnsson R, Ornstein E. Radial tunnel release. Unpredictable outcome in 37 consecutive cases with a 1–5 year follow-up. *Acta Orthop Scand* 1995;66:255–257.

152. Hashizume H, Nishida K, Nanba Y, et al. Non-traumatic paralysis of the posterior interosseous nerve. *J Bone Joint Surg Br* 1996;78:771–776.

153. Sotereanos DG, Varitimidis SE, Giannakopoulos PN, et al. Results of surgical treatment for radial tunnel syndrome. *J Hand Surg Am* 1999;24:566–570.

154. Dellon AL, Mackinnon SE. Radial sensory nerve entrapment in the forearm. *J Hand Surg Am* 1986;11:199–205.

155. Kim DH, Kam AC, Chandika P, et al. Surgical management and outcome in patients with radial nerve lesions. [erratum appears in *J Neurosurg* 2002 Jan;96(1):162]. *J Neurosurg* 2001;95:573–583.

156. Lanzetta M, Foucher G. Entrapment of the superficial branch of the radial nerve (Wartenberg's syndrome). A report of 52 cases. *Int Orthop* 1993;17:342–345.

157. Fritz RC, Helms CA, Steinbach LS, et al. Suprascapular nerve entrapment: evaluation with MR imaging. *Radiology* 1992;182:437–444.

158. Post M, Grinblat E. Nerve entrapment about the shoulder girdle. *Hand Clin* 1992;8:299–306.

159. Rengachary SS, Neff JP, Singer PA, et al. Suprascapular entrapment neuropathy: a clinical, anatomical, and comparative study. Part 1: clinical study. *Neurosurgery* 1979;5:441–446.

160. Zehetgruber H, Noske H, Lang T, et al. Suprascapular nerve entrapment. A meta-analysis. *Int Orthop* 2002;26:339–343.

161. Rengachary SS, Burr D, Lucas S, et al. Suprascapular entrapment neuropathy: a clinical, anatomical, and comparative study. Part 2: anatomical study. *Neurosurgery* 1979;5:447–451.

162. Antoniadis G, Richter HP, Rath S, et al. Suprascapular nerve entrapment: experience with 28 cases. *J Neurosurg* 1996;85:1020–1025.

163. Callahan JD, Scully TB, Shapiro SA, et al. Suprascapular nerve entrapment. A series of 27 cases. *J Neurosurg* 1991;74:893–896.

164. Fabre T, Piton C, Leclouerec G, et al. Entrapment of the suprascapular nerve. *J Bone Joint Surg Br* 1999;81:414–419.

165. Vastamäki M, Göransson H. Suprascapular nerve entrapment. *Clin Orthop Relat Res* 1993:135–143.

166. Post M. Diagnosis and treatment of suprascapular nerve entrapment. *Clin Orthop Relat Res* 1999:92–100.

166b. Novack CB. Thoracic outlet syndrome. *Clin Plast Surg* 2003;30(2):175–188.

167. Atasoy E. Thoracic outlet syndrome: anatomy. *Hand Clin* 2004;20:7–14.

168. Demondion X, Bacqueville E, Paul C, et al. Thoracic outlet: assessment with MR imaging in asymptomatic and symptomatic populations. *Radiology* 2003;227:461–468.

169. Urschel HC Jr. Anatomy of the thoracic outlet. *Thorac Surg Clin* 2007;17:511–520.

170. Urschel HC, Patel A. Thoracic outlet syndromes. *Curr Treat Options Cardiovasc Med* 2003;5:163–168.

171. Urschel HC Jr, Razzuk MA. Neurovascular compression in the thoracic outlet: changing management over 50 years. *Ann Surg* 1998;228:609–617.

172. Sheth RN, Campbell JN. Surgical treatment of thoracic outlet syndrome: a randomized trial comparing two operations. *J Neurosurg Spine* 2005;3:355–363.

173. Qvarfordt PG, Ehrenfeld WK, Stoney RJ. Supraclavicular radical scalenectomy and transaxillary first rib resection for the thoracic outlet syndrome. A combined approach. *Am J Surg* 1984;148:111–116.

174. Dellon AL. The results of supraclavicular brachial plexus neurolysis (without first rib resection) in management of post-traumatic "thoracic outlet syndrome." *J Reconstr Microsurg* 1993;9:11–17.

175. Hempel GK, Rusher AH, Jr., Wheeler CG, et al. Supraclavicular resection of the first rib for thoracic outlet syndrome. *Am J Surg* 1981;141:213–215.

176. Mellière D, Becquemin JP, Etienne G, et al. Severe injuries resulting from operations for thoracic outlet syndrome: can they be avoided? *J Cardiovasc Surg (Torino)* 1991;32:599–603.

177. Pečina M. Contribution to the etiological explanation of the piriformis syndrome. *Acta Anat (Basel)* 1979;105:181–187.

178. Papadopoulos SM, McGillicuddy JE, Albers JW. Unusual cause of 'piriformis muscle syndrome.' *Arch Neurol* 1990;47:1144–1146.

179. Patil PG, Friedman AH. Surgical exposure of the sciatic nerve in the gluteal

region: anatomic and historical comparison of two approaches. *Neurosurgery* 2005;56:165–171.

180. Rask MR. Superior gluteal nerve entrapment syndrome. *Muscle Nerve* 1980; 3:304–307.

181. Russell SM, Kline DG. Complication avoidance in peripheral nerve surgery: injuries, entrapments, and tumors of the extremities—part 2. *Neurosurgery* 2006;59:ONS449–457.

182. Banerjee T, Hall CD. Sciatic entrapment neuropathy. Case report. *J Neurosurg* 1976;45:216–217.

183. Venna N, Bielawski M, Spatz EM. Sciatic nerve entrapment in a child. Case report. *J Neurosurg* 1991;75:652–654.

184. Mozes M, Ouaknine G, Nathan H. Saphenous nerve entrapment simulating vascular disorder. *Surgery* 1975;77:299–303.

185. Mastaglia FL. Tibial nerve entrapment in the popliteal fossa. *Muscle Nerve* 2000;23:1883–1886.

186. Sansone V, Sosio C, da Gama Malchèr M, et al. Two cases of tibial nerve compression caused by uncommon popliteal cysts. *Arthroscopy* 2002;18:E8.

187. Zeiss J, Fenton P, Ebraheim N, et al. Normal magnetic resonance anatomy of the tarsal tunnel. *Foot Ankle* 1990;10:214–218.

188. Kinoshita M, Okuda R, Morikawa J, et al. The dorsiflexion-eversion test for diagnosis of tarsal tunnel syndrome. *J Bone Joint Surg Am* 2001;83-A: 1835–1839.

189. Edwards WG, Lincoln CR, Bassett FH III, et al. The tarsal tunnel syndrome. Diagnosis and treatment. *JAMA* 1969;207:716–720.

190. Frey C, Kerr R. Magnetic resonance imaging and the evaluation of tarsal tunnel syndrome. *Foot Ankle* 1993;14:159–164.

191. Mondelli M, Morana P, Padua L. An electrophysiological severity scale in tarsal tunnel syndrome. *Acta Neurol Scand* 2004;109:284–289.

192. Recht MP, Donley BG. Magnetic resonance imaging of the foot and ankle. *J Am Acad Orthop Surg* 2001;9:187–199.

193. Bailie DS, Kelikian AS. Tarsal tunnel syndrome: diagnosis, surgical technique, and functional outcome. *Foot Ankle Int* 1998;19:65–72.

194. Day FN III, Naples JJ. Endoscopic tarsal tunnel release: update 96. *J Foot Ankle Surg* 1996;35:225–229.

195. Takakura Y, Kitada C, Sugimoto K, et al. Tarsal tunnel syndrome. Causes and results of operative treatment. *J Bone Joint Surg Br* 1991;73:125–128.

196. Pfeiffer WH, Cracchiolo A III. Clinical results after tarsal tunnel decompression. *J Bone Joint Surg Am* 1994;76:1222–1230.

197. Sammarco GJ, Chang L. Outcome of surgical treatment of tarsal tunnel syndrome. *Foot Ankle Int* 2003;24:125–131.

198. Turan I, Rivero-Melián C, Guntner P, et al. Tarsal tunnel syndrome. Outcome of surgery in longstanding cases. *Clin Orthop Relat Res* 1997:151–156.

199. Spinner RJ, Atkinson JL, Scheithauer BW, et al. Peroneal intraneural ganglia: the importance of the articular branch. Clinical series. *J Neurosurg* 2003;99: 319–329.

200. Yang LJ, Gala VC, McGillicuddy JE. Superficial peroneal nerve syndrome: an unusual nerve entrapment. Case report. *J Neurosurg* 2006;104:820–823.

201. Akyuz G, Us O, Türan B, et al. Anterior tarsal tunnel syndrome. *Electromyogr Clin Neurophysiol* 2000;40:123–128.

202. Banerjee T, Koons DD. Superficial peroneal nerve entrapment. Report of two cases. *J Neurosurg* 1981;55:991–992.

203. Borges LF, Hallett M, Selkoe DJ, et al. The anterior tarsal tunnel syndrome. Report of two cases. *J Neurosurg* 1981;54:89–92.

204. Dellon AL. Deep peroneal nerve entrapment on the dorsum of the foot. *Foot Ankle* 1990;11:73–80.

205. Kernohan J, Levack B, Wilson JN. Entrapment of the superficial peroneal nerve. Three case reports. *J Bone Joint Surg Br* 1985;67:60–61.

206. Singh N, Behse F, Buchthal F. Electrophysical study of peroneal palsy. *J Neurol Neurosurg Psychiatry* 1974;37:1202–1213.

207. Kim DH, Kline DG. Management and results of peroneal nerve lesions. *Neurosurgery* 1996;39:312–319; discussion 219–320.

208. Fabre T, Piton C, Andre D, et al. Peroneal nerve entrapment. *J Bone Joint Surg Am* 1998;80:47–53.

209. Mont MA, Dellon AL, Chen F, et al. The operative treatment of peroneal nerve palsy. *J Bone Joint Surg Am* 1996;78:863–869.

210. Abbott R. Sensory rhizotomy for the treatment of childhood spasticity. *J Child Neurol* 1996;11(Suppl 1):S36–42.

211. Groves EWH. On the division of the posterior spinal nerve roots. *Lancet* 1911;2:79–85.

212. White JC, Kjellberg RN. Posterior spinal rhizotomy: a substitute for cordotomy in the relief of localized pain in patients with normal life-expectancy. *Neurochirurgia (Stuttg)* 1973;16:141–170.

213. Sherrington CS. Experiments in examination of the peripheral distribution of the fibers of the posterior roots of some spinal nerves. *Proc R Soc (Lond)* 1896;60:403–411.

214. Foerster O. The dermatomes in man. *Brain* 1933;56:1–39.

215. Liu CN, Chambers WW. Intraspinal sprouting of dorsal root axons; development of new collaterals and preterminals following partial denervation of the spinal cord in the cat. *AMA Arch Neurol Psychiatry* 1958;79:46–61.

216. Hodge CJ Jr, King RB. Medical modification of sensation. *J Neurosurg* 1976; 44:21–28.

217. Sherrington CS. On the anatomical constitution of nerves of skeletal muscles; with remarks on recurrent fibers in the ventral spinal nerve-root. *J Physiol (Lond)* 1894;17:211–258.

218. Coggeshall RE. Law of separation of function of the spinal roots. *Physiol Rev* 1980;60:716–755.

219. Light AR, Metz CB. The morphology of the spinal cord efferent and afferent neurons contributing to the ventral roots of the cat. *J Comp Neurol* 1978; 179:501–515.

220. Hosobuchi Y. The majority of unmyelinated afferent axons in human ventral roots probably conduct pain. *Pain* 1980;8:167–180.

221. North RB, Levy RM. Consensus conference on the neurosurgical management of pain. *Neurosurgery* 1994;34:756–761.

222. Schwartz HG. Anastomoses between cervical nerve roots. *J Neurosurg* 1956; 13:190–194.

223. Felsööry A, Crue BL. Results of 19 years experience with sacral rhizotomy for perineal and perianal cancer pain. *Pain* 1976;2:431–433.

224. Loeser JD. Dorsal rhizotomy for the relief of chronic pain. *J Neurosurg* 1972; 36:745–750.

224b. North RB, Levy RM. *Consensus Conference on the Neurosurgical Management of Pain.* Neurosurgery 1994;34(4):756–760.

225. Barrash JM, Leavens ME. Dorsal rhizotomy for the relief of intractable pain of malignant tumor origin. *J Neurosurg* 1973;38:755–757.

226. Onofrio BM, Campa HK. Evaluation of rhizotomy. Review of 12 years' experience. *J Neurosurg* 1972;36:751–755.

227. Wilkinson HA, Chan AS. Sensory ganglionectomy: theory, technical aspects, and clinical experience. *J Neurosurg* 2001;95:61–66.

228. Dandy WE. Operative relief from pain in lesions of the mouth, tongue, and throat. *Arch Surg* 1929;19:143–148.

229. Hunter CR, Mayfield FH. Role of the upper cervical roots in the production of pain in the head. *Am J Surg* 1949;78:743–751.

230. Hammond SR, Danta G. Occipital neuralgia. *Clin Exp Neurol* 1978;15: 258–270.

231. Stechison MT, Mullin BB. Surgical treatment of greater occipital neuralgia: an appraisal of strategies. *Acta Neurochir (Wien)* 1994;131:236–240.

232. Lozano AM, Vanderlinden G, Bachoo R, et al. Microsurgical C-2 ganglionectomy for chronic intractable occipital pain. *J Neurosurg* 1998;89:359–365.

233. Dubuisson D. Treatment of occipital neuralgia by partial posterior rhizotomy at C1-3. *J Neurosurg* 1995;82:581–586.

234. Kapoor V, Rothfus WE, Grahovac SZ, et al. Refractory occipital neuralgia: preoperative assessment with CT-guided nerve block prior to dorsal cervical rhizotomy. *AJNR Am J Neuroradiol* 2003;24:2105–2110.

235. Acar F, Miller J, Golshani KJ, et al. Pain relief after cervical ganglionectomy (C2 and C3) for the treatment of medically intractable occipital neuralgia. *Stereotact Funct Neurosurg* 2008;86:106–112.

236. Slavin KV, Nersesyan H, Wess C. Peripheral neurostimulation for treatment of intractable occipital neuralgia. *Neurosurgery* 2006;58:112–119.

237. Arbit E, Galicich JH, Burt M, et al. Modified open thoracic rhizotomy for treatment of intractable chest wall pain of malignant etiology. *Ann Thorac Surg* 1989;48:820–823.

238. Smith FP. Trans-spinal ganglionectomy for relief of intercostal pain. *J Neurosurg* 1970;32:574–577.

239. Saris SC, Silver JM, Vieira JF, et al. Sacrococcygeal rhizotomy for perineal pain. *Neurosurgery* 1986;19:789–793.

240. van Kleef M, Liem L, Lousberg R, et al. Radiofrequency lesion adjacent to the dorsal root ganglion for cervicobrachial pain: a prospective double blind randomized study. *Neurosurgery* 1996;38:1127–1131; discussion 1131–1132.

241. North RB, Kidd DH, Campbell JN, et al. Dorsal root ganglionectomy for failed back surgery syndrome: a 5-year follow-up study. *J Neurosurg* 1991; 74:236–242.

242. Taub A, Robinson F, Taub E. Dorsal root ganglionectomy for intractable monoradicular sciatica. A series of 61 patients. *Stereotact Funct Neurosurg* 1995;65:106–110.

243. Falowski S, Celii A, Sharan A. Spinal cord stimulation: an update. *Neurotherapeutics* 2008;5:86–99.

244. Wetzel FT, Phillips FM, Aprill CN, et al. Extradural sensory rhizotomy in the management of chronic lumbar radiculopathy: a minimum 2-year follow-up study. *Spine* 1997;22:2283–2291; discussion 2291–2282.

245. Roberts WJ. A hypothesis on the physiological basis for causalgia and related pains. *Pain* 1986;24:297–311.

246. Smithwick RH. The rationale and technic of sympathectomy for the relief of vascular spasm of the extremities. *N Engl J Med* 1940;222:699–703.

247. Cline MA, Ochoa J, Torebjörk HE. Chronic hyperalgesia and skin warming caused by sensitized C nociceptors. *Brain* 1989;112:621–647.

248. Gracely RH, Lynch SA, Bennett GJ. Painful neuropathy: altered central processing maintained dynamically by peripheral input. *Pain* 1992;51:175–194.

249. Schinkel C, Gaertner A, Zaspel J, et al. Inflammatory mediators are altered in the acute phase of posttraumatic complex regional pain syndrome. *Clin J Pain* 2006;22:235–239.

250. van der Laan L, ter Laak HJ, Gabreëls-Festen A, et al. Complex regional pain syndrome type I (RSD): pathology of skeletal muscle and peripheral nerve. *Neurology* 1998;51:20–25.

251. Mailis A, Wade J. Profile of Caucasian women with possible genetic predisposition to reflex sympathetic dystrophy: a pilot study. *Clin J Pain* 1994;10: 210–217.

252. Walker AE, Nulson F. Electrical stimulation of the upper thoracic portion of the sympathetic chain in man. *Arch Neurol Psych* 1948;59:309–317.

253. Hannington-Kiff JG. Intravenous regional sympathetic block with guanethidine. *Lancet* 1974;1:1019–1020.

254. Davis KD, Treede RD, Raja SN, et al. Topical application of clonidine relieves hyperalgesia in patients with sympathetically maintained pain. *Pain* 1991;47: 309–317.

255. Torebjörk E, Wahren L, Wallin G, et al. Noradrenaline-evoked pain in neuralgia. *Pain* 1995;63:11–20.
256. Abram SE, Lightfoot RW. Treatment of long-standing causalgia with prazosin. *Reg Anaesth* 1981;6:79–81.
257. Arnér S. Intravenous phentolamine test: diagnostic and prognostic use in reflex sympathetic dystrophy. *Pain* 1991;46:17–22.
258. Ghostine SY, Comair YG, Turner DM, et al. Phenoxybenzamine in the treatment of causalgia. Report of 40 cases. *J Neurosurg* 1984;60:1263–1268.
259. Raja SN, Treede RD, Davis KD, et al. Systemic alpha-adrenergic blockade with phentolamine: a diagnostic test for sympathetically maintained pain. *Anesthesiology* 1991;74:691–698.
260. Chabal C, Jacobson L, Russell LC, et al. Pain response to perineuromal injection of normal saline, epinephrine, and lidocaine in humans. *Pain* 1992;49:9–12.
261. Reuben SS. Preventing the development of complex regional pain syndrome after surgery. *Anesthesiology* 2004;101:1215–1224.
262. Reuben SS, Rosenthal EA, Steinberg RB. Surgery on the affected upper extremity of patients with a history of complex regional pain syndrome: a retrospective study of 100 patients. *J Hand Surg Am* 2000;25:1147–1151.
263. Dellemijn PL, Fields HL, Allen RR, et al. The interpretation of pain relief and sensory changes following sympathetic blockade. *Brain* 1994;117(Pt 6):1475–1487.
264. Treede RD, Davis KD, Campbell JN, et al. The plasticity of cutaneous hyperalgesia during sympathetic ganglion blockade in patients with neuropathic pain. *Brain* 1992;115:607–621.
265. Chelimsky TC, Low PA, Naessens JM, et al. Value of autonomic testing in reflex sympathetic dystrophy. *Mayo Clin Proc* 1995;70:1029–1040.
266. Wahren LK, Torebjörk E, Nyström B. Quantitative sensory testing before and after regional guanethidine block in patients with neuralgia in the hand. *Pain* 1991;46:23–30.
267. Shir Y, Cameron LB, Raja SN, et al. The safety of intravenous phentolamine administration in patients with neuropathic pain. *Anesth Analg* 1993;76:1008–1011.
268. Rauck RL, Eisenach JC, Jackson K, et al. Epidural clonidine treatment for refractory reflex sympathetic dystrophy. *Anesthesiology* 1993;79:1163–1169.
269. Galer BS, Rowbotham MC, Von Miller K, et al. Treatment of inflammatory, neuropathic and sympathetically maintained pain in a patient with Sjögren's syndrome. *Pain* 1992;50:205–208.
270. Kirkpatrick AF, Derasari M. Transdermal clonidine: treating reflex sympathetic dystrophy. *Reg Anesth* 1993;18:140–141.
271. DeSalles AAF, Johnson JP. Sympathectomy for pain. In: Winn HR, Youmans JR, eds. *Youmans Neurological Surgery*. 5th ed. Philadelphia: WB Saunders; 2004:3093–3106.
272. Wilkinson HA. Percutaneous radiofrequency upper thoracic sympathectomy. *Neurosurgery* 1996;38:715–725.
273. Hoffert MJ, Greenberg RP, Wolskee PJ, et al. Abnormal and collateral innervations of sympathetic and peripheral sensory fields associated with a case of causalgia. *Pain* 1984;20:1–12.
274. Howng SL, Loh JK. Long-term follow up of upper dorsal sympathetic ganglionectomy for palmar hyperhidrosis—a scale of evaluation. *Gaoxiong Yi Xue Ke Xue Za Zhi* 1987;3:703–707.
275. Ulmer JL, Mayfield FH. Causalgia. A study of 75 cases. *Surg Gynec Obstet* 1946;83:789–796.
276. Manart FD, Sadler TR Jr, Schmitt EA, et al. Upper dorsal sympathectomy. *Am J Surg* 1985;150:762–766.
277. Mockus MB, Rutherford RB, Rosales C, et al. Sympathectomy for causalgia. Patient selection and long-term results. *Arch Surg* 1987;122:668–672.
278. AbuRahma AF, Robinson PA, Powell M, et al. Sympathectomy for reflex sympathetic dystrophy: factors affecting outcome. *Ann Vasc Surg* 1994;8:372–379.
279. Hassantash SA, Afrakhteh M, Maier RV. Causalgia: a meta-analysis of the literature. *Arch Surg* 2003;138:1226–1231.
280. Thompson JE. The diagnosis and management of post-traumatic pain syndromes (causalgia). *Aust N Z J Surg* 1979;49:299–304.
281. Litwin MS. Postsympathectomy neuralgia. *Arch Surg* 1962;84:121–125.
282. Raskin NH, Levinson S, Hoffman PM, et al. Postsympathectomy neuralgia. Amelioration with diphenylhydantoin and carbamazepine. *Am J Surg* 1974;128:75–78.
283. Kramis RC, Roberts WJ, Gillette RG. Post-sympathectomy neuralgia: hypotheses on peripheral and central neuronal mechanisms. *Pain* 1996;64:1–9.
284. Mailis A, Furlan A. Sympathectomy for neuropathic pain. *Cochrane Database Syst Rev* 2003;2:CD002918.

CHAPTER 103 ■ THE SURGICAL MANAGEMENT OF TRIGEMINAL NEURALGIA

WAEL F. ASAAD AND EMAD N. ESKANDAR

INTRODUCTION

Trigeminal neuralgia is the most common of a family of disorders caused by spontaneous (nontraumatic) injury to a cranial nerve. Most cases are believed to result from impingement on the nerve by a vascular structure, usually an artery, causing demyelination and subsequent pathologic electrical activity. Those suffering from this disease report intermittent bouts of sharp, lancinating pain in the distribution of the trigeminal nerve or its three main branches. Hemifacial spasm and glossopharyngeal neuralgia are among the other less common, spontaneous cranial nerve compression diseases, resulting from injury to the seventh and ninth cranial nerves, respectively.

HISTORY

Early descriptions of paroxysms of facial pain reminiscent of the modern conception of trigeminal neuralgia can be found in the works of Aretaeus of Cappadocia in the first century CE, Galen in the second, and Avicenna in the eleventh.[1,2] Although many of these descriptions may resemble toothache, dental caries were relatively rare in those times, and so the connection to trigeminal neuralgia is more plausible.[3] In a letter dated 1677, John Locke, the well-known empiricist philosopher and physician, gave one of the first detailed accounts of a case of trigeminal neuralgia in his patient, the Countess of Northumberland.[4] He described clearly certain features which today are considered classical for this disease: the sudden onset and offset of painful spasms confined to one side of the face, and the characteristic triggering of these symptoms by touch or facial movements.

The label *tic douloureaux* was first applied nearly a century later by Nicolas André,[5] though in retrospect only two of his five cases are likely to have been suffering from trigeminal neuralgia. Shortly thereafter, in 1773, John Fothergill presented a paper to the Medical Society of London entitled, "On a Painful Affliction of the Face." As did Locke before him, he described the key components of true trigeminal neuralgia, including short duration, intensely painful spells occurring at irregular intervals, and elicitation of these symptoms by touch to or motion of the face. His grandnephew, Samuel Fothergill, accurately identified the source of these symptoms as the trigeminal nerve, from whence trigeminal neuralgia was referred to as "Fothergill's Disease."[2]

At that time, the repertoire of available medicines was limited; opium and hemlock extracts were given to patients with inconsistent results. The need for better therapies led to the development of operative strategies. Neurectomy, or the sectioning of peripheral nerves, was the early procedure of choice.[6] However, once it became clear that peripheral nerve lesioning was rarely permanently successful, surgeons devised more invasive methods targeting the trigeminal, or the "Gasserian," ganglion itself for resection or destruction. William Rose[7] developed a procedure in which he approached the trigeminal ganglion by removing the overlying maxilla. As noted by Harvey Cushing,[8] the decision by patients to electively undergo such a disfiguring procedure spoke to the severity of the affliction. In the 1890s, Fedor Krause and Frank Hartley independently developed a transcranial (as opposed to transfacial) procedure for resecting the trigeminal ganglion, which was later adopted by W. W. Keen and refined by Harvey Cushing.[8,9] These operations, in contrast to the retromastoid route in use today, utilized a temporal approach. Before Cushing, uncontrolled bleeding was common, often requiring multiple operative attempts over several days with intervening periods of tamponade, and occasionally necessitating ligation of the carotid artery.[8] Mortality rates often approached 20%. Cushing's technique improved the safety of ganglionectomy substantially, though patients were nevertheless left with sensory loss.

Walter Dandy,[10] in 1925, described a more selective, retromastoid procedure which involved severing only a certain subgroup of the trigeminal nerve roots. This procedure had the advantage of reducing pain while preserving touch. Importantly, based upon his observations across 215 cases, he came to believe that vascular compression of the trigeminal nerve (most often by the superior cerebellar artery, but occasionally by veins) may represent the primary pathophysiology of trigeminal neuralgia.[11] Vilhelm Magnus,[12] a Norwegian surgeon, had made a similar observation in one case (in which a carotid artery aneurysm impinged upon the trigeminal ganglion) in 1927, but Dandy was perhaps the first to suggest that vascular compression was indeed a systematic cause of this disease. Nevertheless, it was not until 1959 that W. James Gardner published the first series of vascular decompression surgeries for trigeminal neuralgia.[13]

Although Gardner reported a 62% success rate (defined as a complete alleviation of pain without recurrence during the follow-up period, which was up to 6 years), just over a quarter of his 200 patients suffered from postoperative sensory loss. Given this and the other risks of surgery, as well as the development of more effective medical therapies, decompressive surgery fell out of favor, giving way to percutaneous ablative methods, which became the last resort of choice.[14]

Recently, microvascular decompression (MVD) has regained prominence as a first-line surgical intervention in those who have failed medical therapy and who are relatively younger, whereas the percutaneous methods are reserved for older or less healthy patients.[15] In addition, the option of radiosurgery has been increasingly utilized. More discussion about these issues is presented below.

PRESENTATION

Typical trigeminal neuralgia is characterized by the following features:

- Paroxysms of pain lasting a few seconds to at most a few minutes
- The pain is intense and usually described as sharp, stabbing, or electrical in nature
- The pain is often precipitated by tactile stimuli to specific and consistent trigger zones or by specific actions (such as chewing or talking)
- Unilateral or asynchronously bilateral

- Involves the V2 > V3 > V1 branches of the trigeminal nerve and does *not* extend behind the ear or into the neck
- If the V1 and V3 branches are affected, so will V2
- Subjective numbness is usually minimal or absent (though it may be a sequela of prior nonmedical treatment)
- The pattern of pain and its manner of elicitation is consistent within an individual, though it may evolve slowly
- Focal neurologic deficits are absent in classic trigeminal neuralgia, though typical symptoms may be elicited by lesions which are also associated with other neurologic findings
- Trigeminal neuralgia may coexist with glossopharyngeal neuralgia, in which case both etiologies require treatment to achieve pain relief

Trigeminal neuralgia typically presents in patients in their late 50s, and is slightly more prevalent in females[16,17]; the bouts of pain may become more frequent with increasing age, and a constant, background pain may appear and slowly worsen.[18] The incidence of trigeminal neuralgia is estimated to be about 3 to 5 persons per 100,000.[16] Risk factors are pre-existing contralateral trigeminal neuralgia and hypertension.[16] Apparent familial forms of this disease have been reported but are very rare.[19,20]

If the pain is described as "throbbing" or "aching" and is associated with a sensation of facial pressure or swelling, the diagnosis is more likely "atypical facial pain."[21] The absence of trigger zones and precipitating actions is characteristic, and subjective numbness may be prominent. This type of pain more often occurs in relatively younger females (<45 years of age), may coexist with a diagnosis of fibromyalgia, and often is associated with psychiatric and social disturbances such as depression, narcotic dependence, and inability to work.

ANATOMY AND PATHOPHYSIOLOGY

The etiology in most cases of trigeminal neuralgia is attributed primarily to compression of the trigeminal nerve by an artery (usually a superior cerebellar artery [SCA]), though in a minority of cases the compressing structure may be a vein.[11,22–24] Other arteries that occasionally seem to compress the nerve, in decreasing order of frequency, are the anterior inferior cerebellar artery, vertebral artery, posterior inferior cerebellar artery, and the basilar artery.[25]

The mechanism by which the pressure of a vascular structure impinging upon a nerve causes injury is likely to be demyelination, at least in part.[26–28] In particular, the root entry zone (REZ), where central oligodendrocytes rather than peripheral Schwann cells give rise to the myelin sheath, is often implicated as being the most vulnerable region of the nerve. Often, the length of the REZ is estimated to be about one-fourth to one-third of the distance along the nerve from its junction with the pons to its exit into Meckel's cave (the "cisternal" portion of the nerve). On histologic examination, this distance averages about 2.5 millimeters and represents usually less than 25% of the total length of the cisternal segment of the trigeminal nerve.[29] The observation that relieving vascular compression more distally along the nerve nevertheless results in the alleviation of pain may reflect abnormalities of the REZ which have been visualized in such cases[30]; these abnormalities may be a result of transmitted mechanical forces to the REZ from the site of distal compression. Therefore, a finding of distal rather than proximal compression of the trigeminal nerve is not generally regarded as a contraindication to decompression, and outcomes after decompressive surgery for distal sites of neurovascular contact do not differ significantly from cases with proximal pathology.[24]

The loss of myelin results in abnormally close apposition of neighboring axons without their proper insulation. Such a situation makes possible the phenomenon of "ephaptic" transmission, whereby action potentials traveling along one axon induce action potentials in neighboring axons.[31,32] Therefore, action potentials within nerve fibers transmitting touch could, through this sort of cross-talk, generate activity in nearby fibers mediating pain.[33] Compounding this, trigeminal nerve injury and associated focal demyelination may lead to the production of ectopic action potentials,[34] further contributing to a sensation of pain.

However, if demyelination is the source of the pathology, how does decompressive surgery result in the often immediate cessation of pain? Two factors are thought to account for this. First, ephaptic conduction may be less effective when a compressive force is removed, allowing relatively more distance between axons. Second, mechanical compression alone can result in the ectopic generation of action potentials, so decompression may reduce the rate of spontaneous, aberrant activity.[35] A third factor, which has an unknown influence on the generation of pain but is likely also an immediate result of nerve decompression, is the release of mechanical conduction block, particularly in larger axons.[33] That some patients have a slower time-course of recovery after decompressive surgery likely reflects a relatively greater contribution of certain more slowly reversible factors over other immediately reversible factors in the etiology of their particular manifestations of the disease.

IMAGING

Imaging is performed in cases of suspected trigeminal neuralgia primarily to rule out multiple sclerosis and cerebello-pontine angle tumors and to assess for vascular malformations and aneurysms. Any of these lesions can mimic the symptoms of trigeminal neuralgia if they result in pressure on the nerve. Suspicion for one of these types of lesions should be especially high when focal neurologic deficits are found on physical exam.

Recently, advances in magnetic resonance (MR) imaging techniques have allowed the possibility that the primary pathology of trigeminal neuralgia, vascular compression, may be visible, thereby confirming the diagnosis. MR angiography (MRA) can demonstrate the presence of relatively larger arteries at the origin of the trigeminal nerve near the pons (Fig. 103.1). One study found that preoperative MRA was accurate in predicting operative findings in 18 of 21 consecutive cases of trigeminal neuralgia.[36] The three cases in which the offending vessel was not visualized included two petrosal veins and a smaller SCA.

In addition to MRA, constructive-interference steady state (CISS, pronounced "kiss") sequences may be useful because of their ability to show cranial nerves in high resolution and with

good contrast. These images may suggest direct contact between the nerve and a vascular structure, as well as demonstrate "kinking" of the nerve (Fig. 103.2). A study examining the relationship between neurovascular proximity on CISS sequences and subsequent radiosurgery found that those with MRA evidence of direct contact had a significantly greater likelihood of responding to radiosurgery.[37] However, other groups are less certain of the relationship between perceived neurovascular contact and symptomatology.[38] Whether these differences are due to different imaging parameters or to differences in image interpretation remains to be clarified.

Another MR technique, diffusion tensor imaging (DTI) has been used to examine demyelinating diseases by measuring the fractional anisotropy (FA) of affected brain tissue. In essence, this technique measures the relative diffusibility of water along different dimensions; the presence of myelin restricts diffusion preferentially in the direction orthogonal to the length of nerve, thereby increasing anisotropy. Because vascular compression may promote a similar end-point, namely a decrease in the integrity of the nerve sheath, DTI has been proposed as a method to corroborate nerve damage in trigeminal neuralgia and other compressive cranial neuropathies by assessing for a decreased FA. So far, however, the sensitivity of this technique[39] is not adequate to recommend this imaging modality for the diagnosis of trigeminal neuralgia.

MEDICAL THERAPY

Anticonvulsant medications are a staple in the medical management of trigeminal neuralgia. Carbamazepine, phenytoin, and lamotrigine are known to be effective, while valproate, gabapentin, and benzodiazepines (among others) have less evidence to support their efficacy, though they may hold promise.[40] Antiepileptic medications such as carbamazepine and phenytoin work, in part, by selectively blocking high-frequency neuronal activity, which in the case of trigeminal neuralgia may limit the degree of ectopic firing.

Based upon current evidence,[41] carbamazepine is considered the first-line therapy. Lamotrigine and baclofen can be added if the pain is still uncontrolled. Oxcarbazine, a derivative of carbamazepine, may be substituted for carbamazepine if the latter is not well-tolerated.

Over time, the efficacy of these medications tends to wane.[42] If the pain becomes refractory to medications, or if the side effects of the medications are intolerable, referral to a surgeon or radiation oncologist is warranted. While MVD is the criterion standard, it is invasive and so requires a healthy and willing patient.

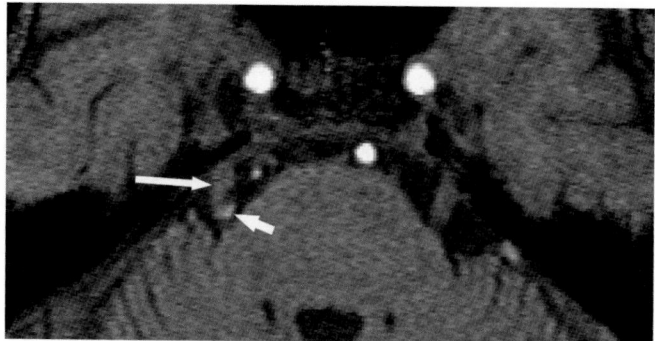
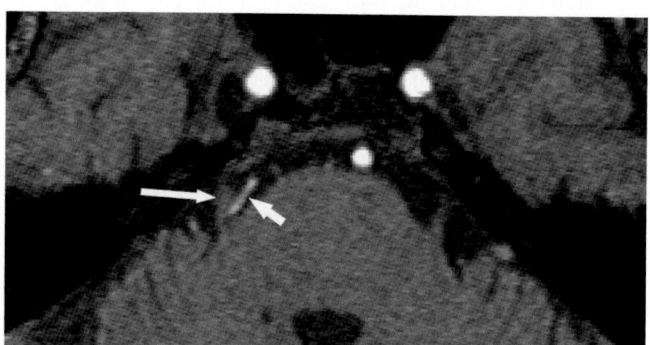

FIGURE 103.1 Images in a 63-year-old man with trigeminal neuralgia, with neurovascular compression caused by the superior cerebellar artery. Two adjacent transverse MRA images (**A,B**) (39/6.5, 20 degrees flip angle) show that the superior cerebellar artery (*short arrow*) has compressed the right trigeminal nerve (*long arrow*) at the medial site. (Reproduced with permission from Yoshino N, Akimoto H, Yamada I, et al. Trigeminal neuralgia: evaluation of neuralgic manifestation and site of neurovascular compression with 3D CISS MR imaging and MR angiography. *Radiology* 2003;228(2):539–545.)

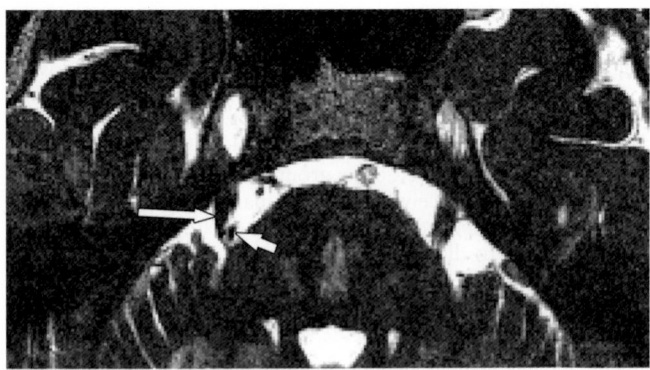
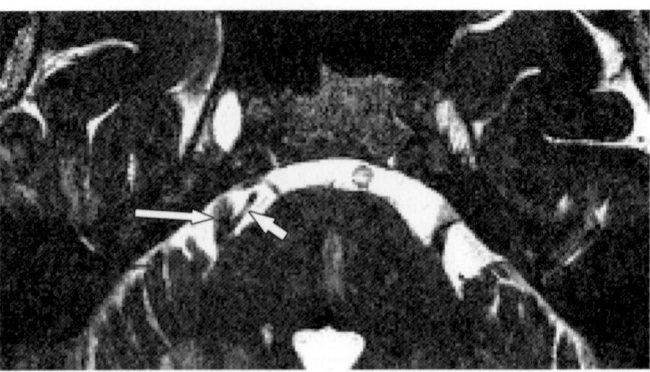

A   B

FIGURE 103.2   Images in a 63-year-old man with trigeminal neuralgia, with neurovascular compression caused by the superior cerebellar artery. Two adjacent transverse three-dimensional CISS MR images (**A,B**) (12.25/ 5.9, 70 degrees flip angle) show that the superior cerebellar artery (*short arrow*) has compressed the REZ of the right trigeminal nerve (*long arrow*) at the medial site. (Reproduced with permission from Yoshino N, Akimoto H, Yamada I, et al. Trigeminal neuralgia: evaluation of neuralgic manifestation and site of neurovascular compression with 3D CISS MR imaging and MR angiography. *Radiology* 2003;228(2):539–545.)

Less invasive options are available, though their efficacies fall short of the long-term, pain-free ideal often achievable with MVD.

MICROVASCULAR DECOMPRESSION SURGERY

MVD is a procedure in which the compressing artery or vein is mobilized away from the nerve. In the case of trigeminal neuralgia, a retrosigmoid craniotomy is performed in order to expose the cisternal portion of the trigeminal nerve, which extends from the pons to the entrance of Meckel's Cave. The patient may be placed in a prone, lateral decubitus, supine and head-tilted, or sitting position, depending on the experience and preference of the surgeon. A short linear or curvilinear incision is made behind the mastoid process such that a small (about 2.5 cm diameter) craniectomy may be performed within the angle of the junction of the sigmoid and transverse sinuses. In order to minimize retraction yet allow proper visualization of the nerve, cerebrospinal fluid is drained from the cisterna magna, thereby relaxing the cerebellum; aggressive retraction can cause potentially serious complications (e.g., venous occlusion, stroke). In addition, auditory evoked potentials can be monitored in order detect early signs of excessive brainstem manipulation or cerebellar retraction.[43]

Once the nerve is exposed, the offending vessel is usually apparent. If so, carefully separating the nerve from this vessel generally requires gentle, blunt spreading with occasional sharp scissoring to break the arachnoid sheets and strands which connect them. A small piece of Teflon may then be interposed between the nerve and vessel to prevent spontaneous reattachment. Rarely, in cases where the problematic vessel was long and ectatic, some surgeons have employed a fenestrated aneurysm clip closed around this vessel and then sutured to the dura, as a means to separate the two structures.[44]

If no compressing vessel is found, some surgeons have advocated dissecting away the possibly thickened arachnoid around the nerve, perhaps placing a small piece of Teflon between the nerve and brainstem, and creating mild neurapraxia by gently squeezing the trigeminal nerve between the tips of the bipolar cautery.[45] At least one group has suggested that the use of a rigid endoscope (tilted at 30 degrees, in their case) may increase the prospect of detecting a compressing vessel.[46]

Overall, MVD has excellent success rates. In one landmark study, nearly three-quarters of patients undergoing MVD were pain-free and off medication after 5 years, and about two-thirds

of those followed for 20 years were still pain-free without medication.[25] Comparable results on long-term pain-free outcomes have been reported by others.[47,48] Despite the initial costs associated with an inpatient neurosurgical procedure, MVD is nevertheless the most cost-effective therapy when considered in light of these long-term benefits.[49] The comparative effectiveness of MVD and percutaneous techniques for treatment of trigeminal neuralgia is shown in Table 103-1.

Several factors are predictive of a good outcome, namely immediate relief of pain postoperatively, male sex, arterial rather than venous compression (at the REZ), and relatively shorter duration of symptoms preoperatively (<8 years).[25,50] In addition, as is the case with other complex surgical procedures, the safety of MVD is dependent to a significant extent on the experience of the surgeon (and the institution at which the procedure is performed); the rates of neurologic complications including stroke, hemorrhage, facial weakness, and the need for ventriculostomy were higher among low-volume surgeons.[51]

The recurrence of facial pain after MVD has been attributed to recurrent vascular compression as well as perhaps granuloma formation around the Teflon[52]; one study found that five of ten MVD reoperations led to the discovery of this condition.[53] The particular techniques best suited to avoid this complication are still a matter of speculation.

RADIOSURGERY

Radiosurgery and its potential for the treatment of a multitude of neurologic disorders have attracted increasing attention over the past several years, though the first radiosurgical procedure for trigeminal neuralgia occurred as far back as 1951.[54] The prospect of a noninvasive and (hopefully) one-time treatment for the affliction of trigeminal neuralgia has obvious appeal to those who suffer from inadequate medical control or unacceptable medication side effects. In general, those who are not satisfied with medical therapy and who refuse or fail MVD (or cannot safely undergo general anesthesia) may be candidates for radiosurgery.

The technical goal of radiosurgery is to impart a focused dose of radiation to the trigeminal nerve or ganglion in such a manner as to create a functional lesion of the pain-mediating structure. The source of radiation is either a gamma knife or a stereotactic radiosurgery system. A gamma knife uses 201 fixed radiation sources that are placed at the ends of collimators which, arranged in a hemisphere, target their energy to a single focal point. Stereotactic radiosurgery systems, by contrast, use a linear accelerator to generate high-energy particles that are then delivered through

TABLE 103.1

RESULTS OF PERCUTANEOUS TECHNIQUES AND POSTERIOR FOSSA EXPLORATION FOR PATIENTS TREATED FOR TRIGEMINAL NEURALGIA

	Patients (%)				
	Percutaneous Techniques			Posterior Fossa Exploration	
	Radiofrequency Rhizotomy (n = 6205)	Glycerol Rhizotomy (n = 1217)	Balloon Compression (n = 759)	Microvascular Decompression (n = 1417)	Partial Trigeminal Rhizotomy (n = 250)
Procedure completed	100	94	99	85	100
Initial pain relief	98	91	93	98	92
Success of procedure	98	85	92	83	92
Pain recurrence	23	54	21	15	18
Facial numbness	98	60	72	2	100
Minor dysesthesia	14	11	14	0.2	5
Major dysesthesia	10	5	5	0.3	5
Anesthesia dolorosa	1.5	1.8	0.1	0	1
Corneal anesthesia	7	3.7	1.5	0.05	3
Keratitis	1	1.8	0	0	0
Trigeminal motor dysfunction	24	1.7	66	0	0
Permanent cranial nerve deficit	0	0	0	3*	
Perioperative morbidity	1.2	1	1.7	10*	
Intracranial hemorrhage or infarction	0	0	0	1*	
Perioperative mortality	0	0	0	0.6*	

*Combined values for microvascular decompression and partial trigeminal rhizotomy.
(Adapted from Taha JM, Tew JM Jr. Comparison of surgical treatments for trigeminal neuralgia: reevaluation of radiofrequency rhizotomy. *Neurosurgery* 1996;38(5):865–871.)

a single source that rotates around the focal point. Both types of radiosurgery have been applied to the treatment of trigeminal neuralgia, and neither appears to hold a significant advantage over the other in terms of efficacy.

The exact target of radiosurgery for trigeminal neuralgia has evolved over time.[55] Currently, the REZ of the trigeminal nerve is considered to be the site which yields the best pain relief.[56,57] Delivering an additional dose to the cisternal portion of the nerve yielded more numbness, but no difference in pain alleviation.[58,59] Similarly, a meta-analysis of recent studies shows that higher doses, while yielding better pain relief, are also associated with increased numbness.[55]

Though radiosurgery does offer the clear benefit of some pain-relief, its application is limited by three main factors: (1) delayed onset of pain-relief; (2) lack of complete pain relief; and (3) poor long-term efficacy.

Radiosurgery has a delayed onset of effect in most patients. One study showed that about 20% of patients responded immediately, but 30 days elapsed before 80% of patients were pain-free. This may be too long for a small number of patients in the midst of a pain crisis, and who therefore require more immediate results.

The lack of consistent, complete, long-term pain relief is a shortcoming which radiosurgery shares with all of the ablative (nondecompressive) techniques. While some initial pain relief is reported by the vast majority of those undergoing these procedures,[60] the percentage of those who are truly pain-free appears to be significantly lower.[61,62] Importantly, the percentage of those who are pain-free and off medications 2 years after radiosurgery has been reported to be 16%,[61] 30%,[63] 50%,[64] ~58%,[65] and just under 60%.[60] In all except the last of these studies, a longer follow-up interval beyond 2 years resulted in finding an increasing proportion of patients relapsing into pain.

Those whose pain is not relieved by radiosurgery are still candidates for MVD. One group reported on six patients who had previously undergone one or two rounds of radiosurgery and

then elected to undergo open decompression.[66] They found that prior irradiation did not technically hamper the operation and that five of these six patients were subsequently pain-free and off medication at last follow-up (about 2 years on average).

PERCUTANEOUS PROCEDURES

A variety of percutaneous options exist for the treatment of trigeminal neuralgia. These procedures typically have the goal of ablating the trigeminal ganglion in order to relieve pain. In general, the degree to which these procedures relieve pain is directly related to the degree of sensory loss observed,[67] reflecting the nonselective methods employed. While immediate pain relief is typical and its frequency may be comparable to that of MVD,[68] the long-term success of these procedures is limited; a meta-analysis of these procedures found that more than 1 in 3 patients will have a recurrence of pain within 3 years, and more time generally yields more recurrences.[69] Nevertheless, these procedures have a role in the operative management of trigeminal neuralgia because the minimally invasive, outpatient nature of the operation makes it suitable for patients who are either unwilling or unable to undergo a craniotomy (i.e., MVD).[15]

The mechanism of ablation is usually radiofrequency thermocoagulation, glycerol rhizolysis, or balloon compression. No single method has been convincingly demonstrated to out-perform the others in terms of either initial pain relief or length of effect.[69] Therefore, the method selected is determined by the experience and comfort of the surgeon. Only one of these procedures (balloon compression) is usually performed under general anesthesia, and all are performed in a day-surgery (outpatient) setting. For radiofrequency gangliolysis and glycerol rhizolysis, a combination of mild to moderate sedation and local anesthesia is employed. In all cases, fluoroscopy is used to guide a needle through the foramen ovale to the trigeminal ganglion (Fig. 103.3). The

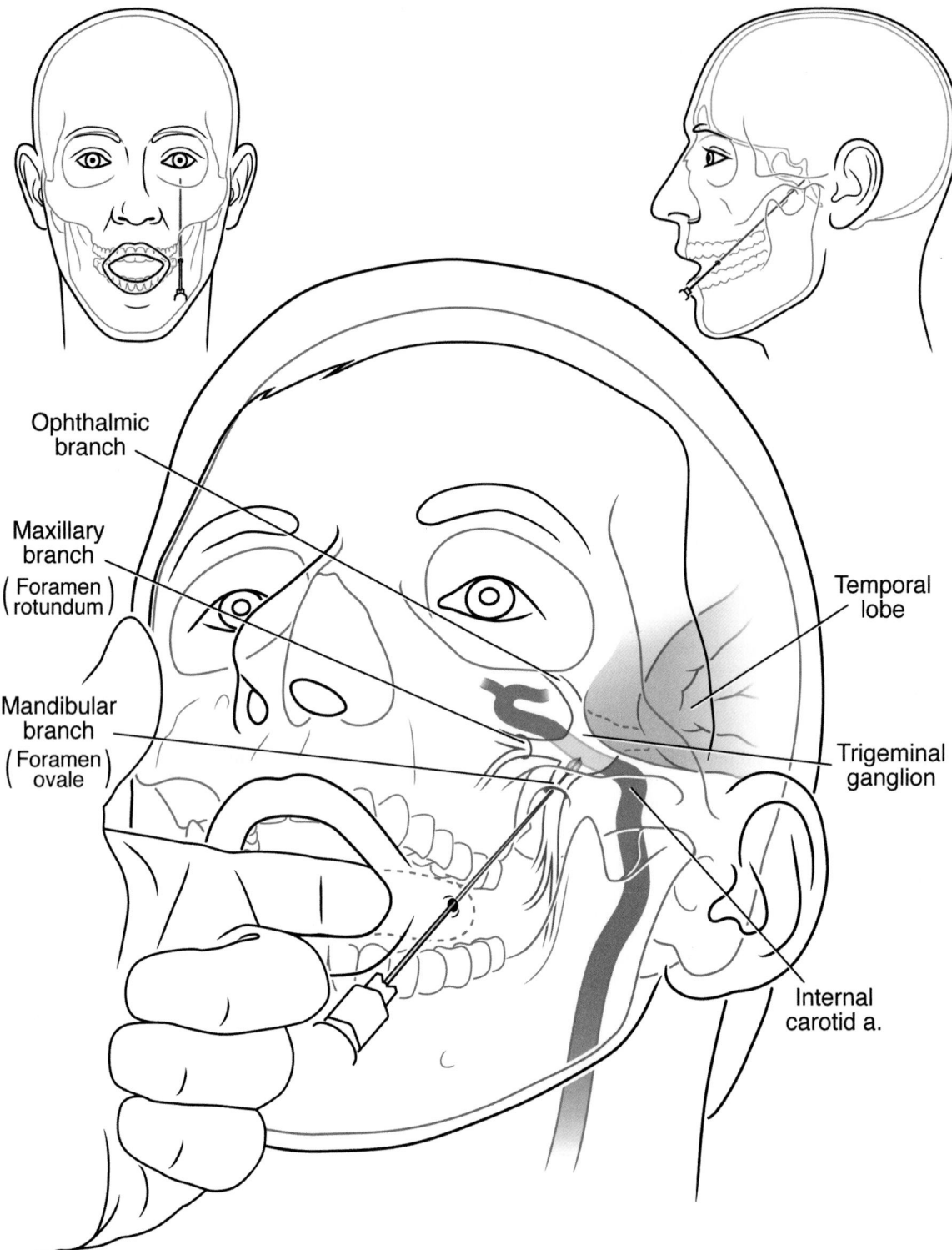

Ophthalmic branch

Maxillary branch
(Foramen rotundum)

Mandibular branch
(Foramen ovale)

Temporal lobe

Trigeminal ganglion

Internal carotid a.

FIGURE 103.3 Radiofrequency treatment of the trigeminal ganglion. The radiofrequency cannula is inserted just lateral to the lateral margin of the lips and advanced medial to the mandible and lateral to the oral mucosa. The index finger of the operator is placed in the patient's mouth to ensure that the tip of the cannula does not penetrate the oral mucosa en route to the foramen ovale. Note the close proximity of the carotid artery, the temporal lobe, and the brainstem to the final position of the cannula. (**Insets**) The proper trajectory of the needle and final needle position are shown in the frontal and axial planes. (Redrawn with permission from Rathmell JP, Borgoy J. Complications associated with radiofrequency treatment for chronic pain. Neal JM, Rathmell JP (eds). Complications in regional anesthesia and pain medicine. Elsevier, Philadelphia; 2007; Figure 29-2, p. 292.)

entry point for the needle should be about 2.5 cm lateral to the angle of the mouth and about 1 cm inferior to the occlusal plane formed by the opposed teeth. The three main branches of the trigeminal nerve are arranged somatotopically such that V1 fibers are the most medial and superior and V3 fibers are the most lateral and inferior. This arrangement means that V3 fibers are encountered first upon entering Meckel's Cave through the foramen ovale and the subsequent divisions are encountered at about 5 mm intervals; as a general guide, on a lateral radiograph, V3 fibers should be encountered at about 5 mm proximal to the clival plane.[70] Advancing more than 7 mm beyond the clival plane may damage the abducens nerve.[71]

Radiofrequency thermocoagulation, or percutaneous radiofrequency trigeminal gangliolysis, replaced electrocoagulation in the 1970s because it allowed a greater degree of control over the heat generated and therefore the size of the lesion.[72] Once the target is located and entered, a temperature of 75° to 85° Celsius for 60 to 90 seconds is used to create the lesion. Short-duration, ~40° stimulation is often first delivered as a test to confirm the correct probe positioning. Because the generation of the lesion can be very painful and result in a profound vagal response, atropine or glycopyrrolate should be on hand to respond to potentially significant drops in heart rate and blood pressure.

Glycerol rhizolysis, meanwhile, entails the injection of a small amount (typically 0.3 mL) of anhydrous glycerol into the cisternal space just posterior to the ganglion[73]; glycerol produces a dose-dependent conduction blockade, inhibiting transmission through C-fibers at lower doses than A-fibers.[74] To aide localization, the same injection needle can be used first to inject contrast, filling the cistern in order to outline the trigeminal ganglion. After the procedure, the patient must remain seated with his or her head tilted forward for about 2 hours in order to minimize the leakage of any excess glycerol toward the brainstem; some have suggested that altering head tilt might bias the lesion toward a particular division. However, because this procedure relies on the use of a fluid which may track through spaces and along nerves and vessels, preferential targeting of individual trigeminal divisions may be difficult to obtain, especially in inexperienced hands.

Balloon compression is a variation of older techniques that applied mechanical force to the trigeminal ganglion in order to produce a functional lesion.[75,76] This technique has been advocated as the preferred method for V1 ablation. Because severe bradycardia and hypotension may follow balloon inflation, general anesthesia is usually employed. The balloon opening pressure may be monitored, and higher values are reported inside Meckel's Cave (~300 cm Hg) as compared with more proximally outside the foramen ovale or more distally into the posterior fossa.[77] The balloon is inflated by the injection of 0.5 to 2.0 mL of radiocontrast, and the visualization of a "pear-shape" formed by the balloon (on lateral radiographs) within trigeminal cistern is typically described.

All ablative techniques (including radiosurgery) entail the possible complication of anesthesia dolorosa (though with radiosurgery the frequency may be less). There are no truly adequate medical therapies for this dreaded condition. Attempted surgical remedies have over the years included a wide variety of procedures from cingulotomy to thalamotomy to REZ lesioning to motor cortex stimulators; the best is yet to be definitively shown.

OTHER PROCEDURES

The ability of subdermal injections of botulinum toxin to achieve adequate, though very temporary (2 to 4 months), relief from the pain of trigeminal neuralgia has been reported.[78,79] Multiple injections are made into the area of pain, and the analgesic effect is observed within 10 to 20 days. Because botulinum toxin has neuromuscular blocking effects as well as antinociceptive effects, many patients will experience some degree of motor palsy. Thus,

while this approach has the advantage of being perhaps the least invasive of the nonmedical options (with the exception of radiosurgery), its disadvantages include short duration of effect and facial weakness.

An even more transient analgesic effect (only about 4 hours) has been reported for the use of intranasal lidocaine spray for second division (V2) trigeminal neuralgia.[80] This strategy succeeds because V2 passes through the sphenopalatine ganglion just behind the middle turbinate. The success of this approach may open the door to longer-lasting medications delivered in the same manner, though its utilization may be limited to the relatively fewer number of patients whose symptoms are restricted to V2.

CONCLUSION

MVD is currently the preferred mode of treatment for medication-refractory patients with typical trigeminal neuralgia and who are able to tolerate a craniotomy. Most patients are pain-free for decades following this procedure. When performed by an experienced surgeon at a capable institution, the risks are relatively low and the treatment will be cost-effective over the long-term. Percutaneous procedures and radiosurgery are preferable for those who may be older or who have significant comorbidities that increase the risk of open surgery under general anesthesia.

References

1. Pearce JM. Trigeminal neuralgia (Fothergill's disease) in the 17th and 18th centuries. *J Neurol Neurosurg Psychiatry* 2003;74(12):1688.
2. Rose FC. Trigeminal neuralgia. *Arch Neurol* 1999;56(9):1163–1164.
3. Harris W. *The Facial Neuralgias.* London: Oxford University Press; 1937.
4. Pearce J. John Locke (1632–1704) and the trigeminal neuralgia of the Countess of Northumberland. *J Neurol Neurosurg Psychiatry* 1993;56:45.
5. Andre N. *Traite sur les maladies de l'urethre.* Paris: Delaguette; 1756.
6. Fowler GR. The operative treatment of facial neuralgia; a comparison of methods and results. *Ann Surg* 1886;3:269–320.
7. Rose W. Removal of the gasserian ganglion for severe neuralgia. *Lancet* 1890; 2:914–915.
8. Cushing H. A Method of total extirpation of the gasserian ganglion for trigeminal neuralgia. *JAMA* 1900;34:1035–1041.
9. Rovit RL, Couldwell WT. A man for all seasons: W.W. Keen. *Neurosurgery* 2002;50(1):181–190.
10. Dandy W. Section of the sensory root of the trigeminal nerve at the pons. Preliminary report of the operative procedure. *Bull Johns Hopkins Hosp* 1925; 36:105–106.
11. Dandy W. Concerning the cause of trigeminal neuralgia. *Am J Surg* 1934;24: 447–455.
12. Magnus V. Aneurysm of the internal carotid artery. *JAMA* 1927;88:1712–1713.
13. Nathoo N, Mayberg MR, Barnett GH. W. James Gardner: pioneer neurosurgeon and inventor. *J Neurosurg* 2004;100(5):965–973.
14. Sweet WH. Percutaneous methods for the treatment of trigeminal neuralgia and other faciocephalic pain; comparison with microvascular decompression. *Semin Neurol* 1988;8(4):272–279.
15. Amirnovin R, Neimat JS, Roberts JA, et al. Multimodality treatment of trigeminal neuralgia. *Stereotact Funct Neurosurg* 2005;83(5–6):197–201.
16. Katusic S, Beard CM, Bergstralh E, et al. Incidence and clinical features of trigeminal neuralgia, Rochester, Minnesota, 1945–1984. *Ann Neurol* 1990; 27(1):89–95.
17. MacDonald BK, Cockerell OC, Sander JW, et al. The incidence and lifetime prevalence of neurological disorders in a prospective community-based study in the UK. *Brain* 2000;123(Pt 4):665–676.
18. Siccoli MM, Bassetti CL, Sandor PS. Facial pain: clinical differential diagnosis. *Lancet Neurol* 2006;5(3):257–267.
19. Savica R, Lagana A, Siracusano R, et al. Idiopathic familial trigeminal neuralgia: a case report. *Neurol Sci* 2007;28(4):196–198.
20. Smyth P, Greenough G, Stommel E. Familial trigeminal neuralgia: case reports and review of the literature. *Headache* 2003;43(8):910–915.
21. Eskandar E, Barker FG 2nd, Rabinov JD. Case records of the Massachusetts General Hospital. Case 21-2006. A 61-year-old man with left-sided facial pain. *N Engl J Med* 2006;355(2):183–188.
22. Gardner WJ, Miklos MV. Response of trigeminal neuralgia to decompression of sensory root; discussion of cause of trigeminal neuralgia. *J Am Med Assoc* 1959;170(15):1773–1776.
23. Jannetta PJ. Microsurgical management of trigeminal neuralgia. *Arch Neurol* 1985;42(8):800.

24. Sindou M, Howeidy T, Acevedo G. Anatomical observations during microvascular decompression for idiopathic trigeminal neuralgia (with correlations between topography of pain and site of the neurovascular conflict). Prospective study in a series of 579 patients. *Acta Neurochir (Wien)* 2002;144(1):1–12, discussion 12–13.

25. Barker FG 2nd, Jannetta PJ, Bissonette DJ, et al. The long-term outcome of microvascular decompression for trigeminal neuralgia. *N Engl J Med* 1996; 334(17):1077–1083.

26. Hilton DA, Love S, Gradidge T, et al. Pathological findings associated with trigeminal neuralgia caused by vascular compression. *Neurosurgery* 1994; 35(2):299–303, discussion 303.

27. Love S, Hilton DA, Coakham HB. Central demyelination of the Vth nerve root in trigeminal neuralgia associated with vascular compression. *Brain Pathol* 1998;8(1):1–11, discussion 11–2.

28. Rappaport ZH, Govrin-Lippmann R, Devor M. An electron-microscopic analysis of biopsy samples of the trigeminal root taken during microvascular decompressive surgery. *Stereotact Funct Neurosurg* 1997;68(1–4 Pt 1):182–186.

29. Peker S, Kurtkaya O, Uzun I, et al. Microanatomy of the central myelin-peripheral myelin transition zone of the trigeminal nerve. *Neurosurgery* 2006;59(2): 354–359, discussion 359.

30. Sindou M. Comment on: microanatomy of the central myelin-peripheral myelin transition zone of the trigeminal nerve. *Neurosurgery* 2006;59(2):358–359.

31. Seltzer Z, Devor M. Ephaptic transmission in chronically damaged peripheral nerves. *Neurology* 1979;29(7):1061–1064.

32. Ramon F, Moore JW. Ephaptic transmission in squid giant axons. *Am J Physiol* 1978;234(5):C162–C169.

33. Love S, Coakham HB. Trigeminal neuralgia: pathology and pathogenesis. *Brain* 2001;124(Pt 12):2347–2360.

34. Burchiel KJ. Abnormal impulse generation in focally demyelinated trigeminal roots. *J Neurosurg* 1980;53(5):674–683.

35. Smith KJ, McDonald WI. Spontaneous and mechanically evoked activity due to central demyelinating lesion. *Nature* 1980;286(5769):154–155.

36. Fukuda H, Ishikawa M, Okumura R. Demonstration of neurovascular compression in trigeminal neuralgia and hemifacial spasm with magnetic resonance imaging: comparison with surgical findings in 60 consecutive cases. *Surg Neurol* 2003;59(2):93–99, discussion 99–100.

37. Erbay SH, Bhadelia RA, Riesenburger R, et al. Association between neurovascular contact on MRI and response to gamma knife radiosurgery in trigeminal neuralgia. *Neuroradiology* 2006;48(1):26–30.

38. Lang E, Naraghi R, Tanrikulu L, et al. Neurovascular relationship at the trigeminal root entry zone in persistent idiopathic facial pain: findings from MRI 3D visualization. *J Neurol Neurosurg Psychiatry* 2005;76(11):1506–1509.

39. Herweh C, Kress B, Rasche D, et al. Loss of anisotropy in trigeminal neuralgia revealed by diffusion tensor imaging. *Neurology* 2007;68(10):776–778.

40. Rogawski MA, Loscher W. The Neurobiology of antiepileptic drugs for the treatment of nonepileptic conditions. *Nat Med* 2004;10(7):685–692.

41. Jorns TP, Zakrzewska JM. Evidence-based approach to the medical management of trigeminal neuralgia. *Br J Neurosurg* 2007;21(3):253–261.

42. Zakrzewska JM, Patsalos PN. Long-term cohort study comparing medical (oxcarbazepine) and surgical management of intractable trigeminal neuralgia. *Pain* 2002;95(3):259–266.

43. Sindou M, Fobe JL, Ciriano D, et al. Hearing prognosis and intraoperative guidance of brainstem auditory evoked potential in microvascular decompression. *Laryngoscope* 1992;102(6):678–682.

44. Attabib N, Kaufmann AM. Use of fenestrated aneurysm clips in microvascular decompression surgery. Technical note and case series. *J Neurosurg* 2007; 106(5):929–931.

45. Revuelta-Gutiérrez R, López-González MA, Sotox-Hernández JL. Surgical treatment of trigeminal neuralgia without vascular compression: 20 years of experience. *Surg Neurol* 2006;66(1):32–36, discussion 36.

46. Teo C, Nakaji P, Mobbs RJ. Endoscope-assisted microvascular decompression for trigeminal neuralgia: technical case report. *Neurosurgery* 2006;59(4 Suppl 2):ONSE489–490, discussion ONSE490.

47. Sindou M, Leston J, Howeidy T, et al. Microvascular decompression for primary Trigeminal Neuralgia (typical or atypical). Long-term effectiveness on pain; prospective study with survival analysis in a consecutive series of 362 patients. *Acta Neurochir (Wien)* 2006;148(12):1235–1245, discussion 1245.

48. Slettebo H, Eide PK. A prospective study of microvascular decompression for trigeminal neuralgia. *Acta Neurochir (Wien)* 1997;139(5):421–425.

49. Pollock BE, Ecker RD. A prospective cost-effectiveness study of trigeminal neuralgia surgery. *Clin J Pain* 2005;21(4):317–322.

50. Li ST, Pan Q, Liu N, et al. Trigeminal neuralgia: what are the important factors for good operative outcomes with microvascular decompression. *Surg Neurol* 2004;62(5):400–404, discussion 404–405.

51. Kalkanis SN, Eskandar EN, Carter BS, et al. Microvascular decompression surgery in the United States, 1996 to 2000: mortality rates, morbidity rates,

and the effects of hospital and surgeon volumes. *Neurosurgery* 2003;52(6): 1251–1261, discussion 1261–1262.

52. Premsagar IC, Moss T, Coakham HB. Teflon-induced granuloma following treatment of trigeminal neuralgia by microvascular decompression. Report of two cases. *J Neurosurg* 1997;87(3):454–457.

53. Chen J, Lee S, Lui T, et al. Teflon granuloma after microvascular decompression for trigeminal neuralgia. *Surg Neurol* 2000;53(3):281–287.

54. Leksell L. Sterotaxic radiosurgery in trigeminal neuralgia. *Acta Chir Scand* 1971;137(4):311–314.

55. Gorgulho AA, De Salles AA. Impact of radiosurgery on the surgical treatment of trigeminal neuralgia. *Surg Neurol* 2006;66(4):350–356.

56. Brisman R, Mooij R. Gamma knife radiosurgery for trigeminal neuralgia: dose-volume histograms of the brainstem and trigeminal nerve. *J Neurosurg* 2000; 93(Suppl 3):155–158.

57. Massager N, Lorenzoni J, Devriendt D, et al. Gamma knife surgery for idiopathic trigeminal neuralgia performed using a far-anterior cisternal target and a high dose of radiation. *J Neurosurg* 2004;100(4):597–605.

58. Flickinger JC, Pollock BE, Kondziolka D, et al. Does increased nerve length within the treatment volume improve trigeminal neuralgia radiosurgery? A prospective double-blind, randomized study. *Int J Radiat Oncol Biol Phys* 2001;51(2):449–454.

59. Pollock BE, Phuong LK, Foote RL, et al. High-dose trigeminal neuralgia radiosurgery associated with increased risk of trigeminal nerve dysfunction. *Neurosurgery* 2001;49(1):58–62, discussion 62–64.

60. Regis J, Metellus P, Hayashi M, et al. Prospective controlled trial of gamma knife surgery for essential trigeminal neuralgia. *J Neurosurg* 2006;104(6): 913–924.

61. Tawk RG, Duffy–Fronckowiak M, Scott BE, et al. Stereotactic gamma knife surgery for trigeminal neuralgia: detailed analysis of treatment response. *J Neurosurg* 2005;102(3):442–449.

62. Pollock BE, Phuong LK, Gorman DA, et al. Stereotactic radiosurgery for idiopathic trigeminal neuralgia. *J Neurosurg* 2002;97(2):347–353.

63. Sheehan J, Pan HC, Stroila M, et al. Gamma knife surgery for trigeminal neuralgia: outcomes and prognostic factors. *J Neurosurg* 2005;102(3):434–441.

64. Dhople A, Kwok Y, Chin L, et al. Efficacy and quality of life outcomes in patients with atypical trigeminal neuralgia treated with gamma-knife radiosurgery. *Int J Radiat Oncol Biol Phys* 2007;69(2):397–403.

65. Pollock BE, Foote RL, Link MJ, et al. Repeat radiosurgery for idiopathic trigeminal neuralgia. *Int J Radiat Oncol Biol Phys* 2005;61(1):192–195.

66. Shetter AG, Zabramski JM, Speiser BL. Microvascular decompression after gamma knife surgery for trigeminal neuralgia: intraoperative findings and treatment outcomes. *J Neurosurg* 2005;102 Suppl:259–261.

67. Burchiel KJ. Percutaneous retrogasserian glycerol rhizolysis in the management of trigeminal neuralgia. *J Neurosurg* 1988;69(3):361–366.

68. Laghmari M, El Ouahabi A, Arkha Y, et al. Are the destructive neurosurgical techniques as effective the microvascular decompression in the management of trigeminal neuralgia? *Surg Neurol* 2007;68(5):505–512.

69. Lopez BC, Hamlyn PJ, Zakrzewska JM. Systematic review of ablative neurosurgical techniques for the treatment of trigeminal neuralgia. *Neurosurgery* 2004;54(4):973–982,discussion 982–983.

70. Taha JM, Tew JM Jr. Treatment of trigeminal neuralgia by percutaneous radiofrequency rhizotomy. *Neurosurg Clin N Am* 1997;8(1):31–39.

71. Tew JM, Tobler WD, Van Loveren H. Percutaneous rhizotomy in the treatment of intractable facial pain (trigeminal, glossopharyngeal and vagal nerves). In: Schmidek HH, Sweet WG, eds. *Operative Neurosurgical Techniques*. New York: Grune & Stratton; 1982:1083–1106.

72. Sweet WH, Wepsic JG. Controlled thermocoagulation of trigeminal ganglion and rootlets for differential destruction of pain fibers. 1. Trigeminal neuralgia. *J Neurosurg* 1974;40(2):143–156.

73. Hakanson S. Trigeminal neuralgia treated by the injection of glycerol into the trigeminal cistern. *Neurosurgery* 1981;9(6):638–646.

74. Burchiel KJ, Russell LC. Glycerol neurolysis: neurophysiological effects of topical glycerol application on rat saphenous nerve. *J Neurosurg* 1985;63(5): 784–788.

75. Shelden CH, Pudenz RH, Fresheater DB, et al. Compression rather than decompression for trigeminal neuralgia. *J Neurosurg* 1955;12(2):123–126.

76. Mullan S, Lichtor T. Percutaneous microcompression of the trigeminal ganglion for trigeminal neuralgia. *J Neurosurg* 1983;59(6):1007–1012.

77. Lee ST, Chen JF. Percutaneous trigeminal ganglion balloon compression for treatment of trigeminal neuralgia—part I: pressure recordings. *Surg Neurol* 2003;59(1):63–66, discussion 66–67.

78. Borodic GE, Acquadro MA. The use of botulinum toxin for the treatment of chronic facial pain. *J Pain* 2002;3(1):21–27.

79. Piovesan EJ, Teive HG, Kowacs PA, et al. An open study of botulinum-A toxin treatment of trigeminal neuralgia. *Neurology* 2005;65(8):1306–1308.

80. Kanai A, Suzuki A, Kobayashi M, et al. Intranasal lidocaine 8% spray for second-division trigeminal neuralgia. *Br J Anaesth* 2006;97(4):559–563.

CHAPTER 104 ■ ABLATIVE NEUROSURGICAL PROCEDURES FOR CHRONIC PAIN

DONALD C. SHIELDS AND EMAD N. ESKANDAR

INTRODUCTION

Chronic pain management often requires pharmacological and/ or surgical approaches for effective symptomatic relief. Neurosurgical interventions have become more efficacious as pain transmission pathways are better understood. In most instances, pharmacological therapies are attempted initially, but invasive approaches are subsequently considered, with appropriate patient selection, if other options are exhausted. Surgical options include anatomic, neuroaugmentative, and ablative approaches which are tailored to the patient's specific needs and comorbidities. Anatomic procedures are designed to alleviate or modify the structural source of pain such as performed in microdiscectomies, laminectomies, or instrumented fusion procedures for metastatic spine disease. Neuroaugmentative techniques include the use of high frequency stimulation or placement of local analgesic administration devices for symptomatic relief. However, in specific patients for whom sequelae such as numbness are acceptable, ablative procedures can be considered in order to interrupt pain signal transmission. Some ablative procedures such as cordotomy have provided initial pain relief with subsequent reemergence of a deafferentation pain. Thus, ablative procedures are often reserved for patients with shortened life expectancies, while more reversible anatomic/neuroaugmentative methods are considered initially in chronic pain patients who require surgical intervention. In recent years, with the emergence of improved pharmacological therapies and high frequency stimulation, the use of stereotactic lesioning for pain has declined considerably. Medial thalamotomy and anterior cingulotomy procedures remain in use by many functional neurosurgeons while mesencephalic tractotomy, trigeminal tractotomy, and hypophysectomy may be occasionally employed by some practitioners.

POSTCENTRAL GYRECTOMY

Resection of sensory cortex was attempted in the 1930s and 1940s for patients with intractable pain.[1,2] Since lateral thalamic nuclei related to spinothalamic tract inputs project directly to primary and secondary sensory cortices, portions of Brodmann's areas 1, 2, and 3 were excised. Procedures performed under local anesthetic for intraoperative cortical mapping resulted in fewer unexpected postoperative deficits. Relatively large craniotomies were required for exposure of the primary motor and sensory cortices. Results from these procedures often demonstrated initial pain relief, but a relapse of the original symptoms upon long-term follow-up.[3] More extensive resections including the postcentral and corresponding precentral gyri resulted in significant pain relief; however, insufficient data is available for a complete assessment of these procedures.[4] As precise sensory and motor functions among different patients vary in these gyri, the resection of cortical grey matter has not emerged as a practical method for pain relief due to the potential for postoperative functional deficits.

CINGULOTOMY

Cingulotomy remains an intracranial ablative procedure in relatively common use. Originally developed to avoid the neurocognitive complications related to frontal lobotomy, anterior cingulotomies have been devised for multiple conditions with generally safe, but variable symptomatic results. Since the 1950s, anterior cingulotomies have been performed in patients with obsessive compulsive disorder, anxiety, depression, chronic pain, and, more recently, acute cancer pain.[5–12] In 1962, Foltz and White employed this technique to uncouple the noxious component of pain from cortical integration.[9] The later anterior bilateral stereotactic "cingulumotomy" was reported in patients with "psychogenic," "organic," or cancer-related pain.[13] With a reported follow-up period from 1 to 9 years, approximately two-thirds of patients with chronic "organic" pain demonstrated significant improvement (Table 104.1). Many lesions (0.2 cm in diameter) were placed 1 to 3 cm posterior to the genu of the corpus callosum.[9,14] Subsequent radiofrequency generated cingulate lesions were reported by Pillay and Hassenbusch with magnetic resonance imaging guidance.[12,15] Favorable results were reported in these studies in patients with chronic pain and Dejerine-Roussy syndrome.

Anatomy and Physiology

The anterior cingulate cortex is a mesocortical structure with crucial roles in affective experience and emotional expression (Fig. 104.1). With multiple connections to limbic structures, nucleus accumbens, thalamus, septum, basal ganglia, and other cortical structures, the anterior cingulate region has been implicated in motor response selection, attention, error detection, and emotional responses.[16–19] Various animal studies have demonstrated the production of complex motor behaviors, vocalization, and

TABLE 104.1

INITIAL RESULTS OF CINGULOTOMY FOR CANCER PAIN

Study	Year	Number of patients	Initial pain relief (% of patients)
Foltz and White[13]	1968	11	82
Turnbull[43]	1972	13	0
Hurt and Ballantine[104]	1973	32	32
Wilson and Chang[105]	1974	19	53
Voris and Whisler[106]	1975	5	100
Pillay and Hassenbusch[15]	1992	10	50
Yen et al.[107]	2005	15	67

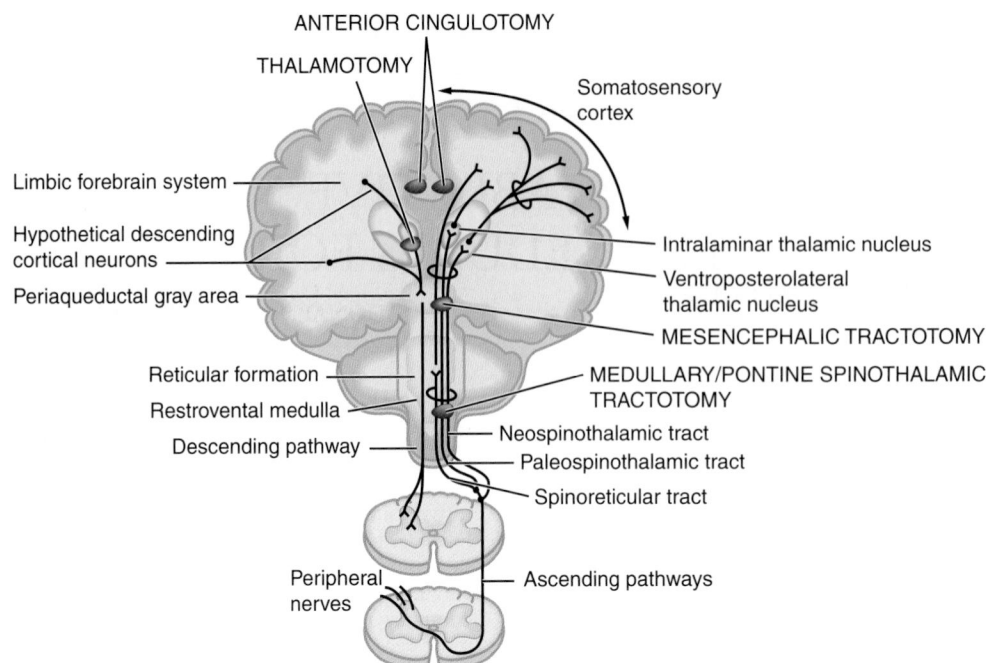

FIGURE 104.1 Specific ablative lesions and their locations relative to the nociceptive pathways.

autonomic responses with cingulate stimulation, although lesions in this area result in impaired problem solving skills and blunted reward responses.[20–26] Human studies have suggested nociceptive stimuli are involved in activation of bilateral anterior cingulate gyri.[27–32] Cutaneous laser stimulation evokes both pain and cerebral potentials although contralateral potentials are more robust than those of the ipsilateral anterior cingulate.[33] Positron emission tomography (PET) and functional magnetic resonance imaging (fMRI) studies suggest that cingulate activation is proportional to the demand for attentional focus and information processing.[34–38] Anterior cingulate activation was most pronounced when patients were required to inhibit competing responses or establish new stimulus–response associations. In studies of patients with bilateral anterior cingulotomies, changes in emotional experience with concomitant derangements in attentional functioning were evident. Focus, persistence, and executive function skills were impaired in tasks requiring sustained attention.[39] Thus, some investigators have proposed the anterior cingulate cortex participates in the integration of sensory inputs, motivational signals, and task demands—such that the subject's attention is focused on the most relevant stimuli for a specific task.[39] As such, the anterior cingulate may reinforce or sustain the perception of pain by amplifying the tendency of patients to emotionally respond to pain or associated inputs.[40,41] Many postcingulotomy patients continue to report pain; however, they are less concerned with or affected by it.

Techniques

Stereotactic frame application and target localization require attachment of the frame on the morning of surgery with subsequent computed tomography (CT) or MRI images prior to the surgical procedure. The frame is typically held in place by four pins tightened against the patient's skull under local anesthesia. After scanning, the projected target can be calculated directly from the imaging data and/or through assessment of the x, y, and z coordinates in relation to the patient's anterior commissure–posterior commissure (AC-PC) line. For the latter, the center point of the frame is compared to the Cartesian coordinates (x, y,

and z) of the subject's anterior/posterior commissures and specific anatomical target. The AC and PC coordinates are entered into a computer program for adjustment of a preloaded Schaltenbrand-Wahren atlas by either shortening or elongating the preset AC-PC distance to accommodate that of the patient. Once adjusted, the projected target coordinates are determined. These coordinates can be compared with coordinates calculated from the MRI and averaged to arrive at the final projected target.

Stereotactic anterior cingulotomies may be performed with local or general anesthesia. MRI localization of the anterior cingulate target approximately 25 mm posterior to the anterior extent of the lateral ventricles is determined. Following attachment of the stereotactic frame to the operating room table, bilateral scalp incisions and burr holes are placed along, or slightly anterior to, the coronal suture 1.5 to 2 cm lateral to the midline. With the coordinates entered on the stereotactic frame, burr holes can be accurately positioned by passing the twist drill through the drill guides set on the frame.

Before the final lesion target is determined, many practitioners employ physiological localization via microelectrode recordings. This technique further confirms the correct target, as discrepancies can often exist between the projected target site from imaging data and that obtained via microelectrode recordings. To begin, a cannula is attached to the arc and aligned to the burr holes. After the cannula passes through the dural opening and into the brain, microelectrodes are inserted into the shaft of the cannula for recording. Many surgeons begin recording 10 to 25 mm above the projected target. Continuous extracellular recordings of single-unit and multiunit neuronal discharges are amplified, displayed on a monitor, and fed into an audio monitor. Neuronal firing/bursting patterns, action potential characteristics, quiet intervals, and background activity provide the surgeon valuable information about anatomical target localization in relation to the measured depth of the microelectrode. One to six electrode tracts, each separated by 2 mm, can be used for target localization. High-frequency stimulation at these sites may also provide information regarding nearby structures. For example, stimulation of lemniscal fibers often results in paresthesias, and that of the internal capsule can cause muscle contractions. Thus, with a

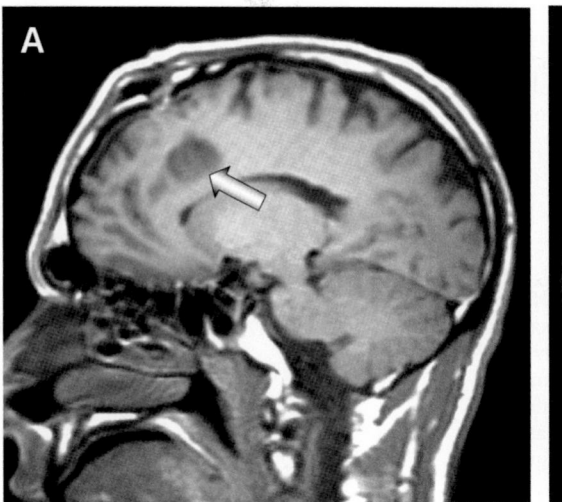
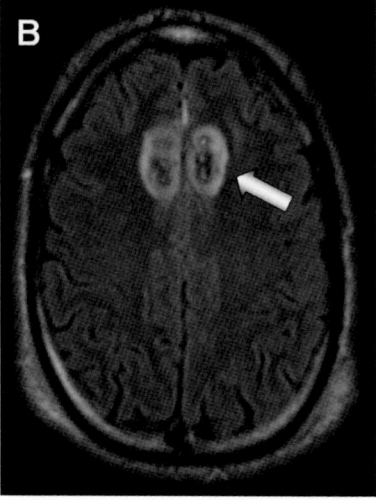

FIGURE 104.2 Representative postoperative ablative lesions. Sagittal (**A**) and axial (**B**) MR images of stereotactic anterior cingulotomy lesions (*arrows*). Three radiofrequency ablations were performed in each cingulate gyrus to form the lesions as shown.

combination of image guidance and physiological localization, lesion targets can often be established with considerable accuracy.

For anterior cingulotomies, lesions are usually positioned in the center of each cingulate gyrus in the medial-lateral plane using a 1 to 2 mm radiofrequency probe (10 mm exposed tip) inserted at the same trajectory as that of the microelectrode. The probe is connected to a radiofrequency generator which monitors tip temperature and electrode impedance during electrical current application. Each lesion can be created in approximately 60 seconds at 85°C. This minimally invasive technique enables the surgeon to reduce the risks of dural bleeding or significant brain shift secondary to cerebrospinal fluid loss. A postoperative MRI before removal of the stereotactic frame allows the surgeon to confirm lesion placement and rule out intracranial hemorrhage (Fig. 104.2).

Results

Patients have reported improvements in their pain scores following cingulotomies from 25% to 80% (average 49%).[10,14,42,43] However, questions remain regarding actual reduction of the sensation of pain or diminution of the patient's emotional and behavioral reactivity to pain.[40,41] In some instances, a bimodal pattern developed wherein patients with mild confusion did not complain of pain and discontinued their use of analgesics without noticeable withdrawal symptoms.[6] Over the ensuing weeks to months, some patients again noted similar but progressively improved pain symptoms as their confusion waned. Some investigators have suggested this alteration of the habituation process deterred patients from fixation on their pain following the procedure.[44]

Complications associated with cingulotomies have been highly variable, but are often self-limited and/or easily treated. Although often transient, seizure onset following this procedure has been reported between 0% to 50% in various series.[8,10,13,14,43,45] Urinary incontinence, short-term hypotension, hemiparesis, aphasia, disorientation, or hemiplegia following hemorrhage have also been described.[8,11–13,43] No operative deaths have been reported; however, postoperative suicide has occurred on occasion. Some series demonstrated improved Wechsler Adult Intelligence Scale scores following cingulotomies, but deficits in the nonverbal sequential tapping test were also observed.[42] Across more recent series, no significant long-term neu-

rological or behavioral changes were reported following bilateral stereotactic cingulotomies.

PREFRONTAL LEUKOTOMY

Cingulotomy procedures were progressively adapted from frontal lobe operations such as the prefrontal leukotomy, designed to treat psychiatric disorders.[46] White matter tracts from thalamic and cingulate structures, representing the rostral extent of the reticular activating system, pass anterior to the lateral ventricular frontal horns. Initial reports of improved pain symptoms in psychiatric patients who underwent resection of these fiber tracts, led to the use of prefrontal leukotomies for chronic pain patients.[47,48] These procedures were largely supplanted by resection of the medial frontal white matter only.[49] Typically, resection of frontal lobe white matter tracts was accomplished via suction under direct vision, injection of sclerosing solutions, or radiofrequency ablation procedures. Results from these procedures varied with regard to pain relief. Of note, noticeable personality changes were often observed in patients with extensive resections who nonetheless received improved pain control. As a result of various cognitive side effects, smaller resections which evolved into the current cingulotomy procedure largely replaced the traditional prefrontal leukotomy.

THALAMOTOMY

As various thalamic nuclei are involved in processing painful stimuli en route to the cingulate gyrus and other cortical structures, the thalamus has historically been targeted in patients with chronic pain.[50,51] Original results with lesions in the ventrocaudal thalamic nucleus were marked by a high incidence of unwanted sensory deficits such as proprioceptive changes and neuropathic pain symptoms.[52,53] Thus, medial thalamotomies which had significantly fewer side effects were considered. Originally, many cancer patients received consideration for medial thalamic lesioning until more advanced pharmacological delivery techniques were adopted. Although less common, patients with tumors which respond poorly to opiate administration, such as head and neck carcinomas, have demonstrated substantial pain reduction from stereotactic thalamotomy procedures. In addition, patients with chronic pain from peripheral deafferentation, stroke, spinal cord injury, arthritis, and Parkinson disease-related neurogenic pain have been treated with thalamotomy procedures.[54–56] Chronic pain patients have also benefited from lesions placed in the pulvinar and anterior thalamus without affecting normal sensation.

Anatomy and Physiology

Medial thalamic structures such as the dorsomedial (DM), centromedian (CM), parafascicular (PF), and centrolateral (CL) nuclei are involved in processing painful stimuli. Axonal projections from the spinothalamic tract ascend in the ventral and ventrolateral spinal cord white matter following decussation. Many of these axons from paleospinothalamic and dorsal spinothalamic tracts terminate in the intralaminar thalamic nuclei such as the CL nucleus. Medial thalamic neurons then project to the cingulate gyrus for further processing.[57] Previous studies have suggested thalamic nociceptive neurons have extensive receptive fields with little discernible somatotopic organization.[58,59] Thus, these cells may play a limited role in localization of painful stimuli; however, they appear to respond to varying stimulus intensities and emotional characterizations of pain.[60] Human studies have demonstrated prolonged thalamic neuronal bursting patterns in subjects with deafferentation pain; lesions colocalized with these patterns in the medial thalamus are reported to substantially improve pain relief.[61]

Neospinothalamic tract axons terminate in the ventral posterolateral thalamic (VPL) nucleus as the corresponding trigeminal fibers project to the ventral posteromedial (VPM) nuclei. Thus, in contradistinction to intralaminar/medial thalamic nuclei, stereotactic lesions in the VPL/VPM (Fig. 104.1) often result in decreased pain and temperature sensation along the contralateral hemibody. In addition, lesions placed in the anterior thalamic nuclei and pulvinar resulted in pain relief in some patients. Since anterior thalamic nuclei project largely to frontal lobe cortical structures, anterior thalamotomies were postulated to play a role in motivational and affective pain components.[62] Pulvinotomy is also rarely performed as exact target sites and electrophysiological data are poorly defined. Although the precise mechanism for pain reduction is not currently understood, previous studies reported long-term pain relief in approximately 25% of patients without evidence of sensory loss.[63]

Techniques

Stereotactic medial thalamotomy procedures are performed after the patient is immobilized in a stereotactic frame with local anesthesia as described previously. MRI sequences are often employed to localize the projected thalamic target and evaluate the anatomical structures unique to each patient. Burr holes can be directed via the stereotactic frame drill guides near the coronal suture approximately 3 cm on each side of the midline. Microelectrode recordings are then commonly used to provide detailed electrophysiological data regarding specific thalamic nuclei, although medial nuclei provide a relatively large target without significant somatotopic arrangement. Thus, without pathognomonic electrophysiological findings, intraoperative testing may not provide definite positioning data in all patients, but deafferentation pain associated with sustained neuronal bursting patterns often responds well to lesioning.[61] Radiofrequency lesions created in or near the dorsomedial nucleus, intralaminar zone, and centromedian nucleus are often most efficacious in relief of chronic pain symptoms. Coordinates from 6 to 10 mm lateral to the AC-PC plane, 7 to 11 mm posterior to the AC-PC midpoint, and from 1 mm below to 2 mm above the AC-PC line have been used in stereotactic thalamotomies[64,65] (Fig. 104.3). Following frame

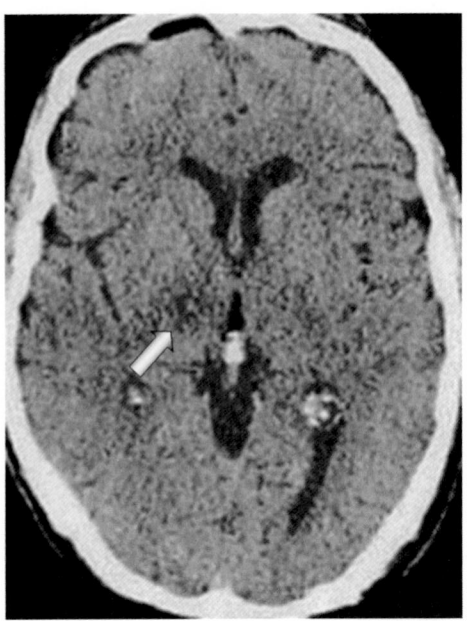

FIGURE 104.3 Postoperative axial CT image following right-sided stereotactic thalamic lesion (*arrow*).

removal, a postoperative MRI can provide the practitioner information regarding the lesion size/position and evidence of intracranial hemorrhage.

Results

Stereotactic medial thalamotomy procedures have been associated with substantial reduction in pain immediately after treatment. Since several medial thalamic nuclei (CM, PF, and CL) are involved in nociceptive pain transmission, an established consensus has not yet emerged regarding a specific nucleus or region to lesion. Nociceptive pain symptoms often respond more favorably than neuropathic pain symptoms to thalamic lesioning. However, long-term follow-up studies have shown recurrence of chronic pain symptoms in many patients.[50] Tasker demonstrated a reduction in nociceptive pain in 46% of subjects while 29% noted neuropathic pain relief[66] (Table 104.2). Frank and colleagues found 60% of patients described pain relief with medial thalamotomies while Jeanmonod et al. reported from 50% to 100% pain relief in approximately two-thirds of patients without production of iatrogenic neurological deficits.[67,68]

RADIOSURGICAL THALAMOTOMIES

Radiosurgical lesions have been documented using both the Leksell gamma knife and linear accelerator systems. With CT and

TABLE 104.2

RESULTS OF THALAMOTOMY FOR CHRONIC PAIN

Study	Year	Initial pain relief (% of patients)
Tasker[66]	198	46
Frank et al.[68]	1987	60
Jeanmonod et al.[67]	1994	67
Young et al.[64]	1995	67

MRI localization techniques, lesion accuracy has been substantially improved in recent years. Some studies demonstrate similar efficacy of radiosurgical and stereotactic thalamotomies.[69] However, pain relief is initially noted by the patient 2 to 3 months after radiosurgical lesioning with stable results 4 to 6 months post-procedure. Thus, radiosurgical thalamotomies may be less efficacious for cancer related pain in patients with shortened life expectancies. In lieu of microelectrode recordings in radiosurgical procedures, fMRI studies may provide anatomical/functional data which can be coregistered with the MRI to provide the investigator more information regarding target size and location.

Using the Leksell stereotaxic system and Cobalt[60] Gamma Unit, Steiner and colleagues described radiosurgical lesioning of the ventromedial thalamus using 160 to 180 Gy. In 24 patients with unilateral lesions placed contralateral to the pain and 26 patients with bilateral lesions, approximately two-thirds of patients noted short-term pain relief.[70] However, with time, only 8 of 52 patients described good pain relief. Later studies by Young et al. found approximately 60% of chronic pain patients with MRI-guided gamma knife lesions retained long-term pain relief using similar radiation dosages.[64] Of note, the latter study used MRI guidance with lesions designed to include intralaminar nuclei, such as the CL nucleus, which project to the cingulate cortex. Frighetto and colleagues reported a smaller population of chronic pain patients who underwent linear accelerator radiosurgical ablation using a 5 mm diameter collimator with 5 to 8 evenly distributed noncoplanar arcs.[71] Maximal radiation dosages varied from 150 to 200 Gy. All of the patients received substantial pain relief, although one patient noted pain recurrence approximately 4 months after treatment. Thus, radiosurgical thalamotomies with MRI target localization may improve safety for patients, although results are delayed by several months.

MESENCEPHALIC TRACTOTOMY

The mesencephalon was considered as a site for lesioning in chronic pain patients in the 1940s (Fig. 104.1).[72] Originally used to treat cancer-related pain, mesencephalic tractotomy was found to be most effective in reducing nociceptive pain of the head, neck, and upper extremities rostral to the C5 dermatome. The lateral spinothalamic and spinoreticular tracts, which lie just beneath the pial surface, are transected at the level of the colliculi while the medial lemniscus is preserved. The lateral spinothalamic tract is more superficial than the spinoreticular tract. These pathways transmit pain information from the contralateral hemibody along with affective and motivational aspects of pain. The procedure has been considered in some patients with partial diaphragm paralysis secondary to lung cancer in which a high cervical cordotomy might result in further diaphragmatic dysfunction. Neuropathic pain related to phantom limb symptoms, postcordotomy dysesthesias, and brachial plexus/lumbosacral plexus avulsion has also been considered for treatment via mesencephalic tractotomy.[73–80]

Techniques

Stereotactic lesioning procedures have described insertion of radiofrequency electrodes through frontal skull burr holes as described previously.[76] This can be achieved under local anesthesia for evaluation of the patient's symptoms intraoperatively. The spinothalamic tracts can be localized with MRI approximately 7 to 9 mm lateral to the midline, 4 to 5 mm inferior to, and 5 mm posterior to the PC. Microelectrode recording data can be used to describe surrounding structures such as the periaqueductal grey or medial lemniscus. Stimulation of the periaqueductal grey region may produce sensations of anxiety, fear, blushing, or piloerection.[81,82] Medial lemniscus stimulation (approximately

9–12 mm lateral to the midline) can result in contralateral paresthesias while spinothalamic tract stimulation usually results in cold or burning sensations.[82] Once the spinothalamic tract is localized, a radiofrequency lesion is created with a radiofrequency electrode. The patient is preferably awake during this period so extraocular movements and sensation can be tested. Once the electrode temperature is above 48°C, the lesion gradually is enlarged over the next 30 to 45 seconds. Typically small lesions are generated initially; after testing the patient's symptoms, the lesion size can be expanded. Practitioners often note a loss of sharp pain sensation which indicates appropriate analgesia, but transient deficits in light touch sensation over the contralateral hemibody have also been described.

Results

Nociceptive pain relief has been described in 60% to 70% of patients, but neuropathic pain results are less favorable.[81] Consistent pain relief has been historically limited by side effects. Because of the close approximation of surrounding structures, it is difficult to create a lesion large enough to encompass the spinothalamic and spinoreticular tracts without encroaching on the medial longitudinal fasciculus, medial lemniscus, and oculomotor nucleus. Thus, ocular motility deficits, sensory loss due to medial lemniscus damage, and dysesthesias can result. Lesions adjacent to the superior colliculus may result in pain relief in 75% of patients, but oculomotor deficits may be present in 87%. Lesions at the level of the inferior colliculus achieve significant pain relief in less than 60% of patients, but oculomotor defects are reduced to around 20%.[80,83]

MEDULLARY AND PONTINE SPINOTHALAMIC TRACTOTOMY

Lesions of the lateral spinothalmic tract at either the pontine or medullary levels (Fig. 104.1) were introduced in 1941 to achieve a more rostral level of analgesia compared to cervical cordotomies.[84,85] At these levels, the lateral spinothalamic tract ascends in the anterolateral white matter. Investigators found painful dysesthesias may develop over time with inconsistent pain relief beyond one year. Resulting sensory loss may also result in tissue injury (i.e., burns) in patients unaware of painful stimuli. Thus, these lesions are typically employed for cancer-related pain in the neck or shoulder in patients with shortened life spans. In addition, lesions in this region can cause interruption of respiratory drive.

Although stereotactic techniques with this procedure have been reported, many medullary and pontine spinothalamic tractotomies were performed with a craniotomy under general anesthesia. The prone or lateral decubitus positions have been employed for creation of a posterior fossa craniotomy and upper cervical laminectomies. Exposure of the medulla allows for tractotomies in the region above or below the obex. Few of these procedures are presently performed due to possible side effects (ipsilateral ataxia or motor deficits) and frequent failure to relieve deep burning/aching pain experienced by many cancer patients.

TRIGEMINAL TRACTOTOMY

Trigeminal tractotomy was developed to disrupt nociceptive pain of the orofacial structures transmitted via the descending trigeminal tract.[86] The most caudal subdivision of the spinal trigeminal nucleus, the nucleus caudalis, is analogous to the spinal cord dorsal horn. This subdivision was selected because it was believed to transmit nociceptive trigeminal inputs, while nonnociceptive sensory information was directed through the rostral subdivisions of the spinal trigeminal nucleus or principal sensory nucleus. More recent studies have refuted this hypothesis, demonstrating nociceptive inputs in the rostral subdivisions as well.[87–89] However, trigeminal tractotomy avoids complete resection of the trigeminal sensory root—leaving tactile and proprioceptive afferents intact. The corneal reflex for instance is lost with complete trigeminal rhizotomy while it is often preserved following a tractotomy.

Trigeminal tractotomy has been considered for relief of cancer-related orofacial pain. The procedure has been combined with cervical rhizotomies for treatment of pain due to head and neck tumors, and has been reported for use in refractory trigeminal neuralgia cases.[90–97] Patients with anesthesia dolorosa or various other types of neuropathic orofacial pain typically have not reported pain relief with this procedure. Both open and stereotactic trigeminal tractotomies have been described for sectioning of the trigeminal tract. In the open procedure, 3–5 mm incisions of the nucleus caudalis have been described. Possible complications include restiform body injury with ipsilateral arm ataxia, dorsal column nuclei injury with ipsilateral proprioception loss, or spinothalamic tract disruption with contralateral pain/temperature loss of the trunk and extremities. Stereotactic trigeminal tractotomy has not gained wide acceptance because target localization in the posterior fossa with most systems is difficult to confirm. Hitchcock reported insertion of an electrode at a 30-degree angle approximately 6 mm from the midline.[98,99] Verification of positioning was confirmed by stimulation at 50 Hz to evaluate for production of facial sensations. Four of five patients with cancer-related pain reported relief of their symptoms.

HYPOTHALAMOTOMY AND HYPOPHYSECTOMY

Patients with violent behavior associated with mental retardation or epilepsy were considered for posterior hypothalamic lesioning in the 1960s.[100] The procedure was also employed with some success in patients with cancer-related pain of the face and postherpetic neuralgia.[101–102] Under local anesthesia, a radiofrequency electrode can be stereotactically placed 2 mm inferior to the AC-PC line and 3 mm lateral to the AC-PC plane in the posterior hypothalamus. Electrical stimulation in this region can cause papillary dilation, hypertension, tachycardia, and a subjective sense of fear or horror. The use of stereotactic hypothalamotomy has not been widely employed since there is no distinct anatomic target, and no clear advantage has been demonstrated versus stereotactic thalamotomy procedures.

Radiosurgical ablation of the pituitary gland has also been effective in treatment of otherwise refractory cancer-related pain.[103] Nine patients in this study with bone metastases underwent Gamma knife radiosurgery with a maximum radiation dose of 160 Gy. The target included the pituitary gland and stalk with either one or two isocenters, 8 mm in total diameter. The optic nerve received a dose no higher than 8 Gy with no resulting visual side effects. Pain relief was reported within several days of treatment, and 1 to 24 month follow-up data revealed no hormonal dysfunction or recurrence of pain. Despite these results, more prospective studies should be completed before radiosurgical ablation of the pituitary can be fully assessed for pain relief.

CONCLUSION

Although deep brain stimulation techniques have supplanted many ablative procedures, the latter provide more cost effective results. Ablative procedures also provide therapy in medically refractory patients such as those with brittle diabetes and others with increased infection risks. Hardware malfunction and skin erosion by stimulator electrodes are also avoided. However, the effects of stereotactic ablative lesions cannot be modulated or reversed as is the case with high frequency stimulation. Thus, ablative procedures for chronic pain have been largely replaced in developed countries by improved pharmacotherapy, intrathecal delivery systems, and high frequency stimulation techniques in patients without contraindications due to underlying medical conditions.

References

1. Leriche R. *La chirurgie de la douleur*. Paris: Masson, 1937.
2. de Gutierrez_Mahoney CG. The treatment of painful phantom limb by removal of postcentral cortex. *J Neurosurg* 1944;1:156–162.
3. White JC, Sweet WH. *Pain and the Neurosurgeon. A Forty-Year Experience*. Springfield, IL: Charles C Thomas, 1969:835–842.
4. Lende RA, Kirsch WM, Druckman R, eds. Relief of facial pain after combined removal of precentral and postcentral cortex. *J Neurosurg* 1971;34:537–543.
5. Ballantine HT Jr. Historical overview of psychosurgery and its problems. *Acta Neurochir Suppl* 1988;44:125–128.
6. Cosgrove GR, Ballantine HT Jr. Cingulotomy in psychotherapy. In: Gildenberg PI, Tasker RR, eds. *Textbook of Stereotactic and Functional Neurosurgery*. New York: McGraw-Hill, 1997:1965–1970.
7. Ballantine HT Jr, Bouckoms AJ, Thomas EK, et al. Treatment of psychiatric illness by stereotactic cingulotomy. *Biol Psychiatry* 1987;22:807–819.
8. Fodstad H, Strandman E, Karlsson B, et al. Treatment of chronic obsessive compulsive states with stereotactic anterior capsulotomy or cingulotomy. *Acta Neurochir* 1982;62:1–23.
9. Foltz EL, White LE Jr. Pain "relief" by frontal cingulumotomy. *J Neurosurg*. 1962;19:89–100.
10. Jenike MA, Baer L, Ballantine HT Jr, et al. Cingulotomy for refractory obsessive-compulsive disorder: a long-term follow-up of 33 patients. *Arch Gen Psychiatry* 1991;48:548–555.
11. Spangler WJ, Cosgrove GR, Ballantine HT Jr, et al. Magnetic resonance image-guided stereotactic cingulotomy for intractable psychiatric disease. *Neurosurgery* 1996;38:1071–1078.
12. Hassenbusch SJ, Pillay Pk, Barnett GH. Radiofrequency cingulotomy for intractable cancer pain using stereotaxis guided by magnetic resonance imaging. *Neurosurgery* 1990;27:220–223.
13. Foltz EL, White LE Jr. The role of rostral cingulumotomy in "pain" relief. *Int J Neurol* 1968;6:353–373.
14. Hurt RW, Ballantine HT Jr. Stereotactic anterior cingulate lesions for persistent pain: a report on 68 cases. *Clin Neurosurg* 1974;21:334–351.
15. Pillay PK, Hassenbusch SJ. Bilateral MRI-guided stereotactic cingulotomy for intractable pain. *Stereotact Funct Neurosurg* 1992;59:33–38.
16. Morecraft RJ, Geula C, Mesulam MM. Architecture of connectivity within a cingulo-fronto-parietal neurocognitive network for directed attention. *Arch Neurol* 1993;50:279–284.
17. Heilman KM, Valenstein E, Watson RT. Localization of neglect. In: Kertesz A, ed. *Localization in Neuropsychology*. New York: Academic Press, 1983: 471–492.
18. Mesulam MM. A cortical network for directed attention and unilateral neglect. *Ann Neurol* 1981;10:309–325.
19. Cohen RA. *Neuropsychology of Attention*. New York: Plenum, 1993.
20. Devinsky O, Morrell MJ, Vogt BA. Contributions of anterior cingulate cortex to behaviour. *Brain* 1995;118:279–306.
21. Woodruff ML, Baisdan RH, Douglas JR. Effect of cingulate and fornix lesions on emotional behavior in rabbits. *Exp Neurol* 1981;74:379–395.
22. Slotnick BM. Disturbances of maternal behavior in the rat following lesions of the cingulate cortex. *Behavior* 1967;29:204–236.
23. Gabriel M. Functions of anterior and posterior cingulate cortex during avoidance learning in rabbits. *Prog Brain Res* 1990;85:467–482.
24. Seamans JK, Floresco SB, Phillips AG. Functional differences between prelimbic and anterior cingulate regions of the rat prefrontal cortex. *Behav Neurosci* 1995;109:1063–1073.
25. Pribram K, Fulton J. An experimental critique of the effects of anterior cingulate ablation in monkey. *Brain* 1954;77:235–246.
26. Bussey TJ, Everitt BJ, Robbins TW. Dissociable effects of cingulate and medial frontal cortex lesions on stimulus-reward learning using a novel pavlovian autoshaping procedure for the rat: implications for the neurobiology of emotion. *Behav Neurosci* 1997;111:908–919.
27. Lenz FA, Rios M, Zirh A, et al. Painful stimuli evoke potentials recorded over the human anterior cingulate gyrus. *J Neurophysiol* 1998;79:2231–2234.
28. Casey KL, Minoshima S, Berger KL, et al. Positron emission tomographic analysis of cerebral structures activated specifically by repetitive noxious heat stimuli. *J Neurophysiol* 1994;71:802–807.
29. Coghill RC, Talbot JD, Evans AC, et al. Distributed processing of pain and vibration by the human brain. *J Neurosci* 1994;14:4095–4108.
30. Craig AD, Reiman EM, Evans A, Bushnell MC. Functional imaging of an illusion of pain. *Nature* 1996;384:258–260.
31. Talbot JD, Marrett S, Evans AC, et al. Multiple representations of pain in human cerebral cortex. *Science* 1991;251:1355–1358.

32. Vogt BA, Derbyshire S, Jones AKP. Pain processing in four regions of human cingulate cortex localized with coregistered PET and MRI. *Eur J Neurosci* 1996;8:1461–1473.

33. Sikes RW, Vogt BA. Nociceptive neurons in area 24 of rabbit cingulate cortex. *J Neurophysiol* 1992;68:1720–1732.

34. Pardo JV, Pardo PJ, Janer KW, et al. The anterior cingulate cortex mediates processing selection in the Stroop attentional conflict paradigm. *Proc Natl Acad Sci* 1990;87:256–259.

35. Posner MI, Petersen SE, Fox PT, et al. Localization of cognitive operations in the human brain. *Science* 1988;240:1627–1631.

36. Paus T, Petrides M, Evans AC, et al. Role of the human anterior cingulate cortex in the control of oculomotor, manual, and speech responses: a positron emission tomography study. *J Neurophysiol* 1993;70:453–469.

37. Paus T, Koski L, Caramanos Z, et al. Regional differences in the effects of task difficulty and motor output on blood flow response in the human anterior cingulate cortex: a review of 107 PET activation studies. *Neuroreport* 1998; 9:R37–R47.

38. Frith CD, Friston K, Liddle PF, et al. Willed action and the prefrontal cortex in man: a study with PET. *Proc R Soc Lond B Biol Sci* 1991;244:241–246.

39. Cohen RA, Kaplan RF, Zuffante P, et al. Alteration of intention and self-initiated action associated with bilateral anterior cingulotomy. *J Neuropsych Clin Neurosci* 1999;11:444–453.

40. Rainville P, Duncan GH, Price DD, et al. Pain affect encoded in human anterior cingulate but not somatosensory cortex. *Science* 1997;277:968–971.

41. Lenz FA, Rios M, Zirh A, et al. Painful stimuli evoke potentials recorded over the human anterior cingulate gyrus. *J Neurophysiol* 1998;79:2231–2234.

42. Faillace LA, Allen RP, McQueen JD, et al. Cognitive deficits from bilateral cingulotomy for intractable pain in man. *Dis Nerv Syst* 1971;32:171–175.

43. Turnbull IM. Bilateral cingulumotomy combined with thalamotomy or mesencephalic tractotomy for pain. *Surg Gynecol Obstet* 1972;134:958–962.

44. Wilkinson HA, Davidson KM, Davidson RI. Bilateral anterior cingulotomy for chronic noncancer pain. *Neurosurgery* 1999;45:1129–1134.

45. Ballantine HT Jr, Cassidy WL, Flanagan NB, et al. Stereotaxic anterior cingulotomy for neuropsychiatric illness and intractable pain. *J Neurosurg* 1967; 27: 488–495.

46. Moniz E. *Tentatives operations dans le traitement de certaines psychoses.* Paris: Masson, 1936.

47. Freeman W, Watts J. Pain mechanisms and the frontal lobes: a study of prefrontal lobotomy for intractable pain. *Ann Intern Med* 1948;28:747–754.

48. Watts JW, Freeman W. Psychosurgery for the relief of unbearable pain. *J Int Coll Surg* 1946;9:679–683.

49. Elithorn A, Glithero E, Slater E. Leucotomy for pain. *J Neurol Neurosurg Psych* 1958:21:249–261.

50. Gorecki JP. Thalamotomy for cancer pain, part I an overview. In: Gildenberg PL, Tasker RR, eds. *Textbook of Stereotactic and Functional Neurosurgery.* New York: McGraw-Hill, 1998:1439–1442.

51. Amano K. Thalamotomy for cancer pain, part II outcome. In: Gildenberg PL, Tasker RR, eds. *Textbook of Stereotactic and Functional Neurosurgery.* New York: McGraw-Hill, 1998:1443–1444.

52. Mark VH, Ervin FR. Role of thalamotomy in treatment of chronic severe pain. *Postgrad Med* 1965;37:563–571.

53. Mark VH, Ervin FR, Yakovlev PI. Correlation of pain relief, sensory loss, and anatomical lesion sites in pain patients treated with stereotactic thalamotomy. *Trans Am Neurol Assoc* 1961;86:86–90.

54. Gorecki J, Hirayama T, Dostrovsky JO, et al. Thalamic stimulation and recording in patients with deafferentation and central pain. *Stereotact Funct Neurosurg* 1989;52:219–226.

55. Davis KD, Kiss ZH, Tasker RR, et al. Thalamic stimulation-evoked sensations in chronic pain patients and in nonpain patients. *J Neurophysiol* 1996;75: 1026–1037.

56. Roth C, Jeanmonod D, Magnin M, et al. Effects of medial thalamotomy and pallido-thalamic tractotomy on sleep and waking EEG in pain and Parkinsonian patients. *Clin Neurophysiol* 2000;111:1266–1275.

57. Kuroda R, Yorimae A, Yamada Y, et al. Frontal cingulotomy reconsidered from a WGA-HRP and c-Fos study in cat. *Acta Neurochir Suppl* 1995;64: 69–73.

58. Giesler GJ, Yeziersky RP, Gerhart KD, et al. Spinothalamic tract neurons that project to medial and/or lateral thalamic nuclei: evidence for a physiologically novel population of spinal cord neurons. *J Neurophysiol* 1981;46:1285–1308.

59. Ammons WS, Girardot MN, Foreman RD. T2-T5 spinothalamic neurons projecting to medial thalamus with viscerosomatic input. *J Neurophysiol* 1985;54:73–89.

60. Bushnell MC, Duncan GH. Sensory and affective aspects of pain perception: is medial thalamus restricted to emotional issues? *Exp Brain Res* 1989;78: 415–418.

61. Jeanmonod D, Magnin M, Morel A. Thalamus and neurogenic pain: physiological, anatomical and clinical data. *Neuroreport* 1993;4:475–478.

62. Gorecki JP. Thalamotomy for cancer pain, part I an overview. In: Gildenberg PL, Tasker RR, eds. *Textbook of Stereotactic and Functional Neurosurgery.* New York: McGraw-Hill, 1998:1417–1424.

63. Yoshii N, Fukuda S. Effects of unilateral and bilateral invasion of thalamic pulvinar for pain relief. *Tohoku J Exp Med* 1979;127:81–84.

64. Young RF, Jacques DS, Rand RW, et al. Technique of stereotactic medial thalamotomy with the Leksell Gamma knife for treatment of chronic pain. *Neurol Res* 1995;17:59–65.

65. Nizuma H, Kwak R, Ikeda S, et al. Follow-up results of centromedian thalamotomy for central pain. *Appl Neurophysiol* 1982;45:324–325.

66. Tasker R. *Stereotactic Surgery.* Edinburgh: Churchill Livingstone, 1984.

67. Jeanmonod D, Magnin M, Morel A. Chronic neurogenic pain and the medial thalamotomy. *Schweiz Rundsch Med Prax* 1994;83:702–707.

68. Frank F, Fabrial AP, Gaist G, et al. Stereotactic mesencephalotomy versus multiple thalamotomies in the treatment of chronic cancer pain syndromes. *Appl Neurophysiol* 1987;50:314–318.

69. Young RF, Jacques DS, Rand RW, et al. Medial thalamotomy with the Leksell gamma knife for treatment of chronic pain. *Acta Naurochir Suppl* 1994;62: 105–110.

70. Steiner L, Forster D, Leksell L, et al. Gammathalamotomy in intractable pain. *Acta Neurochir* 1980;52:173–184.

71. Frighetto L, De Salles A, Wallace R, et al. Linear accelerator thalamotomy. *Surg Neurol* 2004;62:106–114.

72. Walker AE. Releif of pain by mesencephalic tractotomy. *Arch Neurol Psychiatry* 1942;48:865–883.

73. Maxwell RE. Craniofacial pain syndromes: An overview. In: Wilkins R, Rengachary S, eds. *Neurosurgery.* New York: McGraw-Hill, 1983:2327–2336.

74. Wycis HT, Spiegel EA. Long-range results in the treatment of intractable pain by stereotactic midbrain surgery. *J Neurosurg* 1962;19;101–107.

75. Nashold BS Jr, Wilson WP, Slaughter DG. Stereotactic midbrain lesions for central dysesthesia and phantom pain. *J Neurosurg* 1969;30:116–126.

76. Frank F, Tognetti F, Gaist G, et al. Stereotaxic rostral mesencephalotomy in treatment of malignant faciothoracobrachial pain syndromes: a survey of 14 treated patients. *J Neurosurg* 1982;56:807–811.

77. Schieff C, Nashold BS Jr. Stereotactic mesencephalic tractotomy for thalamic pain. *Neurol Res* 1987;9:101–104.

78. Frank F, Fabrizi AP, Gaist G. Stereotactic mesencephalic tractotomy in the treatment of chronic cancer pain. *Acta Neurochir* 1989;99:38–40.

79. Bosch DA. Stereotactic rostral mesencephalotomy in cancer pain and deafferentation pain: a series of 40 cases with follow-up results. *J Neurosurg* 1991; 75:747–751.

80. Gorecki JP. Stereotactic midbrain tractotomy. In: Gildenberg PL, Tasker RR, eds. *Textbook of Stereotactic and Functional Neurosurgery.* New York: McGraw-Hill, 1998:1651–1660.

81. Gybels J, Sweet W. *Neurosurgical Treatment of Persistent Pain.* Vol 11. Basel: Karger, 1989.

82. Nashold BS, Wison WP, Slaughter DG. Sensations evoked by stimulation in the midbrain of man. *J Neurosurg* 1969;30:14–24.

83. Bullard DE, Nashold BS. Mesencephalotomy and other brainstem procedures for pain. In: Youmans JR, ed. *Neurological Surgery.* Vol. 5. Philadelphia: WB Saunders, 1996:3477–3488.

84. Schwartz HG, O'Leary JL. Section of the spinothalamic tract in the medulla with observations of the pathway for pain. *Surgery* 1941;9:183–193.

85. White JC. Spinothalamic tractotomy in the medulla oblongata: an operation for the relief of intractable neuralgias of the occiput, neck, and shoulder. *Arch Surg* 1941;43:113–127.

86. Sjoqvist O. Studies on pain conduction in the trigeminal nerve: a contribution to the surgical treatment of facial pain. *Acta Psychiatry Scand* 1938;17: 1–1139.

87. Nord SG, Young RF. Effects of chronic descending tractotomy on the response patterns of neurons in the trigeminal nuclei principalis and oralis. *Exp Neurol* 1979;65:355–372.

88. Young RF, Oleson TD, Perryman KM. Effect of trigeminal tractotomy on behavioral responses to dental pulp stimulation in monkey. *J Neurosurg* 1981; 55:420–430.

89. Young RF, Oleson TD, Perryman KM. Dental and facial pain sensations in human and non-human primates: effect of trigeminal tractotomy. *Acta Neurochir* 1981;59:276.

90. Kunc Z. Significance of fresh anatomic data on spinal trigeminal tract for possibility of selective tractotomies. In: Knighton RS, Dumke PR, eds. *Pain.* Boston: Little, Brown & Company, 1966:351–366.

91. King RB. Medullary tractotomy for pain relief. In: Wilkins R, Rengachary S, eds. *Neurosurgery.* New York: McGraw-Hill, 1983:2452–2454.

92. Olivecrona H. Trigeminal neuralgia. *Triangle* 1961;5:60–69.

93. Grant FC, Groff RA, Levy FH. Section of the descending spinal root of the fifth cranial nerve. *Arch Neurol Psychiatry* 1940;43:498–509.

94. Olivecrona H. Tractotomy for the relief of trigeminal neuralgia. *Arch Neurol Psychiatry* 1942;47:544–564.

95. Ovelmen-Levitt J, Levitt M, Gorecki J. Pathophysiology of central/neuropathic pain. In: Gildenberg PL, Tasker RR, eds. *Textbook of Stereotactic and Functional Neurosurgery.* New York: McGraw-Hill, 1998:1627–1630.

96. Gorecki JP, Nashold BS. The Duke experience with the nucleus caudalis DREZ operation. *Acta Neurochir Suppl* 1995;64:128–131.

97. Young RF. Stereotactic surgical ablation for pain relief. In: Rengachary SS, Wilkins RH, eds. *Neurosurgical Operative Atlas.* Baltimore: Williams & Wilkins, 1992:177–188.

98. Hitchcock ER. Stereotactic trigeminal tractotomy. *Ann Clin Res* 1970;2: 131–135.

99. Hitchcock ER, Schvarcz JR. Stereotaxic trigeminal tractotomy for postherpetic facial pain. *J Neurosurg* 1972;37:412–417.

100. Sano K. Sedative neurosurgery with special reference to posteromedial hypothalamotomy. *Neurol Med Chir* 1962;4:112–142.

101. Sano K, Sekino H, Hashimoto I, et al. Posteromedial hypothalamotomy in the treatment of intractable pain. *Confin Neurol* 1975;37:285–290.

102. Fairman D. Neurophysiological basis for the hypothalamic lesion in stimulation by chronic implanted electrodes for the relief of intractable pain in cancer. In: Bonical JJ, Albe-Fessard D, eds. *Advances in Pain Research and Therapy.* Vol 1. New York: Raven Press, 1976:843–847.

103. Hayashi M, Taira T, Chernov M, et al. Gamma knife surgery for cancer pain-pituitary gland-stalk ablation: a mulitcenter prospective protocol since 2002. *J Neurosurg* 2004;100:1133–1134.

104. Hurt RW, Ballantine HT. Stereotactic anterior cingulate lesions for persistent pain: a report on 68 cases. *Clin Neurosurg* 1973;21:334–351.

105. Wilson D, Chang E. Bilateral anterior cingulectomy for the relief of intractable pain. *Confin Neurol* 1974;36:61–68.

106. Voris H, Whisler W. Results of stereotaxic surgery for intractable pain. *Confin Neurol* 1975;37:86–96.

107. Yen CP, Kung SS, Su YF, et al. Stereotactic bilateral anterior cingulotomy for intractable pain. *J Clin Neurosci* 2005;12:886–890.

CHAPTER 105 ■ INTERDISCIPLINARY CHRONIC PAIN MANAGEMENT: PERSPECTIVES ON HISTORY, CURRENT STATUS, AND FUTURE VIABILITY

MICHAEL E. SCHATMAN

HISTORY OF INTERDISCIPLINARY CHRONIC PAIN MANAGEMENT

The interdisciplinary approach to chronic pain as it is practiced today represents a relatively new science. In the 1940s, John J. Bonica became the first physician to recognize the complexity of chronic pain syndromes, understanding that they affect patients not only physically but across myriad dimensions of their lives. As chronic pain of nonmalignant origin has been noted to be the most unpredictable type of pain (as compared to acute and chronic pain due to malignancy), it is the most difficult type of pain to treat.[1] Meldrum[2] notes that Bonica found himself frustrated by his inability to effectively treat these patients on his own at Madigan Army Hospital in Washington during World War II and found that consultation with his colleagues seemed to benefit all who were involved. Immediately following the war, Bonica developed the first formal interdisciplinary pain management team at Tacoma General Hospital, with members including an anesthesiologist, orthopedist, neurosurgeon, internist, psychiatrist, and radiation therapist. This team treated all types of pain syndromes, not limiting its practice to patients with chronic pain of nonmalignant origin. Interestingly, unbeknownst to Bonica, F.A.D Alexander was simultaneously developing a similar interdisciplinary pain diagnostic and therapeutic program at a Texas Veterans Administration hospital.[3] Another interdisciplinary program developed in Portland, Oregon, as well as several others in Canada and Europe.[3]

Despite the success achieved by these programs and efforts to promulgate them spearheaded by Bonica, the field of interdisciplinary chronic pain management (ICPM) remained stagnant during the 1950s and the first half of the following decade. Due to a lack of acceptance of the interdisciplinary approach by the medical community, Bonica was "about to give up," and later wrote, "Despite my persistent drum beating, consisting of several hundred lectures and the publication of numerous articles in various parts of the world, the multidisciplinary concept was ignored by the medical profession for two decades."[4] Meldrum[5] has recently suggested that Wilbert Fordyce's integration of a strong behavioral component into Bonica's team in the late 1960s was instrumental in the development of the modern interdisciplinary pain treatment team. With the introduction of this behavioral approach to assessment and treatment, the focus of pain clinics shifted from the eradication of pain to teaching patients how to *manage* their symptoms and restore a positive quality of life.[6] Due to the fact that the purely behavioral approaches to chronic pain were found to be time-consuming and expensive to implement, they were soon replaced in interdisciplinary treatment programs by cognitive-behavioral approaches, which emphasize the patient as an *active participant* in his or her rehabilitation who is able to develop the coping skills necessary to restore independence.[2]

In the 1970s and 1980s, ICPM programs proliferated rapidly to the extent that these clinics were described as "medicine's new growth industry."[7] In addition to providing chronic pain management services, numerous postdoctoral fellowships in pain management developed during this period of time, typically in university-based facilities. Among the most active and prestigious of these facilities was that developed by Bonica at the University of Washington in 1960, where he was succeeded in directorship by the neurosurgeon, John Loeser. Loeser instituted a highly structured inpatient program at the University of Washington that was developed around Fordyce's operant conditioning approach. According to Loeser, the great success of his program was due to the interaction between the various disciplines of the treatment team members rather than to any specific intervention that was applied.[8] By the early 1980s, Aronoff and colleagues[9] suggested that approximately 1000 interdisciplinary treatment centers were in operation in the United States and were becoming more numerous in other parts of the world as well. In 1999, Anooshian and colleagues[10] reported that there were approximately 2000 pain treatment facilities in the United States, with the majority considered multidisciplinary. However, it has been noted that while third party payers were initially enthusiastic regarding these programs, they soon became skeptical. Aronoff states, "By the early 1990s the pain clinic movement was experiencing image problems so serious that some pain programs closed while others changed their names to functional restoration or work-conditioning programs to avoid using the word *pain* as a descriptor."[11] Because of strategic changes in nomenclature, it is difficult to specifically determine the point at which the number of interdisciplinary treatment programs and the availability of this type of pain management began to decline. However, Schatman[12,13] has noted that the number of programs in the United States accredited by the Committee on Accreditation of Rehabilitation Facilities (CARF) declined from 210 in 1998 to 84 in 2005, with a similar but less dramatic decline noted in the number of programs accredited by either CARF, the Joint Commission on Accreditation of Healthcare Organizations, or the American Academy of Pain Management reported between 1997 and 2003. Later in this chapter, the paradox of this decrease in the availability of ICPM programs will be discussed in greater detail.

Theoretical Basis of Interdisciplinary Chronic Pain Management

ICPM, as it is practiced today, is based on the biopsychosocial approach that initially achieved prominence through the work of Engel.[14,15] This model emphasizes the complex and dynamic interaction between physiologic, psychologic, and social factors that serve to perpetuate and potentially worsen pain experience.[16] While considered a relatively new development in medicine, Gilbert[17] notes that the biopsychosocial model was practiced by ancient Greek physicians over 2000 years ago. Certainly, the addition of Wilbert Fordyce to Bonica's treatment team was instrumental in the evolution of the interdisciplinary approach, as it resulted in the consideration of the emotional and behavioral sequelae of chronic pain as well as nociceptive experience. Turk and Melzack[18] suggest that the measurement of pain should involve the motivational-affective and cognitive-evaluative contributions, not just the nociceptive. Undoubtedly, this holds true for the *treatment* of chronic pain as well. Steen and Haugli[19] note that while the biomedical model may be an effective approach to disease states in which the cause is clearly defined, it is not appropriate for conditions such as chronic musculoskeletal pain. Chronic pain is a disease of the *person*, and the person is often obscured by the traditional biomedical approach.[20] The interdisciplinary approach is based on the premise that no one individual can "cure" the patient of all of the ills associated with his or her pain condition. At the time that Bonica was developing his method of treating pain, medicine was becoming progressively more specialized. While specialization serves to enhance expertise, specialization without diversification results in limitations to what the medical field can offer to patients whose conditions are as complex as is chronic pain. This, perhaps, was the greatest wisdom that Bonica contributed to the pain treatment community,

Loeser[8] and numerous others[21–26] have written of the importance of communication between treatment team members. While the terms "multidisciplinary" and "interdisciplinary" are often used interchangeably, it is important to note that "multidisciplinary" suggests only the involvement of multiple disciplines, while "interdisciplinary" suggests the involvement of multiple disciplines *working in concert* to help patients with pain overcome not only nociceptive phenomena, but the emotional and behavioral implications of persistent pain as well. ICPM can be considered the most collaborative approach along the continuum of multidisciplinary models. Because this type of chronic pain treatment requires such close communication among team members, interdisciplinary programs ideally involve treatment teams working in a single setting. In the early days of the discipline, programs were frequently operated in inpatient settings, as the practitioners who developed them believed that inpatient treatment allowed for a higher level of control over contingencies than would outpatient programs. Inpatient treatment, however, was expensive, incurring the criticism of the health insurance industry. In 1990, Peters and Large[27] published a study that found little difference in outcomes between inpatient and outpatient chronic pain management programs. The release of this study coincided with the conversion of many programs from inpatient to outpatient treatment. Currently, there are very few inpatient ICPM programs in the United States, with CARF reporting that as of June of 2007, only 6 of its accredited 83 ICPM programs are inpatient.[28]

The interdisciplinary approach recognizes the bidirectionality of pain and psychosocial factors, considering that emotions and maladaptive behavioral patterns can perpetuate as well as result from persistent physical discomfort. Myriad investigators have made an effort to answer the "chicken-or-the-egg" issue of nociceptive and psychologic factors contributing to the chronic pain experience, with no clear results emerging. In the interdisciplinary model of chronic pain management, this issue is of minimal importance, as patients improve on *multiple* dimensions if they are provided with appropriate guidance and exert maximal effort. As noted earlier in this chapter, the goal of chronic pain management has evolved from "pain elimination" to genuine "pain management," with an emphasis on restoring the patient's independence and overall quality of life. This emphasis is crucial, as a recent analysis[29] suggests that there is little difference in pain relief between common approaches to chronic pain, including medication therapy, surgery, spinal cord stimulation, intrathecal drug delivery, and ICPM programs.

The approaches of ICPM programs vary to a certain degree. However, Okifuji and colleagues[30] suggest that the typical treatment provided includes 3 common elements: (1) medication man-

agement, (2) graded physical exercise, and (3) cognitive and behavioral techniques for pain and stress management. The degree to which each of these elements is emphasized should vary based upon the needs of the specific patient, although is probably more contingent upon the personality of the program and the individual clinicians. While the importance of the cohesiveness and communication between treatment team members cannot be overemphasized, it should be recognized that each team member brings very specific and necessary expertise to the program. Baszanger[31] describes the professionals who treat chronic pain from a team approach as "pluridisciplinary"; each of the disciplines has its own unique training methods and clinical experiences and accordingly is likely to approach the same patient with different assumptions and treatment methods.

Composition of the Interdisciplinary Chronic Pain Management Team and Roles of Members

Authors who have described the composition of treatment teams and the specific roles of their members have tended to rely on the programs that they directed to provide such description.[16,26,32] For the purpose of this chapter, the composition of ICPM treatment teams and the functions that the individual members provide will be described more generically. It is important to note that ICPM treatment team composition varies based on program philosophy and economic factors, although certain "core" members are essential if patients are to be treated through a biopsychosocial model.

- **Medical Director/Physician:** The ICPM program medical director provides medical leadership, and, to a considerable extent, accepts responsibility for the physical well-being of the patients that are treated. While it is important that the physician possesses expertise in the rehabilitation of pain disorders, a survey of programs yields wide variance in the training experience and practice specialties of their medical directors. These specialties include physical medicine and rehabilitation, anesthesiology, neurology, rheumatology, occupational medicine, orthopaedic surgery, neurosurgery, psychiatry, and internal medicine. The physician on an interdisciplinary treatment team is responsible for taking a medical history, evaluating the patient for purposes of providing or confirming a diagnosis, managing medications (which may include detoxification), providing patient education, and guiding other team members in regard to the physical treatment that they provide. Additionally, in some programs, the physician provides interventions such as trigger point injections to patients. While such interventions are not known as a "cure" for chronic pain, Hatzakis and Schatman[33] have advocated for their use in certain situations in order to promote adherence with the physical reconditioning component of an ICPM program. The physician needs to be able to effectively communicate the patient's physical status to other team members. While some medical directors tend to "rule the team with an iron fist," the physician who is seen as warmer and less directive is likely to foster greater team cohesiveness, which is consistent with the literature on small group process.[34] Spoonhour and Schatman[35] have suggested that selflessness is a positive attribute in an ICPM leader, as the most effective medical directors are those who are willing to allow the team member with certain expertise to function in a manner maximizing the benefit of that expertise.

- **Nurse Case Manager:** Nurses on ICPM treatment teams often assume diverse responsibilities and are accordingly invaluable. Because of their medical backgrounds, they can potentially serve as extensions of the physician, obtaining medical histories, monitoring medications, encouraging healthy lifestyles, and providing education to patients and their families. In a role delineation study, Pellino and colleagues[36] determined that assessing, evaluating, and monitoring pain were nurses' most common activities. Nurses are also the multidisciplinary team members that spend the greatest amount of time with patients.[37] Additionally, as many nurses are trained and experienced in case management, a nurse is often the team member responsible for the day-to-day management of the program. Duties may include triaging referred patients, confirming insurance sponsorship, development of policies and procedures, quality assurance, collection and maintenance of patient data, and correspondence with referral sources, employers, attorneys, health insurance providers, and other health care professionals treating a patient.

■ **Psychologist:** Pain psychologists on interdisciplinary treatment teams are responsible for the psychosocial aspects and status of patients' care. As patients become more chronic, their development of maladaptive emotional and behavioral patterns increases, necessitating expert psychologic care if they are to become more functional in their lifestyles. Initially, the psychologist provides a comprehensive psychosocial evaluation, with this evaluation serving multiple purposes. First, the psychologist must determine whether a patient is appropriate for an ICPM program. Psychologic testing routinely used in assessing chronic pain patients can identify conditions such as thought disorders and dramatic personality disorders that would make certain patients inappropriate for admission to a program.[38,39] Through a thorough evaluation, the psychologist can reduce the likelihood that a dramatically disturbed patient will experience yet another failure, while simultaneously protecting the emotional well-being of the rest of the treatment team as well as the therapeutic milieu. The second purpose of the psychosocial evaluation is to identify the specific maladaptive emotional and behavioral patterns that are perpetuating the patient's chronic pain, thereby leading to a treatment plan of cognitive and behavioral interventions that will address these patterns. Like the physician and the nurse, the psychologist is also an educator, although the education that he or she provides is generally focused on psychosocial factors. Typically, the pain psychologist will work with patients on both an individual and group basis, with an emphasis on unlearning maladaptive responses to pain, problem-solving techniques, stress management training, decreasing catastrophization, and enhancing self-efficacy. Through these approaches, reductions in depression and anxiety along with more adaptive behavioral responses to pain are typically evidenced. A pain psychologist will also often work with a patient's family during the course of a program, as the family may unwittingly be reinforcing the "patient role," thereby enabling the patient. Finally, as psychologists are trained as scientist-practitioners, they are likely to coordinate outcomes research for the ICPM team. Such research is of great importance, not only in terms of identifying potential weaknesses of a program, but for marketing purposes as well.

■ **Physical Therapist:** The physical therapist on a pain treatment team is responsible for assessing patients' levels of functioning, and then designing and monitoring programs of graded therapeutic exercise that will safely increase these levels. Areas of focus may include increasing flexibility and range of motion, restoring appropriate posture and body mechanics, ambulation and gait training, development of core strength and stability, cardiovascular fitness, and increasing upper and lower extremity strength and endurance. Treatment is typically provided on both an individual and group basis. Passive modalities such as ultrasound, electrical stimulation, and massage are generally avoided, as the focus of ICPM is on teaching patients *independent* management of their pain. Stretching and strengthening are emphasized, as these exercises have been empirically supported through systematic re-

views as being among the most effective treatments for a number of types of chronic pain.[40-45] It is critical that the treatment team's physical therapist has received specialized training in chronic pain management, and that he or she is *interested* in treating patients with chronic pain. As is true for physicians,[46-48] many physical therapists lack the training and interest necessary to treat patients with chronic pain effectively. Typically, physical therapists are trained in an acute pain model, with an emphasis on passive modalities. The physical therapist who works as a member of an ICPM team must function as a *behaviorist*, demonstrating recognition that the patients have developed emotional sequelae of their pain as well as maladaptive behavioral patterns that must be modified in order to achieve successful outcomes. Training and ongoing supervision of the physical therapist by the treatment team's psychologists is ideal. Rotating potentially disinterested therapists from a hospital's physical therapy department through an ICPM clinic will invariably result in poor outcomes and negatively impact treatment team cohesiveness.

■ **Occupational Therapist:** On many ICPM teams, there is considerable overlap between the duties of physical therapists and occupational therapists. Areas that are considered primarily within the domain of occupational therapist include ergonomic training, upper extremity activities of daily living, work activities, leisure activities, and any other activities that are meaningful and purposeful to the individual patient. Some occupational therapists perform work-site analyses, visiting the work place to which the patient intends to return, observing the specific job-related tasks that he or she will need to perform, and then developing a work simulation component of the ICPM program. Helping patients problem-solve pain management strategies that can be applied in the work place is another critical role of the occupational therapist. As for physical therapists, occupational therapists should have training and experience in applying behavioral interventions as well as traditional occupational therapy training in order to optimize outcomes. Emotional interference with restoration of function should be understood as well, particularly as it relates to return-to-work issues. In some ICPM programs, the occupational therapist serves as the vocational counselor as well.

■ **Vocational Counselor:** The vocational counselor on the treatment team is responsible for a number of important functions, with these functions dictated by the specific goals of the program and the needs of the individual patient. Returning patients to gainful employment is considered a primary goal of many ICPM programs, particularly those that take a *functional restoration* approach.[49] As a large percentage of patients in interdisciplinary treatment programs suffer from pain secondary to work-related injuries,[50,51] vocational issues can become extremely complicated. In such instances, the vocational counselor is responsible for helping the patient understand the benefits of returning to the work force, while simultaneously serving as a case manager who contacts employers, obtains and analyzes job descriptions, and "greases the wheels" to facilitate return to previous employment. In situations in which the previously-held position is no longer available, the vocational counselor may provide a patient with interest and aptitude testing in order to help him or her identify new employment situations that may be realistic given the patient's educational and work histories, economic realities, and any given physical limitations anticipated at the completion of the program. Additionally, there are situations in which a vocational counselor provides testing and counseling in order to prepare a patient for vocational retraining. Like other team members, the vocational counselor needs to be psychologically-minded, understanding issues such as primary and secondary gain as well as the role of psychologic factors in perpetuating perceived disability. Vocational counselors in ICPM programs typically work with patients on both an individual and group basis. At times, the team's vocational specialist will accompany the occupational therapist on a work-site analysis, serving as a "second set of eyes and ears" in order to help understand potential obstacles that may impede efforts to return a patient to the work force.

■ **Biofeedback Therapist:** The biofeedback therapist on the ICPM team is primarily responsible for reducing patients' psychophysiologic reactivity to stress, although also often participates in neuromuscular re-education. Of all the self-management techniques that are taught to a patient through an interdisciplinary program, perhaps those taught by the biofeedback therapist are most important, as they can help shift a patient toward internal locus of control[52] and restore a patient's sense of self-efficacy,[53,54] as well as reduce tension and pain. Biofeedback equipment is utilized to help patients recognize how their bodies respond to stress, as awareness of stress among chronic pain sufferers is often limited.[55] Biofeedback technology provides a patient with visual and/or auditory feedback regarding physiologic functions including muscle tension levels, perspiration, extremity temperature, and brain wave patterns. Once patients gain awareness of how their bodies responds to stress, the biofeedback therapist can teach them to alter these functions through a variety of relaxation techniques, including progressive muscle relaxation, imagery, diaphragmatic breathing, and autogenic techniques. In some ICPM programs, biofeedback training is provided by psychologists, who are often trained in the discipline. However, it is often more cost-efficient to have another team member serve as the biofeedback therapist, with supervision provided by the psychologist. States do not license therapists in biofeedback, although they are eligible for certification through the Biofeedback Certification Institute of America (BCIA). Some physical and occupational therapists are trained in biofeedback, particularly neuromuscular re-education. In certain situations, a physical therapist or occupational therapist will work in tandem with a biofeedback therapist, helping a patient recognize through muscle tension readings the impact of his or her bracing and guarding on levels of function and pain. Biofeedback/relaxation training is generally provided on both an individual and a group basis during the course of an ICPM program. It should be noted that there are some ICPM programs that do not include biofeedback therapy as a core aspect of treatment. However, given the literature on the benefits of biofeedback in the treatment of chronic pain,[52–54] it is likely that this omission relates to reimbursement issues. For example, while the ICPM programs in Pennsylvania (where biofeedback is routinely covered by third party payers) include biofeedback as a central aspect of treatment, biofeedback therapy is *not* reimbursed by third party payers in the state of Washington, thereby essentially precluding its utilization.

■ **Other ICPM team members:** While the "core" treatment team is composed of physicians, psychologists, nurses, physical and occupational therapists, vocational counselors, and biofeedback therapists, some ICPM teams include other disciplines as well. These include therapeutic recreation specialists, social workers, chaplains, dieticians, and non-nurse case managers. However, the functions that these specialized treatment team members fulfill are often performed by other core team members. Although ICPM programs tend to follow a common philosophy of treatment and goals, no two programs are identical. Accordingly, a degree of variance in the composition of the treatment team is to be expected.

The Process of Interdisciplinary Chronic Pain Management

ICPM begins with a referral to the program, which is generally handled by the team member in charge of case management. Re-

ferrals may come from a wide variety of sources, including other physicians and health care providers, attorneys, employers, and insurance carriers. Some ICPM programs are a part of a broader pain management system, in which case triage may be necessary. Due to economic realities, insurance coverage is generally confirmed prior to proceeding. Once this is accomplished, medical records are requested and reviewed in order to ascertain the patient's appropriateness for evaluation.

As ICPM entails comprehensive treatment, the initial evaluation of the patient must be comprehensive as well. Prospective patients are typically evaluated by the physician, psychologist, physical and occupational therapist, biofeedback therapist, and vocational counselor. Following these evaluations, the treatment team members ideally meet in order to discuss the patient's appropriateness for admission, prognosis, and other issues that may have an impact on treatment. As important as the patient's ability to benefit from the *individual components* of the program is the patient's acceptance of and willingness to comply with the program philosophy. For example, a program that emphasizes functional restoration as a means of returning the patient to the work force and closing a disability claim ought not admit a patient who is determined to lack vocational motivation, unless the treatment team is confident that the program will result in a change in this attitude.

One of the biggest mistakes that an ICPM program can make is to simply reject a patient deemed inappropriate for admission and return him or her to the referral source without recommendations. Some patients may be considered physically appropriate for admission, although are not immediately admitted due to psychosocial factors. If the treatment team believes that these factors can be mitigated, delaying admission until the patient has received appropriate psychologic treatment may be in the best interest of the patient and the program. When a patient is determined to never be likely to meet the admission criteria, it behooves the patient and the program to return the patient to the referral source with recommendations for alternative treatment(s). An ICPM clinic is often seen as a "last resort" by referral sources that have a limited understanding of the complexities of chronic pain, and these referral sources may be grateful for ideas regarding managing challenging patients, even if they are not admitted to the program.

ICPM programs tend to be intensive, often requiring patients to participate up to 40 hours per week. While often daunted by the prospect of such a commitment, patients are informed that their day-to-day activities will be varied and that they will not be asked to perform physical tasks that are beyond their functional capacities. Distinguishing between "hurt" and "harm" and assuring patients that the treatment team considers their physical and emotional safety to be of the greatest importance helps build therapeutic trust, thereby enhancing adherence.[33] ICPM programs that are less intensive tend to be of longer duration. A study by Rose and colleagues[56] suggests that outcomes do not relate to program length, and accordingly, the level of intensity of treatment may be based on the personal preferences of the program developers. This is consistent with a more recent study[57] in which the frequency of aggressive spine therapy was determined not to influence clinical outcomes.

Similarly, the specific "mix of services" that patients receive between *and within* programs will vary. Consistency of treatment is considered important,[35] although a "one size fits all" approach is not appropriate given that each patient's circumstances and phenomenologic experience of pain is unique. Typically, patients spend most of their time in the gym engaging in activities that will increase their flexibility, strength, and functional capacities. Early in their programs, patients are likely to require considerable hands-on training by the physical and occupational therapists, as the ineffectiveness of their previous exercise programs is likely the catalyst for referral to an ICPM program. As patients progress, however, they tend to require less of the therapists' attention, with this independence in pain management representing an important milestone in treatment. Patients whose emotional status and behavioral responses to their pain are less dysfunctional will likely require less time with the psychologist than will those patients who are struggling psychosocially. Similarly, patients demonstrating limited psychophysiologic reactivity to stress will require less intensive biofeedback training, and those whose vocational issues are less complex will require less concentrated vocational counseling services. All patients require group education on chronic pain management, and the presenters of the education should make an effort to tailor presented material to the needs and competencies of the group as a whole. The frequency with which a patient sees the physician on an individual basis will vary depending on the specific philosophy of the program. Frequent individual physician appointments are discouraged, particularly as the program progresses, as a goal of ICPM is typically reduction of medical services in lieu of enhanced independent self-management of pain.

The patient-centered nature of ICPM is substantiated by a weekly team conference in which each patient has the opportunity to meet with the entire treatment team in order to discuss his or her progress, any issues that are potentially limiting gains, and goals for the coming week. Feedback should be consistent and coherent. In situations in which patients' adherence is considered good and they are making progress, team conference provides a forum in which they are able to receive much-needed positive reinforcement regarding their attitude and effort. Patients with chronic pain are often unjustifiably blamed for the failures of the primary and secondary care systems to help them recover, making appropriate positive reinforcement even more important. Conversely, in cases in which adherence and progress are considered by the team to be inadequate, the conference provides an opportunity for the treatment team to present a united front in addressing the relevant issues and work with the patients to remedy any problematic aspects of their programs. Numerous studies[58-67] have indicated that characterologically-disturbed patients (i.e., those suffering from personality disorders) are grossly overrepresented in the chronic pain population, and problems associated with treating these patients in ICPM programs have been discussed.[38,39] "Splitting" of treatment team members is not uncommon, particularly in situations in which the patient's agenda is not consistent with that of the team (e.g., a patient in a functional restoration program who would rather continue to collect disability payments than return to active employment may sabotage the efforts of the vocational counselor). Because passively or actively noncompliant patients must face the entire treatment team at the weekly conference, their ability to manipulate the treatment team or individual team members is substantially compromised. While those who treat patients with chronic pain from an ICPM model work to facilitate success for *all* patients, there are those whose inability to make progress necessitates early discharge. Stanos[26] has recently suggested that such premature discharge can potentially encourage enhanced compliance or efforts among other patients in the group. Team conference also provides an excellent opportunity to engage in discharge planning, which should be a holistic process that takes multiple aspects of the patient's long-term pain management planning into consideration. A weekly multidisciplinary progress reported is generated from team conference, with this report sent to the relevant parties. While the attendance of the patient and the core treatment team are mandatory, there are cases in which the presence of other interested parties such as family members, attorneys, insurance company representatives, and employers is also desirable.

Once a patient has completed an ICPM program, he or she can be neither forgotten nor abandoned. Although programs are typically close-ended, follow-up should continue on a quarterly basis for at least a year. For the sake of cost-efficiency, selected measures of patients' emotional and behavioral responses to their pain that are administered at initial evaluation can be sent to them, with the data then analyzed for several purposes. First, if a patient is demonstrating deterioration of pain management skills following discharge, a meeting with the most appropriate team member can be scheduled in order to assess the problem. In effective ICPM programs, such deterioration is uncommon, as patients must meet benchmarks throughout the course of the program indicating assimilation of the central concepts of chronic pain management. However, for example, there are instances in which patients can benefit from adjustment of their home exercise programs. Second, follow-up allows for additional data collection. Outcomes data is of great importance, as even the best ICPM program should consider itself less than perfect and in a process of perpetual evolution. Data from program patients should be analyzed quarterly in order to help the treatment team recognize which elements of the program are succeeding and which need to be reassessed for effectiveness. Positive outcomes data should also be considered a powerful marketing tool, as it is difficult to argue with success. Potential referring physicians may be uninformed regarding the wide range of benefits of interdisciplinary treatment for their patients, and well-organized data may help them understand how a program can make their own lives easier as well as helping their more challenging patients. Additionally, while some health insurance programs may argue against the efficacy of ICPM, data that invalidates their arguments will ideally help convince them of the legitimacy of this treatment approach.

Empirical Support for Interdisciplinary Chronic Pain Management: Clinical Efficacy and Cost-Effectiveness

The methodologically-robust studies supporting not only the clinical efficacy but the cost-effectiveness of ICPM are too numerous to discuss individually. Accordingly, this section of the chapter will focus on the meta-analyses and systematic reviews that provide the discipline with unequivocal empirical support.

The first meta-analysis of ICPM was that performed by Flor and her colleagues[68] in 1992. While their review of 65 studies identified an average pain reduction of only 20%, interdisciplinary treatment programs were found to be effective in reducing medication use, reducing emotional distress, reducing health care utilization, reducing iatrogenic consequences, increasing return to work and physical activity levels, and closing disability claims. Not surprisingly, ICPM programs were determined to be superior to unimodal treatments as well as to no treatment and waiting list controls. The authors also determined that the beneficial effects of the programs appeared to be stable over time. Despite the significance of these findings, Flor and colleagues[68] recommended that they be interpreted with some caution due to inconsistencies in their methodologies and the marginal quality of their research designs and descriptions.

In 1998, Turk and Okifuji[69] performed a comparative analysis of ICPM programs in order to assess their cost-effectiveness as compared to surgery, chronic opioid therapy, and implantable devices. Differences in use of health care services and pain medication along with disability payments were calculated, with the results supporting the strong relative cost-effectiveness of the interdisciplinary approach. Most striking was the finding that ICPM programs were up to 21 times more cost-effective than alternative treatments for chronic pain such as surgery.

Okifuji and colleagues[30] performed a review of the literature on various treatment approaches to chronic pain, analyzing the cost-effectiveness of ICPM in comparison to surgery or conventional medical treatment. ICPM compared favorably to other treatments in terms of pain reduction, management of opioid analgesics, restoration of function as measured by activity levels and return to work, health care utilization, and closure of disability claims. Additionally, the authors dispelled the myth of ICPM representing an expensive approach to pain management, calculating that its use in lieu of the traditional approaches could result in a cost savings of $5 billion per year in the United States. This finding becomes particularly relevant as medicine moves toward "pay for performance" and the controversy regarding the allocation of limited medical resources intensifies.

Turk[70] obtained similar findings in a 2002 review, noting not only that ICPM is comparable to oral medications, surgery, spinal cord stimulation, and intrathecal drug delivery in terms of pain relief, but that interdisciplinary treatment can provide considerable savings in costs for medications and additional health care utilization. The author also noted that the non-ICPM approaches are associated with iatrogenic complications and adverse events, ascertaining the superiority of ICPM in terms of physical functioning, return-to-work rates, and closure of disability claims. Turk's data on cost-effectiveness are dramatic, as he determined that interdisciplinary care is 6.29 times more cost-effective than surgery, 15 times more so than conventional care, and 25 times more cost-effective than spinal cord stimulation.

Hoffman et al.[71] recently performed a meta-analysis of interdisciplinary approaches to chronic pain within the larger context of a meta-analysis of psychologic approaches to chronic low back pain, considering randomized controlled trials from 1982 to 2003. Interdisciplinary treatment was compared to active controls as opposed to passive controls such as waiting lists. Unfortunately, only a small number of outcome measurements were analyzed in this study, although a strength of the meta-analysis was its consideration of posttreatment follow-up (3 to 12 month), and long-term follow-up (more than 12 month) data. Differences between work status of ICPM and active control group patients were statistically significant at follow-up and long-term follow-up, and while pain interference was significantly lower at program completion for patients treated through broad-based approaches, the statistical significance of this difference did not persist through follow-up. Unfortunately, the meta-analysis failed to assess between group differences in work interference at long-term follow-up, which would have been useful given the long-term differences in vocational status that were identified. As a whole, however, this meta-analysis supports the increased function associated with ICPM.

Most recently, Turk and Swanson[29] performed an "analysis and evidence-based synthesis" of the efficacy and cost-effectiveness of medications, surgery, spinal cord stimulation, intrathecal drug delivery systems, and ICPM in the treatment of chronic pain. As was the case in previous reviews, the authors found that all of these approaches resulted in roughly the same amount of pain relief, with only ICPM determined to be essentially free of iatrogenic complications and adverse events, and superior in terms of reducing health care utilization, restoring physical functioning, returning workers to employment, and closing disability claims. Again, ICPM was determined to be numerous times more cost-effective than the other treatments considered in achieving each of these goals.

Perhaps the most compelling empirical support for ICPM is provided by the 2001 and 2002 systematic[72] and Cochrane[73] reviews by Guzman and colleagues and the 2003 Cochrane Review by Schonstein et al.,[74] as these studies involved careful analysis of trial quality. In each of these reviews, the authors determined that ICPM improves pain and function, which was not determined to be the case for less intensive treatments. Not surprisingly, the Cochrane Review by Schonstein and colleagues[74] did not find strong evidence for the efficacy of interdisciplinary treatment for *acute* pain, which is less biopsychosocially-mediated than is chronic pain. Given the complexity of chronic pain, it follows that its treatment requires a more complex, interdisciplinary approach than is necessary for acute pain.[75]

In addition to the meta-analyses and reviews discussed in this section, mention should be made of several individual studies that provide strong support for the efficacy of ICPM, with these investigations examining patients' maintenance of gains achieved through interdisciplinary treatment. Establishment of the long-term efficacy of ICPM is of particular importance given that the duration of the longest randomized controlled trial evaluating chronic opioid therapy is 32 weeks,[76] with the weighted mean duration of such randomized controlled trials determined to be approximately 5 weeks.[70] Reviews of the long-term efficacies of spinal surgery,[77-81] spinal cord stimulation,[82] and intrathecal drug delivery systems[83] have also not been particularly encouraging.

In a 1980 study,[84] severely disabled patients who were treated in an ICPM program were followed for periods ranging from 1 to 8 years. Seventy-seven percent of the treated patients were leading "normal lives" without medication for pain as compared to only 3% of the untreated control groups. Roberts and colleagues[85] performed follow-ups at 8 years on patients treated in an ICPM program. They found that program completers reported significant reductions in pain and higher levels of function at work and at home than those who dropped out of treatment. Lanes et al.[86] followed-up patients with chronic low back pain who were treated in an ICPM at an average of 3.1 years after program completion. They found that 62% of their patients achieved either a good or a fair vocational outcome, and that the majority reported either better or much better general well-being at follow-up than prior to treatment. More recently, Patrick and colleagues[87] performed a 13-year follow up of patients who had been treated at an ICPM program and determined that treatment gains were maintained in all areas assessed (i.e., pain intensity, pain interference, and mood). Additionally, the patients in this study demonstrated levels of general health on most dimensions comparable to peers of similar ages who did not suffer from chronic pain. As a whole, this body of literature suggests that most patients who are treated through an interdisciplinary approach are able to convert short-term learning into long-term lifestyle modification. While the quality of ICPM programs varies, those that strongly emphasize psychoeducational intervention are perhaps more likely to avoid what Turk and Rudy[88] referred to as potential "decay of effect" following completion of treatment.

The Threat to the Viability of Interdisciplinary Chronic Pain Management

As mentioned earlier in this chapter, the number of ICPM programs in the United States has decreased dramatically over the past decade,[28] thereby severely limiting the availability of the treatment for chronic pain for which overall clinical efficacy and cost-efficiency have been most rigorously validated. The demise of the ICPM program is a particularly curious and disturbing phenomenon, particularly given the cost of chronic pain—not only to the individual sufferer, but to society as a whole. In addition to the staggering health care costs associated with chronic pain (estimated at $125 billion annually in 1999),[30] indirect costs such as lost productivity (estimated at $61.2 billion annually in 2003),[89] lost wages, disability compensation, disruption in the work place, and lost productivity of spouses and other caretakers of chronic pain sufferers are also bewildering. For example, it has recently been suggested that disability payments relating to chronic pain may exceed medical costs by a factor of five.[29] Turk[70] estimated that the treatment of chronic pain through ICPM programs in the United States resulted in health care savings of $45 billion annually. As he also noted that only 6% of patients who are treated by pain specialists are fortunate enough to be treated through an interdisciplinary approach, and only 2.5% to 5% of patients with chronic pain are ever treated by a pain specialist,[90] the wholesale development and appropriate utilization of ICPM programs theoretically has the potential to produce savings to society in the *trillions* of dollars annually!

Why would a treatment approach to chronic pain that has been empirically established to be so clinically effective and cost-efficient and that has the potential to help ameliorate suffering on an individual basis and save society as a whole profound sums of money become inaccessible? Schatman[12,13] has examined this paradox from an ethical perspective and identified several potential causes for the demise of the ICPM program.

First, health insurance carriers tend to be "penny wise, pound foolish" in their efforts to contain costs and generate profits. This tendency is somewhat paradoxical, as the insurance industry is certainly aware of the copious body of literature supporting the cost-efficiency of ICPM that has been discussed in this chapter. Aggravating this nonsensical approach is the practice of "carving out" basic treatment components from interdisciplinary programs in an effort to contain costs. Of this practice, Gatchel has recently noted, "This has paradoxically produced the effect of steering patients away from multidisciplinary treatments that demonstrably reduce health-care utilization, and toward more expensive unimodal therapies associated with poorer outcomes."[91] Gatchel and his colleagues[92,93] have performed empirical studies demonstrating the compromised efficacy associated with the carve-out phenomenon. Their research has indicated that physical and psychological functioning as well as vocational outcomes are adversely affected by carve-outs, both at program's completion and at 1-year follow-up. In another study, Gatchel and colleagues[94] conducted a cost-utility analysis of carving-out services from ICPM programs. The authors determined that this "cost-saving" practice of insurers actually resulted in compromised emotional and physical gains, lower reductions in pain, and inferior health-related quality of life, and actually costs more than the intact ICPM program.

Second, it has been noted that, "there is a tendency of third-party payers to expect pain treatment centers to solve all of their (patients') social problems,"[95] not recognizing that even the most effective ICPM program cannot control all outcomes, just as they cannot control all patient and social variables. For example, workers compensation carriers are typically invested in ICPM program patients returning to the work force. In 2000, when the national unemployment rate was below 4%, it was easier to return injured workers to active employment than it was in 2003, when unemployment reached 6%.[96] An example of a patient variable that cannot necessarily be controlled is characterological disturbance. As mentioned earlier in this chapter, a number of studies have identified the overrepresentation of characterologically disturbed patients in the chronic pain population.[58–67] While Schatman[38,39] has elucidated the potential problems associated with treating dramatically characterologically disturbed patients in ICPM programs, the lack of high quality outcome research on the ability of these patients to benefit from interdisciplinary treatment makes their perfunctory exclusion a violation of the bioethical principle of justice. However, experience suggests that personality-disordered chronic pain patients are more likely to experience failure in an ICPM program. Unfortunately, third party payers unrealistically expect interdisciplinary programs to "fix" their patients, regardless of how irreparably "broken" they may be.

Third, pharmaceutical companies have historically marketed medications such as opioids, nonsteroidal anti-inflammatory drugs, and anticonvulsants to health insurance companies as "quick fixes" for chronic pain, despite the lack of empirical evidence supporting monotherapy with medications as more cost-efficient in the long run than ICPM. Similarly, implantable device manufacturers are well-known to market aggressively, despite their lack of an evidence basis for the efficacy and cost-efficiency of their products.

Fourth, the possibility that interventional pain management specialists are becoming progressively less anxious to relinquish control of their patients should be considered. Given decreases in reimbursement for the relatively time-consuming ICPM approach in conjunction with a pattern of higher levels of reimbursement for procedures used to treat chronic pain,[97–99] there exists an increasing fiscal disincentive to refer patients to ICPM programs. Chapman states, "Concurrent with the decline of intensive programs is the rise of procedural interventions and medication, which receives a great deal of support from medical technology and pharmaceutical companies."[100]

Finally, ICPM programs are extremely labor intensive and can only treat a finite number of patients. Accordingly, hospitals in which they are housed do not consider them "cash cows," and accordingly are choosing to discontinue their operation. This is sadly true even in academic medical centers, in which so many of the great ICPM programs once operated. Even "not-for-profit" medical centers have shifted from a professional ethic in which the ethos is amelioration of suffering to the business ethic of cost-containment and profitability. Sadly, it is the patient suffering from chronic pain that is caught between these two "ethical foundations" as ICPM programs continue to close. Schatman[12,13] has addressed the demise of ICPM programs in considerable detail, questioning this unfortunate development from both principle-based and virtue ethics perspectives.

Future Directions: Reviving the Discipline

The quandary with which the field of ICPM is faced is a disturbing and distressing one. In response to perceived helplessness, a number of the top chronic pain management specialists in the United States have chosen to abandon the discipline, while others have chosen to become expatriates, practicing in interdisciplinary settings in the United Kingdom and Canada. Despite criticism regarding these countries' nationalized health care systems, ICPM continues to flourish in these nations, particularly as compared to in the United States. For example, a 2006 study by the British Pain Society[101] indicated that there are 92 ICPM programs in the United Kingdom, serving approximately 60 million inhabitants,[102] thereby producing a ratio of one interdisciplinary clinic for roughly every 650,000 inhabitants. A 2007 study of pain clinics in Canada[103] indicated that there are currently 120 ICPM programs in that country, serving approximately 33 million inhabitants,[104] thereby yielding a ratio of one clinic for every 275,000 inhabitants. While none of the major American pain organizations (e.g., the American Pain Society, the American Academy of Pain Management, the American Society of Pain Educators, the American Academy of Pain Medicine, the American Pain Foundation) was able to provide an estimate in the number of ICPM programs still operating in the United States, a 2005 report aired on ABC's World News Tonight claimed that there were only 200 interdisciplinary clinics in the United States.[105] Based on this number of clinics serving 303 million inhabitants of the United States,[106] the number of inhabitants served by the average ICPM clinic in the United States is approximately 1,500,000. This suggests that access to ICPM in the United States is more than twice as limited as in the United Kingdom, and more than five times as limited as in Canada. Fortifying the argument for superior access to interdisciplinary treatment abroad is the fact that while the number of ICPM clinics in the United States is decreasing rapidly, the number of clinics in the United Kingdom actually increased from 70 in 2001[107] to its 2006 level of 92 such facilities.[101]

Symbolic and specious efforts have been made to improve the quality of pain care in the United States in recent years. For example, the National Pain Care Policy Act[108] was introduced in March of 2005. This bill calls for making adequate treatment, education, and research relating to pain management a national public health priority. One of the bill's provisions is for the development of six government-funded regional pain treatment and research centers. Seemingly, such a program would enhance access to high-quality ICPM. Unfortunately, however, this is not likely to come to fruition. First, the creation of merely six treatment centers when thousands are needed is insufficient. It is true that the National Pain Care Policy Act calls for the development of centers for research as well as for treatment. However, millions of dollars are already being spent at hundreds of institutions across the United States for chronic pain research. Unfortunately, research in the absence of facilities that actually provide treatment that has already been empirically-established as clinically effective and cost-efficient does not serve to solve the chronic pain crisis in the United States. Second, investigation indicates that the bill was referred to the Committees on Energy and Commerce, Ways and Means, Armed Services, and Veterans Affairs, where no action was taken. The National Health Care Policy Act was reintroduced in 2007 as H.R. 2994,[109] and has been referred again to the House Committee on Energy and Commerce. No subsequent action on the bill has been taken, and there is no evidence that this legislation is the top priority of the current (or any) Congress. In an American Pain Society newsletter, Turk[110] suggested that the bill "faces a long and arduous trek through Congress," which is perhaps an understatement. Another spurious and symbolic effort to improve pain care policy in the United States is Congress's declaration of the first decade of the new millennium as the "Decade of Pain Control and Research."[111] It is unlikely that the wholesale closure of ICPM clinics in the United States during this decade represents the most effective effort at pain control. Finally, the campaign to treat pain as "the fifth vital sign" in the current decade by the Joint Commission on Accreditation of Healthcare Organizations has been applied primarily to palliative care, and it is difficult to draw a link between this symptom monitoring practice and the availability of ICPM. Despite these symbolic efforts, the most clinically effective and cost-efficient method for the treatment of chronic pain of benign origin continues to march toward obsolescence.

Accordingly, Schatman[12,13] has suggested that it is the ethical obligation of the federal government to assure that this highest-quality treatment for chronic pain becomes accessible once again—much as the governments of the other "civilized" nations of the world are making efforts to do so. As noted earlier, the cost to society as a whole, as well as to the individual sufferer, is overwhelming. Under the Obama administration, providers of chronic pain care (as well as health care considered more broadly) are hopeful that steps toward nationalized health care will serve to increase the availability of interdisciplinary chronic pain treatment to Americans. Pellegrino[112] has suggested that the moral answer to our health care crisis would be a "mixed economy" in which medical care is removed from the competitive marketplace. He states, "freedom from acute or chronic pain, disability, or disease, is a condition of human flourishing. Human beings cannot attain their fullest potential without some significant measure of health. A good society is one in which each citizen is enabled to flourish, grow, and develop as a human being."[112] Perhaps more so than any other condition, chronic pain robs its victims of the ability to flourish, grow, and develop. ICPM is an approach that cannot become extinct, as it represents the most powerful method that we have to enhance quality of life among those who suffer from chronic pain.

CONCLUSION

The history of ICPM is a rich and distinguished one, as countless patients have experienced relief of their suffering and reclaimed their quality of life through interdisciplinary treatment. Despite substantial and unequivocal empirical support for its clinical utility and cost-efficiency, the number of once abundant programs in the United States has dwindled, resulting in patients being forced to resort to less effective and more expensive treatment

options which tend to focus on body parts as opposed to the person in need. It has been suggested that ICPM needs to be streamlined in order to become consistent with economic realities if the discipline is to survive, with managed care organizations most guilty of advocating "carve-outs."[91] However, practitioners who have seen the dramatic beneficial effects of ICPM programs that are intact question the need to fix a model that is really not broken, as doing so adversely impacts the integrity of the interdisciplinary approach.

Unfortunately, pure capitalism does not necessarily solve every societal problem, and chronic pain is certainly one such example. Despite the opposition to nationalized health care within the medical community,[113–116] no one has offered a realistic proposal other than nationalized health care to solve the growing chronic pain crisis. Government financing and management of ICPM would clearly not be unprecedented, as millions of Americans are treated through Medicare, Medicaid, and the Veteran's Administration systems. It is not surprising that some of the leading ICPM programs in the United States are found within the Veteran's Administration system, which continues to embrace interdisciplinary approaches to medicine.[117–119]

In a presentation at the Eighth World Congress of the International Society for the Study of Pain,[120] the original pioneer of ICPM, John Bonica, was referred to as the "world champion of pain." As chronic pain practitioners, we recognize our fiduciary obligation to advocate on behalf of our individual patients. Unfortunately, doing so in and by itself is no longer necessarily sufficient. Perhaps all of the noble practitioners of the interdisciplinary approach need to become "champions" by sacrificing our time and other available resources to advocate for the preservation of the closest thing to a "cure" for chronic pain that is available to our patients.

References

1. Katz WA. The needs of a patient in pain. *Am J Med* 1998;105:2S–7S.
2. Meldrum ML. A capsule history of pain management. *JAMA* 2003;290: 2470–2475.
3. Bonica JJ. Evolution and current status of pain programs. *J Pain Symptom Manage* 1990;5:368–374.
4. Bonica JJ. Oral history interview. *John C. Liebeskind History of Pain Collection*. Los Angeles, CA: Louise M. Darling Biomedical Library, UCLA; 1993.
5. Meldrum ML. Brief history of multidisciplinary management of chronic pain, 1900–2000. In: Schatman ME, Campbell A, eds. *Chronic Pain Management: Guidelines for Multidisciplinary Program Development*. New York: Informa Healthcare; 2007:1–13.
6. Fordyce WE, Fowler RS, DeLateur B. An application of behavior modification technique to a problem of chronic pain. *Behav Res Ther* 1968;6:105–107.
7. Leff DN. Management of chronic pain: medicine's new growth industry. *Med World News* 1976;54.
8. Loeser JD. Multidisciplinary pain management. In: Merskey H, Loeser JD, Dubner R, eds. *The Paths of Pain, 1975–2005*. Seattle, WA: IASP Press; 2005: 503–511.
9. Aronoff GM, Evans WO, Enders PL. A review of follow-up studies of multidisciplinary pain units. *Pain* 1983;16:1–11.
10. Anooshian J, Streltzer J, Goebert D. Effectiveness of a psychiatric pain clinic. *Psychosomatics* 1999;40:226–232.
11. Aronoff GM. Where have we been? Where are we now? Where are we going? *Clin J Pain* 1997;13:3–5.
12. Schatman ME. The demise of multidisciplinary pain management clinics? *Practical Pain Manage* 2006;6:30–41.
13. Schatman ME. The demise of the multidisciplinary chronic pain management clinic: bioethical perspectives on providing optimal treatment when ethical principles collide. In: Schatman ME, ed. *Ethical Issues in Chronic Pain Management*. New York: Informa Healthcare; 2007:43–62.
14. Engel GL. The need for a new medical model: a challenge for biomedicine. *Science* 1977;196:129–136.
15. Engel GL. The clinical application of the biopsychosocial model. *Am J Psychiatry* 1980;137:535–544.
16. Gatchel RJ, Lou L, Kishino N. Concepts of multidisciplinary pain management. In: Boswell MV, Cole BE, eds. *Weiner's Pain Management: A Practical Guide for Clinicians*. 7th ed. Boca Raton, FL: CRC Press; 2006:1501–1508.
17. Gilbert P. Understanding the biopsychosocial approach: 1. Conceptualisation. *Clin Psych* 2002;14:13–17.
18. Turk DC, Melzack R. The measurement of pain and the assessment of people

experiencing pain. In: Turk DC, Melzack R, eds. *Handbook of Pain Assessment*. 2nd ed. New York: Guildford Press; 2001:3–11.

19. Steen E, Haugli L. Generalised chronic musculoskeletal pain as a rational reaction to a life situation? *Theor Med* 2000;21:581–599.

20. Schatman ME. Psychological assessment of maldynic pain: the need for a phenomenological approach. In: Giordano J, ed. *Maldynia: Inter-disciplinary Perspectives on the Illness of Chronic Pain*. New York: Informa Healthcare; 2009 (in press).

21. Politan PB, Gajraj NM. Integration of pharmacotherapy with psychological treatment of chronic pain. In: Turk DC, Gatchel RJ, eds. *Psychological Approaches to Pain Management: A Practitioner's Handbook*. 2nd ed. New York: Guilford Press; 2002:276–300.

22. Melhorn JM, Kennedy EM. Musculoskeletal disorders, disability, and return-to-work (repetitive strain). In: Schultz IZ, Gatchel RJ, eds. *Handbook of Complex Occupational Disability Claims: Early Risk Identification, Intervention, and Prevention*. New York: Springer Science and Business Media, Inc; 2005: 7–25.

23. Pincus T, Vogel S, Breen A, et al. Persistent back pain—why do physical therapy clinicians continue treatment? A mixed methods study of chiropractors, osteopaths and physiotherapists. *Eur J Pain* 2006;10:67–76.

24. Stanos S, Houle TT. Multidisciplinary and interdisciplinary management of chronic pain. *Phys Med Rehabil Clin N Am* 2006;17:435–450.

25. Costa-Black KM, Durand MJ, Imbeau D, et al. Interdisciplinary team discussion on work environment issues related to low back disability: a multiple case study. *Work* 2007;28:249–265.

26. Stanos S. Developing an interdisciplinary multidisciplinary chronic pain management program: nuts and bolts. In: Schatman ME, Campbell A, eds. *Chronic Pain Management: Guidelines for Multidisciplinary Program Development*. New York: Informa Healthcare; 2007:151–172.

27. Peters JL, Large RG. A randomised control trial evaluating in- and outpatient pain management programmes. *Pain* 1990;41:283–293.

28. Whitney A. Committee on Accreditation of Rehabilitation Facilities. Oral and e-mail personal communication; July 2007.

29. Turk DC, Swanson K. Efficacy and cost-effectiveness treatment for chronic pain: an analysis and evidence-based synthesis. In: Schatman ME, Campbell A, eds. *Chronic Pain Management: Guidelines for Multidisciplinary Program Development*. New York: Informa Healthcare; 2007:15–38.

30. Okifuji A, Turk DC, Kalauoklani D. Clinical outcome and economic evaluation of multidisciplinary pain centers. In: Block AR, Kramer EF, Fernandez E, eds. *Handbook of Pain Syndromes: Biopsychosocial Perspectives*. Mahwah, NJ: Lawrence Erlbaum Associates; 1999:77–97.

31. Baszanger I. Definition of chronic pain and organization of pain centers. *Cah Sociol Demogr Med* 1990;30:75–83.

32. Loeser JD. Multidisciplinary pain programs. In: Loeser JD, Butler SH, Chapman CR, Turk DC eds. *Bonica's Management of Pain*. 2nd ed. Philadelphia: Lippincott Williams & Wilkins; 2001:255–264.

33. Hatzakis M, Schatman ME. The impact of interventional approaches when used within the context of multidisciplinary chronic pain management. In: Schatman ME, Campbell A, eds. *Chronic Pain Management: Guidelines for Multidisciplinary Program Development*. New York: Informa Healthcare; 2007:101–115.

34. Antonuccio DO, Davis C, Lewinsohn PM, et al. Therapist variables related to cohesiveness in a group treatment for depression. *Small Group Behavior* 1987;18:557–564.

35. Spoonhour P, Schatman ME. Development of policies and procedures: assurance of consistent chronic pain management practice. In: Schatman ME, Campbell A, eds. *Chronic Pain Management: Guidelines for Multidisciplinary Program Development*. New York: Informa Healthcare; 2007:189–202.

36. Pellino TA, Willens JS, Polomano RC, et al, and the American Society of Pain Management Nurses. The American Society of Pain Management Nurses role-delineation study. National Association of Orthopaedic Nurses respondents. *Orthop Nurs* 2003;22:289–297.

37. McCaffery M, Ferrell BR, Pasero C. Nurses' personal opinions about patients' pain and their effect on recorded assessments and titration of opioid doses. *Pain Manag Nurs* 2000;1:79–87.

38. Schatman ME. The challenge of the characterologically disturbed chronic pain patient. *Pain Pract* 2003;13:5–7.

39. Schatman ME. Dramatically disturbed patients in interdisciplinary pain programs. *Pract Pain Manage* 2004;4:24–29.

40. Swenson RS. Therapeutic modalities in the management of nonspecific neck pain. *Phys Med Rehabil Clin N Am* 2003:14:605–627.

41. Kay TM, Gross A, Goldsmith C, et al, and the Cervical Overview Group. Exercises for mechanical neck disorders. *Cochrane Database Syst Rev* 2005; 3:CD004250.

42. Arnold LM. Biology and therapy of fibromyalgia. New therapies in fibromyalgia. *Arthritis Res Ther* 2006;8:212.

43. Joines JD. Chronic low back pain: progress in therapy. *Curr Pain Headache Rep* 2006;10:421–425.

44. Gross AR, Goldsmith C, Hoving JL, et al, and the Cervical Overview Group. Conservative management of mechanical neck disorders: a systematic review. *J Rheumatol* 2007;34:1083–1102.

45. Taylor NF, Dodd KJ, Shields N, et al. Therapeutic exercise in physiotherapy practice is beneficial: a summary of systematic reviews 2002–2005. *Aust J Physiother* 2007;53:7–16.

46. Weinstein SM, Laux LF, Thornby JI, et al. Physicians' attitudes toward pain and the use of opioid analgesics: results of a survey from the Texas Cancer Pain Initiative. *South Med J* 2000;93:479–487.

47. Resnick DK. Neuroscience education of undergraduate medical students. Part I: role of neurosurgeons as educators. *J Neurosur* 2000;92:637–641.

48. Potter M, Schafer S, Gonzalez-Mendez E, et al. Opioids for chronic nonmalignant pain: attitudes and practices of primary care physicians in the UCSF/Stanford Collaborative Research Network. University of California, San Francisco. *J Fam Pract* 2001;50:145–151.

49. Mayer TG, Gatchel RJ. *Functional Restoration for Spinal Disorders: The Sports Medicine Approach*. Philadelphia: Lea & Febiger; 1988.

50. Rainville J, Sobel JB, Hartigan C, et al. The effect of compensation involvement on the reporting of pain and disability by patients referred for rehabilitation of chronic low back pain. *Spine,* 1997;22:2016–2024.

51. Wilson KG, Eriksson MY, D'Eon JL, et al. Major depression and insomnia in chronic pain. *Clin J Pain* 2002;18:77–83.

52. Katz RC, Simkin LR, Beauchamp KL, et al. Specific and nonspecific effects of EMG biofeedback. *Biofeedback Self Regul* 1987;12:241–253.

53. Buckelew SP, Conway R, Parker J, et al. Biofeedback/relaxation training and exercise interventions for fibromyalgia: a prospective trial. *Arthritis Care Res* 1998;11:196–209.

54. Nestoriuc Y, Martin A. Efficacy of biofeedback for migraine: a meta-analysis. *Pain* 2007;128:11–127.

55. Haugstad GK, Haugstad TS, Kirste UM, et al. Mensendieck somatocognitive therapy as treatment approach to chronic pelvic pain: results of a randomized controlled intervention study. *Am J Obstet Gynecol* 2006;194:1303–1310.

56. Rose MJ, Reilly JP, Pennie B, et al. Chronic low back pain rehabilitation programs: a study of the optimum duration of treatment and a comparison of group and individual therapy. *Spine* 1997;22:2246–2251.

57. Rainville J, Jouve CA, Hartigan C, et al. Comparison of short- and long-term outcomes for aggressive spine rehabilitation delivered two versus three times per week. *Spine J* 2002;2:402–407.

58. Reich J, Tupin JP, Abramowitz SI. Psychiatric diagnosis of chronic pain patients. *Am J Psychiatry* 1983;140:1495–1498.

59. Fishbain DA, Goldberg M, Meagher BR, et al. Male and female chronic pain patients categorized by DSM-III psychiatric diagnostic criteria. *Pain* 1986;26: 181–197.

60. Polatin PB, Kinney RK, Gatchel RJ, et al. Psychiatric illness and chronic low-back pain. The mind and the spine—which goes first? *Spine* 1993;18:66–71.

61. Gatchel RJ, Garofalo JP, Ellis E, et al. Major psychological disorders in acute and chronic TMD: an initial examination. *J Am Dent Assoc* 1999;127: 1365–1374.

62. Weisberg JN, Keefe FJ. Personality disorders in the chronic pain population: basic concepts, empirical findings, and clinical implications. *Pain Forum* 1997;6:1–9.

63. Monti DA, Herring CL, Schwartzman RJ, et al. Personality assessment of patients with complex regional pain syndrome type I. *Clin J Pain* 1998;14: 295–302.

64. Vittengl JR, Clark LA, Owen-Salters E, et al. Diagnostic change and personality stability following functional restoration treatment in a chronic low back pain patient sample. *Assessment* 1999;6:79–92.

65. Sansone RA, Whitecar P, Meier BP, et al. The prevalence of borderline personality among primary care patients with chronic pain. *Gen Hosp Psychiatry* 2001;23:193–197.

66. Frankenburg FR, Zanarini MC. The association between borderline personality disorder and chronic medical illnesses, poor health-related lifestyle choices, and costly forms of health care utilization. *J Clin Psychiatry* 2004;65:1660–1665.

67. Dersh J, Gatchel RJ, Mayer T, et al. Prevalence of psychiatric disorders in patients with chronic disabling occupational spinal disorders. *Spine* 2006;31: 1156–1162.

68. Flor H, Fydrich T, Turk DC. Efficacy of multidisciplinary pain treatment centers: a meta-analytic review. *Pain* 1992;49:221–230.

69. Turk DC. Okifuji A. Treatment of chronic pain patients: clinical outcomes, cost-effectiveness, and cost-benefits of multidisciplinary pain centers. *Crit Rev Phy Rehab Med* 1998;10:181–208.

70. Turk DC. Clinical effectiveness and cost-effectiveness of treatments for patients with chronic pain. *Clin J Pain* 2002;18:355–365.

71. Hoffman BM, Papas RK, Chatkoff DK, et al. Meta-analysis of psychological interventions for chronic low back pain. *Health Psychology* 2007;26:1–9.

72. Guzmán J, Esmail R, Karjalainen L, et al. Multidisciplinary rehabilitation for chronic low back pain: a systematic review. *BMJ* 2001;322:1511–1516.

73. Guzmán J, Esmail R, Karjalainen L, et al. Multidisciplinary bio-psycho-social rehabilitation for chronic low back pain. *Cochrane Database Syst Rev* 2002; 1:CD000963.

74. Schonstein E, Kenny DT, Keating J, et al. Work conditioning, work hardening and functional restoration for workers with back and neck pain. *Cochrane Database Syst Rev* 2003;1:CD001822.

75. Stanos SP, McLean J, Rader L. Physical medicine rehabilitation approach to pain. *Med Clin North Am* 2007;91:57–95.

76. Ballantyne JC. Problems with chronic opioid therapy and the need for a multidisciplinary approach. In: Schatman ME, Campbell A, eds. *Chronic Pain Management: Guidelines for Multidisciplinary Program Development*. New York: Informa Healthcare; 2007:49–64.

77. Gibson JN, Waddell G, Grant IC. Surgery for degenerative lumbar spondylosis. *Cochrane Database Syst Rev* 2000;3:CD001352.

78. Gibson JN, Grant IC, Waddell G. Surgery for lumbar disc prolapse. *Cochrane Database Syst Rev* 2000;3:CD001350.
79. Fouyas IP, Stratham PF, Sandercock PA, et al. Surgery for cervical radiculomyelopathy. *Cochrane Database Syst Rev* 2001;3:CD001466.
80. Gibson JN, Waddell G. Surgery for degenerative lumbar spondylosis. *Cochrane Database Syst Rev* 2005;4:CD001352.
81. Yi L, Jingping B, Gele J, et al. Operative versus non-operative treatment for thoracolumbar burst fractures without neurological deficit. *Cochrane Database Syst Rev* 2006;4:CD005079.
82. Turner JA, Loeser JD, Deyo RA, et al. Spinal cord stimulation for patients with failed back surgery syndrome or complex regional pain syndrome: a systematic review of effectiveness and complications. *Pain* 2004;108:137–147.
83. Turner JA, Sears JM, Loeser JD. Programmable intrathecal opioid delivery systems for chronic noncancer pain: a systematic review of effectiveness and complications. *Clin J Pain* 2007;23:180–195.
84. Roberts AH, Reinhardt L. The behavioral management of chronic pain: long-term follow-up with comparison groups. *Pain* 1980;8:151–162.
85. Roberts AH Sternbach RA, Polich J. Behavioral management of chronic pain and excess disability: long-term follow-up of an outpatient program. *Clin J Pain* 1993;9:41–48.
86. Lanes TC, Gauron EF, Spratt KF, et al. Long-term follow-up of patients with chronic back pain treated in a multidisciplinary rehabilitation program. *Spine* 1995;20:801–806.
87. Patrick LE, Altmaier EM, Found EM. Long-term outcomes in multidisciplinary treatment of chronic low back pain: results of a 13-year follow-up. *Spine* 2004;29:850–855.
88. Turk DC, Rudy TE. Neglected topics in the treatment of chronic pain patients—relapse, noncompliance, and adherence enhancement. *Pain* 1991;44:5–28.
89. Stewart WF, Ricci JA, Chee E, et al. Lost productive time and cost due to common pain conditions in the US workforce. *JAMA* 2003;290:2443–2454.
90. MarketData Enterprises. *Chronic Pain Management Programs: A Market Analysis.* Valley Stream, NY: MarketData Enterprises; 1995.
91. Gatchel RJ, Kishino ND, Noe C. Carving-out services from multidisciplinary chronic pain management: negative impact on therapeutic efficacy. In: Schatman ME, Campbell A, eds. *Chronic Pain Management: Guidelines for Multidisciplinary Program Development.* New York: Informa Healthcare; 2007: 39–48.
92. Gatchel RJ, Noe CE, Gajraj NM, et al. The negative therapeutic impact on an interdisciplinary pain management program of insurance "treatment carve-out" practices. *J Work Compens* 2001;10:50–63.
93. Robbins H, Gatchel RJ, Noe C, et al. A prospective one-year outcome study of interdisciplinary chronic pain management: compromising its efficacy by managed care policies. *Anesth Analg* 2003;97:156–162.
94. Hatten AL, Gatchel RJ, Polatin PB, et al. A cost-utility analysis of chronic spinal pain treatment outcomes: converting SF-36 data into quality-adjusted life years. *Clin J Pain* 2006;22:700–711.
95. Stieg RL. The cost-effectiveness of pain treatment: who cares? *Clin J Pain* 1990;6:301–304.
96. US Department of Labor. Bureau of Labor Statistics. Available at: http://www.bls.gov/cps/prev_yrs.htm. Accessed October 1, 2007.
97. Lebovits A. Ethics and pain: why and for whom? *Pain Med* 2001;2:92–96.
98. Reiser WS, Brunicardi BO. Assessing the impact of Medicare payment changes. *Health Financ Manage* 2002;56:68–71.
99. Weeks WB, Wallace AE. Long-term financial implications of specialty training for physicians. *Am J Med* 2002;113:393–399.
100. Chapman SL. Chronic pain rehabilitation: lost in a sea of drugs and procedures? *APS Bull* 200;10(Suppl 3):8–9.
101. The British Pain Society. *Pain management programmes SIG secured area.* Available at: http://www.britishpainsociety.org/members_sigs_pmp_secured.htm. Accessed October 1, 2007.
102. World Statesmen. Available at: http://www.worldstatesmen.org/United_Kingdom.html. Accessed October 1, 2007.
103. Peng P, Choiniere M, Dion D, et al, and the STOPPAIN Investigators Group. Challenges in accessing multidisciplinary pain treatment facilities in Canada. *Can J Anaesth* 2007;54:977–984.
104. Statistics Canada. Available at: http://www.statcan.ca/english/edu/clock/population.html. Accessed October 1, 2007.
105. Interstitial Cystitis Association. Café ICA. 2005;5. Available at: http://www.ichelp.org/cafeica/Vol05No04.html. Accessed October 1, 2007.
106. US Census Bureau. US POPClock projection. Available at: http://www.census.gov/population/www/popclockus.html. Accessed October 1, 2007.
107. Peat GM, Moores L, Goldingay S, et al. Pain management program follow-ups: a national survey of current practice in the United Kingdom. *J Pain Symptom Manage* 2001;21:218–226.
108. National Pain Care Policy Act, H.R. 1020. 109th Congress, (2005).
109. National Pain Care Policy Act, H.R. 2994. 110th Congress, (2006).
110. American Pain Society. APS president urges member involvement in grassroots lobbying. *APS E-News* [serial online], 2005;2:4–5. Available at: http://www.ampainsoc.org/enews/september1305/#2. Accessed November 10, 2005.
111. Decade of Pain Control and Research. H.R. 3244. 106th Congress, (2000).
112. Pellegrino ED. The commodification of medical and health care: the moral consequences of a paradigm shift from a professional to a market ethic. *J Med Philos* 1999;24:243–266.
113. Geyman JP. Myths as barriers to health care reform in the United States. *Int J Health Serv* 2003;33:315–329.
114. Gunnar WP. The fundamental law that shapes the United States health care system: is universal health care realistic within the established paradigm? *Ann Health Law* 2006;15:151–181.
115. Menzel P, Light DW. A conservative case for universal access to health care. *Hastings Center Report* 2006;36:36–45.
116. Litow ME. Confronting the fear factor: the coverage/access disparity in universal health care. *Benefits Q,* 2007;23:17–21.
117. Rodin M, Saliba D, Brummel-Smith K, and the American Geriatrics Society Clinical Practice Committee, Department of Veterans Affairs/Department of Defense. Guidelines abstracted from the Department of Veterans Affairs/Department of Defense clinical practice guideline for the management of stroke rehabilitation. *J Am Geriatr Soc* 2006;54:158–162.
118. Howe JL, Witt Sherman D. Interdisciplinary educational approaches to promote team-based geriatrics and palliative care. *Gerontol Geriatr Educ* 2006; 26:1–16.
119. Zilke TM, Morrison RS, Kirby A, et al. Development of an interdisciplinary case management program for combat veterans. *Lippincotts Case Manag* 2006;11:265–270.
120. Liebeskind JC, Meldrum ML. John J. Bonica: world champion of pain. In: Jensen TS, Turner JA, Wiesenfeld-Hallin Z, eds. *Proceeding of the 8th World Congress in Pain Research and Management.* Vol. 8. Seattle, WA: IASP Press; 1997:19–32.

CHAPTER 106 ■ SPINE CLINICS

RALPH F. RASHBAUM, ANDREW R. BLOCK, AND DONNA D. OHNMEISS

INTRODUCTION

Back pain has many different dimensions and is a complex problem. Anatomically, the human spine is a structure of tremendous intricacy, serving functions which, at times, can be contradictory. Consider, for example, the primary roles of the spine—support and flexibility. The spine must be strong enough to keep the body upright. At the same time, the spine must have elastic properties, allowing for broad motion through flexion, extension, and rota-tion. Further, the spine has a protective function, surrounding and cushioning the delicate structures of the spinal cord and nerve roots from damage. The spine is capable of accomplishing these tasks through a conglomeration of bones, joints, tendons, ligaments, discs, nerve tissue, and assorted other structures. Spinal anatomy is complicated by the number of mobile segments, the proximity of the nerve roots, the intricate motions of multiple small joints, and the natural changes that occur with aging. The biomechanics are complex and allow us to perform demanding combined motions such as bending forward and twisting. Also involved in movement are the large muscle groups of the spine. Knowledge of the intricate biochemistry of the intervertebral disc and the role of inflammatory mediators in back pain continues to expand. There is also a significant psychologic component that impacts the behaviors of patients with back pain and their recovery from injury. Considering the complexity of the spine, it is understandable that definitively diagnosing the exact source or sources of symptoms is often difficult or impossible.[1] This task is made even more difficult by the strong impact of personality in reporting and dealing with pain, particularly work-related low back pain.[2]

The spine is continually beset by physical stresses, and, once an individual reaches adulthood, it is in a constant state of degeneration and decline. The very complexity of the human spine creates the conditions that make it so difficult to resolve spine pain. With so many complex and interacting structures, pain can arise from individual structures, multiple structures, or their dynamic interaction. As noted by Jerome Groopman in his best-selling text, *How Doctors Think*,[3] "given all of these structures, the source of the chronic . . . back pain is often a mystery. Doctors can be hard-pressed to identify why a patient is uncomfortable."

Despite its complexity, back pain is a very common problem that severely impacts the lives of many. Using data from the 2002 National Health Interview Survey, Strine and Hootman[4] reported that the 3-month prevalence of back and/or neck pain among adults in the United States was 31%. These subjects generally had more comorbid conditions and greater psychologic distress than did subjects without back or neck pain. As discussed by Fanuele et al.[5] using the SF-36 general health status questionnaire, back pain patients were significantly impaired, even when compared to a variety of other health conditions. In order to effectively treat such patients, one must understand the severity of the problems and appreciate that back pain may often be accompanied by a variety of comorbidities. Chronic back pain is an extremely expensive problem. Many of the patients have failed to gain adequate relief from surgery, and some have suffered injury during the surgery itself. In some patients, the physiologic origin of their pain cannot be definitively determined.

The patient with chronic spine pain is often passed from practitioner to practitioner, often of widely-varying expertise, training, and experience, and each subjecting the patient to their own preferred techniques for palliation. As the patient drifts farther into disability, pain, and medication use, desperation increases, and the cost of single-modality treatments increases in parallel, while the probability of overcoming the pain and of improving function, diminish. It is, according to Groopman, "as though each approach to diagnosis and treatment is essentially a 'franchise' and that too many franchises are battling for control."[3] Such a state of affairs leads to treatments that are increasingly expensive, unfocused, unsubstantiated, and ineffective.

Thus is the complexity of chronic spine pain, and the costly, untenable nature of many treatments. All point to the need for a different approach to chronic spinal pain. The desired approach is no different now from that developed for general chronic pain by Dr. Bonica, and aptly described by Loeser, Turk, and Chapman in the third edition of *Bonica's Management of Pain*.[6] They state that Dr. Bonica:

> . . . brought clinical psychologists, pharmacists and other non-physician providers to the conference table with anesthesiologists, neurologists, physiatrists, neurosurgeons, orthopedic surgeons, psychiatrists and others. This blend of perspectives kept each specialist from exercising specialty-specific tunnel vision, and in conferences a group understanding often emerged that greatly exceeded the understanding that the record would yield after a series of serial consultations.

This is an apt description of the multidisciplinary approach to care. Of course, a multidisciplinary approach alone does not guarantee either efficiency or effectiveness. In order to provide maximally effective and efficient treatment, and to limit treatment costs, a spine treatment facility must include practitioners with the highest levels of training and experience, who follow treatment guidelines that are scientifically-validated yet flexible enough to address the idiosyncrasies of individual patient problems. The care needs to be carefully coordinated to avoid duplication, unnecessary expense, and use of treatments with limited possibility of success. A number of specific principles should guide the multidisciplinary spine facility:

1. Specific algorithms for evaluation and treatment
2. Ongoing multidisciplinary case management and case discussion
3. Active process of continuous quality improvement including outcome measurement, assessment of patient satisfaction, and use of results to improve treatment algorithms
4. Professional education of treatment team members
5. Participation in active research programs

In this chapter, we discuss in the key elements needed to establish and maintain an effective multidisciplinary spine facility.

TREATMENT COMPONENTS

The three major components that comprise the clinical aspects of a multidisciplinary spine center are (1) a group of dedicated, highly-trained physicians and allied health providers with expertise in spine care; (2) a set of treatment algorithms guiding assessment and intervention; and (3) active and aggressive case management, especially when patients fall outside of established treatment algorithms. One of the keys of a successful center is building a team that understands and respects the role and skills of all the other team members.

TREATMENT PROVIDERS

Conservative Care Gatekeepers

Of the many individuals who experience back pain, only about 1% ever undergo spine surgery.[7] It is therefore logical that the initial evaluation of patients presenting to a spine treatment center should be conducted by a "conservative care" physician—one who is specially-trained in the assessment and treatment of spinal disorders. These physicians should be able to triage patients and place them into appropriate assessment and treatment algorithms. Complicated cases and those requiring urgent or emergent intervention can be rapidly identified and referred for appropriate diagnostic procedures and appropriate intervention. However, the majority of cases will be best handled using standard treatment algorithms in which resolution of the injury is expected with minimal intervention. Such physicians may include specialists in anesthesiology, physical medicine and rehabilitation, occupational medicine, or even appropriately-trained and experienced chiropractors.

Pain Management

The most ubiquitous and bothersome indication of spine injury is pain. Unremitting pain, often fluctuating randomly, can decimate both emotional stability and physical capability. As the patient proceeds through treatment at a spine center, it is for pain that the patient most urgently seeks treatment, and it is pain that is most immediately mitigated. Physicians now have a diverse armamentarium of oral and injectable medications that may provide immediate, and at times prolonged, relief. The oral medications are most often opioid analgesics and, even in recently-developed time-release preparations, carry with them both the potential for physical dependence and addiction in up to 40% of chronic pain patients.[8] Targeted injections are of some value in specific conditions (see Chapters 97 and 98 for a detailed discussion), but their use requires sophisticated equipment and advanced training in order to be used safely and effectively. Pain management physicians, often specially-trained anesthesiologists, can effectively use injection therapy, but these treatments must be used in coordination with the other evaluation and treatment efforts, including physical therapy (PT).

Psychology

Patients suffering with spinal injuries and pain experience dramatic emotional and social changes. Up to 80% of patients with persistent spinal pain are diagnosable with clinical depression,[9] and many will express anger as the most common emotion they experience.[10] Fear and avoidance of pain often drive patients into unnecessary functional decline. Marriages and relationships can shatter, and spine injuries often leave economic devastation in their wake. For these reasons, specifically trained psychologists often play a pivotal role within the spine center. Numerous studies have shown that psychosocial factors can complicate recovery from spine surgery (see Block et al.[11] for a review). Thus, one of the major functions played by psychologists is to perform presurgical psychologic screening, providing information to surgeons about the level of psychosocial risk found in patients who are being considered for spine surgery. Such a process allows the surgeon to individualize treatment protocols. In patients who have a high level of identified psychosocial risk, alternatives to spine surgery can be considered. Psychologists often see nonsurgical patients as well, helping them deal with the emotional sequelae of spinal injury and to help them learn new means of coping with pain and its limitations.

Physical Therapy

Many back pain sufferers require little intervention from a physician. Their problems are related to body mechanics and deconditioning. One aspect to PT is that patients often continue the activities they learned during therapy. Many clinics provide patients a home exercise program as their formal treatment period ends. Also, getting into the habit of exercise during PT may encourage patients to continue a more active lifestyle, improving their general health as well as potentially decreasing their back pain.

A conservative approach to the treatment of spine injuries often incorporates PT as a first-line treatment. Frequently, therapists provide the combination of strengthening, stretching, palliative modalities (such as heat or electrical stimulation), and hands-on muscle activation that provide pain relief of such benefit that more intense or even invasive interventions may be avoided. For example, Fritz et al.[12] found that patients with acute spine pain who have high adherence rates to active physical therapy-based exercise programs achieve excellent reductions in disability and pain.

Occupational Therapy

One of the most challenging and costly aspects of back pain is dealing with workplace-related back pain. In many settings, physical therapists take on part of the role of occupational therapists. They can perform structured functional evaluations to determine the patient's current level of performance compared to their job demands.

Spine Surgery

Spine surgery is the topic of many publications, much discussion, and inspiration for developing new implants and operative techniques. Only about 10% of patients seeking care for back pain go on to have surgery. The risks involved, as well as the costs, mandate that surgery is used sparingly and when nonoperative options have failed to provide adequate relief. A spine center of excellence needs a group of well-trained spine specialty surgeons. Although not frequently addressed in the literature, there has been some investigation into the relationship of surgeon experience and complications associated with spine surgery. Wiese et al.[13] found that the complication rate following lumbar microdiscectomy was significantly less among surgeons with a greater level of experience (2.2% vs. 10.7%). In results from a multicenter total disc replacement study, it was reported that among the high-enrolling surgeons and/or centers, the length of hospital stay, operating time, and complication rates were significantly less than among low-enrolling sites.[14] Results of the studies suggest that established spine centers that make use of a team of specialists with varying expertise have an advantage over individual physicians with respect to complication rates. In addition to the spine specialty surgeons, spine specialty operating room staff also contribute to the operative procedure by their familiarity with spinal procedures and instrumentation.

While surgery is sometimes viewed as the "end of the road" in treatment, this should not really be the case. While surgery is a dramatic event, it is only one step in a continuum of care. Treatment does not end with surgery. Most patients who undergo spinal surgery will not have been engaging in typical activities due to pain. Although the surgery may address the structural component of their problem, it cannot address the deconditioning that has occurred. In a spine clinic, there are postoperative rehabilitation protocols for the various types of surgery performed. In this day of escalating surgical options and approaches, physical therapists must gain a clear understanding of each operative intervention and lend their expertise to developing safe and effective rehabilitation protocols that will maximize functional recovery after surgery. For example, a therapist not working closely with spine surgeons may have a difficult time devising the most appropriate and safe program for a patient who has undergone surgery using a nontraditional approach such as the trans-sacral approach to the L5-S1 disc space or extreme lateral interbody fusion for other lumbar discs. Some new procedures require avoidance of specific motions early after surgery with guided progression back to full activity.[15] Without an understanding of the goals and functions of new implants, it is unlikely that a physical therapist working in isolation will be able to design an optimally safe and effective rehabilitation regimen.

One of the advantages of a spine specialty center is the enhanced opportunity for surgeons to participate in clinical trials evaluating new technologies. These centers are often preferred sites due to the expertise of the surgeons and the ability to have a large enough patient population to meet enrollment needs. The benefit to the surgeons is that they can offer patients interventions that would otherwise be unavailable outside of an investigational setting for many years to come. Patients have the benefit of possibly participating in clinical trials if they meet the selection criteria and elect to participate. The multidisciplinary nature of an established spine center offers the optimal atmosphere for testing new and emerging technologies for treating spinal disorders.

Chronic Pain Management Program

The multifaceted nature of spine injuries points to the importance of approaching spine treatment in a multidisciplinary fashion.

After treatment, patients must often resume a life where the very assumptions and boundaries have been greatly distorted, all too often by ongoing pain or marked functional limitations that were not present before illness or injury. With or without surgery for spinal disorders, pain and concomitant limitations often linger and, without proper treatment and planning, these can magnify. The chronic pain management program (CPMP) thus becomes a truly integral component of treatment in most spine centers. Such programs, involving many disciplines (most often physical medicine, physical and occupational therapy, psychology, and others), rely on therapeutic group milieu to assist patients in learning (and helping each other to learn) new ways to deal with pain, minimize its impact on their lives, and to overcome psychosocial barriers. Research on the CPMP approach indicates that patients achieve an average pain reduction of approximately 50%, about 75% are able to get off narcotic medications, and the return to work rate from such programs is approximately 67%.[16] Of course, CPMPs vary widely in terms of their composition and effectiveness. The spine center should, at a minimum, be certified by and adhere to the standards set by the Commission on Accreditation of Rehabilitation Facilities (CARF).

Potential Benefits of a Spine Specialty Clinic

Many components of treating chronic pain of other origins and back pain are similar. What, then, is the advantage of having a spine specialty clinic? Focusing solely on back pain has several potential advantages.

While in the past there may have been more separation between nonsurgical care providers and surgeons, the two can be blended into a comprehensive system. As reported by Rasmussen et al.,[17] the initiation of multidisciplinary "nonsurgical" spine clinics significantly reduced the number of lumbar discectomy surgeries performed. One of the factors that was felt most likely to account for this decline was an improved diagnostic evaluation process.

Considering the wide range of potential pain origins as well as the potential and varying roles of personality factors related to back pain, it is not surprising that patients cover a very broad spectrum of problems and needs. This gives rise to the need for true multidisciplinary care. But also considering these same factors, it is imperative that the care providers have, and maintain, a strong and specific knowledge base regarding spinal disorders. Such skills can only be developed and continually honed by ongoing interaction with back pain patients, continuing professional education, and the cross-training provided by the frequent interaction of professionals from various disciplines caring for similar patients. This is true not only for the physicians involved in the clinic, but also for the physical therapists and other members of the treatment team. By building a strong knowledge base in one area, providers can equip patients with a greater level of education in discussing their spinal problems. With the rapidly increasing knowledge base related to the chemical and biomechanical aspects of back pain, the pain system in chronic pain patients, advances in imaging, the rapid growth of spine surgery treatment options, and the role of diagnostic/therapeutic injections, it will become more and more difficult to keep pace with the current information. As evidenced by the large number of spine-related publications coming into print every month, it may be practically impossible to stay up-to-date if trying to achieve this in a variety of nonspine areas as well.

Specialized spine centers require a large patient population to support all the facets required for the multidisciplinary approach to care. While some painful conditions are relatively rare, back pain is a very common problem. Considering that 80% of people have back pain at some point during their lives and that about 10% go on to develop chronic pain, there are likely to be large enough patient populations in most communities to make a spine center a viable undertaking.

The term "Center of Excellence" is a determination used in several specialties to provide quality assurance for new procedures or technologies or for those surgeries not widely performed, such as video-assisted thoracic surgery.[18] A number of centers of excellence in spine care have emerged in recent years, but there is no uniform set of criteria used to define a spine center of excellence. Such centers have a multidisciplinary treatment philosophy and are committed to providing the highest quality of care. It is these centers of excellence that should be the lead sites in developing treatment guidelines, participating in registries, performing research, and providing education. Implementation of a structured quality assurance program is a critical element of developing a spine center of excellence. Designing and implementing guidelines, assessing outcomes, and implementing changes for improvement may be more manageable in a spine clinic than in a center dealing with multiple problems or in a the setting of an individual practitioner's office. This type of program is becoming increasingly needed in this age of increasing demands for ongoing quality assessment and reimbursement initiatives such as pay for performance.

Within the spine clinic, subspecialization will naturally take place. Based on the interests and skills of the professionals involved with patient care, various physicians will gravitate toward treatment of specific spinal disorders. For example, one may take the majority of patients with unusually challenging cervical spine problems, another may be a leader in one or more areas of spine arthroplasty, and there should be at least one surgeon adept at diagnosing the multiply operated failed back patient who eventually arrives at a spine specialty facility. Some physicians may elect to perform injections while others do not. There is a need for advanced interventions such as spinal cord stimulation for pain management. This type of subspecialization within a spine clinic further provides the care provider the opportunity to hone highly specialized skills as well as allowing them to pursue the interventions they are most interested in providing.

The presence of professionals from multiple disciplines in a spine clinic will also increase awareness about alternate pain mechanisms and approaches to treatment. For example, the addition of chiropractic care providers will increase the awareness of all the care providers of problems arising from the sacroiliac joint and the role of manipulative therapy in treating this group of patients with low back pain.

Coordination of Care

Working one's way through most health care systems can be daunting for patients. A comprehensive spine clinic can reduce confusion and anxiety. Patients can receive a wide variety of services as needed within a single facility. Patients receiving treatment in a single center will become familiar with employees, and they will find less redundant paperwork required for insurance and providing basic history and health data. The best spine centers provide close coordination of care from one provider to another through close communication.

Research and Education

If practicing in a university setting, education and research are built into the framework and environment of patient care. However, the success of programs still depends strongly on the commitment made by the individuals involved. While this is also true in private practice, the challenges are greater. There is no institutional framework or incentive built into the practice that promotes involvement in either research or education. To create a research environment outside the university setting requires a commitment of time and financial resources. However, a practice cannot hope to become a spine care center of excellence without incorporating research and education. The implementation of a research program is becoming easier with the growing use of electronic medical records and registry systems in spine care facilities. Establishing an infrastructure for data collection compliments the current demands for evidence-based medicine and cost-effectiveness information for back pain interventions. Considering the societal costs associated with back pain, these demands may be even greater for spine care specialists than for other disciplines. While in the past, care providers may have been able to be successful without engaging in organized data collection, this is likely to change. Research also provides a venue to gain recognition in the peer group. This is more easily accomplished in a specialty clinic than in one spread across multiple specialties, unless focused efforts can be made in multiple areas.

The increasing use of electronic medical records and national study registries in spine has greatly facilitated tracking treatment outcomes. Although these mechanisms are far superior to traditional paper data collection, they still require time to harvest the data, address unanticipated scenarios, download, analyze, and prepare reports of the data, and write abstracts and manuscripts. One of the greatest advantages of the registries is that some are programmed to contact patients by e-mail up to 24 months after treatment and have patients complete self-assessment forms online without returning to the clinic. Although radiographic follow-up cannot be achieved, the patient's clinical condition can be evaluated.

Another opportunity to become active in spine research is through participation in clinical trials. To do so is a great responsibility for the investigator to ensure that the trials are being conducted in accordance to federal regulations and study protocols. Staff should be hired with experience in conducting clinical trials, regulatory requirements, and experience interacting with institutional review boards or human experimentation ethics committees. Many such trials are financially self-sustaining, as industry sponsors will provide the funding to cover the cost of conducting the trial. Participation in such studies provides the framework for rigorous data collection.

Research is a vital part of quality patient care. Although all care providers want to take the best care of their patients, without measuring and being willing to critically appraise their own outcomes it is impossible for the individual practitioner to assess and improve the quality of care they are delivering. Through the collection of data and ongoing assessment of results, problems, such as spikes in particular complication rates, can be identified and addressed. This is particularly important in a multiple physician group to assess the complications and clinical outcomes of all the care providers in the practice and to ensure that problems are addressed as soon as they are identified.

Accepting the role of serving as faculty for a residency program or establishing a fellowship program can also enhance the intellectual environment of a spine clinic. Such programs often lead to creating lecture series such as grand rounds and journal clubs, which are relatively inexpensive. Creating forums for discussion among all care providers in the group can strengthen the bonds of the practice, allow more insight into what the other team members' discipline offer to overall care, and can enhance care by getting the right patient to the right provider more quickly.

Spine specialty centers have the potential to step to the forefront in shaping the future of spine care on a large-scale basis. Being specialized and focused in one area makes it easier to participate in registry networks and other quality improvement initiatives.

CONCLUSION

The spine is a very complex structure that presents a diagnostic and treatment challenge. The complexity is compounded by the frequent and profound psychologic impact of chronic spinal disorders. A spine center of excellence must be designed to address the complexity of these challenges. One of the primary needs is an organized, deliberately planned approach to the evaluation and treatment of the broad spectrum of back pain patients. The multidisciplinary team must be trained and focused on quality spine care. The use of electronic medical records greatly enhances the ability to track patients and events related to their care. The team of providers must understand the role of the other team members and respect what each has to offer in providing quality care to patients. There must be strong leadership to keep the team focused and functioning well.

Part of developing a center of excellence is incorporating research and education. Research efforts can provide patients and practitioners with the opportunity to participate in clinical trials which can enhance the reputation of the center in the community while at the same time providing a means to assess outcomes of various treatments provided in the clinic. Only through incorporating research can providers have access to the latest technology. Everyone benefits from education. This can take on many forms including lectures, journal clubs, fellowship programs, and conducting research.

References

1. Hazard RG. Low-back and neck pain diagnosis and treatment. *Am J Phys Med Rehabil* 2007;86:S59–S68.
2. Pincus T, Burton AK, Vogel S, Field AP. A systematic review of psychological factors as predictors of chronicity/disability in prospective cohorts of low back pain. *Spine* 2002;27:E109–E120.
3. Groopman J. *How Doctors Think New York*. New York: Houghton Mifflin Company; 2007.
4. Strine TW, Hootman JM. US national prevalence and correlates of low back and neck pain among adults. *Arthritis Rheum* 2007;57:656–665.
5. Fanuele JC, Birkmeyer NJ, Abdu WA, et al. The impact of spinal problems on the health status of patients: have we underestimated the effect? *Spine* 2000; 25:1509–1514.
6. Loeser JD, Butler S, Chapman CR, et al. *Bonica's Management of Pain*. 3rd ed. Philadelphia: Lippincott Williams & Wilkins; 2001.
7. Scientific approach to the assessment and management of activity-related spinal disorders. A monograph for clinicians. Report of the Quebec Task Force on Spinal Disorders. *Spine* 1987;12:S1–S59.
8. Martell BA, O'Connor PG, Kerns RD, et al. Systematic review: opioid treatment for chronic back pain: prevalence, efficacy, and association with addiction. *Ann Intern Med* 2007;146:116–127.
9. Lindsay PG, Wyckoff M. The depression-pain syndrome and its response to antidepressants. *Psychosomatics* 1981;22:571–573, 576–577.
10. Fernandez E, Clark TS, Ruddick-Davis D. A framework for conceptualization and assessment of affective disturbance in pain. In: Block AR, Kremer E, Fernandez E, eds. *Handbook of Pain Syndromes: Biopsychosocial Perspectives*. Mahwah, NJ: Lawrence Erlbaum Associates; 1999.
11. Block AR, Gatchel RJ, Deardorff WW, et al. *The Psychology of Spine Surgery*. Washington, DC: American Psychological Association; 2003.
12. Fritz JM, Cleland JA, Brennan GP. Does adherence to the guideline recommendation for active treatments improve the quality of care for patients with acute low back pain delivered by physical therapists? *Med Care* 2007;45:973–980.
13. Wiese M, Krämer J, Bernsmann K, et al. The related outcome and complication rate in primary lumbar microscopic disc surgery depending on the surgeon's experience: comparative studies. *Spine J* 2004;4:550–556.
14. Regan JJ, McAfee PC, Blumenthal SL, et al. Evaluation of surgical volume and the early experience with lumbar total disc replacement as part of the investigational device exemption study of the Charité Artificial Disc. *Spine* 2006;31:2270–2276.
15. Ozgur BM, Aryan HE, Pimenta L, et al. Extreme Lateral Interbody Fusion (XLIF): a novel surgical technique for anterior lumbar interbody fusion. *Spine J* 2006;6:435–443.
16. Turk DC, Burwinkle TM. Assessment of chronic pain in rehabilitation: Outcomes measures in clinical trials and clinical practice. *Rehabil Psychol* 2005; 50:56–64.
17. Rasmussen C, Nielsen GL, Hansen VK, et al. Rates of lumbar disc surgery before and after implementation of multidisciplinary nonsurgical spine clinics. *Spine* 2005;30:2469–2473.
18. Chin CS, Swanson SJ. Video-assisted thoracic surgery lobectomy: centers of excellence or excellence of centers? *Thorac Surg Clin* 2008;18:263–268.

CHAPTER 107 ■ PAIN MANAGEMENT IN PRIMARY CARE

BILL MCCARBERG

INTRODUCTION

Prevalence of Pain in the United States

Pain is the most common reason cited for patients seeking medical care. Statistics reveal that pain accounts for up to 80% of total visits to physicians' offices.[1,2] In most cases, the patient understands the underlying disease process (e.g., pharyngitis, gastroenteritis, migraine headache). Pain associated with these disorders causes the patient to seek help from his or her physician. Although it is difficult to determine the prevalence of pain in exact numbers, recent surveys suggest that 75–105 million Americans experience pain daily or intermittently.[3–5] Pain management remains an elusive and frustrating goal despite a growing knowledge about the pathophysiology of pain. Taken together, the management of persistent pain in primary care is a complex enterprise.

Financial Implications of Chronic Pain

In 1992, Fishman and colleagues[6] studied a large managed care organization in the Pacific Northwest and followed the costs of medical care for 18 of the most common conditions seen in primary care. Of these 18 conditions, four were described as painful: neck pain, back pain, facial pain, and headache (excluding arthritis). The analysis found stroke to have the highest annual cost at $13,139 per diagnosis, followed by human immunodeficiency virus/acquired immunodeficiency syndrome (HIV/AIDs) ($10,246), dementia ($9824), and cancer ($8992).

Individually, the painful conditions were associated with relatively low annual costs: back and neck pain at $4226, facial pain at $4088, and headache at $4989. Despite these relatively low costs, the group of conditions described as painful were highly prevalent. Taking into account cost and prevalence, pain was the most costly of the 18 conditions with total annual health care costs of $198 million, followed by heart disease ($170 million), hypertension ($112 million), respiratory disease ($90 million), diabetes ($86 million), cancer ($55 million), stroke ($38 million), and HIV/AIDs ($4 million). More than 15 years later, the frequency of these disorders may be similar but the cost is almost certainly much higher.

Care management plans and disease management programs are abundant for other chronic conditions, such as asthma, hypertension, hyperlipidemia, and diabetes mellitus. Treatment strategies include case management, treatment algorithms, provider education, and patient support groups. In contrast, very little emphasis has been placed on studying and developing such initiatives for the group of conditions described as painful. Given the large allocation of U.S. health care dollars for treating patients with these conditions, it is time for the provider, payer, and policy maker communities to take notice.

Chronic Pain Management: The Status Quo

With the onset of pain, most patients attempt self-care with over-the-counter products and/or self-help techniques (e.g., distracting activities, rest). When these methods fail to afford adequate relief, the patient generally seeks help from a medical professional. In many cases, and particularly in health care systems with limited access to specialty care, the gatekeeping primary care provider is the first medical contact. The primary care provider recommends treatment and refers the patient for appropriate specialty care, such as a physical medicine assessment for low back pain.

When pain becomes chronic and specialty care is ineffective in improving the underlying condition, care management becomes more difficult. In a recent survey, only 34% of internists reported that they felt comfortable with their abilities to manage patients with chronic pain.[7] In a related article, Ballantyne wrote that the most difficult issue now facing physicians is, "whether and how to prescribe opioid therapy for chronic pain that is not associated with terminal disease, including pain experienced by the increasing number of patients with cancer in remission."[8] In part, physicians are hesitant to prescribe opioids because they lack both the understanding of how to accurately assess pain and the knowledge of available pain therapies.

Primary care physicians struggle with unexplained variability among pain patients. Physical abnormalities are not predictive of pain severity or dysfunction.[9] Large numbers of patients experience pain that may be constant, over long periods of time, and yet their life functioning is not changed in major ways. Conversely, there are other patients with similar structural abnormalities who suffer substantially more and cannot maintain their usual levels of activity.[10] Patients whose lives are significantly disrupted by pain engage in behaviors that are maladaptive, anticipate more distress, amplify sensations associated with pain, spend more time resting, and complain of less ability to control pain.[11,12]

At the same time, surveys evaluating the adequacy of pain treatment demonstrate that the current system is broken.[13] Patients report that they are not asked about pain, that they are afraid to report pain to their primary care providers, and that they are often not offered treatment. In one recent survey, 22% of pain patients reported being uncomfortable discussing pain with their personal physicians, 13% said they were denied pain medication or referrals to pain specialists, and 70% reported experiencing continued pain despite treatment.[14] Much of this system failure can be attributed to the treatment at the primary care level.

Searching for Solutions

There have been tremendous advances in the knowledge of pain pathophysiology, the understanding of treatments for pain, and recognition of the value in an interdisciplinary approach to pain management. On the scientific front, there has been an explosion in pain research, and new pharmaceutical agents have become available for treating different types of pain. Complementary and alternative therapies for pain management have gained recognition. Novel interventional techniques and surgeries have been introduced. Professional pain societies have sprung up and training is now available to provide physicians and other health care professionals with expertise in pain management. Despite this unprecedented progress, pain care remains grossly inadequate and undertreatment of pain is still considered pandemic. The reasons for this continuing failure are varied, but it is clear that new solutions must focus on primary care.

A NEW APPROACH TO CHRONIC PAIN MANAGEMENT

Primary care is distinguished by familiarity with a wide variety of medical conditions yet proficiency in very few, if any. There are so many different types of pain that it is difficult for a nonexpert provider to become familiar with and comfortable treating pain. Current categories for classifying pain include nociceptive versus neuropathic, acute versus persistent, cancer versus noncancer, and area of the body (headache, abdominal pain, chest pain). These categories are simplistic and helpful only in a general way.

It is also difficult to assess the adequacy of treatment for pain in primary care. We are accustomed to accepted, well-defined, objective measurements. For many other chronic conditions, there are standardized outcome measures. In the diabetic, we can measure hemoglobin A_1C levels. In asthmatics, peak flow and the use of inhaled β agonists guide care. Treatment outcomes for pain are often subjective and confusing. If a patient's pain is better but function is not, is this outcome adequate? If the patient is satisfied with treatment but pain levels remain at 8–9/10, is this treatment sufficient? If the patient returns to work but is on high doses of opioids, is this acceptable? All of these questions, common in a specialty practice, complicate treatment in primary care.

Who Treats Chronic Illness?

When pain becomes chronic, a behavioral syndrome often emerges including depression, anxiety, helplessness, insomnia, deconditioning, and increased reliance on the health care system. At this point, chronic pain becomes a disease process that is amenable to disease management.[15] Chronic back pain is not a diagnosis but rather a description of duration and location. In many cases, it is not possible to be more precise in the diagnosis of low back pain since even experts disagree on the underlying etiology.[16]

Failure to be more precise in the diagnosis should not delay treatment or impede medical management. Treatment in primary care often involves uncertainty, as most of the conditions encountered cannot be diagnosed precisely: viral illness, rash, or headaches are common. Chronic pain falls into the group of conditions that defies definitive diagnosis and is suited to the primary care practice. A patient's suffering can be ameliorated by well-documented, nonpharmacologic interventions including patient education and self-help skills as well as nonspecific analgesics such as nonsteroidal anti-inflammatories and opioids.

All primary care physicians must treat patients with a variety of chronic diseases. In fact, most chronic illness is principally managed at the primary care level (Table 107.1).[17] Improvements in the medical management of asthma, hypertension, and diabetes have arisen from interventions implemented at primary care. Despite lack of expertise, the use of practice guidelines, treatment recommendations, chart reviews, shared experience, and expert assistance, primary care provides excellent medical supervision. Management of persistent pain lends itself to the same paradigm.

TABLE 107.1

CHRONIC CONDITIONS TREATED BY PRIMARY CARE PHYSICIANS VERSUS OTHER SPECIALISTS

Condition	Treated by primary care physicians	Treated by other specialists
Arteriosclerotic Cardiovascular Disease	86%	14%
Stroke	91%	9%
Hypertension	92%	8%
Diabetes Mellitus	90%	10%
Chronic Obstructive Pulmonary Disease	89%	11%
Asthma	94%	6%

A survey of 74 administrators who control the decisions in a variety of health plans representing 2200 to 2.5 million covered lives[18] reflected the widely held belief that chronic pain patients are best treated using a model similar to those used for other chronic conditions. These administrators also felt that primary care was best suited to deal with the majority of patients with chronic pain.

Why Primary Care is Involved

Primary care is based on the elements of trust, advocacy, and quality of life/lifestyle issues. In the primary care setting, patient nonadherence is common and expected. Persuading patients to strive for better health through exercise, diet, stress management, medication adherence, and disease monitoring is a common role for the primary care provider—a role that requires the provider to adopt and maintain a nonjudgmental attitude.

Primary care is uniquely positioned to provide care for patients with chronic pain. Of all specialties, primary care providers have the largest geographic distribution. Rather than clustering around medical centers in the largest cities, they are broadly distributed over diverse communities—from urban clinics to suburban medical centers to private practices in small towns and rural areas.

By its very nature, primary care entails developing a longitudinal experience with patients. Each office visit enables the provider to achieve greater understanding of how individual patients are dealing with their persistent pain. Primary care providers are experienced in providing comfort and disease management for conditions that have no cure. When clinicians are challenged to broaden their definition of pain as a symptom and begin to view it as an illness,[11] primary care is equipped to deal with all aspects of that illness.

When a patient's pain becomes persistent and specialty care becomes less effective as a treatment option, the providers can continue to play a key role by coordinating care, intervening when symptoms change, and constantly encouraging patients on lifestyle choices as they do in all other chronic diseases: weight loss, sleep hygiene, career change, anxiety/depression/anger management, conditioning, acceptance, and judicious use of medications.[19]

From a cost and utilization perspective, primary care is the appropriate setting for chronic pain management. Most types of health insurance, as well as Medicare and Medicaid, cover primary care visits yet may not cover long-term psychosocial treatment or interventional treatment. A 1995 low back pain study looked at 1555 patients cared for by chiropractors, orthopaedic surgeons, or primary care providers. Cost, work status, and time to restoration of baseline status were monitored. All groups achieved similar outcomes yet primary care was the least costly.[20]

Risks of polypharmacy are better managed within the primary care structure since it is accustomed to dealing with multiple diseases in a single patient.

Treating Chronic Pain in the Primary Care Setting—Why a Challenge?

Training in Pain

Much of formal medical training occurs in hospitals where acute symptoms and life-threatening conditions are studied. Very little practice is offered in the management of chronic pain in the outpatient setting. Training in pain management is generally limited to a brief session in a pharmacology or neuroanatomy course.

Medical school and residency fail to include practical pain management (e.g., use of opioids, polypharmacy, behavioral issues) which is essential for effective chronic pain supervision. Many of the issues that are critical to pain management differ from other chronic diseases. These issues—informed consent, nonadherence concerning analgesics, documentation, practice protection—are also not included in most medical curricula. Practical discussions about opioids does occur in the emergency room or on the hospital wards but this is often by word of mouth from supervising physicians, nurses, or other students. Myths and dogma arise from traditions handed down from resident to intern.

As a consequence of this lack in training, most graduating primary care providers are ill-equipped and therefore uncomfortable treating patients with persistent pain.[21] This often leads to undertreatment of the patient's pain.

Disagreement Among Experts—To Treat and Not to Treat

In recognition of the need to improve pain management, the Federation of State Medical Boards issued guidelines on the appropriate work up and treatment of persistent pain.[22] Most states have adopted the Federation recommendations in the form of Intractable Pain Acts. The safe and proper use of opioids is the cornerstone of these acts, encouraging providers to ask patients about pain and use medication when necessary. Increasingly, adequate pain relief is being viewed as a patient's right—and a physician's obligation—sometimes to the point of allowing the patient or family to take legal action against doctors for undertreatment of pain. On the other hand, opioids are now the most prescribed drug in the United States and the most common new drug of abuse.[23] This has led to a rise in new cautions in treating pain.

Despite medical board encouragement and Intractable Pain Acts, providers may be faulted for prescribing opioids. Doctors feel uncertain and uncomfortable caring for persistent pain since underprescribing and overprescribing can lead to legal consequences. The appropriate use of medication is not understood and felt to be risky for all patients.

Barriers to Treating Pain

Many barriers to the management of pain have been well documented in this text and others.[24] These obstacles include relating to the medical system, providers, patients, and regulatory and governmental agencies (Table 107.2).

All of these barriers are operant in primary care practices. At the same time, other obstacles are unique to primary care, making pain management more difficult even for the well-trained, conscientious provider.

Time Constraints. Primary care providers are under constant pressure to do more in less time. With cuts in reimbursement (Medicare, Medicaid, and other types of commercial insurance), a primary care provider's income is only maintained by increasing his or her work load. The 15-minute office visit must include other activities: telephone calls, add-on appointments, emergencies, hospital admissions, serving as preceptor for students or midlevel providers (i.e., interns, residents, nurse practitioners), and reviewing laboratory and x-ray reports.

Patients present with multiple medical complaints at each visit and expect the primary care provider to deal with each one. These complaints range from chronic conditions (diabetes, hypertension, and hypercholesterolemia), situational issues (insomnia, stress at work, menopausal symptoms), preventive care (immunizations, ordering a mammogram), procedures (skin tag removal, knee injections), and other issues (medication refills, disability forms, jury excuses, handicapped parking).

Comprehensive assessment and documentation would be difficult in this setting even if the entire 15 minutes were available for the visit. Because of the need for more documentation as part of the assessment and treatment, effective pain management requires more time than any other chronic disease process.

Lack of Adequate Guidelines. A variety of well-recognized treatment algorithms and evidence-based guidelines exist for treating other chronic conditions encountered by primary care physicians (e.g., cancer,[25] neuropathy,[26] fibromyalgia syndrome[27]). Although guidelines have been developed for some pain problems, there are relatively few specific recommendations for the treatment of persistent pain.

Even when guidelines are available, studies show that often they are not followed.[28] This can be explained in part by the nature of chronic pain. When a patient's chronic pain worsens,

---

TABLE 107.2

BARRIERS TO MANAGEMENT OF PAIN

Medical System	Access to medical care	Access to specialists	Denied coverage of medication or procedures	Denied coverage of CAM therapy*	Preauthorization requirements
Patients	Poor lifestyle choices	Fear to accept proven treatment	Expectation of cure	Stigma of psychiatric care	Beliefs about aging
Providers	Lack of Knowledge	Bias toward treatment	Failure to refer	Nialistic care	Beliefs about aging
Regulatory and Governmental Agencies	Lack of Medicare reimbursement	Oversight of opioid prescribing			

*CAM, complementary and alternative medicine.

the cause is frequently undiscoverable, making it difficult to apply a guideline or to decide on a different treatment when so many therapeutic options have been ineffective.

Patient Nonadherence to Treatment. In other diseases, the consequences of nonadherence are not apparent to the patient. Patients with worsening atherosclerosis, hypertension, or diabetes are very often asymptomatic. In contrast, nonadherence to medical management has serious implications for patients with persistent pain and their physicians. These include:

■ Conflict—Nonadherence to recommended therapy may lead to increases in a patient's need for opioid medication. Conflicts also arise from patients requesting their physician's assistance in such matters as handicapped parking permits, disability claims, and failure to return to work.

■ Risk—A physician's practice may become the target for investigation if patients are identified as overusing or abusing opioid drugs. Physicians are also at risk for enabling patients with persistent pain—facilitating the illness-related behavior rather than consistently encouraging a return to healthy behavior. On the flip side, physicians are not immune to the common suspicion/assumption that an individual's pain complaints are driven by secondary gain (e.g., substance abuse, disability, lawsuits, withdrawal from society, sympathy).

Specialty Referrals. Referrals for patients with persistent pain are unlike any others in primary care practice. A typical referral returns the patient to the primary care provider after the medical issue has resolved or the chronic illness has an understood treatment course. Dysfunctional uterine bleeding is diagnosed and treated before referral back to primary care. The fractured bone is set and stabilized, rehabilitation is arranged, and the patient presents back to primary care with restored function. The congestive heart failure patient has further testing, medication adjustments, and returns to primary care when symptoms have improved and the patient is stable.

The work up and treatment of the persistent pain patient, on the other hand, is very different and varies widely. The acupuncturist diagnoses an imbalance of energy and treats with needles and herbs. The physiatrist may focus on muscle tightness, nerve injury, and offers rehabilitative therapies. The interventionalist uses injections. The chiropractor focuses on structural imbalance of the skeleton and offers manipulation therapy.

Often the diagnoses and procedures for chronic pain are foreign to the primary care provider (e.g., disc disruption, discogram, vertebroplasty, facet arthritis, radiofrequency ablation), instilling a sense that primary care is less than competent in dealing with future patients. Unfamiliar drugs and drug combinations are awkward for physicians to prescribe and monitor. These may include polypharmacy with four or five drugs, combinations of multiple anticonvulsants, multiple opioids, and/or other analgesics, drugs rarely prescribed (e.g., methadone), and doses not used (e.g., high dose opioids or gabapentin).

After referral, patients return to primary care with unclear parameters on what constitutes success. Too often, the patient's pain level is as high as when first referred for specialty care. Psychosocial issues such as depression and anxiety have not been addressed. Monitoring patient behavior associated with opioid use is not well defined. Decisions regarding patient demands for early refills, when to do urine drug testing, how to interpret urine drug test results, and how frequently to schedule follow-up visits can be difficult and uncomfortable.

Comorbid Conditions. The most commonly occurring comorbid conditions in patients with persistent pain are depression, anxiety, insomnia, and substance abuse.[29] These comorbidities complicate care. Patients may resist psychiatric care for many reasons including the perceived stigma, the additional cost, or the belief that their pain is unrelated to the comorbidities.

Pain makes depression worse and depression makes pain worse, both independently.[30] Patients seeking relief from the pain and comorbid conditions may self-medicate with alcohol and other substances such as marijuana, which compounds the problem. They may take prescribed pain medications to treat the comorbid condition, which makes them feel worse.

Failure to address underlying anxiety, depression, insomnia, and substance abuse makes pain treatment more difficult. These comorbid conditions are difficult to treat in stable patients. When persistent pain or a chronic illness is also present, the treatment is even more complicated. It is not likely that a simple, single drug regimen or series of epidural steroid injections will be the long-term solution.

Adversarial Relationship. Medical practice in primary care is built on trust, respect, and advocacy for the patient. The doctor-patient relationship develops over years of providing preventive care, treating acute conditions, and supporting the patient through life transitions such as the birth of a child, the loss of employment, and the death of a close family member. This long-term relationship enables the primary care physician to acquire an understanding of the patient as an individual and allows the physician to better guide the patient through the complexities of medical care.

Persistent pain disrupts the normal pattern and creates an unusual relationship that is not seen in other chronic diseases. The primary care provider may at times feel forced into an uncomfortable adversarial position that he or she is not well trained to manage. Patients with chronic pain ask for many things that at times the physician must argue against or deny. The doctor-patient relationship can become tumultuous on many levels:

■ The patient asks to go on disability and the doctor knows that the longer the patient is out of work the less likely it is that he or she will ever return to gainful employment.

■ The patient asks for a medical excuse from jury duty. The doctor knows that the patient is not working, sitting at home, and is capable of fulfilling his or her civic responsibility.

■ The patient wants to solve his or her problem by getting permanent handicapped license plates. The doctor knows that it is in the patient's best interest to be more active. Parking farther away from the store and walking may provide needed exercise.

■ The patient wants the doctor to order additional or repeated expensive procedures (e.g., magnetic resonance imaging [MRI]) when his or her pain worsens. The doctor refuses because it will not change the treatment or lead to a cure for the persistent pain, and it is disallowed by the patient's health insurance plan.

■ The patient demands more expensive, nonformulary drugs, often the latest new drug being advertised directly to consumers. The doctor argues that the drug is unlikely to be more effective than many generic alternatives and would not be approved by the patient's health insurance.

■ The patient researches "miracle" treatments and cures on the Internet and presents the doctor with printed testimonials. The doctor knows that a majority of these treatments are unproven or perhaps dangerous.

In each of the scenarios described above, the doctor's role is to argue against the patient's wishes. When the doctor is unable to be supportive, the patient begins to question whether his or her "advocate" still wants to help. Often, the patient-doctor relationship becomes strained and the patient may resist potentially beneficial treatment options.

ADDRESSING BARRIERS TO CARE

As mentioned earlier in this chapter, primary care physicians are often uncomfortable treating patients with persistent pain. In addition to a relative lack of knowledge, there are a number of other underlying reasons for this.

Myths and Biases

Patients—Without conscious intention, people attach meaning to all sensory experiences. The smell of a rose may hold a special meaning to someone who received her first bouquet for the high school prom. The sound of the musical tune "Jingle Bells" may signify happiness, family gatherings, and holiday gifts. Pain, especially when it is persistent, often conveys a sense that the person is being punished for some real or perceived infraction. The common idioms associated with pain seem to confirm this understanding: "no pain, no gain," "you need to feel this," and "offer it up."

Too often, patients with chronic pain believe that they suffer because of some mistake they made (i.e., "I had a hard life, Doc. Of course I have pain.") or that pain is to be expected as a part of aging. There is so much meaning attached to pain, sometimes of a religious nature, that it is difficult to convince the patient otherwise. These beliefs about "needing pain" or "deserving pain" complicate treatment.

Providers—Primary care providers are suspicious of patients who complain of pain. Physicians understand certain types of pain—cancer pain, end of life pain, or acute trauma/illness pain—but are less accepting of the persistent pain that has few objective signs of defined conditions. We ask, "Why do some patients complain while others, with the same pathology or anatomy, do not complain?" "What is the secondary gain?" "Is this pain real?"

When pain is not easily explained, bias leads the primary care provider to suspect psychiatric causes. In addition, psychiatric comorbidities are common with persistent pain. Although specialists are more likely to understand the connection between anatomy and psychiatry, the primary care provider may believe that the persistence of the pain relates directly to the depression or anxiety thereby depreciating the pain complaint. Patients perceive this attitude as devaluing their experience.

Patient Resistance

The dichotomy of physical pain versus psychiatric pain is understood by patients. The patient reasons, "If my doctor cannot find anything wrong with me and if there is no fix for my situation, he or she will assume that I must be crazy." For this reason, feelings such as, "You think this is all in my head," are often expressed in patient encounters.

Physical and emotional pain cannot be separated. They coexist and feed on each other. For instance, the most balanced, rational, and accepting patients can still experience high pain levels from fibromyalgia syndrome even when anatomic pathology is lacking. On the other hand, those with extreme mental illness may not complain of pain at all. The best surgeon doing optimal surgery on a patient with low back and leg pain concordant with MRI findings may have surgery fail if an underlying psychiatric comorbid disease is not identified.

Despite wide recognition of the behavioral health comorbidities, patients often resist the suggestion that anxiety and depression may be exacerbating their pain. They equate these diagnoses with hysteria or hypochondria and feel that the physician is depreciating their pain experience. Treating comorbidities is difficult in this setting especially for the nonexpert primary care provider.

Regulatory Scrutiny

Fear of regulatory scrutiny is common in primary care settings although, in reality, very few primary care physician practices are ever monitored. Even fewer practices have had their licensure suspended. These few cases and those covered in the media often involve high profile providers or illegal and immoral activities. Despite this fact, reality does not mitigate perception and regulatory scrutiny, as noted in a previous chapter by Gilson in this text, continues to impede more aggressive pain management in many primary care practices.

Patient Expectations

The paternalistic relationship commonly seen in medical practice is being challenged by consumer activism. Patients have more access to health information than ever before. They have more time and motivation to research their conditions on the Internet, and sometimes know more about treatment options and a particular disease process than their primary care physician. As is often the case, this is a mixed blessing. On the one hand, an informed patient is much more amenable to self-management. On the other hand, an informed patient can present barriers to care.

Most patients with persistent pain do best with self-management skills. Acceptance of their chronic condition, developing strategies including conditioning exercises, and making changes in work or hobbies leads to the best results. However, when information-seeking patients are confronted with "miraculous cures" and daily news articles touting advancements in pain treatment, adapting to pain is difficult for the physician to sell. Too often, patients find themselves on a constant search for the next cure, only to be disappointed when it fails, then moving on to the next "harmless, 100% effective" treatment. As this pattern repeats over and over, the best treatment—acceptance, adaptation, and conditioning—is delayed. The expectations of desperate patients seeking miracle cures create significant barriers to optimum care.

PAIN PRACTITIONER: A PRIMARY CARE MODEL

Training

As in other disciplines, much of the training received by primary care physicians quickly becomes outdated as new knowledge is accumulated and scientific advancements are achieved. Education in all areas of medicine must be lifelong and constantly updated. Medical training provides a knowledge base with courses in neuroanatomy, pathophysiology, and pharmacokinetics. This serves primarily as a foundation and a method for learning and applying new knowledge.

The process of learning and reapplying new knowledge is well accepted in medicine. Despite all the practice management issues and the multilevel barriers to pain care, primary care providers continue to learn and apply new information in their daily clinical practice.

Collaboration with Pain Specialists

Education can occur at formal symposia, professional association meetings, dinner education, through journals, online education, and even the brief encounters with drug representatives. One of the strongest sources of knowledge for primary care is through associations with respected, education-oriented pain specialists.

As primary care physicians, we do not have to know how to operate on a compound fracture, place a cast, or teach the exercises for rehabilitation in order to provide competent aftercare for the patient. In most cases, specialists treat the chief or acute problem until the patient is cured or the condition or is stabilized before referring the patient back to his or her primary care physician. Primary care's task is to understand the treatment provided and continue following the patient's condition to ensure optimal recovery.

Chronic problems rarely result in cure, as the name suggests. Congestive heart failure is not curable and the outpatient care is superbly handled in the primary care setting. Clear understanding of the role of primary care in managing persistent pain as a chronic condition will lead to greater competence in delivering this care.

For their part, pain specialists can greatly improve their communication with primary care. Among the topics which would be helpful are guiding primary care physicians through learning new skills and providing direction regarding when to refer patients back for further specialty care. Such constructive communication can lead to greater self-assurance and competence among primary care physicians as they manage complex pain patients in their practices.

New Focus

Persistent pain patients have similarities and differences from patients with other chronic illnesses. They are both chronic conditions where cure is unlikely. Self-management is the key to success. Denial about the disease and nonadherence to treatment recommendations are common and expected challenges for the provider.

On the other hand, psychiatric issues are more common in persistent pain and interfere with treatment. Patients resist psychosocial diagnosis and interventions. Opioid management that only occurs in persistent pain problems is challenging for the patient and the provider. Nonadherence to treatment recommendations increases morbidity and mortality in diabetes, hypertension, and congestive heart failure. In chronic pain, nonadherence increases the clinicians work stress, thereby requiring more office visits, documentation, and medication surveillance. Although regulatory scrutiny does not occur often, the perception of legal difficulties increases practice discomfort.

In managing pain, it is important for the physician to understand that pain scores are highly subjective and that the focus must be on function. Although measuring pain is important and mandated in a variety of settings,[31] the physician must not lose sight of the twin goals of treatment: function and adaptation.

A new pain complaint or worsening symptoms do not necessarily mandate more medication. In treating diabetes, a worsening $HgbA_1C$ leads the physician to recommend adjustments in diet, exercise, and medication. Similarly, in treating chronic pain, recommendations should take into consideration life stressors, pacing daily activities, depression, anxiety, and worsening of underlying pathology as well as medication. When the primary care provider understands that an increase in pain does not necessarily mean increasing the patient's opioid drug, treatment issues may become easier.

Assessment and Evaluation During Short Visits

Given the typically short office visit and the many pressures on the physician's time, chronic illness management is becoming more difficult. In the typical 15-minute appointment, the patient with low back pain must be evaluated, but he or she may have other conditions requiring assessment, such as hypertension, diabetes, a sleep disorder, and fatigue. Given an hour for the evaluation and adequate support staff, primary care physicians would all be better pain managers. But given a short time, stressed and overworked support staff, and patients with veritable shopping lists of complaints that must be addressed, this is not the case.

Despite the reality of a busy office schedule, primary care is uniquely positioned to take care of the chronic pain patients. We know our patients through associations developed over years of repeated exposure at routine medical care. We understand our patient's coping strategies, family dynamics, and work stresses. The solution to the dilemma lies in making the typical short office visit more effective for patients needing chronic pain management.

The 15-Minute Office Visit

Validating the Patient

Validation is straightforward when a patient presents with an ankle sprain or a sore back. The injury is easily identified by the history and the diagnosis is easily confirmed by physical examination. Diagnostic imaging and/or laboratory reports further support the physician's initial impression, and the patient's chief complaint and the associated pain improve steadily with a short course of uncomplicated therapies—a nonsteroidal anti-inflammatory drug, muscle relaxant, application of cold or heat, and rest.

Validation poses problems for primary care when the patient suffers from chronic pain. We are concerned that the patient will request something we cannot deliver, such as total pain relief, additional MRI studies, or more opioid drugs. The evidence shows that this is not usually the case. In a study of patients with fibromyalgia syndrome, providing the patient with a diagnosis resulted in the patient making fewer visits to the physician's office and becoming more empowered and proactive.[32]

Have you ever asked your patients, "What do you think I can do to help your pain?" Many of us are reluctant to ask because we fear a response that includes a request for long-term disability and opioids. Nonetheless, asking the patient opens a dialogue about expectations and responsibilities perhaps streamlining the office visit.

Once the patient understands that we believe their pain is real, more time can be spent dealing with symptom control, exercise, and other important management issues. At each office visit, make sure that the following steps have been taken:

- Ask about the pain and record the level using a pain score
- Determine the functional status of the patient and whether the treatment is improving function
- Modify the treatment according the patient's response
- Use nonpharmacologic and pharmacologic methods for pain control
- Explain the available options and foster a positive attitude in the patient toward dealing with the pain

Having a set routine with these key goals in mind sets the agenda and can streamline even a difficult, complicated visit.

Assessment Tools

Chronic pain usually starts as an acute pain episode. In most cases, the acute episode resolves and the patient returns to normal function. Even fibromyalgia syndrome, defined as widespread pain for months to years, has a beginning. The work-up and treatment can take months before the correct diagnosis is discovered and the physician becomes aware that the problem is long-term and likely to present problems in management.

At this point, the physician's attention should focus on disease management (i.e., symptom improvement rather than multiple interventions and cure). How can the physician best do this evaluation in a short office visit? Referral may or may not be an option as specialty referral may not be available, too expensive, and time consuming for many patients. Evaluation needs to be focused on the desired outcome of pain reduction, functional improvement, and identification and management of comorbidities. Because such an evaluation can easily take up several visits, handouts and questionnaires can be very useful (i.e., The Initial Pain Assessment Tool, Pain Disability Index, Quality of Life Scale, Zung Self-Rating Depression Scale, and Function and Goal Setting).

Try giving the patient self-assessment forms that measure pain, function, depression, and anxiety, and allow the patient to complete the assignment at home. Patients tend to like these questionnaires since they permit patients to describe in detail issues that the physician may not have the time to elicit during the office visit.

A follow-up visit is designed to review the results with the patient. The handouts direct the follow-up visit to the important outcome variables: pain and function. They are helpful in that they let the patient know which outcomes are most important and what each subsequent office visit will address. The patient who demonstrates anxiety or depression on the self-reported questionnaire is more likely to accept treatment, making discussion and treatment of such comorbidities less time consuming. Assessment is covered in detail elsewhere in this text.

Substance Abuse Screening

Primary care physicians are often hesitant to prescribe opioids. When treating patients with chronic pain, such caution is justified. Substance abuse, particularly involving opioids, is an important comorbidity in chronic pain management. Fortunately, there are multiple questionnaires available to help assess this risk. Commonly used screening tools practical in primary care include The Screener and Opioid Assessment for Patients with Pain,[33] Opioid Risk Tool,[34] and Drug Abuse Screening Test.[35] Patients who score high on any of these scales are more likely to be difficult to manage when treated with opioids. If referral to a pain management specialist is an option, the primary care physician might consider this. Such screening is also covered fully elsewhere in this text.

Goal Setting and Plan of Action

Like other chronic illnesses, patient participation and adherence to treatment recommendations predicts better outcomes. Chronic pain affects many life activities and, in turn, quality of life. Goal-setting discussions direct the patient to improved activity and a targeted outcome. For example, if the patient wants and agrees to spend more time out of bed, walk 10 minutes a day, or work in the garden, any of these might serve as a goal that can be tracked with each visit. As patients begin to anticipate the questions the physician will ask about their goals, visits become more streamlined and focused on a functional outcome.

After the patient has been evaluated and treatment has been initiated, adequate follow-up of a patient with chronic pain can be difficult to accomplish in a 15-minute visit. Follow-up does not take as much time when the physician stays focused on the desired outcome. Consider a routine follow-up for a patient with diabetes. We begin by asking about diet, exercise, foot numbness, vision, and home glucose monitoring. We review the self-monitoring results, then do a physical exam focused on the blood pressure, eyes, heart, and monofilament exam of the feet. We review the $HgbA_1C$, microalbumin, and low-density lipoprotein. We insure that the patient is taking aspirin, a statin, and an ACE inhibitor. We change treatment based on all the information received. All of this is done every day with our diabetics and at each visit; all of this can be accomplished in 15 minutes.

The difference in following chronic pain, and the reason that visits consume more time, is that often it is unclear what to follow, what to ask, and what variables to track at each visit. Too often, the appointment becomes a session wherein the patient complains about pain, disability, and poor quality of life. It is vital that each follow-up session remains focused on symptom management and functional improvement. A patient's pain diary or journal can be helpful in focusing follow-up visits. Pain diaries, available in paper and electronic form, are similar to regular diaries except that the entries focus on pain. Patients record pain-related elements such as the time pain was felt, the type of pain (e.g., burning, stabbing, aching), the location of the pain, what he or she did to alleviate the pain, and whether what they did helped. The patient brings the pain diary to each follow-up session, focusing the visit on a particular pain score and whether the recommended treatment was effective.

Activity and sleep questionnaires are also helpful in concentrating the appointment on these quality of life issues. In a mutual goal-setting discussion with the patient, the questions can revolve around previously agreed upon and previously documented functional outcomes such as the amount of time spent out of bed, the 10-minute walk, or the time spent working in the garden.

Charts reviewed of primary care visits in pain patients frequently demonstrate a failure of adequate documentation.[36] Have the pain score, functional outcome, abuse risk, and side effects been recorded? Given the time pressures, it is no wonder that documentation often is low on our list of priorities. Handouts and questionnaires filed in the patient's chart enhance this record keeping and save time.

Pharmacologic Treatment

There are many pharmacologic treatment options for persistent pain. Pharmacology in primary care is difficult because of the many treatment choices and the lack of agreement among experts. How and why a particular medication is used in a pain patient varies based on pain severity, diagnosis, and many other factors. U.S. Food and Drug Administration-approved drugs or randomized trial results could guide prescribing. Experts are more likely to prescribe based on medical literature and new trends in treatment. Primary care often uses past experience even when this experience is inaccurate or inappropriate. An example of this is the common use of ineffective nonsteroidal anti-inflammatory medications in neuropathic pain treatment in the primary care office.[37] Another example is the use of short-acting hydrocodone compounds by primary care, even though most experts suggest that long-acting opioids are best for persistent pain.[38]

Access to medication is also a major force in pharmacologic options in the primary care setting. Nonformulary drugs or third tier medications requiring high patient copays are a significant factor in prescribing. If the primary care provider has to obtain a preauthorization or justify a prescription, the medication will not be prescribed since this extra step requires excessive time.

As the Ballantyne[8] article points out, opioid prescribing is one of the most difficult decisions facing primary care in managing persistent pain. When prescribing opioids for pain management, physicians are often faced with scenarios that mirror those we associate with addiction: early refills, lost or stolen medication, borrowed medication, and failed urine drug tests. In these cases, documentation is critical. Strategies such as the 4 As of treatment success enable the primary care physician to concentrate on the outcomes that are essential to the patient's overall quality of life (Table 107.3).[39]

Referral to an Addiction Specialist

When to refer a patient to specialty care is always a question and is highly variable among different practitioners. Some providers refer whenever chronic opioid management begins. Others refer only when intervention or surgery is needed. When behavior around the use of an opioid becomes problematic as in the example above, referral is often prudent. At a minimum, documentation of the behavior and an understanding between patient and provider is necessary. The 4 As allow the physician to address the issue and have a treatment strategy. Once the patient learns that early refills will not be tolerated, these requests will stop. It

TABLE 107.3

THE 4 As OF TREATMENT SUCCESS

A-1 = Analgesia or pain score.

A variety of pain scales are available in multiple languages. Pain measurement is the first element in evaluating successful treatment.

A-2 = Activities of daily living or functional outcome that is meaningful to the patient.

At the initial and subsequent visits, work activities, household duties, social activities, hobbies, and physical exercise target are recorded and goal setting is discussed. One important caveat—when treating any chronic condition, a follow-up visit is necessary to evaluate the effectiveness of the treatment.

A-3 = Adverse events.

Anticipating and soliciting feedback from the patient regarding side effects from treatment allows the physician to manage adverse events rather than discontinue otherwise effective pain treatment. Since function is the most important treatment outcome, persistent sleepiness or a cognitive impairment from the opioid must be managed.

A-4 = Aberrant behavior.

If a patient is being treated with opioid analgesics, most primary care physicians worry about the potential for dependence and addiction. Patients on long-term opioid therapy may display behaviors that raise concerns, including early refills, demands for additional medication, and using analgesic medication with other psychoactive drugs such as alcohol.

When such patient behavior occurs, interpretation is difficult. Document the behavior in the patient's chart, discuss it with the patient, and come to a mutual understanding of what action will be taken if the behavior occurs again. With requests for early refills, often the easiest (and least confrontational) response is to refill the medication; however, repeatedly doing what is easiest may lead to repeated requests for refills in the future.

One tactic for dealing with a repeat request for an early refill is to document the request and refuse to refill the medication until the appropriate refill interval. This will prompt a call from the patient at which time the physician can review the agreement about refills, express sympathy, and offer other medication to help the withdrawal. The early refill requests will usually stop. Documenting the behavior helps the physician to focus on setting limits and emphasizing the seriousness of opioid therapy.

---

is important for the physician to recognize the risk and recommend a corrective action (i.e., an abnormal urine drug test may trigger a referral to an addiction medicine provider). The addicted patient will argue and dismiss the risk. If you refuse refills without consultation, the patient looking for access to drugs for diversion or to get high will leave your practice. The patient in need of pain control will comply with the requested consultation.

Motivating Behavior Change in Patients with Chronic Pain

The key message in managing chronic pain is that the way to improve is through changes in lifestyle rather than solely through medication or surgical procedures. It is not an easy message for primary care to deliver because patients expect their physician to give them something to cure their problem. Lifestyle and behavior changes are never easy.

Successful management of chronic pain is much more dependent on what the patient does than on what the physician does

to the patient. The issue becomes one of the patient's readiness to accept responsibility and to adopt a self-management approach. This represents a role reversal for the physician whose task is not to treat but to understand and motivate patients for self-management. On occasion, this may include convincing the patient not to look for another doctor or another procedure.

Because of their unique relationships with patients, primary care physicians are well suited in motivating patients to change. We are motivating patients to lose weight, stop smoking, take their medication, and get flu shots. A patient-centered approach, emphasizing the importance of considering the patient's perspective when making treatment recommendations, has been shown to be a valuable technique.[40] The goals of a patient-centered approach are to:

- Address the patient's concerns
- Enhance a collaborative relationship
- Provide information that the patient is ready to hear
- Refocus the visit from making treatment recommendations to supporting the patient's self-care
- Foster increased patient control of decision-making and responsibility for self-care

It is immediately evident that this technique requires a reorientation of the traditional patient-physician relationship. The physician must learn to view the patient as an autonomous and equal member of the health care team, whose self-knowledge is pivotal to the management of his or her condition (persistent pain).

Reflective listening is a technique that involves making statements that demonstrate the physician's understanding of what the patient has said. There are ways of making reflective statements, including

- Restating what the patient has said
- Paraphrasing what the patient has said
- Anticipating and continuing the patient's thought (i.e., saying what you believe the patient will say next rather than repeating)
- Reflecting the patient's feelings

The patient's readiness to change is the basis of a motivational approach. According to one well-regarded model,[41] patients who strongly believe that their pain only requires a medical or surgical intervention are not ready to accept and adopt self-management. On the other hand, patients who believe that medical and surgical interventions can provide only limited relief from pain are more likely to perceive benefits from self-management techniques. Readiness to self-manage should be assessed on a continuum, and interventions should be tailored to the particular patient's level of readiness to change.

The physician can help the patient to understand the importance of behavior change by guiding him or her through a discussion of the pros and cons, including whether a given change is attainable, how much effort it will take, and how much time it will take given the known obstacles. Motivating the patient involves eliciting the patient's feelings about and reasons for pain self-management, and reflecting back statements that support the premise that self-management is possible. Although time-pressed physicians may balk at the prospect of such a dialogue, the consultation time is usually more efficient (e.g., fewer arguments, less resistance) when a patient is encouraged to speak in a focused manner about a specific problem.

Goals for Pain Self Management. In general, primary care physicians are in agreement about health care goals such as encouraging smoking cessation, maintaining blood pressure within normal limits, and controlling blood sugar. Although the goals for pain self-management are not as clear cut, most pain specialists would advise primary care physicians to consider the following as important when motivating a patient:

1. Beginning or maintaining a regular exercise regimen
2. Using medications as prescribed
3. Returning to normal daily activities given the pain condition
4. Practicing appropriate pain and stress coping strategies (e.g., relaxation techniques, reassuring "self-talk")
5. Returning to or maintaining normal work activities
6. Pacing activities appropriately
7. Monitoring, managing, and/or reporting symptoms of depression as appropriate
8. Practicing good eating habits (e.g., reducing or maintaining an appropriate weight)
9. Engaging in other healthy lifestyle behaviors as necessary (e.g., reducing alcohol consumption, stop smoking)

Importance and Confidence Scales. Patients will change behavior only when they are convinced that it is important and when they have confidence that the change is possible. Assessing patient perceptions of importance and confidence can be helpful when evaluating motivation. For example, patients who give a low rating to the importance of exercise but a high rating to the belief that exercise could be done would need help to change their views of the importance of exercise before adherence could be expected. On the other hand, brainstorming for solutions may be helpful for those who rate importance high and confidence low.

Strategies for Helping Patients Understand the Importance of Change. Information and advice presented in a lecturing style often leads to patient responses of, "Yes, but. . ." and the already too brief visit is taken up with the patient expressing reasons why a recommended change will not work. Social psychology research has shown that, in general, people are more likely to believe what they have said over what others have said to them. It follows that a didactic approach may undermine the physician's attempts to motivate the patient.

Primary care providers are invested in behavior change and motivation. Four strategies have been shown to be effective in helping patients understand the importance of change and increase their confidence to make that change.[42] These uncomplicated strategies are effective because they enable patients to talk themselves into using pain self-management techniques.

1. **Always elicit positive statements from the patient.** Use the "why so high" technique. For example, ask the patient with chronic pain to rate the importance of daily exercise on a scale of 0 (low) to 10 (high). If the patient's answer is 5, ask "Why so high? Why not a 1?" Most patients understand the importance of conditioning and exercise in pain rehabilitation. By asking "why so high," the patient provides the evidence for an exercise program. Once you know the patient's thought process, you can use this to motive a change of behavior.

   "You think it is very important for you to make your muscles stronger to make your pain better" (restating what the patient has expressed).

2. **Examine the pros and cons of behavior change.** Patients will feel ambivalent about self-management. This allows the patient to explore feelings and think through self-management in a judgment-free environment. Bear in mind that although this technique is easy to understand, it can be difficult for the physician to do. He or she must listen, encourage, and provide a summary at the end of the visit.

   "What do you think will happen if you continue to stay in bed?" The patient may steer the conversation back to you: "unless you make me better, I cannot get out of bed" or "unless you give me more pain medication, I will not be able to get out of bed." Be persistent and keep to the same question. The patient has stated earlier that conditioning and exercise are important.

"Your mother was sick all the time. How did that affect you?" Patients may have an environmental background for pain in another family member which impacted them when growing up. Patients may also express concern about the impact of their pain on the other members of the family. The desire to have their pain not have an impact may motivate the patient to different behavior.

3. **Elicit patient concerns about the status quo.** Patients who rate the importance of pain self-management as low may be concerned about their current situation. Ask the patient to talk about the consequences of not making the behavior change. Once the patient has listed as many concerns as he or she can think of, summarize these, using the patient's words if possible. This may help to increase the patient's perception of the importance of the change.

   "If things do not change, what will happen?" The patient may try to guide the discussion back to you and the medical profession, disability, or legal issues. Be persistent about "what will happen with your spouse or children; how will you pay the bills?"

4. **Brainstorm for solutions.** Without giving specific advice, remind the patient that there are usually many ways to achieve self-management. Guide the patient in conceptualizing a number of possibilities. Help the patient to decide which possibilities might work best for him or her. Guide the patient to develop of plan for achieving his or her goal.

   "You spend 16 hours of your day in bed. Any activity makes your pain worse. The last time you tried to exercise, your pain was at a 9/10 and you wanted to go to the hospital. How are you going to get to exercise?" Keep the focus on what the patient can do, or what solutions the patient has. Add suggestions and advice related to the patient's solutions.

Once the patient has adopted a self-management plan with specific goals, the physician can use open-ended questions to encourage the patient to talk about his or her progress. The questions should communicate the physician's interest in the patient's perspective. For instance, "At your last visit, you were thinking about making some changes in pacing your work. I'd be interested in hearing how this is going and whether you've noticed any change in your ability to manage your pain." Such questions enable the physician to conduct an informal assessment of the patient's readiness and also enhance rapport with the patient.

CONCLUSION

Persistent pain, a highly prevalent condition in the United States, has a significant impact on our health and productivity as a society as well as on our medical and financial resources. Primary care is the most appropriate setting for the management of patients with chronic pain because of the mutual understanding that results from a long standing physician-patient relationship. The barriers to managing chronic pain are significant but not insurmountable. Persistent pain is similar to other chronic illness but also has many differences, making management complicated and difficult in the busy primary care office. A new skill set is required by the provider to help the deplorable undertreatment of pain. Available tools (e.g., questionnaires, pain diaries, pain scales) and techniques (e.g., reflective listening, goal setting) make it possible for the primary care physician to provide management for patients with chronic pain in a 15-minute office visit. Diabetes, chronic obstruction pulmonary disease, and other chronic, complicated illnesses require other skills yet have been handled brilliantly in the primary care setting.

Some of the most appreciative patients are those who have a sympathetic provider to help them with chronic pain. Yet treating chronic pain patients is rarely met with enthusiasm in primary care. Patients with chronic pain are complicated and rarely cured. They may have previously made little progress toward normal life functioning, and often have complex psychosocial issues that a physician cannot address. There is never sufficient time to adequately follow-up patients with pain. The primary care provider is accustomed to dealing with chronic problems through short, focused visits and a longitudinal experience. A treatment plan and mutually agreed upon goals allow the physician to conduct a follow-up visit in 15 minutes by focusing discussions on the treatment success that both the physician and patient desire.

References

1. Harstall C. How prevalent is chronic pain? *Pain: Clinical Updates* 2003;X: 1–4.
2. O'Rorke JE, Chen I, Genao I, et al. Physicians' comfort in caring for patients with chronic nonmalignant pain. *Am J Med Sci* 2007;333:93–100.
3. Gallup, Inc. Pain in America: Highlights from a Gallup survey. Arthritis Foundation [Website]. Available at: www.arthritis.org/conditions/speakersofpain/factsheet.asp. Accessed June 9, 1999.
4. Boström BM, Ramberg T, Davis BD, et al. Survey of post-operative patients' pain management. *J Nurs Manag* 1997;5:341–349.
5. Dworkin R, Backonja M, Rowbotham M, et al. Advances in neuropathic pain: diagnosis, mechanisms, and treatment recommendations. *Arch Neurol* 2003; 60:1524–1534.
6. Fishman S, Von Korff M, Lozano P, et al. Chronic care costs in managed care. *Health Aff (Millwood)* 1997;16(3):239–247.
7. O'Rorke JE, Chen I, Genao I, et al. Physicians' comfort in caring for patients with chronic nonmalignant pain. *Am J Med Sci* 2007;333:93–100.
8. Ballantyne JC, Mao J. Opioid therapy for chronic pain. *N Engl J Med* 2003; 349:1943–1953.
9. Flor H, Turk DC. Chronic back pain and rheumatoid arthritis: predicting pain and disability from cognitive variables. *J Behav Med* 1988;11:251–265.
10. Sanders SH, Brena SF, Spier CJ, et al. Chronic back pain patients around the world: cross-cultural similarities and differences. *Clin J Pain* 1992;8:317–323.
11. Reesor KA, Craig KD. Medically incongruent chronic back pain physical limitations, suffering, and ineffective coping. *Pain* 1988;32:35–45.
12. Pinsky J. Chronic pain syndromes and their treatment. In: Brodwin MG, Tellez F, Brodwin SK, eds. *Medical, Psychosocial and Vocational Aspects of Disability*. Athens, GA: Elliott & Fitzpatrick; 1993:179–194.
13. Dahlman GB, Dykes AK, Elander G. Patients' evaluation of pain and nurses' management of analgesics after surgery. The effect of a study day on the subject of pain for nurses working at the thorax surgery department. *J Adv Nurs* 1999; 30:866–874.
14. Drayer R, Henderson J, Reidenberg M. Barriers to better pain control in hospitalized patient. *J Pain Symptom Manage* 1999;17:434–440.
15. Brookoff D. Chronic pain: 1. a new disease: *Hosp Pract (Minneap)* 2000;35(7): 45–59.
16. Deyo R, Rainville J, Kent DL. What can the history and physical examination tell us about low back pain? *JAMA* 1992;268:760–765.
17. Martin JC, Avant RF, Bowman MA, etc. The future of family medicine: a collaborative project of the family medicine community. *Ann Fam Med* 2004; 2(suppl 1):S3–32.
18. Chronic Pain Care Trends: Perspectives from Managed Care, Providers, and Employers. *Managed Care* 2005. MediMedia USA.
19. Bigos SJ, McKee JE. Reliable care through the activity paradigm for back prob-
lems. In: McCarberg B, Passik S, eds. *Expert Guide to Pain Management*. Philadelphia, PA: American College of Physicians; 2005:35–64.
20. Carey TS, Garrett J, Jackman A, et al. The outcomes and costs of care for acute low back pain among patients seen by primary care practitioner, chiropractors, and orthopedic surgeons. The North Carolina Back Pain Project. *New Engl J Med* 1995;333(14):913–917.
21. Cherkin DC, MacCornack FA, Berg AO. Managing low back pain—a comparison of the beliefs and behaviors of family physicians and chiropractors. *West J Med* 1998;149(4):475–480.
22. Federation of State Medical Boards of the United States, Inc. Model Policy for the Use of Controlled Substances for the Treatment of Pain. Available at: www.fsmb.org/pdf/2004_grpol_Controlled_Substances.pdf. Accessed July 8, 2009.
23. SAMHSA. Office of Applied Studies. *Results from the 2005 National Survey on Drug Use and Health*. DHHS Publication No. SMA 06-4194. 2006.
24. *Guideline for the Management of Pain in Osteoarthritis, Rheumatoid Arthritis and Juvenile Chronic Arthritis*. 2nd ed. Glenview, IL: American Pain Society; 2002.
25. *Guideline for the Management of Cancer Pain in Adults and Children*. Glenview, IL: American Pain Society; 2005.
26. Argoff C, Bruckenthal P, Charmichael B, et al. *Consensus Recommendations: Neuropathic Pain*. Charlotte, NC: Primary Care Education Consortium; 2004.
27. *Guideline for the Management of Fibromyalgia Syndrome Pain in Adults and Children*. Glenview, IL: American Pain Society; 2005
28. McCarberg, B. Impact of guidelines on healthcare from the patient and payor perspective: example of the american pain society guidelines. *Dis Manage Health Outcomes* 2004;12(1);73–79.
29. Polatin PB, Kinnedy RK, Gatchel RJ, et al. Psychiatric illness and chronic low-back pain: the mind and the spine—which goes first? *Spine* 1993;18(1):66–71.
30. Fishbain DA, Cutler R, Rosomoff HL, et al. Chronic pain-associated depression: antecedent or consequence of chronic pain? A review. *Clin J Pain* 1997; 13(2):116–137.
31. Jacox AK, CarrDB, Capman CR, et al. Acute pain management: operative or medical procedures and trauma. Clinical Practice Guideline No. 1 AHCPR Publication No. 92-0032; 1992.
32. White KP, Nielson WR, Harth M, et al. Does the label 'fibromyalgia' after health status, function, and health service utilization? A prospective, within-group comparison in a community cohort of adults with chronic widespread pain. *Arthritis Rheum* 2002;47(3):260–265.
33. Butler SF, Budman SH, Fernandez K, et al. Validation of a screener and opioid assessment measure for patient with chronic pain. *Pain* 2004;112:65–75.
34. Webster LR, Webster RM. Predicting aberrant behaviors in opioid-treatment patients: preliminary validation of the Opioid Risk Tool. *Pain Med* 2005;6: 432–442.
35. Skinner HA. The drug abuse screening test. *Addict Behav* 1982;7(4):363–371.
36. Clark JD. Chronic pain prevalence and analgesic prescribing in a general medical population. *J Pain Symptom Manage* 2002;23:131–137.
37. Oster G, Berger A, Dukes E, et al. Use of potentially inappropriate pain-related medications in older adults with painful neuropathic disorders. *Am J Geriatr Pharmacother* 2004;2(3):163–170.
38. McCarberg BH, Barkin RL. Long-acting opioids for chronic pain: pharmacotherapeutic opportunities to enhance compliance, quality of life and analgesia. *Am J Ther* 2001;8(3):181–186.
39. Passik SD, Weinreb HJ. Managing chronic nonmalignant pain: overcoming obstacles to the use of opioids. *Adv Ther* 2000;17:70–83.
40. Stewart MA, McWhinney IR, Weston WW, et al. *Patient-Centered Medicine: Transforming the Clinical Method*. Thousand Oaks, CA: Sage Publications; 1995.
41. Prochaska JO, Diclemente CC, Norcoss JC. In search of how people change: applications to addictive behaviors. *Am Psychol* 1992;47:1102–1114.
42. Rollnick S, Mason P, Butler C. *Health Behavior Change: A Guide for Practitioners*. Edinburgh: Harcourt Publisher; 1999.

CHAPTER 108 ■ PAIN MANAGEMENT AT THE END OF LIFE

JUDITH A. PAICE

Adequate relief of pain at the end of life is an ethical imperative. Studies suggest that although pain may not be the most prevalent symptom during the final days or weeks of life, it is frequently the most distressing.[1-8] In addition to the negative consequences pain has on the patient, inadequate pain control adversely affects the ongoing emotional well-being of family and friends at the bedside. To witness unrelieved pain during the final hours of life leaves long-lasting negative memories of the dying process that can hamper bereavement. The setting of care can dictate whether patients will receive adequate relief during the dying process, and significant change in our systems of care is needed. The majority of end-of-life care is currently provided in institutions, with more than two thirds of individuals dying in hospitals or nursing homes. In a large survey of surviving family members, more than 25% reported that their loved one received inadequate relief of pain in these settings.[9] The challenge for our health care system is to ensure that regardless of setting, pain management at end of life is provided by skilled professionals who understand the special needs of the dying. These skills include assessment of pain in those who might not be able to verbally describe their pain, awareness of pain syndromes common at end of life, as well as familiarity with the pharmacologic and nonpharmacologic management of pain in the dying. Furthermore, clinicians must be aware of the role of suffering and existential distress, as well as management of intractable symptoms.

INTRODUCTION

Currently, death in developed countries is more likely to occur after a long chronic illness. This is in contrast to a century ago when people died a more rapid death, often due to infection. Currently, the most common causes of death in high income countries include ischemic cardiac disease, cerebrovascular disease, and cancer.[10] Globally, 60% of deaths are due to chronic diseases, principally cardiovascular diseases and diabetes, cancers, and chronic respiratory diseases.[11] Thus, people are more likely to die after a long, protracted illness, and pain is a common comorbidity of these illnesses. Several care delivery models exist to address the specialized pain and symptom needs of those with life-threatening illnesses, including palliative care and hospice. Both of these care models focus attention on the patient and family, not unlike the structure of care delivered in truly interdisciplinary pain treatment programs.

Palliative Care

Palliative care strives to relieve suffering and improve the quality of life of those individuals with a life-threatening illness.[12] The palliative care movement in the United States originated in academic medical centers but has moved into community hospitals, outpatient clinics, and other centers of care. In fact, palliative care programs now exist in 31% of hospitals in the United States.[13] Commitment to early identification, thorough assessment, and effective treatment of pain are key components of palliative care, as is attention to other physical, psychosocial, and spiritual concerns. The goal is to neither hasten nor prolong death, but rather affirm life by offering a support system to patients and families. To that end, palliative care is optimally provided by an interdisciplinary group of professionals, including physicians, nurses, social workers, chaplains, and others.

Confusion persists regarding the timing of appropriate referral to palliative care. Previous models of care incorporated palliative care during the final phases of life, once all curative therapy was completed (Fig. 108.1). It is clear that patients and families benefit greatly when palliative care is integrated into the plan of care early during the course of illness (Fig. 108.2). Effective pain management provided during cancer treatment, for example, can allow patients to complete potentially curative or life-prolonging therapies. Attention to other symptoms associated with the underlying illness, including distressing complications of treatment, can provide improved quality of life during this time. Recent research supports the feasibility of integrating palliative and oncology care in ambulatory patients. A study of patients with advanced nonsmall cell lung cancer receiving cancer treatment and palliative care in an outpatient clinic confirmed the high symptom burden experienced by these individuals, despite their newly diagnosed status, and the benefits of early attention to symptom management.[14]

Hospice

The modern concept of hospice care developed from the work of Dame Cicely Saunders and others in the United Kingdom during the 1960s. In this model, free-standing centers of care were developed where patients spent their final days receiving pain and symptom management, along with attention to the emotional and spiritual aspects of the individual's life. A decade later, hospice began in the United States with the same goals of care, but a home-based model quickly took root. In 1982, the Medicare Hospice Benefit was passed to provide reimbursement for these services. A Medicare Part A beneficiary is eligible for this benefit if she or he is determined to have a life expectancy of 6 months or less if the life-limiting disease or combination of comorbid conditions runs its normal course. Studies reveal that patients at end of life and their family members prefer care provided in the home with the support of hospice. Family members of patients receiving hospice services report significantly greater satisfaction with the overall quality of care compared with those dying in institutional settings: 70.7% rated care as "excellent" compared with less than 50%, respectively.[9] Both of these models, palliative care and hospice, provide support to patients and loved ones. As pain is so prevalent, all health care professionals working with people at this time of life must be exceptionally knowledgeable about common pain syndromes as well as appropriate assessment and management.

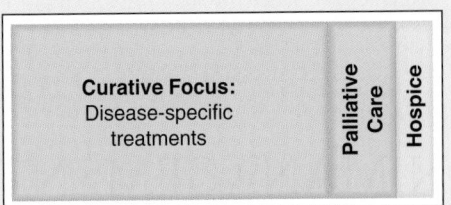

FIGURE 108.1 Previous models of palliative care and hospice.

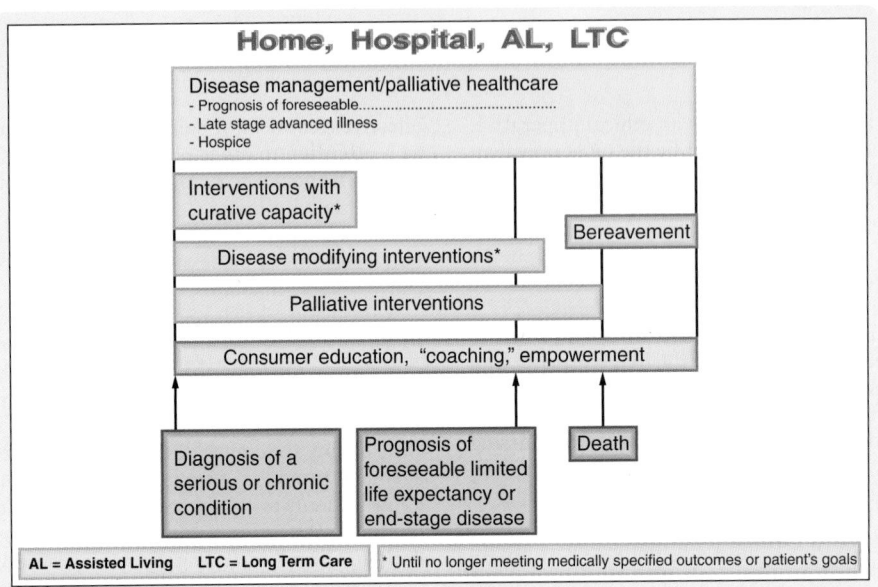

PAIN SYNDROMES COMMON AT THE END OF LIFE

Pain syndromes specific to cancer have been well characterized, yet much research is needed to describe pain associated with other life-threatening illnesses. Furthermore, greater attention is needed to identify pain syndromes most common at the very end of life along with appropriate treatment strategies (Table 108.1).

Cancer

Prevalence rates of pain in advanced cancer vary based upon the settings of care in which the studies were conducted, the instruments used to measure pain and other symptoms, as well as the methods employed in data collection. In general, approximately two thirds of patients with advanced malignant disease experience pain.[2,15–17] Cancer patients referred to palliative care or hospice commonly have a greater prevalence of pain and other symptoms. For example, one study of lung cancer outpatients

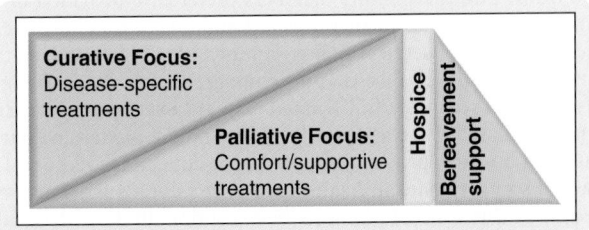

FIGURE 108.2 Proposed model for integration of palliative care.[12]

revealed that 27% had pain, compared with 76% in those referred to palliative care.[18] Regarding the pain trajectory in cancer patients very near the end of life, pain occurred in 54% and 34% at 4 weeks and 1 week prior to death, respectively.[19] Children dying of cancer also are at risk for pain and suffering, yet few studies detail the prevalence and characteristics of pain in this population.[20] The result of unrelieved pain and associated interference may include increased desire for hastened death.[21]

Noncancer Diagnoses

Many life-threatening illnesses are known to cause pain, including human immunodeficiency virus,[22] multiple sclerosis,[23,24] amyotrophic lateral sclerosis,[25] other neurologic disorders,[26] end-stage renal disease,[27] and heart failure.[28–31] At the end of life, it is apparent that many of the pre-existing pain syndromes associated with these disorders can escalate, particularly pain related to progression of disease, immobility, or comorbid complications. Furthermore, many patients with advanced disease are elderly and more likely to have existing chronic pain syndromes, such as osteoarthritis or low back pain.[32] Regrettably, there have been few studies characterizing the prevalence of pain or the types of pain experienced by these individuals with noncancer diagnoses. Greater awareness of the risk and types of pain seen will lead to improved detection, assessment, and treatment.

PAIN ASSESSMENT AT THE END OF LIFE

Challenges in Pain Assessment

Comprehensive assessment of pain at the end of life is imperative. As with all pain, assessment must be conducted upon initial pre-

TABLE 108.1

PAIN SYNDROMES IN PALLIATIVE CARE

Pain Related to Underlying Disease
- Tumor related pain due to pressure or compression
- Chest pain due to end stage cardiac disease
- Ischemia caused by atherosclerotic disease
- Abdominal pain with referral to thorax and shoulder due to liver failure, cirrhosis
- Abdominal pain due to ascites
- Extremity skin pain due to edema
- Back pain and skin discomfort/pruritus due to end-stage renal disease
- Chest pain due to pulmonary fibrosis, emphysema, other advanced lung disorders
- Central nervous system infection (meningitis, cryptosporidium) leading to headache
- Central pain after stroke, particularly affecting thalamus
- Trigeminal neuralgia in multiple sclerosis
- Vaso-occlusion leading to bone, muscle, and visceral pain in sickle cell disease
- Rapid onset of cachexia leading to peripheral neuropathy
- Spasticity due to neuromuscular disorders

Pain Related to Treatment
- Peripheral neuropathy due to chemotherapy, HAART
- Arthralgias and myalgias due to aromatase inhibitors
- Surgically induced phantom pain, chronic neuropathy
- Immunocompromise leading to postherpetic neuropathy
- Aseptic necrosis due to prolonged corticosteroid use

Pain Unrelated to Disease or its Treatment
- Pressure ulcers
- Reduced muscle and fat padding at bony prominences
- Muscle atrophy leading to myalgia
- Immobility leading to joint pain
- Contractures

From Von Roenn JH, Paice JA, Preodor ME. Pain management in palliative care. In: Von Roenn JH, Paice JA, Preodor ME. *Current Diagnosis & Treatment of Pain.* New York: Lange; 2006, with permission.

sentation, regularly throughout the course of care, and during any changes in the patient's pain state.[33] Documentation of and communication about these findings are crucial. Assessment in patients who are cognitively intact and able to verbalize can incorporate standard intensity tools such as the numeric rating scale (NRS), the verbal descriptor scale (VDS), the visual analogue scale (VAS), or the Brief Pain Inventory (BPI) for more comprehensive evaluation. A recent panel of international experts in palliative care rated essential components of pain assessment to include intensity, temporal pattern, treatment and exacerbating/relieving factors, location, and interference with health-related quality of life as essential dimensions.[34] In their content evaluation of more than 64 pain assessment tools, none were found to satisfactorily incorporate all of these domains.

Tools exist that measure multiple symptoms seen in life-threatening illness, and the majority include pain.[35] One study demonstrated that using systematic assessment of symptoms in palliative care yielded a 10-fold greater number than when volunteered by the patient. The investigators conclude that specific detailed symptom investigation is necessary.[36] Examples of tools include the Edmonton Symptom Assessment Scale,[37] the M.D. Anderson Symptom Inventory,[38] the Memorial Symptom Assessment Scale,[39,40] the Rotterdam Symptom Checklist,[41] the Symptom Distress Scale, and others. A limitation is that most of these instruments were developed to assess symptom prevalence and/or

intensity in cancer populations and may not accurately reflect the experience of those with noncancer diagnoses. One exception is the Memorial Symptom Assessment Scale, which has undergone testing in seriously ill cancer and noncancer inpatients.[42] Although symptoms varied between the two groups, there was no significant difference in symptom distress scores, a global measure of symptom burden.[42] Another constraint of these scales for clinical care at end of life is the length of most of these tools, leading to respondent fatigue.[43] The Brief Hospice Inventory[44] was developed specifically to evaluate symptoms, including pain, and satisfaction with hospice care. Initial testing revealed that patients at end of life could complete the instrument.

A wide range of health-related quality of life instruments, such as the European Organization for the Research and Treatment of Cancer QLQ-C30 and the Functional Assessment of Cancer Therapy-General, include symptoms such as pain, but the burden to complete these tools preclude their use in those with advanced disease.[45] Two tools target patients at the end of life: The Hospice Quality of Life Index[46] and McGill Quality of Life Questionnaire.[3] Both instruments include symptoms and can be useful in assessing the global needs of dying patients. Although these tools are appropriate for patients who are cognitively intact, many patients at the end of life develop delirium, some have dementia, and others have limited ability to communicate due to intubation or neurologic disorders.

Pain Assessment in the Cognitively Impaired

Several excellent reviews thoroughly describe tools used to assess pain in cognitively impaired older adults, primarily those with dementia (Table 108.2).[47–50] Although many of these tools may be adapted to assess pain in the dying person with delirium or other disorders, none have undergone extensive testing in these populations. One exception is the Doloplus 2, which has undergone testing in palliative care patients, but investigators found the tool lacked validity and was challenging to use.[51]

Pain Assessment in Those Unable to Communicate

One in five people who die in hospitals have used intensive care unit (ICU) services during their final hospitalization.[52] In a large

TABLE 108.2

PAIN ASSESSMENT TOOLS IN NONVERBAL PATIENTS THAT MAY BE USEFUL IN END OF LIFE CARE

Dementia
Assessment of Discomfort in Dementia Protocol
Checklist of Nonverbal Pain Indicators
Doloplus 2
Nursing Assistant-Administered Instrument to Assess Pain in Demented Individuals
Pain Assessment Scale for Seniors with Severe Dementia
Pain Assessment in Advanced Dementia Scale

Intubated or Unconscious Children (Neonates, Infants, Nonverbal Children)
COMFORT Behavior Scale
Distress Scale for Ventilated Newborn Infants
Faces, Legs, Activity, Cry, Consolability Observational Tool

Intubated or Unconscious Adults
Behavioral Pain Scale
Critical-Care Pain Observational Tool

multicenter study of patients with serious illness, half of those who died during hospitalization had received ICU care.[53] Thus, significant percentages of people with life-threatening illness will be admitted to the ICU prior to death. Yet, one in five patients in ICU lack decision-making capacity and are likely unable to accurately describe their pain.[54] Furthermore, although a number of these patients may be cognitively intact, the use of mechanical ventilation often complicates pain assessment. Some patients may be able to use a NRS, VDS, or VAS, either by pointing to a chart with numbers or a line representing pain or by nodding "yes" when asked sequentially if pain is "mild," "moderate," or "severe." For those patients who cannot use these techniques, several pain assessment tools have been developed to assess pain in the ICU, including the Behavioral Pain Scale[55] and the Critical-Care Pain Observation Tool.[56] For children, several tools exist, including the Faces, Legs, Activity, Cry, Consolability Observational Tool (validated in children 2 months to 7 years and tested in the ICU),[57] Distress Scale for Ventilated Newborn Infants (tested in ventilated newborns), and the COMFORT Behavior Scale (tested in neonates to 3 years of age in ICU).[58]

Although standardized instruments to measure pain at the end of life are needed, several principles can guide clinicians when patients are cognitively impaired and unable to report pain.[50] Behaviors suggestive of pain should be evaluated, including the furrowed brow, guarding, or vocalizing on movement. Consider causes of pain, including the underlying disease and treatments, as well as new complications such as pressure ulcers, constipation, urinary retention, or infection. Ask family members or others who have known the patient if they observe changes in behaviors that might imply discomfort. If any of these indicators suggest that the patient may be in pain, initiate an analgesic trial and reassess. Resolution of the behaviors provides suggestive evidence that pain exists. Regular administration of the analgesic should then be included in the treatment plan.

Pain Measurement in Research Conducted at End of Life

Research in pain at the end of life is hampered by lack of consistency in the use of valid and reliable pain measurement tools. An expert working group convened by the European Association of Palliative Care recommended standardized methods be applied in clinical trials and other pain studies in those with life-threatening illnesses. They recommended unidimensional tools such as the numerical rating scale, VAS or verbal rating scales, or when indicated, multidimensional tools such as the BPI-Short Form or the McGill Pain Questionnaire.[59]

PAIN MANAGEMENT STRATEGIES AT END OF LIFE

The principles employed in treating other patients in pain should be applied to the dying. These include the use of multimodal therapies based upon the underlying pain mechanisms as determined by comprehensive assessment. Of particular challenge at the end of life is the need for alternate routes of administration and a plan of care when pain becomes intractable to standard therapies or adverse effects to the treatment become unmanageable.

Routes of Drug Delivery

Many patients can use the oral route until death. In one study, 43% and 20% of cancer patients were able to take oral opioids at 1 week and 24 hours before death, respectively.[19] When oral delivery is no longer feasible, alternate routes of administration are available. Oral routes, including sublingual, transmucosal, and buccal delivery, as well as enteral, rectal, nasal, parenteral, spinal, topical, and transdermal routes, have all been employed.

Oral, Sublingual, Transmucosal, and Buccal Routes

When patients have difficulty swallowing pills but can take soft food, microsphere formulations of long-acting morphine provide sustained release when the capsule is broken open and the "sprinkles" are placed in applesauce or other soft food. Oral opioid solutions (e.g., morphine, oxycodone, hydromorphone, or methadone) can be swallowed or small volumes (0.5 to 1 mL) of a concentrated solution can be placed sublingually or buccally in patients whose swallowing abilities are limited. Nevertheless, buccal and sublingual uptake of these opioids is slow and not very predictable, particularly with more hydrophilic compounds such as morphine.[60,61] Small studies suggest that most of the analgesic effect of morphine administered in this manner is due to drug dripping down the oropharynx and into the gastrointestinal tract.[62] Conversely, absorption with the use of more lipophilic drugs, such as methadone and fentanyl, is relatively high.[60] Topical morphine mouthwash has been reported to treat chemotherapy-induced oral mucositis and might be useful for other pain syndromes associated with oral lesions.[63,64]

Transmucosal Fentanyl. Oral transmucosal fentanyl citrate (OTFC) is a lipid soluble (lipophilic) synthetic opioid formulation that consists of a lozenge on a stick. Patients must actively rub the fentanyl-containing lozenge against the oral mucosa to provide rapid absorption of the drug, usually experiencing some relief in 5–15 minutes, with a peak effect of 30 minutes.[65,66] This is particularly useful for breakthrough pain that is quick in onset. Unlike other breakthrough pain drugs, the dose of long-acting opioid does not predict the effective dose of OTFC.[67,68] Too rapid application, usually less than 15 minutes, will result in more of the agent being swallowed rather than being absorbed transmucosally. Some patients develop oral candida due to the high sugar content of the compound and others complain of the sweet taste and lack of variety in flavor, particularly with prolonged use.

Buccal Fentanyl. Rapidly dissolving fentanyl buccal tablets (FBT) provide faster onset of effect when compared with oral morphine administration. As with OTFC, peak effect is reported to be 30 minutes.[69] An important difference when comparing FBT with OTFC is that patients do not have to actively rub the applicator within the oral mucosa with buccal administration. This is appreciated by fatigued patients, those with musculoskeletal disorders that make this movement difficult, as well as individuals with oral lesions and those who are embarrassed by public use of the "lollipop"-appearing OTFC formulation. As with OTFC, the dose of long-acting opioid does not predict the effective dose of buccal fentanyl, and one cannot reliably convert from OTFC to FBT since the latter has a greater bioavailability. The rate and extent of fentanyl absorption were greater following FBT compared to OTFC, such that approximately 30% less drug was required when administering FBT to achieve similar OTFC systemic drug levels.[70]

Enteral and Rectal

Pre-existing enteral feeding tubes can be used to deliver medications when patients cannot swallow at the end of life. It is rare that circumstances would require placement of a tube at this time, and doing so may send a contradictory message about the need for enteral nutrition and hydration. The size of the tube and volume of fluid used to mix the "sprinkles" formulation of morphine must be considered when delivering this form long-acting morphine to avoid obstruction of the tube.

Opioids can be delivered via the rectal route using commercially prepared suppositories, compounded suppositories, or microenemas. Studies suggest a larger area under the curve when morphine suppositories are used when compared with oral sustained-release morphine.[71] Sustained-release morphine tablets have also been used rectally, with resultant delayed time to peak plasma level and approximately 90% of the bioavailability achieved by oral administration.[72] Rectal methadone can be used safely and has bioavailability approximately equal to oral methadone.[73,74] Neutropenia and thrombocytopenia are generally considered contraindications to rectal drug administration, but clinicians must consider the goals of care for delivering these drugs as well as the risks and benefits at this time of life. Painful rectal lesions, such as hemorrhoids or fissures, preclude the use of these routes. Attempting to place agents rectally at home may be difficult for family members when caring for loved ones who cannot move or reposition without significant assistance. Case reports of stomal or vaginal administration suggest that these routes can provide effective delivery when other routes are not feasible.[75]

Nasal

Currently, the only commercially available opioid in nasal formulation is the mixed agonist-antagonist butorphanol. This category of opioid is not recommended in end of life care as combining these agents with a pure agonist opioid can result in symptoms of withdrawal or abstinence. Nasal fentanyl, hydromorphone, and morphine have undergone initial investigation, primarily in healthy volunteers.[76-78] Additional research is needed to establish feasibility, tolerability, and efficacy in a population with pain at end of life.

Parenteral

Parenteral administration includes intravenous and subcutaneous delivery of drug. Intramuscular opioid delivery is inappropriate in the palliative care setting due to the pain associated with this route and the variability in systemic uptake of the drug.[33] Intravenous administration of drugs is often used when patients are hospitalized at end of life, as this route provides rapid and predictable drug delivery. For patients being cared for at home, the need for vascular access may be cumbersome. Subcutaneous infusions, including morphine, hydromorphone, and fentanyl, provide an effective and safe alternative.[79] Methadone has been reported to cause local site irritation, although small case reports suggest that lower doses given intermittently are less likely to cause pain.[80] Subcutaneous boluses of morphine have a slower onset and lower peak effect when compared with intravenous boluses, although with continuous infusions they provide similar blood levels and resultant pain relief.[33,81] Subcutaneous infusions may include up to 10 mL/hour, although most patients absorb 2 to 3 mL/hour with the least difficulty. Volumes greater than 10 mL/hour are often poorly absorbed and can lead to pain or leakage of fluid. Hyaluronidase has been reported to speed absorption of subcutaneously administered fluids, although a recent randomized trial yielded no difference in pain or edema between treatment and placebo groups.[82] Despite these findings, these investigators and others suggest that hyaluronidase may have utility when subcutaneous absorption is not well tolerated.

Spinal (Epidural/Intrathecal)

Intraspinal routes, including epidural or intrathecal delivery, allow administration of drugs such as opioids, local anesthetics, and/or alpha-adrenergic agonists more proximate to their respective effector sites.[83,84] A randomized controlled trial demonstrated benefit for ambulatory cancer patients with a life expectancy of at least 3–6 months experiencing pain.[85] However, initiating this therapy during the final hours of life requires the availability of experts to place an external catheter, as well as caregivers with specialized knowledge to safely and effectively

provide care. As with all therapies, the potential risks, including greater caregiver burden, need to be weighed against the benefits. Intraspinal delivery may be considered when patients do not obtain adequate relief from aggressive titration of systemic opioids and other analgesics or they experience intolerable adverse effects.[86] More information regarding the use of intraspinal drug delivery is available in Chapter 99.

Topical

Topical morphine administration to open areas, such as pressure ulcers, burns, malignant skin lesions, and ulcers associated with venous stasis or sickle cell disease, has been reported to be effective in case reports and open label trials.[87-90] However, a recent randomized controlled trial of topical morphine used to treat painful skin ulcers found no benefit when compared with placebo.[91] An analysis of the bioavailability of morphine when delivered to open ulcers found little systemic uptake, a possible explanation for the lack of efficacy.[92] Topical morphine applied to the wrist in a pluronic lecithin organogel (PLO) base for systemic delivery is being used in many hospice settings, yet evidence of its efficacy is lacking. A recent bioavailability study of topical morphine in healthy volunteers revealed that morphine was seldom detected in plasma samples after topical administration, and when values were detected, they were below the level of quantification.[93] These results suggest that topical administration of morphine compounded in a PLO base for topical drug delivery is unlikely to provide relief of pain.

Transdermal

Transdermal fentanyl has been used extensively and a wide range of dosing options (12, 12.5, 25, 50, 75, and 100 mcg/hour patches) makes this route particularly useful in palliative care.[94] Most individuals experience relief for 3 days, although approximately 25% of patients will consistently report increased pain on the third day, despite adequate use of breakthrough medications. These patients benefit from changing the patch more frequently (every 48 hours). Fentanyl is another option when considering opioid rotation, and several reports suggest the resolution of delirium when patients are converted from other opioids to transdermal or intravenous fentanyl.[95,96] Fever, diaphoresis, cachexia, morbid obesity, and ascites may have a significant impact on the absorption, predictability of blood levels, and clinical effects of transdermal fentanyl, although studies are lacking.[97] There is some suggestion in open-label and retrospective studies that transdermal fentanyl may produce less constipation than long-acting morphine. This may be a moot point in patients in palliative care since they are often using significant amounts of supplemental opioids for breakthrough pain.[98-101] A small subset of patients will develop skin irritation due to the adhesive in any patch. Because most topical antihistamines consist of an oil base which would prevent patch adherence, the use of an aqueous based steroid inhaler (intended for the management of asthma) applied prior to patch administration can preclude skin reactions and allows the patch to remain in place.

Intractable Pain or Unmanageable Adverse Effects of Treatment

Although most pain at end of life can be well-managed with available therapies, intractable pain or unmanageable adverse effects can occur that can lead to incredible suffering. In some cases, pain escalates due to rapidly increasing disease burden. At other times, pharmacokinetics of the opioids and other analgesics are altered by organ dysfunction associated with the dying process, leading to inadequate relief.

Effect of Organ Dysfunction on Pharmacokinetics

Organ dysfunction at the end of life will alter the absorption, distribution, metabolism and elimination of analgesic agents, thereby influencing the efficacy of the drug. People with advanced malignancy or other life-threatening illness may undergo changes in any of these phases as a result of extensive disease. Little is known about the alterations in absorption of opioids that occur when people are dying. Factors such as shortened gastrointestinal transit time may delay absorption of oral opioids, particularly long-acting or sustained-release compounds.

Distribution of the drug is in part dependent upon plasma proteins within the vasculature, body fat stores, and total body water.[102] These can all be significantly altered in patients who are cachectic and dehydrated at the end of life. Aging patients are known to have decreased volume of distribution of morphine and fentanyl. Additionally, methadone binds avidly to alpha$_1$ glycoprotein, which is increased in advanced cancer. This leads to decreasing amounts of unbound methadone and a delayed onset of analgesic effect.

Metabolism of drugs can be changed by advanced age, liver dysfunction, and other factors that are widespread in palliative care. Excretion can be altered as renal failure occurs, particularly since most opioids, with the exception being methadone, are mostly excreted by the kidneys. Patients with renal failure or those receiving dialysis might benefit from the use of agents that are more readily dialyzable, such as fentanyl, as opposed to morphine or codeine.[103] Research is needed regarding the effect of advanced disease and the dying process on the pharmacokinetics of analgesics, particularly opioids.

Myoclonus

One consequence of altered pharmacokinetics at the end of life is the development of myoclonus. Myoclonus is a sudden, uncontrollable, nonrhythmic jerking of the extremities. This can be extremely distressing, causing fatigue and sleep disruption, and exacerbating the patient's pain. Furthermore, myoclonus can progress to the development of uncontrolled seizures.[104] Myoclonus has been reported to occur after surgery to the brain,[105] in acquired immunodeficiency syndrome,[106] after hypoxia,[107] and after chlorambucil administration.[108] However, myoclonus at end-of-life care is most commonly associated with opioids. Controversy exists regarding whether this is dose dependent and how much of this effect is from parent drug versus metabolites. Most reports of opioid related myoclonus implicate higher doses, although it has been reported to occur in patients receiving low doses of opioids, particularly hydromorphone.[109,110] Other opioids that have been implicated include methadone[111] and fentanyl.[112] Myoclonus has also been reported during withdrawal from transdermal fentanyl.[113,114]

The underlying mechanism of opioid-induced myoclonus is poorly understood. Myoclonus and seizures have been reported to occur in patients receiving high-dose morphine or hydromorphone administration.[115,116] However, Fainsinger and colleagues[116] describe a case of myoclonus occurring with stable hydromorphone dosing in the face of acute renal failure. A retrospective chart review found that in terminally ill patients receiving parenteral hydromorphone, the dose and duration of drug were associated with the development of myoclonus, while age, gender, and diagnosis were not.[117] These findings point to the role of accumulating neuroexcitatory metabolites that are poorly excreted, either due to prolonged dosing, high doses, or concomitant renal failure. The 3-glucuronide metabolites are implicated as contributing to these neuroexcitatory effects.[118] Both morphine-3-glucuronide (M3G) and hydromorphone-3-glucuronide (H3G) are believed to produce excitatory behaviors, including myoclonus, allodynia, and seizures. In a study of cancer patients who developed allodynia and myoclonus during morphine infusions, M3G levels were elevated.[115] Case reports suggest that

M3G and H3G plasma levels are greatly increased in the presence of renal failure, with the ratio of metabolite to parent compound four times higher than the ratio seen in patients with normal renal function.[119,120] However, one prospective study found no relationship between myoclonus and renal function.[121] In rodent models, H3G has more potent neuroexcitatory effects when compared with M3G.[122]

Regardless of the underlying cause, treatment is imperative. The goal is to significantly reduce the dose of the opioid, and this is usually accomplished by rotation to an alternate opioid.[123,124] Methadone has been used as an alternative agent with success, although other opioids may be easier to titrate and methadone also has been found to produce myoclonus.[111] Other strategies include adding adjuvant analgesics and using interventional techniques (e.g., spinal drug administration, nerve blocks) to potentially reduce the amount of total systemic opioid. Little research is available regarding agents used to reduce myoclonic jerking. Benzodiazepines, including clonazepam, diazepam, and midazolam, have been recommended.[123,125] The mechanism of action of benzodiazepines is through binding to γ-aminobutyric acid type A (GABA$_A$) receptors within the central nervous system, leading to central nervous system depression. At higher doses, benzodiazepines may also limit repetitive neuronal firing, similar to several anticonvulsant compounds. Clonazepam may be useful in patients who can swallow, with doses starting at 0.5 to 1 mg by mouth every 6 or 8 hours, with upward titration as needed. Lorazepam tablets or solution can be placed sublingually if the patient is unable to swallow. Lorazepam and midazolam can be administered parenterally and are often indicated during the final hours of life.

Intractable Pain at End of Life

When pain is poorly managed despite aggressive titration of available therapies, several other options can be employed.[126] First, thorough assessment is needed to rule out potentially reversible etiologies. Because the pain demands immediate attention, titration of the opioid therapy must be aggressive while carefully preventing and treating adverse effects. Additional therapies should be considered, such as corticosteroids, local anesthetics, ketamine, and other therapies. Bringing in a team approach is crucial, including experts in pain and palliative care, as well as chaplains, social workers, psychologists, and others, to address patient and family suffering. When these interventions are unsuccessful, palliative sedation may be considered.

Intravenous Lidocaine. Systemic administration of local anesthetics, such as lidocaine, has been used to treat chronic pain.[127–129] At subanesthetic doses, lidocaine blocks neuronal function in active or depolarized neurons without interfering with the normal function of other sensory or motor neurons. Although historically used as a monthly infusion in chronic pain clinics, similar protocols have been adapted for use in patients at end of life with intractable pain. The dosage is generally 1–3 mg/kg administered intravenously over 20–30 minutes.[130] During the bolus infusion, pain intensity scores often decline significantly. If effective, a continuous infusion of 1–3 mg/kg/hour will be initiated. Immediate signs of toxicity include numbness around the lips or a sensation of thickness of the tongue. Due to the short half-life of lidocaine, the symptoms of toxicity are transient and easily reversible by lowering the infusion rate. However, toxicity has been reported at very low doses of lidocaine.[131]

In concert with the goals of care at this time of life, cardiac monitoring is not usually performed nor are plasma levels of lidocaine obtained. If subcutaneous administration is indicated due to lack of venous access, the initial loading dose is administered over a longer time period (30 minutes to an hour) and the response may be delayed by a few minutes. If subcutaneous infusion is elected, more concentrated lidocaine solutions allow for lower volumes to be infused. If the bolus dose is ineffective or toxicity is unmanageable, the lidocaine challenge is discontinued and other pain relief modalities must be selected.

The lidocaine infusion technique has been reported to be effective in a child with cancer, using 35 mcg/kg per minute initially, with an increase to 50 mcg/kg per minute after several days.[132] The only randomized controlled trial of intravenous lidocaine for neuropathic pain from cancer using 5 mg/kg over 30 minutes found no difference in analgesia.[133] Much more research in this particular area is needed.

Ketamine. Ketamine is an N-methyl-D-aspartate antagonist that can be given by a variety of routes: oral, intravenous, subcutaneous, intranasal, sublingual, epidural, intrathecal, and topical. It has been reported to improve pain relief and reduce opioid requirements in a variety of pain syndromes associated with cancer and other life-threatening illnesses.[134–138] Although it can be used earlier in the course of the disease trajectory, ketamine is most commonly trialed in the face of intractable pain at the end of life.

In a small (n = 10) study of cancer patients who reported pain unrelieved with morphine, a slow bolus of ketamine (0.25 mg/kg or 0.50 mg/kg) was evaluated using a randomized, double-blind, crossover, double-dose design. Ketamine, but not saline solution, significantly reduced the pain intensity in almost all the patients at both doses, with the greatest effect being in those treated with higher doses. Adverse effects included hallucinations in 4 patients and an unpleasant cognitive sensation in 2 patients. These adverse effects responded to diazepam 1 mg intravenously. Drowsiness was also significantly more likely to occur, particularly with the higher dose. The investigators concluded that ketamine improved morphine analgesia in a variety of difficult pain syndromes, yet central adverse effects can limit the use of this therapy.[139]

A study in young children and adolescents who were on high doses of opioids and had uncontrolled cancer pain examined the effect of adding a low-dose ketamine infusion. In 8 of 11 patients, ketamine infusions used as an adjuvant to opioid analgesia provided improvement in pain and was associated with opioid-sparing effects. This allowed reduction in opioid dose that ultimately improved social interaction during this important time.[140]

The usual oral dose of ketamine is 10 to 15 mg every 6 hours. Because oral preparations are not commercially available in the United States, the solution used for injection is administered orally, usually mixed with juice or cola to hide the unpleasant taste. Parenteral dosing is typically 0.04 mg/kg/hour with titration to a maximum of 0.3 mg/kg/hour. When given parenterally or orally, the onset of analgesia is 15–30 minutes with a duration of effect ranging between 15 minutes to 2 hours. A general recommendation is to reduce the opioid dose by approximately 25% when starting ketamine to avoid sedation. Severe side effects are generally associated with doses of parenteral ketamine above 0.5 mg/kg and include psychotomimetic phenomena such as dysphoria, nightmares, hallucinations, excessive salivation, and tachycardia.

Because of the lack of high quality, randomized controlled clinical trials, a recent Cochrane review concluded that there was insufficient evidence to conclude that ketamine improves the effectiveness of opioid treatment in cancer pain.[141,142] Clearly, more research in this area is needed.

Fears of Hastening Death

Pain at the end of life may be poorly managed due to fears of causing respiratory depression. This is particularly true when family members administering opioids at home express fear about causing their loved one's death. It can also occur in institutional settings where clinicians are uncomfortable ordering or administering therapeutic doses of drug. Clinicians and family members also fear "giving the last dose" of an opioid. Education is desper-

ately needed. Respiratory depression is rare in palliative care as most patients are opioid-tolerant. A recent study of cancer patients undergoing parenteral opioid titration for severe pain revealed no change in end-tidal carbon dioxide, oxygen saturation, or respiratory rate.[143] Sykes and Thorns[144] evaluated 17 studies that examined the use of opioids at end of life. None of the five studies that explored opioid use and survival found any relationship. Their own earlier study also found no relationship between the dose or the timing of the opioid administration and the time of death.[145] These authors conclude that the doctrine of double effect, which suggests it is ethical to employ a treatment intending to obtain its beneficial effect (e.g., analgesia) but at the same time recognizing that it may also have harmful effects (e.g., respiratory depression or death), is not relevant. They also argue that it is potentially harmful to invoke this doctrine as it potentiates a myth: one that can lead to greater fear and unrelieved pain. A recent study from the National Hospice Database reported similar results; that the dose of opioid had no appreciable impact on the timing of death in patients with far-advanced disease.[146]

Suffering and Existential Distress

It may be very difficult to distinguish pain from other causes of suffering in dying patients. Although the trend toward greater attention to pain is positive, there is frequently little attention to the role loss, burden, sadness, fear, isolation, and other existential concerns that can play at this time of life.[147] Several studies support the need for more useful definitions and distinctions and to address the role of suffering in the individual's life. For example, one study asked hospice patients about suffering in an open-ended interview, revealing that in the views of the 100 patients included in this study, relief of pain and relief of suffering are not the same.[148] Another study of health care professionals revealed that suffering was viewed quite differently by chaplains, who defined this in spiritual terms, versus pain professionals, who placed existential issues in the context of pain.[149]

Using semistructured interviews, 381 patients with advanced cancer were asked if they felt they were suffering and were also asked about physical symptoms, social concerns, psychologic problems, and existential issues. Approximately 25% reported they were suffering at a moderate-to-extreme level. This suffering was strongly correlated with general malaise, weakness, pain, and depression. Thus, although many patients with advanced cancer do not consider themselves to be suffering, for those who are suffering, it is a multidimensional experience related most strongly to physical symptoms, but with contributions from psychologic distress, existential concerns, and social-relational worries as well.[150] The consequences of unresolved suffering are great, including a wish for hastened death. In a study of 96 terminally ill elders, 15 acknowledged significant suffering that resulted in a wish for a hastened death, and several had even considered strategies to accelerate the dying process. In analyses of the interviews of these individuals, four critical themes emerged: perceived insensitive and uncaring communication of a terminal diagnosis by their health care professional, experiencing unbearable physical pain, unacknowledged feelings regarding undergoing chemotherapy or radiation treatment, and dying in a distressing environment.[151]

Assessment of the whole person should be multidimensional, and an interdisciplinary team is best equipped to address these broad issues. In addition to a thorough pain and symptom assessment, patients should be asked about the meaning of their lives, their sense of hope, the goals they have for this time of their lives, and whether they are suffering. Suffering is a deeply personal experience, accompanied by a wide range of emotions and meanings. Inadequate assessment that only equates pain with suffering can lead to inappropriate increases in opioids, without benefiting their existential concerns, while leading to increased toxicity.[152]

When patients are identified as experiencing suffering, several interventions can be useful. Life review allows the individual to reminisce about life experiences, often leading to self-discovery of meaning in the contributions they have made. Some people benefit by developing letters or videotapes to loved ones, to be read at a later date during anticipated landmark events in the loved one's life, such as college graduation, marriage, or the birth of a child. One novel model to address psychosocial and existential distress in the dying is called dignity therapy.[153] This brief, individualized approach to end-of-life care allows patients to discuss issues that are most important to them and to describe the things they would most want remembered as death draws near. These discussions are recorded, transcribed, and developed into a document, which can be given to family or loved ones. In one study of people with advanced cancer, 76% reported a heightened sense of dignity, 68% reported an increased sense of purpose, 67% reported a heightened sense of meaning, and 47% reported an increased will to live.[154] Family perceptions were also positive, with the majority stating that the document developed by the dying loved one helped during the grieving process and that the document would continue to be a source of comfort for their families and themselves.[155] Those who are suffering often feel voiceless and having professionals witness and listen to their concerns in an empathic manner can be extraordinarily therapeutic.

Nonpharmacologic Techniques

Nonpharmacologic therapies can be particularly useful during the final hours of life. Cognitive-behavioral techniques, physical measures, and education can be used as part of the multimodal treatment plan to reduce pain and suffering. The patient's and caregivers' abilities to participate must be considered when selecting any of these therapies, including their fatigue level, interest, cognition, and other factors.[156] Cognitive-behavioral techniques include guided imagery,[157] meditation,[158] hypnosis,[159] music[160] and art therapy,[161] and other complementary therapies.[162]

Physical measures, including massage,[163,164] reflexology,[165] heat, and other techniques,[166] can produce relaxation and relieve pain. In a small study of massage in hospice patients, reductions in blood pressure, heart rate, and skin temperature were noted, suggestive of a relaxation effect.[167] A potential benefit of all of these therapies is the ability to include family members who are often seeking methods to provide comfort to their loved one.

Family involvement in all aspects of care is crucial. Family caregivers who rate their self-efficacy, or their ability to care for their loved one, as high report much lower levels of strain, as well as decreased negative mood and increased positive mood. Ultimately, the caregiver's self-efficacy in managing the patient's pain related to the patient's physical well-being. In dyads where the family caregiver perceived higher self-efficacy, the patient reported having more energy, feeling less ill, and spending less time in bed.[168] As a result of these findings, Keefe and colleagues[169] developed a partner-guided pain management training intervention that they tested in 78 advanced cancer patients who met criteria for hospice eligibility. Patients and their partners were randomly assigned to the intervention or to usual care as the control condition. The partner-guided pain management training protocol consisted of educational information about cancer pain with systematic training of patients and partners in cognitive and behavioral pain coping skills delivered in the patients' homes over three sessions. The partner-guided pain management protocol significantly increased partners' ratings of their self-efficacy for helping the patient control pain and other symptoms. These family caregivers also showed a trend toward reduced levels of caregiver strain.[169]

Although case reports and open label trials of cognitive-behavioral, physical measures, and educational interventions are reported to be very effective in relieving symptoms, more research is needed.[170] Furthermore, most existing research has been conducted in patients early in the disease trajectory, so more research is needed to determine the potential value, no less the feasibility, of these interventions in the final days and hours of life.

PALLIATIVE SEDATION

Although the majority of individuals with pain at the end of life can obtain relief with available therapies, some dying patients experience distressing symptoms that cannot be controlled. In these cases, palliative sedation may be considered. Several steps are crucial when implementing palliative sedation. First, the team must be confident that all other reasonable options have been explored, the disease is irreversible, and that death would be expected in hours to days.[171] Second, the patient and family should be carefully informed about the risks and benefits of sedation and they should agree with these plans. The entire team (physicians, nurses, respiratory therapy, chaplains, social workers, and others involved in the patient's care) must have the opportunity to discuss this option and agree as a team about the justification for the use of sedation and the details of the care to be provided.[172] These are generally complex cases that are emotionally stressful. All involved can benefit from talking about the complex medical, ethical, and emotional issues they raise.[172-174] Decisions about hydration and nutrition as well as resuscitation status (most centers require that the patient has do not resuscitate orders) should be made prior to initiating sedation. Sedation may be delayed if the patient is awaiting the arrival of a family member from out of town. In some cases, light sedation may be used and reversed once the relative arrives, then restarted and increased once the patient and loved one have had time to say good-bye.[175]

The agent most commonly employed is midazolam, although other benzodiazepines, propofol, or barbiturates can be administered (Table 108.3).[172,176] Benzodiazepines have anxiolytic, muscle relaxant, sedative-hypnotic, anticonvulsant, antiemetic, and amnesic effects. Their mechanism of action is through binding to GABA receptors within the central nervous system leading to central nervous system depression. Midazolam is the shortest acting agent within this class, with an onset of action within 3–5 minutes after intravenous injection and a half life of 1 to 4 hours. These attributes, rapid onset and relatively short duration, as well as the ability to administer it either intravenously or subcutaneously makes this a useful drug in instituting palliative sedation. Furthermore, it is stable with most other agents, but incompatible with corticosteroids such as dexamethasone, betamethasone, or methylprednisolone.

Propofol is an intravenous nonbarbiturate thought to enhance the activity of GABA. The advantages of propofol include rapid onset and short half-life. Although studies are lacking, the recommended dose of propofol to treat refractory pain/suffering is 1–2 mg/kg via intravenous injection over 5 minutes.[177] The bolus may need to be repeated if the first injection ineffective. Bolus doses are followed by a maintenance intravenous infusion of 2–10 mg/kg per hour, using the lowest dose needed to suppress symptoms. Propofol is recommended for intravenous administration; subcutaneous delivery has not been studied. Propofol contains soybean oil and egg yolk phospholipid, and therefore is contraindicated for use in patients with egg hypersensitivity or soya lecithin hypersensitivity.[178]

Family members must be provided sufficient information and support during this time. In a multicenter study conducted in Japan, bereaved family members of cancer patients who received sedation in seven palliative care units were surveyed.[179] The families reported that 69% of the patients were considerably or very distressed before sedation. Although the majority of families were satisfied with the treatment, 25% expressed a high level of emotional distress. The factors associated with high levels of family distress were poor symptom control after sedation, feeling the burden of responsibility for the decision, feeling unprepared for changes in the patient's condition, feeling that the physicians and

TABLE 108.3

DOSES OF AGENTS USED IN PALLIATIVE SEDATION[172,176]

Drug	Route	Bolus dose	Continuous infusion
Midazolam	IV, SQ	5 mg	Starting dose 1 mg/hour; usual maintenance dose 20–120 mg/hour
Lorazepam	IV, SQ, SL, PO	0.5–2 mg PO, SL every 1–2 hours; 2–5 mg SQ or IV	Starting dose 0.5–1.0 mg/hour; usual maintenance dose 4–40 mg/hour
Chlorpromazine	PO, IV, PR	10–25 mg every 2–4 hours	
Haloperidol	PO, IV, SQ	0.5–5 mg PO every 2–4 hours; 1–5 mg IV/SQ bolus	Starting dose 0.2 mg/hour; maintenance 0.2–0.6 mg/hour
Thiopental	IV	5–7 mg/kg/hour	20–80 mg/hour
Pentobarbital	IV	2–3 mg/kg	Starting dose 1 mg/kg/hour; titrate upward as needed
Phenobarbital	IV, SQ	200 mg, can repeat every 10–15 minutes	25 mg/hour; maintenance dose 25–66 mg/hour
Propofol	IV	20–50 mg bolus; may repeat	5–10 mg/hour; may increase dose by 10 mg/hour every 15–20 minutes

IV, intravenous; PO, oral; PR, rectal; SL, sublingual; SQ, subcutaneous.

nurses were not sufficiently compassionate, and a shorter time to their loved one's death. Regular monitoring of patient distress with timely modification of the sedation protocol is vital, as is providing sufficient information and sharing the responsibility for the decision. Family members require emotional support to assist with their anticipatory and ongoing grief.[179] As the use of palliative sedation increases, guidelines should be developed across settings and disciplines to ensure consistency. These guidelines must articulate that this therapy is not euthanasia, but is rather directed toward treatment of symptoms.[180]

CONCLUSION

The relief of pain during the final phase of life is vital for both the patient who is experiencing this pain and for those at the bedside witnessing this distress. All clinicians have the responsibility to learn how to assess pain in the cognitively impaired and how to employ effective pharmacologic and nonpharmacologic treatments. Empathic listening with attention to suffering and existential distress will help improve the quality of life of the dying. When pain remains severe, despite aggressive use of all appropriate options, the team must carefully consider the use of palliative sedation, along with the patient and their loved ones. All of this care involves the skills of a well-functioning interdisciplinary team, combining the expertise of each individual to provide optimal care to the most vulnerable of all of our patients.

References

1. Kutner JS, Bryant LL, Beaty BL, et al. Time course and characteristics of symptom distress and quality of life at the end of life. *J Pain Symptom Manage* 2007;34(3):227–236.
2. Chang VT, Hwang SS, Feuerman M, et al. Symptom and quality of life survey of medical oncology patients at a veterans affairs medical center: a role for symptom assessment. *Cancer* 2000;88(5):1175–1183.
3. Cohen SR, Mount BM. Living with cancer: "good" days and "bad" days—what produces them? Can the McGill quality of life questionnaire distinguish between them? *Cancer* 2000;89(8):1854–1865.
4. Cooley ME, Short TH, Moriarty HJ. Symptom prevalence, distress, and change over time in adults receiving treatment for lung cancer. *Psychooncology* 2003;12(7):694–708.
5. Lo RS, Woo J, Zhoc KC, et al. Quality of life of palliative care patients in the last two weeks of life. *J Pain Symptom Manage* 2002;24(4):388–397.
6. Vainio A, Auvinen A. Prevalence of symptoms among patients with advanced cancer: an international collaborative study. Symptom Prevalence Group. *J Pain Symptom Manage* 1996;12(1):3–10.
7. Hall P, Schroder C, Weaver L. The last 48 hours of life in long-term care: a focused chart audit. *J Am Geriatr Soc* 2002;50(3):501–506.
8. Stromgren AS, Sjögren P, Goldschmidt D, et al. Symptom priority and course of symptomatology in specialized palliative care. *J Pain Symptom Manage* 2006;31(3):199–206.
9. Teno JM, Clarridge BR, Casey V, et al. Family perspectives on end-of-life care at the last place of care. *JAMA* 2004;291(1):88–93.
10. Lopez AD, Mathers CD, Ezzati M, et al. Global and regional burden of disease and risk factors: systematic analysis of population health data. *Lancet* 2001; 367(9524):1747–1757.
11. Abegunde DO, Mathers CD, Adam T, et al. The burden and costs of chronic diseases in low-income and middle-income countries. *Lancet* 2007;370(9603): 1929–1938.
12. WHO Expert Committee. *Cancer Pain Relief and Palliative Care.* 2nd ed. Geneva: World Health Organization; 1996.
13. Center to Advance Palliative Care. New analysis shows hospitals continue to implement palliative care programs at rapid pace. Available at: http://www.capc.org/news-and-events/releases/news-release-4-14-08. Accessed May 3, 2008.
14. Temel JS, Jackson VA, Billings JA, et al. Phase II study: integrated palliative care in newly diagnosed advanced non-small-cell lung cancer patients. *J Clin Oncol* 2007;25(17):2377–2382.
15. Potter J, Hami F, Bryan T, et al. Symptoms in 400 patients referred to palliative care services: prevalence and patterns. *Palliat Med* 2003;17(4):310–314.
16. Wells N. Pain intensity and pain interference in hospitalized patients with cancer. *Oncol Nurs Forum* 2000;27(6):985–991.

17. Meuser T, Pietruck C, Radbruch L, et al. Symptoms during cancer pain treatment following WHO-guidelines: a longitudinal follow-up study of symptom prevalence, severity and etiology. *Pain* 2001;93(3):247–257.

18. Potter J, Higginson IJ. Pain experienced by lung cancer patients: a review of prevalence, causes and pathophysiology. *Lung Cancer* 2004;43(3):247–257.

19. Coyle N, Adelhardt J, Foley KM, et al. Character of terminal illness in the advanced cancer patient: pain and other symptoms during the last four weeks of life. *J Pain Symptom Manage* 1990;5(2):83–93.

20. Wolfe J, Grier HE, Klar N, et al. Symptoms and suffering at the end of life in children with cancer. *N Engl J Med* 2000;342(5):326–333.

21. O'Mahony S, Goulet J, Kornblith A, et al. Desire for hastened death, cancer pain and depression: report of a longitudinal observational study. *J Pain Symptom Manage* 2005;29(5):446–457.

22. Harding R, Easterbrook P, Dinat N, et al. Pain and symptom control in HIV disease: under-researched and poorly managed. *Clin Infect Dis* 2005;40(3):491–492.

23. Higginson IJ, Hart S, Silber E, et al. Symptom prevalence and severity in people severely affected by multiple sclerosis. *J Palliat Care* 2006;22(3):158–165.

24. Ehde DM, Osborne TL, Hanley MA, et al. The scope and nature of pain in persons with multiple sclerosis. *Mult Scler* 2006;12(5):629–638.

25. Ganzini L, Johnston WS, Hoffman WF. Correlates of suffering in amyotrophic lateral sclerosis. *Neurology* 1999;52(7):1434–1440.

26. Saleem T, Leigh PN, Higginson IJ. Symptom prevalence among people affected by advanced and progressive neurological conditions—a systematic review. *J Palliat Care* 2007;23(4):291–299.

27. Murtagh FE, Addington-Hall J, Higginson IJ. The prevalence of symptoms in end-stage renal disease: a systematic review. *Adv Chronic Kidney Dis* 2007;14(1):82–99.

28. Johnson MJ. Management of end stage cardiac failure. *Postgrad Med J* 2007;83(980):395–401.

29. Murray SA, Boyd K, Kendall M, et al. Dying of lung cancer or cardiac failure: prospective qualitative interview study of patients and their carers in the community. *BMJ* 2002;325(7370):929.

30. Anderson H, Ward C, Eardley A, et al. The concerns of patients under palliative care and a heart failure clinic are not being met. *Palliat Med* 2001;15(4):279–286.

31. Nordgren L, Sorensen S. Symptoms experienced in the last six months of life in patients with end-stage heart failure. *Eur J Cardiovasc Nurs* 2003;2(3):213–217.

32. Woolf AD, Pfleger B. Burden of major musculoskeletal conditions. *Bull World Health Organ* 2003;81(9):646–656.

33. Miaskowski C, Cleary J, Burney R, et al. *Guideline for the Management of Cancer Pain in Adults and Children.* Glenview, IL: American Pain Society; 2005:3.

34. Holen JC, Hjermstad MJ, Loge JH, et al. Pain assessment tools: is the content appropriate for use in palliative care? *J Pain Symptom Manage* 2006;32(6):567–580.

35. Paice JA. Assessment of symptom clusters in people with cancer. *J Natl Cancer Inst* 2004;32:98–102.

36. Homsi J, Walsh D, Rivera N, et al. Symptom evaluation in palliative medicine: patient report vs systematic assessment. *Support Care Cancer* 2006;14(5):444–453.

37. Chang VT, Hwang SS, Feuerman M. Validation of the Edmonton Symptom Assessment Scale. *Cancer* 2000;88(9):2164–2171.

38. Cleeland CS, Mendoza TR, Wang XS, et al. Assessing symptom distress in cancer patients: the M.D. Anderson Symptom Inventory. *Cancer* 2000;89(7):1634–1646.

39. Chang VT, Hwang SS, Feuerman M, et al. The Memorial Symptom Assessment Scale short form (MSAS-SF). *Cancer* 2000;89(5):1162–1171.

40. Portenoy RK, Thaler HT, Kornblith AB, et al. The Memorial Symptom Assessment Scale: an instrument for the evaluation of symptom prevalence, characteristics and distress. *Eur J Cancer* 1994;30A(9):1326–1336.

41. Stein KD, Denniston M, Baker F, et al. Validation of a modified Rotterdam Symptom Checklist for use with cancer patients in the United States. *J Pain Symptom Manage* 2003;26(5):975–989.

42. Tranmer JE, Heyland D, Dudgeon D, et al. Measuring the symptom experience of seriously ill cancer and noncancer hospitalized patients near the end of life with the memorial symptom assessment scale. *J Pain Symptom Manage* 2003;25(5):420–429.

43. Hardy JR, Edmonds P, Turner R, et al. The use of the Rotterdam Symptom Checklist in palliative care. *J Pain Symptom Manage* 1999;18(2):79–84.

44. Guo H, Fine PG, Mendoza TR, et al. A preliminary study of the utility of the Brief Hospice Inventory. *J Pain Symptom Manage* 2001;22(2):637–648.

45. Breley DK. Beyond reliability and validity: analysis of selected quality-of-life instruments for use in palliative care. *J Palliat Med* 1992;2(3):299–309.

46. McMillan SC, Mahon M. Measuring quality of life in hospice patients using a newly developed Hospice Quality of Life Index. *Qual Life Res* 1994;3(6):437–447.

47. Herr K, Bjoro K, Decker S. Tools for assessment of pain in nonverbal older adults with dementia: a state-of-the-science review. *J Pain Symptom Manage* 2006;31(2):170–192.

48. Bjoro K, Herr K. Assessment of pain in the nonverbal or cognitively impaired older adult. *Clin Geriatr Med* 2008;24(2):237–262.

49. Hadjistavropoulos T, Herr K, Turk DC, et al. An interdisciplinary expert consensus statement on assessment of pain in older persons. *Clin J Pain* 2007;23(1 Suppl):S1–43.

50. Herr K, Coyne PJ, Key T, et al. Pain assessment in the nonverbal patient: position statement with clinical practice recommendations. *Pain Manag Nurs* 2006;7(2):44–52.

51. Holen JC, Saltvedt I, Fayers PM, et al. Doloplus-2, a valid tool for behavioural pain assessment? *BMC Geriatrics* 2007;7:29.

52. Angus DC, Barnato AE, Linde-Zwirble WT, et al. Use of intensive care at the end of life in the United States: an epidemiologic study. *Crit Care Med* 2004;32(3):638–643.

53. SUPPORT Principal Investigators. A controlled trial to improve care for seriously ill hospitalized patients. The study to understand prognosis and preferences for outcomes and risks of treatment. *JAMA* 1995;274:1591–1598.

54. White DB, Curtis JR, Wolf LE, et al. Life support for patients without a surrogate decision maker: who decides? *Ann Intern Med* 2007;147(1):34–40.

55. Payen JF, Bru O, Bosson JL, et al. Assessing pain in critically ill sedated patients by using a behavioral pain scale. *Crit Care Med* 2001;29(12):2258–2263.

56. Gelinas C, Johnston C. Pain assessment in the critically ill ventilated adult: validation of the critical-care pain observation tool and physiologic indicators. *Clin J Pain* 2007;23(6):497–505.

57. Manworren RC, Hynan LS. Clinical validation of FLACC: preverbal patient pain scale. *Pediatr Nurs* 2003;29(2):140–146.

58. van Dijk M, de Boer JB, Koot HM, et al. The reliability and validity of the COMFORT scale as a postoperative pain instrument in 0 to 3-year-old infants. *Pain* 2000;84(2–3):367–377.

59. Caraceni A, Cherny N, Fainsinger R, et al. Pain measurement tools and methods in clinical research in palliative care: recommendations of an Expert Working Group of the European Association of Palliative Care. *J Pain Symptom Manage* 2002;23(3):239–255.

60. Weinberg DS, Inturrisi CE, Reidenberg B, et al. Sublingual absorption of selected opioid analgesics. *Clin Pharmacol Ther* 1988;44(3):335–342.

61. Reisfield GM, Wilson GR. Rational use of sublingual opioids in palliative medicine. *J Palliat Med* 2007;10(2):465–475.

62. Coluzzi PH. Sublingual morphine: efficacy reviewed. *J Pain Symptom Manage* 1998;16(3):184–192.

63. Cerchietti LC, Navigante AH, Bonomi MR, et al. Effect of topical morphine for mucositis-associated pain following concomitant chemoradiotherapy for head and neck carcinoma. *Cancer* 2002;95(10):2230–2236.

64. Cerchietti LC, Navigante AH, Korte MW, et al. Potential utility of the peripheral analgesic properties of morphine in stomatitis-related pain: a pilot study. *Pain* 2003;105(1–2):265–273.

65. Hanks GW, Nugent M, Higgs CM, et al. Oral transmucosal fentanyl citrate in the management of breakthrough pain in cancer: an open, multicentre, dose-titration and long-term use study. *Palliat Med* 2004;18(8):698–704.

66. Coluzzi PH, Schwartzberg L, Conroy JD, et al. Breakthrough cancer pain: a randomized trial comparing oral transmucosal fentanyl citrate (OTFC) and morphine sulfate immediate release (MSIR). *Pain* 2001;91(1–2):123–130.

67. Payne R, Coluzzi P, Hart L, et al. Long-term safety of oral transmucosal fentanyl citrate for breakthrough cancer pain. *J Pain Symptom Manage* 2001;22(1):575–583.

68. Christie JM, Simmonds M, Patt R, et al. Dose-titration, multicenter study of oral transmucosal fentanyl citrate for the treatment of breakthrough pain in cancer patients using transdermal fentanyl for persistent pain. *J Clin Oncol* 1998;16(10):3238–3245.

69. Portenoy RK, Taylor D, Messina J, et al. A randomized, placebo-controlled study of fentanyl buccal tablet for breakthrough pain in opioid-treated patients with cancer. *Clin J Pain* 2006;22(9):805–811.

70. Darwish M, Kirby M, Robertson P Jr, et al. Absolute and relative bioavailability of fentanyl buccal tablet and oral transmucosal fentanyl citrate. *J Clin Pharmacol* 2007;47(3):343–350.

71. Du X, Skopp G, Aderjan R. The influence of the route of administration: a comparative study at steady state of oral sustained release morphine and morphine sulfate suppositories. *Ther Drug Monit* 1999;21(2):208–214.

72. Gourlay GK. Sustained relief of chronic pain. Pharmacokinetics of sustained release morphine. *Clin Pharmacokinet* 1998;35(3):173–190.

73. Dale O, Sheffels P, Kharasch ED. Bioavailabilities of rectal and oral methadone in healthy subjects. *Br J Clin Pharmacol* 2004;58(2):156–162.

74. Ripamonti C, Zecca E, Brunelli C, et al. Rectal methadone in cancer patients with pain. A preliminary clinical and pharmacokinetic study. *Ann Oncol* 1995;6(8):841–843.

75. McCaffery M, Martin L, Ferrell BR. Analgesic administration via rectum or stoma. *J ET Nurs* 1992;19(4):114–121.

76. Finn J, Wright J, Fong J, et al. A randomised crossover trial of patient controlled intranasal fentanyl and oral morphine for procedural wound care in adult patients with burns. *Burns* 2004;30(3):262–268.

77. Fitzgibbon D, Morgan D, Dockter D, et al. Initial pharmacokinetic, safety and efficacy evaluation of nasal morphine gluconate for breakthrough pain in cancer patients. *Pain* 2003;106(3):309–315.

78. Rudy AC, Coda BA, Archer SM, et al. A multiple-dose phase I study of intranasal hydromorphone hydrochloride in healthy volunteers. *Anesth Analg* 2004;99(5):1379–1386.

79. Watanabe S, Pereira J, Hanson J, et al. Fentanyl by continuous subcutaneous infusion for the management of cancer pain: a retrospective study. *J Pain Symptom Manage* 1998;16(5):323–326.

80. Centeno C, Vara F. Intermittent subcutaneous methadone administration in the management of cancer pain. *J Pain Pall Care Pharmacother* 2005;19(2):7–12.

81. Nelson KA, Glare PA, Walsh D, et al. A prospective, within-patient, crossover study of continuous intravenous and subcutaneous morphine for chronic cancer pain. *J Pain Symptom Manage* 1997;13(5):262–267.

82. Bruera E, Neumann CM, Pituskin E, et al. A randomized controlled trial of local injections of hyaluronidase versus placebo in cancer patients receiving subcutaneous hydration. *Ann Oncol* 1999;10(10):1255–1258.

83. Burton AW, Rajagopal A, Shah HN, et al. Epidural and intrathecal analgesia is effective in treating refractory cancer pain. *Pain Med* 2004;5(3):239–247.

84. Baker L, Lee M, Regnard C, et al. Evolving spinal analgesia practice in palliative care. *Palliat Med* 2004;18(6):507–515.

85. Smith TJ, Staats PS, Deer T, et al. Randomized clinical trial of an implantable drug delivery system compared with comprehensive medical management for refractory cancer pain: impact on pain, drug-related toxicity, and survival. *J Clin Oncol* 2002 ;20(19):4040–4049.

86. Lema MJ. Invasive analgesia techniques for advanced cancer pain. *Surg Oncol Clin N Am* 2001;10(1):127–136.

87. Zeppetella G, Porzio G, Aielli F. Opioids applied topically to painful cutaneous malignant ulcers in a palliative care setting. *J Opioid Manag* 2007; 3(3):161–166.

88. Zeppetella G, Ribeiro MD. Morphine in intrasite gel applied topically to painful ulcers. *J Pain Symptom Manage* 2005;29(2):118–119.

89. Ballas SK. Treatment of painful sickle cell leg ulcers with topical opioids. *Blood* 2002;99(3):1096.

90. Long TD, Cathers TA, Twillman R, et al. Morphine-Infused silver sulfadiazine (MISS) cream for burn analgesia: a pilot study. *J Burn Care Rehabil* 2001; 22(2):118–123.

91. Vernassiere C, Cornet C, Trechot P, et al. Study to determine the efficacy of topical morphine on painful chronic skin ulcers. *J Wound Care* 2005;14(6): 289–293.

92. Ribeiro MD, Joel SP, Zeppetella G. The bioavailability of morphine applied topically to cutaneous ulcers. *J Pain Symptom Manage* 2004;27(5):434–439.

93. Paice JA, Von Roenn JH, Hudgins JC, et al. Morphine bioavailability from a topical gel formulation in volunteers. *J Pain Symptom Manage* 2008;35(3): 314–320.

94. Muijsers RB, Wagstaff AJ. Transdermal fentanyl: an updated review of its pharmacological properties and therapeutic efficacy in chronic cancer pain control. *Drugs* 2001;61(15):2289–2307.

95. Morita T, Takigawa C, Onishi H, et al. Opioid rotation from morphine to fentanyl in delirious cancer patients: an open-label trial. *J Pain Symptom Manage* 2005;30(1):96–103.

96. Mystakidou K, Parpa E, Tsilika E, et al. Pain management of cancer patients with transdermal fentanyl: a study of 1828 step I, II, & III transfers. *J Pain* 2004;5(2):119–132.

97. Hanks GW, Conno F, Cherny N, et al. Morphine and alternative opioids in cancer pain: the EAPC recommendations. *Br J Cancer* 2001;84(5):587–593.

98. Weschules DJ, Bain KT, Reifsnyder J, et al. Toward evidence-based prescribing at end of life: a comparative analysis of sustained-release morphine, oxycodone, and transdermal fentanyl, with pain, constipation, and caregiver interaction outcomes in hospice patients. *Pain Med* 2006;7(4):320–329.

99. Staats PS, Markowitz J, Schein J. Incidence of constipation associated with long-acting opioid therapy: a comparative study. *South Med J* 2004 ;97(2): 129–134.

100. Menten J, Desmedt M, Lossignol D, et al. Longitudinal follow-up of TTS-fentanyl use in patients with cancer-related pain: results of a compassionate-use study with special focus on elderly patients. *Curr Med Res Opin* 2002; 18(8):488–498.

101. Radbruch L, Sabatowski R, Loick G, et al. Constipation and the use of laxatives: a comparison between transdermal fentanyl and oral morphine. *Palliat Med* 2000;14(2):111–119.

102. Jackson K II. Opioid Pharmacokinetics. In: Davis M, Glare P, Hardy J, eds. *Opioids in Cancer Pain*. New York: Oxford University Press; 2005:43–52.

103. Dean M. Opioids in renal failure and dialysis patients. *J Pain Symptom Manage* 2004;28(5):497–504.

104. Golf M, Paice JA, Feulner E, et al. Refractory status epilepticus. *J Palliat Med* 2004;7(1):85–88.

105. Nishigaya K, Kaneko M, Nagaseki Y, et al. Palatal myoclonus induced by extirpation of a cerebellar astrocytoma. Case report. *J Neurosurg* 1998;88(6): 1107–1110.

106. Fontoura P, Vale J, Lima C, et al. Progressive myoclonic ataxia and JC virus encephalitis in an AIDS patient. *J Neurol Neurosurg Psychiatry* 2002;72(5): 653–656.

107. Frucht SJ. The clinical challenge of posthypoxic myoclonus. *Adv Neurol* 2002; 89:85–88.

108. Wyllie AR, Bayliff CD, Kovacs MJ. Myoclonus due to chlorambucil in two adults with lymphoma. *Ann Pharmacother* 1997;31(2):171–174.

109. Patel S, Roshan VR, Lee KC, et al. A myoclonic reaction with low-dose hydromorphone. *Ann Pharmacother* 2006;40(11):2068–2070.

110. Hofmann A, Tangri N, Lafontaine AL, et al. Myoclonus as an acute complication of low-dose hydromorphone in multiple system atrophy. *J Neurol Neurosurg Psychiatry* 2006;77(8):994–995.

111. Sarhill N, Davis MP, Walsh D, et al. Methadone-induced myoclonus in advanced cancer. *Am J Hosp Palliat Care* 2001;18(1):51–53.

112. Bruera E, Pereira J. Acute neuropsychiatric findings in a patient receiving fentanyl for cancer pain. *Pain* 1997;69(1–2):199–201.

113. Andersen G, Jensen NH, Christrup L, et al. Pain, sedation and morphine metabolism in cancer patients during long-term treatment with sustained-release morphine. *Palliat Med* 2002;16(2):107–114.

114. Han PK, Arnold R, Bond G, J et al. Myoclonus secondary to withdrawal from transdermal fentanyl: case report and literature review. *J Pain Symptom Manage* 2002;23(1):66–72.

115. Sjogren P, Thunedborg LP, Christrup L, et al. Is development of hyperalgesia, allodynia and myoclonus related to morphine metabolism during long-term administration? Six case histories. *Acta Anaesthesiol Scand* 1998 ;42(9): 1070–1075.

116. Fainsinger R, Schoeller T, Boiskin M, et al. Palliative care round: cognitive failure and coma after renal failure in a patient receiving captopril and hydromorphone. *J Palliat Care* 1993;9(1):53–55.

117. Thwaites D, McCann S, Broderick P. Hydromorphone neuroexcitation. *J Palliat Med* 2004;7(4):545–550.

118. Smith MT. Neuroexcitatory effects of morphine and hydromorphone: evidence implicating the 3-glucuronide metabolites. *Clin Exper Pharmacol Physiol* 2000;27(7):524–528.

119. Babul N, Darke AC, Hagen N. Hydromorphone metabolite accumulation in renal failure. *J Pain Symptom Manage* 1995;10(3):184–186.

120. Portenoy RK, Foley KM, Stulman J, et al. Plasma morphine and morphine-6-glucuronide during chronic morphine therapy for cancer pain: plasma profiles, steady-state concentrations and the consequences of renal failure. *Pain* 1991;47(1):13–19.

121. Tiseo PJ, Thaler HT, Lapin J, et al. Morphine-6-glucuronide concentrations and opioid-related side effects: a survey in cancer patients. *Pain* 1995;61(1): 47–54.

122. Wright AW, Mather LE, Smith MT. Hydromorphone-3-glucuronide: a more potent neuro-excitant than its structural analogue, morphine-3-glucuronide. *Life Sci* 2001;69(4):409–420.

123. Cherny N, Ripamonti C, Pereira J, et al. Strategies to manage the adverse effects of oral morphine: an evidence-based report. *J Clin Oncol* 2001;19(9): 2542–2554.

124. Sjogren P, Jensen NH, Jensen TS. Disappearance of morphine-induced hyperalgesia after discontinuing or substituting morphine with other opioid agonists. *Pain* 1994;59(2):313–316.

125. Eisele JH Jr, Grigsby EJ, Dea G. Clonazepam treatment of myoclonic contractions associated with high-dose opioids: case report. *Pain* 1992;49(2): 231–232.

126. Moryl N, Coyle N, Foley KM. Managing an acute pain crisis in a patient with advanced cancer: "this is as much of a crisis as a code." *JAMA* 2008; 299(12):1457–1467.

127. Linchitz RM, Raheb JC. Subcutaneous infusion of lidocaine provides effective pain relief for CRPS patients. *Clin J Pain* 1999;15(1):67–72.

128. Wu CL, Tella P, Staats PS, et al. Analgesic effects of intravenous lidocaine and morphine on postamputation pain: a randomized double-blind, active placebo-controlled, crossover trial. *Anesthesiology* 2002;96(4):841–848.

129. Baranowski AP, De Courcey J, Bonello E. A trial of intravenous lidocaine on the pain and allodynia of postherpetic neuralgia. *J Pain Symptom Manage* 1999;17(6):429–433.

130. Ferrini R, Paice JA. How to initiate and monitor infusional lidocaine for severe and/or neuropathic pain. *J Support Oncol* 2004;2(1):90–94.

131. Tei Y, Morita T, Shishido H, et al. Lidocaine intoxication at very small doses in terminally ill cancer patients. J Pain Symptom Manage 2005;30(1):6–7.

132. Massey GV, Pedigo S, Dunn NL, et al. Continuous lidocaine infusion for the relief of refractory malignant pain in a terminally ill pediatric cancer patient. *J Pediatr Hematol Oncol* 2002;24(7):566–568.

133. Bruera E, Ripamonti C, Brenneis C, et al. A randomized double-blind crossover trial of intravenous lidocaine in the treatment of neuropathic cancer pain. *J Pain Symptom Manage* 1992;7(3):138–140.

134. Lossignol DA, Obiols-Portis M, Body JJ. Successful use of ketamine for intractable cancer pain. *Support Care Cancer* 2005;13(3):188–193.

135. Fitzgibbon EJ, Viola R. Parenteral ketamine as an analgesic adjuvant for severe pain: development and retrospective audit of a protocol for a palliative care unit. *J Palliat Med* 2005;8(1):49–57.

136. Kannan TR, Saxena A, Bhatnagar S, et al. Oral ketamine as an adjuvant to oral morphine for neuropathic pain in cancer patients. *J Pain Symptom Manage* 2002;23(1):60–65.

137. Berger JM, Ryan A, Vadivelu N, et al. Ketamine-fentanyl-midazolam infusion for the control of symptoms in terminal life care. *Am J Hosp Palliat Care* 2000;17(2):127–134.

138. Kotlinska-Lemieszek A, Luczak J. Subanesthetic ketamine: an essential adjuvant for intractable cancer pain. *J Pain Symptom Manage* 2004;28(2): 100–102.

139. Mercadante S, Arcuri E, Tirelli W, et al. Analgesic effect of intravenous ketamine in cancer patients on morphine therapy: a randomized, controlled, double-blind, crossover, double-dose study. *J Pain Symptom Manage* 2000;20(4): 246–252.

140. Finkel JC, Pestieau SR, Quezado ZM. Ketamine as an adjuvant for treatment of cancer pain in children and adolescents. *J Pain* 2007;8(6):515–521.

141. Bell RF, Eccleston C, Kalso E. Ketamine as adjuvant to opioids for cancer pain. A qualitative systematic review. *J Pain Symptom Manage* 2003;26(3): 867–875.

142. Bell R, Eccleston C, Kalso E. Ketamine as an adjuvant to opioids for cancer pain. *Cochrane Database Syst Rev* 2003;1:CD003351.

143. Estfan B, Mahmoud F, Shaheen P, et al. Respiratory function during parenteral opioid titration for cancer pain. *Palliat Med* 2007;21(2):81–86.

144. Sykes N, Thorns A. The use of opioids and sedatives at the end of life. *Lancet Oncol* 2003;4(5):312–318.

145. Thorns A, Sykes N. Opioid use in last week of life and implications for end-of-life decision-making. *Lancet* 2000;356(9227):398–399.

146. Portenoy RK, Sibirceva U, Smout R, et al. Opioid use and survival at the end of life: a survey of a hospice population. *J Pain Symptom Manage* 2006;32(6):532–540.

147. Coyle N. The hard work of living in the face of death. *J Pain Symptom Manage* 2006;32(3):266–274.

148. Terry W, Olson LG. Unobvious wounds: the suffering of hospice patients. *Int Med J* 2004;34(11):604–607.

149. Strang P, Strang S, Hultborn R, et al. Existential pain—an entity, a provocation, or a challenge? *J Pain Symptom Manage* 2004;27(3):241–250.

150. Wilson KG, Chochinov HM, McPherson CJ, et al. Suffering with advanced cancer. *J Clin Oncol* 2007;25(13):1691–1697.

151. Schroepfer TA. Critical events in the dying process: the potential for physical and psychosocial suffering. *J Palliat Med* 2007;10(1):136–147.

152. Al-Shahri MZ, Molina EH, Oneschuk D. Medication-focused approach to total pain: poor symptom control, polypharmacy, and adverse reactions. *Am J Hosp Palliat Care* 2003;20(4):307–310.

153. Chochinov HM. Dignity and the essence of medicine: the A, B, C, and D of dignity conserving care. *BMJ* 2007;335(7612):184–187.

154. Chochinov HM, Hack T, Hassard T, et al. Dignity therapy: a novel psychotherapeutic intervention for patients near the end of life. *J Clin Oncol* 2005;23(24):5520–5525.

155. McClement S, Chochinov HM, Hack T, et al. Dignity therapy: family member perspectives. *J Palliat Med* 2007;10(5):1076–1082.

156. Kwekkeboom KL, Bumpus M, Wanta B, et al. Oncology nurses' use of nondrug pain interventions in practice. *J Pain Symptom Manage* 2008;35(1):83–94.

157. Kwekkeboom KL, Kneip J, Pearson L. A pilot study to predict success with guided imagery for cancer pain. *Pain Manag Nurs* 2003;4(3):112–123.

158. Lafferty WE, Downey L, McCarty RL, et al. Evaluating CAM treatment at the end of life: a review of clinical trials for massage and meditation. *Complement Ther Med* 2006;14(2):100–112.

159. Spiegel D, Moore R. Imagery and hypnosis in the treatment of cancer patients. *Oncology (Williston Park)* 1997;11(8):1179–1189.

160. Magill L. The use of music therapy to address the suffering in advanced cancer pain. *J Palliat Care* 2001;17(3):167–172.

161. Nainis N, Paice JA, Ratner J, et al. Relieving symptoms in cancer: innovative use of art therapy. *J Pain Symptom Manage* 2006;31(2):162–169.

162. Deng G, Cassileth BR, Yeung KS. Complementary therapies for cancer-related symptoms. *J Support Oncol* 2004;2(5):419–426.

163. Post-White J, Kinney ME, Savik K, et al. Therapeutic massage and healing touch improve symptoms in cancer. *Integr Canc Ther* 2003;2(4):332–344.

164. Polubinski JP, West L. Implementation of a massage therapy program in the home hospice setting. *J Pain Symptom Manage* 2005;30(1):104–106.

165. Stephenson N, Dalton JA, Carlson J. The effect of foot reflexology on pain in patients with metastatic cancer. *Appl Nurs Res* 2003;16(4):284–286.

166. Zappa SB, Cassileth BR. Complementary approaches to palliative oncological care. *J Nurs Care Qual* 2003;18(1):22–26.

167. Meek SS. Effects of slow stroke back massage on relaxation in hospice clients. *Image J Nurs Sch* 1993;25(1):17–21.

168. Keefe FJ, Ahles TA, Porter LS, et al. The self-efficacy of family caregivers for helping cancer patients manage pain at end-of-life. *Pain* 2003;103(1–2):157–162.

169. Keefe FJ, Ahles TA, Sutton L, et al. Partner-guided cancer pain management at the end of life: a preliminary study. *J Pain Symptom Manage* 2005;29(3):263–272.

170. Kwekkeboom KL, Gretarsdottir E. Systematic review of relaxation interventions for pain. *J Nurs Scholarsh* 2006;38(3):269–277.

171. Muller-Busch HC, Andres I, Jehser T. Sedation in palliative care—A critical analysis of 7 years experience. *BMC Palliat Care* 2003;2:2.

172. Salacz ME, Weissman DE. Controlled sedation for refractory suffering: part I. *J Palliat Med* 2005;8(1):136–137.

173. Lo B, Rubenfeld G. Palliative sedation in dying patients: "we turn to it when everything else hasn't worked." *JAMA* 2005;294(14):1810–1816.

174. de Graeff A, Dean M. Palliative sedation therapy in the last weeks of life: a literature review and recommendations for standards. *J Palliat Med* 2007;10(1):67–85.

175. Hanks-Bell M, Paice J, Krammer L. The use of midazolam hydrochloride continuous infusions in palliative care. *Clin J Oncol Nurs* 2002;6(6):367–369.

176. Rousseau P. Palliative sedation in the management of refractory symptoms. *J Support Oncol* 2004;2:181–186.

177. Lundstrom S, Zachrisson U, Furst CJ. When nothing helps: propofol as sedative and antiemetic in palliative cancer care. *J Pain Symptom Manage* 2005;30(6):570–577.

178. Baker MT, Naguib M. Propofol: the challenges of formulation. *Anesthesiology* 2005;103(4):860–876.

179. Morita T, Ikenaga M, Adachi I, et al. Family experience with palliative sedation therapy for terminally ill cancer patients. *J Pain Symptom Manage* 2004;28(6):557–565.

180. Hawryluck LA, Harvey WR, Lemieux-Charles L, et al. Consensus guidelines on analgesia and sedation in dying intensive care unit patients. *BMC Medical Ethics* 2002;3:E3.

CHAPTER 109 ■ TRAINING PAIN SPECIALISTS

JAMES P. RATHMELL, MICHAEL ZENZ, ROLLIN M. GALLAGHER, AND DAVID L. BROWN

THE EVOLUTION OF PAIN MEDICINE AS A SUBSPECIALTY

It has become impossible for any physician to become an expert in every field. As knowledge expands and the need for detailed skills arises, the natural progression is for specialization to ensue. There has long been a discomfort with specialization despite an unflagging progression in that direction. The urge to both specialize and remain unspecialized dates back to the earliest recorded history of medicine. The first specializations were between the barber-surgeons and the internists, and a rivalry of sorts remains to this day. Writing about Ambrose Paré, the 16th century physician who elevated the role of the barber-surgeons to that of other physicians, the present-day surgeon and historian Sherwin Nuland reflects on the ongoing distinction between internist and surgeon:

> Surgery is an exercise in the use of the intellect. Heckling internists, with tongues barely in check, would prefer that surgical specialists be

viewed merely as dexterous craftsman who carry out the routing errands assigned to them by their more cerebrally endowed medical overseers. I attribute this teasing raillery to a kind of good-natured fraternal envy, not so much of our celebrity status, but rather of the visibility of the cures we surgeons achieve and the particular personal gratification we have while doing it.[1]

In the United States, anesthesiology has progressed toward further specialization, first with the establishment of critical care, then pain management (now pain medicine), and more recently pediatric anesthesiology and cardiothoracic anesthesiology. The addition of pain medicine as a subspecialty of anesthesiology is just one recent example of the growth of medical specialties. With specialization comes a conscious effort to focus practice to become intricately familiar with a more limited realm. The obvious result is a loss of the skills and knowledge needed to practice in the broader parent specialty. In pain medicine, many now view this as a full-time vocation. The scientific meetings and journals that keep pain medicine specialists up-to-date have little overlap with those that are designed to serve anesthesiologists practicing in the operating room. The only common thread between the technical skills needed in the pain clinic and those required for anesthesiology in the operating room is expertise with neural blockade, which is one of several important skill sets needed in pain medicine. The rapid expansion of knowledge in the causes and complications of acute and chronic pain, particularly in the neurobehavioral sciences, has led to a growing recognition that the pain medicine practitioner must acquire a vastly different skill set than those practicing anesthesiology, including expanding their skills as diagnosticians.

Much has been written about the origins of pain medicine as a distinct discipline and anesthesiologists have played a primary role since the start,[2] as have specialists in neurology, psychiatry, neurosurgery, and physical medicine and rehabilitation.[3] Anesthesiology really started with the introduction of effective general anesthetics in the mid-nineteenth century, when surgical pain could be separated from operation. Almost 100 years later, the late John Bonica, an anesthesiologist and recognized father of the specialty we now call pain medicine, developed his career promoting multidisciplinary pain care and formal training of specialists. From his life's work, we now have extensive ongoing efforts to recognize and treat pain effectively, to train subspecialists, and to conduct basic and clinical research to further our understanding of pain and its treatment. The International Association for the Study of Pain (IASP) founded in 1974, its U.S. chapter, the American Pain Society, and the journal *Pain* are legacies left by Dr. Bonica for our patients. Dr. Bonica, beginning his practice with a focus on developing regional anesthesia techniques, soon came to realize that these techniques were inadequate to meet the needs of his patients and that he could not incorporate growing epidemiologic, basic, and clinical scientific evidence of the salience of neurobehavioral factors. This realization evolved to the belief that developing the field of pain as a separate clinical discipline and treating chronic pain competently required the intellectual input and clinical skills of several other specialties. Consequently, he published the first edition of this seminal textbook, *The Management of Pain*, to that end in 1953.[4] It is noteworthy that IASP presidents have backgrounds from anesthesiology, dentistry, neurology, neurophysiology, neurosurgery, psychiatry, and psychology. All share a common intellectual passion and achievement, as well as clinical dedication, to developing pain research, teaching, and clinical care in pain medicine.

Accredited fellowship training in pain medicine is a relatively recent development. Prior to 1992, training was frequently obtained in academic anesthesiology departments, including those of John Bonica, Philip Bridenbaugh, Harold Carron, Daniel Moore, Prithvi Raj, Alon Winnie, and others, and subsequently in programs run by their trainees. These unaccredited programs advanced the specialty, widened interest in pain medicine as a career, and propagated anesthesiology-based pain care in smaller and smaller communities across the country. Other specialists also contributed to the development of the practice model of pain care. Many of the early leaders of pain medicine were from other specialties, and they trained fellows in unaccredited programs as well. Multispecialty entrance into pain medicine training became a tradition in several cities, including Boston, under Daniel Carr (Harvard, Massachusetts General) and Carol Warfield (Harvard, Beth Israel), New York under Kathy Foley, Russ Portenoy, and Bob Breitbart (Sloan-Kettering), and in Seattle under John Loeser, John Bonica's successor (University of Washington), amongst others. For example, one of the authors (Rollin M. Gallagher), provided fellowship training in chronic pain rehabilitation at SUNY Stony Brook and Drexel College of Medicine to doctors with residency backgrounds in neurology, psychiatry, physiatry, and family practice before accreditation was possible. Outside of the United States, with the notable exception of Australia, this type of informal training remains the rule for those seeking expertise in pain medicine. In the United States, the American Board of Anesthesiology (ABA) developed interest in certifying pain medicine training. The failure of coalition of the boards of Anesthesiology, Psychiatry and Neurology, Physical Medicine and Rehabilitation, and Neurosurgery in 1990 to form a conjoint American Board of Medical Specialties (ABMS) board led the ABA, under the leadership of Bill Owens in his roles on both the ABA and the Residency Review Committee (RRC), and through his representations of the subspecialty to the ABMS, to begin accrediting formal training programs and certifying physicians in 1992 through the Accreditation Council for Graduate Medical Education (ACGME). Steve Abram and John Rowlingson were both key members of the group that assisted Dr. Owens in moving the new subspecialty forward.

The number of ACGME-accredited programs (Fig. 109.1) and the number of trainees in accredited programs has grown steadily over the past decade, reaching just under 100 training programs by 1999 that turn out about 250 new pain specialists each year (Fig. 109.2). The ABA working in parallel with the ACGME developed a subspecialty certification examination in pain medicine, first named the "Certificate of Added Qualifications in Pain Management," now titled "Subspecialty Certification in Pain Medicine." The first exam was given in 1993. The number of candidates sitting for the examination has steadily grown since the first exam was given.

Dr. Bonica's original push to develop multidisciplinary pain care recently evolved into collaboration between four specialties agreeing to a single and unified set of program requirements for all ACGME-accredited pain fellowships, regardless of sponsoring specialty. Consequently, in 1999, the ABA invited representatives of the American Board of Psychiatry and Neurology (ABPN) and the American Board of Physical Medicine & Rehabilitation (ABPMR) to join the ABA's Pain Management Examination Committee to broaden the examination beyond its prior focus on

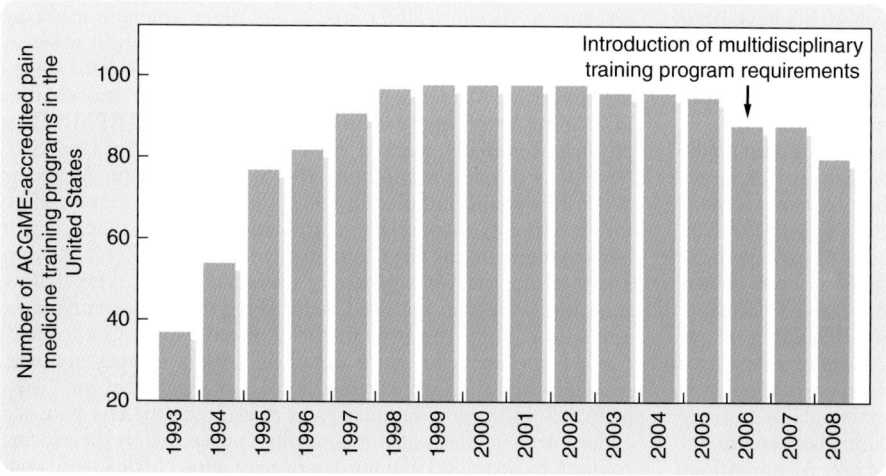

FIGURE 109.1 The number of pain medicine training programs accredited by the ACGME in the United States. The first pain medicine fellowships were accredited in 1993 and the number of programs rose to nearly 100 by 1999; with the introduction of new and more rigorous accreditation standards in the form of Multidisciplinary Training Program Requirements in 2006, the number of programs maintaining accreditation has declined by nearly 20%. (All data were provided by the ABA and are current as of August 2008.)

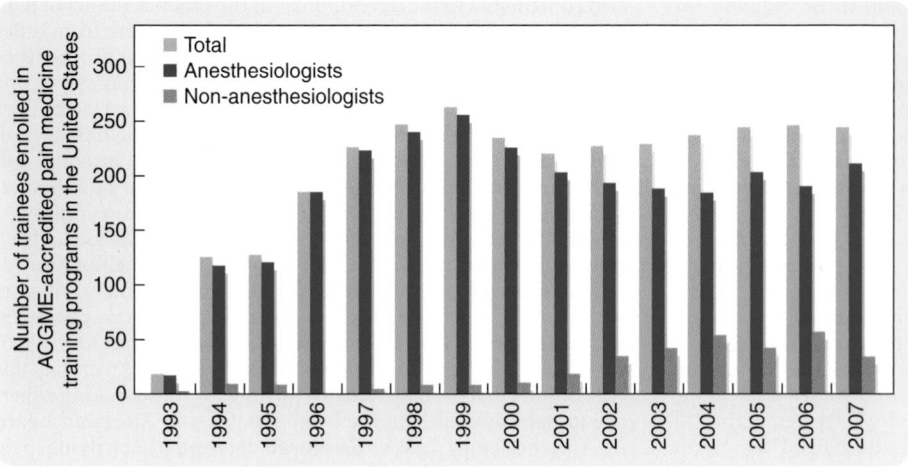

FIGURE 109.2 The number of trainees enrolled in pain medicine training programs accredited by the ACGME in the United States. The first pain medicine fellowships were accredited in 1993 and the number of trainees rose steadily through 1998, leveling off at about 250 trainees each year for the past decade. The number of physicians entering subspecialty training in pain medicine from disciplines other than anesthesiology has risen and these trainees now account for nearly 20% of all trainees. These nonanesthesiologists are primarily from the disciplines of neurology and physical medicine and rehabilitation. (All data were provided by the ABA and are current as of August 2008.)

regional anesthesia, and in 2000, the ABPN and ABPMR began issuing certificates of subspecialty certification in pain management to those diplomates who passed the expanded ABA examination. Between 2002 and 2006, the ACGME working in collaboration with the ABA, ABPN, and ABPMR developed new program requirements for pain fellowship training programs aimed at improving the quality of education in pain medicine and promoting a multidisciplinary approach to care. The new program requirements were adopted in 2006 and the number of programs achieving ongoing accreditation under these broader and more rigorous requirements has declined by nearly 20% (see Fig. 109.2). Equally important in the evolution of the discipline is the creation of academic physicians within the fellowships who undertake research programs to add new knowledge to this needed field of medical practice.

Pain and its consequences draw on resources from all medical disciplines. Dr. Bonica's experiences during World War II suggested that each medical specialist had unique expertise to bring to patients suffering in pain; hence his consistent and effective promotion of a multidisciplinary process for pain care. Also thanks largely to Dr. Bonica, anesthesiology has led the development of formal training programs. Indeed, the majority of currently accredited programs reside within academic anesthesiology departments and most program directors are anesthesiologists. Specialists from other disciplines have also focused their clinical and research efforts on pain. The most obvious example is neurology where the majority of clinical treatment and research about headache and peripheral neuropathy has arisen. Physical medicine and rehabilitation has also long had a focus and expertise in functional restoration, and physiatrists lead many chronic pain rehabilitation programs. And, of course, psychiatrists have been closely involved where pain, illness behavior, stress, depression, anxiety, and substance abuse overlap. During the last decade, specialists from these other disciplines have been seeking subspecialty training in pain medicine with increasing regularity.

The range of practitioners declaring themselves as pain medicine specialists is extraordinary; from clinics that provide largely or solely cognitive-behavioral approaches to chronic pain through functional restoration programs all the way to the type of clinic that offers nothing more than injections of various sorts. "Interventional Pain Medicine" is a term that has been coined for those techniques that involve minimally invasive treatments and minor surgery as part of their application, including neural blockade and implantable analgesic devices. Despite the paucity of scientific evidence to guide pain practitioners, particularly evidence to support the use of many interventional modalities, many techniques appear to have efficacy based on limited observational data and have been adopted into widespread use. As practition-

ers, we are left to choose among available treatment modalities, often with only anecdote and personal experience to guide us in treating a group of desperate patients with intractable pain who are willing to accept almost any treatment, even those which remain unproven. There is no single practice pattern that any pain specialist can point toward as the correct way to treat patients with chronic pain. Training programs vary widely in the scope of what they train practitioners to do. The best pain medicine practitioners strike a reasonable balance between interventional and noninterventional management. This practice pattern is sustainable and those adopting a balanced style of practice will be able to adapt to evolving scientific evidence that appears in support of pain treatment, regardless of the type of treatment. A balance between treatment modalities also allows practitioners to switch from one mode to another or incorporate multiple treatment approaches simultaneously. Use of these interventional modalities is just a small part of the armamentarium of the skilled pain medicine practitioner.

PAIN MEDICINE AS A PRIMARY MEDICAL SCPECIALTY

Dr. Bonica developed his multidisciplinary clinic with the understanding that the expertise of several specialties was necessary to successfully manage chronic pain. A detailed history of the intellectual background of pain medicine, and particularly Bonica's work in the early development of the field can be found in Baszanger's 1998 book, *Inventing Pain Medicine.*[5] Following this trajectory, in 1983, responding to the need to organize the diversity of specialists interested in and practicing pain medicine, and to obtain recognition and representation amongst other established specialists, a multispecialty group of physicians started the American Academy of Algology, whose name was changed in 1986 to American Academy of Pain Medicine (AAPM). These physicians initially worked with their parent ABMS specialty boards to develop a conjoint ABMS Board of Pain Medicine. When this coalition failed in 1989, the ABA took responsibility for developing subspecialty certification in pain management, later changing to the term pain medicine. From 1992–2000, nonanesthesiologists were generally excluded from taking fellowships and were also excluded from taking the ABA-certifying examination. Thus, the large majority of pain specialists formally trained in these fellowships obtained 3 years of anesthesiology residency and then were trained in pain management for 1 year, primarily by anesthesia faculty. As a result, many new pain specialists were intellectually or clinically unprepared by their formal training to assimilate the burden of managing chronic pain comprehensively and longitudinally in a biopsychosocial, chronic disease management model. Accordingly, they focused their efforts on developing interventional pain medicine practices, although many may have learned the additional core skills while managing pain in their practices over years, similar to the experience of the first generation of pain specialists with no formal training. The pattern of regional anesthesia practice was reinforced by the economic structure of health care, which then, and still now, created large incentives for doing procedures rather than emphasizing chronic disease management and functional rehabilitation. Due to these constraints, in 1991, the ABPM was incorporated to provide ABMS-equivalent credentialing for physicians from the primary specialties who were already practicing pain management, and to enable physicians from these other "parent" specialties to enter the practice of pain medicine. The ABPM required a credentialing process that included ABMS certification in anesthesiology, neurology, psychiatry, neurosurgery, or physiatry; documentation of a primary pain medicine practice that was broadly based; valid medical licensure; peer recommendations; and passing of an 8-hour examination in pain medicine that was designed and psychometrically-validated to reflect broadly the multispecialty origins of pain medicine as practiced in the field by experienced pain medicine practitioners, not by specialists or subspecialists in a parent specialty. The ABPM was formed as only a temporary solution to the lack of a credentialing process that was more representative of pain medicine as practiced in the community. The intent of the ABPM since its inception was ultimately to facilitate a separate ABMS Board in Pain Medicine; consequently, it has made two such applications to the ABMS, both which were rejected. Since 1993, the ABPM has credentialed over 2200 physicians as pain medicine specialists from these five specialties and the ABPM is recognized as ABMS equivalent in California, Texas, and Florida.

The rationale for a separate specialty in pain medicine involves the documentation of many factors: public health need[6–8]; a growing consensus of pain treatment as a human right[9]; ethical difficulties that are at the heart of pain medicine practice[10,11]; inadequate education[12] and knowledge[13] and a rapidly growing scientific and practice base[14]; and the need to promote integrated pain medicine with primary care.[15,16] The high costs of inadequately-managed pain reverberate in our society's health care crisis and are well documented. Emblematic of the same, it has been our citizens, the victims of inadequate pain management, who have decried this problem and demanded change through legislation at both a state and national level when organized medicine, itself beset by competition amongst established specialties, cannot act. The rationale is scientific as well. Since the publication of John Bonica's first edition of *Pain Management* in 1953, the problem of pain has challenged some of the best minds in science and medicine. In 1965, Melzack and Wall's[17] seminal paper in *Science* describing the Gate Theory of Pain created a conceptual framework resulting in a relative explosion of science in the physiology, molecular biology, and pharmacology of acute pain and the epidemiology, neurobiology, pathophysiology, genetics, and treatment of chronic pain conditions and diseases at the levels of soma, spinal cord, and brain. For example, a Medline search for titles with the key terms "pain" and "nociception" increased from 30,138 (pain) and 45(nociception) in the decade from 1970–1979 to 146,654 (pain) and 2417(nociception) in the 8 years from 2000–2007. Today's pain medicine physician is potentially armed with this tremendous knowledge base as a foundation for the myriad of effective medications, behavioral therapies, physical therapies, neural blockades, neuromodulatory devices, and cross-cultural complementary and alternative treatments such as acupuncture and meditation. The ABPM, AAPM, and a growing number of pain medicine and other specialists in organized medicine believe that longer training, either a 2-year fellowship or a separate 3-year residency, is needed to learn how, when, and in what combination these tools can be cost-effectively utilized to competently treat patients with chronic pain, to estab-

lish standards for training all physicians, and to lead the development of clinical research and health policy.[18] Although each traditional medical specialty contributes to this knowledge base and skill set, their respective specialists are not trained to manage the entirety of the spectrum of chronic pain contributing to fragmentation not unification of care and failed public health. Table 109.1 outlines the special skills contributed by traditional specialties that converge to define the pain medicine specialist. This specialized knowledge, education, training, and multidisciplinary nature suggest that pain medicine's evolution as a specialty is paralleling that of other disciplines, such as emergency medicine or physical medicine and rehabilitation. Knowledge and skills of the latter disciplines, initially fragmented, later coalesced into primary medical specialties because of the inability of multiple specialties to offer an integrated approach that would best serve patients, medical science, and public health.

Today, the momentum to establish standards for pain medicine as a specialty is now global. For example, in 1998 the government of Australia formally recognized pain medicine as a specialty and endorsed training and credentialing requirements recommended by the newly formed Faculty of Pain Medicine of the Australia New Zealand College of Anaesthetists.[19] In 2007, the Section and Board of Anaesthesiology of the European Union of Medical Specialists (EUMS/UEMS) initiated the establishment of the Multidisciplinary Joint Committee on Pain Medicine of the EUMS/UEMS, which has created a certification examination in pain medicine (see further discussion of training in the European Union later in this chapter). Also in 2007, the Ministry of Health of the People's Republic of China announced the designation of pain medicine as a separate specialty and that there will be a Department of Pain Medicine in all major hospitals in China.[20] In the United States, the ABPM and AAPM have applied jointly to the ACGME for establishing residency training programs in pain medicine under a new residency review committee. The simple rationale is that training for 1 year has proven to be inadequate. Similar to a cardiologist learning the science and clinical practice related to the cardiovascular system, starting with primary prevention of heart disease, by identification and early intervention of risk, and primary and secondary treatment of actual heart disease, the pain medicine specialist will learn about the pain perception and modulation system, from the relatively simple peripheral nociceptor to the system's complex neurobehavioral networks and about the pathophysiologies of this system.[21,22]

TRAINING IN PAIN MEDICINE IN EUROPE

In Europe, there is no systematic training in pain medicine for medical students. The lack of obligatory training leads to later deficiencies in clinical care. Some countries (e.g., Germany) have made efforts in establishing a core curriculum for medical students. However, the worldwide need for a thorough basic education in pain medicine is underestimated by most health care officials.

The postgraduate training varies widely within Europe. This led to guidelines for anesthesiologist specialist training in pain medicine.[23] In these guidelines approved by the EUMS/UEMS, pain medicine is considered to be an area of expertise in anesthesiology. However, simultaneously it is mentioned that pain medicine is not claimed for anesthesiology alone. It is clearly stated that pain medicine is included in anesthesia specialist training on the one side. On the other side, an additional qualification following basic anesthesia training is recommended. The multidisciplinary approach to pain is mentioned and an initiative to set up a multidisciplinary joint committee on pain medicine within the EUMS/UEMS has begun.

The proposed duration of pain medicine training is 3 months during the 5 years of basic anesthetic training required in the European Union. In contrast to this relation representing only

TABLE 109.1

EXAMPLES OF DISEASE AND TREATMENT CONTRIBUTIONS TO PAIN MEDICINE FROM TRADITIONAL SPECIALTIES

Specialty	Illness/Disease Knowledge Contribution	Medical Skill/ Treatment Contribution
Anesthesiology	Acute pain Chronic pain Cancer pain	Regional anesthesia (including neurolytic) Spinal anesthesia Operative anesthesia
Neurology	Peripheral neuropathy Neuropathic pain Central pain Headache	Assessment of neuropathic pain Neuropathic pain analgesia Headache medication
Neurosurgery	Spine disease Central pain	Implantable medication pumps Neurostimulation Spine evaluation and surgery
Orthopaedic Surgery	Low back pain Physical Disability	Spine evaluation and surgery Joint surgery
Palliative Care	Cancer pain	End-of-life symptom management Bioethics
Primary Care	Chronic diseases	Chronic disease management Biopsychosocial medicine
Psychiatry, Behavioral Medicine	Psychiatric comorbidity; Stress, behavior and emotions Fibromyalgia Personality and coping	Antidepressant analgesia Behavioral rehabilitation Biofeedback and relaxation Biopsychosocial formulation Psychotherapies (dynamic, cognitive-behavioral, group, family, hypnosis) Psychiatric diagnosis Psychological and psychometric evaluation Psychopharmacology
Radiological Medicine		Diagnostic imaging Procedure imaging Radiotherapy
Rehabilitation Medicine, Physical Therapy	Musculoskeletal medicine Myofascial pain Physical disability	Physical therapy Physical rehabilitation Transcutaneous electrical nerve stimulation Trigger point therapy
Rheumatology	Joint diseases Fibromyalgia	Joint injections Peripheral nociceptive analgesia (nonsteroidal anti-inflammatory drugs)
Complementary and Alternative Medicine		Acupuncture Massage Meditation Tai Chi

5% of the total time of training, it is recommended to occupy a minimum of 10% of the multiple choice questions in the diploma of the European Academy of Anaesthesia.

Some years ago, the Scandinavian Society of Anaesthesiology and Intensive Care established the Nordic education in advanced pain medicine. The clinical part lasts at least 3 months. The education includes, and this is unique in Europe, a scientific part.[24]

In April 2007, the Royal College of Anaesthetists established a faculty of pain medicine and stressed this as a major way point in the last 50 years.[25] However, the question is rasied: should pain medicine should strive to be a "stand alone speciality" or should it be linked to parent specialties like anesthesiology? Additionally, education is also required for the public and the patients? Both the British and the Irish curriculum in pain medicine require similar training and examination. The candidate has to complete a total of 6 months training in pain medicine before ending up with a 2-day written and oral examination with patient investigation and practical examination. The majority of treatment modalities, where the candidate should have an understanding and experience in the practice, are invasive procedures.

As early as 1992, the German Society of Anaesthesiology started a curriculum and specialist training in pain medicine. This included a 2-week theoretical course and a 1-year practical training requirement in a pain clinic. From this first example, a specialty open for all clinical disciplines has been developed. Since 1996, a specialty called "Specialised Pain Therapy" has been established by the German Medical Assembly. A curriculum has been developed by the German Pain Society and approved by the German Medical Assembly. Similarly to the Society of Anaesthetists, the specialization demands 1 year of clinical training in a certified institution and an 80-hour theoretical course. Additionally, to maintain specialty certification, physicians must attend multidisciplinary pain conferences regularly, where patients are presented and discussed between several disciplines, including at least one psychological discipline. In 2008, Austria introduced a similar specialty, and the German training is approved by the Austrian Medical Assembly.

The dramatic effect of a thorough education and programmatic work has been demonstrated in Catalonia in Spain within a project sponsored by the World Health Organization. Symptom control and patient satisfaction were both improved, and a striking cost savings of many million Euros per year has been demonstrated as compared to the rest of Spain.[26] Europe has lagged behind the United States in developing formal training for pain medicine specialists. In the European Union, training is not uniform, and there remains a long way still to go for a clear and consistent path to specialization and qualification in pain medicine.

TRAINING AND CREDENTIALING IN INTERVENTIONAL PAIN MEDICINE

In our rapidly changing world of modern health care, new technologies are appearing at a dizzying rate. Many of these new treatments require physicians to acquire detailed new knowledge and technical skills. The introduction of new techniques typically extends from centers in the public or private sector, where the ideas are conceived and tested in a limited realm among innovators. From there, anecdote can often take over, and many techniques in pain medicine have blossomed into widespread use with nothing more than word-of-mouth to propagate their use. The use of pulsed radiofrequency treatment for pain is one such example where clinical application has preceded detailed clinical testing.[27]

In the United States and Europe, industry often leads innovation by testing and leading the introduction of new devices. When the innovation appears to have merit in limited trials, many devices have been introduced to the market with approval through the U.S. Food and Drug Administration's (FDA) 510K "substantially similar device" process with little or no data regarding efficacy. Once on the market, the means by which practitioners decide to adopt new technologies, the speed of progression of these new techniques, and—of great importance—the means by which practitioners gain enough expertise to introduce new techniques into their own practices, are all highly variable and seemingly without any rational or consistent approach.

Interventional pain medicine is evolving as a distinct discipline that requires detailed new knowledge and expertise. Familiarity with radiographic anatomy for the conduct of image-guided injection and the minor surgical skills needed to place implanted devices such as spinal cord stimulators and implanted drug delivery systems are just a few of the techniques that practitioners must master. As we set out to introduce new interventional techniques to our own pain practices, we must assure that we have been properly trained to conduct these techniques to ensure safety and success.

Adequate exposure during the fellowship-training period to these newer treatment alternatives is necessary to assure appro-

priate application and optimize patient outcomes. While we do not have scientific data that define the average minimum level of experience that will be necessary to achieve competence, especially for complex procedures that are associated with significant risks, logic dictates that there are a minimum number of these procedures that trainees should be exposed to during a fellowship. The ACGME has established requirements for average minimal numbers of epidural, spinal, and peripheral nerve blocks necessary for accreditation of anesthesiology residency programs. Other medical subspecialties also require a minimum number of specified procedures to achieve and maintain competence: subspecialty training in gastroenterology has a requirement of performing a minimum of 100 esophagogastro-duodenoscopies and 100 colonoscopies with polyp removal[28] during formal training, and subspecialty training in cardiovascular disease requires 100 cardiac catheterizations to demonstrate minimum proficiency.[29] Indeed, the ACGME's RRC for Anesthesiology has accepted revised program requirements for pain medicine training programs that specify minimum exposure of trainees for various techniques, including image-guided spinal injection techniques in the cervical and lumbar spine; sympathetic blockade; neurolytic block, including radiofrequency treatment for pain; intradiscal procedures, including discography; spinal cord stimulation; and placement of permanent spinal drug delivery system. For those techniques that are now widely accepted as a core part of pain practice, we must assure that our trainees gain enough experience to conduct these procedures independently. One key element of the ACGME deliberations about unified pain training is to acknowledge that not all pain fellows will have experience in the wide variety of interventional techniques. Rather, it is hoped that these fellows will gain an understanding of all available options for patients with pain, and yet demonstrate and have competence documented in only those techniques for which formal training is made available during fellowship training.

It is difficult to define the techniques that are core for a pain practitioner, but it does seem that detailed knowledge of radiographic anatomy of the spine and the minor surgical skills required to implant spinal cord stimulators and place permanent spinal drug delivery systems are among those skills most practicing pain physicians would expect a new graduate from a pain fellowship to emerge with. New techniques are appearing at a staggering rate, and we cannot rely on pain fellowship programs to provide all of the technical training that is needed. Stronger standards for minimal training following fellowship are also urgently needed. Some pain practitioners believe that all too many of their colleagues find it perfectly acceptable to attend a brief weekend course and then introduce a highly technical new treatment into practice without additional study, training, or oversight.[30] Intradiscal electrothermal therapy, nucleoplasty, and radiofrequency treatment are among the many techniques that are showing promise and each requires a set of unique knowledge and skills to be used safely and effectively. Practitioners themselves must take the lead in obtaining adequate training *before* proceeding with any new and unfamiliar technique. The weekend workshop is just a start, often a good start—the best will give practitioners a detailed understanding of anatomy, pathophysiology of disease related to the use of the new technique, patient selection, conduct of the procedure, outcomes, and avoidance, management, and recognition of complications. Here we would like to suggest a method for practitioners[31] (Table 109.2): (1) *study the new technique*, the published literature, and gain a detailed knowledge of all aspects of the technique; (2) *attend a workshop*, preferably a hands-on cadaver-based workshop that allows introduction to the technique in as realistic a setting that can be assembled; (3) *plan* adequate time for your initial procedures; (4) *get help* at the bedside during initial conduct of new procedures—perhaps another experienced practitioner at your institution, an invited expert to assist, or team up with a colleague in a related discipline; (5) *inform your patients* that you are intro-

TABLE 109.2

SUGGESTED TRAINING AND EXPERIENCE WHEN INTRODUCING A NEW TECHNIQUE IN TO CLINICAL PRACTICE

1. Study the new technique, the published literature and gain a detailed knowledge of all aspects of the technique
2. Attend a workshop, preferably a hands-on cadaver-based workshop that allows introduction to the technique in as realistic a setting that can be assembled
3. Plan adequate time for your initial procedures
4. Get help at the bedside during initial conduct of new procedures—perhaps another experienced practitioner at your institution, an invited expert to assist, or team up with a colleague in a related discipline
5. Inform your patients that you are introducing a new technique and include this discussion as part of the informed consent process
6. Examine your outcomes carefully in the initial stages of using any new technique and compare them with those of your colleagues and the published literature.

ducing a new technique and include this discussion as part of the informed consent process; (6) *examine your outcomes* carefully in the initial stages of using any new technique and compare them with those of your colleagues and the published literature.

CONCLUSION

The field of evidence-based medicine has emerged as a new paradigm to guide practicing physicians. This field endeavors to educate practitioners about how to frame specific questions based on the clinical problems they are faced with every day. They then venture to the published scientific literature with focused questions about prevention, treatment, and diagnosis of a specific clinical condition. Many evidence-based medicine centers offer concise and periodically updated summaries about specific clinical conditions. The idea is to get the best information available to the practicing clinician. It describes the best available evidence, and if there is no good evidence, it says so. In pain medicine, we are faced with an expanding array of treatment options that strike us as logical developments that *should* provide pain relief for our patients. However, there is a dearth of clinical evidence to guide rational choice and application of the majority of these emerging treatments. So how are we to decide when to apply them?

Merrill[32] recently presented a detailed analysis of the current state of evidence guiding the use of interventional treatments in the field of pain medicine. He points out the frequent flaws in existing studies (largely the lack of valid comparators, such as no treatment) and concludes that, "the practice of invasive pain medicine teeters at a particularly critical juncture . . . crippled by a lack of vigorous self-evaluation of its role in the treatment of chronic pain." Merrill[32] goes on to detail the means by which we, as scientists and clinicians, can proceed to build a better body of evidence for the treatments we are using. But the field of pain medicine is young and early in development, and it is perhaps unreasonable to expect an accumulation of randomized clinical trials just yet.

New treatments evolve slowly in clinical medicine. Applying the scientific method in clinical medicine begins with an observation. Perhaps a chance observation that a certain drug typically used for another purpose provides analgesia to a given patient. If the drug is readily available, a clinician may choose to try treatment on other patients with similar presentations. If an academic sort, the clinician may choose to report the limited success

in a case series. Case series are a valuable beginning: the very beginning of emerging new ideas. If the problem is uniform and prevalent enough, the new treatment may gain the attention of investigators willing to assemble a randomized clinical trial. All too often, sound treatments are never tested for lack of interest or funding. Those that are tested tend to be those under patent where a manufacturer proceeds with these large endeavors understandably in hope of financial return in the event the treatment proves useful. Patients who are suffering from severe and intractable pain are desperate, and they can easily be convinced that desperate measures, however new or unproven, are warranted.

How, then, are we to proceed? Our patients are begging for us to try anything that offers a glimmer of hope in reducing their pain, and we as scientists embrace the rigor of the scientific method and want desperately to do what is best for our patients. We have treatment after treatment that makes logical sense and shows early promise in case series and observational studies, but little data that support an evidence-based approach to practice. Let us take acute low back pain with sciatica as an example. A number of evidence-based reports have emerged to guide clinicians.[33] The only modalities that are rated as "beneficial" or "likely to be beneficial" are advice to stay active, nonsteroidal anti-inflammatory drugs, behavioral therapy, and multidisciplinary treatment programs. Use of opioid analgesics, acupuncture, back schools, epidural steroid injections, and spinal manipulation were all judged to be of "unknown effectiveness." Yet, in actual clinical practice in the United States, a short course of opioid analgesic and early intervention with epidural steroid injections are common. To complicate matters, the use of fluoroscopic guidance and directing injections to the effected level using an interlaminar of transforaminal approach is gaining widespread acceptance, with only uncontrolled case series to guide us as clinicians. To complicate treatment options, those with persistent pain and contained disc herniations now have a dizzying array of treatment options including laser discectomy, thermal disc decompression, and vacuum disc extraction, all using FDA-approved devices with only uncontrolled observational studies that suggest effectiveness.[34] The new devices are as intellectually appealing as they are minimally invasive, yet only open surgical discectomy has proven superior to conservative management in patients with persistent sciatica due to intervertebral disc prolapse.[35]

The evidence-based medicine movement gives little guidance to practitioners whose tools are still under development. They simply remind us that no evidence regarding many of our techniques exists. Without declaring a moratorium on all of interventional pain, Merrill[8] offers the individual practitioner advice: monitor your own outcomes using valid measures, be more reflective and systematic in studying your own outcomes and patterns of care, and provide this information to your patients as part of the decision-making process. As pain practitioners, we have an expanding range of treatment options available to us, few with convincing evidence of efficacy superior to alternate treatments. We must evaluate each patient and use the limited evidence available to us today to guide compassionate and rational, if not evidence-based, use of therapy for our desperate patients.

The urgent need for expanded clinical research in pain medicine, coupled with the recent efforts to improve multidisciplinary training, are straining the ability of training programs to adequately provide the needed education and research experiences for pain medicine fellows in the course of a 1-year fellowship. The ACGME and ABA are currently working toward expanding the pain medicine fellowship to 2 years in order to accomplish these goals. The idea is to provide more comprehensive and multidisciplinary training and to require meaningful research experience during fellowship training. With this approach, we will create a more homogeneous group of pain medicine specialists, who emerge with similar knowledge and skills, regardless of the parent discipline in which they trained. In this way, we can move toward improving the consistency and quality of care for patients with acute, chronic, and cancer-related pain. Will the current approach be enough to train the best pain medicine specialists or will the need to move further toward a primary medical specialty continue? The authors of this chapter have been among those who have worked to craft the changes in education that have emerged from the ACGME (James P. Rathmell and David L. Brown), the ABPM (Rollin M. Gallagher), and the European Union (Michael Zenz). It is our hope in preparing this chapter and other publications of its kind that the major groups working toward improving the education of pain medicine specialists can continue to work together to create the best possible training programs that will ultimately advance the science and practice of pain medicine to the benefit of our patients.

References

1. Nuland SB. The gentle surgeon: Ambrose Paré. In: Nuland SB, ed. *Doctors: The Biography of Medicine*. New York: Knopf; 1988;94.
2. Rathmell JP, Brown DL. The evolution of training in pain medicine in the United States. American Society of Anesthesiologists Newsletter, August 2003.
3. Gallagher RM. Pain education and training: progress or paralysis? *Pain Med* 2002;3(3):196–197.
4. Bonica JJ. *The Management of Pain*. Philadelphia: JB Lippincott; 1953.
5. Baszanger I. *Inventing Pain Medicine: From the Laboratory to the Clinic*. New Brunswick, NJ: Rutgers University Press; 1998.
6. Latham J, Davis BD. The socioeconomic impact of chronic pain. *Disabil Rehabil*. 1994;16:39–44.
7. Burcheil KJ. Social costs of denying access to care. In: Cohen M, Campbell J, eds. *Pain Treatment Centers at Crossroads: A Practical and Conceptual Reappraisal/the Bristol–Myers Squibb Symposium on Pain Research*. Seattle: IASP Press; 1996;125–142.
8. Osterweis M, Kleinman A, Mechanic D. Pain and disability. Clinical, behavioral, and public policy perspectives. In: Institute of Medicine. *Committee on Pain, Disability, and Chronic Illness Behavior*. Washington, DC: National Academy Press; 1987: 280–282.
9. Brennan F, Carr DB, Cousins MJ. Pain management: a fundamental human right. *Anesth Analg* 2007;105:205–221.
10. Gallagher RM. Ethics in pain medicine: good for our health, good for the public health. *Pain Med* 2001;2:87–89.
11. Banja J. Empathy in the physician's pain practice: benefits, barriers, and recommendations. *Pain Med* 2006;7:265–275.
12. Gallagher RM. Pain education and training: progress or paralysis? *Pain Med* 2002;3:196–197.
13. Green CR, Wheeler JR, LaPorte F, et al. How well is pain managed? Who does it well? *Pain Med* 2002;3:56–65.
14. Fishman S, Gallagher RM, Carr D, et al. The case for pain medicine as a medical specialty. *Pain Med* 2004;5:281–286.
15. Gallagher RM. The pain medicine and primary care community rehabilitation model: monitored care for pain disorders in multiple settings. *Clin J Pain* 1999; 15:1–3.
16. Bair MJ. Overcoming fears, frustrations, and competing demands: an effective integration of pain medicine and primary care to treat complex pain patients. *Pain Med* 2007;8:544–545.
17. Melzack R, Wall PD. Pain mechanism: a new theory. *Science* 1965;150: 971–979.
18. Follett K, Dubois K. Program requirements for ACGME training in pain medicine released for the first time. *Pain Med* 2008;9:471–472.
19. Cohen M, Goucke R. Pain medicine recognized as a specialty in Australia. *Pain Med* 2006;7:473.
20. Gallagher RM, Han, J-S. Personal communication. December 15, 2007.
21. Basbaum AI. Distinct neurochemical features of acute and persistent pain. *Proc Natl Acad Sci U S A* 1999;96:7739–7743.
22. Rome HP Jr, Rome JD. Limbically augmented pain syndrome (LAPS): kindling, corticolimbic sensitization, and the convergence of affective and sensory symptoms in chronic pain disorders. *Pain Med* 2000;1:7–23.
23. Cunningham AJ, Knape JTA, Adriaensena H, et al. Guidelines for anaesthesiologist specialist training in pain medicine. Section and Board of Anesthesiology, European Union of Medical Specialists. *Eur J Anaesth* 2007;24:568–570.
24. The Scandanavian Society of Anaesthesiology and Intensive Care Medicine. SSAI's Nordic education in advanced pain medicine. Available at: http://www.ssai.info/Education/pain.html. Accessed February 1, 2009.
25. Justins DM. The Faculty of Pain Medicine of the Royal College of Anaesthetists. *Br J Anaesth* 2008;101:4–7.
26. Gómez-Batiste X, Porta-Sales J, Pascual A, et al, and the Palliative Care Advisory Committee of the Standing Advisory Committee for Socio-Health Affairs, Department of Health, Government of Catalonia. Catalonia WHO palliative care demonstration project at 15 Years (2005). *J Pain Symptom Manage* 2007; 33:584–590.
27. Richebé P, Rathmell JP, Brennan TJ. Immediate early genes after pulsed radiofrequency treatment: neurobiology in need of clinical trials. *Anesthesiology* 2005;102:1–3.
28. Program requirements for residency education in gastroenterology. Accreditation Council for Graduate Medical Education Web site. Available at: http://www.acgme.org/acWebsite/downloads/RRC_progReq/144pr799.pdf. Accessed April 27, 2006.
29. Program requirements for residency education in cardiovascular disease. Accreditation Council for Graduate Medical Education Web site. Available at: http://www.acgme.org/acWebsite/downloads/RRC_progReq/141pr799.pdf. Accessed April 27, 2006.
30. Rathmell JP. The injectionists. *Reg Anesth Pain Med* 2004;29:305–306.
31. Lubenow TR, Rathmell JP. Let's take a rational approach to technical training in pain medicine. *Am Soc Anesth News* 2005;69:6–8.
32. Merrill DG. Hoffman's glasses: evidence-based medicine and the search for quality in the literature of interventional pain medicine. *Reg Anesth Pain Med* 2003;28:547–560.
33. van Tulder M, Koes B. Low back pain and sciatica: acute. In: *Clinical Evidence: Concise 8*. London: BMJ Publishing Group; 2002;226–228.
34. Maroon JC. Current concepts in minimally invasive discectomy. *Neurosurgery*. 2002;51(5 Suppl):S137–S145.
35. Gibson JNA, Grant IC, Wadell G. The Cochrane review of surgery for disc prolapse and degenerative lumbar spondylosis. *Spine* 1999;24:1820–1832.

CHAPTER 110 ■ EMERGENCIES IN THE PAIN CLINIC

CHRISTOPHER GILLIGAN, MILAN STOJANOVIC, AND JAMES P. RATHMELL

This chapter will seek to provide the pain management specialist with an overview of emergencies and complications that may occur in the course of caring for patients with acute and chronic pain. Throughout this review we will also emphasize strategies for decreasing risk; specifically, strategies for identifying specific risks and considering alternatives, understanding rare event analysis, and maintaining a comprehensive view of the patient when prescribing specialty specific interventions. A prudent first step for practitioners who will be managing emergencies related to pain therapies is to understand the incidence of each of these emergencies. However, because complication rates are quite low for serious complications, and because minor complications frequently go unreported, measuring the true incidence of most complications is not generally feasible.

In the United States, the American Society of Anesthesiologists Closed Claims Project offers a relatively comprehensive database of adverse events secondary to pain management interventions, but no incidence can be calculated due to the lack of any knowl-

TABLE 110.1

SPECIFIC PROCEDURES USED FOR THE TREATMENT OF CHRONIC PAIN WITHIN THE AMERICAN SOCIETY OF ANESTHESIOLOGISTS CLOSED CLAIMS PROJECT THAT LED TO MALPRACTICE CLAIMS (n = 284)

	Claims	
	No.	%
Invasive procedures	276	97
Injections	138	49
Epidural steroids ± associated agents	114	
Trigger point	17	
Facet	4	
Other	3	
Blocks	78	27
Peripheral	28	
Stellate ganglion	19	
Other autonomic	9	
Neuraxial	9	
Upper/lower extremity	7	
Axial	4	
Head and neck	2	
Ablative procedures	17	6
Agent	13	
Technique	4	
Implantation or removal of devices	12	4
Implantable pump	5	
Nerve stimulator	4	
Catheter	3	
Device maintenance	20	7
Other interventions	11	4
Noninvasive pain management	8	3
Medication prescription	5	
Opinion/diagnosis	2	
Cupping procedure	1	

(Reproduced with permission from Fitzgibbon DR, Posner KL, Domino KB, et al; American Society of Anesthesiologists. Chronic pain management: American Society of Anesthesiologists Closed Claims Project. *Anesthesiology* 2004;100(1):98–105.)

edge regarding the overall frequency with which the interventions are conducted. A review of the 5475 claims in the American Society Anesthesiologists Closed Claims Project database between 1970 and 1999 showed that claims related to chronic pain management accounted for 10% of all claims in the 1990s. Of the 276 closed claims in the database, epidural steroid injections accounted for 138 (49%) and other peripheral nerve blocks accounted for 78 (27%) of all chronic pain management claims, reflecting the most frequent invasive procedures conducted by anesthesiologists during that time period (Table 110.1). Nerve damage and pneumothorax were the most common adverse events leading to claims in invasive pain management claims (Fig. 110.1). Surprisingly, serious adverse events leading to brain damage or death did occur in association with chronic pain treatment, but at a far lower rate than that seen in surgical and obstetric anesthesia claims. A closer analysis of the subset of claims associated with epidural steroid injections, revealed that death and brain damage occurred only when local anesthetic or opioid (or both) were administered in conjunction with the steroid (Fig. 110.2). This likely reflects unintended delivery of local anesthetic or opioid to the subarachnoid space, or simply the predictable effects of neuraxial opioids; resultant high spinal anesthesia or neuraxial effects of opioid could both have led to respiratory compromise and underscores the need for close observation following neuraxial administration of local anesthetic or opioid. Not infrequently, claims resulted from the maintenance of spinal drug delivery systems (20/276 claims or 7%); these claims often stemmed from refilling of implanted drug reservoirs with potent opioid by nonphysician personnel in the outpatient or home care settings.

BLEEDING COMPLICATIONS

Within one decade of August Bier's discovery of spinal anesthesia, the first known epidural hematoma as a complication of spinal anesthesia occurred in a 36-year-old male following unsuccessful neuraxial blockade for excision of a pilonidal cyst.[1] In that case, repeated lumbar puncture revealed blood tinged cerebrospinal fluid (CSF) and the patient subsequently developed paresthesias and weakness in both lower extremities. The introduction of heparin in 1937 and warfarin in 1941 introduced the possibility of anticoagulation contributing to epidural hematoma formation. Epidural hematoma is a rare but potentially catastrophic complication of spinal or epidural anesthesia or injections. Because the spinal column is an enclosed space, hematoma formation can cause compression and ischemia of neural structures. Bleeding

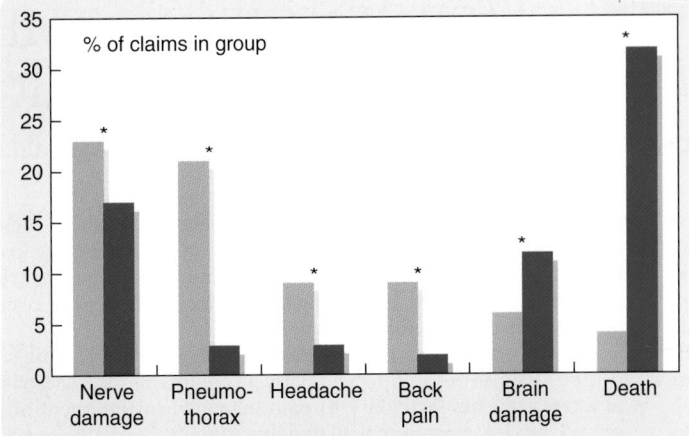

FIGURE 110.1 Primary outcomes within the American Society of Anesthesiologists Closed Claims Project in chronic pain management claims (*yellow bars*) versus surgical/obstetric claims (*green bars*). *p <0.05 (Reproduced with permission Fitzgibbon DR, Posner KL, Domino KB, et al; American Society of Anesthesiologists. Chronic Pain Management: American Society of Anesthesiologists Closed Claims Project. *Anesthesiology* 2004;100(1)98–105.)

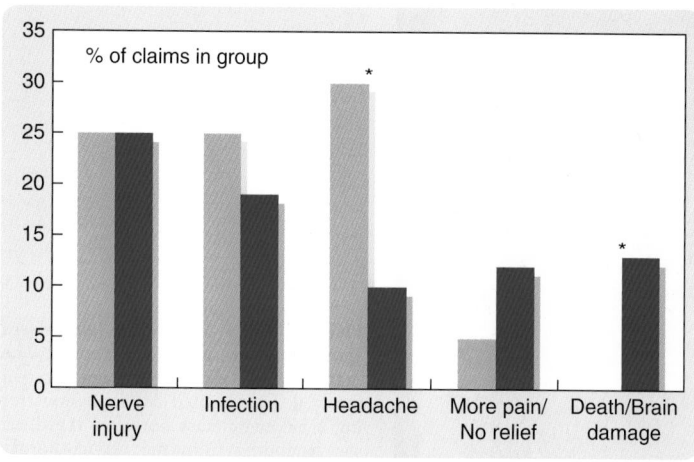

FIGURE 110.2 Most common outcomes within the American Society of Anesthesiologists Closed Claims Project in those claims following epidural steroid injection. *Yellow bars* represent injections with steroids only. *Green bars* indicate injections in which local anesthetic or opioid (or both) were added to the steroid. *$p < 0.05$ between proportion of injection group with that outcome. (Reproduced with permission from Fitzgibbon DR, Posner KL, Domino KB, et al; American Society of Anesthesiologists. Chronic Pain Management: American Society of Anesthesiologists Closed Claims Project. *Anesthesiology* 2004;100(1):98–105.)

may result from injury to the abundant epidural veins or may be arterial. A retrospective study of central neuraxial blocks in Sweden from 1990 to 1999 identified 33 spinal hematomas, during a period when approximately 1,260,000 spinal blocks and 450,000 epidural blocks were administered. In that study, the incidence of spinal hematoma was one in 200,000 after obstetric epidural blockade and one in 3600 among female patients undergoing knee arthroplasty.[2] At a single teaching hospital in Australia, data were collected prospectively over a 16-year period for all epidural catheters placed for postoperative analgesia. During that period, 8210 epidural catheters were inserted and 2 spinal hematomas (1:4105) and 6 epidural abscesses (1:1368) were diagnosed.[3] In rare instances, spinal epidural hematoma has developed following chiropractic manipulation and acupuncture therapy.[4,5] Factors that determine whether epidural hematoma results in injury to neural structures include the location in the spinal column (the level of the cauda equina is relatively resistant to injury, whereas the cervical spinal cord is not), and the rate at which the blood accumulates. Tarlov and colleagues demonstrated in dogs that spinal cord injury due to spinal epidural hematoma depends on both the amount of pressure exerted on the spinal cord and the duration of that pressure elevation.[6] Interestingly, some epidural hematomas cause significant injury despite the fact that their volume is significantly less than that typically used during epidural blood patch placement. Vertebral column neoplasms and vascular malformations are also risk factors. Patients who have an underlying coagulopathy or are being anticoagulated with warfarin, intravenous heparin, subcutaneous low molecular weight heparin, platelet inhibiting medications such as clopidogrel or ticlopidine, platelet glycoprotein IIb/IIIa receptor inhibitors, or fibrinolytic agents are at elevated risk of spinal hematoma formation. In addition, garlic has been shown to inhibit platelet aggregation and has been linked in one case to the development of a spontaneous epidural hematoma. Ginkgo inhibits platelet activating factor and has been linked to several cases of spontaneous intracranial bleeding, and ginseng inhibits platelet aggregation and prolongs both thrombin time and activated partial thromboplastin time, although the clinical significance of these findings remain unclear.[7–9]

Timely diagnosis of spinal epidural hematoma is critical, but in many cases will be challenging. Many patients have few complaints initially, commonly developing progressively worsening back pain as the hematoma expands with or without the immediate or delayed appearance of focal neurologic deficits. A progressive neurologic deficit may develop over a variable interval and with variable severity. Typically, neurologic deficits evolve over the course of several hours but, in some instances, they may develop over several days. In some instances, neurologic deficit rather than pain may be the presenting sign. Physical findings of myelopathy, or the development of the Brown-Sequard syndrome, should be recognized as indicative of spinal cord compression and should prompt emergent diagnostic evaluation and treatment.[10] Intractable leg pain and cauda equina syndrome may develop as well. Urinary retention may precede urinary incontinence. When a spinal epidural hematoma is suspected, a thorough neurologic examination is mandatory. This examination should include evaluation of anal sphincter tone and direct examination in efforts to detect loss of perineal sensation. Furthermore, serial examinations should be performed at short intervals. Findings on physical examination will be variable depending on the level of the lesion. Unilateral or bilateral weakness and/or paresthesias may be present. Hyper- or hyporeflexia may also be present. Depending on the clinical context, the differential diagnosis may include spinal epidural abscess. Urgent laboratory studies should include a complete blood count with platelets as well as a prothrombin time and activated partial thromboplastin time. In addition, a blood bank sample should be sent for type and cross match in preparation for surgery as well as in cases where fresh frozen plasma may be needed to reverse coagulopathies.

Magnetic resonance imaging (MRI) is the preferred radiologic study for diagnosis of spinal epidural hematoma. On sagittal reconstructed computed tomography (CT) or MR images, a spinal epidural hematoma typically appears as a biconvex mass dorsal to the thecal sac, with tapering cephalad and caudad margins (Fig. 110.3). Associated spinal cord edema may also be seen. Acute hemorrhage is characterized by a marked decrease in signal intensity on T2-weighted images. Subacute hematoma is characterized by increased signal intensity on both T1- and T2-weighted images.[11] The dura matter appears as a low signal curvilinear structure separating the hematoma from the spinal cord on T2-weighted gradient echo sequences. In one retrospective study of 17 patients with acute spinal epidural hematoma, 10 patients' T1 weighted images showed isointensity to the spinal cord and, in 7 patients, the hematomas were slightly hyperintense. T2-weighted images showed hyperintensity with areas of hypointensity. Other MRI findings included hematomas showing direct contiguity with the adjacent osseous spine in 13 patients. Posterolateral location of the hematomas was noted in 13 patients. Additional findings were capping of the epidural fat, compression of the epidural fat and ligamentum flavum, and compression of the thecal sac and/or cord.[12] MRI will also help to identify associated spinal cord tumors or arteriovenous malformations. For patients who cannot undergo MRI scanning or in cases where MRI scanning is not immediately available, CT, with or without myelography, is the study of choice. A spinal epidural hematoma appears as a bi-concave dorsal mass typically extending over at least two vertebral levels (Fig. 110.3).[13] Lumbar puncture does not add to

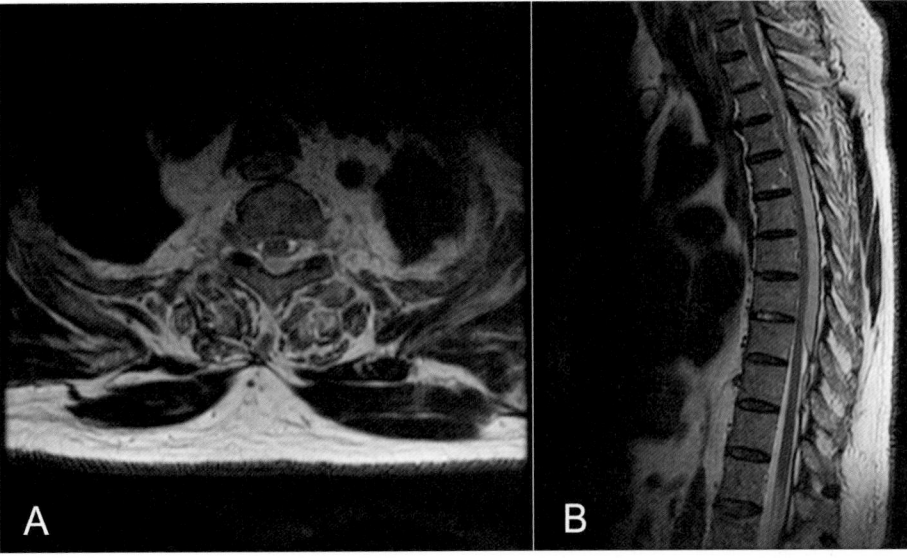

FIGURE 110.3 MRI of the lumbosacral spine demonstrating a lumbar epidural hematoma. (A) Axial and (B) sagittal reconstructed T2-weighted MRIs demonstrating a biconvex mass dorsal to the thecal sac extending from the cervicothoracic junction to the low thoracic area, with tapering cephalad and caudad margins, the typical appearance of an epidural hematoma.

the diagnosis and may worsen the patient's condition in some instances.

When spinal epidural hematoma is entertained as a diagnosis, urgent neurosurgical consultation should be obtained. In a retrospective study of 30 patients who were treated for spinal epidural hematoma between 1979 and 1993, rapidity of surgical decompression of the spinal cord correlated with neurologic outcome.[12] Patients who were taken to surgery within 12 hours of symptom onset fared significantly better than those whose surgery was delayed beyond 12 hours. In this series, the patients' preoperative neurologic status was also predictive of outcome. Of note, in a series of 30 patients, of 8 patients who had complete loss of neurological function (Frankel grade A), 6 improved with surgical decompression and 2 of these regained normal function.[11] Emergent surgical evacuation remains the standard of care and treatment of choice for spinal epidural hematoma. In some instances, spinal epidural hematomas have been successfully conservatively managed, typically in patients whose neurologic examination was spontaneously, steadily improving.[14]

INFECTIOUS COMPLICATIONS

Infectious complications may ensue following either peripheral or central neuraxial blockade, although the latter is more likely to lead to catastrophic sequelae such as meningitis or compression of neural structures. Both superficial and deep infections have been reported following epidural injections, facet joint injections, and trigger point injections. In the case of indwelling catheters, the risk of infection increases with increased duration of catheter therapy. When epidural catheters are left in place for 70 days, the risk of infection reaches 15% with a 1% risk of epidural infection.[15–17] In the case of implanted spinal cord stimulators and intrathecal drug pumps, a review of four prospective trials found 36 infections in 35 patients out of a total of 700 patients who underwent implantation. The overall infection rate was 5% with 57% to 80% of the infections in the trials involving the pump pocket, 13% to 33% involving the lumbar site, and zero to 14% leading to meningitis.[18] All patients undergoing interventional therapies for pain treatment should be given explicit written postprocedural guidelines that include a clear description of the signs and symptoms that may herald an infection and a clear process for contacting pain clinic personnel on an urgent basis if such signs and symptoms develop.

The source of the pathogen may be either external, as in the case of contaminated equipment or breaches in sterile technique, or internal in the case of patients with local or systemic infections such as skin and soft tissue infections or bacteremia. Risk factors for infection include diabetes, alcoholism, smoking, and immunosuppression. Similarly, infections in the epidural space may spread to other areas via hematogenous spread or local extension. Pathogens include skin flora such as *Staphylococcus aureus* and *Staphylococcus epidermis*. In patients with implanted spinal catheters or devices, the incidence of methicillin-resistant *Staphylococcus aureus* epidural infection is particularly high. Injury to the neural structures may occur due to direct compression by an abscess or due to ischemia caused by septic thrombophlebitis.

Initially, patients with epidural abscess present typically with back pain at the affected level of the spine. Subsequently, they may develop radicular pain corresponding to the involved level. They may then progress to development of motor and sensory deficits accompanied by bowel and bladder dysfunction and finally to frank paralysis. Back pain will be present in roughly three quarters of patients, fever in almost half, and neurologic deficits in about one third. Thus, the classic triad of back pain, fever, and neurologic deficit is seen in only a minority of patients.[19] Both the duration of symptoms prior to presentation and the rate of progression of symptoms can be highly variable. Spinal epidural abscesses typically extend over three to four vertebral levels; however, in rare instances they may involve the whole spine. Laboratory studies should include a complete blood count with differential as about two thirds of patients will have leukocytosis. Erythrocyte sedimentation rate and C reactive protein are almost always elevated, although neither of these tests is specific. Blood cultures should be sent prior to the administration of antibiotics and approximately 60% of patients will be bacteremic. When lumbar puncture is performed, CSF analysis shows elevated protein and pleocytosis in three quarters of patients. Gram staining and culture of CSF are negative in the majority of patients. Lumbar puncture adds little to the diagnosis and entails risk of causing meningitis if the needle traverses the epidural abscess en route to the thecal space; CSF should be analyzed if myelography is undertaken.

MRI with intravenous gadolinium is the study of choice to evaluate possible epidural abscess (Fig. 110.4). MRI is highly sensitive for diagnosing epidural abscess and allows evaluation of the dimensions of the abscess which facilitates surgical planning. If MRI is contraindicated or is not readily available, CT myelography is also quite sensitive, but is more invasive. Plain x-rays or CT scan of the spine without myelography may demon-

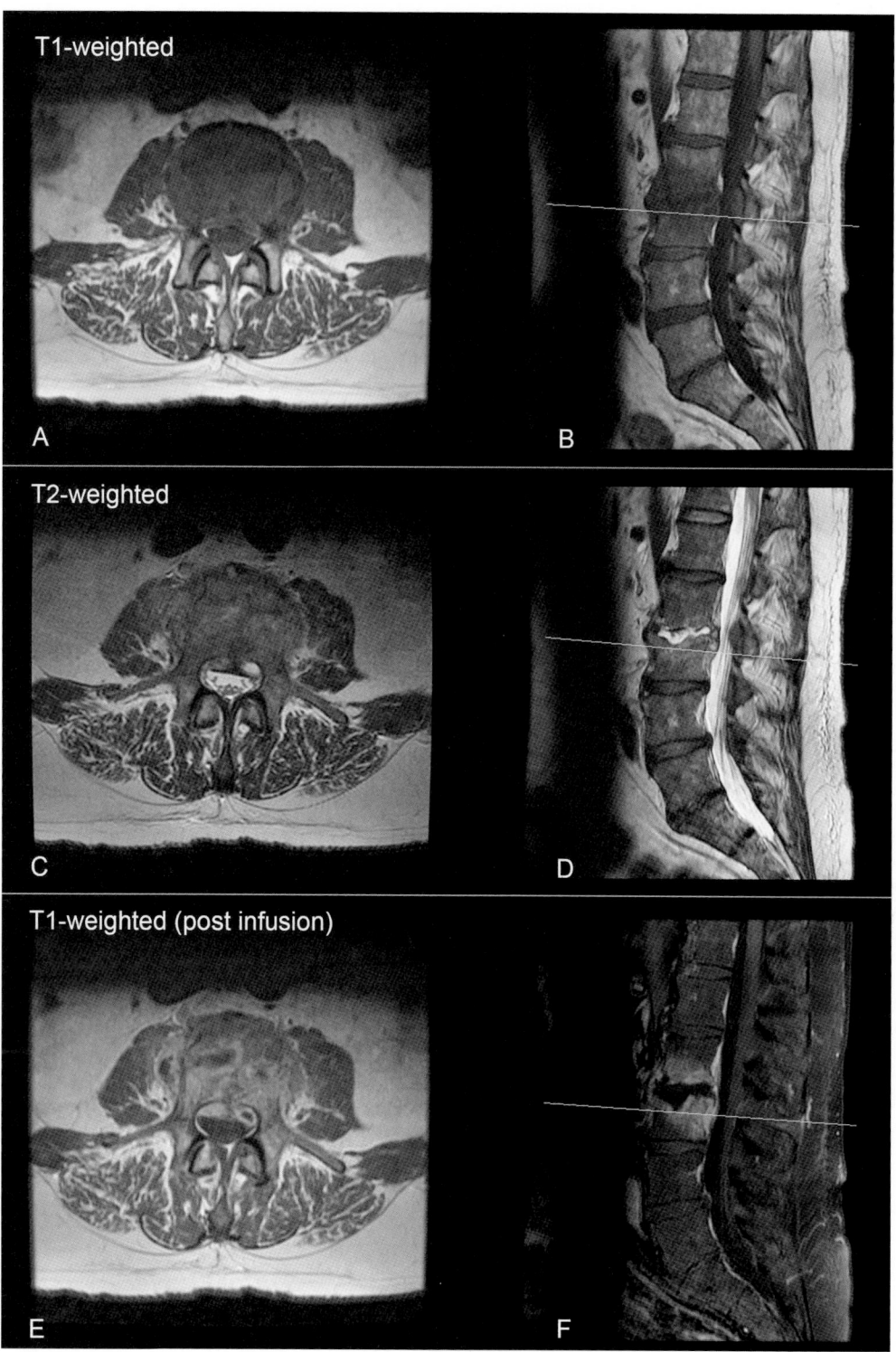

FIGURE 110.4 MRI of the lumbosacral spine demonstrating epidural abscess. This is a 64-year-old who presented with worsening axial low back pain 2 weeks following lumbar epidural injection of steroid for treatment of acute radicular pain. (**A**) Axial and (**B**) sagittal T1-weighted images. (**C**) Axial and (**D**) sagittal T2-weighted images. (**E**) Axial and (**F**) sagittal T1-weighted images following intravenous administration of gadolinium. These findings are compatible with diskitis/osteomyelitis at L2-3, with enhancement of the anterior epidural space and a focus of high T2 and low T1 signal in the left anterior epidural space consistent with epidural abscess.

strate diminished discs space and/or bony destruction suggestive of discitis and osteomyelitis. These conditions coexist with epidural abscess in up to 80% of cases. Urgent surgical drainage accompanied by administration of systemic antibiotics is the standard of care for epidural abscesses.[20] In rare cases, percutaneous drainage with systemic antibiotics or antibiotic treatment in the absence of surgery may be undertaken.[19]

Superficial infections typically present with local erythema, pain, swelling, and, in some cases, purulent discharge. In some instances, superficial infections associated with catheters can be managed with local drainage and antibiotics without removing the catheter.[15] Some cases of superficial infections and pocket site infections following implantations of spinal cord stimulators and intrathecal drug pumps have been successfully managed using oral and parenteral antibiotics that correspond to antimicrobial sensitivities on the basis of wound cultures, while the implanted device has been left in place.[21,22] However, as other authors have noted, device-related infections are rarely completely eradicated without removal of the device in question.[18] This observation mirrors the extensive experience with infected cardiac pacemakers.[23] In all cases, a high degree of vigilance must be maintained in regard to the possibility that a device-related superficial or pocket infection may spread to the neuraxis with catastrophic results. In the event that signs of infection such as erythema, swelling, fluctuance, or tenderness progress along the course of an implanted lead or catheter, the device with all associated hardware should be surgically removed on an urgent basis. Similarly, urgent device removal should be undertaken if the patient displays signs of systemic infection such as fever or chills, or signs of possible meningitis such as fever, neck pain and stiffness, severe headache, or altered mental status. At the time of surgery, separately labeled wound cultures should be sent from all surgical sites and all surgical sites should be extensively irrigated. As with spinal epidural hematoma, the patient's preoperative neurologic function is the best predictor of final neurologic outcome.[24] For any patient where there is a significant concern for systemic infection or meningitis, antibiotics should be administered immediately and should not be delayed until cultures can be obtained. Empiric antibiotic coverage should provide coverage of *Staphylococcus* species, preferably with vancomycin to ensure coverage of methicillin-resistant *Staphylococcus aureus*, and should provide coverage of gram-negative microbes with a third or fourth generation cephalosporin or equivalent.

LOCAL ANESTHETIC SYSTEMIC TOXICITY

Lidocaine and bupivacaine are amide local anesthetics which are widely used in interventional pain management procedures due to their relative safety. Lidocaine is of relatively lower potency and has a rapid onset of action and an intermediate duration of action. Nonetheless, the potential for lidocaine associated systemic toxicity due to excessive dose, inadvertent intravascular administration, or unanticipated rapid absorption is well recognized. Bupivacaine is of higher potency, but has a slower onset and prolonged duration of action. Local anesthetics, including lidocaine and bupivacaine, bind sodium channels and inhibit the sodium permeability that underlies action potentials in both neurons and cardiac myocytes. Local anesthetic inhibition of sodium permeability increases with repeated depolarization. In addition to binding sodium channels, local anesthetics will bind potassium and calcium channels, as well as N-methyl-D-aspartate receptors, beta-adrenergic receptors, and nicotinic acetylcholine receptors. Indeed, local anesthetic toxicity may be mediated in part through binding to these channels and receptors.[25–27] In general, the anesthetic potency of a local anesthetic correlates with its central nervous system (CNS) toxicity. Local anesthetics appear to cause cardiac toxicity through several different mechanisms including inhibition of calcium and potassium channels and inhibition of beta-adrenergic receptors and epinephrine stimulated cAMP formation. Local anesthetics prolong cardiac conduction in a dose dependent fashion. With increasing serum concentration, bupivacaine provokes QT prolongation, ventricular tachycardia, and ventricular fibrillation. Risk factors for the development of local anesthetic toxicity include the extremes of age, reduced hepatic and cardiac function, and pregnancy. The threshold dose of local anesthetic required to provoke seizures is affected by the route and rate of injection, the rate of increase of serum drug concentration, the presence of acidosis, and whether the patient is awake or anesthetized. Local anesthetic toxicity may result from systemic absorption of excessive doses following local infiltration; however, toxicity more commonly occurs due to inadvertent intravascular injection. Intraarterial injection poses a greater risk of CNS and cardiovascular toxicity than intravenous injection because, in the latter case, passage through the lung allows for some clearance of the drug. In the case of intraarterial injection, doses as small as 2.5 mg of bupivacaine or 15 mg of lidocaine have resulted in seizures when injected into the carotid or vertebral arteries, and this is felt to result from direct delivery of the local anesthetic to the brain.[28,29]

In the event of lidocaine toxicity, CNS symptoms typically precede cardiovascular symptoms.[30] CNS symptoms are initially characterized by inhibitory neuronal blockade leading to excitatory manifestations such as perioral numbness, a metallic taste, tinnitus, restlessness, confusion, a sense of impending doom, visual disturbances that are most commonly described as oscillations of objects in the visual fields, shivers, tremors, and tonic-clonic seizures (Fig. 110.5). Sympathetic stimulation is also observed during this phase, with resultant tachycardia and hypertension.[31]

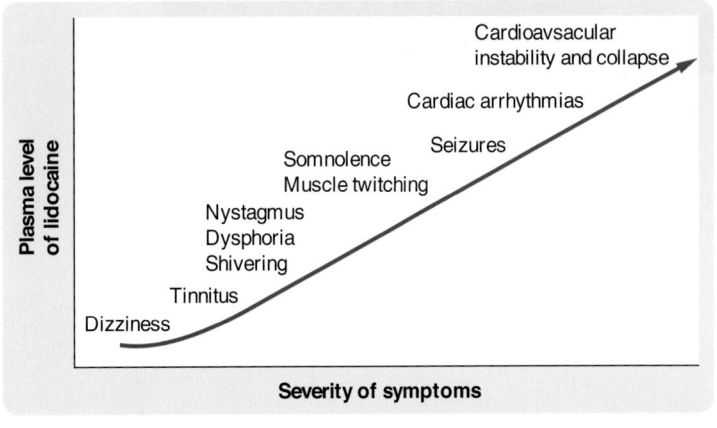

FIGURE 110.5 Relationship between plasma concentration of lidocaine and the development of signs and symptoms of local anesthetic toxicity.

In patients who are receiving procedural sedation with benzodiazepines or other sedatives, the excitatory phase of local anesthetic toxicity may not be apparent. The excitatory phase is followed in episodes of severe toxicity by a depressed phase characterized by coma and respiratory arrest. Cardiovascular toxicity develops at higher serum levels and may include profound bradycardia, arrhythmias, contractile dysfunction, and asystole.[25] In the case of bupivacaine, doses that are insufficient to provoke seizures will provoke cardiac arrhythmias.[32]

Treatment of local anesthetic induced seizures focuses on maintaining the airway and oxygenation. The injection or infusion of local anesthetic must be stopped immediately. Lorazepam, midazolam, thiopental, or propofol may be used to terminate the seizure. Cardiovascular depression with resultant hypotension due to local anesthetic toxicity should be treated with intravenous crystalloids and vasopressors such as norepinephrine, or phenylephrine. In the event of severe contractile dysfunction, epinephrine should be administered. If cardiac arrest occurs, advanced cardiac life support (ACLS) protocol should be pursued, although some authors propose substituting vasopressin for epinephrine. Cardiac arrest due to bupivacaine toxicity has been successfully treated in several cases with intravenous lipid emulsion.[33,34] A 20% lipid emulsion may be administered as a 1.5 mL per kilogram bolus followed by a 0.25 mL per kilogram per minute infusion for 30 to 60 minutes. The mechanism by which lipid infusion is believed to reverse bupivacaine toxicity is by "scavenging" the lipophilic bupivacaine. In the presence of persistent cardiovascular collapse associated with local anesthetic administration, urgent institution of cardiopulmonary bypass can be lifesaving.

Unintended Destinations Following Local Anesthetic Administration

The direct effects of local anesthetics are critically dependent on where they are applied. Inadvertent intrathecal injection of local anesthetic can result in a high thoracic or cervical level of sensory and motor block or total spinal anesthesia, with transient loss of consciousness and respiratory arrest. This is most likely to occur during cervical injections or when a large volume of local anesthetic is used during lumbar injections. Signs and symptoms of a high spinal progress rapidly and most typically include flaccid paralysis, apnea, hypotension, bradycardia, and dilated pupils. They initially include lightheadedness, dizziness, nausea, and vomiting.[29] In addition, the patient may develop air hunger due to loss of intercostal muscle activity, followed by phrenic nerve paralysis and eventually apnea due to blockade of the respiratory center in the brain stem. Blockade of the cardio accelerator fibers at T1 through T4 or of the medulla may produce bradycardia, hypotension, or arrhythmias.[35] Blockade of the Edinger-Westphal nucleus with subsequent loss of efferent parasympathetic activity produces dilated, nonreactive pupils.[36] In the case of subdural injection, symptoms develop more slowly, typically 15 to 30 minutes after injection, and are commonly asymmetric. When symptoms do occur, they may progress to respiratory and cardiovascular collapse as with intrathecal injection. When a high spinal occurs, ventilation with 100% oxygen with a bag valve mask or with endotracheal intubation must be initiated if phrenic nerve blockade or apnea is present. Bradycardia and hypotension should be treated with crystalloids, and atropine, ephedrine, phenylephrine, or epinephrine.[35] The patient may remain awake, but paralyzed during a high spinal, so reassurance that the condition is temporary is warranted, as is consideration of administration of an anxiolytic agent.

Vasovagal Reactions

Vasovagal reactions, which may include frank syncope, are one of the most common emergencies encountered in a pain center.

Fortunately, these episodes typically have a benign natural history. Sir William Gowers first used the term vasovagal in 1907, and vasovagal syncope is now accepted as the most common form of syncope, accounting for two thirds of syncopal episodes presenting to the emergency department.[37] The pathogenesis of vasovagal syncope remains uncertain, but the current understanding is that it results from venous pooling and reduced venous return, and that vigorous contraction of the heart's chambers when they are inadequately filled provokes the Bezold-Jarisch reflex, resulting in paradoxical hypotension and bradycardia. At the onset of a vasovagal reaction patients typically appear pale and diaphoretic and complain of lightheadedness, sweatiness, nausea, and tunnel vision. Myoclonic jerks may accompany vasovagal syncope and may be clinically indistinguishable from seizure activity. If a patient exhibits signs of a vasovagal reaction during an interventional pain treatment procedure, the procedure should be halted, and the patient should be placed supine if not already in that position. Care should be taken to ensure that the patient will not fall and sustain a secondary injury. Randomized trials have demonstrated that leg crossing, and isometric arm exercises can help prevent progression to vasovagal syncope.[38] Most cases of vasovagal syncope will resolve spontaneously and will require only conservative measures. In the event that blood pressure and heart rate continue to decline, an intravenous line should be placed, crystalloids and oxygen administered, the patient should be placed on a cardiac monitor and a vasopressor, such as ephedrine (in 5–10 mg increments) or a chronotrope such as atropine (0.4–1 mg) should be administered.[29]

COMPLICATIONS ASSOCIATED WITH INTRATHECAL DRUG DELIVERY

When drugs are delivered via the intrathecal route, complications may arise either due to withdrawal or due to administration of an excessive dose. In the case of intrathecal baclofen administration, withdrawal may be particularly severe and can even be fatal. Baclofen is an analogue of the inhibitory neurotransmitter gamma-aminobutyric acid. It acts as an agonist of the GABA-b receptors in the brain stem, dorsal horn of the spinal cord, and other CNS regions. Although the mechanism of intrathecal baclofen withdrawal is not established, it may be due to diffuse disinhibition of GABA-b modulated pathways.[39] Although the most common manifestation of under dosage of baclofen is pruritus and return of the patient's spasticity, abrupt baclofen withdrawal may result in a life-threatening syndrome characterized by fever, tachycardia, labile blood pressure or hypotension, malaise, dysphoria, and hallucinations followed by coma, rebound spasticity more severe than the patient's baseline, hyperreflexia or rigidity, paresthesias, priapism in males, and seizures. If not treated adequately and promptly, the patient may develop rhabdomyolysis, brain injury, kidney and liver failure, and disseminated intravascular coagulation.[39,40] In some cases, death ensues.[41] The differential diagnosis of intrathecal baclofen withdrawal includes infection, neuroleptic malignant syndrome, serotonin syndrome, malignant hyperthermia, and autonomic dysreflexia. Paradoxically, the diagnosis may be more difficult to make in more severe cases of withdrawal. Symptoms of intrathecal baclofen withdrawal typically present 1 to 3 days after interruption of baclofen delivery. Interruption of baclofen delivery may be due to an exhausted drug reservoir after missing a scheduled refill, mechanical pump malfunction, catheter kinking or disruption, or mistakes in drug formulation or pump programming. Restoration of adequate intrathecal baclofen delivery by addressing pump problems or by lumbar puncture or drain represents the most definitive therapy.[42] If the pump catheter remains intact, intrathecal baclofen may be administered via the side port. Evaluation of the pump should be performed with the manufacturer's interrogation device. If interrogation of the pump does not reveal the underlying problem, a catheter dye study should be undertaken and the pump should be refilled with medication at the correct concentration. To conduct a catheter dye study, radiographic contrast is administered through the side port of the infusion device to assess the integrity and position of the intrathecal catheter. Oral and enteral baclofen administration (up to 120 mg per day of baclofen in six to eight divided doses in adults), accompanied by intravenous benzodiazepine administration should be undertaken until intrathecal baclofen delivery is restored or if this cannot be accomplished. Oral and enteral baclofen alone are often insufficient to treat withdrawal from intrathecal baclofen. Continuous or intermittent infusions of diazepam or midazolam may be rapidly titrated upward until muscle relaxation, cessation of seizure activity, and normal blood pressure and temperature are restored. Propofol infusion and chemical paralytic agents may also be used in the intubated patient.[43] The patient should be treated in a setting where critical care monitoring and ventilator and cardiovascular support is available. In some cases, patients with hyperthermia have been treated with dantrolene. In case reports, cyproheptadine has proven helpful.[39,44]

In contrast, baclofen overdose typically presents with somnolence, comas, seizures, respiratory depression, hypotonia, and arrhythmias. Treatment consists of intubation and artificial ventilation as indicated, and immediately turning off the pump with the manufacturer's programmer or, if this is not available, emptying the pump reservoir. In cases where the overdose is detected within the first few hours, withdrawal of 30 to 40 cc of CSF via the catheter access port of the pump may reverse the overdose.[45] Physostigmine may reverse drowsiness and respiratory depression (adult dose one to 2 mg IV over 5 to 10 minutes, may repeat every 10 to 30 minutes as required; pediatric dose 0.02 mg per kilogram IV, less than 0.5 mg per minute, may repeat every 5 to 10 minutes as required up to 2 mg maximum).

Opioid Withdrawal

Opioid withdrawal can also occur in patients receiving intrathecal drug delivery or systemic opioids, and typically manifests with anxiety, insomnia, yawning, diaphoresis, lacrimation, rhinorrhea, mydriasis, myalgias, piloerection, nausea, vomiting, diarrhea, and abdominal cramping.[46,47] In patients for whom ongoing opioid therapy is indicated, treatment consists of resuming opioid therapy. In some cases an alternate route of administration may be necessary, such as intravenous and/or transdermal delivery for a patient who is no longer able to take oral medications. In cases where opioid therapy is not indicated, symptoms of opioid withdrawal may be mitigated with alpha-2 adrenergic agonists such as clonidine (0.1 to 0.2 mg per dose increasing to a maximum of 1 mg per day) or lofexidine (0.4 to 0.6 mg per dose increasing to a maximum of 2 mg per day). Alpha-2 adrenergic agonists may cause hypotension, fatigue, lethargy, and dry mouth. Nausea and vomiting may be treated with intravenous fluids and antiemetics such as metoclopramide or prochlorperazine. Diarrhea and colicky abdominal pain may be treated with loperamide or hyoscine butylbromide.[47] Agitation may be treated with benzodiazepines.

ANAPHYLAXIS

At the turn of the 19th century, Charles Richet and Paul Portier coined the term anaphylaxis when they observed that several dogs died following repeat challenges with Physalia extracts during experiments that they reported while guests on Prince Albert of Monaco's yacht in the Mediterranean Sea.[48] In an anaphylactic reaction, the inciting allergen binds to previously formed immu-

noglobulin E (IgE) on the surface of previously sensitized mast cells and basophils. These cells release mediators such as histamine, leukotrienes, prostaglandins, bradykinins, and thromboxanes that cause markedly reduced vascular tone, increased mucous membrane secretions, and increased capillary permeability.[49] Generalized hypersensitivity reactions may be divided into grade 1 or mild reactions, grade 2 or moderate reactions, and grade 3 or severe reactions.[50] Grades two and three correspond with anaphylaxis. Grade one reactions are defined by generalized erythema, urticaria, periorbital edema, or angioedema. Grade two reactions are characterized by dyspnea, stridor, wheezing, nausea and vomiting, dizziness or presyncope, chest or throat tightness, or abdominal pain. Grade 3 reactions are defined by cyanosis or an oxygen saturation less than or equal to 92%, hypotension, confusion, collapse, loss of consciousness, or incontinence. Cutaneous manifestations such as erythema, itch, and urticaria are present in almost all cases, although they may be quite subtle. Therefore, when the diagnosis is unclear, it is crucial to fully undress the patient and carefully examine the skin. In one retrospective study of 1149 cases of generalized hypersensitivity treated in the emergency department, 250 cases were assessed as being due to medications; 145 cases were believed to be due to antibiotics, with the majority being beta-lactam antibiotics. Nonsteroidal antiinflammatory drugs were implicated in 32 cases, narcotics in 11 cases, radiologic contrast in 7 cases, ace inhibitors in 4 cases, vaccines in 4 cases, and other or unclear medications in 47 cases.[50] The median interval between drug administration and fatal collapse is 5 minutes.[51] The differential diagnosis of anaphylactic reaction includes asthma attack, Scombroid poisoning, angioedema either secondary to angiotensin-converting enzyme inhibitors or hereditary, panic attack, and vasovagal syncope (these last two conditions do not cause urticaria, angioedema, or bronchospasm).

There are no randomized trials of therapies for anaphylaxis, so most treatment recommendations are on the basis of consensus. The patient undergoing an anaphylactic reaction should be administered high flow oxygen. Intramuscular epinephrine should be given early to all patients with signs of a systemic reaction such as hypotension, airway edema, or dyspnea (0.3 to 0.5 mg, 1:1000, IM repeated every 15 to 20 minutes if there is no clinical improvement). If anaphylaxis appears to be severe and or imminently life threatening, intravenous epinephrine should be given (0.1 mg, 1:10,000, IV over 5 minutes, followed by an IV infusion of 1 to 4 mcg per minute as needed). Patients receiving epinephrine for anaphylaxis should be monitored in an emergency department or intensive care unit. Aggressive fluid resuscitation with isotonic crystalloids such as normal saline should be undertaken.[52] One to two liters should be rapidly infused. Antihistamines such as diphenhydramine should be given (25–50 mg slowly IV or IM) as well as H2 blockers (e.g., cimetidine 300 mg IM or IV). Bronchospasm should be treated with inhaled beta-adrenergic agents such as albuterol. High-dose intravenous corticosteroids should be administered early, although their therapeutic effects are seen 4 to 6 hours after administration. Other therapies which may be considered in anaphylaxis include vasopressin, which has been beneficial in case reports for severely hypotensive patients, atropine in the setting of severe bradycardia, and glucagon for patients who are unresponsive epinephrine, particularly if they are taking beta-blockers.[49] Pumphrey, who attempted to identify and analyze every fatal anaphylactic reaction in the United Kingdom since 1992, stresses the importance of keeping patients supine with their legs elevated.[51]

Catastrophic Neural Injuries and the Administration of Particulate Steroids

In the cervical spine, the carotid and vertebral arteries lie in close proximity to the stellate ganglion, the cervical facet joints, and the cervical intervertebral foramina. The anterior spinal artery provides the principal vascular supply to the spinal cord. The anterior spinal artery arises rostrally from the vertebral arteries and receives input from 6 to 9 radicular arteries. It is located at the anterior central sulcus and supplies the anterior two thirds of the spinal cord. The posterior spinal arteries supply the posterior one third of the spinal cord. They are paired and run just medial to the dorsal roots. The arteria radicularis magna (the artery of Adamkiewicz) is the largest of the radicular arteries. It is most commonly located at T10 on the left side, but may occur anywhere from T8 to L2 and occurs on the right in 17% of subjects.[53] In addition, the ascending cervical artery and the deep cervical artery each furnish spinal branches that enter the intervertebral foramina. These spinal branches supply the vertebral column but also give rise to radicular arteries that accompany the dorsal and ventral roots of the spinal nerves (Fig. 110.6). In some individuals, the radicular arteries are substantial in size and reinforce the anterior spinal artery. Such reinforcing arteries can occur at any cervical level and those radicular arteries that supply the spinal cord are termed spinal medullary arteries. If reinforcing radicular arteries are compromised by a transforaminal injection, infarction of the cervical spinal cord could ensue. If the vertebral or carotid arteries are entered, infarction of the brain stem and

portions of the brain supplied by the posterior circulation may ensue, causing stroke, often massive stroke resulting in death.

The first report of a complication attributed to cervical transforaminal injection of steroids described a patient who died from a spinal cord infarction.[10] The location of the infarction implied that a radicular artery that reinforced the anterior spinal artery had been compromised, but no evidence was offered about the mechanism by which the artery had been compromised. Images of the placement of the needle were not published.

Reports of spinal cord infarction following cervical[54,55] or lumbar[56,57] transforaminal injection of steroid have appeared, and this topic has been reviewed in detail.[58] Vertebral artery injection with subsequent stroke involving the posterior circulation has also been reported.[59] A similar case of massive infarction involving the posterior cerebral circulation following injection of particulate steroid during attempted intraarticular atlantoaxial joint injection is shown in Figure 110.7.

The exact mechanism of spinal cord injury following transforaminal injections has not been determined. As analyzed using MRI, the pattern of injury strongly implicates a reinforcing radicular artery. Spasm of the artery would seem to be an unlikely mechanism since it is inconsistent with the vasodilatory effect of local anesthetic agents when applied to arterial walls. Embolism

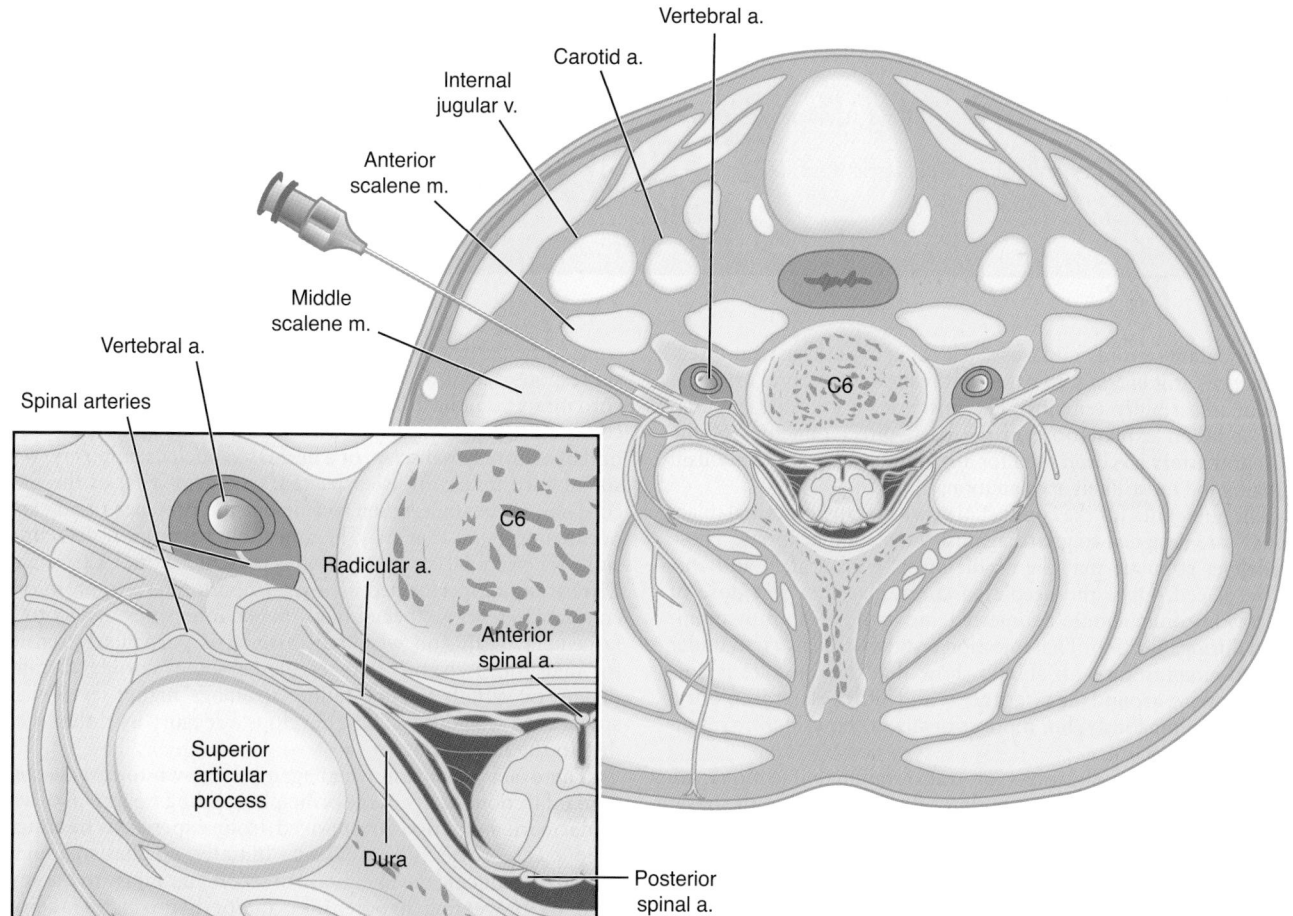

FIGURE 110.6 Axial view of cervical transforaminal injection at the level of C6. The needle has been inserted along the axis of the foramen, and is in final position against the posterior aspect of the intervertebral foramen. Insertion along this axis places the needle behind the spinal nerve, and behind the vertebral artery, which lies anterior to the foramen. *Inset*: A spinal artery arises from the vertebral artery. It supplies the vertebral column. Another spinal artery enters the intervertebral foramen from the ascending cervical artery or deep cervical artery. It furnishes radicular branches that accompany the nerve roots and ultimately reach the anterior and posterior spinal arteries of the spinal cord. (Redrawn after Rathmell JP. Atlas of Image-Guided Intervention in Regional Anesthesia and Pain Medicine. Philadelphia: Lippincott Williams & Wilkins, 2005.)

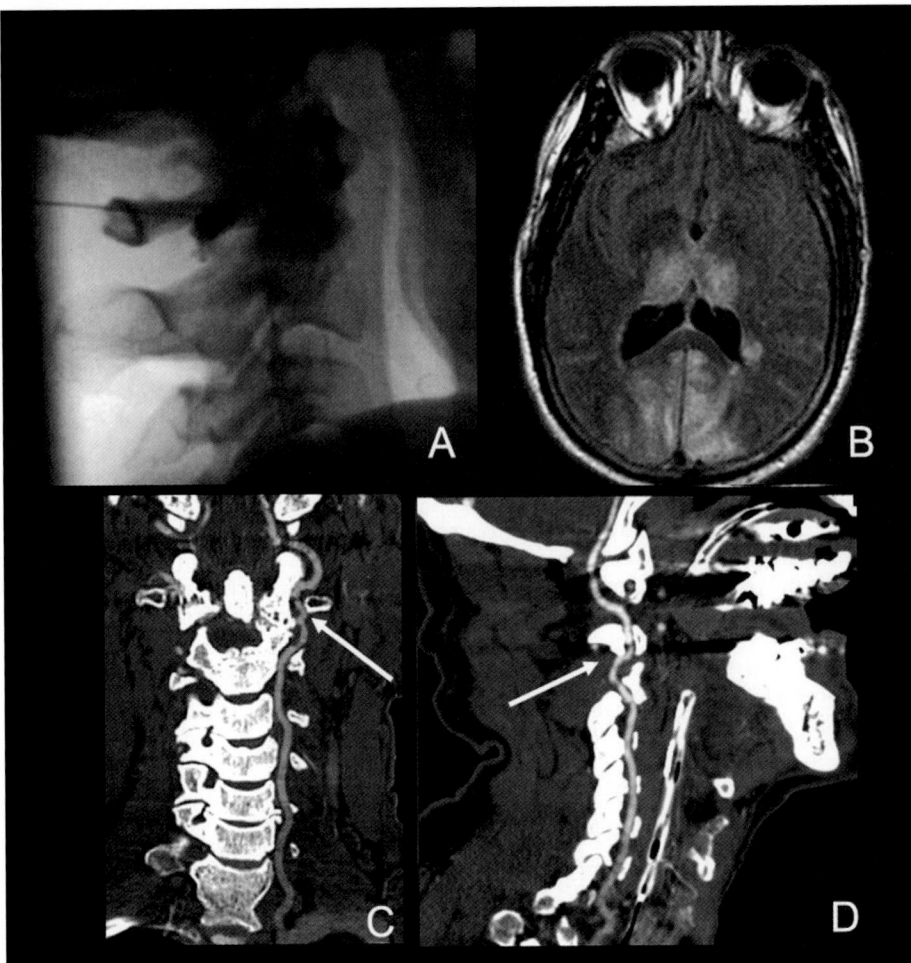

FIGURE 110.7 Cerebrovascular accident following intraarterial injection of particulate steroid during attempted intraarticular atlantoaxial (C1/2) joint injection. (**A**) Lateral fluoroscopy imaging demonstrating needle position adjacent to the C1/2 facet joint. (**B**) Axial MRI (T1 FLAIR sequence) of the brain. (**C**) Frontal and (**D**) axial CT angiography of the vertebral arteries; *arrows* point to a small filling defect within the left vertebral artery adjacent to the left C1/2 facet joint, suggesting the point of needle entry in to the vertebral artery. The proximity of the vertebral artery to the C1/2 facet joint is immediately apparent from the images.

of particulate steroids ranks as the leading hypothesis, but direct evidence is still lacking. In cases involving the vertebral artery, a similar uncertainty remains. The injection of contrast medium cannot be an explanation; in the past, direct puncture of the vertebral artery has been used for angiography. Steroid embolism remains the most likely explanation.

The guidelines for the conduct of cervical transforaminal injections[58] are designed to guard against these complications. These guidelines stipulate that the needle must be accurately and correctly placed. Once the needle has been placed, a test dose of contrast medium should be injected and its flow carefully monitored during injection. That injection tests two things. First, under normal circumstances, it should show that the injectate is correctly flowing around the target nerve and into the lateral epidural space. Simultaneously, but more critically, it shows if intravascular injection occurs.

Neurologic complications of transforaminal injections are typically catastrophic. They are clinically obvious upon the onset of spinal weakness and numbness. Spinal cord infarction due to embolization of a radicular artery is clinically indistinguishable from the anterior spinal artery syndrome, also known as Beck's syndrome. Patients develop abrupt onset of weakness below the level of the infarction, flaccid paralysis, areflexia, loss of pain and temperature perception, and atonic urinary bladder. Position and vibratory sensation will typically be relatively intact. Preserved proprioception at symptom onset has been associated with better outcomes.[60] In contrast to cerebrovascular infarction, spinal cord infarction is frequently painful. Patients may experience a radicular or back pain and, in some cases, spinal cord infarction will mimic angina pectoris.[61] Later in the clinical

course, the patient may develop spasticity, hyperreflexia, Babinski responses, and clonus.[53] In the setting of possible acute spinal cord infarction, the differential diagnosis may include spinal cord compression by a mass lesion such as a spinal epidural or subdural hematoma or abscess, or a herniated nucleus pulposus. When spinal cord infarction is suspected, emergent MRI of the spinal cord should be undertaken to rule out the presence of any space occupying lesion that may be amenable to surgical decompression. When spinal cord infarction is present, sagittal T2-weighted MRI scanning performed at least 4 hours after symptom onset commonly reveals "pencil-like" hyper intensities and cord enlargement. Diffusion weighted imaging is particularly sensitive for detecting ischemic changes in the spinal cord.[62] Common diagnostic pitfalls include failure to image higher levels of the spinal cord when the patient develops a sensory level that is caudad to the infarction.

There is no emergency management known to reverse spinal cord infarction. Many of the principles guiding treatment of acute spinal cord infarction are derived from experience treating ischemic cerebrovascular accidents. Initially, emphasis should be placed on reducing the likelihood of secondary injury to the spinal cord by preventing hypotension and/or hypoxia. In addition, rapid triage and transport to a definitive care facility with appropriate imaging, critical care, and surgical capabilities should be undertaken. In the case of ischemic cerebrovascular accidents, induced hypertension to achieve a mean arterial pressure of 20% to 30% above baseline or to achieve a predefined target mean arterial pressure has been advocated although this therapy remains controversial.[63] Although aspirin has been advocated for the treatment of spinal cord infarction related to atherosclerotic disease or dissection, principally on the basis of its use in the treatment of ischemic stroke, there does not appear to be a role for antiplatelet or anticoagulant therapy in the treatment of spinal cord infarction presumed secondary to embolization of particulate steroids. In a prospective study of 77 patients with acute neurologic deficits secondary to spinal cord injuries, patients treated with 7 days of volume resuscitation with crystalloids, transfusion of blood products to maintain a hematocrit greater than 32, as well as dopamine and Levophed as needed to maintain a mean arterial blood pressure greater than 85 mm Hg had better neurologic outcomes than historical controls.[64] This therapy has not been studied in prospective randomized controlled trials. Treatment of nonpenetrating acute spinal cord injury with methyl prednisolone remains controversial despite evaluation in three large, prospective randomized double blind controlled trials.[65–67] At the current time, there is insufficient evidence to advocate routine administration of methylprednisolone to patients with acute spinal cord infarction. Standard measures to prevent complications of acute paraplegia should be implemented, including measures directed at prevention of deep venous thrombosis and pulmonary embolus, as well as bladder catheterization if indicated. Early consultation with physiatrists should be undertaken in order to optimize functional recovery and prevent development of spasticity and decubiti.

CONCLUSION

Although emergencies in the pain clinic are quite rare, when they do occur they can be catastrophic and even deadly. The pain specialist should be familiar with the most common complications and their mechanisms, as well as techniques that can be used to reduce the risk of said complications. Familiarity with common complications, including their clinical presentations and natural histories, will facilitate prompt recognition and treatment, thereby improving the chances of good outcomes. Pain specialists should educate patients about specific signs and symptoms of complications that may ensue from their treatment and provide them with clear instructions for reaching members of the pain clinic staff in a timely manner, both during clinic hours and on evenings and weekends, in order to achieve prompt identification and treatment of complications when they arise.

References

1. Usubiaga JE. Neurological complications following epidural anesthesia. *Int Anesthesiol Clin* 1975;13(2):1–153.
2. Moen V, Dahlgren N, Irestedt L. Severe neurological complications after central neuraxial blockades in Sweden 1990–1999. *Anesthesiology* 2004;101(4):950–959.
3. Cameron CM, Scott DA, McDonald WM, et al. A review of neuraxial epidural morbidity: experience of more than 8,000 cases at a single teaching hospital. *Anesthesiology* 2007;106(5):997–1002.
4. Segal DH, Lidov MW, Camins MB. Cervical epidural hematoma after chiropractic manipulation in a healthy young woman: case report. *Neurosurgery* 1996;39(5):1043–1045.
5. Keane JR, Ahmadi J, Gruen P. Spinal epidural hematoma with subarachnoid hemorrhage caused by acupuncture. *AJNR Am J Neuroradiol* 1993;14(2):365–366.
6. Tarlov IM. Spinal cord compression studies. III. Time limits for recovery after gradual compression in dogs. *AMA Arch Neurol Psychiatry* 1954;71:588–597.
7. Rose KD, Croissant PD, Parliament CF, et al. Spontaneous spinal epidural hematoma with associated platelet dysfunction from excessive garlic ingestion: a case report. *Neurosurgery* 1990;26(5):880–882.
8. Haemorrhage due to Ginkgo biloba? *Prescrire Int* 2008;17(93):19.
9. Friedman JA, Taylor SA, McDermott W, et al. Multifocal and recurrent subarachnoid hemorrhage due to an herbal supplement containing natural coumarins. *Neurocrit Care* 2007;7(1):76–80.
10. Binder DS, DC; Lawton, MD. Spinal epidural hematoma. *Neurosurgery Quarterly* 2004;14(1):51–59.
11. Lawton MT, Porter RW, Heiserman JE, et al. Surgical management of spinal epidural hematoma: relationship between surgical timing and neurological outcome. *J Neurosurg* 1995;83(1):1–7.
12. Sklar EM, Post JM, Falcone S. MRI of acute spinal epidural hematoma. *J Comput Assist Tomogr* 1999;23(2):238–243.
13. Boukobza M, Guichard JP, Boissonet M, et al. Spinal epidural haematoma: report of 11 cases and review of the literature. *Neuroradiology* 1994;36(6):456–459.
14. Hentschel SJ, Woolfenden AR, Fairholm DJ. Resolution of spontaneous spinal epidural hematoma without surgery: report of two cases. *Spine* 2001;26(22):E525–E527.
15. Rathmell JP, Lake T, Ramundo MB. Infectious risks of chronic pain treatments: injection therapy, surgical implants, and intradiscal techniques. *Regional Anesth Pain Med* 2006;31(4):346–352.
16. de Jong PC, Kansen PJ. A comparison of epidural catheters with or without subcutaneous injection ports for treatment of cancer pain. *Anesth Analg* 1994;78(1):94–100.
17. Mercadante S. Problems of long-term spinal opioid treatment in advanced cancer patients. *Pain* 1999;79(1):1–13.
18. Follett KA, Boortz–Marx RL, Drake JM, et al. Prevention and management of intrathecal drug delivery and spinal cord stimulation system infections. *Anesthesiology* 2004;100(6):1582–1594.
19. Darouiche RO. Spinal epidural abscess. *N Engl J Med* 2006;355(19):2012–2020.
20. Curry WT Jr, Hoh BL, Amin–Hanjani S, et al. Spinal epidural abscess: clinical presentation, management, and outcome. *Surg Neurol* 2005;63(4):364–371; discussion 371.
21. Du Pen S. Complications of neuraxial infusion in cancer patients. *Oncology (Williston Park)* 1999;13(suppl 2):45–51.
22. Du Pen SL, Peterson DG, Williams A, et al. Infection during chronic epidural catheterization: diagnosis and treatment. *Anesthesiology* 1990;73(5):905–909.
23. Wade JS, Cobbs CG. Infections in cardiac pacemakers. *Curr Clin Top Infect Dis* 1988;9:44–61.
24. Lu CH, Chang WN, Lui CC, et al. Adult spinal epidural abscess: clinical features and prognostic factors. *Clin Neurol Neurosurg* 2002;104(4):306–310.
25. Groban L. Central nervous system and cardiac effects from long-acting amide local anesthetic toxicity in the intact animal model. *Reg Anesth Pain Med* 2003;28(1):3–11.
26. Butterworth JF IV, Strichartz GR. Molecular mechanisms of local anesthesia: a review. *Anesthesiology* 1990;72(4):711–734.
27. Hille B. Ionic channels in excitable membranes. Current problems and biophysical approaches. *Biophys J* 1978;22(2):283–294.
28. Kozody R, Ready LB, Barsa JE, et al. Dose requirement of local anaesthetic to produce grand mal seizure during stellate ganglion block. *Can Anaesth Soc J* 1982;29(5):489–491.
29. Mahajan G. Pain clinic emergencies. *Pain Medicine* 2008;9(suppl 1):S113–S120.
30. Sawyer RJ, von Schroeder H. Temporary bilateral blindness after acute lidocaine toxicity. *Anesth Analg* 2002;95(1):224–226.
31. Brown DL, Ransom DM, Hall JA, et al. Regional anesthesia and local anesthetic-induced systemic toxicity: seizure frequency and accompanying cardiovascular changes. *Anesth Analg* 1995;81(2):321–328.
32. de Jong RH, Ronfeld RA, DeRosa RA. Cardiovascular effects of convulsant and supraconvulsant doses of amide local anesthetics. *Anesth Analg* 1982;61(1):3–9.
33. Rosenblatt MA, Abel M, Fischer GW, et al. Successful use of a 20% lipid emulsion to resuscitate a patient after a presumed bupivacaine-related cardiac arrest. *Anesthesiology* 2006;105(1):217–218.
34. Warren JA, Thoma RB, Georgescu A, et al. Intravenous lipid infusion in the successful resuscitation of local anesthetic-induced cardiovascular collapse after supraclavicular brachial plexus block. *Anesth Analg* 2008;106(5):1578–1580.
35. Morgan P. The role of vasopressors in the management of hypotension induced by spinal and epidural anaesthesia. *Can J Anesth* 1994;41(5):404–413.
36. Borgeat A, Blumenthal S. Unintended destinations of local anesthetics. In: Neal JM, Rathmell JP, eds. *Complications in regional anesthesia & pain medicine.* Philadelphia: Saunders; 2007:157–163.
37. Tan MP, Parry SW. Vasovagal syncope in the older patient. *J Am Coll Cardiol* 2008;51(6):599–606.
38. Krediet CT, van Dijk N, Linzer M, et al. Management of vasovagal syncope: controlling or aborting faints by leg crossing and muscle tensing. *Circulation* 2002;106(13):1684–1689.
39. Meythaler JM, Roper JF, Brunner RC. Cyproheptadine for intrathecal baclofen withdrawal. *Arch Phys Med Rehabil* 2003;84(5):638–642.
40. Coffey RJ, Edgar TS, Francisco GE, et al. Abrupt withdrawal from intrathecal baclofen: Recognition and management of a potentially life-threatening syndrome. *Arch Phys Med Rehabil* 2002;83(6):735–741.
41. Green LB, Nelson VS. Death after acute withdrawal of intrathecal baclofen: case report and literature review. *Arch Phys Med Rehabil* 1999;80(12):1600–1604.
42. Duhon BS, Macdonald JD. Infusion of intrathecal baclofen for acute withdrawal. Technical note. *J Neurosurg* 2007;107(4):878–880.
43. Ackland GL, Fox R. Low-dose propofol infusion for controlling acute hyperspasticity after withdrawal of intrathecal baclofen therapy. *Anesthesiology* 2005;103(3):663–665.
44. Zuckerbraun NS, Ferson SS, Albright AL, et al. Intrathecal baclofen withdrawal: emergent recognition and management. *Pediatr Emerg Care* 2004;20(11):759–764.
45. Hsieh JC, Penn RD. Intrathecal baclofen in the treatment of adult spasticity. *Neurosurgical Focus* 2006;21(2):e5.

46. Gowing LR, Farrell M, Ali RL, et al. Alpha2-adrenergic agonists in opioid withdrawal. *Addiction* 2002;97(1):49–58.

47. Armstrong J, Little M, Murray L. Emergency department presentations of naltrexone-accelerated detoxification. *Acad Emerg Med* 2003;10(8):860–866.

48. Brown AF. Anaphylaxis gets the adrenaline going. *Emerg Med J* 2004;21(2):128–129.

49. Part 10.6: Anaphylaxis. *Circulation* 2005;112(suppl 24):IV,143–145.

50. Brown SG. Clinical features and severity grading of anaphylaxis. *J Allergy Clin Immunol* 2004;114(2):371–376.

51. Pumphrey R. Anaphylaxis: can we tell who is at risk of a fatal reaction? *Curr Opin Allergy Clin Immunol* 2004;4(4):285–290.

52. Brown SG, Blackman KE, Stenlake V, et al. Insect sting anaphylaxis: prospective evaluation of treatment with intravenous adrenaline and volume resuscitation. *Emerg Med J* 2004;21(2):149–154.

53. Cheshire WP, Santos CC, Massey EW, et al. Spinal cord infarction: etiology and outcome. *Neurology* 1996;47(2):321–330.

54. Baker R, Dreyfuss P, Mercer S, et al. Cervical transforaminal injection of corticosteroids into a radicular artery: a possible mechanism for spinal cord injury. *Pain* 2003;103(1–2):211–215.

55. Brouwers PJ, Kottink EJ, Simon MA, et al. A cervical anterior spinal artery syndrome after diagnostic blockade of the right C6-nerve root. *Pain* 2001;91(3):397–399.

56. Houten JK, Errico TJ. Paraplegia after lumbosacral nerve root block: report of three cases. *Spine J* 2002;2(1):70–75.

57. Somayaji HS, Saifuddin A, Casey AT, et al. Spinal cord infarction following therapeutic computed tomography-guided left L2 nerve root injection. *Spine* 2005;30(4):E106–E108.

58. Rathmell JP, Aprill C, Bogduk N. Cervical transforaminal injection of steroids. *Anesthesiology* 2004;100(6):1595–600.

59. Rozin L, Rozin R, Koehler SA, et al. Death during transforaminal epidural steroid nerve root block (C7) due to perforation of the left vertebral artery. *Am J Forensic Med Pathol* 2003;24(4):351–355.

60. Masson C, Pruvo JP, Meder JF, et al. Spinal cord infarction: clinical and magnetic resonance imaging findings and short term outcome. *J Neurol Neurosurg Psychiatry* 2004;75(10):1431–1435.

61. Cheshire WP Jr. Spinal cord infarction mimicking angina pectoris. *Mayo Clin Proc* 2000;75(11):1197–1199.

62. Weidauer S, Nichtweiss M, Lanfermann H, et al. Spinal cord infarction: MR imaging and clinical features in 16 cases. *Neuroradiology* 2002;44(10):851–857.

63. Adams HP Jr, del Zoppo G, Alberts MJ, et al. Guidelines for the early management of adults with ischemic stroke: a guideline from the American Heart Association/American Stroke Association Stroke Council, Clinical Cardiology Council, Cardiovascular Radiology and Intervention Council, and the Atherosclerotic Peripheral Vascular Disease and Quality of Care Outcomes in Research Interdisciplinary Working Groups: the American Academy of Neurology affirms the value of this guideline as an educational tool for neurologists. *Stroke* 2007;38(5):1655–1711.

64. Vale FL, Burns J, Jackson AB, et al. Combined medical and surgical treatment after acute spinal cord injury: results of a prospective pilot study to assess the merits of aggressive medical resuscitation and blood pressure management. *J Neurosurg* 1997;87(2):239–246.

65. Miller SM. Methylprednisolone in acute spinal cord injury: a tarnished standard. *J Neurosurg Anesthesiol* 2008;20(2):140–142.

66. Bracken MB, Shepard MJ, Holford TR, et al. Methylprednisolone or tirilazad mesylate administration after acute spinal cord injury: 1-year follow up. Results of the third National Acute Spinal Cord Injury randomized controlled trial. *J Neurosurg* 1998;89(5):699–706.

67. Rozet I. Methylprednisolone in acute spinal cord injury: is there any other ethical choice? *J Neurosurg Anesthesiol* 2008;20(2):137–139.

CHAPTER 111 ■ PAIN MANAGEMENT IN THE EMERGENCY DEPARTMENT

KNOX H. TODD AND JAMES R. MINER

INTRODUCTION

The specialties of both emergency medicine and pain medicine are relatively new members of the modern house of medicine. The first academic department of emergency medicine was established in 1971 and the American Board of Medical Specialties recognized emergency medicine as a distinct specialty by conferring primary board status only 20 years ago. The numbers of visits to U.S. emergency departments (EDs) have increased markedly over the past decade. From 1995 to 2005, annual ED visit volumes increased from 96.5 million to 115.3 million, a 20% increase. During this time, the total number of EDs actually decreased from 4176 to 3795, thus the annual volume for an average-sized ED increased by more than 30%.[1] More than 25,000 emergency physicians are represented by the American College of Emergency Physicians, our specialty's largest physician support organization.

EDs provide care for patients with an extraordinarily broad range of illnesses and injuries associated with both acute and chronic pain. It is commonly believed that injury and trauma are responsible for the majority of ED visits associated with pain; however, this impression is misleading. In a recent multicenter study of adults presenting to EDs in the United States and Canada with moderate to severe pain, two-thirds of presentations resulted from medical, rather than traumatic, conditions.[2] Major categories of discharge diagnoses reported in this study appear in Figure 111.1.

In the United States, the ED serves as a safety net for our fragmented health care system. Pain is but one of many conditions for which emergency physicians treat not only acute clinical presentations, but also care for those with chronic or recurrent painful conditions who are unable to access other parts of the health care system. Emergency physicians also frequently cause pain in the course of performing emergent diagnostic and therapeutic procedures.

This chapter discusses the prevalence of acute and chronic pain in the ED, its assessment, barriers to adequate pain treatment, the influence of substance abuse disorders and aberrant drug-related behaviors on ED pain practices, as well as a variety of commonly employed pain treatment and procedural sedation modalities. Space limits prohibit a discussion of the wide variety of specific painful conditions that present to the ED.

THE PREVALENCE OF PAIN IN THE EMERGENCY DEPARTMENT

Pain is the most frequent reason for seeking ED treatment, and as a presenting complaint, pain accounts for over 70% of visits to U.S. EDs.[3–5] Several single-site ED studies have attempted to define the prevalence of pain more precisely. Over a single week, Johnston et al.[3] conducted a prospective study to determine the incidence and severity of pain among patients presenting to non-

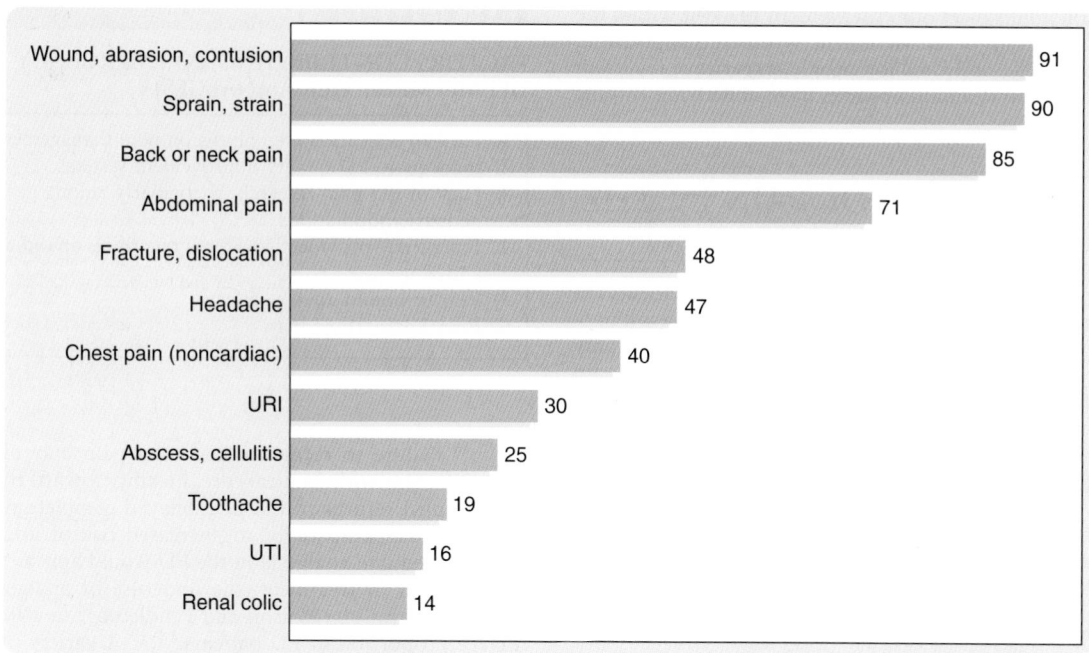

FIGURE 111.1 Major categories of discharge diagnoses among patients presenting to the ED with moderate to severe pain. Note: Other diagnoses present for 243 patients. (Redrawn after Todd KH, Ducharme J, Choiniere M, et al. Pain in the emergency department: results of the Pain and Emergency Medicine Initiative [PEMI] Multicenter Study. *J Pain* 2007;8[6]:460–466.)

critical treatment areas within the EDs of two urban hospitals in Canada. Fifty-eight percent of adults and forty-seven percent of children reported pain on ED arrival. For approximately one-half of both groups reporting pain, the intensity of this pain was considered moderate to severe. At the time of discharge, one-third of both groups continued to experience pain of moderate to severe intensity. In fact, 11% of children and adults in this study actually reported clinically important increases in pain intensity during the ED stay.

A second prospective study, conducted by Tanabe and Buschmann,[4] found that among adults treated at one Chicago ED, 78% presented with a chief complaint related to pain. Of these patients, only 47% received analgesics. For patients receiving analgesics, an average of 74 minutes elapsed from the time of arrival to the time of treatment. Only 15% of patients were treated with opioids, despite high levels of pain intensity. Interestingly, 16% of patients with pain in this study indicated that they would have refused analgesics had they been offered. The principal reported reason for their refusal was the fear of addiction resulting from opioid exposure, even when opioids were indicated for the treatment of pain.

In 2002, Cordell et al.[5] reported an analysis of secondary data from an urban, tertiary-care ED using explicit data abstraction rules to determine the prevalence of pain and to assign painful conditions into standard categories. With inclusion of all age groups, they found evidence of pain in 61% of patients. Pain was the chief complaint for 52% of patient visits. After excluding patients less than 5 years of age for whom chart reviews are obviously less reliable, almost 70% of patient encounters involved pain complaints.

While the high prevalence of pain among ED patients is well-documented, the underlying conditions responsible for pain in this population are less well characterized. In Cordell's[5] retrospective study, 11% of patients presenting to the ED were judged to be suffering from pain that was chronic in nature. In a recent prospective multicenter study conducted in the United States and Canada, 44% of ultimately discharged patients presenting to the ED with pain reported underlying chronic pain syndromes.[2] In

one-half of these cases, the ED visit was prompted by an exacerbation of this chronic pain condition. Importantly, patients with chronic pain reported three to four times the number of annual physician visits when compared to those without chronic pain. Median and mean durations of symptoms for those reporting chronic pain syndromes were 24 and 52 months, respectively. For physicians who view themselves as experts in the management of acute medical and surgical emergencies, chronic pain may represent a less familiar condition with which to contend.

EDs frequently treat patients with chronic or recurrent pain who are often frustrated by a lack of information about ongoing pain management and poor access to specialty-level care. In 2007, we used random digit dial survey methods to interview 500 U.S. adults with chronic or recurrent pain and an ED visit within the past 2 years.[6] Sixty percent were female, their median age was 54, two-thirds were under the care of a physician, and only 14% were uninsured. They reported an average of 4.2 ED visits within the past 2 years. Relatively large proportions reported pain relief during the ED visit and 57% endorsed that "the ED staff understood how to treat my pain" as "definitely true." Although over three-fourths of patients felt receiving that additional information on pain management (82%) or referrals to specialists (74%) was "extremely" or "very" important, only one-half reported receiving such referrals (46%) or information (55%). A significant minority (11%) reported that the "ED staff made me feel like I was just seeking drugs." The majority (55%) were "very" or "completely" satisfied with their medical treatment, while 24% were "neutral" to "completely" dissatisfied. In multivariate models, greater age, male gender, higher level of education, shorter waiting time, use of imaging, and pain relief contributed to patient satisfaction with ED care.

Findings from this survey provide a more precise estimate of the prevalence of ED use associated with chronic and recurrent pain in the United States. The final survey incidence rate of adults reporting a recent ED visit for chronic or recurrent pain was 15% of all those reached by phone. Given the U.S. adult population of approximately 225 million, this survey incidence rate suggests that 34 million adults meet our criteria of an ED visit within the past 2 years for chronic or recurrent pain. Within this population, approximately 43%, or 15 million people, experience recurrent pain, while 57%, or 19 million people, have underlying chronic pain syndromes.[6]

THE ASSESSMENT OF PAIN IN THE EMERGENCY DEPARTMENT

Pain is inherently subjective and inevitably complex. Patients experience pain and suffering as individuals; clinicians assess it only indirectly. The emergency provider's task is to use a commonly understood vocabulary and classification system in assessing pain so that our findings can be communicated consistently. Only by quantifying the pain experience in meaningful ways can we move beyond practices that are influenced by myth and opinion toward a scientific approach to our many questions regarding the pain experience. This challenge is at the root of our difficulties in treating pain and not only in the ED setting, thus issues surrounding pain assessment should have primacy in our attempts to understand our patients' pain experiences.

EDs employ a number of practical unidimensional pain assessment tools. Viewing pain as the "fifth vital sign," as encouraged by The Joint Commission on Accreditation of Health Care Organizations, has fostered the widespread use of such tools. For those without cognitive impairment, pain intensity is routinely assessed with either an 11-point numerical rating scale (NRS) or a graphical rating scale (GRS). The NRS is sensitive to the short-term changes in pain intensity associated with emergency care and is the most commonly employed pain assessment instrument.[7,8] GRS or picture scales are particularly useful for populations with limited literacy, including children.[9,10] The visual analog scale (VAS) is used by some EDs; however, this instrument is more commonly employed in research settings. There is no demonstrated advantage in using a VAS over a NRS in the ED setting; both are reliable and valid measures of pain intensity.[11] In fact, certain patient populations find the NRS easier to complete; therefore, it is preferred over the VAS for routine use.[7,12]

Among nonverbal patients, including infants or those with cognitive impairment and dementia, a number of observational pain scales are available for use. Both the Face, Legs, Activity, Cry, and Consolability observational scale for use in very young children, and the Pain Assessment in Advanced Dementia scale for use in the setting of advanced dementia are used with some frequency in the ED; however, adequate observational pain assessments are less the exception than the rule.[13,14]

No matter the specific pain scale used, assessments should be repeated after therapeutic interventions and at the time of ED discharge. One multicenter study found that relatively few ED patients are reassessed after an initial pain score, reporting that fewer than one-third of ED patients presenting with moderate to severe pain had repeat pain assessments while in the ED.[2] Despite efforts to promote pain intensity as an outcome measure with which to judge the quality of ED pain practice, the finding that pain intensity is measured only once in most EDs may mirrors medicine's traditional view of pain as a diagnostic indicator rather than an outcome deserving of attention in its own right.

OLIGOANALGESIA IN THE EMERGENCY DEPARTMENT

Notwithstanding the clinician's duty to provide compassionate care, pain that is not acknowledged and managed appropriately causes anxiety, depression, sleep disturbances, increased oxygen demands with the potential for end-organ ischemia, and decreased movement with an increased risk of venous thrombo-

TABLE 111.1

FACTORS CONTRIBUTING TO EMERGENCY DEPARTMENT OLIGOANALGESIA

1. Lack of educational emphasis on pain management
2. Inadequate ED quality improvement systems
3. Lack of ED pain research, particularly among geriatric and pediatric populations
4. Emergency providers' concerns regarding opioid addiction and abuse
5. Fear of opioid adverse effects
6. Racial and ethnic bias

sis.[15,16] Failure to recognize and treat pain may also result in dissatisfaction with medical care, hostility toward the physician, unscheduled returns to the ED, delayed complete return to full function, and, potentially, an increased risk of litigation.[17] Although adequate analgesia in the ED would appear to be an important goal of treatment, the underuse of analgesics, termed "oligoanalgesia" by Wilson and Pendleton[18] in 1989, occurs in a large proportion of ED patients.[18-23] A variety of factors are felt to give rise to pain undertreatment and these are listed in Table 111.1.

Emergency medicine investigators have identified a number of risk factors for oligoanalgesia in this setting. As in other settings, the very young or old tend to receive less intensive treatment for pain in ED.[24-26] Studies have documented oligoanalgesia and delays to analgesic administration among those of minority ethnicity for a variety of painful conditions, even when objective evidence for the presence of pain is obvious (e.g., long-bone fractures).[27-30] Although patients' expectations for pain treatment and perceptions of pain intensity do not differ by ethnic groups, when patients are matched for socioeconomic factors, differences have been noted in the manner in which patients of different cultural backgrounds express their pain.[31-33] Differences in the interactions of physicians and patients of different ethnic groups have been described, and subtle differences within these interactions may affect the physician's pain assessment.[34,35] When affect, actual patient-physician interaction, and cultural expressions of ethnicity are removed from a case presentation, such as through written clinical vignettes, patients with similar pain tend to be similarly treated by physicians.[36] Cultural discordance between the patient and the physician may hinder the ability of patients to confer an understanding of their pain to the physician.

Of course, any treatment of pain is dependent on the physician's accurate assessment of the patient's pain. In fact, the only predictor of treatment that Bartfield and colleagues[37] found for ED patients with back pain was the physician's assessment, regardless of the patients' ethnicity, age, or insurance status. Disparities in the treatment of pain are more likely to result from variations in physicians' assessment of pain intensity than variations in treatment among patients judged to have similar degrees of pain.

Although emergency physicians may be reluctant to accept patient report as the most reliable indicator of pain, and disparities between patient's and physician's pain intensity ratings may lead to inadequately treated pain, even patients themselves may be reluctant to report the presence of pain and its intensity. This may be due to low expectations of obtaining pain relief, fear of analgesic side effects, and perhaps the notion that pain is to be expected as part of an underlying disease or from medical treatments. Some patients exhibit an inappropriate fear of addiction when prescribed opioids or fear the stigma associated with opioid use, even in the short term.

PAIN AND OPIOID ABUSE IN THE EMERGENCY DEPARTMENT

ED personnel commonly identify patients who they feel are attempting to obtain opioids for illegitimate purposes. Although drug addiction occurs in all patient populations, it is likely that the ED sees a higher proportion of such patients than a typical office-based practice. Unfortunately, the true prevalence of addiction and aberrant drug seeking behaviors in the ED is unknown and difficult to measure. When the prevalence of such problems is overestimated, oligoanalgesia is the predictable result.

DEFINITIONS

In discussing issues of chemical dependency and aberrant behaviors related to opioid use, a valid system of nomenclature is necessary for clear communication and measurement. Historically, the meaning of different terms has changed, particularly in light of the increased use of chronic opioid therapy for malignant and nonmalignant chronic pain conditions. In treating pain in this population of patients with chronic opioids, confusion over the concepts of physical dependence, tolerance, addiction, and pseudoaddiction may constitute a barrier to understanding and to appropriate treatment. These phenomena are discrete, and standard definitions may be helpful in caring for such patients. Currently accepted definitions of these terms are as follows[38]: *Addiction* is a primary, chronic, neurobiologic disease with genetic, psychosocial, and environmental factors influencing its development and manifestations. It is characterized by behaviors that include one or more of the following: impaired control over drug use, compulsive use, continued use despite harm, and craving. *Physical dependence* is a state of adaptation that often includes tolerance and is manifested by a drug class-specific withdrawal syndrome that can be produced by abrupt cessation, rapid dose reduction, decreasing blood level of the drug, and/or administration of an antagonist. *Tolerance* is a state of adaptation in which exposure to a drug induces changes that result in a diminution of one or more of the drug's effects over time. *Pseudoaddiction* is a term which has been used to describe patient behaviors that may occur when pain is undertreated. Patients with unrelieved pain may become focused on obtaining medications, may "clock watch," and may otherwise seem inappropriately "drug seeking." Even such behaviors as illicit drug use and deception can occur in the patient's efforts to obtain relief. Pseudoaddiction can be distinguished from true addiction in that the behaviors resolve when pain is effectively treated.

The term, "substance abuse" is particularly problematic and resistant to precise definition. The American Psychiatric Association has defined substance abuse as a maladaptive pattern of drug use associated with some manifest harm to the user or others.[39] Other groups using consensus methodology have defined abuse as any use considered to be outside of socially accepted norms.[40] Determining the bounds of "socially accepted norms" within the broad range of social strata treated within any ED is a difficult task. Physicians may believe that they "know abuse when they see it," and its identification may be influenced by subjective judgments that may or may not correspond to socially accepted norms for the index patient's particular social group. Often the term, "substance misuse" is applied to behaviors that are not perceived as particularly extreme (e.g., taking opioid analgesics to relieve symptoms other than pain such as anxiety or boredom).

The difficulty in determining whether a given set of behaviors fall within accepted definitions of substance use, misuse, or abuse has important implications outside the clinical realm. Physicians may prescribe controlled substances for the treatment of pain while patients may use these drugs to treat a broad range of symptoms with varying degrees of relatedness to underlying pain syndromes and may, in fact, use drugs in a manner totally unrelated to the physicians' intent (i.e., to obtain euphoric, rather than analgesic, effects). Given the unclear distinctions between use, misuse, and abuse, and a regulatory climate in which practitioners prescribing patterns are increasingly scrutinized, emergency physicians are understandably reluctant to prescribe controlled substances to patients with whom they expect to have only a transitory relationship.

Using any definition, substance abuse is a highly prevalent problem. The National Survey on Drug Use and Health (formerly the National Household Survey on Drug Abuse) reports that in 2003, an estimated 19.5 million Americans, or 8.2%, of the population aged 12 or older, used an illicit drug during the month prior to the survey interview. Illicit drugs included marijuana, cocaine, heroin, hallucinogens, inhalants, and nonmedical use of prescription-type pain relievers, tranquilizers, stimulants, and sedatives.[41] Importantly, the survey documents an increase in the lifetime reported nonmedical use of pain relievers between 2002 and 2003, from 29.6 million to 31.2 million persons. To be considered nonmedical use, the respondent had to take drugs not prescribed for them or take them only for the "experience or feeling" they caused. Specific analgesics showing statistically significant increases in lifetime use were (in order by magnitude): Vicodin, Lortab, or Lorcet (combination analgesics containing hydrocodone); Percocet, Percodan, or Tylox (combination analgesics containing oxycodone); hydrocodone; OxyContin (extended-release oxycodone); methadone; and tramadol.

In contrast to the prominence of ED-based data collection systems in efforts to monitor deleterious outcomes associated with substance abuse, relatively few studies have systematically assessed substance abuse prevalence and treatment needs in the ED population. As an example, the Drug Abuse Warning Network is a federally financed, public health surveillance system that monitors drug-related ED visits and drug-related deaths investigated by medical examiners and coroners. This reporting system involves hundreds of hospital EDs throughout the United States and provides valuable data with which to monitor drug abuse trends. In contrast to this large monitoring research enterprise, relatively little focus has been given to use of the ED as a setting in which to intervene in substance abuse problems.

In 1997, Soderstrom et al.[42] assessed the prevalence of psychoactive substance use disorders in a large, unselected group of seriously injured patients treated in one Baltimore ED, using standardized diagnostic interviews and explicit criteria. Psychoactive substance use disorders were diagnosed using the Structured Clinical Interview, an instrument based on the Diagnostic and Statistical Manual of Mental Disorders.[43] Of 1118 patients consenting to the study, more than half had one or more lifetime abuse or dependence psychoactive substance use disorders, and 18% were currently considered dependent on drugs other than alcohol.

In 1996, Rockett et al.[44] used direct interviews to ascertain unmet substance abuse treatment needs in a statewide probability sample survey of adults presenting to seven Tennessee EDs. While only 1% of ED medical records indicated a diagnosis of alcohol or drug-related problems, as many as 27% of patients were determined by the researchers to need substance abuse treatment on the basis of explicitly defined case definitions. Less than 10% of patients that were ultimately determined to need substance abuse treatment in this study were actually receiving such care. Thirty-two percent of all patients in this study had a positive saliva or urine assay for psychoactive drugs and 9% screened positive for opioid use. Unmet substance abuse treatment needs varied directly with the frequency of ED visits and inversely with patient age.

A subsequent study by Rockett et al.[45] examined the association between unmet substance abuse treatment needs in the ED and excess utilization of health services in order to estimate the health care costs savings that might result from effective ED-based substance abuse treatment interventions. The researchers estimated that patients with unmet substance abuse treatment needs accounted for an estimated 777 million dollars in extra hospital charges for Tennessee, or 1568 dollars per ED patient when compared to those without substance abuse treatment needs. They suggested that the costs of ED-based screening and intervention efforts targeted to substance abuse disorders would be more than offset by savings from decreased health care utilization and that these programs were likely to be highly cost-effective if implemented.

PAIN AND "DRUG-SEEKING BEHAVIOR" IN THE EMERGENCY DEPARTMENT

The preceding discussion makes clear the high prevalence of both pain and substance abuse disorders in the ED. Although acute and chronic pain is far more common than substance abuse disorders, it is inevitable that emergency physicians will frequently encounter patients presenting with both pain and substance abuse disorders. Professional discussions of pain treatment in the ED frequently center on concerns of being duped by such patients who fabricate painful symptoms in order to obtain opioids, so-called "drug-seeking behavior."[46] Drug-seeking behaviors may represent an entirely appropriate response by those with chronic pains who are routinely undertreated by the medical profession and for whom comprehensive pain treatment centers are in short supply. Although the term drug seeking behavior is poorly defined, it is used in the emergency medicine literature and will be used with acknowledgement of its imprecision.

Only a limited amount of emergency medicine research has addressed this problematic issue. In 1990, Zechnich and Hedges[47] attempted to measure community-wide use of ED services by patients at high risk for drug seeking behavior. In this retrospective, observational study, patients were categorized as exhibiting drug seeking behavior if they sought care at a university hospital in Portland, Oregon, for a specific pain-related diagnosis (i.e., ureteral colic, toothache, back pain, abdominal pain, or headache) and were either independently identified on at least one other local hospital's "patient alert" list or suffered a drug-related death during the year in question. After identifying 33 such patients, they determined the frequency of their ED visits at each of seven local hospitals and conducted detailed chart reviews of their visits at three of these hospitals. The patients identified as drug seeking were generally young and one-half of drug seekers were female. The latter is a surprising finding given that substance abuse disorders are more than twice as common among males.[41] This suggests that drug seeking behaviors are exhibited (or identified) more commonly among female ED patients with substance abuse problems than among males. The 33 patients visited EDs, urgent care clinics, or were hospitalized a total of 379 times over the study period, for an average of 12.6 visits per person annually. Interestingly, although chart reviews identified 17 patients who were told that he or she "would receive no further narcotics" at a given facility, these patients subsequently received controlled substances from another hospital in 93% of cases and from even the same facility in 71%. The authors suggested that information sharing between hospitals could help to identify drug seeking patients and promote more consistent community-wide care and appropriate substance abuse interventions.

The maintenance of lists that include the names and medical information for patients frequently seen in the ED is thought to be a common practice. In a mail survey conducted in 1995, Graber et al.[48] described the use of what were referred to as "problem patient files" in the state of Iowa. Fifty-eight percent of ED medical directors acknowledged the use of such files and responded that the files were consulted an average of 2.6 times per week. Calls between EDs either seeking or responding to requests for information about patients listed in these files were estimated to occur 23 and 20 times per year respectively. Rarely were explicit policies established for limiting access to these files and information was added to the records in an informal fashion.[48]

In 2000, Pope et al.[49] from Vancouver described a case management program for frequent visitors to their inner-city tertiary care ED serving a large number of patients with multiple psychosocial problems, including substance abuse. Of 24 patients described in this study, 5 were said to exhibit drug seeking behavior, and 8 patients suffered from alcohol and drug abuse, personality disorders, and chronic pain. These 24 patients accounted for a staggering 616 visits annually (median 26.5 visits per year). After the implementation of individualized chronic care plans that included social work interventions at the time of the visits, ED use by this group of super-utilizers dropped to a median of 6.5 visits per person per year. In 2003, a publication by Geiderman discussed ethical, legal, and regulatory considerations surrounding the use of what were termed "habitual patient files."[50] The article acknowledged the common and informal use of such files, and set forth standards intended to promote the development of formal policies and procedures to govern their use. The author noted that such files have never been demonstrated to be effective in either reducing ED use by drug seeking patients or in altering care patterns and suggested the need for a research program to explore the impact of their use. Finally, the author called for a coordinated and comprehensive program of physician education to promote the identification and treatment of ED patients with substance abuse disorders.

PAIN AND SUBSTANCE ABUSE IN THE EMERGENCY DEPARTMENT: A BALANCED PERSPECTIVE

In managing pain, emergency physicians are responsible for beneficence as well as nonmaleficence. We must treat pain and ameliorate suffering while minimizing the extent to which our treatment strategies enable substance abuse by our patients. For the vast majority of patients presenting with a first episode of acute pain, whether from trauma, acute medical illness, or procedures performed in the ED, there is little danger of enabling substance abuse and a great deal of room for improvement in the quality of analgesic practices. For a small subset of ED patients, particularly for those presenting with chronic or recurrent pain syndromes, the physician may have legitimate concerns regarding an underlying substance abuse or related disorder. Our task is to balance the often unclear risk of fostering substance abuse, and even diversion, in this subset of patients with the well-known and well-documented risk of under treating painful conditions.

Certainly, the presence of an obvious painful condition (e.g., appendicitis, fracture) should preempt concerns about illegitimate drug-seeking behaviors. Given the high prevalence of chronic pain and the widespread unavailability of chronic pain management resources, particularly for populations served by the ED, pseudoaddiction is the most likely cause for a large proportion of drug-related behaviors deemed aberrant. In particular, patient reports of distress associated with unrelieved symptoms, aggressive complaining about the need for higher doses of analgesics, and unilateral dose escalation by the patient are suggestive of pseudoaddiction. Establishing the diagnosis of pseudoaddiction is particularly difficult if the patient has both pain and a comorbid substance use disorder; however, the two can coexist. The signature of pseudoaddiction is that aberrant behaviors disappear when adequate analgesics are given to control pain.

In dealing with complex chronic pain patients, the emergency physician practicing in isolation may exhibit symptoms of despair and direct his or her anger toward the patient with pain, resulting in more alienation of patients who may have already been abandoned by other sectors of the health care system. This is particularly likely to happen in communities without multidisciplinary treatment centers for either substance abuse disorders or chronic pain and for those with inadequate health care insurance. Thus the patient with chronic pain joins the larger group of those with unmet health care needs that currently crowd our EDs. The hectic nature of emergency medicine practice often does not allow sufficient time for precisely characterizing patients with complex pain complaints and clinicians may lump legitimate pain behaviors with the ploys of those seeking opioids inappropriately. Both groups of patients may be ultimately mistrusted and treated with disdain.

Aside from considerations of pseudoaddiction, chronic pain is often accompanied by mood disorders and psychiatric comorbidities that complicate the management of these challenging patients.[15] The presence of aberrant drug-related behaviors in patients with borderline personality disorders may represent an expression of fear and anger or an attempt to cope with chronic boredom. Patients may use opioids and alcohol in attempts to lessen symptoms of anxiety, panic disorder, depression, or insomnia. Emergency physicians often receive limited training in dealing with such disorders and the specialty's deficiencies in dealing with such problems have been documented.[51] Psychiatric consultation, if available, may be useful in both suggesting alternative causes for aberrant behaviors and tailoring the physician's therapeutic approach to deal with these complicating factors.

For some patients, aberrant drug-related behaviors represent criminal intent to divert or sell controlled substances. The prevalence of behaviors occasioned by such intent is unknown and it is likely that in many cases, multiple etiologies of aberrant behaviors coexist. Certainly, patients with active or past substance use disorders are at increased risk for injuries and illnesses that can lead to chronic pain (e.g., motor vehicle injury).

Finally, although federal regulators and state medical boards do not perceive emergency medicine as a specialty prone to inappropriate prescribing, and investigations of emergency physicians are rare, if not unheard of, many emergency physicians express fears of such scrutiny or sanctions related to prescribing or administering opioids. While this concern is often voiced, it seems likely that this fear represents concern about other, less obvious physician uncertainties related to pain management and substance abuse disorders. Emergency physicians may be concerned about being overburdened by the inherent difficulties of managing patients with complicated pain syndromes and the potential of coexisting substance abuse disorders.

THE EXAMPLE OF SICKLE CELL DISEASE

The condition that best exemplifies the problem of ED-based pseudoaddiction is sickle cell disease. Vaso-occlusive pain crises are the most common reason for ED visits by patients with sickle cell disease and the genetics, molecular biology, and pathophysiology of this disease are relatively well understood. Although the management of sickle cell vaso-occlusive pain crises is viewed as challenging by emergency physicians, it has been a relatively neglected area of research investigation by the specialty.[52] Despite the fact that almost all of the 75,000 annual hospitalizations for pain crises occur after ED treatment, the *Annals of Emergency Medicine*, emergency medicine's premier research journal, has published no clinical research on sickle cell pain management within the past 10 years.

Despite our understanding of the sickle cell disease process, many health professionals are reluctant to prescribe adequate doses of opioids for these patients experiencing pain largely due to addiction concerns.[53] In one survey study, 53% of emergency physicians were of the belief that more than 20% of patients with sickle cell disease were addicted to opioids, while only 23% of hematologists shared this belief.[54] Also, in this survey, 35% of hematologists reported that they followed pain management protocols when treating painful crises as compared to only 17% of emergency physicians.

Nurses' attitudes regarding the prevalence of addiction among this patient population are even more extreme, with 63 respondents reporting that addiction was prevalent.[55] Thirty percent of nurses in this survey reported that they were hesitant to administer high-dose opioids for painful vaso-occlusive crises. A hesitant approach to ED opioid administration in the setting of vaso-occlusive pain crises will predictably lead to continued pain, increased anticipation of pain, and increased patient anxiety. This experience may generate pain-avoidance manifestations by patients that are interpreted by physicians as aberrant drug-related behaviors. Eventually, larger doses of opioids may be administered to control pain that is spiraling out of control with resultant excessive sedation. This apparent sedation in the setting of a painful condition may reinforce the physician's disbelief in the reality of his or her patient's initial pain reports.

It has been demonstrated that this cycle of inadequate care can be broken by the institution of pain management protocols that emphasize continuous opioid infusions and sustained courses of orally administered controlled-release opioids. In 1992, Brookoff and Polomano[56] reported the institution of such a structured analgesic regimen on hospital use by patients with sickle cell disease presenting to the ED of an inner-city university hospital in Philadelphia with remarkable results. After institution of the pain management protocol, the number of hospital admissions for sickle cell pain decreased by 44%, the number of total inpatient days by 57%, the hospital length of stay by 23%, and the number of ED visits by 67%. The authors asserted that these positive results were seen without a subset of patients being "chased away" from the hospital. Others have reported marked decreases in aberrant drug-related behaviors and the number of ED visits by patients with sickle cell disease after instituting long-term management of pain with chronic opioid therapies typically used to treat malignant pain.[57]

PAIN TREATMENT AND PROCEDURAL SEDATION IN THE EMERGENCY DEPARTMENT

Effective pain management involves both pharmacologic and nonpharmacologic modalities. Simply asking about pain and validating the pain reports impacts patients' satisfaction with ED pain management. In one study, patient satisfaction with pain management was predicted more strongly by the perception that ED staff asked about pain than by the actual administration of an analgesic.[58] Other nonpharmacologic modalities, such as reassuring the patient that pain will be addressed, immobilizing and elevating injured extremities, and providing quiet, darkened rooms for patients with migraine headaches are important aspects of quality pain management. Pharmacologic therapies should begin as soon as is practical after presentation to the ED. Analgesic protocols allowing early pain treatment can decrease the time to effective treatment and improve patient outcomes.[59–61]

Analgesics may be administered by a variety of routes; however, the vast majority of medications are administered by the oral or parenteral routes. Oral therapies are most commonly employed as they are convenient and inexpensive for patients who can tolerate oral intake. When pain is severe, analgesics must be given immediately and titrated to effect, generally by parenteral routes. The intravenous, rather than intramuscular, route is indicated in this context. Intramuscular injections are painful, do not allow for rapid titration, exhibit unpredictable absorption, and result in a slower onset of drug action. Unless intravenous access is elusive, there is little to recommend the intramuscular route. In general, it is inappropriate to delay analgesic use until a diagnosis has been made. In the case of acute abdominal pain, for which surgical dogma historically discouraged adequate analgesia, a large series of studies report no deleterious effect of intravenous opioid therapy on our ability to make appropriate diagnoses.[62–68]

SPECIFIC TREATMENT MODALITIES

Analgesics are the most commonly administered class of drug in the ED. The National Center for Health Statistics reports that analgesics account for the top three therapeutic classes of drugs used in the ED (Fig. 111.2).[1] In a recent 20 site survey of ED analgesic practice, a total of 735 doses of 24 different analgesics were administered to 506 patients receiving analgesics while in the ED. Analgesics administered to this cohort of ED patients are listed by prevalence in Table 111.2.[2] The majority of analgesics administered were opioids (59%); morphine being the most commonly used analgesic (20%), followed by ibuprofen (17%).

Nonopioids

Commonly used ED analgesics include opioids, acetaminophen, and nonsteroidal anti-inflammatory drugs (NSAIDs). When opioids are required for pain treatment, nonopioids should be included in order to potentiate the opioid analgesic effect and decrease the severity of side effects. Unfortunately, nonopioid agents exhibit an analgesic ceiling effect and cannot be titrated to effect. This limits their usefulness in the setting of severe or fluctuating pain; however, they should be used as an adjunct to opioid therapies unless otherwise contraindicated.

Acetaminophen is indicated for mild to moderate pain, and is often combined with opioid agents. Acetaminophen, unlike NSAIDs, has no antiplatelet activity or anti-inflammatory effect. Although a great deal of attention has been paid to acetaminophen hepatotoxicity, especially in the setting of chronic malnutrition, alcoholism, or liver disease, such effects are uncommon, particularly when contrasted to the underappreciated high prevalence of NSAID-related adverse effects.

NSAIDs, including salicylates, act to inhibit prostaglandin synthesis by interfering with cyclooxygenase enzymes. They cause platelet dysfunction and can precipitate renal failure in patients with renal insufficiency or volume depletion, a particular concern in the elderly or those presenting to the ED with hemodynamic instability. Ketorolac, the only parenteral available in the United States, is commonly used in the ED and is felt to be particularly

TABLE 111.2

ANALGESICS ADMINISTERED IN THE EMERGENCY DEPARTMENT (735 DOSES GIVEN TO 506 PATIENTS)

Analgesic	N (%)
Morphine	148 (20.1)
Ibuprofen	127 (17.3)
Hydrocodone/acetaminophen	93 (12.7)
Oxycodone/acetaminophen	83 (11.3)
Ketorolac	60 (8.2)
Acetaminophen	53 (7.2)
Hydromorphone	36 (4.9)
Antacid	26 (3.5)
Meperidine	24 (3.3)
Fentanyl	23 (3.1)
Metoclopramide	13 (1.8)
Codeine/acetaminophen	12 (1.6)
Oxycodone	10 (1.4)
Naproxen	9 (1.2)
Other	18 (2.4)
Total	735 (100)

From Todd KH, Ducharme J, Choiniere M, et al. Pain in the emergency department: results of the Pain and Emergency Medicine Initiative (PEMI) Multicenter Study. *J Pain* 2007;8(6):460–466.

useful in the setting of renal colic. One recent study of renal colic in the ED found that a combination or ketorolac and morphine resulted in superior analgesia and reduced adverse effects when compared to the use of either agent alone.[69]

Opioids

Opioid combination analgesics are commonly used for moderate to severe pain. Although the opioid component in these agents does not exhibit ceiling analgesic effects, the nonopioid component dose must be limited; thus, one cannot titrate these analgesics. The convenience of combination therapy must be balanced

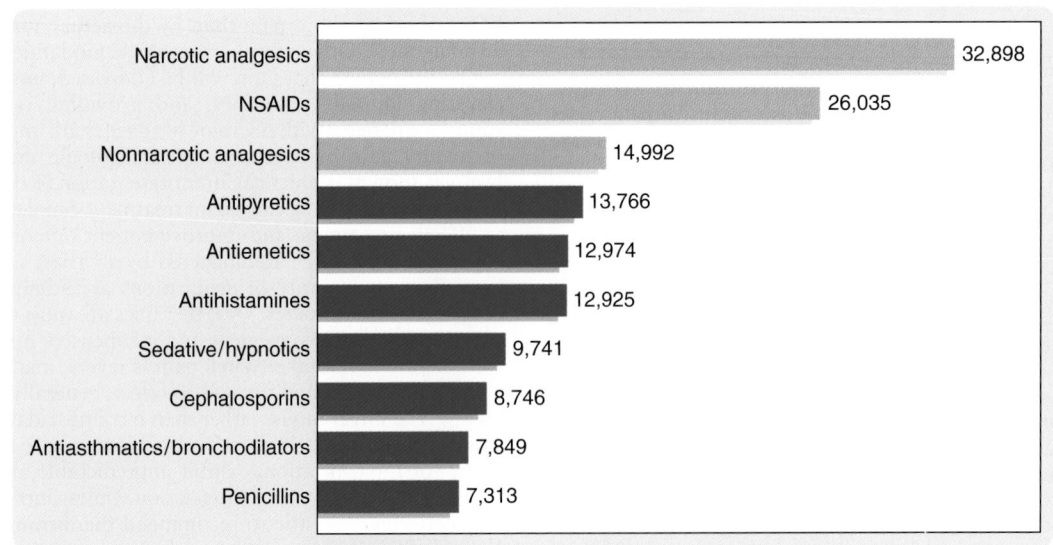

FIGURE 111.2 Top 10 therapeutic drug classes mentioned at emergency department visits. Note: Based on data for 204,851,000 drug mentions in 2005. (Redrawn after Nawar EW, Niska RW, Xu J. National Hospital Ambulatory Medical Care Survey: 2005 Emergency Department Summary. Advance data from vital and health statistics; no. 386. Hyattsville, MD: National Center for Health Statistics; 2007.)

against this limitation. Hydrocodone and oxycodone combination agents are associated with less nausea and vomiting and are preferable to codeine combinations agents. Also, significant proportions of the population are poor metabolizers of codeine, which must be metabolized to morphine in order to manifest analgesic effects, further limiting its effectiveness.

The tramadol/acetaminophen combination agent is indicated for acute pain; however, experience with this agent in the ED setting is limited. In one recent trial of acute ankle sprains presenting to the ED, the tramadol/acetaminophen combination agent had comparable clinical utility to that of hydrocodone with acetaminophen.[70] Tramadol's mechanism of action is unclear: it binds only weakly to opioid receptors and inhibits the reuptake of both norepinephrine and serotonin.

Opioids are the mainstay of ED therapy for moderate to severe pain, and morphine is the standard of comparison for all agents of this class. If contraindicated due to allergy or other sensitivity, hydromorphone or fentanyl may be substituted. These opioids can be rapidly titrated intravenously to control severe pain, allowing early institution of an oral regimen. Fentanyl has the advantage of being relatively short-acting and is preferred in the setting of multiple trauma, head injury, and potential hemodynamic instability. Intravenous morphine is the standard of treatment for severe pain in the ED. Morphine 0.1 mg/kg bolus has been found to be safe but not usually adequate to effect pain relief.[71] Repeat boluses of 0.05 mg/kg every 5 minutes until pain relief represents a safe incremental strategy.

Meperidine is a problematic opioid for a number of reasons. Many EDs have eliminated meperidine completely because of its metabolism to normeperidine, a toxic metabolite causing central excitation and seizures, as well as its contraindication in patients taking monoamine oxidase inhibitors.[72] Historically, subtherapeutic doses of intramuscularly administered meperidine have been used to treat a wide variety of acute pain complaints by generations of physicians. The availability of other opioid agents of equal efficacy with fewer contraindications and less adverse effects argues against its routine use.

Agonist-antagonist opioids, such as nalbuphine and butorphanol, have mixed effects on opioid receptor subtypes, exhibiting ceiling effects on both analgesia and respiratory depression. Because clinically important respiratory depression is distinctly rare in the setting of acute pain treatment, it is difficult to justify their routine use. One possible exception is for patients with advanced pulmonary disease. A particular drawback is that one cannot titrate these drugs to maximal effect because of analgesic ceiling effects. Additionally, these drugs are contraindicated and will induce withdrawal symptoms in patients who are physically dependent on opioids, either because of opioid therapy for chronic pain, methadone maintenance therapy, or active opioid addiction.

Patient-Controlled Analgesia

The use of patient-controlled analgesia (PCA) has been described in emergency medicine for both adults and children.[73,74] While no specific advantage has been found over the titration of opioids, PCA is at least as effective in relieving pain. In the setting of high demands on nursing resources, PCA could serve to ensure that patients' pain treatment needs are addressed in a timely fashion. In addition, patients admitted from the ED to inpatient hospital beds often experience a "pain window" between the last dose of an analgesic in the ED and the first dose administered on the hospital ward. Wider use of ED PCA might obviate this common problem.

Alternative Delivery Routes

Multiple alternative delivery routes for the administration of pain medications have been described. The use of nebulized fentanyl has been described and holds promise as a route of opioid delivery that can be initiated before an intravenous line has been placed.[75-77] Nebulized pain medications, especially for children who have severe pain but have not had an intravenous line placed, could be of use in the ED.

Procedural Sedation and Analgesia

Patients often present to the ED in need of painful or complex procedures that require patient cooperation and must be done emergently. Procedural sedation and analgesia (PSA) practices and policies have evolved rapidly in the ED, and this is a growing area in the practice of emergency medicine. PSA in the ED is complicated by the occurrence of unpredictable concurrent events as well as time and space constraints of the ED. Furthermore, unlike most patients who undergo sedation in other settings, patients in the ED typically have an unpredictable "nothing by mouth" (NPO) status, often have concurrent severe systemic disease, and usually are in severe pain before the procedure begins.

The indications for ED PSA range from pain control for short painful procedures to the need for patient compliance with a complex emergency procedure. The typical target sedation level for ED PSA ranges from minimal through moderate and deep sedation, depending on the demands of specific procedures. Deep sedation can inadvertently result in the patient achieving a level of sedation consistent with general anesthesia, but this is not an intended target level of ED PSA.

Minimal sedation describes a drug-induced state during which patients are sedated but are still able to respond appropriately to verbal commands (according to their developmental age) and whose eyes remain open. Depending on the agent, it is possible to achieve amnesia of the procedure at this level of sedation, but by definition, patients will still respond to their surroundings. It is generally performed for procedures that require patient compliance but are not typically intensely painful when performed with local anesthesia. Minimal sedation is typically used for procedures such as lumbar puncture, evidentiary exams, simple fracture reductions (in combination with local anesthesia), and the incision and drainage of small abscesses.

During minimal sedation, cardiovascular and ventilatory functions are generally maintained, although patients should be monitored for inadvertent over sedation to deeper levels using oxygen saturation monitors and direct observation. Agents typically used for minimal sedation include alfentanil, fentanyl, midazolam, combinations of the two, and low dose ketamine.

Moderate sedation is performed on patients who would benefit from a deeper level of sedation to augment the procedure. Moderate sedation describes patients sedated to the point at which their eyes are closed but they open in response to verbal commands (appropriately to their developmental age) alone or to light tactile stimulation. Patients at this level usually have an intact airway and maintain ventilatory function without support. As with minimal sedation, inadvertent oversedation to deeper levels can occur with moderate sedation. Appropriate monitoring including oxygen saturation, cardiac monitoring, and blood pressure measurements should be done throughout the sedation, and direct observation of the patient's airway should be maintained throughout the procedure. Agents used for moderate sedation in the ED include propofol, etomidate, ketamine, and the combination of fentanyl and midazolam.

Deep sedation is performed on patients who would benefit from a deeper level of sedation, often in order to complete a procedure already begun that requires more patient relaxation than was achieved at a lighter level of sedation. Generally, amnesia of the procedure is similar between moderate and deep sedation, and it is not necessary to sedate patients to a deep level only to obtain amnesia.[78] Deep sedation is achieved in the ED with the same agents as moderate sedation; the difference is in the intended level of sedation. Monitoring requirements for deep sedation are similar to those for moderate sedation.

End tidal carbon dioxide has also been described in ED PSA, but its utility over the direct observation of a patient's ventilatory efforts and airway protection has not been established.[79] Deeply sedated patients can develop respiratory depression but generally maintain a patent airway and adequate ventilation. Patients sedated to this level can progress to a level of sedation consistent with general anesthesia. This can occur after the procedure for which the patient was sedated has been completed. Pain is a powerful stimulant, and after it is removed due to the completion of a procedure or the application of local anesthesia, patients may progress to a deeper level of sedation.[80–82] There is some evidence that the inadvertent progression to general anesthesia occurs more frequently in patients targeted for deep sedation than in those undergoing moderate sedation.[83] For this reason, it is usually safer to use moderate sedation than deep sedation in the ED unless the procedure requires progressively deeper levels of sedation to complete successfully, such as the reduction of hip dislocations.

Patients who progress to an unintended level of sedation consistent with general anesthesia are not arousable, even to pain. The ability to independently maintain ventilatory function is usually impaired, and patients often require assistance in maintaining a patent airway. Patients can quickly progress to the level of general anesthesia using agents commonly employed for moderate and deep sedation, and physicians performing ED PSA must be prepared to provide ventilatory support until the patient's level of consciousness has improved and they are able to protect their airway and ventilate normally.

In order to decrease the likelihood of aspiration, patients who are undergoing moderate or deep sedation in the ED are often kept NPO. Regardless of the target depth of sedation or the agent administered, there is insufficient evidence to support specific fasting requirements prior to procedural sedation. A recent guideline for emergency physicians has made recommendations for the proper risk stratification of patients based of their last oral intake.[84] In general, the risk of aspiration from recent oral intake increases with the depth of sedation and must be balanced with the urgency of the procedure when deciding whether or not to delay sedation due to recent oral intake.

Patients who have not had oral intake other than clear liquids for 3 hours prior to their procedure have a low risk of aspiration at any level of sedation. In patients with recent oral intake in need of an emergent procedure, the risk of aspiration is unlikely to outweigh the risk of delaying the procedure. Since the risk of aspiration likely increases with the depth of sedation, it is prudent to target the lightest level of sedation feasible for the necessary procedure. For nonurgent procedures where a time delay is unlikely to have a negative effect on the patient, patients who have eaten more than clear liquids in the prior 3 hours should have the procedure delayed until 3 hours after their last intake. For urgent procedures falling in between emergency and nonurgent procedures, lighter levels and shorter durations of PSA should be used as the size of oral intake taken within 3 hours of the procedure increases.

Patients who are intoxicated, especially with alcohol, can be especially difficult to sedate. They often have food in their stomachs and the achieved level of sedation can be difficult to predict. In emergent reductions, this increases their risk but does not change the procedure. In patients who can safely have the procedure delayed, intoxicated patients may benefit from a delay in their sedation until the progression of their mental status (getting worse or getting better) can be ascertained through observation.[84–87]

ED PSA is necessarily used for both patients who are medically healthy or have uncomplicated co-existing medical conditions (American Society of Anesthesiologists Physical Class 1 and 2) and those who have more significant or life-threatening co-existing medical conditions (Class 3 and 4). PSA for critically ill children has been described using ketamine[88] and in adults using propofol or etomidate.[89] The degree of respiratory depression noted in these patients was similar to patients with physical status scores of 1 or 2, but an increased rate of hypotension was seen in physical status 3 and 4 patients who received propofol. It may be that ketamine and etomidate are better suited for the emergent sedation of critically ill patients, but there is not yet sufficient data to make a definite recommendation.

The ventilatory status of sedated patients must be monitored. This is generally accomplished with pulse oximetry and direct observation of the patient's respiratory effort. Pulse oximetry is a sensitive measure of oxygenation. If a patient receives supplemental oxygen prior to starting PSA and during the procedure, this monitor may not be as sensitive to changes in the patient's ventilatory status.[79,90,91] End tidal carbon dioxide has been recommended as an additional modality for the monitoring ventilatory status.[87,92] It provides a graphic display of ventilatory status that can be used to detect respiratory depression before it becomes clinically apparent.[79] In the event of hypoventilation, the end tidal carbon dioxide value increases as the respiratory rate decreases. In the event of increasing airway obstruction, the baseline end tidal carbon dioxide value decreases along with a blunting of the waveform due to increased mixing of the nasal expiratory sample with ambient air due to the turbulence from the obstruction.

Ketamine use has been described in adults[93] but is more commonly used for children undergoing ED PSA.[94] Ketamine is a dissociative anesthetic that provides 15–20 minutes of sedation when given intramuscularly, with a return to baseline mental status in 30–60 minutes. It can be given in doses of 1 to 4 mg/kg intramuscularly and should be combined with atropine 0.01 mg/kg to prevent hypersalivation. The 1 mg/kg dose achieves minimal sedation sufficient for such procedures as lumbar puncture, dressing changes, and simple laceration repair. Doses from 2 to 4 mg/kg result in increasingly deeper levels of moderate to deep sedation. Patients sedated with ketamine usually maintain a patent airway and ventilate normally. Patients receiving ketamine should be monitored for respiratory depression and rare occurrences of laryngospasm.[94,95] Emergence phenomena, unpleasant perceptual experiences as patients regain consciousness, have been described in both adults and children.[96–98] The addition of 0.1 mg/kg of midazolam to ketamine has been described to prevent emergence phenomena, but no difference in the occurrence of emergency phenomena has been found with its use.[96] Intravenous ketamine is also used for ED PSA at doses of 1 mg/kg with an onset of 1–2 minutes, followed by moderate sedation lasting 8 to 12 minutes. The adverse effects of intravenous ketamine are similar to those of intramuscular use.

The combination of fentanyl and midazolam has been used for minimal, moderate, and deep sedation in the ED.[79,83,97,99,100] This combination results in longer periods of sedation than other agents and carries a higher rate of respiratory depression than other commonly used agents. While adequate for minimal sedation, the high level of respiratory depression and long duration of action makes this combination less useful for moderate or deep sedation. Dosing for minimal sedation has been described as 0.1 mg/kg intravenous midazolam followed by 0.05 mg/kg intravenous fentanyl, with repeated fentanyl boluses every 1–3 minutes until the patient is adequately sedated. The sedation typically lasts 30–60 minutes with a return to baseline mental status by 45 to 120 minutes. This method of PSA requires direct ventilatory monitoring.

Pentobarbital is a sedative agent typically used for minimal to moderate sedation for radiologic procedures.[101,102] This agent has no analgesic properties and patients who appear sedated after its administration can be aroused with less stimuli than is typical for many of the other agents used in ED PSA, which is an excellent characteristic for preventing over sedation for radiologic procedures, but is of limited utility for painful procedures. The medicine is administered at 2.5 mg/kg intravenously, followed by 1.25

mg/kg every 5 minutes until adequate sedation is achieved. Pulse oximetry should be used; however, the rate of respiratory depression is lower than for other agents.[103]

Methohexital has been used for moderate and deep PSA.[104–106] It is a very short-acting agent with excellent amnestic properties. It is administered at 1 mg/kg intravenously with 0.5 mg/kg repeat boluses every 1–2 minutes as needed. It has an onset of 30 seconds, with sedation lasting 2–4 minutes and returning to baseline within 5–10 minutes. It has been associated with respiratory depression and a quick progression to deeper levels of sedation than intended and can cause over sedation even when carefully titrated. It should therefore be used with close ventilatory monitoring. Compared to propofol, methohexital is similarly effective and safe with single bolus use, but is less safe than propofol when multiple doses are required.[104] It should be used principally for very brief procedures expected to last less than 2–4 minutes, such as the reduction of simple fractures and dislocations.

Propofol is well described for ED PSA.[79–83,89,104,107–112] It is administered as a 1 mg/kg bolus with repeat boluses of 0.5 mg/kg every 2–3 minutes until the patient achieves the desired level of sedation. The sedation persists 2–5 minutes after a single bolus, and longer for patients receiving multiple boluses, with a return to baseline within 10–15 minutes. This medication has been associated with rates of clinically apparent respiratory depression from 4.0% to 7.7% in ED PSA. As with similar agents, close ventilatory monitoring is required. Propofol causes hypotension in critically ill patients and should be used with caution in hemodynamically unstable patients.[89]

Etomidate is also frequently used for ED PSA.[89,113–118] It is given as a single bolus of 0.1 to 0.3 mg/kg, with an onset of sedation in 30–60 seconds, and sedation lasting 7–10 minutes. It is not associated with hypotension and is more commonly used when this is an issue; however, its use is associated with myoclonic jerking in up to 25% of patients. This adverse effect can complicate the procedure for which the patient has been sedated, making it inferior to propofol for the sedation of healthy patients.[89] Etomidate, in single boluses of 0.3 mg/kg, has been shown to cause transient adrenal suppression, but no significant changes in cortisol levels occur, and the significance of this finding remains unclear.[119]

EVOLVING EMERGENCY DEPARTMENT PAIN MANAGEMENT PRACTICE

Pain management practices in the ED continue to evolve. The American College of Emergency Physicians, emergency medicine's principal specialty organization, established its first general policy statement regarding analgesic practices in 2004.[120] Prior to this, data from the National Hospital Ambulatory Medical Care Survey showed that, from 1997 through 2001, there was an impressive 18% increase in analgesic use in U.S. EDs (from 47.2 to 56.2 mentions per 100 visits), with marked increases in both NSAID agents and opioid analgesics.[121]

At the local level, adoptions of pain management guidelines and quality improvement processes have demonstrated dramatic improvements in practices. In one three site study, rates of ED analgesic treatment increased from 54% to 84% over 1 year as a result of individual and group feedback.[122] In a recent study from one Swiss ED, educational programs and guideline implementation led to marked increases in pain intensity documentation, analgesic administration, reduction in pain intensity scores, and improved patient satisfaction over a 4-month period.[123]

We do not know the reasons for the rapid evolution of ED pain management practice. Policy and regulatory initiatives, institutional quality improvement programs, pharmaceutical marketing campaigns, educational efforts, and new knowledge from basic and clinical research are all likely to be influential factors. No matter the cause, emergency medicine pain research is increasing at a rapid pace, and ED pain management practices will continue to evolve.

CONCLUSION

Relieving pain and reducing suffering are primary responsibilities of emergency medicine and much can be done to improve the care of ED patients in pain. Emergency physicians and nurses continue to refine their approach to the problem of pain and, in time, the current large amount of variability in ED pain practices will no doubt lessen. Clinicians, researchers, and policy makers continue to define specialty-specific standards for emergency medicine pain practice. Ongoing quality improvement initiatives are essential to achieving these goals.

References

1. Nawar EW, Niska RW, Xu J, et al. National Hospital Ambulatory Medical Care Survey: 2005 emergency department summary. *Adv Data* 2007;386: 1–32.
2. Todd KH, Ducharme J, Choiniere M, et al. Pain in the emergency department: results of the pain and emergency medicine initiative (PEMI) multicenter study. *J Pain* 2007;8(6):460–466.
3. Johnston CC, Gagnon AJ, Fullerton L, et al. One-week survey of pain intensity on admission to and discharge from the emergency department: a pilot study. *J Emerg Med* 1998;16:377–382.
4. Tanabe P. Buschmann M. A prospective study of ED pain management practices and the patient's perspective. *J Emerg Nurs* 1999;25:171–177.
5. Cordell WH, Keene KK, Giles BK, et al. The high prevalence of pain in emergency medical care. *Am J Emerg Med* 2002;20:165–169.
6. Todd KH, Cowan P, Kelly N. Chronic or recurrent pain in the emergency department: a national telephone survey of patient experience. *Ann Emerg Med* 2007;50(3):S37.
7. Paice JA, Cohen FL. Validity of a verbally administered numeric rating scale to measure cancer pain intensity. *Cancer Nurs* 1997;20:88–93.
8. Farrar JT, Cleary J, Rauck R, et al. Oral transmucosal fentanyl citrate: randomized, double-blinded, placebo-controlled trial for treatment of breakthrough pain in cancer patients. *J Natl Cancer Inst* 1998;90:611–616.
9. Breyer JE, Knott CB. Construct validity estimation for the African-American and Hispanic versions of the Oucher Scale. *J Pediatr Nurs* 1998;13:20–31.
10. Bellamy N, Campbell J, Syrotuik J. Comparative study of self-rating pain scale in osteoarthritis patients. *Curr Med Res Opin* 1999;15:113–119.
11. Todd KH. Pain assessment instruments for use in the emergency department. *Emerg Med Clin N Am* 2005;23(2):285–295.
12. Stahmer SA, Shofer FS, Marino A, et al. Do quantitative changes in pain intensity correlate with pain relief and satisfaction? *Acad Emerg Med* 1998; 5:851–857.
13. Merkel S, Voepel–Lewis T, Shayevitz JR, et al. The FLACC: a behavioral scale for scoring postoperative pain in young children. *Pediatr Nurse* 1997; 23(3):293–297.
14. Warden V, Hurley AC, Volicer L. Development and psychometric evaluation of the pain assessment in advanced dementia (PAINAD) scale. *J Am Med Dir Assoc* 2003;4:9–15.
15. Gureje O, Von Korff M, Simon GE, et al. Persistent pain and well-being: a World Health Organization study in primary care. *JAMA* 1998;280:147–151.
16. Anderson FA Jr, Spencer FA. Risk factors for venous thromboembolism. *Circulation* 2003;107(suppl 1):I9–I16.
17. Furrow BR. Pain management and provider liability: no more excuses. *J Law Med Ethics* 2001;29:28–51.
18. Wilson JE, Pendleton JM. Oligoanalgesia in the emergency department. *Am J Emerg Med* 1989;7:620–621.
19. Stalnikowicz R, Mahamid R, Kaspi S, et al. Undertreatment of acute pain in the emergency department: a challenge. *Int J Qual Health Care* 2005;17(2): 173–176.
20. Pines JM, Perron AD. Oligoanalgesia in ED patients with isolated extremity injury without documented fracture. *Am J Emerg Med* 2005;23(4):580.
21. Neighbor ML, Honner S, Kohn MA. Factors affecting emergency department opioid administration to severely injured patients. *Acad Emerg Med* 2004; 11(12):1290–1296.
22. Fosnocht DE, Swanson ER, Barton ED. Changing attitudes about pain and pain control in emergency medicine. *Emerg Med Clin North Am* 2005;23(2): 297–306.
23. Rupp T, Delaney KA. Inadequate analgesia in emergency medicine. *Ann Emerg Med* 2004;43(4):494–503.
24. Jones JS, Johnson K, McNinch M. Age as a risk factor for inadequate emergency department analgesia. *Am J Emerg Med* 1996;14(2):157–160.

25. Friedland LR, Kulick RM. Emergency department analgesic use in pediatric trauma victims with fractures. *Ann Emerg Med* 1994;23(2):203–207.

26. Selbst SM. Managing pain in the pediatric emergency department. *Pediatr Emerg Care* 1989;5(1):56–63.

27. Todd KH, Samaroo N, Hoffman JR. Ethnicity as a risk factor for inadequate emergency department analgesia. *JAMA* 1993;269(12):1537–1539.

28. Todd KH, Deaton C, D'Adamo AP, et al. Ethnicity and analgesic practice. *Ann Emerg Med* 2000;35(1):11–16.

29. Pletcher MJ, Kertesz SG, Kohn MA, et al. Trends in opioid prescribing by race/ethnicity for patients seeking care in US emergency departments. *JAMA* 2008;299(1):70–78.

30. Epps CD, Ware LJ, Packard A. Ethnic waiting time differences in analgesic administration in the emergency department. *Pain Manag Nurs* 2008;9(1):26–32.

31. Miner J, Biros MH, Trainor A, et al. Patient and physician perceptions as risk factors for oligoanalgesia: a prospective observational study of the relief of pain in the emergency department. *Acad Emerg Med* 2006;13(2):140–146.

32. Pfefferbaum B, Adams J, Aceves J. The influence of culture on pain in Anglo and Hispanic children with cancer. *J Am Acad Child Adolesc Psychiatry* 1990;29(4):642–647.

33. Greenwald HP. Interethnic differences in pain perception. *Pain* 1991;44(2):157–163.

34. Tait RC, Chibnall JT. Physician judgments of chronic pain patients. *Soc Sci Med* 1997;45(8):1199–1205.

35. Cooper-Patrick L, Gallo JJ, Gonzales JJ, et al. Race, gender, and partnership in the patient–physician relationship. *JAMA* 1999;282(6):583–589.

36. Tamayo-Sarver JH, Dawson NV, Hinze SW, et al. The effect of race/ethnicity and desirable social characteristics on physicians' decisions to prescribe opioid analgesics. *Acad Emerg Med* 2003;10(11):1239–1248.

37. Bartfield JM, Salluzzo RF, Raccio-Robak N, et al. Physician and patient factors influencing the treatment of low back pain. *Pain* 1997;73(2):209–211.

38. American Academy of Pain Medicine. Definitions related to the use of opioids for the treatment of pain. Available at: http://www.painmed.org/pdf/definition.pdf. Accessed April 18, 2008.

39. American Psychiatric Association. *Diagnostic and Statistical Manual for Mental Disorders–IV*. Washington, DC: American Psychiatric Association; 1994.

40. Rinaldi RC, Steindler EM, Wilford BB, et al. Clarification and standardization of substance abuse terminology. *JAMA* 1988;259:555–557.

41. Substance Abuse and Mental Health Services Administration. *Overview of Findings from the 2003 National Survey on Drug Use and Health* Rockville, MD: Office of Applied Studies; 2004: NSDUH Series H-24, DHHS Publication No. SMA 04-3963.

42. Soderstrom CA, Smith GS, Dischinger PC, et al. Psychoactive substance use disorders among seriously injured trauma center patients. *JAMA* 1997;277(22):1769–1774.

43. Spitzer RL, Williams JBW, Gibbon M, et al. *Structured Clinical Interview for DSM-III-R, Patient Edition/Non-patient Edition (SCID-P/SCID-NP)*. Washington, DC: American Psychiatric Press; 1990.

44. Rockett IR, Putnam SL, Jia H, et al. Assessing substance abuse treatment need: a statewide hospital emergency department study. *Ann Emerg Med* 2003;41(6):802–813.

45. Rockett IR, Putnam SL, Jia H, et al. Unmet substance abuse treatment need, health services utilization, and cost: a population-based emergency department study. *Ann Emerg Med* 2005;45(2):118–127.

46. Hansen GR. The drug-seeking patient in the emergency room. *Emerg Med Clin N Am* 2005;23(2):349–365.

47. Zechnich AD, Hedges JR. Community-wide emergency department visits by patients suspected of drug-seeking behavior. *Acad Emerg Med* 1996;3(4):312–317.

48. Graber MA, Gjerde C, Bergus G, et al. The use of unofficial "problem patient" files and interinstitutional information transfer in emergency medicine in Iowa. *Am J Emerg Med* 1995;13(5):509–511.

49. Pope D, Fernandes CM, Bouthillette F, et al. Frequent users of the emergency department: a program to improve care and reduce visits. *CMAJ* 2000;162(7):1017–1020.

50. Geiderman JM. Keeping lists and naming names: habitual patient files for suspected nontherapeutic drug-seeking patients. *Ann Emerg Med* 2003;41(6):873–881.

51. Tse SK, Wong TW, Lau CC, et al. How good are accident and emergency doctors in the evaluation of psychiatric patients? *Eur J Emerg Med* 1999;6(4):297–300.

52. Linklater DR, Pemberton L, Taylor S, et al. Painful dilemmas: an evidence-based look at challenging clinical scenarios. *Emerg Med Clin North Am*. 2005;23(2):367–392.

53. Yale SH, Nagib N, Guthrie T. Approach to the vaso-occlusive crisis in adults with sickle cell disease. *Am Fam Phys* 2000;61(5):1349–1356, 1363–1364.

54. Shapiro BS, Benjamin LJ, Payne R, et al. Sickle cell-related pain: perceptions of medical practitioners. *J Pain Symp Manage* 1997;14(3):168–174.

55. Pack-Mabien A, Labbe E, Herbert D, et al. Nurses' attitudes and practices in sickle cell pain management. *Appl Nurs Res* 2001;14(4):187–192.

56. Brookoff D, Polomano R. Treating sickle cell pain like cancer pain. *Ann Int Med* 1992;116(5):364–368.

57. Shaiova L, Wallenstein D. Outpatient management of sickle cell pain with chronic opioid pharmacotherapy. *J Natl Med Assoc* 2004;96(7):984–986.

58. Todd KH, Sloan EP, Chen C, et al. Survey of pain etiology, management,

59. Zohar Z, Eitan A, Halperin P, et al. Pain relief in major trauma patients: an Israeli perspective. *J Trauma* 2001;51(4):767–772.

60. Kelly AM. A process approach to improving pain management in the emergency department: development and evaluation. *J Accid Emerg Med* 2000;17(3):185–187.

61. Fry C, Aholt D. Local anesthesia prior to the insertion of peripherally inserted central catheters. *J Infus Nurs* 2001;24(6):404–408.

62. Attard AR, Corlett MJ, Kidner NJ, et al. Safety of early pain relief for acute abdominal pain. *BMJ* 1992;305:1020–1021.

63. Pace S, Burke TF. Intravenous morphine for early pain relief in patients with acute abdominal pain. *Acad Emerg Med* 1996;3:1086–1092.

64. Vermeulen B, Morabia A, Unger PF, et al. Acute appendicitis: influence of early pain relief on the accuracy of clinical and US findings in the decision to operate—a randomized trial. *Radiology* 1999;210:639–643.

65. Mahadevan M, Graff L. Prospective randomized study of analgesic use for ED patients with right lower quadrant abdominal pain. *Am J Emerg Med* 2000;18:753–756.

66. Kim MK, Strait RT, Sato TT, et al. A randomized clinical trial of analgesia in children with acute abdominal pain. *Acad Emerg Med* 2002;9:281–287.

67. Thomas SH, Silen W, Cheema F, et al. Effects of morphine analgesia on diagnostic accuracy in emergency department patients with abdominal pain: a prospective randomized trial. *J Am Coll Surg* 2003;196:18–31.

68. Gallagher EJ, Esses D, Lee C, et al. Randomized clinical trial of morphine in acute abdominal pain. *Ann Emerg Med* 2006;48:150–160.

69. Safdar B, Degutis LC, Landry K, et al. Intravenous morphine plus ketorolac is superior to either drug alone for treatment of acute renal colic. *Ann Emerg Med* 2006;48:173–181.

70. Hewitt DJ, Todd KH, Xiang J, et al. Tramadol/acetaminophen or hydrocodone/acetaminophen for the treatment of ankle sprain: a randomized, placebo-controlled trial. *Ann Emerg Med* 2007;49(4):468–480.

71. Bijur PE, Kenny MK, Gallagher EJ. Intravenous morphine at 0.1 mg/kg is not effective for controlling severe acute pain in the majority of patients. *Ann Emerg Med* 2005;46(4):362–367.

72. Hershey LA. Meperidine and central neurotoxicity. *Ann Intern Med* 1983;98(4):548–549.

73. Melzer-Lange MD, Walsh-Kelly MD, Lea CM, et al. Patient-controlled analgesia for sickle cell pain crisis in a pediatric emergency department. *Pediatr Emerg Care* 2004;20(1):2–4

74. Evans E, Turley N, Robinson N, et al. Randomised controlled trial of patient controlled analgesia compared with nurse delivered analgesia in an emergency department. *Emerg Med J* 2005;22(1):25–29.

75. Fulda GJ, Giberson F, Fagraeus L. A prospective randomized trial of nebulized morphine compared with patient-controlled analgesia morphine in the management of acute thoracic pain. *J Trauma* 2005;59(2):383–388.

76. Ballas SK, Viscusi ER, Epstein KR. Management of acute chest wall sickle cell pain with nebulized morphine. *Am J Hematol* 2004;76(2):190–191.

77. Bartfield JM, Flint RD, McErlean M, et al. Nebulized fentanyl for relief of abdominal pain. *Acad Emerg Med* 2003;10(3):215–218.

78. Miner JR, Bachman A, Kosman L, et al. Assessment of the onset and persistence of amnesia during procedural sedation with propofol. *Acad Emerg Med* 2005;12(6):491–496.

79. Miner JR, Heegaard W, Plummer D. End-tidal carbon dioxide monitoring during procedural sedation. *Acad Emerg Med* 2002;9(4):275–280.

80. Bassett KE, Anderson JL, Pribble CG, et al. Propofol for procedural sedation in children in the emergency department. *Ann Emerg Med* 2003;42(6):773–782.

81. Frazee BW, Park RS, Lowery D, et al. Propofol for deep procedural sedation in the ED. *Am J Emerg Med* 2005;23(2):190–195.

82. Miner JR, Biros MH, Seigel T, et al. The utility of the bispectral index in procedural sedation with propofol in the emergency department. *Acad Emerg Med* 2005;12(3):190–196.

83. Miner JR, Biros MH, Heegaard W, et al. Bispectral electroencephalographic analysis of patients undergoing procedural sedation in the emergency department. *Acad Emerg Med* 2003;10(6):638–643.

84. Green SM, Roback MG, Miner JR, et al. Fasting and emergency department procedural sedation and analgesia: a consensus-based clinical practice advisory. *Ann Emerg Med* 2007;49(4):454–461.

85. Green SM. Fasting is a consideration—not a necessity—for emergency department procedural sedation and analgesia. *Ann Emerg Med* 2003;42(5):647–650.

86. Agrawal D, Manzi SF, Gupta R, et al. Preprocedural fasting state and adverse events in children undergoing procedural sedation and analgesia in a pediatric emergency department. *Ann Emerg Med* 2003;42(5):636–646.

87. American College of Emergency Physicians. Procedural sedation in the emergency department. *Ann Emerg Med* 2005;46(1):103–104.

88. Green SM, Denmark TK, Cline J, et al. Ketamine sedation for pediatric critical care procedures. *Pediatr Emerg Care* 2001;17(4):244–248.

89. Miner JR, Martel ML, Meyer M, et al. Procedural sedation of critically ill patients in the emergency department. *Acad Emerg Med* 2005;12(2):124–128.

90. Hart LS, Berns SD, Houck CS, et al. The value of end-tidal CO2 monitoring when comparing three methods of conscious sedation for children undergoing painful procedures in the emergency department. *Pediatr Emerg Care* 1997;13(3):189–193.

and satisfaction in two urban emergency departments. *Can J Emerg Med* 2002;4(4):252–256.

91. Bennett J, Peterson T, Burleson JA. Capnography and ventilatory assessment during ambulatory dentoalveolar surgery. *J Oral Maxillofac Surg* 1997;55(9):921–925;discussion 925–926.

92. Levine DA, Platt SL. Novel monitoring techniques for use with procedural sedation. *Curr Opin Pediatr* 2005;17(3):351–354.

93. Chudnofsky CR, Weber JE, Stoyanoff PJ, et al. A combination of midazolam and ketamine for procedural sedation and analgesia in adult emergency department patients. *Acad Emerg Med* 2000;7(3):228–235.

94. Green SM, Krauss B. Clinical practice guideline for emergency department ketamine dissociative sedation in children. *Ann Emerg Med* 2004;44(5):460–471.

95. Green SM, Nakamura R, Johnson NE. Ketamine sedation for pediatric procedures: Part 1, a prospective series. *Ann Emerg Med* 1990;19(9):1024–1032.

96. Wathen JE, Roback MG, Mackenzie T, et al. Does midazolam alter the clinical effects of intravenous ketamine sedation in children? A double-blind, randomized, controlled, emergency department trial. *Ann Emerg Med* 2000;36(6):579–588.

97. Kennedy RM, Porter FL, Miller JP, et al. Comparison of fentanyl/midazolam with ketamine/midazolam for pediatric orthopedic emergencies. *Pediatrics* 1998;102(4 Pt 1):956–963.

98. Green SM, Sherwin TS. Incidence and severity of recovery agitation after ketamine sedation in young adults. *Am J Emerg Med* 2005;23(2):142–144.

99. Peña BM, Krauss B. Adverse events of procedural sedation and analgesia in a pediatric emergency department. *Ann Emerg Med* 1999;34(4 Pt 1):483–491.

100. Dionne RA, Yagiela JA, Moore PA, et al. Comparing efficacy and safety of four intravenous sedation regimens in dental outpatients. *J Am Dent Assoc* 2001;132(6):740–751.

101. Malviya S, Voepel-Lewis T, Tait AR, et al. Pentobarbital vs chloral hydrate for sedation of children undergoing MRI: efficacy and recovery characteristics. *Paediatr Anaesth* 2004;14(7):589–595.

102. Kienstra AJ, Ward MA, Sasan F, et al. Etomidate versus pentobarbital for sedation of children for head and neck CT imaging. *Pediatr Emerg Care* 2004;20(8):499–506.

103. Karian VE, Burrows PE, Zurakowski D, et al. Sedation for pediatric radiological procedures: analysis of potential causes of sedation failure and paradoxical reactions. *Pediatr Radiol* 1999;29(11):869–873.

104. Miner JR, Biros M, Krieg S, et al. Randomized clinical trial of propofol versus methohexital for procedural sedation during fracture and dislocation reduction in the emergency department. *Acad Emerg Med* 2003;10(9):931–937.

105. Zink BJ, Darfler K, Salluzzo RF, et al. The efficacy and safety of methohexital in the emergency department. *Ann Emerg Med* 1991;20(12):1293–1298.

106. Bono JV, Rella JG, Zink BJ, et al. Methohexital for orthopaedic procedures in the emergency department. *Orthop Rev* 1993;22(7):833–838.

107. Pershad J, Godambe SA. Propofol for procedural sedation in the pediatric emergency department. *J Emerg Med* 2004;27(1):11–14.

108. Burton JH, Miner JR, Shipley ER, et al. Propofol for emergency department procedural sedation and analgesia: a tale of three centers. *Acad Emerg Med* 2006;13(1):24–30.

109. Symington L, Thakore S. A review of the use of propofol for procedural sedation in the emergency department. *Emerg Med J* 2006;23(2):89–93.

110. Guenther E, Pribble CG, Junkins EP Jr, et al. Propofol sedation by emergency physicians for elective pediatric outpatient procedures. *Ann Emerg Med* 2003;42(6):783–791.

111. Havel CJ Jr, Strait RT, Hennes H. A clinical trial of propofol vs midazolam for procedural sedation in a pediatric emergency department. *Acad Emerg Med* 1999;6(10):989–997.

112. Miner JR, Burton JH. Clinical practice advisory: Emergency department procedural sedation with propofol. *Ann Emerg Med* 2007;50(2):182–187.

113. Falk J, Zed PJ. Etomidate for procedural sedation in the emergency department. *Ann Pharmacother* 2004;38(7–8):1272–1277.

114. Hunt GS, Spencer MT, Hays DP. Etomidate and midazolam for procedural sedation: prospective, randomized trial. *Am J Emerg Med* 2005;23(3):299–303.

115. Burton JH, Bock AJ, Strout TD, et al. Etomidate and midazolam for reduction of anterior shoulder dislocation: a randomized, controlled trial. *Ann Emerg Med* 2002;40(5):496–504.

116. Vinson DR, Bradbury DR. Etomidate for procedural sedation in emergency medicine. *Ann Emerg Med* 1999;6(10):592–598.

117. Keim SM, Erstad BL, Sakles JC, et al. Etomidate for procedural sedation in the emergency department. *Pharmacotherapy* 2002;22(5):586–592.

118. Ruth WJ, Burton JH, Bock AJ. Intravenous etomidate for procedural sedation in emergency department patients. *Acad Emerg Med* 2001;8(1):13–18.

119. Schenarts CL, Burton JH, Riker RR. Adrenocortical dysfunction following etomidate induction in emergency department patients. *Acad Emerg Med* 2001;8(1):1–7.

120. Pain management in the emergency department. *Ann Emerg Med* 2004;44(2):198.

121. McCaig LF, Burt CW. *National Hospital Ambulatory Medical Care Survey: 2001 emergency department summary. Advance data from vital and health statistics.* Hyattsville, MD: National Center for Health Statistics; 2003:No. 335.

122. Sucov A, Nathanson A, McCormick J, et al. Peer review and feedback can modify pain treatment patterns for emergency department patients with fractures. *Am J Med Qual* 2005;20(3):138–143.

123. Decosterd I, Hugli O, Tamchès E, et al. Oligoanalgesia in the emergency department: short-term beneficial effects of an education program on acute pain. *Ann Emerg Med* 2007;50(4):462–471.

CHAPTER 112 ■ PAIN MANAGEMENT IN THE INTENSIVE CARE UNIT

RICHARD A. MULARSKI, CURTIS N. SESSLER, AND GREGORY A. SCHMIDT

INTRODUCTION

Pain management in the intensive care unit (ICU) has unique characteristics and challenges. Critically ill patients receive state-of-the-art interventions in an aggressive and fast-paced setting with high morbidity and mortality. Concomitant with the life-saving priority of medical management and curative therapy, caregivers in the ICU have a duty to provide equally aggressive assessment and palliation of pain and other distressful symptoms.[1–3] Pain in ICU care is nearly ubiquitous and the challenges of managing pain in this setting are significant.[4–17] Sources of pain include the therapies and treatments used to preserve and restore life, such as invasive procedures, surgery, and monitoring devices, as well as direct nociceptive stimuli from injury, inflammation, and immobility.[4–11,18]

The motivations to treat pain in the ICU include the humane dictum of medicine to relieve suffering as well as the clinical duty to mitigate systemic and physiologic harm that can result from unabated pain, such as altered glucose control, myocardial ischemia, immune system dysfunction, hypercoagulability, ventilator dyssynchrony, restrictive lung physiology, and disrupted sleep.[1,2,19–27] Clinicians who care for the critically ill are obliged to be proficient in the assessment and management of pain. However, barriers to optimizing management of pain in the ICU include a paucity of a high-level evidence-based risk that treatment principles extrapolated from other settings may not be transferable to the ICU, and a challenge of complexity and overlapping needs where unique considerations and patient variability in response can further convolute care delivery.

The delivery of quality pain management must account for the complex critical care setting and is best accomplished using team-directed approaches. The resulting coordinated efforts and different team members with unique specialized skills helps to overcome one major barrier to pain management—multiple competing interests of the clinicians who care for the critically ill patient. This chapter will summarize the science of pain management in the ICU, including pain evaluation and monitoring in the ICU, general pharmacologic treatment of pain, specific ICU syndromes, postoperative pain, regional anesthesia, comanagement of sedation and analgesia, daily awakening and ventilator liberation strategies, proactive interdisciplinary and patient-centered care, and approaches to pain management at the end of life.

INTENSIVE CARE UNIT PAIN MANAGEMENT WITHIN AN INTERDISCIPLINARY MODEL OF CARE

A principled approach to pain management facilitates care for critically ill patients, whether they are enjoying restoration of health or are actively dying. The grounding of pain management in the ICU stems from a broad goal of relieving suffering that is approached from a care model inclusive of palliation as an integral part of the overall care of the critically ill patient.[1,2,27–30] While the evidence-based treatment of pain is guided by technical issues of management and pharmacologic titration, the delivery of optimal pain care requires individualized, patient-centered care with the objective of relieving suffering along a continuum of balanced curative and palliative care.[1,2,13,21,31] In the ICU, the paramount focus on support of vital organ function may lead to the aggressive use of interventions that obscures the holistic perspective of patient-centered goal-directed care.[32] A strategy that incorporates the palliative medicine framework and a holistic care paradigm can facilitate better pain management.

The interdisciplinary paradigm fosters the integration of diverse talents and individual skills and is an appropriate model for aiding the direction of complex ICU care, inclusive of pain management.[33–37] Intensive care medicine is directed and delivered by multiple members of an interdisciplinary team, coordinated by a shared and explicit patient-centered goals for care.[31,32,38] Assessment of pain and the initiation of management strategies begin at the time of admission to the ICU and are guided by pre-existing knowledge of patient's pain experiences and daily reassessment.[1,39,40] The care provided has a foundation of open communication with patients and families to understand how therapies may help achieve an individual's care goals within the reality of illness and disability. The continuity and continuance of care relies on reassessing how the clinical condition, therapies, and symptoms change in lieu of fluid goal-oriented perspectives by patients and families. Such an approach to pain management, within the spectrum of therapeutic modalities used in the ICU, may in itself be one of the most important aspects of healing the suffering that accompanies critical illness.

The key principles that guide pain management in the ICU are that (1) clinicians should be biased toward the provision of analgesia operating from a presumption of pain when objective measures are conflicting or limited, and (2) in general, the prevention of prolonged untreated pain through early recognition and control is preferred to undertreatment and pain escalation. The approach to comprehensive and concurrent palliative treatment in the ICU must be tempered by anticipated side effects and complications, including the ability of pharmacotherapy to prolong the duration of cognitive recovery and mechanical ventilation. Analgesics and sedatives should be interrupted daily in almost all patients, unless the goal of care is comfort only.[41] The balance of palliation and curative therapy requires constant titration and evaluation to optimize the use of sedative and analgesic therapy.

PHYSIOLOGY OF PAIN SPECIFIC TO THE INTENSIVE CARE UNIT

Pain has been defined as "an unpleasant sensory and emotional experience associated with actual or potential tissue damage, or described in terms of such damage."[42] The pathophysiologic mechanism is activation of the nociceptive pathways—neural afferent signals that arise from tissue damage. In the ICU, pain originates from repeated episodes of acute or short-duration stimuli and, frequently, some degree of chronic or sustained pain. Episodic or short duration pain occurs as an immediate experience of localized tissue damage. In critical care settings, acute pain includes both manifestations of underlying illness and iatrogenesis from therapies, such as catheters, surgery, limited procedures, tissue inflammation, and immobility.[4–11,18] Common painful procedures include endotracheal intubation and endotracheal suctioning, phlebotomy, gastric tubes, vascular access devices, and chest tubes. Turning has been shown to be one of the most painful and distressing procedures endured in routine ICU care.[43] Although chronic pain is primarily thought to develop from longstanding processes of tissue injury or sustained pain that include altered tissue responsiveness and subjective sensitivity, chronic pain can be acquired during an ICU stay from prolonged and repeated pain experiences.[4,5,43]

Pain subtypes identified in ICU care include acute postoperative and posttraumatic pain as well as neuropathic pain, and seeking to differentiate types is indicated to guide therapeutic approaches. The major subdivisions include somatic, visceral, neuropathic, and mixed.[19,20] In the ICU, the ability to differentiate the subjective experience of pain is limited by patients' capacity to clearly describe symptoms. For the most part, pain in the ICU is primarily in the somatic domain. Somatic pain is experienced as dull and aching, is often well-localized, and is particularly amenable to opiates and nonsteroidal anti-inflammatory agents that form the mainstay of ICU pain analgesia. Visceral pain that is cramping and colicky can arise from poor bowel care or from underlying gastrointestinal pathology. This type of pain responds well to anticholinergic therapy. Neuropathic pain that manifests with burning and shooting pain along radicular distributions is less well documented in the ICU but deserves consideration along with the potential use of antidepressants and anticonvulsants when appropriate.

Pain produces systemic effects that may add to the critical illness of the ICU patient; these deleterious effects can be lessened by comprehensive pain management.[19,22,23,44–46] Observation and documentation of the physiologic effects of pain both aids its evaluation and titration of pain therapy. Pain affects all systems of the body through neurohormonal mechanisms, catecholamine release, sympathetic outpouring, and the general stress response (Table 112.1).[20,44,47] Pain results in anxiety, tachycardia, diaphoresis, and catabolic metabolism with the resultant effects including increased myocardial oxygen demand, increased bowel motility, tachypnea and altered pulmonary mechanics, water retention as a result of activation of the renin-angiotensin-aldosterone axis, and cytokine production. Untreated pain may result in immune system dysfunction, hypercoagulable states and an increase in thromboembolic disease, altered glucose control, myocardial ischemia, ventilator dyssynchrony, acute restrictive respiratory physiology, and disrupted sleep quality.[19–23] Among the released cytokines are tumor necrosis factor, interleukin-1, and interleukin-6 that may contribute to blood pressure instability in the critically ill.[22,23] Pain also has synergistic effects with anxiety, depression, and sleep disturbances that may compound the detrimental effects on the body and exacerbate the pain experience.[19,21,44,46,48,49] Abatement of pain and treatment effects on the systemic manifestation of pain may be even more important for the tenuous ICU patient. Although a spectrum of excitatory (glutamate, tachykinins, and neurokinins), inhibitory (gamma amino butyric acid), and regulatory (noradrenaline, serotonin,

TABLE 112.1

SYSTEMIC AND PHYSIOLOGIC CONSEQUENCES OF PAIN IN THE INTENSIVE CARE UNIT

Physiologic system and effects	Consequences
Immune: cytokines elaboration and leukocyte dysfunction	Decreased ability to fight infection and hemodynamic instability
Cardiovascular: increased adrenergic tone and increased vascular resistance	Increased myocardial oxygen demand, stress, and ischemia; venous stasis
Renal: activation of renin-angiotensin-aldosterone axis	Water and sodium retention, anasarca
Endocrine: hormonal imbalance, especially cortisol and insulin	Hyperglycemia and hypotension
Respiratory: restrictive physiology, hyperventilation, lowered residual capacity	Ventilator dyssynchrony, atelectasis, hypoxia, increased pneumonia risk, disrupted sleep
Psychological/Neurological: altered sleep stage and serotonergic imbalance	Depression, fatigue, psychosis, sleep deprivation, anxiety
Hematological: hypercoagulability and platelet dysfunction	Gastrointestinal bleeding and thromboembolic disease

opioid) receptors are involved in the complex experience of pain, the mu, kappa, and delta opiate receptors are the prevailing target for pain management in the ICU.[50,51]

EVALUATION AND MONITORING OF PAIN IN THE INTENSIVE CARE UNIT

Pain management in the ICU is based on a universal anticipation for the presence of pain in all patients and the recognition that measurement is requisite for therapeutic guidance.[4,5,52–58] While most patients will require specific therapies to alleviate pain, observational research demonstrates that the minority of patients receive adequate pain assessment and treatment in the ICU.[4,5,16,59–63] Amongst the barriers to measuring pain in the ICU are the paucity of high-level evidence to guide ICU pain management, the lack of valid and reliable instruments for assessing pain when subjective input is not available, the risk that some therapies may potentiate medical problems, and problems with rapid titration and bioavailability. The assessment of pain in the ICU is further complicated by insufficient attention to pain monitoring and lack of subjective patient reports for critically ill patients with altered sensorium.

Despite these limitations, pain management is based on and guided by assessment efforts in the ICU just as in any other practice setting. Professional societies and regulatory bodies have increased efforts to improve the recognition and treatment of pain for hospitalized patients.[25,27,64] The Joint Commission on Accreditation of Health Care Organizations formally requires assessment using standardized techniques, and various groups have proposed quality measures for pain management in the ICU.[65–73] The Veterans Health Administration enacted a directive in 1999 requiring medical providers to assess and record a patient's self-

report of pain using a 10-point numerical or visual rating scale.[74] These policy decisions are based on the concept that to appropriately manage pain, providers need to systematically and serially evaluate the presence and characteristics of pain.

Pain Assessment in the Communicative Patient

Pain assessment begins with the recognition that pain is a subjective interpretation of a unique experience—there is no overt measure of its presence or magnitude. As such, pain is best characterized by a coherent, interactive patient. Although the intensity of pain is a subjective experience, quantifying via rating scales aides in management.[19,66,75–79] In optimal circumstances, formal pain evaluation should assess intensity, duration, site, and type of pain. This evaluation should focus on understanding the cause and prior responses to therapy. In general, more thorough pain assessment is linked to improved pain management.[14,21,23,52,56,80–82]

The intent of asking a patient to rate his or her pain on a valid and reliable scale is to aid therapeutic efforts to relieve the pain. A simple approach for awake and aware patients in the ICU is to quantify pain intensity along a numeric rating scale, particularly assisted with a visual aid. For example, the numerical rating scale shown in Figure 112.1 can aid in serial assessments of pain along a continuum, such as from 0 = no pain to 10 = the worst pain they have ever experienced.[75,77] A pictorial scale, like the Wong-Baker FACES scale (see Fig. 112.1), presents a graphical means of ascribing numbers to a patient's perception and can be used with some reliability even in those with mild alterations of sensorium. While some children may be able to confirm the presence or absence of pain, young children may be limited in their ability to provide additional description when asked. Pain assessment for infants and preverbal toddlers is typically limited to indirect measures similar to other cognitively impaired patients.

Pain Assessment in the Cognitively Impaired Patient

The patient-reported determination of pain intensity is problematic in the ICU since many patients have cognitive impairment. Although pain manifests with various physiologic and behavioral markers, these are relatively poor surrogates for the patient who is unable to express the experience of pain.[19,20,79,81,83] Clinicians, however, can be attentive to patient movement, facial expression, and posturing as a supplementary source of data in patients able to respond but not able to quantify pain with a scale. Methods that combine data from multiple sources are needed to guide evaluation in the cognitively impaired ICU patient.

The earliest pain assessment tools for the noncommunicative ICU patient were developed for infants and young children. The COMFORT Scale[84] and the Face, Legs, Activity, Cry, Consolability (FLACC) Observation tool[85] are two instruments that have confirmed validity and interrater reliability and are in common use today. The COMFORT Scale contains eight behavioral and physiologic factors, each scored 1 to 5.[84] The FLACC Tool assesses pain uses behavioral indicators and body movements, verbal responses (cry), and consolability; it has been validated in a variety of pediatric populations.[85,86]

For adult patients who are marginally conscious or uncommunicative, two behavioral assessment scales have been developed and tested in the ICU with improved psychometric properties over physiologic indicators.[63,87–89] The Behavioral Pain Scale (BPS) has three domains and has been demonstrated to discriminate pain experience distinct from levels of sedation (Table 112.2).[87]

The Critical Care Pain Observation Tool (CPOT) has four domains: facial expression, body movements, muscle tension, and compliance with the ventilator for intubated patients or vocalization for nonintubated patients (Table 112.3).[88,89] Each behavior is rated from 0 to 2 and the total summed for a score ranging

Numeric Rating Scale

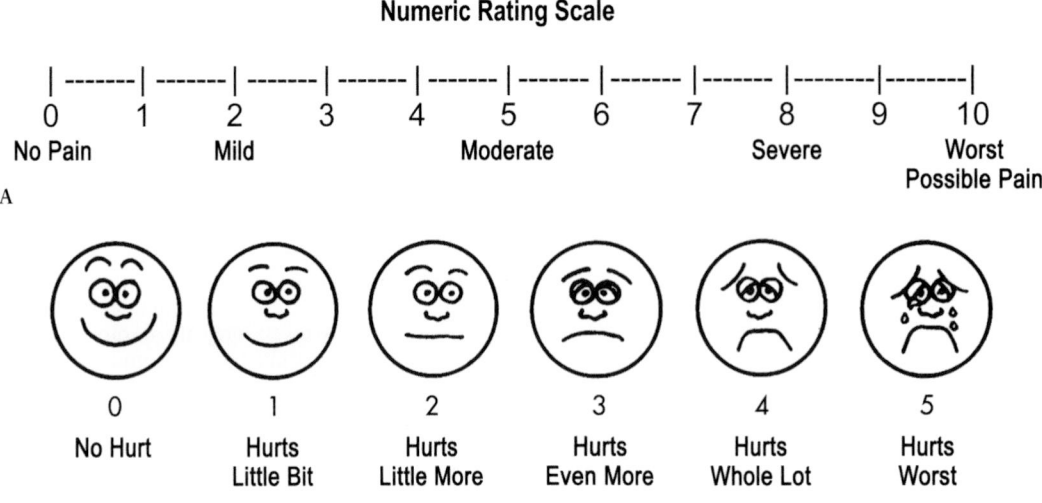

A

B

FIGURE 112.1 The numerical rating scale (**A**) and the Wong-Baker FACES scale (**B**) are advocated as interactive ways for patients in the ICU to rate the intensity of pain. (**A** reproduced from Partners against pain. Available at: www.partnersagainstpain.com/html/assess/scales/as_scale3.htm. Accessed March 6, 2003. with permission. **B** reproduced from Hockenberry MJ, Wilson D, Winkelstein ML. *Wong's Essentials of Pediatric Nursing.* 7th ed. St. Louis: Mosby; 2005:1259, with permission.)

from 0 to 8. A score greater than 3 yielded sensitivity of 67% and specificity of 83% for self-reported pain in conscious ICU patients.[89] The CPOT has been validated in several ICU settings. Gélinas and colleagues[88] studied 105 cardiac surgery patients during periods of rest and during nociceptive and nonnociceptive nursing interventions. Good associations between CPOT and self-reported pain rating were demonstrated for awake patients. Additionally, scores increased significantly during nociceptive, but not nonnociceptive procedures.[88] Responsiveness of CPOT to noxious stimuli suffers somewhat with deepening levels of unconsciousness,[89] much like observations for the BPS.[87] Excellent

TABLE 112.2

THE BEHAVIORAL PAIN SCALE. THREE DOMAINS ARE USED TO APPROXIMATE PAIN INSTENSITY FOR NONCOMMUNICATIVE ICU PATIENTS.

Item	Description	Score
Facial expression	Relaxed	1
	Partially tightened (e.g., brow lowering)	2
	Fully tightened (e.g., eyelid closing)	3
	Grimacing	4
Upper limbs	No movement	1
	Partially bent	2
	Fully bent with finger flexion	3
	Permanently retracted	4
Compliance with ventilation	Tolerating movement	1
	Coughing but tolerating ventilation for most of the time	2
	Fighting ventilator	3
	Unable to control ventilation	4

Reproduced from Payen JF, Bru O, Bosson JL, et al. Assessing pain in critically ill sedated patients by using a behavioral pain scale. *Crit Care Med* 2001;29(12):2258–2263, with permission.

interrater reliability has been demonstrated for both BPS and CPOT.[87–89] These scales can be combined with measurement of sedation (see management section) and confusion/delirium, such as with the Confusion Assessment Method for the Intensive Care Unit[90,91] or the Intensive Care Delirium Screening Checklist,[92] to aid in comprehensive care.

Assessment using multiple sources of physiologic markers and creative interrogation, for example educating patients to signal with hand movements or blinking when pain is inadequately controlled, may improve day-to-day treatment. Changes in physiologic indicators, such as increased heart rate, increased blood pressure, increased respiratory rate, diaphoresis, and mydriasis, especially reductions after analgesic therapy, may provide additional evidence to guide the titration of analgesics, although these are less reliable than behavioral indicators. Family input may be solicited and provide an additional source of data to guide pain care; however, evidence suggests that surrogates lack reliability and should not be the sole source for monitoring.[93–98] Effective strategies are those that are tailored to the capability of an individual patients and are employed frequently and regularly by the care team.

Agitation can have multiple sources in the ICU, but for most ICU patients a preliminary search for pain and a therapeutic trial of analgesia is appropriate prior to sedation. Agitation is characterized by excessive, usually nonpurposeful motor activity associated with internal tension.[99,100] Prospective surveillance indicates that most ICU patients experience some evidence of overt agitation during hospitalization.[101] Agitated behavior can have serious consequences such as patient-initiated removal of critical tubes and catheters or even caregiver injury from combativeness.[101–103] The use of a sedation-agitation scale, such as the Richmond Agitation-Sedation Scale (RASS), Sedation Agitation Scale (SAS), or Adaptation to Intensive Care Environment (ATICE) instrument can promote recognition and documentation of agitation.[104–107] Agitation is often a manifestation of delirium[92] that may arise as a result of many forms of medical illness, alcohol or sedative drug withdrawal, and a variety of medications.[99] It is important to consider that agitation may be a manifestation of unrecognized or undertreated pain. Additionally, agitated behavior may herald life-threatening patient distress from unexpected conditions such as a malpositioned or occluded endotracheal tube, tension pneu-

TABLE 112.3

THE CRITICAL-CARE PAIN OBSERVATION TOOL. FOUR DOMAINS ARE USED TO APPROXIMATE PAIN INTENSITY FOR NONCOMMUNICATIVE ICU PATIENTS.

Indicator	Description	Score	
Facial expression	No muscular tension observed	Relaxed, neutral	0
	Presence of frowning, brow lowering, orbit tightening, and levator contraction	Tense	1
	All of the above facial movements plus eyelid tightly closed	Grimacing	2
Body movements	Does not move at all (does not necessarily mean absence of pain)	Absence of movements	0
	Slow, cautious movements, touching or rubbing the pain site, seeking attention through movements	Protection	1
	Pulling tube, attempting to sit up, moving limbs/thrashing, not following commands, striking at staff, trying to climb out of bed	Restlessness	2
Muscle tension Evaluation by passive flexion and extension of upper extremities	No resistance to passive movements	Relaxed	0
	Resistance to passive movements	Tense, rigid	1
	Strong resistance to passive movements, inability to complete them	Very tense or rigid	2
Compliance with the ventilator (intubated patient)	Alarms not activated, easy ventilation	Tolerating ventilator or movement	0
	Alarms stop spontaneously	Coughing but tolerating	1
OR			
Vocalization (extubated patient)	Asynchrony: blocking ventilation, alarms frequently activated	Fighting ventilator	2
	Talking in normal tone or no sound	Talking in normal tone or no sound	0
	Sighing, moaning	Sighing, moaning	1
	Crying out, sobbing	Crying out, sobbing	2
Total, range			0–8

Reproduced from Gelinas C, Fillion L, Puntillo KA, et al. Validation of the critical-care pain observation tool in adult patients. *Am J Crit Care* 2006;15(4):420–427, with permission.

mothorax, or myocardial ischemia that must be rapidly recognized and treated.

A structured management protocol for agitation and pain can be implemented effectively in the ICU setting and can result in substantial benefits (Fig. 112.2). Chanques and coworkers[108] implemented a protocol for detection of agitation using RASS[104] and pain using a numerical pain scale and the BPS,[87] plus structured management of agitation and pain that included detection of underlying conditions, specific medication selection, and medication de-escalation. They demonstrated significant reductions in the frequency of pain and agitation, as well as a 50% reduction in the duration of mechanical ventilation, compared to prior to protocol. Accordingly, pain and agitation should be routinely sought using validated instruments and managed in a structured logical fashion. In addition to searching for underlying causes, the noncommunicative patient with agitation should be considered to possibly have pain as a causative factor and consideration given to a therapeutic trial of analgesic medication.

PHARMACOLOGIC TREATMENT OF PAIN IN THE INTENSIVE CARE UNIT

General Principles for Pain Management

Pain management is a requisite part of critical care for all ICU patients based on the motivation to attempt to relieve human

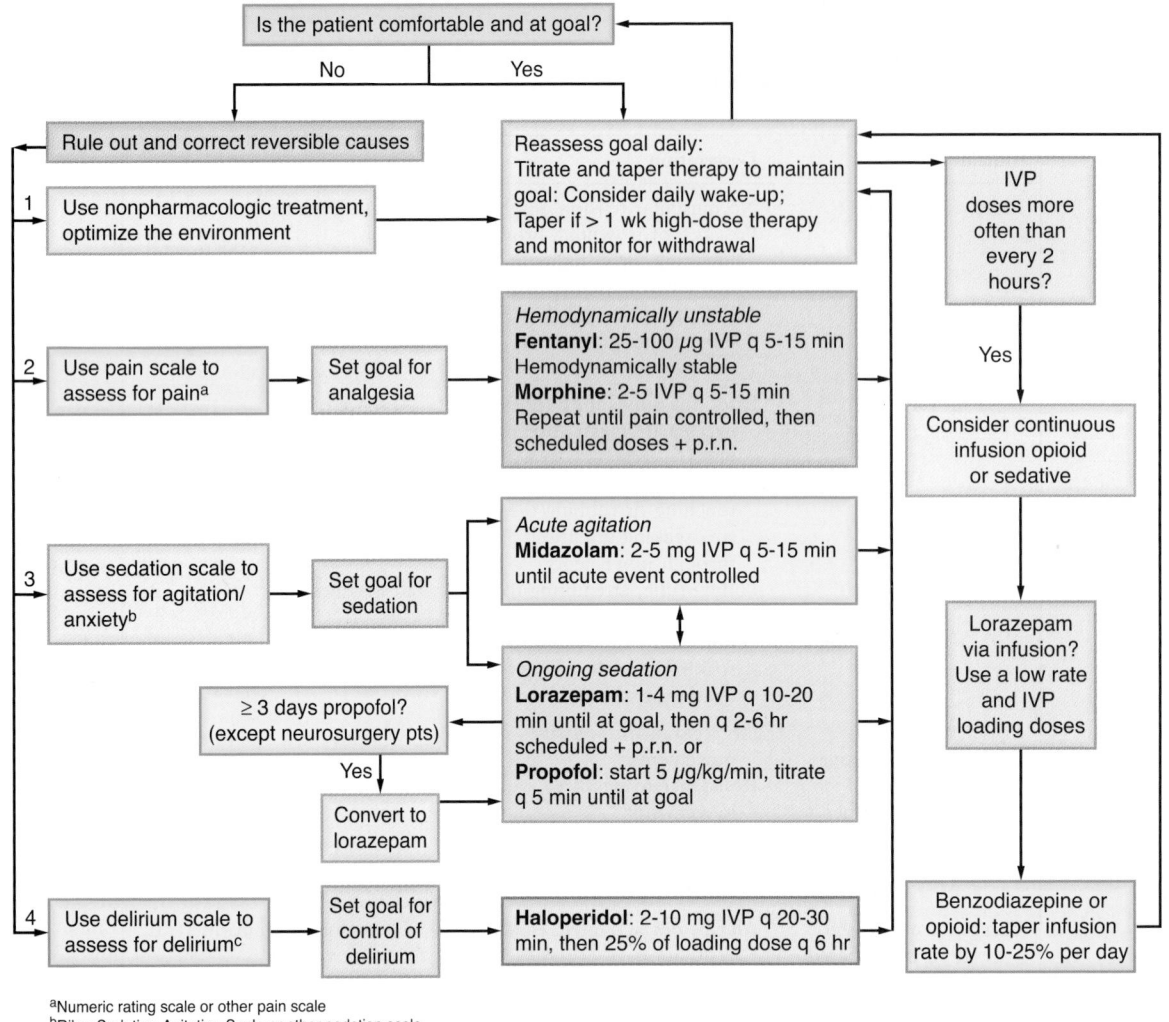

FIGURE 112.2 ACCM/SCCM/ASHP ICU Algorithm for Sedation and Analgesia. This joint statement provides clinical practice guidelines for the sustained use of sedatives and analgesics in the critically ill adult. (Reproduced from Jacobi J, Fraser GL, Coursin DB, et al. Clinical practice guidelines for the sustained use of sedatives and analgesics in the critically ill adult. *Crit Care Med* 2002;30[1]:119–141, with permission.)

suffering and to mitigate systemic physiologic effects engendered by untreated pain. Opiate therapy remains the dominant treatment in the armamentarium for pain therapy in the ICU. Amongst pharmacologic anesthetics, intravenous opiates have the most appropriate potency, absence of a ceiling effect, and usually desirable mild sedative and anxiolytic effects that lead to their dominance in the ICU. Opiates, however, are not without adverse drug effects, including bowel complications, delirium, respiratory suppression, and others. More comprehensive recommendations exist in other chapters of this text (see Chapter 78) and in the general literature for details on opiate therapy.[19,20,52,56,82,109,110] Nonpharmacologic and adjuvant therapies also have a complementary role and should be considered in ICU care.

Opiate Therapy

The objective of administering opiates in the ICU is to improve patient comfort and outcomes for critically ill patients.[19,46,58,110,111] For those with substantial injury, massive surgeries, or severe illness requiring life-support, scheduled or continuous intravenous infusions are part of usual care. For the patient who

is not responding to therapy, consistent analgesia is certainly warranted in those who eventually die of their illness. For many ICU patients, however, opiate therapy may interfere with timely achievement of anticipated outcomes, even when other therapies are resulting in restoration of health. Opiates, like other medications administered for prolonged periods, can manifest protracted durations of effect.[20,41,55,83,109,110,112,113] Analgesia and sedation can persist for days to weeks after sustained infusions are discontinued, and it is common for patients with hepatic or renal disease to experience oversedation. Evidence-based therapeutic recommendations favor bolus dosing and daily interruption of sedative and analgesic medications, except for the dying and those with uncontrolled pain.[1,110,114] For the most part, pain management in the ICU is based on data extrapolated from other settings, and even in existing Society of Critical Care Medicine (SCCM)/American Society of Health-System Pharmacists (ASHP) clinical practice ICU guidelines, no recommendations were based on high level or grade "A" evidence.[25,26,110]

No specific agent has been demonstrated to be preferable in all ICU patients or across all clinical entities. Optimized agent and dosing is a patient-specific quality that is based on the therapeutic balance that pain is relieved without intolerable adverse effects.

Selection of initial analgesic therapy should be based on individual patient characteristics and knowledge of prior opiate exposure, experience, and side effects, when available. Surveys and prospective surveillance studies indicate that morphine and fentanyl are widely used around the world.[63,115–118] For agents like morphine, the intravenous pharmacokinetics include peak effects at 30 minutes and an approximate duration of 2 hours, thus leading to bolus therapy at a frequency of every 30 to 60 minutes. Many critically ill patients' metabolisms are altered, however, which can substantially lengthen the duration of effect.[110]

Morphine and hydromorphone have an active hepatic metabolite in a glucuronide form that accumulates during renal failure.[19,83,119–121] Morphine-6-glucuronide has a half-life greater than 12 hours, has been demonstrated to cross the blood-brain barrier, and has been associated with prolonged sedation after discontinuation of continuous infusions. Caution is warranted in using these drugs in critically ill patients with renal and/or hepatic failure. Vasodilation, cardiovascular instability, and bronchospasm from histamine release are additional side effects that can complicate ICU care. The histaminic response can be differentiated by associated rash or pruritis, response to antihistamines, and short duration (less than a week) if therapy is continued.

Fentanyl has shorter peak and duration of action and can be bolus dosed as often as every 5 minutes, but it has been shown to accumulate when given by continuous infusion based on its lipophilic properties with half-times reported as lasting weeks after steady-state infusion.[19,55,83,109,110,113,122] Fentanyl may produce less hemodynamic instability than other opiates but has a unique side effect of muscle rigidity that appears dose-related.

Remifentanil is a selective mu-opioid receptor agonist approved for use in anesthesia induction and maintenance that may have advantageous properties for ICU care. The novelty in this agent, in contrast to fentanyl, is that remifentanil is metabolized by multiple ubiquitous esterases and its half-life is not known to be protracted by critical illness nor organ dysfunction.[123–127] Due to its pharmacokinetic properties, this agent has a terminal half-life of less than 30 minutes and may reduce the incidence of prolonged sedative complications seen with continuous infusions of other opiates. Preliminary work demonstrates shorter periods of mechanical ventilation when this agent is used over other opiates in short-term studies.[128–130] The agent may adversely produce bradycardia and hypotension, however, which limits it widespread use in the ICU. The agent has been used in traumatic brain injury and neurosurgical settings with favorable effects on neurologic function assessment and a dose-dependent reduction in coughing associated with endotracheal suctioning. Concern remains, however, that the fast offset of this agent may lead to withdrawal and agitated behavior.[131–133]

Other agents may have a role in the ICU, but many possess properties that limit utility in critical care settings. Meperidine is associated with neuroexcitation due to a metabolite, normeperidine. Meperidine has been used in the short term for shivering associated with general anesthesia or to abate drug-induced rigors. It should never be given for more than 1 day or at a cumulative dose over 600 mg in a renal competent patient. Codeine by itself needs conversion to morphine for activity but a proportion of the population lack the enzymatic mechanism. Oxycodone is pharmacologically similar to morphine but only available in oral preparations.

Methadone has many advantages in the non-ICU setting over other agents for the management of chronic pain. However, the oral requirement, slow titration to steady-state, and variable potency limits its utility in the initial unstable period that most ICU patients experience. Methadone is advantageous in those with prior pain syndromes, is inexpensive, and may be preferable for complex pain syndromes due to its N-methyl-D-aspartate antagonism. Methadone can increase the QTc and has been associated with dysrhythmias.

Dosing and frequency are based on providing sufficient and frequent opiates to control underlying and breakthrough pain as well as anticipated prevention from interventions. Reassessment and titration are essential skills for pain management. Patients will have individualistic responses to different opiate medications that cannot be predicted based on underlying characteristics and suggest a role for switching between agents to minimize adverse effects. Changing agents requires skills in equianalgesic dose calculations. Equianalgesic dosing (see Chapter 78) may be estimated by the use of tables, but in general should be decreased in the new agent, especially in the critically ill.[20,109,110,119,134,135] When changing agents, the sum of administered opiates for the prior 24-hour period can be converted to 50% to 80% of the new agent's equivalent dose and then dosed as a continuous infusion or at intervals. Rotation of agents during protracted courses of treatment or combination therapy with different opiates may minimize untoward effects and optimize efficacy.[19,83,136]

Many critically ill patients suffer from chronic progressive diseases and thus do not present opiate naïve to the ICU. Particular care must be taken to avoid withdrawal syndromes and the physiologic consequences that can complicate ICU management. Recognition of withdrawal is crucial to avoid overtreatment with sedative or hypnotic agents. Physical and physiologic dependence can be predicted, and ICU practitioners need to anticipate its occurrence with regular use of opiates, either in the pre-ICU care or during prolonged ICU stays. Acute withdrawal has been shown to occur in ICU patients treated with opiates for greater than a week and may present within 6–12 hours after discontinuation of opiates.[137] The opiate withdrawal syndrome can include sweating, discomfort, agitation, lacrimation, diarrhea, tachycardia, and rebound pain. These symptoms, however, may be blunted in the critically ill patient or in those with concomitant use of sedating medication.

In titrating opiates in those with chronic pain, a breakthrough dose should be provided with a sustained or continuous basal administration. In general, the breakthrough dose can be approximated as 10% to 20% of the 24-hour total opiate requirement. For example, an ICU patient requiring 100 mg of sustained-release oral morphine every 12 hours should have 20–40 mg of oral morphine available every 1–2 hours or 7–14 mg of intravenous morphine available every 30–60 minutes. Breakthrough doses may also be titrated every 30 minutes and by as much as 50% to 100% in subsequent doses if the initial dose did not provide sufficient relief. When increasing opiate needs are sustained, the total daily dose should be adjusted by calculating 24-hour needs and administering approximately to 80% of the daily dose as a basal rate for those with stable syndromes.

For the less severely ill and especially postoperative patients in the ICU, patient-controlled anesthesia (PCA) is often appropriate. In the immediate postinsult period, PCA typically includes three methods of delivering intravenous opiates: a patient-controlled dose that is given on demand using short lockout periods for breakthrough pain,[1] a basal or continuous infusion for patients with higher initial needs or prior tolerance from pre-existing opiate use for chronic pain,[2] and the potential for professional care givers to administer a provider-controlled bolus as needed.[3] Side effects and total dosage is often reduced with PCA and, as a result, less sedation and respiratory depression is experienced.

Nonintravenous administration of opiates is appropriate for some patients in the ICU. A subcutaneous infusion may be beneficial for rare patients, usually those at the end of life following the withdrawal of invasive measures and is dosed similarly to intravenous opiates. In general, the sublingual, buccal, or rectal routes are less desired as palliation can be inconsistent and side effects are increased. The transdermal route is an option for continuous basal opiate therapy, but is less desirable in the ICU, especially early in illness where decreased or variable perfusion may convolute stable absorption. The oral route is ideal for ongoing pain when critical illness is resolving but is often inconsistent early in the ICU process with enteral absorption often compromised.

Epidural routes are advantageous in the postoperative patient and have advantages in reducing systemic side effects.[138,139] For many ICU patients, however, the safe placement and maintenance of epidural anesthesia is limited. When considering analgesia, as in most therapies administered in the ICU, dosing should be responsive to moment-to-moment experiences of pain and proactive in prevention or preemptive treatment of anticipated pain. For example, dosing an opiate at a time interval just shorter than the peak onset is appropriate before painful dressing changes or other planned procedures. The ICU patient often manifests clinical variability and instability that requires frequent intervention, including responsiveness to pain therapy and dosing adjustments based on hemodynamic and metabolic derangements.

In general, there is no upper limit in opiate dosage, and titration is based on pain levels, the patient's tolerance, and adverse effects. Note that for many nonopiate analgesics, toxic metabolites limit this dosing strategy and thus are not the preferred agent to begin treating pain in the ICU. All patients should be anticipated to have predictable and manageable adverse effects with opiate use.

All opiates stimulate intestinal mu receptors and result in dysmotility and constipation. This activity and resultant constipation do not seem to be lessened over time with continued treatment. Thus, prophylaxis with stimulant medications combined with stool softener is appropriate. In the ICU, where enteral routes are not completely compromised, these agents should be administered with the first dose of opiates and titrated to loose stools. Obstipation is not infrequent and requires a digital rectal exam prior and disimpaction before beginning more aggressive bowel routines.

Other common adverse effects of opiate administration include sedation, myoclonus, nausea, and physiologic dependence. Additionally, opiates may have immunomodulating properties that could be worrisome in the ICU where infectious complications are common.[140,141] Nausea and emesis are usually due to stimulation at the chemoreceptor trigger zone, vestibular apparatus, or direct gastrointestinal effects. Antiemetics may be indicated, but the magnitude of this effect often diminishes with continued use. Myoclonus is occasionally seen when high doses of opiates are required and may be tempered by benzodiazepines, neuroleptics, or coadministration of multiple lower dosages of single agents.

Various opiates may produce reactions of varying intensity and types. If adverse effects are intractable and limit appropriate pain management, changing agents or using adjuvant therapies may be advantageous. Sedative side effects of opiates may be desirable when caring for mechanically ventilated patients. Sedation can be minimized, however, by aggressive use of nonopiates and nonpharmacologic agents as well as concurrent administration of central stimulants, such as dextroamphetamine and methylphenidate. Care must be taken to avoid withdrawal reactions once physiologic dependence has developed. Naloxone may be required in some situations where respiratory insufficiency in the spontaneously breathing patient is suspected to be caused by opiates. When used, naloxone should be dosed judiciously and slowly to avoid precipitating withdrawal.

Drug therapy in the ICU is subject to alterations in volume status, plasma protein binding, end-organ dysfunction, and resultant disturbances in bioavailability, clearance, volume of distribution, and pharmacokinetics that, especially for opiate medication, can manifest in protracted durations of effect and other adverse effects.[20,41,55,83,109,110,112,113] Pharmacokinetics and pharmacodynamics for analgesic agents are covered in much detail in other sections of this text (see Chapter 76). In the ICU, therapeutic drug monitoring does not generally apply to the predominant agents used for analgesia and, for the most part, dosing should be reduced and closely monitored for desired and adverse effects.[20,109,110,119,134,135] Specific caution should occur with continuous intravenous dosing of morphine and hydromorphone in the presence of renal insufficiency, as active glucuronide metabolites can accumulate and increase the duration of undesired sedative complications.[19,83,119–121] For the most part, altered pharmacokinetics in the ICU for analgesia and sedative medications are dealt with through proactive assessment and monitoring of clinical end-points (see approaches and details in the subsequent section on management of analgesia and sedation).

Nonopiate and Adjuvant Pain Therapies

Nonopiate pain therapies are less desirable as first-line pain management in all but the least injured or ill ICU patient, but these agents do have roles as adjuvant treatments. Ketorolac is an intravenous nonsteroidal anti-inflammatory medication that may be useful for anti-inflammatory effects, but produces gastrointestinal toxicity and increases the risk for gastrointestinal bleeding that limits its use to less than 5 days at a time or not at all in ICU patients already at risk for bleeding. Corticosteroids, ketamine, and adenosine may have opiate sparing effects as adjuvant therapy, but have not been evaluated in the ICU.[142,143] Lidocaine has also been used as an effective adjuvant for complex or neuropathic syndromes but may be limited in the ICU due to its arrhythmogenic properties.[144] Acetaminophen is a weak analgesic that carries the risk of hepatotoxicity with chronic use that similarly restricts its utility in the ICU except as an intermittently administered antipyretic. Clonidine and its related isomer, dexmedetomidine, are alpha agonists that provide mild sedation and mild analgesia. Dexmedetomidine avoids central respiratory suppression and may be a useful sedative in the spontaneously breathing or weaning ICU patient.[145]

Nonpharmacologic modalities are incompletely studied and infrequently used in the ICU, but have the potential to improve pain management.[19,21,83,146–148] Comprehensive palliative care therapies may include distraction therapies, behavioral modification, touch therapy, meditation, music therapy, palliative radiation or chemotherapy, acupuncture or acupressure, and massage. Epidural strategies, nerve blocks, electrophysiologic options, and specific nonpharmacologic options are receiving increased attention and study in the ICU. Consultation or routine involvement of pain or palliative specialists in interdisciplinary ICU care is expanding and includes the opportunity for mainstream ICU providers to broaden their expertise and experience.

Providers should recognize and anticipate analgesic needs in the ICU, particularly before noxious stimuli such as initiating procedures. Preemptive administration of analgesia improves pain control, decreases sedation and overall dose requirements, decreases catecholamine and stress response, and lessens physiologic complications of pain.[19,82,109,149–151]

TREATMENT OF PAIN—SPECIFIC APPROACHES

The analgesic needs of most critically ill patients are best met with systemic opiate infusion. For some patients, however, there are opportunities to improve analgesic management through more targeted techniques. In large part, the potential advantage of specific analgesic methods is attributable to fewer systemic adverse effects compared to an equivalent degree of analgesia provided intravenously. For example, in a mechanically ventilated patient with multiple, unilateral rib fractures, a paravertebral block or continuous thoracic epidural analgesic infusion might produce better control of pain while simultaneously facilitating an awake patient capable of cooperating with physical therapy and tolerating spontaneous breathing. At the same time, critically ill patients present numerous challenges to the pain practitioner by virtue of increased risk and difficulties in neurologic assessment. The specific techniques for delivering regional anesthesia are delineated more fully in other chapters of this text (see Chapter 51).

Regional Anesthesia

Appropriate use of regional analgesic techniques in the ICU requires four key attributes: (1) an awareness of the range of available methods; (2) technical expertise to deliver a broad array of specialized skills, typically through a "pain service" or an intensivist trained in anesthesiology; (3) high-quality nursing conversant with the unique complications and associated early warning signs[152]; and (4) an organized system for placing catheters aseptically, examining the devices regularly, and recognizing the presence of infections. Because many ICUs do not possess all of these attributes, some specific analgesic techniques are probably underutilized in intensive care. A stronger evidence base, delineating the benefits while determining systematically the magnitude of adverse reactions, could serve to change current practice.

Indications

Regional analgesic approaches should be considered when the nature of the pain is particularly localized anatomically or when systemic administration of narcotics is unduly risky. Surgery and trauma, particularly of the extremities, often cause anatomically localized pain that can be treated regionally. For example, benefits of epidural analgesia have been demonstrated following thoracic surgery, orthopedic procedures of the lower extremities, abdominal operations, cardiac surgery, and multiple rib fractures due to trauma,[153–157] although not all studies have confirmed these findings.[158,159] Epidural analgesia often confers improved pain relief but few studies have been able to demonstrate meaningfully improved outcomes. Nevertheless, in patients with multiple, traumatic rib fractures, a prospective comparison of epidural analgesia (generally bupivacaine, morphine, and fentanyl) and intravenous opioids (morphine, hydromorphone, and fentanyl), showed that the neuraxial approach shortened the duration of mechanical ventilation and reduced the rate of nosocomial pneumonia.[160] Moreover, new evidence emphasizing the importance of vigorously reducing the amount of sedatives and analgesics given to critically ill patients points to an increasing role for regional techniques.[41,161] For brief operative procedures, such as tube thoracostomy, a regional technique provides short-term control of pain with few systemic effects. Localized pain due to severe pancreatitis, malignancy, arterial insufficiency, and cardiac angina may also be amenable to regional techniques. Systemic reasons to avoid or minimize opiates include hemodynamic instability or compromised respirations when intubation is undesirable. One subset of patients in whom regional techniques may be particularly useful is the group with known or suspected sleep-disordered breathing in whom systemic opiates are prone to precipitate respiratory failure from hypoventilation and/or obstructive apnea.

Also, for brief operative procedures, such as tube thoracostomy, a regional technique provides short-term control of pain with few systemic effects. Systemic reasons to avoid or minimize opiates include hemodynamic instability or compromised respirations when intubation is undesirable. One subset of patients in whom regional techniques may be particularly useful is the group with known or suspected sleep-disordered breathing in whom systemic opiates are prone to precipitate respiratory failure from hypoventilation and/or obstructive apnea.

Challenges and Adverse Effects

Critically ill patients, especially outside the postoperative subset, are often poor candidates for regional analgesia. It may be especially difficult to place needles and catheters (difficulties in posi-

tioning, tissue edema, anatomic deformity) or to ascertain their position (which is often judged based on the feedback of an alert and cooperative patient). There is great interest in the potential for ultrasound imaging to improve success rates and decrease complications of regional anesthesia, even extending to patients with coagulopathies.[162,163] Even when a catheter is placed properly, it subsequently may be dislodged related to patient agitation, general nursing activities, performance of radiologic imaging, and other common ICU activities. When malposition is suspected, confirmation may be difficult due to a change in the patient's level of consciousness, coagulation status, or risk of transport. Hazards of placement are higher than in a typical perioperative setting due to coagulopathy, thrombocytopenia, and drugs that impair hemostasis. Attention to measures of clotting function can reduce this risk, but some of these conditions develop during the course of critical illness and after the placement of a potentially risky catheter. Consensus guidelines are available for patients receiving antiplatelet drugs, heparins, oral anticoagulants, thrombolytic drugs, and herbal therapies delineating risk factors, complications, and recommendations for regional anesthesia.[164]

Infection is another consideration when therapy requires catheters. Full barrier precautions during catheter insertion, just as with intravascular catheters, are recommended to lessen the risk of contamination. Sepsis is a daily concern in many critically ill patients. Even when sepsis is absent, systemic inflammation may accompany many illnesses, prompting questions as to the sterility of all invasive devices, including analgesic catheters, possibly necessitating their early withdrawal. Finally, the large number of caregivers of the typically critically ill patients, extending over a number of days, raises the risk of accident related to analgesic catheters. Conspicuous labeling may lower the chances that, for example, an epidural catheter is misidentified as a nephrostomy tube, biliary drain, intravascular device, or pacemaker lead. In addition to hematoma at the site of needle or catheter and infection of the device, regional anesthesia may also be complicated by bradycardia and hypotension (from sympathetic blockade), respiratory depression, itching, nausea, and depressed sensorium. Various factors should be weighed when considering using a regional analgesic technique in the ICU setting (Table 112.4).

TABLE 112.4

CONSIDERATIONS IN THE USE OF REGIONAL ANALGESIC TECHNIQUES

Question	Factors to consider
Can pain be ameliorated simply?	Repositioning or fixation of limb or body
Are there provoking factors?	Fixation, adjustment (e.g., withdrawal of endotracheal tube), or removal of devices
Is pain sufficiently localized to make a regional approach effective?	Postoperative or procedural pain is most amenable
Will it be possible to deliver the analgesia to the proper location and assess its impact?	Patient level of consciousness, limiting anatomic factors
Are there contraindications?	Coagulopathy, sepsis, anatomic concerns
How can risks be minimized?	Tunneled catheters, labeling of catheters, nursing education, repair of coagulopathy

Postoperative Pain

In many regards, postoperative pain presents the ideal conditions for local and regional analgesic techniques. Pain typically arises in a defined anatomic site, catheters can be placed intraoperatively, assuring good placement and reducing complications, surgery is planned, allowing time for full consideration of analgesic options, and most operative patients are not laden initially with systemic inflammation, coagulopathy, and impaired mentation. Further, many studies have compared the addition of local or regional approaches to postoperative analgesia so there is accumulating evidence regarding safety and efficacy.

Pain following median sternotomy is amenable to continuous local anesthetic infusion. In a prospective, randomized, double-blind trial, subjects undergoing open-heart surgery had a pair of infusion catheters inserted at the incision site at the end of the operation.[165] Continuous local infiltration with bupivacaine 0.5% at 4 mL/hour reduced the need for opioids, improved patient satisfaction, facilitated earlier ambulation, and reduced hospital stay. Similar results were reported following coronary artery bypass when ropivacaine was infused locally through a pair of multihole catheters.[166]

Epidural Analgesia and Nerve Blocks

Epidural analgesia has been used extensively for postoperative pain, particularly following thoracic, vascular, and orthopaedic procedures. In one series of patients undergoing thoracoabdominal esophagectomy, thoracic epidural analgesia with bupivacaine plus morphine provided superior analgesia with fewer opioid-related side effects (especially excessive sedation, respiratory depression, hallucinations, and confusion) than intravenous morphine analgesia.[153] There were no differences, however, in length of ICU stay, hospital length of stay, or mortality. Moreover, the

catheter was inadvertently displaced in 18% of subjects and, in many patients in the epidural group, analgesia was insufficient or terminated early.

Some data suggest that epidural analgesia can improve relevant postoperative outcomes, especially in high-risk patients. Potential benefits include reduced thromboembolism and myocardial infarction along with improvements in pulmonary and bowel function.[167] A Cochrane review comparing epidural and systemic anesthesia following elective abdominal surgery concluded that the epidural approach reduced time on the ventilator, the risk of prolonged ventilation, cardiovascular and gastrointestinal complications, and the incidence of acute renal failure, even while improving pain control.[154] For nonsurgical patients, intrathecal approaches are used rarely because of the heightened risk of complications.[168] For pain management in the ICU, clinicians should consider the techniques, indications, and special concerns related to such procedures in the critically ill (Table 112.5).

Procedural and Iatrogenic Pain Episodes

Pain regularly accompanies a wide range of common ICU procedures. Drain and intravascular catheter removal, tracheal suctioning, deep breathing exercises, and turning cause pain and produce measurable increases in pain scores.[169,170] The majority of patients are not premedicated for these procedures despite evidence that patients report significant pain,[63,171] perhaps because clinicians systematically underestimate the pain they cause.[172]

MANAGEMENT OF ANALGESIA AND SEDATION IN THE INTENSIVE CARE UNIT

Core principles of ICU care include providing comfort, relief of distress, and improving tolerance of the ICU environment includ-

---

TABLE 112.5

TECHNIQUES AND INDICATIONS FOR REGIONAL AND EPIDURAL ANALGESIA IN THE INTENSIVE CARE UNIT

Technique	Indication	ICU Considerations
Thoracic epidural	Chest surgery, trauma, refractory angina	Potential for sympathetic blockade with hypotension or bradycardia; epidural hematoma or infection
	Abdominal surgery Pancreatitis	
Lumbar epidural	Lower extremity surgery or trauma	Potential for hypotension
Paravertebral thoracic block	One-sided thoracic surgery, trauma, or chest pain	Potential for pneumothorax
Intercostal nerve block	Chest tube placement, rib pain or fracture	Highly vascular area; potential for pneumothorax
Femoral and sciatic blocks	Thigh and leg pain	Fewer hemodynamic complications than lumbar epidural
Brachial plexus blocks	Arm pain, surgery, trauma	Depending on the particular technique, potential for pneumothorax; epidural, intrathecal, or intra-arterial injection; or phrenic nerve block

ing optimizing acceptance of mechanical ventilation and indwelling tubes and catheters.[99,110] Further, in addition to pain, many patients have anxiety and apprehension related to these experiences. Accordingly, a combination of opioid analgesic and sedative-hypnotic anxiolytic medications are administered to many, if not most, critically ill patients, often by continuous intravenous infusion.[63,172–174]

It is important to employ a structured approach to providing analgesia and sedation in the ICU, with emphasis on interdisciplinary management.[99,110,174] Key concepts include (1) patient assessment and optimizing the ICU environment, (2) evaluation and documentation of pain, agitation, and level of sedation using validated instruments, (3) implementing a patient-focused management strategy that emphasizes matching patient characteristics to appropriate medications, targeting a specific level of sedation, and utilizing algorithms to avoid oversedation, and (4) proper de-escalation of therapy with avoidance of opioid and benzodiazepine withdrawal.[110,175]

Patient assessment should include recognition of underlying medical conditions that might influence analgesic and sedative management, such as chronic pain syndromes, use of analgesic or sedative medications prior to ICU admission, and history of substance abuse. The presence and severity of pain should be sought, preferably by self-reporting and utilizing a numerical pain scale or similar instrument to detect, quantify, and document pain and the patient's response to therapy.[107] Although it is less reliable than self-reporting, the use of a validated tool to infer pain from observed graded patient behaviors may be helpful for the patient who is sedated or otherwise unable to self-report.[173]

The CPOT and the BPS are two of the more thoroughly validated among such tools (see Tables 112.2 and 112.3).[26,87,88] Agitation should be recognized and documented, preferably using a validated tool such as the RASS, the SAS, or the ATICE instruments.[104–106] The level of sedation should be measured and documented regularly (e.g., every 4 hours) using a validated tool that is accurate, simple to use and recall, and has sufficient levels for titration of medications.[173,175] The Ramsay sedation scale (RSS),[176] RASS, and SAS are among the more widely used tools; we favor using RSS, RASS, and the awakeness scale of ATICE since these tools use a logical progression of common actions (eye opening and, in some, following a command) spontaneously, to voice, and if no response to voice, then response to physical stimulation in a stepwise fashion. A sedation level can be targeted and communication is enhanced using a sedation scale.

Selecting the medications best suited to the individual patient is vitally important. Propofol, for example, is preferred when rapid awakening is important.[177] Midazolam and morphine have active metabolites that are subsequently cleared by the kidneys, thus avoidance of these medications in patients who have renal insufficiency is important.[119,174,178] The 2002 *Clinical Practice Guidelines for the Sustained Use of Sedatives and Analgesics in the Critically Ill Adult*, published by SCCM,[110] recommends using fentanyl, hydromorphone, or morphine for intravenous administration (see Fig. 112.2). Prospective surveys from various countries indicate widespread use of fentanyl and morphine, although sufentanil and remifentanil are increasingly used in Europe.[63,115–118] Some clinicians favor emphasizing primary titration of opioids, followed by adjustments in the sedative medication, so-called analgosedation or cosedation.[127,179–180]

Dexmedetomidine is a selective alpha-2-adrenergic receptor agonist with a short half-life of about 2 to 3 hours that has sedative, analgesic, anxiolytic, and sympatholytic effects without depressing respiratory drive. Drug-related adverse effects are primarily cardiovascular, including hypotension and bradycardia, particularly when loading doses are used. In comparative studies, dexmedetomidine is associated with more alert level of consciousness but higher rates of pain and agitation than comparison

drugs.[145,181,182] Although dexmedetomidine is considered to have analgesic properties, these appear insufficient in abating pain in the ICU setting. For example, in a head-to-head comparison with lorazepam in mechanically ventilated adults, the median dose of fentanyl was nearly four-fold higher with dexmedetomidine than with lorazepam.[145]

Continuous infusion of analgesic and sedative medications can provide a smooth course of sedation but has been linked to delayed recovery and longer duration of mechanical ventilation and ICU length of stay.[55] Accordingly, a number of strategies have been demonstrated in prospective randomized controlled studies to result in superior sedation, shorter duration of mechanical ventilation, reduced need for tracheostomy, and/or fewer tests for altered mental status. Strategies include a protocol with preference for intermittent over continuous administration of opioid analgesic and sedative medications,[114] daily interruption of opioid and sedation medications until the patient becomes alert or agitated,[41] preference for using shorter-acting opioid or sedative medications, and systematic approaches to managing sedation, pain, and agitation using repeated measurement and titration of medications to eliminate pain and agitation without inducing oversedation.[108,183] Many hospitals have adopted daily interruption of opioid and sedation (DIS), also referred to as "daily awakening" protocols or a "sedation vacation," in part because organizations such as the Surviving Sepsis Campaign[184] and the Institute for Healthcare Improvement Campaign[185] promote DIS as a component of evidence-based bundled ICU strategies. With DIS, opioid and sedative medications are temporarily discontinued until the patient becomes agitated or is able to follow more than three out of four simple commands, at which time the medications are restarted at half the original dosage. DIS has been demonstrated in prospective trials to be associated with short duration of mechanical ventilation, shorter ICU length of stay, fewer tests for unexplained altered mental status, fewer ICU complications, less posttraumatic stress disorder, and to be safe among patients with risk for coronary artery disease.[41,186] The combination of a daily awakening trial plus a spontaneous breathing trial (SBT) to determine ability to breathe independently is superior to a SBT alone.[161] Safety for patients at high risk for alcohol or analgesic or sedative drug withdrawal syndrome or for having adverse consequence of catecholamine surge remains to be proven.

Preferential use of short-acting agents that have a rapid offset of action has been linked to shorter duration of mechanical ventilation. As discussed above, the use of remifentanil, which is metabolized independently from organ function, has shorter duration of mechanical ventilation in comparison to other opioids.[123–127] Infusion of propofol is associated with shorter duration weaning than midazolam in postoperative patients.[177] In a recent randomized controlled trial, continuous infusion propofol with DIS was associated with shorter duration of mechanical ventilation and, despite its higher acquisition price, cost savings when compared to intermittent lorazepam.[187,188] While dexmedetomidine is regarded as a short-acting agent, no difference in the duration of mechanical ventilation has been noted in randomized controlled trials comparing dexmedetomidine to other sedative hypnotic drugs.[145,182]

Finally, de-escalation of analgesic and sedative medications is important to address carefully as the patient improves and the need for ICU care lessens. Patients who have had a prolonged course of treatment, such as those with acute respiratory distress syndrome, have a higher risk of developing opioid or benzodiazepine withdrawal.[137,189] Clinicians must be alert for possible withdrawal with manifestations such as restlessness, insomnia, delirium, nausea, hypertension, tachycardia, diaphoresis, and fever. It may be necessary to add oral or topical agents to provide a more gradual course.[190,191] Such tapering therapy should be complete prior to discharge unless the use of these medications predated hospitalization.

APPROACHES TO PAIN MANAGEMENT AT THE END OF LIFE

Health care providers play an active role in managing end-of-life care for ICU patients.[192,193] Polling reveals that most people wish to die at home; however, over 50% of deaths continue to occur in the hospital, many with ICU care.[59,194-198] Approximately 15% of patients admitted to the ICU or over 500,000 per year in the United States eventually succumb to advanced illness and die in the ICU setting.[1,71,196,197,199-204] Studies have documented that the majority of dying ICU patients experience moderate to severe pain and distress.[4,5,16,59] Especially at the end of life, pain management should be included within the range of palliative care delivered.[27,29,30] As discussed above, a comprehensive care paradigm that incorporates concurrent palliative management is applicable to all ICU patients. For those dying, an explicit shift in management from curative therapy to comfort-oriented care is indicated.[192,193,205,206]

Although dying in the ICU is frequent, many barriers, including ethical and legal concerns, preclude optimization of pain management at the end of life. Ethical discourse has consistently upheld the appropriateness of withdrawing unwanted or unhelpful therapies to avoid the prolongation of the dying process and the administration of medications with the intent of relieving suffering.[28,207-211] Providers should administer pain medications and other palliative therapies for the dying patient in the ICU, even if the possibility exists that such treatment could possibly hasten death. A doctrine of "double-effect" supports adequate and aggressive palliation of pain to be differentiated from active hastening of death and ethically justifiable, as long as the provider's primary intent is mitigating suffering.[209-211] A clinician should document the reason and titration of agents used for the alleviation of pain well and avoid undertreatment by relying on patient self-report and physiologic responses.

Data suggests that aggressive pain management in the critically ill, contrary to anticipated short-term side effects like transient respiratory depression, may be life-prolonging, as uncontrolled pain can compromise vital organ function (see Table 112.1).[1,212-217] Documentation and physician orders should have specific guidance regarding therapies to avoid ambiguity with medication escalation and delineate the discussions and process that has led to terminal care, such as the observations and reasons for dose escalation of opiates. Dying patients will experience a range of symptoms and other palliative treatments, and a comprehensive care model (Table 112.6) that includes the family and other bereaved acquaintances of the patient are appropriate.[13,19,21,48,83,109]

Guidelines and specialized approaches have been developed for analgesic therapy during the removal of life-sustaining interventions.[12,28,48,52,218] Titration of agents used for the unconscious, dying patient is done by assessing physiologic indicators, such as tachypnea and tachycardia, and observation of behavioral markers, like facial grimacing and restlessness. For some patients at the end of life who are able to have meaningful interactions with loved ones, brief interruption of sedatives and analgesia may be reasonable, maintaining vigilance for the precipitation of withdrawal. An interdisciplinary approach unites the talents of complementary providers to aid in delivering seamless palliative and end-of-life care in the ICU (see Table 112.6). At times, the dying process may be protracted and transition to another setting may be appropriate. As part of the spectrum of good end-of-life care, patients and their families expect pain management to be a central part of quality ICU care.[19,20,28,205,219-222]

TABLE 112.6

END-OF-LIFE CARE AND PAIN MANAGEMENT IN THE DYING INTENSIVE CARE UNIT PATIENT

Clarify and document the goals of care

Notify interested parties (surgeon, oncologist, specialty nurse, outpatient physician, or nurse)

Emphasize to family that care continues, but with new goals (i.e., care is not being "withdrawn," but rather is directed at dignity and comfort)

Discontinue interventions and treatments that do not contribute to comfort (phlebotomy, imaging, remove inessential [not needed for comfort] devices, silence alarms)

Provide sufficient analgesia, generally with systemic narcotics (assure reliable intravenous access, take into account recent and or chronic narcotic use, avoid arbitrary "upper limits" on analgesic dosing, begin with a bolus of drug if planning to remove devices, including the endotracheal tube, that raise the possibility of discomfort)

Educate and reassure family and staff that the purpose of narcotic is to relieve and prevent suffering, not to hasten death

Consider withdrawing the endotracheal tube since this can generally be done with no discomfort to the dying as long as adequately premedicated

Reassess regularly whether the goals of care (comfort) are being met and titrate pharmacologic agents and interventions (clinically examine for signs of discomfort), determine whether vital signs respond to interventions, solicit family input: Do you feel he/she is comfortable?

Invite ministry, palliative care, or pain specialists, where appropriate

Consider transfer out of the ICU for continued comfort care

References

1. Mularski RA. Pain management in the intensive care unit. *Crit Care Clin* 2004;20(3):381–401.
2. Raffin TA. Ethical and legal aspects of forgoing life-sustaining treatments. In: Carlson RW, Geheb MA, eds. *Principles and Practice of Medical Intensive Care*. Philadelphia: WB Saunders; 1993:1731–40.
3. Mularski RA, Osborne ML. The changing ethics of death in the ICU. In: Curtis JR, Rubenfeld GD, eds. *Managing Death in the Intensive Care Unit*. New York: Oxford University Press; 2001:7–18.
4. Desbiens NA, Wu AW, Broste SK, et al. Pain and satisfaction with pain control in seriously ill hospitalized adults: findings from the SUPPORT research investigations. For the SUPPORT investigators. Study to Understand Prognoses and Preferences for Outcomes and Risks of Treatment. *Crit Care Med* 1996; 24(12):1943–1944.
5. Desbiens NA, Wu AW. Pain and suffering in seriously ill hospitalized patients. *J Am Geriatr Soc* 2000;48(5 Suppl):S183–S186.
6. Turner JS, Briggs SJ, Springhorn HE, et al. Patients' recollection of intensive care unit experience. *Crit Care Med* 1990;18(9):966–968.
7. Kwekkeboom KL, Herr K. Assessment of pain in the critically ill. *Crit Care Nurs Clin North Am* 2001;13(2):181–194.
8. Stanik-Hutt JA, Soeken KL, Belcher AE, et al. Pain experiences of traumatically injured patients in a critical care setting. *Am J Crit Care* 2001;10(4): 252–259.
9. Puntillo KA. The phenomenon of pain and critical care nursing. *Heart Lung* 1988;17(3):262–73.
10. Puntillo KA. Dimensions of procedural pain and its analgesic management in critically ill surgical patients. *Am J Crit Care* 1994;3(2):116–122.
11. Novaes MA, Knobel E, Bork AM, et al. Stressors in ICU: perception of the patient, relatives and health care team. *Intensive Care Med* 1999;25(12): 1421–1426.
12. Hawryluck LA, Harvey WR, Lemieux-Charles L, et al. Consensus guidelines on analgesia and sedation in dying intensive care unit patients. *BMC Med Ethics* 2002;12:3:E3.
13. Lanken P. Optimal care for patients dying in the ICU. In: International Consensus Conference in Intensive Care Medicine, Brussels, 2003. Accessed May 23, 2005. Available at: http://europa.eu.int/information_society/activities/intern_ist/IST-international-vademecum.pdf.

14. Caswell DR, Williams JP, Vallejo M, et al. Improving pain management in critical care. *Jt Comm J Qual Improv* 1996;22(10):702–712.

15. Hadorn DC. Setting health care priorities in Oregon. Cost-effectiveness meets the rule of rescue. *JAMA* 1991;265(17):2218–2225.

16. Nelson JE, Meier DE, Oei EJ, et al. Self-reported symptom experience of critically ill cancer patients receiving intensive care. *Crit Care Med* 2001;29(2):277–282.

17. Nelson JE, Meier DE, Litke A, et al. The symptom burden of chronic critical illness. *Crit Care Med* 2004;32(7):1527–1534.

18. Morrison RS, Ahronheim JC, Morrison GR, et al. Pain and discomfort associated with common hospital procedures and experiences. *J Pain Symptom Manage* 1998;15(2):91–101.

19. Doyle D, Hanks GWC, MacDonald N, eds. *Oxford textbook of palliative medicine.* 2nd ed. Oxford England: Oxford University Press; 1998.

20. Jacox A, Carr D, Payne R, et al. *Clinical Practice Guideline Number 9: Management of Cancer Pain.* Rockville, MD: Agency for Health Care Policy and Research, US Dept of Health and Human Services; 1994. AHCPR Publication No. 94–0592.

21. Curtiss CP, Haylock PJ. Managing cancer and noncancer chronic pain in critical care settings. Knowledge and skills every nurse needs to know. *Crit Care Nurs Clin North Am* 2001;13(2):271–280.

22. Epstein J, Breslow MJ. The stress response of critical illness. *Crit Care Clin* 1999;15(1):17–33.

23. Lewis KS, Whipple JK, Michael KA, et al. Effect of analgesic treatment on the physiological consequences of acute pain. *Am J Hosp Pharm* 1994;51(12):1539–1554.

24. Ethical and moral guidelines for the initiation, continuation, and withdrawal of intensive care. American College of Chest Physicians/ Society of Critical Care Medicine Consensus Panel. *Chest* 1990;97(4):949–958.

25. Australian and New Zealand College of Anaesthetists (ANZCA), Faculty of Pain Medicine. *Acute Pain Management: Scientific Evidence.* 2nd ed. Victoria, Australia: Author; 2005. Available at: http://www.anzca.edu.au/resources/books-and-publications. Accessed

26. American Society of Anesthesiologists Task Force on Acute Pain Management (ASATF). Practice guidelines for acute pain management in the perioperative setting: an update report by the American Society of Anesthesiologiests Task Force on Acute Pain Management. *Anesthesiology* 2004;100(6):1573–1581.

27. Selecky PA, Eliasson CA, Hall RI, et al. Palliative and end-of-life care for patients with cardiopulmonary diseases: American College of Chest Physicians position statement. *Chest* 2005;128(5):3599–3610.

28. Consensus report on the ethics of foregoing life-sustaining treatments in the critically ill. Task Force on Ethics of the Society of Critical Care Medicine. *Crit Care Med* 1990;18(12):1435–1439.

29. Lanken PN, Terry PB, Delisser HM, et al. An official American Thoracic Society clinical policy statement: palliative care for patients with respiratory diseases and critical illnesses. *Am J Respir Crit Care Med* 200815;177(8):912–927.

30. Truog RD, Campbell ML, Curtis JR, et al. Recommendations for end-of-life care in the intensive care unit: a consensus statement by the American College [corrected] of Critical Care Medicine. *Crit Care Med* 2008;36(3):953–963.

31. Truog RD, Cist AF, Brackett SE, et al. Recommendations for end-of-life care in the intensive care unit: The Ethics Committee of the Society of Critical Care Medicine. *Crit Care Med* 2001;29(12):2332–2348.

32. Mularski RA, Osborne ML. End-of-life care in the critically ill geriatric population. *Crit Care Clin* 2003;19(4):789–810.

33. Ajemain I. The interdisciplinary team. In: Doyle D, Hanks GWC, MacDonald N, eds. *Oxford Textbook of Palliative Medicine.* 1st ed. New York: Oxford University Press; 1993:18.

34. Cummings I. The interdisciplinary team. In: Doyle D, Hanks GWC, MacDonald N, eds. *Oxford Textbook of Palliative Medicine.* 2nd ed. New York: Oxford University Press; 1998:19–30.

35. Boyle DK, Kochinda C. Enhancing collaborative communication of nurse and physician leadership in two intensive care units. *J Nurs Adm* 2004;34(2):60–70.

36. Baggs JG, Schmitt MH, Mushlin AI, et al. Association between nurse-physician collaboration and patient outcomes in three intensive care units. *Crit Care Med* 1999;27(9):1991–1998.

37. Baggs JG, Ryan SA, Phelps CE, et al. The association between interdisciplinary collaboration and patient outcomes in a medical intensive care unit. *Heart Lung* 1992;21(1):18–24.

38. Mularski RA, Bascom P, Osborne ML. Educational agendas for interdisciplinary end-of-life curricula. *Crit Care Med* 2001;29(2 Suppl):N16–N23.

39. Mularski RA, Osborne ML. Palliative care and intensive care unit care: daily intensive care unit care plan checklist #123. *J Palliat Med* 2006;9(5):1205–1206.

40. Mularski RA, Osborne ML. Palliative care and intensive care unit care: preadmission assessment #122. *J Palliat Med* 2006;9(5):1204–1205.

41. Kress JP, Pohlman AS, O'Connor MF, et al. Daily interruption of sedative infusions in critically ill patients undergoing mechanical ventilation. *N Engl J Med* 2000;342(20):1471–1477.

42. International Association for the Study of Pain. Definitions. Seattle, WA: International Association for the Study of Pain; 2003. Available at: Accessed

43. Pasero C, McCaffery M. Pain in the critically ill. *Am J Nurs* 2002;102(1):59–60.

44. Cross SA. Pathophysiology of pain. *Mayo Clin Proc* 1994;69(4):375–383.

45. Desai PM. Pain management and pulmonary dysfunction. *Crit Care Clin* 1999;15(1):151–166.

46. Gust R, Pecher S, Gust A, et al. Effect of patient-controlled analgesia on pulmonary complications after coronary artery bypass grafting. *Crit Care Med* 1999;27(10):2218–2223.

47. Willis WD, Westlund KN. Neuroanatomy of the pain system and of the pathways that modulate pain. *J Clin Neurophysiol* 1997;14(1):2–31.

48. Cullen L, Greiner J, Titler MG. Pain management in the culture of critical care. *Crit Care Nurs Clin North Am* 2001;13(2):151–166.

49. Ferguson J, Gilroy D, Puntillo K. Dimensions of pain and analgesic administration associated with coronary artery bypass grafting in an Australian intensive care unit. *J Adv Nurs* 1997;26(6):1065–1072.

50. Willis WD. Role of neurotransmitters in sensitization of pain responses. *Ann N Y Acad Sci* 2001;933:142–156.

51. Reisine T, Pasternak G. *Opioid Analgesics and Antagonists.* New York: McGraw-Hill; 1996:521–555.

52. Wilson WC, Smedira NG, Fink C, et al. Ordering and administration of sedatives and analgesics during the withholding and withdrawal of life support from critically ill patients. *JAMA* 1992;267(7):949–953.

53. Dasta JF, Fuhrman TM, McCandles C. Patterns of prescribing and administering drugs for agitation and pain in patients in a surgical intensive care unit. *Crit Care Med* 1994;22(6):974–980.

54. Hansen-Flaschen JH, Brazinsky S, Basile C, et al. Use of sedating drugs and neuromuscular blocking agents in patients requiring mechanical ventilation for respiratory failure. A national survey. *JAMA* 199127;266(20):2870–2875.

55. Kollef MH, Levy NT, Ahrens TS, et al. The use of continuous i.v. sedation is associated with prolongation of mechanical ventilation. *Chest* 1998;114(2):541–548.

56. Lasch K, Carr DB. Pain assessment in seriously ill patients: its importance and need for technical improvement. *Crit Care Med* 1996;24(12):1943–1944.

57. Watling SM, Dasta JF, Seidl EC. Sedatives, analgesics, and paralytics in the ICU. *Ann Pharmacother* 1997;31(2):148–153.

58. Whipple JK, Lewis KS, Quebbeman EJ, et al. Analysis of pain management in critically ill patients. *Pharmacotherapy* 1995;15(5):592–599.

59. A controlled trial to improve care for seriously ill hospitalized patients. The study to understand prognoses and preferences for outcomes and risks of treatments (SUPPORT). The SUPPORT Principal Investigators. *JAMA* 1995;274(20):1591–1598.

60. American Pain Foundation. Fast facts about pain. Available at: http://www.painfoundation.org/page.asp?file=Library/FastFacts.htm. Accessed May 1, 2008.

61. American Pain Society. Chronic pain in American: roadblocks to relief. Available at: http://www.ampainsoc.org/links/roadblocks/. Accessed May 1, 2008.

62. Freire AX, Afessa B, Cawley P, et al. Characteristics associated with analgesia ordering in the intensive care unit and relationships with outcome. *Crit Care Med* 2002;30(11):2468–24672.

63. Payen JF, Chanques G, Mantz J, et al. Current practices in sedation and analgesia for mechanically ventilated critically ill patients: a prospective multicenter patient-based study. *Anesthesiology* 2007;106(4):687–695.

64. Lanken PN, Terry PB, Delisser HM, et al, and the ATS End-of-Life Care Task Force. An Official American Thoracic Society Clinical Policy Statement: palliative care for patients with respiratory diseases and critical illness. *Am J Respir Crit Care Med* 2008;15;177(8):912–927.

65. Joint Commission on Accreditation of Health Care Organization. Pain assessment and management standards. Available at: www.jcaho.org. Accessed May 1, 2008.

66. McCaffery M, Pasero C. *Pain Clinical Manual.* New York: Moseby, Inc; 1999.

67. Palliative care. Guidelines for good practice and audit measures. Report of a Working Group of the Research Unit, Royal College of Physicians. *J R Coll Physicians Lond* 1991;25(4):325–328.

68. Quality improvement guidelines for the treatment of acute pain and cancer pain. American Pain Society Quality of Care Committee. *JAMA* 1995;274(23):1874–1880.

69. Lorenz K, Lynn J, Dy S, et al. Cancer care quality measures: Symptoms and end of life care. *Evid Rep Technol Assess (Full Rep)* 2006;137:1–77.

70. Mularski RA, Curtis JR, Billings JA, et al. Proposed quality measures for palliative care in the critically ill: a consensus from the Robert Wood Johnson Foundation Critical Care Workgroup. *Crit Care Med* 2006;34(11 Suppl):S404–S411.

71. Mularski RA. Defining and measuring quality palliative and end-of-life care in the intensive care unit. *Crit Care Med* 2006;34(11 Suppl):S309–S316.

72. Nelson JE, Mulkerin CM, Adams LL, et al. Improving comfort and communication in the ICU: a practical new tool for palliative care performance measurement and feedback. *Qual Saf Health Care* 2006;15(4):264–271.

73. Wenger NS, Rosenfeld K. Quality indicators for end-of-life care in vulnerable elders. *Ann Intern Med* 2001;135(8 Pt 2):677–685.

74. Kerns RD, Wasse L, Ryan B, et al. *Pain as the 5th Vital Sign Toolkit.* Version 2. Washington, DC: Veterans Health Administration; 2000.

75. Jensen MP, Karoly P, Braver S. The measurement of clinical pain intensity: a comparison of six methods. *Pain* 1986;27(1):117–126.

76. Chapman CR, Casey KL, Dubner R, et al. Pain measurement: an overview. *Pain* 1985;22(1):1–31.

77. Kremer E, Atkinson JH, Ignelzi RJ. Measurement of pain: patient preference does not confound pain measurement. *Pain* 1981;10(2):241–248.

78. Partners against pain. Available at: www.partnersagainstpain.com/html/assess/scales/as_scale3.htm. Accessed March 6, 2003.

79. Ho K, Spence J, Murphy MF. Review of pain-measurement tools. *Ann Emerg Med* 1996;27(4):427–432.

80. Meehan DA, McRae ME, Rourke DA, et al. Analgesic administration, pain intensity, and patient satisfaction in cardiac surgical patients. *Am J Crit Care* 1995;4(6):435–442.

81. Puntillo KA, Miaskowski C, Kehrle K, et al. Relationship between behavioral and physiological indicators of pain, critical care patients' self-reports of pain, and opioid administration. *Crit Care Med* 1997;25(7):1159–1166.

82. Bookbinder M, Coyle N, Kiss M, et al. Implementing national standards for cancer pain management: program model and evaluation. *J Pain Symptom Manage* 1996;12(6):334–347.

83. Foley KM. *Management of Cancer Pain.* 4th ed. Philadelphia: J.B. Lippincott; 1994:2417–2448.

84. Ambuel B, Hamlett KW, Marx CM, et al. Assessing distress in pediatric intensive care environments: the COMFORT scale. *J Pediatr Psychol* 1992;17(1):95–109.

85. Merkel SI, Voepel-Lewis T, Shayevitz JR, et al. The FLACC: a behavioral scale for scoring postoperative pain in young children. *Pediatr Nurs* 1997;23(3):293–297.

86. Manworren RC, Hynan LS. Clinical validation of FLACC: preverbal patient pain scale. *Pediatr Nurs* 2003;29(2):140–146.

87. Payen JF, Bru O, Bosson JL, et al. Assessing pain in critically ill sedated patients by using a behavioral pain scale. *Crit Care Med* 2001;29(12):2258–2263.

88. Gélinas C, FillionL, Puntillo KA, et al. Validation of the critical-care pain observation tool in adult patients. *Am J Crit Care* 2006;15(4):420–427.

89. Gélinas C, Johnston C. Pain assessment in the critically ill ventilated adult: validation of the Critical-Care Pain Observation Tool and physiologic indicators. *Clin J Pain* 2007;23(6):497–505.

90. Ely EW, Inouye SK, Bernard GR, et al. Delirium in mechanically ventilated patients: validity and reliability of the confusion assessment method for the intensive care unit (CAM-ICU). *JAMA* 2001;286(21):2703–2710.

91. Ely EW, Margolin R, Francis J, et al. Evaluation of delirium in critically ill patients: validation of the Confusion Assessment Method for the Intensive Care Unit (CAM-ICU). *Crit Care Med* 2001;29(7):1370–1379.

92. Bergeron N, Dubois MJ, Dumont M, et al. Intensive Care Delirium Screening Checklist: evaluation of a new screening tool. *Intensive Care Med* 2001;27(5):859–864.

93. McPherson CJ, Addington-Hall JM. Judging the quality of care at the end of life: can proxies provide reliable information? *Soc Sci Med* 2003;56(1):95–109.

94. Seckler AB, Meier DE, Mulvihill M, et al. Substituted judgment: how accurate are proxy predictions? *Ann Intern Med* 1991;115(2):92–98.

95. Zweibel NR, Cassel CK. Treatment choices at the end of life: a comparison of decisions by older patients and their physician-selected proxies. *Gerontologist* 1989;29(5):615–621.

96. Uhlmann RF, Pearlman RA, Cain KC. Physicians' and spouses' predictions of elderly patients' resuscitation preferences. *J Gerontol* 1988;43(5):M115–M121.

97. Layde PM, Beam CA, Broste SK, et al. Surrogates' predictions of seriously ill patients' resuscitation preferences. *Arch Fam Med* 1995;4(6):518–523.

98. Sulmasy DP, Haller K, Terry PB. More talk, less paper: predicting the accuracy of substituted judgments. *Am J Med* 1994;96(5):432–438.

99. Sessler CN, Grap MJ, Brophy GM. Multidisciplinary management of sedation and analgesia in critical care. *Semin Respir Crit Care Med* 2001;22(2):211–226.

100. The management of the agitated ICU patient. *Crit Care Med* 2002;30(1 Suppl Management):S97–S123.

101. Fraser GL, Riker RR. Monitoring sedation, agitation, analgesia, and delirium in critically ill adult patients. *Crit Care Clin* 2001;17(4):967–987.

102. Woods JC, Mion LC, Connor JT, et al. Severe agitation among ventilated medical intensive care unit patients: frequency, characteristics and outcomes. *Intensive Care Med* 2004;30(6):1066–1072.

103. Carrión MI, Ayuso D, Marcos M, et al. Accidental removal of endotracheal and nasogastric tubes and intravascular catheters. *Crit Care Med* 2000;28(1):63–66.

104. Sessler CN, Gosnell MS, Grap MJ, et al. The Richmond Agitation-Sedation Scale: validity and reliability in adult intensive care unit patients. *Am J Respir Crit Care Med* 2002;166(10):1338–1344.

105. Riker RR, Picard JT, Fraser GL. Prospective evaluation of the Sedation-Agitation Scale for adult critically ill patients. *Crit Care Med* 1999;27(7):1325–1329.

106. De Jonghe B, Cook D, Griffith L, et al. Adaptation to the Intensive Care Environment (ATICE): development and validation of a new sedation assessment instrument. *Crit Care Med* 2003;31(9):2344–2354.

107. Sessler CN, Jo Grap M, Ramsay MA. Evaluating and monitoring analgesia and sedation in the intensive care unit. *Crit Care* 2008;(12 Suppl 3):S2.

108. Chanques G, Jaber S, Barbotte E, et al. Impact of systematic evaluation of pain and agitation in an intensive care unit. *Crit Care Med* 2006;34(6):1691–1699.

109. World Health Organization. *Cancer Pain Relief and Palliative Care.* Geneva: Author; 1996.

110. Jacobi J, Fraser GL, Coursin DB, et al, and Task Force of the American College of Critical Care Medicine (ACCM) of the Society of Critical Care Medicine (SCCM), American Society of Health-System Pharmacists (ASHP), American College of Chest Physicians. Clinical practice guidelines for the sustained use of sedatives and analgesics in the critically ill adult. *Crit Care Med* 2002;30(1):119–141.

111. Nasraway SA Jr, Jacobi J, Murray MJ, et al, and Task Force of the American College of Critical Care Medicine of the Society of Critical Care Medicine and the American Society of Health-System Pharmacists, American College of Chest Physicians. Sedation, analgesia, and neuromuscular blockade of the critically ill adult: revised clinical practice guidelines for 2002. *Crit Care Med* 2002;30(1):117–118.

112. Bailey JM. Technique for quantifying the duration of intravenous anesthetic effect. *Anesthesiology* 1995;83(5):1095–1103.

113. Kröll W, List WF. Pain treatment in the ICU: intravenous, regional or both? *Eur J Anaesthesiol Suppl* 1997;15:49–52.

114. Brook AD, Ahrens TS, Schaiff R, et al. Effect of a nursing-implemented sedation protocol on the duration of mechanical ventilation. *Crit Care Med* 1999;27(12):2609–2615.

115. Mehta S, Burry L, Fischer S, et al. Canadian survey of the use of sedatives, analgesics, and neuromuscular blocking agents in critically ill patients. *Crit Care Med* 2006;34(2):374–380.

116. Botha J, Le Blanc V. The state of sedation in the nation: results of an Australian survey. *Crit Care Resusc* 2005;7(2):92–96.

117. Rhoney DH, Murry KR. National survey of the use of sedating drugs, neuromuscular blocking agents, and reversal agents in the intensive care unit. *J Intensive Care Med* 2003;18(3):139–145.

118. Soliman HM, Mélot C, Vincent JL. Sedative and analgesic practice in the intensive care unit: the results of a European survey. *Br J Anaesth* 2001;87(2):186–192.

119. Barr J, Donner A. Optimal intravenous dosing strategies for sedatives and analgesics in the intensive care unit. *Crit Care Clin* 1995;11(4):827–847.

120. Tiseo PJ, Thaler HT, Lapin J, et al. Morphine-6-glucuronide concentrations and opioid-related side effects: a survey in cancer patients. *Pain* 1995;61(1):47–54.

121. Mazoit JX, Butscher K, Samii K. Morphine in postoperative patients: pharmacokinetics and pharmacodynamics of metabolites. *Anesth Analg* 2007;105(1):70–78.

122. Shafer A, White PF, Schüttler J, et al. Use of a fentanyl infusion in the intensive care unit: tolerance to its anesthetic effects? *Anesthesiology* 1983;59(3):245–248.

123. Evans TN, Gunning KE, Park GR. Remifentanil for major abdominal surgery. *Anaesthesia* 1997;52(6):606.

124. Westmoreland CL, Hoke JF, Sebel PS, et al. Pharmacokinetics of remifentanil (GI87084B) and its major metabolite (GI90291) in patients undergoing elective inpatient surgery. *Anesthesiology* 1993;79(5):893–903.

125. Wilhelm W, Dorscheid E, Schlaich N, et al. The use of remifentanil in critically ill patients. Clinical findings and early experience [in German]. *Anaesthesist* 1999;48(9):625–629.

126. Scott LJ, Perry CM. Remifentanil: a review of its use during the induction and maintenance of general anaesthesia. *Drugs* 2005;65(13):1793–1823.

127. Breen D, Karabinis A, Malbrain M, et al. Decreased duration of mechanical ventilation when comparing analgesia-based sedation using remifentanil with standard hypnotic-based sedation for up to 10 days in intensive care unit patients: a randomised trial [ISRCTN47583497]. *Crit Care* 2005;9(3):R200–R210.

128. Dahaba AA, Grabner T, Rehak PH, et al. Remifentanil versus morphine analgesia and sedation for mechanically ventilated critically ill patients: a randomized double blind study. *Anesthesiology* 2004;101(3):640–646.

129. Frid I, Haljamäe H, Öhlén J, et al. Brain death: close relatives' use of imagery as a descriptor of experience. *J Adv Nurs* 2007;58(1):63–71.

130. Baillard C, Cohen Y, Le Toumelin P, et al. Remifentanil-midazolam compared to sufentanil-midazolam for ICU long-term sedation [in French]. *Ann Fr Anesth Reanim* 2005;24(5):480–486.

131. Leone M, Albanèse J, Viviand X, et al. The effects of remifentanil on endotracheal suctioning-induced increases in intracranial pressure in head-injured patients. *Anesth Analg* 2004;99(4):1193–1198.

132. Karabinis A, Mandragos K, Stergiopoulos S, et al. Safety and efficacy of analgesia-based sedation with remifentanil versus standard hypnotic-based regimens in intensive care unit patients with brain injuries: a randomised, controlled trial [ISRCTN50308308]. *Crit Care* 2004;8(4):R268–R280.

133. Bauer C, Kreuer S, Ketter R, et al. Remifentanil-propofol versus fentanyl-midazolam combinations for intracranial surgery: influence of anaesthesia technique and intensive sedation on ventilation times and duration of stay in the ICU [in German]. *Anaesthesist* 2007;56(2):128–132.

134. Gordon DB, Stevenson KK, Griffie J, et al. Opioid equianalgesic calculations. *J Palliat Med* 1999;2(2):209–218.

135. American Pain Society. *Principles of Analgesic Use in the Treatment of Acute Pain and Cancer Pain.* Glenview, IL; 1992.

136. Mercadante S. Opioid rotation for cancer pain: rationale and clinical aspects. *Cancer* 1999;86(9):1856–1866.

137. Cammarano WB, Pittet JF, Weitz S, et al. Acute withdrawal syndrome related to the administration of analgesic and sedative medications in adult intensive care unit patients. *Crit Care Med* 1998;26(4):676–684.

138. Block BM, Liu SS, Rowlingson AJ, et al. Efficacy of postoperative epidural analgesia: a meta-analysis. *JAMA* 2003;290(18):2455–2463.

139. Mandabach MG. Perspectives in Pain Management: intrathecal and epidural analgesia. *Crit Care Clin* 1999;15(1):105–118.

140. Chang SL, Beltran JA, Swarup S. Expression of the mu opioid receptor in the

human immunodeficiency virus type 1 transgenic rat model. *J Virol* 2007; 81(16):8406–8411.

141. Feng P, Truant AL, Meissler JJ Jr, et al. Morphine withdrawal lowers host defense to enteric bacteria: spontaneous sepsis and increased sensitivity to oral Salmonella enterica serovar Typhimurium infection. *Infect Immun* 2006; 74(9):5221–5226.

142. Gilron I. Corticosteroids in postoperative pain management: future research directions for a multifaceted therapy. *Acta Anaesthesiol Scand* 2004;48(10): 1221–1222.

143. Pietz B, Lambrecht H, Prien T, et al. The strict separation of clinical and academic budgets: an analysis at a German medical university department of anaesthesia. *Best Pract Res Clin Anaesthesiol* 2002;16(3):371–374.

144. Groudine SB, Fisher HA, Kaufman RP Jr, et al. Intravenous lidocaine speeds the return of bowel function, decreases postoperative pain, and shortens hospital stay in patients undergoing radical retropubic prostatectomy. *Anesth Analg* 1998;86(2):235–239.

145. Pandharipande PP, Pun BT, Herr DL, et al. Effect of sedation with dexmedetomidine vs lorazepam on acute brain dysfunction in mechanically ventilated patients: the MENDS randomized controlled trial. *JAMA* 2007;298(22): 2644–2653.

146. Titler MG, Rakel BA. Nonpharmacologic treatment of pain. *Crit Care Nurs Clin North Am* 2001;13(2):221–232.

147. Mosenthal AC, Lee KF, Huffman J. Palliative care in the surgical intensive care unit. *J Am Coll Surg* 2002;194(1):75–83.

148. Burton AW, Eappen S. Regional anesthesia techniques for pain control in the intensive care unit. *Crit Care Clin* 1999;15(1):77–88.

149. Carr DB. Preempting the memory of pain. *JAMA* 1998;279(14):1114–1115.

150. Tuman KJ, McCarthy RJ, March RJ, et al. Effects of epidural anesthesia and analgesia on coagulation and outcome after major vascular surgery. *Anesth Analg* 1991;73(6):696–704.

151. Summer GJ, Puntillo KA. Management of surgical and procedural pain in a critical care setting. *Crit Care Nurs Clin North Am* 2001;13(2):233–242.

152. Schulz-Stübner S, Boezaart A, Hata JS. Regional analgesia in the critically ill. *Crit Care Med* 2005;33(6):1400–1407.

153. Rudin A, Flisberg P, Johansson J, et al. Thoracic epidural analgesia or intravenous morphine analgesia after thoracoabdominal esophagectomy: a prospective follow-up of 201 patients. *J Cardiothorac Vasc Anesth* 2005;19(3): 350–357.

154. Nishimori M, Ballantyne JC, Low JH. Epidural pain relief versus systemic opioid-based pain relief for abdominal aortic surgery. *Cochrane Database Syst Rev* 2006;3:CD005059.

155. Park WY, Thompson JS, Lee KK. Effect of epidural anesthesia and analgesia on perioperative outcome: a randomized, controlled Veterans Affairs cooperative study. *Ann Surg* 2001;234(4):560–659.

156. Chaney MA. Intrathecal and epidural anesthesia and analgesia for cardiac surgery. *Anesth Analg* 2006;102(1):45–64.

157. Luchette FA, Radafshar SM, Kaiser R, Flynn W, Hassett JM. Prospective evaluation of epidural versus intrapleural catheters for analgesia in chest wall trauma. *J Trauma* 1994;36(6):865–869.

158. Hansdottir V, Philip J, Olsen MF, et al. Thoracic epidural versus intravenous patient-controlled analgesia after cardiac surgery: a randomized controlled trial on length of hospital stay and patient-perceived quality of recovery. *Anesthesiology* 2006;104(1):142–151.

159. Tziavrangos E, Schug SA. Regional anaesthesia and perioperative outcome. *Curr Opin Anaesthesiol* 2006;19(5):521–525.

160. Bulger EM, Edwards T, Klotz P, et al. Epidural analgesia improves outcome after multiple rib fractures. *Surgery* 2004;136(2):426–430.

161. Girard TD, Kress JP, Fuchs BD, et al. Efficacy and safety of a paired sedation and ventilator weaning protocol for mechanically ventilated patients in intensive care (Awakening and Breathing Controlled trial): a randomised controlled trial. *Lancet* 2008;371(9607):126–134.

162. Marhofer P, Chan VW. Ultrasound-guided regional anesthesia: current concepts and future trends. *Anesth Analg* 2007;104(5):1265–1269.

163. Bigeleisen PE. Ultrasound-guided infraclavicular block in an anticoagulated and anesthetized patient. *Anesth Analg* 2007;104(5):1285–1287.

164. Horlocker TT, Wedel DJ, Benzon H, et al. Regional anesthesia in the anticoagulated patient: defining the risks (the second ASRA Consensus Conference on Neuraxial Anesthesia and Anticoagulation). *Reg Anesth Pain Med* 2003; 28(3):172–197.

165. White PF, Rawal S, Latham P, et al. Use of a continuous local anesthetic infusion for pain management after median sternotomy. *Anesthesiology* 2003; 99(4):918–923.

166. Dowling R, Thielmeier K, Ghaly A, et al. Improved pain control after cardiac surgery: results of a randomized, double-blind, clinical trial. *J Thorac Cardiovasc Surg* 2003;126(5):1271–1278.

167. Liu S, Carpenter RL, Neal JM. Epidural anesthesia and analgesia. Their role in postoperative outcome. *Anesthesiology* 1995;82(6):1474–1506.

168. Clark F, Gilbert HC. Regional analgesia in the intensive care unit. Principles and practice. *Crit Care Clin* 2001;17(4):943–966.

169. Puntillo KA, White C, Morris AB, et al. Patients' perceptions and responses to procedural pain: results from Thunder Project II. *Am J Crit Care* 2001; 10(4):238–251.

170. Siffleet J, Young J, Nikoletti S, et al. Patients' self-report of procedural pain in the intensive care unit. *J Clin Nurs* 2007;16(11):2142–2148.

171. Arroyo-Novoa CM, Figueroa-Ramos MI, Puntillo KA, et al. Pain related to

172. tracheal suctioning in awake acutely and critically ill adults: a descriptive study. *Intensive Crit Care Nurs* 2007;24(1):20–27.

172. Arroliga A, Frutos-Vivar F, Hall J, et al. Use of sedatives and neuromuscular blockers in a cohort of patients receiving mechanical ventilation. *Chest* 2005; 128(2):496–506.

173. Sessler CN, Wilhelm W. Analgesia and sedation in the intensive care unit: an overview of the issues. *Crit Care* 2008;(12 Suppl 3):S1.

174. Sessler CN, Varney K. Patient-focused sedation and analgesia in the ICU. *Chest* 2008;133:552–565.

175. Sessler CN. Sedation scales in the ICU. *Chest* 2004;126(6):1727–1730.

176. Ramsay MA, Savege TM, Simpson BR, et al. Controlled sedation with alphaxalone-alphadolone. *Br Med J* 1974;2(5920):656–659.

177. Walder B, Elia N, Henzi I, et al. A lack of evidence of superiority of propofol versus midazolam for sedation in mechanically ventilated critically ill patients: a qualitative and quantitative systematic review. *Anesth Analg* 2001;92(4): 975–983.

178. Bauer TM, Ritz R, Haberthür C, et al. Prolonged sedation due to accumulation of conjugated metabolites of midazolam. *Lancet* 1995;346(8968): 145–147.

179. Richman PS, Baram D, Varela M, Glass PS. Sedation during mechanical ventilation: a trial of benzodiazepine and opiate in combination. *Crit Care Med* 2006;34(5):1395–1401.

180. Shafer A. Complications of sedation with midazolam in the intensive care unit and a comparison with other sedative regimens. *Crit Care Med* 1998; 26(5):947–956.

181. MacLaren R, Forrest LK, Kiser TH. Adjunctive dexmedetomidine therapy in the intensive care unit: a retrospective assessment of impact on sedative and analgesic requirements, levels of sedation and analgesia, and ventilatory and hemodynamic parameters. *Pharmacotherapy* 2007;27(3):351–359.

182. Corbett SM, Rebuck JA, Greene CM, et al. Dexmedetomidine does not improve patient satisfaction when compared with propofol during mechanical ventilation. *Crit Care Med* 2005;33(5):940–945.

183. De Jonghe B, Bastuji-Garin S, Fangio P, et al. Sedation algorithm in critically ill patients without acute brain injury. *Crit Care Med* 2005;33(1):120–127.

184. Dellinger RP, Levy MM, Carlet JM, et al, and the International Surviving Sepsis Campaign Guidelines Committee, American Association of Critical-Care Nurses, American College of Chest Physicians, et al. Surviving Sepsis Campaign: international guidelines for management of severe sepsis and septic shock: 2008. *Crit Care Med* 2008;36(1):296–327.

185. Institute for Healthcare Improvement Campaign (IHI). Available at: http:// www.ihi.org/IHI/Programs/Campaign 2008. Accessed May 5, 2008.

186. Kress JP, Gehlbach B, Lacy M, et al. The long-term psychological effects of daily sedative interruption on critically ill patients. *Am J Respir Crit Care Med* 2003;168(12):1457–1461.

187. Carson SS, Kress JP, Rodgers JE, et al. A randomized trial of intermittent lorazepam versus propofol with daily interruption in mechanically ventilated patients. *Crit Care Med* 2006;34(5):1326–1332.

188. Cox CE, Reed SD, Govert JA, et al. Economic evaluation of propofol and lorazepam for critically ill patients undergoing mechanical ventilation. *Crit Care Med* 2008;36(3):706–714.

189. Korak-Leiter M, Likar R, Oher M, et al. Withdrawal following sufentanil/ propofol and sufentanil/midazolam. Sedation in surgical ICU patients: correlation with central nervous parameters and endogenous opioids. *Intensive Care Med* 2005;31(3):380–387.

190. Tobias JD. Tolerance, withdrawal, and physical dependency after long-term sedation and analgesia of children in the pediatric intensive care unit. *Crit Care Med* 2000;28(6):2122–2132.

191. Berens RJ, Meyer MT, Mikhailov TA, et al. A prospective evaluation of opioid weaning in opioid-dependent pediatric critical care patients. *Anesth Analg* 2006;102(4):1045–1050.

192. Prendergast TJ, Claessens MT, Luce JM. A national survey of end-of-life care for critically ill patients. *Am J Respir Crit Care Med* 1998;158(4):1163–1167.

193. Luce JM, Prendergast TJ. The changing nature of death in the ICU. In: Curtis JR, Rubenfeld GD, eds. *Managing Death in The Intensive Care Unit.* New York: Oxford University Press, 2001:19–29.

194. Field MJ, Cassel CK. *Approaching Death: Improving Care at the End of Life.* Washington DC: National Academy Press; 1997.

195. Deaths by place of death, age, race, and sex: United States; 1999. Centers for Disease Control and Prevention Web site. Available at: www.cdc.gov/nchs/ data/statab/ws00199.table309.pdf. Accessed May 1, 2008.

196. Dartmouth Atlas of Health Care 1999. Center for the Evaluative Clinical Sciences at Dartmouth Medical School. Dartmouth 2002. Available at: www.dartmouthatlas.org/99US. Accessed May 1, 2008.

197. The Leapfrog Group. Factsheet: ICU physician staffing. Available at: http:// www.leapfroggroup.org/media/file/Leapfrog-ICU_Physician_Staffing_Fact_ Sheet.pdf. Accessed May 1, 2008.

198. Linde-Zwirble W, Angus DC, Griffin M, Watson RS, Clermont G. ICU care at the end-of-life in America: an epidemiology study. *Crit Care Med* 2000; 28:A34.

199. Teno JM, Fisher E, Hamel MB, et al. Decision-making and outcomes of prolonged ICU stays in seriously ill patients. *J Am Geriatr Soc* 2000;48(5 Suppl): S70–S74.

200. Zimmerman JE, Wagner DP, Draper EA, et al. Evaluation of acute physiology and chronic health evaluation III predictions of hospital mortality in an independent database. *Crit Care Med* 1998;26(8):1317–1326.

201. Lynn J, Harrell F Jr, Cohn F, et al. Prognoses of seriously ill hospitalized

patients on the days before death: implications for patient care and public policy. New Horiz 1997;5(1):56–61.

202. Knaus WA, Draper EA, Wagner DP, et al. Prognosis in acute organ-system failure. *Ann Surg* 1985;202(6):685–693.

203. Lunney JR, Lynn J, Foley DJ, et al. Patterns of functional decline at the end of life. *JAMA* 2003;289(18):2387–2392.

204. Angus DC, Barnato AE, Linde-Zwirble WT, et al. Use of intensive care at the end of life in the United States: an epidemiologic study. *Crit Care Med* 2004;32(3):638–643.

205. Curtis JR, Rubenfeld GD. *Managing Death in the Intensive Care Unit: The Transition from Cure to Comfort.* New York: Oxford University Press; 2001.

206. Curtis JR, Rubenfeld GD. Improving palliative care for patients in the intensive care unit. *J Palliat Med* 2005;8(4):840–854.

207. American Thoracic Society. Withholding and withdrawing life-sustaining therapy. *Ann Intern Med* 1991;115(6):478–485.

208. President's Commission for the Study of Ethical Problems in Medicine and Biomedical Research and Behavioral Research. *Making Health Care Decisions: A Report on the Ethical and Legal Implications of Informed Consent in the Patient-Practitioner Relationship.* Washington, DC: U.S. Government Printing Office; 1982.

209. Beauchamp TL, Childress JF. *Principles of Biomedical Ethics.* 5th ed. Oxford: Oxford University Press; 2001.

210. Paris JJ, Muir JC, Reardon FE. Ethical and legal issues in intensive care. *J Intensive Care Med* 1997;12(6):298–309.

211. Jonsen AR, Siegler M, Winslade WJ. *Clinical Ethics.* 4th ed. New York: McGraw-Hill; 1998.

212. Bercovitch M, Waller A, Adunsky A. High dose morphine use in the hospice

213. Vella-Brincat J, Macleod AD. Adverse effects of opioids on the central nervous systems of palliative care patients. *J Pain Palliat Care Pharmacother* 2007; 21(1):15–25.

214. Estfan B, Mahmoud F, Shaheen P, et al. Respiratory function during parenteral opioid titration for cancer pain. *Palliat Med* 2007;21(2):81–86.

215. Citron ML, Johnston-Early A, Fossieck BE Jr, et al. Safety and efficacy of continuous intravenous morphine for severe cancer pain. *Am J Med* 1984; 77(2):199–204.

216. Chan JD, Treece PD, Engleberg RA, et al. Narcotic and benzodiazepine use after withdrawal of life support: association with time to death? Chest 2004; 126(1):286–293.

217. Edwards MJ, Richardson RH, Bascom P, et al. Opioids and benzodiazepines appear paradoxically to delay inevitable death after ventilation withdrawal. *J Palliat Care* 2005;21(4):299–302.

218. Rubenfeld GD. Principles and practice of withdrawing life-sustaining treatments. *Crit Care Clin* 2004;20(3):435–451.

219. American Medical Association. Pain Management: the online series. Available at: http://www.ama-ceionline.com. Accessed May 1, 2008.

220. American Medical Association. Education for physicians on end-of-life care. Available at: http://www.ama-assn.org/ama/pub/category/2910.html. Accessed May 1, 2008.

221. Mularski RA, Heine CE, Osborne ML, Ganzini L, Curtis JR. Quality of dying in the ICU: ratings by family members. Chest 2005;128(1):280–287.

222. National Consensus Project. Clinical practice guidelines for palliative care: 2004. Available at: http://www.nationalconsensusproject.org. Accessed January 12, 2007.

setting. A database survey of patient characteristics and effect on life expectancy. *Cancer* 1999;86(5):871–877.

CHAPTER 113 ■ THE FUTURE OF PAIN MEDICINE: AN EPILOGUE

SCOTT M. FISHMAN AND JAMES P. RATHMELL

The creation of this 4th edition of *Bonica's Management of Pain* reflects a major collaboration among many of the world's leading authorities in the basic and clinical sciences. As in prior editions, this text serves as a resource for those who seek to increase their understanding of this aspect of the human condition. However, it also provides an important reference point—an elaboration on how far we have come and how far we have to go in order to prevent, markedly reduce, and perhaps even cure the pervasive problem of pain as a cause of unnecessary suffering, debility, and economic hardship. With this compendium behind us, we now briefly look ahead to where this journey may—and should—lead us before the next edition of this textbook is written.

The future is unpredictable; nonetheless, there are many current trends that portend an optimistic course ahead. Foremost is the pivotal recognition that pain is much more than a symptom and that its consequences, in the acute or chronic form, may be devastating at every level of human health. This profound understanding has begun to transform the perspective of modern medicine, offering greater possibilities for dealing with the burden of disease than ever before. It is reported that the number of patients with chronic pain exceeds that of diabetes, heart disease, and cancer combined.[1] Yet, clinicians remain substantially undereducated about pain and ill-prepared to respond. Nonetheless, significant advances herald great things to come. Prior to the first edition of this textbook, there were no pain specialists, pain journals, pain specialty organizations, pain advocacy groups, pain training programs, or laws or regulations specifically addressing the issues involved in delivering pain relief. At the time that the third and most recent edition of this text was written,

the number of published reports in the realm of pain within the medical literature was a fraction of those today and there was no pain consortium at the National Institutes of Health (NIH). Clinical training of pain specialists was in its infancy, with minimal guidance from accrediting bodies. Certification of pain specialists through the American Board of Medical Specialties (ABMS) was available only to anesthesiologists and the immense problem of pain management in primary care had barely been raised.

Recent unprecedented events suggest that we are on a trajectory toward improved knowledge about pain and increased commitment to pain relief. These events include increasing demands for standards for pain-related assessment and treatment in all health care facilities, mandates for undergraduate medical and continuing education in pain and its management, and the increasing frequency with which administrative and legal complaints are lodged against practitioners who under-treat pain. There is little doubt that the future for pain management is inextricably linked to both science and education. Today, pain has growing representation in the NIH and professional societies are working diligently to further increase this new commitment. As an example of the growing recognition of the need for pain education for all clinicians, the largest state in the U.S., California, legislated mandatory continuing medical education on pain and end of life care for all licensed physicians. Subspecialty clinical training has become much more integrative and multidisciplinary as a result of ground breaking revisions to requirements set by the Accreditation Council of Graduate Medical Education (ACGME.) Previously, such requirements were predominantly directed by the discipline of anesthesiology, but have now been revised through an extraordinary collaboration of multiple disciplines. Unavailable even 10 years ago, training for a physician from any primary clinical discipline is now possible in accredited programs that lead to certification as a pain specialist by the ABMS. Similarly, the multidisciplinary field of palliative medicine is designated as a subspecialty that is intertwined within many ABMS primary specialties, a most recent example of medicine's increasing assimilation of symptom management and quality of life interventions. Although pain medicine has also developed as a broad-based, multidisciplinary subspecialty, its place in the overall structure of the field of medicine as a whole is still in evolution. Reform initiatives are well underway to refine the position of this emerging discipline in effort to advance its research, education, and clinical missions. Great debate remains over whether pain medicine should evolve into a more robust subspecialty that integrates parts of many clinical disciplines or whether it should become a primary specialty in its own right. How pain medicine is ultimately positioned will greatly impact the field of medicine's ability to meet its fundamental obligations to mitigate suffering.

We have recently witnessed unprecedented legislative and regulatory attention to pain and its treatment. Much of this activity relates to the overlap of pain management and prescription drug abuse. Recent developments suggest that states and the federal government remain uncertain how to balance the needs of patients in pain to have appropriate access to controlled substances with safety concerns for the general public. Potential solutions have gained intense scrutiny by the pain and law enforcement communities, respectively. Over time, national policies by the U.S. Drug Enforcement Administration (DEA), Food and Drug Administration (FDA), and the overarching Departments of Justice and Health and Human Services will hopefully evolve into rational approaches that balance compassion and safety. Although many feel that regulators and lawmakers have prioritized prescription drug abuse over undertreated pain, evidence suggests that both public health crises are receiving unprecedented attention and action. With no prior track record of pain related legislative success, 2008 saw the US Congress pass a Veterans Affairs (VA) Pain Care Act (S 2162, HR 6122) and incorporate a military pain care act into the National Defense Authorization Act (H.R. 5658.) Each of these bills mandate increased attention to pain and development of pain services within the VA health system and the Department of Defense. On the heels of this remarkable legislative success, the National Pain Care Policy Act of 2008 was passed by the U.S. House of Representative but failed to emerge from committee within the U.S. Senate. In 2009, this bill was again passed by the U.S. House of Representative and has been subsequently incorporated into a much larger health care reform act by the U.S. Senate. As would seem appropriate, the future of this important national pain legislation is now linked to the overall future of health care reform.

The clinical practice of pain management, now more commonly termed pain medicine, has changed dramatically since the creation of this textbook in 1953. Under the direction of John Bonica, the establishment of specialized centers that focus on pain management arose from anesthesiology roots. These centers were initially based on an intensive multidisciplinary model of care. Despite several decades of research firmly establishing its effectiveness, such care is expensive and has been largely unsustainable. Centers dedicated to this model have faced drastic reorganization or become extinct.

These same anesthesiology roots of pain medicine also shaped another important aspect of the field. With the influx of anesthesiologists came a rise in the use of specific pain treatments that adopted regional anesthetic or injection based techniques. Although any action taken to manage pain should be considered an "intervention," this new clinical arena based on more invasive procedures, such as analgesic injections in the spine or placement

of implantable devices for pain, has been termed "interventional pain medicine." Currently, some experts contend that general pain medicine and interventional pain medicine should be discrete disciplines with practitioners separated based on interventional and noninterventional pain practice. The heightened role of procedural-based pain practices, and some of the drive to isolate this part of care from the rest of pain medicine, has almost certainly been driven by health care reimbursement systems, such as those in the U.S., that reward practitioners with higher payment for procedural care than for almost all other aspects of pain care. Indeed, the reimbursement for pain specialists who perform procedural interventions is often many times that for those who treat the same group of patients and spend the same amount or more time with them, but do not provide such interventions, regardless of the level of evidence of predictive outcomes that might reasonably justify one type of care over another. With lucrative salaries in the private sector, too few of this new breed of interventional pain physician have stayed in the academic realm and fewer still have gone about conducting meaningful clinical trials to examine the efficacy of their interventions.

As major health reform appears imminent in the U.S., pain medicine, and particularly interventional pain medicine, stands at a crossroads as many of the treatments that are part of currently accepted pain practice are expensive but have little or no scientific evidence to support their efficacy. As the forces of health care reform and evidence-based medicine unite to guide clinical practice, many of the treatments that are commonly used today are likely to be used less often. The unbridled growth of interventional pain medicine will incur increasing scrutiny and practice will undoubtedly moderate toward a more balanced form, where practitioners provide a broad range of interventional and noninterventional treatment for common pain conditions. Indeed, for economic, medical, social, and ethical reasons, it seems likely that the field will move toward a more uniform discipline, in which individualized pain care is more similar than dissimilar, based on a relatively broad spectrum of mainstream treatment options, with therapeutic choices based on weighing all available evidence and driven by the best interests of each individual patient.

There is widespread agreement that existing systems are inadequate for training clinicians to treat pain. Despite this, today's clinicians are armed with an unprecedented array of effective tools including pharmacologic, behavioral, and physical therapies; invasive procedures; and cross-cultural complementary and alternative treatments such as acupuncture and meditation. Bringing these and new tools to bear on all cases of pain will be a major challenge, requiring education for nonspecialist clinicians at the professional school and postgraduate levels. Mandating substantive pain education for all clinicians has been a missed opportunity that must be corrected.

If the past predicts the future, pain will continue to be a pervasive problem for mankind, science will continue its exponential growth in knowledge of pain and its treatment, and society will increasingly recognize that pain management is integral to the humane and economically viable practice of medicine. The current economic crisis in health care, if not medicine's covenant to mitigate suffering, demands nothing less than systemic solutions to timely, integrated, and cost-effective pain relief. The current controversies and opportunities in association with better understanding and treatment of pain will likely push us toward a tipping point beyond which the very structure of medicine is likely to have to change.

Currently, medicine possesses greater knowledge and more tools to treat pain than ever before. Despite the undertreatment of pain, undereducation of clinicians, and underfunding of research, medicine is much further along today than it was even a decade ago—a trajectory that bodes well for the future. The optimal organizational structure of science and medicine for advancing understanding and treatment of pain is yet to be defined. But it will most certainly require transcending current barriers that serve to fragment care, such as the illogical separation of the mind and body within the whole person or the splintering of core elements of pain management due to obsolete lines that separate one discipline from another. Change will likely be proportionate to the value we place on reducing suffering along with curing disease. Moreover, how general clinicians and pain scientists of the future are supported and trained, and how the emerging discipline of pain medicine is positioned for continued development and integration throughout health care will greatly impact medicine's ability to meet its mission to understand and treat pain. Looking to the future, we appear to be headed for sweeping change in health care that may well lead to new heights in medical research, education, and clinical care for pain. This, in the light of the remarkable progress that has already been made, is a signal that medicine is rediscovering its fundamental ethos; most assuredly, to cure when possible, but to relieve suffering and provide comfort always.

References

1. National Center for Health Statistics. Health, United States, 2006 with Chartbook on Trends in the Health of Americans. Hyattsville, MD: U.S. Department of Health and Human Services; 2006:68–71.

Page numbers followed by *f* indicate figures; those followed by *t* indicate tables.